MOSBY'S 2004 DRUG GUIDE

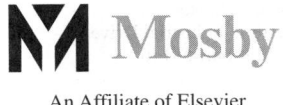

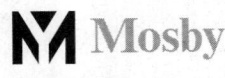

An Imprint of Elsevier

Publishing Director: Linda Duncan
Editor: David Nissen, PharmD
Systems Manager: Robert Norton
Director, Multimedia Production: John Wheeler
Producer, Electronic Publishing: Jeanne Murphy Crook
Assistant Systems Manager: Pete Johnson
Database Publishing Editor: Kathy Dashley
Associate Database Publishing Editor: Amy Rickles
Associate Database Publishing Editor: Randy Francin
Associate Database Publishing Editor: Mary Parton Schierbaum
Consultant Database Publishing Editor: Tanya McDermott
Consultant Database Publishing Editor: Randi Sarsfield
Publishing Services Manager: Linda McKinley
Senior Project Manager: Rich Barber
Senior Book Designer: Julia Dummitt
Consulting Editor, Pharmacy: F. James Grogan, PharmD
Consulting Editor, International Equivalents: Robert E. Pearson, MS
Consulting Editor, Herbal and Supplement Information: Steven Bratman, MD
Consultants, Drug Interactions: Pharmaceutical Information Associates, Ltd.

Drug Consult accepts no payment for listing; inclusion in the publication of any product, company, or individual does not imply endorsement by the editors or publisher.

The information in this edition was obtained from the FDA, from the Health Care Financing Administration, from pharmaceutical supplier catalogs, and from other publicly available sources. While the publisher has attempted to provide accurate information, it freely admits the possibility of error, and will not accept liability for incorrect information, no matter whether the error was from the FDA, from supplier information, or from actual information handling by the publisher, including typographical errors. The publisher does not warrant or guarantee any of the products described herein, and has not performed any independent analysis in connection with any of the product information contained herein. Users should verify important product information with the appropriate supplier.

Pharmacology and knowledge regarding the proper use of herbs and supplements is ever changing. Standard safety precautions must be followed, but as new research and clinical experience broaden our knowledge and understanding, changes in treatment, drug therapy, and use of herbs and supplements may become necessary or appropriate. Readers are advised to check the most current product information provided by the manufacturer of each drug, herbal product, or supplement to be administered to verify the recommended dose, the method and duration of administration, and contraindications. It is the responsibility of the treating licensed prescriber or practitioner, relying on experience and knowledge of the patient, to determine dosages and the best treatment for each individual patient. Neither the Publisher nor the Editor assumes any liability for any injury and/or damage to persons or property arising from this publication.

This publication is not intended as a substitute for medical therapy nor as a manual for self-treatment. Readers should seek professional advice for any specific medical problems.

Rx Equivalents–A Service to International Travelers; Copyright 2003; Robert E. Pearson; Licensed to Drug Consult

Herbal and Supplement Information
Information on herbal drugs and supplements is provided by Prima Health; Copyright © 2001 Prima Communications, Inc.; licensed to Drug Consult.

How Supplied Listings
Information for How supplied listings was obtained, in part, from the MediSource Lexicon Data-base as of June 1, 2003, Copyright 2003 Multum Information Services, Inc. (http://www.multum.com).

Non-FDA Approved Indications
Information on Non-FDA Approved Indications was obtained from the VantageRx Database as of July 1, 2002, Copyright © 2002 Multum Information Services, Inc. (http://www.multum.com).

Disclaimer of Warranties from Multum
THE CUSTOMER ACKNOWLEDGES THAT THE SERVICE IS PROVIDED ON AN "AS IS" BASIS. EXCEPT FOR WARRANTIES WHICH MAY NOT BE DISCLAIMED AS A MATTER OF LAW, MULTUM MAKES NO REPRESENTATIONS OR WARRANTIES WHATSOEVER, EXPRESS OR IMPLIED, INCLUDING BUT NOT LIMITED TO REPRESENTATIONS OR WARRANTIES REGARDING THE ACCURACY OR NATURE OF THE CONTENT OF THE SERVICE, WARRANTIES OF TITLE, NONINFRINGEMENT, MERCHANTABILITY OR FITNESS FOR A PARTICULAR PURPOSE.

The CUSTOMER acknowledges that updates to the Service are at the sole discretion of Multum. Multum makes no representations or warranties whatsoever, express or implied, with respect to the compatibility of the Service, or future releases thereof, with any computer hardware or software, nor does Multum represent or warrant the continuity of the features or the facilities provided by or through the Service as between various releases thereof.

Any warranties expressly provided herein do not apply if: (i) the CUSTOMER alters, mishandles or improperly uses, stores or installs all, or any part, of the Service, (ii) the breach of warranty arises out of or in connection with acts or omissions of persons other than Multum.

Assumption of Risk, Disclaimer of Liability, Indemnity
THE CUSTOMER ASSUMES ALL RISK FOR SELECTION AND USE OF THE SERVICE AND CONTENT PROVIDED. MULTUM SHALL NOT BE RESPONSIBLE FOR ANY ERRORS, MISSTATEMENTS, INACCURACIES OR OMISSIONS REGARDING CONTENT DELIVERED THROUGH THE SERVICE OR ANY DELAYS IN OR INTERRUPTIONS OF SUCH DELIVERY.

THE CUSTOMER ACKNOWLEDGES THAT MULTUM: (A) HAS NO CONTROL OF OR RESPONSIBILITY FOR THE CUSTOMER'S USE OF THE SERVICE OR CONTENT PROVIDED THEREON, (B) HAS NO KNOWLEDGE OF THE SPECIFIC OR UNIQUE CIRCUMSTANCES UNDER WHICH THE SERVICE OR CONTENT PROVIDED THEREON MAY BE USED BY THE CUSTOMER, (C) UNDERTAKES NO OBLIGATION TO SUPPLEMENT OR UPDATE CONTENT OF THE SERVICE, OR (D) HAS NO LIABILITY TO ANY PERSON FOR ANY DATA OR INFORMATION INPUT ON THE SERVICE BY THE CUSTOMER TO THE SERVICE.

MULTUM SHALL NOT BE LIABLE TO ANY PERSON (INCLUDING BUT NOT LIMITED TO THE CUSTOMER AND PERSONS TREATED BY OR ON BEHALF OF THE CUSTOMER) FOR, AND THE CUSTOMER AGREES TO INDEMNIFY AND HOLD MULTUM HARMLESS FROM ANY CLAIMS, LAWSUITS, PROCEEDINGS, COSTS, ATTORNEY'S FEES, DAMAGES OR OTHER LOSSES (COLLECTIVELY, "LOSSES") ARISING OUT OF OR RELATING TO (A) THE CUSTOMER'S USE OF THE SERVICE OR CONTENT PROVIDED THEREON OR ANY EQUIPMENT FURNISHED IN CONNECTION THEREWITH AND (B) ANY DATA OR INFORMATION INPUT ON THE SERVICE BY END-USER, IN ALL CASES INCLUDING BUT NOT LIMITED TO LOSSES FOR TORT, PERSONAL INJURY, MEDICAL MALPRACTICE OR PRODUCT LIABILITY. FURTHER, WITHOUT LIMITING THE FOREGOING, IN NO EVENT SHALL MULTUM BE LIABLE FOR ANY SPECIAL, INCIDENTAL, CONSEQUENTIAL, OR INDIRECT DAMAGES, INCLUDING DAMAGES FOR LOSS OF PROFITS, LOSS OF BUSINESS, OR DOWNTIME, EVEN IF MULTUM HAS BEEN ADVISED OF THE POSSIBILITY OF SUCH DAMAGES. THE INFORMATION CONTAINED WITHIN THE SERVICE IS INTENDED FOR USE ONLY BY PHYSICIANS AND OTHER HEALTHCARE PROFESSIONALS WHO SHOULD RELY ON THEIR CLINICAL DISCRETION AND JUDGMENT IN DIAGNOSIS AND TREATMENT. AS BETWEEN THE CUSTOMER AND MULTUM, THE CUSTOMER HEREBY ASSUMES FULL RESPONSIBILITY FOR INSURING THE APPROPRIATENESS OF USING AND RELYING UPON THE INFORMATION IN VIEW OF ALL ATTENDANT CIRCUMSTANCES, INDICATIONS, AND CONTRAINDICATIONS.

Liability of Multum to the CUSTOMER
Under no circumstances shall Multum be liable to the CUSTOMER or any other person for any direct, indirect, exemplary, special or consequential damages arising out of or relating to the CUSTOMER's use of or inability to use the Service or the Content of the Service provided thereon or any Equipment furnished in connection therewith. Except as set forth in Section 7 below, Multum's total liabilities in connection with this Agreement, whether arising under contract or otherwise, are limited to the fees received by Multum under this Agreement specifically relating to the CUSTOMER's service or product which is the subject of the claim.

Mosby, Inc.
An Imprint of Elsevier
11830 Westline Industrial Drive
St. Louis, Missouri 63146

ISBN 0-323-02872-1

00 01 02 03 04 TG/QV 9 8 7 6 5 4 3 2 1

Contents

Section I

KEYWORD INDEX

Alphabetical listing of generic and U.S. brand names, indications, and FDA Drug Class. The page number is given where the entry appears.

INTERNATIONAL BRANDS INDEX

An alphabetical listing of international brands along with the generic drug name and page number.

Section II

DRUG INFORMATION

Complete manufacturer's package insert supplemented with valuable information, including brand names (U.S. and international), indications, FDA Drug Class, FDA approval date, innovator drug, pregnancy category, cost of therapy, controlled substance schedule, product listing (including therapeutic equivalency ratings and AWP pricing.)

Section III

HERBAL INFORMATION

Complete monographs on the 50 most commonly used herbal drugs and supplements.

Section IV

APPENDICES

Appendix A–Comparative Drug Tables
Appendix B–Additional Information and Tables
Appendix C–Supplier Profiles

Editorial Review Panel

Jennifer L. McQuade, PharmD
Medical Information Consultant
Douglasville, Georgia

Armen Mzrakian, RPh
Director, Facilities Planning and Project Management
Bon Secours and Canterbury Partnership for Care
Jersey City, New Jersey

Leonard L. Naeger, BS, RPh, MS, PhD
Professor of Pharmacology
Saint Louis College of Pharmacy
St. Louis, Missouri

John Nagelhout, PhD, CRNA
Director, Kaiser Permanente School of Anesthesia
California State University, Fullerton
Fullerton, California

Keith Olsen, PharmD, FCCP
Associate Professor
Department of Pharmacy Practice
College of Pharmacy
University of Nebraska Medical Center
Omaha, Nebraska

Clive P. Page, PhD
Professor of Pharmacology
Sackler Institute of Pulmonary Pharmacology
Guy's King's and St. Thomas' School of Biomedical Sciences
King's College
London, United Kingdom

Peter T. Pons, MD, FACEP
Department of Emergency Medicine
Denver Health Medical Center
Professor of Surgery
Division of Emergency Medicine
Department of Surgery
University of Colorado Health Sciences Center
Denver, Colorado

George Safran, MD, MBA
Director
Department of Emergency Medicine
Bon Secours and Canterbury Partnership for Care
Hoboken, New Jersey

Evelyn Salerno, RPh, BS, PharmD, FASCP
Courtesy Professor
School of Nursing
Florida International University
Clinical Assistant Professor
Nova-Southeastern College of Pharmacy
Miami, Florida

Mick J. Sanders, EMT-P, BS, MSA
St. Charles, Missouri
Formerly, Training Specialist
Bureau of Emergency Medical Services
Missouri Department of Health
Jefferson City, Missouri

Roberta J. Secrest, PhD, PharmD, RPh
Scientific Communications Associate Consultant
Global Clinical Information and Communication
Eli Lilly and Company
Indianapolis, Indiana

Richard I. Shader, MD
Professor of Pharmacology and Experimental Therapeutics
Professor of Psychiatry
Tufts University School of Medicine
Boston, Massachusetts

Paula H. Stern, PhD
Professor
Department of Molecular Pharmacology and Biological Chemistry
Northwestern University Medical School
Chicago, Illinois

Greg Susla, PharmD
Clinical Science Specialist
Scientific Affairs Department
Pharmaceutical Division
Bayer Corporation
North Potomac, Maryland

Lynne M. Sylvia, PharmD
Associate Professor of Clinical Pharmacy
Department of Pharmacy Practice
Massachusetts College of Pharmacy and Health Sciences
Boston, Massachusetts

Samuel E. Taylor, PhD
Associate Professor
Director of Pharmacology
Department of Oral and Maxillofacial Surgery and Pharmacology
Baylor College of Dentistry
Texas A&M University System Health Science Center
Dallas, Texas

Peter P. Toth, MD, PhD
Clinical Associate Professor
Southern Illinois University School of Medicine
Springfield, Illinois
Sterling Rock Falls Clinic
Sterling, Illinois

John R. White, Jr., PA-C, PharmD
Associate Professor
Director, Drug Studies Unit
WSU/Sacred Heart Medical Center
Washington State University
Spokane, Washington

John A. Yagiela, DDS, PhD
Professor and Chair
Division of Diagnostic and Surgical Sciences
School of Dentistry
Professor
Department of Anesthesiology
School of Medicine
University of California, Los Angeles
Los Angeles, California

Karen Zaglaniczny, PhD, CRNA, FAAN
Director, Surgical Services Education and Research
Director, Graduate Program
School of Nursing
Oakland University/Beaumont Hospital
Royal Oak, Michigan

How To Use This Professional Drug Reference: An Overview

INTRODUCTION

This represents a compilation of the most current, complete, and unbiased information on prescription pharmaceuticals available today. It is designed for ease of use and is organized in a way that serves the diverse needs of all health care professionals and support staff.

The prescribing information found in this drug reference is for prescription pharmaceuticals and except for a few selected nonprescription drugs those products available without a prescription will not be listed. The intention of this book is not to promote the use of generic drugs over brand name products, or vice versa. Generic drugs are in wide use across the United States. Many state and private health insurance plans promote or mandate generic substitution.

KEYWORD INDEX

The Keyword Index allows the user to find the generic name of a pharmaceutical by looking up any words that might relate to the drug. Each entry within the Keyword Index has a page number where the appropriate monograph and corresponding prescribing information is found in the Drug Information section (Section II). Index terms include generic names, US brand names, FDA-approved indications, and drug class.

FDA-standard names are utilized which are United States Pharmacopoeial Convention, Inc. (USP) approved names for single ingredients. For multiple ingredient drugs each generic chemical is included in alphabetical order, separated by a semicolon (e.g., hydrochlorothiazide; triamterene). This is not necessarily the same order of ingredients used in product names for multiple ingredient drugs; however, since suppliers use different formats, this FDA-standard format allows for easy grouping of identical drugs.

INTERNATIONAL BRAND NAME INDEX

The International Brand Name Index allows the user to quickly find the U.S. equivalent to foreign drugs from 137 countries. Each entry within the International Brand Name Index has a page number where the appropriate monograph for the U.S. equivalent generic drug and corresponding prescribing information is found in the Drug Information Section (Section II).

DRUG INFORMATION

The purpose of the drug monographs is to provide complete information for pharmaceutical decision making. Organized alphabetically by generic name, the core of this information is the FDA-approved labeling for each generic drug. The information is supplemented by data from standard pharmacology texts and peer-reviewed medical journals.

CATEGORIES

The list of categories includes FDA-approved indications, pregnancy category, DEA Controlled Substance Schedule, World Health Organization Formulary, Orphan drugs, and FDA approval date. Indications are listed in alphabetical order, preceding all other categories.

FDA DRUG CLASS

This section is based on drug classes included in the FDA's Center for Drug Evaluation and Research (CDER) National Drug Code Directory Major Drug Class database (http://www.fda.gov/cder/ndc), but is not limited to only this source.

BRAND NAMES

Drug names listed under brand names are U.S. brand names and branded generic names. The primary innovator brand name appears in bold-faced type. Also included among the brand names are international brand equivalents used in 137 countries. All U.S. brand names listed in this section will be found in the keyword index. All international brand names listed in this section will be found in the International Brand Name Index.

COST OF THERAPY

The Cost of Therapy section calculates a net cost based on prescribing information provided in the FDA-approved package insert. The basic assumptions used in calculating therapy cost are provided in the Cost of Therapy section. These include:

- Primary indication for which Cost of Therapy is being calculated.
- Dosage form and strength.
- Dosage rate.
- Total days supply.

In most cases, the dosage rate is based on the lowest oral dosage needed to treat the indication. In cases where drugs are figured on a mg/kg or BSA basis, an average adult weight of 70 kg and BSA of 1.85 m^2 was used to figure dosage rate. In all cases, average wholesale price is applied to these assumptions in order to calculate cost of therapy. When a generic drug is listed, the lowest cost generic available is used.

PRESCRIBING INFORMATION

Each monograph contains complete FDA-approved prescribing information for that drug organized into as many as 17 sections:

- Boxed Warning
- Description
- Clinical Pharmacology
- Clinical Studies
- Indications and Usage
- Contraindications
- Warnings
- Precautions
- Drug Interactions
- Adverse Reactions
- Drug Abuse and Dependence
- Overdosage
- Dosage and Administration
- Animal Pharmacology
- References
- How Supplied
- Product Listing

The prescribing information included in this section is the FDA-approved labeling found in the pharmaceutical manufacturer package inserts. In many cases, the monographs in this section are a combination of the prescribing information for different forms, routes, strengths, and indications.

In some of these combination cases only certain sections of the monograph pertain to all of the products. The first paragraph of the monograph will identify which forms, routes, and strengths are covered within which monograph section. If a drug is available in generic form, the monograph will usually refer to the drug by the generic name, or by an abbreviation of it. In some monographs it is necessary to use the brand name to avoid reader confusion. In other cases, the prescribing information varies so much by route within the same generic drug (e.g., albuterol), that separate; sub-monographs; for each route are required. In these cases, the sub-monographs are preceded by the appropriate route heading (e.g., Oral, Intranasal). All brand names used are the trademark and property of the various manufacturers and suppliers. Inactive ingredients are identified for the innovator brand form of the drug. The brand and their corresponding manufacturers are identified in the Product Listing section.

PRODUCT LISTINGS

Product information is grouped by Dosage Form, and Strength, and sorted by price within package size, giving the brand/product name used by the supplier, the supplier's FDA short name, and the product's official NDC (National Drug Code) number. Much of the information in these listings comes from MediSource Lexicon™.

In making prescribing decisions, and considering generic substitution, physicians can not only identify if generic alternatives are available, but also evaluate whether the cost differential between brands and generics justifies a possible risk in substitution. Furthermore, decisions about alternative drug entities can also be based partially on their economic impact.

Prices are AWP (Average Wholesale Price), a benchmark price used for reimbursement. AWP represents what a retail pharmacist or a dispensing physician might pay for a product, without any special discounts. There are, however, many discounts already in place, so the AWP can often approximate the price that a consumer might pay. The prices listed here are not intended to serve as an up-to-date substitute for supplier price lists. The price listings give the reader a good idea of the range between the high and low prices.

Special Note on AWP: While the AWP price is the closest thing to a benchmark price, and it is commonly used for reimbursement, it has many problems. First of all, no AWP from any source is truly an "average wholesale price." It is a price made up by the marketer of the drug. For example, with brand name drugs most manufacturers set AWP at 25% of their direct price, and the direct price is that published catalog price at which an independent pharmacy could buy before any special discounts. AWP is still commonly used for reimbursement of brand name products. For generic products, AWP will vary in relation to direct price, but the spread is usually greater than the 25% for brand products. As a result AWP greatly overstates the average wholesale costs of drugs. Very few health plans reimburse for generics based on AWP anymore, but instead use the HCFA Upper Limits price.

The HCFA Federal Upper Limits (the Health Care Financing Administration's Federal Financial Participation "upper limits" price for that package size) for each drug is listed along with the other listings by AWP. This is the price reimbursable by Medicare when reimbursement is available. Many states have also adopted this price for use in their Medicaid programs, and many insurance carriers use this price.

AWP is the most common price used for drug reimbursement, but the Federal Upper Limits reimbursement is increasingly being used by many plans to cover generics from any supplier rated equivalent. This is because AWP is usually much higher than the actual acquisition cost for a generic drug by a pharmacy.

In many states, the existence of a Federal Upper Limits price means that substitution is mandatory unless the prescribing physician specifies otherwise, and Medicaid reimburses the dispensing pharmacist at the Federal Upper Limits price plus a dispensing fee. Although the direct price at which pharmacies can purchase a drug is almost always less than the AWP, this difference tends to be much greater for generics than for brands. The Federal Upper Limits price is a better approximation of actual price for generics, and therefore, to estimate the difference in price between the generic and brand, the brand should be compared to the Federal Upper Limits, if one is given.

The NDC number is provided in 5-4-2 format. The labeler code, assigned by the FDA, is the first five digits of all product NDC numbers listed for this supplier. The rest of the NDC number includes four digits assigned by the supplier to identify their unique drug and two digits to identify the package size.

SUPPLIER PROFILES

The supplier profiles section can be used to obtain additional information on a particular supplier. The supplier profiles section serves as an easy reference guide for readers to make further inquiries on their own.

All suppliers in this section are listed alphabetically by their FDA Short Name. Beneath the FDA short name is the full company name, complete address and telephone number (with toll-free numbers where available) for inquiries about their products. Fax numbers and Internet web page addresses are listed, where available.

KEYWORD & INTERNATIONAL BRAND NAME INDEX

This section contains the most comprehensive index found in any drug reference. Information is cross-indexed to allow quick access to drug monographs; the inconvenience of multiple indices is eliminated.

The following features make up the unique Keyword Index:

- Key terms cross-indexed in alphabetical order
- Brand and generic names
- FDA approved indications
- FDA Drug Class

The following features make up the International Brand Name Index:

- Thousands of foreign brand names indexed to the corresponding US-approved generic drug monograph.
- Country of origin for international brand name listed in the monograph.

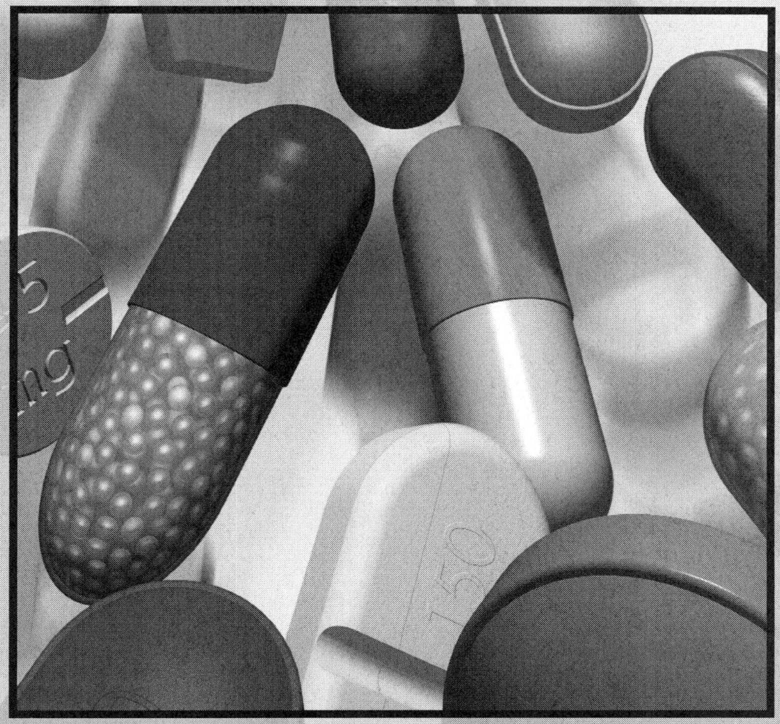

CATEGORY/BRAND Generic name	Page no.

ARTICULOSE-L.A.
Triamcinolone Diacetate II-2711

ASACOL
Mesalamine II-1748

ASCARIASIS
Mebendazole II-1711
Thiabendazole II-2601

ASCITES
Spironolactone II-2483

ASCOMP W/CODEINE
Aspirin; Butalbital; Caffeine; Codeine Phosphate II-208

ASCORBIC ACID
Ascorbic Acid II-203

ASCORBIC ACID DEFICIENCY
Ascorbic Acid II-203

ASENDIN
Amoxapine II-129

ASMALIX
Theophylline II-2593

ASPARAGINASE
Asparaginase II-204

A-SPAS
Dicyclomine Hydrochloride II-763

A-SPAS S L
Hyoscyamine Sulfate II-1404

ASPERGILLOSIS
Amphotericin B II-157
Caspofungin Acetate II-443
Itraconazole II-1517
Voriconazole II-2796

ASPIRIN
Aspirin II-206
Aspirin; Butalbital; Caffeine II-207
Aspirin; Butalbital; Caffeine; Codeine Phosphate II-208
Aspirin; Caffeine; Dihydrocodeine Bitartrate II-208
Aspirin; Caffeine; Propoxyphene Hydrochloride II-209
Aspirin; Codeine Phosphate II-210
Aspirin; Dipyridamole II-210
Aspirin; Hydrocodone Bitartrate II-214
Aspirin; Oxycodone Hydrochloride; Oxycodone Terephthalate II-214

ASPIRIN W/CODEINE
Aspirin; Codeine Phosphate II-210

ASPRO
Aspirin II-206

ASTELIN
Azelastine II-247

ASTHMA
Albuterol II-47
Aminophylline II-106
Beclomethasone Dipropionate II-279
Betamethasone II-298

ASTHMA—cont'd
Betamethasone Acetate; Betamethasone Sodium Phosphate II-299
Bitolterol Mesylate II-327
Budesonide II-347
Cortisone Acetate II-654
Cromolyn Sodium II-656
Dexamethasone II-730
Dexamethasone Acetate II-734
Epinephrine II-934
Flunisolide II-1149
Fluticasone Propionate II-1182
Fluticasone Propionate; Salmeterol Xinafoate II-1197
Formoterol Fumarate II-1214
Hydrocortisone II-1369
Hydrocortisone Sodium Succinate II-1379
Isoetharine Hydrochloride II-1495
Isoproterenol Hydrochloride II-1498
Levalbuterol Hydrochloride II-1595
Metaproterenol Sulfate II-1754
Methylprednisolone II-1787
Methylprednisolone Acetate II-1790
Methylprednisolone Sodium Succinate II-1793
Montelukast Sodium II-1872
Nedocromil Sodium II-1937
Omalizumab II-2032
Pirbuterol Acetate II-2203
Prednisolone II-2233
Prednisolone Sodium Phosphate II-2236
Prednisone II-2240
Salmeterol Xinafoate II-2410
Terbutaline Sulfate II-2574
Theophylline II-2593
Triamcinolone II-2698
Triamcinolone Acetonide II-2701
Triamcinolone Diacetate II-2711
Zafirlukast II-2809
Zileuton II-2830

ASTRAMORPH-PF
Morphine Sulfate II-1877

ASTROCYTOMA
Carmustine II-434
Temozolomide II-2558

ATACAND
Candesartan Cilexetil II-402

ATACAND HCT
Candesartan Cilexetil; Hydrochlorothiazide II-404

ATAMET
Carbidopa; Levodopa II-424

ATARAX
Hydroxyzine II-1398

ATARIN
Acetaminophen; Dichloralphenazone; Isometheptene Mucate II-16

ATAZANAVIR SULFATE
Atazanavir Sulfate II-215

ATELECTASIS, SECONDARY TO MUCUS OBSTRUCTION
Acetylcysteine II-29

ATENOLOL
Atenolol II-222
Atenolol; Chlorthalidone II-226

ATENOLOL W/CHLORTHALIDONE
Atenolol; Chlorthalidone II-226

ATGAM
Lymphocyte Immune Globulin II-1705

ATHERECTOMY, ADJUNCT
Abciximab II-6

ATHEROSCLEROSIS
Fluvastatin Sodium II-1199
Lovastatin II-1688
Pravastatin Sodium II-2224

ATHETOSIS
Diazepam II-740

ATIVAN
Lorazepam II-1678

ATOMOXETINE HYDROCHLORIDE
Atomoxetine Hydrochloride II-227

ATORVASTATIN CALCIUM
Atorvastatin Calcium II-231

ATOVAQUONE
Atovaquone II-234
Atovaquone; Proguanil Hydrochloride II-235

ATRETOL
Carbamazepine II-418

ATROMID-S
Clofibrate II-619

ATROPAIR
Atropine Sulfate II-235

ATROPEN
Atropine Sulfate II-235

ATROPHY, VAGINAL
Estradiol II-986
Estradiol Acetate II-1000
Estradiol; Norethindrone Acetate II-1011
Estradiol-17β; Norgestimate II-1008
Estrogens, Conjugated II-1019
Estrogens, Conjugated; Medroxyprogesterone Acetate II-1027
Estropipate II-1033

ATROPHY, VULVAR
Estradiol II-986
Estradiol Acetate II-1000
Estradiol; Norethindrone Acetate II-1011
Estradiol-17β; Norgestimate II-1008
Estrogens, Conjugated II-1019
Estrogens, Conjugated; Medroxyprogesterone Acetate II-1027
Estropipate II-1033

ATROPINE
Atropine; Hyoscyamine; Phenobarbital; Scopolamine II-239
Atropine Sulfate II-235
Atropine Sulfate; Diphenoxylate Hydrochloride II-238

ATROPISOL
Atropine Sulfate II-235

CATEGORY/BRAND Generic name	Page no.
ATROVENT	
Ipratropium Bromide	II-1480
ATTENTION DEFICIT HYPERACTIVITY DISORDER	
Amphetamine; Dextroamphetamine	II-153
Atomoxetine Hydrochloride	II-227
Dexmethylphenidate Hydrochloride	II-737
Methylphenidate Hydrochloride	II-1781
Pemoline	II-2129
ATTENUVAX	
Measles Virus Vaccine Live	II-1708
AUGMENTIN	
Amoxicillin; Clavulanate Potassium	II-139
AUGMENTIN XR	
Amoxicillin; Clavulanate Potassium	II-139
AURAFAIR	
Antipyrine; Benzocaine	II-187
AURAL ACUTE	
Hydrocortisone; Neomycin Sulfate; Polymyxin B Sulfate	II-1384
AURALGAN	
Antipyrine; Benzocaine	II-187
AURANOFIN	
Auranofin	II-241
AURODEX	
Antipyrine; Benzocaine	II-187
AUROLATE	
Gold Sodium Thiomalate	II-1304
AUROMID	
Antipyrine; Benzocaine	II-187
AUROTHIOGLUCOSE	
Aurothioglucose	II-242
AUROTO	
Antipyrine; Benzocaine	II-187
AVAGE	
Tazarotene	II-2547
AVALIDE	
Hydrochlorothiazide; Irbesartan	II-1351
AVANDAMET	
Metformin Hydrochloride; Rosiglitazone Maleate	II-1764
AVANDIA	
Rosiglitazone Maleate	II-2405
AVAPRO	
Irbesartan	II-1484
AVAXIM	
Hepatitis A Vaccine	II-1339
AVELOX	
Moxifloxacin Hydrochloride	II-1886
AVITA	
Tretinoin	II-2691
AVODART	
Dutasteride	II-897
AVONEX	
Interferon Beta-1a	II-1477
AXERT	
Almotriptan Malate	II-82
AXID	
Nizatidine	II-1992
AZACTAM	
Aztreonam	II-263
AZALINE	
Sulfasalazine	II-2507
AZATADINE MALEATE	
Azatadine Maleate	II-242
AZATHIOPRINE	
Azathioprine	II-243
AZDONE	
Aspirin; Hydrocodone Bitartrate	II-214
AZELAIC ACID	
Azelaic Acid	II-245
AZELASTINE	
Azelastine	II-247
AZELEX	
Azelaic Acid	II-245
AZITHROMYCIN	
Azithromycin	II-250
AZMACORT	
Triamcinolone Acetonide	II-2701
AZOMID	
Acetazolamide	II-28
AZOPT	
Brinzolamide	II-343
AZT	
Zidovudine	II-2822
AZTREONAM	
Aztreonam	II-263
AZULFIDINE	
Sulfasalazine	II-2507
B-12-1000	
Cyanocobalamin	II-661
B-A-C #3	
Aspirin; Butalbital; Caffeine; Codeine Phosphate	II-208
BACLOFEN	
Baclofen	II-266
BACTEREMIA	
Penicillin G Potassium	II-2137
Penicillin G Procaine	II-2140
Piperacillin Sodium	II-2196
Piperacillin Sodium; Tazobactam Sodium	II-2199
Ticarcillin Disodium	II-2616
BACTEREMIA, SECONDARY TO TOOTH EXTRACTION, PREVENTION	
Penicillin G Potassium	II-2137
BACTERIURIA, ASYMPTOMATIC	
Carbenicillin Indanyl Sodium	II-422
BACTICORT	
Hydrocortisone; Neomycin Sulfate; Polymyxin B Sulfate	II-1384
BACTOCILL	
Oxacillin Sodium	II-2053
BACTRIM	
Sulfamethoxazole; Trimethoprim	II-2500
BACTROBAN	
Mupirocin	II-1894
BAL	
Dimercaprol	II-811
BALSALAZIDE DISODIUM	
Balsalazide Disodium	II-272
BANAN	
Cefpodoxime Proxetil	II-484
BANCAP	
Acetaminophen; Butalbital	II-12
BANCAP-HC	
Acetaminophen; Hydrocodone Bitartrate	II-17
BANFLEX	
Orphenadrine Citrate	II-2049
BANOPHEN	
Diphenhydramine Hydrochloride	II-813
BANQUIN	
Hydroquinone	II-1391
BARBIDONNA	
Atropine; Hyoscyamine; Phenobarbital; Scopolamine	II-239
BARBITURATES	
Acetaminophen; Butalbital	II-12
Acetaminophen; Butalbital; Caffeine; Codeine Phosphate	II-12
Methohexital Sodium	II-1770
Pentobarbital Sodium	II-2149
Phenobarbital	II-2167
Secobarbital Sodium	II-2435
Thiopental Sodium	II-2603
BARSTATIN	
Nystatin	II-2005
BARTONELLOSIS	
Doxycycline	II-878
Minocycline Hydrochloride	II-1838
BASILIXIMAB	
Basiliximab	II-273
BCG LIVE	
BCG Live	II-275
BCG VACCINE	
BCG Vaccine	II-276
BECAPLERMIN	
Becaplermin	II-277
BECLOMETHASONE DIPROPIONATE	
Beclomethasone Dipropionate	II-279
BECLOVENT	
Beclomethasone Dipropionate	II-279

CATEGORY/BRAND Generic name	Page no.
BECONASE	
Beclomethasone Dipropionate	II-279
BECONASE AQ	
Beclomethasone Dipropionate	II-279
BECOTIDE	
Beclomethasone Dipropionate	II-279
BEEPEN-VK	
Penicillin V Potassium	II-2142
BEESIX	
Pyridoxine Hydrochloride	II-2297
BEHAVIOR DISORDER	
Thioridazine Hydrochloride	II-2605
BEJEL	
Penicillin G Benzathine	II-2136
Penicillin G Procaine	II-2140
BELDIN	
Diphenhydramine Hydrochloride	II-813
BELIX	
Diphenhydramine Hydrochloride	II-813
BELOC	
Acebutolol Hydrochloride	II-10
BENADRYL	
Diphenhydramine Hydrochloride	II-813
BENAHIST	
Diphenhydramine Hydrochloride	II-813
BENAZEPRIL HYDROCHLORIDE	
Amlodipine Besylate; Benazepril Hydrochloride	II-127
Benazepril Hydrochloride	II-284
Benazepril Hydrochloride; Hydrochlorothiazide	II-288
BENEMID	
Probenecid	II-2248
BENICAR	
Olmesartan Medoxomil	II-2028
BENTYL	
Dicyclomine Hydrochloride	II-763
BENZACLIN	
Benzoyl Peroxide; Clindamycin	II-291
BENZACOT	
Trimethobenzamide Hydrochloride	II-2721
BENZAMYCIN	
Benzoyl Peroxide; Erythromycin	II-292
BENZATHINE BENZYLPENICILLIN	
Penicillin G Benzathine	II-2136
BENZOCAINE	
Antipyrine; Benzocaine	II-187
Benzocaine	II-289
Benzocaine; Butamben Picrate; Tetracaine	II-290
BENZODIAZEPINES	
Alprazolam	II-85
Amitriptyline Hydrochloride; Chlordiazepoxide	II-123
Chlordiazepoxide Hydrochloride	II-539

CATEGORY/BRAND Generic name	Page no.
BENZODIAZEPINES—cont'd	
Chlordiazepoxide Hydrochloride; Clidinium Bromide	II-541
Clonazepam	II-625
Clorazepate Dipotassium	II-638
Diazepam	II-740
Estazolam	II-983
Flurazepam Hydrochloride	II-1175
Lorazepam	II-1678
Midazolam Hydrochloride	II-1823
Oxazepam	II-2063
Quazepam	II-2298
Temazepam	II-2556
Triazolam	II-2715
BENZONATATE	
Benzonatate	II-290
BENZOTIC	
Antipyrine; Benzocaine	II-187
BENZOYL PEROXIDE	
Benzoyl Peroxide; Clindamycin	II-291
Benzoyl Peroxide; Erythromycin	II-292
BENZTROPINE MESYLATE	
Benztropine Mesylate	II-293
BEPRIDIL HYDROCHLORIDE	
Bepridil Hydrochloride	II-295
BERIBERI	
Thiamine Hydrochloride	II-2602
BERUBIGEN	
Cyanocobalamin	II-661
BERYLLIOSIS	
Betamethasone	II-298
Betamethasone Acetate; Betamethasone Sodium Phosphate	II-299
Cortisone Acetate	II-654
Dexamethasone	II-730
Dexamethasone Acetate	II-734
Hydrocortisone	II-1369
Hydrocortisone Sodium Succinate	II-1379
Methylprednisolone	II-1787
Methylprednisolone Acetate	II-1790
Methylprednisolone Sodium Succinate	II-1793
Prednisolone	II-2233
Prednisolone Sodium Phosphate	II-2236
Prednisone	II-2240
Triamcinolone	II-2698
Triamcinolone Acetonide	II-2701
Triamcinolone Diacetate	II-2711
BETA-2	
Isoetharine Hydrochloride	II-1495
BETADERM	
Betamethasone	II-298
Betamethasone Valerate	II-305
BETAFERON	
Interferon Beta-1b, Recombinant	II-1478
BETAGAN	
Levobunolol Hydrochloride	II-1603
BETA-HC	
Hydrocortisone	II-1369
BETALIN 12	
Cyanocobalamin	II-661

CATEGORY/BRAND Generic name	Page no.
BETALIN S	
Thiamine Hydrochloride	II-2602
BETALOC	
Metoprolol	II-1805
BETAMETHACOT	
Betamethasone Valerate	II-305
BETAMETHASONE	
Betamethasone	II-298
Betamethasone Acetate; Betamethasone Sodium Phosphate	II-299
Betamethasone Dipropionate	II-301
Betamethasone Dipropionate; Clotrimazole	II-304
Betamethasone Valerate	II-305
BETANATE	
Betamethasone Dipropionate	II-301
BETAPACE	
Sotalol Hydrochloride	II-2471
BETASERON	
Interferon Beta-1b, Recombinant	II-1478
BETATREX	
Betamethasone Valerate	II-305
BETA-VAL	
Betamethasone Valerate	II-305
BETAXOLOL HYDROCHLORIDE	
Betaxolol Hydrochloride	II-307
BETHANECHOL CHLORIDE	
Bethanechol Chloride	II-312
BETHAPRIM	
Sulfamethoxazole; Trimethoprim	II-2500
BETIMOL	
Timolol	II-2627
Travoprost	II-2685
BETNOVATE	
Betamethasone Valerate	II-305
BETOPTIC	
Betaxolol Hydrochloride	II-307
BETOPTIC S	
Betaxolol Hydrochloride	II-307
BEXAROTENE	
Bexarotene	II-313
BEXTRA	
Valdecoxib	II-2741
BIAMINE	
Thiamine Hydrochloride	II-2602
BIAVAX II	
Mumps and Rubella Virus Vaccine Live	II-1892
BIAXIN	
Clarithromycin	II-597
BICALUTAMIDE	
Bicalutamide	II-318
BICILLIN L-A	
Penicillin G Benzathine	II-2136
BICNU	
Carmustine	II-434

CATEGORY/BRAND
Generic name — Page no.

CATEGORY/BRAND
Generic name — Page no.

CATEGORY/BRAND
Generic name — Page no.

CATEGORY/BRAND
Generic name — Page no.

GEMFIBROZIL
Gemfibrozil II-1269

GEMIFLOXACIN MESYLATE
Gemifloxacin Mesylate II-1273

GEMTUZUMAB OZOGAMICIN
Gemtuzumab Ozogamicin II-1278

GEMZAR
Gemcitabine Hydrochloride II-1265

GENASPORIN H.C.
Hydrocortisone; Neomycin Sulfate; Polymyxin B Sulfate II-1384

GENCEPT
Ethinyl Estradiol; Norethindrone II-1055

GENERALIZED ANXIETY DISORDER
See Anxiety Disorder, Generalized

GENERLAC
Lactulose II-1550

GENITAL ULCER DISEASE
Azithromycin II-250

GENOPTIC
Gentamicin Sulfate II-1279

GENORA
Ethinyl Estradiol; Norethindrone II-1055

GENOX
Tamoxifen Citrate II-2539

GENTACIDIN
Gentamicin Sulfate II-1279

GENTAK
Gentamicin Sulfate II-1279

GENTAMICIN SULFATE
Gentamicin Sulfate II-1279

GENTASOL
Gentamicin Sulfate II-1279

GEN-XENE
Clorazepate Dipotassium II-638

GEODON
Ziprasidone II-2833

GERD
See Gastroesophigeal Reflux Disease

GESTEROL 50
Progesterone II-2262

GIARDIASIS
Nitazoxanide II-1978

GINGIVITIS
Chlorhexidine Gluconate II-542

GLATIRAMER ACETATE
Glatiramer Acetate II-1284

GLAUCOMA, ANGLE-CLOSURE
Acetazolamide II-28
Pilocarpine II-2180

GLAUCOMA, OPEN-ANGLE
Acetazolamide II-28
Apraclonidine Hydrochloride II-188
Betaxolol Hydrochloride II-307
Bimatoprost II-320

CATEGORY/BRAND
Generic name — Page no.

GLAUCOMA, OPEN-ANGLE—cont'd
Brimonidine Tartrate II-340
Brinzolamide II-343
Carteolol Hydrochloride II-435
Dipivefrin Hydrochloride II-820
Dorzolamide Hydrochloride II-858
Dorzolamide Hydrochloride; Timolol Maleate II-860
Epinephrine II-934
Latanoprost II-1574
Levobunolol Hydrochloride II-1603
Pilocarpine II-2180
Timolol II-2627
Travoprost II-2685
Unoprostone Isopropyl II-2732

GLAUCOMA, SECONDARY
Acetazolamide II-28
Unoprostone Isopropyl II-2732

GLAUCON
Epinephrine II-934

GLEEVEC
Imatinib Mesylate II-1421

GLIMEL
Glyburide II-1297

GLIMEPIRIDE
Glimepiride II-1287

GLIOBLASTOMA
Carmustine II-434

GLIOMA, BRAINSTEM
Carmustine II-434

GLIPIZIDE
Glipizide II-1290
Glipizide; Metformin Hydrochloride II-1294

GLUCAGEN
Glucagon (rDNA origin) II-1296

GLUCAGON (RDNA ORIGIN)
Glucagon (rDNA origin) II-1296

GLUCOPHAGE
Metformin Hydrochloride II-1760

GLUCOTROL
Glipizide II-1290

GLUCOTROL XL
Glipizide II-1290

GLUCOVANCE
Glyburide; Metformin Hydrochloride II-1300

GLYBURIDE
Glyburide II-1297
Glyburide; Metformin Hydrochloride II-1300

GLYCOPYRROLATE
Benztropine Mesylate II-293
Glycopyrrolate II-1302

GLYCORT
Hydrocortisone II-1369

GLYNASE
Glyburide II-1297

GLYSET
Miglitol II-1836

CATEGORY/BRAND
Generic name — Page no.

GM-CSF
Sargramostim II-2428

G-MYCIN
Gentamicin Sulfate II-1279

GOITER
Levothyroxine Sodium II-1618

GOLD COMPOUNDS
Auranofin II-241
Aurothioglucose II-242
Gold Sodium Thiomalate II-1304

GOLD SODIUM THIOMALATE
Gold Sodium Thiomalate II-1304

GONORRHEA
Amoxicillin II-131
Ampicillin II-170
Ampicillin Sodium II-172
Cefixime II-466
Cefotaxime Sodium II-474
Cefoxitin Sodium II-482
Cefpodoxime Proxetil II-484
Ceftizoxime Sodium II-500
Ceftriaxone Sodium II-503
Cefuroxime II-507
Ciprofloxacin Hydrochloride II-573
Demeclocycline Hydrochloride II-714
Doxycycline II-878
Gatifloxacin II-1255
Minocycline Hydrochloride II-1838
Norfloxacin II-1997
Ofloxacin II-2015
Penicillin G Potassium II-2137
Penicillin G Procaine II-2140
Piperacillin Sodium II-2196
Piperacillin Sodium; Tazobactam Sodium II-2199
Tetracycline Hydrochloride II-2585
Trovafloxacin Mesylate II-2731

GOSERELIN ACETATE
Goserelin Acetate II-1304

GOUT
Allopurinol II-77
Betamethasone II-298
Betamethasone Acetate; Betamethasone Sodium Phosphate II-299
Colchicine II-649
Cortisone Acetate II-654
Dexamethasone II-730
Dexamethasone Acetate II-734
Hydrocortisone II-1369
Hydrocortisone Acetate II-1373
Hydrocortisone Sodium Succinate II-1379
Indomethacin II-1443
Methylprednisolone II-1787
Methylprednisolone Acetate II-1790
Methylprednisolone Sodium Succinate II-1793
Naproxen II-1924
Naproxen Sodium II-1928
Prednisolone II-2233
Prednisolone Sodium Phosphate II-2236
Prednisone II-2240
Probenecid II-2248
Sulindac II-2512
Triamcinolone II-2698

CATEGORY/BRAND Generic name — Page no.

HEMATINICS—cont'd
Folic Acid II-1208
Sodium Ferric Gluconate II-2464

HEMATOPOIETIC AGENTS
Darbepoetin alfa II-703
Epoetin Alfa II-942
Filgrastim II-1126
Oprelvekin II-2044
Pegfilgrastim II-2120
Sargramostim II-2428

HEMOPHILIA A
Desmopressin Acetate II-723

HEMORRHAGE, POSTPARTUM
Oxytocin II-2082

HEMORRHAGE, SUBARACHNOID
Hemorrhage, Upper Gastrointestinal, Prophylaxis Cimetidine Hydrochloride II-568
Nimodipine II-1974

HEMORRHAGE, UTERINE
Medroxyprogesterone Acetate II-1714
Progesterone II-2262

HEMORRHAGIC DISEASE OF THE NEWBORN
Phytonadione II-2178

HEMORRHEOLOGIC AGENTS
Pentoxifylline II-2154

HEMORRHOIDAL HC
Hydrocortisone Acetate II-1373

HEMORRHOIDS
Hydrocortisone Acetate II-1373

HEMOSTATICS
Phytonadione II-2178

HEMRIL-HC
Hydrocortisone Acetate II-1373

HEMSOL-HC
Hydrocortisone Acetate II-1373

HEPARIN FLUSH
Heparin Sodium II-1334

HEPARIN LOK-PAK
Heparin Sodium II-1334

HEPARIN, LOW WEIGHT
Enoxaparin Sodium II-927

HEPARIN PORCINE
Heparin Sodium II-1334

HEPARIN SODIUM
Heparin Sodium II-1334

HEPATITIS A, IMMUNIZATION
See Immunization, Hepatitis A

HEPATITIS A INACTIVATED
Hepatitis A Inactivated; Hepatitis B (Recombinant) Vaccine II-1338

HEPATITIS A, PROPHYLAXIS
Immune Globulin (Human) II-1434

HEPATITIS A VACCINE
Hepatitis A Vaccine II-1339

HEPATITIS B
Adefovir Dipivoxil II-43
Interferon Alfa-2b, Recombinant II-1471
Lamivudine II-1552

HEPATITIS B IMMUNE GLOBULIN
Hepatitis B Immune Globulin II-1341

HEPATITIS B, IMMUNIZATION
See Immunization, Hepatitis B

HEPATITIS B, POST-EXPOSURE PROPHYLAXIS
Hepatitis B Immune Globulin II-1341

HEPATITIS B (RECOMBINANT) AND INACTIVATED POLIOVIRUS VACCINE COMBINED
Diphtheria and Tetanus Toxoids and Acellular Pertussis Adsorbed; Hepatitis B (Recombinant) and Inactivated Poliovirus Vaccine Combined II-815

HEPATITIS B (RECOMBINANT) VACCINE
Hepatitis A Inactivated; Hepatitis B (Recombinant) Vaccine II-1338

HEPATITIS B VACCINE
Haemophilus B Conjugate Vaccine; Hepatitis B Vaccine II-1326

HEPATITIS B VACCINE, RECOMBINANT
Hepatitis B Vaccine, Recombinant II-1343

HEPATITIS C
Interferon Alfa-2b, Recombinant II-1471
Interferon Alfa-2b; Ribavirin II-1474
Interferon Alfacon-1 II-1477
Peginterferon alfa-2a II-2122
Ribavirin II-2351

HEP-B-GAMMAGEE
Hepatitis B Immune Globulin II-1341

HEPFLUSH
Heparin Sodium II-1334

HEPSERA
Adefovir Dipivoxil II-43

HEPTALAC
Lactulose II-1550

HERCEPTIN
Trastuzumab II-2683

HERPES GENITALIS
Acyclovir II-33
Famciclovir II-1090
Valacyclovir Hydrochloride II-2738

HERPES LABIALIS
Acyclovir II-33
Penciclovir II-2131
Valacyclovir Hydrochloride II-2738

HERPES SIMPLEX ENCEPHALITIS
Acyclovir II-33

HERPES ZOSTER
Acyclovir II-33
Famciclovir II-1090
Valacyclovir Hydrochloride II-2738

HERPES ZOSTER OPHTHALMICUS
Betamethasone II-298
Betamethasone Acetate; Betamethasone Sodium Phosphate II-299
Cortisone Acetate II-654
Dexamethasone II-730
Dexamethasone Acetate II-734
Hydrocortisone II-1369
Hydrocortisone Sodium Succinate II-1379
Methylprednisolone II-1787
Methylprednisolone Acetate II-1790
Methylprednisolone Sodium Succinate II-1793
Prednisolone II-2233
Prednisolone Acetate II-2235
Prednisolone Sodium Phosphate II-2236
Prednisone II-2240
Triamcinolone II-2698
Triamcinolone Acetonide II-2701
Triamcinolone Diacetate II-2711

HEXA-BETALIN
Pyridoxine Hydrochloride II-2297

HEXADROL
Dexamethasone II-730

HEXALEN
Altretamine II-96

HIBTITER
Haemophilus B Conjugate Vaccine II-1325

HICCUPS, INTRACTABLE
Chlorpromazine Hydrochloride II-549

HI-COR
Hydrocortisone II-1369

HIDROMAR
Hydrocortisone II-1369

HISTALET X
Guaifenesin; Pseudoephedrine Hydrochloride II-1316

HISTEX
Chlorpheniramine Maleate II-548

HISTEX PD
Carbinoxamine Maleate II-429

HISTIOCYTOSIS X
Vinblastine Sulfate II-2787

HISTOPLASMOSIS
Amphotericin B II-157
Itraconazole II-1517
Ketoconazole II-1530

HISTOPLASMOSIS, OCULAR
Verteporfin II-2784

HIV INFECTION
See Infection, Human Immunodeficiency Virus

HIVID
Zalcitabine II-2812

HMG COA REDUCTASE INHIBITORS
Atorvastatin Calcium II-231
Fluvastatin Sodium II-1199
Lovastatin II-1688
Lovastatin; Niacin II-1698
Pravastatin Sodium II-2224
Simvastatin II-2454

CATEGORY/BRAND Generic name	Page no.
HODGKIN'S DISEASE	
See Lymphoma, Hodgkin's	
HOLOXAN	
Ifosfamide	II-1420
HOOKWORM	
Mebendazole	II-1711
Thiabendazole	II-2601
HORMONES/HORMONE MODIFIERS	
Anastrozole	II-186
Bicalutamide	II-318
Cabergoline	II-395
Calcitonin (Salmon)	II-397
Chlorotrianisene	II-547
Danazol	II-699
Darbepoetin alfa	II-703
Desmopressin Acetate	II-723
Desogestrel; Ethinyl Estradiol	II-725
Diethylstilbestrol Diphosphate	II-776
Dutasteride	II-897
Epoetin Alfa	II-942
Estradiol	II-986
Estradiol Acetate	II-1000
Estradiol Cypionate; Medroxyprogesterone Acetate	II-1003
Estradiol; Norethindrone Acetate	II-1011
Estradiol-17; Norgestimate	II-1008
Estramustine Phosphate Sodium	II-1017
Estrogens, Conjugated	II-1019
Estrogens, Conjugated; Medroxyprogesterone Acetate	II-1027
Estrogens, Esterified; Methyltestosterone	II-1031
Estropipate	II-1033
Ethinyl Estradiol	II-1040
Ethinyl Estradiol; Ethynodiol Diacetate	II-1042
Ethinyl Estradiol; Ferrous Fumarate; Norethindrone Acetate	II-1042
Ethinyl Estradiol; Levonorgestrel	II-1047
Ethinyl Estradiol; Norelgestromin	II-1050
Ethinyl Estradiol; Norethindrone	II-1055
Ethinyl Estradiol; Norgestimate	II-1059
Ethinyl Estradiol; Norgestrel	II-1068
Exemestane	II-1085
Finasteride	II-1129
Flutamide	II-1181
Fulvestrant	II-1235
Glucagon (rDNA origin)	II-1296
Goserelin Acetate	II-1304
Letrozole	II-1582
Leuprolide Acetate	II-1587
Levonorgestrel	II-1614
Levothyroxine Sodium	II-1618
Medroxyprogesterone Acetate	II-1714
Megestrol Acetate	II-1723
Methimazole	II-1767
Methyltestosterone	II-1796
Nafarelin Acetate	II-1914
Nilutamide	II-1972
Norethindrone	II-1996
Norgestrel	II-2002
Octreotide Acetate	II-2009
Oxytocin	II-2082
Pegvisomant	II-2126
Progesterone	II-2262
Propylthiouracil	II-2293

CATEGORY/BRAND Generic name	Page no.
HORMONES/HORMONE MODIFIERS—cont'd	
Raloxifene Hydrochloride	II-2326
Tamoxifen Citrate	II-2539
Teriparatide (rDNA origin)	II-2578
Testolactone	II-2581
Testosterone Cypionate	II-2581
Toremifene Citrate	II-2669
Triptorelin Pamoate	II-2727
Vasopressin	II-2769
HUMALOG	
Insulin Lispro (Human Analog)	II-1464
HUMAN IMMUNODEFICIENCY VIRUS INFECTION	
See Infection, Human Immunodeficiency Virus	
HUMIBID L.A.	
Guaifenesin	II-1314
HUMIRA	
Adalimumab	II-39
HUMULIN	
Insulin (Human Recombinant)	II-1454
HUMULIN 50 50	
Insulin (Human, Isophane/Regular)	II-1456
HUMULIN 70 30	
Insulin (Human, Isophane/Regular)	II-1456
HUMULIN BR	
Insulin (Human Recombinant)	II-1454
HUMULIN L	
Insulin (Human, Lente)	II-1456
HUMULIN N	
Insulin (Human, Isophane)	II-1455
HUMULIN NPH	
Insulin (Human, Isophane)	II-1455
HUMULIN R	
Insulin (Human Recombinant)	II-1454
HUMULIN U	
Insulin (Human, Lente)	II-1456
HYALURONIC ACID DERIVATIVES	
Hylan G-F 20	II-1403
HYCAMTIN	
Topotecan Hydrochloride	II-2666
HYCO	
Hyoscyamine Sulfate	II-1404
HYCOMED	
Acetaminophen; Hydrocodone Bitartrate	II-17
HYCO-PAP	
Acetaminophen; Hydrocodone Bitartrate	II-17
HYDANTOINS	
Fosphenytoin Sodium	II-1228
Phenytoin Sodium	II-2175
HYDATIDIFORM MOLE	
Methotrexate Sodium	II-1772
HYDELTRASOL	
Prednisolone Sodium Phosphate	II-2236

CATEGORY/BRAND Generic name	Page no.
HYDRALAZINE HYDROCHLORIDE	
Hydralazine Hydrochloride	II-1346
HYDRAMINE	
Diphenhydramine Hydrochloride	II-813
HYDREA	
Hydroxyurea	II-1394
HYDRENE	
Hydrochlorothiazide; Triamterene	II-1362
HYDRIL	
Diphenhydramine Hydrochloride	II-813
HYDRO PAR	
Hydrochlorothiazide	II-1348
HYDROCET	
Acetaminophen; Hydrocodone Bitartrate	II-17
HYDROCHLOROTHIAZIDE	
Amiloride Hydrochloride; Hydrochlorothiazide	II-105
Benazepril Hydrochloride; Hydrochlorothiazide	II-288
Bisoprolol Fumarate; Hydrochlorothiazide	II-326
Candesartan Cilexetil; Hydrochlorothiazide	II-404
Captopril; Hydrochlorothiazide	II-416
Enalapril Maleate; Hydrochlorothiazide	II-923
Eprosartan Mesylate; Hydrochlorothiazide	II-950
Fosinopril Sodium; Hydrochlorothiazide	II-1226
Hydrochlorothiazide	II-1348
Hydrochlorothiazide; Irbesartan	II-1351
Hydrochlorothiazide; Lisinopril	II-1352
Hydrochlorothiazide; Losartan Potassium	II-1354
Hydrochlorothiazide; Metoprolol Tartrate	II-1355
Hydrochlorothiazide; Moexipril Hydrochloride	II-1355
Hydrochlorothiazide; Propranolol Hydrochloride	II-1357
Hydrochlorothiazide; Quinapril Hydrochloride	II-1359
Hydrochlorothiazide; Telmisartan	II-1360
Hydrochlorothiazide; Timolol Maleate	II-1361
Hydrochlorothiazide; Triamterene	II-1362
Hydrochlorothiazide; Valsartan	II-1366
HYDROCODONE BITARTRATE	
Acetaminophen; Hydrocodone Bitartrate	II-17
Aspirin; Hydrocodone Bitartrate	II-214
Hydrocodone Bitartrate; Ibuprofen	II-1367
HYDROCORTEN-A	
Hydrocortisone Acetate	II-1373
HYDROCORTISONE	
Ciprofloxacin Hydrochloride; Hydrocortisone	II-588
Hydrocortisone	II-1369
Hydrocortisone Acetate	II-1373
Hydrocortisone Sodium Succinate	II-1379
Hydrocortisone Valerate	II-1382

CATEGORY/BRAND
Generic name — Page no.

NORIMIN
Ethinyl Estradiol; Norethindrone II-1055
NORINYL
Ethinyl Estradiol; Norethindrone II-1055
NORISODRINE
Isoproterenol Hydrochloride II-1498
NORITATE
Metronidazole II-1812
NORLESTRIN
Ethinyl Estradiol; Norethindrone II-1055
NORLESTRIN FE
Ethinyl Estradiol; Ferrous Fumarate; Norethindrone Acetate II-1042
NORLUTIN
Norethindrone II-1996
NORMODYNE
Labetalol Hydrochloride II-1545
NOROCAINE
Epinephrine; Lidocaine Hydrochloride II-938
Lidocaine Hydrochloride II-1632
NOROXIN
Norfloxacin II-1997
NORPACE
Disopyramide Phosphate II-825
NORPACE CR
Disopyramide Phosphate II-825
NORPHYL
Aminophylline II-106
NORPLANT
Levonorgestrel II-1614
NORPRAMIN
Desipramine Hydrochloride II-716
NOR-PRED S
Prednisolone Sodium Phosphate II-2236
NOR-QD
Norethindrone II-1996
NORQUEST FE
Ethinyl Estradiol; Ferrous Fumarate; Norethindrone Acetate II-1042
NORTRIPTYLINE HYDROCHLORIDE
Nortriptyline Hydrochloride II-2002
NORTRON
Dirithromycin II-824
NORVASC
Amlodipine Besylate II-125
NORVIR
Ritonavir II-2380
NOVANTRONE
Mitoxantrone Hydrochloride II-1856
NOVOCAIN
Procaine Hydrochloride II-2253
NOVOLIN 70 30
Insulin (Human, Isophane/Regular) II-1456

CATEGORY/BRAND
Generic name — Page no.

NOVOLIN 70 30 PENFILL
Insulin (Human Recombinant) II-1454
NOVOLIN L
Insulin (Human, Lente) II-1456
NOVOLIN N
Insulin (Human, Isophane) II-1455
NOVOLIN N PENFILL
Insulin (Human Recombinant) II-1454
NOVOLIN R
Insulin (Human Recombinant) II-1454
NOVOLOG
Insulin Aspart II-1456
NOVOLOG MIX 70/30
Insulin Aspart Protamine; Insulin Aspart II-1459
NOVORAPID
Insulin Aspart II-1456
NUBAIN
Nalbuphine Hydrochloride II-1917
NUCLEOSIDE REVERSE TRANSCRIPTASE INHIBITORS
Abacavir Sulfate; Lamivudine; Zidovudine II-1
Didanosine II-766
Emtricitabine II-910
Lamivudine II-1552
Lamivudine; Zidovudine II-1560
Stavudine II-2486
Zalcitabine II-2812
Zidovudine II-2822
NUCLEOTIDE REVERSE TRANSCRIPTASE INHIBITORS
Tenofovir Disoproxil Fumarate II-2564
NULEV
Hyoscyamine Sulfate II-1404
NUMORPHAN
Oxymorphone Hydrochloride II-2081
NUQUIN HP
Hydroquinone II-1391
NUROFEN
Ibuprofen II-1411
NUTRACORT
Hydrocortisone II-1369
NUTRITION, SUPPLEMENT
Fluoride; Polyvitamin II-1157
NYDRAZID
Isoniazid II-1496
NYEFAX
Nifedipine II-1967
NYSERT
Nystatin II-2005
NYSTATIN
Nystatin II-2005
Nystatin; Triamcinolone Acetonide II-2008
NYSTEX
Nystatin II-2005

CATEGORY/BRAND
Generic name — Page no.

NYSTOP
Nystatin II-2005
OBE-NIX
Phentermine Hydrochloride II-2170
OBESITY, EXOGENOUS
Amphetamine; Dextroamphetamine II-153
Phentermine Hydrochloride II-2170
Sibutramine Hydrochloride II-2447
OBESITY, MANAGEMENT
Orlistat II-2046
OBSESSIVE COMPULSIVE DISORDER
Clomipramine Hydrochloride II-621
Fluoxetine Hydrochloride II-1160
Fluvoxamine Maleate II-1203
Paroxetine Hydrochloride II-2104
Sertraline Hydrochloride II-2439
OBSTRUCTION, PANCREATIC DUCT, SECONDARY TO NEOPLASM
Pancrelipase II-2095
OBSTRUCTIVE PULMONARY DISEASE, CHRONIC
See Chronic Obstructive Pulmonary Disease
OBY-CAP
Phentermine Hydrochloride II-2170
OCCLUSION, ARTERIOVENOUS CANNULA
Streptokinase II-2490
OCCLUSION, CENTRAL VENOUS ACCESS DEVICES
Alteplase, Recombinant II-92
OCCLUSION, INTRAVENOUS CATHETER
Urokinase II-2734
OCTICAIR
Hydrocortisone; Neomycin Sulfate; Polymyxin B Sulfate II-1384
OCTIGEN
Hydrocortisone; Neomycin Sulfate; Polymyxin B Sulfate II-1384
OCTOCAINE
Epinephrine; Lidocaine Hydrochloride II-938
OCTREOTIDE ACETATE
Octreotide Acetate II-2009
OCU-CARPINE
Pilocarpine II-2180
OCU-CHLOR
Chloramphenicol II-536
OCUFEN
Flurbiprofen II-1177
OCUFLOX
Ofloxacin II-2015
OCU-MYCIN
Gentamicin Sulfate II-1279
OCU-PHRIN
Phenylephrine Hydrochloride II-2173
OCU-PRED
Prednisolone Sodium Phosphate II-2236

CATEGORY/BRAND
Generic name — Page no.

OCU-PRED-A
Prednisolone Acetate II-2235

OCUPRESS
Carteolol Hydrochloride II-435

OCUSPORIN HC
Hydrocortisone; Neomycin Sulfate; Polymyxin B Sulfate II-1384

OCU-SUL
Sulfacetamide Sodium II-2497

OCUSULF
Sulfacetamide Sodium II-2497

OCUTRICIN HC
Hydrocortisone; Neomycin Sulfate; Polymyxin B Sulfate II-1384

OCU-TROPINE
Atropine Sulfate II-235

ODRIK
Trandolapril II-2677

OFLOXACIN
Ofloxacin II-2015

OGEN
Estropipate II-1033

OGESTREL
Ethinyl Estradiol; Norgestrel II-1068

OLANZAPINE
Olanzapine II-2022

OLMESARTAN MEDOXOMIL
Olmesartan Medoxomil II-2028

OLOPATADINE HYDROCHLORIDE
Olopatadine Hydrochloride II-2030

OLSALAZINE SODIUM
Olsalazine Sodium II-2030

OMALIZUMAB
Omalizumab II-2032

OMEPRAZOLE
Omeprazole II-2034

OMNICEF
Cefdinir II-455

OMNIHIB
Haemophilus B; Tetanus Toxoid II-1327

OMNIPEN-N
Ampicillin Sodium II-172

ONCASPAR
Pegaspargase II-2118

ONCHOCERCIASIS
Ivermectin II-1528

ONCOVIN
Vincristine Sulfate II-2789

ONDANSETRON HYDROCHLORIDE
Ondansetron Hydrochloride II-2039

ONTAK
Denileukin Diftitox II-715

ONYCHOMYCOSIS
Ciclopirox II-561

CATEGORY/BRAND
Generic name — Page no.

ONY-CLEAR NAIL
Miconazole II-1820

OPHTHACET
Sulfacetamide Sodium II-2497

OPHTHALMIA NEONATORUM
Tetracycline Hydrochloride II-2585

OPHTHALMIA, SYMPATHETIC
Cortisone Acetate II-654
Dexamethasone II-730
Dexamethasone Acetate II-734
Hydrocortisone II-1369
Hydrocortisone Sodium Succinate II-1379
Methylprednisolone II-1787
Methylprednisolone Acetate II-1790
Methylprednisolone Sodium Succinate II-1793
Prednisolone II-2233
Prednisolone Sodium Phosphate II-2236
Prednisone II-2240
Triamcinolone II-2698
Triamcinolone Acetonide II-2701
Triamcinolone Diacetate II-2711

OPHTHALMICS
Apraclonidine Hydrochloride II-188
Atropine Sulfate II-235
Azelastine II-247
Betaxolol Hydrochloride II-307
Bimatoprost II-320
Brimonidine Tartrate II-340
Brinzolamide II-343
Carteolol Hydrochloride II-435
Chloramphenicol II-536
Ciprofloxacin Hydrochloride II-573
Cromolyn Sodium II-656
Dexamethasone II-730
Dexamethasone; Tobramycin II-736
Diclofenac II-748
Dipivefrin Hydrochloride II-820
Dorzolamide Hydrochloride II-858
Dorzolamide Hydrochloride; Timolol Maleate II-860
Emedastine Difumarate II-910
Epinephrine II-934
Erythromycin II-960
Flurbiprofen II-1177
Fomivirsen Sodium II-1210
Gentamicin Sulfate II-1279
Hydrocortisone; Neomycin Sulfate; Polymyxin B Sulfate II-1384
Ketorolac Tromethamine II-1537
Latanoprost II-1574
Levobunolol Hydrochloride II-1603
Levocabastine Hydrochloride II-1606
Levofloxacin II-1607
Lodoxamide Tromethamine II-1657
Loteprednol Etabonate II-1686
Moxifloxacin Hydrochloride II-1886
Norfloxacin II-1997
Ofloxacin II-2015
Olopatadine Hydrochloride II-2030
Pemirolast Potassium II-2128
Phenylephrine Hydrochloride II-2173
Pilocarpine II-2180
Polymyxin B Sulfate; Trimethoprim Sulfate II-2212
Prednisolone Acetate II-2235

CATEGORY/BRAND
Generic name — Page no.

OPHTHALMICS—cont'd
Prednisolone Sodium Phosphate II-2236
Scopolamine II-2432
Sulfacetamide Sodium II-2497
Tetracycline Hydrochloride II-2585
Timolol II-2627
Tobramycin II-2643
Travoprost II-2685
Unoprostone Isopropyl II-2732
Verteporfin II-2784
Vidarabine II-2785

OPHTHOCHLOR
Chloramphenicol II-536

OPIATE DEPENDENCE
Buprenorphine II-363
Naltrexone Hydrochloride II-1920

OPIATE INTOXICATION, DIAGNOSIS
Naloxone Hydrochloride II-1919

OPIATE, WITHDRAWAL
Methadone Hydrochloride II-1766

OPRELVEKIN
Oprelvekin II-2044

OPTICROM
Cromolyn Sodium II-656

OPTIMINE
Azatadine Maleate II-242

OPTIPRESS
Carteolol Hydrochloride II-435

OPTOMYCIN
Chloramphenicol II-536

ORABASE HCA
Hydrocortisone Acetate II-1373

ORACORT
Triamcinolone Acetonide II-2701

ORALONE
Triamcinolone Acetonide II-2701

ORAMORPH SR
Morphine Sulfate II-1877

ORAP
Pimozide II-2189

ORASONE
Prednisone II-2240

ORCHIDECTOMY
Methyltestosterone II-1796

ORCHITIS
Methyltestosterone II-1796

OR-DEX L.A.
Dexamethasone Acetate II-734

ORETIC
Hydrochlorothiazide II-1348

ORETON METHYL
Methyltestosterone II-1796

ORGANIDIN NR
Guaifenesin II-1314

ORIMUNE
Polio Vaccine, Oral Live II-2210

CATEGORY/BRAND Generic name — Page no.

CATEGORY/BRAND Generic name — Page no.

CATEGORY/BRAND Generic name — Page no.

International Brand Names Index

International brand name (Generic name) Page no.

A

International brand name (Generic name)	Page no.
Allerfin (Chlorpheniramine Maleate)	II-548
Allergefon (Carbinoxamine Maleate)	II-429
Allergex (Chlorpheniramine Maleate)	II-548
Allergin (Chlorpheniramine Maleate)	II-548
Allergina (Diphenhydramine Hydrochloride)	II-813
Allerglobuline (Immune Globulin (Human))	II-1434
Allergo-comod (Cromolyn Sodium)	II-656
Allergocrom (Cromolyn Sodium)	II-656
Allergodil (Azelastine)	II-247
Allergyl (Chlorpheniramine Maleate)	II-548
Allerkyn (Chlorpheniramine Maleate)	II-548
Allermax Aqueous (Mometasone Furoate)	II-1866
Allermin (Chlorpheniramine Maleate)	II-548
Allermin (Diphenhydramine Hydrochloride)	II-813
Allerphen (Chlorpheniramine Maleate)	II-548
Allex (Desloratadine)	II-721
Allipen (Ibuprofen)	II-1411
Allnol (Allopurinol)	II-77
Allo 300 (Allopurinol)	II-77
Allo-Basan (Allopurinol)	II-77
Allohex (Loratadine)	II-1675
Allohexal (Allopurinol)	II-77
Allopin (Allopurinol)	II-77
Allopur (Allopurinol)	II-77
Allo-Puren (Allopurinol)	II-77
Allopurinol (Allopurinol)	II-77
Alloril (Allopurinol)	II-77
Allorin (Allopurinol)	II-77
Allozym (Allopurinol)	II-77
Alltec (Cetirizine Hydrochloride)	II-529
Allulose (Aluminum Hydroxide)	II-97
Allurit (Allopurinol)	II-77
Allvoran (Diclofenac)	II-748
Almarion (Theophylline)	II-2593
Almarytm (Flecainide Acetate)	II-1134
Almatol (Spironolactone)	II-2483
Almide (Lodoxamide Tromethamine)	II-1657
Alminth (Albendazole)	II-46
Almiral (Diclofenac)	II-748
Almiral SR (Diclofenac)	II-748
Almodan (Amoxicillin)	II-131
Alna (Tamsulosin Hydrochloride)	II-2544
Alnax (Alprazolam)	II-85
Alodan "Gerot" (Meperidine Hydrochloride)	II-1733
Aloid (Miconazole)	II-1820
Alol (Acebutolol Hydrochloride)	II-10
Alomide SE (Lodoxamide Tromethamine)	II-1657
Alonet (Atenolol)	II-222
Alonix-S (Nifedipine)	II-1967
Alonpin (Diclofenac)	II-748
Alopam (Doxepin Hydrochloride)	II-865
Alopam (Oxazepam)	II-2063
Aloperidin (Haloperidol)	II-1328
Aloperidin (Haloperidol Decanoate)	II-1332
Alopexy (Minoxidil)	II-1845
Alopexyl (Minoxidil)	II-1845
Alopresin (Captopril)	II-411
Alopron (Allopurinol)	II-77
Alorbat (Influenza Virus Vaccine)	II-1451
Alositol (Allopurinol)	II-77
Alostil (Amikacin Sulfate)	II-101
Alotec (Metaproterenol Sulfate)	II-1754
Alovell (Alendronate Sodium)	II-70
Alpain (Mefenamic Acid)	II-1720
Alpaz (Alprazolam)	II-85
Alpha-Baclofen (Baclofen)	II-266
Alpha-Bromocriptine (Bromocriptine Mesylate)	II-344
Alphacort (Betamethasone Valerate)	II-305
Alphadopa (Methyldopa)	II-1778
Alphakinase (Urokinase)	II-2734
Alpha-Lactulose (Lactulose)	II-1550
Alpha-Nifedipine Retard (Nifedipine)	II-1967
Alphapril (Enalapril Maleate)	II-913
Alphexine (Cefaclor)	II-444
Alphrin (Enalapril Maleate)	II-913
Alplax (Alprazolam)	II-85
Alpralid (Alprazolam)	II-85
Alpram (Alprazolam)	II-85
Alpranax (Alprazolam)	II-85
Alprax (Alprazolam)	II-85
Alprocontin (Alprazolam)	II-85
Alpron (Naproxen)	II-1924
Alprostapint (Alprostadil)	II-90
Alprox (Alprazolam)	II-85
Alpurin (Allopurinol)	II-77
Alquingel (Tretinoin)	II-2691
Alrheumat (Ketoprofen)	II-1533
Alrheumun (Ketoprofen)	II-1533
Alrhumat (Ketoprofen)	II-1533
Alsporin (Cephalexin)	II-520
Alsucral (Sucralfate)	II-2493
Altesona (Cortisone Acetate)	II-654
Althocin (Ethambutol Hydrochloride)	II-1039
Altiazem (Diltiazem Hydrochloride)	II-798
Altiazem Retard (Diltiazem Hydrochloride)	II-798
Altiazem RR (Diltiazem Hydrochloride)	II-798
Altol (Atenolol)	II-222
Altran (Captopril)	II-411
Altraxic (Alprazolam)	II-85
Altruline (Sertraline Hydrochloride)	II-2439
Alu-Cap (Aluminum Hydroxide)	II-97
Alucol (Aluminum Hydroxide)	II-97
Aludrox (Aluminum Hydroxide)	II-97
Alugel (Aluminum Hydroxide)	II-97
Alugelibys (Aluminum Hydroxide)	II-97
Alumag (Aluminum Hydroxide)	II-97
Alumigel (Aluminum Hydroxide)	II-97
Aluminox (Aluminum Hydroxide)	II-97
Alunlan (Allopurinol)	II-77
Alurin (Allopurinol)	II-77
Aluron (Allopurinol)	II-77
Alusorb (Aluminum Hydroxide)	II-97
Alu-Tab (Aluminum Hydroxide)	II-97
Alutab (Aluminum Hydroxide)	II-97
Alvadermo Fuerte (Fluocinolone Acetonide)	II-1152
Alvedon (Acetaminophen)	II-11
Alveolex (Acetylcysteine)	II-29
Alviz (Alprazolam)	II-85
Alxil (Cefadroxil Monohydrate)	II-447
Alzac 20 (Fluoxetine Hydrochloride)	II-1160
Alzam (Alprazolam)	II-85
Alzax (Alprazolam)	II-85
Alzental (Albendazole)	II-46
Alzinox (Aluminum Hydroxide)	II-97
Alzol (Albendazole)	II-46
Alzolam (Alprazolam)	II-85
Alzytec (Cetirizine Hydrochloride)	II-529
Amadol (Clofibrate)	II-619
Amagesen Solutab (Amoxicillin)	II-131
Amanda (Amantadine Hydrochloride)	II-97
Amandin (Amantadine Hydrochloride)	II-97
Amantan (Amantadine Hydrochloride)	II-97
Amantix (Amantadine Hydrochloride)	II-97
Amazolon (Amantadine Hydrochloride)	II-97
Ambamida (Erythromycin Ethylsuccinate)	II-965
Amben (Cefadroxil Monohydrate)	II-447
Ambigram (Norfloxacin)	II-1997
Ambilan (Amoxicillin; Clavulanate Potassium)	II-139
Ambramicina (Tetracycline Hydrochloride)	II-2585
Ambutol (Ethambutol Hydrochloride)	II-1039
Amcard (Amlodipine Besylate)	II-125
Amcillin (Ampicillin)	II-170
Amdepin (Amlodipine Besylate)	II-125
Amdipin (Amlodipine Besylate)	II-125
Ameclina (Amoxicillin)	II-131
Ameide (Amiloride Hydrochloride; Hydrochlorothiazide)	II-105
Amelor (Azelastine)	II-247
Ameride (Amiloride Hydrochloride; Hydrochlorothiazide)	II-105
Amermycin (Doxycycline)	II-878
Amerol (Loperamide Hydrochloride)	II-1664
A-Methapred (Methylprednisolone)	II-1787
Ametic (Metoclopramide Hydrochloride)	II-1798
Ametop (Tetracaine Hydrochloride)	II-2584
Ametycine (Mitomycin)	II-1854
Amevan (Metronidazole)	II-1812
Am-Fam 400 (Ibuprofen)	II-1411
Amfipen (Ampicillin)	II-170
Amias (Candesartan Cilexetil)	II-402
Amicacina (Amikacin Sulfate)	II-101
Amicasil (Amikacin Sulfate)	II-101
Amicel (Econazole Nitrate)	II-900
Amicin (Amikacin Sulfate)	II-101
Amicrobin (Norfloxacin)	II-1997
Amidodacore (Amiodarone Hydrochloride)	II-110
Amidryl (Diphenhydramine Hydrochloride)	II-813
Amikafur (Amikacin Sulfate)	II-101
Amikal (Amiloride Hydrochloride)	II-103
Amikan (Amikacin Sulfate)	II-101
Amikayect (Amikacin Sulfate)	II-101
Amiklin (Amikacin Sulfate)	II-101
Amikozit (Amikacin Sulfate)	II-101
Amiktam (Amikacin Sulfate)	II-101
Amil-Co (Amiloride Hydrochloride; Hydrochlorothiazide)	II-105
Amilco (Amiloride Hydrochloride; Hydrochlorothiazide)	II-105
Amilco Mite (Amiloride Hydrochloride; Hydrochlorothiazide)	II-105
Amilit (Amitriptyline Hydrochloride)	II-119
Amilo 5 (Amiloride Hydrochloride)	II-103
Amilocomp beta (Amiloride Hydrochloride; Hydrochlorothiazide)	II-105
Amiloretic (Amiloride Hydrochloride; Hydrochlorothiazide)	II-105
Amiloscan (Amiloride Hydrochloride; Hydrochlorothiazide)	II-105
Amineurin (Amitriptyline Hydrochloride)	II-119
Aminofilina (Aminophylline)	II-106
Aminomal (Aminophylline)	II-106
Aminor (Norethindrone)	II-1996
Amiobeta (Amiodarone Hydrochloride)	II-110
Amiodarex (Amiodarone Hydrochloride)	II-110
Amiodarona (Amiodarone Hydrochloride)	II-110
Amiogamma (Amiodarone Hydrochloride)	II-110
Amiohexal (Amiodarone Hydrochloride)	II-110
Amiorit (Amiodarone Hydrochloride)	II-110
Amipenix (Ampicillin)	II-170
Amiplin (Amitriptyline Hydrochloride)	II-119
Amipress (Labetalol Hydrochloride)	II-1545
Amiprin (Amitriptyline Hydrochloride)	II-119
Amiprol (Diazepam)	II-740
Amisalin (Procainamide Hydrochloride)	II-2250
Amithiazide (Amiloride Hydrochloride; Hydrochlorothiazide)	II-105
Amitrid (Amiloride Hydrochloride; Hydrochlorothiazide)	II-105
Amitrip (Amitriptyline Hydrochloride)	II-119
Amiyodazol (Metronidazole)	II-1812
Amlocar (Amlodipine Besylate)	II-125
Amlodin (Amlodipine Besylate)	II-125
Amlopine (Amlodipine Besylate)	II-125
Amlor (Amlodipine Besylate)	II-125
Amlosyn (Amlodipine Besylate)	II-125
Amminac (Doxorubicin, Liposomal)	II-873
Amocla (Amoxicillin; Clavulanate Potassium)	II-139
Amoclan (Amoxicillin; Clavulanate Potassium)	II-139
Amoclav (Amoxicillin; Clavulanate Potassium)	II-139
Amoclen (Amoxicillin)	II-131
Amodex (Amoxicillin)	II-131
Amo-flamsian (Amoxicillin)	II-131
Amohexal (Amoxicillin)	II-131
Amol (Acetaminophen)	II-11
Amolanic (Amoxicillin; Clavulanate Potassium)	II-139

International brand name (Generic name)	Page no.
Antipres (Guanethidine Monosulfate)	II-1321
Antipressan (Atenolol)	II-222
Antiroid (Propylthiouracil)	II-2293
Antisacer (Phenytoin Sodium)	II-2175
Antisemin (Cyproheptadine Hydrochloride)	II-682
Antizid (Nizatidine)	II-1992
Antizol (Fomepizole)	II-1209
Antodine (Famotidine)	II-1093
Antra (Omeprazole)	II-2034
Antrex (Leucovorin Calcium)	II-1585
Antrimox (Sulfamethoxazole; Trimethoprim)	II-2500
Antroquoril (Betamethasone Valerate)	II-305
Anulax (Bisacodyl)	II-322
Anulette (Ethinyl Estradiol; Levonorgestrel)	II-1047
Anusol + H (Hydrocortisone Acetate)	II-1373
Anxer (Cephalexin)	II-520
Anxidin (Clorazepate Dipotassium)	II-638
Anxiedin (Lorazepam)	II-1678
Anxielax (Clorazepate Dipotassium)	II-638
Anxinil (Buspirone Hydrochloride)	II-382
Anxiolan (Buspirone Hydrochloride)	II-382
Anxiolit (Oxazepam)	II-2063
Anxiolit Retard (Oxazepam)	II-2063
Anxionil (Diazepam)	II-740
Anxipress-D (Amitriptyline Hydrochloride; Perphenazine)	II-124
Anxira (Lorazepam)	II-1678
Anxirid (Alprazolam)	II-85
Anxiron (Buspirone Hydrochloride)	II-382
Anzatax (Paclitaxel)	II-2084
Anzem (Diltiazem Hydrochloride)	II-798
Anzema (Ketoprofen)	II-1533
Anzepam (Lorazepam)	II-1678
Anzief (Allopurinol)	II-77
Anzion (Alprazolam)	II-85
Anzolin (Cefazolin Sodium)	II-452
Apacef (Cefotetan Disodium)	II-478
Apalin (Amikacin Sulfate)	II-101
Apamid (Glipizide)	II-1290
Aparkane (Trihexyphenidyl Hydrochloride)	II-2720
Apdormin (Hydralazine Hydrochloride)	II-1346
Aperon (Acetaminophen; Dichloralphenazone; Isometheptene Mucate)	II-16
Apeton 4 (Cyproheptadine Hydrochloride)	II-682
Aphrodil (Sildenafil Citrate)	II-2451
Apicol (Acyclovir)	II-33
Apigent (Gentamicin Sulfate)	II-1279
Apimid (Flutamide)	II-1181
Apirex (Acetaminophen)	II-11
Apirol (Norfloxacin)	II-1997
Aplacasse (Lorazepam)	II-1678
Aplaket (Ticlopidine Hydrochloride)	II-2622
Aplosyn (Fluocinolone Acetonide)	II-1152
Apo-Acetazolamide (Acetazolamide)	II-28
Apoacor (Verapamil Hydrochloride)	II-2777
Apo-Allopurinol (Allopurinol)	II-77
Apo-Alpraz (Alprazolam)	II-85
Apo-Amitriptyline (Amitriptyline Hydrochloride)	II-119
Apo-Amoxi (Amoxicillin)	II-131
Apo-Ampi (Ampicillin)	II-170
Apo-Atenolol (Atenolol)	II-222
Apo-Benzthropine (Benztropine Mesylate)	II-293
Apo-Bromocriptine (Bromocriptine Mesylate)	II-344
Apo-Cal (Calcium Carbonate)	II-401
Apocanda (Clotrimazole)	II-640
Apo-Carbamazepine (Carbamazepine)	II-418
Apocard (Flecainide Acetate)	II-1134
Apo-Chlorax (Chlordiazepoxide Hydrochloride; Clidinium Bromide)	II-541
Apo-Chlordiazepoxide (Chlordiazepoxide Hydrochloride)	II-539
Apo-Chlorpropamide (Chlorpropamide)	II-554
Apo-Chlorthalidone (Chlorthalidone)	II-555
Apo-Cimetidine (Cimetidine Hydrochloride)	II-568
Apocort (Hydrocortisone Acetate)	II-1373
Apocyclin (Tetracycline Hydrochloride)	II-2585
Apo-diazepam (Diazepam)	II-740
Apo-Diclofenac EC (Diclofenac)	II-748
Apo-diltiazem (Diltiazem Hydrochloride)	II-798
Apo-Dipyridamole FC (Dipyridamole)	II-821
Apo-Erythro-ES (Erythromycin Ethylsuccinate)	II-965
Apo-Erythro-S (Erythromycin Stearate)	II-970
Apo-Ethambutol (Ethambutol Hydrochloride)	II-1039
Apo-Famotidine (Famotidine)	II-1093
Apo-Feno-Micro (Fenofibrate)	II-1105
Apo-Fluphenazine (Fluphenazine Hydrochloride)	II-1172
Apo-Flurazepam (Flurazepam Hydrochloride)	II-1175
Apo-Flurbiprofen (Flurbiprofen)	II-1177
Apo-Folic (Folic Acid)	II-1208
Apo-Frusemide (Furosemide)	II-1237
Apo-Furosemide (Furosemide)	II-1237
Apogastine (Famotidine)	II-1093
Apo-Gemfibrozil (Gemfibrozil)	II-1269
Apo-Glibenclamide (Glyburide)	II-1297
Apo-Haloperidol (Haloperidol)	II-1328
Apo-Hydro (Hydrochlorothiazide)	II-1348
Apo-Hydroxyzine (Hydroxyzine)	II-1398
Apo-Ibuprofen (Ibuprofen)	II-1411
Apo-Imipramine (Imipramine Hydrochloride)	II-1431
Apo-Indomethacin (Indomethacin)	II-1443
APO-ISDN (Isosorbide Dinitrate)	II-1502
Apo-K (Potassium Chloride)	II-2215
Apo-Keto (Ketoprofen)	II-1533
Apolar (Desonide)	II-728
Apo-Lorazepam (Lorazepam)	II-1678
Apo-Meprobamate (Meprobamate)	II-1738
Apo-Methyldopa (Methyldopa)	II-1778
Apo-Metoclop (Metoclopramide Hydrochloride)	II-1798
Apo-Metoprolol (Metoprolol)	II-1805
Apo-Metronidazole (Metronidazole)	II-1812
Apomin (Chlorpheniramine Maleate)	II-548
Apo-Nadol (Nadolol)	II-1911
Apo-Nadolol (Nadolol)	II-1911
Aponal (Doxepin Hydrochloride)	II-865
Apo-Naproxen (Naproxen)	II-1924
Apo-Nicotinic Acid (Niacin)	II-1956
Apo-Nifed (Nifedipine)	II-1967
Apo-Oxazepam (Oxazepam)	II-2063
Apo-Pen-VK (Penicillin V Potassium)	II-2142
APO-Perphenazine (Perphenazine)	II-2162
Apophage (Metformin Hydrochloride)	II-1760
Apo-Pindol (Pindolol)	II-2192
Apo-Pindolol (Pindolol)	II-2192
Apo-Piroxicam (Piroxicam)	II-2205
Apo-Prednisone (Prednisone)	II-2240
Apo-Primidone (Primidone)	II-2247
Apo-Propranolol (Propranolol Hydrochloride)	II-2287
Apo-Ranitidine (Ranitidine Hydrochloride)	II-2334
Apo-Selegiline (Selegiline Hydrochloride)	II-2437
Apo-Sulfatrim (Sulfamethoxazole; Trimethoprim)	II-2500
Apo-Sulin (Sulindac)	II-2512
Apoterin (Clofibrate)	II-619
Apoterin A (Clofibrate)	II-619
Apo-Tetra (Tetracycline Hydrochloride)	II-2585
Apo-Timol (Timolol)	II-2627
Apo-Timolol (Timolol)	II-2627
Apo-Timop (Timolol)	II-2627
Apo-Timop (Travoprost)	II-2685
Apo-triazide (Hydrochlorothiazide; Triamterene)	II-1362
Apo-Triazo (Triazolam)	II-2715
Apo-Trihex (Trihexyphenidyl Hydrochloride)	II-2720
Apovent (Ipratropium Bromide)	II-1480
Apo-Verap (Verapamil Hydrochloride)	II-2777
Apozepam (Diazepam)	II-740
Apo-Zidovudine (Zidovudine)	II-2822
Approvel (Irbesartan)	II-1484
Apranax (Naproxen)	II-1924
Apranax (Naproxen Sodium)	II-1928
Apraxin (Naproxen Sodium)	II-1928
Apresolin (Hydralazine Hydrochloride)	II-1346
Apresolina (Hydralazine Hydrochloride)	II-1346
Aprezin (Hydralazine Hydrochloride)	II-1346
Aprical (Nifedipine)	II-1967
Aprinol (Allopurinol)	II-77
Apronax (Naproxen Sodium)	II-1928
Aprostal (Mefenamic Acid)	II-1720
Aprovel (Irbesartan)	II-1484
Aprovel HCT (Hydrochlorothiazide; Irbesartan)	II-1351
Aproven (Ipratropium Bromide)	II-1480
Apsolol (Propranolol Hydrochloride)	II-2287
Apurin (Allopurinol)	II-77
Aputern (Metoclopramide Hydrochloride)	II-1798
Apuzin (Captopril)	II-411
Aquamycetin (Chloramphenicol)	II-536
Aquanil (Timolol)	II-2627
Aquanil (Travoprost)	II-2685
Aquarid (Furosemide)	II-1237
Aquarius (Ketoconazole)	II-1530
Aquasol E (Vitamin E)	II-2796
Aqucilina (Penicillin G Procaine)	II-2140
Arabitin (Cytarabine)	II-683
Aracytin (Cytarabine)	II-683
Aracytine (Cytarabine)	II-683
Aragest 5 (Medroxyprogesterone Acetate)	II-1714
Arandin (Atenolol)	II-222
Arasemide (Furosemide)	II-1237
Arasena-A (Vidarabine)	II-2785
Arbutol (Ethambutol Hydrochloride)	II-1039
Arcanafenac (Diclofenac)	II-748
Arcanamycin (Erythromycin Stearate)	II-970
Arcasin (Penicillin V Potassium)	II-2142
Arcazol (Metronidazole)	II-1812
Arcental (Ketoprofen)	II-1533
Archifen Eye (Chloramphenicol)	II-536
Arcored (Cyanocobalamin)	II-661
Arcosal (Tolbutamide)	II-2650
Ardin (Loratadine)	II-1675
Ardine (Amoxicillin)	II-131
Aredronet (Pamidronate Disodium)	II-2091
Aremis (Sertraline Hydrochloride)	II-2439
Arendal (Alendronate Sodium)	II-70
Arestal (Loperamide Hydrochloride)	II-1664
Areumatin (Indomethacin)	II-1443
Arfen (Acetaminophen)	II-11
Arflur (Flurbiprofen)	II-1177
Argilex (Indomethacin)	II-1443
Arilin (Metronidazole)	II-1812
Ariline (Metronidazole)	II-1812
Aripax (Lorazepam)	II-1678
Aristocort (Triamcinolone Acetonide)	II-2701
Aristocort A (Triamcinolone Acetonide)	II-2701
Arkamin (Clonidine Hydrochloride)	II-629
Arkine (Trihexyphenidyl Hydrochloride)	II-2720
Armol (Alendronate Sodium)	II-70
Armonil (Diazepam)	II-740
Armophylline (Theophylline)	II-2593
Arodoc (Chlorpropamide)	II-554
Arodoc C (Chlorpropamide)	II-554
Aromasin (Exemestane)	II-1085
Aromasine (Exemestane)	II-1085
Aroxin (Amoxicillin)	II-131
Arpyrox (Piroxicam)	II-2205
Arring (Triazolam)	II-2715
Artagen (Naproxen)	II-1924
Artal (Pentoxifylline)	II-2154
Artamin (Penicillamine)	II-2133
Artensol H (Hydrochlorothiazide; Propranolol Hydrochloride)	II-1357
Arteolol (Carteolol Hydrochloride)	II-435
Arteoptic (Carteolol Hydrochloride)	II-435
Arteoptik (Carteolol Hydrochloride)	II-435

International brand name (Generic name)	Page no.
Axepim (Cefepime Hydrochloride)	II-462
Axetine (Cefuroxime)	II-507
Axialit (Bromocriptine Mesylate)	II-344
Axoban (Ranitidine Hydrochloride)	II-2334
Axone (Ceftriaxone Sodium)	II-503
Ayerogen (Estrogens, Conjugated)	II-1019
Ayerogen Crema Vaginal (Estrogens, Conjugated)	II-1019
Azadose (Azithromycin)	II-250
Azafalk (Azathioprine)	II-243
Azalea (Azelaic Acid)	II-245
Azamedac (Azathioprine)	II-243
Azamun (Azathioprine)	II-243
Azamune (Azathioprine)	II-243
Azanin (Azathioprine)	II-243
Azantac (Ranitidine Hydrochloride)	II-2334
Azapress (Azathioprine)	II-243
Azarten (Losartan Potassium)	II-1682
Azathiodura (Azathioprine)	II-243
Azathioprine (Azathioprine)	II-243
Azatioprina (Azathioprine)	II-243
Azatrilem (Azathioprine)	II-243
Azedipamin (Diazepam)	II-740
Azella (Azelastine)	II-247
Azenil (Azithromycin)	II-250
Azep (Azelastine)	II-247
Azeptin (Azelastine)	II-247
Azide (Chlorothiazide)	II-545
Azillin (Amoxicillin)	II-131
Azimin (Azithromycin)	II-250
Azithral (Azithromycin)	II-250
Azitrocin (Azithromycin)	II-250
Azitromax (Azithromycin)	II-250
Aziwok (Azithromycin)	II-250
Azmacor (Triamcinolone)	II-2698
Azmacort (Triamcinolone)	II-2698
Azmasol (Albuterol)	II-47
Azol (Danazol)	II-699
Azomyne (Azithromycin)	II-250
Azomyr (Desloratadine)	II-721
Azonz (Trazodone Hydrochloride)	II-2686
Azopi (Azathioprine)	II-243
Azor (Alprazolam)	II-85
Azoran (Azathioprine)	II-243
Azoran (Omeprazole)	II-2034
Azovir (Acyclovir)	II-33
Azro (Azithromycin)	II-250
Aztrin (Azithromycin)	II-250
Azucimet (Cimetidine Hydrochloride)	II-568
Azudoxat (Doxycycline)	II-878
Azumon (Estrogens, Conjugated)	II-1019
Azupamil (Verapamil Hydrochloride)	II-2777
Azupentat (Pentoxifylline)	II-2154
Azurogen (Lorazepam)	II-1678
Azutranquil (Oxazepam)	II-2063
B	
B Cort (Budesonide)	II-347
B(6)-Vicotrat (Pyridoxine Hydrochloride)	II-2297
Babel (Naproxen Sodium)	II-1928
Baby Agisten (Clotrimazole)	II-640
Babyspasmil (Dicyclomine Hydrochloride)	II-763
Baccidal (Norfloxacin)	II-1997
Baccidal (Ofloxacin)	II-2015
Bacidal (Sulfamethoxazole; Trimethoprim)	II-2500
Bacin (Sulfamethoxazole; Trimethoprim)	II-2500
Backen (Baclofen)	II-266
Baclan (Baclofen)	II-266
Baclapone (Baclofen)	II-266
Baclo (Baclofen)	II-266
Baclon (Baclofen)	II-266
Baclosal (Baclofen)	II-266
Bacofen (Baclofen)	II-266
Bacquinor (Ciprofloxacin Hydrochloride)	II-573
Bacron (Baclofen)	II-266
Bactacin (Ampicillin Sodium; Sulbactam Sodium)	II-174
Bactamox (Amoxicillin)	II-131
Bacterol (Moxifloxacin Hydrochloride)	II-1886
Bacticel (Sulfamethoxazole; Trimethoprim)	II-2500
Bactiderm (Gentamicin Sulfate)	II-1279
Bactidox (Doxycycline)	II-878
Bactiflox Lactab (Ciprofloxacin Hydrochloride)	II-573
Bactifor (Sulfamethoxazole; Trimethoprim)	II-2500
Bactirel (Clarithromycin)	II-597
Bactocef (Cephradine)	II-526
Bactocin (Ofloxacin)	II-2015
Bactoderm (Mupirocin)	II-1894
Bactoprim (Sulfamethoxazole; Trimethoprim)	II-2500
Bactoscrub (Chlorhexidine Gluconate)	II-542
Bactosept Concentrate (Chlorhexidine Gluconate)	II-542
Bactramin (Sulfamethoxazole; Trimethoprim)	II-2500
Bactrim DS (Sulfamethoxazole; Trimethoprim)	II-2500
Bactrim Forte (Sulfamethoxazole; Trimethoprim)	II-2500
Bactrimel (Sulfamethoxazole; Trimethoprim)	II-2500
Baflox (Ciprofloxacin Hydrochloride)	II-573
Baklofen (Baclofen)	II-266
Baknyl (Erythromycin Ethylsuccinate)	II-965
Baknyl (Erythromycin Stearate)	II-970
Baktar (Sulfamethoxazole; Trimethoprim)	II-2500
Balacon (Dicyclomine Hydrochloride)	II-763
Balance (Chlordiazepoxide Hydrochloride)	II-539
Balcorin (Vancomycin Hydrochloride)	II-2763
Balkaprofen (Ibuprofen)	II-1411
Balminil Expectorant (Guaifenesin)	II-1314
Banan Dry Syrup (Cefpodoxime Proxetil)	II-484
Banndoclin (Doxycycline)	II-878
Bannthrocin (Erythromycin Ethylsuccinate)	II-965
Bannthrocin (Erythromycin Stearate)	II-970
Bantenol (Mebendazole)	II-1711
Barazan (Norfloxacin)	II-1997
Barbilettae (Phenobarbital)	II-2167
Barbiphenyl (Phenobarbital)	II-2167
Barbloc (Pindolol)	II-2192
Barlolin (Bromocriptine Mesylate)	II-344
Barolyn (Metolazone)	II-1802
Baromezole (Omeprazole)	II-2034
Baropan (Baclofen)	II-266
Basal-H-Insulin (Insulin (Human, Isophane))	II-1455
Basaljel (Aluminum Hydroxide)	II-97
Based (Methimazole)	II-1767
Basedillin (Doxycycline)	II-878
Basocef (Cefazolin Sodium)	II-452
Bassado (Doxycycline)	II-878
Baten (Fluconazole)	II-1136
Batrafen (Ciclopirox)	II-561
Batrafen Gel (Ciclopirox)	II-561
Batrafen Nail Lacquer (Ciclopirox)	II-561
Baxan (Cefadroxil Monohydrate)	II-447
Baxima (Cefotaxime Sodium)	II-474
Baxo (Piroxicam)	II-2205
Bay Rho-D (Rho (D) Immune Globulin)	II-2350
Bayaspirina (Aspirin)	II-206
Baycip (Ciprofloxacin Hydrochloride)	II-573
Bayer Aspirin (Aspirin)	II-206
Bayer Aspirin Cardio (Aspirin)	II-206
Bayer Bayrab Rabies Immune Globulin (Rabies Immune Globulin)	II-2323
Baygam (Immune Globulin (Human))	II-1434
Bayhep B (Hepatitis B Immune Globulin)	II-1341
Baymycard (Nisoldipine)	II-1976
Bayrab (Rabies Immune Globulin)	II-2323
BayTet (Tetanus Immune Globulin)	II-2582
BB (Clindamycin)	II-605
Bcnu (Carmustine)	II-434
Beafemic (Mefenamic Acid)	II-1720
Beahexol (Trihexyphenidyl Hydrochloride)	II-2720
Beapen (Penicillin V Potassium)	II-2142
Beapizide (Glipizide)	II-1290
Bearax (Acyclovir)	II-33
Bearcef (Cefuroxime)	II-507
Beartec (Enalapril Maleate)	II-913
Beatacycline (Tetracycline Hydrochloride)	II-2585
Beatizem (Diltiazem Hydrochloride)	II-798
Beatoconazole (Ketoconazole)	II-1530
Beatryl (Fentanyl Citrate)	II-1112
Beavate (Betamethasone Valerate)	II-305
Becanta (Methyldopa)	II-1778
Becardin (Propranolol Hydrochloride)	II-2287
Becenun (Carmustine)	II-434
Beceze (Beclomethasone Dipropionate)	II-279
Beclate (Beclomethasone Dipropionate)	II-279
Beclazone (Beclomethasone Dipropionate)	II-279
Beclazone CFC Free (Beclomethasone Dipropionate)	II-279
Beclo Siozwo Nasenspray (Beclomethasone Dipropionate)	II-279
Beclo-Asma (Beclomethasone Dipropionate)	II-279
Beclocort Nasel (Beclomethasone Dipropionate)	II-279
Becloforte (Beclomethasone Dipropionate)	II-279
Beclomet (Beclomethasone Dipropionate)	II-279
Beclomet Easyhaler (Beclomethasone Dipropionate)	II-279
Beclomet Nasal (Beclomethasone Dipropionate)	II-279
Beclomet Nasal Aqua (Beclomethasone Dipropionate)	II-279
Beclometasone (Beclomethasone Dipropionate)	II-279
Beclone (Beclomethasone Dipropionate)	II-279
Beclo-Rhino (Beclomethasone Dipropionate)	II-279
Beclorhinol (Beclomethasone Dipropionate)	II-279
Becloturmant (Beclomethasone Dipropionate)	II-279
Becodisks (Beclomethasone Dipropionate)	II-279
Bedoc (Cyanocobalamin)	II-661
Bedodeka (Cyanocobalamin)	II-661
Bedrenal (Pindolol)	II-2192
Befar (Alprostadil)	II-90
Begrivac (Influenza Virus Vaccine)	II-1451
Begrivac F (Influenza Virus Vaccine)	II-1451
Behepan (Cyanocobalamin)	II-661
Beknol (Benzonatate)	II-290
Belax (Beclomethasone Dipropionate)	II-279
Bellatram (Tramadol Hydrochloride)	II-2674
Bellpino-Artin (Atropine Sulfate)	II-235
Beloc (Metoprolol)	II-1805
Beloc Comp (Hydrochlorothiazide; Metoprolol Tartrate)	II-1355
Beloc Duriles (Metoprolol)	II-1805
Beloc Zok (Metoprolol)	II-1805
Belustine (Lomustine)	II-1662
Belvas (Lovastatin)	II-1688
Bemedrex Easyhaler (Beclomethasone Dipropionate)	II-279
Bemon (Betamethasone Valerate)	II-305
Benadon (Pyridoxine Hydrochloride)	II-2297
Benadryl N (Diphenhydramine Hydrochloride)	II-813
Benalipril (Enalapril Maleate)	II-913
Benambex (Pentamidine Isethionate)	II-2145
Benapon (Diphenhydramine Hydrochloride)	II-813
Benaxima (Cefotaxime Sodium)	II-474
Benaxona (Ceftriaxone Sodium)	II-503
Bencid (Probenecid)	II-2248
Benclamin (Glyburide)	II-1297
Bencole (Sulfamethoxazole; Trimethoprim)	II-2500
Benda (Mebendazole)	II-1711
Bendapar (Albendazole)	II-46
Bendex-400 (Albendazole)	II-46
Benecid (Probenecid)	II-2248
Beneficat (Trazodone Hydrochloride)	II-2686
Beneflur (Fludarabine Phosphate)	II-1142
Benemide (Probenecid)	II-2248
Benerva (Thiamine Hydrochloride)	II-2602
Beneseron (Interferon Beta-1b, Recombinant)	II-1478

International brand name (Generic name)	Page no.
Beneuril (Thiamine Hydrochloride)	II-2602
Beneuron (Thiamine Hydrochloride)	II-2602
Benhex Cream (Lindane)	II-1642
Bennasone (Betamethasone Valerate)	II-305
Benocid (Indomethacin)	II-1443
Benocten (Diphenhydramine Hydrochloride)	II-813
Benofomin (Metformin Hydrochloride)	II-1760
Benoson (Betamethasone)	II-298
Benoson (Betamethasone Valerate)	II-305
Benoson (500 mcg) (Betamethasone)	II-298
Benostan (Mefenamic Acid)	II-1720
Benoxicam (Piroxicam)	II-2205
Benozil (Flurazepam Hydrochloride)	II-1175
Benpine (Chlordiazepoxide Hydrochloride)	II-539
Bensylate (Benztropine Mesylate)	II-293
Bentylol (Dicyclomine Hydrochloride)	II-763
Ben-U-Ron (Acetaminophen)	II-11
Benuron (Acetaminophen)	II-11
Benuryl (Probenecid)	II-2248
Benzacillin (Penicillin G Benzathine)	II-2136
Benzamycine (Benzoyl Peroxide; Erythromycin)	II-292
Benzanil Simple (Penicillin G Benzathine)	II-2136
Benzetacil (Penicillin G Benzathine)	II-2136
Benzetacil A.P. (Penicillin G Benzathine)	II-2136
Benzetacil L.A. (Penicillin G Benzathine)	II-2136
Benzilfan (Penicillin G Benzathine)	II-2136
Benzodiapin (Chlordiazepoxide Hydrochloride)	II-539
Benzonal (Benzonatate)	II-290
Benzopin (Diazepam)	II-740
Benzotran (Oxazepam)	II-2063
Benzum 2 (Biperiden Hydrochloride)	II-322
Beocid Puroptal (Sulfacetamide Sodium)	II-2497
Beparine (Heparin Sodium)	II-1334
Bepricol (Bepridil Hydrochloride)	II-295
Beprosone (Betamethasone Dipropionate)	II-301
Berifen (Diclofenac)	II-748
Berifen Gel (Diclofenac)	II-748
Beriglobin (Immune Globulin (Human))	II-1434
Beriglobin P (Immune Globulin (Human))	II-1434
Beriglobina (Immune Globulin (Human))	II-1434
Beriglobin-P (Immune Globulin (Human))	II-1434
Berirab P (Rabies Vaccine)	II-2324
Berkamil (Amiloride Hydrochloride)	II-103
Berkatens (Verapamil Hydrochloride)	II-2777
Berkolol (Propranolol Hydrochloride)	II-2287
Berlactone (Spironolactone)	II-2483
Berlicetin (Chloramphenicol Sodium Succinate)	II-537
Berlinsulin Actrapid Normal U-40 (Insulin (Human Recombinant))	II-1454
Berlinsulin H 10 90 (Insulin (Human, Isophane/Regular))	II-1456
Berlinsulin H 20 80 (Insulin (Human, Isophane/Regular))	II-1456
Berlinsulin H 30 70 (Insulin (Human, Isophane/Regular))	II-1456
Berlinsulin H 40 60 (Insulin (Human, Isophane/Regular))	II-1456
Berlinsulin H Basal U-40 (Insulin (Human Recombinant))	II-1454
Berlthyrox (Levothyroxine Sodium)	II-1618
Bernoflox (Ciprofloxacin Hydrochloride)	II-573
Besitran (Sertraline Hydrochloride)	II-2439
Besone (Betamethasone Valerate)	II-305
Bespar (Buspirone Hydrochloride)	II-382
Bessasone (Betamethasone Valerate)	II-305
Best (Diazepam)	II-740
Bestafen (Ibuprofen)	II-1411
Bestalin (Hydroxyzine)	II-1398
Bestasone (Fluocinonide)	II-1156
Bestatin (Simvastatin)	II-2454
Bestelar (Mebendazole)	II-1711
Bestidine (Famotidine)	II-1093
Beta (Betamethasone Valerate)	II-305
Beta cream (Betamethasone Valerate)	II-305
Beta ointment (Betamethasone Valerate)	II-305
Beta Scalp (Betamethasone Valerate)	II-305
Betabion (Thiamine Hydrochloride)	II-2602
Betabloc (Propranolol Hydrochloride)	II-2287
Betablok (Atenolol)	II-222
Betac (Betaxolol Hydrochloride)	II-307
Betacard (Atenolol)	II-222
Beta-Cardone (Sotalol Hydrochloride)	II-2471
Betacin (Indomethacin)	II-1443
Betaclopramide (Metoclopramide Hydrochloride)	II-1798
Betacor (Sotalol Hydrochloride)	II-2471
Betacort (Betamethasone Valerate)	II-305
Betacorten (Betamethasone Valerate)	II-305
Betacrem (Betamethasone Dipropionate)	II-301
Betades (Sotalol Hydrochloride)	II-2471
Betadren (Pindolol)	II-2192
Betagalen (Betamethasone Valerate)	II-305
Betalans (Lansoprazole)	II-1569
Betaloc CR (Metoprolol)	II-1805
Betaloc Zok (Metoprolol)	II-1805
Betamin (Thiamine Hydrochloride)	II-2602
Betanamin (Pemoline)	II-2129
Betanase (Glyburide)	II-1297
Betanese 5 (Glyburide)	II-1297
Betapam (Diazepam)	II-740
Betaperamide (Loperamide Hydrochloride)	II-1664
Betapindol (Pindolol)	II-2192
Betapresin (Penbutolol Sulfate)	II-2131
Betapressin (Penbutolol Sulfate)	II-2131
Betaprofen (Ibuprofen)	II-1411
Betaren (Diclofenac)	II-748
Betaretic (Amiloride Hydrochloride; Hydrochlorothiazide)	II-105
Betarol (Atenolol)	II-222
Betasel (Betaxolol Hydrochloride)	II-307
Betasol (Clobetasol Propionate)	II-617
Betason (Betamethasone)	II-298
Betason (500 mcg) (Betamethasone)	II-298
Betasone (Betamethasone Valerate)	II-305
Betasone DHA (Betamethasone Valerate)	II-305
Betatabs (Thiamine Hydrochloride)	II-2602
Beta-Timelets (Propranolol Hydrochloride)	II-2287
Betaval (Betamethasone Valerate)	II-305
Betavate (Clobetasol Propionate)	II-617
Betaxin (Thiamine Hydrochloride)	II-2602
Betazok (Metoprolol)	II-1805
Betazol (Clobetasol Propionate)	II-617
Betazone (Betamethasone Dipropionate)	II-301
Betim (Timolol)	II-2627
Betlovex (Cyanocobalamin)	II-661
Betnelan (Betamethasone)	II-298
Betnelan (Betamethasone Valerate)	II-305
Betnelan (500 mcg) (Betamethasone)	II-298
Betnelan V (Betamethasone Valerate)	II-305
Betnelan-V (Betamethasone Valerate)	II-305
Betnesol (Betamethasone)	II-298
Betnesol V (Betamethasone Valerate)	II-305
Betnesol-V (Betamethasone Valerate)	II-305
Betneval (Betamethasone Valerate)	II-305
Betnevate (Betamethasone Valerate)	II-305
Betnovat (Betamethasone Valerate)	II-305
Betnovate RD (Betamethasone Valerate)	II-305
Betolvex (Cyanocobalamin)	II-661
Betopic (Betamethasone Valerate)	II-305
Betoprolol (Hydrochlorothiazide; Metoprolol Tartrate)	II-1355
Betoprolol (Metoprolol)	II-1805
Betoptima (Betaxolol Hydrochloride)	II-307
Betoquin (Betaxolol Hydrochloride)	II-307
Betsona (Betamethasone Valerate)	II-305
Bettamousse (Betamethasone Valerate)	II-305
Bevitex (Cyanocobalamin)	II-661
Bevitine (Thiamine Hydrochloride)	II-2602
Bewon (Thiamine Hydrochloride)	II-2602
Bex (Aspirin)	II-206
Bexilona (Diflorasone Diacetate)	II-776
Bexinor (Norfloxacin)	II-1997
Bexivit (Pyridoxine Hydrochloride)	II-2297
Bexon (Clindamycin)	II-605
B.G.B. Norflox (Norfloxacin)	II-1997
Biartac (Diflunisal)	II-777
Biaxin HP (Clarithromycin)	II-597
Bicide (Lindane)	II-1642
Bicillin LA 1.2 (Penicillin G Benzathine)	II-2136
Bicillin LA 2.4 (Penicillin G Benzathine)	II-2136
Biclar (Clarithromycin)	II-597
Biconcor (Bisoprolol Fumarate; Hydrochlorothiazide)	II-326
Bicrolid (Clarithromycin)	II-597
Bideren (Isosorbide Dinitrate)	II-1502
Bidicef (Cefadroxil Monohydrate)	II-447
Bi-Euglucon (Glyburide; Metformin Hydrochloride)	II-1300
Bi-Euglucon M "5" (Glyburide; Metformin Hydrochloride)	II-1300
Bifemelan (Alendronate Sodium)	II-70
Bifen (Ibuprofen)	II-1411
Bifen Cataplasma (Flurbiprofen)	II-1177
Bifinorma (Lactulose)	II-1550
Bifinorma Granulat (Lactulose)	II-1550
Bifiteral (Lactulose)	II-1550
Bifosa (Alendronate Sodium)	II-70
Bifotik (Cefoperazone Sodium)	II-471
Bigafen (Baclofen)	II-266
Bigazol (Ketoconazole)	II-1530
Biklin (Amikacin Sulfate)	II-101
Bildiuretic (Amiloride Hydrochloride; Hydrochlorothiazide)	II-105
Bimaran (Trazodone Hydrochloride)	II-2686
Bimox (Amoxicillin)	II-131
Binaldan (Loperamide Hydrochloride)	II-1664
Binarin (Epirubicin Hydrochloride)	II-938
Binison (Haloperidol)	II-1328
Binoklar (Clarithromycin)	II-597
Binotal (Ampicillin)	II-170
Bintamox (Amoxicillin)	II-131
Biocalcin (Calcitonin (Salmon))	II-397
Biocef (Cefpodoxime Proxetil)	II-484
Biocolyn (Doxycycline)	II-878
Biocort (Hydrocortisone Acetate)	II-1373
Biocoryl (Procainamide Hydrochloride)	II-2250
Biocronil (Enalapril Maleate)	II-913
Biodalgic (Tramadol Hydrochloride)	II-2674
Biodone (Methadone Hydrochloride)	II-1766
Biodone Extra Forte (Methadone Hydrochloride)	II-1766
Biodone Forte (Methadone Hydrochloride)	II-1766
Biodoxi (Doxycycline)	II-878
Biodroxil (Cefadroxil Monohydrate)	II-447
Biofanal (Nystatin)	II-2005
Biofanal Mundgel (Nystatin)	II-2005
Biofaxil (Cefadroxil Monohydrate)	II-447
Bioferon (Interferon Alfa-2b, Recombinant)	II-1471
Biofigran (Filgrastim)	II-1126
Biofloxin (Norfloxacin)	II-1997
Biofurin (Nitrofurantoin, Macrocrystalline)	II-1982
Biogaracin (Gentamicin Sulfate)	II-1279
Biogesic (Acetaminophen)	II-11
Bio-Hep-B (Hepatitis B Vaccine, Recombinant)	II-1343
Biohulin (Insulin (Human Recombinant))	II-1454
Biolincom (Lincomycin Hydrochloride)	II-1640
Biomag (Cimetidine Hydrochloride)	II-568
Biophenicol (Chloramphenicol)	II-536
Biophenicol (Chloramphenicol Sodium Succinate)	II-537
Biorfen (Orphenadrine Citrate)	II-2049
Biorphen (Orphenadrine Citrate)	II-2049
Biosint (Cefotaxime Sodium)	II-474
Biotax (Cefotaxime Sodium)	II-474

International brand name (Generic name)	Page no.
Biotax (Paclitaxel)	II-2084
Biotaxime (Cefotaxime Sodium)	II-474
Biotazol (Metronidazole)	II-1812
Biotrexate (Methotrexate Sodium)	II-1772
Biotriax (Ceftriaxone Sodium)	II-503
Bioxidona (Amoxicillin)	II-131
Bioxyllin (Amoxicillin)	II-131
Bioyl (Bisacodyl)	II-322
Biozolene (Fluconazole)	II-1136
Biozolin (Cefazolin Sodium)	II-452
Biperen (Biperiden Hydrochloride)	II-322
Biperin (Biperiden Hydrochloride)	II-322
Bipiden (Biperiden Hydrochloride)	II-322
Bipro (Betamethasone Valerate)	II-305
Bi-Profenid (Ketoprofen)	II-1533
Bipronyl (Naproxen)	II-1924
Biquinate (Quinine Sulfate)	II-2317
Bi-Rofenid (Ketoprofen)	II-1533
Biron (Buspirone Hydrochloride)	II-382
Birotin (Lovastatin)	II-1688
Bisalax (Bisacodyl)	II-322
Biscosal (Fluocinonide)	II-1156
Bisma (Sucralfate)	II-2493
Bismultin (Econazole Nitrate)	II-900
Biso (Bisoprolol Fumarate)	II-323
BisoABZ (Bisoprolol Fumarate)	II-323
Biso-BASF (Bisoprolol Fumarate)	II-323
Bisobloc (Bisoprolol Fumarate)	II-323
Bisolol (Bisoprolol Fumarate)	II-323
Bisomerck (Bisoprolol Fumarate)	II-323
Bi-Tildiem (Diltiazem Hydrochloride)	II-798
Blanoxan (Bleomycin Sulfate)	II-332
Blastocarb (Carboplatin)	II-430
Blastolem (Cisplatin)	II-589
Blastovin (Vinblastine Sulfate)	II-2787
Blef 10 con Lagrifilm (Sulfacetamide Sodium)	II-2497
Blef-10 (Sulfacetamide Sodium)	II-2497
Blef-30 (Sulfacetamide Sodium)	II-2497
Blend-A-Med (Chlorhexidine Gluconate)	II-542
Bleocin (Bleomycin Sulfate)	II-332
Bleolem (Bleomycin Sulfate)	II-332
Bleomicina (Bleomycin Sulfate)	II-332
Bleomycin (Bleomycin Sulfate)	II-332
Bleomycine (Bleomycin Sulfate)	II-332
Bleomycinum (Bleomycin Sulfate)	II-332
Bleph Liquifilm (Sulfacetamide Sodium)	II-2497
Bleph-30 (Sulfacetamide Sodium)	II-2497
Blocacid (Famotidine)	II-1093
Blocadren (Travoprost)	II-2685
Blocanol (Timolol)	II-2627
Blocanol (Travoprost)	II-2685
Blocard (Propranolol Hydrochloride)	II-2287
Blocaryl (Propranolol Hydrochloride)	II-2287
Blocklin (Pindolol)	II-2192
Bloflex (Cephalexin)	II-520
Blokium (Atenolol)	II-222
Blokium-Diu (Atenolol; Chlorthalidone)	II-226
Blomison (Ethambutol Hydrochloride)	II-1039
Blopress (Candesartan Cilexetil)	II-402
Blopress (Candesartan Cilexetil; Hydrochlorothiazide)	II-404
Blopress Plus (Candesartan Cilexetil; Hydrochlorothiazide)	II-404
Blotex (Atenolol)	II-222
Blucodil (Terbutaline Sulfate)	II-2574
Bluton (Ibuprofen)	II-1411
Bobsule (Hydroxyzine)	II-1398
Bodrex (Acetaminophen)	II-11
Boidan (Amantadine Hydrochloride)	II-97
Bolabomin (Diclofenac)	II-748
Bolutol (Gemfibrozil)	II-1269
Bonabol (Mefenamic Acid)	II-1720
Bonadon N (Pyridoxine Hydrochloride)	II-2297
Bonalerg (Loratadine)	II-1675
Bonalerg - D (Loratadine; Pseudoephedrine Sulfate)	II-1677

International brand name (Generic name)	Page no.
Bonamina (Meclizine Hydrochloride)	II-1713
Bonamine (Meclizine Hydrochloride)	II-1713
Bonatranquan (Lorazepam)	II-1678
Boncalmon (Calcitonin (Salmon))	II-397
Bondigest (Metoclopramide Hydrochloride)	II-1798
Bonidon (Indomethacin)	II-1443
Bonmax (Raloxifene Hydrochloride)	II-2326
Bonnox (Promethazine Hydrochloride)	II-2268
Bonyl (Naproxen)	II-1924
Bonzol (Danazol)	II-699
Boplatex (Carboplatin)	II-430
Borotel (Albendazole)	II-46
Borotropin (Atropine Sulfate)	II-235
Borymycin (Minocycline Hydrochloride)	II-1838
Bosmin (Epinephrine)	II-934
BQL (Enalapril Maleate)	II-913
Braccopiral (Pyrazinamide)	II-2295
Bralifex (Tobramycin)	II-2643
Bralix (Chlordiazepoxide Hydrochloride; Clidinium Bromide)	II-541
Brameston (Bromocriptine Mesylate)	II-344
Brasmatic (Terbutaline Sulfate)	II-2574
Braxan (Amiodarone Hydrochloride)	II-110
Braxidin (Chlordiazepoxide Hydrochloride; Clidinium Bromide)	II-541
Brek (Loperamide Hydrochloride)	II-1664
Bremcillin (Ampicillin)	II-170
Brenal (Acetaminophen)	II-11
Brentan (Miconazole)	II-1820
Bretylate (Bretylium Tosylate)	II-339
Brevimytal (Methohexital Sodium)	II-1770
Brevinor 21 (Ethinyl Estradiol; Norethindrone)	II-1055
Brevinor-1 21 (Ethinyl Estradiol; Norethindrone)	II-1055
Brevital (Methohexital Sodium)	II-1770
Brexic (Piroxicam)	II-2205
Brexicam (Piroxicam)	II-2205
Brexin (Piroxicam)	II-2205
Brexodin (Piroxicam)	II-2205
Bricanyl retard (Terbutaline Sulfate)	II-2574
Bricasma (Terbutaline Sulfate)	II-2574
Bridopen (Ampicillin)	II-170
Brieta (Methohexital Sodium)	II-1770
Brietal Sodium (Methohexital Sodium)	II-1770
Briklin (Amikacin Sulfate)	II-101
Briplatin (Cisplatin)	II-589
Briscotrim (Sulfamethoxazole; Trimethoprim)	II-2500
Brisfirina (Cephapirin Sodium)	II-525
Brispen (Dicloxacillin Sodium)	II-761
Bristaciclina (Tetracycline Hydrochloride)	II-2585
Bristacol (Pravastatin Sodium)	II-2224
Bristamox (Amoxicillin)	II-131
Bristaxol (Paclitaxel)	II-2084
Bristol-Videx EC (Didanosine)	II-766
Bristopen (Oxacillin Sodium)	II-2053
Britapen (Ampicillin)	II-170
Broadced (Ceftriaxone Sodium)	II-503
Broadcef (Cephradine)	II-526
Broadmetz (Amoxicillin)	II-131
Brofesol (Ferrous Sulfate)	II-1122
Brofulin (Griseofulvin, Microcrystalline)	II-1312
Brolin (Famotidine)	II-1093
Bromed (Bromocriptine Mesylate)	II-344
Bromergon (Bromocriptine Mesylate)	II-344
Bromidine (Bromocriptine Mesylate)	II-344
Bromocorn (Bromocriptine Mesylate)	II-344
Bromocrel (Bromocriptine Mesylate)	II-344
Bromohexal (Bromocriptine Mesylate)	II-344
Bromo-Kin (Bromocriptine Mesylate)	II-344
Bromokin (Bromocriptine Mesylate)	II-344
Bromopar (Bromocriptine Mesylate)	II-344
Bronalide (Flunisolide)	II-1149
Broncho D (Diphenhydramine Hydrochloride)	II-813
Bronchocal (Guaifenesin)	II-1314
Bronchodam (Terbutaline Sulfate)	II-2574
Bronchoretard (Theophylline)	II-2593

International brand name (Generic name)	Page no.
Broncho-Spray (Albuterol)	II-47
Bronco Asmo (Terbutaline Sulfate)	II-2574
Bronconox (Beclomethasone Dipropionate)	II-279
Bronconox Forte (Beclomethasone Dipropionate)	II-279
Broncovaleas (Albuterol)	II-47
Bronilide (Flunisolide)	II-1149
Bronmycin (Doxycycline)	II-878
Bronsolvan (Theophylline)	II-2593
Bronter (Albuterol)	II-47
Brospec (Ceftriaxone Sodium)	II-503
Brotopon (Haloperidol)	II-1328
Brozil (Gemfibrozil)	II-1269
Brufanic (Ibuprofen)	II-1411
Brufen 400 (Ibuprofen)	II-1411
Brufen Retard (Ibuprofen)	II-1411
Brufort (Ibuprofen)	II-1411
Brugesic (Ibuprofen)	II-1411
Brulamycin (Tobramycin Sulfate)	II-2646
Brumed (Ibuprofen)	II-1411
Brumetidina (Cimetidine Hydrochloride)	II-568
Brumixol (Ciclopirox)	II-561
Bryterol (Ondansetron Hydrochloride)	II-2039
Brytolin (Albuterol)	II-47
Buburone (Ibuprofen)	II-1411
Bucaine (Bupivacaine Hydrochloride)	II-361
Bucanil (Terbutaline Sulfate)	II-2574
Bucaril (Terbutaline Sulfate)	II-2574
Buccapol Berna (Polio Vaccine, Oral Live)	II-2210
Budecort (Budesonide)	II-347
Budecort Nasal (Budesonide)	II-347
Budecort NT (Budesonide)	II-347
Budeflam (Budesonide)	II-347
Budema (Bumetanide)	II-359
Budenofalk (Budesonide)	II-347
Budeson 3 (Budesonide)	II-347
Budicort Respules (Budesonide)	II-347
Bufect (Ibuprofen)	II-1411
Bufect Forte (Ibuprofen)	II-1411
Buffered Aspirin (Aspirin)	II-206
Bufferin (Aspirin)	II-206
Bufferin Low Dose (Aspirin)	II-206
Bufigen (Nalbuphine Hydrochloride)	II-1917
Bumedyl (Bumetanide)	II-359
Bumet (Bumetanide)	II-359
Bunol (Butorphanol Tartrate)	II-391
Bunolgan (Levobunolol Hydrochloride)	II-1603
Bupirop (Bupivacaine Hydrochloride)	II-361
Bupirop simple sin preservantes (Bupivacaine Hydrochloride)	II-361
Bupivan (Bupivacaine Hydrochloride)	II-361
Bupogesic (Ibuprofen)	II-1411
Buprex (Buprenorphine)	II-363
Buprine (Buprenorphine)	II-363
Burana (Ibuprofen)	II-1411
Burinax (Bumetanide)	II-359
Burten (Ketorolac Tromethamine)	II-1537
Busix (Bumetanide)	II-359
Busphen (Butorphanol Tartrate)	II-391
Buspin (Buspirone Hydrochloride)	II-382
Buspirex (Buspirone Hydrochloride)	II-382
Buspirone (Buspirone Hydrochloride)	II-382
Bustab (Buspirone Hydrochloride)	II-382
Butacort (Budesonide)	II-347
Butacortelone (Ibuprofen)	II-1411
Butahale (Albuterol)	II-47
Butamine (Dobutamine Hydrochloride)	II-834
Butavate (Clobetasol Propionate)	II-617
Butin (Bromocriptine Mesylate)	II-344
Butinat (Bumetanide)	II-359
Butinon (Bumetanide)	II-359
Buto-Asma (Albuterol)	II-47
Butomix (Albuterol)	II-47
Butotal (Albuterol)	II-47
Butylin (Terbutaline Sulfate)	II-2574
Buvacaina (Bupivacaine Hydrochloride)	II-361

International brand name (Generic name)	Page no.
Buvacainas (Bupivacaine Hydrochloride)	II-361
Buventol (Albuterol)	II-47
Buventol Easyhaler (Albuterol)	II-47
B-Vasc (Atenolol)	II-222

C

International brand name (Generic name)	Page no.
C500 (Ascorbic Acid)	II-203
Cabaser (Cabergoline)	II-395
Cadens (Calcitonin (Salmon))	II-397
Cadex (Doxazosin Mesylate)	II-860
Cadicycline (Tetracycline Hydrochloride)	II-2585
Cadil (Doxazosin Mesylate)	II-860
Cadimycetin (Chloramphenicol)	II-536
Cadiquin (Chloroquine)	II-544
Cadistin (Chlorpheniramine Maleate)	II-548
Caelyx (Doxorubicin, Liposomal)	II-873
Caginal (Clotrimazole)	II-640
Calabren (Glyburide)	II-1297
Calacort (Hydrocortisone Acetate)	II-1373
Calapol (Acetaminophen)	II-11
Calaptin (Verapamil Hydrochloride)	II-2777
Calaptin 240 SR (Verapamil Hydrochloride)	II-2777
Calcanate (Calcium Carbonate)	II-401
Calcefor (Calcium Carbonate)	II-401
Calcetat-GRY (Calcium Acetate)	II-400
Calcheck (Nifedipine)	II-1967
Calchek (Amlodipine Besylate)	II-125
Calci Aid (Calcium Carbonate)	II-401
Calcibloc (Nifedipine)	II-1967
Calcibloc OD (Nifedipine)	II-1967
Calcicard (Diltiazem Hydrochloride)	II-798
Calcigard (Nifedipine)	II-1967
Calcigard Retard (Nifedipine)	II-1967
Calcilat (Nifedipine)	II-1967
Calcilos (Calcium Carbonate)	II-401
Calcinin (Calcitonin (Salmon))	II-397
Calcit (Calcium Carbonate)	II-401
Calcitridin (Calcium Carbonate)	II-401
Calcium (Calcium Carbonate)	II-401
Calcium Carbonate (Calcium Carbonate)	II-401
Calcium Dago (Calcium Carbonate)	II-401
Calcium Folinate (Leucovorin Calcium)	II-1585
Calcium Klopfer (Calcium Carbonate)	II-401
Calcium Leucovorin (Leucovorin Calcium)	II-1585
Calciumfolinat-Ebewe (Leucovorin Calcium)	II-1585
Calcium-Sandoz Forte (Calcium Carbonate)	II-401
Calco (Calcitonin (Salmon))	II-397
Calcuren (Calcium Carbonate)	II-401
Caldoral (Calcium Carbonate)	II-401
Calmaril (Thioridazine Hydrochloride)	II-2605
Calmaxid (Nizatidine)	II-1992
Calmlet (Alprazolam)	II-85
Calmpose (Diazepam)	II-740
Calnurs (Diltiazem Hydrochloride)	II-798
Calociclina (Tetracycline Hydrochloride)	II-2585
Calodol (Acetaminophen)	II-11
Calozan (Diclofenac)	II-748
Calpol (Acetaminophen)	II-11
Calsan (Calcium Carbonate)	II-401
Calsynar (Calcitonin (Salmon))	II-397
Caltamol (Carteolol Hydrochloride)	II-435
Calte (Carteolol Hydrochloride)	II-435
Caltine (Calcitonin (Salmon))	II-397
Caltrate 600 (Calcium Carbonate)	II-401
Calypsol (Ketamine Hydrochloride)	II-1528
Camapine (Carbamazepine)	II-418
Cambiex (Bumetanide)	II-359
Camcolit (Lithium Carbonate)	II-1654
Camergan (Promethazine Hydrochloride)	II-2268
Camex (Cefadroxil Monohydrate)	II-447
Camezol (Metronidazole)	II-1812
Camicil (Ampicillin)	II-170
Cam-Kovac (Measles Virus Vaccine Live)	II-1708
Campanex (Cimetidine Hydrochloride)	II-568
Campto (Irinotecan Hydrochloride)	II-1487
Camrox (Piroxicam)	II-2205
Canazol (Clotrimazole)	II-640
Canceren (Methotrexate Sodium)	II-1772
Cancid (Fluconazole)	II-1136
Candazole (Clotrimazole)	II-640
Candesar (Candesartan Cilexetil)	II-402
Candespor (Clotrimazole)	II-640
Candid (Clotrimazole)	II-640
Candida-Lokalicid (Nystatin)	II-2005
Candid-V3 (Clotrimazole)	II-640
Candimon (Clotrimazole)	II-640
Candinox (Clotrimazole)	II-640
Candio-Hermal (Nystatin)	II-2005
Candiplas (Miconazole)	II-1820
Candistat (Itraconazole)	II-1517
Canditral (Itraconazole)	II-1517
Candizol (Miconazole)	II-1820
Candizol oral (Miconazole)	II-1820
Candizole (Clotrimazole)	II-640
Canef (Fluvastatin Sodium)	II-1199
Canesten 1 (Clotrimazole)	II-640
Canestene (Clotrimazole)	II-640
Canifug (Clotrimazole)	II-640
Canstat (Nystatin)	II-2005
Cantacid (Calcium Carbonate)	II-401
Capabiotic (Cefaclor)	II-444
Capace (Captopril)	II-411
Caplenal (Allopurinol)	II-77
Capocard (Captopril)	II-411
Caposan (Captopril)	II-411
Capotena (Captopril)	II-411
Capotril (Captopril)	II-411
Capozid (Captopril; Hydrochlorothiazide)	II-416
Capozide Forte (Captopril; Hydrochlorothiazide)	II-416
Capril (Captopril)	II-411
Caprin (Aspirin)	II-206
Caprysin (Clonidine Hydrochloride)	II-629
Capsoid (Prednisolone)	II-2233
Captace (Captopril)	II-411
Captea (Captopril; Hydrochlorothiazide)	II-416
Captensin (Captopril)	II-411
Capti (Captopril)	II-411
Captoflux (Captopril)	II-411
Captohexal (Captopril)	II-411
Captolane (Captopril)	II-411
Captomax (Captopril)	II-411
Captopren (Captopril)	II-411
Captopril (Captopril)	II-411
Captoprilan (Captopril)	II-411
Captoprilan-D (Captopril; Hydrochlorothiazide)	II-416
Captoril (Captopril)	II-411
Captral (Captopril)	II-411
Capurate (Allopurinol)	II-77
Capxidin (Piroxicam)	II-2205
Carace (Lisinopril)	II-1648
Carace Plus (Hydrochlorothiazide; Lisinopril)	II-1352
Caranil (Isosorbide Dinitrate)	II-1502
Carbac (Loracarbef)	II-1672
Carbachol (Carbenicillin Indanyl Sodium)	II-422
Carbadac (Carbamazepine)	II-418
Carbamann (Carbenicillin Indanyl Sodium)	II-422
Carbametin (Methocarbamol)	II-1768
Carbatol (Carbamazepine)	II-418
Carbazene (Carbamazepine)	II-418
Carbazep (Carbamazepine)	II-418
Carbazina (Carbamazepine)	II-418
Carbilev (Carbidopa; Levodopa)	II-424
Carbinib (Acetazolamide)	II-28
Carbocain (Mepivacaine Hydrochloride)	II-1737
Carbocain Dental (Mepivacaine Hydrochloride)	II-1737
Carbocaina (Mepivacaine Hydrochloride)	II-1737
Carbocaine Caudal 1.5% (Mepivacaine Hydrochloride)	II-1737
Carbocaine Dental (Mepivacaine Hydrochloride)	II-1737
Carbolit (Lithium Carbonate)	II-1654
Carbolith (Lithium Carbonate)	II-1654
Carboplat (Carboplatin)	II-430
Carboplatin a (Carboplatin)	II-430
Carboplatin Abic (Carboplatin)	II-430
Carboplatin DBL (Carboplatin)	II-430
Carboplatin Lederle (Carboplatin)	II-430
Carboplatino (Carboplatin)	II-430
Carbosin (Carboplatin)	II-430
Carbosin Lundbeck (Carboplatin)	II-430
Carbostesin (Bupivacaine Hydrochloride)	II-361
Carbotec (Carboplatin)	II-430
Carbrital (Pentobarbital Sodium)	II-2149
Carcinil (Leuprolide Acetate)	II-1587
Carcinocin (Doxorubicin, Liposomal)	II-873
Cardace (Ramipril)	II-2330
Cardcal (Diltiazem Hydrochloride)	II-798
Cardeloc (Metoprolol)	II-1805
Cardenalin (Doxazosin Mesylate)	II-860
Cardensiel (Bisoprolol Fumarate)	II-323
Cardepine (Nicardipine Hydrochloride)	II-1958
Cardiazem (Diltiazem Hydrochloride)	II-798
Cardiben S.R. (Diltiazem Hydrochloride)	II-798
Cardibloc (Nicardipine Hydrochloride)	II-1958
Cardifen (Nifedipine)	II-1967
Cardigox (Digoxin)	II-780
Cardiject (Dobutamine Hydrochloride)	II-834
Cardil (Diltiazem Hydrochloride)	II-798
Cardil (Doxazosin Mesylate)	II-860
Cardil Retard (Diltiazem Hydrochloride)	II-798
Cardilat (Nifedipine)	II-1967
Cardiloc (Bisoprolol Fumarate)	II-323
Cardina (Timolol)	II-2627
Cardinit (Nitroglycerin)	II-1984
Cardinol (Propranolol Hydrochloride)	II-2287
Cardinol LA (Propranolol Hydrochloride)	II-2287
Cardinor (Amlodipine Besylate)	II-125
Cardioaspirina (Aspirin)	II-206
Cardiocor (Bisoprolol Fumarate)	II-323
Cardiogoxin (Digoxin)	II-780
Cardiomin (Dobutamine Hydrochloride)	II-834
Cardionorm (Nifedipine)	II-1967
Cardiopal (Dopamine Hydrochloride)	II-853
Cardioquinol (Quinidine Sulfate)	II-2314
Cardiorona (Amiodarone Hydrochloride)	II-110
Cardiorytmin (Procainamide Hydrochloride)	II-2250
Cardiosel (Metoprolol)	II-1805
Cardiosta LP (Diltiazem Hydrochloride)	II-798
Cardiostat (Metoprolol)	II-1805
Cardiosteril (Dopamine Hydrochloride)	II-853
Cardioten (Atenolol)	II-222
Cardiover (Verapamil Hydrochloride)	II-2777
Cardioxin (Digoxin)	II-780
Cardipene (Nicardipine Hydrochloride)	II-1958
Cardipril (Captopril)	II-411
Cardium (Diltiazem Hydrochloride)	II-798
Cardivas (Carvedilol)	II-438
Cardizem Retard (Diltiazem Hydrochloride)	II-798
Cardizem SR (Diltiazem Hydrochloride)	II-798
Cardol (Sotalol Hydrochloride)	II-2471
Cardopax (Isosorbide Dinitrate)	II-1502
Cardopax Retard (Isosorbide Dinitrate)	II-1502
Cardoral (Doxazosin Mesylate)	II-860
Cardoxan (Doxazosin Mesylate)	II-860
Cardoxin (Dipyridamole)	II-821
Cardoxin Forte (Dipyridamole)	II-821
Cardular (Doxazosin Mesylate)	II-860
Cardular PP (Doxazosin Mesylate)	II-860
Cardular Uro (Doxazosin Mesylate)	II-860
Cardura XL (Doxazosin Mesylate)	II-860
Carduran (Doxazosin Mesylate)	II-860
Cardura-XL S.R. (Doxazosin Mesylate)	II-860
Carex (Diltiazem Hydrochloride)	II-798
Carexa (Itraconazole)	II-1517

International brand name (Generic name)	Page no.
Caridolin (Carisoprodol)	II-432
Carimycin (Clarithromycin)	II-597
Carisoma (Carisoprodol)	II-432
Carloxan (Cyclophosphamide)	II-666
Carmaz (Carbamazepine)	II-418
Carmol (Methocarbamol)	II-1768
Carmubris (Carmustine)	II-434
Carnosporin (Cephalexin)	II-520
Carnotprim Primperan (Metoclopramide Hydrochloride)	II-1798
Carol (Ibuprofen)	II-1411
Carpaz (Carbamazepine)	II-418
Carpental S.R. (Pentoxifylline)	II-2154
Carplan (Carboplatin)	II-430
Carsodil (Isosorbide Dinitrate)	II-1502
Cartagyl (Clofibrate)	II-619
Carteol (Carteolol Hydrochloride)	II-435
Cartia XT (Diltiazem Hydrochloride)	II-798
Cartrilet (Ticlopidine Hydrochloride)	II-2622
Carvasin (Isosorbide Dinitrate)	II-1502
Carvedlol (Carvedilol)	II-438
Carvisken (Pindolol)	II-2192
Carvrol (Carvedilol)	II-438
Carxin (Methocarbamol)	II-1768
Carzepin (Carbamazepine)	II-418
Carzepine (Carbamazepine)	II-418
Cascor XL (Diltiazem Hydrochloride)	II-798
Cassadan (Alprazolam)	II-85
Catabon (Dopamine Hydrochloride)	II-853
Cataflam DD (Diclofenac)	II-748
Cataflam Drops (Diclofenac)	II-748
Catanac (Diclofenac)	II-748
Catapres Diu (Chlorthalidone; Clonidine Hydrochloride)	II-557
Catapres TTS (Clonidine Hydrochloride)	II-629
Catapresan (Clonidine Hydrochloride)	II-629
Catapresan 100 (Clonidine Hydrochloride)	II-629
Catapresan Depot (Clonidine Hydrochloride)	II-629
Catapresan TTS (Clonidine Hydrochloride)	II-629
Catapressan (Clonidine Hydrochloride)	II-629
Catas (Diclofenac)	II-748
Catelon Eye drop (Carteolol Hydrochloride)	II-435
Catenol (Atenolol)	II-222
Cathejell (Diphenhydramine Hydrochloride)	II-813
Catima (Clotrimazole)	II-640
Catlep (Indomethacin)	II-1443
Catona (Captopril)	II-411
Catoplin (Captopril)	II-411
Caudel (Diazepam)	II-740
Caveril (Verapamil Hydrochloride)	II-2777
Caverject Powder for Injection (Alprostadil)	II-90
Cavumox (Amoxicillin; Clavulanate Potassium)	II-139
CC-Nefro 500 (Calcium Carbonate)	II-401
CCNU (Lomustine)	II-1662
Cebenicol (Chloramphenicol)	II-536
Cebion (Ascorbic Acid)	II-203
Cebutid (Flurbiprofen)	II-1177
CEC (Cefaclor)	II-444
CEC 500 (Cefaclor)	II-444
Cecap (Ascorbic Acid)	II-203
CeCe (Ascorbic Acid)	II-203
Cecenu (Lomustine)	II-1662
Ceclex (Cefaclor)	II-444
Ceclor AF (Cefaclor)	II-444
Ceclor CD (Cefaclor)	II-444
Ceclor MR (Cefaclor)	II-444
Ceclor Retard (Cefaclor)	II-444
Cecon (Ascorbic Acid)	II-203
Cecon Drops (Ascorbic Acid)	II-203
Cedantron (Ondansetron Hydrochloride)	II-2039
Cedar (Hydroxyzine)	II-1398
Cedocard (Isosorbide Dinitrate)	II-1502
Cedocard Retard (Isosorbide Dinitrate)	II-1502
Cedocard SR (Isosorbide Dinitrate)	II-1502
Cedrox (Cefadroxil Monohydrate)	II-447

International brand name (Generic name)	Page no.
Cedroxim (Cefadroxil Monohydrate)	II-447
CEENU (Lomustine)	II-1662
Ceevifil (Ascorbic Acid)	II-203
Cef-3 (Ceftriaxone Sodium)	II-503
Cefa (Cefazolin Sodium)	II-452
Cefabac (Cefaclor)	II-444
Cefabiocin (Cefaclor)	II-444
Cefablan (Cephalexin)	II-520
Cefacar (Cefadroxil Monohydrate)	II-447
Cefacell (Cefadroxil Monohydrate)	II-447
Cefacidal (Cefazolin Sodium)	II-452
Cefacin-M (Cephalexin)	II-520
Cefacle (Cefaclor)	II-444
Cefaclin (Cefaclor)	II-444
Cefaclostad (Cefaclor)	II-444
Cefadal (Cephalexin)	II-520
Cefadin (Cephalexin)	II-520
Cefadin (Cephradine)	II-526
Cefadina (Cephalexin)	II-520
Cefadol (Cefamandole Nafate)	II-449
Cefadril (Cefadroxil Monohydrate)	II-447
Cefadrol (Cefadroxil Monohydrate)	II-447
Cefadrox (Cefadroxil Monohydrate)	II-447
Cefadyl (Cephalexin)	II-520
Cefajet (Cefotaxime Sodium)	II-474
Cefalan (Cefaclor)	II-444
Cefalin (Cephalexin)	II-520
Cefalogen (Ceftriaxone Sodium)	II-503
Cefaloject (Cephapirin Sodium)	II-525
Cefalom (Cefadroxil Monohydrate)	II-447
Cefamezin (Cefazolin Sodium)	II-452
Cefamox (Cefadroxil Monohydrate)	II-447
Cefarad (Cefazolin Sodium)	II-452
Cefaroxil (Cefadroxil Monohydrate)	II-447
Cefaseptin (Cephalexin)	II-520
Cefat (Cefadroxil Monohydrate)	II-447
Cefatrex (Cephapirin Sodium)	II-525
Cefatrexyl (Cephapirin Sodium)	II-525
Cefax (Cephalexin)	II-520
Cefaxil (Cefadroxil Monohydrate)	II-447
Cefaxim (Cefotaxime Sodium)	II-474
Cefaxona (Ceftriaxone Sodium)	II-503
Cefaxone (Ceftriaxone Sodium)	II-503
Cefazin (Cefazolin Sodium)	II-452
Cefazol (Cefazolin Sodium)	II-452
Cefazolina (Cefazolin Sodium)	II-452
Cefazoline Panpharma (Cefazolin Sodium)	II-452
Ceffotan (Ceftazidime)	II-492
Cefin (Ceftriaxone Sodium)	II-503
Cefirad (Cefotaxime Sodium)	II-474
Cefirex (Cephradine)	II-526
Cefix (Cefixime)	II-466
Cefixmycin (Cefixime)	II-466
Cefkor (Cefaclor)	II-444
Cefkor CD (Cefaclor)	II-444
Cefler (Cefaclor)	II-444
Cefmore (Cefoxitin Sodium)	II-482
Cefobactam (Cefoperazone Sodium)	II-471
Cefobis (Cefoperazone Sodium)	II-471
Cefoclin (Cefotaxime Sodium)	II-474
Cefodox (Cefpodoxime Proxetil)	II-484
Cefogen (Cefuroxime)	II-507
Cefogram (Cefoperazone Sodium)	II-471
Cefolatam (Cefoperazone Sodium)	II-471
Cefomic (Cefotaxime Sodium)	II-474
Cefomycin (Cefoperazone Sodium)	II-471
Ceforal (Cefadroxil Monohydrate)	II-447
Ceforal (Cephalexin)	II-520
Ceforin (Cefoperazone Sodium)	II-471
Cefortam (Ceftazidime)	II-492
Cefotal (Ceftriaxone Sodium)	II-503
Cefotax (Cefotaxime Sodium)	II-474
Cefovit (Cephalexin)	II-520
Cefoxil (Cefadroxil Monohydrate)	II-447
Cefoxin (Cefoxitin Sodium)	II-482
Cefozone (Cefoperazone Sodium)	II-471

International brand name (Generic name)	Page no.
Cefpiran (Cefotaxime Sodium)	II-474
Cefpiran (Ceftazidime)	II-492
Cefra (Cephradine)	II-526
Cefradine (Cephradine)	II-526
Cefradur (Cephradine)	II-526
Cefral (Cefaclor)	II-444
Cefra-Om (Cefadroxil Monohydrate)	II-447
Cefrasol (Cephradine)	II-526
Cefriex (Ceftriaxone Sodium)	II-503
Cefril (Cephradine)	II-526
Cefrin (Cephalexin)	II-520
Cefro (Cephradine)	II-526
Cefroxil (Cefadroxil Monohydrate)	II-447
Cefspan (Cefixime)	II-466
Ceftazim (Ceftazidime)	II-492
Ceftenon (Cefotetan Disodium)	II-478
Ceftidin (Ceftazidime)	II-492
Ceftim (Ceftazidime)	II-492
Ceftix (Ceftizoxime Sodium)	II-500
Ceftrex (Ceftriaxone Sodium)	II-503
Ceftrilem (Ceftriaxone Sodium)	II-503
Ceftum (Ceftazidime)	II-492
Cefudura (Cefuroxime)	II-507
Cefuhexal (Cefuroxime)	II-507
Cefuracet (Cefuroxime)	II-507
Cefurax (Cefuroxime)	II-507
Cefuril (Cefuroxime)	II-507
Cefuro-Puren (Cefuroxime)	II-507
Cefurox-wolff (Cefuroxime)	II-507
Cefutil (Cefuroxime)	II-507
Cefxitin (Cefoxitin Sodium)	II-482
Ceglution (Lithium Carbonate)	II-1654
Ceglution 300 (Lithium Carbonate)	II-1654
Celance (Pergolide Mesylate)	II-2155
Celco (Cefaclor)	II-444
Celcox (Celecoxib)	II-515
Celebra (Celecoxib)	II-515
Celeka (Potassium Chloride)	II-2215
Celestamine (Betamethasone)	II-298
Celestan (Betamethasone)	II-298
Celestan Biphase (Betamethasone Acetate; Betamethasone Sodium Phosphate)	II-299
Celestan Depot (Betamethasone Acetate; Betamethasone Sodium Phosphate)	II-299
Celestan V (Betamethasone Valerate)	II-305
Celestan-V (Betamethasone Valerate)	II-305
Celestene (Betamethasone)	II-298
Celestene Chronodose (Betamethasone Acetate; Betamethasone Sodium Phosphate)	II-299
Celestoderm (Betamethasone Valerate)	II-305
Celestoderm V (Betamethasone Valerate)	II-305
Celestoderm-V (Betamethasone Valerate)	II-305
Celeston (Betamethasone)	II-298
Celeston (Betamethasone Acetate; Betamethasone Sodium Phosphate)	II-299
Celeston Chronodose (Betamethasone Acetate; Betamethasone Sodium Phosphate)	II-299
Celeston Valerat (Betamethasone Valerate)	II-305
Celestone (Betamethasone Valerate)	II-305
Celestone (500 mcg) (Betamethasone)	II-298
Celestone Cronodose (Betamethasone Acetate; Betamethasone Sodium Phosphate)	II-299
Celestone-M (Betamethasone Valerate)	II-305
Celestone-Soluspan (Betamethasone Acetate; Betamethasone Sodium Phosphate)	II-299
Celestone-V (Betamethasone Valerate)	II-305
Celex (Cephradine)	II-526
Celexa (Citalopram Hydrobromide)	II-591
Celexil (Cephalexin)	II-520
Celexin (Cephalexin)	II-520
Celib (Celecoxib)	II-515

International brand name (Generic name)	Page no.
Celidin (Atropine Sulfate; Diphenoxylate Hydrochloride)	II-238
Celin (Ascorbic Acid)	II-203
Cellidrin (Allopurinol)	II-77
Cellmustin (Estramustine Phosphate Sodium)	II-1017
Celltop (Etoposide)	II-1080
Celupan (Naltrexone Hydrochloride)	II-1920
Celvista (Raloxifene Hydrochloride)	II-2326
Cemedin 200 (Cimetidine Hydrochloride)	II-568
Cemedin 400 (Cimetidine Hydrochloride)	II-568
Cemedin 800 (Cimetidine Hydrochloride)	II-568
Cementin (Cimetidine Hydrochloride)	II-568
Cemol (Acetaminophen)	II-11
Cendevax (Rubella Virus Vaccine Live)	II-2409
Cendo Carpine (Pilocarpine)	II-2180
Cendo Tropine (Atropine Sulfate)	II-235
Cenilene (Fluphenazine Hydrochloride)	II-1172
Cenlidac (Sulindac)	II-2512
Cenol (Ascorbic Acid)	II-203
Centilax (Hydroxyzine)	II-1398
Centralgin (Meperidine Hydrochloride)	II-1733
Cepacilina (Penicillin G Benzathine)	II-2136
Cepal (Famotidine)	II-1093
Cepan (Cefotetan Disodium)	II-478
Cepastar (Cephalexin)	II-520
Cepazine (Cefuroxime)	II-507
Ceperatam (Cefoperazone Sodium)	II-471
Cepexin (Cephalexin)	II-520
Cephalexyl (Cephalexin)	II-520
Cephanmycin (Cephalexin)	II-520
Cephia (Cephalexin)	II-520
Cephin (Ceftriaxone Sodium)	II-503
Cephin (Cephalexin)	II-520
Cephoral (Cefixime)	II-466
Cephos (Cefadroxil Monohydrate)	II-447
Cepimax (Cefepime Hydrochloride)	II-462
Cepodem (Cefpodoxime Proxetil)	II-484
Cepol (Cephalexin)	II-520
Ceporex Forte (Cephalexin)	II-520
Ceporexin (Cephalexin)	II-520
Ceporexin-E (Cephalexin)	II-520
Ceporexine (Cephalexin)	II-520
Ceprazol (Albendazole)	II-46
Cerax (Hydroxyzine)	II-1398
Cerazine (Cetirizine Hydrochloride)	II-529
Cereen (Haloperidol)	II-1328
Cerepax (Temazepam)	II-2556
Ceretal (Pentoxifylline)	II-2154
Cerexin (Cephalexin)	II-520
Cerixon (Ceftriaxone Sodium)	II-503
Cero (Cefaclor)	II-444
Cerotec (Cetirizine Hydrochloride)	II-529
Cerubidin (Daunorubicin Hydrochloride)	II-708
Cerucal (Metoclopramide Hydrochloride)	II-1798
Cerviprime (Dinoprostone)	II-812
Cerviprost (Dinoprostone)	II-812
C.E.S. (Estrogens, Conjugated)	II-1019
Cesid (Cefaclor)	II-444
Cesol (Praziquantel)	II-2228
Cesplon (Captopril)	II-411
Cesplon Plus (Captopril; Hydrochlorothiazide)	II-416
Cesta (Cetirizine Hydrochloride)	II-529
Cetabrium (Chlordiazepoxide Hydrochloride)	II-539
Cetadexon (Dexamethasone)	II-730
Cetasix (Furosemide)	II-1237
Cetathrocin (Erythromycin Stearate)	II-970
Cetatrex (Sumatriptan Succinate)	II-2516
Cetax (Cefotaxime Sodium)	II-474
Cetazin (Sulfacetamide Sodium)	II-2497
Cetazum (Ceftazidime)	II-492
Ceten (Ceftibuten)	II-496
Cethis (Cetirizine Hydrochloride)	II-529
Cethixim (Cefuroxime)	II-507
Cetilan (Acetylcysteine)	II-29
Cetin (Cetirizine Hydrochloride)	II-529
Cetina (Chloramphenicol)	II-536
Cetina (Chloramphenicol Sodium Succinate)	II-537
Cetirax (Cetirizine Hydrochloride)	II-529
Cetirax D (Cetirizine Hydrochloride; Pseudoephedrine Hydrochloride)	II-532
Ceto (Aspirin)	II-206
Cetoxil (Cefuroxime)	II-507
Cetraxal (Ciprofloxacin Hydrochloride)	II-573
Cetrimed (Cetirizine Hydrochloride)	II-529
Cetrine (Cetirizine Hydrochloride)	II-529
Cetrinets (Ascorbic Acid)	II-203
Cetrizet (Cetirizine Hydrochloride)	II-529
Cetrizin (Cetirizine Hydrochloride)	II-529
Cety (Cetirizine Hydrochloride)	II-529
Ce-Vi-Sol (Ascorbic Acid)	II-203
Cewin (Ascorbic Acid)	II-203
C-Flox (Ciprofloxacin Hydrochloride)	II-573
C-Floxacin (Ciprofloxacin Hydrochloride)	II-573
Check (Cephalexin)	II-520
Chef (Ceftriaxone Sodium)	II-503
Chemacin (Amikacin Sulfate)	II-101
Chemicetina (Chloramphenicol)	II-536
Chemicetina (Chloramphenicol Sodium Succinate)	II-537
Chemitrim (Sulfamethoxazole; Trimethoprim)	II-2500
Chemoprim (Sulfamethoxazole; Trimethoprim)	II-2500
Chibro-Atropine (Atropine Sulfate)	II-235
Chibro-Proscar (Finasteride)	II-1129
Chibro-Timoptol (Timolol)	II-2627
Chibro-Timoptol (Travoprost)	II-2685
Chibroxine (Norfloxacin)	II-1997
Chibroxol (Norfloxacin)	II-1997
Chiclida (Meclizine Hydrochloride)	II-1713
Chilcolan (Dipyridamole)	II-821
Children's Motrin (Ibuprofen)	II-1411
Chinchen (Carisoprodol)	II-432
Chingazol (Clotrimazole)	II-640
Chlobax (Chlordiazepoxide Hydrochloride; Clidinium Bromide)	II-541
Chlomazine (Chlorpromazine Hydrochloride)	II-549
Chloment (Chloramphenicol)	II-536
Chlometon (Chlorpheniramine Maleate)	II-548
Chlomide (Chlorpropamide)	II-554
Chlomy (Chloramphenicol)	II-536
Chloracil (Chloramphenicol)	II-536
Chloracil (Chloramphenicol Sodium Succinate)	II-537
Chloractil (Chlorpromazine Hydrochloride)	II-549
Chloraldurat (Chloral Hydrate)	II-534
Chloralhydrat (Chloral Hydrate)	II-534
Chloralhydrat 500 (Chloral Hydrate)	II-534
Chloralix (Chloral Hydrate)	II-534
Chloramex (Chloramphenicol)	II-536
Chloraminophene (Chlorambucil)	II-535
Chloramno (Chloramphenicol)	II-536
Chloram-P (Chloramphenicol Sodium Succinate)	II-537
Chloramphen (Chloramphenicol Sodium Succinate)	II-537
Chloramphenicol (Chloramphenicol)	II-536
Chloramphenicol (Chloramphenicol Sodium Succinate)	II-537
Chloramphenicol "Agepha" Augensalbe (Chloramphenicol)	II-536
Chloramphenicol "Agepha" Ohrentropfen (Chloramphenicol)	II-536
Chloramphenicol Faure, Ophthadoses (Chloramphenicol)	II-536
Chloramphenicol POS (Chloramphenicol)	II-536
Chloramphenicol PW Ohrentropfen (Chloramphenicol)	II-536
Chloramphenicol RIT (Chloramphenicol)	II-536
Chloramsaar N (Chloramphenicol)	II-536
Chlorazin (Chlorpromazine Hydrochloride)	II-549
Chlorcol (Chloramphenicol)	II-536
Chlordiabet (Chlorpropamide)	II-554
Chlordiazepoxidum (Chlordiazepoxide Hydrochloride)	II-539
Chlorestrol (Gemfibrozil)	II-1269
Chlorhex (Chlorhexidine Gluconate)	II-542
Chlorhexamed (Chlorhexidine Gluconate)	II-542
Chlorhexidine Mouthwash (Chlorhexidine Gluconate)	II-542
Chlorhexidine Obstetric Lotion (Chlorhexidine Gluconate)	II-542
Chlorhexidinium (Chlorhexidine Gluconate)	II-542
Chlorleate (Chlorpheniramine Maleate)	II-548
Chlormide (Chlorpropamide)	II-554
Chlornicol (Chloramphenicol)	II-536
Chlorocide S (Chloramphenicol Sodium Succinate)	II-537
Chlorofoz (Chloroquine)	II-544
Chlorohex gel (Chlorhexidine Gluconate)	II-542
Chlorohex gel Forte (Chlorhexidine Gluconate)	II-542
Chlorohex Mouth Rinse (Chlorhexidine Gluconate)	II-542
Chloromycetin (Chloramphenicol Sodium Succinate)	II-537
Chloromycetin Eye Drops (Chloramphenicol)	II-536
Chloromycetin Eye Ointment (Chloramphenicol)	II-536
Chloromycetin Eye Preparations (Chloramphenicol)	II-536
Chloromycetin Injection (Chloramphenicol Sodium Succinate)	II-537
Chloromycetin Succinate Injection (Chloramphenicol Sodium Succinate)	II-537
Chloromycetine (Chloramphenicol)	II-536
Chloromycetine (Chloramphenicol Sodium Succinate)	II-537
Chlor-Oph (Chloramphenicol)	II-536
Chloroquini Diphosphas (Chloroquine)	II-544
Chlorphen (Chloramphenicol)	II-536
Chlorpheniramine DHA (Chlorpheniramine Maleate)	II-548
Chlorpheno (Chlorpheniramine Maleate)	II-548
Chlorphenon (Chlorpheniramine Maleate)	II-548
Chlorpromanyl (Chlorpromazine Hydrochloride)	II-549
Chlorpromed (Chlorpromazine Hydrochloride)	II-549
Chlorpropamide Medochemie (Chlorpropamide)	II-554
Chlorprosil (Chlorpropamide)	II-554
Chlorpyrimine (Chlorpheniramine Maleate)	II-548
Chlorquin (Chloroquine)	II-544
Chlorsig (Chloramphenicol)	II-536
Chlorsig Eye Preparations (Chloramphenicol)	II-536
Chlortrimeton (Chlorpheniramine Maleate)	II-548
Chlor-Tripolon (Chlorpheniramine Maleate)	II-548
Chlor-Tripolon N.D. (Loratadine; Pseudoephedrine Sulfate)	II-1677
Chlorvescent (Potassium Chloride)	II-2215
Chlothin (Chlorothiazide)	II-545
Chlotride (Chlorothiazide)	II-545
Cholacid (Ursodiol)	II-2737
Cholenal (Clofibrate)	II-619
Choles (Cholestyramine)	II-559
Cholespid (Gemfibrozil)	II-1269
Cholestabyl (Colestipol Hydrochloride)	II-652
Cholestat (Simvastatin)	II-2454
Cholestra (Lovastatin)	II-1688
Chol-Less (Cholestyramine)	II-559
Chooz Antacid Gum 500 (Calcium Carbonate)	II-401
Chronadalate LP (Nifedipine)	II-1967
Chrono-Indocid (Indomethacin)	II-1443
Chrytemin (Imipramine Hydrochloride)	II-1431
Chuichin (Chlordiazepoxide Hydrochloride)	II-539
Ciba Vision Atropine (Atropine Sulfate)	II-235
Cibace (Benazepril Hydrochloride)	II-284
Cibacen (Benazepril Hydrochloride)	II-284
Cibacen Cor (Benazepril Hydrochloride)	II-284

International brand name (Generic name)	Page no.
Cibacen HCT (Benazepril Hydrochloride; Hydrochlorothiazide)	II-288
Cibacene (Benazepril Hydrochloride)	II-284
Cibadrex (Benazepril Hydrochloride; Hydrochlorothiazide)	II-288
Ciclem (Cimetidine Hydrochloride)	II-568
Ciclochem (Ciclopirox)	II-561
Cicloderm (Ciclopirox)	II-561
Cicloferon (Acyclovir)	II-33
Ciclofosfamida (Cyclophosphamide)	II-666
Ciclolen (Cyclophosphamide)	II-666
Ciclopar (Albendazole)	II-46
Ciclotetryl (Tetracycline Hydrochloride)	II-2585
Cicloviral (Acyclovir)	II-33
Ciclovulan (Ethinyl Estradiol; Norethindrone)	II-1055
Cicloxal (Cyclophosphamide)	II-666
Cidanchin (Chloroquine)	II-544
Cidine (Cimetidine Hydrochloride)	II-568
Cidomycin (Gentamicin Sulfate)	II-1279
Ciflox (Ciprofloxacin Hydrochloride)	II-573
Cifloxin (Ciprofloxacin Hydrochloride)	II-573
Cifran (Ciprofloxacin Hydrochloride)	II-573
Cigamet (Cimetidine Hydrochloride)	II-568
Cignatin (Cimetidine Hydrochloride)	II-568
Ciket M (Cimetidine Hydrochloride)	II-568
Cilab (Ciprofloxacin Hydrochloride)	II-573
Cilacil (Penicillin V Potassium)	II-2142
Cilamox (Amoxicillin)	II-131
Cilest (Ethinyl Estradiol; Norgestimate)	II-1059
Cileste (Ethinyl Estradiol; Norgestimate)	II-1059
Cilicaine VK (Penicillin V Potassium)	II-2142
Cillimicina (Lincomycin Hydrochloride)	II-1640
Cillimycin (Lincomycin Hydrochloride)	II-1640
Ciloquin (Ciprofloxacin Hydrochloride)	II-573
Cilosol (Cilostazol)	II-566
Cilotal (Cilostazol)	II-566
Cimal (Cimetidine Hydrochloride)	II-568
Cimbene (Cimetidine Hydrochloride)	II-568
Cimedine (Cimetidine Hydrochloride)	II-568
Cimehexal (Cimetidine Hydrochloride)	II-568
Cimeldine (Cimetidine Hydrochloride)	II-568
Cimet (Cimetidine Hydrochloride)	II-568
Cimetag (Cimetidine Hydrochloride)	II-568
Cimetalgin (Cimetidine Hydrochloride)	II-568
Cimetase (Cimetidine Hydrochloride)	II-568
Cimetid (Cimetidine Hydrochloride)	II-568
Cimetidin (Cimetidine Hydrochloride)	II-568
Cimetidina (Cimetidine Hydrochloride)	II-568
Cimetidine (Cimetidine Hydrochloride)	II-568
Cimetigal (Cimetidine Hydrochloride)	II-568
Cimetin (Cimetidine Hydrochloride)	II-568
Cimetum (Cimetidine Hydrochloride)	II-568
Cimewell (Cimetidine Hydrochloride)	II-568
Cimex (Cimetidine Hydrochloride)	II-568
Cimexillin (Ampicillin)	II-170
Cimlok (Cimetidine Hydrochloride)	II-568
Cimogal (Ciprofloxacin Hydrochloride)	II-573
Cimulcer (Cimetidine Hydrochloride)	II-568
Cinabel (Clotrimazole)	II-640
Cinadine (Cimetidine Hydrochloride)	II-568
Cinaflox (Ciprofloxacin Hydrochloride)	II-573
Cinam (Ampicillin Sodium; Sulbactam Sodium)	II-174
Cincordil (Isosorbide Mononitrate)	II-1507
Cinolon (Fluocinolone Acetonide)	II-1152
CiNU (Lomustine)	II-1662
Cinulcus (Cimetidine Hydrochloride)	II-568
Cipan (Cetirizine Hydrochloride; Pseudoephedrine Hydrochloride)	II-532
Cipaprim (Sulfamethoxazole; Trimethoprim)	II-2500
Cipaprim Forte (Sulfamethoxazole; Trimethoprim)	II-2500
Cipex (Mebendazole)	II-1711
Cipide (Ciprofloxacin Hydrochloride)	II-573
Cipilat (Nifedipine)	II-1967
Ciplactin (Cyproheptadine Hydrochloride)	II-682
Cipladinex 100 (Didanosine)	II-766
Ciplanevimune (Nevirapine)	II-1952
Ciplar (Propranolol Hydrochloride)	II-2287
Ciplar-H (Hydrochlorothiazide; Propranolol Hydrochloride)	II-1357
Ciplox (Ciprofloxacin Hydrochloride)	II-573
Ciplus (Ciprofloxacin Hydrochloride)	II-573
Cipol (Cyclosporine)	II-668
Cipol-N (Cyclosporine)	II-668
Cipralex (Escitalopram Oxalate)	II-973
Cipram (Citalopram Hydrobromide)	II-591
Cipramil (Citalopram Hydrobromide)	II-591
Ciprecu (Ciprofloxacin Hydrochloride)	II-573
Cipril (Lisinopril)	II-1648
Cipril - H (Hydrochlorothiazide; Lisinopril)	II-1352
Ciprinol (Ciprofloxacin Hydrochloride)	II-573
Cipro HC Otic (Ciprofloxacin Hydrochloride; Hydrocortisone)	II-588
Ciprobac (Ciprofloxacin Hydrochloride)	II-573
Ciprobay (Ciprofloxacin Hydrochloride)	II-573
Ciprobay HC (Ciprofloxacin Hydrochloride; Hydrocortisone)	II-588
Ciprobay Uro (Ciprofloxacin Hydrochloride)	II-573
Ciprobid (Ciprofloxacin Hydrochloride)	II-573
Ciprobiotic (Ciprofloxacin Hydrochloride)	II-573
Ciprocan (Ciprofloxacin Hydrochloride)	II-573
Ciprocep (Ciprofloxacin Hydrochloride)	II-573
Ciprocin (Ciprofloxacin Hydrochloride)	II-573
Ciprocinol (Ciprofloxacin Hydrochloride)	II-573
Ciprodar (Ciprofloxacin Hydrochloride)	II-573
Ciprodex (Ciprofloxacin Hydrochloride)	II-573
Ciproflox (Ciprofloxacin Hydrochloride)	II-573
Ciprogis (Ciprofloxacin Hydrochloride)	II-573
Ciproglen (Ciprofloxacin Hydrochloride)	II-573
Ciprok (Ciprofloxacin Hydrochloride)	II-573
Ciprolin (Ciprofloxacin Hydrochloride)	II-573
Ciprolon (Ciprofloxacin Hydrochloride)	II-573
Cipromycin (Ciprofloxacin Hydrochloride)	II-573
Cipropharm (Ciprofloxacin Hydrochloride)	II-573
Ciproquin (Ciprofloxacin Hydrochloride)	II-573
Ciproquinol (Ciprofloxacin Hydrochloride)	II-573
Ciproral (Cyproheptadine Hydrochloride)	II-682
Ciprovit-A (Cyproheptadine Hydrochloride)	II-682
Ciprox (Ciprofloxacin Hydrochloride)	II-573
Ciproxacol (Ciprofloxacin Hydrochloride)	II-573
Ciproxan (Ciprofloxacin Hydrochloride)	II-573
Ciproxin (Ciprofloxacin Hydrochloride)	II-573
Ciproxin (Ciprofloxacin Hydrochloride; Hydrocortisone)	II-588
Ciproxin HC ear drops (Ciprofloxacin Hydrochloride; Hydrocortisone)	II-588
Ciproxina (Ciprofloxacin Hydrochloride)	II-573
Ciproxine (Ciprofloxacin Hydrochloride)	II-573
Ciproxyl (Ciprofloxacin Hydrochloride)	II-573
Ciriax (Ciprofloxacin Hydrochloride)	II-573
Cirilen (Diltiazem Hydrochloride)	II-798
Cirilen AP (Diltiazem Hydrochloride)	II-798
Cirokan (Ciprofloxacin Hydrochloride)	II-573
Ciroxin (Ciprofloxacin Hydrochloride)	II-573
Cirrus (Cetirizine Hydrochloride; Pseudoephedrine Hydrochloride)	II-532
Cismetin (Cimetidine Hydrochloride)	II-568
Cisplatin-Ebewe (Cisplatin)	II-589
Cisplatino (Cisplatin)	II-589
Cisplatinum (Cisplatin)	II-589
Cisplatyl (Cisplatin)	II-589
Cistamine (Cetirizine Hydrochloride)	II-529
Cisticid (Praziquantel)	II-2228
Citanest Adrenalin (Epinephrine Bitartrate; Prilocaine Hydrochloride)	II-937
Citarabina (Cytarabine)	II-683
Citax F (Immune Globulin (Human))	II-1434
Citicil (Ampicillin)	II-170
Citidine (Cimetidine Hydrochloride)	II-568
Citilat (Nifedipine)	II-1967
Citireuma (Sulindac)	II-2512
Citius (Cimetidine Hydrochloride)	II-568
Citoken T (Piroxicam)	II-2205
Citomid (Vincristine Sulfate)	II-2789
Citopam (Citalopram Hydrobromide)	II-591
Citopcin (Ciprofloxacin Hydrochloride)	II-573
Citoplatino (Cisplatin)	II-589
Citosulfan (Busulfan)	II-385
Citravite (Ascorbic Acid)	II-203
Citrec (Leucovorin Calcium)	II-1585
Cityl (Misoprostol)	II-1851
Civeran (Loratadine)	II-1675
Civicor (Verapamil Hydrochloride)	II-2777
Cixa (Ciprofloxacin Hydrochloride)	II-573
Cizoren (Haloperidol)	II-1328
Clacef (Cefotaxime Sodium)	II-474
Clacillin Duo Dry Syrup (Amoxicillin; Clavulanate Potassium)	II-139
Clacine (Clarithromycin)	II-597
Claforan (Cefotaxime Sodium)	II-474
Clafoxim (Cefotaxime Sodium)	II-474
Clamax (Amoxicillin; Clavulanate Potassium)	II-139
Clambiotic (Clarithromycin)	II-597
Clamentin (Amoxicillin; Clavulanate Potassium)	II-139
Clamide (Glyburide)	II-1297
Clamist (Clemastine Fumarate)	II-603
Clamobit (Amoxicillin; Clavulanate Potassium)	II-139
Clamonex (Amoxicillin; Clavulanate Potassium)	II-139
Clamovid (Amoxicillin; Clavulanate Potassium)	II-139
Clamox (Amoxicillin)	II-131
Clamoxin (Amoxicillin; Clavulanate Potassium)	II-139
Clamoxyl (Amoxicillin; Clavulanate Potassium)	II-139
Clamoxyl DuoForte (Amoxicillin; Clavulanate Potassium)	II-139
Clapharma (Clarithromycin)	II-597
Claradol (Acetaminophen)	II-11
Claradol Codeine (Acetaminophen; Codeine Phosphate)	II-13
Claragine (Aspirin)	II-206
Claramax (Desloratadine)	II-721
Claratyne Cold (Loratadine; Pseudoephedrine Sulfate)	II-1677
Claratyne Decongestant (Loratadine; Pseudoephedrine Sulfate)	II-1677
Claraxim (Cefotaxime Sodium)	II-474
Clari (Clarithromycin)	II-597
Claribid (Clarithromycin)	II-597
Claridar (Clarithromycin)	II-597
Clarimac (Clarithromycin)	II-597
Clarinase (Loratadine; Pseudoephedrine Sulfate)	II-1677
Clarinase Repetabs (Loratadine; Pseudoephedrine Sulfate)	II-1677
Clarin-Duo (Amoxicillin; Clavulanate Potassium)	II-139
Claripen (Clarithromycin)	II-597
Clarith (Clarithromycin)	II-597
Claritin Extra (Loratadine; Pseudoephedrine Sulfate)	II-1677
Claritine (Loratadine)	II-1675
Claritrol (Clarithromycin)	II-597
Clarityn (Loratadine)	II-1675
Clarityne (Loratadine)	II-1675
Clarityne D 24H (Loratadine; Pseudoephedrine Sulfate)	II-1677
Clarityne D Pediatrico (Loratadine; Pseudoephedrine Sulfate)	II-1677
Clarityne D Repetabs (Loratadine; Pseudoephedrine Sulfate)	II-1677
Clarityne-D (Loratadine; Pseudoephedrine Sulfate)	II-1677

International brand name (Generic name)	Page no.
Claroma (Clarithromycin)	II-597
Classen (Mercaptopurine)	II-1741
Clatax (Cefotaxime Sodium)	II-474
Clavamox (Amoxicillin; Clavulanate Potassium)	II-139
Claversal (Mesalamine)	II-1748
Clavinex (Amoxicillin; Clavulanate Potassium)	II-139
Clavocef (Cefotaxime Sodium)	II-474
Clavox (Cefotaxime Sodium)	II-474
Clavoxilin Plus (Amoxicillin; Clavulanate Potassium)	II-139
Clavulin (Amoxicillin; Clavulanate Potassium)	II-139
Clavulin Duo Forte (Amoxicillin; Clavulanate Potassium)	II-139
Clavumox (Amoxicillin; Clavulanate Potassium)	II-139
Cleancef (Cefaclor)	II-444
Clearol (Gemfibrozil)	II-1269
Clebudan (Budesonide)	II-347
Cleniderm (Betamethasone Dipropionate)	II-301
Clenil (Beclomethasone Dipropionate)	II-279
Clenil Forte (Beclomethasone Dipropionate)	II-279
Cleo (Tobramycin)	II-2643
Cleridium (Dipyridamole)	II-821
Clesin (Cromolyn Sodium)	II-656
Clexane 40 (Enoxaparin Sodium)	II-927
Clexane Forte (Enoxaparin Sodium)	II-927
Cliacil (Penicillin V Potassium)	II-2142
Cliad (Chlordiazepoxide Hydrochloride; Clidinium Bromide)	II-541
Cliane (Estradiol; Norethindrone Acetate)	II-1011
Clid (Ticlopidine Hydrochloride)	II-2622
Clidol (Sulindac)	II-2512
Climadan (Clindamycin)	II-605
Climaderm (Estradiol)	II-986
Climage (Fenofibrate)	II-1105
Climara Forte (Estradiol)	II-986
Climarest (Estrogens, Conjugated)	II-1019
Climarest plus (Estrogens, Conjugated; Medroxyprogesterone Acetate)	II-1027
Climatrol (Estrogens, Conjugated; Medroxyprogesterone Acetate)	II-1027
Climatrol HT (Estrogens, Conjugated; Medroxyprogesterone Acetate)	II-1027
Climatrol HT Continuo (Estrogens, Conjugated; Medroxyprogesterone Acetate)	II-1027
Climatrol HT Continuo Plus (Estrogens, Conjugated; Medroxyprogesterone Acetate)	II-1027
Climatrol HT Plus (Estrogens, Conjugated; Medroxyprogesterone Acetate)	II-1027
Climopax (Estrogens, Conjugated; Medroxyprogesterone Acetate)	II-1027
Clinacin (Clindamycin)	II-605
Clinbercin (Clindamycin)	II-605
Clincin (Clindamycin)	II-605
Clinda (Clindamycin)	II-605
Clindabeta (Clindamycin)	II-605
Clindacin (Clindamycin)	II-605
Clindal (Clindamycin)	II-605
Clindamax (Clindamycin)	II-605
Clinfol (Clindamycin)	II-605
Clinimycin (Clindamycin)	II-605
Clinofem (Medroxyprogesterone Acetate)	II-1714
Clinovir (Acyclovir)	II-33
Clint (Allopurinol)	II-77
Clobasol (Clobetasol Propionate)	II-617
Clobasone (Clobetasol Propionate)	II-617
Clobenate (Clobetasol Propionate)	II-617
Clobesol (Clobetasol Propionate)	II-617
Clobeson (Clobetasol Propionate)	II-617
Clobet (Clobetasol Propionate)	II-617
Clobutol (Ethambutol Hydrochloride)	II-1039
Clocephen (Acetaminophen)	II-11
Clocreme (Clotrimazole)	II-640
Cloderm (Clobetasol Propionate)	II-617
Cloderm (Clotrimazole)	II-640
Clo-Far (Diclofenac)	II-748
Clofec (Diclofenac)	II-748
Clofeet (Fluocinolone Acetonide)	II-1152
Clofen (Baclofen)	II-266
Clofi ICN (Clofibrate)	II-619
Clofibral (Clofibrate)	II-619
Clofibrato (Clofibrate)	II-619
Clofipront (Clofibrate)	II-619
Clofozine (Clofazimine)	II-619
Clofranil (Clomipramine Hydrochloride)	II-621
Clogesten (Clotrimazole)	II-640
Cloisone (Carbidopa; Levodopa)	II-424
Clo-Kit Junior (Chloroquine)	II-544
Clomacinvag (Clotrimazole)	II-640
Clomaderm (Clotrimazole)	II-640
Clomin (Dicyclomine Hydrochloride)	II-763
Clomizol (Clotrimazole)	II-640
Clonamox (Amoxicillin)	II-131
Clonaren (Diclofenac)	II-748
Clonazine (Chlorpromazine Hydrochloride)	II-549
Clonea (Clotrimazole)	II-640
Clonex (Clonazepam)	II-625
Clonidine (Clonidine Hydrochloride)	II-629
Clonitia (Clotrimazole)	II-640
Clonodifen (Diclofenac)	II-748
Clont (Metronidazole)	II-1812
Clopamon (Metoclopramide Hydrochloride)	II-1798
Clopan (Metoclopramide Hydrochloride)	II-1798
Clopilet (Clopidogrel Bisulfate)	II-635
Clopram (Clomipramine Hydrochloride)	II-621
Clopram (Metoclopramide Hydrochloride)	II-1798
Clopress (Clomipramine Hydrochloride)	II-621
Clopsine (Clozapine)	II-642
Cloracef MR (Cefaclor)	II-444
Clorafen (Chloramphenicol)	II-536
Cloramed (Clorazepate Dipotassium)	II-638
Cloramfeni Ofteno (Chloramphenicol)	II-536
Cloramfeni Ungena (Chloramphenicol)	II-536
Cloran (Doxycycline)	II-878
Cloranfenicol N.T. (Chloramphenicol)	II-536
Clor-K-Zaf (Potassium Chloride)	II-2215
Clormicin (Clarithromycin)	II-597
Cloro (Chlorpheniramine Maleate)	II-548
Cloro Trimeton (Chlorpheniramine Maleate)	II-548
Cloroalergan (Chlorpheniramine Maleate)	II-548
Cloromisan (Chloramphenicol)	II-536
Cloroptic (Chloramphenicol)	II-536
Clorotir (Cefaclor)	II-444
Cloro-Trimeton (Chlorpheniramine Maleate)	II-548
Clorotrimeton (Chlorpheniramine Maleate)	II-548
Clorten (Chlorpheniramine Maleate)	II-548
Clostedal (Carbamazepine)	II-418
Clostet (Tetanus Toxoid)	II-2583
Clostrin (Clotrimazole)	II-640
Clothalton (Chlorthalidone; Clonidine Hydrochloride)	II-557
Clothia (Hydrochlorothiazide)	II-1348
Clotrasone (Betamethasone Dipropionate; Clotrimazole)	II-304
Clotrihexal (Clotrimazole)	II-640
Clotrimaderm (Clotrimazole)	II-640
Clovate (Clobetasol Propionate)	II-617
Clovicin (Acyclovir)	II-33
Cloxy (Clotrimazole)	II-640
Cloxydin (Dicloxacillin Sodium)	II-761
Clozene (Clorazepate Dipotassium)	II-638
Clozol (Clotrimazole)	II-640
Clozole (Clotrimazole)	II-640
Coamoxin (Amoxicillin)	II-131
CoApprovel (Hydrochlorothiazide; Irbesartan)	II-1351
Coaprovel (Hydrochlorothiazide; Irbesartan)	II-1351
Cobalin (Cyanocobalamin)	II-661
Cobalmed (Cyanocobalamin)	II-661
Cobalparen (Cyanocobalamin)	II-661
Cobamin Ophth Soln (Cyanocobalamin)	II-661
Co-Betaloc (Hydrochlorothiazide; Metoprolol Tartrate)	II-1355
Cobutolin (Albuterol)	II-47
Co-Cadamol (Acetaminophen; Codeine Phosphate)	II-13
Codabrol (Acetaminophen; Codeine Phosphate)	II-13
Cod-Acamol Forte (Acetaminophen; Codeine Phosphate)	II-13
Codate (Codeine Phosphate)	II-647
Codeidol (Acetaminophen; Codeine Phosphate)	II-13
Codeidol F (Acetaminophen; Codeine Phosphate)	II-13
Codein Knoll (Codeine Phosphate)	II-647
Codein Kwizda (Codeine Phosphate)	II-647
Codein Phosphate (Codeine Phosphate)	II-647
Codein Slovakofarma (Codeine Phosphate)	II-647
Codeine Linctus (Codeine Phosphate)	II-647
Codeinum Phosphorcum (Codeine Phosphate)	II-647
Codeisan (Codeine Phosphate)	II-647
Codenfan (Codeine Phosphate)	II-647
Codephos (Codeine Phosphate)	II-647
Codicet (Acetaminophen; Codeine Phosphate)	II-13
Codicompren Retard (Codeine Phosphate)	II-647
Codiforton (Codeine Phosphate)	II-647
Codilprane Enfant (Acetaminophen; Codeine Phosphate)	II-13
Codimal (Guaifenesin)	II-1314
Co-Diovan (Hydrochlorothiazide; Valsartan)	II-1366
CoDiovan (Hydrochlorothiazide; Valsartan)	II-1366
Codipar (Acetaminophen; Codeine Phosphate)	II-13
Codiphen (Aspirin; Codeine Phosphate)	II-210
Codipront N (Codeine Phosphate)	II-647
Codis (Aspirin; Codeine Phosphate)	II-210
Codis 500 (Aspirin; Codeine Phosphate)	II-210
Codisal Forte (Acetaminophen; Codeine Phosphate)	II-13
Coditam (Acetaminophen; Codeine Phosphate)	II-13
Codix 5 (Oxycodone Hydrochloride)	II-2076
Codoliprane (Acetaminophen; Codeine Phosphate)	II-13
Codral (Aspirin; Codeine Phosphate)	II-210
Codral Forte (Aspirin; Codeine Phosphate)	II-210
Coforin (Pentostatin)	II-2151
Cogetine (Chloramphenicol)	II-536
Cohistan (Chlorpheniramine Maleate)	II-548
Cokenzen (Candesartan Cilexetil; Hydrochlorothiazide)	II-404
Colace (Docusate Sodium)	II-841
Colain (Chloramphenicol)	II-536
Colastatina (Simvastatin)	II-2454
Colchicin (Colchicine)	II-649
Colchicine (Colchicine)	II-649
Colchicine capsules (Colchicine)	II-649
Colchicine Houde (Colchicine)	II-649
Colchicum-Dispert (Colchicine)	II-649
Colchily (Colchicine)	II-649
Colchimedio (Colchicine)	II-649
Colchiquim (Colchicine)	II-649
Colchisol (Colchicine)	II-649
Colcine (Colchicine)	II-649
Colebron (Clofibrate)	II-619
Coles (Clofibrate)	II-619
Colestepril (Cholestyramine)	II-559
Colestiramina (Cholestyramine)	II-559
Colestrol (Cholestyramine)	II-559
Colfarit (Aspirin)	II-206
Colgout (Colchicine)	II-649
Colifilm (Loperamide Hydrochloride)	II-1664
Colircusi Cloramfenicol (Chloramphenicol)	II-536

International brand name (Generic name)	Page no.
Colirio Sulfacetamido Kriya (Sulfacetamide Sodium)	II-2497
Colitofalk (Mesalamine)	II-1748
Colizole (Sulfamethoxazole; Trimethoprim)	II-2500
Colizole DS (Sulfamethoxazole; Trimethoprim)	II-2500
Colodium (Loperamide Hydrochloride)	II-1664
Colofoam (Hydrocortisone Acetate)	II-1373
Colo-Pleon (Sulfasalazine)	II-2507
Colsancetine (Chloramphenicol)	II-536
Colsor (Acyclovir)	II-33
Colufase (Nitazoxanide)	II-1978
Combantrin-1 (Mebendazole)	II-1711
Combantrin-1 with mebendazole (Mebendazole)	II-1711
Combicyclin (Tetracycline Hydrochloride)	II-2585
Combid (Lamivudine; Zidovudine)	II-1560
Combiflam (Ibuprofen)	II-1411
CombiPatch (Estradiol; Norethindrone Acetate)	II-1011
Combipresan (Chlorthalidone; Clonidine Hydrochloride)	II-557
Combizym (Pancrelipase)	II-2095
Combizym Compositum (Pancrelipase)	II-2095
Combutol (Ethambutol Hydrochloride)	II-1039
Com-Femic (Ferrous Sulfate)	II-1122
Comin (Chlorpheniramine Maleate)	II-548
Comoprin (Aspirin)	II-206
Comox (Sulfamethoxazole; Trimethoprim)	II-2500
Comozol (Ketoconazole)	II-1530
Compensal (Cyanocobalamin)	II-661
Compensal 25,000 (Cyanocobalamin)	II-661
Complement (Naproxen)	II-1924
Compraz (Lansoprazole)	II-1569
Comtade (Entacapone)	II-931
Comtess (Entacapone)	II-931
Conan (Quinapril Hydrochloride)	II-2305
Conazol (Ketoconazole)	II-1530
Conbutol (Ethambutol Hydrochloride)	II-1039
Concerta (Methylphenidate Hydrochloride)	II-1781
Concerta XL (Methylphenidate Hydrochloride)	II-1781
Concor (Bisoprolol Fumarate)	II-323
Concor COR (Bisoprolol Fumarate)	II-323
Concor Plus (Bisoprolol Fumarate; Hydrochlorothiazide)	II-326
Concor Plus Forte (Bisoprolol Fumarate; Hydrochlorothiazide)	II-326
Concordin (Protriptyline Hydrochloride)	II-2294
Concore (Bisoprolol Fumarate)	II-323
Conducil (Isosorbide Dinitrate)	II-1502
Confortid (Indomethacin)	II-1443
Confortid Retard (Indomethacin)	II-1443
Confortid Retardkapseln (Indomethacin)	II-1443
Congex (Naproxen)	II-1924
Conicine (Colchicine)	II-649
Conjugen (Estrogens, Conjugated)	II-1019
Conmy (Terazosin Hydrochloride)	II-2566
Conmycin (Tetracycline Hydrochloride)	II-2585
Conova (Ethinyl Estradiol; Ethynodiol Diacetate)	II-1042
Conpin (Isosorbide Mononitrate)	II-1507
Conpin Retardkaps (Isosorbide Mononitrate)	II-1507
Conprim (Sulfamethoxazole; Trimethoprim)	II-2500
Conquer (Mebendazole)	II-1711
Consec (Ranitidine Hydrochloride)	II-2334
Consolan (Nabumetone)	II-1909
Constan (Alprazolam)	II-85
Consupren (Cyclosporine)	II-668
Contalax (Bisacodyl)	II-322
Contalgin (Morphine Sulfate)	II-1877
Contenton (Amantadine Hydrochloride)	II-97
Contimit (Terbutaline Sulfate)	II-2574
Continue DR (Morphine Sulfate)	II-1877
Contol (Chlordiazepoxide Hydrochloride)	II-539
Contomin (Chlorpromazine Hydrochloride)	II-549
Contramal (Tramadol Hydrochloride)	II-2674
Contramal LP (Tramadol Hydrochloride)	II-2674
Control (Lorazepam)	II-1678
Controlip (Fenofibrate)	II-1105
Controloc (Pantoprazole Sodium)	II-2097
Controlvas (Enalapril Maleate)	II-913
Convertal (Losartan Potassium)	II-1682
Convertal (Nicardipine Hydrochloride)	II-1958
Converten (Enalapril Maleate)	II-913
Convertin (Enalapril Maleate)	II-913
Convulex (Valproate Sodium)	II-2749
Convulex (Valproic Acid)	II-2755
Convuline (Carbamazepine)	II-418
Coochil (Dicyclomine Hydrochloride)	II-763
Copal (Sulindac)	II-2512
Copamide (Chlorpropamide)	II-554
Coquan (Clonazepam)	II-625
Coracten (Nifedipine)	II-1967
Coragoxine (Digoxin)	II-780
Coral (Nifedipine)	II-1967
Coralen (Ranitidine Hydrochloride)	II-2334
Corangin (Isosorbide Mononitrate)	II-1507
Corangin SR (Isosorbide Mononitrate)	II-1507
Coratol (Atenolol)	II-222
Coraver (Verapamil Hydrochloride)	II-2777
Corbeta (Propranolol Hydrochloride)	II-2287
Corbionax (Amiodarone Hydrochloride)	II-110
Cordalat (Nifedipine)	II-1967
Cordalin (Bisoprolol Fumarate)	II-323
Cordarex (Amiodarone Hydrochloride)	II-110
Cordaron (Amiodarone Hydrochloride)	II-110
Cordes H (Hydrocortisone Acetate)	II-1373
Cordil (Isosorbide Dinitrate)	II-1502
Cordil 40 SR (Isosorbide Dinitrate)	II-1502
Cordilox (Verapamil Hydrochloride)	II-2777
Cordilox SR (Verapamil Hydrochloride)	II-2777
Cordipen (Nifedipine)	II-1967
Cordipin (Nifedipine)	II-1967
Cordium (Bepridil Hydrochloride)	II-295
Cordralan (Diclofenac)	II-748
Co-Renitec (Enalapril Maleate; Hydrochlorothiazide)	II-923
Corenitec (Enalapril Maleate; Hydrochlorothiazide)	II-923
Co-Reniten (Enalapril Maleate; Hydrochlorothiazide)	II-923
Coreton (Hydrocortisone)	II-1369
Coreton (Labetalol Hydrochloride)	II-1545
Coric (Lisinopril)	II-1648
Coric Plus (Hydrochlorothiazide; Lisinopril)	II-1352
Corinol (Atenolol; Chlorthalidone)	II-226
Cornaron (Amiodarone Hydrochloride)	II-110
Cornilat (Isosorbide Dinitrate)	II-1502
Corometon (Chlorpheniramine Maleate)	II-548
Coronair (Dipyridamole)	II-821
Coronamole (Dipyridamole)	II-821
Coronex (Isosorbide Dinitrate)	II-1502
Coro-Nitro (Nitroglycerin)	II-1984
Coronovo (Amiodarone Hydrochloride)	II-110
Corosan (Dipyridamole)	II-821
Corosorbide (Isosorbide Dinitrate)	II-1502
Corotenol (Atenolol)	II-222
Corotrend (Nifedipine)	II-1967
Corovliss (Isosorbide Dinitrate)	II-1502
Corovliss Retard (Isosorbide Dinitrate)	II-1502
Corpamil (Verapamil Hydrochloride)	II-2777
Corpril (Ramipril)	II-2330
Corprilor (Enalapril Maleate)	II-913
Correctol (Bisacodyl)	II-322
Corsabutol (Ethambutol Hydrochloride)	II-1039
Corsacin (Ciprofloxacin Hydrochloride)	II-573
Corsaderm (Betamethasone Valerate)	II-305
Corsamet (Cimetidine Hydrochloride)	II-568
Corsazinmid (Pyrazinamide)	II-2295
Corsodyl (Chlorhexidine Gluconate)	II-542
Corsona (Dexamethasone)	II-730
Cortab (Dipyridamole)	II-821
Cortaid (Hydrocortisone Acetate)	II-1373
Cortal (Aspirin)	II-206
Cortamed (Hydrocortisone Acetate)	II-1373
Cortancyl (Prednisone)	II-2240
Cortate (Cortisone Acetate)	II-654
Cortate (Hydrocortisone)	II-1369
Cortef (Hydrocortisone Acetate)	II-1373
Cortef Cream (Hydrocortisone Acetate)	II-1373
Cortes (Hydrocortisone)	II-1369
Cortic Cream (Hydrocortisone Acetate)	II-1373
Corticap (Hydrocortisone Sodium Succinate)	II-1379
Cortidex (Dexamethasone)	II-730
Cortidexason (Dexamethasone)	II-730
Cortilona (Fluocinolone Acetonide)	II-1152
Cortimax (Betamethasone Dipropionate)	II-301
Cortison Ciba (Cortisone Acetate)	II-654
Cortison Nycomed (Cortisone Acetate)	II-654
Cortisone (Cortisone Acetate)	II-654
Cortisone Acetate (Cortisone Acetate)	II-654
Cortisoni Acetas (Cortisone Acetate)	II-654
Cortisporin Ear (Hydrocortisone; Neomycin Sulfate; Polymyxin B Sulfate)	II-1384
Cortixyl (Betamethasone Dipropionate)	II-301
Cortoderm (Hydrocortisone Acetate)	II-1373
Cortogen (Cortisone Acetate)	II-654
Cortone Acetato (Cortisone Acetate)	II-654
Cortone-Azetat (Cortisone Acetate)	II-654
Cortril (Hydrocortisone Acetate)	II-1373
Corubin (Cyanocobalamin)	II-661
Cosflox (Ciprofloxacin Hydrochloride)	II-573
Cosig Forte (Sulfamethoxazole; Trimethoprim)	II-2500
Cosmegen, Lyovac (Dactinomycin)	II-690
Cosmogen Lyovac (Dactinomycin)	II-690
Cosopt (Dorzolamide Hydrochloride; Timolol Maleate)	II-860
Cotareg (Hydrochlorothiazide; Valsartan)	II-1366
Cotazym (Pancrelipase)	II-2095
Cotazym ECS (Pancrelipase)	II-2095
Cotazym-65 B (Pancrelipase)	II-2095
Cotazym-S Forte (Pancrelipase)	II-2095
Cotren (Clotrimazole)	II-640
Cotribase (Sulfamethoxazole; Trimethoprim)	II-2500
Cotrim-Diolan (Sulfamethoxazole; Trimethoprim)	II-2500
Cotrimel (Sulfamethoxazole; Trimethoprim)	II-2500
Cotrix (Sulfamethoxazole; Trimethoprim)	II-2500
Cotronak (Ribavirin)	II-2351
Coumadan Sodico (Warfarin Sodium)	II-2804
Coumadine (Warfarin Sodium)	II-2804
Covarex (Miconazole)	II-1820
Covengar (Clorazepate Dipotassium)	II-638
Covina (Estradiol; Norethindrone Acetate)	II-1011
Covocort (Hydrocortisone)	II-1369
Covospor (Clotrimazole)	II-640
Covosulf (Sulfacetamide Sodium)	II-2497
Coxid (Celecoxib)	II-515
Coxime (Isosorbide Mononitrate)	II-1507
Coxine SR (Isosorbide Mononitrate)	II-1507
Cozole (Sulfamethoxazole; Trimethoprim)	II-2500
CPZ (Cefoperazone Sodium)	II-471
Cranoc (Fluvastatin Sodium)	II-1199
Crasnitin (Asparaginase)	II-204
Cravit (Levofloxacin)	II-1607
Cravit Ophthalmic (Levofloxacin)	II-1607
Crecisan (Minoxidil)	II-1845
Creliverol-12 (Cyanocobalamin)	II-661
Crema Blanca Bustillos (Hydroquinone)	II-1391
Cremicort-H (Hydrocortisone)	II-1369
Cremisona (Fluocinolone Acetonide)	II-1152
Cremosan (Ketoconazole)	II-1530
Crenodyn (Cefadroxil Monohydrate)	II-447
Crinone (Progesterone)	II-2262
Cristapen (Penicillin G Potassium)	II-2137
Crixan (Clarithromycin)	II-597
Croanan Duo Dry Syrup (Amoxicillin; Clavulanate Potassium)	II-139
Crobate (Clobetasol Propionate)	II-617

International brand name (Generic name)	Page no.
Crocin (Acetaminophen)	II-11
Cromabak (Cromolyn Sodium)	II-656
Cromadoses (Cromolyn Sodium)	II-656
Cromal-5 Inhaler (Cromolyn Sodium)	II-656
Cromlex (Cephalexin)	II-520
Cromo-Asma (Cromolyn Sodium)	II-656
Cromogen (Cromolyn Sodium)	II-656
Cromolyn (Cromolyn Sodium)	II-656
Crom-Ophtal (Cromolyn Sodium)	II-656
Cromoptic (Cromolyn Sodium)	II-656
Cronase (Cromolyn Sodium)	II-656
Cronasma (Theophylline)	II-2593
Cronitin (Loratadine)	II-1675
Cronizat (Nizatidine)	II-1992
Cronopen (Loratadine)	II-1675
Cruor (Bepridil Hydrochloride)	II-295
Cryocriptina (Bromocriptine Mesylate)	II-344
Cryopril (Captopril)	II-411
Cryosolona (Methylprednisolone Sodium Succinate)	II-1793
Cryotol (Propofol)	II-2278
Cryptal (Fluconazole)	II-1136
Crysanal (Naproxen)	II-1924
Crystapen V (Penicillin V Potassium)	II-2142
Cuemid (Cholestyramine)	II-559
Cuivasil Spray (Lidocaine)	II-1628
Cumatil (Phenytoin Sodium)	II-2175
Cupripen (Penicillamine)	II-2133
Cuprofen (Ibuprofen)	II-1411
Curacne Ge (Isotretinoin)	II-1510
Curam (Amoxicillin; Clavulanate Potassium)	II-139
Curatane (Isotretinoin)	II-1510
Curazid Forte (Isoniazid)	II-1496
Curinflam (Diclofenac)	II-748
Curisafe (Cefadroxil Monohydrate)	II-447
Curofen (Baclofen)	II-266
Curyken (Loratadine)	II-1675
Cusate (Docusate Sodium)	II-841
Cusicrom (Cromolyn Sodium)	II-656
Cusigel (Fluocinonide)	II-1156
Cusimolol (Timolol)	II-2627
Cusimolol (Travoprost)	II-2685
Cusiviral (Acyclovir)	II-33
Cutacelan (Azelaic Acid)	II-245
Cutaderm (Hydrocortisone)	II-1369
Cutason (Prednisone)	II-2240
Cutter Hyperab (Rho (D) Immune Globulin)	II-2350
Cutter Hyprho-D (Rho (D) Immune Globulin)	II-2350
C-Vex (Pentoxifylline)	II-2154
C-Vimin (Ascorbic Acid)	II-203
Cyben (Cyclobenzaprine Hydrochloride)	II-664
Cycin (Ciprofloxacin Hydrochloride)	II-573
Cyclabid (Tetracycline Hydrochloride)	II-2585
Cyclidox (Doxycycline)	II-878
Cyclimycin (Minocycline Hydrochloride)	II-1838
Cyclivex (Acyclovir)	II-33
Cyclo (Acyclovir)	II-33
Cycloblastine (Cyclophosphamide)	II-666
Cyclo-Cell (Cyclophosphamide)	II-666
Cyclogest (Progesterone)	II-2262
Cyclomed (Acyclovir)	II-33
Cyclomen (Danazol)	II-699
Cyclominol (Dicyclomine Hydrochloride)	II-763
Cyclomycin-K (Cefadroxil Monohydrate)	II-447
Cyclophar (Cyclophosphamide)	II-666
Cyclor (Cefaclor)	II-444
Cyclorax (Acyclovir)	II-33
Cyclostad (Acyclovir)	II-33
Cyclostin (Cyclophosphamide)	II-666
Cyclostin N (Cyclophosphamide)	II-666
Cyclovir (Acyclovir)	II-33
Cygran (Ranitidine Hydrochloride)	II-2334
Cyheptine (Cyproheptadine Hydrochloride)	II-682
Cylat (Cyproheptadine Hydrochloride)	II-682
Cyllanvir (Acyclovir)	II-33
Cymevan (Ganciclovir Sodium)	II-1250
Cymeven (Ganciclovir Sodium)	II-1250
Cynomycin (Minocycline Hydrochloride)	II-1838
Cypercil (Piperacillin Sodium)	II-2196
Cypro H (Cyproheptadine Hydrochloride)	II-682
Cyproatin (Cyproheptadine Hydrochloride)	II-682
Cyprogin (Cyproheptadine Hydrochloride)	II-682
Cypromin (Cyproheptadine Hydrochloride)	II-682
Cyprono (Cyproheptadine Hydrochloride)	II-682
Cyprosian (Cyproheptadine Hydrochloride)	II-682
Cyprostol (Misoprostol)	II-1851
Cyral (Primidone)	II-2247
Cysfec (Ciprofloxacin Hydrochloride)	II-573
Cysin (Lovastatin)	II-1688
Cystagon (Mercaptopurine)	II-1741
Cystonorm (Oxybutynin)	II-2070
Cystrin (Oxybutynin)	II-2070
Cytacon (Cyanocobalamin)	II-661
Cytadine (Cyproheptadine Hydrochloride)	II-682
Cytagon (Glyburide)	II-1297
Cytaman (Cyanocobalamin)	II-661
Cytamen (Cyanocobalamin)	II-661
Cytamid (Flutamide)	II-1181
Cytarabine (Cytarabine)	II-683
Cytarine (Cytarabine)	II-683
Cytine (Cimetidine Hydrochloride)	II-568
Cytoblastin (Vinblastine Sulfate)	II-2787
Cytocristin (Vincristine Sulfate)	II-2789
Cytokan (Cyclophosphamide)	II-666
Cytolog (Misoprostol)	II-1851
Cytonal (Cytarabine)	II-683
Cytophosphan (Cyclophosphamide)	II-666
Cytoplatin (Cisplatin)	II-589
Cytosa U (Cytarabine)	II-683
Cytosar (Cytarabine)	II-683
Cytosar U (Cytarabine)	II-683

D

International brand name (Generic name)	Page no.
D Epifrin (Dipivefrin Hydrochloride)	II-820
Dabex (Metformin Hydrochloride)	II-1760
Dabu (Dexamethasone)	II-730
Dacam (Piroxicam)	II-2205
Dacarbazin (Dacarbazine)	II-687
Dacarbazine DBL (Dacarbazine)	II-687
Dacarbazine Dome (Dacarbazine)	II-687
Dacarbazine For Injection (Dacarbazine)	II-687
Dacarel (Nicardipine Hydrochloride)	II-1958
Dacatic (Dacarbazine)	II-687
Daccorin (Acetaminophen; Dichloralphenazone; Isometheptene Mucate)	II-16
Daclin (Sulindac)	II-2512
Dacmozen (Dactinomycin)	II-690
Dacocilin (Dicloxacillin Sodium)	II-761
Dacorten (Prednisone)	II-2240
Dadcrome (Cromolyn Sodium)	II-656
Dafalgan Codeine (Acetaminophen; Codeine Phosphate)	II-13
Dafloxen (Naproxen Sodium)	II-1928
Daga (Acetaminophen)	II-11
Dagan (Nicardipine Hydrochloride)	II-1958
Dagracycline (Doxycycline)	II-878
Dagynil (Estrogens, Conjugated)	II-1019
Daicefalin (Cephradine)	II-526
Daipres (Clonidine Hydrochloride)	II-629
Daktagold (Ketoconazole)	II-1530
Daktar (Miconazole)	II-1820
Dalacin (Clindamycin)	II-605
Dalacine (Clindamycin)	II-605
Dalcap (Clindamycin)	II-605
Dalmadorm (Flurazepam Hydrochloride)	II-1175
Dalmate (Flurazepam Hydrochloride)	II-1175
Damicine (Clindamycin)	II-605
Damide (Indapamide)	II-1436
Damycin (Idarubicin Hydrochloride)	II-1417
Danasin (Danazol)	II-699
Danasone (Dexamethasone)	II-730
Danatrol (Danazol)	II-699
Danazol (Danazol)	II-699
Danazol Jean Marie (Danazol)	II-699
Danazol-Ratiopharm (Danazol)	II-699
Dancimin C (Ascorbic Acid)	II-203
Danigen (Gentamicin Sulfate)	II-1279
Danilax (Lactulose)	II-1550
Danoclav (Amoxicillin; Clavulanate Potassium)	II-139
Danodiol (Danazol)	II-699
Danoflox (Ofloxacin)	II-2015
Danogen (Danazol)	II-699
Danokrin (Danazol)	II-699
Danol (Danazol)	II-699
Danoval (Danazol)	II-699
Danovir (Acyclovir)	II-33
Dansemid (Sulfacetamide Sodium)	II-2497
Dantamacrin (Dantrolene Sodium)	II-700
Dantrolen (Dantrolene Sodium)	II-700
Daonil (Glyburide)	II-1297
Daono (Glyburide)	II-1297
Dapa (Indapamide)	II-1436
Dapamax (Indapamide)	II-1436
Dapatum D25 (Fluphenazine Decanoate)	II-1170
Dapotum (Fluphenazine Hydrochloride)	II-1172
Dapotum D (Fluphenazine Decanoate)	II-1170
Dapotum Depot (Fluphenazine Decanoate)	II-1170
Dapril (Lisinopril)	II-1648
Daprox (Naproxen)	II-1924
Dapsoderm-X (Dapsone)	II-702
Dapson (Dapsone)	II-702
Dapsone (Dapsone)	II-702
Dapson-Fatol (Dapsone)	II-702
Daquiran (Pramipexole Dihydrochloride)	II-2219
Darax (Hydroxyzine)	II-1398
Dardokef (Cefamandole Nafate)	II-449
Dardum (Cefoperazone Sodium)	II-471
Daren (Emedastine Difumarate)	II-910
Daronal (Amiodarone Hydrochloride)	II-110
Dartobcin (Tobramycin Sulfate)	II-2646
Darvine (Clemastine Fumarate)	II-603
Datril (Acetaminophen)	II-11
Daunoblastin (Daunorubicin Hydrochloride)	II-708
Daunoblastina (Daunorubicin Hydrochloride)	II-708
Daunomycin (Daunorubicin Hydrochloride)	II-708
Daunorubicin Injection (Daunorubicin Hydrochloride)	II-708
Daunoxome (Daunorubicin Citrate Liposome)	II-706
Davesol (Lindane)	II-1642
Daxon (Nitazoxanide)	II-1978
Daxotel (Docetaxel)	II-837
Daypress (Imipramine Hydrochloride)	II-1431
Dayvital (Ascorbic Acid)	II-203
Dazid (Hydrochlorothiazide; Triamterene)	II-1362
Dazil (Diltiazem Hydrochloride)	II-798
DDAVP Desmopressin (Desmopressin Acetate)	II-723
DDL plaster (Diclofenac)	II-748
Deavynfar (Chlorpropamide)	II-554
Debax (Captopril)	II-411
Debetrol (Metronidazole)	II-1812
Debtan (Glyburide)	II-1297
Deca (Fluphenazine Decanoate)	II-1170
Decadran (Dexamethasone)	II-730
Decadron Depot (Dexamethasone Acetate)	II-734
Decadron I.A. (Dexamethasone Acetate)	II-734
Decafen (Fluphenazine Decanoate)	II-1170
Decalogiflox (Lomefloxacin Hydrochloride)	II-1658
Decapeptyl (Triptorelin Pamoate)	II-2727
Decapeptyl CR (Triptorelin Pamoate)	II-2727
Decapeptyl Depot (Triptorelin Pamoate)	II-2727
Decapeptyl L (Triptorelin Pamoate)	II-2727
Decapeptyl LP (Triptorelin Pamoate)	II-2727
Decapeptyl Retard (Triptorelin Pamoate)	II-2727
Decaris (Levamisole Hydrochloride)	II-1598

International brand name (Generic name)	Page no.
Decas (Levamisole Hydrochloride)	II-1598
Decdan (Dexamethasone)	II-730
Decentan (Perphenazine)	II-2162
Decilone (Dexamethasone)	II-730
Declindin (Guanethidine Monosulfate)	II-1321
Decliten (Prazosin Hydrochloride)	II-2229
Decloban (Clobetasol Propionate)	II-617
Declophen (Diclofenac)	II-748
Declot (Ticlopidine Hydrochloride)	II-2622
Decomit (Beclomethasone Dipropionate)	II-279
Decortin (Prednisone)	II-2240
Decortisyl (Prednisone)	II-2240
Decose (Glipizide)	II-1290
Decozol (Miconazole)	II-1820
Decrelip (Gemfibrozil)	II-1269
Decreten (Pindolol)	II-2192
Decrol (Diclofenac)	II-748
Dectancyl (Dexamethasone)	II-730
Dectancyl (Dexamethasone Acetate)	II-734
Dedoxia (Dicyclomine Hydrochloride)	II-763
Dedralen (Doxazosin Mesylate)	II-860
Defanyl (Amoxapine)	II-129
Defense (Cimetidine Hydrochloride)	II-568
Defiltran (Acetazolamide)	II-28
Defirin (Desmopressin Acetate)	II-723
Deflam (Oxaprozin)	II-2059
Deflamon (Metronidazole)	II-1812
Deflamox (Naproxen Sodium)	II-1928
Deflox (Terazosin Hydrochloride)	II-2566
Degranol (Carbamazepine)	II-418
Deherp (Acyclovir)	II-33
Dehidrobenzoperidol (Droperidol)	II-889
Dehychol (Ursodiol)	II-2737
Dehydratin (Acetazolamide)	II-28
Dehydrobenzperidol (Droperidol)	II-889
Dekalax (Bisacodyl)	II-322
Deku (Nabumetone)	II-1909
Delagil (Chloroquine)	II-544
Delcortin (Prednisone)	II-2240
Delice (Lindane)	II-1642
Delifon (Oxybutynin)	II-2070
Delitex (Lindane)	II-1642
Delix (Ramipril)	II-2330
Dellacort A (Prednisone)	II-2240
Delor (Clobetasol Propionate)	II-617
Delphi Creme (Triamcinolone Acetonide)	II-2701
Delphicort (Triamcinolone)	II-2698
Delphicort (Triamcinolone Acetonide)	II-2701
Delta West Carboplatin (Carboplatin)	II-430
Deltabiox (Hydrocortisone; Neomycin Sulfate; Polymyxin B Sulfate)	II-1384
Deltacortene (Prednisone)	II-2240
Deltacortone (Prednisone)	II-2240
Deltazen (Diltiazem Hydrochloride)	II-798
Deltison (Prednisone)	II-2240
Deltisona (Prednisone)	II-2240
Demazin Anti-Allergy (Loratadine)	II-1675
Demil (Bromocriptine Mesylate)	II-344
Demolox (Amoxapine)	II-129
Demulen 50 (Ethinyl Estradiol; Ethynodiol Diacetate)	II-1042
Denan (Simvastatin)	II-2454
Dendri (Betamethasone Valerate)	II-305
Denex (Metoprolol)	II-1805
Denkacort Forte (Triamcinolone Acetonide)	II-2701
Denkaform (Metformin Hydrochloride)	II-1760
Denkifed (Nifedipine)	II-1967
Denosine (Ganciclovir Sodium)	II-1250
Densul (Methyldopa)	II-1778
Dentistar (Doxycycline)	II-878
Denvar (Cefixime)	II-466
Deo-Q Syrup (Theophylline)	II-2593
Deoxymykoin (Doxycycline)	II-878
Depain (Diclofenac)	II-748
Depakene (Valproate Sodium)	II-2749
Depakin (Valproate Sodium)	II-2749
Depakin (Valproic Acid)	II-2755
Depakine (Valproate Sodium)	II-2749
Depakine (Valproic Acid)	II-2755
Depakine Chrono (Valproate Sodium)	II-2749
Depakine Druppels (Valproate Sodium)	II-2749
Depakote (Valproate Sodium)	II-2749
Depalept (Valproate Sodium)	II-2749
Depalept Chrono (Valproate Sodium)	II-2749
Depermide (Indapamide)	II-1436
Depidol (Haloperidol)	II-1328
D'Epifrin (Dipivefrin Hydrochloride)	II-820
Depin (Nifedipine)	II-1967
Depinar (Cyanocobalamin)	II-661
Depizide (Glipizide)	II-1290
Depo Medrol (Methylprednisolone Acetate)	II-1790
Depo-Medrate (Methylprednisolone Acetate)	II-1790
Depo-Medrone (Methylprednisolone Acetate)	II-1790
Depo-Moderin (Methylprednisolone Acetate)	II-1790
Depo-Nisolone (Methylprednisolone Acetate)	II-1790
Deponit NT (Nitroglycerin)	II-1984
Deponit TTS 10 (Nitroglycerin)	II-1984
Deponit TTS 5 (Nitroglycerin)	II-1984
Deponit-5 (Nitroglycerin)	II-1984
Depo-Prodasone (Medroxyprogesterone Acetate)	II-1714
Depot Hormon-M (Testosterone Cypionate)	II-2581
Deprax (Trazodone Hydrochloride)	II-2686
Depresil (Trazodone Hydrochloride)	II-2686
Deprexan (Desipramine Hydrochloride)	II-716
Deprexin (Fluoxetine Hydrochloride)	II-1160
Deprolac (Bromocriptine Mesylate)	II-344
Deproxin (Fluoxetine Hydrochloride)	II-1160
Depsol (Imipramine Hydrochloride)	II-1431
Depsonil (Imipramine Hydrochloride)	II-1431
Deptran (Doxepin Hydrochloride)	II-865
Depyrel (Trazodone Hydrochloride)	II-2686
Depyretin (Acetaminophen)	II-11
Dequaspray (Lidocaine Hydrochloride)	II-1632
Deralbine (Miconazole)	II-1820
Deralin (Propranolol Hydrochloride)	II-2287
Dercason (Desoximetasone)	II-730
Derimine (Oxiconazole Nitrate)	II-2069
Deripen (Ampicillin)	II-170
Deripil (Erythromycin)	II-960
Derm A (Tretinoin)	II-2691
Dermacort (Triamcinolone Acetonide)	II-2701
Derma-Coryl (Econazole Nitrate)	II-900
Dermaid (Hydrocortisone)	II-1369
Dermaid Soft Cream (Hydrocortisone)	II-1369
Dermairol (Tretinoin)	II-2691
Dermalar (Fluocinolone Acetonide)	II-1152
Derma-Mycotral (Miconazole)	II-1820
Dermasten (Clotrimazole)	II-640
Dermatin (Clotrimazole)	II-640
Dermatovate (Clobetasol Propionate)	II-617
Dermazole (Econazole Nitrate)	II-900
Dermestril (Estradiol)	II-986
Dermestril Septem (Estradiol)	II-986
Dermik A (Tretinoin)	II-2691
Dermocortal (Hydrocortisone)	II-1369
Dermoflam (Fluocinolone Acetonide)	II-1152
Dermogen (Gentamicin Sulfate)	II-1279
Dermol (Clobetasol Propionate)	II-617
Dermonilo (Diflorasone Diacetate)	II-776
Dermonistat (Miconazole)	II-1820
Dermoran (Fluocinolone Acetonide)	II-1152
Dermorelle (Vitamin E)	II-2796
Dermosol (Clobetasol Propionate)	II-617
Dermosolon (Prednisolone)	II-2233
Dermotyl (Clobetasol Propionate)	II-617
Dermoval (Clobetasol Propionate)	II-617
Dermovat (Clobetasol Propionate)	II-617
Dermovate (Clobetasol Propionate)	II-617
Dermoxin (Clobetasol Propionate)	II-617
Deroxat (Paroxetine Hydrochloride)	II-2104
Derzid (Betamethasone Valerate)	II-305
Derzid-c (Betamethasone Dipropionate; Clotrimazole)	II-304
Desalark (Dexamethasone)	II-730
Desalex (Desloratadine)	II-721
Desbly (Guaifenesin)	II-1314
Desconet (Diazepam)	II-740
Desconex (Loxapine Succinate)	II-1702
Desec (Omeprazole)	II-2034
Deselazin (Hydralazine Hydrochloride)	II-1346
Desicort (Desoximetasone)	II-730
Desigdron (Dexamethasone)	II-730
Desiken (Ribavirin)	II-2351
Desinflam (Piroxicam)	II-2205
Desiperiden (Biperiden Hydrochloride)	II-322
Desirel (Trazodone Hydrochloride)	II-2686
Desitic (Ticlopidine Hydrochloride)	II-2622
Desitin (Loperamide Hydrochloride)	II-1664
Deslor (Desloratadine)	II-721
Desmin (Desogestrel; Ethinyl Estradiol)	II-725
Desmopressin Nasal Solution (Desmopressin Acetate)	II-723
Desmospray (Desmopressin Acetate)	II-723
Desocort (Desonide)	II-728
Desolett (Desogestrel; Ethinyl Estradiol)	II-725
Deson (Metformin Hydrochloride)	II-1760
Desona Nasal (Budesonide)	II-347
Desonida (Desonide)	II-728
Destrim (Polymyxin B Sulfate; Trimethoprim Sulfate)	II-2212
Desumide (Tolazamide)	II-2649
Detemes Retard (Dihydroergotamine Mesylate)	II-792
Detensiel (Bisoprolol Fumarate)	II-323
Dethasone (Desoximetasone)	II-730
Deticene (Dacarbazine)	II-687
Detimedac (Dacarbazine)	II-687
Detrax 40 (Levamisole Hydrochloride)	II-1598
Detrusitol (Tolterodine Tartrate)	II-2657
Detulin (Vitamin E)	II-2796
Deursil (Ursodiol)	II-2737
Devoxim (Cefixime)	II-466
Dewormis (Levamisole Hydrochloride)	II-1598
Dewormis 50 (Levamisole Hydrochloride)	II-1598
Dexacap (Captopril)	II-411
Dexacortal (Dexamethasone)	II-730
Dexalocal (Dexamethasone)	II-730
Dexame (Dexamethasone)	II-730
Dexamed (Dexamethasone)	II-730
Dexametason (Dexamethasone)	II-730
Dexamethason (Dexamethasone)	II-730
Dexamethasone (Dexamethasone)	II-730
Dexamonozon (Dexamethasone)	II-730
Dexano (Dexamethasone)	II-730
Dexa-P (Dexamethasone)	II-730
Dexasone (Dexamethasone)	II-730
Dexasone S (Dexamethasone)	II-730
Deximune (Cyclosporine)	II-668
Dexmethsone (Dexamethasone)	II-730
Dexona (Dexamethasone)	II-730
Dexotel (Docetaxel)	II-837
Dextin (Metformin Hydrochloride)	II-1760
Dextrasone (Dexamethasone)	II-730
Dextricyl (Guaifenesin)	II-1314
Dezoral (Ketoconazole)	II-1530
Dhabesol (Clobetasol Propionate)	II-617
Dhacillin (Ampicillin)	II-170
DHAcort (Hydrocortisone Acetate)	II-1373
Dhactulose (Lactulose)	II-1550
Dhamotil (Atropine Sulfate; Diphenoxylate Hydrochloride)	II-238
Dhaperazine (Prochlorperazine)	II-2258
Dhatracin (Tetracycline Hydrochloride)	II-2585
Diabecid-R (Tolbutamide)	II-2650
Diabeedol (Chlorpropamide)	II-554
Diabemide (Chlorpropamide)	II-554
Diaben (Glyburide)	II-1297

International brand name (Generic name)	Page no.
Dinazide (Hydrochlorothiazide; Triamterene)	II-1362
Dinisor (Diltiazem Hydrochloride)	II-798
Dinisor (Isosorbide Dinitrate)	II-1502
Dinisor Retard (Diltiazem Hydrochloride)	II-798
Dinol (Etidronate Disodium)	II-1073
Dintoina (Phenytoin Sodium)	II-2175
Diochloram (Chloramphenicol)	II-536
Diocodal (Naproxen)	II-1924
Dioderm (Hydrocortisone)	II-1369
Diondel (Metolazone)	II-1802
Diopine (Dipivefrin Hydrochloride)	II-820
Dioxaflex (Diclofenac)	II-748
Dipaz (Diazepam)	II-740
Dipazide (Glipizide)	II-1290
Dipezona (Diazepam)	II-740
Diphantoine (Phenytoin Sodium)	II-2175
Diphantoine-Z (Phenytoin Sodium)	II-2175
Diphemin (Dipivefrin Hydrochloride)	II-820
Diphensil (Atropine Sulfate; Diphenoxylate Hydrochloride)	II-238
Diphereline (Triptorelin Pamoate)	II-2727
Diphereline PR (Triptorelin Pamoate)	II-2727
Diphereline SR (Triptorelin Pamoate)	II-2727
Dipicin-INH (Isoniazid; Rifampin)	II-1498
Dipinkor (Nifedipine)	II-1967
Diplovax (Measles Virus Vaccine Live)	II-1708
Dipoquin (Dipivefrin Hydrochloride)	II-820
Diporax (Chlordiazepoxide Hydrochloride; Clidinium Bromide)	II-541
Dipot (Clorazepate Dipotassium)	II-638
Diprocel (Betamethasone Dipropionate)	II-301
Diproderm (Betamethasone Dipropionate)	II-301
Diprofol (Propofol)	II-2278
Diprolen (Betamethasone Dipropionate)	II-301
Diprosone-OV (Betamethasone Dipropionate)	II-301
Diprotop (Betamethasone Dipropionate)	II-301
Dipyridan (Dipyridamole)	II-821
Dipyrol (Dipyridamole)	II-821
Diram (Spironolactone)	II-2483
Dirine (Furosemide)	II-1237
Dirinol (Dipyridamole)	II-821
Diroquine (Chloroquine)	II-544
Dirox (Acetaminophen)	II-11
Dirytmin (Disopyramide Phosphate)	II-825
Disal (Salsalate)	II-2418
Disalazin (Sulfasalazine)	II-2507
Disalgesic (Salsalate)	II-2418
Disarim (Chlordiazepoxide Hydrochloride)	II-539
Disatral (Meprobamate)	II-1738
Diseptyl (Sulfamethoxazole; Trimethoprim)	II-2500
Dispal (Orphenadrine Citrate)	II-2049
Dismifen (Acetaminophen)	II-11
Disofarin (Disopyramide Phosphate)	II-825
Disoprivan (Propofol)	II-2278
Disothiazide (Hydrochlorothiazide)	II-1348
Dispamet (Cimetidine Hydrochloride)	II-568
Dispatim (Timolol)	II-2627
Disposef (Clorazepate Dipotassium)	II-638
Dispril (Aspirin)	II-206
Disprin Forte (Aspirin; Codeine Phosphate)	II-210
Disron P (Hydroxyzine)	II-1398
Dissenten (Loperamide Hydrochloride)	II-1664
Dissilax (Bisacodyl)	II-322
Distaclor (Cefaclor)	II-444
Distaclor MR (Cefaclor)	II-444
Distalene (Orphenadrine Citrate)	II-2049
Distalgesic (Acetaminophen; Propoxyphene Napsylate)	II-23
Distamine (Penicillamine)	II-2133
Distaph (Dicloxacillin Sodium)	II-761
Distaquaine V-K (Penicillin V Potassium)	II-2142
Distaxid (Nizatidine)	II-1992
Distocide (Praziquantel)	II-2228
Distoncur (Meprobamate)	II-1738
Ditenaten (Theophylline)	II-2593
DiTePer Anatoxal Berna Vaccine (Diphtheria; Pertussis; Tetanus)	II-818
Ditoin (Phenytoin Sodium)	II-2175
Ditomed (Phenytoin Sodium)	II-2175
Diulo (Metolazone)	II-1802
Diurace (Hydrochlorothiazide)	II-1348
Diuracet-K (Hydrochlorothiazide; Triamterene)	II-1362
Diural (Furosemide)	II-1237
Diuramid (Acetazolamide)	II-28
Diurazide (Chlorothiazide)	II-545
Diuresal (Furosemide)	II-1237
Diuret (Chlorothiazide)	II-545
Diuret-P (Hydrochlorothiazide)	II-1348
Diurex (Hydrochlorothiazide)	II-1348
Diurin (Furosemide)	II-1237
Diurolasa (Furosemide)	II-1237
Diusemide (Furosemide)	II-1237
Diutropin (Oxybutynin)	II-2070
Divigel (Estradiol)	II-986
Dixamid (Indapamide)	II-1436
Dixarit (Clonidine Hydrochloride)	II-629
Dixin (Alprazolam)	II-85
Dixonal (Piroxicam)	II-2205
Dizolam (Alprazolam)	II-85
DNCG Trom (Cromolyn Sodium)	II-656
Dobetin (Cyanocobalamin)	II-661
Doblexan (Piroxicam)	II-2205
Dobuject (Dobutamine Hydrochloride)	II-834
Dobumine (Dobutamine Hydrochloride)	II-834
Dobutamin Giulini (Dobutamine Hydrochloride)	II-834
Dobutamin Hexal (Dobutamine Hydrochloride)	II-834
Dobutamina (Dobutamine Hydrochloride)	II-834
Dobutamin-Ratiopharm (Dobutamine Hydrochloride)	II-834
Docard (Dopamine Hydrochloride)	II-853
Docemine (Cyanocobalamin)	II-661
Dociton (Propranolol Hydrochloride)	II-2287
Dodexen (Diltiazem Hydrochloride)	II-798
Dodexen A.P. (Diltiazem Hydrochloride)	II-798
Dofacef (Cefamandole Nafate)	II-449
Doflex (Diclofenac)	II-748
Doinmycin (Doxycycline)	II-878
Dolac (Ketorolac Tromethamine)	II-1537
Dolan FP (Ibuprofen)	II-1411
Dolana (Tramadol Hydrochloride)	II-2674
Dolantin (Meperidine Hydrochloride)	II-1733
Dolantina (Meperidine Hydrochloride)	II-1733
Dolantine (Meperidine Hydrochloride)	II-1733
Dolaren (Diclofenac)	II-748
Dolazal (Indomethacin)	II-1443
Dolcontin (Morphine Sulfate)	II-1877
Dolcontin Depottab (Morphine Sulfate)	II-1877
Dolestine (Meperidine Hydrochloride)	II-1733
Dolex 500 (Acetaminophen)	II-11
Dolflam-Retard (Diclofenac)	II-748
Dolgit (Ibuprofen)	II-1411
Dolib (Rofecoxib)	II-2396
Dolipol (Tolbutamide)	II-2650
Doliprane (Acetaminophen)	II-11
Dolisec (Sucralfate)	II-2493
Dolitabs (Acetaminophen)	II-11
Dolmed (Methadone Hydrochloride)	II-1766
Dolobis (Diflunisal)	II-777
Dolocid (Diflunisal)	II-777
Dolocyl (Ibuprofen)	II-1411
Dolofen (Acetaminophen)	II-11
Dolofen-F (Ibuprofen)	II-1411
Doloflam (Diclofenac)	II-748
Dologesic (Acetaminophen; Propoxyphene Napsylate)	II-23
Dologesic-32 (Acetaminophen; Propoxyphene Napsylate)	II-23
Dolomax (Ibuprofen)	II-1411
Dolomax (Ketoprofen)	II-1533
Dolomol (Acetaminophen)	II-11
Dolonex (Piroxicam)	II-2205
Dolorex (Ketorolac Tromethamine)	II-1537
Dolorol (Acetaminophen)	II-11
Dolorol Forte (Acetaminophen; Codeine Phosphate)	II-13
Dolostop (Acetaminophen; Propoxyphene Napsylate)	II-23
Dolotemp (Acetaminophen)	II-11
Dolotral (Tramadol Hydrochloride)	II-2674
Dolotren (Diclofenac)	II-748
Dolotren Gel (Diclofenac)	II-748
Doloxene (Propoxyphene Napsylate)	II-2286
Doloxene Compound (Aspirin; Caffeine; Propoxyphene Hydrochloride)	II-209
Doltem (Acetaminophen)	II-11
Doltirol (Ampicillin)	II-170
Dolval (Ibuprofen)	II-1411
Dolviron (Aspirin; Codeine Phosphate)	II-210
Domer (Omeprazole)	II-2034
Dometin (Indomethacin)	II-1443
Dometon (Sulindac)	II-2512
Domical (Amitriptyline Hydrochloride)	II-119
Dominum (Sertraline Hydrochloride)	II-2439
Domnamid (Estazolam)	II-983
Donafan (Loperamide Hydrochloride)	II-1664
Doneurin (Doxepin Hydrochloride)	II-865
Donison (Tolmetin Sodium)	II-2656
Donjust B (Ibuprofen)	II-1411
Donobid (Diflunisal)	II-777
Dopadura (Carbidopa; Levodopa)	II-424
Dopagyt (Methyldopa)	II-1778
Dopamet (Methyldopa)	II-1778
Dopamex (Dopamine Hydrochloride)	II-853
Dopamin (Dopamine Hydrochloride)	II-853
Dopamin AWD (Dopamine Hydrochloride)	II-853
Dopamin Braun (Dopamine Hydrochloride)	II-853
Dopamin Guilini (Dopamine Hydrochloride)	II-853
Dopamin Leopold (Dopamine Hydrochloride)	II-853
Dopamin Natterman (Dopamine Hydrochloride)	II-853
Dopamina (Dopamine Hydrochloride)	II-853
Dopamine (Dopamine Hydrochloride)	II-853
Dopamine Injection (Dopamine Hydrochloride)	II-853
Dopaminex (Dopamine Hydrochloride)	II-853
Dopaminum (Dopamine Hydrochloride)	II-853
Dopasian (Methyldopa)	II-1778
Dopatens (Methyldopa)	II-1778
Dopegyt (Methyldopa)	II-1778
Dophilin (Doxazosin Mesylate)	II-860
Dopicar (Carbidopa; Levodopa)	II-424
Dopinga (Dopamine Hydrochloride)	II-853
Dopmin (Dopamine Hydrochloride)	II-853
Dopmin E (Dopamine Hydrochloride)	II-853
Dopsan (Dapsone)	II-702
Dorbid (Diflunisal)	II-777
Dorink (Danazol)	II-699
Dorival (Ibuprofen)	II-1411
Dormel (Chloral Hydrate)	II-534
Dormicum (Midazolam Hydrochloride)	II-1823
Dormirex (Hydroxyzine)	II-1398
Dormodor (Flurazepam Hydrochloride)	II-1175
Dormonid (Midazolam Hydrochloride)	II-1823
Dormutil (Diphenhydramine Hydrochloride)	II-813
Dosan (Doxazosin Mesylate)	II-860
Dosanac (Diclofenac)	II-748
Dosatropine (Atropine Sulfate)	II-235
Dosil (Doxycycline)	II-878
Dosiseptine (Chlorhexidine Gluconate)	II-542
Dotirol (Ampicillin)	II-170
Dotur (Doxycycline)	II-878
Doval (Diazepam)	II-740
Doxaben (Doxazosin Mesylate)	II-860
Doxacard (Doxazosin Mesylate)	II-860

International brand name (Generic name)	Page no.
Doxaciclin (Doxycycline)	II-878
Doxagamma (Doxazosin Mesylate)	II-860
Doxal (Doxepin Hydrochloride)	II-865
Doxaloc (Doxazosin Mesylate)	II-860
Doxamil (Amoxicillin)	II-131
Doxasyn (Doxazosin Mesylate)	II-860
Doxat (Doxycycline)	II-878
Doxibiotic (Doxycycline)	II-878
Doxilin (Doxycycline)	II-878
Doximed (Doxycycline)	II-878
Doximycin (Doxycycline)	II-878
Doxin (Doxycycline)	II-878
Doxine (Doxycycline)	II-878
Doxi-Sergo (Doxycycline)	II-878
Doxolem (Doxorubicin, Liposomal)	II-873
Doxor Lyo (Doxorubicin, Liposomal)	II-873
Doxorubicin (Doxorubicin, Liposomal)	II-873
Doxorubicin Meiji (Doxorubicin, Liposomal)	II-873
Doxorubin (Doxorubicin, Liposomal)	II-873
Doxsig (Doxycycline)	II-878
Doxy-1 (Doxycycline)	II-878
Doxycin (Doxycycline)	II-878
Doxycline (Doxycycline)	II-878
Doxycycline (Doxycycline)	II-878
Doxylag (Doxycycline)	II-878
Doxylin (Doxycycline)	II-878
Doxymycin (Doxycycline)	II-878
Doxytec (Doxycycline)	II-878
Doxytrim (Doxycycline)	II-878
Dozic (Haloperidol)	II-1328
Dozic (Olanzapine)	II-2022
D-Penil (Penicillamine)	II-2133
DPT (Diphtheria; Pertussis; Tetanus)	II-818
Draconyl (Terbutaline Sulfate)	II-2574
Drafilyn "Z" (Aminophylline)	II-106
Dramine (Meclizine Hydrochloride)	II-1713
Dranolis (Pindolol)	II-2192
Dravyr (Acyclovir)	II-33
Draximox (Amoxicillin)	II-131
Drazine (Hydroxyzine)	II-1398
Drazone (Prednisone)	II-2240
Drenian (Diazepam)	II-740
Drenison (Flurandrenolide)	II-1174
Drenison 1 4 (Flurandrenolide)	II-1174
Drenural (Bumetanide)	II-359
Drenusil (Polythiazide)	II-2213
Dridase (Oxybutynin)	II-2070
Drilan (Acetaminophen)	II-11
Drimpam (Alprazolam)	II-85
Drin (Ibuprofen)	II-1411
Driptane (Oxybutynin)	II-2070
Drix (Bisacodyl)	II-322
Drocef (Cefadroxil Monohydrate)	II-447
Drogenil (Flutamide)	II-1181
Dromadol (Tramadol Hydrochloride)	II-2674
Dromoran (Levorphanol Tartrate)	II-1618
Dronate-OS (Etidronate Disodium)	II-1073
Droperol (Droperidol)	II-889
Drosin (Phenylephrine Hydrochloride)	II-2173
Droxicef (Cefadroxil Monohydrate)	II-447
Droxil (Cefadroxil Monohydrate)	II-447
Droxyl (Cefadroxil Monohydrate)	II-447
Drynalken (Dopamine Hydrochloride)	II-853
Dryptal (Furosemide)	II-1237
D.T. COQ (Diphtheria; Pertussis; Tetanus)	II-818
DTI (Dacarbazine)	II-687
D.T.I.C. (Dacarbazine)	II-687
DTIC (Dacarbazine)	II-687
DTIC Dome (Dacarbazine)	II-687
D.T.I.C.-Dome (Dacarbazine)	II-687
DTIC-Dome (Dacarbazine)	II-687
DTIC-VHB (Dacarbazine)	II-687
DTM (Diltiazem Hydrochloride)	II-798
Duacillin (Ampicillin)	II-170
Duactin 5 (Amlodipine Besylate)	II-125
Duasma (Budesonide)	II-347
Dube Spray (Lidocaine)	II-1628
Dudencer (Omeprazole)	II-2034
Dulco laxo (Bisacodyl)	II-322
Dulcolan (Bisacodyl)	II-322
Dumirox (Fluvoxamine Maleate)	II-1203
Dumocyclin (Tetracycline Hydrochloride)	II-2585
Dumophar (Acyclovir)	II-33
Dumovit (Thiamine Hydrochloride)	II-2602
Dumoxin (Doxycycline)	II-878
Dumozol (Metronidazole)	II-1812
Dumozolam (Triazolam)	II-2715
Dumyrox (Fluvoxamine Maleate)	II-1203
Duncan (Chlorpromazine Hydrochloride)	II-549
Duocide (Sulfamethoxazole; Trimethoprim)	II-2500
duofem (Levonorgestrel)	II-1614
Duogas (Omeprazole)	II-2034
Duolin (Albuterol; Ipratropium Bromide)	II-65
Duoluton (Ethinyl Estradiol; Norgestrel)	II-1068
Duoluton-L (Ethinyl Estradiol; Norgestrel)	II-1068
Duomet (Cimetidine Hydrochloride)	II-568
Duospirel (Albuterol; Ipratropium Bromide)	II-65
Duovir (Lamivudine; Zidovudine)	II-1560
Duphratex (Cephradine)	II-526
Dupin (Diazepam)	II-740
Durabeta (Atenolol)	II-222
Durabiotic (Penicillin G Benzathine)	II-2136
Duracef (Cefadroxil Monohydrate)	II-447
Duractin (Ranitidine Hydrochloride)	II-2334
Durafenat (Fenofibrate)	II-1105
Durafenat Micro (Fenofibrate)	II-1105
Durafungol (Clotrimazole)	II-640
Durafurid (Furosemide)	II-1237
Duralith (Lithium Carbonate)	II-1654
Duralmor (Morphine Sulfate)	II-1877
Duralozam (Lorazepam)	II-1678
Duramesan (Meclizine Hydrochloride)	II-1713
Durametacin (Indomethacin)	II-1443
Duramipress (Prazosin Hydrochloride)	II-2229
Duramycin (Erythromycin Stearate)	II-970
Duranifin (Nifedipine)	II-1967
Duranitrat (Isosorbide Dinitrate)	II-1502
Duranol (Propranolol Hydrochloride)	II-2287
Durantel DS (Cephalexin)	II-520
DuraPenicillin (Penicillin V Potassium)	II-2142
Duraperidol (Haloperidol)	II-1328
Durapindol (Pindolol)	II-2192
Duraprox (Oxaprozin)	II-2059
Durater (Famotidine)	II-1093
Duratrimet (Sulfamethoxazole; Trimethoprim)	II-2500
Durazepam (Oxazepam)	II-2063
Durbis (Disopyramide Phosphate)	II-825
Durbis Retard (Disopyramide Phosphate)	II-825
Durekal (Potassium Chloride)	II-2215
Duroferon (Ferrous Sulfate)	II-1122
Duromorph (Morphine Sulfate)	II-1877
Durules-K (Potassium Chloride)	II-2215
Dusil (Aspirin)	II-206
D-Worm (Mebendazole)	II-1711
Dyalac (Diltiazem Hydrochloride)	II-798
Dyberzide (Hydrochlorothiazide; Triamterene)	II-1362
Dybis (Metformin Hydrochloride)	II-1760
Dymadon (Acetaminophen)	II-11
Dymadon Co (Acetaminophen; Codeine Phosphate)	II-13
Dymadon Forte (Acetaminophen; Codeine Phosphate)	II-13
Dynacef (Cephradine)	II-526
Dynacil (Fosinopril Sodium)	II-1222
Dynacil (Fosinopril Sodium; Hydrochlorothiazide)	II-1226
Dynacirc SRO (Isradipine)	II-1515
Dynatra (Dopamine Hydrochloride)	II-853
Dynexan (Lidocaine)	II-1628
Dynexan (Lidocaine Hydrochloride)	II-1632
Dynos (Dopamine Hydrochloride)	II-853
Dysalfa (Terazosin Hydrochloride)	II-2566
Dyskinon (Biperiden Hydrochloride)	II-322
Dysman (Mefenamic Acid)	II-1720
Dysmenalgit (Naproxen)	II-1924
Dyspamet (Cimetidine Hydrochloride)	II-568
Dyspen (Mefenamic Acid)	II-1720
Dytenzide (Hydrochlorothiazide; Triamterene)	II-1362
Dytide H (Hydrochlorothiazide; Triamterene)	II-1362
D-Zol (Danazol)	II-699
DZP (Diazepam)	II-740
E	
E (Diclofenac)	II-748
E Perle (Vitamin E)	II-2796
E Recordati (Vitamin E)	II-2796
Easifon (Ibuprofen)	II-1411
Ebutol (Ethambutol Hydrochloride)	II-1039
Ecanol (Econazole Nitrate)	II-900
Ecapres (Captopril)	II-411
Ecaprinil-D (Enalapril Maleate; Hydrochlorothiazide)	II-923
Ecaten (Captopril)	II-411
Ecazide (Captopril; Hydrochlorothiazide)	II-416
ECEEZ (Levonorgestrel)	II-1614
Eclaran (Loratadine)	II-1675
Ecobec (Beclomethasone Dipropionate)	II-279
Ecodipin (Nifedipine)	II-1967
Ecofenac (Diclofenac)	II-748
Ecolate (Guaifenesin)	II-1314
Ecomucyl (Acetylcysteine)	II-29
Econ (Econazole Nitrate)	II-900
Economycin (Tetracycline Hydrochloride)	II-2585
Econosone (Prednisone)	II-2240
Ecopan (Mefenamic Acid)	II-1720
Ecotam (Econazole Nitrate)	II-900
Ecotone (Mometasone Furoate)	II-1866
Ecotrin 650 (Aspirin)	II-206
Ecoval (Betamethasone Valerate)	II-305
Ecreme (Econazole Nitrate)	II-900
Ecridoxan (Etodolac)	II-1076
Ectaprim (Sulfamethoxazole; Trimethoprim)	II-2500
Ectiva (Sibutramine Hydrochloride)	II-2447
Ectopal (Danazol)	II-699
Ectosone (Betamethasone Valerate)	II-305
Ecural (Mometasone Furoate)	II-1866
Eczacort (Hydrocortisone)	II-1369
Edamox (Amoxicillin)	II-131
Edegra (Sildenafil Citrate)	II-2451
Edemox (Acetazolamide)	II-28
Edenol (Furosemide)	II-1237
Ederen (Acetazolamide)	II-28
Edicin (Vancomycin Hydrochloride)	II-2763
Ednyt (Enalapril Maleate)	II-913
Eduvir (Acyclovir)	II-33
Edy (Atorvastatin Calcium)	II-231
E.E.S. (Erythromycin Ethylsuccinate)	II-965
EES 400 (Erythromycin Ethylsuccinate)	II-965
EES Granules (Erythromycin Ethylsuccinate)	II-965
EES-200 (Erythromycin Ethylsuccinate)	II-965
EES-400 (Erythromycin Ethylsuccinate)	II-965
Efasedan (Lorazepam)	II-1678
Efavir (Efavirenz)	II-901
Efcortelan (Hydrocortisone)	II-1369
Efcortelan Soluble (Hydrocortisone Sodium Succinate)	II-1379
Eferox (Levothyroxine Sodium)	II-1618
Efexor (Venlafaxine Hydrochloride)	II-2770
Efexor XR (Venlafaxine Hydrochloride)	II-2770
Efexor-XR SR (Venlafaxine Hydrochloride)	II-2770
Effectsal (Norfloxacin)	II-1997
Effederm (Tretinoin)	II-2691
Efferalgan 500 (Acetaminophen)	II-11
Efferalgan Codeine (Acetaminophen; Codeine Phosphate)	II-13
Efferalganodis (Acetaminophen)	II-11
Effexin (Ofloxacin)	II-2015

International brand name (Generic name)	Page no.
Efiken (Ketoprofen)	II-1533
Efosin (Dipyridamole)	II-821
Efotax (Cefotaxime Sodium)	II-474
Efpinex (Amoxicillin)	II-131
Efrin-10 (Phenylephrine Hydrochloride)	II-2173
Efrisel (Phenylephrine Hydrochloride)	II-2173
Efudix (Fluorouracil)	II-1158
E-Gen-C (Ethinyl Estradiol; Levonorgestrel)	II-1047
Eglandin (Alprostadil)	II-90
Egobiotic (Cefadroxil Monohydrate)	II-447
Ehliten (Praziquantel)	II-2228
Einalon S (Haloperidol)	II-1328
Eismycin (Mupirocin)	II-1894
Ejertol (Sildenafil Citrate)	II-2451
Ekzemsalbe (Hydrocortisone Acetate)	II-1373
Elan (Isosorbide Mononitrate)	II-1507
Elanpres (Methyldopa)	II-1778
Elantan (Isosorbide Mononitrate)	II-1507
Elantan Long (Isosorbide Mononitrate)	II-1507
Elantan Retard (Isosorbide Mononitrate)	II-1507
Elatrol (Amitriptyline Hydrochloride)	II-119
Elatrolet (Amitriptyline Hydrochloride)	II-119
Elbrol (Propranolol Hydrochloride)	II-2287
Elcid (Clotrimazole)	II-640
Elcion CR (Diazepam)	II-740
Elcoman (Loperamide Hydrochloride)	II-1664
Elcrit (Clozapine)	II-642
Eldopaque (Hydroquinone)	II-1391
Eldoquin (Hydroquinone)	II-1391
Eldoquin Cream (Hydroquinone)	II-1391
Elebloc (Carteolol Hydrochloride)	II-435
Elegelin (Selegiline Hydrochloride)	II-2437
Elenium (Chlordiazepoxide Hydrochloride)	II-539
Elequine (Levofloxacin)	II-1607
Elfonal (Enalapril Maleate)	II-913
Elica (Mometasone Furoate)	II-1866
Elisor (Pravastatin Sodium)	II-2224
Elixofilina (Theophylline)	II-2593
Elkrip (Bromocriptine Mesylate)	II-344
Ellanco (Lovastatin)	II-1688
Elmego Spray (Indomethacin)	II-1443
Elmetacin (Indomethacin)	II-1443
Elmogan (Gemfibrozil)	II-1269
Elobact (Cefuroxime)	II-507
Elocin (Erythromycin Stearate)	II-970
Elocom (Mometasone Furoate)	II-1866
Elocyn (Mometasone Furoate)	II-1866
Elomet (Mometasone Furoate)	II-1866
Elonton SR (Isosorbide Mononitrate)	II-1507
Elorgan (Pentoxifylline)	II-2154
Eloson (Mometasone Furoate)	II-1866
Elox (Mometasone Furoate)	II-1866
Elpicef (Ceftriaxone Sodium)	II-503
Elstatin (Lovastatin)	II-1688
Eltair (Budesonide)	II-347
Elthyrone (Levothyroxine Sodium)	II-1618
Eltidine (Ranitidine Hydrochloride)	II-2334
Eltroxin (Levothyroxine Sodium)	II-1618
Elyzol (Metronidazole)	II-1812
Emanthal (Albendazole)	II-46
EMB (Ethambutol Hydrochloride)	II-1039
Embutal (Pentobarbital Sodium)	II-2149
Emconcor (Bisoprolol Fumarate)	II-323
Emcor (Bisoprolol Fumarate)	II-323
Emeset (Ondansetron Hydrochloride)	II-2039
Emeside (Ethosuximide)	II-1072
Emestid (Erythromycin Stearate)	II-970
Emetal (Metoclopramide Hydrochloride)	II-1798
Emflam-200 (Ibuprofen)	II-1411
Emforal (Propranolol Hydrochloride)	II-2287
Emitasol (Metoclopramide Hydrochloride)	II-1798
Emo-Cort (Hydrocortisone)	II-1369
Emodin (Ibuprofen)	II-1411
Emopremarin (Estrogens, Conjugated)	II-1019
Emotion (Lorazepam)	II-1678
Emotival (Lorazepam)	II-1678
E-Moxclav (Amoxicillin; Clavulanate Potassium)	II-139
Empecid (Clotrimazole)	II-640
Emperal (Metoclopramide Hydrochloride)	II-1798
Empracet-30 (Acetaminophen; Codeine Phosphate)	II-13
Empracet-60 (Acetaminophen; Codeine Phosphate)	II-13
Empurine (Mercaptopurine)	II-1741
Emquin (Chloroquine)	II-544
Emtexate (Methotrexate Sodium)	II-1772
Emthexat (Methotrexate Sodium)	II-1772
Emthexate (Methotrexate Sodium)	II-1772
Emu-V (Erythromycin)	II-960
Emu-V E (Erythromycin Stearate)	II-970
Emu-Ve (Erythromycin)	II-960
Emuvin (Erythromycin)	II-960
E-Mycin (Erythromycin)	II-960
Emycin (Erythromycin)	II-960
EnaABZ (Enalapril Maleate)	II-913
Enace-D (Enalapril Maleate; Hydrochlorothiazide)	II-923
Enadine (Clorazepate Dipotassium)	II-638
Enafon (Amitriptyline Hydrochloride)	II-119
Enahexal (Enalapril Maleate)	II-913
Enaladil (Enalapril Maleate)	II-913
Enalapril (Enalapril Maleate)	II-913
Enaloc (Enalapril Maleate)	II-913
Enalpapril (Enalapril Maleate)	II-913
Enam (Enalapril Maleate)	II-913
Enanton Depot (Leuprolide Acetate)	II-1587
Enantone (Leuprolide Acetate)	II-1587
Enantone Depot (Leuprolide Acetate)	II-1587
Enantone LP (Leuprolide Acetate)	II-1587
Enantone SR (Leuprolide Acetate)	II-1587
Enap (Enalapril Maleate)	II-913
Enap HL (Enalapril Maleate; Hydrochlorothiazide)	II-923
Enapren (Enalapril Maleate)	II-913
Enapril (Enalapril Maleate)	II-913
Enaprin (Enalapril Maleate)	II-913
Enaril (Enalapril Maleate)	II-913
Enarmon (Methyltestosterone)	II-1796
Enatec (Enalapril Maleate)	II-913
Enbrel (Etanercept)	II-1036
Encine EM (Aspirin)	II-206
Enclor (Chloramphenicol)	II-536
Encore (Acetylcysteine)	II-29
Encorton (Prednisone)	II-2240
Endace (Megestrol Acetate)	II-1723
Endak (Carteolol Hydrochloride)	II-435
Endantadine (Amantadine Hydrochloride)	II-97
Endazole (Metronidazole)	II-1812
Endobulin (Immune Globulin (Human))	II-1434
Endobuline (Immune Globulin (Human))	II-1434
Endometrin (Progesterone)	II-2262
Endone (Oxycodone Hydrochloride)	II-2076
Endoxan (Cyclophosphamide)	II-666
Endoxan Asta (Cyclophosphamide)	II-666
Endoxana (Cyclophosphamide)	II-666
Endoxan-Asta (Cyclophosphamide)	II-666
Endoxon (Cyclophosphamide)	II-666
Endoxon-Asta (Cyclophosphamide)	II-666
Enduxan (Cyclophosphamide)	II-666
Enerzer (Isocarboxazid)	II-1493
Enhancin (Amoxicillin; Clavulanate Potassium)	II-139
Eni (Ciprofloxacin Hydrochloride)	II-573
Enidrel (Oxazepam)	II-2063
Enkacetyn (Chloramphenicol)	II-536
Enkacort (Hydrocortisone Acetate)	II-1373
Enkacyclin (Tetracycline Hydrochloride)	II-2585
Ennamax (Cyproheptadine Hydrochloride)	II-682
Entir (Acyclovir)	II-33
Entocort (Budesonide)	II-347
Entrang (Etodolac)	II-1076
Entrophen (Aspirin)	II-206
Entulic (Guanfacine Hydrochloride)	II-1323
Envas (Enalapril Maleate)	II-913
Enzil (Amantadine Hydrochloride)	II-97
Enzimar (Metoclopramide Hydrochloride)	II-1798
Epamin (Phenytoin Sodium)	II-2175
Epanutin (Phenytoin Sodium)	II-2175
Epaq (Metronidazole)	II-1812
Epaq Inhaler (Albuterol)	II-47
Epatec (Ketoprofen)	II-1533
Epaxal (Hepatitis A Vaccine)	II-1339
Ephynal (Vitamin E)	II-2796
EPI-cell (Epirubicin Hydrochloride)	II-938
Epicordin (Captopril)	II-411
Epicort (Clotrimazole)	II-640
Epicrom (Cromolyn Sodium)	II-656
Epifenac (Diclofenac)	II-748
Epigent (Gentamicin Sulfate)	II-1279
Epikur (Meprobamate)	II-1738
Epilam (Valproate Sodium)	II-2749
Epilan-D (Phenytoin Sodium)	II-2175
Epilantin (Phenytoin Sodium)	II-2175
Epilem (Epirubicin Hydrochloride)	II-938
Epileptin (Phenytoin Sodium)	II-2175
Epileptol (Carbamazepine)	II-418
Epileptol CR (Carbamazepine)	II-418
Epilex (Valproate Sodium)	II-2749
Epilim (Valproic Acid)	II-2755
Epilim Chrono (Valproate Sodium)	II-2749
Epi-Monistat (Miconazole)	II-1820
Epipen Jr. 0.15mg Adrenaline Auto-Injector (Epinephrine)	II-934
Epipen Junior (Epinephrine)	II-934
Epi-Pevaryl (Econazole Nitrate)	II-900
Epiphenicol (Chloramphenicol)	II-536
Epirax (Chlordiazepoxide Hydrochloride; Clidinium Bromide)	II-541
Epirazole (Omeprazole)	II-2034
Epitomax (Topiramate)	II-2661
Epitrim (Sulfamethoxazole; Trimethoprim)	II-2500
Epival (Divalproex Sodium)	II-828
Epival (Valproate Sodium)	II-2749
Epizolone-Depot (Methylprednisolone Acetate)	II-1790
Epoade (Epoetin Alfa)	II-942
Epobron (Ibuprofen)	II-1411
Epocelin (Ceftizoxime Sodium)	II-500
Epokine (Epoetin Alfa)	II-942
Eposal Retard (Carbamazepine)	II-418
Eposerin (Ceftizoxime Sodium)	II-500
Eposin (Etoposide)	II-1080
Epoxide (Chlordiazepoxide Hydrochloride)	II-539
Epoxitin (Epoetin Alfa)	II-942
Eppy (Epinephrine)	II-934
Eppy "N" (Epinephrine)	II-934
Eppystabil (Epinephrine)	II-934
Epsitron (Captopril)	II-411
Eptadone (Methadone Hydrochloride)	II-1766
Eptoin (Phenytoin Sodium)	II-2175
Equibar (Methyldopa)	II-1778
Equilibrium (Chlordiazepoxide Hydrochloride)	II-539
Equin (Estrogens, Conjugated)	II-1019
Equinorm (Clomipramine Hydrochloride)	II-621
Equirex (Chlordiazepoxide Hydrochloride; Clidinium Bromide)	II-541
ERA (Erythromycin Ethylsuccinate)	II-965
ERA (Erythromycin Stearate)	II-970
ERA I.M. (Erythromycin Ethylsuccinate)	II-965
Eracillin (Ampicillin)	II-170
Eraldor (Acetaminophen)	II-11
Eranz (Donepezil Hydrochloride)	II-850
Eraphage (Metformin Hydrochloride)	II-1760
Erbakar (Carboplatin)	II-430
Ercar (Carboplatin)	II-430
Ercestop (Loperamide Hydrochloride)	II-1664
Ercoquin (Hydroxychloroquine Sulfate)	II-1392

International brand name (Generic name)	Page no.
Eremfat (Rifampin)	II-2363
Erganton (Dihydroergotamine Mesylate)	II-792
Ergolactin (Bromocriptine Mesylate)	II-344
Ergont (Dihydroergotamine Mesylate)	II-792
Ergovasan (Dihydroergotamine Mesylate)	II-792
Eribus (Erythromycin Stearate)	II-970
Eridan (Diazepam)	II-740
Eriecu (Erythromycin Ethylsuccinate)	II-965
Eriecu (Erythromycin Stearate)	II-970
Erilax (Orphenadrine Citrate)	II-2049
Erilin (Sildenafil Citrate)	II-2451
Erimit (Erythromycin Stearate)	II-970
Erimycin (Erythromycin Stearate)	II-970
Erimycin-T (Erythromycin)	II-960
Erisul (Erythromycin Ethylsuccinate; Sulfisoxazole Acetyl)	II-968
Eritrazon (Erythromycin Ethylsuccinate)	II-965
Eritrocina (Erythromycin)	II-960
Eritrocina (Erythromycin Ethylsuccinate)	II-965
Eritrocina (Erythromycin Stearate)	II-970
Eritrolag (Erythromycin Ethylsuccinate)	II-965
Eritrolag (Erythromycin Stearate)	II-970
Eritromicina (Erythromycin)	II-960
Eritromicina (Erythromycin Stearate)	II-970
Eritrowel (Erythromycin Ethylsuccinate)	II-965
Erlmetin (Cimetidine Hydrochloride)	II-568
Erloric (Allopurinol)	II-77
Erlvirax (Acyclovir)	II-33
Ermycin (Erythromycin)	II-960
Ermysin (Erythromycin Ethylsuccinate)	II-965
Erocetin (Cephalexin)	II-520
Eromel (Erythromycin Stearate)	II-970
Eros (Erythromycin)	II-960
Erotab (Erythromycin Stearate)	II-970
Eroxim (Sildenafil Citrate)	II-2451
Errolon (Furosemide)	II-1237
Ervevax (Measles Virus Vaccine Live)	II-1708
Ervevax (Rubella Virus Vaccine Live)	II-2409
Erwinase (Asparaginase)	II-204
Ery (Erythromycin Ethylsuccinate)	II-965
Eryacnen (Erythromycin)	II-960
Ery-B (Erythromycin)	II-960
Eryc LD (Erythromycin)	II-960
Eryc-125 (Erythromycin)	II-960
Eryc-250 (Erythromycin)	II-960
Erycen (Erythromycin)	II-960
Erycin (Erythromycin)	II-960
Erycin (Erythromycin Stearate)	II-970
Erycinum (Erythromycin)	II-960
Eryderm (Erythromycin)	II-960
Erydermer (Erythromycin)	II-960
Ery-Diolan (Erythromycin)	II-960
Eryhexal (Erythromycin)	II-960
Erymax (Erythromycin)	II-960
Ery-maxin (Erythromycin)	II-960
Ery-Maxin (Erythromycin Ethylsuccinate)	II-965
Erymed (Erythromycin)	II-960
Erymid (Erythromycin Stearate)	II-970
Erymycin AF (Erythromycin Stearate)	II-970
Erypo (Epoetin Alfa)	II-942
Eryromycen (Erythromycin Ethylsuccinate)	II-965
Erysafe (Erythromycin)	II-960
Eryson (Erythromycin Ethylsuccinate)	II-965
Ery-Tab (Erythromycin)	II-960
Erytab (Erythromycin)	II-960
Erytab-S (Erythromycin Stearate)	II-970
Eryth-Mycin (Erythromycin Stearate)	II-970
Erythrocin (Erythromycin)	II-960
Erythrocin (Erythromycin Ethylsuccinate)	II-965
Erythrocin ES 500 (Erythromycin Ethylsuccinate)	II-965
Erythrocin I.M. (Erythromycin Ethylsuccinate)	II-965
Erythrocine (Erythromycin Ethylsuccinate)	II-965
Erythrocine (Erythromycin Stearate)	II-970
Erythrodar (Erythromycin Ethylsuccinate)	II-965
Erythro-DS (Erythromycin Ethylsuccinate)	II-965
Erythrogenat (Erythromycin Stearate)	II-970
Erythrogenat TS (Erythromycin Ethylsuccinate)	II-965
Erythrogram (Erythromycin Ethylsuccinate)	II-965
Erythrol (Erythromycin Ethylsuccinate)	II-965
Erythromid (Erythromycin)	II-960
Erythromil (Erythromycin Stearate)	II-970
Erythromycin (Erythromycin)	II-960
Erythromycin (Erythromycin Stearate)	II-970
Erythromycine (Erythromycin Stearate)	II-970
Erythromycin-Ratiopharm TS (Erythromycin Ethylsuccinate)	II-965
Erythromycinum (Erythromycin Stearate)	II-970
Erythroped (Erythromycin Ethylsuccinate)	II-965
Erythropen (Erythromycin Stearate)	II-970
Erythro-Teva (Erythromycin)	II-960
Erythro-Teva (Erythromycin Stearate)	II-970
Erytop (Erythromycin)	II-960
Erytral (Pentoxifylline)	II-2154
Erytran (Erythromycin Ethylsuccinate)	II-965
Erytrarco (Erythromycin)	II-960
Erytrociclin (Erythromycin)	II-960
ES (Lisinopril)	II-1648
Esacinone (Fluocinolone Acetonide)	II-1152
Esametone (Methylprednisolone)	II-1787
Esametone (Methylprednisolone Acetate)	II-1790
Esanbutol (Ethambutol Hydrochloride)	II-1039
Esbesul (Sulfamethoxazole; Trimethoprim)	II-2500
Escoflex (Chlorzoxazone)	II-558
Escortin (Miconazole)	II-1820
Esdoxin (Doxycycline)	II-878
ESE (Erythromycin Ethylsuccinate)	II-965
Esgen (Estropipate)	II-1033
Esidrex (Hydrochlorothiazide)	II-1348
Esilgan (Estazolam)	II-983
Esinol (Erythromycin Ethylsuccinate)	II-965
Esiteren (Hydrochlorothiazide; Triamterene)	II-1362
Eskacef (Cephradine)	II-526
Eskazine (Trifluoperazine Hydrochloride)	II-2717
Eskazole (Albendazole)	II-46
Eskotrin (Aspirin)	II-206
Esmino (Chlorpromazine Hydrochloride)	II-549
Esmycin (Erythromycin Ethylsuccinate)	II-965
Esomed (Hydroquinone)	II-1391
Esonide (Budesonide)	II-347
Esoprax (Esomeprazole Magnesium)	II-980
Espa-Formin (Metformin Hydrochloride)	II-1760
Espa-lepsin (Carbamazepine)	II-418
Espazine (Trifluoperazine Hydrochloride)	II-2717
Especlor (Cefaclor)	II-444
Espectrin (Sulfamethoxazole; Trimethoprim)	II-2500
Esperson (Desoximetasone)	II-730
Espo (Epoetin Alfa)	II-942
Esporex (Clotrimazole)	II-640
Esracain Jelly (Lidocaine)	II-1628
Esracain Ointment (Lidocaine)	II-1628
Estalis continuous (Estradiol; Norethindrone Acetate)	II-1011
Estalis Sequi (Estradiol; Norethindrone Acetate)	II-1011
Estazor (Ursodiol)	II-2737
Estima Ge (Progesterone)	II-2262
Estinyl Oestradiol (Ethinyl Estradiol)	II-1040
Esto (Ethinyl Estradiol)	II-1040
Estopein (Ketorolac Tromethamine)	II-1537
Estracomb (Estradiol; Norethindrone Acetate)	II-1011
Estracomb TTS (Estradiol)	II-986
Estracyt (Estramustine Phosphate Sodium)	II-1017
Estraderm MX (Estradiol)	II-986
Estraderm TTS (Estradiol)	II-986
Estragest TTS (Estradiol; Norethindrone Acetate)	II-1011
Estran (Estradiol)	II-986
Estranova (Estrogens, Conjugated)	II-1019
Estrapak 50 (Estradiol)	II-986
Estregur (Chlorotrianisene)	II-547
Estreva (Estradiol)	II-986
Estrifam (Estradiol)	II-986
Estrinor (Ethinyl Estradiol; Norethindrone)	II-1055
Estrofem (Estradiol)	II-986
Estrofem 2 (Estradiol)	II-986
Estrofem Forte (Estradiol)	II-986
Estulic (Guanfacine Hydrochloride)	II-1323
Eszo 2 (Estazolam)	II-983
Etapiam (Ethambutol Hydrochloride)	II-1039
Ethambin-PIN (Ethambutol Hydrochloride)	II-1039
Ethbutol (Ethambutol Hydrochloride)	II-1039
Ethicef (Cefadroxil Monohydrate)	II-447
Ethicol (Simvastatin)	II-2454
Ethinylestradiolum (Ethinyl Estradiol)	II-1040
Ethipramine (Imipramine Hydrochloride)	II-1431
Ethosuximide (Ethosuximide)	II-1072
Ethrine (Dipyridamole)	II-821
Ethymal (Ethosuximide)	II-1072
Etibi (Ethambutol Hydrochloride)	II-1039
Etibon (Etidronate Disodium)	II-1073
Etidoxina (Doxycycline)	II-878
Etimonis (Isosorbide Mononitrate)	II-1507
Etindrax (Allopurinol)	II-77
Etinilestradiolo (Ethinyl Estradiol)	II-1040
Etinycine (Erythromycin)	II-960
Etodin (Etodolac)	II-1076
Etomedec (Etoposide)	II-1080
Etonox (Etodolac)	II-1076
Etopan (Etodolac)	II-1076
Etopan XL (Etodolac)	II-1076
Etophos (Etoposide)	II-1080
Etopos (Etoposide)	II-1080
Etoposido (Etoposide)	II-1080
Etosid (Etoposide)	II-1080
Etosuximida (Ethosuximide)	II-1072
Etrolate (Erythromycin)	II-960
Etromycin (Erythromycin Ethylsuccinate)	II-965
Etrotab (Erythromycin Stearate)	II-970
Eucalen (Alendronate Sodium)	II-70
Eucardic (Carvedilol)	II-438
Eucor (Simvastatin)	II-2454
Eucoran (Amlodipine Besylate)	II-125
Eudigox (Digoxin)	II-780
Eudyna (Tretinoin)	II-2691
Eufilin (Aminophylline)	II-106
Eufilina (Aminophylline)	II-106
Eufilina Mite (Aminophylline)	II-106
Euflex (Flutamide)	II-1181
Eugerial (Nimodipine)	II-1974
Euglim (Glimepiride)	II-1287
Euglucan (Glyburide)	II-1297
Eugynon (Ethinyl Estradiol; Norgestrel)	II-1068
Eugynon 21 (Ethinyl Estradiol; Norgestrel)	II-1068
Eugynon 28 (Ethinyl Estradiol; Norgestrel)	II-1068
Eugynon 30 (Ethinyl Estradiol; Norgestrel)	II-1068
Euhypnos (Temazepam)	II-2556
Eulexine (Flutamide)	II-1181
Eupantol (Pantoprazole Sodium)	II-2097
Eupen (Amoxicillin)	II-131
Euphorin P (Diazepam)	II-740
Euphyllin (Aminophylline)	II-106
Euphyllin Retard (Aminophylline)	II-106
Euphyllin Retard (Theophylline)	II-2593
Euphylong (Theophylline)	II-2593
Euphylong Retardkaps (Theophylline)	II-2593
Euphylong SR (Theophylline)	II-2593
Euradal (Bisoprolol Fumarate)	II-323
Eu-Ran (Ranitidine Hydrochloride)	II-2334
Eureceptor (Cimetidine Hydrochloride)	II-568
Eurex (Prazosin Hydrochloride)	II-2229
Eurocef (Ceftriaxone Sodium)	II-503
Euroclin (Clindamycin)	II-605
Eurodin (Estazolam)	II-983
Euroflox (Norfloxacin)	II-1997
Europlex (Isoniazid)	II-1496
Eurostan (Mefenamic Acid)	II-1720

International brand name (Generic name)	Page no.
Eurythmic (Amiodarone Hydrochloride)	II-110
Eusaprim (Sulfamethoxazole; Trimethoprim)	II-2500
Eutensin (Furosemide)	II-1237
Euthyrox (Levothyroxine Sodium)	II-1618
Eutirox (Levothyroxine Sodium)	II-1618
Eutrim (Sulfamethoxazole; Trimethoprim)	II-2500
Euvax-B (Hepatitis B Immune Globulin)	II-1341
Evacef (Cefadroxil Monohydrate)	II-447
Evafilm (Estradiol)	II-986
Evapause (Progesterone)	II-2262
Evenin (Chlorpheniramine Maleate)	II-548
Eveprem (Estradiol; Norethindrone Acetate)	II-1011
Eviclin (Estradiol; Norethindrone Acetate)	II-1011
Evion (Vitamin E)	II-2796
Evitocor (Atenolol)	II-222
Evorel (Estradiol)	II-986
Evorel Cont (Estradiol; Norethindrone Acetate)	II-1011
Evorel Sequi (Estradiol; Norethindrone Acetate)	II-1011
Evorelconti (Estradiol; Norethindrone Acetate)	II-1011
Evothyl (Fenofibrate)	II-1105
Evrodin (Estazolam)	II-983
Exafil (Albuterol)	II-47
Excaugh 100 (Guaifenesin)	II-1314
Excillin (Ampicillin)	II-170
Exel (Meloxicam)	II-1726
Exipan (Piroxicam)	II-2205
Exiphen (Tamoxifen Citrate)	II-2539
Exirel (Pirbuterol Acetate)	II-2203
Exitane (Chlorhexidine Gluconate)	II-542
Exitop (Etoposide Phosphate)	II-1083
Exocin (Ofloxacin)	II-2015
Exocine (Ofloxacin)	II-2015
Exoderil (Naftifine Hydrochloride)	II-1916
Exomuc (Acetylcysteine)	II-29
Exopen (Tramadol Hydrochloride)	II-2674
Exoseptoplix (Chlorhexidine Gluconate)	II-542
44 Exp (Guaifenesin)	II-1314
Expan (Doxepin Hydrochloride)	II-865
Expandol (Acetaminophen)	II-11
Expanfen (Ibuprofen)	II-1411
Expectorin Cough (Guaifenesin)	II-1314
Extencilline (Penicillin G Benzathine)	II-2136
Extrapen (Ampicillin)	II-170
Extur (Indapamide)	II-1436
Eyebrex (Tobramycin)	II-2643
Eyzu (Estrogens, Conjugated)	II-1019
Ezopta (Ranitidine Hydrochloride)	II-2334
F	
Fabrol (Acetylcysteine)	II-29
Facenol (Tretinoin)	II-2691
Facicam (Piroxicam)	II-2205
Facid (Famotidine)	II-1093
Facort (Triamcinolone Acetonide)	II-2701
Factodin (Clotrimazole)	II-640
Fadin (Famotidine)	II-1093
Fadine (Famotidine)	II-1093
Fafotin (Famotidine)	II-1093
Fagusan N Losung (Guaifenesin)	II-1314
Falergi (Cetirizine Hydrochloride)	II-529
Falexin (Cephalexin)	II-520
Famo (Famotidine)	II-1093
FamoABZ (Famotidine)	II-1093
Famoc (Famotidine)	II-1093
Famocid (Famotidine)	II-1093
Famodar (Famotidine)	II-1093
Famodil (Famotidine)	II-1093
Famodin (Famotidine)	II-1093
Famodine (Famotidine)	II-1093
Famogal (Famotidine)	II-1093
Famogard (Famotidine)	II-1093
Famolta (Famotidine)	II-1093
Famonerton (Famotidine)	II-1093
Famopril (Famotidine)	II-1093
Famopsin (Famotidine)	II-1093
Famos (Famotidine)	II-1093
Famosan (Famotidine)	II-1093
Famotal (Famotidine)	II-1093
Famotep (Famotidine)	II-1093
Famotin (Famotidine)	II-1093
Famotine (Famotidine)	II-1093
Famowal (Famotidine)	II-1093
Famox (Famotidine)	II-1093
Famoxal (Famotidine)	II-1093
Fanox (Famotidine)	II-1093
Farcolin (Albuterol)	II-47
Farconcil (Amoxicillin)	II-131
Farcopril (Captopril)	II-411
Fargan (Promethazine Hydrochloride)	II-2268
Farganesse (Promethazine Hydrochloride)	II-2268
Fargoxin (Digoxin)	II-780
Farin (Warfarin Sodium)	II-2804
Farlutal (Medroxyprogesterone Acetate)	II-1714
Farmablastina (Doxorubicin Hydrochloride)	II-870
Farmacaina (Lidocaine)	II-1628
Farmadiuril (Bumetanide)	II-359
Farmadral (Propranolol Hydrochloride)	II-2287
Farmagard (Nadolol)	II-1911
Farmalex (Cephalexin)	II-520
Farmamide (Ifosfamide)	II-1420
Farmaproina (Penicillin G Procaine)	II-2140
Farmiblastina (Doxorubicin, Liposomal)	II-873
Farmistin CS (Vincristine Sulfate)	II-2789
Farmitrexat (Methotrexate Sodium)	II-1772
Farmorubicin (Epirubicin Hydrochloride)	II-938
Farmorubicin PFS (Epirubicin Hydrochloride)	II-938
Farmorubicina (Epirubicin Hydrochloride)	II-938
Farmorubicina CS (Epirubicin Hydrochloride)	II-938
Farmorubicina R.D. (Epirubicin Hydrochloride)	II-938
Farmorubicine (Epirubicin Hydrochloride)	II-938
Farmoten (Captopril)	II-411
Farmotex (Famotidine)	II-1093
Farmotrex (Methotrexate Sodium)	II-1772
Farnat (Metronidazole)	II-1812
Farnormin (Atenolol)	II-222
Farotin (Famotidine)	II-1093
Farprolol (Propranolol Hydrochloride)	II-2287
Fastum (Ketoprofen)	II-1533
Fatral (Sertraline Hydrochloride)	II-2439
Faverin (Fluvoxamine Maleate)	II-1203
Favorex (Sotalol Hydrochloride)	II-2471
Favoxil (Fluvoxamine Maleate)	II-1203
Faxilen (Cefazolin Sodium)	II-452
Fazol (Ketoconazole)	II-1530
Fazolin (Cefazolin Sodium)	II-452
Febratic (Ibuprofen)	II-1411
Febryn (Ibuprofen)	II-1411
Fectrim (Sulfamethoxazole; Trimethoprim)	II-2500
Fedcor (Nifedipine)	II-1967
Fedipin (Nifedipine)	II-1967
Felantin (Phenytoin Sodium)	II-2175
Felcicam (Piroxicam)	II-2205
Felden (Piroxicam)	II-2205
Feldene Gel (Piroxicam)	II-2205
Felexin (Cephalexin)	II-520
Felison (Flurazepam Hydrochloride)	II-1175
Felo ER (Felodipine)	II-1103
Felo-BASF (Felodipine)	II-1103
Felo-BASF Retardtab (Felodipine)	II-1103
Felo-Bits (Atenolol)	II-222
Felocor (Felodipine)	II-1103
Felocor Retardtab (Felodipine)	II-1103
Felodur ER (Felodipine)	II-1103
Felogard (Felodipine)	II-1103
Felrox (Piroxicam)	II-2205
Felxicam (Piroxicam)	II-2205
Fem 7 (Estradiol)	II-986
Fematrix (Estradiol)	II-986
Femavit (Estrogens, Conjugated)	II-1019
Femen (Mefenamic Acid)	II-1720
Femenal (Ethinyl Estradiol; Norgestrel)	II-1068
Femex (Naproxen)	II-1924
Fempres (Moexipril Hydrochloride)	II-1861
Fempress (Moexipril Hydrochloride)	II-1861
Femsept (Estradiol)	II-986
Femseven (Estradiol)	II-986
Femtran (Estradiol)	II-986
Fenac (Diclofenac)	II-748
Fen-Alcon (Chloramphenicol)	II-536
Fenaler (Chlorpheniramine Maleate)	II-548
Fenamic (Mefenamic Acid)	II-1720
Fenamin (Mefenamic Acid)	II-1720
Fenamol (Mefenamic Acid)	II-1720
Fenamon (Nifedipine)	II-1967
Fenamon SR (Nifedipine)	II-1967
Fenatoin NM (Phenytoin Sodium)	II-2175
Fenazine (Promethazine Hydrochloride)	II-2268
Fenbid (Ibuprofen)	II-1411
Fenemal (Phenobarbital)	II-2167
Fenemal NM Pharma (Phenobarbital)	II-2167
Fenergan (Promethazine Hydrochloride)	II-2268
Fenicol (Chloramphenicol)	II-536
Fenicol oft (Chloramphenicol)	II-536
Fenidantoin S 100 (Phenytoin Sodium)	II-2175
Fenistil hydrocortison (Hydrocortisone Acetate)	II-1373
Fenitron (Phenytoin Sodium)	II-2175
Fenobarbital (Phenobarbital)	II-2167
Fenocin (Penicillin V Potassium)	II-2142
Fenodid (Fentanyl Citrate)	II-1112
Fenofanton (Fenofibrate)	II-1105
Fenogal Lidose (Fenofibrate)	II-1105
Fenoprex (Fenoprofen Calcium)	II-1110
Fenopron (Fenoprofen Calcium)	II-1110
Fenox (Famotidine)	II-1093
Fenoxcillin (Penicillin V Potassium)	II-2142
Fenoxypen (Penicillin V Potassium)	II-2142
Fentanest (Fentanyl Citrate)	II-1112
Fentazin (Perphenazine)	II-2162
Fenytoin (Phenytoin Sodium)	II-2175
Feospan (Ferrous Sulfate)	II-1122
Feprax (Alprazolam)	II-85
Fepron (Fenoprofen Calcium)	II-1110
Ferfacef (Ceftriaxone Sodium)	II-503
Fermagex (Sulfamethoxazole; Trimethoprim)	II-2500
Fermentmycin (Gentamicin Sulfate)	II-1279
Fero-Gradumet Filmtab (Ferrous Sulfate)	II-1122
Ferro-grad (Ferrous Sulfate)	II-1122
Ferrograd (Ferrous Sulfate)	II-1122
Ferrolent (Ferrous Sulfate)	II-1122
Ferronemia (Ferrous Sulfate)	II-1122
Ferrophor (Ferrous Sulfate)	II-1122
Fespan (Ferrous Sulfate)	II-1122
Fetik (Ketoprofen)	II-1533
Fetinor (Gemfibrozil)	II-1269
Fetodrin (Ritodrine Hydrochloride)	II-2379
Fetusin (Oxytocin)	II-2082
Fevarin (Fluvoxamine Maleate)	II-1203
Fexin (Cephalexin)	II-520
Fibonel (Famotidine)	II-1093
Fibralip (Gemfibrozil)	II-1269
Fibrocit (Gemfibrozil)	II-1269
Fibsol (Lisinopril)	II-1648
Ficortril (Hydrocortisone)	II-1369
Ficortril (Hydrocortisone Acetate)	II-1373
Filazem (Diltiazem Hydrochloride)	II-798
Filicine (Folic Acid)	II-1208
Filocot (Hydrocortisone)	II-1369
Fimoflox (Ciprofloxacin Hydrochloride)	II-573
Finallerg (Cetirizine Hydrochloride)	II-529
Finamicina (Rifampin)	II-2363
Fincar (Finasteride)	II-1129
Finired (Finasteride)	II-1129
Finpro (Finasteride)	II-1129
Finska (Loratadine)	II-1675

International brand name (Generic name)	Page no.
Fintal (Cromolyn Sodium)	II-656
Fintel (Albendazole)	II-46
Fiorinal-C 1 2 (Aspirin; Butalbital; Caffeine; Codeine Phosphate)	II-208
Fiorinal-C 1 4 (Aspirin; Butalbital; Caffeine; Codeine Phosphate)	II-208
Firmacort (Methylprednisolone)	II-1787
Fistrin (Finasteride)	II-1129
Fivasa (Mesalamine)	II-1748
Fixef (Cefixime)	II-466
Fixim (Cefixime)	II-466
Fixime (Cefixime)	II-466
Fixiphar (Cefixime)	II-466
Fixoten (Pentoxifylline)	II-2154
Fixx (Cefixime)	II-466
Fladex (Metronidazole)	II-1812
Flagenase (Metronidazole)	II-1812
Flagizole (Metronidazole)	II-1812
Flamaret (Indomethacin)	II-1443
Flamic Gel (Piroxicam)	II-2205
Flamon (Verapamil Hydrochloride)	II-2777
Flanax (Naproxen)	II-1924
Flanax (Naproxen Sodium)	II-1928
Flanax (Rofecoxib)	II-2396
Flanax Forte (Naproxen Sodium)	II-1928
Flasinyl (Metronidazole)	II-1812
Flavettes (Ascorbic Acid)	II-203
Flaxine (Piroxicam)	II-2205
Flazol (Metronidazole)	II-1812
Flebocortid (Hydrocortisone Sodium Succinate)	II-1379
Flecaine (Flecainide Acetate)	II-1134
Flector (Diclofenac)	II-748
Flemex-AC (Acetylcysteine)	II-29
Flemonex (Guaifenesin)	II-1314
Flemoxin (Amoxicillin)	II-131
Flemoxine Ge (Amoxicillin)	II-131
Flexagen (Diclofenac)	II-748
Flexartal (Carisoprodol)	II-432
Flexiban (Cyclobenzaprine Hydrochloride)	II-664
Flexirox (Piroxicam)	II-2205
Flexital (Pentoxifylline)	II-2154
Flixonase (Fluticasone Propionate)	II-1182
Flixonase 24 hour (Fluticasone Propionate)	II-1182
Flixonase Nasal Spray (Fluticasone Propionate)	II-1182
Flixotide (Fluticasone Propionate)	II-1182
Flixotide Disk (Fluticasone Propionate)	II-1182
Flixotide Disks (Fluticasone Propionate)	II-1182
Flixotide Inhaler (Fluticasone Propionate)	II-1182
Flixovate (Fluticasone Propionate)	II-1182
Flobacin (Ofloxacin)	II-2015
Flodil LP (Felodipine)	II-1103
Flodin (Meloxicam)	II-1726
Floginax (Naproxen)	II-1924
Floglugen (Piroxicam)	II-2205
Flogofenac (Diclofenac)	II-748
Flogosan (Piroxicam)	II-2205
Flogozan (Diclofenac)	II-748
Flonax (Naproxen Sodium)	II-1928
Florid (Miconazole)	II-1820
Florid D (Miconazole)	II-1820
Florocycline (Tetracycline Hydrochloride)	II-2585
Floroxin (Ciprofloxacin Hydrochloride)	II-573
Florphen (Flurbiprofen)	II-1177
Flotrin (Terazosin Hydrochloride)	II-2566
Flovacil (Diflunisal)	II-777
Floxacin (Norfloxacin)	II-1997
Floxager (Ciprofloxacin Hydrochloride)	II-573
Floxal (Ofloxacin)	II-2015
Floxantina (Ciprofloxacin Hydrochloride)	II-573
Floxbio (Ciprofloxacin Hydrochloride)	II-573
Floxel (Levofloxacin)	II-1607
Floxil (Ofloxacin)	II-2015
Floxstat (Ofloxacin)	II-2015
Flozet (Fluocinolone Acetonide)	II-1152
Flu-21 (Fluocinonide)	II-1156
Flubason (Desoximetasone)	II-730
Flubiol (Fluocinonide)	II-1156
Flucan (Fluphenazine Decanoate)	II-1170
Flucand (Fluconazole)	II-1136
Flucazol (Fluconazole)	II-1136
Fluciderm (Fluocinolone Acetonide)	II-1152
Flucinom (Flutamide)	II-1181
Flucinome (Flutamide)	II-1181
Flucoral (Fluconazole)	II-1136
Flucort (Fluocinolone Acetonide)	II-1152
Flucozal (Fluconazole)	II-1136
Fluctin (Fluoxetine Hydrochloride)	II-1160
Fluctine (Fluoxetine Hydrochloride)	II-1160
Fludac (Fluoxetine Hydrochloride)	II-1160
Fludecasine (Fluphenazine Decanoate)	II-1170
Fludecate (Fluphenazine Decanoate)	II-1170
Fludecate Multidose (Fluphenazine Decanoate)	II-1170
Fludestrin (Testolactone)	II-2581
Fludex (Indapamide)	II-1436
Fludex SR (Indapamide)	II-1436
Fludizol (Fluconazole)	II-1136
Flufran (Fluoxetine Hydrochloride)	II-1160
Flugerel (Flutamide)	II-1181
Fluimicil (Acetylcysteine)	II-29
Fluimucil (Acetylcysteine)	II-29
Fluken (Flutamide)	II-1181
Flukezol (Fluconazole)	II-1136
Fluleep (Flurazepam Hydrochloride)	II-1175
Flulem (Flutamide)	II-1181
Flulium (Clorazepate Dipotassium)	II-638
Flulone (Fluocinolone Acetonide)	II-1152
Flumach (Spironolactone)	II-2483
Flumeta (Mometasone Furoate)	II-1866
Flunase (Flunisolide)	II-1149
Flunase (Fluticasone Propionate)	II-1182
Flunazine (Fluphenazine Hydrochloride)	II-1172
Flunco (Fluconazole)	II-1136
Flunidor (Diflunisal)	II-777
Fluniget (Diflunisal)	II-777
Flunil (Fluoxetine Hydrochloride)	II-1160
Flunitec (Flunisolide)	II-1149
Flunizol (Fluconazole)	II-1136
Flunolone-V (Fluocinolone Acetonide)	II-1152
Flunox (Flurazepam Hydrochloride)	II-1175
Fluoderm (Fluocinolone Acetonide)	II-1152
Fluoen (Sodium Fluoride)	II-2465
Fluor-A-Day (Sodium Fluoride)	II-2465
Fluoravit (Sodium Fluoride)	II-2465
Fluox (Fluoxetine Hydrochloride)	II-1160
Fluoxac (Fluoxetine Hydrochloride)	II-1160
Fluoxeren (Fluoxetine Hydrochloride)	II-1160
Fluoxil (Fluoxetine Hydrochloride)	II-1160
Fluox-Puren (Fluoxetine Hydrochloride)	II-1160
Flupen (Flurbiprofen)	II-1177
Flurazin (Trifluoperazine Hydrochloride)	II-2717
Flurets (Sodium Fluoride)	II-2465
Flurofen (Flurbiprofen)	II-1177
Fluronin (Fluoxetine Hydrochloride)	II-1160
Flurozin (Flurbiprofen)	II-1177
Flusac (Fluoxetine Hydrochloride)	II-1160
Flusemide (Nicardipine Hydrochloride)	II-1958
Fluseminal (Norfloxacin)	II-1997
Flutamex (Flutamide)	II-1181
Flutan (Flutamide)	II-1181
Flutide (Fluticasone Propionate)	II-1182
Flutin (Fluoxetine Hydrochloride)	II-1160
Flutine (Fluoxetine Hydrochloride)	II-1160
Flutivate (Fluticasone Propionate)	II-1182
Flutol (Flutamide)	II-1181
Fluviral S/F (Influenza Virus Vaccine)	II-1451
Fluvirine (Influenza Virus Vaccine)	II-1451
Fluvohexal (Fluvoxamine Maleate)	II-1203
Fluvoxin (Fluvoxamine Maleate)	II-1203
Fluxen (Fluoxetine Hydrochloride)	II-1160
Fluxetil (Fluoxetine Hydrochloride)	II-1160
Fluxetin (Fluoxetine Hydrochloride)	II-1160
Fluxil (Bumetanide)	II-359
Fluxil (Fluoxetine Hydrochloride)	II-1160
Fluzepam (Flurazepam Hydrochloride)	II-1175
Fluzine (Fluphenazine Hydrochloride)	II-1172
Fluzine-P (Fluphenazine Hydrochloride)	II-1172
Fluzon (Fluocinolone Acetonide)	II-1152
Fluzone (Fluconazole)	II-1136
F-Mon (Perphenazine)	II-2162
Focus (Ibuprofen)	II-1411
Focus (Piroxicam)	II-2205
Folacin (Folic Acid)	II-1208
Folart (Folic Acid)	II-1208
Folasic (Folic Acid)	II-1208
Foliamin (Folic Acid)	II-1208
Folic Acid DHA (Folic Acid)	II-1208
Folicid (Folic Acid)	II-1208
Folico (Folic Acid)	II-1208
Foligan (Allopurinol)	II-77
Folina (Folic Acid)	II-1208
Folinsyre (Folic Acid)	II-1208
Folitab (Folic Acid)	II-1208
Folivit (Folic Acid)	II-1208
Folsan (Folic Acid)	II-1208
Folverlan (Folic Acid)	II-1208
Fondril (Bisoprolol Fumarate)	II-323
Fongistat (Nystatin)	II-2005
Fontego (Bumetanide)	II-359
Fontex (Fluoxetine Hydrochloride)	II-1160
Fonvicol (Cefazolin Sodium)	II-452
Fopou (Methyltestosterone)	II-1796
Foradil P (Formoterol Fumarate)	II-1214
Foradile (Formoterol Fumarate)	II-1214
Forcaltonin (Calcitonin (Salmon))	II-397
Forcan (Fluconazole)	II-1136
Forcanox (Itraconazole)	II-1517
Fordex (Tolbutamide)	II-2650
Fordiuran (Bumetanide)	II-359
Fordrim (Flurazepam Hydrochloride)	II-1175
Forken (Amiodarone Hydrochloride)	II-110
Formin (Metformin Hydrochloride)	II-1760
Formoclean (Formoterol Fumarate)	II-1214
Formulex (Dicyclomine Hydrochloride)	II-763
Formyco (Ketoconazole)	II-1530
Formyxan (Mitoxantrone Hydrochloride)	II-1856
Fornidd (Metformin Hydrochloride)	II-1760
Fortam (Ceftazidime)	II-492
Fortasec (Loperamide Hydrochloride)	II-1664
Fortecortin (Dexamethasone)	II-730
Forterol (Formoterol Fumarate)	II-1214
Fortfen SR (Diclofenac)	II-748
Fortolin (Acetaminophen)	II-11
Forton (Methyltestosterone)	II-1796
Fortum (Ceftazidime)	II-492
Fortum Pro (Ceftazidime)	II-492
Fortumset (Ceftazidime)	II-492
Fortwin (Pentazocine Lactate)	II-2147
Fortzaar (Hydrochlorothiazide; Losartan Potassium)	II-1354
Forzid (Ceftazidime)	II-492
Fosalan (Alendronate Sodium)	II-70
Foscovir (Foscarnet Sodium)	II-1218
Fosicomp (Fosinopril Sodium; Hydrochlorothiazide)	II-1226
Fosinil (Fosinopril Sodium)	II-1222
Fosinorm (Fosinopril Sodium)	II-1222
Fosinorm (Fosinopril Sodium; Hydrochlorothiazide)	II-1226
Fosipres (Fosinopril Sodium)	II-1222
Fositen (Fosinopril Sodium)	II-1222
Fositens (Fosinopril Sodium)	II-1222
Fosmin (Alendronate Sodium)	II-70
Fotax (Cefotaxime Sodium)	II-474
Fotexina (Cefotaxime Sodium)	II-474
Fournox (Ceftazidime)	II-492

International brand name (Generic name)	Page no.
Fovas (Fosinopril Sodium)	II-1222
Foxalepsin (Carbamazepine)	II-418
Foxalepsin Retard (Carbamazepine)	II-418
Foxetin (Fluoxetine Hydrochloride)	II-1160
Foxinon (Norfloxacin)	II-1997
Foxolin (Amoxicillin)	II-131
Foziretic (Fosinopril Sodium; Hydrochlorothiazide)	II-1226
Fozitec (Fosinopril Sodium)	II-1222
Fractal (Fluvastatin Sodium)	II-1199
Fractal LP (Fluvastatin Sodium)	II-1199
Frademicina (Lincomycin Hydrochloride)	II-1640
Fradicilina 600 (Penicillin G Procaine)	II-2140
Fragmin P Forte (Dalteparin Sodium)	II-696
Fragmine (Dalteparin Sodium)	II-696
Franyl (Furosemide)	II-1237
Freejex (Diclofenac)	II-748
Frekven (Propranolol Hydrochloride)	II-2287
Fremet (Cimetidine Hydrochloride)	II-568
Frenal (Cromolyn Sodium)	II-656
Fresofol (Propofol)	II-2278
Frina (Propranolol Hydrochloride)	II-2287
Fristamin (Loratadine)	II-1675
Frixitas (Alprazolam)	II-85
Froben (Flurbiprofen)	II-1177
Froben SR (Flurbiprofen)	II-1177
Fronil (Imipramine Hydrochloride)	II-1431
Frontal (Alprazolam)	II-85
Frotin (Metronidazole)	II-1812
Froxime (Cefuroxime)	II-507
Frumeron (Indapamide)	II-1436
Frusedan (Furosemide)	II-1237
Frusema (Furosemide)	II-1237
Ftazidime (Ceftazidime)	II-492
Ftorocort (Triamcinolone Acetonide)	II-2701
Fudone (Famotidine)	II-1093
Fugacin (Ofloxacin)	II-2015
Fugen (Ketoconazole)	II-1530
Fugentin (Amoxicillin; Clavulanate Potassium)	II-139
Fugerel (Flutamide)	II-1181
Fulcin (Griseofulvin, Microcrystalline)	II-1312
Fulcin Forte (Griseofulvin, Microcrystalline)	II-1312
Fulden (Piroxicam)	II-2205
Fulgram (Norfloxacin)	II-1997
Fullcilina (Amoxicillin)	II-131
Fulsed (Midazolam Hydrochloride)	II-1823
Fulvina P G (Griseofulvin, Ultramicrocrystalline)	II-1313
Fumay (Fluconazole)	II-1136
Funazol (Fluconazole)	II-1136
Funazole Tabs (Ketoconazole)	II-1530
Funcort (Miconazole)	II-1820
Funet (Ketoconazole)	II-1530
Funga (Miconazole)	II-1820
Fungares (Miconazole)	II-1820
Fungarest (Ketoconazole)	II-1530
Fungata (Fluconazole)	II-1136
Fungaway (Ketoconazole)	II-1530
Fungazol (Econazole Nitrate)	II-900
Fungazol Tabs (Ketoconazole)	II-1530
Fungicide (Ketoconazole)	II-1530
Fungicide Tabs (Ketoconazole)	II-1530
Fungicip (Clotrimazole)	II-640
Fungicon (Clotrimazole)	II-640
Fungiderm (Clotrimazole)	II-640
Fungiderm-K (Ketoconazole)	II-1530
Fungilin (Amphotericin B)	II-157
Fungi-M (Miconazole)	II-1820
Fungin (Griseofulvin, Microcrystalline)	II-1312
Funginoc (Ketoconazole)	II-1530
Funginox Tabs (Ketoconazole)	II-1530
Fungiquim (Miconazole)	II-1820
Fungistat (Terconazole)	II-2576
Fungistat 3 (Terconazole)	II-2576
Fungistat 5 (Terconazole)	II-2576
Fungistin (Clotrimazole)	II-640
Fungitrazol (Itraconazole)	II-1517
Fungizid (Clotrimazole)	II-640
Fungizone (Amphotericin B)	II-157
Fungo (Miconazole)	II-1820
Fungo Vaginal Cream (Miconazole)	II-1820
Fungopirox (Ciclopirox)	II-561
Fungoral (Ketoconazole)	II-1530
Fungowas (Ciclopirox)	II-561
Fungtopic (Miconazole)	II-1820
Furadantin Retard (Nitrofurantoin, Macrocrystalline)	II-1982
Furadantina (Nitrofurantoin)	II-1979
Furadantina (Nitrofurantoin, Macrocrystalline)	II-1982
Furadantina MC (Nitrofurantoin, Macrocrystalline)	II-1982
Furadantine (Nitrofurantoin, Macrocrystalline)	II-1982
Furadantine-MC (Nitrofurantoin, Macrocrystalline)	II-1982
Furadoine (Nitrofurantoin)	II-1979
Furanthril (Furosemide)	II-1237
Furantoina (Nitrofurantoin)	II-1979
Furanturil (Furosemide)	II-1237
Furetic (Furosemide)	II-1237
Furix (Furosemide)	II-1237
Furmid (Furosemide)	II-1237
Furobactina (Nitrofurantoin)	II-1979
Furo-Basan (Furosemide)	II-1237
Furolnok (Itraconazole)	II-1517
Furomen (Furosemide)	II-1237
Furomex (Furosemide)	II-1237
Furo-Puren (Furosemide)	II-1237
Furorese (Furosemide)	II-1237
Furoscan (Furosemide)	II-1237
Furosix (Furosemide)	II-1237
Furovite (Furosemide)	II-1237
Furoxime (Cefuroxime)	II-507
Fusalar (Fluocinolone Acetonide)	II-1152
Fusid (Furosemide)	II-1237
Fuweidin (Famotidine)	II-1093
Fuxen (Naproxen)	II-1924
Fytosid (Etoposide Phosphate)	II-1083

G

International brand name (Generic name)	Page no.
GAB (Lindane)	II-1642
Gabatril (Tiagabine Hydrochloride)	II-2612
Gabrilen Retard (Ketoprofen)	II-1533
Gadoserin (Diltiazem Hydrochloride)	II-798
Galentromicina (Erythromycin Stearate)	II-970
Galidrin (Ranitidine Hydrochloride)	II-2334
Gamafine (Immune Globulin (Human))	II-1434
Gamastan Immune Globulin (Immune Globulin (Human))	II-1434
Gamax (Mebendazole)	II-1711
Gambex (Lindane)	II-1642
Gamikal (Amikacin Sulfate)	II-101
Gamma 16 (Immune Globulin (Human))	II-1434
Gammabulin (Immune Globulin (Human))	II-1434
Gammagard S D (Immune Globulin (Human))	II-1434
Gamma-Gel (Aluminum Hydroxide)	II-97
Gammonativ (Immune Globulin (Human))	II-1434
Gantaprim (Sulfamethoxazole; Trimethoprim)	II-2500
Gantin (Gabapentin)	II-1241
Gantrim (Sulfamethoxazole; Trimethoprim)	II-2500
Garabiotic (Gentamicin Sulfate)	II-1279
Garalone (Gentamicin Sulfate)	II-1279
Garamicin (Gentamicin Sulfate)	II-1279
Garamicina (Gentamicin Sulfate)	II-1279
Garamicina Cream (Gentamicin Sulfate)	II-1279
Garamicina Crema (Gentamicin Sulfate)	II-1279
Garamicina Oftalmica (Gentamicin Sulfate)	II-1279
Garasone (Gentamicin Sulfate)	II-1279
Garbilocin (Gentamicin Sulfate)	II-1279
Gardan (Mefenamic Acid)	II-1720
Gardenal (Phenobarbital)	II-2167
Gardenale (Phenobarbital)	II-2167
Gardin (Famotidine)	II-1093
Gascop (Albendazole)	II-46
Gasec (Omeprazole)	II-2034
Gastab (Cimetidine Hydrochloride)	II-568
Gaster (Famotidine)	II-1093
Gastidine (Cimetidine Hydrochloride)	II-568
Gastop (Omeprazole)	II-2034
Gastotec (Misoprostol)	II-1851
Gastracol (Aluminum Hydroxide)	II-97
Gastrax (Nizatidine)	II-1992
Gastrial (Ranitidine Hydrochloride)	II-2334
Gastridin (Famotidine)	II-1093
Gastridin (Ranitidine Hydrochloride)	II-2334
Gastrion (Famotidine)	II-1093
Gastro (Famotidine)	II-1093
Gastrobi (Metoclopramide Hydrochloride)	II-1798
Gastrobitan (Cimetidine Hydrochloride)	II-568
Gastrodin (Cimetidine Hydrochloride)	II-568
Gastrodomina (Famotidine)	II-1093
Gastrodyn Inj (Glycopyrrolate)	II-1302
Gastroloc (Omeprazole)	II-2034
Gastron (Loperamide Hydrochloride)	II-1664
Gastronerton (Metoclopramide Hydrochloride)	II-1798
Gastrosedol (Ranitidine Hydrochloride)	II-2334
Gastrosil (Metoclopramide Hydrochloride)	II-1798
Gastro-Stop (Loperamide Hydrochloride)	II-1664
Gastrul (Misoprostol)	II-1851
Gavistal (Metoclopramide Hydrochloride)	II-1798
Gawei (Cimetidine Hydrochloride)	II-568
G.B.N. (Glyburide)	II-1297
Geangin (Verapamil Hydrochloride)	II-2777
Gelalmin (Aluminum Hydroxide)	II-97
Gelisyn (Fluocinonide)	II-1156
Gelocatil (Acetaminophen)	II-11
Gelox (Aluminum Hydroxide)	II-97
Geluprane 500 (Acetaminophen)	II-11
Gemcite (Gemcitabine Hydrochloride)	II-1265
Gemd (Gemfibrozil)	II-1269
Gemfi (Gemfibrozil)	II-1269
Gemfibril (Gemfibrozil)	II-1269
Gemfibromax (Gemfibrozil)	II-1269
Gemicort (Triamcinolone Acetonide)	II-2701
Gemizol (Gemfibrozil)	II-1269
Gemlipid (Gemfibrozil)	II-1269
Gemnpid (Gemfibrozil)	II-1269
Gemzil (Gemfibrozil)	II-1269
Gencin (Gentamicin Sulfate)	II-1279
Gencolax (Bisacodyl)	II-322
Genephamide (Acetazolamide)	II-28
Genercin (Chloramphenicol)	II-536
Generlog (Triamcinolone Acetonide)	II-2701
Gengraf (Cyclosporine)	II-668
Genin (Quinine Sulfate)	II-2317
Geniquin (Hydroxychloroquine Sulfate)	II-1392
Genlac (Lactulose)	II-1550
Genocin (Chloroquine)	II-544
Genoral (Estropipate)	II-1033
Genoxal (Cyclophosphamide)	II-666
Genrex (Gentamicin Sulfate)	II-1279
Gensil (Metoclopramide Hydrochloride)	II-1798
Gensumycin (Gentamicin Sulfate)	II-1279
Genta Grin (Gentamicin Sulfate)	II-1279
Gentabiotic (Gentamicin Sulfate)	II-1279
Gentabiox (Gentamicin Sulfate)	II-1279
Gentacin (Gentamicin Sulfate)	II-1279
Gentacor (Gentamicin Sulfate)	II-1279
Gentacyl (Gentamicin Sulfate)	II-1279
Gentagram (Gentamicin Sulfate)	II-1279
Gental (Gentamicin Sulfate)	II-1279
Gentalline (Gentamicin Sulfate)	II-1279
Gentalol (Gentamicin Sulfate)	II-1279
Gentalyn (Gentamicin Sulfate)	II-1279
Gentalyn Oftalmico-Otico (Gentamicin Sulfate)	II-1279
Gentamax (Gentamicin Sulfate)	II-1279
Gentamedical (Gentamicin Sulfate)	II-1279

International brand name (Generic name)	Page no.
Grisuvin (Griseofulvin, Microcrystalline)	II-1312
Grivin (Griseofulvin, Microcrystalline)	II-1312
Grospisk (Methyldopa)	II-1778
Grunamox (Amoxicillin)	II-131
Guabeta (Tolbutamide)	II-2650
Guaifenex PSE 60 (Guaifenesin; Pseudoephedrine Hydrochloride)	II-1316
Gubex (Diazepam)	II-740
Gulliostin (Dipyridamole)	II-821
Gunaceta (Acetaminophen)	II-11
Gunevax (Rubella Virus Vaccine Live)	II-2409
Gynatam (Tamoxifen Citrate)	II-2539
Gynatrol (Ethinyl Estradiol; Levonorgestrel)	II-1047
Gyne Lotremin (Clotrimazole)	II-640
Gyne-Lotremin (Clotrimazole)	II-640
Gynesol (Clotrimazole)	II-640
Gynesten-B (Betamethasone Dipropionate; Clotrimazole)	II-304
Gyno Canesten (Clotrimazole)	II-640
Gyno-Canestene (Clotrimazole)	II-640
Gyno-Coryl (Econazole Nitrate)	II-900
Gyno-Daktar (Miconazole)	II-1820
Gyno-Daktarin (Miconazole)	II-1820
Gyno-Monistat (Miconazole)	II-1820
Gyno-neuralgin (Ibuprofen)	II-1411
Gynoplix (Metronidazole)	II-1812
Gynospor (Miconazole)	II-1820
Gyno-Terazol (Terconazole)	II-2576
Gyno-Terazol 3 (Terconazole)	II-2576
GynPolar (Estradiol)	II-986
Gyrablock (Norfloxacin)	II-1997
H	
H-2 (Cimetidine Hydrochloride)	II-568
H2 Bloc (Famotidine)	II-1093
Hadipine S.R. (Nifedipine)	II-1967
Haelan (Flurandrenolide)	II-1174
Haemiton (Clonidine Hydrochloride)	II-629
Haemokion (Phytonadione)	II-2178
Haemoprotect (Ferrous Sulfate)	II-1122
Hagen (Diltiazem Hydrochloride)	II-798
Hairgaine (Minoxidil)	II-1845
Hairgrow (Minoxidil)	II-1845
Hairscience Antidandruff Shampoo (Miconazole)	II-1820
Haldin (Cimetidine Hydrochloride)	II-568
Haldol (Haloperidol Decanoate)	II-1332
Haldol Decanoaat (Haloperidol Decanoate)	II-1332
Haldol Decanoas (Haloperidol Decanoate)	II-1332
Haldol Decanoat (Haloperidol Decanoate)	II-1332
Halidol (Haloperidol)	II-1328
Halidol Decanoas (Haloperidol Decanoate)	II-1332
Halodin (Loratadine)	II-1675
Halojust (Haloperidol)	II-1328
Halomed (Haloperidol)	II-1328
Halomycetin Augensalbe (Chloramphenicol)	II-536
Halo-P (Haloperidol)	II-1328
Haloper (Haloperidol)	II-1328
Haloperil (Haloperidol)	II-1328
Haloperin (Haloperidol)	II-1328
Halopidol (Haloperidol)	II-1328
Halopidol decanoato (Haloperidol Decanoate)	II-1332
Halopol (Haloperidol)	II-1328
Halosten (Haloperidol)	II-1328
Hamarin (Allopurinol)	II-77
H-Ambiotico (Ampicillin)	II-170
Hamitan (Mefenamic Acid)	II-1720
Hamoxillin (Amoxicillin)	II-131
Hansepran (Clofazimine)	II-619
Haricon (Haloperidol)	II-1328
Haridol Decanoate (Haloperidol Decanoate)	II-1332
Haridol-D (Haloperidol)	II-1328
Harine (Pentoxifylline)	II-2154
Harmogen (Estropipate)	II-1033
Harmonet (Estropipate)	II-1033
Harmonin (Meprobamate)	II-1738
Harnal (Tamsulosin Hydrochloride)	II-2544
Hartsorb (Isosorbide Dinitrate)	II-1502
HAVpur (Hepatitis A Vaccine)	II-1339
HBvaxPRO (Hepatitis B Vaccine, Recombinant)	II-1343
3TC-HBV (Lamivudine)	II-1552
H.C.T. (Hydrochlorothiazide)	II-1348
Headlon (Naproxen)	II-1924
Headway (Minoxidil)	II-1845
Hebald (Minoxidil)	II-1845
Heberbiovac HB (Hepatitis B Vaccine, Recombinant)	II-1343
Hecobac (Clarithromycin)	II-597
hefaclor (Cefaclor)	II-444
Heitrin (Terazosin Hydrochloride)	II-2566
Helben (Albendazole)	II-46
Helberina (Heparin Sodium)	II-1334
Heliopar (Chloroquine)	II-544
Helitic (Clarithromycin)	II-597
Helmiben (Praziquantel)	II-2228
Helmindazol (Albendazole)	II-46
Helminzole (Mebendazole)	II-1711
Helocetin (Chloramphenicol)	II-536
Helocetin (Chloramphenicol Sodium Succinate)	II-537
Heloxatin (Oxaliplatin)	II-2056
Helsibon (Diltiazem Hydrochloride)	II-798
Hematolamin (Cyanocobalamin)	II-661
Hemesis (Metoclopramide Hydrochloride)	II-1798
Hemi-Daonil (Glyburide)	II-1297
Hemobion (Ferrous Sulfate)	II-1122
Hemovas (Pentoxifylline)	II-2154
Hepacare (Hepatitis B Vaccine, Recombinant)	II-1343
Hepaflex (Heparin Sodium)	II-1334
Hepalac (Lactulose)	II-1550
Hepalean (Heparin Sodium)	II-1334
Heparin (Heparin Sodium)	II-1334
Heparin Injection B.P. (Heparin Sodium)	II-1334
Heparin Leo (Heparin Sodium)	II-1334
Heparin Novo (Heparin Sodium)	II-1334
Heparin Sodium B Braun (Heparin Sodium)	II-1334
Heparin Subcutaneous (Heparin Sodium)	II-1334
Heparina (Heparin Sodium)	II-1334
Heparina Leo (Heparin Sodium)	II-1334
Heparine (Heparin Sodium)	II-1334
Heparine Choay (Heparin Sodium)	II-1334
Heparine Novo (Heparin Sodium)	II-1334
Hepavax Gene (Hepatitis B Vaccine, Recombinant)	II-1343
Heptasan (Cyproheptadine Hydrochloride)	II-682
Heptodin (Lamivudine)	II-1552
Heptovir (Lamivudine)	II-1552
Hepuman Berna (Hepatitis B Immune Globulin)	II-1341
Herben (Diltiazem Hydrochloride)	II-798
Herbesser (Diltiazem Hydrochloride)	II-798
Herbesser 180 SR (Diltiazem Hydrochloride)	II-798
Herbesser 60 (Diltiazem Hydrochloride)	II-798
Herbesser 90 SR (Diltiazem Hydrochloride)	II-798
Herbesser R100 (Diltiazem Hydrochloride)	II-798
Herbesser R200 (Diltiazem Hydrochloride)	II-798
Herbessor (Diltiazem Hydrochloride)	II-798
Herklin (Lindane)	II-1642
Hermolepsin (Carbamazepine)	II-418
Herpefug (Acyclovir)	II-33
Herpex (Acyclovir)	II-33
Herpoviric Rp Creme (Acyclovir)	II-33
Hesor (Diltiazem Hydrochloride)	II-798
H-Etom (Omeprazole)	II-2034
Hexacycline (Tetracycline Hydrochloride)	II-2585
Hexadent (Chlorhexidine Gluconate)	II-542
Hexadilat (Nifedipine)	II-1967
Hexagastron (Sucralfate)	II-2493
Hexamet (Cimetidine Hydrochloride)	II-568
Hexamycin (Gentamicin Sulfate)	II-1279
Hexapindol (Pindolol)	II-2192
Hexapress (Prazosin Hydrochloride)	II-2229
Hexarone (Amiodarone Hydrochloride)	II-110
Hexasoptin (Verapamil Hydrochloride)	II-2777
Hexasoptin Retard (Verapamil Hydrochloride)	II-2777
Hexastat (Altretamine)	II-96
Hexer (Ranitidine Hydrochloride)	II-2334
Hexinawas (Altretamine)	II-96
Hexit (Lindane)	II-1642
Hexobion 100 (Pyridoxine Hydrochloride)	II-2297
Hexol (Chlorhexidine Gluconate)	II-542
H.G. Dicloxacil (Dicloxacillin Sodium)	II-761
H.G. Metil Dopa (Methyldopa)	II-1778
Hibechin (Promethazine Hydrochloride)	II-2268
Hiberix (Influenza Virus Vaccine)	II-1451
Hiberna (Promethazine Hydrochloride)	II-2268
Hibernal (Chlorpromazine Hydrochloride)	II-549
HIBest (Haemophilus B Conjugate Vaccine)	II-1325
Hibiclens Solution (Chlorhexidine Gluconate)	II-542
Hibident (Chlorhexidine Gluconate)	II-542
Hibidil (Chlorhexidine Gluconate)	II-542
Hibigel (Chlorhexidine Gluconate)	II-542
Hibiguard (Chlorhexidine Gluconate)	II-542
Hibiotic (Amoxicillin; Clavulanate Potassium)	II-139
Hibiscrub (Chlorhexidine Gluconate)	II-542
Hibisol (Chlorhexidine Gluconate)	II-542
Hibitan (Chlorhexidine Gluconate)	II-542
Hibitane (Chlorhexidine Gluconate)	II-542
Hibitane Concentrate (Chlorhexidine Gluconate)	II-542
Hibitane Cream (Chlorhexidine Gluconate)	II-542
Hibitane Dental (Chlorhexidine Gluconate)	II-542
Hibitane Pastillas (Chlorhexidine Gluconate)	II-542
Hibitane Solution (Chlorhexidine Gluconate)	II-542
Hiconcil (Amoxicillin)	II-131
Hidanil (Phenytoin Sodium)	II-2175
Hiderax (Hydroxyzine)	II-1398
Hidil (Gemfibrozil)	II-1269
Hidine (Chlorhexidine Gluconate)	II-542
Hidonac (Acetylcysteine)	II-29
Hidramox (Amoxicillin)	II-131
Hidrazida (Isoniazid)	II-1496
Hidrenox (Hydrochlorothiazide)	II-1348
Hidroaltesona (Hydrocortisone)	II-1369
Hidrosaluretil (Hydrochlorothiazide)	II-1348
Hidrotisona (Hydrocortisone)	II-1369
Highprepin (Methyldopa)	II-1778
Higroton (Chlorthalidone)	II-555
Higrotona (Chlorthalidone)	II-555
Hilong (Oxazepam)	II-2063
Himetin (Cimetidine Hydrochloride)	II-568
Hinicol (Chloramphenicol)	II-536
Hipen (Amoxicillin)	II-131
Hiperil (Captopril)	II-411
Hipoglucin (Metformin Hydrochloride)	II-1760
Hipokinon (Trihexyphenidyl Hydrochloride)	II-2720
Hipolixan (Gemfibrozil)	II-1269
Hislorex (Loratadine)	II-1675
Hissuflux (Furosemide)	II-1237
Histac (Ranitidine Hydrochloride)	II-2334
Histacort (Chlorpheniramine Maleate)	II-548
Histafen (Chlorpheniramine Maleate)	II-548
Histak (Ranitidine Hydrochloride)	II-2334
Histal (Chlorpheniramine Maleate)	II-548
Histalor (Loratadine)	II-1675
Histaloran (Loratadine)	II-1675
Histan (Hydroxyzine)	II-1398
Histar (Chlorpheniramine Maleate)	II-548
Histat (Chlorpheniramine Maleate)	II-548
Histatapp (Chlorpheniramine Maleate)	II-548
Histaton (Chlorpheniramine Maleate)	II-548
Histaverin (Clemastine Fumarate)	II-603
Histavil (Chlorpheniramine Maleate)	II-548
Histazine (Cetirizine Hydrochloride)	II-529
Histergan (Diphenhydramine Hydrochloride)	II-813
Histica (Cetirizine Hydrochloride)	II-529

International brand name (Generic name)	Page no.
Histin (Carbinoxamine Maleate)	II-429
Histin (Chlorpheniramine Maleate)	II-548
Histodil (Cimetidine Hydrochloride)	II-568
Hitrin (Terazosin Hydrochloride)	II-2566
Hizemin (Diclofenac)	II-748
Hizin (Hydroxyzine)	II-1398
H-Loniten (Ibuprofen)	II-1411
H-Next (Ciprofloxacin Hydrochloride)	II-573
Hofcomant (Amantadine Hydrochloride)	II-97
Holfungin (Clotrimazole)	II-640
Honvol (Diethylstilbestrol Diphosphate)	II-776
Hopranolol (Propranolol Hydrochloride)	II-2287
Horizon (Diazepam)	II-740
Hosboral (Amoxicillin)	II-131
Hostaciclina (Tetracycline Hydrochloride)	II-2585
Hostacortin (Prednisone)	II-2240
Hostacyclin (Tetracycline Hydrochloride)	II-2585
Hostacycline (Tetracycline Hydrochloride)	II-2585
Hostacycline-P (Tetracycline Hydrochloride)	II-2585
Hostan (Mefenamic Acid)	II-1720
Hostes (Ampicillin)	II-170
Hotemin (Piroxicam)	II-2205
Huberplex (Chlordiazepoxide Hydrochloride)	II-539
Hulin (Sulfamethoxazole; Trimethoprim)	II-2500
Humalog Lispro (Insulin Lispro (Human Analog))	II-1464
Humalog Mix (Insulin Lispro; Insulin Lispro Protamine)	II-1466
Humalog Mix 25 (Insulin Lispro; Insulin Lispro Protamine)	II-1466
Humalog Mix NPL (Insulin Lispro (Human Analog))	II-1464
Human Actrapid (Insulin (Human Recombinant))	II-1454
Human Insulatard (Insulin (Human, Isophane))	II-1455
Human Monosulin (Insulin (Human, Lente))	II-1456
Human Monotard (Insulin (Human, Lente))	II-1456
Human Nordisulin (Insulin (Human Recombinant))	II-1454
Human Protaphane (Insulin (Human, Isophane))	II-1455
Humedia (Glyburide)	II-1297
Huminsulin Basal (NPH) (Insulin (Human, Isophane))	II-1455
Huminsulin "Lilly" Basal (NPH) (Insulin (Human, Isophane))	II-1455
Huminsulin "Lilly" Long (Insulin (Human, Isophane/Regular))	II-1456
Huminsulin "Lilly" Normal (Insulin (Human Recombinant))	II-1454
Huminsulin Long 100 (Insulin (Human, Lente))	II-1456
Huminsulin Normal (Insulin (Human Recombinant))	II-1454
Huminsulin Profil I (Insulin (Human, Isophane/ Regular))	II-1456
Huminsulin Profil II (Insulin (Human, Isophane/Regular))	II-1456
Huminsulin Profil III (Insulin (Human, Isophane/Regular))	II-1456
Huminsulin Profil IV (Insulin (Human, Isophane/Regular))	II-1456
Humulin 10 90 (Insulin (Human, Isophane/ Regular))	II-1456
Humulin 20 80 (Insulin (Human, Isophane/ Regular))	II-1456
Humulin 30 70 (Insulin (Human, Isophane/ Regular))	II-1456
Humulin 40 60 (Insulin (Human, Isophane/ Regular))	II-1456
Humulin 60 40 (Insulin (Human, Isophane/ Regular))	II-1456
Humulin 80 20 (Insulin (Human, Isophane/ Regular))	II-1456
Humulin 90 10 (Insulin (Human, Isophane/ Regular))	II-1456

International brand name (Generic name)	Page no.
Humulin C (Insulin (Human Recombinant))	II-1454
Humulin I (Insulin (Human, Isophane))	II-1455
Humulin M1 (Insulin (Human, Isophane/ Regular))	II-1456
Humulin M2 (Insulin (Human, Isophane/ Regular))	II-1456
Humulin M3 (Insulin (Human, Isophane/ Regular))	II-1456
Humulin M4 (Insulin (Human, Isophane/ Regular))	II-1456
Humulin (Regular) (Insulin (Human Recombinant))	II-1454
Humulin Regular (Insulin (Human Recombinant))	II-1454
Humulina 10 90 (Insulin (Human, Isophane/ Regular))	II-1456
Humulina 20 80 (Insulin (Human, Isophane/ Regular))	II-1456
Humulina 30 70 (Insulin (Human, Isophane/ Regular))	II-1456
Humulina 40 60 (Insulin (Human, Isophane/ Regular))	II-1456
Humulina 50 50 (Insulin (Human, Isophane/ Regular))	II-1456
Humulina 70 30 (Insulin (Human, Isophane/ Regular))	II-1456
Humulina NPH (Insulin (Human, Isophane))	II-1455
Humulina Regular (Insulin (Human Recombinant))	II-1454
Humuline 20 80 (Insulin (Human, Isophane/ Regular))	II-1456
Humuline 30 70 (Insulin (Human, Isophane/ Regular))	II-1456
Humuline 40 60 (Insulin (Human, Isophane/ Regular))	II-1456
Humuline NPH (Insulin (Human, Isophane))	II-1455
Humuline Regular (Insulin (Human Recombinant))	II-1454
Humulin-R (Insulin (Human Recombinant))	II-1454
Hurusfec (Norfloxacin)	II-1997
Hybloc (Labetalol Hydrochloride)	II-1545
Hycor (Hydrocortisone)	II-1369
Hycor Eye Ointment (Hydrocortisone Acetate)	II-1373
Hycortil (Hydrocortisone Sodium Succinate)	II-1379
Hydac (Felodipine)	II-1103
Hydantin (Phenytoin Sodium)	II-2175
Hydantol (Phenytoin Sodium)	II-2175
Hydcort (Hydrocortisone Valerate)	II-1382
Hyderm (Hydrocortisone Acetate)	II-1373
Hydiphen (Clomipramine Hydrochloride)	II-621
Hydopa (Methyldopa)	II-1778
Hydra (Isoniazid)	II-1496
Hydrapres (Hydralazine Hydrochloride)	II-1346
Hydrazide (Isoniazid)	II-1496
Hydrazin (Isoniazid)	II-1496
Hydrex (Furosemide)	II-1237
Hydrex (Hydrochlorothiazide)	II-1348
Hydrex-semi (Hydrochlorothiazide)	II-1348
Hydrin (Terazosin Hydrochloride)	II-2566
Hydro (Chlorthalidone)	II-555
Hydro Adreson Aquosum (Hydrocortisone Sodium Succinate)	II-1379
Hydro-Adreson Aquosum (Hydrocortisone Sodium Succinate)	II-1379
Hydrochlorzide (Hydrochlorothiazide)	II-1348
Hydrocort (Hydrocortisone Acetate)	II-1373
Hydrocortemel (Hydrocortisone)	II-1369
Hydrocortison (Hydrocortisone)	II-1369
Hydrocortison (Hydrocortisone Acetate)	II-1373
Hydrocortison (Hydrocortisone Sodium Succinate)	II-1379
Hydrocortison Berco (Hydrocortisone Acetate)	II-1373
Hydrocortison Dispersa (Hydrocortisone Acetate)	II-1373
Hydrocortison Streuli (Hydrocortisone Acetate)	II-1373

International brand name (Generic name)	Page no.
Hydrocortisone (Hydrocortisone)	II-1369
Hydrocortisone Astier (Hydrocortisone)	II-1369
Hydrocortisone Roussel (Hydrocortisone Sodium Succinate)	II-1379
Hydrocortisone Upjohn (Hydrocortisone Sodium Succinate)	II-1379
Hydrocortisonum (Hydrocortisone)	II-1369
Hydrocortisyl (Hydrocortisone)	II-1369
Hydrocutan (Hydrocortisone Acetate)	II-1373
Hydroderm (Hydrocortisone)	II-1369
Hydrogalen (Hydrocortisone)	II-1369
Hydrokort (Hydrocortisone)	II-1369
Hydrokortison (Hydrocortisone)	II-1369
Hydrokortison (Hydrocortisone Acetate)	II-1373
Hydro-Less (Indapamide)	II-1436
Hydro-Long (Chlorthalidone)	II-555
Hydromycin (Tetracycline Hydrochloride)	II-2585
Hydrosaluric (Hydrochlorothiazide)	II-1348
Hydrotopic (Hydrocortisone)	II-1369
Hydrotopic (Hydrocortisone Sodium Succinate)	II-1379
Hydrozide (Hydrochlorothiazide)	II-1348
Hygroton 50 (Chlorthalidone)	II-555
Hynorex Retard (Lithium Carbonate)	II-1654
Hypam (Triazolam)	II-2715
Hypatol (Hydralazine Hydrochloride)	II-1346
Hypazon (Spironolactone)	II-2483
Hypen (Etodolac)	II-1076
Hyperchol (Fenofibrate)	II-1105
Hyperetic (Amiloride Hydrochloride; Hydrochlorothiazide)	II-105
Hyperex (Hydralazine Hydrochloride)	II-1346
Hyperilex (Pemoline)	II-2129
Hypermet (Methyldopa)	II-1778
Hypermol (Timolol)	II-2627
Hypernol (Atenolol)	II-222
Hyperphen (Hydralazine Hydrochloride)	II-1346
Hypertol (Chlorthalidone)	II-555
Hyphorin (Estrogens, Conjugated)	II-1019
Hypnomidate (Etomidate)	II-1080
Hypnostan (Thiopental Sodium)	II-2603
Hypnovel (Midazolam Hydrochloride)	II-1823
Hypolag (Methyldopa)	II-1778
Hypomide (Chlorpropamide)	II-554
Hypopress (Captopril)	II-411
Hyposec (Omeprazole)	II-2034
Hypoten (Atenolol)	II-222
Hypotens (Prazosin Hydrochloride)	II-2229
Hypotensor (Captopril)	II-411
Hy-po-tone (Methyldopa)	II-1778
Hypovase (Prazosin Hydrochloride)	II-2229
Hyprosin (Prazosin Hydrochloride)	II-2229
Hytacand (Candesartan Cilexetil; Hydrochlorothiazide)	II-404
Hythalton (Chlorthalidone)	II-555
Hytisone (Hydrocortisone)	II-1369
Hytisone (Hydrocortisone Acetate)	II-1373
Hytone Lotion (Hydrocortisone)	II-1369
Hytracin (Terazosin Hydrochloride)	II-2566
Hytren (Ramipril)	II-2330
Hytrine (Terazosin Hydrochloride)	II-2566
Hytrinex (Terazosin Hydrochloride)	II-2566
Hytrol (Enalapril Maleate)	II-913
Hyzaar DS (Hydrochlorothiazide; Losartan Potassium)	II-1354
Hyzaar forte (Hydrochlorothiazide; Losartan Potassium)	II-1354
Hyzan (Ranitidine Hydrochloride)	II-2334

I

International brand name (Generic name)	Page no.
IB-100 (Ibuprofen)	II-1411
Ibaril (Desoximetasone)	II-730
Iberol Goths (Ferrous Sulfate)	II-1122
Ibiamox (Amoxicillin)	II-131
Ibicyn (Tetracycline Hydrochloride)	II-2585

International brand name (Generic name) Page no.

Insulin Actrapid HM (Insulin (Human Recombinant)) II-1454
Insulin Hoechst-Komb 15 U-100 (Insulin (Human, Isophane/Regular)) II-1456
Insulin Hoechst-Komb 25 U-100 (Insulin (Human, Isophane/Regular)) II-1456
Insulin Hoechst-Komb 50 U-100 (Insulin (Human, Isophane/Regular)) II-1456
Insulin Hoechst-Rapid U-100 (Insulin (Human Recombinant)) II-1454
Insulin Human Actrapid (Insulin (Human Recombinant)) II-1454
Insulin Insulatard HM (Insulin (Human, Isophane)) II-1455
Insulin Insulatard Human (Insulin (Human, Isophane)) II-1455
Insulin Lente MC (Insulin (Human, Lente)) II-1456
Insulin Mixtard 10 HM (Insulin (Human, Isophane/Regular)) II-1456
Insulin Mixtard 15 85 Human (Insulin (Human, Isophane/Regular)) II-1456
Insulin Mixtard 20 HM (Insulin (Human, Isophane/Regular)) II-1456
Insulin Mixtard 30 70 Human (Insulin (Human, Isophane/Regular)) II-1456
Insulin Mixtard 30 HM (Insulin (Human, Isophane/Regular)) II-1456
Insulin Mixtard 40 HM (Insulin (Human, Isophane/Regular)) II-1456
Insulin Mixtard 50 50 HM (Insulin (Human, Isophane/Regular)) II-1456
Insulin Mixtard 50 50 Human (Insulin (Human, Isophane/Regular)) II-1456
Insulin Mixtard 50 HM (Insulin (Human, Isophane/Regular)) II-1456
Insulin Monotard HM (Insulin (Human, Lente)) II-1456
Insulin "Novo Nordisk" Actrapid HM (Insulin (Human Recombinant)) II-1454
Insulin "Novo Nordisk" Insulatard HM (Insulin (Human, Isophane)) II-1455
Insulin "Novo Nordisk" Mixtard HM 15 85 (Insulin (Human, Isophane/Regular)) II-1456
Insulin "Novo Nordisk" Mixtard HM 30 70 (Insulin (Human, Isophane/Regular)) II-1456
Insulin "Novo Nordisk" Mixtard HM 50 50 (Insulin (Human, Isophane/Regular)) II-1456
Insulin "Novo Nordisk" Monotard HM (Insulin (Human, Lente)) II-1456
Insulin "Novo Nordisk" Velosulin HM (Insulin (Human Recombinant)) II-1454
Insulin Protaphane HM (Insulin (Human, Isophane)) II-1455
Insulin Velosulin HM (Insulin (Human Recombinant)) II-1454
Insulina (Insulin (Human Recombinant)) II-1454
Insulina Actrapid HM (Insulin (Human Recombinant)) II-1454
Insulina Combi HM 85 15 (Insulin (Human, Isophane/Regular)) II-1456
Insulina Mixt HM 30 70 (Insulin (Human, Isophane/Regular)) II-1456
Insulina Monotard HM (Insulin (Human, Lente)) II-1456
Insulina Velosulin HM (Insulin (Human Recombinant)) II-1454
Insuline (Insulin (Human, Isophane)) II-1455
Insuline (Insulin (Human Recombinant)) II-1454
Insuline Actrapid (Insulin (Human Recombinant)) II-1454
Insuline Humaan (Insulin (Human, Isophane/Regular)) II-1456
Insuline Humuline 10 90 (Insulin (Human, Isophane/Regular)) II-1456
Insuline Humuline 20 80 (Insulin (Human, Isophane/Regular)) II-1456

International brand name (Generic name) Page no.

Insuline Humuline 30 70 (Insulin (Human, Isophane/Regular)) II-1456
Insuline Humuline 40 60 (Insulin (Human, Isophane/Regular)) II-1456
Insuline Humuline NPH (Insulin (Human, Isophane)) II-1455
Insuline Humuline Regular (Insulin (Human Recombinant)) II-1454
Insuline Humuline Zink (Insulin (Human, Lente)) II-1456
Insuline Insulatard (Insulin (Human, Isophane)) II-1455
Insuline Isuhuman Basal (Insulin (Human, Isophane)) II-1455
Insuline Lispro Humalog (Insulin Lispro (Human Analog)) II-1464
Insuline Velosulin Humaan (Insulin (Human Recombinant)) II-1454
Insuman (Insulin (Human, Isophane/Regular)) II-1456
Insuman (Insulin (Human Recombinant)) II-1454
Insuman Basal (Insulin (Human, Isophane)) II-1455
Insuman Basal (Insulin (Human Recombinant)) II-1454
Insuman Infusat (Insulin (Human Recombinant)) II-1454
Insuman Rapid (Insulin (Human Recombinant)) II-1454
Insumin (Flurazepam Hydrochloride) II-1175
Intaxel (Paclitaxel) II-2084
Integrilin (Eptifibatide) II-951
Interbutol (Ethambutol Hydrochloride) II-1039
Interdoxin (Doxycycline) II-878
Intermox (Amoxicillin) II-131
Internolol (Atenolol) II-222
Intraglobin (Immune Globulin (Human)) II-1434
Intraglobin F (Immune Globulin (Human)) II-1434
Intramed (Ampicillin) II-170
Intraval (Thiopental Sodium) II-2603
Intron-A (Interferon Alfa-2b, Recombinant) II-1471
Introna (Interferon Alfa-2b, Recombinant) II-1471
Intropin IV (Dopamine Hydrochloride) II-853
Invert Plaster (Triamcinolone Acetonide) II-2701
Inviclot (Heparin Sodium) II-1334
Invi-rase (Saquinavir Mesylate) II-2424
Invite (Thiamine Hydrochloride) II-2602
Invoril (Enalapril Maleate) II-913
Invozide (Enalapril Maleate; Hydrochlorothiazide) II-923
Inza (Naproxen) II-1924
Ipamix (Indapamide) II-1436
Ipentol (Pentoxifylline) II-2154
Ipnovel (Midazolam Hydrochloride) II-1823
Ipocol (Mesalamine) II-1748
Ipolab (Labetalol Hydrochloride) II-1545
Ipolina (Hydralazine Hydrochloride) II-1346
Ipolipid (Gemfibrozil) II-1269
Ipra Uni-dose (Ipratropium Bromide) II-1480
Ipravent (Ipratropium Bromide) II-1480
Ipren (Ibuprofen) II-1411
Iprobiot (Chloramphenicol) II-536
Ipvent (Ipratropium Bromide) II-1480
Iqfadina (Ranitidine Hydrochloride) II-2334
Iraxen (Naproxen Sodium) II-1928
Irban (Irbesartan) II-1484
Irban Plus (Hydrochlorothiazide; Irbesartan) II-1351
Irdal (Flurazepam Hydrochloride) II-1175
Iremofar (Hydroxyzine) II-1398
Iremo-pierol (Trifluoperazine Hydrochloride) II-2717
Iretin (Cytarabine) II-683
Irfen (Ibuprofen) II-1411
Irinotel (Irinotecan Hydrochloride) II-1487
Irovel (Irbesartan) II-1484
Irrigor (Nimodipine) II-1974
Irta (Itraconazole) II-1517
Irvell (Irbesartan) II-1484
Isavir (Acyclovir) II-33

International brand name (Generic name) Page no.

Iscotin (Isoniazid) II-1496
Iscover (Clopidogrel Bisulfate) II-635
ISDN (Isosorbide Dinitrate) II-1502
Iselpin (Sucralfate) II-2493
Isephanine (Dipyridamole) II-821
Isimoxin (Amoxicillin) II-131
Iski (Diltiazem Hydrochloride) II-798
Iski-90 SR (Diltiazem Hydrochloride) II-798
Ismeline (Guanethidine Monosulfate) II-1321
Ismexin (Isosorbide Mononitrate) II-1507
Ismipur (Mercaptopurine) II-1741
ISMN (Isosorbide Mononitrate) II-1507
Ismo 20 (Isosorbide Dinitrate) II-1502
Ismo 20 (Isosorbide Mononitrate) II-1507
Ismo-20 (Isosorbide Mononitrate) II-1507
Ismox (Isosorbide Mononitrate) II-1507
Iso Mack (Isosorbide Dinitrate) II-1502
Iso Mack Retard (Isosorbide Dinitrate) II-1502
Isobac (Sulfamethoxazole; Trimethoprim) II-2500
Isobar (Isosorbide Dinitrate) II-1502
Isobid (Isosorbide Mononitrate) II-1507
Isobide (Isosorbide Dinitrate) II-1502
Isobinate (Isosorbide Dinitrate) II-1502
Isocaine 3% (Mepivacaine Hydrochloride) II-1737
Isocard Retard (Isosorbide Dinitrate) II-1502
Iso-Card SR (Verapamil Hydrochloride) II-2777
Isocardide (Isosorbide Dinitrate) II-1502
Isocillin (Penicillin V Potassium) II-2142
Isocord (Isosorbide Dinitrate) II-1502
Isoday 40 (Isosorbide Dinitrate) II-1502
Isodol (Ibuprofen) II-1411
Isogen (Isosorbide Dinitrate) II-1502
Isoket (Isosorbide Dinitrate) II-1502
Isoket Retard (Isosorbide Dinitrate) II-1502
Isoket Spray (Isosorbide Dinitrate) II-1502
Isokin (Isoniazid) II-1496
Isolin (Isoproterenol Hydrochloride) II-1498
Iso-Mack (Isosorbide Dinitrate) II-1502
Isomack (Isosorbide Dinitrate) II-1502
Iso-Mack Retard (Isosorbide Dinitrate) II-1502
Isomack Retard (Isosorbide Dinitrate) II-1502
Isomack Spray (Isosorbide Dinitrate) II-1502
Isomon (Isosorbide Mononitrate) II-1507
Isomonat (Isosorbide Mononitrate) II-1507
Isomonit (Isosorbide Mononitrate) II-1507
Isonep H (Hydrocortisone; Neomycin Sulfate; Polymyxin B Sulfate) II-1384
Isonex (Isoniazid) II-1496
Isoniazid Atlantic (Isoniazid) II-1496
Isoniazida N.T. (Isoniazid) II-1496
Isonit (Isosorbide Dinitrate) II-1502
Isonite (Isosorbide Mononitrate) II-1507
Isopen-20 (Isosorbide Mononitrate) II-1507
Isoprenalin (Isoproterenol Hydrochloride) II-1498
Isopresol (Captopril) II-411
Isoptin Retard (Verapamil Hydrochloride) II-2777
Isoptine (Verapamil Hydrochloride) II-2777
Isoptino (Verapamil Hydrochloride) II-2777
Isopto (Atropine Sulfate) II-235
Isopto Atropin (Atropine Sulfate) II-235
Isopto Atropina (Atropine Sulfate) II-235
Isopto Carpina (Pilocarpine) II-2180
Isopto Cetamida (Sulfacetamide Sodium) II-2497
Isopto Epinal (Epinephrine) II-934
Isopto Fenicol (Chloramphenicol) II-536
Isopto Frin (Phenylephrine Hydrochloride) II-2173
Isopto Karbakolin (Carbenicillin Indanyl Sodium) II-422
Isopto Pilocarpine (Pilocarpine) II-2180
Isopto-Dex (Dexamethasone) II-730
Isopto-Maxidex (Dexamethasone) II-730
Iso-Puren (Isosorbide Dinitrate) II-1502
Isorbide (Isosorbide Dinitrate) II-1502
Isordil (Isosorbide Dinitrate) II-1502
Isoric (Allopurinol) II-77
Isorythm (Disopyramide Phosphate) II-825

International brand name (Generic name)	Page no.
Isostenase (Isosorbide Dinitrate)	II-1502
Isotamine (Isoniazid)	II-1496
Isotard 20 (Isosorbide Dinitrate)	II-1502
Isotard 40 (Isosorbide Dinitrate)	II-1502
Isoten (Bisoprolol Fumarate)	II-323
Isotic (Ciprofloxacin Hydrochloride)	II-573
Isotic Adretor (Timolol)	II-2627
Isotic Adretor (Travoprost)	II-2685
Isotic Salmicol (Chloramphenicol)	II-536
Isotic Tobryne (Tobramycin)	II-2643
Isotren (Isotretinoin)	II-1510
Isotrex (Isotretinoin)	II-1510
Isotrex Gel (Isotretinoin)	II-1510
Isotril ER (Isosorbide Mononitrate)	II-1507
Isotrim (Sulfamethoxazole; Trimethoprim)	II-2500
Isox (Itraconazole)	II-1517
Isoxazine (Sulfisoxazole)	II-2510
Isozid (Isoniazid)	II-1496
Istamex (Chlorpheniramine Maleate)	II-548
Istam-Far (Cyproheptadine Hydrochloride)	II-682
Istaminol (Chlorpheniramine Maleate)	II-548
Istin (Amlodipine Besylate)	II-125
Istubol (Tamoxifen Citrate)	II-2539
Isuprel Mistometer (Isoproterenol Hydrochloride)	II-1498
Isuprel Nebulimetro (Isoproterenol Hydrochloride)	II-1498
Iterax (Hydroxyzine)	II-1398
Itodal (Itraconazole)	II-1517
Itra (Itraconazole)	II-1517
Itracon (Itraconazole)	II-1517
Itranax (Itraconazole)	II-1517
Itrin (Terazosin Hydrochloride)	II-2566
Itrizole (Itraconazole)	II-1517
Iturol (Isosorbide Mononitrate)	II-1507
Itzol (Itraconazole)	II-1517
IV Globulin-S (Immune Globulin (Human))	II-1434
Ivacin (Piperacillin Sodium)	II-2196
Ivemetro (Metronidazole)	II-1812
IVheBex (Hepatitis B Immune Globulin)	II-1341
Iwacillin (Ampicillin)	II-170
Izacef (Cefazolin Sodium)	II-452
Izadima (Ceftazidime)	II-492
Izilox (Moxifloxacin Hydrochloride)	II-1886
Izo (Isosorbide Dinitrate)	II-1502
Izoltil (Amoxicillin)	II-131
J	
Jacutin (Lindane)	II-1642
Jamylene (Docusate Sodium)	II-841
Janacin (Norfloxacin)	II-1997
Jatroneural (Trifluoperazine Hydrochloride)	II-2717
Jatroneural Retard (Trifluoperazine Hydrochloride)	II-2717
Jayacin (Ciprofloxacin Hydrochloride)	II-573
Jellin (Fluocinolone Acetonide)	II-1152
Jenamazol (Clotrimazole)	II-640
Jenampin (Ampicillin)	II-170
Johnstal (Mefenamic Acid)	II-1720
Jonac Gel (Diclofenac)	II-748
Josir (Tamsulosin Hydrochloride)	II-2544
Juformin (Metformin Hydrochloride)	II-1760
Julab (Selegiline Hydrochloride)	II-2437
Julegil (Selegiline Hydrochloride)	II-2437
Julphamox (Amoxicillin)	II-131
Julphapen (Ampicillin)	II-170
Jumex (Selegiline Hydrochloride)	II-2437
Jumexal (Selegiline Hydrochloride)	II-2437
Justpertin (Dipyridamole)	II-821
Justum (Clorazepate Dipotassium)	II-638
Jutabloc (Metoprolol)	II-1805
Jutacor Comp (Captopril; Hydrochlorothiazide)	II-416
Jutadilat (Nifedipine)	II-1967
Jutalar (Doxazosin Mesylate)	II-860
Jutalex (Sotalol Hydrochloride)	II-2471
K	
Kaban (Clocortolone Pivalate)	II-619
Kacinth-A (Amikacin Sulfate)	II-101
Kadolax (Bisacodyl)	II-322
Kainever (Estazolam)	II-983
Kaizem CD (Diltiazem Hydrochloride)	II-798
Kalbrium (Chlordiazepoxide Hydrochloride)	II-539
Kalcef (Cefuroxime)	II-507
Kalcide (Praziquantel)	II-2228
Kaleorid (Potassium Chloride)	II-2215
Kalfoxim (Cefotaxime Sodium)	II-474
Kaliduron (Potassium Chloride)	II-2215
Kaliglutol (Potassium Chloride)	II-2215
Kalilente (Potassium Chloride)	II-2215
Kalinorm (Potassium Chloride)	II-2215
Kalinorm Depottab (Potassium Chloride)	II-2215
Kalinor-Retard P (Potassium Chloride)	II-2215
Kaliolite (Potassium Chloride)	II-2215
Kalipor (Potassium Chloride)	II-2215
Kalipoz (Potassium Chloride)	II-2215
Kalitabs (Potassium Chloride)	II-2215
Kalitrans Retard (Potassium Chloride)	II-2215
Kalium (Potassium Chloride)	II-2215
Kalium Duriles (Potassium Chloride)	II-2215
Kalium Retard (Potassium Chloride)	II-2215
Kalium-Durettes (Potassium Chloride)	II-2215
Kalium-R (Potassium Chloride)	II-2215
Kallmiren (Buspirone Hydrochloride)	II-382
Kalma (Alprazolam)	II-85
Kalmalin (Lorazepam)	II-1678
Kalrifam (Rifampin)	II-2363
Kaltensif (Doxazosin Mesylate)	II-860
Kaltrofen (Ketoprofen)	II-1533
Kaluril (Amiloride Hydrochloride)	II-103
Kaluril (Amiloride Hydrochloride; Hydrochlorothiazide)	II-105
Kalymin (Pyridostigmine Bromide)	II-2296
Kamacaine (Bupivacaine Hydrochloride)	II-361
Kamolas (Acetaminophen)	II-11
Kamoxin (Amoxicillin)	II-131
Kanbine (Amikacin Sulfate)	II-101
Kandistatin (Nystatin)	II-2005
Kanezin (Clotrimazole)	II-640
Kapanol (Morphine Sulfate)	II-1877
Kapanol LP (Morphine Sulfate)	II-1877
Kapodin (Minoxidil)	II-1845
Kaptin (Gabapentin)	II-1241
Karbakolin Isopto (Carbenicillin Indanyl Sodium)	II-422
Karbamazepin (Carbamazepine)	II-418
Kareon (Nortriptyline Hydrochloride)	II-2002
Karison Creme (Clobetasol Propionate)	II-617
Karison Salbe (Clobetasol Propionate)	II-617
Karmoplex (Chlordiazepoxide Hydrochloride)	II-539
Karol (Carteolol Hydrochloride)	II-435
Karteol (Carteolol Hydrochloride)	II-435
Karvea (Irbesartan)	II-1484
Karvezide (Hydrochlorothiazide; Irbesartan)	II-1351
Katopil (Captopril)	II-411
Katrasic (Tramadol Hydrochloride)	II-2674
Kavipen (Penicillin V Potassium)	II-2142
Kay-Cee-L (Potassium Chloride)	II-2215
Kaywan (Phytonadione)	II-2178
K-Cillin (Penicillin G Potassium)	II-2137
KCL Retard (Potassium Chloride)	II-2215
K-Contin (Potassium Chloride)	II-2215
K-Contin Continus (Potassium Chloride)	II-2215
Keal (Sucralfate)	II-2493
Kebanon (Ketoprofen)	II-1533
Keduril (Ketoprofen)	II-1533
Kefacin (Cephalexin)	II-520
Kefaclor (Cefaclor)	II-444
Kefadim (Ceftazidime)	II-492
Kefadol (Cefamandole Nafate)	II-449
Kefalex (Cephalexin)	II-520
Kefalospes (Cephalexin)	II-520
Kefamin (Ceftazidime)	II-492
Kefarin (Cefazolin Sodium)	II-452
Kefaxin (Cephalexin)	II-520
Kefazim (Ceftazidime)	II-492
Kefazin (Cefazolin Sodium)	II-452
Kefdole (Cefamandole Nafate)	II-449
Kefen (Ketoprofen)	II-1533
Kefenid (Ketoprofen)	II-1533
Kefexin (Cephalexin)	II-520
Keflor (Cefaclor)	II-444
Keflor AF (Cefaclor)	II-444
Kefloridina (Cephalexin)	II-520
Kefolor (Cefaclor)	II-444
Keforal (Cephalexin)	II-520
Kefral (Cefaclor)	II-444
Keftriaxon (Ceftriaxone Sodium)	II-503
Kefzim (Ceftazidime)	II-492
Kehancer (Ketoprofen)	II-1533
Keimax (Ceftibuten)	II-496
Kelac (Ketorolac Tromethamine)	II-1537
Kelargine (Chlorpheniramine Maleate)	II-548
Kelatin (Penicillamine)	II-2133
Kelatine (Penicillamine)	II-2133
Kelfex (Cefadroxil Monohydrate)	II-447
Kemicetin (Chloramphenicol Sodium Succinate)	II-537
Kemicetin Augensalbe (Chloramphenicol)	II-536
Kemicetine (Chloramphenicol)	II-536
Kemicetine (Chloramphenicol Sodium Succinate)	II-537
Kemicetine Otologic (Chloramphenicol)	II-536
Kemocarb (Carboplatin)	II-430
Kemocid (Sulfamethoxazole; Trimethoprim)	II-2500
Kemocin (Cefaclor)	II-444
Kemoclin (Tetracycline Hydrochloride)	II-2585
Kemofam (Famotidine)	II-1093
Kemolat (Nifedipine)	II-1967
Kemolexin (Cephalexin)	II-520
Kemopen (Penicillin G Procaine)	II-2140
Kemoplat (Cisplatin)	II-589
Kemoranin (Ranitidine Hydrochloride)	II-2334
Kemorinol (Allopurinol)	II-77
Kemostan (Mefenamic Acid)	II-1720
Kemothrocin (Erythromycin Ethylsuccinate)	II-965
Kemothrocin (Erythromycin Stearate)	II-970
Kemotrim (Sulfamethoxazole; Trimethoprim)	II-2500
Kemzid (Triamcinolone Acetonide)	II-2701
Kenacort (Triamcinolone Acetonide)	II-2701
Kenacort A (Triamcinolone Acetonide)	II-2701
Kenacort A IA ID (Triamcinolone Acetonide)	II-2701
Kenacort A I.A.-I.D. (Triamcinolone Acetonide)	II-2701
Kenacort A I.M. (Triamcinolone Acetonide)	II-2701
Kenacort A in Orabase (Triamcinolone Acetonide)	II-2701
Kenacort E (Triamcinolone Acetonide)	II-2701
Kenacort IM (Triamcinolone Acetonide)	II-2701
Kenacort Retard (Triamcinolone Acetonide)	II-2701
Kenacort T (Triamcinolone Acetonide)	II-2701
Kenacort T Munnsalve (Triamcinolone Acetonide)	II-2701
Kenacort-A IA ID (Triamcinolone Acetonide)	II-2701
Kenacort-A IM (Triamcinolone Acetonide)	II-2701
Kenacort-A in Orabase (Triamcinolone Acetonide)	II-2701
Kenacort-A Intra-articular Intra-dermal (Triamcinolone Acetonide)	II-2701
Kenadion (Phytonadione)	II-2178
Kenalin (Sulindac)	II-2512
Kenalog Dental (Triamcinolone Acetonide)	II-2701
Kenalog-40 (Triamcinolone Acetonide)	II-2701
Kenaprol (Metoprolol)	II-1805
Kenazol (Ketoconazole)	II-1530
Kenazole (Ketoconazole)	II-1530

International brand name (Generic name)	Page no.
Kendaron (Amiodarone Hydrochloride)	II-110
Kendazol (Danazol)	II-699
Kenofen Gel (Ketoprofen)	II-1533
Kenoket (Clonazepam)	II-625
Kenopril (Enalapril Maleate)	II-913
Kenstatin (Pravastatin Sodium)	II-2224
Kentadin (Pentoxifylline)	II-2154
Kenzen (Candesartan Cilexetil)	II-402
Kenzoflex (Ciprofloxacin Hydrochloride)	II-573
Kenzomyl (Mesalamine)	II-1748
Keotsan (Ketoprofen)	II-1533
Kepinol (Sulfamethoxazole; Trimethoprim)	II-2500
Keprofen (Ketoprofen)	II-1533
Keptrix (Ceftriaxone Sodium)	II-503
Kerfenmycin (Cefaclor)	II-444
Kerlon (Betaxolol Hydrochloride)	II-307
Kerlong (Betaxolol Hydrochloride)	II-307
Kerola (Ketorolac Tromethamine)	II-1537
Keromycin (Chloramphenicol)	II-536
Kesnazol (Ketoconazole)	II-1530
Kessar (Tamoxifen Citrate)	II-2539
Ketadom (Ketoprofen)	II-1533
Keta-Hameln (Ketamine Hydrochloride)	II-1528
Ketalin (Ketamine Hydrochloride)	II-1528
Ketamax (Ketamine Hydrochloride)	II-1528
Ketanest (Ketamine Hydrochloride)	II-1528
Ketanine (Captopril)	II-411
Ketanov (Ketorolac Tromethamine)	II-1537
Ketanrift (Allopurinol)	II-77
Ketazol (Ketoconazole)	II-1530
Ketin (Ketoprofen)	II-1533
Ketmin (Ketamine Hydrochloride)	II-1528
Keto Film (Ketoprofen)	II-1533
Ketobun-A (Allopurinol)	II-77
Keto-Comp (Ketoconazole)	II-1530
Ketoconazol (Ketoconazole)	II-1530
Keto-Crema (Ketoconazole)	II-1530
Ketoderm (Ketoconazole)	II-1530
Ketodrol (Ketorolac Tromethamine)	II-1537
Ketofen (Ketoprofen)	II-1533
Ketoflam (Ketoprofen)	II-1533
Ketoisdin (Ketoconazole)	II-1530
Ketolar (Ketamine Hydrochloride)	II-1528
Ketolgin (Ketoprofen)	II-1533
Ketolgin Gel (Ketoprofen)	II-1533
Ketolgin SR (Ketoprofen)	II-1533
Ketomed (Ketoconazole)	II-1530
Ketomex (Ketoprofen)	II-1533
Ketomicin (Ketoconazole)	II-1530
Ketomicol (Ketoconazole)	II-1530
Ketona (Ketoconazole)	II-1530
Ketonal (Ketoprofen)	II-1533
Ketonic (Ketorolac Tromethamine)	II-1537
Ketorac (Ketorolac Tromethamine)	II-1537
Ketorin (Ketoprofen)	II-1533
Keto-Shampoo (Ketoconazole)	II-1530
Ketosolan (Ketoprofen)	II-1533
Ketozal (Ketoconazole)	II-1530
Ketozol (Ketoconazole)	II-1530
Ketrax (Levamisole Hydrochloride)	II-1598
Ketron (Ketorolac Tromethamine)	II-1537
Ketum (Ketoprofen)	II-1533
Kevadon (Ketoprofen)	II-1533
Keval (Lansoprazole)	II-1569
Keyerpril (Captopril)	II-411
Keylyte (Potassium Chloride)	II-2215
Kezon (Ketoconazole)	II-1530
Kiditard (Quinidine Sulfate)	II-2314
Kidrolase (Asparaginase)	II-204
Kimite-patch (Scopolamine)	II-2432
Kimodin (Famotidine)	II-1093
Kinax (Alprazolam)	II-85
Kindoplex (Cefaclor)	II-444
Kinex (Biperiden Hydrochloride)	II-322
Kinflocin (Ofloxacin)	II-2015
Kinidin (Quinidine Sulfate)	II-2314
Kinidin Durules (Quinidine Sulfate)	II-2314
Kinidine (Quinidine Sulfate)	II-2314
Kinidine Durettes (Quinidine Sulfate)	II-2314
Kinilentin (Quinidine Sulfate)	II-2314
Kinin (Quinine Sulfate)	II-2317
Kininh (Quinine Sulfate)	II-2317
Kinline (Selegiline Hydrochloride)	II-2437
Kinoxacin (Ofloxacin)	II-2015
Kinxasen (Doxazosin Mesylate)	II-860
Kinzosin (Terazosin Hydrochloride)	II-2566
Kipres (Montelukast Sodium)	II-1872
Kiradin (Ranitidine Hydrochloride)	II-2334
Klacid (Clarithromycin)	II-597
Klacid XL (Clarithromycin)	II-597
Klacina (Clarithromycin)	II-597
Klamonex (Amoxicillin; Clavulanate Potassium)	II-139
Klaribac (Clarithromycin)	II-597
Klaricid (Clarithromycin)	II-597
Klaricid H.P. (Clarithromycin)	II-597
Klaricid O.D. (Clarithromycin)	II-597
Klaricid Pediatric (Clarithromycin)	II-597
Klaricid XL (Clarithromycin)	II-597
Klariderm (Fluocinonide)	II-1156
Klaridex (Clarithromycin)	II-597
Klaridia (Clarithromycin)	II-597
Klarihist (Loratadine)	II-1675
Klarin (Clarithromycin)	II-597
Klarivitina (Cyproheptadine Hydrochloride)	II-682
Kleotrat (Cefadroxil Monohydrate)	II-447
Klerimed (Clarithromycin)	II-597
Klexane (Enoxaparin Sodium)	II-927
Klidibrax (Chlordiazepoxide Hydrochloride; Clidinium Bromide)	II-541
Klimacobal (Sulindac)	II-2512
Klimonorm (Ethinyl Estradiol; Levonorgestrel)	II-1047
Klinomycin (Minocycline Hydrochloride)	II-1838
Klinset (Loratadine)	II-1675
Kliogest (Estradiol; Norethindrone Acetate)	II-1011
Kliovance (Estradiol; Norethindrone Acetate)	II-1011
Kliovance (Ethinyl Estradiol; Norethindrone)	II-1055
Kloclor BD (Cefaclor)	II-444
Kloderma (Clobetasol Propionate)	II-617
Klometil (Prochlorperazine)	II-2258
Klopoxid (Chlordiazepoxide Hydrochloride)	II-539
Kloral (Chloral Hydrate)	II-534
Kloramfenicol (Chloramphenicol)	II-536
Kloramfenicol (Chloramphenicol Sodium Succinate)	II-537
Kloramfenikol (Chloramphenicol)	II-536
Kloramphenicol (Chloramphenicol)	II-536
Klorheksidos (Chlorhexidine Gluconate)	II-542
Klorhexidin (Chlorhexidine Gluconate)	II-542
Klorhexol (Chlorhexidine Gluconate)	II-542
Klorita (Chloramphenicol)	II-536
Klorokinfosfat (Chloroquine)	II-544
Klorproman (Chlorpromazine Hydrochloride)	II-549
Klorpromazin (Chlorpromazine Hydrochloride)	II-549
Klorzoxazon (Chlorzoxazone)	II-558
Klotaren (Diclofenac)	II-748
Kmoxilin (Amoxicillin; Clavulanate Potassium)	II-139
K-Nase (Streptokinase)	II-2490
Knavon (Ketoprofen)	II-1533
Kobis (Chlorpheniramine Maleate)	II-548
Kodapan (Carbamazepine)	II-418
Kofatol (Cefazolin Sodium)	II-452
Kofuzon (Furosemide)	II-1237
Kolestevan (Simvastatin)	II-2454
Kolkicin (Colchicine)	II-649
Kolyum (Potassium Chloride)	II-2215
Konakion (Phytonadione)	II-2178
Konakion (10 mg) (Phytonadione)	II-2178
Konakion 10 mg (Phytonadione)	II-2178
Konakion MM Paediatric (Phytonadione)	II-2178
Konakion MM Pediatric (Phytonadione)	II-2178
Konaturil (Ketoconazole)	II-1530
Konigen (Gentamicin Sulfate)	II-1279
Konshien (Piroxicam)	II-2205
Korec (Quinapril Hydrochloride)	II-2305
Korticoid (Triamcinolone)	II-2698
K-PE (Dinoprostone)	II-812
Kratium (Diazepam)	II-740
Kratium 2 (Diazepam)	II-740
Krebin (Vincristine Sulfate)	II-2789
Krebsilasi (Pancrelipase)	II-2095
Kredex (Carvedilol)	II-438
Krema-Rosa (Clotrimazole)	II-640
Kriadex (Clonazepam)	II-625
Krisovin (Griseofulvin, Microcrystalline)	II-1312
Kromicin (Azithromycin)	II-250
K-Sacin (Ciprofloxacin Hydrochloride)	II-573
K-SR (Potassium Chloride)	II-2215
KSR (Potassium Chloride)	II-2215
K-Tab (Potassium Chloride)	II-2215
Kulinet (Cyproheptadine Hydrochloride)	II-682
Kutrix (Furosemide)	II-1237
Kydoflam (Piroxicam)	II-2205
Kyofen (Acetaminophen)	II-11
Kyophyllin (Aminophylline)	II-106
Kyypakkaus (Hydrocortisone)	II-1369

L

International brand name (Generic name)	Page no.
La Morph (Morphine Sulfate)	II-1877
Labelol (Labetalol Hydrochloride)	II-1545
Labenda (Albendazole)	II-46
Labesine (Labetalol Hydrochloride)	II-1545
Labijin (Terbinafine Hydrochloride)	II-2570
Lacerol (Diltiazem Hydrochloride)	II-798
Lacin (Clindamycin)	II-605
Lacromycin (Gentamicin Sulfate)	II-1279
Lacson (Lactulose)	II-1550
Lactamox (Amoxicillin; Clavulanate Potassium)	II-139
Lacticare HC (Hydrocortisone)	II-1369
Lactismine (Bromocriptine Mesylate)	II-344
Lactocur (Lactulose)	II-1550
Lactulax (Lactulose)	II-1550
Lactulen (Lactulose)	II-1550
Lactuverlan (Lactulose)	II-1550
Ladazol (Danazol)	II-699
Ladiwin (Lamivudine)	II-1552
Ladogal (Danazol)	II-699
Ladoxillin (Amoxicillin)	II-131
L-Adrenalin (Epinephrine)	II-934
Laevolac (Lactulose)	II-1550
Lagaquin (Chloroquine)	II-544
Lagatrim (Sulfamethoxazole; Trimethoprim)	II-2500
Lagatrim Forte (Sulfamethoxazole; Trimethoprim)	II-2500
Lagavit B12 (Cyanocobalamin)	II-661
Lagur (Clarithromycin)	II-597
Lama (Amlodipine Besylate)	II-125
Lama (Ketoconazole)	II-1530
Lambanol (Docusate Sodium)	II-841
Lambutol (Ethambutol Hydrochloride)	II-1039
Lamictin (Lamotrigine)	II-1561
Lamidac (Lamivudine)	II-1552
Lamidon (Ibuprofen)	II-1411
Lamifen (Terbinafine Hydrochloride)	II-2570
Lamisil Dermgel (Terbinafine Hydrochloride)	II-2570
Lamitol (Labetalol Hydrochloride)	II-1545
Lamodex (Clobetasol Propionate)	II-617
Lamogine (Lamotrigine)	II-1561
Lamoxy (Amoxicillin)	II-131
Lampren (Clofazimine)	II-619
Lamuna (Desogestrel; Ethinyl Estradiol)	II-725
Lamuzid (Lamivudine; Zidovudine)	II-1560
Lanacin (Clindamycin)	II-605
Lanacordin (Digoxin)	II-780
Lanacort (Hydrocortisone Acetate)	II-1373
Lanacrist (Digoxin)	II-780

International brand name (Generic name)	Page no.
Lanaterom (Gemfibrozil)	II-1269
Lancef (Cefotaxime Sodium)	II-474
Lancid (Lansoprazole)	II-1569
Lanclic (Fluoxetine Hydrochloride)	II-1160
Lancopen (Lansoprazole)	II-1569
Landsen (Clonazepam)	II-625
Lanexat (Flumazenil)	II-1146
Langoran (Isosorbide Dinitrate)	II-1502
Langoran LP (Isosorbide Dinitrate)	II-1502
Lanicor (Digoxin)	II-780
Lanikor (Digoxin)	II-780
Lanitop (Digoxin)	II-780
Lanomycin (Amikacin Sulfate)	II-101
Lanorale (Digoxin)	II-780
Lanoxin PG (Digoxin)	II-780
Lanpraz (Lansoprazole)	II-1569
Lanprol (Lansoprazole)	II-1569
Lanproton (Lansoprazole)	II-1569
Lansazol (Lansoprazole)	II-1569
Lansiclav (Amoxicillin; Clavulanate Potassium)	II-139
Lansopep (Lansoprazole)	II-1569
Lanston (Lansoprazole)	II-1569
Lantarel (Methotrexate Sodium)	II-1772
Lanterbine SR (Terbutaline Sulfate)	II-2574
Lantron (Amitriptyline Hydrochloride)	II-119
Lantus (Insulin Glargine)	II-1461
Lanvell (Lansoprazole)	II-1569
Lanximed (Lansoprazole)	II-1569
Lanz (Lansoprazole)	II-1569
Lanzol-30 (Lansoprazole)	II-1569
Lanzopral (Lansoprazole)	II-1569
Lanzor (Lansoprazole)	II-1569
Lapicef (Cefadroxil Monohydrate)	II-447
Lapole (Flurbiprofen)	II-1177
Lapraz (Lansoprazole)	II-1569
Lapren (Clofazimine)	II-619
Lapril (Enalapril Maleate)	II-913
Laproton (Lansoprazole)	II-1569
Laracit (Cytarabine)	II-683
Laractyl (Chlorpromazine Hydrochloride)	II-549
Laraflex (Naproxen)	II-1924
Larapam (Piroxicam)	II-2205
Largactil (Chlorpromazine Hydrochloride)	II-549
Largactil Forte (Chlorpromazine Hydrochloride)	II-549
Lariago (Chloroquine)	II-544
Laricam (Mefloquine Hydrochloride)	II-1721
Larocilin (Amoxicillin)	II-131
Laroxyl (Amitriptyline Hydrochloride)	II-119
Larozyl (Amitriptyline Hydrochloride)	II-119
Larpose (Lorazepam)	II-1678
Larry (Ketoconazole)	II-1530
Laser (Naproxen)	II-1924
Lasiletten (Furosemide)	II-1237
Lasilix (Furosemide)	II-1237
Lasix Retard (Furosemide)	II-1237
Lasma (Theophylline)	II-2593
Laspar (Asparaginase)	II-204
Lastet (Etoposide)	II-1080
Lastrim (Sulfamethoxazole; Trimethoprim)	II-2500
Latotryd (Erythromycin)	II-960
Latycin (Tetracycline Hydrochloride)	II-2585
Laubeel (Lorazepam)	II-1678
Lauzit (Indomethacin)	II-1443
Laver (Triamcinolone Acetonide)	II-2701
Laxacod (Bisacodyl)	II-322
Laxadin (Bisacodyl)	II-322
Laxadine (Docusate Sodium)	II-841
Laxadyl (Bisacodyl)	II-322
Laxamex (Bisacodyl)	II-322
Laxan (Methocarbamol)	II-1768
Laxcodyl (Bisacodyl)	II-322
Laxette (Lactulose)	II-1550
Laximed (Lactulose)	II-1550
Laxitab 5 (Bisacodyl)	II-322
Laxur (Furosemide)	II-1237
Laz (Lansoprazole)	II-1569
Lebic (Baclofen)	II-266
Lecasin (Lidocaine)	II-1628
Leder C (Ascorbic Acid)	II-203
Leder-C (Ascorbic Acid)	II-203
Ledercort (Triamcinolone)	II-2698
Ledercort (Triamcinolone Acetonide)	II-2701
Ledercort A (Triamcinolone Acetonide)	II-2701
Lederderm (Minocycline Hydrochloride)	II-1838
Lederfolin (Leucovorin Calcium)	II-1585
Lederfoline (Leucovorin Calcium)	II-1585
Lederle Leucovorin (Leucovorin Calcium)	II-1585
Ledermicina (Demeclocycline Hydrochloride)	II-714
Ledermycin (Demeclocycline Hydrochloride)	II-714
Lederpax (Erythromycin)	II-960
Lederplatin (Cisplatin)	II-589
Ledertepa (Thiotepa)	II-2609
Ledertrexate (Methotrexate Sodium)	II-1772
Ledervorin Calcium (Leucovorin Calcium)	II-1585
Ledervorin-Calcium (Leucovorin Calcium)	II-1585
Lediamox (Acetazolamide)	II-28
Ledimox (Acetazolamide)	II-28
Ledoxan (Cyclophosphamide)	II-666
Ledoxina (Cyclophosphamide)	II-666
Lefaine (Naproxen Sodium)	II-1928
Lehydan (Phenytoin Sodium)	II-2175
Lembirax (Chlordiazepoxide Hydrochloride; Clidinium Bromide)	II-541
Lemblastine (Vinblastine Sulfate)	II-2787
Lembrol (Diazepam)	II-740
Lemgrip (Acetaminophen)	II-11
Lemnis Fatty Cream HC (Hydrocortisone)	II-1369
Lemocin CX (Chlorhexidine Gluconate)	II-542
Len V.K. (Penicillin V Potassium)	II-2142
Lenal (Temazepam)	II-2556
Lenamet (Cimetidine Hydrochloride)	II-568
Lenamet OTC (Cimetidine Hydrochloride)	II-568
Lencid (Lindane)	II-1642
Lenditro (Oxybutynin)	II-2070
Lenen (Clocortolone Pivalate)	II-619
Leniartil (Naproxen)	II-1924
Lenide-T (Loperamide Hydrochloride)	II-1664
Lenipril (Enalapril Maleate)	II-913
Lenirit (Hydrocortisone)	II-1369
Lenitral (Nitroglycerin)	II-1984
Lenocef (Cephalexin)	II-520
Lenocin (Tetracycline Hydrochloride)	II-2585
Lenovate (Betamethasone Valerate)	II-305
Lenoxicaps (Digoxin)	II-780
Lenoxin (Digoxin)	II-780
Lento-Kalium (Potassium Chloride)	II-2215
Lentolith (Lithium Carbonate)	II-1654
Lentopenil (Penicillin G Benzathine)	II-2136
Lentotran (Chlordiazepoxide Hydrochloride)	II-539
Leo-K (Potassium Chloride)	II-2215
Leostesin Jelly (Lidocaine)	II-1628
Leostesin Ointment (Lidocaine)	II-1628
Lepetan (Buprenorphine)	II-363
Leponex (Clozapine)	II-642
Lepril (Enalapril Maleate)	II-913
Leprim (Sulfamethoxazole; Trimethoprim)	II-2500
Leptanal (Fentanyl Citrate)	II-1112
Leptilan (Valproate Sodium)	II-2749
Leptilan (Valproic Acid)	II-2755
Leptopsique (Perphenazine)	II-2162
Leramex (Acyclovir)	II-33
Lerderfoline (Leucovorin Calcium)	II-1585
Lergia (Loratadine)	II-1675
Lergigan (Promethazine Hydrochloride)	II-2268
Lergium (Cetirizine Hydrochloride)	II-529
Lergium Plus (Cetirizine Hydrochloride; Pseudoephedrine Hydrochloride)	II-532
Lergocil (Azatadine Maleate)	II-242
Leroxacin (Levofloxacin)	II-1607
Lersa (Sulfacetamide Sodium)	II-2497
Lertamine (Loratadine)	II-1675
Lertamine - D (Loratadine; Pseudoephedrine Sulfate)	II-1677
Lesacin (Levofloxacin)	II-1607
Lesaclor (Acyclovir)	II-33
Lescol LP (Fluvastatin Sodium)	II-1199
Lescol XL (Fluvastatin Sodium)	II-1199
Lescot (Sulfamethoxazole; Trimethoprim)	II-2500
Lesefer (Sertraline Hydrochloride)	II-2439
Lespo (Terbinafine Hydrochloride)	II-2570
Lesporina (Cefadroxil Monohydrate)	II-447
Lestid (Colestipol Hydrochloride)	II-652
Lethyl (Phenobarbital)	II-2167
Leucogen (Sargramostim)	II-2428
Leucovorin (Leucovorin Calcium)	II-1585
Leucovorina Calcica (Leucovorin Calcium)	II-1585
Leucovorine Abic (Leucovorin Calcium)	II-1585
Leukerin (Mercaptopurine)	II-1741
Leukosulfan (Busulfan)	II-385
Leuplin (Leuprolide Acetate)	II-1587
Leuplin Depot (Leuprolide Acetate)	II-1587
Leustatine (Cladribine)	II-595
Levanxene (Temazepam)	II-2556
Levanxol (Temazepam)	II-2556
Levaxin (Levothyroxine Sodium)	II-1618
Levodex (Diltiazem Hydrochloride)	II-798
Levokacin (Levofloxacin)	II-1607
Levolac (Lactulose)	II-1550
Levomed (Carbidopa; Levodopa)	II-424
Levomet (Carbidopa; Levodopa)	II-424
Levomycetin (Chloramphenicol)	II-536
Levonelle (Levonorgestrel)	II-1614
Levophta (Levocabastine Hydrochloride)	II-1606
Levothyrox (Levothyroxine Sodium)	II-1618
Levotirox (Levothyroxine Sodium)	II-1618
Levotiroxina (Levothyroxine Sodium)	II-1618
Levox (Levofloxacin)	II-1607
Levoxacin (Levofloxacin)	II-1607
Levozem (Diltiazem Hydrochloride)	II-798
Levsin SL (Hyoscyamine Sulfate)	II-1404
Lexemin (Fenofibrate)	II-1105
Lexfin (Celecoxib)	II-515
Lexin (Carbamazepine)	II-418
Lexin (Cephalexin)	II-520
Lexinor (Norfloxacin)	II-1997
Lexpec (Folic Acid)	II-1208
Libiocid (Lincomycin Hydrochloride)	II-1640
Libnum (Chlordiazepoxide Hydrochloride)	II-539
Libraxin (Chlordiazepoxide Hydrochloride; Clidinium Bromide)	II-541
Libretin (Albuterol)	II-47
Librocol (Chlordiazepoxide Hydrochloride; Clidinium Bromide)	II-541
Librodan (Clindamycin)	II-605
Librofem (Ibuprofen)	II-1411
Licab (Lithium Carbonate)	II-1654
Licarb (Lithium Carbonate)	II-1654
Licarbium (Lithium Carbonate)	II-1654
Licodin (Ticlopidine Hydrochloride)	II-2622
Liconar (Miconazole)	II-1820
Licorax (Naproxen Sodium)	II-1928
Lidemol (Fluocinonide)	II-1156
Lidin (Lithium Carbonate)	II-1654
Lidocain Gel (Lidocaine)	II-1628
Lidocain Ointment (Lidocaine)	II-1628
Lidocain Spray (Lidocaine)	II-1628
Lidonest (Lidocaine)	II-1628
Lidonest (Lidocaine Hydrochloride)	II-1632
Lifaton (Cyanocobalamin)	II-661
Lifaton B12 (Cyanocobalamin)	II-661
Lifibron (Gemfibrozil)	II-1269
Likacin (Amikacin Sulfate)	II-101
Likodin (Cefadroxil Monohydrate)	II-447
Likuden M (Griseofulvin, Microcrystalline)	II-1312
Limas (Lithium Carbonate)	II-1654

International brand name (Generic name)	Page no.
Limbitrol F (Amitriptyline Hydrochloride; Chlordiazepoxide)	II-123
Limbitryl (Amitriptyline Hydrochloride; Chlordiazepoxide)	II-123
Limcee (Ascorbic Acid)	II-203
Linasen (Phenobarbital)	II-2167
Lincil (Nicardipine Hydrochloride)	II-1958
Linco ANB (Lincomycin Hydrochloride)	II-1640
Lincobiotic (Lincomycin Hydrochloride)	II-1640
Lincocine (Lincomycin Hydrochloride)	II-1640
Lincofan (Lincomycin Hydrochloride)	II-1640
Lincomec (Lincomycin Hydrochloride)	II-1640
Lincomed (Lincomycin Hydrochloride)	II-1640
Lincono (Lincomycin Hydrochloride)	II-1640
Lincophar (Lincomycin Hydrochloride)	II-1640
Lincoplus (Lincomycin Hydrochloride)	II-1640
Lindacin (Clindamycin)	II-605
Lindan (Clindamycin)	II-605
Linden Lotion (Lindane)	II-1642
Lindisc (Estradiol)	II-986
Linmycin (Lincomycin Hydrochloride)	II-1640
Linopril (Lisinopril)	II-1648
Linox (Linezolid)	II-1644
Linton (Haloperidol)	II-1328
Lintropsin (Lincomycin Hydrochloride)	II-1640
Linvas (Lisinopril)	II-1648
Liocarpina (Pilocarpine)	II-2180
Liondox (Labetalol Hydrochloride)	II-1545
Liotec (Baclofen)	II-266
Liotropina (Atropine Sulfate)	II-235
Lipanthyl (Fenofibrate)	II-1105
Lipantil (Fenofibrate)	II-1105
Liparison (Fenofibrate)	II-1105
Lipazil (Gemfibrozil)	II-1269
Lipdip (Lovastatin)	II-1688
Lipebin (Lactulose)	II-1550
Lipemol (Pravastatin Sodium)	II-2224
Lipex (Simvastatin)	II-2454
Lipidal (Pravastatin Sodium)	II-2224
Lipidax (Fenofibrate)	II-1105
Lipidys (Gemfibrozil)	II-1269
Lipigem (Gemfibrozil)	II-1269
Lipilim (Clofibrate)	II-619
Lipilo (Fenofibrate)	II-1105
Lipinorm (Simvastatin)	II-2454
Lipira (Gemfibrozil)	II-1269
Lipison (Gemfibrozil)	II-1269
Lipistorol (Gemfibrozil)	II-1269
Lipivas (Lovastatin)	II-1688
Lipizyl (Gemfibrozil)	II-1269
Liplat (Pravastatin Sodium)	II-2224
Liple (Alprostadil)	II-90
Lipocol-Merz (Cholestyramine)	II-559
Lipofen (Fenofibrate)	II-1105
Lipofor (Gemfibrozil)	II-1269
Lipolin (Fenofibrate)	II-1105
Lipolo (Gemfibrozil)	II-1269
Liponorm (Simvastatin)	II-2454
Lipostat (Pravastatin Sodium)	II-2224
Lipovas (Fenofibrate)	II-1105
Lipovas (Lovastatin)	II-1688
Lipovas (Simvastatin)	II-2454
Liprevil (Pravastatin Sodium)	II-2224
Lipril (Lisinopril)	II-1648
Lipsin (Fenofibrate)	II-1105
Liptan (Ibuprofen)	II-1411
Lipur (Gemfibrozil)	II-1269
Liquaemin Sodium (Heparin Sodium)	II-1334
Liquemin (Heparin Sodium)	II-1334
Liquemine (Heparin Sodium)	II-1334
Liquifer (Ferrous Sulfate)	II-1122
Liquipred (Prednisolone)	II-2233
Lirugen Measles (Measles Virus Vaccine Live)	II-1708
Lisa (Cefonicid Sodium)	II-469
Lisacef (Cephradine)	II-526
Lisagent (Gentamicin Sulfate)	II-1279
Lisi ABZ (Lisinopril)	II-1648
Lisibeta (Lisinopril)	II-1648
Lisigamma (Lisinopril)	II-1648
Lisihexal (Lisinopril)	II-1648
Lisiken (Clindamycin)	II-605
Lisino (Loratadine)	II-1675
Lisipril (Lisinopril)	II-1648
Liskantin (Primidone)	II-2247
Liskonum (Lithium Carbonate)	II-1654
Lismol (Cholestyramine)	II-559
Lisodur (Lisinopril)	II-1648
Lisopress (Lisinopril)	II-1648
Lisopril (Lisinopril)	II-1648
Lisoril (Lisinopril)	II-1648
Lisovyr (Acyclovir)	II-33
Lispine (Disopyramide Phosphate)	II-825
Lispril (Lisinopril)	II-1648
Listril (Lisinopril)	II-1648
Litalir (Hydroxyurea)	II-1394
Litax (Cladribine)	II-595
Litheum 300 (Lithium Carbonate)	II-1654
Lithionate (Lithium Carbonate)	II-1654
Lithocap (Lithium Carbonate)	II-1654
Liticon (Pentazocine Lactate)	II-2147
Litilent (Lithium Carbonate)	II-1654
Litinol (Allopurinol)	II-77
Litocarb (Lithium Carbonate)	II-1654
Livesan Ge (Fenofibrate)	II-1105
Livingpherol (Vitamin E)	II-2796
Livo Luk (Lactulose)	II-1550
Livostin ED (Levocabastine Hydrochloride)	II-1606
Llanol (Allopurinol)	II-77
Lobate (Clobetasol Propionate)	II-617
Lobesol (Clobetasol Propionate)	II-617
Lobeta (Loratadine)	II-1675
Lobevat (Clobetasol Propionate)	II-617
Locacid (Tretinoin)	II-2691
Locap (Captopril)	II-411
Locapred (Desonide)	II-728
Locasyn (Flunisolide)	II-1149
Locion EPC (Minoxidil)	II-1845
Lock 2 (Cimetidine Hydrochloride)	II-568
Locol (Fluvastatin Sodium)	II-1199
Locose (Glyburide)	II-1297
Locula (Sulfacetamide Sodium)	II-2497
Lodain (Loratadine)	II-1675
Lodales (Simvastatin)	II-2454
Lodia (Loperamide Hydrochloride)	II-1664
Lodimol (Dipyridamole)	II-821
Lodine LP (Etodolac)	II-1076
Lodine Retard (Etodolac)	II-1076
Lodine SR (Etodolac)	II-1076
Lodoz (Bisoprolol Fumarate; Hydrochlorothiazide)	II-326
Lodulce (Glyburide)	II-1297
Loette (Ethinyl Estradiol; Levonorgestrel)	II-1047
Loette 21 (Ethinyl Estradiol; Levonorgestrel)	II-1047
Lofacol (Lovastatin)	II-1688
Lofarbil (Metoprolol)	II-1805
Lofenac (Diclofenac)	II-748
Lofenoxal (Atropine Sulfate; Diphenoxylate Hydrochloride)	II-238
Lofloquin (Lomefloxacin Hydrochloride)	II-1658
Lofucin (Ciprofloxacin Hydrochloride)	II-573
Logastric (Omeprazole)	II-2034
Logiflox (Lomefloxacin Hydrochloride)	II-1658
Logiparin (Tinzaparin Sodium)	II-2634
Logos (Famotidine)	II-1093
Logynon (Ethinyl Estradiol; Levonorgestrel)	II-1047
Lokilan (Flunisolide)	II-1149
Lokilan Nasal (Flunisolide)	II-1149
Lomac (Omeprazole)	II-2034
Lomar (Lovastatin)	II-1688
Lomebact (Lomefloxacin Hydrochloride)	II-1658
Lomeblastin (Lomustine)	II-1662
Lomeflon (Lomefloxacin Hydrochloride)	II-1658
Lomflox (Lomefloxacin Hydrochloride)	II-1658
Lomilan (Isosorbide Dinitrate)	II-1502
Lomine (Dicyclomine Hydrochloride)	II-763
Lomir (Isradipine)	II-1515
Lomir Retard (Isradipine)	II-1515
Lomir SRO (Isradipine)	II-1515
Lomosol (Aurothioglucose)	II-242
Lomper (Mebendazole)	II-1711
Lomudal (Cromolyn Sodium)	II-656
Lomudal Gastrointestinum (Cromolyn Sodium)	II-656
Lomudal Nasal (Cromolyn Sodium)	II-656
Lomudal Nesespray (Cromolyn Sodium)	II-656
Lomupren-Nasenspray (Cromolyn Sodium)	II-656
Lomusol (Cromolyn Sodium)	II-656
Lomusol Forte (Cromolyn Sodium)	II-656
Lomusol Nasenspray (Cromolyn Sodium)	II-656
Lomustine (Lomustine)	II-1662
Lomy (Loperamide Hydrochloride)	II-1664
Lonazep (Clonazepam)	II-625
Lonene (Etodolac)	II-1076
Lonflex (Cephalexin)	II-520
Longacef (Ceftriaxone Sodium)	II-503
Longopax (Amitriptyline Hydrochloride; Perphenazine)	II-124
Longphine SR (Morphine Sulfate)	II-1877
Lonine (Etodolac)	II-1076
Loniper (Loperamide Hydrochloride)	II-1664
Lonnoten (Minoxidil)	II-1845
Lonolox (Minoxidil)	II-1845
Lonoten (Minoxidil)	II-1845
Lonta (Chlordiazepoxide Hydrochloride; Clidinium Bromide)	II-541
Lonza (Lorazepam)	II-1678
Lop (Loperamide Hydrochloride)	II-1664
Lopam (Lorazepam)	II-1678
Lopamid (Loperamide Hydrochloride)	II-1664
Lopamide (Loperamide Hydrochloride)	II-1664
Lopane (Ibuprofen)	II-1411
Lop-Dia (Loperamide Hydrochloride)	II-1664
Lopedin (Loperamide Hydrochloride)	II-1664
Lopemid (Loperamide Hydrochloride)	II-1664
Lopemin (Loperamide Hydrochloride)	II-1664
Loperacap (Loperamide Hydrochloride)	II-1664
Loperamil (Loperamide Hydrochloride)	II-1664
Loperastat (Loperamide Hydrochloride)	II-1664
Loperhoe (Loperamide Hydrochloride)	II-1664
Loperid (Loperamide Hydrochloride)	II-1664
Loperium (Loperamide Hydrochloride)	II-1664
Lopermide (Loperamide Hydrochloride)	II-1664
Loperol (Loperamide Hydrochloride)	II-1664
Loperyl (Loperamide Hydrochloride)	II-1664
Lopilexin (Cephalexin)	II-520
Lopiretic (Captopril; Hydrochlorothiazide)	II-416
Lopirin (Captopril)	II-411
Lopitrex (Cephapirin Sodium)	II-525
Lopral (Lansoprazole)	II-1569
Lopraz (Omeprazole)	II-2034
Lopresor (Metoprolol)	II-1805
Lopresor Oros (Metoprolol)	II-1805
Lopresor Retard (Metoprolol)	II-1805
Lopresor SR (Metoprolol)	II-1805
Lopress (Prazosin Hydrochloride)	II-2229
Lopril (Captopril)	II-411
Loprox Laca (Ciclopirox)	II-561
Lopurine (Allopurinol)	II-77
Lorabasics (Loratadine)	II-1675
Lorabenz (Lorazepam)	II-1678
Loracert (Loratadine)	II-1675
Loracert P (Loratadine; Pseudoephedrine Sulfate)	II-1677
Loradex (Loratadine)	II-1675
Lorafem (Loracarbef)	II-1672
Lora-Lich (Loratadine)	II-1675
Loram (Lorazepam)	II-1678
Lorano (Loratadine)	II-1675

International brand name (Generic name)	Page no.
Loranox (Loratadine)	II-1675
Lorans (Lorazepam)	II-1678
Lorapam (Lorazepam)	II-1678
Lorastine (Loratadine)	II-1675
Lora-Tabs (Loratadine)	II-1675
Loratadura (Loratadine)	II-1675
Loratrim (Loratadine)	II-1675
Loratyne (Loratadine)	II-1675
Loratyne D (Loratadine; Pseudoephedrine Sulfate)	II-1677
Loravan (Lorazepam)	II-1678
Lorax (Lorazepam)	II-1678
Lorazene (Lorazepam)	II-1678
Lorazep (Lorazepam)	II-1678
Lorazepam (Lorazepam)	II-1678
Lorazin (Loratadine)	II-1675
Lorazin (Lorazepam)	II-1678
Lorazon (Lorazepam)	II-1678
Loreen (Loratadine)	II-1675
Lorelin Depot (Leuprolide Acetate)	II-1587
Lorenin (Lorazepam)	II-1678
Lorfast (Loratadine)	II-1675
Loridem (Lorazepam)	II-1678
Loridin (Loperamide Hydrochloride)	II-1664
Loridin (Loratadine)	II-1675
Lorien (Fluoxetine Hydrochloride)	II-1160
Lorinid (Amiloride Hydrochloride; Hydrochlorothiazide)	II-105
Lorinid Mite (Amiloride Hydrochloride; Hydrochlorothiazide)	II-105
Lorita (Loratadine)	II-1675
Lorivan (Lorazepam)	II-1678
Lorizide (Amiloride Hydrochloride; Hydrochlorothiazide)	II-105
Lorpa (Loperamide Hydrochloride)	II-1664
Lorsedal (Lorazepam)	II-1678
Lorvas (Indapamide)	II-1436
Lorzaar (Losartan Potassium)	II-1682
Lorzem (Lorazepam)	II-1678
Losacar (Losartan Potassium)	II-1682
Losacor (Losartan Potassium)	II-1682
Losec MUPS (Omeprazole)	II-2034
Losmanin (Chlorpheniramine Maleate)	II-548
Lostatin (Lovastatin)	II-1688
Lotadine (Loratadine)	II-1675
Lotemp (Acetaminophen)	II-11
Lo-ten (Atenolol)	II-222
Loten (Atenolol)	II-222
Lotenal (Atenolol)	II-222
Lotirac (Diclofenac)	II-748
Lotramina (Clotrimazole)	II-640
Lotremin (Clotrimazole)	II-640
Lotrial (Enalapril Maleate)	II-913
Lotrial D (Enalapril Maleate; Hydrochlorothiazide)	II-923
Lotricomb (Betamethasone Dipropionate; Clotrimazole)	II-304
Lotriderm (Betamethasone Dipropionate; Clotrimazole)	II-304
Lo-Uric (Allopurinol)	II-77
Louten (Latanoprost)	II-1574
Lovacel (Lovastatin)	II-1688
Lovalip (Lovastatin)	II-1688
Lovalord (Lovastatin)	II-1688
Lovan (Fluoxetine Hydrochloride)	II-1160
Lovastan (Lovastatin)	II-1688
Lovasterol (Lovastatin)	II-1688
Lovastin (Lovastatin)	II-1688
Lovatadin (Lovastatin)	II-1688
Lovecef (Cephradine)	II-526
Loveral (Albendazole)	II-46
Loverine (Dexamethasone)	II-730
Lovina (Desogestrel; Ethinyl Estradiol)	II-725
Lovir (Acyclovir)	II-33
Lovire (Acyclovir)	II-33
Lovium (Diazepam)	II-740
Lowachol (Lovastatin)	II-1688
Lowadina (Loratadine)	II-1675
Lowin (Gemfibrozil)	II-1269
Low-Lip (Gemfibrozil)	II-1269
Lowlipen (Atorvastatin Calcium)	II-231
Lowtril (Enalapril Maleate)	II-913
Loxan (Ciprofloxacin Hydrochloride)	II-573
Loxapac (Loxapine Succinate)	II-1702
Loxen (Nicardipine Hydrochloride)	II-1958
Loxibest (Meloxicam)	II-1726
Loxicam (Meloxicam)	II-1726
Loxinter (Ofloxacin)	II-2015
Lozapin (Clozapine)	II-642
Lozapine (Clozapine)	II-642
Lozence (Cilostazol)	II-566
Lozide (Indapamide)	II-1436
Lozutin (Lovastatin)	II-1688
L-Polamidon (Methadone Hydrochloride)	II-1766
L.P.V. (Penicillin V Potassium)	II-2142
Luci (Fluocinolone Acetonide)	II-1152
Lucostin (Lomustine)	II-1662
Lucostine (Lomustine)	II-1662
Lucrin Depot (Leuprolide Acetate)	II-1587
Lukadin (Amikacin Sulfate)	II-101
Luminal (Phenobarbital)	II-2167
Luminale (Phenobarbital)	II-2167
Luminaletas (Phenobarbital)	II-2167
Luminaletten (Phenobarbital)	II-2167
Luminalettes (Phenobarbital)	II-2167
Lumirelax (Methocarbamol)	II-1768
Lumustine (Lomustine)	II-1662
Lundbeck (Lomustine)	II-1662
Lunetoron (Bumetanide)	II-359
Lunibron-A (Flunisolide)	II-1149
Lunis (Flunisolide)	II-1149
Lupex (Cefazolin Sodium)	II-452
Lupram (Citalopram Hydrobromide)	II-591
Luprolex (Leuprolide Acetate)	II-1587
Lusanoc (Ketoconazole)	II-1530
Lutamidal (Bicalutamide)	II-318
Lutecilina (Penicillin G Benzathine)	II-2136
Lutogynestryl Fuerte (Progesterone)	II-2262
Lyceft (Ceftriaxone Sodium)	II-503
Lyderm (Fluocinonide)	II-1156
Lydin (Ranitidine Hydrochloride)	II-2334
Lydox (Doxycycline)	II-878
Lydroxil (Cefadroxil Monohydrate)	II-447
Lyforan (Cefotaxime Sodium)	II-474
Lygal Kopftinktur N (Prednisolone)	II-2233
Lynoral (Ethinyl Estradiol)	II-1040
Lyogen (Fluphenazine Hydrochloride)	II-1172
Lyogen Depot (Fluphenazine Hydrochloride)	II-1172
Lyo-Hinicol (Chloramphenicol Sodium Succinate)	II-537
Lyophilisate (Cyclophosphamide)	II-666
Lyovac (Dactinomycin)	II-690
Lyple (Alprostadil)	II-90
Lysalgo (Mefenamic Acid)	II-1720
Lyssavac N Berna (Rabies Vaccine)	II-2324
Lystin (Nystatin)	II-2005
Lysuron (Allopurinol)	II-77
Lysuron 300 (Allopurinol)	II-77
Lytelsen (Diltiazem Hydrochloride)	II-798

M

International brand name (Generic name)	Page no.
M S Contin (Morphine Sulfate)	II-1877
MabCampath (Alemtuzumab)	II-69
Mablin (Busulfan)	II-385
Mabron (Tramadol Hydrochloride)	II-2674
Mabthera (Rituximab)	II-2386
Macaine (Bupivacaine Hydrochloride)	II-361
Macladin (Clarithromycin)	II-597
Maclicine (Dicloxacillin Sodium)	II-761
Maclov (Acyclovir)	II-33
Macrepan (Carbamazepine)	II-418
Macrobid (Nitrofurantoin, Macrocrystalline)	II-1982
Macrobiol (Clarithromycin)	II-597
Macrobiol S.R. (Clarithromycin)	II-597
Macrodantina (Nitrofurantoin, Macrocrystalline)	II-1982
Macrofuran (Nitrofurantoin, Macrocrystalline)	II-1982
Macrofurin (Nitrofurantoin, Macrocrystalline)	II-1982
Macroxam (Piroxicam)	II-2205
Macrozit (Azithromycin)	II-250
Madiol (Methyltestosterone)	II-1796
Madiprazole (Omeprazole)	II-2034
Madlexin (Cephalexin)	II-520
Maformin (Metformin Hydrochloride)	II-1760
Magace (Megestrol Acetate)	II-1723
Magdrin (Doxycycline)	II-878
Magesan (Dicyclomine Hydrochloride)	II-763
Magesan P (Dicyclomine Hydrochloride)	II-763
Magicul (Cimetidine Hydrochloride)	II-568
Magluphen (Diclofenac)	II-748
Magnamycin (Cefoperazone Sodium)	II-471
Magnapen (Ampicillin)	II-170
Magnaspor (Cefuroxime)	II-507
Magnimox (Amoxicillin)	II-131
Magniton-R (Indapamide)	II-1436
Magnurol (Terazosin Hydrochloride)	II-2566
Magrilan (Fluoxetine Hydrochloride)	II-1160
Mahaquin (Lomefloxacin Hydrochloride)	II-1658
Maintate (Bisoprolol Fumarate)	II-323
Malaquin (Chloroquine)	II-544
Malaquin (Primaquine Phosphate)	II-2246
Malarex (Chloroquine)	II-544
Malarivon (Chloroquine)	II-544
Malaviron (Chloroquine)	II-544
Malidens (Acetaminophen)	II-11
Malirid (Primaquine Phosphate)	II-2246
Malival (Indomethacin)	II-1443
Malival AP (Indomethacin)	II-1443
Mallorol (Thioridazine Hydrochloride)	II-2605
Malocin (Erythromycin Ethylsuccinate)	II-965
Mamalexin (Cephalexin)	II-520
Mamlexin (Cephalexin)	II-520
Mamofen (Tamoxifen Citrate)	II-2539
Mancef (Cefamandole Nafate)	II-449
Mandokef (Cefamandole Nafate)	II-449
Mandrolax Bisa (Bisacodyl)	II-322
Manegan (Trazodone Hydrochloride)	II-2686
Manic (Mefenamic Acid)	II-1720
Manidon (Verapamil Hydrochloride)	II-2777
Manidon Retard (Verapamil Hydrochloride)	II-2777
Maniprex (Lithium Carbonate)	II-1654
Manlsum (Flurazepam Hydrochloride)	II-1175
Manobaxine (Methocarbamol)	II-1768
Manobrozil (Gemfibrozil)	II-1269
Manodepa (Medroxyprogesterone Acetate)	II-1714
Manoflox (Norfloxacin)	II-1997
Manoglucon (Glyburide)	II-1297
Manolone (Triamcinolone Acetonide)	II-2701
Manomet (Cimetidine Hydrochloride)	II-568
Manorifcin (Rifampin)	II-2363
Manotran (Clorazepate Dipotassium)	II-638
Mantadan (Amantadine Hydrochloride)	II-97
Mantadix (Amantadine Hydrochloride)	II-97
Mantandan (Amantadine Hydrochloride)	II-97
MAO-B (Selegiline Hydrochloride)	II-2437
MAOtil (Selegiline Hydrochloride)	II-2437
Mapin (Naloxone Hydrochloride)	II-1919
Mapluxin (Digoxin)	II-780
Maprostad (Maprotiline Hydrochloride)	II-1706
Maquine (Chloroquine)	II-544
Marcain (Bupivacaine Hydrochloride)	II-361
Marcaina (Bupivacaine Hydrochloride)	II-361
Marcaine Plain (Bupivacaine Hydrochloride)	II-361
Mareen (Doxepin Hydrochloride)	II-865
Marevan (Warfarin Sodium)	II-2804
Marfloxacin (Ofloxacin)	II-2015
Margrilan (Fluoxetine Hydrochloride)	II-1160

International brand name (Generic name)	Page no.
Maril (Metoclopramide Hydrochloride)	II-1798
Maritidine (Cimetidine Hydrochloride)	II-568
Marsemide (Furosemide)	II-1237
Marticil (Ampicillin)	II-170
Martimil (Nortriptyline Hydrochloride)	II-2002
Marvelon (Desogestrel; Ethinyl Estradiol)	II-725
Marvelon 21 (Desogestrel; Ethinyl Estradiol)	II-725
Marvil (Alendronate Sodium)	II-70
Marzolam (Alprazolam)	II-85
Masaton (Allopurinol)	II-77
Maschitt (Hydrochlorothiazide)	II-1348
Masdil (Diltiazem Hydrochloride)	II-798
Masflex (Meloxicam)	II-1726
Matcine (Chlorpromazine Hydrochloride)	II-549
Matrovir (Acyclovir)	II-33
Mavid (Clarithromycin)	II-597
Maviserpin (Reserpine)	II-2346
Maxadol (Acetaminophen; Codeine Phosphate)	II-13
Maxamox (Amoxicillin)	II-131
Maxcef (Cefepime Hydrochloride)	II-462
Maxcil (Amoxicillin)	II-131
Maxeron (Metoclopramide Hydrochloride)	II-1798
MaxiBone (Alendronate Sodium)	II-70
Maxipen (Ampicillin)	II-170
Maxisporin (Cephradine)	II-526
Maxor (Omeprazole)	II-2034
Maxpro (Cefixime)	II-466
Maxtrex (Methotrexate Sodium)	II-1772
Maycor (Isosorbide Dinitrate)	II-1502
Maycor Retard (Isosorbide Dinitrate)	II-1502
Maygace (Megestrol Acetate)	II-1723
Maynor (Acyclovir)	II-33
Mazetol (Carbamazepine)	II-418
MCP-Beta Tropfen (Metoclopramide Hydrochloride)	II-1798
MCR (Morphine Sulfate)	II-1877
M.C.T. (Acetylcysteine)	II-29
Meaverin (Mepivacaine Hydrochloride)	II-1737
Mebex (Mebendazole)	II-1711
Mecid A (Mefenamic Acid)	II-1720
Mecil-N (Ampicillin)	II-170
Meclomid (Metoclopramide Hydrochloride)	II-1798
Meclozine (Meclizine Hydrochloride)	II-1713
Medacinase (Urokinase)	II-2734
Medacter (Miconazole)	II-1820
Medamor (Amiloride Hydrochloride)	II-103
Medepres (Captopril)	II-411
Med-Gastramet (Cimetidine Hydrochloride)	II-568
Med-Glionil (Glyburide)	II-1297
Medianox (Chloral Hydrate)	II-534
Medic Aid Isoniazid (Isoniazid)	II-1496
Mediconcef (Cefaclor)	II-444
Medicyclomine (Dicyclomine Hydrochloride)	II-763
Medifam (Rifampin)	II-2363
Medihaler-Iso (Epinephrine)	II-934
Medikinet (Methylphenidate Hydrochloride)	II-1781
Medilium (Chlordiazepoxide Hydrochloride)	II-539
Medimet (Methyldopa)	II-1778
Medimox (Amoxicillin)	II-131
Medinox Mono (Pentobarbital Sodium)	II-2149
Mediper (Cefoperazone Sodium)	II-471
Medixel (Paclitaxel)	II-2084
Medixin (Sulfamethoxazole; Trimethoprim)	II-2500
Medixon (Methylprednisolone)	II-1787
Medizol (Clotrimazole)	II-640
Mednin (Methylprednisolone)	II-1787
Medobeta (Betamethasone Valerate)	II-305
Medocalum (Chlordiazepoxide Hydrochloride; Clidinium Bromide)	II-541
Medocef (Cefoperazone Sodium)	II-471
Medociprin (Ciprofloxacin Hydrochloride)	II-573
Medoclor (Cefaclor)	II-444
Medocor (Isosorbide Mononitrate)	II-1507
Medocriptine (Bromocriptine Mesylate)	II-344
Medocycline (Tetracycline Hydrochloride)	II-2585
Medoflucon (Fluconazole)	II-1136
Medoglycin (Lincomycin Hydrochloride)	II-1640
Medolin (Albuterol)	II-47
Medomet (Methyldopa)	II-1778
Medomycin (Doxycycline)	II-878
Medopa (Methyldopa)	II-1778
Medopal (Methyldopa)	II-1778
Medopam (Oxazepam)	II-2063
Medoprazole (Omeprazole)	II-2034
Medopren (Methyldopa)	II-1778
Medoric (Allopurinol)	II-77
Medostatin (Lovastatin)	II-1688
Medovir (Acyclovir)	II-33
Medral (Omeprazole)	II-2034
Medrate (Methylprednisolone)	II-1787
Medrate Solubile (Methylprednisolone Sodium Succinate)	II-1793
Medrone (Medroxyprogesterone Acetate)	II-1714
Medrone (Methylprednisolone)	II-1787
Medsavorin (Leucovorin Calcium)	II-1585
Mefac (Mefenamic Acid)	II-1720
Mefacap (Mefenamic Acid)	II-1720
Mefalqic (Mefenamic Acid)	II-1720
Mefanol (Allopurinol)	II-77
Mefast (Mefenamic Acid)	II-1720
Mefliam (Mefloquine Hydrochloride)	II-1721
Mefoxil (Cefoxitin Sodium)	II-482
Mefoxitin (Cefoxitin Sodium)	II-482
Megace OS (Megestrol Acetate)	II-1723
Megacef (Cefazolin Sodium)	II-452
Megacilina Oral (Penicillin V Potassium)	II-2142
Megacillin (Penicillin G Potassium)	II-2137
Megacillin Oral (Penicillin V Potassium)	II-2142
Megafol (Folic Acid)	II-1208
Megalat (Nifedipine)	II-1967
Megaplex (Megestrol Acetate)	II-1723
Megaxin (Moxifloxacin Hydrochloride)	II-1886
Meges (Medroxyprogesterone Acetate)	II-1714
Megestat (Megestrol Acetate)	II-1723
Megion (Ceftriaxone Sodium)	II-503
Meiceral (Omeprazole)	II-2034
Meipril (Enalapril Maleate)	II-913
Meixil (Amoxicillin)	II-131
Me-Korti (Prednisone)	II-2240
Melabon (Aspirin)	II-206
Melanox (Hydroquinone)	II-1391
Melaxan (Bisacodyl)	II-322
Melbin (Metformin Hydrochloride)	II-1760
Meldian (Chlorpropamide)	II-554
Meldopa (Methyldopa)	II-1778
Meleril (Thioridazine Hydrochloride)	II-2605
Melicide (Sucralfate)	II-2493
Melipramine (Imipramine Hydrochloride)	II-1431
Melix (Glyburide)	II-1297
Melizide (Glipizide)	II-1290
Melleretten (Thioridazine Hydrochloride)	II-2605
Melleril (Thioridazine Hydrochloride)	II-2605
Mellerzin (Thioridazine Hydrochloride)	II-2605
Mellitos (Chlorpropamide)	II-554
Mellitos C (Chlorpropamide)	II-554
Melocam (Meloxicam)	II-1726
Mel-OD (Meloxicam)	II-1726
Melodil (Maprotiline Hydrochloride)	II-1706
Melormin (Chlorpropamide)	II-554
Melosteral (Meloxicam)	II-1726
Melox (Meloxicam)	II-1726
Melquin HP (Hydroquinone)	II-1391
Melquine (Hydroquinone)	II-1391
Melrosum (Codeine Phosphate)	II-647
M.Elson (Morphine Sulfate)	II-1877
Melubrin (Chloroquine)	II-544
Melzin (Clonidine Hydrochloride)	II-629
Memorit (Donepezil Hydrochloride)	II-850
Menesit (Carbidopa; Levodopa)	II-424
Menobarb (Phenobarbital)	II-2167
Menocal (Calcitonin (Salmon))	II-397
Meno-MPA (Estradiol)	II-986
Meno-Net (Estradiol; Norethindrone Acetate)	II-1011
Menorest (Estradiol)	II-986
Menoring (Estradiol)	II-986
Menpoz (Estrogens, Conjugated)	II-1019
Mensoton (Ibuprofen)	II-1411
Mentalium (Diazepam)	II-740
Menzol (Norethindrone)	II-1996
Mepem (Meropenem)	II-1743
Mephamycin (Erythromycin)	II-960
Mephanol (Allopurinol)	II-77
Mephaquin (Mefloquine Hydrochloride)	II-1721
Mephaquine (Mefloquine Hydrochloride)	II-1721
Mephenon (Methadone Hydrochloride)	II-1766
Mepicaton 3% (Mepivacaine Hydrochloride)	II-1737
Mepihexal (Mepivacaine Hydrochloride)	II-1737
Mepiozin (Thioridazine Hydrochloride)	II-2605
Mepivastesin (Mepivacaine Hydrochloride)	II-1737
Mepramide (Metoclopramide Hydrochloride)	II-1798
Meprate (Medroxyprogesterone Acetate)	II-1714
Meprin (Meprobamate)	II-1738
Mepro (Meprobamate)	II-1738
Meprodil (Meprobamate)	II-1738
Mepsolone (Methylprednisolone Sodium Succinate)	II-1793
Mepzol (Omeprazole)	II-2034
Merabis (Spironolactone)	II-2483
Meramide (Metoclopramide Hydrochloride)	II-1798
Mercaptopurina (Mercaptopurine)	II-1741
Mercaptyl (Penicillamine)	II-2133
Mercilon (Desogestrel; Ethinyl Estradiol)	II-725
Mereprine (Captopril)	II-411
Merlit (Lorazepam)	II-1678
Meronem (Meropenem)	II-1743
Meropen (Meropenem)	II-1743
Meruvax II (Measles Virus Vaccine Live)	II-1708
Mesacol (Mesalamine)	II-1748
Mesalin (Mesalamine)	II-1748
Mesasal (Mesalamine)	II-1748
M-Eslon (Morphine Sulfate)	II-1877
Meslon (Morphine Sulfate)	II-1877
Mesonta (Betamethasone Dipropionate)	II-301
Mesorin (Mesoridazine Besylate)	II-1752
Mesporin IM (Ceftriaxone Sodium)	II-503
Mesporin IV (Ceftriaxone Sodium)	II-503
Mestacine (Minocycline Hydrochloride)	II-1838
Mestrel (Megestrol Acetate)	II-1723
Metabolin (Thiamine Hydrochloride)	II-2602
Metacen (Indomethacin)	II-1443
Metadate E.R. (Methylphenidate Hydrochloride)	II-1781
Metaderm (Betamethasone Valerate)	II-305
Metadon (Methadone Hydrochloride)	II-1766
Metagesic (Acetaminophen)	II-11
Metagliz (Metoclopramide Hydrochloride)	II-1798
Metalcaptase (Penicillamine)	II-2133
Metamide (Metoclopramide Hydrochloride)	II-1798
Metaoxedrin (Phenylephrine Hydrochloride)	II-2173
Metaryl (Promethazine Hydrochloride)	II-2268
Metasedin (Methadone Hydrochloride)	II-1766
Metaspray (Mometasone Furoate)	II-1866
Metenix 5 (Metolazone)	II-1802
Metex (Methotrexate Sodium)	II-1772
Metfogamma (Metformin Hydrochloride)	II-1760
Metforal (Metformin Hydrochloride)	II-1760
Methacin (Indomethacin)	II-1443
Methaddict (Methadone Hydrochloride)	II-1766
Methaforte Mix (Methadone Hydrochloride)	II-1766
Methocaps (Indomethacin)	II-1443
Methopa (Methyldopa)	II-1778
Methoplain (Methyldopa)	II-1778
Methotrexat Ebewe (Methotrexate Sodium)	II-1772
Methotrexate (Methotrexate Sodium)	II-1772
Methotrexato (Methotrexate Sodium)	II-1772
Methyldopum (Methyldopa)	II-1778
Methyrit (Chlorpheniramine Maleate)	II-548

International brand name (Generic name)	Page no.
Meticon (Cimetidine Hydrochloride)	II-568
Metidrol (Methylprednisolone)	II-1787
Metimazol (Methimazole)	II-1767
Metindol (Indomethacin)	II-1443
Metlazel (Metoclopramide Hydrochloride)	II-1798
Metmic (Mefenamic Acid)	II-1720
Metoclor (Metoclopramide Hydrochloride)	II-1798
Metocobil (Metoclopramide Hydrochloride)	II-1798
Metocyl (Metoclopramide Hydrochloride)	II-1798
Meto-Hennig (Metoprolol)	II-1805
Metohexal (Metoprolol)	II-1805
Metolol (Metoprolol)	II-1805
Metolon (Metoclopramide Hydrochloride)	II-1798
Metomin (Metformin Hydrochloride)	II-1760
Metonate (Betamethasone Dipropionate)	II-301
Metopram (Metoclopramide Hydrochloride)	II-1798
Metopress Retard (Metoprolol)	II-1805
Metoprim (Metoprolol)	II-1805
Metoprogamma (Metoprolol)	II-1805
Metoral (Triamcinolone Acetonide)	II-2701
Metosyn (Fluocinonide)	II-1156
Metram (Metoclopramide Hydrochloride)	II-1798
Metrogyl (Metronidazole)	II-1812
Metrolag (Metronidazole)	II-1812
Metrolex (Metronidazole)	II-1812
Metronidazol McKesson (Metronidazole)	II-1812
Metronide (Metronidazole)	II-1812
Metrozin (Metronidazole)	II-1812
Metrozine (Metronidazole)	II-1812
Metrulen (Ethinyl Estradiol; Ethynodiol Diacetate)	II-1042
Metycortin (Methylprednisolone)	II-1787
Metypred (Methylprednisolone)	II-1787
Mevalotin (Pravastatin Sodium)	II-2224
Meverstin (Lovastatin)	II-1688
Mevilin-L (Measles Virus Vaccine Live)	II-1708
Mevinacor (Lovastatin)	II-1688
Mexalen (Acetaminophen)	II-11
Mexaquin (Chloroquine)	II-544
Mexasone (Dexamethasone)	II-730
Mexate (Methotrexate Sodium)	II-1772
Mexican (Meloxicam)	II-1726
Mexihexal (Mexiletine Hydrochloride)	II-1817
Mexitec (Mexiletine Hydrochloride)	II-1817
Mexpharm (Meloxicam)	II-1726
Mezenol (Sulfamethoxazole; Trimethoprim)	II-2500
Miacalcic (Calcitonin (Salmon))	II-397
Miacin (Amikacin Sulfate)	II-101
Micardis Plus (Hydrochlorothiazide; Telmisartan)	II-1360
Micatin (Miconazole)	II-1820
Miccil (Bumetanide)	II-359
Miclast (Ciclopirox)	II-561
Miclor (Cefaclor)	II-444
Micoffen (Miconazole)	II-1820
Micolak (Econazole Nitrate)	II-900
Micolis (Econazole Nitrate)	II-900
Miconal (Miconazole)	II-1820
Micoral (Itraconazole)	II-1517
Micos (Econazole Nitrate)	II-900
Micosil (Terbinafine Hydrochloride)	II-2570
Micostatin (Nystatin)	II-2005
Micostyl (Econazole Nitrate)	II-900
Micotar Mundgel (Miconazole)	II-1820
Micotef (Miconazole)	II-1820
Micoter (Clotrimazole)	II-640
Micoxolamina (Ciclopirox)	II-561
Micozole (Miconazole)	II-1820
Micreme (Miconazole)	II-1820
Microbanzol (Dipyridamole)	II-821
Microdiol (Desogestrel; Ethinyl Estradiol)	II-725
Microfemin (Ethinyl Estradiol; Levonorgestrel)	II-1047
Microfemin CD (Ethinyl Estradiol; Levonorgestrel)	II-1047
Microfer (Ferrous Sulfate)	II-1122
Microfulvin (Griseofulvin, Microcrystalline)	II-1312
Microfulvin-500 (Griseofulvin, Microcrystalline)	II-1312
Microgest ED (Ethinyl Estradiol; Levonorgestrel)	II-1047
Microgris (Griseofulvin, Microcrystalline)	II-1312
Microgyn (Ethinyl Estradiol; Levonorgestrel)	II-1047
Microgynon (Ethinyl Estradiol; Levonorgestrel)	II-1047
Microgynon 21 (Ethinyl Estradiol; Levonorgestrel)	II-1047
Microgynon 28 (Ethinyl Estradiol; Levonorgestrel)	II-1047
Microgynon CD (Ethinyl Estradiol; Levonorgestrel)	II-1047
Micro-K Extentcaps (Potassium Chloride)	II-2215
Microka (Phytonadione)	II-2178
Micro-Kalium Retard (Potassium Chloride)	II-2215
Microlut (Levonorgestrel)	II-1614
Micromycin (Minocycline Hydrochloride)	II-1838
Micro-Novom (Norethindrone)	II-1996
Micronovum (Norethindrone)	II-1996
Microtid (Ranitidine Hydrochloride)	II-2334
Microtrim (Sulfamethoxazole; Trimethoprim)	II-2500
Microval (Levonorgestrel)	II-1614
Midazol (Midazolam Hydrochloride)	II-1823
Midocil (Tolmetin Sodium)	II-2656
Midolam (Midazolam Hydrochloride)	II-1823
Midorm (Flurazepam Hydrochloride)	II-1175
Midorm AR (Flurazepam Hydrochloride)	II-1175
Midrat (Captopril)	II-411
Miduret (Amiloride Hydrochloride; Hydrochlorothiazide)	II-105
Mifegest (Mifepristone)	II-1834
Mifegyne (Mifepristone)	II-1834
Miflasone (Beclomethasone Dipropionate)	II-279
Miflonide (Budesonide)	II-347
Miflonide Inhaler (Budesonide)	II-347
Miformin (Metformin Hydrochloride)	II-1760
Migaphen (Acetaminophen; Dichloralphenazone; Isometheptene Mucate)	II-16
Miglucan (Glyburide)	II-1297
Migragesin (Sumatriptan Succinate)	II-2516
Migranol (Sumatriptan Succinate)	II-2516
Mikelan (Carteolol Hydrochloride)	II-435
Miketorin (Amitriptyline Hydrochloride)	II-119
Mikrofollin (Ethinyl Estradiol)	II-1040
Milcopen (Penicillin V Potassium)	II-2142
Mildison (Hydrocortisone)	II-1369
Mildison fet krem (Hydrocortisone)	II-1369
Mildison Lipocream (Hydrocortisone)	II-1369
Mildison-Fatty (Hydrocortisone)	II-1369
Milli (Ethinyl Estradiol; Norethindrone)	II-1055
Millibar (Indapamide)	II-1436
Milligon (Chlorpropamide)	II-554
Millsrol (Nitroglycerin)	II-1984
Miltaun (Meprobamate)	II-1738
Milurit (Allopurinol)	II-77
Minaxen (Minocycline Hydrochloride)	II-1838
Minaza (Miconazole)	II-1820
Mindiab (Glipizide)	II-1290
Mindol (Mebendazole)	II-1711
Miniblock (Esmolol Hydrochloride)	II-977
Minidiab (Glipizide)	II-1290
Minidril (Ethinyl Estradiol; Levonorgestrel)	II-1047
Minigynon (Ethinyl Estradiol; Levonorgestrel)	II-1047
Minims Atropine Sulfaat (Atropine Sulfate)	II-235
Minims Atropine Sulfate (Atropine Sulfate)	II-235
Minims Chloramphenicol (Chloramphenicol)	II-536
Minims Eye Drops (Chloramphenicol)	II-536
Minims Hyoscine Hydrobromide (Scopolamine)	II-2432
Minims Phenylephrine HCL 10% (Phenylephrine Hydrochloride)	II-2173
Minims Phenylephrine Hydrochloride (Phenylephrine Hydrochloride)	II-2173
Minims-Atropine (Atropine Sulfate)	II-235
Miniplanor (Allopurinol)	II-77
Minipres (Prazosin Hydrochloride)	II-2229
Minipres SR (Prazosin Hydrochloride)	II-2229
Minipress XL (Prazosin Hydrochloride)	II-2229
Minirin (Desmopressin Acetate)	II-723
Minirin DDAVP (Desmopressin Acetate)	II-723
Minirin Nasal Spray (Desmopressin Acetate)	II-723
Minisiston (Ethinyl Estradiol; Levonorgestrel)	II-1047
Minitent (Captopril)	II-411
Minitran (Amitriptyline Hydrochloride; Perphenazine)	II-124
Minivlar 30 (Ethinyl Estradiol; Levonorgestrel)	II-1047
Mino-50 (Minocycline Hydrochloride)	II-1838
Minobese-Forte (Phentermine Hydrochloride)	II-2170
Minocin G (Minocycline Hydrochloride)	II-1838
Minocin MR (Minocycline Hydrochloride)	II-1838
Minoclin (Minocycline Hydrochloride)	II-1838
Minoclir 50 (Minocycline Hydrochloride)	II-1838
Minomycin (Minocycline Hydrochloride)	II-1838
Minocyclin 50 Stada (Minocycline Hydrochloride)	II-1838
Minodiab (Glipizide)	II-1290
Minogalen (Minocycline Hydrochloride)	II-1838
Minoline (Minocycline Hydrochloride)	II-1838
Minona (Minoxidil)	II-1845
Minopan (Acetaminophen)	II-11
Minotab 50 (Minocycline Hydrochloride)	II-1838
Minotin (Erythromycin Ethylsuccinate)	II-965
Minovlar (Ethinyl Estradiol; Norethindrone)	II-1055
Min-Ovral (Ethinyl Estradiol; Norgestrel)	II-1068
Min-Ovral 21 (Ethinyl Estradiol; Levonorgestrel)	II-1047
Min-Ovral 28 (Ethinyl Estradiol; Levonorgestrel)	II-1047
Mino-Wolff (Minocycline Hydrochloride)	II-1838
Minoxidil Isac (Minoxidil)	II-1845
Minoxidil MK (Minoxidil)	II-1845
Minoximen (Minoxidil)	II-1845
Minoxitrim (Minoxidil)	II-1845
Minoxyl (Minoxidil)	II-1845
Minprog (Alprostadil)	II-90
Minprostin E(2) (Dinoprostone)	II-812
Minrin (Desmopressin Acetate)	II-723
Mintal (Pentobarbital Sodium)	II-2149
Minurin (Desmopressin Acetate)	II-723
Miocardie (Diltiazem Hydrochloride)	II-798
Miocarpine (Pilocarpine)	II-2180
Miocrin (Gold Sodium Thiomalate)	II-1304
Miolene (Ritodrine Hydrochloride)	II-2379
Miopotasio (Potassium Chloride)	II-2215
Miosen (Dipyridamole)	II-821
M.I.R. (Morphine Sulfate)	II-1877
Miracid (Omeprazole)	II-2034
Miraclin (Doxycycline)	II-878
Miracol (Miconazole)	II-1820
Mirafen (Flurbiprofen)	II-1177
Miragenta (Gentamicin Sulfate)	II-1279
Miramycin (Gentamicin Sulfate)	II-1279
Mirapexin (Pramipexole Dihydrochloride)	II-2219
Miravelle (Desogestrel; Ethinyl Estradiol)	II-725
Miravelle Suave (Desogestrel; Ethinyl Estradiol)	II-725
Miroptic (Chloramphenicol)	II-536
Mirpan (Maprotiline Hydrochloride)	II-1706
Mirquin (Chloroquine)	II-544
Miscleron (Clofibrate)	II-619
Misel (Misoprostol)	II-1851
Missile (Sulfamethoxazole; Trimethoprim)	II-2500
Misulban (Busulfan)	II-385
Mitocortyl Demangeaisons (Hydrocortisone)	II-1369
Mitomicina-C (Mitomycin)	II-1854
Mitomycin (Mitomycin)	II-1854
Mitomycin C (Mitomycin)	II-1854
Mitomycin-C (Mitomycin)	II-1854
Mitomycin-C Kyowa (Mitomycin)	II-1854

International brand name (Generic name)	Page no.
Mutabase (Amitriptyline Hydrochloride; Perphenazine)	II-124
Mutabon (Amitriptyline Hydrochloride; Perphenazine)	II-124
Mutabon A (Amitriptyline Hydrochloride; Perphenazine)	II-124
Mutabon D (Amitriptyline Hydrochloride; Perphenazine)	II-124
Mutabon F (Amitriptyline Hydrochloride; Perphenazine)	II-124
Mutabon M (Amitriptyline Hydrochloride; Perphenazine)	II-124
Mutabon-A (Amitriptyline Hydrochloride; Perphenazine)	II-124
Mutabon-D (Amitriptyline Hydrochloride; Perphenazine)	II-124
Mutabon-F (Amitriptyline Hydrochloride; Perphenazine)	II-124
Mutabon-M (Amitriptyline Hydrochloride; Perphenazine)	II-124
Mutagrip (Influenza Virus Vaccine)	II-1451
Mutum (Fluconazole)	II-1136
Mutum CR (Oxybutynin)	II-2070
Muvera (Meloxicam)	II-1726
M-VAC (Measles Virus Vaccine Live)	II-1708
Mycastatin (Nystatin)	II-2005
Mycoban (Clotrimazole)	II-640
Mycobutol (Ethambutol Hydrochloride)	II-1039
Mycocid (Clotrimazole)	II-640
Mycocide (Nystatin)	II-2005
Mycocyst (Fluconazole)	II-1136
Mycofebrin (Ketoconazole)	II-1530
Mycoheal Cream (Miconazole)	II-1820
Mycoheal Oral Gel (Miconazole)	II-1820
Myco-Hermal (Clotrimazole)	II-640
Mycorest (Fluconazole)	II-1136
Mycoril (Clotrimazole)	II-640
Mycoril Spray (Clotrimazole)	II-640
Mycorine (Miconazole)	II-1820
Mycosantin (Nystatin)	II-2005
Mycostatine (Nystatin)	II-2005
Mycoster (Ciclopirox)	II-561
Mycostop (Griseofulvin, Microcrystalline)	II-1312
Mycotel (Albendazole)	II-46
Mycotricide (Praziquantel)	II-2228
Mycozole (Clotrimazole)	II-640
Mycrol (Ethambutol Hydrochloride)	II-1039
Mydopine (Amlodipine Besylate)	II-125
Mydran (Acetaminophen; Dichloralphenazone; Isometheptene Mucate)	II-16
Mydrin (Acetaminophen; Dichloralphenazone; Isometheptene Mucate)	II-16
Myfungar (Oxiconazole Nitrate)	II-2069
Mykoderm (Miconazole)	II-1820
Mykoderm (Nystatin)	II-2005
Mylepsin (Primidone)	II-2247
Mylocort (Hydrocortisone Acetate)	II-1373
Mynocine (Minocycline Hydrochloride)	II-1838
Mynosedin (Ibuprofen)	II-1411
Myo Hermes (Bethanechol Chloride)	II-312
Myocet (Doxorubicin, Liposomal)	II-873
Myocholine (Bethanechol Chloride)	II-312
Myocholine Glenwood (Bethanechol Chloride)	II-312
Myocholine-Glenwood (Bethanechol Chloride)	II-312
Myocin (Methocarbamol)	II-1768
Myocord (Atenolol)	II-222
Myocrisin (Gold Sodium Thiomalate)	II-1304
Myogard (Nifedipine)	II-1967
Myolax (Carisoprodol)	II-432
Myonil (Diltiazem Hydrochloride)	II-798
Myonil Retard (Diltiazem Hydrochloride)	II-798
Myoquin (Quinine Sulfate)	II-2317
Myotonine (Bethanechol Chloride)	II-312
Myotonine Chloride (Bethanechol Chloride)	II-312
Myovin (Nitroglycerin)	II-1984
Myslee (Zolmitriptan)	II-2838
Mysocort (Miconazole)	II-1820
Mysolin (Primidone)	II-2247
Mysteclin (Tetracycline Hydrochloride)	II-2585

N

International brand name (Generic name)	Page no.
Naboal (Diclofenac)	II-748
Nabone (Nabumetone)	II-1909
Nabonet (Nabumetone)	II-1909
Nabuco (Nabumetone)	II-1909
Naburen (Nabumetone)	II-1909
Nabuser (Nabumetone)	II-1909
Nabutil (Loperamide Hydrochloride)	II-1664
Nac Gel (Diclofenac)	II-748
Nacid (Nizatidine)	II-1992
Naclex (Furosemide)	II-1237
Naclof (Diclofenac)	II-748
Nacoflar (Diclofenac)	II-748
Nacton (Nabumetone)	II-1909
Nadic (Nadolol)	II-1911
Nadine (Ranitidine Hydrochloride)	II-2334
Nadipine (Nifedipine)	II-1967
Nadopen-V (Penicillin V Potassium)	II-2142
Nadorex (Nabumetone)	II-1909
Nadostine (Nystatin)	II-2005
Nafasol (Naproxen)	II-1924
Naflex (Nabumetone)	II-1909
Nagifen-D (Ibuprofen)	II-1411
Nail Batrafen (Ciclopirox)	II-561
Nairet (Terbutaline Sulfate)	II-2574
Naixan (Naproxen)	II-1924
Nakacef-A (Cephradine)	II-526
Nakaxone (Ceftriaxone Sodium)	II-503
Nalbix (Clotrimazole)	II-640
Nalcrom (Cromolyn Sodium)	II-656
Nalcryn SP (Nalbuphine Hydrochloride)	II-1917
Nalerona (Naltrexone Hydrochloride)	II-1920
Nalgesic (Fenoprofen Calcium)	II-1110
Nalgesik (Acetaminophen)	II-11
Nalomet (Azatadine Maleate)	II-242
Nalone (Naloxone Hydrochloride)	II-1919
Nalorex (Naltrexone Hydrochloride)	II-1920
Nalox (Metronidazole)	II-1812
Naloxon (Naloxone Hydrochloride)	II-1919
Nametone (Nabumetone)	II-1909
Nansius (Clorazepate Dipotassium)	II-638
Napa (Acetaminophen)	II-11
Napacetin (Ibuprofen)	II-1411
Napamide (Indapamide)	II-1436
Napamol (Acetaminophen)	II-11
Napan (Mefenamic Acid)	II-1720
Napizide (Glipizide)	II-1290
Naplin (Indapamide)	II-1436
Napolon (Naproxen)	II-1924
Naposin (Naproxen)	II-1924
Naprilene (Enalapril Maleate)	II-913
Naprium (Naproxen)	II-1924
Naprius (Naproxen)	II-1924
Naprizide (Enalapril Maleate; Hydrochlorothiazide)	II-923
Naproflam (Naproxen)	II-1924
Naprong (Naproxen)	II-1924
Naprontag (Naproxen)	II-1924
Naprorex (Naproxen)	II-1924
Naprosyn (Naproxen Sodium)	II-1928
Naprosyn LLE (Naproxen)	II-1924
Naprosyn LLE Forte (Naproxen)	II-1924
Naprosyne (Naproxen)	II-1924
Naproxi 250 (Naproxen)	II-1924
Naproxi 500 (Naproxen)	II-1924
Naprux (Naproxen)	II-1924
Napxen (Naproxen)	II-1924
Naramig (Naratriptan Hydrochloride)	II-1932
Narcan Neonatal (Naloxone Hydrochloride)	II-1919
Narcanti (Naloxone Hydrochloride)	II-1919
Narcotan (Naloxone Hydrochloride)	II-1919
Nardelzine (Phenelzine Sulfate)	II-2165
Narfoz (Ondansetron Hydrochloride)	II-2039
Narilet (Ipratropium Bromide)	II-1480
Naritec (Enalapril Maleate)	II-913
Narma (Naproxen)	II-1924
Narocin (Naproxen Sodium)	II-1928
Narol (Buspirone Hydrochloride)	II-382
Narop (Ropivacaine Hydrochloride)	II-2404
Naropeine (Ropivacaine Hydrochloride)	II-2404
Nasacort AQ (Triamcinolone Acetonide)	II-2701
Nasanyl (Nafarelin Acetate)	II-1914
Nasarel (Nafarelin Acetate)	II-1914
Nascobal Intranasal Gel (Cyanocobalamin)	II-661
Naselin (Hydralazine Hydrochloride)	II-1346
Nasocor AQ (Triamcinolone Acetonide)	II-2701
Nasonex Nasal Spray (Mometasone Furoate)	II-1866
Nasotal (Cromolyn Sodium)	II-656
Naspor (Cefotaxime Sodium)	II-474
NAspro (Aspirin)	II-206
Nasterol (Finasteride)	II-1129
Nastil (Ketoconazole)	II-1530
Natam (Flurazepam Hydrochloride)	II-1175
Natead (Rho (D) Immune Globulin)	II-2350
Naticardina (Quinidine Sulfate)	II-2314
Natigoxin (Digoxin)	II-780
Natinate (Niacin)	II-1956
Natralix (Indapamide)	II-1436
Natrilix SR (Indapamide)	II-1436
Natrix (Indapamide)	II-1436
Natrix SR (Indapamide)	II-1436
Natulan (Procarbazine Hydrochloride)	II-2257
Naturogest (Progesterone)	II-2262
Nausil (Metoclopramide Hydrochloride)	II-1798
Nautisol (Prochlorperazine)	II-2258
Navelbin (Vinorelbine Tartrate)	II-2791
Navicalm (Meclizine Hydrochloride)	II-1713
Naxal (Ketoprofen)	II-1533
Naxen (Naproxen)	II-1924
Naxen F (Naproxen)	II-1924
Naxen-F CR (Naproxen)	II-1924
Naxidine (Nizatidine)	II-1992
Naxone (Naloxone Hydrochloride)	II-1919
Naxopren (Naproxen)	II-1924
Naxy (Clarithromycin)	II-597
Naxyn 250 (Naproxen)	II-1924
Naxyn 500 (Naproxen)	II-1924
Nazoderm (Miconazole)	II-1820
Nazol (Danazol)	II-699
Nazole (Ketoconazole)	II-1530
Nazotral (Cromolyn Sodium)	II-656
Nebcina (Tobramycin Sulfate)	II-2646
Nebcine (Tobramycin Sulfate)	II-2646
Nebicina (Tobramycin Sulfate)	II-2646
Nebril (Desipramine Hydrochloride)	II-716
NEBS (Acetaminophen)	II-11
Neciblok (Sucralfate)	II-2493
Necopen (Cefixime)	II-466
Nedipin (Nifedipine)	II-1967
Neekxin (Orphenadrine Citrate)	II-2049
Neexin (Orphenadrine Citrate)	II-2049
Nefadar (Nefazodone Hydrochloride)	II-1939
Nefalox (Cefadroxil Monohydrate)	II-447
Nefoben (Theophylline)	II-2593
Nefrin-Ofteno (Phenylephrine Hydrochloride)	II-2173
Nefryl (Oxybutynin)	II-2070
Nektol 500 (Acetaminophen)	II-11
Nelapine (Nifedipine)	II-1967
Nelapine Retard (Nifedipine)	II-1967
Nemexin (Naltrexone Hydrochloride)	II-1920
Nemozole (Albendazole)	II-46
Neo Atromid (Clofibrate)	II-619
Neo Dopaston (Carbidopa; Levodopa)	II-424
Neobiphyllin (Theophylline)	II-2593
Neobloc (Metoprolol)	II-1805

International brand name (Generic name)	Page no.
Neobon (Alendronate Sodium)	II-70
Neocapil (Minoxidil)	II-1845
Neoceptin-R (Ranitidine Hydrochloride)	II-2334
Neoclarityn (Desloratadine)	II-721
Neocon (Ethinyl Estradiol; Norethindrone)	II-1055
Neocristin (Vincristine Sulfate)	II-2789
Neodrea (Hydroxyurea)	II-1394
Neofloxin (Ciprofloxacin Hydrochloride)	II-573
Neogest (Norgestrel)	II-2002
Neo-Gnostorid (Chlordiazepoxide Hydrochloride)	II-539
Neogram (Amoxicillin)	II-131
Neogynon 21 (Ethinyl Estradiol; Levonorgestrel)	II-1047
Neokef (Cephalexin)	II-520
Neomazine (Chlorpromazine Hydrochloride)	II-549
Neo-Menovar (Estrogens, Conjugated)	II-1019
Neomicol (Miconazole)	II-1820
Neomochin (Meperidine Hydrochloride)	II-1733
Neophyllin (Aminophylline)	II-106
Neoplatin (Carboplatin)	II-430
Neoplatin (Cisplatin)	II-589
Neopramiel (Metoclopramide Hydrochloride)	II-1798
Neorecormon (Epoetin Alfa)	II-942
Neo-Rinactive (Budesonide)	II-347
Neosporin-H (Hydrocortisone; Neomycin Sulfate; Polymyxin B Sulfate)	II-1384
Neosynephrine (Phenylephrine Hydrochloride)	II-2173
Neosynephrine 10% Chibret (Phenylephrine Hydrochloride)	II-2173
Neosynephrine Faure 10% (Phenylephrine Hydrochloride)	II-2173
Neo-Synephrine Ophthalmic Viscous 10% (Phenylephrine Hydrochloride)	II-2173
Neosynephrin-POS (Phenylephrine Hydrochloride)	II-2173
Neotica (Carisoprodol)	II-432
Neotigason (Acitretin)	II-31
Neo-Tigason (Acitretin)	II-31
Neo-Toltinon (Chlorpropamide)	II-554
Neotrexate (Methotrexate Sodium)	II-1772
Neotromax (Filgrastim)	II-1126
Neovulen (Ethinyl Estradiol; Ethynodiol Diacetate)	II-1042
Neoxidil (Minoxidil)	II-1845
NeOxyn (Oxytocin)	II-2082
Nephracet 600 (Calcium Acetate)	II-400
Nephramid (Acetazolamide)	II-28
Nephril (Polythiazide)	II-2213
Nephron (Furosemide)	II-1237
Nepresol (Hydralazine Hydrochloride)	II-1346
Neptal (Acebutolol Hydrochloride)	II-10
Nerbet (Buspirone Hydrochloride)	II-382
Nergadan (Lovastatin)	II-1688
Nergart (Flurazepam Hydrochloride)	II-1175
Neripros (Risperidone)	II-2374
Nerolet (Trifluoperazine Hydrochloride)	II-2717
Nervistop L (Lorazepam)	II-1678
Nesdonal (Thiopental Sodium)	II-2603
Nesontil (Oxazepam)	II-2063
Netaf (Metoclopramide Hydrochloride)	II-1798
Netra (Calcium Carbonate)	II-401
Neufan (Allopurinol)	II-77
Neugeron (Carbamazepine)	II-418
Neulin SA (Theophylline)	II-2593
Neulin-SR (Theophylline)	II-2593
Neupax (Alprazolam)	II-85
Neupax (Fluoxetine Hydrochloride)	II-1160
Neuragon-A (Amitriptyline Hydrochloride; Perphenazine)	II-124
Neuragon-B (Amitriptyline Hydrochloride; Perphenazine)	II-124
Neurodex (Cyanocobalamin)	II-661
Neurotol (Carbamazepine)	II-418
Neurotop (Carbamazepine)	II-418

International brand name (Generic name)	Page no.
Neurotop Retard (Carbamazepine)	II-418
Neutrogena T/Sal (Ketoconazole)	II-1530
Neutromax (Filgrastim)	II-1126
Neutron (Lansoprazole)	II-1569
Neutronorm (Cimetidine Hydrochloride)	II-568
Nevimune (Nevirapine)	II-1952
Newcillin (Penicillin V Potassium)	II-2142
Newkentax (Levamisole Hydrochloride)	II-1598
Newporine (Cefaclor)	II-444
New-Rexan (Methocarbamol)	II-1768
Newspar (Sparfloxacin)	II-2479
Newtaxime (Cefotaxime Sodium)	II-474
Newtock (Formoterol Fumarate)	II-1214
Newtolide (Hydrochlorothiazide)	II-1348
Nex (Nizatidine)	II-1992
Nexxair (Beclomethasone Dipropionate)	II-279
N-Flox (Norfloxacin)	II-1997
Niagestine (Megestrol Acetate)	II-1723
Niar (Selegiline Hydrochloride)	II-2437
Nibromin (Prochlorperazine)	II-2258
NIC (Lorazepam)	II-1678
Nica (Amikacin Sulfate)	II-101
Nicabate (Nicotine)	II-1961
Nicabate TTS (Nicotine)	II-1961
Nicangin (Niacin)	II-1956
Nicardal (Nicardipine Hydrochloride)	II-1958
Nicetal (Isoniazid)	II-1496
Nichogencin (Gentamicin Sulfate)	II-1279
Nicobate CQ Clear (Nicotine)	II-1961
Nicobid (Niacin)	II-1956
Nicodel (Nicardipine Hydrochloride)	II-1958
Nicolan (Nicotine)	II-1961
Nicolan Light (Nicotine)	II-1961
Niconacid (Niacin)	II-1956
Nicopatch (Nicotine)	II-1961
Nicorest (Nicotine)	II-1961
Nicorette Fruit (Nicotine)	II-1961
Nicorette Inhaler (Nicotine)	II-1961
Nicorette Menthe (Nicotine)	II-1961
Nicorette Orange (Nicotine)	II-1961
Nicorette Orange sans sucre (Nicotine)	II-1961
Nicostop (Nicotine)	II-1961
Nicotibine (Isoniazid)	II-1496
Nicotinell (Nicotine)	II-1961
Nicotinell Chewing Gum (Nicotine)	II-1961
Nicotinell Fruit sans sucre (Nicotine)	II-1961
Nicotinell Lozenge (Nicotine)	II-1961
Nicotinell Menthe sans sucre (Nicotine)	II-1961
Nicotinell Mint Lozenge (Nicotine)	II-1961
Nicotinell TTS (Nicotine)	II-1961
Nicotrans (Nicotine)	II-1961
Nicozid (Isoniazid)	II-1496
Nida (Metronidazole)	II-1812
Nidip (Nimodipine)	II-1974
Nifangin (Nifedipine)	II-1967
Nifar (Nifedipine)	II-1967
Nifdemin (Nifedipine)	II-1967
Nifebene (Nifedipine)	II-1967
Nifecard (Nifedipine)	II-1967
Nifecor (Nifedipine)	II-1967
Nifedepat (Nifedipine)	II-1967
Nifedicor (Nifedipine)	II-1967
Nifedilat (Nifedipine)	II-1967
Nifedin (Nifedipine)	II-1967
Nifedine (Nifedipine)	II-1967
Nifedipres (Nifedipine)	II-1967
Nifedirex LP (Nifedipine)	II-1967
Nifehexal (Nifedipine)	II-1967
Nifelat (Nifedipine)	II-1967
Nifelat-Q (Nifedipine)	II-1967
Nifensar (Nifedipine)	II-1967
Nifensar Retard (Nifedipine)	II-1967
Nifestad (Nifedipine)	II-1967
Nificard (Nifedipine)	II-1967
Nifidine (Nifedipine)	II-1967
Nifipen (Nifedipine)	II-1967

International brand name (Generic name)	Page no.
Nifolin (Folic Acid)	II-1208
Nikacid (Niacin)	II-1956
Nikofrenon (Nicotine)	II-1961
Nilapur (Acetaminophen)	II-11
Nilatika (Metoclopramide Hydrochloride)	II-1798
Nilozanoc (Miconazole)	II-1820
Nimaz (Loperamide Hydrochloride)	II-1664
Nimegen (Isotretinoin)	II-1510
Nimicor (Nicardipine Hydrochloride)	II-1958
Nincort (Triamcinolone Acetonide)	II-2701
Nindral (Flurazepam Hydrochloride)	II-1175
Niong Retard (Nitroglycerin)	II-1984
Niotal (Flurazepam Hydrochloride)	II-1175
Niotal (Zolpidem Tartrate)	II-2842
Nipine (Nifedipine)	II-1967
Nipurol (Allopurinol)	II-77
Niquitin (Nicotine)	II-1961
Niquitin CQ (Nicotine)	II-1961
Niquitin sans sucre (Nicotine)	II-1961
Niquitinclear (Nicotine)	II-1961
Nirmadil (Felodipine)	II-1103
Nirulid (Amiloride Hydrochloride)	II-103
Nirvan (Alprazolam)	II-85
Nirvaxal (Chlordiazepoxide Hydrochloride; Clidinium Bromide)	II-541
Nisis (Valsartan)	II-2759
Nisisco (Hydrochlorothiazide; Valsartan)	II-1366
Nisoldin (Nisoldipine)	II-1976
Nisona (Prednisone)	II-2240
Nitan (Nitroprusside, Sodium)	II-1990
Nitorol (Isosorbide Dinitrate)	II-1502
Nitradisc (Nitroglycerin)	II-1984
Nitradisc Pad (Nitroglycerin)	II-1984
Nitradisc TTS (Nitroglycerin)	II-1984
Nitramin (Isosorbide Mononitrate)	II-1507
Nitrest (Zolpidem Tartrate)	II-2842
Nit-Ret (Nitroglycerin)	II-1984
Nitriderm TTS (Nitroglycerin)	II-1984
Nitro Dur TTS (Nitroglycerin)	II-1984
Nitro Mack (Nitroglycerin)	II-1984
Nitro Mack Retard (Nitroglycerin)	II-1984
Nitro Retard (Nitroglycerin)	II-1984
Nitro Rorer (Nitroglycerin)	II-1984
Nitrobaat (Nitroglycerin)	II-1984
Nitrobid (Nitroglycerin)	II-1984
Nitrobid Oint (Nitroglycerin)	II-1984
Nitrocerin (Nitroglycerin)	II-1984
Nitrocine (Nitroglycerin)	II-1984
Nitrocine 5 (Nitroglycerin)	II-1984
Nitrocontin (Nitroglycerin)	II-1984
Nitrocontin Continus (Nitroglycerin)	II-1984
NitroCor (Nitroglycerin)	II-1984
Nitroderm TTS (Nitroglycerin)	II-1984
Nitroderm TTS Ext (Nitroglycerin)	II-1984
Nitroderm TTS-5 (Nitroglycerin)	II-1984
Nitro-Dur 10 (Nitroglycerin)	II-1984
Nitrodyl (Nitroglycerin)	II-1984
Nitrodyl TTS (Nitroglycerin)	II-1984
Nitro-Gesanit Retard (Nitroglycerin)	II-1984
Nitrogesic (Nitroglycerin)	II-1984
Nitroglin (Nitroglycerin)	II-1984
Nitrol (Isosorbide Dinitrate)	II-1502
Nitrol R (Isosorbide Dinitrate)	II-1502
Nitrolong (Nitroglycerin)	II-1984
Nitro-Mack Retard (Nitroglycerin)	II-1984
Nitromack Retard (Nitroglycerin)	II-1984
Nitro-M-Bid (Nitroglycerin)	II-1984
Nitromex (Nitroglycerin)	II-1984
Nitromint (Nitroglycerin)	II-1984
Nitromint Aerosol (Nitroglycerin)	II-1984
Nitromint Retard (Nitroglycerin)	II-1984
Nitrong Retard (Nitroglycerin)	II-1984
Nitrong-SR (Nitroglycerin)	II-1984
Nitropen (Nitroglycerin)	II-1984
Nitro-Pflaster (Nitroglycerin)	II-1984
Nitroplast (Nitroglycerin)	II-1984

International brand name (Generic name)	Page no.
Nitroprol (Nitroglycerin)	II-1984
Nitropront (Nitroglycerin)	II-1984
Nitroprontan (Nitroglycerin)	II-1984
Nitroprusiato de sodio-ecar (Nitroprusside, Sodium)	II-1990
Nitrorectal (Nitroglycerin)	II-1984
Nitrosid (Isosorbide Dinitrate)	II-1502
Nitrosid Retard (Isosorbide Dinitrate)	II-1502
Nitrosorbide (Isosorbide Dinitrate)	II-1502
Nitrosorbon (Isosorbide Dinitrate)	II-1502
Nitrourean (Carmustine)	II-434
Nitrozell Retard (Nitroglycerin)	II-1984
Nitrumon (Carmustine)	II-434
Nivalen (Diazepam)	II-740
Nivalin (Galantamine Hydrobromide)	II-1247
Nivaquine (Chloroquine)	II-544
Nivaquine DP (Chloroquine)	II-544
Nivoflox (Ciprofloxacin Hydrochloride)	II-573
Niyaplat (Cisplatin)	II-589
Niz Creme (Ketoconazole)	II-1530
Niz Shampoo (Ketoconazole)	II-1530
Nizax (Nizatidine)	II-1992
Nizaxid (Nizatidine)	II-1992
Nizoral Cream and Tablets (Ketoconazole)	II-1530
Nizoral Tabs and Cream (Ketoconazole)	II-1530
Noaler (Cromolyn Sodium)	II-656
Noaler Nasal (Cromolyn Sodium)	II-656
Noan (Diazepam)	II-740
Nobec (Beclomethasone Dipropionate)	II-279
Nobfelon (Ibuprofen)	II-1411
Nobgen (Ibuprofen)	II-1411
Nobzol-1 (Fluconazole)	II-1136
Nobzol-2 (Fluconazole)	II-1136
Nocid (Omeprazole)	II-2034
Noctazepam (Oxazepam)	II-2063
Nodiol (Ethinyl Estradiol; Norethindrone)	II-1055
Nofaxin (Levofloxacin)	II-1607
Noglucor (Tolbutamide)	II-2650
Nolcot (Betamethasone Valerate)	II-305
Nolectin (Captopril)	II-411
Noloten (Propranolol Hydrochloride)	II-2287
Noltam (Tamoxifen Citrate)	II-2539
Nolvadex-D (Tamoxifen Citrate)	II-2539
Nomcramp (Dicyclomine Hydrochloride)	II-763
Nonalges (Tramadol Hydrochloride)	II-2674
Nonasma (Metaproterenol Sulfate)	II-1754
Nonpolin (Hydralazine Hydrochloride)	II-1346
Nonspi (Pindolol)	II-2192
Noperten (Lisinopril)	II-1648
Nopil (Sulfamethoxazole; Trimethoprim)	II-2500
Noprenia (Risperidone)	II-2374
Nopres (Fluoxetine Hydrochloride)	II-1160
Noprose (Norfloxacin)	II-1997
Noratin (Loratadine)	II-1675
Norbactin (Norfloxacin)	II-1997
Norbactin Eye Drops (Norfloxacin)	II-1997
Norbiotic (Norfloxacin)	II-1997
Norboral (Glyburide)	II-1297
Norciden (Danazol)	II-699
Norcolut (Norethindrone)	II-1996
Nor-Dacef (Cefadroxil Monohydrate)	II-447
Nordet (Ethinyl Estradiol; Levonorgestrel)	II-1047
Nordette (Ethinyl Estradiol; Levonorgestrel)	II-1047
Nordotol (Carbamazepine)	II-418
Norelut (Norethindrone)	II-1996
Nor-Ethis (Norethindrone)	II-1996
Norexan (Mitoxantrone Hydrochloride)	II-1856
Norfenon (Propafenone Hydrochloride)	II-2274
Norflam-T (Ibuprofen)	II-1411
Norflox (Norfloxacin)	II-1997
Norflox Eye (Norfloxacin)	II-1997
Norflox-AZU (Norfloxacin)	II-1997
Norgalax (Docusate Sodium)	II-841
Norgluc (Chlorpropamide)	II-554
Norglycin (Tolazamide)	II-2649
Noriday (Norethindrone)	II-1996
Noriday 28 (Norethindrone)	II-1996
Norilafin (Sulindac)	II-2512
Noripam (Oxazepam)	II-2063
Noritacin (Norfloxacin)	II-1997
Noritis (Ibuprofen)	II-1411
Noritren (Nortriptyline Hydrochloride)	II-2002
Norivite (Cyanocobalamin)	II-661
Norivite-12 (Cyanocobalamin)	II-661
Norlevo (Levonorgestrel)	II-1614
Norline (Nortriptyline Hydrochloride)	II-2002
Norluten (Norethindrone)	II-1996
Normadate (Labetalol Hydrochloride)	II-1545
Normadil (Nifedipine)	II-1967
Normalin (Guanethidine Monosulfate)	II-1321
Normalip (Fenofibrate)	II-1105
Normalmin (Prochlorperazine)	II-2258
Normalol (Atenolol)	II-222
Normastin (Metoclopramide Hydrochloride)	II-1798
Normaten (Atenolol)	II-222
Normaton (Buspirone Hydrochloride)	II-382
Normax Eye Ear Drops (Norfloxacin)	II-1997
Normelan (Metolazone)	II-1802
Nor-Metrogel (Metronidazole)	II-1812
Normide (Chlordiazepoxide Hydrochloride)	II-539
Normison (Temazepam)	II-2556
Normiten (Atenolol)	II-222
Normodipine (Amlodipine Besylate)	II-125
Normofat (Simvastatin)	II-2454
Normoglic (Chlorpropamide)	II-554
Normolax (Lactulose)	II-1550
Normolip (Fenofibrate)	II-1105
Normolip (Gemfibrozil)	II-1269
Normopresan (Clonidine Hydrochloride)	II-629
Normorytmin (Propafenone Hydrochloride)	II-2274
Norocin (Norfloxacin)	II-1997
Noroxin Oftalmico (Norfloxacin)	II-1997
Noroxin Ophthalmic (Norfloxacin)	II-1997
Noroxine (Norfloxacin)	II-1997
Norpace Retard (Disopyramide Phosphate)	II-825
Norpaso (Disopyramide Phosphate)	II-825
Norphin (Buprenorphine)	II-363
Norpin (Norepinephrine Bitartrate)	II-1994
Norplant 36 (Levonorgestrel)	II-1614
Norpress (Nortriptyline Hydrochloride)	II-2002
Norpurisine (Norfloxacin)	II-1997
Norset (Mirtazapine)	II-1847
Norspor (Itraconazole)	II-1517
Norswel (Naproxen)	II-1924
Nortimil (Desipramine Hydrochloride)	II-716
Norton (Ibuprofen)	II-1411
Nortrilen (Nortriptyline Hydrochloride)	II-2002
Nortrix (Nortriptyline Hydrochloride)	II-2002
Nortyline (Nortriptyline Hydrochloride)	II-2002
Norum (Acyclovir)	II-33
Norvas (Amlodipine Besylate)	II-125
Norvask (Amlodipine Besylate)	II-125
Nor-Vastina (Simvastatin)	II-2454
Norventyl (Nortriptyline Hydrochloride)	II-2002
Nosemin (Cetirizine Hydrochloride)	II-529
Nosim (Isosorbide Dinitrate)	II-1502
Nositrol (Hydrocortisone Sodium Succinate)	II-1379
Nosmin (Cetirizine Hydrochloride)	II-529
Notamin (Loratadine)	II-1675
Noten (Atenolol)	II-222
Notensyl (Dicyclomine Hydrochloride)	II-763
No-Ton (Nabumetone)	II-1909
No-Uric (Allopurinol)	II-77
Novabritine (Amoxicillin)	II-131
Novacef (Cefixime)	II-466
Noval (Timolol)	II-2627
Noval (Travoprost)	II-2685
Novales (Pravastatin Sodium)	II-2224
Novamilor (Amiloride Hydrochloride; Hydrochlorothiazide)	II-105
Novamin (Prochlorperazine)	II-2258
Novamox (Amoxicillin)	II-131
Novamoxin (Amoxicillin)	II-131
Novanaest purum 1% (Procaine Hydrochloride)	II-2253
Novanaest purum 2% (Procaine Hydrochloride)	II-2253
Novantron (Mitoxantrone Hydrochloride)	II-1856
Nova-Pam (Chlordiazepoxide Hydrochloride)	II-539
Novapen (Dicloxacillin Sodium)	II-761
Novasen (Aspirin)	II-206
Novasone Cream (Mometasone Furoate)	II-1866
Novasone Lotion (Mometasone Furoate)	II-1866
Novasone Ointment (Mometasone Furoate)	II-1866
Novastep (Ethinyl Estradiol; Levonorgestrel)	II-1047
Novasulfon (Dapsone)	II-702
Novatec (Lisinopril)	II-1648
Novatrex (Methotrexate Sodium)	II-1772
Novazole (Metronidazole)	II-1812
Novazyd (Hydrochlorothiazide; Lisinopril)	II-1352
Novecin (Ofloxacin)	II-2015
Noveldexis (Cisplatin)	II-589
Novelon (Desogestrel; Ethinyl Estradiol)	II-725
Novenzymin (Amoxicillin)	II-131
Noverme (Mebendazole)	II-1711
Novhepar (Lorazepam)	II-1678
Novidorm (Triazolam)	II-2715
Novitropan (Oxybutynin)	II-2070
Novo Nifedin (Nifedipine)	II-1967
Novo-Ampicillin (Ampicillin)	II-170
Novo-AZT (Zidovudine)	II-2822
Novobutamide (Tolbutamide)	II-2650
Novochlorhydrate (Chloral Hydrate)	II-534
Novocillin (Penicillin G Procaine)	II-2140
Novocimetine (Cimetidine Hydrochloride)	II-568
Novo-Clopate (Clorazepate Dipotassium)	II-638
Novo-Difenac (Diclofenac)	II-748
Novodigal (Digoxin)	II-780
Novodil (Dipyridamole)	II-821
Novodorm (Triazolam)	II-2715
Novofem (Estradiol; Norethindrone Acetate)	II-1011
Novofen (Tamoxifen Citrate)	II-2539
Novogent (Ibuprofen)	II-1411
Novohydroxyzin (Hydroxyzine)	II-1398
Novo-Hylazin (Hydralazine Hydrochloride)	II-1346
Novo-Keto-EC (Ketoprofen)	II-1533
Novolet 30 70 (Insulin (Human, Isophane/ Regular))	II-1456
Novolexin (Cephalexin)	II-520
Novolin ge 30/70 (Insulin (Human, Isophane/ Regular))	II-1456
Novolin ge Lente (Insulin (Human, Lente))	II-1456
Novolin ge NPH (Insulin (Human, Isophane))	II-1455
Novo-lorazem (Lorazepam)	II-1678
Novolten (Diclofenac)	II-748
Novomedopa (Methyldopa)	II-1778
Novomethacin (Indomethacin)	II-1443
NovoMix 30 (Insulin Aspart)	II-1456
Novonaprox (Naproxen)	II-1924
Novoniacin (Niacin)	II-1956
Novonidazole (Metronidazole)	II-1812
NovoNorm (Repaglinide)	II-2343
Novopen-G (Penicillin G Potassium)	II-2137
Novopen-VK (Penicillin V Potassium)	II-2142
Novoperidol (Haloperidol)	II-1328
Novo-Pindol (Pindolol)	II-2192
Novopirocam (Piroxicam)	II-2205
Novopoxide (Chlordiazepoxide Hydrochloride)	II-539
Novopressan (Verapamil Hydrochloride)	II-2777
Novoprofen (Ibuprofen)	II-1411
Novoprotect (Amitriptyline Hydrochloride)	II-119
Novopulmon (Budesonide)	II-347
Novo-ranidine (Ranitidine Hydrochloride)	II-2334
Novosalmol (Albuterol)	II-47
Novosecobarb (Secobarbital Sodium)	II-2435
Novosef (Ceftriaxone Sodium)	II-503
Novosoxazole (Sulfisoxazole)	II-2510
Novospiroton (Spironolactone)	II-2483

International brand name (Generic name)	Page no.
Novo-Sundac (Sulindac)	II-2512
Novoter (Fluocinonide)	II-1156
Novotetra (Tetracycline Hydrochloride)	II-2585
Novo-Timol (Timolol)	II-2627
Novotrimel (Sulfamethoxazole; Trimethoprim)	II-2500
Novo-Veramil (Verapamil Hydrochloride)	II-2777
Novo-VK (Penicillin V Potassium)	II-2142
Novphyllin (Aminophylline)	II-106
Novumtrax (Cytarabine)	II-683
Novynette (Desogestrel; Ethinyl Estradiol)	II-725
Noxraxin (Miconazole)	II-1820
Noxworm (Mebendazole)	II-1711
Nubain SP (Nalbuphine Hydrochloride)	II-1917
Nucotil nasenspray (Desmopressin Acetate)	II-723
Nuctalon (Estazolam)	II-983
Nuctane (Phenytoin Sodium)	II-2175
Nuctane (Triazolam)	II-2715
Nuctulon (Estazolam)	II-983
Nudep (Sertraline Hydrochloride)	II-2439
Nudopa (Methyldopa)	II-1778
Nuelin (Theophylline)	II-2593
Nuelin SA (Theophylline)	II-2593
Nuelin SR (Theophylline)	II-2593
Nufaclapide (Ticlopidine Hydrochloride)	II-2622
Nufaclav (Amoxicillin; Clavulanate Potassium)	II-139
Nufaclind (Clindamycin)	II-605
Nufafloqo (Ofloxacin)	II-2015
Nufatrac (Itraconazole)	II-1517
Nufex (Cephalexin)	II-520
Nuhair (Minoxidil)	II-1845
Nu-K (Potassium Chloride)	II-2215
Nulcer (Cimetidine Hydrochloride)	II-568
Numark (Budesonide)	II-347
Numotac (Isoetharine Hydrochloride)	II-1495
Nu-Pirox (Piroxicam)	II-2205
Nuprafem (Naproxen)	II-1924
Nureflex (Ibuprofen)	II-1411
Nuril (Enalapril Maleate)	II-913
Nu-Seals (Aspirin)	II-206
Nutracort (Hydrocortisone Acetate)	II-1373
Nuvapen (Ampicillin)	II-170
Nuzak (Fluoxetine Hydrochloride)	II-1160
Nyaderm (Nystatin)	II-2005
Nyclin (Niacin)	II-1956
Nycopren (Naproxen)	II-1924
Nyefax Retard (Nifedipine)	II-1967
Nylipton (Trifluoperazine Hydrochloride)	II-2717
Nylol (Timolol)	II-2627
Nylol (Travoprost)	II-2685
Nyogel (Timolol)	II-2627
Nyogel LP (Timolol)	II-2627
Nyolol (Timolol)	II-2627
Nyolol (Travoprost)	II-2685
Nyolol Gel (Timolol)	II-2627
Nyolol Gel (Travoprost)	II-2685
Nyracta (Rosiglitazone Maleate)	II-2405
Nysconitrine (Nitroglycerin)	II-1984
Nystacid (Nystatin)	II-2005
Nystan (Nystatin)	II-2005
Nystatin (Nystatin)	II-2005
Nytol (Diphenhydramine Hydrochloride)	II-813
Nytol Quickgels (Diphenhydramine Hydrochloride)	II-813
O	
Oasil (Chlordiazepoxide Hydrochloride)	II-539
Oasil (Meprobamate)	II-1738
Oasil-Simes (Meprobamate)	II-1738
Obide (Ofloxacin)	II-2015
Obogen (Gentamicin Sulfate)	II-1279
Obracin (Tobramycin Sulfate)	II-2646
Obry (Tobramycin)	II-2643
Occidal (Ofloxacin)	II-2015
Oceral (Oxiconazole Nitrate)	II-2069
Oceral GB (Oxiconazole Nitrate)	II-2069

International brand name (Generic name)	Page no.
Ocid (Omeprazole)	II-2034
O.C.M. (Chlordiazepoxide Hydrochloride)	II-539
Ocsaar (Losartan Potassium)	II-1682
Octagam (Immune Globulin (Human))	II-1434
Octicaina (Benzocaine)	II-289
Octim (Desmopressin Acetate)	II-723
Octostim (Desmopressin Acetate)	II-723
Ocucarpine (Pilocarpine)	II-2180
Ocuchloram (Chloramphenicol)	II-536
Ocuflur (Flurbiprofen)	II-1177
Ocugenta (Gentamicin Sulfate)	II-1279
Ocumicin (Tobramycin)	II-2643
Ocupres (Timolol)	II-2627
Ocupres (Travoprost)	II-2685
Ocuracin (Tobramycin)	II-2643
Ocusert P-20 (Pilocarpine)	II-2180
Ocusert P-40 (Pilocarpine)	II-2180
Ocusert Pilo-20 (Pilocarpine)	II-2180
Ocusert Pilo-40 (Pilocarpine)	II-2180
Ocusert Pilocarpine (Pilocarpine)	II-2180
Odace (Trandolapril)	II-2677
Odemex (Furosemide)	II-1237
Odetol (Ethambutol Hydrochloride)	II-1039
Odipin (Nifedipine)	II-1967
Odoxil (Cefadroxil Monohydrate)	II-447
Odranal (Bupropion Hydrochloride)	II-368
Odyne (Flutamide)	II-1181
Oedemex (Furosemide)	II-1237
Oesclim (Estradiol)	II-986
Oestring (Estradiol)	II-986
Oestrodose (Estradiol)	II-986
Oestro-Feminal (Estrogens, Conjugated)	II-1019
Oestrogel (Estradiol)	II-986
Ofal (Timolol)	II-2627
Ofal (Travoprost)	II-2685
Ofan (Timolol)	II-2627
Ofan (Travoprost)	II-2685
Ofcin (Ofloxacin)	II-2015
Ofenac (Diclofenac)	II-748
Oflin (Ofloxacin)	II-2015
Oflocee (Ofloxacin)	II-2015
Oflocet (Ofloxacin)	II-2015
Oflocin (Ofloxacin)	II-2015
Oflodal (Ofloxacin)	II-2015
Oflodex (Ofloxacin)	II-2015
O-Flox (Ofloxacin)	II-2015
Oflox (Ofloxacin)	II-2015
Ofloxin (Ofloxacin)	II-2015
Oframax (Ceftriaxone Sodium)	II-503
Oftacin (Chloramphenicol)	II-536
Oftagen (Gentamicin Sulfate)	II-1279
Oftalmogenta (Gentamicin Sulfate)	II-1279
Oftalmolosa Cusi Eritromicina (Erythromycin)	II-960
Oftamolets (Erythromycin)	II-960
Oftan Timolol (Timolol)	II-2627
Oftan-Akvakol (Chloramphenicol)	II-536
Oftan-Dexa (Dexamethasone)	II-730
Oftan-Metaoksedrin (Phenylephrine Hydrochloride)	II-2173
Oftan-Pilocarpin (Pilocarpine)	II-2180
Ofticlin (Tetracycline Hydrochloride)	II-2585
Ogast (Lansoprazole)	II-1569
Ogastro (Lansoprazole)	II-1569
Oidisan (Antipyrine; Benzocaine)	II-187
Okacin (Lomefloxacin Hydrochloride)	II-1658
Okavax (Varicella Vaccine)	II-2767
Okinazole (Oxiconazole Nitrate)	II-2069
Olansek (Olanzapine)	II-2022
Oleanz (Olanzapine)	II-2022
Oleomycetin (Chloramphenicol)	II-536
Olexin (Omeprazole)	II-2034
Olfen (Diclofenac)	II-748
Olfen Gel (Diclofenac)	II-748
Olfen Roll-On (Diclofenac)	II-748
Olfen-75 SR (Diclofenac)	II-748
Oliphenicol (Chloramphenicol)	II-536

International brand name (Generic name)	Page no.
Oltens Ge (Captopril)	II-411
Olyster (Terazosin Hydrochloride)	II-2566
Omca (Fluphenazine Hydrochloride)	II-1172
Omed (Omeprazole)	II-2034
Omedar (Omeprazole)	II-2034
Omelon (Omeprazole)	II-2034
OMEP (Omeprazole)	II-2034
Omepral (Omeprazole)	II-2034
Omeprazon (Omeprazole)	II-2034
Omepril (Omeprazole)	II-2034
Omeq (Omeprazole)	II-2034
Omesec (Omeprazole)	II-2034
Omez (Omeprazole)	II-2034
Omezin (Omeprazole)	II-2034
Omezol (Omeprazole)	II-2034
Omezole (Omeprazole)	II-2034
Omezzol (Omeprazole)	II-2034
Omisec (Omeprazole)	II-2034
Omizac (Omeprazole)	II-2034
Omnalio (Chlordiazepoxide Hydrochloride)	II-539
Omnatax (Cefotaxime Sodium)	II-474
Omnaze (Tetracycline Hydrochloride)	II-2585
Omnic (Tamsulosin Hydrochloride)	II-2544
Omnidol (Tramadol Hydrochloride)	II-2674
Omnidrox (Cefadroxil Monohydrate)	II-447
Omnipen (Ampicillin)	II-170
Omniquin (Lomefloxacin Hydrochloride)	II-1658
OMP (Omeprazole)	II-2034
Omsat (Sulfamethoxazole; Trimethoprim)	II-2500
OMZ (Omeprazole)	II-2034
Onaven (Thiothixene)	II-2610
Oncetam (Tamoxifen Citrate)	II-2539
Onco-Carbide (Hydroxyurea)	II-1394
Oncocarbin (Carboplatin)	II-430
Oncodocel (Docetaxel)	II-837
Oncotecan (Topotecan Hydrochloride)	II-2666
OncoTice (BCG Vaccine)	II-276
OncoTICE (BCG Vaccine)	II-276
Oncotron (Mitoxantrone Hydrochloride)	II-1856
Oneflu (Fluconazole)	II-1136
Onemer (Ketorolac Tromethamine)	II-1537
Onikin (Amikacin Sulfate)	II-101
Oniria (Quazepam)	II-2298
Onkotrone (Mitoxantrone Hydrochloride)	II-1856
Onsia (Ondansetron Hydrochloride)	II-2039
Ontop (Lomefloxacin Hydrochloride)	II-1658
Onzayt (Dirithromycin)	II-824
O.P. Pain (Tramadol Hydrochloride)	II-2674
Opal (Omeprazole)	II-2034
Opamox (Oxazepam)	II-2063
O.P.D. (Pilocarpine)	II-2180
Opebrin (Cephradine)	II-526
Opeprim (Mitotane)	II-1855
Operan (Ofloxacin)	II-2015
Operzine (Trifluoperazine Hydrochloride)	II-2717
Opheryl (Orphenadrine Citrate)	II-2049
Ophtagram (Gentamicin Sulfate)	II-1279
Ophtho-Chloram (Chloramphenicol)	II-536
Opistan (Meperidine Hydrochloride)	II-1733
Oplat (Oxaliplatin)	II-2056
Oposim (Propranolol Hydrochloride)	II-2287
Oppvir (Acyclovir)	II-33
Opram (Metoclopramide Hydrochloride)	II-1798
Oprax (Omeprazole)	II-2034
Optamide (Sulfacetamide Sodium)	II-2497
Optanac (Diclofenac)	II-748
Opthaflox (Ciprofloxacin Hydrochloride)	II-573
Opthavir (Acyclovir)	II-33
Opticide (Praziquantel)	II-2228
Opticle (Chloramphenicol)	II-536
Opticron (Cromolyn Sodium)	II-656
Optifen (Ibuprofen)	II-1411
Optigen (Gentamicin Sulfate)	II-1279
Opti-Genta (Gentamicin Sulfate)	II-1279
Optilast (Azelastine)	II-247
Optimin (Loratadine)	II-1675

International brand name (Generic name)	Page no.
Optimol (Timolol)	II-2627
Optimol (Travoprost)	II-2685
Optimycin (Gentamicin Sulfate)	II-1279
Optin (Sulfacetamide Sodium)	II-2497
Optipress (Betaxolol Hydrochloride)	II-307
Optisol (Sulfacetamide Sodium)	II-2497
Optistin (Phenylephrine Hydrochloride)	II-2173
Optisulin (Insulin Glargine)	II-1461
Optium (Amoxicillin)	II-131
Optrex (Cromolyn Sodium)	II-656
Optruma (Raloxifene Hydrochloride)	II-2326
Opturem (Ibuprofen)	II-1411
Opulis (Desloratadine)	II-721
OPV-Merieux (Polio Vaccine, Oral Live)	II-2210
Ora (Lidocaine)	II-1628
Orabet (Metformin Hydrochloride)	II-1760
Orabet (Tolbutamide)	II-2650
Orabetic (Glyburide)	II-1297
Oracef (Cephalexin)	II-520
Oracefal (Cefadroxil Monohydrate)	II-447
Oracillin VK (Penicillin V Potassium)	II-2142
Oraday (Atenolol)	II-222
Oradexon (Dexamethasone)	II-730
Oradroxil (Cefadroxil Monohydrate)	II-447
Orafer (Ferrous Sulfate)	II-1122
Oral Polio Vaccine (Polio Vaccine, Oral Live)	II-2210
Oral Poliomyelitis Vaccine-Sabine (Polio Vaccine, Oral Live)	II-2210
Oral Virelon (Polio Vaccine, Oral Live)	II-2210
Oralten Troche (Clotrimazole)	II-640
Oramedy (Triamcinolone Acetonide)	II-2701
Oramide (Loperamide Hydrochloride)	II-1664
Oramorph (Morphine Sulfate)	II-1877
Oranor (Norfloxacin)	II-1997
Oranyst (Nystatin)	II-2005
Orap (1 mg) (Pimozide)	II-2189
Orap (4 mg) (Pimozide)	II-2189
Orap Forte (4 mg) (Pimozide)	II-2189
Orasthin (Oxytocin)	II-2082
Oratane (Isotretinoin)	II-1510
Oratrol (Acetazolamide)	II-28
Oravir (Famciclovir)	II-1090
Oraxim (Cefuroxime)	II-507
Orbenin (Dicloxacillin Sodium)	II-761
Orbinamon (Thiothixene)	II-2610
Orelox (Cefpodoxime Proxetil)	II-484
Oren (Ibuprofen)	II-1411
Orencyclin F-500 (Tetracycline Hydrochloride)	II-2585
Orfarin (Warfarin Sodium)	II-2804
Orfidal (Lorazepam)	II-1678
Orfil (Valproate Sodium)	II-2749
Orfiril (Valproate Sodium)	II-2749
Orfiril (Valproic Acid)	II-2755
Orfiril Retard (Valproate Sodium)	II-2749
Orgasulin Rapid (Insulin (Human Recombinant))	II-1454
Orgasuline 30/70 (Insulin (Human, Isophane/ Regular))	II-1456
Orgasuline NPH (Insulin (Human, Isophane))	II-1455
Oricef (Cefazolin Sodium)	II-452
Oricyclin (Tetracycline Hydrochloride)	II-2585
Oriphex (Cephalexin)	II-520
Oriprim DS (Sulfamethoxazole; Trimethoprim)	II-2500
Oritaxim (Cefotaxime Sodium)	II-474
Oritaxime (Cefotaxime Sodium)	II-474
Orix (Nifedipine)	II-1967
Orizolin (Cefazolin Sodium)	II-452
Orlest (Ethinyl Estradiol; Norethindrone)	II-1055
Orlobin (Amikacin Sulfate)	II-101
Orocal (Calcium Carbonate)	II-401
Orocin (Ofloxacin)	II-2015
Orodiabin (Chlorpropamide)	II-554
Oroken (Cefixime)	II-466
Oroxine (Levothyroxine Sodium)	II-1618
Orpherin (Orphenadrine Citrate)	II-2049
Orsanac (Norfloxacin)	II-1997
Orsanil (Thioridazine Hydrochloride)	II-2605
Orsinon (Tolbutamide)	II-2650
Orstanorm (Dihydroergotamine Mesylate)	II-792
Ortho 1 35 (Ethinyl Estradiol; Norethindrone)	II-1055
Ortho 7 7 7 (Ethinyl Estradiol; Norethindrone)	II-1055
Ortho-Novum 1 35 (Ethinyl Estradiol; Norethindrone)	II-1055
Ortho-Novum 1 50 (Ethinyl Estradiol; Norethindrone)	II-1055
Ortopsique (Diazepam)	II-740
Ortoton (Methocarbamol)	II-1768
Ortrip (Nortriptyline Hydrochloride)	II-2002
Orucote (Ketoprofen)	II-1533
Orudis E-100 (Ketoprofen)	II-1533
Orudis EC (Ketoprofen)	II-1533
Orudis R-PR (Ketoprofen)	II-1533
Orulop (Loperamide Hydrochloride)	II-1664
Oruvail EC (Ketoprofen)	II-1533
Orvek (Penicillin V Potassium)	II-2142
Oryzanin (Thiamine Hydrochloride)	II-2602
Os-Cal (Calcium Carbonate)	II-401
Osdronat (Alendronate Sodium)	II-70
Oseum (Calcitonin (Salmon))	II-397
Osficar (Alendronate Sodium)	II-70
Oslene (Alendronate Sodium)	II-70
Osmo-Adalat (Nifedipine)	II-1967
Ospamox (Amoxicillin)	II-131
Ospen (Penicillin V Potassium)	II-2142
Ospen 250 (Penicillin V Potassium)	II-2142
Ospexin (Cephalexin)	II-520
Ospronim (Pentazocine Lactate)	II-2147
Ospur Ca 500 (Calcium Carbonate)	II-401
Ossin (Sodium Fluoride)	II-2465
Ostarin (Ibuprofen)	II-1411
Osteluc (Etodolac)	II-1076
Osteocal 500 (Calcium Carbonate)	II-401
Osteofar (Alendronate Sodium)	II-70
Osteoflam (Diclofenac)	II-748
Osteomin (Calcium Carbonate)	II-401
Osteotop (Etidronate Disodium)	II-1073
Osteovan (Alendronate Sodium)	II-70
Osteral (Piroxicam)	II-2205
Osticalcin (Alendronate Sodium)	II-70
Ostofen (Ibuprofen)	II-1411
Ostofen (Ketoprofen)	II-1533
Osyrol (Spironolactone)	II-2483
Otarex (Hydroxyzine)	II-1398
Otised (Antipyrine; Benzocaine)	II-187
Otosec (Ciprofloxacin Hydrochloride)	II-573
Otosec HC (Ciprofloxacin Hydrochloride; Hydrocortisone)	II-588
Otosporin (Hydrocortisone; Neomycin Sulfate; Polymyxin B Sulfate)	II-1384
Otozonbase (Hydrocortisone)	II-1369
Otrasel (Selegiline Hydrochloride)	II-2437
Otreon (Cefpodoxime Proxetil)	II-484
Otrozol (Metronidazole)	II-1812
Ottogenta (Gentamicin Sulfate)	II-1279
Ottovit (Cyanocobalamin)	II-661
Ottovit (Thiamine Hydrochloride)	II-2602
Ovasta (Lovastatin)	II-1688
Oviskin (Betamethasone Dipropionate)	II-301
Ovoplex 30-150 (Ethinyl Estradiol; Levonorgestrel)	II-1047
Ovranette (Ethinyl Estradiol; Levonorgestrel)	II-1047
Ovulen (Ethinyl Estradiol; Ethynodiol Diacetate)	II-1042
Ovulen 1 50 (Ethinyl Estradiol; Ethynodiol Diacetate)	II-1042
Ovulen 50 (Ethinyl Estradiol; Ethynodiol Diacetate)	II-1042
Ovurila (Ketoprofen)	II-1533
Ovurila E (Ketoprofen)	II-1533
Ovysmen (Ethinyl Estradiol; Norethindrone)	II-1055
Ovysmen 0.5 35 (Ethinyl Estradiol; Norethindrone)	II-1055
Ovysmen 1 35 (Ethinyl Estradiol; Norethindrone)	II-1055
Oxahexal (Oxazepam)	II-2063
Oxaline (Oxazepam)	II-2063
Oxaprim (Sulfamethoxazole; Trimethoprim)	II-2500
Oxazole (Sulfisoxazole)	II-2510
Oxedep (Fluoxetine Hydrochloride)	II-1160
Oxepam (Oxazepam)	II-2063
Oxicontin (Oxycodone Hydrochloride)	II-2076
Oxifugol (Fluconazole)	II-1136
Oxiken (Dobutamine Hydrochloride)	II-834
Oxiklorin (Hydroxychloroquine Sulfate)	II-1392
Oxis (Formoterol Fumarate)	II-1214
Oxiton INJ (Oxytocin)	II-2082
Oxitone (Oxytocin)	II-2082
Oxizole (Oxiconazole Nitrate)	II-2069
Oxonazol (Ketoconazole)	II-1530
Oxopurin 400 SR (Pentoxifylline)	II-2154
Ox-Pam (Oxazepam)	II-2063
Oxrate (Oxcarbazepine)	II-2065
Oxy IR (Oxycodone Hydrochloride)	II-2076
Oxyb (Oxybutynin)	II-2070
Oxyban (Oxybutynin)	II-2070
Oxycocet (Acetaminophen; Oxycodone Hydrochloride)	II-21
Oxycod (Oxycodone Hydrochloride)	II-2076
Oxycodan (Aspirin; Oxycodone Hydrochloride; Oxycodone Terephthalate)	II-214
OxyContin (Oxycodone Hydrochloride)	II-2076
Oxycontin CR (Oxycodone Hydrochloride)	II-2076
Oxycontin LP (Oxycodone Hydrochloride)	II-2076
Oxygesic (Oxycodone Hydrochloride)	II-2076
Oxyperazine (Trifluoperazine Hydrochloride)	II-2717
Oxytocin S INJ (Oxytocin)	II-2082
Oyrobin (Oxybutynin)	II-2070
Ozidia (Glipizide)	II-1290
Ozoken (Omeprazole)	II-2034

P

International brand name (Generic name)	Page no.
P Roquine (Chloroquine)	II-544
Paceco (Acetaminophen; Codeine Phosphate)	II-13
Pacedol (Haloperidol)	II-1328
Pacemol (Acetaminophen)	II-11
Paceum (Diazepam)	II-740
Pacifen (Baclofen)	II-266
Pacimol (Acetaminophen)	II-11
Pacinol (Fluphenazine Hydrochloride)	II-1172
Pacinol Prolong (Fluphenazine Hydrochloride)	II-1172
PACIS (BCG Live)	II-275
Pacitane (Trihexyphenidyl Hydrochloride)	II-2720
Pacitran (Diazepam)	II-740
Pactens (Bisoprolol Fumarate)	II-323
Pacyl (Alprazolam)	II-85
Padiken (Amantadine Hydrochloride)	II-97
Paediathrocin (Erythromycin)	II-960
Paediathrocin (Erythromycin Ethylsuccinate)	II-965
Paferxin (Cephalexin)	II-520
Painstop (Diclofenac)	II-748
Palavale (Econazole Nitrate)	II-900
Paldomycin (Doxycycline)	II-878
Paliadon Retardkaps (Hydromorphone Hydrochloride)	II-1388
Palitrex (Cephalexin)	II-520
Palladone (Hydromorphone Hydrochloride)	II-1388
Palladone SR (Hydromorphone Hydrochloride)	II-1388
Palliacol (Aluminum Hydroxide)	II-97
Pallidone (Methadone Hydrochloride)	II-1766
Palum (Primaquine Phosphate)	II-2246
Palux (Alprostadil)	II-90
Pamecil (Ampicillin)	II-170
Pamerex (Quazepam)	II-2298
Pamid (Indapamide)	II-1436
Pamisol (Pamidronate Disodium)	II-2091
Pamocil (Amoxicillin)	II-131
Pamol (Acetaminophen)	II-11

International brand name (Generic name)	Page no.
Pamoxicillin (Amoxicillin)	II-131
Pamoxin (Amoxicillin)	II-131
Panacef (Cefaclor)	II-444
Panacef RM (Cefaclor)	II-444
Panacta (Ampicillin)	II-170
Panadiene (Acetaminophen; Codeine Phosphate)	II-13
Panadeine Co (Acetaminophen; Codeine Phosphate)	II-13
Panadeine Forte (Acetaminophen; Codeine Phosphate)	II-13
Panado-Co Caplets (Acetaminophen; Codeine Phosphate)	II-13
Panafcort (Prednisone)	II-2240
Panafen (Ibuprofen)	II-1411
Panakiron (Dicyclomine Hydrochloride)	II-763
Panaldine (Ticlopidine Hydrochloride)	II-2622
Panamax (Acetaminophen)	II-11
Panamax (Acetaminophen; Codeine Phosphate)	II-13
Panamor (Diclofenac)	II-748
Panaxid (Nizatidine)	II-1992
Panazil (Gemfibrozil)	II-1269
Panbesy (Phentermine Hydrochloride)	II-2170
Panbesyl (Phentermine Hydrochloride)	II-2170
Panbesyl Nyscaps (Phentermine Hydrochloride)	II-2170
Pancrease HL (Pancrelipase)	II-2095
Pancrease MT 10 (Pancrelipase)	II-2095
Pancrease MT 16 (Pancrelipase)	II-2095
Pancrease MT 4 (Pancrelipase)	II-2095
Pancrex (Pancrelipase)	II-2095
Pandiuren (Amiloride Hydrochloride)	II-103
Pandiuren (Amiloride Hydrochloride; Hydrochlorothiazide)	II-105
Pan-Fungex (Clotrimazole)	II-640
Panfungol (Ketoconazole)	II-1530
Pangetan NF (Loperamide Hydrochloride)	II-1664
Panitol (Carbamazepine)	II-418
Panix (Alprazolam)	II-85
Pankrease (Pancrelipase)	II-2095
Panmicol (Clotrimazole)	II-640
Pannocort (Hydrocortisone Acetate)	II-1373
Panodil (Acetaminophen)	II-11
Panolin (Pamidronate Disodium)	II-2091
Panoral (Cefaclor)	II-444
Panoral Forte (Cefaclor)	II-444
Panorin (Pamidronate Disodium)	II-2091
Pantelmin (Mebendazole)	II-1711
Pantemon (Hydrochlorothiazide)	II-1348
Pantocain (Tetracaine Hydrochloride)	II-2584
Pantocycline (Tetracycline Hydrochloride)	II-2585
Pantodac (Pantoprazole Sodium)	II-2097
Pantodar (Pantoprazole Sodium)	II-2097
Pantodrin (Erythromycin)	II-960
Pantoloc (Pantoprazole Sodium)	II-2097
Pantomicina (Erythromycin)	II-960
Pantomicina (Erythromycin Ethylsuccinate)	II-965
Pantomicina (Erythromycin Stearate)	II-970
Pantozol (Pantoprazole Sodium)	II-2097
Pantrop (Ibuprofen)	II-1411
Panuric (Probenecid)	II-2248
Panvilon (Amoxicillin)	II-131
Panwarfin (Warfarin Sodium)	II-2804
Panzid (Ceftazidime)	II-492
Panzytrat (Pancrelipase)	II-2095
Paracefan (Clonidine Hydrochloride)	II-629
Paracet (Acetaminophen)	II-11
Paracod (Acetaminophen; Codeine Phosphate)	II-13
Paracodol (Acetaminophen; Codeine Phosphate)	II-13
Paradine (Acetaminophen; Codeine Phosphate)	II-13
Parafon DSC (Chlorzoxazone)	II-558
Parafon Forte (Chlorzoxazone)	II-558
Paralgin (Acetaminophen)	II-11
Paralief (Acetaminophen)	II-11
Paramol (Acetaminophen)	II-11
Paranthil (Albendazole)	II-46
Paraplatin RTU (Carboplatin)	II-430
Paraplatin-AQ (Carboplatin)	II-430
Paraplatine (Carboplatin)	II-430
Parasma (Albuterol)	II-47
Paratabs (Acetaminophen)	II-11
Paraxin (Chloramphenicol)	II-536
Paraxin (Chloramphenicol Sodium Succinate)	II-537
Parcono (Acetaminophen; Codeine Phosphate)	II-13
Parcoten (Acetaminophen; Codeine Phosphate)	II-13
Parenciclina (Tetracycline Hydrochloride)	II-2585
Parexel (Paclitaxel)	II-2084
Pargitan (Trihexyphenidyl Hydrochloride)	II-2720
Pariet (Rabeprazole Sodium)	II-2319
Parilac (Bromocriptine Mesylate)	II-344
Pariorix (Mumps Virus Vaccine Live)	II-1893
Paritrel (Amantadine Hydrochloride)	II-97
Parixam (Piroxicam)	II-2205
Parizac (Omeprazole)	II-2034
Parkemed (Mefenamic Acid)	II-1720
Parken (Carbidopa; Levodopa)	II-424
Parkin (Carbidopa; Levodopa)	II-424
Parkinane LP (Trihexyphenidyl Hydrochloride)	II-2720
Parkines (Trihexyphenidyl Hydrochloride)	II-2720
Parkintrel (Amantadine Hydrochloride)	II-97
Parkisonal (Trihexyphenidyl Hydrochloride)	II-2720
Parkopan (Trihexyphenidyl Hydrochloride)	II-2720
Parkotil (Pergolide Mesylate)	II-2155
Parotin (Dipyridamole)	II-821
Paroxet (Paroxetine Hydrochloride)	II-2104
Partane (Trihexyphenidyl Hydrochloride)	II-2720
Partobulin (Rho (D) Immune Globulin)	II-2350
Partocon INJ (Oxytocin)	II-2082
Partogloman (Rho (D) Immune Globulin)	II-2350
Parvid (Acetaminophen)	II-11
Parvolex (Acetylcysteine)	II-29
Pasalen (Ketoconazole)	II-1530
Pasconeural-Injektopas 1% (Procaine Hydrochloride)	II-2253
Pasetocin (Amoxicillin)	II-131
Pasotomin (Prochlorperazine)	II-2258
Pasrin (Buspirone Hydrochloride)	II-382
Passton (Mefenamic Acid)	II-1720
Pastimmun (BCG Vaccine)	II-276
Patrex (Sildenafil Citrate)	II-2451
Patsolin (Prazosin Hydrochloride)	II-2229
Pax (Diazepam)	II-740
Paxam (Clonazepam)	II-625
Paxan (Paroxetine Hydrochloride)	II-2104
Paxane (Flurazepam Hydrochloride)	II-1175
Paxene (Paclitaxel)	II-2084
Paxistil (Hydroxyzine)	II-1398
Paxium (Chlordiazepoxide Hydrochloride)	II-539
Paxon (Buspirone Hydrochloride)	II-382
Paxtibi (Nortriptyline Hydrochloride)	II-2002
Paxtine (Paroxetine Hydrochloride)	II-2104
Paxum (Diazepam)	II-740
Paxxet (Paroxetine Hydrochloride)	II-2104
Pazeadin (Diltiazem Hydrochloride)	II-798
P.D.T. Vax Purified (Diphtheria; Pertussis; Tetanus)	II-818
Pebegal (Benzonatate)	II-290
Pectril (Cephalexin)	II-520
Pediakin (Amikacin Sulfate)	II-101
Pediatric Asthcontin for Children SR (Aminophylline)	II-106
Pedi-Dent (Sodium Fluoride)	II-2465
Pedipan (Acetaminophen)	II-11
Pefamic (Mefenamic Acid)	II-1720
Peg-Intron (Interferon Alfa-2b, Recombinant)	II-1471
Pehachlor (Chlorpheniramine Maleate)	II-548
Pehacort (Prednisone)	II-2240
Pehaspas (Chlordiazepoxide Hydrochloride; Clidinium Bromide)	II-541
Pelpica (Promethazine Hydrochloride)	II-2268
Peluces (Haloperidol)	II-1328
Pen V (Penicillin V Potassium)	II-2142
Penadur (Penicillin G Benzathine)	II-2136
Penadur - LA (Penicillin G Benzathine)	II-2136
Penadur L-A (Penicillin G Benzathine)	II-2136
Penadur L.A. (Penicillin G Benzathine)	II-2136
Penadur LA (Penicillin G Benzathine)	II-2136
Penalcol (Mebendazole)	II-1711
Penamox (Amoxicillin)	II-131
Penbeta (Penicillin V Potassium)	II-2142
Penbiosyn (Amoxicillin)	II-131
Penbritin (Ampicillin)	II-170
Pencom (Penicillin G Benzathine)	II-2136
Pencor (Doxazosin Mesylate)	II-860
Pen-Di-Ben (Penicillin G Benzathine)	II-2136
Pendock (Bumetanide)	II-359
Pendramine (Penicillamine)	II-2133
Penedil (Felodipine)	II-1103
Penegra (Sildenafil Citrate)	II-2451
Pengesic (Tramadol Hydrochloride)	II-2674
Penicil (Penicillin G Procaine)	II-2140
Penicillamine (Penicillamine)	II-2133
Penicomb (Econazole Nitrate)	II-900
Penid (Methylphenidate Hydrochloride)	II-1781
Penidural (Penicillin G Benzathine)	II-2136
Penidure LA 12 (Penicillin G Benzathine)	II-2136
Penidure LA 24 (Penicillin G Benzathine)	II-2136
Penidure LA 6 (Penicillin G Benzathine)	II-2136
Penilente (Penicillin G Benzathine)	II-2136
Penilente - LA (Penicillin G Benzathine)	II-2136
Penimadol (Tramadol Hydrochloride)	II-2674
Penodil (Ampicillin)	II-170
Penoral (Penicillin V Potassium)	II-2142
Penphylline (Pentoxifylline)	II-2154
Penrazole (Omeprazole)	II-2034
Pensordil (Isosorbide Dinitrate)	II-1502
Penstabil (Ampicillin)	II-170
Pentacard (Isosorbide Mononitrate)	II-1507
Pentacarinat (Pentamidine Isethionate)	II-2145
Pentacillin (Penicillin V Potassium)	II-2142
Pentafen (Pentazocine Lactate)	II-2147
Pentaglobin (Immune Globulin (Human))	II-1434
Pentamycetin (Chloramphenicol)	II-536
Pentasa Enema (Mesalamine)	II-1748
Pentasa SR (Mesalamine)	II-1748
Pentasa Tab (Mesalamine)	II-1748
Pentasol (Clobetasol Propionate)	II-617
Pentate (Erythromycin Ethylsuccinate)	II-965
Pentawin (Pentazocine Lactate)	II-2147
Pentcillin (Piperacillin Sodium)	II-2196
Pentid (Penicillin V Potassium)	II-2142
Pentids (Penicillin G Potassium)	II-2137
Pentorel (Buprenorphine)	II-363
Pentothal Sodico (Thiopental Sodium)	II-2603
Pentothal Sodium (Thiopental Sodium)	II-2603
Pentox (Pentoxifylline)	II-2154
Pentoxi (Pentoxifylline)	II-2154
Pentoxifilin (Pentoxifylline)	II-2154
Pentoxine (Pentoxifylline)	II-2154
Pentranex (Penicillin V Potassium)	II-2142
Pentrexyl (Ampicillin)	II-170
Pen-Vi-K (Penicillin V Potassium)	II-2142
Pepcid AC (Famotidine)	II-1093
Pepcidac (Famotidine)	II-1093
Pepcidin (Famotidine)	II-1093
Pepcidin Rapitab (Famotidine)	II-1093
Pepcidina (Famotidine)	II-1093
Pepcidine (Famotidine)	II-1093
Pepdif (Famotidine)	II-1093
Pepdine (Famotidine)	II-1093

International brand name (Generic name)	Page no.
Platinol-AQ (Cisplatin)	II-589
Platinoxan (Cisplatin)	II-589
Platistil (Cisplatin)	II-589
Platistin (Cisplatin)	II-589
Plato (Dipyridamole)	II-821
Platof (Pentoxifylline)	II-2154
Platosin (Cisplatin)	II-589
Plegomazine (Chlorpromazine Hydrochloride)	II-549
Plendil Depottab (Felodipine)	II-1103
Plendil Retard (Felodipine)	II-1103
Plentiva (Estrogens, Conjugated; Medroxyprogesterone Acetate)	II-1027
Plentiva Cycle (Estrogens, Conjugated; Medroxyprogesterone Acetate)	II-1027
Plenty (Sibutramine Hydrochloride)	II-2447
Plenur (Lithium Carbonate)	II-1654
Pleon RA (Sulfasalazine)	II-2507
Pletaal (Cilostazol)	II-566
Plewin (Aspirin)	II-206
Plexafer (Ferrous Sulfate)	II-1122
Plidan (Diazepam)	II-740
Plunazol (Fluconazole)	II-1136
Plurimen (Selegiline Hydrochloride)	II-2437
Plurisul Forte (Sulfamethoxazole; Trimethoprim)	II-2500
Plus Kalium Retard (Potassium Chloride)	II-2215
Pluserix (Measles, Mumps and Rubella Virus Vaccine Live)	II-1710
PMQ-INGA (Primaquine Phosphate)	II-2246
PMS Isoniazid (Isoniazid)	II-1496
PMS Lindane (Lindane)	II-1642
Pneumo 23 (Pneumococcal Vaccine)	II-2208
Pneumo 23 Imovax (Pneumococcal Vaccine)	II-2208
Pneumovax (Pneumococcal Vaccine)	II-2208
Pneumovax II (Pneumococcal Vaccine)	II-2208
Pocef (Cefixime)	II-466
Pocin (Erythromycin Stearate)	II-970
Pocin-H (Hydrocortisone; Neomycin Sulfate; Polymyxin B Sulfate)	II-1384
Pocral (Chloral Hydrate)	II-534
Podomexef (Cefpodoxime Proxetil)	II-484
Pofol (Propofol)	II-2278
Polaramine (Chlorpheniramine Maleate)	II-548
Polaratyne (Loratadine)	II-1675
Polaratyne - D (Loratadine; Pseudoephedrine Sulfate)	II-1677
Polarcyclin (Tetracycline Hydrochloride)	II-2585
Polaronil (Chlorpheniramine Maleate)	II-548
Poligot (Dihydroergotamine Mesylate)	II-792
Polinal (Methyldopa)	II-1778
Polio Sabin (Polio Vaccine, Oral Live)	II-2210
Polio Sabin Oral (Polio Vaccine, Oral Live)	II-2210
Polio "Sabin" Oral Vaccine (Polio Vaccine, Oral Live)	II-2210
Polio Sabin OS (Polio Vaccine, Oral Live)	II-2210
Polio Sabin-S (Polio Vaccine, Oral Live)	II-2210
Polio Salk "Sero" (Polio Vaccine, Inactivated)	II-2209
Polio-Kovax (Polio Vaccine, Oral Live)	II-2210
Polioral (Polio Vaccine, Oral Live)	II-2210
Polioral Trivalent (Polio Vaccine, Oral Live)	II-2210
Polistin T-Caps (Carbinoxamine Maleate)	II-429
Polygris (Griseofulvin, Ultramicrocrystalline)	II-1313
Polypress (Prazosin Hydrochloride)	II-2229
Polyquin Forte (Hydroquinone)	II-1391
Polyxit (Gemfibrozil)	II-1269
Ponaltin (Ranitidine Hydrochloride)	II-2334
Poncofen (Mefenamic Acid)	II-1720
Pondactone (Spironolactone)	II-2483
Pondex (Mefenamic Acid)	II-1720
Pondnacef (Cephalexin)	II-520
Pondnadysmen (Mefenamic Acid)	II-1720
Pondtroxin (Levothyroxine Sodium)	II-1618
Ponstan (Mefenamic Acid)	II-1720
Ponstan (500 mg) (Mefenamic Acid)	II-1720
Ponstan Forte (Mefenamic Acid)	II-1720
Ponstan-500 (Mefenamic Acid)	II-1720
Ponstyl (Mefenamic Acid)	II-1720
Pontacid (Mefenamic Acid)	II-1720
Pontal (Mefenamic Acid)	II-1720
Pontyl (Mefenamic Acid)	II-1720
Porazine (Perphenazine)	II-2162
Posanin (Dipyridamole)	II-821
Posid (Etoposide)	II-1080
Posidene (Piroxicam)	II-2205
Posipen (Dicloxacillin Sodium)	II-761
Postadoxin (Meclizine Hydrochloride)	II-1713
Postadoxine (Meclizine Hydrochloride)	II-1713
Postafen (Meclizine Hydrochloride)	II-1713
Postafene (Meclizine Hydrochloride)	II-1713
Postarax (Hydroxyzine)	II-1398
Postinor-2 (Levonorgestrel)	II-1614
Posyd (Etoposide Phosphate)	II-1083
Potarlon (Mefenamic Acid)	II-1720
Potasion (Potassium Chloride)	II-2215
Poten (Atenolol; Chlorthalidone)	II-226
Potendal (Ceftazidime)	II-492
Potensone (Fluphenazine Hydrochloride)	II-1172
Poviral (Acyclovir)	II-33
Powegon (Cimetidine Hydrochloride)	II-568
Poxidium (Chlordiazepoxide Hydrochloride; Clidinium Bromide)	II-541
Pragmarel (Trazodone Hydrochloride)	II-2686
Pragmaten (Fluoxetine Hydrochloride)	II-1160
Pralax (Lactulose)	II-1550
Pramace (Ramipril)	II-2330
Pramidal (Loperamide Hydrochloride)	II-1664
Pramin (Metoclopramide Hydrochloride)	II-1798
Pramotel (Metoclopramide Hydrochloride)	II-1798
Pramur (Ursodiol)	II-2737
Pranadox (Zidovudine)	II-2822
Prandase (Acarbose)	II-9
Prandin E2 (Dinoprostone)	II-812
Praol (Meprobamate)	II-1738
Prascolend (Pravastatin Sodium)	II-2224
Pra-Sec (Omeprazole)	II-2034
Prasig (Prazosin Hydrochloride)	II-2229
Prastan (Pravastatin Sodium)	II-2224
Praten (Captopril)	II-411
Pratisol (Prazosin Hydrochloride)	II-2229
Pratsiol (Prazosin Hydrochloride)	II-2229
Prava (Pravastatin Sodium)	II-2224
Pravacol (Pravastatin Sodium)	II-2224
Pravaselect (Pravastatin Sodium)	II-2224
Pravasin (Pravastatin Sodium)	II-2224
Pravasine (Pravastatin Sodium)	II-2224
Pravastatin Natrium "Mayrho Fer" (Pravastatin Sodium)	II-2224
Pravator (Pravastatin Sodium)	II-2224
Pravidel (Bromocriptine Mesylate)	II-344
Pravyl (Pravastatin Sodium)	II-2224
Praxel (Paclitaxel)	II-2084
Praxiten (Oxazepam)	II-2063
Prayanol (Amantadine Hydrochloride)	II-97
Prazac (Prazosin Hydrochloride)	II-2229
Prazidec (Omeprazole)	II-2034
Prazina (Pyrazinamide)	II-2295
Prazite (Praziquantel)	II-2228
Prazole (Omeprazole)	II-2034
Prazopress (Prazosin Hydrochloride)	II-2229
Preconin (Prednisolone)	II-2233
Predimol (Acetaminophen)	II-11
Prednecort (Prednisolone)	II-2233
Prednicorm (Prednisone)	II-2240
Prednicort (Prednisone)	II-2240
Prednidib (Prednisone)	II-2240
Predni-F (Dexamethasone)	II-730
Prednigalen (Prednisolone Acetate)	II-2235
Predni-Ophtal (Prednisolone Acetate)	II-2235
Prednitone (Prednisone)	II-2240
Prefin (Buprenorphine)	II-363
Prefrin (Phenylephrine Hydrochloride)	II-2173
Premaril Plus (Estrogens, Conjugated; Medroxyprogesterone Acetate)	II-1027
Premarin Crema V (Estrogens, Conjugated)	II-1019
Premarin Crema Vaginal (Estrogens, Conjugated)	II-1019
Premarin Creme (Estrogens, Conjugated)	II-1019
Premarin Pak (Estrogens, Conjugated; Medroxyprogesterone Acetate)	II-1027
Premarin Vaginal Creme (Estrogens, Conjugated)	II-1019
Premarina (Estrogens, Conjugated)	II-1019
Premelle (Estrogens, Conjugated; Medroxyprogesterone Acetate)	II-1027
Premelle Cycle 5 (Estrogens, Conjugated; Medroxyprogesterone Acetate)	II-1027
Premorine (Atenolol)	II-222
Prempak (Estrogens, Conjugated; Medroxyprogesterone Acetate)	II-1027
Prenacid (Desonide)	II-728
Prenalon (Ketoconazole)	II-1530
Prenilone (Prednisolone)	II-2233
Prenolol (Atenolol)	II-222
Prent (Acebutolol Hydrochloride)	II-10
Pre-Par (Ritodrine Hydrochloride)	II-2379
Prepenem (Imipenem; Cilastatin Sodium)	II-1424
Pres (Enalapril Maleate)	II-913
Pres Plus (Enalapril Maleate; Hydrochlorothiazide)	II-923
Prescal (Isradipine)	II-1515
Presil (Enalapril Maleate)	II-913
Presilan (Methyldopa)	II-1778
Presinol (Methyldopa)	II-1778
Presinol 500 (Methyldopa)	II-1778
Presiten (Lisinopril)	II-1648
Presoken (Diltiazem Hydrochloride)	II-798
Presolol (Labetalol Hydrochloride)	II-1545
Presomen (Estrogens, Conjugated)	II-1019
Pressalolo (Labetalol Hydrochloride)	II-1545
Pressin (Prazosin Hydrochloride)	II-2229
Pressyn (Vasopressin)	II-2769
Prestoral (Propranolol Hydrochloride)	II-2287
Pretop (Prednicarbate)	II-2231
Prevagin-Premaril (Estrogens, Conjugated)	II-1019
Preven (Ethinyl Estradiol; Levonorgestrel)	II-1047
Prevenar (Pneumococcal Vaccine)	II-2208
Prevex HC (Hydrocortisone)	II-1369
Prevnar (Pneumococcal Vaccine)	II-2208
Prexan (Naproxen)	II-1924
Prexin (Dipyridamole)	II-821
Priadel (Lithium Carbonate)	II-1654
Priadel Retard (Lithium Carbonate)	II-1654
Priaxen (Naproxen)	II-1924
Pricillin (Ampicillin)	II-170
Primace (Captopril)	II-411
Primacin (Primaquine Phosphate)	II-2246
Primacine (Erythromycin)	II-960
Primafen (Cefotaxime Sodium)	II-474
Primapen (Ampicillin)	II-170
Primax (Ciclopirox)	II-561
Primbactam (Aztreonam)	II-263
Primcillin (Penicillin V Potassium)	II-2142
Primeral (Naproxen)	II-1924
Primex (Bumetanide)	II-359
Primiprost (Dinoprostone)	II-812
Primizum (Oxazepam)	II-2063
Primolut N (Norethindrone)	II-1996
Primolut-N (Norethindrone)	II-1996
Primonil (Imipramine Hydrochloride)	II-1431
Primperan (Metoclopramide Hydrochloride)	II-1798
Primperil (Metoclopramide Hydrochloride)	II-1798
Primulut (Norethindrone)	II-1996
Princol (Lincomycin Hydrochloride)	II-1640
Prinil (Lisinopril)	II-1648
Prinox (Alprazolam)	II-85
Prinparl (Metoclopramide Hydrochloride)	II-1798
Priorheum (Piroxicam)	II-2205

International brand name (Generic name)	Page no.
Priorix (Measles, Mumps and Rubella Virus Vaccine Live)	II-1710
Pristine (Ketoconazole)	II-1530
Pristinex (Ketoconazole)	II-1530
Pritor (Telmisartan)	II-2554
Pritorplus (Hydrochlorothiazide; Telmisartan)	II-1360
Prizma (Fluoxetine Hydrochloride)	II-1160
Proacan D (Loratadine; Pseudoephedrine Sulfate)	II-1677
Proactin (Loratadine)	II-1675
Proartinal (Ibuprofen)	II-1411
Probat (Guaifenesin)	II-1314
Probecid (Probenecid)	II-2248
Probenemid (Probenecid)	II-2248
Probenid (Probenecid)	II-2248
Probi RHO (D) (Rho (D) Immune Globulin)	II-2350
Probiotin (Clindamycin)	II-605
Probiox (Ciprofloxacin Hydrochloride)	II-573
Pro-C (Ascorbic Acid)	II-203
Procadolor N (Procaine Hydrochloride)	II-2253
Procalmadiol (Meprobamate)	II-1738
Procalmidol (Meprobamate)	II-1738
Procapen (Penicillin G Procaine)	II-2140
Proceptin (Omeprazole)	II-2034
Prochlor (Prochlorperazine)	II-2258
Pro-Cid (Probenecid)	II-2248
Procid (Probenecid)	II-2248
Procillin (Penicillin G Procaine)	II-2140
Procimeti (Cimetidine Hydrochloride)	II-568
Proclozine (Prochlorperazine)	II-2258
Procor (Amiodarone Hydrochloride)	II-110
Procren (Leuprolide Acetate)	II-1587
Procren Depot (Leuprolide Acetate)	II-1587
Procrin (Leuprolide Acetate)	II-1587
Proctin (Fluoxetine Hydrochloride)	II-1160
Proctocort (Hydrocortisone Acetate)	II-1373
Pro-Cure (Finasteride)	II-1129
Procuta Ge (Isotretinoin)	II-1510
Procutan (Hydrocortisone)	II-1369
Procythol (Selegiline Hydrochloride)	II-2437
Procytox (Cyclophosphamide)	II-666
Prodac (Nabumetone)	II-1909
Prodafem (Medroxyprogesterone Acetate)	II-1714
Prodep (Fluoxetine Hydrochloride)	II-1160
Prodexin (Naproxen)	II-1924
Prodiabet (Glyburide)	II-1297
Prodilantin (Fosphenytoin Sodium)	II-1228
Prodium (Loperamide Hydrochloride)	II-1664
Prodop (Methyldopa)	II-1778
Prodopa (Methyldopa)	II-1778
Prodren (Dipivefrin Hydrochloride)	II-820
Profenac (Diclofenac)	II-748
Profenid (Ketoprofen)	II-1533
Profenid 50 (Ketoprofen)	II-1533
Profenil (Ketoprofen)	II-1533
Profeno (Ibuprofen)	II-1411
Proflax (Timolol)	II-2627
Proflaxin (Ciprofloxacin Hydrochloride)	II-573
Proflox (Ciprofloxacin Hydrochloride)	II-573
Prof-N-4 (Chlorpheniramine Maleate)	II-548
Profungal (Ketoconazole)	II-1530
Progemzal (Gemfibrozil)	II-1269
Progen (Medroxyprogesterone Acetate)	II-1714
Progering (Progesterone)	II-2262
Progesic (Fenoprofen Calcium)	II-1110
Progest (Progesterone)	II-2262
Progestogel (Progesterone)	II-2262
Progevera (Medroxyprogesterone Acetate)	II-1714
Progout (Allopurinol)	II-77
Progynon (Estradiol)	II-986
Progynon C (Ethinyl Estradiol)	II-1040
Progynova (Estradiol)	II-986
Prohair (Finasteride)	II-1129
Prohibit (Omeprazole)	II-2034
Proksi 250 (Ciprofloxacin Hydrochloride)	II-573
Proksi 500 (Ciprofloxacin Hydrochloride)	II-573

International brand name (Generic name)	Page no.
Prolaken (Metoprolol)	II-1805
Prolanz (Lansoprazole)	II-1569
Prolax (Chlorzoxazone)	II-558
Prolipase (Pancrelipase)	II-2095
Prolixin-D (Fluphenazine Decanoate)	II-1170
Prolol (Propranolol Hydrochloride)	II-2287
Prolol Plus (Propranolol Hydrochloride)	II-2287
Prolongatum (Orphenadrine Citrate)	II-2049
Prolung (Rifampin)	II-2363
Promactil (Chlorpromazine Hydrochloride)	II-549
Prome (Promethazine Hydrochloride)	II-2268
Promedes (Furosemide)	II-1237
Promergan (Promethazine Hydrochloride)	II-2268
Promesan (Promethazine Hydrochloride)	II-2268
Prometax (Rivastigmine Tartrate)	II-2389
Promexin (Chlorpromazine Hydrochloride)	II-549
Promide (Chlorpropamide)	II-554
Promostan (Alprostadil)	II-90
Pronaxen (Naproxen)	II-1924
Proneurin (Promethazine Hydrochloride)	II-2268
Pronicy (Cyproheptadine Hydrochloride)	II-682
Prontamid (Sulfacetamide Sodium)	II-2497
Prontofort (Tramadol Hydrochloride)	II-2674
Propacet (Acetaminophen; Propoxyphene Napsylate)	II-23
Propacil (Propylthiouracil)	II-2293
Propalong (Propranolol Hydrochloride)	II-2287
Propam (Diazepam)	II-740
Propamide (Chlorpropamide)	II-554
Propaphenin (Chlorpromazine Hydrochloride)	II-549
Propax (Oxazepam)	II-2063
Propayerst (Propranolol Hydrochloride)	II-2287
Propeshia (Finasteride)	II-1129
Propess (Dinoprostone)	II-812
Propocam (Propofol)	II-2278
Propofol-Lipuro (Propofol)	II-2278
Propral (Propranolol Hydrochloride)	II-2287
Propycil (Propylthiouracil)	II-2293
Propyl-Thyracil (Propylthiouracil)	II-2293
Proris (Ibuprofen)	II-1411
Proscar 5 (Finasteride)	II-1129
Prosh (Finasteride)	II-1129
Prosogan (Lansoprazole)	II-1569
Prostacare (Finasteride)	II-1129
Prostacom (Finasteride)	II-1129
Prostafilina (Oxacillin Sodium)	II-2053
Prostamid (Flutamide)	II-1181
Prostamustin (Estramustine Phosphate Sodium)	II-1017
Prostandin (Alprostadil)	II-90
Prostap (Leuprolide Acetate)	II-1587
Prostarmon E (Dinoprostone)	II-812
Prostavasin (Alprostadil)	II-90
Prostin 3 (Dinoprostone)	II-812
Prostin E2 Tab (Dinoprostone)	II-812
Prostin E2 Vaginal Cream (Dinoprostone)	II-812
Prostin E2 Vaginal Gel (Dinoprostone)	II-812
Prostin VR Pediatric (Dinoprostone)	II-812
Prostine (Dinoprostone)	II-812
Prostine VR (Alprostadil)	II-90
Prostivas (Alprostadil)	II-90
Prostogenat (Flutamide)	II-1181
Protaphane (Insulin (Human, Isophane))	II-1455
Protaphane HM (Insulin (Human, Isophane))	II-1455
Protector (Atropine Sulfate; Diphenoxylate Hydrochloride)	II-238
Protexin (Amantadine Hydrochloride)	II-97
Protheo (Theophylline)	II-2593
Prothiazine (Promethazine Hydrochloride)	II-2268
Prothyra (Medroxyprogesterone Acetate)	II-1714
Protogen (Dapsone)	II-702
Protopic (Tacrolimus)	II-2532
Protozol (Metronidazole)	II-1812
Protylol (Dicyclomine Hydrochloride)	II-763
Provail CR (Ketoprofen)	II-1533
Provas (Valsartan)	II-2759

International brand name (Generic name)	Page no.
Provasyn (Bromocriptine Mesylate)	II-344
Provon (Ibuprofen)	II-1411
Prowel (Metoclopramide Hydrochloride)	II-1798
Proxalyoc (Piroxicam)	II-2205
Proxen (Naproxen)	II-1924
Proxen LLE (Naproxen)	II-1924
Proxidol (Naproxen Sodium)	II-1928
Proxinor (Norfloxacin)	II-1997
Prox-S (Albuterol)	II-47
Proxuric (Allopurinol)	II-77
Prozac 20 (Fluoxetine Hydrochloride)	II-1160
Prozef (Cefprozil)	II-489
Prozil (Chlorpromazine Hydrochloride)	II-549
Prozin (Chlorpromazine Hydrochloride)	II-549
Prozine (Promethazine Hydrochloride)	II-2268
Prozoladex (Goserelin Acetate)	II-1304
Pryleugan (Imipramine Hydrochloride)	II-1431
Prysoline (Primidone)	II-2247
Psicofar (Chlordiazepoxide Hydrochloride)	II-539
Psiquiwas (Oxazepam)	II-2063
Psychopax (Diazepam)	II-740
Psymion (Maprotiline Hydrochloride)	II-1706
Psynor (Chlorpromazine Hydrochloride)	II-549
Psyrazine (Trifluoperazine Hydrochloride)	II-2717
Ptinolin (Ranitidine Hydrochloride)	II-2334
Puernol (Acetaminophen)	II-11
Pulin (Metoclopramide Hydrochloride)	II-1798
Pulmicort Nasal (Budesonide)	II-347
Pulmicort Nasal Turbohaler (Budesonide)	II-347
Pulmidur (Theophylline)	II-2593
Pulmison (Prednisone)	II-2240
Pulmocodeina (Codeine Phosphate)	II-647
Pulmotide (Budesonide)	II-347
Pulsoton (Methyldopa)	II-1778
Punktyl (Lorazepam)	II-1678
Pupiletto Forte (Phenylephrine Hydrochloride)	II-2173
Purata (Oxazepam)	II-2063
Purbal (Sulfamethoxazole; Trimethoprim)	II-2500
Purgoxin (Digoxin)	II-780
Puricemia (Allopurinol)	II-77
Puricos (Allopurinol)	II-77
Purifam (Famotidine)	II-1093
Purinase (Allopurinol)	II-77
Puri-Nethol (Mercaptopurine)	II-1741
Purinol (Allopurinol)	II-77
Purinox (Allopurinol)	II-77
P-Vate (Clobetasol Propionate)	II-617
P.V. Carpine Liquifilm Ophthalimic Solution (Pilocarpine)	II-2180
Pyassan (Cephalexin)	II-520
Pylor (Loratadine)	II-1675
Pynamic (Mefenamic Acid)	II-1720
Pyndale (Pindolol)	II-2192
Pyogenta (Gentamicin Sulfate)	II-1279
Pyoredol (Phenytoin Sodium)	II-2175
Pyrafat (Pyrazinamide)	II-2295
Pyralin EN (Sulfasalazine)	II-2507
Pyramide (Disopyramide Phosphate)	II-825
Pyramide (Pyrazinamide)	II-2295
Pyrethia (Promethazine Hydrochloride)	II-2268
Pyrocaps (Piroxicam)	II-2205
Pyroxin (Pyridoxine Hydrochloride)	II-2297
Pyroxy (Piroxicam)	II-2205
Pytazen SR (Dipyridamole)	II-821
Pyzamed (Pyrazinamide)	II-2295
P-Zide (Pyrazinamide)	II-2295

Q

International brand name (Generic name)	Page no.
Q Var (Beclomethasone Dipropionate)	II-279
Q200 (Quinine Sulfate)	II-2317
Q300 (Quinine Sulfate)	II-2317
QCef (Cefadroxil Monohydrate)	II-447
Qilaflox (Ciprofloxacin Hydrochloride)	II-573
Qinolon (Ofloxacin)	II-2015
Qipro (Ofloxacin)	II-2015

R

International brand name (Generic name)	Page no.
Rocillin (Amoxicillin)	II-131
Rockamol Plus (Acetaminophen; Codeine Phosphate)	II-13
Rocosgen (Lorazepam)	II-1678
Rocy Gen (Gentamicin Sulfate)	II-1279
Rodatin (Lovastatin)	II-1688
Rofact (Rifampin)	II-2363
Rofcin (Ciprofloxacin Hydrochloride)	II-573
Rofenid (Ketoprofen)	II-1533
Roferon A (Interferon Alfa-2a, Recombinant)	II-1469
Roferon-A HSA Free (Interferon Alfa-2a, Recombinant)	II-1469
Rofetab (Rofecoxib)	II-2396
Rofex (Cephalexin)	II-520
Rofiz Gel (Rofecoxib)	II-2396
Rogasti (Famotidine)	II-1093
Rogitine (Phentolamine Mesylate)	II-2171
Roidenin (Ibuprofen)	II-1411
Rojamin (Cyanocobalamin)	II-661
Rokanite (Aspirin; Codeine Phosphate)	II-210
Rolactin (Diclofenac)	II-748
Rolan (Ranitidine Hydrochloride)	II-2334
Rolesen (Ketorolac Tromethamine)	II-1537
Roletra (Loratadine)	II-1675
Romeda (Estrogens, Conjugated)	II-1019
Romin (Minocycline Hydrochloride)	II-1838
Romoxil (Amoxicillin)	II-131
Ronal (Aspirin)	II-206
Ronalin (Bromocriptine Mesylate)	II-344
Ronemox (Amoxicillin)	II-131
Ropril (Captopril)	II-411
R.O.R. Vax (Measles, Mumps and Rubella Virus Vaccine Live)	II-1710
Rosaced Gel (Metronidazole)	II-1812
Rosacin Eye Drop (Ciprofloxacin Hydrochloride)	II-573
Roscillin (Ampicillin)	II-170
Rosi (Rosiglitazone Maleate)	II-2405
Rosic (Piroxicam)	II-2205
Rosiden (Piroxicam)	II-2205
Rosiden Gel (Piroxicam)	II-2205
Rosig (Piroxicam)	II-2205
Rosig-D (Piroxicam)	II-2205
Rosimol (Ranitidine Hydrochloride)	II-2334
Rosulfant (Sulfasalazine)	II-2507
Rotalin (Carisoprodol)	II-432
Rotopar (Albendazole)	II-46
Roug-mycin (Erythromycin Stearate)	II-970
Rouvax (Measles Virus Vaccine Live)	II-1708
Rovacor (Lovastatin)	II-1688
Rovixida (Gentamicin Sulfate)	II-1279
Rowecef (Ceftriaxone Sodium)	II-503
Roweprazol (Omeprazole)	II-2034
Rowexetina (Fluoxetine Hydrochloride)	II-1160
Roxamol Gelcaps (Acetaminophen)	II-11
Roxcef (Ceftriaxone Sodium)	II-503
Roxen (Naproxen)	II-1924
Roxicaina (Epinephrine; Lidocaine Hydrochloride)	II-938
Roxicaina (Lidocaine)	II-1628
Roxicam (Piroxicam)	II-2205
Roximycin (Doxycycline)	II-878
Roxium (Piroxicam)	II-2205
Roxon (Ceftriaxone Sodium)	II-503
Royen (Calcium Acetate)	II-400
Rozacreme (Metronidazole)	II-1812
Rozagel (Metronidazole)	II-1812
Rozamin (Atenolol)	II-222
Rozex (Metronidazole)	II-1812
Rozex Gel (Metronidazole)	II-1812
Rozide (Pyrazinamide)	II-2295
Rozolex (Albendazole)	II-46
R-Rax (Hydroxyzine)	II-1398
Rubavax (Rubella Virus Vaccine Live)	II-2409
Rubeaten (Rubella Virus Vaccine Live)	II-2409
Rubeaten Berna (Rubella Virus Vaccine Live)	II-2409
Rubidox (Doxorubicin, Liposomal)	II-873
RubieFol (Folic Acid)	II-1208
Rubifen (Methylphenidate Hydrochloride)	II-1781
Rubilem (Daunorubicin Hydrochloride)	II-708
Rubisol (Cyanocobalamin)	II-661
Rubocort (Clobetasol Propionate)	II-617
Rubramin (Cyanocobalamin)	II-661
Rubranova (Cyanocobalamin)	II-661
Rucaina (Lidocaine Hydrochloride)	II-1632
Rucaina Pomada (Lidocaine)	II-1628
Rudi-Rouvax (Measles and Rubella Virus Vaccine Live)	II-1707
Rudivax (Rubella Virus Vaccine Live)	II-2409
Rukasyn (Ampicillin Sodium; Sulbactam Sodium)	II-174
Rumonal (Meloxicam)	II-1726
Rupan (Ibuprofen)	II-1411
Rupenol (Dipyridamole)	II-821
Ruvamed (Piroxicam)	II-2205
Rycarden (Nicardipine Hydrochloride)	II-1958
Rydene (Nicardipine Hydrochloride)	II-1958
Rynacrom M (Cromolyn Sodium)	II-656
Rynconox (Beclomethasone Dipropionate)	II-279
Rythmex (Propafenone Hydrochloride)	II-2274
Rythmical (Disopyramide Phosphate)	II-825
Rythmodan LA (Disopyramide Phosphate)	II-825
Rythmodan Retard (Disopyramide Phosphate)	II-825
Rythmodul (Disopyramide Phosphate)	II-825
Rythocin (Erythromycin Stearate)	II-970
Rytmilen (Disopyramide Phosphate)	II-825
Rytmonorm (Propafenone Hydrochloride)	II-2274
Ryvel (Cetirizine Hydrochloride)	II-529
Ryzen (Cetirizine Hydrochloride)	II-529
S	
S-60 (Cephradine)	II-526
Sabutol (Albuterol)	II-47
Saf Card (Nicardipine Hydrochloride)	II-1958
Safdin (Cephradine)	II-526
Safitex (Tolmetin Sodium)	II-2656
Sagestam eye drops (Gentamicin Sulfate)	II-1279
Sakisozin (Ondansetron Hydrochloride)	II-2039
Salalin (Chlorzoxazone)	II-558
Salazopirina (Sulfasalazine)	II-2507
Salazopyrin Entabs (Sulfasalazine)	II-2507
Salazopyrina (Sulfasalazine)	II-2507
Salazopyrine (Sulfasalazine)	II-2507
Salazopyrine EC (Sulfasalazine)	II-2507
Salbetol (Albuterol)	II-47
Salbron (Albuterol)	II-47
Salbulin (Albuterol)	II-47
Salbutalan (Albuterol)	II-47
Salbutan (Albuterol)	II-47
Salbutin (Albuterol)	II-47
Salbutol (Albuterol)	II-47
Salbutron SR (Albuterol)	II-47
Salbuven (Albuterol)	II-47
Salbuvent (Albuterol)	II-47
Salina (Salsalate)	II-2418
Salinac (Indomethacin)	II-1443
Salipax (Fluoxetine Hydrochloride)	II-1160
Salmagne (Labetalol Hydrochloride)	II-1545
Salmaplon (Albuterol)	II-47
Salmeter (Salmeterol Xinafoate)	II-2410
Salmol (Albuterol)	II-47
Salmundin Retard (Albuterol)	II-47
Salofalk (Mesalamine)	II-1748
Salomol (Albuterol)	II-47
Saltermox (Amoxicillin)	II-131
Salterprim (Allopurinol)	II-77
Saluretil (Chlorothiazide)	II-545
Saluric (Chlorothiazide)	II-545
Salvatrim (Sulfamethoxazole; Trimethoprim)	II-2500
Salzone (Acetaminophen)	II-11
Samixon (Ceftriaxone Sodium)	II-503
Sanatison (Hydrocortisone)	II-1369
Sanaxin (Cephalexin)	II-520
Sancotec (Cetirizine Hydrochloride)	II-529
Sandel (Dipyridamole)	II-821
Sandimmun (Cyclosporine)	II-668
Sandimmun Neoral (Cyclosporine)	II-668
Sandocal (Calcium Carbonate)	II-401
Sandoglobulina (Immune Globulin (Human))	II-1434
Sandoglobuline (Immune Globulin (Human))	II-1434
Sandostatina (Octreotide Acetate)	II-2009
Sandostatina LAR (Octreotide Acetate)	II-2009
Sandostatine (Octreotide Acetate)	II-2009
Sandovac (Influenza Virus Vaccine)	II-1451
Sandrena Gel (Estradiol)	II-986
Sanergal (Flunisolide)	II-1149
Sangcya (Cyclosporine)	II-668
Sanmetidin (Cimetidine Hydrochloride)	II-568
Sanomed (Naproxen Sodium)	II-1928
Sanor (Clorazepate Dipotassium)	II-638
Sanotensin (Guanethidine Monosulfate)	II-1321
Sanpilo (Pilocarpine)	II-2180
Sanpo (Loperamide Hydrochloride)	II-1664
Sans-acne (Erythromycin)	II-960
Santenson (Dexamethasone)	II-730
Santeson (Dexamethasone)	II-730
Sanzol (Cefazolin Sodium)	II-452
Sanzur (Fluoxetine Hydrochloride)	II-1160
Sapilent (Trimipramine Maleate)	II-2726
Sapram (Alprazolam)	II-85
Sapril (Fosinopril Sodium)	II-1222
Sarconyl (Lindane)	II-1642
Saridine (Sulfasalazine)	II-2507
Saridon (Acetaminophen)	II-11
Saril (Salsalate)	II-2418
Saritilron (Naproxen)	II-1924
Saromet (Diazepam)	II-740
Sarotard (Amitriptyline Hydrochloride)	II-119
Saroten (Amitriptyline Hydrochloride)	II-119
Saroten Retard (Amitriptyline Hydrochloride)	II-119
Sarotena (Amitriptyline Hydrochloride)	II-119
Sarotex (Amitriptyline Hydrochloride)	II-119
Sastid Anti-Fungal (Clotrimazole)	II-640
Satoren (Losartan Potassium)	II-1682
Satoren H (Hydrochlorothiazide; Losartan Potassium)	II-1354
Savacol (Chlorhexidine Gluconate)	II-542
Saventrine (Isoproterenol Hydrochloride)	II-1498
Savismin (Diclofenac)	II-748
Savlon (Chlorhexidine Gluconate)	II-542
Savox (Amikacin Sulfate)	II-101
Sawacillin (Amoxicillin)	II-131
Sawamezin (Amoxicillin)	II-131
Sawasone (Dexamethasone)	II-730
Sayomol (Promethazine Hydrochloride)	II-2268
Sburol (Buspirone Hydrochloride)	II-382
Scabecid (Lindane)	II-1642
Scabexyl (Lindane)	II-1642
Scabi (Lindane)	II-1642
Scabisan (Lindane)	II-1642
Scandene (Piroxicam)	II-2205
Scandicain (Mepivacaine Hydrochloride)	II-1737
Scandicaine (Mepivacaine Hydrochloride)	II-1737
Scandinibsa (Mepivacaine Hydrochloride)	II-1737
Scandopa (Methyldopa)	II-1778
Scanicol (Chloramphenicol)	II-536
Scanytin (Nystatin)	II-2005
Schericur (Hydrocortisone)	II-1369
Schericur 0.25% (Hydrocortisone)	II-1369
Scheroson (Cortisone Acetate)	II-654
Schufen (Ibuprofen)	II-1411
Scopoderm Depotplast (Scopolamine)	II-2432
Scopoderm TTS (Scopolamine)	II-2432
Scorbex (Ascorbic Acid)	II-203
Scutamil-C (Carisoprodol)	II-432
Sea-Legs (Meclizine Hydrochloride)	II-1713
Sebizole (Ketoconazole)	II-1530

International brand name (Generic name)	Page no.
Secalip (Fenofibrate)	II-1105
Secanal (Secobarbital Sodium)	II-2435
Secapine (Cimetidine Hydrochloride)	II-568
Secotex (Tamsulosin Hydrochloride)	II-2544
Securon (Verapamil Hydrochloride)	II-2777
Sedacoron (Amiodarone Hydrochloride)	II-110
Sedalin (Albuterol)	II-47
Sedanazin (Gentamicin Sulfate)	II-1279
Sedanium-R (Famotidine)	II-1093
Sedatival (Lorazepam)	II-1678
Sedicel (Selegiline Hydrochloride)	II-2437
Sedistal (Atropine Sulfate; Diphenoxylate Hydrochloride)	II-238
Sedral (Cefadroxil Monohydrate)	II-447
Seduxen (Diazepam)	II-740
Sefac (Estrogens, Conjugated)	II-1019
Sefaretic (Amiloride Hydrochloride; Hydrochlorothiazide)	II-105
Sefasin (Cephalexin)	II-520
Sefdene (Piroxicam)	II-2205
Sefloc (Metoprolol)	II-1805
Sefmal (Tramadol Hydrochloride)	II-2674
Sefmex (Selegiline Hydrochloride)	II-2437
Sefmic (Mefenamic Acid)	II-1720
Sefnor (Norfloxacin)	II-1997
Sefril (Cephradine)	II-526
Seftem (Ceftibuten)	II-496
Seglor (Dihydroergotamine Mesylate)	II-792
Seglor Retard (Dihydroergotamine Mesylate)	II-792
Segurex (Bumetanide)	II-359
Seguril (Furosemide)	II-1237
Selax (Docusate Sodium)	II-841
Selaxa (Amikacin Sulfate)	II-101
Seldiar (Loperamide Hydrochloride)	II-1664
Selectin (Pravastatin Sodium)	II-2224
Selectofur (Furosemide)	II-1237
Selegil (Selegiline Hydrochloride)	II-2437
Selegos (Selegiline Hydrochloride)	II-2437
Selektine (Meloxicam)	II-1726
Selektine (Pravastatin Sodium)	II-2224
Selemycin (Amikacin Sulfate)	II-101
Selepam (Quazepam)	II-2298
Selezyme (Haloperidol)	II-1328
Selgin (Selegiline Hydrochloride)	II-2437
Selipran (Pravastatin Sodium)	II-2224
Selitex (Cetirizine Hydrochloride)	II-529
Selmac (Mefenamic Acid)	II-1720
Selokeen (Metoprolol)	II-1805
Seloken (Metoprolol)	II-1805
Seloken Retard (Metoprolol)	II-1805
Seloken Retard Comp. (Hydrochlorothiazide; Metoprolol Tartrate)	II-1355
Seloken Zoc (Metoprolol)	II-1805
Selokomb (Hydrochlorothiazide; Metoprolol Tartrate)	II-1355
Selokomb 200 (Hydrochlorothiazide; Metoprolol Tartrate)	II-1355
Selokomb Zoc 100 (Hydrochlorothiazide; Metoprolol Tartrate)	II-1355
Selopral (Metoprolol)	II-1805
Selopres Zok (Hydrochlorothiazide; Metoprolol Tartrate)	II-1355
Selo-zok (Metoprolol)	II-1805
Selozok (Metoprolol)	II-1805
Sembrina (Methyldopa)	II-1778
Semicillin (Ampicillin)	II-170
Semi-Daonil (Glyburide)	II-1297
Semi-Euglucon (Glyburide)	II-1297
Sempera (Itraconazole)	II-1517
Sendoxan (Cyclophosphamide)	II-666
Senorm L.A. (Haloperidol Decanoate)	II-1332
Sensaval (Nortriptyline Hydrochloride)	II-2002
Sensibit (Loratadine)	II-1675
Sensibit D (Loratadine; Pseudoephedrine Sulfate)	II-1677
Sensival (Nortriptyline Hydrochloride)	II-2002
Sepamit (Nifedipine)	II-1967
Sepexin (Cephalexin)	II-520
Sephros (Cephradine)	II-526
Sepirone (Buspirone Hydrochloride)	II-382
Sepram (Citalopram Hydrobromide)	II-591
Sepsilem (Cefotaxime Sodium)	II-474
Septalone (Chlorhexidine Gluconate)	II-542
Septicide (Ciprofloxacin Hydrochloride)	II-573
Septilisin (Cephalexin)	II-520
Septol (Chlorhexidine Gluconate)	II-542
Septran (Sulfamethoxazole; Trimethoprim)	II-2500
Septrin (Sulfamethoxazole; Trimethoprim)	II-2500
Septrin DS (Sulfamethoxazole; Trimethoprim)	II-2500
Septrin Familia (Sulfamethoxazole; Trimethoprim)	II-2500
Septrin Forte (Sulfamethoxazole; Trimethoprim)	II-2500
Septrin S (Sulfamethoxazole; Trimethoprim)	II-2500
Sequilar ED (Ethinyl Estradiol; Levonorgestrel)	II-1047
Seralgan (Citalopram Hydrobromide)	II-591
Seranace (Haloperidol)	II-1328
Seranase (Haloperidol)	II-1328
Seren (Chlordiazepoxide Hydrochloride)	II-539
Serenace (Haloperidol)	II-1328
Serenase (Haloperidol)	II-1328
Serenase (Haloperidol Decanoate)	II-1332
Serenase Dekanoat (Haloperidol Decanoate)	II-1332
Serene (Clorazepate Dipotassium)	II-638
Serenelfi (Haloperidol)	II-1328
Serepax (Oxazepam)	II-2063
Seresta (Oxazepam)	II-2063
Seretide (Fluticasone Propionate; Salmeterol Xinafoate)	II-1197
Seretide (Salmeterol Xinafoate)	II-2410
Seretide Accuhaler (Fluticasone Propionate; Salmeterol Xinafoate)	II-1197
Serevent Inhaler and Disks (Salmeterol Xinafoate)	II-2410
Serlain (Sertraline Hydrochloride)	II-2439
Sermonil (Imipramine Hydrochloride)	II-1431
Serobid (Salmeterol Xinafoate)	II-2410
Serocryptin (Bromocriptine Mesylate)	II-344
Serodoxy (Doxycycline)	II-878
Seropram (Citalopram Hydrobromide)	II-591
Serpasil (Reserpine)	II-2346
Serpasol (Reserpine)	II-2346
Serten (Atenolol)	II-222
Sertranex (Sertraline Hydrochloride)	II-2439
Sertranquil (Sertraline Hydrochloride)	II-2439
Servambutol (Ethambutol Hydrochloride)	II-1039
Servamox (Amoxicillin)	II-131
Servicef (Cephalexin)	II-520
Serviclor (Cefaclor)	II-444
Servidapsone (Dapsone)	II-702
Servidone (Chlorthalidone)	II-555
Servidoxine (Doxycycline)	II-878
Servidoxyne (Doxycycline)	II-878
Servigenta (Gentamicin Sulfate)	II-1279
Servipen-V (Penicillin V Potassium)	II-2142
Servispor (Cephalexin)	II-520
Servitet (Tetracycline Hydrochloride)	II-2585
Servitrim (Sulfamethoxazole; Trimethoprim)	II-2500
Servitrocin (Erythromycin Ethylsuccinate)	II-965
Servitrocin (Erythromycin Stearate)	II-970
Serzonil (Nefazodone Hydrochloride)	II-1939
Setamol (Acetaminophen)	II-11
Setin (Metoclopramide Hydrochloride)	II-1798
Setizin (Cetirizine Hydrochloride)	II-529
Setron (Azithromycin)	II-250
Setron (Granisetron Hydrochloride)	II-1308
Severon (Omeprazole)	II-2034
Sevredol (Morphine Sulfate)	II-1877
Shacillin (Ampicillin)	II-170
Shamoxil (Amoxicillin)	II-131
Sharizole (Metronidazole)	II-1812
Sharox-500 (Cefuroxime)	II-507
Shikitan (Amantadine Hydrochloride)	II-97
Shinaderm (Miconazole)	II-1820
Shincort (Triamcinolone Acetonide)	II-2701
Shinfomycin (Cefoperazone Sodium)	II-471
Shintamet (Cimetidine Hydrochloride)	II-568
Shiosol (Gold Sodium Thiomalate)	II-1304
Shiprosyn (Naproxen)	II-1924
Shiton (Norethindrone)	II-1996
Siadocin (Doxycycline)	II-878
Sialexin (Cephalexin)	II-520
Siamdopa (Methyldopa)	II-1778
Siamformet (Metformin Hydrochloride)	II-1760
Siamidine (Cimetidine Hydrochloride)	II-568
Sia-mox (Amoxicillin)	II-131
Sibutral (Sibutramine Hydrochloride)	II-2447
Sibutrex (Sibutramine Hydrochloride)	II-2447
Sicco (Indapamide)	II-1436
Siclidon (Doxycycline)	II-878
Sidenar (Lorazepam)	II-1678
Sideril (Trazodone Hydrochloride)	II-2686
Sidocin (Indomethacin)	II-1443
Sifaclor (Cefaclor)	II-444
Sificrom (Cromolyn Sodium)	II-656
Sifloks (Ciprofloxacin Hydrochloride)	II-573
Sifrol (Pramipexole Dihydrochloride)	II-2219
Sigadoxin (Doxycycline)	II-878
Sigaperidol (Haloperidol)	II-1328
Sigaprim (Sulfamethoxazole; Trimethoprim)	II-2500
Sigillum (Isosorbide Dinitrate)	II-1502
Sigmetadine (Cimetidine Hydrochloride)	II-568
Sil-A-mox (Amoxicillin)	II-131
Silence (Lorazepam)	II-1678
Silmycetin (Chloramphenicol)	II-536
Simaglen (Cimetidine Hydrochloride)	II-568
Simarc-2 (Warfarin Sodium)	II-2804
Simasedan (Diazepam)	II-740
Simbado (Simvastatin)	II-2454
Simchol (Simvastatin)	II-2454
Simcor (Simvastatin)	II-2454
Simetac (Ranitidine Hydrochloride)	II-2334
Simovil (Simvastatin)	II-2454
Simoxil (Amoxicillin)	II-131
Simplene (Epinephrine)	II-934
Simvacor (Simvastatin)	II-2454
Simvatin (Simvastatin)	II-2454
Simvor (Simvastatin)	II-2454
Simvotin (Simvastatin)	II-2454
Sinalgen (Acetaminophen; Hydrocodone Bitartrate)	II-17
Sinalgico (Piroxicam)	II-2205
Sinanin (Meprobamate)	II-1738
Sinapdin (Cyproheptadine Hydrochloride)	II-682
Sinaxar (Methocarbamol)	II-1768
Sindopa (Carbidopa; Levodopa)	II-424
Sinease Repetab (Loratadine; Pseudoephedrine Sulfate)	II-1677
Sinedopa (Carbidopa; Levodopa)	II-424
Sinemet 25 100 (Carbidopa; Levodopa)	II-424
Sinemet Retard (Carbidopa; Levodopa)	II-424
Sinepress (Methyldopa)	II-1778
Sinestron (Lorazepam)	II-1678
Sinflo (Ofloxacin)	II-2015
Singulair Chew (Montelukast Sodium)	II-1872
Sinhistan D (Loratadine; Pseudoephedrine Sulfate)	II-1677
Sinium (Betamethasone Dipropionate; Clotrimazole)	II-304
Sinium (Clotrimazole)	II-640
Sinlex (Cephalexin)	II-520
Sinopril (Lisinopril)	II-1648
Sinotrim (Sulfamethoxazole; Trimethoprim)	II-2500
Sinozol (Itraconazole)	II-1517
Sinquan (Doxepin Hydrochloride)	II-865
Sinquane (Doxepin Hydrochloride)	II-865
Sintec (Enalapril Maleate)	II-913

International brand name (Generic name)	Page no.
Sintelin (Ampicillin)	II-170
Sintesedan (Chlordiazepoxide Hydrochloride)	II-539
Sinthecillin (Cephalexin)	II-520
Sintodian (Droperidol)	II-889
Sintrex (Ceftriaxone Sodium)	II-503
Sinumine (Carbinoxamine Maleate)	II-429
Sinvacor (Simvastatin)	II-2454
Sinzac (Fluoxetine Hydrochloride)	II-1160
Sioban (Albendazole)	II-46
Sipam (Diazepam)	II-740
Sipla (Guaifenesin)	II-1314
Siprogut (Ciprofloxacin Hydrochloride)	II-573
Siqualone (Fluphenazine Decanoate)	II-1170
Siqualone (Fluphenazine Hydrochloride)	II-1172
Siquent Hycor (Hydrocortisone Acetate)	II-1373
Siran 200 (Acetylcysteine)	II-29
Sirdalud (Tizanidine Hydrochloride)	II-2640
Sirdalud MR (Tizanidine Hydrochloride)	II-2640
Sirdalud Retard (Tizanidine Hydrochloride)	II-2640
Sirolax (Lactulose)	II-1550
Sirtal (Carbamazepine)	II-418
Sisare Gel (Estradiol)	II-986
Sistral Hydrocort (Hydrocortisone)	II-1369
Sivastin (Simvastatin)	II-2454
Sivoz (Rofecoxib)	II-2396
Sizopin (Clozapine)	II-642
Skiatropine (Atropine Sulfate)	II-235
Skid Gel E (Erythromycin)	II-960
Skincalm (Hydrocortisone)	II-1369
Skindure (Miconazole)	II-1820
Skinfect (Gentamicin Sulfate)	II-1279
Skinocyclin (Minocycline Hydrochloride)	II-1838
Skinoderm (Azelaic Acid)	II-245
Skinorem (Azelaic Acid)	II-245
Skinoren (Azelaic Acid)	II-245
Skizon (Betamethasone Dipropionate)	II-301
Slaxin (Orphenadrine Citrate)	II-2049
Slo-Theo (Theophylline)	II-2593
Slow Deralin (Propranolol Hydrochloride)	II-2287
Slow-Apresoline (Hydralazine Hydrochloride)	II-1346
Slow-Lopresor (Metoprolol)	II-1805
Smarten (Captopril)	II-411
Sno Pilo (Pilocarpine)	II-2180
Snoffocin (Norfloxacin)	II-1997
Sobelin (Clindamycin)	II-605
Sobile (Oxazepam)	II-2063
Sobril (Oxazepam)	II-2063
Sodipental (Thiopental Sodium)	II-2603
Sofasin (Norfloxacin)	II-1997
Sofden (Piroxicam)	II-2205
Soficlor (Cefaclor)	II-444
Sofidrox (Cefadroxil Monohydrate)	II-447
Sofilex (Cephalexin)	II-520
Sofix (Cefixime)	II-466
Soflax (Docusate Sodium)	II-841
Softon (Docusate Sodium)	II-841
Sohotin (Loratadine)	II-1675
Solanax (Alprazolam)	II-85
Solantin (Dipyridamole)	II-821
Solaquin (Hydroquinone)	II-1391
Solarcaine (Benzocaine)	II-289
Solasic (Mefenamic Acid)	II-1720
Solaskil (Levamisole Hydrochloride)	II-1598
Solavert (Sotalol Hydrochloride)	II-2471
Solaxin (Chlorzoxazone)	II-558
Solcode (Aspirin; Codeine Phosphate)	II-210
Solcodein (Codeine Phosphate)	II-647
Solesorin (Hydralazine Hydrochloride)	II-1346
Solezorin (Hydralazine Hydrochloride)	II-1346
Solganol (Aurothioglucose)	II-242
Solgol (Nadolol)	II-1911
Solmucol (Acetylcysteine)	II-29
Solomet (Methylprednisolone)	II-1787
Solomet (Methylprednisolone Acetate)	II-1790
Solomet (Methylprednisolone Sodium Succinate)	II-1793
Solosa (Glimepiride)	II-1287
Solosin (Theophylline)	II-2593
Solpadeine (Acetaminophen; Codeine Phosphate)	II-13
Solpenox (Amoxicillin)	II-131
Solprin (Aspirin)	II-206
Solpurin (Probenecid)	II-2248
Soltric (Mebendazole)	II-1711
Solu Cortef (Hydrocortisone Sodium Succinate)	II-1379
Solu Cortef M.O.V. (Hydrocortisone Sodium Succinate)	II-1379
Solu Medrol (Methylprednisolone Sodium Succinate)	II-1793
Solufen Lidose (Ibuprofen)	II-1411
Solu-Medrone (Methylprednisolone Sodium Succinate)	II-1793
Solu-Moderin (Methylprednisolone Sodium Succinate)	II-1793
Solu-Paraxin (Chloramphenicol Sodium Succinate)	II-537
Solupred (Prednisolone)	II-2233
Solvetan (Ceftazidime)	II-492
Somac (Pantoprazole Sodium)	II-2097
Somadril (Carisoprodol)	II-432
Sombutol (Pentobarbital Sodium)	II-2149
Somese (Triazolam)	II-2715
Somlan (Flurazepam Hydrochloride)	II-1175
Somnil (Zolpidem Tartrate)	II-2842
Somniton (Triazolam)	II-2715
Somno (Zolpidem Tartrate)	II-2842
Somnox (Chloral Hydrate)	II-534
Somofillina (Theophylline)	II-2593
Somophylin (Aminophylline)	II-106
Sompraz (Esomeprazole Magnesium)	II-980
Sonacon (Diazepam)	II-740
Sonata (Zaleplon)	II-2816
Sone (Prednisone)	II-2240
Songar (Triazolam)	II-2715
Soni-Slo (Isosorbide Dinitrate)	II-1502
Soon-Soon (Ketamine Hydrochloride)	II-1528
Sophidone LP (Hydromorphone Hydrochloride)	II-1388
Sophixin Ofteno (Ciprofloxacin Hydrochloride)	II-573
Soprol (Bisoprolol Fumarate)	II-323
Soproxen (Diclofenac)	II-748
Sorbangil (Isosorbide Dinitrate)	II-1502
Sorbichew (Isosorbide Dinitrate)	II-1502
Sorbid (Isosorbide Dinitrate)	II-1502
Sorbidilat (Isosorbide Dinitrate)	II-1502
Sorbidilat Retard (Isosorbide Dinitrate)	II-1502
Sorbidilat SR (Isosorbide Dinitrate)	II-1502
Sorbidin (Isosorbide Dinitrate)	II-1502
Sorbonit (Isosorbide Dinitrate)	II-1502
Soriflor (Diflorasone Diacetate)	II-776
Sortel (Formoterol Fumarate)	II-1214
Sortis (Atorvastatin Calcium)	II-231
Sosegon (Pentazocine Lactate)	II-2147
Sosser (Sertraline Hydrochloride)	II-2439
Sostril (Ranitidine Hydrochloride)	II-2334
Sotab (Sotalol Hydrochloride)	II-2471
Sotahexal (Sotalol Hydrochloride)	II-2471
Sotalex (Sotalol Hydrochloride)	II-2471
Sotapor (Sotalol Hydrochloride)	II-2471
Sotatic-10 (Metoclopramide Hydrochloride)	II-1798
Sotilen (Piroxicam)	II-2205
Spancef (Cefixime)	II-466
Spara (Sparfloxacin)	II-2479
Sparcort (Diflorasone Diacetate)	II-776
Spardac (Sparfloxacin)	II-2479
Sparlox (Sparfloxacin)	II-2479
Sparos (Sparfloxacin)	II-2479
Sparx (Sparfloxacin)	II-2479
Spasmoten (Chlordiazepoxide Hydrochloride; Clidinium Bromide)	II-541
Spasmotine (Dicyclomine Hydrochloride)	II-763
Spazol (Itraconazole)	II-1517
Spectrum (Ceftazidime)	II-492
Spersacarpine (Pilocarpine)	II-2180
Spersacet (Sulfacetamide Sodium)	II-2497
Spersadex (Dexamethasone)	II-730
Spersanicol (Chloramphenicol)	II-536
Spicline (Minocycline Hydrochloride)	II-1838
Spike (Ketoconazole)	II-1530
Spinax (Baclofen)	II-266
Spiractin (Spironolactone)	II-2483
Spirix (Spironolactone)	II-2483
Spiroctan (Spironolactone)	II-2483
Spirolacton (Spironolactone)	II-2483
Spirolair (Pirbuterol Acetate)	II-2203
Spirolang (Spironolactone)	II-2483
Spiron (Spironolactone)	II-2483
Spirone (Spironolactone)	II-2483
Spironex (Spironolactone)	II-2483
Spirono-Isis (Spironolactone)	II-2483
Spironol (Spironolactone)	II-2483
Spirosine (Cefotaxime Sodium)	II-474
Spirotone (Spironolactone)	II-2483
Spitacin (Ciprofloxacin Hydrochloride)	II-573
Splendil (Felodipine)	II-1103
Splendil ER (Felodipine)	II-1103
Sporacid (Itraconazole)	II-1517
Sporal (Itraconazole)	II-1517
Sporalon (Trifluoperazine Hydrochloride)	II-2717
Sporanox 15 D (Itraconazole)	II-1517
Sporicef (Cephalexin)	II-520
Sporidex (Cephalexin)	II-520
Sporium (Ketoconazole)	II-1530
Sporlab (Itraconazole)	II-1517
Spornar (Itraconazole)	II-1517
Sporostatin P G (Griseofulvin, Ultramicrocrystalline)	II-1313
Sporostatin U F (Griseofulvin, Ultramicrocrystalline)	II-1313
Sporoxyl (Ketoconazole)	II-1530
Sporozol (Ketoconazole)	II-1530
Spren (Aspirin)	II-206
Sprinsol (Chlorpheniramine Maleate)	II-548
Spyrocon (Itraconazole)	II-1517
Squibb-Azactam (Aztreonam)	II-263
Squibb-HC (Hydrocortisone Acetate)	II-1373
Sqworm (Mebendazole)	II-1711
SRM-Rotard (Morphine Sulfate)	II-1877
Srogen (Estrogens, Conjugated)	II-1019
Sroton (Glycopyrrolate)	II-1302
Stabixin (Cefoperazone Sodium)	II-471
Stalene (Fluconazole)	II-1136
Stambutol (Ethambutol Hydrochloride)	II-1039
Stancef (Cefazolin Sodium)	II-452
Standacillin (Ampicillin)	II-170
Stangyl (Trimipramine Maleate)	II-2726
Stapam (Lorazepam)	II-1678
Stapenor (Oxacillin Sodium)	II-2053
Staphcillin (Dicloxacillin Sodium)	II-761
Staphcillin A (Dicloxacillin Sodium)	II-761
Starcef (Cefixime)	II-466
Starcef (Ceftazidime)	II-492
Staren (Diclofenac)	II-748
Staril (Fosinopril Sodium)	II-1222
Starnoc (Zaleplon)	II-2816
Statex (Morphine Sulfate)	II-1877
Statin (Simvastatin)	II-2454
Staurodorm (Flurazepam Hydrochloride)	II-1175
Stavir (Stavudine)	II-2486
Stazol (Cilostazol)	II-566
Stazolin (Cefazolin Sodium)	II-452
Stecin (Acetylcysteine)	II-29
Steclin (Tetracycline Hydrochloride)	II-2585
Steclin V (Tetracycline Hydrochloride)	II-2585
Stediril (Ethinyl Estradiol; Norgestrel)	II-1068
Stediril 30 (Ethinyl Estradiol; Levonorgestrel)	II-1047
Steerometz (Prednisone)	II-2240

International brand name (Generic name)	Page no.
Stemetil (Prochlorperazine)	II-2258
Stemzine (Prochlorperazine)	II-2258
Sterax (Desonide)	II-728
Stermin (Atenolol)	II-222
Sterocort (Triamcinolone)	II-2698
Sterodelta (Diflorasone Diacetate)	II-776
Steroderm (Hydrocortisone Acetate)	II-1373
Steron (Norethindrone)	II-1996
Steronase AQ (Triamcinolone Acetonide)	II-2701
Stesolid (Diazepam)	II-740
Stiedex (Desoximetasone)	II-730
Stiemycin (Erythromycin)	II-960
Stieprox (Ciclopirox)	II-561
Stieva A (Tretinoin)	II-2691
Stieva-A (Tretinoin)	II-2691
Stilnoct (Zolpidem Tartrate)	II-2842
Stilnox (Zolpidem Tartrate)	II-2842
Stimycine (Erythromycin)	II-960
Sting Gel (Diclofenac)	II-748
Stiprox (Ciclopirox)	II-561
Stivate (Clobetasol Propionate)	II-617
Stobrun (Trihexyphenidyl Hydrochloride)	II-2720
Stocrin (Efavirenz)	II-901
Stogamet (Cimetidine Hydrochloride)	II-568
Stolax (Bisacodyl)	II-322
Stomacer (Omeprazole)	II-2034
Stomakon (Cimetidine Hydrochloride)	II-568
Stomax (Famotidine)	II-1093
Stomec (Omeprazole)	II-2034
Stomedine (Cimetidine Hydrochloride)	II-568
Stomet (Cimetidine Hydrochloride)	II-568
Stopan (Sulfamethoxazole; Trimethoprim)	II-2500
Stoparen (Cefotaxime Sodium)	II-474
Stopen (Piroxicam)	II-2205
Stopit (Loperamide Hydrochloride)	II-1664
Stopitch (Hydrocortisone Acetate)	II-1373
Storo (Isosorbide Dinitrate)	II-1502
Storvas (Atorvastatin Calcium)	II-231
Stozole (Omeprazole)	II-2034
Strepfen (Flurbiprofen)	II-1177
Strodin (Glycopyrrolate)	II-1302
Strumazol (Methimazole)	II-1767
Styptin 5 (Norethindrone)	II-1996
Subamycin (Tetracycline Hydrochloride)	II-2585
Subutex (Buprenorphine)	II-363
Succin (Erythromycin Ethylsuccinate)	II-965
Succosa (Sucralfate)	II-2493
Sucef (Cefixime)	II-466
Sucrabest (Sucralfate)	II-2493
Sucralbene (Sucralfate)	II-2493
Sucralfin (Sucralfate)	II-2493
Sucramal (Sucralfate)	II-2493
Sucrazide (Glipizide)	II-1290
Suduvax (Varicella Vaccine)	II-2767
Sufenta Forte (Sufentanil Citrate)	II-2494
Sufortanon (Penicillamine)	II-2133
Sugaprim (Sulfamethoxazole; Trimethoprim)	II-2500
Sugril (Glyburide)	II-1297
Suifac (Omeprazole)	II-2034
Suismycetin (Chloramphenicol)	II-536
Sukingpo (Estrogens, Conjugated)	II-1019
Sul 10 (Sulfacetamide Sodium)	II-2497
Sulbacin (Ampicillin Sodium; Sulbactam Sodium)	II-174
Sulcolon (Sulfasalazine)	II-2507
Sulconar (Carbidopa; Levodopa)	II-424
Sulcran (Sucralfate)	II-2493
Sulcrate (Sucralfate)	II-2493
Suldisyn (Sulconazole Nitrate)	II-2496
Sulen (Sulindac)	II-2512
Sulesorin (Hydralazine Hydrochloride)	II-1346
Sulfa 10 (Sulfacetamide Sodium)	II-2497
Sulfableph (Sulfacetamide Sodium)	II-2497
Sulfacet (Sulfamethoxazole; Trimethoprim)	II-2500
Sulfacetamid Ofteno al 10% (Sulfacetamide Sodium)	II-2497
Sulfacid (Sulfacetamide Sodium)	II-2497
Sulfas-Chinidin (Quinidine Sulfate)	II-2314
Sulfazin (Sulfisoxazole)	II-2510
Sulfazine (Sulfasalazine)	II-2507
Sulfazole (Sulfisoxazole)	II-2510
Sulfex (Sulfacetamide Sodium)	II-2497
Sulfinam (Sulfamethoxazole; Trimethoprim)	II-2500
Sulfona (Dapsone)	II-702
Sulfotrimin (Sulfamethoxazole; Trimethoprim)	II-2500
Sulic (Sulindac)	II-2512
Sulindaco Lisan (Sulindac)	II-2512
Sulindal (Sulindac)	II-2512
Sulindec (Sulindac)	II-2512
Sulinol (Sulindac)	II-2512
Sulmedin (Terbinafine Hydrochloride)	II-2570
Sulmidine (Clonidine Hydrochloride)	II-629
Sulmycin (Gentamicin Sulfate)	II-1279
Sulop (Sulfacetamide Sodium)	II-2497
Suloril (Sulindac)	II-2512
Sulphacalyre (Sulfacetamide Sodium)	II-2497
Sulphafurazole (Sulfisoxazole)	II-2510
Sulreuma (Sulindac)	II-2512
Sultanol (Albuterol)	II-47
Sulthrim (Sulfamethoxazole; Trimethoprim)	II-2500
Sultrex (Estropipate)	II-1033
Sultrona (Estrogens, Conjugated)	II-1019
Sumamed (Azithromycin)	II-250
Sumetropin (Sulfamethoxazole; Trimethoprim)	II-2500
Sumial (Propranolol Hydrochloride)	II-2287
Sumitrex (Sumatriptan Succinate)	II-2516
Summicort (Methylprednisolone)	II-1787
Sumontil (Trimipramine Maleate)	II-2726
Sunflow (Ceftriaxone Sodium)	II-503
Sunolut (Norethindrone)	II-1996
Supedal (Zolpidem Tartrate)	II-2842
Superocin (Ciprofloxacin Hydrochloride)	II-573
Superpeni (Amoxicillin)	II-131
Supertidine (Famotidine)	II-1093
Supeudol (Oxycodone Hydrochloride)	II-2076
Suplac (Bromocriptine Mesylate)	II-344
Supplin (Metronidazole)	II-1812
Supracyclin (Doxycycline)	II-878
Supradol (Ketorolac Tromethamine)	II-1537
Supralan (Fluocinolone Acetonide)	II-1152
Supramycina (Doxycycline)	II-878
Supran (Cefixime)	II-466
Suprarenin (Epinephrine)	II-934
Suprasec (Loperamide Hydrochloride)	II-1664
Suprasma (Albuterol)	II-47
Supra-Vir (Acyclovir)	II-33
Supraviran Creme (Acyclovir)	II-33
Suprecid (Lansoprazole)	II-1569
Suprekof (Guaifenesin)	II-1314
Supres (Hydralazine Hydrochloride)	II-1346
Supressin (Doxazosin Mesylate)	II-860
Suprim (Sulfamethoxazole; Trimethoprim)	II-2500
Suprimal (Meclizine Hydrochloride)	II-1713
Suprin (Sulfamethoxazole; Trimethoprim)	II-2500
Suraben (Glyburide)	II-1297
Surantol (Isosorbide Dinitrate)	II-1502
Surfont (Mebendazole)	II-1711
Surzolin (Cefazolin Sodium)	II-452
Suscard (Nitroglycerin)	II-1984
Susevin (Pentazocine Lactate)	II-2147
Sustac (Nitroglycerin)	II-1984
Sustachlor (Chloramphenicol)	II-536
Sustiva (Efavirenz)	II-901
Sutac (Cetirizine Hydrochloride)	II-529
Sutolin (Naproxen)	II-1924
Sutolin (Naproxen Sodium)	II-1928
Suvalan (Sumatriptan Succinate)	II-2516
Suxilep (Ethosuximide)	II-1072
Suximal (Ethosuximide)	II-1072
Suxinutin (Ethosuximide)	II-1072
Swiflor (Cefaclor)	II-444
Swityl (Dicyclomine Hydrochloride)	II-763
Sycropaz (Meprobamate)	II-1738
Sydepres (Fluphenazine Decanoate)	II-1170
Syklofosfamid (Cyclophosphamide)	II-666
Sylos Vaginal Tab (Oxiconazole Nitrate)	II-2069
Symitec (Cetirizine Hydrochloride)	II-529
Symoron (Methadone Hydrochloride)	II-1766
Synaclyn (Flunisolide)	II-1149
Synalar 25 (Fluocinolone Acetonide)	II-1152
Synalar Simple (Fluocinolone Acetonide)	II-1152
Synarela (Nafarelin Acetate)	II-1914
Synbrozil (Gemfibrozil)	II-1269
Synchlolim (Chloramphenicol Sodium Succinate)	II-537
Syncle (Cephalexin)	II-520
Syndopa (Carbidopa; Levodopa)	II-424
Synecl (Cephalexin)	II-520
Synermox (Amoxicillin; Clavulanate Potassium)	II-139
Syneudon (Amitriptyline Hydrochloride)	II-119
Synflex (Naproxen)	II-1924
Synflex (Naproxen Sodium)	II-1928
Synphase (Ethinyl Estradiol; Norethindrone)	II-1055
Syntaris (Flunisolide)	II-1149
Syntaris Nasal Spray (Flunisolide)	II-1149
Synthetic Oxytocin INJ (Oxytocin)	II-2082
Synthocilin (Ampicillin)	II-170
Synthomycine Succinate (Chloramphenicol Sodium Succinate)	II-537
Synthophyllin (Aminophylline)	II-106
Syntocinon (Oxytocin)	II-2082
Syntocinon INJ (Oxytocin)	II-2082
Syntocinon Spray (Oxytocin)	II-2082
Syntocor (Cefaclor)	II-444
Syntofene (Ibuprofen)	II-1411
Syntovir (Acyclovir)	II-33
Syscan (Fluconazole)	II-1136
Syscor (Nisoldipine)	II-1976
Syscor CC (Nisoldipine)	II-1976
Systen (Estradiol)	II-986
S.Z. (Clobetasol Propionate)	II-617

T

International brand name (Generic name)	Page no.
T4KP (Levothyroxine Sodium)	II-1618
Tabalon (Ibuprofen)	II-1411
Tabalon 400 (Ibuprofen)	II-1411
Tabel (Ketorolac Tromethamine)	II-1537
Tabrin (Ofloxacin)	II-2015
Tacex (Ceftriaxone Sodium)	II-503
Tachydaron (Amiodarone Hydrochloride)	II-110
Tacron (Ticlopidine Hydrochloride)	II-2622
Tadex (Tamoxifen Citrate)	II-2539
Tafil (Alprazolam)	II-85
Tafil D (Alprazolam)	II-85
Tagal (Ceftazidime)	II-492
Taganopain (Acetaminophen)	II-11
Tagonis (Paroxetine Hydrochloride)	II-2104
Tahor (Atorvastatin Calcium)	II-231
Taicefran (Cephradine)	II-526
Taitecin (Clonidine Hydrochloride)	II-629
Takadol (Tramadol Hydrochloride)	II-2674
Takanarumin (Allopurinol)	II-77
Take-C (Ascorbic Acid)	II-203
Takepron (Lansoprazole)	II-1569
Takimetol (Metronidazole)	II-1812
Taks (Diclofenac)	II-748
Talorat D (Loratadine; Pseudoephedrine Sulfate)	II-1677
Taloxa (Felbamate)	II-1099
Talpramin (Imipramine Hydrochloride)	II-1431
Tamaxin (Tamoxifen Citrate)	II-2539
Tambutol (Ethambutol Hydrochloride)	II-1039
Tametin (Cimetidine Hydrochloride)	II-568
Tamifen (Tamoxifen Citrate)	II-2539
Tamik (Dihydroergotamine Mesylate)	II-792

International brand name (Generic name)	Page no.
Tetanogamma (Tetanus Immune Globulin)	II-2582
Tetanol (Tetanus Toxoid)	II-2583
Tetanosson (Tetanus Immune Globulin)	II-2582
Tetatox (Tetanus Toxoid)	II-2583
Tetavax (Tetanus Toxoid)	II-2583
Tetocain (Tetracaine Hydrochloride)	II-2584
Tetocaine (Tetracaine Hydrochloride)	II-2584
Tetra Central (Tetracycline Hydrochloride)	II-2585
Tetra-Atlantis (Tetracycline Hydrochloride)	II-2585
Tetrabioptal (Tetracycline Hydrochloride)	II-2585
Tetrablet (Tetracycline Hydrochloride)	II-2585
Tetracitro S (Tetracycline Hydrochloride)	II-2585
Tetragynon (Ethinyl Estradiol; Levonorgestrel)	II-1047
Tetralen (Tetracycline Hydrochloride)	II-2585
Tetralim (Tetracycline Hydrochloride)	II-2585
Tetralution (Tetracycline Hydrochloride)	II-2585
Tetramig (Tetracycline Hydrochloride)	II-2585
Tetrana (Tetracycline Hydrochloride)	II-2585
Tetranase (Tetracycline Hydrochloride)	II-2585
Tetrano (Tetracycline Hydrochloride)	II-2585
Tetrarco (Tetracycline Hydrochloride)	II-2585
Tetrarco L.A. (Tetracycline Hydrochloride)	II-2585
Tetraseptin (Tetracycline Hydrochloride)	II-2585
Tetrasoline (Hydralazine Hydrochloride)	II-1346
Tetrasuiss (Tetracycline Hydrochloride)	II-2585
Tetrecu (Tetracycline Hydrochloride)	II-2585
Tetrex (Tetracycline Hydrochloride)	II-2585
Tet-Tox (Tetanus Toxoid)	II-2583
Tetuman berna (Tetanus Immune Globulin)	II-2582
Tevacaine (Mepivacaine Hydrochloride)	II-1737
Tevacycline (Tetracycline Hydrochloride)	II-2585
Tevapirin (Aspirin)	II-206
Texate (Methotrexate Sodium)	II-1772
Texate-T (Methotrexate Sodium)	II-1772
Texorate (Methotrexate Sodium)	II-1772
Thacapzol (Methimazole)	II-1767
Thais (Estradiol)	II-986
Thalidone (Chlorthalidone)	II-555
Thelmox (Mebendazole)	II-1711
Theo PA (Theophylline)	II-2593
Theo von CT (Theophylline)	II-2593
Theo-2 (Theophylline)	II-2593
Theo-Bros (Theophylline)	II-2593
Theolair S (Theophylline)	II-2593
Theolan (Theophylline)	II-2593
Theolin (Theophylline)	II-2593
Theolin SR (Theophylline)	II-2593
Theolong (Theophylline)	II-2593
Theomax (Theophylline)	II-2593
Theon (Theophylline)	II-2593
Theoplus (Theophylline)	II-2593
Theoplus Retard (Theophylline)	II-2593
Theospirex Retard (Theophylline)	II-2593
Theostat LP (Theophylline)	II-2593
Theotard (Theophylline)	II-2593
Theotrim (Theophylline)	II-2593
Theourin (Aminophylline)	II-106
Theovent LA (Theophylline)	II-2593
Therabloc (Atenolol)	II-222
Theralite (Lithium Carbonate)	II-1654
Thevier (Levothyroxine Sodium)	II-1618
Thiabet (Metformin Hydrochloride)	II-1760
Thiamazol (Methimazole)	II-1767
Thiasin (Sulfisoxazole)	II-2510
Thidim (Ceftazidime)	II-492
Thilodexine (Dexamethasone)	II-730
Thiomed (Thioridazine Hydrochloride)	II-2605
Thionyl (Thiopental Sodium)	II-2603
Thiopental (Thiopental Sodium)	II-2603
Thioprine (Azathioprine)	II-243
Thioril (Thioridazine Hydrochloride)	II-2605
Thiosia (Thioridazine Hydrochloride)	II-2605
Thixit (Thiothixene)	II-2610
Thombran (Trazodone Hydrochloride)	II-2686
Thosutin (Ethosuximide)	II-1072
Thrombo-Aspilets (Aspirin)	II-206
Thromboliquine (Heparin Sodium)	II-1334
Thrombophob (Heparin Sodium)	II-1334
Thromboreduct (Heparin Sodium)	II-1334
Throxinique (Levothyroxine Sodium)	II-1618
Thycapzol (Methimazole)	II-1767
Thyradin (Levothyroxine Sodium)	II-1618
Thyradin S (Levothyroxine Sodium)	II-1618
Thyrax (Levothyroxine Sodium)	II-1618
Thyrax Duotab (Levothyroxine Sodium)	II-1618
Thyreostat II (Propylthiouracil)	II-2293
Thyrex (Levothyroxine Sodium)	II-1618
Thyro-4 (Levothyroxine Sodium)	II-1618
Thyrosit (Levothyroxine Sodium)	II-1618
Thyroxin (Levothyroxine Sodium)	II-1618
Thyroxine (Levothyroxine Sodium)	II-1618
Thyroxin-Natrium (Levothyroxine Sodium)	II-1618
Thyrozol (Methimazole)	II-1767
Tiabet (Glyburide)	II-1297
Tiaden (Amiloride Hydrochloride; Hydrochlorothiazide)	II-105
Tiadil (Diltiazem Hydrochloride)	II-798
Tialam (Triazolam)	II-2715
Tiamina (Thiamine Hydrochloride)	II-2602
Tiaryt (Amiodarone Hydrochloride)	II-110
Tiazolin (Minoxidil)	II-1845
Tibigon (Ethambutol Hydrochloride)	II-1039
Tibinide (Isoniazid)	II-1496
Tibitol (Ethambutol Hydrochloride)	II-1039
Tibolene (Alendronate Sodium)	II-70
Tibricol (Nifedipine)	II-1967
Tibutol (Ethambutol Hydrochloride)	II-1039
Ticarcin (Ticarcillin Disodium)	II-2616
Ticarpen (Ticarcillin Disodium)	II-2616
Ticdine (Ticlopidine Hydrochloride)	II-2622
Ticlidil (Ticlopidine Hydrochloride)	II-2622
Ticlodix (Ticlopidine Hydrochloride)	II-2622
Ticlodone (Ticlopidine Hydrochloride)	II-2622
Ticlomed (Ticlopidine Hydrochloride)	II-2622
Ticuring (Ticlopidine Hydrochloride)	II-2622
Tidact (Clindamycin)	II-605
Tidilor (Loratadine)	II-1675
Tidomet Forte (Carbidopa; Levodopa)	II-424
Tidomet L.S. (Carbidopa; Levodopa)	II-424
Tidomet Plus (Carbidopa; Levodopa)	II-424
Tienam (Imipenem; Cilastatin Sodium)	II-1424
Tienam 500 (Imipenem; Cilastatin Sodium)	II-1424
Tigen Plaster (Diclofenac)	II-748
Tikleen (Ticlopidine Hydrochloride)	II-2622
Tiklid (Ticlopidine Hydrochloride)	II-2622
Tiklyd (Ticlopidine Hydrochloride)	II-2622
Tikosyn (Dofetilide)	II-842
Tilazem (Diltiazem Hydrochloride)	II-798
Tilazem 90 (Diltiazem Hydrochloride)	II-798
Tildiem (Diltiazem Hydrochloride)	II-798
Tildiem CR (Diltiazem Hydrochloride)	II-798
Tildiem LA (Diltiazem Hydrochloride)	II-798
Tildiem Retard (Diltiazem Hydrochloride)	II-798
Tildopan (Methyldopa)	II-1778
Tilmat (Timolol)	II-2627
Tilodene (Ticlopidine Hydrochloride)	II-2622
Tiloptic (Timolol)	II-2627
Tiloptic (Travoprost)	II-2685
Tim Ophtal (Timolol)	II-2627
Tim Ophtal (Travoprost)	II-2685
Timabak (Timolol)	II-2627
Timacar (Timolol)	II-2627
Timacar (Travoprost)	II-2685
Timacor (Timolol)	II-2627
Timenten (Ticarcillin Disodium; Clavulanate Potassium)	II-2619
Timentine (Ticarcillin Disodium; Clavulanate Potassium)	II-2619
Timet (Cimetidine Hydrochloride)	II-568
Timoftol (Timolol)	II-2627
Timoftol (Travoprost)	II-2685
Timohexal (Timolol)	II-2627
Timohexal (Travoprost)	II-2685
Timol (Timolol)	II-2627
Timol (Travoprost)	II-2685
Timolo (Timolol)	II-2627
Timolol-POS (Timolol)	II-2627
Timolol-POS (Travoprost)	II-2685
Timonil (Carbamazepine)	II-418
Timonil Retard (Carbamazepine)	II-418
Timoptic (Timolol)	II-2627
Timoptic (Travoprost)	II-2685
Timoptic XE (Travoprost)	II-2685
Timoptol (Timolol)	II-2627
Timoptol (Travoprost)	II-2685
Timoptol-XE (Timolol)	II-2627
Timoptol-XE (Travoprost)	II-2685
Timox (Oxcarbazepine)	II-2065
Timozzard (Timolol)	II-2627
Timozzard (Travoprost)	II-2685
Timpilo (Dorzolamide Hydrochloride; Timolol Maleate)	II-860
Tinaderm Extra (Clotrimazole)	II-640
Tinazol (Miconazole)	II-1820
Tinidil (Isosorbide Dinitrate)	II-1502
Tintus (Guaifenesin)	II-1314
Tinza (Nizatidine)	II-1992
Tiodilax (Theophylline)	II-2593
Tiopental Sodico (Thiopental Sodium)	II-2603
Tiotil (Propylthiouracil)	II-2293
Tipidin (Ticlopidine Hydrochloride)	II-2622
Tipidine (Ticlopidine Hydrochloride)	II-2622
Tirlor (Loratadine)	II-1675
Tirodril (Methimazole)	II-1767
Tiroidine (Levothyroxine Sodium)	II-1618
Tirolaxo (Docusate Sodium)	II-841
Tirostat (Propylthiouracil)	II-2293
Tirotax (Cefotaxime Sodium)	II-474
Tiroxin (Levothyroxine Sodium)	II-1618
Tirselon (Tobramycin)	II-2643
Tisamid (Pyrazinamide)	II-2295
Tismalin (Terbutaline Sulfate)	II-2574
Titibe (Prednicarbate)	II-2231
Titol (Timolol)	II-2627
Titol (Travoprost)	II-2685
Titus (Lorazepam)	II-1678
TMS (Sulfamethoxazole; Trimethoprim)	II-2500
Tobacin (Tobramycin)	II-2643
Toberan (Tobramycin)	II-2643
Tobi (Tobramycin)	II-2643
Tobra (Tobramycin Sulfate)	II-2646
Tobradex (Tobramycin)	II-2643
Tobra-gobens (Tobramycin Sulfate)	II-2646
Tobramaxin (Tobramycin)	II-2643
Tobraneg (Tobramycin Sulfate)	II-2646
Tobrimin (Tobramycin)	II-2643
Tobrin (Tobramycin)	II-2643
Tobutol (Ethambutol Hydrochloride)	II-1039
Tobybron (Albuterol)	II-47
Tobyl (Azithromycin)	II-250
Tobymet (Cimetidine Hydrochloride)	II-568
Tocef (Cefixime)	II-466
Tofen (Ibuprofen)	II-1411
Tofranil-PM (Imipramine Hydrochloride)	II-1431
Tohexen (Naproxen)	II-1924
Tohsino (Fluocinonide)	II-1156
Toilax (Bisacodyl)	II-322
Tokiolexin (Cephalexin)	II-520
Tolanase (Tolazamide)	II-2649
Tolbin (Terbutaline Sulfate)	II-2574
Tolbusal (Tolbutamide)	II-2650
Tolbutamida Valdecases (Tolbutamide)	II-2650
Tolchicine (Colchicine)	II-649
Tolexine (Doxycycline)	II-878
Tolexine Ge (Doxycycline)	II-878
Tolimal (Ampicillin)	II-170
Tolisan (Tolazamide)	II-2649
Tolodina (Amoxicillin)	II-131

International brand name (Generic name) Page no.

Tripacel (Diphtheria; Pertussis; Tetanus) II-818
Triphacyclin (Tetracycline Hydrochloride) II-2585
Tripid (Gemfibrozil) II-1269
Tri-Polio (Polio Vaccine, Oral Live) II-2210
Tripress (Trimipramine Maleate) II-2726
Tripta (Amitriptyline Hydrochloride) II-119
Triptafen (Amitriptyline Hydrochloride; Perphenazine) II-124
Triptafen M (Amitriptyline Hydrochloride; Perphenazine) II-124
Triptil (Protriptyline Hydrochloride) II-2294
Triptizol (Amitriptyline Hydrochloride) II-119
Tripvac (Diphtheria; Pertussis; Tetanus) II-818
Triquilar (Ethinyl Estradiol; Levonorgestrel) II-1047
Triquilar ED (Ethinyl Estradiol; Levonorgestrel) II-1047
Tri-Regol (Ethinyl Estradiol; Levonorgestrel) II-1047
Tri-Sequens (Estradiol; Norethindrone Acetate) II-1011
Trisequens (Estradiol; Norethindrone Acetate) II-1011
Trisul (Sulfamethoxazole; Trimethoprim) II-2500
Trisulcom (Sulfamethoxazole; Trimethoprim) II-2500
Tritace (Ramipril) II-2330
Trittico (Trazodone Hydrochloride) II-2686
Triviraten Berna (Measles, Mumps and Rubella Virus Vaccine Live) II-1710
Trixilem (Daunorubicin Hydrochloride) II-708
Trixilem (Methotrexate Sodium) II-1772
Triz (Cetirizine Hydrochloride) II-529
Trizakim (Sulfamethoxazole; Trimethoprim) II-2500
Trizid (Hydrochlorothiazide; Triamterene) II-1362
Trizolin (Norfloxacin) II-1997
Trofentyl (Fentanyl Citrate) II-1112
Trogiar (Metronidazole) II-1812
Trolar (Methocarbamol) II-1768
Trolip (Fenofibrate) II-1105
Trolit (Ethinyl Estradiol; Levonorgestrel) II-1047
Tromalyt (Aspirin) II-206
Tromedal (Ketorolac Tromethamine) II-1537
Tromix (Azithromycin) II-250
Trompersantin (Dipyridamole) II-821
Tronamycin (Tobramycin) II-2643
Tronoxal (Ifosfamide) II-1420
Tropan (Oxybutynin) II-2070
Tropatil (Atropine Sulfate; Diphenoxylate Hydrochloride) II-238
Tropidene (Piroxicam) II-2205
Tropistan (Mefenamic Acid) II-1720
Tropium (Chlordiazepoxide Hydrochloride) II-539
Tropium (Ipratropium Bromide) II-1480
Tropocer (Nimodipine) II-1974
Trozolet (Anastrozole) II-186
Tructum (Ofloxacin) II-2015
Tructum (Terazosin Hydrochloride) II-2566
Trycam (Triazolam) II-2715
Trynol (Amitriptyline Hydrochloride) II-119
Tryptal (Amitriptyline Hydrochloride) II-119
Tryptanol (Amitriptyline Hydrochloride) II-119
Tryptizol (Amitriptyline Hydrochloride) II-119
Trytomer (Amitriptyline Hydrochloride) II-119
Tsudohmin (Diclofenac) II-748
Tsurupioxin (Doxycycline) II-878
Tubilysin (Isoniazid) II-1496
Tums (Calcium Carbonate) II-401
Turfa (Hydrochlorothiazide; Triamterene) II-1362
Turpan (Acetaminophen) II-11
Tusehli (Benzonatate) II-290
Tussol (Methadone Hydrochloride) II-1766
Tybikin (Amikacin Sulfate) II-101
Tyklid (Ticlopidine Hydrochloride) II-2622
Tylenol (Acetaminophen) II-11
Tylenol Extra Fuerte (Acetaminophen) II-11
Tylenol W/Codeine No. 4 (Acetaminophen; Codeine Phosphate) II-13
Tylex (Acetaminophen) II-11
Tylex CD (Acetaminophen; Codeine Phosphate) II-13

International brand name (Generic name) Page no.

Typril-ACE (Captopril) II-411
Tyrex (Theophylline) II-2593
T-Za (Zidovudine) II-2822
Tzoali (Diphenhydramine Hydrochloride) II-813

U

Ubacillin (Ampicillin Sodium; Sulbactam Sodium) II-174
Ubactam (Ampicillin Sodium; Sulbactam Sodium) II-174
Ucefa (Cefadroxil Monohydrate) II-447
Ucholine (Bethanechol Chloride) II-312
Udicil (Cytarabine) II-683
Udicil CS (Cytarabine) II-683
Udrik (Trandolapril) II-2677
Ufarene (Sucralfate) II-2493
Ukidan (Urokinase) II-2734
Ulcaid (Ranitidine Hydrochloride) II-2334
Ulcar (Sucralfate) II-2493
Ulcatif (Famotidine) II-1093
Ulcedin (Cimetidine Hydrochloride) II-568
Ulcedine (Cimetidine Hydrochloride) II-568
Ulcedine (Famotidine) II-1093
Ulcekon (Sucralfate) II-2493
Ulcemet (Cimetidine Hydrochloride) II-568
Ulcenon (Cimetidine Hydrochloride) II-568
Ulcepraz (Pantoprazole Sodium) II-2097
Ulceran (Famotidine) II-1093
Ulceran (Ranitidine Hydrochloride) II-2334
Ulceranin (Ranitidine Hydrochloride) II-2334
Ulcerfen (Cimetidine Hydrochloride) II-568
Ulcerin-P (Aluminum Hydroxide) II-97
Ulcerlmin (Sucralfate) II-2493
Ulcertec (Sucralfate) II-2493
Ulcex (Ranitidine Hydrochloride) II-2334
Ulcidine (Famotidine) II-1093
Ulcim (Cimetidine Hydrochloride) II-568
Ulcimet (Cimetidine Hydrochloride) II-568
Ulcin (Ranitidine Hydrochloride) II-2334
Ulcodina (Cimetidine Hydrochloride) II-568
Ulcofam (Famotidine) II-1093
Ulcogant (Sucralfate) II-2493
Ulcolind H2 (Cimetidine Hydrochloride) II-568
Ulcomedina (Cimetidine Hydrochloride) II-568
Ulcomet (Cimetidine Hydrochloride) II-568
Ulcozol (Omeprazole) II-2034
Ulcumet (Cimetidine Hydrochloride) II-568
Ulcyte (Sucralfate) II-2493
Ulfadin (Famotidine) II-1093
Ulfagel (Famotidine) II-1093
Ulfam (Famotidine) II-1093
Ulfaprim (Sulfamethoxazole; Trimethoprim) II-2500
Ulnor (Omeprazole) II-2034
Ulpax (Lansoprazole) II-1569
Ulped (Famotidine) II-1093
Ulped AR (Famotidine) II-1093
Ulsaheal (Sucralfate) II-2493
Ulsal (Ranitidine Hydrochloride) II-2334
Ulsanic (Sucralfate) II-2493
Ulsen (Omeprazole) II-2034
Ulsidex Forte (Sucralfate) II-2493
Ulsikur (Cimetidine Hydrochloride) II-568
Ultak (Ranitidine Hydrochloride) II-2334
Ultracef (Ceftizoxime Sodium) II-500
Ultracorten (Prednisone) II-2240
Ultracortenol (Prednisolone) II-2233
Ultradol (Etodolac) II-1076
Ultraquin (Hydroquinone) II-1391
Ultraxime (Cefixime) II-466
Ultreon (Azithromycin) II-250
Umbradol (Salsalate) II-2418
Umine (Phentermine Hydrochloride) II-2170
U-Miso (Misoprostol) II-1851
Umprel (Bromocriptine Mesylate) II-344

International brand name (Generic name) Page no.

Umuline Profil 10 (Insulin (Human, Isophane/Regular)) II-1456
Umuline Profil 10 (Insulin (Human Recombinant)) II-1454
Umuline Profil 20 (Insulin (Human, Isophane/Regular)) II-1456
Umuline Profil 20 (Insulin (Human Recombinant)) II-1454
Umuline Profil 30 (Insulin (Human, Isophane/Regular)) II-1456
Umuline Profil 30 (Insulin (Human Recombinant)) II-1454
Umuline Profil 40 (Insulin (Human, Isophane/Regular)) II-1456
Umuline Profil 40 (Insulin (Human Recombinant)) II-1454
Umuline Profil 50 (Insulin (Human Recombinant)) II-1454
Umuline Protamine Isophane (Insulin (Human, Isophane)) II-1455
Umuline Zinc (Insulin (Human, Lente)) II-1456
Unacid (Ampicillin Sodium; Sulbactam Sodium) II-174
Unacim (Ampicillin Sodium; Sulbactam Sodium) II-174
Unamine (Hydroxyzine) II-1398
Unaril (Enalapril Maleate) II-913
Unasyna (Ampicillin Sodium; Sulbactam Sodium) II-174
Unat (Torsemide) II-2671
Undiarrhea (Loperamide Hydrochloride) II-1664
Unex (Ciprofloxacin Hydrochloride) II-573
Unicam (Piroxicam) II-2205
Uniclar (Mometasone Furoate) II-1866
Unicontin-400 Continus (Theophylline) II-2593
Unicordium (Bepridil Hydrochloride) II-295
Unicort (Betamethasone) II-298
Unicort (Hydrocortisone) II-1369
Uniderm (Clobetasol Propionate) II-617
Uniderm (Hydrocortisone) II-1369
Unidipine XL (Nifedipine) II-1967
Unidox (Doxycycline) II-878
Unif (Triamcinolone Acetonide) II-2701
Uniflam (Naproxen Sodium) II-1928
Uniflox (Ciprofloxacin Hydrochloride) II-573
Unifyl Retard (Theophylline) II-2593
Unigo (Metronidazole) II-1812
Unimazole (Methimazole) II-1767
Unimetone (Nabumetone) II-1909
Uniparin (Heparin Sodium) II-1334
Uniphyl CR (Theophylline) II-2593
Uniphyllin (Theophylline) II-2593
Uniphyllin Continus (Theophylline) II-2593
Unipirin (Cephapirin Sodium) II-525
Unipril (Enalapril Maleate) II-913
Unipril (Ramipril) II-2330
Uniquin (Lomefloxacin Hydrochloride) II-1658
Unlren (Diclofenac) II-748
Uniretic (Amiloride Hydrochloride; Hydrochlorothiazide) II-105
Uniretic (Enalapril Maleate; Hydrochlorothiazide) II-923
Unisal (Diflunisal) II-777
Unitimo (Timolol) II-2627
Unitral (Tramadol Hydrochloride) II-2674
Unitrizole (Sulfamethoxazole; Trimethoprim) II-2500
Unival (Sucralfate) II-2493
Univate (Clobetasol Propionate) II-617
UniWarfin (Warfarin Sodium) II-2804
Unizuric 300 (Allopurinol) II-77
Upan (Lorazepam) II-1678
Upfen (Ibuprofen) II-1411
Uphalexin (Cephalexin) II-520
Uprofen (Ibuprofen) II-1411
Upsa C (Ascorbic Acid) II-203
Upsa-C (Ascorbic Acid) II-203

International brand name (Generic name)	Page no.
Uracil (Propylthiouracil)	II-2293
Uramin (Dopamine Hydrochloride)	II-853
Urandil (Chlorthalidone)	II-555
Urantac (Ranitidine Hydrochloride)	II-2334
Urantin (Nitrofurantoin)	II-1979
Urazole (Sulfisoxazole)	II-2510
Urbal (Sucralfate)	II-2493
Urbason (Methylprednisolone)	II-1787
Urbason (Methylprednisolone Acetate)	II-1790
Urbason Retard (Methylprednisolone)	II-1787
Urbason Solubile (Methylprednisolone Sodium Succinate)	II-1793
Urbason Soluble (Methylprednisolone Sodium Succinate)	II-1793
Urdafalk (Ursodiol)	II-2737
Urekacin (Norfloxacin)	II-1997
Urem (Ibuprofen)	II-1411
Urenil (Furosemide)	II-1237
Uresix (Furosemide)	II-1237
Urex-M (Furosemide)	II-1237
Urgendol (Tramadol Hydrochloride)	II-2674
Uric (Allopurinol)	II-77
Uricad (Allopurinol)	II-77
Uriconorm (Allopurinol)	II-77
Uricont (Oxybutynin)	II-2070
Uridoz (Fosfomycin Tromethamine)	II-1222
Uriduct (Doxazosin Mesylate)	II-860
Urinex (Norfloxacin)	II-1997
Urinol (Allopurinol)	II-77
Uripurinol (Allopurinol)	II-77
Urisold (Norfloxacin)	II-1997
U-Ritis (Naproxen)	II-1924
Uritracin (Norfloxacin)	II-1997
Uro Tarivid (Ofloxacin)	II-2015
Urobacid (Norfloxacin)	II-1997
Urobactam (Aztreonam)	II-263
Urobactrim (Sulfamethoxazole; Trimethoprim)	II-2500
Urocef (Cefadroxil Monohydrate)	II-447
Uro-cephoral (Cefixime)	II-466
Urocid (Probenecid)	II-2248
Uroctal (Norfloxacin)	II-1997
Uroflox (Norfloxacin)	II-1997
Urofuran (Nitrofurantoin)	II-1979
Urogquad (Allopurinol)	II-77
Urokine (Urokinase)	II-2734
Urolin (Chlorthalidone)	II-555
Uroquad (Allopurinol)	II-77
Urosin (Allopurinol)	II-77
Urosin (Atenolol)	II-222
Uro-Tablinen (Nitrofurantoin, Macrocrystalline)	II-1982
Urotonine (Bethanechol Chloride)	II-312
Uroxacin (Norfloxacin)	II-1997
Uroxin (Ciprofloxacin Hydrochloride)	II-573
Ursacol (Ursodiol)	II-2737
Ursochol (Ursodiol)	II-2737
Ursodamor (Ursodiol)	II-2737
Ursofalk (Ursodiol)	II-2737
Ursolin (Ursodiol)	II-2737
Ursolit (Ursodiol)	II-2737
Ursolvan (Ursodiol)	II-2737
Urso-Ratiopharm (Ursodiol)	II-2737
Urycin (Erythromycin Stearate)	II-970
U-Save (Cephradine)	II-526
U-Sorbide (Isosorbide Dinitrate)	II-1502
Utemerin (Ritodrine Hydrochloride)	II-2379
UT-in (Norfloxacin)	II-1997
Utinor (Norfloxacin)	II-1997
Utopar (Ritodrine Hydrochloride)	II-2379
Utovlan (Norethindrone)	II-1996
Utrogestan (Progesterone)	II-2262
Utron INJ (Oxytocin)	II-2082
Uvamin (Nitrofurantoin, Macrocrystalline)	II-1982
Uvamin Retard (Nitrofurantoin, Macrocrystalline)	II-1982
Uvamin-E Retard (Nitrofurantoin, Macrocrystalline)	II-1982
Uxen (Amitriptyline Hydrochloride)	II-119
Uzolin (Cefazolin Sodium)	II-452
V	
Vaben (Oxazepam)	II-2063
Vabon (Danazol)	II-699
Vacanyl (Terbutaline Sulfate)	II-2574
Vacillin (Ampicillin)	II-170
Vacolax (Bisacodyl)	II-322
Vacontil (Loperamide Hydrochloride)	II-1664
Vacrovir (Acyclovir)	II-33
Vacuna Antirrabica Humana (Rabies Vaccine)	II-2324
Vagaka (Mebendazole)	II-1711
Vagifem (Estradiol)	II-986
Valaxona (Diazepam)	II-740
Valbet (Betamethasone Dipropionate)	II-301
Valcote (Divalproex Sodium)	II-828
Valcote (Valproate Sodium)	II-2749
Valcyclor (Valacyclovir Hydrochloride)	II-2738
Valdorm (Flurazepam Hydrochloride)	II-1175
Valeans (Alprazolam)	II-85
Valemia (Simvastatin)	II-2454
Valentac (Diclofenac)	II-748
Valeptol (Valproate Sodium)	II-2749
Valeric (Allopurinol)	II-77
Valezone (Betamethasone Valerate)	II-305
Valifol (Isoniazid)	II-1496
Valiquid (Diazepam)	II-740
Valixa (Valganciclovir Hydrochloride)	II-2745
Valoin (Valproate Sodium)	II-2749
Valpakine (Valproate Sodium)	II-2749
Valpam (Diazepam)	II-740
Valparin (Valproate Sodium)	II-2749
Valporal (Valproate Sodium)	II-2749
Valporal (Valproic Acid)	II-2755
Valprax (Valproate Sodium)	II-2749
Valprosid (Valproic Acid)	II-2755
Valsup (Valproate Sodium)	II-2749
Valus (Valdecoxib)	II-2741
Vanafen Otologic (Chloramphenicol)	II-536
Vanafen S (Chloramphenicol)	II-536
Vanauras (Vancomycin Hydrochloride)	II-2763
Vancam (Vancomycin Hydrochloride)	II-2763
Vanccostacin (Vancomycin Hydrochloride)	II-2763
Vanco (Vancomycin Hydrochloride)	II-2763
Vancocina (Vancomycin Hydrochloride)	II-2763
Vancocine (Vancomycin Hydrochloride)	II-2763
Vanco-Teva (Vancomycin Hydrochloride)	II-2763
Vancox (Vancomycin Hydrochloride)	II-2763
Vanesten (Clotrimazole)	II-640
Vanmicina (Vancomycin Hydrochloride)	II-2763
Vanmycetin (Chloramphenicol)	II-536
Vapine (Chlordiazepoxide Hydrochloride)	II-539
Vaqta (Hepatitis A Vaccine)	II-1339
Varitect (Varicella-Zoster Immune Globulin (Human))	II-2768
Varivax II (Varicella Vaccine)	II-2767
Varnoline (Desogestrel; Ethinyl Estradiol)	II-725
Varol (Betamethasone Valerate)	II-305
Varsan (Lindane)	II-1642
V-AS (Aspirin)	II-206
Vascal (Isradipine)	II-1515
Vascard (Nifedipine)	II-1967
Vascardin (Isosorbide Dinitrate)	II-1502
Vascoten (Atenolol)	II-222
Vasdalat (Nifedipine)	II-1967
Vasilcon (Phenytoin Sodium)	II-2175
Vasocardin (Metoprolol)	II-1805
Vasodilat (Isosorbide Dinitrate)	II-1502
Vasodin (Nicardipine Hydrochloride)	II-1958
Vasokor (Dipyridamole)	II-821
Vasolan (Verapamil Hydrochloride)	II-2777
Vasolator (Nitroglycerin)	II-1984
Vasomet (Terazosin Hydrochloride)	II-2566
Vasomil (Verapamil Hydrochloride)	II-2777
Vasopran (Pravastatin Sodium)	II-2224
Vasopress (Enalapril Maleate)	II-913
Vasopril (Fosinopril Sodium)	II-1222
Vasopril Plus (Fosinopril Sodium; Hydrochlorothiazide)	II-1226
Vasopten (Verapamil Hydrochloride)	II-2777
Vasoretic (Enalapril Maleate; Hydrochlorothiazide)	II-923
Vasosan P-Granulat (Cholestyramine)	II-559
Vasosan S-Granulat (Cholestyramine)	II-559
Vasosta (Captopril)	II-411
Vasotenal (Simvastatin)	II-2454
Vasotop (Nimodipine)	II-1974
Vasotrate (Isosorbide Mononitrate)	II-1507
Vastamox (Amoxicillin)	II-131
Vasten (Amlodipine Besylate)	II-125
Vasten (Pravastatin Sodium)	II-2224
Vatran (Diazepam)	II-740
Vaxigrip (Influenza Virus Vaccine)	II-1451
Vaxor (Venlafaxine Hydrochloride)	II-2770
Vazen (Diazepam)	II-740
Vazim (Simvastatin)	II-2454
V-Bloc (Carvedilol)	II-438
V-Cil-K (Penicillin V Potassium)	II-2142
V-Cillin K (Penicillin V Potassium)	II-2142
Veclam (Clarithromycin)	II-597
Vectavir (Penciclovir)	II-2131
Veemycin (Doxycycline)	II-878
Veinobiase (Ascorbic Acid)	II-203
Velamox (Amoxicillin)	II-131
Velamox CL (Amoxicillin; Clavulanate Potassium)	II-139
Velbe (Vinblastine Sulfate)	II-2787
Velexin (Cephalexin)	II-520
Velocef (Cephradine)	II-526
Velodan (Loratadine)	II-1675
Velosef Viol (Cephradine)	II-526
Velosulin (Insulin (Human Recombinant))	II-1454
Velosuline Humaine (Insulin (Human Recombinant))	II-1454
Velsay (Naproxen)	II-1924
Vena (Diphenhydramine Hydrochloride)	II-813
Venalax (Albuterol)	II-47
Venasmin (Diphenhydramine Hydrochloride)	II-813
Vencronyl (Albuterol)	II-47
Venefon (Imipramine Hydrochloride)	II-1431
Venetlin (Albuterol)	II-47
Venitrin (Nitroglycerin)	II-1984
Venix-XR (Venlafaxine Hydrochloride)	II-2770
Venoglobulin S (Immune Globulin (Human))	II-1434
Venoglobulin-I (Immune Globulin (Human))	II-1434
Ventilan (Albuterol)	II-47
Ventimax (Albuterol)	II-47
Ventodisks (Albuterol)	II-47
Ventol (Albuterol)	II-47
Ventolin CFC-Free (Albuterol)	II-47
Ventoline (Albuterol)	II-47
Venvia (Rosiglitazone Maleate)	II-2405
Vepan (Cefadroxil Monohydrate)	II-447
Vepeside (Etoposide)	II-1080
Vepicombin (Penicillin V Potassium)	II-2142
Veracaps SR (Verapamil Hydrochloride)	II-2777
Veracef (Cephradine)	II-526
Veracor (Verapamil Hydrochloride)	II-2777
Veradol (Naproxen)	II-1924
Verahexal (Verapamil Hydrochloride)	II-2777
Veraloc (Verapamil Hydrochloride)	II-2777
Veramex (Verapamil Hydrochloride)	II-2777
Veramil (Verapamil Hydrochloride)	II-2777
Verapin (Verapamil Hydrochloride)	II-2777
Veraplex (Medroxyprogesterone Acetate)	II-1714
Verapress 240 SR (Verapamil Hydrochloride)	II-2777
Veratad (Verapamil Hydrochloride)	II-2777
Verben (Azatadine Maleate)	II-242

International brand name (Generic name)	Page no.
Vercef (Cefaclor)	II-444
Verdilac (Verapamil Hydrochloride)	II-2777
Vericordin (Atenolol)	II-222
Verladyn (Dihydroergotamine Mesylate)	II-792
Verlost (Ranitidine Hydrochloride)	II-2334
Vermin Plus (Albendazole)	II-46
Vermis (Acyclovir)	II-33
Vermisol (Levamisole Hydrochloride)	II-1598
Verpamil (Verapamil Hydrochloride)	II-2777
Versatic (Cefadroxil Monohydrate)	II-447
Versef (Cefaclor)	II-444
Versigen (Gentamicin Sulfate)	II-1279
Verteblan (Dihydroergotamine Mesylate)	II-792
Vertivom (Metoclopramide Hydrochloride)	II-1798
Vesdil (Ramipril)	II-2330
Vesyca (Ranitidine Hydrochloride)	II-2334
Vetrimil (Verapamil Hydrochloride)	II-2777
Vexamet (Dexamethasone)	II-730
Viaclav (Amoxicillin; Clavulanate Potassium)	II-139
Viadoxin (Doxycycline)	II-878
Viarex (Beclomethasone Dipropionate)	II-279
Viarox (Beclomethasone Dipropionate)	II-279
Vibrabiotic (Doxycycline)	II-878
Vibracina (Doxycycline)	II-878
Vibradox (Doxycycline)	II-878
Vibramicina (Doxycycline)	II-878
Vibramycine (Doxycycline)	II-878
Vibramycin-N (Doxycycline)	II-878
Vibra-S (Doxycycline)	II-878
Vibratab (Doxycycline)	II-878
Vibra-Tabs (Doxycycline)	II-878
Vibraveineuse (Doxycycline)	II-878
Vibravenos (Doxycycline)	II-878
Vibravenos SF (Doxycycline)	II-878
Vi-C 500 (Ascorbic Acid)	II-203
Vicapan N (Cyanocobalamin)	II-661
Vicard (Terazosin Hydrochloride)	II-2566
Viccillin (Ampicillin)	II-170
Vicef (Ascorbic Acid)	II-203
Vicorax (Acyclovir)	II-33
Vicrom (Cromolyn Sodium)	II-656
Vidapirocam (Piroxicam)	II-2205
Vidcef (Cefadroxil Monohydrate)	II-447
Viden DDI (Didanosine)	II-766
Videx EC (Didanosine)	II-766
Vidopen (Ampicillin)	II-170
Vigain (Sildenafil Citrate)	II-2451
Vigamox (Moxifloxacin Hydrochloride)	II-1886
Vigil (Modafinil)	II-1858
Vigopen (Nafcillin Sodium)	II-1914
Vikela (Levonorgestrel)	II-1614
Viken (Cefotaxime Sodium)	II-474
Vinafluor (Sodium Fluoride)	II-2465
Vincrisul (Vincristine Sulfate)	II-2789
Vinsen (Naproxen)	II-1924
Vintec (Vincristine Sulfate)	II-2789
Viotisone (Ofloxacin)	II-2015
Vioxx Forte (Rofecoxib)	II-2396
Vipront (Cromolyn Sodium)	II-656
Viraban (Acyclovir)	II-33
Viradoxyl-N (Doxycycline)	II-878
Viraferon (Interferon Alfa-2b, Recombinant)	II-1471
Viralex (Acyclovir)	II-33
Viralex-DS (Acyclovir)	II-33
Virazin (Ribavirin)	II-2351
Vircella (Acyclovir)	II-33
Virdual (Lamivudine; Zidovudine)	II-1560
Virest (Acyclovir)	II-33
Virex (Acyclovir)	II-33
Virgan (Ganciclovir Sodium)	II-1250
Viridal (Alprostadil)	II-90
Virless (Acyclovir)	II-33
Virlix (Cetirizine Hydrochloride)	II-529
Virofral (Amantadine Hydrochloride)	II-97
Virogon (Acyclovir)	II-33
Virolan (Acyclovir)	II-33
Viromed (Acyclovir)	II-33
Vironida (Acyclovir)	II-33
Virormone (Methyltestosterone)	II-1796
Virosol (Amantadine Hydrochloride)	II-97
Virucid (Acyclovir)	II-33
Virucil (Ampicillin)	II-170
Virupos Eye Oint (Acyclovir)	II-33
Visanon (Meprobamate)	II-1738
Viskeen (Pindolol)	II-2192
Viskeen Retard (Pindolol)	II-2192
Viskene (Pindolol)	II-2192
Vistacarpin (Pilocarpine)	II-2180
Vistacrom (Cromolyn Sodium)	II-656
Vistafrin (Phenylephrine Hydrochloride)	II-2173
Vistagan (Levobunolol Hydrochloride)	II-1603
Vistagen (Levobunolol Hydrochloride)	II-1603
Vistosan (Phenylephrine Hydrochloride)	II-2173
Vistrep (Amoxicillin)	II-131
Visudyne (Verteporfin)	II-2784
Visumetazone (Dexamethasone)	II-730
Vitac (Ascorbic Acid)	II-203
Vita-Cedol Orange (Ascorbic Acid)	II-203
Vitacimin (Ascorbic Acid)	II-203
Vitak (Phytonadione)	II-2178
Vitamin A Acid (Tretinoin)	II-2691
Vitamin K (Phytonadione)	II-2178
Vitamina B12-Ecar (Cyanocobalamin)	II-661
Vitamycetin (Chloramphenicol)	II-536
Vitanon (Thiamine Hydrochloride)	II-2602
Vitantial (Thiamine Hydrochloride)	II-2602
Vitapen (Ampicillin)	II-170
Vitaplex (Niacin)	II-1956
Vitarubin (Cyanocobalamin)	II-661
Vitascorbol (Ascorbic Acid)	II-203
Vitazyme (Pancrelipase)	II-2095
Vitralgin (Allopurinol)	II-77
Vitrasert Implant (Ganciclovir Sodium)	II-1250
Vivaquine (Primaquine Phosphate)	II-2246
Vivatec (Lisinopril)	II-1648
Vivazid (Hydrochlorothiazide; Lisinopril)	II-1352
Vividrin (Cromolyn Sodium)	II-656
Vividyl (Nortriptyline Hydrochloride)	II-2002
Vivir (Acyclovir)	II-33
Vivol (Diazepam)	II-740
Vizerul (Ranitidine Hydrochloride)	II-2334
V-Kal-K (Penicillin V Potassium)	II-2142
Voldic (Diclofenac)	II-748
Voldic Emulgel (Diclofenac)	II-748
Volequin (Levofloxacin)	II-1607
Volero (Diclofenac)	II-748
Volfenac (Diclofenac)	II-748
Volon (Triamcinolone)	II-2698
Volon A (Triamcinolone Acetonide)	II-2701
Volon A 10 (Triamcinolone Acetonide)	II-2701
Volon A 40 (Triamcinolone Acetonide)	II-2701
Volon A Antibiotikafrei (Triamcinolone Acetonide)	II-2701
Volon A Spray (Triamcinolone Acetonide)	II-2701
Volta (Diclofenac)	II-748
Voltadex Emulgel (Diclofenac)	II-748
Voltalen (Diclofenac)	II-748
Voltalen Emulgel (Diclofenac)	II-748
Voltaren Emulgel (Diclofenac)	II-748
Voltaren Forte (Diclofenac)	II-748
Voltaren Ofta (Diclofenac)	II-748
Voltaren Oftalmico (Diclofenac)	II-748
Voltaren Ophta (Diclofenac)	II-748
Voltaren Ophtha (Diclofenac)	II-748
Voltaren Rapid (Diclofenac)	II-748
Voltaren Retard (Diclofenac)	II-748
Voltaren SR (Diclofenac)	II-748
Voltarene (Diclofenac)	II-748
Voltarene Emulgel (Diclofenac)	II-748
Voltarol (Diclofenac)	II-748
Voltarol Emulgel (Diclofenac)	II-748
Vomceran (Ondansetron Hydrochloride)	II-2039
Vomitrol (Metoclopramide Hydrochloride)	II-1798
Voncon (Vancomycin Hydrochloride)	II-2763
Vonum (Indomethacin)	II-1443
Vorange (Ascorbic Acid)	II-203
Voren (Diclofenac)	II-748
Voren Emulgel (Diclofenac)	II-748
Voroste (Alendronate Sodium)	II-70
Votalen SR (Diclofenac)	II-748
Voveran (Diclofenac)	II-748
Voveran Emulgel (Diclofenac)	II-748
Voxamin (Fluvoxamine Maleate)	II-1203
Voxxim (Cephalexin)	II-520
V-Pen (Penicillin V Potassium)	II-2142
V-Penicillin Kalium (Penicillin V Potassium)	II-2142
VP-TEC (Etoposide)	II-1080
Vulamox (Amoxicillin; Clavulanate Potassium)	II-139
Vulcasid (Omeprazole)	II-2034
Vurdon (Diclofenac)	II-748
Vypen (Pindolol)	II-2192
V-Z Vax (Varicella Vaccine)	II-2767

W

International brand name (Generic name)	Page no.
Wakazepam (Oxazepam)	II-2063
Wakezepam (Oxazepam)	II-2063
Walacort (Betamethasone)	II-298
Walaphage (Metformin Hydrochloride)	II-1760
Walesolone (Prednisolone)	II-2233
Wanflox (Sparfloxacin)	II-2479
Wanmycin (Doxycycline)	II-878
Waran (Warfarin Sodium)	II-2804
Warfar (Warfarin Sodium)	II-2804
Warfil 5 (Warfarin Sodium)	II-2804
Warfilone (Warfarin Sodium)	II-2804
Warimazol (Clotrimazole)	II-640
Warviron (Acyclovir)	II-33
Waucoton (Propranolol Hydrochloride)	II-2287
Waytrax (Ceftazidime)	II-492
Weichilin (Ranitidine Hydrochloride)	II-2334
Weidos (Ranitidine Hydrochloride)	II-2334
Weimer Adrenaline (Epinephrine)	II-934
Weimok (Famotidine)	II-1093
Weisdin (Cimetidine Hydrochloride)	II-568
Well (Bupropion Hydrochloride)	II-368
Welldorm (Chloral Hydrate)	II-534
Wellvone (Atovaquone)	II-234
Weradren (Epinephrine)	II-934
Wesipin (Atenolol)	II-222
Widecillin (Amoxicillin)	II-131
Winadol (Acetaminophen)	II-11
Winadol Forte (Acetaminophen; Codeine Phosphate)	II-13
Winasorb (Acetaminophen)	II-11
Winlex (Cephalexin)	II-520
Winobanin (Danazol)	II-699
Winpen (Amoxicillin)	II-131
Winpred (Prednisone)	II-2240
WinRho SDF (Rho (D) Immune Globulin)	II-2350
Winsprin (Aspirin)	II-206
Winsumin (Chlorpromazine Hydrochloride)	II-549
Wintermin (Chlorpromazine Hydrochloride)	II-549
Wintrex (Naproxen)	II-1924
Wiretin (Famotidine)	II-1093
Wormgo (Mebendazole)	II-1711
Wormin (Mebendazole)	II-1711
Wycillina A P (Penicillin G Benzathine)	II-2136
Wycort (Hydrocortisone Acetate)	II-1373
Wymesone (Dexamethasone)	II-730
Wypax (Lorazepam)	II-1678
Wytens (Bisoprolol Fumarate; Hydrochlorothiazide)	II-326
Wytens (Guanabenz Acetate)	II-1318

X

International brand name (Generic name)	Page no.
Xacin (Norfloxacin)	II-1997
Xadem (Albendazole)	II-46

Y

Z

DRUG INFORMATION

This Professional Drug Reference provides the complete package insert along with other invaluable pharmaceutical information, including FDA-approved indications, FDA drug class, FDA approval date, innovator drug, pregnancy category, top-selling drugs grouped by top 200, trade names (U.S. and international), benchmark cost of therapy, controlled substance schedule, and hard-to-find pricing for comparisons.

- Monographs are the complete manufacturer's package insert, featuring sections on the following: description, clinical pharmacology, clinical studies, indications and usage, contraindications, warnings, precautions, drug interactions, adverse reactions, drug abuse and dependence, overdose, dosage and administration, animal pharmacology, references, and how supplied.
- Additional value-added information in the Categories section includes FDA-approved indications, drug class, FDA approval date, innovator drug, pregnancy category, brand names (U.S. and international), cost of therapy, and controlled substance schedule.
- The Product Listing section lists products by brand names, strength, package sizes, AWP (average wholesale price), and HCFA (Health Care Financing Administration) pricing.

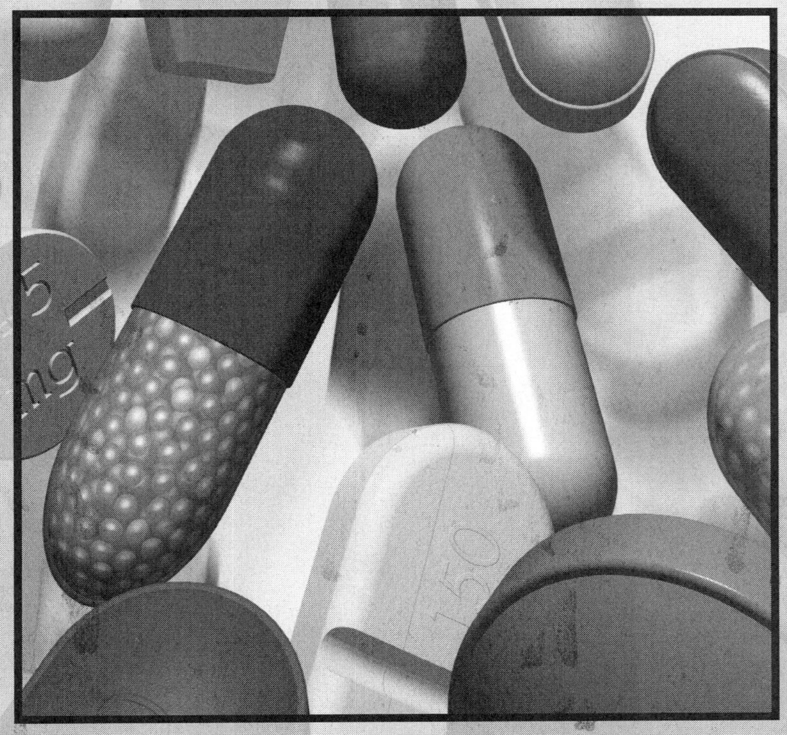

Abacavir Sulfate; Lamivudine; Zidovudine (003512)

For related information, see the comparative table section in Appendix A.

Categories: Infection, human immunodeficiency virus; FDA Approved 2000 Nov; Pregnancy Category C
Drug Classes: Antivirals; Nucleoside reverse transcriptase inhibitors
Brand Names: Trizivir
Cost of Therapy: $1,065.56 (HIV; Trizivir; 300 mg; 150 mg; 300 mg; 2 tablets/day; 30 day supply)

WARNING

Note: The trade names have been used throughout this monograph for clarity.

Trizivir contains 3 nucleoside analogs (abacavir sulfate, lamivudine, and zidovudine) and is intended only for patients whose regimen would otherwise include these 3 components.

Trizivir contains abacavir sulfate (Ziagen), which has been associated with fatal hypersensitivity reactions (see WARNINGS). Patients developing signs or symptoms of hypersensitivity (which include fever; skin rash; fatigue; gastrointestinal symptoms such as nausea, vomiting, diarrhea, or abdominal pain; and respiratory symptoms such as pharyngitis, dyspnea, or cough) should discontinue Trizivir as soon as a hypersensitivity reaction is suspected. To avoid a delay in diagnosis and minimize the risk of a life-threatening hypersensitivity reaction, Trizivir should be permanently discontinued if hypersensitivity cannot be ruled out, even when other diagnoses are possible (*e.g.,* acute onset respiratory diseases, gastroenteritis, or reactions to other medications).

Abacavir (as Trizivir or Ziagen) SHOULD NOT be restarted following a hypersensitivity reaction to abacavir because more severe symptoms will recur within hours and may include life-threatening hypotension and death.

Severe or fatal hypersensitivity reactions can occur within hours after reintroduction of abacavir (as Trizivir or Ziagen) in patients who have no identified history or unrecognized symptoms of hypersensitivity to abacavir therapy (see WARNINGS; PRECAUTIONS, Information for the Patient; and ADVERSE REACTIONS).

Zidovudine has been associated with hematologic toxicity including neutropenia and severe anemia, particularly in patients with advanced HIV disease (see WARNINGS). Prolonged use of zidovudine has been associated with symptomatic myopathy.

Lactic acidosis and severe hepatomegaly with steatosis, including fatal cases, have been reported with the use of nucleoside analogues alone or in combination, including abacavir, lamivudine, zidovudine, and other antiretrovirals (see WARNINGS).

There are limited data on the use of this triple-combination regimen in patients with higher viral load levels (>100,000 copies/ml) at baseline.

DESCRIPTION

TRIZIVIR

Trizivir tablets contain the following 3 synthetic nucleoside analogues: abacavir sulfate (Ziagen), lamivudine (also known as Epivir or 3TC), and zidovudine (also known as Retrovir, azidothymidine, or ZDV) with inhibitory activity against human immunodeficiency virus (HIV).

Trizivir tablets are for oral administration. Each film-coated tablet contains the active ingredients 300 mg of abacavir as abacavir sulfate, 150 mg of lamivudine, and 300 mg of zidovudine, and the inactive ingredients magnesium stearate, microcrystalline cellulose, and sodium starch glycolate. The tablets are coated with a film (Opadry green 03B11434) that is made of FD&C blue no. 2, hydroxypropyl methylcellulose, polyethylene glycol, titanium dioxide, and yellow iron oxide.

ABACAVIR SULFATE

The chemical name of abacavir sulfate is (1*S,cis*)-4-[2-amino-6-(cyclopropylamino)-9*H*-purin-9-yl]-2-cyclopentene-1-methanol sulfate (salt) (2:1). Abacavir sulfate is the enantiomer with *1S,4R* absolute configuration on the cyclopentene ring. It has a molecular formula of $(C_{14}H_{18}N_6O)_2 \cdot H_2SO_4$ and a molecular weight of 670.76 daltons.

Abacavir sulfate is a white to off-white solid with a solubility of approximately 77 mg/ml in distilled water at 25°C.

In vivo, abacavir sulfate dissociates to its free base, abacavir. In this insert, all dosages for Ziagen (abacavir sulfate) are expressed in terms of abacavir.

LAMIVUDINE

The chemical name of lamivudine is (2R,cis)-4-amino-1-(2-hydroxymethyl-1,3-oxathiolan-5-yl)-(1H)-pyrimidin-2-one. Lamivudine is the (-)enantiomer of a dideoxy analogue of cytidine. Lamivudine has also been referred to as (-)2′,3′-dideoxy, 3′-thiacytidine. It has a molecular formula of $C_8H_{11}N_3O_3S$ and a molecular weight of 229.3 daltons.

Lamivudine is a white to off-white crystalline solid with a solubility of approximately 70 mg/ml in water at 20°C.

ZIDOVUDINE

The chemical name of zidovudine is 3′-azido-3′-deoxythymidine. It has a molecular formula of $C_{10}H_{13}N_5O_4$ and a molecular weight of 267.24 daltons.

Zidovudine is a white to beige, crystalline solid with a solubility of 20.1 mg/ml in water at 25°C.

CLINICAL PHARMACOLOGY

MICROBIOLOGY

Mechanism of Action

Abacavir

Abacavir is a carbocyclic synthetic nucleoside analogue. Intracellularly, abacavir is converted by cellular enzymes to the active metabolite, carbovir triphosphate. Carbovir triphosphate is an analogue of deoxyguanosine-5′-triphosphate (dGTP). Carbovir triphosphate inhibits the activity of HIV-1 reverse transcriptase (RT) both by competing with the natural substrate dGTP and by its incorporation into viral DNA. The lack of a 3′-OH group in the incorporated nucleoside analogue prevents the formation of the 5′ to 3′ phosphodiester linkage essential for DNA chain elongation, and therefore, the viral DNA growth is terminated.

Lamivudine

Lamivudine is a synthetic nucleoside analogue. Intracellularly, lamivudine is phosphorylated to its active 5′-triphosphate metabolite, lamivudine triphosphate (L-TP). The principal mode of action of L-TP is inhibition of RT via DNA chain termination after incorporation of the nucleoside analogue. L-TP is a weak inhibitor of mammalian DNA polymerases-α and -β and mitochondrial DNA polymerase-γ.

Zidovudine

Zidovudine is a synthetic nucleoside analogue. Intracellularly, zidovudine is phosphorylated to its active 5′-triphosphate metabolite, zidovudine triphosphate (ZDV-TP). The principal mode of action of ZDV-TP is inhibition of RT via DNA chain termination after incorporation of the nucleoside analogue. ZDV-TP is a weak inhibitor of the mammalian DNA polymerase-α and mitochondrial DNA polymerase-γ and has been reported to be incorporated into the DNA of cells in culture.

Antiviral Activity In Vitro

The relationship between *in vitro* susceptibility of HIV to abacavir, lamivudine, or zidovudine and the inhibition of HIV replication in humans has not been established.

Abacavir

The *in vitro* anti-HIV-1 activity of abacavir was evaluated against a T-cell tropic laboratory strain HIV-1 IIIB in lymphoblastic cell lines, a monocyte/macrophage tropic laboratory strain HIV-1 BaL in primary monocytes/macrophages, and clinical isolates in peripheral blood mononuclear cells. The concentration of drug necessary to inhibit viral replication by 50% (IC_{50}) ranged from 3.7-5.8 μM against HIV-1 IIIB, and was 0.26 ± 0.18 μM (1 μM = 0.28 μg/ml) against 8 clinical isolates. The IC_{50} of abacavir against HIV-1 BaL varied from 0.07-1.0 μM. Abacavir had synergistic activity in combination with amprenavir, nevirapine, and zidovudine, and additive activity in combination with didanosine, lamivudine, stavudine, and zalcitabine *in vitro.* Most of these drug combinations have not been adequately studied in humans.

Lamivudine

In vitro activity of lamivudine against HIV-1 was assessed in a number of cell lines (including monocytes and fresh human peripheral blood lymphocytes). IC_{50} and IC_{90} values (50% and 90% inhibitory concentrations) for lamivudine were 0.0006-0.034 μg/ml and 0.015-0.321 μg/ml, respectively. Lamivudine had anti-HIV-1 activity in all acute virus-cell infections tested.

In HIV-1-infected MT-4 cells, lamivudine in combination with zidovudine had synergistic antiretroviral activity.

Zidovudine

In vitro activity of zidovudine against HIV-1 was assessed in a number of cell lines (including monocytes and fresh human peripheral blood lymphocytes). The IC_{50} and IC_{90} values for zidovudine were 0.003-0.013 μg/ml and 0.03-0.13 μg/ml, respectively. Zidovudine had anti-HIV-1 activity in all acute virus-cell infections tested. However, zidovudine activity was substantially less in chronically infected cell lines. In cell culture drug combination studies, zidovudine demonstrates synergistic activity with delavirdine, didanosine, indinavir, nelfinavir, nevirapine, ritonavir, saquinavir, and zalcitabine, and additive activity with interferon-alpha.

Drug Resistance

HIV-1 isolates with reduced sensitivity to abacavir, lamivudine, or zidovudine have been selected *in vitro* and were also obtained from patients treated with abacavir, lamivudine, zidovudine, or lamivudine plus zidovudine. The clinical relevance of genotypic and phenotypic changes associated with abacavir, lamivudine, or zidovudine therapy is currently under evaluation.

Abacavir

Genetic analysis of isolates from abacavir-treated patients showed point mutations in the reverse transcriptase gene that resulted in amino acid substitutions at positions K65R, L74V, Y115F, and M184V. Phenotypic analysis of HIV-1 isolates that harbored abacavir-associated mutations from 17 patients after 12 weeks of abacavir monotherapy exhibited a 3-fold decrease in susceptibility to abacavir *in vitro.*

Genetic analysis of HIV-1 isolates from 21 previously antiretroviral therapy-naive patients with confirmed virologic failure (plasma HIV-1 RNA ≥400 copies/ml) after 16-48 weeks of abacavir/lamivudine/zidovudine therapy showed that 16/21 isolates had abacavir/lamivudine-associated mutation M184V, either alone (11/21), or in combination with Y115F (1/21) or zidovudine-associated (4/21) mutations at the last time point. Phenotypic data available on isolates from 10 patients showed that 7 of the 10 isolates had 25- to 86-fold decreases in susceptibility to lamivudine *in vitro.* Likewise, isolates from 2 of these 7 patients had 7- to 10-fold decreases in susceptibility to abacavir *in vitro.*

Lamivudine

Genotypic analysis of isolates selected *in vitro* and recovered from lamivudine-treated patients showed that the resistance was due to mutations in the HIV-1 reverse transcriptase gene at codon 184 from methionine to either isoleucine or valine.

Zidovudine

Genotypic analyses of the isolates selected *in vitro* and recovered from zidovudine-treated patients showed mutations, which result in 5 amino acid substitutions (M41L, D67N, K70R, K219Q, T215Y or F) in the HIV-1 reverse transcriptase gene. In general, higher levels of resistance were associated with greater number of mutations. In some patients harboring zidovudine-resistant virus at baseline, phenotypic sensitivity to zidovudine was restored by 12 weeks of treatment with lamivudine and zidovudine. Combination therapy with lamivudine plus zidovudine delayed the emergence of mutations conferring resistance to zidovudine.

Cross-Resistance

Cross-resistance among certain reverse transcriptase inhibitors has been recognized.

Abacavir

Recombinant laboratory strains of HIV-1 (HXB2) containing multiple reverse transcriptase mutations conferring abacavir resistance exhibited cross-resistance to lamivudine, didanosine, and zalcitabine *in vitro*. For clinical information in treatment-experienced patients, see PRECAUTIONS.

Lamivudine

Cross-resistance between lamivudine and zidovudine has not been reported. Cross-resistance to didanosine and zalcitabine has been observed in some patients harboring lamivudine-resistant HIV-1 isolates. In some patients treated with zidovudine plus didanosine or zalcitabine, isolates resistant to multiple drugs, including lamivudine, have emerged (see Zidovudine).

Zidovudine

HIV isolates with multidrug resistance to didanosine, lamivudine, stavudine, zalcitabine, and zidovudine were recovered from a small number of patients treated for ≥1 year with zidovudine plus didanosine or zidovudine plus zalcitabine. The pattern of genotypic resistant mutations with such combination therapies was different (A62V, V75I, F77L, F116Y, Q151M) from the pattern with zidovudine monotherapy, with the 151 mutation being most commonly associated with multidrug resistance. The mutation at codon 151 in combination with the mutations at 62, 75, 77, and 116 results in a virus with reduced susceptibility to didanosine, lamivudine, stavudine, zalcitabine, and zidovudine.

PHARMACOKINETICS IN ADULTS

Trizivir

In a single-dose, 3-way crossover bioavailability study of 1 Trizivir tablet versus 1 Ziagen tablet (300 mg), 1 Epivir tablet (150 mg), plus 1 Retrovir tablet (300 mg) administered simultaneously in healthy subjects (n=24), there was no difference in the extent of absorption, as measured by the area under the plasma concentration-time curve (AUC) and maximal peak concentration (C_{max}), of all 3 components. One Trizivir tablet was bioequivalent to 1 Ziagen tablet (300 mg), 1 Epivir tablet (150 mg), plus 1 Retrovir tablet (300 mg) following single-dose administration to fasting healthy subjects (n=24).

Abacavir

Following oral administration, abacavir is rapidly absorbed and extensively distributed. Binding of abacavir to human plasma proteins is approximately 50%. Binding of abacavir to plasma proteins was independent of concentration. Total blood and plasma drug-related radioactivity concentrations are identical, demonstrating that abacavir readily distributes into erythrocytes. The primary routes of elimination of abacavir are metabolism by alcohol dehydrogenase to form the 5′-carboxylic acid and glucuronyl transferase to form the 5′-glucuronide.

Lamivudine

Following oral administration, lamivudine is rapidly absorbed and extensively distributed. Binding to plasma protein is low. Approximately 70% of an intravenous dose of lamivudine is recovered as unchanged drug in the urine. Metabolism of lamivudine is a minor route of elimination. In humans, the only known metabolite is the trans-sulfoxide metabolite (approximately 5% of an oral dose after 12 hours).

Zidovudine

Following oral administration, zidovudine is rapidly absorbed and extensively distributed. Binding to plasma protein is low. Zidovudine is eliminated primarily by hepatic metabolism. The major metabolite of zidovudine is 3′-azido-3′-deoxy-5′-*O*-β-*D*-glucopyranuronosylthymidine (GZDV). GZDV area under the curve (AUC) is about 3-fold greater than the zidovudine AUC. Urinary recovery of zidovudine and GZDV accounts for 14% and 74% of the dose following oral administration, respectively. A second metabolite, 3′-amino-3′-deoxythymidine (AMT), has been identified in plasma. The AMT AUC was one-fifth of the zidovudine AUC.

In humans, abacavir, lamivudine, and zidovudine are not significantly metabolized by cytochrome P450 enzymes.

The pharmacokinetic properties of abacavir, lamivudine, and zidovudine in fasting patients are summarized in TABLE 1.

EFFECT OF FOOD ON ABSORPTION OF TRIZIVIR

Trizivir may be administered with or without food. Administration with food in a single-dose bioavailability study resulted in lower C_{max}, similar to results observed previously for the reference formulations. The average [90% CI] decrease in abacavir, lamivudine and zidovudine C_{max} was 32% [24-38%], 18% [10-25%], and 28% [13-40%], respectively, when administered with a high-fat meal, compared to administration under fasted conditions. Administration of Trizivir with food did not alter the extent of abacavir, lamivudine, and zidovudine absorption (AUC), as compared to administration under fasted conditions (n=24).

TABLE 1 *Pharmacokinetic Parameters* for Abacavir, Lamivudine, and Zidovudine in Adults*

Parameter		
Abacavir		
Oral bioavailability (%)	86 ± 25	n=6
Apparent volume of distribution (L/kg)	0.86 ± 0.15	n=6
Systemic clearance (L/h/kg)	0.80 ± 0.24	n=6
Renal clearance (L/h/kg)	0.007 ± 0.008	n=6
Elimination half-life (h)†	1.45 ± 0.32	n=20
Lamivudine		
Oral bioavailability (%)	86 ± 16	n=12
Apparent volume of distribution (L/kg)	1.3 ± 0.4	n=20
Systemic clearance (L/h/kg)	0.33 ± 0.06	n=20
Renal clearance (L/h/kg)	0.22 ± 0.06	n=20
Elimination half-life (h)†	5-7	
Zidovudine		
Oral bioavailability (%)	64 ± 10	n=5
Apparent volume of distribution (L/kg)	1.6 ± 0.6	n=8
Systemic clearance (L/h/kg)	1.6 ± 0.6	n=6
Renal clearance (L/h/kg)	0.34 ± 0.05	n=9
Elimination half-life (h)†	0.5 to 3	

* Data presented as mean ± standard deviation except where noted.
† Approximate range.

SPECIAL POPULATIONS

Impaired Renal Function

Trizivir

Because lamivudine and zidovudine require dose adjustment in the presence of renal insufficiency, Trizivir is not recommended for use in patients with creatinine clearance <50 ml/min (see PRECAUTIONS).

Impaired Hepatic Function

Trizivir

A reduction in the daily dose of zidovudine may be necessary in patients with mild to moderate impaired hepatic function or liver cirrhosis. Because Trizivir is a fixed-dose combination that cannot be adjusted for this patient population, Trizivir is not recommended for patients with impaired hepatic function.

Pregnancy

See PRECAUTIONS, Pregnancy Category C.

Zidovudine

Zidovudine pharmacokinetics have been studied in a Phase 1 study of 8 women during the last trimester of pregnancy. As pregnancy progressed, there was no evidence of drug accumulation. The pharmacokinetics of zidovudine were similar to that of nonpregnant adults. Consistent with passive transmission of the drug across the placenta, zidovudine concentrations in neonatal plasma at birth were essentially equal to those in maternal plasma at delivery. Although data are limited, methadone maintenance therapy in 5 pregnant women did not appear to alter zidovudine pharmacokinetics. In a nonpregnant adult population, a potential for interaction has been identified (see CLINICAL PHARMACOLOGY, Drug Interactions).

Abacavir and Lamivudine

No data are available on the pharmacokinetics of abacavir or lamivudine during pregnancy.

Nursing Mothers

See PRECAUTIONS, Nursing Mothers.

Zidovudine

After administration of a single dose of 200 mg zidovudine to 13 HIV-infected women, the mean concentration of zidovudine was similar in human milk and serum.

Abacavir and Lamivudine

No data are available on the pharmacokinetics of abacavir or lamivudine in nursing mothers.

Pediatric Patients

Trizivir

Trizivir is not intended for use in pediatric patients. Trizivir should not be administered to adolescents who weigh less than 40 kg because it is a fixed-dose tablet that cannot be dose adjusted for this patient population (see PRECAUTIONS, Pediatric Use).

Geriatric Patients

The pharmacokinetics of abacavir, lamivudine, and zidovudine have not been studied in patients over 65 years of age.

Gender

Lamivudine and Zidovudine

A pharmacokinetic study in healthy male (n=12) and female (n=12) subjects showed no gender differences in zidovudine exposure (AUC∞) or lamivudine AUC∞ normalized for body weight.

Abacavir

The pharmacokinetics of abacavir with respect to gender have not been determined.

Race

Lamivudine

There are no significant racial differences in lamivudine pharmacokinetics.

Abacavir and Zidovudine

The pharmacokinetics of abacavir and zidovudine with respect to race have not been determined.

DRUG INTERACTIONS

See DRUG INTERACTIONS.

The drug interactions described are based on studies conducted with the individual nucleoside analogues. In humans, abacavir, lamivudine, and zidovudine are not significantly metabolized by cytochrome P450 enzymes; therefore, it is unlikely that clinically significant drug interactions will occur with drugs metabolized through these pathways.

Abacavir

Due to their common metabolic pathways via glucuronyl transferase with zidovudine, 15 HIV-infected patients were enrolled in a crossover study evaluating single doses of abacavir (600 mg), lamivudine (150 mg), and zidovudine (300 mg) alone or in combination. Analysis showed no clinically relevant changes in the pharmacokinetics of abacavir with the addition of lamivudine or zidovudine or the combination of lamivudine and zidovudine. Lamivudine exposure (AUC decreased 15%) and zidovudine exposure (AUC increased 10%) did not show clinically relevant changes with concurrent abacavir.

In a study of 11 HIV-infected subjects receiving methadone-maintenance therapy (40 and 90 mg daily), with 600 mg of Ziagen twice daily (twice the current recommended dose), oral methadone clearance increased 22% (90% CI 6-42%). This alteration will not result in a methadone dose modification in the majority of patients; however, an increased methadone dose may be required in a small number of patients.

Lamivudine and Zidovudine

No clinically significant alterations in lamivudine or zidovudine pharmacokinetics were observed in 12 asymptomatic HIV-infected adult patients given a single dose of zidovudine (200 mg) in combination with multiple doses of lamivudine (300 mg q12h).

TABLE 2 *Effect of Coadministered Drugs on Abacavir, Lamivudine, and Zidovudine AUC**

Coadministered Drug and Dose	Drug Dose	n	Drug Concentrations AUC	Variability	CCD
Drugs That May Alter Lamivudine Blood Concentrations					
Nelfinavir 750 mg q8h × 7-10 days	single 150 mg	11	inc 10%	95% CI: 1-20%	NC
Trimethoprim 160 mg/ sulfamethoxazole 800 mg daily × 5 days	single 300 mg	14	inc 43%	90% CI: 32-55%	NC
Drugs That May Alter Zidovudine Blood Concentrations					
Atovaquone 750 mg q12h with food	200 mg q8h	14	inc 31%	Range 23-78%†	NC
Fluconazole 400 mg daily	200 mg q8h	12	inc 74%	95% CI: 54-98%	Not Reported
Methadone 30-90 mg daily	200 mg q4h	9	inc 43%	Range 16-64%†	NC
Nelfinavir 750 mg q8h × 7-10 days	single 200 mg	11	dec 35%	Range 28-41%	NC
Probenecid 500 mg q6h × 2 days	2 mg/kg q8h × 3 days	3	inc 106%	Range 100-170%†	Not Assessed
Ritonavir 300 mg q6h × 4 days	200 mg q8h × 4 days	9	dec 25%	95% CI: 15-34%	NC
Valproic acid 250 or 500 mg q8h × 4 days	100 mg q8h × 4 days	6	inc 80%	Range 64-130%†	Not Assessed
Drugs That May Alter Abacavir Blood Concentrations					
Ethanol 0.7 g/kg	single 600 mg	24	inc 41%	90% CI: 35-48%	NC

* See DRUG INTERACTIONS for additional information on drug interactions.
† Estimated range of percent difference.
AUC = area under the concentration versus time curve; CCD = Concentration of coadministered drug; CI = confidence interval.
inc = Increase.
dec = Decrease.
NC = no significant change.
Note: ROUTINE DOSE MODIFICATION OF ABACAVIR, LAMIVUDINE, AND ZIDOVUDINE IS NOT WARRANTED WITH COADMINISTRATION OF THE FOLLOWING DRUGS.

INDICATIONS AND USAGE

Trizivir is indicated alone or in combination with other antiretroviral agents for the treatment of HIV-1 infection. The indication for Trizivir is based on 2 controlled trials with abacavir of 16 and 48 weeks in duration that evaluated suppression of HIV RNA and changes in CD4 cell count. At present, there are no results from controlled trials evaluating the effect of abacavir on clinical progression of HIV. There are limited data on the use of this triple-combination regimen in patients with higher viral load levels (>100,000 copies/ml) at baseline.

CONTRAINDICATIONS

Abacavir sulfate, one of the components of Trizivir, has been associated with fatal hypersensitivity reactions. ABACAVIR (as Trizivir or Ziagen) SHOULD NOT BE RESTARTED FOLLOWING A HYPERSENSITIVITY REACTION TO ABACAVIR (see WARNINGS, PRECAUTIONS, and ADVERSE REACTIONS).

Trizivir tablets are contraindicated in patients with previously demonstrated hypersensitivity to any of the components of the product (see WARNINGS).

WARNINGS

HYPERSENSITIVITY REACTION

Trizivir contains abacavir sulfate (Ziagen), which has been associated with fatal hypersensitivity reactions. Patients developing signs or symptoms of hypersensitivity (which include fever; skin rash; fatigue; gastrointestinal symptoms such as nausea, vomiting, diarrhea, or abdominal pain; and respiratory symptoms such as pharyngitis, dyspnea, or cough) should discontinue Trizivir as soon as a hypersensitivity reaction is first suspected, and should seek medical evaluation immediately. To avoid a delay in diagnosis and minimize the risk of a life-threatening hypersensitivity reaction, Trizivir should be permanently discontinued if hypersensitivity cannot be ruled out, even when other diagnoses are possible (*e.g.,* acute onset respiratory diseases, gastroenteritis, or reactions to other medications). Abacavir (as Trizivir or Ziagen) SHOULD NOT be restarted following a hypersensitivity reaction to abacavir because more severe symptoms will recur within hours and may include life-threatening hypotension and death.

Severe or fatal hypersensitivity reactions can occur within hours after reintroduction of abacavir (as Trizivir or Ziagen) in patients who have no identified history or unrecognized symptoms of hypersensitivity to abacavir therapy.

When therapy with abacavir (as Trizivir or Ziagen) has been discontinued for reasons other than symptoms of a hypersensitivity reaction, and if reinitiation of therapy is under consideration, the reason for discontinuation should be evaluated to ensure that the patient did not have symptoms of a hypersensitivity reaction. If hypersensitivity cannot be ruled out, abacavir (as Trizivir or Ziagen) should **NOT** be reintroduced. If symptoms consistent with hypersensitivity are not identified, reintroduction can be undertaken with continued monitoring for symptoms of a hypersensitivity reaction. Patients should be made aware that a hypersensitivity reaction can occur with reintroduction of abacavir (as Trizivir or Ziagen), and that reintroduction of abacavir (as Trizivir or Ziagen) should be undertaken only if medical care can be readily accessed by the patient or others (see ADVERSE REACTIONS).

In clinical trials, hypersensitivity reactions have been reported in approximately 5% of adult and pediatric patients receiving abacavir. Symptoms usually appear within the first 6 weeks of treatment with abacavir although these reactions may occur at any time during therapy (see PRECAUTIONS, Information for the Patient and ADVERSE REACTIONS).

Abacavir Hypersensitivity Reaction Registry: To facilitate reporting of hypersensitivity reactions and collection of information on each case, an Abacavir Hypersensitivity Registry has been established. Physicians should register patients by calling 1-800-270-0425.

LACTIC ACIDOSIS/SEVERE HEPATOMEGALY WITH STEATOSIS

Lactic acidosis and severe hepatomegaly with steatosis, including fatal cases, have been reported with the use of nucleoside analogues alone or in combination, including abacavir, lamivudine, zidovudine, and other antiretrovirals. A majority of these cases have been in women. Obesity and prolonged nucleoside exposure may be risk factors. Particular caution should be exercised when administering Trizivir to any patient with known risk factors for liver disease; however, cases have also been reported in patients with no known risk factors. Treatment with Trizivir should be suspended in any patient who develops clinical or laboratory findings suggestive of lactic acidosis or pronounced hepatotoxicity (which may include hepatomegaly and steatosis even in the absence of marked transaminase elevations).

BONE MARROW SUPPRESSION

Since Trizivir contains zidovudine, Trizivir should be used with caution in patients who have bone marrow compromise evidenced by granulocyte count <1000 cells/mm^3 or hemoglobin <9.5 g/dl. Frequent blood counts are strongly recommended in patients with advanced HIV disease who are treated with Trizivir. For HIV-infected individuals and patients with asymptomatic or early HIV disease, periodic blood counts are recommended.

MYOPATHY

Myopathy and myositis, with pathological changes similar to that produced by HIV disease, have been associated with prolonged use of zidovudine, and therefore may occur with therapy with Trizivir.

POSTTREATMENT EXACERBATIONS OF HEPATITIS

In clinical trials in non-HIV-infected patients treated with lamivudine for chronic hepatitis B (HBV), clinical and laboratory evidence of exacerbations of hepatitis have occurred after discontinuation of lamivudine. These exacerbations have been detected primarily by serum ALT elevations in addition to re-emergence of HBV DNA. Although most events appear to have been self-limited, fatalities have been reported in some cases. Similar events have been reported from post-marketing experience after changes from lamivudine-containing HIV treatment regimens to non-lamivudine-containing regimens in patients infected with both HIV and HBV. The causal relationship to discontinuation of lamivudine treatment is unknown. Patients should be closely monitored with both clinical and laboratory followup for at least several months after stopping treatment. There is insufficient evidence to determine whether re-initiation of lamivudine alters the course of posttreatment exacerbations of hepatitis.

OTHER

Trizivir contains fixed doses of 3 nucleoside analogues: abacavir, lamivudine, and zidovudine and should not be administered concomitantly with abacavir, lamivudine, or zidovudine.

Because Trizivir is a fixed-dose tablet, it should not be prescribed for adults or adolescents who weigh less than 40 kg or other patients requiring dosage adjustment.

The complete prescribing information for all agents being considered for use with Trizivir should be consulted before combination therapy with Trizivir is initiated.

PRECAUTIONS

THERAPY-EXPERIENCED PATIENTS

Abacavir

In clinical trials, patients with prolonged prior nucleoside reverse transcriptase inhibitor (NRTI) exposure or who had HIV-1 isolates that contained multiple mutations conferring resistance to NRTIs had limited response to abacavir. The potential for cross-resistance between abacavir and other NRTIs should be considered when choosing new therapeutic regimens in therapy-experienced patients (see CLINICAL PHARMACOLOGY, Microbiology, Cross-Resistance).

PATIENTS WITH HIV AND HEPATITIS B VIRUS COINFECTION

Lamivudine

Safety and efficacy of lamivudine have not been established for treatment of chronic hepatitis B in patients dually infected with HIV and HBV. In non-HIV-infected patients treated with lamivudine for chronic hepatitis B, emergence of lamivudine-resistant HBV has been detected and has been associated with diminished treatment response (see Epivir-HBV package insert for additional information). Emergence of hepatitis B virus variants associated with resistance to lamivudine has also been reported in HIV-infected patients who have received lamivudine-containing antiretroviral regimens in the presence of concurrent infection with hepatitis B virus.

PATIENTS WITH IMPAIRED RENAL FUNCTION

Trizivir

Since Trizivir is a fixed-dose tablet and the dosage of the individual components cannot be altered, patients with creatinine clearance ≤50 ml/min should not receive Trizivir.

Fat Redistribution

Redistribution/accumulation of body fat including central obesity, dorsocervical fat enlargement (buffalo hump), peripheral wasting, facial wasting, breast enlargement, and "cushingoid appearance" have been observed in patients receiving antiretroviral therapy. The mechanism and long-term consequences of these events are currently unknown. A causal relationship has not been established.

INFORMATION FOR THE PATIENT

Abacavir

Patients should be advised that a Medication Guide and Warning Card summarizing the symptoms of abacavir hypersensitivity reactions should be dispensed by the pharmacist with each new prescription and refill of Trizivir. Patients should be instructed to carry the Warning Card with them.

Patients should be advised of the possibility of a hypersensitivity reaction to abacavir (as Trizivir or Ziagen) that may result in death. Patients developing signs or symptoms of hypersensitivity (which include fever; skin rash; fatigue; gastrointestinal symptoms such as nausea, vomiting, diarrhea, or abdominal pain; and respiratory symptoms such as sore throat, shortness of breath, or cough) should discontinue treatment with Trizivir and seek medical evaluation immediately. **Abacavir (as Trizivir or Ziagen) SHOULD NOT be restarted following a hypersensitivity reaction to abacavir because more severe symptoms will recur within hours and may include life-threatening hypotension and death.** Patients who have interrupted abacavir (as Trizivir or Ziagen) for reasons other than symptoms of hypersensitivity (for example, those who have an interruption in drug supply) should be made aware that a severe or fatal hypersensitivity reaction can occur with reintroduction of abacavir. Patients should be instructed not to reintroduce abacavir (as Trizivir or Ziagen) without medical consultation and that reintroduction of abacavir (as Trizivir or Ziagen) should be undertaken only if medical care can be readily accessed by the patient or others (see ADVERSE REACTIONS and WARNINGS).

Trizivir

Patients should be informed that Trizivir is not a cure for HIV infection and patients may continue to experience illnesses associated with HIV infection, including opportunistic infections. Patients should be advised that the use of Trizivir has not been shown to reduce the risk of transmission of HIV to others through sexual contact or blood contamination.

Patients should be informed that redistribution or accumulation of body fat may occur in patients receiving antiretroviral therapy and that the cause and long-term health effects of these conditions are not known at this time.

Patients should be advised of the importance of taking Trizivir as it is prescribed.

Zidovudine

Patients should be informed that the important toxicities associated with zidovudine are neutropenia and/or anemia. They should be told of the extreme importance of having their blood counts followed closely while on therapy, especially for patients with advanced HIV disease.

CARCINOGENESIS, MUTAGENESIS, AND IMPAIRMENT OF FERTILITY

Carcinogenesis

Abacavir

Abacavir was administered orally at 3 dosage levels to separate groups of mice (60 females and 60 males/group) and rats (56 females and 56 males in each group) in carcinogenicity studies. Single doses were 55, 110, and 330 mg/kg/day in mice and 30, 120, and 600 mg/kg/day in rats. Results showed an increase in the incidence of malignant and non-malignant tumors. Malignant tumors occurred in the preputial gland of males and the clitoral gland of females of both species, and in the liver of female rats. In addition, non-malignant tumors also occurred in the liver and thyroid gland of female rats.

Lamivudine

Long-term carcinogenicity studies with lamivudine in mice and rats showed no evidence of carcinogenic potential at exposures up to 10 times (mice) and 58 times (rats) those observed in humans at the recommended therapeutic dose for HIV infection.

Zidovudine

Zidovudine was administered orally at 3 dosage levels to separate groups of mice and rats (60 females and 60 males in each group). Initial single daily doses were 30, 60, and 120 mg/kg/day in mice and 80, 220, and 600 mg/kg/day in rats. The doses in mice were reduced to 20, 30, and 40 mg/kg/day after day 90 because of treatment-related anemia, whereas in rats only the high dose was reduced to 450 mg/kg/day on Day 91 and then to 300 mg/kg/day on Day 279.

In mice, 7 late-appearing (after 19 months) vaginal neoplasms (5 nonmetastasizing squamous cell carcinomas, 1 squamous cell papilloma, and 1 squamous polyp) occurred in animals given the highest dose. One late-appearing squamous cell papilloma occurred in the vagina of a middle-dose animal. No vaginal tumors were found at the lowest dose.

In rats, 2 late-appearing (after 20 months), nonmetastasizing vaginal squamous cell carcinomas occurred in animals given the highest dose. No vaginal tumors occurred at the low or middle dose in rats. No other drug-related tumors were observed in either sex of either species.

At doses that produced tumors in mice and rats, the estimated drug exposure (as measured by AUC) was approximately 3 times (mouse) and 24 times (rat) the estimated human exposure at the recommended therapeutic dose of 100 mg every 4 hours.

Two transplacental carcinogenicity studies were conducted in mice. One study administered zidovudine at doses of 20 or 40 mg/kg/day from gestation Day 10 through parturition and lactation with dosing continuing in offspring for 24 months postnatally. At these doses, exposures were approximately 3 times the estimated human exposure at the recommended doses. After 24 months at the 40 mg/kg/day dose, an increase in incidence of vaginal tumors was noted with no increase in tumors in the liver or lung or any other organ in either gender. These findings are consistent with results of the standard oral carcinogenicity study in mice, as described earlier. A second study administered zidovudine at maximum tolerated doses of 12.5 or 25 mg/day (~1000 mg/kg nonpregnant body weight or ~450 mg/kg of term body weight) to pregnant mice from Days 12-18 of gestation. There was an increase in the number of tumors in the lung, liver, and female reproductive tracts in the offspring of mice receiving the higher dose level of zidovudine.

It is not known how predictive the results of rodent carcinogenicity studies may be for humans.

Mutagenicity

Abacavir

Abacavir induced chromosomal aberrations both in the presence and absence of metabolic activation in an *in vitro* cytogenetic study in human lymphocytes. Abacavir was mutagenic in the absence of metabolic activation, although it was not mutagenic in the presence of metabolic activation in an L5178Y/TK$^{+/-}$ mouse lymphoma assay. At systemic exposures approximately 9 times higher than that in humans at the therapeutic dose, abacavir was clastogenic in males and not clastogenic in females in an *in vivo* mouse bone marrow micronucleus assay. Abacavir was not mutagenic in bacterial mutagenicity assays in the presence and absence of metabolic activation.

Lamivudine

Lamivudine was mutagenic in a L5178Y/TK$^{+/-}$ mouse lymphoma assay and clastogenic in a cytogenetic assay using cultured human lymphocytes. Lamivudine was negative in a microbial mutagenicity assay, in an *in vitro* cell transformation assay, in a rat micronucleus test, in a rat bone marrow cytogenetic assay, and in an assay for unscheduled DNA synthesis in rat liver.

Zidovudine

Zidovudine was mutagenic in a L5178Y/TK$^{+/-}$ mouse lymphoma assay, positive in an *in vitro* cell transformation assay, clastogenic in a cytogenetic assay using cultured human lymphocytes, and positive in mouse and rat micronucleus tests after repeated doses. It was negative in a cytogenetic study in rats given a single dose.

Impairment of Fertility

Abacavir

Abacavir administered to male and female rats had no adverse effects on fertility judged by conception rates at doses up to approximately 8-fold higher than that in humans at the therapeutic dose based on body surface area comparisons.

Lamivudine

In a study of reproductive performance, lamivudine, administered to male and female rats at doses up to 130 times the usual adult dose based on body surface area considerations, revealed no evidence of impaired fertility judged by conception rates and no effect on the survival, growth, and development to weaning of the offspring.

Zidovudine

Zidovudine, administered to male and female rats at doses up to 7 times the usual adult dose based on body surface area considerations, had no effect on fertility judged by conception rates.

PREGNANCY CATEGORY C

There are no adequate and well-controlled studies of Trizivir in pregnant women. Reproduction studies with abacavir, lamivudine, and zidovudine have been performed in animals (see Abacavir, Lamivudine, and Zidovudine). Trizivir should be used during pregnancy only if the potential benefits outweigh the risks.

Abacavir

Studies in pregnant rats showed that abacavir is transferred to the fetus through the placenta. Developmental toxicity (depressed fetal body weight and reduced crown-rump length) and increased incidences of fetal anasarca and skeletal malformations were observed when rats were treated with abacavir at a dose 35 times higher than the human exposure, based on AUC (1000 mg/kg/day). In a fertility study, evidence of toxicity to the developing embryo and fetuses (increased resorptions, decreased fetal body weights) occurred only at 500 mg/kg/day. The offspring of female rats treated with abacavir at 500 mg/kg/day (beginning at embryo implantation and ending at weaning) showed increased incidence of stillbirth and lower body weights throughout life. In the rabbit, there was no evidence of drug-related developmental toxicity and no increases in fetal malformations at doses up to 8.5 times the human exposure, based on AUC.

Lamivudine

Studies in pregnant rats and rabbits showed that lamivudine is transferred to the fetus through the placenta. Reproduction studies with orally administered lamivudine have been performed in rats and rabbits at doses up to 4000 mg/kg/day and 1000 mg/kg/day, respectively, producing plasma levels up to approximately 35 times that for the adult HIV dose. No evidence of teratogenicity due to lamivudine was observed. Evidence of early embryolethality was seen in the rabbit at exposure levels similar to those observed in humans, but there was no indication of this effect in the rat at exposure levels up to 35 times that in humans.

Zidovudine

Reproduction studies with orally administered zidovudine in the rat and in the rabbit at doses up to 500 mg/kg/day revealed no evidence of teratogenicity with zidovudine. Zidovudine treatment resulted in embryo/fetal toxicity as evidenced by an increase in the incidence of fetal resorptions in rats given 150 or 450 mg/kg/day and rabbits given 500 mg/kg/day. The doses used in the teratology studies resulted in peak zidovudine plasma concentrations (after one-half of the daily dose) in rats 66-226 times, and in rabbits 12-87 times, mean steady-state peak human plasma concentrations (after one-sixth of the daily dose) achieved with the recommended daily dose (100 mg every 4 hours). In an additional teratology study in rats, a dose of 3000 mg/kg/day (very near the oral median lethal dose in rats of approximately 3700 mg/kg) caused marked maternal toxicity and an increase in the incidence of fetal malformations. This dose resulted in peak zidovudine plasma concentrations 350 times peak human plasma concentrations. No evidence of teratogenicity was seen in this experiment at doses of 600 mg/kg/day or less. Two rodent carcinogenicity studies were conducted (see Carcinogenesis, Mutagenesis, and Impairment of Fertility).

Antiretroviral Pregnancy Registry: To monitor maternal-fetal outcomes of pregnant women exposed to Trizivir or other antiretroviral agents, an Antiretroviral Pregnancy Registry has been established. Physicians are encouraged to register patients by calling 1-800-258-4263.

NURSING MOTHERS

The Centers for Disease Control and Prevention recommend that HIV-infected mothers not breastfeed their infants to avoid risking postnatal transmission of HIV infection.

Abacavir, Lamivudine, and Zidovudine

Zidovudine is excreted in breast milk; abacavir and lamivudine are secreted into the milk of lactating rats.

Because of both the potential for HIV transmission and the potential for serious adverse reactions in nursing infants, **mothers should be instructed not to breastfeed if they are receiving Trizivir.**

PEDIATRIC USE

Trizivir is not intended for use in pediatric patients. Trizivir should not be administered to adolescents who weigh less than 40 kg because it is a fixed-dose tablet that cannot be adjusted for this patient population.

GERIATRIC USE

Clinical studies of abacavir, lamivudine, and zidovudine did not include sufficient numbers of patients aged 65 and over to determine whether they respond differently from younger patients. In general, dose selection for an elderly patient should be cautious, reflecting the greater frequency of decreased hepatic, renal, or cardiac function, and of concomitant disease or other drug therapy. Trizivir is not recommended for patients with impaired renal function (*i.e.*, creatinine clearance ≤50 ml/min; see Patients With Impaired Renal Function and DOSAGE AND ADMINISTRATION).

DRUG INTERACTIONS

TRIZIVIR

No clinically significant changes to pharmacokinetic parameters were observed for abacavir, lamivudine, or zidovudine when administered together.

ABACAVIR

Abacavir has no effect on the pharmacokinetic properties of ethanol. Ethanol decreases the elimination of abacavir causing an increase in overall exposure (see CLINICAL PHARMACOLOGY, Drug Interactions).

The addition of methadone has no clinically significant effect on the pharmacokinetic properties of abacavir. In a study of 11 HIV-infected subjects receiving methadone-maintenance therapy (40 and 90 mg daily), with 600 mg of Ziagen twice daily (twice the current recommended dose), oral methadone clearance increased 22% (90% CI 6-42%) This alteration will not result in a methadone dose modification in the majority of patients; however, an increased methadone dose may be required in a small number of patients.

LAMIVUDINE

Trimethoprim (TMP) 160 mg/sulfamethoxazole (SMX) 800 mg once daily has been shown to increase lamivudine exposure (AUC). The effect of higher doses of TMP/SMX on lamivudine pharmacokinetics has not been investigated (see CLINICAL PHARMACOLOGY).

Lamivudine and zalcitabine may inhibit the intracellular phosphorylation of one another. Therefore, use of Trizivir in combination with zalcitabine is not recommended.

ZIDOVUDINE

Coadministration of ganciclovir, interferon-alpha, and other bone marrow suppressive or cytotoxic agents may increase the hematologic toxicity of zidovudine. Concomitant use of zidovudine with stavudine should be avoided since an antagonistic relationship has been demonstrated *in vitro*. In addition, concomitant use of zidovudine with doxorubicin or ribavirin should be avoided because an antagonistic relationship has also been demonstrated *in vitro*.

See CLINICAL PHARMACOLOGY for additional drug interactions.

ADVERSE REACTIONS

ABACAVIR

Hypersensitivity Reaction

Trizivir contains abacavir sulfate (Ziagen), which has been associated with fatal hypersensitivity reactions. Therapy with abacavir (as Trizivir OR Ziagen) SHOULD NOT be restarted following a hypersensitivity reaction because more severe symptoms will recur within hours and may include life-threatening hypotension and death. Patients developing signs or symptoms of hypersensitivity should discontinue treatment as soon as a hypersensitivity reaction is first suspected, and should seek medical evaluation immediately. To avoid a delay in diagnosis and minimize the risk of a life-threatening hypersensitivity reaction, Trizivir should be permanently discontinued if hypersensitivity cannot be ruled out, even when other diagnoses are possible (*e.g.*, acute onset respiratory diseases, gastroenteritis, or reactions to other medications).

Severe or fatal hypersensitivity reactions can occur within hours after reintroduction of abacavir (as Trizivir or Ziagen) in patients who have no identified history or unrecognized symptoms of hypersensitivity to abacavir therapy (see WARNINGS and PRECAUTIONS, Information for the Patient).

When therapy with abacavir (as Trizivir or Ziagen) has been discontinued for reasons other than symptoms of a hypersensitivity reaction, and if reinitiation of therapy is under consideration, the reason for discontinuation should be evaluated to ensure that the patient did not have symptoms of a hypersensitivity reaction. If hypersensitivity cannot be ruled out, abacavir (as Trizivir or Ziagen) should **NOT** be reintroduced. If symptoms consistent with hypersensitivity are not identified, reintroduction can be undertaken with continued monitoring for symptoms of hypersensitivity reaction. Patients should be made aware that a hypersensitivity reaction can occur with reintroduction of abacavir (as Trizivir or Ziagen), and that reintroduction of abacavir (as Trizivir or Ziagen) should be undertaken only if medical care can be readily accessed by the patient or others (see WARNINGS).

In clinical studies, approximately 5% of adult and pediatric patients receiving abacavir developed a hypersensitivity reaction. This reaction is characterized by the appearance of symptoms indicating multi-organ/body system involvement. Symptoms usually appear within the first 6 weeks of treatment with abacavir, although these reactions may occur at any time during therapy. Frequently observed signs and symptoms include fever; skin rash; fatigue; and gastrointestinal symptoms such as nausea, vomiting, diarrhea, or abdominal pain. Other signs and symptoms include malaise, lethargy, myalgia, myolysis, arthralgia, edema, cough, dyspnea, headache, and paresthesia. Some patients who experienced a hypersensitivity reaction were initially thought to have acute onset or worsening respiratory disease. The diagnosis of hypersensitivity reaction should be carefully considered for patients presenting with symptoms of acute onset respiratory diseases, even if alternative respiratory diagnoses (pneumonia, bronchitis, flu-like illness) are possible.

Physical findings include lymphadenopathy, mucous membrane lesions (conjunctivitis and mouth ulcerations), and rash. The rash usually appears maculopapular or urticarial but may be variable in appearance. Hypersensitivity reactions have occurred without rash.

Laboratory abnormalities include elevated liver function tests, increased creatine phosphokinase or creatinine, and lymphopenia. Anaphylaxis, liver failure, renal failure, hypotension, and death have occurred in association with hypersensitivity reactions. Symptoms worsen with continued therapy but often resolve upon discontinuation of abacavir.

Risk factors that may predict the occurrence or severity of hypersensitivity to abacavir have not been identified.

Selected clinical adverse events with a ≥5% frequency during therapy with Ziagen 300 mg twice daily, Epivir 150 mg twice daily, and Retrovir 300 mg twice daily compared with Epivir 150 mg twice daily and Retrovir 300 mg twice daily from CNAAB3003 are listed in TABLE 4.

TABLE 4 *Selected Clinical Adverse Events Grades 1-4 (≥5% Frequency) in Therapy-Naive Adults (CNAAB3003) Through 16 Weeks of Treatment*

Adverse Event	Abacavir/Lamivudine/ Zidovudine (n=83)	Lamivudine/Zidovudine (n=81)
Nausea	47%	41%
Nausea and vomiting	16%	11%
Diarrhea	12%	11%
Loss of appetite/anorexia	11%	10%
Insomnia and other sleep disorders	7%	5%

Selected clinical adverse events with a ≥5% frequency during therapy with Ziagen 300 mg twice daily, lamivudine 150 mg twice daily, and zidovudine 300 mg twice daily compared with indinavir 800 mg 3 times daily, lamivudine 150 mg twice daily, and zidovudine 300 mg twice daily from CNAAB3005 are listed in TABLE 5.

Five subjects in the abacavir arm of study CNAAB3005 experienced worsening of pre-existing depression compared to none in the indinavir arm. The background rates of pre-existing depression were similar in the 2 treatment arms.

Laboratory Abnormalities

Laboratory abnormalities (anemia, neutropenia, liver function test abnormalities, and CPK elevations) were observed with similar frequencies in the 2 treatment groups in studies CNAAB3003 and CNAAB3006. Mild elevations of blood glucose were more frequent in subjects receiving abacavir. In study CNAAB3003, triglyceride elevations (all grades) were more common on the abacavir arm (25%) than on the placebo arm (11%). In study

TABLE 5 *Selected Clinical Adverse Events Grades 1-4 (≥5% Frequency) in Therapy-Naive Adults (CNAAB3005) Through 48 Weeks of Treatment*

Adverse Event	Abacavir/Lamivudine/ Zidovudine (n=262)	Indinavir/Lamivudine/ Zidovudine (n=264)
Nausea	60%	61%
Nausea and vomiting	30%	27%
Diarrhea	26%	27%
Loss of appetite/anorexia	15%	11%
Insomnia and other sleep disorders	13%	12%
Fever and/or chills	20%	13%
Headache	28%	25%
Malaise and/or fatigue	44%	41%

CNAAB3005, hyperglycemia and disorders of lipid metabolism occurred with similar frequency in the abacavir and indinavir treatment arms.

Other Adverse Events

In addition to adverse events in TABLE 4 and TABLE 5, other adverse events observed in the expanded access program for abacavir were pancreatitis and increased GGT.

LAMIVUDINE PLUS ZIDOVUDINE

In 4 randomized, controlled trials of lamivudine 300 mg/day plus zidovudine 600 mg/day, the following selected clinical and laboratory adverse events were observed (see TABLE 6 and TABLE 7).

TABLE 6 *Selected Clinical Adverse Events (≥5% Frequency) in 4 Controlled Clinical Trials With Lamivudine 300 mg/day and Zidovudine 600 mg/day*

Adverse Event	Lamivudine + Zidovudine (n=251)
Body as a Whole	
Headache	35%
Malaise & fatigue	27%
Fever or chills	10%
Digestive	
Nausea	33%
Diarrhea	18%
Nausea & vomiting	13%
Anorexia and/or decreased appetite	10%
Abdominal pain	9%
Abdominal cramps	6%
Dyspepsia	5%
Nervous System	
Neuropathy	12%
Insomnia & other sleep disorders	11%
Dizziness	10%
Depressive disorders	9%
Respiratory	
Nasal signs & symptoms	20%
Cough	18%
Skin	
Skin rashes	9%
Musculoskeletal	
Musculoskeletal pain	12%
Myalgia	8%
Arthralgia	5%

Pancreatitis was observed in 3 of the 656 adult patients (<0.5%) who received lamivudine in controlled clinical trials.

Selected laboratory abnormalities observed during therapy are listed in TABLE 7.

TABLE 7 *Frequencies of Selected Laboratory Abnormalities Among Adults in 4 Controlled Clinical Trials of Lamivudine 300 mg/day plus Zidovudine 600 mg/day**

Test (Abnormal Level)	Lamivudine + Zidovudine % (n)
Neutropenia (ANC <750/mm^3)	7.2% (237)
Anemia (Hgb <8.0 g/dl)	2.9% (241)
Thrombocytopenia (platelets <50,000/mm^3)	0.4% (240)
ALT (>5.0 × ULN)	3.7% (241)
AST (>5.0 × ULN)	1.7% (241)
Bilirubin (>2.5 × ULN)	0.8% (241)
Amylase (>2.0 × ULN)	4.2% (72)

ULN = Upper limit of normal.
ANC = Absolute neutrophil count.
n = Number of patients assessed.
* Frequencies of these laboratory abnormalities were higher in patients with mild laboratory abnormalities at baseline.

Observed During Clinical Practice

The following events have been identified during post-approval use of abacavir, lamivudine and/or zidovudine. Because they are reported voluntarily from a population of unknown size, estimates of frequency cannot be made. These events have been chosen for inclusion due to a combination of their seriousness, frequency of reporting, or potential causal connection to lamivudine and/or zidovudine.

Abacavir

Suspected Stevens-Johnson syndrome (SJS) has been reported in patients receiving abacavir in combination with medications known to be associated with SJS. Because of the overlap of clinical signs and symptoms between hypersensitivity to abacavir and SJS, and the possibility of multiple drug sensitivities in some patients, abacavir should be discontinued and not restarted in such cases.

Abacavir, Lamivudine, and Zidovudine:

Body as a Whole: Redistribution/accumulation of body fat (see PRECAUTIONS, Impaired Renal Function, Fat Redistribution).
Cardiovascular: Cardiomyopathy.
Digestive: Stomatitis.
Endocrine and Metabolic: Gynecomastia, hyperglycemia.
Gastrointestinal: Oral mucosal pigmentation.
General: Vasculitis, weakness.
Hemic and Lymphatic: Aplastic anemia, anemia, lymphadenopathy, pure red cell aplasia, splenomegaly.
Hepatic and Pancreatic: Lactic acidosis and hepatic steatosis, pancreatitis, posttreatment exacerbation of hepatitis B (see WARNINGS).
Hypersensitivity: Sensitization reactions (including anaphylaxis), urticaria.
Musculoskeletal: Muscle weakness, CPK elevation, rhabdomyolysis.
Nervous: Paresthesia, peripheral neuropathy, seizures.
Respiratory: Abnormal breath sounds/wheezing.
Skin: Alopecia, erythema multiforme, Stevens-Johnson syndrome.

DOSAGE AND ADMINISTRATION

A Medication Guide and Warning Card that provide information about recognition of hypersensitivity reactions should be dispensed with each new prescription and refill. To facilitate reporting of hypersensitivity reactions and collection of information on each case, an Abacavir Hypersensitivity Registry has been established. Physicians should register patients by calling 1-800-270-0425.

The recommended oral dose of Trizivir for adults and adolescents is 1 tablet twice daily. Trizivir is not recommended in adults or adolescents who weigh less than 40 kg because it is a fixed-dose tablet.

DOSE ADJUSTMENT

Because it is a fixed-dose tablet, Trizivir should not be prescribed for patients requiring dosage adjustment such as those with creatinine clearance ≤50 ml/min or those experiencing dose-limiting adverse events.

ANIMAL PHARMACOLOGY

Myocardial degeneration was found in mice and rats following administration of abacavir for 2 years. The systemic exposures were equivalent to 7-24 times the expected systemic exposure in humans. The clinical relevance of this finding has not been determined.

HOW SUPPLIED

Trizivir is available as tablets. Each tablet contains 300 mg of abacavir as abacavir sulfate, 150 mg of lamivudine, and 300 mg of zidovudine. The tablets are blue-green, capsule-shaped, film-coated, and imprinted with "GX LL1" on 1 side with no markings on the reverse side.

Storage: Store at 25°C (77°F); excursions permitted to 15-30°C (59-86°F).

PRODUCT LISTING - EQUIVALENTS NOT AVAILABLE

Tablet - Oral - 300 mg;150 mg;300 mg
60's $1109.96 TRIZIVIR, Glaxosmithkline 00173-0691-00

Abciximab (003211)

Categories: Angioplasty, adjunct; Atherectomy, adjunct; Recombinant DNA Origin; FDA Approved 1994 Dec; Pregnancy Category C
Drug Classes: Monoclonal antibodies; Platelet inhibitors
Brand Names: CentoRx
Foreign Brand Availability: ReoPro (Australia; New-Zealand)

DESCRIPTION

Abciximab is the Fab fragment of the chimeric human-murine monoclonal antibody 7E3. Abciximab binds to the glycoprotein (GP) IIb/IIIa receptor of human platelets and inhibits platelet aggregation. Abciximab also binds to the vitronectin ($\alpha_v\beta_3$) receptor found on platelets and vessel wall endothelial and smooth muscle cells.

The chimeric 7E3 antibody is produced by continuous perfusion in mammalian cell culture. The 47,615 dalton Fab fragment is purified from cell culture supernatant by a series of steps involving specific viral inactivation and removal procedures, digestion with papain, and column chromatography.

ReoPro is a clear, colorless, sterile, non-pyrogenic solution for intravenous (IV) use. Each single-use vial contains 2 mg/ml of abciximab in a buffered solution (pH 7.2) of 0.01 M sodium phosphate, 0.15 M sodium chloride, and 0.001% polysorbate 80 in water for injection. No preservatives are added.

CLINICAL PHARMACOLOGY

GENERAL

Abciximab binds to the intact platelet GPIIb/IIIa receptor, which is a member of the integrin family of adhesion receptors and the major platelet surface receptor involved in platelet aggregation. Abciximab inhibits platelet aggregation by preventing the binding of fibrinogen, von Willebrand factor, and other adhesive molecules to GPIIb/IIIa receptor sites on activated platelets. The mechanism of action is thought to involve steric hindrance and/or conformational effects to block access of large molecules to the receptor rather than direct interaction with the RGD (arginine-glycine-aspartic acid) binding site of GPIIb/IIIa.

Abciximab binds with similar affinity to the vitronecton receptor also known as the $\alpha_v\beta_3$ integrin. The vitronection receptor mediates the procoagulant properties of platelets and the proliferative properties of vascular endothelial and smooth muscle cells. In *in vitro* studies using a model cell line derived from melanoma cells, abciximab blocked $\alpha_v\beta_3$-mediated effects including cell adhesion (IC_{50}=0.34 µg/ml). At concentrations which, *in vitro* provide >80% GPIIb/IIIa receptor blockade, but above the *in vivo* therapeutic range, abciximab more effectively blocked the burst of thrombin generation that followed platelet activation than select comparator antibodies which inhibit GPIIb/IIIa alone.[1] The relationship of these *in vitro* data to clinical efficacy is unknown.

PRE-CLINICAL EXPERIENCE

Maximal inhibition of platelet aggregation was observed when ≥80% of GPIIb/IIIa receptors were blocked by abciximab. In non-human primates, abciximab bolus doses of 0.25 mg/kg generally achieved a blockade of at least 80% of platelet receptors and fully inhibited platelet aggregation. Inhibition of platelet function was temporary following a bolus dose, but receptor blockade could be sustained at ≥80% by continuous IV infusion. The inhibitory effects of abciximab were substantially reversed by the transfusion of platelets in monkeys. The antithrombotic efficacy of prototype antibodies [murine 7E3 Fab and $F(ab')_2$] and abciximab was evaluated in dog, monkey and baboon models of coronary, carotid and femoral artery thrombosis. Doses of the murine version of 7E3 or abciximab sufficient to produce high-grade (≥80%) GPIIb/IIIa receptor blockade prevented acute thrombosis and yielded lower rates of thrombosis compared with aspirin and/or heparin.

PHARMACOKINETICS

Following IV bolus administration, free plasma concentrations of abciximab decrease rapidly with an initial half-life of less than 10 minutes and a second phase half-life of about 30 minutes, probably related to rapid binding to the platelet GPIIb/IIIa receptors. Platelet function generally recovers over the course of 48 hours,[2,3] although abciximab remains in the circulation for 15 days or more in a platelet-bound state. Intravenous administration of a 0.25 mg/kg bolus dose of abciximab followed by continuous infusion of 10 µg/min (or a weight-adjusted infusion of 0.125 µg/kg/min to a maximum of 10 µg/min) produces approximately constant free plasma concentrations throughout the infusion. At the termination of the infusion period, free plasma concentrations fall rapidly for approximately 6 hours then decline at a slower rate.

PHARMACODYNAMICS

Intravenous administration in humans of single bolus doses of abciximab from 0.15-0.30 mg/kg produced rapid dose-dependent inhibition of platelet function as measured by *ex vivo* platelet aggregation in response to adenosine diphosphate (ADP) or by prolongation of bleeding time. At the two highest doses (0.25 and 0.30 mg/kg) at 2 hours post injection, over 80% of the GPIIb/IIIa receptors were blocked and platelet aggregation in response to 20 µM ADP was almost abolished. The median bleeding time increased to over 30 minutes at both doses compared with a baseline value of approximately 5 minutes.

Intravenous administration in humans of a single bolus dose of 0.25 mg/kg followed by a continuous infusion of 10 µg/min for periods of 12-96 hours produced sustained high-grade GPIIb/IIIa receptor blockade (≥80%) and inhibition of platelet function (*ex vivo* platelet aggregation in response to 5 or 20 µM ADP less than 20% of baseline and bleeding time greater than 30 minutes) for the duration of the infusion in most patients. Similar results were obtained when a weight-adjusted infusion dose (0.125 µg/kg/min to a maximum of 10 µg/min) was used in patients weighing up to 80 kg. Results in patients who received the 0.25 mg/kg bolus followed by a 5 µg/min infusion for 24 hours showed a similar initial receptor blockade and inhibition of platelet aggregation, but the response was not maintained throughout the infusion period.

Low levels of GPIIb/IIIa receptor blockade are present for up to 10 days following cessation of the infusion. After discontinuation of abciximab infusion, platelet function returns gradually to normal. Bleeding time returned to ≤12 minutes within 12 hours following the end of infusion in 15 of 20 patients (75%), and within 24 hours in 18 of 20 patients (90%). *Ex vivo* platelet aggregation in response to 5 µM ADP returned to ≥50% of baseline within 24 hours following the end of infusion in 11 of 32 patients (34%) and within 48 hours in 23 of 32 patients (72%). In response to 20 µM ADP, *ex vivo* platelet aggregation returned to ≥50% of baseline within 24 hours in 20 of 32 patients (62%) and within 48 hours in 28 of 32 patients (88%).

INDICATIONS AND USAGE

Abciximab is indicated as an adjunct to percutaneous coronary intervention for the prevention of cardiac ischemic complications:

- In patients undergoing percutaneous coronary intervention.
- In patients with unstable angina not responding to conventional medical therapy when percutaneous coronary intervention is planned within 24 hours.

Abciximab use in patients not undergoing percutaneous coronary intervention has not been studied.

Abciximab is intended for use with aspirin and heparin and has been studied only in that setting.

NON-FDA APPROVED INDICATIONS

Abciximab has been used as adjunct therapy in patients with acute myocardial infarction undergoing PTCA, including those with inadequate response to thrombolytic therapy, as well as in patients undergoing elective or unplanned implantation of coronary stents. Results on the use of GP IIb/IIIa inhibitors as adjunct to thrombolytic therapy in patients with ST-elevation have shown an increased incidence of earlier and complete reperfusion (TIMI grade 3 flow). Also, study data suggest the use of abciximab in diabetic patients undergoing percutaneous coronary interventions reduces short and long term complications of ischemic heart disease associated with diabetes. The use of abciximab in these clinical settings has not been approved by the FDA.

CONTRAINDICATIONS

Because abciximab may increase the risk of bleeding, abciximab is contraindicated in the following clinical situations:

- Active internal bleeding.
- Recent (within 6 weeks) gastrointestinal (GI) or genitourinary (GU) bleeding of clinical significance.
- History of cerebrovascular accident (CVA) within 2 years, or CVA with a significant residual neurological deficit.
- Bleeding diathesis.
- Administration of oral anticoagulants within 7 days unless prothrombin time is ≤1.2 times control.
- Thrombocytopenia (<100,000 cells/µl).
- Recent (within 6 weeks) major surgery or trauma.
- Intracranial neoplasm, arteriovenous malformation, or aneurysm.
- Severe uncontrolled hypertension.
- Presumed or documented history of vasculitis.
- Use of IV dextran before PCI, or intent to use it during an intervention.

Abciximab is also contraindicated in patients with known hypersensitivity to any component of this product or to murine proteins.

WARNINGS

Abciximab has the potential to increase the risk of bleeding, particularly in the presence of anticoagulation *e.g.*, from heparin, other anticoagulants, or thrombolytics (see ADVERSE REACTIONS, Bleeding).

The risk of major bleeds due to abciximab therapy may be increased in patients receiving thrombolytics and should be weighed against the anticipated benefits.

Should serious bleeding occur that is not controllable with pressure, the infusion of abciximab and any concomitant heparin should be stopped.

PRECAUTIONS

BLEEDING PRECAUTIONS

To minimize the risk of bleeding with abciximab, it is important to use a low-dose, weight-adjusted heparin regimen, a weight-adjusted abciximab bolus and infusion, strict anticoagulation guidelines, careful vascular access site management, discontinuation of heparin after the procedure and early femoral arterial sheath removal.

Therapy with abciximab requires careful attention to all potential bleeding sites (including catheter insertion sites, arterial and venous puncture sites, cutdown sites, needle puncture sites, and gastrointestinal, genitourinary, and retroperitoneal sites).

Arterial and venous punctures, intramuscular injections, and use of urinary catheters, nasotracheal intubation, nasogastric tubes and automatic blood pressure cuffs should be minimized. When obtaining IV access, non-compressible sites (*e.g.*, subclavian or jugular veins) should be avoided. Saline or heparin locks should be considered for blood drawing. Vascular puncture sites should be documented and monitored. Gentle care should be provided when removing dressings.

Femoral Artery Access Site

Arterial access site care is important to prevent bleeding. Care should be taken when attempting vascular access that only the anterior wall of the femoral artery is punctured, avoiding a Seldinger (through and through) technique for obtaining sheath access. Femoral vein sheath placement should be avoided unless needed. While the vascular sheath is in place, patients should be maintained on complete bed rest with the head of the bed ≤30° and the affected limb restrained in a straight position. Patients may be medicated for back/groin pain as necessary.

Discontinuation of heparin immediately upon completion of the procedure and removal of the arterial sheath within 6 hours is strongly recommended if APTT ≤50 sec or ACT ≤175 sec (see Laboratory Tests). In all circumstances, heparin should be discontinued at least 2 hours prior to arterial sheath removal.

Following sheath removal, pressure should be applied to the femoral artery for at least 30 minutes using either manual compression or a mechanical device for hemostasis. A pressure dressing should be applied following hemostasis. The patient should be maintained on bed rest for 6-8 hours following sheath removal or discontinuation of abciximab, or 4 hours following discontinuation of heparin, whichever is later. The pressure dressing should be removed prior to ambulation. The sheath insertion site and distal pulses of affected leg(s) should be frequently checked while the femoral artery sheath is in place and for 6 hours after femoral artery sheath removal. Any hematoma should be measured and monitored for enlargement.

The following conditions have been associated with an increased risk of bleeding and may be additive with the effect of abciximab in the angioplasty setting: PCI within 12 hours of the onset of symptoms for acute myocardial infarction, prolonged PCI (lasting more than 70 minutes) and failed PCI.

USE OF THROMBOLYTICS, ANTICOAGULANTS AND OTHER ANTIPLATELET AGENTS

In the EPIC, EPILOG, CAPTURE, and EPISTENT trials, abciximab was used concomitantly with heparin and aspirin. Because abciximab inhibits platelet aggregation, caution should be employed when it is used with other drugs that affect hemostasis, including thrombolytics, oral anticoagulants, non-steroidal anti-inflammatory drugs, dipyridamole, and ticlopidine.

In the EPIC trial, there was limited experience with the administration of abciximab with low molecular weight dextran. Low molecular weight dextran was usually given for the deployment of a coronary stent, for which oral anticoagulants were also given. In the 11 patients who received low molecular weight dextran with abciximab, 5 had major bleeding events and 4had minor bleeding events. None of the 5 placebo patients treated with low molecular weight dextran had a major or minor bleeding event (see CONTRAINDICATIONS).

There are limited data on the use of abciximab in patients receiving thrombolytic agents. Because of concern about synergistic effects on bleeding, systemic thrombolytic therapy should be used judiciously.

THROMBOCYTOPENIA

Platelet counts should be monitored prior to treatment, 2-4 hours following the bolus dose of abciximab and at 24 hours or prior to discharge, whichever is first. If a patient experiences an acute platelet decrease (*e.g.*, a platelet decrease to less than 100,000 cells/μl and a decrease of at least 25% from pre-treatment value), additional platelet counts should be determined. These platelet counts should be drawn in 3 separate tubes containing ethylenediaminetetraacetic acid (EDTA), citrate and heparin, respectively, to exclude pseudothrombocytopenia due to *in vitro* anticoagulant interaction. If true thrombocytopenia is verified, abciximab should be immediately discontinued and the condition appropriately monitored and treated. For patients with thrombocytopenia in the clinical trials, a daily platelet count was obtained until it returned to normal. If a patient's platelet count dropped to 60,000 cells/μl, heparin and aspirin were discontinued. If a patient's platelet count dropped below 50,000 cells/μl, platelets were transfused. Most cases of severe thrombocytopenia (<50,000 cells/μl) occurred within the first 24 hours of abciximab administration.

RESTORATION OF PLATELET FUNCTION

In the event of serious uncontrolled bleeding or the need for emergency surgery, abciximab should be discontinued. If platelet function does not return to normal, it may be restored, at least in part, with platelet transfusions.

LABORATORY TESTS

Before infusion of abciximab, platelet count, prothrombin time, ACT and APTT should be measured to identify pre-existing hemostatic abnormalities.

Based on an integrated analysis of data from all studies, the following guidelines may be utilized to minimize the risk for bleeding:

When abciximab is initiated 18-24 hours before PCI, the APTT should be maintained between 60 and 85 seconds during the abciximab and heparin infusion period.

During PCI, the ACT should be maintained between 200 and 300 seconds.

If anticoagulation is continued in these patients following PCI, the APTT should be maintained between 55 and 75 seconds.

The APTT or ACT should be checked prior to arterial sheath removal. The sheath should not be removed unless APTT ≤50 seconds or ACT ≤175 seconds.

READMINISTRATION

Administration of abciximab may result in human anti-chimeric antibody (HACA) formation that could potentially cause allergic or hypersensitivity reactions (including anaphylaxis), thrombocytopenia or diminished benefit upon readministration of abciximab. In the EPIC, EPILOG, and CAPTURE trials, positive HACA responses occurred in approximately 5.8% of the abciximab-treated patients. There was no excess of hypersensitivity or allergic reactions related to abciximab treatment.

Readministration of abciximab to 29 healthy volunteers who had not developed a HACA response after first administration has not led to any change in abciximab pharmacokinetics or to any reduction in antiplatelet potency. However, results in this small group of patients suggest that the incidence of HACA response may be increased after readministration. Readministration to patients who have developed a positive HACA response after initial administration has not been evaluated in clinical trials.

ALLERGIC REACTIONS

Anaphylaxis has not been reported for abciximab-treated patients in any of the Phase 3 clinical trials. However, anaphylaxis may occur. If it does, administration of abciximab should be immediately stopped and standard appropriate resuscitative measures should be initiated.

CARCINOGENESIS, MUTAGENESIS, AND IMPAIRMENT OF FERTILITY

In vitro and *in vivo* mutagenicity studies have not demonstrated any mutagenic effect. Long-term studies in animals have not been performed to evaluate the carcinogenic potential or effects on fertility in male or female animals.

PREGNANCY CATEGORY C

Animal reproduction studies have not been conducted with abciximab. It is also not known whether abciximab can cause fetal harm when administered to a pregnant woman or can affect reproduction capacity. Abciximab should be given to a pregnant woman only if clearly needed.

NURSING MOTHERS

It is not known whether this drug is excreted in human milk or absorbed systemically after ingestion. Because many drugs are excreted in human milk, caution should be exercised when abciximab is administered to a nursing woman.

PEDIATRIC USE

Safety and effectiveness in pediatric patients have not been studied.

GERIATRIC USE

Of the total number of 7860 patients in the four Phase 3 trials, 2933 (37%) were 65 and over, while 653 (8%) were 75 and over. No overall differences in safety or efficacy were observed between patients of age 65 to less than 75 as compared to younger patients. The clinical experience is not adequate to determine whether patients of age 75 or greater respond differently than younger patients.

DRUG INTERACTIONS

Although drug interactions with abciximab have not been studied systematically, abciximab has been administered to patients with ishemic heart disease treated concomitantly with a broad range of medications used in the treatment of angina, myocardial infarction and hypertension. These medications have included heparin, warfarin, beta-adrenergic receptor blockers, calcium channel antagonists, angiotensin converting enzyme inhibitors, IV and oral nitrates, ticlopidine, and aspirin. Heparin, other anticoagulants, thrombolytics, and antiplatelet agents may be associated with an increase in bleeding. Patients with HACA titers may have allergic or hypersensitivity reactions when treated with other diagnostic or therapeutic monoclonal antibodies.

ADVERSE REACTIONS

BLEEDING

Abciximab has the potential to increase the risk of bleeding, particularly in the presence of anticoagulation (*e.g.*, from heparin, other anticoagulants or thrombolytics). Bleeding in the Phase 3 trials was classified as major, minor or insignificant by the criteria of the Thrombolysis in Myocardial Infarction study group.[12] Major bleeding events were defined as either an intracranial hemorrhage or a decrease in hemoglobin greater than 5 g/dl. Minor bleeding events included spontaneous gross hematuria, spontaneous hematemesis, observed blood loss with a hemoglobin decrease of more than 3 g/dl, or a decrease in hemoglobin of at least 4 g/dl without an identified bleeding site. Insignificant bleeding events were defined as a decrease in hemoglobin of less than 3 g/dl or a decrease in hemoglobin between 3-4 g/dl without observed bleeding. In patients who received transfusions, the number of units of blood lost was estimated through an adaptation of the method of Landefeld, *et al.*[13]

In the EPIC trial, in which a non-weight-adjusted, longer-duration heparin dose regimen was used, the most common complication during abciximab therapy was bleeding during the first 36 hours. The incidences of major bleeding, minor bleeding and transfusion of blood products were significantly increased. Major bleeding occurred in 10.6% of patients in the abciximab bolus plus infusion arm compared with 3.3% of patients in the placebo arm. Minor bleeding was seen in 16.8% of abciximab bolus plus infusion patients and 9.2% of placebo patients (4). Approximately 70% of abciximab-treated patients with major bleeding had bleeding at the arterial access site in the groin. Abciximab-treated patients also had a higher incidence of major bleeding events from gastrointestinal, genitourinary, retroperitoneal, and other sites.

Bleeding rates were reduced in the CAPTURE trial, and further reduced in the EPILOG and EPISTENT trials by use of modified dosing regimens and specific patient management techniques. In EPILOG and EPISTENT, using the heparin and abciximab dosing, sheath removal and arterial access site guidelines described under PRECAUTIONS, the incidence of major bleeding in patients treated with abciximab and low-dose, weight-adjusted heparin was not significantly different from that in patients receiving placebo.

Subgroup analyses in the EPIC and CAPTURE trials showed that non-CABG major bleeding was more common in abciximab patients weighing ≤75 kg. In the EPILOG and EPISTENT trials, which used weight-adjusted heparin dosing, the non-CABG major bleeding rates for abciximab-treated patients did not differ substantially by weight subgroup.

Although data are limited, abciximab treatment was not associated with excess major bleeding in patients who underwent CABG surgery. (The range among all treatment arms was 3-5% in EPIC and 1-2% in the CAPTURE, EPILOG, and EPISTENT trials.) Some patients with prolonged bleeding times received platelet transfusions to correct the bleeding time prior to surgery. (See PRECAUTIONS, Restoration of Platelet Function.)

The rates of major bleeding, minor bleeding, and bleeding events requiring transfusions in the CAPTURE, EPILOG, and EPISTENT trials are shown in TABLE 4. The rates of insignificant bleeding events are not included in TABLE 4.

TABLE 4 *Non-CABG Bleeding in Trials of Percutaneous Coronary Intervention (EPILOG, EPISTENT and CAPTURE)*

		Number of Patients With Bleeds (%)		
	n	**Major***	**Minor**	**Requiring Transfusion†**
EPILOG and EPISTENT				
Placebo‡	1748	18 (1.0%)	46 (2.6%)	15 (0.9%)
Abciximab + Low-Dose Heparin§	2525	21 (0.8%)	82 (3.2%)	13 (0.5%)
Abciximab + Standard-Dose Heparin¤	918	17 (1.9%)	70 (7.6%)	7 (0.8%)
CAPTURE				
Placebo¶	635	12 (1.9%)	13 (2.0%)	9 (1.4%)
Abciximab¶	630	24 (3.8%)	30 (4.8%)	15 (2.4%)

* Patients who had bleeding in more than 1 classification are counted only once according to the most severe classification. Patients with multiple bleeding events of the same classification are also counted once within that classification.
† Patients with major non-CABG bleeding who received packed red blood cells or whole blood transfusion.
‡ Standard-dose heparin with or without stent (EPILOG and EPISTENT).
§ Low-dose heparin with or without stent (EPILOG and EPISTENT).
¤ Standard-dose heparin (EPILOG).
¶ Standard-dose heparin (CAPTURE).

INTRACRANIAL HEMORRHAGE AND STROKE

The total incidence of intracranial hemorrhage and non-hemorrhagic stroke across all four trials was not significantly different, 9/3023 for placebo patients and 15/4680 for abciximab-treated patients. The incidence of intracranial hemorrhage was 3/3023 for placebo patients and 7/4680 for abciximab patients.

THROMBOCYTOPENIA

In the clinical trials, patients treated with abciximab were more likely than patients treated with placebo to experience decreases in platelet counts.

Among patients in the EPILOG and EPISTENT trials who were treated with abciximab plus low-dose heparin, the proportion of patients with any thrombocytopenia (platelets less than 100,000 cells/μl) ranged from 2.5-3.0%. The incidence of severe thrombocytopenia (platelets less than 50,000 cells/μl) ranged from 0.4-1.0% and platelet transfusions were required in 0.9-1.1%, respectively. Modestly lower rates were observed among patients treated with placebo plus standard-dose heparin. Overall higher rates were observed among patients in the EPIC and CAPTURE trials treated with abciximab plus longer duration heparin: 2.6-5.2% were found to have any thrombocytopenia, 0.9-1.7% had severe thrombocytopenia, and 2.1-5.5% required platelet transfusion, respectively.

OTHER ADVERSE REACTIONS

TABLE 5 shows adverse events other than bleeding and thrombocytopenia from the combined EPIC, EPILOG and CAPTURE trials which occurred in patients in the bolus plus infusion arm at an incidence of more than 0.5% higher than in those treated with placebo.

TABLE 5 *Adverse Events Among Treated Patients in the EPIC, EPILOG, and CAPTURE Trials*

Event	Placebo (n=2226)	Bolus + Infusion (n=3111)
	Number of Patients (%)	
Cardiovascular System		
Hypotension	230 (10.3%)	447 (14.4%)
Bradycardia	79 (3.5%)	140 (4.5%)
Gastrointestinal System		
Nausea	255 (11.5%)	423 (13.6%)
Vomiting	152 (6.8%)	226 (7.3%)
Abdominal pain	49 (2.2%)	97 (3.1%)
Miscellaneous		
Back pain	304 (13.7%)	546 (17.6%)
Chest pain	208 (9.3%)	356 (11.4%)
Headache	122 (5.5%)	200 (6.4%)
Puncture site pain	58 (2.6%)	113 (3.6%)
Peripheral edema	25 (1.1%)	49 (1.6%)

The following additional adverse events from the EPIC, EPILOG, and CAPTURE trials were reported by investigators for patients treated with a bolus plus infusion of abciximab at incidences which were less than 0.5% higher than for patients in the placebo arm.

Cardiovascular System: Ventricular tachycardia (1.4%), pseudoaneurysm (0.8%), palpitation (0.5%), arteriovenous fistula (0.4%), incomplete AV block (0.3%), nodal arrthythmia (0.2%), complete AV block (0.1%), embolism (limb) (0.1%), thrombophlebitis (0.1%).

Gastrointestinal System: Dyspepsia (2.1%), diarrhea (1.1%), ileus (0.1%), gastroesophogeal reflux (0.1%).

Hemic and Lymphatic System: Anemia (1.3%), leukocytosis (0.5%), petechiae (0.2%).

Nervous System: Dizziness (2.9%), anxiety (1.7%), abnormal thinking (1.3%), agitation (0.7%), hypesthesia (0.6%), confusion (0.5%), muscle contractions (0.4%), coma (0.2%), hypertonia (0.2%), diplopia (0.1%).

Respiratory System: Pneumonia (0.4%), rales (0.4%), pleural effusion (0.3%), bronchitis (0.3%), bronchospasm (0.3%), pleurisy (0.2%), pulmonary embolism (0.2%), rhonchi (0.1%).

Musculoskeletal System: Myalgia (0.2%).

Urogenital System: Urinary retention (0.7%), dysuria (0.4%), abnormal renal function (0.4%), frequent micturition (0.1%), cystalgia (0.1%), urinary incontinence (0.1%), prostatitis (0.1%).

Miscellaneous: Pain (5.4%), sweating increased (1.0%), asthenia (0.7%), incisional pain (0.6%), pruritus (0.5%), abnormal vision (0.3%), edema (0.3%), wound (0.2%), abscess (0.2%), cellulitis (0.2%), peripheral coldness (0.2%), injection site pain (0.1%), dry mouth (0.1%), pallor (0.1%), diabetes mellitus (0.1%), hyperkalemia (0.1%), enlarged abdomen (0.1%), bullous eruption (0.1%), inflammation (0.1%), drug toxicity (0.1%).

DOSAGE AND ADMINISTRATION

The safety and efficacy of abciximab have only been investigated with concomitant administration of heparin and aspirin.

In patients with failed PCI, the continuous infusion of abciximab should be stopped because there is no evidence for abciximab efficacy in that setting.

In the event of serious bleeding that cannot be controlled by compression, abciximab and heparin should be discontinued immediately.

The recommended dosage of abciximab in adults is a 0.25 mg/kg IV bolus administered 10-60 minutes before the start of PCI, followed by a continuous IV infusion of 0.125 μg/kg/min (to a maximum of 10 μg/min) for 12 hours.

Patients with unstable angina not responding to conventional medical therapy and who are planned to undergo PCI within 24 hours may be treated with an abciximab 0.25 mg/kg IV bolus followed by an 18-24 hour IV infusion of 10 μg/min, concluding 1 hour after the PCI.

HOW SUPPLIED

ReoPro 2 mg/ml is supplied in 5 ml vials containing 10 mg abciximab.

Storage: Vials should be stored at 2-8°C (36-46°F). Do not freeze. Do not shake. Do not use beyond the expiration date. Discard any unused portion left in the vial.

PRODUCT LISTING - EQUIVALENTS NOT AVAILABLE

Solution - Intravenous - 2 mg/ml

4 ml $540.02 REOPRO, Lilly, Eli and Company 00002-7140-01

Acarbose *(003262)*

A

For complete prescribing information, refer to the CD-ROM included with the book.

For related information, see the comparative table section in Appendix A.

Categories: Diabetes mellitus; FDA Approved 1995 Sep; Pregnancy Category B

Drug Classes: Alpha glucosidase inhibitors; Antidiabetic agents

Brand Names: Precose

Foreign Brand Availability: Glucobay (Australia; Austria; Bahamas; Bahrain; Barbados; Belgium; Belize; Benin; Bermuda; Bulgaria; Burkina-Faso; Colombia; Costa-Rica; Curacao; Cyprus; Dominican-Republic; Egypt; El-Salvador; England; Ethiopia; Gambia; Germany; Ghana; Greece; Guatemala; Guinea; Guyana; Honduras; Hong-Kong; Hungary; Indonesia; Iran; Iraq; Ivory-Coast; Jamaica; Japan; Jordan; Kenya; Korea; Kuwait; Lebanon; Liberia; Libya; Malawi; Malaysia; Mali; Mauritania; Mauritius; Mexico; Morocco; Netherland-Antilles; Netherlands; New-Zealand; Nicaragua; Niger; Nigeria; Oman; Panama; Philippines; Portugal; Puerto-Rico; Qatar; Republic-of-Yemen; Saudi-Arabia; Senegal; Seychelles; Sierra-Leone; South-Africa; Spain; Sudan; Surinam; Switzerland; Syria; Taiwan; Tanzania; Thailand; Trinidad; Tunia; Uganda; United-Arab-Emirates; Zambia; Zimbabwe); Gluconase (Philippines); Glumida (Spain); Prandase (Canada; Israel)

Cost of Therapy: $65.29 (Diabetes; Precose; 50 mg; 3 tablets/day; 30 day supply)

DESCRIPTION

Acarbose is an oral alpha-glucosidase inhibitor for use in the management of Type 2 diabetes mellitus. Acarbose is an oligosaccharide which is obtained from fermentation processes of a microorganism, *Actinoplanes utahensis,* and is chemically known as *O*-4,6-dideoxy-4-[[(1*S*,4*R*,5*S*,6*S*)-4,5,6-trihydroxy-3-(hydroxymethyl)-2-cyclohexen-1-yl]amino]-α-D-glucopyranosyl-(1→4)-*O*-α-D-glucopyranosyl-(1→4)-D-glucose. It is a white to off-white powder with a molecular weight of 645.6. Acarbose is soluble in water and has a pKa of 5.1. Its empirical formula is $C_{25}H_{43}NO_{18}$.

Precose is available as 25, 50, and 100 mg tablets for oral use. The inactive ingredients are starch, microcrystalline cellulose, magnesium stearate, and colloidal silicon dioxide.

INDICATIONS AND USAGE

Acarbose, as monotherapy, is indicated as an adjunct to diet to lower blood glucose in patients with Type 2 diabetes melitus whose hyperglycemia cannot be managed on diet alone. Acarbose may also be used in combination with a sulfonylurea when diet plus either acarbose or a sulfonylurea do not result in adequate glycemic control. Also, acarbose may be used in combination with insulin or metformin. The effect of acarbose to enhance glycemic control is additive to that of the sulfonylureas, insulin, or metformin when used in combination, presumably because its mechanism of action is different.

In initiating treatment for Type 2 diabetes mellitus, diet should be emphasized as the primary form of treatment. Caloric restriction and weight loss are essential in the obese diabetic patient. Proper dietary management alone may be effective in controlling blood glucose and symptoms of hyperglycemia. The importance of regular physical activity when appropriate should also be stressed. If this treatment program fails to result in adequate glycemic control, the use of acarbose should be considered. The use of acarbose must be viewed by both the physician and patient as a treatment in addition to diet, and not as a substitute for diet or as a convenient mechanism for avoiding dietary restraint.

CONTRAINDICATIONS

Acarbose is contraindicated in patients with known hypersensitivity to the drug and in patients with diabetic ketoacidosis, or cirrhosis.

Acarbose is also contraindicated in patients with inflammatory bowel disease, colonic ulceration, partial intestinal obstruction, or in patients predisposed to intestinal obstruction. In addition, acarbose is contraindicated in patients who have chronic intestinal diseases associated with marked disorders of digestion or absorption and in patients who have conditions that may deteriorate as a result of increased gas formation in the intestine.

DOSAGE AND ADMINISTRATION

There is no fixed dosage regimen for the management of diabetes mellitus with acarbose or any other pharmacologic agent. Dosage of acarbose must be individualized on the basis of both effectiveness and tolerance while not exceeding the maximum recommended dose of 100 mg tid acarbose should be taken 3 times daily at the start (with the first bite) of each main meal. Acarbose should be started at a low dose, with gradual dose escalation as described below, both to reduce gastrointestinal side effects and to permit identification of the minimum dose required for adequate glycemic control of the patient.

During treatment initiation and dose titration (see below), 1 hour postprandial plasma glucose should be used to determine the therapeutic response to acarbose and identify the minimum effective dose for the patient. Thereafter, glycosylated hemoglobin should be measured at intervals of approximately 3 months. The therapeutic goal should be to decrease both postprandial plasma glucose and glycosylated hemoglobin levels to normal or near normal by using the lowest effective dose of acarbose, either as monotherapy or in combination with sulfonylureas, insulin or metformin.

INITIAL DOSAGE

The recommended starting dosage of acarbose is 25 mg given orally 3 times daily at the start (with the first bite) of each main meal. However, some patients may benefit from more gradual dose titration to minimize gastrointestinal side effects. This may be achieved by initiating treatment at 25 mg once per day and subsequently increasing the frequency of administration to achieve 25 mg tid.

MAINTENANCE DOSAGE

Once a 25 mg tid dosage regimen is reached, dosage of acarbose should be adjusted at 4-8 week intervals based on 1 hour postprandial glucose or glycosylated hemoglobin levels, and on tolerance. The dosage can be increased from 25 mg tid to 50 mg tid. Some patients may benefit from further increasing the dosage to 100 mg tid. The maintenance dose ranges from 50-100 mg tid. However, since patients with low body weight may be at increased risk for elevated serum transaminases, only patients with body weight >60 kg should be considered for dose titration above 50 mg tid. If no further reduction in postprandial glucose or glycosylated hemoglobin levels is observed with titration to 100 mg tid, consideration should be given to lowering the dose. Once an effective and tolerated dosage is established, it should be maintained.

MAXIMUM DOSAGE

The maximum recommended dose for patients ≤60 kg is 50 mg tid. The maximum recommended dose for patients >60 kg is 100 mg tid.

PATIENTS RECEIVING SULFONYLUREAS OR INSULIN

Sulfonylurea agents may cause hypoglycemia. Acarbose given in combination with a sulfonylurea or insulin will cause a further lowering of blood glucose and may increase the potential for hypoglycemia. If hypoglycemia occurs, appropriate adjustments in the dosage of these agents should be made.

PRODUCT LISTING - EQUIVALENTS NOT AVAILABLE

Tablet - Oral - 25 mg

84's	$38.31	PRECOSE, Allscripts Pharmaceutical Company	54569-4548-00
100's	$67.35	PRECOSE, Bayer	00026-2863-51

Tablet - Oral - 50 mg

20's	$12.76	PRECOSE, Physicians Total Care	54868-3823-01
42's	$22.80	PRECOSE, Allscripts Pharmaceutical Company	54569-4501-00
100's	$72.54	PRECOSE, Bayer	00026-2861-51
100's	$76.19	PRECOSE, Bayer	00026-2861-48

Tablet - Oral - 100 mg

100's	$70.02	PRECOSE, Bayer	00026-2862-48
100's	$86.86	PRECOSE, Bayer	00026-2862-51

Acebutolol Hydrochloride *(000002)*

For complete prescribing information, refer to the CD-ROM included with the book.

For related information, see the comparative table section in Appendix A.

Categories: Arrhythmia, ventricular; Hypertension, essential; Pregnancy Category B; FDA Approved 1984 Dec
Drug Classes: Antiadrenergics, beta blocking; Antiarrhythmics, class II
Brand Names: ACB; Alol; Beloc; Diasectral; Espesil; Lupar; Neptal; Rhotral; **Sectral**; Sectral LP; Wesfalin
Foreign Brand Availability: Acecor (Italy); Acetanol (Japan); Monitan (Canada); Prent (Argentina; Austria; Chile; Germany; Italy; Netherlands; Portugal; Switzerland); Rhodiasectral (Argentina)
Cost of Therapy: $67.11 (Hypertension; Sectral; 400 mg; 1 capsule/day; 30 day supply)
$29.87 (Hypertension; Generic Capsules; 400 mg; 1 capsule/day; 30 day supply)

DESCRIPTION

Acebutolol hydrochloride is a selective, hydrophilic beta-adrenoreceptor blocking agent with mild intrinsic sympathomimetic activity for use in treating patients with hypertension and ventricular arrhythmias. It is marketed in capsule form for oral administration. Sectral capsules are provided in two dosage strengths which contain 200 or 400 mg of acebutolol as the hydrochloride salt. The inactive ingredients present are D&C red 22, FD&C blue 1, FD&C yellow 6, gelatin, povidone, starch, stearic acid, and titanium dioxide. The 200 mg dosage strength also contains D&C red 28 and the 400 mg dosage strength also contains FD&C red 40.

Acebutolol hydrochloride is a white or slightly off-white powder freely soluble in water, and less soluble in alcohol. Chemically it is defined as the hydrochloride salt of Butanamide, N-[3-acetyl-4-[2-hydroxy-3-[(1-methylethyl)amino]propoxy]phenyl]-,(±)- or (±)-3'-Acetyl-4'-[2- hydroxy-3-(isopropylamino)propoxy] butyranilide.

INDICATIONS AND USAGE

HYPERTENSION

Acebutolol HCl is indicated for the management of hypertension in adults. It may be used alone or in combination with other antihypertensive agents, especially thiazide-type diuretics.

VENTRICULAR ARRHYTHMIAS

Acebutolol HCl is indicated in the management of ventricular premature beats; it reduces the total number of premature beats, as well as the number of paired and multiform ventricular ectopic beats, and R-on-T beats.

CONTRAINDICATIONS

Acebutolol HCl is Contraindicated in:

Persistently severe bradycardia.
Second- and third-degree heart block.
Overt cardiac failure.
Cardiogenic shock.

See WARNINGS.

WARNINGS

CARDIAC FAILURE

Sympathetic stimulation may be essential for support of the circulation in individuals with diminished myocardial contractility, and its inhibition by β-adrenergic receptor blockade may precipitate more severe failure. Although β-blockers should be avoided in overt cardiac failure, acebutolol HCl can be used with caution in patients with a history of heart failure who are controlled with digitalis and/or diuretics. Both digitalis and acebutolol HCl impair AV conduction. If cardiac failure persists, therapy with acebutolol HCl should be withdrawn.

IN PATIENTS WITHOUT A HISTORY OF CARDIAC FAILURE

In patients with aortic or mitral valve disease or compromised left ventricular function, continued depression of the myocardium with β-blocking agents over a period of time may lead to cardiac failure. At the first signs of failure, patients should be digitalized and/or be given a diuretic and the response observed closely. If cardiac failure continues despite adequate digitalization and/or diuretic, acebutolol HCl therapy should be withdrawn.

EXACERBATION OF ISCHEMIC HEART DISEASE FOLLOWING ABRUPT WITHDRAWAL

Following abrupt cessation of therapy with certain β-blocking agents in patients with coronary artery disease, exacerbation of angina pectoris and, in some cases, myocardial infarction and death have been reported. Therefore, such patients should be cautioned against interruption of therapy without a physician's advice. Even in the absence of overt ischemic heart disease, when discontinuation of acebutolol HCl is planned, the patient should be carefully observed, and should be advised to limit physical activity to a minimum while acebutolol HCl is gradually withdrawn over a period of about 2 weeks. (If therapy with an alternative β-blocker is desired, the patient may be transferred directly to comparable doses of another agent without interruption of β-blocking therapy.) If an exacerbation of angina pectoris occurs, antianginal therapy should be restarted immediately in full doses and the patient hospitalized until his condition stabilizes.

PERIPHERAL VASCULAR DISEASE

Treatment with β-antagonists reduces cardiac output and can precipitate or aggravate the symptoms of arterial insufficiency in patients with peripheral or mesenteric vascular disease. Caution should be exercised with such patients, and they should be observed closely for evidence of progression of arterial obstruction.

BRONCHOSPASTIC DISEASES

Patients with bronchospastic disease should, in general, not receive a β-blocker. Because of its relative β_1-selectivity, however, low doses of acebutolol HCl may be used with caution in patients with bronchospastic disease who do not respond to, or who cannot tolerate, alternative treatment. Since β_1-selectivity is not absolute and is dose-dependent, the lowest possible dose of acebutolol HCl should be used initially, preferably in divided doses to avoid the higher plasma levels associated with the longer dose-interval. A bronchodilator, such as theophylline or a β_2-stimulant, should be made available in advance with instructions concerning its use.

ANESTHESIA AND MAJOR SURGERY

The necessity, or desirability, of withdrawal of a β-blocking therapy prior to major surgery is controversial. β-adrenergic receptor blockade impairs the ability of the heart to respond to β-adrenergically mediated reflex stimuli. While this might be of benefit in preventing arrhythmic response, the risk of excessive myocardial depression during general anesthesia may be enhanced and difficulty in restarting and maintaining the heart beat has been reported with beta-blockers. If treatment is continued, particular care should be taken when using anesthetic agents which depress the myocardium, such as ether, cyclopropane, and trichlorethylene, and it is prudent to use the lowest possible dose of acebutolol HCl. Acebutolol HCl, like other β-blockers, is a competitive inhibitor of β-receptor agonists, and its effect on the heart can be reversed by cautious administration of such agents (*e.g.*, dobutamine or isoproterenol).

Manifestations of excessive vagal tone (*e.g.*, profound bradycardia, hypotension) may be corrected with atropine 1-3 mg IV in divided doses.

DIABETES AND HYPOGLYCEMIA

β-blockers may potentiate insulin-induced hypoglycemia and mask some of its manifestations such as tachycardia; however, dizziness and sweating are usually not significantly affected. Diabetic patients should be warned of the possibility of masked hypoglycemia.

THYROTOXICOSIS

β-adrenergic blockade may mask certain clinical signs (tachycardia) of hyperthyroidism. Abrupt withdrawal of β-blockade may precipitate a thyroid storm; therefore, patients suspected of developing thyrotoxicosis from whom acebutolol HCl therapy is to be withdrawn should be monitored closely.

DOSAGE AND ADMINISTRATION

HYPERTENSION

The initial dosage of acebutolol HCl in uncomplicated mild-to-moderate hypertension is 400 mg. This can be given as a single daily dose, but in occasional patients twice daily dosing may be required for adequate 24 hour blood-pressure control. An optimal response is usually achieved with dosages of 400-800 mg/day, although some patients have been maintained on as little as 200 mg/day. Patients with more severe hypertension or who have demonstrated inadequate control may respond to a total of 1200 mg daily (administered bid), or to the addition of a second antihypertensive agent. Beta-1 selectivity diminishes as dosage is increased.

VENTRICULAR ARRYTHMIA

The usual initial dose of acebutolol HCl is 400 mg daily given as 200 mg bid. Dosage should be increased gradually until an optimal clinical response is obtained, generally at 600-1200 mg/day. If treatment is to be discontinued, the dosage should be reduced gradually over a period of about 2 weeks.

USE IN OLDER PATIENTS

Older patients have an approximately 2-fold increase in bioavailability and may require lower maintenance doses. Doses above 800 mg/day should be avoided in the elderly.

PRODUCT LISTING - RATED THERAPEUTICALLY EQUIVALENT

Capsule - Oral - 200 mg

100's	$46.12	FEDERAL UPPER LIMIT, H.C.F.A. F F P	99999-0002-03

100's	$72.74	GENERIC, Esi Lederle Generics	59911-5842-01
100's	$84.05	GENERIC, Qualitest Products Inc	00603-2048-21
100's	$84.11	GENERIC, Moore, H.L. Drug Exchange Inc	00839-8084-06
100's	$85.73	GENERIC, Major Pharmaceuticals Inc	00904-5138-60
100's	$85.91	GENERIC, Ivax Corporation	00182-2629-01
100's	$100.73	GENERIC, Mylan Pharmaceuticals Inc	00378-1200-01
100's	$100.73	GENERIC, Par Pharmaceutical Inc	49884-0587-01
100's	$113.10	GENERIC, Watson Laboratories Inc	52544-0437-01
100's	$210.31	SECTRAL, Wyeth-Ayerst Laboratories	00008-4177-01
Capsule - Oral - 400 mg			
100's	$67.13	FEDERAL UPPER LIMIT, H.C.F.A. F F P	99999-0002-04
100's	$100.95	GENERIC, Qualitest Products Inc	00603-2047-21
100's	$111.88	GENERIC, Ivax Corporation	00182-2630-01
100's	$114.38	GENERIC, Major Pharmaceuticals Inc	00904-5139-60
100's	$121.50	GENERIC, Esi Lederle Generics	59911-5844-01
100's	$133.97	GENERIC, Mylan Pharmaceuticals Inc	00378-1400-01
100's	$133.97	GENERIC, Par Pharmaceutical Inc	49884-0588-01
100's	$150.43	GENERIC, Watson Laboratories Inc	52544-0438-01

PRODUCT LISTING - EQUIVALENTS NOT AVAILABLE

Capsule - Oral - 400 mg			
100's	$223.70	SECTRAL, Wyeth-Ayerst Laboratories	00008-4179-01

Acetaminophen *(000005)*

Categories: Arthritis, osteoarthritis; Cramps, menstrual; Fever; Headache, tension; Pain, mild; WHO Formulary

Drug Classes: Analgesics, non-narcotic; Antipyretics

Brand Names: APAP

Foreign Brand Availability: Acamoli Forte suppositories for Kids (Israel); ACET suppositories (Singapore); Abenol (Canada); Acamol (Chile; Israel); Acetalgin (Switzerland); Acetam (Peru); Acetamol (Italy); Adorem (Colombia); Afebrin (Hong-Kong; Indonesia; Philippines); Algiafin (Chile); Alvedon (Sweden); Amol (Bahrain; Cyprus; Egypt; Iran; Iraq; Jordan; Kuwait; Lebanon; Libya; Oman; Qatar; Republic-of-Yemen; Saudi-Arabia; Syria; United-Arab-Emirates); Anaflon (Germany); Analgiser (Bahrain; Cyprus; Egypt; Iran; Iraq; Jordan; Kuwait; Lebanon; Libya; Oman; Qatar; Republic-of-Yemen; Saudi-Arabia; Syria; United-Arab-Emirates); Apirex (France); Arfen (Benin; Burkina-Faso; Ethiopia; Gambia; Ghana; Guinea; Ivory-Coast; Kenya; Liberia; Malawi; Mali; Mauritania; Mauritius; Morocco; Niger; Nigeria; Senegal; Seychelles; Sierra-Leone; Sudan; Tanzania; Tunia; Uganda; Zambia; Zimbabwe); Atamel (Peru); Ben-U-Ron (Belgium; Germany; Portugal; Switzerland); Benuron (Japan); Biogesic (Indonesia; Philippines; Thailand); Bodrex (Indonesia); Brenal (Philippines); Calapol (Indonesia); Calodol (Philippines); Calpol (Bahamas; Bahrain; Barbados; Belize; Benin; Bermuda; Burkina-Faso; Curacao; Cyprus; Egypt; Ethiopia; Gambia; Ghana; Guinea; Guyana; India; Iran; Iraq; Ireland; Ivory-Coast; Jamaica; Japan; Jordan; Kenya; Kuwait; Lebanon; Liberia; Libya; Malawi; Mali; Mauritania; Mauritius; Morocco; Netherland-Antilles; Niger; Nigeria; Oman; Qatar; Republic-of-Yemen; Saudi-Arabia; Senegal; Seychelles; Sierra-Leone; Sudan; Surinam; Syria; Tanzania; Thailand; Trinidad; Tunia; Uganda; United-Arab-Emirates; Zambia; Zimbabwe); Cemol (Thailand); Claradol (Morocco); Clocephen (Philippines); Crocin (India); Daga (Thailand); Datril (Mexico; Venezuela); Depyretin (Taiwan); Dirox (Argentina); Dismifen (Mexico); Dolex 500 (Colombia); Doliprane (France; Morocco); Dolitabs (France); Dolofen (Colombia); Dolomol (Bahrain; Cyprus; Egypt; Iran; Iraq; Jordan; Kuwait; Lebanon; Libya; Oman; Qatar; Republic-of-Yemen; Saudi-Arabia; Syria; United-Arab-Emirates); Dolorol (South-Africa); Doltem (Peru); Dolotemp (Mexico); Drilan (Philippines); Dymadon (Australia); Efferalgan 500 (Costa-Rica; Dominican-Republic; El-Salvador; Guatemala; Honduras; Israel; Nicaragua; Panama); Efferalganodis (France); Eraldor (Ecuador); Expandol (France); Fortolin (China); Gelocatil (Spain); Geluprane 500 (France); Gunaceta (Indonesia); Kamolas (Indonesia); Kyofen (Colombia); Lemgrip (Belgium); Lotemp (Thailand); Malidens (India); Metagesic (Philippines); Mexalen (Austria; Czech-Republic; Hungary); Minopan (Korea); Nalgesik (Indonesia); Napa (Singapore); Napamol (South-Africa); NEBS (Japan); Nektol 500 (Philippines); Nilapur (Indonesia); Pacemol (Brazil; Singapore); Pacimol (India); Pamol (Denmark; New-Zealand); Panadol (Australia; Bahrain; Benin; Brazil; Bulgaria; Burkina-Faso; Chile; Cyprus; Egypt; England; Ethiopia; Finland; France; Gambia; Ghana; Greece; Guinea; Hong-Kong; Indonesia; Iran; Iraq; Ireland; Israel; Italy; Ivory-Coast; Jordan; Kenya; Korea; Kuwait; Lebanon; Liberia; Libya; Malawi; Mali; Mauritania; Mauritius; Morocco; Netherlands; New-Zealand; Niger; Nigeria; Oman; Qatar; Republic-of-Yemen; Saudi-Arabia; Senegal; Seychelles; Sierra-Leone; Sudan; Switzerland; Syria; Taiwan; Tanzania; Thailand; Tunia; Uganda; United-Arab-Emirates; Zambia; Zimbabwe); Panamax (Australia); Panodil (Denmark; Norway; Sweden); Paracet (Norway); Paralgin (Australia); Paralief (Ireland); Paramol (Taiwan); Paratabs (New-Zealand); Parvid (Philippines); Pedipan (Korea); Pinex (Norway); Predimol (India); Puernol (Italy); Raperon (Korea); Reliv (Sweden); Remedol (Bahamas; Barbados; Belize; Bermuda; Curacao; Guyana; Jamaica; Netherland-Antilles; Surinam; Trinidad); Revanin (Benin; Burkina-Faso; Ethiopia; Gambia; Ghana; Guinea; Ivory-Coast; Kenya; Liberia; Malawi; Mali; Mauritania; Mauritius; Morocco; Niger; Nigeria; Senegal; Seychelles; Sierra-Leone; Sudan; Tanzania; Tunia; Uganda; Zambia; Zimbabwe); Roxamol Gelcaps (Israel); Salzone (Benin; Burkina-Faso; Ethiopia; Gambia; Ghana; Guinea; Ivory-Coast; Kenya; Liberia; Malawi; Mali; Mauritania; Mauritius; Morocco; Niger; Nigeria; Senegal; Seychelles; Sierra-Leone; Sudan; Tanzania; Tunia; Uganda; Zambia; Zimbabwe); Saridon (Colombia); Setamol (Australia); Taganopain (Korea); Tempra (Belgium; Canada; Costa-Rica; Ecuador; El-Salvador; Greece; Guatemala; Honduras; Indonesia; Japan; Mexico; Nicaragua; Panama; Spain; Thailand); Tempte (Taiwan); Temzzard (Mexico); Termofren (Costa-Rica; Dominican-Republic; El-Salvador; Guatemala; Honduras; Nicaragua; Panama); Turpan (Indonesia); Tylenol (Australia; Austria; Brazil; Bulgaria; Canada; China; France; Germany; Hong-Kong; Israel; Japan; Korea; Mexico; Philippines; Portugal; Spain; Switzerland; Thailand); Tylenol Extra Fuerte (Peru); Tylex (Costa-Rica; Dominican-Republic; El-Salvador; Guatemala; Honduras; Nicaragua; Panama); Winadol (Colombia; Venezuela); Winasorb (Costa-Rica; Dominican-Republic; El-Salvador; Guatemala; Honduras; Nicaragua; Panama); Xebramol (Thailand); Zetifen (Philippines); Zolben (Venezuela)

DESCRIPTION

Note: The trade names have been used throughout this monograph for clarity.

Each ***Extra Strength Tylenol Gelcap, Geltab, Caplet, or Tablet*** contains acetaminophen 500 mg.

Each 15 ml (½ fl oz or 1 tablespoonful) of ***Extra Strength Tylenol Adult Liquid Pain Reliever*** contains 500 mg acetaminophen (alcohol 7%).

Each ***Regular Strength Tylenol Caplet or Tablet*** contains acetaminophen 325 mg.

Each ***Tylenol Arthritis Pain Extended Relief Caplet*** contains acetaminophen 650 mg.

INACTIVE INGREDIENTS

Extra Strength Tylenol:

Tablets: Celluose, corn starch, magnesium stearate, sodium starch glycolate.

Caplets: Cellulose, corn starch, FD&C red no. 40, hydroxypropyl methylcellulose, magnesium stearate, polyethylene glycol, sodium starch glycolate.

Gelcaps: Benzyl alcohol, blue no. 1 and no. 2, butylparaben, castor oil, cellulose, corn starch, edetate calcium disodium, gelatin, hydroxypropyl methylcellulose, magnesium stearate, methylparaben, propylparaben, red no. 40, sodium lauryl sulfate, sodium propionate, sodium starch glycolate, titanium dioxide, and yellow no. 10.

Geltabs: Benzyl alcohol, blue no. 1 and 2, butylparaben, castor oil, cellulose, corn starch, edetate calcium disodium, gelatin, hydroxypropyl methylcellulose, magnesium stearate, methylparaben, propylparaben, red no. 40, sodium lauryl sulfate, sodium propionate, sodium starch glycolate, titanium dioxide, and yellow no. 10.

Extra Strength Tylenol Adult Liquid Pain Reliever:

Alcohol (7%), citric acid, D&C yellow no. 10, FD&C blue no. 1, FD&C yellow no. 6, flavor, glycerin, polyethylene glycol, purified water, sodium benzoate, sorbitol, sucrose.

Regular Strength Tylenol:

Tablets: Cellulose, corn starch, magnesium stearate, sodium starch glycolate.

Tylenol Arthritis Pain Extended Relief Caplets:

Corn starch, hydroxyethyl cellulose, hydroxypropyl methylcellulose, magnesium stearate, microcrystalline cellulose, povidone, powdered cellulose, pregelatinized starch, sodium starch glycolate, titanium dioxide, triacetin.

CLINICAL PHARMACOLOGY

Acetaminophen is a clinically proven analgesic and antipyretic. Acetaminophen produces analgesia by elevation of the pain threshold and antipyresis through action on the hypothalamic heat regulating center. Acetaminophen is equal to aspirin in analgesic and antipyretic effectiveness and it is unlikely to produce many of the side effects associated with aspirin and aspirin-containing products.

Tylenol Arthritis Extended Relief uses a unique, patented bilayer caplet. The first layer dissolves quickly to provide prompt relief while the second layer is time released to provide up to 8 hours of relief.

INDICATIONS AND USAGE

For the temporary relief of minor aches and pains associated with headache, muscular aches, backache, minor arthritis pain, common cold, toothache, menstrual cramps and for the reduction of fever.

WARNINGS

EXTRA STRENGTH TYLENOL GELCAPS, GELTABS, CAPLETS, OR TABLETS, EXTRA STRENGTH TYLENOL ADULT LIQUID PAIN RELIEVER, REGULAR STRENGTH TYLENOL TABLETS

Alcohol Warning: If you consume 3 or more alcoholic drinks every day, ask your doctor whether you should take acetaminophen or other pain relievers/fever reducers. Acetaminophen may cause liver damage.

Do not use if carton is opened or red neck wrap or foil seal imprinted with "Safety Seal" is broken.

Do not use:

- With any other product containing acetaminophen.
- For more than 10 days for pain unless directed by a doctor.
- For more than 3 days for fever unless directed by a doctor.

Stop using and ask a doctor if:

- Symptoms do not improve.
- New symptoms occur.
- Pain or fever persists or gets worse.
- Redness or swelling is present.

Do not exceed recommended dose. Keep this and all drugs out of the reach of children. In case of accidental overdose, contact a physician or poison control center immediately. Prompt medical attention is critical for adults as well as for children even if you do not notice any signs or symptoms. As with any drug, if you are pregnant or nursing a baby, seek the advice of a health professional before using this product.

TYLENOL ARTHRITIS PAIN EXTENDED RELIEF CAPLETS

Alcohol Warning: If you consume 3 or more alcoholic drinks every day, ask your doctor whether you should take acetaminophen or other pain relievers/fever reducers. Acetaminophen may cause liver damage.

Do not use if carton is opened or red neck wrap or foil inner seal imprinted with "Safety Seal" is broken. Do not take for pain for more than 10 days or for fever for more than 3 days unless directed by a physician. If pain or fever persists, or gets worse, if new symptoms occur, or if redness or swelling is present, consult a physician because these could be signs of a serious condition. As with any drug, if you are pregnant or nursing a baby, seek the advice of a health professional before using this product. Keep this and all drugs out of the reach of children. In case of accidental overdose, contact a physician or poison control center immediately. Prompt medical attention is critical for adults as well as for children even if you do not notice any signs or symptoms. Do not use with other products containing acetaminophen.

PRECAUTIONS

If a rare sensitivity reaction occurs, the drug should be discontinued.

DOSAGE AND ADMINISTRATION

Extra Strength Tylenol Gelcaps, Geltabs, Caplets, or Tablets:

Adults and children 12 years of age and older: Take 2 gelcaps, geltabs, caplets, or tablets every 4-6 hours as needed. Do not take more than 8 gelcaps, geltabs, caplets or tablets in 24 hours, or as directed by a doctor.

Children under 12 years: Do not use this adult Extra Strength product in children under 12 years of age. This will provide more than the recommended dose (overdose) of Tylenol and could cause serious health problems.

Extra Strength Tylenol Adult Liquid Pain Reliever:

Adults and children 12 years of age and older: Take 2 tablespoons (tbsp) in dose cup provided every 4-6 hours as needed. Do not take more than 8 tablespoons in 24 hours, or as directed by a doctor.

Children under 12 years: Do not use this adult Extra Strength product in children under 12 years of age. This will provide more than the recommended dose (overdose) of Tylenol and could cause serious health problems.

Regular Strength Tylenol Tablets:

Adults and Children 12 years of Age and Older: Take 2 tablets every 4-6 hours as needed. Do not take more than 12 tablets in 24 hours, or as directed by a doctor.

Children 6-11 years of age: Take 1 tablet every 4-6 hours as needed. Do not take more than 5 tablets in 24 hours.

Children under 6 years of age: Do not use this adult Regular Strength product in children under 6 years of age. This will provide more than the recommended dose (overdose) of Tylenol and could cause serious health problems.

Tylenol Arthritis Pain Extended Relief Caplets:

Adults and children 12 years of age and older: Take 2 caplets every 8 hours, not to exceed 6 caplets in any 24 hour period. TAKE 2 CAPLETS WITH WATER, SWALLOW EACH CAPLET WHOLE. DO NOT CRUSH, CHEW, OR DISSOLVE THE CAPLET. Not for use in children under 12 years of age.

HOW SUPPLIED

Extra Strength Tylenol:

Tablets: Colored white, imprinted "TYLENOL" and "500";. Store at room temperature.

Caplets: Colored white, imprinted "TYLENOL 500 mg". Store at room temperature.

Gelcaps: Colored yellow and red, imprinted "Tylenol 500". Store at room temperature; avoid high humidity and excessive heat 40°C (104°F).

Geltabs: Colored yellow and red, imprinted "Tylenol 500". Store at room temperature; avoid high humidity and excessive heat 40°C (104°F).

Extra Strength Tylenol Adult Liquid Pain Reliever:

Mint-flavored liquid (colored green) 8 fl oz tamper-evident bottle with child resistant safety cap and special dosage cup. Store at room temperature.

Regular Strength Tylenol:

Tablets: Colored white, scored, imprinted "TYLENOL" and "325". Store at room temperature.

Tylenol Arthritis Pain Extended Relief:

Caplets: Colored white, engraved "TYLENOL ER". Store at room temperature. Avoid excessive heat (40°C).

Acetaminophen; Butalbital *(000020)*

For complete prescribing information, refer to the CD-ROM included with the book.

Categories: Headache, tension; FDA Approved 1984 Oct; Pregnancy Category C
Drug Classes: Analgesics, non-narcotic; Barbiturates
Brand Names: Bancap; Bucet; Bupap; Butapap; Cephadyn; Conten; Greatab; Indogesic; Isopap; Midrinol; **Phrenilin**; Phrenilin Forte; Sedapap; Tencon; Triaprin
Cost of Therapy: $18.64 (Headache; Phrenilin; 325 mg; 50 mg; 6 tablets/day; 7 day supply)
$10.94 (Headache; Generic Tablets; 325 mg; 50 mg; 6 tablets/day; 7 day supply)

DESCRIPTION

Butalbital (5-allyl-5-isobutylbarbituric acid), a slightly bitter, white, odorless, crystalline powder, is a short to intermediate-acting barbiturate. It has the following empirical formula: $C_{11}H_{16}N_2O_3$. The molecular weight is 224.26.

Acetaminophen (4′-hydroxyacetanalide), a slightly bitter, white, odorless, crystalline powder, is a non-opiate, non-salicylate analgesic and antipyretic. It has the following empirical formula: $C_8H_9NO_2$. The molecular weight is 151.16.

PHRENILIN

Each Phrenilin tablet for oral administration, contains butalbital, 50 mg (*WARNING:* May be habit forming), acetaminophen 325 mg.

In addition each Phrenilin tablet contains the following inactive ingredients: alginic acid, cornstarch, D&C red no. 27 aluminum lake, FD&C blue no. 1 aluminum lake, gelatin, magnesium stearate, microcrystalline cellulose and pregelatinized starch.

PHRENILIN FORTE

Phrenilin Forte capsule for oral administration contains butalbital, 50 mg (*WARNING:* May be habit forming), acetaminophen, 650 mg.

In addition, each Phrenilin Forte capsule may also contain the following inactive ingredients: benzyl alcohol, butylparaben, D&C red no. 28, D&C red no. 33, edetate calcium disodium, FD&C blue no. 1, FD&C red no. 40, gelatin, methylparaben, propylparaben, silicon dioxide, sodium lauryl sulfate, sodium propionate and titanium dioxide.

INDICATIONS AND USAGE

Acetaminophin; butalbital tablets and capsules are indicated for the relief of the symptom complex of tension (or muscle contraction) headache.

Evidence supporting the efficacy and safety of this combination product in the treatment of multiple recurrent headaches is unavailable. Caution in this regard is required because butalbital is habit-forming and potentially abusable.

CONTRAINDICATIONS

This product is contraindicated under the following conditions:

- Hypersensitivity or intolerance to any component of this product.
- Patients with porphyria.

WARNINGS

Butalbital is habit-forming and potentially abusable. Consequently, the extended use of this product is not recommended.

DOSAGE AND ADMINISTRATION

Acetaminophen; Butalbital Tablets: 1 or 2 tablets every four hours. Total daily dosage should not exceed 6 tablets.

Acetaminophen; Butalbital Capsules: 1 capsule every four hours. Total daily dosage should not exceed 6 capsules.

Extended and repeated use of these products is not recommended because of the potential for physical dependence.

PRODUCT LISTING - RATED THERAPEUTICALLY EQUIVALENT

Capsule - Oral - 325 mg;50 mg

100's	$16.50	GENERIC, International Ethical Laboratories Inc	11584-1029-01

Capsule - Oral - 650 mg;50 mg

100's	$43.16	PHRENILIN FORTE, Physicians Total Care	54868-1109-00
100's	$44.43	PHRENILIN FORTE, Carnrick Laboratories Inc	00086-0056-10
100's	$70.63	PHRENILIN FORTE, Amarin Pharmaceuticals	65234-0056-10

Tablet - Oral - 325 mg;50 mg

100's	$28.80	GENERIC, Ecr Pharmaceuticals	00095-0240-01
100's	$31.30	GENERIC, Marnel Pharmaceuticals Inc	00682-1400-01
100's	$36.42	PHRENILIN, Carnrick Laboratories Inc	00086-0050-10
100's	$37.79	GENERIC, Qualitest Products Inc	00603-2540-21
100's	$44.38	PHRENILIN, Amarin Pharmaceuticals	65234-0050-10

Tablet - Oral - 650 mg;50 mg

18's	$13.97	GENERIC, Pd-Rx Pharmaceuticals	55289-0778-18
100's	$34.00	GENERIC, Merz Pharmaceuticals	00259-1278-01
100's	$101.82	GENERIC, Savage Laboratories	00281-0198-17
100's	$101.82	GENERIC, Savage Laboratories	00281-0389-53

PRODUCT LISTING - EQUIVALENTS NOT AVAILABLE

Capsule - Oral - 650 mg;50 mg

100's	$30.45	GENERIC, Qualitest Products Inc	00603-2542-21
100's	$31.56	GENERIC, Forest Pharmaceuticals	00785-2307-01
100's	$33.99	GENERIC, Andrx Pharmaceuticals	62022-0070-01

Tablet - Oral - 650 mg;50 mg

100's	$29.95	GENERIC, Everett Laboratories Inc	00642-0166-10
100's	$33.60	GENERIC, Atley Pharmaceuticals	59702-0650-01
100's	$36.00	GENERIC, Merz Pharmaceuticals	00259-0392-01
100's	$37.71	GENERIC, Andrx Pharmaceuticals	62022-0073-01
100's	$41.60	GENERIC, Mcr/American Pharmaceuticals Inc	58605-0511-01
100's	$61.09	GENERIC, Mcr/American Pharmaceuticals Inc	58605-0524-01

Acetaminophen; Butalbital; Caffeine; Codeine Phosphate *(000022)*

For complete prescribing information, refer to the CD-ROM included with the book.

Categories: Pain, mild to moderate; DEA Class CIII; FDA Approved 1992 Jul; Pregnancy Category C
Drug Classes: Analgesics, narcotic; Barbiturates; Xanthine derivatives
Brand Names: Amaphen W/Codeine; Ezol III; **Fioricet W/Codeine**
Cost of Therapy: $88.12 (Headache; Fioricet w/Codeine; 325 mg; 50 mg; 40 mg; 30 mg; 6 capsules/day; 7 day supply)
$57.12 (Headache; Generic Capsules; 325 mg; 50 mg; 40 mg; 30 mg; 6 capsules/day; 7 day supply)

DESCRIPTION

Fioricet with codeine is supplied in capsule form for oral administration.

Each Capsule Contains:

Acetaminophen: 325 mg
Butalbital: 50 mg (*Warning:* May be habit-forming.)
Caffeine: 40 mg
Codeine Phosphate: 30 mg (½ gr) (*Warning:* May be habit-forming.)

Codeine phosphate [morphine-3-methyl ether phosphate (1:1) (salt) hemihydrate, $C_{18}H_{24}NO_7P$, anhydrous mw 397.37], is a narcotic analgesic and antitussive.

Butalbital (5-allyl-5-isobutylbarbituric acid, $C_{11}H_{16}N_2O_3$, mw 224.26), is a short- to intermediate-acting barbiturate.

Caffeine (1,3,7-trimethylxanthine, $C_8H_{10}N_4O_2$, mw 194.19), is a central nervous system stimulant.

Acetaminophen (4′-hydroxyacetanilide, $C_8H_9NO_2$, mw 151.16), is a non-opiate, non-salicylate analgesic and antipyretic.

Active Ingredients: Codeine phosphate, butalbital, caffeine, and acetaminophen.

Inactive Ingredients: Black iron oxide, colloidal silicon dioxide, D&C red no. 7 (calcium lake), D&C red no. 33, FD&C blue no. 1, FD&C blue no. 1 (aluminum lake), gelatin, magnesium stearate, pregelatinized starch, red iron oxide, sodium lauryl sulfate, and titanium dioxide.

May Also Include: Benzyl alcohol, butylparaben, carboxymethyl-cellulose sodium, edetate calcium disodium, methylparaben, propylparaben, silicon dioxide, and sodium propionate.

INDICATIONS AND USAGE

Acetaminophen; butalbital; caffeine; codeine phosphate is indicated for the relief of the symptom complex of tension (or muscle contraction) headache.

Evidence supporting the efficacy and safety of acetaminophen; butalbital; caffeine; codeine phosphate in the treatment of multiple recurrent headaches is unavailable. Caution in this regard is required because codeine and butalbital are habit-forming and potentially abusable.

CONTRAINDICATIONS

Acetaminophen; butalbital; caffeine; codeine phosphate is contraindicated under the following conditions:

- Hypersensitivity or intolerance to acetaminophen, caffeine, butalbital, or codeine.
- Patients with porphyria.

WARNINGS

In the presence of head injury or other intracranial lesions, the respiratory depressant effects of codeine and other narcotics may be markedly enhanced, as well as their capacity for elevating cerebrospinal fluid pressure. Narcotics also produce other CNS depressant effects, such as drowsiness, that may further obscure the clinical course of the patients with head injuries.

Codeine or other narcotics may obscure signs on which to judge the diagnosis or clinical course of patients with acute abdominal conditions.

Butalbital and codeine are both habit-forming and potentially abusable. Consequently, the extended use of acetaminophen; butalbital; caffeine; codeine phosphate is not recommended.

DOSAGE AND ADMINISTRATION

1 or 2 capsules every 4 hours. Total daily dosage should not exceed 6 capsules.

Extended and repeated use of this product is not recommended because of the potential for physical dependence.

PRODUCT LISTING - RATED THERAPEUTICALLY EQUIVALENT

Capsule - Oral - 325 mg;50 mg;40 mg;30 mg

100's	$137.50	PHRENILIN WITH CAFFEINE AND CODEINE, Amarin Pharmaceuticals	65234-0061-10
100's	$149.00	GENERIC, West Ward Pharmaceutical Corporation	00143-3000-01
100's	$209.82	FIORICET WITH CODEINE, Novartis Pharmaceuticals	00078-0243-05

PRODUCT LISTING - EQUIVALENTS NOT AVAILABLE

Capsule - Oral - 325 mg;50 mg;40 mg;30 mg

100's	$136.00	GENERIC, Qualitest Products Inc	00603-2552-21
100's	$136.00	GENERIC, Qualitest Products Inc	00603-2553-21

Acetaminophen; Codeine Phosphate *(000051)*

Categories: Pain, moderate to severe; Pregnancy Category C; DEA Class CIII; DEA Class CV; FDA Approval Pre 1982

Drug Classes: Analgesics, narcotic

Brand Names: Capital with Codeine; Phenaphen W/Codeine; Pyregesic-C; **Tylenol W Codeine**

Foreign Brand Availability: Algesidal (France); Algimide (Colombia); Algimide F (Colombia); Claradol Codeine (France); Co-Cadamol (Singapore); Codabrol (Israel); Cod-Acamol Forte (Israel); Codalgin (Australia; New-Zealand); Codapane (Australia; New-Zealand); Codeidol (Colombia); Codeidol F (Colombia); Codicet (Thailand); Codilprane Enfant (France); Codipar (England; Ireland); Codisal Forte (Israel); Coditam (Indonesia); Codoliprane (France); Codral Pain Relief (Australia; New-Zealand); Dafalgan Codeine (France); Dolorol Forte (South-Africa); Dymadon Co (Australia; New-Zealand); Dymadon Forte (Australia; New-Zealand); Efferalgan Codeine (Israel); Empracet-30 (Canada); Empracet-60 (Canada); Liquigesic Co (Australia; New-Zealand); Maxadol (South-Africa); Paceco (Malaysia; Singapore); Panadeine (Czech-Republic; Hong-Kong; Hungary; Malaysia); Panadeine Co (Bahrain; Cyprus; Egypt; Iran; Iraq; Israel; Jordan; Kuwait; Lebanon; Libya; Oman; Qatar; Republic-of-Yemen; Saudi-Arabia; Syria; United-Arab-Emirates); Panadeine Forte (Australia; New-Zealand); Panadiene (Australia; Bahamas; Barbados; Belize; Bermuda; Curacao; Guyana; Jamaica; Japan; Netherland-Antilles; New-Zealand; Puerto-Rico; Surinam; Trinidad); Panado-Co Caplets (South-Africa); Panamax (Australia; New-Zealand); Paracod (Israel); Paracodol (South-Africa); Paradine (Malaysia); Parcono (Thailand); Parcoten (Hong-Kong); Rockamol Plus (Israel); Solpadeine (Bahrain; Cyprus; Egypt; Iran; Iraq; Jordan; Kuwait; Lebanon; Libya; Oman; Qatar; Republic-of-Yemen; Saudi-Arabia; Syria; United-Arab-Emirates); Tylenol W/Codeine No. 4 (Canada); Tylex CD (Mexico); Winadol Forte (Colombia); Zapain (England; Ireland)

Cost of Therapy: $0.75 (Pain; Generic Tablets; 300 mg; 30 mg; 6 tablets/day; 7 day supply)
$16.08 (Pain; Tylenol with Codeine #3; 300 mg; 30 mg; 6 tablets/day; 7 day supply)

DESCRIPTION

Acetaminophen, 4′-hydroxyacetanilide, is a nonopiate, non-salicylate analgesic and antipyretic which occurs as a white, odorless, crystalline powder, possessing a slightly bitter taste. It has the following structural formula:

$C_8H_9NO_2$, with a molecular meight of 151.16

Codeine is an alkaloid, obtained from opium or prepared from morphine by methylation. Codeine phosphate occurs as fine, white, needle-shaped crystals, or white, crystalline powder. It is affected by light. Its chemical name is: 7,8-didehydro-4,5α-epoxy-3-methoxy-17-methylmorphinan-6α-ol phosphate (1:1) (salt) hemihydrate. It has the following molecular formula: $C_{18}H_{21}NO_3 \cdot H_3PO_4 \cdot \frac{1}{2}H_2O$ with a molecular weight of 406.37

TABLETS AND ELIXIR

Each Tylenol With Codeine Tablet Contains:

No. 2 Codeine Phosphate: 15 mg (*Warning:* May be habit forming.)
Acetaminophen: 300 mg
No. 3 Codeine Phosphate: 30 mg (*Warning:* May be habit forming.)
Acetaminophen: 300 mg
No. 4 Codeine Phosphate: 60 mg (*Warning:* May be habit forming.)
Acetaminophen: 300 mg

Each 5 ml of Tylenol With Codeine Elixir Contains:

Codeine Phosphate: 12 mg (*Warning:* May be habit forming.)
Acetaminophen: 120 mg
Alcohol 7%

Tylenol Inactive Ingredients: *Tablets:* Powdered cellulose, magnesium stearate, sodium metabisulfite (see WARNINGS), pregelatinized starch, starch (corn); *Elixir:* Alcohol, citric acid, propylene glycol, sodium benzoate, saccharin sodium, sucrose, natural and artificial flavors, FD&C yellow no. 6.

CAPSULES

Phenaphen w/Codeine No. 2 Capsule

Each Phenaphen w/Codeine No. 2 Capsule Contains:

Acetaminophen: 325 mg
Codeine Phosphate: 15 mg (*Warning:* May be habit forming.)

Inactive Ingredients: Corn starch, FD&C yellow no. 10, edible ink, FD&C blue no. 1, FD&C red no. 40, FD&C yellow no. 6, gelatin, magnesium stearate, sodium starch glycolate, stearic acid.

Phenaphen w/Codeine No. 3 Capsule

Each Phenaphen w/Codeine No. 3 Capsule Contains:

Acetaminophen: 325 mg
Codeine Phosphate: 30 mg (*Warning:* May be habit forming.)

Inactive Ingredients: FD&C yellow no. 10, edible ink, FD&C blue no. 1, (FD&C green no. 3 and red no. 40), FD&C yellow no. 6, gelatin, magnesium stearate, sodium starch glycolate, stearic acid.

Phenaphen w/Codeine No. 4 Capsule

Each Phenaphen w/Codeine No. 4 Capsule Contains:

Acetaminophen: 325 mg
Codeine Phosphate: 60 mg (*Warning:* May be habit forming.)

Inactive Ingredients: Corn starch, FD&C yellow no. 10, edible ink, FD&C green no. 3 or blue no. 1, FD&C yellow no. 6, gelatin, lactose, magnesium stearate, sodium starch glycolate stearic acid.

CLINICAL PHARMACOLOGY

Acetaminophen and codeine phosphate tablets, oral solution, and capsules, combine the analgesic effects of a centrally acting analgesic, codeine, with a peripherally acting analgesic, acetaminophen. Both ingrediants are well absorbed orally. The plasma elimination half-life ranges from 1-4 hours for acetaminophen, and from 2.5 to 3 hours for codeine.

PHARMACOKINETICS

The behavior of the individual components is described below:

Codeine: Codeine retains at least one-half of its analgesic activity when administered orally. A reduced first-pass metabolism of codeine by the liver accounts for the greater oral efficacy of codeine when compared to most other morphine-like narcotics. Following absorption, codeine is metabolized by the liver and metabolic products are excreted in the urine. Approximately 10% of the administered codeine is demethylated to morphine, which may account for its analgesic activity.

Acetaminophen: Acetaminophen is distributed throughout most fluids of the body, and is metabolized primarily in the liver. Little unchanged drug is excreted in the urine, but most metabolic products appear in the urine within 24 hours.

INDICATIONS AND USAGE

Acetaminophen and codeine phosphate tablets and capsules are indicated for the relief of mild to moderately severe pain.

Acetaminophen and codeine phosphate oral solution is indicated for the relief of mild to moderate pain.

CONTRAINDICATIONS

Acetaminophen and codeine phosphate tablets, oral solution, or capsules, should not be administered to patients who have previously exhibited hypersensitivity to any component.

WARNINGS

Acetaminophen and codeine phosphate tablets contain sodium metabisulfite, a sulfite that may cause allergic-type reactions including anaphylactic symptoms and life-threatening or less severe asthmatic episodes in certain susceptible people. The overall prevalence of sulfite sensitivity in the general population is unknown and probably low. Sulfite sensitivity is seen more frequently in asthmatic than in nonasthmatic people.

PRECAUTIONS

GENERAL

Head Injury and Increased Intracranial Pressure

The respiratory depressant effects of narcotics and their capacity to elevate cerebrospinal fluid pressure may be markedly exaggerated in the presence of head injury, other intracranial lesions or a pre-existing increase in intracranial pressure. Furthermore, narcotics produce adverse reactions which may obscure the clinical course of patients with head injuries.

Acute Abdominal Conditions

The administration of this product or other narcotics may obscure the diagnosis or clinical course of patients with acute abdominal conditions.

Special Risk Patients

This drug should be given with caution to certain patients such as the elderly or debilitated, and those with severe impairment of hepatic or renal function, hypothyroidism, Addison's disease, and prostatic hypertrophy or urethral stricture.

INFORMATION FOR THE PATIENT

Codeine may impair the mental and/or physical abilities required for the performance of potentially hazardous tasks such as driving a car or operating machinery. The patient using this drug should be cautioned accordingly.

The patient should understand the single-dose and 24 hour dose limits, and the time interval between doses.

CARCINOGENESIS, MUTAGENESIS, AND IMPAIRMENT OF FERTILITY

No long-term studies in animals have been performed with acetaminophen or codeine to determine carcinogenic potential or effects on fertility.

Acetaminophen and codeine have been found to have no mutagenic potential using the Ames Salmonella-Microsomal Activation test, the Basc test on Drosophila germ cells, and the Micronucleus test on mouse bone marrow.

PREGNANCY CATEGORY C

Teratogenic Effects

Codeine

A study in rats and rabbits reported no teratogenic effect of codeine administered during the period of organogenesis in doses ranging from 5 to 120 mg/kg. In the rat, doses at the 120 mg/kg level, in the toxic range for the adult animal, were associated with an increase in embryo resorption at the time of implantation. In another study a single 100 mg/kg dose of codeine administered to pregnant mice reportedly resulted in delayed ossification in the offspring.

There are no studies in humans, and the significance of these findings to humans, if any, is not known.

Acetaminophen and codeine phosphate tablets, oral solution, or capsules, should be used during pregnancy only if the potential benefit justifies the potential risk to the fetus.

Nonteratogenic Effects

Dependence has been reported in newborns whose mothers took opiates regularly during pregnancy. Withdrawal signs include irritability, excessive crying, tremors, hyperreflexia, fever, vomiting, and diarrhea. These signs usually appear during the first few days of life.

LABOR AND DELIVERY

Narcotic analgesics cross the placental barrier. The closer to delivery and the larger the dose used, the greater the possibility of respiratory depression in the newborn. Narcotic analgesics should be avoided during labor if delivery of a premature infant is anticipated. If the mother has received narcotic analgesics during labor, newborn infants should be observed closely for signs of respiratory depression. Resuscitation may be required. The effect of codeine, if any, on the later growth, development, and functional maturation of the child is unknown.

NURSING MOTHERS

Some studies, but not others, have reported detectable amounts of codeine in breast milk. The levels are probably not clinically significant after usual therapeutic dosage. The possibility of clinically important amounts being excreted in breast milk in individuals abusing codeine should be considered.

PEDIATRIC USE

Safe dosage of acetaminophen and codeine phosphate oral solution USP has not been established in children below the age of three years.

DRUG INTERACTIONS

Patients receiving other narcotic analgesics, antipsychotics, antianxiety agents, or other CNS depressants (including alcohol) concomitantly with this drug may exhibit an additive CNS depression. When such combined therapy is contemplated, the dose of one or both agents should be reduced.

The concurrent use of anticholinergics with codeine may produce paralytic ileus.

ADVERSE REACTIONS

The most frequently observed adverse reactions include lightheadedness, dizziness, sedation, shortness of breath, nausea, and vomiting. These effects seem to be more prominent in ambulatory than in non-ambulatory patients, and some of these adverse reactions may be alleviated if the patient lies down. Other adverse reactions include allergic reactions, euphoria, dysphoria, constipation, abdominal pain, and pruritus.

At higher doses, codeine has most of the disadvantages of morphine including respiratory depression.

DOSAGE AND ADMINISTRATION

TABLETS AND CAPSULES

Dosage should be adjusted according to severity of pain and response of the patient.

It should be kept in mind, however, that tolerance to codeine can develop with continued use and that the incidence of untoward effects is dose related. Adult doses of codeine higher than 60 mg fail to give commensurate relief of pain but merely prolong analgesia and are associated with an appreciably increased incidence of undesirable side effects. Equivalently high doses in children would have similar effects.

The usual adult dosage is shown in TABLE 1.

TABLE 1 *Usual Adult Dosage*

	Single Doses (Range)	Maximum 24 Hour Dose
Codeine Phosphate	15-60 mg	360 mg
Acetaminophen	300-1000 mg	4000 mg

Doses may be repeated up to every 4 hours.

The prescriber must determine the number of tablets or capsules per dose and the maximum number of tablets or capsules per 24 hours, based upon the dosage guidance in TABLE 1. This information should be conveyed in the prescription.

For children, the dose of codeine phosphate is 0.5 mg/kg.

ELIXIR

Acetaminophen and codeine phosphate oral solution contains 120 mg of acetaminophen and 12 mg of codeine phosphate/5 ml and is given orally.

The usual doses are:

Children: *7-12 Years:* 10 ml (2 teaspoonfuls) 3 or 4 times daily. *3-6 Years:* 5 ml (1 teaspoonful) 3 or 4 times daily. *Under 3 Years:* Safe dosage has not been established.

Adults: 15 ml (1 tablespoonful) every 4 hours as needed.

HOW SUPPLIED

TYLENOL WITH CODEINE TABLETS

Round, white, imprinted "McNEIL", "TYLENOL CODEINE" and either "2", "3", "4".

Storage: Store tablets ar controlled room temperature (15-30°C, 59-86°F).

Dispense in tight, light-resistant container as defined in the official compendium.

TYLENOL WITH CODEINE ELIXIR

Tylenol with codeine elixir contains 120 mg acetaminophen and 12 mg codeine phosphate/5ml.

Storage: Store elixir at controlled room temperature (15-30°C, 59-86°F). Protect from light. Do not refrigerate. Do not freeze.

Dispense in tight, light-resistant container as defined in the official compendium.

PHENAPHEN WITH CODEINE CAPSULES

No. 2: Black and yellow capsules containing 325 mg acetaminophen and 15 mg codeine phosphate.

No. 3: Black and green capsules containing 325 mg acetaminophen and 30 mg codeine phosphate.

No. 4: Green and white capsules containing 325 mg acetaminophen and 60 mg codeine phosphate.

Storage: Store capsules at controlled room temperature (15-30°C, 59-86°F).

Dispense in tight, light-resistant container.

PRODUCT LISTING - RATED THERAPEUTICALLY EQUIVALENT

Liquid - Oral - 120 mg;12 mg/5 ml

5 ml x 100	$32.40	GENERIC, Pharmaceutical Assoc Inc Div Beach Products	00121-0504-05
5 ml x 100	$55.00	GENERIC, Roxane Laboratories Inc	00054-8013-04
10 ml x 100	$35.65	GENERIC, Pharmaceutical Assoc Inc Div Beach Products	00121-0504-10
12 ml x 100	$39.75	GENERIC, Pharmaceutical Assoc Inc Div Beach Products	00121-0504-12
12 ml x 100	$57.00	GENERIC, Roxane Laboratories Inc	00054-8002-04
15 ml x 100	$42.75	GENERIC, Pharmaceutical Assoc Inc Div Beach Products	00121-0504-15
15 ml x 100	$58.00	GENERIC, Roxane Laboratories Inc	00054-8017-04
120 ml	$2.50	GENERIC, Pharmaceutical Assoc Inc Div Beach Products	00121-0504-04
120 ml	$5.74	GENERIC, Alpharma Uspd Makers Of Barre and Nmc	00472-1419-04
120 ml	$7.30	GENERIC, Morton Grove Pharmaceuticals Inc	60432-0245-04
473 ml	$63.82	TYLENOL WITH CODEINE, Janssen Pharmaceuticals	00045-0508-16
480 ml	$12.95	GENERIC, Geneva Pharmaceuticals	00781-6052-16
480 ml	$12.96	GENERIC, Watson/Schein Pharmaceuticals Inc	00364-7207-16
480 ml	$13.24	GENERIC, Major Pharmaceuticals Inc	00904-0173-16
480 ml	$13.72	GENERIC, Pharmaceutical Assoc Inc Div Beach Products	00121-0504-16
480 ml	$14.00	GENERIC, Mova Pharmaceutical Corporation	55370-0341-48
480 ml	$18.55	GENERIC, Ivax Corporation	00182-1078-40
480 ml	$18.55	GENERIC, Alpharma Uspd Makers Of Barre and Nmc	00472-1419-16
480 ml	$19.82	GENERIC, Mutual/United Research Laboratories	00677-0996-33
480 ml	$19.85	GENERIC, Qualitest Products Inc	00603-1020-58
480 ml	$19.85	GENERIC, Morton Grove Pharmaceuticals Inc	60432-0245-16
500 ml	$20.77	GENERIC, Roxane Laboratories Inc	00054-3005-63
3840 ml	$84.48	GENERIC, Major Pharmaceuticals Inc	00904-0173-28
3840 ml	$84.48	GENERIC, Major Pharmaceuticals Inc	00904-7775-28
3840 ml	$111.28	GENERIC, Alpharma Uspd Makers Of Barre and Nmc	00472-1419-28

Suspension - Oral - 120 mg;12 mg/5 ml

480 ml	$31.49	CAPITAL WITH CODEINE SUSPENSION, Carnrick Laboratories Inc	00086-0046-16
480 ml	$57.81	CAPITAL WITH CODEINE SUSPENSION, Amarin Pharmaceuticals	65234-0046-16

Tablet - Oral - 300 mg;15 mg

15's	$2.92	GENERIC, Pd-Rx Pharmaceuticals	55289-0449-15
100's	$6.30	GENERIC, Warner Chilcott Laboratories	00047-0634-24
100's	$7.43	GENERIC, Interstate Drug Exchange Inc	00814-0246-14
100's	$7.85	GENERIC, Vintage Pharmaceuticals Inc	00254-2063-28
100's	$8.20	GENERIC, Ivax Corporation	00182-1268-01
100's	$8.22	GENERIC, Moore, H.L. Drug Exchange Inc	00839-6717-06
100's	$9.43	GENERIC, Aligen Independent Laboratories Inc	00405-0007-01
100's	$12.61	GENERIC, Major Pharmaceuticals Inc	00904-0571-61
100's	$15.00	FEDERAL UPPER LIMIT, H.C.F.A. F F P	99999-0051-01
100's	$26.92	GENERIC, Major Pharmaceuticals Inc	00904-0571-60
100's	$30.24	GENERIC, Mallinckrodt Medical Inc	00406-0483-01
100's	$30.44	GENERIC, Teva Pharmaceuticals Usa	00093-0050-01
100's	$30.44	GENERIC, Qualitest Products Inc	00603-2337-21
100's	$30.44	GENERIC, Watson/Rugby Laboratories Inc	52544-0850-01

Package	Price	Product, Manufacturer	NDC
100's	$32.29	TYLENOL WITH CODEINE #2, Janssen Pharmaceuticals	00045-0511-60
100's	$33.26	GENERIC, Barr Laboratories Inc	00555-0305-02
100's	$33.26	GENERIC, Mutual/United Research Laboratories	00677-1714-01
100's	$33.26	GENERIC, Duramed Pharmaceuticals Inc	51285-0302-02

Tablet - Oral - 300 mg;30 mg

Package	Price	Product, Manufacturer	NDC
6's	$2.58	GENERIC, Pd-Rx Pharmaceuticals	55289-0005-06
10's	$2.70	GENERIC, Pd-Rx Pharmaceuticals	55289-0005-10
10's	$36.12	GENERIC, Mallinckrodt Medical Inc	00406-0484-62
12's	$2.78	GENERIC, Pd-Rx Pharmaceuticals	55289-0005-12
15's	$2.49	GENERIC, Circle Pharmaceuticals Inc	00659-0416-15
15's	$2.96	GENERIC, Pd-Rx Pharmaceuticals	55289-0005-15
20's	$1.98	GENERIC, Circle Pharmaceuticals Inc	00659-0416-20
20's	$3.90	GENERIC, Pd-Rx Pharmaceuticals	55289-0005-20
24's	$4.32	GENERIC, Pd-Rx Pharmaceuticals	55289-0005-24
25's	$8.25	GENERIC, Pd-Rx Pharmaceuticals	55289-0005-97
30's	$2.97	GENERIC, Circle Pharmaceuticals Inc	00659-0416-30
30's	$4.93	GENERIC, Pd-Rx Pharmaceuticals	55289-0005-30
30's	$7.21	GENERIC, Golden State Medical	60429-0500-30
30's	$10.84	GENERIC, Qualitest Products Inc	00603-2338-16
31 x 10	$56.50	GENERIC, Vangard Labs	00615-0430-63
50's	$18.08	GENERIC, Qualitest Products Inc	00603-2338-19
60's	$21.68	GENERIC, Qualitest Products Inc	00603-2338-20
90's	$32.53	GENERIC, Qualitest Products Inc	00603-2338-02
90's	$60.00	GENERIC, Udl Laboratories Inc	51079-0161-99
100's	$9.38	GENERIC, Century Pharmaceuticals Inc	00436-0182-01
100's	$9.57	GENERIC, Moore, H.L. Drug Exchange Inc	00839-6245-06
100's	$9.75	GENERIC, Interstate Drug Exchange Inc	00814-0248-14
100's	$11.76	GENERIC, Aligen Independent Laboratories Inc	00405-0008-01
100's	$12.60	GENERIC, Ivax Corporation	00182-0948-01
100's	$12.60	GENERIC, Purepac Pharmaceutical Company	00228-2001-10
100's	$14.67	GENERIC, Roxane Laboratories Inc	00054-8022-25
100's	$14.76	GENERIC, Auro Pharmaceutical	55829-0801-10
100's	$16.25	GENERIC, Major Pharmaceuticals Inc	00904-0175-61
100's	$18.24	GENERIC, Ivax Corporation	00182-0948-89
100's	$21.37	FEDERAL UPPER LIMIT, H.C.F.A. F F P	99999-0051-04
100's	$21.41	GENERIC, Vintage Pharmaceuticals Inc	00254-2064-28
100's	$22.13	GENERIC, Roxane Laboratories Inc	00054-8022-24
100's	$22.13	GENERIC, Geneva Pharmaceuticals	00781-1752-13
100's	$25.19	GENERIC, Vangard Labs	00615-0430-29
100's	$26.12	GENERIC, Watson/Rugby Laboratories Inc	52544-0851-01
100's	$28.43	GENERIC, Purepac Pharmaceutical Company	00228-3056-96
100's	$28.43	GENERIC, Major Pharmaceuticals Inc	00904-0175-60
100's	$32.35	GENERIC, Udl Laboratories Inc	51079-0161-20
100's	$33.97	GENERIC, Udl Laboratories Inc	51079-0161-21
100's	$36.10	GENERIC, Purepac Pharmaceutical Company	00228-3020-10
100's	$36.10	GENERIC, Purepac Pharmaceutical Company	00228-3056-11
100's	$36.12	GENERIC, Mallinckrodt Medical Inc	00406-0484-01
100's	$36.14	GENERIC, Teva Pharmaceuticals Usa	00093-0150-01
100's	$36.14	GENERIC, Barr Laboratories Inc	00555-0303-02
100's	$36.14	GENERIC, Qualitest Products Inc	00603-2338-21
100's	$36.14	GENERIC, Mutual/United Research Laboratories	00677-1715-01
100's	$36.14	GENERIC, Duramed Pharmaceuticals Inc	51285-0303-02
100's	$48.75	TYLENOL WITH CODEINE #3, Janssen Pharmaceuticals	00045-0513-60
120's	$43.37	GENERIC, Qualitest Products Inc	00603-2338-22

Tablet - Oral - 300 mg;60 mg

Package	Price	Product, Manufacturer	NDC
100's	$14.72	GENERIC, Warner Chilcott Laboratories	00047-0637-24
100's	$15.75	GENERIC, Interstate Drug Exchange Inc	00814-0250-14
100's	$16.76	GENERIC, Aligen Independent Laboratories Inc	00405-0009-01
100's	$17.39	GENERIC, Vangard Labs	00615-0432-01
100's	$19.10	GENERIC, Purepac Pharmaceutical Company	00228-2003-10
100's	$19.10	GENERIC, Geneva Pharmaceuticals	00781-1654-01
100's	$19.14	GENERIC, Ivax Corporation	00182-1338-01
100's	$19.29	GENERIC, Moore, H.L. Drug Exchange Inc	00839-6499-06
100's	$20.00	GENERIC, Vangard Labs	00615-0432-13
100's	$22.85	GENERIC, Ivax Corporation	00182-1338-89
100's	$26.74	GENERIC, Major Pharmaceuticals Inc	00904-3916-61
100's	$26.96	GENERIC, Auro Pharmaceutical	55829-0802-10
100's	$28.12	FEDERAL UPPER LIMIT, H.C.F.A. F F P	99999-0051-07
100's	$32.48	GENERIC, Vintage Pharmaceuticals Inc	00254-2065-28
100's	$45.93	GENERIC, Mutual/United Research Laboratories	00677-1716-01
100's	$50.92	GENERIC, Major Pharmaceuticals Inc	00904-3916-60
100's	$57.10	GENERIC, Udl Laboratories Inc	51079-0106-20
100's	$59.96	GENERIC, Udl Laboratories Inc	51079-0106-21
100's	$63.80	GENERIC, Purepac Pharmaceutical Company	00228-3021-10
100's	$63.80	GENERIC, Purepac Pharmaceutical Company	00228-3058-11
100's	$63.85	GENERIC, Mallinckrodt Medical Inc	00406-0485-01
100's	$63.87	GENERIC, Teva Pharmaceuticals Usa	00093-0350-01
100's	$63.87	GENERIC, Barr Laboratories Inc	00555-0304-02
100's	$63.87	GENERIC, Duramed Pharmaceuticals Inc	51285-0304-02
100's	$63.87	GENERIC, Watson/Rugby Laboratories Inc	52544-0852-01
100's	$63.88	GENERIC, Qualitest Products Inc	00603-2339-21
100's	$86.15	TYLENOL WITH CODEINE #4, Janssen Pharmaceuticals	00045-0515-60

PRODUCT LISTING - EQUIVALENTS NOT AVAILABLE

Capsule - Oral - 325 mg;30 mg

Package	Price	Product, Manufacturer	NDC
6's	$3.69	PHENAPHEN WITH CODEINE, Southwood Pharmaceuticals Inc	58016-0256-06
60's	$25.81	PHENAPHEN WITH CODEINE, Southwood Pharmaceuticals Inc	58016-0256-60
100's	$47.59	PHENAPHEN WITH CODEINE, Wyeth-Ayerst Laboratories	00031-6257-63

Liquid - Oral - 120 mg;12 mg/5 ml

Package	Price	Product, Manufacturer	NDC
5 ml	$3.48	GENERIC, Prescript Pharmaceuticals	00247-0234-05
10 ml	$3.62	GENERIC, Prescript Pharmaceuticals	00247-0234-10
15 ml	$3.75	GENERIC, Prescript Pharmaceuticals	00247-0234-15
25 ml	$4.02	GENERIC, Prescript Pharmaceuticals	00247-0234-25
30 ml	$4.15	GENERIC, Prescript Pharmaceuticals	00247-0234-30
60 ml	$1.78	GENERIC, Allscripts Pharmaceutical Company	54569-4014-01
60 ml	$4.95	GENERIC, Prescript Pharmaceuticals	00247-0234-60
90 ml	$5.75	GENERIC, Prescript Pharmaceuticals	00247-0234-90
118 ml	$6.49	GENERIC, Prescript Pharmaceuticals	00247-0234-52
120 ml	$3.86	GENERIC, Allscripts Pharmaceutical Company	54569-1001-00
120 ml	$4.60	GENERIC, Physicians Total Care	54868-0378-01
120 ml	$6.54	GENERIC, Prescript Pharmaceuticals	00247-0234-77
120 ml	$6.59	GENERIC, Quality Care Pharmaceuticals Inc	60346-0877-04
120 ml	$7.45	GENERIC, Pharma Pac	52959-1416-03
120 ml	$18.53	GENERIC, Pharma Pac	52959-0141-03
180 ml	$8.14	GENERIC, Prescript Pharmaceuticals	00247-0234-59
200 ml	$8.67	GENERIC, Prescript Pharmaceuticals	00247-0234-79
237 ml	$9.66	GENERIC, Prescript Pharmaceuticals	00247-0234-23
473 ml	$15.94	GENERIC, Prescript Pharmaceuticals	00247-0234-38
480 ml	$10.72	GENERIC, Physicians Total Care	54868-0378-02
480 ml	$12.48	GENERIC, Mikart Inc	46672-0561-16
480 ml	$14.00	GENERIC, Hi-Tech Pharmacal Company Inc	50383-0079-16
480 ml	$14.11	GENERIC, Aligen Independent Laboratories Inc	00405-0012-16
480 ml	$14.21	GENERIC, Allscripts Pharmaceutical Company	54569-4014-00
480 ml	$19.28	GENERIC, Major Pharmaceuticals Inc	00904-7775-16
946 ml	$28.52	GENERIC, Prescript Pharmaceuticals	00247-0234-94

Tablet - Oral - 300 mg;15 mg

Package	Price	Product, Manufacturer	NDC
6's	$3.67	GENERIC, Prescript Pharmaceuticals	00247-0099-06
10's	$3.88	GENERIC, Prescript Pharmaceuticals	00247-0099-10
12's	$0.98	GENERIC, Allscripts Pharmaceutical Company	54569-0311-00
12's	$3.99	GENERIC, Prescript Pharmaceuticals	00247-0099-12
12's	$4.14	GENERIC, Southwood Pharmaceuticals Inc	58016-0269-12
15's	$4.15	GENERIC, Prescript Pharmaceuticals	00247-0099-15
15's	$4.30	GENERIC, Pharma Pac	52959-0208-15
15's	$7.92	GENERIC, Southwood Pharmaceuticals Inc	58016-0269-15
16's	$4.20	GENERIC, Prescript Pharmaceuticals	00247-0099-16
20's	$1.63	GENERIC, Allscripts Pharmaceutical Company	54569-0311-03
20's	$4.41	GENERIC, Prescript Pharmaceuticals	00247-0099-20
20's	$10.60	GENERIC, Southwood Pharmaceuticals Inc	58016-0269-20
24's	$4.62	GENERIC, Prescript Pharmaceuticals	00247-0099-24
24's	$11.50	GENERIC, Southwood Pharmaceuticals Inc	58016-0269-24
30's	$2.44	GENERIC, Allscripts Pharmaceutical Company	54569-0311-02
30's	$4.94	GENERIC, Prescript Pharmaceuticals	00247-0099-30
30's	$15.70	GENERIC, Southwood Pharmaceuticals Inc	58016-0269-30
40's	$3.72	GENERIC, Physicians Total Care	54868-2130-01
50's	$6.00	GENERIC, Prescript Pharmaceuticals	00247-0099-50
100's	$8.65	GENERIC, Prescript Pharmaceuticals	00247-0099-00
100's	$52.33	GENERIC, Southwood Pharmaceuticals Inc	58016-0269-00

Tablet - Oral - 300 mg;30 mg

Package	Price	Product, Manufacturer	NDC
2's	$3.62	GENERIC, Prescript Pharmaceuticals	00247-0078-02
3's	$3.75	GENERIC, Prescript Pharmaceuticals	00247-0078-03
4's	$3.88	GENERIC, Prescript Pharmaceuticals	00247-0078-04
4's	$9.78	GENERIC, Pharma Pac	52959-0003-04
5's	$4.01	GENERIC, Prescript Pharmaceuticals	00247-0078-05
6's	$0.76	GENERIC, Allscripts Pharmaceutical Company	54569-0025-06
6's	$3.58	GENERIC, Southwood Pharmaceuticals Inc	58016-0271-06
6's	$4.15	GENERIC, Prescript Pharmaceuticals	00247-0078-06
6's	$10.21	GENERIC, Pharma Pac	52959-0003-06
8's	$0.86	GENERIC, Allscripts Pharmaceutical Company	54569-2523-03
8's	$4.41	GENERIC, Prescript Pharmaceuticals	00247-0078-08
8's	$4.78	GENERIC, Southwood Pharmaceuticals Inc	58016-0271-08
10's	$1.26	GENERIC, Allscripts Pharmaceutical Company	54569-0025-00
10's	$2.49	GENERIC, Physicians Total Care	54868-0072-09
10's	$4.68	GENERIC, Prescript Pharmaceuticals	00247-0078-10
10's	$5.98	GENERIC, Southwood Pharmaceuticals Inc	58016-0271-10
10's	$10.63	GENERIC, Pharma Pac	52959-0003-10
12's	$1.51	GENERIC, Allscripts Pharmaceutical Company	54569-0025-01
12's	$2.65	GENERIC, Physicians Total Care	54868-0072-00
12's	$4.94	GENERIC, Prescript Pharmaceuticals	00247-0078-12
12's	$7.18	GENERIC, Southwood Pharmaceuticals Inc	58016-0271-12
12's	$11.83	GENERIC, Pharma Pac	52959-0003-12

14's	$8.38	GENERIC, Southwood Pharmaceuticals Inc	58016-0271-14
15's	$1.89	GENERIC, Allscripts Pharmaceutical Company	54569-0025-02
15's	$2.60	GENERIC, Pharmaceutical Corporation Of America	51655-0802-54
15's	$2.89	GENERIC, Physicians Total Care	54868-0072-02
15's	$5.34	GENERIC, Prescript Pharmaceuticals	00247-0078-15
15's	$8.98	GENERIC, Southwood Pharmaceuticals Inc	58016-0271-15
15's	$12.50	GENERIC, Pharma Pac	52959-0003-15
16's	$2.02	GENERIC, Allscripts Pharmaceutical Company	54569-2523-01
16's	$5.47	GENERIC, Prescript Pharmaceuticals	00247-0078-16
16's	$10.34	GENERIC, Southwood Pharmaceuticals Inc	58016-0271-16
16's	$14.03	GENERIC, Pharma Pac	52959-0003-16
18's	$2.27	GENERIC, Allscripts Pharmaceutical Company	54569-2523-02
18's	$10.76	GENERIC, Southwood Pharmaceuticals Inc	58016-0271-18
20's	$2.52	GENERIC, Allscripts Pharmaceutical Company	54569-0025-03
20's	$3.30	GENERIC, Physicians Total Care	54868-0072-03
20's	$6.00	GENERIC, Prescript Pharmaceuticals	00247-0078-20
20's	$11.76	GENERIC, Southwood Pharmaceuticals Inc	58016-0271-20
20's	$17.00	GENERIC, Pharma Pac	52959-0003-20
24's	$3.02	GENERIC, Allscripts Pharmaceutical Company	54569-0025-09
24's	$6.53	GENERIC, Prescript Pharmaceuticals	00247-0078-24
24's	$14.76	GENERIC, Southwood Pharmaceuticals Inc	58016-0271-24
24's	$22.95	GENERIC, Pharma Pac	52959-0003-24
25's	$6.66	GENERIC, Prescript Pharmaceuticals	00247-0078-25
25's	$14.95	GENERIC, Southwood Pharmaceuticals Inc	58016-0271-25
25's	$24.23	GENERIC, Pharma Pac	52959-0003-25
28's	$7.06	GENERIC, Prescript Pharmaceuticals	00247-0078-28
28's	$16.64	GENERIC, Southwood Pharmaceuticals Inc	58016-0271-28
28's	$27.63	GENERIC, Pharma Pac	52959-0003-28
30's	$3.70	GENERIC, Pharmaceutical Corporation Of America	51655-0802-24
30's	$3.78	GENERIC, Allscripts Pharmaceutical Company	54569-0025-04
30's	$4.12	GENERIC, Physicians Total Care	54868-0072-01
30's	$7.33	GENERIC, Prescript Pharmaceuticals	00247-0078-30
30's	$17.94	GENERIC, Southwood Pharmaceuticals Inc	58016-0271-30
30's	$29.16	GENERIC, Pharma Pac	52959-0003-30
36's	$6.40	GENERIC, Allscripts Pharmaceutical Company	54569-0025-08
40's	$4.94	GENERIC, Physicians Total Care	54868-0072-05
40's	$5.04	GENERIC, Allscripts Pharmaceutical Company	54569-2523-00
40's	$23.92	GENERIC, Southwood Pharmaceuticals Inc	58016-0271-40
40's	$32.56	GENERIC, Pharma Pac	52959-0003-40
42's	$25.12	GENERIC, Southwood Pharmaceuticals Inc	58016-0271-42
45's	$9.31	GENERIC, Prescript Pharmaceuticals	00247-0078-45
50's	$5.76	GENERIC, Physicians Total Care	54868-0072-04
50's	$6.30	GENERIC, Allscripts Pharmaceutical Company	54569-0025-05
50's	$9.98	GENERIC, Prescript Pharmaceuticals	00247-0078-50
50's	$29.90	GENERIC, Southwood Pharmaceuticals Inc	58016-0271-50
50's	$36.58	GENERIC, Pharma Pac	52959-0003-50
56's	$33.04	GENERIC, Southwood Pharmaceuticals Inc	58016-0271-56
60's	$6.58	GENERIC, Physicians Total Care	54868-0072-07
60's	$35.88	GENERIC, Southwood Pharmaceuticals Inc	58016-0271-60
60's	$43.76	GENERIC, Pharma Pac	52959-0003-60
90's	$53.82	GENERIC, Southwood Pharmaceuticals Inc	58016-0271-90
100's	$9.85	GENERIC, Physicians Total Care	54868-0072-08
100's	$12.60	GENERIC, Allscripts Pharmaceutical Company	54569-0025-07
100's	$16.59	GENERIC, Prescript Pharmaceuticals	00247-0078-00
100's	$36.14	GENERIC, Ranbaxy Laboratories	63304-0562-01
100's	$41.96	GENERIC, Pharma Pac	52959-0003-00
100's	$59.80	GENERIC, Southwood Pharmaceuticals Inc	58016-0271-00
120's	$71.76	GENERIC, Southwood Pharmaceuticals Inc	58016-0271-02

Tablet - Oral - 300 mg;60 mg

6's	$4.07	GENERIC, Prescript Pharmaceuticals	00247-0085-06
8's	$10.80	GENERIC, Southwood Pharmaceuticals Inc	58016-0272-08
10's	$4.54	GENERIC, Prescript Pharmaceuticals	00247-0085-10
10's	$10.39	GENERIC, Southwood Pharmaceuticals Inc	58016-0272-10
12's	$4.79	GENERIC, Prescript Pharmaceuticals	00247-0085-12
12's	$7.66	GENERIC, Allscripts Pharmaceutical Company	54569-0302-07
12's	$12.46	GENERIC, Southwood Pharmaceuticals Inc	58016-0272-12
15's	$2.87	GENERIC, Allscripts Pharmaceutical Company	54569-0302-06
15's	$3.50	GENERIC, Pharmaceutical Corporation Of America	51655-0816-54
15's	$5.14	GENERIC, Prescript Pharmaceuticals	00247-0085-15
15's	$15.56	GENERIC, Southwood Pharmaceuticals Inc	58016-0272-15
16's	$5.26	GENERIC, Prescript Pharmaceuticals	00247-0085-16
20's	$5.74	GENERIC, Prescript Pharmaceuticals	00247-0085-20
20's	$12.77	GENERIC, Allscripts Pharmaceutical Company	54569-0302-00
20's	$20.40	GENERIC, Southwood Pharmaceuticals Inc	58016-0272-20
20's	$22.50	GENERIC, Pharma Pac	52959-0446-20
24's	$6.21	GENERIC, Prescript Pharmaceuticals	00247-0085-24
24's	$26.52	GENERIC, Pharma Pac	52959-0446-24
28's	$29.09	GENERIC, Southwood Pharmaceuticals Inc	58016-0272-28
30's	$5.45	GENERIC, Pharmaceutical Corporation Of America	51655-0816-24
30's	$6.93	GENERIC, Prescript Pharmaceuticals	00247-0085-30
30's	$19.16	GENERIC, Allscripts Pharmaceutical Company	54569-0302-01
30's	$30.50	GENERIC, Pharma Pac	52959-0446-30
30's	$30.60	GENERIC, Southwood Pharmaceuticals Inc	58016-0272-30
40's	$41.56	GENERIC, Southwood Pharmaceuticals Inc	58016-0272-40
50's	$9.31	GENERIC, Prescript Pharmaceuticals	00247-0085-50
50's	$9.55	GENERIC, Allscripts Pharmaceutical Company	54569-0302-04
50's	$51.96	GENERIC, Southwood Pharmaceuticals Inc	58016-0272-50
60's	$62.34	GENERIC, Southwood Pharmaceuticals Inc	58016-0272-60
60's	$62.50	GENERIC, Pharma Pac	52959-0446-60
100's	$15.27	GENERIC, Prescript Pharmaceuticals	00247-0085-00
100's	$63.87	GENERIC, Allscripts Pharmaceutical Company	54569-0302-03
100's	$96.75	GENERIC, Pharma Pac	52959-0446-00
100's	$103.90	GENERIC, Southwood Pharmaceuticals Inc	58016-0272-00

Tablet - Oral - 650 mg;30 mg

100's	$37.80	EZ III, Stewart-Jackson Pharmaceutical Inc	45985-0625-01

Acetaminophen; Dichloralphenazone; Isometheptene Mucate *(000064)*

Categories: Headache, tension; Headache, vascular; FDA Pre 1938 Drugs

Drug Classes: Adrenergic agonists; Analgesics, non-narcotic; Sedatives/hypnotics

Brand Names: Alidrin; Amidrine; Apap/Isometheptene/Dichlphen; Atarin; Carmid; Drinex; Duradrin; I.D.A.; Iso-Acetazone; Isocom; Isometh/D-Chloralphenaz/Apap; Isopap; Midchlor; **Midrin**; Migain; Migquin; Migraine; Migrapap; Migratine; Migrazone; Migrend; Migrex; Mitride

Foreign Brand Availability: Aperon (Korea); Daccorin (Korea); Migaphen (Korea); Mydran (Korea); Mydrin (Korea)

Cost of Therapy: $20.48 (Headache; Midrin; 325 mg; 100 mg; 65 mg; 6 tablets/day; 7 day supply)
$1.89 (Headache; Generic Tablets; 325 mg; 100 mg; 65 mg; 6 tablets/day; 7 day supply)

DESCRIPTION

Each red Midrin capsule with pink band contains isometheptene mucate 65 mg, dichloralphenazone 100 mg, and acetaminophen 325 mg.

Isometheptene mucate is a white, crystalline powder having a characteristic aromatic odor and bitter taste. It is an unsaturated aliphatic amine with sympathomimetic properties.

Dichloralphenazone is a white, microcrystalline powder, with slight odor and tastes saline at first, becoming acrid. It is a mild sedative.

Acetaminophen, a non-salicylate, occurs as a white, odorless, crystalline powder possessing a slightly bitter taste.

Midrin capsules contain FD&C yellow no. 6 as a color additive.

CLINICAL PHARMACOLOGY

Isometheptene mucate, a sympathomimetic amine, acts by constricting dilated cranial and cerebral arterioles, thus reducing the stimuli that lead to vascular headaches. Dichloralphenazone, a mild sedative, reduces the patient's emotional reaction to the pain of both vascular and tension headaches. Acetaminophen raises the threshold to painful stimuli, thus exerting an analgesic effect against all types of headaches.

INDICATIONS AND USAGE

For relief of tension and vascular headaches.*

***Based on a review of this drug (isometheptene mucate) by the National Academy of Sciences—National Research Council and/or other information, FDA has classified the other indication as "possibly" effective in the treatment of migraine headache. Final classification of the less-than-effective indication requires further investigation.**

CONTRAINDICATIONS

This drug is contraindicated in glaucoma and/or severe cases of renal disease, hypertension, organic heart disease, hepatic disease and in those patients who are on monoamine-oxidase (MAO) inhibitor therapy.

PRECAUTIONS

Caution should be observed in hypertension, peripheral vascular disease and after recent cardiovascular attacks.

ADVERSE REACTIONS

Transient dizziness and skin rash may appear in hypersensitive patients. This can usually be eliminated by reducing the dose.

DOSAGE AND ADMINISTRATION

For Relief of Migraine Headache: The usual adult dosage is 2 capsules at once, followed by 1 capsule every hour until relieved, up to 5 capsules within a 12 hour period.

For Relief of Tension Headache: The usual adult dosage is 1 or 2 capsules every four hours up to 8 capsules a day.

Storage: Store at controlled room temperature 15-30°C (59-86°F) in a dry place.

PRODUCT LISTING - EQUIVALENTS NOT AVAILABLE

Capsule - Oral - 325 mg;100 mg;65 mg

10's	$3.89	GENERIC, Southwood Pharmaceuticals Inc	58016-0288-10
10's	$5.50	GENERIC, Pharmaceutical Corporation Of America	51655-0451-53
10's	$9.31	MIDRIN, Prescript Pharmaceuticals	00247-0145-10
12's	$4.66	GENERIC, Southwood Pharmaceuticals Inc	58016-0288-12
14's	$5.44	GENERIC, Southwood Pharmaceuticals Inc	58016-0322-14

15's	$5.83	GENERIC, Southwood Pharmaceuticals Inc	58016-0288-15
15's	$8.42	MIDRIN, Allscripts Pharmaceutical Company	54569-0343-03
15's	$12.28	MIDRIN, Prescript Pharmaceuticals	00247-0145-15
18's	$6.99	GENERIC, Southwood Pharmaceuticals Inc	58016-0288-18
20's	$7.77	GENERIC, Southwood Pharmaceuticals Inc	58016-0288-20
20's	$7.79	GENERIC, Pd-Rx Pharmaceuticals	55289-0383-20
20's	$7.90	GENERIC, Allscripts Pharmaceutical Company	54569-4665-01
20's	$11.22	MIDRIN, Allscripts Pharmaceutical Company	54569-0343-02
20's	$11.37	GENERIC, Pharma Pac	52959-0447-20
20's	$15.27	MIDRIN, Prescript Pharmaceuticals	00247-0145-20
21's	$8.16	GENERIC, Southwood Pharmaceuticals Inc	58016-0288-21
24's	$9.32	GENERIC, Southwood Pharmaceuticals Inc	58016-0288-24
25's	$9.71	GENERIC, Southwood Pharmaceuticals Inc	58016-0288-25
25's	$18.25	MIDRIN, Prescript Pharmaceuticals	00247-0145-25
28's	$10.88	GENERIC, Southwood Pharmaceuticals Inc	58016-0288-28
28's	$11.51	GENERIC, Pharmaceutical Corporation Of America	51655-0451-29
30's	$6.56	GENERIC, Physicians Total Care	54868-1514-03
30's	$11.85	GENERIC, Allscripts Pharmaceutical Company	54569-4665-02
30's	$14.62	GENERIC, Southwood Pharmaceuticals Inc	58016-0288-30
30's	$15.59	GENERIC, Pharma Pac	52959-0447-30
30's	$16.83	MIDRIN, Allscripts Pharmaceutical Company	54569-0343-00
40's	$15.54	GENERIC, Southwood Pharmaceuticals Inc	58016-0288-40
50's	$8.25	GENERIC, Palisades Pharmaceuticals Inc	51081-0424-05
50's	$9.86	GENERIC, Moore, H.L. Drug Exchange Inc	00839-7561-04
50's	$19.75	GENERIC, Interpharm Inc	53746-0141-50
50's	$19.75	GENERIC, Allscripts Pharmaceutical Company	54569-4665-00
50's	$21.25	GENERIC, Southwood Pharmaceuticals Inc	58016-0288-50
50's	$24.10	GENERIC, Pharma Pac	52959-0447-50
50's	$26.88	GENERIC, Physicians Total Care	54868-1514-04
50's	$28.05	MIDRIN, Carnrick Laboratories Inc	00086-0120-05
50's	$28.05	MIDRIN, Allscripts Pharmaceutical Company	54569-0343-01
50's	$28.05	MIDRIN, Women First Healthcare	64248-0120-05
50's	$28.71	MIDRIN, Physicians Total Care	54868-1435-01
50's	$33.13	MIDRIN, Prescript Pharmaceuticals	00247-0145-50
60's	$10.07	GENERIC, Pd-Rx Pharmaceuticals	55289-0383-60
60's	$11.94	GENERIC, Physicians Total Care	54868-1514-01
60's	$23.31	GENERIC, Southwood Pharmaceuticals Inc	58016-0288-60
90's	$13.40	GENERIC, Pd-Rx Pharmaceuticals	55289-0383-90
100's	$16.00	GENERIC, Palisades Pharmaceuticals Inc	51081-0424-10
100's	$16.75	GENERIC, Breckenridge Inc	51991-0395-01
100's	$16.81	GENERIC, Moore, H.L. Drug Exchange Inc	00839-7561-06
100's	$16.95	GENERIC, Pecos Pharmaceutical	59879-0106-01
100's	$17.02	GENERIC, Physicians Total Care	54868-1514-00
100's	$17.95	GENERIC, Mikart Inc	46672-0253-10
100's	$19.00	GENERIC, Major Pharmaceuticals Inc	00904-1588-60
100's	$19.43	GENERIC, Interstate Drug Exchange Inc	00814-4860-14
100's	$19.71	GENERIC, Vintage Pharmaceuticals Inc	00254-4270-28
100's	$20.85	GENERIC, Aligen Independent Laboratories Inc	00405-4039-01
100's	$22.68	GENERIC, Pd-Rx Pharmaceuticals	55289-0355-17
100's	$26.81	GENERIC, Par Pharmaceutical Inc	49884-0812-01
100's	$38.46	GENERIC, Ivax Corporation	00182-1234-01
100's	$38.85	GENERIC, Southwood Pharmaceuticals Inc	58016-0288-00
100's	$39.55	GENERIC, Major Pharmaceuticals Inc	00904-5491-60
100's	$39.55	GENERIC, Major Pharmaceuticals Inc	00904-7622-60
100's	$40.00	GENERIC, Interpharm Inc	53746-0141-01
100's	$40.75	GENERIC, Mutual/United Research Laboratories	00677-1125-01
100's	$42.90	GENERIC, Barr Laboratories Inc	00555-0364-02
100's	$42.90	GENERIC, Qualitest Products Inc	00603-4664-21
100's	$42.90	GENERIC, Duramed Pharmaceuticals Inc	51285-0364-02
100's	$43.85	GENERIC, Amide Pharmaceutical Inc	52152-0039-02
100's	$43.87	GENERIC, Mutual/United Research Laboratories	00677-1739-01
100's	$48.75	MIDRIN, Carnrick Laboratories Inc	00086-0120-10
100's	$53.63	MIDRIN, Women First Healthcare	64248-0120-10
100's	$55.65	MIDRIN, Physicians Total Care	54868-1435-02
100's	$62.92	MIDRIN, Prescript Pharmaceuticals	00247-0145-00
250's	$30.70	GENERIC, Palisades Pharmaceuticals Inc	51081-0424-25
250's	$31.75	GENERIC, Mikart Inc	46672-0253-25
250's	$37.75	GENERIC, Vintage Pharmaceuticals Inc	00254-4270-33
250's	$42.00	GENERIC, Moore, H.L. Drug Exchange Inc	00839-7561-09
250's	$46.45	GENERIC, Major Pharmaceuticals Inc	00904-1588-70
250's	$46.45	GENERIC, Major Pharmaceuticals Inc	00904-7622-70
250's	$48.95	GENERIC, Par Pharmaceutical Inc	49884-0812-04
250's	$65.14	GENERIC, Breckenridge Inc	51991-0395-02
250's	$75.95	GENERIC, Amide Pharmaceutical Inc	52152-0039-03
250's	$78.75	GENERIC, Interpharm Inc	53746-0141-02
250's	$79.15	GENERIC, Major Pharmaceuticals Inc	00904-5491-70
250's	$79.99	GENERIC, Mutual/United Research Laboratories	00677-1125-03
250's	$94.75	MIDRIN, Carnrick Laboratories Inc	00086-0120-25
250's	$104.03	GENERIC, Qualitest Products Inc	00603-4664-24

Acetaminophen; Hydrocodone Bitartrate *(000070)*

A

Categories: Pain, moderate to severe; Pregnancy Category C; DEA Class CIII; FDA Approved 1982 May
Drug Classes: Analgesics, narcotic
Brand Names: Allay; Anexsia; **Bancap-HC**; Co-Gesic; Dolacet; Dolagesic; Hy-Phen; Hyco-Pap; Hycomed; Hydrocet; Hydrogesic; Lorcet; Lorcet 10/650; Lortab; Margesic; Norco; Polygesic; Stagesic; Vanacet; Vicodin; Vicodin ES; Zydone
Foreign Brand Availability: Sinalgen (Colombia)
Cost of Therapy: $20.97 (Pain; Vicodin; 500 mg; 5 mg; 6 tablets/day; 7 day supply)
$2.06 (Pain; Generic Tablets; 500 mg; 5 mg; 6 tablets/day; 7 day supply)

DESCRIPTION

Hydrocodone bitartrate is an opioid analgesic and antitussive that occurs as fine white crystals or as a crystalline powder. It is affected by light. The chemical name is: 4,5α-Epoxy-3-methoxy-17-methylmorphinan-6-one tartrate (1:1) hydrate (2:5).

Acetaminophen, 4′-hydroxyacetanilide, is a nonopiate, nonsalicylate analgesic, and antipyretic that occurs as a white, odorless crystalline powder possessing a slightly bitter taste.
Storage: Store at controlled room temperature 15-30°C (59-86°F).
Dispense in a tight, light-resistant container with a child-resistant closure.

CLINICAL PHARMACOLOGY

MECHANISM OF ACTION

Hydrocodone is a semisynthetic opioid analgesic and antitussive with multiple actions qualitatively similar to those of codeine. Most of these involve the central nervous system and smooth muscle. The precise mechanism of action of hydrocodone and other opiates is not known, although it is believed to relate to the existence of opiate receptors in the central nervous system. In addition to analgesia, opioids may produce drowsiness, changes in mood, and mental clouding.

Radioimmunoassay techniques have recently been developed for the analysis of hydrocodone in human plasma. After a 10 mg oral dose of hydrocodone bitartrate, a mean peak serum drug level of 23.6 ng/ml and an elimination half-life of 3.8 hours were found.

The analgesic action of acetaminophen involves peripheral influences, but the specific mechanism is as yet undetermined. Antipyretic activity is mediated through hypothalamic heat-regulating centers. Acetaminophen inhibits prostaglandin synthetase. Therapeutic doses of acetaminophen have negligible effects on the cardiovascular or respiratory systems; however, toxic doses may cause circulatory failure and rapid, shallow breathing.

PHARMACOKINETICS

The behavior of the individual components is described below.

Acetaminophen

Acetaminophen is rapidly absorbed from the gastrointestinal tract and is distributed throughout most body tissues. The plasma half-life is 1.25-3 hours but may be increased by liver damage and following overdosage. Elimination of acetaminophen is principally by liver metabolism (conjugation) and subsequent renal excretion of metabolites. Approximately 85% of an oral dose appears in the urine within 24 hours of administration, mostly as the glucuronide conjugate with small amounts of other conjugates and unchanged drug.

Hydrocodone

Following a 10 mg oral dose of hydrocodone administered to 5 adult male subjects, the mean peak concentration was 23.6 ± 5.2 ng/ml. Maximum serum levels were achieved at 1.3 ± 0.3 hours and the half-life was determined to be 3.8 ± 0.3 hours. Hydrocodone exhibits a complex pattern of metabolism including O-demethylation, N-demethylation, and 6-keto reduction to the corresponding 6-α- and 6-β-hydroxymetabolites.

INDICATIONS AND USAGE

Acetaminophen; hydrocodone bitartrate is indicated for the relief of moderate to moderately-severe pain.

CONTRAINDICATIONS

Acetaminophen; hydrocodone bitartrate tablets should not be administered to patients who have previously exhibited hypersensitivity to acetaminophen or hydrocodone.

WARNINGS

RESPIRATORY DEPRESSION

At high doses, or in sensitive patients, hydrocodone may produce dose-related respiratory depression by acting directly on the brain stem respiratory center. Hydrocodone also affects the center that controls respiratory rhythm and may produce irregular and periodic breathing.

HEAD INJURY AND INCREASED INTRACRANIAL PRESSURE

The respiratory depressant effects of opioids and their capacity to elevate cerebrospinal fluid pressure may be markedly exaggerated in the presence of head injury, other intracranial lesions, or a preexisting increase in intracranial pressure. Furthermore, opioids produce adverse reactions which may obscure the clinical course of patients with head injuries.

ACUTE ABDOMINAL CONDITIONS

The administration of opioids may obscure the diagnosis or clinical course of patients with acute abdominal conditions.

PRECAUTIONS

SPECIAL RISK PATIENTS

As with any opioid analgesic agent, acetaminophen; hydrocodone bitartrate tablets should be used with caution in elderly or debilitated patients and in those with severe impairment of hepatic or renal function, hypothyroidism, Addison's disease, prostatic hypertrophy, or

A

urethral stricture. The usual precautions should be observed and the possibility of respiratory depression should be kept in mind.

COUGH REFLEX

Hydrocodone suppresses the cough reflex. As with all opioids, caution should be exercised when acetaminophen; hydrocodone bitartrate tablets are used postoperatively and in patients with pulmonary disease.

INFORMATION FOR THE PATIENT

Hydrocodone, like all opioids, may impair the mental and/or physical abilities required for the performance of potentially hazardous tasks, such as driving a car or operating machinery. Patients should be cautioned accordingly.

Alcohol and other CNS depressants may produce an additive CNS depression when taken with this combination product and should be avoided.

Hydrocodone may be habit forming. Patients should take the drug only for as long as it is prescribed, in the amounts prescribed, and no more frequently than prescribed.

LABORATORY TESTS

In patients with severe hepatic or renal disease, effects of therapy should be monitored with serial liver and/or renal function tests.

DRUG/LABORATORY TEST INTERACTIONS

Acetaminophen may produce false-positive test results for urinary 5-hydroxyindoleacetic acid.

CARCINOGENESIS, MUTAGENESIS, AND IMPAIRMENT OF FERTILITY

No adequate studies have been conducted in animals to determine whether acetaminophen or hydrocodone have a potential for carcinogenesis, mutagenesis, or impairment of fertility.

PREGNANCY CATEGORY C

Teratogenic Effects

Hydrocodone has been shown to be teratogenic in hamsters when given in doses 700 times the human dose. There are no adequate and well-controlled studies in pregnant women. Acetaminophen; hydrocodone bitartrate tablets should be used during pregnancy only if the potential benefit justifies the potential risk to the fetus.

Nonteratogenic Effects

Babies born to mothers who have been taking opioids regularly prior to delivery will be physically dependent. The withdrawal signs include irritability and excessive crying, tremors, hyperactive reflexes, increased respiratory rate, increased stools, sneezing, yawning, vomiting, and fever. The intensity of the syndrome does not always correlate with the duration of maternal opioid use or dose. There is no consensus on the best method of managing withdrawal. Chlorpromazine 0.7-1 mg/kg every 6 hours, and paregoric 2-4 drops/kg every 4 hours, have been used to treat withdrawal symptoms in infants. The duration of therapy is 4-28 days, with the dosage decreased as tolerated.

LABOR AND DELIVERY

As with all opioids, administration of acetaminophen; hydrocodone bitartrate tablets to the mother shortly before delivery may result in some degree of respiratory depression in the newborn, especially if higher doses are used.

NURSING MOTHERS

Acetaminophen is excreted in breast milk in small amounts, but the significance of its effects on nursing infants is not known. It is not known whether hydrocodone is excreted in human milk. Because many drugs are excreted in human milk and because of the potential for serious adverse reactions in nursing infants from acetaminophen and hydrocodone bitartrate tablets, a decision should be made whether to discontinue nursing or to discontinue the drug, taking into account the importance of the drug to the mother.

PEDIATRIC USE

Safety and effectiveness in children have not been established.

DRUG INTERACTIONS

Patients receiving opioids, antihistamines, antipsychotics, antianxiety agents, or other CNS depressants (including alcohol) concomitantly with acetaminophen; hydrocodone bitartrate tablets may exhibit an additive CNS depression. When combined therapy is contemplated, the dose of one or both agents should be reduced.

The use of MAO inhibitors or tricyclic antidepressants with hydrocodone preparations may increase the effect of either the antidepressant or hydrocodone.

The concurrent use of anticholinergics with hydrocodone may produce paralytic ileus.

ADVERSE REACTIONS

The most frequently reported adverse reactions include lightheadedness, dizziness, sedation, nausea, and vomiting. These effects seem to be more prominent in ambulatory than in nonambulatory patients, and some of these adverse reactions may be alleviated if the patient lies down.

Other Adverse Reactions Include:

Central Nervous System: Drowsiness, mental clouding, lethargy, impairment of mental and physical performance, anxiety, fear, dysphoria, psychic dependence, and mood changes.

Gastrointestinal System: The antiemetic phenothiazines are useful in suppression of the nausea and vomiting which may occur; however, some phenothiazine derivatives seem to be antianalgesic and increase the amount of opioid required to produce pain relief, while other phenothiazines reduce the amount of opioid required to produce a given level of analgesia. Prolonged administration of acetaminophen; hydrocodone bitartrate may produce constipation.

Genitourinary System: Ureteral spasm, spasm of vesical sphincters, and urinary retention have been reported with opiates.

Respiratory Depression: Hydrocodone bitartrate may produce dose-related respiratory depression by acting directly on the brain stem respiratory center. Hydrocodone also affects the center that controls respiratory rhythm and may produce irregular and periodic breathing.

If significant respiratory depression occurs, it may be antagonized by the use of naloxone hydrochloride. Apply other supportive measures when indicated.

Dermatological: Skin rash, pruritus.

The following adverse drug events may be borne in mind as potential effects of acetaminophen:

Allergic reactions
Rash
Thrombocytopenia
Agranulocytosis

DOSAGE AND ADMINISTRATION

Dosage should be adjusted according to the severity of pain and the response of the patient. However, it should be kept in mind that tolerance to hydrocodone can develop with continued use and that the incidence of untoward effects is dose-related.

325 mg/5 mg Tablets: The usual adult dosage is 1-2 tablets every 4-6 hours as needed for pain. The total daily dose should not exceed 8 tablets.

325 mg/7.5 mg Tablets: The usual adult dosage is 1 tablet every 4-6 hours as needed for pain. The total daily dose should not exceed 6 tablets.

325 mg/10 mg Tablets: The usual adult dosage is 1 tablet every 4-6 hours as needed for pain. The total daily dose should not exceed 6 tablets.

400 mg/5 mg Tablets: The usual adult dosage is 1-2 tablets every 4-6 hours as needed for pain. The total daily dose should not exceed 8 tablets.

400 mg/7.5 mg Tablets: The usual adult dosage is 1 tablet every 4-6 hours as needed for pain. The total daily dose should not exceed 6 tablets.

400 mg/10 mg Tablets: The usual adult dosage is 1 tablet every 4-6 hours as needed for pain. The total daily dose should not exceed 6 tablets.

500 mg/2.5 mg Tablets: The usual adult dosage is 1-2 tablets every 4-6 hours as needed for pain. The total daily dose should not exceed 8 tablets.

500 mg/5 mg Capsules or Tablets: The usual adult dosage is 1-2 tablets every 4-6 hours as needed for pain. The total daily dose should not exceed 8 capsules or tablets.

500 mg/7.5 mg Tablets: The usual adult dosage is 1 tablet every 4-6 hr as needed for pain. The total daily dose should not exceed 6 tablets.

500 mg/10 mg Tablets: The usual adult dosage is 1 tablet every 4-6 hr as needed for pain. The total daily dose should not exceed 6 tablets.

650 mg/7.5 mg Tablets: The usual adult dosage is 1 tablet every 4-6 hr as needed for pain. The total daily dose should not exceed 6 tablets.

650 mg/10 mg Tablets: The usual adult dosage is 1 tablet every 4-6 hr as needed for pain. The total daily dose should not exceed 6 tablets.

660 mg/10 mg Tablets: The usual adult dosage is 1 tablet every 4-6 hr as needed for pain. The total daily dose should not exceed 6 tablets

750 mg/7.5 mg Tablets: The usual adult dosage is 1 tablet every 4-6 hr as needed for pain. The total daily dose should not exceed 5 tablets.

750 mg/10 mg Tablets: The usual adult dosage is 1 tablet every 4-6 hr as needed for pain. The total daily dose should not exceed 5 tablets.

500 mg/5 mg/15 ml Elixir: The usual adult dosage is 15 ml every 4-6 hours as needed for pain. The total daily dose should not exceed 90 ml.

500 mg/7.5 mg/15 ml Elixir: The usual adult dosage is 15 ml every 4-6 hours as needed for pain. The total daily dose should not exceed 90 ml.

PRODUCT LISTING - RATED THERAPEUTICALLY EQUIVALENT

Capsule - Oral - 500 mg;5 mg

100's	$19.43	FEDERAL UPPER LIMIT, H.C.F.A. F F P	99999-0070-01
100's	$22.61	GENERIC, Mallinckrodt Medical Inc	00406-4357-01
100's	$23.95	GENERIC, Major Pharmaceuticals Inc	00904-3442-60
100's	$25.15	GENERIC, Baker Norton Pharmaceuticals	50732-0786-01
100's	$26.05	GENERIC, Alphagen Laboratories Inc	59743-0011-01
100's	$26.95	GENERIC, Blansett Pharmacal Company Inc	51674-0010-01
100's	$32.22	GENERIC, Marnel Pharmaceuticals Inc	00682-0808-01
100's	$34.14	GENERIC, Roberts Pharmaceutical Corporation	59441-0138-01
100's	$34.64	GENERIC, Carnrick Laboratories Inc	00086-0057-10
100's	$39.05	GENERIC, Ivax Corporation	00182-0156-01
100's	$42.22	GENERIC, Baker Norton Pharmaceuticals	50732-0128-01
100's	$45.50	ZYDONE, Dupont Pharmaceuticals	00056-0091-70
100's	$46.03	GENERIC, Forest Pharmaceuticals	00785-1120-01
100's	$112.22	GENERIC, Forest Pharmaceuticals	00456-0601-01

Elixir - Oral - 500 mg/15 ml;7.5 mg/15 ml

473 ml	$47.96	FEDERAL UPPER LIMIT, H.C.F.A. F F P	99999-0070-22

Elixir - Oral - 500 mg;5 mg/15 ml

480 ml	$58.12	GENERIC, Mallinckrodt Medical Inc	00406-0375-16

Elixir - Oral - 500 mg;7.5 mg/15 ml

15 ml x 40	$124.00	GENERIC, Pharmaceutical Assoc Inc Div Beach Products	00121-0655-15
118 ml	$17.78	GENERIC, Pharmaceutical Assoc Inc Div Beach Products	00121-0655-04
480 ml	$56.79	GENERIC, Cypress Pharmaceutical Inc	60258-0720-16
480 ml	$58.24	GENERIC, Pharmaceutical Assoc Inc Div Beach Products	00121-0655-16
480 ml	$61.85	GENERIC, Ethex Corporation	58177-0909-07

Tablet - Oral - 325 mg;5 mg

9's	$5.85	NORCO, Southwood Pharmaceuticals Inc	58016-0662-09
10's	$6.50	NORCO, Southwood Pharmaceuticals Inc	58016-0662-10
14's	$9.10	NORCO, Southwood Pharmaceuticals Inc	58016-0662-14
15's	$9.75	NORCO, Southwood Pharmaceuticals Inc	58016-0662-15
16's	$10.40	NORCO, Southwood Pharmaceuticals Inc	58016-0662-16

Qty	Price	Product, Manufacturer	NDC
18's	$11.70	NORCO, Southwood Pharmaceuticals Inc	58016-0662-18
20's	$13.00	NORCO, Southwood Pharmaceuticals Inc	58016-0662-20
21's	$13.65	NORCO, Southwood Pharmaceuticals Inc	58016-0662-21
24's	$15.60	NORCO, Southwood Pharmaceuticals Inc	58016-0662-24
25's	$16.25	NORCO, Southwood Pharmaceuticals Inc	58016-0662-25
28's	$18.20	NORCO, Southwood Pharmaceuticals Inc	58016-0662-28
30's	$19.50	NORCO, Southwood Pharmaceuticals Inc	58016-0662-30
40's	$26.00	NORCO, Southwood Pharmaceuticals Inc	58016-0662-40
42's	$27.30	NORCO, Southwood Pharmaceuticals Inc	58016-0662-42
45's	$29.25	NORCO, Southwood Pharmaceuticals Inc	58016-0662-45
50's	$32.50	NORCO, Southwood Pharmaceuticals Inc	58016-0662-50
56's	$36.40	NORCO, Southwood Pharmaceuticals Inc	58016-0662-56
60's	$39.00	NORCO, Southwood Pharmaceuticals Inc	58016-0662-60
75's	$48.75	NORCO, Southwood Pharmaceuticals Inc	58016-0662-75
80's	$52.00	NORCO, Southwood Pharmaceuticals Inc	58016-0662-80
84's	$54.60	NORCO, Southwood Pharmaceuticals Inc	58016-0662-84
90's	$58.50	NORCO, Southwood Pharmaceuticals Inc	58016-0662-90
100's	$54.22	GENERIC, Able Laboratories Inc	53265-0345-10
100's	$65.00	NORCO, Southwood Pharmaceuticals Inc	58016-0662-00
100's	$66.88	NORCO, Watson Laboratories Inc	52544-0913-48
100's	$68.25	NORCO, Watson Laboratories Inc	52544-0913-01
112's	$72.80	NORCO, Southwood Pharmaceuticals Inc	58016-0662-92
120's	$78.00	NORCO, Southwood Pharmaceuticals Inc	58016-0662-02
180's	$117.00	NORCO, Southwood Pharmaceuticals Inc	58016-0662-99
240's	$156.00	NORCO, Southwood Pharmaceuticals Inc	58016-0662-04

Tablet - Oral - 325 mg;7.5 mg

Qty	Price	Product, Manufacturer	NDC
6's	$4.48	NORCO, Southwood Pharmaceuticals Inc	58016-0632-06
9's	$6.71	NORCO, Southwood Pharmaceuticals Inc	58016-0632-09
10's	$7.46	NORCO, Southwood Pharmaceuticals Inc	58016-0632-10
12's	$8.95	NORCO, Southwood Pharmaceuticals Inc	58016-0632-12
14's	$10.44	NORCO, Southwood Pharmaceuticals Inc	58016-0632-14
15's	$11.19	NORCO, Southwood Pharmaceuticals Inc	58016-0632-15
16's	$11.94	NORCO, Southwood Pharmaceuticals Inc	58016-0632-16
18's	$13.43	NORCO, Southwood Pharmaceuticals Inc	58016-0632-18
20's	$14.92	NORCO, Southwood Pharmaceuticals Inc	58016-0632-20
21's	$15.67	NORCO, Southwood Pharmaceuticals Inc	58016-0632-21
24's	$17.90	NORCO, Southwood Pharmaceuticals Inc	58016-0632-24
25's	$18.65	NORCO, Southwood Pharmaceuticals Inc	58016-0632-25
28's	$20.89	NORCO, Southwood Pharmaceuticals Inc	58016-0632-28
30's	$22.38	NORCO, Southwood Pharmaceuticals Inc	58016-0632-30
40's	$29.84	NORCO, Southwood Pharmaceuticals Inc	58016-0632-40
42's	$31.33	NORCO, Southwood Pharmaceuticals Inc	58016-0632-42
45's	$33.57	NORCO, Southwood Pharmaceuticals Inc	58016-0632-45
50's	$37.30	NORCO, Southwood Pharmaceuticals Inc	58016-0632-50
56's	$41.78	NORCO, Southwood Pharmaceuticals Inc	58016-0632-56
60's	$44.76	NORCO, Southwood Pharmaceuticals Inc	58016-0632-60
75's	$55.95	NORCO, Southwood Pharmaceuticals Inc	58016-0632-75
80's	$59.68	NORCO, Southwood Pharmaceuticals Inc	58016-0632-80
84's	$62.66	NORCO, Southwood Pharmaceuticals Inc	58016-0632-84
90's	$67.14	NORCO, Southwood Pharmaceuticals Inc	58016-0632-90
100's	$61.87	GENERIC, Able Laboratories Inc	53265-0335-10
100's	$74.60	NORCO, Southwood Pharmaceuticals Inc	58016-0632-00
100's	$78.33	NORCO, Watson Laboratories Inc	52544-0729-01
112's	$83.55	NORCO, Southwood Pharmaceuticals Inc	58016-0632-92
120's	$89.52	NORCO, Southwood Pharmaceuticals Inc	58016-0632-02
180's	$134.28	NORCO, Southwood Pharmaceuticals Inc	58016-0632-99

Tablet - Oral - 325 mg;10 mg

Qty	Price	Product, Manufacturer	NDC
100's	$69.89	GENERIC, Watson Laboratories Inc	00591-0853-01
100's	$69.89	GENERIC, Watson Laboratories Inc	52544-0853-01
100's	$69.89	GENERIC, Able Laboratories Inc	53265-0328-10
100's	$69.90	GENERIC, Vintage Pharmaceuticals Inc	00254-3601-28
100's	$69.90	GENERIC, Qualitest Products Inc	00603-3887-21
100's	$70.25	GENERIC, Mallinckrodt Medical Inc	00406-0367-01
100's	$104.62	NORCO, Watson Laboratories Inc	52544-0539-01
100's	$110.00	GENERIC, Mallinckrodt Medical Inc	00406-0367-62

Tablet - Oral - 400 mg;5 mg

Qty	Price	Product, Manufacturer	NDC
100's	$56.94	ZYDONE, Endo Laboratories Llc	63481-0668-70

Tablet - Oral - 400 mg;7.5 mg

Qty	Price	Product, Manufacturer	NDC
100's	$62.81	ZYDONE, Endo Laboratories Llc	63481-0669-70

Tablet - Oral - 400 mg;10 mg

Qty	Price	Product, Manufacturer	NDC
100's	$76.50	ZYDONE, Endo Laboratories Llc	63481-0698-70

Tablet - Oral - 500 mg;2.5 mg

Qty	Price	Product, Manufacturer	NDC
100's	$29.95	GENERIC, Major Pharmaceuticals Inc	00904-7630-60
100's	$30.30	GENERIC, Qualitest Products Inc	00603-3880-21
100's	$33.35	GENERIC, Watson Laboratories Inc	00591-0388-01
100's	$33.35	GENERIC, Watson Laboratories Inc	52544-0388-01
100's	$37.08	GENERIC, Royce Laboratories Inc	51875-0386-01
100's	$41.32	GENERIC, Barr Laboratories Inc	00555-0896-02
100's	$85.13	LORTAB, Ucb Pharma Inc	50474-0925-01

Tablet - Oral - 500 mg;5 mg

Qty	Price	Product, Manufacturer	NDC
6's	$13.50	GENERIC, Pd-Rx Pharmaceuticals	55289-0137-06
10's	$13.69	GENERIC, Pd-Rx Pharmaceuticals	55289-0137-10
12's	$13.90	GENERIC, Pd-Rx Pharmaceuticals	55289-0137-12
15's	$14.52	GENERIC, Pd-Rx Pharmaceuticals	55289-0137-15
20's	$5.33	ANEXSIA, Allscripts Pharmaceutical Company	54569-0008-00
20's	$15.38	GENERIC, Pd-Rx Pharmaceuticals	55289-0137-20
24's	$15.83	GENERIC, Pd-Rx Pharmaceuticals	55289-0137-24
25's	$7.86	GENERIC, Pd-Rx Pharmaceuticals	55289-0137-97
30's	$8.00	ANEXSIA, Allscripts Pharmaceutical Company	54569-0008-01
30's	$13.50	GENERIC, Qualitest Products Inc	00603-3881-16
30's	$17.24	GENERIC, Pd-Rx Pharmaceuticals	55289-0137-30
31 x 10	$120.90	GENERIC, Vangard Labs	00615-0400-63
40's	$19.10	GENERIC, Pd-Rx Pharmaceuticals	55289-0137-40
50's	$22.50	GENERIC, Qualitest Products Inc	00603-3881-19
60's	$26.99	GENERIC, Qualitest Products Inc	00603-3881-20
90's	$40.49	GENERIC, Qualitest Products Inc	00603-3881-02
100's	$10.43	GENERIC, Interstate Drug Exchange Inc	00814-0255-14
100's	$11.53	FEDERAL UPPER LIMIT, H.C.F.A. F F P	99999-0070-03
100's	$16.29	GENERIC, Mallinckrodt Medical Inc	00406-0357-63
100's	$16.65	GENERIC, Mikart Inc	46672-0052-10
100's	$17.10	GENERIC, Dey Laboratories	49502-0415-01
100's	$19.50	GENERIC, Creighton Products Corporation	50752-0290-05
100's	$20.50	GENERIC, Vita-Rx Corporation	49727-0957-02
100's	$21.21	GENERIC, Aligen Independent Laboratories Inc	00405-0015-01
100's	$22.75	GENERIC, Ivax Corporation	00182-1765-01
100's	$22.75	GENERIC, Inwood Laboratories Inc	00258-3666-01
100's	$22.75	GENERIC, Moore, H.L. Drug Exchange Inc	00839-7176-06
100's	$22.89	GENERIC, Auro Pharmaceutical	55829-0849-10
100's	$23.88	GENERIC, Mason Pharmaceuticals Inc	12758-0067-01
100's	$25.15	GENERIC, Baker Norton Pharmaceuticals	50732-0785-01
100's	$25.95	GENERIC, Martec Pharmaceuticals Inc	52555-0076-01
100's	$27.45	GENERIC, Ecr Pharmaceuticals	00095-0141-01
100's	$27.54	GENERIC, Ascher, B.F. and Company Inc	00225-0450-15
100's	$28.06	GENERIC, Warner Chilcott Laboratories	00047-0448-24
100's	$31.75	GENERIC, Mallinckrodt Medical Inc	00406-0357-01
100's	$34.09	ANEXSIA, Monarch Pharmaceuticals Inc	61570-0001-01
100's	$36.13	GENERIC, Caremark Inc	00339-4049-12
100's	$39.21	GENERIC, American Health Packaging	62584-0738-01
100's	$39.24	GENERIC, Ivax Corporation	00172-5643-60
100's	$39.94	GENERIC, Barr Laboratories Inc	00555-0915-02
100's	$39.95	GENERIC, Gm Pharmaceuticals	58809-0838-01
100's	$41.55	GENERIC, Watson/Rugby Laboratories Inc	00536-5911-01
100's	$43.00	GENERIC, Schwarz Pharma	00131-2104-37
100's	$43.75	GENERIC, Mallinckrodt Medical Inc	00406-0357-62
100's	$43.96	GENERIC, Major Pharmaceuticals Inc	00904-3440-60
100's	$44.87	LORTAB 5/500, Ucb Pharma Inc	50474-0902-60
100's	$44.99	GENERIC, Vintage Pharmaceuticals Inc	00254-3592-28
100's	$44.99	GENERIC, Qualitest Products Inc	00603-3881-21
100's	$45.65	GENERIC, Par Pharmaceutical Inc	49884-0810-01
100's	$48.84	GENERIC, Major Pharmaceuticals Inc	00904-3440-61
100's	$50.65	GENERIC, Watson Laboratories Inc	00591-0349-01
100's	$50.65	GENERIC, Watson Laboratories Inc	52544-0349-01
100's	$59.00	VICODIN, Knoll Pharmaceutical Company	00044-0727-02
100's	$59.00	VICODIN, Abbott Pharmaceutical	00074-1949-14
100's	$70.19	VICODIN, Knoll Pharmaceutical Company	00044-0727-41
100's	$70.19	VICODIN, Abbott Pharmaceutical	00074-1949-12
100's	$85.13	LORTAB 5/500, Ucb Pharma Inc	50474-0902-01
120's	$53.99	GENERIC, Qualitest Products Inc	00603-3881-22

Tablet - Oral - 500 mg;7.5 mg

Qty	Price	Product, Manufacturer	NDC
30's	$9.60	GENERIC, Medirex Inc	57480-0518-06
100's	$19.13	FEDERAL UPPER LIMIT, H.C.F.A. F F P	99999-0070-07
100's	$32.00	GENERIC, Medirex Inc	57480-0518-01
100's	$33.80	GENERIC, Vintage Pharmaceuticals Inc	00254-3594-28
100's	$37.75	GENERIC, Creighton Products Corporation	50752-0291-05
100's	$39.29	GENERIC, Moore, H.L. Drug Exchange Inc	00839-7781-06
100's	$39.75	GENERIC, Major Pharmaceuticals Inc	00904-7631-60
100's	$40.55	GENERIC, Aligen Independent Laboratories Inc	00405-0016-01
100's	$42.84	GENERIC, Mallinckrodt Medical Inc	00406-0358-01
100's	$43.05	GENERIC, Martec Pharmaceuticals Inc	52555-0652-01
100's	$44.10	GENERIC, Ivax Corporation	00182-0691-01
100's	$45.77	GENERIC, Barr Laboratories Inc	00555-0897-02
100's	$50.50	GENERIC, Mallinckrodt Medical Inc	00406-0358-62
100's	$57.21	GENERIC, Watson Laboratories Inc	00591-0385-01
100's	$57.21	GENERIC, Qualitest Products Inc	00603-3882-21
100's	$57.21	GENERIC, Watson Laboratories Inc	52544-0385-01
100's	$94.28	LORTAB 7.5/500, Ucb Pharma Inc	50474-0907-01
100's	$94.28	LORTAB 7.5/500, Ucb Pharma Inc	50474-0907-60

Tablet - Oral - 500 mg;10 mg

Qty	Price	Product, Manufacturer	NDC
100's	$46.03	FEDERAL UPPER LIMIT, H.C.F.A. F F P	99999-0070-16
100's	$53.27	GENERIC, Mallinckrodt Medical Inc	00406-0363-01
100's	$53.27	GENERIC, Watson Laboratories Inc	00591-0540-01
100's	$53.27	GENERIC, Watson Laboratories Inc	52544-0540-01
100's	$53.75	GENERIC, Mallinckrodt Medical Inc	00406-0363-62
100's	$63.98	ACETAMINOPHEN-HYDROCODONE BITARTRATE, Barr Laboratories Inc	00555-0919-02
100's	$98.85	LORTAB 10, Ucb Pharma Inc	50474-0910-01
100's	$98.85	LORTAB 10, Ucb Pharma Inc	50474-0910-60
100's	$253.03	GENERIC, Watson/Rugby Laboratories Inc	52544-0540-05

Tablet - Oral - 650 mg;7.5 mg

Qty	Price	Product, Manufacturer	NDC
30's	$16.00	ANEXSIA, Pharma Pac	52959-0364-30
40's	$14.96	ANEXSIA, Allscripts Pharmaceutical Company	54569-2292-02
100's	$15.50	FEDERAL UPPER LIMIT, H.C.F.A. F F P	99999-0070-13
100's	$34.25	GENERIC, Vintage Pharmaceuticals Inc	00254-3595-28
100's	$38.35	GENERIC, Major Pharmaceuticals Inc	00904-5022-60
100's	$38.35	GENERIC, Major Pharmaceuticals Inc	00904-5158-60
100's	$43.50	GENERIC, Martec Pharmaceuticals Inc	52555-0653-01
100's	$44.50	ANEXSIA, Pharma Pac	52959-0364-00
100's	$44.72	GENERIC, Ivax Corporation	00182-0692-01
100's	$44.72	GENERIC, Mallinckrodt Medical Inc	00406-0359-01
100's	$49.69	ANEXSIA, Monarch Pharmaceuticals Inc	61570-0002-01
100's	$54.88	GENERIC, Udl Laboratories Inc	51079-0867-21
100's	$58.11	GENERIC, Barr Laboratories Inc	00555-0895-02
100's	$64.57	ANEXSIA, Mallinckrodt Medical Inc	00406-5362-01
100's	$69.50	GENERIC, Watson Laboratories Inc	00591-0502-01
100's	$69.50	GENERIC, Watson Laboratories Inc	52544-0502-01
100's	$69.51	GENERIC, Qualitest Products Inc	00603-3884-21
100's	$99.25	LORCET PLUS, Forest Pharmaceuticals	00785-1122-01
100's	$104.15	LORCET PLUS, Forest Pharmaceuticals	00785-1122-63

Tablet - Oral - 650 mg;10 mg

Qty	Price	Product, Manufacturer	NDC
100's	$18.52	FEDERAL UPPER LIMIT, H.C.F.A. F F P	99999-0070-14

Qty	Price	Product	NDC
100's	$50.72	GENERIC, Vintage Pharmaceuticals Inc	00254-3597-28
100's	$50.78	GENERIC, Moore, H.L. Drug Exchange Inc	00839-8048-06
100's	$50.78	GENERIC, Major Pharmaceuticals Inc	00904-5127-60
100's	$51.80	GENERIC, Martec Pharmaceuticals Inc	52555-0641-01
100's	$53.10	GENERIC, Martec Pharmaceuticals Inc	52555-0672-01
100's	$53.17	GENERIC, Ivax Corporation	00182-0034-01
100's	$53.17	GENERIC, Watson/Rugby Laboratories Inc	00536-5510-01
100's	$53.20	GENERIC, Mallinckrodt Medical Inc	00406-0361-01
100's	$73.77	GENERIC, Barr Laboratories Inc	00555-0898-02
100's	$79.79	GENERIC, Inwood Laboratories Inc	00258-3658-01
100's	$97.76	GENERIC, Watson Laboratories Inc	00591-0503-01
100's	$97.76	GENERIC, Qualitest Products Inc	00603-3885-21
100's	$97.76	GENERIC, Watson Laboratories Inc	52544-0503-01
100's	$115.55	GENERIC, Mallinckrodt Medical Inc	00406-0361-62

Tablet - Oral - 660 mg;10 mg

Qty	Price	Product	NDC
100's	$52.84	FEDERAL UPPER LIMIT, H.C.F.A. F F P	99999-0070-14
100's	$61.17	GENERIC, Mallinckrodt Medical Inc	00406-0362-01
100's	$61.17	GENERIC, Qualitest Products Inc	00603-3886-21
100's	$77.01	VICODIN HP, Knoll Pharmaceutical Company	00044-0725-02
100's	$81.12	ANEXSIA, Mallinckrodt Medical Inc	00406-5363-01

Tablet - Oral - 750 mg;7.5 mg

Qty	Price	Product	NDC
6's	$13.61	GENERIC, Pd-Rx Pharmaceuticals	55289-0360-06
12's	$15.56	GENERIC, Pd-Rx Pharmaceuticals	55289-0360-12
16's	$16.96	GENERIC, Pd-Rx Pharmaceuticals	55289-0360-16
20's	$18.28	GENERIC, Pd-Rx Pharmaceuticals	55289-0360-20
24's	$19.33	GENERIC, Pd-Rx Pharmaceuticals	55289-0360-24
30's	$14.85	GENERIC, Medirex Inc	57480-0519-06
30's	$21.39	GENERIC, Pd-Rx Pharmaceuticals	55289-0360-30
90's	$40.44	GENERIC, Pd-Rx Pharmaceuticals	55289-0360-90
100's	$12.90	GENERIC, Watson Laboratories Inc	52544-0387-01
100's	$15.48	FEDERAL UPPER LIMIT, H.C.F.A. F F P	99999-0070-10
100's	$34.00	GENERIC, Qualitest Products Inc	00603-3883-21
100's	$34.40	GENERIC, Vintage Pharmaceuticals Inc	00254-3596-28
100's	$35.35	GENERIC, Creighton Products Corporation	50752-0292-05
100's	$39.00	GENERIC, Geneva Pharmaceuticals	00781-1532-01
100's	$39.80	GENERIC, Mallinckrodt Medical Inc	00406-0360-01
100's	$39.80	GENERIC, Martec Pharmaceuticals Inc	52555-0654-01
100's	$40.59	GENERIC, Moore, H.L. Drug Exchange Inc	00839-7728-06
100's	$41.66	GENERIC, Aligen Independent Laboratories Inc	00405-0017-01
100's	$42.00	GENERIC, Major Pharmaceuticals Inc	00904-7632-60
100's	$42.50	GENERIC, Ivax Corporation	00182-0681-01
100's	$42.71	GENERIC, Endo Laboratories Llc	60951-0641-70
100's	$43.78	GENERIC, Watson Laboratories Inc	00591-0387-01
100's	$48.10	GENERIC, Udl Laboratories Inc	51079-0748-21
100's	$49.50	GENERIC, Medirex Inc	57480-0519-01
100's	$65.05	VICODIN ES, Knoll Pharmaceutical Company	00044-0728-02
100's	$65.05	VICODIN ES, Abbott Pharmaceutical	00074-1973-14
100's	$69.47	VICODIN ES, Knoll Pharmaceutical Company	00044-0728-41

Tablet - Oral - 750 mg;10 mg

Qty	Price	Product	NDC
100's	$103.57	MAXIDONE, Watson Laboratories Inc	52544-0634-01

PRODUCT LISTING - RATED NOT THERAPEUTICALLY EQUIVALENT

Tablet - Oral - 325 mg;5 mg

Qty	Price	Product	NDC
6's	$3.90	NORCO, Southwood Pharmaceuticals Inc	58016-0662-06
12's	$7.80	NORCO, Southwood Pharmaceuticals Inc	58016-0662-12

Tablet - Oral - 325 mg;7.5 mg

Qty	Price	Product	NDC
240's	$179.04	NORCO, Southwood Pharmaceuticals Inc	58016-0632-04

PRODUCT LISTING - EQUIVALENTS NOT AVAILABLE

Capsule - Oral - 500 mg;5 mg

Qty	Price	Product	NDC
100's	$27.95	GENERIC, Williams,T.E.	51189-0083-01
100's	$29.88	GENERIC, Lunsco Inc	10892-0113-10
100's	$30.49	GENERIC, Seatrace Pharmaceuticals	00551-0180-01
100's	$33.31	GENERIC, Huckaby Pharmacal Inc	58407-0091-01

Elixir - Oral - 500 mg;5 mg/15 ml

Qty	Price	Product	NDC
480 ml	$43.82	ANEXSIA, Monarch Pharmaceuticals Inc	61570-0101-16

Elixir - Oral - 500 mg;7.5 mg/15 ml

Qty	Price	Product	NDC
473 ml	$56.77	GENERIC, Qualitest Products Inc	00603-1295-58
480 ml	$93.80	LORTAB ELIXIR, Ucb Pharma Inc	50474-0909-16

Tablet - Oral - 250 mg;10 mg

Qty	Price	Product	NDC
100's	$69.26	GENERIC, Huckaby Pharmacal Inc	58407-0033-01

Tablet - Oral - 325 mg;5 mg

Qty	Price	Product	NDC
100's	$54.20	GENERIC, Mallinckrodt Medical Inc	00406-0365-01
100's	$67.08	ANEXSIA, Andrx Pharmaceuticals	62022-0563-01

Tablet - Oral - 325 mg;7.5 mg

Qty	Price	Product	NDC
100's	$61.83	GENERIC, Mallinckrodt Medical Inc	00406-0366-01
100's	$76.99	ANEXSIA, Andrx Pharmaceuticals	62022-0663-01

Tablet - Oral - 325 mg;10 mg

Qty	Price	Product	NDC
20's	$15.40	GENERIC, Southwood Pharmaceuticals Inc	58016-0495-20
28's	$21.56	GENERIC, Southwood Pharmaceuticals Inc	58016-0495-28
40's	$30.80	GENERIC, Southwood Pharmaceuticals Inc	58016-0495-40
50's	$38.50	GENERIC, Southwood Pharmaceuticals Inc	58016-0495-50
56's	$43.12	GENERIC, Southwood Pharmaceuticals Inc	58016-0495-56
60's	$46.20	GENERIC, Southwood Pharmaceuticals Inc	58016-0495-60
84's	$64.68	GENERIC, Southwood Pharmaceuticals Inc	58016-0495-84
90's	$69.30	GENERIC, Southwood Pharmaceuticals Inc	58016-0495-90
100's	$77.00	GENERIC, Southwood Pharmaceuticals Inc	58016-0495-00
112's	$86.24	GENERIC, Southwood Pharmaceuticals Inc	58016-0495-99
120's	$92.40	GENERIC, Southwood Pharmaceuticals Inc	58016-0495-02

Tablet - Oral - 500 mg;5 mg

Qty	Price	Product	NDC
1's	$3.41	GENERIC, Prescript Pharmaceuticals	00247-0079-01
2's	$3.46	GENERIC, Prescript Pharmaceuticals	00247-0079-02
3's	$3.52	GENERIC, Prescript Pharmaceuticals	00247-0079-03
4's	$3.56	GENERIC, Prescript Pharmaceuticals	00247-0079-04
4's	$8.24	GENERIC, Pharma Pac	52959-0312-04
5's	$3.62	GENERIC, Prescript Pharmaceuticals	00247-0079-05
6's	$1.40	GENERIC, Allscripts Pharmaceutical Company	54569-0303-07
6's	$3.30	GENERIC, Southwood Pharmaceuticals Inc	58016-0276-06
6's	$3.67	GENERIC, Prescript Pharmaceuticals	00247-0079-06
6's	$11.40	GENERIC, Pharma Pac	52959-0312-06
7's	$3.73	GENERIC, Prescript Pharmaceuticals	00247-0079-07
8's	$3.78	GENERIC, Prescript Pharmaceuticals	00247-0079-08
9's	$4.95	GENERIC, Southwood Pharmaceuticals Inc	58016-0276-09
10's	$2.34	GENERIC, Allscripts Pharmaceutical Company	54569-0303-06
10's	$2.43	GENERIC, Physicians Total Care	54868-0071-03
10's	$3.88	GENERIC, Prescript Pharmaceuticals	00247-0079-10
10's	$5.50	GENERIC, Southwood Pharmaceuticals Inc	58016-0276-10
10's	$16.60	GENERIC, Pharma Pac	52959-0312-10
12's	$2.80	GENERIC, Allscripts Pharmaceutical Company	54569-0303-09
12's	$3.99	GENERIC, Prescript Pharmaceuticals	00247-0079-12
12's	$6.60	GENERIC, Southwood Pharmaceuticals Inc	58016-0276-12
12's	$21.70	GENERIC, Pharma Pac	52959-0312-12
14's	$7.70	GENERIC, Southwood Pharmaceuticals Inc	58016-0276-14
14's	$24.74	GENERIC, Pharma Pac	52959-0312-14
15's	$2.81	GENERIC, Physicians Total Care	54868-0071-05
15's	$3.51	GENERIC, Allscripts Pharmaceutical Company	54569-0303-00
15's	$4.15	GENERIC, Prescript Pharmaceuticals	00247-0079-15
15's	$8.25	GENERIC, Southwood Pharmaceuticals Inc	58016-0276-15
15's	$26.33	GENERIC, Pharma Pac	52959-0312-15
16's	$3.74	GENERIC, Allscripts Pharmaceutical Company	54569-3322-01
16's	$4.20	GENERIC, Prescript Pharmaceuticals	00247-0079-16
16's	$8.80	GENERIC, Southwood Pharmaceuticals Inc	58016-0276-16
16's	$28.08	GENERIC, Pharma Pac	52959-0312-16
18's	$9.90	GENERIC, Southwood Pharmaceuticals Inc	58016-0276-18
20's	$3.18	GENERIC, Physicians Total Care	54868-0071-02
20's	$4.41	GENERIC, Prescript Pharmaceuticals	00247-0079-20
20's	$4.67	GENERIC, Allscripts Pharmaceutical Company	54569-0303-01
20's	$5.65	GENERIC, Pharmaceutical Corporation Of America	51655-0812-52
20's	$11.00	GENERIC, Southwood Pharmaceuticals Inc	58016-0276-20
20's	$34.95	GENERIC, Pharma Pac	52959-0312-20
24's	$4.62	GENERIC, Prescript Pharmaceuticals	00247-0079-24
24's	$5.61	GENERIC, Allscripts Pharmaceutical Company	54569-0303-08
24's	$13.20	GENERIC, Southwood Pharmaceuticals Inc	58016-0276-24
24's	$38.25	GENERIC, Pharma Pac	52959-0312-24
25's	$4.68	GENERIC, Prescript Pharmaceuticals	00247-0079-25
25's	$5.84	GENERIC, Allscripts Pharmaceutical Company	54569-3322-00
25's	$13.75	GENERIC, Southwood Pharmaceuticals Inc	58016-0276-25
25's	$39.85	GENERIC, Pharma Pac	52959-0312-25
27's	$14.85	GENERIC, Southwood Pharmaceuticals Inc	58016-0276-27
28's	$4.84	GENERIC, Prescript Pharmaceuticals	00247-0079-28
28's	$15.40	GENERIC, Southwood Pharmaceuticals Inc	58016-0276-28
30's	$3.94	GENERIC, Physicians Total Care	54868-0071-01
30's	$4.94	GENERIC, Prescript Pharmaceuticals	00247-0079-30
30's	$7.01	GENERIC, Allscripts Pharmaceutical Company	54569-0303-02
30's	$16.50	GENERIC, Southwood Pharmaceuticals Inc	58016-0276-30
30's	$45.97	GENERIC, Pharma Pac	52959-0312-30
36's	$19.80	GENERIC, Southwood Pharmaceuticals Inc	58016-0276-36
40's	$4.70	GENERIC, Physicians Total Care	54868-0071-04
40's	$5.47	GENERIC, Prescript Pharmaceuticals	00247-0079-40
40's	$9.35	GENERIC, Allscripts Pharmaceutical Company	54569-0303-03
40's	$22.00	GENERIC, Southwood Pharmaceuticals Inc	58016-0276-40
40's	$59.59	GENERIC, Pharma Pac	52959-0312-40
42's	$23.10	GENERIC, Southwood Pharmaceuticals Inc	58016-0276-42
45's	$5.74	GENERIC, Prescript Pharmaceuticals	00247-0079-45
45's	$66.98	GENERIC, Pharma Pac	52959-0312-45
50's	$5.46	GENERIC, Physicians Total Care	54868-0071-07
50's	$6.00	GENERIC, Prescript Pharmaceuticals	00247-0079-50
50's	$11.69	GENERIC, Allscripts Pharmaceutical Company	54569-0303-05
50's	$27.50	GENERIC, Southwood Pharmaceuticals Inc	58016-0276-50
50's	$74.27	GENERIC, Pharma Pac	52959-0312-50
56's	$30.80	GENERIC, Southwood Pharmaceuticals Inc	58016-0276-56
58's	$32.77	GENERIC, Pharma Pac	52959-0312-58
60's	$5.66	GENERIC, Physicians Total Care	54868-0071-00
60's	$6.53	GENERIC, Prescript Pharmaceuticals	00247-0079-60
60's	$33.00	GENERIC, Southwood Pharmaceuticals Inc	58016-0276-60
60's	$33.66	GENERIC, Pharma Pac	52959-0312-60
84's	$46.20	GENERIC, Southwood Pharmaceuticals Inc	58016-0276-84
90's	$8.12	GENERIC, Prescript Pharmaceuticals	00247-0079-90
90's	$49.50	GENERIC, Southwood Pharmaceuticals Inc	58016-0276-90
100's	$8.65	GENERIC, Prescript Pharmaceuticals	00247-0079-00
100's	$8.70	GENERIC, Physicians Total Care	54868-0071-08
100's	$42.59	GENERIC, Allscripts Pharmaceutical Company	54569-0303-04
100's	$55.00	GENERIC, Southwood Pharmaceuticals Inc	58016-0276-00

100's	$103.43	GENERIC, Pharma Pac	52959-0312-00
120's	$65.30	GENERIC, Pharma Pac	52959-0312-02
120's	$66.00	GENERIC, Southwood Pharmaceuticals Inc	58016-0276-02

Tablet - Oral - 500 mg;7.5 mg

10's	$15.90	GENERIC, Pharma Pac	52959-0380-10
12's	$7.37	GENERIC, Southwood Pharmaceuticals Inc	58016-0195-12
12's	$17.88	GENERIC, Pharma Pac	52959-0380-12
15's	$9.21	GENERIC, Southwood Pharmaceuticals Inc	58016-0195-15
15's	$20.85	GENERIC, Pharma Pac	52959-0380-15
20's	$9.31	GENERIC, Physicians Total Care	54868-3038-02
20's	$23.80	GENERIC, Pharma Pac	52959-0380-20
24's	$26.16	GENERIC, Pharma Pac	52959-0380-24
25's	$15.35	GENERIC, Southwood Pharmaceuticals Inc	58016-0195-25
30's	$13.97	GENERIC, Physicians Total Care	54868-3038-01
30's	$18.42	GENERIC, Southwood Pharmaceuticals Inc	58016-0195-30
30's	$26.70	GENERIC, Pharma Pac	52959-0380-30
40's	$31.60	GENERIC, Pharma Pac	52959-0380-40
50's	$30.70	GENERIC, Southwood Pharmaceuticals Inc	58016-0195-50
60's	$28.50	GENERIC, Pharma Pac	52959-0380-60
60's	$36.84	GENERIC, Southwood Pharmaceuticals Inc	58016-0195-60
90's	$55.26	GENERIC, Southwood Pharmaceuticals Inc	58016-0195-90
100's	$61.40	GENERIC, Pharma Pac	52959-0380-00
100's	$61.40	GENERIC, Southwood Pharmaceuticals Inc	58016-0195-00
120's	$71.87	GENERIC, Pharma Pac	52959-0380-02
120's	$73.68	GENERIC, Southwood Pharmaceuticals Inc	58016-0195-02

Tablet - Oral - 500 mg;10 mg

10's	$7.21	LORTAB, Southwood Pharmaceuticals Inc	58016-0229-10
10's	$10.50	GENERIC, Pharma Pac	52959-0521-10
14's	$10.09	LORTAB, Southwood Pharmaceuticals Inc	58016-0229-14
20's	$14.42	LORTAB, Southwood Pharmaceuticals Inc	58016-0229-20
20's	$17.90	GENERIC, Pharma Pac	52959-0521-20
21's	$15.14	LORTAB, Southwood Pharmaceuticals Inc	58016-0229-21
28's	$20.19	LORTAB, Southwood Pharmaceuticals Inc	58016-0229-28
30's	$21.63	LORTAB, Southwood Pharmaceuticals Inc	58016-0229-30
30's	$25.80	GENERIC, Pharma Pac	52959-0521-30
40's	$28.84	LORTAB, Southwood Pharmaceuticals Inc	58016-0229-40
40's	$33.70	GENERIC, Pharma Pac	52959-0521-40
50's	$36.05	LORTAB, Southwood Pharmaceuticals Inc	58016-0229-50
50's	$41.00	GENERIC, Pharma Pac	52959-0521-50
60's	$43.26	LORTAB, Southwood Pharmaceuticals Inc	58016-0229-60
60's	$46.60	GENERIC, Pharma Pac	52959-0521-60
80's	$56.60	GENERIC, Pharma Pac	52959-0521-80
80's	$57.68	LORTAB, Southwood Pharmaceuticals Inc	58016-0229-80
90's	$64.89	LORTAB, Southwood Pharmaceuticals Inc	58016-0229-90
100's	$70.00	GENERIC, Pharma Pac	52959-0521-00
100's	$72.10	LORTAB, Southwood Pharmaceuticals Inc	58016-0229-00
120's	$82.20	GENERIC, Pharma Pac	52959-0521-02
120's	$86.40	GENERIC, Southwood Pharmaceuticals Inc	58016-0229-02
180's	$129.60	GENERIC, Southwood Pharmaceuticals Inc	58016-0229-99
240's	$172.80	GENERIC, Southwood Pharmaceuticals Inc	58016-0229-04

Tablet - Oral - 650 mg;7.5 mg

6's	$3.06	GENERIC, Southwood Pharmaceuticals Inc	58016-0239-06
10's	$5.10	GENERIC, Southwood Pharmaceuticals Inc	58016-0239-10
12's	$6.12	GENERIC, Southwood Pharmaceuticals Inc	58016-0239-12
15's	$7.65	GENERIC, Southwood Pharmaceuticals Inc	58016-0239-15
20's	$10.20	GENERIC, Southwood Pharmaceuticals Inc	58016-0239-20
20's	$15.90	GENERIC, Pharma Pac	52959-0372-20
25's	$12.75	GENERIC, Southwood Pharmaceuticals Inc	58016-0239-25
30's	$15.30	GENERIC, Southwood Pharmaceuticals Inc	58016-0239-30
30's	$23.50	GENERIC, Pharma Pac	52959-0372-30
40's	$30.50	GENERIC, Pharma Pac	52959-0372-40
50's	$37.50	GENERIC, Pharma Pac	52959-0372-50
60's	$44.50	GENERIC, Pharma Pac	52959-0372-60
100's	$66.15	GENERIC, Inwood Laboratories Inc	00258-3622-01
100's	$69.50	GENERIC, Pharma Pac	52959-0372-00

Tablet - Oral - 650 mg;10 mg

4's	$6.00	GENERIC, Pharma Pac	52959-0371-04
6's	$7.26	GENERIC, Southwood Pharmaceuticals Inc	58016-0232-06
10's	$12.10	GENERIC, Southwood Pharmaceuticals Inc	58016-0232-10
12's	$14.50	GENERIC, Pharma Pac	52959-0371-12
12's	$14.51	GENERIC, Southwood Pharmaceuticals Inc	58016-0232-12
15's	$18.14	GENERIC, Southwood Pharmaceuticals Inc	58016-0232-15
15's	$18.75	GENERIC, Pharma Pac	52959-0371-15
20's	$24.00	GENERIC, Pharma Pac	52959-0371-20
20's	$24.19	GENERIC, Southwood Pharmaceuticals Inc	58016-0232-20
25's	$30.24	GENERIC, Southwood Pharmaceuticals Inc	58016-0232-25
30's	$15.76	GENERIC, Physicians Total Care	54868-3729-01
30's	$34.50	GENERIC, Pharma Pac	52959-0371-30
30's	$36.29	GENERIC, Southwood Pharmaceuticals Inc	58016-0232-30
40's	$44.00	GENERIC, Pharma Pac	52959-0371-40
40's	$48.38	GENERIC, Southwood Pharmaceuticals Inc	58016-0232-40
50's	$52.50	GENERIC, Pharma Pac	52959-0371-50
50's	$60.48	GENERIC, Southwood Pharmaceuticals Inc	58016-0232-50
60's	$60.00	GENERIC, Pharma Pac	52959-0371-60
60's	$72.57	GENERIC, Southwood Pharmaceuticals Inc	58016-0232-60
90's	$108.86	GENERIC, Southwood Pharmaceuticals Inc	58016-0232-90
100's	$97.76	GENERIC, Pharma Pac	52959-0371-00
100's	$120.95	GENERIC, Southwood Pharmaceuticals Inc	58016-0232-00
100's	$139.63	LORCET 10/650, Forest Pharmaceuticals	00785-6350-01
100's	$144.44	LORCET 10/650, Forest Pharmaceuticals	00785-6350-63
120's	$116.40	GENERIC, Pharma Pac	52959-0371-02
120's	$145.14	GENERIC, Southwood Pharmaceuticals Inc	58016-0232-02
126's	$152.40	GENERIC, Southwood Pharmaceuticals Inc	58016-0232-97

Tablet - Oral - 660 mg;10 mg

100's	$77.01	VICODIN HP, Abbott Pharmaceutical	00074-2274-14

Tablet - Oral - 750 mg;7.5 mg

10's	$5.50	GENERIC, Physicians Total Care	54868-2281-04
12's	$7.26	GENERIC, Southwood Pharmaceuticals Inc	58016-0758-12
12's	$10.76	GENERIC, Pharma Pac	52959-0415-12
14's	$8.47	GENERIC, Southwood Pharmaceuticals Inc	58016-0758-14
15's	$5.85	GENERIC, Allscripts Pharmaceutical Company	54569-3909-01
15's	$8.25	GENERIC, Physicians Total Care	54868-2281-02
15's	$9.08	GENERIC, Southwood Pharmaceuticals Inc	58016-0758-15
16's	$9.68	GENERIC, Southwood Pharmaceuticals Inc	58016-0758-16
20's	$7.80	GENERIC, Allscripts Pharmaceutical Company	54569-3909-00
20's	$9.89	GENERIC, Physicians Total Care	54868-2281-03
20's	$12.10	GENERIC, Southwood Pharmaceuticals Inc	58016-0758-20
20's	$12.28	GENERIC, Southwood Pharmaceuticals Inc	58016-0195-20
20's	$14.74	GENERIC, Pharma Pac	52959-0415-20
25's	$15.13	GENERIC, Southwood Pharmaceuticals Inc	58016-0758-25
28's	$16.94	GENERIC, Southwood Pharmaceuticals Inc	58016-0758-28
30's	$11.70	GENERIC, Allscripts Pharmaceutical Company	54569-3909-02
30's	$14.84	GENERIC, Physicians Total Care	54868-2281-01
30's	$18.15	GENERIC, Southwood Pharmaceuticals Inc	58016-0758-30
30's	$21.47	GENERIC, Pharma Pac	52959-0415-30
40's	$24.20	GENERIC, Southwood Pharmaceuticals Inc	58016-0758-40
42's	$25.41	GENERIC, Southwood Pharmaceuticals Inc	58016-0758-42
45's	$27.23	GENERIC, Southwood Pharmaceuticals Inc	58016-0758-45
45's	$31.80	GENERIC, Pharma Pac	52959-0415-45
50's	$30.25	GENERIC, Southwood Pharmaceuticals Inc	58016-0758-50
50's	$33.78	GENERIC, Pharma Pac	52959-0415-50
56's	$33.88	GENERIC, Southwood Pharmaceuticals Inc	58016-0758-56
60's	$36.30	GENERIC, Southwood Pharmaceuticals Inc	58016-0758-60
60's	$37.73	GENERIC, Pharma Pac	52959-0415-60
70's	$42.35	GENERIC, Southwood Pharmaceuticals Inc	58016-0758-70
75's	$45.38	GENERIC, Southwood Pharmaceuticals Inc	58016-0758-75
84's	$50.82	GENERIC, Southwood Pharmaceuticals Inc	58016-0758-84
90's	$54.45	GENERIC, Southwood Pharmaceuticals Inc	58016-0758-90
100's	$34.69	GENERIC, Physicians Total Care	54868-2281-00
100's	$38.71	GENERIC, Caremark Inc	00339-4051-12
100's	$42.71	GENERIC, Barr Laboratories Inc	00555-0739-02
100's	$60.50	GENERIC, Southwood Pharmaceuticals Inc	58016-0758-00
100's	$62.74	GENERIC, Pharma Pac	52959-0415-01
120's	$71.70	GENERIC, Pharma Pac	52959-0415-02
120's	$72.60	GENERIC, Southwood Pharmaceuticals Inc	58016-0758-02

Acetaminophen; Oxycodone Hydrochloride *(000072)*

Categories: Pain, moderate to severe; Pregnancy Category C; DEA Class CII; FDA Approval Pre 1982
Drug Classes: Analgesics, narcotic
Brand Names: Endocet; Oxycet; **Percocet**; Roxicet; Roxilox; Tylox
Foreign Brand Availability: Oxycocet (Canada); Percocet-Demi (Canada); Percocet-5 (Canada; Israel)
Cost of Therapy: $19.64 (Pain; Percocet; 325 mg; 5 mg; 4 tablets/day; 7 day supply)
$4.31 (Pain; Generic Tablets; 325 mg; 5 mg; 4 tablets/day; 7 day supply)

DESCRIPTION

Acetaminophen, 4′-hydroxyacetanilide, is a non-opiate, nonsalicylate analgesic and antipyretic which occurs as a white, odorless, crystalline powder, possessing a slightly bitter taste. The molecular formula for acetaminophen is $C_8H_9NO_2$ and the molecular weight is 151.17.

Oxycodone, 14-hydroxydihydrocodeinone, is a semisynthetic opioid analgesic which occurs as a white, odorless, crystalline powder having a saline, bitter taste. The molecular formula for oxycodone hydrochloride is $C_{18}H_{21}NO_4 \cdot HCl$ and the molecular weight 351.83. It is derived from the opium alkaloid thebaine.

Each tablet, for oral administration, contains acetaminophen and oxycodone HCl in the following strengths (see TABLE 1).

TABLE 1

7.5/325	
Acetaminophen	325 mg
Oxycodone HCl	7.5 mg
7.5 mg oxycodone HCl is equivalent to 6.7228 mg of oxycodone.	
10/325	
Acetaminophen	325 mg
Oxycodone HCl	10 mg
10 mg oxycodone HCl is equivalent to 8.9637 mg of oxycodone.	
2.5/325	
Acetaminophen	325 mg
Oxycodone HCl	2.5 mg
2.5 mg oxycodone HCl is equivalent to 2.2409 mg of oxycodone.	
5/325	
Acetaminophen	325 mg
Oxycodone HCl	5 mg
5 mg oxycodone HCl is equivalent to 4.4815 mg of oxycodone.	
7.5/500	
Acetaminophen	500 mg
Oxycodone HCl	7.5 mg
7.5 mg oxycodone HCl is equivalent to 6.7228 mg of oxycodone.	
10/650	
Acetaminophen	650 mg
Oxycodone HCl	10 mg
10 mg oxycodone HCl is equivalent to 8.9637 mg of oxycodone.	

All strengths of Percocet also contain the following inactive ingredients: Colloidal silicon dioxide, croscarmellose sodium, crospovidone, microcrystalline cellulose, povidone, pregelatinized starch, and stearic acid. In addition, the 325 mg/2.5 mg strength contains FD&C red no. 40 aluminum lake and the 325 mg/5 mg strength contains FD&C blue no. 1

aluminum lake. The 500 mg/7.5 mg strength contains FD&C yellow no. 6 aluminum lake and the 650 mg/10 mg strength contains D&C yellow no. 10 aluminum lake. The 325 mg/7.5 mg strength contains FD&C yellow no. 6 aluminum lake and the 325 mg/10 mg strength contains D&C yellow no. 10 aluminum lake.

CLINICAL PHARMACOLOGY

The principal ingredient, oxycodone, is a semisynthetic opioid analgesic with multiple actions qualitatively similar to those of morphine; the most prominent involves the central nervous system and organs composed of smooth muscle. The principal actions of therapeutic value of the oxycodone in acetaminophen; oxycodone HCl are analgesia and sedation.

Oxycodone is similar to codeine and methadone in that it retains at least one-half of its analgesic activity when administered orally.

Acetaminophen is a non-opiate, non-salicylate analgesic and antipyretic.

INDICATIONS AND USAGE

Acetaminophen; oxycodone HCl is indicated for the relief of moderate to moderately severe pain.

CONTRAINDICATIONS

Acetaminophen; oxycodone HCl should not be administered to patients who are hypersensitive to oxycodone, acetaminophen, or any other components of this product.

WARNINGS

DRUG DEPENDENCE

Oxycodone can produce drug dependence of the morphine type and, therefore, has the potential for being abused. Psychic dependence, physical dependence and tolerance may develop upon repeated administration of acetaminophen; oxycodone HCl, and it should be prescribed and administered with the same degree of caution appropriate to the use of other oral opioid-containing medications. Like other opioid-containing medications, acetaminophen; oxycodone HCl is subject to the Federal Controlled Substances Act (Schedule II).

PRECAUTIONS

GENERAL

Head Injury and Increased Intracranial Pressure

The respiratory depressant effects of opioids and their capacity to elevate cerebrospinal fluid pressure may be markedly exaggerated in the presence of head injury, other intracranial lesions or a preexisting increase in intracranial pressure. Furthermore, opioids produce adverse reactions which may obscure the clinical course of patients with head injuries.

Acute Abdominal Conditions

The administration of acetaminophen; oxycodone HCl or other opioids may obscure the diagnosis or clinical course in patients with acute abdominal conditions.

Special Risk Patients

Acetaminophen; oxycodone HCl should be given with caution to certain patients such as the elderly or debilitated, and those with severe impairment of hepatic or renal function, hypothyroidism, Addison's disease, and prostatic hypertrophy or urethral stricture.

INFORMATION FOR THE PATIENT

Oxycodone may impair the mental and/or physical abilities required for the performance of potentially hazardous tasks such as driving a car or operating machinery. The patient using acetaminophen; oxycodone HCl should be cautioned accordingly.

USAGE IN PREGNANCY

Teratogenic Effects, Pregnancy Category C

Animal reproductive studies have not been conducted with acetaminophen; oxycodone HCl. It is also not known whether acetaminophen; oxycodone HCl can cause fetal harm when administered to a pregnant woman or can affect reproductive capacity. Acetaminophen; oxycodone HCl should not be given to a pregnant woman unless in the judgment of the physician, the potential benefits outweigh the possible hazards.

Nonteratogenic Effects

Use of opioids during pregnancy may produce physical dependence in the neonate.

Labor and Delivery

As with all opioids, administration of acetaminophen; oxycodone HCl to the mother shortly before delivery may result in some degree of respiratory depression in the newborn and the mother, especially if higher doses are used.

NURSING MOTHERS

It is not known whether acetaminophen; oxycodone HCl is excreted in human milk. Because many drugs are excreted in human milk, caution should be exercised when acetaminophen; oxycodone HCl is administered to a nursing woman.

PEDIATRIC USE

Safety and effectiveness in pediatric patients have not been established.

DRUG INTERACTIONS

Patients receiving other opioid analgesics, general anesthetics, phenothiazines, other tranquilizers, sedative-hypnotics or other CNS depressants (including alcohol) concomitantly with acetaminophen; oxycodone HCl may exhibit an additive CNS depression. When such combined therapy is contemplated, the dose of one or both agents should be reduced.

The concurrent use of anticholinergics with opioids may produce paralytic ileus.

ADVERSE REACTIONS

The most frequently observed adverse reactions include lightheadedness, dizziness, sedation, nausea and vomiting. These effects seem to be more prominent in ambulatory than in nonambulatory patients, and some of these adverse reactions may be alleviated if the patient lies down.

Other adverse reactions include euphoria, dysphoria, constipation, skin rash and pruritus. At higher doses, oxycodone has most of the disadvantages of morphine including respiratory depression.

DOSAGE AND ADMINISTRATION

Dosage should be adjusted according to the severity of the pain and the response of the patient. It may occasionally be necessary to exceed the usual dosage recommended below in cases of more severe pain or in those patients who have become tolerant to the analgesic effect of opioids. Acetaminophen; oxycodone HCl is given orally.

Acetaminophen; oxycodone HCl 325 mg/7.5 mg and 325 mg/10 mg: The usual adult dosage is 1 tablet every 6 hours as needed for pain. The total daily dose of acetaminophen should not exceed 4 g.

Acetaminophen; oxycodone HCl 325 mg/2.5 mg: The usual adult dosage is 1 or 2 tablets every 6 hours. The total daily dose of acetaminophen should not exceed 4 g.

Acetaminophen; oxycodone HCl 325 mg/5 mg, 500 mg/7.5 mg, and 650 mg/10 mg: The usual adult dosage is 1 tablet every 6 hours as needed for pain. The total daily dose of acetaminophen should not exceed 4 g.

TABLE 2

Strength	Maximal Daily Dose
325 mg/7.5 mg	8 tablets
325 mg/10 mg	6 tablets
325 mg/2.5 mg	12 tablets
325 mg/5 mg	12 tablets
500 mg/7.5 mg	8 tablets
650 mg/10 mg	6 tablets

HOW SUPPLIED

Percocet is supplied as follows:

7.5 mg/325 mg: Peach oval-shaped tablet debossed with "PERCOCET" on one side and "7.5/325" on the other.

10 mg/325 mg: Yellow capsule-shaped tablet debossed with "PERCOCET" on one side and "10/325" on the other.

2.5 mg/325 mg: Pink oval tablet embossed with "PERCOCET" on one side and "2.5" on the other.

5 mg/325 mg: Blue, round, tablet, embossed with "PERCOCET" and "5" on one side and bisect on the other.

7.5 mg/500 mg: Peach capsule-shaped tablet embossed with "PERCOCET" on one side and "7.5" on the other.

10 mg/650 mg: Yellow oval tablet embossed with "PERCOCET" on one side and "10" on the other.

STORAGE

Store at controlled room temperature, 15-30°C (59-86°F).

Dispense in a tight, light-resistant container with a child-resistant closure (as required).

PRODUCT LISTING - RATED THERAPEUTICALLY EQUIVALENT

Package	Price	Product	NDC
Capsule - Oral - 500 mg;5 mg			
100's	$21.37	FEDERAL UPPER LIMIT, H.C.F.A. F F P	99999-0072-01
100's	$40.25	GENERIC, Mallinckrodt Medical Inc	00406-0532-01
100's	$41.67	GENERIC, Vintage Pharmaceuticals Inc	00254-4832-28
100's	$41.67	GENERIC, Qualitest Products Inc	00603-4997-21
100's	$46.50	GENERIC, Major Pharmaceuticals Inc	00904-1973-60
100's	$46.61	GENERIC, Aligen Independent Laboratories Inc	00405-0140-01
100's	$49.50	GENERIC, Barr Laboratories Inc	00555-0658-02
100's	$49.50	GENERIC, Duramed Pharmaceuticals Inc	51285-0658-02
100's	$57.00	GENERIC, Barr Laboratories Inc	00555-0651-02
100's	$57.72	ROXILOX, Roxane Laboratories Inc	00054-2795-25
100's	$59.00	GENERIC, Amide Pharmaceutical Inc	52152-0041-02
100's	$79.39	GENERIC, Watson Laboratories Inc	00591-0737-01
100's	$79.39	GENERIC, Watson Laboratories Inc	52544-0737-01
100's	$81.30	GENERIC, Endo Laboratories Llc	60951-0660-70
100's	$115.68	TYLOX, Janssen Pharmaceuticals	00045-0526-60
100's	$152.11	TYLOX, Janssen Pharmaceuticals	00045-0526-79
Tablet - Oral - 325 mg;5 mg			
10's	$6.61	GENERIC, Physicians Total Care	54868-1700-02
20's	$11.01	GENERIC, Physicians Total Care	54868-1700-04
24's	$8.96	GENERIC, Physicians Total Care	54868-1700-03
25 x 4	$83.75	PERCOCET-5/325, Endo Laboratories Llc	63481-0127-75
25 x 4	$120.00	PERCOCET-5/325, Endo Laboratories Llc	63481-0623-75
30's	$15.40	GENERIC, Physicians Total Care	54868-1700-01
100's	$11.92	FEDERAL UPPER LIMIT, H.C.F.A. F F P	99999-0072-03
100's	$19.55	GENERIC, Major Pharmaceuticals Inc	00904-0465-60
100's	$22.50	GENERIC, Parmed Pharmaceuticals Inc	00349-8859-01
100's	$25.73	ROXICET, Roxane Laboratories Inc	00054-4650-25
100's	$27.90	GENERIC, Aligen Independent Laboratories Inc	00405-0139-01
100's	$30.14	ROXICET, Roxane Laboratories Inc	00054-8650-24
100's	$30.14	GENERIC, Endo Laboratories Llc	60951-0602-75
100's	$31.05	GENERIC, Mallinckrodt Medical Inc	00406-0512-01
100's	$31.05	GENERIC, Endo Laboratories Llc	60951-0602-70
100's	$32.00	GENERIC, Amide Pharmaceutical Inc	52152-0075-02
100's	$51.23	GENERIC, Watson Laboratories Inc	00591-0749-01
100's	$51.23	GENERIC, Qualitest Products Inc	00603-4998-21
100's	$51.23	GENERIC, Watson Laboratories Inc	52544-0749-01
100's	$70.13	PERCOCET-5/325, Dupont Pharmaceuticals	00590-0127-75

100's	$83.75	PERCOCET-5/325, Dupont Pharmaceuticals	00590-0127-70
100's	$90.44	PERCOCET-5/325, Endo Laboratories Llc	63481-0127-70
100's	$120.00	PERCOCET-5/325, Endo Laboratories Llc	63481-0623-70
Tablet - Oral - 500 mg;7.5 mg			
100's	$113.25	GENERIC, Endo Laboratories Llc	60951-0796-70
Tablet - Oral - 650 mg;10 mg			
100's	$148.10	GENERIC, Endo Laboratories Llc	60951-0797-70
100's	$181.00	PERCOCET-10/650, Endo Laboratories Llc	63481-0622-70

PRODUCT LISTING - EQUIVALENTS NOT AVAILABLE

Solution - Oral - 325 mg;5 mg/5 ml			
5 ml x 40	$44.55	ROXICET, Roxane Laboratories Inc	00054-8648-16
500 ml	$37.37	ROXICET, Roxane Laboratories Inc	00054-3686-63
Tablet - Oral - 325 mg;2.5 mg			
100's	$55.56	PERCOCET-2.5/325, Endo Laboratories Llc	63481-0627-75
100's	$75.88	PERCOCET-2.5/325, Endo Laboratories Llc	63481-0627-70
Tablet - Oral - 325 mg;7.5 mg			
100's	$129.63	PERCOCET 7.5/325, Endo Laboratories Llc	63481-0628-70
100's	$129.64	PERCOCET 7.5/325, Endo Laboratories Llc	63481-0628-75
Tablet - Oral - 325 mg;10 mg			
100's	$169.50	PERCOCET-10/325, Endo Laboratories Llc	63481-0629-70
100's	$169.52	PERCOCET-10/325, Endo Laboratories Llc	63481-0629-75
Tablet - Oral - 500 mg;5 mg			
100's	$57.60	ROXICET, Roxane Laboratories Inc	00054-4784-25
100's	$63.42	ROXICET, Roxane Laboratories Inc	00054-8784-24
Tablet - Oral - 500 mg;7.5 mg			
100's	$96.88	PERCOCET-7.5/500, Endo Laboratories Llc	63481-0621-75
100's	$105.30	GENERIC, Watson Laboratories Inc	00591-0824-01
100's	$105.30	GENERIC, Watson/Rugby Laboratories Inc	52544-0824-01
100's	$138.44	PERCOCET-7.5/500, Endo Laboratories Llc	63481-0621-70
Tablet - Oral - 650 mg;10 mg			
100's	$137.68	GENERIC, Watson Laboratories Inc	00591-0825-01
100's	$137.68	GENERIC, Watson/Rugby Laboratories Inc	52544-0825-01
100's	$162.72	PERCOCET-10/650, Endo Laboratories Llc	63481-0622-75

Acetaminophen; Propoxyphene Napsylate *(000082)*

Categories: Pain, mild to moderate; DEA Class CIV; FDA Approval Pre 1982; Pregnancy Category C
Drug Classes: Analgesics, narcotic
Brand Names: **Darvocet-N**; Dologesic; Propacet
Foreign Brand Availability: Distalgesic (Hong-Kong; South-Africa); Dologesic-32 (Hong-Kong); Dolostop (Bahrain; Benin; Burkina-Faso; Ethiopia; Gambia; Ghana; Guinea; Iraq; Ivory-Coast; Jordan; Kenya; Liberia; Malawi; Mali; Mauritania; Mauritius; Morocco; Niger; Nigeria; Senegal; Seychelles; Sierra-Leone; South-Africa; Sudan; Tanzania; Tunia; Uganda; Zambia; Zimbabwe)
Cost of Therapy: $13.69 (Pain; Darvocet-N 100; 650 mg; 100 mg; 4 tablets/day; 7 day supply)
$3.57 (Pain; Generic Tablets; 650 mg; 100 mg; 4 tablets/day; 7 day supply)

DESCRIPTION

Propoxyphene napsylate is an odorless, white, crystalline powder with a bitter taste. It is very slightly soluble in water and soluble in methanol, ethanol, chloroform, and acetone. Chemically, it is (αS,1R)-α-[2-(Dimethylamino)-1-methylethyl]-α-phenylphenethyl propionate compound with 2-naphthalenesulfonic acid (1:1) monohydrate. Its molecular weight is 565.72.

Propoxyphene napsylate differs from propoxyphene hydrochloride in that it allows more stable liquid dosage forms and tablet formulations. Because of differences in molecular weight, a dose of 100 mg (176.8 μmol) of propoxyphene napsylate is required to supply an amount of propoxyphene equivalent to that present in 65 mg (172.9 μmol) of propoxyphene hydrochloride.

Each Darvocet-N 50 tablet contains 50 mg (88.4 μmol) propoxyphene napsylate and 325 mg (2,150 μmol) acetaminophen.

Each Darvocet-N 100 tablet contains 100 mg (176.8 μmol) propoxyphene napsylate and 650 mg (4300 μmol) acetaminophen.

Each tablet also contains amberlite, cellulose, FD&C yellow no. 6, magnesium stearate, stearic acid, titanium dioxide, and other inactive ingredients.

Storage: Store at controlled room temperature, 15-30°C (59- 86°F).

CLINICAL PHARMACOLOGY

Propoxyphene is a centrally acting narcotic analgesic agent. Equimolar doses of propoxyphene HCl or napsylate provide similar plasma concentrations. Following administration of 65, 130, or 195 mg of propoxyphene HCl, the bioavailability of propoxyphene is equivalent to that of 100, 200, or 300 mg respectively of propoxyphene napsylate. Peak plasma concentrations of propoxyphene are reached in 2 to 2 ½ hours. After a 100 mg oral dose of propoxyphene napsylate, peak plasma levels of 0.05 to 0.1 μg/ml are achieved. The napsylate salt tends to be absorbed more slowly than the HCl. At or near therapeutic doses, this absorption difference is small when compared with that among subjects and among doses.

Because of this several hundredfold difference in solubility, the absorption rate of very large doses of the napsylate salt is significantly lower than that of equimolar doses of the HCl.

Repeated doses of propoxyphene at 6 hour intervals lead to increasing plasma concentrations with a plateau after the ninth dose at 48 hours.

Propoxyphene is metabolized in the liver to yield norpropoxyphene. Propoxyphene has a half-life of 6-12 hours, whereas that of norpropoxyphene is 30-36 hours.

Norpropoxyphene has substantially less central-nervous-system-depressant effect than propoxyphene but a greater local anesthetic effect, which is similar to that of amitriptyline and antiarrhythmic agents, such as lidocaine and quinidine.

In animal studies in which propoxyphene and norpropoxyphene were continuously infused in large amounts, intracardiac conduction time (PR and QRS intervals) was prolonged. Any intracardiac conduction delay attributable to high concentrations of norpropoxyphene may be of relatively long duration.

Propoxyphene is a mild narcotic analgesic structurally related to methadone. The potency of propoxyphene napsylate is from two thirds to equal that of codeine.

Propoxyphene napsylate and acetaminophen tablets provide the analgesic activity of propoxyphene napsylate and the antipyretic-analgesic activity of acetaminophen.

The combination of propoxyphene and acetaminophen produces greater analgesia than that produced by either propoxyphene or acetaminophen administered alone.

INDICATIONS AND USAGE

These products are indicated for the relief of mild to moderate pain, either when pain is present alone or when it is accompanied by fever.

CONTRAINDICATIONS

Hypersensitivity to propoxyphene or acetaminophen.

WARNINGS

Do not prescribe propoxyphene for patients who are suicidal or addiction-prone.

Prescribe propoxyphene with caution for patients taking tranquilizers or antidepressant drugs and patients who use alcohol in excess.

Tell your patients not to exceed the recommended dose and to limit their intake of alcohol.

Propoxyphene products in excessive doses, either alone or in combination with other CNS depressants, including alcohol, are a major cause of drug-related deaths. Fatalities within the first hour of overdosage are not uncommon. In a survey of deaths due to overdosage conducted in 1975, death occurred within the first hour in approximately 20% of the fatal cases (5% occurred within 15 minutes). Propoxyphene should not be taken in doses higher than those recommended by the physician. The judicious prescribing of propoxyphene is essential to the safe use of this drug. With patients who are depressed or suicidal, consideration should be given to the use of non-narcotic analgesics. Patients should be cautioned about the concomitant use of propoxyphene products and alcohol because of potentially serious CNS-additive effects of these agents. Because of its added depressant effects, propoxyphene should be prescribed with caution for patients whose medical condition requires the concomitant administration of sedatives, tranquilizers, muscle relaxants, antidepressants, or other CNS-depressant drugs. Patients should be advised of the additive depressant effects of these combinations. Many of the propoxyphene-related deaths have occurred in patients with previous histories of emotional disturbances or suicidal ideation or attempts as well as histories of misuse of tranquilizers, alcohol, and other CNS-active drugs. Some deaths have occurred as a consequence of the accidental ingestion of excessive quantities of propoxyphene alone or in combination with other drugs. Patients taking propoxyphene should be warned not to exceed the dosage recommended by the physician.

Usage in Ambulatory Patients: Propoxyphene may impair the mental and/or physical abilities required for the performance of potentially hazardous tasks, such as driving a car or operating machinery. The patient should be cautioned accordingly.

PRECAUTIONS

GENERAL

Propoxyphene should be administered with caution to patients with hepatic or renal impairment since higher serum concentrations or delayed elimination may occur.

PREGNANCY

Safe use in pregnancy has not been established relative to possible adverse effects on fetal development. Instances of withdrawal symptoms in the neonate have been reported following usage during pregnancy. Therefore, propoxyphene should not be used in pregnant women unless, in the judgment of the physician, the potential benefits outweigh the possible hazards.

NURSING MOTHERS

Low levels of propoxyphene have been detected in human milk. In postpartum studies involving nursing mothers who were given propoxyphene, no adverse effects were noted in infants receiving mother's milk.

PEDIATRIC USE

Propoxyphene is not recommended for use in children, because documented clinical experience has been insufficient to establish safety and a suitable dosage regimen in the pediatric age group.

GERIATRIC USE

The rate of propoxyphene metabolism may be reduced in some patients. Increased dosing interval should be considered.

A patient information sheet is available for this product.

DRUG INTERACTIONS

The CNS-depressant effect of propoxyphene is additive with that of other CNS depressants, including alcohol.

As is the case with many medicinal agents, propoxyphene may slow the metabolism of a concomitantly administered drug. Should this occur, the higher serum concentrations of that drug may result in increased pharmacologic or adverse effects of that drug. Such occurrences have been reported when propoxyphene was administered to patients taking antidepressants, anticonvulsants, or warfarin-like drugs. Severe neurologic signs, including coma, have occurred with concurrent use of carbamazepine.

A

ADVERSE REACTIONS

In a survey conducted in hospitalized patients, less than 1% of patients taking propoxyphene HCl at recommended doses experienced side effects. The most frequently reported were dizziness, sedation, nausea, and vomiting. Some of these adverse reactions may be alleviated if the patient lies down.

Other adverse reactions include constipation, abdominal pain, skin rashes, lightheadedness, headache, weakness, euphoria, dysphoria, hallucinations, and minor visual disturbances.

Liver dysfunction has been reported in association with both active components of propoxyphene napsylate and acetaminophen tablets, USP. Propoxyphene therapy has been associated with abnormal liver function tests and more rarely with instances of reversible jaundice (including cholestatic jaundice). Hepatic necrosis may result from acute overdose of acetaminophen. In chronic ethanol abusers, this has been reported rarely with short-term use of acetaminophen dosages of 2.5 to 10 g/day. Fatalities have occurred.

Renal papillary necrosis may result from chronic acetaminophen use, particularly when the dosage is greater than recommended and when combined with aspirin.

Subacute painful myopathy has occurred following chronic propoxyphene overdosage.

DOSAGE AND ADMINISTRATION

These products are given orally. The usual dosage is 100 mg propoxyphene napsylate and 650 mg acetaminophen every 4 hours as needed for pain. The maximum recommended dose of propoxyphene napsylate is 600 mg per day.

Consideration should be given to a reduced total daily dosage in patients with hepatic or renal impairment.

ANIMAL PHARMACOLOGY

The acute lethal doses of the HCl and napsylate salts of propoxyphene were determined in 4 species. The results shown in TABLE 1 indicate that on a molar basis the napsylate salt is less toxic than the HCl. This may be due to the relative insolubility and retarded absorption of propoxyphene napsylate.

TABLE 1 *Acute Oral Toxicity of Propoxyphene*

	LD_{50} (mg/kg) ± SE LD_{50} (mmol/kg)	
Species	**Propoxyphene HCl**	**Propoxyphene Napsylate**
Mouse	282 ± 39 0.75	915 ± 163 1.62
Rat	230 ± 44 0.61	647 ± 95 1.14
Rabbit	ca. 82 0.22	>183 >0.32
Dog	ca. 100 0.27	>183 >0.32

Some indication of the relative insolubility and retarded absorption of propoxyphene napsylate was obtained by measuring plasma propoxyphene levels in 2 groups of 4 dogs following oral administration of equimolar doses of the 2 salts. The peak plasma concentration observed with propoxyphene HCl was much higher than that obtained after administration of the napsylate salt.

Although none of the animals in this experiment died, 3 of the 4 dogs given propoxyphene HCl exhibited convulsive seizures during the time interval corresponding to the peak plasma levels. The 4 animals receiving the napsylate salt were mildly ataxic but not acutely ill.

PRODUCT LISTING - RATED THERAPEUTICALLY EQUIVALENT

Tablet - Oral - Hydrochloride 650 mg;65 mg

100's	$16.75	GENERIC, Major Pharmaceuticals Inc	00904-2171-60
100's	$19.40	GENERIC, Qualitest Products Inc	00603-5463-21
100's	$22.50	GENERIC, Interstate Drug Exchange Inc	00814-6464-14
100's	$28.95	GENERIC, Mylan Pharmaceuticals Inc	00378-0130-01
100's	$28.99	GENERIC, Watson Laboratories Inc	52544-0714-01
100's	$30.40	GENERIC, Watson Laboratories Inc	00591-0714-01
100's	$31.30	GENERIC, Geneva Pharmaceuticals	00781-1378-13
100's	$34.78	GENERIC, Udl Laboratories Inc	51079-0741-20
100's	$35.50	GENERIC, Major Pharmaceuticals Inc	00904-2171-61

Tablet - Oral - Napsylate 325 mg;50 mg

100's	$11.25	GENERIC, Interstate Drug Exchange Inc	00814-6453-14
100's	$41.42	GENERIC, Qualitest Products Inc	00603-5465-21
100's	$48.89	DARVOCET N 50, Lilly, Eli and Company	00002-0351-02

Tablet - Oral - Napsylate 650 mg;100 mg

15 x 6	$60.00	GENERIC, Udl Laboratories Inc	51079-0934-99
30's	$4.87	GENERIC, Med-Pro Inc	53978-5013-05
30's	$6.25	GENERIC, Golden State Medical	60429-0518-30
30's	$25.25	GENERIC, Major Pharmaceuticals Inc	00904-2280-60
31 x 10	$118.35	GENERIC, Vangard Labs	00615-0455-63
60's	$11.23	GENERIC, Golden State Medical	60429-0518-60
60's	$66.70	GENERIC, Ivax Corporation	00172-4980-60
100's	$12.75	GENERIC, Interstate Drug Exchange Inc	00814-6452-14
100's	$12.75	GENERIC, Interstate Drug Exchange Inc	00814-6454-14
100's	$24.53	GENERIC, Aligen Independent Laboratories Inc	00405-0178-01
100's	$33.75	GENERIC, Moore, H.L. Drug Exchange Inc	00839-7330-06
100's	$38.97	GENERIC, Auro Pharmaceutical	55829-0866-10
100's	$50.90	GENERIC, Qualitest Products Inc	00603-5466-21
100's	$50.90	GENERIC, Qualitest Products Inc	00603-5467-21
100's	$50.90	GENERIC, Qualitest Products Inc	00603-5468-21
100's	$51.95	GENERIC, Ivax Corporation	00182-0317-89
100's	$53.50	GENERIC, Mallinckrodt Medical Inc	00406-1721-01
100's	$53.50	GENERIC, Mallinckrodt Medical Inc	00406-1772-01
100's	$54.49	GENERIC, Purepac Pharmaceutical Company	00228-2085-10
100's	$54.50	GENERIC, Teva Pharmaceuticals Usa	00093-0490-01
100's	$54.50	GENERIC, Teva Pharmaceuticals Usa	00093-0890-01
100's	$54.90	GENERIC, Major Pharmaceuticals Inc	00904-2281-60
100's	$55.00	GENERIC, Able Laboratories Inc	53265-0256-10
100's	$55.00	GENERIC, Able Laboratories Inc	53265-0261-10
100's	$56.14	GENERIC, Udl Laboratories Inc	51079-0934-20
100's	$56.14	GENERIC, Udl Laboratories Inc	51079-0934-21
100's	$60.25	GENERIC, Mylan Pharmaceuticals Inc	00378-0155-01
100's	$66.69	GENERIC, Vintage Pharmaceuticals Inc	00254-5112-28
100's	$66.69	GENERIC, Vintage Pharmaceuticals Inc	00254-5113-28
100's	$66.69	GENERIC, Vintage Pharmaceuticals Inc	00254-5114-28
100's	$92.24	DARVOCET N 100, Lilly, Eli and Company	00002-0363-02
100's	$99.54	DARVOCET N 100, Lilly, Eli and Company	00002-0363-33

Tablet - Oral - 650 mg;100 mg

100's	$22.50	FEDERAL UPPER LIMIT, H.C.F.A. F F P	99999-0082-02

PRODUCT LISTING - EQUIVALENTS NOT AVAILABLE

Tablet - Oral - Hydrochloride 650 mg;65 mg

12's	$5.44	GENERIC, Southwood Pharmaceuticals Inc	58016-0279-12
20's	$4.30	GENERIC, Allscripts Pharmaceutical Company	54569-2588-00
20's	$7.59	GENERIC, Southwood Pharmaceuticals Inc	58016-0279-20
30's	$6.29	GENERIC, Pd-Rx Pharmaceuticals	55289-0321-30
30's	$6.45	GENERIC, Allscripts Pharmaceutical Company	54569-2588-01
30's	$8.40	GENERIC, Pharma Pac	52959-0165-30
100's	$16.74	GENERIC, Physicians Total Care	54868-3646-00

Tablet - Oral - Napsylate 650 mg;100 mg

2's	$3.54	GENERIC, Prescript Pharmaceuticals	00247-0086-02
3's	$3.64	GENERIC, Prescript Pharmaceuticals	00247-0086-03
4's	$3.73	GENERIC, Prescript Pharmaceuticals	00247-0086-04
5's	$3.81	GENERIC, Prescript Pharmaceuticals	00247-0086-05
6's	$3.91	GENERIC, Prescript Pharmaceuticals	00247-0086-06
8's	$4.09	GENERIC, Prescript Pharmaceuticals	00247-0086-08
8's	$5.34	GENERIC, Southwood Pharmaceuticals Inc	58016-0212-08
10's	$4.28	GENERIC, Prescript Pharmaceuticals	00247-0086-10
10's	$6.68	GENERIC, Southwood Pharmaceuticals Inc	58016-0212-10
12's	$4.47	GENERIC, Prescript Pharmaceuticals	00247-0086-12
12's	$8.01	GENERIC, Southwood Pharmaceuticals Inc	58016-0212-12
14's	$9.35	GENERIC, Southwood Pharmaceuticals Inc	58016-0212-14
15's	$4.74	GENERIC, Prescript Pharmaceuticals	00247-0086-15
15's	$10.01	GENERIC, Southwood Pharmaceuticals Inc	58016-0212-15
16's	$4.84	GENERIC, Prescript Pharmaceuticals	00247-0086-16
16's	$10.68	GENERIC, Southwood Pharmaceuticals Inc	58016-0212-16
18's	$12.02	GENERIC, Southwood Pharmaceuticals Inc	58016-0212-18
20's	$5.21	GENERIC, Prescript Pharmaceuticals	00247-0086-20
20's	$13.35	GENERIC, Southwood Pharmaceuticals Inc	58016-0212-20
21's	$14.02	GENERIC, Southwood Pharmaceuticals Inc	58016-0212-21
24's	$5.58	GENERIC, Prescript Pharmaceuticals	00247-0086-24
24's	$16.02	GENERIC, Southwood Pharmaceuticals Inc	58016-0212-24
25's	$5.67	GENERIC, Prescript Pharmaceuticals	00247-0086-25
28's	$5.95	GENERIC, Prescript Pharmaceuticals	00247-0086-28
28's	$18.69	GENERIC, Southwood Pharmaceuticals Inc	58016-0212-28
30's	$6.13	GENERIC, Prescript Pharmaceuticals	00247-0086-30
30's	$20.03	GENERIC, Southwood Pharmaceuticals Inc	58016-0212-30
36's	$24.03	GENERIC, Southwood Pharmaceuticals Inc	58016-0212-36
40's	$7.06	GENERIC, Prescript Pharmaceuticals	00247-0086-40
40's	$26.70	GENERIC, Southwood Pharmaceuticals Inc	58016-0212-40
42's	$28.04	GENERIC, Southwood Pharmaceuticals Inc	58016-0212-42
45's	$7.52	GENERIC, Prescript Pharmaceuticals	00247-0086-45
45's	$30.04	GENERIC, Southwood Pharmaceuticals Inc	58016-0212-45
50's	$33.38	GENERIC, Southwood Pharmaceuticals Inc	58016-0212-50
56's	$37.38	GENERIC, Southwood Pharmaceuticals Inc	58016-0212-56
60's	$8.92	GENERIC, Prescript Pharmaceuticals	00247-0086-60
60's	$40.05	GENERIC, Southwood Pharmaceuticals Inc	58016-0212-60
60's	$52.20	GENERIC, Pharma Pac	52959-0335-60
80's	$53.41	GENERIC, Southwood Pharmaceuticals Inc	58016-0212-80
90's	$60.08	GENERIC, Southwood Pharmaceuticals Inc	58016-0212-90
100's	$12.62	GENERIC, Prescript Pharmaceuticals	00247-0086-00
100's	$66.75	GENERIC, Southwood Pharmaceuticals Inc	58016-0212-00
120's	$80.10	GENERIC, Southwood Pharmaceuticals Inc	58016-0212-02

Acetaminophen; Tramadol Hydrochloride (003528)

Categories: Pain; Pregnancy Category C; FDA Approved 2001 Aug
Drug Classes: Analgesics, narcotic-like; Analgesics, non-narcotic
Brand Names: Ultracet
Cost of Therapy: $39.08 (Pain; Ultracet; 325 mg; 37.5 mg; 8 tablets/day; 5 day supply)

DESCRIPTION

Note: The trade name has been used throughout this monograph for clarity.

Ultracet (37.5 mg tramadol hydrochloride/325 mg acetaminophen tablets) combines two analgesics, tramadol and acetaminophen.

The chemical name for tramadol hydrochloride is (±)*cis*-2-[(dimethylamino)methyl]-1-(3-methoxyphenyl) cyclohexanol hydrochloride.

The molecular weight of tramadol hydrochloride is 299.84. Tramadol hydrochloride is a white, bitter, crystalline and odorless powder.

The chemical name for acetaminophen is *N*-acetyl-*p*-aminophenol.

The molecular weight of acetaminophen is 151.17.

Acetaminophen is an analgesic and antipyretic agent which occurs as a white, odorless, crystalline powder, possessing a slightly bitter taste.

Ultracet tablets contain 37.5 mg tramadol hydrochloride and 325 mg acetaminophen and are light yellow in color. Inactive ingredients in the tablet are powdered cellulose, pregelatinized starch, sodium starch glycolate, starch, purified water, magnesium stearate, Opadry Light Yellow, and carnauba wax.

CLINICAL PHARMACOLOGY

The following information is based on studies of tramadol alone or acetaminophen alone, except where otherwise noted:

PHARMACODYNAMICS

Tramadol is a centrally acting synthetic opioid analgesic. Although its mode of action is not completely understood, from animal tests, at least two complementary mechanisms appear applicable: binding of parent and M1 metabolite to μ-opioid receptors and weak inhibition of reuptake of norepinephrine and serotonin.

Opioid activity is due to both low affinity binding of the parent compound and higher affinity binding of the O-demethylated metabolite M1 to μ-opioid receptors. In animal models, M1 is up to 6 times more potent than tramadol in producing analgesia and 200 times more potent in μ-opioid binding. Tramadol-induced analgesia is only partially antagonized by the opiate antagonist naloxone in several animal tests. The relative contribution of both tramadol and M1 to human analgesia is dependent upon the plasma concentrations of each compound (see Pharmacokinetics).

Tramadol has been shown to inhibit reuptake of norepinephrine and serotonin *in vitro*, as have some other opioid analgesics. These mechanisms may contribute independently to the overall analgesic profile of tramadol.

Apart from analgesia, tramadol administration may produce a constellation of symptoms (including dizziness, somnolence, nausea, constipation, sweating and pruritus) similar to that of other opioids.

Acetaminophen is a non-opiate, non-salicylate analgesic.

PHARMACOKINETICS

Tramadol is administered as a racemate and both the [−] and [+] forms of both tramadol and M1 are detected in the circulation. The pharmacokinetics of plasma tramadol and acetaminophen following oral administration of 1 Ultracet tablet are shown in TABLE 1. Tramadol has a slower absorption and longer half-life when compared to acetaminophen.

TABLE 1 *Summary of Mean (±SD) Pharmacokinetic Parameters of the (+)− and (−) Enantiomers of Tramadol and M1 and Acetaminophen Following a Single Oral Dose of 1 Tramadol/Acetaminophen Combination Tablet*

	Parameter*			
	C_{max} (ng/ml)	T_{max} (h)	CL/F (ml/min)	$T_{1/2}$ (h)
(+)−Tramadol	64.3 (9.3)	1.8 (0.6)	588 (226)	5.1 (1.4)
(−)−Tramadol	55.5 (8.1)	1.8 (0.7)	736 (244)	4.7 (1.2)
(+)−M1	10.9 (5.7)	2.1 (0.7)	—	7.8 (3.0)
(−)−M1	12.8 (4.2)	2.2 (0.7)	—	6.2 (1.6)
Acetaminophen	4.2 (0.8)	0.9 (0.7)	365 (84)	2.5 (0.6)

* For acetaminophen, C_{max} was measured as μg/ml.

A single dose pharmacokinetic study of Ultracet in volunteers showed no drug interactions between tramadol and acetaminophen. Upon multiple oral dosing to steady state, however, the bioavailability of tramadol and metabolite M1 was lower for the combination tablets compared to tramadol administered alone. The decrease in AUC was 14% for (+)−tramadol, 10.4% for (−)−tramadol, 11.9% for (+)−M1 and 24.2% for (−)−M1. The cause of this reduced bioavailability is not clear. Following single or multiple dose administration of Ultracet, no significant change in acetaminophen pharmacokinetics was observed when compared to acetaminophen given alone.

Absorption

The absolute bioavailability of tramadol from Ultracet tablets has not been determined. Tramadol HCl has a mean absolute bioavailability of approximately 75% following administration of a single 100 mg oral dose of Ultram (tramadol HCl) tablets. The mean peak plasma concentration of racemic tramadol and M1 after administration of 2 Ultracet tablets occurs at approximately 2 and 3 hours, respectively, post-dose.

Peak plasma concentrations of acetaminophen occur within 1 hour and are not affected by coadministration with tramadol. Oral absorption of acetaminophen following administration of Ultracet occurs primarily in the small intestine.

Food Effects

When Ultracet was administered with food, the time to peak plasma concentration was delayed for approximately 35 minutes for tramadol and almost 1 hour for acetaminophen. However, peak plasma concentration or the extent of absorption of either tramadol or acetaminophen were not affected. The clinical significance of this difference is unknown.

Distribution

The volume of distribution of tramadol was 2.6 and 2.9 L/kg in male and female subjects, respectively, following a 100 mg intravenous dose. The binding of tramadol to human plasma proteins is approximately 20% and binding also appears to be independent of concentration up to 10 μg/ml. Saturation of plasma protein binding occurs only at concentrations outside the clinically relevant range.

Acetaminophen appears to be widely distributed throughout most body tissues except fat. Its apparent volume of distribution is about 0.9 L/kg. A relative small portion (~20%) of acetaminophen is bound to plasma protein.

Metabolism

Following oral administration, tramadol is extensively metabolized by a number of pathways, including CYP2D6 and CYP3A4, as well as by conjugation of parent and metabolites. Approximately 30% of the dose is excreted in the urine as unchanged drug, whereas 60% of the dose is excreted as metabolites. The major metabolic pathways appear to be *N*- and *O*-demethylation and glucuronidation or sulfation in the liver. Metabolite M1 (*O*-desmethyltramadol) is pharmacologically active in animal models. Formation of M1 is dependent on CYP2D6 and as such is subject to inhibition, which may affect the therapeutic response (see DRUG INTERACTIONS).

Approximately 7% of the population has reduced activity of the CYP2D6 isoenzyme of cytochrome P450. These individuals are "poor metabolizers" of debrisoquine, dextromethorphan, tricyclic antidepressants, among other drugs. Based on a population PK analysis of Phase 1 studies in healthy subjects, concentrations of tramadol were approximately 20% higher in "poor metabolizers" versus "extensive metabolizers", while M1 concentrations were 40% lower. *In vitro* drug interaction studies in human liver microsomes indicates that inhibitors of CYP2D6 such as fluoxetine and its metabolite norfluoxetine, amitriptyline and quinidine inhibit the metabolism of tramadol to various degrees. The full pharmacological impact of these alterations in terms of either efficacy or safety is unknown. Concomitant use of SEROTONIN re-uptake INHIBITORS and MAO INHIBITORS may enhance the risk of adverse events, including seizure (see WARNINGS) and serotonin syndrome.

Acetaminophen is primarily metabolized in the liver by first-order kinetics and involves 3 principal separate pathways:

(a) Conjugation with glucuronide;

(b) Conjugation with sulfate; and

(c) Oxidation via the cytochrome, P450-dependent, mixed-function oxidase enzyme pathway to form a reactive intermediate metabolite, which conjugates with glutathione and is then further metabolized to form cysteine and mercapturic acid conjugates. The principal cytochrome P450 isoenzyme involved appears to be CYP2E1, with CYP1A2 and CYP3A4 as additional pathways.

In adults, the majority of acetaminophen is conjugated with glucuronic acid and, to a lesser extent, with sulfate. These glucuronide-, sulfate-, and glutathione-derived metabolites lack biologic activity. In premature infants, newborns, and young infants, the sulfate conjugate predominates.

Elimination

Tramadol is eliminated primarily through metabolism by the liver and the metabolites are eliminated primarily by the kidneys. The plasma elimination half-lives of racemic tramadol and M1 are approximately 5-6 and 7 hours, respectively, after administration of Ultracet. The apparent plasma elimination half-life of racemic tramadol increased to 7-9 hours upon multiple dosing of Ultracet.

The half-life of acetaminophen is about 2-3 hours in adults. It is somewhat shorter in children and somewhat longer in neonates and in cirrhotic patients. Acetaminophen is eliminated from the body primarily by formation of glucuronide and sulfate conjugates in a dose-dependent manner. Less than 9% of acetaminophen is excreted unchanged in the urine.

SPECIAL POPULATIONS

Renal

The pharmacokinetics of Ultracet in patients with renal impairment have not been studied. Based on studies using tramadol alone, excretion of tramadol and metabolite M1 is reduced in patients with creatinine clearance of less than 30 ml/min, adjustment of dosing regimen in this patient population is recommended. (See DOSAGE AND ADMINISTRATION.) The total amount of tramadol and M1 removed during a 4 hour dialysis period is less than 7% of the administered dose based on studies using tramadol alone.

Hepatic

The pharmacokinetics and tolerability of Ultracet in patients with impaired hepatic function has not been studied. Since tramadol and acetaminophen are both extensively metabolized by the liver, the use of Ultracet in patients with hepatic impairment is not recommended (see PRECAUTIONS and DOSAGE AND ADMINISTRATION).

Geriatric

A population pharmacokinetic analysis of data obtained from a clinical trial in patients with chronic pain treated with Ultracet which included 55 patients between 65 and 75 years of age and 19 patients over 75 years of age, showed no significant changes in pharmacokinetics of tramadol and acetaminophen in elderly patients with normal renal and hepatic function (see PRECAUTIONS, Geriatric Use).

Gender

Tramadol clearance was 20% higher in female subjects compared to males on four Phase 1 studies of Ultracet in 50 male and 34 female healthy subjects. The clinical significance of this difference is unknown.

Pediatric

Pharmacokinetics of Ultracet tablets have not been studied in pediatric patients below 16 years of age.

INDICATIONS AND USAGE

Ultracet is indicated for the short-term (5 days or less) management of acute pain.

CONTRAINDICATIONS

Ultracet should not be administered to patients who have previously demonstrated hypersensitivity to tramadol, acetaminophen, any other component of this product or opioids. Ultracet is contraindicated in any situation where opioids are contraindicated, including acute intoxication with any of the following: alcohol, hypnotics, narcotics, centrally acting analgesics, opioids or psychotropic drugs. Ultracet may worsen central nervous system and respiratory depression in these patients.

WARNINGS

SEIZURE RISK

Seizures have been reported in patients receiving tramadol within the recommended dosage range. Spontaneous post-marketing reports indicate that seizure risk is increased with doses of tramadol above the recommended range. Concomitant use of tramadol increases the seizure risk in patients taking:

- **Selective serotonin reuptake inhibitors (SSRI antidepressants or anoretics),**
- **Tricyclic antidepressants (TCAs), and other tricyclic compounds (*e.g.*, cyclobenzaprine, promethazine, etc.), or**
- **Other opioids.**

Administration of tramadol may enhance the seizure risk in patients taking:

- **MAO inhibitors (see also Use With MAO Inhibitors and Serotonin Re-Uptake Inhibitor),**
- **Neuroleptics, or**
- **Other drugs that reduce the seizure threshold.**

Risk of convulsions may also increase in patients with epilepsy, those with a history of seizures, or in patients with a recognized risk for seizure (such as head trauma, metabolic disorders, alcohol and drug withdrawal, CNS infections). In tramadol overdose, naloxone administration may increase the risk of seizure.

ANAPHYLACTOID REACTIONS

Serious and rarely fatal anaphylactoid reactions have been reported in patients receiving therapy with tramadol. When these events do occur it is often following the first dose. Other reported allergic reactions include pruritus, hives, bronchospasm, angioedema, toxic epidermal necrolysis and Stevens-Johnson syndrome. Patients with a history of anaphylactoid reactions to codeine and other opioids may be at increased risk and therefore should not receive Ultracet (see CONTRAINDICATIONS).

RESPIRATORY DEPRESSION

Administer Ultracet cautiously in patients at risk for respiratory depression. In these patients, alternative non-opioid analgesics should be considered. When large doses of tramadol are administered with anesthetic medications or alcohol, respiratory depression may result. Respiratory depression should be treated as an overdose. If naloxone is to be administered, use cautiously because it may precipitate seizures (see Seizure Risk).

INTERACTION WITH CENTRAL NERVOUS SYSTEM (CNS) DEPRESSANTS

Ultracet should be used with caution and in reduced dosages when administered to patients receiving CNS depressants such as alcohol, opioids, anesthetic agents, narcotics, phenothiazines, tranquilizers or sedative hypnotics. Tramadol increases the risk of CNS and respiratory depression in these patients.

INCREASED INTRACRANIAL PRESSURE OR HEAD TRAUMA

Ultracet should be used with caution in patients with increased intracranial pressure or head injury. The respiratory depressant effects of opioids include carbon dioxide retention and secondary elevation of cerebrospinal fluid pressure and may be markedly exaggerated in these patients. Additionally, pupillary changes (miosis) from tramadol may obscure the existence, extent, or course of intracranial pathology. Clinicians should also maintain a high index of suspicion for adverse drug reaction when evaluating altered mental status in these patients if they are receiving Ultracet (see Respiratory Depression).

USE IN AMBULATORY PATIENTS

Tramadol may impair the mental and or physical abilities required for the performance of potentially hazardous tasks such as driving a car or operating machinery. The patient using this drug should be cautioned accordingly.

USE WITH MAO INHIBITORS AND SEROTONIN RE-UPTAKE INHIBITORS

Use Ultracet with great caution in patients taking monoamine oxidase inhibitors. Animal studies have shown increased deaths with combined administration of MAO inhibitors and tramadol. Concomitant use of tramadol with MAO inhibitors or SSRIs increases the risk of adverse events, including seizure and serotonin syndrome.

USE WITH ALCOHOL

Ultracet should not be used concomitantly with alcohol consumption. The use of Ultracet in patients with liver disease is not recommended.

USE WITH OTHER ACETAMINOPHEN-CONTAINING PRODUCTS

Due to the potential for acetaminophen hepatotoxicity at doses higher than the recommended dose, Ultracet should not be used concomitantly with other acetaminophen-containing products.

WITHDRAWAL

Withdrawal symptoms may occur if Ultracet is discontinued abruptly. These symptoms may include: anxiety, sweating, insomnia, rigors, pain, nausea, tremors, diarrhea, upper respiratory symptoms, piloerection, and rarely hallucinations. Clinical experience suggests that withdrawal symptoms may be relieved by tapering the medication.

PHYSICAL DEPENDENCE AND ABUSE

Tramadol may induce psychic and physical dependence of the morphine-type (μ-opioid). Tramadol should not be used in opioid-dependent patients. Tramadol has been shown to reinitiate physical dependence in some patients that have been previously dependent on other opioids. Dependence and abuse, including drug-seeking behavior and taking illicit actions to obtain the drug are not limited to those patients with prior history of opioid dependence.

RISK OF OVERDOSAGE

Serious potential consequences of overdosage with tramadol are central nervous system depression, respiratory depression and death. In treating an overdose, primary attention should be given to maintaining adequate ventilation along with general supportive treatment.

Serious potential consequences of overdosage with acetaminophen are hepatic (centrilobular) necrosis, leading to hepatic failure and death. Emergency help should be sought immediately and treatment initiated immediately if overdose is suspected, even if symptoms are not apparent.

PRECAUTIONS

GENERAL

The recommended dose of Ultracet should not be exceeded.

Do not coadminister Ultracet with other tramadol or acetaminophen-containing products. (See WARNINGS: Use With Other Acetaminophen-Containing Products and Risk of Overdosage.)

PEDIATRIC USE

The safety and effectiveness of Ultracet has not been studied in the pediatric population.

GERIATRIC USE

In general, dose selection for an elderly patient should be cautious, reflecting the greater frequency of decreased hepatic, renal, or cardiac function; of concomitant disease and multiple drug therapy.

ACUTE ABDOMINAL CONDITIONS

The administration of Ultracet may complicate the clinical assessment of patients with acute abdominal conditions.

USE IN RENAL DISEASE

Ultracet has not been studied in patients with impaired renal function. Experience with tramadol suggest that impaired renal function results in a decreased rate and extent of excretion of tramadol and its active metabolite, M1. In patients with creatinine clearances of less than 30 ml/min, it is recommended that the dosing interval of Ultracet be increased not to exceed 2 tablets every 12 hours.

USE IN HEPATIC DISEASE

Ultracet has not been studied in patients with impaired hepatic function. The use of Ultracet in patients with hepatic impairment is not recommended (see WARNINGS, Use With Alcohol).

INFORMATION FOR THE PATIENT

- Ultracet may impair mental or physical abilities required for the performance of potentially hazardous tasks such as driving a car or operating machinery.
- Ultracet should not be taken with alcohol containing beverages.
- The patient should be instructed not to take Ultracet in combination with other tramadol or acetaminophen-containing products, including over-the-counter preparations.
- Ultracet should be used with caution when taking medications such as tranquilizers, hypnotics or other opiate containing analgesics.
- The patient should be instructed to inform the physician if they are pregnant, think they might become pregnant, or are trying to become pregnant (see Labor and Delivery).
- The patient should understand the single-dose and 24 hour dose limit and the time interval between doses, since exceeding these recommendations can result in respiratory depression, seizures, hepatic toxicity and death.

CARCINOGENESIS, MUTAGENESIS, AND IMPAIRMENT OF FERTILITY

There are no animal or laboratory studies on the combination product (tramadol and acetaminophen) to evaluate carcinogenesis, mutagenesis, or impairment of fertility.

A slight but statistically significant increase in two common murine tumors, pulmonary and hepatic, was observed in a mouse carcinogenicity study, particularly in aged mice. Mice were dosed orally up to 30 mg/kg (90 mg/m^2 or 0.5 times the maximum daily human tramadol dosage of 185 mg/m^2) for approximately 2 years, although the study was not done with the Maximum Tolerated Dose. This finding is not believed to suggest risk in humans. No such finding occurred in rat carcinogenicity study (dosing orally up to 30 mg/kg, 180 mg/m^2, or 1 time the maximum daily human tramadol dosage).

Tramadol was not mutagenic in the following assays: Ames *Salmonella* microsomal activation test, CHO/HPRT mammalian cell assay, mouse lymphoma assay (in the absence of metabolic activation), dominant lethal mutation tests in mice, chromosome aberration test in Chinese hamsters, and bone marrow micronucleus tests in mice and Chinese hamsters. Weakly mutagenic results occurred in the presence of metabolic activation in the mouse lymphoma assay and micronucleus test in rats. Overall, the weight of evidence from these tests indicates that tramadol does not pose a genotoxic risk to humans.

No effects on fertility were observed for tramadol at oral dose levels up to 50 mg/kg (350 mg/m^2) in male rats and 75 mg/kg (450 mg/m^2) in female rats. These dosages are 1.6 and 2.4 times the maximum daily human tramadol dosage of 185 mg/m^2.

PREGNANCY CATEGORY C

Teratogenic Effects

No drug-related teratogenic effects were observed in the progeny of rats treated orally with tramadol and acetaminophen. The tramadol/acetaminophen combination product was shown to be embryotoxic and fetotoxic in rats at a maternally toxic dose, 50/434 mg/kg tramadol/acetaminophen (300/2604 mg/m^2 or 1.6 times the maximum daily human tramadol/acetaminophen dosage of 185/1591 mg/m^2), but was not teratogenic at this dose level. Embryo and fetal toxicity consisted of decreased fetal weights and increased supernumerary ribs.

Nonteratogenic Effects

Tramadol alone was evaluated in peri- and post-natal studies in rats. Progeny of dams receiving oral (gavage) dose levels of 50 mg/kg (300 mg/m^2 or 1.6 times the maximum daily human tramadol dosage) or greater had decreased weights, and pup survival was decreased early in lactation at 80 mg/kg (480 mg/m^2 or 2.6 times the maximum daily human tramadol dosage).

There are no adequate and well-controlled studies in pregnant women. Ultracet should be used during pregnancy only if the potential benefit justifies the potential risk to the fetus. Neonatal seizures, neonatal withdrawal syndrome, fetal death and still birth have been reported with tramadol HCl during post-marketing.

LABOR AND DELIVERY

Ultracet should not be used in pregnant women prior to or during labor unless the potential benefits outweigh the risks. Safe use in pregnancy has not been established. Chronic use during pregnancy may lead to physical dependence and post-partum withdrawal symptoms in the newborn. Tramadol has been shown to cross the placenta. The mean ratio of serum tramadol in the umbilical veins compared to maternal veins was 0.83 for 40 women given tramadol during labor.

The effect of Ultracet, if any, on the later growth, development, and functional maturation of the child is unknown.

NURSING MOTHERS

Ultracet is not recommended for obstetrical pre-operative medication or for post-delivery analgesia in nursing mothers because its safety in infants and newborns has not been studied.

Following a single IV 100 mg dose of tramadol, the cumulative excretion in breast milk within 16 hours post-dose was 100 µg of tramadol (0.1% of the maternal dose) and 27 µg of M1.

DRUG INTERACTIONS

In vitro studies indicate that tramadol is unlikely to inhibit the CYP3A4-mediated metabolism of other drugs when tramadol is administered concomitantly at therapeutic doses. Tramadol does not appear to induce its own metabolism in humans, since observed maximal plasma concentrations after multiple oral doses are higher than expected based on single-dose data. Tramadol is a mild inducer of selected drug metabolism pathways measured in animals.

USE WITH CARBAMAZEPINE

Patients taking **carbamazepine** may have a significantly reduced analgesic effect of tramadol. Because carbamazepine increases tramadol metabolism and because of the seizure risk associated with tramadol, concomitant administration of Ultracet and carbamazepine is not recommended.

USE WITH QUINIDINE

Tramadol is metabolized to M1 by CYP2D6. **Quinidine** is a selective inhibitor of that isoenzyme; so that concomitant administration of quinidine and tramadol results in increased concentrations of tramadol and reduced concentrations of M1. The clinical consequences of these findings are unknown. *In vitro* drug interaction studies in human liver microsomes indicate that tramadol has no effect on quinidine metabolism.

USE WITH INHIBITORS OF CYP2D6

In vitro drug interaction studies in human liver microsomes indicate that concomitant administration with inhibitors of CYP2D6 such as fluoxetine, paroxetine, and amitriptyline could result in some inhibition of the metabolism of tramadol.

USE WITH CIMETIDINE

Concomitant administration of Ultracet and **cimetidine** has not been studied. Concomitant administration of tramadol and cimetidine does not result in clinically significant changes in tramadol pharmacokinetics. Therefore, no alteration of the Ultracet dosage regimen is recommended.

USE WITH MAO INHIBITORS

Interactions with **MAO Inhibitors,** due to interference with detoxification mechanisms, have been reported for some centrally acting drugs (see WARNINGS, Use With MAO Inhibitors and Serotonin Re-Uptake Inhibitors).

USE WITH DIGOXIN

Post-marketing surveillance of tramadol has revealed rare reports of **digoxin** toxicity.

USE WITH WARFARIN LIKE COMPOUNDS

Post-marketing surveillance of both tramadol and acetaminophen individual products have revealed rare alterations of warfarin effect, including elevation of prothrombin times.

While such changes have been generally of limited clinical significance for the individual products, periodic evaluation of prothrombin time should be performed when Ultracet and warfarin-like compounds are administered concurrently.

ADVERSE REACTIONS

TABLE 2 reports the incidence rate of treatment-emergent adverse events over 5 days of Ultracet use in clinical trials (subjects took an average of at least 6 tablets/day).

INCIDENCE AT LEAST 1%, CAUSAL RELATIONSHIP AT LEAST POSSIBLE OR GREATER

The following lists adverse reactions that occurred with an incidence of at least 1% in single-dose or repeated-dose clinical trials of Ultracet.

Body as a Whole: Asthenia, fatigue, hot flushes.

Central and Peripheral Nervous System: Dizziness, headache, tremor.

Gastrointestinal System: Abdominal pain, constipation, diarrhea, dyspepsia, flatulence, dry mouth, nausea, vomiting.

TABLE 2 *Incidence of Treatment-Emergent Adverse Events (≥2.0%)*

Body System / Preferred Term	Ultracet (n=142)
Gastrointestinal System	
Constipation	6%
Diarrhea	3%
Nausea	3%
Dry mouth	2%
Psychiatric Disorders	
Somnolence	6%
Anorexia	3%
Insomnia	2%
Central & Peripheral Nervous System	
Dizziness	3%
Skin and Appendages	
Sweating increased	4%
Pruritus	2%
Reproductive Disorders, Male*	
Prostatic disorder	2%

* Number of males = 62.

Psychiatric Disorders: Anorexia, anxiety, confusion, euphoria, insomnia, nervousness, somnolence.

Skin and Appendages: Pruritus, rash, increased sweating.

SELECTED ADVERSE EVENTS OCCURRING AT LESS THAN 1%

The following lists clinically relevant adverse reactions that occurred with an incidence of less than 1% in Ultracet clinical trials.

Body as a Whole: Chest pain, rigors, syncope, withdrawal syndrome.

Cardiovascular Disorders: Hypertension, aggravated hypertension, hypotension.

Central and Peripheral Nervous System: Ataxia, convulsions, hypertonia, migraine, aggravated migraine, involuntary muscle contractions, paraesthesia, stupor, vertigo.

Gastrointestinal System: Dysphagia, melena, tongue edema.

Hearing and Vestibular Disorders: Tinnitus.

Heart Rate and Rhythm Disorders: Arrhythmia, palpitation, tachycardia.

Liver and Biliary System: Hepatic function abnormal.

Metabolic and Nutritional Disorders: Weight decrease.

Psychiatric Disorders: Amnesia, depersonalization, depression, drug abuse, emotional lability, hallucination, impotence, paroniria, abnormal thinking.

Red Blood Cell Disorders: Anemia.

Respiratory System: Dyspnea.

Urinary System: Albuminuria, micturition disorder, oliguria, urinary retention.

Vision Disorders: Abnormal vision.

OTHER CLINICALLY SIGNIFICANT ADVERSE EXPERIENCES PREVIOUSLY REPORTED WITH TRAMADOL HCl

Other events which have been reported with the use of tramadol products and for which a causal association has not been determined include: Vasodilation, orthostatic hypotension, myocardial ischemia, pulmonary edema, allergic reactions (including anaphylaxis and urticaria, Stevens-Johnson syndrome/TENS), cognitive dysfunction, difficulty concentrating, depression, suicidal tendency, hepatitis liver failure and gastrointestinal bleeding. Reported laboratory abnormalities included elevated creatinine and liver function tests. Serotonin syndrome (whose symptoms may include mental status change, hyperreflexia, fever, shivering, tremor, agitation, diaphoresis, seizures and coma) has been reported with tramadol when used concomitantly with other serotonergic agents such as SSRIs and MAOIs.

OTHER CLINICALLY SIGNIFICANT ADVERSE EXPERIENCES PREVIOUSLY REPORTED WITH ACETAMINOPHEN

Allergic reactions (primarily skin rash) or reports of hypersensitivity secondary to acetaminophen are rare and generally controlled by discontinuation of the drug and, when necessary, symptomatic treatment.

DOSAGE AND ADMINISTRATION

For the short-term (5 days or less) management of acute pain, the recommended dose of Ultracet is 2 tablets every 4-6 hours as needed for pain relief up to a maximum of 8 tablets/day.

INDIVIDUALIZATION OF DOSAGE

In patients with creatinine clearances of less than 30 ml/min, it is recommended that the dosing interval of Ultracet be increased not to exceed 2 tablets every 12 hours. Dose selection for an elderly patient should be cautious, in view of the potential for greater sensitivity to adverse events.

HOW SUPPLIED

Ultracet (37.5 mg tramadol HCl/325 mg acetaminophen) tablets (light yellow, film-coated capsule-shaped tablet) debossed "O-M" on one side and "650" on the other.

Dispense in a tight container.

Storage: Store at 25°C (77°F); excursions permitted to 15-30°C (59-86°F).

PRODUCT LISTING - EQUIVALENTS NOT AVAILABLE

Tablet - Oral - 325 mg;37.5 mg

20's	$22.17	ULTRACET, Pharma Pac	52959-0666-20
30's	$27.94	ULTRACET, Southwood Pharmaceuticals Inc	58016-0629-30
60's	$55.88	ULTRACET, Southwood Pharmaceuticals Inc	58016-0629-60

90's	$83.82	ULTRACET, Southwood Pharmaceuticals Inc	58016-0629-90
100's	$93.13	ULTRACET, Southwood Pharmaceuticals Inc	58016-0629-00
100's	$97.71	ULTRACET, Janssen Pharmaceuticals	00045-0650-60
100's	$102.46	ULTRACET, Janssen Pharmaceuticals	00045-0650-10

Acetazolamide *(000086)*

For complete prescribing information, refer to the CD-ROM included with the book.

Categories: Edema; Edema, drug-induced; Glaucoma, angle-closure; Glaucoma, open-angle; Glaucoma, secondary; Hypertension, ocular; Mountain sickness; Seizures, absence; Seizures, unlocalized; Pregnancy Category C; FDA Approved 1953 Jul; WHO Formulary
Drug Classes: Carbonic anhydrase inhibitors
Brand Names: Acetadiazol; Acetamide; Azomid; Dehydratin; **Diamox**; Diamox Sequels; Diamox Sodium; Ederen; Glauconox; Inidrase; Nephramid; Oratrol
Foreign Brand Availability: Albox (Japan); Apo-Acetazolamide (Malaysia); Carbinib (Portugal); Defiltran (Germany); Diamox Sustets (Colombia); Diuramid (Germany); Edemox (Spain); Genephamide (Peru); Glaucomed (Colombia); Glaucomide (New-Zealand); Glaupax (Denmark; Ireland; Japan; Norway; Sweden; Switzerland); Ledimox (Japan); Lediamox (Portugal)
Cost of Therapy: $14.53 (Edema; Diamox; 250 mg; 1 tablet/day; 30 day supply)
$2.69 (Edema; Generic Tablets; 250 mg; 1 tablet/day; 30 day supply)
HCFA JCODE(S): J1120 up to 500 mg IM, IV

DESCRIPTION

Acetazolamide, an inhibitor of the enzyme carbonic anhydrase is a white to faintly yellowish white crystalline, odorless powder, weakly acidic, very slightly soluble in water and slightly soluble in alcohol. The chemical name is *N*-(5-Sulfa-moyl-1,3,4-thiadiazol-2yl)-acetamide.

Acetazolamide is available as oral tablets containing 125 mg and 250 mg of acetazolamide respectively and the following inactive ingredients: Corn Starch, Dibasic Calcium Phosphate, Magnesium Stearate, Povidone, and Sodium Starch Glycolate.

Acetazolamide sustained-release capsules, for oral administration, each containing 500 mg of acetazolamide and the following inactive ingredients: benzoin, ethylcellulose, ethyl vanillin, FD&C blue no. 1, FD&C yellow no. 6, gelatin, glycerin, magnesium stearate, methylparaben, mineral oil, mono- and diglycerides, propylene glycol, propylparaben, silicon dioxide, sucrose, talc, terpene resin, vanillin, and white wax.

Acetazolamide is also available for intravenous use, and is supplied as a sterile powder requiring reconstitution. Each vial contains an amount of acetazolamide sodium equivalent to 500 mg of acetazolamide. The bulk solution is adjusted to pH 9.2 using sodium hydroxide and, if necessary, hydrochloric acid prior to lyophilization.

STORAGE

Store at controlled room temperature 15-30°C (59-86°F).

INDICATIONS AND USAGE

For adjunctive treatment of: edema due to congestive heart failure; drug-induced edema; centrencephalic epilepsies (petit mal, unlocalized seizures); chronic simple (open-angle) glaucoma, secondary glaucoma, and preoperatively in acute angle-closure glaucoma where delay of surgery is desired in order to lower intraocular pressure. Acetazolamide is also indicated for the prevention or amelioration of symptoms associated with acute mountain sickness in climbers attempting rapid ascent and in those who are very susceptible to acute mountain sickness despite gradual ascent.

CONTRAINDICATIONS

Acetazolamide therapy is contraindicated in situations in which sodium and/or potassium blood serum levels are depressed, in cases of marked kidney and liver disease or dysfunction, in suprarenal gland failure, and in hyperchloremic acidosis. It is contraindicated in patients with cirrhosis because of the risk of development of hepatic encephalopathy.

Long-term administration of acetazolamide is contraindicated in patients with chronic noncongestive angle-closure glaucoma since it may permit organic closure of the angle to occur while the worsening glaucoma is masked by lowered intraocular pressure.

WARNINGS

Fatalities have occurred, although rarely, due to severe reactions to sulfonamides including Stevens-Johnson syndrome, toxic epidermal necrolysis, fulminant hepatic necrosis, agranulocytosis, aplastic anemia, and other blood dyscrasias. Sensitizations may recur when a sulfonamide is readministered irrespective of the route of administration. If signs of hypersensitivity or other serious reactions occur, discontinue use of this drug.

Caution is advised for patients receiving concomitant high-dose aspirin and acetazolamide, as anorexia, tachypnea, lethargy, coma and death have been reported.

DOSAGE AND ADMINISTRATION

PREPARATION AND STORAGE OF PARENTERAL SOLUTION

Each 500 mg vial containing sterile acetazolamide sodium parenteral should be reconstituted with at least 5 ml of sterile water for injection prior to use. Reconstituted solutions retain potency for 1 week if refrigerated. Since this product contains no preservative, use within 24 hours of reconstitution is strongly recommended. The direct intravenous route of administration is preferred. Intramuscular administration is not recommended.

TABLETS

Glaucoma

Acetazolamide should be used as an adjunct to the usual therapy. The dosage employed in the treatment of *chronic simple (open-angle) glaucoma* ranges from 250 mg to 1 g of acetazolamide per 24 hours, usually in divided doses for amounts over 250 mg. It has usually been found that a dosage in excess of 1 g per 24 hours does not produce an increased effect. In all cases, the dosage should be adjusted with careful individual attention both to symptomatology and ocular tension. Continuous supervision by a physician is advisable.

In treatment of secondary glaucoma and in the preoperative treatment of some cases of *acute congestive (closed-angle) glaucoma*, the preferred dosage is 250 mg every four hours, although some cases have responded to 250 mg twice daily on short-term therapy. In some acute cases, it may be more satisfactory to administer an initial dose of 500 mg followed by 125 mg every 4 hours depending on the individual case. Intravenous therapy may be used for rapid relief to ocular tension in acute cases. A complementary effect has been noted when acetazolamide has been used in conjunction with miotics or mydriatics as the case demanded.

SUSTAINED-RELEASE CAPSULES

The recommended dosage is 1 capsules (500 mg) two times a day. Usually 1 capsule is administered in the morning and 1 capsule in the evening. It may be necessary to adjust the dose, but it has usually been found that dosage in excess of 2 capsules (1 g) does not produce an increased effect. The dosage should be adjusted with careful individual attention both to symptomatology and intraocular tension. In all cases, continuous supervision by a physician is advisable.

In those unusual instances where adequate control is not obtained by twice-a-day administration of acetazolamide sustained-release capsules the desired control may be established by means of acetazolamide tablets or parenteral. Use tablets or parenteral in accordance with the more frequent dosage schedules recommended for these dosage forms, such as 250 mg every 4 hours, or an initial dose of 500 mg followed by 250 mg or 125 mg every 4 hours, depending on the case in question.

Epilepsy

It is not clearly shown whether the beneficial effects observed in epilepsy are due to direct inhibition of carbonic anhydrase in the central nervous system or whether they are due to the slight degree of acidosis produced by the divided dosage. The best results to date have been seen in petit mal in children. Good results, however, have been seen in patients, both children and adult, in other types of seizures such as grand mal, mixed seizure patterns, myoclonic jerk patterns, etc. The suggested total daily dose is 8-30 mg per kg in divided doses. Although some patients respond to a low dose, the optimum range appears to be from 375-1000 mg daily. However, some investigators feel that daily doses in excess of 1 g do not produce any better results than a 1 g dose. When acetazolamide is given in combination with other anticonvulsants, it is suggested that the starting dose should be 250 mg once daily in addition to the existing medications. This can be increased to levels as indicated above.

The change from other medications to acetazolamide should be gradual and in accordance with usual practice in epilepsy therapy.

Congestive Heart Failure

For diuresis in congestive heart failure, the starting dose in usually 250-375 mg once daily in the morning (5 mg/kg). If, after an initial response, the patient fails to continue to lose edema fluid, do not increase the dose but allow for kidney recovery by skipping medication for a day. Acetazolamide yields best diuretic results when given on alternate days, or for two days alternating with a day of rest.

Failures in therapy may be due to overdosage or too frequent dosage. The use of acetazolamide does not eliminate the need for other therapy such as digitalis, bed rest, and salt restriction.

Drug-Induced Edema

Recommended dosage is 250-375 mg of acetazolamide once a day for 1 or 2 days, alternating with a day of rest.

Acute Mountain Sickness

Dosage is 500-1000 mg daily, in divided doses using tablets or sustained-release capsules as appropriate. In circumstances of rapid ascent, such as in rescue or military operations, the higher dose level of 1000 mg is recommended. It is preferable to initiate dosing 24-48 hours before ascent and to continue for 48 hours while at high altitude, or longer as necessary to control symptoms.

Note: The dosage recommendations for glaucoma and epilepsy differ considerably from those for congestive heart failure, since the first two conditions are not dependent upon carbonic anhydrase inhibition in the kidney which requires intermittent dosage if it is to recover from the inhibitory effect of the therapeutic agent.

Parenteral drug products should be inspected visually for particulate matter and discoloration prior to administration, whenever solution and container permit.

PRODUCT LISTING - RATED THERAPEUTICALLY EQUIVALENT

Powder For Injection - Injectable - 500 mg

1's	$22.50	GENERIC, Bedford Laboratories	55390-0460-01

Tablet - Oral - 125 mg

100's	$34.50	GENERIC, Mutual/United Research Laboratories	00677-1248-01
100's	$34.50	GENERIC, Taro Pharmaceuticals U.S.A. Inc	51672-4022-01
100's	$43.75	DIAMOX, Wyeth-Ayerst Laboratories	00005-4398-23

Tablet - Oral - 250 mg

12's	$1.58	GENERIC, Allscripts Pharmaceutical Company	54569-1697-00
30's	$7.17	GENERIC, Heartland Healthcare Services	61392-0017-63
30's	$7.17	GENERIC, Heartland Healthcare Services	61392-0176-30
30's	$7.17	GENERIC, Heartland Healthcare Services	61392-0176-39
30's	$7.17	GENERIC, Heartland Healthcare Services	61392-0700-30
30's	$7.17	GENERIC, Heartland Healthcare Services	61392-0700-39
30's	$14.57	DIAMOX, Allscripts Pharmaceutical Company	54569-0541-00
31's	$7.41	GENERIC, Heartland Healthcare Services	61392-0176-31
31's	$7.41	GENERIC, Heartland Healthcare Services	61392-0700-31
32's	$7.65	GENERIC, Heartland Healthcare Services	61392-0700-32

45's	$10.76	GENERIC, Heartland Healthcare Services	61392-0700-45
60's	$14.34	GENERIC, Heartland Healthcare Services	61392-0017-66
60's	$14.34	GENERIC, Heartland Healthcare Services	61392-0176-60
60's	$14.34	GENERIC, Heartland Healthcare Services	61392-0176-65
60's	$14.34	GENERIC, Heartland Healthcare Services	61392-0700-60
90's	$21.51	GENERIC, Heartland Healthcare Services	61392-0017-69
90's	$21.51	GENERIC, Heartland Healthcare Services	61392-0176-90
90's	$21.51	GENERIC, Heartland Healthcare Services	61392-0700-90
100's	$4.00	GENERIC, Alra	51641-0153-01
100's	$5.94	GENERIC, Qualitest Products Inc	00603-2070-21
100's	$13.19	GENERIC, Allscripts Pharmaceutical Company	54569-1697-02
100's	$13.80	GENERIC, Aligen Independent Laboratories Inc	00405-4019-01
100's	$24.54	FEDERAL UPPER LIMIT, H.C.F.A. F F P	99999-0086-04
100's	$28.00	GENERIC, Watson/Schein Pharmaceuticals Inc	00364-0400-01
100's	$28.00	GENERIC, Lannett Company Inc	00527-1050-01
100's	$28.00	GENERIC, Watson/Schein Pharmaceuticals Inc	00591-5430-01
100's	$44.50	GENERIC, Taro Pharmaceuticals U.S.A. Inc	51672-4023-01
100's	$48.44	DIAMOX, Storz/Lederle Ophthalmics	57706-0755-23
100's	$56.44	DIAMOX, Wyeth-Ayerst Laboratories	00005-4469-23

PRODUCT LISTING - EQUIVALENTS NOT AVAILABLE

Capsule, Extended Release - Oral - 500 mg

100's	$140.20	DIAMOX SEQUELS, Wyeth-Ayerst Laboratories	00005-0753-23

Powder For Injection - Injectable - 500 mg

1's	$41.63	DIAMOX SODIUM, Wyeth-Ayerst Laboratories	00205-4466-96

Tablet - Oral - 250 mg

5's	$1.74	GENERIC, Allscripts Pharmaceutical Company	54569-1697-01
12's	$5.27	GENERIC, Physicians Total Care	54868-1195-02
100's	$33.47	GENERIC, Physicians Total Care	54868-1195-01

Acetylcysteine *(000101)*

Categories: Amyloidosis, primary; Anesthesia, adjunct; Atelectasis, secondary to mucus obstruction; Bronchiectasis; Bronchitis, chronic; Cystic fibrosis; Emphysema; Overdose, acetaminophen; Pneumonia; Poisoning, acetaminophen; Pulmonary disease, chronic; Tracheobronchitis; Tracheostomy, adjunct; Tuberculosis; Pregnancy Category B; FDA Approved 1963 Sep; WHO Formulary

Drug Classes: Antidotes; Mucolytics

Brand Names: Mucomyst; Mucosil; Mucosol

Foreign Brand Availability: Acerac (Korea); Acetain (Korea); Acypront (Hong-Kong); Alveolex (Ireland); Cetilan (Korea); Ecomucyl (Switzerland); Encore (Taiwan); Exomuc (France); Fabrol (Austria; England; Finland; Greece; Ireland; Sweden); Flemex-AC (Thailand); Fluimicil (Germany; Hungary; Switzerland); Fluimucil (Brazil; China; Colombia; Ecuador; France; Indonesia; Italy; Morocco; Netherlands; Peru; Singapore; Spain; Taiwan; Thailand); Hidonac (Philippines); M.C.T. (Korea); Mucofillin (Japan); Mucolitico (Chile); Mucomiste (Portugal); Mucosof (China); Mucoza (Singapore); Mukolit (Indonesia); Parvolex (Philippines); Siran 200 (Israel); Solmucol (Singapore); Stecin (Korea); Zifluvis (Colombia)

HCFA JCODE(S): J7610 10%, per ml INH; J7615 20%, per ml INH

DESCRIPTION

Acetylcysteine is for inhalation (mucolytic agent) or oral administration (acetaminophen antidote), and available as sterile, unpreserved solutions (not for injection). The solutions contain 20% or 10% acetylcystine, with disodium edetate in purified water. Sodium hydroxide is added to adjust pH to 7. Acetylcystine is the N-acetyl derivative of the N-acetyl derivative of the naturally occurring amino acid, cysteine. The compound is a white crystalline powder with the molecular formula $C_5H_9NO_3S$, a molecular weight of 163.2, and chemical name of N-acetyl-L-cysteine.

This product contains the following inactive ingredients: disodium edetate, sodium hydroxide, and purified water.

CLINICAL PHARMACOLOGY

The viscosity of pulmonary mucous secretions depends on the concentrations of mucoprotein and to a lesser extent deoxyribonucleic acid (DNA). The latter increases with increasing purulence owing to cellular debris. The mucolytic action of acetylcysteine is related to the sulfhydryl group in the molecule. This group probably "opens" disulfide linkages in mucous thereby lowering the viscosity. The mucolytic activity of acetylcysteine is unaltered by the presence of DNA, and increases with increasing pH. Significant mucolysis occurs between pH 7 and 9.

Acetylcysteine undergoes rapid deacetylation *in vivo* to yield cysteine or oxidation to yield diacetylcystine.

Occasionally, patients exposed to the inhalation of an acetylcysteine aerosol respond with the development of increased airways obstruction of varying and unpredictable severity. Those patients who are reactors cannot be identified *a priori* from a random patient population. Even when patients are known to have reacted previously to the inhalation of an acetylcysteine aerosol, they may not react during a subsequent treatment. The converse is also true; patients who have had inhalation treatments of acetylcysteine without incident may still react to a subsequent inhalation with increased airways obstruction. Most patients with bronchospasm are quickly relieved by the use of a bronchodilator given by nebulization. If bronchospasm progresses, the medication should be discontinued immediately.

AS AN ANTIDOTE FOR ACETAMINOPHEN OVERDOSE

(Antidotal) Acetaminophen is rapidly absorbed from the upper gastrointestinal tract with peak plasma levels occurring between 30 and 60 minutes after therapeutic doses and usually within 4 hours following an overdose. The parent compound, which is nontoxic, is extensively metabolized in the liver to form principally the sulfate and glucuronide conjugates which are also nontoxic and are rapidly excreted in the urine. A small fraction of an ingested dose is metabolized in the liver by the cytochrome P-450 mixed function oxidase enzyme system to form a reactive, potentially toxic, intermediate metabolite which preferentially conjugates with hepatic glutathione to form the nontoxic cysteine and mercapturic acid derivatives which are then excreted by the kidney. Therapeutic doses of acetaminophen do not saturate the glucuronide and sulfate conjugation pathways and do not result in the formation of sufficient reactive metabolic to deplete glutathione stores. However, following ingestation of a large overdose (150 mg/kg or greater) the glucuronide and sulfate conjugation pathways are saturated resulting in a larger fraction of the drug being metabolized via the P-450 pathway. The increased formation of reactive metabolite may deplete the hepatic stores of glutathione with subsequent binding of the metabolite to protein molecules within the hepatocyte resulting in cellular necrosis. Acetylcysteine has been shown to reduce the extent of liver injury following acetaminophen overdose. Its effectiveness depends on early administration, with benefit seen principally in patients treated within 16 hours of the overdose. Acetylcysteine probably the liver by maintaining or restoring the glutathione levels, or by acting as an alternate substrate for conjugation with, and thus detoxification of, the reactive metabolite.

INDICATIONS AND USAGE

Acetylcysteine is indicated as adjuvant therapy for patients with abnormal, viscid, or inspissated mucous secretions in such conditions as:

Chronic bronchopulmonary disease (chronic emphysema, emphysema with bronchitis, chronic asthmatic bronchitis, tuberculosis, bronchiectasis and primary amyloidosis of the lung).
Acute bronchopulmonary disease (pneumonia, bronchitis, tracheobronchitis).
Pulmonary complications of cystic fibrosis.
Tracheostomy care.
Pulmonary complications associated with surgery.
Use during anesthesia.
Post-traumatic chest conditions.
Atelectasis due to mucous obstruction.
Diagnostic bronchial studies (bronchograms, bronchospirometry and bronchial wedge catheterization).

ACETYLCYSTEINE AS AN ANTIDOTE FOR ACETAMINOPHEN OVERDOSE

Acetylcysteine, administered orally, is indicated as an antidote to prevent or lessen hepatic injury which may occur following the ingestion of a potentially hepatotoxic quantity of acetaminophen.

It is essential to initiate treatment as soon as possible after the overdose and, in any case, within 24 hours of ingestion.

NON-FDA APPROVED INDICATIONS

Although not approved by the FDA, acetylcysteine has been used as a free radical scavenger to prevent hemorrhagic cystitis caused by alkylating agents such as ifosfamide and cyclophosphamide. It has also been shown to provide some protection against doxorubicin toxicity. Acetylcysteine has been tested as an antineoplastic in various models. It has been tested as an agent to reduce tolerance to cardiovascular nitrates, as an agent to enhance recovery from acute lung injury or pulmonary fibrosis, in the treatment of alcoholic hepatitis, as a glutathione replacement agent in AIDS therapy and to prevent nephropathy induced by nonionic, low-osmolality radiographic contract agents in patient with chronic renal insufficiency.

CONTRAINDICATIONS

Acetylcysteine is contraindicated in those patients who are sensitive to it.

ACETYLCYSTEINE AS AN ANTIDOTE FOR ACETAMINOPHEN OVERDOSE

There are no contraindications to oral administration of acetylcysteine in the treatment of acetaminophen overdose.

WARNINGS

After proper administration of acetylcysteine, an increased volume of liquefied bronchial secretions may occur. When cough is inadequate, the open airway must be maintained by mechanical suction if necessary. When there is a large mechanical block due to foreign body or local accumulation, the airway should be cleared by endotracheal aspiration, with or without bronchoscopy. Asthmatics under treatment with acetylcysteine should be watched carefully. If bronchospasm progresses, the medication should be discontinued immediately.

AS AN ANTIDOTE FOR ACETAMINOPHEN OVERDOSE

Generalized urticaria has been observed rarely in patients receiving oral acetylcysteine for acetaminophen overdose. If this occurs or other allergic symptoms appear, treatment with acetylcysteine should be discontinued unless it is deemed essential and the allergic symptoms can be otherwise controlled.

If encephalopathy due to hepatic failure becomes evident, acetylcysteine treatment should be discontinued to avoid further administration of nitrogenous substances. There are no data indicating that acetylcysteine adversely influences hepatic failure, but this remains a theoretical possibility.

PRECAUTIONS

With the administration of acetylcysteine, the patient may initially notice a slight disagreeable odor which soon is not noticeable. With a face mask there may be a stickiness on the face after nebulization which is easily removed by washing with water.

Under certain conditions, a color change may take place in the solution of acetylcysteine in the opened bottle. The light purple color is the result of a chemical reaction which does not significantly impair the safety or mucolytic effectiveness of acetylcysteine.

A

Continued nebulization of an acetylcysteine solution with a dry gas will result in an increased concentration of the drug in the nebulizer because of evaporation of the solvent. Extreme concentration may impede nebulization and efficient delivery of the drug. Dilution of the nebulizing solutions with sterile water for injection as concentration occurs, will obviate this problem.

AS AN ANTIDOTE FOR ACETAMINOPHEN OVERDOSE

Occasionally severe and persistent vomiting occurs as a symptom of acute acetaminophen overdose. Treatment with oral acetylcysteine may aggravate the vomiting. Patients at risk of gastric hemorrhage (*e.g.*, esophageal varices, peptic ulcers, etc.) should be evaluated concerning the risk of upper gastrointestinal hemorrhage versus the risk of developing hepatic toxicity, and treatment with acetylcysteine given accordingly.

Dilution of the acetylcysteine minimizes the propensity of oral acetylcysteine to aggravate vomiting.

CARCINOGENESIS, MUTAGENESIS, AND IMPAIRMENT OF FERTILITY

Carcinogenesis

Carcinogenicity studies in laboratory animals have not been performed with acetylcysteine in combination with isoproterenol.

Long-term oral studies of acetylcysteine alone in rats (12 months of treatment followed by 6 months of observation) at doses up to 1000 mg/kg/day (5.2 times the human dose) provided no evidence of oncogenic activity.

Mutagenesis

Published data* indicate that acetylcysteine is not mutagenic in the Ames test, both with and without metabolic activation.

Impairment of Fertility

A reproductive toxicity test to assess potential impairment of fertility was performed with acetylcysteine (10%) combined with isoproterenol (0.05%) and administered as an aerosol into a chamber of 12.43 m^3. The combination was administered for 25, 30, or 35 twice a day for 68 days before mating, to 200 male and 150 female rats; no adverse effects were noted in dams or pups. Females after mating were continued on treatment for the next 42 days.

Reproductive toxicity studies of acetylcysteine in the rat given oral doses of acetylcysteine up to 1,000 mg/kg (2.6 or 5.2 times the human dose) in the Segment 1 Study.

PREGNANCY CATEGORY B

Reproduction studies of acetylcysteine with isoproterenol have been performed in rats and of acetylcysteine alone in rabbits at doses up to 2.6 times the human dose. These have revealed no evidence of impaired fertility or harm to the fetus due to acetylcysteine. There are, however, no adequate and well-controlled studies in pregnant women. Because animal reproduction studies may not always be predictiveness of responses, this drug should be used during pregnancy only if clearly needed.

Teratogenic Effects

In a teratology study of acetylcysteine in the rabbit, oral doses of 500 mg/kg/day (2.6 times the human dose) were administered to pregnant does by intubation on days 6 through 16 of gestation. Acetylcysteine was found to be nonteratogenic under the conditions of study.

In the rabbit, two groups (one of 14 and one of 16 pregnant females) were exposed to an aerosol of 10% acetylcysteine and 0.05% isoproterenol HCl for 30 or 35 minutes twice a day from the 6th through the 18th day of pregnancy. No teratogenic effects were observed among the offspring.

Teratology and a perinatal and postnatal toxicity study in rats were performed with a combination of acetylcysteine and isoproterenol administered by the inhalation route. In the rat, two groups of 25 pregnant females each were exposed to the aerosol for 30 and 35 minutes, respectively, twice a day from the 6th through the 15th day of gestation. No teratogenic effects were observed among the offspring.

In the pregnant rat (30 rats per group), twice-daily exposure to an aerosol of acetylcysteine and isoproterenol for 30 or 35 minutes from the 15th day of gestation through the 21th day postpartum was without adverse effect on dams or newborns.

NURSING MOTHERS

It is not known whether this drug is excreted in human milk. Because many drugs are excreted in human milk, caution should be exercised when acetylcysteine is administered to a pregnant woman.

ADVERSE REACTIONS

Adverse effects have included stomatitis, nausea, vomiting, fever, rhinorrhea, drowsiness, clamminess, chest tightness, and bronchoconstriction. Clinically overt acetylasthmatics bronchospasm occurs infrequently and unpredictably even in patients with asthmatic bronchitis or bronchitis complicating bronchial asthma. Acquired sensitization to acetylcysteine has been reported rarely. Reports of sensitization in patients have not been confirmed by patch testing. Sensitization has been confirmed in several inhalation therapists who reported a history of dermal eruptions after frequent and extended exposure to acetylcysteine. Reports of irritation to the tracheal and bronchial tracts have been received and although hemoptysis has occurred in patients receiving acetylcysteine such findings are not uncommon in patients with bronchopulmonary disease and a causal relationship has not been established.

AS AN ANTIDOTE FOR ACETAMINOPHEN OVERDOSE

Oral administration of acetylcysteine, especially in the large doses needed to treat acetaminophen overdose, may result in nausea, vomiting and other gastrointestinal symptoms. Rash with or without mild fever has been observed rarely.

DOSAGE AND ADMINISTRATION

Acetylcysteine Solution 10% and 20%, is available in glass vials containing 4 ml or 30 ml. The 20% solution may be diluted to a lesser concentration with either sodium chloride inhalation solution, sodium chloride injection, or sterile water for injection. The 10% solution may be used undiluted.

Acetylcysteine does not contain an antimicrobial agent, and care must be taken to minimize contamination of the sterile solution. If only a portion of the solution in a vial is used, store the remainder in a refrigerator and use within 96 hours.

Nebulization — face mask, mouth piece, tracheostomy: When nebulized into a face mask, mouth piece or tracheostomy, 1-10 ml of the 20% solution or 2-20 ml of the 10% solution may be given every 2-6 hours; the recommended dose for most patients is 3-5 ml of the 20% solution or 6-10 ml of the 10% solution 3-4 times a day.

Nebulization Tent, Croupette: In special circumstances it may be necessary to nebulize into a tent or Croupette, and this method of use must be individualized to take into account the available equipment and the patient's particular needs. This form of administration requires very large volumes of the solution, occasionally as much as 300 ml during a single treatment period. If a tent or Croupette must be used, the recommended dose is the volume of solution (using 10% or 20% acetylcysteine) that will maintain a very heavy mist in the tent or Croupette for the desired period. Administration for intermittent or continuous prolonged periods, including overnight, may be desirable.

Direct Installation: When used by direct instillation, 1-2 ml of the 10% or 20% solution may then be given as often as every hour.

When used for the routine nursing care of patients with tracheostomy, 1-2 ml of the 10% to 20% solution may be given every 1-4 hours by instillation into the tracheostomy.

Acetylcysteine may be introduced directly into a particular segment of the bronchopulmonary tree by inserting (under local anesthesia and direct vision) a small plastic catheter into the trachea. Two to 5 ml of the 20% solution may then be instilled by means of a syringe connected to the catheter.

Acetylcysteine may also be given through a percutaneous intratracheal catheter. One to 2 ml of the 20% or 2-4 ml of the 10% solution every 1-4 hours may then be given by a syringe attached to the catheter.

Diagnostic Bronchograms: For diagnostic bronchial studies, 2 or 3 administrations of 1-2 ml of the 20% solution or 2-4 ml of the 10% solution should be given by nebulization or by instillation intratracheally, prior to the procedure.

COMPATIBILITY

The physical and chemical compatibility of acetylcysteine solutions with other drugs commonly administered by nebulization, direct instillation, or topical application, has been studied.

Acetylcysteine should not be mixed with all antibiotics. For example, the antibiotics tetracycline HCl, oxytetracycline HCl, and erythromycin lactobionate were found to be incompatible when mixed in the same solution. These agents may be administered from separate solutions if administration of these agents is desirable.

If it is deemed advisable to prepare an admixture, it should be administered as soon as possible after preparation. Do not store unused mixtures.

AS AN ANTIDOTE FOR ACETAMINOPHEN OVERDOSE

Regardless of the quantity of acetaminophen reported to have been ingested, administer acetylcysteine immediately if 24 hours or less have elapsed from the reported time of ingestion of an overdose of acetaminophen. Do not await results of assays for acetaminophen level before initiating treatment with acetylcysteine. The following procedures are recommended:

1. The stomach should be emptied promptly by lavage or by inducing emesis with syrup of ipecac. Syrup of ipecac should be given in a dose of 15 ml for children up to age 12, and 30 ml for adolescents and adults followed immediately by copious quantities of water. The dose should be repeated if emesis does not occur in 20 minutes.
2. In the case of a mixed drug overdose activated charcoal may be indicated. However, if activated charcoal has been administered, lavage before administering acetylcysteine treatment. Activated charcoal adsorbs acetylcysteine *in vitro* and may do so in patients and thereby may reduce in effectiveness.
3. Draw blood for acetaminophen plasma assay and for baseline SGOT, SGPT, bilirubin, prothrombin time, creatinine, BUN, blood sugar and electrolytes. The acetaminophen assay provides a basis for determining the need for continuing with the maintenance doses of acetylcysteine treatment. If an assay cannot be obtained or if the acetaminophen level is clearly in the toxic range (above the dashed line of the nomogram) dosing with acetylcysteine should be continued for the full course of therapy. The laboratory measurements are used to monitor hepatic and renal function and electrolyte and fluid balance.
4. Administer the loading dose of acetylcysteine, 140 mg/kg of body weight. (Prepare acetylcysteine for oral administration as described in TABLE 1).
5. Four hours after the loading dose administer the first maintenance dose (70 mg of acetylcysteine per kg of body weight). The maintenance dose is then repeated at 4 hour intervals for a total of 17 doses unless the acetaminophen assay reveals a nontoxic level as discussed below.
6. If the patient vomits the loading dose or any maintenance dose within 1 hour of administration, repeat the dose.
7. In the occasional instances where the patient is persistently unable to retain the orally administered acetylcysteine, the antidote may be administered by duodenal intubation.
8. Repeat SGOT, SGPT, bilirubin, prothrombin time, creatinine, BUN, blood sugar and electrolytes daily if the acetaminophen plasma level is in the potentially toxic range as discussed below.

SUPPORTIVE TREATMENT OF ACETAMINOPHEN OVERDOSE

1. Maintain fluid and electrolyte balance based on clinical evaluation of state of hydration and serum electrolytes.
2. Treat as necessary for hypoglycemia.

TABLE 1 *Dosage Guide and Preparation*

Body Weight kg	Body Weight lb	Doses in relation to body weight are: Acetylcysteine g	Acetylcysteine ml of 20%	Diluent ml	5% Solution Total ml
			Loading Dose of Acetylcysteine**		
100-109	220-240	15	75	225	300
90-99	198-218	14	70	210	280
80-89	176-196	13	65	195	260
70-79	154-174	11	55	165	220
60-69	132-152	10	50	150	200
50-59	110-130	8	40	120	160
40-49	88-108	7	35	105	140
30-39	66-86	6	30	90	120
20-29	44-64	4	20	60	80
		Maintenance Dose*			
100-109	220-240	7.5	37	113	150
90-99	198-218	7	35	105	140
80-89	176-196	6.5	33	97	130
70-79	154-174	5.5	28	82	110
60-69	132-152	5	25	75	100
50-59	110-130	4	20	60	80
40-49	88-108	3.5	18	52	70
30-39	66-86	3	15	45	60
20-29	44-64	2	10	30	40

* If patient weighs less than 20 kg (usually patients younger than 6 years), calculate the doses of acetylcysteine solution. Each ml of 20% acetylcysteine solution, contains 200 mg of acetylcysteine. The loading dose is 140 mg/kg of body weight. The maintenance dose is 70 mg/kg. Three ml of diluent are added to each ml of 20% acetylcysteine solution. Do not decrease the proportion of diluent.

3. Administer vitamin K_1 if prothrombin time ratio exceeds 1.5 or fresh frozen plasma if the prothrombin time ratio exceeds 3.0.
4. Diuretics and forced diuresis should be avoided (see TABLE 1).

PRODUCT LISTING - RATED THERAPEUTICALLY EQUIVALENT

Solution - Inhalation - 10%

4 ml x 10	$16.88	GENERIC, Faulding Pharmaceutical Company	61703-0203-04
4 ml x 10	$20.28	GENERIC, Abbott Pharmaceutical	00074-3307-01
4 ml x 10	$49.88	GENERIC, Dupont Pharmaceuticals	00590-5214-61
4 ml x 12	$30.74	GENERIC, Roxane Laboratories Inc	00054-8059-05
4 ml x 12	$59.88	GENERIC, Dey Laboratories	49502-0181-04
4 ml x 12	$61.98	MUCOMYST-10, Bristol-Myers Squibb	00087-0572-03
4 ml x 12	$63.72	GENERIC, American Regent Laboratories Inc	00517-7504-12
4 ml x 25	$132.75	GENERIC, American Regent Laboratories Inc	00517-7504-25
10 ml	$7.63	FEDERAL UPPER LIMIT, H.C.F.A. F F P	99999-0101-02
10 ml x 3	$8.76	GENERIC, Abbott Pharmaceutical	00074-3307-02
10 ml x 3	$10.89	GENERIC, Bedford Laboratories	55390-0211-03
10 ml x 3	$19.56	GENERIC, Roxane Laboratories Inc	00054-3027-02
10 ml x 3	$31.25	MUCOMYST-10, Bristol-Myers Squibb	00087-0572-01
10 ml x 3	$39.39	GENERIC, American Regent Laboratories Inc	00517-7510-03
10 ml x 3	$40.26	GENERIC, Dey Laboratories	49502-0181-10
30 ml x 3	$21.00	GENERIC, Bedford Laboratories	55390-0212-03
30 ml x 3	$34.95	GENERIC, Roxane Laboratories Inc	00054-3025-02
30 ml x 3	$39.75	GENERIC, Dey Laboratories	49502-0181-30
30 ml x 3	$52.25	MUCOMYST-10, Bristol-Myers Squibb	00087-0572-02
30 ml x 3	$105.00	GENERIC, American Regent Laboratories Inc	00517-7530-03
30 ml x 3	$182.40	GENERIC, Abbott Pharmaceutical	00074-3307-03
30 ml x 10	$161.88	GENERIC, Dupont Pharmaceuticals	00590-5214-85
30 ml x 10	$184.26	GENERIC, Faulding Pharmaceutical Company	61703-0203-31

Solution - Inhalation - 20%

4 ml x 10	$22.56	GENERIC, Abbott Pharmaceutical	00074-3308-01
4 ml x 10	$51.63	GENERIC, Dupont Pharmaceuticals	00590-5212-61
4 ml x 10	$62.00	GENERIC, Faulding Pharmaceutical Company	61703-0204-04
4 ml x 12	$33.54	GENERIC, Roxane Laboratories Inc	00054-8060-05
4 ml x 12	$63.89	MUCOMYST-20, Bristol-Myers Squibb	00087-0570-07
4 ml x 12	$66.00	GENERIC, Dey Laboratories	49502-0182-04
4 ml x 12	$78.72	GENERIC, American Regent Laboratories Inc	00517-7604-12
10 ml	$9.29	FEDERAL UPPER LIMIT, H.C.F.A. F F P	99999-0101-05
10 ml x 3	$8.91	GENERIC, Abbott Pharmaceutical	00074-3308-02
10 ml x 3	$9.00	GENERIC, Bedford Laboratories	55390-0213-03
10 ml x 3	$24.45	GENERIC, Roxane Laboratories Inc	00054-3028-02
10 ml x 3	$31.68	MUCOMYST-20, Bristol-Myers Squibb	00087-0570-03
10 ml x 3	$45.93	GENERIC, American Regent Laboratories Inc	00517-7610-03
10 ml x 3	$48.66	GENERIC, Dey Laboratories	49502-0182-10
30 ml x 3	$28.50	GENERIC, Abbott Pharmaceutical	00074-3308-03
30 ml x 3	$39.12	GENERIC, Roxane Laboratories Inc	00054-3026-02
30 ml x 3	$43.50	GENERIC, Dey Laboratories	49502-0182-30
30 ml x 3	$53.32	MUCOMYST-20, Bristol-Myers Squibb	00087-0570-09
30 ml x 3	$128.43	GENERIC, American Regent Laboratories Inc	00517-7630-03
30 ml x 3	$133.35	GENERIC, Bedford Laboratories	55390-0214-03
30 ml x 10	$186.39	GENERIC, Dupont Pharmaceuticals	00590-5212-85
30 ml x 10	$217.70	GENERIC, Faulding Pharmaceutical Company	61703-0204-31
100 ml	$92.21	GENERIC, Dey Laboratories	49502-0182-00

PRODUCT LISTING - EQUIVALENTS NOT AVAILABLE

Tablet - Oral - 500 mg

100's	$20.38	ACYS-5, Bio-Tech Pharmacal Inc	53191-0194-01

Acitretin *(003200)*

For complete prescribing information, refer to the CD-ROM included with the book.

Categories: Psoriasis; Pregnancy Category X; FDA Approved 1997 Jun
Drug Classes: Antipsoriatics; Dermatologics; Retinoids
Brand Names: **Soriatane**
Foreign Brand Availability: Neo-Tigason (Thailand); Neotigason (Australia; Austria; Bahamas; Barbados; Belgium; Belize; Benin; Bermuda; Burkina-Faso; China; Colombia; Curacao; Denmark; England; Ethiopia; Finland; Gambia; Germany; Ghana; Guinea; Guyana; Hong-Kong; Ireland; Israel; Ivory-Coast; Jamaica; Kenya; Korea; Liberia; Malawi; Malaysia; Mali; Mauritania; Mauritius; Mexico; Morocco; Netherland-Antilles; Netherlands; New-Zealand; Niger; Nigeria; Norway; Peru; Philippines; Portugal; Puerto-Rico; Senegal; Seychelles; Sierra-Leone; South-Africa; Spain; Sudan; Surinam; Sweden; Switzerland; Taiwan; Tanzania; Trinidad; Tunia; Uganda; Zambia; Zimbabwe)
Cost of Therapy: $351.24 (Psoriasis; Soriatane; 25 mg; 1 tablet/day; 30 day supply)

WARNING

Acitretin must not be used by females who are pregnant, or who intend to become pregnant during therapy or at any time for at least 3 years following discontinuation of therapy. Acitretin also must not be used by females who may not use reliable contraception while undergoing treatment or for at least 3 years following discontinuation of treatment. Acitretin is a metabolite of etretinate, and major human fetal abnormalities have been reported with the administration of etretinate and acitretin. Potentially, any fetus exposed can be affected.

Clinical evidence has shown that concurrent ingestion of acitretin and ethanol has been associated with the formation of etretinate, which has a longer elimination half-life than acitretin. Because the longer elimination half-life of etretinate would increase the duration of teratogenic potential for female patients, ethanol must not be ingested by female patients either during treatment with acitretin or for 2 months after cessation of therapy. This allows for elimination of acitretin, thus removing the substrate for transesterification to etretinate. The mechanism of the metabolic process for conversion of acitretin to etretinate has not been fully defined. It is not known whether substances other than ethanol are associated with transesterification.

Acitretin has been shown to be embryotoxic and/or teratogenic in rabbits, mice, and rats at doses approximately 0.6, 3 and 15 times the maximum recommended therapeutic dose, respectively.

Major human fetal abnormalities associated with etretinate and/or acitretin administration have been reported including meningomyelocele, meningoencephalocele, multiple synostoses, facial dysmorphia, syndactylies, absence of terminal phalanges, malformations of hip, ankle and forearm, low set ears, high palate, decreased cranial volume, cardiovascular malformation and alterations of the skull and cervical vertebrae on x-ray.

Females of reproductive potential must not be given acitretin until pregnancy is excluded. It is contraindicated in females of reproductive potential unless the patient meets ALL of the following conditions:

- **Has severe psoriasis and is unresponsive to other therapies or whose clinical condition contraindicates the use of other treatments;**
- **Has received both oral and written warnings of the hazards of taking acitretin during pregnancy;**
- **Has received both oral and written warnings of the risk of possible contraception failure and of the need to use two reliable forms of contraception simultaneously both during therapy and for at least 3 years *after* discontinuation of therapy and has acknowledged in writing her understanding of these warnings and of the need for using dual contraceptive methods (unless the patient has undergone a hysterectomy or practices abstinence);**
- **Has had a negative serum or urine pregnancy test with a sensitivity of at least 50 mIU/ml within 1 week prior to beginning therapy;**
- **Will begin therapy only on the second or third day of the next normal menstrual period;**
- **Is capable of complying with the mandatory contraceptive measures; and**
- **Is reliable in understanding and carrying out instructions.**

A prescription for acitretin should not be issued by the physician until a report of a negative pregnancy test has been obtained and the patient has begun her menstrual period. Pregnancy testing and contraception counseling should be repeated on a regular basis. To encourage compliance with this recommendation, the physician should prescribe a limited supply of the drug.

Effective contraception must be used for at least 1 month before beginning acitretin therapy, during therapy and for at least 3 years following discontinuation of therapy even where there has been a history of infertility, unless due to hysterectomy. It is recommended that two reliable forms of contraception be used simultaneously unless abstinence is the chosen method. Patients who have undergone tubal ligation should use a second form of contraception.

It is not known whether residual acitretin in seminal fluid poses risk to a fetus while a male patient is taking the drug or after it is discontinued. There have been 5 pregnancies reported in which the male partner was undergoing acitretin treatment. One pregnancy resulted in a normal infant. Two pregnancies ended in spontaneous abortions. In another case, the fetus had bilateral cystic hygromas and multiple cardiopulmonary malformations. The relationship of these malformations to the drug is unknown. The outcome of the fifth case is unknown.

Samples of seminal fluid from 3 male patients treated with acitretin and 6 male patients treated with etretinate have been assayed for the presence of acitretin. The maximum concentration of acitretin observed in the seminal fluid of these men was 12.5 ng/ml. Assuming an ejaculate volume of 10 ml,

A

WARNING — Cont'd

the amount of drug transferred in semen would be 125 ng, which is 1/200,000 of a single 25 mg capsule.

Females who have taken etretinate must continue to follow the contraceptive recommendations for etretinate.

Acitretin, the active metabolite of etretinate, is teratogenic and is contraindicated during pregnancy. The risk of severe fetal malformations is well established when systemic retinoids are taken during pregnancy. Pregnancy must also be prevented after stopping acitretin therapy, while the drug is being eliminated to below a threshold blood concentration that would be associated with an increased incidence of birth defects. Because this threshold has not been established for acitretin in humans and because elimination rates vary among patients, the duration of posttherapy contraception to achieve adequate elimination cannot be calculated precisely. It is strongly recommended that contraception be continued for at least 3 years after stopping treatment with acitretin, based on the following considerations:

- **In the absence of transesterification to form etretinate, greater than 98% of the acitretin would be eliminated within 2 months, assuming a mean elimination half-life of 49 hours.**
- **In cases where etretinate is formed, as has been demonstrated with concomitant administration of acitretin and ethanol, greater than 98% of the etretinate formed would be eliminated: In 2 years, assuming a mean elimination half-life of 120 days; in 3 years, based on the longest demonstrated elimination half-life of 168 days. However, etretinate was found in plasma and subcutaneous fat in 1 patient reported to have had sporadic alcohol intake, 52 months after she stopped acitretin therapy.[1]**
- **An increased incidence of birth defects was estimated based on a limited number of cases which have been reported to Roche, which were identified before the outcome was known, and where pregnancy occurred during the time interval when the patient was being treated with acitretin or etretinate. For cases identified after the outcome was known, severe birth defects have been reported where pregnancy occurred during the time interval when the patient was being treated with acitretin or etretinate.**
- **There have been 202 cases reported before the outcome was known where pregnancy occurred after the last dose of etretinate or acitretin. Fetal outcome remained unknown in approximately one-half of these cases, of which 62 were terminated and 11 were spontaneous abortions. Fetal outcome is known for 103 of these prospectively reported cases. Fifteen of the outcomes were abnormal: hernia, hypocalcemia, hypotonia, undescended testicle, laparoschisis, absent hand/wrist, clubfoot, ichthyosis, apnea/anemia, placental disorder/death and premature birth.[5] Birth defects have also been reported retrospectively (*i.e.,* after the outcome was known). Among the retrospectively reported cases where pregnancy occurred more than 2 years after the last dose of etretinate or acitretin, there are 2 normal outcomes, 3 unknown outcomes and 7 abnormal outcomes. The 7 abnormal outcomes reported are: malformation unspecified, aplasia of the forearm, stillbirth, right ventricular/aortic duct defect, heart malformation unspecified, and chromosomal disorder.[2] For these listed reports, the relationship of the birth defects to the drug is unknown.**

If pregnancy does occur during acitretin therapy or at any time for at least 3 years following discontinuation of acitretin therapy, the physician and patient should discuss the possible effects on the pregnancy.

Acitretin should be prescribed only by physicians who have special competence in the diagnosis and treatment of severe psoriasis, are experienced in the use of systemic retinoids, and understand the risk of teratogenicity.

DESCRIPTION

Soriatane, a retinoid, is available in 10 mg and 25 mg gelatin capsules for oral administration. Chemically, acitretin is all-*trans*-9-(4-methoxy-2,3,6-trimethylphenyl)-3,7-dimethyl-2,4,6,8-nonatetraenoic acid. It is a metabolite of etretinate and is related to both retinoic acid and retinol (vitamin A). It is a yellow to greenish-yellow powder with a molecular weight of 326.44.

Each Soriatane capsule contains acitretin, microcrystalline cellulose, sodium ascorbate, gelatin, black monogramming ink and maltodextrin (a mixture of polysaccharides). Gelatin capsule shells contain gelatin, parabens (methyl and propyl), iron oxide (yellow, black, and red), and titanium dioxide. They may also contain benzyl alcohol, butyl paraben, carboxymethylcellulose sodium, edetate calcium disodium, potassium sorbate and/or sodium propionate.

INDICATIONS AND USAGE

Acitretin is indicated for the treatment of severe psoriasis, including the erythrodermic and generalized pustular types, in adults. Because of significant adverse effects associated with its use, acitretin should be prescribed only by physicians knowledgeable in the systemic use of retinoids. In females of reproductive potential, acitretin should be reserved for patients who are unresponsive to other therapies or whose clinical condition contraindicates the use of other treatments.

Most patients experience relapse of psoriasis after discontinuing therapy. Subsequent courses, when clinically indicated, have produced results similar to the initial course of therapy.

CONTRAINDICATIONS

PREGNANCY CATEGORY X

See BOXED WARNING.

WARNINGS

See also BOXED WARNING.

Hepatotoxicity:

Of the 525 patients treated in US clinical trials, 2 had clinical jaundice with elevated serum bilirubin and transaminases considered related to acitretin treatment. Liver function test results in these patients returned to

Cont'd

normal after acitretin was discontinued. Two (2) of the 1289 patients treated in European clinical trials developed biopsy-confirmed toxic hepatitis. A second biopsy in one of these patients revealed nodule formation suggestive of cirrhosis. One patient in a Canadian clinical trial of 63 patients developed a 3-fold increase of transaminases. A liver biopsy of this patient showed mild lobular disarray, multifocal hepatocyte loss and mild triaditis of the portal tracts compatible with acute reversible hepatic injury. The patient's transaminase levels returned to normal 2 months after acitretin was discontinued.

The potential of acitretin therapy to induce hepatotoxicity was prospectively evaluated using liver biopsies in an open-label study of 128 patients. Pretreatment and posttreatment biopsies were available for 87 patients. A comparison of liver biopsy findings before and after therapy revealed 49 (58%) patients showed no change, 21 (25%) improved and 14 (17%) patients had a worsening of their liver biopsy status. For 6 patients, the classification changed from class 0 (no pathology) to class I (normal fatty infiltration; nuclear variability and portal inflammation; both mild); for 7 patients, the change was from class I to class II (fatty infiltration, nuclear variability, portal inflammation and focal necrosis; all moderate to severe); and for 1 patient, the change was from class II to class IIIb (fibrosis, moderate to severe). No correlation could be found between liver function test result abnormalities and the change in liver biopsy status, and no cumulative dose relationship was found.

Elevations of AST (SGOT), ALT (SGPT), GGT (GGTP) or LDH have occurred in approximately 1 in 3 patients treated with acitretin. Of the 525 patients treated in clinical trials in the US, treatment was discontinued in 20 (3.8%) due to elevated liver function test results. If hepatotoxicity is suspected during treatment with acitretin, the drug should be discontinued and the etiology further investigated.

Ten (10) of 652 patients treated in US clinical trials of etretinate, of which acitretin is the active metabolite, had clinical or histologic hepatitis considered to be possibly or probably related to etretinate treatment. There have been reports of hepatitis-related deaths worldwide; a few of these patients had received etretinate for a month or less before presenting with hepatic symptoms or signs.

Pancreatitis:

Lipid elevations occur in 25-50% of patients treated with acitretin. Triglyceride increases sufficient to be associated with pancreatitis are much less common, although fatal fulminant pancreatitis has been reported for 1 patient.

Pseudotumor cerebri:

Acitretin and other retinoids administered orally have been associated with cases of pseudotumor cerebri (benign intracranial hypertension). Some of these events involved concomitant use of isotretinoin and tetracyclines. However, the event seen in a single acitretin patient was not associated with tetracyline use. Early signs and symptoms include papilledema, headache, nausea and vomiting and visual disturbances. Patients with these signs and symptoms should be examined for papilledema and, if present, should discontinue acitretin immediately and be referred for neurological evaluation and care.

OPHTHALMOLOGIC EFFECTS

The eyes and vision of 329 patients treated with acitretin were examined by ophthalmologists. The findings included dry eyes (23%), irritation of eyes (9%) and brow and lash loss (5%). The following were reported in less than 5% of patients: Bell's Palsy, blepharitis and/or crusting of lids, blurred vision, conjunctivitis, corneal epithelial abnormality, cortical cataract, decreased night vision, diplopia, itchy eyes or eyelids, nuclear cataract, pannus, papilledema, photophobia, posterior subcapsular cataract, recurrent sties and subepithelial corneal lesions.

Any patient treated with acitretin who is experiencing visual difficulties should discontinue the drug and undergo ophthalmologic evaluation.

HYPEROSTOSIS

In clinical trials with acitretin, patients were prospectively evaluated for evidence of development or change in bony abnormalities of the vertebral column, knees and ankles.

Vertebral Results

Of 380 patients treated with acitretin, 15% had preexisting abnormalities of the spine which showed new changes or progression of preexisting findings. Changes included degenerative spurs, anterior bridging of spinal vertebrae, diffuse idiopathic skeletal hyperostosis, ligament calcification and narrowing and destruction of a cervical disc space.

De novo changes (formation of small spurs) were seen in 3 patients after 1½-2½ years.

Skeletal Appendicular Results

Six (6) of 128 patients treated with acitretin showed abnormalities in the knees and ankles before treatment that progressed during treatment. In 5, these changes involved the formation of additional spurs or enlargement of existing spurs. The sixth patient had degenerative joint disease which worsened. No patients developed spurs *de novo.* Clinical complaints did not predict radiographic changes.

LIPIDS

Blood lipid determinations should be performed before acitretin is administered and again at intervals of 1-2 weeks until the lipid response to the drug is established, usually within 4-8 weeks. In patients receiving acitretin during clinical trials, 66% and 33% experienced elevation in triglycerides and cholesterol, respectively. Decreased high density lipoproteins (HDL) occurred in 40%. These effects of acitretin were generally reversible upon cessation of therapy.

Patients with an increased tendency to develop hypertriglyceridemia included those with diabetes mellitus, obesity, increased alcohol intake or a familial history of these conditions.

Hypertriglyceridemia and lowered HDL may increase a patient's cardiovascular risk status. In addition, elevation of serum triglycerides to greater than 800 mg/dl has been associated with fatal fulminant pancreatitis. Therefore, dietary modifications, reduction in acitretin dose, or drug therapy should be employed to control significant elevations of triglycerides.

DOSAGE AND ADMINISTRATION

There is intersubject variation in the pharmacokinetics, clinical efficacy and incidence of side effects with acitretin. A number of the more common side effects are dose related. Individualization of dosage is required to achieve maximum therapeutic response while minimizing side effects. Acitretin therapy should be initiated at 25 or 50 mg/day, given as a single dose with the main meal. Maintenance doses of 25 to 50 mg/day may be given after initial response to treatment; although, in general, therapy should be terminated when lesions have resolved sufficiently. Relapses may be treated as outlined for initial therapy.

Females who have taken etretinate must continue to follow the contraceptive recommendations for etretinate.

PRODUCT LISTING - EQUIVALENTS NOT AVAILABLE

Capsule - Oral - 10 mg

30's	$266.98	SORIATANE, Roche Laboratories	00004-0213-57
30's	$306.63	SORIATANE, Roche Laboratories	00004-0288-57

Capsule - Oral - 25 mg

30's	$351.24	SORIATANE, Roche Laboratories	00004-0214-57
30's	$403.39	SORIATANE, Roche Laboratories	00004-0289-57

Acyclovir (000105)

Categories: Herpes genitalis; Herpes labialis; Herpes simplex encephalitis; Herpes zoster; Infection, herpes simplex virus; Infection, herpes simplex virus, neonatal; Infection, varicella-zoster virus; Varicella; Pregnancy Category C; Pregnancy Category B; FDA Approved 1982 Mar; Patent Expiration 1997 Apr; WHO Formulary

Drug Classes: Antivirals

Brand Names: Zovirax

Foreign Brand Availability: ACERPES (Germany); Acevir (Philippines); Acic Creme (Germany); Aciclofal (Italy); Aciclor (Venezuela); Aciclosina (Peru); Aciclovir-BC IV (Australia); Acihexal (Australia); Acilax cream (Hong-Kong); Acitop (South-Africa); Acivir Cream (India; Israel); Acivir Eye (India); Aclova (Korea); Aclovir (Taiwan; Thailand); Aclovirax (Hong-Kong); Acyclo-V (Australia; New-Zealand); Acyron (Korea); Acyvir (Italy; Korea); Aias (Korea); Apicol (Colombia); Avirax (Canada); Avorax (Hong-Kong; Singapore); Azovir (Indonesia); Bearax (Singapore); Cicloferon (Mexico); Cicloviral (Colombia); Clinovir (Indonesia; Thailand); Clovicin (Taiwan); Colsor (Thailand); Cusiviral (Hong-Kong; Singapore; Spain); Cyclivex (South-Africa); Cyclo (Korea); Cyclomed (Israel); Cyclorax (Hong-Kong); Cyclostad (Philippines); Cyclovir (Benin; Burkina-Faso; Ethiopia; Gambia; Ghana; Guinea; India; Ivory-Coast; Kenya; Liberia; Malawi; Mali; Mauritania; Mauritius; Morocco; Niger; Nigeria; Senegal; Seychelles; Sierra-Leone; Sudan; Tanzania; Tunia; Uganda; Zambia; Zimbabwe); Cyllanvir (Philippines); Danovir (Singapore); Deherp (Taiwan; Thailand); Dravyr (Singapore); Dumophar (Indonesia); Eduvir (Indonesia); Entir (Singapore; Thailand); Erlvirax (Singapore); Herpefug (Germany); Herpex (Bahrain; India; Philippines); Herpoviric Rp Creme (Germany); Inmerax (Chile); Innovirax (Philippines); Isavir (Mexico); Leramex (Thailand); Lesaclor (Mexico); Lisovyr (Argentina); Lovir (Australia; New-Zealand; Singapore); Lovire (South-Africa); Maclov (Mexico); Matrovir (Indonesia); Maynor (Spain); Medovir (Bahrain; Benin; Burkina-Faso; Cyprus; Egypt; Ethiopia; Gambia; Ghana; Guinea; Iran; Iraq; Ivory-Coast; Jordan; Kenya; Kuwait; Lebanon; Liberia; Libya; Malawi; Mali; Mauritania; Mauritius; Morocco; Niger; Nigeria; Oman; Qatar; Republic-of-Yemen; Saudi-Arabia; Senegal; Seychelles; Sierra-Leone; Singapore; South-Africa; Sudan; Syria; Taiwan; Tanzania; Tunia; Uganda; United-Arab-Emirates; Zambia; Zimbabwe); Norum (Thailand); Oppvir (Taiwan; Thailand); Opthavir (Mexico); Poviral (Ecuador; Indonesia); Quavir (Indonesia); Ranvir (Thailand); Raxclo (Philippines); Supra-Vir (Israel); Supraviran Creme (Bahrain; Cyprus; Egypt; Germany; Iran; Iraq; Jordan; Kuwait; Lebanon; Libya; Oman; Qatar; Republic-of-Yemen; Saudi-Arabia; Syria; United-Arab-Emirates); Syntovir (Hong-Kong); Vacrovir (Korea); Vermis (Thailand); Vicorax (Taiwan; Thailand); Viraban (New-Zealand); Viralex (Philippines); Viralex-DS (Philippines); Vircella (Indonesia); Virest (Singapore); Virogon (Thailand); Virolan (Taiwan); Virex (Colombia); Virless (China; Singapore; Taiwan); Viromed (Thailand); Virucid (Hong-Kong); Virupos Eye Oint (Korea); Vivir (Korea); Zetavir (Mexico); Zevin (Thailand); Zodiac (Korea); Vironida (Peru); Warviron (Hong-Kong); Zevin (Hong-Kong); Zoral (Hong-Kong; Singapore); Zorax (Singapore); Zorel (Indonesia); Zoter (Indonesia); Zovir (Denmark); Zyclir (Australia); Zyvir (Kenya)

Cost of Therapy: $267.94 (Herpes Zoster; Zovirax; 800 mg; 5 tablets/day; 10 day supply)
$184.33 (Herpes Zoster; Generic Tablets; 800 mg; 5 tablets/day; 10 day supply)

INTRAVENOUS

DESCRIPTION

Zovirax is the brand name for acyclovir, a synthetic nucleoside analog active against herpes viruses. Acyclovir sodium for injection is a sterile lyophilized powder for intravenous (IV) administration only. Each 500 mg vial contains 500 mg of acyclovir and 49 mg of sodium, and each 1000 mg vial contains 1000 mg acyclovir and 98 mg of sodium. Reconstitution of the 500 mg or 1000 mg vials with 10 ml or 20 ml, respectively, of sterile water for injection results in a solution containing 50 mg/ml of acyclovir. The pH of the reconstituted solution is approximately 11. Further dilution in any appropriate intravenous solution must be performed before infusion (see DOSAGE AND ADMINISTRATION: Method of Preparation and Administration).

Acyclovir sodium is a white, crystalline powder with the molecular formula $C_8H_{10}N_5NaO_3$ and a molecular weight of 247.19. The maximum solubility in water at 25°C exceeds 100 mg/ml. At physiologic pH, acyclovir sodium exists as the un-ionized form with a molecular weight of 225 and a maximum solubility in water at 37°C of 2.5 mg/ml. The pka's of acyclovir are 2.27 and 9.25.

The chemical name of acyclovir sodium is 2-amino-1,9-dihydro-9-[(2-hydroxyethoxy)methyl]-6*H*-purin-6-one monosodium salt.

CLINICAL PHARMACOLOGY

VIROLOGY

Mechanism of Antiviral Action

Acyclovir is a synthetic purine nucleoside analogue with *in vitro* and *in vivo* inhibitory activity against herpes simplex virus types 1 (HSV-1), 2 (HSV-2), and varicella-zoster virus (VZV).

The inhibitory activity of acyclovir is highly selective due to its affinity for the enzyme thymidine kinase (TK) encoded by HSV and VZV. This viral enzyme converts acyclovir into acyclovir monophosphate, a nucleotide analogue. The monophosphate is further converted into diphosphate by cellular guanylate kinase and into triphosphate by a number of cellular enzymes. *In vitro,* acyclovir triphosphate stops replication of herpes viral DNA. This is accomplished in 3 ways: (1) competitive inhibition of viral DNA polymerase, (2) incorporation into and termination of the growing viral DNA chain, and (3) inactivation of the viral DNA polymerase. The greater antiviral activity of acyclovir against HSV compared to VZV is due to its more efficient phosphorylation by the viral TK.

Antiviral Activities

The quantitative relationship between the *in vitro* susceptibility of herpes viruses to antivirals and the clinical response to therapy has not been established in humans, and virus sensitivity testing has not been standardized. Sensitivity testing results, expressed as the concentration of drug required to inhibit by 50% the growth of virus in cell culture (IC_{50}), vary greatly depending upon a number of factors. Using plaque-reduction assays, the IC_{50} against herpes simplex virus isolates ranges from 0.02 to 13.5 μg/ml for HSV-1 and from 0.01 to 9.9 μg/ml for HSV-2. The IC_{50} for acyclovir against most laboratory strains and clinical isolates of VZV ranges from 0.12 to 10.8 μg/ml. Acyclovir also demonstrates activity against the Oka vaccine strain of VZV with a mean IC_{50} of 1.35 μg/ml.

Drug Resistance

Resistance of HSV and VZV to antiviral nucleoside analogues can result from qualitative or quantitative changes in the viral TK and/or DNA polymerase. Clinical isolates of HSV and VZV with reduced susceptibility to acyclovir have been recovered from immunocompromised patients, especially with advanced HIV infection. While most of the acyclovir-resistant mutants isolated thus far from such patients have been found to be TK-deficient mutants, other mutants involving the viral TK gene (TK partial and TK altered) and DNA polymerase have been isolated. TK-negative mutants may cause severe disease in infants and immunocompromised adults. The possibility of viral resistance to acyclovir should be considered in patients who show poor clinical response during therapy.

PHARMACOKINETICS

The pharmacokinetics of acyclovir after IV administration have been evaluated in adult patients with normal renal function during Phase 1/2 studies after single doses ranging from 0.5 to 15 mg/kg and after multiple doses ranging from 2.5 to 15 mg/kg every 8 hours. Proportionality between dose and plasma levels is seen after single doses or at steady state after multiple dosing. Average steady-state peak and trough concentrations from 1 hour infusions administered every 8 hours are given in TABLE 1.

TABLE 1 *Acyclovir Peak and Trough Concentrations at Steady State*

Dosage Regimen	C^{SS}_{max}	C^{SS}_{trough}
5 mg/kg q8h (n=8)	9.8 μg/ml range: 5.5-13.8	0.7 μg/ml range: 0.2-1.0
10 mg/kg q8h (n=7)	22.9 μg/ml range: 14.1-44.1	1.9 μg/ml range: 0.5-2.9

Concentrations achieved in the cerebrospinal fluid are approximately 50% of plasma values. Plasma protein binding is relatively low (9-33%) and drug interactions involving binding site displacement are not anticipated.

Renal excretion of unchanged drug is the major route of acyclovir elimination accounting for 62-91% of the dose. The only major urinary metabolite detected is 9-carboxymethoxymethylguanine accounting for up to 14.1% of the dose in patients with normal renal function.

The half-life and total body clearance of acyclovir are dependent on renal function as shown in TABLE 2.

TABLE 2 *Acyclovir Half-Life and Total Body Clearance*

Creatinine Clearance		Total Body Clearance	
ml/min/1.73 m^2	Half-Life	ml/min/1.73 m^2	ml/min/kg
>80	2.5 hours	327	5.1
50-80	3.0 hours	248	3.9
15-50	3.5 hours	190	3.4
0 (Anuric)	19.5 hours	29	0.5

SPECIAL POPULATIONS

Adults With Impaired Renal Function

Acyclovir was administered at a dose of 2.5 mg/kg to six adult patients with severe renal failure. The peak and trough plasma levels during the 47 hours preceding hemodialysis were 8.5 μg/ml and 0.7 μg/ml, respectively.

Consult DOSAGE AND ADMINISTRATION for recommended adjustments in dosing based upon creatinine clearance.

Pediatrics

Acyclovir pharmacokinetics were determined in 16 pediatric patients with normal renal function ranging in age from 3 months to 16 years at doses of approximately 10 and 20 mg/kg every 8 hours (TABLE 3). Concentrations achieved at these regimens are similar to those in adults receiving 5 mg/kg and 10 mg/kg every 8 hours, respectively (TABLE 1). Acyclovir pharmacokinetics were determined in 12 patients ranging in age from birth to 3 months at doses of 5, 10, and 15 mg/kg every 8 hours (TABLE 3).

TABLE 3 *Acyclovir Pharmacokinetics in Pediatric Patients (Mean ±SD)*

Parameter	Birth to 3 Months of Age (n=12)	3 Months to 12 Years of Age (n=16)
CL (ml/min/kg)	4.46 ± 1.61	8.44 ± 2.92
VDSS (L/kg)	1.08 ± 0.35	1.01 ± 0.28
Elimination half-life (h)	3.80 ± 1.19	2.36 ± 0.97

Drug Interactions

Coadministration of probenecid with acyclovir has been shown to increase the mean acyclovir half-life and the area under the concentration-time curve. Urinary excretion and renal clearance were correspondingly reduced.

INDICATIONS AND USAGE

HERPES SIMPLEX INFECTIONS IN IMMUNOCOMPROMISED PATIENTS

Acyclovir for injection is indicated for the treatment of initial and recurrent mucosal and cutaneous herpes simplex (HSV-1 and HSV-2) in immunocompromised patients.

A

INITIAL EPISODES OF HERPES GENITALIS
Acyclovir for injection is indicated for the treatment of severe initial clinical episodes of herpes genitalis in immunocompetent patients.

HERPES SIMPLEX ENCEPHALITIS
Acyclovir for injection is indicated for the treatment of herpes simplex encephalitis.

NEONATAL HERPES SIMPLEX VIRUS INFECTION
Acyclovir for injection is indicated for the treatment of neonatal herpes infections.

VARICELLA-ZOSTER INFECTIONS IN IMMUNOCOMPROMISED PATIENTS
Acyclovir for injection is indicated for the treatment of varicella-zoster (shingles) infections in immunocompromised patients.

CONTRAINDICATIONS

Acyclovir for injection is contraindicated for patients who develop hypersensitivity to acyclovir or valacyclovir.

WARNINGS

Acyclovir for injection is intended for IV infusion only, and should not be administered topically, intramuscularly, orally, subcutaneously, or in the eye. IV infusions must be given over a period of at least 1 hour to reduce the risk of renal tubular damage (see PRECAUTIONS and DOSAGE AND ADMINISTRATION).

Renal failure, in some cases resulting in death, has been observed with acyclovir therapy (see ADVERSE REACTIONS, Observed During Clinical Practice. Thrombotic thrombocytopenic purpura/hemolytic uremic syndrome (TTP/HUS), which has resulted in death, has occurred in immunocompromised patients receiving acyclovir therapy.

PRECAUTIONS

GENERAL
Precipitation of acyclovir crystals in renal tubules can occur if the maximum solubility of free acyclovir (2.5 mg/ml at 37°C in water) is exceeded or if the drug is administered by bolus injection. Ensuing renal tubular damage can produce acute renal failure.

Abnormal renal function (decreased creatinine clearance) can occur as a result of acyclovir administration and depends on the state of the patient's hydration, other treatments, and the rate of drug administration. Concomitant use of other nephrotoxic drugs, preexisting renal disease, and dehydration make further renal impairment with acyclovir more likely.

Administration of acyclovir by IV infusion must be accompanied by adequate hydration.

When dosage adjustments are required, they should be based on estimated creatinine clearance (see DOSAGE AND ADMINISTRATION).

Approximately 1% of patients receiving intravenous acyclovir have manifested encephalopathic changes characterized by either lethargy, obtundation, tremors, confusion, hallucinations, agitation, seizures, or coma. Acyclovir should be used with caution in those patients who have underlying neurologic abnormalities and those with serious renal, hepatic, or electrolyte abnormalities, or significant hypoxia.

CARCINOGENESIS, MUTAGENESIS, AND IMPAIRMENT OF FERTILITY
The data presented below include references to peak steady-state plasma acyclovir concentrations observed in humans treated with 30 mg/kg/day (10 mg/kg every 8 hours, dosing appropriate for treatment of herpes zoster or herpes encephalitis), or 15 mg/kg/day (5 mg/kg every 8 hours, dosing appropriate for treatment of primary genital herpes or herpes simplex infections in immunocompromised patients). Plasma drug concentrations in animal studies are expressed as multiples of human exposure to acyclovir at the higher and lower dosing schedules (see CLINICAL PHARMACOLOGY, Pharmacokinetics).

Acyclovir was tested in lifetime bioassays in rats and mice at single daily doses of up to 450 mg/kg administered by gavage. There was no statistically significant difference in the incidence of tumors between treated and control animals, nor did acyclovir shorten the latency of tumors. At 450 mg/kg/day, plasma concentrations in both the mouse and rat bioassay were lower than concentrations in humans.

Acyclovir was tested in 16 genetic toxicity assays. No evidence of mutagenicity was observed in 4 microbial assays. Acyclovir demonstrated mutagenic activity in 2 *in vitro* cytogenetic assays (1 mouse lymphoma cell line and human lymphocytes). No mutagenic activity was observed in 5 *in vitro* cytogenetic assays (3 Chinese hamster ovary cell lines and two mouse lymphoma cell lines).

A positive result was demonstrated in 1 of 2 *in vitro* cell transformation assays, and morphologically transformed cells obtained in this assay formed tumors when inoculated into immunosuppressed, syngeneic, weanling mice. No activity was demonstrated in another, possibly less sensitive, *in vitro* cell transformation assay.

Acyclovir caused chromosomal damage in Chinese hamsters at 31-61 times human dose levels. In rats, acyclovir produced a nonsignificant increase in chromosomal damage at 5-10 times human levels. No activity was observed in a dominant lethal study in mice at 3-6 times human levels.

Acyclovir did not impair fertility or reproduction in mice (450 mg/kg/day, PO) or in rats (25 mg/kg/day, SC). In the mouse study, plasma levels were the same as human levels, while in the rat study, they were 1-2 times human levels. At higher doses (50 mg/kg/day, SC) in rats and rabbits (1-2 and 1-3 times human levels, respectively) implantation efficacy, but not litter size, was decreased. In a rat peri- and post-natal study at 50 mg/kg/day, SC, there was a statistically significant decrease in group mean numbers of corpora lutea, total implantation sites, and live fetuses.

No testicular abnormalities were seen in dogs given 50 mg/kg/day, IV for 1 month (1-3 times human levels) or in dogs given 60 mg/kg/day orally for 1 year (the same as human levels). Testicular atrophy and aspermatogenesis were observed in rats and dogs at higher dose levels.

PREGNANCY, TERATOGENIC EFFECTS, PREGNANCY CATEGORY B
Acyclovir was not teratogenic in the mouse (450 mg/kg/day, PO), rabbit (50 mg/kg/day, SC and IV), or rat (50 mg/kg/day, SC). These exposures resulted in plasma levels the same as, 4 and 9, and 1 and 2 times, respectively, human levels.

There are no adequate and well-controlled studies in pregnant women. A prospective epidemiologic registry of acyclovir use during pregnancy was established in 1984 and completed in April 1999. There were 749 pregnancies followed in women exposed to systemic acyclovir during the first trimester of pregnancy resulting in 756 outcomes. The occurrence rate of birth defects approximates that found in the general population. However, the small size of the registry is insufficient to evaluate the risk for less common defects or to permit reliable or definitive conclusions regarding the safety of acyclovir in pregnant women and their developing fetuses. Acyclovir should be used during pregnancy only if the potential benefit justifies the potential risk to the fetus.

NURSING MOTHERS
Acyclovir concentrations have been documented in breast milk in 2 women following oral administration of acyclovir and ranged from 0.6-4.1 times corresponding plasma levels. These concentrations would potentially expose the nursing infant to a dose of acyclovir up to 0.3 mg/kg/day. Acyclovir should be administered to a nursing mother with caution and only when indicated.

GERIATRIC USE
Clinical studies of acyclovir did not include sufficient numbers of patients aged 65 and over to determine whether they respond differently than younger patients. In general, dose selection for an elderly patient should be cautious, usually starting at the low end of the dosing range, reflecting the greater frequency of decreased renal function, and of concomitant disease or other drug therapy.

PEDIATRIC USE
See DOSAGE AND ADMINISTRATION.

DRUG INTERACTIONS

See CLINICAL PHARMACOLOGY, Pharmacokinetics.

ADVERSE REACTIONS

The adverse reactions listed below have been observed in controlled and uncontrolled clinical trials in approximately 700 patients who received acyclovir at ~5 mg/kg (250 mg/m^2) three times daily, and approximately 300 patients who received ~10 mg/kg (500 mg/m^2) three times daily.

The most frequent adverse reactions reported during administration of acyclovir were inflammation or phlebitis at the injection site in approximately 9% of the patients, and transient elevations of serum creatinine or BUN in 5-10% (the higher incidence occurred usually following rapid [less than 10 minutes] IV infusion). Nausea and/or vomiting occurred in approximately 7% of the patients (the majority occurring in nonhospitalized patients who received 10 mg/kg). Itching, rash, or hives occurred in approximately 2% of patients. Elevation of transaminases occurred in 1-2% of patients.

The following hematologic abnormalities occurred at a frequency of less than 1%: Anemia, neutropenia, thrombocytopenia, thrombocytosis, leukocytosis, and neutrophilia. In addition, anorexia and hematuria were observed.

OBSERVED DURING CLINICAL PRACTICE
In addition to adverse events reported from clinical trials, the following events have been identified during post-approval use of acyclovir for injection in clinical practice. Because they are reported voluntarily from a population of unknown size, estimates of frequency cannot be made. These events have been chosen for inclusion due to either their seriousness, frequency of reporting, potential causal connection to acyclovir, or a combination of these factors.

General: Anaphylaxis, angioedema, fever, headache, pain, peripheral edema.
Digestive: Diarrhea, gastrointestinal distress, nausea.
Cardiovascular: Hypotension.
Hematologic and Lymphatic: Disseminated intravascular coagulation, hemolysis, leukopenia, lymphadenopathy.
Hepatobiliary Tract and Pancreas: Elevated liver function tests, hepatitis, hyperbilirubinemia, jaundice.
Musculoskeletal: Myalgia.
Nervous: Aggressive behavior, agitation, ataxia, coma, confusion, delirium, dizziness, hallucinations, obtundation, paresthesia, psychosis, seizure, somnolence. These symptoms may be marked, particularly in older adults (see PRECAUTIONS).
Skin: Alopecia, erythema multiforme, photosensitive rash, pruritus, rash, Stevens-Johnson syndrome, toxic epidermal necrolysis, urticaria. Severe local inflammatory reactions, including tissue necrosis, have occurred following infusion of acyclovir into extravascular tissues.
Special Senses: Visual abnormalities.
Urogenital: Renal failure, elevated blood urea nitrogen, elevated creatinine (see WARNINGS).

DOSAGE AND ADMINISTRATION

CAUTION: RAPID OR BOLUS INTRAVENOUS INJECTION MUST BE AVOIDED (SEE WARNINGS AND PRECAUTIONS).

INTRAMUSCULAR OR SUBCUTANEOUS INJECTION MUST BE AVOIDED (SEE WARNINGS).

Therapy should be initiated as early as possible following onset of signs and symptoms of herpes infections.

A maximum dose equivalent to 20 mg/kg every 8 hours should not be exceeded for any patient.

DOSAGE

Herpes Simplex Infections

Mucosal and Cutaneous Herpes Simplex (HSV-1 and HSV-2) Infections in Immunocompromised Patients

Adults and Adolescents (12 years of age and older): 5 mg/kg infused at a constant rate over 1 hour, every 8 hours for 7 days.

Pediatrics (under 12 years of age): 10 mg/kg infused at a constant rate over 1 hour, every 8 hours for 7 days.

Severe Initial Clinical Episodes of Herpes Genitalis

Adults and Adolescents (12 years of age and older): 5 mg/kg infused at a constant rate over 1 hour, every 8 hours for 5 days.

Herpes Simplex Encephalitis

Adults and Adolescents (12 years of age and older): 10 mg/kg infused at a constant rate over 1 hour, every 8 hours for 10 days.

Pediatrics (3 months to 12 years of age): 20 mg/kg infused at a constant rate over 1 hour, every 8 hours for 10 days.

Neonatal Herpes Simplex Virus Infections

Birth to 3 months: 10 mg/kg infused at a constant rate over 1 hour, every 8 hours for 10 days. In neonatal herpes simplex infections, doses of 15 or 20 mg/kg (infused at a constant rate over 1 hour every 8 hours) have been used; the safety and efficacy of these doses are not known.

Varicella Zoster Infections

Zoster in Immunocompromised Patients

Adults and Adolescents (12 years of age and older): 10 mg/kg infused at a constant rate over 1 hour, every 8 hours for 7 days.

Pediatrics (under 12 years of age): 20 mg/kg infused at a constant rate over 1 hour, every 8 hours for 7 days.

Obese Patients

Obese patients should be dosed at the recommended adult dose using Ideal Body Weight.

Patients With Acute or Chronic Renal Impairment

Refer to DOSAGE AND ADMINISTRATION for recommended doses, and adjust the dosing interval as indicated in TABLE 5.

TABLE 5 *Dosage Adjustments for Patients With Renal Impairment*

Creatinine Clearance (ml/min/1.73 m^2)	Percent of Recommended Dose	Dosing Interval (hours)
>50	100%	8
25-50	100%	12
10-25	100%	24
0-10	50%	24

Hemodialysis

For patients who require dialysis, the mean plasma half-life of acyclovir during hemodialysis is approximately 5 hours. This results in a 60% decrease in plasma concentrations following a 6 hour dialysis period. Therefore, the patient's dosing schedule should be adjusted so that an additional dose is administered after each dialysis.

Peritoneal Dialysis

No supplemental dose appears to be necessary after adjustment of the dosing interval.

METHOD OF PREPARATION

Each 10 ml vial contains acyclovir sodium equivalent to 500 mg of acyclovir. Each 20 ml vial contains acyclovir sodium equivalent to 1000 mg of acyclovir. The contents of the vial should be dissolved in sterile water for injection as described in TABLE 6.

TABLE 6

Contents of Vial	Amount of Diluent
500 mg	10 ml
1000 mg	20 ml

The resulting solution in each case contains 50 mg acyclovir per ml (pH approximately 11). Shake the vial well to assure complete dissolution before measuring and transferring each individual dose. The reconstituted solution should be used within 12 hours. Refrigeration of reconstituted solution may result in the formation of a precipitate which will redissolve at room temperature.

DO NOT USE BACTERIOSTATIC WATER FOR INJECTION CONTAINING BENZYL ALCOHOL OR PARABENS.

ADMINISTRATION

The calculated dose should then be removed and added to any appropriate intravenous solution at a volume selected for administration during each 1 hour infusion. Infusion concentrations of approximately 7 mg/ml or lower are recommended. In clinical studies, the average 70 kg adult received between 60 and 150 ml of fluid per dose. Higher concentrations (*e.g.,* 10 mg/ml) may produce phlebitis or inflammation at the injection site upon inadvertent extravasation. Standard, commercially available electrolyte and glucose solutions are suitable for IV administration; biologic or colloidal fluids (*e.g.,* blood products, protein solutions, etc.) are not recommended.

Once diluted for administration, each dose should be used within 24 hours.

HOW SUPPLIED

Zovirax is supplied in 10 ml sterile vials, each containing acyclovir sodium equivalent to 500 mg of acyclovir, and 20 ml sterile vials, each containing acyclovir sodium equivalent to 1000 mg of acyclovir.

Storage: Store at 15-25°C (59-77°F).

ORAL

DESCRIPTION

Zovirax is the brand name for acyclovir, a synthetic nucleoside analogue active against herpesviruses. Zovirax capsules, tablets, and suspension are formulations for oral administration.

Zovirax 200 mg capsule: Contains 200 mg of acyclovir and the inactive ingredients corn starch, lactose, magnesium stearate, and sodium lauryl sulfate. The capsule shell consists of gelatin, FD&C blue no. 2, and titanium dioxide. May contain one or more parabens. Printed with edible black ink.

Zovirax 400 mg tablet: Contains 400 mg of acyclovir and the inactive ingredients magnesium stearate, microcrystalline cellulose, povidone, and sodium starch glycolate.

Zovirax 800 mg tablet: Contains 800 mg of acyclovir and the inactive ingredients FD&C blue no. 2, magnesium stearate, microcrystalline cellulose, povidone, and sodium starch glycolate.

Each teaspoonful (5 ml) of Zovirax suspension: Contains 200 mg of acyclovir and the inactive ingredients methylparaben 0.1% and propylparaben 0.02% (added as preservatives), carboxymethylcellulose sodium, flavor, glycerin, microcrystalline cellulose, and sorbitol.

Acyclovir is a white, crystalline powder with the molecular formula $C_8H_{11}N_5O_3$ and a molecular weight of 225. The maximum solubility in water at 37°C is 2.5 mg/ml. The pka's of acyclovir are 2.27 and 9.25.

The chemical name of acyclovir is 2-amino-1,9-dihydro-9-[(2-hydroxyethoxy)methyl]-6*H*-purin-6-one.

CLINICAL PHARMACOLOGY

VIROLOGY

Mechanism of Antiviral Action

Acyclovir is a synthetic purine nucleoside analogue with *in vitro* and *in vivo* inhibitory activity against herpes simplex virus types 1 (HSV-1), 2 (HSV-2), and varicella-zoster virus (VZV). The inhibitory activity of acyclovir is highly selective due to its affinity for the enzyme thymidine kinase (TK) encoded by HSV and VZV. This viral enzyme converts acyclovir into acyclovir monophosphate, a nucleotide analogue. The monophosphate is further converted into diphosphate by cellular guanylate kinase and into triphosphate by a number of cellular enzymes. *In vitro,* acyclovir triphosphate stops replication of herpes viral DNA. This is accomplished in three ways: (1) competitive inhibition of viral DNA polymerase; (2) incorporation into and termination of the growing viral DNA chain; and (3) inactivation of the viral DNA polymerase. The greater antiviral activity of acyclovir against HSV compared to VZV is due to its more efficient phosphorylation by the viral TK.

Antiviral Activities

The quantitative relationship between the *in vitro* susceptibility of herpes viruses to antivirals and the clinical response to therapy has not been established in humans, and virus sensitivity testing has not been standardized. Sensitivity testing results, expressed as the concentration of drug required to inhibit by 50% the growth of virus in cell culture (IC_{50}), vary greatly depending upon a number of factors. Using plaque-reduction assays, the IC_{50} against herpes simplex virus isolates ranges from 0.02-13.5 µg/ml for HSV-1 and from 0.01-9.9 µg/ml for HSV-2. The IC_{50} for acyclovir against most laboratory strains and clinical isolates of VZV ranges from 0.12-10.8 µg/ml. Acyclovir also demonstrates activity against the Oka vaccine strain of VZV with a mean IC_{50} of 1.35 µg/ml.

Drug Resistance

Resistance of HSV and VZV to acyclovir can result from qualitative and quantitative changes in the viral TK and/or DNA polymerase. Clinical isolates of HSV and VZV with reduced susceptibility to acyclovir have been recovered from immunocompromised patients, especially with advanced HIV infection. While most of the acyclovir-resistant mutants isolated thus far from immunocompromised patients have been found to be TK-deficient mutants, other mutants involving the viral TK gene (TK partial and TK altered) and DNA polymerase have also been isolated. TK-negative mutants may cause severe disease in infants and immunocompromised adults. The possibility of viral resistance to acyclovir should be considered in patients who show poor clinical response during therapy.

PHARMACOKINETICS

The pharmacokinetics of acyclovir after oral administration have been evaluated in healthy volunteers and in immunocompromised patients with herpes simplex or varicella-zoster virus infection. Acyclovir pharmacokinetic parameters are summarized in TABLE 7.

TABLE 7 *Acyclovir Pharmacokinetic Characteristics*

Parameter	Range
Plasma protein binding	9-33%
Plasma elimination half-life	2.5-3.3 hours
Average oral bioavailability	10-20%*

* Bioavailability decreases with increasing dose.

In one multiple-dose, crossover study in healthy subjects (n=23), it was shown that increases in plasma acyclovir concentrations were less than dose proportional with increasing dose, as shown in TABLE 8. The decrease in bioavailability is a function of the dose and not the dosage form.

TABLE 8 *Acyclovir Peak and Trough Concentrations at Steady State*

Parameter	200 mg	400 mg	800 mg
C^{SS}_{max}	0.83 μg/ml	1.21 μg/ml	1.61 μg/ml
C^{SS}_{trough}	0.46 μg/ml	0.63 μg/ml	0.83 μg/ml

There was no effect of food on the absorption of acyclovir (n=6); therefore, acyclovir capsules, tablets, and suspension may be administered with or without food.

The only known urinary metabolite is 9-[(carboxymethoxy)methyl]guanine.

Special Populations

Adults With Impaired Renal Function

The half-life and total body clearance of acyclovir are dependent on renal function. A dosage adjustment is recommended for patients with reduced renal function (see DOSAGE AND ADMINISTRATION).

Geriatrics

Acyclovir plasma concentrations are higher in geriatric patients compared to younger adults, in part due to age-related changes in renal function. Dosage reduction may be required in geriatric patients with underlying renal impairment (see PRECAUTIONS, Geriatric Use).

Pediatrics

In general, the pharmacokinetics of acyclovir in pediatric patients is similar to that of adults. Mean half-life after oral doses of 300 and 600 mg/m^2 in pediatric patients ages 7 months to 7 years was 2.6 hours (range 1.59-3.74 hours).

Drug Interactions

Coadministration of probenecid with IV acyclovir has been shown to increase the mean acyclovir half-life and the area under the concentration-time curve. Urinary excretion and renal clearance were correspondingly reduced.

INDICATIONS AND USAGE

HERPES ZOSTER INFECTIONS

Acyclovir is indicated for the acute treatment of herpes zoster (shingles).

GENITAL HERPES

Acyclovir is indicated for the treatment of initial episodes and the management of recurrent episodes of genital herpes.

CHICKENPOX

Acyclovir is indicated for the treatment of chickenpox (varicella).

CONTRAINDICATIONS

Acyclovir is contraindicated for patients who develop hypersensitivity to acyclovir or valacyclovir.

WARNINGS

Acyclovir capsules, tablets, and suspension are intended for oral ingestion only. Renal failure, in some cases resulting in death, has been observed with acyclovir therapy (see ADVERSE REACTIONS, Observed During Clinical Practice. Thrombotic thrombocytopenic purpura/hemolytic uremic syndrome (TTP/HUS), which has resulted in death, has occurred in immunocompromised patients receiving acyclovir therapy.

PRECAUTIONS

Dosage adjustment is recommended when administering acyclovir to patients with renal impairment (see DOSAGE AND ADMINISTRATION). Caution should also be exercised when administering acyclovir to patients receiving potentially nephrotoxic agents since this may increase the risk of renal dysfunction and/or the risk of reversible central nervous system symptoms, such as those that have been reported in patients treated with IV acyclovir.

INFORMATION FOR THE PATIENT

Patients are instructed to consult with their physician if they experience severe or troublesome adverse reactions, they become pregnant or intend to become pregnant, they intend to breastfeed while taking orally administered acyclovir, or they have any other questions.

Herpes Zoster

There are no data on treatment initiated more than 72 hours after onset of the zoster rash. Patients should be advised to initiate treatment as soon as possible after a diagnosis of herpes zoster.

Genital Herpes Infections

Patients should be informed that acyclovir is not a cure for genital herpes. There are no data evaluating whether acyclovir will prevent transmission of infection to others. Because genital herpes is a sexually transmitted disease, patients should avoid contact with lesions or intercourse when lesions and/or symptoms are present to avoid infecting partners. Genital herpes can also be transmitted in the absence of symptoms through asymptomatic viral shedding. If medical management of a genital herpes recurrence is indicated, patients should be advised to initiate therapy at the first sign or symptom of an episode.

Chickenpox

Chickenpox in otherwise healthy children is usually a self-limited disease of mild to moderate severity. Adolescents and adults tend to have more severe disease. Treatment was initiated within 24 hours of the typical chickenpox rash in the controlled studies, and there is no information regarding the effects of treatment begun later in the disease course.

CARCINOGENESIS, MUTAGENESIS, AND IMPAIRMENT OF FERTILITY

The data presented below include references to peak steady-state plasma acyclovir concentrations observed in humans treated with 800 mg given orally 5 times a day (dosing appropriate for treatment of herpes zoster) or 200 mg given orally 5 times a day (dosing appropriate for treatment of genital herpes). Plasma drug concentrations in animal studies are expressed as multiples of human exposure to acyclovir at the higher and lower dosing schedules (see CLINICAL PHARMACOLOGY, Pharmacokinetics).

Acyclovir was tested in lifetime bioassays in rats and mice at single daily doses of up to 450 mg/kg administered by gavage. There was no statistically significant difference in the incidence of tumors between treated and control animals, nor did acyclovir shorten the latency of tumors. Maximum plasma concentrations were 3-6 times human levels in the mouse bioassay and 1-2 times human levels in the rat bioassay.

Acyclovir was tested in 16 *in vitro* and *in vivo* genetic toxicity assays. Acyclovir was postive in 5 of the assays.

Acyclovir did not impair fertility or reproduction in mice (450 mg/kg/day, PO) or in rats (25 mg/kg/day, SC). In the mouse study, plasma levels were 9-18 times human levels, while in the rat study, they were 8-15 times human levels. At higher doses (50 mg/kg/day, SC) in rats and rabbits (11-22 and 16-31 times human levels, respectively) implantation efficacy, but not litter size, was decreased. In a rat peri- and post-natal study at 50 mg/kg/day, SC, there was a statistically significant decrease in group mean numbers of corpora lutea, total implantation sites, and live fetuses.

No testicular abnormalities were seen in dogs given 50 mg/kg/day, IV for 1 month (21-41 times human levels) or in dogs given 60 mg/kg/day orally for 1 year (6-12 times human levels). Testicular atrophy and aspermatogenesis were observed in rats and dogs at higher dose levels.

PREGNANCY, TERATOGENIC EFFECTS, PREGNANCY CATEGORY B

Acyclovir administered during organogenesis was not teratogenic in the mouse (450 mg/kg/day, PO), rabbit (50 mg/kg/day, SC and IV), or rat (50 mg/kg/day, SC). These exposures resulted in plasma levels 9 and 18, 16 and 106, and 11 and 22 times, respectively, human levels.

There are no adequate and well-controlled studies in pregnant women. A prospective epidemiologic registry of acyclovir use during pregnancy was established in 1984 and completed in April 1999. There were 749 pregnancies followed in women exposed to systemic acyclovir during the first trimester of pregnancy resulting in 756 outcomes. The occurrence rate of birth defects approximates that found in the general population. However, the small size of the registry is insufficient to evaluate the risk for less common defects or to permit reliable and definitive conclusions regarding the safety of acyclovir in pregnant women and their developing fetuses. Acyclovir should be used during pregnancy only if the potential benefit justifies the potential risk to the fetus.

NURSING MOTHERS

Acyclovir concentrations have been documented in breast milk in 2 women following oral administration of acyclovir and ranged from 0.6 to 4.1 times corresponding plasma levels. These concentrations would potentially expose the nursing infant to a dose of acyclovir up to 0.3 mg/kg/day. Acyclovir should be administered to a nursing mother with caution and only when indicated.

PEDIATRIC USE

Safety and effectiveness of oral formulations of acyclovir in pediatric patients less than 2 years of age have not been established.

GERIATRIC USE

Of 376 subjects who received acyclovir in a clinical study of herpes zoster treatment in immunocompetent subjects greater than or equal to 50 years of age, 244 were 65 and over while 111 were 75 and over. No overall differences in effectiveness for time to cessation of new lesion formation or time to healing were reported between geriatric subjects and younger adult subjects. The duration of pain after healing was longer in patients 65 and over. Nausea, vomiting, and dizziness were reported more frequently in elderly subjects. Elderly patients are more likely to have reduced renal function and require dose reduction. Elderly patients are also more likely to have renal or CNS adverse events. With respect to CNS adverse events observed during clinical practice, somnolence, hallucinations, confusion, and coma were reported more frequently in elderly patients (see CLINICAL PHARMACOLOGY; ADVERSE REACTIONS, Observed During Clinical Practice; and DOSAGE AND ADMINISTRATION).

DRUG INTERACTIONS

See CLINICAL PHARMACOLOGY, Pharmacokinetics.

ADVERSE REACTIONS

HERPES SIMPLEX

Short-Term Administration

The most frequent adverse events reported during clinical trials of treatment of genital herpes with acyclovir 200 mg administered orally 5 times daily every 4 hours for 10 days were nausea and/or vomiting in 8 of 298 patient treatments (2.7%). Nausea and/or vomiting occurred in 2 of 287 (0.7%) patients who received placebo.

Long-Term Administration

The most frequent adverse events reported in a clinical trial for the prevention of recurrences with continuous administration of 400 mg (two 200 mg capsules) 2 times daily for 1 year in 586 patients treated with acyclovir were nausea (4.8%) and diarrhea (2.4%). The 589 control patients receiving intermittent treatment of recurrences with acyclovir for 1 year reported diarrhea (2.7%), nausea (2.4%), and headache (2.2%).

HERPES ZOSTER

The most frequent adverse event reported during 3 clinical trials of treatment of herpes zoster (shingles) with 800 mg of oral acyclovir 5 times daily for 7-10 days in 323 patients was malaise (11.5%). The 323 placebo recipients reported malaise (11.1%).

CHICKENPOX

The most frequent adverse event reported during 3 clinical trials of treatment of chickenpox with oral acyclovir at doses of 10-20 mg/kg four times daily for 5-7 days or 800 mg four times daily for 5 days in 495 patients was diarrhea (3.2%). The 498 patients receiving placebo reported diarrhea (2.2%).

OBSERVED DURING CLINICAL PRACTICE

In addition to adverse events reported from clinical trials, the following events have been identified during post-approval use of acyclovir. Because they are reported voluntarily from a population of unknown size, estimates of frequency cannot be made. These events have been chosen for inclusion due to either their seriousness, frequency of reporting, or potential causal connection to acyclovir, or a combination of these factors.

General: Anaphylaxis, angioedema, fever, headache, pain, peripheral edema.

Nervous: Aggressive behavior, agitation, ataxia, coma, confusion, decreased consciousness, delirium, dizziness, encephalopathy, hallucinations, paresthesia, psychosis, seizure, somnolence, tremors. These symptoms may be marked, particularly in older adults or in patients with renal impairment (see PRECAUTIONS).

Digestive: Diarrhea, gastrointestinal distress, nausea.

Hematologic and Lymphatic: Anemia, leukocytoclastic vasculitis, leukopenia, lymphadenopathy, thrombocytopenia.

Hepatobiliary Tract and Pancreas: Elevated liver function tests, hepatitis, hyperbilirubinemia, jaundice.

Musculoskeletal: Myalgia.

Skin: Alopecia, erythema multiforme, photosensitive rash, pruritus, rash, Stevens-Johnson syndrome, toxic epidermal necrolysis, urticaria.

Special Senses: Visual abnormalities.

Urogenital: Renal failure, elevated blood urea nitrogen, elevated creatinine, hematuria (see WARNINGS).

DOSAGE AND ADMINISTRATION

ACUTE TREATMENT OF HERPES ZOSTER

800 mg every 4 hours orally, 5 times daily for 7-10 days.

GENITAL HERPES

Treatment of Initial Genital Herpes

200 mg every 4 hours, five times daily for 10 days.

Chronic Suppressive Therapy for Recurrent Disease

400 mg two times daily for up to 12 months, followed by re-evaluation. Alternative regimens have included doses ranging from 200 mg three times daily to 200 mg five times daily.

The frequency and severity of episodes of untreated genital herpes may change over time. After 1 year of therapy, the frequency and severity of the patient's genital herpes infection should be re-evaluated to assess the need for continuation of therapy with acyclovir.

Intermittent Therapy

200 mg every 4 hours, five times daily for 5 days. Therapy should be initiated at the earliest sign or symptom (prodrome) of recurrence.

TREATMENT OF CHICKENPOX

Children (2 years of age and older)

20 mg/kg **per dose** orally 4 times daily (80 mg/kg/day) for 5 days. Children over 40 kg should receive the adult dose for chickenpox.

Adults and Children Over 40 kg

800 mg 4 times daily for 5 days.

Intravenous acyclovir is indicated for the treatment of varicella-zoster infections in immunocompromised patients.

When therapy is indicated, it should be initiated at the earliest sign or symptom of chickenpox. There is no information about the efficacy of therapy initiated more than 24 hours after onset of signs and symptoms.

PATIENTS WITH ACUTE OR CHRONIC RENAL IMPAIRMENT

In patients with renal impairment, the dose of acyclovir capsules, tablets, or suspension should be modified as shown in TABLE 9.

TABLE 9 *Dosage Modification for Renal Impairment*

Normal Dosage Regimen	Creatinine Clearance (ml/min/1.73 m^2)	Adjusted Dosage Regimen: Dose	Dosing Interval
200 mg every 4 hours	>10	200 mg	every 4 hours, 5× daily
200 mg every 4 hours	0-10	200 mg	every 12 hours
400 mg every 12 hours	>10	400 mg	every 12 hours
400 mg every 12 hours	0-10	200 mg	every 12 hours
800 mg every 4 hours	>25	800 mg	every 4 hours, 5× daily
800 mg every 4 hours	10-25	800 mg	every 8 hours
800 mg every 4 hours	0-10	800 mg	every 12 hours

HEMODIALYSIS

For patients who require hemodialysis, the mean plasma half-life of acyclovir during hemodialysis is approximately 5 hours. This results in a 60% decrease in plasma concentrations following a 6 hour dialysis period. Therefore, the patient's dosing schedule should be adjusted so that an additional dose is administered after each dialysis.

PERITONEAL DIALYSIS

No supplemental dose appears to be necessary after adjustment of the dosing interval.

BIOEQUIVALENCE OF DOSAGE FORMS

Acyclovir suspension was shown to be bioequivalent to acyclovir capsules (n=20) and one acyclovir 800 mg tablet was shown to be bioequivalent to 4 acyclovir 200 mg capsules (n=24).

HOW SUPPLIED

ZOVIRAX CAPSULES AND TABLETS

Zovirax 200 mg capsules are blue with an opaque cap and body, containing 200 mg acyclovir and printed with "Wellcome ZOVIRAX 200".

Zovirax 400 mg tablets are white, shield-shaped tablets, containing 400 mg acyclovir and engraved with "ZOVIRAX" on one side and a triangle on the other side.

Zovirax 800 mg tablets are light blue, oval tablets containing 800 mg acyclovir and engraved with "ZOVIRAX 800".

Storage: Store at 15-25°C (59-77°F) and protect from moisture.

ZOVIRAX SUSPENSION

Zovirax suspension is an off-white, banana-flavored suspension containing 200 mg acyclovir in each teaspoonful (5 ml).

Storage: Store at 15-25°C (59-77°F).

TOPICAL

DESCRIPTION

Zovirax is the brand name for acyclovir, a synthetic nucleoside analogue active against herpes viruses. Zovirax ointment 5% is a formulation for topical administration. Each gram of Zovirax ointment 5% contains 50 mg of acyclovir in a polyethylene glycol (PEG) base.

Acyclovir is a white, crystalline powder with the molecular formula $C_8H_{11}N_5O_3$ and a molecular weight of 225. The maximum solubility in water at 37°C is 2.5 mg/ml. The pka's of acyclovir are 2.27 and 9.25.

The chemical name of acyclovir is 2-amino-1,9-dihydro-9-[(2-hydroxyethoxy)methyl]-6*H*-purin-6-one.

CLINICAL PHARMACOLOGY

Two clinical pharmacology studies were performed with acyclovir ointment 5% in immunocompromised adults at risk of developing mucocutaneous Herpes simplex virus infections or with localized varicella-zoster infections. These studies were designed to evaluate the dermal tolerance, systemic toxicity, and percutaneous absorption of acyclovir.

In 1 of these studies, which included 16 inpatients, the complete ointment or its vehicle were randomly administered in a dose of 1 cm strips (25 mg acyclovir) 4 times a day for 7 days to an intact skin surface area of 4.5 square inches. No local intolerance, systemic toxicity, or contact dermatitis were observed. In addition, no drug was detected in blood and urine by radioimmunoassay (sensitivity, 0.01 µg/ml).

The other study included 11 patients with localized varicella-zoster infections. In this uncontrolled study, acyclovir was detected in the blood of 9 patients and in the urine of all patients tested. Acyclovir levels in plasma ranged from <0.01 to 0.28 µg/ml in 8 patients with normal renal function, and from <0.01 to 0.78 µg/ml in 1 patient with impaired renal function. Acyclovir excreted in the urine ranged from <0.02% to 9.4% of the daily dose. Therefore, systemic absorption of acyclovir after topical application is minimal.

VIROLOGY

Mechanism of Antiviral Action

Acyclovir is a synthetic purine nucleoside analogue with *in vitro* and *in vivo* inhibitory activity against herpes simplex virus types 1 (HSV-1), 2 (HSV-2), and varicella-zoster virus (VZV).

The inhibitory activity of acyclovir is highly selective due to its affinity for the enzyme thymidine kinase (TK) encoded by HSV and VZV. This viral enzyme converts acyclovir into acyclovir monophosphate, a nucleotide analogue. The monophosphate is further converted into diphosphate by cellular guanylate kinase and into triphosphate by a number of cellular enzymes. *In vitro,* acyclovir triphosphate stops replication of herpes viral DNA. This is accomplished in 3 ways: (1) competitive inhibition of viral DNA polymerase, (2) incorporation into and termination of the growing viral DNA chain, and (3) inactivation of the viral DNA polymerase. The greater antiviral activity of acyclovir against HSV compared to VZV is due to its more efficient phosphorylation by the viral TK.

Antiviral Activities

The quantitative relationship between the *in vitro* susceptibility of herpes viruses to antivirals and the clinical response to therapy has not been established in humans, and virus sensitivity testing has not been standardized. Sensitivity testing results, expressed as the concentration of drug required to inhibit by 50% the growth of virus in cell culture (IC_{50}), vary greatly depending upon a number of factors. Using plaque-reduction assays, the IC_{50} against herpes simplex virus isolates ranges from 0.02 to 13.5 µg/ml for HSV-1 and from 0.01 to 9.9 µg/ml for HSV-2. The IC_{50} for acyclovir against most laboratory strains and clinical isolates of VZV ranges from 0.12 to 10.8 µg/ml. Acyclovir also demonstrates activity against the Oka vaccine strain of VZV with a mean IC_{50} of 1.35 µg/ml.

Drug Resistance

Resistance of HSV and VZV to acyclovir can result from qualitative and quantitative changes in the viral TK and/or DNA polymerase. Clinical isolates of HSV and VZV with reduced susceptibility to acyclovir have been recovered from immunocompromised patients, especially with advanced HIV infection. While most of the acyclovir-resistant mutants isolated thus far from immunocompromised patients have been found to be TK-deficient mutants, other mutants involving the viral TK gene (TK partial and TK altered) and DNA polymerase have been isolated. TK-negative mutants may cause severe disease in infants and immunocompromised adults. The possibility of viral resistance to acyclovir should be considered in patients who show poor clinical response during therapy.

INDICATIONS AND USAGE

Acyclovir ointment 5% is indicated in the management of initial genital herpes and in limited non-life-threatening mucocutaneous Herpes simplex virus infections in immunocompromised patients.

CONTRAINDICATIONS

Acyclovir ointment 5% is contraindicated in patients who develop hypersensitivity to the components of the formulation.

WARNINGS

Acyclovir ointment 5% is intended for cutaneous use only and should not be used in the eye.

PRECAUTIONS

GENERAL

The recommended dosage, frequency of applications, and length of treatment should not be exceeded (see DOSAGE AND ADMINISTRATION). There are no data to support the use of acyclovir ointment 5% to prevent transmission of infection to other persons or prevent recurrent infections when applied in the absence of signs and symptoms. Acyclovir ointment 5% should not be used for the prevention of recurrent HSV infections. Although clinically significant viral resistance associated with the use of acyclovir ointment 5% has not been observed, this possibility exists.

CARCINOGENESIS, MUTAGENESIS, AND IMPAIRMENT OF FERTILITY

Systemic exposure following topical administration of acyclovir is minimal. Dermal carcinogenicity studies were not conducted. Results from the studies of carcinogenesis, mutagenesis, and fertility are not included in the full prescribing information for acyclovir ointment 5% due to the minimal exposures of acyclovir that result from dermal application. Information on these studies is available in the full prescribing information for acyclovir capsules, tablets, and suspension and acyclovir for injection.

PREGNANCY, TERATOGENIC EFFECTS, PREGNANCY CATEGORY B

Acyclovir was not teratogenic in the mouse, rabbit, or rat at exposures greatly in excess of human exposure. There are no adequate and well-controlled studies of systemic acyclovir in pregnant women. A prospective epidemiologic registry of acyclovir use during pregnancy was established in 1984 and completed in April 1999. There were 749 pregnancies followed in women exposed to systemic acyclovir during the first trimester of pregnancy resulting in 756 outcomes. The occurrence rate of birth defects approximates that found in the general population. However, the small size of the registry is insufficient to evaluate the risk for less common defects or to permit reliable or definitive conclusions regarding the safety of acyclovir in pregnant women and their developing fetuses. Systemic acyclovir should be used during pregnancy only if the potential benefit justifies the potential risk to the fetus.

NURSING MOTHERS

It is not known whether topically applied acyclovir is excreted in breast milk. Systemic exposure following topical administration is minimal. After oral administration of acyclovir, acyclovir concentrations have been documented in breast milk in 2 women and ranged from 0.6 to 4.1 times the corresponding plasma levels. These concentrations would potentially expose the nursing infant to a dose of acyclovir up to 0.3 mg/kg/day. Nursing mothers who have active herpetic lesions near or on the breast should avoid nursing.

GERIATRIC USE

Clinical studies of acyclovir ointment did not include sufficient numbers of subjects aged 65 and over to determine whether they respond differently from younger subjects. Other reported clinical experience has not identified differences in responses between the elderly and younger patients. Systemic absorption of acyclovir after topical administration is minimal (see CLINICAL PHARMACOLOGY).

PEDIATRIC USE

Safety and effectiveness in pediatric patients have not been established.

DRUG INTERACTIONS

Clinical experience has identified no interactions resulting from topical or systemic administration of other drugs concomitantly with acyclovir ointment 5%.

ADVERSE REACTIONS

In the controlled clinical trials, mild pain (including transient burning and stinging) was reported by about 30% of patients in both the active and placebo arms; treatment was discontinued in 2 of these patients. Local pruritus occurred in 4% of these patients. In all studies, there was no significant difference between the drug and placebo group in the rate or type of reported adverse reactions nor were there any differences in abnormal clinical laboratory findings.

OBSERVED DURING CLINICAL PRACTICE

Based on clinical practice experience in patients treated with acyclovir ointment in the US, spontaneously reported adverse events are uncommon. Data are insufficient to support an estimate of their incidence or to establish causation. These events may also occur as part of the underlying disease process. Voluntary reports of adverse events that have been received since market introduction include:

General: Edema and/or pain at the application site.

Skin: Pruritus, rash.

DOSAGE AND ADMINISTRATION

Apply sufficient quantity to adequately cover all lesions every 3 hours, 6 times per day for 7 days. The dose size per application will vary depending upon the total lesion area but should approximate a one-half inch ribbon of ointment per 4 square inches of surface area. A finger cot or rubber glove should be used when applying acyclovir to prevent autoinoculation of other body sites and transmission of infection to other persons. **Therapy should be initiated as early as possible following onset of signs and symptoms.**

HOW SUPPLIED

Each gram of Zovirax ointment 5% contains 50 mg acyclovir in a polyethylene glycol base. It is supplied in 15 and 30 g tubes.

Storage: Store at 15-25°C (59-77°F) in a dry place.

PRODUCT LISTING - RATED THERAPEUTICALLY EQUIVALENT

Quantity	Price	Product	NDC
Capsule - Oral - 200 mg			
6's	$12.00	GENERIC, Prescript Pharmaceuticals	00247-0075-06
10's	$7.37	GENERIC, Pd-Rx Pharmaceuticals	55289-0273-10
10's	$22.28	ZOVIRAX, Pd-Rx Pharmaceuticals	55289-0006-10
20's	$32.16	GENERIC, Prescript Pharmaceuticals	00247-0075-20
25's	$9.38	GENERIC, Pd-Rx Pharmaceuticals	55289-0273-25
25's	$17.48	GENERIC, Pharma Pac	52959-0517-25
25's	$37.20	ZOVIRAX, Allscripts Pharmaceutical Company	54569-0091-00
25's	$39.38	GENERIC, Prescript Pharmaceuticals	00247-0075-25
25's	$40.28	ZOVIRAX, Pd-Rx Pharmaceuticals	55289-0006-25
25's	$40.55	ZOVIRAX, Physicians Total Care	54868-0163-02
25's	$72.99	ZOVIRAX, Pharma Pac	52959-0330-25
30's	$20.10	GENERIC, Pharma Pac	52959-0517-30
30's	$46.58	GENERIC, Prescript Pharmaceuticals	00247-0075-30
30's	$48.42	ZOVIRAX, Physicians Total Care	54868-0163-03
35's	$20.79	GENERIC, Pd-Rx Pharmaceuticals	55289-0273-35
35's	$21.00	GENERIC, Pharma Pac	52959-0517-35
35's	$52.08	ZOVIRAX, Allscripts Pharmaceutical Company	54569-0091-02
35's	$53.78	GENERIC, Prescript Pharmaceuticals	00247-0075-35
35's	$53.78	ZOVIRAX, Pd-Rx Pharmaceuticals	55289-0006-35
40's	$60.99	GENERIC, Prescript Pharmaceuticals	00247-0075-40
40's	$64.16	ZOVIRAX, Physicians Total Care	54868-0163-06
42's	$63.87	GENERIC, Prescript Pharmaceuticals	00247-0075-42
48's	$72.51	GENERIC, Prescript Pharmaceuticals	00247-0075-48
50's	$12.75	GENERIC, Pd-Rx Pharmaceuticals	55289-0273-50
50's	$74.40	ZOVIRAX, Allscripts Pharmaceutical Company	54569-0091-01
50's	$74.97	ZOVIRAX, Pd-Rx Pharmaceuticals	55289-0006-50
50's	$75.39	GENERIC, Prescript Pharmaceuticals	00247-0075-50
50's	$79.90	ZOVIRAX, Physicians Total Care	54868-0163-01
50's	$137.50	ZOVIRAX, Pharma Pac	52959-0330-50
60's	$89.80	GENERIC, Prescript Pharmaceuticals	00247-0075-60
100's	$35.25	FEDERAL UPPER LIMIT, H.C.F.A. F F P	99999-0105-01
100's	$97.20	GENERIC, Teva Pharmaceuticals Usa	00093-8940-01
100's	$97.70	GENERIC, Par Pharmaceutical Inc	49884-0460-01
100's	$97.70	GENERIC, Esi Lederle Generics	59911-5831-03
100's	$97.70	GENERIC, Stason Pharmaceuticals Inc	60763-2041-00
100's	$97.70	GENERIC, Boscogen Inc	62033-0204-10
100's	$99.00	GENERIC, Martec Pharmaceuticals Inc	52555-0682-01
100's	$99.15	GENERIC, Udl Laboratories Inc	51079-0876-20
100's	$106.36	GENERIC, Ranbaxy Laboratories	63304-0652-01
100's	$111.29	GENERIC, Roxane Laboratories Inc	00054-8080-25
100's	$111.65	GENERIC, Mova Pharmaceutical Corporation	55370-0557-07
100's	$111.67	GENERIC, Mylan Pharmaceuticals Inc	00378-2200-01
100's	$111.67	GENERIC, Par Pharmaceutical Inc	49884-0565-01
100's	$111.88	GENERIC, Ivax Corporation	00172-4266-60
100's	$111.88	GENERIC, Ivax Corporation	00182-2666-89
100's	$111.92	GENERIC, Purepac Pharmaceutical Company	00228-2605-11
100's	$147.44	GENERIC, Prescript Pharmaceuticals	00247-0075-00
100's	$148.79	ZOVIRAX, Glaxosmithkline	00173-0991-56
100's	$149.85	ZOVIRAX, Physicians Total Care	54868-0163-04
100's	$151.60	ZOVIRAX, Glaxosmithkline	00173-0991-55
100's	$260.00	ZOVIRAX, Pharma Pac	52959-0330-00
120's	$179.58	ZOVIRAX, Physicians Total Care	54868-0163-05
Powder For Injection - Intravenous - 500 mg			
1's	$49.00	GENERIC, Abbott Pharmaceutical	00074-4427-49
10's	$47.50	GENERIC, Abbott Pharmaceutical	00074-4427-01
10's	$120.00	GENERIC, Gensia Sicor Pharmaceuticals Inc	00703-8104-03
10's	$464.38	GENERIC, American Pharmaceutical Partners	63323-0105-10
10's	$528.00	GENERIC, Bedford Laboratories	55390-0612-10
10's	$704.24	ZOVIRAX, Glaxosmithkline	00173-0995-01
Powder For Injection - Intravenous - 1000 mg			
1's	$98.50	GENERIC, Abbott Pharmaceutical	00074-4452-49
10's	$326.92	GENERIC, Abbott Pharmaceutical	00074-4452-01
10's	$884.00	GENERIC, Gensia Sicor Pharmaceuticals Inc	00703-8105-03
10's	$1056.00	GENERIC, Bedford Laboratories	55390-0613-20
10's	$1202.14	ZOVIRAX, Glaxosmithkline	00173-0952-01
Solution - Intravenous - 50 mg/ml			
10 ml	$23.00	GENERIC, Bertek Pharmaceuticals Inc	62794-0401-31
10 ml x 10	$230.00	GENERIC, Bertek Pharmaceuticals Inc	62794-0401-97
20 ml	$43.00	GENERIC, Bertek Pharmaceuticals Inc	62794-0403-31
20 ml x 10	$430.00	GENERIC, Bertek Pharmaceuticals Inc	62794-0403-97
Suspension - Oral - 200 mg/5 ml			
5 ml x 50	$241.20	GENERIC, Alpharma Uspd Makers Of Barre and Nmc	50962-0453-60

Qty	Price	Product	NDC
473 ml	$109.40	GENERIC, Alpharma Uspd Makers Of Barre and Nmc	00472-0082-16
473 ml	$131.89	ZOVIRAX, Glaxosmithkline	00173-0953-96

Tablet - Oral - 400 mg

Qty	Price	Product	NDC
10's	$8.70	GENERIC, Pd-Rx Pharmaceuticals	55289-0462-10
10's	$20.99	GENERIC, Pharma Pac	52959-0544-10
12's	$7.88	GENERIC, Pd-Rx Pharmaceuticals	55289-0462-12
12's	$24.63	GENERIC, Pharma Pac	52959-0544-12
12's	$37.53	ZOVIRAX, Pd-Rx Pharmaceuticals	55289-0691-12
15's	$9.75	GENERIC, Pd-Rx Pharmaceuticals	55289-0462-15
15's	$30.15	GENERIC, Pharma Pac	52959-0544-15
15's	$39.74	ZOVIRAX, Prescript Pharmaceuticals	00247-0336-15
15's	$45.91	ZOVIRAX, Physicians Total Care	54868-3025-00
15's	$57.27	ZOVIRAX, Pd-Rx Pharmaceuticals	55289-0691-15
15's	$245.94	ZOVIRAX, Prescript Pharmaceuticals	00247-0336-00
20's	$50.70	ZOVIRAX, Allscripts Pharmaceutical Company	54569-4192-01
20's	$51.87	ZOVIRAX, Prescript Pharmaceuticals	00247-0336-20
21's	$40.90	GENERIC, Pharma Pac	52959-0544-21
21's	$54.29	ZOVIRAX, Prescript Pharmaceuticals	00247-0336-21
25's	$12.87	GENERIC, Pd-Rx Pharmaceuticals	55289-0462-25
25's	$48.14	GENERIC, Pharma Pac	52959-0544-25
25's	$64.00	ZOVIRAX, Prescript Pharmaceuticals	00247-0336-25
25's	$70.97	ZOVIRAX, Pd-Rx Pharmaceuticals	55289-0691-25
28's	$71.28	ZOVIRAX, Prescript Pharmaceuticals	00247-0336-28
30's	$16.35	GENERIC, Pd-Rx Pharmaceuticals	55289-0462-30
30's	$56.98	GENERIC, Pharma Pac	52959-0544-30
30's	$76.05	ZOVIRAX, Allscripts Pharmaceutical Company	54569-4192-00
30's	$76.13	ZOVIRAX, Prescript Pharmaceuticals	00247-0336-30
50's	$90.46	GENERIC, Pharma Pac	52959-0544-50
100's	$70.48	FEDERAL UPPER LIMIT, H.C.F.A. F F P	99999-0105-02
100's	$188.40	GENERIC, Martec Pharmaceuticals Inc	52555-0683-01
100's	$188.60	GENERIC, Teva Pharmaceuticals Usa	00093-8943-01
100's	$189.60	GENERIC, Mylan Pharmaceuticals Inc	00378-1464-01
100's	$189.60	GENERIC, Carlsbad Technology Inc	61442-0112-01
100's	$189.61	GENERIC, Par Pharmaceutical Inc	49884-0487-01
100's	$189.61	GENERIC, Esi Lederle Generics	59911-3163-04
100's	$194.40	GENERIC, Udl Laboratories Inc	51079-0877-20
100's	$206.40	GENERIC, Ranbaxy Laboratories	63304-0504-01
100's	$216.70	GENERIC, Mova Pharmaceutical Corporation	55370-0555-07
100's	$216.72	GENERIC, Mylan Pharmaceuticals Inc	00378-0253-01
100's	$216.72	GENERIC, Par Pharmaceutical Inc	49884-0566-01
100's	$216.72	GENERIC, Watson/Rugby Laboratories Inc	52544-0335-01
100's	$216.91	GENERIC, Ivax Corporation	00172-4267-60
100's	$216.91	GENERIC, Ivax Corporation	00182-8200-89
100's	$216.97	GENERIC, Purepac Pharmaceutical Company	00228-2606-11
100's	$217.00	GENERIC, Pharma Pac	52959-0544-01
100's	$294.19	ZOVIRAX, Glaxosmithkline	00173-0949-55

Tablet - Oral - 800 mg

Qty	Price	Product	NDC
10's	$49.99	ZOVIRAX, Prescript Pharmaceuticals	00247-0169-10
15's	$93.81	ZOVIRAX, Physicians Total Care	55289-0564-15
20's	$96.61	ZOVIRAX, Prescript Pharmaceuticals	00247-0169-20
20's	$123.03	ZOVIRAX, Physicians Total Care	55289-0564-20
25's	$147.60	ZOVIRAX, Physicians Total Care	54868-2184-03
28's	$133.92	ZOVIRAX, Prescript Pharmaceuticals	00247-0169-28
30's	$143.25	ZOVIRAX, Prescript Pharmaceuticals	00247-0169-30
30's	$167.12	ZOVIRAX, Physicians Total Care	54868-2184-02
35's	$166.55	ZOVIRAX, Prescript Pharmaceuticals	00247-0169-35
48's	$295.80	ZOVIRAX, Physicians Total Care	55289-0564-48
50's	$236.51	ZOVIRAX, Prescript Pharmaceuticals	00247-0169-50
50's	$277.75	ZOVIRAX, Physicians Total Care	54868-2184-04
100's	$121.61	FEDERAL UPPER LIMIT, H.C.F.A. F F P	99999-0105-03
100's	$355.10	GENERIC, Udl Laboratories Inc	51079-0878-20
100's	$366.65	GENERIC, Teva Pharmaceuticals Usa	00093-8947-01
100's	$368.65	GENERIC, Carlsbad Technology Inc	61442-0113-01
100's	$368.68	GENERIC, Mylan Pharmaceuticals Inc	00378-1468-01
100's	$368.70	GENERIC, Par Pharmaceutical Inc	49884-0474-01
100's	$368.70	GENERIC, Esi Lederle Generics	59911-3164-04
100's	$370.60	GENERIC, Martec Pharmaceuticals Inc	52555-0684-01
100's	$401.37	GENERIC, Ranbaxy Laboratories	63304-0505-01
100's	$421.42	GENERIC, Mylan Pharmaceuticals Inc	00378-0302-01
100's	$421.42	GENERIC, Par Pharmaceutical Inc	49884-0567-01
100's	$421.42	GENERIC, Watson/Rugby Laboratories Inc	52544-0336-01
100's	$421.42	GENERIC, Mova Pharmaceutical Corporation	55370-0556-07
100's	$421.60	GENERIC, Ivax Corporation	00172-4268-60
100's	$421.60	GENERIC, Ivax Corporation	00182-2667-89
100's	$421.67	GENERIC, Purepac Pharmaceutical Company	00228-2607-11
100's	$535.88	ZOVIRAX, Physicians Total Care	54868-2184-00
100's	$572.05	ZOVIRAX, Glaxosmithkline	00173-0945-55

PRODUCT LISTING - RATED NOT THERAPEUTICALLY EQUIVALENT

Tablet - Oral - 400 mg

Qty	Price	Product	NDC
35's	$88.26	ZOVIRAX, Prescript Pharmaceuticals	00247-0336-35

PRODUCT LISTING - EQUIVALENTS NOT AVAILABLE

Capsule - Oral - 200 mg

Qty	Price	Product	NDC
15's	$15.68	GENERIC, Allscripts Pharmaceutical Company	54569-4482-02
25's	$14.43	GENERIC, Physicians Total Care	54868-3996-00
25's	$27.99	GENERIC, Allscripts Pharmaceutical Company	54569-4482-00
30's	$17.05	GENERIC, Physicians Total Care	54868-3996-02
35's	$36.58	GENERIC, Allscripts Pharmaceutical Company	54569-4482-03
40's	$22.29	GENERIC, Physicians Total Care	54868-3996-01
50's	$21.36	GENERIC, Physicians Total Care	54868-3996-03
50's	$52.25	GENERIC, Allscripts Pharmaceutical Company	54569-4482-01
100's	$97.70	GENERIC, Watson/Schein Pharmaceuticals Inc	00364-2692-01

Ointment - Topical - 5%

Qty	Price	Product	NDC
3 gm	$20.69	ZOVIRAX TOPICAL, Allscripts Pharmaceutical Company	54569-2047-00
3 gm	$25.62	ZOVIRAX TOPICAL, Physicians Total Care	54868-0165-02
3 gm	$26.51	ZOVIRAX TOPICAL, Biovail Pharmaceuticals Inc	00173-0993-41
3 gm	$26.51	ZOVIRAX TOPICAL, Biovail Pharmaceuticals Inc	64455-0993-41
15 gm	$47.80	ZOVIRAX TOPICAL, Allscripts Pharmaceutical Company	54569-0792-00
15 gm	$58.19	ZOVIRAX TOPICAL, Physicians Total Care	54868-0165-01
15 gm	$68.91	ZOVIRAX TOPICAL, Prescript Pharmaceuticals	00247-0039-15
15 gm	$85.71	ZOVIRAX TOPICAL, Biovail Pharmaceuticals Inc	00173-0993-94
15 gm	$85.71	ZOVIRAX TOPICAL, Biovail Pharmaceuticals Inc	64455-0993-94

Powder For Injection - Intravenous - 500 mg

Qty	Price	Product	NDC
10's	$490.00	GENERIC, Faulding Pharmaceutical Company	61703-0311-21

Powder For Injection - Intravenous - 1000 mg

Qty	Price	Product	NDC
10's	$954.00	GENERIC, Faulding Pharmaceutical Company	61703-0311-43

Solution - Intravenous - 50 mg/ml

Qty	Price	Product	NDC
10 ml x 10	$187.50	GENERIC, American Pharmaceutical Partners	63323-0325-10
20 ml x 10	$350.00	GENERIC, Fujisawa	63323-0325-20

Tablet - Oral - 400 mg

Qty	Price	Product	NDC
2's	$4.08	GENERIC, Allscripts Pharmaceutical Company	54569-4765-00
14's	$28.54	GENERIC, Allscripts Pharmaceutical Company	54569-4765-01
15's	$30.58	GENERIC, Allscripts Pharmaceutical Company	54569-4765-04
25's	$50.96	GENERIC, Allscripts Pharmaceutical Company	54569-4765-02
30's	$14.97	GENERIC, Physicians Total Care	54868-6997-00
45's	$61.16	GENERIC, Allscripts Pharmaceutical Company	54569-4765-05
50's	$101.93	GENERIC, Allscripts Pharmaceutical Company	54569-4765-03
60's	$130.03	GENERIC, Southwood Pharmaceuticals Inc	58016-0112-60
100's	$216.72	GENERIC, Watson/Schein Pharmaceuticals Inc	00364-2689-01

Tablet - Oral - 800 mg

Qty	Price	Product	NDC
20's	$80.27	GENERIC, Southwood Pharmaceuticals Inc	58016-0627-20
30's	$30.71	GENERIC, Physicians Total Care	54686-3998-00
30's	$120.41	GENERIC, Southwood Pharmaceuticals Inc	58016-0627-30
35's	$132.20	GENERIC, Allscripts Pharmaceutical Company	54569-4724-00
50's	$28.97	GENERIC, Physicians Total Care	54686-3998-01
60's	$240.82	GENERIC, Southwood Pharmaceuticals Inc	58016-0627-60
90's	$361.23	GENERIC, Southwood Pharmaceuticals Inc	58016-0627-90
100's	$368.65	GENERIC, Watson/Schein Pharmaceuticals Inc	00364-2690-01
100's	$401.37	GENERIC, Southwood Pharmaceuticals Inc	58016-0627-00

Adalimumab *(003582)*

Categories: Arthritis, rheumatoid; Pregnancy Category B; FDA Approved 2002 Dec
Drug Classes: Disease modifying antirheumatic drugs; Immunomodulators; Monoclonal antibodies; Tumor necrosis factor modulators
Brand Names: Humira
Cost of Therapy: $2,613.20 (Rheumatoid Arthritis; Humira; 40 mg/2 ml; 40 mg every other week; 28 day supply)

WARNING

RISK OF INFECTIONS

Cases of tuberculosis (frequently disseminated or extrapulmonary at clinical presentation) have been observed in patients receiving adalimumab.

Patients should be evaluated for latent tuberculosis infection with a tuberculin skin test. Treatment of latent tuberculosis infection should be initiated prior to therapy with adalimumab.

A

DESCRIPTION

Adalimumab is a recombinant human IgG1 monoclonal antibody specific for human tumor necrosis factor (TNF). Adalimumab was created using phage display technology resulting in an antibody with human derived heavy and light chain variable regions and human IgG1:κ constant regions. Adalimumab is produced by recombinant DNA technology in a mammalian cell expression system and is purified by a process that includes specific viral inactivation and removal steps. It consists of 1330 amino acids and has a molecular weight of approximately 148 kilodaltons.

Humira is supplied in single-use, 1 ml pre-filled glass syringes, and also 2 ml glass vials as a sterile, preservative-free solution for SC administration. The solution of Humira is clear and colorless, with a pH of about 5.2. Each syringe delivers 0.8 ml (40 mg) of drug product. Each vial contains approximately 0.9 ml of solution to deliver 0.8 ml (40 mg) of drug product. Each 0.8 ml Humira contains 40 mg adalimumab, 4.93 mg sodium chloride, 0.69 mg monobasic sodium phosphate dihydrate, 1.22 mg dibasic sodium phosphate dihydrate, 0.24 mg sodium citrate, 1.04 mg citric acid monohydrate, 9.6 mg mannitol, 0.8 mg polysorbate 80 and water for injection. Sodium hydroxide added as necessary to adjust pH.

CLINICAL PHARMACOLOGY

GENERAL

Adalimumab binds specifically to TNF-alpha and blocks its interaction with the p55 and p75 cell surface TNF receptors. Adalimumab also lyses surface TNF expressing cells *in vitro* in the presence of complement. Adalimumab does not bind or inactivate lymphotoxin (TNF-beta). TNF is a naturally occurring cytokine that is involved in normal inflammatory and immune responses. Elevated levels of TNF are found in the synovial fluid of rheumatoid arthritis patients and play an important role in both the pathologic inflammation and the joint destruction that are hallmarks of rheumatoid arthritis.

Adalimumab also modulates biological responses that are induced or regulated by TNF, including changes in the levels of adhesion molecules responsible for leukocyte migration (ELAM-1, VCAM-1, and ICAM-1 with an IC_{50} of 1-2 $\times 10^{-10}$M).

PHARMACODYNAMICS

After treatment with adalimumab, a rapid decrease in levels of acute phase reactants of inflammation (C-reactive protein (CRP) and erythrocyte sedimentation rate (ESR)) and serum cytokines (IL-6) was observed compared to baseline in patients with rheumatoid arthritis. Serum levels of matrix metalloproteinases (MMP-1 and MMP-3) that produce tissue remodeling responsible for cartilage destruction were also decreased after adalimumab administration.

PHARMACOKINETICS

The maximum serum concentration (C_{max}) and the time to reach the maximum concentration (T^{max}) were 4.7 ± 1.6 μg/ml and 131 ± 56 hours respectively, following a single 40 mg SC administration of adalimumab to healthy adult subjects. The average absolute bioavailability of adalimumab estimated from three studies following a single 40 mg SC dose was 64%. The pharmacokinetics of adalimumab were linear over the dose range of 0.5-10.0 mg/kg following a single IV dose.

The single dose pharmacokinetics of adalimumab were determined in several studies with IV doses ranging from 0.25 to 10 mg/kg. The distribution volume (Vss) ranged from 4.7-6.0 L. The systemic clearance of adalimumab is approximately 12 ml/h. The mean terminal half-life was approximately 2 weeks, ranging from 10-20 days across studies. Adalimumab concentrations in the synovial fluid from 5 rheumatoid arthritis patients ranged from 31-96% of those in serum.

Adalimumab mean steady-state trough concentrations of approximately 5 μg/ml and 8-9 μg/ml, were observed without and with methotrexate (MTX) respectively. The serum adalimumab trough levels at steady-state increased approximately proportionally with dose following 20, 40 and 80 mg every other week and every week SC dosing.

In long-term studies with dosing more than 2 years, there was no evidence of changes in clearance over time.

Population pharmacokinetic analyses revealed that there was a trend toward higher apparent clearance of adalimumab in the presence of anti-adalimumab antibodies, and lower clearance with increasing age in patients aged 40 to >75 years.

Minor increases in apparent clearance were also predicted in patients receiving doses lower than the recommended dose and in patients with high rheumatoid factor or CRP concentrations. These increases are not likely to be clinically important.

No gender-related pharmacokinetic differences were observed after correction for a patient's body weight. Healthy volunteers and patients with rheumatoid arthritis displayed similar adalimumab pharmacokinetics.

No pharmacokinetic data are available in patients with hepatic or renal impairment.

Adalimumab has not been studied in children.

DRUG INTERACTIONS

MTX reduced adalimumab apparent clearance after single and multiple dosing by 29% and 44% respectively.

INDICATIONS AND USAGE

Adalimumab is indicated for reducing signs and symptoms and inhibiting the progression of structural damage in adult patients with moderately to severely active rheumatoid arthritis who have had an inadequate response to 1 or more DMARDs. Adalimumab can be used alone or in combination with MTX or other DMARDs.

CONTRAINDICATIONS

Adalimumab should not be administered to patients with known hypersensitivity to adalimumab or any of its components.

WARNINGS

SERIOUS INFECTIONS AND SEPSIS, INCLUDING FATALITIES, HAVE BEEN REPORTED WITH THE USE OF TNF BLOCKING AGENTS INCLUDING ADALIMUMAB. MANY OF THE SERIOUS INFECTIONS HAVE OCCURRED IN PATIENTS ON CONCOMITANT IMMUNOSUPPRESSIVE THERAPY THAT, IN ADDITION TO THEIR RHEUMATOID ARTHRITIS, COULD PREDISPOSE THEM TO INFECTIONS. TUBERCULOSIS AND INVASIVE OPPORTUNISTIC FUNGAL INFECTIONS HAVE BEEN OBSERVED IN PATIENTS TREATED WITH TNF BLOCKING AGENTS INCLUDING ADALIMUMAB.

TREATMENT WITH ADALIMUMAB SHOULD NOT BE INITIATED IN PATIENTS WITH ACTIVE INFECTIONS INCLUDING CHRONIC OR LOCALIZED INFECTIONS. PATIENTS WHO DEVELOP A NEW INFECTION WHILE UNDERGOING TREATMENT WITH ADALIMUMAB SHOULD BE MONITORED CLOSELY. ADMINISTRATION OF ADALIMUMAB SHOULD BE DISCONTINUED IF A PATIENT DEVELOPS A SERIOUS INFECTION. PHYSICIANS SHOULD EXERCISE CAUTION WHEN CONSIDERING THE USE OF ADALIMUMAB IN PATIENTS WITH A HISTORY OF RECURRENT INFECTION OR UNDERLYING CONDITIONS WHICH MAY PREDISPOSE THEM TO INFECTIONS, OR PATIENTS WHO HAVE RESIDED IN REGIONS WHERE TUBERCULOSIS AND HISTOPLASMOSIS ARE ENDEMIC (see PRECAUTIONS, Tuberculosis and ADVERSE REACTIONS, Infections). THE BENEFITS AND RISKS OF ADALIMUMAB TREATMENT SHOULD BE CAREFULLY CONSIDERED BEFORE INITIATION OF ADALIMUMAB THERAPY.

NEUROLOGIC EVENTS

Use of TNF blocking agents, including adalimumab, has been associated with rare cases of exacerbation of clinical symptoms and/or radiographic evidence of demyelinating disease. Prescribers should exercise caution in considering the use of adalimumab in patients with preexisting or recent-onset central nervous system demyelinating disorders.

MALIGNANCIES

Lymphomas have been observed in patients treated with TNF blocking agents including adalimumab. In clinical trials, patients treated with adalimumab had a higher incidence of lymphoma than the expected rate in the general population (see ADVERSE REACTIONS, Malignancies). While patients with rheumatoid arthritis, particularly those with highly active disease, may be at a higher risk (up to several fold) for the development of lymphoma, the role of TNF blockers in the development of malignancy is not known.[4,5]

PRECAUTIONS

GENERAL

Allergic reactions have been observed in approximately 1% of patients receiving adalimumab. If an anaphylactic reaction or other serious allergic reaction occurs, administration of adalimumab should be discontinued immediately and appropriate therapy initiated.

INFORMATION FOR THE PATIENT

The first injection should be performed under the supervision of a qualified health care professional. If a patient or caregiver is to administer adalimumab, he/she should be instructed in injection techniques and their ability to inject subcutaneously should be assessed to ensure the proper administration of adalimumab (see the patient information leaflet that is included with the prescription). A puncture-resistant container for disposal of needles and syringes should be used. Patients or caregivers should be instructed in the technique as well as proper syringe and needle disposal, and be cautioned against reuse of these items.

TUBERCULOSIS

As observed with other TNF blocking agents, tuberculosis associated with the administration of adalimumab in clinical trials has been reported (see WARNINGS). While cases were observed at all doses, the incidence of tuberculosis reactivations was particularly increased at doses of adalimumab that were higher than the recommended dose. All patients recovered after standard antimicrobial therapy. No deaths due to tuberculosis occurred during the clinical trials.

Before initiation of therapy with adalimumab, patients should be evaluated for active or latent tuberculosis infection with a tuberculin skin test. If latent infection is diagnosed, appropriate prophylaxis in accordance with the Centers for Disease Control and Prevention guidelines[6] should be instituted. Patients should be instructed to seek medical advice if signs/symptoms (*e.g.*, persistent cough, wasting/weight loss, low grade fever) suggestive of a tuberculosis infection occur.

IMMUNOSUPPRESSION

The possibility exists for TNF blocking agents, including adalimumab, to affect host defenses against infections and malignancies since TNF mediates inflammation and modulates cellular immune responses. In a study of 64 patients with rheumatoid arthritis treated with adalimumab, there was no evidence of depression of delayed-type hypersensitivity, depression of immunoglobulin levels, or change in enumeration of effector T- and B-cells and NK-cells, monocyte/macrophages, and neutrophils. The impact of treatment with adalimumab on the development and course of malignancies, as well as active and/or chronic infections is not fully understood (see WARNINGS, and ADVERSE REACTIONS: Infections and Malignancies). The safety and efficacy of adalimumab in patients with immunosuppression have not been evaluated.

IMMUNIZATIONS

No data are available on the effects of vaccination in patients receiving adalimumab. Live vaccines should not be given concurrently with adalimumab. No data are available on the secondary transmission of infection by live vaccines in patients receiving adalimumab.

AUTOIMMUNITY

Treatment with adalimumab may result in the formation of autoantibodies and, rarely, in the development of a lupus-like syndrome. If a patient develops symptoms suggestive of a lupus-like syndrome following treatment with adalimumab, treatment should be discontinued (see ADVERSE REACTIONS, Autoantibodies).

CARCINOGENESIS, MUTAGENESIS, AND IMPAIRMENT OF FERTILITY

Long-term animal studies of adalimumab have not been conducted to evaluate the carcinogenic potential or its effect on fertility. No clastogenic or mutagenic effects of adalimumab were observed in the *in vivo* mouse micronucleus test or the *Salmonella-Escherichia coli* (Ames) assay, respectively.

PREGNANCY CATEGORY B

An embryo-fetal perinatal developmental toxicity study has been performed in cynomolgus monkeys at dosages up to 100 mg/kg (266 times human AUC when given 40 mg SC with MTX every week or 373 times human AUC when given 40 mg SC without MTX) and has revealed no evidence of harm to the fetuses due to adalimumab. There are, however, no adequate and well-controlled studies in pregnant women. Because animal reproduction and developmental studies are not always predictive of human response, adalimumab should be used during pregnancy only if clearly needed.

NURSING MOTHERS

It is not known whether adalimumab is excreted in human milk or absorbed systemically after ingestion. Because many drugs and immunoglobulins are excreted in human milk, and because of the potential for serious adverse reactions in nursing infants from adalimumab, a decision should be made whether to discontinue nursing or to discontinue the drug, taking into account the importance of the drug to the mother.

PEDIATRIC USE

Safety and effectiveness of adalimumab in pediatric patients have not been established.

GERIATRIC USE

A total of 519 patients 65 years of age and older, including 107 patients 75 years and older, received adalimumab in clinical studies. No overall difference in effectiveness was observed between these subjects and younger subjects. The frequency of serious infection and malignancy among adalimumab treated subjects over age 65 was higher than for those under age 65. Because there is a higher incidence of infections and malignancies in the elderly population in general, caution should be used when treating the elderly.

DRUG INTERACTIONS

Adalimumab has been studied in rheumatoid arthritis patients taking concomitant MTX (see CLINICAL PHARMACOLOGY, Drug Interations). The data do not suggest the need for dose adjustment of either adalimumab or MTX.

ADVERSE REACTIONS

GENERAL

The most serious adverse reactions were (see WARNINGS):

- Serious infections.
- Neurologic events.
- Malignancies.

The most common adverse reaction with adalimumab was injection site reactions. In placebo-controlled trials, 20% of patients treated with adalimumab developed injection site reactions (erythema and/or itching, hemorrhage, pain or swelling), compared to 14% of patients receiving placebo. Most injection site reactions were described as mild and generally did not necessitate drug discontinuation.

The proportion of patients who discontinued treatment due to adverse events during the double-blind, placebo-controlled portion of Studies I, II, III and IV was 7% for patients taking adalimumab and 4% for placebo-treated patients. The most common adverse events leading to discontinuation of adalimumab were clinical flare reaction (0.7%), rash (0.3%) and pneumonia (0.3%).

Because clinical trials are conducted under widely varying and controlled conditions, adverse reaction rates observed in clinical trials of a drug cannot be directly compared to rates in the clinical trials of another drug and may not predict the rates observed in a broader patient population in clinical practice.

INFECTIONS

In placebo-controlled trials, the rate of infection was 1/patient year in the adalimumab treated patients and 0.9/patient year in the placebo-treated patients. The infections consisted primarily of upper respiratory tract infections, bronchitis and urinary tract infections. Most patients continued on adalimumab after the infection resolved. The incidence of serious infections was 0.04/patient year in adalimumab treated patients and 0.02/patient year in placebo-treated patients. Serious infections observed included pneumonia, septic arthritis, prosthetic and post-surgical infections, erysipelas, cellulitis, diverticulitis, and pyelonephritis (see WARNINGS).

Thirteen (13) cases of tuberculosis, including miliary, lymphatic, peritoneal, and pulmonary were reported in clinical trials. Most of the cases of tuberculosis occurred within the first 8 months after initiation of therapy and may reflect recrudescence of latent disease. Six (6) cases of invasive opportunistic infections caused by histoplasma, aspergillus, and nocardia were also reported in clinical trials (see WARNINGS).

MALIGNANCIES

Among 2468 rheumatoid arthritis patients treated in clinical trials with adalimumab for a median of 24 months, 48 malignancies of various types were observed, including 10 patients with lymphoma. The Standardized Incidence Ratio (SIR) (ratio of observed rate to age-adjusted expected frequency in the general population) for malignancies was 1.0 (95% CI, 0.7, 1.3) and for lymphomas was 5.4 (95% CI, 2.6, 10.0). An increase of up to several fold in the rate of lymphomas has been reported in the rheumatoid arthritis patient population[4], and may be further increased in patients with more severe disease activity[5] (see WARNINGS, Malignancies). The other malignancies observed during use of adalimumab were breast, colon-rectum, uterine-cervical, prostate, melanoma, gallbladder-bile ducts, and other carcinomas.

AUTOANTIBODIES

In the controlled trials, 12% of patients treated with adalimumab and 7% of placebo-treated patients that had negative baseline ANA titers developed positive titers at Week 24. One (1) patient out of 2334 treated with adalimumab developed clinical signs suggestive of new-onset lupus-like syndrome. The patient improved following discontinuation of therapy. No patients developed lupus nephritis or central nervous system symptoms. The impact of long-term treatment with adalimumab on the development of autoimmune diseases is unknown.

IMMUNOGENICITY

Patients in Studies I, II, and III were tested at multiple time points for antibodies to adalimumab during the 6-12 month period. Approximately 5% (58 of 1062) of adult rheumatoid arthritis patients receiving adalimumab developed low-titer antibodies to adalimumab at least once during treatment, which were neutralizing *in vitro*. Patients treated with concomitant MTX had a lower rate of antibody development than patients on adalimumab monotherapy (1% vs 12%). No apparent correlation of antibody development to adverse events was observed. With monotherapy, patients receiving every other week dosing may develop antibodies more frequently than those receiving weekly dosing. In patients receiving the recommended dosage of 40 mg every other week as monotherapy, the ACR 20 response was lower among antibody-positive patients than among antibody-negative patients. The long-term immunogenicity of adalimumab is unknown.

The data reflect the percentage of patients whose test results were considered positive for antibodies to adalimumab in an ELISA assay, and are highly dependent on the sensitivity and specificity of the assay. Additionally the observed incidence of antibody positivity in an assay may be influenced by several factors including sample handling, timing of sample collection, concomitant medications, and underlying disease. For these reasons, comparison of the incidence of antibodies to adalimumab with the incidence of antibodies to other products may be misleading.

OTHER ADVERSE REACTIONS

The data described below reflect exposure to adalimumab in 2334 patients, including 2073 exposed for 6 months, 1497 exposed for greater than 1 year and 1380 in adequate and well-controlled studies (Studies I, II, III, and IV). Adalimumab was studied primarily in placebo-controlled trials and in long-term follow up studies for up to 36 months duration. The population had a mean age of 54 years, 77% were female, 91% were Caucasian and had moderately to severely active rheumatoid arthritis. Most patients received 40 mg adalimumab every other week.

TABLE 4 summarizes events reported at a rate of at least 5% in patients treated with adalimumab 40 mg every other week compared to placebo and with an incidence higher than placebo. Adverse event rates in patients treated with adalimumab 40 mg weekly were similar to rates in patients treated with adalimumab 40 mg every other week.

TABLE 4 *Adverse Events Reported by ≥5% of Patients Treated With Adalimumab During Placebo-Controlled Period of Rheumatoid Arthritis Studies*

	Adalimumab 40 mg Subcutaneous	
Adverse Event (Preferred Term)	**Every Other Week (n=705)**	**Placebo (n=690)**
Respiratory		
Upper respiratory infection	17%	13%
Sinusitis	11%	9%
Flu syndrome	7%	6%
Gastrointestinal		
Nausea	9%	8%
Abdominal pain	7%	4%
Laboratory Tests*		
Laboratory test abnormal	8%	7%
Hypercholesterolemia	6%	4%
Hyperlipidemia	7%	5%
Hematuria	5%	4%
Alkaline phosphatase increased	5%	3%
Other		
Injection site pain	12%	12%
Headache	12%	8%
Rash	12%	6%
Accidental injury	10%	8%
Injection site reaction†	8%	1%
Back pain	6%	4%
Urinary tract infection	8%	5%
Hypertension	5%	3%

* Laboratory test abnormalities were reported as adverse events in European trials.
† Does not include erythema and/or itching, hemorrhage, pain or swelling.

Other Adverse Events

Other infrequent serious adverse events occurring at an incidence of less than 5% in patients treated with adalimumab were:

Body As A Whole: Fever, infection, pain in extremity, pelvic pain, sepsis, surgery, thorax pain, tuberculosis reactivated.

Cardiovascular System: Arrhythmia, atrial fibrillation, cardiovascular disorder, chest pain, congestive heart failure, coronary artery disorder, heart arrest, hypertensive encephalopathy, myocardial infarct, palpitation, pericardial effusion, pericarditis, syncope, tachycardia, vascular disorder.

Collagen Disorder: Lupus erythematosus syndrome.

Digestive System: Cholecystitis, cholelithiasis, esophagitis, gastroenteritis, gastrointestinal disorder, gastrointestinal hemorrhage, hepatic necrosis, vomiting.

Endocrine System: Parathyroid disorder.

Hemic and Lymphatic System: Agranulocytosis, granulocytopenia, leukopenia, lymphoma like reaction, pancytopenia, polycythemia.

Metabolic and Nutritional Disorders: Dehydration, healing abnormal, ketosis, paraproteinemia, peripheral edema.
Musculoskeletal System: Arthritis, bone disorder, bone fracture (not spontaneous), bone necrosis, joint disorder, muscle cramps, myasthenia, pyogenic arthritis, synovitis, tendon disorder.
Neoplasia: Adenoma, carcinomas such as breast, gastrointestinal, skin, urogenital, and others; lymphoma and melanoma.
Nervous System: Confusion, multiple sclerosis, paresthesia, subdural hematoma, tremor.
Respiratory System: Asthma, bronchospasm, dyspnea, lung disorder, lung function decreased, pleural effusion, pneumonia.
Skin and Appendages: Cellulitis, erysipelas, herpes zoster.
Special Senses: Cataract.
Thrombosis: Thrombosis leg.
Urogenital System: Cystitis, kidney calculus, menstrual disorder, pyelonephritis.

DOSAGE AND ADMINISTRATION

The recommended dose of adalimumab for adult patients with rheumatoid arthritis is 40 mg administered every other week as a SC injection. MTX, glucocorticoids, salicylates, nonsteroidal anti-inflammatory drugs (NSAIDs), analgesics or other DMARDs may be continued during treatment with adalimumab. Some patients not taking concomitant MTX may derive additional benefit from increasing the dosing frequency of adalimumab to 40 mg every week.

Adalimumab is intended for use under the guidance and supervision of a physician. Patients may self-inject adalimumab if their physician determines that it is appropriate and with medical follow-up, as necessary, after proper training in injection technique.

The solution in the syringe and in the vial should be carefully inspected visually for particulate matter and discoloration prior to SC administration. If particulates and discolorations are noted, the product should not be used. Adalimumab does not contain preservatives; therefore, unused portions of drug remaining from the syringe or vial should be discarded. NOTE: The needle cover of the syringe contains dry rubber (latex), which should not be handled by persons sensitive to this substance.

Patients using the pre-filled syringes should be instructed to inject the full amount in the syringe (0.8 ml), which provides 40 mg of adalimumab. For patients and institutions using vials, 0.8 ml of solution providing 40 mg of adalimumab should be withdrawn from the vial and administered according to the directions provided in the Patient Information Leaflet.

Injection sites should be rotated and injections should never be given into areas where the skin is tender, bruised, red or hard (see the patient information leaflet that is included with the prescription).

HOW SUPPLIED

Humira is supplied in glass vials and syringes as a preservative-free, sterile solution for SC administration. The following packaging configurations are available:

Patient Use Syringe Carton: Humira is dispensed in a carton containing 2 alcohol preps and 2 dose trays. Each dose tray consists of a single-use, 1 ml pre-filled glass syringe with a fixed 27 gauge ½ inch needle, providing 40 mg (0.8 ml) of adalimumab.
Patient Use Vial Carton: Humira is dispensed in a carton containing 4 alcohol preps and 2 trays. Each dose tray consists of a single-use, 2 ml glass vial providing 40 mg (0.8 ml) of adalimumab and one sterile 1 ml syringe with a fixed 25 gauge 5/8 inch needle.
Institutional Use Syringe Carton: Each carton contains 2 alcohol preps and 1 tray. Each dose tray consists of a single use, 1 ml pre-filled glass syringe with a fixed 27 gauge ½ inch needle (with a needle stick protection device) providing 40 mg (0.8 ml) adalimumab.
Institutional Use Vial Carton: Each carton contains 2 alcohol preps and 1 tray. Each dose tray consists of a 2 ml glass vial providing 40 mg (0.8 ml) of adalimumab, and 1 sterile syringe with a fixed 27 gauge ½ inch needle (with needle stick protection device).

STORAGE AND STABILITY

Do not use beyond the expiration date on the container. Adalimumab must be refrigerated at 2-8°C (36-46°F). DO NOT FREEZE. Protect the vial or/and pre-filled syringe from exposure to light. Store in original carton until time of administration.

PRODUCT LISTING - EQUIVALENTS NOT AVAILABLE

Solution - Subcutaneous - 40 mg
2 ml x 2 $1306.60 HUMIRA, Abbott Pharmaceutical 00074-3799-02

Adapalene *(003292)*

Categories: Acne vulgaris; Pregnancy Category C; FDA Approved 1996 May
Drug Classes: Dermatologics; Retinoids
Brand Names: Differin
Foreign Brand Availability: Adaferin (India; Mexico); Adaferin Gel (Israel); Differin Gel (Austria; Germany; Ireland; Italy; Spain; Sweden; Switzerland); Differine (France)
Cost of Therapy: $27.31 (Acne; Differin Gel; 0.1%; 15 g; 1 application/day; variable day supply)

DESCRIPTION

For topical use only. Not for ophthalmic, oral, or intravaginal use.

Differin (adapalene) cream, 0.1%, contains adapalene 0.1% in an aqueous cream emulsion consisting of carbomer 934P, cyclomethicone, edetate disodium, glycerin, methyl glucose sesquistearate, methylparaben, PEG-20 methyl glucose sesquistearate, phenoxyethanol, propylparaben, purified water, squalane, and trolamine.

Differin (adapalene) gel is used for the topical treatment of acne vulgaris. Each gram of adapalene gel contains adapalene 0.1% (1 mg) in a vehicle consisting of propylene glycol, carbomer 940, poloxamer 182, edelate disodium, methylparaben, sodium hydroxide, and purified water. May contain hydrochloric acid to adjust pH.

The chemical name of adapalene is 6–[3–(1–adamantyl)-4–methoxyphenyl]-2–naphthoic acid. It is a white to off-white powder which is soluble in tetrahydrofuran, sparingly soluble in ethanol, and practically insoluble in water. The molecular formula is $C_{28}H_{28}O_3$ and the molecular weight is 412.52.

CLINICAL PHARMACOLOGY

MECHANISM OF ACTION

Adapalene acts on retinoid receptors. Biochemical and pharmacological profile studies have demonstrated that adapalene is a modulator of cellular differentiation, keratinization, and inflammatory processes — all of which represent important features in the pathology of acne vulgaris.

Mechanistically, adapalene binds to specific retinoic acid nuclear receptors but does not bind to the cytosolic receptor protein. Although the exact mode of action of adapalene is unknown, it is suggested that topical adapalene may normalize the differentiation of follicular epithelial cells resulting in decreased microcomedone formation.

PHARMACOKINETICS

Absorption of adapalene through human skin is low. In a pharmacokinetic study with 6 acne patients treated once daily for 5 days with 2 g of adapalene cream applied to 1000 cm^2 of acne involved skin, there were no quantifiable amounts (limit of quantification = 0.35 ng/ml) of adapalene in the plasma samples from any patient. Excretion appears to be primarily by the biliary route.

INDICATIONS AND USAGE

Adapalene cream and gel are indicated for the topical treatment of acne vulgaris.

CONTRAINDICATIONS

Adapalene cream and gel should not be administered to individuals who are hypersensitive to adapalene or any of the components in the cream vehicle or gel.

WARNINGS

Use of adapalene gel should be discontinued if hypersensitivity to any of the ingredients is noted. Patients with sunburn should be advised not to use this product until fully recovered.

PRECAUTIONS

GENERAL

Certain cutaneous signs and symptoms such as erythema, dryness, scaling, burning, or pruritus may be experienced during treatment. These are most likely to occur during the first 2-4 weeks of treatment, are mostly mild to moderate in intensity, and will usually lessen with continued use of the medication. Depending upon the severity of adverse events, patients should be instructed to reduce the frequency of application or discontinue use.

If a reaction suggesting sensitivity or chemical irritation occurs, use of the medication should be discontinued. Exposure to sunlight, including sunlamps, should be minimized during the use of adapalene. Patients who normally experience high levels of sun exposure, and those with inherent sensitivity to the sun should be warned to exercise caution. Use of sunscreen products and protective clothing over treated areas is recommended when exposure cannot be avoided. Weather extremes, such as wind or cold, also may be irritating to patients under treatment with adapalene.

Avoid contact with eyes, lips, angles of the nose, and mucous membranes. The product should not be applied to cuts, abrasions, eczematous skin, or sunburned skin. As with other retinoids, use of "waxing" as a depilatory method should be avoided on skin treated with adapalene.

INFORMATION FOR THE PATIENT

Patients using adapalene cream should receive the following information and instructions:

1. This medication is to be used only as directed by the physician.
2. It is for external use only.
3. Avoid contact with the eyes, lips, angles of the nose, and mucous membranes.
4. Cleanse area with a mild or soapless cleanser before applying this medication.
5. Moisturizers may be used if necessary; however, products containing alpha hydroxy or glycolic acids should be avoided.
6. Exposure of the eye to this medication may result in reactions such as swelling, conjunctivitis, and eye irritation.
7. This medication should not be applied to cuts, abrasions, eczematous or sunburned skin.
8. Wax epilation should not be performed on treated skin due to the potential for skin erosions.
9. During the early weeks of therapy, an apparent exacerbation of acne may occur. This is due to the action of this medication on previously unseen lesions and should not be considered a reason to discontinue therapy. Overall clinical benefit may be noticed after 2 weeks of therapy, but at least 8 weeks are required to obtain consistent beneficial effects.

CARCINOGENESIS, MUTAGENESIS, AND IMPAIRMENT OF FERTILITY

No photocarcinogenicity studies were conducted. Animal studies have shown an increased risk of skin neoplasms with the use of pharmacologically similar drugs (*e.g.*, retinoids) when exposed to UV irridation in the laboratory or to sunlight. Although the significance of these studies to human use is not clear, patients should be advised to avoid or minimize exposure to either sunlight or artificial UV irridation sources.

Adapalene did not exhibit mutagenic or genotoxic effects *in vivo* (mouse micronucleus test) and *in vitro* (Ames test, Chinese hamster ovary cell assay, mouse lymphoma TK assay) studies.

Cream

Carcinogenicity studies with adapalene have been conducted in mice at topical doses of 0.4, 1.3, and 4.0 mg/kg/day, and in rats at oral doses of 0.15, 0.5, and 1.5 mg/kg/day. These doses are up to 8 times (mice) and 6 times (rats) in terms of mg/m^2/day the maximum potential exposure at the recommended topical human dose (MRHD), assumed to be 2.5 g adapalene cream, which is approximately 1.5 mg/m^2 adapalene. In the oral study, increased incidence of benign and malignant pheochromocytomas in the adrenal medullas of male rats was observed.

Reproductive function and fertility studies were conducted in rats administered oral doses of adapalene in amounts up to 20 mg/kg/day (up to 80 times the MRHD based on mg/m^2 comparisons). No effects of adapalene were found on the reproductive performance or fertility of the F_0 males or females. There were also no detectable effects on the growth, development and subsequent reproductive function of the F_1 generation.

Gel

Carcinogenicity studies have been conducted in mice at topical doses of 0.3, 0.9, and 2.6 mg/kg/day and in rats at oral doses of 0.15, 0.5, and 1.5 mg/kg/day, approximately 4-75 times the maximal daily human topical dose. In the oral study, positive linear trends were observed in the incidence of follicular cell adenomas and carcinomas in the thyroid glands of female rats, and in the incidence of benign and malignant pheochromocytomas in the adrenal medullas of male rats.

PREGNANCY, TERATOGENIC EFFECTS, PREGNANCY CATEGORY C

No teratogenic effects were seen in rats at oral doses of 0.15-5.0 mg/kg/day adapalene (up to 20 times the MRHD based on mg/m^2 comparisons). However, adapalene administered orally at doses of ≥25 mg/kg, (100 times the MRHD for rats or 200 times MRHD for rabbits) has been shown to be teratogenic. Cutaneous teratology studies in rats and rabbits at doses of 0.6, 2.0, and 6.0 mg/kg/day (24 times the MRHD for rats or 48 times the MRHD for rabbits) exhibited no fetotoxicity and only minimal increases in supernumerary ribs in rats. There are no adequate and well-controlled studies in pregnant women. Adapalene should be used during pregnancy only if the potential benefit justifies the potential risk to the fetus.

NURSING MOTHERS

It is not known whether this drug is excreted in human milk. Because many drugs are excreted in human milk, caution should be exercised when adapalene is administered to a nursing woman.

PEDIATRIC USE

Safety and effectiveness in pediatric patients below the age of 12 have not been established.

GERIATRIC USE

Clinical studies of adapalene cream were conducted in patients 12-30 years of age with acne vulgaris and therefore did not include subjects 65 years and older to determine whether they respond differently than younger subjects. Other reported clinical experience has not identified differences in responses between the elderly and younger patients.

DRUG INTERACTIONS

As adapalene has the potential to produce local irritation in some patients, concomitant use of other potentially irritating topical products (medicated or abrasive soaps and cleansers, soaps and cosmetics that have a strong drying effect, and products with high concentrations of alcohol, astringents, spices, or lime rind) should be approached with caution. Particular caution should be exercised in using preparations containing sulfur, resorcinol, or salicylic acid in combination with adapalene. If these preparations have been used, it is advisable not to start therapy with adapalene until the effects of such preparations in the skin have subsided.

ADVERSE REACTIONS

CREAM

In controlled clinical trials, local cutaneous irritation was monitored in 285 acne patients who used adapalene cream once daily for 12 weeks. The frequency and severity of erythema, scaling, dryness, pruritus and burning were assessed during these studies. The incidence of local cutaneous irritation with adapalene cream from the controlled clinical studies is provided in TABLE 2.

TABLE 2 *Incidence of Local Cutaneous Irritation With Adapalene Cream From Controlled Clinical Studies (n=285)*

	None	Mild	Moderate	Severe
Erythema	52% (148)	38% (108)	10% (28)	<1% (1)
Scaling	58% (166)	35% (100)	6% (18)	<1% (1)
Dryness	48% (136)	42% (121)	9% (26)	<1% (2)
Pruritus (persistent)	74% (211)	21% (61)	4% (12)	<1% (1)
Burning/stinging (persistent)	71% (202)	24% (69)	4% (12)	<1% (2)

Other reported local cutaneous adverse events in patients who used adapalene cream once daily included: Sunburn (2%), skin discomfort, burning and stinging (1%), and skin irritation (1%).

Events occurring in less than 1% of patients treated with adapalene cream included: Acne flare, dermatitis and contact dermatitis, eyelid edema, conjunctivitis, erythema, pruritus, skin discoloration, rash, and eczema.

GEL

Some adverse effects such as erythema, scaling, dryness, pruritus, and burning will occur in 10-40% of patients. Pruritus or burning immediately after application also occurs in approximately 20% of patients.

The following adverse experiences were reported in approximately 1% or less of patients: Skin irritation, burning/stinging, erythema, sunburn, and acne flares. These are most commonly seen during the first month of therapy and decrease in frequency and severity thereafter. All adverse effects with use of adapalene gel during clinical trials were reversible upon discontinuation of therapy.

DOSAGE AND ADMINISTRATION

CREAM

Adapalene cream should be applied to affected areas of the skin once daily at nighttime. A thin film of the cream should be applied to the skin areas where acne lesions appear, using enough to cover the entire affected area lightly. A mild transitory sensation of warmth or slight stinging may occur shortly after the application of adapalene cream.

GEL

Adapalene gel should be applied once a day to affected areas after washing in the evening before retiring. A thin film of the gel should be applied, avoiding eyes, lips, and mucous membranes.

During the early weeks of therapy, an apparent exacerbation of acne may occur. This is due to the action of the medication on previously unseen lesions and should not be considered a reason to discontinue therapy. Therapeutic results should be noticed after 8-12 weeks of treatment.

HOW SUPPLIED

Storage: Store at controlled room temperature 20-25°C (68-77°F). Protect from freezing.

PRODUCT LISTING - EQUIVALENTS NOT AVAILABLE

Cream - Topical - 0.1%			
15 gm	$42.19	DIFFERIN, Galderma Laboratories Inc	00299-5915-15
45 gm	$91.06	DIFFERIN, Galderma Laboratories Inc	00299-5915-45
Gel - Topical - 0.1%			
15 gm	$27.31	DIFFERIN, Allscripts Pharmaceutical Company	54569-4640-00
15 gm	$42.19	DIFFERIN, Galderma Laboratories Inc	00299-5910-15
45 gm	$91.06	DIFFERIN, Galderma Laboratories Inc	00299-5910-45
Solution - Topical - 0.1%			
1 ml x 60	$78.56	DIFFERIN, Galderma Laboratories Inc	00299-5905-16
30 ml	$78.56	DIFFERIN, Galderma Laboratories Inc	00299-5905-30

Adefovir Dipivoxil *(003569)*

Categories: Hepatitis B; Pregnancy Category C; FDA Approved 2002 Sep
Drug Classes: Antivirals
Brand Names: Hepsera
Cost of Therapy: $528.00 (Hepatitis B; Hepsera; 10 mg; 1 tablet/day; 30 day supply)

WARNING

SEVERE ACUTE EXACERBATIONS OF HEPATITIS HAVE BEEN REPORTED IN PATIENTS WHO HAVE DISCONTINUED ANTI-HEPATITIS B THERAPY, INCLUDING THERAPY WITH ADEFOVIR DIPIVOXIL. HEPATIC FUNCTION SHOULD BE MONITORED CLOSELY IN PATIENTS WHO DISCONTINUE ANTI-HEPATITIS B THERAPY. IF APPROPRIATE, RESUMPTION OF ANTI-HEPATITIS B THERAPY MAY BE WARRANTED (SEE WARNINGS).

IN PATIENTS AT RISK OF OR HAVING UNDERLYING RENAL DYSFUNCTION, CHRONIC ADMINISTRATION OF ADEFOVIR DIPIVOXIL MAY RESULT IN NEPHROTOXICITY. THESE PATIENTS SHOULD BE MONITORED CLOSELY FOR RENAL FUNCTION AND MAY REQUIRE DOSE ADJUSTMENT (SEE WARNINGS AND DOSAGE AND ADMINISTRATION).

HIV RESISTANCE MAY EMERGE IN CHRONIC HEPATITIS B PATIENTS WITH UNRECOGNIZED OR UNTREATED HUMAN IMMUNODEFICIENCY VIRUS (HIV) INFECTION TREATED WITH ANTI-HEPATITIS B THERAPIES, SUCH AS THERAPY WITH ADEFOVIR DIPIVOXIL, THAT MAY HAVE ACTIVITY AGAINST HIV (SEE WARNINGS).

LACTIC ACIDOSIS AND SEVERE HEPATOMEGALY WITH STEATOSIS, INCLUDING FATAL CASES, HAVE BEEN REPORTED WITH THE USE OF NUCLEOSIDE ANALOGS ALONE OR IN COMBINATION WITH OTHER ANTIRETROVIRALS (SEE WARNINGS).

DESCRIPTION

Hepsera is the tradename for adefovir dipivoxil, a diester prodrug of adefovir. Adefovir is an acyclic nucleotide analog with activity against human hepatitis B virus (HBV).

The chemical name of adefovir dipivoxil is 9-[2-[bis[(pivaloyloxy)methoxy]phosphinyl]-methoxy]ethyl]adenine. It has a molecular formula of $C_{20}H_{32}N_5O_8P$ and a molecular weight of 501.48.

Adefovir dipivoxil is a white to off-white crystalline powder with an aqueous solubility of 19 mg/ml at pH 2.0 and 0.4 mg/ml at pH 7.2. It has an octanol/aqueous phosphate buffer (pH 7) partition coefficient (log p) of 1.91.

Hepsera tablets are for oral administration. Each tablet contains 10 mg of adefovir dipivoxil and the following inactive ingredients: croscarmellose sodium, lactose monohydrate, magnesium stearate, pregelatinized starch, and talc.

CLINICAL PHARMACOLOGY

MICROBIOLOGY

Mechanism of Action

Adefovir is an acyclic nucleotide analog of adenosine monophosphate. Adefovir is phosphorylated to the active metabolite, adefovir diphosphate, by cellular kinases. Adefovir diphosphate inhibits HBV DNA polymerase (reverse transcriptase) by competing with the natural substrate deoxyadenosine triphosphate and by causing DNA chain termination after its incorporation into viral DNA. The inhibition constant (K_i) for adefovir diphosphate for HBV DNA polymerase was 0.1 μM. Adefovir diphosphate is a weak inhibitor of human DNA polymerases α and γ with K_i values of 1.18 μM and 0.97 μM, respectively.

Antiviral Activity

The *in vitro* antiviral activity of adefovir was determined in HBV transfected human hepatoma cell lines. The concentration of adefovir that inhibited 50% of viral DNA synthesis (IC_{50}) varied from 0.2-2.5 μM.

Drug Resistance

Clinical Studies 437 & 438

Genotypic and phenotypic analyses of serum HBV DNA from adefovir dipivoxil (10 mg or 30 mg) treated HBeAg-positive patients (n=215; study 437) and HBAg-negative patients (n=56; study 438) at baseline and week 48 did not identify mutations in the HBV DNA polymerase gene that may confer reduced susceptibility to adefovir. An unconfirmed increase of >1 log_{10} copies/ml in serum HBV DNA was observed in some patients. The molecular basis and/or the clinical significance for the observed unconfirmed increases are not known.

Cross-Resistance

Recombinant HBV variants containing lamivudine-resistance-associated mutations (L528M, M552I, M552V, L528M + M552V) in the HBV DNA polymerase gene were susceptible to adefovir *in vitro*. Adefovir has also demonstrated anti-HBV activity (median reduction in serum HBV DNA of 4.3 log_{10} copies/ml) against clinical isolates of HBV containing lamivudine-resistance-associated mutations (study 435). HBV variants with DNA polymerase mutations T476N and R or W501Q associated with resistance to hepatitis B immunoglobulin were susceptible to adefovir *in vitro*.

PHARMACOKINETICS

The pharmacokinetics of adefovir have been evaluated in healthy volunteers and patients with chronic hepatitis B. Adefovir pharmacokinetics are similar between these populations.

Absorption

Adefovir dipivoxil is a diester prodrug of the active moiety adefovir. Based on a cross study comparison, the approximate oral bioavailability of adefovir from adefovir dipivoxil is 59%.

Following oral administration of a 10 mg single dose of adefovir dipivoxil to chronic hepatitis B patients (n=14), the peak adefovir plasma concentration (C_{max}) was 18.4 ± 6.26 ng/ml (mean ±SD) and occurred between 0.58 and 4.00 hours (median=1.75 hours) post dose. The adefovir area under the plasma concentration-time curve [AUC(0-∞)] was 220 ± 70.0 ng·h/ml. Plasma adefovir concentrations declined in a biexponential manner with a terminal elimination half-life of 7.48 ± 1.65 hours.

The pharmacokinetics of adefovir in subjects with adequate renal function were not affected by once daily dosing of 10 mg adefovir dipivoxil over 7 days. The impact of long-term once daily administration of 10 mg adefovir dipivoxil on adefovir pharmacokinetics has not been evaluated.

Effects of Food on Oral Absorption

Adefovir exposure was unaffected when a 10 mg single dose of adefovir dipivoxil was administered with food (an approximately 1000 kcal high-fat meal). Adefovir dipivoxil may be taken without regard to food.

Distribution

In vitro binding of adefovir to human plasma or human serum proteins is ≤4% over the adefovir concentration range of 0.1 to 25 μg/ml. The volume of distribution at steady-state following intravenous administration of 1.0 or 3.0 mg/kg/day is 392 ± 75 and 352 ± 9 ml/kg, respectively.

Metabolism and Elimination

Following oral administration, adefovir dipivoxil is rapidly converted to adefovir. Forty-five percent (45%) of the dose is recovered as adefovir in the urine over 24 hours at steady state following 10 mg oral doses of adefovir dipivoxil. Adefovir is renally excreted by a combination of glomerular filtration and active tubular secretion (see DRUG INTERACTIONS).

Special Populations

Gender

The pharmacokinetics of adefovir were similar in male and female patients.

Race

Insufficient data are available to determine the effect of race on the pharmacokinetics of adefovir.

Pediatric and Geriatric Patients

Pharmacokinetic studies have not been conducted in children or in the elderly.

Renal Impairment

In subjects with moderately or severely impaired renal function or with end-stage renal disease (ESRD) requiring hemodialysis, C_{max}, AUC, and half-life (T½) were increased compared to subjects with normal renal function. It is recommended that the dosing interval of adefovir dipivoxil be modified in these patients (see DOSAGE AND ADMINISTRATION).

The pharmacokinetics of adefovir in non-chronic hepatitis B patients with varying degrees of renal impairment are described in TABLE 1. In this study, subjects received a 10 mg single dose of adefovir dipivoxil.

***TABLE 1** Pharmacokinetic Parameters (Mean ± SD) of Adefovir in Patients With Varying Degrees of Renal Function*

Renal Function Group	Unimpaired	Mild	Moderate	Severe
Baseline creatinine clearance (ml/min)	>80 (n=7)	50-80 (n=8)	30-49 (n=7)	10-29 (n=10)
C_{max} (ng/ml)	17.8 ± 3.22	22.4 ± 4.04	28.5 ± 8.57	51.6 ± 10.3
AUC(0-∞) (ng·h/ml)	201 ± 40.8	266 ± 55.7	455 ± 176	1240 ± 629
CL/F (ml/min)	469 ± 99.0	356 ± 85.6	237 ± 118	91.7 ± 51.3
CL_{renal} (ml/min)	231 ± 48.9	148 ± 39.3	83.9 ± 27.5	37.0 ± 18.4

A 4 hour period of hemodialysis removed approximately 35% of the adefovir dose. The effect of peritoneal dialysis on adefovir removal has not been evaluated.

Hepatic Impairment

The pharmacokinetics of adefovir following a 10 mg single dose of adefovir dipivoxil have been studied in non-chronic hepatitis B patients with hepatic impairment. There were no substantial alterations in adefovir pharmacokinetics in patients with moderate and severe hepatic impairment compared to unimpaired patients. No change in adefovir dipivoxil dosing is required in patients with hepatic impairment.

Drug Interactions

Adefovir dipivoxil is rapidly converted to adefovir *in vivo*. At concentrations substantially higher (>4000-fold) than those observed *in vivo*, adefovir did not inhibit any of the common human CYP450 enzymes, CYP1A2, CYP2C9, CYP2C19, CYP2D6, and CYP3A4. Adefovir is not a substrate for these enzymes. However, the potential for adefovir to induce CYP450 enzymes is unknown. Based on the results of these *in vitro* experiments and the renal elimination pathway of adefovir, the potential for CYP450 mediated interactions involving adefovir as an inhibitor or substrate with other medicinal products is low.

The pharmacokinetics of adefovir have been evaluated following multiple dose administration of adefovir dipivoxil (10 mg once daily) in combination with lamivudine (100 mg once daily), trimethoprim/sulfamethoxazole (160/800 mg twice daily), acetaminophen (1000 mg four times daily) and ibuprofen (800 mg three times daily) in healthy volunteers (n=18 per study).

Adefovir did not alter the pharmacokinetics of lamivudine, trimethoprim/sulfamethoxazole, acetaminophen and ibuprofen.

The pharmacokinetics of adefovir were unchanged when adefovir dipivoxil was co-administered with lamivudine, trimethoprim/sulfamethoxazole and acetaminophen. When adefovir dipivoxil was co-administered with ibuprofen (800 mg three times daily) increases in adefovir C_{max} (33%), AUC (23%) and urinary recovery were observed. This increase appears to be due to higher oral bioavailability, not a reduction in renal clearance of adefovir.

INDICATIONS AND USAGE

Adefovir dipivoxil is indicated for the treatment of chronic hepatitis B in adults with evidence of active viral replication and either evidence of persistent elevations in serum aminotransferases (ALT or AST) or histologically active disease.

This indication is based on histological, virological, biochemical, and serological responses in adult patients with HBeAg+ and HBeAg-chronic hepatitis B with compensated liver function, and in adult patients with clinical evidence of lamivudine-resistant hepatitis B virus with either compensated or decompensated liver function.

CONTRAINDICATIONS

Adefovir dipivoxil is contraindicated in patients with previously demonstrated hypersensitivity to any of the components of the product.

WARNINGS

EXACERBATIONS OF HEPATITIS AFTER DISCONTINUATION OF TREATMENT

Severe acute exacerbation of hepatitis has been reported in patients who have discontinued antihepatitis B therapy, including therapy with adefovir dipivoxil. Patients who discontinue adefovir dipivoxil should be monitored at repeated intervals over a period of time for hepatic function. If appropriate, resumption of anti-hepatitis B therapy may be warranted.

In clinical trials of adefovir dipivoxil, exacerbations of hepatitis (ALT elevations 10 times the upper limit of normal or greater) occurred in up to 25% of patients after discontinuation of adefovir dipivoxil. Most of these events occurred within 12 weeks of drug discontinuation. These exacerbations generally occurred in the absence of HBeAg seroconversion, and presented as serum ALT elevations in addition to re-emergence of viral replication. In the HBeAg-positive and HBeAg-negative studies in patients with compensated liver function, the exacerbations were not generally accompanied by hepatic decompensation. However, patients with advanced liver disease or cirrhosis may be at higher risk for hepatic decompensation. Although most events appear to have been self-limited or resolved with re-initiation of treatment, severe hepatitis exacerbations, including fatalities, have been reported. Therefore, patients should be closely monitored after stopping treatment.

NEPHROTOXICITY

Nephrotoxicity characterized by a delayed onset of gradual increases in serum creatinine and decreases in serum phosphorus was historically shown to be the treatment-limiting toxicity of adefovir dipivoxil therapy at substantially higher doses in HIV-infected patients (60 and 120 mg daily) and in chronic hepatitis B patients (30 mg daily). Chronic administration of adefovir dipivoxil (10 mg once daily) may result in nephrotoxicity. The overall risk of nephrotoxicity in patients with adequate renal function is low. However, this is of special importance in patients at risk of or having underlying renal dysfunction and patients taking concomitant nephrotoxic agents such as cyclosporine, tacrolimus, aminoglycosides, vancomycin and non-steroidal anti-inflammatory drugs (see ADVERSE REACTIONS).

It is important to monitor renal function for all patients during treatment with adefovir dipivoxil, particularly for those with pre-existing or other risks for renal impairment. Patients with renal insufficiency at baseline or during treatment may require dose adjustment (see DOSAGE AND ADMINISTRATION). The risks and benefits of adefovir dipivoxil treatment should be carefully evaluated prior to discontinuing adefovir dipivoxil in a patient with treatment-emergent nephrotoxicity.

HIV RESISTANCE

Prior to initiating adefovir dipivoxil therapy, HIV antibody testing should be offered to all patients. Treatment with anti-hepatitis B therapies, such as adefovir dipivoxil, that have activity against HIV in a chronic hepatitis B patient with unrecognized or untreated HIV infection may result in emergence of HIV resistance. Adefovir dipivoxil has not been shown to suppress HIV RNA in patients; however, there are limited data on the use of adefovir dipivoxil to treat patients with chronic hepatitis B co-infected with HIV.

LACTIC ACIDOSIS/SEVERE HEPATOMEGALY WITH STEATOSIS

Lactic acidosis and severe hepatomegaly with steatosis, including fatal cases, have been reported with the use of nucleoside analogs alone or in combination with antiretrovirals.

A majority of these cases have been in women. Obesity and prolonged nucleoside exposure may be risk factors. Particular caution should be exercised when administering nucleoside analogs to any patient with known risk factors for liver disease; however, cases have also been reported in patients with no known risk factors. Treatment with adefovir dipivoxil should be suspended in any patient who develops clinical or laboratory findings suggestive of lactic acidosis or pronounced hepatotoxicity (which may include hepatomegaly and steatosis even in the absence of marked transaminase elevations).

PRECAUTIONS

DURATION OF TREATMENT

The optimal duration of adefovir dipivoxil treatment and the relationship between treatment response and long-term outcomes such as hepatocellular carcinoma or decompensated cirrhosis are not known.

CARCINOGENESIS, MUTAGENESIS, AND IMPAIRMENT OF FERTILITY

Carcinogenicity studies in mice and rats receiving adefovir have been conducted. In mice, at dose levels of 1, 3, or 10 mg/kg/day, no treatment-related increases in tumor incidence were found at 10 mg/kg/day (systemic exposure was 10 times that achieved in humans at a therapeutic dose of 10 mg/day). In rats dosed at levels of 0.5, 1.5, or 5 mg/kg/day, no drug-related increase in tumor incidence was observed. The exposure at the high dose was 4 times that at the human therapeutic dose. Adefovir dipivoxil was mutagenic in the *in vitro* mouse lymphoma cell assay (with or without metabolic activation). Adefovir induced chromosomal aberrations in the *in vitro* human peripheral blood lymphocyte assay without metabolic activation. Adefovir was not clastogenic in the *in vivo* mouse micronucleus assay at doses up to 2000 mg/kg and it was not mutagenic in the Ames bacterial reverse mutation assay using *S. typhimurium* and *E. coli* strains in the presence and absence of metabolic activation. In reproductive toxicology studies, no evidence of impaired fertility was seen in male or female rats at doses up to 30 mg/kg/day (systemic exposure 19 times that achieved in humans at the therapeutic dose).

PREGNANCY CATEGORY C

Reproduction studies conducted with adefovir dipivoxil administered orally have shown no embryotoxicity or teratogenicity in rats at doses up to 35 mg/kg/day (systemic exposure approximately 23 times that achieved in humans at the therapeutic dose of 10 mg/day), or in rabbits at 20 mg/kg/day (systemic exposure 40 times human).

When adefovir was administered intravenously to pregnant rats at doses associated with notable maternal toxicity (20 mg/kg/day, systemic exposure 38 times human), embryotoxicity and an increased incidence of fetal malformations (anasarca, depressed eye bulge, umbilical hernia and kinked tail) were observed. No adverse effects on development were seen with adefovir administered intravenously to pregnant rats at 2.5 mg/kg/day (systemic exposure 12 times human).

There are no adequate and well-controlled studies in pregnant women. Because animal reproduction studies are not always predictive of human response, adefovir dipivoxil should be used during pregnancy only if clearly needed and after careful consideration of the risks and benefits.

Pregnancy Registry: To monitor fetal outcomes of pregnant women exposed to adefovir dipivoxil, a pregnancy registry has been established. Healthcare providers are encouraged to register patients by calling 1-800-258-4263.

LABOR AND DELIVERY

There are no studies in pregnant women and no data on the effect of adefovir dipivoxil on transmission of HBV from mother to infant. Therefore, appropriate infant immunizations should be used to prevent neonatal acquisition of hepatitis B virus.

LACTATING WOMEN

It is not known whether adefovir is excreted in human milk. Mothers should be instructed not to breast-feed if they are taking adefovir dipivoxil.

PEDIATRIC USE

Safety and effectiveness in pediatric patients have not been established.

GERIATRIC USE

Clinical studies of adefovir dipivoxil did not include sufficient numbers of patients aged 65 and over to determine whether they respond differently from younger patients. In general, caution should be exercised when prescribing to elderly patients since they have greater frequency of decreased renal or cardiac function due to concomitant disease or other drug therapy.

DRUG INTERACTIONS

Since adefovir is eliminated by the kidney, co-administration of adefovir dipivoxil with drugs that reduce renal function or compete for active tubular secretion may increase serum concentrations of either adefovir and/or these co-administered drugs.

Apart from lamivudine, trimethoprim/sulfamethoxazole and acetaminophen, the effects of coadministration of adefovir dipivoxil with drugs that are excreted renally, or other drugs known to affect renal function have not been evaluated (see CLINICAL PHARMACOLOGY).

Patients should be monitored closely for adverse events when adefovir dipivoxil is co-administered with drugs that are excreted renally or with other drugs known to affect renal function.

Ibuprofen 800 mg three times daily increased adefovir exposure by approximately 23%. The clinical significance of this increase in adefovir exposure is unknown (see CLINICAL PHARMACOLOGY).

While adefovir does not inhibit common CYP450 enzymes, the potential for adefovir to induce CYP450 enzymes is not known.

The effect of adefovir on cyclosporine and tacrolimus concentrations is not known.

ADVERSE REACTIONS

Assessment of adverse reactions is based on two studies (437 and 438) in which 522 patients with chronic hepatitis B received double-blind treatment with adefovir dipivoxil (n=294) or placebo (n=228) for 48 weeks. With extended therapy in the second 48 week treatment period, 492 patients were treated for up to 109 weeks, with a median time on treatment of 49 weeks.

In addition to specific adverse events described under WARNINGS, all treatment-related clinical adverse events that occurred in 3% or greater of adefovir dipivoxil-treated patients compared with placebo are listed in TABLE 6. A summary of Grade 3 and 4 laboratory abnormalities during therapy with adefovir dipivoxil compared with placebo is listed in TABLE 7.

TABLE 6 *Treatment-Related Adverse Events (Grades 1-4) Reported in ≥3% of All Adefovir-Treated Patients in the Pooled 437-438 Studies (0-48 Weeks)*

	Adefovir 10 mg (n=294)	Placebo (n=228)
Asthenia	13%	14%
Headache	9%	10%
Abdominal pain	9%	11%
Nausea	5%	8%
Flatulence	4%	4%
Diarrhea	3%	4%
Dyspepsia	3%	2%

LABORATORY ABNORMALITIES

TABLE 7 *Grade 3-4 Laboratory Abnormalities Reported in ≥1% of All Adefovir Patients in the Pooled 437-438 Studies (0-48 Weeks)*

	Adefovir 10 mg (n=294)	Placebo (n=228)
ALT (>5 × ULN)	20%	41%
Hematuria (≥3+)	11%	10%
AST (>5 × ULN)	8%	23%
Creatine kinase (>4 × ULN)	7%	7%
Amylase (>2 × ULN)	4%	4%
Glycosuria (≥3+)	1%	3%

In patients with adequate renal function, increases in serum creatinine ≥0.3 mg/dl from baseline were observed in 4% of patients treated with adefovir dipivoxil 10 mg daily compared with 2% of patients in the placebo group at week 48. No patients developed a serum creatinine increase ≥0.5 mg/dl from baseline by week 48. By week 96, 10% and 2% of adefovir dipivoxil-treated patients, by Kaplan-Meier estimate, had increases in serum creatinine ≥0.3 mg/dl and ≥0.5 mg/dl from baseline, respectively (no placebo-controlled results were available for comparison beyond week 48). Of the 29 of 492 patients with elevations in serum creatinine ≥0.3 mg/dl from baseline, 20 out of 29 resolved on continued treatment (≤0.2 mg/dl from baseline), 8 of 29 remained unchanged and 1 of 29 resolved on discontinuing treatment **(see Special Risk Patients for changes in serum creatinine in patients with underlying renal insufficiency at baseline).**

SPECIAL RISK PATIENTS

Pre- (n=128) and post-liver transplantation patients (n=196) with chronic hepatitis B and clinical evidence of lamivudine-resistant hepatitis B virus were treated in an open-label study with adefovir dipivoxil for up to 129 weeks, with a median time on treatment of 19 and 56 weeks, respectively. The majority of these patients had some degree of underlying renal insufficiency at baseline or other risk factors for renal dysfunction during treatment. Increases in serum creatinine ≥0.3 mg/dl from baseline were observed in 26% of these patients by week 48 and 37% by week 96 by Kaplan-Meier estimates. Increases in serum creatinine ≥0.5 mg/dl from baseline were observed in 16% of these patients by week 48 and 31% by week 96. Of the 41 of 324 patients with elevations in serum creatinine ≥0.5 mg/dl from baseline, 7 of 41 resolved on continued treatment (≤0.3 mg/dl from baseline), 18 of 41 remained unchanged and 16 of 41 had not resolved. Additionally, decreases in serum phosphorus were observed in 4% of these patients by week 48, and 6% by week 96 by Kaplan-Meier estimates. One percent (3 of 324) of pre- and post-liver transplantation patients discontinued adefovir dipivoxil due to renal events.

Due to the presence of multiple concomitant risk factors for renal dysfunction in these patients, the contributory role of adefovir dipivoxil to these changes in serum creatinine and serum phosphorus is difficult to assess.

A

The most common treatment-related adverse events reported in pre- and post-liver transplantation patients treated with adefovir dipivoxil with a 2% frequency or higher include:

Body as a Whole: Asthenia, abdominal pain, headache, fever.
Gastrointestinal: Nausea, vomiting, diarrhea, flatulence, hepatic failure.
Metabolic and Nutritional: Increases in ALT and AST, abnormal liver function.
Respiratory: Increased cough, pharyngitis, sinusitis.
Skin and Appendages: Pruritus, rash.
Urogenital: Increases in creatinine, renal failure, renal insufficiency.

DOSAGE AND ADMINISTRATION

The recommended dose of adefovir dipivoxil in chronic hepatitis B patients with adequate renal function is 10 mg, once daily, taken orally, without regard to food. The optimal duration of treatment is unknown.

DOSE ADJUSTMENT IN RENAL IMPAIRMENT

Significantly increased drug exposures were seen when adefovir dipivoxil was administered to patients with renal impairment (see CLINICAL PHARMACOLOGY, Pharmacokinetics). Therefore, the dosing interval of adefovir dipivoxil should be adjusted in patients with baseline creatinine clearance <50 ml/min using the following suggested guidelines (see TABLE 8). The safety and effectiveness of these dosing interval adjustment guidelines have not been clinically evaluated. Additionally, it is important to note that these guidelines were derived from data in patients with pre-existing renal impairment at baseline. They may not be appropriate for patients in whom renal insufficiency evolves during treatment with adefovir dipivoxil. Therefore, clinical response to treatment and renal function should be closely monitored in these patients.

TABLE 8 *Dosing Interval Adjustment of Adefovir in Patients With Renal Impairment*

	Creatinine Clearance (ml/min)*			
	≥50	20-49	10-19	Hemodialysis Patients
Recommended dose and dosing interval	10 mg every 24 hours	10 mg every 48 hours	10 mg every 72 hours	10 mg every 7 days following dialysis

* Creatinine clearance calculated by Cockcroft-Gault method using lean or ideal body weight.

The pharmacokinetics of adefovir have not been evaluated in non-hemodialysis patients with creatinine clearance <10 ml/min; therefore, no dosing recommendation is available for these patients.

ANIMAL PHARMACOLOGY

Renal tubular nephropathy characterized by histological alterations and/or increases in BUN and serum creatinine was the primary dose-limiting toxicity associated with administration of adefovir dipivoxil in animals. Nephrotoxicity was observed in animals at systemic exposures approximately 3-10 times higher than those in humans at the recommended therapeutic dose of 10 mg/day.

HOW SUPPLIED

HEPSERA TABLETS

Hepsera is available as tablets. Each tablet contains 10 mg of adefovir dipivoxil. The tablets are white and debossed with "10" and "GILEAD" on one side and the stylized figure of a liver on the other side.

Storage: Store in original container at 25°C (77°F), excursions permitted to 15-30°C (59-86°F).

PRODUCT LISTING - EQUIVALENTS NOT AVAILABLE

Tablet - Oral - 10 mg

30's $528.00 HEPSERA, Gilead Sciences 61958-0501-01

Albendazole (003225)

For complete prescribing information, refer to the CD-ROM included with the book.

Categories: Neurocysticercosis; Tapeworm, dog; Tapeworm, pork; Pregnancy Category C; FDA Approved 1996 Jul; Orphan Drugs; WHO Formulary

Drug Classes: Antihelmintics

Brand Names: Albenza; **Valbazen**

Foreign Brand Availability: Abentel (China); ABZ (India); Adazol (Ecuador); Albatel (Thailand); Albenzol (Ecuador); Albezole (India); Alfuca (Thailand); Alminth (India; Republic-Of-Yemen); Alzental (Bahrain; Cyprus; Egypt; Iran; Iraq; Jordan; Kuwait; Lebanon; Libya; Oman; Qatar; Republic-of-Yemen; Saudi-Arabia; Singapore; Syria; United-Arab-Emirates); Alzol (Thailand); Bendapar (Mexico); Bendex-400 (South-Africa); Borotel (Peru); Ceprazol (Peru); Ciclopar (Colombia); Emanthal (India); Eskazole (Australia; England; Germany; Israel; Japan; Mexico; Netherlands); Fintel (Peru); Gascop (Mexico); Getzol (Colombia); Helben (Indonesia); Helmindazol (Peru); Labenda (Thailand); Loveral (Mexico); Monodox (Colombia); Mycotel (Thailand); Nemozole (India); Paranthil (South-Africa); Rotopar (Ecuador); Rozolex (Costa-Rica; Dominican-Republic; El-Salvador; Guatemala; Honduras; Nicaragua; Panama); Sioban (India); Vermin Plus (Mexico); Xadem (Colombia); Zeben (Thailand); Zentab (Thailand); Zentel (Australia; Bahamas; Bahrain; Barbados; Belize; Benin; Bermuda; Burkina-Faso; Colombia; Costa-Rica; Curacao; Cyprus; Czech-Republic; Dominican-Republic; Ecuador; Egypt; El-Salvador; Ethiopia; France; Gambia; Ghana; Greece; Guatemala; Guinea; Guyana; Honduras; Iran; Iraq; Italy; Ivory-Coast; Jamaica; Jordan; Kenya; Korea; Kuwait; Lebanon; Liberia; Libya; Malawi; Malaysia; Mali; Mauritania; Mauritius; Mexico; Morocco; Netherland-Antilles; Nicaragua; Niger; Nigeria; Oman; Panama; Peru; Philippines; Qatar; Republic-of-Yemen; Saudi-Arabia; Senegal; Seychelles; Sierra-Leone; South-Africa; Sudan; Surinam; Syria; Tanzania; Thailand; Trinidad; Tunia; Uganda; United-Arab-Emirates; Zambia; Zimbabwe)

Cost of Therapy: $160.74 (Helminth Infection; Albenza; 200 mg; 4 tablets/day; 28 day supply)

DESCRIPTION

Albendazole is an orally administered broad-spectrum anthelmintic. Chemically it is methyl 5-(propyl-thio)-2-benzimidazolecarbamate. Its molecular formula is $C_{12}H_{15}N_3O_2S$.

Albendazole is a white to off-white powder. It is soluble in dimethylsulfoxide, strong acids, and strong bases. It is slightly soluble in methanol, chloroform, ethyl acetate and acetonitrile. Albendazole is practically insoluble in water. Each white to off-white, film-coated Albenza tablet contains 200 mg of albendazole.

Albenza inactive ingredients contain: Carnauba wax, hydroxypropyl methylcellulose, lactose monohydrate, magnesium stearate, microcrystalline cellulose, povidone, sodium lauryl sulfate, sodium saccharin, sodium starch glycolate, and starch.

INDICATIONS AND USAGE

Albendazole is indicated for the treatment of the following infections:

Neurocysticercosis: Albendazole is indicated for the treatment of parenchymal neurocysticercosis due to active lesions caused by larval forms of the pork tapeworm, *Taenia solium*.

Lesions considered responsive to albendazole therapy appear as nonenhancing cysts with no surrounding edema on contrast-enhanced computerized tomography. Clinical studies in patients with lesions of this type demonstrate a 74-88% reduction in number of cysts; 40-70% of albendazole-treated patients showed resolution of all active cysts.

Hydatid Disease: Albendazole is indicated for the treatment of cystic hydatid disease of the liver, lung, and peritoneum, caused by the larval form of the dog tapeworm, *Echinococcus granulosus*.

This indication is based on combined clinical studies which demonstrated non-infectious cyst contents in approximately 80-90% of patients given albendazole for 3 cycles of therapy of 28 days each (see DOSAGE AND ADMINISTRATION). Clinical cure (disappearance of cysts) was seen in approximately 30% of these patients, and improvement (reduction in cyst diameter of ≥25%) was seen in an additional 40%.

NOTE: When medically feasible, surgery is considered the treatment of choice for hydatid disease. When administering albendazole in the pre- or post-surgical setting, optimal killing of cyst contents is achieved when three courses of therapy have been given.

NOTE: The efficacy of albendazole in the therapy of alveolar hydatid disease caused by *Echinococcus multiocularis* has not been clearly demonstrated in clinical studies.

CONTRAINDICATIONS

Albendazole is contraindicated in patients with known hypersensitivity to the benzimidazole class of compounds or any components of albendazole tablets.

WARNINGS

Rare fatalities associated with the use of albendazole have been reported due to granulocytopenia or pancytopenia. Blood counts should be monitored at the beginning of each 28 day cycle of therapy, and every 2 weeks while on therapy with albendazole. Albendazole

TABLE 2

Patient Weight	Dose	Duration
Hydatid Disease		
60 kg or greater	400 mg bid, with meals	28 day cycle followed by a 14 day albendazole-free interval, for a total of 3 cycles
Less than 60 kg	15 mg/kg/day given in divided doses bid with meals (maximum total daily dose 800 mg)	
NOTE: When administering albendazole in the pre-or post-surgical setting, optimal killing of cyst contents is achieved when three courses of therapy have been given.		
Neurocysticercosis		
60 kg or greater	400 mg bid, with meals	8-30 days
Less than 60 kg	15 mg/kg/day given in divided doses bid with meals (maximum total daily dose 800 mg)	

may be continued if the total white blood cell count and absolute neutrophil count decrease appear modest and do not progress.

Albandazole should not be used in pregnant women except in clinical circumstances where no alternative management is appropriate. Patients should not become pregnant for at least 1 month following cessation of albendazole therapy. If a patient becomes pregnant while taking this drug, albendazole should be discontinued immediately. If pregancy occurs while taking this drug, the patient should be apprised of the potential hazard to the fetus.

DOSAGE AND ADMINISTRATION

Dosing of albendazole will vary, depending upon which parasitic infections is being treated. (See TABLE 2.)

Patients being treated for neurocysticercosis should receive appropriate steroid and anticonvulsant therapy as required. Oral or intravenous corticosteroids should be considered to prevent cerebral hypertensive episodes during the first week of treatment.

PRODUCT LISTING - EQUIVALENTS NOT AVAILABLE

Tablet - Oral - 200 mg

112's $160.74 ALBENZA, Glaxosmithkline 00007-5500-40

Albuterol (000115)

For related information, see the comparative table section in Appendix A.

Categories: Asthma; Bronchospasm, exercise-induced; Pregnancy Category C; FDA Approval Pre 1982; Patent Expiration 2014 Feb; WHO Formulary

Drug Classes: Adrenergic agonists; Bronchodilators

Brand Names: Airet; Albuterol Sulfate; Proventil; **Ventolin**; Ventolin Rotacaps; Volmax

Foreign Brand Availability: Aerolin (Brazil; Chile; Greece); Airomir (Australia; Canada; France; Hong-Kong; Singapore; Thailand); Asmacaire (Philippines); Asmadil (Benin; Burkina-Faso; Ethiopia; Gambia; Ghana; Guinea; Ivory-Coast; Kenya; Liberia; Malawi; Mali; Mauritania; Mauritius; Morocco; Niger; Nigeria; Senegal; Seychelles; Sierra-Leone; Sudan; Tanzania; Tunia; Uganda; Zambia; Zimbabwe); Asmalin Pulmoneb (Philippines); Asmasal (Thailand); Asmatol (Argentina); Asmaven (England); Asmavent (Canada); Asmidon (Japan); Asmol CFC-Free (Australia); Asmol Uni-Dose (New-Zealand); Assal (Mexico); Asthalin (India); Azmasol (Singapore); Broncho-Spray (Germany); Broncovaleas (Italy); Bronter (Colombia); Brytolin (Philippines); Butahale (Singapore); Buto-Asma (Singapore; Spain; Thailand); Butomix (Peru); Butotal (Chile); Buventol (Singapore; Taiwan); Buventol Easyhaler (France; Indonesia; Thailand); Cobutolin (England); Dilatamol (Indonesia); Epaq Inhaler (Australia); Exafil (Mexico); Farcolin (Bahrain; Cyprus; Egypt; Iran; Iraq; Israel; Jordan; Kuwait; Lebanon; Libya; Oman; Qatar; Republic-of-Yemen; Saudi-Arabia; Syria; United-Arab-Emirates); Glisend (Indonesia); Grafalin (Indonesia); Libretin (Philippines); Medolin (Singapore); Mozal (Taiwan); Novosalmol (Canada); Parasma (Colombia); Prox-S (Philippines); Respax (Australia; New-Zealand); Respreve (Hong-Kong); Sabutol (Singapore); Salbetol (India); Salbron (Indonesia); Salbulin (Costa-Rica; Dominican-Republic; El-Salvador; England; Guatemala; Honduras; Panama); Salbutalan (Mexico); Salbutan (Venezuela); Salbutin (Bahrain; Cyprus; Egypt; Iran; Iraq; Jordan; Kuwait; Lebanon; Libya; Oman; Qatar; Republic-of-Yemen; Saudi-Arabia; Syria; United-Arab-Emirates); Salbutol (Korea; Peru); Salbutron SR (Korea); Salbuven (Indonesia); Salbuvent (Norway); Salmaplon (India); Salmol (China); Salmundin Retard (Germany); Salomol (Taiwan); Sedalin (Philippines); Sultanol (Austria; Germany; Japan); Suprasma (Indonesia); Tobybron (Indonesia); Venalax (Philippines); Vencronyl (Philippines); Venetlin (Japan); Ventilan (Colombia; Portugal); Ventimax (South-Africa); Ventodisks (China); Ventol (Bahrain; Cyprus; Egypt; Iran; Iraq; Jordan; Kuwait; Lebanon; Libya; Oman; Qatar; Republic-of-Yemen; Saudi-Arabia; Syria; United-Arab-Emirates); Ventoline (Denmark; Finland; France; Norway; Sweden); Ventolin CFC-Free (Australia); Zebu (Thailand); Zenmolin (Bahrain; Cyprus; Egypt; Hong-Kong; Iran; Iraq; Israel; Jordan; Kuwait; Lebanon; Libya; Oman; Qatar; Republic-of-Yemen; Saudi-Arabia; Syria; United-Arab-Emirates); Zibil (Mexico)

Cost of Therapy: $26.24 (Asthma; Ventolin Aerosol; 90 μg; 17 g; 8 inhalations/day; 25 day supply)
$19.72 (Asthma; Generic Aerosol; 90 μg; 17 g; 8 inhalations/day; 25 day supply)

HCFA JCODE(S): J7620 0.083%, per ml INH

ORAL

DESCRIPTION

Note: The trade names have been used throughout this monograph for clarity.

VENTOLIN TABLETS

Ventolin tablets contain albuterol sulfate, the racemic form of albuterol and a relatively selective beta$_2$-adrenergic bronchodilator. Albuterol sulfate has the chemical name $(\pm)\alpha^1$-[(*tert*-butylamino)methyl]-4-hydroxy-*m*-xylene-α,α'-diol sulfate (2:1)(salt).

Albuterol sulfate has a molecular weight of 576.7, and the empirical formula is $(C_{13}H_{21}NO_3)_2{\cdot}H_2SO_4$. Albuterol sulfate is a white crystalline powder, soluble in water and slightly soluble in ethanol.

The World Health Organization recommended name for albuterol base is salbutamol.

Each Ventolin tablet contains 2 or 4 mg of albuterol as 2.4 or 4.8 mg, respectively, of albuterol sulfate for oral administration. Each tablet also contains the inactive ingredients corn starch, lactose, and magnesium stearate.

VENTOLIN SYRUP

Ventolin syrup contains albuterol sulfate, the racemic form of albuterol, a relatively selective beta$_2$-adrenergic bronchodilator. Albuterol sulfate has the chemical name α^1-[(*tert*-butylamino)methyl]-4-hydroxy-*m*-xylene-α,α'-diol sulfate (2:1)(salt).

The molecular weight of albuterol sulfate is 576.7, and the empirical formula is $(C_{13}H_{21}NO_3)_2{\cdot}H_2SO_4$. Albuterol sulfate is a white crystalline powder, soluble in water and slightly soluble in ethanol. The World Health Organization's recommended name for albuterol base is salbutamol.

Ventolin syrup for oral administration contains 2 mg of albuterol as 2.4 mg of albuterol sulfate in each teaspoonful (5 ml). The inactive ingredients for Ventolin syrup include: citric acid anhydrous; FD&C yellow no. 6; flavor strawberry artificial F-8636; hydroxypropyl methylcellulose 2906 or 2910; saccharin; sodium benzoate; sodium citrate dihydrate; and water purified. The pH of the syrup is between 3.0 and 4.5.

VOLMAX EXTENDED-RELEASE TABLETS

Volmax (albuterol sulfate) extended-release tablets contain albuterol sulfate, the racemic form of albuterol and a relatively selective beta$_2$-adrenergic bronchodilator, in an extended-release formulation. Albuterol sulfate has the chemical name $(\pm)$ α_1-[(*tert*-butylamino)methyl]-4-hydroxy-*m*-xylene-α,α'-diol sulfate (2:1) (salt).

Albuterol sulfate has a molecular weight of 576.7, and the molecular formula is $(C_{13}H_{21}NO_3)_2{\cdot}H_2SO_4$. Albuterol sulfate is a white crystalline powder, soluble in water and slightly soluble in ethanol.

The World Health Organization recommended name for albuterol base is salbutamol.

Each Volmax extended-release tablet for oral administration contains 4 mg or 8 mg of albuterol as 4.8 mg or 9.6 mg, respectively, of albuterol sulfate in a nondeformable cellulosic material that serves as the rate-controlling membrane. Each tablet also contains the inactive ingredients cellulose acetate, croscarmellose sodium, FD&C blue no. 1 (4 mg tablet only), hydroxypropyl cellulose (8 mg tablet only), hydroxypropyl methylcellulose, magnesium stearate, povidone, silica, sodium chloride, and titanium dioxide.

CLINICAL PHARMACOLOGY

VENTOLIN TABLETS

In vitro studies and *in vivo* pharmacologic studies have demonstrated that albuterol has a preferential effect on beta$_2$-adrenergic receptors compared with isoproterenol. While it is recognized that beta$_2$-adrenergic receptors are the predominant receptors in bronchial smooth muscle, data indicate that there is a population of beta$_2$-receptors in the human heart existing in a concentration between 10 and 50%. The precise function of these receptors has not been established (see WARNINGS).

The pharmacologic effects of beta-adrenergic agonist drugs, including albuterol, are at least in part attributable to stimulation through beta-adrenergic receptors of intracellular adenyl cyclase, the enzyme that catalyzes the conversion of adenosine triphosphate (ATP) to cyclic-3′,5′-adenosine monophosphate (cyclic AMP). Increased cyclic AMP levels are associated with relaxation of bronchial smooth muscle and inhibition of release of mediators of immediate hypersensitivity from cells, especially from mast cells.

Albuterol has been shown in most controlled clinical trials to have more effect on the respiratory tract, in the form of bronchial smooth muscle relaxation, than isoproterenol at comparable doses while producing fewer cardiovascular effects.

Albuterol is longer acting than isoproterenol in most patients by any route of administration because it is not a substrate for the cellular uptake processes for catecholamines nor for catechol-*O*-methyl transferase.

Preclinical

Intravenous (IV) studies in rats with albuterol sulfate have demonstrated that albuterol crosses the blood-brain barrier and reaches brain concentrations amounting to approximately 5.0% of the plasma concentrations. In structures outside the brain barrier (pineal and pituitary glands), albuterol concentrations were found to be 100 times those in the whole brain.

Studies in laboratory animals (minipigs, rodents, and dogs) have demonstrated the occurrence of cardiac arrhythmias and sudden death (with histologic evidence of myocardial necrosis) when beta-agonists and methylxanthines are administered concurrently. The clinical significance of these findings is unknown.

Pharmacokinetics

Albuterol is rapidly absorbed after oral administration of 4 mg Ventolin tablets in normal volunteers. Maximum plasma concentrations of about 18 ng/ml of albuterol are achieved within 2 hours, and the drug is eliminated with a half-life of about 5 hours.

In other studies, the analysis of urine samples of patients given 8 mg of tritiated albuterol orally showed that 76% of the dose was excreted over 3 days, with the majority of the dose being excreted within the first 24 hours. Sixty percent (60%) of this radioactivity was shown to be the metabolite. Feces collected over this period contained 4% of the administered dose.

VENTOLIN SYRUP

The primary action of beta-adrenergic drugs, including albuterol, is to stimulate adenyl cyclase, the enzyme which catalyzes the formation of cyclic-3′,5′-adenosine monophosphate (cyclic AMP) from adenosine triphosphate (ATP) in beta-adrenergic cells. The cyclic AMP thus formed mediates the cellular responses. Increased cyclic AMP levels are associated with relaxation of bronchial smooth muscle and inhibition of release of mediators of immediate hypersensitivity from cells, especially from mast cells.

In vitro studies and *in vivo* pharmacologic studies have demonstrated that albuterol has a preferential effect on beta$_2$-adrenergic receptors compared with isoproterenol. While it is recognized that beta$_2$-adrenergic receptors are the predominant receptors in bronchial smooth muscle, data indicate that there is a population of beta$_2$-receptors in the human heart existing in a concentration between 10 and 50%. The precise function of these receptors has not been established.

In controlled clinical trials, albuterol has been shown to have more effect on the respiratory tract, in the form of bronchial smooth muscle relaxation, than isoproterenol at comparable doses, while producing fewer cardiovascular effects. Controlled clinical studies and other clinical experience have shown that inhaled albuterol, like other beta-adrenergic agonist drugs, can produce a significant cardiovascular effect in some patients, as measured by pulse rate, blood pressure, symptoms, and/or ECG changes.

Albuterol is longer acting than isoproterenol in most patients by any route of administration because it is not a substrate for the cellular uptake processes for catecholamines nor for catechol-*O*-methyl transferase.

Preclinical

Intravenous (IV) studies in rats with albuterol sulfate have demonstrated that albuterol crosses the blood-brain barrier and reaches brain concentrations that are amounting to approximately 5.0% of the plasma concentrations. In structures outside the blood-brain barrier (pineal and pituitary glands), albuterol concentrations were found to be 100 times those in the whole brain.

Studies in laboratory animals (minipigs, rodents, and dogs) have demonstrated the occurrence of cardiac arrhythmias and sudden death (with histologic evidence of myocardial necrosis) when beta-agonists and methylxanthines are administered concurrently. The clinical significance of these findings is unknown.

Pharmacokinetics

Albuterol is rapidly and well absorbed following oral administration. After oral administration of 10 ml of Ventolin syrup (4 mg albuterol) in normal volunteers, maximum plasma albuterol concentrations of about 18 ng/ml are achieved within 2 hours, and the drug is eliminated with a half-life of about 5-6 hours.

In other studies, the analysis of urine samples of patients given 8 mg of tritiated albuterol orally showed that 76% of the dose was excreted over 3 days, with the majority of the dose being excreted within the first 24 hours. Sixty percent (60%) of this radioactivity was shown to be the metabolite. Feces collected over this period contained 4% of the administered dose.

VOLMAX EXTENDED-RELEASE TABLETS

In vitro studies and *in vivo* pharmacologic studies have demonstrated that albuterol has a preferential effect on beta$_2$-adrenergic receptors compared with isoproterenol. While it is recognized that beta$_2$-adrenergic receptors are the predominant receptors in bronchial smooth muscle, data indicates that there is a population of beta$_2$-receptors in the human heart existing in a concentration between 10 and 50%. The precise function of these receptors has not been established. (See WARNINGS, Volmax Extended-Release Tablets.)

The pharmacologic effects of beta-adrenergic agonist drugs, including albuterol, are at least in part attributable to stimulation through beta-adrenergic receptors on intracellular adenyl cyclase, the enzyme that catalyzes the conversion of adenosine triphosphate (ATP) to cyclic-3′,5′-adenosine monophosphate (cyclic AMP). Increased cyclic AMP levels are associated with relaxation of bronchial smooth muscle and inhibition of release of mediators of immediate hypersensitivity from cells, especially from mast cells.

Albuterol has been shown in most controlled clinical trials to have more effect on the respiratory tract, in the form of bronchial smooth muscle relaxation, than isoproterenol at comparable doses while producing fewer cardiovascular effects.

Albuterol is longer acting than isoproterenol in most patients by any route of administration because it is not a substrate for the cellular uptake processes for catecholamines nor for catechol-*O*-methyl transferase.

Preclinical

Intravenous studies in rats with albuterol sulfate have demonstrated that albuterol crosses the blood-brain barrier and reaches brain concentrations amounting to approximately 5.0% of the plasma concentrations. In structures outside the blood-brain barrier (pineal and pituitary glands), albuterol concentrations were found to be 100 times those in the whole brain.

Studies in laboratory animals (minipigs, rodents, and dogs) have demonstrated the occurence of cardiac arrhythmias and sudden death (with histologic evidence of myocardial necrosis) when beta-agonists and methylxanthines were administered concurrently. The clinical significance of these findings is unknown.

Pharmacokinetics and Disposition

In a single-dose study comparing one 8 mg Volmax extended-release tablet with two 4 mg immediate-release Ventolin (albuterol sulfate) tablets in 17 normal adult volunteers, the extent of availability of Volmax extended-release tablets was shown to be about 80% of Ventolin tablets with or without food. In addition, lower mean peak plasma concentration and longer time to reach the peak level were observed with Volmax extended-release tablets as compared with Ventolin tablets. The single-dose study results also showed that food decreases the rate of absorption of albuterol from Volmax extended-release tablets without altering the extent of bioavailability. In addition, the study indicated that food causes a more gradual increase in the fraction of the available dose absorbed from the extended-release formulation as compared with the fasting condition.

In another single-dose study in adults, 8 mg and 4 mg Volmax extended-release tablets were shown to deliver dose-proportional plasma concentrations in the fasting state. Definitive studies for the effect of food on 4 mg Volmax extended-release tablets have not been conducted. However, since food lowers the rate of absorption of 8 mg Volmax extended-release tablets, it is expected that food reduces the rate of absorption of 4 mg Volmax extended-release tablets also.

Volmax extended-release tablets have been formulated to provide duration of action of up to 12 hours. In an 8 day, multiple-dose, crossover study, 15 normal adult male volunteers were given 8 mg Volmax extended-release tablets every 12 hours or 4 mg Ventolin (albuterol sulfate) tablets every 6 hours. Each dose of Volmax extended-release tablets and the corresponding doses of Ventolin tablets were administered in the postprandial state. Steady-state plasma concentrations were reached within 2 days for both formulations. Fluctuations (C_{max}-C_{min}/$C_{average}$) in plasma concentrations were similar for Volmax extended-release tablets administered at 12 hour intervals and Ventolin tablets administered every 6 hours. In addition, the relative bioavailability of Volmax extended-release tablets was approximately 100% of the immediate-release tablet at steady state. A summary of these results is shown in TABLE 1.

TABLE 1 *Mean Values at Steady State*

	Volmax	Ventolin
C_{max}	13.7 ng/ml	13.9 ng/ml
C_{min}	8.1 ng/ml	8.1 ng/ml
T_{max}	6.0 hours	2.6 hours
T½	9.3 hours	7.2 hours
AUC	134 ng·h/ml	132 ng·h/ml

Pharmacokinetic studies of 4 and 8 mg Volmax extended-release tablets have not been conducted in pediatric patients. Bioavailability of 4 and 8 mg Volmax extended-release tablets in pediatric patients relative to 2 and 4 mg immediate-release albuterol has been extrapolated from adult studies showing comparability at steady-state dosing and reduced bioavailability after single dose administration.

INDICATIONS AND USAGE

VENTOLIN TABLETS

Ventolin tablets are indicated for the relief of bronchospasm in adults and children 6 years of age and older with reversible obstructive airway disease.

VENTOLIN SYRUP

Ventolin syrup is indicated for the relief of bronchospasm in adults and children 2 years of age and older with reversible obstructive airway disease.

VOLMAX EXTENDED-RELEASE TABLETS

Volmax extended-release tablets are indicated for the relief of bronchospasm in adults and children 6 years of age and older with reversible obstructive airway disease.

CONTRAINDICATIONS

VENTOLIN TABLETS

Ventolin tablets are contraindicated in patients with a history of hypersensitivity to albuterol or any of its components.

VENTOLIN SYRUP

Ventolin syrup is contraindicated in patients with a history of hypersensitivity to albuterol or any of its components.

VOLMAX EXTENDED-RELEASE TABLETS

Volmax extended-release tablets are contraindicated in patients with a history of hypersensitivity to albuterol or any of its components.

WARNINGS

VENTOLIN TABLETS

Paradoxical Bronchospasm

Ventolin tablets can produce paradoxical bronchospasm, which may be life threatening. If paradoxical bronchospasm occurs, Ventolin tablets should be discontinued immediately and alternative therapy instituted.

Cardiovascular Effects

Ventolin tablets, like all other beta-adrenergic agonists, can produce a clinically significant cardiovascular effect in some patients as measured by pulse rate, blood pressure, and/or symptoms. Although such effects are uncommon after administration of Ventolin tablets at recommended doses, if they occur, the drug may need to be discontinued. In addition, beta-agonists have been reported to produce electrocardiogram (ECG) changes, such as flattening of the T wave, prolongation of the QTc interval, and ST segment depression. The clinical significance of these findings is unknown. Therefore, Ventolin tablets, like all sympathomimetic amines, should be used with caution in patients with cardiovascular disorders, especially coronary insufficiency, cardiac arrhythmias, and hypertension.

Deterioration of Asthma

Asthma may deteriorate acutely over a period of hours or chronically over several days or longer. If the patient needs more doses of Ventolin tablets than usual, this may be a marker of destabilization of asthma and requires reevaluation of the patient and treatment regimen, giving special consideration to the possible need for anti-inflammatory treatment, *e.g.*, corticosteroids.

Use of Anti-Inflammatory Agents

The use of beta-adrenergic agonist bronchodilators alone may not be adequate to control asthma in many patients. Early consideration should be given to adding anti-inflammatory agents, *e.g.*, corticosteroids.

Immediate Hypersensitivity Reactions

Immediate hypersensitivity reactions may occur after administration of albuterol, as demonstrated by rare cases of urticaria, angioedema, rash, bronchospasm, and oropharyngeal edema. Albuterol, like other beta-adrenergic agonists, can produce a significant cardiovascular effect in some patients, as measured by pulse rate, blood pressure, symptoms, and/or electrocardiographic changes.

Rarely, erythema multiforme and Stevens-Johnson syndrome have been associated with the administration of oral albuterol sulfate in children.

VENTOLIN SYRUP

Deterioration of Asthma

Asthma may deteriorate acutely over a period of hours, or chronically over several days or longer. If the patient needs more doses of Ventolin syrup than usual, this may be a marker of destabilization of asthma and requires re-evaluation of the patient and the treatment regimen, giving special consideration to the possible need for anti-inflammatory treatment, *e.g.*, corticosteroids.

Use of Anti-Inflammatory Agents

The use of beta-adrenergic agonist bronchodilators alone may not be adequate to control asthma in many patients. Early consideration should be given to adding anti-inflammatory agents, *e.g.*, corticosteroids.

Cardiovascular Effects

Ventolin syrup, like all other beta-adrenergic agonists, can produce a clinically significant cardiovascular effect in some patients as measured by pulse rate, blood pressure, and/or symptoms. Although such effects are uncommon after administration of Ventolin syrup at recommended doses, if they occur, the drug may need to be discontinued. In addition, beta-agonists have been reported to produce electrocardiogram (ECG) changes, such as flattening of the T wave, prolongation of the QTc interval, and ST segment depression. The clinical significance of these findings is unknown. Therefore, Ventolin syrup, like all sympathomimetic amines, should be used with caution in patients with cardiovascular disorders, especially coronary insufficiency, cardiac arrhythmias, and hypertension.

Paradoxical Bronchospasm

Ventolin syrup can produce paradoxical bronchospasm, which may be life threatening. If paradoxical bronchospasm occurs, Ventolin syrup should be discontinued immediately and alternative therapy instituted.

Immediate Hypersensitivity Reactions

Immediate hypersensitivity reactions may occur after administration of albuterol, as demonstrated by rare cases of urticaria, angioedema, rash, bronchospasm, anaphylaxis, and oropharyngeal edema.

Rarely, erythema multiforme and Stevens-Johnson syndrome have been associated with the administration of oral albuterol sulfate in children.

VOLMAX EXTENDED-RELEASE TABLETS

Immediate hypersensitivity reactions may occur after administration of albuterol, as demonstrated by rare cases of urticaria, angioedema, rash, bronchospasm, and oropharyngeal edema.

Cardiovascular Effects

Volmax extended-release tablets, like all other beta-adrenergic agonists, can produce a clinically significant cardiovascular effect in some patients, as measured by pulse rate, blood pressure, and/or symptoms. Although such effects are uncommon after administration of Volmax extended-release tablets at recommended doses, if they occur, the drug may need to be discontinued. In addition, beta-agonists have been reported to produce electrocardiogram (ECG) changes, such as flattening of the T wave, prolongation of the QTc interval, and ST segment depression. The clinical significance of these findings is unknown. Therefore, Volmax extended-release tablets, like all sympathomimetic amines, should be used with caution in patients with cardiovascular disorders, especially coronary insufficiency, cardiac arrhythmias, and hypertension.

Deterioration of Asthma

Asthma may deteriorate acutely over a period of hours or chronically over several days or longer. If the patient needs more doses of Volmax extended-release tablets than usual, this may be a marker of destabilization of asthma and requires reevaluation of the patient and the treatment regimen, giving special consideration to the possible need for anti-inflammatory treatment, *e.g.*, corticosteroids.

Use of Anti-Inflammatory Agents

The use of beta adrenergic agonist bronchodilators alone may not be adequate to control asthma in many patients. Early consideration should be given to adding anti-inflammatory agents, *e.g.*, corticosteroids.

Paradoxical Bronchospasm

Volmax extended-release tablets can produce paradoxical bronchospasm, which may be life threatening. If paradoxical bronchospasm occurs, Volmax extended-release tablets should be discontinued immediately and alternative therapy instituted.

Rarely, erythema multiforme and Stevens-Johnson syndrome have been associated with the administration of oral albuterol in children.

PRECAUTIONS

VENTOLIN TABLETS

General

Albuterol, as with all sympathomimetic amines, should be used with caution in patients with cardiovascular disorders, especially coronary insufficiency, hypertension, and cardiac arrhythmia; in patients with convulsive disorders, hyperthyroidism, or diabetes mellitus; and in patients who are unusually responsive to sympathomimetic amines. Clinically significant changes in systolic and diastolic blood pressure have been seen in individual patients and could be expected to occur in some patients after use of any beta-adrenergic bronchodilator.

Large doses of IV albuterol have been reported to aggravate preexisting diabetes mellitus and ketoacidosis. As with other beta-agonists, albuterol may produce significant hypokalemia in some patients, possibly through intracellular shunting, which has the potential to produce adverse cardiovascular effects. The decrease is usually transient, not requiring supplementation.

Information for the Patient

The action of Ventolin tablets may last up to 8 hours or longer. Ventolin tablets should not be taken more frequently than recommended. Do not increase the dose or frequency of Ventolin tablets without consulting your physician. If you find that treatment with Ventolin tablets becomes less effective for symptomatic relief, your symptoms get worse, and/or you need to take the product more frequently than usual, you should seek medical attention immediately. While you are taking Ventolin tablets, other asthma medications and inhaled drugs should be taken only as directed by your physician. Common adverse effects include palpitations, chest pain, rapid heart rate, and tremor or nervousness. If you are pregnant or nursing, contact your physician about use of Ventolin tablets. Effective and safe use of Ventolin tablets includes an understanding of the way that it should be administered.

Carcinogenesis, Mutagenesis, and Impairment of Fertility

In a 2 year study in Sprague-Dawley rats, albuterol sulfate caused a significant dose-related increase in the incidence of benign leiomyomas of the mesovarium at dietary doses of 2.0, 10, and 50 mg/kg (approximately ½, 3, and 15 times, respectively, the maximum recommended daily oral dose for adults on a mg/m^2 basis or 2/5, 2, and 10 times, respectively, the maximum recommended daily oral dose for children on a mg/m^2 basis). In another study this effect was blocked by the coadministration of propranolol, a non-selective beta-adrenergic antagonist.

In an 18 month study in CD-1 mice, albuterol sulfate showed no evidence of tumorigenicity at dietary doses of up to 500 mg/kg (approximately 65 times the maximum recommended daily oral dose for adults on a mg/m^2 basis or approximately 50 times the maximum recommended daily oral dose for children on a mg/m^2 basis). In a 22 month study in the Golden hamster, albuterol sulfate showed no evidence of tumorigenicity at dietary doses of up to 50 mg/kg (approximately 8 times the maximum recommended daily oral dose for adults on a mg/m^2 basis or approximately 7 times the maximum recommended daily oral dose for children on a mg/m^2 basis).

Albuterol sulfate was not mutagenic in the Ames test with or without metabolic activation using tester strains *S. typhimurium* TA1537, TA1538, and TA98 or *E. coli* WP2, WP2uvrA, and WP67. No forward mutation was seen in yeast strain *S. cerevisiae* S9 nor any mitotic gene conversion in yeast strain *S. cerevisiae* JD1 with or without metabolic activation. Fluctuation assays in *S. typhimurium* TA98 and *E. coli* WP2, both with metabolic activation, were negative. Albuterol sulfate was not clastogenic in a human peripheral lymphocyte assay or in an AH1 strain mouse micronucleus assay at intraperitoneal doses of up to 200 mg/kg.

Reproduction studies in rats demonstrated no evidence of impaired fertility at oral doses up to 50 mg/kg (approximately 15 times the maximum recommended daily oral dose for adults on a mg/m^2 basis).

Pregnancy, Teratogenic Effects, Pregnancy Category C

Albuterol has been shown to be teratogenic in mice. A study in CD-1 mice at subcutaneous (SC) doses of 0.025, 0.25, and 2.5 mg/kg (approximately 3/1000, 3/100, and 3/10 times, respectively, the maximum recommended daily oral dose for adults on a mg/m^2 basis) showed cleft palate formation in 5 of 111 (4.5%) fetuses at 0.25 mg/kg and in 10 of 108 (9.3%) fetuses at 2.5 mg/kg. The drug did not induce cleft palate formation at the lowest dose, 0.025 mg/kg. Cleft palate also occurred in 22 of 72 (30.5%) fetuses from females treated with 2.5 mg/kg of isoproterenol (positive control) subcutaneously (approximately 3/10 times the maximum recommended daily oral dose for adults on a mg/m^2 basis).

A reproduction study in Stride Dutch rabbits revealed cranioschisis in 7 of 19 (37%) fetuses when albuterol was administered orally at a 50 mg/kg dose (approximately 25 times the maximum recommended daily oral dose for adults on a mg/m^2 basis).

There are no adequate and well-controlled studies in pregnant women. Albuterol should be used during pregnancy only if the potential benefit justifies the potential risk to the fetus.

During worldwide marketing experience, various congenital anomalies, including cleft palate and limb defects, have been rarely reported in the offspring of patients being treated with albuterol. Some of the mothers were taking multiple medications during their pregnancies. No consistent pattern of defects can be discerned, and a relationship between albuterol use and congenital anomalies has not been established.

Use in Labor and Delivery

Because of the potential for beta-agonist interference with uterine contractility, use of Ventolin tablets for relief of bronchospasm during labor should be restricted to those patients in whom the benefits clearly outweigh the risk.

Tocolysis

Albuterol has not been approved for the management of preterm labor. The benefit:risk ratio when albuterol is administered for tocolysis has not been established. Serious adverse reactions, including maternal pulmonary edema, have been reported during or following treatment of premature labor with $beta_2$-agonists, including albuterol.

Nursing Mothers

It is not known whether this drug is excreted in human milk. Because of the potential for tumorigenicity shown for albuterol in some animal studies, a decision should be made whether to discontinue nursing or to discontinue the drug, taking into account the importance of the drug to the mother.

Pediatric Use

Safety and effectiveness in children below 6 years of age have not been established.

VENTOLIN SYRUP

General

Albuterol, as with all sympathomimetic amines, should be used with caution in patients with cardiovascular disorders, especially coronary insufficiency, cardiac arrhythmias, and hypertension; in patients with convulsive disorders, hyperthyroidism, or diabetes mellitus; and in patients who are unusually responsive to sympathomimetic amines. Clinically significant changes in systolic and diastolic blood pressure have been seen and could be expected to occur in some patients after use of any beta-adrenergic bronchodilator.

Large doses of IV albuterol have been reported to aggravate pre-existing diabetes and ketoacidosis. As with other beta-agonists, albuterol may produce significant hypokalemia in some patients, possibly through intracellular shunting, which has the potential to produce adverse cardiovascular effects. The decrease is usually transient, not requiring supplementation.

Information for the Patient

The action of Ventolin syrup may last up to 6 hours or longer. Ventolin syrup should not be taken more frequently than recommended. Do not increase the dose or frequency of doses of Ventolin syrup without consulting your physician. If you find that treatment with Ventolin syrup becomes less effective for symptomatic relief, your symptoms become worse, and/or you need to take the product more frequently than usual, you should seek medical attention immediately. While you are taking Ventolin syrup, other inhaled drugs and asthma medications should be taken only as directed by your physician. Common adverse effects include palpitations, chest pain, rapid heart rate, tremor, or nervousness. If you are pregnant or nursing, contact your physician about the use of Ventolin syrup. Effective use of Ventolin syrup includes an understanding of the way that it should be administered.

A

Carcinogenesis, Mutagenesis, and Impairment of Fertility

In a 2 year study in Sprague-Dawley rats, albuterol sulfate caused a significant dose-related increase in the incidence of benign leiomyomas of the mesovarium at and above dietary doses of 2 mg/kg (corresponding to less than the maximum recommended daily oral dose for adults and children on a mg/m² basis). In another study, this effect was blocked by the coadministration of propranolol, a nonselective beta-adrenergic antagonist.

In an 18 month study in CD-1 mice, albuterol sulfate showed no evidence of tumorigenicity at dietary doses up to 500 mg/kg (approximately 65 times the maximum recommended daily oral dose for adults on a mg/m² basis and approximately 50 times the maximum recommended daily oral dose for children on a mg/m² basis). In a 22 month study in the Golden Hamster, albuterol sulfate showed no evidence of tumorigenicity at dietary doses up to 50 mg/kg (approximately 8 times the maximum recommended daily oral dose for adults and children on a mg/m² basis).

Albuterol sulfate was not mutagenic in the Ames test with or without metabolic activation using tester strains *S. typhimurium* TA1537, TA1538, and TA98 or *E. coli* WP2, WP2uvrA, and WP67. No forward mutation was seen in yeast strain *S. cerevisiae* S9 nor any mitotic gene conversion in yeast strain *S. cerevisiae* JD1 with or without metabolic activation. Fluctuation assays in *S. typhimurium* TA98 and *E. coli* WP2, both with metabolic activation, were negative. Albuterol sulfate was not clastogenic in a human peripheral lymphocyte assay or in an AH1 strain mouse micronucleus assay.

Reproduction studies in rats demonstrated no evidence of impaired fertility at oral doses of albuterol sulfate up to 50 mg/kg (approximately 15 times the maximum recommended daily oral dose for adults on a mg/m² basis).

Pregnancy, Teratogenic Effects, Pregnancy Category C

Albuterol sulfate has been shown to be teratogenic in mice. A study in CD-1 mice at subcutaneous (SC) doses at and above 0.25 mg/kg (corresponding to less than the maximum recommended daily oral dose for adults on a mg/m² basis), induced cleft palate formation in 5 of 111 (4.5%) fetuses. At a SC dose of 2.5 mg/kg (corresponding to less than the maximum recommended daily oral dose for adults on a mg/m² basis), albuterol sulfate induced cleft palate formation in 10 of 108 (9.3%) fetuses. The drug did not induce cleft palate formation when administered at a SC dose of 0.025 mg/kg (significantly less than the maximum recommended daily oral dose for adults on a mg/m² basis). Cleft palate also occurred in 22 of 72 (30.5%) fetuses from females treated with 2.5 mg/kg of isoproterenol (positive control) administered subcutaneously.

A reproduction study in Stride Dutch rabbits revealed cranioschisis in 7 of 19 (37%) fetuses when albuterol was administered orally at a dose of 50 mg/kg (approximately 25 times the maximum recommended daily oral dose for adults on a mg/m² basis).

Studies in pregnant rats with tritiated albuterol demonstrated that approximately 10% of the circulating maternal drug is transferred to the fetus. Disposition in the fetal lungs is comparable to maternal lungs, but fetal liver disposition is 1% of the maternal liver levels.

There are no adequate and well-controlled studies in pregnant women. Because animal reproduction studies are not always predictive of human response, albuterol should be used during pregnancy only if the potential benefit justifies the potential risk to the fetus.

During worldwide marketing experience, various congenital anomalies, including cleft palate and limb defects, have been reported in the offspring of patients being treated with albuterol. Some of the mothers were taking multiple medications during their pregnancies. Because no consistent pattern of defects can be discerned, a relationship between albuterol use and congenital anomalies has not been established.

Use in Labor and Delivery

Use in Labor

Because of the potential for beta-agonist interference with uterine contractility, use of Ventolin syrup for relief of bronchospasm during labor should be restricted to those patients in whom the benefits clearly outweigh the risk.

Tocolysis

Albuterol has not been approved for the management of preterm labor. The benefit:risk ratio when albuterol is administered for tocolysis has not been established. Serious adverse reactions, including maternal pulmonary edema, have been reported during or following treatment of premature labor with beta$_2$-agonists, including albuterol.

Nursing Mothers

It is not known whether this drug is excreted in human milk. Because of the potential for tumorigenicity shown for albuterol in some animal studies, a decision should be made whether to discontinue nursing or to discontinue the drug, taking into account the importance of the drug to the mother.

Pediatric Use

Safety and effectiveness in children below the age of 12 years have not been established.

VOLMAX EXTENDED-RELEASE TABLETS

General

Albuterol, as with all sympathomimetic amines, should be used with caution in patients with cardiovascular disorders, especially coronary insufficiency, cardiac arrhythmias, and hypertension; in patients with convulsive disorders, hyperthyroidism, or diabetes mellitus; and in patients who are unusually responsive to sympathomimetic amines. Clinically significant changes in systolic and diastolic blood pressure have been seen and could be expected to occur in some patients after use of any beta-adrenergic bronchodilator.

In controlled clinical trials in adults, patients treated with Volmax extended-release tablets had increases in selected serum chemistry values and decreases in selected hematologic values. Increases in SGPT were more frequent among patients treated with Volmax extended-release tablets (12 of 247 patients, 4.9%) than among the theophylline (6 of 188 patients, 3.2%) and placebo (1 of 138 patients, 0.7%) groups. Increases in serum glucose concentration were also more frequent among patients treated with Volmax extended-release tablets (23 of 234 patients, 9.8%) than among theothephylline (11 of 173 patients, 6.45%) and placebo (3 of 129 patients, 2.3%) groups. Increases in SGOT were also more frequent among patients treated with Volmax extended-release tablets (10 of 248 patients, 4%) and theophylline (5 of 193, 2.6%) than among patients treated with placebo. Decreases in white blood cell counts were more frequent in patients treated with Volmax extended-release tablets (10 of 247 patients, 4%) compared with patients receiving theophylline (2 of 185 patients, 1.1%) and patients receiving placebo (1 of 141 patients, 0.7%). Decreases in hemoglobin and hematocrit were more frequent in patients receiving Volmax extended-release tablets (16 of 228 patients, 7.0%, and 17 of 230 patients, 7.4%, respectively) than in patients receiving theophylline (5 of 171 patients, 2.9%, and 9 of 173 patients, 5.2%, respectively) and patients receiving placebo (5 of 129 patients, 3.9%, and 3 of 132 patients, 2.3%, respectively). The clinical significance of these results is unknown.

Large doses of intravenous albuterol have been reported to aggravate pre-existing diabetes mellitus and ketoacidosis. As with other beta-agonists, albuterol may produce significant hypokalemia in some patients, possibly through intracellular shunting, which has the potential to produce adverse cardiovascular effects. The decrease is usually transient, not requiring supplementation.

As with any other nondeformable material, caution should be used when administering Volmax extended-release tablets to patients with pre-existing gastrointestinal narrowing from any cause. There have been rare reports of gastrointestinal obstruction in such patients occurring in association with ingestion of products containing delivery systems similar to that contained in Volmax extended-release tablets.

Information for the Patient

Each Volmax extended-release tablet contains a small hole that is part of the unique extended-release system. Volmax extended-release tablets must be swallowed whole with the aid of liquids. DO NOT CHEW OR CRUSH THESE TABLETS.

The outer coating of the tablet is not absorbed and is excreted in the feces; in some instances the empty outer coating may be noticeable in the stool.

The action of Volmax extended-release tablets should last up to 12 hours or longer. Volmax extended-release tablets should not be used more frequently than recommended. Do not increase the dose or frequency of Volmax extended-release tablets without consulting your physician. If you find that treatment with Volmax extended-release tablets becomes less effective for symptomatic relief, your symptoms become worse, and/or you need to use the product more frequently than usual, you should seek medical attention immediately. While you are using Volmax extended-release tablets, other inhaled drugs and asthma medications should be taken only as directed by your physician. Common adverse effects include palpitations, chest pain, rapid heart rate, tremor or nervousness. If you are pregnant or nursing, contact your physician about use of Volmax extended-release tablets. Effective and safe use of Volmax extended-release tablets includes an understanding of the way that it should be administered.

Carcinogenesis, Mutagenesis, and Impairment of Fertility

In a 2 year study in Sprague-Dawley rats, albuterol sulfate caused a significant dose-related increase in the incidence of benign leiomyomas of the mesovarium at dietary doses of 2.0, 10, and 50 mg/kg, (approximately 1/2, 3, and 15 times, respectively, the maximum recommended daily oral dose for adults on a mg/m² basis, or, approximately 2/5, 2, and 10 times, respectively, the maximum recommended daily oral dose for children on a mg/m² basis). In another study this effect was blocked by the coadministration of propranolol, a non-selective beta-adrenergic antagonist. In a 18 month study in CD-1 mice, albuterol sulfate showed no evidence of tumorigenicity at dietary doses of up to 500 mg/kg (approximately 65 times the maximum recommended daily oral dose for adults on a mg/m² basis, or, approximately 50 times the maximum recommended daily oral dose for children on a mg/m² basis). In a 22 month study in the Golden hamster, albuterol sulfate showed no evidence of tumorigenicity at dietary doses of 50 mg/kg (approximately 7 times the maximum recommended daily oral dose for adults and children on a mg/m² basis).

Albuterol sulfate was not mutagenic in the Ames test with or without metabolic activation using tester strains *S. typhimurium* TA 1537, TA 1538, and TA98 or *E. coli* WP2, WP2uvrA, and WP67. No forward mutation was seen in yeast strain *S. cerevisiae* S9 nor any mitotic gene conversion in yeast strain *S. cerevisiae* JD1 with or without metabolic activation. Fluctuation assays in *S. typhimurium* TA98 and *E. coli* WP2, both with metabolic activation, were negative. Albuterol sulfate was not clastogenic in a human peripheral lymphocyte assay or in an AH1 strain mouse micronucleus assay at intraperitoneal doses of up to 200 mg/kg.

Reproduction studies in rats demonstrated no evidence of impaired fertility at oral doses up to 50 mg/kg (approximately 15 times the maximum recommended daily oral dose for adults on a mg/m² basis).

Pregnancy, Teratogenic Effects, Pregnancy Category C

Albuterol Sulfate has been shown to be teratogenic in mice. A study in CD-1 mice at subcutaneous (SC) doses of 0.025, 0.25, and 2.5 mg/kg (approximately 3/1000, 3/100, and 3/10 times the maximum recommended daily oral dose for adults on a mg/m² basis), showed cleft palate formation in 5 of 111 (4.5%) fetuses at 0.25 mg/kg and in 10 of 108 (9.3%) fetuses at 2.5 mg/kg. The drug did not induce cleft palate formation at the lowest dose, 0.025 mg/kg. Cleft palate also occurred in 22 of 72 (30.5%) fetuses of females treated with 2.5 mg/kg of isoproterenol (positive control) subcutaneously (approximately 3/10 times the maximum recommended daily oral dose for adults on a mg/m² basis). A reproduction study in Stride Dutch rabbits revealed cranioschisis in 7/19 fetuses (37%) when albuterol sulfate was administered orally at a 50 mg/kg dose (approximately 25 times the maximum recommended daily oral dose for adults on a mg/m² basis).

There are no adequate and well-controlled studies in pregnant women. Albuterol should be used during pregnancy only if the potential benefit justifies the potential risk to the fetus.

During worldwide marketing experience, various congenital anomalies, including cleft palate and limb defects, have been rarely reported in the offspring of patients being treated with albuterol. Some of the mothers were taking multiple medications during their pregnancies. No consistent pattern of defects can be discerned, and a relationship between albuterol use and congenital anomalies has not been established.

Labor and Delivery

Because of the potential for beta-agonist interference with uterine contractility, use of Volmax extended-release tablets for relief of bronchospasm during labor should be restricted to those patients in whom the benefits clearly outweigh the risks.

Tocolysis

Albuterol has not been approved for the management of pre-term labor. The benefit:risk ratio when albuterol is administered for tocolysis has not been established. Serious adverse reactions, including pulmonary edema, have been reported during or following treatment of premature labor with beta$_2$-agonists, including albuterol.

Nursing Mothers

It is not known whether albuterol is excreted in human milk. Because of the potential for tumorigenicity shown for albuterol in animal studies, a decision should be made whether to discontinue nursing or to discontinue the drug, taking into account the importance of the drug to the mother.

Pediatric Use

The safety and effectiveness of Volmax extended-release tablets have been established in pediatric patients 6 years of age or older. Use of Volmax extended-release tablets in these age groups is supported by evidence from adequate and well-controlled studies of Volmax extended-release tablets in adults; the likelihood that the disease course, pathophysiology, and the drug's effect in pediatric and adult patients are substantially similar; the established safety and effectiveness of immediate-release albuterol tablets in pediatric patients 6 years of age and older; and clinical trials that support the safety of Volmax extended-release tablets in pediatric patients over 6 years of age. The recommended dose of Volmax extended-release tablets for the pediatric population is based upon the recommended pediatric dosing of immediate-release albuterol tablets and pharmacokinetic studies in adults showing comparable bioavailability at steady-state dosing and reduced bioavailability after single dose administration. Safety and effectiveness in pediatric patients below 6 years of age have not been established.

DRUG INTERACTIONS

VENTOLIN TABLETS

The concomitant use of Ventolin tablets and other oral sympathomimetic agents is not recommended since such combined use may lead to deleterious cardiovascular effects. This recommendation does not preclude the judicious use of an aerosol bronchodilator of the adrenergic stimulant type in patients receiving Ventolin tablets. Such concomitant use, however, should be individualized and not given on a routine basis. If regular coadministration is required, then alternative therapy should be considered.

Monoamine Oxidase Inhibitors or Tricyclic Antidepressants

Albuterol should be administered with extreme caution to patients being treated with monoamine oxidase inhibitors or tricyclic antidepressants, or within 2 weeks of discontinuation of such agents, because the action of albuterol on the vascular system may be potentiated.

Beta-Blockers

Beta-adrenergic receptor blocking agents not only block the pulmonary effect of beta-agonists, such as Ventolin tablets, but may produce severe bronchospasm in patients with asthma. Therefore, patients with asthma should not normally be treated with beta-blockers. However, under certain circumstances, *e.g.,* as prophylaxis after myocardial infarction, there may be no acceptable alternatives to the use of beta-adrenergic blocking agents in patients with asthma. In this setting, cardioselective beta-blockers could be considered, although they should be administered with caution.

Diuretics

The ECG changes and/or hypokalemia that may result from the administration of nonpotassium-sparing diuretics (such as loop or thiazide diuretics) can be acutely worsened by beta-agonists, especially when the recommended dose of the beta-agonist is exceeded. Although the clinical significance of these effects is not known, caution is advised in the coadministration of beta-agonists with nonpotassium-sparing diuretics.

Digoxin

Mean decreases of 16-22% in serum digoxin levels were demonstrated after single-dose IV and oral administration of albuterol, respectively, to normal volunteers who had received digoxin for 10 days. The clinical significance of these findings for patients with obstructive airway disease who are receiving albuterol and digoxin on a chronic basis is unclear. Nevertheless, it would be prudent to carefully evaluate the serum digoxin levels in patients who are currently receiving digoxin and albuterol.

VENTOLIN SYRUP

The concomitant use of Ventolin syrup and other oral sympathomimetic agents is not recommended since such combined use may lead to deleterious cardiovascular effects. This recommendation does not preclude the judicious use of an aerosol bronchodilator of the adrenergic stimulant type in patients receiving Ventolin syrup. Such concomitant use, however, should be individualized and not given on a routine basis. If regular coadministration is required, then alternative therapy should be considered.

Beta-Blockers

Beta-adrenergic receptor blocking agents not only block the pulmonary effect of beta-agonists, such as Ventolin syrup, but may produce severe bronchospasm in patients with asthma. Therefore, patients with asthma should not normally be treated with beta-blockers. However, under certain circumstances, *e.g.,* as prophylaxis after myocardial infarction, there may be no acceptable alternatives to the use of beta-adrenergic blocking agents in patients with asthma. In this setting, cardioselective beta-blockers could be considered, although they should be administered with caution.

Diuretics

The ECG changes and/or hypokalemia that may result from the administration of nonpotassium-sparing diuretics (such as loop or thiazide diuretics) can be acutely worsened by beta-agonists, especially when the recommended dose of the beta-agonist is exceeded. Although the clinical significance of these effects is not known, caution is advised in the coadministration of beta-agonists with nonpotassium-sparing diuretics.

Digoxin

Mean decreases of 16-22% in serum digoxin levels were demonstrated after single dose IV and oral administration of albuterol, respectively, to normal volunteers who had received digoxin for 10 days. The clinical significance of these findings for patients with obstructive airway disease who are receiving albuterol and digoxin on a chronic basis is unclear. Nevertheless, it would be prudent to carefully evaluate the serum digoxin levels in patients who are currently receiving digoxin and albuterol.

Monoamine Oxidase Inhibitors or Tricyclic Antidepressants

Albuterol should be administered with extreme caution to patients being treated with monoamine oxidase inhibitors or tricyclic antidepressants, or within 2 weeks of discontinuation of such agents, because the action of albuterol on the vascular system may be potentiated.

VOLMAX EXTENDED-RELEASE TABLETS

The concomitant use of Volmax extended-release tablets and other oral sympathomimetic agents is not recommended since such combined use may lead to deleterious cardiovascular effects. This recommendation does not preclude the judicious use of an aerosol bronchodilator of the adrenergic stimulant type in patients receiving Volmax extended-release tablets. Such concomitant use, however, should be individualized and not given on a routine basis. If regular coadministration is required, then alternative therapy should be considered.

Monoamine Oxidase Inhibitors or Tricyclic Antidepressants

Albuterol should be administered with extreme caution to patients being treated with monoamine oxidase inhibitors or tricyclic antidepressants, or within 2 weeks of discontinuation of such agents, because the action of albuterol on the vascular system may be potentiated.

Beta Blockers

Beta-adrenergic receptor blocking agents not only block the pulmonary effect of beta-agonists, such as Volmax extended-release tablets, but may produce severe bronchospasm in asthmatic patients. Therefore, patients with asthma should not normally be treated with beta-blockers. However, under certain circumstances, *e.g.,* as prophylaxis after myocardial infarction, there may be no acceptable alternatives to the use of beta-adrenergic blocking agents in patients with asthma. In this setting, cardioselective beta-blockers could be considered, although they should be administered with caution.

Diuretics

The ECG changes and/or hypokalemia that may result from the administration of nonpotasssium-sparing diuretics (such as loop or thiazide diuretics) can be acutely worsened by beta-agonists, especially when the recommended dose of the beta-agonist is exceeded. Although the clinical significance of these effects is not known, caution is advised in the coadministration of beta-agonists with non potassium-sparing diuretics.

Digoxin

Mean decreases of 16-22% in serum digoxin levels were demonstrated after single dose intravenous and oral administration of albuterol, respectively, to normal volunteers who had received digoxin for 10 days. The clinical significance of these findings for patients with obstructive airway disease who are receiving albuterol and digoxin on a chronic basis is unclear. Nevertheless, it would be prudent to carefully evaluate the serum digoxin levels in patients who are currently receiving digoxin and albuterol.

ADVERSE REACTIONS

VENTOLIN TABLETS

In clinical trials, the most frequent adverse reactions to Ventolin tablets are shown in TABLE 2.

TABLE 2 *Percent Incidence of Adverse Reactions*

Reaction	Percent Incidence
Central Nervous System	
Nervousness	20%
Tremor	20%
Headache	7%
Sleeplessness	2%
Weakness	2%
Dizziness	2%
Drowsiness	<1%
Restlessness	<1%
Irritability	<1%
Cardiovascular	
Tachycardia	5%
Palpitations	5%
Chest discomfort	<1%
Flushing	<1%
Musculoskeletal	
Muscle cramps	3%
Gastrointestinal	
Nausea	2%
Genitourinary	
Difficulty in micturition	<1%

Cases of urticaria, angioedema, rash, bronchospasm, oropharyngeal edema, and arrhythmias (including atrial fibrillation, supraventricular tachycardia, extrasystoles) have been reported after the use of Ventolin tablets.

In addition, albuterol, like other sympathomimetic agents, can cause adverse reactions such as hypertension, angina, vomiting, vertigo, central nervous system stimulation, unusual taste, and drying or irritation of the oropharynx.

The reactions are generally transient in nature, and it is usually not necessary to discontinue treatment with Ventolin tablets. In selected cases, however, dosage may be reduced temporarily; after the reaction has subsided, dosage should be increased in small increments to the optimal dosage.

VENTOLIN SYRUP

The adverse reactions to albuterol are similar in nature to those of other sympathomimetic agents. In clinical trials, the most frequent adverse reactions to Ventolin syrup in adults and older children are shown in TABLE 3.

TABLE 3 *Percent Incidence of Adverse Reactions in Adults and Children (6-12 Years of Age)*

Adverse Event	Percent Incidence
Central Nervous System	
Tremor	10%
Nervousness	9%
Shakiness	9%
Headache	4%
Dizziness	3%
Excitement	2%
Hyperactivity	2%
Sleeplessness	1%
Disturbed sleep	<1%
Irritable behavior	<1%
Dilated pupils	<1%
Weakness	1%
Cardiovascular	
Tachycardia	1%
Palpitations	<1%
Sweating	<1%
Chest pain	<1%
Ear, Nose, and Throat	
Epistaxis	1%
Gastrointestinal	
Increased appetite	3%
Epigastric pain	<1%
Stomachache	<1%
Musculoskeletal	
Muscle spasm	<1%
Respiratory	
Cough	<1%

In clinical trials, the following adverse reactions to Ventolin syrup were noted more frequently in young children 2-6 years of age than in adults and older children (see TABLE 4).

TABLE 4 *Percent Incidence of Adverse Reactions Noted More Frequently in Children 2-6 Years of Age Than in Older Children and Adults*

Adverse Event	Percent Incidence
Central Nervous System	
Excitement	20%
Nervousness	15%
Hypokinesia	4%
Sleeplessness	2%
Emotional lability	1%
Fatigue	1%
Cardiovascular	
Tachycardia	2%
Pallor	1%
Gastrointestinal	
Gastrointestinal symptoms	2%
Loss of appetite	1%
Ophthalmologic	
Conjunctivitis	1%

Cases of urticaria, angioedema, rash, bronchospasm, oropharyngeal edema, and arrhythmias (including atrial fibrillation, supraventricular tachycardia, and extrasystoles) have been reported after the use of Ventolin syrup.

In addition, albuterol, like other sympathomimetic agents, can cause adverse reactions such as angina, central nervous system stimulation, drying or irritation of the oropharynx, hypertension, nausea, unusual taste, vertigo, and vomiting.

The reactions are generally transient in nature, and it is usually not necessary to discontinue treatment with Ventolin syrup. In selected cases, however, dosage may be reduced temporarily; after the reaction has subsided, dosage should be increased in small increments to the optimal dosage.

VOLMAX EXTENDED-RELEASE TABLETS

The adverse reactions to albuterol are similar in nature to reactions to other sympathomimetic agents. The most frequent adverse reactions to albuterol are nervousness, tremor, headache, tachycardia, and palpitations. Less frequent adverse reactions are muscle cramps, insomnia, nausea, weakness, dizziness, drowsiness, flushing, restlessness, irritability, chest discomfort, and difficulty in micturition.

Rare cases of urticaria, angioedema, rash, bronchospasm, and oropharyngeal edema have been reported after the use of albuterol.

In addition, albuterol, like other sympathomimetic agents, can cause adverse reactions such as hypertension, angina, vomiting, vertigo, central nervous system stimulation, unusual taste, and drying or irritation of the oropharynx.

In controlled clinical trials of adult patients conducted in the US, the following incidence of adverse events was reported (see TABLE 5).

TABLE 5

Event	Volmax (n=330)	Theophylline (n=197)	Other Beta-Agonists (n=20)	Placebo (n=178)
Tremor	24.2%	6.1%	35.0%	1.1%
Headache	18.8%	26.9%	35.0%	20.8%
Nervousness	8.5%	5.1%	10.0%	2.8%
Nausea/vomiting	4.2%	19.8%	5.0%	3.9%
Tachycardia	2.7%	0.5%	5.0%	0%
Muscle cramps	2.7%	0.5%	5.0%	0.6%
Palpitations	2.4%	0.5%	0%	1.1%
Insomnia	2.4%	6.1%	0%	1.7%
Dizziness	1.5%	2.0%	0%	5.1%
Somnolence	0.3%	1.0%	0%	0.6%

A trend was observed among patients treated with Volmax extended-release tablets toward increasing frequency of muscle cramps with increasing patient age (12-20 years, 1.2%; 21-30 years, 2.6%; 31-40 years, 6.9%; 41-50 years, 6.9%), compared with no such events in the placebo group. Also observed was an increasing frequency of tremor with increasing patient age (12-20 years, 29.4%; 21-30 years, 29.9%; 31-40 years, 27.6%; 41-50 years, 37.9%), compared to 2.9% or less in the placebo group.

The reactions are generally transient in nature, and it is usually not necessary to discontinue treatment with Volmax extended-release tablets.

DOSAGE AND ADMINISTRATION

VENTOLIN TABLETS

The following dosages of Ventolin tablets are expressed in terms of albuterol base.

Usual Dosage:

Adults and children over 12 years of age: The usual starting dosage for adults and children 12 years and older is 2 or 4 mg three or four times a day.

Children 6-12 years of age: The usual starting dosage for children 6-12 years of age is 2 mg three or four times a day.

Dose Adjustment:

Adults and children over 12 years of age: For adults and children 12 years and older, a dosage above 4 mg four times a day should be used *only* when the patient fails to respond. If a favorable response does not occur with the 4 mg initial dosage, it should be cautiously increased stepwise up to a maximum of 8 mg four times a day as tolerated.

Children 6-12 years of age who fail to respond to the initial starting dosage of 2 mg four times a day: For children from 6-12 years of age who fail to respond to the initial starting dosage of 2 mg four times a day, the dosage may be cautiously increased stepwise, but not to exceed 24 mg/day (given in divided doses).

The total daily dose should not exceed 32 mg in adults and children 12 years and older.

Elderly Patients and Those Sensitive to Beta-Adrenergic Stimulators

An initial dosage of 2 mg three or four times a day is recommended for elderly patients and for those with a history of unusual sensitivity to beta-adrenergic stimulators. If adequate bronchodilatation is not obtained, dosage may be increased gradually to as much as 8 mg three or four times a day.

VENTOLIN SYRUP

The following dosages of Ventolin syrup are expressed in terms of albuterol base.

Usual Dosage:

Adults and pediatric patients over 12 years of age: The usual starting dosage for adults and children over 12 years of age is 2 mg (1 teaspoonful) or 4 mg (2 teaspoonfuls) 3 or 4 times a day.

Pediatric patients 6-12 years of age: The usual starting dosage for children 6-12 years of age is 2 mg (1 teaspoonful) 3 or 4 times a day.

Pediatric patients 2-6 years of age: Dosing in children 2-6 years of age should be initiated at 0.1 mg/kg of body weight 3 times a day. The starting dosage should not exceed 2 mg (1 teaspoonful) 3 times a day.

Dose Adjustment:

Adults and pediatric patients over 12 years of age: For adults and children over 12 years of age, a dosage above 4 mg four times a day should be used *only* when the patient fails to respond to this dosage. If a favorable response does not occur with the 4 mg initial dosage, it may be cautiously increased stepwise as tolerated, but not to exceed 8 mg four times a day (total daily dose should not exceed 32 mg).

Pediatric patients 6-12 years of age who fail to respond to the initial starting dosage of 2 mg four times a day: For children 6-12 years of age who fail to respond to the initial starting dosage of 2 mg four times a day, the dosage may be cautiously increased stepwise as tolerated but not to exceed 6 mg four times a day (total daily dose should not exceed 24 mg).

Pediatric patients 2-6 years of age who do not respond satisfactorily to the initial dosage: For children 2-6 years of age who do not respond satisfactorily to the initial starting dosage, the dosage may be increased stepwise to 0.2 mg/kg of body weight 3 times a day as tolerated, but not to exceed a maximum of 4 mg (2 teaspoonfuls) given 3 times a day (total daily dose should not exceed 12 mg).

Elderly Patients and Those Sensitive to Beta-Adrenergic Stimulators

The initial dosage should be restricted to 2 mg three or four times a day. If adequate bronchodilation is not obtained, dosage may be increased gradually as tolerated to as much as 8 mg three or four times per day (total daily dose should not exceed 32 mg).

VOLMAX EXTENDED-RELEASE TABLETS

The following dosages of Volmax extended-release tablets are expressed in terms of albuterol base:

Usual Dosage:

Adults and children over 12 years of age: The usual recommended dosage for adults and pediatric patients over 12 years of age is 8 mg every 12 hours. In some patients, 4 mg every 12 hours may be sufficient.

Children 6 to 12 years of age: The usual recommended dosage for children 6 through 12 years of age is 4 mg every 12 hours.

Dosage Adjustment in Adults and Children Over 12 Years of Age

In unusual circumstances, such as adults of low body weight, it may be desirable to use a starting dosage of 4 mg every 12 hours and progress to 8 mg every 12 hours according to response.

If control of reversible airway obstruction is not achieved with the recommended doses in patients on otherwise optimized asthma therapy, the doses may be cautiously increased stepwise under the control of the supervising physician to a maximum dose of 32 mg/day in divided doses (*i.e.*, q12h).

Dosage Adjustment in Children 6–12 Years of Age

If control of reversible airway obstruction is not achieved with the recommended doses in patients on otherwise optimized asthma therapy, the doses may be cautiously increased stepwise under the control of the supervising physician to a maximum dose of 24 mg/day in divided doses (*i.e.*, every 12 hours).

Switching From Oral Ventolin Products

Patients currently maintained on Ventolin (albuterol sulfate) tablets or Ventolin (albuterol sulfate) syrup can be switched to Volmax extended-release tablets. For example, the administration of one 4 mg Volmax extended-release tablet every 12 hours is comparable to one 2 mg Ventolin tablet every 6 hours. Multiples of this regimen up to the maximum recommended daily dose also apply.

Each Volmax extended-release tablet contains a small hole that is part of the unique extended-release system. Volmax extended-release tablets must be swallowed whole with the aid of liquids. DO NOT CHEW OR CRUSH THESE TABLETS.

HOW SUPPLIED

VENTOLIN TABLETS

Ventolin tablets are available as follows:

2 mg of albuterol as the sulfate: White, round, compressed tablets impressed with the product name ("VENTOLIN") and the number "2" on one side and scored on the other with "GLAXO" impressed on each side of the score.

4 mg of albuterol as the sulfate: White, round, compressed tablets impressed with the product name ("VENTOLIN") and the number "4" on one side and scored on the other with "GLAXO" impressed on each side of the score.

Storage: Store between 2 and 25°C (36 and 77°F). Replace cap securely after each opening.

VENTOLIN SYRUP

Ventolin syrup, a clear orange-yellow liquid with a strawberry flavor, contains 2 mg albuterol as the sulfate per 5 ml.

Storage: Store between 2 and 30°C (36 and 86°F). Dispense in tight, light-resistant containers.

VOLMAX EXTENDED-RELEASE TABLETS

Volmax extended-release tablets are available in:

4 mg: Light blue, hexagonal tablets printed with "Volmax" on one side and the number "4" on the other in dark blue ink.

8 mg: White, hexagonal tablets printed with "Volmax" on one side and the number "8" on the other in dark blue ink.

Storage: Store refrigerated, 2-8°C (36-46°F).

INHALATION

DESCRIPTION

Note: The trade name has been used throughout this monograph for clarity.

VENTOLIN INHALATION AEROSOL

Bronchodilator Aerosol.

For Oral Inhalation Only.

The active component of Ventolin inhalation aerosol is albuterol, racemic (α^1-[(*tert*-butylamino)methyl]-4-hydroxy-*m*-xylene-α,α'-diol) and a relatively selective beta$_2$-adrenergic bronchodilator.

Albuterol is the official generic name in the US. The World Health Organization recommended name for the drug is salbutamol. The molecular weight of albuterol is 239.3, and the empirical formula is $C_{13}H_{21}NO_3$. Albuterol is a white to off-white crystalline solid. It is soluble in ethanol, sparingly soluble in water, and very soluble in chloroform.

Ventolin inhalation aerosol is a pressurized metered-dose aerosol unit for oral inhalation. It contains a microcrystalline (95% $\leq$10 μm) suspension of albuterol in propellants (trichloromonofluoromethane and dichlorodifluoromethane) with oleic acid. Each actuation delivers 100 μg of albuterol from the valve and 90 μg of albuterol from the mouthpiece. Each 6.8 g canister provides 80 inhalations and each 17 g canister provides 200 inhalations.

VENTOLIN HFA INHALATION AEROSOL

Bronchodilator Aerosol.

For Oral Inhalation Only.

The active component of Ventolin HFA (albuterol sulfate HFA inhalation aerosol) is albuterol sulfate, the racemic form of albuterol and a relatively selective beta$_2$-adrenergic bronchodilator. Albuterol sulfate has the chemical name α^1-[(*tert*-butylamino)methyl]-4-hydroxy-*m*-xylene-α,α'-diol sulfate (2:1)(salt).

Albuterol sulfate has a molecular weight of 576.7, and the empirical formula is $(C_{13}H_{21}NO_3)_2 \cdot H_2SO_4$. Albuterol sulfate is a white crystalline powder, soluble in water and slightly soluble in ethanol.

The World Health Organization recommended name for albuterol base is salbutamol.

Ventolin HFA is a pressurized metered-dose aerosol unit for oral inhalation. It contains a microcrystalline suspension of albuterol sulfate in propellant HFA-134a (1,1,1,2-tetrafluoroethane). It contains no other excipients.

It is recommended to prime the inhaler before using for the first time and in cases where the inhaler has not been used for more than 2 weeks by releasing 4 test sprays into the air, away from the face. After priming with 4 actuations, each actuation delivers 120 μg of albuterol sulfate in 75 mg of suspension from the valve and 108 μg of albuterol sulfate from the mouthpiece (equivalent to 90 μg of albuterol base from the mouthpiece). Each 18 g canister provides 200 inhalations.

This product does not contain chlorofluorocarbons (CFCs) as the propellant.

VENTOLIN INHALATION SOLUTION, 0.5%

***Potency expressed as albuterol.**

The active component of Ventolin inhalation solution is albuterol sulfate, the racemic form of albuterol and a relatively selective beta$_2$-adrenergic bronchodilator (see CLINICAL PHARMACOLOGY). It has the chemical name α^1-[(*tert*-butylamino)methyl]-4-hydroxy-*m*-xylene-α,α'-diol sulfate (2:1)(salt).

Albuterol sulfate has a molecular weight of 576.7, and the empirical formula is $(C_{13}H_{21}NO_3)_2 \cdot H_2SO_4$. Albuterol sulfate is a white crystalline powder, soluble in water and slightly soluble in ethanol.

The World Health Organization recommended name for albuterol base is salbutamol.

Ventolin inhalation solution, 0.5% is in concentrated form. Dilute the appropriate volume of the solution (see DOSAGE AND ADMINISTRATION) with sterile normal saline solution to a total volume of 3 ml and administer by nebulization.

Each milliliter of Ventolin inhalation solution contains 5 mg of albuterol (as 6 mg of albuterol sulfate) in an aqueous solution containing benzalkonium chloride; sulfuric acid is used to adjust the pH to between 3 and 5. Ventolin inhalation solution contains no sulfiting agents. It is supplied in a 20 ml amber glass bottle.

Ventolin inhalation solution is a clear, colorless to light yellow solution.

VENTOLIN NEBULES INHALATION SOLUTION, 0.083%

***Potency expressed as albuterol.**

Ventolin Nebules inhalation solution is a relatively selective beta$_2$-adrenergic bronchodilator (see CLINICAL PHARMACOLOGY). Albuterol sulfate, the racemic form of albuterol, has the chemical name α^1-[(*tert*-butylamino)methyl]-4-hydroxy-*m*-xylene-α,α'-diol sulfate (2:1)(salt).

Albuterol sulfate has a molecular weight of 576.7, and the empirical formula is $(C_{13}H_{21}NO_3)_2 \cdot H_2SO_4$. Albuterol sulfate is a white crystalline powder, soluble in water and slightly soluble in ethanol.

The World Health Organization recommended name for albuterol base is salbutamol.

Ventolin Nebules inhalation solution requires no dilution before administration by nebulization.

Each milliliter of Ventolin Nebules inhalation solution contains 0.83 mg of albuterol (as 1 mg of albuterol sulfate) in an isotonic, sterile, aqueous solution containing sodium chloride; sulfuric acid is used to adjust the pH to between 3 and 5. Ventolin Nebules inhalation solution contains no sulfiting agents or preservatives.

Ventolin Nebules inhalation solution is a clear, colorless solution.

VENTOLIN ROTACAPS FOR INHALATION

FOR ORAL INHALATION ONLY.

For Use With the Rotahaler Inhalation Device.

Ventolin Rotacaps for inhalation contain a dry powder presentation of albuterol sulfate intended for oral inhalation only. Each light blue and clear, hard gelatin capsule contains a mixture of 200 μg of microfine (95% $\leq$10 μm) albuterol (as the sulfate) with 25 mg of lactose.

The contents of each capsule are inhaled using a specially designed plastic device for inhaling powder called the Rotahaler. When turned, this device opens the capsule and facilitates dispersion of the albuterol sulfate into the airstream created when the patient inhales through the mouthpiece.

Ventolin Rotacaps for inhalation are an alternative inhalation form of albuterol to the metered-dose pressurized inhaler.

The active component of Ventolin Rotacaps for inhalation is albuterol sulfate, the racemic form of albuterol and a relatively selective beta$_2$-adrenergic bronchodilator. It has the chemical name α^1-[(*tert*-butylamino)methyl]-4-hydroxy-*m*-xylene-α,α'-diol sulfate (2:1)(salt).

Albuterol sulfate has a molecular weight of 576.7, and the empirical formula is $(C_{13}H_{21}NO_3)_2 \cdot H_2SO_4$. Albuterol sulfate is a white crystalline powder, soluble in water and slightly soluble in ethanol.

The World Health Organization recommended name for albuterol base is salbutamol.

CLINICAL PHARMACOLOGY

VENTOLIN INHALATION AEROSOL

In vitro studies and *in vivo* pharmacologic studies have demonstrated that albuterol has a preferential effect on beta$_2$-adrenergic receptors compared with isoproterenol. While it is recognized that beta$_2$-adrenergic receptors are the predominant receptors in bronchial smooth muscle, data indicate that there is a population of beta$_2$-receptors in the human heart existing in a concentration between 10 and 50%. The precise function of these receptors has not been established.

The pharmacologic effects of beta-adrenergic agonist drugs, including albuterol, are at least in part attributable to stimulation through beta-adrenergic receptors of intracellular adenyl cyclase, the enzyme that catalyzes the conversion of adenosine triphosphate (ATP) to cyclic-3′,5′-adenosine monophosphate (cyclic AMP). Increased cyclic AMP levels are associated with relaxation of bronchial smooth muscle and inhibition of release of mediators of immediate hypersensitivity from cells, especially from mast cells.

Albuterol has been shown in most controlled clinical trials to have more effect on the respiratory tract, in the form of bronchial smooth muscle relaxation, than isoproterenol at comparable doses while producing fewer cardiovascular effects. Controlled clinical studies and other clinical experience have shown that inhaled albuterol, like other beta-adrenergic agonist drugs, can produce a significant cardiovascular effect in some patients, as measured by pulse rate, blood pressure, symptoms, and/or electrocardiographic changes.

Albuterol is longer acting than isoproterenol in most patients by any route of administration because it is not a substrate for the cellular uptake processes for catecholamines nor for catechol-*O*-methyl transferase.

The effects of rising doses of albuterol and isoproterenol aerosols were studied in volunteers and patients with asthma. Results in normal volunteers indicated that albuterol is one-half to one-quarter as active as isoproterenol in producing increases in heart rate. In patients with asthma similar cardiovascular differentiation between the 2 drugs was also seen.

Preclinical

Intravenous (IV) studies in rats with albuterol sulfate have demonstrated that albuterol crosses the blood-brain barrier and reaches brain concentrations amounting to approximately 5.0% of the plasma concentrations. In structures outside the brain barrier (pineal and pituitary glands), albuterol concentrations were found to be 100 times those in the whole brain.

Studies in laboratory animals (minipigs, rodents, and dogs) have demonstrated the occurrence of cardiac arrhythmias and sudden death (with histologic evidence of myocardial necrosis) when beta-agonists and methylxanthines are administered concurrently. The clinical significance of these findings is unknown.

Pharmacokinetics

Because of its gradual absorption from the bronchi, systemic levels of albuterol are low after inhalation of recommended doses. Studies undertaken with 4 subjects administered tritiated albuterol resulted in maximum plasma concentrations occurring within 2-4 hours. Due to the sensitivity of the assay method, the metabolic rate and half-life of elimination of albuterol in plasma could not be determined. However, urinary excretion provided data indicating that albuterol has an elimination half-life of 3.8 hours. Approximately 72% of the inhaled dose is excreted within 24 hours in the urine, and consists of 28% as unchanged drug and 44% as metabolite.

VENTOLIN HFA INHALATION AEROSOL

Mechanism of Action

In vitro studies and *in vivo* pharmacologic studies have demonstrated that albuterol has a preferential effect on beta$_2$-adrenergic receptors compared with isoproterenol. While it is recognized that beta$_2$-adrenergic receptors are the predominant receptors in bronchial smooth muscle, data indicate that there is a population of beta$_2$-receptors in the human heart existing in a concentration between 10 and 50% of cardiac beta-adrenergic receptors. The precise function of these receptors has not been established (see WARNINGS, Cardiovascular Effects).

Activation of beta$_2$-adrenergic receptors on airway smooth muscle leads to the activation of adenylcyclase and to an increase in the intracellular concentration of cyclic-3′,5′-adenosine monophosphate (cyclic AMP). This increase of cyclic AMP leads to the activation of protein kinase A, which inhibits the phosphorylation of myosin and lowers intracellular ionic calcium concentrations, resulting in relaxation. Albuterol relaxes the smooth muscles of all airways, from the trachea to the terminal bronchioles. Albuterol acts as a functional antagonist to relax the airway irrespective of the spasmogen involved, thus protecting against all bronchoconstrictor challenges. Increased cyclic AMP concentrations are also associated with the inhibition of release of mediators from mast cells in the airway.

Albuterol has been shown in most controlled clinical trials to have more effect on the respiratory tract, in the form of bronchial smooth muscle relaxation, than isoproterenol at comparable doses while producing fewer cardiovascular effects. Controlled clinical studies and other clinical experience have shown that inhaled albuterol, like other beta-adrenergic agonist drugs, can produce a significant cardiovascular effect in some patients, as measured by pulse rate, blood pressure, symptoms, and/or electrocardiographic changes.

Preclinical

Intravenous (IV) studies in rats with albuterol sulfate have demonstrated that albuterol crosses the blood-brain barrier and reaches brain concentrations amounting to approximately 5.0% of the plasma concentrations. In structures outside the blood-brain barrier (pineal and pituitary glands), albuterol concentrations were found to be 100 times those in the whole brain.

Studies in laboratory animals (minipigs, rodents, and dogs) have demonstrated the occurrence of cardiac arrhythmias and sudden death (with histologic evidence of myocardial necrosis) when beta-agonists and methylxanthines are administered concurrently. The clinical significance of these findings is unknown.

Propellant HFA-134a is devoid of pharmacological activity except at very high doses in animals (380-1300 times the maximum human exposure based on comparisons of AUC values), primarily producing ataxia, tremors, dyspnea, or salivation. These are similar to effects produced by the structurally related chlorofluorocarbons (CFCs), which have been used extensively in metered-dose inhalers.

In animals and humans, propellant HFA-134a was found to be rapidly absorbed and rapidly eliminated, with an elimination half-life of 3-27 minutes in animals and 5-7 minutes in humans. Time to maximum plasma concentration (T_{max}) and mean residence time are both extremely short, leading to a transient appearance of HFA-134a in the blood with no evidence of accumulation.

Pharmacokinetics

The systemic levels of albuterol are low after inhalation of recommended doses. A study conducted in 12 healthy male and female subjects using a higher dose (1080 μg of albuterol base) showed that mean peak plasma concentrations of approximately 3 ng/ml occurred after dosing when albuterol was delivered using propellant HFA-134a. The mean time to peak concentrations (T_{max}) was delayed after administration of Ventolin HFA (T_{max} = 0.42 hours) as compared to CFC-propelled albuterol inhaler (T_{max} = 0.17 hours). Apparent terminal plasma half-life of albuterol is approximately 4.6 hours. No further pharmacokinetic studies for Ventolin HFA were conducted in neonates, children, or elderly subjects.

VENTOLIN INHALATION SOLUTION, 0.5%

In vitro studies and *in vivo* pharmacologic studies have demonstrated that albuterol has a preferential effect on beta$_2$-adrenergic receptors compared with isoproterenol. While it is recognized that beta$_2$-adrenergic receptors are the predominant receptors in bronchial smooth muscle, data indicate that there is a population of beta$_2$-receptors in the human heart existing in a concentration between 10 and 50%. The precise function of these receptors has not been established (see WARNINGS).

The pharmacologic effects of beta-adrenergic agonist drugs, including albuterol, are at least in part attributable to stimulation through beta-adrenergic receptors of intracellular adenyl cyclase, the enzyme that catalyzes the conversion of adenosine triphosphate (ATP) to cyclic-3′,5′-adenosine monophosphate (cyclic AMP). Increased cyclic AMP levels are associated with relaxation of bronchial smooth muscle and inhibition of release of mediators of immediate hypersensitivity from cells, especially from mast cells.

Albuterol has been shown in most controlled clinical trials to have more effect on the respiratory tract, in the form of bronchial smooth muscle relaxation, than isoproterenol at comparable doses while producing fewer cardiovascular effects.

Controlled clinical studies and other clinical experience have shown that inhaled albuterol, like other beta-adrenergic agonist drugs, can produce a significant cardiovascular effect in some patients, as measured by pulse rate, blood pressure, symptoms, and/or electrocardiographic changes.

Albuterol is longer acting than isoproterenol in most patients by any route of administration because it is not a substrate for the cellular uptake processes for catecholamines nor for catechol-*O*-methyl transferase.

Pharmacokinetics

Studies in patients with asthma have shown that less than 20% of a single albuterol dose was absorbed following either intermittent positive-pressure breathing (IPPB) or nebulizer administration; the remaining amount was recovered from the nebulizer and apparatus and expired air. Most of the absorbed dose was recovered in the urine within 24 hours after drug administration. Following a 3 mg dose of nebulized albuterol in adults, the maximum albuterol plasma levels at 0.5 hours were 2.1 ng/ml (range, 1.4-3.2 ng/ml). There was a significant dose-related response in FEV_1 (forced expiratory volume in 1 second) and peak flow rate. It has been demonstrated that following oral administration of 4 mg of albuterol, the elimination half-life was 5-6 hours.

Preclinical

Intravenous (IV) studies in rats with albuterol sulfate have demonstrated that albuterol crosses the blood-brain barrier and reaches brain concentrations amounting to approximately 5.0% of the plasma concentrations. In structures outside the brain barrier (pineal and pituitary glands), albuterol concentrations were found to be 100 times those in the whole brain.

Studies in laboratory animals (minipigs, rodents, and dogs) have demonstrated the occurrence of cardiac arrhythmias and sudden death (with histologic evidence of myocardial necrosis) when beta-agonists and methylxanthines are administered concurrently. The clinical significance of these findings is unknown.

VENTOLIN NEBULES INHALATION SOLUTION, 0.083%

In vitro studies and *in vivo* pharmacologic studies have demonstrated that albuterol has a preferential effect on beta$_2$-adrenergic receptors compared with isoproterenol. While it is recognized that beta$_2$-adrenergic receptors are the predominant receptors in bronchial smooth muscle, data indicate that 10-50% of the beta-receptors in the human heart may be beta$_2$-receptors. The precise function of these receptors has not been established.

The pharmacologic effects of beta-adrenergic agonist drugs, including albuterol, are at least in part attributable to stimulation through beta-adrenergic receptors of intracellular adenyl cyclase, the enzyme that catalyzes the conversion of adenosine triphosphate (ATP) to cyclic-3′,5′-adenosine monophosphate (cyclic AMP). Increased cyclic AMP levels are associated with relaxation of bronchial smooth muscle and inhibition of release of mediators of immediate hypersensitivity from cells, especially from mast cells.

Albuterol has been shown in most controlled clinical trials to have more effect on the respiratory tract, in the form of bronchial smooth muscle relaxation, than isoproterenol at comparable doses while producing fewer cardiovascular effects.

Controlled clinical studies and other clinical experience have shown that inhaled albuterol, like other beta-adrenergic agonist drugs, can produce a significant cardiovascular effect in some patients, as measured by pulse rate, blood pressure, symptoms, and/or electrocardiographic changes.

Albuterol is longer acting than isoproterenol in most patients by any route of administration because it is not a substrate for the cellular uptake processes for catecholamines nor for catechol-*O*-methyl transferase.

Pharmacokinetics

Studies in patients with asthma have shown that less than 20% of a single albuterol dose was absorbed following either IPPB (intermittent positive-pressure breathing) or nebulizer administration; the remaining amount was recovered from the nebulizer and apparatus and expired air. Most of the absorbed dose was recovered in the urine 24 hours after drug administration. Following a 3 mg dose of nebulized albuterol in adults, the maximum albuterol plasma levels at 0.5 hours were 2.1 ng/ml (range, 1.4-3.2 ng/ml). There was a significant dose-related response in FEV_1 (forced expiratory volume in 1 second) and peak flow rate. It has been demonstrated that following oral administration of 4 mg of albuterol, the elimination half-life was 5-6 hours.

Preclinical

Intravenous (IV) studies in rats with albuterol sulfate have demonstrated that albuterol crosses the blood-brain barrier and reaches brain concentrations amounting to approximately 5.0% of the plasma concentrations. In structures outside the brain barrier (pineal and pituitary glands), albuterol concentrations were found to be 100 times those in the whole brain.

Studies in laboratory animals (minipigs, rodents, and dogs) have demonstrated the occurrence of cardiac arrhythmias and sudden death (with histologic evidence of myocardial necrosis) when beta-agonists and methylxanthines are administered concurrently. The clinical significance of these findings is unknown.

VENTOLIN ROTACAPS FOR INHALATION

In vitro studies and *in vivo* pharmacologic studies have demonstrated that albuterol has a preferential effect on $beta_2$-adrenergic receptors compared with isoproterenol. While it is recognized that $beta_2$-adrenergic receptors are the predominant receptors in bronchial smooth muscle, data indicate that there is a population of $beta_2$-receptors in the human heart existing in a concentration between 10 and 50%. The precise function of these receptors has not been established (see WARNINGS).

The pharmacologic effects of beta-adrenergic agonist drugs, including albuterol, are at least in part attributable to stimulation through beta-adrenergic receptors of intracellular adenyl cyclase, the enzyme that catalyzes the conversion of adenosine triphosphate (ATP) to cyclic-3′,5′-adenosine monophosphate (cyclic AMP). Increased cyclic AMP levels are associated with relaxation of bronchial smooth muscle and inhibition of release of mediators of immediate hypersensitivity from cells, especially from mast cells.

Albuterol has been shown in most controlled clinical trials to have more effect on the respiratory tract, in the form of bronchial smooth muscle relaxation, than isoproterenol at comparable doses while producing fewer cardiovascular effects. Controlled clinical studies and other clinical experience have shown that inhaled albuterol, like other beta-adrenergic agonist drugs, can produce a significant cardiovascular effect in some patients, as measured by pulse rate, blood pressure, symptoms, and/or electrocardiographic changes.

Albuterol is longer acting than isoproterenol in most patients by any route of administration because it is not a substrate for the normal cellular uptake processes for catecholamines nor for catechol-*O*-methyl transferase.

Pharmacokinetics

Studies undertaken with 4 subjects administered tritiated albuterol from a metered-dose aerosol inhaler resulted in maximum plasma concentrations occurring within 2-4 hours. Due to the sensitivity of the assay method, the metabolic rate and half-life elimination of albuterol in plasma could not be determined. However, urinary excretion provided data indicating that albuterol has an elimination half-life of 3.8 hours. Approximately 72% of the inhaled dose is excreted within 24 hours in the urine, and consists of 28% as unchanged drug and 44% as metabolite.

Preclinical

Intravenous (IV) studies in rats with albuterol sulfate have demonstrated that albuterol crosses the blood-brain barrier and reaches brain concentrations amounting to approximately 5.0% of the plasma concentrations. In structures outside the brain barrier (pineal and pituitary glands), albuterol concentrations were found to be 100 times those in the whole brain.

Studies in laboratory animals (minipigs, rodents, and dogs) have demonstrated the occurrence of cardiac arrhythmias and sudden death (with histologic evidence of myocardial necrosis) when beta-agonists and methylxanthines are administered concurrently. The clinical significance of these findings is unknown.

INDICATIONS AND USAGE

VENTOLIN INHALATION AEROSOL

Ventolin inhalation aerosol is indicated for the prevention and relief of bronchospasm in patients 4 years of age and older with reversible obstructive airway disease and for the prevention of exercise-induced bronchospasm in patients 4 years of age and older.

Ventolin inhalation aerosol can be used with or without concomitant steroid therapy.

VENTOLIN HFA INHALATION AEROSOL

Ventolin HFA is indicated for the treatment or prevention of bronchospasm in adults and children 4 years of age and older with reversible obstructive airway disease and for the prevention of exercise-induced bronchospasm in patients 4 years of age and older.

VENTOLIN INHALATION SOLUTION, 0.5%

Ventolin inhalation solution is indicated for the relief of bronchospasm in patients 2 years of age and older with reversible obstructive airway disease and acute attacks of bronchospasm.

VENTOLIN NEBULES INHALATION SOLUTION, 0.083%

Ventolin Nebules inhalation solution is indicated for the relief of bronchospasm in patients 2 years of age and older with reversible obstructive airway disease and acute attacks of bronchospasm.

VENTOLIN ROTACAPS FOR INHALATION

Ventolin Rotacaps for inhalation are indicated for the prevention and relief of bronchospasm in patients 4 years of age and older with reversible obstructive airway disease and for the prevention of exercise-induced bronchospasm in patients 4 years of age and older. The Ventolin Rotacaps for inhalation formulation is particularly useful in patients who are unable to properly use the pressurized aerosol form of albuterol or who prefer an alternative formulation. Ventolin Rotacaps for inhalation can be used with or without concomitant steroid therapy.

CONTRAINDICATIONS

VENTOLIN INHALATION AEROSOL

Ventolin inhalation aerosol is contraindicated in patients with a history of hypersensitivity to albuterol or any of its components.

VENTOLIN HFA INHALATION AEROSOL

Ventolin HFA is contraindicated in patients with a history of hypersensitivity to albuterol or any other components of Ventolin HFA.

VENTOLIN INHALATION SOLUTION, 0.5%

Ventolin inhalation solution is contraindicated in patients with a history of hypersensitivity to albuterol or any of its components.

VENTOLIN NEBULES INHALATION SOLUTION, 0.083%

Ventolin Nebules inhalation solution is contraindicated in patients with a history of hypersensitivity to albuterol or any of its components.

VENTOLIN ROTACAPS FOR INHALATION

Ventolin Rotacaps for inhalation are contraindicated in patients with a history of hypersensitivity to albuterol or any of its components.

WARNINGS

VENTOLIN INHALATION AEROSOL

Paradoxical Bronchospasm

Ventolin inhalation aerosol can produce paradoxical bronchospasm, which may be life threatening. If paradoxical bronchospasm occurs, Ventolin inhalation aerosol should be discontinued immediately and alternative therapy instituted. It should be recognized that paradoxical bronchospasm, when associated with inhaled formulations, frequently occurs with the first use of a new canister or vial.

Cardiovascular Effects

Ventolin inhalation aerosol, like all other beta-adrenergic agonists, can produce a clinically significant cardiovascular effect in some patients as measured by pulse rate, blood pressure, and/or symptoms. Although such effects are uncommon after administration of Ventolin inhalation aerosol at recommended doses, if they occur, the drug may need to be discontinued. In addition, beta-agonists have been reported to produce electrocardiogram (ECG) changes, such as flattening of the T wave, prolongation of the QTc interval, and ST segment depression. The clinical significance of these findings is unknown. Therefore, Ventolin inhalation aerosol, like all sympathomimetic amines, should be used with caution in patients with cardiovascular disorders, especially coronary insufficiency, cardiac arrhythmias, and hypertension.

Deterioration of Asthma

Asthma may deteriorate acutely over a period of hours or chronically over several days or longer. If the patient needs more doses of Ventolin inhalation aerosol than usual, this may be a marker of destabilization of asthma and requires reevaluation of the patient and treatment regimen, giving special consideration to the possible need for anti-inflammatory treatment, *e.g.*, corticosteroids.

Use of Anti-Inflammatory Agents

The use of beta-adrenergic agonist bronchodilators alone may not be adequate to control asthma in many patients. Early consideration should be given to adding anti-inflammatory agents, *e.g.*, corticosteroids.

Immediate Hypersensitivity Reactions

Immediate hypersensitivity reactions may occur after administration of albuterol inhalation aerosol, as demonstrated by rare cases of urticaria, angioedema, rash, bronchospasm, anaphylaxis, and oropharyngeal edema.

The contents of Ventolin inhalation aerosol are under pressure. Do not puncture. Do not use or store near heat or open flame. Exposure to temperatures above 120°F may cause bursting. Never throw container into fire or incinerator. Keep out of reach of children.

VENTOLIN HFA INHALATION AEROSOL

Paradoxical Bronchospasm

Inhaled albuterol sulfate can produce paradoxical bronchospasm, which may be life threatening. If paradoxical bronchospasm occurs, Ventolin HFA should be discontinued immediately and alternative therapy instituted. It should be recognized that paradoxical bronchospasm, when associated with inhaled formulations, frequently occurs with the first use of a new canister.

Cardiovascular Effects

Ventolin HFA, like all other beta-adrenergic agonists, can produce clinically significant cardiovascular effects in some patients as measured by pulse rate, blood pressure, and/or symptoms. Although such effects are uncommon after administration of Ventolin HFA at recommended doses, if they occur, the drug may need to be discontinued. In addition, beta-agonists have been reported to produce electrocardiogram (ECG) changes, such as flattening of the T wave, prolongation of the QTc interval, and ST segment depression. The clinical significance of these findings is unknown. Therefore, Ventolin HFA, like all sympathomimetic amines, should be used with caution in patients with cardiovascular disorders, especially coronary insufficiency, cardiac arrhythmias, and hypertension.

Deterioration of Asthma

Asthma may deteriorate acutely over a period of hours or chronically over several days or longer. If the patient needs more doses of Ventolin HFA than usual, this may be a marker of destabilization of asthma and requires reevaluation of the patient and treatment regimen, giving special consideration to the possible need for anti-inflammatory treatment, *e.g.*, corticosteroids.

Use of Anti-Inflammatory Agents
The use of beta-adrenergic agonist bronchodilators alone may not be adequate to control asthma in many patients. Early consideration should be given to adding anti-inflammatory agents, *e.g.*, corticosteroids, to the therapeutic regimen.

Immediate Hypersensitivity Reactions
Immediate hypersensitivity reactions may occur after administration of albuterol sulfate inhalation aerosol, as demonstrated by cases of urticaria, angioedema, rash, bronchospasm, anaphylaxis, and oropharyngeal edema.

Do Not Exceed Recommended Dose
Fatalities have been reported in association with excessive use of inhaled sympathomimetic drugs in patients with asthma. The exact cause of death is unknown, but cardiac arrest following an unexpected development of a severe acute asthmatic crisis and subsequent hypoxia is suspected.

VENTOLIN INHALATION SOLUTION, 0.5%
Paradoxical Bronchospasm
Ventolin inhalation solution can produce paradoxical bronchospasm, which may be life threatening. If paradoxical bronchospasm occurs, Ventolin inhalation solution should be discontinued immediately and alternative therapy instituted. It should be recognized that paradoxical bronchospasm, when associated with inhaled formulations, frequently occurs with the first use of a new canister or vial.

Fatalities have been reported in association with excessive use of inhaled sympathomimetic drugs and with the home use of nebulizers. It is therefore essential that the physician instruct the patient in the need for further evaluation if his/her asthma becomes worse.

Cardiovascular Effects
Ventolin inhalation solution, like all other beta-adrenergic agonists, can produce a clinically significant cardiovascular effect in some patients as measured by pulse rate, blood pressure, and/or symptoms. Although such effects are uncommon after administration of Ventolin inhalation solution at recommended doses, if they occur, the drug may need to be discontinued. In addition, beta-agonists have been reported to produce electrocardiogram (ECG) changes, such as flattening of the T wave, prolongation of the QTc interval, and ST segment depression. The clinical significance of these findings is unknown. Therefore, Ventolin inhalation solution, like all sympathomimetic amines, should be used with caution in patients with cardiovascular disorders, especially coronary insufficiency, cardiac arrhythmias, and hypertension.

Deterioration of Asthma
Asthma may deteriorate acutely over a period of hours or chronically over several days or longer. If the patient needs more doses of Ventolin inhalation solution than usual, this may be a marker of destabilization of asthma and requires reevaluation of the patient and treatment regimen, giving special consideration to the possible need for anti-inflammatory treatment, *e.g.*, corticosteroids.

Immediate Hypersensitivity Reactions
Immediate hypersensitivity reactions may occur after administration of albuterol, as demonstrated by rare cases of urticaria, angioedema, rash, bronchospasm, and oropharyngeal edema.

Use of Anti-Inflammatory Agents
The use of beta-adrenergic agonist bronchodilators alone may not be adequate to control asthma in many patients. Early consideration should be given to adding anti-inflammatory agents, *e.g.*, corticosteroids.

Microbial Contamination
To avoid microbial contamination, proper aseptic technique should be used each time the bottle is opened. Precautions should be taken to prevent contact of the dropper tip of the bottle with any surface, including the nebulizer reservoir and associated ventilatory equipment. In addition, if the solution changes color or becomes cloudy, it should not be used.

VENTOLIN NEBULES INHALATION SOLUTION, 0.083%
Paradoxical Bronchospasm
Ventolin Nebules inhalation solution can produce paradoxical bronchospasm, which may be life threatening. If paradoxical bronchospasm occurs, Ventolin Nebules inhalation solution should be discontinued immediately and alternative therapy instituted. It should be recognized that paradoxical bronchospasm, when associated with inhaled formulations, frequently occurs with the first use of a new canister or vial.

Cardiovascular Effects
Ventolin Nebules inhalation solution, like all other beta-adrenergic agonists, can produce a clinically significant cardiovascular effect in some patients as measured by pulse rate, blood pressure, and/or symptoms. Although such effects are uncommon after administration of Ventolin Nebules inhalation solution at recommended doses, if they occur, the drug may need to be discontinued. In addition, beta-agonists have been reported to produce electrocardiogram (ECG) changes, such as flattening of the T wave, prolongation of the QTc interval, and ST segment depression. The clinical significance of these findings is unknown. Therefore, Ventolin Nebules inhalation solution, like all sympathomimetic amines, should be used with caution in patients with cardiovascular disorders, especially coronary insufficiency, cardiac arrhythmias, and hypertension.

Deterioration of Asthma
Asthma may deteriorate acutely over a period of hours or chronically over several days or longer. If the patient needs more doses of Ventolin Nebules inhalation solution than usual, this may be a marker of destabilization of asthma and requires reevaluation of the patient and treatment regimen, giving special consideration to the possible need for anti-inflammatory treatment, *e.g.*, corticosteroids.

Immediate Hypersensitivity Reactions
Immediate hypersensitivity reactions may occur after administration of albuterol, as demonstrated by rare cases of urticaria, angioedema, rash, bronchospasm, and oropharyngeal edema.

Use of Anti-Inflammatory Agents
The use of beta-adrenergic agonist bronchodilators alone may not be adequate to control asthma in many patients. Early consideration should be given to adding anti-inflammatory agents, *e.g.*, corticosteroids.

VENTOLIN ROTACAPS FOR INHALATION
Paradoxical Bronchospasm
Ventolin Rotacaps for inhalation can produce paradoxical bronchospasm, which may be life threatening. If paradoxical bronchospasm occurs, Ventolin Rotacaps for inhalation should be discontinued immediately and alternative therapy instituted.

Cardiovascular Effects
Ventolin Rotacaps for inhalation, like all other beta-adrenergic agonists, can produce a clinically significant cardiovascular effect in some patients as measured by pulse rate, blood pressure, and/or symptoms. Although such effects are uncommon after administration of Ventolin Rotacaps for inhalation at recommended doses, if they occur, the drug may need to be discontinued. In addition, beta-agonists have been reported to produce electrocardiogram (ECG) changes, such as flattening of the T wave, prolongation of the QTc interval, and ST segment depression. The clinical significance of these findings is unknown. Therefore, Ventolin Rotacaps for inhalation, like all sympathomimetic amines, should be used with caution in patients with cardiovascular disorders, especially coronary insufficiency, cardiac arrhythmias, and hypertension.

Deterioration of Asthma
Asthma may deteriorate acutely over a period of hours or chronically over several days or longer. If the patient needs more doses of Ventolin Rotacaps for inhalation than usual, this may be a marker of destabilization of asthma and requires reevaluation of the patient and treatment regimen, giving special consideration to the possible need for anti-inflammatory treatment, *e.g.*, corticosteroids.

Immediate Hypersensitivity Reactions
Immediate hypersensitivity reactions may occur after administration of albuterol, as demonstrated by rare cases of urticaria, angioedema, rash, bronchospasm, anaphylaxis, and oropharyngeal edema.

Use of Anti-Inflammatory Agents
The use of beta-adrenergic agonist bronchodilators alone may not be adequate to control asthma in many patients. Early consideration should be given to adding anti-inflammatory agents, *e.g.*, corticosteroids.

Inhalation of capsule particles may result if damage to the capsule has occurred from handling by the patient.

PRECAUTIONS

VENTOLIN INHALATION AEROSOL
General
Albuterol, as with all sympathomimetic amines, should be used with caution in patients with cardiovascular disorders, especially coronary insufficiency, cardiac arrhythmias, and hypertension; in patients with convulsive disorders, hyperthyroidism, or diabetes mellitus; and in patients who are unusually responsive to sympathomimetic amines. Clinically significant changes in systolic and diastolic blood pressure have been seen in individual patients and could be expected to occur in some patients after use of any beta-adrenergic bronchodilator.

Large doses of IV albuterol have been reported to aggravate preexisting diabetes mellitus and ketoacidosis. As with other beta-agonists, albuterol may produce significant hypokalemia in some patients, possibly through intracellular shunting, which has the potential to produce adverse cardiovascular effects. The decrease is usually transient, not requiring supplementation.

Although there have been no reports concerning the use of Ventolin inhalation aerosol during labor and delivery, it has been reported that high doses of albuterol administered intravenously inhibit uterine contractions. Although this effect is extremely unlikely as a consequence of aerosol use, it should be kept in mind.

Information for the Patient
The action of Ventolin inhalation aerosol may last up to 6 hours or longer. Ventolin inhalation aerosol should not be used more frequently than recommended. Do not increase the dose or frequency of Ventolin inhalation aerosol without consulting your physician. If you find that treatment with Ventolin inhalation aerosol becomes less effective for symptomatic relief, your symptoms become worse, and/or you need to use the product more frequently than usual, you should seek medical attention immediately. While you are using Ventolin inhalation aerosol, other inhaled drugs and asthma medications should be taken only as directed by your physician. Common adverse effects include palpitations, chest pain, rapid heart rate, and tremor or nervousness. If you are pregnant or nursing, contact your physician about use of Ventolin inhalation aerosol. Effective and safe use of Ventolin inhalation aerosol includes an understanding of the way that it should be administered.

In general, the technique for administering Ventolin inhalation aerosol to children is similar to that for adults, since children's smaller ventilatory exchange capacity automatically provides proportionally smaller aerosol intake. Children should use Ventolin inhalation aerosol under adult supervision, as instructed by the patient's physician.

See illustrated Patient's Instructions for Use distributed with the prescription.

Carcinogenesis, Mutagenesis, and Impairment of Fertility
In a 2 year study in Sprague-Dawley rats, albuterol sulfate caused a significant dose-related increase in the incidence of benign leiomyomas of the mesovarium at dietary doses of 2.0,

10, and 50 mg/kg (approximately 15, 70, and 340 times, respectively, the maximum recommended daily inhalation dose for adults on a mg/m^2 basis or approximately 6, 30, and 160 times, respectively, the maximum recommended daily inhalation dose for children on a mg/m^2 basis). In another study this effect was blocked by the coadministration of propranolol, a non-selective beta-adrenergic antagonist. In an 18 month study in CD-1 mice albuterol sulfate showed no evidence of tumorigenicity at dietary doses of up to 500 mg/kg (approximately 1700 times the maximum recommended daily inhalation dose for adults on a mg/m^2 basis or approximately 800 times the maximum recommended daily inhalation dose for children on a mg/m^2 basis). In a 22 month study in the Golden hamster, albuterol sulfate showed no evidence of tumorigenicity at dietary doses of up to 50 mg/kg (approximately 225 times the maximum recommended daily inhalation dose for adults on a mg/m^2 basis or approximately 110 times the maximum recommended daily inhalation dose for children on a mg/m^2 basis).

Albuterol sulfate was not mutagenic in the Ames test with or without metabolic activation using tester strains *S. typhimurium* TA1537, TA1538, and TA98 or *E. coli* WP2, WP2uvrA, and WP67. No forward mutation was seen in yeast strain *S. cerevisiae* S9 nor any mitotic gene conversion in yeast strain *S. cerevisiae* JD1 with or without metabolic activation. Fluctuation assays in *S. typhimurium* TA98 and *E. coli* WP2, both with metabolic activation, were negative. Albuterol sulfate was not clastogenic in a human peripheral lymphocyte assay or in an AH1 strain mouse micronucleus assay at intraperitoneal doses of up to 200 mg/kg.

Reproduction studies in rats demonstrated no evidence of impaired fertility at oral doses up to 50 mg/kg (approximately 340 times the maximum recommended daily inhalation dose for adults on a mg/m^2 basis).

Pregnancy, Teratogenic Effects, Pregnancy Category C

Albuterol sulfate has been shown to be teratogenic in mice. A study in CD-1 mice at subcutaneous doses of 0.025, 0.25, and 2.5 mg/kg (approximately 2/25, 1.0, and 8.0 times, respectively, the maximum recommended daily inhalation dose for adults on a mg/m^2 basis), showed cleft palate formation in 5 of 111 (4.5%) fetuses at 0.25 mg/kg and in 10 of 108 (9.3%) fetuses at 2.5 mg/kg. The drug did not induce cleft palate formation at the lowest dose, 0.025 mg/kg. Cleft palate also occurred in 22 of 72 (30.5%) fetuses from females treated with 2.5 mg/kg of isoproterenol (positive control) subcutaneous (approximately 8 times the maximum recommended daily inhalation dose for adults on a mg/m^2 basis).

A reproduction study in Stride Dutch rabbits revealed cranioschisis in 7 of 19 (37%) fetuses when albuterol sulfate was administered orally at a 50 mg/kg dose (approximately 680 times the maximum recommended daily inhalation dose for adults on a mg/m^2 basis).

There are no adequate and well-controlled studies in pregnant women. Albuterol should be used during pregnancy only if the potential benefit justifies the potential risk to the fetus.

During worldwide marketing experience, various congenital anomalies, including cleft palate and limb defects, have been rarely reported in the offspring of patients being treated with albuterol. Some of the mothers were taking multiple medications during their pregnancies. No consistent pattern of defects can be discerned, and a relationship between albuterol use and congenital anomalies has not been established.

Use in Labor and Delivery

Because of the potential for beta-agonist interference with uterine contractility, use of Ventolin inhalation aerosol for relief of bronchospasm during labor should be restricted to those patients in whom the benefits clearly outweigh the risk.

Tocolysis

Albuterol has not been approved for the management of preterm labor. The benefit:risk ratio when albuterol is administered for tocolysis has not been established. Serious adverse reactions, including maternal pulmonary edema, have been reported during or following treatment of premature labor with beta$_2$-agonists, including albuterol.

Nursing Mothers

It is not known whether this drug is excreted in human milk. Because of the potential for tumorigenicity shown for albuterol in some animal studies, a decision should be made whether to discontinue nursing or to discontinue the drug, taking into account the importance of the drug to the mother.

Pediatric Use

Safety and effectiveness in children below 4 years of age have not been established.

Geriatric Use

Clinical studies of Venolin inhalation aerosol did not include sufficient numbers of subjects aged 65 and over to determine whether they respond differently from younger subjects. Other reported clinical experience has not identified differences in responses between the elderly and younger patients. In general, dose selection for an elderly patient should be cautious, starting at the low end of the dosing range, reflecting the greater frequency of decreased hepatic, renal, or cardiac function, and of concomitant disease or other drug therapy.

VENTOLIN HFA INHALATION AEROSOL

General

Albuterol sulfate, as with all sympathomimetic amines, should be used with caution in patients with cardiovascular disorders, especially coronary insufficiency, hypertension, and cardiac arrhythmia; in patients with convulsive disorders, hyperthyroidism, or diabetes mellitus; and in patients who are unusually responsive to sympathomimetic amines. Clinically significant changes in systolic and diastolic blood pressure have been seen in individual patients and could be expected to occur in some patients after use of any beta-adrenergic bronchodilator.

Large doses of IV albuterol have been reported to aggravate preexisting diabetes mellitus and ketoacidosis. As with other beta-agonists, albuterol may produce significant hypokalemia in some patients, possibly through intracellular shunting, which has the potential to produce adverse cardiovascular effects. The decrease is usually transient, not requiring supplementation.

Information for the Patient

See illustrated Patient's Instructions for Use distributed with the prescription. SHAKE WELL BEFORE USING.

Patients should be given the following information:

It is recommended to prime the inhaler before using for the first time and in cases where the inhaler has not been used for more than 2 weeks by releasing 4 test sprays into the air, away from the face.

KEEPING THE PLASTIC ACTUATOR CLEAN IS VERY IMPORTANT TO PREVENT MEDICATION BUILD-UP AND BLOCKAGE. THE ACTUATOR SHOULD BE WASHED, SHAKEN TO REMOVE EXCESS WATER, AND AIR-DRIED THOROUGHLY AT LEAST ONCE A WEEK. THE INHALER MAY CEASE TO DELIVER MEDICATION IF NOT PROPERLY CLEANED.

The actuator should be cleaned (with the canister removed) by running warm water through the top and bottom for 30 seconds at least once a week. Do not attempt to clean the metal canister or allow the metal canister to become wet. Never immerse the metal canister in water. The actuator must be shaken to remove excess water, then air-dried thoroughly (such as overnight). Blockage from medication build-up or improper medication delivery may result from failure to clean and thoroughly air-dry the actuator.

If the actuator should become blocked (little or no medication coming out of the mouthpiece), the blockage may be removed by washing the actuator as described above.

If it is necessary to use the inhaler before it is completely dry, shake excess water off the plastic actuator, replace canister, shake well, test spray twice away from face, and take the prescribed dose. After such use, the actuator should be rewashed and allowed to air-dry thoroughly.

The action of Ventolin HFA should last up to 4-6 hours. Ventolin HFA should not be used more frequently than recommended. Do not increase the dose or frequency of doses of Ventolin HFA without consulting your physician. If you find that treatment with Ventolin HFA becomes less effective for symptomatic relief, your symptoms become worse, and/or you need to use the product more frequently than usual, you should seek medical attention immediately. While you are using Ventolin HFA, other inhaled drugs and asthma medications should be taken only as directed by your physician.

Common adverse effects of treatment with inhaled albuterol include palpitations, chest pain, rapid heart rate, tremor, and nervousness. If you are pregnant or nursing, contact your physician about use of Ventolin HFA. Effective and safe use of Ventolin HFA includes an understanding of the way that it should be administered.

Use Ventolin HFA only with the actuator supplied with the product. Discard the canister after 200 sprays have been used or 3 months after removal from the moisture-protective foil pouch, whichever comes first. Never immerse the canister into water to determine how full the canister is ("float test").

In general, the technique for administering Ventolin HFA to children is similar to that for adults. Children should use Ventolin HFA under adult supervision, as instructed by the patient's physician. (See Patient's Instructions for Use distributed with the prescription.)

Carcinogenesis, Mutagenesis, and Impairment of Fertility

In a 2 year study in Sprague-Dawley rats, albuterol sulfate caused a dose-related increase in the incidence of benign leiomyomas of the mesovarium at and above dietary doses of 2.0 mg/kg (approximately 14 times the maximum recommended daily inhalation dose for adults on a mg/m^2 basis and approximately 6 times the maximum recommended daily inhalation dose for children on a mg/m^2 basis). In another study this effect was blocked by the coadministration of propranolol, a non-selective beta-adrenergic antagonist. In an 18 month study in CD-1 mice, albuterol sulfate showed no evidence of tumorigenicity at dietary doses of up to 500 mg/kg (approximately 1700 times the maximum recommended daily inhalation dose for adults on a mg/m^2 basis and approximately 800 times the maximum recommended daily inhalation dose for children on a mg/m^2 basis). In a 22 month study in Golden hamsters, albuterol sulfate showed no evidence of tumorigenicity at dietary doses of up to 50 mg/kg (approximately 225 times the maximum recommended daily inhalation dose for adults on a mg/m^2 basis and approximately 110 times the maximum recommended daily inhalation dose for children on a mg/m^2 basis).

Albuterol sulfate was not mutagenic in the Ames test or a mutation test in yeast. Albuterol sulfate was not clastogenic in a human peripheral lymphocyte assay or in an AH1 strain mouse micronucleus assay.

Reproduction studies in rats demonstrated no evidence of impaired fertility at oral doses of albuterol sulfate up to 50 mg/kg (approximately 340 times the maximum recommended daily inhalation dose for adults on a mg/m^2 basis).

Pregnancy, Teratogenic Effects, Pregnancy Category C

Albuterol sulfate has been shown to be teratogenic in mice. A study in CD-1 mice given albuterol sulfate subcutaneously showed cleft palate formation in 5 of 111 (4.5%) fetuses at 0.25 mg/kg (less than the maximum recommended daily inhalation dose for adults on a mg/m^2 basis) and in 10 of 108 (9.3%) fetuses at 2.5 mg/kg (approximately 8 times the maximum recommended daily inhalation dose for adults on a mg/m^2 basis). The drug did not induce cleft palate formation at a dose of 0.025 mg/kg (less than the maximum recommended daily inhalation dose for adults on a mg/m^2 basis). Cleft palate also occurred in 22 of 72 (30.5%) fetuses from females treated subcutaneously with 2.5 mg/kg of isoproterenol (positive control).

A reproduction study in Stride Dutch rabbits revealed cranioschisis in 7 of 19 fetuses (37%) when albuterol sulfate was administered orally at a 50 mg/kg dose (approximately 680 times the maximum recommended daily inhalation dose for adults on a mg/m^2 basis).

In an inhalation reproduction study in New Zealand white rabbits, albuterol sulfate/HFA-134a formulation exhibited enlargement of the frontal portion of the fetal fontanelles at and above inhalation doses of 0.0193 mg/kg (less than the maximum recommended daily inhalation dose for adults on a mg/m^2 basis).

A study in which pregnant rats were dosed with radiolabeled albuterol sulfate demonstrated that drug-related material is transferred from the maternal circulation to the fetus.

There are no adequate and well-controlled studies of Ventolin HFA or albuterol sulfate in pregnant women. Ventolin HFA should be used during pregnancy only if the potential benefit justifies the potential risk to the fetus.

During worldwide marketing experience, various congenital anomalies, including cleft palate and limb defects, have been reported in the offspring of patients being treated with albuterol. Some of the mothers were taking multiple medications during their pregnancies. No consistent pattern of defects can be discerned, and a relationship between albuterol use and congenital anomalies has not been established.

Use in Labor and Delivery

Because of the potential for beta-agonist interference with uterine contractility, use of Ventolin HFA for relief of bronchospasm during labor should be restricted to those patients in whom the benefits clearly outweigh the risk.

Tocolysis

Albuterol has not been approved for the management of preterm labor. The benefit:risk ratio when albuterol is administered for tocolysis has not been established. Serious adverse reactions, including maternal pulmonary edema, have been reported during or following treatment of premature labor with $beta_2$-agonists, including albuterol.

Nursing Mothers

Plasma levels of albuterol sulfate and HFA-134a after inhaled therapeutic doses are very low in humans, but it is not known whether the components of Ventolin HFA are excreted in human milk. Because of the potential for tumorigenicity shown for albuterol in animal studies and lack of experience with the use of Ventolin HFA by nursing mothers, a decision should be made whether to discontinue nursing or to discontinue the drug, taking into account the importance of the drug to the mother. Caution should be exercised when albuterol sulfate is administered to a nursing woman.

Pediatric Use

Results from a 2 week, randomized study in pediatric patients 4-11 years old with mild to moderate asthma have shown that Ventolin HFA is safe and effective in this population. Safety and effectiveness in children below 4 years of age have not been established.

Geriatrics

Clinical studies of Ventolin HFA did not include sufficient numbers of subjects aged 65 and over to determine whether they respond differently from younger subjects. Other reported clinical experience has not identified differences in responses between the elderly and younger patients. In general, dose selection for an elderly patient should be cautious, usually starting at the low end of the dosing range, reflecting the greater frequency of decreased hepatic, renal, or cardiac function, and of concomitant disease or other drug therapy.

VENTOLIN INHALATION SOLUTION, 0.5%

General

Albuterol, as with all sympathomimetic amines, should be used with caution in patients with cardiovascular disorders, especially coronary insufficiency, hypertension, and cardiac arrhythmia; in patients with convulsive disorders, hyperthyroidism, or diabetes mellitus; and in patients who are unusually responsive to sympathomimetic amines. Clinically significant changes in systolic and diastolic blood pressure have been seen in individual patients and could be expected to occur in some patients after use of any beta-adrenergic bronchodilator.

Large doses of IV albuterol have been reported to aggravate preexisting diabetes mellitus and ketoacidosis. As with other beta-agonists, albuterol may produce significant hypokalemia in some patients, possibly through intracellular shunting, which has the potential to produce adverse cardiovascular effects. The decrease is usually transient, not requiring supplementation.

Repeated dosing with 0.15 mg/kg of albuterol inhalation solution in children aged 5-17 years who were initially normokalemic has been associated with an asymptomatic decline of 20-25% in serum potassium levels.

Information for the Patient

The action of Ventolin inhalation solution may last up to 6 hours or longer. Ventolin inhalation solution should not be used more frequently than recommended. Do not increase the dose or frequency of Ventolin inhalation solution without consulting your physician. If you find that treatment with Ventolin inhalation solution becomes less effective for symptomatic relief, your symptoms become worse, and/or you need to use the product more frequently than usual, you should seek medical attention immediately. While you are using Ventolin inhalation solution, other inhaled drugs and asthma medications should be taken only as directed by your physician. Common adverse effects include palpitations, chest pain, rapid heart rate, and tremor or nervousness. If you are pregnant or nursing, contact your physician about use of Ventolin inhalation solution. Effective and safe use of Ventolin inhalation solution includes an understanding of the way that it should be administered.

To avoid microbial contamination, proper aseptic techniques should be used each time the bottle is opened. Precautions should be taken to prevent contact of the dropper tip of the bottle with any surface, including the nebulizer reservoir and associated ventilatory equipment. In addition, if the solution changes color or becomes cloudy, it should not be used.

Drug compatibility (physical and chemical), efficacy, and safety of Ventolin inhalation solution when mixed with other drugs in a nebulizer have not been established.

See illustrated Patient's Instructions for Use distributed with the prescription.

Carcinogenesis, Mutagenesis, and Impairment of Fertility

In a 2 year study in Sprague-Dawley rats, albuterol sulfate caused a significant dose-related increase in the incidence of benign leiomyomas of the mesovarium at dietary doses of 2.0, 10, and 50 mg/kg (approximately 2, 8, and 40 times, respectively, the maximum recommended daily inhalation dose for adults on a mg/m^2 basis or approximately 3/5, 3, and 15 times, respectively, the maximum recommended daily inhalation dose in children on a mg/m^2 basis). In another study this effect was blocked by the coadministration of propranolol, a non-selective beta-adrenergic antagonist. In an 18 month study in CD-1 mice, albuterol sulfate showed no evidence of tumorigenicity at dietary doses of up to 500 mg/kg (approximately 200 times the maximum recommended daily inhalation dose for adults on a mg/m^2 basis or approximately 75 times the maximum recommended daily inhalation dose for children on a mg/m^2 basis). In a 22 month study in the Golden hamster, albuterol sulfate showed no evidence of tumorigenicity at dietary doses of up to 50 mg/kg (approximately 25 times the maximum recommended daily inhalation dose for adults on a mg/m^2 basis or approximately 10 times the maximum recommended daily inhalation dose for children on a mg/m^2 basis).

Albuterol sulfate was not mutagenic in the Ames test with or without metabolic activation using tester strains *S. typhimurium* TA1537, TA1538, and TA98 or *E. coli* WP2, WP2uvrA, and WP67. No forward mutation was seen in yeast strain *S. cerevisiae* S9 nor any mitotic gene conversion in yeast strain *S. cerevisiae* JD1 with or without metabolic activation. Fluctuation assays in *S. typhimurium* TA98 and *E. coli* WP2, both with metabolic activation, were negative. Albuterol sulfate was not clastogenic in a human peripheral lymphocyte assay or in an AH1 strain mouse micronucleus assay at intraperitoneal doses of up to 200 mg/kg.

Reproduction studies in rats demonstrated no evidence of impaired fertility at oral doses up to 50 mg/kg (approximately 40 times the maximum recommended daily inhalation dose for adults on a mg/m^2 basis).

Pregnancy, Teratogenic Effects, Pregnancy Category C

Albuterol has been shown to be teratogenic in mice. A study in CD-1 mice at subcutaneous doses of 0.025, 0.25, and 2.5 mg/kg (approximately 1/100, 1/10, and 1.0 times, respectively, the maximum recommended daily inhalation dose for adults on a mg/m^2 basis) showed cleft palate formation in 5 of 111 (4.5%) fetuses at 0.25 mg/kg and in 10 of 108 (9.3%) fetuses at 2.5 mg/kg. The drug did not induce cleft palate formation at the lowest dose, 0.025 mg/kg. Cleft palate also occurred in 22 of 72 (30.5%) fetuses from females treated with 2.5 mg/kg of isoproterenol (positive control) subcutaneously (approximately 1.0 time the maximum recommended daily inhalation dose for adults on a mg/m^2 basis).

A reproduction study in Stride Dutch rabbits revealed cranioschisis in 7 of 19 (37%) fetuses when albuterol was administered orally at a 50 mg/kg dose (approximately 80 times the maximum recommended daily inhalation dose for adults on a mg/m^2 basis).

There are no adequate and well-controlled studies in pregnant women. Albuterol should be used during pregnancy only if the potential benefit justifies the potential risk to the fetus.

During worldwide marketing experience, various congenital anomalies, including cleft palate and limb defects, have been rarely reported in the offspring of patients being treated with albuterol. Some of the mothers were taking multiple medications during their pregnancies. No consistent pattern of defects can be discerned, and a relationship between albuterol use and congenital anomalies has not been established.

Use in Labor and Delivery

Because of the potential for beta-agonist interference with uterine contractility, use of Ventolin inhalation solution for relief of bronchospasm during labor should be restricted to those patients in whom the benefits clearly outweigh the risk.

Tocolysis

Albuterol has not been approved for the management of preterm labor. The benefit:risk ratio when albuterol is administered for tocolysis has not been established. Serious adverse reactions, including maternal pulmonary edema, have been reported during or following treatment of premature labor with $beta_2$-agonists, including albuterol.

Nursing Mothers

It is not known whether this drug is excreted in human milk. Because of the potential for tumorigenicity shown for albuterol in some animal studies, a decision should be made whether to discontinue nursing or to discontinue the drug, taking into account the importance of the drug to the mother.

Pediatric Use

The safety and effectiveness of Ventolin inhalation solution have been established in children 2 years of age and older. Use of Ventolin inhalation solution in these age-groups is supported by evidence from adequate and well-controlled studies of Ventolin inhalation solution in adults; the likelihood that the disease course, pathophysiology, and the drug's effect in pediatric and adult patients are substantially similar; and published reports of trials in pediatric patients 3 years of age or older. The recommended dose for the pediatric population is based upon three published dose comparison studies of efficacy and safety in children 5-17 years, and on the safety profile in both adults and pediatric patients at doses equal to or higher than the recommended doses. The safety and effectiveness of Ventolin inhalation solution in children below 2 years of age have not been established.

VENTOLIN NEBULES INHALATION SOLUTION, 0.083%

General

Albuterol, as with all sympathomimetic amines, should be used with caution in patients with cardiovascular disorders, especially coronary insufficiency, hypertension, and cardiac arrhythmia; in patients with convulsive disorders, hyperthyroidism, or diabetes mellitus; and in patients who are unusually responsive to sympathomimetic amines. Clinically significant changes in systolic and diastolic blood pressure have been seen in individual patients and could be expected to occur in some patients after use of any beta-adrenergic bronchodilator.

Large doses of IV albuterol have been reported to aggravate preexisting diabetes mellitus and ketoacidosis. As with other beta-agonists, albuterol may produce significant hypokalemia in some patients, possibly through intracellular shunting, which has the potential to produce adverse cardiovascular effects. The decrease is usually transient, not requiring supplementation.

Repeated dosing with 0.15 mg/kg of albuterol inhalation solution in children aged 5-17 years who were initially normokalemic has been associated with an asymptomatic decline of 20-25% in serum potassium levels.

Information for the Patient

The action of Ventolin Nebules inhalation solution may last up to 6 hours or longer. Ventolin Nebules inhalation solution should not be used more frequently than recommended. Do not increase the dose or frequency of Ventolin Nebules inhalation solution without consulting your physician. If you find that treatment with Ventolin Nebules inhalation solution becomes less effective for symptomatic relief, your symptoms become worse, and/or you need to use the product more frequently than usual, you should seek medical attention immediately. While you are using Ventolin Nebules inhalation solution, other inhaled drugs and asthma medications should be taken only as directed by your physician. Common adverse effects include palpitations, chest pain, rapid heart rate, and tremor or nervousness. If you are pregnant or nursing, contact your physician about use of Ventolin Nebules inhalation solution. Effective and safe use of Ventolin Nebules inhalation solution includes an understanding of the way that it should be administered.

Drug compatibility (physical and chemical), efficacy, and safety of Ventolin Nebules inhalation solution when mixed with other drugs in a nebulizer have not been established.

See illustrated Patient's Instructions for Use distributed with the prescription.

Carcinogenesis, Mutagenesis, and Impairment of Fertility

In a 2 year study in Sprague-Dawley rats, albuterol sulfate caused a significant dose-related increase in the incidence of benign leiomyomas of the mesovarium at dietary doses of 2.0, 10, and 50 mg/kg (approximately 2, 8, and 40 times, respectively, the maximum recommended daily inhalation dose for adults on a mg/m^2 basis or approximately 3/5, 3, and 150 times, respectively, the maximum recommended daily inhalation dose in children on a mg/m^2 basis). In another study this effect was blocked by the coadministration of propranolol, a non-selective beta-adrenergic antagonist. In an 18 month study in CD-1 mice, albuterol sulfate showed no evidence of tumorigenicity at dietary doses up to 500 mg/kg (approximately 200 times the maximum recommended daily inhalation dose for adults on a mg/m^2 basis or approximately 75 times the maximum recommended daily inhalation dose for children on a mg/m^2 basis). In a 22 month study in the Golden hamster, albuterol sulfate showed no evidence of tumorigenicity at dietary doses up to 50 mg/kg (approximately 25 times the maximum recommended daily inhalation dose for adults on a mg/m^2 basis or approximately 10 times the maximum recommended daily inhalation dose for children on a mg/m^2 basis).

Albuterol sulfate was not mutagenic in the Ames test with or without metabolic activation using tester strains *S. typhimurium* TA1537, TA1538, and TA98 or *E. coli* WP2, WP2uvrA, and WP67. No forward mutation was seen in yeast strain *S. cerevisiae* S9 nor any mitotic gene conversion in yeast strain *S. cerevisiae* JD1 with or without metabolic activation. Fluctuation assays in *S. typhimurium* TA98 and *E. coli* WP2, both with metabolic activation, were negative. Albuterol sulfate was not clastogenic in a human peripheral lymphocyte assay or in an AH1 strain mouse micronucleus assay at intraperitoneal doses of up to 200 mg/kg.

Reproduction studies in rats demonstrated no evidence of impaired fertility at oral doses up to 50 mg/kg (approximately 40 times the maximum recommended daily inhalation dose for adults on a mg/m^2 basis).

Pregnancy, Teratogenic Effects, Pregnancy Category C

Albuterol has been shown to be teratogenic in mice. A study in CD-1 mice at subcutaneous doses of 0.025, 0.25, and 2.5 mg/kg (approximately 1/100, 1/10, and 1.0 times, respectively, the maximum recommended daily inhalation dose for adults on a mg/m^2 basis) showed cleft palate formation in 5 of 111 (4.5%) fetuses at 0.25 mg/kg and in 10 of 108 (9.3%) fetuses at 2.5 mg/kg. The drug did not induce cleft palate formation at the lowest dose, 0.025 mg/kg. Cleft palate also occurred in 22 of 72 (30.5%) fetuses from females treated with 2.5 mg/kg of isoproterenol (positive control) subcutaneously (approximately 1.0 time the maximum recommended daily inhalation dose for adults on a mg/m^2 basis).

A reproduction study in Stride Dutch rabbits revealed cranioschisis in 7 of 19 (37%) fetuses when albuterol was administered orally at a 50 mg/kg dose (approximately 80 times the maximum recommended daily inhalation dose for adults on a mg/m^2 basis).

There are no adequate and well-controlled studies in pregnant women. Albuterol should be used during pregnancy only if the potential benefit justifies the potential risk to the fetus.

During worldwide marketing experience, various congenital anomalies, including cleft palate and limb defects, have been rarely reported in the offspring of patients being treated with albuterol. Some of the mothers were taking multiple medications during their pregnancies. No consistent pattern of defects can be discerned, and a relationship between albuterol use and congenital anomalies has not been established.

Use in Labor and Delivery

Because of the potential for beta-agonist interference with uterine contractility, use of Ventolin Nebules inhalation solution for relief of bronchospasm during labor should be restricted to those patients in whom the benefits clearly outweigh the risk.

Tocolysis

Albuterol has not been approved for the management of preterm labor. The benefit:risk ratio when albuterol is administered for tocolysis has not been established. Serious adverse reactions, including maternal pulmonary edema, have been reported during or following treatment of premature labor with $beta_2$-agonists, including albuterol.

Nursing Mothers

It is not known whether this drug is excreted in human milk. Because of the potential for tumorigenicity shown for albuterol in some animal studies, a decision should be made whether to discontinue nursing or to discontinue the drug, taking into account the importance of the drug to the mother.

Pediatric Use

The safety and effectiveness of Ventolin Nebules inhalation solution have been established in children 2 years of age and older. Use of Ventolin Nebules inhalation solution in these age-groups is supported by evidence from adequate and well-controlled studies of Ventolin Nebules inhalation solution in adults; the likelihood that the disease course, pathophysiology, and the drug's effect in pediatric and adult patients are substantially similar; and published reports of trials in pediatric patients 3 years of age or older. The recommended dose for the pediatric population is based upon 3 published dose comparison studies of efficacy and safety in children 5-17 years, and on the safety profile in both adults and pediatric patients at doses equal to or higher than the recommended doses. The safety and effectiveness of Ventolin Nebules inhalation solution in children below 2 years of age have not been established.

VENTOLIN ROTACAPS FOR INHALATION

General

Albuterol, as with all sympathomimetic amines, should be used with caution in patients with cardiovascular disorders, especially coronary insufficiency, hypertension, and cardiac arrhythmia; in patients with convulsive disorders, hyperthyroidism, or diabetes mellitus; and in patients who are unusually responsive to sympathomimetic amines. Clinically significant changes in systolic and diastolic blood pressure have been seen in individual patients and could be expected to occur in some patients after use of any beta-adrenergic bronchodilator. As with other beta-agonists, albuterol may produce significant hypokalemia in some patients, possibly through intracellular shunting, which has the potential to produce adverse cardiovascular effects. The decrease is usually transient, not requiring supplementation.

Information for the Patient

The action of Ventolin Rotacaps for inhalation may last for up to 6 hours or longer. Ventolin Rotacaps for inhalation should not be used more frequently than recommended. Do not increase the dose or frequency of Ventolin Rotacaps for inhalation without consulting your physician. If you find that treatment with Ventolin Rotacaps for inhalation becomes less effective for symptomatic relief, your symptoms become worse, and/or you need to use the product more frequently than usual, you should seek medical attention immediately. While you are using Ventolin Rotacaps for inhalation, other inhaled drugs and asthma medications should be taken only as directed by your physician. Common adverse effects include palpitations, chest pain, rapid heart rate, and tremor or nervousness. If you are pregnant or nursing, contact your physician about use of Ventolin Rotacaps for inhalation. Effective and safe use of Ventolin Rotacaps for inhalation includes an understanding of the way that it should be administered.

Children should use Ventolin Rotacaps for inhalation under adult supervision, as instructed by the patient's physician.

See illustrated Patient's Instructions for Use distributed with the prescription.

Carcinogenesis, Mutagenesis, and Impairment of Fertility

In a 2 year study in Sprague-Dawley rats, albuterol sulfate caused a significant dose-related increase in the incidence of benign leiomyomas of the mesovarium at dietary doses of 2.0, 10, and 50 mg/kg (approximately 7, 35, and 170 times, respectively, the maximum recommended daily inhalation dose for adults on a mg/m^2 basis or approximately 3, 15, and 80 times, respectively, the maximum recommended daily inhalation dose in children on a mg/m^2 basis). In another study this effect was blocked by the coadministration of propranolol, a non-selective beta-adrenergic antagonist. In an 18 month study in CD-1 mice, albuterol sulfate showed no evidence of tumorigenicity at dietary doses of up to 500 mg/kg (approximately 850 times the maximum recommended daily inhalation dose for adults on a mg/m^2 basis or approximately 400 times the maximum recommended daily inhalation dose for children on a mg/m^2 basis). In a 22 month study in the Golden hamster, albuterol sulfate showed no evidence of tumorigenicity at dietary doses of up to 50 mg/kg (approximately 120 times the maximum recommended daily inhalation dose for adults on a mg/m^2 basis or approximately 55 times the maximum recommended daily inhalation dose for children on a mg/m^2 basis).

Albuterol sulfate was not mutagenic in the Ames test with or without metabolic activation using tester strains *S. typhimurium* TA1537, TA1538, and TA98 or *E. coli* WP2, WP2uvrA, and WP67. No forward mutation was seen in yeast strain *S. cerevisiae* S9 nor any mitotic gene conversion in yeast strain *S. cerevisiae* JD1 with or without metabolic activation. Fluctuation assays in *S. typhimurium* TA98 and *E. coli* WP2, both with metabolic activation, were negative. Albuterol sulfate was not clastogenic in a human peripheral lymphocyte assay or in an AH1 strain mouse micronucleus assay at intraperitoneal doses of up to 200 mg/kg.

Reproduction studies in rats demonstrated no evidence of impaired fertility at oral doses up to 50 mg/kg (approximately 170 times the maximum recommended daily inhalation dose for adults on a mg/m^2 basis).

Pregnancy, Teratogenic Effects, Pregnancy Category C

Albuterol has been shown to be teratogenic in mice. A study in CD-1 mice at subcutaneous doses of 0.025, 0.25, and 2.5 mg/kg (approximately 1/25, 2/5, and 4 times, respectively, the maximum recommended daily inhalation dose for adults on a mg/m^2 basis) showed cleft palate formation in 5 of 111 (4.5%) fetuses at 0.25 mg/kg and in 10 of 108 (9.3%) fetuses at 2.5 mg/kg. The drug did not induce cleft palate formation at the lowest dose, 0.025 mg/kg. Cleft palate also occurred in 22 of 72 (30.5%) fetuses from females treated with 2.5 mg/kg of isoproterenol (positive control) subcutaneously, approximately 4 times the maximum recommended daily inhalation dose for adults on a mg/m^2 basis.

A reproduction study in Stride Dutch rabbits revealed cranioschisis in 7 of 19 (37%) fetuses when albuterol was administered orally at a 50 mg/kg dose (approximately 340 times the maximum recommended daily inhalation dose for adults on a mg/m^2 basis).

There are no adequate and well-controlled studies in pregnant women. Albuterol should be used during pregnancy only if the potential benefit justifies the potential risk to the fetus.

During worldwide marketing experience, various congenital anomalies, including cleft palate and limb defects, have been rarely reported in the offspring of patients being treated with albuterol. Some of the mothers were taking multiple medications during their pregnancies. No consistent pattern of defects can be discerned, and a relationship between albuterol use and congenital anomalies has not been established.

Use in Labor and Delivery

Because of the potential for beta-agonist interference with uterine contractility, use of Ventolin Rotacaps for inhalation for relief of bronchospasm during labor should be restricted to those patients in whom the benefits clearly outweigh the risk.

Tocolysis
Albuterol has not been approved for the management of preterm labor. The benefit:risk ratio when albuterol is administered for tocolysis has not been established. Serious adverse reactions, including maternal pulmonary edema, have been reported during or following treatment of premature labor with $beta_2$-agonists, including albuterol.

Nursing Mothers
It is not known whether this drug is excreted in human milk after inhalation of recommended doses. Because of the potential for tumorigenicity shown for albuterol in some animal studies, a decision should be made whether to discontinue nursing or to discontinue the drug, taking into account the importance of the drug to the mother.

Pediatric Use
Safety and effectiveness in children below 4 years of age have not been established.

DRUG INTERACTIONS

VENTOLIN INHALATION AEROSOL

Other short-acting sympathomimetic aerosol bronchodilators should not be used concomitantly with albuterol. If additional adrenergic drugs are to be administered by any route, they should be used with caution to avoid deleterious cardiovascular effects.

Monoamine Oxidase Inhibitors or Tricyclic Antidepressants
Albuterol should be administered with extreme caution to patients being treated with monoamine oxidase inhibitors or tricyclic antidepressants, or within 2 weeks of discontinuation of such agents, because the action of albuterol on the vascular system may be potentiated.

Beta-Blockers
Beta-adrenergic receptor blocking agents not only block the pulmonary effect of beta-agonists, such as Ventolin inhalation aerosol, but may produce severe bronchospasm in patients with asthma. Therefore, patients with asthma should not normally be treated with beta-blockers. However, under certain circumstances, *e.g.,* as prophylaxis after myocardial infarction, there may be no acceptable alternatives to the use of beta-adrenergic blocking agents in patients with asthma. In this setting, cardioselective beta-blockers could be considered, although they should be administered with caution.

Diuretics
The ECG changes and/or hypokalemia that may result from the administration of nonpotassium-sparing diuretics (such as loop or thiazide diuretics) can be acutely worsened by beta-agonists, especially when the recommended dose of the beta-agonist is exceeded. Although the clinical significance of these effects is not known, caution is advised in the coadministration of beta-agonists with nonpotassium-sparing diuretics.

Digoxin
Mean decreases of 16-22% in serum digoxin levels were demonstrated after single-dose IV and oral administration of albuterol, respectively, to normal volunteers who had received digoxin for 10 days. The clinical significance of these findings for patients with obstructive airway disease who are receiving albuterol and digoxin on a chronic basis is unclear. Nevertheless, it would be prudent to carefully evaluate the serum digoxin levels in patients who are currently receiving digoxin and albuterol.

VENTOLIN HFA INHALATION AEROSOL

Other short-acting sympathomimetic aerosol bronchodilators should not be used concomitantly with albuterol. If additional adrenergic drugs are to be administered by any route, they should be used with caution to avoid deleterious cardiovascular effects.

Monoamine Oxidase Inhibitors or Tricyclic Antidepressants
Ventolin HFA should be administered with extreme caution to patients being treated with monoamine oxidase inhibitors or tricyclic antidepressants, or within 2 weeks of discontinuation of such agents, because the action of albuterol on the vascular system may be potentiated.

Beta-Blockers
Beta-adrenergic receptor blocking agents not only block the pulmonary effect of beta-agonists, such as Ventolin HFA, but may produce severe bronchospasm in patients with asthma. Therefore, patients with asthma should not normally be treated with beta-blockers. However, under certain circumstances, *e.g.,* as prophylaxis after myocardial infarction, there may be no acceptable alternatives to the use of beta-adrenergic blocking agents in patients with asthma. In this setting, cardioselective beta-blockers should be considered, although they should be administered with caution.

Diuretics
The ECG changes and/or hypokalemia that may result from the administration of nonpotassium-sparing diuretics (such as loop or thiazide diuretics) can be acutely worsened by beta-agonists, especially when the recommended dose of the beta-agonist is exceeded. Although the clinical significance of these effects is not known, caution is advised in the coadministration of beta-agonists with nonpotassium-sparing diuretics.

Digoxin
Mean decreases of 16-22% in serum digoxin levels were demonstrated after single-dose IV and oral administration of albuterol, respectively, to normal volunteers who had received digoxin for 10 days. The clinical significance of these findings for patients with obstructive airway disease who are receiving albuterol and digoxin on a chronic basis is unclear. Nevertheless, it would be prudent to carefully evaluate the serum digoxin levels in patients who are currently receiving digoxin and albuterol.

VENTOLIN INHALATION SOLUTION, 0.5%

Other short-acting sympathomimetic aerosol bronchodilators or epinephrine should not be used concomitantly with albuterol. If additional adrenergic drugs are to be administered by any route, they should be used with caution to avoid deleterious cardiovascular effects.

Monoamine Oxidase Inhibitors or Tricyclic Antidepressants
Albuterol should be administered with extreme caution to patients being treated with monoamine oxidase inhibitors or tricyclic antidepressants, or within 2 weeks of discontinuation of such agents, because the action of albuterol on the vascular system may be potentiated.

Beta-Blockers
Beta-adrenergic receptor blocking agents not only block the pulmonary effect of beta-agonists, such as Ventolin inhalation solution, but may produce severe bronchospasm in patients with asthma. Therefore, patients with asthma should not normally be treated with beta-blockers. However, under certain circumstances, *e.g.,* as prophylaxis after myocardial infarction, there may be no acceptable alternatives to the use of beta-adrenergic blocking agents in patients with asthma. In this setting, cardioselective beta-blockers could be considered, although they should be administered with caution.

Diuretics
The ECG changes and/or hypokalemia that may result from the administration of nonpotassium-sparing diuretics (such as loop or thiazide diuretics) can be acutely worsened by beta-agonists, especially when the recommended dose of the beta-agonist is exceeded. Although the clinical significance of these effects is not known, caution is advised in the coadministration of beta-agonists with nonpotassium-sparing diuretics.

Digoxin
Mean decreases of 16-22% in serum digoxin levels were demonstrated after single-dose IV and oral administration of albuterol, respectively, to normal volunteers who had received digoxin for 10 days. The clinical significance of these findings for patients with obstructive airway disease who are receiving albuterol and digoxin on a chronic basis is unclear. Nevertheless, it would be prudent to carefully evaluate the serum digoxin levels in patients who are currently receiving digoxin and albuterol.

VENTOLIN NEBULES INHALATION SOLUTION, 0.083%

Other short-acting sympathomimetic aerosol bronchodilators or epinephrine should not be used concomitantly with albuterol. If additional adrenergic drugs are to be administered by any route, they should be used with caution to avoid deleterious cardiovascular effects.

Monoamine Oxidase Inhibitors or Tricyclic Antidepressants
Albuterol should be administered with extreme caution to patients being treated with monoamine oxidase inhibitors or tricyclic antidepressants, or within 2 weeks of discontinuation of such agents, because the action of albuterol on the vascular system may be potentiated.

Beta-Blockers
Beta-adrenergic receptor blocking agents not only block the pulmonary effect of beta-agonists, such as Ventolin Nebules inhalation solution, but may produce severe bronchospasm in patients with asthma. Therefore, patients with asthma should not normally be treated with beta-blockers. However, under certain circumstances, *e.g.,* as prophylaxis after myocardial infarction, there may be no acceptable alternatives to the use of beta-adrenergic blocking agents in patients with asthma. In this setting, cardioselective beta-blockers could be considered, although they should be administered with caution.

Diuretics
The ECG changes and/or hypokalemia that may result from the administration of nonpotassium-sparing diuretics (such as loop or thiazide diuretics) can be acutely worsened by beta-agonists, especially when the recommended dose of the beta-agonist is exceeded. Although the clinical significance of these effects is not known, caution is advised in the coadministration of beta-agonists with nonpotassium-sparing diuretics.

Digoxin
Mean decreases of 16-22% in serum digoxin levels were demonstrated after single-dose IV and oral administration of albuterol, respectively, to normal volunteers who had received digoxin for 10 days. The clinical significance of these findings for patients with obstructive airway disease who are receiving albuterol and digoxin on a chronic basis is unclear. Nevertheless, it would be prudent to carefully evaluate the serum digoxin levels in patients who are currently receiving digoxin and albuterol.

VENTOLIN ROTACAPS FOR INHALATION

Other short-acting sympathomimetic aerosol bronchodilators should not be used concomitantly with albuterol. If additional adrenergic drugs are to be administered by any route, they should be used with caution to avoid deleterious cardiovascular effects.

Monoamine Oxidase Inhibitors or Tricyclic Antidepressants
Albuterol should be administered with extreme caution to patients being treated with monoamine oxidase inhibitors or tricyclic antidepressants, or within 2 weeks of discontinuation of such agents, because the action of albuterol on the vascular system may be potentiated.

Beta-Blockers
Beta-adrenergic receptor blocking agents not only block the pulmonary effect of beta-agonists, such as Ventolin Rotacaps for inhalation, but may produce severe bronchospasm in patients with asthma. Therefore, patients with asthma should not normally be treated with beta-blockers. However, under certain circumstances, *e.g.,* as prophylaxis after myocardial infarction, there may be no acceptable alternatives to the use of beta-adrenergic blocking

agents in patients with asthma. In this setting, cardioselective beta-blockers could be considered, although they should be administered with caution.

Diuretics

The ECG changes and/or hypokalemia that may result from the administration of nonpotassium-sparing diuretics (such as loop or thiazide diuretics) can be acutely worsened by beta-agonists, especially when the recommended dose of the beta-agonist is exceeded. Although the clinical significance of these effects is not known, caution is advised in the coadministration of beta-agonists with nonpotassium-sparing diuretics.

Digoxin

Mean decreases of 16-22% in serum digoxin levels were demonstrated after single-dose IV and oral administration of albuterol, respectively, to normal volunteers who had received digoxin for 10 days. The clinical significance of these findings for patients with obstructive airway disease who are receiving albuterol and digoxin on a chronic basis is unclear. Nevertheless, it would be prudent to carefully evaluate the serum digoxin levels in patients who are currently receiving digoxin and albuterol.

ADVERSE REACTIONS

VENTOLIN INHALATION AEROSOL

The adverse reactions to albuterol are similar in nature to reactions to other sympathomimetic agents, although the incidence of certain cardiovascular effects is lower with albuterol (see TABLE 6 and TABLE 7).

TABLE 6 *Percent Incidence of Adverse Reactions in Patients ≥12 Years of Age in a 13 Week Clinical Trial**

Reaction	Albuterol	Isoproterenol
Tremor	<15%	<15%
Nausea	<15%	<15%
Tachycardia	10%	10%
Palpitations	<10%	<15%
Nervousness	<10%	<15%
Increased blood pressure	<5%	<5%
Dizziness	<5%	<5%
Heartburn	<5%	<5%

* A 13 week double-blind study compared albuterol and isoproterenol inhalation aerosols in 147 patients with asthma.

TABLE 7 *Percent Incidence of Adverse Reactions in Children 4-11 Years of Age in a 12 Week Trial**

Reaction	Percent Incidence
Central Nervous System	
Headache	3%
Nervousness	1%
Lightheadedness	<1%
Tremor	<1%
Agitation	1%
Nightmares	1%
Hyperactivity	1%
Aggressive behavior	1%
Gastrointestinal	
Nausea and/or vomiting	6%
Stomachache	3%
Diarrhea	1%
Oropharyngeal	
Throat irritation	6%
Discoloration of teeth	1%
Respiratory	
Epistaxis	3%
Cough	2%
Musculoskeletal	
Muscle cramp	1%

* A 12 week double-blind trial in 104 patients aged 4-11 years.

Cases of urticaria, angioedema, rash, bronchospasm, hoarseness, oropharyngeal edema, and arrhythmias (including atrial fibrillation, supraventricular tachycardia, extrasystoles) have been reported after the use of Ventolin inhalation aerosol.

In addition, albuterol, like other sympathomimetic agents, can cause adverse reactions such as hypertension, angina, vertigo, central nervous system stimulation, sleeplessness, and unusual taste.

VENTOLIN HFA INHALATION AEROSOL

Adverse reaction information concerning Ventolin HFA is derived from two 12 week, randomized, double-blind studies in 610 adolescent and adult patients with asthma that compared Ventolin HFA, a CFC 11/12-propelled albuterol inhaler, and an HFA-134a placebo inhaler. TABLE 8 lists the incidence of all adverse events (whether considered by the investigator to be related or unrelated to drug) from these studies that occurred at a rate of 3% or greater in the group treated with Ventolin HFA and more frequently in the group treated with Ventolin HFA than in the HFA-134a placebo inhaler group. Overall, the incidence and nature of the adverse events reported for Ventolin HFA and a CFC 11/12-propelled albuterol inhaler were comparable. Results in a 2 week pediatric clinical study (n=135) showed that the adverse event profile was generally similar to that of the adult.

Adverse events reported by less than 3% of the adolescent and adult patients receiving Ventolin HFA and by a greater proportion of patients receiving Ventolin HFA than receiving HFA-134a placebo inhaler and that have the potential to be related to Ventolin HFA include diarrhea, laryngitis, oropharyngeal edema, cough, lung disorders, tachycardia, and extrasystoles. Palpitation and dizziness have also been observed with Ventolin HFA.

TABLE 8 *Adverse Experience Incidence (% of Patients) in 2 Large 12 Week Adolescent and Adult Clinical Trials**

Adverse Event Type	Ventolin HFA (n=202)	CFC 11/12-Propelled Albuterol Inhaler (n=207)	Placebo HFA-134a (n=201)
Ear, Nose, and Throat			
Throat irritation	10%	6%	7%
Upper respiratory inflammation	5%	5%	2%
Lower Respiratory			
Viral respiratory infections	7%	4%	4%
Cough	5%	2%	2%
Musculoskeletal			
Musculoskeletal pain	5%	5%	4%

* This table includes all adverse events (whether considered by the investigator to be drug-related or unrelated to drug) that occurred at an incidence rate of at least 3.0% in the group treated with Ventolin HFA and more frequently in the group treated with Ventolin HFA than in the HFA-134a placebo inhaler group.

Cases of urticaria, angioedema, rash, bronchospasm, hoarseness, and arrhythmias (including atrial fibrillation, supraventricular tachycardia, extrasystoles) have been reported after the use of albuterol.

In addition, albuterol, like other sympathomimetic agents, can cause adverse reactions such as hypertension, angina, vertigo, central nervous system stimulation, sleeplessness, headache, and drying or irritation of the oropharynx.

VENTOLIN INHALATION SOLUTION, 0.5%

The results of clinical trials with Ventolin inhalation solution in 135 patients showed the following side effects that were considered probably or possibly drug related (see TABLE 9).

TABLE 9 *Percent Incidence of Adverse Reactions*

Reaction	n=135
Central Nervous System	
Tremors	20%
Dizziness	7%
Nervousness	4%
Headache	3%
Sleeplessness	1%
Gastrointestinal	
Nausea	4%
Dyspepsia	1%
Ear, Nose, and Throat	
Nasal congestion	1%
Pharyngitis	<1%
Cardiovascular	
Tachycardia	1%
Hypertension	1%
Respiratory	
Bronchospasm	8%
Cough	4%
Bronchitis	4%
Wheezing	1%

No clinically relevant laboratory abnormalities related to Ventolin inhalation solution administration were determined in these studies.

Cases of urticaria, angioedema, rash, bronchospasm, hoarseness, oropharyngeal edema, and arrhythmias (including atrial fibrillation, supraventricular tachycardia, extrasystoles) have been reported after the use of Ventolin inhalation solution.

VENTOLIN NEBULES INHALATION SOLUTION, 0.083%

The results of clinical trials with Ventolin (albuterol sulfate) inhalation solution, 0.5% in 135 patients showed the following side effects that were considered probably or possibly drug related (see TABLE 10).

TABLE 10 *Percent Incidence of Adverse Reactions*

Reaction	n=135
Central Nervous System	
Tremors	20%
Dizziness	7%
Nervousness	4%
Headache	3%
Sleeplessness	1%
Gastrointestinal	
Nausea	4%
Dyspepsia	1%
Ear, Nose, and Throat	
Nasal congestion	1%
Pharyngitis	<1%
Cardiovascular	
Tachycardia	1%
Hypertension	1%
Respiratory	
Bronchospasm	8%
Cough	4%
Bronchitis	4%
Wheezing	1%

No clinically relevant laboratory abnormalities related to Ventolin inhalation solution administration were determined in these studies.

Cases of urticaria, angioedema, rash, bronchospasm, hoarseness, oropharyngeal edema, and arrhythmias (including atrial fibrillation, supraventricular tachycardia, extrasystoles) have been reported after the use of Ventolin Nebules inhalation solution.

VENTOLIN ROTACAPS FOR INHALATION

The adverse reactions to albuterol are similar in nature to reactions to other sympathomimetic agents, although the incidence of certain cardiovascular effects is lower with albuterol. Results of clinical trials with Ventolin Rotacaps for inhalation 200 μg in 172 patients aged 12 years and older (adults) and 129 patients aged 4-12 years (children) are shown in TABLE 11 and TABLE 12.

TABLE 11 *Percent Incidence of Adverse Reactions in Patients ≥12 Years of Age*

Reaction	Percent Incidence
Central Nervous System	
Headache	2%
Nervousness	1%
Tremor	1%
Sleeplessness	<1%
Dizziness	<1%
Lightheadedness	<1%
Digestive System	
Throat irritation	2%
Burning in the stomach	<1%
Dry mouth	<1%
Bad taste	<1%
Respiratory System	
Coughing	5%
Bronchospasm	1%

TABLE 12 *Percent Incidence of Adverse Reactions in Children 4-12 Years of Age*

Reaction	Percent Incidence
Central Nervous System	
Headache	5%
Dizziness	<1%
Hyperactivity	<1%
Gastrointestinal	
Nausea and/or vomiting	4%
Stomachache	2%
Diarrhea	<1%
Respiratory System	
Epistaxis	2%
Hoarseness	2%
Nasal congestion	2%
Cough	2%
Oropharyngeal	
Throat irritation	2%
Unusual taste	2%

Cases of urticaria, angioedema, rash, bronchospasm, hoarseness, oropharyngeal edema, and arrhythmias (including atrial fibrillation, supraventricular tachycardia, extrasystoles) have been reported after the use of Ventolin Rotacaps for inhalation.

In addition, albuterol, like other sympathomimetic agents, can cause adverse reactions such as hypertension, angina, vertigo, and CNS stimulation.

DOSAGE AND ADMINISTRATION

VENTOLIN INHALATION AEROSOL

For treatment of acute episodes of bronchospasm or prevention of asthmatic symptoms, the usual dosage for adults and children 4 years of age and older is 2 inhalations repeated every 4-6 hours; in some patients, 1 inhalation every 4 hours may be sufficient. More frequent administration or a larger number of inhalations are not recommended. It is recommended to "test spray" Ventolin inhalation aerosol. Do this by spraying 4 times into the air before using for the first time and when the inhaler has not been used for a prolonged period of time (*i.e.*, more than 4 weeks).

The use of Ventolin inhalation aerosol can be continued as medically indicated to control recurring bouts of bronchospasm. During this time most patients gain optimal benefit from regular use of the inhaler. Safe usage for periods extending over several years has been documented.

If a previously effective dosage regimen fails to provide the usual response, this may be a marker of destabilization of asthma and requires reevaluation of the patient and the treatment regimen, giving special consideration to the possible need for anti-inflammatory treatment, *e.g.*, corticosteroids.

Exercise-Induced Bronchospasm Prevention

The usual dosage for adults and children 4 years and older is 2 inhalations 15 minutes before exercise.

For treatment, see above.

VENTOLIN HFA INHALATION AEROSOL

Adult and Pediatric Asthma

For treatment of acute episodes of bronchospasm or prevention of asthmatic symptoms, the usual dosage for adults and children 4 years of age and older is 2 inhalations repeated every 4-6 hours; in some patients, 1 inhalation every 4 hours may be sufficient. More frequent administration or a larger number of inhalations is not recommended. It is recommended to prime the inhaler before using for the first time and in cases where the inhaler has not been used for more than 2 weeks by releasing 4 test sprays into the air, away from the face.

Ventolin HFA can also be used to relieve acute symptoms of asthma. The use of Ventolin HFA can be continued as medically indicated to control recurring bouts of bronchospasm. If a previously effective dosage regimen fails to provide the usual response, this may be a marker of destabilization of asthma and requires reevaluation of the patient and the treatment regimen, giving special consideration to the possible need for anti-inflammatory treatment, *e.g.*, corticosteroids.

Safe usage of albuterol for periods extending over several years has been documented.

Exercise-Induced Bronchospasm Prevention

The usual dosage for adults and children 4 years and older is 2 inhalations 15-30 minutes before exercise. For treatment, see above.

Cleaning

To maintain proper use of this product, it is important that the actuator be washed and dried thoroughly at least once a week. The inhaler may cease to deliver medication if not properly cleaned and dried thoroughly. **See PRECAUTIONS, Information for the Patient.** Keeping the plastic actuator clean is very important to prevent medication build-up and blockage. If the actuator becomes blocked with drug, washing the actuator will remove the blockage.

VENTOLIN INHALATION SOLUTION, 0.5%

To avoid microbial contamination, proper aseptic techniques should be used each time the bottle is opened. Precautions should be taken to prevent contact of the dropper tip of the bottle with any surface, including the nebulizer reservoir and associated ventilatory equipment. In addition, if the solution changes color or becomes cloudy, it should not be used.

Children 2-12 Years of Age

For children 2-12 years of age, initial dosing should be based upon body weight (0.1-0.15 mg/kg/dose), with subsequent dosing titrated to achieve the desired clinical response. Dosing should not exceed 2.5 mg three to four times daily by nebulization. TABLE 13 outlines approximate dosing according to body weight.

TABLE 13

Approximate Weight		Dose	Volume of Inhalation Solutions
10-15 kg	22-33 lb	1.25 mg	0.25 ml
>15 kg	>33 lb	2.5 mg	0.5 ml

The appropriate volume of the 0.5% inhalation solution should be diluted in sterile normal saline solution to a total volume of 3 ml prior to administration via nebulization.

Adults and Children Over 12 Years of Age

The usual dosage for adults and children over 12 years of age is 2.5 mg of albuterol administered 3-4 times daily by nebulization. More frequent administration or higher doses are not recommended. To administer 2.5 mg of albuterol, dilute 0.5 ml of the 0.5% inhalation solution with 2.5 ml of sterile normal saline solution. The flow rate is regulated to suit the particular nebulizer so that Ventolin inhalation solution will be delivered over approximately 5-15 minutes.

The use of Ventolin inhalation solution can be continued as medically indicated to control recurring bouts of bronchospasm. During this time most patients gain optimal benefit from regular use of the inhalation solution.

If a previously effective dosage regimen fails to provide the usual relief, medical advice should be sought immediately as this is often a sign of seriously worsening asthma that would require reassessment of therapy.

Drug compatibility (physical and chemical), efficacy, and safety of Ventolin inhalation solution when mixed with other drugs in a nebulizer have not been established.

VENTOLIN NEBULES INHALATION SOLUTION, 0.083%

Adults and Children 2-12 Years of Age

The usual dosage for adults and for children weighing at least 15 kg is 2.5 mg of albuterol (1 nebule) administered 3-4 times daily by nebulization. Children weighing less than 15 kg who require less than 2.5 mg/dose (*i.e.*, less than a full nebule) should use Ventolin inhalation solution instead of Ventolin Nebules inhalation solution. More frequent administration or higher doses are not recommended. To administer 2.5 mg of albuterol, administer the entire contents of 1 sterile unit dose nebule (3 ml of 0.083% inhalation solution) by nebulization. The flow rate is regulated to suit the particular nebulizer so that Ventolin Nebules inhalation solution will be delivered over approximately 5-15 minutes.

The use of Ventolin Nebules inhalation solution can be continued as medically indicated to control recurring bouts of bronchospasm. During this time most patients gain optimal benefit from regular use of the inhalation solution.

If a previously effective dosage regimen fails to provide the usual relief, medical advice should be sought immediately as this is often a sign of seriously worsening asthma that would require reassessment of therapy.

Drug compatibility (physical and chemical), efficacy, and safety of Ventolin Nebules inhalation solution when mixed with other drugs in a nebulizer have not been established.

VENTOLIN ROTACAPS FOR INHALATION

The usual dosage of Ventolin Rotacaps for inhalation for adults and children 4 years of age and older is the contents of one 200 μg capsule inhaled every 4-6 hours using a Rotahaler inhalation device. In some patients, the contents of two 200 μg capsules inhaled every 4-6 hours may be required. Larger doses or more frequent administration is not recommended.

The use of Ventolin Rotacaps for inhalation can be continued as medically indicated to control recurring bouts of bronchospasm. During this time most patients gain optimal benefit from regular use of the Ventolin Rotacaps for inhalation formulation.

If a previously effective dosage regimen fails to provide the usual relief, medical advice should be sought immediately as this is often a sign of seriously worsening asthma that would require reassessment of therapy.

Exercise-Induced Bronchospasm Prevention

The usual dosage of Ventolin Rotacaps for inhalation for adults and children 4 years of age and older is the contents of one 200 μg capsule inhaled using a Rotahaler 15 minutes before exercise.

HOW SUPPLIED

VENTOLIN INHALATION AEROSOL

Ventolin inhalation aerosol is supplied in 6.8 g canisters containing 80 metered inhalations and in 17 g canisters containing 200 metered inhalations. Each actuation delivers 100 μg of albuterol from the valve and 90 μg of albuterol from the mouthpiece. Each canister is supplied with a blue oral adapter and patient's instructions. Also available, Ventolin inhalation aerosol refill 17 g canister only with patient's instructions.

The blue adapter supplied with Ventolin inhalation aerosol should not be used with any other product canisters, and adapters from other products should not be used with a Ventolin inhalation aerosol canister. The correct amount of medication in each canister cannot be assured after 80 actuations from the 6.8 g canister and 200 actuations from the 17.0 g canister, even though the canister is not completely empty. The canister should be discarded when the labeled number of actuations have been used.

Storage

Store between 15 and 30°C (59 and 86°F). As with most inhaled medications in aerosol canisters, the therapeutic effect of this medication may decrease when the canister is cold; for best results, the canister should be at room temperature before use. Shake well before using.

Note: The statement below is required by the Federal government Clean Air Act for all products containing chlorofluorocarbons.

WARNING: This product contains trichloromonofluoromethane and dichlorodifluoromethane, substances which harm public health and environment by destroying ozone in the upper atmosphere.

A notice similar to the above warning has been placed in the patient instruction leaflet pursuant to regulations of the US Environmental Protection Agency (EPA). The patient's warning states that the patient should consult his or her physician if there are questions about alternatives.

VENTOLIN HFA INHALATION AEROSOL

Ventolin HFA (albuterol sulfate HFA inhalation aerosol) is supplied as a pressurized aluminum canister with a blue plastic actuator and a blue strapcap packaged within a moisture-protective foil pouch. The moisture-protective foil pouch also contains a desiccant that should be discarded when the pouch is opened.

It is recommended to prime the inhaler before using for the first time and in cases where the inhaler has not been used for more than 2 weeks by releasing 4 test sprays into the air, away from the face. After priming with 4 actuations, each actuation delivers 120 μg of albuterol sulfate in 75 mg of suspension from the valve and 108 μg of albuterol sulfate from the mouthpiece (equivalent to 90 μg of albuterol base from the mouthpiece). The canister is labeled with a net weight of 18 g and contains 200 metered inhalations.

The blue actuator supplied with Ventolin HFA should not be used with any other product canisters, and actuators from other products should not be used with a Ventolin HFA canister. The correct amount of medication in each canister cannot be assured after 200 actuations, even though the canister is not completely empty. The canister should be discarded when 200 actuations have been used or 3 months after removal from the moisture-protective foil pouch, whichever comes first. Never immerse the canister into water to determine how full the canister is ("float test").

Contents Under Pressure: Do not puncture. Do not use or store near heat or open flame. Exposure to temperatures above 120°F may cause bursting. Never throw container into fire or incinerator. Keep out of reach of children. Avoid spraying in eyes.

Storage

Store between 15 and 25°C (59 and 77°F). Store canister with mouthpiece down. For best results, the canister should be at room temperature before use. SHAKE WELL BEFORE USING.

Ventolin HFA does not contain chlorofluorocarbons (CFCs) as the propellant.

VENTOLIN INHALATION SOLUTION, 0.5%

Ventolin inhalation solution 0.5% is supplied in bottles of 20 ml with accompanying calibrated dropper.

Storage: Store between 2 and 25°C (36 and 77°F).

VENTOLIN NEBULES INHALATION SOLUTION, 0.083%

Ventolin Nebules inhalation solution, 0.083% is contained in plastic, sterile, unit dose Nebules of 3 ml each supplied in foil pouches.

Storage: Protect from light. Store in refrigerator between 2 and 8°C (36 and 46°F). Ventolin Nebules inhalation solution may be held at room temperature for up to 2 weeks before use. (Nebules must be used within 2 weeks of removal from refrigerator; record date the Nebules are removed from the refrigerator in the space provided on the product carton.) Discard if solution becomes discolored.

Note: Ventolin Nebules inhalation solution is colorless.

VENTOLIN ROTACAPS FOR INHALATION

Ventolin Rotacaps for inhalation, 200 μg, are light blue and clear, with "Ventolin 200" printed on the blue cap and "GLAXO" printed on the clear body.

Also available, Ventolin Rotacaps for inhalation refill.

Storage: Store between 2 and 30°C (36 and 86°F). Replace cap securely after each opening.

PRODUCT LISTING - RATED THERAPEUTICALLY EQUIVALENT

Size	Price	Product	NDC
Aerosol - Inhalation - 90 mcg/Inh			
7 gm	$18.40	VENTOLIN, Glaxosmithkline	00173-0463-00
17 gm	$19.79	GENERIC, Dey Laboratories	49502-0333-27
17 gm	$20.00	GENERIC, Alpharma Uspd Makers Of Barre and Nmc	00472-1264-63
17 gm	$20.00	GENERIC, Sidmak Laboratories Inc	50111-0801-32
17 gm	$21.50	GENERIC, Major Pharmaceuticals Inc	00904-5079-34
17 gm	$23.10	GENERIC, Pharma Pac	52959-0094-03
17 gm	$29.85	GENERIC, Andrx Pharmaceuticals	62037-0794-44
17 gm	$35.09	VENTOLIN, Physicians Total Care	54868-1903-00
17 gm	$35.35	VENTOLIN, Glaxosmithkline	00173-0321-98
17 gm	$37.30	VENTOLIN, Pharma Pac	52959-0588-01
17 gm	$38.39	VENTOLIN, Physicians Total Care	54868-0730-01
Aerosol with Adapter - Inhalation - 90 mcg/Inh			
17 gm	$10.95	GENERIC, Dey Laboratories	49502-0333-17
17 gm	$29.79	GENERIC, Ivax Corporation	00172-4390-18
17 gm	$29.79	GENERIC, Sidmak Laboratories Inc	50111-0801-31
17 gm	$30.00	VENTOLIN, Southwood Pharmaceuticals Inc	58016-6099-01
17 gm	$32.12	VENTOLIN, Allscripts Pharmaceutical Company	54569-1003-00
17 gm	$38.35	VENTOLIN, Glaxosmithkline	00173-0321-88
Solution - Inhalation - 0.083%			
3 ml	$0.43	FEDERAL UPPER LIMIT, H.C.F.A. F F P	99999-0115-11
3 ml x 24	$29.04	GENERIC, Warrick Pharmaceuticals Corporation	59930-1517-01
3 ml x 25	$30.00	GENERIC, Copley	38245-0669-17
3 ml x 25	$30.25	GENERIC, Dey Laboratories	49502-0697-03
3 ml x 25	$30.25	GENERIC, Hi-Tech Pharmacal Company Inc	50383-0742-25
3 ml x 25	$30.25	GENERIC, Novopharm Usa Inc	55953-0209-25
3 ml x 25	$30.25	GENERIC, Warrick Pharmaceuticals Corporation	59930-1500-08
3 ml x 25	$30.50	GENERIC, Qualitest Products Inc	00603-1005-40
3 ml x 25	$30.87	GENERIC, Ivax Corporation	00172-6405-44
3 ml x 25	$31.00	GENERIC, Alpharma Uspd Makers Of Barre and Nmc	00472-0831-23
3 ml x 25	$31.00	GENERIC, Nephron	00487-9501-25
3 ml x 25	$31.25	GENERIC, Major Pharmaceuticals Inc	00904-7731-17
3 ml x 25	$32.20	GENERIC, Aligen Independent Laboratories Inc	00405-2131-25
3 ml x 25	$32.31	GENERIC, Moore, H.L. Drug Exchange Inc	00839-7860-18
3 ml x 25	$32.60	GENERIC, Geneva Pharmaceuticals	00781-9150-93
3 ml x 25	$51.25	PROVENTIL, Schering Corporation	00085-0209-01
3 ml x 25	$56.09	PROVENTIL, Schering Corporation	00085-1806-01
3 ml x 30	$24.00	GENERIC, Nephron	00487-9501-01
3 ml x 30	$24.00	GENERIC, Nephron	00487-9501-03
3 ml x 30	$36.30	GENERIC, Dey Laboratories	49502-0697-33
3 ml x 30	$37.06	GENERIC, Alpharma Uspd Makers Of Barre and Nmc	00472-0831-30
3 ml x 60	$48.00	GENERIC, Nephron	00487-9501-60
3 ml x 60	$72.60	GENERIC, Dey Laboratories	49502-0697-60
3 ml x 60	$72.60	GENERIC, Warrick Pharmaceuticals Corporation	59930-1500-06
3 ml x 60	$72.60	GENERIC, Warrick Pharmaceuticals Corporation	59930-1517-02
3 ml x 60	$73.17	GENERIC, Moore, H.L. Drug Exchange Inc	00839-7860-35
3 ml x 60	$73.80	GENERIC, Ivax Corporation	00172-6405-49
3 ml x 60	$74.40	GENERIC, Alpharma Uspd Makers Of Barre and Nmc	00472-0831-60
3 ml x 60	$75.00	GENERIC, Morton Grove Pharmaceuticals Inc	60432-0094-06
Solution - Inhalation - 0.5%			
0.50 ml x 30	$27.00	GENERIC, Nephron	00487-9901-30
20 ml	$6.72	FEDERAL UPPER LIMIT, H.C.F.A. F F P	99999-0115-12
20 ml	$12.50	GENERIC, Qualitest Products Inc	00603-1006-43
20 ml	$14.65	GENERIC, Major Pharmaceuticals Inc	00904-7658-55
20 ml	$14.99	GENERIC, Ivax Corporation	00182-6014-65
20 ml	$14.99	GENERIC, Dey Laboratories	49502-0105-01
20 ml	$14.99	GENERIC, Novopharm Usa Inc	55953-0212-20
20 ml	$14.99	GENERIC, Warrick Pharmaceuticals Corporation	59930-1515-04
20 ml	$14.99	GENERIC, Warrick Pharmaceuticals Corporation	59930-1647-02
20 ml	$16.48	GENERIC, Moore, H.L. Drug Exchange Inc	00839-7861-97
20 ml	$16.50	GENERIC, Hi-Tech Pharmacal Company Inc	50383-0741-20
20 ml	$16.71	GENERIC, Alpharma Uspd Makers Of Barre and Nmc	00472-0832-20
20 ml	$16.71	GENERIC, Alpharma Uspd Makers Of Barre and Nmc	00472-0832-30
20 ml	$17.00	GENERIC, Bausch and Lomb	24208-0347-20
20 ml	$20.58	PROVENTIL, Allscripts Pharmaceutical Company	54569-1989-00
20 ml	$22.05	VENTOLIN, Pharma Pac	52959-0589-00
20 ml	$22.50	PROVENTIL, Schering Corporation	00085-0208-02
20 ml	$23.58	VENTOLIN, Physicians Total Care	54868-3479-00
Syrup - Oral - 2 mg/5 ml			
5 ml x 50	$62.60	GENERIC, Udl Laboratories Inc	51079-0761-10
120 ml	$11.07	GENERIC, Alpharma Uspd Makers Of Barre and Nmc	00472-0825-04

A

Size	Price	Product	NDC
120 ml	$18.00	VENTOLIN, Southwood Pharmaceuticals Inc	58016-0482-24
180 ml	$29.20	GENERIC, Pharma Pac	52959-0153-06
240 ml	$19.38	GENERIC, Alpharma Uspd Makers Of Barre and Nmc	00472-0825-08
240 ml	$36.00	VENTOLIN, Southwood Pharmaceuticals Inc	58016-0482-48
473 ml	$26.25	GENERIC, Moore, H.L. Drug Exchange Inc	00839-7746-69
473 ml	$30.79	GENERIC, Teva Pharmaceuticals Usa	00093-0661-16
480 ml	$24.77	GENERIC, Aligen Independent Laboratories Inc	00405-2135-16
480 ml	$26.23	GENERIC, Mova Pharmaceutical Corporation	55370-0315-48
480 ml	$26.40	GENERIC, Watson Laboratories Inc	52544-0419-16
480 ml	$27.90	GENERIC, Major Pharmaceuticals Inc	00904-7681-16
480 ml	$30.79	GENERIC, Qualitest Products Inc	00603-1007-58
480 ml	$34.99	GENERIC, Par Pharmaceutical Inc	49884-0411-33
480 ml	$39.60	GENERIC, Hi-Tech Pharmacal Company Inc	50383-0740-16
480 ml	$40.15	GENERIC, Alpharma Uspd Makers Of Barre and Nmc	00472-0825-16

Tablet - Oral - 2 mg

Size	Price	Product	NDC
20's	$6.72	GENERIC, Pd-Rx Pharmaceuticals	55289-0363-20
20's	$8.95	GENERIC, Pharma Pac	52959-0425-20
24's	$8.06	GENERIC, Pd-Rx Pharmaceuticals	55289-0363-24
30's	$8.10	GENERIC, Heartland Healthcare Services	61392-0567-30
30's	$8.10	GENERIC, Heartland Healthcare Services	61392-0567-39
30's	$8.55	GENERIC, Pd-Rx Pharmaceuticals	55289-0363-30
30's	$15.59	PROVENTIL, Pd-Rx Pharmaceuticals	55289-0009-30
30's	$17.31	VENTOLIN, Pd-Rx Pharmaceuticals	55289-0809-30
30's	$23.84	GENERIC, Medirex Inc	57480-8422-06
31's	$8.37	GENERIC, Heartland Healthcare Services	61392-0567-31
32's	$8.64	GENERIC, Heartland Healthcare Services	61392-0567-32
45's	$12.15	GENERIC, Heartland Healthcare Services	61392-0567-45
60's	$16.20	GENERIC, Heartland Healthcare Services	61392-0567-60
60's	$16.20	GENERIC, Heartland Healthcare Services	61392-0567-65
60's	$31.19	PROVENTIL, Pd-Rx Pharmaceuticals	55289-0009-60
90's	$24.30	GENERIC, Heartland Healthcare Services	61392-0567-90
90's	$24.30	GENERIC, Heartland Healthcare Services	61392-0567-95
100's	$4.77	FEDERAL UPPER LIMIT, H.C.F.A. F F P	99999-0115-15
100's	$7.55	GENERIC, Raway Pharmacal Inc	00686-0657-20
100's	$23.07	GENERIC, Moore, H.L. Drug Exchange Inc	00839-7867-06
100's	$23.50	GENERIC, Mova Pharmaceutical Corporation	55370-0111-07
100's	$23.65	GENERIC, Warrick Pharmaceuticals Corporation	59930-1520-01
100's	$24.00	GENERIC, Aligen Independent Laboratories Inc	00405-4030-01
100's	$24.50	GENERIC, Moore, H.L. Drug Exchange Inc	00839-7611-06
100's	$24.90	GENERIC, Major Pharmaceuticals Inc	00904-2876-60
100's	$25.38	GENERIC, Major Pharmaceuticals Inc	00904-2876-61
100's	$27.75	GENERIC, Medirex Inc	57480-0422-01
100's	$27.90	GENERIC, Martec Pharmaceuticals Inc	52555-0581-01
100's	$28.05	GENERIC, Geneva Pharmaceuticals	00781-1671-01
100's	$28.25	GENERIC, Warner Chilcott Laboratories	00047-0956-24
100's	$31.14	GENERIC, Mylan Pharmaceuticals Inc	00378-0255-01
100's	$31.14	GENERIC, Mutual Pharmaceutical Co Inc	53489-0176-01
100's	$32.07	GENERIC, Udl Laboratories Inc	51079-0657-20
100's	$48.92	PROVENTIL, Schering Corporation	00085-0252-02
120's	$22.50	GENERIC, Martec Pharmaceuticals Inc	52555-0491-01

Tablet - Oral - 4 mg

Size	Price	Product	NDC
30's	$10.05	GENERIC, Pd-Rx Pharmaceuticals	55289-0045-30
30's	$11.87	GENERIC, Heartland Healthcare Services	61392-0570-30
30's	$11.87	GENERIC, Heartland Healthcare Services	61392-0570-39
30's	$25.61	VENTOLIN, Pd-Rx Pharmaceuticals	55289-0810-30
31's	$12.26	GENERIC, Heartland Healthcare Services	61392-0570-31
32's	$12.66	GENERIC, Heartland Healthcare Services	61392-0570-32
45's	$17.80	GENERIC, Heartland Healthcare Services	61392-0570-45
60's	$23.73	GENERIC, Heartland Healthcare Services	61392-0570-60
60's	$23.73	GENERIC, Heartland Healthcare Services	61392-0570-65
90's	$35.60	GENERIC, Heartland Healthcare Services	61392-0570-90
90's	$35.60	GENERIC, Heartland Healthcare Services	61392-0570-95
100's	$8.00	GENERIC, Raway Pharmacal Inc	00686-0658-20
100's	$9.00	FEDERAL UPPER LIMIT, H.C.F.A. F F P	99999-0115-16
100's	$35.00	GENERIC, Mova Pharmaceutical Corporation	55370-0112-07
100's	$35.20	GENERIC, Warrick Pharmaceuticals Corporation	59930-1530-01
100's	$35.25	GENERIC, Martec Pharmaceuticals Inc	52555-0492-01
100's	$35.30	GENERIC, Major Pharmaceuticals Inc	00904-2877-60
100's	$35.51	GENERIC, Moore, H.L. Drug Exchange Inc	00839-7612-06
100's	$36.38	GENERIC, Major Pharmaceuticals Inc	00904-2877-61
100's	$38.05	GENERIC, Aligen Independent Laboratories Inc	00405-4031-01
100's	$39.90	GENERIC, Martec Pharmaceuticals Inc	52555-0582-01
100's	$41.30	GENERIC, Geneva Pharmaceuticals	00781-1672-01
100's	$43.50	GENERIC, Medirex Inc	57480-0423-01
100's	$45.76	GENERIC, Mylan Pharmaceuticals Inc	00378-0572-01
100's	$45.76	GENERIC, Mutual Pharmaceutical Co Inc	53489-0177-01
100's	$47.13	GENERIC, Udl Laboratories Inc	51079-0658-20
100's	$74.40	PROVENTIL, Schering Corporation	00085-0573-02
100's	$86.77	PROVENTIL, Physicians Total Care	54868-0308-01

Tablet, Extended Release - Oral - 8 mg

Size	Price	Product	NDC
100's	$218.42	VOLMAX, Muro Pharmaceuticals Inc	00451-0399-50

PRODUCT LISTING - RATED NOT THERAPEUTICALLY EQUIVALENT

Aerosol - Inhalation - 90 mcg/Inh

Size	Price	Product	NDC
17 gm	$19.79	GENERIC, Warrick Pharmaceuticals Corporation	59930-1560-02
17 gm	$19.98	GENERIC, Moore, H.L. Drug Exchange Inc	00839-7608-80
17 gm	$31.49	PROVENTIL, Schering Corporation	00085-0614-03
17 gm	$32.66	PROVENTIL, Allscripts Pharmaceutical Company	54569-0052-00
17 gm	$36.41	PROVENTIL, Physicians Total Care	54868-1041-01
17 gm	$36.83	PROVENTIL, Pharma Pac	52959-0293-00

Aerosol with Adapter - Inhalation - 90 mcg/Inh

Size	Price	Product	NDC
6 gm	$14.96	GENERIC, Prescript Pharmaceuticals	00247-0084-86
17 gm	$21.41	GENERIC, Warrick Pharmaceuticals Corporation	59930-1560-01
17 gm	$21.67	GENERIC, Moore, H.L. Drug Exchange Inc	00839-7608-07
17 gm	$22.48	GENERIC, Martec Pharmaceuticals Inc	52555-0594-17
17 gm	$22.95	GENERIC, Major Pharmaceuticals Inc	00904-5078-34
17 gm	$32.39	GENERIC, Prescript Pharmaceuticals	00247-0084-17
17 gm	$41.81	PROVENTIL, Schering Corporation	00085-0614-02

Aerosol with Adapter - Inhalation - 108 mcg/Inh

Size	Price	Product	NDC
6.70 gm	$34.65	PROVENTIL HFA, Pharma Pac	52959-0569-01
6.70 gm	$41.05	PROVENTIL HFA, Schering Corporation	00085-1132-01
18 gm	$37.63	VENTOLIN HFA, Glaxosmithkline	00173-0682-00

Tablet, Extended Release - Oral - 4 mg

Size	Price	Product	NDC
15's	$17.21	PROVENTIL REPETABS, Pd-Rx Pharmaceuticals	55289-0634-15
20's	$20.12	PROVENTIL REPETABS, Allscripts Pharmaceutical Company	54569-0387-02
30's	$41.75	VOLMAX, Physicians Total Care	55289-0498-30
60's	$49.84	VOLMAX, Allscripts Pharmaceutical Company	54569-4178-01
60's	$70.70	PROVENTIL REPETABS, Pd-Rx Pharmaceuticals	55289-0634-60
100's	$91.45	PROVENTIL REPETABS, Schering Corporation	00085-0431-02
100's	$109.21	VOLMAX, Muro Pharmaceuticals Inc	00451-0398-50
100's	$114.55	PROVENTIL REPETABS, Schering Corporation	00085-0431-04
180's	$113.96	PROVENTIL REPETABS, Allscripts Pharmaceutical Company	54569-8589-00

PRODUCT LISTING - EQUIVALENTS NOT AVAILABLE

Aerosol - Inhalation - 90 mcg/Inh

Size	Price	Product	NDC
17 gm	$11.99	GENERIC, Physicians Total Care	54868-3739-00
17 gm	$26.67	GENERIC, Prescript Pharmaceuticals	00247-0348-17
17 gm	$28.75	GENERIC, Allscripts Pharmaceutical Company	54569-4245-00

Aerosol with Adapter - Inhalation - 90 mcg/Inh

Size	Price	Product	NDC
17 gm	$9.24	GENERIC, Physicians Total Care	54868-3709-00
17 gm	$21.35	GENERIC, Southwood Pharmaceuticals Inc	58016-6569-01

Capsule - Inhalation - 200 mcg

Size	Price	Product	NDC
24's	$24.55	VENTOLIN ROTACAPS, Glaxosmithkline	00173-0389-03
96's	$42.66	VENTOLIN ROTACAPS, Physicians Total Care	54868-2649-01
100's	$32.15	VENTOLIN ROTACAPS, Glaxo Wellcome	00173-0389-02
100's	$37.92	VENTOLIN ROTACAPS, Allscripts Pharmaceutical Company	54569-3741-00

Solution - Inhalation - 0.021%

Size	Price	Product	NDC
3 ml x 25	$40.00	ACCUNEB, Dey Laboratories	49502-0692-03

Solution - Inhalation - 0.042%

Size	Price	Product	NDC
3 ml x 25	$40.00	ACCUNEB, Dey Laboratories	49502-0693-03

Solution - Inhalation - 0.083%

Size	Price	Product	NDC
3 ml x 25	$30.50	GENERIC, Rxelite	66794-0001-25
3 ml x 25	$34.63	GENERIC, Allscripts Pharmaceutical Company	54569-3899-00
3 ml x 30	$36.60	GENERIC, Rxelite	66794-0001-30
3 ml x 60	$73.20	GENERIC, Rxelite	66794-0001-60

Solution - Inhalation - 0.5%

Size	Price	Product	NDC
3 ml x 25	$14.21	GENERIC, Physicians Total Care	54868-2472-01
20 ml	$9.98	GENERIC, Physicians Total Care	54868-3407-00
20 ml	$14.99	GENERIC, Allscripts Pharmaceutical Company	54569-3900-00
20 ml	$15.53	GENERIC, Southwood Pharmaceuticals Inc	58016-6404-01
20 ml	$21.20	GENERIC, Southwood Pharmaceuticals Inc	58016-5018-20
20 ml	$22.64	GENERIC, Pharma Pac	52959-0741-20
20 ml	$23.69	GENERIC, Southwood Pharmaceuticals Inc	58016-5018-01

Syrup - Oral - 2 mg/5 ml

Size	Price	Product	NDC
118 ml	$10.00	GENERIC, Allscripts Pharmaceutical Company	54569-4899-00
118.25 ml	$6.65	GENERIC, Allscripts Pharmaceutical Company	54569-3700-01
120 ml	$7.90	GENERIC, Alpharma Uspd Makers Of Barre and Nmc	63874-0709-12
120 ml	$19.97	GENERIC, Pharma Pac	52959-0153-03
480 ml	$8.24	GENERIC, Physicians Total Care	54868-2887-00
480 ml	$10.96	GENERIC, Alpharma Uspd Makers Of Barre and Nmc	63874-0709-48
480 ml	$33.10	GENERIC, Pharma Pac	52959-0153-09

Tablet - Oral - 2 mg

4's	$3.52	GENERIC, Prescript Pharmaceuticals	00247-0264-04
6's	$3.59	GENERIC, Prescript Pharmaceuticals	00247-0264-06
12's	$4.34	GENERIC, Southwood Pharmaceuticals Inc	58016-0473-12
15's	$3.95	GENERIC, Prescript Pharmaceuticals	00247-0264-15
15's	$5.42	GENERIC, Southwood Pharmaceuticals Inc	58016-0473-15
15's	$13.77	GENERIC, Alpharma Uspd Makers Of Barre and Nmc	63874-0377-15
20's	$3.78	GENERIC, Alpharma Uspd Makers Of Barre and Nmc	63874-0377-20
20's	$4.15	GENERIC, Prescript Pharmaceuticals	00247-0264-20
20's	$7.23	GENERIC, Southwood Pharmaceuticals Inc	58016-0473-20
24's	$4.82	GENERIC, Alpharma Uspd Makers Of Barre and Nmc	63874-0377-24
24's	$8.68	GENERIC, Southwood Pharmaceuticals Inc	58016-0473-24
30's	$2.30	GENERIC, Physicians Total Care	54868-1073-03
30's	$4.54	GENERIC, Prescript Pharmaceuticals	00247-0264-30
30's	$7.90	GENERIC, Allscripts Pharmaceutical Company	54569-3409-00
30's	$10.85	GENERIC, Southwood Pharmaceuticals Inc	58016-0473-30
32's	$4.62	GENERIC, Prescript Pharmaceuticals	00247-0264-32
50's	$2.94	GENERIC, Physicians Total Care	54868-1073-06
60's	$3.27	GENERIC, Physicians Total Care	54868-1073-04
90's	$32.55	GENERIC, Southwood Pharmaceuticals Inc	58016-0473-90
100's	$3.89	GENERIC, Physicians Total Care	54868-1073-02
100's	$5.62	GENERIC, Alpharma Uspd Makers Of Barre and Nmc	63874-0377-01
100's	$36.17	GENERIC, Southwood Pharmaceuticals Inc	58016-0473-00
120's	$5.20	GENERIC, Physicians Total Care	54868-1073-05

Tablet - Oral - 4 mg

4's	$3.67	GENERIC, Prescript Pharmaceuticals	00247-0265-04
10's	$3.87	GENERIC, Allscripts Pharmaceutical Company	54569-2874-02
12's	$6.47	GENERIC, Southwood Pharmaceuticals Inc	58016-0603-12
15's	$4.54	GENERIC, Prescript Pharmaceuticals	00247-0265-15
15's	$8.09	GENERIC, Southwood Pharmaceuticals Inc	58016-0603-15
20's	$4.94	GENERIC, Prescript Pharmaceuticals	00247-0265-20
20's	$10.79	GENERIC, Southwood Pharmaceuticals Inc	58016-0603-20
24's	$6.08	GENERIC, Alpharma Uspd Makers Of Barre and Nmc	63874-0378-24
24's	$12.94	GENERIC, Southwood Pharmaceuticals Inc	58016-0603-24
30's	$2.74	GENERIC, Physicians Total Care	54868-1074-03
30's	$5.74	GENERIC, Prescript Pharmaceuticals	00247-0265-30
30's	$11.60	GENERIC, Allscripts Pharmaceutical Company	54569-2874-00
30's	$16.17	GENERIC, Southwood Pharmaceuticals Inc	58016-0603-30
60's	$4.14	GENERIC, Physicians Total Care	54868-1074-07
60's	$23.20	GENERIC, Allscripts Pharmaceutical Company	54569-2874-01
100's	$5.34	GENERIC, Physicians Total Care	54868-1074-05
100's	$11.19	GENERIC, Alpharma Uspd Makers Of Barre and Nmc	63874-0378-01
100's	$53.92	GENERIC, Southwood Pharmaceuticals Inc	58016-0603-00
120's	$6.95	GENERIC, Physicians Total Care	54868-1074-06

Tablet, Extended Release - Oral - 4 mg

100's	$83.95	GENERIC, Odyssey Pharmaceutical	65473-0754-01

Tablet, Extended Release - Oral - 8 mg

60's	$106.87	VOLMAX, Allscripts Pharmaceutical Company	54569-4172-01
100's	$167.90	GENERIC, Odyssey Pharmaceutical	65473-0758-01

Albuterol; Ipratropium Bromide *(003214)*

For complete prescribing information, refer to the CD-ROM included with the book.

For related information, see the comparative table section in Appendix A.

Categories: Emphysema; Chronic obstructive pulmonary disease; Bronchitis, chronic; Pregnancy Category C; FDA Approved 1996 Oct
Drug Classes: Adrenergic agonists; Anticholinergics; Bronchodilators
Brand Names: Combivent
Foreign Brand Availability: Albugenol TR (Dominican-Republic; El-Salvador; Guatemala; Honduras); Combivent Aerosol (Australia; New-Zealand); Duolin (Australia; India); Duospirel (Austria)
Cost of Therapy: $54.71 (Asthma; Combivent Inhalation Aerosol; 103 µg;18 µg; 8 inhalations/day; 25 day supply)

DESCRIPTION

Combivent inhalation aerosol is a combination of albuterol sulfate and ipratropium bromide. Ipratropium bromide is an anticholinergic bronchodilator chemically described as 8-azoniabicyclo[3.2.1]octane, 3-(3-hydroxy-1-oxo-2-phenylpropoxy)-8-methyl-8-(1-methylethyl)-, bromide, monohydrate (endo,syn)-, (±): a synthetic quaternary ammonium compound chemically related to atropine. Ipratropium bromide is a white to off-white crystalline substance soluble in water and lower alcohols but insoluble in lipophilic solvents such as ether, chloroform and fluorocarbons. The chemical formula is $C_{20}H_{30}BrNO_3{\cdot}H_2O$, and the molecular weight is 430.4.

Albuterol sulfate, chemically known as (1,3-benzenedimethanol, a'-[[(1,1-dimethylethyl)amino]methyl]-4-hydroxy, sulfate (2:1)(salt), (±)-, is a relatively selective beta$_2$-adrenergic bronchodilator. Albuterol is the official generic name in the US. The World Health Organization's recommended name for the drug is salbutamol. Albuterol sulfate is a white to off-white crystalline powder soluble in water and slightly soluble in ethanol. The chemical formula is $(C_{13}H_{21}NO_3)_2{\cdot}H_2SO_4$, and the molecular weight is 576.7.

Combivent Inhalation Aerosol contains a microcrystalline suspension of albuterol sulfate; ipratropium bromide in a pressurized metered-dose aerosol unit for oral inhalation administration. The 200 inhalation unit has a net weight of 14.7 grams. Each actuation meters 120 µg of albuterol sulfate and 21 µg of ipratropium bromide from the valve and delivers 103 µg of albuterol sulfate (equivalent to 90 µg albuterol base) and 18 µg of ipratropium bromide from the mouthpiece. The excipients are dichlorodifluoromethane, dichlorotetrafluoroethane, and trichloromonofluoromethane as propellants and soya lecithin.

INDICATIONS AND USAGE

Albuterol sulfate; ipratropium bromide inhalation aerosol is indicated for use in patients with chronic obstructive pulmonary disease (COPD) on a regular aerosol bronchodilator who continue to have evidence of bronchospasm and require a second bronchodilator.

CONTRAINDICATIONS

Albuterol sulfate; ipratropium bromide inhalation aerosol is contraindicated in patients with a history of hypersensitivity to soya lecithin or related food products, such as soybean and peanut. Albuterol sulfate; ipratropium bromide inhalation aerosol is also contraindicated in patients hypersensitive to any other components of the drug product or to atropine and/or its derivatives.

WARNINGS

PARADOXICAL BRONCHOSPASM

Albuterol sulfate; ipratropium bromide inhalation aerosol can produce paradoxical bronchospasm that can be life-threatening. If it occurs, the preparation should be discontinued immediately and alternative therapy instituted. It should be recognized that paradoxical bronchospasm, when associated with inhaled formulations, frequently occurs with the first use of a new canister.

CARDIOVASCULAR EFFECT

The albuterol sulfate contained in albuterol sulfate; ipratropium bromide inhalation aerosol, like other beta-adrenergic agonists, can produce a clinically significant cardiovascular effect in some patients, as measured by pulse rate, blood pressure, and/or symptoms. Although such effects are uncommon after administration of albuterol sulfate; ipratropium bromide inhalation aerosol at recommended doses, if they occur, discontinuation of the drug may be indicated. In addition, beta-adrenergic agents have been reported to produce ECG changes, such as flattening of the T wave, prolongation of the QTc interval, and ST segment depression. Therefore, albuterol sulfate; ipratropium bromide inhalation aerosol should be used with caution in patients with cardiovascular disorders, especially coronary insufficiency, cardiac arrhythmias, and hypertension.

DO NOT EXCEED RECOMMENDED DOSE

Fatalities have been reported in association with excessive use of inhaled sympathomimetic drugs in patients with asthma. The exact cause of death is unknown, but cardiac arrest following an unexpected development of a severe acute asthmatic crisis and subsequent hypoxia is suspected.

IMMEDIATE HYPERSENSITIVITY REACTIONS

Immediate hypersensitivity reactions may occur after administration of albuterol sulfate or ipratropium bromide, as demonstrated by rare cases of urticaria, angioedema, rash, bronchospasm, anaphylaxis and oropharyngeal edema.

STORAGE CONDITIONS

The contents of albuterol sulfate; ipratropium bromide inhalation aerosol are under pressure. Do not puncture. Do not use or store near heat or open flame. Exposure to temperatures above 120°F may cause bursting. Never throw the container into a fire or incinerator. Keep out of reach of children.

DOSAGE AND ADMINISTRATION

The dose of albuterol sulfate; ipratropium bromide inhalation aerosol is 2 inhalations 4 times a day. Patients may take additional inhalations as required; however, the total number of inhalations should not exceed 12 in 24 hours. Safety and efficacy of additional doses of albuterol sulfate; ipratropium bromide inhalation aerosol beyond 12 puffs/24 hours have not been studied. Also, safety and efficacy of extra doses of ipratropium or albuterol in addition to the recommended doses of albuterol sulfate; ipratropium bromide inhalation aerosol have not been studied. It is recommended to "test-spray" three times before using for the first time and in cases where the aerosol has not been used for more than 24 hours.

PRODUCT LISTING - EQUIVALENTS NOT AVAILABLE

Aerosol with Adapter - Inhalation - 103 mcg;18 mcg/Inh

14.70 gm	$40.40	COMBIVENT, Allscripts Pharmaceutical Company	54569-4600-00
14.70 gm	$54.71	COMBIVENT, Boehringer-Ingelheim	00597-0013-14

Solution - Inhalation - 3 mg;0.5 mg/3 ml

3 ml x 30	$60.00	DUONEB, Dey Laboratories	49502-0672-30
3 ml x 60	$120.00	DUONEB, Dey Laboratories	49502-0672-60

A

Aldesleukin (003125)

For complete prescribing information, refer to the CD-ROM included with the book.

Categories: Carcinoma, renal; Melanoma, malignant; Recombinant DNA Origin; FDA Approved 1992 May; Pregnancy Category C; Orphan Drugs
Drug Classes: Antineoplastics, biological response modifiers
Brand Names: Interleukin-2; **Proleukin**
HCFA JCODE(S): J9015 per single use vial IM, IV

WARNING

Therapy with aldesleukin should be restricted to patients with normal cardiac and pulmonary functions as defined by thallium stress testing and formal pulmonary function testing. Extreme caution should be used in patients with normal thallium stress tests and a normal pulmonary function test who have a history of prior cardiac or pulmonary disease.

Aldesleukin for injection should be administered only in a hospital setting under the supervision of a qualified physician experienced in the use of anticancer agents. An intensive care facility and specialists skilled in cardiopulmonary or intensive care medicine must be available.

Aldesleukin administration has been associated with capillary leak syndrome (CLS) which is characterized by a loss of vascular tone and extravasation of plasma proteins and fluid into the extravascular space. CLS results in hypotension and reduced organ perfusion which may be severe and can result in death. CLS may be associated with cardiac arrhythmias (supraventricular and ventricular), angina, myocardial infarction, respiratory insufficiency requiring intubation, gastrointestinal bleeding or infarction, renal insuffiency, edema, and mental status changes.

Aldesleukin treatment is associated with impaired neutrophil function (reduced chemotaxis) and with an increased risk of disseminated infection, including sepsis and bacterial endocarditis. Consequently, preexisting bacterial infections should be adequately treated prior to initiation of aldesleukin therapy. Patients with indwelling central lines are particularly at risk for infection with gram positive microorganisms. Antibiotic prophylaxis with oxacillin, nafcillin, ciprofloxacin, or vancomycin has been associated with a reduced incidence of staphylococcal infections.

Aldesleukin administration should be withheld in patients developing moderate to severe lethargy or somnolence; continued administration may result in coma.

DESCRIPTION

Aldesleukin for injection, a human recombinant interleukin-2 product, is a highly purified protein with a molecular weight of approximately 15,300 daltons. The chemical name is des-alanyl-1, serine-125 human interleukin-2. Aldesleukin, a lymphokine, is produced by recombinant DNA technology using a genetically engineered *E. coli* strain containing an analog of the human interleukin-2 gene. Genetic engineering techniques were used to modify the human IL-2 gene, and the resulting expression clone encodes a modified human interleukin-2. This recombinant form differs from native interleukin-2 in the following ways: a) aldesleukin is not glycosylated because it is derived from *E. coli*; b) the molecule has no N-terminal alanine; the codon for this amino acid was deleted during the genetic engineering procedure; c) the molecule has serine substituted for cysteine at amino acid position 125; this was accomplished by site specific manipulation during the genetic engineering procedure; and d) the aggregation state of aldesleukin is likely to be different from that of native interleukin-2.

The *in vitro* biological activities of the native nonrecombinant molecule have been reproduced with aldesleukin.[1,2]

Aldesleukin is supplied as a sterile, white to off-white, lyophilized cake in single-use vials intended for intravenous (IV) administration. When reconstituted with 1.2 ml sterile water for injection, each ml contains 18 million IU (1.1 mg) aldesleukin, 50 mg mannitol, and 0.18 mg sodium dodecyl sulfate, buffered with approximately 0.17 mg monobasic and 0.89 mg dibasic sodium phosphate to a pH of 7.5 (range 7.2-7.8). The manufacturing process for aldesleukin involves fermentation in a defined medium containing tetracycline hydrochloride. The presence of the antibiotic is not detectable in the final product. Aldesleukin contains no preservatives in the final product.

Aldesleukin biological potency is determined by a lymphocyte proliferation bioassay and is expressed in International Units (IU) as established by the World Health Organization 1st International Standard for Interleukin-2 (human). The relationship between potency and protein mass is as follows:

18 million (18×10^6) IU aldesleukin=1.1 mg protein

INDICATIONS AND USAGE

Aldesleukin is indicated for the treatment of adults with metastatic renal cell carcinoma (metastatic RCC).

Aldesleukin is indicated for the treatment of adults with metastatic melanoma.

Careful patient selection is mandatory prior to the administration of aldesleukin. See CONTRAINDICATIONS and WARNINGS regarding patient screening, including recommended cardiac and pulmonary function tests and laboratory tests.

Evaluation of clinical studies to date reveals that patients with more favorable ECOG performance status (ECOG PS O) at treatment initiation respond better to aldesleukin, with a higher response rate and lower toxicity. Therefore, selection of patients for treatment should include assessment of performance status.

Experience in patients with PS >1 is extremely limited.

NON-FDA APPROVED INDICATIONS

Aldesleukin has been used without FDA approval in the treatment of HIV-infected patients and patients with leukemia.

CONTRAINDICATIONS

Aldesleukin is contraindicated in patients with a known history of hypersensitivity to interleukin-2 or any component of the aldesleukin formulation.

Aldesleukin is contraindicated in patients with an abnormal thallium stress test or abnormal pulmonary function tests and those with organ allografts. Retreatment with aldesleukin is contraindicated in patients who have experienced the following drug-related toxicities while receiving an earlier course of therapy:

- Sustained ventricular tachycardia (≥5 beats).
- Cardiac arrhythmias not controlled or unresponsive to management.
- Chest pain with ECG changes, consistent with angina or myocardial infarction.
- Cardiac tamponade.
- Intubation required >72 hours.
- Renal failure requiring dialysis >72 hours.
- Coma or toxic psychosis lasting >48 hours.
- Repetitive or difficult to control seizures.
- Bowel ischemia/perforation.
- GI bleeding requiring surgery.

WARNINGS

See BOXED WARNING.

Because of the severe adverse events which generally accompany aldesleukin therapy at the recommended dosages, thorough clinical evaluation should be performed to identify patients with significant cardiac, pulmonary, renal, hepatic, or CNS impairment in whom aldesleukin is contraindicated. Patients with normal cardiovascular, pulmonary, hepatic, and CNS function may experience serious, life threatening or fatal adverse events. Adverse events are frequent, often serious, and sometimes fatal.

Should adverse events which require dose modification occur, dosage should be withheld rather than reduced (See DOSAGE AND ADMINISTRATION, Dose Modification.)

Aldesleukin has been associated with exacerbation of pre-existing or initial presentation of autoimmune disease and inflammatory disorders. Exacerbation of Crohn's disease, scleroderma thyroiditis, inflammatory arthritis, diabetes mellitus, oculo-bulbar myasthenia gravis, crescentic IgA glomerulonephritis, cholecystitis, cerebral vasculitis, Stevens-Johnson syndrome and bulbous phemphigoid, has been reported following treatment with IL-2.

All patients should have thorough evaluation and treatment of CNS metastases and have a negative scan prior to receiving aldesleukin therapy. New neurologic signs, symptoms, and anatomic lesions following aldesleukin therapy have been reported in patients without evidence of CNS metastases. Clinical manifestations included changes in mental status, speech difficulties, cortical blindness, limb or gait ataxia, hallucinations, agitation, obtundation, and coma. Radiological findings included multiple and, less commonly, single cortical lesions on MRI and evidence of demyelination. Neurologic signs and symptoms associated with aldesleukin therapy usually improve after discontinuation of aldesleukin therapy; however, there are reports of permanent neurologic defects. One case of possible cerebral vasculitis, responsive to dexamethasone, has been reported. In patients with known seizure disorders, extreme caution should be exercised as aldesleukin may cause seizures.

DOSAGE AND ADMINISTRATION

The recommended aldesleukin for injection treatment regimen is administered by a 15 minute IV infusion every 8 hours. Before initiating treatment, carefully review INDICATIONS AND USAGE, CONTRAINDICATIONS, and WARNINGS, particularly regarding patient selection, possible serious adverse events, patient monitoring and withholding dosage. The following schedule has been used to treat adult patients with renal cell carcinoma (metastatic RCC) or metastatic melanoma. Each course of treatment consists of two 5 day treatment cycles separated by a rest period.

600,000 IU/kg (0.037 mg/kg) dose administered every 8 hours by a 15 minute IV infusion for a maximum of 14 doses. Following 9 days of rest, the schedule is repeated for another 14 doses, for a maximum of 28 doses per course, as tolerated. During clinical trials, doses were frequently held for toxicity (see Dose Modification). Metastatic RCC patients treated with this schedule received a median of 20 of the 28 doses during the first course of therapy. Metastatic melanoma patients received a median of 18 doses during the first course of therapy.

RETREATMENT

Patients should be evaluated for response approximately 4 weeks after completion of a course of therapy and again immediately prior to the scheduled start of the next treatment course. Additional courses of treatment should be given to patients only if there is some tumor shrinkage following the last course and retreatment is not contraindicated (see CONTRAINDICATIONS). Each treatment course should be separated by a rest period of at least 7 weeks from the date of hospital discharge.

DOSE MODIFICATION

Dose modification for toxicity should be accomplished by withholding or interrupting a dose rather than reducing the dose to be given. Decisions to stop, hold, or restart aldesleukin therapy must be made after a global assessment of the patient. With this in mind, the guidelines in TABLE 5 and TABLE 6 should be used.

RECONSTITUTION AND DILUTION DIRECTIONS

Reconstitution and dilution procedures other than those recommended may alter the delivery and/or pharmacology of aldesleukin and thus should be avoided.

1. Aldesleukin is a sterile, white to off-white, preservative-free, lyophilized powder suitable for IV infusion upon reconstitution and dilution. **EACH VIAL CONTAINS 22 MILLION IU (1.3 MG) OF ALDESLEUKIN AND SHOULD BE RECONSTITUTED ASEPTICALLY WITH 1.2 ML OF STERILE WATER FOR INJECTION. WHEN RECONSTITUTED AS DIRECTED, EACH ML CONTAINS 18 MILLION IU (1.1 MG) OF ALDESLEUKIN.** The resulting solution should be a clear, colorless to slightly yellow liquid. The vial is for single-use only and any unused portion should be discarded.

TABLE 5 *Retreatment With Aldesleukin is Contraindicated in Patients Who Have Experienced the Following Toxicities*

Body System	
Cardiovascular	Sustained ventricular tachycardia (≥5 beats)
	Cardiac rhythm disturbances not controlled or unresponsive to management
	Chest pain with ECG changes, consistent with angina or myocardial infarction
	Cardiac tamponade
Respiratory	Intubation required >72 hours
Urogenital	Renal failure requiring dialysis >72 hours
Nervous	Coma or toxic psychosis lasting >48 hours
	Repetitive or difficult to control seizures
Gastrointestinal	Bowel ischemia/perforation
	GI bleeding requiring surgery

TABLE 6 *Doses Should Be Held and Restarted According to the Following*

Organ System	Hold Dose For	Subsequent Doses May Be Given if
Cardiovascular	Atrial fibrillation, supraventricular tachycardia, or bradycardia that requires treatment or is recurrent or persistent	Patient is asymptomatic with full recovery to normal sinus rhythm
	Systolic bp <90 mm Hg with increasing requirements for pressors	Systolic bp ≥90 mm Hg and stable or improving requirements for pressors
	Any ECG change consistent with MI, ischemia or myocarditis with or without chest pain; suspicion of cardiac ischemia	Patient is asymptomatic, MI and myocarditis have been ruled out, clinical suspicion of angina is low; there is no evidence of ventricular hypokinesa
Respiratory	O_2 saturation <94% on room air or <90% with 2 liters O_2 by nasal prongs	O_2 saturation ≥94% on room air or ≥90% with 2 liters O_2 by nasal prongs
Nervous	Mental status changes, including moderate confusion or agitation	Mental status changes completely resolved
Body as a Whole	Sepsis syndrome, patient is clinically unstable	Sepsis syndrome has resolved, patient is clinically stable, infection is under treatment
Urogenital	Serum creatinine >4.5 mg/dl or a serum creatinine of ≥4 mg/dl in the presence of severe volume overload, acidosis, or hyperkalemia	Serum creatinine <4 mg/dl and fluid and electrolyte status is stable
	Persistent oliguria, urine output of <10 ml/hour for 16 to 24 hours with rising serum creatinine	Urine output >10 ml/hour with a decrease of serum creatinine >1.5 mg/dl or normalization of serum creatinine
Digestive	Signs of hepatic failure including encephalopathy, increasing ascites, liver pain, hypoglycemia	All signs of hepatic failure have resolved*
	Stool guaiac repeatedly >3-4+	Stool guaiac negative
Skin	Bullous dermatitis or marked worsening of preexisting skin condition, avoid topical steroid therapy	Resolution of all signs of bullous dermatitis

* Discontinue all further treatment for that course. A new course of treatment, if warranted, should be initiated no sooner than 7 weeks after cessation of adverse event and hospital discharge.

2. During reconstitution, the sterile water for injection should be directed at the side of the vial and the contents gently swirled to avoid excess foaming. DO NOT SHAKE.
3. The dose of aldesleukin, reconstituted in sterile water for injection (without preservative) should be diluted aseptically in 50 ml of 5% dextrose injection (D5W) and infused over a 15 minute period.

In cases where the total dose of aldesleukin is 1.5 mg or less (*e.g.*, a patient with a body weight of less than 40 kilograms), the dose of aldesleukin should be diluted in a smaller volume of D5W. Concentrations of aldesleukin below 30 μg/ml and above 70 μg/ml have shown increased variability in drug delivery. Dilution and delivery of aldesleukin outside of this concentration range should be avoided.

4. Glass bottles and plastic (polyvinyl chloride) bags have been used in clinical trials with comparable results. It is recommended that plastic bags be used as the dilution container since experimental studies suggest that use of plastic containers results in more consistent drug delivery. **In-line filters should not be used when administering aldesleukin.**
5. Before and after reconstitution and dilution, store in a refrigerator at 2-8°C (36-46°F). Do not freeze. Administer aldesleukin within 48 hours of reconstitution. The solution should be brought to room temperature prior to infusion in the patient.
6. Reconstitution or dilution with bacteriostatic water for injection or 0.9% sodium chloride injection should be avoided because of increased aggregation. Aldesleukin should not be coadministered with other drugs in the same container.
7. Parenteral drug products should be inspected visually for particulate matter and discoloration prior to administration, whenever solution and container permit.

PRODUCT LISTING - RATED THERAPEUTICALLY EQUIVALENT

Powder For Injection - Injectable - 22000000 IU

1's $773.13 PROLEUKIN, Chiron Therapeutics 53905-0991-01

Alefacept

(003586)

A

Categories: Psoriasis; Pregnancy Category B; FDA Approved 2003 Jan
Drug Classes: Immunosuppressives
Brand Names: Amevive
Cost of Therapy: $3,980.00 (Psoriasis; Amevive; 15 mg/vial; 15 mg/week; 28 day supply)

DESCRIPTION

Amevive (alefacept) is an immunosuppressive dimeric fusion protein that consists of the extracellular CD2-binding portion of the human leukocyte function antigen-3 (LFA-3) linked to the Fc (hinge, C_H2 and C_H3 domains) portion of human IgG1. Alefacept is produced by recombinant DNA technology in a Chinese Hamster Ovary (CHO) mammalian cell expression system. The molecular weight of alefacept is 91.4 kilodaltons.

Amevive is supplied as a sterile, white-to-off-white, preservative-free, lyophilized powder for parenteral administration. After reconstitution with 0.6 ml of the supplied sterile water for injection, the solution of Amevive is clear, with a pH of approximately 6.9.

Amevive is available in 2 formulations. Amevive for intramuscular (IM) injection contains 15 mg alefacept per 0.5 ml of reconstituted solution. Amevive for intravenous (IV) injection contains 7.5 mg alefacept per 0.5 ml of reconstituted solution. Both formulations also contain 12.5 mg sucrose, 5.0 mg glycine, 3.6 mg sodium citrate dihydrate, and 0.06 mg citric acid monohydrate per 0.5 ml.

CLINICAL PHARMACOLOGY

Alefacept interferes with lymphocyte activation by specifically binding to the lymphocyte antigen, CD2, and inhibiting LFA-3/CD2 interaction. Activation of T lymphocytes involving the interaction between LFA-3 on antigen-presenting cells and CD2 on T lymphocytes plays a role in the pathophysiology of chronic plaque psoriasis. The majority of T lymphocytes in psoriatic lesions are of the memory effector phenotype characterized by the presence of the CD45RO marker,[1] express activation markers (*e.g.,* CD25, CD69) and release inflammatory cytokines, such as interferon γ.

Alefacept also causes a reduction in subsets of CD2+ T lymphocytes (primarily CD45RO+), presumably by bridging between CD2 on target lymphocytes and immunoglobulin Fc receptors on cytotoxic cells, such as natural killer cells. Treatment with alefacept results in a reduction in circulating total CD4+ and CD8+ T lymphocyte counts. CD2 is also expressed at low levels on the surface of natural killer cells and certain bone marrow B lymphocytes. Therefore, the potential exists for alefacept to affect the activation and numbers of cells other than T lymphocytes. In clinical studies of alefacept, minor changes in the numbers of circulating cells other than T lymphocytes have been observed.

PHARMACOKINETICS

In patients with moderate to severe plaque psoriasis, following a 7.5 mg IV administration, the mean volume of distribution of alefacept was 94 ml/kg, the mean clearance was 0.25 ml/h/kg, and the mean elimination half-life was approximately 270 hours. Following an IM injection, bioavailability was 63%.

The pharmacokinetics of alefacept in pediatric patients have not been studied. The effects of renal or hepatic impairment on the pharmacokinetics of alefacept have not been studied.

PHARMACODYNAMICS

At doses tested in clinical trials, alefacept therapy resulted in a dose-dependent decrease in circulating total lymphocytes.[2] This reduction predominantly affected the memory effector subset of the CD4+ and CD8+ T lymphocyte compartments (CD4+CD45RO+ and CD8+CD45RO+), the predominant phenotype in psoriatic lesions. Circulating naïve T lymphocyte and natural killer cell counts appeared to be only minimally susceptible to alefacept treatment, while circulating B lymphocyte counts appeared not to be affected by alefacept (see ADVERSE REACTIONS, Effect on Lymphocyte Counts).

INDICATIONS AND USAGE

Alefacept is indicated for the treatment of adult patients with moderate to severe chronic plaque psoriasis who are candidates for systemic therapy or phototherapy.

CONTRAINDICATIONS

Alefacept should not be administered to patients with known hypersensitivity to alefacept or any of its components.

WARNINGS

LYMPHOPENIA

AMEVIVE INDUCES DOSE-DEPENDENT REDUCTIONS IN CIRCULATING CD4+ AND CD8+ T LYMPHOCYTE COUNTS.

A COURSE OF AMEVIVE THERAPY SHOULD NOT BE INITIATED IN PATIENTS WITH A CD4+ T LYMPHOCYTE COUNT BELOW NORMAL. THE CD4+ T LYMPHOCYTE COUNTS OF PATIENTS RECEIVING AMEVIVE SHOULD BE MONITORED WEEKLY THROUGHOUT THE COURSE OF THE 12 WEEK DOSING REGIMEN. DOSING SHOULD BE WITHHELD IF CD4+ T LYMPHOCYTE COUNTS ARE BELOW 250 CELLS/μl. THE DRUG SHOULD BE DISCONTINUED IF THE COUNTS REMAIN BELOW 250 CELLS/μl FOR 1 MONTH (SEE DOSAGE AND ADMINISTRATION).

MALIGNANCIES

Alefacept may increase the risk of malignancies. Some patients who received alefacept in clinical studies developed malignancies (see ADVERSE REACTIONS, Malignancies). In preclinical studies, animals developed B cell hyperplasia, and 1 animal developed a lymphoma (see PRECAUTIONS, Carcinogenesis, Mutagenesis, and Impairment of Fertility). Alefacept should not be administered to patients with a history of systemic malignancy. Caution should be exercised when considering the use of alefacept in patients at high risk for malignancy. If a patient develops a malignancy, alefacept should be discontinued.

SERIOUS INFECTIONS

Alefacept is an immunosuppressive agent and, therefore, has the potential to increase the risk of infection and reactivate latent, chronic infections. Alefacept should not be administered to patients with a clinically important infection. Caution should be exercised when considering the use of alefacept in patients with chronic infections or a history of recurrent infection. Patients should be monitored for signs and symptoms of infection during or after a course of alefacept. New infections should be closely monitored. If a patient develops a serious infection, alefacept should be discontinued (see ADVERSE REACTIONS, Infections).

PRECAUTIONS

EFFECTS ON THE IMMUNE SYSTEM

Patients receiving other immunosuppressive agents or phototherapy should not receive concurrent therapy with alefacept because of the possibility of excessive immunosuppression. The duration of the period following treatment with alefacept before one should consider starting other immunosuppressive therapy has not been evaluated.

The safety and efficacy of vaccines, specifically live or live-attenuated vaccines, administered to patients being treated with alefacept have not been studied. In a study of 46 patients with chronic plaque psoriasis, the ability to mount immunity to tetanus toxoid (recall antigen) and an experimental neo-antigen was preserved in those patients undergoing alefacept therapy.

ALLERGIC REACTIONS

Hypersensitivity reactions (urticaria, angioedema) were associated with the administration of alefacept. If an anaphylactic reaction or other serious allergic reaction occurs, administration of alefacept should be discontinued immediately and appropriate therapy initiated.

INFORMATION FOR THE PATIENT

Patients should be informed of the need for regular monitoring of white blood cell (lymphocyte) counts during therapy and that alefacept must be administered under the supervision of a physician. Patients should also be informed that alefacept reduces lymphocyte counts, which could increase their chances of developing an infection or a malignancy. Patients should be advised to inform their physician promptly if they develop any signs of an infection or malignancy while undergoing a course of treatment with alefacept.

Female patients should also be advised to notify their physicians if they become pregnant while taking alefacept (or within 8 weeks of discontinuing alefacept) and be advised of the existence of and encouraged to enroll in the Pregnancy Registry. Call 1-866-Amevive (1-866-263-8483) to enroll into the Registry (see Pregnancy Category B).

LABORATORY TESTS

CD4+ T lymphocyte counts should be monitored weekly during the 12 week dosing period and used to guide dosing. Patients should have normal CD4+ T lymphocyte counts prior to an initial or a subsequent course of treatment with alefacept. Dosing should be withheld if CD4+ T lymphocyte counts are below 250 cells/μl. Alefacept should be discontinued if CD4+ T lymphocyte counts remain below 250 cells/μl for 1 month.

CARCINOGENESIS, MUTAGENESIS, AND IMPAIRMENT OF FERTILITY

In a chronic toxicity study, cynomolgus monkeys were dosed weekly for 52 weeks with IV alefacept at 1 mg/kg/dose or 20 mg/kg/dose. One animal in the high dose group developed a B-cell lymphoma that was detected after 28 weeks of dosing. Additional animals in both dose groups developed B-cell hyperplasia of the spleen and lymph nodes.

All animals in the study were positive for an endemic primate gammaherpes virus also known as lymphocryptovirus (LCV). Latent LCV infection is generally asymptomatic, but can lead to B-cell lymphomas when animals are immune suppressed.

In a separate study, baboons given 3 doses of alefacept at 1 mg/kg every 8 weeks were found to have centroblast proliferation in B-cell dependent areas in the germinal centers of the spleen following a 116 day washout period.

The role of alefacept in the development of the lymphoid malignancy and the hyperplasia observed in non-human primates and the relevance to humans is unknown. Immunodeficiency-associated lymphocyte disorders (plasmacytic hyperplasia, polymorphic proliferation, and B-cell lymphomas) occur in patients who have congenital or acquired immunodeficiencies including those resulting from immunosuppressive therapy.

No carcinogenicity or fertility studies were conducted.

Mutagenicity studies were conducted *in vitro* and *in vivo;* no evidence of mutagenicity was observed.

PREGNANCY CATEGORY B

Women of childbearing potential make up a considerable segment of the patient population affected by psoriasis. Since the effect of alefacept on pregnancy and fetal development, including immune system development, is not known, health care providers are encouraged to enroll patients currently taking alefacept who become pregnant into the Biogen Pregnancy Registry by calling 1-866-Amevive (1-866-263-8483).

Reproductive toxicology studies have been performed in cynomolgus monkeys at doses up to 5 mg/kg/week (about 62 times the human dose based on body weight) and have revealed no evidence of impaired fertility or harm to the fetus due to alefacept. No abortifacient or teratogenic effects were observed in cynomolgus monkeys following IV bolus injections of alefacept administered weekly during the period of organogenesis to gestation. Alefacept underwent trans-placental passage and produced *in utero* exposure in the developing monkeys. *In utero,* serum levels of exposure in these monkeys were 23% of maternal serum levels. No evidence of fetal toxicity including adverse effects on immune system development was observed in any of these animals.

Animal reproduction studies, however, are not always predictive of human response and there are no adequate and well-controlled studies in pregnant women. Because the risk to the development of the fetal immune system and postnatal immune function in humans is unknown, alefacept should be used during pregnancy only if clearly needed. If pregnancy occurs while taking alefacept, continued use of the drug should be assessed.

NURSING MOTHERS

It is not known whether alefacept is excreted in human milk. Because many drugs are excreted in human milk, and because there exists the potential for serious adverse reactions in nursing infants from alefacept, a decision should be made whether to discontinue nursing while taking the drug or to discontinue the use of the drug, taking into account the importance of the drug to the mother.

GERIATRIC USE

Of the 1357 patients who received alefacept in clinical trials, a total of 100 patients were ≥65 years of age and 13 patients were ≥75 years of age. No differences in safety or efficacy were observed between older and younger patients, but there were not sufficient data to exclude important differences. Because the incidence of infections and certain malignancies is higher in the elderly population, in general, caution should be used in treating the elderly.

PEDIATRIC USE

The safety and efficacy of alefacept in pediatric patients have not been studied. Alefacept is not indicated for pediatric patients.

DRUG INTERACTIONS

No formal interaction studies have been performed. The duration of the period following treatment with alefacept before one should consider starting other immunosuppressive therapy has not been evaluated.

ADVERSE REACTIONS

The most serious adverse reactions were:

- Lymphopenia (see WARNINGS).
- Malignancies (see WARNINGS).
- Serious infections requiring hospitalization (see WARNINGS).
- Hypersensitivity reactions (see PRECAUTIONS, Allergic Reactions).

Commonly observed adverse events seen in the first course of placebo-controlled clinical trials with at least a 2% higher incidence in the alefacept-treated patients compared to placebo-treated patients were: pharyngitis, dizziness, increased cough, nausea, pruritus, myalgia, chills, injection site pain, injection site inflammation, and accidental injury. The only adverse event that occurred at a 5% or higher incidence among alefacept-treated patients compared to placebo-treated patients was chills (1% placebo versus 6% alefacept), which occurred predominantly with IV administration.

The adverse reactions which most commonly resulted in clinical intervention were cardiovascular events including coronary artery disorder in <1% of patients and myocardial infarct in <1% of patients. These events were not observed in any of the 413 placebo-treated patients. The total number of patients hospitalized for cardiovascular events in the alefacept-treated group was 1.2% (11/876).

The most common events resulting in discontinuation of treatment with alefacept were CD4+ T lymphocyte levels below 250 cells/μl (see WARNINGS and ADVERSE REACTIONS, Effect on Lymphocyte Counts), headache (0.2%), and nausea (0.2%).

Because clinical trials are conducted under widely varying conditions, adverse event rates observed in the clinical trials of a drug cannot be directly compared to rates in the clinical trials of another drug and may not reflect the rates observed in practice. The adverse reaction information does, however, provide a basis for identifying the adverse events that appear to be related to drug use and a basis for approximating rates.

The data described below reflect exposure to alefacept in a total of 1357 psoriasis patients, 85% of whom received 1-2 courses of therapy and the rest received 3-6 courses and were followed for up to 3 years. Of the 1357 total patients, 876 received their first course in placebo-controlled studies. The population studied ranged in age from 16-84 years, and included 69% men and 31% women. The patients were mostly Caucasian (89%), reflecting the general psoriatic population. Disease severity at baseline was moderate to severe psoriasis.

EFFECT ON LYMPHOCYTE COUNTS

In the IM study (Study 2), 4% of patients temporarily discontinued treatment and no patients permanently discontinued treatment due to CD4+ T lymphocyte counts below the specified threshold of 250 cells/μl. In Study 2, 10%, 28%, and 42% of patients had total lymphocyte, CD4+, and CD8+ T lymphocyte counts below normal, respectively. Twelve weeks after a course of therapy (12 weekly doses), 2%, 8%, and 21% of patients had total lymphocyte, CD4+, and CD8+ T cell counts below normal.

In the first course of the IV study (Study 1), 10% of patients temporarily discontinued treatment and 2% permanently discontinued treatment due to CD4+ T lymphocyte counts below the specified threshold of 250 cells/μl. During the first course of Study 1, 22% of patients had total lymphocyte counts below normal, 48% had CD4+ T lymphocyte counts below normal and 59% had CD8+ T lymphocyte counts below normal. The maximal effect on lymphocytes was observed within 6-8 weeks of initiation of treatment. Twelve weeks after a course of therapy (12 weekly doses), 4% of patients had total lymphocyte counts below normal, 19% had CD4+ T lymphocyte counts below normal, and 36% had CD8+ T lymphocyte counts below normal.

For patients receiving a second course of alefacept in Study 1, 17% of patients had total lymphocyte counts below normal, 44% had CD4+ T lymphocyte counts below normal, and 56% had CD8+ T lymphocyte counts below normal. Twelve weeks after completing dosing, 3% of patients had total lymphocyte counts below normal, 17% had CD4+ T lymphocyte counts below normal, and 35% had CD8+ T lymphocyte counts below normal (see WARNINGS, and PRECAUTIONS, Laboratory Tests).

MALIGNANCIES

In the 24 week period constituting the first course of placebo-controlled studies, 13 malignancies were diagnosed in 11 alefacept-treated patients. The incidence of malignancies was 1.3% (11/876) for alefacept-treated patients compared to 0.5% (2/413) in the placebo group.

Among 1357 patients who received alefacept, 25 patients were diagnosed with 35 treatment-emergent malignancies. The majority of these malignancies (23 cases) were basal (6) or squamous cell cancers (17) of the skin. Three cases of lymphoma were observed; 1

was classified as non-Hodgkin's follicle-center cell lymphoma and 2 were classified as Hodgkin's disease.

INFECTIONS

In the 24 week period constituting the first course of placebo-controlled studies, serious infections (infections requiring hospitalization) were seen at a rate of 0.9% (8/876) in alefacept-treated patients and 0.2% (1/413) in the placebo group. In patients receiving repeated courses of alefacept therapy, the rates of serious infections were 0.7% (5/756) and 1.5% (3/199) in the second and third course of therapy, respectively. Serious infections among 1357 alefacept-treated patients included necrotizing cellulitis, peritonsillar abscess, post-operative and burn wound infection, toxic shock, pneumonia, appendicitis, pre-septal cellulitis, cholecystitis, gastroenteritis and herpes simplex infection.

HYPERSENSITIVITY REACTIONS

In clinical studies 2 patients were reported to experience angioedema, 1 of whom was hospitalized. In the 24 week period constituting the first course of placebo-controlled studies, urticaria was reported in 6 (<1%) alefacept-treated patients versus 1 patient in the control group. Urticaria resulted in discontinuation of therapy in 1 of the alefacept-treated patients.

INJECTION SITE REACTIONS

In the IM study (Study 2), 16% of alefacept-treated patients and 8% of placebo-treated patients reported injection site reactions. Reactions at the site of injection were generally mild, typically occurred on single occasions, and included either pain (7%), inflammation (4%), bleeding (4%), edema (2%), non-specific reaction (2%), mass (1%), or skin hypersensitivity (<1%). In the clinical trials, a single case of injection site reaction led to the discontinuation of alefacept.

IMMUNOGENICITY

Approximately 3% (35/1306) of patients receiving alefacept developed low-titer antibodies to alefacept. No apparent correlation of antibody development and clinical response or adverse events was observed. The long-term immunogenicity of alefacept is unknown.

The data reflect the percentage of patients whose test results were considered positive for antibodies to alefacept in an ELISA assay, and are highly dependent on the sensitivity and specificity of the assay. Additionally, the observed incidence of antibody positivity in an assay may be influenced by several factors including sample handling, timing of sample collection, concomitant medications, and underlying disease. For these reasons, comparison of the incidence of antibodies to alefacept with the incidence of antibodies to other products may be misleading.

OTHER OBSERVED ADVERSE REACTIONS FROM CLINICAL TRIALS

Less common events that were observed at a higher rate in alefacept-treated patients include rare cases (9) of transaminase elevations to 5-10 times the upper limit of normal.

DOSAGE AND ADMINISTRATION

Alefacept should only be used under the guidance and supervision of a physician.

The recommended dose of alefacept is 7.5 mg given once weekly as an IV bolus or 15 mg given once weekly as an IM injection. The recommended regimen is a course of 12 weekly injections. Retreatment with an additional 12 week course may be initiated provided that CD4+ T lymphocyte counts are within the normal range, and a minimum of a 12 week interval has passed since the previous course of treatment. Data on retreatment beyond 2 cycles are limited.

The CD4+ T lymphocyte counts of patients receiving alefacept should be monitored weekly before initiating dosing and throughout the course of the 12 week dosing regimen. Dosing should be withheld if CD4+ T lymphocyte counts are below 250 cells/μl. The drug should be discontinued if the counts remain below 250 cells/μl for 1 month (see PRECAUTIONS, Laboratory Tests).

PREPARATION INSTRUCTIONS

Alefacept should be reconstituted by a health care professional using aseptic technique. Each vial is intended for single patient use only.

Do not add other medications to solutions containing alefacept. Do not reconstitute alefacept with other diluents. Do not filter reconstituted solution during preparation or administration.

Following reconstitution, the product should be used immediately or within 4 hours if stored in the vial at 2-8°C (36-46°F). ALEFACEPT NOT USED WITHIN 4 HOURS OF RECONSTITUTION SHOULD BE DISCARDED.

ADMINISTRATION INSTRUCTIONS

For IM use, inject the full 0.5 ml of solution. Rotate injection sites so that a different site is used for each new injection. New injections should be given at least 1 inch from an old site and never into areas where the skin is tender, bruised, red, or hard.

HOW SUPPLIED

Amevive for IV administration is supplied in either a carton containing 4 administration dose packs, or in a carton containing 1 administration dose pack. Each dose pack contains one 7.5 mg single-use vial of Amevive, one 10 ml single-use diluent vial (sterile water for injection), 1 syringe, one 23 gauge, ¾ inch winged infusion set, and two 23 gauge, 1¼ inch needles.

Amevive for IM administration is supplied in either a carton containing 4 administration dose packs, or in a carton containing 1 administration dose pack. Each dose pack contains one 15 mg single-use vial of Amevive, one 10 ml single-use diluent vial (sterile water for injection), 1 syringe, and two 23 gauge, 1¼ inch needles.

Amevive is reconstituted with 0.6 ml of the 10 ml single-use diluent.

Storage: The dose tray containing Amevive (lyophilized powder) should be stored at controlled room temperature (15-30°C; 59-86°F). PROTECT FROM LIGHT. Retain in carton until time of use.

PRODUCT LISTING - EQUIVALENTS NOT AVAILABLE

Powder For Injection - Intramuscular - 15 mg

1's	$995.00	AMEVIVE, Biogen	59627-0021-04
4's	$3980.00	AMEVIVE, Biogen	59627-0021-03

Powder For Injection - Intravenous - 7.5 mg

1's	$700.00	AMEVIVE, Biogen	59627-0020-02
4's	$2800.00	AMEVIVE, Biogen	59627-0020-01

Alemtuzumab *(003522)*

For complete prescribing information, refer to the CD-ROM included with the book.

Categories: Leukemia, chronic lymphocytic; Pregnancy Category C; FDA Approved 2001 May; Orphan Drugs
Drug Classes: Antineoplastics, monoclonal antibodies; Monoclonal antibodies
Brand Names: Campath
Foreign Brand Availability: MabCampath (Austria; Belgium; Bulgaria; Czech-Republic; Denmark; England; Finland; France; Germany; Greece; Hungary; Ireland; Israel; Italy; Netherlands; Norway; Poland; Portugal; Slovenia; Spain; Sweden; Switzerland; Turkey)

WARNING

Alemtuzumab should be administered under the supervision of a physician experienced in the use of antineoplastic therapy.

Hematologic Toxicity: **Serious and, in rare instances fatal, pancytopenia/marrow hypoplasia, autoimmune idiopathic thrombocytopenia, and autoimmune hemolytic anemia have occurred in patients receiving alemtuzumab therapy. Single doses of alemtuzumab greater than 30 mg or cumulative doses greater than 90 mg/week should not be administered because these doses are associated with a higher incidence of pancytopenia.**

Infusion Reactions: **Campath can result in serious infusion reactions. Patients should be carefully monitored during infusions and alemtuzumab discontinued if indicated. (See DOSAGE AND ADMINISTRATION.) Gradual escalation to the recommended maintenance dose is required at the initiation of therapy and after interruption of therapy for 7 or more days.**

Infections, Opportunistic Infections: **Serious, sometimes fatal bacterial, viral, fungal, and protozoan infections have been reported in patients receiving alemtuzumab therapy. Prophylaxis directed against *Pneumocystis carinii* pneumonia (PCP) and herpes virus infections has been shown to decrease, but not eliminate, the occurrence of these infections.**

DESCRIPTION

Campath (alemtuzumab) is a recombinant DNA-derived humanized monoclonal antibody (Campath-1H) that is directed against the 21-28 kD cell surface glycoprotein, CD52. CD52 is expressed on the surface of normal and malignant B and T lymphocytes, NK cells, monocytes, macrophages, and tissues of the male reproductive system. The Campath-1H antibody is an IgG1 kappa with human variable framework and constant regions, and complementarity-determining regions from a murine (rat) monoclonal antibody (Campath-1G). The Campath-1H antibody has an approximate molecular weight of 150 kD.

Campath is produced in mammalian cell (Chinese hamster ovary) suspension culture in a medium containing neomycin. Neomycin is not detectable in the final product. Campath is a sterile, clear, colorless, isotonic pH 6.8-7.4 solution for injection. Each single use ampoule of Campath contains 30 mg alemtuzumab, 24.0 mg sodium chloride, 3.5 mg dibasic sodium phosphate, 0.6 mg potassium chloride, 0.6 mg monobasic potassium phosphate, 0.3 mg polysorbate 80, and 0.056 mg disodium edetate. No preservatives are added.

INDICATIONS AND USAGE

Alemtuzumab is indicated for the treatment of B-cell chronic lymphocytic leukemia (B-CLL) in patients who have been treated with alkylating agents and who have failed fludarabine therapy. Determination of the effectiveness of alemtuzumab is based on overall response rates. Comparative, randomized trials demonstrating increased survival or clinical benefits such as improvement in disease-related symptoms have not yet been conducted.

NON-FDA APPROVED INDICATIONS

Preliminary trials have studied alemtuzumab in non-Hodgkin's lymphoma, rheumatoid arthritis, severe resistant autoimmune neutropenia, refractory autoimmune thrombocytopenia purpura, T-cell prolymphocytic leukemia, cutaneous scleroderma, multiple sclerosis, refractory ocular inflammatory disease, and as an immunosuppressant in renal and bone marrow transplantation. None of these uses is approved by the FDA and comparative efficacy and safety studies have not been performed.

CONTRAINDICATIONS

Alemtuzumab is contraindicated in patients who have active systemic infections, underlying immunodeficiency (*e.g.*, seropositive for HIV), or known Type I hypersensitivity or anaphylactic reactions to alemtuzumab or to any one of its components.

WARNINGS

See BOXED WARNING.

INFUSION-RELATED EVENTS

Alemtuzumab has been associated with infusion-related events including hypotension, rigors, fever, shortness of breath, bronchospasm, chills, and/or rash. In order to ameliorate or avoid infusion-related events, patients should be premedicated with an oral antihistamine and acetaminophen prior to dosing and monitored closely for infusion-related adverse events. In addition, alemtuzumab should be initiated at a low dose with gradual escalation to the effective dose. Careful monitoring of blood pressure and hypotensive symptoms is recommended especially in patients with ischemic heart disease and in patients on antihypertensive medications. If therapy is interrupted for 7 or more days, alemtuzumab should be reinstituted with gradual dose escalation. (See DOSAGE AND ADMINISTRATION.)

IMMUNOSUPPRESSION/OPPORTUNISTIC INFECTIONS

Alemtuzumab induces profound lymphopenia. A variety of opportunistic infections have been reported in patients receiving alemtuzumab therapy. If a serious infection occurs, alemtuzumab therapy should be interrupted and may be reinitiated following the resolution of the infection.

Anti-infective prophylaxis is recommended upon initiation of therapy and for a minimum of 2 months following the last dose of alemtuzumab or until $CD4^+$ counts are ≥200 cells/µl. The median time to recovery of $CD4^+$ counts to ≥200/µl was 2 months, however, full recovery (to baseline) of $CD4^+$ and $CD8^+$ counts may take more than 12 months. (See BOXED WARNING and DOSAGE AND ADMINISTRATION.)

Because of the potential for Graft versus Host Disease (GVHD) in severely lymphopenic patients, irradiation of any blood products administered prior to recovery from lymphopenia is recommended.

HEMATOLOGIC TOXICITY

Severe, prolonged, and in rare instances fatal, myelosuppression has occurred in patients with leukemia and lymphoma receiving alemtuzumab. Bone marrow aplasia and hypoplasia were observed in the clinical studies at the recommended dose. The incidence of these complications increased with doses above the recommended dose. In addition, severe and fatal autoimmune anemia and thrombocytopenia were observed in patients with CLL. Alemtuzumab should be discontinued for severe hematologic toxicity (see TABLE 3) or in any patient with evidence of autoimmune hematologic toxicity. Following resolution of transient, non-immune myelosuppression, alemtuzumab may be reinitiated with caution. (See DOSAGE AND ADMINISTRATION.) There is no information on the safety of resumption of alemtuzumab in patients with autoimmune cytopenias or marrow aplasia.

DOSAGE AND ADMINISTRATION

Alemtuzumab should be administered under the supervision of a physician experienced in the use of antineoplastic therapy.

DOSING SCHEDULE AND ADMINISTRATION

Alemtuzumab therapy should be initiated at a dose of 3 mg administered as a 2 hour IV infusion daily. When the alemtuzumab 3 mg daily dose is tolerated (*e.g.*, infusion-related toxicities are ≤Grade 2), the daily dose should be escalated to 10 mg and continued until tolerated. When the 10 mg dose is tolerated, the maintenance dose of alemtuzumab 30 mg may be initiated. The maintenance dose of alemtuzumab is 30 mg/day administered 3 times/week on alternate days (*i.e.*, Monday, Wednesday, and Friday) for up to 12 weeks. In most patients, escalation to 30 mg can be accomplished in 3-7 days. **Dose escalation to the recommended maintenance dose of 30 mg administered 3 times/week is required. Single doses of alemtuzumab greater than 30 mg or cumulative weekly doses of greater than 90 mg should not be administered since higher doses are associated with an increased incidence of pancytopenia.** (See BOXED WARNING.) Alemtuzumab should be administered intravenously only. The infusion should be administered over a 2 hour period. **DO NOT ADMINISTER AS AN IV PUSH OR BOLUS.**

RECOMMENDED CONCOMITANT MEDICATIONS

Premedication should be given prior to the first dose, at dose escalations, and as clinically indicated. The premedication used in clinical studies was diphenhydramine 50 mg and acetaminophen 650 mg administered 30 minutes prior to alemtuzumab infusion. In cases where severe infusion-related events occur, treatment with hydrocortisone 200 mg was used in decreasing the infusion-related events.

Patients should receive anti-infective prophylaxis to minimize the risks of serious opportunistic infections. (See BOXED WARNING.) The anti-infective regimen used on Study 1 consisted of trimethoprim/sulfamethoxazole DS twice daily (bid) 3 times/week and famciclovir or equivalent 250 mg twice a day (bid) upon initiation of alemtuzumab therapy. Prophylaxis should be continued for 2 months after completion of alemtuzumab therapy or until the $CD4^+$ count is ≥200 cells/µl, whichever occurs later.

DOSE MODIFICATION AND REINITIATION OF THERAPY

Alemtuzumab therapy should be discontinued during serious infection, serious hematologic toxicity, or other serious toxicity until the event resolves. (See WARNINGS.) Alemtuzumab therapy should be permanently discontinued if evidence of autoimmune anemia or thrombocytopenia appears. TABLE 3 includes recommendations for dose modification for severe neutropenia or thrombocytopenia.

INCOMPATIBILITIES

No incompatibilities between alemtuzumab and polyvinylchloride (PVC) bags, PVC or polyethylene-lined PVC administration sets, or low-protein binding filters have been observed. No data are available concerning the incompatibility of alemtuzumab with other drug substances. Other drug substances should not be added or simultaneously infused through the same IV line.

TABLE 3 *Dose Modification and Reinitiation of Therapy for Hematologic Toxicity*

Hematologic Toxicity	Dose Modification and Reinitiation of Therapy
For first occurrence of ANC <250/µl and/or platelet count ≤25,000/µl	Withhold alemtuzumab therapy. When ANC ≥500/µl and platelet count ≥50,000/µl, resume alemtuzumab therapy at same dose. If delay between dosing is ≥7 days, initiate therapy at alemtuzumab 3 mg and escalate to 10 mg and then to 30 mg as tolerated.
For second occurrence of ANC <250/µl and/or platelet count ≤25,000/µl	Withhold alemtuzumab therapy. When ANC ≥500/µl and platelet count ≥50,000/µl, resume alemtuzumab therapy at **10 mg.** If delay between dosing is ≥7 days, initiate therapy at alemtuzumab 3 mg and escalate to **10 mg only.**
For third occurrence of ANC <250/µl and/or platelet count ≤25,000/µl	Discontinue alemtuzumab therapy permanently.
For a decrease of ANC and/or platelet count to ≤50% of the baseline value in patients initiating therapy with a baseline ANC ≤500/µl and/or a baseline platelet count ≤25,000/µl	Withhold alemtuzumab therapy. When ANC and/or platelet count return to baseline value(s), resume alemtuzumab therapy. If the delay between dosing ≥7 days, initiate therapy at alemtuzumab 3 mg and escalate to 10 mg and then to 30 mg as tolerated.

PRODUCT LISTING - EQUIVALENTS NOT AVAILABLE

Injection - Intravenous - 10 mg/ml

3 ml x 3	$5537.69	CAMPATH, Berlex Laboratories	50419-0355-10
3 ml x 12	$19372.50	CAMPATH, Berlex Laboratories	50419-0355-12

Alendronate Sodium *(003232)*

Categories: Osteoporosis, glucocorticoid-induced; Osteoporosis; Paget's disease; FDA Approved 1995 Sep; Pregnancy Category C
Drug Classes: Bisphosphonates
Brand Names: Fosamax
Foreign Brand Availability: Alend (Korea); Alovell (Indonesia); Arendal (Peru); Armol (Colombia); Bifemelan (Colombia); Bifosa (India); Eucalen (Colombia); Fosalan (Israel); Fosmin (Peru); Marvil (Peru); MaxiBone (Israel); Neobon (Colombia); Oslene (Indonesia); Osteovan (Costa-Rica); Osdronat (Colombia); Osficar (Colombia); Osteofar (Indonesia); Osticalcin (Colombia); Tibolene (Colombia); Voroste (Indonesia)
Cost of Therapy: $73.47 (Osteoporosis; Fosamax ; 10 mg; 1 tablet/day; 30 day supply)

DESCRIPTION

Alendronate sodium is a bisphosphonate that acts as a specific inhibitor of osteoclast-mediated bone resorption. Bisphosphonates are synthetic analogs of pyrophosphate that bind to the hydroxyapatite found in bone.

Alendronate sodium is chemically described as (4-amino-1-hydroxybutylidene)bisphosphonic acid monosodium salt trihydrate.

The empirical formula of alendronate sodium is $C_4H_{12}NNaO_7P_2{\cdot}3H_2O$ and its formula weight is 325.12.

Alendronate sodium is a white, crystalline, nonhygroscopic powder. It is soluble in water, very slightly soluble in alcohol, and practically insoluble in chloroform.

Fosamax for oral administration contains 6.53, 13.05, 45.68, 52.21, or 91.37 mg of alendronate monosodium salt trihydrate, which is the molar equivalent of 5, 10, 35, 40, and 70 mg, respectively, of free acid, and the following inactive ingredients: microcrystalline cellulose, anhydrous lactose, croscarmellose sodium, and magnesium stearate. Fosamax tablets 10 mg also contain carnauba wax.

CLINICAL PHARMACOLOGY

MECHANISM OF ACTION

Animal studies have indicated the following mode of action. At the cellular level, alendronate shows preferential localization to sites of bone resorption, specifically under osteoclasts. The osteoclasts adhere normally to the bone surface but lack the ruffled border that is indicative of active resorption. Alendronate does not interfere with osteoclast recruitment or attachment, but it does inhibit osteoclast activity. Studies in mice on the localization of radioactive [^{3}H]alendronate in bone showed about 10-fold higher uptake on osteoclast surfaces than on osteoblast surfaces. Bones examined 6 and 49 days after [^{3}H]alendronate administration in rats and mice, respectively, showed that normal bone was formed on top of the alendronate, which was incorporated inside the matrix. While incorporated in bone matrix, alendronate is not pharmacologically active. Thus, alendronate must be continuously administered to suppress osteoclasts on newly formed resorption surfaces. Histomorphometry in baboons and rats showed that alendronate treatment reduces bone turnover (*i.e.*, the number of sites at which bone is remodeled). In addition, bone formation exceeds bone resorption at these remodeling sites, leading to progressive gains in bone mass.

PHARMACOKINETICS

Absorption

Relative to an intravenous (IV) reference dose, the mean oral bioavailability of alendronate in women was 0.64% for doses ranging from 5-70 mg when administered after an overnight fast and 2 hours before a standardized breakfast. Oral bioavailability of the 10 mg tablet in men (0.59%) was similar to that in women when administered after an overnight fast and 2 hours before breakfast.

A study examining the effect of timing of a meal on the bioavailability of alendronate was performed in 49 postmenopausal women. Bioavailability was decreased (by approximately 40%) when 10 mg alendronate was administered either 0.5 or 1 hour before a standardized breakfast, when compared to dosing 2 hours before eating. In studies of treatment and prevention of osteoporosis, alendronate was effective when administered at least 30 minutes before breakfast.

Bioavailability was negligible whether alendronate was administered with or up to 2 hours after a standardized breakfast. Concomitant administration of alendronate with coffee or orange juice reduced bioavailability by approximately 60%.

Distribution

Preclinical studies (in male rats) show that alendronate transiently distributes to soft tissues following 1 mg/kg IV administration but is then rapidly redistributed to bone or excreted in the urine. The mean steady-state volume of distribution, exclusive of bone, is at least 28 L in humans. Concentrations of drug in plasma following therapeutic oral doses are too low (less than 5 ng/ml) for analytical detection. Protein binding in human plasma is approximately 78%.

Metabolism

There is no evidence that alendronate is metabolized in animals or humans.

Excretion

Following a single IV dose of [^{14}C]alendronate, approximately 50% of the radioactivity was excreted in the urine within 72 hours and little or no radioactivity was recovered in the feces. Following a single 10 mg IV dose, the renal clearance of alendronate was 71 ml/min (64, 78; 90% confidence interval [CI]), and systemic clearance did not exceed 200 ml/min. Plasma concentrations fell by more than 95% within 6 hours following IV administration. The terminal half-life in humans is estimated to exceed 10 years, probably reflecting release of alendronate from the skeleton. Based on the above, it is estimated that after 10 years of oral treatment with alendronate sodium tablets (10 mg daily) the amount of alendronate released daily from the skeleton is approximately 25% of that absorbed from the gastrointestinal tract.

Special Populations

Pediatric

Alendronate pharmacokinetics have not been investigated in patients <18 years of age.

Gender

Bioavailability and the fraction of an IV dose excreted in urine were similar in men and women.

Geriatric

Bioavailability and disposition (urinary excretion) were similar in elderly and younger patients. No dosage adjustment is necessary (see DOSAGE AND ADMINISTRATION).

Race

Pharmacokinetic differences due to race have not been studied.

Renal Insufficiency

Preclinical studies show that, in rats with kidney failure, increasing amounts of drug are present in plasma, kidney, spleen, and tibia. In healthy controls, drug that is not deposited in bone is rapidly excreted in the urine. No evidence of saturation of bone uptake was found after 3 weeks dosing with cumulative IV doses of 35 mg/kg in young male rats. Although no clinical information is available, it is likely that, as in animals, elimination of alendronate via the kidney will be reduced in patients with impaired renal function. Therefore, somewhat greater accumulation of alendronate in bone might be expected in patients with impaired renal function.

No dosage adjustment is necessary for patients with mild-to-moderate renal insufficiency (creatinine clearance 35-60 ml/min). **Alendronate sodium is not recommended for patients with more severe renal insufficiency (creatinine clearance <35 ml/min) due to lack of experience with alendronate in renal failure.**

Hepatic Insufficiency

As there is evidence that alendronate is not metabolized or excreted in the bile, no studies were conducted in patients with hepatic insufficiency. No dosage adjustment is necessary.

Drug Interactions

Also see DRUG INTERACTIONS.

Intravenous ranitidine was shown to double the bioavailability of oral alendronate. The clinical significance of this increased bioavailability and whether similar increases will occur in patients given oral H_2-antagonists is unknown.

In healthy subjects, oral prednisone (20 mg three times daily for 5 days) did not produce a clinically meaningful change in the oral bioavailability of alendronate (a mean increase ranging from 20-44%).

Products containing calcium and other multivalent cations are likely to interfere with absorption of alendronate.

PHARMACODYNAMICS

Alendronate is a bisphosphonate that binds to bone hydroxyapatite and specifically inhibits the activity of osteoclasts, the bone-resorbing cells. Alendronate reduces bone resorption with no direct effect on bone formation, although the latter process is ultimately reduced because bone resorption and formation are coupled during bone turnover.

Osteoporosis in Postmenopausal Women

Osteoporosis is characterized by low bone mass that leads to an increased risk of fracture. The diagnosis can be confirmed by the finding of low bone mass, evidence of fracture on x-ray, a history of osteoporotic fracture, or height loss or kyphosis, indicative of vertebral (spinal) fracture. Osteoporosis occurs in both males and females but is most common among women following the menopause, when bone turnover increases and the rate of bone resorption exceeds that of bone formation. These changes result in progressive bone loss and lead to osteoporosis in a significant proportion of women over age 50. Fractures, usually of the spine, hip, and wrist, are the common consequences. From age 50-90, the risk of hip fracture in white women increases 50-fold and the risk of vertebral fracture 15- to 30-fold. It is estimated that approximately 40% of 50-year-old women will sustain 1 or more osteoporosis-related fractures of the spine, hip, or wrist during their remaining lifetimes. Hip fractures, in particular, are associated with substantial morbidity, disability, and mortality.

Daily oral doses of alendronate (5, 20, and 40 mg for 6 weeks) in postmenopausal women produced biochemical changes indicative of dose-dependent inhibition of bone resorption, including decreases in urinary calcium and urinary markers of bone collagen degradation (such as deoxypyridinoline and cross-linked N-telopeptides of Type 1 collagen). These biochemical changes tended to return toward baseline values as early as 3 weeks following the discontinuation of therapy with alendronate and did not differ from placebo after 7 months.

Long-term treatment of osteoporosis with alendronate sodium 10 mg/day (for up to 5 years) reduced urinary excretion of markers of bone resorption, deoxypyridinoline and cross-linked N-telopeptides of Type 1 collagen, by approximately 50% and 70%, respectively, to reach levels similar to those seen in healthy premenopausal women. Similar decreases were seen in patients in osteoporosis prevention studies who received alendronate sodium 5 mg/day. The decrease in the rate of bone resorption indicated by these markers was evident as early as 1 month and at 3-6 months reached a plateau that was maintained for the entire duration of treatment with alendronate sodium. In osteoporosis treatment studies alendronate sodium 10 mg/day decreased the markers of bone formation, osteocalcin and bone specific alkaline phosphatase by approximately 50%, and total serum alkaline phosphatase, by approximately 25-30% to reach a plateau after 6-12 months. In osteoporosis prevention studies alendronate sodium 5 mg/day decreased osteocalcin and total serum alkaline phosphatase by approximately 40% and 15%, respectively. Similar reductions in the rate of bone turnover were observed in postmenopausal women during 1 year studies with once weekly alendronate sodium 70 mg for the treatment of osteoporosis and once weekly alendronate sodium 35 mg for the prevention of osteoporosis. These data indicate that the rate of bone turnover reached a new steady-state, despite the progressive increase in the total amount of alendronate deposited within bone.

As a result of inhibition of bone resorption, asymptomatic reductions in serum calcium and phosphate concentrations were also observed following treatment with alendronate sodium. In the long-term studies, reductions from baseline in serum calcium (approximately 2%) and phosphate (approximately 4-6%) were evident the first month after the initiation of alendronate sodium 10 mg. No further decreases in serum calcium were observed for the 5 year duration of treatment, however, serum phosphate returned toward prestudy levels during years 3-5. Similar reductions were observed with alendronate sodium 5 mg/day. In 1 year studies with once weekly alendronate sodium 35 and 70 mg, similar reductions were observed at 6 and 12 months. The reduction in serum phosphate may reflect not only the positive bone mineral balance due to alendronate sodium but also a decrease in renal phosphate reabsorption.

Osteoporosis in Men

Treatment of men with osteoporosis with alendronate sodium 10 mg/day for 2 years reduced urinary excretion of cross-linked N-telopeptides of Type 1 collagen by approximately 60% and bone-specific alkaline phosphatase by approximately 40%.

Glucocorticoid-Induced Osteoporosis

Sustained use of glucocorticoids is commonly associated with development of osteoporosis and resulting fractures (especially vertebral, hip, and rib). It occurs both in males and females of all ages. Osteoporosis occurs as a result of inhibited bone formation and increased bone resorption resulting in net bone loss. Alendronate decreases bone resorption without directly inhibiting bone formation.

In clinical studies of up to 2 years' duration, alendronate sodium 5 and 10 mg/day reduced cross-linked N-telopeptides of Type 1 collagen (a marker of bone resorption) by approximately 60% and reduced bone-specific alkaline phosphatase and total serum alkaline phosphatase (markers of bone formation) by approximately 15-30% and 8-18%, respectively. As a result of inhibition of bone resorption, alendronate sodium 5 and 10 mg/day induced asymptomatic decreases in serum calcium (approximately 1-2%) and serum phosphate (approximately 1-8%).

Paget's Disease of Bone

Paget's disease of bone is a chronic, focal skeletal disorder characterized by greatly increased and disorderly bone remodeling. Excessive osteoclastic bone resorption is followed by osteoblastic new bone formation, leading to the replacement of the normal bone architecture by disorganized, enlarged, and weakened bone structure.

Clinical manifestations of Paget's disease range from no symptoms to severe morbidity due to bone pain, bone deformity, pathological fractures, and neurological and other complications. Serum alkaline phosphatase, the most frequently used biochemical index of disease activity, provides an objective measure of disease severity and response to therapy.

Alendronate sodium decreases the rate of bone resorption directly, which leads to an indirect decrease in bone formation. In clinical trials, alendronate sodium 40 mg once daily for 6 months produced significant decreases in serum alkaline phosphatase as well as in urinary markers of bone collagen degradation. As a result of the inhibition of bone resorption, alendronate sodium induced generally mild, transient, and asymptomatic decreases in serum calcium and phosphate.

INDICATIONS AND USAGE

Alendronate sodium is indicated for:

Treatment and prevention of osteoporosis in postmenopausal women.

For the treatment of osteoporosis, alendronate sodium increases bone mass and reduces the incidence of fractures, including those of the hip and spine (vertebral compression fractures). Osteoporosis may be confirmed by the finding of low bone mass (for example, at least 2 standard deviations below the premenopausal mean) or by the presence or history of osteoporotic fracture. (See CLINICAL PHARMACOLOGY, Pharmacodynamics.)

For the prevention of osteoporosis, alendronate sodium may be considered in postmenopausal women who are at risk of developing osteoporosis and for whom the desired clinical outcome is to maintain bone mass and to reduce the risk of future fracture. Bone loss is particularly rapid in postmenopausal women younger than age 60. Risk factors often associated with the development of postmenopausal osteoporosis include early menopause; moderately low bone mass (for example, at least 1 standard deviation below the mean for healthy young adult women); thin body build; Caucasian or Asian race; and family history of osteoporosis. The presence of such risk factors may be important when considering the use of alendronate sodium for prevention of osteoporosis.

Treatment to increase bone mass in men with osteoporosis.

Treatment of glucocorticoid-induced osteoporosis in men and women receiving glucocorticoids in a daily dosage equivalent to 7.5 mg or greater of prednisone and who have low bone mineral density (see PRECAUTIONS, Glucocorticoid-Induced Osteoporosis). Patients treated with glucocorticoids should receive adequate amounts of calcium and vitamin D.

Treatment of Paget's disease of bone in men and women.

Treatment is indicated in patients with Paget's disease of bone having alkaline phosphatase at least 2 times the upper limit of normal, or those who are symptomatic, or those at risk for future complications from their disease.

NON-FDA APPROVED INDICATIONS

Preliminary data have shown alendronate to reduce bone turnover in early rheumatoid arthritis. Alendronate has been used in patients with severe secondary hyperparathyroidism to prevent post parathyroidectomy induced hypocalcemia.

CONTRAINDICATIONS

Abnormalities of the esophagus which delay esophageal emptying such as stricture or achalasia.

Inability to stand or sit upright for at least 30 minutes.

Hypersensitivity to any component of this product.

Hypocalcemia (see PRECAUTIONS, General).

WARNINGS

Alendronate sodium, like other bisphosphonates, may cause local irritation of the upper gastrointestinal mucosa.

Esophageal adverse experiences, such as esophagitis, esophageal ulcers and esophageal erosions, occasionally with bleeding and rarely followed by esophageal stricture or perforation, have been reported in patients receiving treatment with alendronate sodium. In some cases these have been severe and required hospitalization. Physicians should therefore be alert to any signs or symptoms signaling a possible esophageal reaction and patients should be instructed to discontinue alendronate sodium and seek medical attention if they develop dysphagia, odynophagia, retrosternal pain or new or worsening heartburn.

The risk of severe esophageal adverse experiences appears to be greater in patients who lie down after taking alendronate sodium and/or who fail to swallow it with a full glass (6-8 oz) of water, and/or who continue to take alendronate sodium after developing symptoms suggestive of esophageal irritation. Therefore, it is very important that the full dosing instructions are provided to, and understood by, the patient (see DOSAGE AND ADMINISTRATION). In patients who cannot comply with dosing instructions due to mental disability, therapy with alendronate sodium should be used under appropriate supervision.

Because of possible irritant effects of alendronate sodium on the upper gastrointestinal mucosa and a potential for worsening of the underlying disease, caution should be used when alendronate sodium is given to patients with active upper gastrointestinal problems (such as dysphagia, esophageal diseases, gastritis, duodenitis, or ulcers).

There have been postmarketing reports of gastric and duodenal ulcers, some severe and with complications, although no increased risk was observed in controlled clinical trials.

PRECAUTIONS

GENERAL

Causes of osteoporosis other than estrogen deficiency, aging, and glucocorticoid use should be considered.

Hypocalcemia must be corrected before initiating therapy with alendronate sodium (see CONTRAINDICATIONS). Other disturbances of mineral metabolism (such as vitamin D deficiency) should also be effectively treated. Presumably due to the effects of alendronate sodium on increasing bone mineral, small, asymptomatic decreases in serum calcium and phosphate may occur, especially in patients with Paget's disease, in whom the pretreatment rate of bone turnover may be greatly elevated and in patients receiving glucocorticoids, in whom calcium absorption may be decreased.

Ensuring adequate calcium and vitamin D intake is especially important in patients with Paget's disease of bone and in patients receiving glucocorticoids.

RENAL INSUFFICIENCY

Alendronate sodium is not recommended for patients with renal insufficiency (creatinine clearance <35 ml/min). (See DOSAGE AND ADMINISTRATION.)

GLUCOCORTICOID-INDUCED OSTEOPOROSIS

The risk versus benefit of alendronate sodium for treatment at daily dosages of glucocorticoids less than 7.5 mg of prednisone or equivalent has not been established (see INDICATIONS AND USAGE). Before initiating treatment, the hormonal status of both men and women should be ascertained and appropriate replacement considered.

A bone mineral density measurement should be made at the initiation of therapy and repeated after 6-12 months of combined alendronate sodium and glucocorticoid treatment.

The efficacy of alendronate sodium for the treatment of glucocorticoid-induced osteoporosis has been shown in patients with a median bone mineral density which was 1.2 standard deviations below the mean for healthy young adults.

The efficacy of alendronate sodium has been established in studies of 2 years' duration. The greatest increase in bone mineral density occurred in the first year with maintenance or smaller gains during the second year. Efficacy of alendronate sodium beyond 2 years has not been studied.

The efficacy of alendronate sodium in respect to fracture prevention has been demonstrated for vertebral fractures. However, this finding was based on very few fractures that occurred primarily in postmenopausal women. The efficacy for prevention of nonvertebral fractures has not been demonstrated.

INFORMATION FOR THE PATIENT

General

Physicians should instruct their patients to read the patient package insert before starting therapy with alendronate sodium and to reread it each time the prescription is renewed.

Patients should be instructed to take supplemental calcium and vitamin D, if daily dietary intake is inadequate. Weight-bearing exercise should be considered along with the modification of certain behavioral factors, such as cigarette smoking and/or excessive alcohol consumption, if these factors exist.

Dosing Instructions

Patients should be instructed that the expected benefits of alendronate sodium may only be obtained when each tablet is swallowed with plain water the first thing upon arising for the day at least 30 minutes before the first food, beverage, or medication of the day. Even dosing with orange juice or coffee has been shown to markedly reduce the absorption of alendronate sodium (see CLINICAL PHARMACOLOGY, Pharmacokinetics, Absorption).

To facilitate delivery to the stomach and thus reduce the potential for esophageal irritation patients should be instructed to swallow alendronate sodium with a full glass of water (6-8 oz) and not to lie down for at least 30 minutes and until after their first food of the day. Patients should not chew or suck on the tablet because of a potential for oropharyngeal ulceration. Patients should be specifically instructed not to take alendronate sodium at bedtime or before arising for the day. Patients should be informed that failure to follow these instructions may increase their risk of esophageal problems. Patients should be instructed that if they develop symptoms of esophageal disease (such as difficulty or pain upon swallowing, retrosternal pain or new or worsening heartburn) they should stop taking alendronate sodium and consult their physician.

Patients should be instructed that if they miss a dose of once weekly alendronate sodium, they should take 1 tablet on the morning after they remember. They should not take 2 tablets on the same day but should return to taking 1 tablet once a week, as originally scheduled on their chosen day.

CARCINOGENESIS, MUTAGENESIS, AND IMPAIRMENT OF FERTILITY

Harderian gland (a retro-orbital gland not present in human) adenomas were increased in high-dose female mice (p=0.003) in a 92 week oral carcinogenicity study at doses of alendronate of 1, 3, and 10 mg/kg/day (males) or 1, 2, and 5 mg/kg/day (females). These doses are equivalent to 0.12 to 1.2 times a maximum recommended daily dose of 40 mg (Paget's disease) based on surface area, mg/m^2. The relevance of this finding to humans is unknown.

Parafollicular cell (thyroid) adenomas were increased in high-dose male rats (p=0.003) in a 2 year carcinogenicity study at doses of 1 and 3.75 mg/kg body weight. These doses are equivalent to 0.26 and 1 times a 40 mg human daily dose based on surface area, mg/m^2. The relevance of this finding to humans is unknown.

Alendronate was not genotoxic in the *in vitro* microbial mutagenesis assay with and without metabolic activation, in an *in vitro* mammalian cell mutagenesis assay, in an *in vitro* alkaline elution assay in rat hepatocytes, and in an *in vivo* chromosomal aberration assay in mice. In an *in vitro* chromosomal aberration assay in Chinese hamster ovary cells, however, alendronate gave equivocal results.

Alendronate had no effect on fertility (male or female) in rats at oral doses up to 5 mg/kg/day (1.3 times a 40 mg human daily dose based on surface area, mg/m^2).

PREGNANCY CATEGORY C

Reproduction studies in rats showed decreased postimplantation survival at 2 mg/kg/day and decreased body weight gain in normal pups at 1 mg/kg/day. Sites of incomplete fetal ossification were statistically significantly increased in rats beginning at 10 mg/kg/day in vertebral (cervical, thoracic, and lumbar), skull, and sternebral bones. The above doses ranged from 0.26 times (1 mg/kg) to 2.6 times (10 mg/kg) a maximum recommended daily dose of 40 mg (Paget's disease) based on surface area, mg/m^2. No similar fetal effects were seen when pregnant rabbits were treated at doses up to 35 mg/kg/day (10.3 times the 40 mg human daily dose based on surface area, mg/m^2).

Both total and ionized calcium decreased in pregnant rats at 15 mg/kg/day (3.9 times a 40 mg human daily dose based on surface area, mg/m^2) resulting in delays and failures of delivery. Protracted parturition due to maternal hypocalcemia occurred in rats at doses as low as 0.5 mg/kg/day (0.13 times a 40 mg human daily dose based on surface area, mg/m^2) when rats were treated from before mating through gestation. Maternotoxicity (late pregnancy deaths) occurred in the female rats treated with 15 mg/kg/day for varying periods of time ranging from treatment only during pre-mating to treatment only during early, middle, or late gestation; these deaths were lessened but not eliminated by cessation of treatment. Calcium supplementation either in the drinking water or by minipump could not ameliorate the hypocalcemia or prevent maternal and neonatal deaths due to delays in delivery; calcium supplementation IV prevented maternal, but not fetal deaths.

There are no studies in pregnant women. Alendronate sodium should be used during pregnancy only if the potential benefit justifies the potential risk to the mother and fetus.

NURSING MOTHERS

It is not known whether alendronate is excreted in human milk. Because many drugs are excreted in human milk, caution should be exercised when alendronate is administered to nursing women.

PEDIATRIC USE

Safety and effectiveness in pediatric patients have not been established.

GERIATRIC USE

Of the patients receiving alendronate sodium in the Fracture Intervention Trial (FIT), 71% (n=2302) were ≥65 years of age and 17% (n=550) were ≥75 years of age. Of the patients receiving alendronate sodium in the US and Multinational osteoporosis treatment studies in women, the osteoporosis study in men, glucocorticoid-induced osteoporosis studies, and Paget's disease studies, 45%, 50%, 37%, and 70%, respectively, were 65 years of age or over. No overall differences in efficacy or safety were observed between these patients and younger patients, but greater sensitivity of some older individuals cannot be ruled out.

DRUG INTERACTIONS

Also see CLINICAL PHARMACOLOGY, Pharmacokinetics, Drug Interactions.

ESTROGEN/HORMONE REPLACEMENT THERAPY (HRT)

Concomitant use of HRT (estrogen ± progestin) and alendronate sodium was assessed in two clinical studies of 1 or 2 years' duration in postmenopausal osteoporotic women. In these studies, the safety and tolerability profile of the combination was consistent with those of the individual treatments; however, the degree of suppression of bone turnover (as assessed by mineralizing surface) was significantly greater with the combination than with either component alone. The long-term effects of combined alendronate sodium and HRT on fracture occurrence have not been studied (see ADVERSE REACTIONS, Clinical Studies, Concomitant Use With Estrogen/Hormone Replacement Therapy).

CALCIUM SUPPLEMENTS/ANTACIDS

It is likely that calcium supplements, antacids, and some oral medications will interfere with absorption of alendronate sodium. Therefore, patients must wait at least one-half hour after taking alendronate sodium before taking any other oral medications.

ASPIRIN

In clinical studies, the incidence of upper gastrointestinal adverse events was increased in patients receiving concomitant therapy with doses of alendronate sodium greater than 10 mg and aspirin-containing products.

NONSTEROIDAL ANTI-INFLAMMATORY DRUGS (NSAIDS)

Alendronate sodium may be administered to patients taking NSAIDs. In a 3 year, controlled, clinical study (n=2027) during which a majority of patients received concomitant NSAIDs, the incidence of upper gastrointestinal adverse events was similar in patients taking alendronate sodium 5 or 10 mg/day compared to those taking placebo. However, since NSAID use is associated with gastrointestinal irritation, caution should be used during concomitant use with alendronate sodium.

ADVERSE REACTIONS

CLINICAL STUDIES

In clinical studies of up to 5 years in duration adverse experiences associated with alendronate sodium usually were mild, and generally did not require discontinuation of therapy.

Alendronate sodium has been evaluated for safety in approximately 8000 postmenopausal women in clinical studies.

Treatment of Osteoporosis

Postmenopausal Women

In two identically designed, 3 year, placebo-controlled, double-blind, multicenter studies (US and Multinational; n=994), discontinuation of therapy due to any clinical adverse experience occurred in 4.1% of 196 patients treated with alendronate sodium 10 mg/day and 6.0% of 397 patients treated with placebo. In the Fracture Intervention Trial (n=6459), discontinuation of therapy due to any clinical adverse experience occurred in 9.1% of 3236 patients treated with alendronate sodium 5 mg/day for 2 years and 10 mg/day for either 1 or 2 additional years and 10.1% of 3223 patients treated with placebo. Discontinuations due to upper gastrointestinal adverse experiences were: alendronate sodium, 3.2%; placebo, 2.7%. In these study populations, 49-54% had a history of gastrointestinal disorders at baseline and 54-89% used nonsteroidal anti-inflammatory drugs or aspirin at some time during the studies. Adverse experiences from these studies considered by the investigators as possibly, probably, or definitely drug related in ≥1% of patients treated with either alendronate sodium or placebo are presented in TABLE 3.

Rarely, rash and erythema have occurred.

One patient treated with alendronate sodium (10 mg/day), who had a history of peptic ulcer disease and gastrectomy and who was taking concomitant aspirin developed an anastomotic ulcer with mild hemorrhage, which was considered drug related. Aspirin and alendronate sodium were discontinued and the patient recovered.

The adverse experience profile was similar for the 401 patients treated with either 5 or 20 mg doses of alendronate sodium in the US and Multinational studies. The adverse experience profile for the 296 patients who received continued treatment with either 5 or 10 mg doses of alendronate sodium in the 2 year extension of these studies (treatment years 4 and 5) was similar to that observed during the 3 year placebo-controlled period. During the extension period, of the 151 patients treated with alendronate sodium 10 mg/day, the proportion of patients who discontinued therapy due to any clinical adverse experience was similar to that during the first 3 years of the study.

In a 1 year, double-blind multicenter study, the overall safety and tolerability profiles of once weekly alendronate sodium 70 mg and alendronate sodium 10 mg daily were similar. The adverse experiences considered by the investigators as possibly, probably, or definitely drug related in ≥1% of patients in either treatment group are presented in TABLE 4.

Men

In a 2 year, placebo-controlled, double-blind, multicenter study, discontinuation of therapy due to any clinical adverse experience occurred in 2.7% of men treated with alendronate sodium 10 mg/day and 10.5% of men treated with placebo. The adverse experiences considered by the investigators as possibly, probably, or definitely drug related in ≥2% of patients treated with either alendronate sodium 10 mg/day or placebo are presented in TABLE 5.

Prevention of Osteoporosis in Postmenopausal Women

The safety of alendronate sodium 5 mg/day in postmenopausal women 40-60 years of age has been evaluated in three double-blind, placebo-controlled studies involving over 1400 patients randomized to receive alendronate sodium for either 2 or 3 years. In these studies the overall safety profiles of alendronate sodium 5 mg/day and placebo were similar. Discontinuation of therapy due to any clinical adverse experience occurred in 7.5% of 642 patients treated with alendronate sodium 5 mg/day and 5.7% of 648 patients treated with placebo.

In a 1 year, double-blind multicenter study, the overall safety and tolerability profiles of once weekly alendronate sodium 35 mg and alendronate sodium 5 mg daily were similar.

The adverse experiences from these studies considered by the investigators as possibly, probably, or definitely drug related in ≥1% of patients treated with either once weekly alendronate sodium 35 mg, alendronate sodium 5 mg/day, or placebo are presented in TABLE 6.

TABLE 3 *Osteoporosis Treatment Studies in Postmenopausal Women — Adverse experiences considered possibly, probably, or definitely drug related by the investigators and reported in ≥1% of patients*

	US/Multinational Studies		Fracture Intervention Trial	
	Alendronate Sodium* (n=196)	Placebo (n=397)	Alendronate Sodium† (n=3236)	Placebo (n=3223)
Gastrointestinal				
Abdominal pain	6.6%	4.8%	1.5%	1.5%
Nausea	3.6%	4.0%	1.1%	1.5%
Dyspepsia	3.6%	3.5%	1.1%	1.2%
Constipation	3.1%	1.8%	0.0%	0.2%
Diarrhea	3.1%	1.8%	0.6%	0.3%
Flatulence	2.6%	0.5%	0.2%	0.3%
Acid regurgitation	2.0%	4.3%	1.1%	0.9%
Esophageal ulcer	1.5%	0.0%	0.1%	0.1%
Vomiting	1.0%	1.5%	0.2%	0.3%
Dysphagia	1.0%	0.0%	0.1%	0.1%
Abdominal distention	1.0%	0.8%	0.0%	0.0%
Gastritis	0.5%	1.3%	0.6%	0.7%
Musculoskeletal				
Musculoskeletal (bone, muscle, or joint) pain	4.1%	2.5%	0.4%	0.3%
Muscle cramp	0.0%	1.0%	0.2%	0.1%
Nervous System/Psychiatric				
Headache	2.6%	1.5%	0.2%	0.2%
Dizziness	0.0%	1.0%	0.0%	0.1%
Special Senses				
Taste perversion	0.5%	1.0%	0.1%	0.0%

* 10 mg/day for 3 years.
† 5 mg/day for 2 years and 10 mg/day for either 1 or 2 additional years.

TABLE 4 *Osteoporosis Treatment Studies in Postmenopausal Women — Adverse experiences considered possibly, probably, or definitely drug related by the investigators and reported in ≥1% of patients*

	Alendronate Sodium	
	Once Weekly 70 mg (n=519)	10 mg/day (n=370)
Gastrointestinal		
Abdominal pain	3.7%	3.0%
Dyspepsia	2.7%	2.2%
Acid regurgitation	1.9%	2.4%
Nausea	1.9%	2.4%
Abdominal distension	1.0%	1.4%
Constipation	0.8%	1.6%
Flatulence	0.4%	1.6%
Gastritis	0.2%	1.1%
Gastric ulcer	0.0%	1.1%
Musculoskeletal		
Musculoskeletal (bone, muscle, joint) pain	2.9%	3.2%
Muscle cramp	0.2%	1.1%

TABLE 5 *Osteoporosis Study in Men — Adverse experiences considered possibly, probably, or definitely drug related by the investigators and reported in ≥2% of patients*

	Alendronate Sodium 10 mg/day (n=146)	Placebo (n=95)
Gastrointestinal		
Acid regurgitation	4.1%	3.2%
Flatulence	4.1%	1.1%
Dyspepsia	3.4%	0.0%
Abdominal pain	2.1%	1.1%
Nausea	2.1%	0.0%

Concomitant Use With Estrogen/Hormone Replacement Therapy

In two studies (of 1 and 2 years' duration) of postmenopausal osteoporotic women (total: n=853), the safety and tolerability profile of combined treatment with alendronate sodium 10 mg once daily and estrogen ± progestin (n=354) was consistent with those of the individual treatments.

Treatment of Glucocorticoid-Induced Osteoporosis

In two, 1 year, placebo-controlled, double-blind, multicenter studies in patients receiving glucocorticoid treatment, the overall safety and tolerability profiles of alendronate sodium 5 and 10 mg/day were generally similar to that of placebo. The adverse experiences con-

TABLE 6 *Osteoporosis Prevention Studies in Postmenopausal Women — Adverse experiences considered possibly, probably, or definitely drug related by the investigators and reported in ≥1% of patients*

	2 and 3 Year Studies		1 Year Study	
	Alendronate Sodium 5 mg/day (n=642)	Placebo (n=648)	Alendronate Sodium 5 mg/day (n=361)	Once Weekly Alendronate Sodium 35 mg (n=362)
Gastrointestinal				
Dyspepsia	1.9%	1.4%	2.2%	1.7%
Abdominal pain	1.7%	3.4%	4.2%	2.2%
Acid regurgitation	1.4%	2.5%	4.2%	4.7%
Nausea	1.4%	1.4%	2.5%	1.4%
Diarrhea	1.1%	1.7%	1.1%	0.6%
Constipation	0.9%	0.5%	1.7%	0.3%
Abdominal distension	0.2%	0.3%	1.4%	1.1%
Musculoskeletal				
Musculoskeletal (bone, muscle, or joint) pain	0.8%	0.9%	1.9%	2.2%

sidered by the investigators as possibly, probably, or definitely drug related in ≥1% of patients treated with either alendronate sodium 5 or 10 mg/day or placebo are presented in TABLE 7.

TABLE 7 *One Year Studies in Glucocorticoid-Treated Patients — Adverse experiences considered possibly, probably, or definitely drug related by the investigators and reported in ≥1% of patients*

	Alendronate Sodium		
	10 mg/day (n=157)	5 mg/day (n=161)	Placebo (n=159)
Gastrointestinal			
Abdominal pain	3.2%	1.9%	0.0%
Acid regurgitation	2.5%	1.9%	1.3%
Constipation	1.3%	0.6%	0.0%
Melena	1.3%	0.0%	0.0%
Nausea	0.6%	1.2%	0.6%
Diarrhea	0.0%	0.0%	1.3%
Nervous System/Psychiatric			
Headache	0.6%	0.0%	1.3%

The overall safety and tolerability profile in the glucocorticoid-induced osteoporosis population that continued therapy for the second year of the studies (alendronate sodium: n=147) was consistent with that observed in the first year.

Paget's Disease of Bone

In clinical studies (osteoporosis and Paget's disease), adverse experiences reported in 175 patients taking alendronate sodium 40 mg/day for 3-12 months were similar to those in postmenopausal women treated with alendronate sodium 10 mg/day. However, there was an apparent increased incidence of upper gastrointestinal adverse experiences in patients taking alendronate sodium 40 mg/day (17.7% alendronate sodium vs 10.2% placebo). One case of esophagitis and 2 cases of gastritis resulted in discontinuation of treatment.

Additionally, musculoskeletal (bone, muscle, or joint) pain, which has been described in patients with Paget's disease treated with other bisphosphonates, was considered by the investigators as possibly, probably, or definitely drug related in approximately 6% of patients treated with alendronate sodium 40 mg/day versus approximately 1% of patients treated with placebo, but rarely resulted in discontinuation of therapy. Discontinuation of therapy due to any clinical adverse experience occurred in 6.4% of patients with Paget's disease treated with alendronate sodium 40 mg/day and 2.4% of patients treated with placebo.

Laboratory Test Findings

In double-blind, multicenter, controlled studies, asymptomatic, mild, and transient decreases in serum calcium and phosphate were observed in approximately 18% and 10%, respectively, of patients taking alendronate sodium versus approximately 12% and 3% of those taking placebo. However, the incidences of decreases in serum calcium to <8.0 mg/dl (2.0 mM) and serum phosphate to ≤2.0 mg/dl (0.65 mM) were similar in both treatment groups.

POSTMARKETING EXPERIENCE

The following adverse reactions have been reported in postmarketing use:

Body as a Whole: Hypersensitivity reactions including urticaria and rarely angioedema.

Gastrointestinal: Esophagitis, esophageal erosions, esophageal ulcers, rarely esophageal stricture or perforation, and oropharyngeal ulceration. Gastric or duodenal ulcers, some severe and with complications have also been reported (see WARNINGS; PRECAUTIONS, Information for the Patient; and DOSAGE AND ADMINISTRATION).

Skin: Rash (occasionally with photosensitivity).

Special Senses: Rarely uveitis.

DOSAGE AND ADMINISTRATION

Alendronate sodium must be taken *at least* one-half hour before the first food, beverage, or medication of the day with plain water only (see PRECAUTIONS, Information for the Patient). Other beverages (including mineral water), food, and some medications are likely to reduce the absorption of alendronate sodium (see DRUG INTERACTIONS). Waiting less than 30 minutes, or taking alendronate sodium with food, beverages (other than plain water) or other medications will lessen the effect of alendronate sodium by decreasing its absorption into the body.

To facilitate delivery to the stomach and thus reduce the potential for esophageal irritation, alendronate sodium should only be swallowed upon arising for the day with a full glass of water (6-8 oz) and patients should not lie down for at least 30 minutes and until after their first food of the day. Alendronate sodium should not be taken at bedtime or before arising for the day. Failure to follow these instructions may increase the risk of esophageal adverse experiences (see WARNINGS and PRECAUTIONS, Information for the Patient).

Patients should receive supplemental calcium and vitamin D, if dietary intake is inadequate (see PRECAUTIONS, General).

No dosage adjustment is necessary for the elderly or for patients with mild-to-moderate renal insufficiency (creatinine clearance 35-60 ml/min). Alendronate sodium is not recommended for patients with more severe renal insufficiency (creatinine clearance <35 ml/min) due to lack of experience.

TREATMENT OF OSTEOPOROSIS IN POSTMENOPAUSAL WOMEN

See INDICATIONS AND USAGE.

The recommended dosage is:

- One 70 mg tablet once weekly; or
- One 10 mg tablet once daily.

TREATMENT TO INCREASE BONE MASS IN MEN WITH OSTEOPOROSIS

The recommended dosage is one 10 mg tablet once daily.

Alternatively, one 70 mg tablet once weekly may be considered.

PREVENTION OF OSTEOPOROSIS IN POSTMENOPAUSAL WOMEN

See INDICATIONS AND USAGE.

The recommended dosage is:

- One 35 mg tablet once weekly; or
- One 5 mg tablet once daily.

The safety of treatment and prevention of osteoporosis with alendronate sodium has been studied for up to 7 years.

TREATMENT OF GLUCOCORTICOID-INDUCED OSTEOPOROSIS IN MEN AND WOMEN

The recommended dosage is one 5 mg tablet once a day, except for postmenopausal women not receiving estrogen, for whom the recommended dosage is one 10 mg tablet once a day.

PAGET'S DISEASE OF BONE IN MEN AND WOMEN

The recommended treatment regimen is 40 mg once a day for 6 months.

RETREATMENT OF PAGET'S DISEASE

In clinical studies in which patients were followed every 6 months, relapses during the 12 months following therapy occurred in 9% (3 out of 32) of patients who responded to treatment with alendronate sodium. Specific retreatment data are not available, although responses to alendronate sodium were similar in patients who had received prior bisphosphonate therapy and those who had not. Retreatment with alendronate sodium may be considered, following a 6 month post-treatment evaluation period in patients who have relapsed, based on increases in serum alkaline phosphatase, which should be measured periodically. Retreatment may also be considered in those who failed to normalize their serum alkaline phosphatase.

ANIMAL PHARMACOLOGY

The relative inhibitory activities on bone resorption and mineralization of alendronate and etidronate were compared in the Schenk assay, which is based on histological examination of the epiphyses of growing rats. In this assay, the lowest dose of alendronate that interfered with bone mineralization (leading to osteomalacia) was 6000-fold the antiresorptive dose. The corresponding ratio for etidronate was 1 to 1. These data suggest that alendronate administered in therapeutic doses is highly unlikely to induce osteomalacia.

HOW SUPPLIED

Fosamax Tablets are available in:

5 mg: White, round, uncoated tablets with an outline of a bone image on one side and code "MRK 925" on the other.

10 mg: White, oval, wax-polished tablets with code "MRK" on one side and "936" on the other.

35 mg: White, oval, uncoated tablets with code "77" on one side and a bone image on the other.

40 mg: White, triangular-shaped, uncoated tablets with code "MRK 212" on one side and "FOSAMAX" on the other.

70 mg: White, oval, uncoated tablets with code "31" on one side and an outline of a bone image on the other.

Storage: Store in a well-closed container at controlled room temperature 15-30°C (59-86°F).

PRODUCT LISTING - EQUIVALENTS NOT AVAILABLE

Tablet - Oral - 5 mg

30's	$73.47	FOSAMAX, Merck & Company Inc	00006-0925-31
100's	$244.91	FOSAMAX, Merck & Company Inc	00006-0925-58

Tablet - Oral - 10 mg

30's	$66.15	FOSAMAX, Allscripts Pharmaceutical Company	54569-4866-00
30's	$73.47	FOSAMAX, Merck & Company Inc	00006-0936-31
31 x 25	$1441.01	FOSAMAX, Merck & Company Inc	00006-0936-72
100's	$244.91	FOSAMAX, Merck & Company Inc	00006-0936-28
100's	$244.91	FOSAMAX, Merck & Company Inc	00006-0936-58

Tablet - Oral - 35 mg

4's	$68.58	FOSAMAX, Merck & Company Inc	00006-0077-44
20's	$342.93	FOSAMAX, Merck & Company Inc	00006-0077-21

Tablet - Oral - 40 mg

30's	$165.64	FOSAMAX, Merck & Company Inc	00006-0212-31

Tablet - Oral - 70 mg

4's	$68.58	FOSAMAX, Merck & Company Inc	00006-0031-44
4's	$68.58	FOSAMAX, Southwood Pharmaceuticals Inc	58016-0613-04
20's	$342.93	FOSAMAX, Merck & Company Inc	00006-0031-21

Alfentanil Hydrochloride *(000122)*

For complete prescribing information, refer to the CD-ROM included with the book.

For related information, see the comparative table section in Appendix A.

Categories: Anesthesia, adjunct; Anesthesia, general; Pregnancy Category C; DEA Class CII; FDA Approved 1986 Dec
Drug Classes: Analgesics, narcotic
Brand Names: Alfenta
Foreign Brand Availability: Rapifen (Australia; Austria; Belgium; Czech-Republic; Denmark; England; Finland; France; Germany; Greece; Hong-Kong; Hungary; Israel; Italy; Mexico; Netherlands; New-Zealand; Norway; Portugal; South-Africa; Sweden; Switzerland; Taiwan)

DESCRIPTION

Alfentanil HCl injection is an opioid analgesic chemically designated as N-[1-[2-(4-ethyl-4,5-dihydro-5-oxo-1H-tetrazol-1-yl)ethyl]-4-(methoxymethyl)-4-piperidinyl]-N-phenylpropanamide monohydrochloride (1:1) with a molecular weight of 452.98.

Alfenta is a sterile, non-pyrogenic, preservative free aqueous solution containing alfentanil HCl equivalent to 500 µg/ml of alfentanil base for intravenous injection. The solution, which contains sodium chloride for isotonicity, has a pH range of 4.0-6.0.

INDICATIONS AND USAGE

Alfentanil HCl is Indicated:

- As an analgesic adjunct given in incremental doses in the maintenance of anesthesia with barbiturate/nitrous oxide/oxygen.
- As an analgesic administered by continuous infusion with nitrous oxide/oxygen in the maintenance of general anesthesia.
- As a primary anesthetic agent for the induction of anesthesia in patients undergoing general surgery in which endotracheal intubation and mechanical ventilation are required.
- As the analgesic component for monitored anesthesia care (MAC).

SEE TABLE 1 FOR MORE COMPLETE INFORMATION ON THE USE OF ALFENTANIL.

NON-FDA APPROVED INDICATIONS

Alfentanil has also been used as a continuous epidural infusion or epidural bolus injection for postoperative pain relief and in combination with bupivacaine for pain associated with labor. Alfentanil has also been used for patient controlled analgesia during procedures such as wound dressing changes, vaginal ovum pickup procedure, and extracorporeal shock wave lithotripsy. These uses are not currently approved by the FDA.

CONTRAINDICATIONS

Alfentanil HCl is contraindicated in patients with known hypersensitivity to the drug.

WARNINGS

ALFENTANIL SHOULD BE ADMINISTERED ONLY BY PERSONS SPECIFICALLY TRAINED IN THE USE OF INTRAVENOUS AND GENERAL ANESTHETIC AGENTS AND IN THE MANAGEMENT OF RESPIRATORY EFFECTS OF POTENT OPIOIDS.

AN OPIOID ANTAGONIST, RESUSCITATIVE AND INTUBATION EQUIPMENT AND OXYGEN SHOULD BE READILY AVAILABLE.

BECAUSE OF THE POSSIBILITY OF DELAYED RESPIRATORY DEPRESSION, MONITORING OF THE PATIENT MUST CONTINUE WELL AFTER SURGERY.

Alfentanil HCl administered in initial dosages up to 20 µg/kg may cause skeletal muscle rigidity, particularly of the truncal muscles. The incidence and severity of muscle rigidity is usually dose- related. Administration of alfentanil at anesthetic induction dosages (above 130 µg/kg) will consistently produce muscular rigidity with an immediate onset. The onset of muscular rigidity occurs earlier than with other opioids. Alfentanil may produce muscular rigidity that involves all skeletal muscles, including those of the neck and extremities. The incidence may be reduced by: 1) routine methods of administration of neuromuscular blocking agents for balanced opioid anesthesia; 2) administration of up to 1/4 of the full paralyzing dose of a neuromuscular blocking agent just prior to administration of alfentanil at dosages up to 130 µg/kg; following loss of consciousness, a full paralyzing dose of a neuromuscular blocking agent should be administered; or 3) simultaneous administration of alfentanil and a full paralyzing dose of a neuromuscular blocking agent when alfentanil is used in rapidly administered anesthetic dosages (above 130 µg/kg).

The neuromuscular blocking agent used should be appropriate for the patient's cardiovascular status. Adequate facilities should be available for postoperative monitoring and ventilation of patients administered alfentanil. It is essential that these facilities be fully equipped to handle all degrees of respiratory depression.

PATIENTS RECEIVING MONITORED ANESTHESIA CARE (MAC) SHOULD BE CONTINUOUSLY MONITORED BY PERSONS NOT INVOLVED IN THE CONDUCT OF THE SURGICAL OR DIAGNOSTIC PROCEDURE; OXYGEN SUPPLEMENTATION SHOULD BE IMMEDIATELY AVAILABLE AND PROVIDED WHERE CLINICALLY INDICATED; OXYGEN SATURATION SHOULD BE CONTINUOUSLY MONITORED; THE PATIENT SHOULD BE OBSERVED FOR EARLY SIGNS OF HYPOTENSION, APNEA, UPPER AIRWAY OBSTRUCTION AND/OR OXYGEN DESATURATION.

Severe and unpredictable potentiation of monoamine oxidase (MAO) inhibitors has been reported for other opioid analgesics, and rarely with alfentanil. Therefore when alfentanil is administered to patients who have received MAO inhibitors within 14 days, appropriate monitoring and ready availability of vasodilators and beta-blockers for the treatment of hypertension is recommended.

DOSAGE AND ADMINISTRATION

The dosage of alfentanil HCl should be individualized in each patient according to body weight, physical status, underlying pathological condition, use of other drugs, and type and duration of surgical procedure and anesthesia. In obese patients (more than 20% above ideal total body weight), the dosage of alfentanil should be determined on the basis of lean body weight. The dose of alfentanil should be reduced in elderly or debilitated patients.

Vital signs should be monitored routinely.

See Dosage Guidelines in TABLE 1 for the use of alfentanil: (1) by incremental injection as an analgesic adjunct to anesthesia with barbiturate/nitrous oxide/oxygen for short surgical procedures (expected duration of less than one hour); (2) by continuous infusion as a maintenance analgesic with nitrous oxide/oxygen for general surgical procedures; and (3) by intravenous injection in anesthetic doses for the induction of anesthesia for general surgical procedures with a minimum expected duration of 45 minutes; and (4) by intravenous injection as the analgesic component for monitored anesthesia care (MAC).

TABLE 1 *Dosage Guidelines*

Dosage should be individualized And titrated for use during general anesthesia

Spontaneous Breathing/Assisted Ventilation	Induction of Analgesia: 8-20 µg/kg Maintenance of Analgesia: 3-5 µg/kg q 5-20 min or 0.5 to 1 µg/kg/min Total dose: 8-40 µg/kg
Assisted or Controlled Ventilation Incremental Injection (To attenuate response to laryngoscopy and intubation)	Induction of Analgesia: 20-50 µg/kg Maintenance of Analgesia: 5-15 µg/kg q 5-20 min Total dose: Up to 75 µg/kg
Continuous Infusion (To provide attenuation of response to intubation and incision)	Infusion rates are variable and should be titrated to the desired clinical effect. See Infusion Dosage Guidelines Below. Induction of Analgesia: 50-75 µg/kg Maintenance of Analgesia: 0.5 to 3 µg/kg/min (Average rate 1 to 1.5 µg/kg/min) Total dose: Dependent on duration of procedure
Anesthetic Induction	Induction of Anesthesia: 130-245 µg/kg Maintenance of Anesthesia: 0.5 to 1.5 µg/kg/min or general anesthetic Total dose: Dependent on duration of procedure At these doses, truncal rigidity should be expected and a muscle relaxant should be utilized. Administer slowly (over 3 minutes). Concentration of inhalation agents reduced by 30-50% for initial hour.
Monitored Anesthesia Care (MAC) (For sedated and responsive, spontaneously breathing patients)	Induction of MAC: 3-8 µg/kg Maintenance of MAC: 3-5 µg/kg q 5-20 min or 0.25 to 1 µg/kg/min Total dose: 3-40 µg/kg

INFUSION DOSAGE

Continuous Infusion

0.5-3.0 µg/kg/min administered with nitrous oxide/oxygen in patients undergoing general surgery. Following an anesthetic induction dose of alfentanil, infusion rate requirements are reduced by 30-50% for the first hour of maintenance.

Changes in vital signs that indicate a response to surgical stress or lightening of anesthesia may be controlled by increasing the rate up to a maximum of 4.0 µg/kg/min and/or administration of bolus doses of 7 µg/kg. If changes are not controlled after three bolus doses given over a 5 minute period, a barbiturate, vasodilator, and/or inhalation agent should be used. Infusion rates should always be adjusted downward in the absence of these signs until there is some response to surgical stimulation.

Rather than an increase in infusion rate, 7 µg/kg bolus doses of alfentanil or a potent inhalation agent should be administered in response to signs of lightening of anesthesia within the last 15 minutes of surgery. Administration of alfentanil infusion should be discontinued at least 10-15 minutes prior to the end of surgery.

Usage in Children: Clinical data to support the use of alfentanil in patients under 12 years of age are not presently available. Therefore, such use is not recommended.

Premedication: The selection of preanesthetic medications should be based upon the needs of the individual patient.

Neuromuscular Blocking Agents: The neuromuscular blocking agent selected should be compatible with the patient's condition, taking into account the hemodynamic effects of a particular muscle relaxant and the degree of skeletal muscle relaxation required (see WARNINGS.

In patients administered anesthetic (induction) dosages of alfentanil, it is essential that qualified personnel and adequate facilities are available for the management of intraoperative and postoperative respiratory depression.

Also see WARNINGS.

For purposes of administering small volumes of alfentanil accurately, the use of a tuberculin syringe or equivalent is recommended.

The physical and chemical compatibility of alfentanil have been demonstrated in solution with normal saline, 5% dextrose in normal saline, 5% dextrose in water and lactated Ringer's. Clinical studies of alfentanil infusion have been conducted with alfentanil diluted to a concentration range of 25-80 µg/ml.

As an example of the preparation of alfentanil for infusion, 20 ml of alfentanil added to 230 ml of diluent provides a 40 µg/ml solution of alfentanil.

Parenteral drug products should be inspected visually for particulate matter and discoloration prior to administration, whenever solution and container permit.

SAFETY AND HANDLING

Alfentanil HCl is supplied in individually sealed dosage forms which pose no known risk to health-care providers having incidental contact. Accidental dermal exposure to alfentanil should be treated by rinsing the affected area with water.

PRODUCT LISTING - RATED THERAPEUTICALLY EQUIVALENT

Solution - Injectable - 0.5 mg/ml

Size	Price	Product	NDC
2 ml x 10	$73.68	GENERIC, Abbott Pharmaceutical	10019-0060-01
2 ml x 10	$87.28	GENERIC, Abbott Pharmaceutical	00074-2266-02
2 ml x 10	$105.20	ALFENTA, Taylor Pharmaceuticals	11098-0060-02
5 ml x 10	$132.00	GENERIC, Abbott Pharmaceutical	10019-0060-02
5 ml x 10	$156.51	GENERIC, Abbott Pharmaceutical	00074-2266-05
5 ml x 10	$188.60	ALFENTA, Taylor Pharmaceuticals	11098-0060-05
5 ml x 10	$387.50	ALFENTA, Baxter Pharmaceutical Products, Inc	10019-0050-06
10 ml x 5	$152.25	ALFENTA, Taylor Pharmaceuticals	11098-0060-10
20 ml x 5	$266.50	ALFENTA, Taylor Pharmaceuticals	11098-0060-20

Alitretinoin *(003472)*

Categories: Sarcoma, Kaposi's; FDA Approved 1999 Feb; Pregnancy Category D; Orphan Drugs
Drug Classes: Dermatologics; Retinoids
Brand Names: Panretin
Cost of Therapy: $2,562.50 (Kaposi's sarcoma; Panretin; 0.1%; 60 g; 2 applications/day; variable day supply)

DESCRIPTION

Panretin gel 0.1% contains alitretinoin and is intended for topical application only. The chemical name is 9-*cis*-retinoic acid.

Chemically, alitretinoin is related to vitamin A. It is a yellow powder with a molecular weight of 300.44 and a molecular formula of $C_{20}H_{28}O_2$. It is slightly soluble in ethanol (7.01 mg/g at 25°C) and insoluble in water. Panretin gel is a clear, yellow gel containing 0.1% (w/w) alitretinoin in a base of dehydrated alcohol, polyethylene glycol 400, hydroxypropyl cellulose, and butylated hydroxytoluene.

CLINICAL PHARMACOLOGY

MECHANISM OF ACTION

Alitretinoin (9-*cis*-retinoic acid) is a naturally-occurring endogenous retinoid that binds to and activates all known intracellular retinoid receptor subtypes (RARα, RARβ, RARγ, RXRα, RXRβ, and RXRγ). Once activated these receptors function as transcription factors that regulate the expression of genes that control the process of cellular differentiation and proliferation in both normal and neoplastic cells. Alitretinoin inhibits the growth of Kaposi's sarcoma (KS) cells *in vitro.*

PHARMACOKINETICS

No studies have examined plasma 9-*cis*-retinoic acid concentrations before and after treatment with alitretinoin gel. There is, however, indirect evidence that absorption is not extensive. Plasma concentrations of 9-*cis*-retinoic acid were evaluated during clinical studies in patients with cutaneous lesions of AIDS-related KS after repeated multiple-daily dose application of alitretinoin gel for up to 60 weeks. The range of 9-*cis*-retinoic acid plasma concentrations in these patients was similar to the range of circulating, naturally-occurring 9-*cis*-retinoic acid plasma concentrations in untreated healthy volunteers.

Although there are no detectable plasma concentrations of 9-*cis*-retinoic acid metabolites after topical application of alitretinoin gel, *in vitro* studies indicate that the drug is metabolized to 4-hydroxy-9-*cis*-retinoic acid and 4-oxo-9-*cis*-retinoic acid by CYP 2C9, 3A4, 1A1, and 1A2 enzymes. *In vivo,* 4-oxo-9-*cis*-retinoic acid is the major circulating metabolite following oral administration of 9-*cis*-retinoic acid.

No formal pharmacokinetic drug interaction studies between alitretinoin gel and antiretroviral agents have been conducted.

INDICATIONS AND USAGE

Alitretinoin gel is indicated for topical treatment of cutaneous lesions in patients with AIDS-related Kaposi's sarcoma. Alitretinoin gel is not indicated when systemic anti-KS therapy is required (*e.g.,* more than 10 new KS lesions in the prior month, symptomatic lymphedema, symptomatic pulmonary KS, or symptomatic visceral involvement). There is no experience to date using alitretinoin gel with systemic anti-KS treatment.

CONTRAINDICATIONS

Alitretinoin gel is contraindicated in patients with a known hypersensitivity to retinoids or to any of the ingredients of the product.

WARNINGS

PREGNANCY

Alitretinoin gel could cause fetal harm if significant absorption were to occur in a pregnant woman. 9-*cis*-Retinoic acid has been shown to be teratogenic in rabbits and mice. An increased incidence of fused sternebrae and limb and craniofacial defects occurred in rabbits given oral doses of 0.5 mg/kg/day (about 5 times the estimated daily human topical dose on a mg/m^2 basis, assuming complete systemic absorption of 9-*cis*-retinoic acid, when alitretinoin gel is administered as a 60 g tube over 1 month in a 60 kg human) during the period of organogenesis. Limb and craniofacial defects also occurred in mice given a single oral dose of 50 mg/kg on day 11 of gestation (about 127 times the estimated daily human topical dose on a mg/m^2 basis). Oral 9-*cis*-retinoic acid was also embryocidal, as indicated by early resorptions and post-implantation loss when it was given during the period of organogenesis to rabbits at doses of 1.5 mg/kg/day (about 15 times the estimated daily human topical dose on a mg/m^2 basis) and to rats at doses of 5 mg/kg/day (about 25 times the estimated daily human topical dose on a mg/m^2 basis). Animal reproduction studies with topical 9-*cis*-retinoic acid have not been conducted. It is not known whether topical alitretinoin gel can modulate endogenous 9-*cis*-retinoic acid levels in a pregnant woman nor whether systemic exposure is increased by application to ulcerated lesions or by duration of treatment. There are no adequate and well-controlled studies in pregnant women. If alitretinoin gel is used during pregnancy, or if the patient becomes pregnant while taking it, the patient should be apprised of the potential hazard to the fetus. Women of child-bearing potential should be advised to avoid becoming pregnant.

PRECAUTIONS

Alitretinoin gel is indicated for topical treatment of Kaposi's sarcoma. Patients with cutaneous T-cell lymphoma were less tolerant of topical alitretinoin gel; 5 of 7 patients had 6 episodes of treatment-limiting toxicities — Grade 3 dermal irritation — with alitretinoin gel (0.01 or 0.05%).

PHOTOSENSITIVITY

Retinoids as a class have been associated with photosensitivity. There were no reports of photosensitivity associated with the use of alitretinoin gel in the clinical studies. Nonetheless, because *in vitro* data indicate that 9-*cis*-retinoic acid may have a weak photosensitizing effect, patients should be advised to minimize exposure of treated areas to sunlight and sunlamps during the use of alitretinoin gel.

DRUG/LABORATORY TEST INTERACTIONS

No interference with laboratory tests has been observed.

CARCINOGENESIS, MUTAGENESIS, AND IMPAIRMENT OF FERTILITY

Long-term studies in animals to assess the carcinogenic potential of 9-*cis*-retinoic acid have not been conducted. 9-*cis*-Retinoic acid was not mutagenic *in vitro* (bacterial assays, Chinese hamster ovary cell HGPRT mutation assay) and was not clastogenic *in vitro* (chromosome aberration test in human lymphocytes) nor *in vivo* (mouse micronucleus test).

PREGNANCY CATEGORY D

See WARNINGS.

NURSING MOTHERS

It is not known whether alitretinoin or its metabolites are excreted in human milk. Because many drugs are excreted in human milk and because of the potential for adverse reactions from alitretinoin gel in nursing infants, mothers should discontinue nursing prior to using the drug.

PEDIATRIC USE

Safety and effectiveness in pediatric patients have not been established.

GERIATRIC USE

Inadequate information is available to assess safety and efficacy in patients age 65 years or older.

DRUG INTERACTIONS

Patients who are applying alitretinoin gel should not concurrently use products that contain DEET (N,N-diethyl-m-toluamide), a common component of insect repellent products. Animal toxicity studies showed increased DEET toxicity when DEET was included as part of the formulation.

Although there was no clinical evidence in the vehicle-controlled studies of drug interactions with systemic antiretroviral agents, including protease inhibitors, macrolide antibiotics, and azole antifungals, the effect of alitretinoin gel on the steady-state concentrations of these drugs is not known. No drug interaction data are available on concomitant administration of alitretinoin gel and systemic anti-KS agents.

ADVERSE REACTIONS

The safety of alitretinoin gel has been assessed in clinical studies of 385 patients with AIDS-related KS. Adverse events associated with the use of alitretinoin gel in patients with AIDS-related KS occurred almost exclusively at the site of application. The dermal toxicity begins as erythema; with continued application of alitretinoin gel, erythema may increase and edema may develop. Dermal toxicity may become treatment-limiting, with intense erythema, edema, and vesiculation. Usually, however, adverse events are mild to moderate in severity; they led to withdrawal from the study in only 7% of the patients. Severe local (application site) skin adverse events occurred in about 10% of patients in the US study (vs 0% in the vehicle control). TABLE 2 lists the adverse events that occurred at the application site with an incidence of at least 5% during the double-blind phase in the alitretinoin gel-treated group and in the vehicle control group in either of the two controlled studies. Adverse events were reported at other sites but generally were similar in the two groups.

DOSAGE AND ADMINISTRATION

Alitretinoin gel should initially be applied 2 times a day to cutaneous KS lesions. The application frequency can be gradually increased to 3 or 4 times a day according to individual lesion tolerance. If application site toxicity occurs, the application frequency can be reduced. Should severe irritation occur, application of drug can be temporarily discontinued for a few days until the symptoms subside.

Sufficient gel should be applied to cover the lesion with a generous coating. The gel should be allowed to dry for 3-5 minutes before covering with clothing. Because unaffected skin may become irritated, application of the gel to normal skin surrounding the lesions should be avoided. In addition, do not apply the gel on or near mucosal surfaces of the body.

A response of KS lesions may be seen as soon as 2 weeks after initiation of therapy but most patients require longer application. With continued application, further benefit may be attained. Some patients have required over 14 weeks to respond. In clinical trials, alitret-

TABLE 2 *Adverse Events With an Incidence of at Least 5% at the Application Site in Either Controlled Study in Patients Receiving Alitretinoin Gel or Vehicle Control*

	Study 1		Study 2	
	Alitretinoin Gel	Vehicle Gel	Alitretinoin Gel	Vehicle Gel
Adverse Event Term	n=134	n=134	n=36	n=46
Rash*	77%	11%	25%	4%
Pain†	34%	7%	0%	4%
Pruritus‡	11%	4%	8%	4%
Exfoliative dermatitis§	9%	2%	3%	0%
Skin disorder¤	8%	1%	0%	0%
Paresthesia¶	3%	0%	22%	7%
Edema**	8%	3%	3%	0%

Includes Investigator terms:
* Erythema, scaling, irritation, redness, rash, dermatitis.
† Burning, pain.
‡ Itching, pruritus.
§ Flaking, peeling, desquamation, exfoliation.
¤ Excoriation, cracking, scab, crusting, drainage, eschar, fissure or oozing.
¶ Stinging, tingling.
** Edema, swelling, inflammation.

inoin gel was applied for up to 96 weeks. Alitretinoin gel should be continued as long as the patient is deriving benefit.

Occlusive dressings should not be used with alitretinoin gel.

HOW SUPPLIED

Storage: Store at 25°C (77°F); excursions permitted to 15-30°C (59-86°F).

PRODUCT LISTING - EQUIVALENTS NOT AVAILABLE

Gel - Topical - 0.1%

60 gm $2562.50 PANRETIN, Ligand Pharmaceuticals 64365-0501-01

Allopurinol *(000133)*

Categories: Arthritis, gouty; Calculus, oxalate; Calculus, renal; Hyperuricemia; Hyperuricemia, secondary to leukemia; Hyperuricemia, secondary to lymphoma; Leukemia, adjunct; Lymphoma, adjunct; Pregnancy Category C; FDA Approved 1974 Jan; WHO Formulary; Orphan Drugs

Drug Classes: Antigout agents; Purine analogs

Brand Names: Lopurin; Lysuron; **Zyloprim**

Foreign Brand Availability: Adenock (Japan); Alinol (Thailand); Allnol (Hong-Kong); Allo 300 (Germany); Allo-Basan (Switzerland); Allohexal (Australia); Allo-Puren (Germany); Allopin (Thailand); Allopur (Norway; Switzerland); Allopurinol (Malaysia); Alloril (Israel); Allorin (New-Zealand); Allozym (Japan); Allurit (Italy); Alopron (Bahamas; Barbados; Belize; Bermuda; Curacao; Guyana; Jamaica; Netherland-Antilles; Surinam; Trinidad); Alositol (Japan); Alpurin (Philippines); Alunlan (Philippines; Taiwan); Alurin (Guatemala); Aluron (Venezuela); Anoprolin (Japan); Anzief (Japan); Apo-Allopurinol (Canada); Aprinol (Japan); Apurin (Denmark; Finland; Greece; Netherlands); Atisuril (Mexico); Caplenal (England; Ireland); Capurate (Australia; Taiwan); Cellidrin (Germany); Clint (Benin; Burkina-Faso; Ethiopia; Gambia; Ghana; Guinea; Ivory-Coast; Kenya; Liberia; Malawi; Mali; Mauritania; Mauritius; Morocco; Niger; Nigeria; Senegal; Seychelles; Sierra-Leone; Sudan; Tanzania; Tunia; Uganda; Zambia; Zimbabwe); Erloric (Singapore); Etindrax (Mexico); Foligan (Germany; Switzerland); Gichtex (Austria); Hamarin (England); Isoric (Indonesia); Kemorinol (Indonesia); Ketanrift (Japan); Ketobun-A (Japan); Litinol (Venezuela); Llanol (Indonesia; Philippines); Lo-Uric (South-Africa); Lopurine (Philippines); Lysuron 300 (Switzerland); Masaton (Japan); Medoric (Thailand); Mefanol (Ecuador); Mephanol (Bahrain; Benin; Burkina-Faso; Cyprus; Egypt; Ethiopia; Gambia; Ghana; Guinea; Hong-Kong; Iran; Iraq; Ivory-Coast; Jordan; Kenya; Kuwait; Lebanon; Liberia; Libya; Malawi; Malaysia; Mali; Mauritania; Mauritius; Morocco; Niger; Nigeria; Oman; Qatar; Republic-of-Yemen; Saudi-Arabia; Senegal; Seychelles; Sierra-Leone; Sudan; Switzerland; Syria; Tanzania; Tunia; Uganda; United-Arab-Emirates; Zambia; Zimbabwe); Milurit (Bulgaria; Hong-Kong; Hungary); Miniplanor (Japan); Neufan (Japan); Nipurol (Venezuela); No-Uric (Bahrain; Cyprus; Egypt; Iran; Iraq; Jordan; Kuwait; Lebanon; Libya; Oman; Qatar; Republic-of-Yemen; Saudi-Arabia; Syria; United-Arab-Emirates); Progout (Australia; China; Hong-Kong; New-Zealand; Singapore); Proxuric (Indonesia); Puricemia (Indonesia); Puricos (South-Africa); Purinase (Philippines); Purinol (Ireland; Malaysia); Purinox (Costa-Rica; Dominican-Republic; El-Salvador; Guatemala; Honduras; Nicaragua; Panama); Ranpuric (South-Africa); Remid (Germany); Riball (Japan); Rinolic (Indonesia); Salterprim (South-Africa); Takanarumin (Japan); Tonsaric (Taiwan); Unizuric 300 (Mexico); Uric (Japan); Uricad (Thailand); Uriconorm (Switzerland); Urinol (Malaysia); Uripurinol (Germany); Urogquad (Argentina); Uroquad (Bahamas; Barbados; Belize; Benin; Bermuda; Burkina-Faso; Curacao; Ethiopia; Gambia; Ghana; Guinea; Guyana; Indonesia; Ivory-Coast; Jamaica; Kenya; Liberia; Malawi; Mali; Mauritania; Mauritius; Morocco; Netherland-Antilles; Niger; Nigeria; Senegal; Seychelles; Sierra-Leone; Sudan; Surinam; Tanzania; Trinidad; Tunia; Uganda; Zambia; Zimbabwe); Urosin (Austria; Ecuador; Germany); Valeric (Singapore); Vitralgin (Peru); Xanturic (France); Xylonol (Taiwan); Zylapour (Greece); Zylol (Israel); Zyloric (Argentina; Bahrain; Belgium; Benin; Brazil; Bulgaria; Burkina-Faso; Chile; China; Cyprus; Czech-Republic; Denmark; Egypt; England; Ethiopia; Finland; France; Gambia; Germany; Ghana; Guinea; Hong-Kong; Hungary; India; Indonesia; Iran; Iraq; Ireland; Israel; Italy; Ivory-Coast; Jordan; Kenya; Korea; Kuwait; Lebanon; Liberia; Libya; Malawi; Malaysia; Mali; Mauritania; Mauritius; Morocco; Netherlands; Niger; Nigeria; Norway; Oman; Peru; Portugal; Qatar; Republic-of-Yemen; Saudi-Arabia; Senegal; Seychelles; Sierra-Leone; Spain; Sudan; Sweden; Switzerland; Syria; Taiwan; Tanzania; Thailand; Tunia; Uganda; United-Arab-Emirates; Zambia; Zimbabwe); Zyroric (Korea)

Cost of Therapy: $22.85 (Gout; Zyloprim; 300 mg; 1 tablet/day; 30 day supply)
$3.26 (Gout; Generic Tablets; 300 mg; 1 tablet/day; 30 day supply)

DESCRIPTION

Allopurinol is known chemically as 1,5-dihydro-4*H*-pyrazolo [3,4-*d*]pyrimidin-4-one. It is a xanthine oxidase inhibitor which is administered orally and intravenously.

TABLETS

Each scored white tablet contains 100 mg allopurinol and the inactive ingredients lactose, magnesium stearate, potato starch, and povidone. Each scored peach tablet contains 300 mg allopurinol and the inactive ingredients corn starch, FD&C yellow no. 6 lake, lactose, magnesium stearate, and povidone. Its solubility in water at 37°C is 80.0 mg/dl and is greater in an alkaline solution.

INJECTION

The injection is a sterile solution for intravenous infusion only. It is available in vials as the sterile lyophilized sodium salt of allopurinol equivalent to 500 mg of allopurinol. Allopurinol for injection contains no preservatives. It is a white amorphous mass with a molecular weight of 158.09 and molecular formula $C_5H_3N_4NaO$. The pKa of allopurinol sodium is 9.31.

CLINICAL PHARMACOLOGY

Allopurinol acts on purine catabolism, without disrupting the biosynthesis of purines. It reduces the production of uric acid by inhibiting the biochemical reactions immediately preceding its formation. The degree of this decrease is dose dependent.

Allopurinol is a structural analogue of the natural purine base, hypoxanthine. It is an inhibitor of xanthine oxidase, the enzyme responsible for the conversion of hypoxanthine to xanthine and of xanthine to uric acid, the end product of purine metabolism in man. Allopurinol is metabolized to the corresponding xanthine analogue, oxipurinol (alloxanthine), which also is an inhibitor of xanthine oxidase.

Reutilization of both hypoxanthine and xanthine for nucleotide and nucleic acid synthesis is markedly enhanced when their oxidations are inhibited by allopurinol and oxipurinol. This reutilization does not disrupt normal nucleic acid anabolism, however, because feedback inhibition is an integral part of purine biosynthesis. As a result of xanthine oxidase inhibition, the serum concentration of hypoxanthine plus xanthine in patients receiving allopurinol for treatment of hyperuricemia is usually in the range of 0.3-0.4 mg/dl compared to a normal level of approximately 0.15 mg/dl. A maximum of 0.9 mg/dl of these oxypurines has been reported when the serum urate was lowered to less than 2 mg/dl by high doses of allopurinol. These values are far below the saturation levels at which point their precipitation would be expected to occur (above 7 mg/dl).

The renal clearance of hypoxanthine and xanthine is at least 10 times greater than that of uric acid. The increased xanthine and hypoxanthine in the urine have not been accompanied by problems of nephrolithiasis. There are isolated case reports of xanthine crystalluria in patients who were treated with oral allopurinol. Xanthine crystalluria has been reported in only three patients. Two of the patients had Lesch-Nyhan syndrome, which is characterized by excessive uric acid production combined with a deficiency of the enzyme, hypoxanthineguanine phosphoribosyltransferase (HGPRTase). This enzyme is required for the conversion of hypoxanthine, xanthine, and guanine to their respective nucleotides. The third patient had lymphosarcoma and produced an extremely large amount of uric acid because of rapid cell lysis during chemotherapy.

The action of allopurinol differs from that of uricosuric agents, which lower the serum uric acid level by increasing urinary excretion of uric acid. Allopurinol reduces both the serum and urinary uric acid levels by inhibiting the formation of uric acid. The use of allopurinol to block the formation of urates avoids the hazard of increased renal excretion of uric acid posed by uricosuric drugs.

FOR TABLETS ONLY

Allopurinol is approximately 90% absorbed from the gastrointestinal tract. Peak plasma levels generally occur at 1.5 hours and 4.5 hours for allopurinol and oxipurinol respectively, and after a single oral dose of 300 mg allopurinol, maximum plasma levels of about 3 μg/ml of allopurinol and 6.5 μg/ml of oxipurinol are produced.

Approximately 20% of the ingested allopurinol is excreted in the feces. Because of its rapid oxidation to oxipurinol and a renal clearance rate approximately that of glomerular filtration rate, allopurinol has a plasma half-life of about 1-2 hours. Oxipurinol, however, has a longer plasma half-life (approximately 15.0 hours) and therefore effective xanthine oxidase inhibition is maintained over a 24 hour period with single daily doses of allopurinol. Whereas allopurinol is cleared essentially by glomerular filtration, oxipurinol is reabsorbed in the kidney tubules in a manner similar to the reabsorption of uric acid.

The clearance of oxipurinol is increased by uricosuric drugs, and as a consequence, the addition of a uricosuric agent reduces to some degree the inhibition of xanthine oxidase by oxipurinol and increases to some degree the urinary excretion of uric acid. In practice, the net effect of such combined therapy may be useful in some patients in achieving minimum serum uric acid levels provided the total urinary uric acid load does not exceed the competence of the patient's renal function.

Hyperuricemia may be primary, as in gout, or secondary to diseases such as acute and chronic leukemia, polycythemia vera, multiple myeloma, and psoriasis. It may occur with the use of diuretic agents, during renal dialysis, in the presence of renal damage, during starvation or reducing diets and in the treatment of neoplastic disease where rapid resolution of tissue masses may occur. Asymptomatic hyperuricemia is not an indication for treatment with allopurinol (see INDICATIONS AND USAGE).

Gout is a metabolic disorder which is characterized by hyperuricemia and resultant deposition of monosodium urate in the tissues, particularly the joints and kidneys. The etiology of this hyperuricemia is the overproduction of uric acid in relation to the patient's ability to excrete it. If progressive deposition of urates is to be arrested or reversed, it is necessary to reduce the serum uric acid level below the saturation point to suppress urate precipitation.

Administration of allopurinol generally results in a fall in both serum and urinary uric acid within 2-3 days. The degree of this decrease can be manipulated almost at will since it is dose-dependent. A week or more of treatment with allopurinol may be required before its full effects are manifested; likewise, uric acid may return to pretreatment levels slowly (usually after a period of 7-10 days following cessation of therapy). This reflects primarily the accumulation and slow clearance of oxipurinol. In some patients a dramatic fall in urinary uric acid excretion may not occur, particularly in those with severe tophaceous gout. It has been postulated that this may be due to the mobilization of urate from tissue deposits as the serum uric acid level begins to fall.

The action of oral allopurinol differs from that of uricosuric agents, which lower the serum uric acid level by increasing urinary excretion of uric acid. Allopurinol reduces both the serum and urinary uric acid levels by inhibiting the formation of uric acid. The use of allopurinal to block the formation of urates avoids the hazard of increased renal excretion of uric acid posed by uricosuric drugs.

Allopurinol can substantially reduce serum and urinary uric acid levels in previously refractory patients even in the presence of renal damage serious enough to render uricosuric drugs virtually ineffective. Salicylates may be given conjointly for their antirheumatic effect without compromising the action of allopurinol. This is in contrast to the nullifying effect of salicylates on uricosuric drugs.

Allopurinol also inhibits the enzymatic oxidation of mercaptopurine, the sulfur-containing analogue of hypoxanthine, to 6-thiouric acid. This oxidation, which is catalyzed by xanthine oxidase, inactivates mercaptopurine. Hence, the inhibition of such oxidation by allopurinol may result in as much as a 75% reduction in the therapeutic dose requirement of mercaptopurine when the two compounds are given together.

FOR INJECTION ONLY

Pharmacokinetics

Following intravenous administration in 6 healthy male and female subjects, allopurinol was rapidly eliminated from the systemic circulation primarily via oxidative metabolism to oxypurinol, with no detectable plasma concentration of allopurinol after 5 hours post dosing. Approximately 12% of the allopurinol intravenous dose was excreted unchanged, 76% excreted as oxypurinol, and the remaining dose excreted as riboside conjugates in the urine. The rapid conversion of allopurinol to oxypurinol was not significantly different after repeated allopurinol dosing. Oxypurinol was present in systemic circulation in much higher concentrations and for a much longer period than allopurinol; thus, it is generally believed that the pharmacological action of allopurinol is mediated via oxypurinol. Oxypurinol was primarily eliminated unchanged in urine by glomerular filtration and tubular reabsorption, with a net renal clearance of about 30 ml/min.

To compare the pharmacokinetics of allopurinol and oxypurinol between intravenous (IV) and oral (PO) administration of allopurinol sodium for injection, a well-controlled, four-way crossover study was conducted in 16 healthy male volunteers. Allopurinol sodium for injection was administered via an intravenous infusion over 30 minutes. Pharmacokinetic parameter estimates of allopurinol (mean ± SD) following single IV and PO administration of allopurinol sodium for injection are summarized in TABLE 1.

TABLE 1 *Administration of Allopurinol Sodium for Injection*

Allopurinol Parameters	100 mg IV	300 mg IV	100 mg PO*	300 mg PO
C_{max} (μg/ml)	158 ± 0.22	5.12 ± 0.82	0.53 ± 0.10	1.35 ± 0.49
T_{max} (h)	0.50	0.50	1.00 ± 0.39	1.67 ± 0.96
T½ (h)	1.00 ± 0.46	1.21 ± 0.33	0.98 ± 0.43	1.32 ± 0.32
AUC(0→∞) (hr·μg/ml)	1.99 ± 0.63	7.10 ± 1.28	1.03 ± 0.24	3.69 ± 0.96
CL (ml/min/kg)	12.2 ± 3.11	9.94 ± 2.36		
Vss (L/kg)†	0.84 ± 0.13	0.87 ± 0.13		
$F_{absolute}$ (%)‡			48.8 ± 19.7	52.7 ± 13.1

* n=7.
† Volume of distribution (steady-state).
‡ Absolute bioavailability.

Oxypurinol was measurable in the plasma within 10-15 minutes following the administration of allopurinol sodium for injection. Pharmacokinetic parameter estimates of oxypurinol following IV and PO administration of allopurinol sodium for injection are shown in TABLE 2.

TABLE 2 *Administration of Allopurinol Sodium for Injection*

Oxypurinol Parameters	100 mg IV	300 mg IV	100 mg PO	300 mg PO
C_{max} (μg/ml)	2.20 ± 0.31	6.18 ± 0.78	2.36 ± 0.30	6.36 ± 0.83
T_{max} (h)	3.89 ± 1.41	4.16 ± 1.2	3.10 ± 1.49	4.13 ± 1.35
T½ (h)	24.1 ± 5.4	23.5 ± 4.5	24.9 ± 8.4	23.7 ± 3.4
AUC(0→∞) (hr·μg/ml)	80 ± 24	231 ± 54	83 ± 22	245 ± 49
$F_{relative}$ (%)*			107 ± 25	108 ± 9

* Relative bioavailability.

In general, the ratio of the area under the plasma concentration versus. time curve [AUC(0→∞)] for between oxyupurinol and allopurinol was in the magnitude of 30-40. The C_{max} and AUC(0→∞) for both allopurinol and oxypurinol following IV administration of allopurinol sodium for injection were dose proportional in the dose range of 100-300 mg. The half-life of allopurinol and oxypurinol was not influenced by the route of allopurinol sodium for injection administration. Oral and intravenous administration of allopurinol sodium for injection at equal doses produced nearly superimposable oxypurinol plasma concentration versus time profiles, and the relative bioavailability of oxypurinol ($F_{relative}$) was approximately 100%. Thus, the pharmacokinetics and plasma profiles of oxypurinol, the major pharmacological component derived form allopurinol, are similar after intravenous and oral administration of allopurinol sodium for injection.

INDICATIONS AND USAGE

TABLETS

THIS IS NOT AN INNOCUOUS DRUG. IT IS NOT RECOMMENDED FOR THE TREATMENT OF ASYMPTOMATIC HYPERURICEMIA.

Allopurinol reduces serum and urinary uric acid concentrations. Its use should be individualized for each patient and requires an understanding of its mode of action and pharmacokinetics (see CLINICAL PHARMACOLOGY, CONTRAINDICATIONS, WARNINGS and PRECAUTIONS).

Allopurinol is Indicated in:

1. The management of patients with signs and symptoms of primary or secondary gout (acute attacks, tophi, joint destruction, uric acid lithiasis and/or nephropathy).
2. The management of patients with leukemia, lymphoma and malignancies who are receiving cancer therapy which causes elevations of serum and urinary uric acid levels. Treatment with allopurinol should be discontinued when the potential for overproduction of uric acid is no longer present.
3. The management of patients with recurrent calcium oxalate calculi whose daily uric acid excretion exceeds 800 mg/day in male patients and 750 mg/day in female patients. Therapy in such patients should be carefully assessed initially and reassessed periodically to determine in each case that treatment is beneficial and that the benefits outweigh the risks.

INJECTION

Allopurinol sodium for injection is indicated for the management of patients with leukemia, lymphoma, and solid tumor malignancies who are receiving cancer therapy which causes elevations of serum and urinary uric acid levels and who cannot tolerate oral therapy.

NON-FDA APPROVED INDICATIONS

Non-FDA approved indications include use in the treatment of old world cutaneous leishmaniasis and Zahorsky's herpangina.

CONTRAINDICATIONS

Patients who have developed a severe reaction to allopurinol should not be restarted on the drug.

WARNINGS

ALLOPURINOL SHOULD BE DISCONTINUED AT THE FIRST APPEARANCE OF SKIN RASH OR OTHER SIGNS WHICH MAY INDICATE AN ALLERGIC REACTION. In some instances with oral allopurinol, a skin rash may be followed by more severe hypersensitivity reactions such as exfoliative, urticarial and purpuric lesions as well as Stevens-Johnson syndrome (erythema multiform exudativum), and/or generalized vasculitis, irreversible hepatotoxicity and on rare occasions, death.

In patients receiving mercaptopurine or azathioprine, the concomitant administration of 300-600 mg of allopurinol per day will require a reduction in dose to approximately one-third to one-fourth of the usual dose of mercaptopurine or azathioprine. Subsequent adjustment of doses of mercaptopurine or azathioprine should be made on the basis of therapeutic response and the appearance of toxic effects (see CLINICAL PHARMACOLOGY and DRUG INTERACTIONS).

A few cases of reversible clinical hepatotoxicity have been noted in patients taking allopurinol, and in some patients asymptomatic rises in serum alkaline phosphatase or serum transaminase have been observed. If anorexia, weight loss or pruritus develop in patients on allopurinol, evaluation of liver function should be part of their diagnostic workup. In patients with pre-existing liver disease, periodic liver function tests are recommended during the early stages of therapy.

Due to the occasional occurrence of drowsiness, patients should be alerted to the need for due precaution when engaging in activities where alertness is mandatory.

The occurrence of hypersensitivity reactions to allopurinol may be increased in patients with decreased renal function receiving thiazides and allopurinol concurrently. For this reason, in patients with decreased renal function, such combinations should be administered with caution and patients should be observed closely.

PRECAUTIONS

GENERAL

An increase in acute attacks of gout has been reported during the early stages of allopurinol administration, even when normal or subnormal serum uric acid levels have been attained. Accordingly, maintenance doses of colchicine generally should be given prophylactically when allopurinol is begun. In addition, it is recommended that the patient start with a low dose of allopurinol (100 mg daily) and increase at weekly intervals by 100 mg until a serum uric acid level of 6 mg/dl or less is attained but without exceeding the maximum recommended dose (800 mg/day). The use of colchicine or anti-inflammatory agents may be required to suppress gouty attacks in some cases. The attacks usually become shorter and less severe after several months of therapy. The mobilization of urates from tissue deposits which cause fluctuations in the serum uric acid levels may be a possible explanation for these episodes. Even with adequate allopurinol therapy, it may require several months to deplete the uric acid pool sufficiently to achieve control of the acute attacks.

A fluid intake sufficient to yield a daily urinary output of at least two liters for adults and the maintenance of a neutral or, preferably, slightly alkaline urine are desirable to (1) avoid the theoretical possibility of formation of xanthine calculi under the influence of allopurinol therapy and (2) help prevent renal precipitation of urates in patients receiving concomitant uricosuric agents.

Some patients with pre-existing renal disease or poor urate clearance have shown a rise in BUN during allopurinol administration, although a decrease in BUN has also been observed with allopurinol for injection. In patients with hyperuricemia due to malignancy, the vast majority of changes in renal function are attributable to the underlying malignancy rather than to therapy with allopurinol. Although the mechanism responsible for this has not been established, patients with impaired renal function should be carefully observed during the early stages of allopurinol administration so that the dosage can be appropriately adjusted for renal function.

Renal failure in association with allopurinol administration has been observed among patients with hyperuricemia secondary to neoplastic diseases. Concurrent conditions such as multiple myeloma and congestive myocardial disease were present among those patients whose renal dysfunction increased after allopurinol was begun. Renal failure is also frequently associated with gouty nephropathy and rarely with allopurinol-associated hypersensitivity reactions. Albuminuria has been observed among patients who developed clinical gout following chronic glomerulonephritis and chronic pyelonephritis.

Patients with decreased renal function require lower doses of allopurinol than those with normal renal function. Lower than recommended doses should be used to initiate therapy in any patients with decreased renal function and they should be observed closely during the early stages of allopurinol administration. In patients with severely impaired renal function or decreased urate clearance, the half-life of oxipurinol in the plasma is greatly prolonged. Therefore, a dose of 100 mg/day or 300 mg/day of oral allopurinol twice a week, or perhaps less, may be sufficient to maintain adequate xanthine oxidase inhibition to reduce serum urate levels. The appropriate dose of allopurinol sodium for injection for patients with a creatinine clearance ≤10 ml/min is 100 mg/day. for patients with creatinine clearance between 10 and 20 ml/min, a dose of 200 mg/day is recommended. With extreme renal impairment (creatinine clearance less than 3 ml/min), the interval between doses may also need to be extended.

Bone marrow depression has been reported in patients receiving allopurinol, most of whom received concomitant drugs with the potential for causing this reaction. This has occurred as early as 6 weeks to as long as 6 years after the initiation of allopurinol therapy. Rarely a patient may develop varying degrees of bone marrow depression, affecting one or more cell lines, while receiving allopurinol alone.

INFORMATION FOR THE PATIENT

Patients taking allopurinol tablets should be informed of the following:

1. They should be cautioned to discontinue allopurinol and to consult their physician immediately at the first sign of a skin rash, painful urination, blood in the urine, irritation of the eyes, or swelling of the lips or mouth.
2. They should be reminded to continue drug therapy prescribed for gouty attacks since optimal benefit of allopurinol may be delayed for 2-6 weeks.
3. They should be encouraged to increase fluid intake during therapy to prevent renal stones.
4. If a single dose of allopurinol is occasionally forgotten, there is no need to double the dose at the next scheduled time.
5. There may be certain risks associated with the concomitant use of allopurinol and dicumarol, sulfinpyrazone, mercaptopurine, azathioprine, ampicillin, amoxicillin and thiazide diuretics, and they should follow the instructions of their physician.
6. Due to the occasional occurrence of drowsiness, patients should take precautions when engaging in activities where alertness is mandatory.
7. Patients may wish to take allopurinol after meals to minimize gastric irritation.

LABORATORY TESTS

The correct dosage and schedule for maintaining the serum uric acid within the normal range is best determined by using the serum uric acid as an index.

In patients with pre-existing liver disease, periodic liver function tests are recommended during the early stages of therapy (see WARNINGS).

Allopurinol and its primary active metabolite, oxipurinol, are eliminated by the kidneys; therefore, changes in renal function have a profound effect on dosage. In patients with decreased renal function or who have concurrent illnesses which can affect renal function such as hypertension and diabetes mellitus, periodic laboratory parameters of renal function, particularly BUN and serum creatinine or creatinine clearance, should be performed and the patient's allopurinol dosage reassessed.

The prothrombin time should be reassessed periodically in the patients receiving dicumarol who are given allopurinol.

DRUG/LABORATORY TEST INTERACTIONS

Allopurinol is not known to alter the accuracy of laboratory tests.

PREGNANCY, TERATOGENIC EFFECTS, PREGNANCY CATEGORY C

Tablets

Reproductive studies have been performed in rats and rabbits at doses of oral allopurinol up to 20 times the usual human dose (5 mg/kg/day), and it was concluded that there was no impaired fertility or harm to the fetus due to allopurinol. There is a published report of a study in pregnant mice given 50 or 100 mg/kg allopurinol intraperitoneally on gestation days 10 or 13. There were increased numbers of dead fetuses in dams given 100 mg/kg allopurinol but not in those given 50 mg/kg. There were increased numbers of external malformations in fetuses at both doses of allopurinol on gestation day 10 and increased numbers of skeletal malformations in fetuses at both doses on gestation day 13. It cannot be determined whether this represented a fetal effect or an effect secondary to maternal toxicity. There are, however, no adequate or well-controlled studies in pregnant women. Because animal reproduction studies are not always predictive of human response, this drug should be used during pregnancy only if clearly needed.

Injection

There was no evidence of fetotoxicity or teratogenicity in rats or rabbits treated during the period of organogenesis with oral allopurinol at doses up to 200 mg/kg/day and up to 100 mg/kg/day, respectively (about three times the human dose on a mg/m^2 basis). However, there is a published report in pregnant mice that single intraperitoneal doses of 50 or 100 mg/kg (about 1/3 or 3/4 the human dose on a mg/m^2 basis) of allopurinol on gestation days 10 or 13 produced significant increases in fetal deaths and teratogenic effects (cleft palate, harelip, and digital defects). It is uncertain whether these findings represented a fetal effect or an effect secondary to maternal toxicity. There are, however, no adequate or well-controlled studies in pregnant women. Because animal reproduction studies are not always predictive of human response, this drug should be used during pregnancy only if the potential benefit justifies the potential risk to the fetus.

Experience with allopurinol during human pregnancy has been limited partly because women of reproductive age rarely require treatment with allopurinol. There are two unpublished reports and one published paper describing women giving birth to normal offspring after receiving allopurinol during pregnancy.

There have been no pregnancies reported in patients receiving allopurinol sodium for injection, but it assumed that the same risks would apply.

NURSING MOTHERS

Allopurinol and oxipurinol have been found in the milk of a mother who was receiving allopurinol. Since the effect of allopurinol on the nursing infant is unknown, caution should be exercised when allopurinol is administered to a nursing woman.

PEDIATRIC USE

Tablets

Allopurinol is rarely indicated for use in children with the exception of those with hyperuricemia secondary to malignancy or to certain rare inborn errors of purine metabolism. Patients may wish to take allopurinol after meals to minimize gastric irritation (see INDICATIONS AND USAGE and DOSAGE AND ADMINISTRATION).

Injection

Clinical data are available on approximately 200 pediatric patients treated with allopurinol sodium for injection. The efficacy and safety profile observed in this patient population were similar to that observed in adults (see INDICATIONS AND USAGE and DOSAGE AND ADMINISTRATION).

GERIATRIC USE

Injection

Clinical studies of allopurinol sodium for injection did not include sufficient numbers of patients aged 65 and over to determine whether they respond differently than younger patients. Other reported clinical experience has not identified differences in responses between the elderly and younger patients. In general, dose selection for an elderly patient should be cautious, usually starting at the low end of the dosing range, reflecting the greater frequency of decreased hepatic, renal, or cardiac function, and of concomitant disease or other drug therapy.

DRUG INTERACTIONS

The following drug interactions were observed in some patients undergoing treatment with oral allopurinol. Although the pattern of use for oral allopurinol includes longer term therapy, particularly for gout and renal calculi, the experience gained may be relevant.

Mercaptopurine/Azathioprine: Allopurinol inhibits the enzymatic oxidation of mercaptopurine and azathioprine to 6-thiouric acid. This oxidation, which is catalyzed by xanthine oxidase, inactivates mercaptopurine. In patients receiving mercaptopurine or azathioprine, the concomitant administration of 300-600 mg/day of allopurinol will require a reduction in dose to approximately one third to one fourth of the usual dose of mercaptopurine or azathioprine. Subsequent adjustment of doses of mercaptopurine or azathioprine should be made on the basis of therapeutic response and the appearance of toxic effects (see CLINICAL PHARMACOLOGY).

Dicumarol: It has been reported that allopurinol prolongs the half-life of the anticoagulant, dicumarol. The clinical basis of this drug interaction has not been established but should be noted when allopurinol is given to patients already on dicumarol therapy. Consequently, prothrombin time should be reassessed periodically in patients receiving both drugs.

Uricosuric Agents: Since the excretion of oxipurinol is similar to that of urate, uricosuric agents, which increase the excretion of urate, are also likely to increase the excretion of oxipurinol and thus lower the degree of inhibition of xanthine oxidase. The concomitant administration of uricosuric agents and allopurinol has been associated with a decrease in the excretion of oxypurines (hypoxanthine and xanthine) for oral allopurinol and decreases the inhibition of xanthine oxidase by oxypurinol for the allopurinol sodium for injection. There was an increase in urinary uric acid excretion compared with that observed with allopurinol alone. Although clinical evidence to date has not demonstrated renal precipitation of oxypurines in patients either on allopurinol alone or in combination with uricosuric agents, the possibility should be kept in mind.

Thiazide Diuretics: The reports that the concomitant use of allopurinol and thiazide diuretics may contribute to the enhancement of allopurinol toxicity in some patients have been reviewed in an attempt to establish a cause-and-effect relationship and a mechanism of causation. Review of these case reports indicates that the patients were mainly receiving thiazide diuretics for hypertension and that tests to rule out decreased renal function secondary to hypertensive nephropathy were not often performed. In those patients in whom renal insufficiency was documented, however, the recommendation to lower the dose of allopurinol was not followed. Although a causal mechanism and a cause-and-effect relationship have not been established, current evidence suggests that renal function should be monitored in patients on thiazide diuretics and allopurinol even in the absence of renal failure, and dosage levels should be even more conservatively adjusted in those patients on such combined therapy if diminished renal function is detected. (See WARNINGS).

Ampicillin/Amoxicillin: An increase in the frequency of skin rash has been reported among patients receiving ampicillin or amoxicillin concurrently with allopurinol compared to patients who are not receiving both drugs. The cause of the reported association has not been established.

Cytotoxic Agents: Enhanced bone marrow suppression by cyclophosphamide and other cytotoxic agents has been reported among patients with neoplastic disease, except leukemia, in the presence of allopurinol. However, in a well-controlled study of patients with lymphoma on combination therapy, allopurinol did not increase the marrow toxicity of patients treated with cyclophosphamide, doxorubicin, bleomycin, procarbazine and/or mechlorethamine.

Chlorpropamide: Chlorpropamide's plasma half-life may be prolonged by allopurinol, since allopurinol and chlorpropamide may compete for excretion in the renal tubule. The risk of hypoglycemia secondary to this mechanism may be increased if allopurinol and chlorpropamide are given concomitantly in the presence of renal insufficiency.

Cyclosporin: Reports indicate that cyclosporine levels may be increased during concomitant treatment with allopurinol sodium for injection. Monitoring of cyclosporine levels and possible adjustment of cyclosporine dosage should be considered when these drugs are co-administered.

Tolbutamide's conversion to inactive metabolites has been shown to be catalyzed by xanthine oxidase from rat liver. The clinical significance, if any, of these observations is unknown.

ADVERSE REACTIONS

The most frequent adverse reaction to allopurinol is skin rash. Skin reactions can be severe and sometimes fatal. Therefore, treatment with allopurinol should be discontinued immediately if a rash develops (see WARNINGS).

TABLETS

Data upon which the following estimates of incidence of adverse reactions are made are derived from experiences reported in the literature, unpublished clinical trials and voluntary reports since marketing of allopurinol began. Past experience suggested that the most frequent event following the initiation of allopurinol treatment was an increase in acute attacks of gout (average 6% in early studies). An analysis of current usage suggests that the incidence of acute gouty attacks has diminished to less than 1%. The explanation for this decrease has not been determined but may be due in part to initiating therapy more gradually (see PRECAUTIONS and DOSAGE AND ADMINISTRATION).

Some patients with the most severe reaction also had fever, chills, arthralgias, cholestatic jaundice, eosinophilia and mild leukocytosis or leukopenia. Among 55 patients with gout treated with allopurinol for 3-34 months (average greater than 1 year) and followed prospectively, Rundles observed that 3% of patients developed a type of drug reaction which was predominantly a pruritic maculopapular skin eruption, sometimes scaly or exfoliative. However, with current usage, skin reactions have been observed less frequently than 1%. The explanation for this decrease is not obvious. The incidence of skin rash may be increased in the presence of renal insufficiency. The frequency of skin rash among patients receiving ampicillin or amoxicillin concurrently with allopurinol has been reported to be increased (see PRECAUTIONS).

Most Common Reactions* Probably Causally Related:

Gastrointestinal: Diarrhea, nausea, alkaline phosphatase increase, SGOT/SGPT increase.

Metabolic and Nutritional: Acute attacks of gout.

Skin and Appendages: Rash, maculopapular rash.

*Early clinical studies and incidence rates from early clinical experience with allopurinol suggested that these adverse reactions were found to occur at a rate of greater than 1%. The most frequent event observed was acute attacks of gout following the initiation of therapy. Analyses of current usage suggest that the incidence of these adverse reactions is now less than 1%. The explanation for this decrease has not been determined, but it may be due to following recommended usage (see ADVERSE REACTIONS, INDICATIONS AND USAGE, PRECAUTIONS and DOSAGE AND ADMINISTRATION).

Incidence Less Than 1% Probably Causally Related:

Body as a Whole: Ecchymosis, fever, headache.

Cardiovascular: Necrotizing angiitis, vasculitis.

Gastrointestinal: Hepatic necrosis, granulomatous hepatitis, hepatomegaly, hyperbilirubinemia, cholestatic jaundice, vomiting, intermittent abdominal pain, gastritis, dyspepsia.

Hemic and Lymphatic: Thrombocytopenia, eosinophilia, leukocytosis, leukopenia.

Musculoskeletal: Myopathy, arthralgias.

Nervous: Peripheral neuropathy, neuritis, paresthesia, somnolence.

Respiratory: Epistaxis.

Skin and Appendages: Erythema multiform exudativum (Stevens-Johnson syndrome), toxic epidermal necrolysis (Lyell's syndrome), hypersensitivity vasculitis, purpura, vesicular bullous dermatitis, exfoliative dermatitis, eczematoid dermatitis, pruritus, urticaria, alopecia, onycholysis, lichen planus.

Special Senses: Taste loss/perversion.

Urogenital: Renal failure, uremia (see PRECAUTIONS).

Incidence Less Than 1% Causal Relationship Unknown:

Body as a Whole: Malaise.

Cardiovascular: Pericarditis, peripheral vascular disease, thrombophlebitis, bradycardia, vasodilation.

Endocrine: Infertility (male), hypercalcemia, gynecomastia (male).

Gastrointestinal: Hemorrhagic pancreatitis, gastrointestinal bleeding, stomatitis, salivary gland swelling, hyperlipidemia, tongue edema, anorexia.

Hemic and Lymphatic: Aplastic anemia, agranulocytosis, eosinophilic fibrohistiocytic lesion of bone marrow, pancytopenia, prothrombin decrease, anemia, hemolytic anemia, reticulocytosis, lymphadenopathy, lymphocytosis.

Musculoskeletal: Myalgia.

Nervous: Optic neuritis, confusion, dizziness, vertigo, foot drop, decrease in libido, depression, amnesia, tinnitus, asthenia, insomnia.

Respiratory: Bronchospasm, asthma, pharyngitis, rhinitis.

Skin and Appendages: Furunculosis, facial edema, sweating, skin edema.

Special Senses: Cataracts, macular retinitis, iritis, conjunctivitis, amblyopia.

Urogenital: Nephritis, impotence, primary hematuria, albuminuria.

INJECTION

In an uncontrolled, compassionate plea protocol, 125 or 1378 patients reported a total of 301 adverse reactions while receiving allopurinol sodium for injection. Most of the patients had advanced malignancies or serious underlying diseases and were taking multiple concomitant medications. Side effects directly attributable to allopurinol sodium for injection were reported in 19 patients. Fifteen of these adverse experiences were allergic in nature (rash, eosinophilia, local injection site reaction). One adverse experience of severe diarrhea and one incidence of nausea were also reported as being possibly attributable to allopurinol sodium for injection. Two patients had serious adverse experiences (decreased renal function and generalized seizure) reported as being possibly attributable to allopurinol sodium for injection.

A listing of the adverse reactions regardless of causality reported from clinical trials follows.

Incidence Greater Than 1%:

Cutaneous/Dermatologic: Rash (1.5%).

Genitourinary: Renal failure/insufficiency (1.2%).

Gastrointestinal: Nausea (1.3%), vomiting (1.2%).

Incidence Less Than 1%:

Body as a Whole: Fever, pain, chills, alopecia, infection, sepsis, enlarged abdomen, mucositis/pharyngitis, blast crisis, cellulitis, hypervolemia.

Cardiovascular: Heart failure, cardiorespiratory arrest, hypertension, pulmonary embolus, hypotension, decreased venous pressure, flushing, headache, stroke, septic shock, cardiovascular disorder, ECG abnormality, hemorrhage, bradycardia, thrombophlebitis, ventricular fibrillation.

Cutaneous/Dermatologic: Urticaria, pruritus, local injection site reaction.

Gastrointestinal: Diarrhea, gastrointestinal bleeding, hyperbilirubinemia, splenomegaly, hepatomegaly, intestinal obstruction, jaundice, flatulence, constipation, liver failure, procititis.

Genitourinary: Hematuria, increased creatinine, oliguria, kidney function abnormality, urinary tract infection.

Hematologic: Leukopenia, marrow aplasia, thrombocytopenia, eosinophilia, neutropenia, anemia, pancytopenia, ecchymosis, bone marrow suppression, disseminated intravascular coagulation.

Metabolic: Hypocalcemia, hyperphosphatemia, hypokalemia, hyperuricemia, electrolyte abnormality, hypercalcemia, hyperglycemia, hypernatremia, hyponatremia, metabolic acidosis, edema, glycosuria, hyperkalemia, lactic acidosis, water intoxication, hypomagnesemia.

Neurologic: Seizure, status epilepticus, myoclonus, twitching, agitation, mental status changes, cerebral infarction, coma, dystonia, paralysis, tremor.

Pulmonary: Respiratory failure/insufficiency, ARDS, increased respiration rate, apnea.

Musculoskeletal: Arthralgia.

Other: Hypotonia, diaphoresis, tumor lysis syndrome.

DOSAGE AND ADMINISTRATION

TABLETS

The dosage of allopurinol to accomplish full control of gout and to lower serum uric acid to normal or near-normal levels varies with the severity of the disease. The average is 200-300 mg/day for patients with mild gout and 400-600 mg/day for those with moderately severe tophaceous gout. The appropriate dosage may be administered in divided doses or as a single equivalent dose with the 300 mg tablet. Dosage requirements in excess of 300 mg should be administered in divided doses. The minimal effective dosage is 100/200 mg daily and the maximal recommended dosage is 800 mg daily. To reduce the possibility of flare-up of acute gouty attacks, it is recommended that the patient start with a low dose of allopurinol (100 mg daily) and increase at weekly intervals by 100 mg until a serum uric acid level of 6 mg/dl or less is attained but without exceeding the maximal recommended dosage.

Normal serum urate levels are usually achieved in 1-3 weeks. The upper limit of normal is about 7 mg/dl for men and postmenopausal women and 6 mg/dl for premenopausal women. Too much reliance should not be placed on a single serum uric acid determination since, for technical reasons, estimation of uric acid may be difficult. By selecting the appropriate dosage and, in certain patients, using uricosuric agents concurrently, it is possible to reduce serum uric acid to normal or, if desired, to as low as 2-3 mg/dl and keep it there indefinitely.

While adjusting the dosage of allopurinol in patients who are being treated with colchicine and/or anti-inflammatory agents, it is wise to continue the latter therapy until serum uric acid has been normalized and there has been freedom from acute gouty attacks for several months.

In transferring a patient from a uricosuric agent to allopurinol, the dose of the uricosuric agent should be gradually reduced over a period of several weeks and the dose of allopurinol gradually increased to the required dose needed to maintain a normal serum uric acid level.

It should also be noted that allopurinol is generally better tolerated if taken following meals. A fluid intake sufficient to yield a daily urinary output of at least two liters and the maintenance of a neutral or, preferably, slightly alkaline urine are desirable.

Since allopurinol and its metabolites are primarily eliminated only by the kidney, accumulation of the drug can occur in renal failure, and the dose of allopurinol should consequently be reduced. With a creatinine clearance of 10-20 ml/min, a daily dosage of 200 mg of allopurinol is suitable. When the creatinine clearance is less than 10 ml/min the daily dosage should not exceed 100 mg. With extreme renal impairment (creatinine clearance less than 3 ml/min) the interval between doses may also need to be lengthened.

The correct size and frequency of dosage for maintaining the serum uric acid just within the normal range is best determined by using the serum uric acid level as an index.

For the prevention of uric acid nephropathy during the vigorous therapy of neoplastic disease, treatment with 600-800 mg daily for 2-3 days is advisable together with a high fluid intake. Otherwise similar considerations to the above recommendations for treating patients with gout govern the regulation of dosage for maintenance purposes in secondary hyperuricemia.

The dose of allopurinol recommended for management of recurrent calcium oxalate stones in hyperuricosuric patients is 200-300 mg/day in divided doses or as the single equivalent. This dose may be adjusted up or down depending upon the resultant control of the hyperuricosuria based upon subsequent 24 hour urinary urate determinations. Clinical experience suggests that patients with recurrent calcium oxalate stones may also benefit from dietary changes such as the reduction of animal protein, sodium, refined sugars, oxalate-rich foods, and excessive calcium intake as well as an increase in oral fluids and dietary fiber.

Children, 6-10 years of age, with secondary hyperuricemia associated with malignancies may be given 300 mg allopurinol daily while those under 6 years are generally given 150 mg daily. The response is evaluated after approximately 48 hours of therapy and a dosage adjustment is made if necessary.

INJECTION

Children and Adults: The dosage of allopurinol sodium for injection to lower serum uric acid to normal or near-normal varies with the severity of the disease. The amount and frequency of dosage for maintaining the serum uric acid just within the normal range is best determined by using the serum uric acid level as an index. In adults, in one clinical trial, doses over 600 mg a day did not appear to be more effective. The recommended daily dose of allopurinol sodium for injection is as follows:

The Recommended Daily Dose of Allopurinol Sodium for Injection

Adult: 200-400 mg/m^2/day (maximum 600 mg/day).

Child: Starting dose 200 mg/m^2/day.

Hydration: A fluid intake sufficient to yield a daily urinary output of at least two liters in adults and the maintenance of a neutral or, preferably, slightly alkaline urine are desirable.

Impaired Renal Function: The dose of allopurinol sodium for injection should be reduced in patients with impaired renal function to avoid accumulation of allopurinol and its metabolites (see TABLE 3).

TABLE 3

Creatinine Clearance	Recommended Daily Dose
10-20 ml/min	200 mg/day
3-10 ml/min	100 mg/day
<3 ml/min	100 mg/day at extended intervals

Administration: In both adults and children, the daily dose can be given as single infusion or in equally divided infusions at 6, 8, or 12 hour intervals at the recommended final concentration of not greater than 6 mg/ml (see Preparation of Solution). The rate of infusion depends on the volume of infusate. Whenever possible, therapy with allopurinol sodium for injection should be initiated 24-48 hours before the start of chemotherapy known to cause tumor cell lysis (including adrenocorticosteroids).

Allopurinol sodium for injection should not be mixed with or administered through the same intravenous port with agents which are incompatible in solution with allopurinol sodium for injection (see Preparation for Solution).

Preparation of Solution: Allopurinol sodium for injection must be reconstituted and diluted. The contents of each 30 ml vial should be dissolved with 25 ml of sterile water for injection. Reconstitution yields a clear, almost colorless solution with no more than a slight opalescence. This concentrated solution has a pH of 11.1-11.8. It should be diluted to the desired concentration with 0.9% sodium chloride injection or 5% dextrose for injection. Sodium bicarbonate-containing solutions should not be used. A final concentration of no greater than 6 mg/ml is recommended. The solution should be stored at 20-25°C (68-77°F) and administration should begin with 10 hours after reconstitution. Do not refrigerate the reconstituted and/or diluted product.

Parenteral drug products should be inspected visually for particulate matter and discoloration prior to administration, whenever solution and container permit. Do not use this product if particulate matter or discoloration is present.

Drugs that are physically incompatible in solution with allopurinol sodium for injection include:

Amikacin sulfate, amphotericin B, carmustine, cefotaxime sodium, chlorpromazine HCl, cimetidine HCl, clinicamycin phosphate, cytarabine, dacarbazine, daunorubicin HCl, diphenhydramine HCl, doxorubicin HCl, doxycycline hyclate, droperidol, floxuridine, gentamicin sulfate, haloperidol lactate, hydroxyzine HCl, idarubicin HCl, imipenem-cilastatin sodium, mechlorethamine HCl, meperidine HCl, metoclopramide HCl, methylprednisolone sodium succinate, minocycline HCl, nalbuphine HCl, netilmicin sulfate, ondansetron HCl, prochlorperazine edisylate, promethazine HCl, sodium bicarbonate, streptozocin, tobramycin sulfate, vinorelbine tartrate.

HOW SUPPLIED

TABLETS

100 mg: Tablets are white, scored, flat cylindrical tablets imprinted with "Zyloprim 100" on a raised hexagon.

300 mg: Tablets are peach, scored, flat cylindrical tablets imprinted with "Zyloprim 100" on a raised hexagon.

Storage: Store at 15-25°C (59-77°F) in a dry place and protect from light.

INJECTION

STERILE SINGLE USE VIAL FOR INTRAVENOUS INFUSION.

Allopurinol sodium for injection is supplied as white lyophilized powder equivalent to 500 mg of allopurinol.

Storage: Store unconstituted powder at 25°C (77°F); excursions permitted to 15-30°C (59-86°F).

PRODUCT LISTING - RATED THERAPEUTICALLY EQUIVALENT

Tablet - Oral - 100 mg

Qty	Price	Product	NDC
15's	$1.92	GENERIC, Heartland Healthcare Services	61392-0103-15
25's	$3.10	GENERIC, Udl Laboratories Inc	51079-0205-19
30's	$3.83	GENERIC, Heartland Healthcare Services	61392-0103-30
30's	$3.83	GENERIC, Heartland Healthcare Services	61392-0103-39
30's	$5.99	GENERIC, Pharma Pac	52959-0473-30
31 x 10	$57.24	GENERIC, Vangard Labs	00615-1592-53
31 x 10	$57.24	GENERIC, Vangard Labs	00615-1592-63
31's	$3.83	GENERIC, Heartland Healthcare Services	61392-0103-31
32's	$4.09	GENERIC, Heartland Healthcare Services	61392-0103-32
45's	$5.75	GENERIC, Heartland Healthcare Services	61392-0103-45
60's	$7.67	GENERIC, Heartland Healthcare Services	61392-0103-60
60's	$7.67	GENERIC, Heartland Healthcare Services	61392-0103-65
90's	$11.50	GENERIC, Heartland Healthcare Services	61392-0103-90
100's	$5.70	GENERIC, Interstate Drug Exchange Inc	00814-0510-14
100's	$7.75	GENERIC, Mova Pharmaceutical Corporation	55370-0527-07
100's	$7.84	FEDERAL UPPER LIMIT, H.C.F.A. F F P	99999-0133-01
100's	$9.20	GENERIC, Aligen Independent Laboratories Inc	00405-4036-01
100's	$9.69	GENERIC, Parmed Pharmaceuticals Inc	00349-8911-01
100's	$9.79	GENERIC, Moore, H.L. Drug Exchange Inc	00839-7713-06
100's	$11.24	GENERIC, Auro Pharmaceutical	55829-0121-10
100's	$13.97	GENERIC, Vangard Labs	00615-1592-13
100's	$16.63	GENERIC, Ivax Corporation	00182-1481-89
100's	$17.99	GENERIC, Qualitest Products Inc	00603-2117-21
100's	$18.36	GENERIC, Geneva Pharmaceuticals	00781-1080-01
100's	$18.50	GENERIC, Watson/Schein Pharmaceuticals Inc	00364-0632-01
100's	$19.36	GENERIC, Geneva Pharmaceuticals	00781-1080-13
100's	$19.70	GENERIC, Par Pharmaceutical Inc	49884-0602-01
100's	$21.72	GENERIC, Mylan Pharmaceuticals Inc	00378-0137-01
100's	$22.37	GENERIC, Udl Laboratories Inc	51079-0205-20
100's	$24.18	GENERIC, Major Pharmaceuticals Inc	00904-2613-60
100's	$24.24	GENERIC, Watson/Schein Pharmaceuticals Inc	00591-5543-01
100's	$24.24	GENERIC, Mutual Pharmaceutical Co Inc	53489-0156-01
100's	$24.42	GENERIC, Mutual/United Research Laboratories	00677-0870-01
100's	$24.42	GENERIC, Par Pharmaceutical Inc	49884-0104-01
100's	$26.87	GENERIC, Major Pharmaceuticals Inc	00904-2613-61
100's	$29.30	ZYLOPRIM, Faro Pharmaceuticals Inc	60976-0996-55
100's	$33.28	ZYLOPRIM, Prometheus Inc	65483-0991-10
100's	$60.50	GENERIC, Pharma Pac	52959-0311-00
200 x 5	$184.63	GENERIC, Vangard Labs	00615-1592-43

Tablet - Oral - 300 mg

Qty	Price	Product	NDC
3's	$2.82	GENERIC, Pd-Rx Pharmaceuticals	55289-0010-03
30's	$5.88	GENERIC, Pd-Rx Pharmaceuticals	55289-0010-30
30's	$14.30	GENERIC, Heartland Healthcare Services	61392-0104-30
30's	$14.30	GENERIC, Heartland Healthcare Services	61392-0104-39
30's	$21.43	GENERIC, Golden State Medical	60429-0014-30
30's	$23.67	ZYLOPRIM, Physicians Total Care	54868-0678-02
31 x 10	$156.18	GENERIC, Vangard Labs	00615-1593-53
31 x 10	$156.18	GENERIC, Vangard Labs	00615-1593-63
31's	$14.78	GENERIC, Heartland Healthcare Services	61392-0104-31
32's	$15.26	GENERIC, Heartland Healthcare Services	61392-0104-32
45's	$21.46	GENERIC, Heartland Healthcare Services	61392-0104-45
60's	$28.61	GENERIC, Heartland Healthcare Services	61392-0104-60
60's	$28.61	GENERIC, Heartland Healthcare Services	61392-0104-65
90's	$8.60	GENERIC, Pd-Rx Pharmaceuticals	55289-0010-90
90's	$42.91	GENERIC, Heartland Healthcare Services	61392-0104-90
90's	$74.90	GENERIC, Golden State Medical	60429-0014-90
100's	$10.05	FEDERAL UPPER LIMIT, H.C.F.A. F F P	99999-0133-04
100's	$10.88	GENERIC, Pd-Rx Pharmaceuticals	55289-0010-01
100's	$13.05	GENERIC, Interstate Drug Exchange Inc	00814-0511-14
100's	$18.10	GENERIC, Mova Pharmaceutical Corporation	55370-0529-07
100's	$22.30	GENERIC, Aligen Independent Laboratories Inc	00405-4037-01
100's	$22.75	GENERIC, Martec Pharmaceuticals Inc	52555-0210-01
100's	$22.94	GENERIC, Parmed Pharmaceuticals Inc	00349-8912-01
100's	$23.69	GENERIC, Moore, H.L. Drug Exchange Inc	00839-7714-06
100's	$29.44	GENERIC, Auro Pharmaceutical	55829-0122-10
100's	$33.23	GENERIC, Ivax Corporation	00182-1482-89
100's	$35.75	GENERIC, Vangard Labs	00615-1593-13
100's	$35.75	GENERIC, Geneva Pharmaceuticals	00781-1082-13
100's	$44.48	GENERIC, Watson/Schein Pharmaceuticals Inc	00364-0633-01
100's	$49.25	GENERIC, Qualitest Products Inc	00603-2118-21
100's	$50.29	GENERIC, Geneva Pharmaceuticals	00781-1082-01
100's	$53.55	GENERIC, Par Pharmaceutical Inc	49884-0603-01
100's	$58.45	GENERIC, Major Pharmaceuticals Inc	00904-2614-60
100's	$59.04	GENERIC, Mylan Pharmaceuticals Inc	00378-0181-01
100's	$60.81	GENERIC, Udl Laboratories Inc	51079-0206-20
100's	$64.40	GENERIC, Mutual Pharmaceutical Co Inc	53489-0157-01
100's	$64.50	GENERIC, Watson Laboratories Inc	00591-5544-01
100's	$66.89	GENERIC, Par Pharmaceutical Inc	49884-0105-01
100's	$73.53	GENERIC, Major Pharmaceuticals Inc	00904-2614-61
100's	$76.15	ZYLOPRIM, Physicians Total Care	54868-0678-01
100's	$80.27	ZYLOPRIM, Faro Pharmaceuticals Inc	60976-0998-55
100's	$91.14	ZYLOPRIM, Prometheus Inc	65483-0993-10
100's	$352.64	ZYLOPRIM, Faro Pharmaceuticals Inc	60976-0998-70
200 x 5	$503.82	GENERIC, Vangard Labs	00615-1593-43

PRODUCT LISTING - EQUIVALENTS NOT AVAILABLE

Powder For Injection - Intravenous - 500 mg

Qty	Price	Product	NDC
1's	$500.00	ALOPRIM, Nabi	59730-5601-01

Tablet - Oral - 100 mg

Qty	Price	Product	NDC
12's	$2.33	GENERIC, Southwood Pharmaceuticals Inc	58016-0941-12
20's	$3.89	GENERIC, Southwood Pharmaceuticals Inc	58016-0941-20
30's	$5.84	GENERIC, Southwood Pharmaceuticals Inc	58016-0941-30
30's	$6.52	GENERIC, Allscripts Pharmaceutical Company	54569-0233-03
60's	$5.10	GENERIC, Physicians Total Care	54868-0075-03
100's	$7.38	GENERIC, Physicians Total Care	54868-0075-04
100's	$9.75	GENERIC, Cmc-Consolidated Midland Corporation	00223-0114-01
100's	$19.45	GENERIC, Southwood Pharmaceuticals Inc	58016-0941-00
100's	$21.72	GENERIC, Allscripts Pharmaceutical Company	54569-0233-00

Tablet - Oral - 300 mg

Qty	Price	Product	NDC
12's	$4.01	GENERIC, Alpharma Uspd Makers Of Barre and Nmc	63874-0755-12
12's	$6.93	GENERIC, Southwood Pharmaceuticals Inc	58016-0942-12
20's	$5.39	GENERIC, Alpharma Uspd Makers Of Barre and Nmc	63874-0755-20
20's	$10.65	GENERIC, Southwood Pharmaceuticals Inc	58016-0942-20
30's	$5.96	GENERIC, Alpharma Uspd Makers Of Barre and Nmc	63874-0755-30
30's	$6.67	GENERIC, Physicians Total Care	54868-0076-06
30's	$15.40	GENERIC, Pharmaceutical Corporation Of America	51655-0038-24
30's	$15.98	GENERIC, Southwood Pharmaceuticals Inc	58016-0942-30

A

30's	$16.25	GENERIC, Allscripts Pharmaceutical Company	54569-0235-01
50's	$10.00	GENERIC, Physicians Total Care	54868-0076-05
60's	$11.67	GENERIC, Physicians Total Care	54868-0076-02
100's	$18.33	GENERIC, Physicians Total Care	54868-0076-03
100's	$21.00	GENERIC, Cmc-Consolidated Midland Corporation	00223-0115-01
100's	$53.27	GENERIC, Southwood Pharmaceuticals Inc	58016-0942-00
100's	$54.16	GENERIC, Allscripts Pharmaceutical Company	54569-0235-00
100's	$56.47	GENERIC, Alpharma Uspd Makers Of Barre and Nmc	63874-0755-01

Almotriptan Malate *(003243)*

For related information, see the comparative table section in Appendix A.

Categories: Headache, migraine; Pregnancy Category C; FDA Approved 2001 May
Drug Classes: Serotonin receptor agonists
Brand Names: Axert
Cost of Therapy: $11.75 (Migraine Headache; Axert; 12.5 mg; 1 tablet/day; 1 day supply)

DESCRIPTION

Axert tablets contain almotriptan malate, a selective 5-hydroxytryptamine$_{1B/1D}$ (5-HT$_{1B/1D}$) receptor agonist. Almotriptan malate is chemically designated as 1-[[[3-[2-(Dimethylamino)ethyl]-1H-indol-5-yl]methyl]sulfonyl] pyrrolidine (±)-hydroxybutane-dioate (1:1).

Its empirical formula is $C_{17}H_{25}N_3O_2S{\cdot}C_4H_6O_5$, representing a molecular weight of 469.56. Almotriptan is a white to slightly yellow crystalline powder that is soluble in water. Axert tablets for oral administration contain almotriptan malate equivalent to 6.25 or 12.5 mg of almotriptan. Each compressed tablet contains the following inactive ingredients: mannitol, cellulose, povidone, sodium starch glycolate, sodium stearyl fumarate, titanium dioxide, hydroxypropyl methylcellulose, polyethylene glycol, propylene glycol, iron oxide (6.25 mg only), FD&C blue no. 2 (12.5 mg only), and carnauba wax.

CLINICAL PHARMACOLOGY

MECHANISM OF ACTION

Almotriptan binds with high affinity to 5-HT$_{1D}$, 5-HT$_{1B}$, and 5-HT$_{1F}$ receptors. Almotriptan has weak affinity for 5-HT$_{1A}$ and 5-HT$_7$ receptors, but has no significant affinity or pharmacological activity at 5-HT$_2$, 5-HT$_3$, 5-HT$_4$, 5-HT$_6$; alpha or beta adrenergic; adenosine (A_1, A_2); angiotensin (AT_1, AT_2); dopamine (D_1, D_2); endothelin (ET_A, ET_B); or tachykinin (NK_1, NK_2, NK_3) binding sites.

Current theories on the etiology of migraine headache suggest that symptoms are due to local cranial vasodilatation and/or to the release of vasoactive and proinflammatory peptides from sensory nerve endings in an activated trigeminal system. The therapeutic activity of almotriptan in migraine can most likely be attributed to agonist effects at 5-HT$_{1B/1D}$ receptors on the extracerebral, intracranial blood vessels that become dilated during a migraine attack, and on nerve terminals in the trigeminal system. Activation of these receptors results in cranial vessel constriction, inhibition of neuropeptide release, and reduced transmission in trigeminal pain pathways.

PHARMACOKINETICS

General

Almotriptan is well absorbed after oral administration (absolute bioavailability about 70%) with peak plasma levels 1-3 hours after administration; food does not affect pharmacokinetics. Almotriptan has a mean half-life of 3-4 hours. It is eliminated primarily by renal excretion (about 75% of the oral dose). Almotriptan is minimally protein bound (approximately 35%) and the mean apparent volume of distribution is approximately 180-200 liters.

Metabolism and Excretion

Almotriptan is metabolized by one minor and two major pathways. Monoamine oxidase (MAO)-mediated oxidative deamination (approximately 27% of the dose), and cytochrome P450-mediated oxidation (approximately 12% of the dose) are the major routes of metabolism, while flavin monooxygenase is the minor route. MAO-A is responsible for the formation of the indoleacetic acid metabolite, whereas cytochrome P450 (3A4 and 2D6) catalyzes the hydroxylation of the pyrrolidine ring to an intermediate that is further oxidized by aldehyde dehydrogenase to the gamma-aminobutyric acid derivative. Both metabolites are inactive.

Approximately 40% of an administered dose is excreted unchanged in urine. Renal clearance exceeds the glomerular filtration rate by approximately 3-fold, indicating an active mechanism. Approximately 13% of the administered dose is excreted via feces, both unchanged and metabolized.

SPECIAL POPULATIONS

Geriatric

Renal and total clearance, and amount of drug excreted in the urine were lower in elderly healthy volunteers (age 65-76 years) than in younger healthy volunteers (age 19-34 years), resulting in longer terminal half-life (3.7 hours vs 3.2 hours) and a 25% higher area under the plasma concentration-time curve in the elderly subjects. The differences, however, do not appear to be clinically significant.

Pediatric

The pharmacokinetics of almotriptan in pediatric patients have not been evaluated.

Gender

No significant gender differences have been observed in pharmacokinetic parameters.

Race

No significant differences have been observed in pharmacokinetic parameters between Caucasian and African-American volunteers.

Hepatic Impairment

The pharmacokinetics of almotriptan have not been assessed in this population. Based on the known mechanisms of clearance of almotriptan, the maximum decrease expected in almotriptan clearance due to hepatic impairment would be 60% (see DOSAGE AND ADMINISTRATION).

Renal Impairment

The clearance of almotriptan was approximately 65% lower in patients with severe renal impairment (CL/F = 19.8 L/h; creatinine clearance between 10 and 30 ml/min) and approximately 40% lower in patients with moderate renal impairment (CL/F = 34.2 L/h; creatinine clearance between 31 and 71 ml/min) than in healthy volunteers (CL/F = 57 L/h). Maximal plasma concentrations of almotriptan increased by approximately 80% in these patients (see DOSAGE AND ADMINISTRATION).

DRUG INTERACTIONS

See also DRUG INTERACTIONS.

All drug interaction studies were performed in healthy volunteers using a single 12.5 mg dose of almotriptan and multiple doses of the other drug.

Monoamine Oxidase Inhibitors: Coadministration of almotriptan and moclobemide (150 mg bid for 8 days) resulted in a 27% decrease in almotriptan clearance.

Propranolol: Coadministration of almotriptan and propranolol (80 mg bid for 7 days) resulted in no significant changes in the pharmacokinetics of almotriptan.

Selective Serotonin Reuptake Inhibitors: Coadministration of almotriptan and fluoxetine (60 mg daily for 8 days), a potent inhibitor of CYP4502D6, had no effect on almotriptan clearance, but maximal concentrations of almotriptan were increased 18%. This difference is not clinically significant.

Verapamil: Coadministration of almotriptan and verapamil (120 mg sustained release tablets bid for 7 days), an inhibitor of CYP4503A4, resulted in a 20% increase in the area under the plasma concentration-time curve, and in a 24% increase in maximal plasma concentrations of almotriptan. Neither of these changes is clinically significant.

Ketoconazole and Other Potent CYP3A4 Inhibitors: Coadministration of almotriptan and the potent CYP3A4 inhibitor ketoconazole (400 mg qd for 3 days) resulted in an approximately 60% increase in the area under the plasma concentration-time curve and maximal plasma concentrations of almotriptan. Although the interaction between almotriptan and other potent CYP3A4 inhibitors (*e.g.*, itraconazole, ritonavir, and erythromycin) has not been studied, increased exposures to almotriptan may be expected when almotriptan is used concomitantly with these medications.

INDICATIONS AND USAGE

Almotriptan malate tablets are indicated for the acute treatment of migraine with or without aura in adults.

Almotriptan malate is not intended for the prophylactic therapy of migraine or for use in the management of hemiplegic or basilar migraine (see CONTRAINDICATIONS). Safety and effectiveness of almotriptan malate have not been established for cluster headache, which is present in an older, predominantly male population.

CONTRAINDICATIONS

Almotriptan malate tablets should not be given to patients with ischemic heart disease (angina pectoris, history of myocardial infarction, or documented silent ischemia), or to patients who have symptoms or findings consistent with ischemic heart disease, coronary artery vasospasm, including Prinzmetal's variant angina, or other significant underlying cardiovascular disease (see WARNINGS).

Because almotriptan malate may increase blood pressure, it should not be given to patients with uncontrolled hypertension (see WARNINGS).

Almotriptan malate should not be administered within 24 hours of treatment with another 5-HT$_1$ agonist, or an ergotamine-containing or ergot-type medication like dihydroergotamine or methysergide.

Almotriptan malate should not be given to patients with hemiplegic or basilar migraine.

Almotriptan malate is contraindicated in patients who are hypersensitive to almotriptan or any of its ingredients.

WARNINGS

Almotriptan malate tablets should only be used where a clear diagnosis of migraine has been established.

RISK OF MYOCARDIAL ISCHEMIA AND/OR INFARCTION AND OTHER ADVERSE CARDIAC EVENTS

Because of the potential of this class of compounds (5-HT$_{1B/1D}$ agonists) to cause coronary vasospasm, almotriptan malate should not be given to patients with documented ischemic or vasospastic coronary artery disease (see CONTRAINDICATIONS). It is strongly recommended that 5-HT$_1$ agonists (including almotriptan malate) not be given to patients in whom unrecognized coronary artery disease (CAD) is predicted by the presence of risk factors (*e.g.*, hypertension, hypercholesterolemia, smoker, obesity, diabetes, strong family history of CAD, female with surgical or physiological menopause, or male over 40 years of age) unless a cardiovascular evaluation provides satisfactory clinical evidence that the patient is reasonably free of coronary artery and ischemic myocardial disease or other significant underlying cardiovascular disease. The sensitivity of cardiac diagnostic procedures to detect cardiovascular diseases or predisposition to coronary artery vasospasm is modest at best. If, during the cardiovascular evaluation, the patient's medical history, electrocardiogram (ECG), or other investigations reveal findings indicative of, or consistent with, coronary artery vasospasm or myocardial ischemia, almotriptan malate should not be administered (see CONTRAINDICATIONS). For patients with risk factors predictive of CAD, who are determined to have a satisfactory cardiovascular evaluation, it is strongly recommended that administration of the first dose of almotriptan malate take place in the setting of a physician's office or similar medically staffed and equipped facility, unless the patient has previously received almotriptan. Because cardiac ischemia can occur in the absence of clinical symptoms, consideration should be given to obtaining an ECG during the interval immediately following the first use of almotriptan malate in a patient with risk factors.

It is recommended that patients who are intermittent long-term users of almotriptan malate and who have or acquire risk factors predictive of CAD, as described above, undergo periodic interval cardiovascular evaluation as they continue to use almotriptan malate.

The systematic approach described above is intended to reduce the likelihood that patients with unrecognized cardiovascular disease will be inadvertently exposed to almotriptan malate.

CARDIAC EVENTS AND FATALITIES ASSOCIATED WITH 5-HT_1 AGONISTS

Serious adverse cardiac events, including acute myocardial infarction, life-threatening disturbances of cardiac rhythm, and death have been reported within a few hours following the administration of other 5-HT_1 agonists. Considering the extent of use of 5-HT_1 agonists in patients with migraine, the incidence of these events is extremely low. Among the 3865 subjects/patients who received almotriptan malate in premarketing clinical trials, one patient was hospitalized for observation after a scheduled ECG was found to be abnormal (negative T-waves on the left leads) 48 hours after taking a single 6.25 mg dose of almotriptan.The patient, a 48-year-old female, had previously taken 3 other doses for earlier migraine attacks. Myocardial enzymes at the time of the abnormal ECG were normal. The patient was diagnosed as having had myocardial ischemia, and it was also found that she had a family history of coronary disease. An ECG performed 2 days later was normal, as was a follow-up coronary angiography. The patient recovered without incident.

CEREBROVASCULAR EVENTS AND FATALITIES WITH 5-HT_1 AGONISTS

Cerebral hemorrhage, subarachnoid hemorrhage, stroke, and other cerebrovascular events have been reported in patients treated with other 5-HT_1 agonists, and some have resulted in fatalities. In a number of cases, it appears possible that the cerebrovascular events were primary, the agonist having been administered in the incorrect belief that the symptoms experienced were a consequence of migraine, when they were not. It should be noted that patients with migraine may be at increased risk of certain cerebrovascular events (*e.g.*, stroke, hemorrhage, transient ischemic attack).

OTHER VASOSPASM-RELATED EVENTS

5-HT_1 agonists may cause vasospastic reactions other than coronary artery vasospasm. Both peripheral vascular ischemia and colonic ischemia with abdominal pain and bloody diarrhea have been reported with 5-HT_1 agonists.

INCREASES IN BLOOD PRESSURE

Significant elevations in systemic blood pressure, including hypertensive crisis, have been reported on rare occasions in patients with and without a history of hypertension treated with other 5-HT_1 agonists. Almotriptan malate is contraindicated in patients with uncontrolled hypertension (see CONTRAINDICATIONS). In volunteers, small increases in mean systolic and diastolic blood pressure relative to placebo were seen over the first 4 hours after administration of 12.5 mg of almotriptan (0.21 and 1.35 mm Hg, respectively). The effect of almotriptan on blood pressure was also assessed in patients with hypertension controlled by medication. In this population, mean increases in systolic and diastolic blood pressure relative to placebo over the first 4 hours after administration of 12.5 mg of almotriptan were 4.87 and 0.26 mm Hg, respectively. The slight increases in blood pressure in both volunteers and controlled hypertensive patients were not considered clinically significant.

An 18% increase in mean pulmonary artery pressure was seen following dosing with another 5-HT_1 agonist in a study evaluating subjects undergoing cardiac catheterization.

PRECAUTIONS

GENERAL

As with other 5-$HT_{1B/1D}$ agonists, sensations of tightness, pain, pressure, and heaviness in the precordium, throat, neck, and jaw have been reported after treatment with almotriptan malate tablets. These events have not been associated with arrhythmias or ischemic ECG changes in clinical trials. Because drugs in this class may cause coronary artery vasospasm, patients who experience signs or symptoms suggestive of angina following dosing should be evaluated for the presence of CAD or a predisposition to Prinzmetal's variant angina before receiving additional doses of medication, and should be monitored electrocardiographically if dosing is resumed and similar symptoms recur. Similarly, patients who experience other symptoms or signs suggestive of decreased arterial flow, such as ischemic bowel syndrome or Raynaud's syndrome following the use of any 5-HT_1 agonist are candidates for further evaluation (see WARNINGS).

Almotriptan malate should also be administered with caution to patients with diseases that may alter the absorption, metabolism, or excretion of drugs, such as those with impaired hepatic or renal function (see CLINICAL PHARMACOLOGY, Special Populations).

For a given attack, if a patient does not respond to the first dose of almotriptan malate, the diagnosis of migraine headache should be reconsidered before the administration of a second dose.

BINDING TO MELANIN-CONTAINING TISSUES

When pigmented rats were given a single oral dose of 5 mg/kg of radiolabeled almotriptan, the elimination half-life of radioactivity from the eye was 22 days. This finding suggests that almotriptan and/or its metabolites may bind to the melanin of the eye. Because almotriptan could accumulate in melanin-rich tissues over time, there is the possibility that it could cause toxicity in these tissues over extended use. However, no adverse retinal effects related to treatment with almotriptan were noted in a 52 week toxicity study in dogs given up to 12.5 mg/kg/day (resulting in systemic exposure [plasma AUC] to parent drug approximately 20 times that in humans receiving the maximum recommended daily dose of 25 mg). Although no systematic monitoring of ophthalmologic function was undertaken in clinical trials, and no specific recommendations for ophthalmologic monitoring are offered, prescribers should be aware of the possibility of long-term ophthalmologic effects.

CORNEAL OPACITIES

Three (3) male dogs (out of a total of 14 treated) in a 52 week toxicity study of oral almotriptan, developed slight corneal opacities that were noted after 51, but not after 25, weeks of treatment. The doses at which this occurred were 2, 5, and 12.5 mg/kg/day. The opacity reversed in the affected dog at 12.5 mg/kg/day after a 4 week drug-free period. Systemic exposure (plasma AUC) to parent drug at 2 mg/kg/day was approximately 2.5 times the exposure in humans receiving the maximum recommended daily dose of 25 mg. A no-effect dose was not established.

INFORMATION FOR THE PATIENT

Refer to the PATIENT INFORMATION that is distributed with the prescription for complete information.

LABORATORY TESTS

No specific laboratory tests are recommended for monitoring patients.

DRUG/LABORATORY TEST INTERACTIONS

Almotriptan malate is not known to interfere with commonly employed clinical laboratory tests.

CARCINOGENESIS, MUTAGENESIS, AND IMPAIRMENT OF FERTILITY

Carcinogenesis

The carcinogenic potential of almotriptan was evaluated by oral gavage for up to 103 weeks in mice at doses up to 250 mg/kg/day and in rats for up to 104 weeks at doses up to 75 mg/kg/day. These doses were associated with plasma exposures (AUC) to parent drug that were approximately 40 and 78 times, in mice and rats respectively, the plasma AUC observed in humans receiving the maximum recommended daily dose (MRDD) of 25 mg. Because of high mortality rates in both studies, which reached statistical significance in high dose female mice, all female rats, all male mice, and high dose female mice were terminated between weeks 96 and 98. There was no increase in tumors related to almotriptan administration.

Mutagenesis

Almotriptan was not mutagenic, with or without metabolic activation, in two *in vitro* gene mutation assays, the Ames test and the thymidine locus mouse lymphoma assay. Almotriptan was not clastogenic in an *in vivo* mouse micronucleus assay. Almotriptan produced an equivocal weakly positive response in *in vitro* cytogenetics assays in human lymphocytes.

Impairment of Fertility

When female rats received almotriptan by oral gavage prior to and during mating and up to implantation at doses of 25, 100, and 400 mg/kg/day, prolongation of the estrous cycle was observed at a dose of 100 mg/kg/day (40 times the maximum recommended daily dose [MRDD] of 25 mg on a mg/m^2 basis). No effects on fertility were noted in female rats at 25 mg/kg/day (approximately 10 times the MRDD on a mg/m^2 basis).

PREGNANCY CATEGORY C

When almotriptan was administered by oral gavage to pregnant rats throughout the period of organogenesis at doses of 125, 250, 500, and 1000 mg/kg/day, an increase in embryolethality was seen at the highest dose (maternal exposure, based on plasma AUC of parent drug, was approximately 958 times the human exposure at the maximum recommended daily dose [MRDD] of 25 mg). Increased incidences of fetal skeletal variations (decreased ossification) were noted at doses greater than 125 mg/kg/day (maternal exposure 80 times human exposure at MRDD). Similar studies in rabbits conducted with almotriptan at doses of 5, 20, and 60 mg/kg/day demonstrated increases in embryolethality at the high dose (50 times the MRDD on a mg/m^2 basis). When almotriptan was administered to rats throughout the periods of gestation and lactation at doses of 25, 100, and 400 mg/kg/day, gestation length was increased and litter size and offspring body weight were decreased at the high dose (160 times the MRDD on a mg/m^2 basis). The decrease in pup weight persisted throughout lactation.The no-observed-effect level in this study was 100 mg/kg/day (40 times the MRDD on a mg/m^2 basis).

There are no adequate and well-controlled studies in pregnant women; therefore almotriptan malate should be used during pregnancy only if the potential benefit justifies the potential risk to the fetus.

NURSING MOTHERS

It is not known whether almotriptan is excreted in human milk. Because many drugs are excreted in human milk, caution should be exercised when almotriptan malate is administered to a nursing woman.Lactating rats dosed with almotriptan had milk levels equivalent to maternal plasma levels at 0.5 hours and 7 times higher than plasma levels at 6 hours after dosing.

PEDIATRIC USE

Safety and effectiveness of almotriptan malate in pediatric patients have not been established; therefore, almotriptan malate is not recommended for use in patients under 18 years of age.

Postmarketing experience with other triptans include a limited number of reports that describe pediatric patients who have experienced clinically serious adverse events that are similar in nature to those reported rarely in adults. The long-term safety of almotriptan in pediatric patients has not been studied.

GERIATRIC USE

Clinical studies of almotriptan malate did not include sufficient numbers of subjects aged 65 and over to determine whether they respond differently from younger subjects. Clearance of almotriptan was lower in elderly volunteers than in younger individuals but there were no observed differences in the safety and tolerability between the two populations (see CLINICAL PHARMACOLOGY, Special Populations). In general, dose selection for an elderly patient should be cautious, usually starting at the low end of the dosing range, reflecting the greater frequency of decreased hepatic, renal or cardiac function, and of concomitant disease or other drug therapy. The recommended dose of almotriptan malate for elderly patients with normal renal function for their age is the same as that recommended for younger adults.

DRUG INTERACTIONS

See also CLINICAL PHARMACOLOGY, Drug Interactions.

Ergot-Containing Drugs: These drugs have been reported to cause prolonged vasospastic reactions. Because there is a theoretical basis that these effects may be additive, use of ergotamine-containing or ergot-type medications (like dihydroergotamine or methysergide) and almotriptan malate within 24 hours of each other should be avoided (see CONTRAINDICATIONS).

Monoamine Oxidase Inhibitors: Coadministration of moclobemide resulted in a 27% decrease in almotriptan clearance and an increase in C_{max} of approximately 6%. No dose adjustment is necessary.

Other 5-HT$_{1B/1D}$ Agonists: Concomitant use of other 5-HT$_{1B/1D}$ agonists within 24 hours of treatment with almotriptan malate is contraindicated (see CONTRAINDICATIONS).

Propranolol: The pharmacokinetics of almotriptan were not affected by coadministration of propranolol.

Selective Serotonin Reuptake Inhibitors (SSRIs): SSRIs (*e.g.,* fluoxetine, fluvoxamine, paroxetine, sertraline) have been rarely reported to cause weakness, hyperreflexia, and incoordination when coadministered with 5-HT$_1$ agonists. If concomitant treatment with almotriptan malate and an SSRI is clinically warranted, appropriate observation of the patient is advised.

Verapamil: Coadministration of almotriptan and verapamil resulted in a 24% increase in plasma concentrations of almotriptan. No dose adjustment is necessary.

Ketoconazole and Other Potent CYP3A4 Inhibitors: Coadministration of almotriptan and the potent CYP3A4 inhibitor ketoconazole (400 mg qd for 3 days) resulted in an approximately 60% increase in the area under the plasma concentration-time curve and maximal plasma concentrations of almotriptan. Although the interaction between almotriptan and other potent CYP3A4 inhibitors (*e.g.,* itraconazole, ritonavir, and erythromycin) has not been studied, increased exposures to almotriptan may be expected when almotriptan is used concomitantly with these medications.

ADVERSE REACTIONS

Serious cardiac events, including some that have been fatal, have occurred following use of 5-HT$_1$ agonists. These events are extremely rare and most have been reported in patients with risk factors predictive of CAD. Events reported have included coronary artery vasospasm, transient myocardial ischemia, myocardial infarction, ventricular tachycardia, and ventricular fibrillation (see CONTRAINDICATIONS, WARNINGS and PRECAUTIONS).

INCIDENCE IN CONTROLLED CLINICAL TRIALS

Adverse events were assessed in controlled clinical trials that included 1840 patients who received one or two doses of almotriptan malate tablets and 386 patients who received placebo.

The most common adverse events during treatment with almotriptan malate were nausea, somnolence, headache, paresthesia, and dry mouth. In long-term open-label studies where patients were allowed to treat multiple attacks for up to 1 year, 5% (63 out of 1347 patients) withdrew due to adverse experiences.

TABLE 2 lists the adverse events that occurred in at least 1% of the patients treated with almotriptan malate, and at an incidence greater than in patients treated with placebo, regardless of drug relationship. These events reflect experience gained under closely monitored conditions of clinical trials in a highly selected patient population. In actual clinical practice or in other clinical trials, these frequency estimates may not apply, as the conditions of use, reporting behavior, and the kinds of patients treated may differ.

TABLE 2 *Incidence of Adverse Events in Controlled Clinical Trials*

(Reported in at least 1% of patients treated with almotriptan malate, and at an incidence greater than placebo)

	Percent of Patients Reporting the Event		
	Almotriptan Malate		
Adverse Event	6.25 mg (n=527)	12.5 mg (n=1313)	Placebo (n=386)
Digestive			
Nausea	1%	2%	1%
Dry mouth	1%	1%	0.5%
Nervous			
Paresthesia	1%	1%	0.5%

Almotriptan malate is generally well tolerated. Most adverse events were mild in intensity and were transient, and did not lead to long-lasting effects. The incidence of adverse events in controlled clinical trials was not affected by gender, weight, age, presence of aura, or use of prophylactic medications or oral contraceptives. There were insufficient data to assess the effect of race on the incidence of adverse events.

OTHER EVENTS

In this section, the frequencies of less commonly reported adverse events are presented. However, the role of almotriptan malate in their causation cannot be reliably determined. Furthermore, variability associated with adverse event reporting, the terminology used to describe adverse events, etc., limit the value of the quantitative frequency estimates provided. Event frequencies are calculated as the number of patients who used almotriptan malate in controlled clinical trials and reported an event, divided by the total number of patients exposed to almotriptan malate in these studies. All reported events are included, except the ones already listed in TABLE 2, those unlikely to be drug-related, and those poorly characterized. Events are further classified within body system categories and enumerated in order of decreasing frequency using the following definitions: *frequent* adverse events are those occurring in at least 1/100 patients; *infrequent* adverse events are those occurring in 1/100 to 1/1000 patients; and *rare* adverse events are those occurring in fewer than 1/1000 patients.

Body: *Frequent:* Headache. *Infrequent:* Abdominal cramp or pain, asthenia, chills, back pain, chest pain, neck pain, fatigue, and rigid neck. *Rare:* Fever and photosensitivity reaction.

Cardiovascular: *Infrequent:* Vasodilation, palpitations, and tachycardia. *Rare:* Hypertension and syncope.

Digestive: *Infrequent:* Diarrhea, vomiting, and dyspepsia. *Rare:* Colitis, gastritis, gastroenteritis, esophageal reflux, increased thirst, and increased salivation.

Metabolic: *Infrequent:* Hyperglycemia and increased serum creatine phosphokinase. *Rare:* Increased gamma glutamyl transpeptidase and hypercholesteremia.

Musculoskeletal: *Infrequent:* Myalgia and muscular weakness. *Rare:* Arthralgia, arthritis, and myopathy.

Nervous: *Frequent:* Dizziness and somnolence. *Infrequent:* Tremor, vertigo, anxiety, hypesthesia, restlessness, CNS stimulation, insomnia, and shakiness. *Rare:* Change in dreams, impaired concentration, abnormal coordination, depressive symptoms, euphoria, hyperreflexia, hypertonia, nervousness, neuropathy, nightmares, and nystagmus.

Respiratory: *Infrequent:* Pharyngitis, rhinitis, dyspnea, laryngismus, sinusitis, bronchitis, and epistaxis. *Rare:* Hyperventilation, laryngitis, and sneezing.

Skin: *Infrequent:* Diaphoresis, dermatitis, erythema, pruritus, and rash.

Special Senses: *Infrequent:* Ear pain, conjunctivitis, eye irritation, hyperacusis, and taste alteration. *Rare:* Diplopia, dry eyes, eye pain, otitis media, parosmia, scotoma, and tinnitus.

Urogenital: *Infrequent:* Dysmenorrhea.

DOSAGE AND ADMINISTRATION

In controlled clinical trials, single doses of 6.25 and 12.5 mg of almotriptan malate tablets were effective for the acute treatment of migraines in adults, with the 12.5 mg dose tending to be a more effective dose. Individuals may vary in response to doses of almotriptan malate. The choice of dose should therefore be made on an individual basis.

If the headache returns, the dose may be repeated after 2 hours, but no more than two doses should be given within a 24 hour period. Controlled trials have not adequately established the effectiveness of a second dose if the initial dose is ineffective.

The safety of treating an average of more than four headaches in a 30 day period has not been established.

HEPATIC IMPAIRMENT

The pharmacokinetics of almotriptan have not been assessed in this population. The maximum decrease expected in the clearance of almotriptan due to hepatic impairment is 60%. Therefore, the maximum daily dose should not exceed 12.5 mg over a 24 hour period, and a starting dose of 6.25 mg should be used (see CLINICAL PHARMACOLOGY, Pharmacokinetics).

RENAL IMPAIRMENT

In patients with severe renal impairment, the clearance of almotriptan was decreased. Therefore, the maximum daily dose should not exceed 12.5 mg over a 24 hour period, and a starting dose of 6.25 mg should be used (see CLINICAL PHARMACOLOGY, Pharmacokinetics).

HOW SUPPLIED

Axert tablets are available as follows:

6.25 mg: White, circular, biconvex tablet, printed in red with the code "2080".

12.5 mg: White, circular, biconvex tablet, printed in blue with a stylized A.

Storage: Store at 25°C (77°F); excursions permitted to 15-30°C (59-86°F).

PRODUCT LISTING - EQUIVALENTS NOT AVAILABLE

Tablet - Oral - 6.25 mg

6's	$70.48	AXERT, Pharmacia and Upjohn	00025-2080-06

Tablet - Oral - 12.5 mg

6's	$70.48	AXERT, Pharmacia and Upjohn	00025-2085-06

Alprazolam (000140)

Categories: Anxiety disorder, generalized; Panic disorder; Pregnancy Category D; DEA Class CIV; FDA Approved 1981 Oct; Top 200 Drugs
Drug Classes: Anxiolytics; Benzodiazepines; Sedatives/hypnotics
Brand Names: Alprazolam Intensol; **Xanax**
Foreign Brand Availability: Alcelam (Thailand); Alganax (Indonesia); Alnax (Thailand); Alpaz (Peru); Alplax (Argentina); Alpralid (Israel); Alpram (Korea); Alpranax (Bahrain; Cyprus; Egypt; Iran; Iraq; Jordan; Kuwait; Lebanon; Libya; Oman; Qatar; Republic-of-Yemen; Saudi-Arabia; Syria; United-Arab-Emirates); Alprax (India); Alprocontin (India); Alprox (Israel; Taiwan); Altraxic (Philippines); Alviz (Indonesia); Alzam (South-Africa); Alzax (Korea); Alzolam (India); Anpress (Thailand); Ansiopax (Chile); Anxirid (South-Africa); Anzion (Thailand); Apo-Alpraz (Canada; Singapore); Azor (South-Africa); Calmlet (Indonesia); Cassadan (Germany); Constan (Japan); Dixin (Colombia); Dizolam (Singapore); Drimpam (South-Africa); Feprax (Indonesia); Frixitas (Indonesia); Frontal (Brazil); Kalma (Australia; New-Zealand; Taiwan); Kinax (Taiwan); Marzolam (Thailand); Neupax (Mexico); Nirvan (Colombia); Pacyl (India); Panix (South-Africa); Pharnax (Thailand); Prinox (Argentina); Restyl (Bahrain; Cyprus; Egypt; Iran; Iraq; Jordan; Kuwait; Lebanon; Libya; Oman; Qatar; Republic-of-Yemen; Saudi-Arabia; Syria; United-Arab-Emirates); Sapram (Korea); Solanax (Japan); Tafil (Costa-Rica; Denmark; El-Salvador; Germany; Guatemala; Honduras; Mexico; Nicaragua; Panama; Venezuela); Tafil D (Mauritius); Tensivan (Colombia); Trankimazin (Spain); Tranquinal (Ecuador; Peru); Tricalma (Chile; Peru); Valeans (Italy); Xanacine (Thailand); Xanagis (Israel); Xanax TS (Canada); Xanolam (South-Africa); Xanor (Austria; Finland; Norway; Philippines; South-Africa; Sweden); Zacetin (Korea); Zanapam (Bahrain; Cyprus; Egypt; Iran; Iraq; Israel; Jordan; Korea; Kuwait; Lebanon; Libya; Oman; Qatar; Republic-of-Yemen; Saudi-Arabia; Syria; United-Arab-Emirates); Zolarem (Bahrain; Benin; Burkina-Faso; Cyprus; Egypt; Ethiopia; Gambia; Ghana; Guinea; Iran; Iraq; Israel; Ivory-Coast; Jordan; Kenya; Kuwait; Lebanon; Liberia; Libya; Malawi; Mali; Mauritania; Mauritius; Morocco; Niger; Nigeria; Oman; Qatar; Republic-of-Yemen; Saudi-Arabia; Senegal; Seychelles; Sierra-Leone; South-Africa; Sudan; Syria; Tanzania; Tunia; Uganda; United-Arab-Emirates; Zambia; Zimbabwe); Zoldac (Benin; Burkina-Faso; Ethiopia; Gambia; Ghana; Guinea; Ivory-Coast; Kenya; Liberia; Malawi; Mali; Mauritania; Mauritius; Morocco; Niger; Nigeria; Senegal; Seychelles; Sierra-Leone; South-Africa; Sudan; Tanzania; Tunia; Uganda; Zambia; Zimbabwe); Zolam (India); Zopax (South-Africa); Zotran (Chile); Zypraz (Indonesia)
Cost of Therapy: \$96.26 (Anxiety; Xanax; 0.25 mg; 3 tablets/day; 30 day supply)
\$41.76 (Anxiety; Generic Tablets; 0.25 mg; 3 tablets/day; 30 day supply)

DESCRIPTION

Xanax tablets contain alprazolam which is a triazolo analog of the 1,4 benzodiazepine class of central nervous system-active compounds.

The chemical name of alprazolam is 8-Chloro-1-methyl-6-phenyl-4H-s-triazolo [4,3-α][1,4] benzodiazepine.

Alprazolam is a white crystalline powder, which is soluble in methanol or ethanol but which has no appreciable solubility in water at physiological pH.

Each Xanax tablet, for oral administration, contains 0.25, 0.5, 1 or 2 mg of alprazolam. **Inactive Ingredients:** Cellulose, corn starch, docusate sodium, lactose, magnesium stearate, silicon dioxide, and sodium benzoate. In addition, the 0.5 mg tablet contains FD&C yellow no. 6 and the 1 mg tablet contains FD&C blue no. 2.

CLINICAL PHARMACOLOGY

CNS agents of the 1,4 benzodiazepine class presumably exert their effects by binding at stereo specific receptors at several sites within the central nervous system. Their exact mechanism of action is unknown. Clinically, all benzodiazepines cause a dose-related central nervous system depressant activity varying from mild impairment of task performance to hypnosis.

Following oral administration, alprazolam is readily absorbed. Peak concentrations in the plasma occur in 1-2 hours following administration. Plasma levels are proportionate to the dose given; over the dose range of 0.5-3.0 mg, peak levels of 8.0-37 ng/ml were observed. Using a specific assay methodology, the mean plasma elimination half-life of alprazolam has been found to be about 11.2 hours (range: 6.3-26.9 hours) in healthy adults.

The predominant metabolites are α-hydroxy-alprazolam and a benzophenone derived from alprazolam. The biological activity of α-hydroxy-alprazolam is approximately one-half that of alprazolam. The benzophenone metabolite is essentially inactive. Plasma levels of these metabolites are extremely low, thus precluding precise pharmacokinetic description. However, their half-lives appear to be of the same order of magnitude as that of alprazolam. Alprazolam and its metabolites are excreted primarily in the urine.

The ability of alprazolam to induce human hepatic enzyme systems has not yet been determined. However, this is not a property of benzodiazepines in general. Further, alprazolam did not affect the prothrombin or plasma warfarin levels in male volunteers administered sodium warfarin orally.

In vitro, alprazolam is bound (80%) to human serum protein.

Changes in the absorption, distribution, metabolism, and excretion of benzodiazepines have been reported in a variety of disease states including alcoholism, impaired hepatic function, and impaired renal function. Changes have also been demonstrated in geriatric patients. A mean half-life of alprazolam of 16.3 hours has been observed in healthy elderly subjects (range: 9.0-26.9 hours, n=16) compared to 11.0 hours (range: 6.3-15.8 hours, n=16) in healthy adult subjects. In patients with alcoholic liver disease the half-life of alprazolam ranged between 5.8 and 65.3 hours (mean: 19.7 hours, n=17) as compared to between 6.3 and 26.9 hours (mean=11.4 hours, n=17) in healthy subjects. In an obese group of subjects the half-life of alprazolam ranged between 9.9 and 40.4 hours (mean=21.8 hours, n=12) as compared to between 6.3 and 15.8 hours (mean=10.6 hours, n=12) in healthy subjects.

Because of its similarity to other benzodiazepines, it is assumed that alprazolam undergoes transplacental passage and that it is excreted in human milk.

INDICATIONS AND USAGE

Alprazolam is indicated for the management of anxiety disorder (a condition corresponding most closely to the APA Diagnostic and Statistical Manual [DSM-III-R] diagnosis of generalized anxiety disorder) or the short-term relief of symptoms of anxiety. Anxiety or tension associated with the stress of everyday life usually does not require treatment with an anxiolytic.

Generalized anxiety disorder is characterized by unrealistic or excessive anxiety and worry (apprehensive expectation) about two or more life circumstances, for a period of six months or longer, during which the person has been bothered more days than not by these concerns. At least 6 of the following 18 symptoms are often present in these patients: *Motor Tension:* Trembling, twitching, or feeling shaky; muscle tension, aches, or soreness; restlessness; easy fatigability. *Autonomic Hyperactivity:* Shortness of breath or smothering sensations; palpitations or accelerated heart rate; sweating, or cold clammy hands; dry mouth; dizziness or lightheadedness; nausea, diarrhea, or other abdominal distress; flushes or chills; frequent urination; trouble swallowing or 'lump in throat'). *Vigilance and Scanning:* Feeling keyed up or on edge; exaggerated startle response; difficulty concentrating or "mind going blank" because of anxiety; trouble falling or staying asleep; irritability. These symptoms must not be secondary to another psychiatric disorder or caused by some organic factor.

Anxiety associated with depression is responsive to alprazolam.

Alprazolam is also indicated for the treatment of panic disorder, with or without agoraphobia.

Studies supporting this claim were conducted in patients whose diagnoses corresponded closely to the DSM-III-R criteria for panic disorder.

Panic disorder is an illness characterized by recurrent panic attacks. The panic attacks, at least initially, are unexpected. Later in the course of this disturbance certain situations (*e.g.,* driving a car or being in a crowded place) may become associated with having a panic attack. These panic attacks are not triggered by situations in which the person is the focus of others' attention (as in social phobia). The diagnosis requires 4 such attacks within a 4-week period, or one or more attacks followed by at least a month of persistent fear of having another attack. The panic attacks must be characterized by at least 4 off the following symptoms: dyspnea or smothering sensations; dizziness, unsteady feelings, or faintness; palpitations or tachycardia; trembling or shaking; sweating; choking; nausea or abdominal distress; depersonalization or derealization; paresthesias; hot flashes or chills; chest pain or discomfort; fear of dying; fear of going crazy or of doing something uncontrolled. At least some of the panic attack symptoms must develop suddenly, and the panic attack symptoms must not be attributable to some known organic factors. Panic disorder is frequently associated with some symptoms of agoraphobia.

Demonstrations of the effectiveness of alprazolam by systematic clinical study are limited to 4 months duration for anxiety disorder and 4-10 weeks duration for panic disorder; however, patients with panic disorder have been treated on an open basis for up to 8 months without apparent loss of benefit. The physician should periodically reassess the usefulness of the drug for the individual patient.

NON-FDA APPROVED INDICATIONS

Alprazolam is currently under study for use in depression, but is not FDA approved for treatment of this condition alone. Studies have also found the drug to have a role in the treatment of premenstrual syndrome. However, further study is needed for this indication.

CONTRAINDICATIONS

Alprazolam tablets are contraindicated in patients with known sensitivity to this drug or other benzodiazepines. Alprazolam may be used in patients with open angle glaucoma who are receiving appropriate therapy, but is contraindicated in patients with acute narrow angle glaucoma.

Alprazolam is contraindicated with ketaconazole and itraconzole, since these medications significantly impair the oxidative metabolism mediated by cytochrome P450 3A (CYP 3A) (see WARNINGS and DRUG INTERACTIONS).

WARNINGS

DEPENDENCE AND WITHDRAWAL REACTIONS, INCLUDING SEIZURES

Certain adverse clinical events, some life-threatening, are a direct consequence of physical dependence to alprazolam. These include a spectrum of withdrawal symptoms; the most important is seizure. Even after relatively short-term use at the doses recommended for the treatment of transient anxiety and anxiety disorder (*i.e.,* 0.75-4.0 mg per day), there is some risk of dependence. Spontaneous reporting system data suggest that the risk of dependence and its severity appear to be greater in patients treated with doses greater than 4 mg/day and for long periods (more than 12 weeks). However, in a controlled postmarketing discontinuation study of panic disorder patients, the duration of treatment (3 months compared to 6 months) had no effect on the ability of patients to taper to zero dose. In contrast, patients treated with doses of alprazolam greater than 4 mg/day had more difficulty tapering to zero dose than those treated with less than 4 mg/day.

THE IMPORTANCE OF DOSE AND THE RISKS OF ALPRAZOLAM AS A TREATMENT FOR PANIC DISORDER

Because the management of panic disorder often requires the use of average daily doses of alprazolam above 4 mg, the risk of dependence among panic disorder patients may be higher than that among those treated for less severe anxiety. Experience in randomized placebo-controlled discontinuation studies of patients with panic disorder showed a high rate of rebound and withdrawal symptoms in patients treated with alprazolam compared to placebo treated patients.

Relapse or return of illness was defined as a return of symptoms characteristic of panic disorder (primarily panic attacks) to levels approximately equal to those seen at baseline before active treatment was initiated. Rebound refers to a return of symptoms of panic disorder to a level substantially greater in frequency, or more severe in intensity than seen at baseline. Withdrawal symptoms were identified as those which were generally not characteristic of panic disorder and which occurred for the first time more frequently during discontinuation than at baseline.

In a controlled clinical trial in which 63 patients were randomized to alprazolam and where withdrawal symptoms were specifically sought, the following were identified as symptoms of withdrawal: heightened sensory perception, impaired concentration, dysosmia, clouded sensorium, paresthesias, muscle cramps, muscle twitch, diarrhea, blurred vision, appetite decrease and weight loss. Other symptoms, such as anxiety and insomnia, were frequently seen during discontinuation, but it could not be determined if they were due to return of illness, rebound or withdrawal.

In a larger database comprised of both controlled and uncontrolled studies in which 641 patients received alprazolam, discontinuation-emergent symptoms which occurred at a rate of over 5% in patients treated with alprazolam and at a greater rate than the placebo treated group were as follows:

Discontinuation-Emergent Symptom Incidence: Percentage of 641 Alprazolam-Treated Panic Disorder Patients Reporting Events.

Neurologic: Insomnia (29.5), light-headedness (19.3), abnormal involuntary movement (17.3), headache (17.0), muscular twitching (6.9), impaired coordination (6.6), muscle tone disorders (5.9), weakness (5.8).
Psychiatric: Anxiety (19.2), fatigue and tiredness (18.4), irritability (10.5), cognitive disorder (10.3), memory impairment (5.5), depression (5.1), confusional state (5.0).
Gastrointestinal: Nausea/vomiting (16.5), diarrhea (13.6), decreased salivation (10.6).
Metabolic-Nutritional: Weight loss (13.3), decreased appetite (12.8).
Dermatological: Sweating (14.4).
Cardiovascular: Tachycardia (12.2).
Special Senses: Blurred vision (10.0).

From the studies cited, it has not been determined whether these symptoms are clearly related to the dose and duration of therapy with alprazolam in patients with panic disorder.

In two controlled trials of 6-8 weeks duration where the ability of patients to discontinue medication was measured, 71-93% of alprazolam treated patients tapered completely off therapy compared to 89-96% of placebo treated patients. In a controlled postmarketing discontinuation study of panic disorder patients, the duration of treatment (3 months compared to 6 months) had no effect on the ability of patients to taper to zero dose.

Seizures attributable to alprazolam were seen after drug discontinuance or dose reduction in 8 of 1980 patients with panic disorder or in patients participating in clinical trials where doses of alprazolam greater than 4 mg daily for over 3 months were permitted. Five of these cases clearly occurred during abrupt dose reduction, or discontinuation from daily doses of 2-10 mg. Three cases occurred in situations where there was not a clear relationship to abrupt dose reduction or discontinuation. In one instance, seizure occurred after discontinuation from a single dose of 1 mg after tapering at a rate of 1 mg every 3 days from 6 mg daily. In two other instances, the relationship to taper is indeterminate; in both of these cases the patients had been receiving doses of 3 mg daily prior to seizure. The duration of use in the above 8 cases ranged from 4-22 weeks. There have been occasional voluntary reports of patients developing seizures while apparently tapering gradually from alprazolam. The risk of seizure seems to be greatest 24-72 hours after discontinuation (see DOSAGE AND ADMINISTRATION for recommended tapering and discontinuation schedule).

STATUS EPILEPTICUS AND ITS TREATMENT

The medical event voluntary reporting system shows that withdrawal seizures have been reported in association with the discontinuation of alprazolam. In most cases, only a single seizure was reported; however, multiple seizures and status epilepticus were reported as well. Ordinarily, the treatment of status epilepticus of any etiology involves use of intravenous benzodiazepines plus phenytoin or barbiturates, maintenance of a patent airway and adequate hydration. For additional details regarding therapy, consultation with an appropriate specialist may be considered.

INTERDOSE SYMPTOMS

Early morning anxiety and emergence of anxiety symptoms between doses of alprazolam have been reported in patients with panic disorder taking prescribed maintenance doses of alprazolam. These symptoms may reflect the development of tolerance or a time interval between doses which is longer than the duration of clinical action of the administered dose. In either case, it is presumed that the prescribed dose is not sufficient to maintain plasma levels above those needed to prevent relapse, rebound or withdrawal symptoms over the entire course of the interdosing interval. In these situations, it is recommended that the same total daily dose be given divided as more frequent administrations (see DOSAGE AND ADMINISTRATION).

RISK OF DOSE REDUCTION

Withdrawal reactions may occur when dosage reduction occurs for any reason. This includes purposeful tapering, but also inadvertent reduction of dose (*e.g.*, the patient forgets, the patient is admitted to a hospital, etc.). Therefore, the dosage of alprazolam should be reduced or discontinued gradually (see DOSAGE AND ADMINISTRATION).

Alprazolam tablets are not of value in the treatment of psychotic patients and should not be employed in lieu of appropriate treatment for psychosis. Because of its CNS depressant effects, patients receiving alprazolam should be cautioned against engaging in hazardous occupations or activities requiring complete mental alertness such as operating machinery or driving a motor vehicle. For the same reason, patients should be cautioned about the simultaneous ingestion of alcohol and other CNS depressant drugs during treatment with alprazolam.

Benzodiazepines can potentially cause fetal harm when administered to pregnant women. If alprazolam is used during pregnancy, or if the patient becomes pregnant while taking this drug, the patient should be apprised of the potential hazard to the fetus. Because of experience with other members of the benzodiazepine class, alprazolam is assumed to be capable of causing an increased risk of congenital abnormalities when administered to a pregnant woman during the first trimester. Because use of these drugs is rarely a matter of urgency, their use during the first trimester should almost always be avoided. The possibility that a woman of childbearing potential may be pregnant at the time of institution of therapy should be considered. Patients should be advised that if they become pregnant during therapy or intend to become pregnant they should communicate with their physicians about the desirability of discontinuing the drug.

ALPRAZOLAM INTERACTION WITH DRUGS THAT INHIBIT METABOLISM VIA CYTOCHROME P450 3A

The initial step in alprazolam metabolism is hydroxylation catalyzed by cytochrome P450 3A (CYP 3A). Drugs that inhibit this metabolic pathway may have a profound effect on the clearance of alprazolam. Consequently, alprazolam should be avoided in patients receiving very potent inhibitors in CYP 3A. With drugs inhibiting CYP 3A to a lesser but still significant degree, alprazolam should be used only with caution and consideration of appropriate dosage reduction. For some drugs, an interaction with alprazolam has been quantified with clinical data; for other drugs, interactions are predicted from *in vitro* data and/or experience with similar drugs in the same pharmacologic class.

The following are examples of drugs known to inhibit the metabolism of alpraxzolam and/or related benzodiazepines, presumably through inhibition of CYP 3A.

Potent CYP 3A Inhibitors: *Azole Antifungal Agents:* Although *in vivo* interaction data with alprazolam are not available, ketoconazole and itraconazole are potent CYP 3A inhibitors and the coadministration of alprazolam with them is not recommended. Other azole-type antifungal agents should also be considered potent CYP 3A inhibitors and the coadministration of alprazolam with them is not recommended (see CONTRAINDICATIONS).

Drugs demonstrated to be CYP 3A inhibitors on the basis of clinical studies involving alprazolam (caution and consideration of appropriate alprazolam dose reduction are recommended during coadministration with the following drugs):

- ***Nefazodone:*** Coadministration of nefazodone increased alprazolam concentration two-fold.
- ***Fluvoxamine:*** Coadministration of fluvoxamine approximately doubled the maximum plasma concentration of alprazolam, decreased clearance by 49%, increased half-life by 71%, and decreased measured psychomotor performance.
- ***Cimetidine:*** Coadministration of cimetidine increased the maximum plasma concentration of alprazolam by 86%, decreased clearance by 42%, and increased half-life by 16%.

Other drugs possibly affecting alprazolam metabolism by inhibition of CYP 3A are discussed in DRUG INTERACTIONS.

PRECAUTIONS

GENERAL

If alprazolam tablets are to be combined with other psychotropic agents or anticonvulsant drugs, careful consideration should be given to the pharmacology of the agents to be employed, particularly with compounds which might potentiate the action of benzodiazepines (see DRUG INTERACTIONS).

As with other psychotropic medications, the usual precautions with respect to administration of the drug and size of the prescription are indicated for severely depressed patients or those in whom there is reason to expect concealed suicidal ideation or plans.

It is recommended that the dosage be limited to the smallest effective dose to preclude the development of ataxia or oversedation which may be a particular problem in elderly or debilitated patients (see DOSAGE AND ADMINISTRATION). The usual precautions in treating patients with impaired renal, hepatic or pulmonary function should be observed. There have been rare reports of death in patients with severe pulmonary disease shortly after the initiation of treatment with alprazolam. A decreased systemic alprazolam elimination rate (*e.g.*, increased plasma half-life) has been observed in both alcoholic liver disease patients and obese patients receiving alprazolam (see CLINICAL PHARMACOLOGY).

Episodes of hypomania and mania have been reported in association with the use of alprazolam in patients with depression.

Alprazolam has a weak uricosuric effect. Although other medications with weak uricosuric effect have been reported to cause acute renal failure, there have been no reported instances of acute renal failure attributable to therapy with alprazolam.

INFORMATION FOR THE PATIENT

For All Users of Alprazolam

To assure safe and effective use of benzodiazepines, all patients prescribed alprazolam should be provided with the following guidance. In addition, panic disorder patients, for whom doses greater than 4 mg/day are typically prescribed, should be advised about the risks associated with the use of higher doses.

1. Inform your physician about any alcohol consumption and medicine you are taking now, including medication you may buy without a prescription. Alcohol should generally not be used during treatment with benzodiazepines.
2. Not recommended for use in pregnancy. Therefore, inform your physician if you are pregnant, if you are planning to have a child, or if you become pregnant while you are taking this medication.
3. Inform your physician if you are nursing.
4. Until you experience how this medication affects you, do not drive a car or operate potentially dangerous machinery, etc.
5. Do not increase the dose even if you think the medication "does not work anymore" without consulting your physician. Benzodiazepines, even when used as recommended, may produce emotional and/or physical dependence.
6. Do not stop taking this medication abruptly or decrease the dose without consulting your physician, since withdrawal symptoms can occur.

Additional Advice for Panic Disorder Patients

The use of alprazolam at doses greater than 4 mg/day, often necessary to treat panic disorder, is accompanied by risks that you need to carefully consider. When used at high doses greater than 4 mg/day, which may or may not be required for your treatment, alprazolam has the potential to cause severe emotional and physical dependence in some patients and these patients may find it exceedingly difficult to terminate treatment. In two controlled trials of 6-8 weeks duration where the ability of patients to discontinue medication was measured, 7-29% of patients treated with alprazolam did not completely taper off therapy. In a controlled postmarketing discontinuation study of panic disorder patients, the patients treated with doses of alprazolam greater than 4 mg/day had more difficulty tapering to zero dose than patients treated with less than 4 mg/day. In all cases, it is important that your physician help you discontinue this medication in a careful and safe manner to avoid overly extended use of alprazolam.

In addition, the extended use at doses greater than 4 mg/day appears to increase the incidence and severity of withdrawal reactions when alprazolam is discontinued. These are generally minor but seizure can occur, especially if you reduce the dose too rapidly or discontinue the medication abruptly. Seizure can be life-threatening.

LABORATORY TESTS

Laboratory tests are not ordinarily required in otherwise healthy patients.

DRUG/LABORATORY TEST INTERACTIONS

Although interactions between benzodiazepines and commonly employed clinical laboratory tests have occasionally been reported, there is no consistent pattern for a specific drug or specific test.

CARCINOGENESIS, MUTAGENESIS, AND IMPAIRMENT OF FERTILITY

No evidence of carcinogenic potential was observed during 2-year bioassay studies of alprazolam in rats at doses up to 30 mg/kg/day (150 times the maximum recommended daily human dose of 10 mg/day) and in mice at doses up to 10 mg/kg/day (50 times the maximum recommended daily human dose).

Alprazolam was not mutagenic in the rat micronucleus test at doses up to 100 mg/kg, which is 500 times the maximum recommended daily human dose of 10 mg/day. Alprazolam also was not mutagenic *in vitro* in the DNA Damage/Alkaline Elution Assay or the Ames Assay.

Alprazolam produced no impairment of fertility in rats at doses up to 5 mg/kg/day, which is 25 times the maximum recommended daily human dose of 10 mg/day.

PREGNANCY CATEGORY D

Teratogenic Effects

See WARNINGS.

Nonteratogenic Effects

It should be considered that the child born of a mother who is receiving benzodiazepines may be at some risk for withdrawal symptoms from the drug during the postnatal period. Also, neonatal flaccidity and respiratory problems have been reported in children born of mothers who have been receiving benzodiazepines.

LABOR AND DELIVERY

Alprazolam has no established use in labor or delivery.

NURSING MOTHERS

Benzodiazepines are known to be excreted in human milk. It should be assumed that alprazolam is as well. Chronic administration of diazepam to nursing mothers has been reported to cause their infants to become lethargic and to lose weight. As a general rule, nursing should not be undertaken by mothers who must use alprazolam.

PEDIATRIC USE

Safety and effectiveness of alprazolam in individuals below 18 years of age have not been established.

DRUG INTERACTIONS

The benzodiazepines, including alprazolam, produce additive CNS depressant effects when co-administered with other psychotropic medications, anticonvulsants, antihistaminics, ethanol, and other drugs which themselves produce CNS depression.

The steady state plasma concentrations of imipramine and desipramine have been reported to be increased an average of 31% and 20%, respectively, by the concomitant administration of alprazolam tablets in doses up to 4 mg/day. The clinical significance of these changes is unknown.

Drugs That Inhibit Alprazolam Metabolism Via Cytochrome P450 3A: The initial step in alprazolam metabolism is hydroxylation catalyzed by cytochrome P450 3A (CYP 3A). Drugs which inhibit this metabolic pathway may have a profound effect on the clearance of alprazolam (see CONTRAINDICATIONS and WARNINGS for additional drugs of this type).

Drugs Demonstrated to be CYP 3A Inhibitors of Possible Clinical Significance on the Basis of Clinical Studies Involving Alprazolam (caution is recommended during coadministration with alprazolam):

Fluoxetine: Coadministration of fluoxetine with alprazolam increased the maximum plasma concentration of alprazolam by 46%, decreased clearance by 21%, increased half-life by 17%, and decreased measured psychomotor performance.

Propoxyphene: Coadministration of propoxyphene decreased the maximum plasma concentration of alprazolam by 6%, decreased clearance by 38%, and increased half-life by 58%.

Oral Contraceptives: Coadministration of oral contraceptives increased the maximum plasma concentration of alprazolam by 18%, decreased clearance by 22%, and increased half-life by 29%.

Drugs and other substances demonstrated to be CYP 3A inhibitors on the basis of clinical studies involving benzodiazepines metabolized similarly to alprazolam or on the basis of *in vitro* studies with alprazolam or other benzodiazepines (caution is recommended during coadministration with alprazolam): Available data from clinical studies of benzodiazepines other than alprazolam suggest a possible drug interaction with alprazolam for the following: diltiazem, isoniazid, macrolide antibiotics such as erythromycin and clarithromycin, and grapefruit juice. Data from *in vitro* studies of alprazolam suggest a possible drug interaction with alprazolam for the following: sertraline and paroxetine. Data from *in vitro* studies of benzodiazepines other than alprazolam suggest a possible drug interaction for the following: ergotamine, cyclosporine, amiodarone, nicardipine, and nifedipine. Caution is recommended during the coadministration of any of these with alprazolam (see WARNINGS).

ADVERSE REACTIONS

Side effects to alprazolam tablets, if they occur, are generally observed at the beginning of therapy and usually disappear upon continued medication. In the usual patient, the most frequent side effects are likely to be an extension of the pharmacological activity of alprazolam (*e.g.,* drowsiness or light-headedness).

The data cited in TABLE 1 and TABLE 2 are estimates of untoward clinical event incidence among patients who participated under the following clinical conditions: relatively short duration (*i.e.,* 4 weeks) placebo-controlled clinical studies with dosages up to 4 mg/day of alprazolam (for the management of anxiety disorders or for the short-term relief of the symptoms of anxiety) and short-term (up to 10 weeks) placebo-controlled clinical studies with dosages up to 10 mg/day of alprazolam in patients with panic disorder, with or without agoraphobia.

These data cannot be used to predict precisely the incidence of untoward events in the course of usual medical practice where patient characteristics, and other factors often differ from those in clinical trials. These figures cannot be compared with those obtained from other clinical studies involving related drug products and placebo as each group of drug trials are conducted under a different set of conditions.

Comparison of the cited figures, however, can provide the prescriber with some basis for estimating the relative contributions of drug and non-drug factors to the untoward event incidence in the population studied. Even this use must be approached cautiously, as a drug may relieve a symptom in one patient but induce it in others. (For example, an anxiolytic drug may relieve dry mouth [a symptom of anxiety] in some subjects but induce it [an untoward event] in others.)

Additionally, for anxiety disorders the cited figures can provide the prescriber with an indication as to the frequency with which physician intervention (*e.g.,* increased surveillance, decreased dosage or discontinuation of drug therapy) may be necessary because of the untoward clinical event (see TABLE 1).

TABLE 1 *Anxiety Disorders*

	Treatment-Emergent Symptom Incidence*		Incidence of Intervention Because of Symptom
	Alprazolam	Placebo	Alprazolam
Number of Patients	565	505	565
Central Nervous System			
Drowsiness	41.0%	21.6%	15.1%
Light-headedness	20.8%	19.3%	1.2%
Depression	13.9%	18.1%	2.4%
Headache	12.9%	19.6%	1.1%
Confusion	9.9%	10.0%	0.9%
Insomnia	8.9%	18.4%	1.3%
Nervousness	4.1%	10.3%	1.1%
Syncope	3.1%	4.0%	†
Dizziness	1.8%	0.8%	2.5%
Akathisia	1.6%	1.2%	†
Tiredness/sleepiness	†	†	1.8%
Gastrointestinal			
Dry mouth	14.7%	13.3%	0.7%
Constipation	10.4%	11.4%	0.9%
Diarrhea	10.1%	10.3%	1.2%
Nausea/vomiting	9.6%	12.8%	1.7%
Increased salivation	4.2%	2.4%	†
Cardiovascular			
Tachycardia/palpitations	7.7%	15.6%	0.4%
Hypotension	4.7%	2.2%	†
Sensory			
Blurred vision	6.2%	6.2%	0.4%
Musculoskeletal			
Rigidity	4.2%	5.3%	†
Tremor	4.0%	8.8%	0.4%
Cutaneous			
Dermatitis/allergy	3.8%	3.1%	0.6%
Other			
Nasal congestion	7.3%	9.3%	†
Weight gain	2.7%	2.7%	†
Weight loss	2.3%	3.0%	†

* Events reported by 1% or more of alprazolam patients are included.
† None reported.

In addition to the relatively common (*i.e.,* greater than 1%) untoward events enumerated in TABLE 1, the following adverse events have been reported in association with the use of benzodiazepines: dystonia, irritability, concentration difficulties, anorexia, transient amnesia or memory impairment, loss of coordination, fatigue, seizures, sedation, slurred speech, jaundice, musculoskeletal weakness, pruritus, diplopia, dysarthria, changes in libido, menstrual irregularities, incontinence, and urinary retention (see TABLE 2).

In addition to the relatively common (*i.e.,* greater than 1%) untoward events enumerated in TABLE 2, the following adverse events have been reported in association with the use of alprazolam: seizures, hallucinations, depersonalization, taste alterations, diplopia, elevated bilirubin, elevated hepatic enzymes, and jaundice.

There have also been reports of withdrawal seizures upon rapid decrease or abrupt discontinuation of alprazolam tablets (see WARNINGS).

To discontinue treatment in patients taking alprazolam, the dosage should be reduced slowly in keeping with good medical practice. It is suggested that the daily dosage of alprazolam be decreased by no more than 0.5 mg every 3 days (see DOSAGE AND ADMINISTRATION). Some patients may benefit from an even slower dosage reduction. In a controlled postmarketing discontinuation study of panic disorder patients which compared this recommended taper schedule with a slower taper schedule, no difference was observed between the groups in the proportion of patients who tapered to zero dose; however, the slower schedule was associated with a reduction in symptoms associated with a withdrawal syndrome.

Panic disorder has been associated with primary and secondary major depressive disorders and increased reports of suicide among untreated patients. Therefore, the same precaution must be exercised when using doses of alprazolam greater than 4 mg/day in treating patients with panic disorders as is exercised with the use of any psychotropic drug in treating depressed patients or those in whom there is reason to expect concealed suicidal ideation or plans.

As with all benzodiazepines, paradoxical reactions such as stimulation, increased muscle spasticity, sleep disturbances, hallucinations, and other adverse behavioral effects such as agitation, rage, irritability, and aggressive or hostile behavior have been reported rarely. In many of the spontaneous case reports of adverse behavioral effects, patients were receiving other CNS drugs concomitantly and/or were described as having underlying psychiatric conditions. Should any of the above events occur, alprazolam should be discontinued. Isolated published reports involving small numbers of patients have suggested that patients who have borderline personality disorder, a prior history of violent or aggressive behavior, or alcohol or substance abuse may be at risk for such events. Instances of irritability, hos-

A

TABLE 2 *Panic Disorders*

	Treatment-Emergent Symptom Incidence*	
	Alprazolam	**Placebo**
Number of Patients	**1388**	**1231**
Central Nervous System		
Drowsiness	76.8%	42.7%
Fatigue and tiredness	48.6%	42.3%
Impaired coordination	40.1%	17.9%
Irritability	33.1%	30.1%
Memory impairment	33.1%	22.1%
Light-headedness/dizziness	29.8%	36.9%
Insomnia	29.4%	41.8%
Headache	29.2%	35.6%
Cognitive disorder	28.8%	20.5%
Dysarthria	23.3%	6.3%
Anxiety	16.6%	24.9%
Abnormal involuntary movement	14.8%	21.0%
Decreased libido	14.4%	8.0%
Depression	13.8%	14.0%
Confusional state	10.4%	8.2%
Muscular twitching	7.9%	11.8%
Increased libido	7.7%	4.1%
Change in libido (not specified)	7.1%	5.6%
Weakness	7.1%	8.4%
Muscle tone disorders	6.3%	7.5%
Syncope	3.8%	4.8%
Akathisia	3.0%	4.3%
Agitation	2.9%	2.6%
Disinhibition	2.7%	1.5%
Paresthesia	2.4%	3.2%
Talkativeness	2.2%	1.0%
Vasomotor disturbances	2.0%	2.6%
Derealization	1.9%	1.2%
Dream abnormalities	1.8%	1.5%
Fear	1.4%	1.0%
Feeling warm	1.3%	0.5%
Gastrointestinal		
Decreased salivation	32.8%	34.2%
Constipation	26.2%	15.4%
Nausea/vomiting	22.0%	31.8%
Diarrhea	20.6%	22.8%
Abdominal distress	18.3%	21.5%
Increased salivation	5.6%	4.4%
Cardio–Respiratory		
Nasal congestion	17.4%	16.5%
Tachycardia	15.4%	26.8%
Chest pain	10.6%	18.1%
Hyperventilation	9.7%	14.5%
Upper respiratory infection	4.3%	3.7%
Sensory		
Blurred vision	21.0%	21.4%
Tinnitus	6.6%	10.4%
Musculoskeletal		
Muscular cramps	2.4%	2.4%
Muscle stiffness	2.2%	3.3%
Cutaneous		
Sweating	15.1%	23.5%
Rash	10.8%	8.1%
Other		
Increased appetite	32.7%	22.8%
Decreased appetite	27.8%	24.1%
Weight gain	27.2%	17.9%
Weight loss	22.6%	16.5%
Micturition difficulties	12.2%	8.6%
Menstrual disorders	10.4%	8.7%
Sexual dysfunction	7.4%	3.7%
Edema	4.9%	5.6%
Incontinence	1.5%	0.6%
Infection	1.3%	1.7%

* Events reported by 1% or more of alprazolam patients are included.

tility, and intrusive thoughts have been reported during discontinuation of alprazolam in patients with post—traumatic stress disorder.

Laboratory analyses were performed on patients participating in the clinical program for alprazolam. The following incidences of abnormalities shown in TABLE 3 were observed in patients receiving alprazolam and in patients in the corresponding placebo group. Few of these abnormalities were considered to be of physiological significance.

When treatment with alprazolam is protracted, periodic blood counts, urinalysis, and blood chemistry analyses are advisable.

Minor changes in EEG patterns, usually low-voltage fast activity have been observed in patients during therapy with alprazolam and are of no known significance.

Post Introduction Reports: Various adverse drug reactions have been reported in association with the use of alprazolam since market introduction. The majority of these reactions were reported through the medical event voluntary reporting system. Because of the spontaneous nature of the reporting of medical events and the lack of controls, a causal relationship to the use of alprazolam cannot be readily determined. Reported events include: liver enzyme elevations, hepatitis, hepatic failure, Stevens—Johnson syndrome, hyperprolactinemia, gynecomastia, and galactorrhea.

DOSAGE AND ADMINISTRATION

Dosage should be individualized for maximum beneficial effect. While the usual daily dosages given below will meet the needs of most patients, there will be some who require doses greater than 4 mg/day. In such cases, dosage should be increased cautiously to avoid adverse effects.

TABLE 3

	Alprazolam		Placebo	
	Low	**High**	**Low**	**High**
Hematology				
Hematocrit	*	*	*	*
Hemoglobin	*	*	*	*
Total WBC count	1.4	2.3	1.0	2.0
Neutrophil count	2.3	3.0	4.2	1.7
Lymphocyte count	5.5	7.4	5.4	9.5
Monocyte count	5.3	2.8	6.4	*
Eosinophil count	3.2	9.5	3.3	7.2
Basophil count	*	*	*	*
Urinalysis				
Albumin	—	*	—	*
Sugar	—	*	—	*
RBC/HPF	—	3.4	—	5.0
WBC/HPF	—	25.7	—	25.9
Blood Chemistry				
Creatinine	2.2	1.9	3.5	1.0
Bilirubin	*	1.6	*	*
SGOT	*	3.2	1.0	1.8
Alkaline phosphatase	*	1.7	*	1.8

* Less than 1%.

ANXIETY DISORDERS AND TRANSIENT SYMPTOMS OF ANXIETY

Treatment for patients with anxiety should be initiated with a dose of 0.25-0.5 mg given 3 times daily. The dose may be increased to achieve a maximum therapeutic effect, at intervals of 3-4 days, to a maximum daily dose of 4 mg, given in divided doses. The lowest possible effective dose should be employed and the need for continued treatment reassessed frequently. The risk of dependence may increase with dose and duration of treatment.

In elderly patients, in patients with advanced liver disease or in patients with debilitating disease, the usual starting dose is 0.25 mg, given 2 or 3 times daily. This may be gradually increased if needed and tolerated. The elderly may be especially sensitive to the effects of benzodiazepines.

If side effects occur at the recommended starting dose, the dose may be lowered.

In all patients, dosage should be reduced gradually when discontinuing therapy or when decreasing the daily dosage. Although there are no systematically collected data to support a specific discontinuation schedule, it is suggested that the daily dosage be decreased by no more than 0.5 mg every 3 days. Some patients may require an even slower dosage reduction.

PANIC DISORDER

The successful treatment of many panic disorder patients has required the use of alprazolam at doses greater than 4 mg daily. In controlled trials conducted to establish the efficacy of alprazolam in panic disorder, doses in the range of 1-10 mg daily were used. The mean dosage employed was approximately 5-6 mg daily. Among the approximately 1700 patients participating in the panic disorder development program, about 300 received alprazolam in dosages of greater than 7 mg/day, including approximately 100 patients who received maximum dosages of greater than 9 mg/day. Occasional patients required as much as 10 mg a day to achieve a successful response.

Generally, therapy should be initiated at a low dose to minimize the risk of adverse responses in patients especially sensitive to the drug. Thereafter, the dose can be increased at intervals equal to at least 5 times the elimination half-life (about 11 hours in young patients, about 16 hours in elderly patients). Longer titration intervals should probably be used because the maximum therapeutic response may not occur until after the plasma levels achieve steady state. Dose should be advanced until an acceptable therapeutic response (*i.e.*, a substantial reduction in or total elimination of panic attacks) is achieved, intolerance occurs, or the maximum recommended dose is attained. For patients receiving doses greater than 4 mg/day, periodic reassessment and consideration of dosage reduction is advised. In a controlled postmarketing dose-response study, patients treated with doses of alprazolam greater than 4 mg/day for 3 months were able to taper to 50% of their total maintenance dose without apparent loss of clinical benefit. Because of the danger of withdrawal, abrupt discontinuation of treatment should be avoided (see WARNINGS and PRECAUTIONS).

THE FOLLOWING REGIMEN IS ONE THAT FOLLOWS THE PRINCIPLES OUTLINED ABOVE

Treatment may be initiated with a dose of 0.5 mg three 3 daily. Depending on the response, the dose may be increased at intervals of 3-4 days in increments of no more than 1 mg per day. Slower titration to the dose levels greater than 4 mg/day may be advisable to allow full expression of the pharmacodynamic effect of alprazolam. To lessen the possibility of interdose symptoms, the times of administration should be distributed as evenly as possible throughout the waking hours, that is, on a 3 or 4 times per day schedule.

The necessary duration of treatment for panic disorder patients responding to alprazolam is unknown. After a period of extended freedom from attacks, a carefully supervised tapered discontinuation may be attempted, but there is evidence that this may often be difficult to accomplish without recurrence of symptoms and/or the manifestation of withdrawal phenomena.

In any case, reduction of dose must be undertaken under close supervision and must be gradual. If significant withdrawal symptoms develop, the previous dosing schedule should be reinstituted and, only after stabilization, should a less rapid schedule of discontinuation be attempted. In a controlled postmarketing discontinuation study of panic disorder patients which compared this recommended taper schedule with a slower taper schedule, no difference was observed between the groups in the proportion of patients who tapered to zero dose; however, the slower schedule was associated with a reduction in symptoms associated with a withdrawl syndrome. It is suggested that the dose be reduced by no more than 0.5 mg every 3 days, with the understanding that some patients may benefit from an even more gradual discontinuation. Some patients may prove resistant to all discontinuation regimens.

ANIMAL PHARMACOLOGY

When rats were treated with alprazolam at 3, 10, and 30 mg/kg/day (15-150 times the maximum recommended human dose) orally for 2 years, a tendency for a dose related increase in the number of cataracts was observed in females and a tendency for a dose related increase in corneal vascularization was observed in males. These lesions did not appear until after 11 months of treatment.

HOW SUPPLIED

Xanax Tablets are Available as Follows:

0.25 mg: White, oval, scored, imprinted "XANAX 0.25".

0.5 mg: Peach, oval, scored, imprinted "XANAX 0.5".

1 mg: Blue, oval, scored, imprinted "XANAX 1.0".

2 mg: White, oblong, multi-scored, imprinted "XANAX" on one side and "2" on the reverse side.

Storage: Store at controlled room temperature 20-25°C (68-77°F).

PRODUCT LISTING - RATED THERAPEUTICALLY EQUIVALENT

Concentrate - Oral - 1 mg/ml

30 ml	$37.50	GENERIC, Roxane Laboratories Inc	00054-3068-44

Solution - Oral - 0.5 mg/5 ml

500 ml	$51.75	GENERIC, Roxane Laboratories Inc	00054-3067-63

Tablet - Oral - 0.25 mg

2's	$1.25	GENERIC, Allscripts Pharmaceutical Company	54569-3755-03
5's	$8.71	GENERIC, Pd-Rx Pharmaceuticals	55289-0962-05
14's	$8.73	GENERIC, Allscripts Pharmaceutical Company	54569-3755-02
15's	$16.31	XANAX, Allscripts Pharmaceutical Company	54569-0953-06
15's	$17.88	XANAX, Physicians Total Care	54868-0992-03
30's	$3.35	GENERIC, Medirex Inc	57480-0520-06
30's	$10.62	GENERIC, Pd-Rx Pharmaceuticals	55289-0962-30
30's	$17.18	GENERIC, Heartland Healthcare Services	61392-0034-30
30's	$17.18	GENERIC, Heartland Healthcare Services	61392-0034-39
30's	$18.51	GENERIC, Allscripts Pharmaceutical Company	54569-3755-00
30's	$28.51	XANAX, Pharma Pac	52959-0322-30
30's	$29.36	XANAX, Pd-Rx Pharmaceuticals	55289-0346-30
30's	$32.62	XANAX, Allscripts Pharmaceutical Company	54569-0953-00
30's	$33.95	XANAX, Physicians Total Care	54868-0992-01
31 x 10	$193.66	GENERIC, Vangard Labs	00615-0426-53
31 x 10	$193.66	GENERIC, Vangard Labs	00615-0426-63
31's	$17.76	GENERIC, Heartland Healthcare Services	61392-0034-31
32's	$18.33	GENERIC, Heartland Healthcare Services	61392-0034-32
45's	$25.77	GENERIC, Heartland Healthcare Services	61392-0034-45
50's	$55.39	XANAX, Physicians Total Care	54868-0992-02
60's	$12.90	GENERIC, Pd-Rx Pharmaceuticals	55289-0962-60
60's	$34.37	GENERIC, Heartland Healthcare Services	61392-0034-60
60's	$34.37	GENERIC, Heartland Healthcare Services	61392-0034-65
60's	$37.41	GENERIC, Allscripts Pharmaceutical Company	54569-3755-01
90's	$15.18	GENERIC, Pd-Rx Pharmaceuticals	55289-0962-90
90's	$51.55	GENERIC, Heartland Healthcare Services	61392-0034-90
90's	$51.55	GENERIC, Heartland Healthcare Services	61392-0034-95
90's	$56.12	GENERIC, Allscripts Pharmaceutical Company	54569-3755-04
100's	$4.80	FEDERAL UPPER LIMIT, H.C.F.A. F F P	99999-0140-06
100's	$46.40	GENERIC, Major Pharmaceuticals Inc	00904-7791-60
100's	$46.40	GENERIC, Major Pharmaceuticals Inc	00904-7918-60
100's	$48.23	GENERIC, West Point Pharma	59591-0051-68
100's	$50.55	GENERIC, Qualitest Products Inc	00603-2346-21
100's	$51.00	GENERIC, Roxane Laboratories Inc	00054-4104-25
100's	$51.95	GENERIC, Novopharm Usa Inc	55953-0126-40
100's	$52.06	GENERIC, Aligen Independent Laboratories Inc	00405-4043-01
100's	$52.50	GENERIC, Martec Pharmaceuticals Inc	52555-0589-01
100's	$53.00	GENERIC, Roxane Laboratories Inc	00054-8104-25
100's	$53.46	GENERIC, Moore, H.L. Drug Exchange Inc	00839-7851-06
100's	$53.50	GENERIC, Ivax Corporation	00172-4835-60
100's	$53.50	GENERIC, Ivax Corporation	00182-0027-01
100's	$53.55	GENERIC, Geneva Pharmaceuticals	00781-1326-01
100's	$57.00	GENERIC, Roxane Laboratories Inc	00054-8104-24
100's	$57.15	GENERIC, Medirex Inc	57480-0520-01
100's	$61.67	GENERIC, Greenstone Limited	59762-3719-01
100's	$61.94	GENERIC, Purepac Pharmaceutical Company	00228-2027-10
100's	$62.50	GENERIC, Ivax Corporation	00182-0027-89
100's	$63.54	GENERIC, Udl Laboratories Inc	51079-0788-20
100's	$69.50	GENERIC, Mylan Pharmaceuticals Inc	00378-4001-01
100's	$69.52	GENERIC, Geneva Pharmaceuticals	00781-1061-01
100's	$73.82	GENERIC, Udl Laboratories Inc	51079-0788-21
100's	$80.20	GENERIC, Watson Laboratories Inc	52544-0682-01
100's	$106.95	XANAX, Pharmacia Corporation	00009-0029-01
100's	$338.91	GENERIC, Geneva Pharmaceuticals	00781-1061-05
120's	$17.46	GENERIC, Pd-Rx Pharmaceuticals	55289-0962-98
150's	$100.14	GENERIC, Sky Pharmaceuticals Packaging, Inc	63739-0010-15

Tablet - Oral - 0.5 mg

12's	$15.90	XANAX, Allscripts Pharmaceutical Company	54569-0954-00
15's	$5.92	GENERIC, Pd-Rx Pharmaceuticals	55289-0945-15
20's	$14.75	GENERIC, Allscripts Pharmaceutical Company	54569-3756-01
20's	$22.78	XANAX, Pharma Pac	52959-0162-20
20's	$28.51	XANAX, Physicians Total Care	54868-0522-01
30's	$4.05	GENERIC, Medirex Inc	57480-0521-06
30's	$11.00	GENERIC, Pd-Rx Pharmaceuticals	55289-0945-30
30's	$20.37	GENERIC, Heartland Healthcare Services	61392-0035-30
30's	$20.37	GENERIC, Heartland Healthcare Services	61392-0035-39
30's	$22.13	GENERIC, Allscripts Pharmaceutical Company	54569-3756-00
30's	$34.51	XANAX, Pd-Rx Pharmaceuticals	55289-0011-30
30's	$41.86	XANAX, Physicians Total Care	54868-0522-03
31 x 10	$233.43	GENERIC, Vangard Labs	00615-0401-53
31 x 10	$233.43	GENERIC, Vangard Labs	00615-0401-63
31's	$21.05	GENERIC, Heartland Healthcare Services	61392-0035-31
32's	$21.73	GENERIC, Heartland Healthcare Services	61392-0035-32
45's	$30.56	GENERIC, Heartland Healthcare Services	61392-0035-45
50's	$68.56	XANAX, Physicians Total Care	54868-0522-02
60's	$12.00	GENERIC, Pd-Rx Pharmaceuticals	55289-0945-60
60's	$40.75	GENERIC, Heartland Healthcare Services	61392-0035-60
60's	$40.75	GENERIC, Heartland Healthcare Services	61392-0035-65
60's	$49.69	GENERIC, Allscripts Pharmaceutical Company	54569-3756-02
60's	$81.91	XANAX, Physicians Total Care	54868-0522-05
90's	$6.00	GENERIC, Pd-Rx Pharmaceuticals	55289-0945-90
90's	$61.12	GENERIC, Heartland Healthcare Services	61392-0035-90
90's	$61.12	GENERIC, Heartland Healthcare Services	61392-0035-95
100's	$4.93	FEDERAL UPPER LIMIT, H.C.F.A. F F P	99999-0140-02
100's	$10.65	GENERIC, Vangard Labs	00615-0401-13
100's	$57.75	GENERIC, Major Pharmaceuticals Inc	00904-7792-60
100's	$57.75	GENERIC, Major Pharmaceuticals Inc	00904-7919-60
100's	$60.08	GENERIC, West Point Pharma	59591-0052-68
100's	$63.00	GENERIC, Roxane Laboratories Inc	00054-4105-25
100's	$63.50	GENERIC, Qualitest Products Inc	00603-2347-21
100's	$64.88	GENERIC, Novopharm Usa Inc	55953-0127-40
100's	$65.21	GENERIC, Aligen Independent Laboratories Inc	00405-4044-01
100's	$65.80	GENERIC, Martec Pharmaceuticals Inc	52555-0590-01
100's	$66.62	GENERIC, Ivax Corporation	00172-4836-60
100's	$66.62	GENERIC, Ivax Corporation	00182-0028-01
100's	$68.51	GENERIC, Moore, H.L. Drug Exchange Inc	00839-7852-06
100's	$69.65	GENERIC, Medirex Inc	57480-0521-01
100's	$70.00	GENERIC, Roxane Laboratories Inc	00054-8105-24
100's	$74.01	GENERIC, Purepac Pharmaceutical Company	00228-2029-10
100's	$74.25	GENERIC, Ivax Corporation	00182-0028-89
100's	$74.29	GENERIC, Greenstone Limited	59762-3720-01
100's	$75.97	GENERIC, Udl Laboratories Inc	51079-0789-20
100's	$86.02	GENERIC, Udl Laboratories Inc	51079-0789-21
100's	$86.61	GENERIC, Geneva Pharmaceuticals	00781-1077-01
100's	$95.85	GENERIC, Mylan Pharmaceuticals Inc	00378-4003-01
100's	$95.89	GENERIC, Watson Laboratories Inc	52544-0683-01
100's	$127.30	XANAX, Physicians Total Care	54868-0522-04
100's	$133.24	XANAX, Pharmacia Corporation	00009-0055-01
100's	$144.28	XANAX, Pharmacia Corporation	00009-0055-46
120's	$6.93	GENERIC, Pd-Rx Pharmaceuticals	55289-0945-91

Tablet - Oral - 1 mg

30's	$5.31	GENERIC, Medirex Inc	57480-0522-06
30's	$10.65	GENERIC, Pd-Rx Pharmaceuticals	55289-0920-30
30's	$25.40	GENERIC, Heartland Healthcare Services	61392-0036-30
30's	$25.40	GENERIC, Heartland Healthcare Services	61392-0036-39
30's	$35.40	XANAX, Allscripts Pharmaceutical Company	54569-1769-00
30's	$38.17	XANAX, Pd-Rx Pharmaceuticals	55289-0345-30
31's	$26.25	GENERIC, Heartland Healthcare Services	61392-0036-31
32's	$27.10	GENERIC, Heartland Healthcare Services	61392-0036-32
45's	$38.10	GENERIC, Heartland Healthcare Services	61392-0036-45
60's	$12.96	GENERIC, Pd-Rx Pharmaceuticals	55289-0920-60
60's	$50.80	GENERIC, Heartland Healthcare Services	61392-0036-60
90's	$76.20	GENERIC, Heartland Healthcare Services	61392-0036-90
100's	$6.00	FEDERAL UPPER LIMIT, H.C.F.A. F F P	99999-0140-10
100's	$77.05	GENERIC, Major Pharmaceuticals Inc	00904-7793-60
100's	$77.05	GENERIC, Major Pharmaceuticals Inc	00904-7920-60
100's	$80.13	GENERIC, West Point Pharma	59591-0053-68
100's	$84.00	GENERIC, Roxane Laboratories Inc	00054-4107-25
100's	$85.12	GENERIC, Qualitest Products Inc	00603-2348-21
100's	$87.63	GENERIC, Aligen Independent Laboratories Inc	00405-4045-01
100's	$87.66	GENERIC, Novopharm Usa Inc	55953-0131-40
100's	$88.00	GENERIC, Roxane Laboratories Inc	00054-8107-25
100's	$88.40	GENERIC, Martec Pharmaceuticals Inc	52555-0508-01
100's	$88.40	GENERIC, Martec Pharmaceuticals Inc	52555-0591-01
100's	$88.87	GENERIC, Ivax Corporation	00172-4837-60
100's	$88.87	GENERIC, Ivax Corporation	00182-0029-01
100's	$88.90	GENERIC, Moore, H.L. Drug Exchange Inc	00839-7853-06
100's	$90.25	GENERIC, Medirex Inc	57480-0522-01
100's	$92.00	GENERIC, Roxane Laboratories Inc	00054-8107-24
100's	$92.50	GENERIC, Ivax Corporation	00182-0029-89
100's	$98.42	GENERIC, Greenstone Limited	59762-3721-01
100's	$98.65	GENERIC, Purepac Pharmaceutical Company	00228-2031-10
100's	$101.35	GENERIC, Udl Laboratories Inc	51079-0790-20
100's	$110.07	GENERIC, Udl Laboratories Inc	51079-0790-21
100's	$115.55	GENERIC, Mylan Pharmaceuticals Inc	00378-4005-01
100's	$115.56	GENERIC, Geneva Pharmaceuticals	00781-1079-01
100's	$117.99	XANAX, Pharmacia and Upjohn	00009-0090-17
100's	$127.92	GENERIC, Watson Laboratories Inc	52544-0684-01
100's	$177.78	XANAX, Pharmacia Corporation	00009-0090-01

Tablet - Oral - 2 mg

30's	$18.73	GENERIC, Pd-Rx Pharmaceuticals	55289-0523-30
30's	$36.00	GENERIC, Heartland Healthcare Services	61392-0037-30
30's	$36.00	GENERIC, Heartland Healthcare Services	61392-0037-39
31's	$37.20	GENERIC, Heartland Healthcare Services	61392-0037-31
32's	$38.40	GENERIC, Heartland Healthcare Services	61392-0037-32
45's	$54.00	GENERIC, Heartland Healthcare Services	61392-0037-45
60's	$29.13	GENERIC, Pd-Rx Pharmaceuticals	55289-0523-60
60's	$72.00	GENERIC, Heartland Healthcare Services	61392-0037-60
90's	$108.00	GENERIC, Heartland Healthcare Services	61392-0037-90
100's	$15.63	FEDERAL UPPER LIMIT, H.C.F.A. F F P	99999-0140-13
100's	$136.28	GENERIC, West Point Pharma	59591-0054-68
100's	$151.10	GENERIC, Ivax Corporation	00172-4845-60
100's	$151.10	GENERIC, Ivax Corporation	00182-0030-01
100's	$169.36	GENERIC, Greenstone Limited	59762-3722-01
100's	$169.60	GENERIC, Purepac Pharmaceutical Company	00228-2039-10
100's	$196.45	GENERIC, Mylan Pharmaceuticals Inc	00378-4007-01
100's	$196.47	GENERIC, Geneva Pharmaceuticals	00781-1089-01
100's	$198.50	GENERIC, Southwood Pharmaceuticals Inc	58016-0379-00
100's	$302.26	XANAX, Pharmacia and Upjohn	00009-0094-01

PRODUCT LISTING - EQUIVALENTS NOT AVAILABLE

Tablet - Oral - 0.25 mg

1's	$3.42	GENERIC, Prescript Pharmaceuticals	00247-0208-01
2's	$3.48	GENERIC, Prescript Pharmaceuticals	00247-0208-02
3's	$3.55	GENERIC, Prescript Pharmaceuticals	00247-0208-03
4's	$3.62	GENERIC, Prescript Pharmaceuticals	00247-0208-04
7's	$3.81	GENERIC, Prescript Pharmaceuticals	00247-0208-07
10's	$4.01	GENERIC, Prescript Pharmaceuticals	00247-0208-10
12's	$4.15	GENERIC, Prescript Pharmaceuticals	00247-0208-12
12's	$7.02	GENERIC, Southwood Pharmaceuticals Inc	58016-0198-12
14's	$4.28	GENERIC, Prescript Pharmaceuticals	00247-0208-14
15's	$3.09	GENERIC, Physicians Total Care	54868-2929-00
15's	$8.77	GENERIC, Southwood Pharmaceuticals Inc	58016-0198-15
20's	$2.45	GENERIC, Physicians Total Care	54868-2929-05
20's	$11.70	GENERIC, Southwood Pharmaceuticals Inc	58016-0198-20
20's	$17.88	GENERIC, Pharma Pac	52959-0321-20
30's	$3.68	GENERIC, Physicians Total Care	54868-2929-02
30's	$5.34	GENERIC, Prescript Pharmaceuticals	00247-0208-30
30's	$15.60	GENERIC, Pharmaceutical Corporation Of America	51655-0861-24
30's	$17.55	GENERIC, Southwood Pharmaceuticals Inc	58016-0198-30
30's	$18.05	GENERIC, Pharma Pac	52959-0321-30
50's	$4.46	GENERIC, Physicians Total Care	54868-2929-01
60's	$4.02	GENERIC, Physicians Total Care	54868-2929-06
60's	$16.60	GENERIC, Pharmaceutical Corporation Of America	51655-0861-25
60's	$35.10	GENERIC, Southwood Pharmaceuticals Inc	58016-0198-60
90's	$24.40	GENERIC, Pharmaceutical Corporation Of America	51655-0861-26
100's	$6.42	GENERIC, Physicians Total Care	54868-2929-03
100's	$58.50	GENERIC, Southwood Pharmaceuticals Inc	58016-0198-00
100's	$108.74	XANAX, Pharmacia and Upjohn	00009-0029-46

Tablet - Oral - 0.5 mg

2's	$3.44	GENERIC, Prescript Pharmaceuticals	00247-0209-02
6's	$5.25	GENERIC, Southwood Pharmaceuticals Inc	58016-0197-06
7's	$3.64	GENERIC, Prescript Pharmaceuticals	00247-0209-07
8's	$3.67	GENERIC, Prescript Pharmaceuticals	00247-0209-08
9's	$7.88	GENERIC, Southwood Pharmaceuticals Inc	58016-0197-09
10's	$8.75	GENERIC, Southwood Pharmaceuticals Inc	58016-0197-10
12's	$3.84	GENERIC, Prescript Pharmaceuticals	00247-0209-12
12's	$10.50	GENERIC, Southwood Pharmaceuticals Inc	58016-0197-12
14's	$3.91	GENERIC, Prescript Pharmaceuticals	00247-0209-14
14's	$12.25	GENERIC, Southwood Pharmaceuticals Inc	58016-0197-14
15's	$13.13	GENERIC, Southwood Pharmaceuticals Inc	58016-0197-15
16's	$3.99	GENERIC, Prescript Pharmaceuticals	00247-0209-16
18's	$15.75	GENERIC, Southwood Pharmaceuticals Inc	58016-0197-18
20's	$3.32	GENERIC, Physicians Total Care	54868-2930-07
20's	$4.15	GENERIC, Prescript Pharmaceuticals	00247-0209-20
20's	$17.50	GENERIC, Southwood Pharmaceuticals Inc	58016-0197-20
24's	$21.00	GENERIC, Southwood Pharmaceuticals Inc	58016-0197-24
25's	$3.52	GENERIC, Physicians Total Care	54868-2930-06
30's	$3.72	GENERIC, Physicians Total Care	54868-2930-03
30's	$4.54	GENERIC, Prescript Pharmaceuticals	00247-0209-30
30's	$21.70	GENERIC, Pharmaceutical Corporation Of America	51655-0860-24
30's	$22.20	GENERIC, Southwood Pharmaceuticals Inc	58016-0197-30
30's	$23.45	GENERIC, Pharma Pac	52959-0457-30
50's	$4.54	GENERIC, Physicians Total Care	54868-2930-02
50's	$43.73	GENERIC, Southwood Pharmaceuticals Inc	58016-0197-50
60's	$4.95	GENERIC, Physicians Total Care	54868-2930-04
60's	$42.40	GENERIC, Pharmaceutical Corporation Of America	51655-0860-25
60's	$52.50	GENERIC, Southwood Pharmaceuticals Inc	58016-0197-60
90's	$6.17	GENERIC, Physicians Total Care	54868-2930-05
90's	$63.10	GENERIC, Pharmaceutical Corporation Of America	51655-0860-26
100's	$6.58	GENERIC, Physicians Total Care	54868-2930-01
100's	$7.33	GENERIC, Prescript Pharmaceuticals	00247-0209-00
100's	$87.50	GENERIC, Southwood Pharmaceuticals Inc	58016-0197-00
120's	$83.80	GENERIC, Pharmaceutical Corporation Of America	51655-0860-82
150's	$124.75	GENERIC, Sky Pharmaceuticals Packaging, Inc	63739-0011-15

Tablet - Oral - 1 mg

2's	$5.34	GENERIC, Prescript Pharmaceuticals	00247-0210-02
4's	$7.33	GENERIC, Prescript Pharmaceuticals	00247-0210-04
7's	$10.31	GENERIC, Prescript Pharmaceuticals	00247-0210-07
8's	$11.29	GENERIC, Prescript Pharmaceuticals	00247-0210-08
10's	$11.65	GENERIC, Southwood Pharmaceuticals Inc	58016-0840-10
12's	$13.98	GENERIC, Southwood Pharmaceuticals Inc	58016-0840-12
14's	$16.31	GENERIC, Southwood Pharmaceuticals Inc	58016-0840-14
14's	$17.25	GENERIC, Prescript Pharmaceuticals	00247-0210-14
15's	$17.48	GENERIC, Southwood Pharmaceuticals Inc	58016-0840-15
18's	$20.97	GENERIC, Southwood Pharmaceuticals Inc	58016-0840-18
20's	$3.33	GENERIC, Physicians Total Care	54868-3005-04
20's	$23.30	GENERIC, Southwood Pharmaceuticals Inc	58016-0840-20
21's	$24.46	GENERIC, Southwood Pharmaceuticals Inc	58016-0840-21
24's	$27.96	GENERIC, Southwood Pharmaceuticals Inc	58016-0840-24
25's	$29.13	GENERIC, Southwood Pharmaceuticals Inc	58016-0840-25
28's	$32.62	GENERIC, Southwood Pharmaceuticals Inc	58016-0840-28
30's	$4.04	GENERIC, Physicians Total Care	54868-3005-02
30's	$26.90	GENERIC, Pharmaceutical Corporation Of America	51655-0863-24
30's	$29.97	GENERIC, Allscripts Pharmaceutical Company	54569-4619-01
30's	$30.17	GENERIC, Pharma Pac	52959-0524-30
30's	$33.13	GENERIC, Prescript Pharmaceuticals	00247-0210-30
30's	$34.95	GENERIC, Southwood Pharmaceuticals Inc	58016-0840-30
40's	$46.60	GENERIC, Southwood Pharmaceuticals Inc	58016-0840-40
60's	$5.58	GENERIC, Physicians Total Care	54868-3005-03
60's	$52.80	GENERIC, Pharmaceutical Corporation Of America	51655-0863-25
60's	$59.93	GENERIC, Allscripts Pharmaceutical Company	54569-4619-02
60's	$69.90	GENERIC, Southwood Pharmaceuticals Inc	58016-0840-60
90's	$78.70	GENERIC, Pharmaceutical Corporation Of America	51655-0863-26
90's	$89.90	GENERIC, Allscripts Pharmaceutical Company	54569-4619-00
100's	$25.75	GENERIC, Physicians Total Care	54868-3005-01
100's	$114.11	XANAX, Pharmacia and Upjohn	00009-0090-46
100's	$116.50	GENERIC, Southwood Pharmaceuticals Inc	58016-0840-00
120's	$104.60	GENERIC, Pharmaceutical Corporation Of America	51655-0863-82
150's	$166.43	GENERIC, Sky Pharmaceuticals Packaging, Inc	63739-0012-15

Tablet - Oral - 2 mg

10's	$19.86	GENERIC, Southwood Pharmaceuticals Inc	58016-0379-10
12's	$23.82	GENERIC, Southwood Pharmaceuticals Inc	58016-0379-12
14's	$27.79	GENERIC, Southwood Pharmaceuticals Inc	58016-0379-14
15's	$29.78	GENERIC, Southwood Pharmaceuticals Inc	58016-0379-15
20's	$39.70	GENERIC, Southwood Pharmaceuticals Inc	58016-0379-20
21's	$41.69	GENERIC, Southwood Pharmaceuticals Inc	58016-0379-21
24's	$47.64	GENERIC, Southwood Pharmaceuticals Inc	58016-0379-24
25's	$49.63	GENERIC, Southwood Pharmaceuticals Inc	58016-0379-25
28's	$55.58	GENERIC, Southwood Pharmaceuticals Inc	58016-0379-28
30's	$59.55	GENERIC, Southwood Pharmaceuticals Inc	58016-0379-30
40's	$67.80	GENERIC, Allscripts Pharmaceutical Company	54569-4900-02
40's	$79.40	GENERIC, Southwood Pharmaceuticals Inc	58016-0379-40
60's	$101.70	GENERIC, Allscripts Pharmaceutical Company	54569-4900-00
60's	$119.10	GENERIC, Southwood Pharmaceuticals Inc	58016-0379-60
90's	$152.55	GENERIC, Allscripts Pharmaceutical Company	54569-4900-01

Alprostadil *(000141)*

For complete prescribing information, refer to the CD-ROM included with the book.

Categories: Ductus arteriosus; Erectile dysfunction; FDA Approved 1981 Oct
Drug Classes: Impotence agents; Prostaglandins; Vasodilators
Brand Names: **Caverject**; Edex; Muse; **Prostin VR**
Foreign Brand Availability: Alprostapint (Israel); Befar (Hong-Kong); Caverject Powder for Injection (Australia); Eglandin (Korea; Singapore); Liple (Japan); Lyple (Japan); Minprog (Austria; Germany); Palux (Japan); Promostan (Taiwan); Prostandin (Japan; Korea); Prostavasin (China; Hong-Kong; Philippines); Prostine VR (France); Prostivas (Denmark; Finland; Norway; Sweden); Viridal (Germany)
Cost of Therapy: $24.24 (Impotence; Caverject Powder for Injection; 20 µg; 1 injection; variable day supply)
HCFA JCODE(S): J0270 1.25 µg OTH

INTRAVASCULAR

WARNING

Apnea is experienced by about 10–12% of neonates with congenital heart defects treated with alprostadil solution. Apnea is most often seen in neonates weighing less than 2 kg at birth and usually appears during the first hour of drug infusion. Therefore, respiratory status should be monitored throughout treatment, and alprostadil VR pediatric should be used where ventilatory assistance is immediately available.

DESCRIPTION

Prostin VR pediatric sterile solution for intravascular infusion contains 500 µg alprostadil, more commonly known as prostaglandin E_1, in 1.0 ml dehydrated alcohol.

The chemical name for alprostadil is (11α, 13E, 15S)-11,15dihydroxy-9-oxoprost-13-en-1-oic acid, and the molecular weight is 354.49.

Alprostadil is a white to off-white crystalline powder with a melting point between 110° and 116°C. Its solubility at 35°C is 8000 μg per 100 ml double distilled water.

INDICATIONS AND USAGE

Alprostadil solution is indicated for palliative, not definitive, therapy to temporarily maintain the patency of the ductus arteriosus until corrective or palliative surgery can be performed in neonates who have congenital heart defects and who depend upon the patent ductus for survival. Such congenital heart defects include pulmonary atresia, pulmonary stenosis, tricuspid atresia, tetralogy of Fallot, interruption of the aortic arch, coarctation of the aorta, or transposition of the great vessels with or without other defects.

In infants with restricted pulmonary blood flow, the increase in blood oxygenation is inversely proportional to pretreatment pO_2 values; that is, patients with low pO_2 values respond best, and patients with pO_2 values of 40 torr or more usually have little response.

Alprostadil VR pediatric should be administered only by trained personnel in facilities that provide pediatric intensive care.

CONTRAINDICATIONS

None.

WARNINGS

See BOXED WARNING.

NOTE: Alprostadil VR pediatric sterile solution must be diluted before it is administered. (See DOSAGE AND ADMINISTRATION, Dilution Instructions.)

The administration of alprostadil VR pediatric to neonates may result in gastric outlet obstruction secondary to antral hyperplasia. This effect appears to be related to duration of therapy and cumulative dose of the drug. Neonates receiving alprostadil VR pediatric at recommended doses for more than 120 hours should be closely monitored for evidence of antral hyperplasia and gastric outlet obstruction.

Alprostadil VR pediatric should be infused for the shortest time and at the lowest dose that will produce the desired effects. The risks of long-term infusion of alprostadil VR pediatric should be weighed against the possible benefits that critically ill infants may derive from its administration.

DOSAGE AND ADMINISTRATION

The preferred route of administration for alprostadil solution is continuous intravenous infusion into a large vein. Alternatively, alprostadil VR pediatric may be administered through an umbilical artery catheter placed at the ductal opening. Increases in blood pO_2 have been the same in neonates who received the drug by either route of administration.

Begin infusion with 0.05-0.1 μg alprostadil per kg of body weight per minute. A starting dose of 0.1 μg/kg of body weight per minute is the recommended starting dose based on clinical studies; however, adequate clinical response has been reported using a starting dose of 0.05 μg/kg of body weight per minute. After a therapeutic response is achieved (increased pO_2 in infants with restricted pulmonary blood flow or increased systemic blood pressure and blood pH in infants with restricted systemic blood flow), reduce the infusion rate to provide the lowest possible dosage that maintains the response. This may be accomplished by reducing the dosage from 0.1 to 0.05 to 0.025 to 0.01 μg/kg of body weight per minute. If response to 0.05 μg per kg of body weight per minute is inadequate, dosage can be increased up to 0.4 μg/kg of body weight per minute although, in general, higher infusion rates do not produce greater effects.

Dilution Instructions: To prepare infusion solutions, dilute 1 ml of alprostadil VR pediatric sterile solution with sodium chloride injection or dextrose injection. Undiluted alprostadil VR pediatric sterile solution may interact with the plastic sidewalls of volumetric infusion chambers causing a change in the appearance of the chamber and creating a hazy solution. Should this occur, the solution and the volumetric infusion chamber should be replaced.

When using a volumetric infusion chamber, the appropriate amount of intravenous infusion solution, avoiding direct contact of the undiluted solution with the walls of the volumetric infusion chamber.

Dilute to volumes appropriate for the pump delivery system available. Prepare fresh infusion solutions every 24 hours. *Discard any solution more than 24 hours old.* (See TABLE 1.)

TABLE 1 *Sample Dilutions and Infusion Rates to Provide a Dosage of 0.1 μg per Kilogram of Body Weight per Minute*

Add 1 Ampoule (500 μg) Alprostadil to:	Approximate Concentration of Resulting Solution (μg/ml)	Infusion Rate (ml/min/kg of Body Weight)
250 ml	2	0.05
100 ml	5	0.02
50 ml	10	0.01
25 ml	20	0.005

Example: To provide 0.1 μg/kg of body weight per minute to an infant weighing 2.8 kg using a solution of 1 ampoule:

Alprostadil VR Pediatric in 100 ml of Saline or Dextrose:

INFUSION RATE: 0.02 ml/min/kg × 2.8 kg = 0.056 ml/min or 3.36 ml/h.

INTRACAVERNOSAL

DESCRIPTION

Caverject: For Intracavernosal Use.

Caverject sterile powder contains alprostadil as the naturally occurring form of prostaglandin E_1 (PGE_1) and designated chemically as (11α, 13E, 15S)-11,15-dihydroxy-9-oxoprost-13-en-1-oic acid. The molecular weight is 354.49.

Alprostadil is a white to off-white crystalline powder with a melting point between 115° and 116°C. Its solubility at 35°C is 8000 μg per 100 ml double distilled water. Caverject is available as a sterile freeze-dried powder for intracavernosal use in four sizes: 5, 10, 20, and 40 μg vial. When reconstituted as directed with 1 ml of bacteriostatic water for injection or sterile water, both preserved with benzyl alcohol 0.945% w/v, gives 1.13 ml of reconstituted solution. Each ml of Caverject contains 5.4, 10.5, 20.5 or 41.1 μg of alprostadil depending on vial strength, 172 mg lactose, 47 μg sodium citrate, and 8.4 mg benzyl alcohol. The deliverable amount of alprostadil is 5, 10, 20 or 40 μg/ml because approximately 0.4 μg for the 5 μg strength, 0.5 μg for the 10 and 20 μg strengths and 1.1 μg for the 40 μg strength is lost due to absorption to the vial and syringe. When necessary, the pH of alprostadil for injection was adjusted with hydrochloric acid and/or sodium hydroxide before lyophilization.

INDICATIONS AND USAGE

Alprostadil is indicated for the treatment of erectile dysfunction due to neurogenic, vasculogenic, psychogenic, or mixed etiology.

Intracavernosal alprostadil may be a useful adjunct to other diagnostic tests in the diagnosis of erectile dysfunction.

CONTRAINDICATIONS

Alprostadil should not be used in patients who have a known hypersensitivity to the drug, in patients who have conditions that might predispose them to priapism, such as sickle cell anemia or trait, multiple myeloma, or leukemia, or in patients with anatomical deformation of the penis, such as angulation, cavernosal fibrosis, or Peyronie's disease. Patients with penile implants should not be treated with alprostadil.

Alprostadil should not be used in women or children and is not for use in newborns.

Alprostadil should not be used in men for whom sexual activity is inadvisable or contraindicated.

DOSAGE AND ADMINISTRATION

CAVERJECT

The dose of alprostadil should be individualized for each patient by careful titration under supervision by the physician. In clinical studies, patients were treated with alprostadil in doses ranging from 0.2-140 μg; however, since 99% of patients received doses of 60 μg or less, doses of greater than 60 μg are not recommended. In general, the lowest possible effective dose should always be employed. In clinical studies, over 80% of patients experienced an erection sufficient for sexual intercourse after intracavernosal injection of alprostadil. A ½-inch, 27- to 30-gauge needle is generally recommended.

Initial Titration in Physician's Office

Erectile Dysfunction of Vasculogenic, Psychogenic, or Mixed Etiology: Dosage titration should be initiated at 2.5 μg of alprostadil. If there is a partial response, the dose may be increased by 2.5 μg to a dose of 5 μg and then in increments of 5-10 μg, depending upon erectile response, until the dose that produces an erection suitable for intercourse and not exceeding a duration of 1 hour is reached. If there is no response to the initial 2.5 μg dose, the second dose may be increased to 7.5 μg, followed by increments of 5-10 μg. The patient must stay in the physician's office until complete detumescence occurs. If there is no response, then the next higher dose should be given within 1 hour. If there is a response, then there should be at least a 1 day interval before the next dose is given.

Erectile Dysfunction of Pure Neurogenic Etiology (Spinal Cord Injury): Dosage titration should initiated at 1.25 μg of alprostadil. The dose may be increased by 1.25 μg to a dose of 2.5 μg, followed by an increment of 2.5 μg to a dose of 5 μg, and then in 5-μg increments until the dose that produces an erection suitable for intercourse and not exceeding a duration of 1 hour is reached. The patient must stay in the physician's office until complete detumescence occurs. If there is no response, then the next higher dose may be given within 1 hour. If there is a response, then there should be at least a 1 day interval before the next dose is given.

The majority of patients (56%) in one clinical study involving 579 patients were titrated to doses of greater than 5 μg but less than or equal to 20 μg. The mean dose at the end of the titration phase was 17.8 μg of alprostadil.

Maintenance Therapy

The first injections of alprostadil must be done at the physician's office by medically trained personnel. Self-injection therapy by the patient can be started only after the patient is properly instructed and well-trained in the self-injection technique. The physician should make a careful assessment of the patient's skills and competence with this procedure. This intracavernosal injection must be done under sterile conditions. The site of injection is usually along the dorso-lateral aspect of the proximal third of the penis. Visible veins should be avoided. The side of the penis that is injected and the site of the injection must be alternated; the injection site must be cleansed with an alcohol swab.

The dose of alprostadil that is selected for self-injection treatment should provide the patient with an erection that is satisfactory for sexual intercourse and that is maintained for no longer than 1 hour. If the duration of the erection is longer than 1 hour, the dose of alprostadil should be reduced. Self-injection therapy for use at home should be initiated at the dose that was determined in the physician's office; however, dose adjustment, if required (up to 57% of patients in one clinical study), should be made only after consultation with the physician. The dose should be adjusted in accordance with the titration guidelines described above. The effectiveness of alprostadil for long-term use of up to 6 months has been documented in an uncontrolled, self-injection study. The mean dose of alprostadil at the end of 6 months was 20.7 μg in this study.

Careful and continuous follow-up of the patient while in the self-injection program must be exercised. This is especially true for the initial self-injections, since adjustments in the dose of alprostadil may be needed. This recommended frequency of injection is no more than 3 times weekly, with at least 24 hours between each dose. The reconstituted vial of alprostadil is intended for single use only and should be discarded after use. The user should be instructed in the proper disposal of the syringe, needle, and vial.

A

While on self-injection treatment, it is recommended that the patient visit the prescribing physician's office every 3 months. At that time, the efficacy and safety of the therapy should be assessed, and the dose of alprostadil should be adjusted, if needed.

Alprostadil as an Adjunct to the Diagnosis of Erectile Dysfunction

In the simplest diagnostic test for erectile dysfunction (pharmacologic testing), patients are monitored for the occurrence of an erection after an intracavernosal injection of alprostadil. Extensions of this testing are the use of alprostadil as an adjunct to laboratory investigations, such as duplex or Doppler imaging[133], Xenon washout tests, radioisotope penogram, and penile arteriography, to allow visualization and assessment of penile vasculature. For any less of these tests, a single dose of alprostadil that induces an erection with firm rigidity should be used.

General Procedure for Solution Preparation

Alprostadil is packaged in a 5 ml glass vial. Bacteriostatic water for injection or sterile water, both preserved with benzyl alcohol 0.945% w/v, must be used as the diluent for reconstitution. After reconstitution with 1 ml of diluent, the volume of the resulting solution is 1.13 ml. One ml of this solution will contain 5.4, 10.5, 20.5 or 41.1 µg of alprostadil depending on vial strength, 172 mg of lactose, and 47 µg of sodium citrate and 8.4 mg of benzyl alcohol. The deliverable amount of alprostadil is 5, 10, 20 or 40 µg per ml because approximately 0.4 µg for the 5 µg strength, 0.5 µg for the 10 and 20 µg strengths and 1.1 µg for the 40 µg strength is lost due to absorption to the vial and syringe. After reconstitution, the solution of alprostadil should be used within 24 hours when stored at or below 25°C (77°F) and not refrigerated or frozen. Parenteral drug products should be inspected visually for particulate matter and discoloration prior to administration whenever the solution and container permit.

EDEX

The dosage range of alprostadil for the treatment of erectile dysfunction is 1-40 µg. The intracavernous injection should be given over a 5-10 second interval. In a study with a dose range of 1-20 µg of alprostadil, the mean dose was 10.7 µg at the end of the dose titration period. In 2 studies with a dose range of 1-40 µg of alprostadil, the mean dose was 21.9 µg at the end of the dose titration period. Doses greater than 40 µg have not been studied. The patient is advised not to exceed the optimum alprostadil dose which was determined in the doctor's office. The lowest possible effective dose should always be used.

Preparation of Solution: The Edex vial is intended for intracavernous injection only after reconstitution of the powder with 1.2 ml of sterile 0.9% sodium chloride. The alprostadil diluent (sterile 0.9% sodium chloride) in the pre-filled syringe supplied in the kit is only for reconstitution of the dry powder in the alprostadil vial.

Prepare the alprostadil solution immediately before use. The Edex vial should be reconstituted with 1.2 ml of sterile 0.9% sodium chloride. Do not administer unless solution is clear. Do not add any drugs or solutions to the alprostadil solution. Discard unused drug solution. The reconstituted solution should not be stored.

Parenteral drug products should be inspected visually for particulate matter and discoloration prior to administration.

CAUTION: Do not re-use any remaining drug solution due to the possibility of bacterial contamination.

Administration: Alprostadil is given as an intracavernous injection over a 5-10 second interval.

Stability: The single dose vials should be reconstituted only when it is certain that the patient is ready to administer the drug. The reconstituted drug solution should be used immediately after reconstitution. Any remaining solution should be discarded.

PRODUCT LISTING - RATED THERAPEUTICALLY EQUIVALENT

Powder For Injection - Injectable - 5 mcg

1's	$225.00	GENERIC, Bedford Laboratories	55390-0506-10
5's	$1125.00	GENERIC, Bedford Laboratories	55390-0506-05

Powder For Injection - Injectable - 10 mcg

1's	$18.10	CAVERJECT, Pharmacia Corporation	00009-3778-04
1's	$21.33	CAVERJECT, Pharmacia Corporation	00009-3778-13
1's	$42.18	EDEX, Schwarz Pharma	00091-1110-11
2's	$39.38	EDEX REFILL, Schwarz Pharma	00091-1027-22
4's	$92.96	EDEX, Schwarz Pharma	00091-1410-44
6's	$107.60	EDEX, Schwarz Pharma	00091-1010-06
6's	$131.53	CAVERJECT, Pharmacia Corporation	00009-3778-05
6's	$154.95	CAVERJECT, Pharmacia Corporation	00009-3778-08

Powder For Injection - Injectable - 20 mcg

1's	$24.24	CAVERJECT, Pharmacia Corporation	00009-3701-08
1's	$27.46	CAVERJECT, Pharmacia Corporation	00009-3701-13
1's	$56.99	EDEX, Schwarz Pharma	00091-1120-11
2's	$50.19	EDEX REFILL, Schwarz Pharma	00091-1029-22
4's	$119.70	EDEX, Schwarz Pharma	00091-1420-44
6's	$158.49	EDEX, Schwarz Pharma	00091-1020-06
6's	$176.11	CAVERJECT, Pharmacia Corporation	00009-3701-05
6's	$199.55	CAVERJECT, Pharmacia Corporation	00009-3701-01

Powder For Injection - Injectable - 40 mcg

2's	$72.34	EDEX, Schwarz Pharma	00091-1032-22
2's	$78.71	EDEX REFILL, Schwarz Pharma	00091-1140-11
4's	$135.99	EDEX, Schwarz Pharma	00091-1040-44
4's	$149.93	EDEX, Schwarz Pharma	00091-1440-44
6's	$206.66	EDEX, Schwarz Pharma	00091-1040-06
6's	$221.25	CAVERJECT, Pharmacia Corporation	00009-7686-04

Solution - Injectable - 0.5 mg/ml

1 ml	$216.00	GENERIC, Bedford Laboratories	55390-0503-10
1 ml x 5	$937.50	GENERIC, Gensia Sicor Pharmaceuticals Inc	00703-1501-02

PRODUCT LISTING - EQUIVALENTS NOT AVAILABLE

Powder For Injection - Injectable - 5 mcg

4's	$49.79	EDEX, Schwarz Pharma	00091-1005-44
6's	$116.49	CAVERJECT, Pharmacia and Upjohn	00009-7212-03

Powder For Injection - Injectable - 10 mcg

2's	$48.78	CAVERJECT, Pharmacia and Upjohn	00009-5181-01

Powder For Injection - Injectable - 20 mcg

2's	$62.81	CAVERJECT, Pharmacia Corporation	00009-5182-01

Solution - Injectable - 0.5 mg/ml

1 ml x 5	$2511.15	PROSTIN VR PEDIATRIC, Pharmacia and Upjohn	00009-3169-06

Solution - Injectable - 20 mcg/ml

2 ml x 5	$182.41	CAVERJECT, Pharmacia and Upjohn	00009-7650-02

Suppository - Transurethral - 125 mcg

1's	$19.00	MUSE, Vivus Inc	62541-0110-01
6's	$118.50	MUSE, Allscripts Pharmaceutical Company	54569-4423-00
6's	$128.25	MUSE, Vivus Inc	62541-0110-06

Suppository - Transurethral - 250 mcg

1's	$19.88	MUSE, Vivus Inc	62541-0120-01
6's	$124.13	MUSE, Allscripts Pharmaceutical Company	54569-4424-00
6's	$134.25	MUSE, Vivus Inc	62541-0120-06

Suppository - Transurethral - 500 mcg

1's	$21.25	MUSE, Vivus Inc	62541-0130-01
6's	$132.75	MUSE, Allscripts Pharmaceutical Company	54569-4425-00
6's	$143.63	MUSE, Vivus Inc	62541-0130-06

Suppository - Transurethral - 1000 mcg

1's	$22.94	MUSE, Vivus Inc	62541-0140-01
6's	$143.25	MUSE, Allscripts Pharmaceutical Company	54569-4426-00
6's	$154.88	MUSE, Vivus Inc	62541-0140-06

Alteplase, Recombinant *(000143)*

Categories: Embolism, pulmonary; Myocardial infarction; Occlusion, central venous access devices; Pregnancy Category C; FDA Approved 1987 Nov

Drug Classes: Thrombolytics

Brand Names: **Activase**; Cathflo Activase; TPA

Foreign Brand Availability: Actilyse (Australia; Austria; Bahrain; Colombia; Cyprus; Denmark; Egypt; England; Finland; France; Germany; Greece; Hong-Kong; India; Indonesia; Iran; Iraq; Israel; Italy; Jordan; Korea; Kuwait; Lebanon; Libya; Malaysia; Mexico; Netherlands; New-Zealand; Norway; Oman; Philippines; Portugal; Qatar; Republic-of-Yemen; Saudi-Arabia; South-Africa; Spain; Sweden; Switzerland; Syria; Taiwan; Thailand; United-Arab-Emirates); Activacin (Japan)

HCFA JCODE(S): J2996 per 10 mg IV

DESCRIPTION

Alteplase is a tissue plasminogen activator (t-PA) produced by recombinant DNA technology. It is a sterile, purified glycoprotein of 527 amino acids. It is synthesized using the complementary DNA (cDNA) for natural human tissue-type plasminogen activator (t-PA) obtained from a human melanoma cell line. The manufacturing process involves the secretion of the enzyme alteplase into the culture medium by an established mammalian cell line (Chinese Hamster Ovary cells) into which the cDNA for alteplase has been genetically inserted. Fermentation is carried out in a nutrient medium containing the antibiotic gentamicin, 100 mg/L. However, the presence of the antibiotic is not detectable in the final product.

Phosphoric acid and/or sodium hydroxide may be used prior to lyophilization for pH adjustment.

Activase is a sterile, white to off-white, lyophilized powder for intravenous (IV) administration after reconstitution with sterile water for injection.

TABLE 1 *Quantitative Composition of the Lyophilized Product*

	100 mg Vial	50 mg Vial
Alteplase	100 mg (58 million IU)	50 mg (29 million IU)
L-arginine	3.5 g	1.7 g
Phosphoric acid	1 g	0.5 g
Polysorbate 80	≤11 mg	≤4 mg
Vacuum	No	Yes

Biological potency is determined by an *in vitro* clot lysis assay and is expressed in international units as tested against the WHO standard. The specific activity of alteplase is 580,000 IU/mg.

Cathflo Activase is a sterile, white to pale yellow, lyophilized powder for intracatheter instillation for restoration of function to central venous access devices following reconstitution with sterile water for injection.

Each vial of Cathflo Activase contains 2.2 mg of alteplase (which includes a 10% overfill), 77 mg of L-arginine, 0.2 mg of polysorbate 80, and phosphoric acid for pH adjustment. Each reconstituted vial will deliver 2 mg of Cathflo Activase, at a pH of approximately 7.3.

CLINICAL PHARMACOLOGY

Alteplase is an enzyme (serine protease) which has the property of fibrin-enhanced conversion of plasminogen to plasmin. It produces limited conversion of plasminogen in the absence of fibrin. When introduced into the systemic circulation at pharmacologic concentration, alteplase binds to fibrin in a thrombus and converts the entrapped plasminogen to plasmin. This initiates local fibrinolysis with limited systemic proteolysis. Following administration of 100 mg alteplase, there is a decrease (16%-36%) in circulating fibrinogen.[1,2] In a controlled trial, 8 of 73 patients (11%) receiving alteplase (1.25 mg/kg body weight over 3 hours) experienced a decrease in fibrinogen to below 100 mg/dl.[2]

In patients with acute myocardial infarction administered 100 mg of alteplase as an accelerated IV infusion over 90 minutes, plasma clearance occurred with an initial half-life of less than 5 minutes and a terminal half-life of 72 minutes. There is no difference in the dominant initial plasma half-life between the 3 hour and accelerated regimens for AMI. The plasma clearance of alteplase is 380-570 ml/min.[3,4] The clearance is mediated primarily by the liver. The initial volume of distribution approximates plasma volume.

When alteplase is administered for restoration of function to central venous access devices according to the instructions in DOSAGE AND ADMINISTRATION, circulating plasma levels of alteplase are not expected to reach pharmacologic concentrations. If a 2 mg dose of alteplase were administered by bolus injection directly into the systemic circulation (rather than instilled into the catheter), the concentration of circulating alteplase would be expected to return to endogenous circulating levels of 5-10 ng/ml within 30 minutes.[20]

INDICATIONS AND USAGE

ACUTE MYOCARDIAL INFARCTION

Alteplase is indicated for use in the management of acute myocardial infarction in adults for the improvement of ventricular function following AMI, the reduction of the incidence of congestive heart failure, and the reduction of mortality associated with AMI. Treatment should be initiated as soon as possible after the onset of AMI symptoms (see CLINICAL PHARMACOLOGY).

ACUTE ISCHEMIC STROKE

Alteplase is indicated for the management of acute ischemic stroke in adults for improving neurological recovery and reducing the incidence of disability. **Treatment should only be initiated within 3 hours after the onset of stroke symptoms, and after exclusion of intracranial hemorrhage by a cranial computerized tomography (CT) scan or other diagnostic imaging method sensitive for the presence of hemorrhage (see CONTRAINDICATIONS).**

PULMONARY EMBOLISM

Alteplase is indicated in the management of acute massive pulmonary embolism (PE) in adults:

For the lysis of acute pulmonary emboli, defined as obstruction of blood flow to a lobe or multiple segments of the lungs.

For the lysis of pulmonary emboli accompanied by unstable hemodynamics, *e.g.*, failure to maintain blood pressure without supportive measures.

The diagnosis should be confirmed by objective means, such as pulmonary angiography or noninvasive procedures such as lung scanning.

CENTRAL VENOUS ACCESS DEVICES

Alteplase is indicated for the restoration of function to central venous access devices as assessed by the ability to withdraw blood.

NON-FDA APPROVED INDICATIONS

Although not FDA approved, alteplase has been used in select patients with deep vein thrombosis. Treatment of unstable angina pectoris with thrombolytic agents has been relatively unsuccessful or complicated by side effects. Results on the use of a reduced thrombolytic dosage combined with a GP IIb/IIIa inhibitor in patients with ST-elevation have shown an increased incidence of earlier and complete reperfusion (TIMI grade 3 flow). No increased risk of bleeding complications was observed. Alteplase has also been used in selective patients to treat hematomas that have formed in the ventricular system of the brain as a result of intraventricular hemorrhage (IVH), however, this use has not been approved by the FDA.

CONTRAINDICATIONS

ACUTE MYOCARDIAL INFARCTION OR PULMONARY EMBOLISM

Alteplase therapy in patients with acute myocardial infarction or pulmonary embolism is contraindicated in the following situations because of an increased risk of bleeding:

- Active internal bleeding.
- History of cerebrovascular accident.
- Recent (within 2 months) intracranial or intraspinal surgery or trauma (see WARNINGS).
- Intracranial neoplasm, arteriovenous malformation, or aneurysm.
- Known bleeding diathesis.
- Severe uncontrolled hypertension.

ACUTE LSCHEMIC STROKE

Alteplase therapy in patients with acute ischemic stroke is contraindicated in the following situations because of an increased risk of bleeding, which could result in significant disability or death:

- Evidence of intracranial hemorrhage on pretreatment evaluation.
- Suspicion of subarachnoid hemorrhage on pretreatment evaluation.
- Recent (within 3 months) intracranial or intraspinal surgery, serious head trauma, or previous stroke.
- History of intracranial hemorrhage.
- Uncontrolled hypertension at time of treatment (*e.g.*, >185 mm Hg systolic or >110 mm Hg diastolic).
- Seizure at the onset of stroke.
- Active internal bleeding.
- Intracranial neoplasm, arteriovenous malformation, or aneurysm.
- ***Known bleeding diathesis including but not limited to:***

  Current use of oral anticoagulants (*e.g.*, warfarin sodium) or an International Normalized Ratio (INR) >1.7 or a prothrombin time (PT) >15 seconds.

  Administration of heparin within 48 hours preceding the onset of stroke and have an elevated activated partial thromboplastin time (aPTT) at presentation.

  Platelet count <100,000/mm^3.

CENTRAL VENOUS ACCESS DEVICES

Alteplase should not be administered to patients with known hyper-sensitivity to alteplase or any component of the formulation (see DESCRIPTION).

WARNINGS

BLEEDING

The most common complication encountered during alteplase therapy is bleeding. The type of bleeding associated with thrombolytic therapy can be divided into 2 broad categories:

- Internal bleeding, involving intracranial and retroperitoneal sites, or the gastrointestinal, genitourinary, or respiratory tracts.
- Superficial or surface bleeding, observed mainly at invaded or disturbed sites (*e.g.*, venous cutdowns, arterial punctures, sites of recent surgical intervention).

The concomitant use of heparin anticoagulation may contribute to bleeding. Some of the hemorrhagic episodes occurred 1 or more days after the effects of alteplase had dissipated, but while heparin therapy was continuing.

As fibrin is lysed during alteplase therapy, bleeding from recent puncture sites may occur. Therefore, thrombolytic therapy requires careful attention to all potential bleeding sites (including catheter insertion sites, arterial and venous puncture sites, cutdown sites, and needle puncture sites).

Intramuscular injections and nonessential handling of the patient should be avoided during treatment with alteplase. Venipunctures should be performed carefully and only as required.

Should an arterial puncture be necessary during an infusion of alteplase, it is preferable to use an upper extremity vessel that is accessible to manual compression. Pressure should be applied for at least 30 minutes, a pressure dressing applied, and the puncture site checked frequently for evidence of bleeding.

Should serious bleeding (not controllable by local pressure) occur, the infusion of alteplase and any concomitant heparin should be terminated immediately.

Each patient being considered for therapy with alteplase should be carefully evaluated and anticipated benefits weighed against potential risks associated with therapy.

In the following conditions, the risks of alteplase for all approved indications may be increased and should be weighed against the anticipated benefits:

- Recent major surgery, *e.g.*, coronary artery bypass graft, obstetrical delivery, organ biopsy, previous puncture of noncompressible vessels.
- Cerebrovascular disease.
- Recent gastrointestinal or genitourinary bleeding.
- Recent trauma.
- ***Hypertension:*** Systolic BP ≥175 mm Hg and/or diastolic BP ≥110 mm Hg.
- High likelihood of left heart thrombus, *e.g.*, mitral stenosis with atrial fibrillation.
- Acute pericarditis.
- Subacute bacterial endocarditis.
- Hemostatic defects including those secondary to severe hepatic or renal disease.
- Significant hepatic dysfunction.
- Pregnancy.
- Diabetic hemorrhagic retinopathy, or other hemorrhagic ophthalmic conditions.
- Septic thrombophlebitis or occluded AV cannula at seriously infected site.
- Advanced age (*e.g.*, over 75 years old).
- Patients currently receiving oral anticoagulants, *e.g.*, warfarin sodium.
- Any other condition in which bleeding constitutes a significant hazard or would be particularly difficult to manage because of its location.

CHOLESTEROL EMBOLIZATION

Cholesterol embolism has been reported rarely in patients treated with all types of thrombolytic agents; the true incidence is unknown. This serious condition, which can be lethal, is also associated with invasive vascular procedures (*e.g.*, cardiac catheterization, angiography, vascular surgery) and/or anticoagulant therapy. Clinical features of cholesterol embolism may include livedo reticularis, "purple toe" syndrome, acute renal failure, gangrenous digits, hypertension, pancreatitis, myocardial infarction, cerebral infarction, spinal cord infarction, retinal artery occlusion, bowel infarction, and rhabdomyolysis.

USE IN ACUTE MYOCARDIAL INFARCTION

In a small subgroup of AMI patients who are at low risk for death from cardiac causes (*i.e.*, no previous myocardial infarction, Killip class I) and who have high blood pressure at the time of presentation, the risk for stroke may offset the survival benefit produced by thrombolytic therapy.[14]

ARRHYTHMIAS

Coronary thrombolysis may result in arrhythmias associated with reperfusion. These arrhythmias (such as sinus bradycardia, accelerated idioventricular rhythm, ventricular premature depolarizations, ventricular tachycardia) are not different from those often seen in the ordinary course of acute myocardial infarction and may be managed with standard antiarrhythmic measures. It is recommended that antiarrhythmic therapy for bradycardia and/or ventricular irritability be available when infusions of alteplase, recombinant are administered.

USE IN ACUTE LSCHEMIC STROKE

In addition to the previously listed conditions, the risks of alteplase therapy to treat acute ischemic stroke may be increased in the following conditions and should be weighed against the anticipated benefits:

- Patients with severe neurological deficit (*e.g.*, NIHSS >22) at presentation. There is an increased risk of intracranial hemorrhage in these patients.
- Patients with major early infarct signs on a computerized cranial tomography (CT) scan (*e.g.*, substantial edema, mass effect, or midline shift).

In patients without recent use of oral anticoagulants or heparin, alteplase treatment can be initiated prior to the availability of coagulation study results. However, infusion should be discontinued if either a pre-treatment International Normalized Ratio (INR) >1.7 or a prothrombin time (PT) >15 seconds or an elevated activated partial thromboplastin time (aPTT) is identified.

Treatment should be limited to facilities that can provide appropriate evaluation and management of ICH.

In acute ischemic stroke, neither the incidence of intracranial hemorrhage nor the benefits of therapy are known in patients treated with alteplase more than 3 hours after the onset of

A

symptoms. **Therefore, treatment of patients with acute ischemic stroke more than 3 hours after symptom onset is not recommended.**

Due to the increased risk for misdiagnosis of acute ischemic stroke, special diligence is required in making this diagnosis in patients whose blood glucose values are <50 mg/dl or >400 mg/dl. The safety and efficacy of treatment with alteplase in patients with minor neurological deficit or with rapidly improving symptoms prior to the start of alteplase administration has not been evaluated. **Therefore, treatment of patients with minor neurological deficit or with rapidly improving symptoms is not recommended.**

USE IN PULMONARY EMBOLISM

It should be recognized that the treatment of pulmonary embolism with alteplase has not been shown to constitute adequate clinical treatment of underlying deep vein thrombosis. Furthermore, the possible risk of reembolization due to the lysis of underlying deep venous thrombi should be considered.

USE IN CENTRAL VENOUS ACCESS DEVICES

There are no warnings when alteplase is used in CVADs.

PRECAUTIONS

GENERAL

Standard management of myocardial infarction or pulmonary embolism should be implemented concomitantly with alteplase treatment. Noncompressible arterial puncture must be avoided and internal jugular and subclavian venous punctures should be avoided to minimize bleeding from noncompressible sites. Arterial and venous punctures should be minimized. In the event of serious bleeding, alteplase and heparin should be discontinued immediately. Heparin effects can be reversed by protamine.

Orolingual angioedema has been observed in post-market experience in patients treated for acute ischemic stroke and in patients treated for acute myocardial infarction (see DRUG INTERACTIONS and ADVERSE REACTIONS, Allergic Reactions). Onset of angioedema occurred during and up to 2 hours after infusion of alteplase. In many cases, patients were receiving concomitant angiotensin-converting enzyme inhibitors. Patients treated with alteplase should be monitored during and for several hours after infusion for signs of orolingual angioedema. If angioedema is noted, promptly institute appropriate therapy (*e.g.,* antihistamines, IV corticosteroids or epinephrine) and consider discontinuing the alteplase infusion. Rare fatal cases of hemorrhage associated with traumatic intubation in patients administered alteplase have been reported.

Catheter dysfunction may be caused by a variety of conditions other than thrombus formation, such as catheter malposition, mechanical failure, constriction by a suture, and lipid deposits or drug precipitates within the catheter lumen. These types of conditions should be considered before treatment with alteplase for use in CVADs.

Because of the risk of damage to the vascular wall or collapse of soft-walled catheters, vigorous suction should not be applied during attempts to determine catheter occlusion.

Excessive pressure should be avoided when alteplase is instilled into the catheter. Such force could cause rupture of the catheter or expulsion of the clot into the circulation.

BLEEDING

The most frequent adverse reaction associated with all thrombolytics in all approved indications is bleeding.[15,16] Alteplase for use in CVADs has not been studied in patients known to be at risk for bleeding events that may be associated with the use of thrombolytics. Caution should be exercised with patients who have active internal bleeding or who have had any of the following within 48 hours: surgery, obstetrical delivery, percutaneous biopsy of viscera or deep tissues, or puncture of non-compressible vessels. In addition, caution should be exercised with patients who have thrombocytopenia, other hemostatic defects (including those secondary to severe hepatic or renal disease), or any condition for which bleeding constitutes a significant hazard or would be particularly difficult to manage because of its location, or who are at high risk for embolic complications (*e.g.,* venous thrombosis in the region of the catheter). Death and permanent disability have been reported in patients who have experienced stroke and other serious bleeding episodes when receiving pharmacologic doses of a thrombolytic.

Should serious bleeding in a critical location (*e.g.,* intracranial, gastrointestinal, retroperitoneal, pericardial) occur, treatment with alteplase should be stopped and the drug should be withdrawn from the catheter.

INFECTIONS

Alteplase for use in CVADs should be used with caution in the presence of known or suspected infection in the catheter. Using alteplase in patients with infected catheters may release a localized infection into the systemic circulation (see ADVERSE REACTIONS). As with all catheterization procedures, care should be used to maintain aseptic technique.

READMINISTRATION

There is no experience with readministration of alteplase for IV use. If an anaphylactoid reaction occurs, the infusion should be discontinued immediately and appropriate therapy initiated.

Although sustained antibody formation in patients receiving 1 dose of alteplase has not been documented, readministration should be undertaken with caution. Detectable levels of antibody (a single point measurement) were reported in 1 patient, but subsequent antibody test results were negative.

In clinical trials, patients received up to two 2 mg/2 ml doses (4 mg total) of alteplase for use in CVADs. Additional readministration of alteplase has not been studied. Antibody formation in patients receiving 1 or more doses of alteplase for restoration of function to CVADs has not been studied.

DRUG/LABORATORY TEST INTERACTIONS

During alteplase therapy, if coagulation tests and/or measures of fibrinolytic activity are performed, the results may be unreliable unless specific precautions are taken to prevent *in vitro* artifacts. Alteplase is an enzyme that when present in blood in pharmacologic concentrations remains active under *in vitro* conditions. This can lead to degradation of fibrinogen in blood samples removed for analysis. Collection of blood samples in the presence of aprotinin (150-200 U/ml) can to some extent mitigate this phenomenon.

Potential interactions between alteplase for use in CVADs and laboratory tests have not been studied.

USE OF ANTITHROMBOTICS

Aspirin and heparin have been administered concomitantly with and following infusions of alteplase in the management of acute myocardial infarction or pulmonary embolism. Because heparin, aspirin, or alteplase may cause bleeding complications, careful monitoring for bleeding is advised, especially at arterial puncture sites.

The concomitant use of heparin or aspirin during the first 24 hours following symptom onset were prohibited in The NINDS t-PA Stroke Trial. The safety of such concomitant use with alteplase for the management of acute ischemic stroke is unknown.

BLOOD PRESSURE CONTROL

Blood pressure should be monitored frequently and controlled during and following alteplase administration in the management of acute ischemic stroke. In the NINDS t-PA Stroke Trial, blood pressure was actively controlled (≤185/110 mm Hg) for 24 hours. Blood pressure was monitored during the hospital stay.

CARCINOGENESIS, MUTAGENESIS, AND IMPAIRMENT OF FERTILITY

Long-term studies in animals have not been performed to evaluate the carcinogenic potential or the effect on fertility. Short-term studies, which evaluated tumorigenicity of alteplase and effect on tumor metastases in rodents, were negative.

Studies to determine mutagenicity (Ames test) and chromosomal aberration assays in human lymphocytes were negative at all concentrations tested. Cytotoxicity, as reflected by a decrease in mitotic index, was evidenced only after prolonged exposure and only at the highest concentrations tested.

PREGNANCY CATEGORY C

Alteplase has been shown to have an embryocidal effect in rabbits when intravenously administered in doses of approximately 2 times (3 mg/kg) the human dose for AMI and approximately 100 times (3 mg/kg) the human dose for restoration of function to occluded CVADs. No maternal or fetal toxicity was evident at 0.65 times (1 mg/kg) the human dose for AMI and 33 times (1 mg/kg) the human dose for restoration of function to occluded CVADs in pregnant rats and rabbits dosed during the period of organogenesis. There are no adequate and well controlled studies in pregnant women. Alteplase should be used during pregnancy only if the potential benefit justifies the potential risk to the fetus.

NURSING MOTHERS

It is not known whether alteplase is excreted in human milk. Because many drugs are excreted in human milk, caution should be exercised when alteplase is administered to a nursing woman.

PEDIATRIC USE

Safety and effectiveness of alteplase for IV use in pediatric patients have not been established.

Alteplase for use in CVADs has not been studied in patients who are younger than 2 years of age or who weigh less than 10 kg. In Trials 1 and 2, 126 (11%) of 1135 patients treated were from 2-16 years of age. No study drug-related adverse events were observed in these patients. A total of 65 patients (6% of all patients treated in the studies) weighed ≥10 kg and <30 kg. These low body weight patients received up to 2 doses of Alteplase, with each dose equal to 110% of the internal lumen volume of the catheter (to a maximum dose of 2 mg). The rates of catheter function restoration in these subsets of patients were similar to those observed in adult patients. However, there was insufficient enrollment of pediatric patients to draw any conclusions regarding relative efficacy in the pediatric or low weight subgroups, relative efficacy related to catheter types used in these patients, or relative rates of adverse events.

GERIATRIC USE

In 312 patients enrolled in the improperly functioning CVAD trials who were age 65 years and over, no incidents of intracranial hemorrhage (ICH), embolic events, or major bleeding events were observed. One hundred three (103) of these patients were age 75 years and over, and 12 were age 85 years and over. The effect of alteplase on common age-related comorbidities has not been studied. In general, caution should be used in geriatric patients with conditions known to increase the risk of bleeding (see PRECAUTIONS, Bleeding).

DRUG INTERACTIONS

The interaction of alteplase with other cardioactive or cerebroactive drugs has not been studied. In addition to bleeding associated with heparin and vitamin K antagonists, drugs that alter platelet function (such as acetylsalicylic acid, dipyridamole and abciximab) may increase the risk of bleeding if administered prior to, during, or after alteplase therapy.

There have been post-marketing reports of orolingual angioedema associated with the use of alteplase. Many patients, primarily acute ischemic stroke patients, were receiving concomitant angiotensin-converting enzyme inhibitors. (See PRECAUTIONS, General and ADVERSE REACTIONS, Allergic Reactions.)

The interaction of alteplase for use in CVADs with other drugs has not been formally studied. Concomitant use of drugs affecting coagulation and/or platelet function has not been studied.

ADVERSE REACTIONS

BLEEDING

The most frequent adverse reaction associated with alteplase for IV use in all approved indications is bleeding (see WARNINGS).[15,18]

Should serious bleeding in a critical location (intracranial, gastrointestinal, retroperitoneal, pericardial) occur, alteplase therapy should be discontinued immediately, along with any concomitant therapy with heparin. Death and permanent disability are not uncommonly reported in patients that have experienced stroke (including intracranial bleeding) and other serious bleeding episodes.

In the GUSTO trial for the treatment of acute myocardial infarction, using the accelerated infusion regimen the incidence of all strokes for the alteplase-treated patients was 1.6%, while the incidence of nonfatal stroke was 0.9%. The incidence of hemorrhagic stroke was 0.7%, not all of which were fatal. The incidence of all strokes, as well as that for hemorrhagic stroke, increased with increasing age. Data from previous trials utilizing a 3 hour infusion of (≤100 mg indicated that the incidence of total stroke in six randomized double-blind placebo controlled trials[2,7-11,17] was 1.2% (37/3161) in alteplase-treated patients compared with 0.9% (27/3092) in placebo-treated patients.

For the 3 hour infusion regimen, the incidence of significant internal bleeding (estimated as >250 cc blood loss) has been reported in studies in over 800 patients. These data do not include patients treated with the alteplase accelerated infusion.

TABLE 6

	Total Dose ≤100 mg
Gastrointestinal	5%
Genitourinary	4%
Ecchymosis	1%
Retroperitoneal	<1%
Epistaxis	<1%
Gingival	<1%

The incidence of intracranial hemorrhage (ICH) in acute myocardial infarction patients treated with alteplase is shown in TABLE 7.

TABLE 7

Dose	Number of Patients	ICH
100 mg, 3 hours	3,272	0.4%
≤100 mg, accelerated	10,396	0.7%
150 mg	1,779	1.3%
1-1.4 mg/kg	237	0.4%

These data indicate that a dose of 150 mg of alteplase should not be used in the treatment of AMI because it has been associated with an increase in intracranial bleeding.[18]

For acute massive pulmonary embolism, bleeding events were consistent with the general safety profile observed with alteplase in acute myocardial infarction patients receiving the 3 hour infusion regimen.

The incidence of ICH, especially symptomatic ICH, in patients with acute ischemic stroke was higher in alteplase-treated patients than placebo patients (see CLINICAL PHARMACOLOGY).

A study of another alteplase product, Actilyse, in acute ischemic stroke, suggested that doses greater than 0.9 mg/kg may be associated with an increased incidence of ICH.[19] **Doses greater than 0.9 mg/kg (maximum 90 mg) should not be used in the management of acute ischemic stroke.**

Bleeding events other than ICH were noted in the studies of acute ischemic stroke and were consistent with the general safety profile of alteplase. In The NINDS t-PA Stroke Trial (Parts 1 and 2), the frequency of bleeding requiring red blood cell transfusions was 6.4% for alteplase-treated patients compared to 3.8% for placebo (p=0.19, using Mantel-Haenszel Chi-Square).

Fibrin, which is part of the hemostatic plug formed at needle puncture sites will be lysed during alteplase therapy. Therefore, alteplase therapy requires careful attention to potential bleeding sites, *e.g.*, catheter insertion sites, and arterial puncture sites.

In the improperly functioning CVAD trials, the most serious adverse events reported after treatment were sepsis (see PRECAUTIONS, Infections), gastrointestinal bleeding, and venous thrombosis.

Because clinical trials are conducted under widely varying conditions, adverse reaction rates observed in the clinical trials of a drug cannot be directly compared to rates in the clinical trials of another drug and may not reflect the rates observed in practice.

The data described below reflect exposure to alteplase for use in CVADs in 1122 patients, of whom 880 received a single dose and 242 received 2 sequential doses of alteplase.

In the alteplase for use in CVADs clinical trials, only limited, focused types of serious adverse events were recorded, including death, major hemorrhage, intracranial hemorrhage, pulmonary or arterial emboli, and other serious adverse events not thought to be attributed to underlying disease or concurrent illness. Major hemorrhage was defined as severe blood loss (>5 ml/kg), blood loss requiring transfusion, or blood loss causing hypotension. Non-serious adverse events and serious events thought to be due to underlying disease or concurrent illness were not recorded. Patients were observed for serious adverse events until catheter function was deemed to be restored or for a maximum of 4 or 6 hours depending on study. For most patients the observation period was 30 minutes to 2 hours. Spontaneously reported deaths and serious adverse events that were not thought to be related to the patient's underlying disease were also recorded during the 30 days following treatment.

Four catheter-related sepsis events occurred from 15 minutes to 1 day after treatment with alteplase, and a fifth sepsis event occurred on Day 3 after alteplase treatment. All 5 patients had positive catheter or peripheral blood cultures within 24 hours after symptom onset.

Three patients had a major hemorrhage from a gastrointestinal source from 2-3 days after alteplase treatment. One case of injection site hemorrhage was observed at 4 hours after treatment in a patient with pre-existing thrombocytopenia. These events may have been related to underlying disease and treatments for malignancy, but a contribution to occurrence of the events from alteplase cannot be ruled out. There were no reports of intracranial hemorrhage.

Three cases of subclavian and upper extremity deep venous thrombosis were reported 3-7 days after treatment. These events may have been related to underlying disease or to the long-term presence of an indwelling catheter, but a contribution to occurrence of the events from alteplase treatment cannot be ruled out. There were no reports of pulmonary emboli.

There were no gender-related differences observed in the rates of adverse reactions. Adverse reactions profiles were similar across age subgroups, but there was insufficient enrollment of pediatric patients to draw any conclusions regarding relative adverse event rates (see PRECAUTIONS, Pediatric Use).

ALLERGIC REACTIONS

Allergic-type reactions, *e.g.*, anaphylactoid reaction, laryngeal edema, orolingual angioedema, rash, and urticaria have been reported. A cause and effect relationship to alteplase therapy has not been established. When such reactions occur, they usually respond to conventional therapy.

There have been post-marketing reports of orolingual angioedema, associated with the use of alteplase. Most reports were of patients treated for acute ischemic stroke, some reports were of patients treated for acute myocardial infarctions (see PRECAUTIONS, General). Many of these patients received concomitant angiotensin-converting enzyme inhibitors (see DRUG INTERACTIONS).

Most cases resolved with prompt treatment; there have been rare fatalities as a result of upper airway hemorrhage from intubation trauma.

No allergic-type reactions were observed in the trials in patients treated with alteplase for use in CVADs. If an anaphylactic reaction occurs, appropriate therapy should be administered.

OTHER ADVERSE REACTIONS

The following adverse reactions have been reported among patients receiving alteplase, recombinant in clinical trials and in post marketing experience. These reactions are frequent sequelae of the underlying disease and the effect of alteplase, recombinant on the incidence of these events is unknown.

Use in Acute Myocardial Infarction: Arrhythmias, AV block, cardiogenic shock, heart failure, cardiac arrest, recurrent ischemia, myocardial reinfarction, myocardial rupture, electromechanical dissociation, pericardial effusion, pericarditis, mitral regurgitation, cardiac tamponade, thromboembolism, pulmonary edema. These events may be life threatening and may lead to death. Nausea and/or vomiting, hypotension and fever have also been reported.

Use in Pulmonary Embolism: Pulmonary reembolization, pulmonary edema, pleural effusion, thromboembolism, hypotension. These events may be life threatening and may lead to death. Fever has also been reported.

Use in Acute Ischemic Stroke: Cerebral edema, cerebral herniation, seizure, new ischemic stroke. These events may be life threatening and may lead to death.

DOSAGE AND ADMINISTRATION

Alteplase is for IV administration only. Extravasation of alteplase infusion can cause ecchymosis and/or inflammation. Management consists of terminating the infusion at that IV site and application of local therapy.

ACUTE MYOCARDIAL INFARCTION

Administer alteplase as soon as possible after the onset of symptoms.

There are two alteplase dose regimens for use in the management of acute myocardial infarction; controlled studies to compare clinical outcomes with these regimens have not been conducted.

A DOSE OF 150 mg OF ALTEPLASE SHOULD NOT BE USED FOR THE TREATMENT OF ACUTE MYOCARDIAL INFARCTION BECAUSE IT HAS BEEN ASSOCIATED WITH AN INCREASE IN INTRACRANIAL BLEEDING.

ACCELERATED INFUSION

The recommended total dose is based upon patient weight, not to exceed 100 mg. For patients weighing >67 kg, the recommended dose administered is 100 mg as a 15 mg IV bolus, followed by 50 mg infused over the next 30 minutes, and then 35 mg infused over the next 60 minutes.

For patients weighing ≤67 kg, the recommended dose is administered as a 15 mg IV bolus, followed by 0.75 mg/kg infused over the next 30 minutes not to exceed 50 mg, and then 0.50 mg/kg over the next 60 minutes not to exceed 35 mg.

The safety and efficacy of this accelerated infusion of alteplase regimen has only been investigated with concomitant administration of heparin and aspirin as described in CLINICAL PHARMACOLOGY.

a. ***The bolus dose may be prepared in one of the following ways:***

1. By removing 15 ml from the vial of reconstituted (1 mg/ml) alteplase using a syringe and needle. If this method is used with the 50 mg vials, the syringe should not be primed with air and the needle should be inserted into the alteplase vial stopper. If the 100 mg vial is used, the needle should be inserted away from the puncture mark made by the transfer device.
2. By removing 15 ml from a port (second injection site) on the infusion line after the infusion set is primed.
3. By programming an infusion pump to deliver a 15 ml (1 mg/ml) bolus at the initiation of the infusion.

b. ***The remainder of the alteplase dose may be administered as follows:***

50 mg Vials: Administer using either a polyvinyl chloride bag or glass vial and infusion set.

100 mg Vials: Insert the spike end of an infusion set through the same puncture site created by the transfer device in the stopper of the vial of reconstituted alteplase. Hang the alteplase vial from the plastic molded capping attached to the bottom of the vial.

3 HOUR INFUSION

The recommended dose is 100 mg administered as 60 mg in the first hour (of which 6-10 mg is administered as a bolus), 20 mg over the second hour, and 20 mg over the third hour. For smaller patients (<65 kg), a dose of 1.25 mg/kg administered over 3 hours, as described above, may be used.[15]

Although the value of the use of anticoagulants during and following administration of alteplase has not been fully studied, heparin has been administered concomitantly for 24 hours or longer in more than 90% of patients.

Aspirin and/or dipyridamole have been given to patients receiving alteplase during and/or following heparin treatment.

a. ***The bolus dose may be prepared in one of the following ways:***

1. By removing 6-10 ml from the vial of reconstituted (1 mg/ml) alteplase using a syringe and needle. If this method is used with the 50 mg vials, the syringe should not be primed with air and the needle should be inserted into the alteplase vial stopper. If the 100 mg vial is used, the needle should be inserted away from the puncture mark made by the transfer device.
2. By removing 6-10 ml from a port (second injection site) on the infusion line after the infusion set is primed.
3. By programming an infusion pump to deliver a 6-10 ml (1 mg/ml) bolus at the initiation of the infusion.

b. ***The remainder of the alteplase dose may be administered as follows:***

50 mg Vials: Administer using either a polyvinyl chloride bag or glass vial and infusion set.

100 mg Vials: Insert the spike end of an infusion set through the same puncture site created by the transfer device in the stopper of the vial of reconstituted alteplase. Hang the alteplase vial from the plastic molded capping attached to the bottom of the vial.

ACUTE ISCHEMIC STROKE

THE TOTAL DOSE FOR TREATMENT OF ACUTE ISCHEMIC STROKE SHOULD NOT EXCEED 90 mg.

The recommended dose is 0.9 mg/kg (not to exceed 90 mg total dose) infused over 60 minutes with 10% of the total dose administered as an initial IV bolus over 1 minute.

The safety and efficacy of this regimen with concomitant administration of heparin and aspirin during the first 24 hours after symptom onset has not been investigated.

a. ***The bolus dose may be prepared in one of the following ways:***

1. By removing the appropriate volume from the vial of reconstituted (1 mg/ml) alteplase using a syringe and needle. If this method is used with the 50 mg vials, the syringe should not be primed with air and the needle should be inserted into the alteplase vial stopper. If the 100 mg vial is used, the needle should be inserted away from the puncture mark made by the transfer device.
2. By removing the appropriate volume from a port (second injection site) on the infusion line after the infusion set is primed.
3. By programming an infusion pump to deliver the appropriate volume as a bolus at the initiation of the infusion.

b. ***The remainder of the alteplase dose may be administered as follows:***

50 mg Vials: Administer using either a polyvinyl chloride bag or glass vial and infusion set.

100 mg Vials: Remove from the vial any quantity of drug in excess of that specified for patient treatment. Insert the spike end of an infusion set through the same puncture site created by the transfer device in the stopper of the vial of reconstituted alteplase. Hang the alteplase vial from the plastic molded capping attached to the bottom of the vial.

PULMONARY EMBOLISM

The recommended dose is 100 mg administered by IV infusion over 2 hours. Heparin therapy should be instituted or reinstituted near the end of or immediately following the alteplase infusion when the partial thromboplastin time or thrombin time returns to twice normal or less.

The alteplase dose may be administered as follows:

50 mg Vials: Administer using either a polyvinyl chloride bag or glass vial and infusion set.

100 mg Vials: Insert the spike end of an infusion set through the same puncture site created by the transfer device in the stopper of the vial of reconstituted alteplase. Hang the alteplase vial from the plastic molded capping attached to the bottom of the vial.

RECONSTITUTION AND DILUTION

Alteplase should be reconstituted by aseptically adding the appropriate volume of the accompanying sterile water for injection to the vial. It is important that alteplase be reconstituted only with sterile water for injection without preservatives. Do not use bacteriostatic water for injection. The reconstituted preparation results in a colorless to pale yellow transparent solution containing alteplase 1 mg/ml at approximately pH 7.3. The osmolality of this solution is approximately 215 mOsm/kg.

Because alteplase contains no antibacterial preservatives, it should be reconstituted immediately before use. The solution may be used for IV administration within 8 hours following reconstitution when stored between 2-30°C (36-86°F). Before further dilution or administration, the product should be visually inspected for particulate matter and discoloration prior to administration whenever solution and container permit.

Alteplase may be administered as reconstituted at 1 mg/ml. As an alternative, the reconstituted solution may be diluted further immediately before administration in an equal volume of 0.9% sodium chloride injection or 5% dextrose injection to yield a concentration of 0.5 mg/ml. Either polyvinyl chloride bags or glass vials are acceptable. Alteplase is stable for up to 8 hours in these solutions at room temperature. Exposure to light has no effect on the stability of these solutions. Excessive agitation during dilution should be avoided; mixing should be accomplished with gentle swirling and/or slow inversion. Do not use other infusion solutions, *e.g.*, sterile water for injection or preservative-containing solutions for further dilution.

No other medication should be added to infusion solutions containing alteplase. Any unused infusion solution should be discarded.

IMPROPERLY FUNCTIONING CVADS

Alteplase is for instillation into the dysfunctional catheter at a concentration of 1 mg/ml.

- ***Patients weighing ≥30 kg:*** 2 mg in 2 ml.
- ***Patients weighing ≥10 to <30 kg:*** 110% of the internal lumen volume of the catheter, not to exceed 2 mg in 2 ml.

If catheter function is not restored at 120 minutes after 1 dose of alteplase, a second dose may be instilled (see Instructions for Administration). There is no efficacy or safety information on dosing in excess of 2 mg/dose for this indication. Studies have not been performed with administration of total doses greater than 4 mg (two 2 mg doses).

INSTRUCTIONS FOR ADMINISTRATION

Alteplase contains no antibacterial preservatives and should be reconstituted immediately before use. The solution may be used for intracatheter instillation within 8 hours following reconstitution when stored at 2-30°C (36-86°F).

No other medication should be added to solutions containing alteplase.

Instillation of solution into the catheter

1. Inspect the product prior to administration for foreign matter and discoloration.
2. Withdraw 2.0 ml (2.0 mg) of solution from the reconstituted vial.
3. Instill the appropriate dose of alteplase (see DOSAGE AND ADMINISTRATION) into the occluded catheter.
4. After 30 minutes of dwell time, assess catheter function by attempting to aspirate blood. If the catheter is functional, go to Step 7. If the catheter is not functional, go to Step 5.
5. After 120 minutes of dwell time, assess catheter function by attempting to aspirate blood and catheter contents. If the catheter is functional, go to Step 7. If the catheter is not functional, go to Step 6.
6. If catheter function is not restored after 1 dose of alteplase, a second dose may be instilled.
7. If catheter function has been restored, aspirate 4-5 ml of blood to remove alteplase and residual clot, and gently irrigate the catheter with 0.9% sodium chloride.

Any unused solution should be discarded.

HOW SUPPLIED

Activase: Activase is supplied as a sterile, lyophilized powder in 50 mg vials containing vacuum and in 100 mg vials without vacuum.

Cathflo Activase: Cathflo Activase is supplied as a sterile, lyophilized powder in 2 mg vials.

STABILITY AND STORAGE

Activase: Store lyophilized Activase at controlled room temperature not to exceed 30°C (86°F), or under refrigeration 2-8°C (36-46°F).

Cathflo Activase: Store lyophilized Cathflo Activase at refrigerated temperature 2-8°C (36-46°F).

Protect the lyophilized material during extended storage from excessive exposure to light.

Do not use beyond the expiration date stamped on the vial.

PRODUCT LISTING - EQUIVALENTS NOT AVAILABLE

Powder For Injection - Injectable - 50 mg
1's $1487.06 ACTIVASE, Genentech 50242-0044-13

Powder For Injection - Injectable - 100 mg
1's $2974.13 ACTIVASE, Genentech 50242-0085-27

Powder For Injection - Intravenous - 2 mg
1's $77.25 CATHFLO ACTIVASE, Genentech 50242-0041-64

Altretamine (003001)

For complete prescribing information, refer to the CD-ROM included with the book.

Categories: Carcinoma, ovarian; Pregnancy Category D; FDA Approved 1990 Dec; Orphan Drugs
Drug Classes: Antineoplastics, alkylating agents
Brand Names: **Hexalen**
Foreign Brand Availability: Hexastat (Denmark; Finland; France; Italy; Norway; Portugal); Hexinawas (Spain)
Cost of Therapy: $1520.06 (Ovarian Carcinoma; Hexalen ; 50 mg; 8 capsules/day; 21 day supply)

WARNING

1. **Hexalen should only be given under the supervision of a physician experienced in the use of antineoplastic agents.**
2. **Peripheral blood counts should be monitored at least monthly, prior to the initiation of each course of altretamine, and as clinically indicated.**
3. **Because of the possibility of altretamine-related neurotoxicity, neurologic examination should be performed regularly during altretamine administration.**

DESCRIPTION

Altretamine, is a synthetic cytotoxic antineoplastic s-triazine derivative. Altretamine capsules contain 50 mg of altretamine for oral administration. Inert ingredients include lactose, anhydrous and calcium stearate. Altretamine is known chemically as N, N,N', N',N", N"-hexamethyl-1,3,5-triazine-2,4,6-triamine.

Its empirical formula is $C_9H_{18}N_6$ with a molecular weight of 210.28. Altretamine is a white crystalline powder, melting at 172° ± 1°C. Altretamine is practically insoluble in water but is increasingly soluble at pH3 and below.

INDICATIONS AND USAGE

Altretamine is indicated for use as a single agent in the palliative treatment of patients with persistent or recurrent ovarian cancer following first-line therapy with a cisplatin and/or alkylating agent-based combination.

CONTRAINDICATIONS

Altretamine is contraindicated in patients who have shown hypersensitivity to it. Altretamine should not be employed in patients with preexisting severe bone marrow depression or severe neurologic toxicity. Altretamine has been administered safely, however, to patients heavily pretreated with cisplatin and/or alkylating agents, including patients with preexisting cisplatin neuropathies. Careful monitoring of neurologic function in these patients is essential.

WARNINGS

(See BOXED WARNING.)

Concurrent administration of altretamine and antidepressants of the monoamine oxidase (MAO) inhibitor class may cause severe orthostatic hypotension. Four (4) patients, all over 60 years of age, were reported to have experienced symptomatic hypotension after 4-7 days of concomitant therapy with altretamine and MAO inhibitors.

Altretamine causes mild to moderate myelosuppression and neurotoxicity. Blood counts and a neurologic examination should be performed prior to the initiation of each course of therapy and the dose of altretamine adjusted as clinically indicated (see DOSAGE AND ADMINISTRATION.)

PREGNANCY CATEGORY D

Altretamine has been shown to be embryotoxic and teratogenic in rats and rabbits when given at doses 2 and 10 times the human dose. Altretamine may cause fetal damage when administered to a pregnant woman. If altretamine is used during pregnancy, or if the patient becomes pregnant while taking the drug, the patient should be apprised of the potential hazard to the fetus. Women of childbearing potential should be advised to avoid becoming pregnant.

DOSAGE AND ADMINISTRATION

Altretamine is administered orally. Doses are calculated on the basis of body surface area.

Altretamine may be administered either for 14 or 21 consecutive days in a 28 day cycle at a dose of 260 mg/m^2/day. The total daily dose should be given as 4 divided oral doses after meals and at bedtime. There is no pharmacokinetic information supporting this dosing regimen and the effect of food on altretamine bioavailability or pharmacokinetics has not been evaluated.

Altretamine should be temporarily discontinued (for 14 days or longer) and subsequently restarted at 200 mg/m^2/day for any of the following situations:

1) Gastrointestinal intolerance unresponsive to symptomatic measures;
2) White blood count $<2000/mm^3$ or granulocyte count $<1000/mm^3$;
3) Platelet count $<75{,}000/mm^3$;
4) Progressive neurotoxicity.

If neurologic symptoms fail to stabilize on the reduced dose schedule, altretamine should be discontinued indefinitely.

Procedures for proper handling and disposal of anticancer drugs should be considered. Several guidelines on this subject have been published.[2-8] There is no general agreement that all of the procedures recommended in the guidelines are necessary or appropriate.

PRODUCT LISTING - EQUIVALENTS NOT AVAILABLE

Capsule - Oral - 50 mg

100's	$760.00	HEXALEN, Us Bioscience	58178-0001-70
100's	$904.80	HEXALEN, Mgi Pharma Inc	58063-0001-70

Aluminum Hydroxide *(000159)*

Categories: Gastric hyperacidity; Gastritis; Ulcer, peptic; FDA Pre 1938 Drugs; WHO Formulary
Drug Classes: Gastrointestinals; Vitamins/minerals
Brand Names: Acidex; Algel; Allulose; Alumag; Aluminox; Alusorb; Gamma-Gel; Gelalmin; Gelox; Palliacol
Foreign Brand Availability: Aldrox (Argentina; Belgium); Algeldraat (Netherlands); Alu-Cap (Bahrain; Benin; Burkina-Faso; Cyprus; Egypt; Ethiopia; Gambia; Ghana; Guinea; Iran; Iraq; Ivory-Coast; Jordan; Kenya; Kuwait; Lebanon; Liberia; Libya; Malawi; Mali; Mauritania; Mauritius; Morocco; Niger; Nigeria; Oman; Qatar; Republic-of-Yemen; Saudi-Arabia; Senegal; Seychelles; Sierra-Leone; Sudan; Syria; Tanzania; Tunia; Uganda; United-Arab-Emirates; Zambia; Zimbabwe); Alucol (Italy); Aludrox (Germany; India); Alugel (Germany); Alugelibys (Spain); Alumigel (Japan); Alu-Tab (Australia; Hong-Kong; Philippines); Alutab (Malaysia; New-Zealand); Alzinox (Philippines); Amphogel (Australia); Amphojel (Canada; Korea; New-Zealand; South-Africa); Basaljel (Canada); Gastracol (Switzerland); Pepsamar (Benin; Brazil; Burkina-Faso; Chile; Colombia; Ethiopia; Gambia; Ghana; Greece; Guinea; Ivory-Coast; Kenya; Liberia; Malawi; Mali; Mauritania; Mauritius; Morocco; Niger; Nigeria; Peru; Portugal; Senegal; Seychelles; Sierra-Leone; Spain; Sudan; Tanzania; Tunia; Uganda; Venezuela; Zambia; Zimbabwe); Rocgel (France); Ulcerin-P (Taiwan)

DESCRIPTION

SUSPENSION

Peppermint Flavored

Each teaspoonful (5 ml) contains 320 mg of aluminum hydroxide [$Al(OH)_3$] as a gel, and not more than 0.10 mEq of sodium. The inactive ingredients present are calcium benzoate, glycerin, hydroxypropyl methylcellulose, menthol, peppermint oil, potassium butylparaben, potassium propylparaben, saccharin, simethicone, sorbitol solution, and water.

Without Flavor

Each teaspoonful (5 ml) contains 320 mg of aluminum hydroxide [$Al(OH)_3$] as a gel. The inactive ingredients present are butylparaben, calcium benzoate, glycerin, hydroxypropyl methylcellulose, methylparaben, propylparaben, saccharin, simethicone, sorbitol solution, and water.

TABLETS

Tablets available in 0.3 and 0.6 g strengths. Each contains, respectively, the equivalent of 300 and 600 mg aluminum hydroxide as a dried gel. The inactive ingredients present are artificial and natural flavors, cellulose, hydrogenated vegetable oil, magnesium stearate, polacrilin potassium, saccharin, starch, and talc. The 0.3 g strength is equivalent to about 1 teaspoonful of the suspension and the 0.6 g strength is equivalent to about 2 teaspoonfuls. Each 0.3 g tablet contains 0.08 mEq of sodium and each 0.6 g tablet contains 0.13 mEq of sodium.

INDICATIONS AND USAGE

For the symptomatic relief of hyperacidity associated with the diagnosis of peptic ulcer, gastritis, peptic esophagitis, gastric hyperacidity, and hiatal hernia.

WARNINGS

Patients are advised not to take more than 1 teaspoonfuls (60 ml) or twelve 0.3 g tablets or six 0.6 g tablets in a 24 hour period or use this maximum dosage for more than 2 weeks except under the advice and supervision of a physician. Prolonged use of aluminum-containing antacids in patients with renal failure may result in or worsen dialysis osteomalacia. Elevated tissue aluminum levels contribute to the development of dialysis encephalopathy and osteomalacia syndromes. Also, a number of cases of dialysis encephalopathy have been associated with elevated aluminum levels in the dialysate water. Small amounts of aluminum are absorbed from the gastrointestinal tract and renal excretion of aluminum is impaired in renal failure. Prolonged use of aluminum-containing antacids in such patients may contribute to increased plasma levels of aluminum. Aluminum is not well removed by dialysis because it is bound to albumin and transferrin, which do not cross dialysis membranes. As a result, aluminum is deposited in bone, and dialysis osteomalacia may develop when large amounts of aluminum are ingested orally by patients with impaired renal function. Pregnant women and nursing mothers are advised to seek the advice of a health professional before using this product.

PRECAUTIONS

May cause constipation.

DRUG INTERACTIONS

Antacids may interact with certain prescription drugs.

This product must not be taken if the patient is presently taking a prescription antibiotic drug containing any form of tetracycline.

If patients are presently taking a prescription drug, they are advised to check with their physicians before taking this product.

DOSAGE AND ADMINISTRATION

SUSPENSION

Two (2) teaspoonfuls followed by a sip of water if desired, 5 or 6 times daily, between meals and on retiring. Two (2) teaspoonfuls have the capacity to neutralize 20 mEq of acid.

TABLETS

Two (2) tablets of the 0.3 g strength, or 1 tablet of the 0.6 g strength, 5 or 6 times daily between meals and on retiring. Two (2) tablets have the capacity to neutralize 16 mEq of acid.

It is unnecessary to chew the 0.3 g tablet before swallowing with water. After chewing the 0.6 g tablet, one-half glass of water should be sipped.

Amantadine Hydrochloride *(000174)*

Categories: Extrapyramidal disorder, drug-induced; Influenza A; Influenza A, prophylaxis; Parkinson's disease; Pregnancy Category C; FDA Approved 1966 Oct
Drug Classes: Antiparkinson agents; Antivirals; Dopaminergics
Brand Names: Contenton; Mantandan; Shikitan; **Symmetrel**; Topharmin
Foreign Brand Availability: Aldinam (Chile); Amanda (Taiwan); Amandin (Taiwan); Amantan (Belgium); Amantix (Colombia); Amazolon (Japan); a.m.t. (Germany); Atarin (Finland); Boidan (Japan); Endantadine (Canada); Enzil (Taiwan); Hofcomant (Austria; Finland); Infectoflu (Germany); Mantadan (Italy); Mantadix (Belgium); Padiken (Mexico); Parkintrel (Korea); Paritrel (Israel); PK-Merz (Austria; Bahrain; Benin; Burkina-Faso; Cyprus; Czech-Republic; Egypt; Ethiopia; Gambia; Germany; Ghana; Guinea; Hong-Kong; Hungary; Iran; Iraq; Ivory-Coast; Jordan; Kenya; Korea; Kuwait; Lebanon; Liberia; Libya; Malawi; Malaysia; Mali; Mauritania; Mauritius; Morocco; Niger; Nigeria; Oman; Portugal; Qatar; Republic-of-Yemen; Saudi-Arabia; Senegal; Seychelles; Sierra-Leone; Sudan; Switzerland; Syria; Taiwan; Tanzania; Tunia; Uganda; United-Arab-Emirates; Zambia; Zimbabwe); Prayanol (Chile); Protexin (Spain); Tregor (Germany); Virofral (Sweden); Virosol (Argentina)
Cost of Therapy: $79.58 (Parkinsonism; Symmetrel; 100 mg; 2 tablets/day; 30 day supply)
$13.94 (Parkinsonism; Generic Tablets; 100 mg; 2 tablets/day; 30 day supply)

DESCRIPTION

Symmetrel is designated generically as amantadine hydrochloride and chemically as 1-adamantanamine hydrochloride.

Amantadine hydrochloride is a stable white or nearly white crystalline powder, freely soluble in water and soluble in alcohol and in chloroform.

Amantadine hydrochloride has pharmacological actions as both an anti-Parkinson and an antiviral drug.

Amantadine hydrochloride is available in tablets, capsules, and syrup.

Symmetrel Tablets: *Active Ingredients:* 100 mg amantadine HCl. *Inactive Ingredients:* Hydroxypropyl methylcellulose, magnesium stearate, microcrystalline cellulose, sodium starch glycolate, FD&C yellow no. 6.

Symmetrel Syrup: *Active Ingredients:* Syrup contains 50 mg of amantadine HCl per 5 ml. *Inactive Ingredients:* Artificial raspberry flavor, citric acid, methylparaben, propylparaben, and sorbitol sodium.

Amantadine Hydrochloride Capsules: *Active Ingredients:* 100 mg of amantadine HCl. *Inactive Ingredients:* D&C yellow no. 10, FD&C blue no. 1, FD&C yellow no. 6, gelatin, glycerin, hydrogenated vegetable oil, lecithin, partially hydrogenated soybean and palm oils, simethicone, soybean oil, titanium dioxide, white wax, and other ingredients.

CLINICAL PHARMACOLOGY

PHARMACODYNAMICS

Mechanism of Action

Parkinson's Disease

The mechanism of action of amantadine in the treatment of Parkinson's disease and drug-induced extrapyramidal reactions is not known. Data from animal studies have either shown or suggested amantadine HCl:

To enhance extracellular concentrations of dopamine by increasing dopamine release or decreasing reuptake of dopamine into presynaptic neurons;

To stimulate the dopamine receptor itself or drive the post synaptic dopaminergic system to a more dopamine sensitive status.

However, doses employed in the animal studies were often of a magnitude greater than the clinically therapeutic range (low μM) showed amantadine to inhibit the N-methyl-D-aspartic acid (NMDA) receptor-mediated stimulation of acetylcholine release from rat striatum, mostly likely at the MK-801 site.

It has been shown to cause an increase in dopamine release in the animal brain. Although the drug does not possess anticholinergic activity in dogs at doses of 31.5 mg/kg, equivalent to an approximate human dose of 15.8 mg/kg (based on body surface area conversions), clinically it exhibits anticholinergic-like side effects such as dry mouth, urinary retention, and constipation.

Antiviral

The mechanism by which amantadine exerts its antiviral activity is not clearly understood. It appears to mainly prevent the release of infectious viral nucleic acid into the host cell by interfering with the function of the transmembrane domain of the viral M2 protein. In certain cases, amantadine is also known to prevent virus assembly during virus replication. It does not appear to interfere with the immunogenicity of inactivated influenza A virus vaccine.

Antiviral Activity

Amantadine inhibits the replication of influenza A virus isolates from each of the subtypes, *i.e.,* H1N1, H2N2 and H3N2. It has very little or no activity against influenza B virus isolates. A quantitative relationship between the *in vitro* susceptibility of influenza A virus to amantadine and the clinical response to therapy has not been established in man. Sensitivity test results, expressed as the concentration of amantadine required to inhibit by 50% the growth of virus (ED_{50}) in tissue culture vary greatly (0.1-25.0 μg/ml) depending upon the assay protocol used, size of virus inoculum, isolates of influenza A virus strains tested, and the cell type used. Host cells in tissue culture readily tolerated amantadine up to a concentration of 100 μg/ml.

Drug Resistance

Influenza A variants with reduced *in vitro* sensitivity to amantadine have been isolated from epidemic strains in areas where adamantine derivatives are being used. Influenza viruses with reduced *in vitro* sensitivity have been shown to be transmissible and to cause typical influenza illness. The quantitative relationship between the *in vitro* sensitivity of influenza A variants to amantadine and the clinical response to therapy has not been established.

PHARMACOKINETICS

Amantadine is well absorbed orally. Maximum plasma concentrations are directly related to dose for doses up to 200 mg/day. Doses above 200 mg/day may result in a greater than proportional increase in maximum plasma concentrations. It is primarily excreted unchanged in the urine by glomerular filtration and tubular secretion. Eight metabolites of amantadine have been identified in human urine. One metabolite, an N-acetylated compound, was quantified in human urine and accounted for 5-15% of the administered dose. Plasma acetylamantadine accounted for up to 80% of the concurrent amantadine plasma concentration in 5 of 12 healthy volunteers following the ingestion of a 200 mg dose of amantadine. Acetylamantadine was not detected in the plasma of the 7 volunteers. The contribution of this metabolite to efficacy or toxicity is not known.

There appears to be a relationship between plasma amantadine concentrations and toxicity. As concentration increases toxicity seems to be more prevalent, however absolute values of amantadine concentrations associated with adverse effects have not been fully defined.

Amantadine pharmacokinetics were determined in 24 normal adult male volunteers after the oral administration of a single amantadine 100 mg soft-gel capsule. The mean ± SD maximum plasma concentration was 0.22 ± 0.03 μg/ml (range: 0.18-0.32 μg/ml). The time to peak concentration was 3.3 ± 1.5 hours (range: 1.5-8.0 hours). The apparent oral clearance was 0.28 ± 0.11 L/h/kg (range: 0.14-0.62 L/h/kg). The half-life was 17 ± 4 hours (range: 10-25 hours). Across other studies, amantadine plasma half-life has averaged 16 ± 6 hours (range: 9-31 hours) in 19 healthy volunteers.

After the oral administration of a single 100 mg capsule, several studies showed mean maximum plasma concentrations of 0.2-0.4 μg/ml and mean times to peak concentration of 2.5-4 hours. Mean half-lives ranged from 10-14 hours.

After oral administration of a single dose of 100 mg amantadine syrup to 5 healthy volunteers, the mean ± SD maximum plasma concentration C_{max} was 0.24 ± 0.04 μg/ml and ranged from 0.18-0.28 μg/ml. After 15 days of amantadine 100 mg bid., the C_{max} was 0.47 ± 0.11 μg/ml in 4 of the 5 volunteers. The administration of amantadine tablets as a 200 mg single dose to 6 healthy subjects resulted in a C_{max} of 0.51 ± 0.14 μg/ml. Across studies, the time to C_{max} (T_{max}) averaged about 2-4 hours.

Plasma amantadine clearance ranged from 0.2-0.3 L/h/kg after the administration of 5-25 mg intravenous doses of amantadine to 15 healthy volunteers.

In 6 healthy volunteers, the ratio of amantadine clearance to apparent oral plasma clearance was 0.79 ± 0.17 (mean ± SD).

The volume of distribution determined after the intravenous administration of amantadine to 15 healthy subjects was 3-8 L/kg, suggesting tissue binding. Amantadine, after single oral 200 mg doses to 6 healthy young subjects and to 6 healthy elderly subjects has been found in nasal mucus at mean ± SD concentrations of 0.15 ± 0.16, 0.28 ± 0.26, and 0.39 ± 0.34 μg/g at 1, 4, and 8 hours after dosing, respectively. These concentrations represented 31 ± 33%, 59 ± 61%, and 95 ± 86% of the corresponding plasma amantadine concentrations. Amantadine is approximately 67% bound to plasma proteins over a concentration range of 0.1-2.0 μg/ml. Following the administration of amantadine 100 mg as a single dose, the mean ± SD red blood cell to plasma ratio ranged from 2.7 ± 0.5 in 6 healthy subjects to 1.4 ± 0.2 in 8 patients with renal insufficiency.

The apparent oral plasma clearance of amantadine is reduced and the plasma half-life and plasma concentrations are increased in healthy elderly individuals age 60 and older. After single dose administration of 25-75 mg to 7 healthy, elderly male volunteers, the apparent plasma clearance of amantadine was 0.10 ± 0.04 L/h/kg (range 0.06-0.17 L/h/kg) and the half-life was 29 ± 7 hours (range 20-41 hours). Whether these changes are due to decline in renal function or other age-related factors is not known.

In a study of young healthy subjects (n=20), mean renal clearance of amantadine, normalized for body mass index, was significantly higher in males compared to females ($p < 0.032$).

Compared with otherwise healthy adult individuals, the clearance of amantadine is significantly reduced in adult patients with renal insufficiency. The elimination half-life increases 2- to 3-fold or greater when creatinine clearance is less than 40 ml/min/1.73m^2 and averages 8 days in patients on chronic maintenance hemodialysis. Amantadine is removed in negligible amounts by hemodialysis.

The pH of the urine has been reported to influence the excretion rate of amantadine. Since the excretion rate of amantadine increases rapidly when the urine is acidic, the administration of urine acidifying drugs may increase the elimination of the drug from the body.

INDICATIONS AND USAGE

Amantadine HCl is indicated for the prophylaxis and treatment of signs and symptoms of infection caused by various strains of influenza A virus. Amantadine HCl is also indicated in the treatment of parkinsonism and drug-induced extrapyramidal reactions.

INFLUENZA A PROPHYLAXIS

Amantadine HCl is indicated for chemoprophylaxis against signs and symptoms of influenza A virus infection when early vaccination is not feasible or when the vaccine is contraindicated or not available. In the prophylaxis of influenza, early vaccination on an annual basis as recommended by the Centers for Disease Control's Immunization Practices Advisory Committee is the method of choice. Because amantadine does not completely prevent the host immune response to influenza A infection, individuals who take this drug may still develop immune responses to natural disease or vaccination and may be protected when later exposed to antigenically related viruses. Following vaccination during an influenza A outbreak, amantadine prophylaxis should be considered for the 2-4 week time period required to develop an antibody response.

INFLUENZA A TREATMENT

Amantadine HCl is also indicated in the treatment of uncomplicated respiratory tract illness caused by influenza A virus strains especially when administered early in the course of illness. There are no well-controlled clinical studies demonstrating that treatment with amantadine will avoid the development of influenza A virus pneumonitis or other complications in high risk patients.

There is no clinical evidence indicating that amantadine is effective in the prophylaxis or treatment of viral respiratory tract illnesses other than those caused by influenza A strains.

PARKINSON'S DISEASE/SYNDROME

Amantadine HCl is indicated in the treatment of idiopathic Parkinson's disease (Paralysis Agitans), postencephalitic parkinsonism, and symptomatic parkinsonism which may follow injury to the nervous system by carbon monoxide intoxication. It is indicated in those elderly patients believed to develop parkinsonism in association with cerebral arteriosclerosis. In the treatment of Parkinson's disease, amantadine is less effective than levodopa, (-)-3-(3,4-dihydroxyphenyl)-L-alanine, and its efficacy in comparison with the anticholinergic antiparkinson drugs has not yet been established.

DRUG-INDUCED EXTRAPYRAMIDAL REACTIONS

Amantadine HCl is indicated in the treatment of drug-induced extrapyramidal reactions. Although anticholinergic-type side effects have been noted with amantadine HCl when used in patients with drug-induced extrapyramidal reactions, there is a lower incidence of these side effects than that observed with anticholinergic antiparkinson drugs.

CONTRAINDICATIONS

Amantadine HCl is contraindicated in patients with known hypersensitivity to the drug.

WARNINGS

DEATHS

Deaths have been reported from overdose with amantadine HCl. The lowest reported acute lethal dose was 2 grams. Acute toxicity may be attributable to the anticholinergic effects of amantadine. Drug overdose has resulted in cardiac, respiratory, renal or central nervous system (CNS) toxicity. Cardiac dysfunction includes arrhythmia, tachycardia and hypertension.

SUICIDE ATTEMPTS

Suicide attempts, some of which have been fatal, have been reported in patients treated with amantadine HCl, many of whom received short courses for influenza treatment or prophylaxis. The incidence of suicide attempts is not known and the pathophysiologic mechanism is not understood. Suicide attempts and suicidal ideation have been reported in patients with and without prior history of psychiatric illness. Amantadine HCl can exacerbate mental problems in patients with a history of psychiatric disorders or substance abuse. Patients who attempt suicide may exhibit abnormal mental states which include disorientation, confusion, depression, personality changes, agitation, aggressive behavior, hallucinations, paranoia, other psychotic reactions, and somnolence or insomnia. Because of the possibility of serious adverse effects, caution should be observed when prescribing amantadine HCl to patients being treated with drugs having CNS effects, or for whom the potential risks outweigh the benefit of treatment. Because some patients have attempted suicide by overdosing with amantadine, prescriptions should be written for the smallest quantity consistent with good patient management.

CNS EFFECTS

Patients with a history of epilepsy or other "seizures" should be observed closely for possible increased seizure activity.

Patients receiving amantadine HCl who note CNS effects or blurring of vision should be cautioned against driving or working in situations where alertness and adequate motor coordination are important.

OTHER

Patients with a history of congestive heart failure or peripheral edema should be followed closely as there are patients who developed congestive heart failure while receiving amantadine HCl.

Patients with Parkinson's disease improving on amantadine HCl should resume normal activities gradually and cautiously, consistent with other medical considerations, such as the presence of osteoporosis or phlebothrombosis.

Because amantadine HCl has anticholinergic effects and may cause mydriasis, it should not be given to patients with untreated angle closure glaucoma.

PRECAUTIONS

Amantadine HCl should not be discontinued abruptly in patients with Parkinson's disease since a few patients have experienced a parkinsonian crisis, *i.e.*, a sudden marked clinical deterioration, when this medication was suddenly stopped. The dose of anticholinergic drug or of amantadine HCl should be reduced if atropine-like effects appear when these drugs are used concurrently.

NEUROLEPTIC MALIGNANT SYNDROME (NMS)

Sporadic cases of possible Neuroleptic Malignant Syndrome (NMS) have been reported in association with dose reduction or withdrawal of amantadine HCl therapy. Therefore, patients should be observed carefully when the dosage of amantadine HCl is reduced abruptly or discontinued, especially if the patient is receiving neuroleptics.

NMS is an uncommon but life-threatening syndrome characterized by fever or hyperthermia; neurologic findings include muscle rigidity, involuntary movements, altered consciousness; mental status changes; other disturbances, such as autonomic dysfunction, tachycardia, tachypnea, hyper- or hypotension; and laboratory findings such as creatine phosphokinase elevation, leukocytosis and increased serum myoglobin.

The early diagnosis of this condition is important for the appropriate management of these patients. Considering NMS as a possible diagnosis and ruling out other acute illnesses (*e.g.*, pneumonia, systemic infection, etc.) is essential. This may be especially complex if the clinical presentation includes both serious medical illness and untreated or inadequately treated extrapyramidal signs and symptoms (EPS). Other important considerations in the differential diagnosis include central anticholinergic toxicity, heat stroke, drug fever and primary central nervous system (CNS) pathology.

The management of NMS should include: (1) intensive symptomatic treatment and medical monitoring, and (2) treatment of any concomitant serious medical problems for which specific treatments are available. Dopamine agonists, such as bromocriptine, and muscle relaxants, such as dantrolene are often used in the treatment of NMS, however, their effectiveness has not been demonstrated in controlled studies.

RENAL DISEASE

Because amantadine HCl is mainly excreted in the urine, it accumulates in the plasma and in the body when renal function declines. Thus, the dose of amantadine HCl should be reduced in patients with renal impairment and in individuals who are 65 years of age or older.

LIVER DISEASE

Care should be exercised when administering amantadine HCl to patients with liver disease. Rare instances of reversible elevation of liver enzymes have been reported in patients receiving amantadine HCl, though a specific relationship between the drug and such changes has not been established.

OTHER

The dose of amantadine HCl may need careful adjustment in patients with congestive heart failure, peripheral edema, or orthostatic hypotension. Care should be exercised when administering amantadine HCl to patients with a history of recurrent eczematoid rash, or to patients with psychosis or severe psychoneurosis not controlled by chemotherapeutic agents.

CARCINOGENESIS, MUTAGENESIS, AND IMPAIRMENT OF FERTILITY

Long-term *in vivo* animal studies designed to evaluate the carcinogenic potential of amantadine HCl have not been performed. In several *in vitro* assays for gene mutation, amantadine HCl did not increase the number of spontaneously observed mutations in 4 strains of *Salmonella typhumunum* (Ames Test) or in a mammalian cell line (Chinese Hamster Ovary cells) when incubations were performed either with or without a liver metabolic activation extract. Further, there was no evidence of chromosome damage observed in an *in vitro* test using freshly derived and stimulated human peripheral blood lymphocytes (with and without metabolic activation) or in an *in vivo* mouse bone marrow micronucleus test (140-550 mg/kg; estimated human equivalent doses of 11.7-45.8 mg/kg based on body surface area conversion).

In a three litter reproduction study in rats, amantadine at a dose of 32 mg/kg/day (estimated human equivalent dose of 4.5 mg/kg/day, based on body surface area conversions) administered to both males and females slightly impaired fertility. There were no effects on fertility at a dose level of 10 mg/kg/day (estimated human equivalent dose of 1.4 mg/kg/day); intermediate doses were not tested.

Failed fertility has been reported during human *in vitro* fertilization (IVF) when the sperm donor ingested amantadine 2 weeks prior to, and during, the IVF cycle.

PREGNANCY, TERATOGENIC EFFECTS, PREGNANCY CATEGORY C

Amantadine HCl has been shown to be embryotoxic and teratogenic in rats at 50 mg/kg/day (estimated human equivalent dose of 7.1 mg/kg/day based on body surface area conversion), while a dose of 37 mg/kg/day (estimated human equivalent dose of 5.3 mg/kg/day) was without effect. Embryotoxic and teratogenic drug effects were not seen in rabbits that received 32 mg/kg/day (estimated human equivalent dose of 9.6 mg/kg/day, based on body surface area conversion). There are no adequate and well-controlled studies in pregnant women. Human data regarding teratogenicity after maternal use of amantadine is scarce. Tetralogy of Fallot and tibial hemimelia (normal karyotype) occurred in an infant exposed to amantadine during the first trimester of pregnancy (100 mg po for 7 days during the 6th and 7th week of gestation). Cardiovascular maldevelopment (single ventricle with pulmonary atresia) was associated with maternal exposure to amantadine (100 mg/d) administered during the first 2 weeks of pregnancy. Amantadine HCl should be used during pregnancy only if the potential benefit justifies the potential risk to the embryo or the fetus.

NURSING MOTHERS

Amantadine HCl is excreted in human milk. Use is not recommended in nursing mothers.

PEDIATRIC USE

The safety and efficacy of amantadine HCl in newborn infants and infants below the age of 1 year have not been established.

GERIATRIC USE

Because amantadine HCl is primarily excreted in the urine, it accumulates in the plasma and in the body when renal function declines. Thus, the dose of amantadine HCl should be reduced in patients with renal impairment and in individuals who are 65 years of age or older. The dose of amantadine HCl may need reduction in patients with congestive heart failure, peripheral edema, or orthostatic hypotension (see DOSAGE AND ADMINISTRATION).

INFORMATION FOR THE PATIENT

Patients should be advised of the following information:

Blurry vision and/or impaired mental acuity may occur.

Gradually increase physical activity as the symptoms of Parkinson's disease improve.

Avoid excessive alcohol usage, since it may increase the potential for CNS effects such as dizziness, confusion, lightheadedness, and orthostatic hypotension.

Avoid getting up suddenly from a sitting or lying position. If dizziness or lightheadedness occurs, notify physician.

Notify physician of mood/mental changes, swelling of extremities, difficulty urinating and/or shortness of breath occur.

Do not take more medication than prescribed because of the risk of overdose. If there is no improvement in a few days, or if medication appears less effective after a few weeks, discuss with a physician.

Consult physician before discontinuing medication.

Seek medical attention immediately if it is suspected that an overdose of medication has been taken.

DRUG INTERACTIONS

Careful observation is required when amantadine HCl is administered concurrently with CNS stimulants.

Agents with anticholinergic properties may potentiate the anticholinergic-like side effects of amantadine.

Coadministration of thioridazine has been reported to worsen the tremor in elderly patients with Parkinson's disease; however, it is not known if other phenothiazines produce a similar response.

Coadministration of Dyazide (triamterene/hydrochlorothiazide) resulted in a higher plasma amantadine concentration in a 61-year-old man receiving amantadine HCl 100 mg tid for Parkinson's disease. It is not known which of the components of Dyazide contributed to the observation or if related drugs produce a similar response.

Coadministration of trimethoprim-sulfamethoxazole may impair renal clearance of amantadine resulting in higher plasma concentrations.

Coadministration of quinine or quinidine with amantadine was shown to reduce the renal clearance of amantadine.

ADVERSE REACTIONS

The adverse reactions reported most frequently at the recommended dose of amantadine HCl (5-10%) are: Nausea, dizziness (lightheadedness), and insomnia.

Less frequently (1-5%) reported adverse reactions are: Depression, anxiety and irritability, hallucinations, confusion, anorexia, dry mouth, constipation, ataxia, livedo reticularis, peripheral edema, orthostatic hypotension, headache, somnolence, nervousness, dream abnormality, agitation, dry nose, diarrhea and fatigue.

Infrequently (0.1-1%) occurring adverse reactions are: Congestive heart failure, psychosis, urinary retention, dyspnea, fatigue, skin rash, vomiting, weakness, slurred speech, euphoria, confusion, thinking abnormality, amnesia, hyperkinesia, hypertension, decreased libido, and visual disturbance, including punctate subepithelial or other corneal opacity, corneal edema, decreased visual acuity, sensitivity to light, and optic nerve palsy.

Rare (<0.1%) occurring adverse reactions are: Instances of convulsion, leukopenia, neutropenia, eczematoid dermatitis, oculogyric episodes, unsuccessful suicide attempt, suicide, and suicidal ideation (see WARNINGS).

Other adverse reactions reported during postmarketing experience with amantadine HCl usage include:

Nervous System/Psychiatric: Coma, stupor, delirium, hypokinesia, hypertonia, delusions, aggressive behavior, paranoid reaction, manic reaction, involuntary muscle contractions, gait abnormalities, paresthesia, EEG changes, and tremor.

Cardiovascular: Cardiac arrest, arrhythmias including malignant arrhythmias, hypotension, and tachycardia.

Respiratory: Acute respiratory failure, pulmonary edema, and tachypnea.

Gastrointestinal: Dysphagia.

Hematologic: Leukocytosis.

Special Senses: Keratitis and mydriasis.

Skin and Appendages: Pruritus and diaphoresis.

Miscellaneous: Neuroleptic malignant syndrome (see WARNINGS), allergic reactions including anaphylactic reactions, edema, and fever.

Laboratory Test: Elevated CPK, BUN, serum creatinine, alkaline phosphatase, LDH, bilirubin, GGT, SGOT, and SGPT.

DOSAGE AND ADMINISTRATION

The dose of amantadine HCl may need reduction in patients with congestive heart failure, peripheral edema, orthostatic hypotension, or impaired renal function (see Dosage for Renal Impairment).

DOSAGE FOR PROPHYLAXIS AND TREATMENT OF UNCOMPLICATED INFLUENZA A VIRUS ILLNESS

Adults: The adult daily dosage of amantadine is 200 mg; two 100 mg capsules (or 4 teaspoonfuls of syrup) as a single daily dose. The daily dosage may be split into 1 capsule of 100 mg (or 2 teaspoonfuls of syrup) twice a day. If CNS effects develop in once-a-day dosage, a split dosage schedule may reduce such complaints. In persons 65 years of age or older, the daily dosage of amantadine HCl is 100 mg.

A 100 mg daily dose has also been shown in experimental challenge studies to be effective as prophylaxis in healthy adults who are not at high risk for influenza-related complications. However, it has not been demonstrated that a 100 mg daily dose is as effective as a 200 mg daily dose for prophylaxis, nor has the 100 mg daily dose been studied in the treatment of acute influenza illness. In recent clinical trials, the incidence of CNS side effects associated with the 100 mg daily dose was at or near the level of placebo. The 100 mg dose is recommended for persons who have demonstrated intolerance to 200 mg of amantadine daily because of CNS or other toxicities.

Children 1-9 Years of Age: The total daily dose should be calculated on the basis of 2-4 mg/lb/day (4.4-8.8 mg/kg/day), but not to exceed 150 mg per day.

Children 9-12 Years of Age: The total daily dose is 200 mg given as 1 capsule of 100 mg (or 2 teaspoonfuls of syrup) twice a day. The 100 mg daily dose has not been studied in children. Therefore, there are no data which demonstrate that this dose is as effective as or safer than the 200 mg daily dose in this patient population.

Prophylactic dosing should be started in anticipation of an influenza A outbreak and before or after contact with individuals with influenza A virus respiratory tract illness.

Amantadine HCl should be continued daily for at least 10 days following a known exposure. If amantadine HCl is used chemoprophylactically in conjunction with inactivated influenza A virus vaccine until protective antibody responses develop, then it should be administered for 2-4 weeks after the vaccine has been given. When inactivated influenza A virus vaccine is unavailable or contraindicated, amantadine HCl should be administered for the duration of known influenza A in the community because of repeated and unknown exposure.

Treatment of influenza A virus illness should be started as soon as possible, preferably within 24-48 hours after onset of signs and symptoms, and should be continued for 24-48 hours after the disappearance of signs and symptoms.

DOSAGE FOR PARKINSONISM

Adults: The usual dose of amantadine HCl is 100 mg twice a day when used alone. Amantadine HCl has an onset of action usually within 48 hours.

The initial dose of amantadine HCl is 100 mg daily for patients with serious associated medical illness or who are receiving high doses of other antiparkinson drugs. After one to several weeks at 100 mg once daily, the dose may be increased to 100 mg twice daily, if necessary.

Occasionally, patients whose responses are not optimal with amantadine HCl at 200 mg daily may benefit from an increase up to 400 mg daily in divided doses. However, such patients should be supervised closely by their physicians.

Patients initially deriving benefit from amantadine HCl not uncommonly experience a fall-off of effectiveness after a few months. Benefit may be regained by increasing the dose to 300 mg daily. Alternatively, temporary discontinuation of amantadine HCl for several weeks, followed by reinitiation of the drug, may result in regaining benefit in some patients. A decision to use other antiparkinson drugs may be necessary.

DOSAGE FOR CONCOMITANT THERAPY

Some patients who do not respond to anticholinergic antiparkinson drugs may respond to amantadine HCl. When amantadine HCl or anticholinergic antiparkinson drugs are each used with marginal benefit, concomitant use may produce additional benefit.

When amantadine HCl and levodopa are initiated concurrently, the patient can exhibit rapid therapeutic benefits. Amantadine HCl should be held constant at 100 mg daily or twice daily while the daily dose of levodopa is gradually increased to optimal benefit.

When amantadine HCl is added to optimal well-tolerated doses of levodopa, additional benefit may result, including smoothing out the fluctuations in improvement which sometimes occur in patients on levodopa alone. Patients who require a reduction in their usual dose of levodopa because of development of side effects may possibly regain lost benefit with the addition of amantadine HCl.

DOSAGE FOR DRUG-INDUCED EXTRAPYRAMIDAL REACTIONS

Adults: The usual dose of amantadine HCl is 100 mg twice a day. Occasionally, patients whose responses are not optimal with amantadine HCl at 200 mg daily may benefit from an increase up to 300 mg daily in divided doses.

DOSAGE FOR RENAL IMPAIRMENT

Depending upon creatinine clearance, the following dosage adjustments are recommended. The recommended dosage for patients on hemodialysis is 200 mg every 7 days.

TABLE 1

Creatinine Clearance (ml/min/1.73 m^2)	Amantadine HCl Dosage
30-50	200 mg 1st day and 100 mg each day thereafter
15-29	200 mg 1st day followed by 100 mg on alternate days
<15	200 mg every 7 days

HOW SUPPLIED

Symmetrel Tablets: Available in light orange, convex curved, triangular shaped 100 mg tablets with "SYMMETREL" debossed on one side and plain on the other side.

Symmetrel Syrup: Available as a clear, colorless syrup [each 5 ml (1 teaspoonful) contains 50 mg amantadine hydrochloride].

Amantadine HCl Capsules: Available as capsules (each yellow, soft gelatin capsule contains 100 mg of amantadine HCl).

Storage: Store at controlled room temperature 15-30°C (59-86°F). Protect from moisture. Dispense in a tight, light-resistant container.

PRODUCT LISTING - RATED THERAPEUTICALLY EQUIVALENT

Capsule - Oral - 100 mg			
6's	$3.77	GENERIC, Pd-Rx Pharmaceuticals	55289-0012-06
10's	$6.44	GENERIC, Pd-Rx Pharmaceuticals	55289-0012-10
10's	$9.06	GENERIC, Dhs Inc	55887-0767-10
10's	$9.73	GENERIC, Pharma Pac	52959-0007-10
14's	$7.65	GENERIC, Pd-Rx Pharmaceuticals	55289-0012-14
14's	$11.26	GENERIC, Dhs Inc	55887-0767-14
14's	$12.96	GENERIC, Pharma Pac	52959-0007-14
15's	$13.88	GENERIC, Pharma Pac	52959-0007-15
20's	$10.79	GENERIC, Pd-Rx Pharmaceuticals	55289-0012-20
20's	$12.22	GENERIC, Dhs Inc	55887-0767-20
20's	$18.01	GENERIC, Pharma Pac	52959-0007-20
25's	$10.47	GENERIC, Pd-Rx Pharmaceuticals	55289-0012-97
30's	$16.94	GENERIC, Heartland Healthcare Services	61392-0042-39
30's	$16.94	GENERIC, Heartland Healthcare Services	61392-0105-30
30's	$16.94	GENERIC, Heartland Healthcare Services	61392-0105-39
30's	$26.70	GENERIC, Pharma Pac	52959-0007-30
31's	$17.50	GENERIC, Heartland Healthcare Services	61392-0042-31
31's	$17.50	GENERIC, Heartland Healthcare Services	61392-0105-31
32's	$18.07	GENERIC, Heartland Healthcare Services	61392-0042-32
32's	$18.07	GENERIC, Heartland Healthcare Services	61392-0105-32
45's	$25.41	GENERIC, Heartland Healthcare Services	61392-0105-45
60's	$33.87	GENERIC, Heartland Healthcare Services	61392-0042-65
60's	$33.87	GENERIC, Heartland Healthcare Services	61392-0105-60
90's	$50.81	GENERIC, Heartland Healthcare Services	61392-0105-90
100's	$15.72	FEDERAL UPPER LIMIT, H.C.F.A. F F P	99999-0174-02
100's	$25.00	GENERIC, Raway Pharmacal Inc	00686-2291-10
100's	$30.00	GENERIC, Chase Laboratories Inc	54429-3185-01
100's	$30.59	GENERIC, Qualitest Products Inc	00603-2163-21
100's	$30.59	GENERIC, Qualitest Products Inc	00603-2164-21
100's	$31.00	GENERIC, Raway Pharmacal Inc	00686-0481-20
100's	$31.50	GENERIC, Geneva Pharmaceuticals	00781-2105-01
100's	$31.50	GENERIC, Geneva Pharmaceuticals	00781-2105-13
100's	$31.50	GENERIC, Major Pharmaceuticals Inc	00904-3430-60
100's	$31.50	GENERIC, Major Pharmaceuticals Inc	00904-3431-60
100's	$32.95	GENERIC, Geneva Pharmaceuticals	00781-2106-01
100's	$33.50	GENERIC, Watson/Rugby Laboratories Inc	00536-3043-01
100's	$34.24	GENERIC, Purepac Pharmaceutical Company	00228-2291-10
100's	$34.82	GENERIC, Dixon-Shane Inc	17236-0849-01
100's	$36.00	GENERIC, Martec Pharmaceuticals Inc	52555-0122-01
100's	$36.20	GENERIC, Aligen Independent Laboratories Inc	00405-4042-01
100's	$36.58	GENERIC, Invamed Inc	52189-0211-24
100's	$36.59	GENERIC, Ivax Corporation	00182-1258-01
100's	$36.59	GENERIC, Moore, H.L. Drug Exchange Inc	00839-7250-06
100's	$36.59	GENERIC, Moore, H.L. Drug Exchange Inc	00839-7471-06
100's	$37.10	GENERIC, Martec Pharmaceuticals Inc	52555-0675-01
100's	$59.78	GENERIC, Udl Laboratories Inc	51079-0481-20
100's	$60.10	GENERIC, Dixon-Shane Inc	17236-0849-11
100's	$62.17	GENERIC, Rosemont Pharmaceutical Corporation	00832-1015-00
100's	$62.19	GENERIC, Geneva Pharmaceuticals	00781-2048-01
100's	$68.39	GENERIC, Major Pharmaceuticals Inc	00904-3430-61
Syrup - Oral - 50 mg/5 ml			
10 ml x 100	$100.00	GENERIC, Pharmaceutical Assoc Inc Div Beach Products	00121-0646-10
20 ml x 100	$174.63	GENERIC, Pharmaceutical Assoc Inc Div Beach Products	00121-0646-20
473 ml	$63.98	GENERIC, Hi-Tech Pharmacal Company Inc	50383-0807-16
480 ml	$31.49	FEDERAL UPPER LIMIT, H.C.F.A. F F P	99999-0174-04

Size	Price	Product	NDC
480 ml	$34.35	GENERIC, Pharmaceutical Assoc Inc Div Beach Products	00121-0646-16
480 ml	$59.95	GENERIC, Qualitest Products Inc	00603-1010-58
480 ml	$63.02	GENERIC, Ivax Corporation	00182-6016-40
480 ml	$63.12	GENERIC, Aligen Independent Laboratories Inc	00405-2140-16
480 ml	$70.00	GENERIC, Major Pharmaceuticals Inc	00904-3432-16
480 ml	$70.70	GENERIC, Morton Grove Pharmaceuticals Inc	60432-0093-16
480 ml	$71.00	GENERIC, Alpharma Uspd Makers Of Barre and Nmc	00472-0833-16
480 ml	$74.27	GENERIC, Endo Laboratories Llc	60951-0656-16
480 ml	$125.75	SYMMETREL, Endo Laboratories Llc	63481-0205-16

PRODUCT LISTING - EQUIVALENTS NOT AVAILABLE

Size	Price	Product	NDC
Capsule - Oral - 100 mg			
4's	$4.05	GENERIC, Prescript Pharmaceuticals	00247-0133-04
7's	$4.55	GENERIC, Prescript Pharmaceuticals	00247-0133-07
9's	$4.91	GENERIC, Prescript Pharmaceuticals	00247-0133-09
10's	$3.48	GENERIC, Allscripts Pharmaceutical Company	54569-0084-03
10's	$3.52	GENERIC, Physicians Total Care	54868-0800-01
10's	$5.07	GENERIC, Prescript Pharmaceuticals	00247-0133-10
10's	$8.47	GENERIC, Southwood Pharmaceuticals Inc	58016-0153-10
14's	$4.87	GENERIC, Allscripts Pharmaceutical Company	54569-0084-02
14's	$5.76	GENERIC, Prescript Pharmaceuticals	00247-0133-14
14's	$11.86	GENERIC, Southwood Pharmaceuticals Inc	58016-0153-14
15's	$4.62	GENERIC, Physicians Total Care	54868-0800-07
15's	$5.93	GENERIC, Prescript Pharmaceuticals	00247-0133-15
15's	$12.71	GENERIC, Southwood Pharmaceuticals Inc	58016-0153-15
16's	$6.11	GENERIC, Prescript Pharmaceuticals	00247-0133-16
20's	$5.71	GENERIC, Physicians Total Care	54868-0800-02
20's	$6.80	GENERIC, Prescript Pharmaceuticals	00247-0133-20
20's	$6.96	GENERIC, Allscripts Pharmaceutical Company	54569-0084-04
20's	$16.94	GENERIC, Southwood Pharmaceuticals Inc	58016-0153-20
21's	$6.96	GENERIC, Prescript Pharmaceuticals	00247-0133-21
30's	$7.91	GENERIC, Physicians Total Care	54868-0800-03
30's	$8.52	GENERIC, Prescript Pharmaceuticals	00247-0133-30
30's	$20.68	GENERIC, Southwood Pharmaceuticals Inc	58016-0153-30
60's	$13.68	GENERIC, Prescript Pharmaceuticals	00247-0133-60
90's	$18.84	GENERIC, Prescript Pharmaceuticals	00247-0133-90
100's	$23.24	GENERIC, Physicians Total Care	54868-0800-04
100's	$50.53	GENERIC, Apothecon Inc	62269-0211-24
100's	$84.72	GENERIC, Southwood Pharmaceuticals Inc	58016-0153-00
Syrup - Oral - 50 mg/5 ml			
150 ml	$43.25	GENERIC, Southwood Pharmaceuticals Inc	58016-0331-30
480 ml	$62.50	GENERIC, Mikart Inc	46672-0606-16
480 ml	$70.85	GENERIC, Moore, H.L. Drug Exchange Inc	00839-7667-69
480 ml	$90.56	SYMMETREL, Dupont Pharmaceuticals	00056-0205-16
Tablet - Oral - 100 mg			
100's	$132.63	SYMMETREL, Endo Laboratories Llc	63481-0108-70

Ambenonium Chloride (000175)

Categories: Myasthenia gravis; FDA Approved 1956 May; Pregnancy Category C
Drug Classes: Cholinesterase inhibitors; Musculoskeletal agents; Stimulants, muscle
Brand Names: **Mytelase**
Cost of Therapy: $110.83 (Myasthenia Gravis; Mytelase; 10 mg; 3 tablets/day; 30 day supply)

DESCRIPTION

Ambenonium chloride is a white crystalline powder soluble in water to 20% weight/volume.

CLINICAL PHARMACOLOGY

A cholinesterase inhibitor with all the pharmacologic actions of acetylcholine, both of muscarinic & nicotinic types. Cholinesterase inactivates acetylcholine. Myasthenia gravis is a pathologic exhaustion of voluntary muscles, resulting in a state resembling paralysis, due either to an underproduction of acetylcholine or to an overproduction and activity of cholinesterase at the myoneural junction. Like neostigmine, ambenonium suppresses cholinesterase but it has the advantage of a longer duration of action and fewer side effects on the gastro-intestinal tract. Because its action is longer, administration of ambenonium is necessary only every 3 or 4 hours, depending upon the clinical response. Usually medication is not required throughout the night so that the patient can sleep uninterruptedly.

INDICATIONS AND USAGE

Myasthenia gravis.

CONTRAINDICATIONS

Since belladonna derivatives (atropine, etc.) may suppress the parasympathomimetic (muscarinic) symptoms of excessive gastrointestinal stimulation, leaving only the more serious symptoms of fasciculation and paralysis of voluntary muscle as signs of overdosage, routine administration of atropine with ambenonium is contraindicated.

Because ambenonium has a more prolonged action than other antimyasthenic drugs, simultaneous administration with other cholinergics is contraindicated except under strict medical supervision. The overlap in duration of action of several drugs complicates dosage schedules. Thus, when transferring to ambenonium chloride all other cholinergics should be suspended until the patient has been stabilized. In most instances the myasthenic symptoms are effectively controlled by ambenonium alone.

Ambenonium should be used with caution in patients with asthma or in patients with mechanical intestinal or urinary obstruction.

DOSAGE AND ADMINISTRATION

The oral dose must be individualized according to the patient's response because the disease varies widely in its severity in different patients, and patients vary in their sensitivity to cholinergic drugs. There is a highly critical point of maximum therapeutic effectiveness with optimum muscle strength and no gastrointestinal disturbances requiring close supervision of a physician familiar with the disease.

Since the warning of overdosage is minimal and the requirements of patients vary tremendously, great care and supervision are required. That a narrow margin exists between the first appearance of side effects and serious toxic effects must be borne in mind constantly. Caution in increasing dosage is essential.

For the moderately severe myasthenic patient from 5-25 mg ambenonium chloride 3 or 4 times daily is an effective dose. Some patients do well with as little as 5 mg per dose, while others require as much as from 50-75 mg per dose. The physician should start with a 5 mg dose, carefully observing the effect of the drug in each patient. The dosage may be gradually increased to determine the effective and safe dose for each patient. In addition to individual variations in dosage requirements, the amount of cholinergic medication necessary to control symptoms may fluctuate in each patient, depending upon his activity and the current status of the disease, including spontaneous remission. A few patients have required greater doses for adequate control of the myasthenic symptoms, but increasing the dosage above 200 mg daily requires exacting supervision of a physician well aware of the signs and treatment of overdosage with cholinergic medication.

PRODUCT LISTING - EQUIVALENTS NOT AVAILABLE

Size	Price	Product	NDC
Tablet - Oral - 10 mg			
100's	$123.14	MYTELASE CHLORIDE, Sanofi Winthrop Pharmaceuticals	00024-1287-04

Amikacin Sulfate (000178)

For complete prescribing information, refer to the CD-ROM included with the book.

Categories: Burns; Infection, bone; Infection, central nervous system; Infection, intra-abdominal; Infection, joint; Infection, postoperative; Infection, respiratory tract; Infection, skin and skin structures; Infection, urinary tract; Peritonitis; Septicemia; Septicemia, neonatal; Pregnancy Category D; FDA Approved 1981 Jan
Drug Classes: Antibiotics, aminoglycosides
Brand Names: **Amikin**
Foreign Brand Availability: Akacin (Thailand); Akicin (Korea; Thailand); Akim (Ecuador); Alostil (Indonesia); Amicacina (Spain); Amicasil (Italy); Amicin (India); Amikafur (Mexico); Amikan (Italy); Amikayect (Mexico); Amiklin (France); Amikozit (Bahrain; Cyprus; Egypt; Iran; Iraq; Jordan; Kuwait; Lebanon; Libya; Oman; Qatar; Republic-of-Yemen; Saudi-Arabia; Syria; United-Arab-Emirates); Amiktam (Korea); Amukin (Belgium; Netherlands); Apalin (Hong-Kong); Biklin (Austria; Denmark; Finland; Germany; Philippines; Sweden); Briklin (Greece); Chemacin (Italy); Gamikal (Mexico); Glukamin (Ecuador); Kacinth-A (South-Africa); Kanbine (Spain); Lanomycin (Greece); Likacin (Bahrain; Cyprus; Egypt; Iran; Iraq; Israel; Jordan; Kuwait; Lebanon; Libya; Oman; Qatar; Republic-of-Yemen; Saudi-Arabia; Syria; Thailand; United-Arab-Emirates); Lukadin (Italy); Miacin (Bahrain; Cyprus; Egypt; Iran; Iraq; Jordan; Kuwait; Lebanon; Libya; Oman; Qatar; Republic-of-Yemen; Saudi-Arabia; Syria; United-Arab-Emirates); Nica (Philippines); Onikin (Philippines); Orlobin (Greece); Pediakin (Philippines); Pierami (Taiwan); Savox (Taiwan); Selaxa (Greece); Selemycin (Bahrain; Cyprus; Egypt; Hong-Kong; Iran; Iraq; Jordan; Kuwait; Lebanon; Libya; Oman; Qatar; Republic-of-Yemen; Saudi-Arabia; Syria; United-Arab-Emirates); Tybikin (Thailand); Yectamid (Mexico)
Cost of Therapy: $477.78 (Infection; Amikin Injection; 250 mg/ml; 1050 mg/day; 7 day supply)
$64.31 (Infection; Generic Injection; 250 mg/ml; 1050 mg/day; 7 day supply)

WARNING

Patients treated with parenteral aminoglycosides should be under close clinical observation because of the potential ototoxicity and nephrotoxicity associated with their use. Safety for treatment periods which are longer than 14 days has not been established.

Neurotoxicity, manifested as vestibular and permanent bilateral auditory ototoxicity can occur in patients with preexisting renal damage and in patients with normal renal function treated at higher doses and/or for periods longer than those recommended. The risk of aminoglycoside-induced ototoxicity is greater in patients with renal damage. High frequency deafness usually occurs first and can be detected only by audiometric testing. Vertigo may occur and may be evidence of vestibular injury. Other manifestations of neurotoxicity may include numbness, skin tingling, muscle twitching, and convulsions. The risk of hearing loss due to aminoglycosides increases with the degree of exposure to either high peak or high trough serum concentrations. Patients developing cochlear damage may not have symptoms during therapy to warn them of developing eighth-nerve toxicity, and total or partial irreversible bilateral deafness may occur after the drug has been discontinued. Aminoglycoside-induced ototoxicity is usually irreversible.

Aminoglycosides are potentially nephrotoxic. The risk of nephrotoxicity is greater in patients with impaired renal function and in those who receive high doses or prolonged therapy.

Neuromuscular blockade and respiratory paralysis have been reported following parenteral injection, topical instillation (as in orthopedic and abdominal irritation or in local treatment of empyema), and following oral use of aminoglycosides. The possibility of these phenomena should be considered if aminoglycosides are administered by any route, especially in patients receiving anesthetics, neuromuscular blocking agents such as tubocurarine, succinylcholine, decamethonium, or in patients receiving massive transfusions of citrate-anticoagulated blood. If blockade occurs, calcium salts may reverse these phenomena, but mechanical respiratory assistance may be necessary. Renal and eight-nerve function should be closely monitored especially in patients with known or suspected renal impairment at the onset of therapy and also in those whose renal function is initially normal but who develop signs of renal dysfunction during therapy. Serum concentrations of amikacin should be monitored when feasible to assure adequate levels and to avoid potentially toxic levels and prolonged peak concentrations above micrograms per ml. Urine should be examined for decreased specific gravity, increased excretion of proteins, and the presence of cells or casts. Blood urea nitrogen, serum creatinine, or creatinine

WARNING — Cont'd

clearance should be measured periodically. Serial audiograms should be obtained where feasible in patients old enough to be tested, particularly high risk patients. Evidence of ototoxicity (dizziness, vertigo, tinnitus, roaring in the ears, and hearing loss) or nephrotoxicity requires discontinuation of the drug or dosage adjustment.

Concurrent and/or sequential systemic, oral, or topical use of other neurotoxic or nephrotoxic products, particularly bacitracin, cisplatin, amphotericin B, cephaloridine, paromomycin, viomycin, polymyxin B, colistin, vancomycin, or other aminoglycosides should be avoided. Other factors that may increase risk of toxicity are advanced age and dehydration.

The concurrent use of Amikin with potent diuretics (ethacrynic acid, or furosemide) should be avoided since diuretics by themselves may cause ototoxicity. In addition, when administered intravenously, diuretics may enhance aminoglycoside toxicity by altering antibiotic concentrations in serum and tissue.

DESCRIPTION

Amikacin sulfate is a semi-synthetic aminoglycoside antibiotic derived from kanamycin. It is $C_{22}H_{43}N_5O_{13}{\cdot}2H_2SO_4$. D-Streptamine, O-3-amino-3-deoxy-α-D-glucopyranosyl-(1→6)-O-(6-amino-6-deoxy-α-D-glucopyranosyl-(1→4))-N[1]-(4-amino-2-hydroxyl-1-oxobutyl)-2-deoxy-,(S)-,sulfate (1:2) (salt).

The dosage form is supplied as a sterile, colorless to light straw colored solution. The 100 mg/2 ml vial contains, in addition to amikacin sulfate, 0.13% sodium bisulfite and 0.5% sodium citrate with pH adjusted to 4.5 with sulfuric acid. The 500 mg/2 ml vial and the 1 g/4 ml vial contain 0.66% sodium bisulfite and 2.5% sodium citrate with pH adjusted to 4.5 with sulfuric acid.

Vial headspace contains nitrogen.

INDICATIONS AND USAGE

Amikin is indicated in the short-term treatment of serious infections due to susceptible strains of Gram-negative bacteria, including *Pseudomonas* species, *Escherichia coli,* species of indole-positive and indole-negative *Proteus, Providencia* species, *Klebsiella-Enterobacter-Serratia* species, and *Acinetobacter (Mima-Herellea)* species.

Clinical studies have shown Amikin to be effective in bacterial septicemia (including neonatal sepsis); in serious infections of the respiratory tract, bones and joints, central nervous system (including meningitis) and skin and soft tissue intra-abdominal infections (including peritonitis); and in burns and postoperative infections (including postvascular surgery). Clinical studies have shown Amikin also to be effective in serious complicated and recurrent urinary tract infections due to these organisms. Aminoglycosides, including Amikin injectable, are not indicated in uncomplicated initial episodes of urinary tract infections unless the causative organisms are not susceptible to antibiotics having less potential toxicity.

Bacteriologic studies should be performed to identify causative organisms and their susceptibilities to amikacin. Amikin may be considered as initial therapy in suspected Gram-negative infections and therapy may be instituted before obtaining the results of susceptibility testing. Clinical trials demonstrated that Amikin was ineffective in infections caused by gentamicin and/or tobramycin-resistant strains of Gram-negative organisms, particularly *Proteus rettgeri, Providencia stuartii, Serratia marcescens,* and *Pseudomonas aeruginosa.* The decision to continue therapy with the drug should be based on results of the susceptibility tests, the severity of the infection, the response of the patient and the important additional considerations contained in BOXED WARNING .

Amikin has also been shown to be effective in staphylococcal infections and may be considered as initial therapy under certain conditions in the treatment of known or suspected staphylococcal disease such as, severe infections where the causative organism may be either a Gram-negative bacterium or a *Staphylococcus,* infections due to susceptible strains of staphylococci in patients allergic to other antibiotics, and in mixed staphylococcal/Gram-negative infections.

In certain severe infections such as neonatal sepsis, concomitant therapy with a penicillin-type drug may be indicated because of the possibility of infections due to Gram-positive organisms such as streptococci or pneumococci.

CONTRAINDICATIONS

A history of hypersensitivity to amikacin is a contraindication for its use. A history of hypersensitivity or serious toxic reactions to aminoglycosides may contraindicate the use of any other aminoglycosides because of the known cross-sensitivities of patients to drugs in this class.

WARNINGS

See BOXED WARNING.

Aminoglycosides can cause fetal harm when administered to a pregnant woman. Aminoglycosides cross the placenta and there have been several reports of total irreversible, bilateral congenital deafness in children whose mothers received streptomycin during pregnancy. Although serious side effects to the fetus or newborns have not been reported in the treatment of pregnant women with other aminoglycosides, the potential for harm exists. Reproduction studies of amikacin have been performed in rats and mice and revealed no evidence of impaired fertility or harm to the fetus due to amikacin. There are no well controlled studies in pregnant women, but investigational experience does not include any positive evidence of adverse effects to the fetus. If this drug is used during pregnancy, or if the patient becomes pregnant while taking this drug, the patient should be apprised of the potential hazard to the fetus.

Contains sodium bisulfite, a sulfite that may cause allergic-type reactions including anaphylactic symptoms and life-threatening or less severe asthmatic episodes in certain susceptible people. The overall prevalence of sulfite sensitivity in the general population is unknown and probably low. Sulfite sensitivity is seen more frequently in asthmatic than nonasthmatic people.

DOSAGE AND ADMINISTRATION

The patient's pretreatment body weight should be obtained for calculation of correct dosage. Amikin may be given intramuscularly or intravenously.

The status of renal function should be estimated by measurement of the serum creatinine concentration or calculation of the endogenous creatinine clearance rate. The blood urea nitrogen (BUN) is much less reliable for this purpose. Reassessment of renal function should be made periodically during therapy.

Whenever possible, amikacin concentrations in serum should be measured to assure adequate but not excessive levels. It is desirable to measure both peak and tough serum concentrations intermittently during therapy. Peak concentrations (30-90 minutes after injection) above 35 μg/ml and trough concentrations (just prior to the next dose) above 10 μg/ml should be avoided. Dosage should be adjusted as indicated.

INTRAMUSCULAR ADMINISTRATION FOR PATIENTS WITH NORMAL RENAL FUNCTION

The recommended dosage for adults, children and older infants (see BOXED WARNING) with normal renal function is 15 mg/kg/day divided into 2 or 3 equal doses administered at equally-divided intervals *i.e.,* 7.5 mg/kg q12h or 5 mg/kg q8h. Treatment of patients in the heavier weight classes should not exceed 1.5 g/day.

When amikacin is indicated is newborns (see BOXED WARNING), it is recommended that a loading dose of 10 mg/kg be administered initially to be followed with 7.5 mg/kg every 12 hours.

The usual duration of treatment is 7-10 days. It is desirable to limit the duration of treatment to short term whenever feasible. The total daily dose by all routes of administration should not exceed 15 mg/kg/day. In difficult and complicated infections where treatment beyond 10 days is considered, the use of Amikin should be reevaluated. It continued, amikacin serum levels, and renal, auditory, and vestibular functions should be monitored. At the recommended dosage level, uncomplicated infections due to amikacin-sensitive organisms should respond in 24-48 hours, If definite clinical response does not occur within 3-5 days, therapy should be stopped and the antibiotic susceptibility patterns of the invading organism should be rechecked. Failure of the infection to respond may be due to resistance of the organism or to the presence of septic foci requiring surgical drainage.

When Amikin is indicated in uncomplicated urinary tract infections, a dose of 250 mg twice daily may be used (TABLE 1):

TABLE 1 *Dosage Guidelines — Adult and Children With Normal Renal Function*

Patient Weight		Dosage	
		7.5 mg/kg	5 mg/kg
lbs	kg	q12h OR	q8h
99	45	337.5 mg	225 mg
110	50	375 mg	250 mg
121	55	412.5 mg	275 mg
132	60	450 mg	300 mg
143	65	487.5 mg	325 mg
154	70	525 mg	350 mg
165	75	562.6 mg	375 mg
176	80	600 mg	400 mg
187	85	637.5 mg	425 mg
198	90	675 mg	450 mg
209	95	712.5 mg	475 mg
220	100	750 mg	500 mg

Available as: 100 mg/2 ml vial, 500 mg/2 ml vial, 1 g/4 ml vial, 500 mg/2 ml disposable syringe.

INTRAMUSCULAR ADMINISTRATION FOR PATIENTS WITH IMPAIRED RENAL FUNCTION

Whenever possible, serum amikacin concentrations should be monitored by appropriate assay procedures. Doses may be adjusted in patients with impaired renal function either by administering normal doses at prolonged intervals or by administering reduced doses at a fixed interval.

Both methods are based on the patient's creatinine clearance or serum creatinine values since these have been found to correlate with aminoglycoside half-lives in patients with diminished renal function. These dosage schedules must be used in conjunction with careful clinical and laboratory observations of the patient and should be modified as necessary. Neither method should be used when dialysis is being performed.

NORMAL DOSAGE AT PROLONGED INTERVALS

If the creatinine clearance rate is not available and the patient's condition is stable, a dosage interval in hours for the normal dose can be calculated by multiplying the patient's serum creatinine by 9, *e.g.,* if the serum creatinine concentration is 2 mg/100 ml, the recommended single dose (7.5 mg/kg) should be administered every 18 hours.

REDUCED DOSAGE AT FIXED TIME INTERVALS

When renal function is impaired and it is desirable to administer Amikin at a fixed time interval, dosage must be reduced. In these patients, serum Amikin concentrations should be measured to assure accurate administration of Amikin and to avoid concentrations above 35 μg/ml. If serum assay determinations are not available and the patient's condition is stable, serum creatinine and creatinine clearance values are the most readily available indicators of the degree of renal impairment to use as a guide for dosage.

First, initiate therapy by administering a normal dose, 7.5 mg/kg, as a loading dose. This loading dose is the same as the normally recommended dose which would be calculated for a patient with normal renal function as described above.

To determine the size of maintenance doses administered every 12 hours, the loading dose should be reduced in proportion to the reduction in the patient's creatinine clearance rate.

Maintenance Dose Every 12 Hours = [(observed CC in ml/min) ÷ (normal CC in ml/min)] × calculated loading dose in mg

(CC = creatinine clearance rate)

An alternate rough guide for determining reduced dosage at 12-hours intervals (for patients whose steady state serum creatinine values are known) is to divide the normally recommended dose by the patient's serum creatinine.

The above dosage schedules are not intended to be rigid recommendations but are provided as guides to dosage when the measurement of amikacin serum levels is not feasible.

INTRAVENOUS ADMINISTRATION

The individual dose, the total daily dose, and the total cumulative dose of Amikin are identical to the dose recommended for intramuscular administration. The solution of intravenous use is prepared by adding the contents of a 500 mg vial to 100 or 200 ml of sterile diluent such as normal saline or 5% dextrose in water or any of the compatible solutions listed below.

The solution is administered to adults over a 30-60 minute period. The total daily dose should not exceed 15 mg/kg/day and may be divided into either 2 or 3 equally-divided doses at equally-divided intervals.

In pediatric patients the amount of fluid used will depend on the amount of Amikin ordered for the patient. It should be a sufficient amount to infuse the Amikin over a 30-60 minute period. Infants should receive a 1-2 hour infusion.

STABILITY IN IV FLUIDS

Amikin is stable for 24 hours at room temperature at concentrations of 0.25 and 5.0 mg/ml in the following solutions:

5% dextrose injection.
5% dextrose and 0.2% sodium chloride injection.
5% dextrose and 0.45% sodium chloride injection.
0.9% sodium chloride injection.
Lactated Ringer's injection.
NormosolM in 5% dextrose injection (or Plasma-Lyte 56 injection in 5% dextrose in water).
NormosolR in 5% dextrose injection (or Plasma-Lyte 148 injection in 5% dextrose in water).

In the above solutions with Amikin concentrations of 0.25 and 5.0 mg/ml, solutions aged for 60 days at 4°C and then stored at 25°C had utility times of 24 hours.

At the same concentrations, solutions frozen and aged for 30 days at -15°C, thawed, and stored at 25°C had utility times of 24 hours.

Parenteral drug products should be inspected visually for particulate matter and discoloration prior to administration whenever the solution and container permit.

Aminoglycosides administered by any of the above routes should not be physically premixed with other drugs but should be administered separately.

Because of the potential toxicity of aminoglycosides, "fixed dosage" recommendations which are not based upon body weight are not advised. Rather, it is essential to calculate the dosage to fit the needs of each patient.

PRODUCT LISTING - RATED THERAPEUTICALLY EQUIVALENT

Solution - Intravenous - 50 mg/ml

Package	Price	Product	NDC
2 ml x 10	$87.50	GENERIC, Gensia Sicor Pharmaceuticals Inc	00703-9022-03
2 ml x 10	$155.92	GENERIC, Abbott Pharmaceutical	00074-1955-01
2 ml x 10	$325.00	GENERIC, Vha Supply	55390-0223-02
2 ml x 10	$325.00	GENERIC, Bedford Laboratories	55390-0225-02
2 ml x 10	$330.38	AMIKIN PEDIATRIC, Bristol-Myers Squibb	00015-3015-20
2 ml x 10	$330.38	AMIKIN PEDIATRIC, Bristol-Myers Squibb	00015-3015-97
2 ml x 10	$440.50	GENERIC, Faulding Pharmaceutical Company	61703-0201-07
2 ml x 10	$450.00	GENERIC, Solo Pak Medical Products Inc	39769-0236-02

Solution - Intravenous - 62.5 mg/ml

Package	Price	Product	NDC
8 ml x 25	$3139.75	GENERIC, Abbott Pharmaceutical	00074-2434-03

Solution - Intravenous - 250 mg/ml

Package	Price	Product	NDC
2 ml x 10	$87.50	GENERIC, Gensia Sicor Pharmaceuticals Inc	00703-9032-03
2 ml x 10	$165.45	GENERIC, Sanofi Winthrop Pharmaceuticals	00024-0016-11
2 ml x 10	$187.03	GENERIC, Abbott Pharmaceutical	00074-1956-01
2 ml x 10	$195.94	GENERIC, Abbott Pharmaceutical	00074-1958-01
2 ml x 10	$342.60	AMIKIN, Bristol-Myers Squibb	00015-3020-97
2 ml x 10	$437.50	GENERIC, Vha Supply	55390-0224-02
2 ml x 10	$437.50	GENERIC, Bedford Laboratories	55390-0226-02
2 ml x 10	$637.50	GENERIC, Esi Lederle Generics	00641-0123-23
2 ml x 10	$685.44	AMIKIN, Bristol-Myers Squibb	00015-3020-96
2 ml x 10	$734.30	GENERIC, Faulding Pharmaceutical Company	61703-0202-07
3 ml x 10	$1132.40	GENERIC, Faulding Pharmaceutical Company	61703-0202-08
4 ml x 10	$175.00	GENERIC, Gensia Sicor Pharmaceuticals Inc	00703-9040-03
4 ml x 10	$330.88	GENERIC, Sanofi Winthrop Pharmaceuticals	00024-0016-12
4 ml x 10	$399.00	GENERIC, Abbott Pharmaceutical	00074-1957-01
4 ml x 10	$677.10	AMIKIN, Bristol-Myers Squibb	00015-3023-97
4 ml x 10	$875.00	GENERIC, Bedford Laboratories	55390-0224-04
4 ml x 10	$875.00	GENERIC, Bedford Laboratories	55390-0226-04
4 ml x 10	$1200.00	GENERIC, Esi Lederle Generics	00641-2357-43
4 ml x 10	$1509.90	GENERIC, Faulding Pharmaceutical Company	61703-0202-04

Solution - Intravenous - 500 mg/100 ml

Package	Price	Product	NDC
100 ml x 24	$2783.00	AMIKACIN SULFATE-SODIUM CHLORIDE, Abbott Pharmaceutical	00074-5795-23

PRODUCT LISTING - EQUIVALENTS NOT AVAILABLE

Solution - Intravenous - 250 mg/ml

Package	Price	Product	NDC
2 ml x 10	$329.00	AMIKIN, Bristol-Myers Squibb	00015-3020-20
2 ml x 10	$685.44	AMIKIN, Bristol-Myers Squibb	00015-3020-21
4 ml x 10	$650.10	AMIKIN, Bristol-Myers Squibb	00015-3023-20

Amiloride Hydrochloride *(000179)*

Categories: Heart failure, congestive; Hypertension, essential; Pregnancy Category B; FDA Approved 1981 Oct; WHO Formulary
Drug Classes: Diuretics, potassium sparing
Brand Names: Midamor
Foreign Brand Availability: Amikal (Denmark; Sweden); Amilo 5 (Korea); Berkamil (Ireland); Kaluril (Australia; Taiwan); Medamor (Finland); Modamide (France); Nirulid (Denmark); Pandiuren (Argentina)
Cost of Therapy: $17.30 (Hypertension; Midamor; 5 mg; 1 tablet/day; 30 day supply)
$8.40 (Hypertension; Generic Tablets; 5 mg; 1 tablet/day; 30 day supply)

DESCRIPTION

Amiloride HCl, an antikaliuretic-diuretic agent, is a pyrazine-carbonyl-guanidine that is unrelated chemically to other known antikaliuretic or diuretic agents. It is the salt of a moderately strong base (pKa 8.7). It is designated chemically as 3,5-diamino-6-chloro-*N*-(diaminomethylene)pyrazinecarboxamide monohydrochloride, dihydrate and has a molecular weight of 302.12. Its empirical formula is $C_6H_8ClN_7O{\cdot}HCl{\cdot}2H_2O$.

Midamor is available for oral use as tablets containing 5 mg of anhydrous amiloride HCl. Each tablet contains the following inactive ingredients: calcium phosphate, D&C yellow 10, iron oxide, lactose, magnesium stearate and starch.

CLINICAL PHARMACOLOGY

Amiloride HCl is a potassium-conserving (antikaliuretic) drug that possesses weak (compared with thiazide diuretics) natriuretic, diuretic, and antihypertensive activity. These effects have been partially additive to the effects of thiazide diuretics in some clinical studies. When administered with a thiazide or loop diuretic, amiloride HCl has been shown to decrease the enhanced urinary excretion of magnesium which occurs when a thiazide or loop diuretic is used alone. Amiloride HCl has potassium-conserving activity in patients receiving kaliuretic-diuretic agents.

Amiloride HCl is not an aldosterone antagonist and its effects are seen even in the absence of aldosterone.

Amiloride HCl exerts its potassium sparing effect through the inhibition of sodium reabsorption at the distal convoluted tubule, cortical collecting tubule and collecting duct; this decreases the net negative potential of the tubular lumen and reduces both potassium and hydrogen secretion and their subsequent excretion. This mechanism accounts in large part for the potassium sparing action of amiloride.

Amiloride HCl usually begins to act within 2 hours after an oral dose. Its effect on electrolyte excretion reaches a peak between 6 and 10 hours and lasts about 24 hours. Peak plasma levels are obtained in 3-4 hours and the plasma half-life varies from 6-9 hours. Effects on electrolytes increase with single doses of amiloride HCl up to approximately 15 mg.

Amiloride HCl is not metabolized by the liver but is excreted unchanged by the kidneys. About 50% of a 20 mg dose of amiloride HCl is excreted in the urine and 40% in the stool within 72 hours. Amiloride HCl has little effect on glomerular filtration rate or renal blood flow. Because amiloride HCl is not metabolized by the liver, drug accumulation is not anticipated in patients with hepatic dysfunction, but accumulation can occur if the hepatorenal syndrome develops.

INDICATIONS AND USAGE

Amiloride HCl is indicated as adjunctive treatment with thiazide diuretics or other kaliuretic-diuretic agents in congestive heart failure or hypertension to:

- Help restore normal serum potassium levels in patients who develop hypokalemia on the kaliuretic diuretic.
- Prevent development of hypokalemia in patients who would be exposed to particular risk if hypokalemia were to develop, *e.g.*, digitalized patients or patients with significant cardiac arrhythmias.

The use of potassium-conserving agents is often unnecessary in patients receiving diuretics for uncomplicated essential hypertension when such patients have a normal diet. Amiloride HCl has little additive diuretic or antihypertensive effect when added to a thiazide diuretic.

Amiloride HCl should rarely be used alone. It has weak (compared with thiazides) diuretic and antihypertensive effects. Used as single agents, potassium sparing diuretics, including amiloride HCl, result in an increased risk of hyperkalemia (approximately 10% with amiloride). Amiloride HCl should be used alone only when persistent hypokalemia has been documented and only with careful titration of the dose and close monitoring of serum electrolytes.

CONTRAINDICATIONS

HYPERKALEMIA

Amiloride HCl should not be used in the presence of elevated serum potassium levels (greater than 5.5 mEq/L).

ANTIKALIURETIC THERAPY OR POTASSIUM SUPPLEMENTATION

Amiloride HCl should not be given to patients receiving other potassium-conserving agents, such as spironolactone or triamterene. Potassium supplementation in the form of medication, potassium-containing salt substitutes or a potassium-rich diet should not be used with amiloride HCl except in severe and/or refractory cases of hypokalemia. Such concomitant therapy can be associated with rapid increases in serum potassium levels. If potassium supplementation is used, careful monitoring of the serum potassium level is necessary.

IMPAIRED RENAL FUNCTION

Anuria, acute or chronic renal insufficiency, and evidence of diabetic nephropathy are contraindications to the use of amiloride HCl. Patients with evidence of renal functional impairment (blood urea nitrogen [BUN] levels over 30 mg/100 ml or serum creatinine levels over 1.5 mg/100 ml) or diabetes mellitus should not receive the drug without careful, frequent and continuing monitoring of serum electrolytes, creatinine, and BUN levels. Potassium retention associated with the use of an antikaliuretic agent is accentuated in the presence of renal impairment and may result in the rapid development of hyperkalemia.

HYPERSENSITIVITY

Amiloride HCl is contraindicated in patients who are hypersensitive to this product.

WARNINGS

HYPERKALEMIA

Like other potassium-conserving agents, amiloride may cause hyperkalemia (serum potassium levels greater than 5.5 mEq/L) which, if uncorrected, is potentially fatal. Hyperkalemia occurs commonly (about 10%) when amiloride is used without a kaliuretic diuretic. This incidence is greater in patients with renal impairment, diabetes mellitus (with or without recognized renal insufficiency), and in the elderly. When amiloride HCl is used concomitantly with a thiazide diuretic in patients without these complications, the risk of hyperkalemia is reduced to about 1-2%. It is thus essential to monitor serum potassium levels carefully in any patient receiving amiloride, particularly when it is first introduced, at the time of diuretic dosage adjustments, and during any illness that could affect renal function.

The risk of hyperkalemia may be increased when potassium-conserving agents, including amiloride HCl, are administered concomitantly with an angiotensin-converting enzyme inhibitor, cyclosporine or tacrolimus. (See DRUG INTERACTIONS.) Warning signs or symptoms of hyperkalemia include paresthesias, muscular weakness, fatigue, flaccid paralysis of the extremities, bradycardia, shock, and ECG abnormalities. Monitoring of the serum potassium level is essential because mild hyperkalemia is not usually associated with an abnormal ECG.

When abnormal, the ECG in hyperkalemia is characterized primarily by tall, peaked T waves or elevations from previous tracings. There may also be lowering of the R wave and increased depth of the S wave, widening and even disappearance of the P wave, progressive widening of the QRS complex, prolongation of the PR interval, and ST depression.

Treatment of Hyperkalemia

If hyperkalemia occurs in patients taking amiloride HCl, the drug should be discontinued immediately. If the serum potassium level exceeds 6.5 mEq/L, active measures should be taken to reduce it. Such measures include the intravenous administration of sodium bicarbonate solution or oral or parenteral glucose with a rapid-acting insulin preparation. If needed, a cation exchange resin such as sodium polystyrene sulfonate may be given orally or by enema. Patients with persistent hyperkalemia may require dialysis.

DIABETES MELLITUS

In diabetic patients, hyperkalemia has been reported with the use of all potassium-conserving diuretics, including amiloride HCl, even in patients without evidence of diabetic nephropathy. Therefore, amiloride HCl should be avoided, if possible, in diabetic patients and, if it is used, serum electrolytes and renal function must be monitored frequently.

Amiloride HCl should be discontinued at least 3 days before glucose tolerance testing.

METABOLIC OR RESPIRATORY ACIDOSIS

Antikaliuretic therapy should be instituted only with caution in severely ill patients in whom respiratory or metabolic acidosis may occur, such as patients with cardiopulmonary disease or poorly controlled diabetes. If amiloride HCl is given to these patients, frequent monitoring of acid-base balance is necessary. Shifts in acid-base balance alter the ratio of extracellular/intracellular potassium, and the development of acidosis may be associated with rapid increases in serum potassium levels.

PRECAUTIONS

GENERAL

Electrolyte Imbalance and BUN Increases

Hyponatremia and hypochloremia may occur when amiloride HCl is used with other diuretics and increases in BUN levels have been reported. These increases usually have accompanied vigorous fluid elimination, especially when diuretic therapy was used in seriously ill patients, such as those who had hepatic cirrhosis with ascites and metabolic alkalosis, or those with resistant edema. Therefore, when amiloride HCl is given with other diuretics to such patients, careful monitoring of serum electrolytes and BUN levels is important. In patients with pre-existing severe liver disease, hepatic encephalopathy, manifested by tremors, confusion, and coma, and increased jaundice, have been reported in association with diuretics, including amiloride HCl.

CARCINOGENESIS, MUTAGENESIS, AND IMPAIRMENT OF FERTILITY

There was no evidence of a tumorigenic effect when amiloride HCl was administered for 92 weeks to mice at doses up to 10 mg/kg/day (25 times the maximum daily human dose). Amiloride HCl has also been administered for 104 weeks to male and female rats at doses up to 6 and 8 mg/kg/day (15 and 20 times the maximum daily dose for humans, respectively) and showed no evidence of carcinogenicity.

Amiloride HCl was devoid of mutagenic activity in various strains of *Salmonella typhimurium* with or without a mammalian liver microsomal activation system (Ames test).

PREGNANCY CATEGORY B

Teratogenicity studies with amiloride HCl in rabbits and mice given 20 and 25 times the maximum human dose, respectively, revealed no evidence of harm to the fetus, although studies showed that the drug crossed the placenta in modest amounts. Reproduction studies in rats at 20 times the expected maximum daily dose for humans showed no evidence of impaired fertility. At approximately 5 or more times the expected maximum daily dose for humans, some toxicity was seen in adult rats and rabbits and a decrease in rat pup growth and survival occurred.

There are, however, no adequate and well-controlled studies in pregnant women. Because animal reproduction studies are not always predictive of human response, this drug should be used during pregnancy only if clearly needed.

NURSING MOTHERS

Studies in rats have shown that amiloride is excreted in milk in concentrations higher than those found in blood, but it is not known whether amiloride HCl is excreted in human milk. Because many drugs are excreted in human milk and because of the potential for serious adverse reactions in nursing infants from amiloride HCl, a decision should be made whether to discontinue nursing or to discontinue the drug, taking into account the importance of the drug to the mother.

PEDIATRIC USE

Safety and effectiveness in pediatric patients have not been established.

GERIATRIC USE

Clinical studies of amiloride HCl did not include sufficient numbers of subjects aged 65 and over to determine whether they respond differently from younger subjects. Other reported clinical experience has not identified differences in responses between the elderly and younger patients. In general, dose selection for an elderly patient should be cautious, usually starting at the low end of the dosing range, reflecting the greater frequency of decreased hepatic, renal or cardiac function, and of concomitant disease or other drug therapy.

This drug is known to be substantially excreted by the kidney, and the risk of toxic reactions to this drug may be greater in patients with impaired renal function. Because elderly patients are more likely to have decreased renal function, care should be taken in dose selection, and it may be useful to monitor renal function. (See CONTRAINDICATIONS, Impaired Renal Function.)

DRUG INTERACTIONS

When amiloride HCl is administered concomitantly with an angiotensin-converting enzyme inhibitor, cyclosporine or tacrolimus, the risk of hyperkalemia may be increased. Therefore, if concomitant use of these agents is indicated because of demonstrated hypokalemia, they should be used with caution and with frequent monitoring of serum potassium. (See WARNINGS.)

Lithium generally should not be given with diuretics because they reduce its renal clearance and add a high risk of lithium toxicity. Read circulars for lithium preparations before use of such concomitant therapy.

In some patients, the administration of a non-steroidal anti-inflammatory agent can reduce the diuretic, natriuretic, and antihypertensive effects of loop, potassium-sparing and thiazide diuretics. Therefore, when amiloride HCl and non-steroidal anti-inflammatory agents are used concomitantly, the patient should be observed closely to determine if the desired effect of the diuretic is obtained. Since indomethacin and potassium-sparing diuretics, including amiloride HCl, may each be associated with increased serum potassium levels, the potential effects on potassium kinetics and renal function should be considered when these agents are administered concurrently.

ADVERSE REACTIONS

Amiloride HCl is usually well tolerated and, except for hyperkalemia (serum potassium levels greater than 5.5 mEq/L — see WARNINGS), significant adverse effects have been reported infrequently. Minor adverse reactions were reported relatively frequently (about 20%) but the relationship of many of the reports to amiloride HCl is uncertain and the overall frequency was similar in hydrochlorothiazide treated groups. Nausea/anorexia, abdominal pain, flatulence, and mild skin rash have been reported and probably are related to amiloride. Other adverse experiences that have been reported with amiloride are generally those known to be associated with diuresis, or with the underlying disease being treated.

The adverse reactions for amiloride HCl listed in TABLE 1 have been arranged into two groups: (1) incidence greater than 1%; and (2) incidence 1% or less. The incidence for group (1) was determined from clinical studies conducted in the US (837 patients treated with amiloride HCl). The adverse effects listed in group (2) include reports from the same clinical studies and voluntary reports since marketing. The probability of a causal relationship exists between amiloride HCl and these adverse reactions, some of which have been reported only rarely.

CAUSAL RELATIONSHIP UNKNOWN

Other reactions have been reported but occurred under circumstances where a causal relationship could not be established. However, in these rarely reported events, that possibility cannot be excluded. Therefore, these observations are listed to serve as alerting information to physicians.

Activation of probable pre-existing peptic ulcer;
Aplastic anemia;
Neutropenia;
Abnormal liver function.

DOSAGE AND ADMINISTRATION

Amiloride HCl should be administered with food.

Amiloride HCl, one 5 mg tablet daily, should be added to the usual antihypertensive or diuretic dosage of a kaliuretic diuretic. The dosage may be increased to 10 mg/day, if necessary. More than two 5 mg tablets of amiloride HCl daily usually are not needed, and there is little controlled experience with such doses. If persistent hypokalemia is documented with 10 mg, the dose can be increased to 15 mg, then 20 mg, with careful monitoring of electrolytes.

In treating patients with congestive heart failure after an initial diuresis has been achieved, potassium loss may also decrease and the need for amiloride HCl should be re-evaluated. Dosage adjustment may be necessary. Maintenance therapy may be on an intermittent basis.

If it is necessary to use amiloride HCl alone (see INDICATIONS AND USAGE), the starting dosage should be one 5 mg tablet daily. This dosage may be increased to 10 mg/day,

TABLE 1

Incidence >1%	Incidence ≤1%
Body as a Whole	
Headache*	Back pain
Weakness	Chest pain
Fatigability	Neck/shoulder ache
	Pain, extremities
Cardiovascular	
None	Angina pectoris
	Orthostatic hypotension
	Arrhythmia
	Palpitation
Digestive	
Nausea/anorexia*	Jaundice
Diarrhea*	GI bleeding
Vomiting*	Abdominal fullness
Abdominal pain	GI disturbance
Gas pain	Thirst
Appetite changes	Heartburn
Constipation	Flatulence
	Dyspepsia
Metabolic	
Elevated serum potassium levels (>5.5 mEq/L)†	None
Skin	
None	Skin rash
	Itching
	Dryness of mouth
	Pruritus
	Alopecia
Musculoskeletal	
Muscle cramps	Joint pain
	Leg ache
Nervous	
Dizziness	Paresthesia
Encephalopathy	Tremors
	Vertigo
Psychiatric	
None	Nervousness
	Mental confusion
	Insomnia
	Decreased libido
	Depression
	Somnolence
Respiratory	
Cough	Shortness of breath
Dyspnea	
Special Senses	
None	Visual disturbances
	Nasal congestion
	Tinnitus
	Increased intraocular pressure
Urogenital	
Impotence	Polyuria
	Dysuria
	Urinary frequency
	Bladder spasms
	Gynecomastia

* Reactions occurring in 3-8% of patients treated with amiloride HCl. (Those reactions occurring in less than 3% of the patients are unmarked.)
† See WARNINGS.

if necessary. More than two 5 mg tablets usually are not needed, and there is little controlled experience with such doses. If persistent hypokalemia is documented with 10 mg, the dose can be increased to 15 mg, then 20 mg, with careful monitoring of electrolytes.

HOW SUPPLIED

MIDAMOR TABLETS

5 mg: Yellow, diamond-shaped, compressed tablets, coded "MSD 92" on one side and "MIDAMOR" on the other.

Storage: Protect from moisture, freezing and excessive heat.

PRODUCT LISTING - RATED THERAPEUTICALLY EQUIVALENT

Tablet - Oral - 5 mg

100's	$28.00	GENERIC, Major Pharmaceuticals Inc	00904-2111-60
100's	$41.45	GENERIC, Ivax Corporation	00182-1828-01
100's	$47.57	GENERIC, Par Pharmaceutical Inc	49884-0117-01
100's	$57.65	MIDAMOR, Merck & Company Inc	00006-0092-68

A

Amiloride Hydrochloride; Hydrochlorothiazide *(000180)*

For complete prescribing information, refer to the CD-ROM included with the book.

Categories: Heart failure, congestive; Hypertension, essential; Pregnancy Category B; FDA Approval Pre 1982

Drug Classes: Diuretics, potassium sparing

Brand Names: Ameide; Amiloride Hcl W/Hctz; Amiloscan; Lorizide; **Moduretic**; Pandiuren

Foreign Brand Availability: Adco-Retic (South-Africa); Add-Acten (Bahrain; Benin; Burkina-Faso; Cyprus; Egypt; Ethiopia; Gambia; Ghana; Guinea; Iran; Iraq; Ivory-Coast; Jordan; Kenya; Kuwait; Lebanon; Liberia; Libya; Malawi; Mali; Mauritania; Mauritius; Morocco; Niger; Nigeria; Oman; Qatar; Republic-of-Yemen; Saudi-Arabia; Senegal; Seychelles; Sierra-Leone; Sudan; Syria; Tanzania; Tunia; Uganda; United-Arab-Emirates; Zambia; Zimbabwe); Ameride (Spain); Amil-Co (England); Amilco (Denmark); Amilco Mite (Denmark); Amilocomp beta (Germany); Amiloretic (South-Africa); Amithiazide (Hong-Kong); Amitrid (Taiwan); Amizide (Australia; New-Zealand; South-Africa; Taiwan); Amuretic (Bahrain; Cyprus; Egypt; Iran; Iraq; Jordan; Kuwait; Lebanon; Libya; Oman; Qatar; Republic-of-Yemen; Saudi-Arabia; Syria; United-Arab-Emirates); Betaretic (South-Africa); Bildiuretic (Thailand); Hyperetic (Thailand); Kaluril (Israel); Lorinid (Indonesia); Lorinid Mite (Indonesia); Miduret (Thailand); Moduret (Canada); Moduretic Mite (Norway); Moure-M (Thailand); Novamilor (Canada); Rhefluin (Mexico); Sefaretic (Hong-Kong); Tiaden (Taiwan); Uniretic (Bahrain; Cyprus; Egypt; Iran; Iraq; Jordan; Kuwait; Lebanon; Libya; Oman; Qatar; Republic-of-Yemen; Saudi-Arabia; Syria; United-Arab-Emirates); Yostiretic (Bahrain; Cyprus; Egypt; Iran; Iraq; Jordan; Kuwait; Lebanon; Libya; Oman; Qatar; Republic-of-Yemen; Saudi-Arabia; Syria; United-Arab-Emirates)

Cost of Therapy: $19.66 (Hypertension; Moduretic 5–50; 5 mg; 50 mg; 1 tablet/day; 30 day supply)
$2.04 (Hypertension; Generic Tablets; 5 mg; 50 mg; 1 tablet/day; 30 day supply)

DESCRIPTION

Moduretic combines the potassium-conserving action of amiloride hydrochloride with the natriuretic action of hydrochlorothiazide.

Amiloride HCl is designated chemically as 3,5-diamino-6-chloro-*N*-(diaminomethylene)pyrazinecarboxamide monohydrochloride, dihydrate and has a molecular weight of 302.12. Its empirical formula is $C_6H_8ClN_7O \cdot HCl \cdot 2H_2O$.

Hydrochlorothiazide is designated chemically as 6-chloro-3,4-dihydro-2*H*-1,2,4-benzothiadiazine-7-sulfonamide 1,1-dioxide. Its empirical formula is $C_7H_8ClN_3O_4S_2$.

It is a white, or practically white, crystalline powder with a molecular weight of 297.74, which is slightly soluble in water, but freely soluble in sodium hydroxide solution.

Moduretic is available for oral use as tablets containing 5 mg of anhydrous amiloride HCl and 50 mg of hydrochlorothiazide. Each tablet contains the following inactive ingredients: calcium phosphate, FD&C yellow 6, guar gum, lactose, magnesium stearate and starch.

INDICATIONS AND USAGE

Amiloride HCl; hydrochlorothiazide is indicated in those patients with hypertension or with congestive heart failure who develop hypokalemia when thiazides or other kaliuretic diuretics are used alone, or in whom maintenance of normal serum potassium levels is considered to be clinically important, *e.g.*, digitalized patients, or patients with significant cardiac arrhythmias.

The use of potassium-conserving agents is often unnecessary in patients receiving diuretics for uncomplicated essential hypertension when such patients have a normal diet.

Amiloride HCl; hydrochlorothiazide may be used alone or as an adjunct to other antihypertensive drugs, such as methyldopa or beta blockers. Since amiloride HCl; hydrochlorothiazide enhances the action of these agents, dosage adjustments may be necessary to avoid an excessive fall in blood pressure and other unwanted side effects.

This fixed combination drug is not indicated for the initial therapy of edema or hypertension except in individuals in whom the development of hypokalemia cannot be risked.

CONTRAINDICATIONS

HYPERKALEMIA

Amiloride HCl; hydrochlorothiazide should not be used in the presence of elevated serum potassium levels (greater than 5.5 mEq/L).

ANTIKALIURETIC THERAPY OR POTASSIUM SUPPLEMENTATION

Amiloride HCl; hydrochlorothiazide should not be given to patients receiving other potassium-conserving agents, such as spironolactone or triamterene. Potassium supplementation in the form of medication, potassium-containing salt substitutes or a potassium-rich diet should not be used with amiloride HCl; hydrochlorothiazide except in severe and/or refractory cases of hypokalemia. Such concomitant therapy can be associated with rapid increases in serum potassium levels. If potassium supplementation is used, careful monitoring of the serum potassium level is necessary.

IMPAIRED RENAL FUNCTION

Anuria, acute or chronic renal insufficiency, and evidence of diabetic nephropathy are contraindications to the use of amiloride HCl; hydrochlorothiazide. Patients with evidence of renal functional impairment [blood urea nitrogen (BUN) levels over 30 mg/100 ml or serum creatinine levels over 1.5 mg/100 ml] or diabetes mellitus should not receive the drug without careful, frequent and continuing monitoring of serum electrolytes, creatinine, and BUN levels. Potassium retention associated with the use of an antikaliuretic agent is accentuated in the presence of renal impairment and may result in the rapid development of hyperkalemia.

HYPERSENSITIVITY

Amiloride HCl; hydrochlorothiazide is contraindicated in patients who are hypersensitive to this product, or to other sulfonamide-derived drugs.

A

WARNINGS

HYPERKALEMIA

Like other potassium-conserving diuretic combinations, amiloride HCl; hydrochlorothiazide may cause hyperkalemia (serum potassium levels greater than 5.5 mEq/L). In patients without renal impairment or diabetes mellitus, the risk of hyperkalemia with amiloride HCl; hydrochlorothiazide is about 1-2%. This risk is higher in patients with renal impairment or diabetes mellitus (even without recognized diabetic nephropathy). Since hyperkalemia, if uncorrected, is potentially fatal, it is essential to monitor serum potassium levels carefully in any patient receiving amiloride HCl; hydrochlorothiazide, particularly when it is first introduced, at the time of dosage adjustments, and during any illness that could affect renal function.

The risk of hyperkalemia may be increased when potassium-conserving agents, including amiloride HCl; hydrochlorothiazide, are administered concomitantly with an angiotensin-converting enzyme inhibitor, an angiotensin II receptor antagonist, cyclosproine or tacrolimus. Warning signs or symptoms of hyperkalemia include paresthesias, muscular weakness, fatigue, flaccid paralysis of the extremities, bradycardia, shock, and ECG abnormalities. Monitoring of the serum potassium level is essential because mild hyperkalemia is not usually associated with an abnormal ECG.

When abnormal, the ECG in hyperkalemia is characterized primarily by tall, peaked T waves or elevations from previous tracings. There may also be lowering of the R wave and increased depth of the S wave, widening and even disappearance of the P wave, progressive widening of the QRS complex, prolongation of the PR interval, and ST depression.

Treatment of Hyperkalemia

If hyperkalemia occurs in patients taking amiloride HCl; hydrochlorothiazide, the drug should be discontinued immediately. If the serum potassium level exceeds 6.5 mEq/L, active measures should be taken to reduce it. Such measures include the intravenous (IV) administration of sodium bicarbonate solution or oral or parenteral glucose with a rapid-acting insulin preparation. If needed, a cation exchange resin such as sodium polystyrene sulfonate may be given orally or by enema. Patients with persistent hyperkalemia may require dialysis.

DIABETES MELLITUS

In diabetic patients, hyperkalemia has been reported with the use of all potassium-conserving diuretics, including amiloride HCl, even in patients without evidence of diabetic nephropathy. Therefore, amiloride HCl; hydrochlorothiazide should be avoided, if possible, in diabetic patients and, if it is used, serum electrolytes and renal function must be monitored frequently.

Amiloride HCl; hydrochlorothiazide should be discontinued at least 3 days before glucose tolerance testing.

METABOLIC OR RESPIRATORY ACIDOSIS

Antikaliuretic therapy should be instituted only with caution in severely ill patients in whom respiratory or metabolic acidosis may occur, such as patients with cardiopulmonary disease or poorly controlled diabetes. If amiloride HCl; hydrochlorothiazide is given to these patients, frequent monitoring of acid-base balance is necessary. Shifts in acid-base balance alter the ratio of extracellular/intracellular potassium, and the development of acidosis may be associated with rapid increases in serum potassium levels.

DOSAGE AND ADMINISTRATION

Amiloride HCl; hydrochlorothiazide should be administered with food.

The usual starting dosage is 1 tablet a day. The dosage may be increased to 2 tablets a day, if necessary. More than 2 tablets of amiloride HCl; hydrochlorothiazide daily usually are not needed and there is no controlled experience with such doses. Hydrochlorothiazide can be given at doses of 12.5 to 50 mg/day when used alone. Patients usually do not require doses of hydrochlorothiazide in excess of 50 mg daily when combined with other antihypertensive agents.

The daily dose is usually given as a single dose but may be given in divided doses. Once an initial diuresis has been achieved, dosage adjustment may be necessary. Maintenance therapy may be on an intermittent basis.

PRODUCT LISTING - RATED THERAPEUTICALLY EQUIVALENT

Tablet - Oral - 5 mg;50 mg

100's	$6.59	FEDERAL UPPER LIMIT, H.C.F.A. F F P	99999-0180-01
100's	$15.50	GENERIC, Raway Pharmacal Inc	00686-0421-20
100's	$28.90	GENERIC, Teva Pharmaceuticals Usa	00332-2205-09
100's	$30.44	GENERIC, Moore, H.L. Drug Exchange Inc	00839-7446-06
100's	$32.55	GENERIC, Major Pharmaceuticals Inc	00904-2113-60
100's	$32.75	GENERIC, West Point Pharma	59591-0162-68
100's	$32.86	GENERIC, Barr Laboratories Inc	00555-0483-02
100's	$33.90	GENERIC, Aligen Independent Laboratories Inc	00405-4053-01
100's	$34.97	GENERIC, Vangard Labs	00615-3516-13
100's	$35.56	GENERIC, Udl Laboratories Inc	51079-0421-20
100's	$36.30	GENERIC, Major Pharmaceuticals Inc	00904-2113-61
100's	$37.95	GENERIC, Martec Pharmaceuticals Inc	52555-0338-01
100's	$38.00	GENERIC, Ivax Corporation	00182-1877-01
100's	$38.00	GENERIC, Geneva Pharmaceuticals	00781-1119-01
100's	$38.69	GENERIC, Endo Laboratories Llc	60951-0764-70
100's	$42.45	GENERIC, Mylan Pharmaceuticals Inc	00378-0577-01
100's	$54.65	GENERIC, Major Pharmaceuticals Inc	00904-2114-60
100's	$55.19	GENERIC, Watson Laboratories Inc	52544-0685-01
100's	$65.53	MODURETIC 5-50, Merck & Company Inc	00006-0917-68

PRODUCT LISTING - EQUIVALENTS NOT AVAILABLE

Tablet - Oral - 5 mg;50 mg

30's	$3.47	GENERIC, Physicians Total Care	54868-0667-01
100's	$6.79	GENERIC, Physicians Total Care	54868-0667-00

Aminophylline *(000207)*

Categories: Asthma; Pregnancy Category C; FDA Approved 1981 Feb; WHO Formulary
Drug Classes: Bronchodilators; Xanthine derivatives
Brand Names: **Aminophylline**; Inophyline; Norphyl; Novphyllin; Somophyllin; Synthophyllin; Theourin; Truphylline (G&W)
Foreign Brand Availability: Aminofilina (Ecuador; Guatemala); Aminomal (Czech-Republic; Italy); Anephyllin (Japan); Asiphyl-line (Taiwan); Asthcontin (Korea); Drafilyn "Z" (Mexico); Eufilin (Brazil); Eufilina (Spain); Eufilina Mite (Portugal); Euphyllin (Austria; Belgium; Bulgaria; Czech-Republic; Finland; Germany; Netherlands; Norway); Euphyllin Retard (Benin; Burkina-Faso; Ethiopia; Gambia; Ghana; Guinea; Ivory-Coast; Kenya; Liberia; Malawi; Mali; Mauritania; Mauritius; Morocco; Niger; Nigeria; Senegal; Seychelles; Sierra-Leone; South-Africa; Sudan; Tanzania; Tunia; Uganda; Zambia; Zimbabwe); Kyophyllin (Japan); Neo-phyllin (Malaysia); Pediatric Asthcontin for Children SR (Korea); Peterphyllin (South-Africa); Phyllotemp (Germany; Greece); Tefamin (Italy); Teofylamin (Denmark)
HCFA JCODE(S): J0280 up to 250 mg IV

INTRAVENOUS

DESCRIPTION

Aminophylline injection is a sterile, nonpyrogenic solution of theophylline in water for injection. Aminophylline (dihydrate) is approximately 79% of anhydrous theophylline by weight. Aminophylline injection is administered by slow intravenous (IV) injection or diluted and administered by intravenous infusion.

Each milliliter contains aminophylline (calculated as the dihydrate) 25 mg (equivalent to 19.7 mg anhydrous theophylline) prepared with the aid of ethylenediamine. The solution may contain an excess of ethylenediamine for pH adjustment. pH is 8.8 (8.6-9.0). The osmolar concentration is 0.17 mOsmol/ml (calc.). Headspace nitrogen gassed.

The solution contains no bacteriostat or antimicrobial agent and is intended for use only as a single-dose injection. When smaller doses are required the unused portion should be discarded.

Aminophylline, a xanthine bronchodilator, is a 2:1 complex of theophylline and ethylenediamine and has the chemical name 1H-Purine-2,6,-dione,3,7-dihydro-1,3-dimethyl-, compounded with 1,2-ethanediamine (2:1).

STORAGE

Store at controlled room temperature 15-30°C (59-86°F).

PROTECT FROM LIGHT. Keep syringes in carton until time of use.

SINGLE DOSE CONTAINER. Discard unused portion.

CLINICAL PHARMACOLOGY

AMINOPHYLLINE SHOULD BE CONSIDERED A MIXTURE OF THEOPHYLLINE AND BASE. THE ACTIVITY IS THAT OF THEOPHYLLINE ALONE.

Theophylline directly relaxes the smooth muscle of the bronchial airway and pulmonary blood vessels, thus acting mainly as a bronchodilator and smooth muscle relaxant. It has also been demonstrated that aminophylline has a potent effect on diaphragmatic contractility in normal persons and may then be capable of reducing fatigability and therapy improve contractility in patients with chronic obstructive airway disease. The exact mode of action remains unsettled. Although theophylline does cause inhibition of phosphodiesterase with a resultant increase in intracellular cyclic AMP, other agents similarly inhibit the enzyme producing a rise of cyclic AMP but are unassociated with any demonstrable bronchodilation. Other mechanisms proposed include an effect on translocation of intracellular calcium; prostaglandin antagonism; stimulation of catecholamines endogenously; inhibition of cyclic guanosine monophosphate metabolism and adenosine receptor antagonism. None of these mechanisms has been proved, however.

In vitro, theophylline has been shown to act synergistically with beta agonists and there are now available data which do demonstrate an additive effect *in vivo* with combined use.

PHARMACOKINETICS

The half-life of theophylline is influenced by a number of known variables. It may be prolonged in chronic alcoholics, particularly those with liver disease (cirrhosis or alcoholic liver disease), in patients with congestive heart failure, and in those patients taking certain other drugs (see DRUG INTERACTIONS). Newborns and neonates have extremely slow clearance rates compared to older infants and children, *i.e.,* those over 1 year. Older children have rapid clearance rates while most non-smoking adults have clearance rates between these two extremes. In premature neonates the decreased clearance is related to oxidative pathways that have yet to be established.

TABLE 1 *Theophylline Elimination Characteristics*

	Half-Life	
	Range	Mean
Children	1-9 hours	3.7 hours
Adults	3-15 hours	7.7 hours

In cigarette smokers (1-2 packs/day) the mean half-life is 4-5 hours, much shorter than in non-smokers. The increase in clearance associated with smoking is presumably due to stimulation of the hepatic metabolic pathway by components of cigarette smoke. The duration of this effect after cessation of smoking is unknown but may require 6 months to 2 years before the rate approaches that of the non-smoker.

INDICATIONS AND USAGE

For the relief of acute bronchial asthma and reversible bronchospasm associated with chronic bronchitis and emphysema.

CONTRAINDICATIONS

This product is contraindicated in individuals who have shown hypersensitivity to its components, including ethylenediamine.

It is also contraindicated in patients with active peptic ulcer disease, and in individuals with underlying seizure disorders (unless receiving appropriate anticonvulsant medications).

WARNINGS

Serum levels above 20 μg/ml are rarely found after appropriate administration of the recommended doses. However, in individuals in whom theophylline plasma clearance in reduced *for any reason,* even conventional doses may result in increased serum levels and potential toxicity. Reduced theophylline clearance has been documented in the following readily identifiable groups: (1) patients with impaired liver function; (2) patients over 55 years of age, particularly males and those with chronic lung disease; (3) those with cardiac failure from any cause; (4) patients with sustained high fever; (5) neonates and infants under 1 year of age; and (6) those patients taking certain drugs (see DRUG INTERACTIONS). Frequently, such patients have markedly prolonged theophylline serum levels following discontinuation of the drug.

Reduction of dosage and laboratory monitoring is especially appropriate in the above individuals.

Serious side effects such as ventricular arrhythmias, convulsions or even death may appear as the first sign of toxicity without any previous warning. Less serious signs of theophylline toxicity (*i.e.,* nausea and restlessness) may occur frequently when initiating therapy, but are usually transient; when such signs are persistent during maintenance therapy, they are often associated with serum concentrations above 20 μg/ml. Stated differently; *serious toxicity is not reliably preceded by less severe side effects.* A serum concentration measurement is the only reliable method of predicting potentially life-threatening toxicity.

Many patients who require theophylline exhibit tachycardia due to their underlying disease process so that the cause/effect relationship to elevated serum theophylline concentrations may not be appreciated.

Theophylline products may cause or worsen arrhythmias and any significant change in rate and/or rhythm warrants monitoring and further investigation.

Studies in laboratory animals (minipigs, rodents, and dogs) recorded the occurrence of cardiac arrhythmias and sudden death (with histologic evidence of myocardial necrosis) when beta-agonists and methylxanthines were administered concurrently. The significance of these findings when applied to humans is currently unknown.

PRECAUTIONS

GENERAL

On the average, theophylline half-life is shorter in cigarette and marijuana smokers than in non-smokers, but smokers can have half-lives as long as non-smokers. Theophylline should not be administered concurrently with other xanthines. Use with caution in patients with hypoxemia, hypertension, or those with a history of peptic ulcer. Theophylline may occasionally act as a local irritant to GI tract when administered orally, although gastrointestinal symptoms are more commonly centrally mediated and associated with serum drug concentrations over 20 μg/ml.

LABORATORY TESTS

Serum levels should be monitored periodically to determine the theophylline level associated with observed clinical response and as the method of predicting toxicity.

DRUG/LABORATORY TEST INTERACTIONS

Currently available analytical methods, including high pressure liquid chromatography and immunoassay techniques, for measuring serum theophylline levels are specific. Metabolites and other drugs generally do not affect the results. Other new analytic methods are also now in use. The physician should be aware of the laboratory method used and whether other drugs will interfere with the assay for theophylline.

CARCINOGENESIS, MUTAGENESIS, AND IMPAIRMENT OF FERTILITY

Long-term carcinogenicity studies have not been performed with theophylline.

Chromosome-breaking activity was detected in human cell cultures at concentrations of theophylline up to 50 times the therapeutic serum concentration in humans. Theophylline was not mutagenic in the dominant lethal assay in male mice given theophylline intraperitoneally in doses up to 30 times the maximum daily human oral dose.

Studies to determine the effect on fertility have not been performed with theophylline.

PREGNANCY CATEGORY C

Animal reproduction studies have not been conducted with theophylline. It is also not known whether theophylline can cause fetal harm when administered to a pregnant woman or can affect reproduction capacity. Xanthines should be given to a pregnant woman only if clearly needed.

NURSING MOTHERS

Theophylline is distributed into breast milk and may cause irritability or other signs of toxicity in nursing infants. Because of the potential for serious adverse reactions in nursing infants from theophylline, a decision should be made whether to discontinue nursing or to discontinue the drug, taking into account the importance of the drug to the mother.

PEDIATRIC USE

Sufficient numbers of infants under the age of 1 year have not been studied in clinical trials to support use in this age group; however, there is evidence recorded that the use of dosage recommendations for older infants and young children (16 mg/kg/24 hours) may result in the development of toxic serum levels. Such findings very probably reflect differences in the metabolic handling of the drug related to absent or undeveloped enzyme systems. Consequently, the use of the drug in this age group should carefully consider the associated benefits and risks. If used, the maintenance dose must be conservative and in accord with the following guidelines:

Initial Maintenance Dosage of Theophylline:

1.0 mg theophylline (anhydrous) = 1.3 mg aminophylline (dihydrate)

Premature Infants:

Up to 24 days postnatal age — 1.0 mg/kg q12h

Beyond 24 days postnatal age — 1.5 mg/kg q12h

Infants 6-52 Weeks:

[(0.2 × age in weeks) + 5.0] × kg body wt = 24 hour dose in mg

Up to 26 weeks, divide into q8h dosing intervals.

From 26-52 weeks, divide into q6h dosing intervals.

Final dosage should be guided by serum concentration after a steady state (no further accumulation of drug) has been acheived.

DRUG INTERACTIONS

Toxic synergism with ephedrine has been documented and may occur with other sympathomimetic bronchodilators. In addition, the following drug interactions have been demonstrated (see TABLE 2).

TABLE 2

Theophylline With:	
Allopurinol (high-dose)	Increased serum theophylline levels
Cimetidine	Increased serum theophylline levels
Ciprofloxacin	Increased serum theophylline levels
Erythromycin, troleandomycin	Increased serum theophylline levels
Lithium carbonate	Increased renal excretion of lithium
Oral contraceptives	Increased serum theophylline levels
Phenytoin	Decreased theophylline and phenytoin serum levels
Propranolol	Increased serum theophylline levels
Rifampin	Decreased serum theophylline levels

ADVERSE REACTIONS

The following adverse reactions have been observed, but there has not been enough systematic collection of data to support an estimate of their frequency. The most consistent adverse reactions are usually due to overdosage.

Gastrointestinal: Nausea, vomiting, epigastric pain, hematemesis, diarrhea.

Central Nervous System: Headaches, irritability, restlessness, insomnia, reflex hyperexcitability, muscle twitching, clonic and tonic generalized convulsions.

Cardiovascular: Palpitation, tachycardia, extrasystoles, flushing, hypotension, circulatory failure, ventricular arrhythmias.

Respiratory: Tachypnea.

Renal: Potentiation of diuresis.

Others: Alopecia, hyperglycemia and inappropriate ADH syndrome, rash (consider ethylenediamine).

DOSAGE AND ADMINISTRATION

Effective use of theophylline (*i.e.,* the concentration of drug in the serum associated with optimal benefit and minimal risk of toxicity) is considered to occur when the theophylline concentration is maintained from 10-20 μg/ml. The early studies from which these levels were derived were carried out in patients immediately or shortly after recovery from acute exacerbations of their disease (some hospitalized with status asthmaticus).

Although the 20 μg/ml level remains appropriate as a critical value (above which toxicity is more likely to occur) for safety purposes, additional data are now available which indicate that the serum theophylline concentrations required to produce maximum physiologic benefit may, in fact, fluctuate with the degree of bronchospasm present and are variable. Therefore, the physician should individualize the range appropriate to the patient's requirements, based on both symptomatic response and improvement in pulmonary function. It should be stressed that serum theophylline concentrations maintained at the upper level of the 10-20 μg/ml range may be associated with potential toxicity when factors known to reduce theophylline clearance are operative. (See WARNINGS.)

Theophylline does not distribute into fatty tissue. Dosage should be calculated on the basis of lean (ideal) body weight where mg/kg doses are presented.

Caution should be exercised for younger children who cannot complain of minor side effects. Older adults, those with cor pulmonale, congestive heart failure, and/or liver disease may have usually low dosage requirements and thus may experience toxicity at the maximal dosage recommended below.

DOSAGE GUIDELINES

Acute Symptoms of Bronchospasm Requiring Rapid Attainment of Theophylline Serum Levels for Bronchodilation

NOTE: Status asthmaticus should be considered a medical emergency and defined as that degree of bronchospasm which is not rapidly responsive to usual doses of conventional bronchodilators. Optimal therapy for such patients frequently requires both *additional medication,* parenterally administered, and *close monitoring,* preferably in an intensive care setting.

Patients not Currently Receiving Theophylline Products

Patients Currently Receiving Theophylline Products

Determine, where possible, the time, amount, dosage form, and route of administration of the last dose the patient received.

The loading dose for theophylline is based on the principle that each 0.5 mg/kg of theophylline administered as a loading dose will result in a 1 μg/ml increase in serum theophylline concentration. Ideally, the loading dose should be deferred if a serum theophylline concentration can be obtained rapidly.

If this is not possible, the clinician must exercise judgement in selecting a dose based on the potential for benefit and risk. When there is sufficient respiratory distress to warrant a small risk, then 2.5 mg/kg or theophylline administered in rapidly absorbed form is likely

TABLE 3 *Aminophylline Dosage*

	Loading	Maintenance
Children age 1 to under 9 years	6.3 mg/kg *(5.0)	1.0 mg/kg/h *(0.79)
Children age 9 to under 16 years and smokers	6.3 mg/kg *(5.0)	0.8 mg/kg/h *(0.63)
Otherwise healthy non-smoking adults	6.3 mg/kg *(5.0)	0.5 mg/kg/h *(0.40)
Older patients and patients with cor pulmonale	6.3 mg/kg *(5.0)	0.3 mg/kg/h *(0.24)
Patients with congestive heart failure	6.3 mg/kg *(5.0)	0.1-0.2 mg/kg/h *(0.08-0.16)

* = Equivalent dosage of theophylline.

to increase the serum concentration by approximately 5 μg/ml. If the patient is not experiencing theophylline toxicity, this is unlikely to result in dangerous adverse effects.

Subsequent to the decision regarding modification of the loading dose for this group of patients, the maintenance dosage recommendations are the same as those described above.

PRINCIPLES OF IV THERAPY

The loading dose of aminophylline can be given by very slow IV push, or more conveniently, may be infused in a small quantity (usually 100-200 ml) of 5% dextrose injection or 0.9% sodium chloride injection. Do not exceed the rate of 25 mg/min.

Thereafter, maintenance therapy can be administered by a large volume infusion to deliver the desired amount of drug each hour. Aminophylline is compatible with the most commonly used IV solutions.

Oral therapy should be substituted for IV aminophylline as soon as adequate improvement is achieved.

INTRAVENOUS ADMIXTURE INCOMPATIBILITY

Although there have been reports of aminophylline precipitating in acidic media, these reports do not apply to the dilute solutions found in IV infusions. Aminophylline injection should not be mixed in a syringe with other drugs but should be added separately to the IV solution.

When an IV solution containing aminophylline is given "piggyback," the IV system already in place should be turned off while the aminophylline is infused if there is a potential problem with admixture incompatibility.

Because of the alkalinity of aminophylline containing solutions, drugs known to be alkali labile should be avoided in admixtures. These included epinephrine HCl, norepinephrine bitartrate, isoproterenol HCl and penicillin G potassium. It is suggested that specialized literature be consulted before preparing admixtures with aminophylline and other drugs.

Parenteral drug products should be inspected visually for particulate matter discoloration prior to administration, whenever solution and container permit. Do not administer unless solution is clear and container is undamaged. Discard unused portion. Do not use if crystals have separated from solution.

ORAL

DESCRIPTION

Aminophylline, a xanthine bronchodilator, is a 2:1 complex of theophylline and ethylenediamine. Aminophylline dihydrate contains approximately 79% of anhydrous theophylline, whereas aminophylline anhydrous contains approximately 86% anhydrous theophylline. Aminophylline occurs as white or slightly yellowish granules or powder, having a slight ammoniacal odor and a bitter taste.

AMINOPHYLLINE ORAL SOLUTION

Each 5 ml of oral solution contains: Aminophylline anhydrous 105 mg (equivalent to 91 mg theophylline anhydrous).

Inactive ingredients: The oral solution contains ethylenediamine, flavoring, FD&C yellow no. 6, glycerin, methylparaben, propylparaben, saccharin sodium, sorbitol, and water.

AMINOPHYLLINE TABLETS

Each tablet for oral administration contains: Aminophylline (dihydrate) 100 mg (equivalent to 79 mg theophylline anhydrous) or aminophylline (dihydrate) 200 mg (equivalent to 158 mg theophylline anhydrous).

Inactive ingredients: The tablets contain colloidal silicon dioxide, calcium phosphate dibasic, magnesium stearate, and sodium starch glycolate.

CLINICAL PHARMACOLOGY

AMINOPHYLLINE SHOULD BE CONSIDERED AS A MIXTURE OF THEOPHYLLINE AND BASE. THE ACTIVITY IS THAT OF THEOPHYLLINE ALONE.

Theophylline directly relaxes the smooth muscle of the bronchial airway and pulmonary blood vessels, thus acting mainly as a bronchodilator and smooth muscle relaxant. It has also been demonstrated that aminophylline has a potent effect on diaphragmatic contractility in normal persons and may then be capable of reducing fatigability and therapy improve contractility in patients with chronic obstructive airway disease. The exact mode of action remains unsettled. Although theophylline does cause inhibition of phosphodiesterase with a resultant increase in intracellular cyclic AMP, other agents similarly inhibit the enzyme producing a rise of cyclic AMP but are unassociated with any demonstrable bronchodilation. Other mechanisms proposed include an effect on translocation of intracellular calcium; prostaglandin antagonism; stimulation of catecholamines endogenously; inhibition of cyclic guanosine monophosphate metabolism and adenosine receptor antagonism. None of these mechanisms has been proved, however.

In vitro, theophylline has been shown to act synergistically with beta agonists and there are now available data which do demonstrate an additive effect *in vivo* with combined use.

PHARMACOKINETICS

The half-life of theophylline is influenced by a number of known variables. It may be prolonged in chronic alcoholics, particularly those with liver disease (cirrhosis or alcoholic liver disease), in patients with congestive heart failure, and in those patients taking certain other drugs (see DRUG INTERACTIONS). Newborns and neonates have extremely slow clearance rates compared to older infants and children, *i.e.,* those over 1 year. Older children have rapid clearance rates while most non-smoking adults have clearance rates between these two extremes. In premature neonates the decreased clearance is related to oxidative pathways that have yet to be established.

TABLE 4 *Theophylline Elimination Characteristics*

	Half-Life	
	Range	Mean
Children	1-9 hours	3.7 hours
Adults	3-15 hours	7.7 hours

In cigarette smokers (1-2 packs/day) the mean half-life is 4-5 hours, much shorter than in non-smokers. The increase in clearance associated with smoking is presumably due to stimulation of the hepatic metabolic pathway by components of cigarette smoke. The duration of this effect after cessation of smoking is unknown but may require 6 months to 2 years before the rate approaches that of the non-smoker.

INDICATIONS AND USAGE

For relief and/or prevention of symptoms from asthma and reversible bronchospasm associated with chronic bronchitis and emphysema.

CONTRAINDICATIONS

This product is contraindicated in individuals who have shown hypersensitivity to its components. It is also contraindicated in patients with active peptic ulcer disease, and in individuals with underlying seizure disorders (unless receiving appropriate anticonvulsant medications).

WARNINGS

Serum levels above 20 μg/ml are rarely found after appropriate administration of the recommended doses. However, in individuals in whom theophylline plasma clearance in reduced *for any reason,* even conventional doses may result in increased serum levels and potential toxicity. Reduced theophylline clearance has been documented in the following readily identifiable groups: (1) patients with impaired liver function; (2) patients over 55 years of age, particularly males and those with chronic lung disease; (3) those with cardiac failure from any cause; (4) patients with sustained high fever; (5) neonates and infants under 1 year of age; and (6) those patients taking certain drugs (see DRUG INTERACTIONS). Frequently, such patients have markedly prolonged theophylline serum levels following discontinuation of the drug.

Reduction of dosage and laboratory monitoring is especially appropriate in the above individuals.

Serious side effects such as ventricular arrhythmias, convulsions or even death may appear as the first sign of toxicity without any previous warning. Less serious signs of theophylline toxicity (*i.e.,* nausea and restlessness) may occur frequently when initiating therapy, but are usually transient; when such signs are persistent during maintenance therapy, they are often associated with serum concentrations above 20 μg/ml. Stated differently; *serious toxicity is not reliably preceded by less severe side effects.* A serum concentration measurement is the only reliable method of predicting potentially life-threatening toxicity.

Many patients who require theophylline exhibit tachycardia due to their underlying disease process so that the cause/effect relationship to elevated serum theophylline concentrations may not be appreciated.

Theophylline products may cause or worsen arrhythmias and any significant change in rate and/or rhythm warrants monitoring and further investigation.

Studies in laboratory animals (minipigs, rodents, and dogs) recorded the occurrence of cardiac arrhythmias and sudden death (with histologic evidence of myocardial necrosis) when beta-agonists and methylxanthines were administered concurrently. The significance of these findings when applied to humans is currently unknown.

PRECAUTIONS

GENERAL

On the average, theophylline half-life is shorter in cigarette and marijuana smokers than in non-smokers, but smokers can have half-lives as long as non-smokers. Theophylline should not be administered concurrently with other xanthines. Use with caution in patients with hypoxemia, hypertension, or those with a history of peptic ulcer. Theophylline may occasionally act as a local irritant to GI tract although gastrointestinal symptoms are more commonly centrally mediated and associated with serum drug concentrations over 20 μg/ml.

INFORMATION FOR THE PATIENT

The importance of taking only the prescribed dose and time interval between doses should be reinforced.

LABORATORY TESTS

Serum levels should be monitored periodically to determine the theophylline level associated with observed clinical response and as the method of predicting toxicity. For such measurements, the serum sample should be obtained at the time of peak concentration, 1-2 hours after administration for immediate release products. It is important that the patient will not have missed or taken additional doses during the previous 48 hours and that dosing intervals will have been reasonably equally spaced. DOSAGE ADJUSTMENT BASED ON SERUM THEOPHYLLINE MEASUREMENTS WHEN THESE INSTRUCTIONS HAVE NOT BEEN FOLLOWED MAY RESULT IN RECOMMENDATIONS THAT PRESENT RISK OF TOXICITY TO THE PATIENT.

DRUG/LABORATORY TEST INTERACTIONS

Currently available analytical methods, including high pressure liquid chromatography and immunoassay techniques, for measuring serum theophylline levels are specific. Metabolites and other drugs generally do not affect the results. Other new analytic methods are also now in use. The physician should be aware of the laboratory method used and whether other drugs will interfere with the assay for theophylline.

CARCINOGENESIS, MUTAGENESIS, AND IMPAIRMENT OF FERTILITY

Long-term carcinogenicity studies have not been performed with theophylline.

Chromosome-breaking activity was detected in human cell cultures at concentrations of theophylline up to 50 times the therapeutic serum concentrations in humans. Theophylline was not mutagenic in the dominant lethal assay in male mice given theophylline intraperitoneally in doses up to 30 times the maximum daily human oral dose.

Studies to determine the effect on fertility have not been performed with theophylline.

PREGNANCY CATEGORY C

Animal reproduction studies have not been conducted with theophylline. It is also not known whether theophylline can cause fetal harm when administered to a pregnant woman or can affect reproduction capacity. Xanthines should be given to a pregnant woman only if clearly needed.

NURSING MOTHERS

Theophylline is distributed into breast milk and may cause irritability or other signs of toxicity in nursing infants. Because of the potential for serious adverse reactions in nursing infants from theophylline, a decision should be made whether to discontinue nursing or to discontinue the drug, taking into account the importance of the drug to the mother.

PEDIATRIC USE

Sufficient numbers of infants under the age of 1 year have not been studied in clinical trials to support use in this age group; however, there is evidence recorded that the use of dosage recommendations for older infants and young children (16 mg/kg/24 hours) may result in the development of toxic serum levels. Such findings very probably reflect differences in the metabolic handling of the drug related to absent or undeveloped enzyme systems. Consequently, the use of the drug in this age group should carefully consider the associated benefits and risks. If used, the maintenance dose must be conservative and in accord with the following guidelines:

Initial Maintenance Dosage (of theophylline anhydrous):

1 mg theophylline anhydrous = 1.3 mg aminophylline dihydrate

Premature Infants:

Up to 24 days postnatal age — 1.0 mg/kg q12h

Beyond 24 days postnatal age — 1.5 mg/kg q12h

Infants 6-52 Weeks:

[(0.2 × age in weeks) + 5.0] × kg body wt = 24 hour dose in mg

Up to 26 Weeks, divide into q8h dosing intervals.

From 26-52 Weeks, divide into q6h dosing intervals.

Final dosage should be guided by serum concentration after a steady state (no further accumulation of drug) has been acheived.

DRUG INTERACTIONS

Toxic synergism with ephedrine has been documented and may occur with other sympathomimetic bronchodilators. In addition, the following drug interactions have been demonstrated (see TABLE 5).

TABLE 5

Aminophylline With:	Effect
Allopurinol (high-dose)	Increased serum theophylline levels
Cimetidine	Increased serum theophylline levels
Ciprofloxacin	Increased serum theophylline levels
Erythromycin, troleandomycin	Increased serum theophylline levels
Lithium carbonate	Increased renal excretion of lithium
Oral contraceptives	Increased serum theophylline levels
Phenytoin	Decreased theophylline and phenytoin serum levels
Propranolol	Increased serum theophylline levels
Rifampin	Decreased serum theophylline levels

ADVERSE REACTIONS

The following adverse reactions have been observed, but there has not been enough systematic collection of data to support an estimate of their frequency. The most consistent adverse reactions are usually due to overdosage.

Gastrointestinal: Nausea, vomiting, epigastric pain, hematemesis, diarrhea.

Central Nervous System: Headaches, irritability, restlessness, insomnia, reflex hyperexcitability, muscle twitching, clonic and tonic generalized convulsions.

Cardiovascular: Palpitation, tachycardia, extrasystoles, flushing, hypotension, circulatory failure, ventricular arrhythmias.

Respiratory: Tachypnea.

Renal: Potentiation of diuresis.

Others: Alopecia, hyperglycemia and inappropriate ADH syndrome, rash (consider ethylenediamine).

DOSAGE AND ADMINISTRATION

Effective use of theophylline (*i.e.,* the concentration of drug in the serum associated with optimal benefit and minimal risk of toxicity) is considered to occur when the theophylline concentration is maintained from 10-20 µg/ml. The early studies from which these levels were derived were carried out in patients immediately or shortly after recovery from acute exacerbations of their disease (some hospitalized with status asthmaticus).

Although the 20 µg/ml level remains appropriate as a critical value (above which toxicity is more likely to occur) for safety purposes, additional data are now available which indicate that the serum theophylline concentrations required to produce maximum physiologic benefit may, in fact, fluctuate with the degree of bronchospasm present and are variable. Therefore, the physician should individualize the range appropriate to the patient's requirements, based on both symptomatic response and improvement in pulmonary function. It should be stressed that serum theophylline concentrations maintained at the upper level of the 10-20 µg/ml range may be associated with potential toxicity when factors known to reduce theophylline clearance are operative. (See WARNINGS.)

If it is not possible to obtain serum level determinations, restriction of the daily dose (in otherwise healthy adults) to not greater than 13 mg/kg/day, to a maximum of 900 mg, in divided doses will result in relatively few patients exceeding serum levels of 20 µg/ml and the resultant greater risk of toxicity.

Caution should be exercised for younger children who cannot complain of minor side effects. Older adults, those with cor pulmonale, congestive heart failure, and/or liver disease may have unusually low dosage requirements and thus may experience toxicity at the maximal dosage recommended below.

Theophylline does not distribute into fatty tissue. Dosage should be calculated on the basis of lean (ideal) body weight where mg/kg doses are presented.

FREQUENCY OF DOSING

When immediate release products with rapid absorption are used, dosing to maintain serum levels generally requires administration every 6 hours. This is particularly true in children, but dosing intervals up to 8 hours may be satisfactory in adults since they eliminate the drug at a slower rate. Some children, and adults requiring higher than average doses (those having rapid rates of clearance, *e.g.,* half-lives of under 6 hours) may benefit and be more effectively controlled during chronic therapy when given products with sustained-release characteristics since these provide longer dosing intervals and/or less fluctuation in serum concentration between dosing.

Dosage guidelines are approximations only and the wide range of theophylline clearance between individuals (particularly those with concomitant disease) makes indiscriminate usage hazardous.

DOSAGE GUIDELINES

*All dosages expressed in terms of theophylline. For conversion to mg aminophylline, the following equivalents apply:

1 mg theophylline equivalent to:

a. 1.16 mg aminophylline anhydrous (as contained in oral solution).

b. 1.27 mg aminophylline dihydrate (as contained in the tablets).

Acute Symptoms of Bronchospasm Requiring Rapid Attainment of Theophylline Serum Levels for Bronchodilation

Note: Status asthmaticus should be considered a medical emergency and is defined as that degree of bronchospasm which is not rapidly responsive to usual doses of conventional bronchodilators. Optimal therapy for such patients frequently requires both *additional medication,* parenterally administered, and *close monitoring,* preferably in an intensive care setting.

Patients not Currently Receiving Theophylline Products

TABLE 6

	Theophylline Oral Loading	Dosage Maintenance
Children age 1 to under 9 years	5 mg/kg	4 mg/kg q6h
Children age 9 to under 16 years; and smokers	5 mg/kg	3 mg/kg q6h
Otherwise healthy non-smoking adults	5 mg/kg	3 mg/kg q8h
Older patients and patients with cor pulmonale	5 mg/kg	2 mg/kg q8h
Patients with congestive heart failure	5 mg/kg	1-2 mg/kg q12h

Patients Currently Receiving Theophylline Products

Determine, where possible, the time, amount, dosage form, and route of administration of the last dose the patient received.

The loading dose for theophylline is based on the principle that each 0.5 mg/kg of theophylline administered as a loading dose will result in a 1.0 µg/ml increase in serum theophylline concentration. Ideally, the loading dose should be deferred if a serum theophylline concentration can be obtained rapidly.

If this is not possible, the clinician must exercise judgement in selecting a dose based on the potential for benefit and risk. When there is sufficient respiratory distress to warrant a small risk, then 2.5 mg/kg or theophylline administered in rapidly absorbed form is likely to increase serum concentration by approximately 5 µg/ml. If the patient is not experiencing theophylline toxicity, this is unlikely to result in dangerous adverse reactions.

Subsequent to the decision regarding use of a loading dose for this group of patients, the maintenance dosage recommendations are the same as those described above.

Chronic Therapy

Theophylline is a treatment for the management of reversible bronchospasm (asthma, chronic bronchitis and emphysema) to prevent symptoms and maintain patent airways. A dosage form which allows small incremental doses is desirable for initiating therapy. A liquid preparation should be considered for children to permit both greater ease of and more accurate dosage adjustment. Slow clinical titration is generally preferred to assure acceptance and safety of the medication, and to allow the patient to develop tolerance to transient caffeine-like side effects.

Initial Dose

16 mg/kg/24 hours or 400 mg/24 hours (whichever is less) of theophylline in divided doses at 6-8 hour intervals.

Increasing Dose

The above dosage may be increased in approximately 25% increments at 3 day intervals so long as the drug is tolerated; until clinical response is satisfactory or the maximum dose as indicated in Maximum Dose of Theophylline Where the Serum Concentration is not Measured is reached. The serum concentration may be checked at these intervals, but at a minimum, should be determined at the end of this adjustment period.

It is important that no patient be maintained on any dosage that is not tolerated. When instructing patients to increase dosage according to the schedule above, they should be told not to take a subsequent dose if apparent side effects occur and to resume therapy at a lower dose once adverse effects have disappeared.

Maximum Dose of Theophylline Where the Serum Concentration is not Measured

WARNING: DO NOT ATTEMPT TO MAINTAIN ANY DOSE THAT IS NOT TOLERATED.

Not to exceed the following (or 900 mg, whichever is less) (see TABLE 7).

TABLE 7

Age 1 to under 9 years	24 mg/kg/day
Age 9 to under 12 years	20 mg/kg/day
Age 12 to under 16 years	18 mg/kg/day
Age 16 years and older	13 mg/kg/day

Measurement of Serum Theophylline Concentrations During Chronic Therapy

If the above maximum doses are to be maintained or exceeded, serum theophylline measurement is essential. See PRECAUTIONS, Laboratory Tests for guidance.

Final Adjustment of Dosage

Dosage adjustment after serum theophylline measurement (see TABLE 8).

TABLE 8

If Serum Theophylline Is:	Directions:
Within desired range	Maintain dosage if tolerated.
Too high: 20-25 μg/ml	Decrease doses by about 10% and recheck serum level after 3 days.
20-30 μg/ml	Skip the next dose and decrease subsequent doses by about 25%. Recheck serum level after 3 days.
Over 30 μg/ml	Skip next 2 doses and decrease subsequent doses by 50%. Recheck serum level after 3 days.
Too low	Increase dosage by 25% at 3 day intervals until either the desired serum concentration and/or clinical response is achieved. The total daily dose may need to be administered at more frequent intervals if symptoms occur repeatedly at the end of a dosing interval.

The serum concentration may be rechecked at appropriate intervals, but at least at the end of any adjustment period. When the patient's condition is otherwise clinically stable and none of the recognized factors which alter elimination are present, measurement of serum levels need be repeated only every 6-12 months.

HOW SUPPLIED

AMINOPHYLLINE ORAL SOLUTION

Aminophylline oral solution is apricot flavored with 105 mg (anhydrous) per 5 ml oral solution.

Storage: Store at controlled room temperature 15-30°C (59-86°F).

Do not refrigerate oral solution.

AMINOPHYLLINE TABLETS

Aminophylline tablets are supplied as:

100 mg: White, scored tablets, identified "54 859" (equivalent to 79 mg theophylline anhydrous).

200 mg: White, scored tablets, identified "54 930" (equivalent to 158 mg theophylline anhydrous).

Storage: Store at controlled room temperature 15-30°C (59-86°F).

PRODUCT LISTING - RATED THERAPEUTICALLY EQUIVALENT

Solution - Intravenous - 25 mg/ml

10 ml	$1.20	GENERIC, Moore, H.L. Drug Exchange Inc	00839-5673-30
10 ml x 10	$38.24	GENERIC, Abbott Pharmaceutical	00074-4909-18
10 ml x 10	$157.08	GENERIC, Abbott Pharmaceutical	00074-4909-03
10 ml x 25	$19.75	GENERIC, American Regent Laboratories Inc	00517-3810-25
10 ml x 25	$20.48	GENERIC, Abbott Pharmaceutical	00074-7385-01
10 ml x 25	$22.27	GENERIC, Abbott Pharmaceutical	00074-5921-01
20 ml x 10	$47.62	GENERIC, Abbott Pharmaceutical	00074-4906-19
20 ml x 10	$166.68	GENERIC, Abbott Pharmaceutical	00074-4906-03
20 ml x 25	$22.25	GENERIC, American Regent Laboratories Inc	00517-3820-25
20 ml x 25	$26.13	GENERIC, Abbott Pharmaceutical	00074-5922-01
20 ml x 25	$31.47	GENERIC, Abbott Pharmaceutical	00074-7386-01

Solution - Oral - 105 mg/5 ml

10 ml x 40	$23.20	GENERIC, Roxane Laboratories Inc	00054-8049-16
15 ml x 40	$24.00	GENERIC, Roxane Laboratories Inc	00054-8050-16
240 ml	$11.90	GENERIC, Major Pharmaceuticals Inc	00904-2616-09
240 ml	$14.80	GENERIC, Alpharma Uspd Makers Of Barre and Nmc	00472-0873-08
500 ml	$18.01	GENERIC, Roxane Laboratories Inc	00054-3045-63

Suppository - Rectal - 250 mg

10's	$13.12	GENERIC, Qualitest Products Inc	00603-8020-10

Tablet - Oral - 100 mg

100's	$0.74	GENERIC, Global Pharmaceutical Corporation	00115-2150-01
100's	$2.78	FEDERAL UPPER LIMIT, H.C.F.A. F F P	99999-0207-01
100's	$3.45	GENERIC, Watson/Schein Pharmaceuticals Inc	00364-0004-01
100's	$3.45	GENERIC, Geneva Pharmaceuticals	00781-1214-01
100's	$3.50	GENERIC, Roxane Laboratories Inc	00054-4025-25
100's	$4.20	GENERIC, Major Pharmaceuticals Inc	00904-2273-60
100's	$5.01	GENERIC, Vangard Labs	00615-1608-01
100's	$5.57	GENERIC, Vangard Labs	00615-1608-13
100's	$6.05	GENERIC, West Ward Pharmaceutical Corporation	00143-1020-01
100's	$8.26	GENERIC, Roxane Laboratories Inc	00054-8025-25

Tablet - Oral - 200 mg

100's	$1.00	GENERIC, Global Pharmaceutical Corporation	00115-2158-01
100's	$3.90	FEDERAL UPPER LIMIT, H.C.F.A. F F P	99999-0207-03
100's	$4.03	GENERIC, Roxane Laboratories Inc	00054-4026-25
100's	$4.35	GENERIC, Geneva Pharmaceuticals	00781-1318-01
100's	$4.90	GENERIC, Moore, H.L. Drug Exchange Inc	00839-1011-06
100's	$5.99	GENERIC, Watson/Schein Pharmaceuticals Inc	00364-0005-01
100's	$6.69	GENERIC, Vangard Labs	00615-1606-01
100's	$6.79	GENERIC, Major Pharmaceuticals Inc	00904-2283-60
100's	$7.44	GENERIC, Vangard Labs	00615-1606-13
100's	$7.54	GENERIC, Major Pharmaceuticals Inc	00904-2283-61
100's	$7.55	GENERIC, West Ward Pharmaceutical Corporation	00143-1025-01
100's	$9.66	GENERIC, Roxane Laboratories Inc	00054-8026-25

PRODUCT LISTING - RATED NOT THERAPEUTICALLY EQUIVALENT

Tablet - Oral - 100 mg

100's	$6.05	GENERIC, Mutual/United Research Laboratories	00677-0003-01

Tablet - Oral - 200 mg

100's	$7.55	GENERIC, Mutual/United Research Laboratories	00677-0007-01

PRODUCT LISTING - EQUIVALENTS NOT AVAILABLE

Solution - Intravenous - 25 mg/ml

10 ml x 25	$42.04	GENERIC, Physicians Total Care	54868-0004-00
10 ml x 100	$85.00	GENERIC, Raway Pharmacal Inc	00686-3810-25
20 ml	$4.08	GENERIC, Allscripts Pharmaceutical Company	54569-3130-01
20 ml x 100	$105.00	GENERIC, Raway Pharmacal Inc	00686-3820-25

Suppository - Rectal - 250 mg

10's	$14.34	GENERIC, Watson/Rugby Laboratories Inc	00536-1301-19
10's	$17.33	GENERIC, G and W Laboratories Inc	00713-0125-09
25's	$34.65	GENERIC, G and W Laboratories Inc	00713-0125-25

Suppository - Rectal - 500 mg

10's	$19.25	GENERIC, G and W Laboratories Inc	00713-0103-09
25's	$36.58	GENERIC, G and W Laboratories Inc	00713-0103-25
50's	$57.75	GENERIC, G and W Laboratories Inc	00713-0103-50

Amiodarone Hydrochloride *(000212)*

Categories: Arrhythmia, ventricular; Fibrillation, ventricular; Tachycardia, ventricular; Pregnancy Category D; FDA Approved 1985 Dec; Orphan Drugs

Drug Classes: Antiarrhythmics, class III

Brand Names: **Cordarone**; Cordarone I.V.

Foreign Brand Availability: Aldarin (Benin; Burkina-Faso; Ethiopia; Gambia; Ghana; Guinea; Ivory-Coast; Kenya; Liberia; Malawi; Mali; Mauritania; Mauritius; Morocco; Niger; Nigeria; Senegal; Seychelles; Sierra-Leone; Sudan; Tanzania; Tunia; Uganda; Zambia; Zimbabwe); Aldarone (India); Amidodacore (Israel); Amiobeta (Germany); Amiogamma (Germany); Amiorit (Colombia); Amiodarex (Germany); Amiodarona (Chile); Amiohexal (Germany); Ancaron (Japan); Angoron (Greece); Aratac (Australia; New-Zealand; Singapore; Taiwan; Thailand); Arycor (Colombia); Atlansil (Argentina; Brazil; Ecuador; Peru); Braxan (Costa-Rica; El-Salvador; Guatemala; Honduras; Mexico; Nicaragua; Panama); Cardiorona (Mexico); Corbionax (France); Cordarex (Germany); Cordaron (Bulgaria); Cordarone X (Australia; England; Ireland; New-Zealand; South-Africa); Cornaron (Germany); Coronovo (Argentina); Daronal (Colombia); Eurythmic (India); Forken (Mexico); Hexarone (South-Africa); Kendaron (Indonesia); Procor (Israel); Sedacoron (Austria; Hong-Kong; Taiwan); Tachydaron (Germany); Tiaryt (Indonesia); Trangorex (Spain)

Cost of Therapy: $235.39 (Arrhythmia; Cordarone; 200 mg; 2 tablets/day; 30 day supply)
$118.76 (Arrhythmia; Generic Tablets; 200 mg; 2 tablets/day; 30 day supply)

INTRAVENOUS

DESCRIPTION

Cordarone intravenous (IV) contains amiodarone HCl ($C_{25}H_{29}I_2NO_3 \cdot HCl$), a Class III antiarrhythmic drug. Amiodarone HCl is (2-butyl-3-benzofuranyl)[4-[2-(diethylamino)ethoxy]-3,5-diiodophenyl]methanone hydrochloride.

Amiodarone HCl is a white to slightly yellow crystalline powder, and is very slightly soluble in water. It has a molecular weight of 681.78 and contains 37.3% iodine by weight. Cordarone IV is a sterile clear, pale-yellow solution visually free from particulates. Each milliliter of the Cordarone IV formulation contains 50 mg of amiodarone HCl, 20.2 mg of benzyl alcohol, 100 mg of polysorbate 80, and water for injection.

CLINICAL PHARMACOLOGY

MECHANISM OF ACTION

Amiodarone is generally considered a Class III antiarrhythmic drug, but it possesses electrophysiologic characteristics of all four Vaughan Williams classes. Like Class I drugs, amiodarone blocks sodium channels at rapid pacing frequencies, and like Class II drugs, it exerts a noncompetitive antisympathetic action. One of its main effects, with prolonged administration, is to lengthen the cardiac action potential, a Class III effect. The negative chronotropic effect of amiodarone in nodal tissues is similar to the effect of Class IV drugs. In addition to blocking sodium channels, amiodarone blocks myocardial potassium channels, which contributes to slowing of conduction and prolongation of refractoriness. The antisympathetic action and the block of calcium and potassium channels are responsible for the negative dromotropic effects on the sinus node and for the slowing of conduction and prolongation of refractoriness in the atrioventricular (AV) node. Its vasodilatory action can decrease cardiac workload and consequently myocardial oxygen consumption.

Amiodarone HCl IV administration prolongs intranodal conduction (Atrial-His, AH) and refractoriness of the atrioventricular node (ERP AVN), but has little or no effect on sinus cycle length (SCL), refractoriness of the right atrium and right ventricle (ERP RA and ERP RV), repolarization (QTc), intraventricular conduction (QRS), and infranodal conduction (His-ventricular, HV). A comparison of the electrophysiologic effects of amiodarone HCl IV and oral amiodarone HCl is shown in TABLE 1.

TABLE 1 *Effects of IV and Oral Amiodarone HCl on Electrophysiologic Parameters*

Formulation	SCL	QRS	QTc	AH	HV	ERP RA	ERP RV	ERP AVN
IV	NC	NC	NC	Inc	NC	NC	NC	Inc
Oral	Inc	NC	Inc	Inc	NC	Inc	Inc	Inc

Inc Increases.
NC No Change.

At higher doses (>10 mg/kg) of amiodarone HCl IV, prolongation of the ERP RV and modest prolongation of the QRS have been seen. These differences between oral and IV administration suggest that the initial acute effects of amiodarone HCl IV may be predominantly focused on the AV node, causing an intranodal conduction delay and increased nodal refractoriness due to slow channel blockade (Class IV activity) and noncompetitive adrenergic antagonism (Class II activity).

PHARMACOKINETICS AND METABOLISM

Amiodarone exhibits complex disposition characteristics after IV administration. Peak serum concentrations after single 5 mg/kg 15 minute IV infusions in healthy subjects range between 5 and 41 mg/L. Peak concentrations after 10 minute infusions of 150 mg amiodarone HCl IV in patients with ventricular fibrillation (VF) or hemodynamically unstable ventricular tachycardia (VT) range between 7 and 26 mg/L. Due to rapid distribution, serum concentrations decline to 10% of peak values within 30-45 minutes after the end of the infusion. In clinical trials, after 48 hours of continued infusions (125, 500, or 1000 mg/day) plus supplemental (150 mg) infusions (for recurrent arrhythmias), amiodarone mean serum concentrations between 0.7-1.4 mg/L were observed (n=260).

N-desethylamiodarone (DEA) is the major active metabolite of amiodarone in humans. DEA serum concentrations above 0.05 mg/L are not usually seen until after several days of continuous infusion but with prolonged therapy reach approximately the same concentration as amiodarone. The enzymes responsible for the N-deethylation are believed to be the cytochrome P-450 3A (CYP3A) subfamily, principally CYP3A4. This isozyme is present in both the liver and intestines. The highly variable systemic availability of oral amiodarone may be attributed potentially to large interindividual variability in CYP3A4 activity.

Amiodarone is eliminated primarily by hepatic metabolism and biliary excretion and there is negligible excretion of amiodarone or DEA in urine. Neither amiodarone nor DEA is dialyzable. Amiodarone and DEA cross the placenta and both appear in breast milk.

No data are available on the activity of DEA in humans, but in animals, it has significant electrophysiologic and antiarrhythmic effects generally similar to amiodarone itself. DEA's precise role and contribution to the antiarrhythmic activity of oral amiodarone are not certain. The development of maximal ventricular Class III effects after oral amiodarone HCl administration in humans correlates more closely with DEA accumulation over time than with amiodarone accumulation. On the other hand, after amiodarone HCl IV administration, there is evidence of activity well before significant concentrations of DEA are attained.

TABLE 2 summarizes the mean ranges of pharmacokinetic parameters of amiodarone reported in single dose IV (5 mg/kg over 15 min) studies of healthy subjects.

TABLE 2 *Pharmacokinetic Profile After IV Amiodarone Administration*

Drug	Clearance (ml/h/kg)	Vc (L/kg)	Vss (L/kg)	$T_{½}$ (days)
Amiodarone	90-158	0.2	40-84	20-47
Desethylamiodarone	197-290	—	68-168	≥AMI $T_{½}$

Notes: Vc and Vss denote the central and steady-state volumes of distribution from IV studies.
— Denotes not available.

Desethylamiodarone clearance and volume involve an unknown biotransformation factor.

The systemic availability of ***oral*** amiodarone in healthy subjects ranges between 33 and 65%. From *in vitro* studies, the protein binding of amiodarone is >96%.

In clinical studies of 2-7 days, clearance of amiodarone after IV administration in patients with VT and VF ranged between 220 and 440 ml/h/kg. Age, sex, renal disease, and hepatic disease (cirrhosis) do not have marked effects on the disposition of amiodarone or DEA. Renal impairment does not influence the pharmacokinetics of amiodarone. After a single dose of amiodarone HCl IV in cirrhotic patients, significantly lower C_{max} and average concentration values are seen for DEA, but mean amiodarone levels are unchanged. Normal subjects over 65 years of age show lower clearances (about 100 ml/h/kg) than younger subjects (about 150 ml/h/kg) and an increase in $T_{½}$ from about 20-47 days. In patients with severe left ventricular dysfunction, the pharmacokinetics of amiodarone are not significantly altered but the terminal disposition $T_{½}$ of DEA is prolonged. Although no dosage adjustment for patients with renal, hepatic, or cardiac abnormalities has been defined during chronic treatment with ***oral*** amiodarone HCl, close clinical monitoring is prudent for elderly patients and those with severe left ventricular dysfunction.

There is no established relationship between drug concentration and therapeutic response for short-term IV use. Steady-state amiodarone concentrations of 1 to 2.5 mg/L have been associated with antiarrhythmic effects and acceptable toxicity following chronic ***oral*** amiodarone HCl therapy.

PHARMACODYNAMICS

Amiodarone HCl IV has been reported to produce negative inotropic and vasodilatory effects in animals and humans. In clinical studies of patients with refractory VF or hemodynamically unstable VT, treatment-emergent, drug-related hypotension occurred in 288 of 1836 patients (16%) treated with amiodarone HCl IV. No correlations were seen between the baseline ejection fraction and the occurrence of clinically significant hypotension during infusion of amiodarone HCl IV.

INDICATIONS AND USAGE

Amiodarone HCl IV is indicated for initiation of treatment and prophylaxis of frequently recurring ventricular fibrillation and hemodynamically unstable ventricular tachycardia in patients refractory to other therapy. Amiodarone HCl IV also can be used to treat patients with VT/VF for whom oral amiodarone HCl is indicated, but who are unable to take oral medication. During or after treatment with amiodarone HCl IV, patients may be transferred to oral amiodarone HCl therapy (see DOSAGE AND ADMINISTRATION).

Amiodarone HCl IV should be used for acute treatment until the patient's ventricular arrhythmias are stabilized. Most patients will require this therapy for 48-96 hours, but amiodarone HCl IV may be safely administered for longer periods if necessary.

NON-FDA APPROVED INDICATIONS

Although not FDA approved, amiodarone is used to treat paroxysmal supraventricular tachycardia, atrial fibrillation, and atrial flutter.

CONTRAINDICATIONS

Amiodarone HCl IV is contraindicated in patients with known hypersensitivity to any of the components of amiodarone HCl IV, or in patients with cardiogenic shock, marked sinus bradycardia, and second- or third-degree AV block unless a functioning pacemaker is available.

WARNINGS

HYPOTENSION

Hypotension is the most common adverse effect seen with amiodarone HCl IV. In clinical trials, treatment-emergent, drug-related hypotension was reported as an adverse effect in 288 (16%) of 1836 patients treated with amiodarone HCl IV. Clinically significant hypotension during infusions was seen most often in the first several hours of treatment and was not dose related, but appeared to be related to the rate of infusion. Hypotension necessitating alterations in amiodarone HCl IV therapy was reported in 3% of patients, with permanent discontinuation required in less than 2% of patients.

Hypotension should be treated initially by slowing the infusion; additional standard therapy may be needed, including the following: vasopressor drugs, positive inotropic agents, and volume expansion. ***The initial rate of infusion should be monitored closely and should not exceed that prescribed in*** DOSAGE AND ADMINISTRATION.

In some cases, hypotension may be refractory resulting in fatal outcome (see ADVERSE REACTIONS, Postmarketing Reports).

BRADYCARDIA AND AV BLOCK

Drug-related bradycardia occurred in 90 (4.9%) of 1836 patients in clinical trials while they were receiving amiodarone HCl IV for life-threatening VT/VF; it was not dose-related. Bradycardia should be treated by slowing the infusion rate or discontinuing amiodarone HCl IV. In some patients, inserting a pacemaker is required. Despite such measures, bradycardia was progressive and terminal in 1 patient during the controlled trials. Patients with a known predisposition to bradycardia or AV block should be treated with amiodarone HCl IV in a setting where a temporary pacemaker is available.

LONG-TERM USE

See labeling for oral amiodarone HCl. There has been limited experience in patients receiving amiodarone HCl IV for longer than 3 weeks.

NEONATAL HYPO- OR HYPERTHYROIDISM

Although amiodarone HCl use during pregnancy is uncommon, there have been a small number of published reports of congenital goiter/hypothyroidism and hyperthyroidism associated with its oral administration. If amiodarone HCl IV is administered during pregnancy, the patient should be apprised of the potential hazard to the fetus.

PRECAUTIONS

Amiodarone HCl IV should be administered only by physicians who are experienced in the treatment of life-threatening arrhythmias, who are thoroughly familiar with the risks and benefits of amiodarone HCl therapy, and who have access to facilities adequate for monitoring the effectiveness and side effects of treatment.

LIVER ENZYME ELEVATIONS

Elevations of blood hepatic enzyme values — alanine aminotransferase (ALT), aspartate aminotransferase (AST), and gamma-glutamyl transferase (GGT) — are seen commonly in patients with immediately life-threatening VT/VF. Interpreting elevated AST activity can be difficult because the values may be elevated in patients who have had recent myocardial infarction, congestive heart failure, or multiple electrical defibrillations. Approximately 54% of patients receiving amiodarone HCl IV in clinical studies had baseline liver enzyme elevations, and 13% had clinically significant elevations. In 81% of patients with both baseline and on-therapy data available, the liver enzyme elevations either improved during therapy or remained at baseline levels. Baseline abnormalities in hepatic enzymes are not a contraindication to treatment.

Rare cases of fatal hepatocellular necrosis after treatment with amiodarone HCl IV have been reported. Two patients, one 28 years of age and the other 60 years of age, were treated for atrial arrhythmias with an initial infusion of 1500 mg over 5 hours, a rate much higher than recommended. Both patients developed hepatic and renal failure within 24 hours after the start of amiodarone HCl IV treatment and died on Day 14 and Day 4, respectively. Because these episodes of hepatic necrosis may have been due to the rapid rate of infusion with possible rate-related hypotension, ***the initial rate of infusion should be monitored closely and should not exceed that prescribed in DOSAGE AND ADMINISTRATION.***

In patients with life-threatening arrhythmias, the potential risk of hepatic injury should be weighed against the potential benefit of amiodarone HCl IV therapy, but patients receiving amiodarone HCl IV should be monitored carefully for evidence of progressive hepatic injury. Consideration should be given to reducing the rate of administration or withdrawing amiodarone HCl IV in such cases.

PROARRHYTHMIA

Like all antiarrhythmic agents, amiodarone HCl IV may cause a worsening of existing arrhythmias or precipitate a new arrhythmia. Proarrhythmia, primarily torsades de pointes, has been associated with prolongation by amiodarone HCl IV of the QTc interval to 500 milliseconds or greater. Although QTc prolongation occurred frequently in patients receiving amiodarone HCl IV, torsades de pointes or new-onset VF occurred infrequently (less than 2%). Patients should be monitored for QTc prolongation during infusion with amiodarone HCl IV. Combination of amiodarone with other antiarrythmic therapy that prolongs the QTc should be reserved for patients with life-threatening ventricular arrhythmias who are incompletely responsive to a single agent.

The need to coadminister amiodarone with any other drug known to prolong the QTc interval must be based on a careful assessment of the potential risks and benefits of doing so for each patient.

A careful assessment of the potential risks and benefits of administering amiodarone HCl IV must be made in patients with thyroid dysfunction due to the possibility of arrhythmia breakthrough or exacerbation of arrhythmia, which may result in death, in these patients.

PULMONARY DISORDERS

ARDS

Two percent (2%) of patients were reported to have adult respiratory distress syndrome (ARDS) during clinical studies. ARDS is a disorder characterized by bilateral, diffuse pulmonary infiltrates with pulmonary edema and varying degrees of respiratory insufficiency. The clinical and radiographic picture can arise after a variety of lung injuries, such as those resulting from trauma, shock, prolonged cardiopulmonary resuscitation, and aspiration pneumonia, conditions present in many of the patients enrolled in the clinical studies. It is not possible to determine what role, if any, amiodarone HCl IV played in causing or exacerbating the pulmonary disorder in those patients.

Postoperatively, occurrences of ARDS have been reported in patients receiving ***oral*** amiodarone HCl therapy who have undergone either cardiac or noncardiac surgery. Although patients usually respond well to vigorous respiratory therapy, in rare instances the outcome has been fatal. Until further studies have been performed, it is recommended that FiO_2 and the determinants of oxygen delivery to the tissues (*e.g.*, SaO_2, PaO_2) be closely monitored in patients on amiodarone HCl.

Pulmonary Fibrosis

Only 1 of more than 1000 patients treated with amiodarone HCl IV in clinical studies developed pulmonary fibrosis. In that patient, the condition was diagnosed 3 months after treatment with amiodarone HCl IV, during which time she received ***oral*** amiodarone HCl. Pulmonary toxicity is a well-recognized complication of long-term amiodarone HCl use (see labeling for oral amiodarone HCl).

SURGERY

Close perioperative monitoring is recommended in patients undergoing general anesthesia who are on amiodarone therapy as they may be more sensitive to the myocardial depressant and conduction defects of halogenated inhalational anesthetics.

ELECTROLYTE DISTURBANCES

Patients with hypokalemia or hypomagnesemia should have the condition corrected whenever possible before being treated with amiodarone HCl IV, as these disorders can exaggerate the degree of QTc prolongation and increase the potential for torsades de pointes. Special attention should be given to electrolyte and acid-base balance in patients experiencing severe or prolonged diarrhea or in patients receiving concomitant diuretics.

CARCINOGENESIS, MUTAGENESIS, AND IMPAIRMENT OF FERTILITY

No carcinogenicity studies were conducted with amiodarone HCl IV. However, ***oral*** amiodarone HCl caused a statistically significant, dose-related increase in the incidence of thyroid tumors (follicular adenoma and/or carcinoma) in rats. The incidence of thyroid tumors in rats was greater than the incidence in controls even at the lowest dose level tested, *i.e.*, 5 mg/kg/day (approximately 0.08 times the maximum recommended human maintenance dose*).

Mutagenicity studies conducted with amiodarone HCl (Ames, micronucleus, and lysogenic induction tests) were negative.

No fertility studies were conducted with amiodarone HCl IV. However, in a study in which amiodarone HCl was orally administered to male and female rats, beginning 9 weeks prior to mating, reduced fertility was observed at a dose level of 90 mg/kg/day (approximately 1.4 times the maximum recommended human maintenance dose*).

*600 mg in a 50 kg patient (dose compared on a body surface area basis).

PREGNANCY CATEGORY D

See WARNINGS, Neonatal Hypo- or Hyperthyroidism. In addition to causing infrequent congenital goiter/hypothyroidism and hyperthyroidism, amiodarone has caused a variety of adverse effects in animals.

In a reproductive study in which amiodarone was given intravenously to rabbits at dosages of 5, 10, or 25 mg/kg/day (about 0.1, 0.3, and 0.7 times the maximum recommended human dose [MRHD] on a body surface area basis), maternal deaths occurred in all groups, including controls. Embryotoxicity (as manifested by fewer full-term fetuses and increased resorptions with concomitantly lower litter weights) occurred at dosages of 10 mg/kg and above. No evidence of embryotoxicity was observed at 5 mg/kg and no teratogenicity was observed at any dosages.

In a teratology study in which amiodarone was administered by continuous IV infusion to rats at dosages of 25, 50, or 100 mg/kg/day (about 0.4, 0.7, and 1.4 times the MRHD when compared on a body surface area basis), maternal toxicity (as evidenced by reduced weight gain and food consumption) and embryotoxicity (as evidenced by increased resorptions, decreased live litter size, reduced body weights, and retarded sternum and metacarpal ossification) were observed in the 100 mg/kg group.

Amiodarone HCl IV should be used during pregnancy only if the potential benefit to the mother justifies the risk to the fetus.

NURSING MOTHERS

Amiodarone is excreted in human milk, suggesting that breast-feeding could expose the nursing infant to a significant dose of the drug. Nursing offspring of lactating rats administered amiodarone have demonstrated reduced viability and reduced body weight gains. The risk of exposing the infant to amiodarone should be weighed against the potential benefit of arrhythmia suppression in the mother. The mother should be advised to discontinue nursing.

LABOR AND DELIVERY

It is not known whether the use of amiodarone HCl during labor or delivery has any immediate or delayed adverse effects. Preclinical studies in rodents have not shown any effect on the duration of gestation or on parturition.

PEDIATRIC USE

The safety and efficacy of amiodarone HCl in the pediatric population have not been established; therefore, its use in pediatric patients is not recommended.

Amiodarone HCl IV contains the preservative benzyl alcohol (see DESCRIPTION). There have been reports of fatal "gasping syndrome" in neonates (children less than 1 month of age) following the administration of IV solutions containing the preservative benzyl alcohol. Symptoms include a striking onset of gasping respiration, hypotension, bradycardia, and cardiovascular collapse.

GERIATRIC USE

Clinical studies of amiodarone HCl IV did not include sufficient numbers of subjects aged 65 and over to determine whether they respond differently from younger subjects. Other reported clinical experience has not identified differences in responses between the elderly and younger patients. In general, dose selection for an elderly patient should be cautious, usually starting at the low end of the dosing range, reflecting the greater frequency of decreased hepatic, renal, or cardiac function, and of concomitant disease or other drug therapy.

DRUG INTERACTIONS

Amiodarone is metabolized to desethylamiodarone by the cytochrome P450 (CYP450) enzyme group, specifically cytochrome P450 3A4 (CYP3A4). This isoenzyme is present in both the liver and intestines (see CLINICAL PHARMACOLOGY, Pharmacokinetics and Metabolism). Amiodarone is also known to be an inhibitor of CYP3A4. Therefore, amiodarone has the **potential** for interactions with drugs or substances that may be substrates, inhibitors or inducers of CYP3A4. While only a limited number of *in vivo* drug-drug interactions with amiodarone have been reported, chiefly with the oral formulation, the potential for other interactions should be anticipated. This is especially important for drugs associated with serious toxicity, such as other antiarrhythmics. If such drugs are needed, their dose should be reassessed and, where appropriate, plasma concentration measured. In view of the long and variable half-life of amiodarone, potential for drug interactions exists not only with concomitant medication but also with drugs administered after discontinuation of amiodarone.

Since amiodarone is a substrate for CYP3A4, drugs/substances that inhibit CYP3A4 may decrease the metabolism and increase serum concentrations of amiodarone, with the potential for toxic effects. Reported examples of this interaction include the following:

Protease inhibitors: Protease inhibitors are known to inhibit CYP3A4 to varying degrees. Inhibition of CYP3A4 by **indinavir** has been reported to result in increased serum concentrations of amiodarone. Monitoring for amiodarone toxicity and serial measurement of amiodarone serum concentration during concomitant protease inhibitor therapy should be considered.

Histamine H_2 antagonists: **Cimetidine** inhibits CYP3A4 and can increase serum amiodarone levels.

Other substances: Grapefruit juice inhibits CYP3A4-mediated metabolism of oral amiodarone in the intestinal mucosa, resulting in increased plasma levels of amiodarone; therefore, grapefruit juice should not be taken during treatment with oral amiodarone. This information should be considered when changing from IV amiodarone to oral amiodarone (see DOSAGE AND ADMINISTRATION, Intravenous to Oral Transition).

Amiodarone may suppress certain CYP450 enzymes (enzyme inhibition). This can result in unexpectedly high plasma levels of other drugs which are metabolized by those CYP450 enzymes and may lead to toxic effects. Reported examples of this interaction include the following:

Immunosuppressives: **Cyclosporine** (CYP3A4 substrate) administered in combination with oral amiodarone has been reported to produce persistently elevated plasma concentrations of cyclosporine resulting in elevated creatinine, despite reduction in dose of cyclosporine.

HMG-CoA Reductase Inhibitors: Simvastatin (CYP3A4 substrate) in combination with amiodarone has been associated with reports of myopathy/rhabdomyolysis.

Cardiovasculars:

Cardiac glycosides: In patients receiving **digoxin** therapy, administration of oral amiodarone regularly results in an increase in serum digoxin concentration that may reach toxic levels with resultant clinical toxicity. Amiodarone taken concomitantly with digoxin increases the serum digoxin concentration by 70% after 1 day. **On administration of oral amiodarone, the need for digitalis therapy should be reviewed and the dose reduced by approximately 50% or discontinued.** If digitalis treatment is continued, serum levels should be closely monitored and patients observed for clinical evidence of toxicity. These precautions probably should apply to digitoxin administration as well.

Antiarrhythmics: Other antiarrhythmic drugs, such as **quinidine, procainamide, disopyramide,** and **phenytoin,** have been used concurrently with amiodarone. There have been case reports of increased steady-state levels of quinidine, procainamide, and phenytoin during concomitant therapy with amiodarone. Phenytoin decreases serum amiodarone levels. Amiodarone taken concomitantly with quinidine increases quinidine serum concentration by 33% after 2 days. Amiodarone taken concomitantly with procainamide for less than 7 days increases plasma concentrations of procainamide and n-acetyl procainamide by 55% and 33%, respectively. Quinidine and procainamide doses should be reduced by one-third when either is administered with amiodarone. Plasma levels of **flecainide** have been reported to increase in the presence of oral amiodarone; because of this, the dosage of flecainide should be adjusted when these drugs are administered concomitantly. In general, any added antiarrhythmic drug should be initiated at a lower than usual dose with careful monitoring. Combination of amiodarone with other antiarrhythmic therapy should be reserved for patients with life-threatening ventricular arrhythmias who are incompletely responsive to a single agent or incompletely responsive to amiodarone. During transfer to oral amiodarone, the dose levels of previously administered agents should be reduced by 30-50% several days after the addition of oral amiodarone (see DOSAGE AND ADMINISTRATION, Intravenous to Oral Transition). The continued need for the other antiarrhythmic agent should be reviewed after the effects of amiodarone have been established, and discontinuation ordinarily should be attempted. If the treatment is continued, these patients should be particularly carefully monitored for adverse effects, especially conduction disturbances and exacerbation of tachyarrhythmias, as amiodarone is continued. In amiodarone-treated patients who require additional antiarrhythmic therapy, the initial dose of such agents should be approximately half of the usual recommended dose.

Antihypertensives: Amiodarone should be used with caution in patients receiving **β-receptor blocking agents** (*e.g.,* propanolol, a CYP3A4 inhibitor) or **calcium channel antagonists** (*e.g.,* verapamil, a CYP3A4 substrate, and diltiazem, a CYP3A4 inhibitor) because of the possible potentiation of bradycardia, sinus arrest, and AV block; if necessary, amiodarone can continue to be used after insertion of a pacemaker in patients with severe bradycardia or sinus arrest.

Anticoagulants: Potentiation of **warfarin**-type (CYP2C9 and CYP3A4 substrate) anticoagulant response is almost always seen in patients receiving amiodarone and can result in serious or fatal bleeding. Since the concomitant administration of warfarin with amiodarone increases the prothrombin time by 100% after 3-4 days, **the dose of the anticoagulant should be reduced by one-third to one-half, and prothrombin times should be monitored closely.**

Some drugs/substances are known to accelerate the metabolism of amiodarone by stimulating the synthesis of CYP3A4 (enzyme induction). This may lead to low amiodarone serum levels and potential decrease in efficacy. Reported examples of this interaction include the following:

Antibiotics: **Rifampin** is a potent inducer of CYP3A4. Administration of rifampin concomitantly with oral amiodarone has been shown to result in decreases in serum concentrations of amiodarone and desethylamiodarone.

Other substances, including herbal preparations: **St. John's Wort** (Hypericum perforatum) induces CYP3A4. Since amiodarone is a substrate for CYP3A4, there is the potential that the use of St. John's Wort in patients receiving amiodarone could result in reduced amiodarone levels.

Other reported interactions with amiodarone:

Fentanyl (CYP3A4 substrate) in combination with amiodarone may cause hypotension, bradycardia, decreased cardiac output.

Sinus bradycardia has been reported with oral amiodarone in combination with **lidocaine** (CYP3A4 substrate) given for local anesthesia. Seizure, associated with increased lidocaine concentrations, has been reported with concomitant administration of IV amiodarone.

Dextromethorphan is a substrate for both CYP2D6 and CYP3A4. Amiodarone inhibits CYP2D6.

Cholestyramine increases enterohepatic elimination of amiodarone and may reduce serum levels and T½.

Disopyramide increases QT prolongation which could cause arrhythmia.

Hemodynamic and electrophysiologic interactions have also been observed after concomitant administration with **propranolol, diltiazem,** and **verapamil.**

VOLATILE ANESTHETIC AGENTS

See PRECAUTIONS, Surgery.

In addition to the interactions noted above, chronic (>2 weeks) ***oral*** amiodarone HCl administration impairs metabolism of phenytoin, dextromethorphan, and methotrexate.

ADVERSE REACTIONS

In a total of 1836 patients in controlled and uncontrolled clinical trials, 14% of patients received amiodarone HCl IV for at least 1 week, 5% received it for at least 2 weeks, 2% received it for at least 3 weeks, and 1% received it for more than 3 weeks, without an increased incidence of severe adverse reactions. The mean duration of therapy in these studies was 5.6 days; median exposure was 3.7 days.

The most important treatment-emergent adverse effects were hypotension, asystole/cardiac arrest/electromechanical dissociation (EMD), cardiogenic shock, congestive heart failure, bradycardia, liver function test abnormalities, VT, and AV block. Overall, treatment was discontinued for about 9% of the patients because of adverse effects. The most common adverse effects leading to discontinuation of amiodarone HCl IV therapy were hypotension (1.6%), asystole/cardiac arrest/EMD (1.2%), VT (1.1%), and cardiogenic shock (1%).

TABLE 3 lists the most common (incidence ≥2%) treatment-emergent adverse events during amiodarone HCl IV therapy considered at least possibly drug-related. These data were collected from the Wyeth-Ayerst clinical trials involving 1836 patients with life-threatening VT/VF. Data from all assigned treatment groups are pooled because none of the adverse events appeared to be dose-related.

TABLE 3 *Summary Tabulation of Treatment-Emergent Drug-Related Study Events in Patients Receiving Amiodarone HCl IV in Controlled and Open-Label Studies (≥2% Incidence)*

Study Event	Controlled Studies (n=814)	Open-Label Studies (n=1022)	Total (n=1836)
Body as a Whole			
Fever	24 (2.9%)	13 (1.2%)	37 (2.0%)
Cardiovascular System			
Bradycardia	49 (6.0%)	41 (4.0%)	90 (4.9%)
Congestive heart failure	18 (2.2%)	21 (2.0%)	39 (2.1%)
Heart arrest	29 (3.5%)	26 (2.5%)	55 (2.9%)
Hypotension	165 (20.2%)	123 (12.0%)	288 (15.6%)
Ventricular tachycardia	15 (1.8%)	30 (2.9%)	45 (2.4%)
Digestive System			
Liver function tests abnormal	35 (4.2%)	29 (2.8%)	64 (3.4%)
Nausea	29 (3.5%)	43 (4.2%)	72 (3.9%)

Other treatment-emergent possibly drug-related adverse events reported in less than 2% of patients receiving amiodarone HCl IV in Wyeth-Ayerst controlled and uncontrolled studies included the following: Abnormal kidney function, atrial fibrillation, diarrhea, increased ALT, increased AST, lung edema, nodal arrhythmia, prolonged QT interval, respiratory disorder, shock, sinus bradycardia, Stevens-Johnson syndrome, thrombocytopenia, VF, and vomiting.

POSTMARKETING REPORTS

In postmarketing surveillance, hypotension (sometimes fatal), sinus arrest, pseudotumor cerebri, toxic epidermal necrolysis, exfoliative dermatitis, pancytopenia, neutropenia, erythema multiforme, angioedema, bronchospasm, and anaphylactic shock also have been reported with amiodarone therapy.

Also, in patients receiving recommended dosages, there have been postmarketing reports of the following injection site reactions: pain, erythema, edema, pigment changes, venous thrombosis, phlebitis, thrombophlebitis, cellulitis, necrosis, and skin sloughing (see DOSAGE AND ADMINISTRATION).

DOSAGE AND ADMINISTRATION

Amiodarone shows considerable interindividual variation in response. Thus, although a starting dose adequate to suppress life-threatening arrhythmias is needed, close monitoring with adjustment of dose as needed is essential. The recommended starting dose of amiodarone HCl IV is about 1000 mg over the first 24 hours of therapy, delivered by the following infusion regimen (see TABLE 4).

TABLE 4 *Amiodarone HCl IV Dose Recommendations — First 24 Hours*

Loading Infusions	
First **Rapid:**	**150 mg over the FIRST 10 minutes (15 mg/min).** Add 3 ml of amiodarone HCl IV (150 mg) to 100 ml D_5W (concentration = 1.5 mg/ml). Infuse 100 ml over 10 minutes.
Followed by **Slow:**	**360 mg over the NEXT 6 hours (1 mg/min).** Add 18 ml of amiodarone HCl IV (900 mg) to 500 ml D_5W (concentration = 1.8 mg/ml).
Maintenance Infusion	**540 mg over the REMAINING 18 hours (0.5 mg/min).** Decrease the rate of the slow loading infusion to 0.5 mg/min.

After the first 24 hours, the maintenance infusion rate of 0.5 mg/min (720 mg/24 hours) should be continued utilizing a concentration of 1-6 mg/ml (amiodarone HCl IV concentrations greater than 2 mg/ml should be administered via a central venous catheter). In the event of breakthrough episodes of VF or hemodynamically unstable VT, 150 mg supplemental infusions of amiodarone HCl IV mixed in 100 ml of D_5W may be administered. Such infusions should be administered over 10 minutes to minimize the potential for hypotension. The rate of the maintenance infusion may be increased to achieve effective arrhythmia suppression.

The first 24 hour dose may be individualized for each patient; however, in controlled clinical trials, mean daily doses above 2100 mg were associated with an increased risk of hypotension. The initial infusion rate should not exceed 30 mg/min.

Based on the experience from clinical studies of amiodarone HCl IV, a maintenance infusion of up to 0.5 mg/min can be cautiously continued for 2-3 weeks regardless of the patient's age, renal function, or left ventricular function. There has been limited experience in patients receiving amiodarone HCl IV for longer than 3 weeks.

The surface properties of solutions containing injectable amiodarone are altered such that the drop size may be reduced. This reduction may lead to underdosage of the patient by up to 30% if drop counter infusion sets are used. Amiodarone HCl IV must be delivered by a volumetric infusion pump.

Amiodarone HCl IV should, whenever possible, be administered through a central venous catheter dedicated to that purpose. An in-line filter should be used during administration.

Amiodarone HCl IV concentrations greater than 3 mg/ml in D_5W have been associated with a high incidence of peripheral vein phlebitis; however, concentrations of 2.5 mg/ml or less appear to be less irritating. Therefore, for infusions longer than 1 hour, amiodarone HCl IV concentrations should not exceed 2 mg/ml unless a central venous catheter is used (see ADVERSE REACTIONS, Postmarketing Reports).

Amiodarone HCl IV infusions exceeding 2 hours must be administered in glass or polyolefin bottles containing D_5W. Use of **evacuated glass containers** for admixing amiodarone HCl IV is not recommended as incompatibility with a buffer in the container may cause precipitation.

It is well known that amiodarone adsorbs to polyvinyl chloride (PVC) tubing and the clinical trial dose administration schedule was designed to account for this adsorption. All of the clinical trials were conducted using PVC tubing and its use is therefore recommended. The concentrations and rates of infusion provided in DOSAGE AND ADMINISTRATION reflect doses identified in these studies. It is important that the recommended infusion regimen be followed closely.

Amiodarone HCl IV has been found to leach out plasticizers, including DEHP [di-(2-ethylhexyl)phthalate] from IV tubing (including PVC tubing). The degree of leaching increases when infusing amiodarone HCl IV at higher concentrations and lower flow rates than provided in DOSAGE AND ADMINISTRATION.

Amiodarone HCl IV does not need to be protected from light during administration.

TABLE 5 *Amiodarone HCl Solution Stability*

Solution	Concentration	Container	Comments
D_5W*	1.0-6.0 mg/ml	PVC	Physically compatible, with amiodarone loss <10% at 2 hours
D_5W*	1.0-6.0 mg/ml	Polyolefin, glass	Physically compatible, with no amiodarone loss at 24 hours

* 5% Dextrose in water.

ADMIXTURE INCOMPATIBILITY

Amiodarone HCl IV in D_5W is incompatible with the drugs shown in TABLE 6.

TABLE 6 *Y-Site Injection Incompatibility*

Drug	Vehicle	Amiodarone Concentration	Comments
Aminophylline	D_5W	4 mg/ml	Precipitate
Cefamandole nafate	D_5W	4 mg/ml	Precipitate
Cefazolin sodium	D_5W	4 mg/ml	Precipitate
Mezlocillin sodium	D_5W	4 mg/ml	Precipitate
Heparin sodium	D_5W	—	Precipitate
Sodium bicarbonate	D_5W	3 mg/ml	Precipitate

INTRAVENOUS TO ORAL TRANSITION

Patients whose arrhythmias have been suppressed by amiodarone HCl IV may be switched to oral amiodarone HCl. The optimal dose for changing from IV to oral administration of amiodarone HCl will depend on the dose of amiodarone HCl IV already administered, as well as the bioavailability of oral amiodarone HCl. When changing to oral amiodarone HCl therapy, clinical monitoring is recommended, particularly for elderly patients.

Since there are some differences between the safety and efficacy profiles of the IV and oral formulations, the prescriber is advised to review the package insert for oral amiodarone when switching from IV to oral amiodarone therapy.

Since grapefruit juice is known to inhibit CYP3A4-mediated metabolism of oral amiodarone in the intestinal mucosa, resulting in increased plasma levels of amiodarone; grapefruit juice should not be taken during treatment with oral amiodarone (see DRUG INTERACTIONS).

TABLE 7 provides suggested doses of oral amiodarone HCl to be initiated after varying durations of amiodarone HCl IV administration. These recommendations are made on the basis of a comparable total body amount of amiodarone delivered by the IV and oral routes, based on 50% bioavailability of oral amiodarone.

TABLE 7 *Recommendations for Oral Dosage After IV Infusion*

Duration of Amiodarone HCl IV Infusion*	Initial Daily Dose of Oral Amiodarone HCl
<1 week	800-1600 mg
1-3 weeks	600-800 mg
>3 weeks†	400 mg

* Assuming a 720 mg/day infusion (0.5 mg/min).
† Amiodarone HCl IV is not intended for maintenance treatment.

HOW SUPPLIED

Cordarone IV (amiodarone HCl) is available in ampuls containing 3 ml (50 mg/ml) each.

STORAGE

Store at room temperature, 15-25°C (59-77°F).

Protect from light and excessive heat.

Use carton to protect contents from light until used.

ORAL

DESCRIPTION

Cordarone is a member of a new class of antiarrhythmic drugs with predominantly Class III (Vaughan Williams' classification) effects, available for oral administration as pink, scored tablets containing 200 mg of amiodarone hydrochloride. The inactive ingredients present are colloidal silicon dioxide, lactose, magnesium stearate, povidone, starch, and FD&C red 40. Amiodarone hydrochloride is a benzofuran derivative: 2-butyl-3-benzofuranyl 4-[2-(diethylamino)-ethoxy]-3,5-diiodophenyl ketone hydrochloride. It is not chemically related to any other available antiarrhythmic drug.

It has a molecular formula of $C_{25}H_{29}I_2NO_3 \cdot HCl$ and molecular weight of 681.8.

Amiodarone HCl is a white to cream-colored crystalline powder. It is slightly soluble in water, soluble in alcohol, and freely soluble in chloroform. It contains 37.3% iodine by weight.

CLINICAL PHARMACOLOGY

ELECTROPHYSIOLOGY/MECHANISM OF ACTION

In animals, amiodarone HCl is effective in the prevention or suppression of experimentally-induced arrhythmias. The antiarrhythmic effect of amiodarone HCl may be due to at least two major properties: (1) a prolongation of the myocardial cell-action potential duration and refractory period and (2) noncompetitive α- and β-adrenergic inhibition.

Amiodarone HCl prolongs the duration of the action potential of all cardiac fibers while causing minimal reduction of dV/dt (maximal upstroke velocity of the action potential). The refractory period is prolonged in all cardiac tissues. Amiodarone HCl increases the cardiac refractory period without influencing resting membrane potential, except in automatic cells where the slope of the prepotential is reduced, generally reducing automaticity. These electrophysiologic effects are reflected in a decreased sinus rate of 15-20%, increased PR and QT intervals of about 10%, the development of U-waves, and changes in T-wave contour. These changes should not require discontinuation of amiodarone HCl as they are evidence of its pharmacological action, although amiodarone HCl can cause marked sinus bradycardia or sinus arrest and heart block. On rare occasions, QT prolongation has been associated with worsening of arrhythmia (see WARNINGS).

HEMODYNAMICS

In animal studies and after IV administration in man, amiodarone HCl relaxes vascular smooth muscle, reduces peripheral vascular resistance (afterload), and slightly increases cardiac index. After oral dosing, however, amiodarone HCl produces no significant change in left ventricular ejection fraction (LVEF), even in patients with depressed LVEF. After acute IV dosing in man, amiodarone HCl may have a mild negative inotropic effect.

PHARMACOKINETICS

Following oral administration in man, amiodarone HCl is slowly and variably absorbed. The bioavailability of amiodarone HCl is approximately 50%, but has varied between 35 and 65% in various studies. Maximum plasma concentrations are attained 3-7 hours after a single dose. Despite this, the onset of action may occur in 2-3 days, but more commonly takes 1-3 weeks, even with loading doses. Plasma concentrations with chronic dosing at 100-600 mg/day are approximately dose proportional, with a mean 0.5 mg/L increase for each 100 mg/day. These means, however, include considerable individual variability. Food increases the rate and extent of absorption of amiodarone HCl. The effects of food upon the bioavailability of amiodarone HCl have been studied in 30 healthy subjects who received a single 600 mg dose immediately after consuming a high fat meal and following an overnight fast. The area under the plasma concentration-time curve (AUC) and the peak plasma concentration (C_{max}) of amiodarone increased by 2.3 (range 1.7-3.6) and 3.8 (range 2.7-4.4) times, respectively, in the presence of food. Food also increased the rate of absorption of amiodarone, decreasing the time to peak plasma concentration (T_{max}) by 37%. The mean AUC and mean C_{max} of desethylamiodarone increased by 55% (range 58-101%) and 32% (range 4-84%), respectively, but there was no change in the T_{max} in the presence of food.

Amiodarone HCl has a very large but variable volume of distribution, averaging about 60 L/kg, because of extensive accumulation in various sites, especially adipose tissue and highly perfused organs, such as the liver, lung, and spleen. One major metabolite of amiodarone HCl, desethylamiodarone (DEA), has been identified in man; it accumulates to an even greater extent in almost all tissues. No data are available on the activity of DEA in humans, but in animals, it has significant electrophysiologic and antiarrhythmic effects generally similar to amiodarone itself. DEA's precise role and contribution to the antiarrhythmic activity of oral amiodarone are not certain. The development of maximal ventricular Class III effects after oral amiodarone HCl administration in humans correlates more closely with DEA accumulation over time than with amiodarone accumulation.

Amiodarone is eliminated primarily by hepatic metabolism and biliary excretion and there is negligible excretion of amiodarone or DEA in urine. Neither amiodarone nor DEA is dialyzable.

In clinical studies of 2-7 days, clearance of amiodarone after IV administration in patients with VT and VF ranged between 220 and 440 ml/h/kg. Age, sex, renal disease, and hepatic disease (cirrhosis) do not have marked effects on the disposition of amiodarone or DEA. Renal impairment does not influence the pharmacokinetics of amiodarone. After a single dose of IV amiodarone in cirrhotic patients, significantly lower C_{max} and average concentration values are seen for DEA, but mean amiodarone levels are unchanged. Normal subjects over 65 years of age show lower clearances (about 100 ml/h/kg) than younger subjects (about 150 ml/h/kg) and an increase in $T_{1/2}$ from about 20-47 days. In patients with severe left ventricular dysfunction, the pharmacokinetics of amiodarone are not significantly altered but the terminal disposition $T_{1/2}$ of DEA is prolonged. Although no dosage adjustment for patients with renal, hepatic, or cardiac abnormalities has been defined during chronic treatment with amiodarone HCl, close clinical monitoring is prudent for elderly patients and those with severe left ventricular dysfunction.

Following single dose administration in 12 healthy subjects, amiodarone HCl exhibited multi-compartmental pharmacokinetics with a mean apparent plasma terminal elimination half-life of 58 days (range 15-142 days) for amiodarone and 36 days (range 14-75 days) for the active metabolite (DEA). In patients, following discontinuation of chronic oral therapy, amiodarone HCl has been shown to have a biphasic elimination with an initial one-half reduction of plasma levels after 2.5 to 10 days. A much slower terminal plasma-elimination phase shows a half-life of the parent compound ranging from 26-107 days, with a mean of approximately 53 days and most patients in the 40-55 day range. In the absence of a loading-dose period, steady-state plasma concentrations, at constant oral dosing, would therefore be reached between 130 and 535 days, with an average of 265 days. For the metabolite, the mean plasma-elimination half-life was approximately 61 days. These data probably reflect an initial elimination of drug from well-perfused tissue (the 2.5 to 10 day half-life phase), followed by a terminal phase representing extremely slow elimination from poorly perfused tissue compartments such as fat.

The considerable intersubject variation in both phases of elimination, as well as uncertainty as to what compartment is critical to drug effect, requires attention to individual responses once arrhythmia control is achieved with loading doses because the correct maintenance dose is determined, in part, by the elimination rates. Daily maintenance doses of amiodarone HCl should be based on individual patient requirements (see DOSAGE AND ADMINISTRATION).

Amiodarone HCl and its metabolite have a limited transplacental transfer of approximately 10-50%. The parent drug and its metabolite have been detected in breast milk.

Amiodarone HCl is highly protein-bound (approximately 96%).

Although electrophysiologic effects, such as prolongation of QTc, can be seen within hours after a parenteral dose of amiodarone HCl, effects on abnormal rhythms are not seen before 2-3 days and usually require 1-3 weeks, even when a loading dose is used. There may be a continued increase in effect for longer periods still. There is evidence that the time to effect is shorter when a loading-dose regimen is used.

Consistent with the slow rate of elimination, antiarrhythmic effects persist for weeks or months after amiodarone HCl is discontinued, but the time of recurrence is variable and unpredictable. In general, when the drug is resumed after recurrence of the arrhythmia, control is established relatively rapidly compared to the initial response, presumably because tissue stores were not wholly depleted at the time of recurrence.

PHARMACODYNAMICS

There is no well-established relationship of plasma concentration to effectiveness, but it does appear that concentrations much below 1 mg/L are often ineffective and that levels above 2.5 mg/L are generally not needed. Within individuals dose reductions and ensuing decreased plasma concentrations can result in loss of arrhythmia control. Plasma-concentration measurements can be used to identify patients whose levels are unusually low, and who might benefit from a dose increase, or unusually high, and who might have dosage reduction in the hope of minimizing side effects. Some observations have suggested a plasma concentration, dose, or dose/duration relationship for side effects such as pulmonary fibrosis, liver-enzyme elevations, corneal deposits and facial pigmentation, peripheral neuropathy, gastrointestinal and central nervous system effects.

MONITORING EFFECTIVENESS

Predicting the effectiveness of any antiarrhythmic agent in long-term prevention of recurrent ventricular tachycardia and ventricular fibrillation is difficult and controversial, with highly qualified investigators recommending use of ambulatory monitoring, programmed electrical stimulation with various stimulation regimens, or a combination of these, to assess response. There is no present consensus on many aspects of how best to assess effectiveness, but there is a reasonable consensus on some aspects:

If a patient with a history of cardiac arrest does not manifest a hemodynamically unstable arrhythmia during electrocardiographic monitoring prior to treatment, assessment of the effectiveness of amiodarone HCl requires some provocative approach, either exercise or programmed electrical stimulation (PES).

Whether provocation is also needed in patients who do manifest their life-threatening arrhythmia spontaneously is not settled, but there are reasons to consider PES or other provocation in such patients. In the fraction of patients whose PES-inducible arrhythmia can be made noninducible by amiodarone HCl (a fraction that has varied widely in various series from less than 10% to almost 40%, perhaps due to different stimulation criteria), the prognosis has been almost uniformly excellent, with very low recurrence (ventricular tachycardia or sudden death) rates. More controversial is the meaning of continued inducibility. There has been an impression that continued inducibility in amiodarone HCl patients may not foretell a poor prognosis but, in fact, many observers have found greater recurrence rates in patients who remain inducible than in those who do not. A number of criteria have been proposed, however, for identifying patients who remain inducible but who seem likely nonetheless to do well on amiodarone HCl. These criteria include increased difficulty of induction (more stimuli or more rapid stimuli), which has been reported to predict a lower rate of recurrence, and ability to tolerate the induced ventricular tachycardia without severe symptoms, a finding that has been reported to correlate with better survival but not with lower recurrence rates. While these criteria require confirmation and further study in general, *easier* inducibility or *poorer* tolerance of the induced arrhythmia should suggest consideration of a need to revise treatment.

Several predictors of success not based on PES have also been suggested, including complete elimination of all nonsustained ventricular tachycardia on ambulatory monitoring and very low premature ventricular-beat rates (less than 1 VPB/1000 normal beats).

While these issues remain unsettled for amiodarone HCl, as for other agents, the prescriber of amiodarone HCl should have access to (direct or through referral), and familiarity with, the full range of evaluatory procedures used in the care of patients with life-threatening arrhythmias.

It is difficult to describe the effectiveness rates of amiodarone HCl, as these depend on the specific arrhythmia treated, the success criteria used, the underlying cardiac disease of the patient, the number of drugs tried before resorting to amiodarone HCl, the duration of follow-up, the dose of amiodarone HCl, the use of additional antiarrhythmic agents, and many other factors. As amiodarone HCl has been studied principally in patients with refractory life-threatening ventricular arrhythmias, in whom drug therapy must be selected on the basis of response and cannot be assigned arbitrarily, randomized comparisons with other agents or placebo have not been possible. Reports of series of treated patients with a history of cardiac arrest and mean follow-up of 1 year or more have given mortality (due to arrhythmia) rates that were highly variable, ranging from less than 5% to over 30%, with most series in the range of 10-15%. Overall arrhythmia-recurrence rates (fatal and nonfatal) also were highly variable (and, as noted above, depended on response to PES and other measures), and depend on whether patients who do not seem to respond initially are included. In most cases, considering only patients who seemed to respond well enough to be placed on long-term treatment, recurrence rates have ranged from 20-40% in series with a mean follow-up of a year or more.

INDICATIONS AND USAGE

Because of its life-threatening side effects and the substantial management difficulties associated with its use (see WARNINGS), amiodarone HCl is indicated only for the treatment of the following documented, life-threatening recurrent ventricular arrhythmias when these have not responded to documented adequate doses of other available antiarrhythmics or when alternative agents could not be tolerated.

Recurrent ventricular fibrillation.

Recurrent hemodynamically unstable ventricular tachycardia.

As is the case for other antiarrhythmic agents, there is no evidence from controlled trials that the use of amiodarone HCl tablets favorably affects survival.

Amiodarone HCl should be used only by physicians familiar with and with access to (directly or through referral) the use of all available modalities for treating recurrent life-threatening ventricular arrhythmias, and who have access to appropriate monitoring facilities, including in-hospital and ambulatory continuous electrocardiographic monitoring and electrophysiologic techniques. Because of the life-threatening nature of the arrhythmias treated, potential interactions with prior therapy, and potential exacerbation of the arrhythmia, initiation of therapy with amiodarone HCl should be carried out in the hospital.

NON-FDA APPROVED INDICATIONS

Although not FDA approved, amiodarone is used to treat paroxysmal supraventricular tachycardia, atrial fibrillation, and atrial flutter.

CONTRAINDICATIONS

Amiodarone HCl is contraindicated in severe sinus-node dysfunction, causing marked sinus bradycardia; second- and third-degree atrioventricular block; and when episodes of bradycardia have caused syncope (except when used in conjunction with a pacemaker).

Amiodarone HCl is contraindicated in patients with a known hypersensitivity to the drug.

WARNINGS

Amiodarone HCl is intended for use only in patients with the indicated life-threatening arrhythmias because its use is accompanied by substantial toxicity.

Amiodarone HCl has several potentially fatal toxicities, the most important of which is pulmonary toxicity (hypersensitivity pneumonitis or interstitial/alveolar pneumonitis) that has resulted in clinically manifest disease at rates as high as 10-17% in some series of patients with ventricular arrhythmias given doses around 400 mg/day, and as abnormal diffusion capacity without symptoms in a much higher percentage of patients. Pulmonary toxicity has been fatal about 10% of the time. Liver injury is common with amiodarone HCl, but is usually mild and evidenced only by abnormal liver enzymes. Overt liver disease can occur, however, and has been fatal in a few cases. Like other antiarrhythmics, amiodarone HCl can exacerbate the arrhythmia, *e.g.*, by making the arrhythmia less well tolerated or more difficult to reverse. This has occurred in 2-5% of patients in various series, and significant heart block or sinus bradycardia has been seen in 2-5%. All of these events should be manageable in the proper clinical setting in most cases. Although the frequency of such proarrhythmic events does not appear greater with amiodarone HCl than with many other agents used in this population, the effects are prolonged when they occur.

Even in patients at high risk of arrhythmic death, in whom the toxicity of amiodarone HCl is an acceptable risk, amiodarone HCl poses major management problems that could be life-threatening in a population at risk of sudden death, so that every effort should be made to utilize alternative agents first.

The difficulty of using amiodarone HCl effectively and safely itself poses a significant risk to patients. Patients with the indicated arrhythmias must be hospitalized while the loading dose of amiodarone HCl is given, and a response generally requires at least 1 week, usually 2 or more. Because absorption and elimination are variable, maintenance-dose selection is difficult, and it is not unusual to require dosage decrease or discontinuation of treatment. In a retrospective survey of 192 patients with ventricular tachyarrhythmias, 84 required dose reduction and 18 required at least temporary discontinuation because of adverse effects, and several series have reported 15-20% overall frequencies of discontinuation due to adverse reactions. The time at which a previously controlled life-threatening arrhythmia will recur after discontinuation or dose adjustment is unpredictable, ranging from weeks to months. The patient is obviously at great risk during this time and may need prolonged hospitalization. Attempts to substitute other antiarrhythmic agents when amiodarone HCl must be stopped will be made difficult by the gradually, but unpredictably, changing amiodarone body burden. A similar problem exists when amiodarone HCl is not effective; it still poses the risk of an interaction with whatever subsequent treatment is tried.

MORTALITY

In the National Heart, Lung and Blood Institute's Cardiac Arrhythmia Suppression Trial (CAST), a long-term, multi-centered, randomized, double-blind study in patients with asymptomatic non-life-threatening ventricular arrhythmias who had had myocardial infarctions more than 6 days but less than 2 years previously, an excessive mortality or non-fatal cardiac arrest rate was seen in patients treated with encainide or flecainide (56/730) compared with that seen in patients assigned to matched placebo-treated groups (22/725). The average duration of treatment with encainide or flecainide in this study was 10 months.

Amiodarone HCl therapy was evaluated in two multi-centered, randomized, double-blind, placebo-controlled trials involving 1202 (Canadian Amiodarone Myocardial Infarction Arrhythmia Trial; CAMIAT) and 1486 (European Myocardial Infarction Amiodarone Trial; EMIAT) post-MI patients followed for up to 2 years. Patients in CAMIAT qualified with ventricular arrhythmias, and those randomized to amiodarone received weight- and response-adjusted doses of 200-400 mg/day. Patients in EMIAT qualified with ejection fraction <40%, and those randomized to amiodarone received fixed doses of 200 mg/day. Both studies had weeks-long loading dose schedules. Intent-to-treat all-cause mortality results were as follows (see TABLE 8).

These data are consistent with the results of a pooled analysis of smaller, controlled studies involving patients with structural heart disease (including myocardial infarction).

PULMONARY TOXICITY

Amiodarone HCl tablets may cause a clinical syndrome of cough and progressive dyspnea accompanied by functional, radiographic, gallium-scan, and pathological data consistent with pulmonary toxicity, the frequency of which varies from 2-7% in most published re-

TABLE 8

	Placebo		Amiodarone		Relative Risk	
	n	Deaths	n	Deaths		95% CI
EMIAT	743	102	743	103	0.99	0.76-1.31
CAMIAT	596	68	606	57	0.88	0.58-1.16

ports, but is as high as 10-17% in some reports. Therefore, when amiodarone HCl therapy is initiated, a baseline chest X-ray and pulmonary-function tests, including diffusion capacity, should be performed. The patient should return for a history, physical exam, and chest X-ray every 3-6 months.

Preexisting pulmonary disease does not appear to increase the risk of developing pulmonary toxicity; however, these patients have a poorer prognosis if pulmonary toxicity does develop.

Pulmonary toxicity secondary to amiodarone HCl seems to result from either indirect or direct toxicity as represented by hypersensitivity pneumonitis or interstitial/alveolar pneumonitis, respectively.

Hypersensitivity pneumonitis usually appears earlier in the course of therapy, and rechallenging these patients with amiodarone HCl results in a more rapid recurrence of greater severity. Bronchoalveolar lavage is the procedure of choice to confirm this diagnosis, which can be made when a T suppressor/cytotoxic (CD8-positive) lymphocytosis is noted. Steroid therapy should be instituted and amiodarone HCl therapy discontinued in these patients.

Interstitial/alveolar pneumonitis may result from the release of oxygen radicals and/or phospholipidosis and is characterized by findings of diffuse alveolar damage, interstitial pneumonitis or fibrosis in lung biopsy specimens. Phospholipidosis (foamy cells, foamy macrophages), due to inhibition of phospholipase, will be present in most cases of amiodarone HCl-induced pulmonary toxicity; however, these changes also are present in approximately 50% of all patients on amiodarone HCl therapy. These cells should be used as markers of therapy, but not as evidence of toxicity. A diagnosis of amiodarone HCl-induced interstitial/alveolar pneumonitis should lead, at a minimum, to dose reduction or, preferably, to withdrawal of the amiodarone HCl to establish reversibility, especially if other acceptable antiarrhythmic therapies are available. Where these measures have been instituted, a reduction in symptoms of amiodarone-induced pulmonary toxicity was usually noted within the first week, and a clinical improvement was greatest in the first 2-3 weeks. Chest X-ray changes usually resolve within 2-4 months. According to some experts, steroids may prove beneficial. Prednisone in doses of 40-60 mg/day or equivalent doses of other steroids have been given and tapered over the course of several weeks depending upon the condition of the patient. In some cases rechallenge with amiodarone HCl at a lower dose has not resulted in return of toxicity. Recent reports suggest that the use of lower loading and maintenance doses of amiodarone HCl are associated with a decreased incidence of amiodarone HCl-induced pulmonary toxicity.

In a patient receiving amiodarone HCl, any new respiratory symptoms should suggest the possibility of pulmonary toxicity, and the history, physical exam, chest X-ray, and pulmonary-function tests (with diffusion capacity) should be repeated and evaluated. A 15% decrease in diffusion capacity has a high sensitivity but only a moderate specificity for pulmonary toxicity; as the decrease in diffusion capacity approaches 30%, the sensitivity decreases but the specificity increases. A gallium-scan also may be performed as part of the diagnostic workup.

Fatalities, secondary to pulmonary toxicity, have occurred in approximately 10% of cases. However, in patients with life-threatening arrhythmias, discontinuation of amiodarone HCl therapy due to suspected drug-induced pulmonary toxicity should be undertaken with caution, as the most common cause of death in these patients is sudden cardiac death. Therefore, every effort should be made to rule out other causes of respiratory impairment (*i.e.*, congestive heart failure with Swan-Ganz catheterization if necessary, respiratory infection, pulmonary embolism, malignancy, etc.) before discontinuing amiodarone HCl in these patients. In addition, bronchoalveolar lavage, transbronchial lung biopsy and/or open lung biopsy may be necessary to confirm the diagnosis, especially in those cases where no acceptable alternative therapy is available.

If a diagnosis of amiodarone HCl-induced hypersensitivity pneumonitis is made, amiodarone HCl should be discontinued, and treatment with steroids should be instituted. If a diagnosis of amiodarone HCl-induced interstitial/alveolar pneumonitis is made, steroid therapy should be instituted and, preferably, amiodarone HCl discontinued or, at a minimum, reduced in dosage. Some cases of amiodarone HCl-induced interstitial/alveolar pneumonitis may resolve following a reduction in amiodarone HCl dosage in conjunction with the administration of steroids. In some patients, rechallenge at a lower dose has not resulted in return of interstitial/alveolar pneumonitis; however, in some patients (perhaps because of severe alveolar damage) the pulmonary lesions have not been reversible.

WORSENED ARRHYTHMIA

Amiodarone HCl, like other antiarrhythmics, can cause serious exacerbation of the presenting arrhythmia, a risk that may be enhanced by the presence of concomitant antiarrhythmics. Exacerbation has been reported in about 2-5% in most series, and has included new ventricular fibrillation, incessant ventricular tachycardia, increased resistance to cardioversion, and polymorphic ventricular tachycardia associated with QTc prolongation (Torsade de Pointes). In addition, amiodarone HCl has caused symptomatic bradycardia or sinus arrest with suppression of escape foci in 2-4% of patients.

The need to coadminister amiodarone with any other drug known to prolong the QTc interval must be based on a careful assessment of the potential risks and benefits of doing so for each patient.

A careful assessment of the potential risks and benefits of administering amiodarone HCl must be made in patients with thyroid dysfunction due to the possibility of arrhythmia breakthrough or exacerbation of arrhythmia in these patients.

LIVER INJURY

Elevations of hepatic enzyme levels are seen frequently in patients exposed to amiodarone HCl and in most cases are asymptomatic. If the increase exceeds 3 times normal, or doubles in a patient with an elevated baseline, discontinuation of amiodarone HCl or dosage reduction should be considered. In a few cases in which biopsy has been done, the histology has resembled that of alcoholic hepatitis or cirrhosis. Hepatic failure has been a rare cause of death in patients treated with amiodarone HCl.

LOSS OF VISION

Cases of optic neuropathy and/or optic neuritis, usually resulting in visual impairment, have been reported in patients treated with amiodarone. In some cases, visual impairment has progressed to permanent blindness. Optic neuropathy and/or neuritis may occur at any time following initiation of therapy. A causal relationship to the drug has not been clearly established. If symptoms of visual impairment appear, such as changes in visual acuity and decreases in peripheral vision, prompt ophthalmic examination is recommended. Appearance of optic neuropathy and/or neuritis calls for re-evaluation of amiodarone HCl therapy. The risks and complications of antiarrhythmic therapy with amiodarone HCl must be weighed against its benefits in patients whose lives are threatened by cardiac arrhythmias. Regular ophthalmic examination, including fundoscopy and slit-lamp examination, is recommended during administration of amiodarone HCl. (See ADVERSE REACTIONS.)

NEONATAL HYPO- OR HYPERTHYROIDISM

Amiodarone HCl can cause fetal harm when administered to a pregnant woman. Although amiodarone HCl use during pregnancy is uncommon, there have been a small number of published reports of congenital goiter/hypothyroidism and hyperthyroidism. If amiodarone HCl is used during pregnancy, or if the patient becomes pregnant while taking amiodarone HCl, the patient should be apprised of the potential hazard to the fetus.

In general, amiodarone HCl tablets should be used during pregnancy only if the potential benefit to the mother justifies the unknown risk to the fetus.

In pregnant rats and rabbits, amiodarone HCl in doses of 25 mg/kg/day (approximately 0.4 and 0.9 times, respectively, the maximum recommended human maintenance dose*) had no adverse effects on the fetus. In the rabbit, 75 mg/kg/day (approximately 2.7 times the maximum recommended human maintenance dose*) caused abortions in greater than 90% of the animals. In the rat, doses of 50 mg/kg/day or more were associated with slight displacement of the testes and an increased incidence of incomplete ossification of some skull and digital bones; at 100 mg/kg/day or more, fetal body weights were reduced; at 200 mg/kg/day, there was an increased incidence of fetal resorption. (These doses in the rat are approximately 0.8, 1.6 and 3.2 times the maximum recommended human maintenance dose.*) Adverse effects on fetal growth and survival also were noted in one of two strains of mice at a dose of 5 mg/kg/day (approximately 0.04 times the maximum recommended human maintenance dose*).

*600 mg in a 50 kg patient (doses compared on a body surface area basis).

PRECAUTIONS

IMPAIRMENT OF VISION

Optic Neuropathy and/or Neuritis

Cases of optic neuropathy and optic neuritis have been reported (see WARNINGS).

Corneal Microdeposits

Corneal microdeposits appear in the majority of adults treated with amiodarone HCl. They are usually discernible only by slit-lamp examination, but give rise to symptoms such as visual halos or blurred vision in as many as 10% of patients. Corneal microdeposits are reversible upon reduction of dose or termination of treatment. Asymptomatic microdeposits alone are not a reason to reduce dose or discontinue treatment (see ADVERSE REACTIONS).

NEUROLOGIC

Chronic administration of oral amiodarone in rare instances may lead to the development of peripheral neuropathy that may resolve when amiodarone is discontinued, but this resolution has been slow and incomplete.

PHOTOSENSITIVITY

Amiodarone HCl has induced photosensitization in about 10% of patients; some protection may be afforded by the use of sun-barrier creams or protective clothing. During long-term treatment, a blue-gray discoloration of the exposed skin may occur. The risk may be increased in patients of fair complexion or those with excessive sun exposure, and may be related to cumulative dose and duration of therapy.

THYROID ABNORMALITIES

Amiodarone HCl inhibits peripheral conversion of thyroxine (T_4) to triiodothyronine (T_3) and may cause increased thyroxine levels, decreased T_3 levels, and increased levels of inactive reverse T_3 (rT_3) in clinically euthyroid patients. It is also a potential source of large amounts of inorganic iodine. Because of its release of inorganic iodine, or perhaps for other reasons, amiodarone HCl can cause either hypothyroidism or hyperthyroidism. Thyroid function should be monitored prior to treatment and periodically thereafter, particularly in elderly patients, and in any patient with a history of thyroid nodules, goiter, or other thyroid dysfunction. Because of the slow elimination of amiodarone HCl and its metabolites, high plasma iodide levels, altered thyroid function, and abnormal thyroid-function tests may persist for several weeks or even months following amiodarone HCl withdrawal.

Hypothyroidism has been reported in 2-4% of patients in most series, but in 8-10% in some series. This condition may be identified by relevant clinical symptoms and particularly by elevated serum TSH levels. In some clinically hypothyroid amiodarone-treated patients, free thyroxine index values may be normal. Hypothyroidism is best managed by amiodarone HCl dose reduction and/or thyroid hormone supplement. However, therapy must be individualized, and it may be necessary to discontinue amiodarone HCl tablets in some patients.

Hyperthyroidism occurs in about 2% of patients receiving amiodarone HCl, but the incidence may be higher among patients with prior inadequate dietary iodine intake. Amiodarone HCl-induced hyperthyroidism usually poses a greater hazard to the patient than hypothyroidism because of the possibility of arrhythmia breakthrough or aggravation, which may result in death. In fact, IF ANY NEW SIGNS OF ARRHYTHMIA APPEAR, THE POSSIBILITY OF HYPERTHYROIDISM SHOULD BE CONSIDERED. Hyperthyroidism is best identified by relevant clinical symptoms and signs, accompanied usually by abnormally elevated levels of serum T_3 RIA, and further elevations of serum T_4, and a subnormal serum TSH level (using a sufficiently sensitive TSH assay). The finding of a flat TSH response to TRH is confirmatory of hyperthyroidism and may be sought in equivocal cases. Since arrhythmia breakthroughs may accompany amiodarone HCl-induced hyperthyroidism, aggressive medical treatment is indicated, including, if possible, dose reduction or withdrawal of amiodarone HCl. The institution of antithyroid drugs, β-adrenergic blockers and/or temporary corticosteroid therapy may be necessary. The action of antithyroid drugs may be especially delayed in amiodarone-induced thyrotoxicosis because of substantial quantities of preformed thyroid hormones stored in the gland. Radioactive iodine therapy is contraindicated because of the low radioiodine uptake associated with amiodarone-induced hyperthyroidism. Experience with thyroid surgery in this setting is extremely limited, and this form of therapy runs the theoretical risk of inducing thyroid storm. Amiodarone HCl-induced hyperthyroidism may be followed by a transient period of hypothyroidism.

SURGERY

Volatile Anesthetic Agents

Close perioperative monitoring is recommended in patients undergoing general anesthesia who are on amiodarone therapy as they may be more sensitive to the myocardial depressant and conduction effects of halogenated inhalational anesthetics.

Hypotension Postbypass

Rare occurrences of hypotension upon discontinuation of cardiopulmonary bypass during open-heart surgery in patients receiving amiodarone HCl have been reported. The relationship of this event to amiodarone HCl therapy is unknown.

Adult Respiratory Distress Syndrome (ARDS)

Postoperatively, occurrences of ARDS have been reported in patients receiving amiodarone HCl therapy who have undergone either cardiac or noncardiac surgery. Although patients usually respond well to vigorous respiratory therapy, in rare instances the outcome has been fatal. Until further studies have been performed, it is recommended that FiO_2 and the determinants of oxygen delivery to the tissues (*e.g.*, SaO_2, PaO_2) be closely monitored in patients on amiodarone HCl.

LABORATORY TESTS

Elevations in liver enzymes (SGOT and SGPT) can occur. Liver enzymes in patients on relatively high maintenance doses should be monitored on a regular basis. Persistent significant elevations in the liver enzymes or hepatomegaly should alert the physician to consider reducing the maintenance dose of amiodarone HCl or discontinuing therapy.

Amiodarone HCl alters the results of thyroid-function tests, causing an increase in serum T_4 and serum reverse T_3, and a decline in serum T_3 levels. Despite these biochemical changes, most patients remain clinically euthyroid.

ELECTROLYTE DISTURBANCES

Since antiarrhythmic drugs may be ineffective or may be arrhythmogenic in patients with hypokalemia, any potassium or magnesium deficiency should be corrected before instituting and during amiodarone HCl therapy. Use caution when coadministering amiodarone HCl with drugs which may induce hypokalemia and/or hypomagnesemia.

CARCINOGENESIS, MUTAGENESIS, AND IMPAIRMENT OF FERTILITY

Amiodarone HCl was associated with a statistically significant, dose-related increase in the incidence of thyroid tumors (follicular adenoma and/or carcinoma) in rats. The incidence of thyroid tumors was greater than control even at the lowest dose level tested, *i.e.*, 5 mg/kg/day (approximately 0.08 times the maximum recommended human maintenance dose*).

Mutagenicity studies (Ames, micronucleus, and lysogenic tests) with amiodarone HCl were negative.

In a study in which amiodarone HCl was administered to male and female rats, beginning 9 weeks prior to mating, reduced fertility was observed at a dose level of 90 mg/kg/day (approximately 1.4 times the maximum recommended human maintenance dose*).

*600 mg in a 50 kg patient (dose compared on a body surface area basis).

PREGNANCY CATEGORY D

See WARNINGS, Neonatal Hypo- or Hyperthyroidism.

LABOR AND DELIVERY

It is not known whether the use of amiodarone HCl during labor or delivery has any immediate or delayed adverse effects. Preclinical studies in rodents have not shown any effect of amiodarone HCl on the duration of gestation or on parturition.

NURSING MOTHERS

Amiodarone HCl is excreted in human milk, suggesting that breast-feeding could expose the nursing infant to a significant dose of the drug. Nursing offspring of lactating rats administered amiodarone HCl have been shown to be less viable and have reduced body-weight gains. Therefore, when amiodarone HCl therapy is indicated, the mother should be advised to discontinue nursing.

PEDIATRIC USE

The safety and effectiveness of amiodarone HCl tablets in pediatric patients have not been established.

GERIATRIC USE

Clinical studies of amiodarone HCl tablets did not include sufficient numbers of subjects aged 65 and over to determine whether they respond differently from younger subjects. Other reported clinical experience has not identified differences in responses between the elderly and younger patients. In general, dose selection for an elderly patient should be cautious, usually starting at the low end of the dosing range, reflecting the greater frequency of decreased hepatic, renal, or cardiac function, and of concomitant disease or other drug therapy.

DRUG INTERACTIONS

Amiodarone is metabolized to desethylamiodarone by the cytochrome P450 (CYP450) enzyme group, specifically cytochrome P450 3A4 (CYP3A4). This isoenzyme is present in both the liver and intestines (see CLINICAL PHARMACOLOGY, Pharmacokinetics and Metabolism). Amiodarone is also known to be an inhibitor of CYP3A4. Therefore, amiodarone has the **potential** for interactions with drugs or substances that may be substrates, inhibitors or inducers of CYP3A4. While only a limited number of *in vivo* drug-drug interactions with amiodarone have been reported, the potential for other interactions should be anticipated. This is especially important for drugs associated with serious toxicity, such as other antiarrhythmics. If such drugs are needed, their dose should be reassessed and, where appropriate, plasma concentration measured.

In view of the long and variable half-life of amiodarone, potential for drug interactions exists not only with concomitant medication but also with drugs administered after discontinuation of amiodarone.

Since amiodarone is a substrate for CYP3A4, drugs/substances that inhibit CYP3A4 may decrease the metabolism and increase serum concentrations of amiodarone, with the potential for toxic effects. Reported examples of this interaction include the following:

Protease inhibitors: Protease inhibitors are known to inhibit CYP3A4 to varying degrees. Inhibition of CYP3A4 by **indinavir** has been reported to result in increased serum concentrations of amiodarone. Monitoring for amiodarone toxicity and serial measurement of amiodarone serum concentration during concomitant protease inhibitor therapy should be considered.

Histamine H_2 antagonists: **Cimetidine** inhibits CYP3A4 and can increase serum amiodarone levels.

Other substances: Grapefruit juice inhibits CYP3A4-mediated metabolism of oral amiodarone in the intestinal mucosa, resulting in increased plasma levels of amiodarone; therefore, grapefruit juice should not be taken during treatment with oral amiodarone (see DOSAGE AND ADMINISTRATION).

Amiodarone may suppress certain CYP450 enzymes (enzyme inhibition). This can result in unexpectedly high plasma levels of other drugs which are metabolized by those CYP450 enzymes and may lead to toxic effects. Reported examples of this interaction include the following:

Immunosuppressives: **Cyclosporine** (CYP3A4 substrate) administered in combination with oral amiodarone has been reported to produce persistently elevated plasma concentrations of cyclosporine resulting in elevated creatinine, despite reduction in dose of cyclosporine.

HMG-CoA reductase inhibitors: Simvastin (CYP3A4 substrate) in combination with amiodarone has been associated with reports of myopathy/rhabdomyolysis.

Cardiovasculars:

Cardiac glycosides: In patients receiving **digoxin** therapy, administration of oral amiodarone regularly results in an increase in the serum digoxin concentration that may reach toxic levels with resultant clinical toxicity. Amiodarone taken concomitantly with digoxin increases the serum digoxin concentration by 70% after 1 day. **On initiation of oral amiodarone, the need for digitalis therapy should be reviewed and the dose reduced by approximately 50% or discontinued.** If digitalis treatment is continued, serum levels should be closely monitored and patients observed for clinical evidence of toxicity. These precautions probably should apply to digitoxin administration as well.

Antiarrhythmics: Other antiarrhythmic drugs, such as **quinidine, procainamide, disopyramide,** and **phenytoin,** have been used concurrently with oral amiodarone.

There have been case reports of increased steady-state levels of quinidine, procainamide, and phenytoin during concomitant therapy with amiodarone. Phenytoin decreases serum amiodarone levels. Amiodarone taken concomitantly with quinidine increases quinidine serum concentration by 33% after 2 days. Amiodarone taken concomitantly with procainamide for less than 7 days increases plasma concentrations of procainamide and n-acetyl procainamide by 55% and 33%, respectively. Quinidine and procainamide doses should be reduced by one-third when either is administered with amiodarone. Plasma levels of **flecainide** have been reported to increase in the presence of oral amiodarone; because of this, the dosage of flecainide should be adjusted when these drugs are administered concomitantly. In general, any added antiarrhythmic drug should be initiated at a lower than usual dose with careful monitoring.

Combination of amiodarone with other antiarrhythmic therapy should be reserved for patients with life-threatening ventricular arrhythmias who are incompletely responsive to a single agent or incompletely responsive to amiodarone. During transfer to amiodarone the dose levels of previously administered agents should be reduced by 30-50% several days after the addition of amiodarone, when arrhythmia suppression should be beginning. The continued need for the other antiarrhythmic agent should be reviewed after the effects of amiodarone have been established, and discontinuation ordinarily should be attempted. If the treatment is continued, these patients should be particularly carefully monitored for adverse effects, especially conduction disturbances and exacerbation of tachyarrhythmias, as amiodarone is continued. In amiodarone-treated patients who require additional antiarrhythmic therapy, the initial dose of such agents should be approximately half of the usual recommended dose.

Antihypertensives: Amiodarone should be used with caution in patients receiving **β-receptor blocking agents** (*e.g.*, propanolol, a CYP3A4 inhibitor) or **calcium channel antagonists** (*e.g.*, verapamil, a CYP3A4 substrate, and diltiazem, a CYP3A4 inhibitor) because of the possible potentiation of bradycardia, sinus arrest, and AV block; if necessary, amiodarone can continue to be used after insertion of a pacemaker in patients with severe bradycardia or sinus arrest.

Anticoagulants: Potentiation of **warfarin**-type (CYP2C9 and CYP3A4 substrate) anticoagulant response is almost always seen in patients receiving amiodarone and can result in serious or fatal bleeding. Since the concomitant administration of warfarin with amiodarone increases the prothrombin time by 100% after 3-4 days, **the dose of the anticoagulant should be reduced by one-third to one-half, and prothrombin times should be monitored closely.**

Some drugs/substances are known to accelerate the metabolism of amiodarone by stimulating the synthesis of CYP3A4 (enzyme induction). This may lead to low amiodarone serum levels and potential decrease in efficacy. Reported examples of this interaction include the following:

Antibiotics: **Rifampin** is a potent inducer of CYP3A4. Administration of rifampin concomitantly with oral amiodarone has been shown to result in decreases in serum concentrations of amiodarone and desethylamiodarone.

Other substances, including herbal preparations: **St. John's Wort** (Hypericum perforatum) induces CYP3A4. Since amiodarone is a substrate for CYP3A4, there is the potential that the use of St. John's Wort in patients receiving amiodarone could result in reduced amiodarone levels.

Other reported interactions with amiodarone:

Fetanyl (CYP3A4 substrate) in combination with amiodarone may cause hypotension, bradycardia, decreased cardiac output.

Sinus bradycardia has been reported with oral amiodarone in combination with **lidocaine** (CYP3A4 substrate) given for local anesthesia. Seizure, associated with increased lidocaine concentrations, has been reported with concomitant administration of IV amiodarone.

Dextromethorphan is a substrate for both CYP2D6 and CYP3A4. Amiodarone inhibits CYP2D6.

Cholestyramine increases enterohepatic elimination of amiodarone and may reduce serum levels and T½.

Disopyramide increases QT prolongation which could cause arrhythmia.

Hemodynamic and electrophysiologic interactions have also been observed after concomitant administration with **propranolol, diltiazem,** and **verapamil.**

VOLATILE ANESTHETIC AGENTS

See PRECAUTIONS, Surgery, Volatile Anesthetic Agents.

In addition to the interactions noted above, chronic (>2 weeks) ***oral*** amiodarone HCl administration impairs metabolism of phenytoin, dextromethorphan, and methotrexate.

ADVERSE REACTIONS

Adverse reactions have been very common in virtually all series of patients treated with amiodarone HCl for ventricular arrhythmias with relatively large doses of drug (400 mg/day and above), occurring in about three-fourths of all patients and causing discontinuation in 7-18%. The most serious reactions are pulmonary toxicity, exacerbation of arrhythmia, and rare serious liver injury (see WARNINGS), but other adverse effects constitute important problems. They are often reversible with dose reduction or cessation of amiodarone HCl treatment. Most of the adverse effects appear to become more frequent with continued treatment beyond 6 months, although rates appear to remain relatively constant beyond 1 year. The time and dose relationships of adverse effects are under continued study.

Neurologic problems are extremely common, occurring in 20-40% of patients and including malaise and fatigue, tremor and involuntary movements, poor coordination and gait, and peripheral neuropathy; they are rarely a reason to stop therapy and may respond to dose reductions or discontinuation (see PRECAUTIONS).

Gastrointestinal complaints, most commonly nausea, vomiting, constipation, and anorexia, occur in about 25% of patients but rarely require discontinuation of drug. These commonly occur during high-dose administration (*i.e.,* loading dose) and usually respond to dose reduction or divided doses.

Ophthalmic abnormalities including optic neuropathy and/or optic neuritis, in some cases progressing to permanent blindness, papilledema, corneal degeneration, photosensitivity, eye discomfort, scotoma, lens opacities, and macular degeneration have been reported. (See WARNINGS.)

Asymptomatic corneal microdeposits are present in virtually all adult patients who have been on drug for more than 6 months. Some patients develop eye symptoms of halos, photophobia, and dry eyes. Vision is rarely affected and drug discontinuation is rarely needed.

Dermatological adverse reactions occur in about 15% of patients, with photosensitivity being most common (about 10%). Sunscreen and protection from sun exposure may be helpful, and drug discontinuation is not usually necessary. Prolonged exposure to amiodarone HCl occasionally results in a blue-gray pigmentation. This is slowly and occasionally incompletely reversible on discontinuation of drug but is of cosmetic importance only.

Cardiovascular adverse reactions, other than exacerbation of the arrhythmias, include the uncommon occurrence of congestive heart failure (3%) and bradycardia. Bradycardia usually responds to dosage reduction but may require a pacemaker for control. CHF rarely requires drug discontinuation. Cardiac conduction abnormalities occur infrequently and are reversible on discontinuation of drug.

The following side-effect rates are based on a retrospective study of 241 patients treated for 2-1515 days (mean 441.3 days).

The following side effects were each reported in 10-33% of patients:

Gastrointestinal: Nausea and vomiting.

The following side effects were each reported in 4-9% of patients:

Dermatologic: Solar dermatitis/photosensitivity.

Neurologic: Malaise and fatigue, tremor/abnormal involuntary movements, lack of coordination, abnormal gait/ataxia, dizziness, paresthesias.

Gastrointestinal: Constipation, anorexia.

Ophthalmologic: Visual disturbances.

Hepatic: Abnormal liver-function tests.

Respiratory: Pulmonary inflammation or fibrosis.

The following side effects were each reported in 1-3% of patients:

Thyroid: Hypothyroidism, hyperthyroidism.

Neurologic: Decreased libido, insomnia, headache, sleep disturbances.

Cardiovascular: Congestive heart failure, cardiac arrhythmias, SA node dysfunction.

Gastrointestinal: Abdominal pain.

Hepatic: Nonspecific hepatic disorders.

Other: Flushing, abnormal taste and smell, edema, abnormal salivation, coagulation abnormalities.

The following side effects were each reported in less than 1% of patients:

Blue skin discoloration, rash, spontaneous ecchymosis, alopecia, hypotension, and cardiac conduction abnormalities.

In surveys of almost 5000 patients treated in open US studies and in published reports of treatment with amiodarone HCl, the adverse reactions most frequently requiring discontinuation of amiodarone HCl included pulmonary infiltrates or fibrosis, paroxysmal ventricular tachycardia, congestive heart failure, and elevation of liver enzymes. Other symptoms causing discontinuations less often included visual disturbances, solar dermatitis, blue skin discoloration, hyperthyroidism, and hypothyroidism.

POSTMARKETING REPORTS

In postmarketing surveillance, sinus arrest, hepatitis, cholestatic hepatitis, cirrhosis, epididymitis, impotence, vasculitis, pseudotumor cerebri, syndrome of inappropriate antidiuretic hormone secretion (SIADH), thrombocytopenia, angioedema, bronchiolitis obliterans organizing pneumonia (possibly fatal), bronchospasm, pleuritis, pancreatitis, toxic epidermal necrolysis, myopathy, rhabdomyolysis, hemolytic anemia, aplastic anemia, pancytopenia, neutropenia, erythema multiforme, Stevens-Johnson syndrome, and exfoliative dermatitis, also have been reported in patients receiving amiodarone HCl.

DOSAGE AND ADMINISTRATION

BECAUSE OF THE UNIQUE PHARMACOKINETIC PROPERTIES, DIFFICULT DOSING SCHEDULE, AND SEVERITY OF THE SIDE EFFECTS IF PATIENTS ARE IMPROPERLY MONITORED, AMIODARONE HCl SHOULD BE ADMINISTERED ONLY BY PHYSICIANS WHO ARE EXPERIENCED IN THE TREATMENT OF LIFE-THREATENING ARRHYTHMIAS WHO ARE THOROUGHLY FAMILIAR WITH THE RISKS AND BENEFITS OF AMIODARONE HCl THERAPY, AND WHO HAVE ACCESS TO LABORATORY FACILITIES CAPABLE OF ADEQUATELY MONITORING THE EFFECTIVENESS AND SIDE EFFECTS OF TREATMENT.

In order to insure that an antiarrhythmic effect will be observed without waiting several months, loading doses are required. A uniform, optimal dosage schedule for administration of amiodarone HCl has not been determined. Because of the food effect on absorption, amiodarone HCl should be administered consistently with regard to meals (see CLINICAL PHARMACOLOGY). Individual patient titration is suggested according to the following guidelines.

For life-threatening ventricular arrhythmias, such as ventricular fibrillation or hemodynamically unstable ventricular tachycardia: Close monitoring of the patients is indicated during the loading phase, particularly until risk of recurrent ventricular tachycardia or fibrillation has abated. Because of the serious nature of the arrhythmia and the lack of predictable time course of effect, loading should be performed in a hospital setting. Loading doses of 800-1600 mg/day are required for 1-3 weeks (occasionally longer) until initial therapeutic response occurs. (Administration of amiodarone HCl in divided doses with meals is suggested for total daily doses of 1000 mg or higher, or when gastrointestinal intolerance occurs.) If side effects become excessive, the dose should be reduced. Elimination of recurrence of ventricular fibrillation and tachycardia usually occurs within 1-3 weeks, along with reduction in complex and total ventricular ectopic beats.

Since grapefruit juice is known to inhibit CYP3A4-mediated metabolism of oral amiodarone in the intestinal mucosa, resulting in increased plasma levels of amiodarone; grapefruit juice should not be taken during treatment with oral amiodarone (see DRUG INTERACTIONS).

Upon starting amiodarone HCl therapy, an attempt should be made to gradually discontinue prior antiarrhythmic drugs (see DRUG INTERACTIONS). When adequate arrhythmia control is achieved, or if side effects become prominent, amiodarone HCl dose should be reduced to 600-800 mg/day for 1 month and then to the maintenance dose, usually 400 mg/day (see CLINICAL PHARMACOLOGY, Monitoring Effectiveness). Some patients may require larger maintenance doses, up to 600 mg/day, and some can be controlled on lower doses. Amiodarone HCl may be administered as a single daily dose, or in patients with severe gastrointestinal intolerance, as a bid dose. In each patient, the chronic maintenance dose should be determined according to antiarrhythmic effect as assessed by symptoms, Holter recordings, and/or programmed electrical stimulation and by patient tolerance. Plasma concentrations may be helpful in evaluating nonresponsiveness or unexpectedly severe toxicity (see CLINICAL PHARMACOLOGY).

The lowest effective dose should be used to prevent the occurrence of side effects. In all instances, the physician must be guided by the severity of the individual patient's arrhythmia and response to therapy.

When dosage adjustments are necessary, the patient should be closely monitored for an extended period of time because of the long and variable half-life of amiodarone HCl and the difficulty in predicting the time required to attain a new steady-state level of drug. Dosage suggestions are summarized in TABLE 9.

TABLE 9

	Loading Dose (daily)	Adjustment and Maintenance Dose (daily)	
Ventricular arrhythmias	1-3 weeks	~1 month	Usual maintenance
	800-1600 mg	600-800 mg	400 mg

HOW SUPPLIED

Cordarone (amiodarone HCl) tablets are available in 200 mg, round, convex-faced, pink tablets with a raised "C" and marked "200" on one side, with reverse side scored and marked "WYETH" and "4188".

STORAGE

Keep tightly closed.

Store at room temperature, approximately 25°C (77°F).

Protect from light.

Dispense in a light-resistant, tight container.
Use carton to protect contents from light.

PRODUCT LISTING - RATED THERAPEUTICALLY EQUIVALENT

Package	Price	Labeler	NDC
Solution - Intravenous - 50 mg/ml			
3 ml x 10	$344.40	GENERIC, Abbott Pharmaceutical	00074-4348-35
Tablet - Oral - 200 mg			
60's	$119.44	FEDERAL UPPER LIMIT, H.C.F.A. F F P	99999-0212-01
60's	$198.15	GENERIC, Teva Pharmaceuticals Usa	00093-9133-06
60's	$198.15	GENERIC, Par Pharmaceutical Inc	49884-0458-02
60's	$198.16	GENERIC, Taro Pharmaceuticals U.S.A. Inc	51672-4025-04
60's	$202.91	GENERIC, Eon Labs Manufacturing Inc	00185-0144-60
60's	$211.85	GENERIC, Upsher-Smith Laboratories Inc	00245-0147-60
60's	$235.39	CORDARONE, Wyeth-Ayerst Laboratories	00008-4188-04
90's	$290.96	GENERIC, Geneva Pharmaceuticals	00781-1203-92
90's	$317.78	GENERIC, Upsher-Smith Laboratories Inc	00245-0147-90
100's	$197.93	GENERIC, Geneva Pharmaceuticals	00781-1203-60
100's	$200.66	GENERIC, Barr Laboratories Inc	00555-0917-09
100's	$277.20	GENERIC, Novopharm Usa Inc	55953-0214-40
100's	$329.00	GENERIC, Udl Laboratories Inc	51079-0906-20
100's	$353.08	GENERIC, Upsher-Smith Laboratories Inc	00245-0147-01
100's	$392.31	CORDARONE, Wyeth-Ayerst Laboratories	00008-4188-06
250's	$825.00	GENERIC, Teva Pharmaceuticals Usa	00093-9133-52
250's	$826.07	GENERIC, Par Pharmaceutical Inc	49884-0458-04

PRODUCT LISTING - EQUIVALENTS NOT AVAILABLE

Package	Price	Labeler	NDC
Solution - Intravenous - 50 mg/ml			
3 ml x 10	$337.50	GENERIC, Baxter I.V. Systems Division	10019-0131-01
3 ml x 10	$837.50	GENERIC, Baxter Pharmaceutical Products, Inc	62086-0153-03
3 ml x 10	$869.10	GENERIC, Bedford Laboratories	55390-0058-10
3 ml x 10	$1022.50	GENERIC, Faulding Pharmaceutical Company	61703-0241-03
3 ml x 10	$1057.10	CORDARONE I.V., Wyeth-Ayerst Laboratories	00008-0814-01
3 ml x 25	$2109.25	GENERIC, American Pharmaceutical Partners	63323-0616-13
3 ml x 25	$2109.50	GENERIC, American Pharmaceutical Partners	63323-0616-03
18 ml	$521.40	GENERIC, Bedford Laboratories	55390-0057-01
Tablet - Oral - 200 mg			
60's	$181.40	GENERIC, Allscripts Pharmaceutical Company	54569-5140-00
Tablet - Oral - 400 mg			
30's	$211.85	GENERIC, Upsher-Smith Laboratories Inc	00245-0145-30
100's	$458.93	GENERIC, Upsher-Smith Laboratories Inc	00245-0145-01

Amitriptyline Hydrochloride *(000213)*

For related information, see the comparative table section in Appendix A.

Categories: Depression; WHO Formulary; FDA Approved 1961 Apr; Pregnancy Category C
Drug Classes: Antidepressants, tricyclic
Brand Names: **Elavil**; Larozyl; Vanatrip
Foreign Brand Availability: Adepril (Italy); Amilit (Italy); Amineurin (Germany); Amiplin (Taiwan); Amiprin (Japan); Amitrip (New-Zealand); Amyline (Ireland); Anapsique (Mexico); Apo-Amitriptyline (Canada); Domical (England); Elatrol (Israel); Elatrolet (Israel); Enafon (Korea); Endep (Australia; New-Zealand); Lantron (Japan); Laroxyl (Benin; Burkina-Faso; Ethiopia; France; Gambia; Germany; Ghana; Guinea; Italy; Ivory-Coast; Kenya; Liberia; Malawi; Mali; Mauritania; Mauritius; Morocco; Niger; Nigeria; Senegal; Seychelles; Sierra-Leone; South-Africa; Sudan; Tanzania; Tunia; Uganda; Zambia; Zimbabwe); Miketorin (Japan); Novoprotect (Germany); Pinsaun (Taiwan); Redomex (Belgium); Sarotard (Korea); Saroten Retard (Malaysia); Saroten (Benin; Burkina-Faso; Cyprus; Denmark; Ethiopia; Finland; Gambia; Germany; Ghana; Greece; Guinea; Iran; Ivory-Coast; Kenya; Liberia; Malawi; Mali; Mauritania; Mauritius; Morocco; Niger; Nigeria; Portugal; Senegal; Seychelles; Sierra-Leone; South-Africa; Sudan; Sweden; Switzerland; Tanzania; Tunia; Uganda; Zambia; Zimbabwe); Sarotena (India); Sarotex (Netherlands; Norway); Syneudon (Germany); Teperin (Hungary; Iraq; Jordan); Trepiline (South-Africa); Tridep (India); Tripta (Malaysia; Thailand); Triptizol (Italy); Trynol (Taiwan); Tryptal (Israel); Tryptanol (Argentina; Hong-Kong; Japan; Malaysia; Mexico; New-Zealand; South-Africa; Thailand); Tryptizol (Austria; Belgium; Denmark; England; Netherlands; Norway; Portugal; Spain; Sweden; Switzerland); Trytomer (India); Uxen (Argentina)
Cost of Therapy: $28.29 (Depression; Elavil; 50 mg; 1 tablet/day; 30 day supply)
$0.98 (Depression; Generic Tablets; 50 mg; 1 tablet/day; 30 day supply)
HCFA JCODE(S): J1320 up to 20 mg IM

DESCRIPTION

Amitriptyline HCl is 3-(10,11-dihydro-5*H*-dibenzo [*a,d*] cycloheptene-5-ylidene)-*N,N*-dimethyl-1-propanamine hydrochloride. Its empirical formula is $C_{20}H_{23}N{\cdot}HCl$.

Amitriptyline HCl, a dibenzocycloheptadiene derivative, has a molecular weight of 313.87. It is a white, odorless, crystalline compound which is freely soluble in water.

Elavil (amitriptyline HCl) is supplied as 10, 25, 50, 75, 100, and 150 mg tablets and as a sterile solution for intramuscular use. Inactive ingredients of the tablets are calcium phosphate, cellulose, colloidal silicon dioxide, hydroxypropyl cellulose, hydroxypropyl methylcellulose, lactose, magnesium stearate, starch, stearic acid, talc, and titanium dioxide. *Elavil 10 mg tablets* also contain FD&C blue 1. *Elavil 25 mg tablets* also contain D&C yellow 10, FD&C blue 1, and FD&C yellow 6. *Elavil 50 mg tablets* also contain D&C yellow 10, FD&C yellow 6 and iron oxide. *Elavil 75 mg tablets* also contain FD&C yellow 6. *Elavil 100 mg tablets* also contain FD&C blue 2 and FD&C red 40. *Elavil 150 mg tablets* also contain FD&C blue 2 and FD&C yellow 6.

Each milliliter of the sterile solution contains: Amitriptyline hydrochloride: 10 mg; dextrose: 44 mg; water for injection, qs: 1 ml. *Added as Preservatives:* Methylparaben: 1.5 mg; propylparaben: 0.2 mg.

CLINICAL PHARMACOLOGY

Amitriptyline HCl is an antidepressant with sedative effects. Its mechanism of action in man is not known. It is not a monoamine oxidase inhibitor and it does not act primarily by stimulation of the central nervous system.

Amitriptyline inhibits the membrane pump mechanism responsible for uptake of norepinephrine and serotonin in adrenergic and serotonergic neurons. Pharmacologically this action may potentiate or prolong neuronal activity since reuptake of these biogenic amines is important physiologically in terminating transmitting activity. This interference with the reuptake of norepinephrine and/or serotonin is believed by some to underlie the antidepressant activity of amitriptyline.

METABOLISM

Studies in man following oral administration of ^{14}C-labeled drug indicated that amitriptyline is rapidly absorbed and metabolized. Radioactivity of the plasma was practically negligible, although significant amounts of radioactivity appeared in the urine by 4-6 hours and one-half to one-third of the drug was excreted within 24 hours.

Amitriptyline is metabolized by N-demethylation and bridge hydroxylation in man, rabbit, and rat. Virtually the entire dose is excreted as glucuronide or sulfate conjugate of metabolites, with little unchanged drug appearing in the urine. Other metabolic pathways may be involved.

INDICATIONS AND USAGE

For the relief of symptoms of depression. Endogenous depression is more likely to be alleviated than are other depressive states.

NON-FDA APPROVED INDICATIONS

Amitriptyline has also been used in the treatment of dysthymia, neuropathic and chronic pain, somatoform pain disorder, migraine and post traumatic stress disorder, although these uses are not explicitly approved by the FDA.

CONTRAINDICATIONS

Amitriptyline HCl is contraindicated in patients who have shown prior hypersensitivity to it.

It should not be given concomitantly with monoamine oxidase inhibitors. Hyperpyretic crises, severe convulsions, and deaths have occurred in patients receiving tricyclic antidepressant and monoamine oxidase inhibiting drugs simultaneously. When it is desired to replace a monoamine oxidase inhibitor with amitriptyline HCl, a minimum of 14 days should be allowed to elapse after the former is discontinued. Amitriptyline HCl should then be initiated cautiously with gradual increase in dosage until optimum response is achieved.

Amitriptyline HCl should not be given with cisapride due to the potential for increased QT interval and increased risk for arrhythmia.

This drug is not recommended for use during the acute recovery phase following myocardial infarction.

WARNINGS

Amitriptyline HCl may block the antihypertensive action of guanethidine or similarly acting compounds.

It should be used with caution in patients with a history of seizures and, because of its atropine-like action, in patients with a history of urinary retention, angle-closure glaucoma or increased intraocular pressure. In patients with angle-closure glaucoma, even average doses may precipitate an attack.

Patients with cardiovascular disorders should be watched closely. Tricyclic antidepressant drugs, including amitriptyline HCl, particularly when given in high doses, have been reported to produce arrhythmias, sinus tachycardia, and prolongation of the conduction time. Myocardial infarction and stroke have been reported with drugs of this class.

Close supervision is required when amitriptyline HCl is given to hyperthyroid patients or those receiving thyroid medication.

Amitriptyline HCl may enhance the response to alcohol and the effects of barbiturates and other CNS depressants. In patients who may use alcohol excessively, it should be borne in mind that the potentiation may increase the danger inherent in any suicide attempt or overdosage. Delirium has been reported with concurrent administration of amitriptyline and disulfiram.

USE IN PREGNANCY, PREGNANCY CATEGORY C

Teratogenic effects were not observed in mice, rats, or rabbits when amitriptyline was given orally at doses of 2-40 mg/kg/day (up to 13 times the maximum recommended human amitriptyline dose of 150 mg/day or 3 mg/kg/day for a 50 kg patient). Studies in literature have shown amitriptyline to be teratogenic in mice and hamsters when given by various routes of administration at doses of 28-100 mg/kg/day (9-33 times the maximum recommended human dose), producing multiple malformations. Another study in the rat reported that an oral dose of 25 mg/kg/day (8 times the maximum recommended human dose) produced delays in ossification of fetal vertebral bodies without other signs of embryotoxicity. In rabbits, an oral dose of 60 mg/kg/day (20 times the maximum recommended human dose) was reported to cause incomplete ossification of the cranial bones.

Amitriptyline has been shown to cross the placenta. Although a causal relationship has not been established, there have been a few reports of adverse events, including CNS effects, limb deformities, or developmental delay, in infants whose mothers had taken amitriptyline during pregnancy.

There are no adequate and well-controlled studies in pregnant women. Amitriptyline HCl should be used during pregnancy only if the potential benefit to the mother justifies the potential risk to the fetus.

NURSING MOTHERS

Amitriptyline is excreted into breast milk. In one report in which a patient received amitriptyline 100 mg/day while nursing her infant, levels of 83-141 ng/ml were detected in the mother's serum. Levels of 135-151 ng/ml were found in the breast milk, but no trace of the drug could be detected in the infant's serum.

Because of the potential for serious adverse reactions in nursing infants from amitriptyline, a decision should be made whether to discontinue nursing or to discontinue the drug, taking into account the importance of the drug to the mother.

USEAGE IN PEDIATRIC PATIENTS

In view of the lack of experience with the use of this drug in pediatric patients, it is not recommended at the present time for patients under 12 years of age.

PRECAUTIONS

Schizophrenic patients may develop increased symptoms of psychosis; patients with paranoid symptomatology may have an exaggeration of such symptoms. Depressed patients, particularly those with known manic-depressive illness, may experience a shift to mania or hypomania. In these circumstances the dose of amitriptyline may be reduced or a major tranquilizer such as perphenazine may be administered concurrently.

The possibility of suicide in depressed patients remains until significant remission occurs. Potentially suicidal patients should not have access to large quantities of this drug. Prescriptions should be written for the smallest amount feasible.

Concurrent administration of amitriptyline HCl and electroshock therapy may increase the hazards associated with such therapy. Such treatment should be limited to patients for whom it is essential.

When possible, the drug should be discontinued several days before elective surgery.

Both elevation and lowering of blood sugar levels have been reported.

Amitriptyline HCl should be used with caution in patients with impaired liver function.

INFORMATION FOR THE PATIENT

While on therapy with amitriptyline HCl, patients should be advised as to the possible impairment of mental and/or physical abilities required for performance of hazardous tasks, such as operating machinery or driving a motor vehicle.

GERIATRIC USE

Clinical experience has not identified differences in responses between elderly and younger patients. In general, dose selection for an elderly patient should be cautious, usually starting at the low end of the dosing range, reflecting the greater frequency of decreased hepatic function, concomitant disease and other drug therapy in elderly patients.

Geriatric patients are particularly sensitive to the anticholinergic side effects of tricyclic antidepressants including amitriptyline HCl. Peripheral anticholinergic effects include tachycardia, urinary retention, constipation, dry mouth, blurred vision, and exacerbation of narrow-angle glaucoma. Central nervous system anticholinergic effects include cognitive impairment, psychomotor slowing, confusion, sedation, and delirium. Elderly patients taking amitriptyline HCl may be at increased risk for falls. Elderly patients should be started on low doses of amitriptyline HCl and observed closely (see DOSAGE AND ADMINISTRATION).

DRUG INTERACTIONS

DRUGS METABOLIZED BY P450 2D6

The biochemical activity of the drug metabolizing isozyme cytochrome P450 2D6 (debrisoquin hydroxylase) is reduced in a subset of the Caucasian population (about 7-10% of Caucasians are so called "poor metabolizers"); reliable estimates of the prevalence of reduced P450 2D6 isozyme activity among Asian, African and other populations are not yet available. Poor metabolizers have higher than expected plasma concentrations of tricyclic antidepressants (TCAs) when given usual doses. Depending on the fraction of drug metabolized by P450 2D6, the increase in plasma concentration may be small, or quite large (8-fold increase in plasma AUC of the TCA).

In addition, certain drugs inhibit the activity of this isozyme and make normal metabolizers resemble poor metabolizers. An individual who is stable on a given dose of TCA may become abruptly toxic when given one of these inhibiting drugs as concomitant therapy. The drugs that inhibit cytochrome P450 2D6 include some that are not metabolized by the enzyme (quinidine; cimetidine) and many that are substrates for P450 2D6 (many other antidepressants, phenothiazines, and the Type 1C antiarrhythmics propafenone and flecainide). While all the selective serotonin reuptake inhibitors (SSRIs), *e.g.*, fluoxetine, sertraline, and paroxetine, inhibit P450 2D6, they may vary in the extent of inhibition. The extent to which SSRI-TCA interactions may pose clinical problems will depend on the degree of inhibition and the pharmacokinetics of the SSRI involved. Nevertheless, caution is indicated in the coadministration of TCAs with any of the SSRIs and also in switching from one class to the other. Of particular importance, sufficient time must elapse before initiating TCA treatment in a patient being withdrawn from fluoxetine, given the long half-life of the parent and active metabolite (at least 5 weeks may be necessary).

Concomitant use of tricyclic antidepressants with drugs that can inhibit cytochrome P450 2D6 may require lower doses than usually prescribed for either the tricyclic antidepressant or the other drug. Furthermore, whenever one of these other drugs is withdrawn from cotherapy, an increased dose of tricyclic antidepressant may be required. It is desirable to monitor TCA plasma levels whenever a TCA is going to be coadministered with another drug known to be an inhibitor of P450 2D6.

MONOAMINE OXIDASE INHIBITORS

(See CONTRAINDICATIONS.) Guanethidine or similarly acting compounds; thyroid medication; alcohol, barbiturates and other CNS depressants; and disulfiram (see WARNINGS).

When amitriptyline HCl is given with anticholinergic agents or sympathomimetic drugs, including epinephrine combined with local anesthetics, close supervision and careful adjustment of dosages are required.

Hyperpyrexia has been reported when amitriptyline HCl is administered with anticholinergic agents or with neuroleptic drugs, particularly during hot weather.

Paralytic ileus may occur in patients taking tricyclic antidepressants in combination with anticholinergic-type drugs.

Cimetidine is reported to reduce hepatic metabolism of certain tricyclic antidepressants, thereby delaying elimination and increasing steady-state concentrations of these drugs. Clinically significant effects have been reported with the tricyclic antidepressants when used concomitantly with cimetidine. Increases in plasma levels of tricyclic antidepressants, and in the frequency and severity of side effects, particularly anticholinergic, have been reported when cimetidine was added to the drug regimen. Discontinuation of cimetidine in well-controlled patients receiving tricyclic antidepressants and cimetidine may decrease the plasma levels and efficacy of the antidepressants.

Caution is advised if patients receive large doses of ethchlorvynol concurrently. Transient delirium has been reported in patients who were treated with 1 g of ethchlorvynol and 75-150 mg of amitriptyline HCl.

ADVERSE REACTIONS

Within each category the following adverse reactions are listed in order of decreasing severity. Included in the listing are a few adverse reactions which have not been reported with this specific drug. However, pharmacological similarities among the tricyclic antidepressant drugs require that each of the reactions be considered when amitriptyline is administered.

Cardiovascular: Myocardial infarction; stroke; nonspecific ECG changes and changes in AV conduction; heart block; arrhythmias; hypotension, particularly orthostatic hypotension; syncope; hypertension; tachycardia; palpitation.

CNS and Neuromuscular: Coma; seizures; hallucinations; delusions; confusional states; disorientation; incoordination; ataxia; tremors; peripheral neuropathy; numbness, tingling, and paresthesias of the extremities; extrapyramidal symptoms including abnormal involuntary movements and tardive dyskinesia; dysarthria; disturbed concentration; excitement; anxiety; insomnia; restlessness; nightmares; drowsiness; dizziness; weakness; fatigue; headache; syndrome of inappropriate ADH (antidiuretic hormone) secretion; tinnitus; alteration in EEG patterns.

Anticholinergic: Paralytic ileus; hyperpyrexia; urinary retention; dilatation of the urinary tract; constipation; blurred vision, disturbance of accommodation, increased ocular pressure, mydriasis; dry mouth.

Allergic: Skin rash; urticaria; photosensitization; edema of face and tongue.

Hematologic: Bone marrow depression including agranulocytosis, leukopenia, thrombocytopenia; purpura; eosinophilia.

Gastrointestinal: Rarely hepatitis (including altered liver function and jaundice); nausea; epigastric distress; vomiting; anorexia; stomatitis; peculiar taste; diarrhea; parotid swelling; black tongue.

Endocrine: Testicular swelling and gynecomastia in the male; breast enlargement and galactorrhea in the female; increased or decreased libido; impotence; elevation and lowering of blood sugar levels.

Other: Alopecia; edema; weight gain or loss; urinary frequency; increased perspiration.

WITHDRAWAL SYMPTOMS

After prolonged administration, abrupt cessation of treatment may produce nausea, headache, and malaise. Gradual dosage reduction has been reported to produce, within 2 weeks, transient symptoms including irritability, restlessness, and dream and sleep disturbance.

These symptoms are not indicative of addiction. Rare instances have been reported of mania or hypomania occurring within 2-7 days following cessation of chronic therapy with tricyclic antidepressants.

CAUSAL RELATIONSHIP UNKNOWN

Other reactions, reported under circumstances where a causal relationship could not be established, are listed to serve as alerting information to physicians:

Body as a Whole: Lupus-like syndrome (migratory arthritis, positive ANA and rheumatoid factor).

Digestive: Hepatic failure, ageusia.

POSTMARKETING ADVERSE EVENTS

A syndrome resembling neuroleptic malignant syndrome (NMS) has been very rarely reported after starting or increasing the dose of amitriptyline HCl, with and without concomitant medications known to cause NMS. Symptoms have included muscle rigidity, fever, mental status changes, diaphoresis, tachycardia, and tremor.

Very rare cases of serotonin syndrome (SS) have been reported with amitriptyline HCl in combination with other drugs that have a recognized association with SS.

DOSAGE AND ADMINISTRATION

ORAL DOSAGE

Dosage should be initiated at a low level and increased gradually, noting carefully the clinical response and any evidence of intolerance.

Initial Dosage for Adults

For outpatients 75 mg of amitriptyline HCl a day in divided doses is usually satisfactory. If necessary, this may be increased to a total of 150 mg/day. Increases are made preferably in the late afternoon and/or bedtime doses. A sedative effect may be apparent before the antidepressant effect is noted, but an adequate therapeutic effect may take as long as 30 days to develop.

An alternate method of initiating therapy in outpatients is to begin with 50-100 mg amitriptyline HCl at bedtime. This may be increased by 25 or 50 mg as necessary in the bedtime dose to a total of 150 mg/day.

Hospitalized patients may require 100 mg a day initially. This can be increased gradually to 200 mg a day if necessary. A small number of hospitalized patients may need as much as 300 mg a day.

Adolescent and Elderly Patients

In general, lower dosages are recommended for these patients. Ten (10) mg three times a day with 20 mg at bedtime may be satisfactory in adolescent and elderly patients who do not tolerate higher dosages.

Maintenance

The usual maintenance dosage of amitriptyline HCl is 50-100 mg/day. In some patients 40 mg/day is sufficient. For maintenance therapy the total daily dosage may be given in a single dose preferably at bedtime. When satisfactory improvement has been reached, dosage should be reduced to the lowest amount that will maintain relief of symptoms. It is appropriate to continue maintenance therapy 3 months or longer to lessen the possibility of relapse.

INTRAMUSCULAR ADMINISTRATION

Initially, 20-30 mg (2-3 ml) four times a day.

When amitriptyline HCl injection is administered intramuscularly, the effects may appear more rapidly than with oral administration.

When amitriptyline HCl injection is used for initial therapy in patients unable or unwilling to take amitriptyline HCl tablets, the tablets should replace the injection as soon as possible.

USAGE IN PEDIATRIC PATIENTS

In view of the lack of experience with the use of this drug in pediatric patients, it is not recommended at the present time for patients under 12 years of age.

PLASMA LEVELS

Because of the wide variation in the absorption and distribution of tricyclic antidepressants in body fluids, it is difficult to directly correlate plasma levels and therapeutic effect. However, determination of plasma levels may be useful in identifying patients who appear to have toxic effects and may have excessively high levels, or those in whom lack of absorption or noncompliance is suspected. Because of increased intestinal transit time and decreased hepatic metabolism in elderly patients, plasma levels are generally higher for a given oral dose of amitriptyline HCl than in younger patients. Elderly patients should be monitored carefully and quantitative serum levels obtained as clinically appropriate. Adjustments in dosage should be made according to the patient's clinical response and not on the basis of plasma levels.[14]

HOW SUPPLIED

TABLETS

Elavil tablets are available in:

10 mg: Blue, round, film coated tablets, identified with "40" debossed on one side and "ELAVIL" on the other side.

25 mg: Yellow, round, film coated tablets, identified with "45" debossed on one side and "ELAVIL" on the other side.

50 mg: Beige, round, film coated tablets, identified with "41" debossed on one side and "ELAVIL" on the other side.

75 mg: Orange, round, film coated tablets, identified with "42" debossed on one side and "ELAVIL" on the other side.

100 mg: Mauve, round, film coated tablets, identified with "43" debossed on one side and "ELAVIL" on the other side.

150 mg: Blue, capsule shaped, film coated tablets, identified with "47" debossed on one side and "ELAVIL" on the other side.

Storage: Store amitriptyline HCl tablets in a well-closed container. Avoid storage at temperatures above 30°C (86°F). In addition, amitriptyline HCl tablets 10 mg must be protected from light and stored in a well-closed, light-resistant container.

INJECTION

Elavil, 10 mg/ml: Is a clear, colorless solution, and is supplied in 10 ml vials.

Storage: Protect amitriptyline HCl injection from freezing and avoid storage above 30°C (86°F).

PRODUCT LISTING - RATED THERAPEUTICALLY EQUIVALENT

Solution - Intramuscular - 10 mg/ml

Quantity	Price	Product	NDC
10 ml	$4.50	GENERIC, Cmc-Consolidated Midland Corporation	00223-7162-10

Tablet - Oral - 10 mg

Quantity	Price	Product	NDC
10's	$1.86	GENERIC, Southwood Pharmaceuticals Inc	58016-0813-10
12's	$2.23	GENERIC, Southwood Pharmaceuticals Inc	58016-0813-12
14's	$0.76	GENERIC, Allscripts Pharmaceutical Company	54569-0172-04
15's	$2.79	GENERIC, Southwood Pharmaceuticals Inc	58016-0813-15
20's	$1.51	GENERIC, Physicians Total Care	54868-0064-03
20's	$3.72	GENERIC, Southwood Pharmaceuticals Inc	58016-0813-20
20's	$4.15	GENERIC, Prescript Pharmaceuticals	00247-0614-20
24's	$4.46	GENERIC, Southwood Pharmaceuticals Inc	58016-0813-24
30's	$1.64	GENERIC, Allscripts Pharmaceutical Company	54569-0172-00
30's	$1.67	GENERIC, Circle Pharmaceuticals Inc	00659-3027-30
30's	$1.72	GENERIC, Physicians Total Care	54868-0064-07
30's	$3.60	GENERIC, Pd-Rx Pharmaceuticals	55289-0124-30
30's	$3.79	GENERIC, Heartland Healthcare Services	61392-0143-30
30's	$3.80	GENERIC, Heartland Healthcare Services	61392-0143-39
30's	$4.54	GENERIC, Prescript Pharmaceuticals	00247-0614-30
30's	$5.58	GENERIC, Southwood Pharmaceuticals Inc	58016-0813-30
30's	$5.73	GENERIC, St. Mary'S Mpp	60760-0212-30
30's	$15.38	ELAVIL, Pharma Pac	52959-0396-30
31 x 10	$43.40	GENERIC, Vangard Labs	00615-0828-53
31 x 10	$43.40	GENERIC, Vangard Labs	00615-0828-63
31's	$3.92	GENERIC, Heartland Healthcare Services	61392-0143-31
32's	$4.05	GENERIC, Heartland Healthcare Services	61392-0143-32
45's	$5.69	GENERIC, Heartland Healthcare Services	61392-0143-45
50's	$2.12	GENERIC, Physicians Total Care	54868-0064-04
50's	$2.73	GENERIC, Allscripts Pharmaceutical Company	54569-0172-02
50's	$5.34	GENERIC, Prescript Pharmaceuticals	00247-0614-50
50's	$9.30	GENERIC, Southwood Pharmaceuticals Inc	58016-0813-50
50's	$13.94	ELAVIL, Prescript Pharmaceuticals	00247-1059-50
60's	$2.32	GENERIC, Physicians Total Care	54868-0064-02
60's	$5.74	GENERIC, Prescript Pharmaceuticals	00247-0614-60
60's	$7.59	GENERIC, Heartland Healthcare Services	61392-0143-60
60's	$7.59	GENERIC, Heartland Healthcare Services	61392-0143-65
60's	$11.15	GENERIC, Southwood Pharmaceuticals Inc	58016-0813-60
60's	$16.06	ELAVIL, Prescript Pharmaceuticals	00247-1059-60
90's	$6.93	GENERIC, Prescript Pharmaceuticals	00247-0614-90
90's	$11.38	GENERIC, Heartland Healthcare Services	61392-0143-90
90's	$11.38	GENERIC, Heartland Healthcare Services	61392-0143-95
90's	$16.73	GENERIC, Southwood Pharmaceuticals Inc	58016-0813-90
100's	$2.25	GENERIC, Cmc-Consolidated Midland Corporation	00223-0195-01
100's	$3.13	GENERIC, Physicians Total Care	54868-0064-05
100's	$3.74	GENERIC, Teva Pharmaceuticals Usa	00332-2120-09
100's	$4.25	GENERIC, Raway Pharmacal Inc	00686-0131-20
100's	$5.40	GENERIC, Moore, H.L. Drug Exchange Inc	00839-6191-06
100's	$5.45	GENERIC, Allscripts Pharmaceutical Company	54569-0172-01
100's	$5.70	FEDERAL UPPER LIMIT, H.C.F.A. F F P	99999-0213-01
100's	$5.95	GENERIC, Purepac Pharmaceutical Company	00228-2131-10
100's	$12.62	GENERIC, Ivax Corporation	00182-1018-89
100's	$13.99	GENERIC, Geneva Pharmaceuticals	00781-1486-13
100's	$15.18	GENERIC, Major Pharmaceuticals Inc	00904-0200-61
100's	$17.50	GENERIC, Qualitest Products Inc	00603-2212-21
100's	$17.90	GENERIC, Major Pharmaceuticals Inc	00904-0200-60
100's	$18.03	GENERIC, Udl Laboratories Inc	51079-0131-20
100's	$18.05	GENERIC, Mylan Pharmaceuticals Inc	00378-2610-01
100's	$18.08	GENERIC, Mutual/United Research Laboratories	00677-0475-01
100's	$18.08	GENERIC, Geneva Pharmaceuticals	00781-1486-01
100's	$18.08	GENERIC, Mutual Pharmaceutical Co Inc	53489-0104-01
100's	$18.59	GENERIC, Southwood Pharmaceuticals Inc	58016-0813-00
100's	$26.43	ELAVIL, Astra-Zeneca Pharmaceuticals	00310-0040-10
120's	$15.18	GENERIC, Heartland Healthcare Services	61392-0143-34

Tablet - Oral - 25 mg

Quantity	Price	Product	NDC
4's	$3.56	GENERIC, Prescript Pharmaceuticals	00247-0615-04
7's	$3.73	GENERIC, Prescript Pharmaceuticals	00247-0615-07
10's	$3.88	GENERIC, Prescript Pharmaceuticals	00247-0615-10
10's	$5.11	GENERIC, Pharma Pac	52959-0348-10
12's	$3.99	GENERIC, Prescript Pharmaceuticals	00247-0615-12
12's	$6.02	GENERIC, Pharma Pac	52959-0348-12
12's	$7.92	GENERIC, Pd-Rx Pharmaceuticals	55289-0730-12
14's	$7.02	GENERIC, Pharma Pac	52959-0348-14
15's	$4.15	GENERIC, Prescript Pharmaceuticals	00247-0615-15
15's	$7.47	GENERIC, Pharma Pac	52959-0348-15
15's	$9.71	ELAVIL, Physicians Total Care	54868-0409-00
15's	$10.49	GENERIC, Southwood Pharmaceuticals Inc	58016-0814-15
20's	$1.60	GENERIC, Physicians Total Care	54868-0065-04
20's	$9.90	GENERIC, Pharma Pac	52959-0348-20
20's	$13.99	GENERIC, Southwood Pharmaceuticals Inc	58016-0814-20
25's	$3.12	GENERIC, Udl Laboratories Inc	51079-0107-19
25's	$9.28	GENERIC, Pd-Rx Pharmaceuticals	55289-0730-25
25's	$17.49	GENERIC, Southwood Pharmaceuticals Inc	58016-0814-25
30's	$1.79	GENERIC, Circle Pharmaceuticals Inc	00659-3028-30
30's	$2.15	GENERIC, Pharmaceutical Corporation Of America	51655-0121-24
30's	$2.33	GENERIC, Physicians Total Care	54868-0065-02
30's	$3.28	GENERIC, Golden State Medical	60429-0016-30
30's	$4.46	GENERIC, Heartland Healthcare Services	61392-0140-30
30's	$4.46	GENERIC, Heartland Healthcare Services	61392-0140-39
30's	$4.94	GENERIC, Prescript Pharmaceuticals	00247-0615-30
30's	$6.77	GENERIC, St. Mary'S Mpp	60760-0367-30
30's	$12.26	GENERIC, Pd-Rx Pharmaceuticals	55289-0730-30
30's	$14.77	GENERIC, Pharma Pac	52959-0348-30
30's	$14.89	ELAVIL, Allscripts Pharmaceutical Company	54569-0174-00
30's	$20.98	GENERIC, Southwood Pharmaceuticals Inc	58016-0814-30
31 x 10	$50.04	GENERIC, Vangard Labs	00615-0829-53
31 x 10	$50.04	GENERIC, Vangard Labs	00615-0829-63
31's	$4.60	GENERIC, Heartland Healthcare Services	61392-0140-31
32's	$4.75	GENERIC, Heartland Healthcare Services	61392-0140-32
45's	$6.68	GENERIC, Heartland Healthcare Services	61392-0140-45
50's	$2.33	GENERIC, Physicians Total Care	54868-0065-05
50's	$22.81	GENERIC, Pharma Pac	52959-0348-50
50's	$27.18	ELAVIL, Prescript Pharmaceuticals	00247-1060-50
60's	$2.58	GENERIC, Physicians Total Care	54868-0065-03
60's	$5.90	GENERIC, Golden State Medical	60429-0016-60
60's	$6.53	GENERIC, Prescript Pharmaceuticals	00247-0615-60
60's	$7.80	GENERIC, St. Mary'S Mpp	60760-0367-60
60's	$8.91	GENERIC, Heartland Healthcare Services	61392-0140-60
60's	$8.91	GENERIC, Heartland Healthcare Services	61392-0140-65
60's	$12.93	GENERIC, Pd-Rx Pharmaceuticals	55289-0730-60
60's	$12.93	GENERIC, Pd-Rx Pharmaceuticals	58864-0022-60
60's	$27.84	GENERIC, Pharma Pac	52959-0348-60
60's	$31.94	ELAVIL, Prescript Pharmaceuticals	00247-1060-60
90's	$3.31	GENERIC, Physicians Total Care	54868-0065-07
90's	$8.12	GENERIC, Prescript Pharmaceuticals	00247-0615-90
90's	$8.53	GENERIC, Golden State Medical	60429-0016-90
90's	$13.37	GENERIC, Heartland Healthcare Services	61392-0140-90
90's	$13.37	GENERIC, Heartland Healthcare Services	61392-0140-95
90's	$13.59	GENERIC, Pd-Rx Pharmaceuticals	58864-0022-90
90's	$35.58	GENERIC, Pharma Pac	52959-0348-90
100's	$1.96	GENERIC, Purepac Pharmaceutical Company	00228-2132-10

100's	$2.75	GENERIC, Cmc-Consolidated Midland Corporation	00223-0196-01
100's	$3.56	GENERIC, Physicians Total Care	54868-0065-08
100's	$4.55	GENERIC, Raway Pharmacal Inc	00686-0107-20
100's	$5.48	FEDERAL UPPER LIMIT, H.C.F.A. F F P	99999-0213-05
100's	$6.00	GENERIC, Teva Pharmaceuticals Usa	00332-2122-09
100's	$8.65	GENERIC, Prescript Pharmaceuticals	00247-0615-00
100's	$10.46	GENERIC, Moore, H.L. Drug Exchange Inc	00839-6192-06
100's	$14.80	GENERIC, Ivax Corporation	00182-1019-89
100's	$16.15	GENERIC, Geneva Pharmaceuticals	00781-1487-13
100's	$17.10	GENERIC, Pd-Rx Pharmaceuticals	55289-0730-01
100's	$17.41	GENERIC, Major Pharmaceuticals Inc	00904-0201-61
100's	$33.78	GENERIC, Pharma Pac	52959-0348-00
100's	$35.50	GENERIC, Qualitest Products Inc	00603-2213-21
100's	$36.10	GENERIC, Mylan Pharmaceuticals Inc	00378-2625-01
100's	$36.11	GENERIC, Mutual/United Research Laboratories	00677-0476-01
100's	$36.11	GENERIC, Geneva Pharmaceuticals	00781-1487-01
100's	$36.11	GENERIC, Mutual Pharmaceutical Co Inc	53489-0105-01
100's	$36.57	GENERIC, Udl Laboratories Inc	51079-0107-20
100's	$43.80	GENERIC, Major Pharmaceuticals Inc	00904-0201-60
100's	$49.64	ELAVIL, Astra-Zeneca Pharmaceuticals	00310-0045-39
100's	$53.01	ELAVIL, Astra-Zeneca Pharmaceuticals	00310-0045-10
100's	$69.95	GENERIC, Southwood Pharmaceuticals Inc	58016-0814-00
118's	$9.60	GENERIC, Prescript Pharmaceuticals	00247-0615-52
120's	$11.10	GENERIC, Golden State Medical	60429-0016-12
120's	$17.82	GENERIC, Heartland Healthcare Services	61392-0140-34
180's	$16.30	GENERIC, Golden State Medical	60429-0016-18
200 x 5	$161.42	GENERIC, Vangard Labs	00615-0829-43

Tablet - Oral - 50 mg

10's	$9.65	GENERIC, Pharma Pac	52959-0514-10
12's	$1.49	GENERIC, Allscripts Pharmaceutical Company	54569-1519-03
15's	$17.47	GENERIC, Southwood Pharmaceuticals Inc	58016-0815-15
20's	$23.29	GENERIC, Southwood Pharmaceuticals Inc	58016-0815-20
30's	$2.01	GENERIC, Physicians Total Care	54868-0066-05
30's	$2.10	GENERIC, Major Pharmaceuticals Inc	00904-0202-46
30's	$4.15	GENERIC, Golden State Medical	60429-0017-30
30's	$4.54	GENERIC, Prescript Pharmaceuticals	00247-1201-30
30's	$5.48	GENERIC, Pd-Rx Pharmaceuticals	55289-0016-30
30's	$7.27	GENERIC, Heartland Healthcare Services	61392-0141-30
30's	$7.27	GENERIC, Heartland Healthcare Services	61392-0141-39
30's	$18.90	GENERIC, Allscripts Pharmaceutical Company	54569-1519-01
30's	$24.45	GENERIC, Pharma Pac	52959-0514-30
30's	$34.94	GENERIC, Southwood Pharmaceuticals Inc	58016-0815-30
30's	$236.60	GENERIC, Medirex Inc	57480-0303-06
31's	$7.52	GENERIC, Heartland Healthcare Services	61392-0141-31
32's	$7.76	GENERIC, Heartland Healthcare Services	61392-0141-32
45's	$10.91	GENERIC, Heartland Healthcare Services	61392-0141-45
50's	$2.62	GENERIC, Physicians Total Care	54868-0066-03
60's	$2.92	GENERIC, Physicians Total Care	54868-0066-02
60's	$6.80	GENERIC, Pd-Rx Pharmaceuticals	55289-0016-60
60's	$7.50	GENERIC, Golden State Medical	60429-0017-60
60's	$14.55	GENERIC, Heartland Healthcare Services	61392-0141-60
60's	$14.55	GENERIC, Heartland Healthcare Services	61392-0141-65
60's	$37.80	GENERIC, Allscripts Pharmaceutical Company	54569-1519-02
60's	$42.90	GENERIC, Pharma Pac	52959-0514-60
60's	$69.87	GENERIC, Southwood Pharmaceuticals Inc	58016-0815-60
90's	$11.00	GENERIC, Golden State Medical	60429-0017-90
90's	$21.82	GENERIC, Heartland Healthcare Services	61392-0141-90
90's	$21.82	GENERIC, Heartland Healthcare Services	61392-0141-95
100's	$3.25	GENERIC, Cmc-Consolidated Midland Corporation	00223-0197-01
100's	$4.12	GENERIC, Physicians Total Care	54868-0066-06
100's	$4.95	GENERIC, Raway Pharmacal Inc	00686-0133-20
100's	$6.66	FEDERAL UPPER LIMIT, H.C.F.A. F F P	99999-0213-09
100's	$7.33	GENERIC, Prescript Pharmaceuticals	00247-1201-00
100's	$10.68	GENERIC, Teva Pharmaceuticals Usa	00332-2124-09
100's	$11.19	GENERIC, Moore, H.L. Drug Exchange Inc	00839-6193-06
100's	$11.40	GENERIC, Martec Pharmaceuticals Inc	52555-0977-01
100's	$12.95	GENERIC, Purepac Pharmaceutical Company	00228-2133-10
100's	$18.30	GENERIC, Sidmak Laboratories Inc	50111-0368-01
100's	$18.92	GENERIC, Ivax Corporation	00182-1020-89
100's	$20.07	GENERIC, Major Pharmaceuticals Inc	00904-0202-61
100's	$24.49	GENERIC, Geneva Pharmaceuticals	00781-1488-13
100's	$59.08	GENERIC, Gm Pharmaceuticals	58809-0717-01
100's	$63.00	GENERIC, Qualitest Products Inc	00603-2214-21
100's	$63.00	GENERIC, Allscripts Pharmaceutical Company	54569-1519-00
100's	$63.50	GENERIC, Major Pharmaceuticals Inc	00904-0202-60
100's	$64.14	GENERIC, Mutual/United Research Laboratories	00677-0477-01
100's	$64.14	GENERIC, Geneva Pharmaceuticals	00781-1488-01
100's	$64.14	GENERIC, Mutual Pharmaceutical Co Inc	53489-0106-01
100's	$64.15	GENERIC, Mylan Pharmaceuticals Inc	00378-2650-01
100's	$64.89	GENERIC, Udl Laboratories Inc	51079-0133-20
100's	$74.62	ELAVIL, Astra-Zeneca Pharmaceuticals	00310-0041-39
100's	$94.30	ELAVIL, Astra-Zeneca Pharmaceuticals	00310-0041-10
100's	$116.45	GENERIC, Southwood Pharmaceuticals Inc	58016-0815-00
150's	$46.87	GENERIC, Pharma Pac	52959-0514-00
250's	$15.20	GENERIC, Md Pharmaceutical Inc	43567-0540-10

Tablet - Oral - 75 mg

30's	$4.54	GENERIC, Prescript Pharmaceuticals	00247-1242-30
60's	$52.20	GENERIC, Allscripts Pharmaceutical Company	54569-1864-02
100's	$2.45	GENERIC, Physicians Total Care	54868-2357-00
100's	$3.75	GENERIC, Cmc-Consolidated Midland Corporation	00223-0198-01
100's	$4.64	GENERIC, Purepac Pharmaceutical Company	00228-2134-10
100's	$7.25	GENERIC, Cmc-Consolidated Midland Corporation	00223-0199-01
100's	$7.41	FEDERAL UPPER LIMIT, H.C.F.A. F F P	99999-0213-13
100's	$8.90	GENERIC, Raway Pharmacal Inc	00686-0147-20
100's	$13.70	GENERIC, Moore, H.L. Drug Exchange Inc	00839-6194-06
100's	$14.62	GENERIC, Teva Pharmaceuticals Usa	00332-2126-09
100's	$16.92	GENERIC, Allscripts Pharmaceutical Company	54569-1864-01
100's	$23.00	GENERIC, Ivax Corporation	00182-1021-89
100's	$23.00	GENERIC, Pharma Pac	52959-0284-00
100's	$24.36	GENERIC, Major Pharmaceuticals Inc	00904-0203-61
100's	$25.81	GENERIC, Vangard Labs	00615-0831-13
100's	$25.87	GENERIC, Geneva Pharmaceuticals	00781-1489-13
100's	$87.00	GENERIC, Qualitest Products Inc	00603-2215-21
100's	$87.25	GENERIC, Major Pharmaceuticals Inc	00904-0203-60
100's	$88.10	GENERIC, Mylan Pharmaceuticals Inc	00378-2675-01
100's	$88.13	GENERIC, Mutual/United Research Laboratories	00677-0478-01
100's	$88.13	GENERIC, Geneva Pharmaceuticals	00781-1489-01
100's	$88.13	GENERIC, Mutual Pharmaceutical Co Inc	53489-0107-01
100's	$89.61	GENERIC, Udl Laboratories Inc	51079-0147-20
100's	$129.13	ELAVIL, Astra-Zeneca Pharmaceuticals	00310-0042-10

Tablet - Oral - 100 mg

14's	$25.48	GENERIC, Pharma Pac	52959-0542-14
28's	$36.41	GENERIC, Pharma Pac	52959-0542-28
30's	$2.45	GENERIC, Physicians Total Care	54868-2433-02
30's	$4.94	GENERIC, Prescript Pharmaceuticals	00247-1243-30
30's	$13.43	GENERIC, Heartland Healthcare Services	61392-0153-30
30's	$13.43	GENERIC, Heartland Healthcare Services	61392-0153-39
30's	$32.40	GENERIC, Allscripts Pharmaceutical Company	54569-2146-01
30's	$39.25	GENERIC, Pharma Pac	52959-0542-30
31's	$13.87	GENERIC, Heartland Healthcare Services	61392-0153-31
32's	$14.32	GENERIC, Heartland Healthcare Services	61392-0153-32
40's	$52.03	GENERIC, Pharma Pac	52959-0542-40
45's	$20.14	GENERIC, Heartland Healthcare Services	61392-0153-45
60's	$26.85	GENERIC, Heartland Healthcare Services	61392-0153-60
90's	$40.28	GENERIC, Heartland Healthcare Services	61392-0153-90
100's	$6.00	GENERIC, Cmc-Consolidated Midland Corporation	00223-0201-01
100's	$9.95	GENERIC, Raway Pharmacal Inc	00686-0563-20
100's	$15.00	FEDERAL UPPER LIMIT, H.C.F.A. F F P	99999-0213-16
100's	$18.48	GENERIC, Teva Pharmaceuticals Usa	00332-2128-09
100's	$19.70	GENERIC, Moore, H.L. Drug Exchange Inc	00839-6223-06
100's	$19.95	GENERIC, Purepac Pharmaceutical Company	00228-2135-10
100's	$19.95	GENERIC, Sidmak Laboratories Inc	50111-0370-01
100's	$27.90	GENERIC, Ivax Corporation	00182-1063-89
100's	$29.15	GENERIC, Major Pharmaceuticals Inc	00904-0204-61
100's	$40.19	GENERIC, Geneva Pharmaceuticals	00781-1490-13
100's	$108.00	GENERIC, Qualitest Products Inc	00603-2216-21
100's	$108.00	GENERIC, Allscripts Pharmaceutical Company	54569-2146-00
100's	$110.00	GENERIC, Major Pharmaceuticals Inc	00904-0204-60
100's	$111.10	GENERIC, Mylan Pharmaceuticals Inc	00378-2685-01
100's	$111.11	GENERIC, Mutual/United Research Laboratories	00677-0568-01
100's	$111.11	GENERIC, Geneva Pharmaceuticals	00781-1490-01
100's	$111.11	GENERIC, Mutual Pharmaceutical Co Inc	53489-0108-01
100's	$111.24	GENERIC, Udl Laboratories Inc	51079-0563-20
100's	$133.50	GENERIC, Southwood Pharmaceuticals Inc	58016-0858-00
100's	$163.31	ELAVIL, Astra-Zeneca Pharmaceuticals	00310-0043-10

Tablet - Oral - 150 mg

30's	$71.10	ELAVIL, Astra-Zeneca Pharmaceuticals	00310-0047-30
100's	$7.75	GENERIC, Cmc-Consolidated Midland Corporation	00223-0200-01
100's	$16.50	GENERIC, Raway Pharmacal Inc	00686-0564-20
100's	$22.13	GENERIC, Moore, H.L. Drug Exchange Inc	00839-6401-06
100's	$22.99	GENERIC, Ivax Corporation	00182-1486-01
100's	$23.96	FEDERAL UPPER LIMIT, H.C.F.A. F F P	99999-0213-19
100's	$26.62	GENERIC, Major Pharmaceuticals Inc	00904-0205-60
100's	$37.80	GENERIC, Geneva Pharmaceuticals	00781-1491-13
100's	$113.00	GENERIC, Qualitest Products Inc	00603-2217-21
100's	$116.15	GENERIC, Mylan Pharmaceuticals Inc	00378-2695-01
100's	$116.16	GENERIC, Mutual/United Research Laboratories	00677-0645-01
100's	$116.16	GENERIC, Geneva Pharmaceuticals	00781-1491-01
100's	$116.16	GENERIC, Mutual Pharmaceutical Co Inc	53489-0109-01
100's	$118.45	GENERIC, Udl Laboratories Inc	51079-0564-20
100's	$232.34	ELAVIL, Astra-Zeneca Pharmaceuticals	00310-0047-10

PRODUCT LISTING - EQUIVALENTS NOT AVAILABLE

Solution - Intramuscular - 10 mg/ml

10 ml	$12.66	ELAVIL, Astra-Zeneca Pharmaceuticals	00310-0049-10

Tablet - Oral - 10 mg			
15's	$5.85	GENERIC, Pharma Pac	52959-0008-15
20's	$7.52	GENERIC, Pharma Pac	52959-0008-20
30's	$6.10	GENERIC, Pharmaceutical Corporation Of America	51655-0633-24
30's	$6.78	GENERIC, Alpharma Uspd Makers Of Barre and Nmc	63874-0311-30
30's	$9.82	GENERIC, Pharma Pac	52959-0008-30
40's	$12.68	GENERIC, Pharma Pac	52959-0008-40
60's	$20.00	GENERIC, Pharma Pac	52959-0008-60
90's	$29.84	GENERIC, Pharma Pac	52959-0008-90
100's	$21.60	GENERIC, Alpharma Uspd Makers Of Barre and Nmc	63874-0311-01
120's	$39.60	GENERIC, Pharma Pac	52959-0008-02
Tablet - Oral - 25 mg			
12's	$1.26	GENERIC, Allscripts Pharmaceutical Company	54569-0175-03
14's	$1.47	GENERIC, Allscripts Pharmaceutical Company	54569-0175-05
15's	$2.37	GENERIC, Physicians Total Care	54868-0065-09
15's	$5.33	GENERIC, Allscripts Pharmaceutical Company	54569-0175-02
20's	$6.17	GENERIC, Alpharma Uspd Makers Of Barre and Nmc	63874-0430-20
30's	$10.65	GENERIC, Allscripts Pharmaceutical Company	54569-0175-00
30's	$14.67	GENERIC, Alpharma Uspd Makers Of Barre and Nmc	63874-0430-30
40's	$27.98	GENERIC, Southwood Pharmaceuticals Inc	58016-0814-40
50's	$17.75	GENERIC, Allscripts Pharmaceutical Company	54569-0175-06
50's	$34.97	GENERIC, Southwood Pharmaceuticals Inc	58016-0814-50
60's	$21.20	GENERIC, Pharmaceutical Corporation Of America	51655-0121-25
60's	$21.30	GENERIC, Allscripts Pharmaceutical Company	54569-0175-04
60's	$41.97	GENERIC, Southwood Pharmaceuticals Inc	58016-0814-60
90's	$31.95	GENERIC, Allscripts Pharmaceutical Company	54569-0175-08
90's	$62.96	GENERIC, Southwood Pharmaceuticals Inc	58016-0814-90
100's	$35.50	GENERIC, Allscripts Pharmaceutical Company	54569-0175-01
100's	$41.10	GENERIC, Alpharma Uspd Makers Of Barre and Nmc	63874-0430-01
120's	$83.94	GENERIC, Southwood Pharmaceuticals Inc	58016-0814-02
Tablet - Oral - 50 mg			
15's	$10.55	GENERIC, Alpharma Uspd Makers Of Barre and Nmc	63874-0359-15
20's	$14.22	GENERIC, Alpharma Uspd Makers Of Barre and Nmc	63874-0359-20
28's	$32.61	GENERIC, Southwood Pharmaceuticals Inc	58016-0815-28
30's	$5.89	GENERIC, Pharmaceutical Corporation Of America	51655-0082-24
30's	$21.08	GENERIC, Alpharma Uspd Makers Of Barre and Nmc	63874-0359-30
50's	$35.14	GENERIC, Alpharma Uspd Makers Of Barre and Nmc	63874-0359-50
60's	$42.18	GENERIC, Alpharma Uspd Makers Of Barre and Nmc	63874-0359-60
90's	$104.80	GENERIC, Southwood Pharmaceuticals Inc	58016-0815-90
100's	$70.27	GENERIC, Alpharma Uspd Makers Of Barre and Nmc	63874-0359-01
Tablet - Oral - 75 mg			
30's	$3.43	GENERIC, Physicians Total Care	54868-2357-02
30's	$9.40	GENERIC, Pharmaceutical Corporation Of America	51655-0062-24
Tablet - Oral - 100 mg			
14's	$18.69	GENERIC, Southwood Pharmaceuticals Inc	58016-0858-14
28's	$37.38	GENERIC, Southwood Pharmaceuticals Inc	58016-0858-28
30's	$40.05	GENERIC, Southwood Pharmaceuticals Inc	58016-0858-30
40's	$53.40	GENERIC, Southwood Pharmaceuticals Inc	58016-0858-40
50's	$66.75	GENERIC, Southwood Pharmaceuticals Inc	58016-0858-50
60's	$80.10	GENERIC, Southwood Pharmaceuticals Inc	58016-0858-60
100's	$8.93	GENERIC, Physicians Total Care	54868-2433-00
Tablet - Oral - 150 mg			
30's	$62.00	GENERIC, Southwood Pharmaceuticals Inc	58016-0710-30
60's	$124.00	GENERIC, Southwood Pharmaceuticals Inc	58016-0710-60
90's	$186.00	GENERIC, Southwood Pharmaceuticals Inc	58016-0710-90
100's	$10.91	GENERIC, Physicians Total Care	54868-2434-00
100's	$206.67	GENERIC, Southwood Pharmaceuticals Inc	58016-0710-00

Amitriptyline Hydrochloride; Chlordiazepoxide *(000214)*

For complete prescribing information, refer to the CD-ROM included with the book.

Categories: Anxiety; Depression; DEA Class CIV; FDA Approval Pre 1982; Pregnancy Category D
Drug Classes: Antidepressants, tricyclic; Anxiolytics; Benzodiazepines
Brand Names: **Limbitrol**
Foreign Brand Availability: Limbitrol F (South-Africa); Limbitryl (Italy)
Cost of Therapy: $144.31 (Depression; Limbitrol DS; 25 mg; 10 mg; 3 tablets/day; 30 day supply)
$53.40 (Depression; Generic Tablets; 25 mg; 10 mg; 3 tablets/day; 30 day supply)

DESCRIPTION

Note: The trade name has been used throughout this monograph for clarity.

Limbitrol combines for oral administration, chlordiazepoxide, an agent for the relief of anxiety and tension, and amitriptyline, an antidepressant. It is available in DS (double strength) white, film-coated tablets, each containing 10 mg chlordiazepoxide and 25 mg amitriptyline (as the hydrochloride salt); and in blue, film-coated tablets, each containing 5 mg chlordiazepoxide and 12.5 mg amitriptyline (as the hydrochloride salt). Each tablet also contains corn starch, hydroxypropyl cellulose, hydroxypropyl methylcellulose, lactose, magnesium stearate, polyethylene glycol, povidone and propylene glycol; Limbitrol tablets contain the following colorant system: FD&C blue no. 1 aluminum lake and titanium dioxide; Limbitrol DS tablets contain titanium dioxide.

Chlordiazepoxide is a benzodiazepine with the formula 7-chloro-2-(methylamino)-5-phenyl-3*H*-1,4-benzodiazepine 4-oxide. It is a slightly yellow crystalline material and is insoluble in water. The molecular weight is 299.76.

Amitriptyline is a dibenzocycloheptadiene derivative. The formula is 10,11-dihydro-*N,N*-dimethyl-5H-dibenzo[a,d]cycloheptene-$\Delta^{5,\gamma}$-propylamine hydrochloride. It is a white or practically white crystalline compound that is freely soluble in water. The molecular weight is 313.87.

INDICATIONS AND USAGE

Limbitrol is indicated for the treatment of patients with moderate to severe depression associated with moderate to severe anxiety.

The therapeutic response to Limbitrol occurs earlier and with fewer treatment failures than when either amitriptyline or chlordiazepoxide is used alone.

Symptoms likely to respond in the first week of treatment include: Insomnia, feelings of guilt or worthlessness, agitation, psychic and somatic anxiety, suicidal ideation and anorexia.

CONTRAINDICATIONS

Limbitrol is contraindicated in patients with hypersensitivity to either benzodiazepines or tricyclic antidepressants. It should not be given concomitantly with a monoamine oxidase inhibitor. Hyperpyretic crises, severe convulsions and deaths have occurred in patients receiving a tricyclic antidepressant and a monoamine oxidase inhibitor simultaneously. When it is desired to replace a monoamine oxidase inhibitor with Limbitrol, a minimum of 14 days should be allowed to elapse after the former is discontinued. Limbitrol should then be initiated cautiously with gradual increase in dosage until optimum response is achieved.

This drug is contraindicated during the acute recovery phase following myocardial infarction.

WARNINGS

Because of the atropine-like action of the amitriptyline component, great care should be used in treating patients with a history of urinary retention or angle-closure glaucoma. In patients with glaucoma, even average doses may precipitate an attack. Severe constipation may occur in patients taking tricyclic antidepressants in combination with anticholinergic-type drugs.

Patients with cardiovascular disorders should be watched closely. Tricyclic antidepressant drugs, particularly when given in high doses, have been reported to produce arrhythmias, sinus tachycardia and prolongation of conduction time. Myocardial infarction and stroke have been reported in patients receiving drugs of this class.

Because of the sedative effects of Limbitrol, patients should be cautioned about combined effects with alcohol or other CNS depressants. The additive effects may produce a harmful level of sedation and CNS depression.

Patients receiving Limbitrol should be cautioned against engaging in hazardous occupations requiring complete mental alertness, such as operating machinery or driving a motor vehicle.

Usage in Pregnancy

Safe use of Limbitrol during pregnancy and lactation has not been established. Because of the chlordiazepoxide component, please note the following:

An increased risk of congenital malformations associated with the use of minor tranquilizers (chlordiazepoxide, diazepam and meprobamate) during the first trimester of pregnancy has been suggested in several studies. Because use of these drugs is rarely a matter of urgency, their use during this period should almost always be avoided. The possibility that a woman of childbearing potential may be pregnant at the time of institution of therapy should be considered. Patients should be advised that if they become pregnant during therapy or intend to become pregnant they should communicate with their physicians about the desirability of discontinuing the drug.

Withdrawal symptoms of the barbiturate type have occurred after the discontinuation of benzodiazepines.

DOSAGE AND ADMINISTRATION

Optimum dosage varies with the severity of the symptoms and the response of the individual patient. When a satisfactory response is obtained, dosage should be reduced to the smallest

A

amount needed to maintain the remission. The larger portion of the total daily dose may be taken at bedtime. In some patients, a single dose at bedtime may be sufficient. In general, lower dosages are recommended for elderly patients.

Limbitrol DS (double strength) tablets are recommended in an initial dosage of 3 or 4 tablets daily in divided doses; this may be increased to 6 tablets daily as required. Some patients respond to smaller doses and can be maintained on 2 tablets daily.

Limbitrol tablets in an initial dosage of 3 or 4 tablets daily in divided doses may be satisfactory in patients who do not tolerate higher doses.

PRODUCT LISTING - RATED THERAPEUTICALLY EQUIVALENT

Tablet - Oral - 12.5 mg;5 mg

Size	Price	Product	NDC
14's	$18.42	LIMBITROL, Pd-Rx Pharmaceuticals	55289-0508-14
100's	$23.90	GENERIC, Major Pharmaceuticals Inc	00904-1700-60
100's	$39.49	GENERIC, Moore, H.L. Drug Exchange Inc	00839-7279-06
100's	$42.70	GENERIC, Qualitest Products Inc	00603-2690-21
100's	$68.62	LIMBITROL, Roche Laboratories	00140-0070-49
100's	$79.17	GENERIC, Mylan Pharmaceuticals Inc	00378-0211-01
100's	$82.38	LIMBITROL, Allscripts Pharmaceutical Company	54569-0173-00
100's	$113.71	LIMBITROL, Roche Laboratories	00140-0070-01
100's	$132.73	LIMBITROL, Physicians Total Care	54868-0501-00

Tablet - Oral - 25 mg;10 mg

Size	Price	Product	NDC
100's	$59.33	GENERIC, Moore, H.L. Drug Exchange Inc	00839-7280-06
100's	$62.50	GENERIC, Qualitest Products Inc	00603-2691-21
100's	$96.03	LIMBITROL DS, Roche Laboratories	00140-0071-49
100's	$111.72	GENERIC, Mylan Pharmaceuticals Inc	00378-0277-01
100's	$160.34	LIMBITROL DS, Roche Laboratories	00140-0071-01

PRODUCT LISTING - EQUIVALENTS NOT AVAILABLE

Tablet - Oral - 12.5 mg;5 mg

Size	Price	Product	NDC
100's	$24.37	GENERIC, Physicians Total Care	54868-2206-01
100's	$113.71	LIMBITROL, Icn Pharmaceuticals Inc	00187-3805-10

Tablet - Oral - 25 mg;10 mg

Size	Price	Product	NDC
100's	$160.34	LIMBITROL DS, Icn Pharmaceuticals Inc	00187-3806-10

Amitriptyline Hydrochloride; Perphenazine *(000215)*

Categories: Anxiety; Depression; Schizophrenia; FDA Approval Pre 1982; Pregnancy Category D
Drug Classes: Antidepressants, tricyclic; Antipsychotics; Anxiolytics; Phenothiazines
Brand Names: Etrafon; **Triavil**
Foreign Brand Availability: Anxipress-D (Thailand); Longopax (Germany); Minitran (Greece); Mutabase (Spain); Mutabon (Italy); Mutabon-A (Bahamas; Barbados; Belize; Bermuda; Curacao; Guyana; Jamaica; Netherland-Antilles; Surinam; Trinidad); Mutabon-D (Bahamas; Barbados; Belize; Bermuda; Curacao; Guyana; Jamaica; Netherland-Antilles; Surinam; Trinidad); Mutabon-F (Bahamas; Barbados; Belize; Bermuda; Curacao; Guyana; Jamaica; Netherland-Antilles; Surinam; Trinidad); Mutabon-M (Bahamas; Barbados; Belize; Bermuda; Curacao; Guyana; Jamaica; Netherland-Antilles; Surinam; Trinidad); Mutabon A (Bahrain; Cyprus; Egypt; Iran; Iraq; Israel; Jordan; Libya; Mexico; Netherlands; Oman; Qatar; Saudi-Arabia; Syria; United-Arab-Emirates); Mutabon D (Bahrain; Cyprus; Egypt; Indonesia; Iran; Iraq; Israel; Jordan; Libya; Mexico; Netherlands; Oman; Qatar; Saudi-Arabia; Syria; United-Arab-Emirates); Mutabon F (Bahrain; Cyprus; Egypt; Iran; Iraq; Israel; Jordan; Libya; Netherlands; Oman; Qatar; Saudi-Arabia; Syria; United-Arab-Emirates); Mutabon M (Bahrain; Cyprus; Egypt; Indonesia; Iran; Iraq; Israel; Jordan; Libya; Oman; Qatar; Saudi-Arabia; Syria; United-Arab-Emirates); Neuragon-A (Thailand); Neuragon-B (Thailand); Pertriptyl (Finland); Triptafen (England; Ireland); Triptafen M (England)
Cost of Therapy: $67.64 (Depression; Triavil; 25 mg; 2 mg; 2 tablets/day; 30 day supply)
$17.25 (Depression; Generic Tablets; 25 mg; 2 mg; 2 tablets/day; 30 day supply)

DESCRIPTION

Perphenazine and amitriptyline hydrochloride tablets are available in multiple strengths to afford dosage flexibility for optimum management. They are available as perphenazine and amitriptyline hydrochloride 2-10 tablets, 2 mg perphenazine and 10 mg amitriptyline hydrochloride; perphenazine and amitriptyline hydrochloride 2-25 tablets , 2 mg perphenazine and 25 mg amitriptyline hydrochloride; perphenazine and amitriptyline hydrochloride 4-25 tablets, 4 mg perphenazine and 25 mg amitriptyline hydrochloride.

FOR COMPLETE PRESCRIBING INFORMATION, REFER TO THE INDIVIDUAL DRUG MONOGRAPHS (AMITRIPTYLINE HYDROCHLORIDE; PERPHENAZINE).

INDICATIONS AND USAGE

Perphenazine and amitriptyline HCl tablets are indicated for the treatment of patients with moderate to severe anxiety and/or agitation and depressed mood; patients with depression in whom anxiety and/or agitation are moderate or severe; patients with anxiety and depression associated with chronic physical disease; patients in whom depression and anxiety cannot be clearly differentiated.

Schizophrenic patients who have associated symptoms of depression should be considered for therapy with perphenazine and amitriptyline HCl.

DOSAGE AND ADMINISTRATION

INITIAL DOSAGE

In psychoneurotic patients whose anxiety and depression warrant combined therapy, one perphenazine and amitriptyline HCl tablet (2-25) or one perphenazine and amitriptyline HCl tablet (4-25) three or four times a day is recommended.

In elderly patients and adolescents, a lower initial dosage may be needed. The dosage may then be adjusted cautiously to produce an adequate response.

In more severely ill patients with schizophrenia, two perphenazine and amitriptyline HCl tablets (4-25) three times a day are recommended as the initial dosage. If necessary, a fourth dose may be given at bedtime. The total daily dosage should not exceed 8 tablets of any strength.

MAINTENANCE DOSAGE

Depending on the condition being treated, the onset of therapeutic response may vary from a few days to a few weeks or even longer. After a satisfactory response is noted, dosage should be reduced to the smallest dose which is effective for relief of the symptoms for which perphenazine and amitriptyline HCl tablets are being administered. A useful maintenance dosage is one perphenazine and amitriptyline HCl tablet (2-25) or one perphenazine and amitriptyline HCl tablet (4-25) two to four times a day. In some patients, maintenance dosage is required for many months.

Perphenazine and amitriptyline hydrochloride 2-10 tablets can be used to increase flexibility in adjusting maintenance dosage to the lowest amount consistent with relief of symptoms.

Storage: Store perphenazine and amitriptyline hydrochloride 2-10, 2-25, and 4-25 tablets between 2°C and 25°C (36°F and 77°F). In addition, protect unit-dose packages from excessive moisture.

PRODUCT LISTING - RATED THERAPEUTICALLY EQUIVALENT

Tablet - Oral - 10 mg;2 mg

Size	Price	Product	NDC
30's	$15.15	GENERIC, Heartland Healthcare Services	61392-0071-30
30's	$15.15	GENERIC, Heartland Healthcare Services	61392-0071-39
31's	$15.65	GENERIC, Heartland Healthcare Services	61392-0071-31
32's	$16.16	GENERIC, Heartland Healthcare Services	61392-0071-32
45's	$22.72	GENERIC, Heartland Healthcare Services	61392-0071-45
60's	$30.30	GENERIC, Heartland Healthcare Services	61392-0071-60
90's	$45.44	GENERIC, Heartland Healthcare Services	61392-0071-90
100's	$7.04	FEDERAL UPPER LIMIT, H.C.F.A. F F P	99999-0215-01
100's	$15.00	GENERIC, Aligen Independent Laboratories Inc	00405-4787-01
100's	$17.68	GENERIC, Qualitest Products Inc	00603-5115-21
100's	$18.40	GENERIC, Major Pharmaceuticals Inc	00904-1820-60
100's	$18.95	GENERIC, Watson Laboratories Inc	52544-0706-01
100's	$19.24	GENERIC, Moore, H.L. Drug Exchange Inc	00839-6225-06
100's	$24.75	GENERIC, Martec Pharmaceuticals Inc	52555-0460-01
100's	$24.95	GENERIC, Ivax Corporation	00182-1235-01
100's	$24.95	GENERIC, Mylan Pharmaceuticals Inc	00378-0330-01
100's	$29.13	GENERIC, Major Pharmaceuticals Inc	00904-1820-61
100's	$38.84	GENERIC, Major Pharmaceuticals Inc	00904-7636-61
100's	$54.86	TRIAVIL, Lotus Biochemical Corporation	59417-0401-71

Tablet - Oral - 10 mg;4 mg

Size	Price	Product	NDC
100's	$19.00	GENERIC, Aligen Independent Laboratories Inc	00405-4789-01
100's	$19.54	GENERIC, Qualitest Products Inc	00603-5117-21
100's	$20.30	GENERIC, Major Pharmaceuticals Inc	00904-1840-60
100's	$21.20	GENERIC, Watson Laboratories Inc	52544-0708-01
100's	$24.30	GENERIC, Moore, H.L. Drug Exchange Inc	00839-6226-06
100's	$28.20	GENERIC, Martec Pharmaceuticals Inc	52555-0462-01
100's	$28.50	GENERIC, Ivax Corporation	00182-1237-01
100's	$28.50	GENERIC, Mylan Pharmaceuticals Inc	00378-0042-01
100's	$52.88	GENERIC, Major Pharmaceuticals Inc	00904-7638-61

Tablet - Oral - 25 mg;2 mg

Size	Price	Product	NDC
30's	$20.49	GENERIC, Heartland Healthcare Services	61392-0072-30
30's	$20.49	GENERIC, Heartland Healthcare Services	61392-0072-39
31's	$21.17	GENERIC, Heartland Healthcare Services	61392-0072-31
32's	$21.86	GENERIC, Heartland Healthcare Services	61392-0072-32
45's	$30.74	GENERIC, Heartland Healthcare Services	61392-0072-45
60's	$40.98	GENERIC, Heartland Healthcare Services	61392-0072-60
90's	$61.47	GENERIC, Heartland Healthcare Services	61392-0072-90
100's	$8.69	FEDERAL UPPER LIMIT, H.C.F.A. F F P	99999-0215-05
100's	$14.25	GENERIC, Interstate Drug Exchange Inc	00814-5956-14
100's	$19.50	GENERIC, Aligen Independent Laboratories Inc	00405-4788-01
100's	$22.61	GENERIC, Qualitest Products Inc	00603-5116-21
100's	$23.40	GENERIC, Major Pharmaceuticals Inc	00904-1825-60
100's	$24.50	GENERIC, Moore, H.L. Drug Exchange Inc	00839-6217-06
100's	$28.75	GENERIC, Martec Pharmaceuticals Inc	52555-0461-01
100's	$28.89	GENERIC, Geneva Pharmaceuticals	00781-1273-01
100's	$28.95	GENERIC, Ivax Corporation	00182-1236-01
100's	$28.95	GENERIC, Mylan Pharmaceuticals Inc	00378-0442-01
100's	$28.95	GENERIC, Watson Laboratories Inc	52544-0707-01
100's	$33.64	GENERIC, Major Pharmaceuticals Inc	00904-1825-61
100's	$44.85	GENERIC, Major Pharmaceuticals Inc	00904-7637-61
100's	$70.42	TRIAVIL, Lotus Biochemical Corporation	59417-0402-71

Tablet - Oral - 25 mg;4 mg

Size	Price	Product	NDC
100's	$14.38	GENERIC, Pd-Rx Pharmaceuticals	55289-0185-17
100's	$21.00	GENERIC, Aligen Independent Laboratories Inc	00405-4790-01
100's	$25.11	GENERIC, Qualitest Products Inc	00603-5118-21
100's	$25.80	GENERIC, Major Pharmaceuticals Inc	00904-1845-60
100's	$25.83	GENERIC, Geneva Pharmaceuticals	00781-1267-01
100's	$26.99	GENERIC, Moore, H.L. Drug Exchange Inc	00839-6227-06
100's	$31.00	GENERIC, Martec Pharmaceuticals Inc	52555-0464-01
100's	$31.30	GENERIC, Ivax Corporation	00182-1238-01
100's	$31.30	GENERIC, Mylan Pharmaceuticals Inc	00378-0574-01
100's	$31.30	GENERIC, Watson Laboratories Inc	52544-0709-01
100's	$40.39	GENERIC, Major Pharmaceuticals Inc	00904-1845-61
100's	$48.00	GENERIC, Geneva Pharmaceuticals	00781-1267-13
100's	$76.39	TRIAVIL, Lotus Biochemical Corporation	59417-0404-71

Tablet - Oral - 50 mg;4 mg

Size	Price	Product	NDC
100's	$35.55	GENERIC, Major Pharmaceuticals Inc	00904-1850-60
100's	$42.40	GENERIC, Qualitest Products Inc	00603-5119-21
100's	$43.27	GENERIC, Moore, H.L. Drug Exchange Inc	00839-7233-06

100's	$61.14	GENERIC, Major Pharmaceuticals Inc	00904-1850-61
100's	$74.25	GENERIC, Mylan Pharmaceuticals Inc	00378-0073-01

PRODUCT LISTING - RATED NOT THERAPEUTICALLY EQUIVALENT

Tablet - Oral - 10 mg;2 mg			
100's	$77.93	ETRAFON 2-10, Schering Corporation	00085-0287-08
100's	$88.66	ETRAFON 2-10, Schering Corporation	00085-0287-04
Tablet - Oral - 25 mg;2 mg			
100's	$97.92	ETRAFON 2-25, Schering Corporation	00085-0598-08
100's	$112.74	ETRAFON 2-25, Schering Corporation	00085-0598-04
Tablet - Oral - 25 mg;4 mg			
100's	$122.44	ETRAFON FORTE, Schering Corporation	00085-0720-04
100's	$127.28	ETRAFON FORTE, Schering Corporation	00085-0720-08

PRODUCT LISTING - EQUIVALENTS NOT AVAILABLE

Tablet - Oral - 10 mg;2 mg			
50's	$5.14	GENERIC, Physicians Total Care	54868-0124-02
100's	$8.62	GENERIC, Physicians Total Care	54868-0124-03
Tablet - Oral - 10 mg;4 mg			
30's	$4.59	GENERIC, Physicians Total Care	54868-1483-01
Tablet - Oral - 25 mg;2 mg			
30's	$3.87	GENERIC, Physicians Total Care	54868-0125-02
50's	$5.33	GENERIC, Physicians Total Care	54868-0125-03
100's	$8.17	GENERIC, Physicians Total Care	54868-0125-04
100's	$28.89	GENERIC, Allscripts Pharmaceutical Company	54569-3270-00
200's	$16.33	GENERIC, Physicians Total Care	54868-0125-05
Tablet - Oral - 50 mg;4 mg			
100's	$24.21	GENERIC, Physicians Total Care	54868-3927-00

Amlodipine Besylate *(003072)*

For related information, see the comparative table section in Appendix A.

Categories: Angina, chronic stable; Angina, variant; Hypertension, essential; Pregnancy Category C; FDA Approved 1992 Jul
Drug Classes: Calcium channel blockers
Brand Names: Norvasc
Foreign Brand Availability: Amcard (India); Amdepin (Benin; Burkina-Faso; Ethiopia; Gambia; Ghana; Guinea; Ivory-Coast; Kenya; Liberia; Malawi; Mali; Mauritania; Mauritius; Morocco; Niger; Nigeria; Senegal; Seychelles; Sierra-Leone; Sudan; Tanzania; Tunia; Uganda; Zambia; Zimbabwe); Amdipin (Colombia); Amlocar (Peru); Amlodin (Japan); Amlopine (Thailand); Amlor (Belgium; France; Israel); Amlosyn (Colombia); Calchek (India); Cardinor (Colombia); Duactin 5 (Bahrain; Cyprus; Egypt; Iran; Iraq; Jordan; Kuwait; Lebanon; Libya; Oman; Qatar; Republic-of-Yemen; Saudi-Arabia; Syria; United-Arab-Emirates); Eucoran (Colombia); Istin (England; Ireland); Lama (India); Mydopine (Bahrain; Cyprus; Egypt; Iran; Iraq; Jordan; Kuwait; Lebanon; Libya; Oman; Qatar; Republic-of-Yemen; Saudi-Arabia; Syria; United-Arab-Emirates); Normodipine (Singapore); Norvas (Colombia; Mexico; Spain); Norvask (Bulgaria; Indonesia); Tensivask (Indonesia); Vasten (Colombia)
Cost of Therapy: $43.88 (Hypertension; Norvasc; 5 mg; 1 tablet/day; 30 day supply)

DESCRIPTION

Norvasc is the besylate salt of amlodipine, and is a long-acting calcium channel blocker.

Norvasc is chemically described as (R.S.) 3-ethyl-5-methyl-2-(2-aminoethoxymethyl)-4-(2-chlorophenyl)-1,4-dihydro-6-methyl-3,5-pyridinedicarboxylate benzenesulphonate. Its empirical formula is $C_{20}H_{25}ClN_2O_5 \cdot C_6H_6O_3S$.

Amlodipine besylate is a white crystalline powder with a molecular weight of 567.1. It is slightly soluble in water and sparingly soluble in ethanol. Norvasc tablets are formulated as white tablets equivalent to 2.5, 5 and 10 mg of amlodipine for oral administration. In addition to the active ingredient, amlodipine besylate, each tablet contains the following inactive ingredients: microcrystalline cellulose, dibasic calcium phosphate anhydrous, sodium starch glycolate, and magnesium stearate.

CLINICAL PHARMACOLOGY

MECHANISM OF ACTION

Amlodipine besylate is a dihydropyridine calcium antagonist (calcium ion antagonist or slow-channel blocker) that inhibits the transmembrane influx of calcium ions into vascular smooth muscle and cardiac muscle. Experimental data suggest that amlodipine besylate binds to both dihydropyridine and nondihydropyridine binding sites. The contractile processes of cardiac muscle and vascular smooth muscle are dependent upon the movement of extracellular calcium ions into these cells through specific ion channels. Amlodipine besylate inhibits calcium ion influx across cell membranes selectively, with a greater effect on vascular smooth muscle cells than on cardiac muscle cells. Negative inotropic effects can be detected *in vitro* but such effects have not been seen in intact animals at therapeutic doses. Serum calcium concentration is not affected by amlodipine besylate. Within the physiologic pH range, amlodipine besylate is an ionized compound (pKa = 8.6), and its kinetic interaction with the calcium channel receptor is characterized by a gradual rate of association and dissociation with the receptor binding site, resulting in a gradual onset of effect.

Amlodipine besylate is a peripheral arterial vasodilator that acts directly on vascular smooth muscle to cause a reduction in peripheral vascular resistance and reduction in blood pressure.

The precise mechanisms by which amlodipine besylate relieves angina have not been fully delineated, but are thought to include the following:

Exertional Angina: In patients with exertional angina, amlodipine besylate reduces the total peripheral resistance (afterload) against which the heart works and reduces the rate pressure product, and thus myocardial oxygen demand, at any given level of exercise.

Vasospastic Angina: Amlodipine besylate has been demonstrated to block constriction and restore blood flow in coronary arteries and arterioles in response to calcium, potassium epinephrine, serotonin, and thromboxane A_2 analog in experimental animal models and in human coronary vessels *in vitro*. This inhibition of coronary spasm is responsible for the effectiveness of amlodipine besylate in vasospastic (Prinzmetal's or variant) angina.

PHARMACOKINETICS AND METABOLISM

After oral administration of therapeutic doses of amlodipine besylate, absorption produces peak plasma concentrations between 6 and 12 hours. Absolute bioavailability has been estimated to be between 64 and 90%. The bioavailability of amlodipine besylate is not altered by the presence of food.

Amlodipine besylate is extensively (about 90%) converted to inactive metabolites via hepatic metabolism with 10% of the parent compound and 60% of the metabolites excreted in the urine. *Ex vivo* studies have shown that approximately 93% of the circulating drug is bound to plasma proteins in hypertensive patients. Elimination from the plasma is biphasic with a terminal elimination half-life of about 30-50 hours. Steady-state plasma levels of amlodipine besylate are reached after 7-8 days of consecutive daily dosing.

The pharmacokinetics of amlodipine besylate are not significantly influenced by renal impairment. Patients with renal failure may therefore receive the usual initial dose.

Elderly patients and patients with hepatic insufficiency have decreased clearance of amlodipine with a resulting increase in AUC of approximately 40-60%, and a lower initial dose may be required. A similar increase in AUC was observed in patients with moderate to severe heart failure.

PHARMACODYNAMICS

Hemodynamics

Following administration of therapeutic doses to patients with hypertension, amlodipine besylate produces vasodilation resulting in a reduction of supine and standing blood pressures. These decreases in blood pressure are not accompanied by a significant change in heart rate or plasma catecholamine levels with chronic dosing. Although the acute intravenous administration of amlodipine decreases arterial blood pressure and increases heart rate in hemodynamic studies of patients with chronic stable angina, chronic administration of oral amlodipine in clinical trials did not lead to clinically significant changes in heart rate or blood pressures in normotensive patients with angina.

With chronic once daily oral administration, antihypertensive effectiveness is maintained for at least 24 hours. Plasma concentrations correlate with effect in both young and elderly patients. The magnitude of reduction in blood pressure with amlodipine besylate is also correlated with the height of pretreatment elevation; thus, individuals with moderate hypertension (diastolic pressure 105-114 mm Hg) had about a 50% greater response than patients with mild hypertension (diastolic pressure 90-104 mm Hg). Normotensive subjects experienced no clinically significant change in blood pressures (+1/-2 mm Hg).

In hypertensive patients with normal renal function, therapeutic doses of amlodipine besylate resulted in a decrease in renal vascular resistance and an increase in glomerular filtration rate and effective renal plasma flow without change in filtration fraction or proteinuria.

As with other calcium channel blockers, hemodynamic measurements of cardiac function at rest and during exercise (or pacing) in patients with normal ventricular function treated with amlodipine besylate have generally demonstrated a small increase in cardiac index without significant influence on dP/dt or on left ventricular end diastolic pressure or volume. In hemodynamic studies, amlodipine besylate has not been associated with a negative inotropic effect when administered in the therapeutic dose range to intact animals and man, even when coadministered with beta-blockers to man. Similar findings, however, have been observed in normals or well-compensated patients with heart failure with agents possessing significant negative inotropic effects.

STUDIES IN PATIENTS WITH CONGESTIVE HEART FAILURE

Amlodipine besylate has been compared to placebo in four 8-12 week studies of patients with NYHA class II/III heart failure, involving a total of 697 patients. In these studies, there was no evidence of worsened heart failure based on measures of exercise tolerance, NYHA classification, symptoms, or LVEF. In a long-term (follow-up at least 6 months, mean 13.8 months) placebo-controlled mortality/morbidity study of amlodipine besylate 5-10 mg in 1153 patients with NYHA classes III (n=931) or IV (n=222) heart failure on stable doses of diuretics, digoxin, and ACE inhibitors, amlodipine besylate had no effect on the primary endpoint of the study which was the combined endpoint of all-cause mortality and cardiac morbidity (as defined by life-threatening arrhythmia, acute myocardial infarction, or hospitalization for worsened heart failure), or on NYHA classification, or symptoms of heart failure. Total combined all-cause mortality and cardiac morbidity events were 222/571 (39%) for patients on amlodipine besylate and 246/583 (42%) for patients on placebo; the cardiac morbid events represented about 25% of the endpoints in the study.

ELECTROPHYSIOLOGIC EFFECTS

Amlodipine besylate does not change sinoatrial nodal function or atrioventricular conduction in intact animals or man. In patients with chronic stable angina, intravenous administration of 10 mg did not significantly alter A-H and H-V conduction and sinus node recovery time after pacing. Similar results were obtained in patients receiving amlodipine besylate and concomitant beta blockers. In clinical studies in which amlodipine besylate was administered in combination with beta-blockers to patients with either hypertension or angina, no adverse effects on electrocardiographic parameters were observed. In clinical trials with angina patients alone, amlodipine besylate therapy did not alter electrocardiographic intervals or produce higher degrees of AV blocks.

EFFECTS IN HYPERTENSION

The antihypertensive efficacy of amlodipine besylate has been demonstrated in a total of 15 double-blind, placebo-controlled, randomized studies involving 800 patients on amlodipine besylate and 538 on placebo. Once daily administration produced statistically significant placebo-corrected reductions in supine and standing blood pressures at 24 hours postdose, averaging about 12/6 mm Hg in the standing position and 13/7 mm Hg in the supine position in patients with mild to moderate hypertension. Maintenance of the blood pressure effect over the 24 hour dosing interval was observed, with little difference in peak and trough effect. Tolerance was not demonstrated in patients studied for up to 1 year. The 3 parallel, fixed dose, dose response studies showed that the reduction in supine and standing blood pressures was dose-related within the recommended dosing range. Effects on diastolic pressure were similar in young and older patients. The effect on systolic pressure was greater in older patients, perhaps because of greater baseline systolic pressure. Effects were similar in black and white patients.

EFFECTS IN CHRONIC STABLE ANGINA

The effectiveness of 5-10 mg/day of amlodipine besylate in exercise-induced angina has been evaluated in 8 placebo-controlled, double-blind clinical trials of up to 6 weeks duration involving 1038 patients (684 amlodipine besylate, 354 placebo) with chronic stable angina. In 5 of the 8 studies significant increases in exercise time (bicycle or treadmill) were seen with the 10 mg dose. Increases in symptom-limited exercise time averaged 12.8% (63 sec) for amlodipine besylate 10 mg, and averaged 7.9% (38 sec) for amlodipine besylate 5 mg. Amlodipine besylate 10 mg also increased time to 1 mm ST segment deviation in several studies and decreased angina attack rate. The sustained efficacy of amlodipine besylate in angina patients has been demonstrated over long-term dosing. In patients with angina there were no clinically significant reductions in blood pressures (4/1 mm Hg) or changes in heart rate (+0.3 bpm).

EFFECTS IN VASOSPASTIC ANGINA

In a double-blind, placebo-controlled clinical trial of 4 weeks duration in 50 patients, amlodipine besylate therapy decreased attacks by approximately 4/week compared with a placebo decrease of approximately 1/week ($p < 0.01$). Two (2) of 23 amlodipine besylate and 7 of 27 placebo patients discontinued from the study due to lack of clinical improvement.

INDICATIONS AND USAGE

Hypertension: Amlodipine besylate is indicated for the treatment of hypertension. It may be used alone or in combination with other antihypertensive agents.

Chronic Stable Angina: Amlodipine besylate is indicated for the treatment of chronic stable angina. Amlodipine besylate may be used alone or in combination with other antianginal agents.

Vasospastic Angina (Prinzmetal's or variant angina): Amlodipine besylate is indicated for the treatment of confirmed or suspected vasospastic angina. Amlodipine besylate may be used as monotherapy or in combination with other antianginal drugs.

NON-FDA APPROVED INDICATIONS

Recent data have shown that the use of amlodipine is associated with a significant decrease in left ventricular (LV) mass in hypertensive patients with LV hypertrophy, a significant decrease in urinary albumin excretory rate in hypertensive patients with non-insulin dependent diabetes mellitus, and significant pulmonary artery vasodilation in patients with pulmonary hypertension.

CONTRAINDICATIONS

Amlodipine besylate is contraindicated in patients with known sensitivity to amlodipine.

WARNINGS

INCREASED ANGINA AND/OR MYOCARDIAL INFARCTION

Rarely, patients, particularly those with severe obstructive coronary artery disease, have developed documented increased frequency, duration and/or severity of angina or acute myocardial infarction on starting calcium channel blocker therapy or at the time of dosage increase. The mechanism of this effect has not been elucidated.

PRECAUTIONS

GENERAL

Since the vasodilation induced by amlodipine besylate is gradual in onset, acute hypotension has rarely been reported after oral administration of amlodipine besylate. Nonetheless, caution should be exercised when administering amlodipine besylate as with any other peripheral vasodilator particularly in patients with severe aortic stenosis.

USE IN PATIENTS WITH CONGESTIVE HEART FAILURE

In general, calcium channel blockers should be used with caution in patients with heart failure. Amlodipine besylate (5-10 mg/day) has been studied in a placebo-controlled trial of 1153 patients with NYHA Class III or IV heart failure (see CLINICAL PHARMACOLOGY) on stable doses of ACE inhibitor, digoxin, and diuretics. Follow-up was at least 6 months, with a mean of about 14 months. There was no overall adverse effect on survival or cardiac morbidity (as defined by life-threatening arrhythmia, acute myocardial infarction, or hospitalization for worsened heart failure). Amlodipine besylate has been compared to placebo in four 8-12 week studies of patients with NYHA class II/III heart failure, involving a total of 697 patients. In these studies, there was no evidence of worsened heart failure based on measures of exercise tolerance, NYHA classification, symptoms, or LVEF.

BETA-BLOCKER WITHDRAWAL

Amlodipine besylate is not a beta-blocker and therefore gives no protection against the dangers of abrupt beta-blocker withdrawal; any such withdrawal should be by gradual reduction of the dose of beta-blocker.

PATIENTS WITH HEPATIC FAILURE

Since amlodipine besylate is extensively metabolized by the liver and the plasma elimination half-life ($T_{1/2}$) is 56 hours in patients with impaired hepatic function, caution should be exercised when administering amlodipine besylate to patients with severe hepatic impairment.

DRUG/LABORATORY TEST INTERACTIONS

None known.

CARCINOGENESIS, MUTAGENESIS, AND IMPAIRMENT OF FERTILITY

Rats and mice treated with amlodipine in the diet for 2 years, at concentrations calculated to provide daily dosage levels of 0.5, 1.25, and 2.5 mg/kg/day showed no evidence of carcinogenicity. The highest dose (for mice, similar to, and for rats twice [based on patient weight of 50 kg] the maximum recommended clinical dose of 10 mg on a mg/m^2 basis), was close to the maximum tolerated dose for mice but not for rats.

Mutagenicity studies revealed no drug related effects at either the gene or chromosome levels.

There was no effect on the fertility of rats treated with amlodipine (males for 64 days and females 14 days prior to mating) at doses up to 10 mg/kg/day (8 times [based on patient weight of 50 kg] the maximum recommended human dose of 10 mg on a mg/m^2 basis).

PREGNANCY CATEGORY C

No evidence of teratogenicity or other embryo/fetal toxicity was found when pregnant rats or rabbits were treated orally with up to 10 mg/kg amlodipine (respectively 8 times and 23 times [based on patient weight of 50 kg] the maximum recommended human dose of 10 mg on a mg/m^2 basis) during their respective periods of major organogenesis. However, litter size was significantly decreased (by about 50%) and the number of intrauterine deaths was significantly increased (about 5-fold) in rats administered 10 mg/kg amlodipine for 14 days before mating and throughout mating and gestation. Amlodipine has been shown to prolong both the gestation period and the duration of labor in rats at this dose. There are no adequate and well-controlled studies in pregnant women. Amlodipine should be used during pregnancy only if the potential benefit justifies the potential risk to the fetus.

NURSING MOTHERS

It is not known whether amlodipine is excreted in human milk. In the absence of this information, it is recommended that nursing be discontinued while amlodipine besylate is administered.

PEDIATRIC USE

Safety and effectiveness of amlodipine besylate in children have not been established.

GERIATRIC USE

Clinical studies of amlodipine besylate did not include sufficient numbers of subjects aged 65 and over to determine whether they respond differently from younger subjects. Other reported clinical experience has not identified differences in responses between the elderly and younger patients. In general, dose selection for an elderly patient should be cautious, usually starting at the low end of the dosing range, reflecting the greater frequency of decreased hepatic, renal, or cardiac function, and of concomitant disease or other drug therapy. Elderly patients have decreased clearance of amlodipine with a resulting increase of AUC of approximately 40-60%, and a lower initial dose may be required (see DOSAGE AND ADMINISTRATION).

DRUG INTERACTIONS

In vitro data in human plasma indicate that amlodipine besylate has no effect on the protein binding of drugs tested (digoxin, phenytoin, warfarin, and indomethacin).

SPECIAL STUDIES — EFFECT OF OTHER AGENTS ON AMLODIPINE BESYLATE

Cimetidine: Coadministration of amlodipine besylate with cimetidine did not alter the pharmacokinetics of amlodipine besylate.

Grapefruit Juice: Coadministration of 240 ml of grapefruit juice with a single oral dose of amlodipine 10 mg in 20 healthy volunteers had no significant effect on the pharmacokinetics of amlodipine.

Maalox (antacid): Coadministration of the antacid Maalox with a single dose of amlodipine besylate had no significant effect on the pharmacokinetics of amlodipine besylate.

Sildenafil: A single 100 mg dose of sildenafil (Viagra) in subjects with essential hypertension had no effect on the pharmacokinetic parameters of amlodipine besylate. When amlodipine besylate and sildenafil were used in combination, each agent independently exerted its own blood pressure lowering effect.

SPECIAL STUDIES — EFFECT OF AMLODIPINE BESYLATE ON OTHER AGENTS

Atorvastatin: Coadministration of multiple 10 mg doses of amlodipine besylate with 80 mg of atorvastatin resulted in no significant change in the steady state pharmacokinetic parameters of atorvastatin.

Digoxin: Coadministration of amlodipine besylate with digoxin did not change serum digoxin levels or digoxin renal clearance in normal volunteers.

Ethanol (alcohol): Single and multiple 10 mg doses of amlodipine besylate had no significant effect on the pharmacokinetics of ethanol.

Warfarin: Coadministration of amlodipine besylate with warfarin did not change the warfarin prothrombin response time.

In clinical trials, amlodipine besylate has been safely administered with thiazide diuretics, beta-blockers, angiotensin-converting enzyme inhibitors, long-acting nitrates, sublingual nitroglycerin, digoxin, warfarin, non-steroidal anti-inflammatory drugs, antibiotics, and oral hypoglycemic drugs.

ADVERSE REACTIONS

Amlodipine besylate has been evaluated for safety in more than 11,000 patients in US and foreign clinical trials. In general, treatment with amlodipine besylate was well-tolerated at doses up to 10 mg daily. Most adverse reactions reported during therapy with amlodipine besylate were of mild or moderate severity. In controlled clinical trials directly comparing amlodipine besylate (n=1730) in doses up to 10 mg to placebo (n=1250), discontinuation of amlodipine besylate due to adverse reactions was required in only about 1.5% of patients and was not significantly different from placebo (about 1%). The most common side effects are headache and edema. The incidence (%) of side effects which occurred in a dose related manner are found in TABLE 1.

TABLE 1

Adverse Event	2.5 mg n=275	5.0 mg n=296	10.0 mg n=268	Placebo n=520
Edema	1.8%	3.0%	10.8%	0.6%
Dizziness	1.1%	3.4%	3.4%	1.5%
Flushing	0.7%	1.4%	2.6%	0.0%
Palpitation	0.7%	1.4%	4.5%	0.6%

Other adverse experiences which were not clearly dose related but which were reported with an incidence greater than 1.0% in placebo-controlled clinical trials can be found in TABLE 2.

TABLE 2 *Placebo-Controlled Studies*

Adverse Event	Amlodipine Besylate (n=1730)	Placebo (n=1250)
Headache	7.3%	7.8%
Fatigue	4.5%	2.8%
Nausea	2.9%	1.9%
Abdominal pain	1.6%	0.3%
Somnolence	1.4%	0.6%

For several adverse experiences that appear to be drug and dose related, there was a greater incidence in women than men associated with amlodipine treatment as shown in TABLE 3.

TABLE 3

	Amlodipine Besylate		Placebo	
ADR	M=% (n=1218)	F=% (n=512)	M=% (n=914)	F=% (n=336)
Edema	5.6%	14.6%	1.4%	5.1%
Flushing	1.5%	4.5%	0.3%	0.9%
Palpitations	1.4%	3.3%	0.9%	0.9%
Somnolence	1.3%	1.6%	0.8%	0.3%

The following events occurred in ≤1% but >0.1% of patients in controlled clinical trials or under conditions of open trials or marketing experience where a causal relationship is uncertain; they are listed to alert the physician to a possible relationship:

Cardiovascular: Arrhythmia (including ventricular tachycardia and atrial fibrillation), bradycardia, chest pain, hypotension, peripheral ischemia, syncope, tachycardia, postural dizziness, postural hypotension, vasculitis.

Central and Peripheral Nervous System: Hypoesthesia, neuropathy peripheral, paresthesia, tremor, vertigo.

Gastrointestinal: Anorexia, constipation, dyspepsia,† dysphagia, diarrhea, flatulence, pancreatitis, vomiting, gingival hyperplasia.

General: Allergic reaction, asthenia,† back pain, hot flushes, malaise, pain, rigors, weight gain, weight decrease.

Musculoskeletal System: Arthralgia, arthrosis, muscle cramps,† myalgia.

Psychiatric: Sexual dysfunction (male† and female), insomnia, nervousness, depression, abnormal dreams, anxiety, depersonalization.

Respiratory System: Dyspnea,† epistaxis.

Skin and Appendages: Angioedema, erythema multiforme, pruritus,† rash,† rash erythematous, rash maculopapular.

Special Senses: Abnormal vision, conjunctivitis, diplopia, eye pain, tinnitus.

Urinary System: Micturition frequency, micturition disorder, nocturia.

Autonomic Nervous System: Dry mouth, increased sweating.

Metabolic and Nutritional: Hyperglycemia, thirst.

Hemopoietic: Leukopenia, purpura, thrombocytopenia.

†These events occurred in less than 1% in placebo-controlled trials, but the incidence of these side effects was between 1 and 2% in all multiple dose studies.

The following events occurred in ≤0.1% of patients: Cardiac failure, pulse irregularity, extrasystoles, skin discoloration, urticaria, skin dryness, alopecia, dermatitis, muscle weakness, twitching, ataxia, hypertonia, migraine, cold and clammy skin, apathy, agitation, amnesia, gastritis, increased appetite, loose stools, coughing, rhinitis, dysuria, polyuria, parosmia, taste perversion, abnormal visual accommodation, and xerophthalmia.

Other reactions occurred sporadically and cannot be distinguished from medications or concurrent disease states such as myocardial infarction and angina.

Amlodipine besylate therapy has not been associated with clinically significant changes in routine laboratory tests. No clinically relevant changes were noted in serum potassium, serum glucose, total triglycerides, total cholesterol, HDL cholesterol, uric acid, blood urea nitrogen, or creatinine.

The following postmarketing event has been reported infrequently where a causal relationship is uncertain: gynecomastia. In postmarketing experience, jaundice and hepatic enzyme elevations (mostly consistent with cholestasis or hepatitis) in some cases severe enough to require hospitalization have been reported in association with use of amlodipine.

Amlodipine besylate has been used safely in patients with chronic obstructive pulmonary disease, well-compensated congestive heart failure, peripheral vascular disease, diabetes mellitus, and abnormal lipid profiles.

DOSAGE AND ADMINISTRATION

The usual initial antihypertensive oral dose of amlodipine besylate is 5 mg once daily with a maximum dose of 10 mg once daily. Small, fragile, or elderly individuals, or patients with hepatic insufficiency may be started on 2.5 mg once daily and this dose may be used when adding amlodipine besylate to other antihypertensive therapy.

Dosage should be adjusted according to each patient's need. In general, titration should proceed over 7-14 days so that the physician can fully assess the patient's response to each dose level. Titration may proceed more rapidly, however, if clinically warranted, provided the patient is assessed frequently.

The recommended dose for chronic stable or vasospastic angina is 5-10 mg, with the lower dose suggested in the elderly and in patients with hepatic insufficiency. Most patients will require 10 mg for adequate effect. See ADVERSE REACTIONS for information related to dosage and side effects.

Coadministration with other antihypertensive and/or antianginal drugs: Amlodipine besylate has been safely administered with thiazides, ACE inhibitors, beta-blockers, long-acting nitrates, and/or sublingual nitroglycerin.

HOW SUPPLIED

Norvasc 2.5 mg Tablets: (Amlodipine besylate equivalent to 2.5 mg of amlodipine per tablet.) White, diamond, flat-faced, beveled edged engraved with "NORVASC" on one side and "2.5" on the other side.

Norvasc 5 mg Tablets: (Amlodipine besylate equivalent to 5 mg of amlodipine per tablet.) White, elongated octagon, flat-faced, beveled edged engraved with both "NORVASC" and "5" on one side and plain on the other side.

Norvasc 10 mg Tablets: (Amlodipine besylate equivalent to 10 mg of amlodipine per tablet.) White, round, flat-faced, beveled edged engraved with both "NORVASC" and "10" on one side and plain on the other side.

Storage: Store bottles at controlled room temperature, 15-30°C (59-86°F) and dispense in tight, light-resistant containers.

PRODUCT LISTING - EQUIVALENTS NOT AVAILABLE

Tablet - Oral - 2.5 mg

30's	$47.43	NORVASC, Physicians Total Care	54868-3853-01
90's	$135.30	NORVASC, Pfizer U.S. Pharmaceuticals	00069-1520-68

Tablet - Oral - 5 mg

30's	$37.70	NORVASC, Allscripts Pharmaceutical Company	54569-3866-01
30's	$43.75	NORVASC, Physicians Total Care	54868-2873-01
30's	$51.15	NORVASC, Pd-Rx Pharmaceuticals	55289-0103-30
60's	$86.33	NORVASC, Physicians Total Care	54868-2873-03
90's	$113.10	NORVASC, Allscripts Pharmaceutical Company	54569-3866-00
90's	$131.65	NORVASC, Physicians Total Care	54868-2873-04
90's	$135.30	NORVASC, Pfizer U.S. Pharmaceuticals	00069-1530-68
100's	$130.73	NORVASC, Physicians Total Care	54868-2873-00
100's	$136.00	NORVASC, Allscripts Pharmaceutical Company	54569-3866-02
100's	$150.34	NORVASC, Pfizer U.S. Pharmaceuticals	00069-1530-41

Tablet - Oral - 10 mg

30's	$65.24	NORVASC, Allscripts Pharmaceutical Company	54569-4472-00
30's	$72.71	NORVASC, Physicians Total Care	54868-3464-01
30's	$104.94	NORVASC, Pd-Rx Pharmaceuticals	55289-0549-30
90's	$195.70	NORVASC, Pfizer U.S. Pharmaceuticals	00069-1540-68
100's	$217.45	NORVASC, Pfizer U.S. Pharmaceuticals	00069-1540-41

Amlodipine Besylate; Benazepril Hydrochloride *(003212)*

Categories: Hypertension, essential; Pregnancy Category C, 1st Trimester; Pregnancy Category D, 2nd & 3rd Trimesters; FDA Approved 1995 Mar
Drug Classes: Angiotensin converting enzyme inhibitors; Calcium channel blockers
Brand Names: Lotrel
Cost of Therapy: $63.82 (Hypertension; Lotrel; 2.5 mg; 10 mg; 1 capsule/day; 30 day supply)

DESCRIPTION

Lotrel is a combination of amlodipine besylate and benazepril hydrochloride. The capsules are formulated for oral administration with a combination of amlodipine besylate equivalent to 2.5 or 5 mg of amlodipine and 10 or 20 mg of benazepril hydrochloride. The inactive ingredients of the capsules are calcium phosphate, cellulose compounds, colloidal silicon dioxide, crospovidone, gelatin, hydrogenated castor oil, iron oxides, lactose, magnesium stearate, polysorbate 80, silicon dioxide, sodium lauryl sulfate, sodium starch glycolate, starch, talc, and titanium dioxide.

FOR COMPLETE PRESCRIBING INFORMATION REFER TO AMLODIPINE BESYLATE AND BENAZEPRIL HYDROCHLORIDE.

INDICATIONS AND USAGE

Amlodipine besylate; benazepril HCl in indicated for the treatment of hypertension.

This fixed combination drug is not indicated for the initial therapy of hypertension. See DOSAGE AND ADMINISTRATION.

In using amlodipine besylate; benazepril HCl, consideration should be given to the fact that an ACE inhibitor, captopril, has caused agranulocytosis, particularly in patients with renal impairment or collagen-vascular disease. Available data are insufficient to show that benazepril does not have a similar risk.

DOSAGE AND ADMINISTRATION

Amlodipine is an effective treatment of hypertension in once-daily doses of 2.5-10 mg while benazepril is effective in doses of 10-80 mg. In clinical trials of amlodipine/benazepril combination therapy using amlodipine doses of 2.5-5 mg and benazepril doses of 10-20 mg, the

A

antihypertensive effects increased with increasing dose of amlodipine in all patient groups, and the effects increased with increasing dose of benazepril in nonblack groups. All patient groups benefited from the reduction in amlodipine-induced edema.

The hazards of benazepril are generally independent of dose; those of amlodipine are a mixture of dose-dependent phenomena (primarily peripheral edema) and dose-independent phenomena, the former much more common than the latter. When benazepril is added to a regimen of amlodipine, the incidence of edema is substantially reduced. Therapy with any combination of amlodipine and benazepril will thus be associated with both sets of dose-independent hazards, but the incidence of edema will generally be less than that seen with similar (or higher) doses of amlodipine monotherapy.

Rarely, the dose-independent hazards of benazepril are serious. To minimize dose-independent hazards, it is usually appropriate to begin therapy with amlodipine besylate; benazepril HCl only after a patient has either (a) failed to achieve the desired antihypertensive effect with one or the other monotherapy, or (b) demonstrated inability to achieve adequate antihypertensives effect with amlodipine therapy without developing edema.

DOSE TITRATION GUIDED BY CLINICAL EFFECT

A patient whose blood pressure is not adequately controlled with amlodipine (or another dihydropyridine) alone or with benazepril (or another ACE inhibitor) alone may be switched to combination therapy with amlodipine besylate;benazepril HCl. The addition of benazepril to a regimen of amlodipine should not be expected to provide additional antihypertensive effect in African-Americans. However, all patient groups benefit from the reduction in amlodipine-induced edema. Dosage must be guided by clinical response; steady-state levels of benazepril and amlodipine will be reached after approximately 2 and 7 days of dosing, respectively.

In patients whose blood pressures are adequately controlled with amlodipine but who experience unacceptable edema, combination therapy may achieve similar (or better) blood-pressure control without edema. Especially in nonblacks, it may be prudent to minimize the risk of excessive response by reducing the dose of amlodipine as benazepril is added to the regimen.

REPLACEMENT THERAPY

For convenience, patients receiving amlodipine and benazepril from separate tablets may instead wish to receive capsules of amlodipine besylate; benazepril HCl containing the same component doses.

USE IN PATIENTS WITH METABOLIC IMPAIRMENTS

Regimens of therapy with Lotrel need not take account of renal function as long as the patient's creatinine clearance is >30 ml/min/1.73 m^2 (serum creatinine roughly ≤3 mg/dl or 265 μmol/l). In patients with more severe renal impairment, the recommended initial dose of benazepril is 5 mg. Amlodipine besylate; benazepril HCl is not recommended in these patients.

In small, elderly, frail, or hepatically impaired patients, the recommended initial dose of amlodipine, as monotherapy or as a component of combination therapy, is 2.5 mg.

HOW SUPPLIED

Lotrel is available as capsules containing amlodipine/benazepril HCl 2.5/10 mg, 5/10 mg, and 5/20 mg.

Capsules are imprinted with "Lotrel" and a portion of the NDC code.

STORAGE

Do not store above 30°C (86°F). Protect from moisture and light.

Dispense in tight, light-resistant container.

PRODUCT LISTING - EQUIVALENTS NOT AVAILABLE

Capsule - Oral - 2.5 mg;10 mg

100's	$212.74	LOTREL, Novartis Pharmaceuticals	00083-2255-30

Capsule - Oral - 5 mg;10 mg

30's	$62.88	LOTREL, Physicians Total Care	54868-4073-00
100's	$216.96	LOTREL, Novartis Pharmaceuticals	00083-2260-30

Capsule - Oral - 5 mg;20 mg

100's	$229.10	LOTREL, Novartis Pharmaceuticals	00083-2265-30

Capsule - Oral - 10 mg;20 mg

100's	$266.16	LOTREL, Novartis Pharmaceuticals	00078-0364-05

Ammonium Lactate *(000223)*

Categories: Ichthyosis vulgaris; Xerosis; Pregnancy Category C; FDA Approved 1985 Apr
Drug Classes: Dermatologics
Brand Names: Lac-Hydrin

DESCRIPTION

Lac-Hydrin is a formulation of 12% lactic acid neutralized with ammonium hydroxide, as ammonium lactate, with a pH of 4.4-5.4. Lac-Hydrin cream also contains water, light mineral oil, glyceryl stearate, polyoxyl 100 stearate, propylene glycol, polyoxyl 40 stearate, glycerin, cetyl alcohol, magnesium aluminum silicate, laureth-4, methyl and propyl parabens, and methylcellulose. Lactic acid is a racemic mixture of 2-hydroxypropanoic acid.

CLINICAL PHARMACOLOGY

Lactic acid is an alpha-hydroxy acid. It is a normal constituent of tissues and blood. The alpha-hydroxy acids (and their salts) are felt to act as humectants when applied to the skin. This property may influence hydration of the stratum corneum. In addition, lactic acid, when applied to the skin, may act to decrease corneocyte cohesion. The mechanism(s) by which this is accomplished is not yet known.

An *in vitro* study of percutaneous absorption of ammonium lactate cream using human cadaver skin indicates that approximately 6.1% of the material was absorbed after 68 hours.

INDICATIONS AND USAGE

Ammonium lactate cream is indicated for the treatment of ichthyosis vulgaris and xerosis.

CONTRAINDICATIONS

None known.

WARNINGS

Use of this product should be discontinued if hypersensitivity to any of the ingredients is noted. Sun exposure (natural or artificial sunlight) to areas of the skin treated with ammonium lactate cream should be minimized or avoided (see PRECAUTIONS).

PRECAUTIONS

GENERAL

For external use only. Stinging or burning may occur when applied to skin with fissures, erosions, or that is otherwise abraded (for example, after shaving the legs). Caution is advised when used on the face because of the potential for irritation. The potential for post-inflammatory hypo- or hyperpigmentation has not been studied.

INFORMATION FOR THE PATIENT

Patients using ammonium lactate cream should receive the following information and instructions:

1. This medication is to be used as directed by the physician, and should not be used for any disorder other than for which it was prescribed. Caution is advised when used on the face because of the potential for irritation. It is for external use only. Avoid contact with eyes, lips, or mucous membranes.
2. Patients should minimize or avoid use of this product on areas of the skin that may be exposed to natural or artificial sunlight, including the face. If sun exposure is unavoidable, clothing should be worn to protect the skin.
3. This medication may cause stinging or burning when applied to skin with fissures, erosions, or abrasions (for example, after shaving the legs).
4. If the skin condition worsens with treatment, the medication should be promptly discontinued.

CARCINOGENESIS, MUTAGENESIS, AND IMPAIRMENT OF FERTILITY

A long-term photocarcinogenicity study in hairless albino mice suggested that topically applied 12% ammonium lactate cream enhanced the rate of ultraviolet light-induced skin tumor formation. Although the biologic significance of these results to humans is not clear, patients should minimize or avoid use of this product on areas of the skin that may be exposed to natural or artificial sunlight, including the face. Long-term dermal carcinogenicity studies in animals have not been conducted to evaluate the carcinogenic potential of ammonium lactate.

PREGNANCY, TERATOGENIC EFFECTS, PREGNANCY CATEGORY C

Animal reproduction studies have not been conducted with ammonium lactate cream. It is also not known whether ammonium lactate cream can cause fetal harm when administered to a pregnant woman or can affect reproduction capacity. Ammonium lactate cream should be given to a pregnant woman only if clearly needed.

NURSING MOTHERS

Although lactic acid is a normal constituent of blood and tissues, it is not known to what extent this drug affects normal lactic acid levels in human milk. Because many drugs are excreted in human milk, caution should be exercised when ammonium lactate cream is administered to a nursing woman.

PEDIATRIC USE

The safety and effectiveness of ammonium lactate cream have not been established in pediatric patients less than 12 years old. Potential systemic toxicity from percutaneous absorption has not been studied. Because of the increased surface area to body weight ratio in pediatric patients, the systemic burden of lactic acid may be increased.

ADVERSE REACTIONS

In controlled clinical trials of patients with ichthyosis vulgaris, the most frequent adverse reactions in patients treated with ammonium lactate cream were rash (including erythema and irritation) and burning/stinging. Each was reported in approximately 10-15% of patients. In addition, itching was reported in approximately 5% of patients.

In controlled clinical trials of patients with xerosis, the most frequent adverse reactions in patients treated with ammonium lactate cream were transient burning, in about 3% of patients, stinging, dry skin and rash, each reported in approximately 2% of patients.

DOSAGE AND ADMINISTRATION

Apply to the affected areas and rub in thoroughly. Use twice daily or as directed by a physician.

HOW SUPPLIED

Lac-Hydrin Cream 12% is available in 140 g plastic tubes and 385 g plastic bottle.
Storage: Store at controlled room temperature, 15-30°C (59-86°F).

PRODUCT LISTING - RATED THERAPEUTICALLY EQUIVALENT

Lotion - Topical - 12%

225 ml	$38.13	GENERIC, Paddock Laboratories Inc	00574-2021-08
400 ml	$60.00	GENERIC, Paddock Laboratories Inc	00574-2021-16

PRODUCT LISTING - EQUIVALENTS NOT AVAILABLE

Cream - Topical - 12%

140 gm	$9.21	AMLACTIN, Upsher-Smith Laboratories Inc	00245-0024-14
140 gm	$19.95	GENERIC, Clay-Park Laboratories Inc	45802-0513-77

140 gm x 2	$37.90	LAC-HYDRIN, Allscripts Pharmaceutical Company	54569-4645-00
140 gm x 2	$44.35	LAC-HYDRIN, Bristol-Myers Squibb	00072-5730-28
266 gm	$38.30	GENERIC, Clay-Park Laboratories Inc	45802-0493-83
385 gm	$58.06	LAC-HYDRIN, Bristol-Myers Squibb	00072-5730-38
Lotion - Topical - 12%			
225 ml	$10.23	AMLACTIN, Upsher-Smith Laboratories Inc	00245-0023-22
225 ml	$18.24	GENERIC, Clay-Park Laboratories Inc	45802-0525-55
225 ml	$36.19	LAC-HYDRIN, Allscripts Pharmaceutical Company	54569-3883-00
225 ml	$40.75	LAC-HYDRIN, Physicians Total Care	54868-2262-03
225 ml	$42.36	LAC-HYDRIN, Bristol-Myers Squibb	00072-5712-08
400 ml	$16.89	AMLACTIN, Upsher-Smith Laboratories Inc	00245-0023-40
400 ml	$28.51	GENERIC, Clay-Park Laboratories Inc	45802-0525-26
400 ml	$63.83	LAC-HYDRIN, Physicians Total Care	54868-2262-00
400 ml	$66.67	LAC-HYDRIN, Bristol-Myers Squibb	00072-5712-14

Amoxapine *(000230)*

For related information, see the comparative table section in Appendix A.

Categories: Depression; Pregnancy Category C; FDA Approved 1980 Sep
Drug Classes: Antidepressants, tricyclic
Brand Names: Asendin
Foreign Brand Availability: Amoxan (Japan); Asendis (England; Ireland); Defanyl (France); Demolox (Denmark; India; Portugal; Spain)
Cost of Therapy: $116.09 (Depression; Generic Tablets; 100 mg; 3 tablets/day; 30 day supply)

DESCRIPTION

Amoxapine is an antidepressant of the dibenzoxazepine class, chemically distinct from the dibenzazepines, dibenzocycloheptenes, and dibenzoxepines.

It is designated chemically as 2-chloro-11-(1-piperazinyl)dibenz-[*b,f*][1,4]oxazepine. The molecular weight is 313.8. The empirical formula is $C_{17}H_{16}ClN_3O$.

Asendin is supplied for oral administration as 25, 50, 100, and 150 mg tablets.

Inactive ingredients: All tablets contain corn starch, dibasic calcium phosphate, magnesium stearate, pregelatinized starch and stearic acid. Additionally, the 50 and 150 mg tablets contain FD&C yellow no. 6 and the 100 mg tablet contains blue 2.

CLINICAL PHARMACOLOGY

Amoxapine is an antidepressant with a mild sedative component to its action. The mechanism of its clinical action in man is not well understood. In animals, amoxapine reduced the uptake of norepinephrine and serotonin and blocked the response of dopamine receptors to dopamine. Amoxapine is not a monoamine oxidase inhibitor.

Amoxapine is absorbed rapidly and reaches peak blood levels approximately 90 minutes after ingestion. It is almost completely metabolized. The main route of excretion is the kidney. *In vitro* tests show that amoxapine binding to human serum is approximately 90%.

In man, amoxapine serum concentration declines with a half-life of 8 hours. However, the major metabolite, 8-hydroxyamoxapine, has a biologic half-life of 30 hours. Metabolites are excreted in the urine in conjugated form as glucuronides.

Clinical studies have demonstrated that amoxapine has a more rapid onset of action than either amitriptyline or imipramine. The initial clinical effect may occur within 4-7 days and occurs within 2 weeks in over 80% of responders.

INDICATIONS AND USAGE

Amoxapine is indicated for the relief of symptoms of depression in patients with neurotic or reactive depressive disorders as well as endogenous and psychotic depressions. It is indicated for depression accompanied by anxiety or agitation.

CONTRAINDICATIONS

Amoxapine is contraindicated in patients who have shown prior hypersensitivity to dibenzoxazepine compounds. It should not be given concomitantly with monoamine oxidase inhibitors. Hyperpyretic crises, severe convulsions and deaths have occurred in patients receiving tricyclic antidepressants and monoamine oxidase inhibitors simultaneously. When it is desired to replace a monoamine oxidase inhibitor with amoxapine, a minimum of 14 days should be allowed to elapse after the former is discontinued. Amoxapine should then be initiated cautiously with gradual increase in dosage until optimum response is achieved. The drug is not recommended for use during the acute recovery phase following myocardial infarction.

WARNINGS

TARDIVE DYSKINESIA

Tardive dyskinesia, a syndrome consisting of potentially irreversible, involuntary, dyskinetic movements may develop in patients treated with neuroleptic (*i.e.,* antipsychotics) drugs. (Amoxapine is not an antipsychotic, but it has substantive neuroleptic activity). Although the prevalence of the syndrome appears to be highest among the elderly, especially elderly women, it is impossible to rely upon prevalence estimates to predict, at the inception of neuroleptic treatment, which patients are likely to develop the syndrome. Whether neuroleptic drug products differ in their potential to cause tardive dyskinesia is unknown.

Both the risk of developing the syndrome and the likelihood that it will become irreversible are believed to increase as the duration of treatment and the total cumulative dose of neuroleptic drugs administered to the patient increase. However, the syndrome can develop, although much less commonly, after relatively brief treatment periods at low doses.

There is no known treatment for established cases of tardive dyskinesia, although the syndrome may remit, partially or completely, if neuroleptic treatment is withdrawn. Neuroleptic treatment itself, however, may suppress (or partially suppress) the signs and symptoms of the syndrome and thereby may possibly mask the underlying disease process. The effect that symptomatic suppression has upon the long-term course of the syndrome is unknown.

Given these considerations, neuroleptics should be prescribed in a manner that is most likely to minimize the occurrence of tardive dyskinesia. Chronic neuroleptic treatment should generally be reserved for patients who suffer from a chronic illness that, (1) is known to respond to neuroleptic drugs, and (2) for whom alternative, equally effective, but potentially less harmful treatments are not available or appropriate. In patients who do require chronic treatment, the smallest dose and the shortest duration of treatment producing a satisfactory clinical response should be sought. The need for continued treatment should be reassessed periodically.

If signs and symptoms of tardive dyskinesia appear in a patient on neuroleptics, drug discontinuation should be considered. However, some patients may require treatment despite the presence of the syndrome.

(For further information about the description of tardive dyskinesia and its clinical detection, please refer to PRECAUTIONS, Information for the Patient and ADVERSE REACTIONS.)

NEUROLEPTIC MALIGNANT SYNDROME (NMS)

A potentially fatal symptom complex sometimes referred to as Neuroleptic Malignant Syndrome (NMS) has been reported in association with antipsychotic drugs and with amoxapine. Clinical manifestations of NMS are hyperpyrexia, muscle rigidity, altered mental status and evidence of autonomic instability (irregular pulse or blood pressure, tachycardia, diaphoresis, and cardiac dysrhythmias).

The diagnostic evaluation of patients with this syndrome is complicated. In arriving at a diagnosis, it is important to identify cases where the clinical presentation includes both serious medical illness (*e.g.,* pneumonia, systemic infection, etc.) and untreated or inadequately treated extrapyramidal signs and symptoms (EPS). Other important considerations in the differential diagnosis include central anticholinergic toxicity, heat stroke, drug fever and primary central nervous system (CNS) pathology.

The management of NMS should include (1) immediate discontinuation of antipsychotic drugs and other drugs not essential to concurrent therapy, (2) intensive symptomatic treatment and medical monitoring, and (3) treatment of any concomitant serious medical problems for which specific treatments are available. There is no general agreement about specific pharmacological treatment regimens for uncomplicated NMS.

If a patient requires antipsychotic drug treatment after recovery from NMS, the potential reintroduction of drug therapy should be carefully considered. The patient should be carefully monitored since recurrences of NMS have been reported.

Amoxapine should be used with caution in patients with a history of urinary retention, angle-closure glaucoma or increased intraocular pressure. Patients with cardiovascular disorders should be watched closely. Tricyclic antidepressant drugs, particularly when given in high doses, can induce sinus tachycardia, changes in conduction time, and arrhythmias. Myocardial infarction and stroke have been reported with drugs of this class.

Extreme caution should be used in treating patients with a history of convulsive disorder or those with overt or latent seizure disorders.

PRECAUTIONS

GENERAL

In prescribing the drug it should be borne in mind that the possibility of suicide is inherent in any severe depression, and persists until a significant remission occurs; the drug should be dispensed in the smallest suitable amount. Manic depressive patients may experience a shift to the manic phase. Schizophrenic patients may develop increased symptoms of psychosis; patients with paranoid symptomatology may have an exaggeration of such symptoms. This may require reduction of dosage or the addition of a major tranquilizer to the therapeutic regimen. Antidepressant drugs can cause skin rashes and/or "drug fever" in susceptible individuals. These allergic reactions may, in rare cases, be severe. They are more likely to occur during the first few days of treatment, but may also occur later. Amoxapine should be discontinued if rash and/or fever develop. Amoxapine possesses a degree of dopamine-blocking activity which may cause extrapyramidal symptoms in <1% of patients. Rarely, symptoms indicative of tardive dyskinesia have been reported.

INFORMATION FOR THE PATIENT

Given the likelihood that some patients exposed chronically to neuroleptics will develop tardive dyskinesia, it is advised that all patients in whom chronic use is contemplated be given, if possible, full information about this risk. The decision to inform patients and/or their guardians must obviously take into account the clinical circumstances and the competency of the patient to understand the information provided.

Patients should be warned of the possibility of drowsiness that may impair performance of potentially hazardous tasks such as driving an automobile or operating machinery.

THERAPEUTIC INTERACTIONS

Concurrent administration with electroshock therapy may increase the hazards associated with such therapy.

CARCINOGENESIS, MUTAGENESIS, AND IMPAIRMENT OF FERTILITY

In a 21 month toxicity study at 3 dose levels in rats, pancreatic islet cell hyperplasia occurred with slightly increased incidence at doses 5-10 times the human dose. Pancreatic adeno-carcinoma was detected in low incidence in the mid-dose group only, and may possibly have resulted from endocrine-mediated organ hyperfunction. The significance of these findings to man is not known.

Treatment of male rats with 5-10 times the human dose resulted in a slight decrease in the number of fertile matings. Female rats receiving oral doses within the therapeutic range displayed a reversible increase in estrous cycle length.

PREGNANCY CATEGORY C

Studies performed in mice, rats, and rabbits have demonstrated no evidence of teratogenic effect due to amoxapine. Embryotoxicity was seen in rats and rabbits given oral doses approximating the human dose. Fetotoxic effects (intrauterine death, stillbirth, decreased birth weight) were seen in animals studied at oral doses 3-10 times the human dose. Decreased postnatal survival (between days 0-4) was demonstrated in the offspring of rats at 5-10 times the human dose. There are no adequate and well-controlled studies in pregnant women. Amoxapine should be used during pregnancy only if the potential benefit justifies the potential risk to the fetus.

NURSING MOTHERS

Amoxapine, like many other systemic drugs, is excreted in human milk. Because effects of the drug on infants are unknown, caution should be exercised when amoxapine is administered to nursing women.

PEDIATRIC USE

Safety and effectiveness in children below the age of 16 have not been established.

DRUG INTERACTIONS

See CONTRAINDICATIONS about concurrent usage of tricyclic antidepressants and monoamine oxidase inhibitors. Paralytic ileus may occur in patients taking tricyclic antidepressants in combination with anticholinergic drugs. Amoxapine may enhance the response to alcohol and the effects of barbiturates and other CNS depressants. Serum levels of several tricyclic antidepressants have been reported to be significantly increased when cimetidine is administered concurrently. Although such an interaction has not been reported to date with amoxapine, specific interaction studies have not been done, and the possibility should be considered.

DRUGS METABOLIZED BY P450 2D6

The biochemical activity of the drug metabolizing isozyme cytochrome P450 2D6 (debrisoquin hydroxylase) is reduced in a subset of the caucasian population (about 7-10% of caucasians are so called "poor metabolizers"); reliable estimates of the prevalence of reduced P450 2D6 isozyme activity among Asian, African, and other populations are not yet available. Poor metabolizers have higher than expected plasma concentrations of tricyclic antidepressants (TCAs) when given usual doses. Depending on the fraction of drug metabolizers by P450 2D6, the increase in plasma concentration may be small, or quite large (8-fold increase in plasma AUC of the TCA).

In addition, certain drugs inhibit the activity of this isozyme and make normal metabolizers resemble poor metabolizers. An individual who is stable on a given dose of TCA may become abruptly toxic when given 1 of these inhibiting drugs as concomitant therapy. The drugs that inhibit cytochrome P450 2D6 include some that are not metabolized by the enzyme (quinidine; cimetidine) and many that are substrates for P450 2D6 (many other antidepressants, phenothiazines, and the Type 1C antiarrhythmics propafenone and flecainide). While all the selective serotonin reuptake inhibitors (SSRIs), *e.g.*, fluoxetine, sertraline, and paroxetine, inhibit P450 2D6, they may vary in the extent of inhibition. The extent to which SSRI TCA interactions may pose clinical problems will depend on the degree of inhibition and the pharmacokinetics of the SSRI involved. Nevertheless, caution is indicated in the co-administration of TCAs with any of the SSRIs and also in switching from 1 class to the other. Of particular importance, sufficient time must elapse before initiating TCA treatment in a patient being withdrawn from fluoxetine, given the long half-life of the parent and active metabolite (at least 5 weeks may be necessary).

Concomitant use of tricyclic antidepressants with drugs that can inhibit cytochrome P450 2D6 may require lower doses than usually prescribed for either the tricyclic antidepressant or the other drug. Furthermore, whenever 1 of these other drugs is withdrawn from co-therapy, an increased dose of tricyclic antidepressant may be required. It is desirable to monitor TCA plasma levels whenever a TCA is going to be co-administered with another drug known to be an inhibitor of P450 2D6.

ADVERSE REACTIONS

Adverse reactions reported in controlled studies in the US are categorized with respect to incidence below. Following this is a listing of reactions known to occur with other antidepressant drugs of this class.

INCIDENCE GREATER THAN 1%

The most frequent types of adverse reactions occurring with amoxapine tablets in controlled clinical trials were sedative and anticholinergic: these included drowsiness (14%), dry mouth (14%), constipation (12%), and blurred vision (7%).

Less Frequently Reported Reactions Are:

CNS and Neuromuscular: Anxiety, insomnia, restlessness, nervousness, palpitations, tremors, confusion, excitement, nightmares, ataxia, alterations in EEG patterns.

Allergic: Edema, skin rash.

Endocrine: Elevation of prolactin levels.

Gastrointestinal: Nausea.

Other: Dizziness, headache, fatigue, weakness, excessive appetite, increased perspiration.

INCIDENCE LESS THAN 1%

Anticholinergic: Disturbances of accommodation, mydriasis, delayed micturition, urinary retention, nasal stuffiness.

Cardiovascular: Hypotension, hypertension, syncope, tachycardia.

Allergic: Drug fever, urticaria, photosensitization, pruritus, vasculitis, hepatitis.

CNS and Neuromuscular: Tingling, paresthesias of the extremities, tinnitus, disorientation, seizures, hypomania, numbness, incoordination, disturbed concentration, hyperthermia, extrapyramidal symptoms, including tardive dyskinesia. Neuroleptic malignant syndrome has been reported (see WARNINGS).

Hematologic: Leukopenia, agranulocytosis.

Gastrointestinal: Epigastric distress, vomiting, flatulence, abdominal pain, peculiar taste, diarrhea.

Endocrine: Increased or decreased libido, impotence, menstrual irregularity, breast enlargement and galactorrhea in the female, syndrome of inappropriate antidiuretic hormone secretion.

Other: Lacrimation, weight gain or loss, altered liver function, painful ejaculation.

DRUG RELATIONSHIP UNKNOWN

The following reactions have been reported rarely, and occurred under uncontrolled circumstances where a drug relationship was difficult to assess. These observations are listed to serve as alerting information to physicians:

Anticholinergic: Paralytic ileus.

Cardiovascular: Atrial arrhythmias (including atrial fibrillation), myocardial infarction, stroke, heart block.

CNS and Neuromuscular: Hallucinations.

Hematologic: Thrombocytopenia, eosinophilia, purpura, petechiae.

Gastrointestinal: Parotid swelling.

Endocrine: Change in blood glucose levels.

Other: Pancreatitis, hepatitis, jaundice, urinary frequency, testicular swelling, anorexia, alopecia.

ADDITIONAL ADVERSE REACTIONS

The following reactions have been reported with other antidepressant drugs:

Anticholinergic: Sublingual adenitis, dilation of the urinary tract.

CNS and Neuromuscular: Delusions.

Gastrointestinal: Stomatitis, black tongue.

Endocrine: Gynecomastia.

DOSAGE AND ADMINISTRATION

Effective dosage of amoxapine tablets may vary from 1 patient to another. Usual effective dosage is 200-300 mg daily. Three weeks constitutes an adequate period of trial providing dosage has reached 300 mg daily (or lower level of tolerance) for at least 2 weeks. If no response is seen at 300 mg, dosage may be increased, depending upon tolerance, up to 400 mg daily. Hospitalized patients who have been refractory to antidepressant therapy and who have no history of convulsive seizures may have dosage raised cautiously up to 600 mg daily in divided doses.

Amoxapine tablets may be given in a single daily dose, not to exceed 300 mg, preferably at bedtime. If the total daily dose exceeds 300 mg, it should be given in divided doses.

INITIAL DOSAGE FOR ADULTS

Usual starting dosage is 50 mg 2 or 3 times daily. Depending upon tolerance, dosage may be increased to 100 mg 2 or 3 times daily by the end of the first week. (Initial dosage of 300 mg daily may be given, but notable sedation may occur in some patients during the first few days of therapy at this level.) Increases above 300 mg daily should be made only if 300 mg daily has been ineffective during a trial period of at least 2 weeks. When effective dosage is established, the drug may be given in a single dose (not to exceed 300 mg) at bedtime.

ELDERLY PATIENTS

In general, lower dosages are recommended for these patients. Recommended starting dosage of amoxapine tablets is 25 mg 2 or 3 times daily. If no intolerance is observed, dosage may be increased by the end of the first week to 50 mg 2 or 3 times daily. Although 100-150 mg daily may be adequate for many elderly patients, some may require higher dosage. Careful increases up to 300 mg daily are indicated in such cases.

Once an effective dosage is established, amoxapine tablets may conveniently be given in a single bedtime dose, not to exceed 300 mg.

MAINTENANCE

Recommended maintenance dosage of amoxapine tablets is the lowest dose that will maintain remission. If symptoms reappear, dosage should be increased to the earlier level until they are controlled.

For maintenance therapy at dosages of 300 mg or less, a single dose at bedtime is recommended.

HOW SUPPLIED

Asendin amoxapine tablets are supplied as follows:

25 mg tablets: White, heptagon-shaped tablets, engraved on 1 side with "LL" above "25" and with "A13" on the other scored side.

50 mg tablets: Orange, heptagon-shaped tablets, engraved on 1 side with "LL" above "50" and with "A15" on the other scored side.

100 mg tablets: Blue, heptagon-shaped tablets, engraved on 1 side with "LL" above "100" and with "A17" on the other scored side.

150 mg tablets: Peach, heptagon-shaped tablets, engraved on 1 side with "LL" above "150" and with "A18" on the other scored side.

Storage: Store at controlled room temperature, 15-30°C (59-86°F).

PRODUCT LISTING - RATED THERAPEUTICALLY EQUIVALENT

Package	Price	Source	NDC
Tablet - Oral - 25 mg			
100's	$46.70	GENERIC, Moore, H.L. Drug Exchange Inc	00839-7604-06
100's	$49.20	GENERIC, Qualitest Products Inc	00603-2240-21
100's	$49.22	GENERIC, Dixon-Shane Inc	17236-0888-01
100's	$49.76	GENERIC, Major Pharmaceuticals Inc	00904-3994-61
100's	$52.95	GENERIC, Major Pharmaceuticals Inc	00904-3994-60
100's	$61.45	GENERIC, Geneva Pharmaceuticals	00781-1844-01
100's	$61.48	GENERIC, Ivax Corporation	00182-1043-01
100's	$61.51	GENERIC, Watson/Schein Pharmaceuticals Inc	00364-2432-01
100's	$61.51	GENERIC, Watson Laboratories Inc	00591-0379-01
100's	$61.51	GENERIC, Watson Laboratories Inc	52544-0379-01
Tablet - Oral - 50 mg			
100's	$54.25	FEDERAL UPPER LIMIT, H.C.F.A. F F P	99999-0230-02

100's	$76.48	GENERIC, Moore, H.L. Drug Exchange Inc	00839-7605-06
100's	$78.94	GENERIC, Major Pharmaceuticals Inc	00904-3995-61
100's	$84.20	GENERIC, Major Pharmaceuticals Inc	00904-3995-60
100's	$99.89	GENERIC, Watson/Schein Pharmaceuticals Inc	00364-2433-01
100's	$99.89	GENERIC, Watson Laboratories Inc	52544-0380-01
100's	$99.90	GENERIC, Geneva Pharmaceuticals	00781-1845-01
100's	$99.95	GENERIC, Dixon-Shane Inc	17236-0889-01
100's	$99.95	GENERIC, Martec Pharmaceuticals Inc	52555-0540-01
Tablet - Oral - 100 mg			
100's	$128.99	GENERIC, Moore, H.L. Drug Exchange Inc	00839-7606-06
100's	$134.80	GENERIC, Qualitest Products Inc	00603-2242-21
100's	$135.70	GENERIC, Major Pharmaceuticals Inc	00904-3996-60
100's	$139.95	GENERIC, Parmed Pharmaceuticals Inc	00349-8709-01
100's	$166.80	GENERIC, Geneva Pharmaceuticals	00781-1846-01
100's	$166.83	GENERIC, Dixon-Shane Inc	17236-0890-01
100's	$166.83	GENERIC, Martec Pharmaceuticals Inc	52555-0541-01
100's	$166.95	GENERIC, Watson/Schein Pharmaceuticals Inc	00364-2434-01
100's	$166.95	GENERIC, Watson Laboratories Inc	00591-0381-01
100's	$166.95	GENERIC, Watson Laboratories Inc	52544-0381-01
Tablet - Oral - 150 mg			
30's	$60.95	GENERIC, Moore, H.L. Drug Exchange Inc	00839-7607-19
30's	$62.95	GENERIC, Major Pharmaceuticals Inc	00904-3997-46
30's	$63.15	GENERIC, Qualitest Products Inc	00603-2243-16
30's	$66.83	GENERIC, Mutual/United Research Laboratories	00677-1380-07
30's	$70.00	GENERIC, Geneva Pharmaceuticals	00781-1847-31
30's	$78.90	GENERIC, Dixon-Shane Inc	17236-0891-01
30's	$78.90	GENERIC, Dixon-Shane Inc	17236-0891-03
30's	$78.99	GENERIC, Watson/Schein Pharmaceuticals Inc	00364-2435-30
30's	$78.99	GENERIC, Watson Laboratories Inc	00591-0382-30
30's	$78.99	GENERIC, Watson Laboratories Inc	52544-0382-30
100's	$249.85	GENERIC, Watson Laboratories Inc	52544-0382-01

Amoxicillin *(000231)*

A

For related information, see the comparative table section in Appendix A.

Categories: Gonorrhea; Infection, ear, middle; Infection, genital tract; Infection, lower respiratory tract; Infection, upper respiratory tract; Infection, skin and skin structures; Infection, sinus; Infection, urinary tract; Pharyngitis; Pneumonia; Tonsilitis; Ulcer, H. pylori associated; Pregnancy Category B; FDA Approved 1979 Aug; WHO Formulary

Drug Classes: Antibiotics, penicillins

Brand Names: **Amoxil**; Biomox; Larotid; Polymox; Senox; Trimox; Wymox; Yisulon

Foreign Brand Availability: Abdimox (Indonesia); Acimox (Mexico); Acticillin (Thailand); Actimoxi (Spain); Adbiotin (Colombia); Agerpen (Spain); A-Gram (France); Alfamox (Italy); Almodan (England); Alphamox (Australia; New-Zealand); Amagesen Solutab (Germany); Ameclina (Mexico); Amoclen (Czech-Republic); Amodex (France); Amo-flamsian (Spain); Amohexal (Australia); Amolin (Japan; Taiwan); Amophar GE (France); Amosine (Indonesia); Amoval (Peru); Amox (Bahrain; Cyprus; Egypt; Iran; Iraq; Israel; Italy; Jordan; Kuwait; Lebanon; Libya; Oman; Qatar; Republic-of-Yemen; Saudi-Arabia; Syria; United-Arab-Emirates); Amoxa (Hong-Kong; Singapore); Amoxal (Colombia); Amoxapen (Bahamas; Barbados; Belize; Bermuda; Curacao; Guyana; Hong-Kong; Jamaica; Korea; Netherland-Antilles; Puerto-Rico; Singapore; Surinam; Trinidad); Amoxaren (Spain); Amoxcillin (Thailand); Amoxi (Israel); Amoxibasan (Germany); Amoxicilina (Colombia; Ecuador); Amoxiclin (Peru); Amoxidal (Argentina); Amoxidin (Bahamas; Bahrain; Barbados; Belize; Benin; Bermuda; Burkina-Faso; Curacao; Cyprus; Egypt; Ethiopia; Gambia; Ghana; Guinea; Guyana; Iran; Iraq; Israel; Ivory-Coast; Jamaica; Jordan; Kenya; Kuwait; Lebanon; Liberia; Libya; Malawi; Mali; Mauritania; Mauritius; Morocco; Netherland-Antilles; Niger; Nigeria; Oman; Puerto-Rico; Qatar; Republic-of-Yemen; Saudi-Arabia; Senegal; Seychelles; Sierra-Leone; South-Africa; Sudan; Surinam; Syria; Tanzania; Trinidad; Tunia; Uganda; United-Arab-Emirates; Zambia; Zimbabwe); Amoxihexal (Germany); Amoxillin (Israel; Italy; Norway); Amoxipen (Italy; Peru); Amoxisol (Mexico); Amoxivan (India); Amoxivet (Mexico); Amoxy (Thailand); Amoxy-diolan (Germany); Amoxypen (Germany; Peru); Apo-Amoxi (Malaysia); Ardine (Mexico; Spain); Aroxin (Singapore); Azillin (Switzerland); Bactamox (Costa-Rica; Dominican-Republic; El-Salvador; Guatemala; Honduras; Nicaragua; Panama); Bimox (Colombia); Bintamox (Indonesia); Bioxidona (Spain); Bioxyllin (Indonesia); Bristamox (Ecuador; France; Peru; Sweden); Broadmetz (Philippines); Cilamox (Australia; New-Zealand; Philippines); Clamox (Finland); Clamoxyl (Australia; Austria; Bahamas; Barbados; Belgium; Belize; Bermuda; Curacao; France; Germany; Guyana; Jamaica; Japan; Netherland-Antilles; Netherlands; New-Zealand; Peru; Portugal; Puerto-Rico; Spain; Surinam; Switzerland; Trinidad); Clonamox (China); Coamoxin (Spain); Doxamil (Mexico); Draximox (Denmark); Edamox (Hong-Kong); Efpinex (Japan); Eupen (Dominican-Republic; El-Salvador; Guatemala; Honduras; Nicaragua; Panama; Spain); Farconcil (Bahrain; Cyprus; Egypt; Iran; Iraq; Israel; Jordan; Kuwait; Lebanon; Libya; Oman; Qatar; Republic-of-Yemen; Saudi-Arabia; Syria; United-Arab-Emirates); Fisamox (Australia; New-Zealand); Flemoxin (Bahrain; China; Cyprus; Egypt; Iran; Iraq; Israel; Jordan; Kuwait; Lebanon; Libya; Oman; Qatar; Republic-of-Yemen; Saudi-Arabia; Syria; United-Arab-Emirates); Flemoxine Ge (France); Foxolin (Korea); Fullcilina (Argentina); Gexcil (Philippines); Gimalxina (Mexico); Gomcillin (Korea); Grinsul (Argentina); Grunamox (Ecuador); Hamoxillin (Hong-Kong); Hiconcil (Belgium; Bulgaria; France; Indonesia; Israel; Netherlands); Hidramox (Mexico); Hipen (Benin; Burkina-Faso; Ethiopia; Gambia; Ghana; Guinea; Ivory-Coast; Kenya; Liberia; Malawi; Mali; Mauritania; Mauritius; Morocco; Niger; Nigeria; Senegal; Seychelles; Sierra-Leone; South-Africa; Sudan; Tanzania; Tunia; Uganda; Zambia; Zimbabwe); Hosboral (Spain); Ibiamox (Bahrain; Cyprus; Egypt; Iran; Iraq; Jordan; Kuwait; Lebanon; Libya; Oman; Qatar; Republic-of-Yemen; Saudi-Arabia; Syria; Taiwan; Thailand; United-Arab-Emirates); Ikamoxil (Indonesia); Imacillin (Denmark; Norway; Sweden); Imaxilin (Colombia); Intermox (Philippines); Isimoxin (Italy); Izoltil (Bahrain; Benin; Burkina-Faso; Cyprus; Egypt; Ethiopia; Gambia; Ghana; Guinea; Iran; Iraq; Israel; Ivory-Coast; Jordan; Kenya; Kuwait; Lebanon; Liberia; Libya; Malawi; Mali; Mauritania; Mauritius; Morocco; Niger; Nigeria; Oman; Qatar; Republic-of-Yemen; Saudi-Arabia; Senegal; Seychelles; Sierra-Leone; South-Africa; Sudan; Syria; Tanzania; Tunia; Uganda; United-Arab-Emirates; Zambia; Zimbabwe); Julphamox (Peru); Kamoxin (Thailand); Ladoxillin (Philippines); Lamoxy (India); Larocilin (Argentina); Magnimox (Peru); Maxamox (Australia); Maxcil (South-Africa); Medimox (Indonesia); Meixil (Thailand); Mopen (Italy); Morgenxil (Spain); Mox (India); Moxacin (Australia); Moxaline (Belgium); Moxarin (Bahrain; Cyprus; Egypt; Iran; Iraq; Israel; Jordan; Kuwait; Lebanon; Libya; Oman; Qatar; Republic-of-Yemen; Saudi-Arabia; Syria; United-Arab-Emirates); Moxilen (Benin; Burkina-Faso; Ethiopia; Gambia; Ghana; Guinea; Hong-Kong; Ivory-Coast; Kenya; Liberia; Malawi; Mali; Mauritania; Mauritius; Morocco; Niger; Nigeria; Senegal; Seychelles; Sierra-Leone; South-Africa; Sudan; Taiwan; Tanzania; Tunia; Uganda; Zambia; Zimbabwe); Moximar (Philippines); Moxtid (Indonesia); Moxylin (Ecuador); Moxypen (Israel; South-Africa); Moxyvit (Israel); Neogram (Colombia); Novabritine (Belgium); Novamox (Philippines); Novamoxin (Canada); Novenzymin (Argentina); Optium (Argentina); Ospamox (Austria; Bahrain; Bulgaria; Costa-Rica; Cyprus; Dominican-Republic; Egypt; El-Salvador; Guatemala; Honduras; Hong-Kong; Indonesia; Iran; Iraq; Israel; Jordan; Kuwait; Lebanon; Libya; Malaysia; New-Zealand; Nicaragua; Oman; Panama; Peru; Portugal; Qatar; Republic-of-Yemen; Saudi-Arabia; Syria; United-Arab-Emirates); Pamocil (Italy); Pamoxicillin (Taiwan); Pamoxin (Korea); Panvilon (Philippines); Pasetocin (Japan); Penamox (Argentina; China; Mexico; Peru); Penbiosyn (Philippines); Piramox (Bahrain; Benin; Burkina-Faso; Cyprus; Egypt; Ethiopia; Gambia; Ghana; Guinea; Iran; Iraq; Israel; Ivory-Coast; Jordan; Kenya; Kuwait; Lebanon; Liberia; Libya; Malawi; Mali; Mauritania; Mauritius; Morocco; Niger; Nigeria; Oman; Qatar; Republic-of-Yemen; Saudi-Arabia; Senegal; Seychelles; Sierra-Leone; South-Africa; Sudan; Syria; Tanzania; Tunia; Uganda; United-Arab-Emirates; Zambia; Zimbabwe); Rancil (Thailand); Ranmoxy (South-Africa); Ranoxyl (Malaysia); Robamox (Indonesia); Rocillin (South-Africa); Romoxil (Philippines); Ronemox (India); Saltermox (South-Africa); Sawacillin (Japan); Sawamezin (Japan); Servamox (Taiwan); Shamoxil (Bahrain; Cyprus; Egypt; Iran; Iraq; Jordan; Kuwait; Lebanon; Libya; Oman; Qatar; Republic-of-Yemen; Saudi-Arabia; Syria; United-Arab-Emirates); Sia-mox (Thailand); Sil-A-mox (Thailand); Simoxil (Italy); Solpenox (Indonesia); Superpeni (Spain); Teramoxyl (Philippines); Tolodina (Spain); Tormoxin (Republic-Of-Yemen); Triafamox (Argentina); Triamoxil (Argentina); Vastamox (Philippines); Velamox (Peru); Vistrep (Philippines); Widecillin (Indonesia); Winpen (Benin; Burkina-Faso; Ethiopia; Gambia; Ghana; Guinea; Ivory-Coast; Kenya; Liberia; Malawi; Mali; Mauritania; Mauritius; Morocco; Niger; Nigeria; Senegal; Seychelles; Sierra-Leone; Sudan; Tanzania; Tunia; Uganda; Zambia; Zimbabwe); Xiltrop (Indonesia); Zamox (Colombia); Zamoxil (Malaysia); Zerrsox (Philippines); Zimox (Italy)

Cost of Therapy: $27.13 (Infection; Amoxil; 875 mg; 2 tablets/day; 14 day supply)
$10.48 (Infection; Generic Capsules; 500 mg; 3 capsules/day; 14 day supply)

DESCRIPTION

Amoxicillin is a semisynthetic antibiotic, an analog of ampicillin, with a broad spectrum of bactericidal activity against many gram-positive and gram-negative microorganisms. Chemically it is (2*S*,5*R*,6*R*)-6-[(*R*)-(-)-2-amino-2-(*p*-hydroxyphenyl)acetamido]-3,3-dimethyl-7-oxo-4-thia-1-azabicyclo[3.2.0]heptane-2-carboxylic acid trihydrate.

The amoxicillin molecular formula is $C_{16}H_{19}N_3O_5S \cdot 3H_2O$, and the molecular weight is 419.45.

Amoxil capsules, tablets, and powder for oral suspension are intended for oral administration.

CAPSULES

Each Amoxil capsule, with royal blue opaque cap and pink opaque body, contains 250 or 500 mg amoxicillin as the trihydrate. *Inactive Ingredients:* D&C red no. 28, FD&C blue no. 1, FD&C red no. 40, gelatin, magnesium stearate, and titanium dioxide.

TABLETS

Each tablet contains 500 or 875 mg amoxicillin as the trihydrate. *Inactive Ingredients:* Colloidal silicon dioxide, crospovidone, FD&C red no. 30 aluminum lake, hydroxypropyl methylcellulose, magnesium stearate, microcrystalline cellulose, polyethylene glycol, sodium starch glycolate, and titanium dioxide.

CHEWABLE TABLETS

Each cherry-banana-peppermint-flavored tablet contains 200 or 400 mg amoxicillin as the trihydrate.

Each 200 mg chewable table contains 0.0005 mEq (0.0107 mg) of sodium; the 400 mg chewable tablet contains 0.0009 mEq (0.0215 mg) of sodium. *200 and 400 mg Inactive Ingredients:* Aspartame, crospovidone, FD&C red no. 40 aluminum lake, flavorings, magnesium stearate, and mannitol.

See PRECAUTIONS.

POWDER FOR ORAL SUSPENSION

Each 5 millileter of reconstituted suspension contains 125, 200, 250, or 400 mg amoxicillin as the trihydrate. Each 5 ml of the 125 mg reconstituted suspension contains 0.11 mEq (2.51 mg) of sodium; each 5 ml of the 250 mg reconstituted suspension contains 0.15 mEq (3.36 mg) of sodium. Each 5 ml of the 200 mg reconstituted suspension contains 0.15 mEq (3.39 mg) of sodium; each 5 ml of the 400 mg reconstituted suspension contains 0.19 mEq (4.33 mg) of sodium.

PEDIATRIC DROPS FOR ORAL SUSPENSION

Each ml of reconstituted suspension contains 50 mg amoxicillin as the trihydrate and 0.03 mEq (0.69 mg) of sodium.

Amoxicillin trihydrate for oral suspension 125 mg/5 ml (reconstituted) is a strawberry-flavored pink suspension; the 200, 250 (or 50 mg/ml), and 400 mg/5 ml are bubble-gum-flavored pink suspensions. *Inactive Ingredients:* FD&C red no. 3, flavorings, silica gel, sodium benzoate, sodium citrate, sucrose, and xanthan gum.

CLINICAL PHARMACOLOGY

Amoxicillin is stable in the presence of gastric acid and is rapidly absorbed after oral administration. The effect of food on the absorption of amoxicillin from amoxicillin tablets and suspension has been partially investigated. The 400 and 875 mg formulations have been studied only when administered at the start of a light meal. However, food effect studies have not been performed with the 200 and 500 mg formulations. Amoxicillin diffuses readily into most body tissues and fluids, with the exception of brain and spinal fluid, except when meninges are inflamed. The half-life of amoxicillin is 61.3 minutes. Most of the amoxicillin is excreted unchanged in the urine; its excretion can be delayed by concurrent administration of probenecid. In blood serum, amoxicillin is approximately 20% protein-bound.

Orally administered doses of 250 and 500 mg amoxicillin capsules result in average peak blood levels 1-2 hours after administration in the range of 3.5-5.0 µg/ml and 5.5-7.5 µg/ml, respectively.

Mean amoxicillin pharmacokinetic parameters from an open, two-part, single-dose crossover bioequivalence study in 27 adults comparing 875 mg of amoxicillin with 875 mg of amoxicillin/clavulanate potassium showed that the 875 mg tablet of amoxicillin produces an AUC(0-∞) of 35.4 ± 8.1 µg·h/ml and a C_{max} of 13.8 ± 4.1 µg/ml. Dosing was at the start of a light meal following an overnight fast.

Orally administered doses of amoxicillin suspension, 125 and 250 mg/5 ml, result in average peak blood levels 1-2 hours after administration in the range of 1.5-3.0 µg/ml and 3.5-5.0 µg/ml, respectively.

Oral administration of single doses of 400 mg amoxicillin chewable tablets and 400 mg/5 ml suspension to 24 adult volunteers yielded comparable pharmacokinetic data (see TABLE 1).

TABLE 1

Amoxicillin Dose*	Amoxicillin (±SD) AUC(0-∞) (µg·h/ml)	C_{max}† (µg/ml)
400 mg (5 ml of suspension)	17.1 (3.1)	5.92 (1.62)
400 mg (one chewable tablet)	17.9 (2.4)	5.18 (1.64)

* Administered at the start of a light meal.
† Mean values of 24 normal volunteers. Peak concentrations occurred approximately 1 hour after the dose.

Detectable serum levels are observed up to 8 hours after an orally administered dose of amoxicillin. Following a 1 g dose and utilizing a special skin window technique to determine levels of the antibiotic, it was noted that therapeutic levels were found in the interstitial fluid. Approximately 60% of an orally administered dose of amoxicillin is excreted in the urine within 6-8 hours.

MICROBIOLOGY

Amoxicillin is similar to ampicillin in its bactericidal action against susceptible organisms during the stage of active multiplication. It acts through the inhibition of biosynthesis of cell wall mucopeptide. Amoxicillin has been shown to be active against most strains of the following microorganisms, both *in vitro* and in clinical infections as described in INDICATIONS AND USAGE.

Aerobic Gram-Positive Microorganisms:

Enterococcus faecalis.
Staphylococcus spp.* (β-lactamase-negative strains only).
Streptococcus pneumoniae.
Streptococcus spp. (α- and β-hemolytic strains only).

*Staphylococci which are susceptible to amoxicillin but resistant to methicillin/oxacillin should be considered as resistant to amoxicillin.

Aerobic Gram-Negative Microorganisms:

Escherichia coli (β-lactamase-negative strains only).
Haemophilus influenzae (β-lactamase-negative strains only).
Neisseria gonorrhoeae (β-lactamase-negative strains only).
Proteus mirabilis (β-lactamase-negative strains only).

Helicobacter:

Helicobacter pylori.

SUSCEPTIBILITY TESTING

Dilution Techniques

Quantitative methods are used to determine antimicrobial minimum inhibitory concentrations (MICs). These MICs provide estimates of the susceptibility of bacteria to antimicrobial compounds. The MICs should be determined using a standardized procedure. Standardized procedures are based on a dilution method[1] (broth or agar) or equivalent with standardized inoculum concentrations and standardized concentrations of **ampicillin** powder. Ampicillin is sometimes used to predict susceptibility of *Streptococcus pneumoniae* to amoxicillin; however, some intermediate strains have been shown to be susceptible to amoxicillin. Therefore, *Streptococcus pneumoniae* susceptibility should be tested using amoxicillin powder. The MIC values should be interpreted according to the criteria in TABLE 2 and TABLE 3.

TABLE 2 *For Gram-Positive Aerobes*

	MIC	Interpretation
Enterococcus		
	≤8 µg/ml	Susceptible (S)
	≥16 µg/ml	Resistant (R)
*Staphylococcus**		
	≤0.25 µg/ml	Susceptible (S)
	≥0.5 µg/ml	Resistant (R)
Streptococcus (except *S. pneumoniae*)		
	≤0.25 µg/ml	Susceptible (S)
	0.5 to 4 µg/ml	Intermediate (I)
	≥8 µg/ml	Resistant (R)
S. pneumoniae† from non-meningitis sources (**Amoxicillin** powder should be used to determine susceptibility)		
	≤2.0 µg/ml	Susceptible (S)
	4.0 µg/ml	Intermediate (I)
	≥8.0 µg/ml	Resistant (R)

* Staphylococci which are susceptible to amoxicillin but resistant to methicillin/oxacillin should be considered as resistant to amoxicillin.
† These interpretive standards are applicable only to broth microdilution susceptibility tests using cation-adjusted Mueller-Hinton broth with 2-5% lysed horse blood.
Note: These criteria are based on the recommended doses for respiratory tract infections.

TABLE 3 *For Gram-Negative Aerobes*

	MIC	Interpretation
Enterobacteriaceae		
	≤8 µg/ml	Susceptible (S)
	16 µg/ml	Intermediate (I)
	≥32 µg/ml	Resistant (R)
*H. influenzae**		
	≤1 µg/ml	Susceptible (S)
	2 µg/ml	Intermediate (I)
	≥4 µg/ml	Resistant (R)

* These interpretive standards are applicable only to broth microdilution test with *Haemophilus influenzae* using *Haemophilus* Test Medium (HTM).[1]

A report of "Susceptible" indicates that the pathogen is likely to be inhibited if the antimicrobial compound in the blood reaches the concentrations usually achievable. A report of "Intermediate" indicates that the result should be considered equivocal, and, if the microorganism is not fully susceptible to alternative, clinically feasible drugs, the test should be repeated. This category implies possible clinical applicability in body sites where the drug is physiologically concentrated or in situations where high dosage of drug can be used. This category also provides a buffer zone which prevents small uncontrolled technical factors from causing major discrepancies in interpretation. A report of "Resistant" indicates that the pathogen is not likely to be inhibited if the antimicrobial compound in the blood reaches the concentrations usually achievable; other therapy should be selected.

Standardized susceptibility test procedures require the use of laboratory control microorganisms to control the technical aspects of the laboratory procedures. Standard **ampicillin** powder should provide the MIC values found in TABLE 4 and TABLE 5.

TABLE 4

Microorganism	MIC
E. coli ATCC 25922	2-8 µg/ml
E. faecalis ATCC 29212	0.5-2 µg/ml
H. influenzae ATCC 49247*	2-8 µg/ml
S. aureus ATCC 29213	0.25-1 µg/ml

* This quality control range is applicable to only *H. influenzae* ATCC 49247 tested by a broth microdilution procedure using HTM.[1]

TABLE 5 *Using Amoxicillin to Determine Susceptibility*

Microorganism	MIC Range
S. pneumoniae ATCC 49619*	0.03-0.12 µg/ml

* This quality control range is applicable to only *S. pneumoniae* ATCC 49619 tested by the broth microdilution procedure using cation-adjusted Mueller-Hinton broth with 2-5% lysed horse blood.

Diffusion Techniques

Quantitative methods that require measurement of zone diameters also provide reproducible estimates of the susceptibility of bacteria to antimicrobial compounds. One such standardized procedure[2] requires the use of standardized inoculum concentrations. This procedure uses paper disks impregnated with 10 µg ampicillin to test the susceptibility of microorganisms, except *S. pneumoniae,* to amoxicillin. Interpretation involves correlation of the diameter obtained in the disk test with the MIC for **ampicillin.**

Reports from the laboratory providing results of the standard single-disk susceptibility test with a 10 µg ampicillin disk should be interpreted according to the criteria found in TABLE 6 and TABLE 7.

TABLE 6 *For Gram-Positive Aerobes*

	Zone Diameter	Interpretation
Enterococcus		
	≥17 mm	Susceptible (S)
	≤16 mm	Resistant (R)
*Staphylococcus**		
	≥29 mm	Susceptible (S)
	≤28 mm	Resistant (R)
β-hemolytic streptococci		
	≥26 mm	Susceptible (S)
	19-25 mm	Intermediate (I)
	≤18 mm	Resistant (R)

* Staphylococci which are susceptible to amoxicillin but resistant to methicillin/oxacillin should be considered as resistant to amoxicillin.

Note: For streptococci (other than β-hemolytic streptococci and *S. pneumoniae*), an ampicillin MIC should be determined.

S. pneumoniae

S. pneumoniae should be tested using a 1 µg oxacillin disk. Isolates with oxacillin zone sizes of ≥20 mm are susceptible to amoxicillin. An amoxicillin MIC should be determined on isolates of *S. pneumoniae* with oxacillin zone sizes of ≤19 mm.

TABLE 7 *For Gram-Negative Aerobes*

	Zone Diameter	Interpretation
Enterobacteriaceae		
	≥17 mm	Susceptible (S)
	14-16 mm	Intermediate (I)
	≤13 mm	Resistant (R)
*H. influenzae**		
	≥22 mm	Susceptible (S)
	19-21 mm	Intermediate (I)
	≤18 mm	Resistant (R)

* These interpretive standards are applicable only to disk diffusion susceptibility tests with *H. influenzae* using *Haemophilus* Test Medium (HTM).[2]

Interpretation should be as stated above for results using dilution techniques.

As with standard dilution techniques, disk diffusion susceptibility test procedures require the use of laboratory control microorganisms. The 10 µg **ampicillin** disk should provide the following zone diameters in these laboratory test quality control strains (see TABLE 8 and TABLE 9).

TABLE 8

Microorganism	Zone Diameter
E. coli ATCC 25922	16-22 mm
H. influenzae ATCC 49247*	13-21 mm
S. aureus ATCC 25923	27-35 mm

* This quality control range is applicable to only *H. influenzae* ATCC 49247 tested by a disk diffusion procedure using HTM.[2]

TABLE 9 *Using 1 µg Oxacillin Disk*

Microorganism	Zone Diameter
S. pneumoniae ATCC 49619*	8-12 mm

* This quality control range is applicable to only *S. pneumoniae* ATCC 49619 tested by a disk diffusion procedure using Mueller-Hinton agar supplemented with 5% sheep blood and incubated in 5% CO_2.

Susceptibility Testing for Helicobacter pylori

In vitro susceptibility testing methods and diagnostic products currently available for determining minimum inhibitory concentrations (MICs) and zone sizes have not been standardized, validated, or approved for testing *H. pylori* microorganisms.

Culture and susceptibility testing should be obtained in patients who fail triple therapy. If clarithromycin resistance is found, a non-clarithromycin-containing regimen should be used.

INDICATIONS AND USAGE

Amoxicillin is indicated in the treatment of infections due to susceptible (ONLY β-lactamase-negative) strains of the designated microorganisms in the conditions listed below:

Infections of the ear, nose, and throat due to *Streptococcus* spp. (α- and β-hemolytic strains only), *Streptococcus pneumoniae, Staphylococcus* spp., or *H. influenzae.*

Infections of the genitourinary tract due to *E. coli, P. mirabilis,* or *E. faecalis.*

Infections of the skin and skin structure due to *Streptococcus* spp. (α- and β-hemolytic strains only), *Staphylococcus* spp., or *E. coli.*

Infections of the lower respiratory tract due to *Streptococcus* spp. (α- and β-hemolytic strains only), *Streptococcus pneumoniae, Staphylococcus* spp., or *H. influenzae.*

Gonorrhea, acute uncomplicated (ano-genital and urethral infections) due to *N. gonorrhoeae* (males and females).

Therapy may be instituted prior to obtaining results from bacteriological and susceptibility studies to determine the causative organisms and their susceptibility to amoxicillin.

Indicated surgical procedures should be performed.

H. PYLORI ERADICATION TO REDUCE THE RISK OF DUODENAL ULCER RECURRENCE

Triple Therapy

Amoxicillin/Clarithromycin/Lansoprazole

Amoxicillin, in combination with clarithromycin plus lansoprazole as triple therapy, is indicated for the treatment of patients with *H. pylori* infection and duodenal ulcer disease (active or 1 year history of a duodenal ulcer) to eradicate *H. pylori.* Eradication of *H. pylori* has been shown to reduce the risk of duodenal ulcer recurrence (see DOSAGE AND ADMINISTRATION).

Dual Therapy

Amoxicillin/Lansoprazole

Amoxicillin, in combination with lansoprazole delayed-release capsules as dual therapy, is indicated for the treatment of patients with *H. pylori* infection and duodenal ulcer disease (active or 1 year history of a duodenal ulcer) **who are either allergic or intolerant to clarithromycin or in whom resistance to clarithromycin is known or suspected.** (See the CLINICAL PHARMACOLOGY, Microbiology section of the clarithromycin product information.) Eradication of *H. pylori* has been shown to reduce the risk of duodenal ulcer recurrence. (See DOSAGE AND ADMINISTRATION.)

NON-FDA APPROVED INDICATIONS

In addition, amoxicillin may be used for the treatment of actinomycosis and Lyme disease, although these uses have not been approved by the FDA.

CONTRAINDICATIONS

A history of allergic reaction to any of the penicillins is a contraindication.

WARNINGS

SERIOUS AND OCCASIONALLY FATAL HYPERSENSITIVITY (ANAPHYLACTIC) REACTIONS HAVE BEEN REPORTED IN PATIENTS ON PENICILLIN THERAPY. ALTHOUGH ANAPHYLAXIS IS MORE FREQUENT FOLLOWING PARENTERAL THERAPY, IT HAS OCCURRED IN PATIENTS ON ORAL PENICILLINS. THESE REACTIONS ARE MORE LIKELY TO OCCUR IN INDIVIDUALS WITH A HISTORY OF PENICILLIN HYPERSENSITIVITY AND/OR A HISTORY OF SENSITIVITY TO MULTIPLE ALLERGENS. THERE HAVE BEEN REPORTS OF INDIVIDUALS WITH A HISTORY OF PENICILLIN HYPERSENSITIVITY WHO HAVE EXPERIENCED SEVERE REACTIONS WHEN TREATED WITH CEPHALOSPORINS. BEFORE INITIATING THERAPY WITH *AMOXICILLIN,* CAREFUL INQUIRY SHOULD BE MADE CONCERNING PREVIOUS HYPERSENSITIVITY REACTIONS TO PENICILLINS, CEPHALOSPORINS, OR OTHER ALLERGENS. IF AN ALLERGIC REACTION OCCURS, *AMOXICILLIN* SHOULD BE DISCONTINUED AND APPROPRIATE THERAPY INSTITUTED. **SERIOUS ANAPHYLACTIC REACTIONS REQUIRE IMMEDIATE EMERGENCY TREATMENT WITH EPINEPHRINE. OXYGEN, IV STEROIDS, AND AIRWAY MANAGEMENT, INCLUDING INTUBATION, SHOULD ALSO BE ADMINISTERED AS INDICATED.**

Pseudomembranous colitis has been reported with nearly all antibacterial agents, including amoxicillin, and may range in severity from mild to life-threatening. Therefore, it is important to consider this diagnosis in patients who present with diarrhea subsequent to the administration of antibacterial agents.

Treatment with antibacterial agents alters the normal flora of the colon and may permit overgrowth of clostridia. Studies indicate that a toxin produced by *Clostridium difficile* is a primary cause of "antibiotic-associated colitis".

After the diagnosis of pseudomembranous colitis has been established, appropriate therapeutic measures should be initiated. Mild cases of pseudomembranous colitis usually respond to drug discontinuation alone. In moderate to severe cases, consideration should be given to management with fluids and electrolytes, protein supplementation, and treatment with an antibacterial drug clinically effective against *Clostridium difficile* colitis.

PRECAUTIONS

GENERAL

The possibility of superinfections with mycotic or bacterial pathogens should be kept in mind during therapy. If superinfections occur, amoxicillin should be discontinued and appropriate therapy instituted.

PHENYLKETONURICS

Each 200 mg amoxicillin chewable tablet contains 1.82 mg phenylalanine; each 400 mg chewable tablet contains 3.64 phenylalanine. The amoxicillin suspensions do not contain phenylalanine and can be used by phenylketonurics.

LABORATORY TESTS

As with any potent drug, periodic assessment of renal, hepatic, and hematopoietic function should be made during prolonged therapy.

All patients with gonorrhea should have a serologic test for syphilis at the time of diagnosis. Patients treated with amoxicillin should have a follow-up serologic test for syphilis after 3 months.

DRUG/LABORATORY TEST INTERACTIONS

High urine concentrations of ampicillin may result in false-positive reactions when testing for the presence of glucose in urine using Clinitest, Benedict's Solution or Fehling's Solu-

A

tion. Since this effect may also occur with amoxicillin, it is recommended that glucose tests based on enzymatic glucose oxidase reactions (such as Clinistix or Tes-Tape) be used.

Following administration of ampicillin to pregnant women, a transient decrease in plasma concentration of total conjugated estriol, estriol-glucuronide, conjugated estrone, and estradiol has been noted. This effect may also occur with amoxicillin.

CARCINOGENESIS, MUTAGENESIS, AND IMPAIRMENT OF FERTILITY

Long-term studies in animals have not been performed to evaluate carcinogenic potential. Studies to detect mutagenic potential of amoxicillin alone have not been conducted; however, the following information is available from tests on a 4:1 mixture of amoxicillin and potassium clavulanate. Amoxicillin; potassium clavulanate was non-mutagenic in the Ames bacterial mutation assay, and the yeast gene conversion assay. Amoxicillin; potassium clavulanate was weakly positive in the mouse lymphoma assay, but the trend toward increased mutation frequencies in this assay occurred at doses that were also associated with decreased cell survival. Amoxicillin; potassium clavulanate was negative in the mouse micronucleus test, and in the dominant lethal assay in mice. Potassium clavulanate alone was tested in the Ames bacterial mutation assay and in the mouse micronucleus test, and was negative in each of these assays. In a multi-generation reproduction study in rats, no impairment of fertility or other adverse reproductive effects were seen at doses up to 500 mg/kg (approximately 3 times the human dose in mg/m^2).

PREGNANCY, TERATOGENIC EFFECTS, PREGNANCY CATEGORY B

Reproduction studies have been performed in mice and rats at doses up to 10 times the human dose and have revealed no evidence of impaired fertility or harm to the fetus due to amoxicillin. There are, however, no adequate and well-controlled studies in pregnant women. Because animal reproduction studies are not always predictive of human response, this drug should be used during pregnancy only if clearly needed.

LABOR AND DELIVERY

Oral ampicillin-class antibiotics are poorly absorbed during labor. Studies in guinea pigs showed that IV administration of ampicillin slightly decreased the uterine tone and frequency of contractions but moderately increased the height and duration of contractions. However, it is not known whether use of amoxicillin in humans during labor or delivery has immediate or delayed adverse effects on the fetus, prolongs the duration of labor, or increases the likelihood that forceps delivery or other obstetrical intervention or resuscitation of the newborn will be necessary.

NURSING MOTHERS

Penicillins have been shown to be excreted in human milk. Amoxicillin use by nursing mothers may lead to sensitization of infants. Caution should be exercised when amoxicillin is administered to a nursing woman.

PEDIATRIC USE

Because of incompletely developed renal function in neonates and young infants, the elimination of amoxicillin may be delayed. Dosing of amoxicillin should be modified in pediatric patients 12 weeks or younger (≤3 months). [See DOSAGE AND ADMINISTRATION, Neonates and Infants Aged ≤12 Weeks (≤3 months).]

DRUG INTERACTIONS

Probenecid decreases the renal tubular secretion of amoxicillin. Concurrent use of amoxicillin and probenecid may result in increased and prolonged blood levels of amoxicillin.

Chloramphenicol, macrolides, sulfonamides, and tetracyclines may interfere with the bactericidal effects of penicillin. This has been demonstrated *in vitro;* however, the clinical significance of this interaction is not well documented.

ADVERSE REACTIONS

As with other penicillins, it may be expected that untoward reactions will be essentially limited to sensitivity phenomena. They are more likely to occur in individuals who have previously demonstrated hypersensitivity to penicillins and in those with a history of allergy, asthma, hay fever, or urticaria.

The following adverse reactions have been reported as associated with the use of penicillins:

Gastrointestinal: Nausea, vomiting, diarrhea, and hemorrhagic/pseudomembranous colitis.

Onset of pseudomembranous colitis symptoms may occur during or after antibiotic treatment. (See WARNINGS.)

Hypersensitivity Reactions: Serum sickness like reactions, erythematous maculopapular rashes, erythema multiforme, Stevens-Johnson Syndrome, exfoliative dermatitus, toxic epidermal necrolysis, acute generalized exanthematous pustulosis, hypersensitivity vasculitis and urticaria have been reported. *NOTE:* These hypersensitivity reactions may be controlled with antihistamines and, if necessary, systemic corticosteroids. Whenever such reactions occur, amoxicillin should be discontinued unless, in the opinion of the physician, the condition being treated is life-threatening and amenable only to amoxicillin therapy.

Liver: A moderate rise in AST (SGOT) and/or ALT (SGPT) has been noted, but the significance of this finding is unknown. Hepatic dysfunction including cholestatic jaundice, hepatic cholestasis and acute cytolytic hepatitis have been reported.

Hemic and Lymphatic Systems: Anemia, including hemolytic anemia, thrombocytopenia, thrombocytopenic purpura, eosinophilia, leukopenia, and agranulocytosis have been reported during therapy with penicillins. These reactions are usually reversible on discontinuation of therapy and are believed to be hypersensitivity phenomena.

Central Nervous System: Reversible hyperactivity, agitation, anxiety, insomnia, confusion, convulsions, behavioral changes, and/or dizziness have been reported rarely.

Miscellaneous: Superficial tooth discoloration has been reported very rarely in children. Good oral hygiene may help to prevent tooth discoloration as it can usually be removed by brushing.

COMBINATION THERAPY WITH CLARITHROMYCIN AND LANSOPRAZOLE

In clinical trials using combination therapy with amoxicillin plus clarithromycin and lansoprazole, and amoxicillin plus lansoprazole, no adverse reactions peculiar to these drug combinations were observed. Adverse reactions that have occurred have been limited to those that had been previously reported with amoxicillin, clarithromycin, or lansoprazole.

Triple Therapy

Amoxicillin/Clarithromycin/Lansoprazole

The most frequently reported adverse events for patients who received triple therapy were diarrhea (7%), headache (6%), and taste perversion (5%). No treatment-emergent adverse events were observed at significantly higher rates with triple therapy than with any dual therapy regimen.

Dual Therapy

Amoxicillin/Lansoprazole

The most frequently reported adverse events for patients who received amoxicillin tid plus lansoprazole tid dual therapy were diarrhea (8%) and headache (7%). No treatment-emergent adverse events were observed at significantly higher rates with amoxicillin tid plus lansoprazole tid dual therapy than with lansoprazole alone.

For more information on adverse reactions with clarithromycin or lansoprazole, refer to the ADVERSE REACTIONS section of their respective product information.

DOSAGE AND ADMINISTRATION

Amoxicillin capsules, chewable tablets, and oral suspensions may be given without regard to meals. The 400 mg suspension, 400 mg chewable tablet, and the 875 mg tablet have been studied only when administered at the start of a light meal. However, food effect studies have not been performed with the 200 and 500 mg formulations.

NEONATES AND INFANTS AGED ≤12 WEEKS (≤3 MONTHS)

Due to incompletely developed renal function affecting elimination of amoxicillin in this age group, the recommended upper dose of amoxicillin is 30 mg/kg/day divided q12h.

TABLE 12

Infection	Severity*	Usual Adult Dose	Usual Dose for Children >3 months†‡
Ear/nose/throat	Mild/moderate	500 mg q12h or 250 mg q8h	25 mg/kg/day in divided doses q12h **or** 20 mg/kg/day in divided doses q8h
	Severe	875 mg q12h or 500 mg q8h	45 mg/kg/day in divided doses q12h **or** 40 mg/kg/day in divided doses q8h
Lower respiratory tract	Mild/moderate or severe	875 mg q12h or 500 mg q8h	45 mg/kg/day in divided doses q12h **or** 40 mg/kg/day in divided doses q8h
Skin/skin structure	Mild/moderate	500 mg q12h or 250 mg q8h	25 mg/kg/day in divided doses q12h **or** 20 mg/kg/day in divided doses q8h
	Severe	875 mg q12h or 500 mg q8h	45 mg/kg/day in divided doses q12h **or** 40 mg/kg/day in divided doses q8h
Genitourinary tract	Mild/moderate	500 mg q12h or 250 mg q8h	25 mg/kg/day in divided doses q12h **or** 20 mg/kg/day in divided doses q8h
	Severe	875 mg q12h or 500 mg q8h	45 mg/kg/day in divided doses q12h **or** 40 mg/kg/day in divided doses q8h
Gonorrhea acute, uncomplicated ano-genital and urethral infections in males and females		3 g as single oral dose	Prepubertal children: 50 mg/kg amoxicillin, combined with 25 mg/kg probenecid as a single dose§

* Dosing for infections caused by less susceptible organisms should follow the recommendations for severe infections.

† The children's dosage is intended for individuals whose weight is less than 40 kg. Children weighing 40 kg or more should be dosed according to the adult recommendations.

‡ Each strength of amoxicillin suspension is available as a chewable tablet for use by older children.

§ **NOTE: SINCE PROBENECID IS CONTRAINDICATED IN CHILDREN UNDER 2 YEARS, DO NOT USE THIS REGIMEN IN THESE CASES.**

ADULTS AND PEDIATRIC PATIENTS >3 MONTHS

After reconstitution, the required amount of suspension should be placed directly on the child's tongue for swallowing. Alternate means of administration are to add the required amount of suspension to formula, milk, fruit juice, water, ginger ale, or cold drinks. These preparations should then be taken immediately. To be certain the child is receiving full dosage, such preparations should be consumed in entirety.

All patients with gonorrhea should be evaluated for syphilis (see PRECAUTIONS, Laboratory Tests).

Larger doses may be required for stubborn or severe infections.

GENERAL

It should be recognized that in the treatment of chronic urinary tract infections, frequent bacteriological and clinical appraisals are necessary. Smaller doses than those recommended above should not be used. Even higher doses may be needed at times. In stubborn infections, therapy may be required for several weeks. It may be necessary to continue clinical and/or bacteriological follow-up for several months after cessation of therapy. Except for gonorrhea, treatment should be continued for a minimum of 48-72 hours beyond the time that the patient becomes asymptomatic or evidence of bacterial eradication has been obtained. It is recommended that there be at least 10 days' treatment for any infection caused by *Streptococcus pyogenes* to prevent the occurrence of acute rheumatic fever.

H. pylori Eradication to Reduce the Risk of Duodenal Ulcer Recurrence

Triple Therapy

Amoxicillin/Clarithromycin/Lansoprazole: The recommended adult oral dose is 1 g amoxicillin, 500 mg clarithromycin, and 30 mg lansoprazole, all given twice daily (q12h) for 14 days (see INDICATIONS AND USAGE).

Dual Therapy

Amoxicillin/Lansoprazole: The recommended adult oral dose is 1 g amoxicillin and 30 mg lansoprazole, each given 3 times daily (q8h) for 14 days. (See INDICATIONS AND USAGE.)

Please refer to the CONTRAINDICATIONS and WARNINGS sections of the clarithromycin and the lansoprazole product information, and for information regarding dosing in elderly and renally impaired patients.

DOSING RECOMMENDATIONS FOR ADULTS WITH IMPAIRED RENAL FUNCTION

Patients with impaired renal function do not generally require a reduction in dose unless the impairment is severe. Severely impaired patients with a glomerular filtration rate of <30 ml/min should not receive the 875 mg tablet. Patients with a glomerular filtration rate of 10-30 ml/min should receive 500 or 250 mg every 12 hours, depending on the severity of the infection. Patients with a less than 10 ml/min glomerular filtration rate should receive 500 or 250 mg every 24 hours, depending on severity of the infection.

Hemodialysis patients should receive 500 or 250 mg every 24 hours, depending on severity of the infection. They should receive an additional dose both during and at the end of dialysis.

There are currently no dosing recommendations for pediatric patients with impaired renal function.

HOW SUPPLIED

AMOXIL CAPSULES

Each capsule contains 250 or 500 mg amoxicillin as the trihydrate. The cap and body of the 250 mg capsule are imprinted with the product name "AMOXIL" and "250"; the cap and body of the 500 mg capsule are imprinted with "AMOXIL" and "500".

Storage: Store at or below 20°C (68°F). Dispense in a tight container.

AMOXIL TABLETS

Each tablet contains 500 or 875 mg amoxicillin as the trihydrate. Each film-coated, capsule-shaped, pink tablet is debossed with "AMOXIL" centered over "500" or "875," respectively. The 875 mg tablet is scored on the reverse side.

Storage: Store at or below 25°C (77°F). Dispense in a tight container.

AMOXIL CHEWABLE TABLETS

Each cherry-banana-peppermint-flavored tablet contains 200 or 400 mg amoxicillin as the trihydrate. The 200 and 400 mg pale pink round tablets are imprinted with the product name "AMOXIL" and "200" or "400" along the edge of one side.

Storage: Store at or below 25°C (77°F). Dispense in a tight container.

AMOXIL FOR ORAL SUSPENSION

Each 5 milliliter of reconstituted strawberry-flavored suspension contains 125 mg amoxicillin as the trihydrate. Each 5 ml of reconstituted bubble-gum-flavored suspension contains 200, 250, or 400 mg amoxicillin as the trihydrate.

Storage: Store unreconstituted powder at or below 20°C (68°F).

Note: SHAKE WELL BEFORE USING. Keep bottle tightly closed. Any unused portion of the reconstituted suspension must be discarded after 14 days. Refrigeration preferable, but not required.

AMOXIL PEDIATRIC DROPS FOR ORAL SUSPENSION

Each ml of bubble-gum-flavored reconstituted suspension contains 50 mg amoxicillin as the trihydrate.

Storage: Store at or below 20°C (68°F).

Note: SHAKE WELL BEFORE USING. Keep bottle tightly closed. Any unused portion of the reconstituted suspension must be discarded after 14 days. Refrigeration preferable, but not required.

PRODUCT LISTING - RATED THERAPEUTICALLY EQUIVALENT

Capsule - Oral - 250 mg

Size	Price	Manufacturer	NDC
6's	$7.00	GENERIC, Pd-Rx Pharmaceuticals	55289-0019-06
15's	$2.55	GENERIC, Circle Pharmaceuticals Inc	00659-0103-15
15's	$9.60	GENERIC, Pd-Rx Pharmaceuticals	55289-0019-15
20's	$8.06	GENERIC, Pharma Pac	52959-0011-20
21's	$3.15	GENERIC, Circle Pharmaceuticals Inc	00659-0103-21
21's	$8.37	GENERIC, Pharma Pac	52959-0011-21
21's	$9.12	GENERIC, Dhs Inc	55887-0993-21
21's	$9.80	GENERIC, Pd-Rx Pharmaceuticals	55289-0019-21
24's	$9.36	GENERIC, Pharma Pac	52959-0011-24
24's	$10.30	GENERIC, Pd-Rx Pharmaceuticals	55289-0019-24
25's	$12.00	GENERIC, Pd-Rx Pharmaceuticals	55289-0019-97
30 x 12	$94.20	GENERIC, Geneva Pharmaceuticals	00003-0101-20
30's	$2.98	GENERIC, Circle Pharmaceuticals Inc	00659-0103-30
30's	$3.94	GENERIC, Pd-Rx Pharmaceuticals	55289-0028-30
30's	$4.67	AMOXIL, Physicians Total Care	54868-0193-01
30's	$6.70	GENERIC, Allscripts Pharmaceutical Company	54569-1508-00
30's	$7.00	GENERIC, Teva Pharmaceuticals Usa	00332-3107-04
30's	$7.99	GENERIC, Golden State Medical	60429-0021-30
30's	$9.66	GENERIC, Dhs Inc	55887-0993-30
30's	$10.98	GENERIC, Pd-Rx Pharmaceuticals	55289-0019-30
30's	$11.55	GENERIC, Pharma Pac	52959-0011-30
30's	$29.70	GENERIC, Med-Pro Inc	53978-5002-05
40's	$4.60	GENERIC, Circle Pharmaceuticals Inc	00659-0103-40
40's	$14.48	GENERIC, Pd-Rx Pharmaceuticals	55289-0019-40
40's	$15.20	GENERIC, Pharma Pac	52959-0011-40
50's	$5.34	GENERIC, Pd-Rx Pharmaceuticals	55289-0028-50
60's	$18.75	GENERIC, Pd-Rx Pharmaceuticals	55289-0019-60
100's	$6.36	FEDERAL UPPER LIMIT, H.C.F.A. F F P	99999-0231-02
100's	$9.00	GENERIC, International Ethical Laboratories Inc	11584-0391-00
100's	$9.95	GENERIC, Raway Pharmacal Inc	00686-3107-09
100's	$10.46	GENERIC, Pd-Rx Pharmaceuticals	55289-0028-01
100's	$12.25	GENERIC, Raway Pharmacal Inc	00686-0600-20
100's	$13.88	GENERIC, Interstate Drug Exchange Inc	00814-0690-14
100's	$15.95	GENERIC, Major Pharmaceuticals Inc	00904-2617-60
100's	$16.33	GENERIC, Mylan Pharmaceuticals Inc	00378-0204-01
100's	$19.50	GENERIC, Martec Pharmaceuticals Inc	52555-0148-01
100's	$19.80	GENERIC, Geneva Pharmaceuticals	00781-2020-01
100's	$20.25	GENERIC, Watson/Schein Pharmaceuticals Inc	00364-2040-01
100's	$20.95	GENERIC, Teva Pharmaceuticals Usa	00332-3107-09
100's	$21.95	GENERIC, Teva Pharmaceuticals Usa	00332-3107-05
100's	$22.05	GENERIC, Aligen Independent Laboratories Inc	00405-4083-01
100's	$22.38	GENERIC, Pd-Rx Pharmaceuticals	55289-0019-01
100's	$23.95	GENERIC, Major Pharmaceuticals Inc	00904-2617-61
100's	$23.99	GENERIC, Ivax Corporation	00182-1070-01
100's	$24.89	GENERIC, Bristol-Myers Squibb	00003-0101-51
100's	$24.91	GENERIC, Moore, H.L. Drug Exchange Inc	00839-6037-06
100's	$24.94	GENERIC, Mova Pharmaceutical Corporation	55370-0884-07
100's	$24.97	GENERIC, Ranbaxy Laboratories	63304-0654-01
100's	$25.00	GENERIC, Teva Pharmaceuticals Usa	00093-3107-01
100's	$25.00	GENERIC, Purepac Pharmaceutical Company	00228-2688-11
100's	$26.10	GENERIC, Udl Laboratories Inc	51079-0600-20
100's	$26.10	GENERIC, Medirex Inc	57480-0455-01
100's	$27.00	GENERIC, Ivax Corporation	00182-1070-89
100's	$33.25	GENERIC, Bristol-Myers Squibb	00015-7278-73
100's	$35.71	GENERIC, Bristol-Myers Squibb	00015-7278-62

Capsule - Oral - 500 mg

Size	Price	Manufacturer	NDC
4's	$4.45	GENERIC, Pd-Rx Pharmaceuticals	55289-0020-04
6's	$5.36	GENERIC, Pharma Pac	52959-0020-06
6's	$6.25	GENERIC, Pd-Rx Pharmaceuticals	55289-0020-06
9's	$7.25	GENERIC, Pd-Rx Pharmaceuticals	55289-0020-09
14's	$8.30	GENERIC, Pd-Rx Pharmaceuticals	55289-0020-14
15's	$9.03	GENERIC, Pd-Rx Pharmaceuticals	55289-0020-15
20's	$5.62	AMOXIL, Physicians Total Care	54868-0348-02
20's	$11.70	GENERIC, Ranbaxy Laboratories	63304-0762-20
20's	$13.74	GENERIC, Pharma Pac	52959-0020-20
21's	$4.50	GENERIC, Circle Pharmaceuticals Inc	00659-0104-21
21's	$5.30	GENERIC, Pd-Rx Pharmaceuticals	55289-0029-21
21's	$12.62	GENERIC, Dhs Inc	55887-0982-21
21's	$14.26	GENERIC, Pharma Pac	52959-0020-21
24's	$13.90	GENERIC, Pd-Rx Pharmaceuticals	55289-0020-24
28's	$16.23	GENERIC, Pd-Rx Pharmaceuticals	55289-0020-28
28's	$18.92	GENERIC, Pharma Pac	52959-0020-28
30 x 12	$402.00	GENERIC, Bristol-Myers Squibb	00003-0109-20
30 x 30	$167.47	GENERIC, Bristol-Myers Squibb	00003-0109-30
30's	$4.58	GENERIC, Circle Pharmaceuticals Inc	00659-0104-30
30's	$5.76	GENERIC, Pd-Rx Pharmaceuticals	55289-0029-30
30's	$7.82	AMOXIL, Physicians Total Care	54868-0348-01
30's	$13.95	GENERIC, Teva Pharmaceuticals Usa	55953-0716-27
30's	$14.75	GENERIC, Golden State Medical	60429-0022-30
30's	$17.43	GENERIC, Pd-Rx Pharmaceuticals	55289-0020-30
30's	$18.06	GENERIC, Dhs Inc	55887-0982-30
30's	$20.99	GENERIC, Pharma Pac	52959-0020-30
30's	$43.00	GENERIC, Med-Pro Inc	53978-5003-05
40's	$8.19	GENERIC, Circle Pharmaceuticals Inc	00659-0104-40
40's	$24.84	GENERIC, Pharma Pac	52959-0020-40
42's	$18.88	GENERIC, Pd-Rx Pharmaceuticals	55289-0020-42
50's	$9.50	GENERIC, Raway Pharmacal Inc	00686-3109-07
50's	$12.40	GENERIC, Novopharm Usa Inc	55953-0716-33
50's	$13.95	GENERIC, Interstate Drug Exchange Inc	00814-0692-08
50's	$16.95	GENERIC, Major Pharmaceuticals Inc	00904-2618-51
50's	$19.60	GENERIC, Martec Pharmaceuticals Inc	52555-0149-00
50's	$20.35	GENERIC, Pd-Rx Pharmaceuticals	55289-0020-50
50's	$21.60	GENERIC, Watson/Schein Pharmaceuticals Inc	00364-2041-50
50's	$22.30	GENERIC, Mutual/United Research Laboratories	00677-0661-02
50's	$23.00	GENERIC, Ivax Corporation	00182-1071-19
50's	$23.35	GENERIC, Teva Pharmaceuticals Usa	00093-3109-53
50's	$23.35	GENERIC, Mylan Pharmaceuticals Inc	00378-0205-89
50's	$23.35	GENERIC, Aligen Independent Laboratories Inc	00405-4084-50

50's $23.35 GENERIC, Moore, H.L. Drug Exchange Inc 00839-6038-04
56's $20.63 GENERIC, Pd-Rx Pharmaceuticals 55289-0020-56
60's $21.88 GENERIC, Pd-Rx Pharmaceuticals 55289-0020-60
63's $24.63 GENERIC, Pd-Rx Pharmaceuticals 55289-0020-63
100's $12.72 FEDERAL UPPER LIMIT, H.C.F.A. F F P 99999-0231-07
100's $16.50 GENERIC, Raway Pharmacal Inc 00686-0601-20
100's $16.80 GENERIC, International Ethical Laboratories Inc 11584-0401-00
100's $24.95 GENERIC, Warner Chilcott Laboratories 00047-0731-24
100's $36.35 GENERIC, Novopharm Usa Inc 55953-0716-40
100's $39.00 GENERIC, Mutual/United Research Laboratories 00677-0661-01
100's $39.00 GENERIC, Geneva Pharmaceuticals 00781-2613-01
100's $39.36 GENERIC, Purepac Pharmaceutical Company 00228-2689-11
100's $43.41 GENERIC, Bristol-Myers Squibb 00003-0109-55
100's $43.41 GENERIC, Ranbaxy Laboratories 63304-0655-01
100's $45.50 GENERIC, Ivax Corporation 00182-1071-89
100's $46.53 GENERIC, Bristol-Myers Squibb 00003-0109-51
100's $49.00 GENERIC, Udl Laboratories Inc 51079-0601-20
100's $49.00 GENERIC, Medirex Inc 57480-0456-01
100's $58.75 GENERIC, Mova Pharmaceutical Corporation 55370-0885-07

Powder For Reconstitution - Oral - 50 mg/ml

15 ml $1.80 AMOXIL PEDIATRIC DROPS, Glaxosmithkline 00029-6035-20
15 ml $2.44 GENERIC, Bristol-Myers Squibb 00003-1738-15
15 ml $2.65 AMOXIL PEDIATRIC DROPS, Physicians Total Care 54868-3016-00
30 ml $3.45 AMOXIL PEDIATRIC DROPS, Glaxosmithkline 00029-6038-39

Powder For Reconstitution - Oral - 125 mg/5 ml

5 ml x 25 $51.50 GENERIC, Bristol-Myers Squibb 00015-7276-75
80 ml $2.69 GENERIC, Moore, H.L. Drug Exchange Inc 00839-6115-71
80 ml $3.09 GENERIC, Mova Pharmaceutical Corporation 55370-0886-80
80 ml $3.10 GENERIC, Bristol-Myers Squibb 00003-1737-30
80 ml $3.12 GENERIC, Teva Pharmaceuticals Usa 00093-4150-79
80 ml $7.82 AMOXIL, Pharma Pac 52959-1005-02
80's $2.55 GENERIC, Major Pharmaceuticals Inc 00904-2619-06
80's $2.70 GENERIC, Interstate Drug Exchange Inc 00814-0700-52
80's $3.75 GENERIC, Interstate Drug Exchange Inc 00814-0701-52
100 ml $2.33 AMOXIL, Physicians Total Care 54868-0195-02
100 ml $2.82 GENERIC, Moore, H.L. Drug Exchange Inc 00839-6115-73
100 ml $2.95 GENERIC, Major Pharmaceuticals Inc 00904-2619-04
100 ml $3.47 GENERIC, Martec Pharmaceuticals Inc 52555-0141-01
100 ml $3.56 GENERIC, Bristol-Myers Squibb 00003-1737-40
100 ml $3.59 GENERIC, Teva Pharmaceuticals Usa 00093-4150-73
100 ml $3.59 GENERIC, Ivax Corporation 00182-1072-70
100 ml $3.59 GENERIC, Qualitest Products Inc 00603-6500-84
100 ml $3.61 GENERIC, Mova Pharmaceutical Corporation 55370-0886-13
100 ml $3.76 GENERIC, Mylan Pharmaceuticals Inc 00378-0206-02
100 ml $6.39 GENERIC, Pharma Pac 52959-0181-01
100 ml $8.72 AMOXIL, Pharma Pac 52959-1005-03
100's $2.85 GENERIC, Interstate Drug Exchange Inc 00814-0700-54
100's $2.95 GENERIC, Geneva Pharmaceuticals 00781-6195-46
100's $4.43 GENERIC, Interstate Drug Exchange Inc 00814-0701-54
100's $4.73 GENERIC, Geneva Pharmaceuticals 00781-6191-46
150 ml $2.49 AMOXIL, Physicians Total Care 54868-0195-01
150 ml $3.02 FEDERAL UPPER LIMIT, H.C.F.A. F F P 99999-0231-27
150 ml $3.55 AMOXIL, Glaxosmithkline 00029-6008-22
150 ml $3.70 GENERIC, Major Pharmaceuticals Inc 00904-2619-07
150 ml $3.71 GENERIC, Moore, H.L. Drug Exchange Inc 00839-6115-75
150 ml $4.11 GENERIC, Bristol-Myers Squibb 00003-1737-45
150 ml $4.14 GENERIC, Ivax Corporation 00182-1072-72
150 ml $4.64 AMOXIL, Allscripts Pharmaceutical Company 54569-0093-00
150 ml $4.69 GENERIC, Mova Pharmaceutical Corporation 55370-0886-14
150 ml $4.71 GENERIC, Teva Pharmaceuticals Usa 00093-4150-80
150 ml $4.72 GENERIC, Mylan Pharmaceuticals Inc 00378-0206-06
150 ml $4.72 GENERIC, Martec Pharmaceuticals Inc 52555-0141-07
150 ml $9.55 AMOXIL, Pharma Pac 52959-1005-01
150's $3.37 GENERIC, Interstate Drug Exchange Inc 00814-0700-58
150's $3.58 GENERIC, Geneva Pharmaceuticals 00781-6195-55
150's $5.25 GENERIC, Interstate Drug Exchange Inc 00814-0701-58
200 ml $5.88 GENERIC, Novopharm Usa Inc 55953-0149-53

Powder For Reconstitution - Oral - 250 mg/5 ml

5 ml x 10 $8.00 AMOXIL, Glaxosmithkline 00029-6009-18
5 ml x 25 $56.50 GENERIC, Bristol-Myers Squibb 00015-7277-75
80 ml $4.31 GENERIC, Moore, H.L. Drug Exchange Inc 00839-6116-71
80 ml $4.72 GENERIC, Watson/Rugby Laboratories Inc 00536-0105-71
80 ml $5.31 GENERIC, Bristol-Myers Squibb 00003-1738-30
80 ml $5.35 GENERIC, Teva Pharmaceuticals Usa 00093-4155-79
80 ml $5.42 GENERIC, Mova Pharmaceutical Corporation 55370-0887-80
80 ml $7.85 AMOXIL, Pharma Pac 52959-1006-02
80's $3.95 GENERIC, Major Pharmaceuticals Inc 00904-2620-06
100 ml $2.46 GENERIC, International Ethical Laboratories Inc 11584-0381-00
100 ml $3.48 AMOXIL, Physicians Total Care 54868-0196-02
100 ml $4.80 GENERIC, Major Pharmaceuticals Inc 00904-2620-04
100 ml $4.85 GENERIC, Moore, H.L. Drug Exchange Inc 00839-6116-73
100 ml $5.15 GENERIC, Martec Pharmaceuticals Inc 52555-0142-01
100 ml $5.30 AMOXIL, Glaxosmithkline 00029-6009-23
100 ml $6.09 GENERIC, Bristol-Myers Squibb 00003-1738-40
100 ml $6.09 GENERIC, Mova Pharmaceutical Corporation 55370-0887-13
100 ml $6.13 GENERIC, Teva Pharmaceuticals Usa 00093-4155-73
100 ml $6.13 GENERIC, Ivax Corporation 00182-1073-70
100 ml $6.13 GENERIC, Mylan Pharmaceuticals Inc 00378-0207-02
100 ml $7.06 GENERIC, Consolidated Pharmaceutical Group 61423-0835-15
100 ml $8.99 AMOXIL, Pharma Pac 52959-1006-03
150 ml $2.82 GENERIC, International Ethical Laboratories Inc 11584-0381-05
150 ml $3.86 AMOXIL, Physicians Total Care 54868-0196-01
150 ml $5.85 GENERIC, Major Pharmaceuticals Inc 00904-2620-07
150 ml $6.06 GENERIC, Moore, H.L. Drug Exchange Inc 00839-6116-75
150 ml $6.10 AMOXIL, Glaxosmithkline 00029-6009-22
150 ml $6.34 GENERIC, Martec Pharmaceuticals Inc 52555-0142-07
150 ml $6.83 AMOXIL, Allscripts Pharmaceutical Company 54569-0094-00
150 ml $7.06 GENERIC, Bristol-Myers Squibb 00003-1738-45
150 ml $7.08 GENERIC, Mova Pharmaceutical Corporation 55370-0887-14
150 ml $7.11 GENERIC, Teva Pharmaceuticals Usa 00093-4155-80
150 ml $7.11 GENERIC, Ivax Corporation 00182-1073-72
150 ml $7.11 GENERIC, Novopharm Usa Inc 55953-0673-47
150 ml $7.12 GENERIC, Mylan Pharmaceuticals Inc 00378-0207-06
150 ml $9.15 GENERIC, Pharma Pac 52959-1463-03
150 ml $10.36 AMOXIL, Pharma Pac 52959-1006-01
150 ml $10.43 GENERIC, Bristol-Myers Squibb 00015-7277-60
150's $5.35 GENERIC, Geneva Pharmaceuticals 00781-6191-55
200 ml $7.70 GENERIC, Novopharm Usa Inc 55953-0130-53

Tablet - Oral - 500 mg

100's $49.81 GENERIC, Teva Pharmaceuticals Usa 00093-2263-01

Tablet - Oral - 875 mg

20's $20.45 GENERIC, Ranbaxy Laboratories 63304-0763-20
100's $87.21 GENERIC, Teva Pharmaceuticals Usa 00093-2264-01
100's $96.90 GENERIC, Ranbaxy Laboratories 63304-0763-01

Tablet, Chewable - Oral - 125 mg

30's $6.18 AMOXIL, Physicians Total Care 54868-1044-01
30's $10.40 GENERIC, Pd-Rx Pharmaceuticals 55289-0398-30
60's $7.85 GENERIC, Warrick Pharmaceuticals Corporation 59930-1573-01
100's $11.00 GENERIC, Purepac Pharmaceutical Company 00228-2639-11
100's $11.00 GENERIC, Warrick Pharmaceuticals Corporation 59930-1573-02
100's $11.95 GENERIC, Qualitest Products Inc 00603-2273-21
100's $22.50 GENERIC, Teva Pharmaceuticals Usa 00093-2267-01
100's $24.65 GENERIC, Ranbaxy Laboratories 63304-0514-01

Tablet, Chewable - Oral - 200 mg

20's $8.93 GENERIC, Ranbaxy Laboratories 63304-0760-20
20's $10.15 AMOXIL, Sk Beecham Pharmaceuticals 00029-6044-12
20's $10.15 AMOXIL, Allscripts Pharmaceutical Company 54569-4790-00
100's $50.75 AMOXIL, Sk Beecham Pharmaceuticals 00029-6044-20

Tablet, Chewable - Oral - 250 mg

6's $3.30 GENERIC, Pd-Rx Pharmaceuticals 55289-0182-06
15's $3.43 GENERIC, Allscripts Pharmaceutical Company 54569-3689-02
19's $16.53 GENERIC, Pharma Pac 52959-0246-19
21's $17.01 GENERIC, Pharma Pac 52959-0246-21
30's $8.12 AMOXIL, Physicians Total Care 54868-0807-01
30's $10.89 GENERIC, Med-Pro Inc 53978-1257-05
30's $11.10 GENERIC, Pd-Rx Pharmaceuticals 55289-0182-30
30's $22.77 GENERIC, Pharma Pac 52959-0246-30
30's $23.39 AMOXIL, Pharma Pac 52959-0012-30
45's $10.30 GENERIC, Allscripts Pharmaceutical Company 54569-3689-03
60's $13.75 GENERIC, Warrick Pharmaceuticals Corporation 59930-1611-01
100's $15.95 FEDERAL UPPER LIMIT, H.C.F.A. F F P 99999-0231-24
100's $22.82 GENERIC, Qualitest Products Inc 00603-2274-21
100's $22.85 GENERIC, Moore, H.L. Drug Exchange Inc 00839-7776-06
100's $22.85 GENERIC, Warrick Pharmaceuticals Corporation 59930-1611-02
100's $22.92 GENERIC, Mova Pharmaceutical Corporation 55370-0892-07
100's $23.02 GENERIC, Aligen Independent Laboratories Inc 00405-4086-01
100's $23.05 GENERIC, Purepac Pharmaceutical Company 00228-2640-11
100's $23.07 GENERIC, Geneva Pharmaceuticals 00781-1098-01
100's $27.00 GENERIC, Major Pharmaceuticals Inc 00904-7713-60
100's $45.00 GENERIC, Teva Pharmaceuticals Usa 00093-2268-01
100's $45.00 GENERIC, Ranbaxy Laboratories 63304-0515-01
200's $57.82 GENERIC, Ranbaxy Laboratories 63304-0515-04
250's $57.00 GENERIC, Purepac Pharmaceutical Company 00228-2640-25

Tablet, Chewable - Oral - 400 mg

20's	$10.91	GENERIC, Ranbaxy Laboratories	63304-0761-20
20's	$12.40	AMOXIL, Sk Beecham Pharmaceuticals	00029-6045-12
20's	$12.40	AMOXIL, Allscripts Pharmaceutical Company	54569-4791-00
30's	$18.60	AMOXIL, Allscripts Pharmaceutical Company	54569-4791-01
100's	$54.56	GENERIC, Ranbaxy Laboratories	63304-0761-01
100's	$62.00	AMOXIL, Sk Beecham Pharmaceuticals	00029-6045-20

PRODUCT LISTING - EQUIVALENTS NOT AVAILABLE

Capsule - Oral - 250 mg

1's	$3.39	GENERIC, Prescript Pharmaceuticals	00247-0001-01
2's	$3.44	GENERIC, Prescript Pharmaceuticals	00247-0001-02
3's	$0.75	GENERIC, Allscripts Pharmaceutical Company	54569-3876-00
3's	$3.47	GENERIC, Prescript Pharmaceuticals	00247-0001-03
4's	$3.52	GENERIC, Prescript Pharmaceuticals	00247-0001-04
5's	$3.55	GENERIC, Prescript Pharmaceuticals	00247-0001-05
6's	$1.30	GENERIC, Allscripts Pharmaceutical Company	54569-3986-01
6's	$1.82	GENERIC, Physicians Total Care	54868-3107-08
6's	$3.59	GENERIC, Prescript Pharmaceuticals	00247-0001-06
8's	$3.67	GENERIC, Prescript Pharmaceuticals	00247-0001-08
9's	$1.89	GENERIC, Southwood Pharmaceuticals Inc	58016-0103-09
9's	$2.25	GENERIC, Allscripts Pharmaceutical Company	54569-1746-09
9's	$3.71	GENERIC, Prescript Pharmaceuticals	00247-0001-09
10's	$3.75	GENERIC, Prescript Pharmaceuticals	00247-0001-10
12's	$2.52	GENERIC, Southwood Pharmaceuticals Inc	58016-0103-12
12's	$3.84	GENERIC, Prescript Pharmaceuticals	00247-0001-12
14's	$8.99	GENERIC, Dhs Inc	55887-0993-14
15's	$2.54	GENERIC, Physicians Total Care	54868-3107-09
15's	$3.15	GENERIC, Southwood Pharmaceuticals Inc	58016-0103-15
15's	$3.75	GENERIC, Allscripts Pharmaceutical Company	54569-1746-05
15's	$3.95	GENERIC, Prescript Pharmaceuticals	00247-0001-15
18's	$5.98	GENERIC, Southwood Pharmaceuticals Inc	58016-0103-18
20's	$2.95	GENERIC, Physicians Total Care	54868-3107-07
20's	$4.15	GENERIC, Prescript Pharmaceuticals	00247-0001-20
20's	$6.65	GENERIC, Southwood Pharmaceuticals Inc	58016-0103-20
20's	$6.75	GENERIC, Alpharma Uspd Makers Of Barre and Nmc	63874-0101-20
21's	$4.19	GENERIC, Prescript Pharmaceuticals	00247-0001-21
21's	$5.24	GENERIC, Allscripts Pharmaceutical Company	54569-1746-01
21's	$6.98	GENERIC, Southwood Pharmaceuticals Inc	58016-0103-21
21's	$6.98	GENERIC, Alpharma Uspd Makers Of Barre and Nmc	63874-0101-21
24's	$4.31	GENERIC, Prescript Pharmaceuticals	00247-0001-24
24's	$7.98	GENERIC, Southwood Pharmaceuticals Inc	58016-0103-24
25's	$4.34	GENERIC, Prescript Pharmaceuticals	00247-0001-25
28's	$4.47	GENERIC, Prescript Pharmaceuticals	00247-0001-28
30's	$3.75	GENERIC, Physicians Total Care	54868-3107-01
30's	$4.54	GENERIC, Prescript Pharmaceuticals	00247-0001-30
30's	$7.49	GENERIC, Allscripts Pharmaceutical Company	54569-1746-00
30's	$8.85	GENERIC, Pharmaceutical Corporation Of America	51655-0075-24
30's	$8.92	GENERIC, Alpharma Uspd Makers Of Barre and Nmc	63874-0101-30
30's	$9.97	GENERIC, Southwood Pharmaceuticals Inc	58016-0103-30
40's	$4.56	GENERIC, Physicians Total Care	54868-3107-03
40's	$4.94	GENERIC, Prescript Pharmaceuticals	00247-0001-40
40's	$9.24	GENERIC, Pharmaceutical Corporation Of America	51655-0075-51
40's	$10.24	GENERIC, Alpharma Uspd Makers Of Barre and Nmc	63874-0101-40
40's	$13.27	GENERIC, Southwood Pharmaceuticals Inc	58016-0103-40
42's	$5.02	GENERIC, Prescript Pharmaceuticals	00247-0001-42
42's	$10.49	GENERIC, Allscripts Pharmaceutical Company	54569-1746-08
45's	$10.91	GENERIC, Alphagen Laboratories Inc	63874-0101-45
100's	$7.33	GENERIC, Prescript Pharmaceuticals	00247-0001-00
100's	$8.73	GENERIC, Physicians Total Care	54868-3107-00
100's	$14.40	AMOXICOT, C.O. Truxton Inc	00463-5019-01
100's	$24.94	GENERIC, Alpharma Uspd Makers Of Barre and Nmc	63874-0101-01
100's	$33.24	GENERIC, Southwood Pharmaceuticals Inc	58016-0103-00
250's	$13.28	GENERIC, Prescript Pharmaceuticals	00247-0001-69

Capsule - Oral - 500 mg

1's	$3.41	GENERIC, Prescript Pharmaceuticals	00247-0002-01
2's	$3.46	GENERIC, Prescript Pharmaceuticals	00247-0002-02
3's	$1.40	GENERIC, Allscripts Pharmaceutical Company	54569-1861-04
3's	$3.52	GENERIC, Prescript Pharmaceuticals	00247-0002-03
4's	$1.87	GENERIC, Allscripts Pharmaceutical Company	54569-3335-05
4's	$3.56	GENERIC, Prescript Pharmaceuticals	00247-0002-04
5's	$3.62	GENERIC, Prescript Pharmaceuticals	00247-0002-05
6's	$3.67	GENERIC, Prescript Pharmaceuticals	00247-0002-06
8's	$3.78	GENERIC, Prescript Pharmaceuticals	00247-0002-08
9's	$2.76	GENERIC, Physicians Total Care	54868-3109-06
9's	$3.84	GENERIC, Prescript Pharmaceuticals	00247-0002-09
9's	$4.20	GENERIC, Allscripts Pharmaceutical Company	54569-1861-08
9's	$5.28	GENERIC, Southwood Pharmaceuticals Inc	58016-0104-09
10's	$3.88	GENERIC, Prescript Pharmaceuticals	00247-0002-10
12's	$3.99	GENERIC, Prescript Pharmaceuticals	00247-0002-12
12's	$7.04	GENERIC, Southwood Pharmaceuticals Inc	58016-0104-12
14's	$4.09	GENERIC, Prescript Pharmaceuticals	00247-0002-14
14's	$8.22	GENERIC, Southwood Pharmaceuticals Inc	58016-0104-14
15's	$3.71	GENERIC, Physicians Total Care	54868-3109-08
15's	$4.15	GENERIC, Prescript Pharmaceuticals	00247-0002-15
15's	$7.01	GENERIC, Allscripts Pharmaceutical Company	54569-1861-05
15's	$8.80	GENERIC, Southwood Pharmaceuticals Inc	58016-0104-15
16's	$4.20	GENERIC, Prescript Pharmaceuticals	00247-0002-16
18's	$4.31	GENERIC, Prescript Pharmaceuticals	00247-0002-18
18's	$10.56	GENERIC, Southwood Pharmaceuticals Inc	58016-0104-18
20's	$4.41	GENERIC, Prescript Pharmaceuticals	00247-0002-20
20's	$4.50	GENERIC, Physicians Total Care	54868-3109-07
20's	$11.74	GENERIC, Southwood Pharmaceuticals Inc	58016-0104-20
21's	$4.47	GENERIC, Prescript Pharmaceuticals	00247-0002-21
21's	$9.81	GENERIC, Allscripts Pharmaceutical Company	54569-1861-02
21's	$12.32	GENERIC, Southwood Pharmaceuticals Inc	58016-0104-21
21's	$13.84	GENERIC, Alpharma Uspd Makers Of Barre and Nmc	63874-0102-21
22's	$4.52	GENERIC, Prescript Pharmaceuticals	00247-0002-22
24's	$4.62	GENERIC, Prescript Pharmaceuticals	00247-0002-24
24's	$14.09	GENERIC, Southwood Pharmaceuticals Inc	58016-0104-24
25's	$4.68	GENERIC, Prescript Pharmaceuticals	00247-0002-25
27's	$4.79	GENERIC, Prescript Pharmaceuticals	00247-0002-27
28's	$4.84	GENERIC, Prescript Pharmaceuticals	00247-0002-28
28's	$16.43	GENERIC, Southwood Pharmaceuticals Inc	58016-0104-28
28's	$18.02	GENERIC, Alpharma Uspd Makers Of Barre and Nmc	63874-0102-28
30's	$4.94	GENERIC, Prescript Pharmaceuticals	00247-0002-30
30's	$6.09	GENERIC, Physicians Total Care	54868-3109-01
30's	$12.40	GENERIC, Pharmaceutical Corporation Of America	51655-0157-24
30's	$14.01	GENERIC, Allscripts Pharmaceutical Company	54569-1861-00
30's	$17.61	GENERIC, Southwood Pharmaceuticals Inc	58016-0104-30
30's	$19.45	GENERIC, Alpharma Uspd Makers Of Barre and Nmc	63874-0102-30
32's	$5.05	GENERIC, Prescript Pharmaceuticals	00247-0002-32
36's	$5.26	GENERIC, Prescript Pharmaceuticals	00247-0002-36
40's	$2.16	GENERIC, Alpharma Uspd Makers Of Barre and Nmc	63874-0102-40
40's	$5.47	GENERIC, Prescript Pharmaceuticals	00247-0002-40
40's	$18.68	GENERIC, Allscripts Pharmaceutical Company	54569-1861-01
40's	$23.48	GENERIC, Southwood Pharmaceuticals Inc	58016-0104-40
42's	$5.58	GENERIC, Prescript Pharmaceuticals	00247-0002-42
42's	$19.61	GENERIC, Allscripts Pharmaceutical Company	54569-1861-09
42's	$26.08	GENERIC, Pharma Pac	52959-0020-42
45's	$27.55	GENERIC, Alpharma Uspd Makers Of Barre and Nmc	63874-0102-45
50's	$6.00	GENERIC, Prescript Pharmaceuticals	00247-0002-50
50's	$9.59	GENERIC, Physicians Total Care	54868-3109-04
50's	$15.00	AMOXICOT, C.O. Truxton Inc	00463-5020-55
100's	$8.65	GENERIC, Prescript Pharmaceuticals	00247-0002-00
100's	$17.19	GENERIC, Physicians Total Care	54868-3109-02
100's	$46.70	GENERIC, Allscripts Pharmaceutical Company	54569-3335-07
100's	$58.69	GENERIC, Southwood Pharmaceuticals Inc	58016-0104-00
250's	$16.59	GENERIC, Prescript Pharmaceuticals	00247-0002-69

Powder For Reconstitution - Oral - 125 mg/5 ml

80 ml	$3.12	GENERIC, Allscripts Pharmaceutical Company	45469-2953-00
80 ml	$3.12	GENERIC, Allscripts Pharmaceutical Company	54569-2953-00
80 ml	$4.04	GENERIC, Prescript Pharmaceuticals	00247-0021-80
100 ml	$3.00	AMOXICOT, C.O. Truxton Inc	00463-5015-01
100 ml	$3.59	GENERIC, Allscripts Pharmaceutical Company	45469-2928-00
100 ml	$3.59	GENERIC, Allscripts Pharmaceutical Company	54569-2928-00
100 ml	$4.19	GENERIC, Alpharma Uspd Makers Of Barre and Nmc	63874-0143-10
100 ml	$4.20	GENERIC, Prescript Pharmaceuticals	00247-0021-00
100's	$2.70	GENERIC, Physicians Total Care	54868-4150-02
150 ml	$3.90	AMOXICOT, C.O. Truxton Inc	00463-5015-15
150 ml	$4.62	GENERIC, Prescript Pharmaceuticals	00247-0021-78
150 ml	$4.71	GENERIC, Allscripts Pharmaceutical Company	45469-2930-00
150 ml	$4.71	GENERIC, Allscripts Pharmaceutical Company	54569-2930-00
150 ml	$4.95	GENERIC, Alpharma Uspd Makers Of Barre and Nmc	63874-0143-15
150's	$2.78	GENERIC, Physicians Total Care	54868-4150-01

Powder For Reconstitution - Oral - 200 mg/5 ml

5 ml x 10	$20.00	AMOXIL, Sk Beecham Pharmaceuticals	00029-6048-18
50 ml	$5.10	AMOXIL, Sk Beecham Pharmaceuticals	00029-6048-54
75 ml	$7.60	AMOXIL, Sk Beecham Pharmaceuticals	00029-6048-55
100 ml	$9.14	AMOXIL, Ranbaxy Laboratories	63304-0969-04
100 ml	$10.15	AMOXIL, Sk Beecham Pharmaceuticals	00029-6048-59
100 ml	$10.15	AMOXIL, Allscripts Pharmaceutical Company	54569-4796-00

Powder For Reconstitution - Oral - 250 mg/5 ml

Size	Price	Product	NDC
5 ml	$3.45	GENERIC, Prescript Pharmaceuticals	00247-0022-05
10 ml	$3.53	GENERIC, Prescript Pharmaceuticals	00247-0022-10
80 ml	$4.80	GENERIC, Prescript Pharmaceuticals	00247-0022-80
80 ml	$5.35	GENERIC, Allscripts Pharmaceutical Company	54569-2954-00
80 ml	$5.35	GENERIC, Southwood Pharmaceuticals Inc	58016-1007-01
100 ml	$3.62	GENERIC, Physicians Total Care	54868-4155-02
100 ml	$4.80	AMOXICOT, C.O. Truxton Inc	00463-5016-01
100 ml	$5.16	GENERIC, Prescript Pharmaceuticals	00247-0022-00
100 ml	$6.13	GENERIC, Allscripts Pharmaceutical Company	54569-2929-00
100 ml	$6.83	GENERIC, Alpharma Uspd Makers Of Barre and Nmc	63874-0144-10
150 ml	$4.26	GENERIC, Physicians Total Care	54868-4155-01
150 ml	$6.00	AMOXICOT, C.O. Truxton Inc	00463-5016-15
150 ml	$6.07	GENERIC, Prescript Pharmaceuticals	00247-0022-78
150 ml	$7.11	GENERIC, Allscripts Pharmaceutical Company	54569-2931-00
150 ml	$7.11	GENERIC, Southwood Pharmaceuticals Inc	58016-1006-01
150 ml	$8.05	GENERIC, Alpharma Uspd Makers Of Barre and Nmc	63874-0144-15
200 ml	$6.10	GENERIC, Physicians Total Care	54868-4155-03
200 ml	$6.98	GENERIC, Prescript Pharmaceuticals	00247-0022-79
200 ml	$12.23	GENERIC, R.I.D. Inc Distributor	54807-0251-20

Powder For Reconstitution - Oral - 400 mg/5 ml

Size	Price	Product	NDC
5 ml x 10	$25.00	AMOXIL, Sk Beecham Pharmaceuticals	00029-6049-18
50 ml	$5.45	AMOXIL, Sk Beecham Pharmaceuticals	00029-6049-54
75 ml	$8.15	AMOXIL, Sk Beecham Pharmaceuticals	00029-6049-55
100 ml	$9.81	AMOXIL, Ranbaxy Laboratories	63304-0970-04
100 ml	$10.90	AMOXIL, Sk Beecham Pharmaceuticals	00029-6049-59
100 ml	$10.90	AMOXIL, Allscripts Pharmaceutical Company	54569-4797-00

Tablet - Oral - 500 mg

Size	Price	Product	NDC
20's	$11.70	AMOXIL, Sk Beecham Pharmaceuticals	00029-6046-12
100's	$55.35	AMOXIL, Sk Beecham Pharmaceuticals	00029-6046-20

Tablet - Oral - 875 mg

Size	Price	Product	NDC
20's	$19.38	AMOXIL, Allscripts Pharmaceutical Company	54569-4608-00
20's	$20.45	AMOXIL, Sk Beecham Pharmaceuticals	00029-6047-12
100's	$96.90	AMOXIL, Sk Beecham Pharmaceuticals	00029-6047-20

Tablet, Chewable - Oral - 125 mg

Size	Price	Product	NDC
20's	$10.91	GENERIC, Alpharma Uspd Makers Of Barre and Nmc	63874-0239-20
30's	$13.34	GENERIC, Alpharma Uspd Makers Of Barre and Nmc	63874-0239-30
100's	$23.10	GENERIC, Alpharma Uspd Makers Of Barre and Nmc	63874-0239-01

Tablet, Chewable - Oral - 250 mg

Size	Price	Product	NDC
2's	$0.47	GENERIC, Allscripts Pharmaceutical Company	54569-3689-06
2's	$3.94	GENERIC, Prescript Pharmaceuticals	00247-0023-02
4's	$4.52	GENERIC, Prescript Pharmaceuticals	00247-0023-04
6's	$5.11	GENERIC, Prescript Pharmaceuticals	00247-0023-06
8's	$5.68	GENERIC, Prescript Pharmaceuticals	00247-0023-08
9's	$2.10	GENERIC, Allscripts Pharmaceutical Company	54569-3689-04
15's	$7.72	GENERIC, Prescript Pharmaceuticals	00247-0023-15
20's	$9.18	GENERIC, Prescript Pharmaceuticals	00247-0023-20
20's	$12.02	GENERIC, Alpharma Uspd Makers Of Barre and Nmc	63874-0240-20
21's	$9.47	GENERIC, Prescript Pharmaceuticals	00247-0023-21
28's	$11.51	GENERIC, Prescript Pharmaceuticals	00247-0023-28
30's	$6.99	GENERIC, Allscripts Pharmaceutical Company	54569-3689-00
30's	$7.57	GENERIC, Physicians Total Care	54868-3105-00
30's	$12.09	GENERIC, Prescript Pharmaceuticals	00247-0023-30
30's	$15.32	GENERIC, Alpharma Uspd Makers Of Barre and Nmc	63874-0240-30
40's	$9.32	GENERIC, Allscripts Pharmaceutical Company	54569-3689-05
40's	$15.00	GENERIC, Prescript Pharmaceuticals	00247-0023-40
100's	$29.59	GENERIC, Alpharma Uspd Makers Of Barre and Nmc	63874-0240-01
100's	$32.47	GENERIC, Prescript Pharmaceuticals	00247-0023-00

Amoxicillin; Clarithromycin; Lansoprazole *(003412)*

For complete prescribing information, refer to the CD-ROM included with the book.

Categories: Ulcer, duodenal; FDA Approved 1997 Dec; Pregnancy Category C
Drug Classes: Antibiotics, macrolides; Antibiotics, penicillins; Gastrointestinals; Proton pump inhibitors
Brand Names: Prevpac
Cost of Therapy: $240.58 (Ulcer; Prevpac Kit; 500 mg; 500 mg; 30 mg; 1 kit/day; 14 day supply)

DESCRIPTION

THESE PRODUCTS ARE INTENDED ONLY FOR USE AS DESCRIBED. The individual products contained in this package should not be used alone or in combination for other purposes. The information described in this labeling concerns only the use of these products as indicated in this daily administration pack. For information on use of the individual components when dispensed as individual medications outside this combined use for treating *Helicobacter pylori (H. pylori)*, please see the package inserts for each individual product.

Prevpac consists of a daily administration pack containing two lansoprazole 30 mg capsules, four amoxicillin 500 mg capsules, and two clarithromycin 500 mg tablets, for oral administration.

PREVACID DELAYED-RELEASE CAPSULES

The active ingredient in Prevacid capsules is a substituted benzimidazole, 2-[[[3-methyl-4-(2,2,2-trifluoroethoxy)-2-pyridyl]methyl]sulfinyl] benzimidazole, a compound that inhibits gastric acid secretion. Its empirical formula is $C_{16}H_{14}F_3N_3O_2S$ with a molecular weight of 369.37.

Lansoprazole is a white to brownish-white odorless crystalline powder which melts with decomposition at approximately 166°C. Lansoprazole is freely soluble in dimethylformamide; soluble in methanol; sparingly soluble in ethanol; slightly soluble in ethyl acetate, dichloromethane and acetonitrile; very slightly soluble in ether; and practically insoluble in hexane and water.

Each delayed-release capsule contains enteric-coated granules consisting of lansoprazole (30 mg), hydroxypropyl cellulose, low substituted hydroxypropyl cellulose, colloidal silicon dioxide, magnesium carbonate, methacrylic acid copolymer, starch, talc, sugar sphere, sucrose, polyethylene glycol, polysorbate 80, and titanium dioxide. Components of the gelatin capsule include gelatin, titanium dioxide, D&C red no. 28, FD&C blue no. 1, and FD&C red no. 40.

TRIMOX

Amoxicillin, (2*S*,5*R*,6*R*)-6-[(*R*)-(-)-2-Amino-2-(*p*-hydroxyphenyl)acetamido]-3,3-dimethyl-7-oxo-4-thia-1-azabicyclo[3.2.0]heptane-2-carboxylic acid trihydrate, is a semi-synthetic penicillin, an analogue of ampicillin.

The empirical formula is $C_{16}H_{19}N_3O_5S{\cdot}3H_2O$, and the molecular weight is 419.45.

The flesh body/maroon cap capsules contain amoxicillin trihydrate equivalent to 500 mg of amoxicillin. The inactive ingredient in the capsules is magnesium stearate.

BIAXIN FILMTAB

Clarithromycin is a semi-synthetic macrolide antibiotic. Chemically, it is 6-*O*-methylerythromycin. The molecular formula is $C_{38}H_{69}NO_{13}$, and the molecular weight is 747.96.

Clarithromycin is a white to off-white crystalline powder. It is soluble in acetone, slightly soluble in methanol, ethanol, and acetonitrile, and practically insoluble in water. Each yellow oval film-coated immediate-release tablet contains 500 mg of clarithromycin and the following inactive ingredients: hydroxypropyl methylcellulose, hydroxypropyl cellulose, colloidal silicon dioxide, croscarmellose sodium, D&C yellow no. 10, magnesium stearate, microcrystalline cellulose, povidone, propylene glycol, sorbic acid, sorbitan monooleate, titanium dioxide, and vanillin.

INDICATIONS AND USAGE

H. PYLORI ERADICATION TO REDUCE THE RISK OF DUODENAL ULCER RECURRENCE

The components in Prevpac (lansoprazole, amoxicillin, and clarithromycin) are indicated for the treatment of patients with *H. pylori* infection and duodenal ulcer disease (active or 1 year history of a duodenal ulcer) to eradicate *H. pylori*. Eradication of *H. pylori* has been shown to reduce the risk of duodenal ulcer recurrence (see DOSAGE AND ADMINISTRATION).

CONTRAINDICATIONS

Prevpac is contraindicated in patients with known hypersensitivity to any component of the formulation of lansoprazole, any macrolide antibiotic, or any penicillin.

Concomitant administration of amoxicillin; clarithromycin; lansoprazole with cisapride, pimozide, astemizole, or terfenadine is contraindicated. There have been post-marketing reports of drug interactions when clarithromycin and/or erythromycin are coadministered with cisapride, pimozide, astemizole , or terfenadine resulting in cardiac arrhythmias (QT prolongation, ventricular tachycardia, ventricular fibrillation, and torsades de pointes) most likely due to inhibition of metabolism of these drugs by erythromycin and clarithromycin. Fatalities have been reported.

Please refer to full prescribing information for amoxicillin and clarithromycin before prescribing.

WARNINGS

AMOXICILLIN

Serious and occasionally fatal hypersensitivity (anaphylactic) reactions have been reported in patients on penicillin therapy. Although anaphylaxis is more frequent following parenteral therapy, it has occurred in patients on oral penicillins. These reactions are more likely to occur in individuals with a history of penicillin hypersensitivity and/or a history of sensitivity to multiple allergens.

There have been reports of individuals with a history of penicillin hypersensitivity who have experienced severe reactions when treated with cephalosporins. Before initiating therapy with amoxicillin, careful inquiry should be made concerning previous hypersensitivity reactions to penicillins, cephalosporins, or other allergens. If an allergic reaction occurs, amoxicillin should be discontinued and appropriate therapy instituted.

SERIOUS ANAPHYLACTIC REACTIONS REQUIRE IMMEDIATE EMERGENCY TREATMENT WITH EPINEPHRINE. OXYGEN, INTRAVENOUS STEROIDS, AND AIRWAY MANAGEMENT, INCLUDING INTUBATION, SHOULD ALSO BE ADMINISTERED AS INDICATED.

CLARITHROMYCIN

CLARITHROMYCIN SHOULD NOT BE USED IN PREGNANT WOMEN EXCEPT IN CLINICAL CIRCUMSTANCES WHERE NO ALTERNATIVE THERAPY IS APPROPRIATE. IF PREGNANCY OCCURS WHILE TAKING CLARITHRO-

MYCIN, THE PATIENT SHOULD BE APPRISED OF THE POTENTIAL HAZARD TO THE FETUS. CLARITHROMYCIN HAS DEMONSTRATED ADVERSE EFFECTS OF PREGNANCY OUTCOME AND/OR EMBRYO-FETAL DEVELOPMENT IN MONKEYS, RATS, MICE, AND RABBITS AT DOSES THAT PRODUCED PLASMA LEVELS 2-17 TIMES THE SERUM LEVELS ACHIEVED IN HUMANS TREATED AT THE MAXIMUM RECOMMENDED HUMAN DOSES.

AMOXICILLIN AND/OR CLARITHROMYCIN

Pseudomembranous colitis has been reported with nearly all antibacterial agents, including clarithromycin and amoxicillin, and may range in severity from mild to life threatening. Therefore, it is important to consider this diagnosis in patients who present with diarrhea subsequent to the administration of antibacterial agents.

Treatment with antibacterial agents alters the normal flora of the colon and may permit overgrowth of clostridia. Studies indicate that a toxin produced by *Clostridium difficile* is a primary cause of "antibiotic-associated colitis."

After the diagnosis of pseudomembranous colitis has been established, therapeutic measures should be initiated. Mild cases of pseudomembranous colitis usually respond to discontinuation of the drug alone. In moderate to severe cases, consideration should be given to management with fluids and electrolytes, protein supplementation, and treatment with an antibacterial drug clinically effective against *Clostridium difficile* colitis.

DOSAGE AND ADMINISTRATION

H. PYLORI ERADICATION TO REDUCE THE RISK OF DUODENAL ULCER RECURRENCE

The recommended adult oral dose is 30 mg lansoprazole, 1 g amoxicillin, and 500 mg clarithromycin administered together twice daily (morning and evening) for 10 or 14 days. (See INDICATIONS AND USAGE.)

Amoxicillin; clarithromycin; lansoprazole is not recommended in patients with creatinine clearance less than 30 ml/min.

PRODUCT LISTING - EQUIVALENTS NOT AVAILABLE

Kit - Oral - Strength n/a

14's	$252.36	PREVPAC, Allscripts Pharmaceutical Company	54569-4592-00
14's	$294.93	PREVPAC, Tap Pharmaceuticals Inc	00300-3702-01

Amoxicillin; Clavulanate Potassium *(000232)*

For related information, see the comparative table section in Appendix A.

Categories: Infection, ear, middle; Infection, lower respiratory tract; Infection, sinus; Infection, skin and skin structures; Infection, urinary tract; Infection, upper respiratory tract; Pregnancy Category B; FDA Approved 1984 Aug; WHO Formulary

Drug Classes: Antibiotics, penicillins

Brand Names: **Augmentin**; Augmentin XR

Foreign Brand Availability: Aclam (Indonesia); Ambilan (Peru); Amocla (Korea); Amoclan (Bahrain; Cyprus; Egypt; Iran; Iraq; Jordan; Korea; Kuwait; Lebanon; Libya; Oman; Qatar; Republic-of-Yemen; Saudi-Arabia; Syria; United-Arab-Emirates); Amoclav (Germany); Amolanic (Korea); Amolanic Duo (Korea); Amometin (Korea); Amoxiclav (Mexico); Amoxiclav-BID (Mexico); Amoxiclav-Teva (Israel); Amoxsiklav (Thailand); Amoxsiklav 3X (Thailand); Amoxsiklav Forte (Thailand); Ancla (Indonesia); Auclatin Duo Dry Syrup (Korea); AugMaxcil (South-Africa); Augmentan (Germany); Augmentine (Spain); Augucillin Duo (Korea); Ausclav (Australia); Ausclav Duo Forte (Australia); Ausclav Duo 400 (Australia); Auspilic (Indonesia); Cavumox (Thailand); Clacillin Duo Dry Syrup (Korea); Clamax (Korea); Clamentin (South-Africa); Clamobit (Indonesia); Clamonex (Korea; Singapore); Clamovid (Singapore); Clamoxin (Mexico); Clamoxyl (Australia); Clamoxyl DuoForte (Australia); Clarin-Duo (Korea); Clavamox (Israel); Clavinex (Chile; Peru); Clavoxilin Plus (Peru); Clavulin (Benin; Burkina-Faso; Canada; Colombia; Costa-Rica; Dominican-Republic; El-Salvador; Ethiopia; Gambia; Ghana; Guatemala; Guinea; Honduras; Ivory-Coast; Kenya; Liberia; Malawi; Mali; Mauritania; Mauritius; Morocco; Nicaragua; Niger; Nigeria; Panama; Senegal; Seychelles; Sierra-Leone; Sudan; Tanzania; Tunia; Uganda; Zambia; Zimbabwe); Clavulin Duo Forte (Australia); Clavamox (Germany; India; Indonesia); Clavumox (Peru; South-Africa); Croanan Duo Dry Syrup (Korea); Curam (Colombia; Peru; Singapore; Taiwan; Thailand); Danoclav (Indonesia); E-Moxclav (Bahrain; Cyprus; Egypt; Iran; Iraq; Jordan; Kuwait; Lebanon; Libya; Oman; Qatar; Republic-of-Yemen; Saudi-Arabia; Syria; United-Arab-Emirates); Enhancin (Singapore); Fugentin (Singapore); Hibiotic (Bahrain; Cyprus; Egypt; Iran; Iraq; Jordan; Kuwait; Lebanon; Libya; Oman; Qatar; Republic-of-Yemen; Saudi-Arabia; Syria; United-Arab-Emirates); Inciclav (Indonesia); Klamonex (Korea); Kmoxilin (Korea); Lactamox (Korea); Lansiclav (Indonesia); Moxiclav (Bahrain; Cyprus; Egypt; Iran; Iraq; Jordan; Kuwait; Lebanon; Libya; Oman; Qatar; Republic-of-Yemen; Saudi-Arabia; Singapore; Syria; United-Arab-Emirates); Moxicle (Korea); Moxyclav (South-Africa); Nufaclav (Indonesia); Ranclav (South-Africa; Thailand); Synermox (New-Zealand); Velamox CL (Peru); Viaclav (Indonesia); Vulamox (Colombia); Xiclav (Indonesia)

Cost of Therapy: $93.05 (Infection; Augmentin; 500 mg; 125 mg; 2 tablets/day; 14 day supply)

DESCRIPTION

Note: The trade name has been used throughout this monograph for clarity.

AUGMENTIN POWDER FOR ORAL SUSPENSION AND CHEWABLE TABLETS

Augmentin is an oral antibacterial combination consisting of the semisynthetic antibiotic amoxicillin and the β-lactamase inhibitor, clavulanate potassium (the potassium salt of clavulanic acid). Amoxicillin is an analog of ampicillin, derived from the basic penicillin nucleus, 6-aminopenicillanic acid. The amoxicillin molecular formula is $C_{16}H_{19}N_3O_5S{\cdot}3H_2O$ and the molecular weight is 419.46. Chemically, amoxicillin is (*2S,5R,6R*)-6-[(*R*)-(-)-2-Amino-2-(*p*-hydroxyphenyl) acetamido]-3,3-dimethyl-7-oxo-4-thia-1-azabicyclo[3.2.0]heptane-2-carboxylic acid trihydrate.

Clavulanic acid is produced by the fermentation of *Streptomyces clavuligerus.* It is a β-lactam structurally related to the penicillins and possesses the ability to inactivate a wide variety of β-lactamases by blocking the active sites of these enzymes. Clavulanic acid is particularly active against the clinically important plasmid mediated β-lactamases frequently responsible for transferred drug resistance to penicillins and cephalosporins. The clavulanate potassium molecular formula is $C_8H_8KNO_5$ and the molecular weight is 237.25. Chemically clavulanate potassium is potassium (Z)-(*2R,5R*)-3-(2-hydroxyethylidene)-7-oxo-4-oxa-1-azabicyclo[3.2.0]-heptane-2-carboxylate.

Inactive Ingredients

Powder for Oral Suspension: Colloidal silicon dioxide, flavorings (see HOW SUPPLIED, Augmentin Powder for Oral Suspension and Chewable Tablets), succinic acid, xanthan gum, and one or more of the following: aspartame (see PRECAUTIONS, Augmentin Powder for Oral Suspension and Chewable Tablets, Information for the Patient), hydroxypropyl methylcellulose, mannitol, silica gel, silicon dioxide and sodium saccharin.

Chewable Tablets: Colloidal silicon dioxide, flavorings (see HOW SUPPLIED, Augmentin Powder for Oral Suspension and Chewable Tablets), magnesium stearate, mannitol and one or more of the following: aspartame (see PRECAUTIONS, Augmentin Powder for Oral Suspension and Chewable Tablets, Information for the Patient), D&C yellow no. 10, FD&C red no. 40, glycine, sodium saccharin and succinic acid.

Each 125 mg chewable tablet and each 5 ml of reconstituted Augmentin 125 mg/5 ml oral suspension contains 0.16 mEq potassium. Each 250 mg chewable tablet and each 5 ml of reconstituted Augmentin 250 mg/5 ml oral suspension contains 0.32 mEq potassium. Each 200 mg chewable tablet and each 5 ml of reconstituted Augmentin 200 mg/5 ml oral suspension contains 0.14 mEq potassium. Each 400 mg chewable tablet and each 5 ml of reconstituted Augmentin 400 mg/5 ml oral suspension contains 0.29 mEq of potassium.

AUGMENTIN TABLETS

Augmentin is an oral antibacterial combination consisting of the semisynthetic antibiotic amoxicillin and the β-lactamase inhibitor, clavulanate potassium (the potassium salt of clavulanic acid). Amoxicillin is an analog of ampicillin, derived from the basic penicillin nucleus, 6-aminopenicillanic acid. The amoxicillin molecular formula is $C_{16}H_{19}N_3O_5S{\cdot}3H_2O$ and the molecular weight is 419.46. Chemically, amoxicillin is (*2S,5R,6R*)-6-[(*R*)-(-)-2-Amino-2-(*p*-hydroxyphenyl) acetamido]-3,3-dimethyl-7-oxo-4-thia-1-azabicyclo[3.2.0]heptane-2-carboxylic acid trihydrate.

Clavulanic acid is produced by the fermentation of *Streptomyces clavuligerus.* It is a β-lactam structurally related to the penicillins and possesses the ability to inactivate a wide variety of β-lactamases by blocking the active sites of these enzymes. Clavulanic acid is particularly active against the clinically important plasmid mediated β-lactamases frequently responsible for transferred drug resistance to penicillins and cephalosporins. The clavulanate potassium molecular formula is $C_8H_8KNO_5$ and the molecular weight is 237.25. Chemically clavulanate potassium is potassium (Z)-(*2R,5R*)-3-(2-hydroxyethylidene)-7-oxo-4-oxa-1-azabicyclo[3.2.0]-heptane-2-carboxylate.

Inactive Ingredients

Tablets: Colloidal silicon dioxide, hydroxypropyl methylcellulose, magnesium stearate, microcrystalline cellulose, polyethylene glycol, sodium starch glycolate and titanium dioxide.

Each Augmentin tablet contains 0.63 mEq potassium.

AUGMENTIN ES-600 POWDER FOR ORAL SUSPENSION

Augmentin ES-600 is an oral antibacterial combination consisting of the semisynthetic antibiotic amoxicillin and the β-lactamase inhibitor, clavulanate potassium (the potassium salt of clavulanic acid). Amoxicillin is an analog of ampicillin, derived from the basic penicillin nucleus, 6-aminopenicillanic acid. The amoxicillin molecular formula is $C_{16}H_{19}N_3O_5S{\cdot}3H_2O$ and the molecular weight is 419.46. Chemically, amoxicillin is (*2S,5R,6R*)-6-[(*R*)-(-)-2-Amino-2-(*p*-hydroxyphenyl) acetamido]-3,3-dimethyl-7-oxo-4-thia-1-azabicyclo[3.2.0]heptane-2-carboxylic acid trihydrate.

Clavulanic acid is produced by the fermentation of *Streptomyces clavuligerus.* It is a β-lactam structurally related to the penicillins and possesses the ability to inactivate a wide variety of β-lactamases by blocking the active sites of these enzymes. Clavulanic acid is particularly active against the clinically important plasmid mediated β-lactamases frequently responsible for transferred drug resistance to penicillins and cephalosporins. The clavulanate potassium molecular formula is $C_8H_8KNO_5$ and the molecular weight is 237.25. Chemically clavulanate potassium is potassium (Z)-(*2R,5R*)-3-(2-hydroxyethylidene)-7-oxo-4-oxa-1-azabicyclo[3.2.0]-heptane-2-carboxylate.

Inactive Ingredients

Powder for Oral Suspension: Colloidal silicon dioxide, orange-raspberry flavor, succinic acid, xanthan gum, aspartame (see PRECAUTIONS, Augmentin ES-600 Powder for Oral Suspension, Phenylketonurics), hydroxypropyl methylcellulose, and silicon dioxide.

Each 5 ml of reconstituted 600 mg/5 ml Augmentin ES-600 oral suspension contains 0.23 mEq potassium.

AUGMENTIN XR EXTENDED-RELEASE TABLETS

Augmentin XR is an oral antibacterial combination consisting of the semisynthetic antibiotic amoxicillin (present as amoxicillin trihydrate and amoxicillin sodium) and the β-lactamase inhibitor, clavulanate potassium (the potassium salt of clavulanic acid). Amoxicillin is an analog of ampicillin, derived from the basic penicillin nucleus, 6-aminopenicillanic acid. The amoxicillin trihydrate molecular formula is $C_{16}H_{19}N_3O_5S{\cdot}3H_2O$ and the molecular weight is 419.45. Chemically, amoxicillin trihydrate is (*2S,5R,6R*)-6-[(*R*)-(-)-2-Amino-2-(*p*-hydroxyphenyl)acetamido]-3,3-dimethyl-7-oxo-4-thia-1-azabicyclo[3.2.0]heptane-2-carboxylic acid trihydrate.

The amoxicillin sodium molecular formula is $C_{16}H_{18}N_3NaO_5S$ and the molecular weight is 387.39. Chemically, amoxicillin sodium is [2S-[2α,5α,6β(S*)]]-6-[[Amino(4-hydroxyphenyl)acetyl]amino]-3,3-dimethyl-7-oxo-4-thia-1-azabicyclo[3.2.0]heptane-2-carboxylic acid monosodium salt.

Clavulanic acid is produced by the fermentation of *Streptomyces clavuligerus.* It is a β-lactam structurally related to the penicillins and possesses the ability to inactivate a wide variety of β-lactamases by blocking the active sites of these enzymes. Clavulanic acid is particularly active against the clinically important plasmid mediated β-lactamases frequently responsible for transferred drug resistance to penicillins and cephalosporins. The clavulanate potassium molecular formula is $C_8H_8KNO_5$ and the molecular weight is 237.25.

Chemically clavulanate potassium is potassium (Z)-(2*R*, 5*R*)-3-(2-hydroxyethylidene)-7-oxo-4-oxa-1-azabicyclo[3.2.0]-heptane-2-carboxylate.

Inactive Ingredients

Extended-Release Tablets: Citric acid, colloidal silicon dioxide, hydroxypropyl methylcellulose, magnesium stearate, microcrystalline cellulose, polyethylene glycol, sodium starch glycolate, titanium dioxide, xanthan gum.

Each Augmentin XR tablet contains 12.6 mg (0.32 mEq) of potassium and 29.3 mg (1.27 mEq) of sodium.

CLINICAL PHARMACOLOGY

AUGMENTIN POWDER FOR ORAL SUSPENSION AND CHEWABLE TABLETS

Amoxicillin and clavulanate potassium are well absorbed from the gastrointestinal tract after oral administration of Augmentin. Dosing in the fasted or fed state has minimal effect on the pharmacokinetics of amoxicillin. While Augmentin can be given without regard to meals, absorption of clavulanate potassium when taken with food is greater relative to the fasted state.

In one study, the relative bioavailability of clavulanate was reduced when Augmentin was dosed at 30 and 150 minutes after the start of a high fat breakfast. The safety and efficacy of Augmentin have been established in clinical trials where Augmentin was taken without regard to meals. Oral administration of single doses of 400 mg Augmentin chewable tablets and 400 mg/5 ml suspension to 28 adult volunteers yielded comparable pharmacokinetic data.

TABLE 1

Dose*	AUC(0-∞) (µg·h/ml)		C_{max} (µg/ml)†	
Amoxicillin/ Clavulanate Potassium	Amoxicillin (±SD)	Clavulanate Potassium (±SD)	Amoxicillin (±SD)	Clavulanate Potassium (±SD)
400/57 mg (5 ml of suspension)	17.29 ± 2.28	2.34 ± 0.94	6.94 ± 1.24	1.10 ± 0.42
400/57 mg (1 chewable tablet)	17.24 ± 2.64	2.17 ± 0.73	6.67 ± 1.37	1.03 ± 0.33

* Administered at the start of a light meal.
† Mean values of 28 normal volunteers. Peak concentrations occurred approximately 1 hour after the dose.

Oral administration of 5 ml of Augmentin 250 mg/5 ml suspension or the equivalent dose of 10 ml Augmentin 125 mg/5 ml suspension provides average peak serum concentrations approximately 1 hour after dosing of 6.9 µg/ml for amoxicillin and 1.6 µg/ml for clavulanic acid. The areas under the serum concentration curves obtained during the first 4 hours after dosing were 12.6 µg·h/ml for amoxicillin and 2.9 µg·h/ml for clavulanic acid when 5 ml of Augmentin 250 mg/5 ml suspension or equivalent dose of 10 ml of Augmentin 125 mg/5 ml suspension was administered to adult volunteers. One Augmentin 250 mg chewable tablet or 2 Augmentin 125 mg chewable tablets are equivalent to 5 ml of Augmentin 250 mg/5 ml suspension and provide similar serum levels of amoxicillin and clavulanic acid.

Amoxicillin serum concentrations achieved with Augmentin are similar to those produced by the oral administration of equivalent doses of amoxicillin alone. The half-life of amoxicillin after the oral administration of Augmentin is 1.3 hours and that of clavulanic acid is 1.0 hour. Time above the minimum inhibitory concentration of 1.0 µg/ml for amoxicillin has been shown to be similar after corresponding q12h and q8h dosing regimens of Augmentin in adults and children.

Approximately 50-70% of the amoxicillin and approximately 25-40% of the clavulanic acid are excreted unchanged in urine during the first 6 hours after administration of 10 ml of Augmentin 250 mg/5 ml suspension.

Concurrent administration of probenecid delays amoxicillin excretion but does not delay renal excretion of clavulanic acid.

Neither component in Augmentin is highly protein-bound; clavulanic acid has been found to be approximately 25% bound to human serum and amoxicillin approximately 18% bound.

Amoxicillin diffuses readily into most body tissues and fluids with the exception of the brain and spinal fluid. The results of experiments involving the administration of clavulanic acid to animals suggest that this compound, like amoxicillin, is well distributed in body tissues.

Two hours after oral administration of a single 35 mg/kg dose of Augmentin suspension to fasting children, average concentrations of 3.0 µg/ml of amoxicillin and 0.5 µg/ml of clavulanic acid were detected in middle ear effusions.

Microbiology

Amoxicillin is a semisynthetic antibiotic with a broad spectrum of bactericidal activity against many gram-positive and gram-negative microorganisms. Amoxicillin is, however, susceptible to degradation by β-lactamases and, therefore, the spectrum of activity does not include organisms which produce these enzymes. Clavulanic acid is a β-lactam, structurally related to the penicillins, which possesses the ability to inactivate a wide range of β-lactamase enzymes commonly found in microorganisms resistant to penicillins and cephalosporins. In particular, it has good activity against the clinically important plasmid mediated β-lactamases frequently responsible for transferred drug resistance.

The formulation of amoxicillin and clavulanic acid in Augmentin protects amoxicillin from degradation by β-lactamase enzymes and effectively extends the antibiotic spectrum of amoxicillin to include many bacteria normally resistant to amoxicillin and other β-lactam antibiotics. Thus, Augmentin possesses the distinctive properties of a broad-spectrum antibiotic and a β-lactamase inhibitor.

Amoxicillin/clavulanic acid has been shown to be active against most strains of the following microorganisms, both *in vitro* and in clinical infections as described in INDICATIONS AND USAGE, Augmentin Powder for Oral Suspension and Chewable Tablets.

Gram-Positive Aerobes

Staphylococcus aureus (β-lactamase and non-β-lactamase producing).

Staphylococci which are resistant to methicillin/oxacillin must be considered resistant to amoxicillin/clavulanic acid.

Gram-Negative Aerobes

Enterobacter species. (Although most strains of *Enterobacter* species are resistant *in vitro*, clinical efficacy has been demonstrated with Augmentin in urinary tract infections caused by these organisms.)

Escherichia coli (β-lactamase and non-β-lactamase producing).

Haemophilus influenzae (β-lactamase and non-β-lactamase producing).

Klebsiella species (all known strains are β-lactamase producing).

Moraxella catarrhalis (β-lactamase and non-β-lactamase producing).

The following *in vitro* data are available, **but their clinical significance is unknown.**

Amoxicillin/clavulanic acid exhibits *in vitro* minimal inhibitory concentrations (MICs) of 2 µg/ml or less against most (≥90%) strains of *Streptococcus pneumoniae**; MICs of 0.06 µg/ml or less against most (≥90%) strains of *Neisseria gonorrhoeae*; MICs of 4 µg/ml or less against most (≥90%) strains of staphylococci and anaerobic bacteria; and MICs of 8 µg/ml or less against most (≥90%) strains of other listed organisms. However, with the exception of organisms shown to respond to amoxicillin alone, the safety and effectiveness of amoxicillin/clavulanic acid in treating clinical infections due to these microorganisms have not been established in adequate and well-controlled clinical trials.

*Because amoxicillin has greater *in vitro* activity against *Streptococcus pneumoniae* than does ampicillin or penicillin, the majority of *S. pneumoniae* strains with intermediate susceptibility to ampicillin or penicillin are fully susceptible to amoxicillin.

Gram-Positive Aerobes

*Enterococcus faecalis**.

Staphylococcus epidermidis (β-lactamase and non-β-lactamase producing).

Staphylococcus saprophyticus (β-lactamase and non-β-lactamase producing).

*Streptococcus pneumoniae**†.

*Streptococcus pyogenes**†.

Viridans group Streptococcus*†.

Gram-Negative Aerobes

Eikenella corrodens (β-lactamase and non-β-lactamase producing).

*Neisseria gonorrhoeae** (β-lactamase and non-β-lactamase producing).

*Proteus mirabilis** (β-lactamase and non-β-lactamase producing).

Anaerobic Bacteria

Bacteroides species, including *Bacteroides fragilis* (β-lactamase and non-β-lactamase producing).

Fusobacterium species (β-lactamase and non-β-lactamase producing).

Peptostreptococcus species†.

*Adequate and well-controlled clinical trials have established the effectiveness of amoxicillin alone in treating certain clinical infections due to these organisms.

†These are non-β-lactamase-producing organisms and, therefore, are susceptible to amoxicillin alone.

Susceptibility Testing

Dilution Techniques

Quantitative methods are used to determine antimicrobial minimal inhibitory concentrations (MICs). These MICs provide estimates of the susceptibility of bacteria to antimicrobial compounds. The MICs should be determined using a standardized procedure. Standardized procedures are based on a dilution method[1] (broth or agar) or equivalent with standardized inoculum concentrations and standardized concentrations of amoxicillin/clavulanate potassium powder.

The recommended dilution pattern utilizes a constant amoxicillin/clavulanate potassium ratio of 2 to 1 in all tubes with varying amounts of amoxicillin. MICs are expressed in terms of the amoxicillin concentration in the presence of clavulanic acid at a constant 2 parts amoxicillin to 1 part clavulanic acid. The MIC values should be interpreted according to the criteria in TABLE 2, TABLE 3, TABLE 4, and TABLE 5.

Recommended Ranges for Amoxicillin/Clavulanic Acid Susceptibility Testing

For gram-negative enteric aerobes see TABLE 2.

TABLE 2

MIC	Interpretation
≤8/4 µg/ml	Susceptible (S)
16/8 µg/ml	Intermediate (I)
≥32/16 µg/ml	Resistant (R)

For *Staphylococcus** and *Haemophilus* species see TABLE 3.

TABLE 3

MIC	Interpretation
≤4/2 µg/ml	Susceptible (S)
≥8/4 µg/ml	Resistant (R)

* Staphylococci which are susceptible to amoxicillin/clavulanic acid but resistant to methicillin/oxacillin must be considered as resistant.

For *Streptococcus pneumoniae* from non-meningitis sources: Isolates should be tested using amoxicillin/clavulanic acid and the following criteria should be used see TABLE 4. **Note:** These interpretive criteria are based on the recommended doses for respiratory tract infections.

A report of "Susceptible" indicates that the pathogen is likely to be inhibited if the antimicrobial compound in the blood reaches the concentration usually achievable. A report of "Intermediate" indicates that the result should be considered equivocal, and, if the micro-

TABLE 4

MIC	Interpretation
≤2/1 µg/ml	Susceptible (S)
4/2 µg/ml	Intermediate (I)
≥8/4 µg/ml	Resistant (R)

organism is not fully susceptible to alternative, clinically feasible drugs, the test should be repeated. This category implies possible clinical applicability in body sites where the drug is physiologically concentrated or in situations where high dosage of drug can be used. This category also provides a buffer zone that prevents small uncontrolled technical factors from causing major discrepancies in interpretation. A report of "Resistant" indicates that the pathogen is not likely to be inhibited if the antimicrobial compound in the blood reaches the concentrations usually achievable; other therapy should be selected.

Standardized susceptibility test procedures require the use of laboratory control microorganisms to control the technical aspects of the laboratory procedures. Standard amoxicillin/clavulanate potassium powder should provide the MIC values in TABLE 5.

TABLE 5

Microorganism		MIC Range*
Escherichia coli	ATCC 25922	2-8 µg/ml
Escherichia coli	ATCC 35218	4-16 µg/ml
Enterococcus faecalis	ATCC 29212	0.25-1.0 µg/ml
Haemophilus influenzae	ATCC 49247	2-16 µg/ml
Staphylococcus aureus	ATCC 29213	0.12-0.5 µg/ml
Streptococcus pneumoniae	ATCC 49619	0.03-0.12 µg/ml

* Expressed as concentration of amoxicillin in the presence of clavulanic acid at a constant 2 parts amoxicillin to 1 part clavulanic acid.

Diffusion Techniques

Quantitative methods that require measurement of zone diameters also provide reproducible estimates of the susceptibility of bacteria to antimicrobial compounds. One such standardized procedure$_2$ requires the use of standardized inoculum concentrations. This procedure uses paper disks impregnated with 30 µg of amoxicillin/clavulanate potassium (20 µg amoxicillin plus 10 µg clavulanate potassium) to test the susceptibility of microorganisms to amoxicillin/clavulanic acid.

Reports from the laboratory providing results of the standard single-disk susceptibility test with a 30 µg amoxicillin/clavulanate potassium (20 µg amoxicillin plus 10 µg clavulanate potassium) disk should be interpreted according to the criteria in TABLE 6, TABLE 7, and TABLE 8.

Recommended Ranges for Amoxicillin/Clavulanic Acid Susceptibility Testing

For *Staphylococcus** species and *H. influenzae*† see TABLE 6.

TABLE 6

Zone Diameter	Interpretation
≥20 mm	Susceptible (S)
≤19 mm	Resistant (R)

* Staphylococci which are resistant to methicillin/oxacillin must be considered as resistant to amoxicillin/clavulanic acid.
† A broth microdilution method should be used for testing *H. influenzae*. β-lactamase negative, ampicillin-resistant strains must be considered resistant to amoxicillin/clavulanic acid.

For other organisms except *S. pneumoniae** and *N. gonorrhoeae*† see TABLE 7.

TABLE 7

Zone Diameter	Interpretation
≥18 mm	Susceptible (S)
14-17 mm	Intermediate (I)
≤13 mm	Resistant (R)

* Susceptibility of *S. pneumoniae* should be determined using a 1 µg oxacillin disk. Isolates with oxacillin zone sizes of ≥20 mm are susceptible to amoxicillin/clavulanic acid. An amoxicillin/clavulanic acid MIC should be determined on isolates of *S. pneumoniae* with oxacillin zone sizes of ≤19 mm.
† A broth microdilution method should be used for testing *N. gonorrhoeae* and interpreted according to penicillin breakpoints.

Interpretation should be as stated above for results using dilution techniques. Interpretation involves correlation of the diameter obtained in the disk test with the MIC for amoxicillin/clavulanic acid.

As with standardized dilution techniques, diffusion methods require the use of laboratory control microorganisms that are used to control the technical aspects of the laboratory procedures. For the diffusion technique, the 30 µg amoxicillin/clavulanate potassium (20 µg amoxicillin plus 10 µg clavulanate potassium) disk should provide the zone diameters in these laboratory quality control strains (see TABLE 8).

TABLE 8

Microorganism		Zone Diameter
Escherichia coli	ATCC 25922	19-25 mm
Escherichia coli	ATCC 35218	18-22 mm
Staphylococcus aureus	ATCC 25923	28-36 mm

AUGMENTIN TABLETS

Amoxicillin and clavulanate potassium are well absorbed from the gastrointestinal tract after oral administration of Augmentin. Dosing in the fasted or fed state has minimal effect on the pharmacokinetics of amoxicillin. While Augmentin can be given without regard to meals, absorption of clavulanate potassium when taken with food is greater relative to the fasted state. In one study, the relative bioavailability of clavulanate was reduced when Augmentin was dosed at 30 and 150 minutes after the start of a high fat breakfast. The safety and efficacy of Augmentin have been established in clinical trials where Augmentin was taken without regard to meals.

TABLE 9 *Mean* Amoxicillin and Clavulanate Potassium Pharmacokinetic Parameters*

Dose† and Regimen	AUC(0-∞) (µg·h/ml)		C_{max} (µg/ml)†	
Amoxicillin/ Clavulanate Potassium	Amoxicillin (±SD)	Clavulanate Potassium (±SD)	Amoxicillin (±SD)	Clavulanate Potassium (±SD)
250/125 mg q8h	26.7 ± 4.56	12.6 ± 3.25	3.3 ± 1.12	1.5 ± 0.70
500/125 mg q12h	33.4 ± 6.76	8.6 ± 1.95	6.5 ± 1.41	1.8 ± 0.61
500/125 mg q8h	53.4 ± 8.87	15.7 ± 3.86	7.2 ± 2.26	2.4 ± 0.83
875/125 mg q12h	53.5 ± 12.31	10.2 ± 3.04	11.6 ± 2.78	2.2 ± 0.99

* Mean values of 14 normal volunteers (n=15 for clavulanate potassium in the low-dose regimens). Peak concentrations occurred approximately 1.5 hours after the dose.
† Administered at the start of a light meal.

Amoxicillin serum concentrations achieved with Augmentin are similar to those produced by the oral administration of equivalent doses of amoxicillin alone. The half-life of amoxicillin after the oral administration of Augmentin is 1.3 hours and that of clavulanic acid is 1.0 hour.

Approximately 50-70% of the amoxicillin and approximately 25-40% of the clavulanic acid are excreted unchanged in urine during the first 6 hours after administration of a single Augmentin 250 or 500 mg tablet.

Concurrent administration of probenecid delays amoxicillin excretion but does not delay renal excretion of clavulanic acid.

Neither component in Augmentin is highly protein-bound; clavulanic acid has been found to be approximately 25% bound to human serum and amoxicillin approximately 18% bound.

Amoxicillin diffuses readily into most body tissues and fluids with the exception of the brain and spinal fluid. The results of experiments involving the administration of clavulanic acid to animals suggest that this compound, like amoxicillin, is well distributed in body tissues.

Microbiology

Amoxicillin is a semisynthetic antibiotic with a broad spectrum of bactericidal activity against many gram-positive and gram-negative microorganisms. Amoxicillin is, however, susceptible to degradation by β-lactamases and, therefore, the spectrum of activity does not include organisms which produce these enzymes. Clavulanic acid is a β-lactam, structurally related to the penicillins, which possesses the ability to inactivate a wide range of β-lactamase enzymes commonly found in microorganisms resistant to penicillins and cephalosporins. In particular, it has good activity against the clinically important plasmid mediated β-lactamases frequently responsible for transferred drug resistance.

The formulation of amoxicillin and clavulanic acid in Augmentin protects amoxicillin from degradation by β-lactamase enzymes and effectively extends the antibiotic spectrum of amoxicillin to include many bacteria normally resistant to amoxicillin and other β-lactam antibiotics. Thus, Augmentin possesses the properties of a broad-spectrum antibiotic and a β-lactamase inhibitor.

Amoxicillin/clavulanic acid has been shown to be active against most strains of the following microorganisms, both *in vitro* and in clinical infections as described in INDICATIONS AND USAGE, Augmentin Tablets.

Gram-Positive Aerobes

*Staphylococcus aureus** (β-lactamase and non-β-lactamase producing).
*Staphylococci which are resistant to methicillin/oxacillin must be considered resistant to amoxicillin/clavulanic acid.

Gram-Negative Aerobes

Enterobacter species. (Although most strains of *Enterobacter* species are resistant *in vitro,* clinical efficacy has been demonstrated with Augmentin in urinary tract infections caused by these organisms.)
Escherichia coli (β-lactamase and non-β-lactamase producing).
Haemophilus influenzae (β-lactamase and non-β-lactamase producing).
Klebsiella species (all known strains are β-lactamase producing).
Moraxella catarrhalis (β-lactamase and non-β-lactamase producing).

The following *in vitro* data are available, **but their clinical significance is unknown.**

Amoxicillin/clavulanic acid exhibits *in vitro* minimal inhibitory concentrations (MICs) of 2 µg/ml or less against most (≥90%) strains of *Streptococcus pneumoniae**; MICs of 0.06 µg/ml or less against most (≥90%) strains of *Neisseria gonorrhoeae;* MICs of 4 µg/ml or

A

less against most (≥90%) strains of staphylococci and anaerobic bacteria; and MICs of 8 μg/ml or less against most (≥90%) strains of other listed organisms. However, with the exception of organisms shown to respond to amoxicillin alone, the safety and effectiveness of amoxicillin/clavulanic acid in treating clinical infections due to these microorganisms have not been established in adequate and well-controlled clinical trials.

*Because amoxicillin has greater *in vitro* activity against *Streptococcus pneumoniae* than does ampicillin or penicillin, the majority of *S. pneumoniae* strains with intermediate susceptibility to ampicillin or penicillin are fully susceptible to amoxicillin.

Gram-Positive Aerobes

*Enterococcus faecalis**.
Staphylococcus epidermidis (β-lactamase and non-β-lactamase producing).
Staphylococcus saprophyticus (β-lactamase and non-β-lactamase producing).
*Streptococcus pneumoniae**†.
*Streptococcus pyogenes**†.
viridans group *Streptococcus**†.

Gram-Negative Aerobes

Eikenella corrodens (β-lactamase and non-β-lactamase producing).
*Neisseria gonorrhoeae** (β-lactamase and non-β-lactamase producing).
*Proteus mirabilis** (β-lactamase and non-β-lactamase producing).

Anaerobic Bacteria

Bacteroides species, including *Bacteroides fragilis* (β-lactamase and non-β-lactamase producing).
Fusobacterium species (β-lactamase and non-β-lactamase producing).
Peptostreptococcus species†.

*Adequate and well-controlled clinical trials have established the effectiveness of amoxicillin alone in treating certain clinical infections due to these organisms.

†These are non-β-lactamase-producing organisms and, therefore, are susceptible to amoxicillin alone.

Susceptibility Testing

Dilution Techniques

Quantitative methods are used to determine antimicrobial minimal inhibitory concentrations (MICs). These MICs provide estimates of the susceptibility of bacteria to antimicrobial compounds. The MICs should be determined using a standardized procedure. Standardized procedures are based on a dilution method[1] (broth or agar) or equivalent with standardized inoculum concentrations and standardized concentrations of amoxicillin/clavulanate potassium powder.

The recommended dilution pattern utilizes a constant amoxicillin/clavulanate potassium ratio of 2 to 1 in all tubes with varying amounts of amoxicillin. MICs are expressed in terms of the amoxicillin concentration in the presence of clavulanic acid at a constant 2 parts amoxicillin to 1 part clavulanic acid. The MIC values should be interpreted according to the criteria in TABLE 10, TABLE 11, TABLE 12, and TABLE 13.

Recommended Ranges for Amoxicillin/Clavulanic Acid Susceptibility Testing

For gram-negative enteric aerobes see TABLE 10.

TABLE 10

MIC	Interpretation
≤8/4 μg/ml	Susceptible (S)
16/8 μg/ml	Intermediate (I)
≥32/16 μg/ml	Resistant (R)

For *Staphylococcus* and *Haemophilus* species see TABLE 11.

TABLE 11

MIC	Interpretation
≤4/2 μg/ml	Susceptible (S)
≥8/4 μg/ml	Resistant (R)

* Staphylococci which are susceptible to amoxicillin/clavulanic acid but resistant to methicillin/oxacillin must be considered as resistant.

For *Streptococcus pneumoniae* from non-meningitis sources: Isolates should be tested using amoxicillin/clavulanic acid and the criteria in TABLE 12 should be used.

TABLE 12

MIC	Interpretation
≤2/1 μg/ml	Susceptible (S)
4/2 μg/ml	Intermediate (I)
≥8/4 μg/ml	Resistant (R)

Note: These interpretive criteria are based on the recommended doses for respiratory tract infections.

A report of "Susceptible" indicates that the pathogen is likely to be inhibited if the antimicrobial compound in the blood reaches the concentration usually achievable. A report of "Intermediate" indicates that the result should be considered equivocal, and, if the microorganism is not fully susceptible to alternative, clinically feasible drugs, the test should be repeated. This category implies possible clinical applicability in body sites where the drug is physiologically concentrated or in situations where high dosage of drug can be used. This category also provides a buffer zone which prevents small uncontrolled technical factors from causing major discrepancies in interpretation. A report of "Resistant" indicates that the pathogen is not likely to be inhibited if the antimicrobial compound in the blood reaches the concentrations usually achievable; other therapy should be selected.

Standardized susceptibility test procedures require the use of laboratory control microorganisms to control the technical aspects of the laboratory procedures. Standard amoxicillin/clavulanate potassium powder should provide the MIC values in TABLE 13.

TABLE 13

Microorganism		MIC Range*
Escherichia coli	ATCC 25922	2-8 μg/ml
Escherichia coli	ATCC 35218	4-16 μg/ml
Enterococcus faecalis	ATCC 29212	0.25-1.0 μg/ml
Haemophilus influenzae	ATCC 49247	2-16 μg/ml
Staphylococcus aureus	ATCC 29213	0.12-0.5 μg/ml
Streptococcus pneumoniae	ATCC 49619	0.03-0.12 μg/ml

* Expressed as concentration of amoxicillin in the presence of clavulanic acid at a constant 2 parts amoxicillin to 1 part clavulanic acid.

Diffusion Techniques

Quantitative methods that require measurement of zone diameters also provide reproducible estimates of the susceptibility of bacteria to antimicrobial compounds. One such standardized procedure[2] requires the use of standardized inoculum concentrations. This procedure uses paper disks impregnated with 30 μg of amoxicillin/clavulanate potassium (20 μg amoxicillin plus 10 μg clavulanate potassium) to test the susceptibility of microorganisms to amoxicillin/clavulanic acid.

Reports from the laboratory providing results of the standard single-disk susceptibility test with a 30 μg amoxicillin/clavulanate acid (20 μg amoxicillin plus 10 μg clavulanate potassium) disk should be interpreted according to the criteria in TABLE 14, TABLE 15, and TABLE 16.

Recommended Ranges for Amoxicillin/Clavulanic Acid Susceptibility Testing

For *Staphylococcus** species and *H. influenzae*† see TABLE 14.

TABLE 14

Zone Diameter	Interpretation
≥20 mm	Susceptible (S)
≤19 mm	Resistant (R)

* Staphylococci which are resistant to methicillin/oxacillin must be considered as resistant to amoxicillin/clavulanic acid.
† A broth microdilution method should be used for testing *H. influenzae*. β-lactamase negative, ampicillin-resistant strains must be considered resistant to amoxicillin/clavulanic acid.

For other organisms except *S. pneumoniae** and *N. gonorrhoeae*† see TABLE 15.

TABLE 15

Zone Diameter	Interpretation
≥18 mm	Susceptible (S)
14-17 mm	Intermediate (I)
≤13 mm	Resistant (R)

* Susceptibility of *S. pneumoniae* should be determined using a 1 μg oxacillin disk. Isolates with oxacillin zone sizes of ≥20 mm are susceptible to amoxicillin/clavulanic acid. An amoxicillin/clavulanic acid MIC should be determined on isolates of *S. pneumoniae* with oxacillin zone sizes of ≤19 mm.
† A broth microdilution method should be used for testing *N. gonorrhoeae* and interpreted according to penicillin breakpoints.

Interpretation should be as stated above for results using dilution techniques. Interpretation involves correlation of the diameter obtained in the disk test with the MIC for amoxicillin/clavulanic acid.

As with standardized dilution techniques, diffusion methods require the use of laboratory control microorganisms that are used to control the technical aspects of the laboratory procedures. For the diffusion technique, the 30 μg amoxicillin/clavulanate potassium (20 μg amoxicillin plus 10 μg clavulanate potassium) disk should provide the zone diameters in TABLE 16 in these laboratory quality control strains.

TABLE 16

Microorganism		Zone Diameter
Escherichia coli	ATCC 25922	19-25 mm
Escherichia coli	ATCC 35218	18-22 mm
Staphylococcus aureus	ATCC 25923	28-36 mm

AUGMENTIN ES-600 POWDER FOR ORAL SUSPENSION

The pharmacokinetics of amoxicillin and clavulanate were determined in a study of 19 pediatric patients, aged 8 months to 11 years, given Augmentin ES-600 at an amoxicillin dose of 45 mg/kg q12h with snack or meal. The mean plasma amoxicillin and clavulanate pharmacokinetic parameter values are listed in TABLE 17.

The effect of food on the oral absorption of Augmentin ES-600 has not been studied.

Approximately 50-70% of the amoxicillin and approximately 25-40% of the clavulanic acid are excreted unchanged in urine during the first 6 hours after administration of 10 ml of Augmentin 250 mg/5 ml suspension.

Concurrent administration of probenecid delays amoxicillin excretion but does not delay renal excretion of clavulanic acid.

Neither component in Augmentin ES-600 is highly protein-bound; clavulanic acid has been found to be approximately 25% bound to human serum and amoxicillin approximately 18% bound.

TABLE 17 *Mean (±SD) Plasma Amoxicillin and Clavulanate Pharmacokinetic Parameter Values**

Parameter†	Amoxicillin	Clavulanate
C_{max} (μg/ml)	15.7 ± 7.7	1.7 ± 0.9
T_{max} (h)	2.0 (1.0-4.0)	1.1 (1.0-4.0)
AUC(0-t) (μg·h/ml)	59.8 ± 20.0	4.0 ± 1.9
T½ (h)	1.4 ± 0.3	1.1 ± 0.3
CL/F (L/h/kg)	0.9 ± 0.4	1.1 ± 1.1

* Following administration of 45 mg/kg of Augmentin ES-600 every 12 hours to pediatric patients.
† Arithmetic mean ± standard deviation, except T_{max} values which are medians (ranges).

Oral administration of a single dose of Augmentin ES-600 at 45 mg/kg (based on the amoxicillin component) to pediatric patients, aged 9 months to 8 years, yielded the pharmacokinetic data shown in TABLE 18 for amoxicillin in plasma and middle ear fluid (MEF).

TABLE 18 *Amoxicillin Concentrations in Plasma and Middle Ear Fluid Following Administration of 45 mg/kg of Augmentin ES-600 to Pediatric Patients*

	Amoxicillin Concentration	
Timepoint	**In Plasma**	**In MEF**
1 Hour		
Mean	7.7 μg/ml	3.2 μg/ml
Median	9.3 μg/ml	3.5 μg/ml
Range	1.5-14.0 μg/ml	0.2-5.5 μg/ml
n	5	4
2 Hour		
Mean	15.7 μg/ml	3.3 μg/ml
Median	13.0 μg/ml	2.4 μg/ml
Range	11.0-25.0 μg/ml	1.9-6 μg/ml
n	7	5
3 Hour		
Mean	13.0 μg/ml	5.8 μg/ml
Median	12.0 μg/ml	6.5 μg/ml
Range	5.5-21.0 μg/ml	3.9-7.4 μg/ml
n	5	5

Dose administered immediately prior to eating.

Amoxicillin diffuses readily into most body tissues and fluids with the exception of the brain and spinal fluid. The results of experiments involving the administration of clavulanic acid to animals suggest that this compound, like amoxicillin, is well distributed in body tissues.

Microbiology

Amoxicillin is a semisynthetic antibiotic with a broad spectrum of bactericidal activity against many gram-positive and gram-negative microorganisms. Amoxicillin is, however, susceptible to degradation by β-lactamases and, therefore, the spectrum of activity does not include organisms which produce these enzymes. Clavulanic acid is a β-lactam, structurally related to the penicillins, which possesses the ability to inactivate a wide range of β-lactamase enzymes commonly found in microorganisms resistant to penicillins and cephalosporins. In particular, it has good activity against the clinically important plasmid mediated β-lactamases frequently responsible for transferred drug resistance.

The clavulanic acid component in Augmentin ES-600 protects amoxicillin from degradation by β-lactamase enzymes and effectively extends the antibiotic spectrum of amoxicillin to include many bacteria normally resistant to amoxicillin and other β-lactam antibiotics. Thus, Augmentin ES-600 possesses the distinctive properties of a broad-spectrum antibiotic and a β-lactamase inhibitor.

Amoxicillin/clavulanic acid has been shown to be active against most strains of the following microorganisms, both *in vitro* and in clinical infections as described in INDICATIONS AND USAGE, Augmentin ES-600 Powder for Oral Suspension.

Aerobic Gram-Positive Microorganisms

Streptococcus pneumoniae (including isolates with penicillin MICs = 2 μg/ml).

Aerobic Gram-Negative Microorganisms

Haemophilus influenzae (including β-lactamase-producing strains).

Moraxella catarrhalis (including β-lactamase-producing strains).

The following *in vitro* data are available, but their clinical significance is unknown.

At least 90% of the following microorganisms exhibit an *in vitro* minimum inhibitory concentration (MIC) less than or equal to the susceptible breakpoint for amoxicillin/clavulanic acid. However, with the exception of organisms shown to respond to amoxicillin alone, the safety and effectiveness of amoxicillin/clavulanic acid in treating clinical infections due to these microorganisms have not been established in adequate and well-controlled clinical trials.

Aerobic Gram-Positive Microorganisms

Staphylococcus aureus (including β-lactamase-producing strains).

Streptococcus pyogenes.

Note: Staphylococci which are resistant to methicillin/oxacillin must be considered resistant to amoxicillin/clavulanic acid.

Note: *S. pyogenes* do not produce β-lactamase and, therefore, are susceptible to amoxicillin alone. Adequate and well-controlled clinical trials have established the effectiveness of amoxicillin alone in treating certain clinical infections due to *S. pyogenes.*

Susceptibility Testing

Dilution Techniques

Quantitative methods are used to determine antimicrobial minimum inhibitory concentrations (MICs). These MICs provide estimates of the susceptibility of bacteria to antimicrobial compounds. The MICs should be determined using a standardized procedure.[3,4]

Standardized procedures are based on a dilution method (broth for *S. pneumoniae* and *H. influenzae*) or equivalent with standardized inoculum concentrations and standardized concentrations of amoxicillin/clavulanate potassium powder.

The recommended dilution pattern utilizes a constant amoxicillin/clavulanate potassium ratio of 2 to 1 in all tubes with varying amounts of amoxicillin. MICs are expressed in terms of the amoxicillin concentration in the presence of clavulanic acid at a constant 2 parts amoxicillin to 1 part clavulanic acid. The MIC values should be interpreted according to the criteria in TABLE 19 and TABLE 20.

For testing *Streptococcus pneumoniaea** see TABLE 19.

TABLE 19

MIC	Interpretation
≤2/1 μg/ml	Susceptible (S)
4/2 μg/ml	Intermediate (I)
≥8/4 μg/ml	Resistant (R)

* These interpretive standards are applicable only to broth microdilution susceptibility tests using cation-adjusted Mueller-Hinton broth with 2-5% lysed horse blood.[4]

For testing *Haemophilus influenzae** see TABLE 20.

TABLE 20

MIC	Interpretation
≤4/2 μg/ml	Susceptible (S)
≥8/4 μg/ml	Resistant (R)

* These interpretive standards are applicable only to broth microdilution susceptibility tests with *Haemophilus* spp. using *Haemophilus* Test Medium (HTM).[4]

A report of "Susceptible" indicates that the pathogen is likely to be inhibited if the antimicrobial compound in the blood reaches the concentration usually achievable. A report of "Intermediate" indicates that the result should be considered equivocal, and, if the microorganism is not fully susceptible to alternative, clinically feasible drugs, the test should be repeated. This category implies possible clinical applicability in body sites where the drug is physiologically concentrated or in situations where high dosage of drug can be used. This category also provides a buffer zone that prevents small uncontrolled technical factors from causing major discrepancies in interpretation. A report of "Resistant" indicates that the pathogen is not likely to be inhibited if the antimicrobial compound in the blood reaches the concentrations usually achievable; other therapy should be selected.

Standardized susceptibility test procedures require the use of laboratory control microorganisms to control the technical aspects of the laboratory procedures. Standard amoxicillin/clavulanate potassium powder should provide the MIC values shown in TABLE 21.

TABLE 21

Microorganism		MIC Range*
Escherichia coli	ATCC 35218†	4-16 μg/ml
Haemophilus influenzae‡	ATCC 49247	2-16 μg/ml
Streptococcus pneumoniae§	ATCC 49619	0.03-0.12 μg/ml

* Expressed as concentration of amoxicilli μg/mln in the presence of clavulanic acid at a constant 2 parts amoxicillin to 1 part clavulanic acid.
† *H. influenzae* quality control.
‡ This quality control range is applicable to *H. influenzae* ATCC 49247 tested by a broth microdilution procedure using HTM.[4]
§ This quality control range is applicable to *S. pneumoniae* ATCC 49619 tested by a broth microdilution procedure using cation-adjusted Mueller-Hinton broth with 2-5% lysed horse blood.[4]

Diffusion Techniques

Quantitative methods that require measurement of zone diameters also provide reproducible estimates of the susceptibility of bacteria to antimicrobial compounds. One such standardized procedure[5] requires the use of standardized inoculum concentrations. This procedure uses paper disks impregnated with 30 μg of amoxicillin/clavulanate potassium (20 μg amoxicillin plus 10 μg clavulanate potassium) to test the susceptibility of microorganisms to amoxicillin/clavulanic acid.

Reports from the laboratory providing results of the standard single-disk susceptibility test with a 30 μg amoxicillin/clavulanate potassium (20 μg amoxicillin plus 10 μg clavulanate potassium) disk should be interpreted according to the following criteria.

For *H. influenzae** see TABLE 22.

TABLE 22

Zone Diameter	Interpretation
≥20 mm	Susceptible (S)
≤19 mm	Resistant (R)

* These zone diameter standards are applicable only to tests conducted with *Haemophilus* spp. using HTM.[4]

Note: β-lactamase-negative, ampicillin-resistant *H. influenzae* strains must be considered resistant to amoxicillin/clavulanic acid.

A

For *Streptococcus pneumoniae:*

Susceptibility of *S. pneumoniae* should be determined using a 1 μg oxacillin disk. Isolates with an oxacillin zone sizes of ≥20 mm are susceptible to amoxicillin/clavulanic acid.* An amoxicillin/clavulanic acid MIC should be determined on isolates of *S. pneumoniae* with oxacillin zone sizes of ≤19 mm.

*These zone diameter standards for *S. pneumoniae* apply only to tests performed using Mueller-Hinton agar supplemented with 5% sheep blood incubated in 5% CO_2.[4]

Interpretation should be as stated above for results using dilution techniques. Interpretation involves correlation of the diameter obtained in the disk test with the MIC for amoxicillin/clavulanic acid.

As with standardized dilution techniques, diffusion methods require the use of laboratory control microorganisms that are used to control the technical aspects of the laboratory procedures. For the diffusion technique, the 30 μg amoxicillin/clavulanate potassium (20 μg amoxicillin plus 10 μg clavulanate potassium) disk should provide the zone diameters shown in TABLE 23 in these laboratory quality control strains.

TABLE 23

Microorganism		Zone Diameter
*Escherichia coli**	ATCC 35218	18-22 mm
Haemophilus influenzae†	ATCC 49247	15-23 mm

* *H. influenzae* quality control.
† This quality control limit applies only to tests conducted with *H. influenzae* ATCC 49247 using HTM.

AUGMENTIN XR EXTENDED-RELEASE TABLETS

Amoxicillin and clavulanate potassium are well absorbed from the gastrointestinal tract after oral administration of Augmentin XR.

Augmentin XR is an extended-release formulation which provides sustained plasma concentrations of amoxicillin. Amoxicillin systemic exposure achieved with Augmentin XR is similar to that produced by the oral administration of equivalent doses of amoxicillin alone. In a study of healthy adult volunteers, the pharmacokinetics of Augmentin XR were compared when administered in a fasted state, at the start of a standardized meal (612 kcal, 89.3 g carb, 24.9 g fat, 14.0 g protein), or 30 minutes after a high-fat meal. When the systemic exposure to both amoxicillin and clavulanate is taken into consideration, Augmentin XR is optimally administered at the start of a standardized meal. Absorption of amoxicillin is decreased in the fasted state. Augmentin XR is not recommended to be taken with a high fat meal, because clavulanate absorption is decreased. The pharmacokinetics of the components of Augmentin XR following administration of 2 Augmentin XR tablets at the start of a standardized meal are presented in TABLE 24.

TABLE 24 *Mean (SD) Pharmacokinetic Parameters for Amoxicillin and Clavulanate Following Oral Administration of 2 Augmentin XR Tablets (2000/125 mg) to Healthy Adult Volunteers [n=55] Fed a Standardized Meal*

Parameter (Units)	Amoxicillin	Clavulanate
AUC(0-∞) (μg·h/ml)	71.6 (16.5)	5.29 (1.55)
C_{max} (μg/ml)	17.0 (4.0)	2.05 (0.80)
T_{max} (hours)*	1.50 (1.00-6.00)	1.03 (0.75-3.00)
T½ (hours)	1.27 (0.20)	1.03 (0.17)

* Median (range).

The half-life of amoxicillin after the oral administration of Augmentin XR is approximately 1.3 hours, and that of clavulanate is approximately 1.0 hour.

Clearance of amoxicillin is predominantly renal, with approximately 60-80% of the dose being excreted unchanged in urine, whereas clearance of clavulanate has both a renal (30-50%) and a non-renal component.

Concurrent administration of probenecid delays amoxicillin excretion but does not delay renal excretion of clavulanate.

In a study of adults, the pharmacokinetics of amoxicillin and clavulanate were not affected by administration of an antacid, either simultaneously with or 2 hours after Augmentin XR.

Neither component in Augmentin XR is highly protein-bound; clavulanate has been found to be approximately 25% bound to human serum and amoxicillin approximately 18% bound.

Amoxicillin diffuses readily into most body tissues and fluids with the exception of the brain and spinal fluid. The results of experiments involving the administration of clavulanic acid to animals suggest that this compound, like amoxicillin, is well distributed in body tissues.

Microbiology

Amoxicillin is a semisynthetic antibiotic with a broad spectrum of bactericidal activity against many gram-positive and gram-negative microorganisms. Amoxicillin is, however, susceptible to degradation by β-lactamases, and therefore, the spectrum of activity does not include organisms which produce these enzymes. Clavulanic acid is a β-lactam, structurally related to the penicillins, which possesses the ability to inactivate a wide range of β-lactamase enzymes commonly found in microorganisms resistant to penicillins and cephalosporins. In particular, it has good activity against the clinically important plasmid mediated β-lactamases frequently responsible for transferred drug resistance.

The clavulanic acid component in Augmentin XR protects amoxicillin from degradation by β-lactamase enzymes and effectively extends the antibiotic spectrum of amoxicillin to include many bacteria normally resistant to amoxicillin and other β-lactam antibiotics.

Amoxicillin/clavulanic acid has been shown to be active against most strains of the following microorganisms, both *in vitro* and in clinical infections as described in INDICATIONS AND USAGE, Augmentin XR Extended-Release Tablets.

Aerobic Gram-Positive Microorganisms

Streptococcus pneumoniae (including isolates with penicillin MICs ≤2 μg/ml).
Staphylococcus aureus (including β-lactamase producing strains).

NOTE: Staphylococci which are resistant to methicillin/oxacillin must be considered resistant to amoxicillin/clavulanic acid.

Aerobic Gram-Negative Microorganisms

Haemophilus influenzae (including β-lactamase producing strains).
Moraxella catarrhalis (including β-lactamase producing strains).
Haemophilus parainfluenzae (including β-lactamase producing strains).
Klebsiella pneumoniae (all known strains are β-lactamase producing).

The following *in vitro* data are available, **but their clinical significance is unknown.**

Amoxicillin/clavulanic acid exhibits *in vitro* minimal inhibitory concentrations (MICs) of 2.0 μg/ml or less against most (≥90%) strains of Streptococcus pyogenes and MICs of 4.0 μg/ml or less against most (≥90%) strains of the anaerobic bacteria listed below.

Aerobic Gram-Positive Microorganisms

Streptococcus pyogenes.

Anaerobic Microorganisms

Bacteroides fragilis (including β-lactamase producing strains).
Fusobacterium nucleatum (including β-lactamase producing strains).
Peptostreptococcus magnus.
Peptostreptococcus micros.

NOTE: *S. pyogenes, P. magnus* and *P. micros* do not produce β-lactamase, and therefore, are susceptible to amoxicillin alone. Adequate and well-controlled clinical trials have established the effectiveness of amoxicillin alone in treating certain clinical infections due to *S. pyogenes.*

Susceptibility Testing

Dilution Techniques

Quantitative methods are used to determine antimicrobial minimum inhibitory concentrations (MICs). These MICs provide estimates of the susceptibility of bacteria to antimicrobial compounds. The MICs should be determined using a standardized procedure.[3,6] Standardized procedures are based on a dilution method (broth or agar; broth for *S. pneumoniae* and *Haemophilus* species) or equivalent with standardized inoculum concentrations and standardized concentrations of amoxicillin/clavulanate potassium powder.

The recommended dilution pattern utilizes a constant amoxicillin/clavulanate potassium ratio of 2 to 1 in all tubes with varying amounts of amoxicillin. MICs are expressed in terms of the amoxicillin concentration in the presence of clavulanic acid at a constant 2 parts amoxicillin to 1 part clavulanic acid.

The MIC values should be interpreted according to the criteria in TABLE 25, TABLE 26, and TABLE 27.

For testing *Klebsiella pneumoniae* see TABLE 25.

TABLE 25

MIC	Interpretation
≤8/4 μg/ml	Susceptible (S)
16/8 μg/ml	Intermediate (I)
≥32/16 μg/ml	Resistant (R)

For testing *Streptococcus pneumoniaea** see TABLE 26.

TABLE 26

MIC	Interpretation
≤2/1 μg/ml	Susceptible (S)
4/2 μg/ml	Intermediate (I)
≥8/4 μg/ml	Resistant (R)

* These interpretive standards are applicable only to broth microdilution susceptibility tests using cation-adjusted Mueller-Hinton broth with 2-5% lysed horse blood.[6]

For testing *Staphylococcus* species and Haemophilus species* see TABLE 27.

TABLE 27

MIC	Interpretation
≤4/2 μg/ml	Susceptible (S)
≥8/4 μg/ml	Resistant (R)

* These interpretive standards are applicable only to broth microdilution susceptibility tests with *Haemophilus* spp. using *Haemophilus* Test Medium (HTM).[6]

NOTE: Staphylococci which are resistant to methicillin/oxacillin must be considered resistant to amoxicillin/clavulanic acid.

A report of "Susceptible" indicates that the pathogen is likely to be inhibited if the antimicrobial compound in the blood reaches the concentration usually achievable. A report of "Intermediate" indicates that the result should be considered equivocal, and if the microorganism is not fully susceptible to alternative, clinically feasible drugs, the test should be repeated. This category implies possible clinical applicability in body sites where the drug is physiologically concentrated or in situations where high dosage of drug can be used. This category also provides a buffer zone which prevents small uncontrolled technical factors from causing major discrepancies in interpretation. A report of "Resistant" indicates that the pathogen is not likely to be inhibited if the antimicrobial compound in the blood reaches the concentrations usually achievable; other therapy should be selected.

Standardized susceptibility test procedures require the use of laboratory control microorganisms to control the technical aspects of the laboratory procedures. Standard amoxicillin/clavulanate potassium powder should provide the MIC values in TABLE 28.

TABLE 28

Microorganism		MIC Range*
Escherichia coli	ATCC 35218	4-16 µg/ml
Escherichia coli	ATCC 25922	2-8 µg/ml
Haemophilus influenzae†	ATCC 49247	2-16 µg/ml
Staphylococcus aureus	ATCC 29213	0.12-0.5 µg/ml
Streptococcus pneumoniae‡	ATCC 49619	0.03-0.12 µg/ml

* Expressed as concentration of amoxicillin in the presence of clavulanic acid at a constant 2 parts amoxicillin to 1 part clavulanic acid.
† This quality control range is applicable to *H. influenzae* ATCC 49247 tested by a broth microdilution procedure using HTM.[6]
‡ This quality control range is applicable to *S. pneumoniae* ATCC 49619 tested by a broth microdilution procedure using cation-adjusted Mueller-Hinton broth with 2-5% lysed horse blood.[6]

Diffusion Techniques
Quantitative methods that require measurement of zone diameters also provide reproducible estimates of the susceptibility of bacteria to antimicrobial compounds. One such standardized procedure[5] requires the use of standardized inoculum concentrations. This procedure uses paper disks impregnated with 30 µg of amoxicillin/clavulanate potassium (20 µg amoxicillin plus 10 µg clavulanate potassium) to test the susceptibility of microorganisms to amoxicillin/clavulanic acid.

Reports from the laboratory providing results of the standard single-disk susceptibility test with a 30 µg amoxicillin/clavulanate potassium (20 µg amoxicillin plus 10 µg clavulanate potassium) disk should be interpreted according to the criteria in TABLE 29 and TABLE 30.

For testing *Klebsiella pneumoniae* see TABLE 29.

TABLE 29

Zone Diameter	Interpretation
≥18 mm	Susceptible (S)
14-17 mm	Intermediate (I)
≤13 mm	Resistant (R)

For testing *Staphylococcus* and *Haemophilus* species* see TABLE 30.

TABLE 30

Zone Diameter	Interpretation
≥20 mm	Susceptible (S)
≤19 mm	Resistant (R)

* These zone diameter standards are applicable only to tests conducted with *Haemophilus* spp. using HTM.[6]

NOTE: Staphylococci which are resistant to methicillin/oxacillin must be considered resistant to amoxicillin/clavulanic acid.

NOTE: β-lactamase negative, ampicillin-resistant *H. influenzae* strains must be considered resistant to amoxicillin/clavulanic acid.

For testing *Streptococcus pneumoniae:*

Susceptibility of *S. pneumoniae* should be determined using a 1 µg oxacillin disk. Isolates with oxacillin zone sizes of ≥20 mm are susceptible to amoxicillin/clavulanic acid.* An amoxicillin/clavulanic acid MIC should be determined on isolates of *S. pneumoniae* with oxacillin zone sizes of ≤19 mm.

*These zone diameter standards for *S. pneumoniae* apply only to tests performed using Mueller-Hinton agar supplemented with 5% sheep blood incubated in 5% CO_2.[6]

Interpretation should be as stated above for results using dilution techniques.

Interpretation involves correlation of the diameter obtained in the disk test with the MIC for amoxicillin/clavulanic acid.

As with standardized dilution techniques, diffusion methods require the use of laboratory control microorganisms that are used to control the technical aspects of the laboratory procedures. For the diffusion technique, the 30 µg amoxicillin/clavulanate potassium (20 µg amoxicillin plus 10 µg clavulanate potassium) disk should provide the zone diameters TABLE 31 in these laboratory quality control strains.

TABLE 31

Microorganism		Zone Diameter
Escherichia coli	ATCC 35218	19-25 mm
Escherichia coli	ATCC 25922	18-22 mm
Staphylococcus aureus	ATCC 25923	28-36 mm
*Haemophilus influenzae**	ATCC 49247	15-23 mm

* This quality control limit applies only to tests conducted with *H. influenzae* ATCC 49247 using HTM.[6]

INDICATIONS AND USAGE

AUGMENTIN POWDER FOR ORAL SUSPENSION AND CHEWABLE TABLETS

Augmentin is indicated in the treatment of infections caused by susceptible strains of the designated organisms in the conditions listed below:

Lower Respiratory Tract Infections caused by β-lactamase-producing strains of *Haemophilus influenzae* and *Moraxella (Branhamella) catarrhalis.*

Otitis Media caused by β-lactamase-producing strains of *Haemophilus influenzae* and *Moraxella (Branhamella) catarrhalis.*

Sinusitis caused by β-lactamase-producing strains of *Haemophilus influenzae* and *Moraxella (Branhamella) catarrhalis.*

Skin and Skin Structure Infections caused by β-lactamase-producing strains of *Staphylococcus aureus, Escherichia coli* and *Klebsiella* spp.

Urinary Tract Infections caused by β-lactamase-producing strains of *Escherichia coli, Klebsiella* spp. and *Enterobacter* spp.

While Augmentin is indicated only for the conditions listed above, infections caused by ampicillin-susceptible organisms are also amenable to Augmentin treatment due to its amoxicillin content. Therefore, mixed infections caused by ampicillin-susceptible organisms and β-lactamase-producing organisms susceptible to Augmentin should not require the addition of another antibiotic. Because amoxicillin has greater *in vitro* activity against *Streptococcus pneumoniae* than does ampicillin or penicillin, the majority of *S. pneumoniae* strains with intermediate susceptibility to ampicillin or penicillin are fully susceptible to amoxicillin and Augmentin. (See CLINICAL PHARMACOLOGY, Augmentin Powder for Oral Suspension and Chewable Tablets, Microbiology.)

Bacteriological studies, to determine the causative organisms and their susceptibility to Augmentin, should be performed together with any indicated surgical procedures.

Therapy may be instituted prior to obtaining the results from bacteriological and susceptibility studies to determine the causative organisms and their susceptibility to Augmentin when there is reason to believe the infection may involve any of the β-lactamase-producing organisms listed above. Once the results are known, therapy should be adjusted, if appropriate.

AUGMENTIN TABLETS

Augmentin is indicated in the treatment of infections caused by susceptible strains of the designated organisms in the conditions listed below:

Lower Respiratory Tract Infections caused by β-lactamase-producing strains of *Haemophilus influenzae* and *Moraxella (Branhamella) catarrhalis.*

Otitis Media caused by β-lactamase-producing strains of *Haemophilus influenzae* and *Moraxella (Branhamella) catarrhalis.*

Sinusitis caused by β-lactamase-producing strains of *Haemophilus influenzae* and *Moraxella (Branhamella) catarrhalis.*

Skin and Skin Structure Infections caused by β-lactamase-producing strains of *Staphylococcus aureus, Escherichia coli* and *Klebsiella* spp.

Urinary Tract Infections caused by β-lactamase-producing strains of *Escherichia coli, Klebsiella* spp. and *Enterobacter* spp.

While Augmentin is indicated only for the conditions listed above, infections caused by ampicillin-susceptible organisms are also amenable to Augmentin treatment due to its amoxicillin content. Therefore, mixed infections caused by ampicillin-susceptible organisms and β-lactamase-producing organisms susceptible to Augmentin should not require the addition of another antibiotic. Because amoxicillin has greater *in vitro* activity against *Streptococcus pneumoniae* than does ampicillin or penicillin, the majority of *S. pneumoniae* strains with intermediate susceptibility to ampicillin or penicillin are fully susceptible to amoxicillin and Augmentin. (See CLINICAL PHARMACOLOGY, Augmentin Tablets, Microbiology.)

Bacteriological studies, to determine the causative organisms and their susceptibility to Augmentin, should be performed together with any indicated surgical procedures. Therapy may be instituted prior to obtaining the results from bacteriological and susceptibility studies to determine the causative organisms and their susceptibility to Augmentin when there is reason to believe the infection may involve any of the β-lactamase-producing organisms listed above. Once the results are known, therapy should be adjusted, if appropriate.

AUGMENTIN ES-600 POWDER FOR ORAL SUSPENSION

Augmentin ES-600 is indicated for the treatment of pediatric patients with recurrent or persistent acute otitis media due to *S. pneumoniae* (penicillin MICs ≤2 µg/ml), *H. influenzae* (including β-lactamase-producing strains), or *M. catarrhalis* (including β-lactamase-producing strains) characterized by the following risk factors: antibiotic exposure for acute otitis media within the preceding 3 months, and either of the following:

- Age ≤2 years.
- Daycare attendance.

See CLINICAL PHARMACOLOGY, Augmentin ES-600 Powder for Oral Suspension, Microbiology.

Note: Acute otitis media due to *S. pneumoniae* alone can be treated with amoxicillin. Augmentin ES-600 is not indicated for the treatment of acute otitis media due to *S. pneumoniae* with penicillin MIC ≥4 µg /ml.

Bacteriological studies to determine the causative organisms and their susceptibility to Augmentin ES-600 should be performed, when indicated. Therapy may be instituted prior to obtaining the results from these studies when there is reason to believe the infection may involve both *S. pneumoniae* (penicillin MIC ≤2 µg/ml) and the β-lactamase-producing organisms listed above. Once the results are known, therapy should be adjusted appropriately.

AUGMENTIN XR EXTENDED-RELEASE TABLETS

Augmentin XR extended-release tablets are indicated for the treatment of patients with community-acquired pneumonia or acute bacterial sinusitis due to confirmed, or suspected β-lactamase-producing pathogens (*i.e., H. influenzae, M. catarrhalis, H. parainfluenzae, K. pneumoniae,* or methicillin-susceptible *S. aureus*) and *S. pneumoniae* with reduced susceptibility to penicillin (*i.e.,* penicillin MICs = 2 µg/ml). Augmentin XR is not indicated for the treatment of infections due to *S. pneumoniae* with penicillin MIC ≥4 µg/ml. Data are limited with regard to infections due to *S. pneumoniae* with penicillin MICs ≥4 µg/ml.

Of the common epidemiological risk factors for patients with resistant pneumococcal infections, only age >65 years was studied. Patients with other common risk factors for resistant pneumococcal infections (*e.g.,* alcoholism, immune-suppressive illness, and presence of multiple co-morbid conditions) were not studied.

In patients with community-acquired pneumonia in whom penicillin-resistant *S. pneumoniae* is suspected, bacteriological studies should be performed to determine the causative organisms and their susceptibility when Augmentin XR is prescribed. Once the results are known, therapy should be adjusted appropriately.

Acute bacterial sinusitis or community-acquired pneumonia due to a penicillin-susceptible strain of *S. pneumoniae* plus a β-lactamase-producing pathogen can be treated with another Augmentin product containing lower daily doses of amoxicillin (*i.e.,* 500 mg q8h or 875 mg q12h). Acute bacterial sinusitis or community-acquired pneumonia due to *S. pneumoniae* alone can be treated with amoxicillin.

NON-FDA APPROVED INDICATIONS

It has been used without FDA approval in combination with ciprofloxacin for the treatment of low-risk febrile neutropenia.

CONTRAINDICATIONS

AUGMENTIN POWDER FOR ORAL SUSPENSION AND CHEWABLE TABLETS

Augmentin is contraindicated in patients with a history of allergic reactions to any penicillin. It is also contraindicated in patients with a previous history of Augmentin-associated cholestatic jaundice/hepatic dysfunction.

AUGMENTIN TABLETS

Augmentin is contraindicated in patients with a history of allergic reactions to any penicillin. It is also contraindicated in patients with a previous history of Augmentin-associated cholestatic jaundice/hepatic dysfunction.

AUGMENTIN ES-600 POWDER FOR ORAL SUSPENSION

Augmentin ES-600 is contraindicated in patients with a history of allergic reactions to any penicillin. It is also contraindicated in patients with a previous history of Augmentin-associated cholestatic jaundice/hepatic dysfunction.

AUGMENTIN XR EXTENDED-RELEASE TABLETS

Augmentin XR is contraindicated in patients with a history of allergic reactions to any penicillin. It is also contraindicated in patients with a previous history of cholestatic jaundice/hepatic dysfunction associated with treatment with amoxicillin/clavulanate.

Augmentin XR is contraindicated in patients with severe renal impairment (creatinine clearance <30 ml/min) and in hemodialysis patients.

WARNINGS

AUGMENTIN POWDER FOR ORAL SUSPENSION AND CHEWABLE TABLETS

SERIOUS AND OCCASIONALLY FATAL HYPERSENSITIVITY (ANAPHYLACTIC) REACTIONS HAVE BEEN REPORTED IN PATIENTS ON PENICILLIN THERAPY. THESE REACTIONS ARE MORE LIKELY TO OCCUR IN INDIVIDUALS WITH A HISTORY OF PENICILLIN HYPERSENSITIVITY AND/OR A HISTORY OF SENSITIVITY TO MULTIPLE ALLERGENS. THERE HAVE BEEN REPORTS OF INDIVIDUALS WITH A HISTORY OF PENICILLIN HYPERSENSITIVITY WHO HAVE EXPERIENCED SEVERE REACTIONS WHEN TREATED WITH CEPHALOSPORINS. BEFORE INITIATING THERAPY WITH AUGMENTIN, CAREFUL INQUIRY SHOULD BE MADE CONCERNING PREVIOUS HYPERSENSITIVITY REACTIONS TO PENICILLINS, CEPHALOSPORINS OR OTHER ALLERGENS. IF AN ALLERGIC REACTION OCCURS, AUGMENTIN SHOULD BE DISCONTINUED AND THE APPROPRIATE THERAPY INSTITUTED. **SERIOUS ANAPHYLACTIC REACTIONS REQUIRE IMMEDIATE EMERGENCY TREATMENT WITH EPINEPHRINE. OXYGEN, INTRAVENOUS STEROIDS AND AIRWAY MANAGEMENT, INCLUDING INTUBATION, SHOULD ALSO BE ADMINISTERED AS INDICATED.**

Pseudomembranous colitis has been reported with nearly all antibacterial agents, including Augmentin, and has ranged in severity from mild to life-threatening. Therefore, it is important to consider this diagnosis in patients who present with diarrhea subsequent to the administration of antibacterial agents.

Treatment with antibacterial agents alters the normal flora of the colon and may permit overgrowth of clostridia. Studies indicate that a toxin produced by *Clostridium difficile* is one primary cause of "antibiotic associated colitis".

After the diagnosis of pseudomembranous colitis has been established, appropriate therapeutic measures should be initiated. Mild cases of pseudomembranous colitis usually respond to drug discontinuation alone. In moderate to severe cases, consideration should be given to management with fluids and electrolytes, protein supplementation and treatment with an antibacterial drug clinically effective against *Clostridium difficile* colitis.

Augmentin should be used with caution in patients with evidence of hepatic dysfunction. Hepatic toxicity associated with the use of Augmentin is usually reversible. On rare occasions, deaths have been reported (less than 1 death reported per estimated 4 million prescriptions worldwide). These have generally been cases associated with serious underlying diseases or concomitant medications. (See CONTRAINDICATIONS, Augmentin Powder for Oral Suspension and Chewable Tablets and ADVERSE REACTIONS, Augmentin Powder for Oral Suspension and Chewable Tablets, Liver.)

AUGMENTIN TABLETS

SERIOUS AND OCCASIONALLY FATAL HYPERSENSITIVITY (ANAPHYLACTIC) REACTIONS HAVE BEEN REPORTED IN PATIENTS ON PENICILLIN THERAPY. THESE REACTIONS ARE MORE LIKELY TO OCCUR IN INDIVIDUALS WITH A HISTORY OF PENICILLIN HYPERSENSITIVITY AND/OR A HISTORY OF SENSITIVITY TO MULTIPLE ALLERGENS. THERE HAVE BEEN REPORTS OF INDIVIDUALS WITH A HISTORY OF PENICILLIN HYPERSENSITIVITY WHO HAVE EXPERIENCED SEVERE REACTIONS WHEN TREATED WITH CEPHALOSPORINS. BEFORE INITIATING THERAPY WITH AUGMENTIN, CAREFUL INQUIRY SHOULD BE MADE CONCERNING PREVIOUS HYPERSENSITIVITY REACTIONS TO PENICILLINS, CEPHALOSPORINS OR OTHER ALLERGENS. IF AN ALLERGIC REACTION OCCURS, AUGMENTIN SHOULD BE DISCONTINUED AND THE APPROPRIATE THERAPY INSTITUTED. **SERIOUS ANAPHYLACTIC REACTIONS REQUIRE IMMEDIATE EMERGENCY TREATMENT WITH EPINEPHRINE. OXYGEN, INTRAVENOUS STEROIDS AND AIRWAY MANAGEMENT, INCLUDING INTUBATION, SHOULD ALSO BE ADMINISTERED AS INDICATED.**

Pseudomembranous colitis has been reported with nearly all antibacterial agents, including Augmentin, and has ranged in severity from mild to life-threatening. Therefore, it is important to consider this diagnosis in patients who present with diarrhea subsequent to the administration of antibacterial agents.

Treatment with antibacterial agents alters the normal flora of the colon and may permit overgrowth of clostridia. Studies indicate that a toxin produced by *Clostridium difficile* is one primary cause of "antibiotic associated colitis".

After the diagnosis of pseudomembranous colitis has been established, appropriate therapeutic measures should be initiated. Mild cases of pseudomembranous colitis usually respond to drug discontinuation alone. In moderate to severe cases, consideration should be given to management with fluids and electrolytes, protein supplementation and treatment with an antibacterial drug clinically effective against *Clostridium difficile* colitis.

Augmentin should be used with caution in patients with evidence of hepatic dysfunction. Hepatic toxicity associated with the use of Augmentin is usually reversible. On rare occasions, deaths have been reported (less than 1 death reported per estimated 4 million prescriptions worldwide). These have generally been cases associated with serious underlying diseases or concomitant medications. (See CONTRAINDICATIONS, Augmentin Tablets and ADVERSE REACTIONS, Augmentin Tablets, Liver.)

AUGMENTIN ES-600 POWDER FOR ORAL SUSPENSION

SERIOUS AND OCCASIONALLY FATAL HYPERSENSITIVITY (ANAPHYLACTIC) REACTIONS HAVE BEEN REPORTED IN PATIENTS ON PENICILLIN THERAPY. THESE REACTIONS ARE MORE LIKELY TO OCCUR IN INDIVIDUALS WITH A HISTORY OF PENICILLIN HYPERSENSITIVITY AND/OR A HISTORY OF SENSITIVITY TO MULTIPLE ALLERGENS. THERE HAVE BEEN REPORTS OF INDIVIDUALS WITH A HISTORY OF PENICILLIN HYPERSENSITIVITY WHO HAVE EXPERIENCED SEVERE REACTIONS WHEN TREATED WITH CEPHALOSPORINS. BEFORE INITIATING THERAPY WITH AUGMENTIN ES-600, CAREFUL INQUIRY SHOULD BE MADE CONCERNING PREVIOUS HYPERSENSITIVITY REACTIONS TO PENICILLINS, CEPHALOSPORINS OR OTHER ALLERGENS. IF AN ALLERGIC REACTION OCCURS, AUGMENTIN ES-600 SHOULD BE DISCONTINUED AND THE APPROPRIATE THERAPY INSTITUTED. **SERIOUS ANAPHYLACTIC REACTIONS REQUIRE IMMEDIATE EMERGENCY TREATMENT WITH EPINEPHRINE. OXYGEN, INTRAVENOUS STEROIDS AND AIRWAY MANAGEMENT, INCLUDING INTUBATION, SHOULD ALSO BE ADMINISTERED AS INDICATED.**

Pseudomembranous colitis has been reported with nearly all antibacterial agents, including amoxicillin/clavulanate potassium, and has ranged in severity from mild to life-threatening. Therefore, it is important to consider this diagnosis in patients who present with diarrhea subsequent to the administration of antibacterial agents.

Treatment with antibacterial agents alters the normal flora of the colon and may permit overgrowth of clostridia. Studies indicate that a toxin produced by *Clostridium difficile* is one primary cause of "antibiotic associated colitis".

After the diagnosis of pseudomembranous colitis has been established, appropriate therapeutic measures should be initiated. Mild cases of pseudomembranous colitis usually respond to drug discontinuation alone. In moderate to severe cases, consideration should be given to management with fluids and electrolytes, protein supplementation and treatment with an antibacterial drug clinically effective against *Clostridium difficile* colitis.

Augmentin ES-600 should be used with caution in patients with evidence of hepatic dysfunction. Hepatic toxicity associated with the use of amoxicillin/clavulanate potassium is usually reversible. On rare occasions, deaths have been reported (less than 1 death reported per estimated 4 million prescriptions worldwide). These have generally been cases associated with serious underlying diseases or concomitant medications. (See CONTRAINDICATIONS, Augmentin ES-600 Powder for Oral Suspension and ADVERSE REACTIONS, Augmentin ES-600 Powder for Oral Suspension, Liver.)

AUGMENTIN XR EXTENDED-RELEASE TABLETS

SERIOUS AND OCCASIONALLY FATAL HYPERSENSITIVITY (ANAPHYLACTIC) REACTIONS HAVE BEEN REPORTED IN PATIENTS ON PENICILLIN THERAPY. THESE REACTIONS ARE MORE LIKELY TO OCCUR IN INDIVIDUALS WITH A HISTORY OF PENICILLIN HYPERSENSITIVITY AND/OR A HISTORY OF SENSITIVITY TO MULTIPLE ALLERGENS. THERE HAVE BEEN REPORTS OF INDIVIDUALS WITH A HISTORY OF PENICILLIN HYPERSENSITIVITY WHO HAVE EXPERIENCED SEVERE REACTIONS WHEN TREATED WITH CEPHALOSPORINS. BEFORE INITIATING THERAPY WITH AUGMENTIN XR, CAREFUL INQUIRY SHOULD BE MADE CONCERNING PREVIOUS HYPERSENSITIVITY REACTIONS TO PENICILLINS, CEPHALOSPORINS OR OTHER ALLERGENS. IF AN ALLERGIC REACTION OCCURS, AUGMENTIN XR SHOULD BE DISCONTINUED AND THE APPROPRIATE THERAPY INSTITUTED. **SERIOUS ANAPHYLACTIC REACTIONS REQUIRE IMMEDIATE EMERGENCY TREATMENT WITH EPINEPHRINE. OXYGEN, INTRAVENOUS STEROIDS AND AIRWAY MANAGEMENT, INCLUDING INTUBATION, SHOULD ALSO BE ADMINISTERED AS INDICATED.**

Pseudomembranous colitis has been reported with nearly all antibacterial agents, including amoxicillin/clavulanate potassium, and has ranged in severity from mild to life-threatening. Therefore, it is important to consider this diagnosis in patients who present with diarrhea subsequent to the administration of antibacterial agents.

Treatment with antibacterial agents alters the normal flora of the colon and may permit overgrowth of clostridia. Studies indicate that a toxin produced by *Clostridium difficile* is one primary cause of "antibiotic associated colitis".

After the diagnosis of pseudomembranous colitis has been established, appropriate therapeutic measures should be initiated. Mild cases of pseudomembranous colitis usually respond to drug discontinuation alone. In moderate to severe cases, consideration should be given to management with fluids and electrolytes, protein supplementation and treatment with an antibacterial drug clinically effective against *Clostridium difficile* colitis.

Augmentin XR should be used with caution in patients with evidence of hepatic dysfunction. Hepatic toxicity associated with the use of amoxicillin/clavulanate potassium is usually reversible. On rare occasions, deaths have been reported (less than 1 death reported per estimated 4 million prescriptions worldwide). These have generally been cases associated with serious underlying diseases or concomitant medications. (See CONTRAINDICATIONS, Augmentin XR Extended-Release Tablets and ADVERSE REACTIONS, Augmentin XR Extended-Release Tablets, Liver.)

PRECAUTIONS

AUGMENTIN POWDER FOR ORAL SUSPENSION AND CHEWABLE TABLETS

General

While Augmentin possesses the characteristic low toxicity of the penicillin group of antibiotics, periodic assessment of organ system functions, including renal, hepatic and hematopoietic function, is advisable during prolonged therapy.

A high percentage of patients with mononucleosis who receive ampicillin develop an erythematous skin rash. Thus, ampicillin class antibiotics should not be administered to patients with mononucleosis.

The possibility of superinfections with mycotic or bacterial pathogens should be kept in mind during therapy. If superinfections occur (usually involving *Pseudomonas* or *Candida*), the drug should be discontinued and/or appropriate therapy instituted.

Information for the Patient

Augmentin may be taken every 8 hours or every 12 hours, depending on the strength of the product prescribed. Each dose should be taken with a meal or snack to reduce the possibility of gastrointestinal upset. Many antibiotics can cause diarrhea. If diarrhea is severe or lasts more than 2 or 3 days, call your doctor.

Make sure your child completes the entire prescribed course of treatment, even if he/she begins to feel better after a few days. Keep suspension refrigerated. Shake well before using. When dosing a child with Augmentin suspension (liquid), use a dosing spoon or medicine dropper. Be sure to rinse the spoon or dropper after each use. Bottles of Augmentin suspension may contain more liquid than required. Follow your doctor's instructions about the amount to use and the days of treatment your child requires. Discard any unused medicine.

Phenylketonurics

Each 200 mg Augmentin chewable tablet contains 2.1 mg phenylalanine; each 400 mg chewable tablet contains 4.2 mg phenylalanine; each 5 ml of either the 200 mg/5 ml or 400 mg/5 ml oral suspension contains 7 mg phenylalanine. The other Augmentin products do not contain phenylalanine and can be used by phenylketonurics. Contact your physician or pharmacist.

Drug/Laboratory Test Interactions

Oral administration of Augmentin will result in high urine concentrations of amoxicillin. High urine concentrations of ampicillin may result in false-positive reactions when testing for the presence of glucose in urine using Clinitest, Benedict's Solution or Fehling's Solution. Since this effect may also occur with amoxicillin and therefore Augmentin, it is recommended that glucose tests based on enzymatic glucose oxidase reactions (such as Clinistix or Tes-Tape) be used.

Following administration of ampicillin to pregnant women a transient decrease in plasma concentration of total conjugated estriol, estriol-glucuronide, conjugated estrone and estradiol has been noted. This effect may also occur with amoxicillin and therefore Augmentin.

Carcinogenesis, Mutagenesis, and Impairment of Fertility

Long-term studies in animals have not been performed to evaluate carcinogenic potential.

Mutagenesis

The mutagenic potential of Augmentin was investigated *in vitro* with an Ames test, a human lymphocyte cytogenetic assay, a yeast test and a mouse lymphoma forward mutation assay, and *in vivo* with mouse micronucleus tests and a dominant lethal test. All were negative apart from the *in vitro* mouse lymphoma assay where weak activity was found at very high, cytotoxic concentrations.

Impairment of Fertility

Augmentin at oral doses of up to 1200 mg/kg/day (5.7 times the maximum human dose, 1480 mg/m^2/day, based on body surface area) was found to have no effect on fertility and reproductive performance in rats, dosed with a 2:1 ratio formulation of amoxicillin:clavulanate.

Pregnancy, Teratogenic Effects, Pregnancy Category B

Reproduction studies performed in pregnant rats and mice given Augmentin at oral dosages up to 1200 mg/kg/day, equivalent to 7200 and 4080 mg/m^2/day, respectively (4.9 and 2.8 times the maximum human oral dose based on body surface area), revealed no evidence of harm to the fetus due to Augmentin. There are, however, no adequate and well-controlled studies in pregnant women. Because animal reproduction studies are not always predictive of human response, this drug should be used during pregnancy only if clearly needed.

Labor and Delivery

Oral ampicillin class antibiotics are generally poorly absorbed during labor. Studies in guinea pigs have shown that intravenous administration of ampicillin decreased the uterine tone, frequency of contractions, height of contractions and duration of contractions. However, it is not known whether the use of Augmentin in humans during labor or delivery has immediate or delayed adverse effects on the fetus, prolongs the duration of labor, or increases the likelihood that forceps delivery or other obstetrical intervention or resuscitation of the newborn will be necessary. In a single study in women with premature rupture of fetal membranes, it was reported that prophylactic treatment with Augmentin may be associated with an increased risk of necrotizing enterocolitis in neonates.

Nursing Mothers

Ampicillin class antibiotics are excreted in the milk; therefore, caution should be exercised when Augmentin is administered to a nursing woman.

Pediatric Use

Because of incompletely developed renal function in neonates and young infants, the elimination of amoxicillin may be delayed. Dosing of Augmentin should be modified in pediatric patients younger than 12 weeks (3 months). (See DOSAGE AND ADMINISTRATION, Augmentin Powder for Oral Suspension and Chewable Tablets, Dosage, Pediatric Patients.)

AUGMENTIN TABLETS

General

While Augmentin possesses the characteristic low toxicity of the penicillin group of antibiotics, periodic assessment of organ system functions, including renal, hepatic and hematopoietic function, is advisable during prolonged therapy.

A high percentage of patients with mononucleosis who receive ampicillin develop an erythematous skin rash. Thus, ampicillin class antibiotics should not be administered to patients with mononucleosis.

The possibility of superinfections with mycotic or bacterial pathogens should be kept in mind during therapy. If superinfections occur (usually involving *Pseudomonas* or *Candida*), the drug should be discontinued and/or appropriate therapy instituted.

Drug/Laboratory Test Interactions

Oral administration of Augmentin will result in high urine concentrations of amoxicillin. High urine concentrations of ampicillin may result in false-positive reactions when testing for the presence of glucose in urine using Clinitest, Benedict's Solution or Fehling's Solution. Since this effect may also occur with amoxicillin and therefore Augmentin, it is recommended that glucose tests based on enzymatic glucose oxidase reactions (such as Clinistix or Tes-Tape) be used.

Following administration of ampicillin to pregnant women a transient decrease in plasma concentration of total conjugated estriol, estriol-glucuronide, conjugated estrone and estradiol has been noted. This effect may also occur with amoxicillin and therefore Augmentin.

Carcinogenesis, Mutagenesis, and Impairment of Fertility

Long-term studies in animals have not been performed to evaluate carcinogenic potential.

Mutagenesis

The mutagenic potential of Augmentin was investigated *in vitro* with an Ames test, a human lymphocyte cytogenetic assay, a yeast test and a mouse lymphoma forward mutation assay, and *in vivo* with mouse micronucleus tests and a dominant lethal test. All were negative apart from the *in vitro* mouse lymphoma assay where weak activity was found at very high, cytotoxic concentrations.

Impairment of Fertility

Augmentin at oral doses of up to 1200 mg/kg/day (5.7 times the maximum human dose, 1480 mg/m^2/day, based on body surface area) was found to have no effect on fertility and reproductive performance in rats, dosed with a 2:1 ratio formulation of amoxicillin:clavulanate.

Pregnancy, Teratogenic Effects, Pregnancy Category B

Reproduction studies performed in pregnant rats and mice given Augmentin at oral dosages up to 1200 mg/kg/day, equivalent to 7200 and 4080 mg/m^2/day, respectively (4.9 and 2.8 times the maximum human oral dose based on body surface area), revealed no evidence of harm to the fetus due to Augmentin. There are, however, no adequate and well-controlled studies in pregnant women. Because animal reproduction studies are not always predictive of human response, this drug should be used during pregnancy only if clearly needed.

Labor and Delivery

Oral ampicillin class antibiotics are generally poorly absorbed during labor. Studies in guinea pigs have shown that intravenous administration of ampicillin decreased the uterine tone, frequency of contractions, height of contractions and duration of contractions. However, it is not known whether the use of Augmentin in humans during labor or delivery has immediate or delayed adverse effects on the fetus, prolongs the duration of labor, or increases the likelihood that forceps delivery or other obstetrical intervention or resuscitation of the newborn will be necessary. In a single study in women with premature rupture of fetal membranes, it was reported that prophylactic treatment with Augmentin may be associated with an increased risk of necrotizing enterocolitis in neonates.

Nursing Mothers

Ampicillin class antibiotics are excreted in the milk; therefore, caution should be exercised when Augmentin is administered to a nursing woman.

AUGMENTIN ES-600 POWDER FOR ORAL SUSPENSION

General

While amoxicillin/clavulanate possesses the characteristic low toxicity of the penicillin group of antibiotics, periodic assessment of organ system functions, including renal, hepatic and hematopoietic function, is advisable if therapy is for longer than the drug is approved for administration.

A high percentage of patients with mononucleosis who receive ampicillin develop an erythematous skin rash. Thus, ampicillin class antibiotics should not be administered to patients with mononucleosis.

The possibility of superinfections with mycotic or bacterial pathogens should be kept in mind during therapy. If superinfections occur (usually involving *Pseudomonas* or *Candida*), the drug should be discontinued and/or appropriate therapy instituted.

Information for the Patient

Augmentin ES-600 should be taken every 12 hours with a meal or snack to reduce the possibility of gastrointestinal upset. If diarrhea develops and is severe or lasts more than 2 or 3 days, call your doctor.

The entire prescribed course of treatment should be completed, even if your child begins to feel better after a few days. Keep suspension refrigerated. Shake well before using. When dosing a child with Augmentin ES-600 suspension (liquid), use a dosing spoon or medicine dropper. Be sure to rinse the spoon or dropper after each use. Bottles of Augmentin ES-600 suspension may contain more liquid than required. Follow your doctor's instructions about the amount to use and the days of treatment your child requires. Discard any unused medicine.

Phenylketonurics

Each 5 ml of the 600 mg/5 ml Augmentin ES-600 suspension contains 7 mg phenylalanine.

Drug/Laboratory Test Interactions

Oral administration of Augmentin will result in high urine concentrations of amoxicillin. High urine concentrations of ampicillin may result in false-positive reactions when testing for the presence of glucose in urine using Clinitest, Benedict's Solution or Fehling's Solution. Since this effect may also occur with amoxicillin and therefore Augmentin ES-600, it is recommended that glucose tests based on enzymatic glucose oxidase reactions (such as Clinistix or Tes-Tape) be used.

Following administration of ampicillin to pregnant women a transient decrease in plasma concentration of total conjugated estriol, estriol-glucuronide, conjugated estrone and estradiol has been noted. This effect may also occur with amoxicillin and therefore Augmentin ES-600.

Carcinogenesis, Mutagenesis, and Impairment of Fertility

Long-term studies in animals have not been performed to evaluate carcinogenic potential. The mutagenic potential of Augmentin was investigated *in vitro* with an Ames test, a human lymphocyte cytogenetic assay, a yeast test and a mouse lymphoma forward mutation assay, and *in vivo* with mouse micronucleus tests and a dominant lethal test. All were negative apart from the *in vitro* mouse lymphoma assay where weak activity was found at very high, cytotoxic concentrations. Augmentin at oral doses of up to 1200 mg/kg/day (5.7 times the maximum adult human dose based on body surface area) was found to have no effect on fertility and reproductive performance in rats, dosed with a 2:1 ratio formulation of amoxicillin:clavulanate.

Pregnancy, Teratogenic Effects, Pregnancy Category B

Reproduction studies performed in pregnant rats and mice given Augmentin at oral dosages up to 1200 mg/kg/day (4.9 and 2.8 times the maximum adult human oral dose based on body surface area, respectively), revealed no evidence of harm to the fetus due to Augmentin. There are, however, no adequate and well-controlled studies in pregnant women. Because animal reproduction studies are not always predictive of human response, this drug should be used during pregnancy only if clearly needed.

Labor and Delivery

Oral ampicillin class antibiotics are generally poorly absorbed during labor. Studies in guinea pigs have shown that intravenous administration of ampicillin decreased the uterine tone, frequency of contractions, height of contractions and duration of contractions. However, it is not known whether the use of Augmentin in humans during labor or delivery has immediate or delayed adverse effects on the fetus, prolongs the duration of labor, or increases the likelihood that forceps delivery or other obstetrical intervention or resuscitation of the newborn will be necessary. In a single study in women with premature rupture of fetal membranes, it was reported that prophylactic treatment with Augmentin may be associated with an increased risk of necrotizing enterocolitis in neonates.

Nursing Mothers

Ampicillin class antibiotics are excreted in human milk; therefore, caution should be exercised when Augmentin is administered to a nursing woman.

Pediatric Use

Safety and efficacy of Augmentin ES-600 in infants younger than 3 months of age have not been established. Safety and efficacy of Augmentin ES-600 have been demonstrated for treatment of acute otitis media in infants and children 3 months of age to 12 years of age.

AUGMENTIN XR EXTENDED-RELEASE TABLETS

General

While amoxicillin/clavulanate possesses the characteristic low toxicity of the penicillin group of antibiotics, periodic assessment of organ system functions, including renal, hepatic and hematopoietic function, is advisable if therapy is for longer than the drug is approved for administration.

A high percentage of patients with mononucleosis who receive ampicillin develop an erythematous skin rash. Thus, ampicillin class antibiotics should not be administered to patients with mononucleosis.

The possibility of superinfections with mycotic or bacterial pathogens should be kept in mind during therapy. If superinfections occur (usually involving *Pseudomonas* or *Candida*), the drug should be discontinued and/or appropriate therapy instituted.

Information for the Patient

Augmentin XR should be taken every 12 hours with a meal or snack to reduce the possibility of gastrointestinal upset. If diarrhea develops and is severe or lasts more than 2 or 3 days, call your doctor. The entire prescribed course of treatment should be completed, even if you begin to feel better after a few days. Discard any unused medicine.

Drug/Laboratory Test Interactions

Oral administration of Augmentin XR will result in high urine concentrations of amoxicillin. High urine concentrations of ampicillin may result in false-positive reactions when testing for the presence of glucose in urine using Clinitest, Benedict's Solution or Fehling's Solution. Since this effect may also occur with amoxicillin and therefore Augmentin XR, it is recommended that glucose tests based on enzymatic glucose oxidase reactions (such as Clinistix or Tes-Tape) be used.

Following administration of ampicillin to pregnant women a transient decrease in plasma concentration of total conjugated estriol, estriol-glucuronide, conjugated estrone and estradiol has been noted. This effect may also occur with amoxicillin and therefore Augmentin XR.

Carcinogenesis, Mutagenesis, and Impairment of Fertility

Long-term studies in animals have not been performed to evaluate carcinogenic potential. The mutagenic potential of Augmentin was investigated *in vitro* with an Ames test, a human lymphocyte cytogenetic assay, a yeast test and a mouse lymphoma forward mutation assay, and *in vivo* with mouse micronucleus tests and a dominant lethal test. All were negative apart from the *in vitro* mouse lymphoma assay where weak activity was found at very high, cytotoxic concentrations. Augmentin at oral doses of up to 1200 mg/kg/day (1.9 times the maximum human dose of amoxicillin and 15 times the maximum human dose of clavulanate based on body surface area) was found to have no effect on fertility and reproductive performance in rats dosed with a 2:1 ratio formulation of amoxicillin:clavulanate.

Pregnancy, Teratogenic Effects, Pregnancy Category B

Reproduction studies performed in pregnant rats and mice given Augmentin at oral doses up to 1200 mg/kg/day revealed no evidence of harm to the fetus due to Augmentin. In terms of body surface area, the doses in rats were 1.6 times the maximum human oral dose of amoxicillin and 13 times the maximum human dose for clavulanate. For mice, these doses were 0.9 and 7.4 times the maximum human oral dose of amoxicillin and clavulanate, respectively. There are, however, no adequate and well-controlled studies in pregnant women. Because animal reproduction studies are not always predictive of human response, this drug should be used during pregnancy only if clearly needed.

Labor and Delivery

Oral ampicillin class antibiotics are generally poorly absorbed during labor. Studies in guinea pigs have shown that intravenous administration of ampicillin decreased the uterine tone, frequency of contractions, height of contractions and duration of contractions. However, it is not known whether the use of Augmentin XR in humans during labor or delivery has immediate or delayed adverse effects on the fetus, prolongs the duration of labor, or increases the likelihood that forceps delivery or other obstetrical intervention or resuscitation of the newborn will be necessary.

Nursing Mothers

Ampicillin class antibiotics are excreted in the milk; therefore, caution should be exercised when Augmentin XR is administered to a nursing woman.

Pediatric Use

Safety and effectiveness in pediatric patients below the age of 16 years have not been established.

Geriatric Use

Of the total number of subjects in clinical studies of Augmentin XR, 19.2% were 65 and over and 7.9% were 75 and older. No overall differences in safety and effectiveness were observed between these subjects and younger subjects, and other clinical experience has not reported differences in responses between the elderly and younger patients, but a greater sensitivity of some older individuals cannot be ruled out.

This drug is known to be substantially excreted by the kidney, and the risk of dose-dependent toxic reactions to this drug may be greater in patients with impaired renal function. Because elderly patients are more likely to have decreased renal function, it may be useful to monitor renal function.

Each Augmentin XR tablet contains 29.3 mg (1.27 mEq) of sodium.

DRUG INTERACTIONS

AUGMENTIN POWDER FOR ORAL SUSPENSION AND CHEWABLE TABLETS

Probenecid decreases the renal tubular secretion of amoxicillin. Concurrent use with Augmentin may result in increased and prolonged blood levels of amoxicillin. Co-administration of probenecid cannot be recommended.

The concurrent administration of allopurinol and ampicillin increases substantially the incidence of rashes in patients receiving both drugs as compared to patients receiving ampicillin alone. It is not known whether this potentiation of ampicillin rashes is due to allopurinol or the hyperuricemia present in these patients. There are no data with Augmentin and allopurinol administered concurrently.

In common with other broad-spectrum antibiotics, Augmentin may reduce the efficacy of oral contraceptives.

AUGMENTIN TABLETS

Probenecid decreases the renal tubular secretion of amoxicillin. Concurrent use with Augmentin may result in increased and prolonged blood levels of amoxicillin. Co-administration of probenecid cannot be recommended.

The concurrent administration of allopurinol and ampicillin increases substantially the incidence of rashes in patients receiving both drugs as compared to patients receiving ampicillin alone. It is not known whether this potentiation of ampicillin rashes is due to allopurinol or the hyperuricemia present in these patients. There are no data with Augmentin and allopurinol administered concurrently.

In common with other broad-spectrum antibiotics, Augmentin may reduce the efficacy of oral contraceptives.

AUGMENTIN ES-600 POWDER FOR ORAL SUSPENSION

Probenecid decreases the renal tubular secretion of amoxicillin. Concurrent use with Augmentin ES-600 may result in increased and prolonged blood levels of amoxicillin. Co-administration of probenecid cannot be recommended.

The concurrent administration of allopurinol and ampicillin increases substantially the incidence of rashes in patients receiving both drugs as compared to patients receiving ampicillin alone. It is not known whether this potentiation of ampicillin rashes is due to allopurinol or the hyperuricemia present in these patients. There are no data with Augmentin ES-600 and allopurinol administered concurrently.

In common with other broad-spectrum antibiotics, amoxicillin/clavulanate may reduce the efficacy of oral contraceptives.

AUGMENTIN XR EXTENDED-RELEASE TABLETS

Probenecid decreases the renal tubular secretion of amoxicillin. Concurrent use with Augmentin XR may result in increased and prolonged blood levels of amoxicillin. Coadministration of probenecid cannot be recommended.

The concurrent administration of allopurinol and ampicillin increases substantially the incidence of rashes in patients receiving both drugs as compared to patients receiving ampicillin alone. It is not known whether this potentiation of ampicillin rashes is due to allopurinol or the hyperuricemia present in these patients. In Augmentin XR controlled clinical trials, 22 patients received concomitant allopurinol and Augmentin XR. No rashes were reported in these patients. However, this sample size is too small to allow for any conclusions to be drawn regarding the risk of rashes with concomitant Augmentin XR and allopurinol use.

In common with other broad-spectrum antibiotics, Augmentin XR may reduce the efficacy of oral contraceptives.

ADVERSE REACTIONS

AUGMENTIN POWDER FOR ORAL SUSPENSION AND CHEWABLE TABLETS

Augmentin is generally well tolerated. The majority of side effects observed in clinical trials were of a mild and transient nature and less than 3% of patients discontinued therapy because of drug-related side effects. From the original premarketing studies, where both pediatric and adult patients were enrolled, the most frequently reported adverse effects were diarrhea/loose stools (9%), nausea (3%), skin rashes and urticaria (3%), vomiting (1%) and vaginitis (1%). The overall incidence of side effects, and in particular diarrhea, increased with the higher recommended dose. Other less frequently reported reactions include: abdominal discomfort, flatulence and headache.

In pediatric patients (aged 2 months to 12 years), one US/Canadian clinical trial was conducted which compared Augmentin 45/6.4 mg/kg/day (divided q12h) for 10 days versus Augmentin 40/10 mg/kg/day (divided q8h) for 10 days in the treatment of acute otitis media. A total of 575 patients were enrolled, and only the suspension formulations were used in this trial. Overall, the adverse event profile seen was comparable to that noted above. However, there were differences in the rates of diarrhea, skin rashes/urticaria, and diaper area rashes.

The following adverse reactions have been reported for ampicillin class antibiotics:

Gastrointestinal: Diarrhea, nausea, vomiting, indigestion, gastritis, stomatitis, glossitis, black "hairy" tongue, mucocutaneous candidiasis, enterocolitis, and hemorrhagic/pseudomembranous colitis. Onset of pseudomembranous colitis symptoms may occur during or after antibiotic treatment. (See WARNINGS, Augmentin Powder for Oral Suspension and Chewable Tablets.)

Hypersensitivity Reactions: Skin rashes, pruritus, urticaria, angioedema, serum sickness-like reactions (urticaria or skin rash accompanied by arthritis, arthralgia, myalgia and frequently fever), erythema multiforme (rarely Stevens-Johnson syndrome), acute generalized exanthematous pustulosis and an occasional case of exfoliative dermatitis (including toxic epidermal necrolysis) have been reported. These reactions may be controlled with antihistamines and, if necessary, systemic corticosteroids. Whenever such reactions occur, the drug should be discontinued, unless the opinion of the physician dictates otherwise. Serious and occasional fatal hypersensitivity (anaphylactic) reactions can occur with oral penicillin. (See WARNINGS, Augmentin Powder for Oral Suspension and Chewable Tablets.)

Liver: A moderate rise in AST (SGOT) and/or ALT (SGPT) has been noted in patients treated with ampicillin class antibiotics but the significance of these findings is unknown. Hepatic dysfunction, including increases in serum transaminases (AST and/or ALT), serum bilirubin and/or alkaline phosphatase, has been infrequently reported with Augmentin. It has been reported more commonly in the elderly, in males, or in patients on prolonged treatment. The histologic findings on liver biopsy have consisted of predominantly cholestatic, hepatocellular, or mixed cholestatic-hepatocellular changes. The onset of signs/symptoms of hepatic dysfunction may occur during or several weeks after therapy has been discontinued. The hepatic dysfunction, which may be severe, is usually reversible. On rare occasions, deaths have been reported (less than 1 death reported per estimated 4 million prescriptions worldwide). These have generally been cases associated with serious underlying diseases or concomitant medications.

Renal: Interstitial nephritis and hematuria have been reported rarely.

Hemic and Lymphatic Systems: Anemia, including hemolytic anemia, thrombocytopenia, thrombocytopenic purpura, eosinophilia, leukopenia and agranulocytosis have been reported during therapy with penicillins. These reactions are usually reversible on discontinuation of therapy and are believed to be hypersensitivity phenomena. A slight thrombocytosis was noted in less than 1% of the patients treated with Augmentin. There have been reports of increased prothrombin time in patients receiving Augmentin and anticoagulant therapy concomitantly.

Central Nervous System: Agitation, anxiety, behavioral changes, confusion, convulsions, dizziness, insomnia, and reversible hyperactivity have been reported rarely.

Miscellaneous: Tooth discoloration has been reported very rarely in children. Good oral hygiene may help to prevent tooth discoloration as it can usually be removed by brushing.

AUGMENTIN TABLETS

Augmentin is generally well tolerated. The majority of side effects observed in clinical trials were of a mild and transient nature and less than 3% of patients discontinued therapy because of drug-related side effects. The most frequently reported adverse effects were diarrhea/loose stools (9%), nausea (3%), skin rashes and urticaria (3%), vomiting (1%) and vaginitis (1%). The overall incidence of side effects, and in particular diarrhea, increased with the higher recommended dose. Other less frequently reported reactions include: abdominal discomfort, flatulence and headache.

The following adverse reactions have been reported for ampicillin class antibiotics:

Gastrointestinal: Diarrhea, nausea, vomiting, indigestion, gastritis, stomatitis, glossitis, black "hairy" tongue, mucocutaneous candidiasis, enterocolitis, and hemorrhagic/pseudomembranous colitis. Onset of pseudomembranous colitis symptoms may occur during or after antibiotic treatment. (See WARNINGS, Augmentin Tablets.)

Hypersensitivity Reactions: Skin rashes, pruritus, urticaria, angioedema, serum sickness-like reactions (urticaria or skin rash accompanied by arthritis, arthralgia, myalgia and frequently fever), erythema multiforme (rarely Stevens-Johnson syndrome), acute generalized exanthematous pustulosis and an occasional case of exfoliative dermatitis (including toxic epidermal necrolysis) have been reported. These reactions may be controlled with antihistamines and, if necessary, systemic corticosteroids. Whenever such reactions occur, the drug should be discontinued, unless the opinion of the physician dictates otherwise. Serious and occasional fatal hypersensitivity (anaphylactic) reactions can occur with oral penicillin. (See WARNINGS, Augmentin Tablets.)

Liver: A moderate rise in AST (SGOT) and/or ALT (SGPT) has been noted in patients treated with ampicillin class antibiotics but the significance of these findings is unknown. Hepatic dysfunction, including increases in serum transaminases (AST and/or ALT), serum bilirubin and/or alkaline phosphatase, has been infrequently reported with Augmentin. It has been reported more commonly in the elderly, in males, or in patients on prolonged treatment. The histologic findings on liver biopsy have consisted of predominantly cholestatic, hepatocellular, or mixed cholestatic-hepatocellular changes. The onset of signs/symptoms of hepatic dysfunction may occur during or several weeks after therapy has been discontinued. The hepatic dysfunction, which may be severe, is usually reversible. On rare occasions, deaths have been reported (less than 1 death reported per estimated 4 million prescriptions worldwide). These have generally been cases associated with serious underlying diseases or concomitant medications.

Renal: Interstitial nephritis and hematuria have been reported rarely.

Hemic and Lymphatic Systems: Anemia, including hemolytic anemia, thrombocytopenia, thrombocytopenic purpura, eosinophilia, leukopenia and agranulocytosis have been reported during therapy with penicillins. These reactions are usually reversible on discontinuation of therapy and are believed to be hypersensitivity phenomena. A slight thrombocytosis was noted in less than 1% of the patients treated with Augmentin. There have been reports of increased prothrombin time in patients receiving Augmentin and anticoagulant therapy concomitantly.

Central Nervous System: Agitation, anxiety, behavioral changes, confusion, convulsions, dizziness, insomnia, and reversible hyperactivity have been reported rarely.

AUGMENTIN ES-600 POWDER FOR ORAL SUSPENSION

Augmentin ES-600 is generally well tolerated. The majority of side effects observed in pediatric clinical trials of acute otitis media were either mild or moderate, and transient in nature; 4.4% of patients discontinued therapy because of drug-related side effects. The most commonly reported side effects with probable or suspected relationship to Augmentin ES-600 were contact dermatitis, *i.e.,* diaper rash (3.5%), diarrhea (2.9%), vomiting (2.2%), moniliasis (1.4%), and rash (1.1%). The most common adverse experiences leading to withdrawal that were of probable or suspected relationship to Augmentin ES-600 were diarrhea (2.5%) and vomiting (1.4%).

The following adverse reactions have been reported for ampicillin class antibiotics:

Gastrointestinal: Diarrhea, nausea, vomiting, indigestion, gastritis, stomatitis, glossitis, black "hairy" tongue, mucocutaneous candidiasis, enterocolitis, and hemorrhagic/pseudomembranous colitis. Onset of pseudomembranous colitis symptoms may occur during or after antibiotic treatment. (See WARNINGS, Augmentin ES-600 Powder for Oral Suspension.)

Hypersensitivity Reactions: Skin rashes, pruritus, urticaria, angioedema, serum sickness-like reactions (urticaria or skin rash accompanied by arthritis, arthralgia, myalgia and frequently fever), erythema multiforme (rarely Stevens-Johnson syndrome), acute generalised exanthematous pustulosis and an occasional case of exfoliative dermatitis (including toxic epidermal necrolysis) have been reported. These reactions may be controlled with antihistamines and, if necessary, systemic corticosteroids. Whenever such reactions occur, the drug should be discontinued, unless the opinion of the physician dictates otherwise. Serious and occasional fatal hypersensitivity (anaphylactic) reactions can occur with oral penicillin. (See WARNINGS, Augmentin ES-600 Powder for Oral Suspension.)

Liver: A moderate rise in AST (SGOT) and/or ALT (SGPT) has been noted in patients treated with ampicillin class antibiotics but the significance of these findings is unknown. Hepatic dysfunction, including increases in serum transaminases (AST and/or ALT), serum bilirubin and/or alkaline phosphatase, has been infrequently reported with Augmentin. It has been reported more commonly in the elderly, in males, or in patients on prolonged treatment. The histologic findings on liver biopsy have consisted of predominantly cholestatic, hepatocellular, or mixed cholestatic-hepatocellular changes. The onset of signs/symptoms of hepatic dysfunction may occur during or several weeks after therapy has been discontinued. The hepatic dysfunction, which may be severe, is usually reversible. On rare occasions, deaths have been reported (less than 1 death reported per estimated 4 million prescriptions worldwide). These have generally been cases associated with serious underlying diseases or concomitant medications.

Renal: Interstitial nephritis and hematuria have been reported rarely.

Hemic and Lymphatic Systems: Anemia, including hemolytic anemia, thrombocytopenia, thrombocytopenic purpura, eosinophilia, leukopenia and agranulocytosis have been reported during therapy with penicillins. These reactions are usually reversible on discontinuation of therapy and are believed to be hypersensitivity phenomena. A slight thrombocytosis was noted in less than 1% of the patients treated with Augmentin. There have been reports of increased prothrombin time in patients receiving Augmentin and anticoagulant therapy concomitantly.

Central Nervous System: Agitation, anxiety, behavioral changes, confusion, convulsions, dizziness, insomnia, and reversible hyperactivity have been reported rarely.

Miscellaneous: Tooth discoloration has been reported very rarely in children. Good oral hygiene may help to prevent tooth discoloration as it can usually be removed by brushing.

AUGMENTIN XR EXTENDED-RELEASE TABLETS

In clinical trials, 4144 patients have been treated with Augmentin XR. The majority of side effects observed in clinical trials were of a mild and transient nature; 2% of patients discontinued therapy because of drug-related side effects. The most frequently reported adverse effects which were suspected or probably drug-related were diarrhea (15.6%), nausea (2.2%), genital moniliasis (2.1%) and abdominal pain (1.6%). Augmentin XR had a higher rate of diarrhea which required corrective therapy (4.0% vs 2.4% for Augmentin XR and all comparators, respectively).

The following adverse reactions have been reported for ampicillin class antibiotics:

Gastrointestinal: Diarrhea, nausea, vomiting, indigestion, gastritis, stomatitis, glossitis, black "hairy" tongue, mucocutaneous candidiasis, enterocolitis, and hemorrhagic/pseudomembranous colitis. Onset of pseudomembranous colitis symptoms may occur during or after antibiotic treatment. (See WARNINGS, Augmentin XR Extended-Release Tablets.)

Hypersensitivity Reactions: Skin rashes, pruritus, urticaria, angioedema, serum sickness-like reactions (urticaria or skin rash accompanied by arthritis, arthralgia, myalgia and frequently fever), erythema multiforme (rarely Stevens-Johnson Syndrome), acute generalized exanthematous pustulosis, and an occasional case of exfoliative dermatitis (including toxic epidermal necrolysis) have been reported. Whenever such reactions occur, the drug should be discontinued, unless the opinion of the physician dictates otherwise. Serious and occasional fatal hypersensitivity (anaphylactic) reactions can occur with oral penicillin. (See WARNINGS, Augmentin XR Extended-Release Tablets.)

Liver: A moderate rise in AST (SGOT) and/or ALT (SGPT) has been noted in patients treated with ampicillin class antibiotics but the significance of these findings is unknown. Hepatic dysfunction, including increases in serum transaminases (AST and/or ALT), serum bilirubin and/or alkaline phosphatase, has been infrequently reported with Augmentin or Augmentin XR. It has been reported more commonly in the elderly, in males, or in patients on prolonged treatment. The histologic findings on liver biopsy have consisted of predominantly cholestatic, hepatocellular, or mixed cholestatichepatocellular changes. The onset of signs/symptoms of hepatic dysfunction may occur during or several weeks after therapy has been discontinued. The hepatic dysfunction, which may be severe, is usually reversible. On rare occasions, deaths have been reported (less than 1 death reported per estimated 4 million prescriptions worldwide). These have generally been cases associated with serious underlying diseases or concomitant medications.

Renal: Interstitial nephritis and hematuria have been reported rarely.

Hemic and Lymphatic Systems: Anemia, including hemolytic anemia, thrombocytopenia, thrombocytopenic purpura, eosinophilia, leukopenia and agranulocytosis have been reported during therapy with penicillins. These reactions are usually reversible on discontinuation of therapy and are believed to be hypersensitivity phenomena. Mild to moderate thrombocytosis was noted in <1% of patients treated with Augmentin and 3.6% of patients treated with Augmentin XR. There have been reports of increased prothrombin time in patients receiving Augmentin and anticoagulant therapy concomitantly.

Central Nervous System: Agitation, anxiety, behavioral changes, confusion, convulsions, dizziness, headache, insomnia, and reversible hyperactivity have been reported rarely.

DOSAGE AND ADMINISTRATION

AUGMENTIN POWDER FOR ORAL SUSPENSION AND CHEWABLE TABLETS

Dosage

Pediatric Patients

Based on the amoxicillin component, Augmentin should be dosed as follows.

Neonates and Infants Aged <12 Weeks (3 Months)

Due to incompletely developed renal function affecting elimination of amoxicillin in this age group, the recommended dose of Augmentin is 30 mg/kg/day divided q12h, based on the amoxicillin component. Clavulanate elimination is unaltered in this age group. Experience with the 200 mg/5 ml formulation in this age group is limited and, thus, use of the 125 mg/5 ml oral suspension is recommended.

Patients Aged 12 Weeks (3 Months) and Older

Pediatric Patients Weighing 40 kg and More

Pediatric patients weighing 40 kg and more should be dosed according to the following adult recommendations: The usual adult dose is 1 Augmentin 500 mg tablet every 12 hours or 1 Augmentin 250 mg tablet every 8 hours. For more severe infections and infections of the respiratory tract, the dose should be 1 Augmentin 875 mg tablet every 12 hours or 1 Augmentin 500 mg tablet every 8 hours. Among adults treated with 875 mg every 12 hours, significantly fewer experienced severe diarrhea or withdrawals with diarrhea versus adults treated with 500 mg every 8 hours. For detailed adult dosage recommendations, please see complete prescribing information for Augmentin tablets.

Hepatically impaired patients should be dosed with caution and hepatic function monitored at regular intervals. (See WARNINGS, Augmentin Powder for Oral Suspension and Chewable Tablets.)

Adults

Adults who have difficulty swallowing may be given the 125 mg/5 ml or 250 mg/5 ml suspension in place of the 500 mg tablet. The 200 mg/5 ml suspension or the 400 mg/5 ml suspension may be used in place of the 875 mg tablet. See dosage recommendations in

TABLE 38

Infections	Dosing Regimen q12h* 200 or 400 mg/5 ml oral suspension†	Dosing Regimen q8h 125 or 250 mg/5 ml oral suspension†
Otitis media‡, sinusitis, lower respiratory tract infections, and more severe infections	45 mg/kg/day q12h	40 mg/kg/day q8h
Less severe infections	25 mg/kg/day q12h	20 mg/kg/day q8h

* The q12h regimen is recommended as it is associated with significantly less diarrhea. However, the q12h formulations (200 and 400 mg) contain aspartame and should not be used by phenylketonurics.

† Each strength of Augmentin suspension is available as a chewable tablet for use by older children.

‡ Duration of therapy studied and recommended for acute otitis media is 10 days.

Augmentin Powder for Oral Suspension and Chewable Tablets, Pediatric Patients Weighing 40 kg and More for children weighing 40 kg or more.

The Augmentin 250 mg tablet and the 250 mg chewable tablet do not contain the same amount of clavulanic acid (as the potassium salt). The Augmentin 250 mg tablet contains 125 mg of clavulanic acid, whereas the 250 mg chewable tablet contains 62.5 mg of clavulanic acid. Therefore, the Augmentin 250 mg tablet and the 250 mg chewable tablet should not be substituted for each other, as they are not interchangeable.

Due to the different amoxicillin to clavulanic acid ratios in the Augmentin 250 mg tablet (250/125) versus the Augmentin 250 mg chewable tablet (250/62.5), the Augmentin 250 mg tablet should not be used until the child weighs at least 40 kg and more.

Note: SHAKE ORAL SUSPENSION WELL BEFORE USING.

Reconstituted suspension must be stored under refrigeration and discarded after 10 days.

Administration

Augmentin may be taken without regard to meals; however, absorption of clavulanate potassium is enhanced when Augmentin is administered at the start of a meal. To minimize the potential for gastrointestinal intolerance, Augmentin should be taken at the start of a meal.

AUGMENTIN TABLETS

Since both the Augmentin 250 mg and 500 mg tablets contain the same amount of clavulanic acid (125 mg, as the potassium salt), 2 Augmentin 250 mg tablets are not equivalent to 1 Augmentin 500 mg tablet. Therefore, 2 Augmentin 250 mg tablets should not be substituted for 1 Augmentin 500 mg tablet.

Dosage

Adults

The usual adult dose is 1 Augmentin 500 mg tablet every 12 hours or 1 Augmentin 250 mg tablet every 8 hours. For more severe infections and infections of the respiratory tract, the dose should be 1 Augmentin 875 mg tablet every 12 hours or 1 Augmentin 500 mg tablet every 8 hours.

Patients with impaired renal function do not generally require a reduction in dose unless the impairment is severe. Severely impaired patients with a glomerular filtration rate of <30 ml/min should not receive the 875 mg tablet. Patients with a glomerular filtration rate of 10-30 ml/min should receive 500 mg or 250 mg every 12 hours, depending on the severity of the infection. Patients with a less than 10 ml/min glomerular filtration rate should receive 500 mg or 250 mg every 24 hours, depending on severity of the infection.

Hemodialysis patients should receive 500 mg or 250 mg every 24 hours, depending on severity of the infection. They should receive an additional dose both during and at the end of dialysis. Hepatically impaired patients should be dosed with caution and hepatic function monitored at regular intervals. (See WARNINGS, Augmentin Tablets.)

Pediatric Patients

Pediatric patients weighing 40 kg or more should be dosed according to the adult recommendations.

Due to the different amoxicillin to clavulanic acid ratios in the Augmentin 250 mg tablet (250/125) versus the Augmentin 250 mg chewable tablet (250/62.5), the Augmentin 250 mg tablet should not be used until the pediatric patient weighs at least 40 kg or more.

Administration

Augmentin may be taken without regard to meals; however, absorption of clavulanate potassium is enhanced when Augmentin is administered at the start of a meal. To minimize the potential for gastrointestinal intolerance, Augmentin should be taken at the start of a meal.

AUGMENTIN ES-600 POWDER FOR ORAL SUSPENSION

Augmentin ES-600, 600 mg/5 ml, does not contain the same amount of clavulanic acid (as the potassium salt) as any of the other Augmentin suspensions. Augmentin ES-600 contains 42.9 mg of clavulanic acid per 5 ml whereas Augmentin 200 mg/5 ml suspension contains 28.5 mg of clavulanic acid per 5 ml and the 400 mg/5 ml suspension contains 57 mg of clavulanic acid per 5 ml. Therefore, the Augmentin 200 mg/5 ml and 400 mg/5 ml suspensions should not be substituted for Augmentin ES-600, as they are not interchangeable.

Dosage

Pediatric Patients 3 Months and Older

Based on the amoxicillin component (600 mg/5 ml), the recommended dose of Augmentin ES-600 is 90 mg/kg/day divided every 12 hours, administered for 10 days (see TABLE 39).

TABLE 39

Body Weight	Volume of Augmentin ES-600 Providing 90 mg/kg/day
8 kg	3.0 ml twice daily
12 kg	4.5 ml twice daily
16 kg	6.0 ml twice daily
20 kg	7.5 ml twice daily
24 kg	9.0 ml twice daily
28 kg	10.5 ml twice daily
32 kg	12.0 ml twice daily
36 kg	13.5 ml twice daily

Pediatric Patients Weighing 40 kg and More

Experience with Augmentin ES-600 (600 mg/5 ml formulation) in this group is not available.

Adults

Experience with Augmentin ES-600 (600 mg/5 ml formulation) in adults is not available and adults who have difficulty swallowing should not be given Augmentin ES-600 (600 mg/5 ml) in place of the Augmentin 500 mg or 875 mg tablet.

Hepatically impaired patients should be dosed with caution and hepatic function monitored at regular intervals. (See WARNINGS, Augmentin ES-600 Powder for Oral Suspension.)

Note: SHAKE ORAL SUSPENSION WELL BEFORE USING.

Administration

To minimize the potential for gastrointestinal intolerance, Augmentin ES-600 should be taken at the start of a meal. Absorption of clavulanate potassium may be enhanced when Augmentin ES-600 is administered at the start of a meal.

AUGMENTIN XR EXTENDED-RELEASE TABLETS

Augmentin XR should be taken at the start of a meal to enhance the absorption of amoxicillin and to minimize the potential for gastrointestinal intolerance. Absorption of the amoxicillin component is decreased when Augmentin XR is taken on an empty stomach (see CLINICAL PHARMACOLOGY, Augmentin XR Extended-Release Tablets).

The recommended dose of Augmentin XR is 4000 mg/250 mg daily according to TABLE 40.

TABLE 40

Indication	Dose	Duration
Acute bacterial sinusitis	2 tablets q12h	10 days
Community acquired pneumonia	2 tablets q12h	7-10 days

Augmentin tablets (250 mg or 500 mg) CANNOT be used to provide the same dosages as Augmentin XR extended-release tablets. This is because Augmentin XR contains 62.5 mg of clavulanic acid, while the Augmentin 250 mg and 500 mg tablets each contain 125 mg of clavulanic acid. In addition, the extended-release tablet provides an extended time course of plasma amoxicillin concentrations compared to immediate release tablets. Thus, 2 Augmentin 500 mg tablets are not equivalent to 1 Augmentin XR tablet.

Renally Impaired Patients: The pharmacokinetics of Augmentin XR have not been studied in patients with renal impairment. Augmentin XR is contraindicated in severely impaired patients with a creatinine clearance of <30 ml/min and in hemodialysis patients (see CONTRAINDICATIONS, Augmentin XR Extended-Release Tablets).

Hepatically Impaired Patients: Hepatically impaired patients should be dosed with caution and hepatic function monitored at regular intervals (see WARNINGS, Augmentin XR Extended-Release Tablets).

Pediatric Use: Safety and effectiveness in pediatric patients below the age of 16 have not been established.

Geriatric Use: No dosage adjustment is required for the elderly (see PRECAUTIONS, Augmentin XR Extended-Release Tablets).

HOW SUPPLIED

AUGMENTIN POWDER FOR ORAL SUSPENSION AND CHEWABLE TABLETS

Augmentin for Oral Suspension

125 mg/5 ml: Each 5 ml of reconstituted banana-flavored suspension contains 125 mg amoxicillin and 31.25 mg clavulanic acid as the potassium salt.

200 mg/5 ml: Each 5 ml of reconstituted orange-raspberry-flavored suspension contains 200 mg amoxicillin and 28.5 mg clavulanic acid as the potassium salt.

250 mg/5 ml: Each 5 ml of reconstituted orange-flavored suspension contains 250 mg amoxicillin and 62.5 mg clavulanic acid as the potassium salt.

400 mg/5 ml: Each 5 ml of reconstituted orange-raspberry-flavored suspension contains 400 mg amoxicillin and 57 mg clavulanic acid as the potassium salt.

Augmentin Chewable Tablets

125 mg: Each mottled yellow, round, lemon-lime-flavored tablet, debossed with "BMP 189", contains 125 mg amoxicillin as the trihydrate and 31.25 mg clavulanic acid as the potassium salt.

200 mg: Each mottled pink, round, biconvex, cherry-banana-flavored tablet contains 200 mg amoxicillin as the trihydrate and 28.5 mg clavulanic acid as the potassium salt.

250 mg: Each mottled yellow, round, lemon-lime-flavored tablet, debossed with "BMP 190", contains 250 mg amoxicillin as the trihydrate and 62.5 mg clavulanic acid as the potassium salt.

400 mg: Each mottled pink, round, biconvex, cherry-banana-flavored tablet contains 400 mg amoxicillin as the trihydrate and 57.0 mg clavulanic acid as the potassium salt.

Storage: Store tablets and dry powder at or below 25°C (77°F). Dispense in original containers. Store reconstituted suspension under refrigeration. Discard unused suspension after 10 days.

AUGMENTIN TABLETS

250 mg: Each white oval filmcoated tablet, debossed with "AUGMENTIN" on 1 side and "250/125" on the other side, contains 250 mg amoxicillin as the trihydrate and 125 mg clavulanic acid as the potassium salt.

500 mg: Each white oval filmcoated tablet, debossed with "AUGMENTIN" on 1 side and "500/125" on the other side, contains 500 mg amoxicillin as the trihydrate and 125 mg clavulanic acid as the potassium salt.

875 mg: Each scored white capsule-shaped tablet, debossed with "AUGMENTIN 875" on 1 side and scored on the other side, contains 875 mg amoxicillin as the trihydrate and 125 mg clavulanic acid as the potassium salt.

Storage: Store tablets and dry powder at or below 25°C (77°F). Dispense in original container.

AUGMENTIN ES-600 POWDER FOR ORAL SUSPENSION

600 mg/5 ml: Each 5 ml of reconstituted orange-raspberry-flavored suspension contains 600 mg amoxicillin and 42.9 mg clavulanic acid as the potassium salt.

Storage: Store reconstituted suspension under refrigeration. Discard unused suspension after 10 days. Store dry powder for oral suspension at or below 25°C (77°F). Dispense in original container.

AUGMENTIN XR EXTENDED-RELEASE TABLETS

Each white, oval filmcoated bilayer tablet, debossed with "AC 1000/62.5", contains amoxicillin trihydrate and amoxicillin sodium equivalent to a total of 1000 mg of amoxicillin and clavulanate potassium equivalent to 62.5 mg of clavulanic acid.

Storage: Store tablets at or below 25°C (77°F). Dispense in original container.

PRODUCT LISTING - RATED THERAPEUTICALLY EQUIVALENT

Powder For Reconstitution - Oral - 200 mg;28.5 mg/5 ml			
100 ml	$36.17	GENERIC, Geneva Pharmaceuticals	00781-6102-46
Powder For Reconstitution - Oral - 400 mg;57 mg/5 ml			
100 ml	$68.93	GENERIC, Geneva Pharmaceuticals	00781-6104-46
Tablet - Oral - 500 mg;125 mg			
20's	$75.69	GENERIC, Teva Pharmaceuticals Usa	00093-2274-34
20's	$75.69	GENERIC, Geneva Pharmaceuticals	00781-1831-20
Tablet - Oral - 875 mg;125 mg			
20's	$101.03	GENERIC, Teva Pharmaceuticals Usa	00093-2275-34
20's	$101.03	GENERIC, Geneva Pharmaceuticals	00781-1852-20
Tablet, Chewable - Oral - 200 mg;28.5 mg			
20's	$36.17	GENERIC, Geneva Pharmaceuticals	00781-1619-66
Tablet, Chewable - Oral - 400 mg;57 mg			
20's	$68.93	GENERIC, Geneva Pharmaceuticals	00781-1643-66

PRODUCT LISTING - EQUIVALENTS NOT AVAILABLE

Powder For Reconstitution - Oral - 125 mg;31.25 mg/5 ml			
75 ml	$13.30	AUGMENTIN, Compumed Pharmaceuticals	00403-0363-18
75 ml	$14.00	AUGMENTIN, Southwood Pharmaceuticals Inc	58016-1009-03
75 ml	$15.40	AUGMENTIN, Allscripts Pharmaceutical Company	54569-1019-00
75 ml	$17.02	AUGMENTIN, Physicians Total Care	54868-0199-03
75 ml	$17.68	AUGMENTIN, Cheshire Drugs	55175-1221-07
75 ml	$21.20	AUGMENTIN, Glaxosmithkline	00029-6085-39
75 ml	$21.56	AUGMENTIN, Prescript Pharmaceuticals	00247-0035-75
75 ml	$35.52	AUGMENTIN, Cheshire Drugs	55175-1223-07
100 ml	$21.84	AUGMENTIN, Alpharma Uspd Makers Of Barre and Nmc	63874-0148-10
100 ml	$27.64	AUGMENTIN, Prescript Pharmaceuticals	00247-0035-00
100 ml	$28.24	AUGMENTIN, Glaxosmithkline	00029-6085-23
150 ml	$27.00	AUGMENTIN, Compumed Pharmaceuticals	00403-0361-18
150 ml	$32.00	AUGMENTIN, Allscripts Pharmaceutical Company	54569-0137-00
150 ml	$32.24	AUGMENTIN, Alpharma Uspd Makers Of Barre and Nmc	63874-0148-15
150 ml	$32.80	AUGMENTIN, Physicians Total Care	54868-0199-02
150 ml	$38.11	AUGMENTIN, Cheshire Drugs	55175-1221-05
150 ml	$39.78	AUGMENTIN, Prescript Pharmaceuticals	00247-0035-78
150 ml	$41.54	AUGMENTIN, Glaxosmithkline	00029-6085-22
Powder For Reconstitution - Oral - 200 mg;28.5 mg/5 ml			
50 ml	$18.45	GENERIC, Lek Pharmaceutical and Chemical Company	66685-1011-00
50 ml	$20.50	AUGMENTIN, Glaxosmithkline	00029-6087-29
75 ml	$24.63	GENERIC, Lek Pharmaceutical and Chemical Company	66685-1011-01
75 ml	$27.36	AUGMENTIN, Glaxosmithkline	00029-6087-39
100 ml	$30.95	AUGMENTIN, Allscripts Pharmaceutical Company	54569-4352-00
100 ml	$36.17	GENERIC, Lek Pharmaceutical and Chemical Company	66685-1011-02
100 ml	$40.19	AUGMENTIN, Glaxosmithkline	00029-6087-51
100 ml	$40.91	AUGMENTIN, Physicians Total Care	54868-4208-00
100 ml	$44.46	AUGMENTIN, Cheshire Drugs	55175-6020-01

A

Powder For Reconstitution - Oral - 250 mg;62.5 mg/5 ml

75 ml	$25.15	AUGMENTIN, Compumed Pharmaceuticals	00403-0367-18
75 ml	$29.35	AUGMENTIN, Allscripts Pharmaceutical Company	54569-0120-00
75 ml	$33.54	AUGMENTIN, Pharma Pac	52959-1012-01
75 ml	$40.40	AUGMENTIN, Glaxosmithkline	00029-6090-39
75 ml	$45.29	AUGMENTIN, Prescript Pharmaceuticals	00247-0025-75
100 ml	$34.50	AUGMENTIN, Compumed Pharmaceuticals	00403-5183-18
100 ml	$43.37	AUGMENTIN, Alpharma Uspd Makers Of Barre and Nmc	63874-0147-10
100 ml	$53.93	AUGMENTIN, Glaxosmithkline	00029-6090-23
100 ml	$59.27	AUGMENTIN, Prescript Pharmaceuticals	00247-0025-00
150 ml	$51.40	AUGMENTIN, Compumed Pharmaceuticals	00403-0365-18
150 ml	$61.00	AUGMENTIN, Allscripts Pharmaceutical Company	54569-0117-00
150 ml	$61.98	AUGMENTIN, Physicians Total Care	54868-0200-01
150 ml	$63.44	AUGMENTIN, Alpharma Uspd Makers Of Barre and Nmc	63874-0147-15
150 ml	$64.84	AUGMENTIN, Pharma Pac	52959-1012-00
150 ml	$79.22	AUGMENTIN, Glaxosmithkline	00029-6090-22
150 ml	$80.88	AUGMENTIN, Cheshire Drugs	55175-1223-05
150 ml	$87.24	AUGMENTIN, Prescript Pharmaceuticals	00247-0025-78

Powder For Reconstitution - Oral - 400 mg;57 mg/5 ml

50 ml	$34.70	AUGMENTIN, Allscripts Pharmaceutical Company	54569-4892-00
50 ml	$35.15	GENERIC, Lek Pharmaceutical and Chemical Company	66685-1012-00
50 ml	$39.05	AUGMENTIN, Glaxosmithkline	00029-6092-29
75 ml	$46.25	AUGMENTIN, Allscripts Pharmaceutical Company	54569-4889-00
75 ml	$46.82	GENERIC, Lek Pharmaceutical and Chemical Company	66685-1012-01
75 ml	$52.02	AUGMENTIN, Glaxosmithkline	00029-6092-39
100 ml	$56.15	AUGMENTIN, Pharma Pac	52959-1431-00
100 ml	$58.95	AUGMENTIN, Allscripts Pharmaceutical Company	54569-4353-00
100 ml	$68.93	GENERIC, Lek Pharmaceutical and Chemical Company	66685-1012-02
100 ml	$70.25	AUGMENTIN, Pharma Pac	52959-1430-00
100 ml	$76.59	AUGMENTIN, Glaxosmithkline	00029-6092-51
100 ml	$77.50	AUGMENTIN, Physicians Total Care	54868-4080-00

Powder For Reconstitution - Oral - 600 mg;42.9 mg/5 ml

50 ml	$39.05	AUGMENTIN ES-600, Glaxosmithkline	00029-6094-29
75 ml	$39.05	AUGMENTIN ES-600, Glaxosmithkline	00029-6094-39
100 ml	$52.03	AUGMENTIN ES-600, Glaxosmithkline	00029-6094-51
150 ml	$76.59	AUGMENTIN ES-600, Glaxosmithkline	00029-6094-22

Tablet - Oral - 250 mg;125 mg

2's	$9.41	AUGMENTIN, Prescript Pharmaceuticals	00247-0026-02
3's	$12.45	AUGMENTIN, Prescript Pharmaceuticals	00247-0026-03
4's	$8.51	AUGMENTIN, Allscripts Pharmaceutical Company	54569-1962-03
4's	$15.48	AUGMENTIN, Prescript Pharmaceuticals	00247-0026-04
4's	$18.12	AUGMENTIN, Quality Care Pharmaceuticals Inc	60346-0082-44
6's	$21.54	AUGMENTIN, Prescript Pharmaceuticals	00247-0026-06
8's	$27.60	AUGMENTIN, Prescript Pharmaceuticals	00247-0026-08
9's	$27.26	AUGMENTIN, Pharma Pac	52959-0343-09
10's	$21.80	AUGMENTIN, Southwood Pharmaceuticals Inc	59016-0134-10
12's	$21.00	AUGMENTIN, Southwood Pharmaceuticals Inc	59016-0134-12
14's	$28.72	AUGMENTIN, Southwood Pharmaceuticals Inc	59016-0134-14
15's	$30.75	AUGMENTIN, Southwood Pharmaceuticals Inc	59016-0134-15
15's	$31.92	AUGMENTIN, Allscripts Pharmaceutical Company	54569-1962-00
15's	$41.82	AUGMENTIN, Pd-Rx Pharmaceuticals	55289-0242-15
15's	$42.22	AUGMENTIN, Pharma Pac	52959-0343-15
15's	$48.81	AUGMENTIN, Prescript Pharmaceuticals	00247-0026-15
20's	$59.00	AUGMENTIN, Drx Pharmaceutical Consultants	55045-1478-07
20's	$63.98	AUGMENTIN, Prescript Pharmaceuticals	00247-0026-20
21's	$39.00	AUGMENTIN, Compumed Pharmaceuticals	00403-0369-21
21's	$44.69	AUGMENTIN, Allscripts Pharmaceutical Company	54569-1962-01
21's	$54.86	AUGMENTIN, Pharma Pac	52959-0343-21
21's	$58.98	AUGMENTIN, Pd-Rx Pharmaceuticals	55289-0242-21
21's	$65.02	AUGMENTIN, Alpharma Uspd Makers Of Barre and Nmc	63874-0103-21
21's	$67.00	AUGMENTIN, Prescript Pharmaceuticals	00247-0026-21
24's	$76.09	AUGMENTIN, Prescript Pharmaceuticals	00247-0026-24
30's	$56.00	AUGMENTIN, Compumed Pharmaceuticals	00403-0369-30
30's	$67.67	AUGMENTIN, Allscripts Pharmaceutical Company	54569-0142-01
30's	$70.49	AUGMENTIN, Pharma Pac	52959-0343-30
30's	$82.97	AUGMENTIN, Alpharma Uspd Makers Of Barre and Nmc	63874-0103-30
30's	$85.73	AUGMENTIN, Glaxosmithkline	00029-6075-27
30's	$85.73	AUGMENTIN, Southwood Pharmaceuticals Inc	58016-0106-30
30's	$91.00	AUGMENTIN, Drx Pharmaceutical Consultants	55045-1478-08
30's	$94.28	AUGMENTIN, Prescript Pharmaceuticals	00247-0026-30
42's	$89.38	AUGMENTIN, Allscripts Pharmaceutical Company	54569-1962-02
100's	$255.48	AUGMENTIN, Alpharma Uspd Makers Of Barre and Nmc	63874-0103-01
100's	$292.84	AUGMENTIN, Glaxosmithkline	00029-6075-31

Tablet - Oral - 500 mg;125 mg

1's	$7.81	AUGMENTIN, Prescript Pharmaceuticals	00247-0027-01
2's	$8.29	AUGMENTIN, Allscripts Pharmaceutical Company	54569-1959-08
2's	$12.27	AUGMENTIN, Prescript Pharmaceuticals	00247-0027-02
3's	$16.73	AUGMENTIN, Prescript Pharmaceuticals	00247-0027-03
3's	$19.64	AUGMENTIN, Quality Care Pharmaceuticals Inc	60346-0364-03
4's	$12.52	AUGMENTIN, Allscripts Pharmaceutical Company	54569-1959-03
4's	$21.20	AUGMENTIN, Prescript Pharmaceuticals	00247-0027-04
4's	$21.45	AUGMENTIN, Quality Care Pharmaceuticals Inc	60346-0364-44
4's	$28.03	AMOXICILLIN-CLAVULANATE, Pharma Pac	52959-0702-04
7's	$34.58	AUGMENTIN, Prescript Pharmaceuticals	00247-0027-07
9's	$28.18	AUGMENTIN, Allscripts Pharmaceutical Company	54569-1959-05
9's	$42.26	AUGMENTIN, Quality Care Pharmaceuticals Inc	60346-0364-09
9's	$43.49	AUGMENTIN, Prescript Pharmaceuticals	00247-0027-09
9's	$44.45	AMOXICILLIN-CLAVULANATE, Pharma Pac	52959-0702-09
10's	$46.17	AUGMENTIN, Physicians Total Care	54868-0388-00
10's	$47.95	AUGMENTIN, Prescript Pharmaceuticals	00247-0027-10
12's	$56.66	AMOXICILLIN-CLAVULANATE, Pharma Pac	52959-0702-12
14's	$53.63	AUGMENTIN, Allscripts Pharmaceutical Company	54569-1959-04
14's	$64.44	AMOXICILLIN-CLAVULANATE, Pharma Pac	52959-0702-14
14's	$65.80	AUGMENTIN, Prescript Pharmaceuticals	00247-0027-14
14's	$75.88	AUGMENTIN, Pharma Pac	52959-0021-14
15's	$46.97	AUGMENTIN, Allscripts Pharmaceutical Company	54569-1959-00
15's	$55.21	AUGMENTIN, Cheshire Drugs	55175-1220-05
15's	$60.92	AUGMENTIN, Quality Care Pharmaceuticals Inc	60346-0364-15
15's	$64.90	AUGMENTIN, Physicians Total Care	54868-0388-02
15's	$69.00	AMOXICILLIN-CLAVULANATE, Pharma Pac	52959-0702-15
15's	$70.26	AUGMENTIN, Prescript Pharmaceuticals	00247-0027-15
15's	$80.99	AUGMENTIN, Pd-Rx Pharmaceuticals	55289-0296-15
15's	$81.25	AUGMENTIN, Pharma Pac	52959-0021-15
20's	$66.38	AUGMENTIN, Allscripts Pharmaceutical Company	54569-0136-03
20's	$67.71	AUGMENTIN, Cheshire Drugs	55175-1220-02
20's	$69.68	AUGMENTIN, Alpharma Uspd Makers Of Barre and Nmc	63874-0115-20
20's	$75.69	GENERIC, Lek Pharmaceutical and Chemical Company	66685-1002-00
20's	$82.42	GENERIC, Southwood Pharmaceuticals Inc	58016-1002-20
20's	$84.10	AUGMENTIN, Glaxosmithkline	00029-6080-12
20's	$84.10	AUGMENTIN, Southwood Pharmaceuticals Inc	58016-0107-20
20's	$85.79	AMOXICILLIN-CLAVULANATE, Pharma Pac	52959-0702-20
20's	$86.13	AUGMENTIN, Physicians Total Care	54868-0388-01
20's	$92.56	AUGMENTIN, Prescript Pharmaceuticals	00247-0027-20
20's	$102.10	AUGMENTIN, Pharma Pac	52959-0021-20
21's	$69.70	AUGMENTIN, Allscripts Pharmaceutical Company	54569-1959-01
21's	$70.94	AUGMENTIN, Cheshire Drugs	55175-1220-01
21's	$72.80	AUGMENTIN, Alpharma Uspd Makers Of Barre and Nmc	63874-0115-21
21's	$83.31	AUGMENTIN, Quality Care Pharmaceuticals Inc	60346-0364-21
21's	$89.18	AMOXICILLIN-CLAVULANATE, Pharma Pac	52959-0702-21
21's	$97.02	AUGMENTIN, Prescript Pharmaceuticals	00247-0027-21
21's	$105.21	AUGMENTIN, Pharma Pac	52959-0021-21
28's	$90.54	AUGMENTIN, Physicians Total Care	54868-0388-05
30's	$86.45	AUGMENTIN, Glaxosmithkline	00029-6080-27
30's	$86.45	AUGMENTIN, Allscripts Pharmaceutical Company	54569-0136-01
30's	$96.45	AUGMENTIN, Cheshire Drugs	55175-1220-00
30's	$99.57	AUGMENTIN, Allscripts Pharmaceutical Company	54569-1959-06
30's	$107.12	AUGMENTIN, Alpharma Uspd Makers Of Barre and Nmc	63874-0115-30
30's	$126.23	AMOXICILLIN-CLAVULANATE, Pharma Pac	52959-0702-30
30's	$127.99	AUGMENTIN, Physicians Total Care	54868-0388-04
30's	$137.16	AUGMENTIN, Prescript Pharmaceuticals	00247-0027-30
30's	$146.52	AUGMENTIN, Pd-Rx Pharmaceuticals	55289-0296-30

30's	$149.10	AUGMENTIN, Pharma Pac	52959-0021-30
40's	$167.86	AMOXICILLIN-CLAVULANATE, Pharma Pac	52959-0702-40
100's	$332.32	AUGMENTIN, Alpharma Uspd Makers Of Barre and Nmc	63874-0115-01
100's	$430.91	AUGMENTIN, Glaxosmithkline	00029-6080-31
Tablet - Oral - 875 mg;125 mg			
2's	$10.23	AUGMENTIN, Allscripts Pharmaceutical Company	54569-4458-01
10's	$44.30	AUGMENTIN, Allscripts Pharmaceutical Company	54569-4458-00
10's	$53.20	AUGMENTIN, Cheshire Drugs	55175-1222-01
10's	$54.41	AUGMENTIN, Physicians Total Care	54868-3903-00
10's	$67.53	AUGMENTIN, Pd-Rx Pharmaceuticals	55289-0512-10
10's	$77.87	AUGMENTIN, Pharma Pac	52959-0478-10
14's	$71.59	AUGMENTIN, Allscripts Pharmaceutical Company	54569-4458-02
14's	$95.38	AUGMENTIN, Pharma Pac	52959-0478-14
15's	$104.43	AUGMENTIN, Pharma Pac	52959-0478-15
20's	$88.60	AUGMENTIN, Allscripts Pharmaceutical Company	54569-4325-00
20's	$97.75	AUGMENTIN, Cheshire Drugs	55175-1222-02
20's	$101.03	GENERIC, Lek Pharmaceutical and Chemical Company	66685-1001-00
20's	$107.63	AUGMENTIN, Physicians Total Care	54868-3903-01
20's	$110.01	GENERIC, Southwood Pharmaceuticals Inc	58016-1000-01
20's	$112.26	AUGMENTIN, Glaxosmithkline	00029-6086-12
20's	$112.26	AUGMENTIN, Southwood Pharmaceuticals Inc	58016-0512-20
20's	$117.97	AUGMENTIN, Pharma Pac	52959-0478-20
100's	$575.20	AUGMENTIN, Glaxosmithkline	00029-6086-21
Tablet, Chewable - Oral - 125 mg;31.25 mg			
15's	$16.16	AUGMENTIN, Alpharma Uspd Makers Of Barre and Nmc	63874-0116-15
15's	$21.12	AUGMENTIN, Pd-Rx Pharmaceuticals	55289-0240-15
20's	$18.27	AUGMENTIN, Allscripts Pharmaceutical Company	54569-0298-00
20's	$22.86	AUGMENTIN, Alpharma Uspd Makers Of Barre and Nmc	63874-0116-20
21's	$25.19	AUGMENTIN, Alpharma Uspd Makers Of Barre and Nmc	63874-0116-21
30's	$27.50	AUGMENTIN, Compumed Pharmaceuticals	00403-0357-30
30's	$30.20	AUGMENTIN, Allscripts Pharmaceutical Company	54569-0298-01
30's	$33.00	AUGMENTIN, Pharma Pac	52959-0470-30
30's	$37.93	AUGMENTIN, Cheshire Drugs	55175-1850-00
30's	$38.04	AUGMENTIN, Alpharma Uspd Makers Of Barre and Nmc	63874-0116-30
30's	$41.54	AUGMENTIN, Glaxosmithkline	00029-6073-47
Tablet, Chewable - Oral - 200 mg;28.5 mg			
20's	$30.95	AUGMENTIN, Allscripts Pharmaceutical Company	54569-4337-00
20's	$40.19	AUGMENTIN, Glaxosmithkline	00029-6071-12
Tablet, Chewable - Oral - 250 mg;62.5 mg			
2's	$3.84	AUGMENTIN, Allscripts Pharmaceutical Company	54569-0121-00
3's	$15.74	AUGMENTIN, Quality Care Pharmaceuticals Inc	60346-0074-03
9's	$29.87	AUGMENTIN, Quality Care Pharmaceuticals Inc	60346-0074-09
10's	$24.61	AUGMENTIN, Physicians Total Care	54868-0387-00
14's	$31.84	AUGMENTIN, Alpharma Uspd Makers Of Barre and Nmc	63874-0117-14
15's	$28.77	AUGMENTIN, Allscripts Pharmaceutical Company	54569-0121-03
15's	$34.08	AUGMENTIN, Alpharma Uspd Makers Of Barre and Nmc	63874-0117-15
15's	$40.53	AUGMENTIN, Cheshire Drugs	55175-1219-05
15's	$41.43	AUGMENTIN, Quality Care Pharmaceuticals Inc	60346-0074-15
20's	$37.60	AUGMENTIN, Southwood Pharmaceuticals Inc	58016-0134-20
20's	$42.18	AUGMENTIN, Alpharma Uspd Makers Of Barre and Nmc	63874-0117-20
20's	$62.32	AUGMENTIN, Physicians Total Care	54868-0387-02
21's	$50.39	AUGMENTIN, Physicians Total Care	54868-0387-03
21's	$53.12	AUGMENTIN, Quality Care Pharmaceuticals Inc	60346-0590-21
21's	$57.02	AUGMENTIN, Cheshire Drugs	55175-1219-01
21's	$57.47	AUGMENTIN, Quality Care Pharmaceuticals Inc	60346-0074-21
30's	$51.70	AUGMENTIN, Compumed Pharmaceuticals	00403-0359-18
30's	$52.51	AUGMENTIN, Prescript Pharmaceuticals	00247-0077-30
30's	$53.37	AUGMENTIN, Southwood Pharmaceuticals Inc	58016-0134-30
30's	$57.55	AUGMENTIN, Allscripts Pharmaceutical Company	54569-0121-01
30's	$70.36	AUGMENTIN, Cheshire Drugs	55175-1745-00
30's	$70.74	AUGMENTIN, Cheshire Drugs	55175-1219-00
30's	$71.66	AUGMENTIN, Pharma Pac	52959-0022-30
30's	$79.13	AUGMENTIN, Alpharma Uspd Makers Of Barre and Nmc	63874-0117-30
30's	$79.22	AUGMENTIN, Glaxosmithkline	00029-6074-47
30's	$92.27	AUGMENTIN, Physicians Total Care	54868-0387-01
Tablet, Chewable - Oral - 400 mg;57 mg			
20's	$58.95	AUGMENTIN, Allscripts Pharmaceutical Company	54569-4338-00
20's	$76.59	AUGMENTIN, Glaxosmithkline	00029-6072-12
Tablet, Extended Release - Oral - 1000 mg;62.5 mg			
28's	$78.59	AUGMENTIN XR, Glaxosmithkline	00029-6096-28
40's	$112.26	AUGMENTIN XR, Glaxosmithkline	00029-6096-40

Amphetamine; Dextroamphetamine *(003289)*

Categories: Attention deficit hyperactivity disorder; Narcolepsy; Obesity, exogenous; DEA Class CII; FDA Approved 1996 Feb; Pregnancy Category C
Drug Classes: Adrenergic agonists; Anorexiants; Amphetamines; Stimulants, central nervous system
Brand Names: Adderall
Cost of Therapy: $47.62 (Attention Deficit Disorder; Adderall; 5 mg; 1 tablet/day; 30 day supply)
$38.45 (Attention Deficit Disorder; Generic Capsules; 5 mg; 1 tablet/day; 30 day supply)
$78.24 (Attention Deficit Disorder; Adderall XR; 10 mg; 1 tablet/day; 30 day supply)

WARNING

Note: The trade names have been used throughout this monograph for clarity.

Adderall

AMPHETAMINES HAVE A HIGH POTENTIAL FOR ABUSE. ADMINISTRATION OF AMPHETAMINES FOR PROLONGED PERIODS OF TIME MAY LEAD TO DRUG DEPENDENCE AND MUST BE AVOIDED. PARTICULAR ATTENTION SHOULD BE PAID TO THE POSSIBILITY OF SUBJECTS OBTAINING AMPHETAMINES FOR NON-THERAPEUTIC USE OR DISTRIBUTION TO OTHERS, AND THE DRUGS SHOULD BE PRESCRIBED OR DISPENSED SPARINGLY.

Adderall XR

AMPHETAMINES HAVE A HIGH POTENTIAL FOR ABUSE. ADMINISTRATION OF AMPHETAMINES FOR PROLONGED PERIODS OF TIME MAY LEAD TO DRUG DEPENDENCE. PARTICULAR ATTENTION SHOULD BE PAID TO THE POSSIBILITY OF SUBJECTS OBTAINING AMPHETAMINES FOR NON-THERAPEUTIC USE OR DISTRIBUTION TO OTHERS AND THE DRUGS SHOULD BE PRESCRIBED OR DISPENSED SPARINGLY.

DESCRIPTION

ADDERALL

A single entity amphetamine product combining the neutral sulfate salts of dextroamphetamine and amphetamine, with the dextro isomer of amphetamine saccharate and d,l-amphetamine aspartate.

Active Ingredients:

5 mg: Each tablet contains 1.25 mg of dextroamphetamine saccharate, amphetamine aspartate, dextroamphetamine sulfate, and amphetamine sulfate for a total amphetamine base equivalence of 3.13 mg.

7.5 mg: Each tablet contains 1.875 mg of dextroamphetamine saccharate, amphetamine aspartate, dextroamphetamine sulfate, and amphetamine sulfate for a total amphetamine base equivalence of 4.7 mg.

10 mg: Each tablet contains 2.5 mg of dextroamphetamine saccharate, amphetamine aspartate, dextroamphetamine sulfate, and amphetamine sulfate for a total amphetamine base equivalence of 6.3 mg.

12.5 mg: Each tablet contains 3.125 mg of dextroamphetamine saccharate, amphetamine aspartate, dextroamphetamine sulfate, and amphetamine sulfate for a total amphetamine base equivalence of 7.8 mg.

15 mg: Each tablet contains 3.75 mg of dextroamphetamine saccharate, amphetamine aspartate, dextroamphetamine sulfate, and amphetamine sulfate for a total amphetamine base equivalence of 9.4 mg.

20 mg: Each tablet contains 5 mg of dextroamphetamine saccharate, amphetamine aspartate, dextroamphetamine sulfate, and amphetamine sulfate for a total amphetamine base equivalence of 12.6 mg.

30 mg: Each tablet contains 7.5 mg of dextroamphetamine saccharate, amphetamine aspartate, dextroamphetamine sulfate, and amphetamine sulfate for a total amphetamine base equivalence of 18.8 mg.

Inactive Ingredients: Sucrose, lactose, corn starch, acacia and magnesium stearate.

Colors:

Adderall 5, 7.5, and 10 mg contain FD&C blue no. 1.

Adderall 12.5, 15, 20, and 30 mg contain FD&C yellow no. 6 as a color additive.

ADDERALL XR

Adderall XR is a once daily extended-release, single-entity amphetamine product. Adderall XR combines the neutral sulfate salts of dextroamphetamine and amphetamine, with the dextro isomer of amphetamine saccharate and d,l-amphetamine aspartate monohydrate. The Adderall XR capsule contains two types of drug-containing beads designed to give a double-pulsed delivery of amphetamines, which prolongs the release of amphetamine from Adderall XR compared to the conventional Adderall (immediate-release) tablet formulation.

Active Ingredients:

10 mg: Each tablet contains 2.5 mg of dextroamphetamine saccharate, amphetamine aspartate monohydrate, dextroamphetamine sulfate, and amphetamine sulfate for a total amphetamine base equivalence of 6.3 mg.

20 mg: Each tablet contains 5.0 mg of dextroamphetamine saccharate, amphetamine aspartate monohydrate, dextroamphetamine sulfate, and amphetamine sulfate for a total amphetamine base equivalence of 12.5 mg.

30 mg: Each tablet contains 7.5 mg of dextroamphetamine saccharate, amphetamine aspartate monohydrate, dextroamphetamine sulfate, and amphetamine sulfate for a total amphetamine base equivalence of 18.8 mg.

Inactive Ingredients and Colors: The inactive ingredients in Adderall XR capsules include: gelatin capsules, hydroxypropyl methylcellulose, methacrylic acid copolymer, opadry beige, sugar spheres, talc, and triethyl citrate. Gelatin capsules contain edible inks, kosher gelatin, and titanium dioxide. The 10 mg capsules also contain FD&C blue no. 2. The 20 and 30 mg capsules also contain red iron oxide and yellow iron oxide.

CLINICAL PHARMACOLOGY

ADDERALL

Amphetamines are non-catecholamine sympathomimetic amines with CNS stimulant activity. Peripheral actions include elevation of systolic and diastolic blood pressures and weak bronchodilator and respiratory stimulant action.

There is neither specific evidence which clearly establishes the mechanism whereby amphetamine produces mental and behavioral effects in children, nor conclusive evidence regarding how these effects relate to the condition of the central nervous system.

ADDERALL XR

Pharmacodynamics

Amphetamines are non-catecholamine sympathomimetic amines with CNS stimulant activity. The mode of therapeutic action in Attention Deficit Hyperactivity Disorder (ADHD) is not known. Amphetamines are thought to block the reuptake of norepinephrine and dopamine into the presynaptic neuron and increase the release of these monoamines into the extraneuronal space.

Pharmacokinetics

Pharmacokinetic studies of Adderall XR have been conducted in healthy adult and pediatric (6-12 years) subjects, and pediatric patients with ADHD. Both Adderall (immediate-release) tablets and Adderall XR capsules contain d-amphetamine and l-amphetamine salts in the ratio of 3:1. Following administration of Adderall (immediate-release), the peak plasma concentrations occurred in about 3 hours for both d-amphetamine and l-amphetamine.

The time to reach maximum plasma concentration (T_{max}) for Adderall XR is about 7 hours, which is about 4 hours longer compared to Adderall (immediate-release). This is consistent with the extended-release nature of the product.

A single dose of Adderall XR 20 mg capsules provided comparable plasma concentration profiles of both d-amphetamine and l-amphetamine to Adderall (immediate-release) 10 mg bid administered 4 hours apart.

The mean elimination half-life is 1 hour shorter for d-amphetamine and 2 hours shorter for l-amphetamine in children aged 6-12 years compared to that in adults ($T_{1/2}$ is 10 hours for d-amphetamine and 13 hours for l-amphetamine in adults, and 9 hours and 11 hours, respectively, for children). Adderall XR demonstrates linear pharmacokinetics over the dose range of 10-30 mg. There is no unexpected accumulation at steady state.

Food does not affect the extent of absorption of Adderall XR capsules, but prolongs T_{max} by 2.5 hours (from 5.2 hours at fasted state to 7.7 hours after a high-fat meal). Opening the capsule and sprinkling the contents on applesauce results in comparable absorption to the intact capsule taken in the fasted state.

Special Populations

Pediatric Patients

Children eliminated amphetamine faster than adults. The elimination half-life ($T_{1/2}$) is approximately 1 hour shorter for d-amphetamine and 2 hours shorter for l-amphetamine in children than in adults. However, children had higher systemic exposure to amphetamine (C_{max} and AUC) than adults for a given dose of Adderall XR, which was attributed to the higher dose administered to children on a mg/kg body weight basis compared to adults. Upon dose normalization on a mg/kg basis, children showed 30% less systemic exposure compared to adults.

Gender

Systemic exposure to amphetamine was 20-30% higher in women (n=20) than in men (n=20) due to the higher dose administered to women on a mg/kg body weight basis. When the exposure parameters (C_{max} and AUC) were normalized by dose (mg/kg), these differences diminished.

Race

Formal pharmacokinetic studies for race have not been conducted. However, amphetamine pharmacokinetics appeared to be comparable among Caucasians (n=33), Blacks (n=8) and Hispanics (n=10).

INDICATIONS AND USAGE

ADDERALL

Attention Deficit Disorder With Hyperactivity: Adderall is indicated as an integral part of a total treatment program which typically includes other remedial measures (psychological, educational, social) for a stabilizing effect in children with behavioral syndrome characterized by the following group of developmentally inappropriate symptoms: moderate to severe distractibility, short attention span, hyperactivity, emotional lability, and impulsivity. The diagnosis of this syndrome should not be made with finality when these symptoms are only of comparatively recent origin. Nonlocalizing (soft) neurological signs, learning disability and abnormal EEG may or may not be present, and a diagnosis of central nervous system dysfunction may or may not be warranted.

In Narcolepsy.

ADDERALL XR

Adderall XR is indicated for the treatment of Attention Deficit Hyperactivity Disorder (ADHD).

The efficacy of Adderall XR in the treatment of ADHD was established on the basis of two controlled trials of children aged 6-12 who met DSM-IV criteria for ADHD (see CLINICAL PHARMACOLOGY, Adderall XR), along with extrapolation from the known efficacy of Adderall, the immediate-release formulation of this substance.

A diagnosis of Attention Deficit Hyperactivity Disorder (ADHD; DSM-IV) implies the presence of hyperactive-impulsive or inattentive symptoms that caused impairment and were present before age 7 years. The symptoms must cause clinically significant impairment, *e.g.,* in social, academic, or occupational functioning, and be present in two or more settings, *e.g.,* school (or work) and at home. The symptoms must not be better accounted for by another mental disorder. For the Inattentive Type, at least 6 of the following symptoms must have persisted for at least 6 months: lack of attention to details/careless mistakes; lack of sustained attention; poor listener; failure to follow through on tasks; poor organization; avoids tasks requiring sustained mental effort; loses things; easily distracted; forgetful. For the Hyperactive-Impulsive Type, at least 6 of the following symptoms must have persisted for at least 6 month: fidgeting/squirming; leaving seat; inappropriate running/climbing; difficulty with quiet activities; "on the go"; excessive talking; blurting answers; can't wait turn; intrusive. The Combined Type requires both inattentive and hyperactive-impulsive criteria to be met.

Special Diagnostic Considerations

Specific etiology of this syndrome is unknown, and there is no single diagnostic test. Adequate diagnosis requires the use not only of medical but of special psychological, educational, and social resources. Learning may or may not be impaired. The diagnosis must be based upon a complete history and evaluation of the child and not solely on the presence of the required number of DSM-IV characteristics.

Need for Comprehensive Treatment Program

Adderall XR is indicated as an integral part of a total treatment program for ADHD that may include other measures (psychological, educational, social) for patients with this syndrome. Drug treatment may not be indicated for all children with this syndrome. Stimulants are not intended for use in the child who exhibits symptoms secondary to environmental factors and/or other primary psychiatric disorders, including psychosis. Appropriate educational placement is essential and psychosocial intervention is often helpful. When remedial measures alone are insufficient, the decision to prescribe stimulant medication will depend upon the physician's assessment of the chronicity and severity of the child's symptoms.

Long-Term Use

The effectiveness of Adderall XR for long-term use, *i.e.,* for more than 3 weeks, has not been systematically evaluated in controlled trials. Therefore, the physician who elects to use Adderall XR for extended periods should periodically re-evaluate the long-term usefulness of the drug for the individual patient.

CONTRAINDICATIONS

ADDERALL

Advanced arteriosclerosis, symptomatic cardiovascular disease, moderate to severe hypertension, hyperthyroidism, known hypersensitivity or idiosyncrasy to the sympathomimetic amines, glaucoma.

Agitated states.

Patients with a history of drug abuse.

During or within 14 days following the administration of monoamine oxidase inhibitors (hypertensive crises may result).

ADDERALL XR

Advanced arteriosclerosis, symptomatic cardiovascular disease, moderate to severe hypertension, hyperthyroidism, known hypersensitivity or idiosyncrasy to the sympathomimetic amines, glaucoma.

Agitated states.

Patients with a history of drug abuse.

During or within 14 days following the administration of monoamine oxidase inhibitors (hypertensive crises may result).

WARNINGS

ADDERALL

Clinical experience suggests that in psychotic children, administration of amphetamine may exacerbate symptoms of behavior disturbance and thought disorder. Data are inadequate to determine whether chronic administration of amphetamine may be associated with growth inhibition; therefore, growth should be monitored during treatment.

Usage in Nursing Mothers

Amphetamines are excreted in human milk. Mothers taking amphetamines should be advised to refrain from nursing.

ADDERALL XR

Psychosis

Clinical experience suggests that, in psychotic patients, administration of amphetamine may exacerbate symptoms of behavior disturbance and thought disorder.

Long-Term Suppression of Growth

Data are inadequate to determine whether chronic use of stimulants in children, including amphetamine, may be causally associated with suppression of growth. Therefore, growth should be monitored during treatment, and patients who are not growing or gaining weight as expected should have their treatment interrupted.

PRECAUTIONS

ADDERALL

General

Caution is to be exercised in prescribing amphetamines for patients with even mild hypertension.

The least amount feasible should be prescribed or dispensed at one time in order to minimize the possibility of overdosage.

Information for the Patient

Amphetamines may impair the ability of the patient to engage in potentially hazardous activities such as operating machinery or vehicles; the patient should therefore be cautioned accordingly.

Drug/Laboratory Test Interactions

Amphetamines can cause a significant elevation in plasma corticosteroid levels. This increase is greatest in the evening.

Amphetamines may interfere with urinary steroid determinations.

Carcinogenesis/Mutagenesis

Mutagenicity studies and long-term studies in animals to determine the carcinogenic potential of amphetamine, have not been performed.

Pregnancy, Teratogenic Effects, Pregnancy Category C

Amphetamine has been shown to have embryotoxic and teratogenic effects when administered to A/Jax mice and C57BL mice in doses approximately 41 times the maximum human dose. Embryotoxic effects were not seen in New Zealand white rabbits given the drug in doses 7 times the human dose nor in rats given 12.5 times the maximum human dose.While there are no adequate and well-controlled studies in pregnant women, there has been one report of severe congenital bony deformity, tracheoesophageal fistula, and anal atresia (vater association) in a baby born to a woman who took dextroamphetamine sulfate with lovastatin during the first trimester of pregnancy. Amphetamines should be used during pregnancy only if the potential benefit justifies the potential risk to the fetus.

Nonteratogenic Effects

Infants born to mothers dependent on amphetamines have an increased risk of premature delivery and low birth weight. Also, these infants may experience symptoms of withdrawal as demonstrated by dysphoria, including agitation, and significant lassitude.

Pediatric Use

Long-term effects of amphetamines in children have not been well established. Amphetamines are not recommended for use in children under 3 years of age with Attention Deficit Disorder with Hyperactivity described under INDICATIONS AND USAGE, Adderall.

Amphetamines have been reported to exacerbate motor and phonic tics and Tourette's syndrome. Therefore, clinical evaluation for tics and Tourette's syndrome in children and their families should precede use of stimulant medications.

Drug treatment is not indicated in all cases of Attention Deficit Disorder with Hyperactivity and should be considered only in light of the complete history and evaluation of the child. The decision to prescribe amphetamines should depend on the physician's assessment of the chronicity and severity of the child's symptoms and their appropriateness for his/her age. Prescription should not depend solely on the presence of one or more of the behavioral characteristics. When these symptoms are associated with acute stress reactions, treatment with amphetamines is usually not indicated.

ADDERALL XR

General

The least amount of amphetamine feasible should be prescribed or dispensed at one time in order to minimize the possibility of overdosage.

Hypertension and Other Cardiovascular Conditions

Caution is to be exercised in prescribing amphetamines for patients with even mild hypertension (see CONTRAINDICATIONS, Adderall XR). Blood pressure and pulse should be monitored at appropriate intervals in patients taking Adderall XR, especially patients with hypertension.

Tics

Amphetamines have been reported to exacerbate motor and phonic tics and Tourette's syndrome. Therefore, clinical evaluation for tics and Tourette's syndrome in children and their families should precede use of stimulant medications.

Information for the Patient

Amphetamines may impair the ability of the patient to engage in potentially hazardous activities such as operating machinery or vehicles; the patient should therefore be cautioned accordingly.

Drug/Laboratory Test Interactions

Amphetamines can cause a significant elevation in plasma corticosteroid levels. This increase is greatest in the evening.

Amphetamines may interfere with urinary steroid determinations.

Carcinogenesis, Mutagenesis, and Impairment of Fertility

No evidence of carcinogenicity was found in studies in which d,l-amphetamine (enantiomer ratio of 1:1) was administered to mice and rats in the diet for 2 years at doses of up to 30 mg/kg/day in male mice, 19 mg/kg/day in female mice, and 5 mg/kg/day in male and female rats. These doses are approximately 2.4, 1.5, and 0.8 times, respectively, the maximum recommended human dose of 30 mg/day on a mg/m^2 body surface area basis.

Amphetamine, in the enantiomer ratio present in Adderall (immediate-release) (d- to l-ratio of 3:1), was not clastogenic in the mouse bone marrow micronucleus test *in vivo* and was negative when tested in the *E. coli* component of the Ames test *in vitro.* d,l-Amphetamine (1:1 enantiomer ratio) has been reported to produce a positive response in the mouse bone marrow micronucleus test, an equivocal response in the Ames test, and negative responses in the *in vitro* sister chromatid exchange and chromosomal aberration assays.

Amphetamine, in the enantiomer ratio present in Adderall (immediate-release) (d- to l-ratio of 3:1), did not adversely affect fertility or early embryonic development in the rat at doses of up to 20 mg/kg/day (approximately 5 times the maximum recommended human dose of 30 mg/day on a mg/m^2 body surface area basis).

Pregnancy Category C

Amphetamine, in the enantiomer ratio present in Adderall (d- to l- ratio of 3:1), had no apparent effects on embryofetal morphological development or survival when orally administered to pregnant rats and rabbits throughout the period of organogenesis at doses of up to 6 and 16 mg/kg/day, respectively. These doses are approximately 1.5 and 8 times, respectively, the maximum recommended human dose of 30 mg/day on a mg/m^2 body surface area basis. Fetal malformations and death have been reported in mice following parenteral administration of d-amphetamine doses of 50 mg/kg/day (approximately 6 times the maximum recommended human dose of 30 mg/day on a mg/m^2 basis) or greater to pregnant animals. Administration of these doses was also associated with severe maternal toxicity.

A number of studies in rodents indicate that prenatal or early postnatal exposure to amphetamine (d- or d,l-), at doses similar to those used clinically, can result in long-term neurochemical and behavioral alterations. Reported behavioral effects include learning and memory deficits, altered locomotor activity, and changes in sexual function.

There are no adequate and well-controlled studies in pregnant women. There has been one report of severe congenital bony deformity, tracheo-esophageal fistula, and anal atresia (vater association) in a baby born to a woman who took dextroamphetamine sulfate with lovastatin during the first trimester of pregnancy. Amphetamines should be used during pregnancy only if the potential benefit justifies the potential risk to the fetus.

Nonteratogenic Effects

Infants born to mothers dependent on amphetamines have an increased risk of premature delivery and low birth weight. Also, these infants may experience symptoms of withdrawal as demonstrated by dysphoria, including agitation, and significant lassitude.

Usage in Nursing Mothers

Amphetamines are excreted in human milk. Mothers taking amphetamines should be advised to refrain from nursing.

Pediatric Use

Adderall XR is indicated for use in children 6 years of age and older.

Use in Children Under 6 Years of Age

Effects of Adderall XR in 3- to 5-year-olds have not been studied. Long-term effects of amphetamines in children have not been well established. Amphetamines are not recommended for use in children under 3 years of age.

Geriatric Use

Adderall XR has not been studied in the geriatric population.

DRUG INTERACTIONS

ADDERALL

Acidifying Agents: Gastrointestinal acidifying agents (guanethidine, reserpine, glutamic acid HCl, ascorbic acid, fruit juices, etc.) lower absorption of amphetamines.

Urinary Acidifying Agents: (ammonium chloride, sodium acid phosphate, etc.) Increase the concentration of the ionized species of the amphetamine molecule, thereby increasing urinary excretion. Both groups of agents lower blood levels and efficacy of amphetamines.

Adrenergic Blockers: Adrenergic blockers are inhibited by amphetamines.

Alkalinizing Agents: Gastrointestinal alkalinizing agents (sodium bicarbonate, etc.) increase absorption of amphetamines. Urinary alkalinizing agents (acetazolamide, some thiazides) increase the concentration of the non-ionized species of the amphetamine molecule, thereby decreasing urinary excretion. Both groups of agents increase blood levels and therefore potentiate the actions of amphetamines.

Antidepressants, Tricyclic: Amphetamines may enhance the activity of tricyclic or sympathomimetic agents; d-amphetamine with desipramine or protriptyline and possibly other tricyclics cause striking and sustained increases in the concentration of d-amphetamine in the brain; cardiovascular effects can be potentiated.

MAO Inhibitors: MAOI antidepressants, as well as a metabolite of furazolidone, slow amphetamine metabolism. This slowing potentiates amphetamines, increasing their effect on the release of norepinephrine and other monoamines from adrenergic nerve endings; this can cause headaches and other signs of hypertensive crisis. A variety of neurological toxic effects and malignant hyperpyrexia can occur, sometimes with fatal results.

Antihistamines: Amphetamines may counteract the sedative effect of antihistamines.

Antihypertensives: Amphetamines may antagonize the hypotensive effects of antihypertensives.

Chlorpromazine: Chlorpromazine blocks dopamine and norepinephrine receptors, thus inhibiting the central stimulant effects of amphetamines, and can be used to treat amphetamine poisoning.

Ethosuximide: Amphetamines may delay intestinal absorption of ethosuximide.

Haloperidol: Haloperidol blocks dopamine receptors, thus inhibiting the central stimulant effects of amphetamines.

Lithium Carbonate: The anorectic and stimulatory effects of amphetamines may be inhibited by lithium carbonate.

Meperidine: Amphetamines potentiate the analgesic effect of meperidine.

Methenamine Therapy: Urinary excretion of amphetamines is increased, and efficacy is reduced, by acidifying agents used in methenamine therapy.

Norepinephrine: Amphetamines enhance the adrenergic effect of norepinephrine.

Phenobarbital: Amphetamines may delay intestinal absorption of phenobarbital; co-administration of phenobarbital may produce a synergistic anticonvulsant action.

Phenytoin: Amphetamines may delay intestinal absorption of phenytoin; co-administration of phenytoin may produce a synergistic anticonvulsant action.

Propoxyphene: In cases of propoxyphene overdosage, amphetamine CNS stimulation is potentiated and fatal convulsions can occur.

Veratrum Alkaloids: Amphetamines inhibit the hypotensive effect of veratrum alkaloids.

ADDERALL XR

Acidifying Agents: Gastrointestinal acidifying agents (guanethidine, reserpine, glutamic acid HCl, ascorbic acid, etc.) lower absorption of amphetamines.

Urinary Acidifying Agents: These agents (ammonium chloride, sodium acid phosphate, etc.) increase the concentration of the ionized species of the amphetamine molecule, thereby increasing urinary excretion. Both groups of agents lower blood levels and efficacy of amphetamines.

Adrenergic Blockers: Adrenergic blockers are inhibited by amphetamines.

Alkalinizing Agents: Gastrointestinal alkalinizing agents (sodium bicarbonate, etc.) increase absorption of amphetamines. Coadministration of Adderall XR and gastrointestinal alkalinizing agents, such as antacids, should be avoided. Urinary alkalinizing agents (acetazolamide, some thiazides) increase the concentration of the non-ionized species of the amphetamine molecule, thereby decreasing urinary excretion. Both groups of agents increase blood levels and therefore potentiate the actions of amphetamines.

Antidepressants, Tricyclic: Amphetamines may enhance the activity of tricyclic antidepressants or sympathomimetic agents; d-amphetamine with desipramine or protriptyline and possibly other tricyclics cause striking and sustained increases in the concentration of d-amphetamine in the brain; cardiovascular effects can be potentiated.

MAO Inhibitors: MAOI antidepressants, as well as a metabolite of furazolidone, slow amphetamine metabolism. This slowing potentiates amphetamines, increasing their effect on the release of norepinephrine and other monoamines from adrenergic nerve endings; this can cause headaches and other signs of hypertensive crisis. A variety of toxic neurological effects and malignant hyperpyrexia can occur, sometimes with fatal results.

Antihistamines: Amphetamines may counteract the sedative effect of antihistamines.

Antihypertensives: Amphetamines may antagonize the hypotensive effects of antihypertensives.

Chlorpromazine: Chlorpromazine blocks dopamine and norepinephrine receptors, thus inhibiting the central stimulant effects of amphetamines, and can be used to treat amphetamine poisoning.

Ethosuximide: Amphetamines may delay intestinal absorption of ethosuximide.

Haloperidol: Haloperidol blocks dopamine receptors, thus inhibiting the central stimulant effects of amphetamines.

Lithium Carbonate: The anorectic and stimulatory effects of amphetamines may be inhibited by lithium carbonate.

Meperidine: Amphetamines potentiate the analgesic effect of meperidine.

Methenamine Therapy: Urinary excretion of amphetamines is increased, and efficacy is reduced, by acidifying agents used in methenamine therapy.

Norepinephrine: Amphetamines enhance the adrenergic effect of norepinephrine.

Phenobarbital: Amphetamines may delay intestinal absorption of phenobarbital; coadministration of phenobarbital may produce a synergistic anticonvulsant action.

Phenytoin: Amphetamines may delay intestinal absorption of phenytoin; coadministration of phenytoin may produce a synergistic anticonvulsant action.

Propoxyphene: In cases of propoxyphene overdosage, amphetamine CNS stimulation is potentiated and fatal convulsions can occur.

Veratrum Alkaloids: Amphetamines inhibit the hypotensive effect of veratrum alkaloids.

ADVERSE REACTIONS

ADDERALL

Cardiovascular: Palpitations, tachycardia, elevation of blood pressure. There have been isolated reports of cardiomyopathy associated with chronic amphetamine use.

Central Nervous System: Psychotic episodes at recommended doses (rare), overstimulation, restlessness, dizziness, insomnia, euphoria, dyskinesia, dysphoria, tremor, headache, exacerbation of motor and phonic tics and Tourette's syndrome.

Gastrointestinal: Dryness of the mouth, unpleasant taste, diarrhea, constipation, other gastrointestinal disturbances. Anorexia and weight loss may occur as undesirable effects when amphetamines are used for other than the anorectic effect.

Allergic: Urticaria.

Endocrine: Impotence, changes in libido.

ADDERALL XR

The premarketing development program for Adderall XR included exposures in a total of 685 participants in clinical trials (615 patients, 70 healthy adults subjects). These participants received Adderall XR at daily doses up to 30 mg. The 615 patients (ages 6-12) were evaluated in two controlled clinical studies, one open-label clinical study, and one single-dose clinical pharmacology study (n=20). Safety data on all patients are included in the discussion that follows. Adverse reactions were assessed by collecting adverse events, results of physical examinations, vital signs, weights, laboratory analyses, and ECGs.

Adverse events during exposure were obtained primarily by general inquiry and recorded by clinical investigators using terminology of their own choosing. Consequently, it is not possible to provide a meaningful estimate of the proportion of individuals experiencing adverse events without first grouping similar types of events into a smaller number of standardized event categories. In the tables and listings that follow, COSTART terminology has been used to classify reported adverse events.

The stated frequencies of adverse events represent the proportion of individuals who experienced, at least once, a treatment-emergent adverse event of the type listed.

Adverse Events Associated With Discontinuation of Treatment

In two placebo-controlled studies of up to 5 weeks duration, 2.4% (10/425) of Adderall XR treated patients discontinued due to adverse events (including 3 patients with loss of appetite, 1 of whom also reported insomnia) compared to 2.7% (7/259) receiving placebo. The most frequent adverse events associated with discontinuation of Adderall XR in controlled and uncontrolled, multiple-dose clinical trials (n=595) are presented in TABLE 1. Over half of these patients were exposed to Adderall XR for 12 months or more.

TABLE 1

Adverse Event	Patients Discontinuing (n=595)
Anorexia (loss of appetite)	2.9%
Insomnia	1.5%
Weight loss	1.2%
Emotional lability	1.0%
Depression	0.7%

Adverse Events Occurring in a Controlled Trial

Adverse events reported in a 3 week clinical trial of pediatric patients treated with Adderall XR or placebo are presented in TABLE 2.

The prescriber should be aware that these figures cannot be used to predict the incidence of adverse events in the course of usual medical practice where patient characteristics and other factors differ from those which prevailed in the clinical trials. Similarly, the cited frequencies cannot be compared with figures obtained from other clinical investigations involving different treatments, uses, and investigators. The cited figures, however, do provide the prescribing physician with some basis for estimating the relative contribution of drug and non-drug factors to the adverse event incidence rate in the population studied.

TABLE 2 *Adverse Events Reported by More Than 1% of Patients Receiving Adderall XR With Higher Incidence Than on Placebo in a 584 Patient Clinical Study*

Body System Preferred Term	Adderall XR (n=374)	Placebo (n=210)
General		
Abdominal pain (stomachache)	14%	10%
Accidental injury	3%	2%
Asthenia (fatigue)	2%	0%
Fever	5%	2%
Infection	4%	2%
Viral infection	2%	0%
Digestive System		
Loss of appetite	22%	2%
Diarrhea	2%	1%
Dyspepsia	2%	1%
Nausea	5%	3%
Vomiting	7%	4%
Nervous System		
Dizziness	2%	0%
Emotional lability	9%	2%
Insomnia	17%	2%
Nervousness	6%	2%
Metabolic/Nutritional		
Weight loss	4%	0%

The following adverse reactions have been associated with amphetamine use:

Cardiovascular: Palpitations, tachycardia, elevation of blood pressure. There have been isolated reports of cardiomyopathy associated with chronic amphetamine use.

Central Nervous System: Psychotic episodes at recommended doses, overstimulation, restlessness, dizziness, insomnia, euphoria, dyskinesia, dysphoria, tremor, headache, exacerbation of motor and phonic tics and Tourette's syndrome.

Gastrointestinal: Dryness of the mouth, unpleasant taste, diarrhea, constipation, other gastrointestinal disturbances. Anorexia and weight loss may occur as undesirable effects.

Allergic: Urticaria.

Endocrine: Impotence, changes in libido.

DOSAGE AND ADMINISTRATION

ADDERALL

Regardless of indication, amphetamines should be administered at the lowest effective dosage and dosage should be individually adjusted. Late evening doses should be avoided because of the resulting insomnia.

Attention Deficit Disorder With Hyperactivity

Not recommended for children under 3 years of age. In children from 3-5 years of age, start with 2.5 mg daily; daily dosage may be raised in increments of 2.5 mg at weekly intervals until optimal response is obtained.

In children 6 years of age and older, start with 5 mg once or twice daily; daily dosage may be raised in increments of 5 mg at weekly intervals until optimal response is obtained. Only in rare cases will it be necessary to exceed a total of 40 mg per day. Give first dose on awakening; additional doses (1 or 2) at intervals of 4-6 hours.

Where possible, drug administration should be interrupted occasionally to determine if there is a recurrence of behavioral symptoms sufficient to require continued therapy.

Narcolepsy

Usual dose 5-60 mg per day in divided doses, depending on the individual patient response.

Narcolepsy seldom occurs in children under 12 years of age; however, when it does, dextroamphetamine sulfate may be used. The suggested initial dose for patients aged 6-12 is 5 mg daily; daily dose may be raised in increments of 5 mg at weekly intervals until optimal response is obtained. In patients 12 years of age and older, start with 10 mg daily; daily dosage may be raised in increments of 10 mg at weekly intervals until optimal response is obtained. If bothersome adverse reactions appear (*e.g.,* insomnia or anorexia), dosage should be reduced. Give first dose on awakening; additional doses (1 or 2) at intervals of 4-6 hours.

ADDERALL XR

In children with ADHD who are 6 years of age and older and are either starting treatment for the first time or switching from another medication, start with 10 mg once daily in the morning; daily dosage may be raised in increments of 10 mg at weekly intervals. Dosage should be individualized according to the needs and response of the patient. Amphetamines should be administered at the lowest effective dosage. The maximum recommended dose is 30 mg/day; doses greater than 30 mg/day of Adderall XR have not been studied.

Amphetamines are not recommended for children under 3 years of age. Adderall XR has not been studied in children under 6 years of age.

Patients Currently Using Adderall: Based on bioequivalence data, patients taking divided doses of immediate-release Adderall, for example twice a day, may be switched to Adderall XR at the same total daily dose taken once daily. Titrate at weekly intervals to appropriate efficacy and tolerability as indicated.

Adderall XR capsules may be taken whole, or the capsule may be opened and the entire contents sprinkled on applesauce. If the patient is using the sprinkle administration method, the sprinkled applesauce should be consumed immediately; it should not be stored. Patients should take the applesauce with sprinkled beads in its entirety without chewing. The dose of a single capsule should not be divided. The contents of the entire capsule should be taken, and patients should not take anything less than 1 capsule per day.

Adderall XR should be given upon awakening. Afternoon doses should be avoided because of the potential for insomnia.

Where possible, drug administration should be interrupted occasionally to determine if there is a recurrence of behavioral symptoms sufficient to require continued therapy.

ANIMAL PHARMACOLOGY

ADDERALL XR

Acute administration of high doses of amphetamine (d- or d,l-) has been shown to produce long-lasting neurotoxic effects, including irreversible nerve fiber damage, in rodents. The significance of these findings to humans is unknown.

HOW SUPPLIED

ADDERALL

Adderall tablets are available as follows:

- ***5 mg:*** Blue double-scored tablet, debossed "AD" on one side and "5" on the other side.
- ***7.5 mg:*** Blue double-scored tablet, debossed "AD" on one side and "7.5" on the other side.
- ***10 mg:*** Blue double-scored tablet, debossed "AD" on one side and "10" on the other side.
- ***12.5 mg:*** Orange double-scored tablet, debossed "AD" on one side and "12.5" on the other side.
- ***15 mg:*** Orange double-scored tablet, debossed "AD" on one side and "15" on the other side.
- ***20 mg:*** Orange double-scored tablet, debossed "AD" on one side and "20" on the other side.
- ***30 mg:*** Orange double-scored tablet, debossed "AD" on one side and "30" on the other side.

Dispense in a tight, light-resistant container.

Storage: Store at controlled room temperature 15-30°C (59-86°F).

ADDERALL XR

Adderall XR capsules are available as follows:

- ***10 mg:*** Blue/blue (imprinted "SHIRE 381 10 mg").
- ***20 mg:*** Orange/orange (imprinted "SHIRE 381 20 mg").
- ***30 mg:*** Natural/orange (imprinted "SHIRE 381 30 mg").

Dispense in a tight, light-resistant container.

Storage: Store at 25°C (77°F). Excursions permitted to 15-30°C (59-86°F).

PRODUCT LISTING - RATED THERAPEUTICALLY EQUIVALENT

Tablet - Oral - 5 mg

100's	$137.16	GENERIC, Barr Laboratories Inc	00555-0971-02
100's	$158.74	ADDERALL, Shire Richwood Pharmaceutical Company Inc	58521-0031-01

Tablet - Oral - 7.5 mg

100's	$142.85	GENERIC, Barr Laboratories Inc	00555-0775-02

Tablet - Oral - 10 mg

100's	$137.16	GENERIC, Eon Labs Manufacturing Inc	00185-0111-01
100's	$137.16	GENERIC, Barr Laboratories Inc	00555-0972-02
100's	$158.74	ADDERALL, Shire Richwood Pharmaceutical Company Inc	58521-0032-01

Tablet - Oral - 12.5 mg

100's	$142.85	GENERIC, Barr Laboratories Inc	00555-0776-02

Tablet - Oral - 15 mg

100's	$142.85	GENERIC, Barr Laboratories Inc	00555-0777-02

Tablet - Oral - 20 mg

100's	$137.16	GENERIC, Eon Labs Manufacturing Inc	00185-0401-01
100's	$137.16	GENERIC, Barr Laboratories Inc	00555-0973-02
100's	$158.74	ADDERALL, Shire Richwood Pharmaceutical Company Inc	58521-0033-01

Tablet - Oral - 30 mg

100's	$137.16	GENERIC, Eon Labs Manufacturing Inc	00185-0404-01
100's	$137.16	GENERIC, Barr Laboratories Inc	00555-0974-02
100's	$158.74	ADDERALL, Shire Richwood Pharmaceutical Company Inc	58521-0034-01

PRODUCT LISTING - EQUIVALENTS NOT AVAILABLE

Capsule, Extended Release - Oral - 5 mg

100's	$260.81	ADDERALL XR, Shire Richwood Pharmaceutical Company Inc	54092-0381-01

Capsule, Extended Release - Oral - 10 mg

100's	$260.81	ADDERALL XR, Shire Richwood Pharmaceutical Company Inc	54092-0383-01

Capsule, Extended Release - Oral - 15 mg

100's	$260.81	ADDERALL XR, Shire Richwood Pharmaceutical Company Inc	54092-0385-01

Capsule, Extended Release - Oral - 20 mg

100's	$260.81	ADDERALL XR, Shire Richwood Pharmaceutical Company Inc	54092-0387-01

Capsule, Extended Release - Oral - 25 mg

100's	$260.81	ADDERALL XR, Shire Richwood Pharmaceutical Company Inc	54092-0389-01

Capsule, Extended Release - Oral - 30 mg

100's	$260.81	ADDERALL XR, Shire Richwood Pharmaceutical Company Inc	54092-0391-01

Tablet - Oral - 5 mg

100's	$137.16	GENERIC, Eon Labs Manufacturing Inc	00185-0084-01
100's	$142.87	GENERIC, Ranbaxy Laboratories	63304-0908-01

Tablet - Oral - 7.5 mg

100's	$158.74	ADDERALL, Shire Richwood Pharmaceutical Company Inc	58521-0075-01

Tablet - Oral - 10 mg

100's	$142.87	GENERIC, Ranbaxy Laboratories	63304-0909-01

Tablet - Oral - 12.5 mg

100's	$158.74	ADDERALL, Shire Richwood Pharmaceutical Company Inc	58521-0125-01

Tablet - Oral - 15 mg

100's	$158.74	ADDERALL, Shire Richwood Pharmaceutical Company Inc	58521-0150-01

Tablet - Oral - 20 mg

100's	$142.87	GENERIC, Ranbaxy Laboratories	63304-0910-01

Tablet - Oral - 30 mg

100's	$142.87	GENERIC, Ranbaxy Laboratories	63304-0911-01

Amphotericin B *(000235)*

For related information, see the comparative table section in Appendix A.

Categories: Aspergillosis; Blastomycosis; Candidiasis; Coccidioidomycosis; Cryptococcosis; Histoplasmosis; Infection, fungal; Leishmaniasis; Mucormycosis; Sporotrichosis; Zygomycosis; Pregnancy Category B; FDA Approved 1964 Nov; Orphan Drugs; WHO Formulary

Drug Classes: Antifungals

Brand Names: Abelcet; Ambisome; Amphocin; Amphotec; Fungilin; **Fungizone IV**; **Fungizone Topical**

Foreign Brand Availability: Ampho-Moronal (Germany); Fungizone (Canada; France)

HCFA JCODE(S): J0285 50 mg IV

INTRAVENOUS

WARNING

This drug should be used *primarily* for treatment of patients with progressive and potentially life-threatening fungal infections; it should not be used to treat noninvasive forms of fungal disease such as oral thrush, vaginal candidiasis and esophageal candidiasis, in patients with normal neutrophil counts.

EXERCISE CAUTION to prevent inadvertent overdose with amphotericin B injection. Verify the product name and dosage if dose exceeds 1.5 mg/kg.

DESCRIPTION

Amphotericin B is an antifungal polyene antibiotic obtained from a strain of *Streptomyces nodosus.* Amphotericin B is designated chemically as [1R-(1R*,3S*,5R*,6R*,9R*,11R*,15S*,16R*,17R*,18S*,19E,21E,23E,25E,27E,29E,31E,33R*,35S*,36R*,37S*)]-33-[(3-Amino-3,6-dideoxy-β-D-mannopyranosyl)-oxy]-1,3,5,6,9,11,17,37-octahydroxy-15,16,18-trimethyl-13-oxo-14,39-dioxabicyclo[33.3.1]nonatriaconta-19,21,23,25,27,29,31-heptaene-36-carboxylic acid. The empirical formula is $C_{47}H_{73}NO_{17}$. The molecular weight is 924.10.

Each vial of Fungizone contains a sterile, nonpyrogenic, lyophilized cake (which may partially reduce to powder following manufacture) providing 50 mg amphotericin B and 41 mg sodium desoxycholate with 20.2 mg sodium phosphates as a buffer.

Crystalline amphotericin B is insoluble in water; therefore, the antibiotic is solubilized by the addition of sodium desoxycholate to form a mixture which provides a colloidal dispersion for intravenous infusion following reconstitution.

At the time of manufacture the air in the vial is replaced by nitrogen.

CLINICAL PHARMACOLOGY

Microbiology: Amphotericin B shows a high order of *in vitro* activity against many species of fungi. *Histoplasma capsulatum, Coccidioides immitis, Candida* species, *Blastomyces dermatitidis, Rhodotorula, Cryptococcus neoformans, Sporothrix schenckii, Mucor mucedo,* and *Aspergillus fumigatus* are all inhibited by concentrations of amphotericin B ranging from 0.03–1.0 µg/ml *in vitro*. While *Candida albicans* is generally quite susceptible to amphotericin B, non-*albicans* species may be less susceptible. *Pseudallescheria boydii* and *Fusarium* sp. are often resistant to amphotericin B. The antibiotic is without effect on bacteria, rickettsiae, and viruses.

Susceptibility Testing: Standardized techniques for susceptibility testing for antifungal agents have not been established and results of susceptibility studies have not been correlated with clinical outcomes.

Pharmacokinetics: Amphotericin B is fungistatic or fungicidal depending on the concentration obtained in body fluids and the susceptibility of the fungus. The drug acts by binding to sterols in the cell membrane of susceptible fungi with a resultant change in membrane permeability allowing leakage of intercellular components. Mammalian cell membranes also contain sterols and it has been suggested that the damage to human cells and fungal cells may share common mechanisms.

An initial intravenous infusion of 1–5 mg of amphotericin B per day, gradually increased to 0.4 and 0.6 mg/kg daily, produces peak plasma concentrations ranging from approximately 0.5 to 2 µg/ml. Following a rapid initial fall, plasma concentrations plateau at about 0.5 µg/ml. An elimination half-life of approximately 15 days follows an initial plasma half-life of about 24 hours. Amphotericin B circulating in plasma is highly (>90%) to plasma proteins and is poorly dialyzable. Approximately two thirds of concurrent plasma concentrations have been detected in fluids from inflamed pleura, peritoneum, synovium, and aqueous humor. Concentrations in the cerebrospinal fluid seldom exceed 2.5% of those in the plasma. Little amphotericin B penetrates into vitreous humor or normal amniotic fluid. Complete details of tissue distribution are not known.

Amphotericin B is excreted very slowly (over weeks to months) by the kidneys with 2–5% of a given dose being excreted in the biologically active form. Details of possible metabolic pathways are not known. After treatment is discontinued, the drug can be detected in the urine for at least 7 weeks due to the slow disappearance of the drug. The cumulative urinary output over a 7-day period amounts to approximately 40% of the amount of drug infused.

INDICATIONS AND USAGE

Amphotericin B for injection should be administered primarily to patients with progressive, potentially-life-threatening fungal infections. This potent drug should not be used to threat noninvasive fungal infections, such as oral thrush, vaginal candidiasis, and esophageal candidiasis in patients with normal neutrophil counts.

Amphotericin B for injection is specifically intended to treat potentially life-threatening fungal infection: aspergillosis, cryptococcosis (torulosis). North American blastomycosis, systemic candidiasis, coccidioidomycosis, histoplasmosis, zygomycosis including mucormycosis due to susceptible species of the genera *Absidia, Mucor,* and *Rhizopus,* and infections due to related susceptible species of *Conidiobolus, Basidiobolus,* and sporotrichosis.

Amphotericin B may be useful in the treatment of American mucocutaneous leishmaniasis, but it is not the drug of choice as primary therapy.

CONTRAINDICATIONS

This product is contraindicated in those patients who have shown hypersensitivity to amphotericin B or any other component in the formulation unless, in the opinion of the physician, the condition requiring treatment is life-threatening and amenable only to amphotericin B therapy.

WARNINGS

Amphotericin B is frequently the only effective treatment available for potentially life-threatening fungal disease. In each case, its possible life-saving benefit must be balanced against its untoward and dangerous side effects.

PRECAUTIONS

GENERAL

Amphotericin B should be administered intravenously under close clinical observation by medically trained personnel. It should be reserved for treatment of patients with progressive, potentially life-threatening fungal infections due to susceptible organisms (see INDICATIONS AND USAGE).

Acute reactions including fever, shaking chills, hypotension, anorexia, nausea, vomiting, headache, and tachypnea are common 1–3 hours after starting an intravenous infusion. These reactions are usually more severe with the first few doses of amphotericin B and usually diminish with subsequent doses.

Rapid intravenous infusion has been associated with hypotension, hypokalemia, arrhythmias, and shock and should, therefore, be avoided (see DOSAGE AND ADMINISTRATION).

Amphotericin B should be used with care in patients with reduced renal function; frequent monitoring of renal function is recommended (see Laboratory Tests) and ADVERSE REACTIONS). In some patients hydration and sodium repletion prior to amphotericin B administration may reduce the risk of developing nephrotoxicity. Supplemental alkali medication may decrease renal tubular acidosis complications.

Since acute pulmonary reactions have been reported in patients given amphotericin B during or shortly after leukocyte transfusion, it is advisable to temporally separate these infusions as far as possible and to monitor pulmonary function (see DRUG INTERACTIONS).

Leukoencephalopathy has been reported following use of amphotericin B. Literature reports have suggested that total body irradiation may be a predisposition.

Whenever medication is interrupted for a period longer than 7 days, therapy should be resumed by starting with the lowest dosage level (*e.g.,* 0.25 mg/kg of body weight), and increased gradually as outlined in DOSAGE AND ADMINISTRATION.

LABORATORY TESTS

Renal function should be monitored frequently during amphotericin B therapy (see ADVERSE REACTIONS). It is also advisable to monitor on a regular basis liver function, serum electrolytes (particularly magnesium and potassium), blood counts, and hemoglobin concentrations. Laboratory test results should be used as a guide to subsequent dosage adjustments.

CARCINOGENESIS, MUTAGENESIS, AND IMPAIRMENT OF FERTILITY

No long-term studies in animals have been performed to evaluate carcinogenic potential. There also have been no studies to determine mutagenicity or whether this medication affects fertility in males or females.

PREGNANCY, TERATOGENIC EFFECTS, PREGNANCY CATEGORY B

Reproduction studies in animals have revealed no evidence of harm to the fetus due to amphotericin B for injection. Systemic fungal infections have been successfully treated in pregnant women with amphotericin B for injection without obvious effects to the fetus, but the number of cases reported has been small. Because animal reproduction studies are not always predictive of human response, and adequate and well-controlled studies have not been conducted in pregnant women, this drug should be used during pregnancy only if clearly indicated.

NURSING MOTHERS

It is not known whether amphotericin B is excreted in human milk. Because many drugs are excreted in human milk and considering the potential toxicity of amphotericin B, it is prudent to advise a nursing mother to discontinue nursing.

PEDIATRIC USE

Safety and effectiveness in pediatric patients have not been established through adequate and well-controlled studies. Systemic fungal infections have been successfully treated in pediatric patients without reports of unusual side effects. Amphotericin B for injection when administered to pediatric patients should be limited to the smallest dose compatible with an effective therapeutic regimen.

DRUG INTERACTIONS

When administered concurrently, the following drugs may interact with amphotericin B:

Antineoplastic Agents: May enhance the potential for renal toxicity, bronchospasm, and hypotension. Antineoplastic agents (*e.g.,* nitrogen mustard, etc.) should be given concomitantly only with great caution.

Corticosteroids and Corticotropin (ACTH): May potentiate amphotericin B-induced hypokalemia which may predispose the patient to cardiac dysfunction. Avoid concomitant use unless necessary to control side effects of amphotericin B. If used concomitantly, closely monitor serum electrolytes and cardiac function (see ADVERSE REACTIONS).

Digitalis Glycosides: Amphotericin B-induced hypokalemia may potentiate digitalis toxicity. Serum potassium levels and cardiac function should be closely monitored and any deficit promptly corrected.

Flucytosine: While a synergistic relationship with amphotericin B has been reported, concomitant use may increase the toxicity of flucytosine by possible increasing its cellular uptake and/or impairing its renal excretion.

Imidazoles (e.g., Ketoconazole, Miconazole, Clotrimazole, Fluconazole, etc.): *In vitro* and animal studies with the combination of amphotericin B and imidazoles suggest that imidazoles may induce fungal resistance to amphotericin B. Combination therapy should be administered with caution, especially in immunocompromised patients.

Other Nephrotoxic Medications: Agents such as aminoglycosides, cyclosporine, and pentamidine may enhance the potential for drug-induced renal toxicity, and should be used concomitantly only with great caution. Intensive monitoring of renal function is recommended in patients requiring any combination of nephrotoxic medications (see PRECAUTIONS, Laboratory Tests).

Skeletal Muscle Relaxants: Amphotericin B-induced hypokalemia may enhance the curariform effect of skeletal muscle relaxants (*e.g.,* tubocurarine). Serum potassium levels should be monitored and deficiencies corrected.

Leukocyte Transfusions: Acute pulmonary toxicity has been reported in patients receiving intravenous amphotericin B and leukocyte transfusions (see PRECAUTIONS, General).

ADVERSE REACTIONS

Although some patients may tolerate full intravenous doses of amphotericin B without difficulty, most will exhibit some intolerance, often at less than the full therapeutic dose.

Tolerance may be improved by treatment with aspirin, antipyretics (*e.g.,* acetaminophen), antihistamines, or antiemetics. Meperidine (25–50 mg IV) has been shown in some patients to decrease the duration of shaking chills and fever that may accompany the infusion of amphotericin B.

Administration of amphotericin B on alternate days may decrease anorexia and phlebitis.

Intravenous administration of small doses of adrenal corticosteroids just prior to or during the amphotericin B infusion may help decrease febrile reactions. Dosage and duration of such corticosteroid therapy should be kept to a minimum (see DRUG INTERACTIONS).

Addition of heparin (1000 units per infusion), and the use of a pediatric scalp-vein needle may lessen the incidence of thrombophlebitis. Extravasation may cause chemical irritation.

The adverse reactions most commonly observed are:

General (Body as a Whole): Fever (sometimes accompanied by shaking chills usually occurring within 15–20 minutes after initiation of treatment); malaise; weight loss.

Cardiopulmonary: Hypotension; tachypnea.

Gastrointestinal: Anorexia, nausea; vomiting; diarrhea; dyspepsia; cramping epigastric pain.

Hematologic: Normochromic, normocytic anemia.

Local: Pain at the injection site with or without phlebitis or thrombophlebitis.

Musculoskeletal: Generalized pain, including muscle and joint pains.

Neurologic: Headache.

Renal: **Decreased** renal function and renal function abnormalities including: azotemia, hypokalemia, hyposthenuria, renal tubular acidosis; and nephrocalcinosis. These usually improve with interruption of therapy. However, some permanent impairment often occurs, especially in those patients receiving large amounts (over 5 g) of amphotericin B or receiving other nephrotoxic agents. In some patients hydration and sodium repletion prior to amphotericin B administration may reduce the risk of developing nephrotoxicity. Supplemental alkali medication may decrease renal tubular acidosis.

The following adverse reactions have also been reported:

General (Body as a Whole): Flushing.

Allergic: Anaphylactoid and other allergic reactions; bronchospasm; wheezing.

Cardiopulmonary: Cardiac arrest; shock; cardiac failure; pulmonary edema; hypersensitivity pneumonitis; arrhythmias, including ventricular fibrillation; dyspnea; hypertension.

Dermatologic: Rash, in particular maculopapular; pruritus.

Gastrointestinal: Acute liver failure; hepatitis; jaundice; hemorrhagic gastroenteritis; melena.

Hematologic: Agranulocytosis; coagulation defects; thrombocytopenia; leukopenia; eosinophilia; leukocytosis.

Neurologic: Convulsions; hearing loss; tinnitus; transient vertigo; visual impairment; diplopia; peripheral neuropathy; other neurologic symptoms.

Renal: Acute renal failure, anuria; oliguria.

Altered Laboratory Findings:

Serum Electrolytes: Hypomagnesemia; hypo- and hyperkalemia; hypocalcemia.

Liver Function Tests: Elevations of AST, ALT, GGT, bilirubin, and alkaline phosphatase.

Renal Function Tests: Elevations of BUN and serum creatinine.

DOSAGE AND ADMINISTRATION

CAUTION: Under no circumstances should a total daily dose of 1.5 mg/kg be exceeded. Amphotericin B overdoses can result in cardio-respiratory arrest.

Amphotericin B should be administered by *slow* intervenous infusion. Intravenous infusion should be given over a period of approximately 2–6 hours (depending on the dose) observing the usual precautions for intravenous therapy (see PRECAUTIONS, General). The recommended concentration for intravenous infusion is 0.1 mg/ml (1 mg/10 ml).

Since patient tolerance varies greatly, the dosage of amphotericin B must be individualized and adjusted according to the patient's clinical status (*e.g.,* site and severity of infection, etiologic agent, cardio-renal function, etc.).

A single intravenous **test dose** (1 mg in 20 ml of 5% dextrose solution) administered over 20-30 minutes may be preferred. The patient's temperature, pulse, respiration, and blood pressure should be recorded every 30 minutes for 2–4 hours.

In patients with **good cardio-renal function** and a **well tolerated test dose,** therapy is usually initiated with a daily dose of 0.25 mg/kg of body weight. However, in those patients having **severe and rapidly progressive fungal infection,** therapy may be initiated with a daily dose of 0.3 mg/kg of body weight. In patients with **impaired cardio-renal function** or a **severe reaction to the test dose,** therapy should be initiated with smaller daily doses (*i.e.,* 5–10 mg).

Depending on the patient's cardio-renal status (see PRECAUTIONS, Laboratory Tests), doses may gradually be increased by 5–10 mg/day to final daily dosage of 0.5–0.7 mg/kg.

There are insufficient data presently available to define total dosage requirements and duration of treatment necessary for eradication of specific mycoses. The optimal dose is unknown. Total daily dosage may range up to 1.0 mg/kg/day or up to 1.5 mg/kg when given on alternate days.

Sporotrichosis: Therapy with intravenous amphotericin B for sporotrichosis has ranged up to 9 months with a total dose up to 2.5 g.

Aspergillosis: Aspergillosis has been treated with amphotericin B intravenously for a period up to 11 months with a total dose up to 3.6 g.

Rhinocerebral Phycomycosis: This fulminating disease, generally occurs in association with diabetic ketoacidosis. It is, therefore, imperative that diabetic control be restored in order for treatment with amphotericin B intravenous injection to be successful. In contradistinction, pulmonary phycomycosis, which is more common in association with hematologic malignancies, is often an incidental finding at autopsy. A cumulative dose of at least 3 g of amphotericin B is recommended to treat rhinocerebral phycomycosis. Although a total dose of 3–4 g will infrequently cause lasting renal impairment, this would seem a reasonable minimum where there is clinical evidence of invasion of deep tissue. Since rhinocerebral phycomycosis usually follows a rapidly fatal course, the therapeutic approach must necessarily be more aggressive than that used in more indolent mycoses.

PREPARATION OF SOLUTIONS

Reconstitute as Follows: An initial concentrate of 5 mg amphotericin B per ml is first prepared by rapidly expressing 10 ml sterile water for injection *without a bacteriostatic agent* directly into the lyophilized cake, using a sterile needle (minimum diameter: 20 gauge) and syringe. Shake the vial immediately until the colloidal solution is clear. The infusion solution, providing 0.1 mg amphotericin B per ml, is then obtained by further dilution (1:50) with 5% dextrose injection *of pH above 4.2.* The pH of each container of dextrose injection should be ascertained before use. Commercial dextrose injection usually has a pH above 4.2; however, if it is below 4.2., then 1 or 2 ml of buffer should be added to the dextrose injection before it is used to dilute the concentrated solution of amphotericin B. The recommended buffer has the following composition:

Dibasic Sodium Phosphate (Anhydrous): 1.59 g

Monobasic Sodium Phosphate (Anhydrous): 0.96 g

Water for Injection: qs 100 ml

The buffer should be sterilized before it is added to the dextrose injection, either by filtration through a bacterial retentive stone, mat, or membrane, or by autoclaving for 30 minutes at 15 lb pressure (121°C).

CAUTION: Aseptic technique must be strictly observed in all handling, since no preservative or bacteriostatic agent is present in the antibiotic or in the materials used to prepare it for administration. **All entries into the vial or into the diluents must be made with a sterile needle. Do not reconstitute with saline solutions. The use of any diluent other than the ones recommended or the presence of a bacteriostatic agent (*e.g.,* benzyl alcohol) in the diluent may cause precipitation of the antibiotic. Do not use the initial concentrate or the infusion solution if there is any evidence of precipitation or foreign matter in either one.**

An in-line membrane filter may be used for intravenous infusion of amphotericin B; **however, the mean pore diameter of the filter should not be less than 1.0 micron in order to assure passage of the antibiotic dispersion.**

HOW SUPPLIED

Available as single vials providing 50 mg amphotericin B as a yellow to orange lyophilized cake (which may partially reduce to powder following manufacture).

Storage: Prior to reconstitution Amphocin should be stored under refrigeration 2–8°C (36–46°F), protected against exposure to light. Retain in carton until time of use. The concentrate (5 mg amphotericin B per ml after reconstitution with 10 ml sterile water for injection) may be stored in the dark, at room temperature for 24 hours, or at refrigerator temperatures for one week with minimal loss of potency and clarity. Any unused material should then be discarded. Solutions prepared for intravenous infusion (0.1 mg or less amphotericin B per ml) should be used promptly after preparation and should be protected from light during administration.

ORAL

DESCRIPTION

Fungizone oral suspension contains amphotericin B, an antifungal polyene antibiotic obtained from a strain of *Streptomyces nodosus.* Amphotericin B is designated chemically as [1R-1R*,3S*,5R*,6R*,9R*,11R*,15S*,16R*,17R*,18S*,19E,21E,23E,25E,27E,29E,31E, 33R*,35S*,36R*,37S*)]-33-[(3-Amino-3,6-dideoxy-β-(O-mannopyranosyl)oxy]-1,3,5,6, 9,11,17,37-octahydroxy-15, 16, 18-trimethyl-13-oxo-14, 39-dioxabicyclo[33.3.1]nonatriaconta-19,21,23,25,27,29,31-heptaene-36-carboxylic acid.

The structural formula is $C_{47}H_{73}NO_{17}$. The molecular weight is 924.10.

Fungizone oral suspension is a flavored aqueous suspension providing 100 mg amphotericin B per ml. Inactive ingredients: not more than 0.55 percent alcohol, carboxymethylcellulose sodium, citric acid, flavors, glycerin, methyl- and propylparaben, mono- and dibasic sodium phosphate, potassium chloride, sodium benzoate, sodium metabisulfite, and purified water.

CLINICAL PHARMACOLOGY

MICROBIOLOGY

Mechanism of Action: Amphotericin B exhibits antifungal activity by binding to sterols in the cell membrane of susceptible fungi with a resultant change of membrane permeability allowing leakage of intracellular components.

Anti-Candida Activity *In Vitro*: *Candida* species are inhibited by concentrations of amphotericin B ranging from 0.03–2.0 μg/ml *in vitro.* While *Candida albicans* is generally quite susceptible to amphotericin B, non-*albicans* species may be less susceptible. The activity of amphotericin B is fungistatic or fungicidal depending on the concentration at the site of infection and the susceptibility of the fungal organism. However, standardized techniques for susceptibility testing of antifungal agents have not been established and results of susceptibility studies have not been correlated with clinical outcomes. The antibiotic is without effect against bacteria, rickettsiae and viruses.

Drug Resistance: Mutants with decreased susceptibility to amphotericin B have been isolated from several fungal species after serial passage *in vitro* in the presence of the drug, and from some patients receiving prolonged therapy. However, the clinical relevance of drug resistance to clinical outcome has not been established.

PHARMACOKINETICS

Amphotericin B administered as amphotericin B oral suspension is poorly absorbed from the gastrointestinal tract. In limited studies conducted in both pediatric and adult patients administered amphotericin B oral suspension (dose 100 mg 4–6 times a day), the average amphotericin B serum concentration measured by microbiological assay following at least 14 days of therapy was 0.05 μg/ml (range <0.01-0.15). Serum concentrations did not show evidence of significant antibiotic accumulation over a period of two weeks. Metabolic pathways have not been elucidated.

INDICATIONS AND USAGE

Amphotericin B oral suspension is indicated for the treatment of oral candidiasis caused by susceptible strains of *Candida albicans.*

When appropriate, it is recommended that identification of the causative pathogen be obtained by means of suitable mycologic techniques before the initiation of treatment.

CONTRAINDICATIONS

Amphotericin B oral suspension is contraindicated in patients with a history of hypersensitivity to any of its components.

PRECAUTIONS

GENERAL

Amphotericin B oral suspension is not to be used for the treatment of systemic mycoses. If a systemic mycosis is suspected or documented, appropriate therapy should be instituted. Superficial candidal lesions present in addition to the oral infection should be treated concomitantly with an appropriate topical anti-candidal preparation.

If irritation or hypersensitivity develops with amphotericin B oral suspension, treatment should be discontinued and appropriate therapy instituted.

INFORMATION FOR THE PATIENT

Patients taking this medication should be provided the following information:

1. Use as directed by your physician. This medication is only for the treatment of oral candidiasis and should not be used for any other diseases or symptoms.

2. The medication works by direct contact with the oral *Candida* lesions; you should try to swish the medication around in your mouth as long as reasonably possible before swallowing.
3. If symptoms of local irritation develop, preexisting symptoms worsen, or new symptoms develop, your physician should be notified promptly.
4. Notify your physician if symptoms recur after discontinuation of medication.

CARCINOGENESIS, MUTAGENESIS, AND IMPAIRMENT OF FERTILITY

No long-term studies have been performed to evaluate carcinogenic or mutagenic potential of amphotericin B oral suspension. Animal studies of amphotericin B oral suspension have shown effects on reproduction.

PREGNANCY CATEGORY C

Amphotericin B oral suspension has been shown to cause a significantly higher incidence of stillborn fetuses when administered to pregnant rats at a dose of 200 mg/kg/day (4× the human dose, based on body surface area considerations). No signs of fetal abnormalities were observed. An increased number of deaths occurred in pregnant rabbits administered 50 mg/kg/day (2× the human dose) and 100 mg/kg/day (4× the human dose). The number of births were also reduced at those doses and one stillbirth occurred at the lower dose. No fetal abnormalities were observed. There are no adequate and well-controlled studies in pregnant women. Amphotericin B oral suspension should be used during pregnancy only if the potential benefit justifies the potential risk to the fetus.

NURSING MOTHERS

Though systematic absorption is poor, it is not known whether amphotericin B is excreted in human milk. Because many drugs are excreted in human milk and because of the potential for serious adverse reactions in nursing infants from amphotericin B oral suspension, a decision should be made whether to discontinue nursing or to discontinue the drug taking into account the importance of the drug to the mother.

PEDIATRIC USE

There has been limited study of amphotericin B oral suspension in pediatric patients, although studies have included premature infants. Doses used have been 100 mg four times per day regardless of age. Mycological eradication of oral *Candida* in these studies has been in the range of 10–20%, although clinical responses are more frequent.

DRUG INTERACTIONS

Antagonism between amphotericin B and imidazole derivatives, such as miconazole, and ketoconazole, which inhibit ergosterol synthesis, has been reported. However, the clinical significance of this phenomenon has not been demonstrated.

ADVERSE REACTIONS

Rash, gastrointestinal symptoms, including nausea, vomiting, steatorrhea, and diarrhea have been reported following administration of amphotericin B oral suspension. Rare occurrences of urticaria, angioedema, Stevens-Johnson Syndrome and toxic epidermal necrolysis have also been reported.

DOSAGE AND ADMINISTRATION

The recommended dosage for amphotericin B oral suspension in adults and pediatric patients is 1 ml (100 mg), four times daily. If possible, the suspension should be administered between meals to permit prolonged contact with the oral lesions.

Shake well before using. The suspension should be dropped directly on the tongue with the calibrated dropper. Patients should be directed to swish the medication in the mouth for as long as is reasonably possible before swallowing. If application by swabbing is desired, a non-absorbent swab should be used in applying medication.

The recommended duration of therapy is 2 weeks, although longer treatment may be necessary based on clinical response. Recurrence of oral candidiasis may be common depending on patient risk factors.

HOW SUPPLIED

Storage: Store at controlled room temperature 15–30°C (59–86°F); avoid freezing. Protect from direct sunlight. Keep tightly closed.

TOPICAL

DESCRIPTION

Lotion: Amphotericin B lotion contains the antifungal antibiotic amphotericin B at a concentration of 3% (30 mg/ml) in a tinted, unscented aqueous lotion vehicle with thimerosal, titanium dioxide, guar gum, propylene glycol, cetyl alcohol, stearyl alcohol, sorbitan monopalmitate, polysorbate 20, glyceryl monostearate, polyethylene glycol monostearate, simethicone, sorbic acid, sodium citrate, methylparaben, and propylparaben.
Ointment: Amphotericin B ointment contains the antifungal antibiotic Amphotericin B at a concentration of 3% (30 mg/g) in a tinted form of Plastibase (plasticized hydrocarbon gel), a polyethylene and mineral oil gel base with titanium dioxide.

CLINICAL PHARMACOLOGY

Amphotericin B is an antibiotic with antifungal activity produced by a strain of *Streptomyces nodosus.* It has been shown to exhibit greater *in vitro* activity than nystatin against *Candida (Monilia) albicans.* In clinical studies involving cutaneous and mucocutaneous candidal infections, results with topical preparations of amphotericin B were comparable to those obtained with nystatin in similar formulations.

Although amphotericin B exhibits some *in vitro* activity against the superficial dermatophytes (ringworm organisms), it has not demonstrated an effectiveness *in vivo* on topical application. Amphotericin B has no significant effect either *in vitro* or clinically against gram-positive or gram-negative bacteria, or viruses.

INDICATIONS AND USAGE

Amphotericin B lotion and ointment are indicated in the treatment of cutaneous and mucocutaneous mycotic infections caused by *Candida (Monilia)* species.

CONTRAINDICATIONS

The preparations are contraindicated in patients with a history of hypersensitivity to any of its components.

PRECAUTIONS

Should a reaction of hypersensitivity occur the drug should be immediately withdrawn and appropriate measures taken.

The lotion preparation is not for ophthalmic use.

ADVERSE REACTIONS

No evidence of any systemic toxicity or side effects has been observed during or following even prolonged, intensive and extensive application of amphotericin B lotion or ointment.
Lotion: The preparation is extremely well tolerated by all age groups, including infants, even when therapy must be continued for many months. It is not a primary irritant and apparently has only a slight sensitizing potential. Local intolerance, which seldom occurs, has included increased pruritus with or without other subjective or objective evidence of local irritation, or exacerbation of preexisting candidal lesions. Allergic contact dermatitis is rare.
Ointment: The preparation is usually well tolerated by all age groups. It is not a primary irritant and apparently has only a slight sensitizing potential. However, it is well to remember that any oleaginous ointment vehicle may occasionally irritate when applied to moist, intertriginous areas.

DOSAGE AND ADMINISTRATION

Amphotericin B lotion or ointment should be applied liberally to the candidal lesions 2–4 times daily. Duration of therapy depends on individual patient response. Intertriginous lesions usually respond within a few days, and treatment may be completed in 1–3 weeks. Similarly, candidiasis of the diaper area, perleche, and glabrous skin lesions usually clear in 1–2 weeks. Interdigital (erosio) lesions may require 2–4 weeks of intensive therapy, paronychias also require relatively prolonged therapy, and those onychomycoses which respond may require several months or more of treatment. (Relapses are frequently encountered in the last three clinical conditions.)
Note: The preparation does not stain the skin when thoroughly rubbed into the lesion, although nail lesions may be stained.
The patient should be informed that any discoloration of fabrics is readily removed with soap and warm water or a standard cleaning fluid.

HOW SUPPLIED

Storage: Store at room temperature, avoid freezing.

PRODUCT LISTING - RATED THERAPEUTICALLY EQUIVALENT

Powder For Injection - Intravenous - 50 mg

1's	$10.00	GENERIC, Pharma-Tek	39822-1055-05
1's	$11.64	GENERIC, Abbott Pharmaceutical	00074-9785-01
1's	$20.45	FUNGIZONE, Bristol-Myers Squibb	00003-0437-30
1's	$25.00	GENERIC, Raway Pharmacal Inc	00686-0363-20
1's	$30.94	GENERIC, Chiron Therapeutics	00702-2330-91
1's	$36.26	GENERIC, Pharmacia and Upjohn	00013-1405-44
1's	$38.60	FUNGIZONE, Bristol-Myers Squibb	00003-0437-32

Powder For Reconstitution - Compounding - 50 mg

1's	$45.48	FUNGIZONE FOR TISSUE CULTURE, Bristol-Myers Squibb	00003-0437-60

PRODUCT LISTING - EQUIVALENTS NOT AVAILABLE

Cream - Topical - 3%

20 gm	$32.71	FUNGIZONE CREAM, Bristol-Myers Squibb	00003-0411-20

Lotion - Topical - 3%

30 ml	$44.86	FUNGIZONE LOTION, Bristol-Myers Squibb	00003-0412-30

Suspension - Oral - 100 mg/ml

24 ml	$30.24	FUNGIZONE, Physicians Total Care	54868-3845-00

Amphotericin B Lipid Complex *(003277)*

For related information, see the comparative table section in Appendix A.

Categories: Infection, fungal; Pregnancy Category C; FDA Approved 1995 Nov; Orphan Drugs
Drug Classes: Antifungals
Brand Names: **Abelcet**; ABLC
Foreign Brand Availability: Ambisome (Australia; France; Hong-Kong; Israel; Korea; New-Zealand)
HCFA JCODE(S): J0286 50 mg IV

DESCRIPTION

Amphotericin B Lipid Complex (ABLC) is a sterile, pyrogen-free suspension for intravenous infusion. ABLC consists of amphotericin B complexed with two phospholipids in a 1:1 drug-to-lipid molar ratio. The two phospholipids, L-α-dimyristoylphosphatidylcholine (DMPC) and L-α-dimyristoylphosphatidylglycerol (DMPG), are present in a 7:3 molar ratio. ABLC is yellow and opaque in appearance, with a pH of 5.0-7.0
NOTE: Liposomal encapsulation or incorporation in a lipid complex can substantially affect a drug's functional properties relative to those of the unencapsulated or

nonlipid-associated drug. In addition, different liposomal or lipid-complexed products with a common active ingredient may vary from one another in the chemical composition and physical form of the lipid component. Such differences may affect functional properties of these drug products.

Amphotericin B is a polygene, antifungal antibiotic produced from a strain of *Streptomyces nodosus*. Amphotericin B is designated chemically as [1R-(1R*,3S*,5R*,6R*,9R*, 11R*,15S*,16R*,17R*,18S*,19E,21E,23E,25E,27E,29E,31E,33R*,35S*,36R*,37S*)]-33-[(3-Amino-3,6-dideoxy-β-D-mannopyranosyl) oxy]-1,3,5,6,9,11,17,37-octahydroxy-15, 16,18-trimethyl-13-oxo-14,39-dioxabicyclo[33.3.1] nonatriaconta-19,21,23,25,27,29,31-heptaene-36-carboxylic acid.

It has a molecular weight of 924.09 and a molecular formula of $C_{47}H_{73}NO_{17}$.

ABLC is provided as a sterile, opaque suspension in 20 ml glass, single-use vials. Each vial of ABLC contains 100 mg of amphotericin B (see DOSAGE AND ADMINISTRATION), and each ml of ABLC contains:

Amphotericin B: 5.0 mg
L-α-dimyristoylphosphatidylcholine (DMPC): 3.4 mg
L-α-dimyristoylphosphatidylglycerol (DMPG): 1.5 mg
Sodium Chloride: 9.0 mg
Water for Injection: q.s. 1.0 ml

CLINICAL PHARMACOLOGY

MICROBIOLOGY

Mechanism of Action

The active component of ABLC, amphotericin B, acts by binding to sterols in the cell membrane of susceptible fungi, with a resultant change in the permeability of the membrane. Mammalian cell membranes also contain sterols, and damage to human cells is believed to occur through the same mechanism of action.

Activity In Vitro and In Vivo

ABLC shows *in vitro* activity against *Aspergillus* sp. (n=3) and *Candida* sp. (n=10), with MICs generally <1 μg/ml. Depending upon the species and strain of *Aspergillus* and *Candida* tested, significant *in vitro* differences in susceptibility to amphotericin B have been reported (MICs ranging from 0.1 to >10 μg/ml). However, standardized techniques for susceptibility testing for antifungal agents have not been established, and results of susceptibility studies do not necessarily correlate with clinical outcome.

ABLC is active in animal models against *Aspergillus fumigatus, Candida albicans, C. guillermondii, C. stellatoideae, C. tropicalis, Cryptococcus sp., Coccidioidomyces sp., Histoplasma sp.,*, and *Blastomyces sp.* in which end-points were clearance of microorganisms from target organ(s) and/or prolonged survival of infected animals.

Drug Resistance

Fungal species with decreased susceptibility to amphotericin B have been isolated after serial passage in culture media containing the drug, and from some patients receiving prolonged therapy. Although the relevance of drug resistance to clinical outcome has not been established, fungal species which are resistant to amphotericin B may also be resistant to ABLC.

PHARMACOKINETICS

The assay used to measure amphotericin B in the blood after the administration of ABLC does not distinguish amphotericin B that is complexed with the phospholipids of ABLC from amphotericin B that is uncomplexed.

The pharmacokinetics of amphotericin B after the administration of ABLC are nonlinear. Volume of distribution and clearance from blood increase with increasing dose of ABLC, resulting in less than proportional increases in blood concentrations of amphotericin B over a dose range of 0.6-5.0 mg/kg/day. The pharmacokinetics of amphotericin B in whole blood after the administration of ABLC and amphotericin B desoxycholate are in TABLE 1.

TABLE 1 *Pharmacokinetic Parameters of Amphotericin B in Whole Blood in Patients Administered Multiple Doses of ABLC or Amphotericin B Desoxycholate*

Pharmacokinetic Parameter	ABLC 5 mg/kg/day for 5-7 days Mean ±SD	Amphotericin B 0.6 mg/kg/day for 42 days* Mean ±SD
Peak concentration (μg/ml)	1.7 ± 0.8 (n=10)†	1.1 ± 0.2 (n=5)
Concentration at end of dosing interval (μg/ml)	0.6 ± 0.3 (n=10)†	0.4 ± 0.2 (n=5)
Area under blood concentration-time curve (AUC(0-24h)) (μg·h/ml)	14 ± 7 (n=14)†‡	17.1 ± 5 (n=5)
Clearance (ml/h*/kg)	436 ± 188.5 (n=14)†‡	38 ± 15 (n=5)
Apparent volume of distribution (Vd_{area}) (L/kg)	131 ± 57.7 (n=8)‡	5 ± 2.8 (n=5)
Terminal elimination half-life (h)	173.4 ± 78 (n=8)‡	91.1 ± 40.9 (n=5)
Amount excreted in urine over 24h after last dose (% of dose)§	0.9 ± 0.4 (n=8)‡	9.6 ± 2.5 (n=8)

* Data from patients with mucocutaneous leishmaniasis. Infusion rate was 0.25 mg/kg/h.
† Data from studies in patients with cytologically proven cancer being treated with chemotherapy or neutropenic patients with presumed or proven fungal infection. Infusion rate was 2.5 mg/kg/h.
‡ Data from patients with mucocutaneous leishmaniasis. Infusion rate was 4.0 mg/kg/h.
§ Percentage of dose excreted in 24 hours after last dose.

The large volume of distribution and high clearance from blood of amphotericin B after the administration of ABLC probably reflect uptake by tissues. The long terminal elimination half-life probably reflects a slow redistribution from tissues. Although amphotericin B is excreted slowly, there is little accumulation in the blood after repeated dosing. AUC of amphotericin B increased approximately 34% from day 1 after the administration of ABLC 5 mg/kg/day for 7 days. The effect of gender or ethnicity on the pharmacokinetics of ABLC has not been studied.

Tissue concentrations of amphotericin B have been obtained at autopsy from one heart transplant patient who received three doses of ABLC at 5.3 mg/kg/day (see TABLE 2).

TABLE 2 *Concentration in Human Tissues*

Organ	Amphotericin B Tissue Concentration
Spleen	290 μg/g
Lung	222 μg/g
Liver	196 μg/g
Lymph node	7.6 μg/g
Kidney	6.9 μg/g
Heart	5.0 μg/g
Brain	1.6 μg/g

This pattern of distribution is consistent with that observed in preclinical studies in dogs in which greatest concentrations of amphotericin B after ABLC administration were observed in the liver, spleen, and lung; however, the relationship of tissue concentrations of amphotericin B to its biological activity when administered as ABLC is unknown.

SPECIAL POPULATIONS

Hepatic Impairment

The effect of hepatic impairment on the disposition of ABLC is not known.

Renal Impairment

The effect of renal impairment on the disposition of ABLC is not known. The effect of dialysis on the elimination of ABLC has not been studied; however, amphotericin B is not removed by hemodialysis when administered as amphotericin B desoxycholate.

Pediatric and Elderly Patients

The pharmacokinetics and pharmacodynamics of pediatric patients (≤16 years of age) and elderly patients (≥65 years of age) have not been studied.

INDICATIONS AND USAGE

ABLC is indicated for the treatment of invasive fungal infections in patients who are refractory to or intolerant of conventional amphotericin B therapy. This is based on open-label treatment of patients judged by their physicians to be intolerant to or failing conventional amphotericin B therapy.

CONTRAINDICATIONS

ABLC is contraindicated in patients who have shown hypersensitivity to amphotericin B or any other component in the formulation.

WARNINGS

Anaphylaxis has been reported with amphotericin B desoxycholate and other amphotericin B-containing drugs. Anaphylaxis has been reported with ABLC with an incidence rate of <0.1%. If severe respiratory distress occurs, the infusion should be immediately discontinued. The patient should not receive further infusions of ABLC.

PRECAUTIONS

GENERAL

As with any amphotericin B-containing product, during the initial dosing of ABLC, the drug should be administered under close clinical observation by medically trained personnel.

Acute reactions including fever and chills may occur 1-2 hours after starting an intravenous infusion of ABLC. These reactions are usually more common with the first few doses of ABLC and generally diminish with subsequent doses. Infusion has been rarely associated with hypotension, brochospasm, arrhythmias, and shock.

LABORATORY TESTS

Serum creatinine should be monitored frequently during ABLC therapy (see ADVERSE REACTIONS). It is also advisable to regularly monitor liver function, serum electrolytes (particularly magnesium and potassium), and complete blood counts.

CARCINOGENESIS, MUTAGENESIS, AND IMPAIRMENT OF FERTILITY

No long-term studies in animals have been performed to evaluate the carcinogenic potential of ABLC. The following *in vitro* (with and without metabolic activation) and *in vivo* studies to assess ABLC for mutagenic potential were conducted: bacterial reverse mutation assay, mouse lymphoma forward mutation assay, chromosomal aberration assay in CHO cells, and *in vivo* mouse micronucleus assay. ABLC was found to be without mutagenic effects in all assay systems. Studies demonstrated that ABLC had no impact on fertility in male and female rats at doses up to 0.32 times the recommended human dose (based on body surface area considerations).

PREGNANCY, TERATOGENIC EFFECTS, PREGNANCY CATEGORY B

There are no reports of pregnant women having been treated with ABLC. Reproductive studies in rats and rabbits at doses of ABLC up to 0.64 times the human dose revealed no harm to the fetus. Because animal reproductive studies are not always predictive of human response, and adequate and well-controlled studies have not been conducted in pregnant women, ABLC should be used during pregnancy only after taking into account the importance of the drug to the mother.

NURSING MOTHERS

It is not known whether ABLC is excreted in human milk. Because many drugs are excreted in human milk, and because of the potential for serious adverse reactions in breastfed infants from ABLC, a decision should be made whether to discontinue nursing or to discontinue the drug, taking into account the importance of the drug to the mother.

A

PEDIATRIC USE

One hundred eleven (111) children (2 were enrolled twice and counted as separate patients), age 16 years and under, of whom 11 were less than 1 year, have been treated with ABLC at 5 mg/kg/day in two open-label studies and one small, prospective, single-arm study. In one single-center study, 5 children with hepatosplenic candidiasis were effectively treated with 2.5 mg/kg/day of ABLC. No serious unexpected adverse events have been reported.

GERIATRIC USE

Forty-nine (49) elderly patients, age 65 years or over, have been treated with ABLC at 5 mg/kg/day in two open-label studies and one small, prospective, single-arm study. No serious unexpected adverse events have been reported.

DRUG INTERACTIONS

No formal clinical studies of drug interactions have been conducted with ABLC. However, when administered concomitantly, the following drugs are known to interact with amphotericin B; therefore, the following drugs may interact with ABLC:

Antineoplastic Agents: Concurrent use of antineoplastic agents and amphotericin B may enhance the potential for renal toxicity, bronchospasm, and hypotension. Antineoplastic agents should be given concomitantly with ABLC with great caution.

Corticosteroids and Corticotropin (ACTH): Concurrent use of corticosteroids and corticotropin (ACTH) with amphotericin B may potentiate hypokalemia which could predispose the patient to cardiac dysfunction. If used concomitantly with ABLC, serum electrolytes and cardiac function should be closely monitored.

Cyclosporin A: Data from a prospective study of prophylactic ABLC in 22 patients undergoing bone marrow transplantation suggested that concurrent initiation of cyclosporin A and ABLC within several days of bone marrow ablation may be associated with increased nephrotoxicity.

Digitalis Glycosides: Concurrent use of amphotericin B may induce hypokalemia and may potentiate digitalis toxicity. When administered concomitantly with ABLC, serum potassium levels should be closely monitored.

Flucytosine: Concurrent use of flucytosine with amphotericin B-containing preparations may increase the toxicity of flucytosine by possibly increasing its cellular uptake and/or impairing its renal excretion. Flucytosine should be given concomitantly with ABLC with caution.

Imidazoles (e.g., ketoconazole, miconazole, clotrimazole, fluconazole, etc.): Antagonism between amphotericin B and imidazole derivatives such as miconazole and ketoconazole, which inhibit ergosterol synthesis, has been reported in both *in vitro* and *in vivo* animal studies. The clinical significance of these findings has not been determined.

Leukocyte Transfusions: Acute pulmonary toxicity has been reported in patients receiving intravenous amphotericin B and leukocyte transfusions. Leukocyte transfusions and ABLC should not be given concurrently.

Other Nephrotoxic Medications: Concurrent use of amphotericin B and agents such as aminoglycosides and pentamidine may enhance the potential for drug-induced renal toxicity. Aminoglycosides and pentamidine should be used concomitantly with ABLC only with great caution. Intensive monitoring of renal function is recommend in patients requiring any combination of nephrotoxic medications.

Skeletal Muscle Relaxants: Amphotericin B-induced hypokalemia may enhance the curariform effect of skeletal muscle relaxants (*e.g.,* tubocurarine) due to hypokalemia. When administered concomitantly with ABLC, serum potassium levels should be closely monitored.

Zidovudine: Increased myelotoxicity and nephrotoxicity were observed in dogs when either ABLC (at doses 0.16 or 0.5 times the recommended human dose) or amphotericin B desoxycholate (at 0.5 times the recommended human dose) were administered concomitantly with zidovudine for 30 days. If zidovudine is used concomitantly with ABLC, renal and hematologic function should be closely monitored.

ADVERSE REACTIONS

The total safety data base is composed of 921 patients treated with ABLC (5 patients were enrolled twice and counted as separate patients), of whom 775 were treated with 5 mg/kg/day. Of these 775 patients, 194 patients were treated in four comparative studies; 25 were treated in open-label, non-comparative studies; and 556 patients were treated in an open-label, emergency-use program. Most had underlying hematologic neoplasms, and many were receiving multiple concomitant medications. Of the 556 patients treated with ABLC, 9% discontinued treatment due to adverse events regardless of presumed relationship to study drug.

In general, the adverse events most commonly reported with ABLC were transient chills and/or fever during infusion of the drug.

The following adverse events have also been reported in patients using ABLC in open-label, uncontrolled clinical studies. The causal association between these adverse events and ABLC is uncertain.

Body as a Whole: Malaise, weight loss, deafness, injection site reaction including inflammation.

Allergic: Bronchospasm, wheezing, asthma, anaphylactoid and other allergic reactions.

Cardiopulmonary: Cardiac failure, pulmonary edema, shock, myocardial infarction, hemoptysis, tachypnea, thrombophlebitis, pulmonary embolus, cardiomyopathy, pleural effusion, arrhythmias including ventricular fibrillation.

Dermatological: Maculopapular rash, pruritus, exfoliative dermatitis, erythema multiforme.

Gastrointestinal: Acute liver failure, hepatitis, jaundice, melena, anorexia, dyspepsia, cramping, epigastric pain, veno-occlusive liver disease, diarrhea, hepatomegaly, cholangitis, cholecystitis.

Hematologic: Coagulation defects, leukocytosis, blood dyscrasias including eosinophilia.

Musculoskeletal: Myasthenia, including bone, muscle, and joint pains.

TABLE 3 *Adverse Events* With an Incidence of ≥3% (n=556)*

Adverse Event	
Chills	18%
Fever	14%
Increased serum creatinine	11%
Multiple organ failure	11%
Nausea	9%
Hypotension	8%
Respiratory failure	8%
Vomiting	8%
Dyspnea	7%
Sepsis	7%
Diarrhea	6%
Headache	6%
Heart Arrest	6%
Hypertension	5%
Hypokalemia	5%
Infection	5%
Kidney failure	5%
Pain	5%
Thrombocytopenia	5%
Abdominal pain	4%
Anemia	4%
Bilirubinemia	4%
Gastrointestinal hemorrhage	4%
Leukopenia	4%
Rash	4%
Respiratory disorder	4%
Chest pain	3%
Nausea and vomiting	3%

* The causal association between these adverse events and ABLC is uncertain.

Neurologic: Convulsions, tinnitus, visual impairment, hearing loss, peripheral neuropathy, transient vertigo, diplopia, encephalopathy, cerebral vascular accident, extrapyramidal syndrome and other neurologic symptoms.

Urogenital: Oliguria, decreased renal function, anuria, renal tubular acidosis, impotence, dysuria.

Serum Electrolyte Abnormalities: Hypomagnesemia, hyperkalemia, hypocalcemia, hypercalcemia.

Liver Function Test Abnormalities: Increased AST, ALT, alkaline phosphatase, LDH.

Renal Function Test Abnormalities: Increased BUN.

Other Test Abnormalities: Acidosis, hyperamylasemia, hypoglycemia, hyperglycemia, hyperuricemia, hypophosphatemia.

DOSAGE AND ADMINISTRATION

The recommended daily dosage for adults and children is 5.0 mg/kg given as a single infusion. ABLC should be administered by intravenous infusion at a rate of 2.5 mg/kg/h. If the infusion time exceeds 2 hours, mix the contents by shaking the infusion bag every 2 hours.

Renal toxicity of ABLC, as measured by serum creatinine levels, has been shown to be dose dependent. Decisions about dose adjustments should be made only after taking into account the overall clinical condition of the patient.

DO NOT DILUTE WITH SALINE SOLUTIONS OR MIX WITH OTHER DRUGS OR ELECTROLYTES as the compatibility of ABLC with these materials has not been established. An existing intravenous line should be flushed with 5.0% dextrose injection before infusion of ABLC, or a separate infusion line should be used. DO NOTE USE AN IN-LINE FILTER.

The diluted ready-for-use admixture is stable for up to 48 hours at 2-8°C (36-46°F) and an additional 6 hours at room temperature.

HOW SUPPLIED

Each vial contains 100 mg of Abelcet in 20 ml of suspension. Single-use vials along with 5 micron filter needles are individually packaged.

STORAGE

Prior to admixture, Abelcet should be stored at 2-8°C (36-46°F) and protected from exposure to light. Do not freeze. Abelcet should be retained in the carton until time of use.

The admixed Abelcet and 5.0% dextrose injection may be stored for up to 48 hours at 2-8°C (36-46°F) and an additional 6 hours at room temperature. Do not freeze. Any unused material should be discarded.

PRODUCT LISTING - EQUIVALENTS NOT AVAILABLE

Powder For Injection - Intravenous - 50 mg

1's	$196.25	AMBISOME, Fujisawa	00469-3051-30

Suspension - Intravenous - 5 mg/ml

10 ml	$134.66	ABELCET, Liposome Company Inc, The	61799-0101-31
20 ml	$230.00	ABELCET, Liposome Company Inc, The	61799-0101-41

Amphotericin B Liposome *(003513)*

For related information, see the comparative table section in Appendix A.

Categories: Infection, fungal; Leishmaniasis; Meningitis, cryptococcal; FDA Approved 1997 Aug; Pregnancy Category B
Drug Classes: Antifungals
Brand Names: **AmBisome**

DESCRIPTION

Note: The trade name was left in this monograph for clarification.

AmBisome for injection is a sterile, nonpyrogenic lyophilized product for intravenous (IV) infusion. Each vial contains 50 mg of amphotericin B, intercalated into a liposomal membrane consisting of approximately 213 mg hydrogenated soy phosphatidylcholine; 52 mg cholesterol; 84 mg distearoylphosphatidylglycerol; 0.64 mg alpha tocopherol; together with 900 mg sucrose; and 27 mg disodium succinate hexahydrate as buffer. Following reconstitution with sterile water for injection, the resulting pH of the suspension is between 5.0-6.0.

AmBisome is a true single bilayer liposomal drug delivery system. Liposomes are closed, spherical vesicles created by mixing specific proportions of amphophilic substances such as phospholipids and cholesterol so that they arrange themselves into multiple concentric bilayer membranes when hydrated in aqueous solutions. Single bilayer liposomes are then formed by microemulsification of multilamellar vesicles using a homogenizer. AmBisome consists of these unilamellar bilayer liposomes with amphotericin B intercalated within the membrane. Due to the nature and quantity of amphophilic substances used, and the lipophilic moiety in the amphotericin B molecule, the drug is an integral part of the overall structure of the AmBisome liposomes. AmBisome contains true liposomes that are less than 100 nm in diameter.

Note: Liposomal encapsulation or incorporation into a lipid complex can substantially affect a drug's functional properties relative to those of the unencapsulated drug or nonlipid associated drug. In addition, different liposomal or lipid-complex products with a common active ingredient may vary from one another in the chemical composition and physical form of the lipid component. Such differences may affect the functional properties of these drug products.

Amphotericin B is a macrocyclic, polyene, antifungal antibiotic produced from a strain of *Streptomyces nodosus*. Amphotericin B is designated chemically as:

[1R-(1R*,3S*,5R*,6R*,9R*,11R*,15S*,16R*,17R*,18S*,19E,21E,23E,25E,27E,29E, 31E,33R*,35S*,36R*,37S*)]-33-[(3-Amino-3,6-dideoxy-β-D- mannopyranosyl)oxy]-1,3, 5,6,9,11,17,37-octahydroxy-15,16,18-trimethyl-13-oxo-14,39- dioxabicyclo[33.3.1]nonatriaconta-19,21,23,25,27,29,31-heptaene-36-carboxylic acid.

Amphotericin B has a molecular formula of $C_{47}H_{73}NO_{17}$ and a molecular weight of 924.09.

CLINICAL PHARMACOLOGY

MICROBIOLOGY

Mechanism of Action

Amphotericin B, the active ingredient of AmBisome, acts by binding to the sterol component of a cell membrane leading to alterations in cell permeability and cell death. While amphotericin B has a higher affinity for the ergosterol component of the fungal cell membrane, it can also bind to the cholesterol component of the mammalian cell leading to cytotoxicity. AmBisome, the liposomal preparation of amphotericin B, has been shown to penetrate the cell wall of both extracellular and intracellular forms of susceptible fungi.

Activity In Vitro and In Vivo

AmBisome has shown *in vitro* activity comparable to amphotericin B against the following organisms: *Aspergillus* species *(A. fumigatus, A. flavus), Candida* species *(C. albicans, C. krusei, C. lusitaniae, C. parapsilosis, C. tropicalis), Cryptococcus neoformans,* and *Blastomyces dermatitidis.* However, standardized techniques for susceptibility testing of antifungal agents have not been established and results of such studies do not necessarily correlate with clinical outcome.

AmBisome is active in animal models against *Aspergillus fumigatus, Candida albicans, Candida krusei, Candida lusitaniae, Cryptococcus neoformans, Blastomyces dermatitidis, Coccidioides immitis, Histoplasma capsulatum, Paracoccidioides brasiliensis, Leishmania donovani,* and *Leishmania infantum.* The administration of AmBisome in these animal models demonstrated prolonged survival of infected animals, reduction of microorganisms from target organs, or a decrease in lung weight.

Drug Resistance

Mutants with decreased susceptibility to amphotericin B have been isolated from several fungal species after serial passage in culture media containing the drug, and from some patients receiving prolonged therapy. Drug combination studies *in vitro* and *in vivo* suggest that imidazoles may induce resistance to amphotericin B. However, the clinical relevance of drug resistance has not been established.

PHARMACOKINETICS

The assay used to measure amphotericin B in the serum after administration of AmBisome does not distinguish amphotericin B that is complexed with the phospholipids of AmBisome from amphotericin B that is uncomplexed. The pharmacokinetic profile of amphotericin B after administration of AmBisome is based upon total serum concentrations of amphotericin B. The pharmacokinetic profile of amphotericin B was determined in febrile neutropenic cancer and bone marrow transplant patients who received 1-2 hour infusions of 1.0-5.0 mg/kg/day AmBisome for 3-20 days.

The pharmacokinetics of amphotericin B after administration of AmBisome are nonlinear such that there is a greater than proportional increase in serum concentrations with an increase in dose from 1.0-5.0 mg/kg/day. The pharmacokinetic parameters of total amphotericin B (mean ± SD) after the first dose and at steady state are shown in TABLE 1.

Distribution

Based on total amphotericin B concentrations measured within a dosing interval (24 hours) after administration of AmBisome, the mean half-life was 7-10 hours. However, based on total amphotericin B concentration measured up to 49 days after dosing of AmBisome, the mean half-life was 100-153 hours. The long terminal elimination half-life is probably a slow redistribution from tissues. Steady state concentrations were generally achieved within 4 days of dosing.

Although variable, mean trough concentrations of amphotericin B remained relatively constant with repeated administration of the same dose over the range of 1.0-5.0 mg/kg/day, indicating no significant drug accumulation in the serum.

***TABLE 1** Pharmacokinetic Parameters of AmBisome*

	Dose (mg/kg/day)					
	1.0		2.5		5.0	
	Day 1	Last Day	Day 1	Last Day	Day 1	Last Day
	n=8	n=7	n=7	n=7	n=12	n=9
Parameters						
C_{max} (μg/ml)	7.3 ± 3.8	12.2 ± 4.9	17.2 ± 7.1	31.4 ± 17.8	57.6 ± 21.0	83.0 ± 35.2
AUC(0-24) (μg·h/ml)	27 ± 14	60 ± 20	65 ± 33	197 ± 183	269 ± 96	555 ± 311
T½ (h)	10.7 ± 6.4	7.0 ± 2.1	8.1 ± 2.3	6.3 ± 2.0	6.4 ± 2.1	6.8 ± 2.1
Vss (L/kg)	0.44 ± 0.27	0.14 ± 0.05	0.40 ± 0.37	0.16 ± 0.09	0.16 ± 0.10	0.10 ± 0.07
Cl (ml/h/kg)	39 ± 22	17 ± 6	51 ± 44	22 ± 15	21 ± 14	11 ± 6

Metabolism

The metabolic pathways of amphotericin B after administration of AmBisome are not known.

Excretion

The mean clearance at steady state was independent of dose. The excretion of amphotericin B after administration of AmBisome has not been studied.

Pharmacokinetics in Special Populations

Renal Impairment

The effect of renal impairment on the disposition of amphotericin B after administration of AmBisome has not been studied. However, AmBisome has been successfully administered to patients with pre-existing renal impairment.

Hepatic Impairment

The effect of hepatic impairment on the disposition of amphotericin B after administration of AmBisome is not known.

Pediatric and Elderly Patients

The pharmacokinetics of amphotericin B after administration of AmBisome in pediatric and elderly patients have not been studied; however, AmBisome has been used in pediatric and elderly patients.

Gender and Ethnicity

The effect of gender or ethnicity on the pharmacokinetics of amphotericin B after administration of AmBisome is not known.

INDICATIONS AND USAGE

AmBisome is indicated for the following:

- Empirical therapy for presumed fungal infection in febrile, neutropenic patients.
- Treatment of cryptococcal meningitis in HIV infected patients.
- Treatment of patients with *Aspergillus* species, *Candida* species and/or *Cryptococcus* species infections (see above for the treatment of cryptococcal meningitis) refractory to amphotericin B deoxycholate, or in patients where renal impairment or unacceptable toxicity precludes the use of amphotericin B deoxycholate.
- Treatment of visceral leishmaniasis. In immunocompromised patients with visceral leishmaniasis treated with AmBisome, relapse rates were high following initial clearance of parasites.

See DOSAGE AND ADMINISTRATION for recommended doses by indication.

CONTRAINDICATIONS

AmBisome is contraindicated in those patients who have demonstrated or have known hypersensitivity to amphotericin B deoxycholate or any other constituents of the product unless, in the opinion of the treating physician, the benefit of therapy outweighs the risk.

WARNINGS

Anaphylaxis has been reported with amphotericin B deoxycholate and other amphotericin B-containing drugs, including AmBisome. If a severe anaphylactic reaction occurs, the infusion should be immediately discontinued and the patient should not receive further infusions of AmBisome.

PRECAUTIONS

GENERAL

As with any amphotericin B-containing product the drug should be administered by medically trained personnel. During the initial dosing period, patients should be under close clinical observation. AmBisome has been shown to be significantly less toxic than amphotericin B deoxycholate; however, adverse events may still occur.

LABORATORY TESTS

Patient management should include laboratory evaluation of renal, hepatic and hematopoietic function, and serum electrolytes (particularly magnesium and potassium).

CARCINOGENESIS, MUTAGENESIS, AND IMPAIRMENT OF FERTILITY

No long term studies in animals have been performed to evaluate carcinogenic potential of AmBisome. AmBisome has not been tested to determine its mutagenic potential. A Segment I Reproductive Study in rats found an abnormal estrous cycle (prolonged diestrus) and decreased number of corpora lutea in the high dose groups (10 and 15 mg/kg, doses equivalent to human doses of 1.6 and 2.4 mg/kg based on body surface area considerations). AmBisome did not affect fertility or days to copulation. There were no effects on male reproductive function.

A

PREGNANCY CATEGORY B

There have been no adequate and well-controlled studies of AmBisome in pregnant women. Systemic fungal infections have been successfully treated in pregnant women with amphotericin B deoxycholate, but the number of cases reported has been small.

Segment II studies in both rats and rabbits have concluded that AmBisome had no teratogenic potential in these species. In rats, the maternal nontoxic dose of AmBisome was estimated to be 5 mg/kg (equivalent to 0.16-0.8 times the recommended human clinical dose range of 1-5 mg/kg) and in rabbits, 3 mg/kg (equivalent to 0.2-1 times the recommended human clinical dose range), based on body surface area correction. Rabbits receiving the higher doses, (equivalent to 0.5-2 times the recommended human dose) of AmBisome experienced a higher rate of spontaneous abortions than did the control groups. AmBisome should only be used during pregnancy if the possible benefits to be derived outweigh the potential risks involved.

NURSING MOTHERS

Many drugs are excreted in human milk. However, it is not known whether AmBisome is excreted in human milk. Due to the potential for serious adverse reactions in breast-fed infants, a decision should be made whether to discontinue nursing or whether to discontinue the drug, taking into account the importance of the drug to the mother.

PEDIATRIC USE

Pediatric patients, age 1 month to 16 years, with presumed fungal infection (empirical therapy), confirmed systemic fungal infections or with visceral leishmaniasis have been successfully treated with AmBisome. In studies which included 302 pediatric patients administered AmBisome, there was no evidence of any differences in efficacy or safety of AmBisome compared to adults. Since pediatric patients have received AmBisome at doses comparable to those used in adults on a per kilogram body weight basis, no dosage adjustment is required in this population. Safety and effectiveness in pediatric patients below the age of 1 month have not been established.

(See DOSAGE AND ADMINISTRATION.)

GERIATRIC USE

Experience with AmBisome in the elderly (65 years or older) comprised 72 patients. It has not been necessary to alter the dose of AmBisome for this population. As with most other drugs, elderly patients receiving AmBisome should be carefully monitored.

DRUG INTERACTIONS

No formal clinical studies of drug interactions have been conducted with AmBisome. However, the following drugs are known to interact with amphotericin B and may interact with AmBisome:

Antineoplastic Agents: Concurrent use of antineoplastic agents may enhance the potential for renal toxicity, bronchospasm, and hypotension. Antineoplastic agents should be given concomitantly with caution.

Corticosteroids and Corticotropin (ACTH): Concurrent use of corticosteroids and ACTH may potentiate hypokalemia which could predispose the patient to cardiac dysfunction. If used concomitantly, serum electrolytes and cardiac function should be closely monitored.

Digitalis Glycosides: Concurrent use may induce hypokalemia and may potentiate digitalis toxicity. When administered concomitantly, serum potassium levels should be closely monitored.

Flucytosine: Concurrent use of flucytosine may increase the toxicity of flucytosine by possibly increasing its cellular uptake and/or impairing its renal excretion.

Azoles (e.g., Ketoconazole, Miconazole, Clotrimazole, Fluconazole, etc.): *In vitro* and *in vivo* animal studies of the combination of amphotericin B and imidazoles suggest that imidazoles may induce fungal resistance to amphotericin B. Combination therapy should be administered with caution, especially in immunocompromised patients.

Leukocyte Transfusions: Acute pulmonary toxicity has been reported in patients simultaneously receiving IV amphotericin B and leukocyte transfusions.

Other Nephrotoxic Medications: Concurrent use of amphotericin B and other nephrotoxic medications may enhance the potential for drug-induced renal toxicity. Intensive monitoring of renal function is recommended in patients requiring any combination of nephrotoxic medications.

Skeletal Muscle Relaxants: Amphotericin B-induced hypokalemia may enhance the curariform effect of skeletal muscle relaxants (*e.g.*, tubocurarine) due to hypokalemia. When administered concomitantly, serum potassium levels should be closely monitored.

ADVERSE REACTIONS

The following adverse events are based on the experience of 592 adult patients (295 treated with AmBisome and 297 treated with amphotericin B deoxycholate) and 95 pediatric patients (48 treated with AmBisome and 47 treated with amphotericin B deoxycholate) in Study 94-0-002, a randomized double-blind, multi-center study in febrile, neutropenic patients. AmBisome and amphotericin B were infused over 2 hours.

The incidence of common adverse events (incidence of 10% or greater) occurring with AmBisome compared to amphotericin B deoxycholate, regardless of relationship to study drug, is shown in TABLE 7.

AmBisome was well tolerated. AmBisome had a lower incidence of chills, hypertension, hypotension, tachycardia, hypoxia, hypokalemia, and various events related to decreased kidney function as compared to amphotericin B deoxycholate.

In pediatric patients (16 years of age or less) in this double-blind study, AmBisome compared to amphotericin B deoxycholate had a lower incidence of hypokalemia (37% vs 55%), chills (29% vs 68%), vomiting (27% vs 55%), and hypertension (10% vs 21%). Similar trends, although with a somewhat lower incidence, were observed in open-label, randomized Study 104-14 involving 205 febrile neutropenic pediatric patients (141 treated with AmBisome and 64 treated with amphotericin B deoxycholate). Pediatric patients appear to have more tolerance than older individuals for the nephrotoxic effects of amphotericin B deoxycholate.

TABLE 7 *Empirical Therapy Study 94-0-002*

	Common adverse events	
	AmBisome	**Amphotericin B**
Adverse Event by Body System	**n=343**	**n=344**
Body as a Whole		
Abdominal pain	19.8%	21.8%
Asthenia	13.1%	10.8%
Back pain	12.0%	7.3%
Blood product transfusion reaction	18.4%	18.6%
Chills	47.5%	75.9%
Infection	11.1%	9.3%
Pain	14.0%	12.8%
Sepsis	14.0%	11.3%
Cardiovascular System		
Chest pain	12.0%	11.6%
Hypertension	7.9%	16.3%
Hypotension	14.3%	21.5%
Tachycardia	13.4%	20.9%
Digestive System		
Diarrhea	30.3%	27.3%
Gastrointestinal hemorrhage	9.9%	11.3%
Nausea	39.7%	38.7%
Vomiting	31.8%	43.9%
Metabolic and Nutritional Disorders		
Alkaline phosphatase increased	22.2%	19.2%
ALT (SGPT) increased	14.6%	14.0%
AST (SGOT) increased	12.8%	12.8%
Bilirubinemia	18.1%	19.2%
BUN increased	21.0%	31.1%
Creatinine increased	22.4%	42.2%
Edema	14.3%	14.8%
Hyperglycemia	23.0%	27.9%
Hypernatremia	4.1%	11.0%
Hypervolemia	12.2%	15.4%
Hypocalcemia	18.4%	20.9%
Hypokalemia	42.9%	50.6%
Hypomagnesemia	20.4%	25.6%
Peripheral edema	14.6%	17.2%
Nervous System		
Anxiety	13.7%	11.0%
Confusion	11.4%	13.4%
Headache	19.8%	20.9%
Insomnia	17.2%	14.2%
Respiratory System		
Cough increased	17.8%	21.8%
Dyspnea	23.0%	29.1%
Epistaxis	14.9%	20.1%
Hypoxia	7.6%	14.8%
Lung disorder	17.8%	17.4%
Pleural effusion	12.5%	9.6%
Rhinitis	11.1%	11.0%
Skin and Appendages		
Pruritus	10.8%	10.2%
Rash	24.8%	24.4%
Sweating	7.0%	10.8%
Urogenital System		
Hematuria	14.0%	14.0%

The following adverse events are based on the experience of 244 patients (202 adult and 42 pediatric patients) of whom 85 patients were treated with AmBisome 3 mg/kg, 81 patients were treated with AmBisome 5 mg/kg and 78 patients treated with amphotericin B lipid complex 5 mg/kg in Study 97-0-034, a randomized double-blind, multi-center study in febrile, neutropenic patients. AmBisome and amphotericin B lipid complex were infused over 2 hours. The incidence of adverse events occurring in more than 10% of subjects in 1 or more arms regardless of relationship to study drug are summarized in TABLE 8.

The following adverse events are based on the experience of 267 patients (266 adult patients and 1 pediatric patient) of whom 86 patients were treated with AmBisome 3 mg/kg, 94 patients were treated with AmBisome 6 mg/kg and 87 patients treated with amphotericin B deoxycholate 0.7 mg/kg in Study 94-0-013 a randomized, double-blind, comparative multi-center trial, in the treatment of cryptococcal meningitis in HIV positive patients. The incidence of adverse events occurring in more than 10% of subjects in 1 or more arms regardless of relationship to study drug are summarized in TABLE 9.

INFUSION RELATED REACTIONS

In Study 94-0-002, the large, double-blind study of pediatric and adult febrile neutropenic patients, no premedication to prevent infusion related reaction was administered prior to the first dose of study drug (Day 1). AmBisome-treated patients had a lower incidence of infusion related fever (17% vs 44%), chills/rigors (18% vs 54%) and vomiting (6% vs 8%) on Day 1 as compared to amphotericin B deoxycholate-treated patients.

The incidence of infusion related reactions on Day 1 in pediatric and adult patients is summarized in TABLE 10.

Cardiorespiratory events, except for vasodilatation (flushing), during all study drug infusions were more frequent in amphotericin B-treated patients as summarized in TABLE 11.

The percentage of patients who received drugs either for the treatment or prevention of infusion related reactions (*e.g.*, acetaminophen, diphenhydramine, meperidine and hydrocortisone) was lower in AmBisome-treated patients compared with amphotericin B deoxycholate-treated patients.

In the empirical therapy study 97-0-034, on Day 1, where no premedication was administered, the overall incidence of infusion related events of chills/rigors was significantly lower for patients administered AmBisome compared with amphotericin B lipid complex. Fever, chills/rigors and hypoxia were significantly lower for each AmBisome group compared with the amphotericin B lipid complex group. The infusion related event hypoxia was reported for 11.5% of amphotericin B lipid complex- treated patients compared with 0% of

TABLE 8 *Empirical Therapy Study 97-0-034*

Common Adverse Events

Adverse Event by Body System	AmBisome 3 mg/kg/day	AmBisome 5 mg/kg/day	Amphotericin B Lipid Complex 5 mg/kg/day
	n=85	n=81	n=78
Body as a Whole			
Abdominal pain	12.9%	9.9%	11.5%
Asthenia	8.2%	6.2%	11.5%
Chills/rigors	40.0%	48.1%	89.7%
Sepsis	12.9%	7.4%	11.5%
Transfusion reaction	10.6%	8.6%	5.1%
Cardiovascular System			
Chest pain	8.2%	11.1%	6.4%
Hypertension	10.6%	19.8%	23.1%
Hypotension	10.6%	7.4%	19.2%
Tachycardia	9.4%	18.5%	23.1%
Digestive System			
Diarrhea	15.3%	17.3%	14.1%
Nausea	25.9%	29.6%	37.2%
Vomiting	22.4%	25.9%	30.8%
Metabolic and Nutritional Disorders			
Alkaline phosphatase increased	7.1%	8.6%	12.8%
Bilirubinemia	16.5%	11.1%	11.5%
BUN increased	20.0%	18.5%	28.2%
Creatinine increased	20.0%	18.5%	48.7%
Edema	12.9%	12.3%	12.8%
Hyperglycemia	8.2%	8.6%	14.1%
Hypervolemia	8.2%	11.1%	14.1%
Hypocalcemia	10.6%	4.9%	5.1%
Hypokalemia	37.6%	43.2%	39.7%
Hypomagnesemia	15.3%	25.9%	15.4%
Liver function tests abnormal	10.6%	7.4%	11.5%
Nervous System			
Anxiety	10.6%	7.4%	9.0%
Confusion	12.9%	8.6%	3.8%
Headache	9.4%	17.3%	10.3%
Respiratory System			
Dyspnea	17.6%	22.2%	23.1%
Epistaxis	10.6%	8.6%	14.1%
Hypoxia	7.1%	6.2%	20.5%
Lung disorder	14.1%	13.6%	15.4%
Skin and Appendages			
Rash	23.5%	22.2%	14.1%

TABLE 9 *Cryptococcal Meningitis Therapy Study 94-0-013*

Common Adverse Events

Adverse Event by Body System	AmBisome 3 mg/kg/day	AmBisome 6 mg/kg/day	Amphotericin B Lipid Complex 0.7 mg/kg/day
	n=86	n=94	n=87
Body as a Whole			
Abdominal pain	7.0%	7.4%	10.3%
Infection	12.8%	11.7%	6.9%
Procedural complication	8.1%	9.6%	10.3%
Cardiovascular System			
Phlebitis	9.3%	10.6%	25.3%
Digestive System			
Anorexia	14.0%	9.6%	11.5%
Constipation	15.1%	14.9%	20.7%
Diarrhea	10.5%	16.0%	10.3%
Nausea	16.3%	21.3%	25.3%
Vomiting	10.5%	21.3%	20.7%
Hemic and Lymphatic System			
Anemia	26.7%	47.9%	43.7%
Leukopenia	15.1%	17.0%	17.2%
Thrombocytopenia	5.8%	12.8%	6.9%
Metabolic and Nutritional Disorders			
Bilirubinemia	0%	8.5%	12.6%
BUN increased	9.3%	7.4%	10.3%
Creatinine increased	18.6%	39.4%	43.7%
Hyperglycemia	9.3%	12.8%	17.2%
Hypocalcemia	12.8%	17.0%	13.8%
Hypokalemia	31.4%	51.1%	48.3%
Hypomagnesemia	29.1%	48.9%	40.2%
Hyponatremia	11.6%	8.5%	9.2%
Liver function tests abnormal	12.8%	4.3%	9.2%
Nervous System			
Dizziness	7.0%	8.5%	10.3%
Insomnia	22.1%	17.0%	20.7%
Respiratory System			
Cough increased	8.1%	2.1%	10.3%
Skin and Appendages			
Rash	4.7%	11.7%	4.6%

patients administered 3 mg/kg/day AmBisome and 1.2% of patients treated with 5 mg/kg/day AmBisome.

TABLE 10 *Incidence of Day 1 Infusion Related Reactions (IRR) by Patient Age*

	Pediatric Patients† AmBisome	Pediatric Patients† Amphotericin B	Adult Patients‡ AmBisome	Adult Patients‡ Amphotericin B
Total number of patients receiving at least 1 dose of study drug	48	47	295	297
Patients with fever* Increase ≤1.0°C	6 (13%)	22 (47%)	52 (18%)	128 (43%)
Patients with chills/rigors	4 (8%)	22 (47%)	59 (20%)	165 (56%)
Patients with nausea	4(8%)	4 (9%)	38 (13%)	31 (10%)
Patients with vomiting	2 (4%)	7 (15%)	19 (6%)	21 (7%)
Patients with other reactions	10 (21%)	13 (28%)	47 (16%)	69 (23%)

* Day 1 body temperature increased above the temperature taken within 1 hour prior to infusion (preinfusion temperature) or above the lowest infusion value (no preinfusion temperature recorded).
† ≤16 years of age.
‡ >16 years of age.

TABLE 11 *Incidence of Infusion Related Cardiorespiratory Events*

Event	AmBisome n=343	Amphotericin B n=344
Hypotension	12 (3.5%)	28 (8.1%)
Tachycardia	8 (2.3%)	43 (12.5%)
Hypertension	8 (2.3%)	39 (11.3%)
Vasodilatation	18 (5.2%)	2 (0.6%)
Dyspnea	16 (4.7%)	25 (7.3%)
Hyperventilation	4 (1.2%)	17 (4.9%)
Hypoxia	1 (0.3%)	22 (6.4%)

TABLE 12 *Incidence of Day 1 Infusion Related Reactions (IRR) Chills/Rigors Empirical Therapy Study 97-0-034*

	AmBisome 3 mg/kg/day	AmBisome 5 mg/kg/day	AmBisome BOTH	Amphotericin B Lipid Complex 5 mg/kg/day
Total number of patients	85	81	166	78
Patients with chills/rigors (Day 1*)	16 (18.8%)	19 (23.5%)	35 (21.1%)	62 (79.5%)
Patients with other notable reactions:				
Fever (≥1.0°C increase in temperature)	20 (23.5%)	16 (19.8%)	36 (21.7%)	45 (57.7%)
Nausea	9 (10.6%)	7 (8.6%)	16 (9.6%)	9 (11.5%)
Vomiting	5 (5.9%)	5 (6.2%)	10 (6.0%)	11 (14.1%)
Hypertension	4 (4.7%)	7 (8.6%)	11 (6.6%)	12 (15.4%)
Tachycardia	2 (2.4%)	8 (9.9%)	10 (6.0%)	14 (17.9%)
Dyspnea	4 (4.7%)	8 (9.9%)	12 (7.2%)	8 (10.3%)
Hypoxia	0	1 (1.2%)	1 (<1%)	9 (11.5%)

* Day 1 body temperature increased above the temperature taken within 1 hour prior to infusion (preinfusion temperature) or above the lowest infusion value (no preinfusion temperature recorded). Patients were not administered premedications to prevent infusion related reactions prior to the Day 1 study drug infusion.

In Study 94-0-013, a randomized double-blind multicenter trial comparing AmBisome and amphotericin B deoxycholate as initial therapy for cryptococcal meningitis, premedications to prevent infusion related reactions were permitted. AmBisome treated patients had a lower incidence of fever, chill/rigors and respiratory adverse events as summarized in TABLE 13.

TABLE 13 *Incidence of Infusion-Related Reactions Study 94-0-013*

	AmBisome 3 mg/kg	AmBisome 6 mg/kg	Amphotericin B
Total number of patients receiving at least 1 dose of study drug	86	94	87
Patients with fever increase >1°C	6 (7%)	8 (9%)	24 (28%)
Patients with chills/rigors	5 (6%)	8 (9%)	42 (48%)
Patients with nausea	11 (13%)	13 (14%)	18 (20%)
Patients with vomiting	14 (16%)	13 (14%)	16 (18%)
Respiratory adverse events	0	1 (1%)	8 (9%)

There have been a few reports of flushing, back pain with or without chest tightness, and chest pain associated with AmBisome administration; on occasion this has been severe. Where these symptoms were noted, the reaction developed within a few minutes after the start of infusion and disappeared rapidly when the infusion was stopped. The symptoms do not occur with every dose and usually do not recur on subsequent administrations when the infusion rate is slowed.

A

TOXICITY AND DISCONTINUATION OF DOSING

In Study 94-0-002, a significantly lower incidence of grade 3 or 4 toxicity was observed in the AmBisome group compared with the amphotericin B group. In addition, nearly 3 times as many patients administered amphotericin B required a reduction in dose due to toxicity or discontinuation of study drug due to an infusion related reaction compared with those administered AmBisome.

In empirical therapy study 97-0-034, a greater proportion of patients in the amphotericin B lipid complex group discontinued the study drug due to an adverse event than in the AmBisome groups.

LESS COMMON ADVERSE EVENTS

The following adverse events also have been reported in 2-10% of AmBisome-treated patients receiving chemotherapy or bone marrow transplantation, or had HIV disease in six comparative, clinical trials:

Body as a Whole: Abdomen enlarged, allergic reaction, cellulitis, cell mediated immunological reaction, face edema, graft vs host disease, malaise, neck pain, and procedural complication.

Cardiovascular System: Arrhythmia, atrial fibrillation, bradycardia, cardiac arrest, cardiomegaly, hemorrhage, postural hypotension, valvular heart disease, vascular disorder, and vasodilatation (flushing).

Digestive System: Anorexia, constipation, dry mouth/nose, dyspepsia, dysphagia, eructation, fecal incontinence, flatulence, hemorrhoids, gum/oral hemorrhage, hematemesis, hepatocellular damage, hepatomegaly, liver function test abnormal, ileus, mucositis, rectal disorder, stomatitis, ulcerative stomatitis, and veno-occlusive liver disease.

Hemic & Lymphatic System: Anemia, coagulation disorder, ecchymosis, fluid overload, petechia, prothrombin decreased, prothrombin increased, and thrombocytopenia.

Metabolic & Nutritional Disorders: Acidosis, amylase increased, hyperchloremia, hyperkalemia, hypermagnesemia, hyperphosphatemia, hyponatremia, hypophosphatemia, hypoproteinemia, lactate dehydrogenase increased, nonprotein nitrogen (NPN) increased, and respiratory alkalosis.

Musculoskeletal System: Arthralgia, bone pain, dystonia, myalgia, and rigors.

Nervous System: Agitation, coma, convulsion, cough, depression, dysesthesia, dizziness, hallucinations, nervousness, paresthesia, somnolence, thinking abnormality, and tremor.

Respiratory System: Asthma, atelectasis, hemoptysis, hiccup, hyperventilation, influenza-like symptoms, lung edema, pharyngitis, pneumonia, respiratory insufficiency, respiratory failure, and sinusitis.

Skin & Appendages: Alopecia, dry skin, herpes simplex, injection site inflammation, maculopapular rash, purpura, skin discoloration, skin disorder, skin ulcer, urticaria, and vesiculobullous rash.

Special Senses: Conjunctivitis, dry eyes, and eye hemorrhage.

Urogenital System: Abnormal renal function, acute kidney failure, acute renal failure, dysuria, kidney failure, toxic nephropathy, urinary incontinence, and vaginal hemorrhage.

The following infrequent adverse experiences have been reported in postmarketing surveillance, in addition to those mentioned above: Angioedema, erythema, urticaria, cyanosis/hypoventilation, pulmonary edema, agranulocytosis, hemorrhagic cystitis.

CLINICAL LABORATORY VALUES

The effect of AmBisome on renal and hepatic function and on serum electrolytes was assessed from laboratory values measured repeatedly in Study 94-0-002. The frequency and magnitude of hepatic test abnormalities were similar in the AmBisome and amphotericin B groups. Nephrotoxicity was defined as creatinine values increasing 100% or more over pretreatment levels in pediatric patients, and creatinine values increasing 100% or more over pretreatment levels in adult patients provided the peak creatinine concentration was >1.2 mg/dl. Hypokalemia was defined as potassium levels ≤2.5 mmol/L any time during treatment.

Incidence of nephrotoxicity, mean peak serum creatinine concentration, mean change from baseline in serum creatinine, and incidence of hypokalemia in the double-blind randomized study were lower in the AmBisome group as summarized in TABLE 14.

TABLE 14 *Study 94-0-002 Laboratory Evidence of Nephrotoxicity*

	AmBisome	Amphotericin B
Total number of patients receiving at least 1 dose of study drug	343	344
Nephrotoxicity	64 (18.7%)	116 (33.7%)
Mean peak creatinine	1.24 mg/dl	1.52 mg/dl
Mean change from baseline in creatinine	0.48 mg/dl	0.77 mg/dl
Hypokalemia	23 (6.7%)	40 (11.6%)

In empirical therapy study 97-0-034, the incidence of nephrotoxicity as measured by increases of serum creatinine from baseline was significantly lower for patients administered AmBisome (individual dose groups and combined) compared with amphotericin B lipid complex.

The incidence of nephrotoxicity in Study 94-0-013, comparative trial in cryptococcal meningitis was lower in the AmBisome groups as shown in TABLE 16.

DOSAGE AND ADMINISTRATION

AmBisome should be administered by IV infusion, using a controlled infusion device, over a period of approximately 120 minutes.

An inline membrane filter may be used for the IV infusion of AmBisome; provided **THE MEAN PORE DIAMETER OF THE FILTER IS NOT LESS THAN 1.0 MICRON. Note: An existing IV line must be flushed with 5% dextrose injection prior to infusion of AmBisome. If this is not feasible, AmBisome must be administered through a separate line.**

TABLE 15 *Incidence of Nephrotoxicity*

Empirical Therapy Study 97-0-034

	AmBisome			Amphotericin B Lipid Complex
	3 mg/kg/day	5 mg/kg/day	BOTH	5 mg/kg/day
Total number of patients	85	81	166	78
Number With Nephrotoxicity				
1.5 × baseline serum creatinine value	25 (29.4%)	21 (25.9%)	46 (27.7%)	49 (62.8%)
2 × baseline serum creatinine value	12 (14.1%)	12 (14.8%)	24 (14.5%)	33 (42.3%)

TABLE 16 *Laboratory Evidence of Nephrotoxicity Study 94-0-013*

	AmBisome		
	3 mg/kg/day	5 mg/kg/day	Amphotericin B
Total number of patients at least 1 dose of study drug	86	94	87
Number With Nephrotoxicity			
1.5 × baseline serum creatinine	30 (35%)	44 (47%)	52 (60%)
2 × baseline serum creatinine	12 (14%)	20 (21%)	29 (33%)

Infusion time may be reduced to approximately 60 minutes in patients in whom the treatment is well-tolerated. If the patient experiences discomfort during infusion, the duration of infusion may be increased.

The recommended initial dose of AmBisome for each indication for adult and pediatric patients is listed in TABLE 17.

TABLE 17

Indication	Dose
Empirical therapy	3.0 mg/kg/day
Systemic fungal infections: *Aspergillus, Candida, Cryptococcus*	3.0 - 5.0 mg/kg/day
Cryptococcal meningitis in HIV infected patients	6.0 mg/kg/day

Dosing and rate of infusion should be individualized to the needs of the specific patient to ensure maximum efficacy while minimizing systemic toxicities or adverse events.

Doses recommended for visceral leishmaniasis are presented in TABLE 18.

TABLE 18

Visceral Leishmaniasis	Dose (mg/kg/day)
Immunocompetent patients	3.0 (days 1-5) and 3.0 on days 14, 21
Immunocompromised patients	4.0 (days 1-5) and 4.0 on days 10, 17, 24, 31, 38

For immunocompetent patients who do not achieve parasitic clearance with the recommended dose, a repeat course of therapy may be useful.

For immunocompromised patients who do not clear parasites or who experience relapses, expert advice regarding further treatment is recommended.

HOW SUPPLIED

AmBisome for injection is available in 50 mg vials.

STORAGE

Unopened vials of lyophilized material must be stored under refrigeration at 2-8°C (36-46°F).

Storage of Reconstituted Product Concentrate

The reconstituted product concentrate may be stored for up to 24 hours at 2-8°C (36-46°F) following reconstitution with sterile water for injection. Do not freeze.

Storage of Diluted Product

Injection of AmBisome should commence within 6 hours of dilution with 5% dextrose injection.

As with all parenteral drug products, the reconstituted AmBisome should be inspected visually for particulate matter and discoloration prior to administration, whenever solution and container permit. Do not use material if there is any evidence of precipitation or foreign matter. Aseptic technique must be strictly observed in all handling since no preservative or bacteriostatic agent is present in AmBisome or in the materials specified for reconstitution and dilution.

Amphotericin B; Cholesteryl Sulfate *(003399)*

Categories: Infection, fungal; Pregnancy Category B; FDA Approved 1997 Aug
Drug Classes: Antifungals
Brand Names: Amphotec
Foreign Brand Availability: Amphocil (Hong-Kong; Israel; Mexico; Philippines)

DESCRIPTION

Amphotericin B is a sterile, pyrogen-free, lyophilized powder for reconstitution and intravenous (IV) administration. Amphotec consists of a 1:1 (molar ratio) complex of amphotericin B and cholesteryl sulfate. Upon reconstitution, amphotericin forms a colloidal dispersion of microscopic disc-shaped particles.

Note: Liposomal encapsulation or incorporation into a lipid complex can substantially affect a drug's functional properties relative to those of the unencapsulated drug or non-lipid associated drug. In addition, different liposomal or lipid-complex products with a common active ingredient may vary from one another in the chemical composition and physical form of the lipid component. Such differences may affect the functional properties of these drug products.

Amphotericin B is an antifungal polyene antibiotic produced by a strain of *Streptomyces nodosus.*

Amphotericin B, which is the established name for [1R-(1*R**,3*S**,5*R**,6*R**,9*R**,11*R**,15*S**,16*R**,17*R**,18*S**,19*E*,21*E*,23*E*,25*E*,27*E*,29*E*,31*E*,33*R**,35*S**,36*R**,37*S**)]-33-[(3-Amino-3,6-dideoxy-β-D-mannopyranosyl)oxy]-1,3,5,6,9,11,17,37-octahydroxy-15,16,18-trimethyl-13-oxo-14,39-dioxabicyclo[33.3.1] nonatriaconta-19,21,23,25,27,29,31-heptaene-36-carboxylic acid.

The molecular formula of the drug is $C_{47}H_{73}NO_{17}$; its molecular weight is 924.10.

Amphotec is available in 50 and 100 mg single dose vials. Each 50 mg single dose vial contains amphotericin B, 50 mg; sodium cholesteryl sulfate, 26.4 mg; tromethamine, 5.64 mg; disodium edetate dihydrate, 0.372 mg; lactose monohydrate, 950 mg; and hydrochloric acid, qs, as a sterile, nonpyrogenic, lyophilized powder. Each 100 mg single dose vial contains amphotericin B, 100 mg; sodium cholesteryl sulfate, 52.8 mg; tromethamine, 11.28 mg; disodium edetate dihydrate, 0.744 mg; lactose monohydrate, 1900 mg; and hydrochloric acid, qs, as a sterile, nonpyrogenic, lyophilized powder.

CLINICAL PHARMACOLOGY

MICROBIOLOGY

Mechanism of Action

Amphotericin B is a polyene antibiotic that acts by binding to sterols (primarily ergosterol) in cell membranes of sensitive fungi, with subsequent leakage of intracellular contents and cell death due to changes in membrane permeability. Amphotericin B also binds to the sterols (primarily cholesterol) in mammalian cell membranes, which is believed to account for its toxicity in animals and humans.

Activity In Vitro and In Vivo

Amphotericin B is active *in vitro* against *Aspergillus* and *Candida* species. One hundred and twelve (112) clinical isolates of four different *Aspergillus* species and 88 clinical isolates of five different *Candida* species were tested, with a majority of minimum inhibitory concentrations (MICs) <1 μg/ml. Amphotericin B is also active *in vitro* against other fungi. *In vitro,* amphotericin B is fungistatic or fungicidal, depending upon the concentration of the drug and the susceptibility of the fungal organism. However, standardized techniques for susceptibility testing for antifungal agents have not been established, and results of susceptibility studies do not necessarily correlate with clinical outcome.

Amphotericin B is active in murine models against *Aspergillus fumigatus, Candida albicans, Coccidioides immitis* and *Cryptococcus neoformans,* and in an immunosuppressed rabbit model of aspergillosis in which endpoints were prolonged survival of infected animals and clearance of microorganisms from target organ(s). Amphotericin B also was active in a hamster model of visceral leishmaniasis, a disease caused by infection of macrophages of the mononuclear phagocytic system by a protozoal parasite of the genus *Leishmania.* In this hamster model the endpoints were also prolonged survival of infected animals and clearance of microorganisms from target organ(s).

Drug Resistance

Variants with reduced susceptibility to amphotericin B have been isolated from several fungal species after serial passage in cell culture media containing the drug and from some patients receiving prolonged therapy with amphotericin B deoxycholate. Although the relevance of drug resistance to clinical outcome has not been established, fungal organisms that are resistant to amphotericin B may also be resistant to amphotericin B.

PHARMACOKINETICS

The pharmacokinetics of amphotericin B, administered as amphotericin B, were studied in 51 bone marrow transplant patients with systemic fungal infections. The median (range) age and weight of those patients were 32 (3-52) years and 69.5 (14-116) kg, respectively. Amphotericin B doses ranged from 0.5-8.0 mg/kg/day. The assay used in this study to measure amphotericin B in plasma does not distinguish amphotericin B that is complexed with cholesteryl sulfate from uncomplexed amphotericin B.

A population modeling approach was used to estimate pharmacokinetic parameters (see TABLE 1). The pharmacokinetics of amphotericin B, were best described by an open, two-compartment structural model. The pharmacokinetics of amphotericin B, administered as amphotericin B, were nonlinear. Steady state volume of distribution (Vss) and total plasma clearance (CLt) increased with escalating doses, resulting in less than proportional increases in plasma concentration over a dose range of 0.5-8.0 mg/kg/day. The increased volume of distribution probably reflected uptake by tissues. The covariates of body weight and dose level accounted for a substantial portion of the variability of the pharmacokinetic estimates between patients. The unexplained variability in clearance was 26%. Based on the population model developed for these patients, pharmacokinetic parameters were predicted for four doses of amphotericin B and are provided in the TABLE 1.

***TABLE 1** Predicted Pharmacokinetic Parameters of Amphotericin B after Administration of Multiple Doses of Amphotericin B**

Mean Pharmacokinetic Parameter†	Amphotericin B 3 mg/kg/day	Amphotericin B 4 mg/kg/day
Vss (L/kg)	3.8	4.1
CLt (L/h/kg)	0.105	0.112
Distribution Half-Life (minutes)	3.5	3.5
Elimination Half-Life (hours)	27.5	28.2
C_{max} (μg/ml)	2.6	2.9
AUCss (μg/ml·h)	29	36

* Data obtained using population modeling in 51 bone marrow transplant patients. The modeling assumes amphotericin B pharmacokinetics after administration of AMPHOTEC is best described by a 2-compartment model. Infusion rate = 1 mg/kg/hour.
† Definitions: Vss - Volume of distribution at steady state, CLt - Total plasma clearance, C_{max} - Maximum plasma concentration achieved at the end of an infusion, AUCss - Area under the plasma concentration time curve at steady-state.

In addition, the pharmacokinetics of amphotericin B, administered as amphotericin B deoxycholate, were studied in 15 patients in whom amphotericin B deoxycholate was administered for the treatment of aspergillus infections or empirical therapy. The median (range) age and weight for these patients were 21 (4-66) years and 60 (19-117) kg, respectively. A population modeling approach was used to estimate the pharmacokinetic parameters. The pharmacokinetics of amphotericin B, administered as amphotericin B deoxycholate, was best described as an open, two-compartment model with linear elimination.

The predicted pharmacokinetic parameters are provided in TABLE 2.

***TABLE 2** Predicted Pharmacokinetic Parameters of Amphotericin B after Administration of Multiple Doses of 1 mg/kg Amphotericin B Deoxycholate**

Mean Pharmacokinetic Parameter†	Values
Vss (L/kg)	1.1
CLt (L/h/kg)	0.028
Distribution Half-Life (minutes)	38
Elimination Half-Life (hours)	39
C_{max} (μg/ml)	2.9
AUCss (μg/ml·h)	36

* Data obtained using population modeling in 15 patients in whom amphotericin B deoxycholate was administered for treatment of aspergillus infection or empiric therapy. The modeling assumes amphotericin B pharmacokinetics after administration of amphotericin B deoxycholate are best described by a 2-compartment model. Infusion rate = 0.25 mg/kg/hour.
† Definitions: Vss - Volume of distribution at steady state, CLt - Total plasma clearance, C_{max} - Maximum plasma concentration achieved at the end of an infusion, AUCss - Area under the plasma concentration time curve at steady-state.

An analytical assay that is able to distinguish between amphotericin B in the Amphotec complex and amphotericin B which is not complexed to cholesteryl sulfate was used to analyze samples from a study of 25 patients who were either immunocompromised with aspergillosis or both febrile and neutropenic. Following a 1 mg/kg/hour infusion, 25 ± 18% (mean ±SD) of the total amphotericin B concentration measured in plasma was in the Amphotec complex, dropping to 9.3 ± 7.9% at 1 hour and 7.5 ± 9.3% at 24 hours after the end of the infusion.

PHARMACOKINETICS IN SPECIAL POPULATIONS

A population modeling approach was used to assess the effect of renal function, hepatic function, and age on the pharmacokinetics of amphotericin B in 51 patients receiving bone marrow transplants as described earlier.

Renal Impairment

The pharmacokinetics of amphotericin B were not related to baseline serum creatinine clearance in the population studied; the median (range) creatinine clearance for this population was 74.0 (range: 35-202) ml/min/70 kg. The effect of more severe renal impairment on the pharmacokinetics of amphotericin B has not been studied.

Hepatic Impairment

The pharmacokinetics of amphotericin B were not related to baseline liver function, as determined by liver enzymes and total bilirubin. For the population tested, the mean ±SD values for AST and total bilirubin were 59.4 ± 70.0 IU/ml and 3.5 ± 3.7 mg/dl, respectively. The effect of more severe hepatic impairment on the pharmacokinetics of amphotericin B has not been studied.

Age

The pharmacokinetics of amphotericin B were not related to the age of the patient. The median (range) age for the population in this study was 32 (3-52) years.

INDICATIONS AND USAGE

Amphotericin B is indicated for the treatment of invasive aspergillosis in patients where renal impairment or unacceptable toxicity precludes the use of amphotericin B deoxycholate in effective doses, and in patients with invasive aspergillosis where prior amphotericin B deoxycholate therapy has failed.

NON-FDA APPROVED INDICATIONS

Amphotericin B cholesteryl sulfate has also been used to treat other invasive fungal infections in immunosuppressed patients, as empirical therapy in patients with neutropenia and fever, and as treatment of visceral leishmaniasis.

CONTRAINDICATIONS

Amphotericin B should not be administered to patients who have documented hypersensitivity to any of its components, unless, in the opinion of the physician, the advantages of using amphotericin B outweigh the risks of hypersensitivity.

WARNINGS

Anaphylaxis has been reported with amphotericin B deoxycholate and other amphotericin B-containing drugs. Immediate treatment of anaphylaxis or anaphylactoid reactions is required. Epinephrine, oxygen, intravenous steroids, and airway management should be administered as indicated. If severe respiratory distress occurs, the infusion should be immediately discontinued. The patient should not receive further infusions of amphotericin B.

PRECAUTIONS

GENERAL

Amphotericin B should be administered intravenously. Acute infusion-related reactions including fever, chills, hypoxia, hypotension, nausea, or tachypnea, may occur 1 to 3 hours after starting intravenous infusion. These reactions are usually more sever or more frequent with the initial doses of amphotericin B and usually diminish with subsequent doses. Acute infusion-related reactions can be managed by pretreatment with antihistamines and corticosteroids and/or by reducing the rate of infusion and by prompt administration of antihistamines and corticosteroids. (See ADVERSE REACTIONS.)

Rapid intravenous infusion should be avoided.

LABORATORY TESTS

particularly tests of renal and hepatic function, serum electrolytes, complete blood count and prothrombin time should be monitored as medically indicated.

CARCINOGENESIS, MUTAGENESIS, AND IMPAIRMENT OF FERTILITY

No long-term studies in animals have been performed with amphotericin B or amphotericin B deoxycholate to evaluate carcinogenic potential. Amphotericin B and/or amphotericin B deoxycholate were not mutagenic *in vitro* with and without an exogenous mammalian microsomal metabolic activation system when assayed in the *Salmonella* reverse mutation assay, the CHO chromosomal aberration assay and the mouse lymphoma forward mutation assay. Amphotericin B was also negative *in vivo* in the mouse bone marrow micronucleus assay. No studies have been conducted to determine if amphotericin B affects fertility or if it produces adverse effects when administered peri- or post-natally in animals. In multiple dose toxicity studies of up to 13 weeks in rats at doses up to 0.5 times the recommended human dose and in dogs at doses up to 0.4 times the recommended human dose (based on body surface area), ovarian and testicular histology were unaffected.

PREGNANCY, TERATOGENIC EFFECTS, PREGNANCY CATEGORY B

There are no reports of pregnant women having been treated with amphotericin B. Reproductive studies with amphotericin B in rats at doses up to 0.4 times the recommended human dose and in rabbits at doses up to 1.1 times the recommended human dose have revealed no evidence of harm to the fetus due to treatment with amphotericin B. Because animal reproduction studies are not always predictive of human response and because adequate and well controlled studies have not been conducted in pregnant women, amphotericin B should be used during pregnancy only if the anticipated benefit to the patient outweighs the potential risk to the fetus.

NURSING MOTHERS

It is not known whether amphotericin B is excreted in milk. Because of the potential for serious adverse reactions in nursing infants from amphotericin B, a decision should be made to discontinue nursing or discontinue treatment with amphotericin B, taking into account the importance of the drug to the mother.

PEDIATRIC USE

Ninety-seven (97) pediatric patients with systemic fungal infections have been treated with amphotericin B, at daily doses (mg/kg) similar to those given to adults. No unexpected adverse events have been reported. In the same empiric, multicenter trial, pediatric patients (<16 years) treated with amphotericin B had significantly less renal toxicity than amphotericin B deoxycholate patients. Only 12% (3/25) of pediatric patients treated with amphotericin B developed nephrotoxicity compared to 52% (11/21) of pediatric patients receiving amphotericin B deoxycholate. Renal toxicity defined as either a doubling or an increase of 1.0 mg/dl or more from baseline serum creatinine, or ≥50% decrease from baseline calculated creatinine clearance.

GERIATRIC USE

Sixty-eight (68) patients at least 65 years of age have been treated with amphotericin B. No unexpected adverse events have been reported.

DRUG INTERACTIONS

No formal drug interaction studies have been conducted with amphotericin B. When administered concomitantly, the following drugs are known to interact with amphotericin B; therefore the following drugs may interact with Amphotec.

Corticosteroids and Corticotropin (ACTH): Concurrent use of corticosteroids and corticotropin (ACTH) with amphotericin B may potentiate hypokalemia which could predispose the patient to cardiac dysfunction. If corticosteroids or corticotropin are used concomitantly with amphotericin B, serum electrolytes and cardiac function should be monitored.

Cyclosporine and Tacrolimus: In the same randomized, double-blind, empiric trial to compare amphotericin B and amphotericin B deoxycholate, patients with normal baseline serum creatinine were prospectively enrolled into four strata: adults receiving cyclosporine or tacrolimus (n=89); or pediatric patients (<16 years old) receiving cyclosporine or tacrolimus (n=15); adults not receiving cyclosporine or tacrolimus (n=75); or pediatric patients not receiving cyclosporine or tacrolimus (n=34). Patients were assessed for renal toxicity defined as either a doubling or an increase of 1.0 mg/dl or more from baseline serum creatinine, or ≥50% decrease from baseline calculated creatinine clearance. Adults and pediatric patients receiving cyclosporine or tacrolimus in addition to amphotericin B had a significantly lower rate of renal toxicity (31%, 16/51), compared to the amphotericin B deoxycholate patients receiving cyclosporine or tacrolimus (68%, 34/50). In the adults and pediatric patients not receiving cyclosporine or tacrolimus, only 8% (4/51) of the amphotericin B patients experienced renal toxicity compared to 35% (17/49) of the amphotericin B deoxycholate patients.

Digitalis Glycosides: Concurrent use of amphotericin B may induce hypokalemia and may potentiate digitalis toxicity. If digitalis glycosides are administered concomitantly with amphotericin B, serum potassium levels should be closely monitored.

Flucytosine: Concurrent use of flucytosine with amphotericin B-containing preparations may increase the toxicity of flucytosine by possibly increasing its cellular uptake and/or impairing its renal excretion. Caution is urged when flucytosine is given concomitantly with amphotericin B.

Imidazoles (e.g., Ketoconazole, Miconazole, Clotrimazole, Fluconazole, etc.): Antagonism between amphotericin B and imidazole derivatives such as miconazole and ketoconazole which inhibit ergosterol synthesis, has been reported in both *in vitro* and *in vivo* animal studies. The clinical significance of these findings has not been determined.

Other Nephrotoxic Medications: Concurrent use of amphotericin B and agents such as aminoglycosides and pentamidine may enhance the potential for drug-induced renal toxicity. Caution is urged if aminoglycosides or pentamidine are used concomitantly with amphotericin B. Intensive monitoring of renal function is recommended in patients requiring any combination of nephrotoxic medications.

Skeletal Muscle Relaxants: Amphotericin B-induced hypokalemia may enhance the curariform effect of skeletal muscle relaxants (*e.g.,* tubocurarine) due to hypokalemia. If skeletal muscle relaxants are administered concomitantly with amphotericin B, serum potassium levels should be closely monitored.

ADVERSE REACTIONS

The following adverse events are based on the experience of 572 amphotericin B patients from 5 open studies of patients with systemic fungal infections, of whom 526 were treated with a daily dose of 3-6 mg/kg. Additionally, comparative adverse event data from 150 amphotericin B (4 or 6 mg/kg/day) and 146 amphotericin B deoxycholate (0.8 or 1 mg/kg/day) patients in prospectively randomized double-blinded studies of empiric treatment of febrile and neutropenic patients or treatment of aspergillosis are also provided.

INFUSION-RELATED ADVERSE EVENTS

Infusion-related adverse events (1-3 hours after starting intravenous infusion) occurred most frequently in association with the first infusion of amphotericin B. Their frequency and severity decreased with subsequent dosing. Based on the combined non-comparative studies, 35% (197/569) of the patients reported chills or chills and fever, possibly or probably related to amphotericin B, on the first day of dosing, compared to 14% (58/422) by the seventh dose. In the comparative studies, a similar decreasing trend was noted for amphotericin B and amphotericin B deoxycholate.

Adverse events that were considered to be possibly or probably related to amphotericin B and that occurred in 5% or more of the patients are summarized in TABLE 4.

Additionally, the following adverse events also occurred in 5% or more of amphotericin B patients; however, the causal relationship of these adverse events is uncertain:

Cardiovascular System: Cardiovascular disorder, hemorrhage, postural hypotension.

Digestive System: Diarrhea, dry mouth, hematemesis, jaundice, stomatitis.

Hemic and Lymphatic System: Anemia, coagulation disorder, prothrombin decreased.

Metabolic and Nutritional Disorders: Edema, generalized edema, hypocalcemia, hypophosphatemia, peripheral edema, weight gain.

Nervous System: Confusion, dizziness, insomnia, somnolence, thinking abnormal, tremor.

Respiratory System: Apnea, asthma, cough increased, epistaxis, hyperventilation, lung disorder, rhinitis.

Skin and Appendages: Maculopapular rash, pruritus, rash, sweating.

Special Senses: Eye hemorrhage.

Urogenital: Hematuria.

The following adverse events occurred in 1% to less than 5% of amphotericin B patients. The causal association between these adverse events and amphotericin B is uncertain.

General (body as a whole): Accidental injury, allergic reaction, asthenia, death, hypothermia, immune system disorder, infection, injection site pain, injection site reaction, neck pain.

Cardiovascular System: Arrhythmia, atrial fibrillation, bradycardia, congestive heart failure, heart arrest, phlebitis, shock, supraventricular tachycardia, syncope, vasodilatation, venoocclusive liver disease, ventricular extrasystoles.

TABLE 4 *Summary of Probably and Possibly Related Adverse Events Reported by ≥5% of Amphotericin B Patients*

	Non-Comparative Studies		Comparative Studies*	
Adverse Event	Amphotericin B (n=572) %	Amphotericin B Aspergillosis Patients (n=161) %	Amphotericin B (n=150) %	Amphotericin B Deoxycholate (n=146) %
Body as a Whole				
Chills	50%	55%	77%	56%
Fever	33%	34%	55%	47%
Headache	5%	8%	4%	3%
Chills and fever	3%	3%	7%	2%
Cardiovascular System				
Hypotension	10%	9%	12%	5%
Tachycardia	10%	12%	9%	5%
Hypertension	7%	9%	7%	6%
Digestive System				
Nausea	8%	12%	7%	7%
Nausea and vomiting	7%	11%	4%	7%
Vomiting	6%	8%	11%	8%
Liver function test abnormal	4%	4%	11%	8%
Hemic and Lymphatic System				
Thrombocytopenia	6%	7%	1%	1%
Metabolic/Nutritional Disorders				
Creatinine increased†	12%	12%	21%	34%
Hypokalemia	8%	7%	26%	29%
Hypomagnesemia	4%	7%	6%	11%
Hyperbilirubinemia	3%	2%	19%	17%
Alkaline phosphatase increased	3%	3%	7%	8%
Hyperglycemia	1%	1%	6%	9%
Respiratory System				
Dyspnea	5%	4%	9%	4%
Hypoxia	5%	6%	9%	5%

* From amphotericin B (4 or 6 mg/kg/day) and amphotericin B deoxycholate (0.8 or 1 mg/kg/day) patients in prospectively randomized double-blinded studies of empiric treatment of febrile and neutropenic patients or treatment of first-line aspergillosis, respectively.
† Includes patients with "kidney function abnormal" which was associated with an increase in creatinine.

Digestive System: Anorexia, bloody diarrhea, constipation, dyspepsia, fecal incontinence, gamma glutamyl transpeptidase increased, gastrointestinal disorder, gastrointestinal hemorrhage, gingivitis, glossitis, hepatic failure, melena, mouth ulceration, oral moniliasis, rectal disorder.

Hemic and Lymphatic system: Ecchymosis, fibrinogen increased, hypochromic anemia, leukocytosis, leukopenia, petechia, thromboplastin decreased.

Metabolic and Nutritional Disorders: Acidosis, BUN increased, dehydration, hyponatremia, hyperkalemia, hyperlipemia, hypernatremia, hypervolemia, hypoglycemia, hypoproteinemia, lactic dehydrogenase increased, AST (SGOT) increased, ALT (SGPT) increased, weight loss.

Musculoskeletal System: Arthralgia, myalgia.

Nervous System: Agitation, anxiety, convulsion, depression, hallucinations, hypertonia, nervousness, neuropathy, paresthesia, psychosis, speech disorder, stupor.

Respiratory System: Hemoptysis, lung edema, pharyngitis, pleural effusion, respiratory disorder, sinusitis.

Skin and Appendages: Acne, alopecia, petechial rash, skin discoloration, skin disorder, skin nodule, skin ulcer, urticaria, vesiculobullous rash.

Special Senses: Amblyopia, deafness, ear disorder, tinnitus.

Urogenital System: Albuminuria, dysuria, glycosuria, kidney failure, oliguria, urinary incontinence, urinary retention, urinary tract disorder.

DOSAGE AND ADMINISTRATION

The recommended dose for adults and pediatric patients is 3-4 mg/kg as required, once a day.

Amphotericin B, reconstituted in Sterile Water for Injection, is administered diluted in 5% Dextrose for Injection by intravenous infusion at a rate of 1 mg/kg/hour. A test dose immediately preceding the first dose is advisable when commencing all new courses of treatment. A small amount of drug (*e.g.,* 10 ml of the final preparation containing between 1.6-8.3 mg) should be infused over 15-30 minutes and the patient carefully observed for the next 30 minutes.

The infusion time may be shortened to a minimum of 2 hours for patients who show no evidence of intolerance or infusion-related reactions. If the patient experiences acute reactions or cannot tolerate the infusion volume, the infusion time may be extended.

DIRECTIONS FOR RECONSTITUTION AND PREPARATION OF INFUSION ADMIXTURE

Amphotericin B must be reconstituted by addition of sterile water for injection. Using sterile syringe and a 20-gauge needle, rapidly add the following volumes to the vial to provide a liquid containing 5 mg of amphotericin B per ml. Shake gently by hand, rotating the vial until all solids have dissolved. Note that the fluid may be opalescent or clear. For the 50 mg/vial add 10 ml sterile water for injection. For the 100 mg/vial add 20 ml sterile water for injection.

For infusion, further dilute the reconstituted liquid to a final concentration of approximately 0.6 mg/ml (range 0.16 mg/ml to 0.83 mg/ml). TABLE 5 provides dilution recommendations.

Do not reconstitute the lyophilized powder with saline or dextrose solutions, or admix the reconstituted liquid with saline or electrolytes. The use of any solution other than those recommended, or the presence of a bacteriostatic agent (*e.g.,* benzyl alcohol) in the solution may cause precipitation of amphotericin B. **Do not filter or use an in-line filter with amphotericin B.**

TABLE 5

Dose of Amphotec	Volume of Reconstituted Aamphotec	Infusion Bag Size for 5% Dextrose for Injection
10-35 mg	2-7 ml	50 ml
35-70 mg	7-14 ml	100 ml
70-175 mg	14-35 ml	250 ml
175-350 mg	35-70 ml	500 ml
350-1000 mg	70-200 ml	1000 ml

Do not mix the infusion admixture with other drugs. If administered through an existing intravenous line, flush with 5% Dextrose for Injection prior to, and following, infusion of amphotericin B, otherwise administer via a separate line.

Parenteral drug products should be inspected visually for particulate matter and discoloration prior to administration whenever solution and container permit. Do not use if a precipitate or foreign matter is present, or if the seal is not intact. Strict aseptic technique always should be observed during reconstitution and dilution since no preservatives are present in the lyophilized drug or in the solutions used for reconstitution and dilution.

After reconstitution, the drug should be refrigerated at 2-8°C (36-46°F) and used within 24 hours. **Do not freeze.** After further dilution with 5% dextrose for injection, the infusion should be stored in a refrigerator (2-8°C) and used within 24 hours. Partially used vials should be discarded.

HOW SUPPLIED

Amphotec Cholesteryl Sulfate Complex for Injection is a sterile lyophilized powder supplied in single use glass vials. Each vial is individually packaged.

Storage: Store unopened vials of amphotericin B at 15-30°C (59-86°F). Amphotericin B should be retained in the carton until time of use.

PRODUCT LISTING - EQUIVALENTS NOT AVAILABLE

Powder For Injection - Intravenous - 50 mg

1's	$84.00	AMPHOTEC, Sequus Pharmaceuticals Inc	61471-0115-12
1's	$93.33	AMPHOTEC, Intermune Pharmaceuticals	64116-0025-01

Powder For Injection - Intravenous - 100 mg

1's	$160.00	AMPHOTEC, Sequus Pharmaceuticals Inc	61471-0110-12
1's	$160.00	AMPHOTEC, Intermune Pharmaceuticals	64116-0021-01

A

Ampicillin (000239)

For related information, see the comparative table section in Appendix A.

Categories: Gonorrhea; Infection, ear, middle; Infection, gastrointestinal tract; Infection, lower respiratory tract; Infection, sinus; Infection, upper respiratory tract; Pregnancy Category B; FDA Approval Pre 1982

Drug Classes: Antibiotics, penicillins

Brand Names: Ampicillin; Marcillin; Pfizerpen; **Principen**; Totacillin

Foreign Brand Availability: Aldribid (Philippines); Aletmicina (Argentina); Alphacin (Australia; New-Zealand); Amcillin (Indonesia; Thailand); Amfipen (Bahrain; Cyprus; Egypt; England; Iran; Iraq; Ireland; Israel; Jordan; Kuwait; Lebanon; Libya; Oman; Qatar; Republic-of-Yemen; Saudi-Arabia; Syria; United-Arab-Emirates); Amipenix (Japan); Ampecu (Ecuador); Ampenolet (Greece); Ampex (Indonesia); Ampexin (Malaysia); Ampibex (Colombia); Ampiblan (Colombia); Ampicher (Ecuador); Ampicilina (Ecuador); Ampicin (Canada; Philippines); Ampiclox (Singapore); Ampicyn (Taiwan); Ampidar (Bahrain; Cyprus; Egypt; Iran; Iraq; Israel; Jordan; Kuwait; Lebanon; Libya; Oman; Qatar; Republic-of-Yemen; Saudi-Arabia; Syria; United-Arab-Emirates); Ampifen (Netherlands); Ampiflex (Peru); Ampilag (Bahamas; Barbados; Belize; Benin; Bermuda; Burkina-Faso; Curacao; Ethiopia; Gambia; Ghana; Guinea; Guyana; Ivory-Coast; Jamaica; Kenya; Liberia; Malawi; Mali; Mauritania; Mauritius; Morocco; Netherland-Antilles; Niger; Nigeria; Puerto-Rico; Senegal; Seychelles; Sierra-Leone; South-Africa; Sudan; Surinam; Tanzania; Trinidad; Tunia; Uganda; Zambia; Zimbabwe); Ampilin (India); Ampillin (Malaysia); Ampipen (India; South-Africa); Ampivral (Colombia); Ampliblan (Colombia); Amplibin (Peru); Ampolin (Taiwan); Amsapen (Mexico); Anglopen (Mexico); Apo-Ampi (Canada); Binotal (Austria; Colombia; Ecuador; Germany; Mexico; Peru); Bremcillin (Indonesia); Bridopen (Philippines); Britapen (Spain); Camicil (Benin; Burkina-Faso; Ethiopia; Gambia; Ghana; Guinea; Ivory-Coast; Kenya; Liberia; Malawi; Mali; Mauritania; Mauritius; Morocco; Niger; Nigeria; Senegal; Seychelles; Sierra-Leone; South-Africa; Sudan; Tanzania; Tunia; Uganda; Zambia; Zimbabwe); Cimexillin (Switzerland); Citicil (Italy); Deripen (Ecuador); Dhacillin (Hong-Kong; Malaysia); Diferin (Mexico); Doltirol (Argentina); Dotirol (Peru); Duacillin (Malaysia); Eracillin (Thailand); Excillin (Philippines); Extrapen (Bahrain; Benin; Burkina-Faso; Cyprus; Egypt; Ethiopia; Gambia; Ghana; Guinea; Iran; Iraq; Israel; Ivory-Coast; Jordan; Kenya; Kuwait; Lebanon; Liberia; Libya; Malawi; Mali; Mauritania; Mauritius; Morocco; Niger; Nigeria; Oman; Qatar; Republic-of-Yemen; Saudi-Arabia; Senegal; Seychelles; Sierra-Leone; South-Africa; Sudan; Syria; Tanzania; Tunia; Uganda; United-Arab-Emirates; Zambia; Zimbabwe); H-Ambiotico (Colombia); Hostes (Argentina); Ikacillin (Indonesia); Intramed (South-Africa); Iwacillin (Japan); Jenampin (Germany); Julphapen (Peru); Magnapen (Peru); Marticil (Philippines); Maxipen (Colombia); Mecil-N (Philippines); Novo-Ampicillin (Canada); Nuvapen (Spain); Omnipen (Bahrain; Cyprus; Ecuador; Egypt; Iran; Iraq; Israel; Jordan; Kuwait; Lebanon; Libya; Mexico; Oman; Qatar; Republic-of-Yemen; Saudi-Arabia; Syria; United-Arab-Emirates); Pamecil (Benin; Burkina-Faso; Ethiopia; Gambia; Ghana; Guinea; Hong-Kong; Ivory-Coast; Kenya; Liberia; Malawi; Malaysia; Mali; Mauritania; Mauritius; Morocco; Niger; Nigeria; Senegal; Seychelles; Sierra-Leone; South-Africa; Sudan; Tanzania; Tunia; Uganda; Zambia; Zimbabwe); Panacta (Singapore); Penbritin (Bahamas; Bahrain; Barbados; Belgium; Belize; Benin; Bermuda; Burkina-Faso; Curacao; Cyprus; Ecuador; Egypt; England; Ethiopia; Gambia; Ghana; Guinea; Guyana; Hong-Kong; Indonesia; Iran; Iraq; Ireland; Israel; Ivory-Coast; Jamaica; Jordan; Kenya; Kuwait; Lebanon; Liberia; Libya; Malawi; Malaysia; Mali; Mauritania; Mauritius; Mexico; Morocco; Netherland-Antilles; Niger; Nigeria; Oman; Peru; Philippines; Puerto-Rico; Qatar; Republic-of-Yemen; Saudi-Arabia; Senegal; Seychelles; Sierra-Leone; South-Africa; Sudan; Surinam; Syria; Tanzania; Trinidad; Tunia; Uganda; United-Arab-Emirates; Zambia; Zimbabwe); Penodil (Bahamas; Barbados; Belize; Bermuda; Curacao; Guyana; Jamaica; Netherland-Antilles; Puerto-Rico; Surinam; Trinidad); Penstabil (Germany); Pentrexyl (Belgium; Benin; Burkina-Faso; Denmark; Ecuador; England; Ethiopia; Gambia; Ghana; Greece; Guinea; Hong-Kong; Israel; Ivory-Coast; Kenya; Liberia; Malawi; Mali; Mauritania; Mauritius; Mexico; Morocco; Niger; Nigeria; Peru; Senegal; Seychelles; Sierra-Leone; South-Africa; Sudan; Tanzania; Thailand; Tunia; Uganda; Zambia; Zimbabwe); Petercillin (South-Africa); Pricillin (Singapore); Primapen (Indonesia); Radiocillina (Bahrain; Benin; Burkina-Faso; Cyprus; Egypt; Ethiopia; Gambia; Ghana; Guinea; Iran; Iraq; Israel; Ivory-Coast; Jordan; Kenya; Kuwait; Lebanon; Liberia; Libya; Malawi; Mali; Mauritania; Mauritius; Morocco; Niger; Nigeria; Oman; Qatar; Republic-of-Yemen; Saudi-Arabia; Senegal; Seychelles; Sierra-Leone; South-Africa; Sudan; Syria; Tanzania; Tunia; Uganda; United-Arab-Emirates; Zambia; Zimbabwe); Rimacillin (Bahamas; Bahrain; Barbados; Belize; Benin; Bermuda; Burkina-Faso; Curacao; Cyprus; Egypt; Ethiopia; Gambia; Ghana; Guinea; Guyana; Iran; Iraq; Israel; Ivory-Coast; Jamaica; Jordan; Kenya; Kuwait; Lebanon; Liberia; Libya; Malawi; Mali; Mauritania; Mauritius; Morocco; Netherland-Antilles; Niger; Nigeria; Oman; Puerto-Rico; Qatar; Republic-of-Yemen; Saudi-Arabia; Senegal; Seychelles; Sierra-Leone; South-Africa; Sudan; Surinam; Syria; Tanzania; Trinidad; Tunia; Uganda; United-Arab-Emirates; Zambia; Zimbabwe); Roscillin (India); Semicillin (Hungary); Shacillin (Bahrain; Cyprus; Egypt; Iran; Iraq; Jordan; Kuwait; Lebanon; Libya; Oman; Qatar; Republic-of-Yemen; Saudi-Arabia; Syria; United-Arab-Emirates); Sintelin (Peru); Standacillin (Bahrain; Cyprus; Egypt; Iran; Iraq; Israel; Jordan; Kuwait; Lebanon; Libya; Oman; Qatar; Republic-of-Yemen; Saudi-Arabia; Syria; United-Arab-Emirates); Synthocilin (India); Tolimal (Argentina); Totapen (France); Tricil (Benin; Burkina-Faso; Ethiopia; Gambia; Ghana; Guinea; Ivory-Coast; Kenya; Liberia; Malawi; Mali; Mauritania; Mauritius; Morocco; Niger; Nigeria; Senegal; Seychelles; Sierra-Leone; Sudan; Tanzania; Tunia; Uganda; Zambia; Zimbabwe); Trifalicina (Argentina); Trihypen (Thailand); Trilaxin (Philippines); Vacillin (Thailand); Viccillin (Indonesia); Vidopen (England; Ireland); Virucil (Colombia); Vitapen (Israel)

Cost of Therapy: $80.16 (Infection; Omnipen-N Powder for Injection; 1000 mg; 2 g/day; 14 day supply)
$42.00 (Infection; Generic Powder for Injection; 1000 mg; 2 g/day; 14 day supply)

HCFA JCODE(S): J0290 up to 500 mg IM, IV

DESCRIPTION

Ampicillin is a semisynthetic penicillin derived from the basic penicillin nucleus, 6-aminopenicillanic acid.

Ampicillin capsules contain 250 or 500 mg ampicillin. The inactive ingredients are magnesium stearate and FD&C yellow no. 6.

Ampicillin for oral suspension is a powder that; when reconstituted as directed, yields a suspension of 125 or 250 mg ampicillin per 5 ml. The inactive ingredients are FD&C red 3, flavoring, silica gel, sodium benzoate, sodium citrate, sucrose, and xanthan gum.

CLINICAL PHARMACOLOGY

MICROBIOLOGY

Ampicillin is similar to benzyl penicillin in its bactericidal action against sensitive organisms during the stage of active multiplication. It acts through the inhibition of biosynthesis of cell wall mucopeptide. Ampicillin differs *in vitro* spectrum. It exerts high *in vitro* activity against many strains of *Haemophilus influenzae, Neisseria gonorrhoeae, Neisseria meningitidis, Neisseria catarrhalis, Escherichia coli, Proteus mirabilis, Bacteroides funduliformis,* and *Salmonella* and *Shigella* organisms.

In vitro studies have also demonstrated the sensitivity of many strains of the following gram-positive bacteria: alpha-hemolytic *streptococci, Diplococcus pneumoniae,* nonpenicillinase-producing staphylococci, *Bacillus anthracis,* and most strains of enterococci and clostridia. Ampicillin generally provides less *in vitro* activity than penicillin G does against gram-positive bacteria. Because it does not resist destruction by penicillinase, it is not effective against penicillin-producing bacteria, particularly resistant staphylococci. All strains of *Pseudomonas* and most strains of *Klebsiella* and *Aerobacter* organisms are resistant.

PHARMACOKINETICS

Ampicillin is acid stable and therefore well absorbed. Food, however, retards absorption. Blood serum levels of approximately 2 μg/ml are attained within 1-2 hours following a 250 mg oral dose given to fasting adults. Detectable amounts persist for about 6 hours.

Ampicillin diffuses readily into all body tissues and fluids with the exception of brain and spinal fluid except when meninges are inflamed. Higher serum levels are obtained following IM injection. Most of the ampicillin is excreted unchanged in the urine; and this excretion can be delayed by concurrent administration of probenecid. The active form appears in the bile in higher concentrations than those found in the serum. Ampicillin is one of the least serum bound of all the penicillins; averaging about 20% compared to approximately 60-90% for other penicillins.

INDICATIONS AND USAGE

Ampicillin is indicated primarily in the treatment of infections due to susceptible strains of the following:

Gram-Negative Organisms: *Shigella, Salmonella* (including *S. typhosa*), *H. influenzae, E. coli, P. mirabilis, N. gonorrhoeae,* and *N. meningitidis.*

Gram-Positive Organisms: *Streptococci, S. pneumoniae,* and nonpenicillinase-producing staphylococci.

Because of its wide spectrum and bactericidal action, ampicillin may be useful in instituting therapy; however, bacteriologic studies to determine the causative organisms and their sensitivity to ampicillin should be performed.

NON-FDA APPROVED INDICATIONS

Although not approved by the FDA, ampicillin has been used for prophylaxis against group B streptococcal infections in obstetrical patients.

CONTRAINDICATIONS

A history of an allergic reaction to any of the penicillins is a contraindication.

WARNINGS

SERIOUS AND OCCASIONALLY FATAL HYPERSENSITIVITY (ANAPHYLACTOID) REACTIONS HAVE BEEN REPORTED IN PATIENTS ON PENICILLIN THERAPY. ALTHOUGH ANAPHYLAXIS IS MORE FREQUENT FOLLOWING PARENTERAL THERAPY, IT HAS OCCURRED IN PATIENTS ON ORAL PENICILLINS. THESE REACTIONS ARE MORE APT TO OCCUR IN INDIVIDUALS WITH A HISTORY OF SENSITIVITY TO MULTIPLE ALLERGENS. THERE HAVE BEEN REPORTS OF INDIVIDUALS WITH A HISTORY OF PENICILLIN HYPERSENSITIVITY WHO EXPERIENCED SEVERE REACTIONS WHEN TREATED WITH CEPHALOSPORINS. BEFORE THERAPY WITH A PENICILLIN, CAREFUL INQUIRY SHOULD BE MADE CONCERNING PREVIOUS HYPERSENSITIVITY REACTIONS TO PENICILLINS, CEPHALOSPORINS, AND OTHER ALLERGENS. IF AN ALLERGIC REACTION OCCURS, THE DRUG SHOULD BE DISCONTINUED AND THE APPROPRIATE THERAPY SHOULD BE INSTITUTED. SERIOUS ANAPHYLACTOID REACTIONS REQUIRE IMMEDIATE EMERGENCY TREATMENT WITH EPINEPHRINE. OXYGEN, INTRAVENOUS STEROIDS, AND AIRWAY MANAGEMENT, INCLUDING INTUBATION, SHOULD ALSO BE ADMINISTERED AS INDICATED.

USAGE IN PREGNANCY

Safety for use in pregnancy has not been established.

PRECAUTIONS

As with any antibiotic preparation, constant observation for signs of overgrowth of nonsusceptible organisms, including fungi, is essential. If superinfection should occur (usually involving *Aerobacter, Pseudomonas,* or *Candida* organisms), the drug should be discontinued and/or appropriate therapy instituted. As with any potent agent, it is advisable to check periodically for organ system dysfunction during prolonged therapy; this includes renal, hepatic, and hematopoietic systems. This is particularly important in premature infants, neonates, and other infants.

ADVERSE REACTIONS

As with other penicillins, it may be expected that untoward reactions will be essentially limited to sensitivity phenomena. These reactions are more likely to occur in individuals who have previously demonstrated hypersensitivity to penicillins and in those with a history of allergy, asthma, hay fever, or urticaria. The following adverse reactions have been reported as associated with the use of ampicillin:

Gastrointestinal: Glossitis, stomatitis, black "hairy" tongue, nausea, vomiting, enterocolitis, pseudomembranous colitis, and diarrhea. (These reactions are usually associated with oral dosage forms.)

Hypersensitivity Reactions: An erythematous maculopapular rash has been reported fairly frequently. Urticaria and erythema multiforme have been reported occasionally. A few cases of exfoliative dermatitis have been reported. Anaphylaxis is the most serious reaction experienced and has usually been associated with the parenteral dosage form.

Liver: A moderate rise in serum glutamic-oxaloacetic transaminase (SGOT) has been noted, particularly in infants, but the significance of this finding is unknown.

Hemic and Lymphatic Systems: Anemia, thrombocytopenia, thrombocytopenic purpura, eosinophilia, leukopenia, and agranulocytosis have been reported during therapy with the penicillins. These reactions are usually reversible on discontinuation of therapy and are believed to be sensitivity reactions.

Note: Urticaria, other skin rashes, and serum sickness-like reactions may be controlled with antihistamines and, if necessary, systemic corticosteroids. Whenever such reactions occur, ampicillin should be discontinued unless, in the opinion of the physician, the condition being treated is life-threatening and amenable only to ampicillin therapy.

DOSAGE AND ADMINISTRATION

INFECTIONS OF THE EAR, NOSE, AND THROAT

Infections of the ear, nose, throat, and lower respiratory tract due to streptococci, pneumococci, and nonpenicillinase-producing staphylococci and also those infections of the upper and lower respiratory tract due to *H. influenzae.*

Adults: 250 mg every 6 hours.

Children: 50 mg/kg/day in divided doses every 6 or 8 hours.

INFECTIONS OF THE GENITOURINARY TRACT CAUSED BY SENSITIVE GRAM-NEGATIVE AND GRAM-POSITIVE BACTERIA

Adults: 500 mg every 6 hours.
Larger doses may be required for severe infections.
Children: 100 mg/kg/day in divided doses every 6 hours.

UNCOMPLICATED URETHRITIS DUE TO N. GONORRHOEAE

Adult Males and Females: 3.5 g single oral dose administered simultaneously with 1 g of probenecid.
Cases of gonorrhea with a suspected lesion of syphilis should have dark-field examinations before receiving ampicillin and monthly serologic tests for a minimum of 4 months.

INFECTIONS OF THE GASTROINTESTINAL TRACT

Adults: 500 mg every 6 hours.
Children: 100 mg/kg/day in divided doses every 6 hours.
Larger doses may be required for stubborn or severe infections. The children's dosage is intended for individuals whose weight will not cause a dosage to be calculated greater than that recommended for adults. Children weighing more than 20 kg should be dosed according to the adult recommendations.

It should be recognized that in the treatment of chronic urinary tract and intestinal infections, frequent bacteriologic follow-up is required for several months after cessation of therapy.

Treatment should be continued for a minimum of 48-72 hours beyond the time that the patient becomes asymptomatic or evidence of bacterial eradication has been obtained. It is recommended that there be at least 10 days of treatment for any infection caused by hemolytic streptococci to help prevent the occurrence of acute rheumatic fever to glomerulonephritis.

DIRECTIONS FOR MIXING ORAL SUSPENSION

Prepare suspension at time of dispensing as follows: Tap bottle until all powder flows freely. Add approximately ½ of the total amount of water for reconstitution (see TABLE 1), and shake vigorously to wet powder. Add the remainder of the water and again shake vigorously.

TABLE 1

Bottle Size	Amount of Water Required for Reconstitution
125 mg/ 5 ml*	
100 ml	78 ml
200 ml	155 ml
250 mg/5 ml†	
100 ml	74 ml
200 ml	148 ml

* Each teaspoonful (5 ml) will contain 125 mg ampicillin.
† Each teaspoonful (5 ml) will contain 250 mg ampicillin.

SHAKE WELL BEFORE USING. Keep bottle tightly closed. Any unused portion of the reconstituted suspension must be discarded after 14 days under refrigeration.

PRODUCT LISTING - RATED THERAPEUTICALLY EQUIVALENT

Capsule - Oral - 250 mg

Qty	Price	Product	NDC
10's	$3.88	GENERIC, Pd-Rx Pharmaceuticals	55289-0023-10
20's	$6.25	GENERIC, Pd-Rx Pharmaceuticals	55289-0023-20
28's	$2.85	GENERIC, Circle Pharmaceuticals Inc	00659-0127-28
28's	$7.08	GENERIC, Pd-Rx Pharmaceuticals	55289-0023-28
30's	$5.75	GENERIC, Teva Pharmaceuticals Usa	00332-3111-04
30's	$7.50	GENERIC, Pd-Rx Pharmaceuticals	55289-0023-30
40's	$3.65	GENERIC, Circle Pharmaceuticals Inc	00659-0127-40
40's	$5.31	GENERIC, Golden State Medical	60429-0023-40
40's	$8.75	GENERIC, Pd-Rx Pharmaceuticals	55289-0023-40
40's	$22.10	GENERIC, Med-Pro Inc	53978-5018-06
100's	$5.95	GENERIC, Raway Pharmacal Inc	00686-3111-09
100's	$7.43	GENERIC, Vangard Labs	00615-0120-01
100's	$7.50	GENERIC, C.O. Truxton Inc	00463-5011-01
100's	$8.51	FEDERAL UPPER LIMIT, H.C.F.A. F F P	99999-0239-02
100's	$10.00	GENERIC, Raway Pharmacal Inc	00686-0602-20
100's	$11.00	GENERIC, Moore, H.L. Drug Exchange Inc	00839-5087-06
100's	$11.55	GENERIC, Interstate Drug Exchange Inc	00814-0720-14
100's	$11.75	GENERIC, Major Pharmaceuticals Inc	00904-2017-60
100's	$11.76	GENERIC, Mylan Pharmaceuticals Inc	00378-0115-01
100's	$11.76	GENERIC, Geneva Pharmaceuticals	00781-2555-01
100's	$11.93	GENERIC, Ivax Corporation	00182-0163-01
100's	$11.93	GENERIC, Teva Pharmaceuticals Usa	00332-3111-01
100's	$11.93	GENERIC, Qualitest Products Inc	00603-2290-21
100's	$12.11	GENERIC, Aligen Independent Laboratories Inc	00405-4089-01
100's	$18.55	GENERIC, Pd-Rx Pharmaceuticals	55289-0023-01
100's	$18.57	GENERIC, Bristol-Myers Squibb	00015-7992-65
100's	$18.85	GENERIC, Ivax Corporation	00182-0163-89
100's	$20.98	GENERIC, Bristol-Myers Squibb	00015-7992-68
100's	$21.11	GENERIC, Mova Pharmaceutical Corporation	55370-0880-07
100's	$23.46	GENERIC, Bristol-Myers Squibb	00003-0122-50
100's	$23.46	GENERIC, Teva Pharmaceuticals Usa	00093-5145-01

Capsule - Oral - 500 mg

Qty	Price	Product	NDC
4's	$6.20	GENERIC, Pd-Rx Pharmaceuticals	55289-0024-04
7's	$7.13	GENERIC, Pd-Rx Pharmaceuticals	55289-0024-07
10's	$8.05	GENERIC, Pd-Rx Pharmaceuticals	55289-0024-10
20's	$11.50	GENERIC, Pd-Rx Pharmaceuticals	55289-0024-20
25's	$16.25	GENERIC, Pd-Rx Pharmaceuticals	55289-0024-97
28's	$4.10	GENERIC, Circle Pharmaceuticals Inc	00659-0128-28
28's	$5.84	GENERIC, Pd-Rx Pharmaceuticals	55289-0033-28
28's	$13.53	GENERIC, Pd-Rx Pharmaceuticals	55289-0024-28
30's	$14.15	GENERIC, Pd-Rx Pharmaceuticals	55289-0024-30
40's	$5.20	GENERIC, Circle Pharmaceuticals Inc	00659-0128-40
40's	$7.54	GENERIC, Pd-Rx Pharmaceuticals	55289-0033-40
40's	$17.20	GENERIC, Pd-Rx Pharmaceuticals	55289-0024-40
40's	$32.60	GENERIC, Med-Pro Inc	53978-5019-06
100's	$10.95	GENERIC, Raway Pharmacal Inc	00686-3313-09
100's	$15.80	FEDERAL UPPER LIMIT, H.C.F.A. F F P	99999-0239-06
100's	$17.55	GENERIC, Raway Pharmacal Inc	00686-0603-20
100's	$19.44	GENERIC, Moore, H.L. Drug Exchange Inc	00839-5130-06
100's	$19.95	GENERIC, Major Pharmaceuticals Inc	00904-2073-60
100's	$20.80	GENERIC, Geneva Pharmaceuticals	00781-2999-01
100's	$20.85	GENERIC, Interstate Drug Exchange Inc	00814-0722-14
100's	$21.29	GENERIC, Mylan Pharmaceuticals Inc	00378-2116-01
100's	$21.29	GENERIC, Qualitest Products Inc	00603-2291-21
100's	$21.50	GENERIC, Ivax Corporation	00182-0641-01
100's	$22.00	GENERIC, Mylan Pharmaceuticals Inc	00378-0116-01
100's	$24.19	GENERIC, Aligen Independent Laboratories Inc	00405-4090-01
100's	$25.92	GENERIC, Marnel Pharmaceuticals Inc	00682-9113-01
100's	$32.00	GENERIC, Ivax Corporation	00182-0641-89
100's	$35.55	GENERIC, Bristol-Myers Squibb	00015-7993-68
100's	$35.89	GENERIC, Mova Pharmaceutical Corporation	55370-0881-07
100's	$39.88	GENERIC, Bristol-Myers Squibb	00003-0134-50
100's	$39.88	GENERIC, Teva Pharmaceuticals Usa	00093-5146-01

Powder For Injection - Injectable - 1 Gm

Qty	Price	Product	NDC
1's	$1.59	GENERIC, Bristol-Myers Squibb	00015-7404-20
1's	$1.71	GENERIC, Bristol-Myers Squibb	00015-7404-18
1's	$3.88	OMNIPEN-N, Wyeth-Ayerst Laboratories	00008-0315-04
1's	$4.76	OMNIPEN-N, Wyeth-Ayerst Laboratories	00008-0315-23
1's	$18.75	TOTACILLIN-N, Glaxosmithkline	00029-6610-40
10 each	$48.75	GENERIC, American Pharmaceutical Partners	63323-0389-10
10's	$14.88	TOTACILLIN-N, Glaxosmithkline	00029-6610-25
10's	$22.13	TOTACILLIN-N, Glaxosmithkline	00029-6610-21
10's	$23.60	GENERIC, Bristol-Myers Squibb	00015-7404-99
10's	$24.50	GENERIC, Bristol-Myers Squibb	00015-7404-36
10's	$24.50	GENERIC, Bristol-Myers Squibb	00015-7404-94
10's	$27.90	GENERIC, Bristol-Myers Squibb	00015-7404-89
10's	$48.50	GENERIC, Bristol-Myers Squibb	00015-7404-28
10's	$88.90	GENERIC, Bristol-Myers Squibb	00015-7404-29

Powder For Injection - Injectable - 2 Gm

Qty	Price	Product	NDC
1's	$2.45	GENERIC, Bristol-Myers Squibb	00015-7405-20
1's	$2.51	GENERIC, Bristol-Myers Squibb	00015-7405-28
1's	$2.56	GENERIC, Bristol-Myers Squibb	00015-7405-18
1's	$6.83	OMNIPEN-N, Wyeth-Ayerst Laboratories	00008-0315-09
1's	$7.74	OMNIPEN-N, Wyeth-Ayerst Laboratories	00008-0315-25
1's	$35.88	TOTACILLIN-N, Glaxosmithkline	00029-6612-40
10's	$24.25	TOTACILLIN-N, Glaxosmithkline	00029-6612-22
10's	$25.63	GENERIC, Bristol-Myers Squibb	00015-7405-29
10's	$38.40	TOTACILLIN-N, Glaxosmithkline	00029-6612-21
10's	$68.20	OMNIPEN-N, Wyeth-Ayerst Laboratories	00008-0315-10
10's	$68.93	GENERIC, Geneva Pharmaceuticals	00781-3714-46
10's	$97.50	GENERIC, American Pharmaceutical Partners	63323-0399-23

Powder For Injection - Injectable - 10 Gm

Qty	Price	Product	NDC
10's	$147.60	GENERIC, Bristol-Myers Squibb	00015-7100-98
10's	$173.28	TOTACILLIN-N, Glaxosmithkline	00029-6613-21

Powder For Injection - Injectable - 125 mg

Qty	Price	Product	NDC
1's	$6.80	GENERIC, Bristol-Myers Squibb	00015-7401-20
10's	$13.48	GENERIC, Geneva Pharmaceuticals	00781-3700-76
10's	$15.80	GENERIC, Bristol-Myers Squibb	00015-7401-99

Powder For Injection - Injectable - 250 mg

Qty	Price	Product	NDC
1's	$8.00	GENERIC, Bristol-Myers Squibb	00015-7402-20
10's	$7.88	TOTACILLIN-N, Glaxosmithkline	00029-6600-24
10's	$16.13	GENERIC, American Pharmaceutical Partners	63323-0387-10
10's	$16.20	GENERIC, Bristol-Myers Squibb	00015-7402-99

Powder For Injection - Injectable - 500 mg

Qty	Price	Product	NDC
1's	$4.18	OMNIPEN-N, Wyeth-Ayerst Laboratories	00008-0315-27
1's	$10.40	GENERIC, Bristol-Myers Squibb	00015-7403-20
10's	$10.38	TOTACILLIN-N, Glaxosmithkline	00029-6605-24
10's	$17.40	GENERIC, Bristol-Myers Squibb	00015-7403-99
10's	$21.70	GENERIC, Bristol-Myers Squibb	00015-7403-94
10's	$29.75	GENERIC, American Pharmaceutical Partners	63323-0388-10
10's	$37.90	GENERIC, Bristol-Myers Squibb	00015-7403-30
10's	$43.05	GENERIC, Geneva Pharmaceuticals	00781-3706-46
40's	$7.70	GENERIC, Golden State Medical	60429-0024-40
100's	$13.79	GENERIC, Vangard Labs	00615-0121-01
100's	$22.29	GENERIC, Teva Pharmaceuticals Usa	00332-3113-05

Powder For Reconstitution - Oral - 125 mg/5 ml

Qty	Price	Product	NDC
100 ml	$2.35	GENERIC, Major Pharmaceuticals Inc	00904-4010-04
100 ml	$2.48	GENERIC, Interstate Drug Exchange Inc	00814-0725-54
100 ml	$2.76	GENERIC, Mylan Pharmaceuticals Inc	00378-0117-02
100 ml	$2.87	GENERIC, Ivax Corporation	00182-0274-70
100 ml	$4.60	GENERIC, Bristol-Myers Squibb	00003-0969-09
100 ml	$4.77	GENERIC, Mova Pharmaceutical Corporation	55370-0882-13
200 ml	$3.96	GENERIC, Major Pharmaceuticals Inc	00904-4010-08
200 ml	$4.64	GENERIC, Ivax Corporation	00182-0274-73
200 ml	$4.64	GENERIC, Mylan Pharmaceuticals Inc	00378-0117-04

Size	Price	Product / Manufacturer	NDC
200 ml	$4.64	GENERIC, Aligen Independent Laboratories Inc	00405-2275-70
200 ml	$5.78	GENERIC, Bristol-Myers Squibb	00015-7988-67
200 ml	$8.28	GENERIC, Mova Pharmaceutical Corporation	55370-0882-40
200 ml	$9.20	GENERIC, Bristol-Myers Squibb	00003-0969-61

Powder For Reconstitution - Oral - 250 mg/5 ml

Size	Price	Product / Manufacturer	NDC
100 ml	$3.90	GENERIC, Ivax Corporation	00182-0275-70
100 ml	$4.12	GENERIC, Mylan Pharmaceuticals Inc	00378-0118-02
100 ml	$7.04	GENERIC, Mova Pharmaceutical Corporation	55370-0883-13
100 ml	$7.82	GENERIC, Bristol-Myers Squibb	00003-0972-52
100's	$3.75	GENERIC, Interstate Drug Exchange Inc	00814-0728-54
100's	$3.90	GENERIC, Major Pharmaceuticals Inc	00904-4014-04
200 ml	$6.50	GENERIC, Mylan Pharmaceuticals Inc	00378-0118-04
200 ml	$6.70	GENERIC, Ivax Corporation	00182-0275-73
200 ml	$10.95	GENERIC, Pharma Pac	52959-0130-03
200 ml	$14.08	GENERIC, Mova Pharmaceutical Corporation	55370-0883-40
200 ml	$15.64	GENERIC, Bristol-Myers Squibb	00003-0972-61
200's	$4.94	GENERIC, Moore, H.L. Drug Exchange Inc	00839-6445-78
200's	$5.26	GENERIC, Interstate Drug Exchange Inc	00814-0728-60
200's	$6.50	GENERIC, Major Pharmaceuticals Inc	00904-4014-08

PRODUCT LISTING - EQUIVALENTS NOT AVAILABLE

Capsule - Oral - 250 mg

Size	Price	Product / Manufacturer	NDC
1's	$3.41	GENERIC, Prescript Pharmaceuticals	00247-0156-01
3's	$3.52	GENERIC, Prescript Pharmaceuticals	00247-0156-03
4's	$3.56	GENERIC, Prescript Pharmaceuticals	00247-0156-04
8's	$1.49	GENERIC, Southwood Pharmaceuticals Inc	58016-0148-08
9's	$1.67	GENERIC, Southwood Pharmaceuticals Inc	58016-0148-09
10's	$1.86	GENERIC, Southwood Pharmaceuticals Inc	58016-0148-10
12's	$2.23	GENERIC, Southwood Pharmaceuticals Inc	58016-0148-12
12's	$3.99	GENERIC, Prescript Pharmaceuticals	00247-0156-12
14's	$2.60	GENERIC, Southwood Pharmaceuticals Inc	58016-0148-14
15's	$2.78	GENERIC, Southwood Pharmaceuticals Inc	58016-0148-15
15's	$4.15	GENERIC, Prescript Pharmaceuticals	00247-0156-15
16's	$4.20	GENERIC, Prescript Pharmaceuticals	00247-0156-16
20's	$3.71	GENERIC, Southwood Pharmaceuticals Inc	58016-0148-20
20's	$4.41	GENERIC, Prescript Pharmaceuticals	00247-0156-20
21's	$4.47	GENERIC, Prescript Pharmaceuticals	00247-0156-21
21's	$6.29	GENERIC, Alpharma Uspd Makers Of Barre and Nmc	63874-0113-21
24's	$4.45	GENERIC, Southwood Pharmaceuticals Inc	58016-0148-24
28's	$3.28	GENERIC, Allscripts Pharmaceutical Company	54569-1719-02
28's	$4.84	GENERIC, Prescript Pharmaceuticals	00247-0156-28
28's	$4.86	GENERIC, Prescript Pharmaceuticals	00247-0156-29
28's	$5.20	GENERIC, Southwood Pharmaceuticals Inc	58016-0148-28
28's	$7.60	GENERIC, Alpharma Uspd Makers Of Barre and Nmc	63874-0113-28
30's	$3.81	GENERIC, Physicians Total Care	54868-3111-03
30's	$4.94	GENERIC, Prescript Pharmaceuticals	00247-0156-30
30's	$5.57	GENERIC, Southwood Pharmaceuticals Inc	58016-0148-30
40's	$4.69	GENERIC, Allscripts Pharmaceutical Company	54569-1719-00
40's	$4.89	GENERIC, Physicians Total Care	54868-3111-01
40's	$5.47	GENERIC, Prescript Pharmaceuticals	00247-0156-40
40's	$5.73	GENERIC, Pharmaceutical Corporation Of America	51655-0104-51
40's	$7.42	GENERIC, Southwood Pharmaceuticals Inc	58016-0148-40
40's	$9.78	GENERIC, Alpharma Uspd Makers Of Barre and Nmc	63874-0113-40
50's	$9.28	GENERIC, Southwood Pharmaceuticals Inc	58016-0148-50
100's	$10.24	GENERIC, Physicians Total Care	54868-3111-05
100's	$18.56	GENERIC, Southwood Pharmaceuticals Inc	58016-0148-00

Capsule - Oral - 500 mg

Size	Price	Product / Manufacturer	NDC
3's	$3.71	GENERIC, Prescript Pharmaceuticals	00247-0157-03
4's	$3.84	GENERIC, Prescript Pharmaceuticals	00247-0157-04
7's	$2.32	GENERIC, Southwood Pharmaceuticals Inc	58016-0149-07
7's	$2.36	GENERIC, Physicians Total Care	54868-3113-01
7's	$4.19	GENERIC, Prescript Pharmaceuticals	00247-0157-07
8's	$4.31	GENERIC, Prescript Pharmaceuticals	00247-0157-08
10's	$3.31	GENERIC, Southwood Pharmaceuticals Inc	58016-0149-10
16's	$5.26	GENERIC, Prescript Pharmaceuticals	00247-0157-16
18's	$5.49	GENERIC, Prescript Pharmaceuticals	00247-0157-18
20's	$4.28	GENERIC, Physicians Total Care	54868-3113-07
20's	$5.74	GENERIC, Prescript Pharmaceuticals	00247-0157-20
20's	$6.62	GENERIC, Southwood Pharmaceuticals Inc	58016-0149-20
20's	$9.05	GENERIC, Pharma Pac	52959-0389-20
21's	$5.86	GENERIC, Prescript Pharmaceuticals	00247-0157-21
21's	$6.96	GENERIC, Southwood Pharmaceuticals Inc	58016-0149-21
21's	$7.99	GENERIC, Alpharma Uspd Makers Of Barre and Nmc	63874-0114-21
24's	$7.95	GENERIC, Southwood Pharmaceuticals Inc	58016-0149-24
25's	$8.28	GENERIC, Southwood Pharmaceuticals Inc	58016-0149-25
28's	$6.00	GENERIC, Allscripts Pharmaceutical Company	54569-2411-01
28's	$6.69	GENERIC, Prescript Pharmaceuticals	00247-0157-28
28's	$9.27	GENERIC, Southwood Pharmaceuticals Inc	58016-0149-28
28's	$10.80	GENERIC, Pharma Pac	52959-0389-28
28's	$11.00	GENERIC, Alpharma Uspd Makers Of Barre and Nmc	63874-0114-28
30's	$5.75	GENERIC, Physicians Total Care	54868-3113-05
30's	$6.93	GENERIC, Prescript Pharmaceuticals	00247-0157-30
30's	$9.94	GENERIC, Southwood Pharmaceuticals Inc	58016-0149-30
30's	$11.30	GENERIC, Pharma Pac	52959-0389-30
30's	$11.58	GENERIC, Alpharma Uspd Makers Of Barre and Nmc	63874-0114-30
40's	$7.21	GENERIC, Physicians Total Care	54868-3113-03
40's	$8.12	GENERIC, Prescript Pharmaceuticals	00247-0157-40
40's	$8.57	GENERIC, Allscripts Pharmaceutical Company	54569-2411-00
40's	$13.25	GENERIC, Southwood Pharmaceuticals Inc	58016-0149-40
40's	$13.50	GENERIC, Pharma Pac	52959-0389-40
40's	$13.80	GENERIC, Alpharma Uspd Makers Of Barre and Nmc	63874-0114-40
60's	$10.16	GENERIC, Physicians Total Care	54868-3113-08
100's	$16.04	GENERIC, Physicians Total Care	54868-3113-00
100's	$33.12	GENERIC, Southwood Pharmaceuticals Inc	58016-0149-00

Powder For Injection - Injectable - 1 Gm

Size	Price	Product / Manufacturer	NDC
10's	$15.00	GENERIC, Raway Pharmacal Inc	00686-3708-70
10's	$27.23	GENERIC, Physicians Total Care	54868-3481-00
10's	$28.63	TOTACILLIN-N, Abbott Pharmaceutical	00074-6612-07

Powder For Injection - Injectable - 2 Gm

Size	Price	Product / Manufacturer	NDC
10's	$23.00	GENERIC, Raway Pharmacal Inc	00686-3712-80
10's	$34.56	GENERIC, Bristol-Myers Squibb	00015-7405-95
10's	$45.90	GENERIC, Bristol-Myers Squibb	00015-7405-99
10's	$46.90	GENERIC, Bristol-Myers Squibb	00015-7405-89

Powder For Injection - Injectable - 10 Gm

Size	Price	Product / Manufacturer	NDC
1's	$13.35	GENERIC, Bristol-Myers Squibb	00015-7100-28

Powder For Injection - Injectable - 250 mg

Size	Price	Product / Manufacturer	NDC
10's	$10.00	GENERIC, Raway Pharmacal Inc	00686-3702-76

Powder For Injection - Injectable - 500 mg

Size	Price	Product / Manufacturer	NDC
10's	$12.00	GENERIC, Raway Pharmacal Inc	00686-3704-76
10's	$19.42	GENERIC, Physicians Total Care	54868-4047-00

Powder For Reconstitution - Oral - 125 mg/5 ml

Size	Price	Product / Manufacturer	NDC
100 ml	$3.90	GENERIC, Southwood Pharmaceuticals Inc	58016-1031-01
100 ml	$4.36	GENERIC, Physicians Total Care	54868-4129-01
100 ml	$7.49	GENERIC, Alpharma Uspd Makers Of Barre and Nmc	63874-0145-10
200 ml	$7.00	GENERIC, Southwood Pharmaceuticals Inc	58016-1032-01
200 ml	$7.47	GENERIC, Physicians Total Care	54868-4129-02
200 ml	$9.69	GENERIC, Alpharma Uspd Makers Of Barre and Nmc	63874-0145-20

Powder For Reconstitution - Oral - 250 mg/5 ml

Size	Price	Product / Manufacturer	NDC
100 ml	$6.71	GENERIC, Southwood Pharmaceuticals Inc	58016-1033-01
100 ml	$10.87	GENERIC, Alpharma Uspd Makers Of Barre and Nmc	63874-0146-10
150 ml	$7.70	GENERIC, Southwood Pharmaceuticals Inc	58016-1062-01
200 ml	$5.43	GENERIC, Physicians Total Care	54868-4131-01
200 ml	$9.10	GENERIC, Southwood Pharmaceuticals Inc	58016-1034-01
200 ml	$12.59	GENERIC, Alpharma Uspd Makers Of Barre and Nmc	63874-0146-20

Ampicillin Sodium *(000237)*

For related information, see the comparative table section in Appendix A.

Categories: Gonorrhea; Infection, ear, middle; Infection, gastrointestinal tract; Infection, genital tract; Infection, lower respiratory tract; Infection, sinus; Infection, upper respiratory tract; Infection, urinary tract; Pregnancy Category B; FDA Approved 1967 Apr; WHO Formulary

Drug Classes: Antibiotics, penicillins

Brand Names: Omnipen-N; Totacillin-N

HCFA JCODE(S): J0290 up to 500 mg IM, IV

DESCRIPTION

Ampicillin sodium is derived from the penicillin nucleus, 6-aminopenicillanic acid (6-APA), isolated by Beecham. Chemically it is D (-) α-aminobenzyl penicillin sodium salt.

CLINICAL PHARMACOLOGY

MICROBIOLOGY

Ampicillin sodium is similar to benzyl penicillin in its bactericidal action against sensitive organisms during the stage of active multiplication. It acts through the inhibition of biosynthesis of cell wall mucopeptide. Ampicillin sodium differs in *in vitro* spectrum from benzyl penicillin in the Gram-negative spectrum. It exerts high *in vitro* activity against many strains of *Haemophilus influenzae, Neisseria gonorrhoeae, Neisseria meningitidis, Neisseria catarrhalis, Escherichia coli, Proteus mirabilis, Bacteroides funduliformis, Salmonellae* and *Shigellae*.

In vitro studies have also demonstrated the sensitivity of many strains of the following Gram-positive bacteria: alpha- and beta-hemolytic streptococci, *Diplococcus pneumoniae,* nonpenicillinase-producing staphylococci, *Bacillus anthracis,* and most strains of enterococci and clostridia. Ampicillin generally provides less *in vitro* activity than penicillin G against Gram-positive bacteria. Because it does not resist destruction by penicillinase, it is not effective against penicillinase-producing bacteria, particularly resistant staphylococci. All strains of *Pseudomonas* and most strains of *Klebsiella* and *Aerobacter* are resistant.

PHARMACOKINETICS

Ampicillin sodium diffuses readily into all body tissues and fluids with the exception of brain and spinal fluid except when meninges are inflamed. It produces high and persistent blood levels. Most of the ampicillin is excreted unchanged in the urine and this excretion can be delayed by concurrent administration of probenecid. The active form appears in the bile in higher concentrations than found in the serum. Ampicillin sodium is one of the least serum bound of all the penicillins, averaging about 20% compared to approximately 60-90% for other penicillins.

INDICATIONS AND USAGE

Ampicillin sodium is indicated in the treatment of infections due to susceptible strains of the following:

Gram-Negative Organisms: *Shigellae, Salmonellae* (including *S. typhosa*), *H. influenzae, E. coli, P. mirabilis, N. gonorrhoeae,* and *N. meningitidis.*

Gram-Positive Organisms: Streptococci, *S. pneumoniae,* and nonpenicillinase-producing staphylococci.

Because of its wide spectrum and bactericidal action, it may be useful in instituting therapy; however, bacteriological studies to determine the causative organisms and their sensitivity to ampicillin should be performed.

Indicated surgical procedures should be performed.

CONTRAINDICATIONS

A history of allergic reaction to any of the penicillins is a contraindication.

WARNINGS

SERIOUS AND OCCASIONALLY FATAL HYPERSENSITIVITY (ANAPHYLACTOID) REACTIONS HAVE BEEN REPORTED IN PATIENTS ON PENICILLIN THERAPY. ALTHOUGH ANAPHYLAXIS IS MORE FREQUENT FOLLOWING PARENTERAL THERAPY, IT HAS OCCURRED IN PATIENTS ON ORAL PENICILLINS. THESE REACTIONS ARE MORE APT TO OCCUR IN INDIVIDUALS WITH A HISTORY OF PENICILLIN HYPERSENSITIVITY AND/OR HYPERSENSITIVITY REACTIONS TO MULTIPLE ALLERGENS. THERE HAVE BEEN REPORTS OF INDIVIDUALS WITH A HISTORY OF PENICILLIN HYPERSENSITIVITY WHO HAVE EXPERIENCED SEVERE REACTIONS WHEN TREATED WITH CEPHALOSPORINS. BEFORE THERAPY WITH A PENICILLIN, CAREFUL INQUIRY SHOULD BE MADE CONCERNING PREVIOUS HYPERSENSITIVITY REACTIONS TO PENICILLINS, CEPHALOSPORINS, AND OTHER ALLERGENS. IF AN ALLERGIC REACTION OCCURS, THE DRUG SHOULD BE DISCONTINUED AND THE APPROPRIATE THERAPY INSTITUTED. **SERIOUS ANAPHYLACTOID REACTIONS REQUIRE IMMEDIATE EMERGENCY TREATMENT WITH EPINEPHRINE. OXYGEN, INTRAVENOUS STEROIDS, AND AIRWAY MANAGEMENT, INCLUDING INTUBATION, SHOULD ALSO BE ADMINISTERED AS INDICATED.**

USAGE IN PREGNANCY: SAFETY FOR USE IN PREGNANCY HAS NOT BEEN ESTABLISHED.

PRECAUTIONS

As with any antibiotic preparation, constant observation for signs of overgrowth of nonsusceptible organisms, including fungi, is essential. Should superinfection occur (usually involving *Aerobacter, Pseudomonas,* or *Candida*), the drug should be discontinued and/or appropriate therapy instituted. As with any potent agent, it is advisable to check periodically for organ system dysfunction during prolonged therapy; this includes renal, hepatic, and hematopoietic systems. This is particularly important in prematures, neonates and other infants.

ADVERSE REACTIONS

As with other penicillins, it may be expected that untoward reactions will be essentially limited to sensitivity phenomena. They are more likely to occur in individuals who have previously demonstrated hypersensitivity to penicillins and in those with a history of allergy, asthma, hay fever, or urticaria.

The following adverse reactions have been reported as associated with the use of ampicillin:

Gastrointestinal: Glossitis, stomatitis, black "hairy" tongue, nausea, vomiting, and diarrhea. (These reactions are usually associated with oral dosage forms.)

Hypersensitivity Reactions: An erythematous maculopapular rash has been reported fairly frequently. Urticaria and erythema multiforme have been reported occasionally. A few cases of exfoliative dermatitis have been reported. Anaphylaxis is the most serious reaction experienced and has usually been associated with the parenteral dosage form.

Note: Urticaria, other skin rashes, and serum sicknesslike reactions may be controlled with antihistamines and, if necessary, systemic corticosteroids. Whenever such reactions occur, ampicillin should be discontinued unless, in the opinion of the physician, the condition being treated is life-threatening and amenable only to ampicillin therapy.

Liver: A moderate rise in serum glutamic oxaloacetic transaminase (SGOT) has been noted, particularly in infants, but the significance of this finding is unknown.

Hemic and Lymphatic Systems: Anemia, thrombocytopenia, thrombocytopenic purpura, eosinophilia, leukopenia, and agranulocytosis have been reported during therapy with the penicillins. These reactions are usually reversible on discontinuation of therapy and are believed to be sensitivity reactions.

DOSAGE AND ADMINISTRATION

Infections of the ear, nose, throat, and lower respiratory tract: Due to streptococci, pneumococci, and nonpenicillinase-producing staphylococci, and also those infections of **the upper and lower respiratory tract** due to *H. influenzae:Adults:* 250-500 mg every 6 hours. *Children:* 12.5 mg/kg every 6 hours.

Infection of the genitourinary tract: Caused by sensitive gram-negative and gram-positive bacteria: *Adults:* 500 mg every 6 hours. *Children:* 12.5 mg/kg every 6 hours.

Urethritis: Due to *N. gonorrhoeae* in adult males: 500 mg every 12 hours for 1 day. Treatment may be repeated if necessary.

Cases of gonorrhea with a suspected lesion of syphilis should have dark-field examinations before receiving Ampicillin, and monthly serological tests for a minimum of 4 months.

Infections of the gastrointestinal tract: *Adults:* 500 mg every 6 hours. *Children:* 12.5 mg/kg every 6 hours.

Larger doses may be required for stubborn or severe infections. The children's dosage is intended for individuals whose weight will not cause a dosage to be calculated greater than that recommended for adults. Children weighing more than 20 kg should be dosed according to the adult recommendations.

It should be recognized that in the treatment of chronic urinary tract and intestinal infections, frequent bacteriological and clinical appraisals are necessary. Smaller doses than those recommended above should not be used. Even higher doses may be needed at times. In stubborn infections, therapy may be required for several weeks. It may be necessary to continue clinical and/or bacteriological follow-up for several months after cessation of therapy.

Treatment should be continued for a minimum of 48-72 hours beyond the time that the patient becomes asymptomatic or evidence of bacterial eradication has been obtained. It is recommended that there be at least 10 days' treatment for any infection caused by hemolytic streptococci to help prevent the occurrence of acute rheumatic fever or glomerulonephritis.

Bacterial meningitis: Children with bacterial meningitis caused by *N. meningitidis* or *H. influenzae* have been successfully treated with doses of 150-200 mg/kg/day. A few adults have been successfully treated for bacterial meningitis with doses ranging from 8-14 g daily. Treatment was initiated with intravenous drip therapy for at least 3 days, and continued with frequent (every 3-4 hours) intramuscular therapy.

Septicemia: For adults, a dosage of 8-14 g daily is recommended, starting with IV administration for at least 3 days and continuing with the IM route every 3-4 hours. For children, a dosage of 150-200 mg/kg/day is recommended, starting with IV administration for at least 3 days and continuing with the IM route every 3-4 hours.

As with other parenteral drugs, ampicillin sodium should be inspected visually for particulate matter and discoloration.

DIRECTIONS FOR USE — INTRAMUSCULAR ADMINISTRATION

250 mg, 500 mg, 1 g and 2 g Standard Vials

(Concentrations of approximately 125 and 250 mg/ml). For initial reconstitution, use sterile water for injection.

TABLE 1

Vial Size	Amount of Diluent to be Added	Volume After Reconstitution	Concentration
250 mg	0.9 ml	1.0 ml	250 mg/ml
	1.9 ml	2.0 ml	125 mg/ml
500 mg	1.7 ml	2.0 ml	250 mg/ml
1 g	3.4 ml	4.0 ml	250 mg/ml
	7.4 ml	8.0 ml	125 mg/ml
2 g	6.8 ml	8.0 ml	250 mg/ml

Add the required amount of sterile water for injection and shake vigorously to reconstitute. As with all intramuscular preparations, ampicillin sodium should be injected well within the body of a relatively large muscle using usual techniques and precautions.

Stability: Use solutions within one hour after reconstitution. Stability studies demonstrate that ampicillin sodium at 125 and 250 mg/ml concentrations maintain their potencies up to 1 hour.

Intravenous Therapy: Intravenous therapy is recommended in serious infections when prompt, effective levels of the antibiotic must reach the site of the infection. Such infections include meningitis, subacute bacterial endocarditis, peritonitis, septicemia, severe forms of chronic bronchitis, osteomyelitis, pneumonia and pyelonephritis due to susceptible organisms.

The 1 g and 2 g in the standard vials and the piggyback bottles may be given either intravenous drip or by direct intravenous injection. For direct intravenous injection, dissolve 1 g or 2 g in at least 7.4 ml sterile water for injection and administer slowly over 10-15 minutes.

CAUTION: More rapid administration may result in convulsive seizures.

Direct Intravenous Injection: Concentrations of 50 and 100 mg/ml.

Reconstitute 250 or 500 mg in 5 ml of sterile water for injection. Administer every 6 hours by slow injection (3-4 minutes).

Stability: The resulting solutions must be used within 2 hours at room temperature (70-75°F) or within 4 hours if kept under refrigeration (40°F).

Continuous Intravenous Infusion: Concentration of $\leq$30 mg/ml.

Reconstitute as directed under Directions for Use — Intramuscular Administration (as described above), withdraw the entire contents, then further dilute to a concentration of $\leq$30 mg/ml.

Stability: For IV solutions, see TABLE 5.

500 mg, 1 g and 2 g Piggyback Bottles

For initial reconstitution, use sterile water for injection, sodium chloride injection or 5% dextrose in water*.

Intravenous Drip Infusion: Concentrations of approximately 5 mg/ml to 20 mg/ml.

500 mg Piggyback Bottle: Reconstitute with a minimum of 50 ml of sterile water for injection, sodium chloride injection., or 5% dextrose in water* and shake well.

TABLE 2

Amount of Diluent to be Added	Concentration
50 ml	10 mg/ml
100 ml	5 mg/ml

1 gm Piggyback Bottle: Reconstitute with a minimum of 49 ml of sterile water for injection, sodium chloride injection, or 5% dextrose in water* and shake well.

2 gm Piggyback Bottle: Reconstitute with 99 ml of sterile water for injection, sodium chloride injection, 5% dextrose in water* and shake well.

Stability: For IV solutions, see TABLE 5.

A

TABLE 3

Amount of Diluent to be Added	Concentration
49 ml	20 mg/ml
99 ml	10 mg/ml

TABLE 4

Amount of Diluent to be Added	Concentration
99 ml	20 mg/ml

*If the piggyback bottle is reconstituted using 5% dextrose in water to a concentration of ≤20 mg/ml, the resulting solution is stable for 2 hours at room temperature (70-75°F) or 3 hours under refrigeration (40°F).

TABLE 5 *Stability Period*

Intravenous Solution	Concentration	Room Temperature (70-75°F)	Refrigeration (40°F)
Sterile water for injection	≤30 mg/ml	8 hours	48 hours
	≤20 mg/ml	8 hours	72 hours
Sodium chloride injection	≤30 mg/ml	8 hours	48 hours
	≤20 mg/ml	8 hours	72 hours
5% Dextrose in water	≤20 mg/ml	2 hours	3 hours
5% Dextrose in 0.45% sodium chloride solution	≤10 mg/ml	2 hours	3 hours
Lactated Ringer's solution	≤30 mg/ml	8 hours	24 hours

Unused portions of any solution must be discarded after the time periods listed above. **Store dry powder at room temperature (70-75°F) or below.**

CDC GUIDELINES FOR TREATMENT OF SEXUALLY TRANSMITTED DISEASES

Gonococcal Infections:[1]Disseminated Gonococcal Infection (hospitalization recommended): When the infecting organism is proven to be penicillin-sensitive, parenteral treatment may be switched to ampicillin 1 g every 6 hours (or equivalent).

Rape Victims (prophylaxis of infection) — alternative regimen for pregnant women or when tetracycline is contraindicated: 3.5 g orally with 1 g probenecid.

Ampicillin Sodium; Sulbactam Sodium *(000238)*

For related information, see the comparative table section in Appendix A.

Categories: Infection, gynecologic; Infection, intra-abdominal; Infection, skin and skin structures; Pregnancy Category B; FDA Approved 1986 Dec
Drug Classes: Antibiotics, penicillins
Brand Names: **Unasyn**
Foreign Brand Availability: Ansulina (Taiwan); Bactacin (Korea); Cinam (Indonesia); Dibacin (Korea); Rukasyn (Korea); Sulbacin (India; Korea); Ubacillin (Korea); Ubactam (Korea); Unacid (Germany; Switzerland); Unacim (France); Unasyna (Mexico)
Cost of Therapy: $859.88 (Infection; Unasyn Powder for Injection; 2 g; 1 g; 12 g/day; 14 day supply)
$825.50 (Infection; Generic Powder for Injection; 2 g; 1 g; 12 g/day; 14 day supply)
HCFA JCODE(S): J0295 1.5 gm IM, IV

DESCRIPTION

Unasyn is an injectable antibacterial combination consisting of the semisynthetic antibiotic ampicillin sodium and the beta-lactamase inhibitor sulbactam sodium for intravenous and intramuscular administration.

Ampicillin sodium is derived from the penicillin nucleus, 6-aminopenicillanic acid. Chemically, it is monosodium (2S,5R,6R)-6-[(R)-2-amino-2-phenylacetamido]-3,3-dimethyl-7-oxo-4-thia-1-aza-bicyclo(3.2.0)heptane-2-carboxylate and has a molecular weight of 371.39. Its chemical formula is $C_{16}H_{18}N_3NaO_4S$.

Sulbactam sodium is a derivative of the basic penicillin nucleus. Chemically, sulbactam sodium is sodium penicillinate sulfone; sodium (2S,5R)-3,3-dimethyl-7-oxo-4-thia-1-azabicyclo(3.2.0)heptane-2-carboxylate 4,4-dioxide. Its chemical formula is $C_8H_{10}NNaO_5S$ with a molecular weight of 255.22.

Ampicillin sodium; sulbactam sodium parenteral combination, is available as a white to off-white dry powder for reconstitution. Ampicillin sodium; sulbactam sodium dry powder is freely soluble in aqueous diluents to yield pale yellow to yellow solutions containing ampicillin sodium and sulbactam sodium equivalent to 250 mg ampicillin per ml and 125 mg sulbactam per ml. The pH of the solutions is between 8.0 and 10.0.

Dilute solutions (up to 30 mg ampicillin and 15 mg sulbactam per ml) are essentially colorless to pale yellow. The pH of dilute solutions remains the same.

1.5 g of Unasyn (1 g ampicillin as the sodium salt plus 0.5 g sulbactam as the sodium salt) parenteral contains approximately 115 mg (5 mEq) of sodium.

3 g of Unasyn (2 g ampicillin as the sodium salt plus 1 g sulbactam as the sodium salt) parenteral contains approximately 230 mg (10 mEq) of sodium.

Ampicillin sodium; sulbactam sodium pharmacy bulk package is a vial containing a sterile preparation of ampicillin sodium and sulbactam sodium for parenteral use that contains many single doses. The pharmacy bulk package is for use in pharmacy admixture setting; it provides many single doses of ampicillin sodium; sulbactam sodium for addition to suitable parenteral fluids in preparation of admixtures for intravenous infusion.

CLINICAL PHARMACOLOGY

GENERAL

Immediately after completion of a 15 minute intravenous infusion of ampicillin sodium; sulbactam sodium, peak serum concentrations of ampicillin and sulbactam are attained. Ampicillin serum levels are similar to those produced by the administration of equivalent amounts of ampicillin alone. Peak ampicillin serum levels ranging from 109-150 µg/ml are attained after administration of 2000 mg of ampicillin plus 1000 mg sulbactam and 40-71 µg/ml after administration of 1000 mg ampicillin plus 500 mg sulbactam. The corresponding mean peak serum levels for sulbactam range from 48-88 µg/ml and 21-40 µg/ml, respectively. After an intramuscular injection of 1000 mg ampicillin plus 500 mg sulbactam, peak ampicillin serum levels ranging from 8-37 µg/ml and peak sulbactam serum levels ranging from 6-24 µg/ml are attained.

The mean serum half-life of both drugs is approximately 1 hour in healthy volunteers.

Approximately 75-85% of both ampicillin and sulbactam is excreted unchanged in the urine during the first 8 hours after administration of ampicillin sodium; sulbactam sodium to individuals with normal renal function. Somewhat higher and more prolonged serum levels of ampicillin and sulbactam can be achieved with the concurrent administration of probenecid.

In patients with impaired renal function, the elimination kinetics of ampicillin and sulbactam are similarly affected; hence the ratio of one to the other will remain constant whatever the renal function. The dose of ampicillin sodium; sulbactam sodium in such patients should be administered less frequently in accordance with the usual practice for ampicillin (see DOSAGE AND ADMINISTRATION).

Ampicillin has been found to be approximately 28% reversibly bound to human serum protein and sulbactam approximately 38% reversibly bound.

The average levels (see TABLE 1) of ampicillin and sulbactam were measured in the tissues and fluids listed.

TABLE 1 *Concentration of Unasyn in Various Body Tissues and Fluids*

Fluid or Tissue	Dose (g) Ampicillin;Sulbactam	Concentration (µg/ml or µg/g) Ampicillin;Sulbactam
Peritoneal fluid	0.5/0.5 IV	7/14
Blister fluid (cantharides)	0.5/0.5 IV	8/20
Tissue fluid	1/0.5 IV	8/4
Intestinal mucosa	0.5/0.5 IV	11/18
Appendix	2/1 IV	3/40

Penetration of both ampicillin and sulbactam into cerebrospinal fluid in the presence of inflamed meninges has been demonstrated after IV administration of Unasyn.

MICROBIOLOGY

Ampicillin is similar to benzyl penicillin in its bactericidal action against susceptible organisms during the stage of active multiplication. It acts through the inhibition of cell wall mucopeptide biosynthesis. Ampicillin has a broad spectrum of bactericidal activity against many gram-positive and gram-negative aerobic and anaerobic bacteria. (Ampicillin is, however, degraded by beta-lactamases; and therefore the spectrum of activity does not normally include organisms that produce these enzymes.)

A wide range of beta-lactamases found in microorganisms resistant to penicillins and cephalosporins have been shown in biochemical studies with cell free bacterial systems to be irreversibly inhibited by sulbactam. Although sulbactam alone possesses little useful antibacterial activity except against *Neisseriaceae* organisms; whole organism studies have shown that sulbactam restores ampicillin activity against beta-lactamase–producing strains. In particular, sulbactam has good inhibitory activity against the clinically important plasmid-mediated beta-lactamases most frequently responsible for transferred drug resistance. Sulbactam has no effect on the activity of ampicillin against ampicillin susceptible strains.

The presence of sulbactam in the ampicillin sodium; sulbatcam sodium formulation effectively extends the antibiotic spectrum of ampicillin to include many bacteria normally resistant to it and to other beta-lactam antibiotics. Thus ampicillin sodium; sulbatctam sodium possesses the properties of a broad-spectrum antibiotic and a beta-lactamase inhibitor.

While *in vitro* studies have demonstrated the susceptibility of most strains of the following organisms, clinical efficacy for infections other than those included in INDICATIONS AND USAGE has not been documented.

Gram-Positive Bacteria: *Staphylococcus aureus* (beta-lactamase and non–beta-lactamase producing), *Staphylococcus epidermidis* (beta-lactamase and non–beta-lactamase producing), *Staphylococcus saprophyticus* (beta-lactamase and non–beta-lactamase producing), *Streptococcus faecalis** (*Enterococcus*), *Streptococcus pneumoniae** (formerly *D. pneumoniae*), *Streptococcus pyogenes*†, *Streptococcus viridans*.*

Gram-Negative Bacteria: *Haemophilus influenzae* (beta-lactamase and non–beta-lactamase producing), *Moraxella catarrhalis* (beta-lactamase and non–beta-lactamase producing), *Escherichia coli* (beta-lactamase and non–beta-lactamase producing), *Klebsiella* species (all known strains are beta-lactamase producing), *Proteus mirabilis* (beta-lactamase and non–beta-lactamase producing), *Proteus vulgaris, Providencia rettgeri, Providencia stuartii, Morganella morganii,* and *Neisseria gonorrhoeae* (beta-lactamase and non–beta-lactamase producing).

Anaerobes: *Clostridium* spp.,* *Peptococcus* spp.,* *Peptostreptococcus* spp., *Bacteroides* spp., including *B. fragilis*.

*These are not beta-lactamase producing strains and therefore are susceptible to ampicillin alone.

SUSCEPTIBILITY TESTING

Diffusion Technique: For the Kirby-Bauer method of susceptibility testing, a 20 µg (10 µg ampicillin + 10 µg sulbactam) diffusion disk should be used. The method is one outlined in the NCCLS publication M 2-A 3*. With this procedure, a report from the laboratory of "Susceptible" indicates that the infecting organism is likely to respond to ampicillin sodium; sulbatctam sodium therapy; and a report of "Resistant" indicates that the infecting organism is not likely to respond to therapy. An "Intermediate" susceptibility report suggests that the infecting organism would be susceptible to ampicillin sodium; sulbatctam sodium if a higher dosage is used or if the infection is confined to tissues or fluids (*e.g.,* urine) in which high antibiotic levels are attained.

Dilution Techniques: Broth or agar dilution methods may be used to determine the minimal inhibitory concentration (MIC) value for susceptibility of bacterial isolates to ampicillin-;sulbactam. The method used is one outlined in the NCCLS publication M 7-A.** Tubes should be inoculated to contain 10^5 to 10^6 organisms/ml or plates "spotted" with 10^4 organisms.

The recommended dilution method employs a constant ampicillin/sulbactam ratio of 2:1 in all tubes with increasing concentrations of ampicillin. MICs are reported in terms of ampicillin concentration in the presence of sulbactam at a constant 2 parts ampicillin to 1 part sulbactam (see TABLE 2)

TABLE 2 *Recommended Ampicillin;Sulbactam, Susceptibility Ranges*†‡*

	Resistant (mm)	Intermediate (mm)	Susceptible (mm)
Gram(-) and Staphylococcus			
Kirby-Bauer Zone sizes	≤11 mm	12-13 mm	≥14 mm
MIC (μg of ampicillin/ml)	≥32	16	≤8
Haemophilus influenzae			
Bauer/Kirby Zones sizes	≤19	—	≥20
MIC (μg of ampicillin/ml)	≥4	—	≤2

* The non-beta-lactamase producing organisms that are normally susceptible to ampicillin, such as streptococci, will have similar zone sizes as for ampicillin disks.

† Staphylococci resistant to methicillin, oxacillin, or nafcillin must be considered resistant to Unasyn.

‡ The quality-control cultures should have the assigned daily ranges for ampicillin; sulbactam (see TABLE 3).

TABLE 3

	Disks (mm)	Mode MIC (μg/ml ampicillin;μg/ml sulbactam)
E. coli	(ATCC 25922) 20-24	2/1
S. aureus	(ATCC 25923) 29-37	0.12/0.06
E. coli	(ATCC 35218) 13-19	8/4

INDICATIONS AND USAGE

Ampicillin sodium; sulbactam sodium is indicated for the treatment of infections due to susceptible strains of the designated microorganisms in the conditions listed.

Skin and Skin Structure Infections: Caused by beta-lactamase producing strains of *Staphylococcus aureus, Escherichia coli,*† Klebsiella spp.† (including *K. pneumoniae*†), *Proteus mirabilis*†, *Bacteroides fragilis*†, *Enterobacter* spp.†, and *Acinetobacter calcoaceticus*†.

Intra-Abdominal Infections: Caused by beta-lactamase producing strains of *Escherichia coli, Klebsiella* spp. (including *K. pneumoniae*†), *Bacteroides* spp. (including *B. fragilis*), and *Enterobacter* spp.†.

Gynecologic Infections: Caused by beta-lactamase producing strains of *Escherichia coli*†, and *Bacteroides* spp.† (including *B. fragilis*†).

†Efficacy for this organism in this organ system was studied in fewer than 10 infections.

While ampicillin sodium; sulbactam sodium is indicated only for the conditions listed, infections caused by ampicillin-susceptible organisms are also amenable to treatment with ampicillin sodium; sulbatctam sodium due to its ampicillin content. Therefore mixed infections caused by ampicillin-susceptible organisms and beta-lactamase producing organisms susceptible to ampicillin sodium/sulbactam sodium should not require the addition of another antibiotic.

Appropriate culture and susceptibility tests should be performed before treatment in order to isolate and identify the organisms causing infection and to determine their susceptibility to ampicillin sodium; sulbactam sodium.

When there is reason to believe the infection may involve any of the beta-lactamase producing organisms listed in the indicated organ systems; therapy may be instituted prior to obtaining the results from bacteriologic and susceptibility studies. Once the results are known, therapy should be adjusted if appropriate.

CONTRAINDICATIONS

The use of ampicillin sodium/sulbactam sodium is contraindicated in individuals with a history of hypersensitivity reactions to any of the penicillins.

WARNINGS

SERIOUS AND OCCASIONALLY FATAL HYPERSENSITIVITY (ANAPHYLACTIC) REACTIONS HAVE BEEN REPORTED IN PATIENTS ON PENICILLIN THERAPY. THESE REACTIONS ARE MORE APT TO OCCUR IN INDIVIDUALS WITH A HISTORY OF PENICILLIN HYPERSENSITIVITY AND/OR HYPERSENSITIVITY REACTIONS TO MULTIPLE ALLERGENS. THERE HAVE BEEN REPORTS OF INDIVIDUALS WITH A HISTORY OF PENICILLIN HYPERSENSITIVITY WHO HAVE EXPERIENCED SEVERE REACTIONS WHEN TREATED WITH CEPHALOSPORINS. BEFORE THERAPY WITH A PENICILLIN, CAREFUL INQUIRY SHOULD BE MADE CONCERNING PREVIOUS HYPERSENSITIVITY REACTIONS TO PENICILLINS, CEPHALOSPORINS, AND OTHER ALLERGENS. IF AN ALLERGIC REACTION OCCURS, AMPICILLIN SODIUM; SULBATCTAM SODIUM SHOULD BE DISCONTINUED AND THE APPROPRIATE THERAPY INSTITUTED.

Pseudomembranous colitis has been reported with nearly all antibacterial agents, including ampicillin sodium; sulbactam sodium and has ranged in severity from mild to life threatening. Therefore it is important to consider this diagnosis in patients who present with diarrhea subsequent to the administration of antibacterial agents.

Treatment with antibacterial agents alters the normal flora of the colon and may permit overgrowth of clostridia. Studies indicate that toxin produced by *Clostridium difficile* is one primary cause of "antibiotic-associated colitis."

Mild cases of pseudomembranous colitis usually respond to drug discontinuation alone. In moderate to severe cases, consideration should be given to management with fluids and electrolytes, protein supplementation; and treatment with an antibacterial drug clinically effective against *C. difficile* colitis.

SERIOUS ANAPHYLACTOID REACTIONS REQUIRE IMMEDIATE EMERGENCY TREATMENT WITH EPINEPHRINE. OXYGEN, INTRAVENOUS STEROIDS, AND AIRWAY MANAGEMENT, INCLUDING INTUBATION, SHOULD ALSO BE ADMINISTERED AS INDICATED.

PRECAUTIONS

GENERAL

A high percentage of patients with mononucleosis who receive ampicillin develop a skin rash. Thus ampicillin-class antibiotics should not be administered to patients with mononucleosis. In patients treated with ampicillin sodium; sulbactam sodium the possibility of superinfections with mycotic or bacterial pathogens should be kept in mind during therapy. If superinfections occur (usually involving *Pseudomonas* or *Candida* organisms), the drug should be discontinued and/or appropriate therapy instituted.

DRUG/LABORATORY TEST INTERACTIONS

Administration of ampicillin sodium; sulbactam sodium will result in high urine concentration of ampicillin. High urine concentrations of ampicillin may result in false-positive reactions in testing for the presence of glucose in urine using Clinitest, Benedict's solution or Fehling's solution. It is recommended that glucose tests based on enzymatic glucose oxidase reactions (such as Clinistix or Tes-Tape) be used. Following administration of ampicillin to pregnant women, a transient decrease in plasma concentration of total conjugated estriol, estriol-glucuronide, and conjugated estrone and estradiol has been noted. This effect may also occur with ampicillin sodium; sulbactam sodium.

CARCINOGENESIS, MUTAGENESIS, AND IMPAIRMENT OF FERTILITY

Long-term studies in animals have not been performed to evaluate carcinogenic or mutagenic potential.

PREGNANCY CATEGORY B

Reproduction studies have been performed in mice, rats, and rabbits at doses up to ten (10) times the human dose and have revealed no evidence of impaired fertility or harm to the fetus due to ampicillin sodium; sulbactam sodium. There are, however, no adequate and well-controlled studies in pregnant women. Because animal reproduction studies are not always predictive of human response, this drug should be used during pregnancy only if clearly needed. (See Drug/Laboratory Test Interactions.)

LABOR AND DELIVERY

Studies in guinea pigs have shown that intravenous administration of ampicillin decreased the uterine tone, frequency of contractions, height of contractions, and duration of contractions. However, it is not known whether the use of ampicillin sodium; sulbactam sodium in humans during labor or delivery has immediate or delayed adverse effects on the fetus, prolongs the duration of labor, or increases the likelihood that forceps delivery or other obstetric intervention or resuscitation of the newborn will be necessary.

NURSING MOTHERS

Low concentrations of ampicillin and sulbactam are excreted in the milk; therefore caution should be exercised when ampicillin sodium;sulbatctam sodium is administered to a nursing woman.

PEDIATRIC USE

The efficacy and safety of ampicillin sodium; sulbactam sodium have not been established in infants and children under the age of 12.

DRUG INTERACTIONS

Probenecid decreases the renal tubular secretion of ampicillin and sulbactam. Concurrent use of probenecid and ampicillin sodium/sulbactam sodium may result in increased and prolonged blood levels of ampicillin and sulbactam. The concurrent administration of allopurinol and ampicillin substantially increases the incidence of rashes in patients receiving both drugs as compared to patients receiving ampicillin alone. It is not known whether this potentiation of ampicillin rashes is due to allopurinol or the hyperuricemia present in these patients. There are no data with ampicillin sodium; sulbactam sodium and allopurinol administered concurrently. Ampicillin sodium; sulbactam sodium and aminoglycosides should not be reconstituted together due to the *in vitro* inactivation of aminoglycosides by the ampicillin component of ampicillin sodium; sulbactam sodium.

ADVERSE REACTIONS

Ampicillin sodium; sulbactam sodium is generally well tolerated. These adverse reactions have been reported.

LOCAL ADVERSE REACTIONS

Pain at IM Injection Site: 16%
Pain at IV Injection Site: 3%
Thrombophlebitis: 3%

SYSTEMIC ADVERSE REACTIONS

The most frequently reported adverse reactions were diarrhea in 3% of the patients and rash in less than 2% of the patients.

Additional systemic reactions reported in less than 1% of the patients were: Itching, nausea, vomiting, candidiasis, fatigue, malaise, headache, chest pain, flatulence, abdominal distention, glossitis, urine retention, dysuria, edema, facial swelling, erythema, chills, tightness in throat, substernal pain, epistaxis, and mucosal bleeding.

ADVERSE LABORATORY CHANGES

Adverse laboratory changes without regard to drug relationship that were reported during clinical trials were:

Hepatic: Increased AST (SGOT), ALT (SGPT), alkaline phosphatase, and LDH.

Hematologic: Decreased hemoglobin, hematocrit, RBC, WBC, neutrophils, lymphocytes, platelets and increased lymphocytes, monocytes, basophils, eosinophils, and platelets.

Blood Chemistry: Decreased serum albumin and total proteins.

Renal: Increased BUN and creatinine.

Urinalysis: Presence of RBCs and hyaline casts in urine.

These adverse reactions have been reported with ampicillin-class antibiotics and can also occur with ampicillin sodium; sulbactam sodium.

Gastrointestinal: Gastritis, stomatitis, black "hairy" tongue, and enterocolitis. Onset of postmembranous colitis symptoms may occur during or after antibiotic treatment. (See WARNINGS.)

Hypersensitivity Reactions: Urticaria, erythema multiforme, and an occasional case of exfoliative dermatitis have been reported. These reactions may be controlled with antihistamines and, if necessary, systemic corticosteroids. Whenever such reactions occur, the drug should be discontinued, unless the opinion of the physician dictates otherwise. Serious and occasionally fatal hypersensitivity (anaphylactic) reactions can occur with a penicillin. (See WARNINGS.)

Hematologic: In addition to the adverse laboratory changes listed above for ampicillin sodium; sulbactam sodium, agranulocytosis has been reported during therapy with penicillins. All of these reactions are usually reversible on discontinuation of therapy and are believed to be hypersensitivity phenomena. Some individuals have developed a positive direct Coombs' test during treatment with ampicillin sodium; sulbactam sodium, as with other beta-lactam antibiotics.

DOSAGE AND ADMINISTRATION

Ampicillin sodium; sulbactam sodium may be administered by either the IV or IM routes. The intent of the pharmacy bulk package is for preparation of solutions for IV infusion only.

For IV administration, the dose can be given by slow IV injection over at least 10-15 minutes or can also be delivered, in greater dilutions, with 50-100 ml of a compatible diluent as an IV infusion over 15-30 minutes.

Ampicillin sodium; sulbactam sodium may be administered by deep IM injection. (See Preparation for Intramuscular Injection.)

The recommended adult dosage of ampicillin sodium; sulbactam sodium is 1.5 g (1 g ampicillin as the sodium salt plus 0.5 g sulbactam as the sodium salt) to 3 g (2 g ampicillin as the sodium salt plus 1 g sulbactam as the sodium salt) every 6 hours. This 1.5 to 3 g range represents the total of ampicillin content plus the sulbactam content of ampicillin sodium; sulbactam sodium, and corresponds to a range of 1 g ampicillin/0.5 g sulbactam to 2 g ampicillin/1 g sulbactam. The total dose of sulbactam should not exceed 4 g/day.

IMPAIRED RENAL FUNCTION

In patients with impairment of renal function, the elimination kinetics of ampicillin and sulbactam are similarly affected, hence the ration of one to the other will remain constant whatever the renal function. The dose of ampicillin sodium; sulbactam sodium in such patients should be administered less frequently in accordance with the usual practice for ampicillin and according to the recommendations found in TABLE 4.

TABLE 4 *Dosage Guide for Patients With Renal Impairment*

Creatinine Clearance (ml/min/1.73m²)	Ampicillin/Sulbactam Half-Life (H)	Recommended Ampicillin Sodium; Sulbactam Sodium Dosage
≥30	1	1.5-3.0 g q6h-q8h
15-29	5	1.5-3.0 g q12h
5-14	9	1.5-3.0 g q24h

When only serum creatinine is available, a specific formula (based on sex, weight, and age of the patient) may be used to convert this value into creatinine clearance. The serum creatinine should represent a steady state of renal function.

Males: [Weight (kg) × (140 - Age)] ÷ [72 × Serum creatinine]

Females: 0.85 × above value

COMPATIBILITY, RECONSTITUTION, AND STABILITY

Ampicillin sodium; sulbactam sodium sterile powder is to be stored at or below 30°C (86°F) prior to reconstitution.

When concomitant therapy with aminoglycosides is indicated, ampicillin sodium; sulbactam sodium and aminoglycosides should be reconstituted and administered separately, due to the *in vitro* inactivation of aminoglycosides by any of the aminopenicillins.

DIRECTIONS FOR USE

General Dissolution Procedures: Ampicillin sodium; sulbactam sodium sterile powder for intravenous and intramuscular use may be reconstituted with any of the compatible diluents described in this insert. Solutions should be allowed to stand after dissolution to allow any foaming to dissipate in order to permit visual inspection for complete solubilization.

Preparation for Intravenous Use

1.5 g and 3.0 g Bottles: Ampicillin sodium; sulbactam sodium sterile powder in piggyback units may be reconstituted directly to the desired concentrations using any of the following parenteral diluents. Reconstitution of ampicillin sodium; sulbactam sodium, at the specified concentrations, with these diluents provide stable solutions for the time periods are indicated in TABLE 5. (After the indicated time periods, any unused portions of solutions should be discarded.)

TABLE 5

Diluent	Maximum Concentrations (mg/ml) Ampicillin/Sulbactam	Use Periods
Sterile water for injection	45 (30/15)	8 h 25°C
	45 (30/15)	48 h 4°C
	30 (20/10)	72 h 4°C
0.9% Sodium chloride injection	45 (30/15)	8 h 25°C
	45 (30/15)	48 h 4°C
	30 (20/10)	72 h 4°C
5% Dextrose injection	30 (20/10)	2 h 25°C
	30 (20/10)	4 h 4°C
	3 (2/1)	4 h 25°C
Lacated Ringer's injection	45 (30/15)	8 h 25°C
	45 (30/15)	24 h 4°C
M/6 Sodium lactate injection	45 (30/15)	8 h 25°C
	45 (30/15)	8 h 4°C
5% Dextrose in 0.45% saline	3 (2/1)	4 h 25°C
	15 (10/5)	4 hr 4°C
10% Invert sugar	3 (2/1)	4 h 25°C
	30 (20/10)	3 h 4°C

If piggyback bottles are unavailable, standard vials of ampicillin sodium; sulbactam sodium sterile powder may be used. Initially, the vials may be reconstituted with sterile water for injection to yield solutions containing 375 mg ampicillin sodium; sulbactam sodium per ml (250 mg ampicillin/125 mg sulbactam per ml). An appropriate volume should then be immediately diluted with a suitable parenteral diluent to yield solutions containing 3-45 mg ampicillin sodium; sulbactam sodium per ml (2-30 mg ampicillin/1-15 mg sulbactam/per ml).

1.5 g ADD-Vantage Vials: Ampicillin sodium; sulbatctam sodium in the ADD-Vantage system is intended as a single dose for intravenous administration after dilution with the ADD-Vantage Flexible Diluent Container containing 50, 100, or 250 ml of 0.9% sodium chloride injection.

3 g ADD-Vantage Vials: Ampicillin sodium; sulbatctam sodium in the ADD-Vantage system is intended as a single dose for intravenous administration after dilution with the ADD-Vantage Flexible Diluent Container containing 100 or 250 ml of 0.9% sodium chloride injection.

Ampicillin sodium; sulbatctam sodium in the ADD-Vantage system is to be reconstituted with 0.9% sodium chloride injection, only. Reconstitution of ampicillin sodium; sulbatctam sodium, at the specified concentration, with 0.9% sodium chloride injection, provides stable solutions for the time period indicated below:

Diluent: 0.9% sodium chloride injection.

Maximum Concentration (mg/ml) Unasyn (Ampicillin; Sulbactam): 30 (20/10).

Use Period: 8 hours 25°C.

In 0.9% Sodium Chloride Injection

The final diluted solution of ampicillin sodium; sulbactam sodium should be completely administered *within 8 hours* in order to assure proper potency.

Preparation for Intramuscular Injection

1.5 and 3.0 g Standard Vials: Vials for intramuscular use may be reconstituted with sterile water for injection, 05% lidocaine HCl injection, or 2% lidocaine HCl injection. Consult TABLE 6 for recommended volumes to be added to obtain solutions containing 375 mg ampicillin sodium; sulbatctam sodium per ml (250 mg ampicillin/125 mg sulbactam per ml). *Note: Use only freshly prepared solutions and administer within 1 hour after preparation.*

Directions for Proper Use of Pharmacy Bulk Package

The 15 g vial may be reconstituted with either 92 ml sterile water for injection or 0.9% sodium chloride injection. The diluent should be added in two seperate aliquots in a suitable work area, such as a laminar flow hood. Add 50 ml of solution; shake to dissolve. Then add an additional 42 ml and shake. The solution should be allowed to stand after dissolution to allow any foaming to dissipate in order to permit visual inspection for complete solubilization. The resultant solution will have a final concentration of approximately 100 mg/ml ampicillin and 50 mg/ml sulbactam. The closure may be penetrated only one time after reconstitution, if needed, using a suitable sterile transfer device or dispensing set that allows for measured dispensing of the contents.

After reconstitution, use within 2 hours (if stored at room temperature) or within 4 hours (if stored under refrigeration).

TABLE 6

Unasyn Vial Size(g)	Volume of Diluent to be Added (ml)	Withdrawal Volume (ml)*
1.5	3.2	4.0
3.0	6.4	8.0

* There is sufficient excess present to allow withdrawal and administration of the stated volumes.

ANIMAL PHARMACOLOGY

While reversible glycogenosis was observed in laboratory animals, this phenomenon was dose- and time-dependent and is not expected to develop at the therapeutic doses and corresponding plasma levels attained during the relatively short periods of combined ampicillin/sulbactam therapy in man.

HOW SUPPLIED

Unasyn is supplied as a sterile off-white dry powder in glass vials and piggyback bottles.
Storage: Ampicillin sodium; sulbatctam sodium sterile powder is to be stored at or below 30°C (86°F) prior to reconstitution.

PRODUCT LISTING - RATED THERAPEUTICALLY EQUIVALENT

Powder For Injection - Injectable - 10 Gm;5 Gm

1's	$73.71	GENERIC, Esi Lederle Generics	59911-5900-01

PRODUCT LISTING - EQUIVALENTS NOT AVAILABLE

Powder For Injection - Injectable - 1 Gm;0.5 Gm

10's	$78.09	GENERIC, Esi Lederle Generics	59911-5901-02
10's	$81.35	UNASYN, Pfizer U.S. Pharmaceuticals	00049-0013-83
10's	$86.31	UNASYN, Pfizer U.S. Pharmaceuticals	00049-0031-83
10's	$94.29	UNASYN, Pfizer U.S. Pharmaceuticals	00049-0022-83

Powder For Injection - Injectable - 2 Gm;1 Gm

10's	$147.41	GENERIC, Esi Lederle Generics	59911-5902-02
10's	$153.55	UNASYN, Pfizer U.S. Pharmaceuticals	00049-0014-83
10's	$158.50	UNASYN, Pfizer U.S. Pharmaceuticals	00049-0032-83
10's	$162.36	UNASYN, Pfizer U.S. Pharmaceuticals	00049-0023-83

Powder For Injection - Injectable - 10 Gm;5 Gm

1's	$76.79	UNASYN, Pfizer U.S. Pharmaceuticals	00049-0024-28

Amprenavir (003433)

For related information, see the comparative table section in Appendix A.

Categories: Infection, human immunodeficiency virus; FDA Approved 1999 April; Pregnancy Category C
Drug Classes: Antivirals; Protease inhibitors
Brand Names: Agenerase
Cost of Therapy: $634.44 (HIV; Agenerase; 150 mg; 16 capsules/day; 30 day supply)

WARNING

Because of the potential risk of toxicity from the large amount of the excipient, propylene glycol, amprenavir oral solution is contraindicated in infants and children below the age of 4 years, pregnant women, patients with hepatic or renal failure, and patients treated with disulfiram or metronidazole (see CONTRAINDICATIONS and WARNINGS).

Amprenavir oral solution should be used only when amprenavir capsules or other protease inhibitor formulations are not therapeutic options.

DESCRIPTION

Amprenavir is an inhibitor of the human immunodeficiency virus (HIV) protease. The chemical name of amprenavir is (3*S*)-tetrahydro-3-furyl *N*-[(1*S*,2*R*)-3-(4-amino-*N*-isobutylbenzenesulfonamido)-1-benzyl-2-hydroxypropyl]carbamate. Amprenavir is a single stereoisomer with the (3*S*)(1*S*,2*R*) configuration. It has a molecular formula of $C_{25}H_{35}N_3O_6S$ and a molecular weight of 505.64.

Amprenavir is a white to cream-colored solid with a solubility of approximately 0.04 mg/ml in water at 25°C.

AGENERASE CAPSULES

Agenerase capsules are available for oral administration in strengths of 50 and 150 mg. Each 50 mg capsule contains the inactive ingredients d-alpha tocopheryl polyethylene glycol 1000 succinate (TPGS), polyethylene glycol 400 (PEG 400) 246.7 mg, and propylene glycol 19 mg. Each 150 mg capsule contains the inactive ingredients TPGS, PEG 400 740 mg, and propylene glycol 57 mg. The capsule shell contains the inactive ingredients d-sorbitol and sorbitans solution, gelatin, glycerin, and titanium dioxide. The soft gelatin capsules are printed with edible red ink. Each 150 mg Agenerase capsule contains 109 IU vitamin E in the form of TPGS. The total amount of vitamin E in the recommended daily adult dose of Agenerase is 1744 IU.

AGENERASE ORAL SOLUTION

Agenerase oral solution is for oral administration. One milliliter (1 ml) of Agenerase oral solution contains 15 mg of amprenavir in solution and the inactive ingredients acesulfame potassium, artificial grape bubblegum flavor, citric acid (anhydrous), d-alpha tocopheryl polyethylene glycol 1000 succinate (TPGS), menthol, natural peppermint flavor, polyethylene glycol 400 (PEG 400) (170 mg), propylene glycol (550 mg), saccharin sodium, sodium chloride, and sodium citrate (dihydrate). Solutions of sodium hydroxide and/or diluted hydrochloric acid may have been added to adjust pH. Each ml of Agenerase oral solution contains 46 IU vitamin E in the form of TPGS. Propylene glycol is in the formulation to achieve adequate solubility of amprenavir. The recommended daily dose of amprenavir oral solution of 22.5 mg/kg twice daily corresponds to a propylene glycol intake of 1650 mg/kg/day. Acceptable intake of propylene glycol for pharmaceuticals has not been established.

CLINICAL PHARMACOLOGY

MICROBIOLOGY

Mechanism of Action

Amprenavir is an inhibitor of HIV-1 protease. Amprenavir binds to the active site of HIV-1 protease and thereby prevents the processing of viral gag and gag-pol polyprotein precursors, resulting in the formation of immature non-infectious viral particles.

Antiviral Activity In Vitro

The *in vitro* antiviral activity of amprenavir was evaluated against HIV-1 IIIB in both acutely and chronically infected lymphoblastic cell lines (MT-4, CEM-CCRF, H9) and in peripheral blood lymphocytes. The 50% inhibitory concentration (IC_{50}) of amprenavir ranged from 0.012-0.08 μM in acutely infected cells and was 0.41 μM in chronically infected cells (1 μM = 0.50 μg/ml). Amprenavir exhibited synergistic anti-HIV-1 activity in combination with abacavir, zidovudine, didanosine, or saquinavir, and additive anti-HIV-1 activity in combination with indinavir, nelfinavir, and ritonavir *in vitro*. These drug combinations have not been adequately studied in humans. The relationship between *in vitro* anti-HIV-1 activity of amprenavir and the inhibition of HIV-1 replication in humans has not been defined.

Resistance

HIV-1 isolates with a decreased susceptibility to amprenavir have been selected *in vitro* and obtained from patients treated with amprenavir. Genotypic analysis of isolates from amprenavir-treated patients showed mutations in the HIV-1 protease gene resulting in amino acid substitutions primarily at positions V32I, M46I/L, I47V, I50V, I54L/M, and I84V as well as mutations in the p7/p1 and p1/p6 gag cleavage sites. Phenotypic analysis of HIV-1 isolates from 21 nucleoside reverse transcriptase inhibitor- (NRTI-) experienced, protease inhibitor-naïve patients treated with amprenavir in combination with NRTIs for 16-48 weeks identified isolates from 15 patients who exhibited a 4- to 17-fold decrease in susceptibility to amprenavir *in vitro* compared to wild-type virus. Clinical isolates that exhibited a decrease in amprenavir susceptibility harbored one or more amprenavir-associated mutations. The clinical relevance of the genotypic and phenotypic changes associated with amprenavir therapy is under evaluation.

Cross-Resistance

Varying degrees of HIV-1 cross-resistance among protease inhibitors have been observed. Five (5) of 15 amprenavir-resistant isolates exhibited 4- to 8-fold decrease in susceptibility to ritonavir. However, amprenavir-resistant isolates were susceptible to either indinavir or saquinavir.

PHARMACOKINETICS IN ADULTS

The pharmacokinetic properties of amprenavir have been studied in asymptomatic, HIV-infected adult patients after administration of single oral doses of 150-1200 mg and multiple oral doses of 300-1200 mg twice daily.

Absorption and Bioavailability

Amprenavir was rapidly absorbed after oral administration in HIV-1-infected patients with a time to peak concentration (T_{max}) typically between 1 and 2 hours after a single oral dose. The absolute oral bioavailability of amprenavir in humans has not been established.

Increases in the area under the plasma concentration versus time curve (AUC) after single oral doses between 150 and 1200 mg were slightly greater than dose-proportional. Increases in AUC were dose-proportional after 3 weeks of dosing with doses from 300-1200 mg twice daily. The pharmacokinetic parameters after administration of amprenavir 1200 mg bid for 3 weeks to HIV-infected subjects are shown in TABLE 1.

TABLE 1 *Average (%CV) Pharmacokinetic Parameters After 1200 mg bid of Amprenavir Capsules (n=54)*

C_{max} (μg/ml)	T_{max} (hours)	AUC(0-12) (μg·h/ml)	C_{avg} (μg/ml)	C_{min} (μg/ml)	CL/F (ml/min/kg)
7.66 (54%)	1.0 (42%)	17.7 (47%)	1.48 (47%)	0.32 (77%)	19.5 (46%)

The relative bioavailability of amprenavir capsules and oral solution was assessed in healthy adults. Amprenavir oral solution was 14% less bioavailable compared to the capsules.

Food Effect on Absorption

The relative bioavailability of amprenavir capsules was assessed in the fasting and fed states in healthy volunteers (standardized high-fat meal: 967 kcal, 67 g fat, 33 g protein, 58 g carbohydrate). Administration of a single 1200 mg dose of amprenavir in the fed state compared to the fasted state was associated with changes in C_{max} (fed: 6.18 ± 2.92 μg/ml, fasted: 9.72 ± 2.75 μg/ml), T_{max} (fed: 1.51 ± 0.68, fasted: 1.05 ± 0.63), and AUC(0-∞) (fed: 22.06 ± 11.6 μg·h/ml, fasted: 28.05 ± 10.1 μg·h/ml). Amprenavir may be taken with or without food, but should not be taken with a high-fat meal (see DOSAGE AND ADMINISTRATION).

Distribution

The apparent volume of distribution (Vz/F) is approximately 430 L in healthy adult subjects. *In vitro* binding is approximately 90% to plasma proteins. The high affinity binding protein for amprenavir is alpha$_1$-acid glycoprotein (AAG). The partitioning of amprenavir into erythrocytes is low, but increases as amprenavir concentrations increase, reflecting the higher amount of unbound drug at higher concentrations.

Metabolism

Amprenavir is metabolized in the liver by the cytochrome P4503A4 (CYP3A4) enzyme system. The 2 major metabolites result from oxidation of the tetrahydrofuran and aniline moieties. Glucuronide conjugates of oxidized metabolites have been identified as minor metabolites in urine and feces.

Amprenavir oral solution contains a large amount of propylene glycol, which is hepatically metabolized by the alcohol and aldehyde dehydrogenase enzyme pathway. Alcohol dehydrogenase (ADH) is present in the human fetal liver at 2 months of gestational age, but at only 3% of adult activity. Although the data are limited, it appears that by 12-30 months of postnatal age, ADH activity is equal to or greater than that observed in adults. Additionally, certain patient groups (females, Asians, Eskimos, Native Americans) may be at increased risk of propylene glycol-associated adverse events due to diminished ability to metabolize propylene glycol (see Special Populations: Gender and Race).

Elimination

Excretion of unchanged amprenavir in urine and feces is minimal. Approximately 14% and 75% of an administered single dose of ^{14}C-amprenavir can be accounted for as radiocarbon in urine and feces, respectively. Two metabolites accounted for >90% of the radiocarbon in fecal samples. The plasma elimination half-life of amprenavir ranged from 7.1-10.6 hours.

SPECIAL POPULATIONS

Hepatic Insufficiency

Amprenavir oral solution is contraindicated in patients with hepatic failure.

Patients with hepatic impairment are at increased risk of propylene glycol-associated adverse events (see WARNINGS). Amprenavir oral solution should be used with caution in patients with hepatic impairment. Amprenavir capsules have been studied in adult patients with impaired hepatic function using a single 600 mg oral dose. The AUC(0-∞) was significantly greater in patients with moderate cirrhosis (25.76 ± 14.68 μg·h/ml) compared with healthy volunteers (12.00 ± 4.38 μg·h/ml). The AUC(0-∞) and C_{max} were significantly greater in patients with severe cirrhosis [AUC(0-∞): 38.66 ± 16.08 μg·h/ml; C_{max}: 9.43 ± 2.61 μg/ml] compared with healthy volunteers [AUC(0-∞): 12.00 ± 4.38 μg·h/ml; C_{max}: 4.90 ± 1.39 μg/ml]. Patients with impaired hepatic function require dosage adjustment (see DOSAGE AND ADMINISTRATION).

Renal Insufficiency

Amprenavir oral solution is contraindicated in patients with renal failure.

Patients with renal impairment are at increased risk of propylene glycol-associated adverse events. Additionally, because metabolites of the excipient propylene glycol in amprenavir oral solution may alter acid-base balance, patients with renal impairment should be monitored for potential adverse events (see WARNINGS). Amprenavir oral solution should be used with caution in patients with renal impairment. The impact of renal impairment on amprenavir elimination has not been studied. The renal elimination of unchanged amprenavir represents <3% of the administered dose.

Pediatric Patients

Amprenavir oral solution is contraindicated in infants and children below 4 years of age (see CONTRAINDICATIONS and WARNINGS).

The pharmacokinetics of amprenavir have been studied after either single or repeat doses of amprenavir capsules or oral solution in 84 pediatric patients. Twenty (20) HIV-1-infected children ranging in age from 4-12 years received single doses from 5-20 mg/kg using 25 or 150 mg capsules. The C_{max} of amprenavir increased less than proportionally with dose. The AUC(0-∞) increased proportionally at doses between 5 and 20 mg/kg. Amprenavir is 14% less bioavailable from the liquid formulation than from the capsules; therefore **amprenavir capsules and amprenavir oral solution are not interchangeable on a milligram-per-milligram basis.**

TABLE 2 *Average (%CV) Pharmacokinetic Parameters in Children Ages 4-12 Years Receiving 20 mg/kg bid or 15 mg/kg tid of Amprenavir Oral Solution*

Dose	n	C_{max} (μg/ml)	T_{max} (hours)	AUC(ss)* (μg·h/ml)	C_{avg} (μg/ml)	C_{min} (μg/ml)	CL/F (ml/min/kg)
20 mg/kg bid	20	6.77 (51%)	1.1 (21%)	15.46 (59%)	1.29 (59%)	0.24 (98%)	29 (58%)
15 mg/kg tid	17	3.99 (37%)	1.4 (90%)	8.73 (36%)	1.09 (36%)	0.27 (95%)	32 (34%)

* AUC is 0-12 hours for bid and 0-8 hours for tid, therefore the C_{avg} is a better comparison of the exposures.

Geriatric Patients

The pharmacokinetics of amprenavir have not been studied in patients over 65 years of age.

Gender

The pharmacokinetics of amprenavir do not differ between males and females. Females may have a lower amount of alcohol dehydrogenase compared with males and may be at increased risk of propylene glycol-associated adverse events; no data are available on propylene glycol metabolism in females.

Race

The pharmacokinetics of amprenavir do not differ between blacks and non-blacks. Certain ethnic populations (Asians, Eskimos, and Native Americans) may be at increased risk of propylene glycol-associated adverse events because of alcohol dehydrogenase polymorphisms; no data are available on propylene glycol metabolism in these groups.

DRUG INTERACTIONS

See also CONTRAINDICATIONS, WARNINGS, and DRUG INTERACTIONS.

Amprenavir is metabolized in the liver by the cytochrome P450 enzyme system. Amprenavir inhibits CYP3A4. Caution should be used when coadministering medications that are substrates, inhibitors, or inducers of CYP3A4, or potentially toxic medications that are metabolized by CYP3A4. Amprenavir does not inhibit CYP2D6, CYP1A2, CYP2C9, CYP2C19, CYP2E1, or uridine glucuronosyltransferase (UDPGT).

Drug interaction studies were performed with amprenavir capsules and other drugs likely to be coadministered or drugs commonly used as probes for pharmacokinetic interactions. The effects of coadministration of amprenavir on the AUC, C_{max}, and C_{min} are summarized in TABLE 3 (effect of other drugs on amprenavir) and TABLE 4 (effect of amprenavir on other drugs). For information regarding clinical recommendations, see PRECAUTIONS.

TABLE 3 *Drug Interactions: Pharmacokinetic Parameters for Amprenavir in the Presence of the Coadministered Drug*

				% Change in Amprenavir Pharmacokinetic Parameters* (90% CI)		
Coadministered Drug	Dose of Coadministered Drug	Dose of Amprenavir	n	C_{max}	AUC	C_{min}
Abacavir	300 mg bid for 3 weeks	900 mg bid for 3 weeks	4	inc 47 (dec 15 to inc 154)	inc 29 (dec 18 to inc 103)	inc 27 (dec 46 to inc 197)
Clarithromycin	500 mg bid for 4 days	1200 mg bid for 4 days	12	inc 15 (inc 1 to inc 31)	inc 18 (inc 8 to inc 29)	inc 39 (inc 31 to inc 47)
Delavirdine	600 mg bid for 10 days	600 mg bid for 10 days	9	inc 40‡	inc 130‡	inc 125‡
Ethinyl estradiol/ norethindrone	0.035 mg/1 mg for 1 cycle	1200 mg bid for 28 days	10	NC (dec 20 to inc 3	dec 22 (dec 35 to dec 8)	dec 20 (dec 41 to inc 8)
Indinavir	800 mg tid for 2 weeks (fasted)	750 or 800 mg tid for 2 weeks (fasted)	9	inc 18 (dec 13 to inc 58)	inc 33 (inc 2 to inc 73)	inc 25 (dec 27 to inc 116)
Ketoconazole	400 mg single dose	1200 mg single dose	12	dec 16 (dec 25 to dec 6)	inc 31 (inc 20 to inc 42)	NA
Lamivudine	150 mg single dose	600 mg single dose	11	NC (dec 17 to inc 9)	NC (dec 15 to inc 14)	NA
Nelfinavir	750 mg tid for 2 weeks (fed)	750 or 800 mg tid for 2 weeks (fed)	6	dec 14 (dec 38 to inc 20)	NC (dec 19 to inc 47)	inc 189 (inc 52 to inc 448)
Rifabutin	300 mg qd for 10 days	1200 mg bid for 10 days	5	NC (dec 21 to inc 10)	dec 15 (dec 28 to 0)	dec 15 (dec 38 to inc 17)
Rifampin	300 mg qd for 4 days	1200 mg bid for 4 days	11	dec 70 (dec 76 to dec 62)	dec 82 (dec 84 to dec 78)	dec 92 (dec 95 to dec 89)
Ritonavir	100 mg bid for 2-4 weeks	600 mg bid	18	dec 30† (dec 44 to dec 14)	inc 64† (inc 37 to inc 97)	inc 508† (inc 394 to inc 649)
Ritonavir	200 mg qd for 2-4 weeks	1200 md qd	12	NC† (dec 17 to inc 30)	inc 62† (inc 35 to inc 94)	inc 319† (inc 190 to inc 508)
Saquinavir	800 mg tid for 2 weeks (fed)	750 or 800 mg tid for 2 weeks (fed)	7	dec 37 (dec 54 to dec 14)	dec 32 (dec 49 to dec 9)	dec 14 (dec 52 to inc 54)
Zidovudine	300 mg single dose	600 mg single dose	12	NC (dec 5 to inc 24)	inc 13 (dec 2 to inc 31)	NA

* Based on total-drug concentrations.
† Compared to amprenavir capsules 1200 mg bid in the same patients.
‡ Median percent change; confidence interval not reported.
inc = Increase.
dec = Decrease.
NC = No change (inc or dec <10%).
NA = C_{min} not calculated for single-dose study.

Nucleoside Reverse Transcriptase Inhibitors (NRTIs)

There was no effect of amprenavir on abacavir in subjects receiving both agents based on historical data.

HIV Protease Inhibitors

Concurrent use of amprenavir oral solution and ritonavir oral solution is not recommended because the large amount of propylene glycol in amprenavir oral solution and ethanol in ritonavir oral solution may compete for the same metabolic pathway for elimination. This combination has not been studied in pediatric patients.

The effect of amprenavir on total drug concentrations of other HIV protease inhibitors in subjects receiving both agents was evaluated using comparisons to historical data. Indinavir steady-state C_{max}, AUC, and C_{min} were decreased by 22%, 38%, and 27%, respectively, by concomitant amprenavir. Similar decreases in C_{max} and AUC were seen after the first dose. Saquinavir steady-state C_{max}, AUC, and C_{min} were increased 21%, decreased 19%, and decreased 48%, respectively, by concomitant amprenavir. Nelfinavir steady-state C_{max}, AUC, and C_{min} were increased by 12%, 15%, and 14%, respectively, by concomitant amprenavir.

Methadone

Coadministration of amprenavir and methadone can decrease plasma levels of methadone.

Coadministration of amprenavir and methadone as compared to a non-matched historical control group resulted in a 30%, 27%, and 25% decrease in serum amprenavir AUC, C_{max}, and C_{min}, respectively.

For information regarding clinical recommendations, see DRUG INTERACTIONS.

INDICATIONS AND USAGE

Amprenavir is indicated in combination with other antiretroviral agents for the treatment of HIV-1 infection.

The following points should be considered when initiating therapy with amprenavir:

In a study of NRTI-experienced, protease inhibitor-naive patients, amprenavir was found to be significantly less effective than indinavir.

TABLE 4 *Drug Interactions: Pharmacokinetic Parameters for Coadministered Drug in the Presence of Amprenavir*

Coadministered Drug	Dose of Coadministered Drug	Dose of Amprenavir	n	% Change in Pharmacokinetic Parameters of Coadministered Drug (90% CI) C_{max}	AUC	C_{min}
Clarithromycin	500 mg bid for 4 days	1200 mg bid for 4 days	12	dec 10 (dec 24 to inc 7)	NC (dec 17 to inc 11)	NC (dec 13 to inc 20)
Delavirdine	600 mg bid for 10 days	600 mg bid for 10 days	9	dec 47*	dec 61*	dec 88*
Ethinyl estradiol	0.035 mg for 1 cycle	1200 mg bid for 28 days	10	NC (dec 25 to inc 15)	NC (dec 14 to inc 38)	inc 32 (dec 3 to inc 79)
Norethindrone	1.0 mg for 1 cycle	1200 mg bid for 28 ays	10	NC (dec 20 to inc 18)	inc 18 (inc 1 to inc 38)	inc 45 (inc 13 to inc 88)
Ketoconazole	400 mg single dose	1200 mg single dose	12	inc 19 (inc 8 to inc 33)	inc 44 (inc 31 to inc 59)	NA
Lamivudine	150 mg single dose	600 mg single dose	11	NC (dec 17 to inc 3)	NC (dec 11 to 0)	NA
Methadone						
R-methadone (active)	44-100 mg qd for >30 days	1200 mg bid for 10 days	16	dec 25 (dec 32 to dec 18)	dec 13 (dec 21 to dec 5)	dec 21 (dec 32 to dec 9)
S-methadone (inactive)	44-100 mg qd for >30 days	1200 mg bid for 10 days	16	dec 48 (dec 55 to dec 40)	dec 40 (dec 46 to dec 32)	dec 53 (dec 60 to dec 43)
Rifabutin	300 mg qd for 10 days	1200 mg bid for 10 days	5	inc 119 (inc 82 to inc 164)	inc 193 (inc 156 to inc 235)	inc 271 (inc 171 to inc 409)
Rifampin	300 mg qd for 4 days	1200 mg bid for 4 days	11	NC (dec 13 to inc 12)	NC (dec 10 to inc 13)	ND
Zidovudine	300 mg single dose	600 mg single dose	12	inc 40 (inc 14 to inc 71)	inc 31 (inc 19 to inc 45)	NA

* Median percent change; confidence interval not reported.
inc = Increase.
dec = Decrease.
NC = No change (inc or dec <10%).
NA = C_{min} not calculated for single-dose study.
ND = Interaction cannot be determined as C_{min} was below the lower limit of quantitation.

Mild to moderate gastrointestinal adverse events led to discontinuation of amprenavir primarily during the first 12 weeks of therapy (see ADVERSE REACTIONS).

There are no data on response to therapy with amprenavir in protease inhibitor-experienced patients.

Amprenavir oral solution should be used only when amprenavir capsules or other protease inhibitor formulations are not therapeutic options.

CONTRAINDICATIONS

Because of the potential risk of toxicity from the large amount of the excipient propylene glycol, amprenavir oral solution is contraindicated in infants and children below the age of 4 years, pregnant women, patients with hepatic or renal failure, and patients treated with disulfiram or metronidazole (see WARNINGS and PRECAUTIONS).

Coadministration of amprenavir is contraindicated with drugs that are highly dependent on CYP3A4 for clearance and for which elevated plasma concentrations are associated with serious and/or life-threatening events. These drugs are listed in TABLE 6.

TABLE 6 *Drugs That Are Contraindicated With Amprenavir*

Drug Class	Drugs Within Class That Are Contraindicated With Amprenavir
Oral Solution	
Alcohol-dependence treatment	Disulfiram
Antibiotic	Metronidazole
Capsules and Oral Solution	
Ergot derivatives	Dihydroergotamine, ergonovine, ergotamine, methylergonovine
GI motility agent	Cisapride
Neuroleptic	Pimozide
Sedatives/hyponotics	Midazolam, triazolam

If amprenavir capsules are coadministered with ritonavir capsules, the antiarrhythmic agents flecainide and propafenone are also contraindicated.

Amprenavir is contraindicated in patients with previously demonstrated clinically significant hypersensitivity to any of the components of this product.

WARNINGS

ALERT: Find out about medicines that should not be taken with amprenavir.

Because of the potential risk of toxicity from the large amount of the excipient propylene glycol, amprenavir oral solution is contraindicated in infants and children below the age of 4 years, pregnant women, patients with hepatic or renal failure, and patients treated with disulfiram or metronidazole (see CLINICAL PHARMACOLOGY, CONTRAINDICATIONS, and PRECAUTIONS).

Because of the possible toxicity associated with the large amount of propylene glycol and the lack of information on chronic exposure to large amounts of propylene glycol, amprenavir oral solution should be used only when amprenavir capsules or other protease inhibitor formulations are not therapeutic options. Certain ethnic populations (Asians, Eskimos, Native Americans) and women may be at increased risk of propylene glycol-associated adverse events due to diminished ability to metabolize propylene glycol; no data are available on propylene glycol metabolism in these groups (see CLINICAL PHARMACOLOGY, Special Populations: Gender and Race).

If patients require treatment with amprenavir oral solution, they should be monitored closely for propylene glycol-associated adverse events, including seizures, stupor, tachycardia, hyperosmolality, lactic acidosis, renal toxicity, and hemolysis. Patients should be switched from amprenavir oral solution to amprenavir capsules as soon as they are able to take the capsule formulation.

Concurrent use of amprenavir oral solution and ritonavir oral solution is not recommended because the large amount of propylene glycol in amprenavir oral solution and ethanol in ritonavir oral solution may compete for the same metabolic pathway for elimination.

Use of alcoholic beverages is not recommended in patients treated with amprenavir oral solution.

Serious and/or life-threatening drug interactions could occur between amprenavir and amiodarone, lidocaine (systemic), tricyclic antidepressants, and quinidine. Concentration monitoring of these agents is recommended if these agents are used concomitantly with amprenavir (see CONTRAINDICATIONS).

Rifampin should not be used in combination with amprenavir because it reduces plasma concentrations and AUC of amprenavir by about 90%.

Concomitant use of amprenavir and St. John's wort (hypericum perforatum) or products containing St. John's wort is not recommended. Coadministration of protease inhibitors, including amprenavir, with St. John's wort is expected to substantially decrease protease inhibitor concentrations and may result in suboptimal levels of amprenavir and lead to loss of virologic response and possible resistance to amprenavir or to the class of protease inhibitors.

Concomitant use of amprenavir with lovastatin or simvastatin is not recommended. Caution should be exercised if HIV protease inhibitors, including amprenavir, are used concurrently with other HMG-CoA reductase inhibitors that are also metabolized by the CYP3A4 pathway (*e.g.*, atorvastatin). The risk of myopathy, including rhabdomyolysis, may be increased when HIV protease inhibitors, including amprenavir, are used in combination with these drugs.

Particular caution should be used when prescribing sildenafil in patients receiving amprenavir. Coadministration of amprenavir with sildenafil is expected to substantially increase sildenafil concentrations and may result in an increase in sildenafil-associated adverse events, including hypotension, visual changes, and priapism (see PRECAUTIONS, Information for the Patient; DRUG INTERACTIONS; and the complete prescribing information for sildenafil).

Severe and life-threatening skin reactions, including Stevens-Johnson syndrome, have occurred in patients treated with amprenavir (see ADVERSE REACTIONS).

Acute hemolytic anemia has been reported in a patient treated with amprenavir.

New onset diabetes mellitus, exacerbation of pre-existing diabetes mellitus, and hyperglycemia have been reported during post-marketing surveillance in HIV-infected patients receiving protease inhibitor therapy. Some patients required either initiation or dose adjustments of insulin or oral hypoglycemic agents for treatment of these events. In some cases, diabetic ketoacidosis has occurred. In those patients who discontinued protease inhibitor therapy, hyperglycemia persisted in some cases. Because these events have been reported voluntarily during clinical practice, estimates of frequency cannot be made and causal relationships between protease inhibitor therapy and these events have not been established.

PRECAUTIONS

GENERAL

Amprenavir capsules and oral solution are not interchangeable on a milligram-per-milligram basis (see CLINICAL PHARMACOLOGY, Special Populations, Pediatric Patients and CONTRAINDICATIONS).

Amprenavir is a sulfonamide. The potential for cross-sensitivity between drugs in the sulfonamide class and amprenavir is unknown. Amprenavir should be used with caution in patients with a known sulfonamide allergy.

Amprenavir is principally metabolized by the liver. Amprenavir, when used alone and in combination with low-dose ritonavir, has been associated with elevations of SGOT (AST) and SGPT (ALT) in some patients. Caution should be exercised when administering amprenavir to patients with hepatic impairment (see DOSAGE AND ADMINISTRATION). Appropriate laboratory testing should be conducted prior to initiating therapy with amprenavir and at periodic intervals during treatment.

Formulations of amprenavir provide high daily doses of vitamin E (see Information for the Patient, DESCRIPTION, and DOSAGE AND ADMINISTRATION). The effects of long-term, high-dose vitamin E administration in humans is not well characterized and has not been specifically studied in HIV-infected individuals. High vitamin E doses may exacerbate the blood coagulation defect of vitamin K deficiency caused by anticoagulant therapy or malabsorption.

PATIENTS WITH HEMOPHILIA

There have been reports of spontaneous bleeding in patients with hemophilia A and B treated with protease inhibitors. In some patients, additional factor VIII was required. In many of the reported cases, treatment with protease inhibitors was continued or restarted. A causal relationship between protease inhibitor therapy and these episodes has not been established.

FAT REDISTRIBUTION

Redistribution/accumulation of body fat, including central obesity, dorsocervical fat enlargement (buffalo hump), peripheral wasting, facial wasting, breast enlargement, and "cushingoid appearance," have been observed in patients receiving antiretroviral therapy. The mechanism and long-term consequences of these events are currently unknown. A causal relationship has not been established.

LIPID ELEVATIONS

Treatment with amprenavir alone or in combination with ritonavir capsules has resulted in increases in the concentration of total cholesterol and triglycerides. Triglyceride and cholesterol testing should be performed prior to initiation of therapy with amprenavir and at periodic intervals during treatment. Lipid disorders should be managed as clinically appropriate. See DRUG INTERACTIONS, Established and Other Potentially Significant Drug Interactions for additional information on potential drug interactions with amprenavir and HMG-CoA reductase inhibitors.

RESISTANCE/CROSS-RESISTANCE

Because the potential for HIV cross-resistance among protease inhibitors has not been fully explored, it is unknown what effect amprenavir therapy will have on the activity of subsequently administered protease inhibitors. It is also unknown what effect previous treatment with other protease inhibitors will have on the activity of amprenavir (see CLINICAL PHARMACOLOGY, Microbiology).

INFORMATION FOR THE PATIENT

A statement to patients and health care providers is included on the product's bottle label: **ALERT: Find out about medicines that should NOT be taken with amprenavir.** See the Patient Instructions that are distributed with the prescription.

Amprenavir oral solution is contraindicated in infants and children below the age of 4 years, pregnant women, patients with hepatic or renal failure, and patients treated with disulfiram or metronidazole. Amprenavir oral solution should be used only when amprenavir capsules or other protease inhibitor formulations are not therapeutic options.

Patients treated with amprenavir capsules should be cautioned against switching to amprenavir oral solution because of the increased risk of adverse events from the large amount of propylene glycol in amprenavir oral solution.

Women, Asians, Eskimos, or Native Americans, as well as patients who have hepatic or renal insufficiency, should be informed that they may be at increased risk of adverse events from the large amount of propylene glycol in amprenavir oral solution.

Patients should be informed that amprenavir is not a cure for HIV infection and that they may continue to develop opportunistic infections and other complications associated with HIV disease. The long-term effects of amprenavir are unknown at this time. Patients should be told that there are currently no data demonstrating that therapy with amprenavir can reduce the risk of transmitting HIV to others through sexual contact.

Patients should remain under the care of a physician while using amprenavir. Patients should be advised to take amprenavir every day as prescribed. Amprenavir must always be used in combination with other antiretroviral drugs. Patients should not alter the dose or discontinue therapy without consulting their physician. If a dose is missed, patients should take the dose as soon as possible and then return to their normal schedule. However, if a dose is skipped, the patient should not double the next dose.

Patients should inform their doctor if they have a sulfa allergy. The potential for cross-sensitivity between drugs in the sulfonamide class and amprenavir is unknown.

Amprenavir may interact with some drugs; therefore, patients should be advised to report to their doctor the use of any other prescription or nonprescription medication or herbal products, particularly St. John's wort.

Patients taking antacids (or the buffered formulation of didanosine) should take amprenavir at least 1 hour before or after antacid (or the buffered formulation of didanosine) use.

Patients should be advised that drinking alcoholic beverages is not recommended while taking amprenavir oral solution.

Patients receiving sildenafil should be advised that they may be at an increased risk of sildenafil-associated adverse events including hypotension, visual changes, and priapism, and should promptly report any symptoms to their doctor.

Patients taking amprenavir should be instructed **not** to use hormonal contraceptives because some birth control pills (those containing ethinyl estradiol/norethindrone) have been found to decrease the concentration of amprenavir. Therefore, patients receiving hormonal contraceptives should be instructed to use alternate contraceptive measures during therapy with amprenavir.

High-fat meals may decrease the absorption of amprenavir and should be avoided. Amprenavir may be taken with meals of normal fat content.

Patients should be informed that redistribution or accumulation of body fat may occur in patients receiving antiretroviral therapy and that the cause and long-term health effects of these conditions are not known at this time.

Adult and pediatric patients should be advised not to take supplemental vitamin E since the vitamin E content of amprenavir capsules and oral solution exceeds the Reference Daily Intake (adults 30 IU, pediatrics approximately 10 IU).

LABORATORY TESTS

The combination of amprenavir and low-dose ritonavir has been associated with elevations of cholesterol and triglycerides, SGOT (AST), and SGPT (ALT) in some patients. Appropriate laboratory testing should be considered prior to initiating combination therapy with amprenavir and ritonavir capsules and at periodic intervals or if any clinical signs or symptoms of hyperlipidemia or elevated liver function tests occur during therapy. For comprehensive information concerning laboratory test alterations associated with ritonavir, physicians should refer to the complete prescribing information for ritonavir.

CARCINOGENESIS AND MUTAGENESIS

Amprenavir was evaluated for carcinogenic potential by oral gavage administration to mice and rats for up to 104 weeks. Daily doses of 50, 275-300, and 500-600 mg/kg/day were administered to mice and doses of 50, 190, and 750 mg/kg/day were administered to rats. Results showed an increase in the incidence of benign hepatocellular adenomas and an increase in the combined incidence of hepatocellular adenomas plus carcinoma in males of both species at the highest doses tested. Female mice and rats were not affected. These observations were made at systemic exposures equivalent to approximately 2 times (mice) and 4 times (rats) the human exposure [based on $AUC_{(0-24h)}$ measurement] at the recommended dose of 1200 mg twice daily. Administration of amprenavir did not cause a statistically significant increase in the incidence of any other benign or malignant neoplasm in mice or rats. It is not known how predictive the results of rodent carcinogenicity studies may be for humans. However, amprenavir was not mutagenic or genotoxic in a battery of *in vitro* and *in vivo* assays including bacterial reverse mutation (Ames), mouse lymphoma, rat micronucleus, and chromosome aberrations in human lymphocytes.

FERTILITY

The effects of amprenavir on fertility and general reproductive performance were investigated in male rats (treated for 28 days before mating, at doses producing up to twice the expected clinical exposure based on AUC comparisons) and female rats (treated for 15 days before mating through Day 17 of gestation at doses producing up to 2 times the expected clinical exposure). Amprenavir did not impair mating or fertility of male or female rats and did not affect the development and maturation of sperm from treated rats. The reproductive performance of the F1 generation born to female rats given amprenavir was not different from control animals.

PREGNANCY AND REPRODUCTION

Capsules

Pregnancy Category C

Embryo/fetal development studies were conducted in rats (dosed from 15 days before pairing to Day 17 of gestation) and rabbits (dosed from Day 8 to Day 20 of gestation). In pregnant rabbits, amprenavir administration was associated with abortions and an increased incidence of 3 minor skeletal variations resulting from deficient ossification of the femur, humerus trochlea, and humerus. Systemic exposure at the highest tested dose was approximately one-twentieth of the exposure seen at the recommended human dose. In rat fetuses, thymic elongation and incomplete ossification of bones were attributed to amprenavir. Both findings were seen at systemic exposures that were one-half of that associated with the recommended human dose.

Pre- and post-natal developmental studies were performed in rats dosed from Day 7 of gestation to Day 22 of lactation. Reduced body weights (10-20%) were observed in the offspring. The systemic exposure associated with this finding was approximately twice the exposure in humans following administration of the recommended human dose. The subsequent development of these offspring, including fertility and reproductive performance, was not affected by the maternal administration of amprenavir.

There are no adequate and well-controlled studies in pregnant women. Amprenavir should be used during pregnancy only if the potential benefit justifies the potential risk to the fetus. **Antiretroviral Pregnancy Registry:** To monitor maternal-fetal outcomes of pregnant women exposed to amprenavir, an Antiretroviral Pregnancy Registry has been established. Physicians are encouraged to register patients by calling 1-800-258-4263.

Oral Solution

Amprenavir oral solution is contraindicated during pregnancy due to the potential risk of toxicity to the fetus from the high propylene glycol content. Therefore, if amprenavir is used in pregnant women, the amprenavir capsules formulation should be used (see Capsules).

NURSING MOTHERS

The Centers for Disease Control and Prevention recommend that HIV-infected mothers not breastfeed their infants to avoid risking postnatal transmission of HIV. Although it is not known if amprenavir is excreted in human milk, amprenavir is secreted into the milk of lactating rats. Because of both the potential for HIV transmission and the potential for serious adverse reactions in nursing infants, **mothers should be instructed not to breastfeed if they are receiving amprenavir.**

PEDIATRIC USE

Amprenavir oral solution is contraindicated in infants and children below the age of 4 years due to the potential risk of toxicity from the excipient propylene glycol (see CONTRAINDICATIONS and WARNINGS). Alcohol dehydrogenase (ADH), which metabolizes propylene glycol, is present in the human fetal liver at 2 months gestational age, but only at 3% of adult activity. Although the data are limited, it appears that by 12-30 months of postnatal age, ADH activity is equal to or greater than that observed in adults.

Two hundred fifty-one (251) patients aged 4 and above have received amprenavir as single or multiple doses in studies. An adverse event profile similar to that seen in adults was seen in pediatric patients.

Amprenavir capsules have not been evaluated in pediatric patients below the age of 4 years (see CLINICAL PHARMACOLOGY and DOSAGE AND ADMINISTRATION).

Concurrent use of amprenavir oral solution and ritonavir oral solution is not recommended because the large amount of propylene glycol in amprenavir oral solution and ethanol in ritonavir oral solution may compete for the same metabolic pathway for elimination. This combination has not been studied in pediatric patients.

GERIATRIC USE

Clinical studies of amprenavir did not include sufficient numbers of patients aged 65 and over to determine whether they respond differently from younger adults. In general, dose selection for an elderly patient should be cautious, reflecting the greater frequency of decreased hepatic, renal, or cardiac function, and of concomitant disease or other drug therapy.

DRUG INTERACTIONS

See also CONTRAINDICATIONS; WARNINGS; and CLINICAL PHARMACOLOGY, Drug Interactions.

Amprenavir is an inhibitor of cytochrome P450 3A4 metabolism and therefore should not be administered concurrently with medications with narrow therapeutic windows that are substrates of CYP3A4. There are other agents that may result in serious and/or life-threatening drug interactions (see CONTRAINDICATIONS and WARNINGS).

Use of alcoholic beverages is not recommended in patients treated with amprenavir oral solution.

TABLE 7 *Drugs That Should Not Be Coadministered With Amprenavir*

Drug Class/Drug Name	Clinical Comment
Alcohol-Dependence Treatment:	
Disulfiram	**CONTRAINDICATED** due to potential risk of toxicity from the large amount of the expient, propylene glycol, in amprenavir oral solution.
Antibiotic:	
Metronidazole	**CONTRAINDICATED** due to potential risk of toxicity from the large amount of the expient, propylene glycol, in amprenavir oral solution.
Antimycobacterials:	
Rifampin†	May lead to loss of virologic response and possible resistance to amprenavir or to the class of protease inhibitors.
Ergot Derivatives:	
Dihydroergotamine, ergonovine, ergotamine, methylergonovine	**CONTRAINDICATED** due to potential for serious and/or life-threatening reactions such as acute ergot toxicity characterized by peripheral vasospasm and ischemia of the extremities and other tissues.
GI Motility Agents:	
Cisapride	**CONTRAINDICATED** due to potential for serious and/or life-threatening reactions such as cardiac arrhythmias.
Herbal Products:	
St. John's wort (hypericum perforatum)	May lead to loss of virologic response and possible resistance to amprenavir or to the class of protease inhibitors.
HIV-Protease Inhibitor:	
Ritonavir oral solution	Concurrent use of amprenavir oral solution and ritonavir oral solution is not recommended because the large amount of propylene glycol in amprevanir oral solution in ritonivir oral solution may compete for the same metobolic pathway for elimination.o
HMG Co-Reductase Inhibitors:	
Lovastatin, simvastatin	Potential for serious reactions such as risk of myopathy including rhabdomyolysis.
Neuroleptic:	
Pimozide	**CONTRAINDICATED** due to potential for serious and/or life-threatening reactions such as cardiac arrhythmias.
Non-Nucleoside Reverse Transcriptase Inhibitor:	
Delavirdine†	May lead to loss of virologic response and possible resistance to delavirdine.
Oral Contraceptives:	
Ethinyl estradiol/norethindrone	May lead to loss of virologic response and possible resistance to amprenavir. Alternative methods of non-hormal contraception are recommended.
Sedative/Hypnotics:	
Midazolam, triazolam	**CONTRAINDICATED** due to potential for serious and/or life-threatening reactions such as prolonged or increased sedation or respiratory depression.

† See TABLE 3 and TABLE 4 for magnitude of interaction.

ESTABLISHED AND OTHER POTENTIALLY SIGNIFICANT DRUG INTERACTIONS

Alteration in dose or regimen may be recommended based on drug interaction studies or predicted interaction.

HIV-Antiviral Agents

Non-Nucleoside Reverse Transcriptase Inhibitors

Efavirenz, nevirapine.

Effect: Decreases amprenavir concentration.

Clinical Comment: Appropriate doses of the combinations with respect to safety and efficacy have not been established.

Nucleoside Reverse Transcriptase Inhibitor

Didanosine (buffered formulation only).

Effect: Decreases amprenavir concentration.

Clinical Comment: Take amprenavir at least 1 hour before or after the buffered formulation of didanosine.

HIV-Protease Inhibitors

Indinavir,* lopinavir/ritonavir, nelfinavir.*

Effect: Increases amprenavir concentration. Amprenavir's effect on other protease inhibitors is not well established.

Clinical Comment: Appropriate doses of the combinations with respect to safety and efficacy have not been established.

HIV-Protease Inhibitor

Ritonavir capsules.*

Effect: Increases amprenavir concentration.

Clinical Comment: The dose of amprenavir should be reduced when used in combination with ritonavir capsules (see DOSAGE AND ADMINISTRATION). Also, see the full prescribing information for ritonavir for additional drug interaction information. Concurrent use of amprenavir oral solution and ritonavir oral solution is not recommended because the large amount of propylene glycol in amprenavir oral solution and ethanol in ritonavir oral solution may compete for the same metabolic pathway for elimination.

HIV-Protease Inhibitor

Saquinavir.*

Effect: Decreases amprvnavir concentration. Amprenavir's effect on saquinavir is not well established.

Clinical Comment: Appropriate doses of the combination with respect to safety and efficacy have not been established.

*See TABLE 3 and TABLE 4 for magnitude of interaction.

Other Agents

Antacids

Effect: Decreases amprenavir concentration.

Clinical Comment: Take amprenavir at least 1 hour before or after antacids.

Antiarrhythmics

Amiodarone, lidocaine (systemic), and quinidine.

Effect: Increases antiarrhythmics concentration.

Clinical Comment: Caution is warranted and therapeutic concentration monitoring is recommended for antiarrhythmics when coadministered with amprenavir, if available.

Antiarrhythmic

Bepridil.

Effect: Increases bepridil concentration.

Clinical Comment: Use with caution. Increased bepridil exposure may be associated with life-threatening reactions such as cardiac arrhythmias.

Anticoagulant

Warfarin.

Clinical Comment: Concentrations of warfarin may be affected. It is recommended that INR (international normalized ratio) be monitored.

Anticonvulsants

Carbamazepine, phenobarbital, phenytoin.

Effect: Decreases amprenavir concentration.

Clinical Comment: Use with caution. Amprenavir may be less effective due to decreased amprenavir plasma concentrations in patients taking these agents concomitantly.

Antifungals

Ketoconazole, itraconazole.

Effect: Increases ketoconazole concentration. Increases itraconazole concentration.

Clinical Comment: Increase monitoring for adverse events due to ketoconazole or itraconazole. Dose reduction of ketoconazole or itraconazole may be needed for patients receiving more than 400 mg ketoconazole or itraconazole per day.

Antimycobacterial

Rifabutin.*

Effect: Increases rifabutin and rifabutin metabolite concentration.

Clinical Comment: A dosage reduction of rifabutin to at least half the recommended dose is required when amprenavir and rifabutin are coadministered.* A complete blood count should be performed weekly and as clinically indicated in order to monitor for neutropenia in patients receiving amprenavir and rifabutin.

Benzodiazepines

Alprazolam, clorazepate, diazepam, flurazepam.

Effect: Increases benzodiazepines concentration.

Clinical Comment: Clinical significance is unknown; however, a decrease in benzodiazepine dose may be needed.

Calcim Channel Blockers

Diltiazem, felodipine, nifedipine, nicardipine, nimodipine, verapamil, amlodipine, nisoldipine, isradipine.

Effect: Increases calcim channel blockers concentration.

Clinical Comment: Caution is warranted and clinical monitoring of patients is recommended.

Corticosteroid

Dexamethasone.

Effect: Decreases amprenavir concentration.

Clinical Comment: Use with caution. Amprenavir may be less effective due to decreased amprenavir plasma concentrations in patients taking these agents concomitantly.

Erectile Dysfunction Agent

Sildenafil.

Effect: Increases sildenafil concentration.

Clinical Comment: Use with caution at reduced doses of 25 mg every 48 hours with increased monitoring for adverse events.

HMG-CoA Reductase Inhibitors

Atorvastatin.

Effect: Increases atorvastatin concentration.

Clinical Comment: Use lowest possible dose of atorvastatin with careful monitoring or consider other HMG-CoA reductase inhibitors such as pravastatin or fluvastatin in combination with amprenavir.

Immunosuppressants
Cyclosporine, tacrolimus, rapamycin.
Effect: Increases immunosuppressants concentration.
Clinical Comment: Therapeutic concentration monitoring is recommended for immunosuppressant agents when coadministered with amprenavir.

Narcotic Analgesics
Methadone.*
Effect: Decreases amprenavir concentration. Decreases methadone concentration.
Clinical Comment: Amprenavir may be less effective due to decreased amprenavir plasma concentrations in patients taking these agents concomitantly. Alternative antiretroviral therapy should be considered. Dosage of methadone may need to be increased when coadministered with amprenavir.

Tricyclic Antidepressants
Amitriptyline, imipramine.
Effect: Increases tricyclics concentration.
Clinical Comment: Therapeutic concentration monitoring is recommended for tricyclic antidepressants when coadministered with amprenavir.
*See TABLE 3 and TABLE 4 for magnitude of interaction.

ADVERSE REACTIONS

In clinical studies, adverse events leading to amprenavir discontinuation occurred primarily during the first 12 weeks of therapy, and were mostly due to gastrointestinal events (nausea, vomiting, diarrhea, and abdominal pain/discomfort), which were mild to moderate in severity.

Skin rash occurred in 22% of patients treated with amprenavir in studies PROAB3001 and PROAB3006. Rashes were usually maculopapular and of mild or moderate intensity, some with pruritus. Rashes had a median onset of 11 days after amprenavir initiation and a median duration of 10 days. Skin rashes led to amprenavir discontinuation in approximately 3% of patients. In some patients with mild or moderate rash, amprenavir dosing was often continued without interruption; if interrupted, reintroduction of amprenavir generally did not result in rash recurrence.

Severe or life-threatening rash (Grade 3 or 4), including cases of Stevens-Johnson syndrome, occurred in approximately 1% of recipients of amprenavir (see WARNINGS). Amprenavir therapy should be discontinued for severe or life-threatening rashes and for moderate rashes accompanied by systemic symptoms.

TABLE 8 *Selected Clinical Adverse Events of All Grades Reported in >5% of Adult Patients*

	PROAB3001		PROAB3006	
	Therapy-Naive Patients		NRTI-Experienced Patients	
Adverse Event	Amprenavir*/ Lamivudine/ Zidovudine (n=113)	Lamivudine/ Zidovudine (n=109)	Amprenavir*/ NRTI (n=245)	Indinavir/ NRTI (n=241)
Digestive				
Nausea	74%	50%	43%	35%
Vomiting	34%	17%	24%	20%
Diarrhea or loose stools	39%	35%	60%	41%
Taste disorders	10%	6%	2%	8%
Skin				
Rash	27%	6%	20%	15%
Nervous				
Paresthesia, oral/perioral	26%	6%	31%	2%
Paresthesia, peripheral	10%	4%	14%	10%
Psychiatric				
Depressive or mood disorders	16%	4%	9%	13%

* Amprenavir capsules.

Among amprenavir-treated patients in Phase 3 studies, 2 patients developed *de novo* diabetes mellitus, 1 patient developed a dorsocervical fat enlargement (buffalo hump), and 9 patients developed fat redistribution.

TABLE 9 *Selected Laboratory Abnormalities of All Grades Reported in ≥5% of Adult Patients*

	PROAB3001		PROAB3006	
	Therapy-Naive Patients		NRTI-Experienced Patients	
Laboratory Abnormality (non-fasting specimens)	Amprenavir*/ Lamivudine/ Zidovudine (n=111)	Lamivudine/ Zidovudine (n=108)	Amprenavir*/ NRTI (n=237)	Indinavir/ NRTI (n=239)
Hyperglycemia (>116 mg/dl)	45%	31%	53%	58%
Hypertriglyceridemia (>213 mg/dl)	41%	27%	56%	52%
Hypercholesterolemia (>283 mg/dl)	7%	3%	13%	15%

* Amprenavir capsules.

In studies PROAB3001 and PROAB3006, no increased frequency of Grade 3 or 4 AST, ALT, amylase, or bilirubin elevations was seen compared to controls.

Pediatric Patients: An adverse event profile similar to that seen in adults was seen in pediatric patients.

CONCOMITANT THERAPY WITH RITONAVIR

TABLE 10 *Selected Clinical Adverse Events of All Grades Reported in ≥5% of Adult Patients in Ongoing, Open-Label Clinical Trials of Amprenavir Capsules in Combination With Ritonavir Capsules*

Adverse Event	Amprenavir 1200 mg Plus Ritonavir 200 mg qd* (n=101)	Amprenavir 600 mg Plus Ritonavir 100 mg bid† (n=215)
Diarrhea/loose stools	25%	7%
Nausea	23%	7%
Vomiting	10%	4%
Adbominal symptoms	13%	3%
Headache	15%	3%
Parasthesias	8%	2%
Rash	9%	2%
Fatigue	5%	4%

* Data from 2 ongoing, open-label studies in treatment-naive patients also receiving abacavir/lamivudine.
† Data from 3 ongoing, open-label studies in treatment-naive and treatment-experienced patients receiving combination antiretroviral therapy.

Treatment with amprenavir in combination with ritonavir capsules has resulted in increases in the concentration of total cholesterol and triglycerides (see PRECAUTIONS: Lipid Elevations and Laboratory Tests).

DOSAGE AND ADMINISTRATION

Amprenavir may be taken with or without food; however, a high-fat meal decreases the absorption of amprenavir and should be avoided (see CLINICAL PHARMACOLOGY, Pharmacokinetics in Adults, Food Effect on Absorption). **Adult and pediatric patients should be advised not to take supplemental vitamin E since the vitamin E content of amprenavir capsules and oral solution exceeds the Reference Daily Intake (adults 30 IU, pediatrics approximately 10 IU) (see DESCRIPTION).**

Amprenavir capsules and amprenavir oral solution are not interchangeable on a milligram-per-milligram basis (see CLINICAL PHARMACOLOGY).

CAPSULES

Adults

The recommended oral dose of amprenavir capsules for adults is 1200 mg (eight 150 mg capsules) twice daily in combination with other antiretroviral agents.

Concomitant Therapy

If amprenavir and ritonavir are used in combination, the recommended dosage regimens are: amprenavir 1200 mg with ritonavir 200 mg once daily or Agenerase 600 mg with ritonavir 100 mg twice daily.

Pediatric Patients

For adolescents (13-16 years), the recommended oral dose of amprenavir capsules is 1200 mg (eight 150 mg capsules) twice daily in combination with other antiretroviral agents. For patients between 4 and 12 years of age or for patients 13-16 years of age with weight of <50 kg, the recommended oral dose of amprenavir capsules is 20 mg/kg twice daily or 15 mg/kg three times daily (to a maximum daily dose of 2400 mg) in combination with other antiretroviral agents.

Patients With Hepatic Impairment

Amprenavir capsules should be used with caution in patients with moderate or severe hepatic impairment. Patients with a Child-Pugh score ranging from 5-8 should receive a reduced dose of amprenavir capsules of 450 mg twice daily, and patients with a Child-Pugh score ranging from 9-12 should receive a reduced dose of amprenavir capsules of 300 mg twice daily (see CLINICAL PHARMACOLOGY, Special Populations, Hepatic Insufficiency).

ORAL SOLUTION

The recommended dose of amprenavir oral solution based on body weight and age is shown in TABLE 11. **Consideration should be given to switching patients from amprenavir oral solution to amprenavir capsules as soon as they are able to take the capsule formulation (see WARNINGS).**

TABLE 11 *Recommended Dosages of Amprenavir Oral Solution*

Age/Weight Criteria	Dose bid	Dose tid
4-12 years or 13-16 years and <50 kg	22.5 mg/kg (1.5 ml/kg) (max. dose 2800 mg/day)	17 mg/kg (1.1 ml/kg) (max. dose 2800 mg/day)
13-16 years and ≥50 kg or >16 years	1400 mg	NA

Concomitant Therapy

Concurrent use of amprenavir oral solution and ritonavir oral solution is not recommended because the large amount of propylene glycol in amprenavir oral solution and ethanol in ritonavir oral solution may compete for the same metabolic pathway for elimination.

Patients With Hepatic Impairment
Amprenavir oral solution is contraindicated in patients with hepatic failure (see CONTRAINDICATIONS).

Patients with hepatic impairment are at increased risk of propylene glycol-associated adverse events (see WARNINGS). Amprenavir oral solution should be used with caution in patients with hepatic impairment. Based on a study with amprenavir capsules, adult patients with a Child-Pugh score ranging from 5-8 should receive a reduced dose of amprenavir oral solution of 513 mg (34 ml) twice daily, and adult patients with a Child-Pugh score ranging from 9-12 should receive a reduced dose of amprenavir oral solution of 342 mg (23 ml) twice daily (see CLINICAL PHARMACOLOGY, Special Populations, Hepatic Insufficiency).

Amprenavir oral solution has not been studied in children with hepatic impairment.

Renal Insufficiency
Amprenavir oral solution is contraindicated in patients with renal failure (see CONTRAINDICATIONS).

Patients with renal impairment are at increased risk of propylene glycol-associated adverse events. Amprenavir oral solution should be used with caution in patients with renal impairment (see WARNINGS).

HOW SUPPLIED

AGENERASE CAPSULES

50 mg: Oblong, opaque off-white to cream-colored soft gelatin capsules printed with "GX CC1" on one side.
100 mg: Oblong, opaque off-white to cream-colored soft gelatin capsules printed with "GX CC2" on one side.
Storage: Store at controlled room temperature of 25°C (77°F).

AGENERASE ORAL SOLUTION

A clear, pale yellow to yellow, grape-bubblegum-peppermint-flavored liquid, contains 15 mg of amprenavir in each 1 ml.

This product does not require reconstitution.
Storage: Store at controlled room temperature of 25°C (77°F).

PRODUCT LISTING - EQUIVALENTS NOT AVAILABLE

Capsule - Oral - 150 mg			
240's	$317.22	AGENERASE, Allscripts Pharmaceutical Company	54569-4813-00
240's	$367.77	AGENERASE, Glaxosmithkline	00173-0672-00
Solution - Oral - 15 mg/ml			
240 ml	$36.77	AGENERASE, Glaxosmithkline	00173-0687-00

Anagrelide Hydrochloride *(003327)*

Categories: Thrombocythemia; Pregnancy Category C; FDA Approved 1997 Jan; Orphan Drugs
Drug Classes: Platelet inhibitors
Brand Names: **Agrylin**
Cost of Therapy: $680.71 (Thrombocythemia; Agrylin; 1 mg; 2 capsules/day; 30 day supply)

DESCRIPTION

Dosage Form: 0.5 mg and 1 mg capsules for oral administration.
Active Ingredient: Agrylin capsules contain either 0.5 mg or 1 mg of anagrelide base (as anagrelide HCl).
Inactive Ingredients: Povidone, anhydrous lactose, lactose monohydrate, microcrystalline cellulose, crospovidone, magnesium stearate.
Chemical Name: 6,7-dichloro-1, 5-dihydroimidazo(2,1-b)quinazolin-2(3H)-one monohydrochloride monohydrate.
Molecular Formula: $C_{10}H_7Cl_2N_3O \cdot HCl \cdot H_2O$
Molecular Weight: 310.55
Appearance: Off-white powder.
Solubility: Anagrelide HCl is very slightly soluble in water, sparingly soluble in dimethyl sulfoxide and sparingly soluble in dimethylformamide.

CLINICAL PHARMACOLOGY

The mechanism by which anagrelide reduces blood platelet count is still under investigation. Studies in patients support a hypothesis of dose-related reduction in platelet production resulting from a decrease in megakaryocyte hypermaturation. In blood withdrawn from normal volunteers treated with anagrelide, a disruption was found in the postmitotic phase of megakaryocyte development and a reduction in megakaryocyte size and plaidy. At therapeutic doses, anagrelide does not produce significant changes in white cell counts or coagulation parameters, and may have a small, but clinically insignificant effect on red cell parameters. Platelet aggregation is inhibited in people at doses higher than those required to reduce platelet count. Anagrelide inhibits cyclic AMP phosphodiesterase, as well as ADP- and collagen-induced platelet aggregation.

Following oral administration of ^{14}C-anagrelide in people, more than 70% of radioactivity was recovered in urine. Based on limited data, there appears to be a trend toward dose linearity between doses of 0.5 mg and 2.0 mg. At fasting and at a dose of 0.5 mg of anagrelide, the plasma half-life is 1.3 hours. The available plasma concentration time data at steady state in patients showed that anagrelide does not accumulate in plasma after repeated administration. The drug is extensively metabolized; less than 1% is recovered in the urine as anagrelide.

When a 0.5 mg dose of anagrelide was taken after food, its bioavailability (based on AUC values) was modestly reduced by an average of 13.8% and its plasma half-life slightly increased (to 1.8 hours), when compared with drug administered to the same subjects in the fasted state. The peak plasma level was lowered by an average of 45% and delayed by 2 hours.

INDICATIONS AND USAGE

Anagrelide HCl capsules are indicated for the treatment of patients with Essential Thrombocythemia to reduce the elevated platelet count and the risk of thrombosis and to ameliorate associated symptoms (see DOSAGE AND ADMINISTRATION).

WARNINGS

CARDIOVASCULAR

Anagrelide should be used with caution in patients with known or suspected heart disease, and only if the potential benefits of therapy outweigh the potential risks. Because of the positive inotropic effects and side-effects of anagrelide, a pre-treatment cardiovascular examination is recommended along with careful monitoring during treatment in humans, therapeutic doses of anagrelide may cause cardiovascular effects, including vasodilation, tachycardia, palpitations, and congestive heart failure.

RENAL

It is recommended that patients with renal insufficiency (creatinine ≥2 mg/dl) receive anagrelide when, in the physician's judgment, the potential benefits of therapy outweigh the potential risks. These patients should be monitored closely for signs of renal toxicity while receiving anagrelide (see ADVERSE REACTIONS, Urogenital System).

HEPATIC

It is recommended that patients with evidence of hepatic dysfunction (bilirubin, SGOT, or measures of liver function >1.5 times the upper limit of normal) receive anagrelide when, in the physician's judgment, the potential benefits of therapy outweigh the potential risks. These patients should be monitored closely for signs of hepatic toxicity while receiving anagrelide (see ADVERSE REACTIONS, Hepatic System).

PRECAUTIONS

LABORATORY TESTS

Anagrelide therapy requires close clinical supervision of the patient. While the platelet count is being lowered (usually during the first 2 weeks of treatment), blood counts (hemoglobin, white blood cells), liver function (SGOT, SGPT) and renal function (serum creatinine, BUN) should be monitored.

In 9 subjects receiving a single 5 mg dose of anagrelide, standing blood pressure fell an average of 22/15 mm Hg, usually accompanied by dizziness. Only minimal changes in blood pressure were observed following a dose of 2 mg.

CESSATION OF ANAGRELIDE HCl TREATMENT

In general, interruption of anagrelide treatment is followed by an increase in platelet count. After sudden stoppage of anagrelide therapy, the increase in platelet count can be observed within 4 days.

CARCINOGENESIS, MUTAGENESIS, AND IMPAIRMENT OF FERTILITY

No long-term studies in animals have been performed to evaluate carcinogenic potential of anagrelide HCl. Anagrelide HCl was not genotoxic in the Ames test, the mouse lymphoma cell (L5178Y, TK) forward mutation test, the human lymphocyte chromosome aberration test, or the mouse micronucleus test. Anagrelide HCl at oral doses up to 240 mg/kg/day (1440 mg/m^2 /day, 195 times the recommended maximum human dose based on body surface area) was found to have no effect on fertility and reproductive performance of male rats. However, in female rats, at oral doses of 60 mg/kg/day (360 mg/m^2/day, 49 times the recommended maximum human dose based on body surface area) or higher, it disrupted implantation when administered in early pregnancy and retarded or blocked parturition when administered in late pregnancy.

PREGNANCY CATEGORY C

Teratogenic Effects

Teratology studies have been performed in pregnant rats at oral doses up to 900 mg/kg/day (5400 mg/m^2/day, 730 times the recommended maximum human dose based on body surface area) and in pregnant rabbits at oral doses up to 20 mg/kg/day (240 mg/m^2/day, 32 times the recommended maximum human dose based on body surface area) and have revealed no evidence of impaired fertility or harm to the fetus due to anagrelide HCl.

Nonteratogenic Effects

A fertility and reproductive performance study performed in female rats revealed that anagrelide HCl at oral doses of 60 mg/kg/day (360 mg/m^2/day, 49 times the recommended maximum human dose based on body surface area) or higher disrupted implantation and exerted adverse effect on embryo/fetal survival.

A perinatal and postnatal study performed in female rats revealed that anagrelide HCl at oral doses of 60 mg/kg/day (360 mg/m^2/day, 49 times the recommended maximum human dose based on body surface area) or higher produced delay or blockage of parturition, deaths of nondelivering pregnant dams and their fully developed fetuses, and increased mortality in the pups born.

Five (5) women became pregnant while on anagrelide treatment at doses of 1-4 mg/day. Treatment was stopped as soon as it was realized that they were pregnant. All delivered normal, healthy babies. There are no adequate and well-controlled studies in pregnant women. Anagrelide HCl should be used during pregnancy only if the potential benefit justifies the potential risk to the fetus.

Anagrelide is not recommended in women who are or may become pregnant. If this drug is used during pregnancy, or if the patient becomes pregnant while taking this drug, the patient should be apprised of the potential harm to the fetus. Women of child-bearing potential should be instructed that they must not be pregnant and that they should use contraception while taking anagrelide. Anagrelide may cause fetal harm when administered to a pregnant woman.

A

NURSING MOTHERS

It is not know whether this drug is excreted in human milk. Because many drugs are excreted in human milk and because of the potential or serious adverse reaction in nursing infants from anagrelide HCl a decision should be made whether to discontinue nursing or discontinue the drug, taking into account the importance of the drug to the mother.

PEDIATRIC USE

The safety and efficacy of anagrelide in patients under the age of 16 years have not been established. Anagrelide has been used successfully in 8 pediatric patients (age range 8-17 years), including 3 patients with essential thrombocythemia who were treated at a dose of 1-4 mg/day.

DRUG INTERACTIONS

Bioavailability studies evaluating possible interactions between anagrelide and other drugs have not been conducted. The most common medications used concomitantly with anagrelide have been aspirin, acetaminophen, furosemide, iron, ranitidine, hydroxyurea, and allopurinol. The most frequently used concomitant cardiac medication has been digoxin. Although drug-to-drug interaction studies have not been conducted, there is no clinical evidence to suggest that anagrelide interacts with any of these compounds.

There is a single report which suggests that sucralfate may interfere with anagrelide absorption.

Food has no clinically significant effect on the bioavailability of anagrelide.

ADVERSE REACTIONS

While most reported adverse events during anagrelide therapy have been mild in intensity and have decreased in frequency with continued therapy, serious adverse events reported in patients with ET and/or in patients with thrombocythemia of other etiologies include: congestive heart failure, myocardial infarction, cardiomyopathy, cardiomegaly, complete heart block, atrial fibrillation, cerebrovascular accident, pericarditis, pulmonary infiltrates, pulmonary fibrosis, pulmonary hypertension, pancreatitis, gastric/duodenal.

Of the 551 ET patients treated with anagrelide for a mean duration of 65 weeks, 82 (15%) were discontinued from the study because of adverse events or abnormal laboratory test results. The most common adverse events for treatment discontinuation were headache, diarrhea, edema, palpitation, and abdominal pain. Overall, the occurrence rate of all adverse events was 17.9 per 1000 treatment days. The occurrence rate of adverse events increased at higher doses of anagrelide.

TABLE 2 *Most Frequently Reported Adverse Reactions to Anagrelide (in 5% or greater of 551 patients with ET) in Clinical Trials*

Adverse Reaction	
Headache	44.5%
Palpitations	27.2%
Diarrhea	24.3%
Asthenia	22.1%
Edema, other	19.8%
Abdominal pain	17.4%
Nausea	15.1%
Pain, other	14.7%
Dizziness	14.5%
Dyspnea	10.5%
Flatulence	10.5%
Chest pain	7.8%
Rash, including urticaria	7.8%
Vomiting	7.4%
Paresthesia	7.3%
Tachycardia	7.3%
Peripheral edema	7.1%
Dyspepsia	6.4%
Back pain	6.4%
Anorexia	5.8%
Malaise	5.8%

Adverse events with an incidence of 1% to <5% included:

Body as a Whole System: Fever, flu symptoms, chills, neck pain, photosensitivity.

Cardiovascular System: Arrhythmia, hemorrhage, cardiovascular disease, cerebrovascular accident, angina pectoris, heart failure, postural hypotension, vasodilatation, migraine, syncope.

Digestive System: Constipation, GI distress, GI hemorrhage, gastritis, melena, aphthous stomatitis, eructation, nausea, vomiting.

Hemic and Lymphatic System: Anemia, thrombocytopenia, ecchymosis, lymphadenoma. Platelet counts below 1000,000/µl occurred in 35 patients and reduction below 50,000/µl occurred in 7 of the 551 ET patients while on anagrelide therapy. Thrombocythemia promptly recovered upon discontinuation of anagrelide.

Hepatic System: Elevated liver enzymes were observed in 2 of 551 patients during therapy.

Musculoskeletal System: Arthralgia, myalgia, leg cramps.

Nervous System: Depression, somnolence, confusion, insomnia, hypertension, nervousness, amnesia.

Nutritional Disorders: Dehydration

Respiratory System: Rhinitis, epistaxis, respiratory disease, sinusitis, pneumonia, bronchitis, asthma.

Skin and Appendages System: Pruritus, skin disease, alopecia.

Special Senses: Amblyopia, abnormal vision, tinnitus, visual field abnormality, diplopia.

Urogenital System: Dysuria, hematuria.

Of the 551 ET patients, 10 were found to have renal abnormalities. Six (6) of the 10 experienced renal failure (approximately 1%) while on anagrelide treatment. In 2, the renal failure was considered to be possibly related to anagrelide treatment.. The remaining 4 were found to have pre-existing renal impairment and were successfully treated with anagrelide. Doses ranged from 1.5-6.0 mg/day with exposure periods of 2-12 months. Serum creatinine remained within normal limits and no dose adjustment was required because of renal insufficiency.

DOSAGE AND ADMINISTRATION

Treatment with anagrelide HCl capsules should be initiated under close medical supervision. The recommended starting dosage of anagrelide HCl is 0.5 mg 4 times daily or 1 mg twice daily, which should be maintained for at least 1 week. Dosage should then be adjusted to the lowest effective dosage required to reduce and maintain platelet count below 600,000/µl and ideally to the normal range. The dosage should be increased by not more than 0.5 mg/day in any one week. Dosage should not exceed 10 mg/day or 2.5 mg in a single dose (see PRECAUTIONS). The decision to treat asymptomatic young adults with essential for thrombocythemia should be individualized.

To monitor the effect of anagrelide and prevent the occurrence of thrombocytopenia, platelet counts should be performed every 2 days during the first week of treatment and at least weekly thereafter until the maintenance dosage is reached.

Typically, platelet count begins to respond with 7-14 days at the proper dosage. Most patients will experience an adequate response at a dose of 1.5-3.0 mg/day. Patients with known or suspected heart disease, renal insufficiency, or hepatic dysfunction should be monitored closely.

HOW SUPPLIED

Agrylin is available as 0.5 mg, opaque white capsules imprinted "ROBERTS 063" in black ink. 1 mg, opaque, gray capsules imprinted "ROBERTS 064" in black ink.
Storage: Store from 15-25°C (59-77°F), in a light-resistant container.

PRODUCT LISTING - EQUIVALENTS NOT AVAILABLE

Capsule - Oral - 0.5 mg

100's	$567.26	AGRYLIN, Roberts Pharmaceutical Corporation	54092-0063-01

Capsule - Oral - 1 mg

100's	$1134.52	AGRYLIN, Roberts Pharmaceutical Corporation	54092-0064-01

Anakinra *(003534)*

Categories: Arthritis, rheumatoid; FDA Approved 2001 Nov; Pregnancy Category B
Drug Classes: Disease modifying antirheumatic drugs; Interleukin receptor antagonists
Brand Names: Kineret
Cost of Therapy: $1,311.90 (Rheumatoid Arthritis; Kineret Injection; 100 mg; 1 injection/day; 30 day supply)

DESCRIPTION

Kineret (anakinra) is a recombinant, nonglycosylated form of the human interleukin-1 receptor antagonist (IL-1Ra). Kineret differs from native human IL-1Ra in that it has the addition of a single methionine residue at its amino terminus. Kineret consists of 153 amino acids and has a molecular weight of 17.3 kilodaltons. It is produced by recombinant DNA technology using an *E. coli* bacterial expression system.

Kineret is supplied in single use 1 ml prefilled glass syringes with 27 gauge needles as a sterile, clear, colorless-to-white, preservative-free solution for daily subcutaneous (SC) administration. Each 1 ml prefilled glass syringe contains: 0.67 ml (100 mg) of anakinra in a solution (pH 6.5) containing sodium citrate (1.29 mg), sodium chloride (5.48 mg), disodium EDTA (0.12 mg), and polysorbate 80 (0.70 mg) in water for injection.

CLINICAL PHARMACOLOGY

Anakinra blocks the biologic activity of IL-1 by competitively inhibiting IL-1 binding to the interleukin-1 type I receptor (IL-1RI), which is expressed in a wide variety of tissues and organs.[1]

IL-1 production is induced in response to inflammatory stimuli and mediates various physiologic responses including inflammatory and immunological responses. IL-1 has a broad range of activities including cartilage degradation by its induction of the rapid loss of proteoglycans, as well as stimulation of bone resorption.[2] The levels of the naturally occurring IL-1Ra in synovium and synovial fluid from rheumatoid arthritis (RA) patients are not sufficient to compete with the elevated amount of locally produced IL-1.[3,4,5]

PHARMACOKINETICS

The absolute bioavailability of anakinra after a 70 mg SC bolus injection in healthy subjects (n=11) is 95%. In subjects with RA, maximum plasma concentrations of anakinra occurred 3-7 hours after SC administration of anakinra at clinically relevant doses (1-2 mg/kg; n=18); the terminal half-life ranged from 4-6 hours. In RA patients, no unexpected accumulation of anakinra was observed after daily SC doses for up to 24 weeks.

The influence of demographic covariates on the pharmacokinetics of anakinra was studied using population pharmacokinetic analysis encompassing 341 patients receiving daily SC injection of anakinra at doses of 30, 75, and 150 mg for up to 24 weeks. The estimated anakinra clearance increased with increasing creatinine clearance and body weight. After adjusting for creatinine clearance and body weight, gender and age were not significant factors for mean plasma clearance.

Patients With Renal Impairment

The mean plasma clearance of anakinra decreased 70-75% in normal subjects with severe or end stage renal disease (defined as creatinine clearance less than 30 ml/minute, as estimated from serum creatinine levels[6]). No formal studies have been conducted examining the pharmacokinetics of anakinra administered subcutaneously in rheumatoid arthritis patients with renal impairment.

Patients With Hepatic Dysfunction

No formal studies have been conducted examining the pharmacokinetics of anakinra administered subcutaneously in rheumatoid arthritis patients with hepatic impairment.

INDICATIONS AND USAGE

Anakinra is indicated for the reduction in signs and symptoms of moderately to severely active rheumatoid arthritis, in patients 18 years of age or older who have failed 1 or more disease modifying antirheumatic drugs (DMARDs). Anakinra can be used alone or in combination with DMARDs other than Tumor Necrosis Factor (TNF) blocking agents (see WARNINGS).

CONTRAINDICATIONS

Anakinra is contraindicated in patients with known hypersensitivity to *E. coli*-derived proteins, anakinra, or any components of the product.

WARNINGS

ANAKINRA HAS BEEN ASSOCIATED WITH AN INCREASED INCIDENCE OF SERIOUS INFECTIONS (2%) vs PLACEBO (<1%). ADMINISTRATION OF ANAKINRA SHOULD BE DISCONTINUED IF A PATIENT DEVELOPS A SERIOUS INFECTION. TREATMENT WITH ANAKINRA SHOULD NOT BE INITIATED IN PATIENTS WITH ACTIVE INFECTIONS. THE SAFETY AND EFFICACY OF ANAKINRA IN IMMUNOSUPPRESSED PATIENTS OR IN PATIENTS WITH CHRONIC INFECTIONS HAVE NOT BEEN EVALUATED. THE SAFETY OF ANAKINRA USED IN COMBINATION WITH TNF BLOCKING AGENTS HAS NOT BEEN ESTABLISHED. PRELIMINARY DATA SUGGEST A HIGHER RATE OF SERIOUS INFECTIONS (7%, 4/58) WHEN ANAKINRA AND ETANERCEPT ARE USED IN COMBINATION COMPARED WITH WHEN ANAKINRA IS USED ALONE. IN THIS COMBINATION STUDY NEUTROPENIA (NEUTROPHIL COUNT ≤1000/mm^3) WAS OBSERVED IN 3% OF PATIENTS (2/58). USE OF ANAKINRA WITH TNF BLOCKING AGENTS SHOULD ONLY BE DONE WITH EXTREME CAUTION AND WHEN NO SATISFACTORY ALTERNATIVES EXIST.

PRECAUTIONS

GENERAL

Hypersensitivity reactions associated with anakinra administration are rare. If a severe hypersensitivity reaction occurs, administration of anakinra should be discontinued and appropriate therapy initiated.

IMMUNOSUPPRESSION

The impact of treatment with anakinra on active and/or chronic infections and the development of malignancies is not known. (See WARNINGS and ADVERSE REACTIONS, Infections and ADVERSE REACTIONS, Malignancies.)

IMMUNIZATIONS

No data are available on the effects of vaccination in patients receiving anakinra. Live vaccines should not be given concurrently with anakinra. No data are available on the secondary transmission of infection by live vaccines in patients receiving anakinra (see Immunosuppression). Since anakinra interferes with normal immune response mechanisms to new antigens such as vaccines, vaccination may not be effective in patients receiving anakinra.

INFORMATION FOR THE PATIENT

If a physician has determined that a patient can safely and effectively receive anakinra at home, patients and their caregivers should be instructed on the proper dosage and administration of anakinra. All patients should be provided with the "Information for Patients and Caregivers" insert. While this "Information for Patients and Caregivers" insert provides information about the product and its use, it is not intended to take the place of regular discussions between the patient and healthcare provider.

Patients should be informed of the signs and symptoms of allergic and other adverse drug reactions and advised of appropriate actions. Patients and their caregivers should be thoroughly instructed in the importance of proper disposal and cautioned against the reuse of needles, syringes, and drug product. A puncture-resistant container for the disposal of used syringes should be available to the patient. The full container should be disposed of according to the directions provided by the healthcare professional.

LABORATORY TESTS

Patients receiving anakinra may experience a decrease in neutrophil counts. In the placebo-controlled studies, 8% of patients receiving anakinra had decreases in neutrophil counts of at least 1 World Health Organization (WHO) toxicity grade compared with 2% in the placebo control group. Six anakinra-treated patients (0.3%) experienced neutropenia (ANC $\leq 1 \times 10^9$/L). This is discussed in more detail in the ADVERSE REACTIONS, Hematologic Events section. Neutrophil counts should be assessed prior to initiating anakinra treatment, and while receiving anakinra, monthly for 3 months, and thereafter quarterly for a period up to 1 year.

CARCINOGENESIS, MUTAGENESIS, AND IMPAIRMENT OF FERTILITY

Anakinra has not been evaluated for its carcinogenic potential in animals. Using a standard *in vivo* and *in vitro* battery of mutagenesis assays, anakinra did not induce gene mutations in either bacteria or mammalian cells. In rats and rabbits, anakinra at doses of up to 100-fold greater than the human dose had no adverse effects on male or female fertility.

PREGNANCY CATEGORY B

Reproductive studies have been conducted with anakinra on rats and rabbits at doses up to 100 times the human dose and have revealed no evidence of impaired fertility or harm to the fetus. There are, however, no adequate and well-controlled studies in pregnant women. Because animal reproduction studies are not always predictive of human response, anakinra should be used during pregnancy only if clearly needed.

NURSING MOTHERS

It is not known whether anakinra is secreted in human milk. Because many drugs are secreted in human milk, caution should be exercised if anakinra is administered to nursing women.

PEDIATRIC USE

The safety and efficacy of anakinra in patients with juvenile rheumatoid arthritis (JRA) have not been established.

GERIATRIC USE

A total of 653 patients ≥65 years of age, including 135 patients ≥75 years of age, were studied in clinical trials. No differences in safety or effectiveness were observed between these patients and younger patients, but greater sensitivity of some older individuals cannot be ruled out. Because there is a higher incidence of infections in the elderly population in general, caution should be used in treating the elderly.

This drug is known to be substantially excreted by the kidney, and the risk of toxic reactions to this drug may be greater in patients with impaired renal function.

DRUG INTERACTIONS

No drug-drug interaction studies in human subjects have been conducted. Toxicologic and toxicokinetic studies in rats did not demonstrate any alterations in the clearance or toxicologic profile of either methotrexate or anakinra when the two agents were administered together.

ADVERSE REACTIONS

The most serious adverse reactions were:

Serious Infections — see WARNINGS.

Neutropenia, particularly when used in combination with TNF blocking agents — see WARNINGS.

The most common adverse reaction with anakinra is injection site reactions. These reactions were the most common reason for withdrawing from studies.

Because clinical trials are conducted under widely varying and controlled conditions, adverse reaction rates observed in clinical trials of a drug cannot be directly compared to rates in the clinical trials of another drug and may not predict the rates observed in a broader patient population in clinical practice.

The data described herein reflect exposure to anakinra in 2606 patients, including 1812 exposed for at least 6 months and 570 exposed for at least 1 year. Studies 1 and 4 used the recommended dose of 100 mg/day. The patients studied were representative of the general population of patients with rheumatoid arthritis.

INJECTION-SITE REACTIONS

The most common and consistently reported treatment-related adverse event associated with anakinra is injection-site reaction (ISR). The majority of ISRs were reported as mild. These typically lasted for 14-28 days and were characterized by 1 or more of the following: erythema, ecchymosis, inflammation, and pain. In Studies 1 and 4, 71% of patients developed an ISR, which was typically reported within the first 4 weeks of therapy. The development of ISRs in patients who had not previously experienced ISRs was uncommon after the first month of therapy.

INFECTIONS

In Studies 1 and 4 combined, the incidence of infection was 40% in the anakinra-treated patients and 35% in placebo-treated patients. The incidence of serious infections in studies 1 and 4 was 1.8% in anakinra-treated patients and 0.6% in placebo-treated patients over 6 months. These infections consisted primarily of bacterial events such as cellulitis, pneumonia, and bone and joint infections, rather than unusual, opportunistic, fungal, or viral infections. Patients with asthma appeared to be at higher risk of developing serious infections; anakinra 5% vs placebo <1%. Most patients continued on study drug after the infection resolved. There were no on-study deaths due to serious infectious episodes in either study.

In a study in which patients were receiving both etanercept and anakinra for up to 24 weeks, the incidence of serious infections was 7%. These infections consisted of bacterial pneumonia (2 cases) and cellulitis (2 cases), which recovered with antibiotic treatment.

MALIGNANCIES

Twenty-one malignancies of various types were observed in 2531 RA patients treated in clinical trials with anakinra for up to 50 months. The observed rates and incidences were similar to those expected for the population studied.

HEMATOLOGIC EVENTS

In placebo-controlled studies with anakinra, treatment was associated with small reductions in the mean values for total white blood count, platelets, and absolute neutrophil blood count (ANC), and a small increase in the mean eosinophil differential percentage.

In all placebo-controlled studies, 8% of patients receiving anakinra had decreases in ANC of at least 1 WHO toxicity grade, compared with 2% of placebo patients. Six anakinra-treated patients (0.3%) developed neutropenia (ANC $\leq 1 \times 10^9$/L). Additional patients treated with anakinra plus etanercept (2/58, 3%) developed ANC $\leq 1 \times 10^9$/L. While neutropenic, one patient developed cellulitis and the other patient developed pneumonia. Both patients recovered with antibiotic therapy.

IMMUNOGENICITY

In Study 4, 28% of patients tested positively for anti-anakinra antibodies at month 6 in a highly sensitive, anakinra-binding biosensor assay. Of the 1274 subjects with available data, <1% (n=9) were seropositive in a cell-based bioassay for antibodies capable of neutralizing the biologic effects of anakinra. None of these 9 subjects were positive for neutralizing antibodies at more than 1 time point, and all of these subjects were negative for neutralizing antibodies by 9 months. No correlation between antibody development and clinical response or adverse events was observed. The long-term immunogenicity of anakinra is unknown.

Antibody assay results are highly dependent on the sensitivity and specificity of the assays. Additionally, the observed incidence of antibody positivity in an assay may be influenced by several factors, including sample handling, concomitant medications, and underlying disease. For these reasons, comparison of the incidence of antibodies to anakinra with the incidence of antibodies to other products may be misleading.

OTHER ADVERSE EVENTS

TABLE 3 reflects adverse events in Studies 1 and 4, that occurred with a frequency of ≥5% and a higher frequency in anakinra-treated patients.

***TABLE 3** Percent of RA Patients Reporting Adverse Events (Studies 1 and 4)*

Preferred Term	Placebo (n=534)	Anakinra 100 mg/day (n=1366)
Injection site reaction	28%	71%
Infection	35%	40%
URI	13%	13%
Sinusitis	4%	6%
Influenza-like symptoms	4%	5%
Other	23%	26%
Headache	9%	12%
Nausea	6%	8%
Dizziness	5%	7%
Sinusitis	6%	7%
Influenza-like symptoms	5%	6%
Pain abdominal	4%	5%

DOSAGE AND ADMINISTRATION

The recommended dose of anakinra for the treatment of patients with rheumatoid arthritis is 100 mg/day administered daily by subcutaneous injection. Higher doses did not result in a higher response. The dose should be administered at approximately the same time every day. Anakinra is provided in single-use 1 ml prefilled glass syringes. Instructions on appropriate use should be given by the health care professional to the patient or care provider. Patients or care providers should not be allowed to administer anakinra until he/she has demonstrated a thorough understanding of procedures and an ability to inject the product. After administration of anakinra, it is essential to follow the proper procedure for disposal of syringes and needles. See the "Information for Patients and Caregivers" leaflet for detailed instructions on the handling and injection of anakinra.

Visually inspect the solution for particulate matter and discoloration before administration. If particulates or discoloration are observed, the prefilled syringe should not be used.

Administer only 1 dose (the entire contents of 1 prefilled glass syringe) per day. Discard any unused portions; anakinra contains no preservative. Do not save unused drug for later administration.

HOW SUPPLIED

Kineret is supplied in single-use preservative free, 1 ml prefilled glass syringes with 27 gauge needles. Each prefilled glass syringe contains 0.67 ml (100 mg) of anakinra.

STORAGE

Do not use Kineret beyond the expiration date shown on the carton. Kineret should be stored in the refrigerator at 2-8°C (36-46°F). **DO NOT FREEZE OR SHAKE.** Protect from light.

PRODUCT LISTING - EQUIVALENTS NOT AVAILABLE

Solution - Subcutaneous - 100 mg/0.67 ml

0.67 ml	$41.25	KINERET, Amgen	55513-0177-01
0.67 ml x 7	$306.11	KINERET, Amgen	55513-0177-07

Anastrozole *(003272)*

For complete prescribing information, refer to the CD-ROM included with the book.

Categories: Carcinoma, breast; Pregnancy Category D; FDA Approved 1995 Dec
Drug Classes: Antineoplastics, aromatase inhibitors; Hormones/hormone modifiers
Brand Names: **Arimidex**
Foreign Brand Availability: Trozolet (Colombia)
Cost of Therapy: $227.23 (Breast Cancer; Arimidex; 1 mg; 1 tablet/day; 30 day supply)

DESCRIPTION

Arimidex (anastrozole) tablets for oral administration contain 1 mg of anastrozole, a nonsteroidal aromatase inhibitor. It is chemically described as 1,3-Benzenediacentonitrile, α,α,α′,α′-tetramethyl-5-(1H-1,2,4-triazol-1-ylmethyl). Its molecular formula is $C_{17}H_{19}N_5$.

Anastrozole is an off-white powder with a molecular weight of 293.4. Anastrozole has moderate aqueous solubility (0.5 mg/ml at 25°C); solubility is independent of pH in the physiological range. Anastrozole is freely soluble in methanol, acetone, ethanol, and tetrahydrofuran, and very soluble in acetonitrite.

Inactive Ingredients: Lactose, magnesium stearate, hydroxypropylmethylcellulose, polyethylene glycol, povidone, sodium starch glycolate, and titanium dioxide.

INDICATIONS AND USAGE

Anastrozole is indicated for adjuvant treatment of postmenopausal women with hormone receptor early breast cancer.

The effectiveness of anastrozole in early breast cancer is based on an analysis of recurrence-free survival in patients treated for a median of 31 months. Further follow-up of study patients will be required to determine long-term outcomes.

Anastrozole is indicated for the first-line treatment of postmenopausal women with hormone receptor positive or hormone receptor unknown locally advanced or metastatic breast cancer.

Anastrozole is indicated for the treatment of advanced breast cancer in postmenopausal women with disease progression following tamoxifen therapy. Patients with ER-negative disease and patients who did not respond to previous tamoxifen therapy rarely responded to anastrozole.

CONTRAINDICATIONS

Anastrozole is contraindicated in any patient who has shown a hypersensitivity reaction to the drug or to any of the excipients.

WARNINGS

Anastrozole can cause fetal harm when administered to a pregnant woman. Anastrozole has been found to cross the placenta following oral administration of 0.1 mg/kg in rats and rabbits (about 1 and 1.9 times the recommended human dose, respectively, on a mg/m^2 basis). Studies in both rats and rabbits at doses equal to or greater than 0.1 and 0.02 mg/kg/day, respectively (about 1 and one-third, respectively, the recommended human dose on a mg/m^2 basis), administered during the period of organogenesis showed that anastrozole increased pregnancy loss (increased pre- and/or post-implantation loss, increased resorption, and decreased numbers of live fetuses); effects were dose-related in rats. Placental weights were significantly increased in rats at doses of 0.1 mg/kg/day or more.

Evidence of fetotoxicity, including delayed fetal development (*i.e.,* incomplete ossification and depressed fetal body weights), was observed in rats administered doses of 1 mg/kg/day [which produced plasma anastrozole $C_{ss,max}$ and AUC(0-24h)] that were 19 and 9 times higher than the respective values found in healthy postmenopausal volunteers at the recommended dose). There was no evidence of teratogenicity in rats administered doses of up to 1.0 mg/kg/day. In rabbits, anastrozole caused pregnancy failure at doses equal to or greater than 1.0 mg/kg/day (about 16 times the recommended human dose on a mg/m^2 basis); there was no evidence of teratogenicity in rabbits administered 0.2 mg/kg/day (about 3 times the recommended human dose on a mg/m^2 basis).

There are no adequate and well-controlled studies in pregnant women using anastrozole. If anastrozole is used during pregnancy, or if the patient becomes pregnant while receiving this drug, the patient should be apprised of the potential hazard to the fetus or potential risk for loss of the pregnancy.

DOSAGE AND ADMINISTRATION

The dose of anastrozole is one 1 mg tablet taken once a day. For patients with advanced breast cancer, anastrozole should be continued until tumor progression.

For adjuvant treatment of early breast cancer in postmenopausal women, the optimal duration of therapy is unknown. The median duration of therapy at the time of data analysis was 31 months; the ongoing ATAC trial is planned for 5 years of treatment.

PATIENTS WITH HEPATIC IMPAIRMENT

Hepatic metabolism accounts for approximately 85% of anastrozole elimination. Although clearance of anastrozole was decreased in patients with cirrhosis due to alcohol abuse, plasma anastrozole concentrations stayed in the usual range seen in patients without liver disease. Therefore, no changes in dose are recommended for patients with mild-to-moderate hepatic impairment, although patients should be monitored for side effects. Anastrozole has not been studied in patients with severe hepatic impairment.

PATIENTS WITH RENAL IMPAIRMENT

No changes in dose are necessary for patients with renal impairment.

USE IN THE ELDERLY

No dosage adjustment is necessary.

PRODUCT LISTING - EQUIVALENTS NOT AVAILABLE

Tablet - Oral - 1 mg

30's	$227.23	ARIMIDEX, Astra-Zeneca Pharmaceuticals	00310-0201-30

Anthrax Vaccine Adsorbed *(003549)*

For complete prescribing information, refer to the CD-ROM included with the book.

Categories: Immunization, anthrax; FDA Approved 2002 Jan; Pregnancy Category D
Drug Classes: Vaccines
Brand Names: **BioThrax**

DESCRIPTION

Note: The trade name has been used throughout this monograph for clarity.

Anthrax Vaccine Adsorbed, (BioThrax) is a sterile, milky-white suspension (when mixed) made from cell-free filtrates of microaerophilic cultures of an avirulent, nonencapsulated strain of *Bacillus anthracis.* The production cultures are grown in a chemically defined protein-free medium consisting of a mixture of amino acids, vitamins, inorganic salts and sugars. The final product, prepared from the sterile filtrate culture fluid contains proteins, including the 83 kDa protective antigen protein, released during the growth period. The final product contains no dead or live bacteria. The final product is formulated to contain 1.2 mg/ml aluminum, added as aluminum hydroxide in 0.85% sodium chloride. The product is formulated to contain 25 μg/ml benzethonium chloride and 100 μg/ml formaldehyde, added as preservatives.

INDICATIONS AND USAGE

BioThrax is indicated for the active immunization against *Bacillus anthracis* of individuals between 18 and 65 years of age who come in contact with animal products such as hides, hair or bones that come from anthrax endemic areas, and that may be contaminated with *Bacillus anthracis* spores. BioThrax is also indicated for individuals at high risk of exposure to *Bacillus anthracis* spores such as veterinarians, laboratory workers and others whose occupation may involve handling potentially infected animals or other contaminated materials.

Since the risk of anthrax infection in the general population is low, routine immunization is not recommended.

The safety and efficacy of BioThrax in a post-exposure setting has not been established.

CONTRAINDICATIONS

The use of BioThrax is contraindicated in subjects with a history of anaphylactic or anaphylactic-like reaction following a previous dose of BioThrax, or any of the vaccine components.

WARNINGS

Preliminary results of a recent unpublished retrospective study of infants born to women in the US military service worldwide in 1998 and 1999 suggest that the vaccine may be linked with an increase in the number of birth defects when given during pregnancy (unpublished data, Department of Defense). Although these data are unconfirmed, pregnant women should not be vaccinated against anthrax unless the potential benefits of vaccination have been determined to outweigh the potential risk to the fetus.

Animal reproduction studies have not been conducted with BioThrax.

DOSAGE AND ADMINISTRATION

DOSAGE

Immunization consists of three subcutaneous injections, 0.5 ml each, given 2 weeks apart followed by three additional subcutaneous injections, 0.5 ml each, given at 6, 12, and 18 months. Subsequent booster injections of 0.5 ml of BioThrax at 1 year intervals are recommended.

ADMINISTRATION

Use a separate 5/8 inch, 25 to 27 gauge sterile needle and syringe for each patient to avoid transmission of viral hepatitis and other infectious agents. Use a different site for each sequential injection of this vaccine and do not mix with any other product in the syringe.

Antipyrine; Benzocaine *(000263)*

Categories: Cerumen, inspissated; Infection, ear, middle; Pregnancy Category C; FDA Pre 1938 Drugs
Drug Classes: Analgesics, topical; Anesthetics, topical; Otics
Brand Names: A B Otic; Allergen; Antipyrine W/Benzocaine; Aurafair; **Auralgan**; Auralgicin; Auraltone; Aurodex; Auromid; Auroto; Benzotic; Dec-Agesic A.B.; Decon Otic; Dolotic; Ear Drops; Ear Drops Rx; Earocol; Lanaurine; Otipyrin; Oto; Otocalm
Foreign Brand Availability: Auralgan (non-prescription) (Australia); Auralgan Otic (Philippines); Auralyt (Colombia; Ecuador; Mexico); Oidisan (Colombia); Otised (South-Africa)

DESCRIPTION

Each ml Contains:

Antipyrine: 54.0 mg
Benzocaine: 14.0 mg
Glycerin dehydrated q.s. to 1.0 ml

Contains not more than 0.6% moisture (also contains oxyquinoline sulfate).

TOPICAL DECONGESTANT AND ANALGESIC

Antipyrine; benzocaine is an otic solution containing antipyrine, benzocaine, and dehydrated glycerin. The solution congeals at 0°C (32°F) but returns to normal consistency, unchanged, at room temperature.

CLINICAL PHARMACOLOGY

Antipyrine; benzocaine combines the hygroscopic property of dehydrated glycerin with the analgesic action of antipyrine and benzocaine to relieve pressure, reduce inflammation and congestion, and alleviate pain and discomfort in acute otitis media.

Antipyrine; benzocaine does not blanch the tympanic membrane or mask the landmarks and, therefore, does not distort the otoscopic picture.

INDICATIONS AND USAGE

ACUTE OTITIS MEDIA OF VARIOUS ETIOLOGIES

- Prompt relief of pain and reduction of inflammation in the congestive and serous stages.
- Adjuvant therapy during systemic antibiotic administration for resolution of the infection.

Because of the close anatomical relationship of the eustachian tube to the nasal cavity, otitis media is a frequent problem, especially in children in whom the tube is shorter, wider, and more horizontal than in adults.

REMOVAL OF CERUMEN

Facilitates the removal of excessive or impacted cerumen.

CONTRAINDICATIONS

Hypersensitivity to any of the components or substances related to them.

Perforated tympanic membrane is considered a contraindication to the use of any medication in the external ear canal.

WARNINGS

Discontinue promptly if sensitization or irritation occurs.

PRECAUTIONS

CARCINOGENESIS, MUTAGENESIS, AND IMPAIRMENT OF FERTILITY

No long-term studies in animals or humans have been conducted.

PREGNANCY CATEGORY C

Animal reproduction studies have not been conducted with antipyrine; benzocaine. It is also not known whether antipyrine; benzocaine can cause fetal harm when administered to a pregnant woman, or can affect reproduction capacity. Antipyrine; benzocaine should be given to a pregnant woman only if clearly needed.

NURSING MOTHERS

It is not known whether this drug is excreted in human milk. Because many drugs are excreted in human milk, caution should be exercised when antipyrine; benzocaine is administered to a nursing woman.

DOSAGE AND ADMINISTRATION

ACUTE OTITIS MEDIA

Instill antipyrine; benzocaine permitting the solution to run along the wall of the canal until it is filled. Avoid touching the ear with dropper. Then moisten a cotton pledget with antipyrine; benzocaine and insert into meatus. Repeat every 1-2 hours until pain and congestion are relieved.

REMOVAL OF CERUMEN

Before: Instill antipyrine; benzocaine three times daily for two or three days to help detach cerumen from wall of canal and facilitate removal.
After: Antipyrine; benzocaine is useful for drying out the canal or relieving discomfort.
Before and after removal of cerumen, a cotton pledget moistened with antipyrine; benzocaine should be inserted into the meatus following instillation.
NOTE: Do not rinse dropper after use. Replace dropper in bottle after each use. Hold dropper assembly by screw cap and, without compressing the rubber bulb, insert into drug container and screw down tightly.
Protect the solution from light and heat, and do not use if it is brown or contains a precipitate.

DISCARD THIS PRODUCT 6 MONTHS AFTER DROPPER IS FIRST PLACED IN THE DRUG SOLUTION

Storage: Store at room temperature (approximately 25°C).

PRODUCT LISTING - EQUIVALENTS NOT AVAILABLE

Solution - Otic - 54 mg;14 mg/ml

10 ml	$1.47	GENERIC, Moore, H.L. Drug Exchange Inc	00839-6342-30
10 ml	$1.75	GENERIC, Raway Pharmacal Inc	00686-0561-62
10 ml	$1.80	GENERIC, Clay-Park Laboratories Inc	45802-0311-68
10 ml	$2.04	GENERIC, Aligen Independent Laboratories Inc	00405-2025-51
10 ml	$2.25	GENERIC, Thames Pharmacal Company Inc	49158-0178-43
10 ml	$2.92	GENERIC, Physicians Total Care	54868-2034-00
10 ml	$3.10	GENERIC, Liquipharm Inc	54198-0132-99
10 ml	$4.12	GENERIC, Prescript Pharmaceuticals	00247-0349-10
10 ml	$5.05	GENERIC, Southwood Pharmaceuticals Inc	58016-6444-01
10 ml	$17.96	AURALGAN, Allscripts Pharmaceutical Company	54569-0884-00
10 ml	$19.29	AURALGAN, Physicians Total Care	54868-0549-01
10 ml	$19.86	AURALGAN, Wyeth-Ayerst Laboratories	00046-1000-10
14 ml	$4.44	GENERIC, Prescript Pharmaceuticals	00247-0349-41
14 ml	$4.48	GENERIC, Prescript Pharmaceuticals	00247-0349-73
15 ml	$1.73	GENERIC, Moore, H.L. Drug Exchange Inc	00839-6342-61
15 ml	$2.10	GENERIC, Liquipharm Inc	54198-0132-15
15 ml	$2.30	GENERIC, Thames Pharmacal Company Inc	49158-0178-30
15 ml	$2.65	AURODEX, Major Pharmaceuticals Inc	00904-0793-35
15 ml	$2.95	GENERIC, Clay-Park Laboratories Inc	45802-0311-56
15 ml	$3.00	GENERIC, Ivax Corporation	00182-1175-33
15 ml	$3.04	GENERIC, Physicians Total Care	54868-2034-01
15 ml	$3.08	GENERIC, Vintage Pharmaceuticals Inc	00254-9010-43
15 ml	$3.08	GENERIC, Alpharma Uspd Makers Of Barre and Nmc	00472-0016-99
15 ml	$3.08	GENERIC, Qualitest Products Inc	00603-7020-73
15 ml	$3.37	GENERIC, Bausch and Lomb	24208-0420-15
15 ml	$4.49	GENERIC, Prescript Pharmaceuticals	00247-0349-15
15 ml	$5.50	GENERIC, Marlop Pharmaceuticals Inc	12939-0230-15
15 ml	$5.62	GENERIC, Alpharma Uspd Makers Of Barre and Nmc	63874-0719-15
15 ml	$6.17	GENERIC, Allscripts Pharmaceutical Company	54569-2113-00
15 ml	$6.51	GENERIC, Southwood Pharmaceuticals Inc	58016-6003-01
15 ml	$7.03	AURODEX, Pharma Pac	52959-0135-03
15 ml	$12.27	GENERIC, Qualitest Products Inc	00603-7240-73

A

Apraclonidine Hydrochloride *(000276)*

Categories: Glaucoma, open-angle; Surgery, ophthalmic, adjunct; Pregnancy Category C; FDA Approved 1987 Dec
Drug Classes: Adrenergic agonists; Ophthalmics
Brand Names: Iopidine
Cost of Therapy: $53.94 (Ocular Hypertension; Iopidine Ophthalmic Solution; 0.5%; 5 ml; 3 drops/day; variable day supply)

DESCRIPTION

This monograph contains prescribing information for both Iopidine ophthalmic solution and Iopidine 0.5% ophthalmic solution.

BOTH FORMS

Iopidine ophthalmic solution and Iopidine 0.5% ophthalmic solution contain apraclonidine hydrochloride, an alpha adrenergic agonist, in a sterile isotonic solution for topical application to the eye. Apraclonidine hydrochloride is a white to off-white powder and is highly soluble in water. Its chemical name is 2-[(4-amino-2,6 dichlorophenyl)imino]imidazolidine monohydrochloride with an empirical formula of $C_9H_{11}Cl_3N_4$.

IOPIDINE

The molecular weight is 281.60.

Each ml of Iopidine ophthalmic solution contains: *Actives:* Apraclonidine hydrochloride 11.5 mg equivalent to apraclonidine base 10 mg. *Preservative:* Benzalkonium chloride 0.01%. *Inactives:* Sodium chloride, sodium acetate, sodium hydroxide and/or hydrochloric acid (pH 4.4-7.8) and purified water.

IOPIDINE 0.5%

The molecular weight is 281.57.

Each ml of Iopidine 0.5% ophthalmic solution contains: *Active:* Apraclonidine hydrochloride 5.75 mg equivalent to apraclonidine base 5 mg. *Preservative:* Benzalkonium chloride 0.01%. *Inactive:* Sodium chloride, sodium acetate, sodium hydroxide and/or hydrochloric acid (pH 4.4-7.8) and purified water.

CLINICAL PHARMACOLOGY

APRACLONIDINE HCl OPHTHALMIC SOLUTION

Apraclonidine is a relatively selective, alpha adrenergic agonist and does not have significant membrane stabilizing (local anesthetic) activity. When instilled into the eye, apraclonidine HCl ophthalmic solution has the action of reducing intraocular pressure. Ophthalmic apraclonidine has minimal effect of cardiovascular parameters.

Optic nerve head damage and visual field loss may result from an acute elevation in intraocular pressure that can occur after argon or Nd:YAG laser surgical procedures. Elevated intraocular pressure, whether acute or chronic in duration, is a major risk factor in the pathogenesis of visual field loss. The higher the peak or spike of intraocular pressure, the greater the likelihood of visual field loss and optic nerve damage especially in patients with previously compromised optic nerves. The onset of action with apraclonidine HCl ophthalmic solution can usually be noted within 1 hour and the maximum intraocular pressure reduction usually occurs 3-5 hours after application of a single dose. The precise mechanism of the ocular hypotensive action of apraclonidine HCl ophthalmic solution is not completely established at this time. Aqueous fluorophotometry studies in man suggest that its predominant action may be related to a reduction of aqueous formation. Controlled clinical studies of patients requiring argon laser trabeculoplasty, argon laser iridotomy or Nd:YAG posterior capsulotomy showed that apraclonidine HCl ophthalmic solution controlled or prevented the postsurgical intraocular pressure rise typically observed in patients after undergoing those procedures. After surgery, the mean intraocular pressure was 1.2 to 4 mm Hg below the corresponding presurgical baseline pressure before apraclonidine HCl ophthalmic solution treatment. With placebo treatment, postsurgical pressures were 2.5-8.4 mm Hg higher than their corresponding presurgical baselines. Overall, only 2% of patients treated with apraclonidine HCl ophthalmic solution had severe intraocular pressure elevations (spike ≥10 mm Hg) during the first 3 hours after laser surgery, whereas 23% of placebo-treated patients responded with severe pressure spikes (TABLE 1). Of the patients that experienced a pressure spike after surgery, the peak intraocular pressure was above 30 mm Hg in most patients (TABLE 2) and was above 50 mm Hg in 7 placebo-treated patients and 1 apraclonidine HCl ophthalmic solution-treated patient.

TABLE 1 *Incidence of Intraocular Pressure Spikes ≥10 mm Hg*

Laser Procedure	P-Value	Apraclonidine HCl *n (%)	Placebo *n (%)
Trabeculoplasty			
Study 1	<0.05	0/40 (0%)	6/35 (17%)
Study 2	-0.06	2/41 (5%)	8/42 (19%)
Iridotomy			
Study 1	<0.05	0/11 (0%)	4/10 (40%)
Study 2	-0.05	0/17 (0%)	4/19 (21%)
Nd:YAG Capsulotomy			
Study 1	<0.05	3/80 (4%)	19/83 (23%)
Study 2	<0.05	0/83 (0%)	22/81 (27%)

* Number spikes/number eyes.

APRACLONIDINE HCl 0.5% OPHTHALMIC SOLUTION

Apraclonidine hydrochloride is a relatively selective alpha-2-adrenergic agonist. When instilled in the eye, apraclonidine 0.5% ophthalmic solution, has the action of reducing elevated, as well as normal, intraocular pressure (IOP), whether or not accompanied by glaucoma. Ophthalmic apraclonidine has minimal effect on cardiovascular parameters.

Elevated IOP presents a major risk factor in glaucomatous field loss. The higher the level of IOP, the greater the likelihood of optic nerve damage and visual field loss. Apraclonidine

TABLE 2 *Magnitude of Postsurgical Intraocular Pressure in Trabeculoplasty, Iridotomy and Nd:YAG Capsulotomy Patients With Severe Pressure Spikes ≥10 mm Hg*

Treatment	Total Spikes	Maximum Postsurgical Intraocular Pressure 20-29 mm Hg	30-39 mm Hg	40-49 mm Hg	>50 mm Hg
Apraclonidine HCl	8	1	4	2	1
Placebo	78	16	47	8	7

HCl 0.5% ophthalmic solution has the action of reducing IOP. The onset of action of apraclonidine can usually be noted within 1 hour, and maximum IOP reduction occurs about 3 hours after installation. Aqueous flurophotometry studies demonstrate that apraclonidine's predominant mechanism of action is reduction of aqueous flow via stimulation of the alpha-adrenergic system. Repeated dose-response and comparative studies (0.125-1.0% apraclonidine) demonstrate that 0.5% apraclonidine is at the top of the dose/response IOP reduction curve.

The clinical utility of apraclonidine HCl 0.5% ophthalmic solution is most apparent for those glaucoma patients on maximally tolerated medical therapy. Patients on maximally tolerated medical therapy with uncontrolled IOP and scheduled to undergo laster trabeculoplasty or trabeculectomy surgery were enrolled into a double-masked, placebo-controlled, multi-center clinical trial to determine if apraclonidine HCl 0.5% ophthalmic solution, dosed 3 times daily (tid), could delay the need for surgery for up to 3 months.

All patients enrolled into this trial had advanced glaucoma and were undergoing maximally tolerated medical therapy, *i.e.,* patients were using combinations of a topical beta blocker, sympathomimetics, parasympathomimetics and oral carbonic anhydrase inhibitors. Patients were considered to be treatment failures in this study if, in the opinion of the investigators, their IOP was uncontrolled by the masked study medication or there was evidence of further optic nerve damage or visual field loss, and surgery was indicated. Of 171 patients receiving masked medication, 84 were treated with apraclonidine HCl 0.5% ophthalmic solution and 87 were treated with placebo (apraclonidine vehicle).

Apraclonidine treatment resulted in a significantly greater percentage of treatment successes compared to patients treated with placebo. In this placebo-controlled maximum therapy trial, 14.3% of patients treated with apraclonidine HCl 0.5% ophthalmic solution were discontinued due to adverse events, primarily allergic-like reactions (12.9%).

The IOP lowering efficacy of apraclonidine HCl 0.5% ophthalmic solution diminishes over time in some patients. This loss of effect, or tachyphylaxis, appears to be an individual occurrence with a variable time of onset and should be closely monitored.

An unpredictable decrease of IOP control in some patients and incidence of ocular allergic responses and systemic side effects may limit the utility of apraclonidine HCl 0.5% ophthalmic solution. However, patients on maximally tolerated medical therapy may still benefit from the additional IOP reduction provided by the short-term use of apraclonidine HCl 0.5% ophthalmic solution.

Topical use of apraclonidine HCl 0.5% ophthalmic solution leads to systemic absorption. Studies of apraclonidine HCl 0.5% ophthalmic solution dosed 1 drop three times a day in both eyes for 10 days in normal volunteers yielded mean peak and trough concentrations of 0.9 ng/ml and 0.5 ng/ml, respectively. The half-life of apraclonidine HCl 0.5% ophthalmic solution was calculated to be 8 hours.

Apraclonidine HCl 0.5% ophthalmic solution, because of its alpha adrenergic activity, is a vasoconstrictor. Single dose ocular blood flow studies in monkeys, using the microsphere technique, demonstrated a reduced blood flow for the anterior segment; however, no reduction in blood flow was observed in the posterior segment of the eye after a topical dose of apraclonidine HCl 0.5% ophthalmic solution. Ocular blood flow studies have not been conducted in humans.

INDICATIONS AND USAGE

APRACLONIDINE HCl OPHTHALMIC SOLUTION

Apraclonidine HCl ophthalmic solution is indicated to control or prevent postsurgical elevations in intraocular pressure that occur in patients after argon laser trabeculoplasty, argon laser iridotomy or Nd:YAG posterior capsulotomy.

APRACLONIDINE HCl 0.5% OPHTHALMIC SOLUTION

Apraclonidine HCl 0.5% ophthalmic solution is indicated for short-term adjunctive therapy in patients on maximally tolerated medical therapy who require additional IOP reduction. Patients on maximally tolerated medical therapy who are treated with apraclonidine HCl 0.5% ophthalmic solution to delay surgery should have frequent followup examinations and treatment should be discontinued if the intraocular pressure rises significantly.

The addition of apraclonidine HCl 0.5% ophthalmic solution to patients already using two aqueous suppressing drugs (*i.e.,* beta-blocker plus carbonic anhydrase inhibitor) as part of their maximally tolerated medical therapy may not provide additional benefit. This is because apraclonidine HCl 0.5% ophthalmic solution is an aqueous suppressing drug and the addition of a third aqueous suppressant may not significantly reduce IOP.

The IOP lowering efficacy of apraclonidine HCl 0.5% ophthalmic solution diminishes over time in some patients. This loss of effect, or tachyphylaxis, appears to be an individual occurrence with a variable time of onset and should be closely monitored. The benefit for most patients is less than 1 month.

CONTRAINDICATIONS

APRACLONIDINE HCl OPHTHALMIC SOLUTION

Apraclonidine HCl ophthalmic solution is contraindicated in patients receiving monoamine oxidase inhibitor therapy and for patients with hypersensitivity to any component of this medication or to clonidine.

APRACLONIDINE HCl 0.5% OPHTHALMIC SOLUTION

Apraclonidine HCl 0.5% ophthalmic solution is contraindicated in patients with hypersensitivity to apraclonidine or any other component of this medication, as well as systemic clonidine. It is also contraindicated in patients receiving monoamine oxidase inhibitors (MAO inhibitors).

WARNINGS

APRACLONIDINE HCl OPHTHALMIC SOLUTION

FOR TOPICAL OPHTHALMIC USE ONLY.

APRACLONIDINE HCl 0.5% OPHTHALMIC SOLUTION

Not for injection or oral ingestion. Topical ophthalmic use only.

PRECAUTIONS

APRACLONIDINE HCl OPHTHALMIC SOLUTION

General

Since apraclonidine HCl ophthalmic solution is a potent depressor of intraocular pressure, patients who develop exaggerated reductions in intraocular pressure should be closely monitored.

Although the acute administration of 2 drops of apraclonidine HCl ophthalmic solution has minimal effect on heart rate or blood pressure in clinical studies, evaluating patients undergoing anterior segment laser surgery, the preclinical pharmacologic profile of this drug suggests that caution should be observed in treating patients with severe cardiovascular disease including hypertension.

The possibility of a vasovagal attack occurring during laser surgery should be considered and caution used in patients with history of such episodes.

Topical ocular administration of 2 drops of 0.5%, 1% and 1.5% apraclonidine HCl ophthalmic solution to New Zealand Albino rabbits 3 times daily for 1 month resulted in sporadic and transient instances of minimal corneal cloudiness in the 1.5% group only. No histopathological changes were noted in those eyes. No adverse ocular effects were observed in cynomolgus monkeys treated with 2 drops of 1.5% apraclonidine HCl ophthalmic solution applied 3 times daily for 3 months. No corneal changes were observed in 320 humans given at least one dose of 1% apraclonidine HCl ophthalmic solution.

Carcinogenesis, Mutagenesis, and Impairment of Fertility

No significant change in tumor incidence or type was observed following 2 years of oral administration of apraclonidine HCl to rats and mice at dosages of 1 and 0.6 mg/kg/day, up to 50 and 30 times, respectively, the maximum dose recommended for human topical ocular use.

Apraclonidine HCl was not mutagenic in a series of *in vitro* mutagenicity assays, including the Ames test, a mouse lymphoma forward mutation assay, a chromosome aberration assay in cultured Chinese hamster ovary (CHO) cells, a sister chromatid exchange assay in (CHO) cells, and a cell transformation assay. An *in vivo* mouse micronucleous assay conducted with apraclonidine HCl also provided no evidence of mutagenicity. Reproduction and fertility studies in rats showed no adverse effect on male or female fertility at a dose of 0.5 mg/kg (25 times the maximum recommended human dose).

Pregnancy Category C

Apraclonidine HCl has been shown to have an embryocidal effect in rabbits when given in an oral dose of 3 mg/kg (150 times the maximum recommended human dose). Dose related maternal toxicity was observed in pregnant rats at 0.3 mg/kg (15 times the maximum recommended human dose). There are no adequate and well controlled studies in pregnant women. Apraclonidine HCl 1% ophthalmic solution should be used during pregnancy only if the potential benefit justifies the potential risk to the fetus.

Nursing Mothers

It is not known if topically applied apraclonidine HCl ophthalmic solution is excreted in human milk. A decision should be considered to discontinue nursing temporarily for the 1 day on which apraclonidine HCl ophthalmic solution is used.

Pediatric Use

Safety and effectiveness in pediatric patients have not been established.

APRACLONIDINE HCl 0.5% OPHTHALMIC SOLUTION

General

Glaucoma patients on maximally tolerated medical therapy who are treated with apraclonidine HCl 0.5% ophthalmic solution to delay surgery should have their visual fields monitored periodically.

Although the topical use of apraclonidine HCl 0.5% ophthalmic solution has not been studied in renal failure patients, structurally related clonidine undergoes a significant increase in half-life in patients with severe renal impairment. Close monitoring of cardiovascular parameters in patients with impaired renal function is advised if they are candidates for topical apraclonidine therapy. Close monitoring of cardiovascular parameters in patients with impaired liver function is also advised as the systemic dosage form of clonidine is partly metabolized in the liver.

While the topical administration of apraclonidine HCl 0.5% ophthalmic solution had minimal effect on heart rate or blood pressure in clinical studies evaluating glaucoma patients, the preclinical pharmacology profile of this drug suggests that caution should be observed in treating patients with severe, uncontrolled cardiovascular disease, including hypertension.

Apraclonidine HCl 0.5% ophthalmic solution should be used with caution in patients with coronary insufficiency, recent myocardial infarction, cerebrovascular disease, chronic renal failure, Raynaud's disease, or thromboangiitis obliterans. Caution and monitoring of depressed patients are advised since apraclonidine has been infrequently associated with depression.

Apraclonidine HCl can cause dizziness and somnolence. Patients who engage in hazardous activities requiring mental alertness should be warned of the potential for a decrease in mental alertness while using apraclonidine. Topical ocular administration of two drops of 0.5%, 1% and 1.5% apraclonidine HCl ophthalmic solution to New Zealand Albino rabbits 3 times daily for 1 month resulted in sporadic and transient instances of minimal corneal edema in the 1.5% group only; no histopathological changes were noted in those eyes.

Use of apraclonidine HCl 0.5% ophthalmic solution can lead to an allergic-like reaction characterized wholly or in part by the symptoms of hyperemia, pruritus, discomfort, tearing, foreign body sensation, and edema of the lids and conjunctiva. If ocular allergic-like symptoms occur, apraclonidine HCl 0.5% ophthalmic solution therapy should be discontinued.

Information for the Patient

Do not touch dropper tip to any surface as this may contaminate the contents.

Carcinogenesis, Mutagenesis, and Impairment of Fertility

No significant change in tumor incidence or type was observed following 2 years of oral administration of apraclonidine HCl to rats and mice at dosages of 1.0 and 0.6 mg/kg, up to 20 and 12 times, respectively, the maximum dose recommended for human topical ocular use.

Apraclonidine HCl was not mutagenic in a series of *in vitro* mutagenicity tests, including the Ames test, a mouse lymphoma forward mutation assay, a chromosome aberration assay in cultured Chinese hamster ovary (CHO) cells, a sister chromatid exchange assay in (CHO) cells, and a cell transformation assay. An *in vivo* mouse micronucleus assay conducted with apraclonidine HCl also provided no evidence of mutagenicity.

Reproduction and fertility studies in rats showed no adverse effect on male or female fertility at a dose of 0.5 mg/kg (5-10 times the maximum recommended human dose).

Pregnancy Category C

Apraclonidine HCl has been shown to have an embryocidal effect in rabbits when given in an oral dose of 3.0 mg/kg (60 times the maximum recommended human dose). Dose related maternal toxicity was observed in pregnant rats at 0.3 mg/kg (6 times the maximum recommended human dose). There are no adequate and well controlled studies in pregnant women. Apraclonidine HCl 0.5% ophthalmic solution should be used during pregnancy only if the potential benefit justifies the potential risk to the fetus.

Nursing Mothers

It is not known whether this drug is excreted in human milk. Because many drugs are excreted in human milk, caution should be exercised when apraclonidine HCl 0.5% ophthalmic solution is administered to a nursing woman.

Pediatric Use

Safety and effectiveness in pediatric patients have not been established.

DRUG INTERACTIONS

APRACLONIDINE HCl OPHTHALMIC SOLUTION

Interactions with other agents have not been investigated.

APRACLONIDINE HCl 0.5% OPHTHALMIC SOLUTION

Apraclonidine should not be used in patients receiving MAO inhibitors. (See CONTRAINDICATIONS.) Although no specific drug interactions with topical glaucoma drugs or systemic medications were identified in clinical studies of apraclonidine HCl 0.5% ophthalmic solution, the possibility of an additive or potentiating effect with CNS depressants (alcohol, barbiturates, opiates, sedatives, anesthetics) should be considered. Tricyclic antidepressants have been reported to blunt the hypotensive effect of systemic clonidine. It is not known whether the concurrent use of these agents with apraclonidine can lead to a reduction in IOP lowering effect. No data on the level of circulating catecholamines after apraclonidine withdrawal are available. Caution, however, is advised in patients taking tricyclic antidepressants which can affect the metabolism and uptake of circulating amines.

An additive hypotensive effect has been reported with the combination of systemic clonidine and neuroleptic therapy. Systemic clonidine may inhibit the production of catecholamines in response to insulin-induced hypoglycemia and mask the signs and symptoms of hypoglycemia.

Since apraclonidine may reduce pulse and blood pressure, caution in using drugs such as beta-blockers (ophthalmic and systemic), antihypertensives, and cardiac glycosides is advised. Patients using cardiovascular drugs concurrently with apraclonidine 0.5% ophthalmic solution should have pulse and blood pressures frequently monitored. Caution should be exercised with simultaneous use of clonidine and other similar pharmacologic agents.

ADVERSE REACTIONS

APRACLONIDINE HCl OPHTHALMIC SOLUTION

The following adverse events, occurring in less than 2% of patients, were reported in association with the use of apraclonidine HCl ophthalmic solution in laser surgery: Ocular injection, upper lid elevation, irregular heart rate, nasal decongestion, ocular inflammation, conjunctival blanching, and mydriasis.

The following adverse events were observed in investigational studies dosing apraclonidine HCl ophthalmic solution once or twice daily for up to 28 days in nonlaser studies:

Ocular: Conjunctival blanching, upper lid elevation, mydriasis, burning, discomfort, foreign body sensation, dryness, itching, hypotony, blurred or dimmed vision, allergic response, conjunctival microhemorrhage.

Gastrointestinal: Abdominal pain, diarrhea, stomach discomfort, emesis.

Cardiovascular: Bradycardia, vasovagal attack, palpitations, orthostatic episode.

Central Nervous System: Insomnia, dream disturbances, irritability, decreased libido.

Other: Taste abnormalities, dry mouth, nasal burning or dryness, headache, head cold sensation, chest heaviness or burning, clammy or sweaty palms, body heat sensation, shortness of breath, increased pharyngeal secretion, extremity pain or numbness, fatigue, paresthesia, pruritus not associated with rash.

APRACLONIDINE HCl 0.5% OPHTHALMIC SOLUTION

Use of apraclonidine HCl 0.5% ophthalmic solution can lead to an allergic-like reaction characterized wholly or in part by the symptoms of hyperemia, pruritus, discomfort, tearing, foreign body sensation, and edema of the lids and conjunctiva. If ocular allergic-like symptoms occur, apraclonidine HCl 0.5% ophthalmic solution therapy should be discontinued.

In clinical studies the overall discontinuation rate related to apraclonidine HCl 0.5% ophthalmic solution was 15%. The most commonly reported events leading to discontinuation included (in decreasing order of frequency) hyperemia, pruritus, tearing, discomfort, lid edema, dry mouth, and foreign body sensation.

The following adverse reactions (incidences) were reported in clinical studies of apraclonidine HCl 0.5% ophthalmic solution as being possibly, probably, or definitely related to therapy:

Ocular: Hyperemia (13%), pruritus (10%), discomfort (6%), tearing (4%). *The following adverse reactions were reported in less than 3% of the patients:* Lid edema, blurred vision, foreign body sensation, dry eye, conjunctivitis, discharge, blanching. *The following adverse reactions were reported in less than 1% of the patients:* Lid margin crusting, conjunctival follicles, conjunctival edema, edema, abnormal vision, pain, lid disorder, keratitis, blepharitis, photophobia, corneal staining, lid erythema, blepharoconjunctivitis, irritation, corneal erosion, corneal infiltrate, keratopathy, lid scales, lid retraction.

Nonocular — Body as a Whole: *The following adverse reactions were reported in less than 3% of the patients:* Headache, asthenia. *The following adverse reactions (incidences) were reported in less than 1% of the patients:* Chest pain, abnormal coordination, malaise, facial edema.

Nonocular — Cardiovascular: *The following adverse reactions were reported in less than 1% of the patients:* Peripheral edema, arrhythmia. Although no reports of bradycardia related to apraclonidine HCl 0.5% ophthalmic solution were available from clinical studies, the possibility of its occurrence based on apraclonidine's alpha-2-agonist effect should be considered (see CLINICAL PHARMACOLOGY).

Central Nervous System: *The following adverse reactions were reported in less than 1% of the patients:* Somnolence, dizziness, nervousness, depression, insomnia, paresthesia.

Digestive System: Dry mouth (10%). *The following adverse reactions were reported in less than 1% of the patients:* Constipation, nausea.

Musculoskeletal: Myalgia (0.2%).

Respiratory System: Dry nose (2%). *The following adverse reactions were reported in less than 1% of the patients:* Rhinitis, dyspnea, pharyngitis, asthma.

Skin: *The following adverse reactions were reported in less than 1% of the patients:* Contact dermatitis, dermatitis.

Special Senses: Taste perversion (3%), parosmia (0.2%).

DOSAGE AND ADMINISTRATION

APRACLONIDINE HCl OPHTHALMIC SOLUTION

One drop of apraclonidine HCl ophthalmic solution should be instilled in the scheduled operative eye 1 hour before initiating anterior segment laser surgery and a second drop should be instilled to the same eye immediately upon completion of the laser surgical procedure. Use a separate container for each single-drop dose and discard each container after use.

APRACLONIDINE HCl 0.5% OPHTHALMIC SOLUTION

One (1) to 2 drops of apraclonidine HCl 0.5% ophthalmic solution should be instilled in the affected eye(s) 3 times daily. Since apraclonidine HCl 0.5% ophthalmic solution will be used with other ocular glaucoma therapies, an approximate 5 minute interval between instillation of each medication should be practiced to prevent washout of the previous dose.

NOT FOR INJECTION INTO THE EYE. NOT FOR ORAL INGESTION.

HOW SUPPLIED

IOPIDINE OPHTHALMIC SOLUTION

Iopidine ophthalmic solution 1% as base is a sterile, isotonic, aqueous solution containing apraclonidine HCl.

Supplied as follows: 0.1 ml in plastic ophthlamic dispensers, packaged 2 per pouch. These dispensers are enclosed in a foil overwrap as an added barrier to evaporation.

Storage: Store at 2-25°C (34-77°F).

Protect from light.

IOPIDINE 0.5% OPHTHALMIC SOLUTION

Iopidine 0.5% ophthalmic solution as base in a sterile, isotonic, aqueous solution containing apraclonidine HCl.

Supplied in plastic ophthalmic Drop-Tainer 5 and 10 ml dispensers.

Storage: Store between 2-27°C (36-80°F).

Protect from freezing and light.

PRODUCT LISTING - EQUIVALENTS NOT AVAILABLE

Solution - Ophthalmic - 0.5%

Size	Price	Product	NDC
5 ml	$34.68	IOPIDINE, Southwood Pharmaceuticals Inc	58016-6508-05
5 ml	$53.94	IOPIDINE, Allscripts Pharmaceutical Company	54569-4405-00
5 ml	$64.69	IOPIDINE, Alcon Laboratories Inc	00065-0665-05
10 ml	$104.94	IOPIDINE, Allscripts Pharmaceutical Company	54569-4296-00
10 ml	$128.06	IOPIDINE, Alcon Laboratories Inc	00065-0665-10

Solution - Ophthalmic - 1%

Size	Price	Product	NDC
0.10 ml x 24	$258.00	IOPIDINE, Alcon Laboratories Inc	00065-0660-10

Aprepitant *(003590)*

Categories: Nausea, secondary to cancer chemotherapy; Vomiting, secondary to cancer chemotherapy; Pregnancy Category B; FDA Approved 2003 Mar

Drug Classes: Antiemetics/antivertigo; Substance P antagonists

Brand Names: **Emend**

DESCRIPTION

Emend is a substance P/neurokinin 1 (NK_1) receptor antagonist, chemically described as 5-[[(2*R*,3*S*)-2-[(1*R*)-1-[3,5-bis(trifluoromethyl)phenyl]ethoxy]-3-(4-fluorophenyl)-4-morpholinyl]methyl]-1,2-dihydro-3*H*-1,2,4-triazol-3-one.

Its empirical formula is $C_{23}H_{21}F_7N_4O_3$.

Aprepitant is a white to off-white crystalline solid, with a molecular weight of 534.43. It is practically insoluble in water. Aprepitant is sparingly soluble in ethanol and isopropyl acetate and slightly soluble in acetonitrile.

Each capsule of Emend for oral administration contains either 80 or 125 mg of aprepitant and the following inactive ingredients: sucrose, microcrystalline cellulose, hydroxypropyl cellulose and sodium lauryl sulfate. The capsule shell excipients are gelatin and titanium dioxide. The 125 mg capsule also contains red ferric oxide and yellow ferric oxide.

CLINICAL PHARMACOLOGY

MECHANISM OF ACTION

Aprepitant is a selective high-affinity antagonist of human substance P/neurokinin 1 (NK_1) receptors. Aprepitant has little or no affinity for serotonin ($5\text{-}HT_3$), dopamine, and corticosteroid receptors, the targets of existing therapies for chemotherapy-induced nausea and vomiting (CINV).

Aprepitant has been shown in animal models to inhibit emesis induced by cytotoxic chemotherapeutic agents, such as cisplatin, via central actions. Animal and human Positron Emission Tomography (PET) studies with aprepitant have shown that it crosses the blood brain barrier and occupies brain NK_1 receptors. Animal and human studies show that aprepitant augments the antiemetic activity of the $5\text{-}HT_3$-receptor antagonist ondansetron and the corticosteroid dexamethasone and inhibits both the acute and delayed phases of cisplatin-induced emesis.

PHARMACOKINETICS

Absorption

The mean absolute oral bioavailability of aprepitant is approximately 60-65% and the mean peak plasma concentration (C_{max}) of aprepitant occurred at approximately 4 hours (T_{max}). Oral administration of the capsule with a standard breakfast had no clinically meaningful effect on the bioavailability of aprepitant.

The pharmacokinetics of aprepitant are non-linear across the clinical dose range. In healthy young adults, the increase in AUC(0-∞) was 26% greater than dose proportional between 80 and 125 mg single doses administered in the fed state.

Following oral administration of a single 125 mg dose of aprepitant on Day 1 and 80 mg once daily on Days 2 and 3, the AUC(0-24h) was approximately 19.6 μg·h/ml and 21.2 μg·h/ml on Day 1 and Day 3, respectively. The C_{max} of 1.6 μg/ml and 1.4 μg/ml were reached in approximately 4 hours (T_{max}) on Day 1 and Day 3, respectively.

Distribution

Aprepitant is greater than 95% bound to plasma proteins. The mean apparent volume of distribution at steady state (Vd_{ss}) is approximately 70 L in humans.

Aprepitant crosses the placenta in rats and rabbits and crosses the blood brain barrier in humans (see Mechanism of Action).

Metabolism

Aprepitant undergoes extensive metabolism. *In vitro* studies using human liver microsomes indicate that aprepitant is metabolized primarily by CYP3A4 with minor metabolism by CYP1A2 and CYP2C19. Metabolism is largely via oxidation at the morpholine ring and its side chains. No metabolism by CYP2D6, CYP2C9, or CYP2E1 was detected. In healthy young adults, aprepitant accounts for approximately 24% of the radioactivity in plasma over 72 hours following a single oral 300 mg dose of [^{14}C]-aprepitant, indicating a substantial presence of metabolites in the plasma. Seven metabolites of aprepitant, which are only weakly active, have been identified in human plasma.

Excretion

Following administration of a single IV 100 mg dose of [^{14}C]-aprepitant prodrug to healthy subjects, 57% of the radioactivity was recovered in urine and 45% in feces. A study was not conducted with radiolabeled capsule formulation. The results after oral administration may differ.

Aprepitant is eliminated primarily by metabolism; aprepitant is not renally excreted. The apparent plasma clearance of aprepitant ranged from approximately 62-90 ml/min. The apparent terminal half-life ranged from approximately 9-13 hours.

SPECIAL POPULATIONS

Gender

Following oral administration of a single 125 mg dose of aprepitant, no difference in AUC(0-24h) was observed between males and females. The C_{max} for aprepitant is 16% higher in females as compared with males. The half-life of aprepitant is 25% lower in females as compared with males and T_{max} occurs at approximately the same time. These differences are not considered clinically meaningful. No dosage adjustment for aprepitant is necessary based on gender.

Geriatric

Following oral administration of a single 125 mg dose of aprepitant on Day 1 and 80 mg once daily on Days 2-5, the AUC(0-24h) of aprepitant was 21% higher on Day 1 and 36% higher on Day 5 in elderly (≥65 years) relative to younger adults. The C_{max} was 10% higher on Day 1 and 24% higher on Day 5 in elderly relative to younger adults. These differences are not considered clinically meaningful. No dosage adjustment for aprepitant is necessary in elderly patients.

Pediatric

The pharmacokinetics of aprepitant have not been evaluated in patients below 18 years of age.

Race

Following oral administration of a single 125 mg dose of aprepitant, the AUC(0-24h) is approximately 25% and 29% higher in Hispanics as compared with Whites and Blacks, respectively. The C_{max} is 22% and 31% higher in Hispanics as compared with Whites and Blacks, respectively. These differences are not considered clinically meaningful. There was no difference in AUC(0-24h) or C_{max} between Whites and Blacks. No dosage adjustment for aprepitant is necessary based on race.

Hepatic Insufficiency

Aprepitant was well tolerated in patients with mild to moderate hepatic insufficiency. Following administration of a single 125 mg dose of aprepitant on Day 1 and 80 mg once daily on Days 2 and 3 to patients with mild hepatic insufficiency (Child-Pugh score 5-6), the AUC(0-24h) of aprepitant was 11% lower on Day 1 and 36% lower on Day 3, as compared with healthy subjects given the same regimen. In patients with moderate hepatic insufficiency (Child-Pugh score 7-9), the AUC(0-24h) of aprepitant was 10% higher on Day 1 and 18% higher on Day 3, as compared with healthy subjects given the same regimen. These differences in AUC(0-24h) are not considered clinically meaningful; therefore, no dosage adjustment for aprepitant is necessary in patients with mild to moderate hepatic insufficiency.

There are no clinical or pharmacokinetic data in patients with severe hepatic insufficiency (Child-Pugh score >9) (see PRECAUTIONS).

Renal Insufficiency

A single 240 mg dose of aprepitant was administered to patients with severe renal insufficiency (CRCL <30 ml/min) and to patients with end stage renal disease (ESRD) requiring hemodialysis.

In patients with severe renal insufficiency, the AUC(0-∞) of total aprepitant (unbound and protein bound) decreased by 21% and C_{max} decreased by 32%, relative to healthy subjects. In patients with ESRD undergoing hemodialysis, the AUC(0-∞) of total aprepitant decreased by 42% and C_{max} decreased by 32%. Due to modest decreases in protein binding of aprepitant in patients with renal disease, the AUC of pharmacologically active unbound drug was not significantly affected in patients with renal insufficiency compared with healthy subjects. Hemodialysis conducted 4 or 48 hours after dosing had no significant effect on the pharmacokinetics of aprepitant; less than 0.2% of the dose was recovered in the dialysate.

No dosage adjustment for aprepitant is necessary for patients with renal insufficiency or for patients with ESRD undergoing hemodialysis.

INDICATIONS AND USAGE

Aprepitant, in combination with other antiemetic agents, is indicated for the prevention of acute and delayed nausea and vomiting associated with initial and repeat courses of highly emetogenic cancer chemotherapy, including high-dose cisplatin (see DOSAGE AND ADMINISTRATION).

CONTRAINDICATIONS

Aprepitant is a moderate CYP3A4 inhibitor. Aprepitant should not be used concurrently with pimozide, terfenadine, astemizole, or cisapride. Inhibition of cytochrome P450 isoenzyme 3A4 (CYP3A4) by aprepitant could result in elevated plasma concentrations of these drugs, potentially causing serious or life-threatening reactions (see DRUG INTERACTIONS).

Aprepitant is contraindicated in patients who are hypersensitive to any component of the product.

PRECAUTIONS

GENERAL

Aprepitant should be used with caution in patients receiving concomitant medicinal products, including chemotherapy agents that are primarily metabolized through CYP3A4. Inhibition of CYP3A4 by aprepitant could result in elevated plasma concentrations of these concomitant medicinal products. The effect of aprepitant on the pharmacokinetics of orally administered CYP3A4 substrates is expected to be greater than the effect of aprepitant on the pharmacokinetics of intravenously administered CYP3A4 substrates (see DRUG INTERACTIONS).

Chemotherapy agents that are known to be metabolized by CYP3A4 include docetaxel, paclitaxel, etoposide, irinotecan, ifosfamide, imatinib, vinorelbine, vinblastine and vincristine. In clinical studies, aprepitant was administered commonly with etoposide, vinorelbine, or paclitaxel. The doses of these agents were not adjusted to account for potential drug interactions.

Due to the small number of patients in clinical studies who received the CYP3A4 substrates docetaxel, vinblastine, vincristine, or ifosfamide, particular caution and careful monitoring are advised in patients receiving these agents or other chemotherapy agents metabolized primarily by CYP3A4 that were not studied (see DRUG INTERACTIONS).

Chronic continuous use of aprepitant for prevention of nausea and vomiting is not recommended because it has not been studied and because the drug interaction profile may change during chronic continuous use.

Coadministration of aprepitant with warfarin may result in a clinically significant decrease in International Normalized Ratio (INR) of prothrombin time. In patients on chronic warfarin therapy, the INR should be closely monitored in the 2 week period, particularly at 7-10 days, following initiation of the 3 day regimen of aprepitant with each chemotherapy cycle (see DRUG INTERACTIONS).

The efficacy of oral contraceptives during administration of aprepitant may be reduced. Although effects on contraception with a 3 day regimen of aprepitant given concomitantly with oral contraceptives has not been studied, alternative or back-up methods of contraception should be used (see DRUG INTERACTIONS).

There are no clinical or pharmacokinetic data in patients with severe hepatic insufficiency (Child-Pugh score >9). Therefore, caution should be exercised when aprepitant is administered in these patients (see CLINICAL PHARMACOLOGY, Special Populations, Hepatic Insufficiency and DOSAGE AND ADMINISTRATION).

INFORMATION FOR THE PATIENT

Physicians should instruct their patients to read the patient package insert before starting therapy with aprepitant and to reread it each time the prescription is renewed.

Patients should be instructed to take aprepitant only as prescribed. Patients should be advised to take their first dose (125 mg) of aprepitant 1 hour prior to chemotherapy treatment.

Aprepitant may interact with some drugs including chemotherapy; therefore, patients should be advised to report to their doctor the use of any other prescription, non-prescription medication or herbal products.

Patients on chronic warfarin therapy should be instructed to have their clotting status closely monitored in the 2 week period, particularly at 7-10 days, following initiation of the 3 day regimen of aprepitant with each chemotherapy cycle.

Administration of aprepitant may reduce the efficacy of oral contraceptives. Patients should be advised to use alternative or back-up methods of contraception.

CARCINOGENESIS, MUTAGENESIS, AND IMPAIRMENT OF FERTILITY

Three 2 year carcinogenicity studies of aprepitant (two in Sprague-Dawley rats and one in CD-1 mice) were conducted with aprepitant. Dose selection for the studies was based on saturation of absorption in both species. In the rat carcinogenicity studies, animals were treated with oral doses of 0.05, 0.25, 1, 5, 25, 125 mg/kg twice daily. The highest dose tested produced a systemic exposure to aprepitant [plasma AUC(0-24h)] of 0.4-1.4 times the human exposure [AUC(0-24h) = 19.6 µg·h/ml] at the recommended dose of 125 mg/day. Treatment with aprepitant at doses of 5-125 mg/kg twice per day produced thyroid follicular cell adenomas and carcinomas in male rats. In female rats, it produced increased incidences of hepatocellular adenoma at 25 and 125 mg/kg twice daily, and thyroid follicular adenoma at the 125 mg/kg twice daily dose. In the mouse carcinogenicity study, animals were treated with oral doses of 2.5, 25, 125, and 500 mg/kg/day. The highest tested dose produced a systemic exposure of about 2.2-2.7 times the human exposure at the recommended dose. Treatment with aprepitant produced skin fibrosarcomas in male mice of 125 and 500 mg/kg/day groups.

Aprepitant was not genotoxic in the Ames test, the human lymphoblastoid cell (TK6) mutagenesis test, the rat hepatocyte DNA strand break test, the Chinese hamster ovary (CHO) cell chromosome aberration test and the mouse micronucleus test.

Aprepitant did not affect the fertility or general reproductive performance of male or female rats at doses up to the maximum feasible dose of 1000 mg/kg twice daily (providing exposure in male rats lower than the exposure at the recommended human dose and exposure in female rats at about 1.6 times the human exposure).

PREGNANCY, TERATOGENIC EFFECTS, PREGNANCY CATEGORY B

Teratology studies have been performed in rats at oral doses up to 1000 mg/kg twice daily [plasma AUC(0-24h) of 31.3 µg·h/ml, about 1.6 times the human exposure at the recommended dose] and in rabbits at oral doses up to 25 mg/kg/day [plasma AUC(0-24h) of 26.9 µg·h/ml, about 1.4 times the human exposure at the recommended dose] and have revealed no evidence of impaired fertility or harm to the fetus due to aprepitant. There are, however, no adequate and well-controlled studies in pregnant women. Because animal reproduction studies are not always predictive of human response, this drug should be used during pregnancy only if clearly needed.

NURSING MOTHERS

Aprepitant is excreted in the milk of rats. It is not known whether this drug is excreted in human milk. Because many drugs are excreted in human milk and because of the potential for possible serious adverse reactions in nursing infants from aprepitant and because of the potential for tumorigenicity shown for aprepitant in rodent carcinogenicity studies, a decision should be made whether to discontinue nursing or to discontinue the drug, taking into account the importance of the drug to the mother.

PEDIATRIC USE

Safety and effectiveness of aprepitant in pediatric patients have not been established.

GERIATRIC USE

In 2 well-controlled clinical studies, of the total number of patients (n=544) treated with aprepitant, 31% were 65 and over, while 5% were 75 and over. No overall differences in safety or effectiveness were observed between these subjects and younger subjects. Greater sensitivity of some older individuals cannot be ruled out. Dosage adjustment in the elderly is not necessary.

DRUG INTERACTIONS

Aprepitant is a substrate, a moderate inhibitor, and an inducer of CYP3A4. Aprepitant is also an inducer of CYP2C9.

EFFECT OF APREPITANT ON THE PHARMACOKINETICS OF OTHER AGENTS

As a moderate inhibitor of CYP3A4, aprepitant can increase plasma concentrations of coadministered medicinal products that are metabolized through CYP3A4 (see CONTRAINDICATIONS).

Aprepitant has been shown to induce the metabolism of S(-) warfarin and tolbutamide, which are metabolized through CYP2C9. Coadministration of aprepitant with these drugs or other drugs that are known to be metabolized by CYP2C9, such as phenytoin, may result in lower plasma concentrations of these drugs.

Aprepitant is unlikely to interact with drugs that are substrates for the P-glycoprotein transporter, as demonstrated by the lack of interaction of aprepitant with digoxin in a clinical drug interaction study.

5-HT$_3$ Antagonists

In clinical drug interaction studies, aprepitant did not have clinically important effects on the pharmacokinetics of ondansetron or granisetron. No clinical or drug interaction study was conducted with dolasetron.

Corticosteroids

Dexamethasone: Aprepitant, when given as a regimen of 125 mg with dexamethasone coadministered orally as 20 mg on Day 1, and aprepitant when given as 80 mg/day with dexamethasone coadministered orally as 8 mg on Days 2 through 5, increased the AUC of dexamethasone, a CYP3A4 substrate by 2.2-fold, on Days 1 and 5. The oral dexamethasone doses should be reduced by approximately 50% when coadministered with aprepitant, to achieve exposures of dexamethasone similar to those obtained when it is given without aprepitant. The daily dose of dexamethasone administered in clinical studies with aprepitant reflects an approximate 50% reduction of the dose of dexamethasone (see DOSAGE AND ADMINISTRATION).

Methylprednisolone: Aprepitant, when given as a regimen of 125 mg on Day 1 and 80 mg/day on Days 2 and 3, increased the AUC of methylprednisolone, a CYP3A4 substrate, by 1.34-fold on Day 1 and by 2.5-fold on Day 3, when methylprednisolone was coadministered intravenously as 125 mg on Day 1 and orally as 40 mg on Days 2 and 3. The IV methylprednisolone dose should be reduced by approximately 25%, and the oral methylprednisolone dose should be reduced by approximately 50% when coadministered with aprepitant to achieve exposures of methylprednisolone similar to those obtained when it is given without aprepitant.

Chemotherapeutic Agents

See PRECAUTIONS, General.

Warfarin

A single 125 mg dose of aprepitant was administered on Day 1 and 80 mg/day on Days 2 and 3 to healthy subjects who were stabilized on chronic warfarin therapy. Although there was no effect of aprepitant on the plasma AUC of R(+) or S(-) warfarin determined on Day 3, there was a 34% decrease in S(-) warfarin (a CYP2C9 substrate) trough concentration accompanied by a 14% decrease in the prothrombin time (reported as International Normalized Ratio or INR) 5 days after completion of dosing with aprepitant. In patients on chronic warfarin therapy, the prothrombin time (INR) should be closely monitored in the 2 week period, particularly at 7-10 days, following initiation of the 3 day regimen of aprepitant with each chemotherapy cycle.

Tolbutamide

Aprepitant, when given as 125 mg on Day 1 and 80 mg/day on Days 2 and 3, decreased the AUC of tolbutamide (a CYP2C9 substrate) by 23% on Day 4, 28% on Day 8, and 15% on Day 15, when a single dose of tolbutamide 500 mg was administered orally prior to the administration of the 3 day regimen of aprepitant and on Days 4, 8, and 15.

Oral Contraceptives

Aprepitant, when given once daily for 14 days as a 100 mg capsule with an oral contraceptive containing 35 μg of ethinyl estradiol and 1 mg of norethindrone, decreased the AUC of ethinyl estradiol by 43%, and decreased the AUC of norethindrone by 8%; therefore, the efficacy of oral contraceptives during administration of aprepitant may be reduced. Although a 3 day regimen of aprepitant given concomitantly with oral contraceptives has not been studied, alternative or back-up methods of contraception should be used.

Midazolam

Aprepitant increased the AUC of midazolam, a sensitive CYP3A4 substrate, by 2.3-fold on Day 1 and 3.3-fold on Day 5, when a single oral dose of midazolam 2 mg was coadministered on Day 1 and Day 5 of a regimen of aprepitant 125 mg on Day 1 and 80 mg/day on Days 2-5. The potential effects of increased plasma concentrations of midazolam or other benzodiazepines metabolized via CYP3A4 (alprazolam, triazolam) should be considered when coadministering these agents with aprepitant.

In another study with IV administration of midazolam, aprepitant was given as 125 mg on Day 1 and 80 mg/day on Days 2 and 3, and midazolam 2 mg IV was given prior to the administration of the 3 day regimen of aprepitant and on Days 4, 8, and 15. Aprepitant increased the AUC of midazolam by 25% on Day 4 and decreased the AUC of midazolam by 19% on Day 8 relative to the dosing of aprepitant on Days 1-3. These effects were not considered clinically important. The AUC of midazolam on Day 15 was similar to that observed at baseline.

EFFECT OF OTHER AGENTS ON THE PHARMACOKINETICS OF APREPITANT

Aprepitant is a substrate for CYP3A4; therefore, coadministration of aprepitant with drugs that inhibit CYP3A4 activity may result in increased plasma concentrations of aprepitant. Consequently, concomitant administration of aprepitant with strong CYP3A4 inhibitors (*e.g.*, ketoconazole, itraconazole, nefazodone, troleandomycin, clarithromycin, ritonavir, nelfinavir) should be approached with caution. Because moderate CYP3A4 inhibitors (*e.g.*, diltiazem) result in 2-fold increase in plasma concentrations of aprepitant, concomitant administration should also be approached with caution.

Aprepitant is a substrate for CYP3A4; therefore, coadministration of aprepitant with drugs that strongly induce CYP3A4 activity (*e.g.*, rifampin, carbamazepine, phenytoin) may result in reduced plasma concentrations of aprepitant that may result in decreased efficacy of aprepitant.

Ketoconazole: When a single 125 mg dose of aprepitant was administered on Day 5 of a 10 day regimen of 400 mg/day of ketoconazole, a strong CYP3A4 inhibitor, the AUC of aprepitant increased approximately 5-fold and the mean terminal half-life of aprepitant increased approximately 3-fold. Concomitant administration of aprepitant with strong CYP3A4 inhibitors should be approached cautiously.

Rifampin: When a single 375 mg dose of aprepitant was administered on Day 9 of a 14 day regimen of 600 mg/day of rifampin, a strong CYP3A4 inducer, the AUC of aprepitant decreased approximately 11-fold and the mean terminal half-life decreased approximately 3-fold.

Coadministration of aprepitant with drugs that induce CYP3A4 activity may result in reduced plasma concentrations and decreased efficacy of aprepitant.

ADDITIONAL INTERACTIONS

Diltiazem: In patients with mild to moderate hypertension, administration of aprepitant once daily, as a tablet formulation comparable to 230 mg of the capsule formulation, with diltiazem 120 mg 3 times daily for 5 days, resulted in a 2-fold increase of aprepitant AUC and a simultaneous 1.7-fold increase of diltiazem AUC. These pharmacokinetic effects did not result in clinically meaningful changes in ECG, heart rate or blood pressure beyond those changes induced by diltiazem alone.

Paroxetine: Coadministration of once daily doses of aprepitant, as a tablet formulation comparable to 85 mg or 170 mg of the capsule formulation, with paroxetine 20 mg once daily, resulted in a decrease in AUC by approximately 25% and C_{max} by approximately 20% of both aprepitant and paroxetine.

ADVERSE REACTIONS

The overall safety of aprepitant was evaluated in approximately 3300 individuals.

In 2 well-controlled clinical trials in patients receiving highly emetogenic cancer chemotherapy, 544 patients were treated with aprepitant during Cycle 1 of chemotherapy and 413 of these patients continued into the Multiple-Cycle extension for up to 6 cycles of chemotherapy. Aprepitant was given in combination with ondansetron and dexamethasone and was generally well tolerated. Most adverse experiences reported in these clinical studies were described as mild to moderate in intensity.

In Cycle 1, clinical adverse experiences were reported in approximately 69% of patients treated with the aprepitant regimen compared with approximately 68% of patients treated with standard therapy. TABLE 4 shows the percent of patients with clinical adverse experiences reported at an incidence ≥3% during Cycle 1 of the 2 combined Phase III studies.

TABLE 4 *Percent of Patients With Clinical Adverse Experiences (Incidence ≥3%) in CINV Phase III Studies (Cycle 1)*

	Aprepitant Regimen (n=544)	Standard Therapy (n=550)
Body as a Whole/Site Unspecified		
Abdominal pain	4.6%	3.3%
Asthenia/fatigue	17.8%	11.8%
Dehydration	5.9%	5.1%
Dizziness	6.6%	4.4%
Fever	2.9%	3.5%
Mucous membrane disorder	2.6%	3.1%
Digestive System		
Constipation	10.3%	12.2%
Diarrhea	10.3%	7.5%
Epigastric discomfort	4.0%	3.1%
Gastritis	4.2%	3.1%
Heartburn	5.3%	4.9%
Nausea	12.7%	11.8%
Vomiting	7.5%	7.6%
Eyes, Ears, Nose, and Throat		
Tinnitus	3.7%	3.8%
Hemic and Lymphatic System		
Neutropenia	3.1%	2.9%
Metabolism and Nutrition		
Anorexia	10.1%	9.5%
Nervous System		
Headache	8.5%	8.7%
Insomnia	2.9%	3.1%
Respiratory System		
Hiccups	10.8%	5.6%

The following additional clinical adverse experiences (incidence >0.5% and greater than standard therapy), regardless of causality, were reported in patients treated with aprepitant regimen:

Body as a Whole: Diaphoresis, edema, flushing, malaise, malignant neoplasm, pelvic pain, septic shock, upper respiratory infection.

Cardiovascular System: Deep venous thrombosis, hypertension, hypotension, myocardial infarction, pulmonary embolism, tachycardia.

Digestive System: Acid reflux, deglutition disorder, dysgeusia, dyspepsia, dysphagia, flatulence, obstipation, salivation increased, taste disturbance.

Endocrine System: Diabetes mellitus.

Eyes, Ears, Nose, and Throat: Nasal secretion, pharyngitis, vocal disturbance.

Hemic and Lymphatic System: Anemia, febrile neutropenia, thrombocytopenia.

Metabolism and Nutrition: Appetite decreased, hypokalemia, weight loss.

Musculoskeletal System: Muscular weakness, musculoskeletal pain, myalgia.

Nervous System: Peripheral neuropathy, sensory neuropathy.

Psychiatric Disorder: Anxiety disorder, confusion, depression.

Respiratory System: Cough, dyspnea, lower respiratory infection, non-small cell lung carcinoma, pneumonitis, respiratory insufficiency.

Skin and Skin Appendages: Alopecia, rash.

Urogenital System: Dysuria, renal insufficiency.

LABORATORY ADVERSE EXPERIENCES

TABLE 5 shows the percent of patients with laboratory adverse experiences reported at an incidence ≥3% during Cycle 1 of the 2 combined Phase III studies.

The following additional laboratory adverse experiences (incidence >0.5% and greater than standard therapy), regardless of causality, were reported in patients treated with aprepi-

TABLE 5 *Percent of Patients With Laboratory Adverse Experiences (Incidence ≥3%) in CINV Phase III Studies (Cycle 1)*

	Aprepitant Regimen (n=544)	Standard Therapy (n=550)
ALT increased	6.0%	4.3%
AST increased	3.0%	1.3%
Blood urea nitrogen increased	4.7%	3.5%
Sermu creatine increased	3.7%	4.3%
Proteinuria	6.8%	5.3%

tant regimen: alkaline phosphatase increased, hyperglycemia, hyponatremia, leukocytes increased, erythrocyturia, leukocyturia.

The adverse experiences of increased AST and ALT were generally mild and transient.

The adverse experience profile in the Multiple-Cycle extension for up to 6 cycles of chemotherapy was generally similar to that observed in Cycle 1.

In addition, isolated cases of serious adverse experiences, regardless of causality, of bradycardia, disorientation, and perforating duodenal ulcer were reported in CINV clinical studies.

Stevens-Johnson syndrome was reported in a patient receiving aprepitant with cancer chemotherapy in another CINV study. Angioedema and urticaria were reported in a patient receiving aprepitant in a non-CINV study.

DOSAGE AND ADMINISTRATION

Aprepitant is given for 3 days as part of a regimen that includes a corticosteroid and a 5-HT_3 antagonist. The recommended dose of aprepitant is 125 mg orally 1 hour prior to chemotherapy treatment (Day 1) and 80 mg once daily in the morning on Days 2 and 3. Aprepitant has not been studied for the treatment of established nausea and vomiting.

In clinical studies, the regimen shown in TABLE 6 was used.

TABLE 6

	Day 1	Day 2	Day 3	Day 4
Aprepitant*	125 mg	80 mg	80 mg	none
Dexamethasone†	12 mg orally	8 mg orally	8 mg orally	8 mg orally
Ondansetron‡	32 mg IV	none	none	none

* Aprepitant was administered orally 1 hour prior to chemotherapy treatment on Day 1 and in the morning on Days 2 and 3.
† Dexamethasone was administered 30 minutes prior to chemotherapy treatment on Day 1 and in the morning on Days 2 through 4. The dose of dexamethasone was chosen to account for drug interactions.
‡ Ondansetron was administered 30 minutes prior to chemotherapy treatment on Day 1.

Chronic continuous administration is not recommended (see PRECAUTIONS).

See DRUG INTERACTIONS for additional information on dose adjustment for corticosteroids when coadministered with aprepitant.

Refer to the full prescribing information for coadministered antiemetic agents.

Aprepitant may be taken with or without food.

No dosage adjustment is necessary for the elderly.

No dosage adjustment is necessary for patients with renal insufficiency or for patients with end stage renal disease undergoing hemodialysis.

No dosage adjustment is necessary for patients with mild to moderate hepatic insufficiency (Child-Pugh score 5-9). There are no clinical data in patients with severe hepatic insufficiency (Child-Pugh score >9).

HOW SUPPLIED

EMEND CAPSULES

80 mg: White, opaque, hard gelatin capsule with "461" and "80 mg" printed radially in black ink on the body.

125 mg: Opaque, hard gelatin capsule with white body and pink cap with "462" and "125 mg" printed radially in black ink on the body.

Unit-of-use tri-fold pack containing one 125 mg capsule and two 80 mg capsules.

Storage

Bottles: Store at 20-25°C (68-77°F) The desiccant should remain in the original bottle.

Blisters: Store at 20-25°C (68-77°F).

Argatroban *(003499)*

Categories: Thrombocytopenia, heparin-induced; Pregnancy Category B; FDA Approved 2000 Jul
Drug Classes: Anticoagulants; Thrombin inhibitors
Brand Names: Acova

DESCRIPTION

Argatroban is a synthetic direct thrombin inhibitor derived from L-arginine. The chemical name for argatroban is 1-[5-[(aminoiminomethyl)amino]-1-oxo-2-[[(1,2,3,4-tetrahydro-3-methyl-8-quinolinyl)sulfonyl]amino]pentyl]-4-methyl-2-piperidinecarboxylic acid, monohydrate. Argatroban has 4 asymmetric carbons. One of the asymmetric carbons has an *R* configuration (stereoisomer Type I) and an *S* configuration (stereoisomer Type II). Argatroban consists of a mixture of *R* and *S* stereoisomers in a ratio of approximately 65:35.

The molecular formula of argatroban is $C_{23}H_{36}N_6O_5S{\cdot}H_2O$. Its molecular weight is 526.66.

Argatroban is a white, odorless crystalline powder that is freely soluble in glacial acetic acid, slightly soluble in ethanol, and insoluble in acetone, ethyl acetate and ether. Acova injection is a sterile clear, colorless to pale yellow, slightly viscous solution. Acova is available in 250 mg (in 2.5 ml) single-use amber vials, with gray flip-top caps. Each ml of sterile, nonpyrogenic solution contains 100 mg argatroban. *Inert Ingredients:* 750 mg D-sorbitol, 1000 mg dehydrated alcohol.

CLINICAL PHARMACOLOGY

MECHANISM OF ACTION

Argatroban is a direct thrombin inhibitor that reversibly binds to the thrombin active site. Argatroban does not require the co-factor antithrombin III for antithrombotic activity. Argatroban exerts its anticoagulant effects by inhibiting thrombin-catalyzed or-induced reactions, including fibrin formation; activation of coagulation factors V, VIII, and XIII; protein C; and platelet aggregation.

Argatroban is highly selective for thrombin with an inhibitory constant (Ki) of 0.04 μM. At therapeutic concentrations, argatroban has little or no effect on related serine proteases (trypsin, factor Xa, plasmin, and kallikrein).

Argatroban is capable of inhibiting the action of both free and clot-associated thrombin.

Argatroban does not interact with heparin-induced antibodies. Evaluation of sera in 12 healthy subjects and 8 patients who received multiple doses of argatroban did not reveal antibody formation to argatroban.

PHARMACOKINETICS

Distribution

Argatroban distributes mainly in the extracellular fluid as evidenced by an apparent steady-state volume of distribution of 174 ml/kg (12.18 L in a 70 kg adult). Argatroban is 54% bound to human serum proteins, with binding to albumin and α_1-acid glycoprotein being 20% and 34%, respectively.

Metabolism

The main route of argatroban metabolism is hydroxylation and aromatization of the 3-methyltetrahydroquinoline ring in the liver. The formation of each of the 4 known metabolites is catalyzed *in vitro* by the human liver microsomal cytochrome P450 enzymes CYP3A4/5. The primary metabolite (M1) exerts 3- to 5-fold weaker anticoagulant effects than argatroban. Unchanged argatroban is the major component in plasma. The plasma concentrations of M1 range between 0-20% of that of the parent drug. The other metabolites (M2-4) are found only in very low quantities in the urine and have not been detected in plasma or feces. These data, together with the lack of effect of erythromycin (a potent CYP3A4/5 inhibitor) on argatroban pharmacokinetics suggest that CYP3A4/5 mediated metabolism is not an important elimination pathway *in vivo*.

Total body clearance is approximately 5.1 ml/min/kg (0.31 L/kg/h) for infusion doses up to 40 μg/kg/min. The terminal elimination half-life of argatroban ranges between 39 and 51 minutes.

There is no interconversion of the 21-(R): 21-(S) diastereoisomers. The plasma ratio of these diastereoisomers is unchanged by metabolism or hepatic impairment, remaining constant at 65:35 (±2%).

Excretion

Argatroban is excreted primarily in the feces, presumably through biliary secretion. In a study in which ^{14}C-argatroban (5 μg/kg/min) was infused for 4 hours into healthy subjects, approximately 65% of the radioactivity was recovered in the feces within 6 days of the start of infusion with little or no radioactivity subsequently detected. Approximately 22% of the radioactivity appeared in the urine within 12 hours of the start of infusion. Little or no additional urinary radioactivity was subsequently detected. Average percent recovery of unchanged drug, relative to total dose, was 16% in urine and at least 14% in feces.

PHARMACOKINETIC/PHARMACODYNAMIC RELATIONSHIP

When argatroban is administered by continuous infusion, anticoagulant effects and plasma concentrations of argatroban follow similar, predictable temporal response profiles, with low intersubject variability. Immediately upon initiation of argatroban infusion, anticoagulant effects are produced as plasma argatroban concentrations begin to rise. Steady-state levels of both drug and anticoagulant effect are typically attained within 1-3 hours and are maintained until the infusion is discontinued or the dosage adjusted. Steady-state plasma argatroban concentrations increase proportionally with dose (for infusion doses up to 40 μg/kg/min in healthy subjects) and are well correlated with steady-state anticoagulant effects. For infusion doses up to 40 μg/kg/min, argatroban increases in a dose-dependent fashion, the activated partial thromboplastin time (aPTT), the activated clotting time (ACT), the prothrombin time (PT) and International Normalized Ratio (INR), and the thrombin time (TT) in healthy volunteers and cardiac patients.

EFFECT ON INTERNATIONAL NORMALIZED RATIO (INR)

Because argatroban is a direct thrombin inhibitor, co-administration of argatroban and warfarin produces a combined effect on the laboratory measurement of the INR. However, concurrent therapy, compared to warfarin monotherapy, exerts no additional effect on vitamin K dependent factor Xa activity.

The relationship between INR on co-therapy and warfarin alone is dependent on both the dose of argatroban and the thromboplastin reagent used. This relationship is influenced by the International Sensitivity Index (ISI) of the thromboplastin. (See DOSAGE AND ADMINISTRATION, Conversion to Oral Anticoagulant Therapy.)

SPECIAL POPULATIONS

Renal Impairment

No dosage adjustment is necessary in patients with renal dysfunction. The effect of renal disease on the pharmacokinetics of argatroban was studied in 6 subjects with normal renal function (mean CLCR = 95 ± 16 ml/min) and in 18 subjects with mild (mean CLCR = 64 ± 10 ml/min), moderate (mean CLCR = 41 ± 5.8 ml/min), and severe (mean CLCR = 5 ± 7 ml/min) renal impairment. The pharmacokinetics and pharmacodynamics of argatroban at dosages up to 5 μg/kg/min were not significantly affected by renal dysfunction.

A

Hepatic Impairment

The dosage of argatroban should be decreased in patients with hepatic impairment (see PRECAUTIONS and DOSAGE AND ADMINISTRATION). Patients with hepatic impairment were not studied in percutaneous coronary intervention (PCI) trials. At a dose of 2.5 μg/kg/min, hepatic impairment is associated with decreased clearance and increased elimination half-life of argatroban (to 1.9 ml/min/kg and 181 minutes, respectively, for patients with a Child-Pugh score >6).

Age, Gender

There are no clinically significant effects of age or gender on the pharmacokinetics or pharmacodynamics (*e.g.,* aPTT) of argatroban.

DRUG-DRUG INTERACTIONS

Digoxin: In 12 healthy volunteers, intravenous infusion of argatroban (2 μg/kg/min) over 5 days (study days 11-15) did not affect the steady-state pharmacokinetics of oral digoxin (0.375 mg daily for 15 days).

Erythromycin: In 10 healthy subjects, orally administered erythromycin (a potent inhibitor of CYP3A4/5) at 500 mg 4 times daily for 7 days had no effect on the pharmacokinetics of argatroban at a dose of 1 μg/kg/min for 5 hours. These data suggest oxidative metabolism by CYP3A4/5 is not an important elimination pathway *in vivo* for argatroban.

INDICATIONS AND USAGE

Argatroban is indicated as an anticoagulant for prophylaxis or treatment of thrombosis in patients with heparin-induced thrombocytopenia.

Argatroban is indicated as an anticoagulant in patients with or at risk for heparin-induced thrombocytopenia undergoing percutaneous coronary interventions (PCI).

CONTRAINDICATIONS

Argatroban is contraindicated in patients with overt major bleeding, or in patients hypersensitive to this product or any of its components (see WARNINGS).

WARNINGS

Argatroban is intended for intravenous administration. All parenteral anticoagulants should be discontinued before administration of argatroban.

HEMORRHAGE

Hemorrhage can occur at any site in the body in patients receiving argatroban. An unexplained fall in hematocrit, fall in blood pressure, or any other unexplained symptom should lead to consideration of a hemorrhagic event. Argatroban should be used with extreme caution in disease states and other circumstances in which there is an increased danger of hemorrhage. These include severe hypertension; immediately following lumbar puncture; spinal anesthesia; major surgery, especially involving the brain, spinal cord, or eye; hematologic conditions associated with increased bleeding tendencies such as congenital or acquired bleeding disorders and gastrointestinal lesions such as ulcerations.

PRECAUTIONS

HEPATIC IMPAIRMENT

Caution should be exercised when administering argatroban to patients with hepatic disease, by starting with a lower dose and carefully titrating until the desired level of anticoagulation is achieved. Also, upon cessation of argatroban infusion in the hepatically impaired patient, full reversal of anticoagulant effects may require longer than 4 hours due to decreased clearance and increased elimination half-life of argatroban (see DOSAGE AND ADMINISTRATION).

Use of high doses of argatroban in PCI patients with clinically significant hepatic disease or AST/ALT levels ≥3 times the upper limit of normal should be avoided. Such patients were not studied in PCI trials.

LABORATORY TESTS

Anticoagulation effects associated with argatroban infusion at doses up to 40 μg/kg/min correlate with increases of the activated partial thromboplastin time (aPTT).

Although other global clot-based tests including prothrombin time (PT), the International Normalized Ratio (INR) and thrombin time (TT) are affected by argatroban; the therapeutic ranges for these tests have not been identified for argatroban therapy. Plasma argatroban concentrations also correlate well with anticoagulant effects (see CLINICAL PHARMACOLOGY).

In clinical trials in PCI, the activated clotting time (ACT) was used for monitoring argatroban activity during the procedure.

The concomitant use of argatroban and warfarin results in prolongation of the PT and INR beyond that produced by warfarin alone. Alternative approaches for monitoring concurrent argatroban and warfarin therapy are described in a subsequent section (see DOSAGE AND ADMINISTRATION).

CARCINOGENESIS, MUTAGENESIS, AND IMPAIRMENT OF FERTILITY

No long-term studies in animals have been performed to evaluate the carcinogenic potential of argatroban.

Argatroban was not genotoxic in the Ames test, the Chinese hamster ovary cell (CHO/HGPRT) forward mutation test, the Chinese hamster lung fibroblast chromosome aberration test, the rat hepatocyte and WI-38 human fetal lung cell unscheduled DNA synthesis (UDS) tests, or the mouse micronucleus test.

Argatroban at intravenous doses up to 27 mg/kg/day (0.3 times the recommended maximum human dose based on body surface area) was found to have no effect on fertility and reproductive performance of male and female rats.

PREGNANCY, TERATOGENIC EFFECTS, PREGNANCY CATEGORY B

Teratology studies have been performed in rats with intravenous doses up to 27 mg/kg/day (0.3 times the recommended maximum human dose based on body surface area) and rabbits at intravenous doses up to 10.8 mg/kg/day (0.2 times the recommended maximum human dose based on body surface area) and have revealed no evidence of impaired fertility or harm to the fetus due to argatroban. There are however, no adequate and well-controlled studies in pregnant women. Because animal reproduction studies are not always predictive of human response, this drug should be used during pregnancy only if clearly needed.

NURSING MOTHERS

Experiments in rats show that argatroban is detected in milk. It is not known whether this drug is excreted in human milk. Because many drugs are excreted in human milk and because of the potential for serious adverse reactions in nursing infants from argatroban, a decision should be made whether to discontinue nursing or to discontinue the drug, taking into account the importance of the drug to the mother.

GERIATRIC USE

In the clinical studies of adult patients with HIT or HITTS, the effectiveness of argatroban was not affected by age.

PEDIATRIC USE

The safety and effectiveness of argatroban in patients below the age of 18 years have not been established.

DRUG INTERACTIONS

Heparin: Since heparin is contraindicated in patients with heparin-induced thrombocytopenia, the co-administration of argatroban and heparin is unlikely for this indication. However, if argatroban is to be initiated after cessation of heparin therapy, allow sufficient time for heparin's effect on the aPTT to decrease prior to initiation of argatroban therapy.

Aspirin/Acetaminophen: Pharmacokinetic or pharmacodynamic drug-drug interactions have not been demonstrated between argatroban and concomitantly administered aspirin (162.5 mg orally given 26 and 2 hours prior to initiation of argatroban 1 μg/kg/min over 4 hours) or acetaminophen (1000 mg orally given 12, 6 and 0 hours prior to, and 6 and 12 hours subsequent to, initiation of argatroban 1.5 μg/kg/min over 18 hours).

Oral Anticoagulant Agents: Pharmacokinetic drug-drug interactions between argatroban and warfarin (7.5 mg single oral dose) have not been demonstrated. However, the concomitant use of argatroban and warfarin (5-7.5 mg initial oral dose followed by 2.5-6 mg/day orally for 6-10 days) results in prolongation of the prothrombin time (PT) and International Normalized Ratio (INR) (see CLINICAL PHARMACOLOGY and DOSAGE AND ADMINISTRATION).

Thrombolytic Agents: The safety and effectiveness of argatroban with thrombolytic agents have not been established (see ADVERSE REACTIONS, Adverse Events Reported in Other Populations, Intracranial Bleeding).

Glycoprotein IIb/IIIa Antagonists: The safety and effectiveness of argatroban with glycoprotein IIb/IIIa antagonists have not been established.

Co-Administration: Concomitant use of argatroban with antiplatelet agents, thrombolytics, and other anticoagulants may increase the risk of bleeding (see WARNINGS). Drug-drug interactions have not been observed between argatroban and digoxin or erythromycin (see CLINICAL PHARMACOLOGY, Drug-Drug Interactions).

ADVERSE REACTIONS

ADVERSE EVENTS REPORTED IN HIT/HITTS PATIENTS

The following safety information is based on all 568 patients treated with argatroban in Study 1 and Study 2. The safety profile of the patients from these studies is compared with that of 193 historical controls in which the adverse events were collected retrospectively. The adverse events reported in this section include all events regardless of relationship to treatment. Adverse events are separated into hemorrhagic and non-hemorrhagic events.

Major bleeding was defined as bleeding that was overt and associated with a hemoglobin decrease ≥2 g/dl, that led to a transfusion of ≥2 units, or that was intracranial, retroperitoneal, or into a major prosthetic joint. Minor bleeding was overt bleeding that did not meet the criteria for major bleeding.

TABLE 3 gives an overview of the most frequently observed hemorrhagic events, presented separately by major and minor bleeding, sorted by decreasing occurrence among argatroban-treated HIT/HITTS patients.

TABLE 4 gives an overview of the most frequently observed non-hemorrhagic events sorted by decreasing frequency of occurrence (≥2%) among argatroban-treated HIT/HITTS patients.

ADVERSE EVENTS REPORTED IN HIT/HITTS PATIENTS UNDERGOING PCI

The following safety information is based on 91 patients initially treated with argatroban and 21 patients subsequently re-exposed to argatroban for a total of 112 PCIs with argatroban anticoagulation. The adverse events reported in this section include all events regardless of relationship to treatment. Adverse events are separated into hemorrhagic (TABLE 5) and non-hemorrhagic (TABLE 6) events.

Major bleeding was defined as bleeding that was overt and associated with a hemoglobin decrease ≥5 g/dl, that led to a transfusion of ≥2 units, or that was intracranial, retroperitoneal, or into a major prosthetic joint.

The rate of major bleeding events and intracranial hemorrhage in the PCI trials was 1.8% and in the placebo arm of the EPILOG trial (placebo plus standard dose, weight-adjusted heparin) was 3.1%.

TABLE 6 gives an overview of the most frequently observed non-hemorrhagic events (>2%), sorted by decreasing frequency of occurrence among argatroban-treated PCI patients.

There were 22 serious adverse events in 17 PCI patients (19.6% in 112 interventions). The types of events, which are listed regardless of relationship to treatment, are shown in TABLE 7. TABLE 7 lists the serious adverse events occurring in argatroban-treated HIT/HITTS patients undergoing PCI.

TABLE 3 *Major and Minor Hemorrhagic Adverse Events in HIT/HITTS Patients*

	Study 1 & 2† (n=568)	Historical Control (n=193)
Major Hemorrhagic Events*		
Overall bleeding	5.3%	6.7%
Gastrointestinal	2.3%	1.6%
Genitourinary and hematuria	0.9%	0.5%
Decrease in hemoglobin/hematocrit	0.7%	0%
Multisystem hemorrhage and DIC	0.5%	1%
Limb and BKA stump	0.5%	0%
Intracranial hemorrhage	0%‡	0.5%
Minor Hemorrhagic Events*		
Gastrointestinal	14.4%	18.1%
Genitourinary and hematuria	11.6%	0.8%
Decrease in hemoglobin and hematocrit	10.4%	0%
Groin	5.4%	3.1%
Hemoptysis	2.9%	0.8%
Brachial	2.4%	0.8%

* Patients may have experienced more than one event.
† Argatroban-treated patients.
‡ One patient experienced intracranial hemorrhage 4 days after discontinuation of argatroban and following therapy with urokinase and oral anticoagulation.
DIC = Disseminated intravascular coagulation.
BKA = Below the knee amputation.

TABLE 4 *Non-Hemorrhagic Adverse Events in HIT/HITTS Patients**

	Study 1 & 2† (n=568)	Historical Control (n=193)
Dyspnea	8.1%	8.8%
Hypotension	7.2%	2.6%
Fever	6.9%	2.1%
Diarrhea	6.2%	1.6%
Sepsis	6.0%	12.4%
Cardiac arrest	5.8%	3.1%
Nausea	4.8%	0.5%
Ventricular tachycardia	4.8%	3.1%
Pain	4.6%	3.1%
Urinary tract infection	4.6%	5.2%
Vomiting	4.2%	0%
Infection	3.7%	3.6%
Pneumonia	3.3%	9.3%
Atrial fibrillation	3.0%	11.4%
Coughing	2.8%	1.6%
Abnormal renal function	2.8%	4.7%
Abdominal pain	2.6%	1.6%
Cerebrovascular disorder	2.3%	4.1%

* Patients may have experienced more than one event.
† All argatroban-treated patients.

TABLE 5 *Major and Minor Hemorrhagic Adverse Events in HIT/HITTS Patients Undergoing PCI*

	Argatroban-Treated Patients (n=112)†
Major Hemorrhagic Events*	
Retroperitoneal	0.9%
Gastrointestinal	0.9%
Intracranial hemorrhage	0%
Minor Hemorrhagic Events*	
Groin (bleeding or hematoma)	3.6%
Gastrointestinal (includes hematemesis)	2.6%
Genitourinary (includes hematuria)	1.8%
Decrease in hemoglobin and/or hematocrit	1.8%
CABG (coronary arteries)	1.8%
Access site	0.9%
Hemoptysis	0.9%
Other	0.9%

* Patients may have experienced more than one adverse event.
† 91 patients who underwent 112 interventions.
CABG = coronary artery bypass graft.

ADVERSE EVENTS REPORTED IN OTHER POPULATIONS

The following safety information is based on a total of 1127 individuals who were treated with argatroban in clinical pharmacology studies (n=211) or for other clinical indications (n=916).

Intracranial Bleeding

Intracranial bleeding only occurred in patients with acute myocardial infarction who were started on both argatroban and thrombolytic therapy with streptokinase. The overall frequency of this potentially life-threatening complication among patients receiving both argatroban and thrombolytic therapy (streptokinase or tissue plasminogen activator) was 1% (8 out of 810 patients). Intracranial bleeding was not observed in 317 subjects or patients who did not receive concomitant thrombolysis (see WARNINGS).

Allergic Reactions

156 allergic reactions or suspected allergic reactions were observed in 1127 individuals who were treated with argatroban in clinical pharmacology studies or for various clinical indications. About 95% (148/156) of these reactions occurred in patients who concomitantly received thrombolytic therapy (*e.g.*, streptokinase) for acute myocardial infarction and/or contrast media for coronary angiography.

Allergic reactions or suspected allergic reactions in populations other than HIT patients include (in descending order of frequency*):

- ***Airway Reactions (coughing, dyspnea):*** 10% or more
- ***Skin Reactions (rash, bullous eruption):*** 1 to <10%
- ***General Reactions (vasodilation):*** 1-10%
- *The CIOMS (Council for International Organization of Medical Sciences) III standard categories are used for classification of frequencies.

Table 6 *Non-Hemorrhagic Adverse Events* in HIT/HITTS Patients Undergoing PCI*

	Argatroban Procedures* (n=112)†	Controls (n=2226)‡
Chest pain	15.2%	9.3%
Hypotension	10.7%	10.3%
Back pain	8.0%	13.7%
Nausea	7.1%	11.5%
Vomiting	6.3%	6.8%
Headache	5.4%	5.5%
Bradycardia	4.5%	3.5%
Abdominal pain	3.6%	2.2%
Fever	3.6%	<0.5%
Myocardial infarction	3.6%	NR

* Patients may have experienced more than one adverse event.
† 91 patients who underwent 112 interventions.
‡ Controls from EPIC (Evaluation of c7E3 Fab in the Prevention of Ischemic Complications), EPILOG (Evaluation in PTCA to Improve Long-Term Outcome with Abciximab GP IIb/IIIa Blockade Study) and CAPTURE (Chimeric 7E3 Antiplatelet Therapy in Unstable angina Refractory to standard treatment) trials. Source: ReoPro Prescribing Information.
NR = Not reported.

TABLE 7 *Serious Adverse Events in HIT/HITTS Patients Undergoing PCI**

Coded Term	Argatroban Procedures† (n=112)
Chest pain	1 (0.9%)
Fever	1 (0.9%)
Retroperitoneal hemorrhage	1 (0.9%)
Angina pectoris	2 (1.8%)
Aortic stenosis	1 (0.9%)
Coronary thrombosis	2 (1.8%)
Arterial thrombosis	1 (0.9%)
Myocardial infarction	4 (3.5%)
Myocardial ischemia	2 (1.8%)
Occlusion coronary	2 (1.8%)
Gastrointestinal hemorrhage	1 (0.9%)
Gastrointestinal disorder (GERD)	1 (0.9%)
Cerebrovascular disorder	1 (0.9%)
Lung edema	1 (0.9%)
Vascular disorder	1 (0.9%)

* Individual events may also have been reported elsewhere (see TABLE 5 and TABLE 6).
† 91 patients underwent 112 procedures. Some patients may have experienced more than one event.

DOSAGE AND ADMINISTRATION

Argatroban, as supplied, is a concentrated drug (100 mg/ml) which must be diluted 100-fold prior to infusion. Argatroban should not be mixed with other drugs prior to dilution in a suitable intravenous fluid.

PREPARATION FOR INTRAVENOUS ADMINISTRATION

Argatroban should be diluted in 0.9% sodium chloride injection, 5% dextrose injection, or lactated Ringer's injection to a final concentration of 1 mg/ml. The contents of each 2.5 ml vial should be diluted 100-fold by mixing with 250 ml of diluent. Use 250 mg (2.5 ml) per 250 ml of diluent or 500 mg (5 ml) per 500 ml of diluent. The constituted solution must be mixed by repeated inversion of the diluent bag for 1 minute. Upon preparation, the solution may show slight but brief haziness due to the formation of microprecipitates that rapidly dissolve upon mixing. The pH of the intravenous solution prepared as recommended is 3.2-7.5.

HEPARIN-INDUCED THROMBOCYTOPENIA (HIT/HITTS)

Initial Dosage

Before administering argatroban, discontinue heparin therapy and obtain a baseline aPTT. The recommended initial dose of argatroban for adult patients without hepatic impairment is 2 μg/kg/min, administered as a continuous infusion (see TABLE 8).

Monitoring Therapy

In general, therapy with argatroban is monitored using the aPTT. Tests of anticoagulant effects (including the aPTT) typically attain steady-state levels within 1-3 hours following initiation of argatroban. Dose adjustment may be required to attain the target aPTT. Check the aPTT 2 hours after initiation of therapy to confirm that the patient has allowed the desired therapeutic range.

Dosage Adjustment

After the initial dose of argatroban, the dose can be adjusted as clinically indicated (not to exceed 10 μg/kg/min), until the steady-state aPTT is 1.5 to 3 times the initial baseline value (not to exceed 100 seconds) for mean values of aPTT obtained after initial doses of argatroban).

A

TABLE 8 *Standard Infusion Rates for 2 μg/kg/min Dose (1 mg/ml final concentration)*

Body Weight	Infusion Rate
50 kg	6 ml/h
60 kg	7 ml/h
70 kg	8 ml/h
80 kg	10 ml/h
90 kg	11 ml/h
100 kg	12 ml/h
110 kg	13 ml/h
120 kg	14 ml/h
130 kg	16 ml/h
140 kg	17 ml/h

PERCUTANEOUS CORONARY INTERVENTIONS (PCI) IN HIT/HITTS PATIENTS

Initial Dosage

An infusion of argatroban should be started at 25 μg/kg/min and a bolus of 350 μg/kg administered via a large bore intravenous (IV) line over 3-5 minutes. Activated clotting time (ACT) should be checked 5-10 minutes after the bolus dose is completed. The procedure may proceed if the ACT is greater than 300 seconds.

Dosage Adjustment

If the ACT is less than 300 seconds, an additional IV bolus dose of 150 μg/kg should be administered, the infusion dose increased to 30 μg/kg/min, and the ACT checked 5-10 minutes later. If the ACT is greater than 450 seconds, the infusion rate should be decreased to 15 μg/kg/min, and the ACT checked 5-10 minutes later. Once a therapeutic ACT (between 300 and 450 seconds) has been achieved, this infusion dose should be continued for the duration of the procedure.

In case of dissection, impending abrupt closure, thrombus formation during the procedure, or inability to achieve or maintain an ACT over 300 seconds, additional bolus doses of 150 μg/kg may be administered and the infusion dose increased to 40 μg/kg/min. The ACT should be checked after each additional bolus or change in the rate of infusion.

Monitoring Therapy

Therapy with argatroban is monitored using ACT. ACTs should be obtained before dosing, 5-10 minutes after bolus dosing and after change in the infusion rate, and at the end of the PCI procedure. Additional ACTs should be drawn about every 20-30 minutes during a prolonged procedure.

Continued Anticoagulation After PCI

If a patient requires anticoagulation after the procedure, argatroban may be continued, but at a lower infusion dose [see Heparin-Induced Thrombocytopenia (HIT/HITTS)].

DOSING IN SPECIAL POPULATIONS

Hepatic Impairment

For patients with heparin-induced thrombocytopenia with hepatic impairment, the initial dose of argatroban should be reduced. For patients with moderate hepatic impairment, an initial dose of 0.5 μg/kg/min is recommended, based on the approximate 4-fold decrease in argatroban clearance relative to those with normal hepatic function. The aPTT should be monitored closely and the dosage should be adjusted as clinically indicated (see PRECAUTIONS).

Hepatic Impairment in HIT/HITTS Patients Undergoing PCI

For hepatically impaired HIT/HITTS patients undergoing PCI, refer to PRECAUTIONS, Hepatic Impairment.

Renal Impairment

No dosage adjustment is necessary in patients with renal impairment (see PRECAUTIONS).

CONVERSION TO ORAL ANTICOAGULANT THERAPY

Initiating Oral Anticoagulant Therapy

Once the decision is made to initiate oral anticoagulant therapy, recognize the potential for combined effects on INR with co-administration of argatroban and warfarin. A loading dose of warfarin should not be used. Initiate therapy using the expected daily dose of warfarin.

Co-Administration of Warfarin and Argatroban at Doses up to 2 μg/kg/min

Use of argatroban with warfarin results in prolongation of INR beyond that produced by warfarin alone. The previously established relationship between INR and bleeding risk is altered. The combination of argatroban and warfarin does not cause further reduction in the vitamin K dependent factor Xa activity than that which is seen with warfarin alone. The relationship between INR obtained on combined therapy and INR obtained on warfarin alone is dependent on both the dose of argatroban and the thromboplastin reagent used.

INR should be measured daily while argatroban and warfarin are co-administered. In general, with doses of argatroban up to 2 μg/kg/min, argatroban can be discontinued when the INR is >4 on combined therapy. After argatroban is discontinued, repeat the INR measurement in 4-6 hours. If the repeat INR is below the desired therapeutic range, resume the infusion of argatroban and repeat the procedure daily until the desired therapeutic range on warfarin alone is reached.

Co-Administration of Warfarin and Argatroban at Doses Greater Than 2 μg/kg/min

For doses greater than 2 μg/kg/min, the relationship of INR on warfarin alone to the INR on warfarin plus argatroban is less predictable. In this case, in order to predict the INR on warfarin alone, temporarily reduce the dose of argatroban to a dose of 2 μg/kg/min. Repeat the INR on argatroban and warfarin 4-6 hours after reduction of the argatroban dose and follow the process outlined above for administering argatroban at doses up to 2 μg/kg/min.

STABILITY/COMPATIBILITY

Argatroban is a clear, colorless to pale yellow, slightly viscous solution. If the solution is cloudy, or if an insoluble precipitate is noted, the vial should be discarded.

Solutions prepared as recommended are stable at 25°C (77°F) with excursions permitted to 15-30°C (59-86°F) in ambient indoor light for 24 hours; therefore, light resistant measures such as foil protection for intravenous lines are unnecessary. Solutions are physically and chemically stable for up to 48 hours when stored at 2-8°C in the dark. Prepared solutions should not be exposed to direct sunlight. No significant potency losses have been noted following simulated delivery of the solution through intravenous tubing.

HOW SUPPLIED

Acova injection is supplied in 2.5 ml solution in single-use vials at the concentration of 100 mg/ml. Each vial contains 250 mg of argatroban.

Storage: Store the vials in original cartons at room temperature [25°C (77°F) excursion permitted to 15-30°C (59-86°F)]. Do not freeze. Retain in the original carton to protect from light.

PRODUCT LISTING - EQUIVALENTS NOT AVAILABLE

Solution - Intravenous - 100 mg/ml

2.50 ml	$896.31	ACOVA, Glaxosmithkline	00007-4407-01
2.50 ml x 10	$7500.00	ACOVA, Glaxosmithkline	00007-4407-10

Aripiprazole *(003577)*

Categories: Schizophrenia; Pregnancy Category C; FDA Approved 2002 Nov
Drug Classes: Antipsychotics
Brand Names: Abilify
Cost of Therapy: $316.88 (Schizophrenia; Abilify; 10 mg; 1 tablet/day; 30 day supply)

DESCRIPTION

Abilify (aripiprazole) is a psychotropic drug that is available as tablets for oral administration. Aripiprazole is 7-[4-[4-(2,3-dichlorophenyl)-1-piperazinyl]butoxy]-3,4-dihydrocarbostyril. The empirical formula is $C_{23}H_{27}Cl_2N_3O_2$ and its molecular weight is 448.38.

Abilify tablets are available in 2, 5, 10, 15, 20, and 30 mg strengths. Inactive ingredients include lactose monohydrate, cornstarch, microcrystalline cellulose, hydroxypropyl cellulose, and magnesium stearate. Colorants include ferric oxide (yellow or red) and FD&C blue no. 2 aluminum lake.

CLINICAL PHARMACOLOGY

PHARMACODYNAMICS

Aripiprazole exhibits high affinity for dopamine D_2 and D_3, serotonin 5-HT_{1A} and 5-HT_{2A} receptors (Ki values of 0.34, 0.8, 1.7, and 3.4 nM, respectively), moderate affinity for dopamine D_4, serotonin 5-HT_{2C} and 5-HT_7, alpha$_1$-adrenergic and histamine H_1 receptors (Ki values of 44, 15, 39, 57, and 61 nM, respectively), and moderate affinity for serotonin reuptake site (Ki = 98 nM). Aripiprazole has no appreciable affinity for cholinergic muscarinic receptors (IC_{50} >1000 nM). Aripiprazole functions as a partial agonist at the dopamine D_2 and the serotonin 5-HT_{1A} receptors, and as an antagonist at serotonin 5-HT_{2A} receptor.

The mechanism of action of aripiprazole, as with other drugs having efficacy in schizophrenia, is unknown. However, it has been proposed that the efficacy of aripiprazole is mediated through a combination of partial agonist activity at D_2 and 5-HT_{1A} receptors and antagonist activity at 5-HT_{2A} receptors. Actions at receptors other than D_2, 5-HT_{1A}, and 5-HT_{2A} may explain some of the other clinical effects of aripiprazole, *e.g.*, the orthostatic hypotension observed with aripiprazole may be explained by its antagonist activity at adrenergic alpha$_1$ receptors.

PHARMACOKINETICS

Aripiprazole activity is presumably primarily due to the parent drug, aripiprazole, and to a lesser extent, to its major metabolite dehydro-aripiprazole, which has been shown to have affinities for D_2 receptors similar to the parent drug and represents 40% of the parent drug exposure in plasma. The mean elimination half-lives are about 75 hours and 94 hours for aripiprazole and dehydro-aripiprazole, respectively. Steady-state concentrations are attained within 14 days of dosing for both active moieties. Aripiprazole accumulation is predictable from single-dose pharmacokinetics. At steady state, the pharmacokinetics of aripiprazole are dose-proportional. Elimination of aripiprazole is mainly through hepatic metabolism involving two P450 isozymes, CYP2D6 and CYP3A4.

Absorption

Aripiprazole is well absorbed, with peak plasma concentrations occurring within 3-5 hours; the absolute oral bioavailability of the tablet formulation is 87%. Aripiprazole can be administered with or without food. Administration of a 15 mg aripiprazole tablet with a standard high-fat meal did not significantly affect the C_{max} or AUC of aripiprazole or its active metabolite, dehydro-aripiprazole, but delayed T_{max} by 3 hours for aripiprazole and 12 hours for dehydro-aripiprazole.

Distribution

The steady-state volume of distribution of aripiprazole following intravenous administration is high (404 L or 4.9 L/kg), indicating extensive extravascular distribution. At therapeutic concentrations, aripiprazole and its major metabolite are greater than 99% bound to serum proteins, primarily to albumin. In healthy human volunteers administered 0.5 to 30 mg/day aripiprazole for 14 days, there was dose-dependent D_2-receptor occupancy indicating brain penetration of aripiprazole in humans.

Metabolism and Elimination

Aripiprazole is metabolized primarily by 3 biotransformation pathways: dehydrogenation, hydroxylation, and N-dealkylation. Based on *in vitro* studies, CYP3A4 and CYP2D6 enzymes are responsible for dehydrogenation and hydroxylation of aripiprazole, and N-dealkylation is catalyzed by CYP3A4. Aripiprazole is the predominant drug moiety in the systemic circulation. At steady state, dehydroaripiprazole, the active metabolite, represents about 40% of aripiprazole AUC in plasma.

Approximately 8% of Caucasians lack the capacity to metabolize CYP2D6 substrates and are classified as poor metabolizers (PM), whereas the rest are extensive metabolizers (EM). PMs have about an 80% increase in aripiprazole exposure and about a 30% decrease in exposure to the active metabolite compared to EMs, resulting in about a 60% higher exposure to the total active moieties from a given dose of aripiprazole compared to EMs. Coadministration of aripiprazole with known inhibitors of CYP2D6, like quinidine in EMs results in a 112% increase in aripiprazole plasma exposure, and dosing adjustment is needed (see DRUG INTERACTIONS). The mean elimination half-lives are about 75 hours and 146 hours for aripiprazole in EMs and PMs, respectively. Aripiprazole does not inhibit or induce the CYP2D6 pathway.

Following a single oral dose of [^{14}C]-labeled aripiprazole, approximately 25% and 55% of the administered radioactivity was recovered in the urine and feces, respectively. Less than 1% of unchanged aripiprazole was excreted in the urine and approximately 18% of the oral dose was recovered unchanged in the feces.

SPECIAL POPULATIONS

In general, no dosage adjustment for aripiprazole is required on the basis of a patient's age, gender, race, smoking status, hepatic function, or renal function (see DOSAGE AND ADMINISTRATION, Dosing in Special Populations). The pharmacokinetics of aripiprazole in special populations are described below.

Hepatic Impairment

In a single-dose study (15 mg of aripiprazole) in subjects with varying degrees of liver cirrhosis (Child-Pugh Classes A, B, and C), the AUC of aripiprazole, compared to healthy subjects, increased 31% in mild HI, increased 8% in moderate HI, and decreased 20% in severe HI. None of these differences would require dose adjustment.

Renal Impairment

In patients with severe renal impairment (creatinine clearance <30 ml/min), C_{max} of aripiprazole (given in a single dose of 15 mg) and dehydro-aripiprazole increased by 36% and 53%, respectively, but AUC was 15% lower for aripiprazole and 7% higher for dehydro-aripiprazole. Renal excretion of both unchanged aripiprazole and dehydroaripiprazole is less than 1% of the dose. No dosage adjustment is required in subjects with renal impairment.

Elderly

In formal single-dose pharmacokinetic studies (with aripiprazole given in a single dose of 15 mg), aripiprazole clearance was 20% lower in elderly (≥65 years) subjects compared to younger adult subjects (18-64 years). There was no detectable age effect, however, in the population pharmacokinetic analysis in schizophrenia patients. Also, the pharmacokinetics of aripiprazole after multiple doses in elderly patients appeared similar to that observed in young healthy subjects. No dosage adjustment is recommended for elderly patients. (See PRECAUTIONS, Geriatric Use.)

Gender

C_{max} and AUC of aripiprazole and its active metabolite, dehydro-aripiprazole, are 30-40% higher in women than in men, and correspondingly, the apparent oral clearance of aripiprazole is lower in women. These differences, however, are largely explained by differences in body weight (25%) between men and women. No dosage adjustment is recommended based on gender.

Race

Although no specific pharmacokinetic study was conducted to investigate the effects of race on the disposition of aripiprazole, population pharmacokinetic evaluation revealed no evidence of clinically significant race-related differences in the pharmacokinetics of aripiprazole. No dosage adjustment is recommended based on race.

Smoking

Based on studies utilizing human liver enzymes *in vitro*, aripiprazole is not a substrate for CYP1A2 and also does not undergo direct glucuronidation. Smoking should, therefore, not have an effect on the pharmacokinetics of aripiprazole. Consistent with these *in vitro* results, population pharmacokinetic evaluation did not reveal any significant pharmacokinetic differences between smokers and nonsmokers. No dosage adjustment is recommended based on smoking status.

DRUG-DRUG INTERACTIONS

Potential for Other Drugs to Affect Aripiprazole

Aripiprazole is not a substrate of CYP1A1, CYP1A2, CYP2A6, CYP2B6, CYP2C8, CYP2C9, CYP2C19, or CYP2E1 enzymes. Aripiprazole also does not undergo direct glucuronidation. This suggests that an interaction of aripiprazole with inhibitors or inducers of these enzymes, or other factors, like smoking, is unlikely.

Both CYP3A4 and CYP2D6 are responsible for aripiprazole metabolism. Agents that induce CYP3A4 (*e.g.*, carbamazepine) could cause an increase in aripiprazole clearance and lower blood levels. Inhibitors of CYP3A4 (*e.g.*, ketoconazole) or CYP2D6 (*e.g.*, quinidine, fluoxetine, or paroxetine) can inhibit aripiprazole elimination and cause increased blood levels.

Potential for Aripiprazole to Affect Other Drugs

Aripiprazole is unlikely to cause clinically important pharmacokinetic interactions with drugs metabolized by cytochrome P450 enzymes. In *in vivo* studies, 10-30 mg/day doses of aripiprazole had no significant effect on metabolism by CYP2D6 (dextromethorphan), CYP2C9 (warfarin), CYP2C19 (omeprazole, warfarin), and CYP3A4 (dextromethorphan) substrates. Additionally, aripiprazole and dehydroaripiprazole did not show potential for altering CYP1A2-mediated metabolism *in vitro* (see DRUG INTERACTIONS).

Aripiprazole had no clinically important interactions with the following drugs:

Famotidine: Coadministration of aripiprazole (given in a single dose of 15 mg) with a 40 mg single dose of the H_2 antagonist famotidine, a potent gastric acid blocker, decreased the solubility of aripiprazole and, hence, its rate of absorption, reducing by 37% and 21% the C_{max} of aripiprazole and dehydro-aripiprazole, respectively, and by 13% and 15%, respectively, the extent of absorption (AUC). No dosage adjustment of aripiprazole is required when administered concomitantly with famotidine.

Valproate: When valproate (500-1500 mg/day) and aripiprazole (30 mg/day) were coadministered at steady state, the C_{max} and AUC of aripiprazole were decreased by 25%. No dosage adjustment of aripiprazole is required when administered concomitantly with valproate.

Lithium: A pharmacokinetic interaction of aripiprazole with lithium is unlikely because lithium is not bound to plasma proteins, is not metabolized, and is almost entirely excreted unchanged in urine. Coadministration of therapeutic doses of lithium (1200-1800 mg/day) for 21 days with aripiprazole (30 mg/day) did not result in clinically significant changes in the pharmacokinetics of aripiprazole or its active metabolite, dehydro-aripiprazole (C_{max} and AUC increased by less than 20%). No dosage adjustment of aripiprazole is required when administered concomitantly with lithium.

Dextromethorphan: Aripiprazole at doses of 10-30 mg/day for 14 days had no effect on dextromethorphan's O-dealkylation to its major metabolite, dextrorphan, a pathway known to be dependent on CYP2D6 activity. Aripiprazole also had no effect on dextromethorphan's N-demethylation to its metabolite 3-methyoxymorphan, a pathway known to be dependent on CYP3A4 activity. No dosage adjustment of dextromethorphan is required when administered concomitantly with aripiprazole.

Warfarin: Aripiprazole 10 mg/day for 14 days had no effect on the pharmacokinetics of R- and S-warfarin or on the pharmacodynamic end point of International Normalized Ratio, indicating the lack of a clinically relevant effect of aripiprazole on CYP2C9 and CYP2C19 metabolism or the binding of highly protein-bound warfarin. No dosage adjustment of warfarin is required when administered concomitantly with aripiprazole.

Omeprazole: Aripiprazole 10 mg/day for 15 days had no effect on the pharmacokinetics of a single 20 mg dose of omeprazole, a CYP2C19 substrate, in healthy subjects. No dosage adjustment of omeprazole is required when administered concomitantly with aripiprazole.

INDICATIONS AND USAGE

Aripiprazole is indicated for the treatment of schizophrenia. The efficacy of aripiprazole in the treatment of schizophrenia was established in short-term (4 and 6 week) controlled trials of schizophrenic inpatients.

The long-term efficacy of aripiprazole in the treatment of schizophrenia has not been established. The physician who elects to use aripiprazole for extended periods should periodically re-evaluate the long-term usefulness of the drug for the individual patient.

CONTRAINDICATIONS

Aripiprazole is contraindicated in patients with a known hypersensitivity to the product.

WARNINGS

NEUROLEPTIC MALIGNANT SYNDROME (NMS)

A potentially fatal symptom complex sometimes referred to as Neuroleptic Malignant Syndrome (NMS) has been reported in association with administration of antipsychotic drugs, including aripiprazole. Two possible cases of NMS occurred during aripiprazole treatment in the premarketing worldwide clinical database. Clinical manifestations of NMS are hyperpyrexia, muscle rigidity, altered mental status, and evidence of autonomic instability (irregular pulse or blood pressure, tachycardia, diaphoresis, and cardiac dysrhythmia). Additional signs may include elevated creatine phosphokinase, myoglobinuria (rhabdomyolysis), and acute renal failure.

The diagnostic evaluation of patients with this syndrome is complicated. In arriving at a diagnosis, it is important to exclude cases where the clinical presentation includes both serious medical illness (*e.g.*, pneumonia, systemic infection, etc.) and untreated or inadequately treated extrapyramidal signs and symptoms (EPS). Other important considerations in the differential diagnosis include central anticholinergic toxicity, heat stroke, drug fever, and primary central nervous system pathology.

The management of NMS should include: (1) immediate discontinuation of antipsychotic drugs and other drugs not essential to concurrent therapy; (2) intensive symptomatic treatment and medical monitoring; and (3) treatment of any concomitant serious medical problems for which specific treatments are available. There is no general agreement about specific pharmacological treatment regimens for uncomplicated NMS.

If a patient requires antipsychotic drug treatment after recovery from NMS, the potential reintroduction of drug therapy should be carefully considered. The patient should be carefully monitored, since recurrences of NMS have been reported.

TARDIVE DYSKINESIA

A syndrome of potentially irreversible, involuntary, dyskinetic movements may develop in patients treated with antipsychotic drugs. Although the prevalence of the syndrome appears to be highest among the elderly, especially elderly women, it is impossible to rely upon prevalence estimates to predict, at the inception of antipsychotic treatment, which patients are likely to develop the syndrome. Whether antipsychotic drug products differ in their potential to cause tardive dyskinesia is unknown.

The risk of developing tardive dyskinesia and the likelihood that it will become irreversible are believed to increase as the duration of treatment and the total cumulative dose of antipsychotic drugs administered to the patient increase. However, the syndrome can develop, although much less commonly, after relatively brief treatment periods at low doses.

There is no known treatment for established cases of tardive dyskinesia, although the syndrome may remit, partially or completely, if antipsychotic treatment is withdrawn. Antipsychotic treatment, itself, however, may suppress (or partially suppress) the signs and symptoms of the syndrome and, thereby, may possibly mask the underlying process. The effect that symptomatic suppression has upon the long-term course of the syndrome is unknown.

Given these considerations, aripiprazole should be prescribed in a manner that is most likely to minimize the occurrence of tardive dyskinesia. Chronic antipsychotic treatment should generally be reserved for patients who suffer from a chronic illness that (1) is known to respond to antipsychotic drugs, and (2) for whom alternative, equally effective, but potentially less harmful treatments are not available or appropriate. In patients who do require chronic treatment, the smallest dose and the shortest duration of treatment producing a satisfactory clinical response should be sought. The need for continued treatment should be reassessed periodically.

If signs and symptoms of tardive dyskinesia appear in a patient on aripiprazole, drug discontinuation should be considered. However, some patients may require treatment with aripiprazole despite the presence of the syndrome.

PRECAUTIONS

GENERAL

Orthostatic Hypotension

Aripiprazole may be associated with orthostatic hypotension, perhaps due to its α1-adrenergic receptor antagonism. The incidence of orthostatic hypotension associated events from five short-term, placebo-controlled trials in schizophrenia (n=926) on aripiprazole included: orthostatic hypotension (placebo 1%, aripiprazole 1.9%), orthostatic lightheadedness (placebo 1%, aripiprazole 0.9%), and syncope (placebo 1%, aripiprazole 0.6%). The incidence of a significant orthostatic change in blood pressure (defined as a decrease of at least 30 mm Hg in systolic blood pressure when changing from a supine to standing position) for aripiprazole was not statistically different from placebo (14% among aripiprazole-treated patients and 12% among placebo-treated patients).

Aripiprazole should be used with caution in patients with known cardiovascular disease (history of myocardial infarction or ischemic heart disease, heart failure or conduction abnormalities), cerebrovascular disease, or conditions which would predispose patients to hypotension (dehydration, hypovolemia, and treatment with antihypertensive medications).

Seizure

Seizures occurred in 0.1% (1/926) of aripiprazole-treated patients in short-term, placebo-controlled trials. As with other antipsychotic drugs, aripiprazole should be used cautiously in patients with a history of seizures or with conditions that lower the seizure threshold, *e.g.*, Alzheimer's dementia. Conditions that lower the seizure threshold may be more prevalent in a population of 65 years or older.

Potential for Cognitive and Motor Impairment

In short-term, placebo-controlled trials, somnolence was reported in 11% of patients on aripiprazole compared to 8% of patients on placebo; somnolence led to discontinuation in 0.1% (1/926) of patients on aripiprazole in short-term, placebo-controlled trials. Despite the relatively modest increased incidence of somnolence compared to placebo, aripiprazole, like other antipsychotics, may have the potential to impair judgment, thinking, or motor skills. Patients should be cautioned about operating hazardous machinery, including automobiles, until they are reasonably certain that therapy with aripiprazole does not affect them adversely.

Body Temperature Regulation

Disruption of the body's ability to reduce core body temperature has been attributed to antipsychotic agents. Appropriate care is advised when prescribing aripiprazole for patients who will be experiencing conditions which may contribute to an elevation in core body temperature, *e.g.*, exercising strenuously, exposure to extreme heat, receiving concomitant medication with anticholinergic activity, or being subject to dehydration.

Dysphagia

Esophageal dysmotility and aspiration have been associated with antipsychotic drug use. Aspiration pneumonia is a common cause of morbidity and mortality in elderly patients, in particular those with advanced Alzheimer's dementia. Aripiprazole and other antipsychotic drugs should be used cautiously in patients at risk for aspiration pneumonia (see Use in Patients With Concomitant Illness).

Suicide

The possibility of a suicide attempt is inherent in psychotic illnesses, and close supervision of high-risk patients should accompany drug therapy. Prescriptions for aripiprazole should be written for the smallest quantity of tablets consistent with good patient management in order to reduce the risk of overdose.

Use in Patients With Concomitant Illness

Safety Experience in Elderly Patients With Psychosis Associated With Alzheimer's Disease

In a flexible dose (2-15 mg/day), 10 week, placebo-controlled study of aripiprazole in elderly patients (mean age: 81.5 years; range: 56-95) with psychosis associated with Alzheimer's dementia, 4 of 105 patients (3.8%) who received aripiprazole died compared to no deaths among 102 patients who received placebo during or within 30 days after termination of the double-blind portion of the study. Three of the patients (age 92, 91, and 87 years) died following the discontinuation of aripiprazole in the double-blind phase of the study (causes of death were pneumonia, heart failure, and shock). The fourth patient (age 78 years) died following hip surgery while in the double-blind portion of the study. The treatment-emergent adverse events that were reported at an incidence of $\geq$5% and having a greater incidence than placebo in this study were accidental injury, somnolence, and bronchitis. Eight percent (8%) of the aripiprazole treated patients reported somnolence compared to 1% of placebo patients. In a small pilot, open-label, ascending-dose, cohort study (n=30) in elderly patients with dementia, aripiprazole was associated in a dose-related fashion with somnolence.

The safety and efficacy of aripiprazole in the treatment of patients with psychosis associated with dementia has not been established. If the prescriber elects to treat such patients with aripiprazole, vigilance should be exercised, particularly for the emergence of difficulty swallowing or excessive somnolence, which could predispose to accidental injury or aspiration.

Clinical experience with aripiprazole in patients with certain concomitant systemic illnesses (see CLINICAL PHARMACOLOGY, Special Populations: Renal Impairment and Hepatic Impairment) is limited.

Aripiprazole has not been evaluated or used to any appreciable extent in patients with a recent history of myocardial infarction or unstable heart disease. Patients with these diagnoses were excluded from premarketing clinical studies.

INFORMATION FOR THE PATIENT

Physicians are advised to discuss the following issues with patients for whom they prescribe Aripiprazole:

Interference with cognitive and motor performance: Because aripiprazole may have the potential to impair judgment, thinking, or motor skills, patients should be cautioned about operating hazardous machinery, including automobiles, until they are reasonably certain that aripiprazole therapy does not affect them adversely.

Pregnancy: Patients should be advised to notify their physician if they become pregnant or intend to become pregnant during therapy with aripiprazole.

Nursing: Patients should be advised not to breast-feed an infant if they are taking aripiprazole.

Concomitant medication: Patients should be advised to inform their physicians if they are taking, or plan to take, any prescription or over-the-counter drugs, since there is a potential for interactions.

Alcohol: Patients should be advised to avoid alcohol while taking aripiprazole.

Heat exposure and dehydration: Patients should be advised regarding appropriate care in avoiding overheating and dehydration.

CARCINOGENESIS, MUTAGENESIS, AND IMPAIRMENT OF FERTILITY

Carcinogenesis

Lifetime carcinogenicity studies were conducted in ICR mice and in Sprague-Dawley (SD) and F344 rats. Aripiprazole was administered for 2 years in the diet at doses of 1, 3, 10, and 30 mg/kg/day to ICR mice and 1, 3, and 10 mg/kg/day to F344 rats (0.2 to 5 and 0.3 to 3 times the maximum recommended human dose [MRHD] based on mg/m^2, respectively). In addition, SD rats were dosed orally for 2 years at 10, 20, 40, and 60 mg/kg/day (3-19 times the MRHD based on mg/m^2). Aripiprazole did not induce tumors in male mice or rats. In female mice, the incidences of pituitary gland adenomas and mammary gland adenocarcinomas and adenoacanthomas were increased at dietary doses of 3-30 mg/kg/day (0.1-0.9 times human exposure at MRHD based on AUC and 0.5 to 5 times the MRHD based on mg/m^2). In female rats, the incidence of mammary gland fibroadenomas was increased at a dietary dose of 10 mg/kg/day (0.1 times human exposure at MRHD based on AUC and 3 times the MRHD based on mg/m^2); and the incidences of adrenocortical carcinomas and combined adrenocortical adenomas/carcinomas were increased at an oral dose of 60 mg/kg/day (14 times human exposure at MRHD based on AUC and 19 times the MRHD based on mg/m^2).

Proliferative changes in the pituitary and mammary gland of rodents have been observed following chronic administration of other antipsychotic agents and are considered prolactin-mediated. Serum prolactin was not measured in the aripiprazole carcinogenicity studies. However, increases in serum prolactin levels were observed in female mice in a 13 week dietary study at the doses associated with mammary gland and pituitary tumors. Serum prolactin was not increased in female rats in 4 and 13 week dietary studies at the dose associated with mammary gland tumors. The relevance for human risk of the findings of prolactin-mediated endocrine tumors in rodents is unknown.

Mutagenesis

The mutagenic potential of aripiprazole was tested in the *in vitro* bacterial reverse-mutation assay, the *in vitro* bacterial DNA repair assay, the *in vitro* forward gene mutation assay in mouse lymphoma cells, the *in vitro* chromosomal aberration assay in Chinese hamster lung (CHL) cells, the *in vivo* micronucleus assay in mice, and the unscheduled DNA synthesis assay in rats. Aripiprazole and a metabolite (2,3-DCPP) were clastogenic in the *in vitro* chromosomal aberration assay in CHL cells with and without metabolic activation. The metabolite, 2,3-DCPP, produced increases in numerical aberrations in the *in vitro* assay in CHL cells in the absence of metabolic activation. A positive response was obtained in the *in vivo* micronucleus assay in mice, however, the response was shown to be due to a mechanism not considered relevant to humans.

Impairment of Fertility

Female rats were treated with oral doses of 2, 6, and 20 mg/kg/day (0.6, 2, and 6 times the maximum recommended human dose [MRHD] on a mg/m^2 basis) of aripiprazole from 2 weeks prior to mating through Day 7 of gestation. Estrus cycle irregularities and increased corpora lutea were seen at all doses, but no impairment of fertility was seen. Increased pre-implantation loss was seen at 6 and 20 mg/kg, and decreased fetal weight was seen at 20 mg/kg.

Male rats were treated with oral doses of 20, 40, and 60 mg/kg/day (6, 13, and 19 times the MRHD on a mg/m^2 basis) of aripiprazole from 9 weeks prior to mating through mating. Disturbances in spermatogenesis were seen at 60 mg/kg, and prostate atrophy was seen at 40 and 60 mg/kg, but no impairment of fertility was seen.

PREGNANCY CATEGORY C

In animal studies aripiprazole demonstrated developmental toxicity, including possible teratogenic effects in rats and rabbits.

Pregnant rats were treated with oral doses of 3, 10, and 30 mg/kg/day (1, 3, and 10 times the maximum recommended human dose [MRHD] on a mg/m^2 basis) of aripiprazole during the period of organogenesis. Gestation was slightly prolonged at 30 mg/kg. Treatment caused a slight delay in fetal development as evidenced by decreased fetal weight (30 mg/kg), undescended testes (30 mg/kg), and delayed skeletal ossification (10 and 30 mg/kg). There were no adverse effects on embryofetal or pup survival. Delivered offspring had decreased bodyweights (10 and 30 mg/kg), and increased incidences of hepatodiaphragmatic nodules and diaphragmatic hernia at 30 mg/kg (the other dose groups were not examined for these findings). (A low incidence of diaphragmatic hernia was also seen in the fetuses exposed to 30 mg/kg.) Postnatally, delayed vaginal opening was seen at 10 and 30 mg/kg and impaired reproductive performance (decreased fertility rate, corpora lutea, implants, and live fetuses, and increased post-implantation loss, likely mediated through effects on female offspring) was seen at 30 mg/kg. Some maternal toxicity was seen at 30 mg/kg, however, there was no evidence to suggest that these developmental effects were secondary to maternal toxicity.

Pregnant rabbits were treated with oral doses of 10, 30, and 100 mg/kg/day (2, 3, and 11 times human exposure at MRHD based on AUC and 6, 19, and 65 times the MRHD based on mg/m^2) of aripiprazole during the period of organogenesis. Decreased maternal food consumption and increased abortions were seen at 100 mg/kg. Treatment caused increased fetal mortality (100 mg/kg), decreased fetal weight (30 and 100 mg/kg), increased incidence of a skeletal abnormality (fused sternebrae at 30 and 100 mg/kg) and minor skeletal variations (100 mg/kg).

In a study in which rats were treated with oral doses of 3, 10, and 30 mg/kg/day (1, 3, and 10 times the MRHD on a mg/m^2 basis) of aripiprazole perinatally and postnatally (from Day 17 of gestation through Day 21 postpartum), slight maternal toxicity and slightly prolonged gestation were seen at 30 mg/kg. An increase in stillbirths, and decreases in pup weight (persisting into adulthood) and survival, were seen at this dose.

There are no adequate and well-controlled studies in pregnant women. It is not known whether aripiprazole can cause fetal harm when administered to a pregnant woman or can affect reproductive capacity. Aripiprazole should be used during pregnancy only if the potential benefit outweighs the potential risk to the fetus.

LABOR AND DELIVERY

The effect of aripiprazole on labor and delivery in humans is unknown.

NURSING MOTHERS

Aripiprazole was excreted in milk of rats during lactation. It is not known whether aripiprazole or its metabolites are excreted in human milk. It is recommended that women receiving aripiprazole should not breast-feed.

PEDIATRIC USE

Safety and effectiveness in pediatric and adolescent patients have not been established.

GERIATRIC USE

Of the 5592 patients treated with aripiprazole in premarketing clinical trials, 659 (12%) were ≥65 years old and 525 (9%) were ≥75 years old. The majority (91%) of the 659 patients were diagnosed with dementia of the Alzheimer's type.

Placebo-controlled studies of aripiprazole in schizophrenia did not include sufficient numbers of subjects aged 65 and over to determine whether they respond differently from younger subjects. There was no effect of age on the pharmacokinetics of a single 15 mg dose of aripiprazole. Aripiprazole clearance was decreased by 20% in elderly subjects (≥65 years) compared to younger adult subjects (18-64 years), but there was no detectable effect of age in the population pharmacokinetic analysis in schizophrenia patients.

Studies of elderly patients with psychosis associated with Alzheimer's disease have suggested that there may be a different tolerability profile in this population compared to younger patients with schizophrenia (see Use in Patients With Concomitant Illness). The safety and efficacy of aripiprazole in the treatment of patients with psychosis associated with Alzheimer's disease has not been established. If the prescriber elects to treat such patients with aripiprazole, vigilance should be exercised.

DRUG INTERACTIONS

Given the primary CNS effects of aripiprazole, caution should be used when aripiprazole is taken in combination with other centrally acting drugs and alcohol. Due to its α_1-adrenergic receptor antagonism, aripiprazole has the potential to enhance the effect of certain antihypertensive agents.

POTENTIAL FOR OTHER DRUGS TO AFFECT ARIPIPRAZOLE

Aripiprazole is not a substrate of CYP1A1, CYP1A2, CYP2A6, CYP2B6, CYP2C8, CYP2C9, CYP2C19, or CYP2E1 enzymes. Aripiprazole also does not undergo direct glucuronidation. This suggests that an interaction of aripiprazole with inhibitors or inducers of these enzymes, or other factors, like smoking, is unlikely.

Both CYP3A4 and CYP2D6 are responsible for aripiprazole metabolism. Agents that induce CYP3A4 (*e.g.*, carbamazepine) could cause an increase in aripiprazole clearance and lower blood levels. Inhibitors of CYP3A4 (*e.g.*, ketoconazole) or CYP2D6 (*e.g.*, quinidine, fluoxetine, or paroxetine) can inhibit aripiprazole elimination and cause increased blood levels.

Ketoconazole: Coadministration of ketoconazole (200 mg/day for 14 days) with a 15 mg single dose of aripiprazole increased the AUC of aripiprazole and its active metabolite by 63% and 77%, respectively. The effect of a higher ketoconazole dose (400 mg/day) has not been studied. When concomitant administration of ketoconazole with aripiprazole occurs, aripiprazole dose should be reduced to one-half of its normal dose. Other strong inhibitors of CYP3A4 (itraconazole) would be expected to have similar effects and need similar dose reductions; weaker inhibitors (erythromycin, grapefruit juice) have not been studied. When the CYP3A4 inhibitor is withdrawn from the combination therapy, aripiprazole dose should then be increased.

Quinidine: Coadministration of a 10 mg single dose of aripiprazole with quinidine (166 mg/day for 13 days), a potent inhibitor of CYP2D6, increased the AUC of aripiprazole by 112% but decreased the AUC of its active metabolite, dehydroaripiprazole, by 35%. Aripiprazole dose should be reduced to one-half of its normal dose when concomitant administration of quinidine with aripiprazole occurs. Other significant inhibitors of CYP2D6, such as fluoxetine or paroxetine, would be expected to have similar effects and, therefore, should be accompanied by similar dose reductions. When the CYP2D6 inhibitor is withdrawn from the combination therapy, aripiprazole dose should then be increased.

Carbamazepine: Coadministration of carbamazepine (200 mg bid), a potent CYP3A4 inducer, with aripiprazole (30 mg qd) resulted in an approximate 70% decrease in C_{max} and AUC values of both aripiprazole and its active metabolite, dehydro-aripiprazole. When carbamazepine is added to aripiprazole therapy, aripiprazole dose should be doubled. Additional dose increases should be based on clinical evaluation. When carbamazepine is withdrawn from the combination therapy, aripiprazole dose should then be reduced.

No clinically significant effect of famotidine, valproate, or lithium was seen on the pharmacokinetics of aripiprazole (see CLINICAL PHARMACOLOGY, Drug-Drug Interactions).

POTENTIAL FOR ARIPIPRAZOLE TO AFFECT OTHER DRUGS

Aripiprazole is unlikely to cause clinically important pharmacokinetic interactions with drugs metabolized by cytochrome P450 enzymes. In *in vivo* studies, 10-30 mg/day doses of aripiprazole had no significant effect on metabolism by CYP2D6 (dextromethorphan), CYP2C9 (warfarin), CYP2C19 (omeprazole, warfarin), and CYP3A4 (dextromethorphan) substrates. Additionally, aripiprazole and dehydroaripiprazole did not show potential for altering CYP1A2-mediated metabolism *in vitro* (see CLINICAL PHARMACOLOGY, Drug-Drug Interactions).

Alcohol: There was no significant difference between aripiprazole coadministered with ethanol and placebo coadministered with ethanol on performance of gross motor skills or stimulus response in healthy subjects. As with most psychoactive medications, patients should be advised to avoid alcohol while taking aripiprazole.

ADVERSE REACTIONS

Aripiprazole has been evaluated for safety in 5592 patients who participated in multiple-dose, premarketing trials in schizophrenia, bipolar mania, and dementia of the Alzheimer's type, and who had approximately 3639 patient-years of exposure. A total of 1887 aripiprazole-treated patients were treated for at least 180 days and 1251 aripiprazole-treated patients had at least 1 year of exposure.

The conditions and duration of treatment with aripiprazole included (in overlapping categories) double-blind and comparative and noncomparative open-label studies, inpatient and outpatient studies, fixed- and flexible-dose studies, and short- and longer-term exposure.

Adverse events during exposure were obtained by collecting volunteered adverse events, as well as results of physical examinations, vital signs, weights, laboratory analyses, and ECG. Adverse experiences were recorded by clinical investigators using terminology of their own choosing. In the tables and tabulations that follow, modified COSTART dictionary terminology has been used initially to classify reported adverse events into a smaller number of standardized event categories, in order to provide a meaningful estimate of the proportion of individuals experiencing adverse events.

The stated frequencies of adverse events represent the proportion of individuals who experienced at least once, a treatment-emergent adverse event of the type listed. An event was considered treatment emergent if it occurred for the first time or worsened while receiving therapy following baseline evaluation. There was no attempt to use investigator causality assessments; *i.e.*, all reported events are included.

The prescriber should be aware that the figures in the tables and tabulations cannot be used to predict the incidence of side effects in the course of usual medical practice where patient characteristics and other factors differ from those that prevailed in the clinical trials. Similarly, the cited frequencies cannot be compared with figures obtained from other clinical investigations involving different treatment, uses, and investigators. The cited figures, however, do provide the prescribing physician with some basis for estimating the relative contribution of drug and nondrug factors to the adverse event incidence in the population studied.

ADVERSE FINDINGS OBSERVED IN SHORT-TERM, PLACEBO-CONTROLLED TRIALS OF PATIENTS WITH SCHIZOPHRENIA

The following findings are based on a pool of five placebo-controlled trials (four 4-week and one 6-week) in which aripiprazole was administered in doses ranging from 2-30 mg/day.

Adverse Events Associated With Discontinuation of Treatment in Short-Term, Placebo-Controlled Trials

Overall, there was no difference in the incidence of discontinuation due to adverse events between aripiprazole-treated (7%) and placebo-treated (9%) patients. The types of adverse events that led to discontinuation were similar between the aripiprazole and placebo-treated patients.

Adverse Events Occurring at an Incidence of 2% or More Among Aripiprazole-Treated Patients and Greater Than Placebo in Short-Term Placebo-Controlled Trials

TABLE 1 enumerates the incidence, rounded to the nearest percent, of treatment-emergent adverse events that occurred during acute therapy (up to 6 weeks), including only those events that occurred in 2% or more of patients treated with aripiprazole (doses ≥2 mg/day) and for which the incidence in patients treated with aripiprazole was greater than the incidence in patients treated with placebo.

An examination of population subgroups did not reveal any clear evidence of differential adverse event incidence on the basis of age, gender, or race.

Dose-Related Adverse Events

Dose response relationships for the incidence of treatment-emergent adverse events were evaluated from four trials comparing various fixed doses (2, 10, 15, 20, and 30 mg/day) of aripiprazole to placebo. This analysis, stratified by study, indicated that the only adverse event to have a possible dose response relationship, and then most prominent only with 30 mg, was somnolence (placebo, 7.7%; 15 mg, 8.7%; 20 mg, 7.5%; 30 mg, 15.3%).

TABLE 1 *Treatment-Emergent Adverse Events in Short-Term, Placebo-Controlled Trials**

Body System / Adverse Event	Aripiprazole (n=926)	Placebo (n=413)
Body as a Whole		
Headache	32%	25%
Asthenia	7%	5%
Fever	2%	1%
Digestive System		
Nausea	14%	10%
Vomiting	12%	7%
Constipation	10%	8%
Nervous System		
Anxiety	25%	24%
Insomnia	24%	19%
Lightheadedness	11%	7%
Somnolence	11%	8%
Akathisia	10%	7%
Tremor	3%	2%
Repiratory System		
Rhinitis	4%	3%
Coughing	3%	2%
Skin and Appendages		
Rash	6%	5%
Special Senses		
Blurred vision	3%	1%

* Events reported by at least 2% of patients treated with aripiprazole, except the following events, which had an incidence equal to or less than placebo: abdominal pain, accidental injury, back pain, dental pain, dyspepsia, diarrhea, dry mouth, myalgia, agitation, psychosis, extrapyramidal syndrome, hypertonia, pharyngitis, upper respiratory tract infection, dysmenorrhea, vaginitis.

Extrapyramidal Symptoms

In the short-term, placebo-controlled trials, the incidence of reported EPS for aripiprazole-treated patients was 6% vs 6% for placebo. Objectively collected data from those trials on the Simpson Angus Rating Scale (for EPS), the Barnes Akathisia Scale (for akathisia), and the Assessments of Involuntary Movement Scales (for dyskinesias) also did not show a difference between aripiprazole and placebo, with the exception of the Barnes Akathisia Scale (aripiprazole, 0.08; placebo, -0.05).

Laboratory Test Abnormalities

A between group comparison for 4-6 week placebo-controlled trials revealed no medically important differences between the aripiprazole and placebo groups in the proportions of patients experiencing potentially clinically significant changes in routine serum chemistry, hematology, or urinalysis parameters. Similarly, there were no aripiprazole/placebo differences in the incidence of discontinuations for changes in serum chemistry, hematology, or urinalysis.

Weight Gain

In short-term trials, there was a slight difference in mean weight gain between aripiprazole and placebo patients (+0.7 kg vs -0.05 kg, respectively), and also a difference in the proportion of patients meeting a weight gain criterion of >7% of body weight [aripiprazole (8%) compared to placebo (3%)]. TABLE 2 provides the weight change results from a long-term (52 week) study of aripiprazole, both mean change from baseline and proportions of patients meeting a weight gain criterion of >7% of body weight relative to baseline, categorized by BMI at baseline (see TABLE 2).

TABLE 2 *Weight Change Results Categorized by BMI at Baseline*

	BMI <23	BMI 23-27	BMI >27
Mean change from baseline	2.6 kg	1.4 kg	-1.2 kg
% With ≥7% increase BW	30%	19%	8%

ECG Changes

Between group comparisons for pooled, placebo-controlled trials revealed no significant differences between aripiprazole and placebo in the proportion of patients experiencing potentially important changes in ECG parameters; in fact, within the dose range of 10-30 mg/day, aripiprazole tended to slightly shorten the QTc interval. Aripiprazole was associated with a median increase in heart rate of 4 beats/min compared to a 1 beat/min increase among placebo patients.

OTHER ADVERSE EVENTS OBSERVED DURING THE PREMARKETING EVALUATION OF ARIPIPRAZOLE

Following is a list of modified COSTART terms that reflect treatment-emergent adverse events as defined in the introduction to ADVERSE REACTIONS reported by patients treated with aripiprazole at multiple doses ≥2 mg/day during any phase of a trial within the database of 5592 patients. All reported events are included except those already listed in TABLE 1, or other parts of ADVERSE REACTIONS, those considered in WARNINGS or PRECAUTIONS, those event terms which were so general as to be uninformative, events reported with an incidence of <0.05% and which did not have a substantial probability of being acutely life-threatening, events that are otherwise common as background events, and events considered unlikely to be drug related. It is important to emphasize that, although the events reported occurred during treatment with aripiprazole, they were not necessarily caused by it.

Events are further categorized by body system and listed in order of decreasing frequency according to the following definitions: *Frequent* adverse events are those occurring in at least 1/100 patients (only those not already listed in the tabulated results from placebo-controlled trials appear in this listing); *infrequent* adverse events are those occurring in 1/100 to 1/1000 patients; *rare* events are those occurring in fewer than 1/1000 patients.

Body as a Whole: *Frequent:* Flu syndrome, peripheral edema, chest pain, neck pain, neck rigidity; *Infrequent:* Pelvic pain, suicide attempt, face edema, malaise, photosensitivity, arm rigidity, jaw pain, chills, bloating, jaw tightness, enlarged abdomen, chest tightness; *Rare:* Throat pain, back tightness, head heaviness, moniliasis, throat tightness, leg rigidity, neck tightness, Mendelson's syndrome, heat stroke.

Cardiovascular System: *Frequent:* Hypertension, tachycardia, hypotension, bradycardia; *Infrequent:* Palpitation, hemorrhage, myocardial infarction, prolonged QT interval, cardiac arrest, atrial fibrillation, heart failure, AV block, myocardial ischemia, phlebitis, deep vein thrombosis, angina pectoris, extrasystoles; *Rare:* Vasovagal reaction, cardiomegaly, atrial flutter, thrombophlebitis.

Digestive System: *Frequent:* Anorexia, nausea and vomiting; *Infrequent:* Increased appetite, gastroenteritis, dysphagia, flatulence, gastritis, tooth caries, gingivitis, hemorrhoids, gastroesophageal reflux, gastrointestinal hemorrhage, periodontal abscess, tongue edema, fecal incontinence, colitis, rectal hemorrhage, stomatitis, mouth ulcer, cholecystitis, fecal impaction, oral monliasis, cholelithiasis, eructation, intestinal obstruction, peptic ulcer; *Rare:* Esophagitis, gum hemorrhage, glossitis, hematemesis, melena, duodenal ulcer, cheilitis, hepatitis, hepatomegaly, pancreatitis, intestinal perforation.

Endocrine System: *Infrequent:* Hypothyroidism; *Rare:* Goiter, hyperthyroidism.

Hemic/Lymphatic System: *Frequent:* Ecchymosis, anemia; *Infrequent:* Hypochromic anemia, leukopenia, leukocytosis, lymphadenopathy, thrombocytopenia; *Rare:* Eosinophilia, thrombocythemia, macrocytic anemia.

Metabolic and Nutritional Disorders: *Frequent:* Weight loss, creatine phosphokinase increased; *Infrequent:* Dehydration, edema, hypercholesteremia, hyperglycemia, hypokalemia, diabetes mellitus, SGPT increased, hyperlipemia, hypoglycemia, thirst, BUN increased, hyponatremia, SGOT increased, alkaline phosphatase increased, iron deficiency anemia, creatinine increased, bilirubinemia, lactic dehydrogenase increased, obesity; *Rare:* Hyperkalemia, gout, hypernatremia, cyanosis, hyperuricemia, hypoglycemic reaction.

Musculoskeletal System: *Frequent:* Muscle cramp; *Infrequent:* Arthralgia, bone pain, myasthenia, arthritis, arthrosis, muscle weakness, spasm, bursitis; *Rare:* Rhabdomyolysis, tendonitis, tenosynovitis, rheumatoid arthritis, myopathy.

Nervous System: *Frequent:* Depression, nervousness, increased salivation, hostility, suicidal thought, manic reaction, abnormal gait, confusion, cogwheel rigidity; *Infrequent:* Dystonia, twitch, impaired concentration, paresthesia, vasodilation, hypesthesia, extremity tremor, impotence, bradykinesia, decreased libido, panic attack, apathy, dyskinesia, hypersomnia, vertigo, dysarthria, tardive dyskinesia, ataxia, impaired memory, stupor, increased libido, amnesia, cerebrovascular accident, hyperactivity, depersonalization, hypokinesia, restless leg, myoclonus, dysphoria, neuropathy, increased reflexes, slowed thinking, hyperkinesia, hyperesthesia, hypotonia, oculogyric crisis; *Rare:* Delirium, euphoria, buccoglossal syndrome, akinesia, blunted affect, decreased consciousness, incoordination, cerebral ischemia, decreased reflexes, obsessive thought, intracranial hemorrhage.

Respiratory System: *Frequent:* Dyspnea, pneumonia; *Infrequent:* Asthma, epistaxis, hiccup, laryngitis; *Rare:* Hemoptysis, aspiration pneumonia, increased sputum, dry nasal passages, pulmonary edema, pulmonary embolism, hypoxia, respiratory failure, apnea.

Skin and Appendages: *Frequent:* Dry skin, pruritus, sweating, skin ulcer; *Infrequent:* Acne, vesiculobullous rash, eczema, alopecia, psoriasis, seborrhea; *Rare:* Maculopapular rash, exfoliative dermatitis, urticaria.

Special Senses: *Frequent:* Conjunctivitis, ear pain; *Infrequent:* Dry eye, eye pain, tinnitus, otitis media, cataract, altered taste, blepharitis; *Rare:* Increased lacrimation, frequent blinking, otitis externa, amblyopia, deafness, diplopia, eye hemorrhage, photophobia.

Urogenital System: *Frequent:* Urinary incontinence; *Infrequent:* Cystitis, urinary frequency, leukorrhea, urinary retention, hematuria, dysuria, amenorrhea, abnormal ejaculation, vaginal hemorrhage, vaginal moniliasis, kidney failure, uterus hemorrhage, menorrhagia, albuminuria, kidney calculus, nocturia, polyuria, urinary urgency; *Rare:* Breast pain, cervicitis, female lactation, anorgasmy, urinary burning, glycosuria, gynecomastia, urolithiasis, priapism.

DOSAGE AND ADMINISTRATION

USUAL DOSE

The recommended starting and target dose for aripiprazole is 10 or 15 mg/day administered on a once-a-day schedule without regard to meals. Aripiprazole has been systematically evaluated and shown to be effective in a dose range of 10-30 mg/day, however, doses higher than 10 or 15 mg/day, the lowest doses in these trials, were not more effective than 10 or 15 mg/day. Dosage increases should not be made before 2 weeks, the time needed to achieve steady state.

DOSING IN SPECIAL POPULATIONS

Dosage adjustments are not routinely indicated on the basis of age, gender, race, or renal or hepatic impairment status (see CLINICAL PHARMACOLOGY, Special Populations).

Dosage adjustment for patients taking aripiprazole concomitantly with potential CYP3A4 inhibitors: When concomitant administration of ketoconazole with aripiprazole occurs, aripiprazole dose should be reduced to one-half of the usual dose. When the CYP3A4 inhibitor is withdrawn from the combination therapy, aripiprazole dose should then be increased.

Dosage adjustment for patients taking aripiprazole concomitantly with potential CYP2D6 inhibitors: When concomitant administration of potential CYP2D6 inhibitors such as quinidine, fluoxetine, or paroxetine with aripiprazole occurs, aripiprazole dose should be reduced at least to one-half of its normal dose. When the

CYP2D6 inhibitor is withdrawn from the combination therapy, aripiprazole dose should then be increased.

Dosage adjustment for patients taking potential CYP3A4 inducers: When potential CYP3A4 inducer such as carbamazepine is added to aripiprazole therapy, aripiprazole dose should be doubled (to 20 or 30 mg). Additional dose increases should be based on clinical evaluation. When carbamazepine is withdrawn from the combination therapy, aripiprazole dose should be reduced to 10-15 mg.

MAINTENANCE THERAPY

There is no body of evidence available from controlled trials to answer the question of how long a patient treated with aripiprazole should remain on it. It is generally agreed, however, that pharmacological treatment for episodes of acute schizophrenia should continue for up to 6 months or longer. Patients should be periodically reassessed to determine the need for maintenance treatment.

SWITCHING FROM OTHER ANTIPSYCHOTICS

There are no systematically collected data to specifically address switching patients with schizophrenia from other antipsychotics to aripiprazole or concerning concomitant administration with other antipsychotics. While immediate discontinuation of the previous antipsychotic treatment may be acceptable for some patients with schizophrenia, more gradual discontinuation may be most appropriate for others. In all cases, the period of overlapping antipsychotic administration should be minimized.

ANIMAL PHARMACOLOGY

Aripiprazole produced retinal degeneration in albino rats in a 26 week chronic toxicity study at a dose of 60 mg/kg and in a 2 year carcinogenicity study at doses of 40 and 60 mg/kg. The 40 and 60 mg/kg doses are 13 and 19 times the maximum recommended human dose (MRHD) based on mg/m^2 and 7-14 times human exposure at MRHD based on AUC. Evaluation of the retinas of albino mice and of monkeys did not reveal evidence of retinal degeneration. Additional studies to further evaluate the mechanism have not been performed. The relevance of this finding to human risk is unknown.

HOW SUPPLIED

Abilify (aripiprazole) tablets are available in the following strengths and packages:

2 mg: Green, modified rectangular, scored tablets, debossed on one side with "A-006" and "2".
5 mg: Blue, modified rectangular, scored tablets, debossed on one side with "A-007" and "5".
10 mg: Pink, modified rectangular tablets, debossed on one side with "A-008" and "10".
15 mg: Yellow, round tablets, debossed on one side with "A-009" and "15".
20 mg: White, round tablets, debossed on one side with "A-010" and "20".
30 mg: Pink, round tablets, debossed on one side with "A-011" and "30".

Storage: Store at 25°C (77°F); excursions permitted to 15-30°C (59-86°F).

PRODUCT LISTING - EQUIVALENTS NOT AVAILABLE

Tablet - Oral - 10 mg			
10 x 10	$1056.25	ABILIFY, Bristol-Myers Squibb	59148-0008-35
30's	$316.88	ABILIFY, Bristol-Myers Squibb	59148-0008-13
Tablet - Oral - 15 mg			
10 x 10	$1056.25	ABILIFY, Bristol-Myers Squibb	59148-0009-35
30's	$316.88	ABILIFY, Bristol-Myers Squibb	59148-0009-13
Tablet - Oral - 20 mg			
10 x 10	$1493.75	ABILIFY, Bristol-Myers Squibb	59148-0010-35
30's	$448.13	ABILIFY, Bristol-Myers Squibb	59148-0010-13
Tablet - Oral - 30 mg			
10 x 10	$1493.75	ABILIFY, Bristol-Myers Squibb	59148-0011-35
30's	$448.13	ABILIFY, Bristol-Myers Squibb	59148-0011-13

Arsenic Trioxide *(003509)*

For complete prescribing information, refer to the CD-ROM included with the book.

Categories: Leukemia, acute promyelocytic; FDA Approved 2000 Sep; Pregnancy Category D; Orphan Drugs
Drug Classes: Antineoplastics, miscellaneous
Brand Names: Trisenox

WARNING

Experienced Physician and Institution:

Arsenic trioxide injection should be administered under the supervision of a physician who is experienced in the management of patients with acute leukemia.

APL Differentiation Syndrome:

Some patients with APL treated with arsenic trioxide have experienced symptoms similar to a syndrome called the retinoic-acid-Acute Promyelocytic Leukemia (RA-APL) or APL differentiation syndrome, characterized by fever, dyspnea, weight gain, pulmonary infiltrates and pleural or pericardial effusions, with or without leukocytosis. This syndrome can be fatal. The management of the syndrome has not been fully studied, but high-dose steroids have been used at the first suspicion of the APL differentiation syndrome and appear to mitigate signs and symptoms. At the first signs that could suggest the syndrome (unexplained fever, dyspnea and/or weight gain, abnormal chest auscultatory findings or radiographic abnormalities), high-dose steroids (dexamethasone 10 mg intravenously bid) should be immediately initiated, irrespective of the leukocyte count, and continued for at least 3 days or longer until signs and symptoms have abated. The majority of patients do not require termination of arsenic trioxide therapy during treatment of the APL differentiation syndrome.

WARNING — *Cont'd*

ECG Abnormalities:

Arsenic trioxide can cause QT interval prolongation and complete atrioventricular block. QT prolongation can lead to a torsade de pointes-type ventricular arrhythmia, which can be fatal. The risk of torsade de pointes is related to the extent of QT prolongation, concomitant administration of QT prolonging drugs, a history of torsade de pointes, pre-existing QT interval prolongation, congestive heart failure, administration of potassium-wasting diuretics, or other conditions that result in hypokalemia or hypomagnesemia. One patient (also receiving amphotericin B) had torsade de pointes during induction therapy for relapsed APL with arsenic trioxide.

ECG and Electrolyte Monitoring Recommendations:

Prior to initiating therapy with arsenic trioxide, a 12-lead ECG should be performed and serum electrolytes (potassium, calcium, and magnesium) and creatinine should be assessed; pre-existing electrolyte abnormalities should be corrected and, if possible, drugs that are known to prolong the QT interval should be discontinued. For QTc greater than 500 milliseconds, corrective measures should be completed and the QTc reassessed with serial ECGs prior to considering using arsenic trioxide. During therapy with arsenic trioxide, potassium concentrations should be kept above 4 mEq/dl and magnesium concentrations should be kept above 1.8 mg/dl. Patients who reach an absolute QT interval value >500 milliseconds should be reassessed and immediate action should be taken to correct concomitant risk factors, if any, while the risk/benefit of continuing versus suspending arsenic trioxide therapy should be considered. If syncope, rapid or irregular heartbeat develops, the patient should be hospitalized for monitoring, serum electrolytes should be assessed, arsenic trioxide therapy should be temporarily discontinued until the QTc interval regresses to below 460 milliseconds, electrolyte abnormalities are corrected, and the syncope and irregular heartbeat cease. There are no data on the effect of arsenic trioxide on the QTc interval during the infusion.

DESCRIPTION

Trisenox is a sterile injectable solution of arsenic trioxide. The molecular formula of the drug substance in the solid state is As_2O_3, with a molecular weight of 197.8 g.

Trisenox is available in 10 ml, single-use ampules containing 10 mg of arsenic trioxide. Trisenox is formulated as a sterile, nonpyrogenic, clear solution of arsenic trixoide in water for injection using sodium hydroxide and dilute hydrochloric acid to adjust to pH 8. Trisenox is preservative-free. Arsenic trioxide, the active ingredient, is present at a concentration of 1.0 mg/ml. Inactive ingredients and their respective approximate concentrations are sodium hydroxide (1.2 mg/ml) and hydrochloric acid, which is used to adjust the pH to 7.0-9.0.

INDICATIONS AND USAGE

Arsenic trioxide is indicated for induction of remission and consolidation in patients with acute promyelocytic leukemia (APL) who are refracroty to, or have relapsed from, retinoid and anthracycline chemotherapy, and whose APL is characterized by the presence of t(15;17) translocation or PML/RAR-alpha gene expression.

The response rate of other acute myelogenous leukemia subtypes to arsenic trioxide has not been examined.

CONTRAINDICATIONS

Arsenic trioxide is contraindicated in patients who are hypersensitive to arsenic.

WARNINGS

See BOXED WARNING.

Arsenic trioxide should be administered under the supervision of a physician who is experienced in the management of patients with acute leukemia.

APL DIFFERENTIATION SYNDROME

Nine (9) of 40 patients with APL treated with arsenic trioxide, at a dose of 0.15 mg/kg, experienced the APL differentiation syndrome (see BOXED WARNING).

HYPERLEUKOCYTOSIS

Treatment with arsenic trioxide has been associated with the development of hyperleukocytosis ($\geq 10 \times 10^3/\mu l$) in 20 of 40 patients. A relationship did not exist between baseline WBC counts and development of hyperleukocytosis nor baseline WBC counts and peak WBC counts. Hyperleukocytosis was not treated with additional chemotherapy. WBC counts during consolidation were not as high as during induction treatment.

QT PROLONGATION

See BOXED WARNING.

QT/QTc prolongation should be expected during treatment with arsenic trioxide and torsades de pointes as well as complete heart block has been reported. Over 460 ECG tracings from 40 patients with refractory or relapsed APL treated with arsenic trioxide were evaluated for QTc prolongation. Sixteen of 40 patients (40%) had at least one ECG tracing with a QTc interval greater than 500 milliseconds. Prolongation of the QTc was observed between 1 and 5 weeks after arsenic trioxide infusion, and then returned towards baseline by the end of 8 weeks after arsenic trioxide infusion. In these ECG evaluations, women did not experience more pronounced QT prolongation than men, and there was no correlation with age.

Complete AV Block: Complete AV block has been reported with arsenic trioxide in the published literature including a case of a patient with APL.

CARCINOGENESIS

Carcinogenicity studies have not been conducted with arsenic trioxide by intravenous administration. The active ingredient of arsenic trioxide, arsenic trioxide, is a human carcinogen.

A

PREGNANCY

Arsenic trioxide may cause fetal harm when administered to a pregnant woman. Studies in pregnant mice, rats, hamsters, and primates have shown that inorganic arsenicals cross the placental barrier when given orally or by injection. The reproductive toxicity of arsenic trioxide has been studied in a limited manner. An increase in resorptions, neural-tube defects, anophthalmia and microphthalmia were observed in rats administered 10 mg/kg of arsenic trioxide on gestation day 9 (approximately 10 times the recommended human daily dose on a mg/m^2 basis). Similar findings occurred in mice administered a 10 mg/kg dose of a related trivalent arsenic, sodium arsenite, (approximately 5 times the projected human dose on a mg/m^2 basis) on gestation days 6, 7, 8 or 9. Intravenous injection of 2 mg/kg sodium arsenite (approximately equivalent to the projected human daily dose on a mg/m^2 basis) on gestation day 7 (the lowest dose tested) resulted in neural-tube defects in hamsters.

There are no studies in pregnant women using arsenic trioxide. If this drug is used during pregnancy or if the patient becomes pregnant while taking this drug, the patient should be apprised of the potential harm to the fetus. One patient who became pregnant while receiving arsenic trioxide had a miscarriage. Women of childbearing potential should be advised to avoid becoming pregnant.

DOSAGE AND ADMINISTRATION

Arsenic trioxide should be diluted with 100-250 ml 5% dextrose injection or 0.9% sodium chloride injection, using proper aseptic technique, immediately after withdrawal from the ampule. The arsenic trioxide ampule is single-use and does not contain any preservatives. Unused portions of each ampule should be discarded properly. Do not save any unused portions for later administration. Do not mix arsenic trioxide with other medications.

Arsenic trioxide should be administered intravenously over 1-2 hours. The infusion duration may be extended up to 4 hours if acute vasomotor reactions are observed. A central venous catheter is not required.

STABILITY

After dilution, arsenic trioxide is chemically and physically stable when stored for 24 hours at room temperature and 48 hours when refrigerated.

DOSING REGIMEN

Arsenic trioxide is recommended to be given according to the following schedule:

Induction Treatment Schedule: Arsenic trioxide should be administered intravenously at a dose of 0.15 mg/kg daily until bone marrow remission. Total induction dose should not exceed 60 doses.

Consolidation Treatment Schedule: Consolidation treatment should begin 3-6 weeks after completion of induction therapy. Arsenic trioxide should be administered intravenously at a dose of 0.15 mg/kg daily for 25 doses over a period up to 5 weeks.

HANDLING AND DISPOSAL

Procedures for proper handling and disposal of anticancer drugs should be considered. Several guidelines on this subject have been published.[1-7] There is no general agreement that all of the procedures recommended in the guidelines are necessary or appropriate.

PRODUCT LISTING - EQUIVALENTS NOT AVAILABLE

Solution - Intravenous - 1 mg/ml

10 ml x 10 $3300.00 TRISENOX, Cell Therapeutics, Inc 60553-0111-10

Articaine Hydrochloride; Epinephrine Bitartrate *(003525)*

For complete prescribing information, refer to the CD-ROM included with the book.

Categories: Anesthesia, local; Anesthesia, regional; Anesthesia, infiltration; FDA Approved 2000 Apr; Pregnancy Category C
Drug Classes: Anesthetics, local
Brand Names: Septocaine

DESCRIPTION

Note: The trade name has been used throughout this monograph for clarity.

Septocaine injection is a sterile, aqueous solution that contains articaine hydrochloride 4% (40 mg/ml) with epinephrine bitartrate in a 1:100,000 strength. Articaine hydrochloride is a local anesthetic, which is chemically designated as 4-methyl-3-[2-(propylamino)-propionamido]-2-thiophene-carboxylic acid, methyl ester hydrochloride and is a racemic mixture. Articaine hydrochloride has a molecular weight of 320.84 and the molecular formula $C_{13}H_{20}N_2O_3S \cdot HCl$.

Articaine hydrochloride has a partition coefficient in n-octanol/Soerensen buffer (pH: 7.35) of 17 and a pKa of 7.8.

Epinephrine bitartrate, (-)-1-(3,4-Dihydroxyphenyl)-2-methylamino-ethanol (+) tartrate (1:1) salt, is a vasoconstrictor that is added to articaine HCl in a concentration of 1:100,000 as the free base. It has a molecular weight of 333.3. The molecular formula is $C_9H_{13}NO_3 \cdot C_4H_6O_6$.

Septocaine contains articaine HCl (40 mg/ml), epinephrine as bitartrate (1:100,000), sodium chloride (1.6 mg/ml), and sodium metabisulfite (0.5 mg/ml). The product is formulated with a 15% overage of epinephrine. The pH is adjusted to 5.0 with sodium hydroxide.

INDICATIONS AND USAGE

Septocaine is indicated for local, infiltrative, or conductive anesthesia in both simple and complex dental and periodontal procedures.

CONTRAINDICATIONS

Septocaine is contraindicated in patients with a known history of hypersensitivity to local anesthetics of the amide type, or in patients with known hypersensitivity to sodium metabisulfite.

WARNINGS

ACCIDENTAL INTRAVASCULAR INJECTION MAY BE ASSOCIATED WITH CONVULSIONS, FOLLOWED BY CENTRAL NERVOUS SYSTEM OR CARDIORESPIRATORY DEPRESSION AND COMA, PROGRESSING ULTIMATELY TO RESPIRATORY ARREST. DENTAL PRACTITIONERS AND/OR CLINICIANS WHO EMPLOY LOCAL ANESTHETIC AGENTS SHOULD BE WELL VERSED IN DIAGNOSIS AND MANAGEMENT OF EMERGENCIES THAT MAY ARISE FROM THEIR USE. RESUSCITATIVE EQUIPMENT, OXYGEN, AND OTHER RESUSCITATIVE DRUGS SHOULD BE AVAILABLE FOR IMMEDIATE USE.

Intravascular injections should be avoided. To avoid intravascular injection, aspiration should be performed before Septocaine is injected. The needle must be repositioned until no return of blood can be elicited by aspiration. Note, however, that the absence of blood in the syringe does not guarantee that intravascular injection has been avoided.

Septocaine contains epinephrine that can cause local tissue necrosis or systemic toxicity. Usual precautions for epinephrine administration should be observed.

Septocaine contains sodium metabisulfite, a sulfite that may cause allergic-type reactions including anaphylactic symptoms and life-threatening or less severe asthmatic episodes in certain susceptible people. The overall prevalence of sulfite sensitivity in the general population is unknown. Sulfite sensitivity is seen more frequently in asthmatic than in non-asthmatic people.

DOSAGE AND ADMINISTRATION

TABLE 3 summarizes the recommended volumes and concentrations of Septocaine for various types of anesthetic procedures. The dosages suggested in TABLE 3 are for normal healthy adults, administered by submucosal infiltration and/or nerve block.

TABLE 3 *Recommended Dosages*

	Septocaine Injection	
Procedure	**Volume**	**Total Dose of Articaine HCl**
Infiltration	0.5-2.5 ml	20-100 mg
Nerve block	0.5-3.4 ml	20-136 mg
Oral surgery	1.0-5.1 ml	40-204 mg

The above suggested volumes serve only as a guide. Other volumes may be used provided the total maximum recommended dose is not exceeded.

These recommended doses serve only as a guide to the amount of anesthetic required for most routine procedures. The actual volumes to be used depend on a number of factors such as type and extent of surgical procedure, depth of anesthesia, degree of muscular relaxation, and condition of the patient. In all cases, the smallest dose that will produce the desired result should be given. Dosages should be reduced for pediatric patients, elderly patients, and patients with cardiac and/or liver disease.

The onset of anesthesia, and the duration of anesthesia are proportional to the volume and concentration (*i.e.*, total dose) of local anesthetic used. Caution should be exercised when employing large volumes since the incidence of side effects may be dose-related.

MAXIMUM RECOMMENDED DOSAGES

Adults

For normal healthy adults, the maximum dose of articaine HCl administered by submucosal infiltration and/or nerve block should not exceed 7 mg/kg (0.175 ml/kg) or 3.2 mg/lb (0.0795 ml/lb) of body weight.

Pediatric Patients

Use in pediatric patients under 4 years of age is not recommended. The quantity to be injected should be determined by the age and weight of the child and the magnitude of the operation. Do not exceed the equivalent of 7 mg/kg (0.175 ml/kg) or 3.2 mg/lb (0.0795 ml/lb) of body weight.

STERILIZATION, STORAGE, AND TECHNICAL PROCEDURES

For chemical disinfection of the carpule, either isopropyl alcohol (91%) or ethyl alcohol (70%) is recommended. Many commercially available brands of isopropyl (rubbing) alcohol, as well as solutions of ethyl alcohol not of USP grade, contain denaturants that are injurious to rubber and therefore are not to be used.

Parenteral drug products should be inspected visually for particulate matter and discoloration prior to administration, whenever solution and container permit.

PRODUCT LISTING - EQUIVALENTS NOT AVAILABLE

Solution - Injectable - 4%;1:100000

1.70 ml x 50 $27.30 SEPTOCAINE, Septodont Incorporated 12862-1050-02

Ascorbic Acid *(000290)*

Categories: Ascorbic acid deficiency; Scurvy; Urinary acidification; FDA Pre 1938 Drugs; WHO Formulary
Drug Classes: Vitamins/minerals
Brand Names: C-Tym; Cebid; Cecore 500; Cee-500; Cetane; **Cevalin**; Mega C A Plus; Vitamin C
Foreign Brand Availability: Acidylina (Italy); Agrumina (Italy); Ascorbin (Malaysia); Askorbin (Indonesia); C500 (Israel); C-Vimin (Finland; Sweden); Cebion (Austria; Bahrain; Chile; Colombia; Cyprus; Czech-Republic; Ecuador; Egypt; Germany; Greece; Iran; Iraq; Italy; Jordan; Kuwait; Lebanon; Libya; Oman; Peru; Portugal; Qatar; Republic-of-Yemen; Saudi-Arabia; Spain; Syria; United-Arab-Emirates); CeCe (Korea); Cecap (Hong-Kong); Cecon (Bahamas; Barbados; Belize; Bermuda; Curacao; Guyana; Jamaica; Netherland-Antilles; Surinam; Trinidad); Cecon Drops (Australia); Celin (India); Cenol (Belgium); Ceevifil (Philippines); Cetrinets (Malaysia); Ce-Vi-Sol (Mexico); Cewin (Brazil); Citravite (India; New-Zealand); Dancimin C (Indonesia); Dayvital (Netherlands); Flavettes (Hong-Kong); Ikacee (Indonesia); Leder C (Taiwan); Leder-C (Ecuador); Limcee (India); Pro-C (Australia); Redoxon (Argentina; Australia; Austria; Bahrain; Brazil; Colombia; Cyprus; Egypt; Finland; Greece; Hong-Kong; Iran; Iraq; Ireland; Israel; Italy; Jordan; Kuwait; Lebanon; Libya; New-Zealand; Oman; Peru; Portugal; Qatar; Republic-of-Yemen; Saudi-Arabia; Spain; Switzerland; Syria; United-Arab-Emirates; Venezuela); Redoxon C (Bahamas; Barbados; Belize; Benin; Bermuda; Burkina-Faso; Curacao; Ethiopia; Gambia; Ghana; Guinea; Guyana; Ivory-Coast; Jamaica; Kenya; Liberia; Malawi; Mali; Mauritania; Mauritius; Morocco; Netherland-Antilles; Niger; Nigeria; Senegal; Seychelles; Sierra-Leone; Sudan; Surinam; Tanzania; Trinidad; Tunia; Uganda; Zambia; Zimbabwe); Redoxon Forte (India; Mexico); Scorbex (South-Africa); Take-C (Taiwan); Tanvimil-C (Argentina); Upsa-C (Bahrain; Cyprus; Egypt; Iran; Iraq; Israel; Jordan; Kuwait; Lebanon; Libya; Oman; Qatar; Republic-of-Yemen; Saudi-Arabia; Syria; United-Arab-Emirates); Upsa C (Costa-Rica; Dominican-Republic; El-Salvador; Guatemala; Honduras; Nicaragua; Panama); Vi-C 500 (Israel); Vicef (Benin; Burkina-Faso; Ethiopia; Gambia; Ghana; Guinea; Ivory-Coast; Kenya; Liberia; Malawi; Mali; Mauritania; Mauritius; Morocco; Niger; Nigeria; Senegal; Seychelles; Sierra-Leone; Sudan; Tanzania; Tunia; Uganda; Zambia; Zimbabwe); Veinobiase (Costa-Rica; Dominican-Republic; El-Salvador; Guatemala; Honduras; Nicaragua; Panama); Vita-Cedol Orange (Bahamas; Barbados; Belize; Bermuda; Curacao; Guyana; Jamaica; Netherland-Antilles; Surinam; Trinidad); Vitac (Chile); Vitacimin (Peru); Vitascorbol (France); Vorange (Malaysia); Xon-ce (Indonesia)

IM-IV-SC

DESCRIPTION

Cenolate (ascorbic acid injection) is a sterile, nonpyrogenic solution of sodium ascorbate prepared from ascorbic acid with the aid of sodium bicarbonate in water for injection. Cenolate is indicated for injection by the intravenous, intramuscular, and subcutaneous routes. Each ml contains 562.5 mg of sodium ascorbate, equivalent to 500 mg ascorbic acid; sodium hydrosulfite, 5 mg added as an antioxidant. Contains sodium bicarbonate and may contain additional ascorbic acid for pH adjustment. pH 6.1 (5.5-7.0). 8.6 mOsmol/ml (calc.). It contains no bacteriostat, antimicrobial agent or added buffer.

Protect from light. Keep ampuls in tray until time of use.

Sodium ascorbate (sodium derivative of ascorbic acid) is chemically designated $C_6H_7NaO_6$, minute crystals freely soluble in water.

CLINICAL PHARMACOLOGY

Ascorbic acid (vitamin C) has few strictly pharmacological actions. Administration in amounts greatly in excess of physiologic requirements causes no demonstrable effects. The vitamin is an essential coenzyme for collagen formation, tissue repair and synthesis of lipids and proteins. It acts both as a reducing agent and as an antioxidant and is necessary for many physiologic functions, *e.g.*, metabolism of iron and folic acid, resistance to infection, and preservation of blood vessel integrity. Signs and symptoms of early vitamin C deficiency include malaise, irritability, arthralgia, hyperkeratosis of hair follicles, nosebleed, and petechial hemorrhages. Prolonged deficiency leads to clinical scurvy.

Ascorbic acid is normally present in both plasma and cells. The absorbed vitamin is ubiquitous in all body tissues. The highest concentrations are found in glandular tissue, the lowest in muscle and stored fat. Ascorbic acid is partially destroyed and partially excreted by the body. There is a renal threshold for vitamin C; the vitamin is excreted by the kidney in large amounts only when the plasma concentration exceeds this threshold, which is approximately 1.4 mg/100 ml. When the body is saturated with ascorbic acid, the plasma concentration will be about the same as that of the renal threshold; if further amounts are then administered, most of it escapes into the urine. When body tissues are not saturated and plasma concentration is low, administration of ascorbic acid results in little or no renal excretion.

A major route of metabolism of ascorbic acid involves its conversion to urinary oxalate, presumably through intermediate formation of its oxidized product, dehydroascorbic acid.

INDICATIONS AND USAGE

Ascorbic acid injection is indicated for ascorbic acid deficiency.

Parenteral ascorbic acid supplementation may be necessary in the treatment of scurvy for patients with gastric disorders, for patients with extensive injuries, for surgical patients and others who cannot take oral vitamins. Acute ascorbic acid deficiency may be associated with extensive injuries and other states of extreme stress. Vitamin C requirements are also significantly increased in certain diseases and conditions such as tuberculosis, hyperthyroidism, peptic ulcer, neoplastic disease, pregnancy and lactation.

CONTRAINDICATIONS

None known.

WARNINGS

Ascorbic acid injection contains sodium hydrosulfite, a sulfite that may cause allergic-type reactions including anaphylactic symptoms and life-threatening or less severe asthmatic episodes in certain susceptible people. The overall prevalence of sulfite sensitivity in the general population is unknown and probably low. Sulfite sensitivity is seen more frequently in asthmatic than in nonasthmatic people.

PRECAUTIONS

CAUTION: Since high internal pressure may develop on long storage, precautions should be taken to wrap the ampul in a protective covering while it is being opened.

Do not administer unless solution is clear and container is intact. Discard unused portion.

Acidification of the urine by ascorbic acid may cause precipitation of cystine, urate or oxalate stones and will alter the excretion of certain other drugs administered concurrently. Large doses interfere with the anticoagulant effect of warfarin and the presence of ascorbic acid in the urine can interfere with tests for glycosuria.

As ascorbic acid has on occasion been used as a specific antidote for symptoms resulting from interaction between ethanol and disulfiram, it may be expected that the concurrent administration of ascorbic acid injection will interfere with the effectiveness of disulfiram given to patients to encourage abstention from alcohol.

PREGNANCY CATEGORY C

Animal reproduction studies have not been conducted with ascorbic acid injection. It is also not known whether ascorbic acid injection can cause fetal harm when administered to a pregnant woman or can affect reproduction capacity. Ascorbic acid injection should be given to a pregnant woman only if clearly needed.

NONTERATOGENIC EFFECTS

High doses of vitamin C taken during pregnancy have been reported to cause scurvy in infants removed from this environment at birth.

ADVERSE REACTIONS

Pain and swelling at the site of injection have been reported in some patients.

Large doses may cause diarrhea. Also see PRECAUTIONS.

DOSAGE AND ADMINISTRATION

Ascorbic acid injection is usually injected intramuscularly or subcutaneously. The solution has a pH of 5.5-7.0 and is not usually irritating to tissues. The solution also may be injected intravenously, but a higher percentage of the drug will be excreted in the urine than when the subcutaneous or intramuscular route is employed. When administered intravenously, ascorbic acid injection should be slowly infused with large volume solutions. Ascorbic acid injection should be added to such solutions shortly before venoclysis; any of the mixture remaining after administration should be discarded.

It is difficult to establish an exact dosage of ascorbic acid suitable for the treatment of deficiencies. In general, therapeutic doses should substantially exceed the recommended daily dietary allowances for healthy persons: Adults, 55-60 mg; infants, 35 mg; children, 40 mg; adolescents, 45-60 mg; pregnant and lactating women, 60 mg. The blood level of ascorbic acid in normal persons ranges from 0.4-1.5 mg/100 ml.

The usual therapeutic parenteral dose ranges from 100-250 mg (0.2-0.5 ml of ascorbic acid injection), once or twice daily. If the deficiency is extreme, 1-2 g (2-4 ml) may be given. There is no appreciable danger from excessive dosage because superfluous amounts of the vitamin are rapidly excreted in the urine.

When extensive injuries are treated, ascorbic acid may be given if any doubt exists regarding previous nutrition with the vitamin. Patients with deep and extensive burns may require 200-500 mg (0.4-1.0 ml) daily to maintain measurable blood concentrations. Doses of 1 g daily for 4-7 days may be given before operation in gastrectomy patients. Similar doses also have been used postoperatively to aid wound healing following extensive surgical procedures.

Parenteral drug products should be inspected visually for particulate matter and discoloration prior to administration, whenever solution and container permit. See PRECAUTIONS.

HOW SUPPLIED

Cenolate (ascorbic acid injection) (500 mg/ml) is supplied in single-dose 1 and 2 ml ampuls.

Protect from exposure to light.

CAUTION: Cenolate ampuls should be stored in a refrigerator and should not be allowed to stand at room temperature before use. Failure to follow this caution may lead to excessive pressure inside the ampul. Since pressure may develop on long storage, precautions should be taken to wrap the container in a protective covering while it is being opened.

ORAL

CLINICAL PHARMACOLOGY

Ascorbic acid is needed by the body for:

- Wound healing.
- Collagen synthesis.
- Carbohydrate metabolism.

PHARMACOKINETICS

Ascorbic acid is readily absorbed by the gastrointestinal system after oral administration. It is metabolized in the liver by oxidation and sulfation. Unused amounts are excreted in the urine as unchanged drug and its metabolites.

Ascorbic acid is an antioxidant.

INDICATIONS AND USAGE

Ascorbic acid is indicated:

- For the prevention and treatment of scurvy.
- For urinary acidification.
- As a dietary supplement.

CONTRAINDICATIONS

Ascorbic acid is contraindicated in:

- Tartrazine sensitivity.
- Sulfite sensitivity.
- G-6-PD deficiency.

PRECAUTIONS

Excessive doses for prolonged periods of time should not be taken by diabetics, patients with renal calculi, patients undergoing anticoagulant therapy or patients with a history of gout.

A

LABORATORY TEST INTERACTIONS

False Negative: Amine-dependent stool occult blood, urine bilirubin, blood, leukocyte determinations.

False Positive: Urine glucose.

Decrease: Urine amphetamine, serum AST, urine barbiturate, serum bicarbonate, serum bilirubin, serum cholesterol, serum CK, serum creatinine, urine glucose, serum HDL-cholesterol, urine oxalate, urine porphobilinogen, serum triglycerides, serum urea nitrogen, serum uric acid, urine uric acid.

Increase: Serum amylase (only at toxic ascorbic acid levels), serum AST, serum bilirubin, serum glucose, serum HbA1c, urine β-hydroxybutyrate, urine 17-hydroxy corticosteroids, urine iodide, urine 17-ketosteroids, urine oxalate, serum phosphate, CSF and urine protein, serum uric acid.

PREGNANCY

Pregnancy Category A if doses do not exceed the recommended daily allowance.

Pregnancy Category C if doses exceed the recommended daily allowance.

NURSING MOTHERS

Ascorbic acid is excreted in breast milk. The recommended daily allowance in lactating mothers is 90-100 mg.

DRUG INTERACTIONS

Antacids: Ascorbic acid increases the amount of aluminum absorbed from aluminum-containing antacids.

ADVERSE REACTIONS

CNS: Dizziness, fatigue, flushing, headache, insomnia.

GI: Anorexia, cramps, diarrhea, heartburn, nausea, vomiting.

Genitourinary: Crystalluria, oxalate or urate renal stones, polyuria, urine acidification.

Hematologic: Hemolysis (after large doses in patients with G-6-PD deficiency), sickle cell crisis.

DOSAGE AND ADMINISTRATION

ADULTS

Scurvy: 100-500 mg qd for at least 2 weeks, then 50 mg or more qd.

Urinary Acidification: 4-12 g qd in divided doses.

Dietary Supplementation: 50-200 mg qd.

PEDIATRIC PATIENTS

Scurvy: 100-300 mg qd for at least 2 weeks, then 35 mg or more qd.

Urinary Acidification: 500 mg q6-8h.

Dietary Supplementation: 35-100 mg qd.

PRODUCT LISTING - RATED THERAPEUTICALLY EQUIVALENT

Tablet - Oral - 250 mg

30's	$2.03	GENERIC, Heartland Healthcare Services	61392-0155-30
30's	$2.03	GENERIC, Heartland Healthcare Services	61392-0155-39
30's	$2.03	GENERIC, Heartland Healthcare Services	61392-0156-30
31's	$2.09	GENERIC, Heartland Healthcare Services	61392-0155-31
60's	$4.05	GENERIC, Heartland Healthcare Services	61392-0155-60
60's	$4.05	GENERIC, Heartland Healthcare Services	61392-0155-65
90's	$6.08	GENERIC, Heartland Healthcare Services	61392-0155-90

Tablet - Oral - 500 mg

30's	$2.23	GENERIC, Heartland Healthcare Services	61392-0156-39
31's	$2.30	GENERIC, Heartland Healthcare Services	61392-0156-31
32's	$2.38	GENERIC, Heartland Healthcare Services	61392-0156-32
60's	$4.46	GENERIC, Heartland Healthcare Services	61392-0156-60
60's	$4.46	GENERIC, Heartland Healthcare Services	61392-0156-65
90's	$6.68	GENERIC, Heartland Healthcare Services	61392-0156-90

PRODUCT LISTING - EQUIVALENTS NOT AVAILABLE

Solution - Injectable - 222 mg/ml

30 ml	$4.20	GENERIC, Merit Pharmaceuticals	30727-0340-80
30 ml	$4.60	GENERIC, Torrance Company	00389-0080-30
30 ml	$6.90	GENERIC, Merit Pharmaceuticals	30727-0645-80
50 ml	$12.95	GENERIC, Merit Pharmaceuticals	30727-0339-90

Solution - Injectable - 250 mg/ml

2 ml x 25	$60.00	GENERIC, Cmc-Consolidated Midland Corporation	00223-8875-02
30 ml	$3.95	GENERIC, Keene Pharmaceuticals Inc	00588-5261-90
30 ml	$6.00	GENERIC, Cmc-Consolidated Midland Corporation	00223-7185-30
30 ml	$6.00	GENERIC, Cmc-Consolidated Midland Corporation	00223-8873-30
30 ml	$9.40	GENERIC, Pasadena Research Laboratories Inc	00418-2721-30
50 ml	$7.90	GENERIC, Merit Pharmaceuticals	30727-0399-90
100 ml	$12.95	GENERIC, Merit Pharmaceuticals	30727-0399-95

Solution - Injectable - 500 mg/ml

1 ml x 50	$34.44	CENOLATE, Abbott Pharmaceutical	00074-3118-31
1 ml x 100	$106.25	CENOLATE, Abbott Pharmaceutical	00074-3118-02
2 ml x 50	$40.97	CENOLATE, Abbott Pharmaceutical	00074-3397-32
2 ml x 100	$62.50	CENOLATE, Abbott Pharmaceutical	00074-3397-02
50 ml	$3.00	GENERIC, Pegasus Laboratories Inc	10974-0709-50
50 ml	$3.79	GENERIC, Mcguff Company	49072-0037-50
50 ml	$4.25	GENERIC, Torrance Company	00389-0486-50
50 ml	$4.25	GENERIC, Pegasus Laboratories Inc	10974-0080-30
50 ml	$6.45	GENERIC, Mcguff Company	49072-0039-50
50 ml	$7.45	GENERIC, Major Pharmaceuticals Inc	00904-0945-50
50 ml	$7.50	GENERIC, Cmc-Consolidated Midland Corporation	00223-7186-50
50 ml	$9.95	GENERIC, Legere Pharmaceuticals	25332-0086-50
50 ml	$10.53	GENERIC, Pasadena Research Laboratories Inc	00418-3460-50
50 ml	$12.50	GENERIC, American Regent Laboratories Inc	00517-5050-01
50 ml	$21.59	GENERIC, Physicians Total Care	54868-4115-00
50 ml x 10	$65.00	GENERIC, Raway Pharmacal Inc	00686-5050-01

Asparaginase *(000297)*

For complete prescribing information, refer to the CD-ROM included with the book.

Categories: Leukemia, acute lymphoblastic; Pregnancy Category C; FDA Pre 1938 Drugs; WHO Formulary

Drug Classes: Antineoplastics, enzymes

Brand Names: Elspar; L-Asparaginase

Foreign Brand Availability: Crasnitin (Austria; Germany; Hungary; Netherlands; Portugal; Switzerland); Erwinase (New-Zealand; Singapore; Thailand); Kidrolase (Canada; Czech-Republic; France; Peru); Laspar (South-Africa); Leunase (Australia; Hong-Kong; India; Indonesia; Japan; Korea; Malaysia; New-Zealand; Taiwan; Thailand)

HCFA JCODE(S): J9020 10,000 units IV, IM

WARNING

IT IS RECOMMENDED THAT ASPARAGINASE BE ADMINISTERED TO PATIENTS ONLY IN A HOSPITAL SETTING UNDER THE SUPERVISION OF A PHYSICIAN WHO IS QUALIFIED BY TRAINING AND EXPERIENCE TO ADMINISTER CANCER CHEMOTHERAPEUTIC AGENTS, BECAUSE OF THE POSSIBILITY OF SEVERE REACTIONS, INCLUDING ANAPHYLAXIS AND SUDDEN DEATH. THE PHYSICIAN MUST BE PREPARED TO TREAT ANAPHYLAXIS AT EACH ADMINISTRATION OF THE DRUG.

IN THE TREATMENT OF EACH PATIENT THE PHYSICIAN MUST WEIGH CAREFULLY THE POSSIBILITY OF ACHIEVING THERAPEUTIC BENEFIT VERSUS THE RISK OF TOXICITY. THE FOLLOWING DATA SHOULD BE THOROUGHLY REVIEWED BEFORE ADMINISTERING THE COMPOUND.

DESCRIPTION

Elspar contains the enzyme L-asparagine amidohydrolase, type EC-2, derived from *Escherichia coli*. It is a white crystalline powder that is freely soluble in water and practically insoluble in methanol, acetone and chloroform. Its activity is expressed in terms of International Units (I.U.) according to the recommendation of the International Union of Biochemistry. The specific activity of Asparaginase is at least 225 I.U. per milligram of protein and each vial contains 10,000 I.U. of asparaginase and 80 mg of mannitol, an inactive ingredient, as a sterile, white lyophilized plug or powder for intravenous or intramuscular injection after reconstitution.

INDICATIONS AND USAGE

Asparaginase is indicated in the therapy of patients with acute lymphocytic leukemia. This agent is useful primarily in combination with other chemotherapeutic agents in the induction of remissions of the disease in children.[3,4] Asparaginase should not be used as the sole induction agent unless combination therapy is deemed inappropriate. Asparaginase is not recommended for maintenance therapy.

NON-FDA APPROVED INDICATIONS

Asparaginase has also been used in the treatment of adult lymphoblastic leukemia. However, this specific use has not been approved by the FDA.

CONTRAINDICATIONS

Asparaginase is contraindicated in patients with pancreatitis or a history of pancreatitis. Acute hemorrhagic pancreatitis, in some instances fatal, has been reported following asparaginase administration.[4-7] Asparaginase is also contraindicated in patients who have had previous anaphylactic reactions to it.

WARNINGS

Allergic reactions to asparaginase are frequent and may occur during the primary course of therapy. They are not completely predictable on the basis of the intradermal skin test. Anaphylaxis and death have occurred in a hospital setting with experienced observers.

Once a patient has received asparaginase as part of a treatment regimen, retreatment with this agent at a later time is associated with increased risk of hypersensitivity reactions. In patients found by skin testing to be hypersensitive to asparaginase, and in any patient who has received a previous course of therapy with asparaginase, therapy with this agent should be instituted or reinstituted only after the successful desensitization, and then only if in the judgement of the physician the possible benefit is greater than the increased risk. Desensitization itself may be hazardous. (See DOSAGE AND ADMINISTRATION.)

In view of the unpredictability of the adverse reactions to asparaginase, it is recommended that this product be used in a hospital setting. Asparaginase has an adverse effect on liver function in the majority of patients. Therapy with asparaginase may increase preexisting liver impairment caused by prior therapy or the underlying disease. Because of this there is a possibility that asparaginase may increase the toxicity of other medications.[3,7]

The administration of Asparaginase *intravenously concurrently with or immediately before* a course of vincristine and prednisone may be associated with increased toxicity.[3] (See DOSAGE AND ADMINISTRATION, Recommended Induction Regimens.)

DOSAGE AND ADMINISTRATION

As a component of selected multiple agent induction regimens, asparaginase may be administered by either the intravenous or the intramuscular route. When administered intravenously this enzyme should be given over a period of not less than thirty minutes through the side arm of an already running infusion of Sodium Chloride Injection or Dextrose Injection 5% (D_5W). Asparaginase has little tendency to cause phlebitis when given intravenously. Anaphylactic reactions require the immediate use of epinephrine, oxygen, and intravenous steroids.

When administering asparaginase intramuscularly, the volume at a single injection site should be limited to 2 ml. If a volume greater than 2 ml is to be administered, two injection sites should be used.

Unfavorable interactions of asparaginase with some antitumor agents have been demonstrated. It is recommended therefore, that asparaginase be used in combination regimens only by physicians familiar with the benefits and risks of a given regimen. During the period of its inhibition of protein synthesis and cell replication asparaginase may interfere with the action of drugs such as methotrexate which require cell replication for their lethal effect. Asparaginase may interfere with the enzymatic detoxification of other drugs, particularly in the liver.

RECOMMENDED INDUCTION REGIMENS

When using chemotherapeutic agents in combination for the induction of remissions in patients with acute lymphocytic leukemia, regimens are sought which provide maximum chance of success while avoiding excessive cumulative toxicity or negative drug interactions.

One of the following combination regimens incorporating asparaginase is recommended for acute lymphocytic leukemia in children: (In the regimens below, Day 1 is considered to be the first day of therapy.)

Regimen I[3]:

Prednisone: 40 mg/square meter of body surface area per day orally in three divided doses for 15 days, followed by tapering of the dosage as follows: 20 mg/square meter for 2 days, 10 mg/square meter for 2 days, 5 mg/square meter for 2 days, 2.5 mg/square meter for 2 days and then discontinue.

Vincristine Sulfate: 2 mg/square meter of body surface area intravenously once weekly on Days 1,8, and 15 of the treatment period. The maximum single dose should not exceed 2.0 mg.

Asparaginase: 1,000 I.U./kg/day intravenously for ten successive days beginning on Day 22 of the treatment period.

Regimen II[4]:

Prednisone: 40 mg/square meter of body surface area per day orally in three divided doses for 28 days (the total daily dose should be to the nearest 2.5 mg), following which the dosage of prednisone should be discontinued gradually over a 14 day period.

Vincristine Sulfate: 1.5 mg/square meter of body surface area intravenously weekly for four doses, on Days 1,8,15, and 22 of the treatment period. The maximum single dose should not exceed 2.0 mg.

Asparaginase: 6,000 I.U./square meter of body surface area intramuscularly on Days 4,7,10,13,16,19,22,25, and 28 of the treatment period.

When a remission is obtained with either of the above regimens, appropriate maintenance therapy must be instituted. Asparaginase should not be used as part of a maintenance regimen. The above regimens do not preclude a need for special therapy directed toward the prevention of central nervous system leukemia.

It should be noted that asparaginase has been used in combination regimens other than those recommended above. It is important to keep in mind that asparaginase administered intravenously concurrently with or immediately before a course of vincristine and prednisone may be associated with increased toxicity. Physicians using a given regimen should be thoroughly familiar with its benefits and risks. Clinical data are insufficient for a recommendation concerning the use of combination regimens in adults. Asparaginase toxicity is reported to be greater in adults than in children.

Use of asparaginase as the sole induction agent should be undertaken only in an unusual situation when a combined regimen is inappropriate because of toxicity or other specific patient-related factors, or in cases refractory to other therapy. When asparaginase is to be used as the sole induction agent for children or adults the recommended dosage regimen is 200 I.U./kg/day intravenously for 28 days.[5, 7,21, 22] When complete remissions were obtained with this regimen, they were of short duration, 1 or 3 months. Asparaginase has been used as the sole induction agent in other regimens.[6,21, 24] Physicians using a given regimen should be thoroughly familiar with its benefits and risks.

Patients undergoing induction therapy must be carefully monitored and the therapeutic regimen adjusted according to response and toxicity.

Such adjustments should always involve decreasing dosages of one or more agents of discontinuation depending on the degree of toxicity. Patients who have received a course of asparaginase, if retreated, have an increased risk of hypersensitivity reactions. Therefore, retreatment should be undertaken only when the benefit of such therapy is weighed against the increased risk.

INTRADERMAL SKIN TEST

Because of the occurrence of allergic reactions, an intradermal skin test should be performed prior to the initial administration of asparaginase and when asparaginase is given after an interval of a week or more has elapsed between doses. The skin test solution may be prepared as follows: Reconstitute the contents of a 10,000 I.U. vial with 5.0 ml of diluent. From this solution (2,000 I.U./ml) withdraw 0.1 ml and inject it into another vial containing 9.9 ml of diluent, yielding a skin test solution of approximately 20.01 I.U./ml. Use 0.1 ml of this solution (about 2.0 I.U.) for the intradermal skin test. The skin test site should be observed for at least one hour for the appearance of a wheal or erythema either of which indicates a positive reaction. An allergic reaction even to the skin test dose in certain sensitized individuals may rarely occur. A negative skin test reaction does not preclude the possibility of the development of an allergic reaction.

DESENSITIZATION

Desensitization should be performed before administering the first dose of asparaginase on initiation of therapy in positive reactors, and on retreatment of any patient in whom such therapy is deemed necessary after carefully weighing the increased risk of hypersensitivity reactions. Rapid desensitization of the patient may be attempted with progressively increasing amounts of intravenously administered asparaginase provided adequate

Cont'd

precautions are taken to treat an allergic reaction should it occur. One reported schedule[21,22] begins with a total of 1 I.U. given intravenously and doubles the dose every 10 minutes, provided no reaction has occurred, until the accumulated total amount given the planned doses for that day.

For convenience TABLE 1 is included to calculate the number of doses necessary to reach the patient's total dose that day.

***TABLE 1** Asparaginase, DOSAGE AND ADMINISTRATION*

Injection Number	Asparaginase Dose in I.U.	Accumulated Total Dose
1	1	1
2	2	3
3	4	7
4	8	15
5	16	31
6	32	63
7	64	127
8	128	255
9	256	511
10	512	1023
11	1024	2047
12	2048	4095
13	4096	8191
14	8192	16383
15	16384	32767
16	32768	65535
17	65536	131071
18	131072	262143

For example: A patient weighing 20 kg who is to receive 200 I.U./kg (total dose 4000 I.U.) would receive injections 1 through 12 during desensitization.

DIRECTIONS FOR RECONSTITUTION

Parenteral drug products should be inspected visually for particulate matter and discoloration prior to administration whenever solution and container permit. When reconstituted, asparaginase should be a clear, colorless solution. If the solution becomes cloudy, discard.

FOR INTRAVENOUS USE

Reconstitute with Sterile Water for Injection or with Sodium Chloride Injection. The volume recommended for reconstitution is 5 ml for the 10,000 unit vials. Ordinary shaking during reconstitution does not inactivate the enzyme. This solution may be used for direct intravenous administration within an eight hour period following restoration. For administration by infusion, solutions should be diluted with the isotonic solutions, Sodium Chloride or Dextrose Injection 5%. These solutions should be infused within eight hours and only if clear.

Occasionally, a very small number of gelatinous fiber-like particles may develop on standing. Filtration through a 5.0 micron filter during administration will remove the particles with no resultant loss in potency. Some loss of potency has been observed with the use of a 0.2 micron filter.

FOR INTRAMUSCULAR USE

When asparaginase is administered intramuscularly according to the schedule cited in the induction regimen, reconstitution is carried out by adding 2 ml Sodium Chloride Injection to the 10,000 unit vial. The resulting solution should be used within eight hours and only if clear.

STORAGE

Store at 2-8°C (36-46°F). Asparaginase does not contain a preservative. Unused, reconstituted solution should be stored at 2 to 8°C (36-46°F) and discarded after eight hours, or sooner if it becomes cloudy.

PRODUCT LISTING - EQUIVALENTS NOT AVAILABLE

Powder For Injection - Injectable - 10000 IU

1's $65.91 ELSPAR, Merck & Company Inc 00006-4612-00

A

Aspirin (000299)

For related information, see the comparative table section in Appendix A.

Categories: Arthritis, rheumatoid; Inflammation; Pain, mild to moderate; Pregnancy Category D; FDA Pre 1938 Drugs; WHO Formulary

Drug Classes: Analgesics, non-narcotic; Antipyretics; Salicylates

Brand Names: Acetylsalicylic Acid; Amiprine; Ascriptin; Buffered Aspirin; Dasprin; Easprin; Entaprin; Megaprin; Or-Prin; Salicylic Acid; Sloprin; Trinprin; Winsprin; **Zorprin**

Foreign Brand Availability: AAS (Argentina; Brazil; Spain); ASS (Germany); Acesal (Italy); Acetard (Denmark; Finland; Sweden); Acetosal (Israel); Adiro (Mexico; Venezuela); Albyl-E (Norway); Anacin (Israel); Anasprin (Brazil); Ansin (Taiwan); Anthrom (Philippines); Asaphen E.C. (Canada); Asapor (Finland); Asatard (South-Africa); Asawin (Colombia; Mexico; Peru); Aspa (Taiwan); Aspec (New-Zealand); Aspent (Thailand); Aspex (Israel); Aspilets (Indonesia); Aspirem (Bahamas; Barbados; Belize; Bermuda; Curacao; Guyana; Jamaica; Netherland-Antilles; Surinam; Trinidad); Aspirin (Bahrain; Benin; Burkina-Faso; Cyprus; Egypt; Ethiopia; Gambia; Ghana; Guinea; Iran; Iraq; Israel; Ivory-Coast; Jordan; Kenya; Kuwait; Lebanon; Liberia; Libya; Malawi; Mali; Mauritania; Mauritius; Morocco; Niger; Nigeria; Oman; Qatar; Republic-of-Yemen; Saudi-Arabia; Senegal; Seychelles; Sierra-Leone; Sudan; Syria; Tanzania; Tunia; Uganda; United-Arab-Emirates; Zambia; Zimbabwe); Aspirin Bayer (Hong-Kong); Aspirina (Chile; Colombia; Ecuador); Aspirisucre (France); Aspro (Australia; Austria; Belgium; Czech-Republic; England; Germany; Hungary; Ireland; Israel; Italy; Malaysia; Netherlands; New-Zealand; Portugal; Spain; Switzerland); Bayaspirina (Argentina); Bayer Aspirin (Australia); Bayer Aspirin Cardio (South-Africa); Bex (Australia); Bufferin (Italy); Bufferin Low Dose (Singapore); Caprin (England); Cardioaspirina (Colombia); Ceto (Indonesia); Claragine (France); Colfarit (Austria; Czech-Republic; Germany; Hungary; Switzerland); Comoprin (Thailand); Cortal (Philippines); Dispril (Bahrain; Belgium; Cyprus; Egypt; Iran; Iraq; Jordan; Kuwait; Lebanon; Libya; Oman; Qatar; Republic-of-Yemen; Saudi-Arabia; Sweden; Syria; United-Arab-Emirates); Disprin (Australia; Bahamas; Barbados; Belize; Benin; Bermuda; Burkina-Faso; Curacao; England; Ethiopia; Gambia; Ghana; Guinea; Guyana; Hong-Kong; India; Ireland; Ivory-Coast; Jamaica; Kenya; Liberia; Malawi; Malaysia; Mali; Mauritania; Mauritius; Morocco; Netherland-Antilles; New-Zealand; Niger; Nigeria; Senegal; Seychelles; Sierra-Leone; South-Africa; Sudan; Surinam; Tanzania; Trinidad; Tunia; Uganda; Zambia; Zimbabwe); Dusil (Malaysia); Ecotrin (Argentina; Chile; Costa-Rica; Dominican-Republic; El-Salvador; Guatemala; Honduras; New-Zealand; Nicaragua; Panama; Taiwan); Ecotrin 650 (Hong-Kong); Encine EM (Taiwan); Entrophen (Canada); Eskotrin (Venezuela); Globentyl (Denmark; Norway); Idotyl (Denmark); Melabon (Germany); NAspro (Indonesia); Novasen (Canada); Nu-Seals (Bahrain; Benin; Burkina-Faso; Cyprus; Egypt; Ethiopia; Gambia; Ghana; Guinea; Iran; Iraq; Ivory-Coast; Jordan; Kenya; Kuwait; Lebanon; Liberia; Libya; Malawi; Mali; Mauritania; Mauritius; Morocco; Niger; Nigeria; Oman; Qatar; Republic-of-Yemen; Saudi-Arabia; Senegal; Seychelles; Sierra-Leone; Sudan; Syria; Tanzania; Tunia; Uganda; United-Arab-Emirates; Zambia; Zimbabwe); Plewin (Chile); Rhonal (Argentina; Belgium; Bulgaria; Ecuador; Netherlands; Peru; Spain; Switzerland; Venezuela); Ronal (Brazil); Solprin (Australia); Spren (Australia); Tevapirin (Israel); Thrombo-Aspilets (Indonesia); Tromalyt (Colombia); V-AS (Thailand)

DESCRIPTION

Aspirin delayed-release enteric-coated tablets contain 15 grains (975 mg) aspirin for oral administration. *Also Contain:* Candelilla wax; colloidal silicon dioxide; corn starch 1500; dusty rose Opaspray; hydroxypropyl methylcellulose (15 cps); methylparaben; microcrystalline cellulose; mistron spray talc; polyethylene glycol 3350; propylparaben; stearic acid powder; vanillin; zinc stearate. The enteric coating is designed to prevent the release of aspirin in the stomach and thereby reduce gastric irritation and total occult blood loss. The pharmacologic effects of aspirin include analgesia, antipyresis, antiinflammatory activity, and antirheumatic activity.

CLINICAL PHARMACOLOGY

Aspirin is a salicylate that has demonstrated antiinflammatory, analgesic, antipyretic, and antirheumatic activity.

Aspirin's mode of action as an antiinflammatory and antirheumatic agent may be due to inhibition of synthesis and release of prostaglandins.

Aspirin appears to produce analgesia by virtue of both a peripheral and CNS effect.

Peripherally, aspirin acts by inhibiting the synthesis and release of prostaglandins. Acting centrally, it would appear to produce analgesia at a hypothalamic site in the brain, although the mode of action is not known.

Aspirin also acts on the hypothalamus to produce antipyresis; heat dissipation is increased as a result of vasodilation and increased peripheral blood flow. Aspirin's antipyretic activity may also be related to inhibition of synthesis and release of prostaglandins.

In a crossover study, aspirin at a dose of one tablet (15 grains) three times a day produced an average fecal blood loss of 1.54 ml/day. Uncoated aspirin at a dosage of three 5 grain tablets given three times a day caused an average fecal blood loss of 4.33 ml/day.

Aspirin tablets are enteric-coated. This coating acts to prevent the release of aspirin in the stomach but permits the tablet to dissolve with resultant absorption in the upper portion of the small intestine. This reduces any gastric irritation that may occur with uncoated aspirin but does delay the onset of action. Aspirin is rapidly hydrolyzed primarily in the liver to salicylic acid, which is conjugated with glycine (forming salicyluric acid) and glucuronic acid and excreted largely in the urine. As a result of the rapid hydrolysis, plasma concentrations of aspirin are always low and rarely exceed 20 mcg/ml at ordinary therapeutic doses. The peak salicylate level for uncoated aspirin occurs in about 2 hours; however with enteric-coated aspirin tablets this is delayed. A direct correlation between salicylate plasma levels and clinical analgesic effectiveness has not been definitely established, but effective analgesia is usually achieved at plasma levels of 15-30 mg/100 ml. Effective antiinflammatory activity is usually achieved at salicylate plasma levels of 20-30 mg/100 ml. There is also poor correlation between toxic symptoms and plasma salicylate concentrations, but most patients exhibit symptoms of salicylism at plasma salicylate levels of 35 mg/100 ml. The plasma half-life for aspirin is approximately 15 minutes; that for salicylate lengthens as the dose increases: Doses of 300-650 mg have a half-life of 3.1-3.2 hours; with doses of 1 g, the half-life is increased to 5 hours and with 2 g it is increased to about 9 hours.

Salicylates are excreted mainly by the kidney. Studies in man indicate that salicylate is excreted in the urine as free salicylic acid (10%), salicyluric acid (75%), salicylic phenolic (10%) and acyl (5%) glucuronides and gentisic acid (<1%).

INDICATIONS AND USAGE

Aspirin, delayed-release, enteric-coated tablets, are indicated in patients who need the higher 15 grain dose of aspirin in the long-term palliative treatment of mild to moderate pain and inflammation of arthritic and other inflammatory conditions.

NON-FDA APPROVED INDICATIONS

Aspirin is commonly used for the symptomatic treatment of pain and fever, rheumatic fever, preeclampsia, and Kawasaki's Syndrome in children, however, the FDA has approved none of these uses.

Conflicting data are available for the use of aspirin as a chemoprotective agent against colorectal cancer. Varied dosing regimens, duration of therapy, and follow-up times have been reported. An appropriate dose and duration of aspirin therapy has not been determined.

CONTRAINDICATIONS

Aspirin should not be used in patients who have previously exhibited hypersensitivity to aspirin and/or nonsteroidal antiinflammatory agents.

Aspirin should not be given to patients with a recent history of gastrointestinal bleeding or in patients with bleeding disorders (*e.g.,* hemophilia).

WARNINGS

Aspirin tablets should be used with caution when anticoagulants are prescribed concurrently, for aspirin may depress the concentration of prothrombin in plasma and thereby increase bleeding time. Large doses of salicylates have a hypoglycemic action and may enhance the effect of the oral hypoglycemics. Consequently, they should not be given concomitantly; if however, this is necessary, the dosage of the hypoglycemic agent must be reduced while the salicylate is given. This hypoglycemic action may also affect the insulin requirements of diabetics.

Although salicylates in large doses are uricosuric agents, smaller amounts may decrease the uricosuric effects of probenecid, sulfinpyrazone, and phenylbutazone.

PRECAUTIONS

GENERAL

Aspirin tablets should be administered with caution to patients with asthma, nasal polyps, or nasal allergies.

Consult a physician before giving this medicine to children, including teenagers, with chicken pox or flu.

In patients receiving large doses of aspirin and/or prolonged therapy, mild salicylate intoxication (salicylism) may develop that may be reversed by reduction in dosage.

Although the fecal blood loss with enteric-coated aspirin is less than that with uncoated aspirin tablets, enteric-coated aspirin tablets should be administered with caution to patients with a history of gastric distress, ulcer, or bleeding problems. Occult gastrointestinal bleeding occurs in many patients but is not correlated with gastric distress. The amount of blood lost is usually insignificant clinically, but with prolonged administration, it may result in iron deficiency anemia.

Sodium excretion produced by spironolactone may be decreased in the presence of salicylates.

Salicylates can produce changes in thyroid function tests.

Salicylates should be used with caution in patients with severe hepatic damage, preexisting hypoprothrombinemia, or vitamin K deficiency, and in those undergoing surgery.

USAGE IN PREGNANCY

It has been reported that adverse effects were increased in the mother and fetus following chronic ingestion of aspirin. Prolonged pregnancy and labor with increased bleeding before and after delivery, as well as decreased birth weight and increased rate of stillbirth were correlated with high blood salicylate levels. Because of possible adverse effects on the neonate and the potential for increased maternal blood loss, aspirin should be avoided during the last three months of pregnancy.

DRUG INTERACTIONS

Anticoagulants: See WARNINGS.

Hypoglycemic Agents: See WARNINGS.

Uricosuric Agents: Aspirin may decrease the effects of probenecid, sulfinpyrazone, and phenylbutazone.

Spironolactone: See PRECAUTIONS.

Alcohol: Has a synergistic effect with aspirin in causing gastrointestinal bleeding.

Corticosteroids: Concomitant administration with aspirin may increase the risk of gastrointestinal ulceration and may reduce serum salicylate levels.

Pyrazolone Derivatives (phenylbutazone, oxyphenbutazone, and possibly dipyrone): Concomitant administration with aspirin may increase the risk of gastrointestinal ulceration.

Nonsteroidal Antiinflammatory Agents: Aspirin is contraindicated in patients who are hypersensitive to nonsteroidal antiinflammatory agents.

Urinary Alkalinizers: Decrease aspirin effectiveness by increasing the rate of salicylate renal excretion.

Phenobarbital: Decreases aspirin effectiveness by enzyme induction.

Phenytoin: Serum phenytoin levels may be increased by aspirin.

Propranolol: May decrease aspirin's antiinflammatory action by competing for the same receptors.

Antacids: Enteric-coated aspirin should not be given concurrently with antacids, since an increase in the pH of the stomach may effect the enteric coating of the tablets.

ADVERSE REACTIONS

Gastrointestinal: Dyspepsia, thirst, nausea, vomiting, diarrhea, acute reversible hepatotoxicity, gastrointestinal bleeding, and/or ulceration.

Special Senses: Tinnitus, vertigo, reversible hearing loss, and dimness of vision.

Hematologic: Prolongation of bleeding time, leukopenia, thrombocytopenia, purpura, decreased plasma iron concentration and shortened erythrocyte survival time.

Dermatologic and Hypersensitivity: Urticaria, angioedema, pruritus, sweating, various skin eruptions, asthma, and anaphylaxis.

Neurologic: Mental confusion, drowsiness, and dizziness.

Body as a Whole: Headache and fever.

DOSAGE AND ADMINISTRATION

Usual Adult Dosage: One tablet 3-4 times daily.

Patients who have displayed no significant adverse effects on a long term qid regimen and who receive a total daily dosage of aspirin no greater than 3.9 g may be considered for a bid regimen (2 tablets of enteric-coated aspirin twice daily). Patients on the bid enteric-coated aspirin regimen should be closely monitored for serum salicylate levels, increased incidence of CNS-related adverse effects, increased fecal blood loss, or any other signs or symptoms suggestive of significant blood loss.

If necessary, dosage may be increased until relief is obtained, but dosage should be maintained slightly below that which produces tinnitus. Plasma salicylate levels may also be helpful in determining proper dosage (see CLINICAL PHARMACOLOGY).

Storage: Store at controlled room temperature 15-30°C (59-86°F).

PRODUCT LISTING - RATED THERAPEUTICALLY EQUIVALENT

Tablet - Oral - Buffered 325 mg

30's	$2.00	GENERIC, Heartland Healthcare Services	61392-0033-30
30's	$2.00	GENERIC, Heartland Healthcare Services	61392-0033-39
31's	$2.07	GENERIC, Heartland Healthcare Services	61392-0033-31
32's	$2.14	GENERIC, Heartland Healthcare Services	61392-0033-32
60's	$4.00	GENERIC, Heartland Healthcare Services	61392-0033-60
60's	$4.00	GENERIC, Heartland Healthcare Services	61392-0033-65
90's	$6.00	GENERIC, Heartland Healthcare Services	61392-0033-95

Tablet, Chewable - Oral - 81 mg

30's	$2.07	GENERIC, Heartland Healthcare Services	61392-0032-30
30's	$2.07	GENERIC, Heartland Healthcare Services	61392-0032-39
31's	$2.14	GENERIC, Heartland Healthcare Services	61392-0032-31
32's	$2.20	GENERIC, Heartland Healthcare Services	61392-0032-32
60's	$4.13	GENERIC, Heartland Healthcare Services	61392-0032-60
60's	$4.13	GENERIC, Heartland Healthcare Services	61392-0032-65

Tablet, Enteric Coated - Oral - 81 mg

30's	$2.43	GENERIC, Heartland Healthcare Services	61392-0096-30
30's	$2.43	GENERIC, Heartland Healthcare Services	61392-0096-39
31's	$2.51	GENERIC, Heartland Healthcare Services	61392-0096-31
32's	$2.59	GENERIC, Heartland Healthcare Services	61392-0096-32
60's	$4.86	GENERIC, Heartland Healthcare Services	61392-0096-60

Tablet, Enteric Coated - Oral - 975 mg

100's	$59.15	EASPRIN, Lotus Biochemical Corporation	59417-0975-71

PRODUCT LISTING - EQUIVALENTS NOT AVAILABLE

Tablet, Enteric Coated - Oral - 975 mg

50's	$1.76	GENERIC, Time Cap Laboratories Inc	49483-0224-05
100's	$8.19	GENERIC, Time Cap Laboratories Inc	49483-0224-01
100's	$12.84	GENERIC, Marlex Pharmaceuticals	10135-0174-01
100's	$15.32	GENERIC, Caraco Pharmaceutical Laboratories	57664-0186-08

Tablet, Extended Release - Oral - 800 mg

100's	$7.66	GENERIC, Major Pharmaceuticals Inc	00904-0585-60
100's	$8.03	GENERIC, Moore, H.L. Drug Exchange Inc	00839-7269-06
100's	$9.00	GENERIC, Aligen Independent Laboratories Inc	00405-4100-01
100's	$13.49	GENERIC, Cheshire Drugs	55175-1693-00
100's	$58.68	ZORPRIN, Par Pharmaceutical Inc	49884-0057-01
100's	$80.64	GENERIC, Mutual/United Research Laboratories	00677-1799-01
100's	$98.49	ZORPRIN, Par Pharmaceutical Inc	49884-0657-01

Tablet, Extended Release - Oral - 975 mg

100's	$11.48	GENERIC, Moore, H.L. Drug Exchange Inc	00839-7404-06
100's	$13.20	GENERIC, Ivax Corporation	00182-1065-01
100's	$13.31	GENERIC, Invamed Inc	52189-0220-24
100's	$13.40	GENERIC, Major Pharmaceuticals Inc	00904-5212-60
100's	$14.50	GENERIC, Major Pharmaceuticals Inc	00904-0582-60

Aspirin; Butalbital; Caffeine (000304)

For complete prescribing information, refer to the CD-ROM included with the book.

Categories: Headache, tension; DEA Class CIII; Pregnancy Category C; FDA Approved 1983 Aug
Drug Classes: Analgesics, non-narcotic
Brand Names: Butal Compound; Farbital; **Fiorinal**; Fiormor; Fiortal; Fortabs; Idenal; Isollyl; Laniroif; Lanorinal; Tecnal; Trianal
Cost of Therapy: $24.36 (Headache; Fiorinal; 325 mg; 50 mg; 40 mg; 6 tablets/day; 7 day supply)
$1.55 (Headache; Generic Tablets; 325 mg; 50 mg; 40 mg; 6 tablets/day; 7 day supply)

DESCRIPTION

Each Fiorinal tablet/capsule for oral administration contains: Butalbital 50 mg (*Warning:* May be habit-forming); aspirin, 325 mg; caffeine, 40 mg.

Butalbital, 5-allyl-5-isobutyl-barbituric acid, has an empirical formula of $C_{11}H_{16}N_2O_3$ and a molecular weight of 224.26.

Aspirin, benzoic acid, 2-(acetyloxy)-, has an empirical formula of $C_9H_8O_4$ and a molecular weight of 180.16.

Caffeine, 1, 3, 7-trimethylxanthine, has an empirical formula of $C_8H_{10}N_4O_2$ and a molecular weight of 194.19.

TABLETS

Active Ingredients: Aspirin, butalbital, and caffeine.

Inactive Ingredients: Alginic acid, lactose, microcrystalline cellulose, povidone, stearic acid, and another ingredient.

CAPSULES

Active Ingredients: Aspirin, butalbital, and caffeine.

Inactive Ingredients: D&C yellow no. 10, gelatin, microcrystalline cellulose, sodium lauryl sulfate, starch, and talc.

May Also Include: Benzyl alcohol, butylparaben, color additives including FD&C blue no. 1, FD&C green no. 3, FD&C yellow no. 6, edetate calcium disodium, methylparaben, propylparaben, silicon dioxide, and sodium propionate.

INDICATIONS AND USAGE

Butalbital; aspirin; caffeine is indicated for the relief of the symptom complex of tension (or muscle contraction) headache. Evidence supporting the efficacy and safety of butalbital; aspirin; caffeine in the treatment of multiple recurrent headaches is unavailable. Caution in this regard is required because butalbital is habit-forming and potentially abusable.

CONTRAINDICATIONS

Butalbital; Aspirin; Caffeine is Contraindicated Under the Following Conditions:

1. Hypersensitivity or intolerance to aspirin, caffeine, or butalbital.
2. Patients with a hemorrhagic diathesis (*e.g.,* hemophilia, hypoprothrombinemia, von Willebrand's disease, the thrombocytopenias, thrombasthenia and other ill-defined hereditary platelet dysfunctions, severe vitamin K deficiency and severe liver damage).
3. Patients with the syndrome of nasal polyps, angioedema and bronchospastic reactivity to aspirin or other nonsteroidal anti-inflammatory drugs. Anaphylactoid reactions have occurred in such patients.
4. Peptic ulcer or other serious gastrointestinal lesions.
5. Patients with porphyria.

WARNINGS

Therapeutic doses of aspirin can cause anaphylactic shock and other severe allergic reactions. It should be ascertained if the patient is allergic to aspirin, although a specific history of allergy may be lacking.

Significant bleeding can result from aspirin therapy in patients with peptic ulcer or other gastrointestinal lesions, and in patients with bleeding disorders. Aspirin administered preoperatively may prolong the bleeding time. Butalbital is habit-forming and potentially abusable. Consequently, the extended use of butalbital; aspirin; caffeine is not recommended. Results from epidemiologic studies indicate an association between aspirin and Reye's Syndrome. Caution should be used in administering this product to children, including teenagers, with chicken pox or flu.

DOSAGE AND ADMINISTRATION

One (1) or 2 tablets or capsules every 4 hours. Total daily dose should not exceed 6 tablets or capsules.

Extended and repeated use of this product is not recommended because of the potential for physical dependence.

PRODUCT LISTING - RATED THERAPEUTICALLY EQUIVALENT

Capsule - Oral - 325 mg;50 mg;40 mg

100's	$37.13	GENERIC, Moore, H.L. Drug Exchange Inc	00839-7047-06
100's	$37.99	GENERIC, Ivax Corporation	00182-0140-01
100's	$38.90	GENERIC, Creighton Products Corporation	50752-0278-05
100's	$39.70	GENERIC, Aligen Independent Laboratories Inc	00405-0029-01
100's	$75.92	GENERIC, Major Pharmaceuticals Inc	00904-3934-60
100's	$89.00	GENERIC, Lannett Company Inc	00527-1552-01
100's	$100.12	FIORINAL, Novartis Pharmaceuticals	00078-0103-05

Tablet - Oral - 325 mg;50 mg;40 mg

100's	$4.46	GENERIC, Geneva Pharmaceuticals	00781-1435-01
100's	$4.58	GENERIC, Aligen Independent Laboratories Inc	00405-0028-01
100's	$5.63	GENERIC, Interstate Drug Exchange Inc	00814-3822-14
100's	$6.75	GENERIC, Watson/Schein Pharmaceuticals Inc	00364-0677-01
100's	$6.95	GENERIC, Moore, H.L. Drug Exchange Inc	00839-6733-06
100's	$7.10	GENERIC, Creighton Products Corporation	50752-0277-05
100's	$15.00	GENERIC, Auro Pharmaceutical	55829-0815-10
100's	$15.25	GENERIC, Ivax Corporation	00182-1631-01
100's	$64.20	GENERIC, Major Pharmaceuticals Inc	00904-3892-60
100's	$70.25	GENERIC, West Ward Pharmaceutical Corporation	00143-1785-01
100's	$71.27	GENERIC, Qualitest Products Inc	00603-2550-21
100's	$79.40	GENERIC, Qualitest Products Inc	00603-2548-21
100's	$103.60	GENERIC, Purepac Pharmaceutical Company	00228-2023-10

PRODUCT LISTING - EQUIVALENTS NOT AVAILABLE

Tablet - Oral - 325 mg;50 mg;40 mg

6's	$4.94	GENERIC, Prescript Pharmaceuticals	00247-0214-06
9's	$5.74	GENERIC, Prescript Pharmaceuticals	00247-0214-09
10's	$4.78	GENERIC, Southwood Pharmaceuticals Inc	58016-0233-10
12's	$5.73	GENERIC, Southwood Pharmaceuticals Inc	58016-0233-12
12's	$6.53	GENERIC, Prescript Pharmaceuticals	00247-0214-12
14's	$6.69	GENERIC, Southwood Pharmaceuticals Inc	58016-0233-14
15's	$7.16	GENERIC, Southwood Pharmaceuticals Inc	58016-0233-15
15's	$7.33	GENERIC, Prescript Pharmaceuticals	00247-0214-15
20's	$8.65	GENERIC, Prescript Pharmaceuticals	00247-0214-20
20's	$9.55	GENERIC, Southwood Pharmaceuticals Inc	58016-0233-20
21's	$10.03	GENERIC, Southwood Pharmaceuticals Inc	58016-0233-21
24's	$11.46	GENERIC, Southwood Pharmaceuticals Inc	58016-0233-24
25's	$9.98	GENERIC, Prescript Pharmaceuticals	00247-0214-25
25's	$11.94	GENERIC, Southwood Pharmaceuticals Inc	58016-0233-25

28's	$10.76	GENERIC, Prescript Pharmaceuticals	00247-0214-28
28's	$13.37	GENERIC, Southwood Pharmaceuticals Inc	58016-0233-28
30's	$11.29	GENERIC, Prescript Pharmaceuticals	00247-0214-30
30's	$14.33	GENERIC, Southwood Pharmaceuticals Inc	58016-0233-30
40's	$19.10	GENERIC, Southwood Pharmaceuticals Inc	58016-0233-40
50's	$23.25	GENERIC, Southwood Pharmaceuticals Inc	58016-0233-50
60's	$28.66	GENERIC, Southwood Pharmaceuticals Inc	58016-0233-60
100's	$29.82	GENERIC, Prescript Pharmaceuticals	00247-0214-00
100's	$46.50	GENERIC, Southwood Pharmaceuticals Inc	58016-0233-00

Aspirin; Butalbital; Caffeine; Codeine Phosphate *(000302)*

For complete prescribing information, refer to the CD-ROM included with the book.

Categories: Headache, tension; DEA Class CIII; FDA Approved 1990 Oct; Pregnancy Category C
Drug Classes: Analgesics, narcotic
Brand Names: Ascomp W/Codeine; B-A-C #3; **Fiorinal W Codeine**; Idenal; Isobutal; Tecnal C 1/4; Tecnal C 1/2; Trianal C 1/4; Trianal C 1/2
Foreign Brand Availability: Fiorinal-C 1 4 (Canada); Fiorinal-C 1 2 (Canada)
Cost of Therapy: $88.12 (Headache; Fiorinal with Codeine; 325 mg; 50 mg; 40 mg; 30 mg; 6 capsules/day; 7 day supply)
$39.37 (Headache; Generic Capsules; 325 mg; 50 mg; 40 mg; 30 mg; 6 capsules/day; 7 day supply)

DESCRIPTION

Fiorinal with Codeine is supplied in capsule form for oral administration.

Each capsule contains:

Codeine Phosphate: 30 mg.
Butalbital: 50 mg.
Caffeine: 40 mg.
Aspirin: 325 mg.

Codeine phosphate [morphine-3-methyl ether phosphate (1:1) (salt) hemihydrate. $C_{18}H_{24}NO_7P$, anhydrous mw 397.37], is a narcotic analgesic and antitussive.

Butalbital (5-allyl-5-isobutylbarbituric acid, $C_{11}H_{16}N_2O_3$, mw 224.26), is a short- to intermediate-acting barbiturate.

Caffeine (1,3,7-trimethylxanthine, $C_8H_{10}N_4O_2$, mw 194.19), is a central nervous system stimulant.

Aspirin is benzoic acid, 2-(acetyloxy)-, $C_9H_8O_4$, mw 180.16, is an analgesic, antipyretic, anti-inflammatory.

Inactive Ingredients: D&C yellow no. 10, FD&C blue no. 1, FD&C red no. 3, FD&C yellow no. 6, gelatin, microcrystalline cellulose, sodium lauryl sulfate, starch, talc, titanium dioxide.

May Also Include: Benzyl alcohol, butylparaben, edetate calcium disodium, glycerin, methylparaben, propylparaben, silicon dioxide, sodium propionate.

INDICATIONS AND USAGE

Aspirin; butalbital; caffeine; codeine phosphate is indicated for the relief of the symptom complex of tension (or muscle contraction) headache.

Evidence supporting the efficacy of aspirin; butalbital; caffeine; codeine phosphate is derived from 2 multi-clinic trials that compared patients with tension headache randomly assigned to 4 parallel treatments: Fiorinal (aspirin, butalbital, caffeine, codeine phosphate), codeine, Fiorinal with Codeine (aspirin, butalbital, and caffeine), and placebo. Response was assessed over the course of the first 4 hours of each of 2 distinct headaches, separated by at least 24 hours. Aspirin; butalbital; caffeine; codeine phosphate proved statistically significantly superior to each of its components [(aspirin; butalbital; caffeine), codeine] and to placebo on measures of pain relief.

Evidence supporting the efficacy and safety of aspirin; butalbital; caffeine; codeine phosphate in the treatment of multiple recurrent headaches is unavailable. Caution in this regard is required because codeine and butalbital are habit-forming and potentially abusable.

CONTRAINDICATIONS

Aspirin; Butalbital; Caffeine; Codeine Phosphate is contraindicated under the following conditions:

- Hypersensitivity or intolerance to aspirin, caffeine, butalbital or codeine.
- Patients with a hemorrhagic diathesis (*e.g.,* hemophilia, hypoprothrombinemia, von Willebrand's disease, the thrombocytopenias, thrombasthenia and other ill-defined hereditary platelet dysfunctions, severe vitamin K deficiency and severe liver damage).
- Patients with the syndrome of nasal polyps, angioedema and bronchospastic reactivity to aspirin or other non-steroidal anti-inflammatory drugs. Anaphylactoid reactions have occurred in such patients.
- Peptic ulcer or other serious gastrointestinal lesions.
- Patients with porphyria.

WARNINGS

Therapeutic doses of aspirin can cause anaphylactic shock and other severe allergic reactions. It should be ascertained if the patient is allergic to aspirin, although a specific history of allergy may be lacking.

Significant bleeding can result from aspirin therapy in patients with peptic ulcer or other gastrointestinal lesions, and in patients with bleeding disorders.

Aspirin administered pre-operatively may prolong the bleeding time.

In the presence of head injury or other intracranial lesions, the respiratory depressant effects of codeine and other narcotics may be markedly enhanced, as well as their capacity for elevating cerebrospinal fluid pressure. Narcotics also produce other CNS depressant effects, such as drowsiness, that may further obscure the clinical course of patients with head injuries.

Codeine or other narcotics may obscure signs on which to judge the diagnosis or clinical course of patients with acute abdominal conditions.

Butalbital and codeine are both habit-forming and potentially abusable. Consequently, the extended use of aspirin; butalbital; caffeine; codeine phosphate is not recommended.

Results from epidemiologic studies indicate an association between aspirin and Reye's Syndrome. Caution should be used in administering this product to children, including teenagers, with chicken pox or flu.

DOSAGE AND ADMINISTRATION

One (1) or 2 capsules every 4 hours. Total daily dosage should not exceed 6 capsules.

Extended and repeated use of this product is not recommended because of the potential for physical dependence.

PRODUCT LISTING - RATED THERAPEUTICALLY EQUIVALENT

Capsule - Oral - 325 mg;50 mg;40 mg;30 mg

100's	$93.61	GENERIC, Qualitest Products Inc	00603-2549-21
100's	$93.74	GENERIC, Ivax Corporation	00182-0036-01
100's	$93.74	GENERIC, Major Pharmaceuticals Inc	00904-5140-60
100's	$133.13	GENERIC, Duramed Pharmaceuticals Inc	51285-0684-02
100's	$138.00	GENERIC, Lannett Company Inc	00527-1312-01
100's	$140.16	GENERIC, Watson Laboratories Inc	00591-0425-01
100's	$140.16	GENERIC, Watson Laboratories Inc	52544-0425-01
100's	$141.03	GENERIC, Endo Laboratories Llc	60951-0675-70
100's	$209.82	FIORINAL WITH CODEINE, Novartis Pharmaceuticals	00078-0107-05

PRODUCT LISTING - EQUIVALENTS NOT AVAILABLE

Capsule - Oral - 325 mg;50 mg;40 mg;30 mg

6's	$10.42	GENERIC, Prescript Pharmaceuticals	00247-0337-06
10's	$15.13	GENERIC, Prescript Pharmaceuticals	00247-0337-10
12's	$17.49	GENERIC, Prescript Pharmaceuticals	00247-0337-12
15's	$21.02	GENERIC, Prescript Pharmaceuticals	00247-0337-15
16's	$22.20	GENERIC, Prescript Pharmaceuticals	00247-0337-16
20's	$26.92	GENERIC, Prescript Pharmaceuticals	00247-0337-20
24's	$31.62	GENERIC, Prescript Pharmaceuticals	00247-0337-24
25's	$32.80	GENERIC, Prescript Pharmaceuticals	00247-0337-25
30's	$38.69	GENERIC, Prescript Pharmaceuticals	00247-0337-30
50's	$62.25	GENERIC, Prescript Pharmaceuticals	00247-0337-50
100's	$121.15	GENERIC, Prescript Pharmaceuticals	00247-0337-00
100's	$139.95	GENERIC, Breckenridge Inc	51991-0074-01

Aspirin; Caffeine; Dihydrocodeine Bitartrate *(000306)*

Categories: Pain, moderate to moderately severe; DEA Class CIII; FDA Approved 1983 Sep; Pregnancy Category C
Drug Classes: Analgesics, narcotic; Salicylates
Brand Names: Dihydrocodeine Compound; Synalgos-Dc
Cost of Therapy: $100.50 (Pain; Synalgos DC; 356.4 mg; 30 mg; 16 mg; 12 capsules/day; 7 day supply)

DESCRIPTION

Note: The trade name has been used throughout this monograph for clarity.

Each Synalgos-DC capsule contains 16 mg drocode (dihydrocodeine) bitartrate (Warning — may be habit-forming), 356.4 mg aspirin, and 30 mg caffeine.

The inactive ingredients present are alginic acid, cellulose, D&C red 28, FD&C blue 1, gelatin, iron oxides, stearic acid, and titanium dioxide.

CLINICAL PHARMACOLOGY

Dihydrocodeine is a semisynthetic narcotic analgesic, related to codeine, with multiple actions qualitatively similar to those of codeine; the most prominent of these involve the central nervous system and organs with smooth-muscle components. The principal action of therapeutic value is analgesia.

Synalgos-DC also contains the nonnarcotic antipyreticanalgesic, aspirin.

INDICATIONS AND USAGE

For the relief of moderate to moderately severe pain.

CONTRAINDICATIONS

Hypersensitivity to dihydrocodeine, codeine, or aspirin.

WARNINGS

Salicylates should be used with extreme caution in the presence of peptic ulcer or coagulation abnormalities.

DRUG DEPENDENCE

Dihydrocodeine can produce drug dependence of the codeine type and therefore has the potential of being abused. Psychic dependence, physical dependence, and tolerance may develop upon repeated administration of dihydrocodeine, and it should be prescribed and administered with the same degree of caution appropriate to the use of other oral narcotic-containing medications.

Like other narcotic-containing medications, dihydrocodeine is subject to the provisions of the Federal Controlled Substances Act.

USAGE IN AMBULATORY PATIENTS

Dihydrocodeine may impair the mental and/or physical abilities required for the performance of potentially hazardous tasks, such as driving a car or operating machinery. The patient using Synalgos-DC should be cautioned accordingly.

INTERACTIONS WITH OTHER CENTRAL NERVOUS SYSTEM DEPRESSANTS

Patients receiving other narcotic analgesics, general anesthetics, tranquilizers, sedative-hypnotics, or other CNS depressants (including alcohol) concomitantly with Synalgos-DC may exhibit an additive CNS depression. When such combined therapy is contemplated, the dose of 1 or both agents should be reduced.

USE IN PREGNANCY

Reproduction studies have not been performed in animals. There is no adequate information on whether this drug may affect fertility in human males and females or has a teratogenic potential or other adverse effect on the fetus.

USE IN CHILDREN

Preparations containing aspirin should be kept out of the reach of children. Synalgos-DC is not recommended for patients 12 years of age and under. Since there is no experience in children who have received this drug, safety and efficacy in children have not been established.

PRECAUTIONS

Synalgos-DC should be given with caution to certain patients, such as the elderly or debilitated.

DRUG INTERACTIONS

The CNS-depressant effects of Synalgos-DC may be additive with that of other CNS depressants.

See WARNINGS.

Aspirin may enhance the effects of anticoagulants and inhibit the uricosuric effects of uricosuric agents.

GERIATRIC USE

Clinical studies of Synalgos-DC did not include sufficient numbers of subjects aged 65 and over to determine whether elderly subjects respond differently from younger subjects.

In general, dose selection for an elderly patient should be cautious, starting at the low end of the dosing range, reflecting the greater frequency of decreased hepatic, renal, or cardiac function, and of concomitant disease or other drug therapy.

ADVERSE REACTIONS

The most frequently observed reactions include light-headedness, dizziness, drowsiness, sedation, nausea, vomiting, constipation, pruritus, and skin reactions.

DOSAGE AND ADMINISTRATION

Dosage should be adjusted according to the severity of the pain and the response of the patient. Synalgos-DC is given orally. The usual adult dose is 2 capsules every 4 hours as needed for pain.

HOW SUPPLIED

Synalgos-DC capsules are blue and gray, marked "WFHC" and "4191".

Storage: Store at room temperature, approx. 25°C (77°F).

Keep tightly closed.

Dispense in tight container.

PRODUCT LISTING - EQUIVALENTS NOT AVAILABLE

Capsule - Oral - 356.4 mg;30 mg;16 mg

12 x 3	$41.33	SYNALGOS-DC, Women First Healthcare	64248-0419-12
15's	$14.19	GENERIC, Southwood Pharmaceuticals Inc	58016-0262-16
100's	$119.64	SYNALGOS-DC, Wyeth-Ayerst Laboratories	00008-4191-01
100's	$131.60	SYNALGOS-DC, Women First Healthcare	64248-0419-10

Aspirin; Caffeine; Propoxyphene Hydrochloride (000311)

For complete prescribing information, refer to the CD-ROM included with the book.

Categories: Fever with pain; Pain, mild to moderate; DEA Class CIV; FDA Approved 1983 Mar; Pregnancy Category C; Pregnancy Category D, 3rd Trimester

Drug Classes: Analgesics, narcotic; Salicylates

Brand Names: 692; Cotanal-65; **Darvon Compound**; Dibagesic; Doloxene Compound; Propoxyphene Compound

Cost of Therapy: $25.28 (Pain; Darvon Compound-65; 389 mg; 32.4 mg; 65 mg; 6 capsules/day; 7 day supply)
$9.68 (Pain; Generic Capsules; 389 mg; 32.4 mg; 65 mg; 6 capsules/day; 7 day supply)

DESCRIPTION

Propoxyphene hydrochloride is an odorless, white crystalline powder with a bitter taste. It is freely soluble in water. Chemically, it is (2*S*,3*R*)-(+) -4-(Dimethylamino)-3-methyl-1,2-diphenyl-2-butanol propionate (ester) hydrochloride.

Its molecular weight is 375.94.

Each Pulvule contains 65 mg (172.9 μmol) propoxyphene hydrochloride, 389 mg (2159 μmol) aspirin, and 32.4 mg (166.8 μmol) caffeine.

It also contains FD&C red no. 3, FD&C yellow no. 6, gelatin, glutamic acid hydrochloride, iron oxide, kaolin, silicone, titanium dioxide, and other inactive ingredients.

INDICATIONS AND USAGE

This product is indicated for the relief of mild to moderate pain, either when pain is present alone or when it is accompanied by fever.

CONTRAINDICATIONS

Hypersensitivity to propoxyphene, aspirin, or caffeine.

WARNINGS

Do not prescribe propoxyphene for patients who are suicidal or addiction-prone.

Prescribe propoxyphene with caution for patients taking tranquilizers or antidepressant drugs and patients who use alcohol in excess.

Tell your patients not to exceed the recommended dose and to limit their intake of alcohol.

Propoxyphene products in excessive doses, either alone or in combination with other CNS depressants, including alcohol, are a major cause of drug-related deaths. Fatalities within the first hour of overdosage are not uncommon. In a survey of deaths due to overdosage conducted in 1975, in approximately 20% of the fatal cases, death occurred within the first hour (5% occurred within 15 minutes). Propoxyphene should not be taken in doses higher than those recommended by the physician. The judicious prescribing of propoxyphene is essential to the safe use of this drug. With patients who are depressed or suicidal, consideration should be given to the use of non-narcotic analgesics. Patients should be cautioned about the concomitant use of propoxyphene products and alcohol because of potentially serious CNS-additive effects of these agents. Because of its added depressant effects, propoxyphene should be prescribed with caution for those patients whose medical condition requires the concomitant administration of sedatives, tranquilizers, muscle relaxants, antidepressants, or other CNS-depressant drugs. Patients should be advised of the additive depressant effects of these combinations.

Many of the propoxyphene-related deaths have occurred in patients with previous histories of emotional disturbances or suicidal ideation or attempts as well as histories of misuse of tranquilizers, alcohol, and other CNS-active drugs. Some deaths have occurred as a consequence of the accidental ingestion of excessive quantities of propoxyphene alone or in combination with other drugs. Patients taking propoxyphene should be warned not to exceed the dosage recommended by the physician.

Drug Dependence: Propoxyphene, when taken in higher-than-recommended doses over long periods of time, can produce drug dependence characterized by psychic dependence and, less frequently, physical dependence and tolerance. Propoxyphene will only partially suppress the withdrawal syndrome in individuals physically dependent on morphine or other narcotics. The abuse liability of propoxyphene is qualitatively similar to that of codeine although quantitatively less, and propoxyphene should be prescribed with the same degree of caution appropriate to the use of codeine.

Usage in Ambulatory Patients: Propoxyphene may impair the mental and/or physical abilities required for the performance of potentially hazardous tasks, such as driving a car or operating machinery. The patients should be cautioned accordingly.

Warning: Reye Syndrome is a rare but serious disease which can follow flu or chicken pox in children and teenagers. While the cause of Reye Syndrome is unknown, some reports claim aspirin (or salicylates) may increase the risk of developing this disease.

DOSAGE AND ADMINISTRATION

This product is given orally. The usual dosage is 65 mg propoxyphene HCl, 389 mg aspirin, and 32.4 mg caffeine every 4 hours as needed for pain.

The maximum recommended dose of propoxyphene HCl is 390 mg/day.

Consideration should be given to a reduced total daily dosage in patients with hepatic or renal impairment.

PRODUCT LISTING - RATED THERAPEUTICALLY EQUIVALENT

Capsule - Oral - 389 mg;32.4 mg;65 mg

12's	$4.13	GENERIC, Southwood Pharmaceuticals Inc	58016-0215-12
15's	$4.88	GENERIC, Southwood Pharmaceuticals Inc	58016-0215-15
20's	$6.88	GENERIC, Southwood Pharmaceuticals Inc	58016-0215-20
28's	$6.61	GENERIC, Southwood Pharmaceuticals Inc	58016-0215-28
30's	$10.31	GENERIC, Southwood Pharmaceuticals Inc	58016-0215-30
100's	$12.23	GENERIC, Interstate Drug Exchange Inc	00814-6460-14
100's	$13.50	GENERIC, Alra	51641-0323-01
100's	$20.30	GENERIC, Geneva Pharmaceuticals	00781-2367-01
100's	$23.10	GENERIC, Qualitest Products Inc	00603-5460-21
100's	$23.20	GENERIC, Major Pharmaceuticals Inc	00904-7701-60
100's	$23.27	GENERIC, Moore, H.L. Drug Exchange Inc	00839-1561-06
100's	$25.00	GENERIC, Alra	51641-0323-11
100's	$25.79	GENERIC, Aligen Independent Laboratories Inc	00405-0173-01
100's	$25.95	GENERIC, Ivax Corporation	00182-1673-01
100's	$34.38	GENERIC, Southwood Pharmaceuticals Inc	58016-0215-00
100's	$60.18	DARVON COMPOUND-65, Lilly, Eli and Company	00002-3111-02

PRODUCT LISTING - EQUIVALENTS NOT AVAILABLE

Capsule - Oral - 389 mg;32.4 mg;65 mg

100's	$39.10	GENERIC, Mylan Pharmaceuticals Inc	00378-0131-01

A

Aspirin; Codeine Phosphate *(000317)*

For complete prescribing information, refer to the CD-ROM included with the book.

Categories: Pain, mild; Pain, moderate; Pain, moderate to severe; Pregnancy Category C; DEA Class CIII; FDA Pre 1938 Drugs
Drug Classes: Analgesics, narcotic; Salicylates
Brand Names: Aspirin W/Codeine; Codral; Dolviron; Emcodeine; **Empirin W Codeine**
Foreign Brand Availability: Aspalgin (Australia); Codiphen (Australia); Codis (Australia; Bahamas; Bahrain; Barbados; Belize; Bermuda; Curacao; Cyprus; Egypt; Guyana; Iran; Iraq; Jamaica; Jordan; Kuwait; Lebanon; Libya; Netherland-Antilles; Oman; Qatar; Republic-of-Yemen; Saudi-Arabia; Surinam; Syria; Trinidad; United-Arab-Emirates); Codis 500 (Bahrain; Cyprus; Egypt; Iran; Iraq; Jordan; Kuwait; Lebanon; Libya; Oman; Qatar; Republic-of-Yemen; Saudi-Arabia; Syria; United-Arab-Emirates); Codral Forte (Australia); Disprin Forte (Australia); Rokanite (Israel); Solcode (Australia)
Cost of Therapy: $3.34 (Pain; Generic Tablets; 325 mg; 30 mg; 6 tablets/day; 7 day supply)

DESCRIPTION

Empirin with Codeine is supplied in tablet form for oral administration. Each tablet contains aspirin 325 mg, codeine phosphate in one of the following strengths: no. 3, 30 mg and no. 4, 60 mg (*Warning:* may be habit-forming), and the inactive ingredients colloidal silicon dioxide, microcrystalline cellulose, potato starch, and stearic acid.

Empirin with Codeine has analgesic, antipyretic and anti-inflammatory effects.

The components of Empirin with Codeine have the following chemical names:

a. Aspirin: 2-(acetyloxy)benzoic acid
b. Codeine phosphate: (5α,6α)-7,8-didehydro-4,5-epoxy-3-methoxy-17-methylmorphinan-6-ol phosphate (1:1) (salt) hemihydrate

INDICATIONS AND USAGE

Aspirin; codeine phosphate is indicated for the relief of mild, moderate, and moderate to severe pain.

CONTRAINDICATIONS

Aspirin; codeine phosphate is contraindicated under the following conditions:

1. Hypersensitivity or intolerance to aspirin or codeine.
2. Severe bleeding, disorders of coagulation or primary hemostasis, including hemophilia, hypoprothrombinemia, von Willebrand's disease, the thrombocytopenias, thrombasthenia and other ill-defined hereditary platelet dysfunctions, as well as such associated conditions as severe vitamin K deficiency and severe liver damage.
3. Anticoagulant therapy.
4. Peptic ulcer, or other serious gastrointestinal lesions.
5. Children or teenagers with the symptoms of chicken pox or influenza. Reye's Syndrome has been reported to be associated with aspirin use in this population.

WARNINGS

Therapeutic doses of aspirin can cause anaphylactic shock and other severe allergic reactions. A history of allergy is often lacking.

Significant bleeding can result from aspirin therapy in patients with peptic ulcer or other gastrointestinal lesions, and in patients with bleeding disorders. Aspirin administered preoperatively may prolong the bleeding time.

In the presence of head injury or other intracranial lesions, the respiratory depressant effects of codeine and other narcotics may be markedly enhanced, as well as their capacity for elevating cerebrospinal fluid pressure. Narcotics also produce other CNS depressant effects, such as drowsiness that may further obscure the clinical course of patients with head injuries.

Codeine or other narcotics may obscure signs on which to judge the diagnosis or clinical course of patients with acute abdominal conditions.

DOSAGE AND ADMINISTRATION

Dosage is adjusted according to the severity of pain and the response of the patient. It may occasionally be necessary to exceed the usual dosage recommended below when pain is severe or the patient has become tolerant to the analgesic effect of codeine. Aspirin; codeine phosphate is given orally. The usual adult dose for aspirin; codeine phosphate No. 3 is 1 or 2 tablets every 4 hours as required. The usual adult dose for aspirin; codeine phosphate No. 4 is 1 tablet every 4 hours as required.

Aspirin; codeine phosphate should be taken with food or a full glass of milk or water to lessen gastric irritation.

PRODUCT LISTING - EQUIVALENTS NOT AVAILABLE

Tablet - Oral - 325 mg;15 mg

100's	$8.25	GENERIC, Interstate Drug Exchange Inc	00814-0925-14

Tablet - Oral - 325 mg;30 mg

4's	$3.62	GENERIC, Prescript Pharmaceuticals	00247-0125-04
6's	$3.75	GENERIC, Prescript Pharmaceuticals	00247-0125-06
10's	$4.01	GENERIC, Prescript Pharmaceuticals	00247-0125-10
12's	$1.35	GENERIC, Allscripts Pharmaceutical Company	54569-0300-00
12's	$4.15	GENERIC, Prescript Pharmaceuticals	00247-0125-12
15's	$2.70	GENERIC, Pharmaceutical Corporation Of America	51655-0817-54
15's	$4.34	GENERIC, Prescript Pharmaceuticals	00247-0125-15
15's	$5.25	GENERIC, Southwood Pharmaceuticals Inc	58016-0226-15
16's	$4.41	GENERIC, Prescript Pharmaceuticals	00247-0125-16
20's	$2.26	GENERIC, Allscripts Pharmaceutical Company	54569-0300-01
20's	$4.68	GENERIC, Prescript Pharmaceuticals	00247-0125-20
20's	$7.00	GENERIC, Southwood Pharmaceuticals Inc	58016-0226-20
24's	$4.94	GENERIC, Prescript Pharmaceuticals	00247-0125-24
24's	$6.73	GENERIC, Southwood Pharmaceuticals Inc	58016-0226-24
28's	$5.22	GENERIC, Prescript Pharmaceuticals	00247-0125-28
30's	$3.39	GENERIC, Allscripts Pharmaceutical Company	54569-0300-02
30's	$4.55	GENERIC, Pharmaceutical Corporation Of America	51655-0817-24
30's	$5.34	GENERIC, Prescript Pharmaceuticals	00247-0125-30
30's	$10.50	GENERIC, Southwood Pharmaceuticals Inc	58016-0226-30
50's	$6.66	GENERIC, Prescript Pharmaceuticals	00247-0125-50
100's	$7.95	GENERIC, Vangard Labs	00615-0445-01
100's	$9.40	GENERIC, Major Pharmaceuticals Inc	00904-3900-60
100's	$9.71	GENERIC, Moore, H.L. Drug Exchange Inc	00839-6435-06
100's	$9.98	GENERIC, Prescript Pharmaceuticals	00247-0125-00
100's	$10.50	GENERIC, Interstate Drug Exchange Inc	00814-0926-14
100's	$10.80	GENERIC, Geneva Pharmaceuticals	00781-1660-01
100's	$13.09	GENERIC, Ivax Corporation	00182-1225-01
100's	$13.09	GENERIC, Vintage Pharmaceuticals Inc	00254-2120-28
100's	$13.10	GENERIC, Moore, H.L. Drug Exchange Inc	00839-7857-06
100's	$13.40	GENERIC, Qualitest Products Inc	00603-2361-21
100's	$13.44	GENERIC, Aligen Independent Laboratories Inc	00405-0021-01
100's	$13.95	GENERIC, Martec Pharmaceuticals Inc	52555-0333-01
100's	$16.95	GENERIC, Ivax Corporation	00172-3984-60
100's	$16.97	GENERIC, Mutual/United Research Laboratories	00677-0647-01
100's	$35.00	GENERIC, Southwood Pharmaceuticals Inc	58016-0226-00

Tablet - Oral - 325 mg;60 mg

15's	$2.74	GENERIC, Allscripts Pharmaceutical Company	54569-0280-02
15's	$3.80	GENERIC, Pharmaceutical Corporation Of America	51655-0818-54
30's	$5.40	GENERIC, Pharmaceutical Corporation Of America	51655-0818-24
100's	$18.00	GENERIC, Interstate Drug Exchange Inc	00814-0927-14
100's	$18.25	GENERIC, Geneva Pharmaceuticals	00781-1875-01
100's	$19.00	GENERIC, Qualitest Products Inc	00603-2362-21
100's	$19.10	GENERIC, Moore, H.L. Drug Exchange Inc	00839-7858-06
100's	$20.67	GENERIC, Aligen Independent Laboratories Inc	00405-0022-01
100's	$23.40	GENERIC, Martec Pharmaceuticals Inc	52555-0334-01
100's	$26.45	GENERIC, Vintage Pharmaceuticals Inc	00254-2121-28
100's	$26.48	GENERIC, Ivax Corporation	00172-3985-60
100's	$38.94	GENERIC, Major Pharmaceuticals Inc	00904-3907-60
100's	$81.70	GENERIC, Southwood Pharmaceuticals Inc	58016-0227-00

Aspirin; Dipyridamole *(003456)*

Categories: Stroke, prophylaxis; FDA Approved 1999 Nov; Pregnancy Category B, Dipyridamole; Pregnancy Category D, Aspirin
Drug Classes: Platelet inhibitors; Salicylates
Brand Names: **Aggrenox**
Foreign Brand Availability: Asasantin SR (Australia)
Cost of Therapy: $119.24 (Stroke; Aggrenox; 25 mg; 200 mg; 2 capsules/day; 30 day supply)

DESCRIPTION

Aggrenox is a combination antiplatelet agent intended for oral administration. Each hard gelatin capsule contains 200 mg dipyridamole in an extended-release form and 25 mg aspirin, as an immediate-release sugar-coated tablet. In addition, each capsule contains the following inactive ingredients: acacia, aluminum stearate, colloidal silicon dioxide, corn starch, dimethicone, hydroxypropyl methylcellulose, hydroxypropyl methylcellulose phthalate, lactose monohydrate, methacrylic acid copolymer, microcrystalline cellulose, povidone, stearic acid, sucrose, talc, tartaric acid, titanium dioxide, and triacetin.

Each capsule shell contains gelatin, red iron oxide and yellow iron oxide, titanium dioxide, and water.

ASPIRIN

The antiplatelet agent aspirin (acetylsalicylic acid) is chemically known as benzoic acid, 2-(acetyloxy)-.

Aspirin is an odorless white needle-like crystalline or powdery substance. When exposed to moisture, aspirin hydrolyzes into salicylic and acetic acids, and gives off a vinegary odor. It is highly lipid soluble and slightly soluble in water.

DIPYRIDAMOLE

Dipyridamole is an antiplatelet agent chemically described as 2,6-bis(diethanolamino)-4,8-dipiperidino-pyrimido(5,4-d) pyrimidine (= dipyridamole).

Dipyridamole is an odorless yellow crystalline substance, having a bitter taste. It is soluble in dilute acids, methanol and chloroform, and is practically insoluble in water.

CLINICAL PHARMACOLOGY

MECHANISM OF ACTION

The antithrombotic action of aspirin; dipyridamole is the result of the additive antiplatelet effects of dipyridamole and aspirin.

Aspirin

Aspirin inhibits platelet aggregation by irreversible inhibition of platelet cyclo-oxygenase and thus inhibits the generation of thromboxane A_2, a powerful inducer of platelet aggregation and vasoconstriction.

Dipyridamole

Dipyridamole inhibits the uptake of adenosine into platelets, endothelial cells and erythrocytes *in vitro* and *in vivo*; the inhibition occurs in a dose-dependent manner at therapeutic concentrations (0.5-1.9 μg/ml). This inhibition results in an increase in local concentrations of adenosine which acts on the platelet A_2-receptor thereby stimulating platelet adenylate cyclase and increasing platelet cyclic-3′,5′-adenosine monophosphate (cAMP) levels. Via this mechanism, platelet aggregation is inhibited in response to various stimuli such as platelet activating factor (PAF), collagen, and adenosine diphosphate (ADP).

Dipyridamole inhibits phosphodiesterase (PDE) in various tissues. While the inhibition of cAMP-PDE is weak, therapeutic levels of dipyridamole inhibit cyclic-3′,5′-guanosine monophosphate-PDE (cGMP-PDE), thereby augmenting the increase in cGMP produced by EDRF (endothelium-derived relaxing factor, now identified as nitric oxide).

PHARMACOKINETICS

There are no significant interactions between aspirin and dipyridamole. The kinetics of the components are unchanged by their coadministration as aspirin; dipyridamole.

ASPIRIN

Absorption

Peak plasma levels of aspirin are achieved 0.63 hours (0.5 to 1 hour) after administration of a 50 mg aspirin daily dose from aspirin; dipyridamole (given as 25 mg bid). The peak plasma concentration at steady-state is 319 ng/ml (175-463 ng/ml). Aspirin undergoes moderate hydrolysis to salicylic acid in the liver and the gastrointestinal wall, with 50-75% of an administered dose reaching the systemic circulation as intact aspirin.

Effect of Food

When aspirin; dipyridamole capsules were taken with a high fat meal, there was no difference for aspirin in AUC at steady-state, and the approximaetly 50% decrease in C_{max} was not considered clinically relevant based on a similar degree of cyclo-oxygenase inhibition comparing the fed and fasted state.

Distribution

Aspirin is poorly bound to plasma proteins and its apparent volume of distribution is low (10 L). Its metabolite, salicylic acid, is highly bound to plasma proteins, but its binding is concentration-dependent (nonlinear). At low concentrations (<100 μg/ml), approximately 90% of salicylic acid is bound to albumin. Salicylic acid is widely distributed to all tissues and fluids in the body, including the central nervous system, breast milk, and fetal tissues. Early signs of salicylate overdose (salicylism), including tinnitus (ringing in the ears), occur at plasma concentrations approximating 200 μg/ml (see ADVERSE REACTIONS).

Metabolism and Elimination

Aspirin is rapidly hydrolyzed in plasma to salicylic acid, with a half-life of 20 minutes. Plasma levels of aspirin are essentially undetectable 2 to 2.5 hours after dosing and peak salicylic acid concentrations occur 1 hour (range: 0.5 to 2 hours) after administration of aspirin. Salicylic acid is primarily conjugated in the liver to form salicyluric acid, a phenolic glucuronide, an acyl glucuronide, and a number of minor metabolites. Salicylate metabolism is saturable and total body clearance decreases at higher serum concentrations due to the limited ability of the liver to form both salicyluric acid and phenolic glucuronide. Following toxic doses (10-20 g), the plasma half-life may be increased to over 20 hours.

The elimination of acetylsalicylic acid follows first-order kinetics with aspirin; dipyridamole and has a half-life of 0.33 hours. The half-life of salicylic acid is 1.71 hours. Both values correspond well with data from the literature at lower doses which state a resultant half-life of approximately 2-3 hours. At higher doses, the elimination of salicylic acid follows zero-order kinetics (*i.e.,* the rate of elimination is constant in relation to plasma concentration), with an apparent half-life of 6 hours or higher. Renal excretion of unchanged drug depends upon urinary pH. As urinary pH rises above 6.5, the renal clearance of free salicylate increases from <5% to >80%. Alkalinization of the urine is a key concept in the management of salicylate overdose. Following therapeutic doses, about 10% is excreted as salicylic acid and 75% as salicyluric acid, as the phenolic and acyl glucuronides, in urine.

Special Populations

Hepatic Dysfunction

Aspirin is to be avoided in patients with severe hepatic insufficiency.

Renal Dysfunction

Aspirin is to be avoided in patients with severe renal failure (glomerular filtration rate less than 10 ml/min).

DIPYRIDAMOLE

Absorption

Peak plasma levels of dipyridamole are achieved 2 hours (range 1-6 hours) after administration of a daily dose of 400 mg aspirin; dipyridamole (given as 200 mg bid). The peak plasma concentration at steady-state is 1.98 μg/ml (1.01-3.99 μg/ml) and the steady state trough concentration is 0.53 μg/ml (0.18-1.01 μg/ml).

Effect of Food

When aspirin; dipyridamole capsules were taken with a high fat meal, dipyridamole peak plasma levels (C_{max}) and total absorption (AUC) were decreased at steady-state by 20-30% compared to fasting. Due to the similar degree of inhibition of adenosine uptake at these plasma concentrations, this food effect is not considered clinically relevant.

Distribution

Dipyridamole is highly lipophilic (log P=3.71, pH=7); however, it has been shown that the drug does not cross the blood-brain barrier to any significant extent in animals. The steady-state volume of distribution of dipyridamole is about 92 L. Approximately 99% of dipyridamole is bound to plasma proteins, predominantly to alpha 1-acid glycoprotein and albumin.

Metabolism and Elimination

Dipyridamole is metabolized in the liver, primarily by conjugation with glucuronic acid, of which monoglucuronide which has low pharmacodynamic activity is the primary metabolite. In plasma, about 80% of the total amount is present as parent compound and 20% as monoglucuronide. Most of the glucuronide metabolite (about 95%) is excreted via bile into the feces, with some evidence of enterohepatic circulation. Renal excretion of parent compound is negligible and urinary excretion of the glucuronide metabolite is low (about 5%). With intravenous (IV) treatment of dipyridamole, a triphasic profile is obtained: a rapid alpha phase, with a half-life of about 3.4 minutes, a beta phase, with a half-life of about 39 minutes, (which, together with the alpha phase accounts for about 70% of the total area under the curve, AUC) and a prolonged elimination phase λ_z with a half-life of about 15.5 hours. Due to the extended absorption phase of the dipyridamole component, only the terminal phase is apparent from oral treatment with aspirin; dipyridamole which, in trial 9.123 was 13.6 hours.

Special Populations

Geriatric Patients

In ESPS2, plasma concentrations (determined as AUC) of dipyridamole in healthy elderly subjects (>65 years) were about 40% higher than in subjects younger than 55 years receiving treatment with aspirin; dipyridamole.

Hepatic Dysfunction

No study has been conducted with the aspirin; dipyridamole formulation in patients with hepatic dysfunction.

In a study conducted with an intravenous formulation of dipyridamole, patients with mild to severe hepatic insufficiency showed no change in plasma concentrations of dipyridamole but showed an increase in the pharmacologically inactive monoglucuronide metabolite.

Dipyridamole can be dosed without restriction as long as there is no evidence of hepatic failure.

Renal Dysfunction

No study has been conducted with the aspirin; dipyridamole formulation in patients with renal dysfunction.

In ESPS2 patients, with creatinine clearances ranging from about 15 to >100 ml/min, no changes were observed in the pharmacokinetics of dipyridamole or its glucuronide metabolite if data were corrected for differences in age.

INDICATIONS AND USAGE

Aspirin; dipyridamole is indicated to reduce the risk of stroke in patients who have had transient ischemia of the brain or completed ischemic stroke due to thrombosis.

CONTRAINDICATIONS

Aspirin; dipyridamole is contraindicated in patients with hypersensitivity to dipyridamole, aspirin or any of the other product components.

ALLERGY

Aspirin is contraindicated in patients with known allergy to nonsteroidal anti-inflammatory drug products and in patients with the syndrome of asthma, rhinitis, and nasal polyps. Aspirin may cause severe urticaria, angioedema or bronchospasm (asthma).

REYE'S SYNDROME

Aspirin should not be used in children or teenagers for viral infections, with or without fever, because of the risk of Reye's syndrome with concomitant use of aspirin in certain viral illnesses.

WARNINGS

ALCOHOL WARNING

Patients who consume 3 or more alcoholic drinks every day should be counseled about the bleeding risks involved with chronic, heavy alcohol use while taking aspirin.

COAGULATION ABNORMALITIES

Even low doses of aspirin can inhibit platelet function leading to an increase in bleeding time. This can adversely affect patients with inherited or acquired (liver disease or vitamin K deficiency) bleeding disorders.

GASTROINTESTINAL (GI) SIDE EFFECTS

GI side effects include stomach pain, heartburn, nausea, vomiting, and gross GI bleeding. Although minor upper GI symptoms, such as dyspepsia, are common and can occur anytime during therapy, physicians should remain alert for signs of ulceration and bleeding, even in the absence of previous GI symptoms. Physicians should inform patients about the signs and symptoms of GI side effects and what steps to take if they occur.

PEPTIC ULCER DISEASE

Patients with a history of active peptic ulcer disease should avoid using aspirin, which can cause gastric mucosal irritation and bleeding.

PRECAUTIONS

GENERAL

Aspirin; dipyridamole is not interchangeable with the individual components of aspirin and dipyridamole tablets.

Coronary Artery Disease

Dipyridamole has a vasodilatory effect and should be used with caution in patients with severe coronary artery disease (*e.g.,* unstable angina or recently sustained myocardial infarction). Chest pain may be aggravated in patients with underlying coronary artery disease who are receiving dipyridamole.

A

For stroke or TIA patients for whom aspirin is indicated to prevent recurrent myocardial infarction (MI) or angina pectoris, the aspirin in this product may not provide adequate treatment for the cardiac indications.

Hepatic Insufficiency

Elevations of hepatic enzymes and hepatic failure have been reported in association with dipyridamole administration.

Hypotension

Dipyridamole should be used with caution in patients with hypotension since it can produce peripheral vasodilation.

Renal Failure

Avoid aspirin in patients with severe renal failure (glomerular filtration rate less than 10 ml/min).

Risk of Bleeding

In ESPS2 the incidence of gastrointestinal bleeding was 68 patients (4.1%) in the aspirin; dipyridamole group, 36 patients (2.2%) in the dipyridamole group, 52 patients (3.2%) in the aspirin group, and 34 patients (2.1%) in the placebo groups.

The incidence of intracranial hemorrhage was 9 patients (0.6%) in the aspirin; dipyridamole group, 6 patients (0.5%) in the dipyridamole group, 6 patients (0.4%) in the aspirin group, and 7 patients (0.4%) in the placebo groups.

LABORATORY TESTS

Aspirin has been associated with elevated hepatic enzymes, blood urea nitrogen and serum creatinine, hyperkalemia, proteinuria, and prolonged bleeding time.

Dipyridamole has been associated with elevated hepatic enzymes.

CARCINOGENESIS, MUTAGENESIS, AND IMPAIRMENT OF FERTILITY

Carcinogenesis

Dipyridamole

In a 111 week oral study in mice and in a 128-142 week oral study in rats, dipyridamole produced no significant carcinogenic effects at doses of 8, 25, and 75 mg/kg. For a 50 kg person of average height (1.46 m^2 body surface area), the dose of dipyridamole at 75 mg/kg/day (225 mg/m^2/day in mice or 450 mg/m^2/day in rats) represents 0.76 or 1.5 times the recommended human dose (8 mg/kg/day or 296 mg/m^2/day) on a body surface area basis.

Mutagenicity

Combination of Aspirin and Dipyridamole

Mutagenicity testing with combination of dipyridamole and aspirin in a ratio of 1:5 revealed no mutagenic potential in the Ames test, *in vivo* chromosome aberration tests in mice and hamsters, oral micronucleus tests in mice and hamsters and dominant lethal test in mice. Aspirin induced chromosome aberrations in cultured human fibroblasts.

Fertility

Aspirin

Aspirin inhibits ovulation in rats.

Dipyridamole

Reproduction studies with dipyridamole revealed no evidence of impaired fertility in rats at oral dosages of up to 500 mg/kg/day or 3000 mg/m^2/day (~10 times the recommended human dose on a body surface area basis). A significant reduction in number of corpora lutea with consequent reduction in implantations and live fetuses was, however, observed at dose of dipyridamole of 1250 mg/kg/day or 7500 mg/m^2/day in rats (~25 times the recommended human dose on a body surface area basis).

Combination of Aspirin and Dipyridamole

Combination of dipyridamole and aspirin was not tested for effect on fertility and reproductive performance.

PREGNANCY CATEGORY D

Aspirin

Aspirin may produce adverse maternal effects: anemia, ante- or postpartum hemorrhage, prolonged gestation and labor. Maternal aspirin use during later stages of pregnancy may cause adverse fetal effects: low birth weight, increased incidence of intracranial hemorrhage in premature infants, stillbirths, neonatal death. Aspirin should be avoided 1 week prior to and during labor and delivery because it can result in excessive blood loss at delivery.

Reproduction studies have been performed with combination of dipyridamole and aspirin in a ratio of 1:4.4 in rats and rabbits and have revealed no teratogenic evidence at doses of up to 405 mg/kg/day in rats and 135 mg/kg/day in rabbits. However, treatment with combination of dipyridamole and aspirin at 405 mg/kg/day induced abortion in rats. The doses of dipyridamole at 75 mg/kg/day represent 1.5 times the recommended human dose on a body surface area basis. In these studies, aspirin itself was teratogenic at doses of 330 mg/kg/day (1980 mg/m^2/day) in rats (spina bifida, exencephaly, microphthalmia, and coelosomia) and 110 mg/kg/day (1320 mg/m^2/day) in rabbits (congested fetuses, agenesis of skull and upper jaw, generalized edema with malformation of the head, and diaphanous skin). The doses of aspirin at 330 mg/kg/day in rats and at 110 mg/kg/day in rabbits were ~54 and 36 times the recommended human dose, respectively, on a body surface area basis.

There were no adequate and well-controlled studies in pregnant women. Aspirin; dipyridamole should be used during pregnancy only if the potential benefit justifies the potential risk to the fetus. Due to the aspirin component, aspirin; dipyridamole should be avoided in the third trimester of pregnancy.

PREGNANCY CATEGORY B

Dipyridamole

Reproduction studies with dipyridamole have been performed in mice at doses up to 125 mg/kg (375 mg/m^2, ~1.3 times the recommended human dose), in rats at doses up to 1000 mg/kg (6000 mg/m^2, 20 times the recommended human dose) and in rabbits at doses up to 40 mg/kg (480 mg/m^2, ~1.6 times the recommended human dose) and have revealed no evidence of harm to the fetus.

NURSING MOTHERS

Dipyridamole (n=1) and aspirin are excreted in human breast milk in low concentrations. Therefore, caution should be exercised when aspirin; dipyridamole is administered to a nursing woman.

PEDIATRIC USE

Safety and effectiveness of aspirin; dipyridamole in pediatric patients have not been studied. Due to the aspirin component, use of this product in the pediatric population is not recommended (see CONTRAINDICATIONS).

DRUG INTERACTIONS

No pharmacokinetic drug-drug interaction studies were conducted with the aspirin; dipyridamole formulation.

The following information was obtained from the literature.

Adenosine: Dipyridamole has been reported to increase the plasma levels and cardiovascular effects of adenosine. Adjustment of adenosine dosage may be necessary.

Angiotensin Converting Enzyme (ACE) Inhibitors: Due to the indirect effect of aspirin on the renin-angiotensin conversion pathway, the hyponatremic and hypotensive effects of ACE inhibitors may be diminished by concomitant administration of aspirin.

Acetazolamide: Concurrent use of aspirin and acetazolamide can lead to high serum concentrations of acetazolamide (and toxicity) due to competition at the renal tubule for secretion.

Anticoagulant Therapy (heparin and warfarin): Patients on anticoagulation therapy are at increased risk for bleeding because of drug-drug interactions and effects on platelets. Aspirin can displace warfarin from protein binding sites, leading to prolongation of both the prothrombin time and the bleeding time. Aspirin can increase the anticoagulant activity of heparin, increasing bleeding risk.

Anticonvulsants: Salicylic acid can displace protein-bound phenytoin and valproic acid, leading to a decrease in the total concentration of phenytoin and an increase in serum valproic acid levels.

Beta Blockers: The hypotensive effects of beta blockers may be diminished by the concomitant administration of aspirin due to inhibition of renal prostaglandins, leading to decreased renal blood flow and salt and fluid retention.

Cholinesterase Inhibitors: Dipyridamole may counteract the anticholinesterase effect of cholinesterase inhibitors, thereby potentially aggravating myasthenia gravis.

Diuretics: The effectiveness of diuretics in patients with underlying renal or cardiovascular disease may be diminished by the concomitant administration of aspirin due to inhibition of renal prostaglandins, leading to decreased renal blood flow and salt and fluid retention.

Methotrexate: Salicylate can inhibit renal clearance of methotrexate, leading to bone marrow toxicity, especially in the elderly or renal impaired.

Nonsteroidal Anti-Inflammatory Drugs (NSAIDs): The concurrent use of aspirin with other NSAIDs may increase bleeding or lead to decreased renal function.

Oral Hypoglycemics: Moderate doses of aspirin may increase the effectiveness of oral hypoglycemic drugs, leading to hypoglycemia.

Uricosuric Agents (probenecid and sulfinpyrazone): Salicylates antagonize the uricosuric action of uricosuric agents.

ADVERSE REACTIONS

A 24 month, multicenter, double-blind, randomized study (ESPS2) was conducted to compare the efficacy and safety of aspirin; dipyridamole with placebo, extended-release dipyridamole alone and aspirin alone. The study was conducted in a total of 6602 male and female patients who had experienced a previous ischemic stroke or transient ischemia of the brain within 3 months prior to randomization.

TABLE 2A and TABLE 2B present the incidence of adverse events that occurred in 1% or more of patients treated with aspirin; dipyridamole where the incidence was also greater than in those patients treated with placebo. There is no clear benefit of aspirin; dipyridamole over aspirin with respect to safety.

Discontinuation due to adverse events in ESPS2 was 25% for aspirin; dipyridamole, 25% for extended-release dipyridamole, 19% for aspirin, and 21% for placebo (see TABLE 3).

OTHER ADVERSE EVENTS

Adverse reactions that occurred in less than 1% of patients treated with aspirin; dipyridamole in the ESPS2 study and that were medically judged to be possibly related to either dipyridamole or aspirin are listed below (see WARNINGS).

Body as a Whole: Allergic reaction, fever.

Cardiovascular: Hypotension.

Central Nervous System: Coma, dizziness, paresthesia, cerebral hemorrhage, intracranial hemorrhage, subarachnoid hemorrhage.

Gastrointestinal: Gastritis, ulceration, and perforation.

Hearing and Vestibular Disorders: Tinnitus and deafness. Patients with high frequency hearing loss may have difficulty perceiving tinnitus. In these patients, tinnitus cannot be used as a clinical indicator of salicylism.

Heart Rate and Rhythm Disorders: Tachycardia, palpitation, arrhythmia, supraventricular tachycardia.

Liver and Biliary System Disorders: Cholelithiasis, jaundice, hepatic function abnormal.

Metabolic and Nutritional Disorders: Hyperglycemia, thirst.

Platelet, Bleeding, and Clotting Disorders: Hematoma, gingival bleeding.

Psychiatric Disorders: Agitation.

TABLE 2A *Incidence of Adverse Events in ESPS2**

Body System / Preferred Term	Aspirin; Dipyridamole n=1650	ER-DP Alone n=1654
Total no. (%) of patients with at least one on-treatment adverse event	1319 (79.9%)	1305 (78.9%)
Central & Peripheral Nervous System Disorders		
Headache	647 (39.2%)	634 (38.3%)
Convulsions	28 (1.7%)	15 (0.9%)
Gastrointestinal System Disorders		
Dyspepsia	303 (18.4%)	288 (17.4%)
Abdomina pain	289 (17.5%)	255 (15.4%)
Nausea	264 (16.0%)	254 (15.4%)
Diarrhea	210 (12.7%)	257 (15.5%)
Vomiting	138 (8.4%)	129 (7.8%)
Hemorrhage rectum	26 (1.6%)	22 (1.3%)
Melena	31 (1.9%)	10 (0.6%)
Hemorrhoids	16 (1.0%)	13 (0.8%)
GI hemorrhage	20 (1.2%)	5 (0.3%)
Body as a Whole — General Disorders		
Pain	105 (6.4%)	88 (5.3%)
Fatigue	95 (5.8%)	93 (5.6%)
Back pain	76 (4.6%)	77 (4.7%)
Accidental injury	42 (2.5%)	24 (1.5%)
Malaise	27 (1.6%)	23 (1.4%)
Asthenia	29 (1.8%)	19 (1.1%)
Syncope	17 (1.0%)	13 (0.8%)
Psychiatric Disorders		
Amnesia	39 (2.4%)	40 (2.4%)
Confusion	18 (1.1%)	9 (0.5%)
Anorexia	19 (1.2%)	17 (1.0%)
Somnolence	20 (1.2%)	13 (0.8%)
Musculoskeletal System Disorders		
Arthralgia	91 (5.5%)	75 (4.5%)
Arthritis	34 (2.1%)	25 (1.5%)
Arthrosis	18 (1.1%)	22 (1.3%)
Myalgia	20 (1.2%)	16 (1.0%)
Respiratory System Disorders		
Coughing	25 (1.5%)	18 (1.1%)
Upper respiratory tract infection	16 (1.0%)	9 (0.5%)
Cardiovascular Disorders, General		
Cardiac failure	26 (1.6%)	17 (1.0%)
Platelet, Bleeding & Clotting Disorders		
Hemorrhage NOS	52 (3.2%)	24 (1.5%)
Epistaxis	39 (2.4%)	16 (1.0%)
Purpura	23 (1.4%)	8 (0.5%)
Neoplasm		
Neoplasm NOS	28 (1.7%)	16 (1.0%)
Red Blood Cell Disorders		
Anemia	27 (1.6%)	16 (1.0%)

* Reported by ≥1% of patients during aspirin; dipyridamole treatment where the incidence was greater than in those treated with placebo.
Note: ER-DP = extended-release dipyridamole 200 mg; ASA = aspirin 25 mg.
Note: The dosage regimen for all treatment groups is bid.
Note: NOS = not otherwise specified.

TABLE 2B *Incidence of Adverse Events in ESPS2**

Body System / Preferred Term	ASA Alone n=1649	Placebo n=1649
Total no. (%) of patients with at least one on-treatment adverse event	1323 (80.2%)	1304 (79.1%)
Central & Peripheral Nervous System Disorders		
Headache	585 (33.8%)	543 (32.9%)
Convulsions	28 (1.7%)	26 (1.6%)
Gastrointestinal System Disorders		
Dyspepsia	299 (18.1%)	275 (16.7%)
Abdomina pain	262 (15.9%)	239 (14.5%)
Nausea	210 (12.7%)	323 (14.1%)
Diarrhea	112 (6.8%)	161 (9.8%)
Vomiting	101 (6.1%)	118 (7.2%)
Hemorrhage rectum	16 (1.0%)	13 (0.8%)
Melena	20 (1.2%)	13 (0.8%)
Hemorrhoids	10 (0.6%)	10 (0.6%)
GI hemorrhage	15 (0.9%)	7 (0.4%)
Body as a Whole — General Disorders		
Pain	103 (6.2%)	99 (6.0%)
Fatigue	97 (5.9%)	90 (5.5%)
Back pain	74 (4.5%)	65 (3.9%)
Accidental injury	51 (3.1%)	37 (2.2%)
Malaise	26 (1.6%)	22 (1.3%)
Asthenia	17 (1.0%)	18 (1.1%)
Syncope	16 (1.0%)	8 (0.5%)
Psychiatric Disorders		
Amnesia	57 (3.5%)	34 (2.1%)
Confusion	22 (1.3%)	15 (0.9%)
Anorexia	10 (0.6%)	15 (0.9%)
Somnolence	18 (1.1%)	9 (0.5%)
Musculoskeletal System Disorders		
Arthralgia	91 (5.5%)	76 (4.6%)
Arthritis	17 (1.0%)	19 (1.2%)
Arthrosis	16 (0.8%)	14 (0.8%)
Myalgia	11 (0.7%)	11 (0.7%)
Respiratory System Disorders		
Coughing	32 (1.9%)	21 (1.3%)
Upper respiratory tract infection	16 (1.0%)	14 (0.8%)
Cardiovascular Disorders, General		
Cardiac failure	30 (1.8%)	25 (1.5%)
Platelet, Bleeding & Clotting Disorders		
Hemorrhage NOS	46 (2.8%)	24 (1.5%)
Epistaxis	45 (2.7%)	25 (1.5%)
Purpura	9 (0.5%)	7 (0.4%)
Neoplasm		
Neoplasm NOS	23 (1.4%)	20 (1.2%)
Red Blood Cell Disorders		
Anemia	19 (1.2%)	9 (0.5%)

* Reported by ≥1% of patients during aspirin; dipyridamole treatment where the incidence was greater than in those treated with placebo.
Note: ER-DP = extended-release dipyridamole 200 mg; ASA = aspirin 25 mg.
Note: The dosage regimen for all treatment groups is bid.
Note: NOS = not otherwise specified.

Reproductive: Uterine hemorrhage.
Respiratory: Hyperpnea, asthma, bronchospasm, hemoptysis, pulmonary edema.
Special Senses, Other Disorders: Taste loss.
Skin and Appendages Disorders: Pruritus, urticaria.
Urogenital: Renal insufficiency and failure, hematuria.
Vascular (extracardiac) Disorders: Flushing.

The following is a list of additional adverse reactions that have been reported either in the literature or are from postmarketing spontaneous reports for either dipyridamole or aspirin.

Body as a Whole: Hypothermia, chest pain.
Cardiovascular: Angina pectoris.
Central Nervous System: Cerebral edema.
Fluid and Electrolyte: Hyperkalemia, metabolic acidosis, respiratory alkalosis, hypokalemia.
Gastrointestinal: Pancreatitis, Reye's syndrome, hematemesis.
Hearing and Vestibular Disorders: Hearing loss.
Hypersensitivity: Acute anaphylaxis, laryngeal edema.
Liver and Biliary System Disorders: Hepatitis, hepatic failure.
Musculoskeletal: Rhabdomyolysis.
Metabolic and Nutritional Disorders: Hypoglycemia, dehydration.
Platelet, Bleeding, and Clotting Disorders: Prolongation of the prothrombin time, disseminated intravascular coagulation, coagulopathy, thrombocytopenia.
Reproductive: Prolonged pregnancy and labor, stillbirths, lower birth weight infants, antepartum and postpartum bleeding.
Respiratory: Tachypnea, dyspnea.
Skin and Appendages Disorders: Rash, alopecia, angioedema, Stevens-Johnson syndrome.
Urogenital: Interstitial nephritis, papillary necrosis, proteinuria.
Vascular (extracardiac disorders): Allergic vasculitis.

The following is a list of adverse events that have been reported either in the literature or are from postmarketing spontaneous reports for either dipyridamole or aspirin. The causal relationship of these adverse events has not been established: anorexia, aplastic anemia, pancytopenia, thrombocytosis.

LABORATORY CHANGES

Over the course of the 24 month study (ESPS2), patients treated with aspirin; dipyridamole showed a decline (mean change from baseline) in hemoglobin of 0.25 g/dl, hematocrit of 0.75%, and erythrocyte count of $0.13 \times 10^6/mm^3$.

TABLE 3 *Incidence of Adverse Events That Led to the Discontinuation of Treatment**

	Treatment Groups			
	ASA; DP n=1650	**ER-DP n=1654**	**ASA n=1649**	**Placebo n=1649**
Patients with at least one adverse event that led to treatment discontinuation	417 (25%)	419 (25%)	318 (19%)	352 (21%)
Headache	165 (10%)	166 (10%)	57 (3%)	69 (4%)
Dizziness	85 (5%)	97 (6%)	69 (4%)	68 (4%)
Nausea	91 (6%)	95 (6%)	51 (3%)	53 (3%)
Abdominal pain	74 (4%)	64 (4%)	56 (3%)	52 (3%)
Dyspepsia	59 (4%)	61 (4%)	49 (3%)	46 (3%)
Vomiting	53 (3%)	52 (3%)	28 (2%)	24 (1%)
Diarrhea	35 (2%)	41 (2%)	9 (<1%)	16 (<1%)
Stroke	39 (2%)	48 (3%)	57 (3%)	73 (4%)
Transient ischemic attack	35 (2%)	40 (2%)	26 (2%)	48 (3%)
Angina pectoris	23 (1%)	20 (1%)	16 (<1%)	26 (2%)

* Adverse events with an incidence of ≥1% in the aspirin; dipyridamole group.
ER-DP = Extended-release dipyridamole 200 mg.
ASA = Aspirin 25 mg.
ASA; DP = Aspirin; dipyridamole.
Note: The dosage regimen for all treatment groups is bid.

DOSAGE AND ADMINISTRATION

The recommended dose of aspirin; dipyridamole is 1 capsule given orally twice daily, 1 in the morning and 1 in the evening. The capsules should be swallowed whole without chewing.

Aspirin; dipyridamole capsules may be administered with or without food.

Aspirin; dipyridamole is not interchangeable with the individual components of aspirin and dipyridamole tablets.

HOW SUPPLIED

Aggrenox is available as a hard gelatin capsule, with a red cap and an ivory-colored body, 24.0 mm in length, containing yellow extended-release pellets incorporating dipyridamole and a round white tablet incorporating immediate-release aspirin. The capsule body is imprinted in red with the Boehringer Ingelheim logo and with "01A".

STORAGE

Store at 25°C (77°F); excursions permitted to 15-30°C (59-86°F).

Protect from excessive moisture.

PRODUCT LISTING - EQUIVALENTS NOT AVAILABLE

Capsule, Extended Release - Oral - 25 mg;200 mg

60's $119.24 AGGRENOX, Boehringer-Ingelheim 00597-0001-60

Aspirin; Hydrocodone Bitartrate *(000319)*

For complete prescribing information, refer to the CD-ROM included with the book.

Categories: Pain, moderate to moderately severe; Pregnancy Category C; DEA Class CIII; FDA Approved 1988 Jan
Drug Classes: Analgesics, narcotic; Salicylates
Brand Names: Alor; **Azdone**; Damason-P; Lortab Asa; Panasal
Cost of Therapy: $15.83 (Pain; Generic Tablets; 500 mg; 5 mg; 6 tablets/day; 7 day supply)

DESCRIPTION

Each Tablet Contains:

***Hydrocodone Bitartrate**:** 5 mg

Aspirin: 500 mg

**Warning:* May be habit forming.

Hydrocodone bitartrate is an opioid analgesic and antitussive and occurs as fine, white crystals or as a crystalline powder. It is affected by light. The chemical name is: 4,5 α-epoxy-3-methoxy-17-methylmorphinan-6-one tartrate (1:1) hydrate (2:5).

Aspirin, salicylic acid acetate, is a non-opiate, salicylate analgesic, anti-inflammatory, and antipyretic which occurs as a white, crystalline tabular or needle-like powder and is odorless or has a faint odor.

Inactive Ingredients: Corn starch, D&C red no. 7 (calcium lake), sodium starch glycolate, and stearic acid.

INDICATIONS AND USAGE

For the relief of moderate to moderately severe pain.

CONTRAINDICATIONS

Aspirin; hydrocodone bitartrate tablets are contraindicated under the following conditions:

(1) Hypersensitivity or intolerance to hydrocodone or aspirin.
(2) Severe bleeding, disorders of coagulation or primary hemostasis including hemophilia, hypoprothrombinemia, von Willebrand's disease, thrombocytopenias, thrombasthenia and other ill-defined hereditary platelet dysfunctions, severe vitamin K deficiency and severe liver damage.
(3) Anticoagulant therapy.
(4) Peptic ulcer, or other serious gastrointestinal lesions.

WARNINGS

HYDROCODONE

Respiratory Depression: At high doses or in sensitive patients, hydrocodone may produce dose-related respiratory depression by acting directly on the brain stem respiratory center. Hydrocodone also affects the center that controls respiratory rhythm, and may produce irregular and periodic breathing.

Head Injury and Increased Intracranial Pressure: The respiratory depressant effects of narcotics and their capacity to elevate cerebrospinal fluid pressure may be markedly exaggerated in the presence of head injury, other intracranial lesions or a pre-existing increase in intracranial pressure. Furthermore, narcotics produce adverse reactions which may obscure the clinical course of patients with head injuries.

Acute Abdominal Conditions: The administration of narcotics may obscure the diagnosis or clinical course of patients with acute abdominal conditions.

ASPIRIN

Allergic Reactions: Therapeutic doses of aspirin can cause anaphylactic shock and other severe allergic reactions. A history of allergy is often lacking.

Bleeding: Significant bleeding can result from aspirin therapy in patients with peptic ulcer or other gastrointestinal lesions, and in patients with bleeding disorders. Aspirin administered preoperatively may prolong the bleeding time.

DOSAGE AND ADMINISTRATION

Dosage should be adjusted according to the severity of the pain and the response of the patient. However, tolerance to hydrocodone can develop with continued use and the incidence of untoward effects is dose related.

The usual adult dosage is 1 or 2 tablets every four to six hours as needed for pain. The total 24 hour dose should not exceed 8 tablets.

Aspirin; hydrocodone bitartrate tablets should be taken with food or a full glass of milk or water to lessen gastric irritation.

Storage: Store at controlled room temperature 15-30°C (59-86°F). Protect from moisture. Dispense in a tight, light-resistant container with a child-resistant closure.

PRODUCT LISTING - EQUIVALENTS NOT AVAILABLE

Tablet - Oral - 500 mg;5 mg

100's $37.68 GENERIC, Mason Pharmaceuticals Inc 12758-0057-01

Aspirin; Oxycodone Hydrochloride; Oxycodone Terephthalate *(000322)*

Categories: Pain, moderate to moderately severe; DEA Class CII; FDA Approval Pre 1982; Pregnancy Category C; Pregnancy Category D, 3rd Trimester
Drug Classes: Analgesics, narcotic; Salicylates
Brand Names: Endodan; **Percodan**; Roxiprin
Foreign Brand Availability: Oxycodan (Canada); Percodan-Demi (Canada)
Cost of Therapy: $24.26 (Pain; Percodan; 325 mg; 4.5 mg; 0.38 mg; 4 tablets/day; 7 day supply)
$6.41 (Pain; Generic Tablets; 325 mg; 4.5 mg; 0.38 mg; 4 tablets/day; 7 day supply)

DESCRIPTION

Note: This prescribing information pertains to both Percodan and Percodan-Demi. (The innovator brand name has been left in so as to avoid confusion.)

PERCODAN

Each Tablet of Percodan Contains:

Oxycodone Hydrochloride: 4.50 mg (equivalent to 4.0338 mg of oxycodone). *Warning:* May be habit forming.

Oxycodone Terephthalate: 0.38 mg (equivalent to 0.3008 mg of oxycodone). *Warning:* May be habit forming.

Aspirin: 325 mg

Percodan Tablets Also Contain: D&C yellow 10, FD&C yellow 6, microcrystalline cellulose and starch.

The oxycodone component is 14-hydroxydihydrocodeinone, a white odorless crystalline powder which is derived from the opium alkaloid, thebaine.

PERCODAN-DEMI

Each Tablet of Percodan-Demi Contains:

Oxycodone Hydrochloride: 2.25 mg (equivalent to 2.0169 mg of oxycodone). *Warning:* May be habit forming.

Oxycodone Terephthalate: 0.19 mg (equivalent to 0.1504 mg of oxycodone). *Warning:* May be habit forming.

Aspirin: 325 mg

Percodan-Demi Tablets Also Contain: Microcrystalline cellulose and starch.

The oxycodone component is 14-hydroxydihydrocodeinone, a white odorless crystalline powder which is derived from the opium alkaloid, thebaine.

CLINICAL PHARMACOLOGY

The principal ingredient, oxycodone, is a semisynthetic narcotic analgesic with multiple actions qualitatively similar to those of morphine; the most prominent of these involve the central nervous system and organs composed of smooth muscle. The principle actions of therapeutic value of the oxycodone in Percodan are analgesia and sedation.

Oxycodone is similar to codeine and methadone in that it retains at least one half of its analgesic activity when administered orally.

Percodan also contains the non-narcotic antipyretic-analgesic, aspirin.

INDICATIONS AND USAGE

For the relief of moderate to moderately severe pain.

CONTRAINDICATIONS

Hypersensitivity to oxycodone or aspirin.

WARNINGS

Drug Dependence: Oxycodone can produce drug dependence of the morphine type and, therefore, has the potential for being abused. Psychic dependence, physical dependence and tolerance may develop upon repeated administration of Percodan, and it should be prescribed and administered with the same degree of caution appropriate to the use of other oral narcotic-containing medications. Like other narcotic-containing medications, Percodan is subject to the Federal Controlled Substances Act.

Usage in Ambulatory Patients: Oxycodone may impair the mental and/or physical abilities required for the performance of potentially hazardous tasks such as driving a car or operating machinery. The patient using Percodan should be cautioned accordingly.

Interaction with Other Central Nervous System Depressants: Patients receiving other narcotic analgesics, general anesthetics, phenothiazines, other tranquilizers, sedative-hypnotics or other CNS depressants (including alcohol) concomitantly with Percodan may exhibit an additive CNS depression. When such combined therapy is contemplated, the dose of one or both agents should be reduced.

Usage in Pregnancy: Safe use in pregnancy has not been established relative to possible adverse effects on fetal development. Therefore, Percodan should not be used in pregnant women unless, in the judgment of the physician, the potential benefits outweigh the possible hazards.

Use in Children: Percodan should not be administered to children. Percodan-Demi, containing half the amount of oxycodone, can be considered.

Reye Syndrome: Reye Syndrome is a rare but serious disease which can follow flu or chicken pox in children and teenagers. While the cause of Reye Syndrome is unknown, some reports claim aspirin (or salicylates) may increase the risk of developing this disease. Salicylates should be used with caution in the presence of peptic ulcer or coagulation abnormalities.

PRECAUTIONS

Head Injury and Increased Intracranial Pressure: The respiratory depressant effects of narcotics and their capacity to elevate cerebrospinal fluid pressure may be markedly exaggerated in the presence of head injury, other intracranial lesions or a pre-existing increase in intracranial pressure. Furthermore, narcotics produce adverse reactions which may obscure the clinical course of patients with head injuries.

Acute Abdominal Conditions: The administration of Percodan or other narcotics may obscure the diagnosis or clinical course in patients with acute abdominal conditions.

Special Risk Patients: Percodan should be given with caution to certain patients such as the elderly or debilitated, and those with severe impairment of hepatic or renal function, hypothyroidism, Addison's disease, and prostatic hypertrophy or urethral stricture.

DRUG INTERACTIONS

The CNS depressant effects of Percodan may be additive with that of other CNS depressants. (See WARNINGS.)

Aspirin may enhance the effect of anticoagulants and inhibit the uricosuric effects of uricosuric agents.

ADVERSE REACTIONS

The most frequently observed adverse reactions include lightheadedness, dizziness, sedation, nausea and vomiting. These effects seem to be more prominent in ambulatory than in nonambulatory patients, and some of these adverse reactions may be alleviated if the patient lies down.

Other adverse reactions include euphoria, dysphoria, constipation and pruritus.

DOSAGE AND ADMINISTRATION

Dosage should be adjusted according to the severity of the pain and the response of the patient. It may occasionally be necessary to exceed the usual dosage recommended below in cases of more severe pain or in those patients who have become tolerant to the analgesic effect of narcotics.

PERCODAN

Percodan is given orally. The usual adult dose is 1 tablet every 6 hours as needed for pain.

PERCODAN-DEMI

Percodan-Demi is given orally:

Adults: One (1) or 2 tablets every 6 hours.
Children 12 Years and Older: One-half tablet every 6 hours.
Children 6 to 12 Years: One quarter tablet every 6 hours.

Percodan-Demi is not indicated for children under 6 years of age.

HOW SUPPLIED

Percodan: Supplied as a yellow tablet, with one face scored and inscribed "PERCODAN" and the other face plain.

Percodan-Demi: Supplied as white, scored tablets.

Storage: Store at contolled room temperature (15-30°C, 59-86°F).

PRODUCT LISTING - RATED THERAPEUTICALLY EQUIVALENT

Tablet - Oral - 325 mg;4.5 mg;0.38 mg

100's	$19.55	GENERIC, Major Pharmaceuticals Inc	00904-0464-60
100's	$22.28	ROXIPRIN, Roxane Laboratories Inc	00054-4653-25
100's	$22.95	GENERIC, Ivax Corporation	00182-1508-01
100's	$33.08	ROXIPRIN, Roxane Laboratories Inc	00054-8653-24
100's	$34.43	GENERIC, Watson Laboratories Inc	52544-0820-01
100's	$51.65	GENERIC, Endo Laboratories Llc	60951-0610-70
100's	$120.38	PERCODAN, Endo Laboratories Llc	63481-0135-70

PRODUCT LISTING - EQUIVALENTS NOT AVAILABLE

Tablet - Oral - 325 mg;2.25 mg;0.19 mg

100's	$66.13	PERCODAN-DEMI, Dupont Pharmaceuticals	00590-0166-70

Tablet - Oral - 325 mg;4.5 mg;0.38 mg

25 x 4	$120.38	PERCODAN, Endo Laboratories Llc	63481-0135-75
100's	$86.63	PERCODAN, Dupont Pharmaceuticals	00590-0135-70

Atazanavir Sulfate *(003603)*

Categories: Infection, human immunodeficiency virus; Pregnancy Category B; FDA Approved 2003 Jun
Drug Classes: Antivirals; Protease Inhibitors
Brand Names: **Reyataz**

DESCRIPTION

Reyataz (atazanavir sulfate) is an azapeptide inhibitor of HIV-1 protease.

The chemical name for atazanavir sulfate is (3*S*,8*S*,9*S*,12*S*)-3,12-Bis(1,1-dimethylethyl)-8-hydroxy-4,11-dioxo-9-(phenylmethyl)-6-[[4-(2-pyridinyl)phenyl]methyl]-2,5,6,10,13-pentaazatetradecanedioic acid dimethyl ester, sulfate (1:1). Its molecular formula is $C_{38}H_{52}N_6O_7 \cdot H_2SO_4$, which corresponds to a molecular weight of 802.9 (sulfuric acid salt). The free base molecular weight is 704.9.

Atazanavir sulfate is a white to pale yellow crystalline powder. It is slightly soluble in water (4-5 mg/ml, free base equivalent) with the pH of a saturated solution in water being about 1.9 at 24 ± 3°C.

Reyataz capsules are available for oral administration in strengths containing the equivalent of 100, 150, or 200 mg of atazanavir as atazanavir sulfate and the following inactive ingredients: crospovidone, lactose monohydrate, and magnesium stearate. The capsule shells contain the following inactive ingredients: gelatin, FD&C blue no. 2, and titanium dioxide. The capsules are printed with ink containing shellac, titanium dioxide, FD&C blue no. 2, isopropyl alcohol, ammonium hydroxide, propylene glycol, n-butyl alcohol, simethicone, and dehydrated alcohol.

CLINICAL PHARMACOLOGY

MICROBIOLOGY

Mechanism of Action

Atazanavir is an azapeptide HIV-1 protease inhibitor. The compound selectively inhibits the virus-specific processing of viral Gag and Gag-Pol polyproteins in HIV-1 infected cells, thus preventing formation of mature virions.

Antiviral Activity In Vitro

Atazanavir exhibits anti-HIV-1 activity with a mean 50% effective concentration (EC_{50}) in the absence of human serum of 2-5 nM against a variety of laboratory and clinical HIV-1 isolates grown in peripheral blood mononuclear cells, macrophages, CEMSS cells, and MT-2 cells. Two-drug combination studies with atazanavir showed additive to antagonistic antiviral activity *in vitro* with abacavir and the NNRTIs (delavirdine, efavirenz, and nevirapine) and additive antiviral activity *in vitro* with the protease inhibitors (amprenavir, indinavir, lopinavir, nelfinavir, ritonavir, and saquinavir) and NRTIs (didanosine, lamivudine, stavudine, tenofovir, zalcitabine, and zidovudine) without enhanced cytotoxicity.

Resistance In Vitro

HIV-1 isolates with reduced susceptibility to atazanavir (93- to 183-fold resistant) from three different viral strains were selected *in vitro* by 5 months. The mutations in these HIV-1 viruses that appeared to contribute to atazanavir resistance included N88S, I50L, I84V, A71V, and M46I. Changes were also observed at the protease cleavage sites following drug selection. The I50L substitution, with or without an A71V substitution, conferred atazanavir resistance in recombinant viral clones in a variety of genetic backgrounds. Recombinant viruses containing the I50L mutation were growth impaired and showed increased susceptibility to other protease inhibitors (amprenavir, indinavir, lopinavir, nelfinavir, ritonavir, and saquinavir).

Cross-Resistance In Vitro

Atazanavir susceptibility was evaluated *in vitro* using a diverse panel of 551 clinical isolates from patients without prior atazanavir exposure. These isolates exhibited resistance to at least one approved protease inhibitor, with resistance defined as ≥2.5-fold change in EC_{50} relative to a reference strain. Greater than 80% of the isolates resistant to 1 or 2 protease inhibitors (with the majority resistant to nelfinavir) retained susceptibility to atazanavir despite the presence of key mutations (*e.g.,* D30N) associated with protease inhibitor resistance. Of 104 isolates displaying nelfinavir-specific resistance, 84 retained susceptibility to atazanavir. There was a clear trend toward decreased atazanavir susceptibility as isolates exhibited resistance to multiple protease inhibitors. Baseline phenotypic and genotypic analyses of clinical isolates from atazanavir clinical trials of protease inhibitor-experienced subjects showed that isolates cross-resistant to multiple protease inhibitors were also highly cross-resistant (61-95%) to atazanavir. Greater than 90% of the isolates containing mutations I84V or G48V were resistant to atazanavir. Greater than 60% of isolates containing L90M, A71V/T, M46I, or a change at V82 were resistant to atazanavir, and 38% of isolates containing a D30N mutation in addition to other changes were resistant to atazanavir. Atazanavir-resistant isolates were highly cross-resistant (51-100%) to other protease inhibitors (amprenavir, indinavir, lopinavir, nelfinavir, ritonavir, and saquinavir). The I50L and I50V substitutions yielded selective resistance to atazanavir and amprenavir, respectively, and did not appear to confer cross-resistance.

Resistance In Vivo

Atazanavir-resistant isolates have been obtained from patients experiencing virologic failure on atazanavir therapy. There were 14 atazanavir-resistant isolates from studies of treatment-naive patients (n=96 evaluable isolates) that showed decreases in susceptibility levels from baseline, and all had an I50L substitution emerge on atazanavir therapy (after an average of 50 weeks of therapy) often in combination with an A71V mutation. Phenotypic analysis of the isolates containing the signature mutation I50L showed atazanavir-specific resistance, which coincided with increased susceptibility to other protease inhibitors (amprenavir, indinavir, lopinavir, nelfinavir, ritonavir, and saquinavir). In contrast, 89% (32 of 36) of atazanavir-resistant isolates from studies of treatment- experienced patients (n=67 evaluable isolates) treated with atazanavir (n=26) or atazanavir plus saquinavir (n=10) showed no evidence of the emergence of the I50L substitution. Instead, these isolates displayed decreased susceptibility to multiple protease inhibitors and contained mutations associated with resistance to multiple protease inhibitors. These mutations included I84V, L90M, A71V/T, N88S/D, and M46I, which conferred atazanavir resistance and reduced the clinical response to atazanavir. Generally, if protease inhibitor mutations were present in the HIV-1 of the patient at baseline, atazanavir resistance developed through mutations associated with resistance to other protease inhibitors instead of the I50L mutation. These mutations conferred high cross-resistance to other protease inhibitors with 100% of the isolates resistant to nelfinavir, >80% of the isolates resistant to indinavir, ritonavir, and saquinavir, and >35% of the isolates resistant to amprenavir and lopinavir. Genotypic and/or phenotypic analysis of baseline virus may aid in determining atazanavir susceptibility before initiation of atazanavir therapy.

PHARMACOKINETICS

The pharmacokinetics of atazanavir were evaluated in healthy adult volunteers and in HIV-infected patients (see TABLE 1).

Absorption

Atazanavir is rapidly absorbed with a T_{max} of approximately 2.5 hours. Atazanavir demonstrates nonlinear pharmacokinetics with greater than dose-proportional increases in AUC and C_{max} values over the dose range of 200-800 mg once daily. Steady-state is achieved between Days 4 and 8, with an accumulation of approximately 2.3-fold.

Food Effect

Administration of atazanavir sulfate with food enhances bioavailability and reduces pharmacokinetic variability. Administration of a single 400 mg dose of atazanavir sulfate with a light meal (357 kcal, 8.2 g fat, 10.6 g protein) resulted in a 70% increase in AUC and 57% increase in C_{max} relative to the fasting state. Administration of a single 400 mg dose of

A

TABLE 1 *Steady-State Pharmacokinetics of Atazanavir in Healthy Subjects or HIV-Infected Patients in the Fed State After Atazanavir 400 mg Once Daily*

Parameter	Healthy Subjects (n=14)	HIV-Infected Patients (n=13)
C_{max} (ng/ml)		
Geometric mean (CV%)	5199 (26)	2298 (71)
Mean (SD)	5358 (1371)	3152 (2231)
T_{max} (h)		
Median	2.5	2.0
AUC (ng·h/ml)		
Geometric mean (CV%)	28132 (28)	14874 (91)
Mean (SD)	29303 (8263)	22262 (20159)
T½ (h)		
Mean (SD)	7.9 (2.9)	6.5 (2.6)
C_{min} (ng/ml)		
Geometric mean (CV%)	159 (88)	120 (109)
Mean (SD)	218 (191)	273 (298)*

* n=12.

atazanavir sulfate with a high-fat meal (721 kcal, 37.3 g fat, 29.4 g protein) resulted in a mean increase in AUC of 35% with no change in C_{max} relative to the fasting state. Administration of atazanavir sulfate with either a light meal or high-fat meal decreased the coefficient of variation of AUC and C_{max} by approximately one half compared to the fasting state.

Distribution

Atazanavir is 86% bound to human serum proteins and protein binding is independent of concentration. Atazanavir binds to both alpha-1-acid glycoprotein (AAG) and albumin to a similar extent (89% and 86%, respectively). In a multiple-dose study in HIV-infected patients dosed with atazanavir sulfate 400 mg once daily with a light meal for 12 weeks, atazanavir was detected in the cerebrospinal fluid and semen. The cerebrospinal fluid/plasma ratio for atazanavir (n=4) ranged between 0.0021 and 0.0226 and seminal fluid/plasma ratio (n=5) ranged between 0.11 and 4.42.

Metabolism

Atazanavir is extensively metabolized in humans. The major biotransformation pathways of atazanavir in humans consisted of monooxygenation and dioxygenation. Other minor biotransformation pathways for atazanavir or its metabolites consisted of glucuronidation, N-dealkylation, hydrolysis, and oxygenation with dehydrogenation. Two minor metabolites of atazanavir in plasma have been characterized. Neither metabolite demonstrated *in vitro* antiviral activity. *In vitro* studies using human liver microsomes suggested that atazanavir is metabolized by CYP3A.

Elimination

Following a single 400 mg dose of ^{14}C-atazanavir, 79% and 13% of the total radioactivity was recovered in the feces and urine, respectively. Unchanged drug accounted for approximately 20% and 7% of the administered dose in the feces and urine, respectively. The mean elimination half-life of atazanavir in healthy volunteers (n=214) and HIV-infected adult patients (n=13) was approximately 7 hours at steady state following a dose of 400 mg daily with a light meal.

Effects on Electrocardiogram

Concentration- and dose-dependent prolongation of the PR interval in the electrocardiogram has been observed in healthy volunteers receiving atazanavir. In a placebo-controlled study (AI424-076), the mean (±SD) maximum change in PR interval from the predose value was 24 (±15) msec following oral dosing with 400 mg of atazanavir (n=65) compared to 13 (±11) msec following dosing with placebo (n=67). The PR interval prolongations in this study were asymptomatic. There is limited information on the potential for a pharmacodynamic interaction in humans between atazanavir and other drugs that prolong the PR interval of the electrocardiogram. (See WARNINGS.)

Electrocardiographic effects of atazanavir were determined in a clinical pharmacology study of 72 healthy subjects. Oral doses of 400 and 800 mg were compared with placebo; there was no concentration-dependent effect of atazanavir on the QTc interval (using Fridericia's correction). In 1793 HIV-infected patients receiving antiretroviral regimens, QTc prolongation was comparable in the atazanavir and comparator regimens. No atazanavir-treated healthy subject or HIV-infected patient had a QTc interval >500 msec.

SPECIAL POPULATIONS

Age/Gender

A study of the pharmacokinetics of atazanavir was performed in young (n=29; 18-40 years) and elderly (n=30; ≥65 years) healthy subjects. There were no clinically important pharmacokinetic differences observed due to age or gender.

Race

There are insufficient data to determine whether there are any effects of race on the pharmacokinetics of atazanavir.

Pediatrics

The pharmacokinetics of atazanavir in pediatric patients are under investigation. There are insufficient data at this time to recommend a dose.

Impaired Renal Function

In healthy subjects, the renal elimination of unchanged atazanavir was approximately 7% of the administered dose. There are no pharmacokinetic data available on patients with impaired renal function.

Impaired Hepatic Function

Atazanavir is metabolized and eliminated primarily by the liver. Atazanavir sulfate has been studied in adult subjects with moderate to severe hepatic impairment (14 Child-Pugh B and 2 Child-Pugh C subjects) after a single 400 mg dose. The mean AUC(0-∞) was 42% greater in subjects with impaired hepatic function than in healthy volunteers. The mean half-life of atazanavir in hepatically impaired subjects was 12.1 hours compared to 6.4 hours in healthy volunteers. Increased concentrations of atazanavir are expected in patients with moderately or severely impaired hepatic function (see PRECAUTIONS and DOSAGE AND ADMINISTRATION).

DRUG-DRUG INTERACTIONS

See also CONTRAINDICATIONS, WARNINGS, and DRUG INTERACTIONS.

Atazanavir is metabolized in the liver by CYP3A. Atazanavir inhibits CYP3A and UGT1A1 at clinically relevant concentrations with Ki of 2.35 μM (CYP3A4 isoform) and 1.9 μM. Atazanavir sulfate should not be administered concurrently with medications with narrow therapeutic windows that are substrates of CYP3A or UGT1A1 (see CONTRAINDICATIONS).

Atazanavir competitively inhibits CYP1A2 and CYP2C9 with Ki values of 12 μM and a C_{max}/Ki ratio of ~0.25. There is a potential drug-drug interaction between atazanavir and CYP1A2 or CYP2C9 substrates. Atazanavir does not inhibit CYP2C19 or CYP2E1 at clinically relevant concentrations.

Atazanavir has been shown *in vivo* not to induce its own metabolism, nor to increase the biotransformation of some drugs metabolized by CYP3A. In a multiple-dose study, atazanavir sulfate decreased the urinary ratio of endogenous 6β-OH cortisol to cortisol versus baseline, indicating that CYP3A production was not induced.

Drugs that induce CYP3A activity may increase the clearance of atazanavir, resulting in lowered plasma concentrations. Coadministration of atazanavir sulfate and other drugs that inhibit CYP3A may increase atazanavir plasma concentrations.

Drug interaction studies were performed with atazanavir sulfate and other drugs likely to be coadministered and some drugs commonly used as probes for pharmacokinetic interactions. The effects of coadministration of atazanavir sulfate on the AUC, C_{max}, and C_{min} are summarized in TABLE 2 and TABLE 3. For information regarding clinical recommendations, see TABLE 8 and DRUG INTERACTIONS, Established and Other Potentially Significant Drug Interactions.

INDICATIONS AND USAGE

Atazanavir sulfate is indicated in combination with other antiretroviral agents for the treatment of HIV-1 infection.

This indication is based on analyses of plasma HIV-1 RNA levels and CD4 cell counts from controlled studies of 48 weeks duration in antiretroviral-naive patients and a controlled study of 24 weeks duration in antiretroviral-treatment-experienced patients.

In antiretroviral-treatment-experienced patients, the use of atazanavir sulfate may be considered for adults with HIV strains that are expected to be susceptible to atazanavir sulfate as assessed by genotypic and/or phenotypic testing. (See CLINICAL PHARMACOLOGY, Microbiology.)

CONTRAINDICATIONS

Atazanavir sulfate is contraindicated in patients with known hypersensitivity to any of its ingredients, including atazanavir.

Coadministration of atazanavir sulfate is contraindicated with drugs that are highly dependent on CYP3A for clearance and for which elevated plasma concentrations are associated with serious and/or life-threatening events. These drugs are listed in TABLE 7.

WARNINGS

ALERT: Find out about medicines that should NOT be taken with atazanavir sulfate. This statement is included on the product's bottle label. (See CONTRAINDICATIONS, WARNINGS, Drug Interactions, and DRUG INTERACTIONS.)

DRUG INTERACTIONS

Atazanavir is an inhibitor of CYP3A and UGT1A1. Coadministration of atazanavir sulfate and drugs primarily metabolized by CYP3A (*e.g.,* calcium channel blockers, HMG-CoA reductase inhibitors, immunosuppressants, and sildenafil) or UGT1A1 (*e.g.,* irinotecan) may result in increased plasma concentrations of the other drug that could increase or prolong its therapeutic and adverse effects. (See TABLE 8 and DRUG INTERACTIONS, Established and Other Potentially Significant Drug Interactions.)

Particular caution should be used when prescribing sildenafil in patients receiving protease inhibitors, including atazanavir sulfate. Coadministration of a protease inhibitor with sildenafil is expected to substantially increase sildenafil concentrations and may result in an increase in sildenafil-associated adverse events, including hypotension, visual changes, and priapism. (See DRUG INTERACTIONS; PRECAUTIONS, Information for the Patient; and the complete prescribing information for sildenafil.)

Concomitant use of atazanavir sulfate with lovastatin or simvastatin is not recommended. Caution should be exercised if HIV protease inhibitors, including atazanavir sulfate, are used concurrently with other HMG-CoA reductase inhibitors that are also metabolized by the CYP3A pathway (*e.g.,* atorvastatin). The risk of myopathy, including rhabdomyolysis, may be increased when HIV protease inhibitors, including atazanavir sulfate, are used in combination with these drugs.

Concomitant use of atazanavir sulfate and St. John's wort *(Hypericum perforatum),* or products containing St. John's wort, is not recommended. Coadministration of protease inhibitors, including atazanavir sulfate, with St. John's wort is expected to substantially decrease concentrations of the protease inhibitor and may result in suboptimal levels of atazanavir and lead to loss of virologic response and possible resistance to atazanavir or to the class of protease inhibitors.

PR INTERVAL PROLONGATION

Atazanavir has been shown to prolong the PR interval of the electrocardiogram in some patients. In healthy volunteers and in patients, abnormalities in atrioventricular (AV) conduction were asymptomatic and limited to first-degree AV block with rare exceptions. In

TABLE 2 *Drug Interactions: Pharmacokinetic Parameters for Atazanavir in the Presence of Coadministered Drugs*

Coadministered Drug Dose/Schedule of Coadministered Drug	Atazanavir Dose/Schedule	n	Ratio (90% Confindence Interval) of Atazanavir Pharmacokinetic Parameters With/Without Coadministered Drug; No Effect = 1.00 C_{max}	AUC	C_{min}
Atenolol					
50 mg qd, d 7-11 and d 19-23	400 mg qd, d 1-11	19	1.00 (0.89, 1.12)	0.93 (0.85, 1.01)	0.74 (0.65, 0.86)
Clarithromycin					
500 mg qd, d 7-10 and d 18-21	400 mg qd, d 1-10	29	1.06 (0.93, 1.20)	1.28 (1.16, 1.43)	1.91 (1.66, 2.21)
Didanosine (ddl) (buffered tablets) plus Stavudine (d4T)					
ddl: 200 mg × 1 dose, d4T: 40 mg × 1 dose	400 mg × 1 dose simultaneously with ddl and d4T	32*	0.11 (0.06, 0.18)	0.13 (0.08, 0.21)	0.16 (0.10, 0.27)
ddl: 200 mg × 1 dose, d4T: 40 mg × 1 dose	400 mg × 1 dose 1 h after ddl + d4T	32*	1.12 (0.67, 1.18)	1.03 (0.64, 1.67)	1.03 (0.61, 1.73)
Diltiazem					
180 mg qd, d 7-11 and d 19-23	400 mg qd, d 1-11	30	1.04 (0.96, 1.11)	1.00 (0.95, 1.05)	0.98 (0.90, 1.07)
Efavirenz					
600 mg qd, d 7-20	400 mg qd, d 1-20	27	0.41 (0.33, 0.51)	0.26 (0.22, 0.32)	0.07 (0.05, 0.10)
Efavirenz and Ritonavir					
Efavirenz 600 mg qd 2 h after atazanavir sulfate and ritonavir 100 mg qd simultaneously with atazanavir sulfate, d 7-20	400 mg qd, d 1-6 then 300 mg qd d 7-20	13	1.14 (0.83, 1.58)	1.39 (1.02, 1.88)	1.48 (1.24, 1.76)
Ketoconazole					
200 mg qd, d 7-13	400 mg qd, d 1-13	14	0.99 (0.77, 1.28)	1.10 (0.89, 1.37)	1.03 (0.53, 2.01)
Rifabutin					
150 mg qd, d 15-28	400 mg qd, d 1-28	7	1.34 (1.14, 1.59)	1.15 (0.98, 1.34)	1.13 (0.68, 1.87)
Ritonavir†					
100 mg qd, d 11-20	300 mg qd, d 1-20	28	1.86 (1.69, 2.05)	3.38 (3.13, 3.63)	11.89 (10.23, 13.82)

* One subject did not receive atazanavir sulfate.
† Compared with atazanavir 400 mg qd historical data, administration of atazanavir/ritonavir 300/100 mg qd increased the atazanavir geometric mean values of C_{max}, AUC, and C_{min} by 18%, 103%, and 671%, respectively. The geometric mean values of atazanavir pharmacokinetic parameters when coadministered with ritonavir were: C_{max} = 6129 ng/ml, AUC = 57039 ng·h/ml, and C_{min} = 1227 ng/ml.

clinical trials, asymptomatic first-degree AV block was observed in 5.9% of atazanavir-treated patients (n=920), 5.2% of lopinavir/ritonavir-treated patients (n=252), 10.4% of nelfinavir-treated patients (n=48), and in 3.0% of efavirenz-treated patients (n=329). There has been no second- or third-degree AV block. Because of limited clinical experience, atazanavir should be used with caution in patients with preexisting conduction system disease (*e.g.,* marked first-degree AV block or secondor third-degree AV block). (See CLINICAL PHARMACOLOGY, Pharmacokinetics, Effects on Electrocardiogram.)

In a pharmacokinetic study between atazanavir 400 mg once daily and diltiazem 180 mg once daily, a CYP3A substrate, there was a 2-fold increase in the diltiazem plasma concentration and an additive effect on the PR interval. When used in combination with atazanavir, a dose reduction of diltiazem by one half should be considered and ECG monitoring is recommended. In a pharmacokinetic study between atazanavir 400 mg once daily and atenolol 50 mg once daily, there was no substantial additive effect of atazanavir and atenolol on the PR interval. When used in combination with atazanavir, there is no need to adjust the dose of atenolol. (See DRUG INTERACTIONS.)

Pharmacokinetic studies between atazanavir and other drugs that prolong the PR interval including beta blockers (other than atenolol), verapamil, and digoxin have not been performed. An additive effect of atazanavir and these drugs cannot be excluded; therefore, caution should be exercised when atazanavir is given concurrently with these drugs, especially those that are metabolized by CYP3A (*e.g.,* verapamil). (See DRUG INTERACTIONS.)

DIABETES MELLITUS/HYPERGLYCEMIA

New-onset diabetes mellitus, exacerbation of preexisting diabetes mellitus, and hyperglycemia have been reported during post-marketing surveillance in HIV-infected patients receiving protease inhibitor therapy. Some patients required either initiation or dose adjustments of insulin or oral hypoglycemic agents for treatment of these events. In some cases, diabetic ketoacidosis has occurred. In those patients who discontinued protease inhibitor therapy, hyperglycemia persisted in some cases. Because these events have been reported voluntarily during clinical practice, estimates of frequency cannot be made and a causal relationship between protease inhibitor therapy and these events has not been established.

TABLE 3 *Drug Interactions: Pharmacokinetic Parameters for Coadministered Drugs in the Presence of Atazanavir Sulfate*

Coadministered Drug Dose/Schedule of Coadministered Drug	Atazanavir Dose/Schedule	n	Ratio (90% Confindence Interval) of Coadministered Drug Pharmacokinetic Parameters With/Without Atazanavir; No Effect = 1.00 C_{max}	AUC	C_{min}
Atenolol					
50 mg qd, d 7-11 and d 19-23	400 mg qd, d 1-11	19	1.34 (1.26, 1.42)	1.25 (1.16, 1.34)	1.02 (0.88, 1.19)
Clarithromycin					
500 mg qd, d 7-10 and d 18-21	400 mg qd, d 1-10	21	1.50 (1.32, 1.71)	1.94 (1.75, 2.16)	0.38 (0.35, 0.43)
			OH-clarithromycin:		
			0.28 (0.24, 0.33)	0.30 (0.26, 0.34)	2.64 (2.36, 2.94)
Didanosine (ddl) (buffered tablets) plus Stavudine (d4T)					
ddl: 200 mg × 1 dose, d4T: 40 mg × 1 dose	400 mg × 1 dose simultaneous with ddl and d4T	32*	ddl: 0.92 (0.84, 1.02)	ddl: 0.98 (0.92, 1.05)	NA
			d4T: 1.08 (0.96, 1.22)	d4T: 1.00 (0.97, 1.03)	d4T: 1.04 (0.94, 1.16)
Diltiazem					
180 mg qd, d 7-11 and d 19-23	400 mg qd, d 1-11	28	1.98 (1.78, 2.19)	2.25 (2.09, 2.16)	0.41 (0.37, 0.47)
			Desacetyl-diltiazem:		
			2.72 (2.44, 3.03)	2.65 (2.45, 2.87)	0.45 (0.41, 0.49)
Ethinyl Estradiol & Norethindrone					
Ortho-Novum 7/7/7 qd, d 1-29	400 mg qd, d 16-29	19	Ethinyl estradiol:		
			1.15 (0.99, 1.32)	1.48 (1.31, 1.68)	1.91 (1.57, 2.33)
			Norethindrone:		
			1.67 (1.42, 1.96)	2.10 (1.68, 2.62)	3.62 (2.57, 5.09)
Rifabutin					
300 mg qd, d 1-10 then 150 mg qd, d 11-20	600 mg qd†, d 11-20	3	1.18 (0.94, 1.48)	2.10 (1.57, 2.79)	3.43 (1.98, 5.96)
			25-O-desacetyl-rifabutin:		
			8.20 (5.90, 11.40)	22.01 (15.97, 30.34)	75.6 (30.1, 190.0)
Saquinavir (soft gelatin capsules)‡					
1200 mg qd, d 1-13	400 mg qd, d 7-13	7	4.39 (3.24, 5.95)	5.49 (4.04, 7.47)	6.86 (5.29, 8.91)
Lamivudine + Zidovudine					
150 mg lamivudine + 300 mg zidovudine bid, d 1-12	400 mg qd, d 7-12	19	Lamivudine:		
			1.04 (0.92, 1.16)	1.03 (0.98, 1.08)	1.12 (1.04, 1.21)
			Zidovudine:		
			1.05 (0.88, 1.24)	1.05 (0.96, 1.14)	0.69 (0.57, 0.84)
			Zidovudine glucuronide:		
			0.95 (0.88, 1.02)	1.00 (0.97, 1.03)	0.82 (0.62, 1.08)

* One subject did not receive atazanavir sulfate.
† Not the recommended therapeutic dose of atazanavir.
‡ The combination of atazanavir and saquinavir 1200 mg qd produced daily saquinavir exposures similar to the values produced by the standard therapeutic dosing of saquinavir at 1200 mg tid. However, the C_{max} is about 79% higher than that for the standard dosing of saquinavir (soft gelatin capsules) alone at 1200 mg tid.
NA=not available.

TABLE 7 *Drugs That Are Contraindicated With Atazanavir Sulfate Due to Potential CYP450-Mediated Interactions**

Drug Class	Drugs Within Class That Are Contraindicated With Atazanavir Sulfate
Benzodiazepines	Midazolam, triazolam
Ergot derivatives	Dihydroegotamine, ergotamine, ergonovine, methylergonovine
GI motility agent	Cisapride
Neuroleptic	Pimozide

* Please see TABLE 8 for additional drugs that should not be coadministered with atazanavir sulfate.

PRECAUTIONS

GENERAL

Hyperbilirubinemia

Most patients taking atazanavir sulfate experience asymptomatic elevations in indirect (unconjugated) bilirubin related to inhibition of UDP-glucuronosyl transferase (UGT). This hyperbilirubinemia is reversible upon discontinuation of atazanavir sulfate. Hepatic transaminase elevations that occur with hyperbilirubinemia should be evaluated for alternative etiologies. No long-term safety data are available for patients experiencing persistent elevations in total bilirubin >5 times ULN. Alternative antiretroviral therapy to atazanavir sulfate may be considered if jaundice or scleral icterus associated with bilirubin elevations presents cosmetic concerns for patients. Dose reduction of atazanavir is not recommended since long-term efficacy of reduced doses has not been established. (See TABLE 11A, TABLE 11B, TABLE 13A, and TABLE 13B.)

Hepatic Impairment and Toxicity

Atazanavir is principally metabolized by the liver; caution should be exercised when administering this drug to patients with hepatic impairment because atazanavir concentrations may be increased (see DOSAGE AND ADMINISTRATION). Patients with underlying hepatitis B or C viral infections or marked elevations in transaminases prior to treatment may be at increased risk for developing further transaminase elevations or hepatic decompensation.

Resistance/Cross-Resistance

Various degrees of cross-resistance among protease inhibitors have been observed. Resistance to atazanavir may not preclude the subsequent use of other protease inhibitors. (See CLINICAL PHARMACOLOGY, Microbiology.)

Hemophilia

There have been reports of increased bleeding, including spontaneous skin hematomas and hemarthrosis, in patients with hemophilia type A and B treated with protease inhibitors. In some patients, additional factor VIII was given. In more than half of the reported cases, treatment with protease inhibitors was continued or reintroduced. A causal relationship between protease inhibitor therapy and these events has not been established.

Lactic Acidosis Syndrome

Cases of lactic acidosis syndrome (LAS), sometimes fatal, and symptomatic hyperlactatemia have been reported in patients receiving atazanavir sulfate in combination with nucleoside analogues, which are known to be associated with increased risk of LAS. Female gender and obesity are also known risk factors for LAS. The contribution of atazanavir sulfate to the risk of development of LAS has not been established.

Fat Redistribution

Redistribution/accumulation of body fat, including central obesity, dorsocervical fat enlargement (buffalo hump), peripheral wasting, facial wasting, breast enlargement, and "cushingoid appearance" have been observed in patients receiving antiretroviral therapy. The mechanism and long-term consequences of these events are currently unknown. A causal relationship has not been established.

INFORMATION FOR THE PATIENT

A statement to patients and healthcare providers is included on the product's bottle label: **ALERT: Find out about medicines that should NOT be taken with atazanavir sulfate.** A Patient Package Insert (PPI) for atazanavir sulfate is available for patient information.

Patients should be told that sustained decreases in plasma HIV RNA have been associated with a reduced risk of progression to AIDS and death. Patients should remain under the care of a physician while using atazanavir sulfate. Patients should be advised to take atazanavir sulfate with food every day and take other concomitant antiretroviral therapy as prescribed. Atazanavir sulfate must always be used in combination with other antiretroviral drugs. Patients should not alter the dose or discontinue therapy without consulting with their doctor. If a dose of atazanavir sulfate is missed, patients should take the dose as soon as possible and then return to their normal schedule. However, if a dose is skipped, the patient should not double the next dose.

Patients should be informed that atazanavir sulfate is not a cure for HIV infection and that they may continue to develop opportunistic infections and other complications associated with HIV disease. Patients should be told that there are currently no data demonstrating that therapy with atazanavir sulfate can reduce the risk of transmitting HIV to others through sexual contact.

Atazanavir sulfate may interact with some drugs; therefore, patients should be advised to report to their doctor the use of any other prescription, nonprescription medication, or herbal products, particularly St. John's wort.

Patients receiving sildenafil and atazanavir should be advised that they may be at an increased risk of sildenafil-associated adverse events including hypotension, visual changes, and prolonged penile erection, and should promptly report any symptoms to their doctor.

Patients should be informed that atazanavir may produce changes in the electrocardiogram (PR prolongation). Patients should consult their physician if they are experiencing symptoms such as dizziness or lightheadedness.

Atazanavir sulfate should be taken with food to enhance absorption.

Patients should be informed that asymptomatic elevations in indirect bilirubin have occurred in patients receiving atazanavir sulfate. This may be accompanied by yellowing of the skin or whites of the eyes and alternative antiretroviral therapy may be considered if the patient has cosmetic concerns.

Patients should be informed that redistribution or accumulation of body fat may occur in patients receiving antiretroviral therapy including protease inhibitors and that the cause and long-term health effects of these conditions are not known at this time. It is unknown whether long-term use of atazanavir sulfate will result in a lower incidence of lipodystrophy than with other protease inhibitors.

CARCINOGENESIS, MUTAGENESIS, AND IMPAIRMENT OF FERTILITY

Long-term carcinogenicity studies of atazanavir in animals have not been completed. Atazanavir tested positive in an *in vitro* clastogenicity test using primary human lymphocytes, in the absence and presence of metabolic activation. Atazanavir tested negative in the *in vitro* Ames reverse-mutation assay, *in vivo* micronucleus and DNA repair tests in rats, and *in vivo* DNA damage test in rat duodenum (comet assay).

At the systemic drug exposure levels (AUC) equal to (in male rats) or 2 times (in female rats) those at the human clinical dose (400 mg/daily), atazanavir did not produce significant effects on mating, fertility, or early embryonic development.

PREGNANCY CATEGORY B

At maternal doses producing the systemic drug exposure levels equal to (in rabbits) or 2 times (in rats) those at the human clinical dose (400 mg once daily), atazanavir did not produce teratogenic effects. In the pre- and post-natal development assessment in rats, atazanavir, at maternally toxic drug exposure levels 2 times those at the human clinical dose, caused body weight loss or weight gain suppression in the offspring. Offspring were unaffected at a lower dose that produced maternal exposure equivalent to that observed in humans given 400 mg once daily.

Hyperbilirubinemia occurred frequently during treatment with atazanavir sulfate. It is not known whether atazanavir sulfate administered to the mother during pregnancy will exacerbate physiological hyperbilirubinemia and lead to kernicterus in neonates and young infants. In the prepartum period, additional monitoring and alternative therapy to atazanavir sulfate should be considered.

There are no adequate and well-controlled studies in pregnant women. Cases of lactic acidosis syndrome, sometimes fatal, and symptomatic hyperlactatemia have been reported in patients (including pregnant women) receiving atazanavir sulfate in combination with nucleoside analogues, which are known to be associated with increased risk of lactic acidosis syndrome. Atazanavir sulfate should be used during pregnancy only if the potential benefit justifies the potential risk to the fetus. (See General, Lactic Acidosis Syndrome.)

Antiretroviral Pregnancy Registry: To monitor maternal-fetal outcomes of pregnant women exposed to atazanavir sulfate, an Antiretroviral Pregnancy Registry has been established. Physicians are encouraged to register patients by calling 1-800-258-4263.

NURSING MOTHERS

The Centers for Disease Control and Prevention recommend that HIV-infected mothers not breast-feed their infants to avoid risking postnatal transmission of HIV. It is not known whether atazanavir is secreted in human milk. A study in lactating rats has demonstrated that atazanavir is secreted in milk. Because of both the potential for HIV transmission and the potential for serious adverse reactions in nursing infants, **mothers should be instructed not to breast-feed if they are receiving atazanavir sulfate.**

PEDIATRIC USE

The optimal dosing regimen for use of atazanavir sulfate in pediatric patients has not been established. Atazanavir sulfate should not be administered to pediatric patients below the age of 3 months due to the risk of kernicterus.

GERIATRIC USE

Clinical studies of atazanavir sulfate did not include sufficient numbers of patients aged 65 and over to determine whether they respond differently from younger patients. Based on a comparison of mean single dose pharmacokinetic values for C_{max} and AUC, a dose adjustment based upon age is not recommended. In general, appropriate caution should be exercised in the administration and monitoring of atazanavir sulfate in elderly patients reflecting the greater frequency of decreased hepatic, renal, or cardiac function, and of concomitant disease or other drug therapy.

DRUG INTERACTIONS

Atazanavir is an inhibitor of CYP3A and UGT1A1. Coadministration of atazanavir sulfate and drugs primarily metabolized by CYP3A (*e.g.*, calcium channel blockers, HMG-CoA reductase inhibitors, immunosuppressants, and sildenafil) or UGT1A1 (*e.g.*, irinotecan) may result in increased plasma concentrations of the other drug that could increase or prolong both its therapeutic and adverse effects, (see TABLE 8 and Established and Other Potentially Significant Drug Interactions). Atazanavir is metabolized in the liver by the cytochrome P450 enzyme system. Coadministration of atazanavir sulfate and drugs that induce CYP3A, such as rifampin, may decrease atazanavir plasma concentrations and reduce its therapeutic effect. Coadministration of atazanavir sulfate and drugs that inhibit CYP3A may increase atazanavir plasma concentrations.

Atazanavir solubility decreases as pH increases. Reduced plasma concentrations of atazanavir are expected if antacids, buffered medications, H_2-receptor antagonists, and proton-pump inhibitors are administrated with atazanavir.

Atazanavir has the potential to prolong the PR interval of the electrocardiogram in some patients. Caution should be used when coadministering atazanavir sulfate with medicinal products known to induce PR interval prolongation [*e.g.*, atenolol, diltiazem (see Established and Other Potentially Significant Drug Interactions)].

Drugs that are contraindicated or not recommended for coadministration with atazanavir sulfate are included in TABLE 8. These recommendations are based on either drug interaction studies or predicted interactions due to the expected magnitude of interaction and potential for serious events or loss of efficacy.

ESTABLISHED AND OTHER POTENTIALLY SIGNIFICANT DRUG INTERACTIONS

Alteration in dose or regimen may be recommended based on drug interaction studies or predicted interactions. (For magnitude of interactions, see TABLE 2 and TABLE 3.)

HIV-Antiviral Agents

Nucleoside Reverse Transcriptase Inhibitors (NRTIs)

Didanosine Buffered Formulations

Effect: Decreases atazanavir concentration.

Clinical Comments: Coadministration with atazanavir sulfate did not alter exposure to didanosine; however, exposure to atazanavir was markedly decreased by coadmin-

TABLE 8 *Drugs That Should Not Be Administered With Atazanavir Sulfate*

Drug Class: Specific Drugs	Clinical Comment
Antimycobacterials: Rifampin	Decreases plasma concentrations and AUC of most protease inhibitors by about 90%. This may result in loss of therapeutic effect and development of resistance.
Antineoplastics: Irinotecan	Atazanavir inhibits UGT and may interfere with the metabolism of irinotecan, resulting in increased irinotecan toxicities.
Benzodiazepines: Midazolam, triazolam	CONTRAINDICATED due to potential for serious and/or life-threatening events such as prolonged or increased sedation or respiratory depression.
Calcium Channel Blockers: Bepridil	Potential for serious and/or life-threatening adverse events.
Ergot Derivatives: Dihydroergotamine, ergotamine, ergonovine, methylergonovine	CONTRAINDICATED due to potential for serious and/or life-threatening events such as acute ergot toxicity characterized by peripheral vasospasm and ischemia of the extremities and other tissues.
GI Motility Agent: Cisapride	CONTRAINDICATED due to potential for serious and/or life-threatening reactions such as cardiac arrhythmias.
HMG-CoA Reductase Inhibitors: Lovastatin, simvastatin	Potential for serious reactions such as myopathy including rhabdomyolysis.
Neuroleptic: Pimozide	CONTRAINDICATED due to potential for serious and/or life-threatening reactions such as cardiac arrhythmias.
Protease Inhibitors: Indinavir	Both atazanavir sulfate and indinavir are associated with indirect (unconjugated) hyperbilirubinemia. Combinations of these drugs have not been studied and coadministration of atazanavir sulfate and indinavir is not recommended.
Proton-Pump Inhibitors	Concomitant use of atazanavir sulfate and proton-pump inhibitors is not recommended. Coadministration of atazanavir sulfate with proton-pump inhibitors is expected to substantially decrease atazanavir sulfate plasma concentrations and reduce its therapeutic effect.
Herbal Products: St. John's wort *(Hypericum perforatum)*	Patients taking atazanavir sulfate should not use products containing St. John's wort *(Hypericum perforatum)* because coadministration may be expected to reduce plasma concentrations of atazanavir. This may result in loss of therapeutic effect and development of resistance.

istration of atazanavir sulfate with didanosine buffered tablets (presumably due to the increase in gastric pH caused by buffers in the didanosine tablets). In addition, it is recommended that didanosine be administered on an empty stomach; therefore, atazanavir sulfate should be given (with food) 2 hours before or 1 hour after didanosine buffered formulations (see CLINICAL PHARMACOLOGY, Drug-Drug Interactions). (Although no interaction is expected with didanosine EC capsules, because didanosine EC capsules are to be given on an empty stomach and atazanavir sulfate is to be given with food, they should be administered at different times.)

Non-Nucleoside Reverse Transcriptase Inhibitors (NNRTIs)

Efavirenz:

Effect: Decreases atazanavir concentration.

Clinical Comments: If atazanavir sulfate is to be coadministered with efavirenz, which decreases atazanavir exposure, it is recommended that atazanavir sulfate 300 mg with ritonavir 100 mg be coadministered with efavirenz 600 mg (all as a single daily dose with food), as this combination results in atazanavir exposure that approximates the mean exposure to atazanavir produced by 400 mg of atazanavir sulfate alone. Atazanavir sulfate without ritonavir should not be coadministered with efavirenz.

Protease Inhibitors

Saquinavir (soft gelatin capsules):

Effect: Increases saquinavir concentration.

Clinical Comments: Appropriate dosing recommendations for this combination, with respect to efficacy and safety, have not been established.

Ritonavir:

Effect: Increases atazanavir concentration.

Clinical Comments: Coadministration of atazanavir sulfate and ritonavir is currently under clinical investigation. If atazanavir sulfate is coadministered with ritonavir, it is recommended that atazanavir sulfate 300 mg once daily be given with ritonavir 100 mg once daily with food.

Other Agents

Antacids and Buffered Medications

Effect: Decreases atazanavir concentration.

Clinical Comments: Reduced plasma concentrations of atazanavir are expected if antacids, including buffered medications, are administered with atazanavir sulfate. Atazanavir sulfate should be administered 2 hours before or 1 hour after these medications.

Antiarrhythmics

Amiodarone, Lidocaine (systemic), and Quinidine:

Effect: Increases amiodarone, lidocaine (systemic), and quinidine concentrations.

Clinical Comments: Coadministration with atazanavir sulfate has the potential to produce serious and/or life-threatening adverse events and has not been studied. Concentration monitoring of these drugs is recommended if they are used concomitantly with atazanavir sulfate.

Anticoagulants

Warfarin:

Effect: Increases warfarin concentration.

Clinical Comments: Coadministration with atazanavir sulfate has the potential to produce serious and/or life-threatening bleeding and has not been studied. It is recommended that INR (International Normalization Ratio) be monitored.

Antidepressants

Tricyclic Antidepressants:

Effect: Increases tricyclic antidepressants concentration.

Clinical Comments: Coadministration with atazanavir sulfate has the potential to produce serious and/or life-threatening adverse events and has not been studied. Concentration monitoring of these drugs is recommended if they are used concomitantly with atazanavir sulfate.

Antimycobacterials

Rifabutin:

Effect: Increases rifabutin concentrations.

Clinical Comments: A rifabutin dose reduction of up to 75% (*e.g.,* 150 mg every other day or 3 times/week) is recommended.

Calcium Channel Blockers

Diltiazem:

Effect: Increases diltiazem and desacetyl-diltiazem concentration.

Clinical Comments: Caution is warranted. A dose reduction of diltiazem by 50% should be considered. ECG monitoring is recommended.

e.g., **Felodipine, Nifedipine, Nicardipine, and Verapamil:**

Effect: Increases calcium channel blocker concentration.

Clinical Comments: Caution is warranted. Dose titration of the calcium channel blocker should be considered. ECG monitoring is recommended.

Erectile Dysfunction Agents

Sildenafil:

Effect: Increases sildenafil concentration.

Clinical Comments: Coadministration may result in an increase in sildenafil-associated adverse events, including hypotension, visual changes, and priapism. Use sildenafil with caution at a reduced dose of 25 mg every 48 hours and monitor for adverse events.

HMG-CoA Reductase Inhibitors

Atorvastatin:

Effect: Increases atorvastatin concentration.

Clinical Comments: The risk of myopathy including rhabdomyolysis may be increased when protease inhibitors, including atazanavir sulfate, are used in combination with atorvastatin. Caution should be exercised.

H_2-Receptor Antagonists

Effect: Decreases atazanavir concentration.

Clinical Comments: Reduced plasma concentrations of atazanavir are expected if H_2-receptor antagonists are administered with atazanavir sulfate. This may result in loss of therapeutic effect and development of resistance. To lessen the effect of H_2-receptor antagonists on atazanavir exposure, it is recommended that an H_2-receptor antagonist and atazanavir sulfate be administered as far apart as possible, preferably 12 hours apart.

Immunosuppresants

Cyclosporine, Sirolimus, Tacrolimus:

Effect: Increases immunosuppressants concentration.

Clinical Comments: Therapeutic concentration monitoring is recommended for immunosuppressant agents when coadministered with atazanavir sulfate.

Macrolide Antibiotics

Clarithromycin:

Effect: Increases clarithromycin, decreases 14-OH clarithromycin, and increases atazanavir concentrations.

Clinical Comments: Increased concentrations of clarithromycin may cause QTc prolongations; therefore, a dose reduction of clarithromycin by 50% should be considered when it is coadministered with atazanavir sulfate. In addition, concentrations of the active metabolite 14-OH clarithromycin are significantly reduced; consider alternative therapy for indications other than infections due to *Mycobacterium avium* complex.

Oral Contraceptives

Ethinyl Estradiol and Norethindrone:

Effect: Increases ethinyl estradiol and norethindrone concentrations.

Clinical Comments: Mean concentrations of ethinyl estradiol, when coadministered as a 35 μg dose with atazanavir sulfate, are increased to a level between mean concentrations produced by a 35 and a 50 μg ethinyl estradiol dose. Decreased HDL or increased insulin resistance may be associated with increased mean concentrations of norethindrone, when coadministered with atazanavir sulfate, particularly in diabetic women. Caution should be exercised. It is recommended that the lowest effective dose of each oral contraceptive component be used.

Based on known metabolic profiles, clinically significant drug interactions are not expected between atazanavir sulfate and fluvastatin, pravastatin, dapsone, trimethoprim/

sulfamethoxazole, azithromycin, erythromycin, itraconazole, or fluconazole. Atazanavir sulfate does not interact with substrates of CYP2D6 (*e.g.*, nortriptyline, desipramine, metoprolol).

ADVERSE REACTIONS

ADULT PATIENTS

Treatment-Emergent Adverse Events in Treatment-Naive Patients

Selected clinical adverse events of moderate or severe intensity in ≥3% of treatment-naive patients receiving combination therapy including atazanavir sulfate are presented in TABLE 10A and TABLE 10B. For other information regarding observed or potentially serious adverse events, see WARNINGS and PRECAUTIONS.

TABLE 10A *Selected Treatment-Emergent Adverse Events of Moderate or Severe Intensity Reported in ≥3% of Adult Treatment-Naive Patients**

	Phase III Study AI424-034	
	64 Weeks†	
	Atazanavir Sulfate 400 mg Once Daily + Lamivudine + Zidovudine‡ (n=404)	Efavirenz 600 mg Once Daily + Lamivudine + Zidovudine‡ (n=401)
Body as a Whole		
Headache	14	13
Fever	4	6
Pain	3	2
Fatigue	2	2
Back pain	2	5
Digestive System		
Nausea	16	13
Jaundice/scleral icterus	7	<1
Abdominal pain	6	5
Vomiting	6	8
Diarrhea	6	7
Metabolic and Nutritional System		
Lipodystrophy	1	1
Musculoskeletal System		
Arthralgia	<1	2
Nervous System		
Depression	4	5
Insomnia	3	5
Dizziness	3	8
Peripheral neurologic symptoms	1	2
Respiratory System		
Increased cough	3	4
Skin and Appendages		
Rash	9	13

* Based on regimen(s) containing atazanavir sulfate.
† Median time on therapy.
‡ As a fixed dose combination: 150 mg lamivudine, 300 mg zidovudine twice daily.

TABLE 10B *Selected Treatment-Emergent Adverse Events of Moderate or Severe Intensity Reported in ≥3% of Adult Treatment-Naive Patients**

	Phase II Studies AI424-007, -008	
	120 Weeks†‡	73 Weeks†‡
	Atazanavir Sulfate 400 mg Once Daily + Stavudine + Lamivudine or Stavudine + Didanosine (n=279)	Nelfinavir 750 mg tid or 1250 mg bid + Stavudine + Lamivudine or Stavudine + Didanosine (n=191)
Body as a Whole		
Headache	10	8
Fever	5	5
Pain	1	2
Fatigue	3	2
Back pain	6	3
Digestive System		
Nausea	10	6
Jaundice/scleral icterus	8	§
Abdominal pain	10	8
Vomiting	8	7
Diarrhea	8	25
Metabolic and Nutritional System		
Lipodystrophy	8	3
Musculoskeletal System		
Arthralgia	4	4
Nervous System		
Depression	8	3
Insomnia	1	<1
Dizziness	1	§
Peripheral neurologic symptoms	8	7
Respiratory System		
Increased cough	5	1
Skin and Appendages		
Rash	10	3

* Based on regimen(s) containing atazanavir sulfate.
† Median time on therapy.
‡ Includes long-term follow-up.
§ None reported in this treatment arm.

Treatment-Emergent Adverse Events in Treatment-Experienced Patients

In Phase III clinical trials, atazanavir sulfate has been studied in 144 treatment-experienced patients in combination with two NRTIs (AI424-043) and in 229 treatment-experienced patients in combination with either ritonavir, tenofovir, and one NRTI or saquinavir, tenofovir, and one NRTI (AI424-045). Treatment-emergent adverse events of moderate or severe intensity were comparable between these patients and treatment-naive patients (TABLE 10A and TABLE 10B).

Treatment-Emergent Adverse Events in All Atazanavir Sulfate-Treated Patients

Treatment-emergent adverse events of at least moderate intensity occurring in less than 3% of adult patients receiving atazanavir sulfate in all Phase II/III clinical trials (n=1597) and considered of possible, probable, certain, or unknown relationship to treatment with atazanavir sulfate-containing regimens, and not listed in TABLE 10A and TABLE 10B are listed below by body system.

Body as a Whole: Allergic reaction, angioedema, asthenia, burning sensation, chest pain, dysplasia, edema, facial atrophy, generalized edema, heat sensitivity, infection, malaise, overdose, pallor, peripheral edema, photosensitivity, substernal chest pain, sweating.

Cardiovascular System: Heart arrest, heart block, hypertension, myocarditis, palpitation, syncope, vasodilatation.

Digestive System: Acholia, anorexia, aphthous stomatitis, colitis, constipation, dental pain, dyspepsia, enlarged abdomen, esophageal ulcer, esophagitis, flatulence, gastritis, gastroenteritis, gastrointestinal disorder, hepatitis, hepatomegaly, hepatosplenomegaly, increased appetite, liver damage, liver fatty deposit, mouth ulcer, pancreatitis, peptic ulcer.

Endocrine System: Decreased male fertility.

Hemic and Lymphatic System: Ecchymosis, purpura.

Metabolic and Nutritional Disorders: Buffalo hump, dehydration, diabetes mellitus, dyslipidemia, gout, lactic acidosis, lipohypertrophy, obesity, weight decrease, weight gain.

Musculoskeletal System: Bone pain, extremity pain, muscle atrophy, myalgia, myasthenia, myopathy.

Nervous System: Abnormal dream, abnormal gait, agitation, amnesia, anxiety, confusion, convulsion, decreased libido, emotional lability, hallucination, hostility, hyperkinesia, hypesthesia, increased reflexes, nervousness, psychosis, sleep disorder, somnolence, suicide attempt, twitch.

Respiratory System: Dyspnea, hiccup, hypoxia.

Skin and Appendages: Alopecia, cellulitis, dermatophytosis, dry skin, eczema, nail disorder, pruritus, seborrhea, urticaria, vesiculobullous rash.

Special Senses: Otitis, taste perversion, tinnitus.

Urogenital System: Abnormal urine, amenorrhea, crystalluria, gynecomastia, hematuria, impotence, kidney calculus, kidney failure, kidney pain, menstrual disorder, oliguria, pelvic pain, polyuria, proteinuria, urinary frequency, urinary tract infection.

LABORATORY ABNORMALITIES

The percentages of adult treatment-naive patients treated with combination therapy including atazanavir sulfate with Grade 3-4 laboratory abnormalities are presented in TABLE 11A and TABLE 11B.

TABLE 11A *Selected Grade 3-4 Laboratory Abnormalities Reported in ≥2% of Adult Treatment-Naive Patients**

		Phase III Study AI424-034	
		64 Weeks†	
Variable	Limit§	Atazanavir Sulfate 400 mg Once Daily + Lamivudine + Zidovudine‡ (n=404)	Efavirenz 600 mg Once Daily + Lamivudine + Zidovudine‡ (n=401)
Chemistry	**High**		
SGOT/AST	≥5.1 × ULN	2%	2%
SGPT/ALT	≥5.1 × ULN	4%	3%
Total bilirubin	≥2.6 × ULN	35%	<1%
Amylase	≥2.1 × ULN	¤	¤
Lipase	≥2.1 × ULN	<1%	1%
Hematology	**Low**		
Hemoglobin	<8.0 g/dl	5%	3%
Neutophils	<750 cells/mm^3	7%	9%

* Based on regimen(s) containing atazanavir sulfate.
† Median time on therapy.
‡ As a fixed-dose combination: 150 mg lamivudine, 300 mg zidovudine twice daily.
§ ULN=upper limit of normal.
¤ None reported in this treatment arm.

Patients Co-Infected With Hepatitis B and/or Hepatitis C Virus

Liver function tests should be monitored in patients with a history of hepatitis B or C. In studies AI424-008 and AI424-034, 74 patients treated with 400 mg of atazanavir sulfate once daily, 58 who received efavirenz, and 12 who received nelfinavir were seropositive for hepatitis B and/or C at study entry. AST levels >5 times the upper limit of normal (ULN) developed in 9% of the atazanavir sulfate-treated patients, 5% of the efavirenz-treated patients, and 17% of the nelfinavir-treated patients. ALT levels >5 times ULN developed in 15% of the atazanavir sulfate-treated patients, 14% of the efavirenz-treated patients, and 17% of the nelfinavir-treated patients. Within atazanavir and control regimens, no difference in frequency of bilirubin elevations was noted between seropositive and seronegative patients (see PRECAUTIONS, General).

TABLE 11B *Selected Grade 3-4 Laboratory Abnormalities Reported in ≥2% of Adult Treatment-Naive Patients**

		Phase II Studies AI424-007, -008	
		120 Weeks†‡	73 Weeks†‡
		Atazanavir Sulfate 400 mg Once Daily +	Nelfinavir 750 mg tid or 1250 mg bid +
		Stavudine + Lamivudine or Stavudine + Didanosine	Stavudine + Lamivudine or Stavudine + Didanosine
Variable	**Limit§**	**(n=279)**	**(n=191)**
Chemistry	**High**		
SGOT/AST	≥5.1 × ULN	7%	5%
SGPT/ALT	≥5.1 × ULN	9%	7%
Total bilirubin	≥2.6 × ULN	47%	3%
Amylase	≥2.1 × ULN	14%	10%
Lipase	≥2.1 × ULN	4%	5%
Hematology	**Low**		
Hemoglobin	<8.0 g/dl	<1%	4%
Neutophils	<750 cells/mm^3	3%	7%

* Based on regimen(s) containing atazanavir sulfate.
† Median time on therapy.
‡ Includes long-term follow-up.
§ ULN=upper limit of normal.

Lipids — Study AI424-034

For Study AI424-034, changes from baseline in fasting LDL-cholesterol, HDL-cholesterol, total cholesterol, and fasting triglycerides are shown in TABLE 12.

TABLE 12 *Lipid Values, Mean Change From Baseline, Study AI424-034*

	n§	LDL-Cholesterol¤	HDL-Cholesterol	Total cholesterol	Triglycerides¤
		Atazanavir Sulfate*			
Baseline	383	98 mg/dl	39 mg/dl	164 mg/dl	138 mg/dl
Week 48	283	98 mg/dl	43 mg/dl	168 mg/dl	124 mg/dl
Change‡	272	+1%	+13%	+2%	-9%
		Efavirenz†			
Baseline	378	98 mg/dl	38 mg/dl	162 mg/dl	129 mg/dl
Week 48	264	114 mg/dl	46 mg/dl	195 mg/dl	168 mg/dl
Change‡	253	+18%	+24%	+21%	+23%

* Atazanavir sulfate 400 mg once daily with the fixed-dose combination: 150 mg lamivudine, 300 mg zidovudine twice daily.
† Efavirenz 600 mg once daily with the fixed-dose combination: 150 mg lamivudine, 300 mg zidovudine twice daily.
‡ The change from baseline is the mean of within-patient changes from baseline for patients with both baseline and Week 48 values and is not a simple difference of the baseline and Week 48 mean values.
§ Number of patients with LDL-cholesterol measured.
¤ Fasting.

The percentages of adult treatment-experienced patients treated with combination therapy including atazanavir sulfate with Grade 3-4 laboratory abnormalities are presented in TABLE 13A and TABLE 13B.

TABLE 13A *Selected Grade 3-4 Laboratory Abnormalities Reported in ≥2% of Adult Treatment-Experienced Patients**

		Phase III Study AI424-043	
		24 Weeks†	
		Atazanavir Sulfate 400 mg Once Daily	Lopinavir + Ritonavir (400/100 mg) bid‡
		+ 2 NRTIs	+ 2 NRTIs
Variable	**Limit§**	**(n=144)**	**(n=146)**
Chemistry	**High**		
SGOT/AST	≥5.1 × ULN	3%	1%
SGPT/ALT	≥5.1 × ULN	6%	1%
Total bilirubin	≥2.6 × ULN	22%	¤
Lipase	≥2.1 × ULN	4%	3%
Hematology	**Low**		
Platelets	<50,000 cells/mm^3	¤	¤
Neutophils	<750 cells/mm^3	5%	3%

* Based on regimen(s) containing atazanavir sulfate.
† Median time on therapy.
‡ As a fixed-dose combination.
§ ULN=upper limit of normal.
¤ None reported in this treatment arm.

Lipids — Study AI424-043

For Study AI424-043, changes from baseline in fasting LDL-cholesterol, HDL-cholesterol, total cholesterol, and fasting triglycerides are shown in TABLE 14.

DOSAGE AND ADMINISTRATION

ADULTS

The recommended dose of atazanavir sulfate is 400 mg (two 200 mg capsules) once daily taken with food.

TABLE 13B *Selected Grade 3-4 Laboratory Abnormalities Reported in ≥2% of Adult Treatment-Experienced Patients**

		Phase II Study AI424-045		
		15 Weeks†	12 Weeks†	13 Weeks†
		Atazanavir Sulfate 300 mg Once Daily +	Atazanavir Sulfate 400 mg Once Daily +	Lopinavir + Ritonavir
		Ritonavir 100 mg Once Daily +	Saquinavir‡ 1200 mg Once Daily +	(400/100 mg) bid§ +
		Tenofovir + NRTI	Tenofovir + NRTI	Tenofovir + NRTI
Variable	**Limit¤**	**(n=119)**	**(n=110)**	**(n=118)**
Chemistry	**High**			
SGOT/AST	≥5.1 × ULN	<1%	2%	<1%
SGPT/ALT	≥5.1 × ULN	3%	3%	3%
Total bilirubin	≥2.6 × ULN	40%	13%	¶
Lipase	≥2.1 × ULN	4%	<1%	6%
Hematology	**Low**			
Platelets	<50,000 cells/mm^3	<1%	4%	<1%
Neutophils	<750 cells/mm^3	4%	5%	4%

* Based on regimen(s) containing atazanavir sulfate.
† Median time on therapy.
‡ Soft gelatin capsules.
§ As a fixed-dose combination.
¤ ULN=upper limit of normal.
¶ None reported in this treatment arm.

TABLE 14 *Lipid Values, Mean Change From Baseline, Study AI424-043*

	n§	LDL-Cholesterol¤¶	HDL-Cholesterol	Total cholesterol	Triglycerides¶
		Atazanavir Sulfate*			
Baseline	143	106 mg/dl	39 mg/dl	181 mg/dl	192 mg/dl
Week 24	123	95 mg/dl	41 mg/dl	170 mg/dl	193 mg/dl
Change‡	123	-6%	+12%	-2%	-2%
		Lopinavir + Ritonavir†			
Baseline	144	103 mg/dl	37 mg/dl	175 mg/dl	192 mg/dl
Week 24	107	107 mg/dl	45 mg/dl	201 mg/dl	262 mg/dl
Change‡	106	+5%	+18%	+17%	+55%

* Atazanavir sulfate 400 mg once daily + 2 NRTIs.
† Lopinavir + ritonavir (400/100 mg) bid + 2 NRTIs.
‡ The change from baseline is the mean of within-patient changes from baseline for patients with both baseline and Week 24 values and is not a simple difference of the baseline and Week 24 mean values.
§ Number of patients with LDL-cholesterol measured.
¤ Protocol-defined co-primary safety outcome measure.
¶ Fasting.

Important Dosing Information:

Efavirenz: When coadministered with efavirenz, it is recommended that atazanavir sulfate 300 mg and ritonavir 100 mg be given with efavirenz 600 mg (all as a single daily dose with food). Atazanavir sulfate without ritonavir should not be coadministered with efavirenz.

Didanosine: When coadministered with didanosine buffered formulations, atazanavir sulfate should be given (with food) 2 hours before or 1 hour after didanosine.

For these drugs and other antiretroviral agents (*e.g.,* ritonavir, saquinavir) for which dosing modification may be appropriate, see CLINICAL PHARMACOLOGY, Drug-Drug Interactions and DRUG INTERACTIONS, Established and Other Potentially Significant Drug Interactions.

PATIENTS WITH RENAL IMPAIRMENT

There are insufficient data to recommend a dosage adjustment for patients with renal impairment (see CLINICAL PHARMACOLOGY, Special Populations, Impaired Renal Function).

PATIENTS WITH HEPATIC IMPAIRMENT

Atazanavir sulfate should be used with caution in patients with mild to moderate hepatic insufficiency. A dose reduction to 300 mg once daily should be considered for patients with moderate hepatic insufficiency (Child-Pugh Class B). Atazanavir sulfate should not be used in patients with severe hepatic insufficiency (Child-Pugh Class C). (See PRECAUTIONS and CLINICAL PHARMACOLOGY, Special Populations, Impaired Hepatic Function.)

HOW SUPPLIED

Reyataz (atazanavir sulfate) capsules are available in the following strengths* and configurations:

100 mg: Blue/white cap/body with "BMS 100 mg" in white ink and "3623" in blue ink.
150 mg: Blue/powder blue cap/body with "BMS 150 mg" in white ink and "3624" in blue ink.
200 mg: Blue/blue cap/body with "BMS 200 mg" in white ink and "3631" in white ink.
*Atazanavir equivalent as atazanavir sulfate.

Storage: Reyataz (atazanavir sulfate) capsules should be stored at 25°C (77°F); excursions permitted to 15-30°C (59-86°F).

Atenolol (000333)

For related information, see the comparative table section in Appendix A.

Categories: Angina pectoris; Hypertension, essential; Myocardial infarction; Pregnancy Category C; FDA Approved 1981 Aug; WHO Formulary

Drug Classes: Antiadrenergics, beta blocking

Brand Names: **Tenormin**

Foreign Brand Availability: Alonet (Singapore); Altol (India); Anolene (Korea); Anselol (New-Zealand); Antipressan (England; Ireland); Apo-Atenolol (Israel); Arandin (Korea); Asten (Korea); Atcardil (Philippines); Atecard (India); AteHexal (Australia; Germany); Atelol (Benin; Burkina-Faso; Ethiopia; Gambia; Ghana; Guinea; Ivory-Coast; Kenya; Liberia; Malawi; Mali; Mauritania; Mauritius; Morocco; Niger; Nigeria; Senegal; Seychelles; Sierra-Leone; South-Africa; Sudan; Tanzania; Tunia; Uganda; Zambia; Zimbabwe); Atenblock (Finland); Atendol (Germany); Atenet (Denmark); Ateni (Israel); Atenil (Switzerland); Ateno (Bahrain; Cyprus; Egypt; Iran; Iraq; Jordan; Kuwait; Lebanon; Libya; Oman; Qatar; Republic-of-Yemen; Saudi-Arabia; Syria; United-Arab-Emirates); Atenogamma (Germany); Atenol (Italy); Atereal (Germany); Aterol (South-Africa); Atinol (Taiwan); Atolmin (Korea); Betablok (Indonesia); Betacard (Bahrain; India); Betarol (Korea); Blokium (Bahrain; Benin; Burkina-Faso; Chile; Costa-Rica; Cyprus; Dominican-Republic; Egypt; El-Salvador; Ethiopia; Gambia; Ghana; Guatemala; Guinea; Honduras; Iran; Iraq; Israel; Ivory-Coast; Jordan; Kenya; Kuwait; Lebanon; Liberia; Libya; Malawi; Mali; Mauritania; Mauritius; Morocco; Nicaragua; Niger; Nigeria; Oman; Panama; Qatar; Republic-of-Yemen; Saudi-Arabia; Senegal; Seychelles; Sierra-Leone; South-Africa; Sudan; Syria; Tanzania; Tunia; Uganda; United-Arab-Emirates; Venezuela; Zambia; Zimbabwe); Blotex (Mexico); B-Vasc (South-Africa); Cardioten (Philippines); Catenol (Benin; Burkina-Faso; Ethiopia; Gambia; Ghana; Guinea; Ivory-Coast; Kenya; Liberia; Malawi; Mali; Mauritania; Mauritius; Morocco; Niger; Nigeria; Senegal; Seychelles; Sierra-Leone; South-Africa; Sudan; Tanzania; Tunia; Uganda; Zambia; Zimbabwe); Coratol (Malaysia; Thailand); Corotenol (Bahrain; Cyprus; Egypt; Iran; Iraq; Israel; Jordan; Kuwait; Lebanon; Libya; Oman; Qatar; Republic-of-Yemen; Saudi-Arabia; Syria; United-Arab-Emirates); Durabeta (Philippines); Evitocor (Germany); Farnormin (Indonesia); Felo-Bits (Argentina); Hypernol (Singapore); Hypoten (Bahrain; Cyprus; Egypt; Iran; Iraq; Israel; Jordan; Kuwait; Lebanon; Libya; Oman; Qatar; Republic-of-Yemen; Saudi-Arabia; Syria; United-Arab-Emirates); Internolol (Indonesia); Lo-ten (Hong-Kong; New-Zealand; Taiwan); Loten (Malaysia); Lotenal (Korea); Myocord (Argentina); Normalol (Israel); Normaten (Hong-Kong); Normiten (Israel); Noten (Australia; Malaysia; New-Zealand; Singapore); Oraday (Malaysia; Thailand); Premorine (Argentina); Prenolol (Singapore; Thailand); Rozamin (Korea); Serten (Philippines); Stermin (Taiwan); Temoret (Korea); Tenidon (Denmark); Tenoblock (Finland); Tenocor (Thailand); Tenolin (Canada); Tenolol (Benin; Burkina-Faso; Ethiopia; Gambia; Ghana; Guinea; Ivory-Coast; Kenya; Liberia; Malawi; Mali; Mauritania; Mauritius; Morocco; Niger; Nigeria; Senegal; Seychelles; Sierra-Leone; Singapore; South-Africa; Sudan; Tanzania; Thailand; Tunia; Uganda; Zambia; Zimbabwe); Tenopress (Bahrain; Cyprus; Egypt; Iran; Iraq; Jordan; Kuwait; Lebanon; Libya; Oman; Qatar; Republic-of-Yemen; Saudi-Arabia; Syria; United-Arab-Emirates); Tenoprin (Finland); Tenormine (France); Tensig (Australia); Therabloc (Philippines); Tredol (Bahrain; Cyprus; Egypt; Iran; Iraq; Israel; Jordan; Kuwait; Lebanon; Libya; Oman; Qatar; Republic-of-Yemen; Saudi-Arabia; Syria; United-Arab-Emirates); Urosin (Taiwan); Vascoten (Hong-Kong; Thailand); Vericordin (Argentina); Wesipin (Taiwan)

Cost of Therapy: $38.50 (Hypertension; Tenormin; 50 mg; 1 tablet/day; 30 day supply)
$1.59 (Hypertension; Generic Tablets; 50 mg; 1 tablet/day; 30 day supply)

DESCRIPTION

Atenolol, a synthetic, $beta_1$-selective (cardioselective) adrenoreceptor blocking agent, may be chemically described as benzeneacetamide, 4 -[2′-hydroxy-3′-[(1- methylethyl) amino] propoxy]-.

Atenolol (free base) has a molecular weight of 266.34. It is a relatively polar hydrophilic compound with a water solubility of 26.5 mg/ml at 37°C and a log partition coefficient (octanol/water) of 0.23. It is freely soluble in 1N HCl (300 mg/ml at 25°C) and less soluble in chloroform (3 mg/ml at 25°C). The molecular formula of atenolol is $C_{14}H_{22}N_2O_3$.

TABLETS

Tenormin is available as 25, 50 and 100 mg tablets for oral administration.

Tenormin Inactive Ingredients: Magnesium stearate, microcrystalline cellulose, povidone, sodium starch glycolate.

IV INJECTION

Atenolol for parenteral administration contains 5 mg atenolol in 10 ml sterile, isotonic, citrate-buffered, aqueous solution. The pH of the solution is 5.5-6.5.

Tenormin Inactive Ingredients: Sodium chloride for isotonicity and citric acid and sodium hydroxide to adjust pH.

CLINICAL PHARMACOLOGY

Atenolol is a $beta_1$-selective (cardioselective) beta-adrenergic receptor blocking agent without membrane stabilizing or intrinsic sympathomimetic (partial agonist) activities. This preferential effect is not absolute, however, and at higher doses, atenolol inhibits $beta_2$-adrenoreceptors, chiefly located in the bronchial and vascular musculature.

PHARMACOKINETICS AND METABOLISM

In man, absorption of an oral dose is rapid and consistent but incomplete. Approximately 50% of an oral dose is absorbed from the gastrointestinal tract, the remainder being excreted unchanged in the feces. Peak blood levels are reached between 2 and 4 hours after ingestion. Unlike propranolol or metoprolol, but like nadolol, atenolol undergoes little or no metabolism by the liver, and the absorbed portion is eliminated primarily by renal excretion. Over 85% of an intravenous dose is excreted in urine within 24 hours compared with approximately 50% for an oral dose. Atenolol also differs from propranolol in that only a small amount (6-16%) is bound to proteins in the plasma. This kinetic profile results in relatively consistent plasma drug levels with about a 4-fold interpatient variation.

The elimination half-life of oral atenolol is approximately 6-7 hours, and there is no alteration of the kinetic profile of the drug by chronic administration. Following intravenous administration, peak plasma levels are reached within 5 minutes. Declines from peak levels are rapid (5- to 10-fold) during the first 7 hours; thereafter, plasma levels decay with a half-life similar to that of orally administered drug. Following oral doses of 50 or 100 mg, both beta-blocking and antihypertensive effects persist for at least 24 hours. When renal function is impaired, elimination of atenolol is closely related to the glomerular filtration rate; significant accumulation occurs when the creatinine clearance falls below 35 ml/min/1.73 m^2. (See DOSAGE AND ADMINISTRATION.)

PHARMACODYNAMICS

In standard animal or human pharmacological tests, beta-adrenoreceptor blocking activity of atenolol has been demonstrated by:

1. Reduction in resting and exercise heart rate and cardiac output.
2. Reduction of systolic and diastolic blood pressure at rest and on exercise.
3. Inhibition of isoproterenol induced tachycardia.
4. Reduction in reflex orthostatic tachycardia.

A significant beta-blocking effect of atenolol, as measured by reduction of exercise tachycardia, is apparent within 1 hour following oral administration of a single dose. This effect is maximal at about 2-4 hours, and persists for at least 24 hours. Maximum reduction in exercise tachycardia occurs within 5 minutes of an intravenous dose. For both orally and intravenously administered drug, the duration of action is dose related and also bears a linear relationship to the logarithm of plasma atenolol concentration. The effect on exercise tachycardia of a single 10 mg intravenous dose is largely dissipated by 12 hours, whereas beta-blocking activity of single oral doses of 50 and 100 mg is still evident beyond 24 hours following administration. However, as has been shown for all beta-blocking agents, the antihypertensive effect does not appear to be related to plasma level.

In normal subjects, the $beta_1$ selectivity of atenolol has been shown by its reduced ability to reverse the $beta_2$-mediated vasodilating effect of isoproterenol as compared to equivalent beta-blocking doses of propranolol. In asthmatic patients, a dose of atenolol producing a greater effect on resting heart rate than propranolol resulted in much less increase in airway resistance. In a placebo controlled comparison of approximately equipotent oral doses of several beta-blockers, atenolol produced a significantly smaller decrease of FEV_1 than nonselective beta-blockers such as propranolol and, unlike those agents, did not inhibit bronchodilation in response to isoproterenol.

Consistent with its negative chronotropic effect due to beta blockade of the SA node, atenolol increases sinus cycle length and sinus node recovery time. Conduction in the A-V node is also prolonged. Atenolol is devoid of membrane stabilizing activity, and increasing the dose well beyond that producing beta blockade does not further depress myocardial contractility. Several studies have demonstrated a moderate (approximately 10%) increase in stroke volume at rest and during exercise.

In controlled clinical trials, atenolol, given as a single daily oral dose, was an effective antihypertensive agent providing 24 hour reduction of blood pressure. Atenolol has been studied in combination with thiazide-type diuretics, and the blood pressure effects of the combination are approximately additive. Atenolol is also compatible with methyldopa, hydralazine, and prazosin, each combination resulting in a larger fall in blood pressure than with the single agents. The dose range of atenolol is narrow and increasing the dose beyond 100 mg once daily is not associated with increased antihypertensive effect. The mechanisms of the antihypertensive effects of beta-blocking agents have not been established. Several possible mechanisms have been proposed and include:

1. Competitive antagonism of catecholamines at peripheral (especially cardiac) adrenergic neuron sites, leading to decreased cardiac output.
2. A central effect leading to reduced sympathetic outflow to the periphery.
3. Suppression of renin activity.

The results from long-term studies have not shown any diminution of the antihypertensive efficacy of atenolol with prolonged use.

By blocking the positive chronotropic and inotropic effects of catecholamines and by decreasing blood pressure, atenolol generally reduces the oxygen requirements of the heart at any given level of effort, making it useful for many patients in the long-term management of angina pectoris. On the other hand, atenolol can increase oxygen requirements by increasing left ventricular fiber length and end diastolic pressure, particularly in patients with heart failure.

In a multicenter clinical trial (ISIS-1) conducted in 16,027 patients with suspected myocardial infarction, patients presenting within 12 hours (mean = 5 hours) after the onset of pain were randomized to either conventional therapy plus atenolol (n=8037), or conventional therapy alone (n=7990). Patients with a heart rate of <50 bpm or systolic blood pressure <100 mm Hg, or with other contraindications to beta blockade were excluded. Thirty-eight percent of each group were treated within 4 hours of onset of pain. The mean time from onset of pain to entry was 5.0 ± 2.7 hours in both groups. Patients in the atenolol group were to receive atenolol IV injection 5-10 mg given over 5 minutes plus atenolol tablets 50 mg every 12 hours orally on the first study day (the first oral dose administered about 15 minutes after the IV dose) followed by either atenolol tablets 100 mg once daily or atenolol tablets 50 mg twice daily on days 2-7. The groups were similar in demographic and medical history characteristics and in electrocardiographic evidence of myocardial infarction, bundle branch block, and first degree atrioventricular block at entry.

During the treatment period (days 0-7), the vascular mortality rates were 3.89% in the atenolol group (313 deaths) and 4.57% in the control group (365 deaths). This absolute difference in rates, 0.68%, is statistically significant at the P<0.05 level. The absolute difference translates into a proportional reduction of 15% (3.89 -4.57/4.57 = -0.15). The 95% confidence limits are 1-27%. Most of the difference was attributed to mortality in days 0-1 (atenolol: 121 deaths; control: 171 deaths).

Despite the large size of the ISIS-1 trial, it is not possible to identify clearly subgroups of patients most likely or least likely to benefit from early treatment with atenolol. Good clinical judgment suggests, however, that patients who are dependent on sympathetic stimulation for maintenance of adequate cardiac output and blood pressure are not good candidates for beta blockade. Indeed, the trial protocol reflected that judgment by excluding patients with blood pressure consistently below 100 mm Hg systolic. The overall results of the study are compatible with the possibility that patients with borderline blood pressure (less than 120 mm Hg systolic), especially if over 60 years of age, are less likely to benefit.

The mechanism through which atenolol improves survival in patients with definite or suspected acute myocardial infarction is unknown, as is the case for other beta-blockers in the postinfarction setting. Atenolol, in addition to its effects on survival, has shown other clinical benefits including reduced frequency of ventricular premature beats, reduced chest pain, and reduced enzyme elevation.

INDICATIONS AND USAGE

ACUTE MYOCARDIAL INFARCTION

Atenolol is indicated in the management of hemodynamically stable patients with definite or suspected acute myocardial infarction to reduce cardiovascular mortality. Treatment can be initiated as soon as the patient's clinical condition allows. (See DOSAGE AND ADMINISTRATION, CONTRAINDICATIONS, and WARNINGS.) In general, there is no basis for treating patients like those who were excluded from the ISIS-1 trial (blood pressure less than 100 mm Hg systolic, heart rate less than 50 bpm) or have other reasons to avoid beta blockade. As noted above, some subgroups (*e.g.*, elderly patients with systolic blood pressure below 120 mm Hg) seemed less likely to benefit.

TABLETS

Hypertension: Atenolol is indicated in the management of hypertension. It may be used alone or concomitantly with other antihypertensive agents, particularly with a thiazide-type diuretic.

Angina Pectoris Due to Coronary Atherosclerosis: Atenolol is indicated for the long-term management of patients with angina pectoris.

CONTRAINDICATIONS

Atenolol is contraindicated in sinus bradycardia, heart block greater than first degree, cardiogenic shock, and overt cardiac failure. (See WARNINGS.)

WARNINGS

CARDIAC FAILURE

Sympathetic stimulation is necessary in supporting circulatory function in congestive heart failure, and beta blockade carries the potential hazard of further depressing myocardial contractility and precipitating more severe failure. In patients who have congestive heart failure controlled by digitalis and/or diuretics, atenolol should be administered cautiously. Both digitalis and atenolol slow A-V conduction.

In patients with acute myocardial infarction, cardiac failure which is not promptly and effectively controlled by 80 mg of intravenous furosemide or equivalent therapy is a contraindication to beta-blocker treatment.

In patients without a history of cardiac failure: Continued depression of the myocardium with beta-blocking agents over a period of time can, in some cases, lead to cardiac failure. At the first sign or symptom of impending cardiac failure, patients should be fully digitalized and/or be given a diuretic and the response observed closely. If cardiac failure continues despite adequate digitalization and diuresis, atenolol should be withdrawn. (See DOSAGE AND ADMINISTRATION.)

Cessation of therapy with atenolol: Patients with coronary artery disease, who are being treated with atenolol, should be advised against abrupt discontinuation of therapy. Severe exacerbation of angina and the occurrence of myocardial infarction and ventricular arrhythmias have been reported in angina patients following the abrupt discontinuation of therapy with beta-blockers. The last two complications may occur with or without preceding exacerbation of the angina pectoris. As with other beta-blockers, when discontinuation of atenolol is planned, the patients should be carefully observed and advised to limit physical activity to a minimum. If the angina worsens or acute coronary insufficiency develops, it is recommended that atenolol be promptly reinstituted, at least temporarily. Because coronary artery disease is common and may be unrecognized, it may be prudent not to discontinue atenolol therapy abruptly even in patients treated only for hypertension. (See DOSAGE AND ADMINISTRATION.)

CONCOMITANT USE OF CALCIUM CHANNEL BLOCKERS

Bradycardia and heart block can occur and the left ventricular end diastolic pressure can rise when beta-blockers are administered with verapamil or diltiazem. Patients with pre-existing conduction abnormalities or left ventricular dysfunction are particularly susceptible. (See PRECAUTIONS.)

BRONCHOSPASTIC DISEASES

PATIENTS WITH BRONCHOSPASTIC DISEASE SHOULD, IN GENERAL, NOT RECEIVE BETA-BLOCKERS. Because of its relative beta$_1$ selectivity, however, atenolol may be used with caution in patients with bronchospastic disease who do not respond to, or cannot tolerate, other antihypertensive treatment. Since beta$_1$ selectivity is not absolute, the lowest possible dose of atenolol should be used with therapy initiated at 50 mg and a beta$_2$-stimulating agent (bronchodilator) should be made available. If dosage must be increased, dividing the dose should be considered in order to achieve lower peak blood levels.

ANESTHESIA AND MAJOR SURGERY

It is not advisable to withdraw beta-adrenoreceptor blocking drugs prior to surgery in the majority of patients. However, care should be taken when using anesthetic agents such as those which may depress the myocardium. Vagal dominance, if it occurs, may be corrected with atropine (1-2 mg IV).

Atenolol, like other beta-blockers, is a competitive inhibitor of beta-receptor agonists and its effects on the heart can be reversed by administration of such agents (*e.g.*, dobutamine or isoproterenol with caution).

DIABETES AND HYPOGLYCEMIA

Atenolol should be used with caution in diabetic patients if a beta-blocking agent is required. Beta-blockers may mask tachycardia occurring with hypoglycemia, but other manifestations such as dizziness and sweating may not be significantly affected. At recommended doses atenolol does not potentiate insulin-induced hypoglycemia and, unlike nonselective beta-blockers, does not delay recovery of blood glucose to normal levels.

THYROTOXICOSIS

Beta-adrenergic blockade may mask certain clinical signs (*e.g.*, tachycardia) of hyperthyroidism. Abrupt withdrawal of beta blockade might precipitate a thyroid storm; therefore, patients suspected of developing thyrotoxicosis from whom atenolol therapy is to be withdrawn should be monitored closely. (See DOSAGE AND ADMINISTRATION.)

PREGNANCY AND FETAL INJURY

Atenolol can cause fetal harm when administered to a pregnant woman. Atenolol crosses the placental barrier and appears in cord blood. Administration of atenolol, starting in the second trimester of pregnancy, has been associated with the birth of infants that are small for gestational age. No studies have been performed on the use of atenolol in the first trimester, and the possibility of fetal injury cannot be excluded. If this drug is used during pregnancy, or if the patient becomes pregnant while taking this drug, the patient should be apprised of the potential hazard to the fetus.

Atenolol has been shown to produce a dose-related increase in embryo/fetal resorptions in rats at doses equal to or greater than 50 mg/kg/day or 25 or more times when maximum recommended human antihypertensive dose.* Although similar effects were not seen in rabbits, the compound was not evaluated in rabbits at doses above 25 mg/kg/day or 12.5 times the maximum recommended human antihypertensive dose.*

*Based on the maximum dose of 100 mg/day in a 50 kg patient.

PRECAUTIONS

GENERAL

Patients already on a beta-blocker must be evaluated carefully before atenolol is administered. Initial and subsequent atenolol dosages can be adjusted downward depending on clinical observations including pulse and blood pressure. Atenolol may aggravate peripheral arterial circulatory disorders.

IMPAIRED RENAL FUNCTION

The drug should be used with caution in patients with impaired renal function (see DOSAGE AND ADMINISTRATION).

CARCINOGENESIS, MUTAGENESIS, AND IMPAIRMENT OF FERTILITY

Two long-term (maximum dosing duration of 18 or 24 months) rat studies and one long-term (maximum dosing duration of 18 months) mouse study, each employing dose levels as high as 300 mg/kg/day or 150 times the maximum recommended human antihypertensive dose,* did not indicate a carcinogenic potential of atenolol. A third (24 month) rat study, employing doses of 500 and 1500 mg/kg/day (250 and 750 times the maximum recommended human antihypertensive dose*) resulted in increased incidences of benign adrenal medullary tumors in males and females, mammary fibroadenomas in females, and anterior pituitary adenomas and thyroid parafollicular cell carcinomas in males. No evidence of a mutagenic potential of atenolol was uncovered in the dominant lethal test (mouse), *in vivo* cytogenetics test (Chinese hamster) or Ames test (*S. typhimurium*).

Fertility of male or female rats (evaluated at dose levels as high as 200 mg/kg/day or 100 times the maximum recommended human dose*) was unaffected by atenolol administration.

*Based on the maximum dose of 100 mg/day in a 50 kg patient.

PREGNANCY, TERATOGENIC EFFECTS, PREGNANCY CATEGORY D

See WARNINGS, Pregnancy and Fetal Injury.

NURSING MOTHERS

Atenolol is excreted in human breast milk at a ratio of 1.5-6.8 when compared to the concentration in plasma. Caution should be exercised when atenolol is administered to a nursing woman. Clinically significant bradycardia has been reported in breast fed infants. Premature infants, or infants with impaired renal function, may be more likely to develop adverse effects.

PEDIATRIC USE

Safety and effectiveness in pediatric patients have not been established.

DRUG INTERACTIONS

Catecholamine-depleting drugs (*e.g.*, reserpine) may have an additive effect when given with beta-blocking agents. Patients treated with atenolol plus a catecholamine depletor should therefore be closely observed for evidence of hypotension and/or marked bradycardia which may produce vertigo, syncope, or postural hypotension.

Calcium channel blockers may also have an additive effect when given with atenolol. (See WARNINGS.)

Beta-blockers may exacerbate the rebound hypertension which can follow the withdrawal of clonidine. If the two drugs are coadministered, the beta-blocker should be withdrawn several days before the gradual withdraw of clonidine. If replacing clonidine by beta-blocker therapy, the introduction of beta-blockers should be delayed for several days after clonidine administration has stopped.

Information on concurrent usage of atenolol and aspirin is limited. Data from several studies, *i.e.*, TIMI-II, ISIS-2, currently do not suggest any clinical interaction between aspirin and beta-blockers in the acute myocardial infarction setting.

While taking beta-blockers, patients with a history of anaphylactic reaction to a variety of allergens may have a more severe reaction on repeated challenge, either accidental, diagnostic or therapeutic. Such patients may be unresponsive to the usual doses of epinephrine used to treat the allergic reaction.

Additional Information for the IV Injection: Caution should be exercised with atenolol IV when given in close proximity with drugs that may also have depressant effect on myocardial contractility. On rare occasions, concomitant use of IV beta-blockers and IV verapamil has resulted in serious adverse reactions, especially in patients with severe cardiomyopathy, congestive heart failure, or recent myocardial infarction.

ADVERSE REACTIONS

Most adverse effects have been mild and transient.

The frequency estimates in TABLE 1 were derived from controlled studies in hypertensive patients in which adverse reactions were either volunteered by the patient (US studies) or elicited, *e.g.*, by checklist (foreign studies). The reported frequency of elicited adverse effects was higher for both atenolol and placebo-treated patients than when these reactions were volunteered. Where frequency of adverse effects of atenolol and placebo is similar, causal relationship to atenolol is uncertain.

ACUTE MYOCARDIAL INFARCTION

In a series of investigations in the treatment of acute myocardial infarction, bradycardia and hypotension occurred more commonly, as expected for any beta-blocker, in atenolol-treated

TABLE 1 *Adverse Effects*

	Volunteered (US Studies)		Total - Volunteered and Elicited (Foreign + US Studies)	
	Atenolol (n=164)	Placebo (n=206)	Atenolol (n=399)	Placebo (n=407)
Cardiovascular				
Bradycardia	3%	0%	3%	0%
Cold extremities	0%	0.5%	12%	5%
Postural hypotension	2%	1%	4%	5%
Leg pain	0%	0.5%	3%	1%
Central Nervous System/Neuromuscular				
Dizziness	4%	1%	13%	6%
Vertigo	2%	0.5%	2%	0.2%
Light headedness	1%	0%	3%	0.7%
Tiredness	0.6%	0.5%	26%	13%
Fatigue	3%	1%	6%	5%
Lethargy	1%	0%	3%	0.7%
Drowsiness	0.6%	0%	2%	0.5%
Depression	0.6%	0.5%	12%	9%
Dreaming	0%	0%	3%	1%
Gastrointestinal				
Diarrhea	2%	0%	3%	2%
Nausea	4%	1%	3%	1%
Respiratory (see WARNINGS)				
Wheeziness	0%	0%	3%	3%
Dyspnea	0.6%	1%	6%	4%

patients than in control patients. However, these usually responded to atropine and/or to withholding further dosage of atenolol. The incidence of heart failure was not increased by atenolol. Inotropic agents were infrequently used. The reported frequency of these and other events occurring during these investigations is given in TABLE 2.

In a study of 477 patients, the following adverse events were reported during either intravenous and/or oral atenolol administration (see TABLE 2).

TABLE 2 *Adverse Effects*

	Conventional Therapy Plus Atenolol (n=244)	Conventional Therapy Alone (n=233)
Bradycardia	43 (18%)	24 (10%)
Hypotension	60 (25%)	34 (15%)
Bronchospasm	3 (1.2%)	2 (0.9%)
Heart failure	46 (19%)	56 (24%)
Heart block	11 (4.5%)	10 (4.3%)
BBB + Major axis deviation	16 (6.6%)	28 (12%)
Supraventricular tachycardia	28 (11.5%)	45 (19%)
Atrial fibrillation	12 (5%)	29 (11%)
Atrial flutter	4 (1.6%)	7 (3%)
Ventricular tachycardia	39 (16%)	52 (22%)
Cardiac reinfarction	0 (0%)	6 (2.6%)
Total cardiac arrests	4 (1.6%)	16 (6.9%)
Nonfatal cardiac arrests	4 (1.6%)	12 (5.1%)
Deaths	7 (2.9%)	16 (6.9%)
Cardiogenic shock	1 (0.4%)	4 (1.7%)
Development of ventricular septal defect	0 (0%)	2 (0.9%)
Development of mitral regurgitation	0 (0%)	2 (0.9%)
Renal failure	1 (0.4%)	0 (0%)
Pulmonary emboli	3 (1.2%)	0 (0%)

In the subsequent International Study of Infarct Survival (ISIS-1) including over 16,000 patients of whom 8037 were randomized to receive atenolol treatment, the dosage of intravenous and subsequent oral atenolol was either discontinued or reduced for the following reasons (see TABLE 3).

TABLE 3 *Reasons for Reduced Dosage*

	IV Atenolol Reduced Dose (<5 mg)*		Oral Partial Dose	
Hypotension/bradycardia	105	(1.3%)	1168	(14.5%)
Cardiogenic shock	4	(0.04%)	35	(0.44%)
Reinfarction	0	(0%)	5	(0.06%)
Cardiac arrest	5	(0.06%)	28	(0.34%)
Heart block (> first degree)	5	(0.06%)	143	(1.7%)
Cardiac failure	1	(0.01%)	233	(2.9%)
Arrhythmias	3	(0.04%)	22	(0.27%)
Bronchospasm	1	(0.01%)	50	(0.62%)

* Full dosage was 10 mg and some patients received less than 10 mg but more than 5 mg.

During postmarketing experience with atenolol, the following have been reported in temporal relationship to the use of the drug: Elevated liver enzymes and/or bilirubin, hallucinations, headache, impotence, Peyronie's disease, postural hypotension which may be associated with syncope, psoriasiform rash or exacerbation of psoriasis, psychoses, purpura, reversible alopecia, thrombocytopenia and visual disturbances. Atenolol, like other beta-blockers, has been associated with the development of antinuclear antibodies (ANA), and lupus syndrome.

POTENTIAL ADVERSE EFFECTS

In addition, a variety of adverse effects have been reported with other beta-adrenergic blocking agents, and may be considered potential adverse effects of atenolol.

Hematologic: Agranulocytosis.

Allergic: Fever, combined with aching and sore throat, laryngospasm, and respiratory distress.

Central Nervous System: Reversible mental depression progressing to catatonia; an acute reversible syndrome characterized by disorientation of time and place; short-term memory loss; emotional lability with slightly clouded sensorium; and, decreased performance on neuropsychometrics.

Gastrointestinal: Mesenteric arterial thrombosis, ischemic colitis.

Other: Erythematous rash, Raynaud's phenomenon.

Miscellaneous: There have been reports of skin rashes and/or dry eyes associated with the use of beta-adrenergic blocking drugs. The reported incidence is small, and in most cases, the symptoms have cleared when treatment was withdrawn. Discontinuance of the drug should be considered if any such reaction is not otherwise explicable. Patients should be closely monitored following cessation of therapy. (See DOSAGE AND ADMINISTRATION.)

The oculomucocutaneous syndrome associated with the beta-blocker practolol has not been reported with atenolol. Furthermore, a number of patients who had previously demonstrated established practolol reactions were transferred to atenolol therapy with subsequent resolution or quiescence of the reaction.

DOSAGE AND ADMINISTRATION

TABLETS

Hypertension

The initial dose of atenolol is 50 mg given as one tablet a day either alone or added to diuretic therapy. The full effect of this dose will usually be seen within 1-2 weeks. If an optimal response is not achieved, the dosage should be increased to atenolol 100 mg given as 1 tablet a day. Increasing the dosage beyond 100 mg a day is unlikely to produce any further benefit.

Atenolol may be used alone or concomitantly with other antihypertensive agents including thiazide-type diuretics, hydralazine, prazosin, and alpha-methyldopa.

Angina Pectoris

The initial dose of atenolol is 50 mg given as 1 tablet a day. If an optimal response is not achieved within 1 week, the dosage should be increased to atenolol 100 mg given as 1 tablet a day. Some patients may require a dosage of 200 mg once a day for optimal effect.

Twenty-four (24) hour control with once daily dosing is achieved by giving doses larger than necessary to achieve an immediate maximum effect. The maximum early effect on exercise tolerance occurs with doses of 50-100 mg, but at these doses the effect at 24 hours is attenuated, averaging about 50-75% of that observed with once a day oral doses of 200 mg.

Elderly Patients or Patients with Renal Impairment

Atenolol is excreted by the kidneys; consequently dosage should be adjusted in cases of severe impairment of renal function. Some reduction in dosage may also be appropriate for the elderly, since decreased kidney function is a physiologic consequence of aging. Atenolol excretion would be expected to decrease with advancing age.

No significant accumulation of atenolol occurs until creatinine clearance falls below 35 ml/min/1.73 m^2. Accumulation of atenolol and prolongation of its half-life were studied in subjects with creatinine clearance between 5 and 105 ml/min. Peak plasma levels were significantly increased in subjects with creatinine clearances below 30 ml/min.

The following maximum oral dosages are recommended for elderly, renally-impaired patients and for patients with renal impairment due to other causes. (See TABLE 4.)

TABLE 4 *Dosage and Renal Impairment*

Creatinine Clearance (ml/min/1.73 m^2)	Atenolol Elimination Half-Life (h)	Maximum Dosage
15-35	16-27	50 mg daily
<15	>27	25 mg daily

Some renally-impaired or elderly patients being treated for hypertension may require a lower starting dose of atenolol: 25 mg given as 1 tablet a day. If this 25 mg dose is used, assessment of efficacy must be made carefully. This should include measurement of blood pressure just prior to the next dose ("trough" blood pressure) to ensure that the treatment effect is present for a full 24 hours.

Although a similar dosage reduction may be considered for elderly and/or renally-impaired patients being treated for indications other than hypertension, data are not available for these patient populations.

Patients on hemodialysis should be given 25 or 50 mg after each dialysis; this should be done under hospital supervision as marked falls in blood pressure can occur.

Cessation of Therapy in Patients with Angina Pectoris

If withdrawal of atenolol therapy is planned, it should be achieved gradually and patients should be carefully observed and advised to limit physical activity to a minimum.

TABLETS AND IV INJECTION

Acute Myocardial Infarction

In patients with definite or suspected acute myocardial infarction, treatment with atenolol IV injection should be initiated as soon as possible after the patient's arrival in the hospital and after eligibility is established. Such treatment should be initiated in a coronary care or similar unit immediately after the patient's hemodynamic condition has stabilized. Treatment should begin with the intravenous administration of 5 mg atenolol over 5 minutes followed by another 5 mg intravenous injection 10 minutes later. Atenolol IV injection should be administered under carefully controlled conditions including monitoring of blood pressure, heart rate, and electrocardiogram. Dilutions of atenolol IV injection in dextrose injection, sodium chloride injection, or sodium chloride and dextrose injection may be used. These admixtures are stable for 48 hours if they are not used immediately.

In patients who tolerate the full intravenous dose (10 mg), atenolol tablets 50 mg should be initiated 10 minutes after the last intravenous dose followed by another 50 mg oral dose 12 hours later. Thereafter, atenolol can be given orally either 100 mg once daily or 50 mg twice a day for a further 6-9 days or until discharge from the hospital. If bradycardia or hypotension requiring treatment or any other untoward effects occur, atenolol should be discontinued.

Data from other beta-blocker trials suggest that if there is any question concerning the use of IV beta-blocker or clinical estimate that there is a contraindication, the IV beta-blocker may be eliminated and patients fulfilling the safety criteria may be given atenolol tablets 50 mg twice daily or 100 mg once a day for at least seven days (if the IV dosing is excluded).

Although the demonstration of efficacy of atenolol is based entirely on data from the first 7 postinfarction days, data from other beta-blocker trials suggest that treatment with beta-blockers that are effective in the postinfarction setting may be continued for 1-3 years if there are no contraindications.

Atenolol is an additional treatment to standard coronary care unit therapy.

ANIMAL PHARMACOLOGY

Chronic studies employing oral atenolol performed in animals have revealed the occurrence of vacuolation of epithelial cells of Brunner's glands in the duodenum of both male and female dogs at all tested dose levels of atenolol (starting at 15 mg/kg/day or 7.5 times the maximum recommended human antihypertensive dose*) and increased incidence of atrial degeneration of hearts of male rats at 300 but not 150 mg atenolol/kg/day (150 and 75 times the maximum recommended human antihypertensive dose,* respectively).

*Based on the maximum dose of 100 mg/day in a 50 kg patient.

HOW SUPPLIED

TABLETS

25 mg Tenormin: Round, flat, uncoated white tablets identified with "T" debossed on one side and "107" debossed on the other side.

50 mg Tenormin: Round, flat, uncoated white tablets identified with with "TENORMIN" debossed on one side and "105" debossed on the other side, bisected.

100 mg Tenormin: Round, flat, uncoated white tablets identified with "TENORMIN" debossed on one side and "101" debossed on the other side.

STORAGE

Tablets: Store at controlled room temperature, 20-25°C (68-77°F). Dispense in well-closed, light resistant containers.

IV Injection: Protect from light. Keep ampules in outer packaging until time of use. Store at room temperature.

Parenteral drug products should be inspected visually for particulate matter and discoloration prior to administration, whenever solution and container permit.

PRODUCT LISTING - RATED THERAPEUTICALLY EQUIVALENT

Tablet - Oral - 25 mg

15's	$7.02	GENERIC, Southwood Pharmaceuticals Inc	58016-0582-15
20's	$14.05	GENERIC, Southwood Pharmaceuticals Inc	58016-0582-20
25 x 30	$453.38	GENERIC, Sky Pharmaceuticals Packaging, Inc	63739-0027-03
25's	$8.67	GENERIC, Pd-Rx Pharmaceuticals	55289-0227-97
25's	$20.00	GENERIC, Udl Laboratories Inc	51079-0759-19
30 x 25	$453.38	GENERIC, Sky Pharmaceuticals Packaging, Inc	63739-0027-01
30's	$14.16	GENERIC, Pd-Rx Pharmaceuticals	55289-0227-30
30's	$20.40	GENERIC, Heartland Healthcare Services	61392-0542-30
30's	$20.40	GENERIC, Heartland Healthcare Services	61392-0542-39
30's	$21.07	GENERIC, Southwood Pharmaceuticals Inc	58016-0582-30
31 x 10	$217.78	GENERIC, Vangard Labs	00615-3544-53
31 x 10	$217.78	GENERIC, Vangard Labs	00615-3544-63
31's	$21.08	GENERIC, Heartland Healthcare Services	61392-0542-31
32's	$21.76	GENERIC, Heartland Healthcare Services	61392-0542-32
45's	$30.60	GENERIC, Heartland Healthcare Services	61392-0542-45
60's	$40.80	GENERIC, Heartland Healthcare Services	61392-0542-60
60's	$40.80	GENERIC, Heartland Healthcare Services	61392-0542-65
60's	$42.14	GENERIC, Southwood Pharmaceuticals Inc	58016-0582-60
90's	$61.20	GENERIC, Heartland Healthcare Services	61392-0542-90
90's	$63.82	GENERIC, Golden State Medical	60429-0211-90
100's	$6.14	FEDERAL UPPER LIMIT, H.C.F.A. F F P	99999-0333-01
100's	$6.88	GENERIC, Esi Lederle Generics	00005-3218-43
100's	$63.75	GENERIC, Invamed Inc	52189-0259-24
100's	$63.85	GENERIC, Ipr Pharmaceuticals Inc	54921-0107-10
100's	$68.57	GENERIC, Moore, H.L. Drug Exchange Inc	00839-7951-06
100's	$70.20	GENERIC, Major Pharmaceuticals Inc	00904-5392-60
100's	$70.23	GENERIC, Southwood Pharmaceuticals Inc	58016-0582-00
100's	$70.25	GENERIC, Ivax Corporation	00182-1001-01
100's	$70.25	GENERIC, West Point Pharma	59591-0007-68
100's	$70.25	GENERIC, Apothecon Inc	62269-0259-24
100's	$70.55	GENERIC, Aligen Independent Laboratories Inc	00405-4106-01
100's	$71.25	GENERIC, Pharma Pac	52959-0463-01
100's	$73.98	GENERIC, Mutual Pharmaceutical Co Inc	53489-0536-01
100's	$78.10	GENERIC, Ivax Corporation	00182-1001-89
100's	$80.03	GENERIC, Udl Laboratories Inc	51079-0759-20
100's	$81.75	GENERIC, Mylan Pharmaceuticals Inc	00378-0218-01
100's	$81.76	GENERIC, Geneva Pharmaceuticals	00781-1078-01
100's	$81.77	GENERIC, Mutual/United Research Laboratories	00677-1633-01
100's	$125.79	TENORMIN, Astra-Zeneca Pharmaceuticals	00310-0107-10
200 x 5	$702.52	GENERIC, Vangard Labs	00615-3544-43

Tablet - Oral - 50 mg

3's	$2.76	GENERIC, Pd-Rx Pharmaceuticals	55289-0228-03
6's	$4.45	GENERIC, Allscripts Pharmaceutical Company	54569-3432-03
7's	$5.19	GENERIC, Allscripts Pharmaceutical Company	54569-3432-05
25 x 30	$529.95	GENERIC, Sky Pharmaceuticals Packaging, Inc	63739-0028-03
25's	$8.67	GENERIC, Pd-Rx Pharmaceuticals	55289-0228-97
25's	$24.34	GENERIC, Udl Laboratories Inc	51079-0684-19
30's	$8.25	GENERIC, Pd-Rx Pharmaceuticals	55289-0228-30
30's	$21.10	GENERIC, Heartland Healthcare Services	61392-0543-30
30's	$21.10	GENERIC, Heartland Healthcare Services	61392-0543-39
30's	$22.08	GENERIC, Golden State Medical	60429-0025-30
30's	$22.23	GENERIC, Allscripts Pharmaceutical Company	54569-3432-01
30's	$28.50	GENERIC, Pharma Pac	52959-0253-30
30's	$38.56	GENERIC, Medirex Inc	57480-0446-06
30's	$41.06	TENORMIN, Pharma Pac	52959-0280-30
30's	$61.35	TENORMIN, Pd-Rx Pharmaceuticals	55289-0254-30
31 x 10	$261.55	GENERIC, Vangard Labs	00615-3532-53
31 x 10	$261.55	GENERIC, Vangard Labs	00615-3532-63
31's	$21.81	GENERIC, Heartland Healthcare Services	61392-0543-31
32's	$22.51	GENERIC, Heartland Healthcare Services	61392-0543-32
40's	$34.70	GENERIC, Pharma Pac	52959-0253-40
45's	$31.65	GENERIC, Heartland Healthcare Services	61392-0543-45
60's	$15.96	GENERIC, Pd-Rx Pharmaceuticals	55289-0228-60
60's	$42.21	GENERIC, Heartland Healthcare Services	61392-0543-60
60's	$42.21	GENERIC, Heartland Healthcare Services	61392-0543-65
60's	$44.45	GENERIC, Allscripts Pharmaceutical Company	54569-3432-04
90's	$63.31	GENERIC, Heartland Healthcare Services	61392-0543-90
90's	$65.19	GENERIC, Golden State Medical	60429-0025-90
100's	$4.64	FEDERAL UPPER LIMIT, H.C.F.A. F F P	99999-0333-05
100's	$5.31	GENERIC, Esi Lederle Generics	00005-3219-43
100's	$13.43	GENERIC, Pd-Rx Pharmaceuticals	55289-0228-01
100's	$24.95	GENERIC, Seneca Pharmaceuticals	47028-0054-01
100's	$61.25	GENERIC, Mova Pharmaceutical Corporation	55370-0122-07
100's	$61.50	GENERIC, Aligen Independent Laboratories Inc	00405-4107-01
100's	$65.00	GENERIC, Major Pharmaceuticals Inc	00904-7634-60
100's	$65.02	GENERIC, Ipr Pharmaceuticals Inc	54921-0105-10
100's	$65.02	GENERIC, Ipr Pharmaceuticals Inc	54921-0105-39
100's	$65.38	GENERIC, Invamed Inc	52189-0256-24
100's	$67.49	GENERIC, Moore, H.L. Drug Exchange Inc	00839-7723-06
100's	$67.49	GENERIC, Moore, H.L. Drug Exchange Inc	00839-7741-06
100's	$67.50	GENERIC, Martec Pharmaceuticals Inc	52555-0006-01
100's	$67.50	GENERIC, Martec Pharmaceuticals Inc	52555-0531-01
100's	$67.53	GENERIC, Watson/Schein Pharmaceuticals Inc	00364-2513-01
100's	$68.10	GENERIC, Rexall Group	60814-0710-01
100's	$69.69	GENERIC, Apothecon Inc	62269-0256-24
100's	$71.75	GENERIC, West Point Pharma	59591-0263-68
100's	$71.90	GENERIC, Pharma Pac	52959-0253-00
100's	$73.50	GENERIC, Martec Pharmaceuticals Inc	52555-0673-01
100's	$73.97	GENERIC, Allscripts Pharmaceutical Company	54569-3432-00
100's	$75.99	GENERIC, Watson/Schein Pharmaceuticals Inc	00364-2513-90
100's	$75.99	GENERIC, Geneva Pharmaceuticals	00781-1506-13
100's	$78.16	GENERIC, Major Pharmaceuticals Inc	00904-7634-61
100's	$83.42	GENERIC, Teva Pharmaceuticals Usa	00093-0752-01
100's	$83.42	GENERIC, Geneva Pharmaceuticals	00781-1506-01
100's	$84.70	GENERIC, Mylan Pharmaceuticals Inc	00378-0231-01
100's	$89.15	GENERIC, Udl Laboratories Inc	51079-0684-20
100's	$89.84	GENERIC, Mutual Pharmaceutical Co Inc	53489-0529-01
100's	$90.01	GENERIC, Par Pharmaceutical Inc	49884-0456-01
100's	$128.34	TENORMIN, Astra-Zeneca Pharmaceuticals	00310-0105-10
100's	$129.46	TENORMIN, Physicians Total Care	54868-0701-00
200 x 5	$843.71	GENERIC, Vangard Labs	00615-3532-43

Tablet - Oral - 100 mg

30's	$7.79	GENERIC, Pd-Rx Pharmaceuticals	55289-0653-30
30's	$28.35	GENERIC, Heartland Healthcare Services	61392-0546-30
30's	$28.35	GENERIC, Heartland Healthcare Services	61392-0546-39
30's	$31.08	GENERIC, Golden State Medical	60429-0026-30
30's	$31.83	GENERIC, Allscripts Pharmaceutical Company	54569-3654-00
30's	$58.06	GENERIC, Medirex Inc	57480-0447-06
30's	$65.12	TENORMIN, Pd-Rx Pharmaceuticals	55289-0587-30
31's	$29.30	GENERIC, Heartland Healthcare Services	61392-0546-31
32's	$30.24	GENERIC, Heartland Healthcare Services	61392-0546-32
45's	$42.53	GENERIC, Heartland Healthcare Services	61392-0546-45
60's	$56.70	GENERIC, Heartland Healthcare Services	61392-0546-60
60's	$64.40	GENERIC, Allscripts Pharmaceutical Company	54569-3654-03
90's	$85.05	GENERIC, Heartland Healthcare Services	61392-0546-90
100's	$7.50	FEDERAL UPPER LIMIT, H.C.F.A. F F P	99999-0333-09
100's	$8.38	GENERIC, Esi Lederle Generics	00005-3220-43
100's	$91.85	GENERIC, Mova Pharmaceutical Corporation	55370-0124-07
100's	$94.50	GENERIC, Major Pharmaceuticals Inc	00904-7635-60
100's	$94.94	GENERIC, Ipr Pharmaceuticals Inc	54921-0101-10
100's	$94.94	GENERIC, Ipr Pharmaceuticals Inc	54921-0101-39
100's	$95.45	GENERIC, Rexall Group	60814-0711-01

100's	$96.80	GENERIC, Aligen Independent Laboratories Inc	00405-4108-01
100's	$96.95	GENERIC, Invamed Inc	52189-0257-24
100's	$97.65	GENERIC, West Point Pharma	59591-0265-68
100's	$98.55	GENERIC, Watson/Schein Pharmaceuticals Inc	00364-2514-01
100's	$98.55	GENERIC, Watson/Schein Pharmaceuticals Inc	00591-5778-01
100's	$98.60	GENERIC, Martec Pharmaceuticals Inc	52555-0007-01
100's	$98.60	GENERIC, Martec Pharmaceuticals Inc	52555-0534-01
100's	$100.25	GENERIC, Apothecon Inc	62269-0257-24
100's	$101.24	GENERIC, Moore, H.L. Drug Exchange Inc	00839-7742-06
100's	$103.95	GENERIC, Martec Pharmaceuticals Inc	52555-0674-01
100's	$105.00	GENERIC, Major Pharmaceuticals Inc	00904-7635-61
100's	$105.75	GENERIC, Watson/Schein Pharmaceuticals Inc	00364-2514-90
100's	$109.33	GENERIC, Moore, H.L. Drug Exchange Inc	00839-7724-06
100's	$121.75	GENERIC, Geneva Pharmaceuticals	00781-1507-13
100's	$121.80	GENERIC, Mylan Pharmaceuticals Inc	00378-0757-01
100's	$125.15	GENERIC, Teva Pharmaceuticals Usa	00093-0753-01
100's	$125.15	GENERIC, Geneva Pharmaceuticals	00781-1507-01
100's	$137.03	GENERIC, Par Pharmaceutical Inc	49884-0457-01
100's	$143.43	GENERIC, Mutual Pharmaceutical Co Inc	53489-0530-01
100's	$149.25	GENERIC, Udl Laboratories Inc	51079-0685-20
100's	$192.54	TENORMIN, Astra-Zeneca Pharmaceuticals	00310-0101-10

PRODUCT LISTING - EQUIVALENTS NOT AVAILABLE

Solution - Injectable - 0.5 mg/ml			
10 ml	$50.28	TENORMIN, Astra-Zeneca Pharmaceuticals	00310-0108-10
Tablet - Oral - 25 mg			
30's	$3.00	GENERIC, Physicians Total Care	54868-2349-02
30's	$21.44	GENERIC, Allscripts Pharmaceutical Company	54569-3885-00
60's	$4.25	GENERIC, Physicians Total Care	54868-2349-03
100's	$6.23	GENERIC, Physicians Total Care	54868-2349-01
Tablet - Oral - 50 mg			
15's	$13.42	GENERIC, Southwood Pharmaceuticals Inc	58016-0333-15
30's	$2.47	GENERIC, Physicians Total Care	54868-1871-01
30's	$26.80	GENERIC, Southwood Pharmaceuticals Inc	58016-0333-30
60's	$4.30	GENERIC, Physicians Total Care	54868-1871-00
60's	$53.70	GENERIC, Southwood Pharmaceuticals Inc	58016-0333-60
100's	$6.28	GENERIC, Physicians Total Care	54868-1871-02
100's	$89.50	GENERIC, Southwood Pharmaceuticals Inc	58016-0333-00
Tablet - Oral - 100 mg			
12's	$18.90	GENERIC, Southwood Pharmaceuticals Inc	58016-0771-12
15's	$23.63	GENERIC, Southwood Pharmaceuticals Inc	58016-0771-15
20's	$31.50	GENERIC, Southwood Pharmaceuticals Inc	58016-0771-20
30's	$3.39	GENERIC, Physicians Total Care	54868-1971-03
30's	$30.07	GENERIC, Pharmaceutical Corporation Of America	51655-0532-24
30's	$47.25	GENERIC, Southwood Pharmaceuticals Inc	58016-0771-30
60's	$5.44	GENERIC, Physicians Total Care	54868-1971-00
100's	$8.18	GENERIC, Physicians Total Care	54868-1971-01
100's	$157.50	GENERIC, Southwood Pharmaceuticals Inc	58016-0771-00

Atenolol; Chlorthalidone *(000334)*

Categories: Hypertension, essential; Pregnancy Category C; FDA Approved 1984 Jun
Drug Classes: Antiadrenergics, beta blocking; Diuretics, thiazide and derivatives
Brand Names: Atenolol W/Chlorthalidone; **Tenoretic**
Foreign Brand Availability: Atecard-D (India); Atel (Germany); Atenigron (Italy); Ateno-Basan (Switzerland); Atenoblok - Co (South-Africa); Atenogamma (Germany); Blokium-Diu (Bahrain; Benin; Burkina-Faso; Costa-Rica; Cyprus; Dominican-Republic; Egypt; El-Salvador; Ethiopia; Gambia; Ghana; Guatemala; Guinea; Honduras; Iran; Iraq; Ivory-Coast; Jordan; Kenya; Kuwait; Lebanon; Liberia; Libya; Malawi; Mali; Mauritania; Mauritius; Morocco; Nicaragua; Niger; Nigeria; Oman; Panama; Qatar; Republic-of-Yemen; Saudi-Arabia; Senegal; Seychelles; Sierra-Leone; Sudan; Syria; Tanzania; Tunia; Uganda; United-Arab-Emirates; Zambia; Zimbabwe); Corinol (Korea); Poten (Korea); Target (Hong-Kong; Taiwan); Teneretic (Germany); Tenolone (Italy); Tenoret (Bahrain; Benin; Burkina-Faso; Cyprus; Egypt; England; Ethiopia; Gambia; Ghana; Guinea; Iran; Iraq; Ivory-Coast; Jordan; Kenya; Kuwait; Lebanon; Liberia; Libya; Malawi; Mali; Mauritania; Mauritius; Morocco; Niger; Nigeria; Oman; Qatar; Republic-of-Yemen; Saudi-Arabia; Senegal; Seychelles; Sierra-Leone; Sudan; Syria; Tanzania; Tunia; Uganda; United-Arab-Emirates; Zambia; Zimbabwe); Tenoret 50 (Hong-Kong; Indonesia; Malaysia; Thailand); Tenoretic Co (Peru); Tenoric (India); Teridon (Korea)
Cost of Therapy: $43.96 (Hypertension; Tenoretic 50; 50 mg; 25 mg; 1 tablet/day; 30 day supply)
$3.67 (Hypertension; Generic Tablets; 50 mg; 25 mg; 1 tablet/day; 30 day supply)

DESCRIPTION

Atenolol; chlorthalidone is for the treatment of hypertension. It combines the antihypertensive activity of two agents: a beta$_1$-selective (cardioselective) hydrophilic blocking agent (atenolol) and a monosulfonamyl diuretic (chlorthalidone). Atenolol is benzeneacetamide, 4-[2'-hydroxy-3'-[(1-methylethyl) amino] propoxy]-.

FOR COMPLETE PRESCRIBING INFORMATION REFER TO THE INDIVIDUAL DRUG MONOGRAPHS (ATENOLOL; CHLORTHALIDONE).

INDICATIONS AND USAGE

Atenolol; chlorthalidone is indicated in the treatment of hypertension. This fixed dose combination drug is not indicated for initial therapy of hypertension. If the fixed dose combination represents the dose appropriate to the individual patient's needs, it may be more convenient than the separate components.

DOSAGE AND ADMINISTRATION

DOSAGE MUST BE INDIVIDUALIZED (see INDICATIONS AND USAGE).

Chlorthalidone is usually given at a dose of 25 mg daily; the usual initial dose of atenolol is 50 mg daily. Therefore, the initial dose should be one Atenolol; chlorthalidone 50 tablet given once a day. If an optimal response is not achieved, the dosage should be increased to one Atenolol; chlorthalidone 100 tablet given once a day.

When necessary, another antihypertensive agent may be added gradually beginning with 50% of the usual recommended starting dose to avoid an excessive fall in blood pressure.

Since atenolol is excreted via the kidneys, dosage should be adjusted in cases of severe impairment of renal function. No significant accumulation of atenolol occurs until creatinine clearance falls below 35 ml/min/1.73m^2 (normal range is 100-150 ml/min/1.73m^2); therefore, the maximum dosages found in TABLE 1 are recommended for patients with renal impairment.

TABLE 1

Creatinine Clearance (ml/min/1.73m^2)	Atenolol Elimination Half-Life (h)	Maximum Dosage
15-35	16-27	50 mg daily
<15	>27	50 mg every other day

Tenoretic 50 mg Tablets (atenolol 50 mg and chlorthalidone 25 mg): White, round, biconvex, uncoated tablets with "Tenoretic" on one side and "115" on the other side, bisected.
Tenoretic 100 mg Tablets (atenolol 100 mg and chlorthalidone 25 mg): White, round, biconvex, uncoated tablets with "Tenoretic" on one side and "117" on the other side.
Storage: Store at controlled room temperature, 20-25°C (68-77°F). Dispense in well-closed, light-resistant containers.

PRODUCT LISTING - RATED THERAPEUTICALLY EQUIVALENT

Tablet - Oral - 50 mg;25 mg			
12's	$12.35	TENORETIC 50, Southwood Pharmaceuticals Inc	58016-0600-12
15's	$15.44	TENORETIC 50, Southwood Pharmaceuticals Inc	58016-0600-15
20's	$20.58	TENORETIC 50, Southwood Pharmaceuticals Inc	58016-0600-20
30's	$17.43	GENERIC, Pd-Rx Pharmaceuticals	55289-0993-30
30's	$30.87	TENORETIC 50, Southwood Pharmaceuticals Inc	58016-0600-30
30's	$39.02	TENORETIC 50, Allscripts Pharmaceutical Company	54569-0596-00
30's	$43.07	TENORETIC 50, Physicians Total Care	54868-0321-00
100's	$17.62	FEDERAL UPPER LIMIT, H.C.F.A. F F P	99999-0334-01
100's	$79.80	GENERIC, Qualitest Products Inc	00603-2374-21
100's	$80.12	GENERIC, Ipr Pharmaceuticals Inc	54921-0115-10
100's	$80.57	GENERIC, Moore, H.L. Drug Exchange Inc	00839-7807-06
100's	$85.65	GENERIC, Major Pharmaceuticals Inc	00904-7881-60
100's	$85.90	GENERIC, Watson/Rugby Laboratories Inc	00536-3332-01
100's	$92.00	GENERIC, Geneva Pharmaceuticals	00781-1315-01
100's	$92.14	GENERIC, Aligen Independent Laboratories Inc	00405-4103-01
100's	$92.40	GENERIC, Martec Pharmaceuticals Inc	52555-0547-01
100's	$92.50	GENERIC, Watson/Schein Pharmaceuticals Inc	00364-2527-01
100's	$92.50	GENERIC, Watson/Schein Pharmaceuticals Inc	00591-5782-01
100's	$92.58	GENERIC, Martec Pharmaceuticals Inc	52555-0450-01
100's	$97.15	GENERIC, Mutual/United Research Laboratories	00677-1480-01
100's	$97.15	GENERIC, Mutual Pharmaceutical Co Inc	53489-0531-01
100's	$97.21	GENERIC, Mylan Pharmaceuticals Inc	00378-2063-01
100's	$146.54	TENORETIC 50, Astra-Zeneca Pharmaceuticals	00310-0115-10
Tablet - Oral - 100 mg;25 mg			
30's	$25.73	GENERIC, Pd-Rx Pharmaceuticals	55289-0988-30
100's	$25.49	FEDERAL UPPER LIMIT, H.C.F.A. F F P	99999-0334-02
100's	$111.45	GENERIC, Qualitest Products Inc	00603-2375-21
100's	$112.45	GENERIC, Ipr Pharmaceuticals Inc	54921-0117-10
100's	$113.09	GENERIC, Moore, H.L. Drug Exchange Inc	00839-7808-06
100's	$120.25	GENERIC, Major Pharmaceuticals Inc	00904-7882-60
100's	$129.00	GENERIC, Martec Pharmaceuticals Inc	52555-0548-01
100's	$129.03	GENERIC, Aligen Independent Laboratories Inc	00405-4104-01
100's	$129.94	GENERIC, Geneva Pharmaceuticals	00781-1316-01
100's	$129.95	GENERIC, Watson/Schein Pharmaceuticals Inc	00364-2528-01
100's	$129.95	GENERIC, Watson/Schein Pharmaceuticals Inc	00591-5783-01
100's	$130.05	GENERIC, Ivax Corporation	00182-1943-01
100's	$130.05	GENERIC, Martec Pharmaceuticals Inc	52555-0451-01
100's	$136.49	GENERIC, Mutual/United Research Laboratories	00677-1481-01
100's	$136.49	GENERIC, Mutual Pharmaceutical Co Inc	53489-0532-01
100's	$136.55	GENERIC, Mylan Pharmaceuticals Inc	00378-2064-01
100's	$205.66	TENORETIC 100, Astra-Zeneca Pharmaceuticals	00310-0117-10

PRODUCT LISTING - EQUIVALENTS NOT AVAILABLE

Tablet - Oral - 50 mg;25 mg			
30's	$5.61	GENERIC, Physicians Total Care	54868-2683-01
100's	$12.24	GENERIC, Physicians Total Care	54868-2683-00

Atomoxetine Hydrochloride (003578)

Categories: Attention deficit hyperactivity disorder; Pregnancy Category C; FDA Approved 2002 Nov
Drug Classes: Selective norepinephrine reuptake inhibitor
Brand Names: Strattera
Cost of Therapy: $187.50 (Hyperactivity Disorder; Strattera; 40 mg; 2 tablets/day; 30 day supply)

DESCRIPTION

Strattera (atomoxetine hydrochloride) is a selective norepinephrine reuptake inhibitor. Atomoxetine hydrochloride is the *R*(-) isomer as determined by x-ray diffraction. The chemical designation is (-)-*N*-Methyl-3-phenyl-3-(*o*-tolyloxy)-propylamine hydrochloride. The molecular formula is $C_{17}H_{21}NO \cdot HCl$, which corresponds to a molecular weight of 291.82.

Atomoxetine hydrochloride is a white to practically white solid, which has a solubility of 27.8 mg/ml in water.

Strattera capsules are intended for oral administration only.

Each capsule contains atomoxetine hydrochloride equivalent to 10, 18, 25, 40, or 60 mg of atomoxetine. The capsules also contain pregelatinized starch and dimethicone. The capsule shells contain gelatin, sodium lauryl sulfate, and other inactive ingredients. The capsule shells also contain 1 or more of the following: FD&C blue no. 2, synthetic yellow iron oxide, titanium dioxide. The capsules are imprinted with edible black ink.

CLINICAL PHARMACOLOGY

PHARMACODYNAMICS AND MECHANISM OF ACTION

The precise mechanism by which atomoxetine produces its therapeutic effects in Attention-Deficit/Hyperactivity Disorder (ADHD) is unknown, but is thought to be related to selective inhibition of the pre-synaptic norepinephrine transporter, as determined in *ex vivo* uptake and neurotransmitter depletion studies.

HUMAN PHARMACOKINETICS

Atomoxetine is well-absorbed after oral administration and is minimally affected by food. It is eliminated primarily by oxidative metabolism through the cytochrome P450 2D6 (CYP2D6) enzymatic pathway and subsequent glucuronidation. Atomoxetine has a half-life of about 5 hours. A fraction of the population (about 7% of Caucasians and 2% of African Americans) are poor metabolizers (PMs) of CYP2D6 metabolized drugs. These individuals have reduced activity in this pathway resulting in 10-fold higher AUCs, 5-fold higher peak plasma concentrations, and slower elimination (plasma half-life of about 24 hours) of atomoxetine compared with people with normal activity [extensive metabolizers (EMs)]. Drugs that inhibit CYP2D6, such as fluoxetine, paroxetine, and quinidine, cause similar increases in exposure.

The pharmacokinetics of atomoxetine have been evaluated in more than 400 children and adolescents in selected clinical trials, primarily using population pharmacokinetic studies. Single-dose and steady-state individual pharmacokinetic data were also obtained in children, adolescents, and adults. When doses were normalized to a mg/kg basis, similar half-life, C_{max}, and AUC values were observed in children, adolescents, and adults. Clearance and volume of distribution after adjustment for body weight were also similar.

Absorption and Distribution

Atomoxetine is rapidly absorbed after oral administration, with absolute bioavailability of about 63% in EMs and 94% in PMs. Maximal plasma concentrations (C_{max}) are reached approximately 1-2 hours after dosing.

Atomoxetine HCl can be administered with or without food. Administration of atomoxetine HCl with a standard high-fat meal in adults did not affect the extent of oral absorption of atomoxetine (AUC), but did decrease the rate of absorption, resulting in a 37% lower C_{max}, and delayed T_{max} by 3 hours. In clinical trials with children and adolescents, administration of atomoxetine HCl with food resulted in a 9% lower C_{max}.

The steady-state volume of distribution after intravenous administration is 0.85 L/kg indicating that atomoxetine distributes primarily into total body water. Volume of distribution is similar across the patient weight range after normalizing for body weight.

At therapeutic concentrations, 98% of atomoxetine in plasma is bound to protein, primarily albumin.

Metabolism and Elimination

Atomoxetine is metabolized primarily through the CYP2D6 enzymatic pathway. People with reduced activity in this pathway (PMs) have higher plasma concentrations of atomoxetine compared with people with normal activity (EMs). For PMs, AUC of atomoxetine is approximately 10-fold and $C_{ss,max}$ is about 5-fold greater than EMs. Laboratory tests are available to identify CYP2D6 PMs. Coadministration of atomoxetine HCl with potent inhibitors of CYP2D6, such as fluoxetine, paroxetine, or quinidine, results in a substantial increase in atomoxetine plasma exposure, and dosing adjustment may be necessary (see Drug-Drug Interactions). Atomoxetine did not inhibit or induce the CYP2D6 pathway.

The major oxidative metabolite formed, regardless of CYP2D6 status, is 4-hydroxyatomoxetine, which is glucuronidated. 4-Hydroxyatomoxetine is equipotent to atomoxetine as an inhibitor of the norepinephrine transporter but circulates in plasma at much lower concentrations (1% of atomoxetine concentration in EMs and 0.1% of atomoxetine concentration in PMs). 4-Hydroxyatomoxetine is primarily formed by CYP2D6, but in PMs, 4-hydroxyatomoxetine is formed at a slower rate by several other cytochrome P450 enzymes. N-desmethylatomoxetine is formed by CYP2C19 and other cytochrome P450 enzymes, but has substantially less pharmacological activity compared with atomoxetine and circulates in plasma at lower concentrations (5% of atomoxetine concentration in EMs and 45% of atomoxetine concentration in PMs).

Mean apparent plasma clearance of atomoxetine after oral administration in adult EMs is 0.35 L/h/kg and the mean half-life is 5.2 hours. Following oral administration of atomoxetine to PMs, mean apparent plasma clearance is 0.03 L/h/kg and mean half-life is 21.6 hours. For PMs, AUC of atomoxetine is approximately 10-fold and $C_{ss,max}$ is about 5-fold greater than EMs. The elimination half-life of 4-hydroxyatomoxetine is similar to that of N-desmethylatomoxetine (6-8 hours) in EM subjects, while the half-life of N-desmethylatomoxetine is much longer in PM subjects (34-40 hours).

Atomoxetine is excreted primarily as 4-hydroxyatomoxetine-*O*-glucuronide, mainly in the urine (greater than 80% of the dose) and to a lesser extent in the feces (less than 17% of the dose). Only a small fraction of the atomoxetine HCl dose is excreted as unchanged atomoxetine (less than 3% of the dose), indicating extensive biotransformation.

SPECIAL POPULATIONS

Hepatic Insufficiency

Atomoxetine exposure (AUC) is increased, compared with normal subjects, in EM subjects with moderate (Child-Pugh Class B) (2-fold increase) and severe (Child-Pugh Class C) (4-fold increase) hepatic insufficiency. Dosage adjustment is recommended for patients with moderate or severe hepatic insufficiency (see DOSAGE AND ADMINISTRATION).

Renal Insufficiency

EM subjects with end stage renal disease had higher systemic exposure to atomoxetine than healthy subjects (about a 65% increase), but there was no difference when exposure was corrected for mg/kg dose. Atomoxetine HCl can therefore be administered to ADHD patients with end stage renal disease or lesser degrees of renal insufficiency using the normal dosing regimen.

Geriatric

The pharmacokinetics of atomoxetine have not been evaluated in the geriatric population.

Pediatric

The pharmacokinetics of atomoxetine in children and adolescents are similar to those in adults. The pharmacokinetics of atomoxetine have not been evaluated in children under 6 years of age.

Gender

Gender did not influence atomoxetine disposition.

Ethnic Origin

Ethnic origin did not influence atomoxetine disposition (except that PMs are more common in Caucasians).

DRUG-DRUG INTERACTIONS

CYP2D6 Activity and Atomoxetine Plasma Concentration

Atomoxetine is primarily metabolized by the CYP2D6 pathway to 4-hydroxyatomoxetine. In EMs, inhibitors of CYP2D6 increase atomoxetine steady-state plasma concentrations to exposures similar to those observed in PMs. Dosage adjustment of atomoxetine HCl in EMs may be necessary when coadministered with CYP2D6 inhibitors, *e.g.*, paroxetine, fluoxetine, and quinidine (see DRUG INTERACTIONS). *In vitro* studies suggest that coadministration of cytochrome P450 inhibitors to PMs will not increase the plasma concentrations of atomoxetine.

Effect of Atomoxetine on P450 Enzymes

Atomoxetine did not cause clinically important inhibition or induction of cytochrome P450 enzymes, including CYP1A2, CYP3A, CYP2D6, and CYP2C9.

Albuterol

Albuterol (600 μg IV over 2 hours) induced increases in heart rate and blood pressure. These effects were potentiated by atomoxetine (60 mg bid for 5 days) and were most marked after the initial coadministration of albuterol and atomoxetine (see DRUG INTERACTIONS).

Alcohol

Consumption of ethanol with atomoxetine HCl did not change the intoxicating effects of ethanol.

Desipramine

Coadministration of atomoxetine HCl (40 or 60 mg bid for 13 days) with desipramine, a model compound for CYP2D6 metabolized drugs (single dose of 50 mg), did not alter the pharmacokinetics of desipramine. No dose adjustment is recommended for drugs metabolized by CYP2D6.

Methylphenidate

Coadministration of methylphenidate with atomoxetine HCl did not increase cardiovascular effects beyond those seen with methylphenidate alone.

Midazolam

Coadministration of atomoxetine HCl (60 mg bid for 12 days) with midazolam, a model compound for CYP3A4 metabolized drugs (single dose of 5 mg), resulted in 15% increase in AUC of midazolam. No dose adjustment is recommended for drugs metabolized by CYP3A.

Drugs Highly Bound to Plasma Protein

In vitro drug-displacement studies were conducted with atomoxetine and other highly bound drugs at therapeutic concentrations. Atomoxetine did not affect the binding of warfarin, acetylsalicylic acid, phenytoin, or diazepam to human albumin. Similarly, these compounds did not affect the binding of atomoxetine to human albumin.

Drugs That Affect Gastric pH

Drugs that elevate gastric pH (magnesium hydroxide/aluminum hydroxide, omeprazole) had no effect on atomoxetine HCl bioavailability.

INDICATIONS AND USAGE

Atomoxetine HCl is indicated for the treatment of Attention-Deficit/Hyperactivity Disorder (ADHD).

The effectiveness of atomoxetine HCl in the treatment of ADHD was established in 2 placebo-controlled trials in children, 2 placebo-controlled trials in children and adolescents, and 2 placebo-controlled trials in adults who met DSM-IV criteria for ADHD.

A diagnosis of ADHD (DSM-IV) implies the presence of hyperactive-impulsive or inattentive symptoms that cause impairment and that were present before age 7 years. The symptoms must be persistent, must be more severe than is typically observed in individuals at a comparable level of development, must cause clinically significant impairment, *e.g.*, in social, academic, or occupational functioning, and must be present in 2 or more settings, *e.g.*, school (or work) and at home. The symptoms must not be better accounted for by another mental disorder. For the Inattentive Type, at least 6 of the following symptoms must have persisted for at least 6 months: lack of attention to details/careless mistakes, lack of sustained attention, poor listener, failure to follow through on tasks, poor organization, avoids tasks requiring sustained mental effort, loses things, easily distracted, forgetful. For the Hyperactive-Impulsive Type, at least 6 of the following symptoms must have persisted for at least 6 months: fidgeting/squirming, leaving seat, inappropriate running/climbing, difficulty with quiet activities, "on the go," excessive talking, blurting answers, can't wait turn, intrusive. For a Combined Type diagnosis, both inattentive and hyperactive-impulsive criteria must be met.

SPECIAL DIAGNOSTIC CONSIDERATIONS

The specific etiology of ADHD is unknown, and there is no single diagnostic test. Adequate diagnosis requires the use not only of medical but of special psychological, educational, and social resources. Learning may or may not be impaired. The diagnosis must be based upon a complete history and evaluation of the patient and not solely on the presence of the required number of DSM-IV characteristics.

NEED FOR COMPREHENSIVE TREATMENT PROGRAM

Atomoxetine HCl is indicated as an integral part of a total treatment program for ADHD that may include other measures (psychological, educational, social) for patients with this syndrome. Drug treatment may not be indicated for all patients with this syndrome. Drug treatment is not intended for use in the patient who exhibits symptoms secondary to environmental factors and/or other primary psychiatric disorders, including psychosis. Appropriate educational placement is essential in children and adolescents with this diagnosis and psychosocial intervention is often helpful. When remedial measures alone are insufficient, the decision to prescribe drug treatment medication will depend upon the physician's assessment of the chronicity and severity of the patient's symptoms.

LONG-TERM USE

The effectiveness of atomoxetine HCl for long-term use, *i.e.*, for more than 9 weeks in child and adolescent patients and 10 weeks in adult patients, has not been systematically evaluated in controlled trials. Therefore, the physician who elects to use atomoxetine HCl for extended periods should periodically reevaluate the long-term usefulness of the drug for the individual patient (see DOSAGE AND ADMINISTRATION).

CONTRAINDICATIONS

HYPERSENSITIVITY

Atomoxetine HCl is contraindicated in patients known to be hypersensitive to atomoxetine or other constituents of the product (see WARNINGS).

MONOAMINE OXIDASE INHIBITORS (MAOI)

Atomoxetine HCl should not be taken with an MAOI, or within 2 weeks after discontinuing an MAOI. Treatment with an MAOI should not be initiated within 2 weeks after discontinuing atomoxetine HCl. With other drugs that affect brain monoamine concentrations, there have been reports of serious, sometimes fatal, reactions (including hyperthermia, rigidity, myoclonus, autonomic instability with possible rapid fluctuations of vital signs, and mental status changes that include extreme agitation progressing to delirium and coma) when taken in combination with an MAOI. Some cases presented with features resembling neuroleptic malignant syndrome. Such reactions may occur when these drugs are given concurrently or in close proximity.

NARROW ANGLE GLAUCOMA

In clinical trials, atomoxetine HCl use was associated with an increased risk of mydriasis and therefore its use is not recommended in patients with narrow angle glaucoma.

WARNINGS

ALLERGIC EVENTS

Although uncommon, allergic reactions, including angioneurotic edema, urticaria, and rash, have been reported in patients taking atomoxetine HCl.

GROWTH

Growth should be monitored during treatment with atomoxetine HCl . During acute treatment studies (up to 9 weeks), atomoxetine HCl-treated patients lost an average of 0.4 kg, while placebo patients gained an average of 1.5 kg. In a controlled trial that randomized patients to placebo or 1 of 3 atomoxetine doses, 1.3%, 7.1%, 19.3%, and 29.1% of patients lost at least 3.5% of their body weight in the placebo, 0.5, 1.2, and 1.8 mg/kg/day atomoxetine HCl dose groups, respectively. During acute treatment studies, atomoxetine HCl-treated patients grew an average of 0.9 cm, while placebo-treated patients grew an average of 1.1 cm. There are no long-term, placebo-controlled data to evaluate the effect of atomoxetine HCl on growth. Weight and height were assessed during open-label studies of 12 and 18 months, and mean rates of growth were compared to normal growth curves. Patients treated with atomoxetine HCl for at least 18 months gained an average of 6.5 kg while mean weight percentile decreased slightly from 68 to 60. For this same group of patients, the average gain in height was 9.3 cm with a slight decrease in mean height percentile from 54 to 50. Among patients treated for at least 6 months, mean weight gain was lower for poor metabolizer (PM) patients compared with extensive metabolizer (EM) patients (+0.7 kg compared with +3.0 kg), while mean growth for PM patients was 4.3 cm and mean growth for EM patients was 4.4 cm. Whether final adult height or weight is affected by treatment with atomoxetine HCl is unknown. Patients requiring long-term therapy should be monitored and consideration should be given to interrupting therapy in patients who are not growing or gaining weight satisfactorily.

PRECAUTIONS

GENERAL

Effects on Blood Pressure and Heart Rate

Atomoxetine HCl should be used with caution in patients with hypertension, tachycardia, or cardiovascular or cerebrovascular disease because it can increase blood pressure and heart rate. Pulse and blood pressure should be measured at baseline, following atomoxetine HCl dose increases, and periodically while on therapy.

In pediatric placebo-controlled trials, atomoxetine HCl-treated subjects experienced a mean increase in heart rate of about 6 beats/min compared with placebo subjects. At the final study visit before drug discontinuation, 3.6% (12/335) of atomoxetine HCl-treated subjects had heart rate increases of at least 25 beats/min and a heart rate of at least 110 beats/min, compared with 0.5% (1/204) of placebo subjects. No pediatric subject had a heart rate increase of at least 25 beats/min and a heart rate of at least 110 beats/min on more than 1 occasion. Tachycardia was identified as an adverse event for 1.5% (5/340) of these pediatric subjects compared with 0.5% (1/207) of placebo subjects. The mean heart rate increase in extensive metabolizer (EM) patients was 6.7 beats/min, and in poor metabolizer (PM) patients 10.4 beats/min.

Atomoxetine HCl-treated pediatric subjects experienced mean increases of about 1.5 mm Hg in systolic and diastolic blood pressures compared with placebo. At the final study visit before drug discontinuation, 6.8% (22/324) of atomoxetine HCl-treated pediatric subjects had high systolic blood pressure measurements compared with 3.0% (6/197) of placebo subjects. High systolic blood pressures were measured on 2 or more occasions in 8.6% (28/324) of atomoxetine HCl-treated subjects and 3.6% (7/197) of placebo subjects. At the final study visit before drug discontinuation, 2.8% (9/326) of atomoxetine HCl-treated pediatric subjects had high diastolic blood pressure measurements compared with 0.5% (1/200) of placebo subjects. High diastolic blood pressures were measured on 2 or more occasions in 5.2% (17/326) of atomoxetine HCl-treated subjects and 1.5% (3/200) placebo subjects. (High systolic and diastolic blood pressure measurements were defined as those exceeding the 95th percentile, stratified by age, gender, and height percentile — National High Blood Pressure Education Working Group on Hypertension Control in Children and Adolescents.)

In adult placebo-controlled trials, atomoxetine HCl-treated subjects experienced a mean increase in heart rate of 5 beats/min compared with placebo subjects. Tachycardia was identified as an adverse event for 3% (8/269) of these adult atomoxetine subjects compared with 0.8% (2/263) of placebo subjects.

Atomoxetine HCl-treated adult subjects experienced mean increases in systolic (about 3 mm Hg) and diastolic (about 1 mm Hg) blood pressures compared with placebo. At the final study visit before drug discontinuation, 1.9% (5/258) of atomoxetine HCl-treated adult subjects had systolic blood pressure measurements ≥150 mm Hg compared with 1.2% (3/256) of placebo subjects. At the final study visit before drug discontinuation, 0.8% (2/257) of atomoxetine HCl-treated adult subjects had diastolic blood pressure measurements ≥100 mm Hg compared with 0.4% (1/257) of placebo subjects. No adult subject had a high systolic or diastolic blood pressure detected on more than 1 occasion.

Orthostatic hypotension has been reported in subjects taking atomoxetine HCl. In short-term child- and adolescent-controlled trials, 1.8% (6/340) of atomoxetine HCl-treated subjects experienced symptoms of postural hypotension compared with 0.5% (1/207) of placebo-treated subjects. Atomoxetine HCl should be used with caution in any condition that may predispose patients to hypotension.

Effects on Urine Outflow From the Bladder

In adult ADHD controlled trials, the rates of urinary retention (3%, 7/269) and urinary hesitation (3%, 7/269) were increased among atomoxetine subjects compared with placebo subjects (0%, 0/263). Two adult atomoxetine subjects and no placebo subjects discontinued from controlled clinical trials because of urinary retention. A complaint of urinary retention or urinary hesitancy should be considered potentially related to atomoxetine.

INFORMATION FOR THE PATIENT

Patients should consult a physician if they are taking or plan to take any prescription or over-the-counter medicines, dietary supplements, or herbal remedies.

Patients should consult a physician if they are nursing, pregnant, or thinking of becoming pregnant while taking atomoxetine HCl.

Patients may take atomoxetine HCl with or without food.

If patients miss a dose, they should take it as soon as possible, but should not take more than the prescribed total daily amount of atomoxetine HCl in any 24 hour period.

Patients should use caution when driving a car or operating hazardous machinery until they are reasonably certain that their performance is not affected by atomoxetine.

LABORATORY TESTS

Routine laboratory tests are not required.

CYP2D6 Metabolism: Poor metabolizers (PMs) of CYP2D6 have a 10-fold higher AUC and a 5-fold higher peak concentration to a given dose of atomoxetine HCl compared with extensive metabolizers (EMs). Approximately 7% of a Caucasian population are PMs. Laboratory tests are available to identify CYP2D6 PMs. The blood levels in PMs are similar to those attained by taking strong inhibitors of CYP2D6. The higher blood levels in PMs lead to a higher rate of some adverse effects of atomoxetine HCl (see ADVERSE REACTIONS).

CARCINOGENESIS, MUTAGENESIS, AND IMPAIRMENT OF FERTILITY

Carcinogenesis

Atomoxetine HCl was not carcinogenic in rats and mice when given in the diet for 2 years at time-weighted average doses up to 47 and 458 mg/kg/day, respectively. The highest dose used in rats is approximately 8 and 5 times the maximum human dose in children and adults, respectively, on a mg/m^2 basis. Plasma levels (AUC) of atomoxetine at this dose in rats are estimated to be 1.8 times (extensive metabolizers) or 0.2 times (poor metabolizers) those in humans receiving the maximum human dose. The highest dose used in mice is approximately 39 and 26 times the maximum human dose in children and adults, respectively, on a mg/m^2 basis.

Mutagenesis

Atomoxetine HCl was negative in a battery of genotoxicity studies that included a reverse point mutation assay (Ames Test), an *in vitro* mouse lymphoma assay, a chromosomal aberration test in Chinese hamster ovary cells, an unscheduled DNA synthesis test in rat hepatocytes, and an *in vivo* micronucleus test in mice. However, there was a slight increase in the percentage of Chinese hamster ovary cells with diplochromosomes, suggesting endoreduplication (numerical aberration).

The metabolite N-desmethylatomoxetine HCl was negative in the Ames Test, mouse lymphoma assay, and unscheduled DNA synthesis test.

Impairment of Fertility

Atomoxetine HCl did not impair fertility in rats when given in the diet at doses of up to 57 mg/kg/day, which is approximately 6 times the maximum human dose on a mg/m^2 basis.

PREGNANCY CATEGORY C

Pregnant rabbits were treated with up to 100 mg/kg/day of atomoxetine by gavage throughout the period of organogenesis. At this dose, in 1 of 3 studies, a decrease in live fetuses and an increase in early resorptions was observed. Slight increases in the incidences of atypical origin of carotid artery and absent subclavian artery were observed. These findings were observed at doses that caused slight maternal toxicity. The no-effect dose for these findings was 30 mg/kg/day. The 100 mg/kg dose is approximately 23 times the maximum human dose on a mg/m^2 basis; plasma levels (AUC) of atomoxetine at this dose in rabbits are estimated to be 3.3 times (extensive metabolizers) or 0.4 times (poor metabolizers) those in humans receiving the maximum human dose.

Rats were treated with up to approximately 50 mg/kg/day of atomoxetine (approximately 6 times the maximum human dose on a mg/m^2 basis) in the diet from 2 (females) or 10 (males) weeks prior to mating through the periods of organogenesis and lactation. In 1 of 2 studies, decreases in pup weight and pup survival were observed. The decreased pup survival was also seen at 25 mg/kg (but not at 13 mg/kg). In a study in which rats were treated with atomoxetine in the diet from 2 (females) or 10 (males) weeks prior to mating throughout the period of organogenesis, a decrease in fetal (female only) weight and an increase in the incidence of incomplete ossification of the vertebral arch in fetuses were observed at 40 mg/kg/day (approximately 5 times the maximum human dose on a mg/m^2 basis) but not at 20 mg/kg/day.

No adverse fetal effects were seen when pregnant rats were treated with up to 150 mg/kg/day (approximately 17 times the maximum human dose on a mg/m^2 basis) by gavage throughout the period of organogenesis.

No adequate and well-controlled studies have been conducted in pregnant women. Atomoxetine HCl should not be used during pregnancy unless the potential benefit justifies the potential risk to the fetus.

LABOR AND DELIVERY

Parturition in rats was not affected by atomoxetine. The effect of atomoxetine HCl on labor and delivery in humans is unknown.

NURSING MOTHERS

Atomoxetine and/or its metabolites were excreted in the milk of rats. It is not known if atomoxetine is excreted in human milk. Caution should be exercised if atomoxetine HCl is administered to a nursing woman.

PEDIATRIC USE

The safety and efficacy of atomoxetine HCl in pediatric patients less than 6 years of age have not been established. The efficacy of atomoxetine HCl beyond 9 weeks and safety of atomoxetine HCl beyond 1 year of treatment have not been systematically evaluated.

A study was conducted in young rats to evaluate the effects of atomoxetine on growth and neurobehavioral and sexual development. Rats were treated with 1, 10, or 50 mg/kg/day (approximately 0.2, 2, and 8 times, respectively, the maximum human dose on a mg/m^2 basis) of atomoxetine given by gavage from the early postnatal period (Day 10 of age) through adulthood. Slight delays in onset of vaginal patency (all doses) and preputial separation (10 and 50 mg/kg), slight decreases in epididymal weight and sperm number (10 and 50 mg/kg), and a slight decrease in corpora lutea (50 mg/kg) were seen, but there were no effects on fertility or reproductive performance. A slight delay in onset of incisor eruption was seen at 50 mg/kg. A slight increase in motor activity was seen on Day 15 (males at 10 and 50 and females at 50 mg/kg) and on Day 30 (females at 50 mg/kg) but not on Day 60 of age. There were no effects on learning and memory tests. The significance of these findings to humans is unknown.

GERIATRIC USE

The safety and efficacy of atomoxetine HCl in geriatric patients have not been established.

DRUG INTERACTIONS

ALBUTEROL

Atomoxetine HCl should be administered with caution to patients being treated with albuterol (or other beta$_2$ agonists) because the action of albuterol on the cardiovascular system can be potentiated.

CYP2D6 INHIBITORS

Atomoxetine is primarily metabolized by the CYP2D6 pathway to 4-hydroxyatomoxetine. In EMs, selective inhibitors of CYP2D6 increase atomoxetine steady-state plasma concentrations to exposures similar to those observed in PMs. Dosage adjustment of atomoxetine HCl may be necessary when coadministered with CYP2D6 inhibitors, *e.g.*, paroxetine, fluoxetine, and quinidine (see DOSAGE AND ADMINISTRATION). In EM individuals treated with paroxetine or fluoxetine, the AUC of atomoxetine is approximately 6- to 8-fold and $C_{ss,max}$ is about 3- to 4-fold greater than atomoxetine alone.

In vitro studies suggest that coadministration of cytochrome P450 inhibitors to PMs will not increase the plasma concentrations of atomoxetine.

MONOAMINE OXIDASE INHIBITORS

See CONTRAINDICATIONS.

PRESSOR AGENTS

Because of possible effects on blood pressure, atomoxetine HCl should be used cautiously with pressor agents.

ADVERSE REACTIONS

Atomoxetine HCl was administered to 2067 children or adolescent patients with ADHD and 270 adults with ADHD in clinical studies. During the ADHD clinical trials, 169 patients were treated for longer than 1 year and 526 patients were treated for over 6 months.

The data in the following tables and text cannot be used to predict the incidence of side effects in the course of usual medical practice where patient characteristics and other factors differ from those that prevailed in the clinical trials. Similarly, the cited frequencies cannot be compared with data obtained from other clinical investigations involving different treatments, uses, or investigators. The cited data provide the prescribing physician with some basis for estimating the relative contribution of drug and non-drug factors to the adverse event incidence in the population studied.

CHILD AND ADOLESCENT CLINICAL TRIALS

Reasons for Discontinuation of Treatment Due to Adverse Events in Child and Adolescent Clinical Trials

In acute child and adolescent placebo-controlled trials, 3.5% (15/427) of atomoxetine subjects and 1.4% (4/294) placebo subjects discontinued for adverse events. For all studies, (including open-label and long-term studies), 5% of extensive metabolizer (EM) patients and 7% of poor metabolizer (PM) patients discontinued because of an adverse event. Among atomoxetine HCl-treated patients, aggression (0.5%, n=2); irritability (0.5%, n=2); somnolence (0.5%, n=2); and vomiting (0.5%, n=2) were the reasons for discontinuation reported by more than 1 patient.

Commonly Observed Adverse Events in Acute Child and Adolescent, Placebo-Controlled Trials

Commonly observed adverse events associated with the use of atomoxetine HCl (incidence of 2% or greater) and not observed at an equivalent incidence among placebo-treated patients (atomoxetine HCl incidence greater than placebo) are listed in TABLE 1 for the bid trials. Results were similar in the qd trial except as shown in TABLE 2, which shows both bid and qd results for selected adverse events. The most commonly observed adverse events in patients treated with atomoxetine HCl (incidence of 5% or greater and at least twice the incidence in placebo patients, for either bid or qd dosing) were: dyspepsia, nausea, vomiting, fatigue, appetite decreased, dizziness, and mood swings (see TABLE 1 and TABLE 2).

The following adverse events occurred in at least 2% of PM patients and were either twice as frequent or statistically significantly more frequent in PM patients compared with EM patients: decreased appetite (23% of PMs, 16% of EMs); insomnia (13% of PMs, 7% of EMs); sedation (4% of PMs, 2% of EMs); depression (6% of PMs, 2% of EMs); tremor (4%

TABLE 1 *Common Treatment-Emergent Adverse Events Associated With the Use of Atomoxetine HCl in Acute (Up to 9 Weeks) Child and Adolescent Trials*

	% of Patients Reporting Events From bid Trials	
	Atomoxetine HCl	Placebo
Adverse Event*	(n=340)	(n=207)
Gastrointestinal Disorders		
Abdominal pain upper	20%	16%
Constipation	3%	1%
Dyspepsia	4%	2%
Vomiting	11%	9%
Infections		
Ear infection	3%	1%
Influenza	3%	1%
Investigations		
Weight decreased	2%	0%
Metabolism and Nutritional Disorders		
Appetite decreased	14%	6%
Nervous System Disorders		
Dizziness (except vertigo)	6%	3%
Headache	27%	25%
Somnolence	7%	5%
Psychiatric Disorders		
Crying	2%	1%
Irritability	8%	5%
Mood swings	2%	0%
Respiratory, Thoracic, and Mediastinal Disorders		
Cough	11%	7%
Rhinorrhea	4%	3%
Skin and Subcutaneous Tissue Disorders		
Dermatitis	4%	1%

* Events reported by at least 2% of patients treated with atomoxetine, and greater than placebo. The following events did not meet this criterion but were reported by more atomoxetine-treated patients than placebo-treated patients and are possibly related to atomoxetine treatment: anorexia, blood pressure increased, early morning awakening, flushing, mydriasis, sinus tachycardia, tearfulness. The following events were reported by at least 2% of patients treated with atomoxetine, and equal to or less than placebo: arthralgia, gastroenteritis viral, insomnia, sore throat, nasal congestion, nasopharyngitis, pruritus, sinus congestion, upper respiratory tract infection.

TABLE 2 *Common Treatment-Emergent Adverse Events Associated With the Use of Atomoxetine HCl in Acute (Up to 9 Weeks) Child and Adolescent Trials*

	bid Trials		qd Trials	
	Atomoxetine HCl	Placebo	Atomoxetine HCl	Placebo
Adverse Event	(n=340)	(n=207)	(n=85)	(n=85)
Gastrointestinal Disorders				
Abdominal pain upper	20%	16%	16%	9%
Constipation	3%	1%	0%	0%
Diarrhea	3%	6%	4%	1%
Dry mouth	1%	2%	4%	1%
Dyspepsia	4%	2%	8%	0%
Nausea	7%	8%	12%	2%
Vomiting	11%	9%	15%	1%
General Disorders				
Fatigue	4%	5%	9%	1%
Psychiatric Disorders				
Mood swings	2%	0%	5%	2%

of PMs, 1% of EMs); early morning awakening (3% of PMs, 1% of EMs); pruritus (2% of PMs, 1% of EMs); mydriasis (2% of PMs, 1% of EMs).

ADULT CLINICAL TRIALS

Reasons for Discontinuation of Treatment Due to Adverse Events in Acute Adult Placebo-Controlled Trials

In the acute adult placebo-controlled trials, 8.5% (23/270) atomoxetine subjects and 3.4% (9/266) placebo subjects discontinued for adverse events. Among atomoxetine HCl-treated patients, insomnia (1.1%, n=3); chest pain (0.7%, n=2); palpitations (0.7%, n=2); and urinary retention (0.7%, n=2) were the reasons for discontinuation reported by more than 1 patient.

Commonly Observed Adverse Events in Acute Adult Placebo-Controlled Trials

Commonly observed adverse events associated with the use of atomoxetine HCl (incidence of 2% or greater) and not observed at an equivalent incidence among placebo-treated patients (atomoxetine HCl incidence greater than placebo) are listed in TABLE 3. The most commonly observed adverse events in patients treated with atomoxetine HCl (incidence of 5% or greater and at least twice the incidence in placebo patients) were: constipation, dry mouth, nausea, appetite decreased, dizziness, insomnia, decreased libido, ejaculatory problems, impotence, urinary hesitation and/or urinary retention and/or difficulty in micturition, and dysmenorrhea (see TABLE 3).

Male and Female Sexual Dysfunction

Atomoxetine appears to impair sexual function in some patients. Changes in sexual desire, sexual performance, and sexual satisfaction are not well assessed in most clinical trials because they need special attention and because patients and physicians may be reluctant to discuss them. Accordingly, estimates of the incidence of untoward sexual experience and performance cited in product labeling are likely to underestimate the actual incidence. TABLE 4 displays the incidence of sexual side effects reported by at least 2% of adult patients taking atomoxetine HCl in placebo-controlled trials.

There are no adequate and well-controlled studies examining sexual dysfunction with atomoxetine HCl treatment. While it is difficult to know the precise risk of sexual dysfunction associated with the use of atomoxetine HCl, physicians should routinely inquire about such possible side effects.

DOSAGE AND ADMINISTRATION

INITIAL TREATMENT

Dosing of Children and Adolescents Up to 70 kg Body Weight

Atomoxetine HCl should be initiated at a total daily dose of approximately 0.5 mg/kg and increased after a minimum of 3 days to a target total daily dose of approximately 1.2 mg/kg administered either as a single daily dose in the morning or as evenly divided doses in the morning and late afternoon/early evening. No additional benefit has been demonstrated for doses higher than 1.2 mg/kg/day.

The total daily dose in children and adolescents should not exceed 1.4 mg/kg or 100 mg, whichever is less.

Dosing of Children and Adolescents Over 70 kg Body Weight and Adults

Atomoxetine HCl should be initiated at a total daily dose of 40 mg and increased after a minimum of 3 days to a target total daily dose of approximately 80 mg administered either as a single daily dose in the morning or as evenly divided doses in the morning and late afternoon/early evening. After 2-4 additional weeks, the dose may be increased to a maximum of 100 mg in patients who have not achieved an optimal response. There are no data that support increased effectiveness at higher doses.

The maximum recommended total daily dose in children and adolescents over 70 kg and adults is 100 mg.

MAINTENANCE/EXTENDED TREATMENT

There is no evidence available from controlled trials to indicate how long the patient with ADHD should be treated with atomoxetine HCl. It is generally agreed, however, that pharmacological treatment of ADHD may be needed for extended periods. Nevertheless, the physician who elects to use atomoxetine HCl for extended periods should periodically re-evaluate the long-term usefulness of the drug for the individual patient.

GENERAL DOSING INFORMATION

Atomoxetine HCl may be taken with or without food.

The safety of single doses over 120 mg and total daily doses above 150 mg have not been systematically evaluated.

TABLE 3 *Common Treatment-Emergent Adverse Events Associated With the Use of Atomoxetine HCl in Acute (up to 10 weeks) Adult Trials*

Adverse Event*	Atomoxetine HCl	Placebo
System Organ Class/Adverse Event	(n=269)	(n=263)
Cardiac Disorders		
Palpitations	4%	1%
Gastrointestinal Disorders		
Constipation	10%	4%
Dry mouth	21%	6%
Dyspepsia	6%	4%
Flatulence	2%	1%
Nausea	12%	5%
General Disorders and Administration Site Conditions		
Fatigue and/or lethargy	7%	4%
Pyrexia	3%	2%
Rigors	3%	1%
Infections		
Sinusitis	6%	4%
Investigations		
Weight decreased	2%	1%
Metabolism and Nutritional Disorders		
Appetite decreased	10%	3%
Musculoskeletal, Connective Tissue, and Bone Disorders		
Myalgia	3%	2%
Nervous System Disorders		
Dizziness	6%	2%
Headache	17%	17%
Insomnia and/or middle insomnia	16%	8%
Paraesthesia	4%	2%
Sinus headache	3%	1%
Psychiatric Disorders		
Abnormal dreams	4%	3%
Libido decreased	6%	2%
Sleep disorder	4%	2%
Renal and Urinary Disorders		
Urinary hesitation and/or urinary retention and/or difficulty in micturition	8%	0%
Reproductive System and Breast Disorders		
Dysmenorrhoea‡	7%	3%
Ejaculation failure† and/or ejaculation disorder†	5%	2%
Erectile disturbance†	7%	1%
Impotence†	3%	0%
Menses delayed‡	2%	1%
Menstrual disorder‡	3%	2%
Menstruation irregular‡	2%	0%
Orgasm abnormal	2%	1%
Prostatitis†	3%	0%
Skin and Subcutaneous Tissue Disorders		
Dermatitis	2%	1%
Sweating increased	4%	1%
Vascular Disorders		
Hot flushes	3%	1%

* Events reported by at least 2% of patients treated with atomoxetine, and greater than placebo. The following events did not meet this criterion but were reported by more atomoxetine-treated patients than placebo-treated patients and are possibly related to atomoxetine treatment: early morning awakening, peripheral coldness, tachycardia. The following events were reported by at least 2% of patients treated with atomoxetine, and equal to or less than placebo: abdominal pain upper, arthralgia, back pain, cough, diarrhea, influenza, irritability, nasopharyngitis, sore throat, upper respiratory tract infection, vomiting.
† Based on total number of males (atomoxetine HCl, n=174; placebo, n=172).
‡ Based on total number of females (atomoxetine HCl, n=95; placebo, n=91).

TABLE 4

	Atomoxetine HCl	Placebo
Erectile disturbance*	7%	1%
Impotence*	3%	0%
Orgasm abnormal	2%	1%

* Males only.

Dosing Adjustment for Hepatically Impaired Patients

For those ADHD patients who have hepatic insufficiency (HI), dosage adjustment is recommended as follows: For patients with moderate HI (Child-Pugh Class B), initial and target doses should be reduced to 50% of the normal dose (for patients without HI). For patients with severe HI (Child-Pugh Class C), initial dose and target doses should be reduced to 25% of normal (see CLINICAL PHARMACOLOGY, Special Populations).

Dosing Adjustment for Use With a Strong CYP2D6 Inhibitor

In children and adolescents up to 70 kg body weight administered strong CYP2D6 inhibitors, *e.g.*, paroxetine, fluoxetine, quinidine, atomoxetine HCl should be initiated at 0.5 mg/kg/day and only increased to the usual target dose of 1.2 mg/kg/day if symptoms fail to improve after 4 weeks and the initial dose is well tolerated.

In children and adolescents over 70 kg body weight and adults administered strong CYP2D6 inhibitors, *e.g.*, paroxetine, fluoxetine, quinidine, atomoxetine HCl should be initiated at 40 mg/day and only increased to the usual target dose of 80 mg/day if symptoms fail to improve after 4 weeks and the initial dose is well tolerated.

Atomoxetine can be discontinued without being tapered.

HOW SUPPLIED

Strattera capsules are supplied in:

10 mg:* Opaque white capsules imprinted with "Lilly 3227".
18 mg:* Gold and opaque white capsules imprinted with "Lilly 3238".
25 mg:* Opaque blue and opaque white capsules imprinted with "Lilly 3228".
40 mg:* Opaque blue capsules imprinted with "Lilly 3229".
60 mg:* Opaque blue and gold capsules imprinted with "Lilly 3239".
*Atomoxetine base equivalent.

Storage: Store at 25°C (77°F); excursions permitted to 15-30°C (59-86°F).

PRODUCT LISTING - EQUIVALENTS NOT AVAILABLE

Capsule - Oral - 10 mg
30's $93.75 STRATTERA, Lilly, Eli and Company 00002-3227-30
Capsule - Oral - 18 mg
30's $93.75 STRATTERA, Lilly, Eli and Company 00002-3238-30
Capsule - Oral - 25 mg
30's $93.75 STRATTERA, Lilly, Eli and Company 00002-3228-30
Capsule - Oral - 40 mg
30's $93.75 STRATTERA, Lilly, Eli and Company 00002-3229-30
Capsule - Oral - 60 mg
30's $93.75 STRATTERA, Lilly, Eli and Company 00002-3239-30

Atorvastatin Calcium (003318)

For related information, see the comparative table section in Appendix A.

Categories: Hypercholesterolemia; Hyperlipidemia; Hypertriglyceridemia; FDA Approved 1996 Dec; Pregnancy Category X
Drug Classes: Antihyperlipidemics; HMG CoA reductase inhibitors
Brand Names: Lipitor
Foreign Brand Availability: Ator (Bahrain; Cyprus; Egypt; Iran; Iraq; Jordan; Kuwait; Lebanon; Libya; Oman; Qatar; Republic-of-Yemen; Saudi-Arabia; Syria; United-Arab-Emirates); Atorlip (Colombia); Atovarol (Colombia); Edy (Colombia); Glustar (Colombia); Lowlipen (Colombia); Sortis (Germany); Storvas (India); Tahor (France; Mauritius)
Cost of Therapy: $59.12 (Hypercholesterolemia; Lipitor; 10 mg; 1 tablet/day; 30 day supply)

DESCRIPTION

Atorvastatin calcium is a synthetic lipid-lowering agent. Atorvastatin is an inhibitor of 3-hydroxy-3-methylglutaryl-coenzyme A (HMG-CoA) reductase. This enzyme catalyzes the conversion of HMG-CoA to mevalonate, an early and rate-limiting step in cholesterol biosynthesis.

Atorvastatin calcium is [R-(R*,R*)]-2-(4-fluorophenyl)-β,δ-dihydroxy-5-(1-methylethyl)-3-phenyl-4-[(phenylamino)carbonyl]-lH-pyrrole-1-heptanoic acid, calcium salt (2:1) trihydrate. The empirical formula of atorvastatin calcium is $(C_{33}H_{34}FN_2O_5)_2Ca{\cdot}3H_2O$ and its molecular weight is 1209.42.

Atorvastatin calcium is a white to off-white crystalline powder that is insoluble in aqueous solutions of pH 4 and below. Atorvastatin calcium is very slightly soluble in distilled water, pH 7.4 phosphate buffer, and acetonitrile, slightly soluble in ethanol, and freely soluble in methanol.

Lipitor tablets for oral administration contain 10, 20, 40 or 80 mg atorvastatin and the following inactive ingredients: calcium carbonate, candelilla wax, croscarmellose sodium, hydroxypropyl cellulose, lactose monohydrate, magnesium stearate, microcrystalline cellulose, Opadry White YS-1-7040 (hydroxypropylmethylcellulose, polyethylene glycol, talc, titanium dioxide), polysorbate 80, simethicone emulsion.

CLINICAL PHARMACOLOGY

MECHANISM OF ACTION

Atorvastatin is a selective, competitive inhibitor of HMG-CoA reductase, the rate-limiting enzyme that converts 3-hydroxy-3-methylglutaryl-coenzyme A to mevalonate, a precursor of sterols, including cholesterol. Cholesterol and triglycerides circulate in the bloodstream as part of lipoprotein complexes. With ultracentrifugation, these complexes separate into HDL (high-density lipoprotein), IDL (intermediate-density lipoprotein), LDL (low-density lipoprotein), and VLDL (very-low-density lipoprotein) fractions. Triglycerides (TG) and cholesterol in the liver are incorporated into VLDL and released into the plasma for delivery to peripheral tissues. LDL is formed from VLDL and is catabolized primarily through the high-affinity LDL receptor. Clinical and pathologic studies show that elevated plasma levels of total cholesterol (total-C), LDL-cholesterol (LDL-C), and apolipoprotein B (apo B) promote human atherosclerosis and are risk factors for developing cardiovascular disease, while increased levels of HDL-C are associated with a decreased cardiovascular risk.

In animal models, atorvastatin calcium lowers plasma cholesterol and lipoprotein levels by inhibiting HMG-CoA reductase and cholesterol synthesis in the liver and by increasing the number of hepatic LDL receptors on the cell-surface to enhance uptake and catabolism of LDL; atorvastatin calcium also reduces LDL production and the number of LDL particles. Atorvastatin calcium reduces LDL-C in some patients with homozygous familial hypercholesterolemia (FH), a population that rarely responds to other lipid-lowering medication(s).

A variety of clinical studies have demonstrated that elevated levels of total-C, LDL-C, and apo B (a membrane complex for LDL-C) promote human atherosclerosis. Similarly, decreased levels of HDL-C (and its transport complex, apo A) are associated with the development of atherosclerosis. Epidemiologic investigations have established that cardiovascular morbidity and mortality vary directly with the level of total-C and LDL-C, and inversely with the level of HDL-C.

Atorvastatin calcium reduces total-C, LDL-C, and apo B in patients with homozygous and heterozygous FH, nonfamilial forms of hypercholesterolemia, and mixed dyslipidemia. Atorvastatin calcium also reduces VLDL-C and TG and produces variable increases in HDL-C and apolipoprotein A-1. Atorvastatin calcium reduces total-C, LDL-C, VLDL-C, apo B, TG, and non-HDL-C, and increases HDL-C in patients with isolated hypertriglyceridermia. Atorvastatin calcium reduces intermediate density lipoprotein cholesterol (IDL-C) in patients with dysbetalipoproteinemia. The effect of atorvastatin calcium on cardiovascular morbidity and mortality has not been determined.

Like LDL, cholesterol-enriched triglyceride-rich lipoproteins, including VLDL, intermediate density lipoprotein (IDL), and remnants, can also promote atherosclerosis. Elevated plasma triglycerides are frequently found in a triad with low HDL-C levels and small LDL particles, as well as in association with non-lipid metabolic risk factors for coronary heart disease. As such, total plasma TG has not consistently been shown to be an independent risk factor for CHD. Furthermore, the independent effect of raising HDL or lowering TG on the risk of coronary and cardiovascular morbidity and mortality has not been determined.

PHARMACODYNAMICS

Atorvastatin as well as some of its metabolites are pharmacologically active in humans. The liver is the primary site of action and the principal site of cholesterol synthesis and LDL clearance. Drug dosage rather than systemic drug concentration correlates better with LDL-C reduction. Individualization of drug dosage should be based on therapeutic response (see DOSAGE AND ADMINISTRATION).

PHARMACOKINETICS AND DRUG METABOLISM

Absorption

Atorvastatin is rapidly absorbed after oral administration; maximum plasma concentrations occur within 1-2 hours. Extent of absorption increases in proportion to atorvastatin dose. The absolute bioavailability of atorvastatin (parent drug) is approximately 14% and the systemic availability of HMG-CoA reductase inhibitory activity is approximately 30%. The low systemic availability is attributed to presystemic clearance in gastrointestinal mucosa and/or hepatic first-pass metabolism. Although food decreases the rate and extent of drug absorption by approximately 25% and 9%, respectively, as assessed by C_{max} and AUC, LDL-C reduction is similar whether atorvastatin is given with or without food. Plasma atorvastatin concentrations are lower (approximately 30% for C_{max} and AUC) following evening drug administration compared with morning. However, LDL-C reduction is the same regardless of the time of day of drug administration (see DOSAGE AND ADMINISTRATION).

Distribution

Mean volume of distribution of atorvastatin is approximately 381 L. Atorvastatin is ≥98% bound to plasma proteins. A blood/plasma ratio of approximately 0.25 indicates poor drug penetration into red blood cells. Based on observations in rats, atorvastatin is likely to be secreted in human milk (see CONTRAINDICATIONS, Pregnancy and Lactation and PRECAUTIONS, Nursing Mothers).

Metabolism

Atorvastatin is extensively metabolized to ortho- and parahydroxylated derivatives and various beta-oxidation products. *In vitro* inhibition of HMG-CoA reductase by ortho- and parahydroxylated metabolites is equivalent to that of atorvastatin. Approximately 70% of circulating inhibitory activity for HMG-CoA reductase is attributed to active metabolites. *In vitro* studies suggest the importance of atorvastatin metabolism by cytochrome P450 3A4, consistent with increased plasma concentrations of atorvastatin in humans following coadministration with erythromycin, a known inhibitor of this isozyme (see DRUG INTERACTIONS). In animals, the ortho-hydroxy metabolite undergoes further glucuronidation.

Excretion

Atorvastatin and its metabolites are eliminated primarily in bile following hepatic and/or extra-hepatic metabolism; however, the drug does not appear to undergo enterohepatic recirculation. Mean plasma elimination half-life of atorvastatin in humans is approximately 14 hours, but the half-life of inhibitory activity for HMG-CoA reductase is 20-30 hours due to the contribution of active metabolites. Less than 2% of a dose of atorvastatin is recovered in urine following oral administration.

SPECIAL POPULATIONS

Geriatric

Plasma concentrations of atorvastatin are higher (approximately 40% for C_{max} and 30% for AUC) in healthy elderly subjects (age ≥65 years) than in young adults. Clinical data suggest a greater degree of LDL-lowering at any dose of drug in the elderly patient population compared to younger adults (see PRECAUTIONS, Geriatric Use).

Pediatric

Pharmacokinetic data in the pediatric population are not available.

Gender

Plasma concentrations of atorvastatin in women differ from those in men (approximately 20% higher for C_{max} and 10% lower for AUC); however, there is no clinically significant difference in LDL-C reduction with atorvastatin calcium between men and women.

Renal Insufficiency

Renal disease has no influence on the plasma concentrations or LDL-C reduction of atorvastatin; thus, dose adjustment in patients with renal dysfunction is not necessary (see DOSAGE AND ADMINISTRATION).

Hemodialysis

While studies have not been conducted in patients with end-stage renal disease, hemodialysis is not expected to significantly enhance clearance of atorvastatin since the drug is extensively bound to plasma proteins.

Hepatic Insufficiency

In patients with chronic alcoholic liver disease, plasma concentrations of atorvastatin are markedly increased. C_{max} and AUC are each 4-fold greater in patients with Childs-Pugh A disease. C_{max} and AUC are approximately 16-fold and 11-fold increased, respectively, in patients with Childs-Pugh B disease (see CONTRAINDICATIONS).

A

INDICATIONS AND USAGE

Atorvastatin calcium is indicated:

As an adjunct to diet to reduce elevated total-C, LDL-C, apo B, and TG levels and to increase HDL-C in patients with primary hypercholesterolemia (heterozygous familial and nonfamilial) and mixed dyslipidemia (*Fredrickson* Types IIa and IIb).

As an adjunct to diet for the treatment of patients with elevated serum TG levels (*Fredrickson* Type IV).

For the treatment of patients with primary dysbetalipoproteinemia (*Fredrickson* Type III) who do not respond adequately to diet.

To reduce total-C and LDL-C in patients with homozygous familial hypercholesterolemia as an adjunct to other lipid-lowering treatments (*e.g.,* LDL apheresis) or if such treatments are unavailable.

As an adjunct to diet to reduce total-C, LDL-C, and apo B levels in boys and postmenarchal girls, 10-17 years of age, with heterozygous familial hypercholesterolemia if after an adequate trial of diet therapy the following findings are present:

a. LDL-C remains ≥190 mg/dl or
b. LDL-C remains ≥160 mg/dl and:
- There is a positive family history of premature cardiovascular disease or
- Two or more other CVD risk factors are present in the pediatric patient.

Therapy with lipid-altering agents should be a component of multiple-risk-factor intervention in individuals at increased risk for atherosclerotic vascular disease due to hypercholesterolemia. Lipid-altering agents should be used in addition to a diet restricted in saturated fat and cholesterol only when the response to diet and other nonpharmacological measures has been inadequate [see *National Cholesterol Education Program (NCEP) Guidelines,* summarized in TABLE 6].

***TABLE 6** NCEP Treatment Guidelines: LDL-C Goals and Cutpoints for Therapeutic Lifestyle Changes and Drug Therapy in Different Risk Categories*

Risk Category	LDL Goal (mg/dl)	LDL Level at Which to Initiate Therapeutic Lifestyle Changes (mg/dl)	LDL Level at Which to Consider Drug Therapy (mg/dl)
CHD* or CHD risk equivalents (10 y risk >20%)	<100	≥100	≥130 (100-129: drug optional)†
2+ Risk factors (10 y risk ≤20%)	<130	≥130	10 y risk 10-20%: ≥130 10 y risk <10%: ≥160
0-1 Risk factor‡	<160	≥160	≥190 (160-189: LDL-lowering drug optional)

* CHD, coronary heart disease.
† Some authorities recommend use of LDL-lowering drugs in this category if an LDL-C level of <100 mg/dl cannot be achieved by therapeutic lifestyle changes. Others prefer use of drugs that primarily modify triglycerides and HDL-C, *e.g.,* nicominic acid or fibrate. Clinical judgement also may call for deferring drug therapy in this subcategory.
‡ Almost all people with 0-1 risk factor have 10 year risk <10%; thus, 10 year risk assessment in people with 0-1 risk factor is not necessary.

After the LDL-C goal has been achieved, if the TG is still ≥200 mg/dl, non HDL-C (total-C minus HDL-C) becomes a secondary target of therapy. Non-HDL-C goals are set 30 mg/dl higher than LDL-C goals for each risk category.

Prior to initiating therapy with atorvastatin calcium, secondary causes for hypercholesterolemia (*e.g.,* poorly controlled diabetes mellitus, hypothyroidism, nephrotic syndrome, dysproteinemias, obstructive liver disease, other drug therapy, and alcoholism) should be excluded, and a lipid profile performed to measure total-C, LDL-C, HDL-C, and TG. For patients with TG <400 mg/dl (<4.5 mmol/L), LDL-C can be estimated using the following equation: LDL-C = total-C - (0.20 × [TG] + HDL-C). For TG levels >400 mg/dl (>4.5 mmol/L), this equation is less accurate and LDL-C concentrations should be determined by ultracentrifugation.

Atorvastatin calcium has not been studied in conditions where the major lipoprotein abnormality is elevation of chylomicrons (*Fredrickson* Types I and V).

The NCEP classification of cholesterol levels in pediatric patients with a familial history of hypercholesterolemia or premature cardiovascular disease is summarized in TABLE 7.

TABLE 7

Category	Total-C (mg/dl)	LDL-C (mg/dl)
Acceptable	<170	<110
Borderline	170-199	110-129
High	≥200	≥130

NON-FDA APPROVED INDICATIONS

HMG-CoA reductase inhibitors are also used in patients without clinical signs of coronary heart disease as part of a treatment regimen to decrease total and LDL cholesterol, slow the development of coronary atherosclerosis, and prevent primary coronary events. No conclusions have been drawn regarding the effect of atorvastatin on cardiovascular morbidity and mortality, although HMG-CoA reductase inhibitors have been associated with markedly beneficial effects.

CONTRAINDICATIONS

Active liver disease or unexplained persistent elevations of serum transaminases.

Hypersensitivity to any component of this medication.

PREGNANCY AND LACTATION

Atherosclerosis is a chronic process and discontinuation of lipid-lowering drugs during pregnancy should have little impact on the outcome of long-term therapy of primary hypercholesterolemia. Cholesterol and other products of cholesterol biosynthesis are essential components for fetal development (including synthesis of steroids and cell membranes). Since HMG-CoA reductase inhibitors decrease cholesterol synthesis and possibly the synthesis of other biologically active substances derived from cholesterol, they may cause fetal harm when administered to pregnant women. Therefore, HMG-CoA reductase inhibitors are contraindicated during pregnancy and in nursing mothers. ATORVASTATIN SHOULD BE ADMINISTERED TO WOMEN OF CHILDBEARING AGE ONLY WHEN SUCH PATIENTS ARE HIGHLY UNLIKELY TO CONCEIVE AND HAVE BEEN INFORMED OF THE POTENTIAL HAZARDS. If the patient becomes pregnant while taking this drug, therapy should be discontinued and the patient apprised of the potential hazard to the fetus.

WARNINGS

LIVER DYSFUNCTION

HMG-CoA reductase inhibitors, like some other lipid-lowering therapies, have been associated with biochemical abnormalities of liver function. **Persistent elevations (>3 times the upper limit of normal [ULN] occurring on 2 or more occasions) in serum transaminases occurred in 0.7% of patients who received atorvastatin in clinical trials. The incidence of these abnormalities was 0.2%, 0.2%, 0.6%, and 2.3% for 10, 20, 40, and 80 mg, respectively.**

One patient in clinical trials developed jaundice. Increases in liver function tests (LFT) in other patients were not associated with jaundice or other clinical signs or symptoms. Upon dose reduction, drug interruption, or discontinuation, transaminase levels returned to or near pretreatment levels without sequelae. Eighteen (18) of 30 patients with persistent LFT elevations continued treatment with a reduced dose of atorvastatin.

It is recommended that liver function tests be performed prior to and at 12 weeks following both the initiation of therapy and any elevation of dose, and periodically (*e.g.,* semiannually) thereafter. Liver enzyme changes generally occur in the first 3 months of treatment with atorvastatin. Patients who develop increased transaminase levels should be monitored until the abnormalities resolve. Should an increase in ALT or AST of >3 times ULN persist, reduction of dose or withdrawal of atorvastatin is recommended.

Atorvastatin should be used with caution in patients who consume substantial quantities of alcohol and/or have a history of liver disease. Active liver disease or unexplained persistent transaminase elevations are contraindications to the use of atorvastatin (see CONTRAINDICATIONS).

SKELETAL MUSCLE

Rare cases of rhabdomyolysis with acute renal failure secondary to myoglobinuria have been reported with atorvastatin and with other drugs in this class.

Uncomplicated myalgia has been reported in atorvastatin-treated patients (see ADVERSE REACTIONS). Myopathy, defined as muscle aches or muscle weakness in conjunction with increases in creatine phosphokinase (CPK) values >10 times ULN, should be considered in any patient with diffuse myalgias, muscle tenderness or weakness, and/or marked elevation of CPK. Patients should be advised to report promptly unexplained muscle pain, tenderness or weakness, particularly if accompanied by malaise or fever. Atorvastatin therapy should be discontinued if markedly elevated CPK levels occur or myopathy is diagnosed or suspected.

The risk of myopathy during treatment with drugs in this class is increased with concurrent administration of cyclosporine, fibric acid derivatives, erythromycin, niacin, or azole antifungals. Physicians considering combined therapy with atorvastatin and fibric acid derivatives, erythromycin, immunosuppressive drugs, azole antifungals, or lipid-lowering doses of niacin should carefully weigh the potential benefits and risks and should carefully monitor patients for any signs or symptoms of muscle pain, tenderness, or weakness, particularly during the initial months of therapy and during any periods of upward dosage titration of either drug. Periodic creatine phosphokinase (CPK) determinations may be considered in such situations, but there is no assurance that such monitoring will prevent the occurence of severe myopathy.

Atorvastatin therapy should be temporarily withheld or discontinued in any patient with an acute, serious condition suggestive of a myopathy or having a risk factor predisposing to the development of renal failure secondary to rhabdomyolysis (*e.g.,* severe acute infection, hypotension, major surgery, trauma, severe metabolic, endocrine and electrolyte disorders, and uncontrolled seizures).

PRECAUTIONS

GENERAL

Before instituting therapy with atorvastatin, an attempt should be made to control hypercholesterolemia with appropriate diet, exercise, and weight reduction in obese patients, and to treat other underlying medical problems (see INDICATIONS AND USAGE).

INFORMATION FOR THE PATIENT

Patients should be advised to report promptly unexplained muscle pain, tenderness, or weakness, particularly if accompanied by malaise or fever.

ENDOCRINE FUNCTION

HMG-CoA reductase inhibitors interfere with cholesterol synthesis and theoretically might blunt adrenal and/or gonadal steroid production. Clinical studies have shown that atorvastatin does not reduce basal plasma cortisol concentration or impair adrenal reserve. The effects of HMG-CoA reductase inhibitors on male fertility have not been studied in adequate numbers of patients. The effects, if any, on the pituitary-gonadal axis in premenopausal women are unknown. Caution should be exercised if an HMG-CoA reductase inhibitor is administered concomitantly with drugs that may decrease the levels or activity of endogenous steroid hormones, such as ketoconazole, spironolactone, and cimetidine.

A

CNS TOXICITY

Brain hemorrhage was seen in a female dog treated for 3 months at 120 mg/kg/day. Brain hemorrhage and optic nerve vacuolation were seen in another female dog that was sacrificed in moribund condition after 11 weeks of escalating doses up to 280 mg/kg/day. The 120 mg/kg dose resulted in a systemic exposure approximately 16 times the human plasma area-under-the curve (AUC, 0-24 hours) based on the maximum human dose of 80 mg/day. A single tonic convulsion was seen in each of 2 male dogs (1 treated at 10 mg/kg/day and 1 at 120 mg/kg/day) in a 2 year study. No CNS lesions have been observed in mice after chronic treatment for up to 2 years at doses up to 400 mg/kg/day or in rats at doses up to 100 mg/kg/day. These doses were 6-11 times (mouse) and 8-16 times (rat) the human AUC(0-24) based on the maximum recommended human dose of 80 mg/day.

CNS vascular lesions, characterized by perivascular hemorrhages, edema, and mononuclear cell infiltration of perivascular spaces, have been observed in dogs treated with other members of this class. A chemically similar drug in this class produced optic nerve degeneration (Wallerian degeneration of retinogeniculate fibers) in clinically normal dogs in a dose-dependent fashion at a dose that produced plasma drug levels about 30 times higher than the mean drug level in humans taking the highest recommended dose.

CARCINOGENESIS, MUTAGENESIS, AND IMPAIRMENT OF FERTILITY

In a 2 year carcinogenicity study in rats at dose levels of 10, 30, and 100 mg/kg/day, 2 rare tumors were found in muscle in high-dose females: in 1, there was a rhabdomyosarcoma and, in another, there was a fibrosarcoma. This dose represents a plasma AUC(0-24) value of approximately 16 times the mean human plasma drug exposure after an 80 mg oral dose.

A 2 year carcinogenicity study in mice given 100, 200, or 400 mg/kg/day resulted in a significant increase in liver adenomas in high-dose males and liver carcinomas in high-dose females. These findings occurred at plasma AUC(0-24) values of approximately 6 times the mean human plasma drug exposure after an 80 mg oral dose.

In vitro, atorvastatin was not mutagenic or clastogenic in the following tests with and without metabolic activation: the Ames test with *Salmonella typhimurium* and *Escherichia coli,* the HGPRT forward mutation assay in Chinese hamster lung cells, and the chromosomal aberration assay in Chinese hamster lung cells. Atorvastatin was negative in the *in vivo* mouse micronucleus test.

Studies in rats performed at doses up to 175 mg/kg (15 times the human exposure) produced no changes in fertility. There was aplasia and aspermia in the epididymis of 2 of 10 rats treated with 100 mg/kg/day of atorvastatin for 3 months (16 times the human AUC at the 80 mg dose); testis weights were significantly lower at 30 and 100 mg/kg and epididymal weight was lower at 100 mg/kg. Male rats given 100 mg/kg/day for 11 weeks prior to mating had decreased sperm motility, spermatid head concentration, and increased abnormal sperm. Atorvastatin caused no adverse effects on semen parameters, or reproductive organ histopathology in dogs given doses of 10, 40, or 120 mg/kg for 2 years.

PREGNANCY CATEGORY X

See CONTRAINDICATIONS.

Safety in pregnant women has not been established. Atorvastatin crosses the rat placenta and reaches a level in fetal liver equivalent to that of maternal plasma. Atorvastatin was not teratogenic in rats at doses up to 300 mg/kg/day or in rabbits at doses up to 100 mg/kg/day. These doses resulted in multiples of about 30 times (rat) or 20 times (rabbit) the human exposure based on surface area (mg/m^2).

In a study in rats given 20, 100, or 225 mg/kg/day, from gestation Day 7 through to lactation Day 21 (weaning), there was decreased pup survival at birth, neonate, weaning, and maturity in pups of mothers dosed with 225 mg/kg/day. Body weight was decreased on Days 4 and 21 in pups of mothers dosed at 100 mg/kg/day; pup body weight was decreased at birth and at Days 4, 21, and 91 at 225 mg/kg/day. Pup development was delayed (rotorod performance at 100 mg/kg/day and acoustic startle at 225 mg/kg/day; pinnae detachment and eye opening at 225 mg/kg/day). These doses correspond to 6 times (100 mg/kg) and 22 times (225 mg/kg) the human AUC at 80 mg/day.

Rare reports of congenital anomalies have been received following intrauterine exposure to HMG-CoA reductase inhibitors. There has been one report of severe congenital bony deformity, tracheo-esophageal fistula, and anal atresia (VATER association) in a baby born to a woman who took lovastatin with dextroamphetamine sulfate during the first trimester of pregnancy. Atorvastatin calcium should be administered to women of child-bearing potential only when such patients are highly unlikely to conceive and have been informed of the potential hazards. If the woman becomes pregnant while taking atorvastatin calcium, it should be discontinued and the patient advised again as to the potential hazards to the fetus.

NURSING MOTHERS

Nursing rat pups had plasma and liver drug levels of 50% and 40%, respectively, of that in their mother's milk. Because of the potential for adverse reactions in nursing infants, women taking atorvastatin calcium should not breast-feed (see CONTRAINDICATIONS).

PEDIATRIC USE

Safety and effectiveness in patients 10-17 years of age with heterozygous familial hypercholesterolemia have been evaluated in controlled clinical trials for 6 months duration in adolescent boys and postmenarchal girls. Patients treated with atorvastatin calcium had an adverse experience profile generally similar to that of patients treated with placebo, the most common adverse experiences observed in both groups, regardless of causality assessment, were infections. **Doses greater than 20 mg have not been studied in this patient population.** In this limited controlled study, there was no detectable effect on growth or sexual maturation in boys or on menstrual cycle length in girls. See ADVERSE REACTIONS, Pediatric Patients; and DOSAGE AND ADMINISTRATION, Heterozygous Familial Hypercholesterolemia in Pediatric Patients (10-17 years of age). Adolescent females should be counseled on appropriate contraceptive methods while on atorvastatin calcium therapy (see CONTRAINDICATIONS and PRECAUTIONSPregnancy Category X). **Atorvastatin calcium has not been studied in controlled clinical trials involving pre-pubertal patients or patients younger than 10 years of age.**

Clinical efficacy with doses up to 80 mg/day for 1 year have been evaluated in an uncontrolled study of patients with homozygous FH including 8 pediatric patients.

GERIATRIC USE

The safety and efficacy of atorvastatin (10-80 mg) in the geriatric population (≥65 years of age) was evaluated in the ACCESS study. In this 54 week open-label trial 1958 patients initiated therapy with atorvastatin 10 mg. Of these, 835 were elderly (≥65 years) and 1123 were non-elderly. The mean change in LDL-C from baseline after 6 weeks of treatment with atorvastatin 10 mg was -38.2% in the elderly patients versus -34.6% in the non-elderly group.

The rates of discontinuation due to adverse events were similar between the two age groups. There were no differences in clinically relevant laboratory abnormalities between the age groups.

DRUG INTERACTIONS

The risk of myopathy during treatment with other drugs of this class is increased with concurrent administration of cyclosporine, fibric acid derivatives, niacin (nicotinic acid), erythromycin, azole antifungals (see WARNINGS, Skeletal Muscle).

Antacid: When atorvastatin and Maalox TC suspension were coadministered, plasma concentrations of atorvastatin decreased approximately 35%. However, LDL-C reduction was not altered.

Antipyrine: Because atorvastatin does not affect the pharmacokinetics of antipyrine, interactions with other drugs metabolized via the same cytochrome isozymes are not expected.

Colestipol: Plasma concentrations of atorvastatin decreased approximately 25% when colestipol and atorvastatin were coadministered. However, LDL-C reduction was greater when atorvastatin and colestipol were coadministered than when either drug was given alone.

Cimetidine: Atorvastatin plasma concentrations and LDL-C reduction were not altered by coadministration of cimetidine.

Digoxin: When multiple doses of atorvastatin and digoxin were coadministered, steady-state plasma digoxin concentrations increased by approximately 20%. Patients taking digoxin should be monitored appropriately.

Erythromycin: In healthy individuals, plasma concentrations of atorvastatin increased approximately 40% with coadministration of atorvastatin and erythromycin, a known inhibitor of cytochrome P450 3A4 (see WARNINGS, Skeletal Muscle).

Oral Contraceptives: Coadministration of atorvastatin and an oral contraceptive increased AUC values for norethindrone and ethinyl estradiol by approximately 30% and 20%. These increases should be considered when selecting an oral contraceptive for a woman taking atorvastatin.

Warfarin: Atorvastatin had no clinically significant effect on prothrombin time when administered to patients receiving chronic warfarin treatment.

ADVERSE REACTIONS

Atorvastatin calcium is generally well-tolerated. Adverse reactions have usually been mild and transient. In controlled clinical studies of 2502 patients, <2% of patients were discontinued due to adverse experiences attributable to atorvastatin. The most frequent adverse events thought to be related to atorvastatin were constipation, flatulence, dyspepsia, and abdominal pain.

CLINICAL ADVERSE EXPERIENCES

Adverse experiences reported in ≥2% of patients in placebo-controlled clinical studies of atorvastatin, regardless of causality assessment, are shown in TABLE 8.

TABLE 8 *Adverse Events in Placebo-Controlled Studies*

Body System	Placebo	Atorvastatin			
		10 mg	20 mg	40 mg	80 mg
Adverse Event	n=270	n=863	n=36	n=79	n=94
Body as a Whole					
Infection	10.0%	10.3%	2.8%	10.1%	7.4%
Headache	7.0%	5.4%	16.7%	2.5%	6.4%
Accidental injury	3.7%	4.2%	0.0%	1.3%	3.2%
Flu syndrome	1.9%	2.2%	0.0%	2.5%	3.2%
Abdominal pain	0.7%	2.8%	0.0%	3.8%	2.1%
Back pain	3.0%	2.8%	0.0%	3.8%	1.1%
Allergic reaction	2.6%	0.9%	2.8%	1.3%	0.0%
Asthenia	1.9%	2.2%	0.0%	3.8%	0.0%
Digestive System					
Constipation	1.8%	2.1%	0.0%	2.5%	1.1%
Diarrhea	1.5%	2.7%	0.0%	3.8%	5.3%
Dyspepsia	4.1%	2.3%	2.8%	1.3%	2.1%
Flatulence	3.3%	2.1%	2.8%	1.3%	1.1%
Respiratory System					
Sinusitis	2.6%	2.8%	0.0%	2.5%	6.4%
Pharyngitis	1.5%	2.5%	0.0%	1.3%	2.1%
Skin and Appendages					
Rash	0.7%	3.9%	2.8%	3.8%	1.1%
Musculoskeletal System					
Arthralgia	1.5%	2.0%	0.0%	5.1%	0.0%
Myalgia	1.1%	3.2%	5.6%	1.3%	0.0%

The following adverse events were reported, regardless of causality assessment in patients treated with atorvastatin in clinical trials. The events in *italics* occurred in ≥2% of patients and the events in plain type occurred in <2% of patients.

Body as a Whole: *Chest pain,* face edema, fever, neck rigidity, malaise, photosensitivity reaction, generalized edema.

Digestive System: *Nausea,* gastroenteritis, liver function tests abnormal, colitis, vomiting, gastritis, dry mouth, rectal hemorrhage, esophagitis, eructation, glossitis, mouth ulceration, anorexia, increased appetite, stomatitis, biliary pain, cheilitis, duodenal ulcer, dysphagia, enteritis, melena, gum hemorrhage, stomach ulcer, tenesmus, ulcerative stomatitis, hepatitis, pancreatitis, cholestatic jaundice.

Respiratory System: *Bronchitis, rhinitis,* pneumonia, dyspnea, asthma, epistaxis.

Nervous System: *Insomnia, dizziness,* paresthesia, somnolence, amnesia, abnormal dreams, libido decreased, emotional lability, incoordination, peripheral neuropathy, torticollis, facial paralysis, hyperkinesia, depression, hypesthesis, hypertonia.

Musculoskeletal System: *Arthritis,* leg cramps, bursitis, tenosynovitis, myasthenia, tendinous contracture, myositis.

Skin and Appendages: Pruritus, contact dermatitis, alopecia, dry skin, sweating, acne, urticaria, eczema, seborrhea, skin ulcer.

Urogenital System: *Urinary tract infection,* urinary frequency, cystitis, hematuria, impotence, dysuria, kidney calculus, nocturia, epididymitis, fibrocystic breast, vaginal hemorrhage, albuminuria, breast enlargement, metrorrhagia, nephritis, urinary incontinence, urinary retention, urinary urgency, abnormal ejaculation, uterine hemorrhage.

Special Senses: Amblyopia, tinnitus, dry eyes, refraction disorder, eye hemorrhage, deafness, glaucoma, parosmia, taste loss, taste perversion.

Cardiovascular System: Palpitation, vasodilatation, syncope, migraine, postural hypotension, phlebitis, arrhythmia, angina pectoris, hypertension.

Metabolic and Nutrtional Disorders: *Peripheral edema,* hyperglycemia, creatine phosphokinase increased, gout, weight gain, hypoglycemia.

Hemic and Lymphatic System: Ecchymosis, anemia, lymphadenopathy, thrombocytopenia, petechia.

POSTINTRODUCTION REPORTS

Adverse events associated with atorvastatin calcium therapy reported since market introduction, that are not listed above, regardless of causality assessment, include the following: anaphylaxis, angioneurotic edema, bullous rashes (including erythema multiforme, Stevens-Johnson syndrome, and toxic epidermal necrolysis), and rhabdomyolysis.

PEDIATRIC PATIENTS (AGES 10-17 YEARS)

In a 26 week controlled study in boys and postmenarchal girls (n=140), the safety and tolerability profile of atorvastatin calcium 10-20 mg daily was generally similar to that of placebo (see PRECAUTIONS, Pediatric Use).

DOSAGE AND ADMINISTRATION

The patient should be placed on a standard cholesterol-lowering diet before receiving atorvastatin calcium and should continue on this diet during treatment with atorvastatin calcium.

HYPERCHOLESTEROLEMIA (HETEROZYGOUS FAMILIAL AND NONFAMILIAL) AND MIXED DYSLIPIDEMIA (FREDRICKSON TYPES IIA AND IIB)

The recommended starting dose of atorvastatin calcium is 10 or 20 mg once daily. Patients who require a large reduction in LDL-C (more than 45%) may be started at 40 mg once daily. The dosage range of atorvastatin calcium is 10-80 mg once daily. Atorvastatin calcium can be administered as a single dose at any time of the day, with or without food. The starting dose and maintenance doses of atorvastatin calcium should be individualized according to patient characteristics such as goal of therapy and response (see *NCEP Guidelines,* summarized in TABLE 6). After initiation and/or upon titration of atorvastatin calcium, lipid levels should be analyzed within 2-4 weeks and dosage adjusted accordingly.

Since the goal of treatment is to lower LDL-C, the NCEP recommends that LDL-C levels be used to initiate and assess treatment response. Only if LDL-C levels are not available, should total-C be used to monitor therapy.

HETEROZYGOUS FAMILIAL HYPERCHOLESTEROLEMIA IN PEDIATRIC PATIENTS (10-17 YEARS OF AGE)

The recommended starting dose of atorvastatin calcium is 10 mg/day; the maximum recommended dose is 20 mg/day (doses greater than 20 mg have not been studied in this patient population). Doses should be individualized according to the recommended goal of therapy (see NCEP Pediatric Panel Guidelines[1], CLINICAL PHARMACOLOGY, and INDICATIONS AND USAGE). Adjustments should be made at intervals of 4 weeks or more.

HOMOZYGOUS FAMILIAL HYPERCHOLESTEROLEMIA

The dosage of atorvastatin calcium in patients with homozygous FH is 10-80 mg daily. Atorvastatin calcium should be used as an adjunct to other lipid-lowering treatments (*e.g.,* LDL apheresis) in these patients or if such treatments are unavailable.

CONCOMITANT THERAPY

Atorvastatin may be used in combination with a bile acid binding resin for additive effect. The combination of HMG-CoA reductase inhibitors and fibrates should generally be avoided (see WARNINGS, Skeletal Muscle and DRUG INTERACTIONS for other drug-drug interactions).

DOSAGE IN PATIENTS WITH RENAL INSUFFICIENCY

Renal disease does not affect the plasma concentrations nor LDL-C reduction of atorvastatin; thus, dosage adjustment in patients with renal dysfunction is not necessary (see CLINICAL PHARMACOLOGY, Pharmacokinetics and Drug Metabolism).

HOW SUPPLIED

LIPITOR TABLETS

Lipitor is supplied as white, elliptical, film-coated tablets of atorvastatin calcium containing 10, 20, 40 and 80 mg atorvastatin.

10 mg: Coded "PD 155" on one side and "10" on the other.
20 mg: Coded "PD 156" on one side and "20" on the other.
40 mg: Coded "PD 157" on one side and "40" on the other.
80 mg: Coded "PD 158" on one side and "80" on the other.

Storage: Store at controlled room temperature 20-25°C (68-77°F).

PRODUCT LISTING - EQUIVALENTS NOT AVAILABLE

Tablet - Oral - 10 mg

30's	$59.12	LIPITOR, Allscripts Pharmaceutical Company	54569-4466-00
30's	$66.87	LIPITOR, Physicians Total Care	54868-3934-00
90's	$214.70	LIPITOR, Parke-Davis	00071-0155-23
100's	$197.08	LIPITOR, Allscripts Pharmaceutical Company	54569-4466-01
100's	$250.49	LIPITOR, Parke-Davis	00071-0155-40

Tablet - Oral - 20 mg

30's	$91.41	LIPITOR, Allscripts Pharmaceutical Company	54569-4467-00
30's	$102.74	LIPITOR, Physicians Total Care	54868-3946-00
90's	$327.93	LIPITOR, Parke-Davis	00071-0156-23
100's	$382.58	LIPITOR, Parke-Davis	00071-0156-40

Tablet - Oral - 40 mg

30's	$117.77	LIPITOR, Physicians Total Care	54868-4229-00
90's	$327.93	LIPITOR, Parke-Davis	00071-0157-23

Tablet - Oral - 80 mg

90's	$327.93	LIPITOR, Parke-Davis	00071-0158-23

Atovaquone (003136)

For complete prescribing information, refer to the CD-ROM included with the book.

Categories: Pneumonia, pneumocystis carinii; Pregnancy Category C; FDA Approved 1992 Nov; Orphan Drugs
Drug Classes: Antiprotozoals
Brand Names: **Mepron**
Foreign Brand Availability: Wellvone (Australia; Denmark; England; France; Germany; Netherlands; Sweden; Switzerland)
Cost of Therapy: $738.64 (Pneumocystis carinii Pneumonia; Mepron Suspension; 750 mg/5 ml; 10 ml/day; 21 day supply)

DESCRIPTION

Mepron (atovaquone) is an antiprotozoal agent. The chemical name of atovaquone is *trans*-2-[4-(4-chlorophenyl)cyclohexyl]-3-hydroxy-1,4-naphthalenedione. Atovaquone is a yellow crystalline solid that is practically insoluble in water. It has a molecular weight of 366.84 and the molecular formula $C_{22}H_{19}ClO_3$.

Mepron suspension is a formulation of micro-fine particles of atovaquone. The atovaquone particles, reduced in size to facilitate absorption, are significantly smaller than those in the previously marketed tablet formulation. Mepron suspension is for oral administration and is bright yellow with a citrus flavor. Each teaspoonful (5 ml) contains 750 mg of atovaquone and the inactive ingredients benzyl alcohol, flavor, poloxamer 188, purified water, saccharin sodium, and xanthan gum.

INDICATIONS AND USAGE

Atovaquone suspension is indicated for the prevention of *Pneumocystis carinii* pneumonia in patients who are intolerant to trimethoprim-sulfamethoxazole (TMP-SMX).

Atovaquone suspension is also indicated for the acute oral treatment of mild-to-moderate PCP in patients who are intolerant to TMP-SMX.

NON-FDA APPROVED INDICATIONS

Atovaquone is not approved by the FDA for the treatment and maintenance therapy of toxoplasmosis or for the treatment of malaria, although some efficacy has been reported. Atovaquone has also shown some efficacy in the treatment of the symptoms associated with gastrointestinal microsporidiosis in AIDS patients, although larger clinical trials are needed.

CONTRAINDICATIONS

Atovaquone suspension is contraindicated for patients who develop or have a history of potentially life-threatening allergic reactions to any of the components of the formulation.

WARNINGS

Clinical experience with atovaquone for the treatment of PCP has been limited to patients with mild-to-moderate PCP [(A-a)DO_2 ≤45 mm Hg]. Treatment of more severe episodes of PCP has not been systematically studied with this agent. Also, the efficacy of atovaquone in patients who are failing therapy with TMP-SMX has not been systematically studied.

DOSAGE AND ADMINISTRATION

DOSAGE

Prevention of PCP

Adults and Adolescents (13-16 years): The recommended oral dose is 1500 mg (10 ml) once daily administered with a meal.

Treatment of Mild-to-Moderate PCP

Adults and Adolescents (13-16 years): The recommended oral dose is 750 mg (5 ml) administered with meals twice daily for 21 days (total daily dose 1500 mg).

Note: Failure to administer atovaquone suspension with meals may result in lower plasma atovaquone concentrations and may limit response to therapy.

ADMINISTRATION

Foil Pouch: Open pouch by removing tab at perforation and tear at notch. Take entire contents by mouth. Can be discharged into a dosing spoon or cup or directly into the mouth.

Bottle: SHAKE BOTTLE GENTLY BEFORE USING.

PRODUCT LISTING - EQUIVALENTS NOT AVAILABLE

Suspension - Oral - 750 mg/5 ml

5 ml x 42	$703.50	MEPRON, Glaxosmithkline	00173-0547-00

10 ml x 30	$553.98	MEPRON, Glaxosmithkline	00173-0548-00
210 ml	$738.64	MEPRON, Glaxosmithkline	00173-0665-18

Atovaquone; Proguanil Hydrochloride (003498)

For complete prescribing information, refer to the CD-ROM included with the book.

Categories: Malaria; Malaria, prophylaxis; FDA Approved 2000 Jul; Pregnancy Category C
Drug Classes: Antiprotozoals
Brand Names: Malarone
Cost of Therapy: $56.45 (Malaria Treatment; Malarone; 250 mg; 100 mg; 4 tablets/day; 3 day supply)

DESCRIPTION

Malarone (atovaquone and proguanil hydrochloride) is a fixed-dose combination of the antimalarial agents atovaquone and proguanil hydrochloride. The chemical name of atovaquone is *trans*-2-[4-(4-chlorophenyl)cyclohexyl]-3-hydroxy-1,4-naphthalenedione. Atovaquone is a yellow crystalline solid that is practically insoluble in water. It has a molecular weight of 366.84 and the molecular formula $C_{22}H_{19}ClO_3$.

The chemical name of proguanil hydrochloride is 1-(4-chlorophenyl)-5-isopropyl-biguanide hydrochloride. Proguanil hydrochloride is a white crystalline solid that is sparingly soluble in water. It has a molecular weight of 290.22 and the molecular formula $C_{11}H_{16}ClN_5{\cdot}HCl$.

Malrone tablets and Malrone pediatric tablets are for oral administration. Each Malrone tablet contains 250 mg of atovaquone and 100 mg of proguanil hydrochloride and each Malrone pediatric tablet contains 62.5 mg of atovaquone and 25 mg of proguanil hydrochloride. The inactive ingredients in both tablets are low-substituted hydroxypropyl cellulose, magnesium stearate, microcrystalline cellulose, poloxamer 188, povidone K30, and sodium starch glycolate. The tablet coating contains red iron oxide, polyethylene glycol 400, hydroxypropyl methylcellulose, polyethylene glycol 8000, and titanium dioxide.

INDICATIONS AND USAGE

PREVENTION OF MALARIA

Atovaquone; proguanil HCl is indicated for the prophylaxis of *P. falciparum* malaria, including in areas where chloroquine resistance has been reported.

TREATMENT OF MALARIA

Atovaquone; proguanil HCl is indicated for the treatment of acute, uncomplicated *P. falciparum* malaria. Atovaquone; proguanil HCl has been shown to be effective in regions where the drugs chloroquine, halofantrine, mefloqine, and amodiaquine may have unacceptable failure rates, presumably due to drug resistance.

CONTRAINDICATIONS

Atovaquone; proguanil HCl is contraindicated in individuals with known hypersensitivity to atovaquone or proguanil HCl or any component of the formulation. During clinical trials, 1 case of anaphylaxis following treatment with atovaquone/proguanil was observed.

Atovaquone; proguanil HCl is contraindicated for prophylaxis of *P. falciparum* malaria in patients with severe renal impairment (creatinine clearance <30 ml/min).

DOSAGE AND ADMINISTRATION

The daily dose should be taken at the same time each day with food or a milky drink. In the event of vomiting within 1 hour after dosing, a repeat dose should be taken.

PREVENTION OF MALARIA

Prophylactic treatment with atovaquone; proguanil HCl should be started 1 or 2 days before entering a malaria-endemic area and continued daily during the stay and for 7 days after return.

Adults

One atovaquone; proguanil HCl tablet (adult strength = 250 mg atovaquone/100 mg proguanil HCl) per day.

Pediatric Patients

The dosage for prevention of malaria in pediatric patients is based upon body weight (see TABLE 7).

TABLE 7 *Dosage for Prevention of Malaria in Pediatric Patients*

Weight	Atovaquone/Proguanil HCl Total Daily Dose	Dosage Regimen
11-20 kg	62.5 mg/25 mg	1 atovaquone; proguanil HCl pediatric tablet daily.
21-30 kg	125 mg/50 mg	2 atovaquone; proguanil HCl pediatric tablets as a single dose daily.
31-40 kg	187.5 mg/75 mg	3 atovaquone; proguanil HCl pediatric tablets as a single dose daily.
>40 kg	250 mg/100 mg	1 atovaquone; proguanil HCl tablet (adult strength) as a single dose daily.

TREATMENT OF ACUTE MALARIA

Adults

Four aqvaquone; proguanil HCl tablets (adult strength; total daily dose 1 g atovaquone/400 mg proguanil HCl) as a single dose daily for 3 consecutive days.

Pediatric Patients

The dosage for treatment of acute malaria in pediatric patients is based upon body weight (see TABLE 8).

TABLE 8 *Dosage for Treatment of Acute Malaria in Pediatric Patients*

Weight	Atovaquone/Proguanil HCl Total Daily Dose	Dosage Regimen
11-20 kg	250 mg/100 mg	1 atovaquone; proguanil HCl tablet (adult strength) daily for 3 consecutive days.
21-30 kg	500 mg/200 mg	2 atovaquone; proguanil HCl tablets (adult strenght) as a single dose daily for 3 consecutive days.
31-40 kg	750 mg/300 mg	3 atovaquone; proguanil HCl tablets (adult strength) as a single dose daily for 3 consecutive days.
>40 kg	1 g/400 mg	4 atovaquone; proguanil HCl tablets (adult strength) as a single dose daily for 3 consecutive days.

PATIENTS WITH RENAL IMPAIRMENT

Atovaquone; proguanil HCl should not be used for malaria prophylaxis in patients with severe renal impairment (creatinine clearance <30 ml/min), and alternatives to atovaquone; proguanil HCl should be recommended for treatment of acute *P. falciparum* malaria whenever possible (see CONTRAINDICATIONS). No dosage adjustments are needed in patients with mild to moderate renal impairment.

PATIENTS WITH HEPATIC IMPAIRMENT

No dosage adjustments are needed in patinets with mild to moderate hepatic impairment. No studies have been conducted in patients with severe hepatic impairment.

PRODUCT LISTING - EQUIVALENTS NOT AVAILABLE

Tablet - Oral - 62.5 mg;25 mg

100's	$174.00	MALARONE PEDIATRIC, Glaxosmithkline	00173-0676-01

Tablet - Oral - 250 mg;100 mg

24's	$120.00	MALARONE, Glaxosmithkline	00173-0675-02
100's	$470.40	MALARONE, Glaxosmithkline	00173-0675-01

Atropine Sulfate (000336)

Categories: Anesthesia, adjunct; Bradycardia; Cycloplegia; Heart block; Mydriasis; Toxicity, cholinergic drugs; Toxicity, mushroom; Toxicity, organophosphate; Inflamation, uvea, adjunct; Pylorospasm; Suppression, vagal activity; Spasm, gastrointestinal; Colic, biliary; Colic, ureteral; FDA Approval Pre 1982; Pregnancy Category B; WHO Formulary
Drug Classes: Antiarrhythmics; Anticholinergics; Antidotes; Cycloplegics; Mydriatics; Ophthalmics; Preanesthetics
Brand Names: Atro Ofteno; Atropair; Atropen; Atropinol; Atropisol; Borotropin; Dosatropine; I-Tropine; **Isopto Atropine**; Isotic cycloma; Liotropina; Minims-Atropine; Ocu-Tropine; Sal-Tropine; Spectro-Atropine
Foreign Brand Availability: Atropin (Germany; Sweden); Atropin "Dak" (Denmark); Atropin Dispersa (Switzerland); Atropin Minims (Norway); Atropina (Italy); Atropina Llorens (Spain); Atropine (Greece); Atropine Dispersa (Hong-Kong); Atropine Martinet (France); Atropine Sulfate (Israel); Atropine Sulfate Tablets (England); Atropini Sulfas (Bulgaria); Atropt (Australia; New-Zealand); Atrospan (Israel); Bellpino-Artin (India); Cendo Tropine (Indonesia); Chibro-Atropine (France); Ciba Vision Atropine (Thailand); Isopto (England); Isopto Atropin (Sweden); Isopto Atropina (Ecuador); Minims Atropine Sulfaat (Netherlands); Minims Atropine Sulfate (Bahrain; Cyprus; Egypt; England; Hong-Kong; Iran; Iraq; Jordan; Kuwait; Lebanon; Libya; Oman; Qatar; Republic-of-Yemen; Saudi-Arabia; Syria; United-Arab-Emirates); Skiatropine (Switzerland); Ximex Optidrop (Indonesia)
HCFA JCODE(S): J0460 up to 0.3 mg IV, IM, SC

OPHTHALMIC

DESCRIPTION

Atropine sulfate sterile ophthalmic solution is a topical anticholinergic for ophthalmic use.
Chemical Name: Benzeneacetic acid, α-(hydroxymethyl)-,8-methyl-8-azabicyclo-(3,2,1) oct-3-yl ester, endo-(±)-, sulfate (2:1)(salt), monohydate.
Atropine Sulfate Sterile Ophthalmic Solution Contains: Atropine sulfate 1% with chlorobutanol (chloral deriv.) 0.5%; boric acid; sodium citrate; hydrochloric acid and/or sodium hydroxide to adjust the pH; and purified water.

CLINICAL PHARMACOLOGY

Anticholinergics act directly on the smooth muscles and secretory glands innervated by postganglionic cholinergic nerves. They act by blocking the parasympathomimetic (muscarinic) effects of acetylcholine and parasympathomimetic drugs at these sites.

INDICATIONS AND USAGE

Atropine sulfate is used to produce mydriasis and cycloplegia for refraction, or for iris dilation and relaxation of the ciliary muscle desirable in acute inflammatory conditions of the anterior uveal tract.

CONTRAINDICATIONS

Should not be used in patients with glaucoma or predisposition to narrow-angle glaucoma. Should not be used in children who have previously had a severe systemic reaction to atropine.

WARNINGS

Excessive use in children and certain susceptible individuals may produce general toxic symptoms. If this occurs, discontinue medication and use appropriate therapy.

PRECAUTIONS

INFORMATION FOR THE PATIENT

Keep out of reach of children.

CARCINOGENESIS, MUTAGENESIS, AND IMPAIRMENT OF FERTILITY

No studies have been conducted in animals or in humans to evaluate the potential of these effects.

PREGNANCY CATEGORY B

See Injection, Pregnancy, Teratogenic Effects, Pregnancy Category B.

PEDIATRIC USE

See CONTRAINDICATIONS and WARNINGS.

ADVERSE REACTIONS

Prolonged use may cause general systemic reactions, allergic lid reactions, local irritation, hyperemia, edema, follicular, conjunctivitis or dermatitis.

DOSAGE AND ADMINISTRATION

1 or 2 drops in the eyes 3 times a day or as directed by physician.

IM-IV-SC

DESCRIPTION

Atropine is chemically 1 α H, 5 α H - Tropan-3 α-ol ($\pm$)-tropate (ester).

Atropine rarely occurs as such in any of the plants and has been prepared by synthesis. It is usually employed in the form of atropine sulfate (the sulfate [2:1] monohydrate salt of atropine), which has much greater solubility in water.

Atropine sulfate injection is a sterile aqueous solution of atropine sulfate. Each ml contains atropine sulfate, 0.1 mg; sodium chloride, 7 mg, for isotonicity; citric acid, 6.3 mg, and sodium citrate, 2.9 mg, as buffers. May contain additional citric acid and/or sodium citrate for pH adjustment (3.0-6.5). The air above the liquid in the container has been displaced by nitrogen gas.

CLINICAL PHARMACOLOGY

Atropine inhibits the muscarinic actions of acetylcholine at postganglionic parasympathetic neuroeffector sites including smooth muscle, secretory glands, and CNS sites. Large doses may block nicotinic receptors at the autonomic ganglia and at the neuromuscular junction.

Specific anticholinergic responses are dose-related. Small doses of atropine inhibit salivary and bronchial secretions and sweating; moderate doses dilate the pupil, inhibit accommodation and increase the heart rate (vagolytic effect); larger doses will decrease motility of the GI and urinary tracts; very large doses will inhibit gastric acid secretion.

INDICATIONS AND USAGE

Atropine sulfate injection may be given parenterally as a pre-anesthetic medication in surgical patients to reduce salivation and bronchial secretions. It may also be used to suppress vagal activity associated with the use of halogenated hydrocarbons during inhalation anesthesia and reflex excitation arising from mechanical stimulation during surgery.

The antispasmodic action of atropine is useful in pylorospasm and other spastic conditions of the gastrointestinal tract. For ureteral and biliary colic, atropine concomitantly with morphine may be indicated.

Atropine relaxes the upper GI tract and colon during hypotonic radiography.

In poisoning by the organic phosphate cholinesterase inhibitors found in certain insecticides and by chemical warfare nerve gases, large doses of atropine relieve the muscarine-like symptoms and some of the central nervous system manifestations. It is also used as an antidote for mushroom poisoning due to muscarine in certain species such as *Amanita muscaria.*

CONTRAINDICATIONS

Atropine sulfate is contraindicated in patients with a history of *hypersensitivity* to this drug.

Ocular: Narrow-angle glaucoma; adhesions (synechiae) between the iris and lens of the eye.

Cardiovascular: Tachycardia; unstable cardiovascular status in acute hemorrhage.

GI: Obstructive disease (*e.g.,* achalasia, pyloroduodenal stenosis or pyloric obstruction, cardiospasm, etc.); paralytic ileus; intestinal atony of the elderly or debilitated patient; severe ulcerative colitis; toxic megacolon complicating ulcerative colitis; hepatic disease.

GU: Obstructive uropathy (*e.g.,* bladder neck obstruction due to prostatic hypertrophy); renal disease.

Musculoskeletal: Myasthenia gravis.

WARNINGS

Heat prostration can occur with anticholinergic drug use (fever and heat stroke due to decreased sweating) in the presence of a high environmental temperature.

Diarrhea may be an early symptom of incomplete intestinal obstruction, especially in patients with ileostomy or colostomy. Treatment of diarrhea with these drugs is inappropriate and possibly harmful.

USAGE IN THE ELDERLY

Elderly patients may react with excitement, agitation, drowsiness, and other untoward manifestations to even small doses of anticholinergic drugs.

Usage in gastric ulcer may produce a delay in gastric emptying time and may complicate such therapy (antral stasis).

PRECAUTIONS

GENERAL

Potentially Hazardous Tasks: Atropine may produce drowsiness, dizziness or blurred vision; patients should observe caution while driving or performing other tasks requiring alertness.

Atropine Should Be Used With Caution in:

CNS: Autonomic neuropathy.

Ocular: Glaucoma, light irides. If there is mydriasis and photophobia, dark glasses should be worn. Atropine should be used with caution in patients over 40 years of age because of the increased incidence of glaucoma.

GI: Hepatic disease; early evidence of ileus, as in peritonitis; ulcerative colitis (large doses may suppress intestinal motility and precipitate or aggravate toxic megacolon); hiatal hernia associated with reflux esophagitis (anticholinergics may aggravate it).

GU: Renal disease; prostatic hypertrophy. Patients with prostatism can have dysuria and may require catheterization.

Endocrine: Hyperthyroidism.

Cardiovascular: Coronary heart disease; congestive heart failure; cardiac arrhythmias; tachycardia; hypertension.

Usage in Biliary Tract Disease: The use of atropine should not be relied upon in the presence of complication of biliary tract disease.

Special Risk Patients: Atropine should be used cautiously in infants, small children and persons with Down's syndrome, brain damage or spasticity.

Pulmonary: Debilitated patients with chronic lung disease; reduction in bronchial secretions can lead to inspissation and formation of bronchial plugs.

Atropine should be used cautiously in patients with asthma or allergies.

PREGNANCY, TERATOGENIC EFFECTS, PREGNANCY CATEGORY B

Reproduction studies performed in mice at doses of 50 mg per kg of body weight have revealed no evidence of impaired fertility or harm to the fetus due to atropine. There are, however, no adequate and well-controlled studies in pregnant women. Because animal reproduction studies are not always predictive of human response, this drug should be used during pregnancy only if clearly needed.

NURSING MOTHERS

Atropine may be excreted in milk, causing infant toxicity, and may reduce breast milk production. Documentation is lacking or conflicting. Safety for use in nursing mothers has not been established.

PEDIATRIC USE

(See DOSAGE AND ADMINISTRATION, Usual Pediatric Dosage.)

DRUG INTERACTIONS

Antihistamines, antipsychotics, antiparkinson drugs, alphaprodine, buclizine, meperidine, orphenadrine, benzodiazepines and **tricyclic antidepressants** may enhance the anticholinergic effects of atropine and its derivatives. **Nitrates, nitrites, alkalinizing agents, primidone, thioxanthenes, methylphenidate, disopyramide, procainamide** and **quinidine** may also potentiate side effects. **Monoamine oxidase inhibitors** block detoxification of atropine, and thus, potentiate its actions. Concurrent long-term therapy with **corticosteroids** or **haloperidol** may increase intraocular pressure. Atropine may antagonize the miotic actions of cholinesterase inhibitors.

The bronchial relaxation produced by **sympathomimetics** is enhanced by atropine.

Inhibition of gastric acid secretion by atropine is antagonized by **guanethidine, histamine** and **reserpine.**

Because of the potential for adverse effects, atropine should be used cautiously with **digitalis, slow release digoxin tablets, cholinergics** and **neostigmine.**

The IV administration of atropine in the presence of **cyclopropane anesthesia** can result in ventricular arrhythmias.

Atropine may enhance **nitrofurantoin** and **thiazide-diuretic** bioavailability by slowing GI motility.

The effects of **metoclopramide** on GI motility are antagonized by atropine.

ADVERSE REACTIONS

GI: Xerostomia; altered taste perception; nausea; vomiting; dysphagia; heartburn, constipation; bloated feeling; paralytic ileus; gastroesophageal reflux.

GU: Urinary hesitancy and retention; impotence.

Ocular: Blurred vision; mydriasis; photophobia; cycloplegia; increased intraocular pressure.

Cardiovascular: Palpitations; bradycardia (following low doses of atropine); tachycardia (after higher doses).

CNS: Headache; flushing; nervousness; drowsiness; weakness; dizziness; insomnia; fever. Elderly patients may exhibit mental confusion or excitement to even small doses. Large doses may produce CNS stimulation (restlessness, tremor).

Dermatologic — Hypersensitivity: Severe allergic reactions including anaphylaxis, urticaria, and other dermal manifestations.

Other: Suppression of lactation; nasal congestion; decreased sweating. Complete anhidrosis cannot occur because large doses would be required, producing severe side effects from parasympathetic paralysis.

DOSAGE AND ADMINISTRATION

Please note that the optional STICK-GARD Safety Needle, featured with stock numbers 2038 and 2039 and the optional InterLink Syringe Cannula featured with stock numbers 3038 and 3039 are interchangeable with a standard needle. InterLink Syringe Cannula are specifically designed for use with InterLink injection sites, identified by a colored alert ring around the septum and are not compatible with conventional injection sites.

USUAL ADULT DOSAGE

Antimuscarinic: Intramuscular, intravenous, or subcutaneous, 400-600 µg (0.4-0.6 mg) every 4-6 hours.
Arrhythmias: Intravenous, 400 µg (0.4 mg) to 1 mg every 1-2 hours as needed, up to a maximum of 2 mg.
Gastrointestinal Radiography: Intramuscular, 1 mg.
Preanesthesia (Antisialagogue): Intramuscular, 200-600 µg (0.2-0.6 mg) ½ — 1 hour before surgery.
Cholinergic Adjunct (Curariform Block): Intravenous, 600 µg (0.6 mg) to 1.2 mg administered a few minutes before or concurrently with 500 µg (0.5 mg) to 2 mg of neostigmine methylsulfate, using separate syringes.
Antidote (to Cholinesterase Inhibitors): Intravenous, 2-4 mg initially, then 2 mg repeated every 5-10 minutes until muscarinic symptoms disappear or signs of atropine toxicity appear.
Antidote (to Muscarine in Mushroom Poisoning): Intramuscular or intravenous, 1-2 mg every hour until respiratory effects subside.
Antidote (to Organophosphate Pesticides): Intramuscular or intravenous, 1-2 mg, repeated in 20-30 minutes as soon as cyanosis has cleared. Continue dosage until definite improvement occurs and is maintained, sometimes for 2 days or more.

USUAL PEDIATRIC DOSAGE

Antimuscarinic: Subcutaneous, 10 µg (0.01 mg) per kg of body weight, not to exceed 400 µg (0.4 mg), or 300 µg (0.3 mg) per square meter of body surface, every 4 to 6 hours.
Arrhythmias: Intravenous, 10-30 µg (0.01-0.03 mg) per kg of body weight.
Preanesthesia (Antisialagogue) or Preanesthesia (Antiarrhythmic): *Subcutaneous:*
Children Weighing up to 3 kg: 100 µg (0.1 mg)
Children Weighing 7-9 kg: 200 µg (0.2 mg)
Children Weighing 12-16 kg: 300 µg (0.3 mg)
Children Weighing 20-27 kg: 400 µg (0.4 mg)
Children Weighing 32 kg: 500 µg (0.5 mg)
Children Weighing 41 kg: 600 µg (0.6 mg)
Antidote (to Cholinesterase Inhibitors): Intravenous or intramuscular, 1 mg initially, then 0.5 to 1 mg every 5-10 minutes until muscarinic symptoms disappear or signs of atropine toxicity appear.
NOTE: Parenteral drug products should be inspected visually for particulate matter and discoloration prior to administration, whenever solution and container permit.

HOW SUPPLIED

Syringe Assembly Directions: The Mini-Jet syringe with needle is the basic unit upon which all the other syringe systems are built; slight adaptations and/or additional auxiliary parts create the other syringe systems. Assembly directions remain essentially the same.

1. Remove protective caps.
2. Thread vial into injector 3½ turns, or until needle penetrates stopper. *CAUTION:* IMPROPER ENGAGING MAY CAUSE GLASS BREAKAGE AND SUBSEQUENT INJURY.
3. Remove needle cap and expel air.

Storage: Store at controlled room temperature 15-30°C (59-86°F).

PRODUCT LISTING - RATED THERAPEUTICALLY EQUIVALENT

Ointment - Ophthalmic - 1%			
3.50 gm	$3.30	GENERIC, Qualitest Products Inc	00603-7071-70
Solution - Injectable - 0.05 mg/ml			
5 ml x 10	$62.50	GENERIC, Abbott Pharmaceutical	00074-7897-15
Solution - Injectable - 0.1 mg/ml			
5 ml x 10	$32.30	GENERIC, Abbott Pharmaceutical	00074-4910-15
5 ml x 10	$52.37	GENERIC, Abbott Pharmaceutical	00074-4910-34
5 ml x 10	$123.48	GENERIC, Abbott Pharmaceutical	00074-4910-01
5 ml x 25	$342.30	GENERIC, Abbott Pharmaceutical	00074-4910-33
10 ml x 10	$26.30	GENERIC, Abbott Pharmaceutical	00074-4911-34
10 ml x 10	$34.44	GENERIC, Abbott Pharmaceutical	00074-4911-18
10 ml x 10	$127.44	GENERIC, Abbott Pharmaceutical	00074-4911-01
10 ml x 25	$352.20	GENERIC, Abbott Pharmaceutical	00074-4911-33
Solution - Injectable - 0.4 mg/ml			
1 ml x 25	$20.00	GENERIC, American Pharmaceutical Partners	63323-0234-01
Solution - Injectable - 0.5 mg/ml			
1 ml x 25	$59.50	GENERIC, American Pharmaceutical Partners	63323-0243-01
Solution - Injectable - 1 mg/ml			
1 ml x 25	$49.50	GENERIC, American Pharmaceutical Partners	63323-0246-01
Solution - Ophthalmic - 1%			
15 ml	$4.46	GENERIC, Fougera	00168-0172-15

PRODUCT LISTING - EQUIVALENTS NOT AVAILABLE

Ointment - Ophthalmic - 1%			
3.50 gm	$1.35	GENERIC, Ocumed Inc	51944-3555-00
3.50 gm	$1.35	GENERIC, Ocumed Inc	51944-3555-30
3.50 gm	$2.42	GENERIC, Aligen Independent Laboratories Inc	00405-0500-08
3.50 gm	$2.42	GENERIC, Bausch and Lomb	24208-0825-55
3.50 gm	$2.75	GENERIC, Raway Pharmacal Inc	00686-0825-55
3.50 gm	$3.80	GENERIC, Fougera	00168-0065-38
Solution - Injectable - 0.1 mg/ml			
5 ml	$12.35	GENERIC, Allscripts Pharmaceutical Company	54569-3588-00
5 ml x 10	$37.50	GENERIC, International Medication Systems, Limited	00548-3338-00
10 ml	$5.77	GENERIC, Physicians Total Care	54868-0006-00
10 ml	$12.74	GENERIC, Allscripts Pharmaceutical Company	54569-2236-00
10 ml x 10	$50.00	GENERIC, International Medication Systems, Limited	00548-3339-00
30 ml	$3.00	GENERIC, C.O. Truxton Inc	00463-1006-20
Solution - Injectable - 0.4 mg/ml			
1 ml x 10	$6.00	GENERIC, Pro Metic Pharma	62174-0405-07
1 ml x 25	$11.00	GENERIC, American Regent Laboratories Inc	00517-0401-25
1 ml x 25	$15.00	GENERIC, Cmc-Consolidated Midland Corporation	00223-7193-25
1 ml x 25	$16.25	GENERIC, Cmc-Consolidated Midland Corporation	00223-7191-25
1 ml x 25	$16.50	GENERIC, Baxter Pharmaceutical Products, Inc	10019-0250-12
1 ml x 100	$45.75	GENERIC, Cmc-Consolidated Midland Corporation	00223-7192-00
1 ml x 100	$95.00	GENERIC, Raway Pharmacal Inc	00686-0805-25
20 ml	$1.61	GENERIC, Physicians Total Care	54868-0740-00
20 ml	$5.34	GENERIC, Lilly, Eli and Company	00002-1675-01
20 ml x 10	$11.13	GENERIC, Physicians Total Care	54868-0740-01
20 ml x 10	$19.10	GENERIC, Baxter Pharmaceutical Products, Inc	10019-0250-20
20 ml x 25	$33.25	GENERIC, Allscripts Pharmaceutical Company	54569-2192-00
20 ml x 25	$75.00	GENERIC, American Pharmaceutical Partners	63323-0234-20
25 ml	$10.19	GENERIC, Allscripts Pharmaceutical Company	54569-3947-00
Solution - Injectable - 0.5 mg/ml			
30 ml	$2.00	GENERIC, C.O. Truxton Inc	00463-1006-30
Solution - Injectable - 0.8 mg/ml			
0.50 ml x 25	$12.25	GENERIC, American Regent Laboratories Inc	00517-0805-25
Solution - Injectable - 1 mg/ml			
1 ml x 10	$8.80	GENERIC, Pro Metic Pharma	62174-0408-07
1 ml x 25	$12.25	GENERIC, American Regent Laboratories Inc	00517-0101-25
1 ml x 25	$12.25	GENERIC, American Regent Laboratories Inc	00517-1010-25
1 ml x 25	$16.00	GENERIC, Baxter Pharmaceutical Products, Inc	10019-0251-12
1 ml x 25	$16.25	GENERIC, Cmc-Consolidated Midland Corporation	00223-7206-01
1 ml x 25	$21.69	GENERIC, Physicians Total Care	54868-3893-00
1 ml x 100	$83.00	GENERIC, Raway Pharmacal Inc	00686-1010-25
Solution - Ophthalmic - 1%			
1 ml x 12	$29.06	ATROPISOL, Ciba Vision Ophthalmics	00058-0770-12
2 ml	$2.98	GENERIC, Martec Pharmaceuticals Inc	52555-0992-01
2 ml	$3.07	GENERIC, Allscripts Pharmaceutical Company	54569-2460-00
2 ml	$3.25	GENERIC, Raway Pharmacal Inc	00686-0750-60
2 ml	$4.05	GENERIC, Akorn Inc	17478-0214-20
2 ml x 12	$57.72	GENERIC, Alcon Laboratories Inc	00065-0702-12
4 ml	$2.35	GENERIC, Moore, H.L. Drug Exchange Inc	00839-5492-43
4 ml	$2.75	GENERIC, Cmc-Consolidated Midland Corporation	00223-4105-03
5 ml	$1.60	GENERIC, Paco Pharmaceutical Services, Inc	52967-0503-35
5 ml	$2.52	GENERIC, Apotex Usa Inc	60505-7484-02
5 ml	$2.94	GENERIC, Bausch and Lomb	24208-0750-60
5 ml	$3.00	GENERIC, Falcon Pharmaceuticals, Ltd.	61314-0303-01
5 ml	$3.10	GENERIC, Advanced Remedies Inc	57685-0050-07
5 ml	$3.16	GENERIC, Martec Pharmaceuticals Inc	52555-0992-05
5 ml	$3.48	GENERIC, Aligen Independent Laboratories Inc	00405-6010-05
5 ml	$3.77	GENERIC, Allscripts Pharmaceutical Company	54569-2784-00
5 ml	$8.31	ATROPISOL, Ciba Vision Ophthalmics	00058-0705-05
5 ml	$18.31	ISOPTO ATROPINE, Alcon Laboratories Inc	00998-0303-05
10 ml	$3.40	GENERIC, Falcon Pharmaceuticals, Ltd.	61314-0303-02
15 ml	$1.95	GENERIC, Paco Pharmaceutical Services, Inc	52967-0503-45
15 ml	$2.25	GENERIC, Ocumed Inc	51944-4480-02
15 ml	$2.25	GENERIC, Ocumed Inc	51944-4480-42
15 ml	$3.00	GENERIC, Cmc-Consolidated Midland Corporation	00223-6101-15
15 ml	$3.10	ATROSULF-1, Miza Pharmaceutcials Dba Optopics Laboratories Corporation	52238-0913-16
15 ml	$3.25	GENERIC, Raway Pharmacal Inc	00686-0750-06
15 ml	$3.36	GENERIC, Bausch and Lomb	24208-0750-06
15 ml	$3.75	GENERIC, Interstate Drug Exchange Inc	00814-0964-42
15 ml	$3.80	GENERIC, Martec Pharmaceuticals Inc	52555-0992-10
15 ml	$3.84	GENERIC, Steris Laboratories Inc	00402-0796-15
15 ml	$4.21	GENERIC, Aligen Independent Laboratories Inc	00405-6010-15
15 ml	$5.19	GENERIC, Allscripts Pharmaceutical Company	54569-2112-00
15 ml	$5.50	GENERIC, Major Pharmaceuticals Inc	00904-0824-35
15 ml	$6.84	GENERIC, Prescript Pharmaceuticals	00247-0042-15
15 ml	$8.54	GENERIC, Allergan Inc	11980-0002-15
15 ml	$23.81	ISOPTO ATROPINE, Alcon Laboratories Inc	00998-0303-15

Solution - Ophthalmic - 2%
2 ml x 12 $57.08 GENERIC, Alcon Laboratories Inc 00065-0703-12
Tablet - Oral - 0.4 mg
100's $29.95 GENERIC, Hope Pharmaceuticals 60267-0742-30

Atropine Sulfate; Diphenoxylate Hydrochloride *(000339)*

Categories: Diarrhea; Pregnancy Category C; DEA Class CV; FDA Approval Pre 1982
Drug Classes: Anticholinergics; Antidiarrheals
Brand Names: Celidin; Diarphen; Diphenatol; Diphensil; Lomocot; **Lomotil**; Lonox; Lotab; Reasac; Vi-Atro
Foreign Brand Availability: Dhamotil (Hong-Kong; Malaysia); Diarase (Malaysia); Diarsed (France); Diastop (New-Zealand); Dilomil (Thailand); Lofenoxal (Australia); Protector (Spain); Reasec (Belgium; Bulgaria; Czech-Republic; Germany; Greece; Hungary; Italy; Switzerland); Retardin (Denmark); Sedistal (Israel); Tropatil (Mexico)
Cost of Therapy: $87.04 (Diarrhea; Lomotil; 0.025 mg; 2.5 mg; 12 tablets/day; 10 day supply)
$3.78 (Diarrhea; Generic Tablets; 0.025 mg; 2.5 mg; 12 tablets/day; 10 day supply)

DESCRIPTION

Each Lomotil tablet and each 5 ml of Lomotil liquid for oral use contains diphenoxylate hydrochloride (abbreviated here as HCl: 2.5 mg) and atropine sulfate: 0.025 mg. (Warning—May be habit forming.)

Inactive ingredients of diphenoxylate hydrochloride and atropine sulfate include confectioner's sugar, corn starch, lactose monohydrate, magnesium stearate, and sodium starch glycolate. Each tablet may also include the following: acacia, sorbitol, sucrose, and talc. Inactive ingredients of Lomotil liquid include cherry flavor, citric acid, ethyl alcohol 15%, FD&C yellow no. 6, glycerin, sodium phosphate, sorbitol, and water.

Diphenoxylate hydrochloride, an antidiarrheal, is ethyl 1-(3-cyano-3,3-diphenylpropyl)-4-phenylisonipecotate monohydrochloride. Its chemical formula is $C_{30}H_{32}N_2O_2 \cdot HCl$, with a molecular weight of 489.06.

Atropine sulfate, an anticholinergic, is endo-(±)-α-(hydroxymethyl) benzeneacetic acid 8-methyl-8-azabicyclo(3.2.1) oct-3-yl ester sulfate (2:1) (salt) monohydrate. Its chemical formula is $(C_{17}H_{23}NO_3)_2 \cdot H_2SO_4 \cdot H_2O$, with a molecular weight of 694.85.

IMPORTANT INFORMATION

Lomotil is classified as a Schedule V controlled substance by federal law. Diphenoxylate hydrochloride is chemically related to the narcotic meperidine. Therefore, in case of overdosage, treatment is similar to that for meperidine or morphine intoxication, in which prolonged and careful monitoring is essential. Respiratory depression may be evidenced as late as 30 hours after ingestion and may recur in spite of an initial response to narcotic antagonists. A subtherapeutic amount of atropine sulfate is present to discourage deliberate overdosage. LOMOTIL IS *NOT* AN INNOCUOUS DRUG AND DOSAGE RECOMMENDATIONS SHOULD BE STRICTLY ADHERED TO, ESPECIALLY IN CHILDREN. KEEP THIS AND ALL MEDICATIONS OUT OF REACH OF CHILDREN.

CLINICAL PHARMACOLOGY

Diphenoxylate is rapidly and extensively metabolized in man by ester hydrolysis to diphenoxylic acid (difenoxine), which is biologically active and the major metabolite in the blood. After a 5 mg oral dose of carbon-14 labeled diphenoxylate HCl in ethanolic solution was given to 3 healthy volunteers, an average of 14% of the drug plus its metabolites was excreted in the urine and 49% in the feces over a 4 day period. Urinary excretion of the unmetabolized drug constituted less than 1% of the dose, and diphenoxylic acid plus its glucuronide conjugate constituted about 6% of the dose. In a 16-subject crossover bioavailability study, a liner relationship in the dose range of 2.5 to 10 mg was found between the dose of diphenoxylate HCl (given as atropine sulfate; diphenoxylate HCl oral solution) and the peak plasma concentration, the area under the plasma concentration-time curve, and the amount of diphenoxylic acid excreted in the urine. In the same study the bioavailability of the tablet compared with an equal dose of the liquid was approximately 90%. The average peak plasma concentration of diphenoxylic acid following ingestion of four 2.5 mg tablets was 163 ng/ml at about 2 hours, and the elimination half-life of diphenoxylic acid was approximately 12-14 hours.

In dogs, diphenoxylate HCl has a direct effect on circular smooth muscle of the bowel, that conceivably results in segmentation and prolongation of gastrointestinal transit time. The clinical antidiarrheal action of diphenoxylate HCl may thus be a consequence of enhanced segmentation that allows increased contact of the intraluminal contents with the intestinal mucosa.

INDICATIONS AND USAGE

Atropine sulfate; diphenoxylate HCl is effective as adjunctive therapy in the management of diarrhea.

CONTRAINDICATIONS

Atropine sulfate; diphenoxylate HCl is contraindicated in patients with:

1. Known hypersensitivity to diphenoxylate or atropine.
2. Obstructive jaundice.
3. Diarrhea associated with pseudomembranous enterocolitis or enterotoxin-producing bacteria.

WARNINGS

ATROPINE SULFATE; DIPHENOXYLATE HCl IS *NOT* AN INNOCUOUS DRUG AND DOSAGE RECOMMENDATIONS SHOULD BE STRICTLY ADHERED TO, ESPECIALLY IN CHILDREN. ATROPINE SULFATE; DIPHENOXYLATE HCl IS NOT RECOMMENDED FOR CHILDREN UNDER 2 YEARS OF AGE. OVERDOSAGE MAY RESULT IN SEVERE RESPIRATORY DEPRESSION AND COMA, POSSIBLY LEADING TO PERMANENT BRAIN DAMAGE OR DEATH. THEREFORE, KEEP THIS MEDICATION OUT OF THE REACH OF CHILDREN.

THE USE OF ATROPINE SULFATE; DIPHENOXYLATE HCl SHOULD BE ACCOMPANIED BY APPROPRIATE FLUID AND ELECTROLYTE THERAPY, WHEN INDICATED. IF SEVERE DEHYDRATION OR ELECTROLYTE IMBALANCE IS PRESENT, ATROPINE SULFATE; DIPHENOXYLATE HCl SHOULD BE WITHHELD UNTIL APPROPRIATE CORRECTIVE THERAPY HAS BEEN INITIATED. DRUG-INDUCED INHIBITION OF PERISTALSIS MAY RESULT IN FLUID RETENTION IN THE INTESTINE, WHICH MAY FURTHER AGGRAVATE DEHYDRATION AND ELECTROLYTE IMBALANCE.

ATROPINE SULFATE; DIPHENOXYLATE HCl SHOULD BE USED WITH SPECIAL CAUTION IN YOUNG CHILDREN BECAUSE THIS AGE GROUP MAY BE PREDISPOSED TO DELAYED DIPHENOXYLATE TOXICITY AND BECAUSE OF THE GREATER VARIABILITY OF RESPONSE IN THIS AGE GROUP.

Antiperistaltic agents may prolong and/or worsen diarrhea associated with organisms that penetrate the intestinal mucosa (toxigenic *E. coli, Salmonella, Shigella*), and pseudomembranous enterocolitis associated with broad-spectrum antibiotics. Antiperistaltic agents should not be used in these conditions.

In some patients with acute ulcerative colitis, agents that inhibit intestinal motility or prolong intestinal transit time have been reported to induce toxic megacolon. Consequently, patients with acute ulcerative colitis should be carefully observed and atropine sulfate; diphenoxylate HCl therapy should be discontinued promptly if abdominal distention occurs or if other untoward symptoms develop.

Since the chemical structure of diphenoxylate HCl is similar to that of meperidine HCl, the concurrent use of atropine sulfate; diphenoxylate HCl with monoamine oxidase (MAO) inhibitors may, in theory, precipitate hypertensive crisis.

Atropine sulfate; diphenoxylate HCl should be used with extreme caution in patients with advanced hepatorenal disease and in all patients with abnormal liver function since hepatic coma may be precipitated.

Diphenoxylate HCl may potentiate the action of barbiturates, tranquilizers, and alcohol. Therefore, the patient should be closely observed when any of these are used concomitantly.

PRECAUTIONS

GENERAL

Since a subtherapeutic dose of atropine has been added to the diphenoxylate HCl, consideration should be given to the precautions relating to the use of atropine. In children, atropine sulfate; diphenoxylate HCl should be used with caution since signs of atropinism may occur even with recommended doses, particularly in patients with Down's syndrome.

INFORMATION FOR THE PATIENT

INFORM THE PATIENT (PARENT OR GUARDIAN) NOT TO EXCEED THE RECOMMENDED DOSAGE AND TO KEEP ATROPINE SULFATE; DIPHENOXYLATE HCl OUT OF THE REACH OF CHILDREN AND IN A CHILD-RESISTANT CONTAINER. INFORM THE PATIENT OF THE CONSEQUENCES OF OVERDOSAGE, INCLUDING SEVERE RESPIRATORY DEPRESSION AND COMA, POSSIBLY LEADING TO PERMANENT BRAIN DAMAGE OR DEATH. Atropine sulfate; diphenoxylate HCl may produce drowsiness or dizziness. The patient should be cautioned regarding activities requiring mental alertness, such as driving or operating dangerous machinery. Potentiation of the action of alcohol, barbiturates, and tranquilizers with concomitant use of atropine sulfate; diphenoxylate HCl should be explained to the patient. The physician should also provide the patient with other information in this labeling, as appropriate.

CARCINOGENESIS, MUTAGENESIS, AND IMPAIRMENT OF FERTILITY

No long-term study in animals has been performed to evaluate carcinogenic potential. Diphenoxylate HCl was administered to male and female rats in their diets to provide dose levels of 4-20 mg/kg/day throughout a three-litter reproduction study. At 50 times the human dose (20 mg/kg/day), female weight gain was reduced and there was a marked effect on fertility as only 4 of 27 females became pregnant in three test breedings. The relevance of this finding to usage of atropine sulfate; diphenoxylate HCl in humans is unknown.

PREGNANCY CATEGORY C

Diphenoxylate HCl has been shown to have an effect on fertility in rats when given in doses 50 times the human dose (see Carcinogenesis, Mutagenesis, and Impairment of Fertility). Other findings in this study include a decrease in maternal weight gain of 30% at 20 mg/kg/day and of 10% at 4 mg/kg/day. At 10 times the human dose (4 mg/kg/day), average litter size was slightly reduced.

Teratology studies were conducted in rats, rabbits, and mice with diphenoxylate HCl at oral doses of 0.4 to 20 mg/kg/day. Due to experimental design and small numbers of litters, embryotoxic, fetotoxic, or teratogenic effects cannot be adequately assessed. However, examination of the available fetuses did not reveal any indication of teratogenicity.

There are no adequate and well-controlled studies in pregnant women. Atropine sulfate; diphenoxylate HCl should be used during pregnancy only if the anticipated benefit justifies the potential risk to the fetus.

NURSING MOTHERS

Caution should be exercised when atropine sulfate; diphenoxylate HCl is administered to a nursing woman, since the physicochemical characteristics of the major metabolite, diphenoxylic acid, are such that it may be excreted in breast milk and since it is known that atropine is excreted in breast milk.

PEDIATRIC USE

Atropine sulfate; diphenoxylate HCl may be used as an adjunct to the treatment of diarrhea but should be accompanied by appropriate fluid and electrolyte therapy, if needed. ATROPINE SULFATE; DIPHENOXYLATE HCl IS NOT RECOMMENDED FOR PEDIATRIC PATIENTS UNDER 2 YEARS OF AGE. Atropine sulfate; diphenoxylate HCl should be used with special caution in young children because of the greater variability of response in this age group. See WARNINGS and DOSAGE AND ADMINISTRATION.

A

DRUG INTERACTIONS

Known drug interactions include barbiturates, tranquilizers and alcohol. Atropine sulfate; diphenoxylate HCl may interact with MAO inhibitors (see WARNINGS).

In studies with male rats diphenoxylate HCl was found to inhibit the hepatic microsomal enzyme system at a dose of 2 mg/kg/day. Therefore, diphenoxylate has the potential to prolong the biological half-life of drugs for which the rate of elimination is dependent on the microsomal drug metabolizing enzyme system.

ADVERSE REACTIONS

At therapeutic doses, the following have been reported; they are listed in decreasing order of severity, but not of frequency:

Nervous System: Numbness of extremities, euphoria, depression, malaise/lethargy, confusion, sedation/drowsiness, dizziness, restlessness, headache.

Allergic: Anaphylaxis, angioneurotic edema, urticaria, swelling of the gums, pruritus.

Gastrointestinal System: Toxic megacolon, paralytic ileus, pancreatitis, vomiting, nausea, anorexia, abdominal discomfort.

The following atropine sulfate effects are listed in decreasing order of severity, but not of frequency: Hyperthermia, tachycardia, urinary retention, flushing, dryness of the skin and mucous membranes. These effects may occur, especially in children.

THIS MEDICATION SHOULD BE KEPT IN A CHILD-RESISTANT CONTAINER AND OUT OF THE REACH OF CHILDREN SINCE AN OVERDOSAGE MAY RESULT IN SEVERE RESPIRATORY DEPRESSION AND COMA, POSSIBLY LEADING TO PERMANENT BRAIN DAMAGE OR DEATH.

DOSAGE AND ADMINISTRATION

DO NOT EXCEED RECOMMENDED DOSAGE.

ADULTS

The recommended initial dosage is two atropine sulfate; diphenoxylate HCl tablets 4 times daily (20 mg per day) or 10 ml (two regular teaspoonfuls) of atropine sulfate; diphenoxylate HCl liquid 4 times daily. Most patients will require this dosage until initial control has been achieved, after which the dosage may be reduced to meet individual requirements. Control may often be maintained with as little as 5 mg (two tablets or 10 ml of liquid) daily.

Clinical improvement of acute diarrhea is usually observed within 48 hours. If clinical improvement of chronic diarrhea after treatment with a maximum daily dose of 20 mg of diphenoxylate HCl is not observed within 10 days, symptoms are unlikely to be controlled by further administration.

CHILDREN

Atropine sulfate; diphenoxylate HCl is not recommended in children under 2 years of age and should be used with special caution in young children (see WARNINGS and PRECAUTIONS). The nutritional status and degree of dehydration must be considered. In children under 13 years of age, use oral solution. Do not use the tablets for this age group.

FOR ORAL SOLUTION ONLY

Only the plastic dropper should be used when measuring atropine sulfate; diphenoxylate HCl liquid for administration to children.

Dosage Schedule for Children: The recommended initial total daily dosage of atropine sulfate; diphenoxylate HCl liquid for children is 0.3-0.4 mg/kg administered in four divided doses. TABLE 1 provides an *approximate* initial daily dosage recommendation for children. These pediatric schedules are the best approximation of an average dose recommendation

TABLE 1

Age (years)	Approximate (kg)	Weight (lb)	Dosage in ml (4 times daily)
2	11-14	24-31	1.5-3.0
3	12-16	26-35	2.0-3.0
4	14-20	31-44	2.0-4.0
5	16-23	35-51	2.5-4.5
6-8	17-32	38-71	2.5-5.0
9-12	23-55	51-121	3.5-5.0

which may be adjusted downward according to the overall nutritional status and degree of dehydration encountered in the sick child. Reduction of dosage may be made as soon as initial control of symptoms has been achieved. Maintenance dosage may be as low as one-fourth of the initial dosage. If no response occurs within 48 hours, atropine sulfate; diphenoxylate HCl is unlikely to be effective.

KEEP THIS AND ALL MEDICATIONS OUT OF THE REACH OF CHILDREN.

HOW SUPPLIED

Diphenoxylate hydrochloride and atropine sulfate tablets are available as white, round "3966" containing 2.5 mg diphenoxylate hydrochloride (WARNING: May be habit-forming).

Lomotil Tablets: Lomotil tablets are round, white, with "SEARLE" debossed on one side and "61" on the other side.

Lomotil Oral Solution: Lomotil oral solution should be dispensed only in original container. Only the enclosed plastic dropper should be used when measuring Lomotil oral solution for administration to children.

STORAGE

Store at controlled room temperature 15-30°C (59-86°F).

Dispense in a well-closed, light-resistant container. Use child-resistant closure.

PRODUCT LISTING - RATED THERAPEUTICALLY EQUIVALENT

Liquid - Oral - 0.025 mg;2.5 mg/5 ml

5 ml x 40	$35.60	GENERIC, Roxane Laboratories Inc	00054-8191-16
10 ml x 40	$58.80	GENERIC, Roxane Laboratories Inc	00054-8171-16
60 ml	$6.28	GENERIC, Roxane Laboratories Inc	00054-3194-46
60 ml	$21.44	LOMOTIL, Searle	00025-0066-02

Tablet - Oral - 0.025 mg;2.5 mg

15's	$1.86	GENERIC, Circle Pharmaceuticals Inc	00659-1611-15
20's	$1.86	GENERIC, Circle Pharmaceuticals Inc	00659-1611-20
30's	$2.34	GENERIC, Circle Pharmaceuticals Inc	00659-1611-30
100's	$3.15	GENERIC, Major Pharmaceuticals Inc	00904-0032-60
100's	$3.44	GENERIC, Vita-Rx Corporation	49727-0266-02
100's	$4.46	GENERIC, Moore, H.L. Drug Exchange Inc	00839-6120-06
100's	$4.68	GENERIC, Caremark Inc	00339-4037-12
100's	$6.35	GENERIC, Md Pharmaceutical Inc	43567-0535-07
100's	$37.43	FEDERAL UPPER LIMIT, H.C.F.A. F F P	99999-0339-01
100's	$45.45	GENERIC, Mallinckrodt Medical Inc	00406-0463-01
100's	$45.95	GENERIC, Eon Labs Manufacturing Inc	00185-0024-01
100's	$47.80	GENERIC, Udl Laboratories Inc	51079-0067-20
100's	$47.90	GENERIC, Ivax Corporation	00172-3966-60
100's	$47.90	GENERIC, Geneva Pharmaceuticals	00781-1262-01
100's	$48.00	GENERIC, Mylan Pharmaceuticals Inc	00378-0415-01
100's	$48.00	GENERIC, Qualitest Products Inc	00603-3360-21
100's	$48.00	GENERIC, Par Pharmaceutical Inc	49884-0771-01
100's	$50.73	GENERIC, Geneva Pharmaceuticals	00781-1262-13
100's	$72.53	LOMOTIL, Searle	00025-0061-31
100's	$76.80	LOMOTIL, Searle	00025-0061-34

PRODUCT LISTING - EQUIVALENTS NOT AVAILABLE

Tablet - Oral - 0.025 mg;2.5 mg

3's	$3.59	GENERIC, Prescript Pharmaceuticals	00247-0095-03
4's	$3.67	GENERIC, Prescript Pharmaceuticals	00247-0095-04
6's	$2.34	GENERIC, Southwood Pharmaceuticals Inc	58016-0713-06
6's	$3.84	GENERIC, Prescript Pharmaceuticals	00247-0095-06
8's	$3.99	GENERIC, Prescript Pharmaceuticals	00247-0095-08
10's	$4.15	GENERIC, Prescript Pharmaceuticals	00247-0095-10
10's	$4.25	GENERIC, Southwood Pharmaceuticals Inc	58016-0713-10
12's	$4.31	GENERIC, Prescript Pharmaceuticals	00247-0095-12
12's	$5.10	GENERIC, Southwood Pharmaceuticals Inc	58016-0713-12
14's	$5.95	GENERIC, Southwood Pharmaceuticals Inc	58016-0713-14
15's	$4.54	GENERIC, Prescript Pharmaceuticals	00247-0095-15
15's	$6.37	GENERIC, Southwood Pharmaceuticals Inc	58016-0713-15
16's	$4.62	GENERIC, Prescript Pharmaceuticals	00247-0095-16
16's	$7.03	GENERIC, Southwood Pharmaceuticals Inc	58016-0713-16
18's	$4.79	GENERIC, Prescript Pharmaceuticals	00247-0095-18
20's	$4.94	GENERIC, Prescript Pharmaceuticals	00247-0095-20
20's	$8.79	GENERIC, Southwood Pharmaceuticals Inc	58016-0713-20
21's	$8.93	GENERIC, Southwood Pharmaceuticals Inc	58016-0713-21
24's	$10.20	GENERIC, Southwood Pharmaceuticals Inc	58016-0713-24
28's	$11.90	GENERIC, Southwood Pharmaceuticals Inc	58016-0713-28
30's	$5.74	GENERIC, Prescript Pharmaceuticals	00247-0095-30
30's	$12.75	GENERIC, Southwood Pharmaceuticals Inc	58016-0713-30
40's	$6.53	GENERIC, Prescript Pharmaceuticals	00247-0095-40
40's	$17.00	GENERIC, Southwood Pharmaceuticals Inc	58016-0713-40
50's	$7.33	GENERIC, Prescript Pharmaceuticals	00247-0095-50
60's	$25.50	GENERIC, Southwood Pharmaceuticals Inc	58016-0713-60
100's	$3.75	GENERIC, Interstate Drug Exchange Inc	00814-2600-14
100's	$4.78	GENERIC, Vangard Labs	00615-0429-01
100's	$11.29	GENERIC, Prescript Pharmaceuticals	00247-0095-00
100's	$42.50	GENERIC, Southwood Pharmaceuticals Inc	58016-0713-00
100's	$48.50	GENERIC, Able Laboratories Inc	53265-0237-10

Atropine; Hyoscyamine; Phenobarbital; Scopolamine *(000383)*

Categories: Enterocolitis; Irritable bowel syndrome; Ulcer, duodenal, adjunct; Pregnancy Category C; FDA Pre 1938 Drugs
Drug Classes: Anticholinergics; Gastrointestinals
Brand Names: Antispasmodic; Barbidonna; Chardonna-2; **Donnatal**; Donnatal Extentabs; Spasmolin

DESCRIPTION

Note: The trade name has been used throughout this monograph for clarity.

DONNATAL EXTENTABS

Each Donnatal Extentabs tablet contains: Phenobarbital* (3/4 gr), 48.6 mg; hyoscyamine sulfate, 0.3111 mg; atropine sulfate, 0.0582 mg; scopolamine hydrobromide, 0.0195 mg.

***Warning:** May be habit forming.

Each Donnatal Extentabs tablet contains the equivalent of three Donnatal tablets. Extentabs are designed to release the ingredients gradually to provide effects for up to 12 hours.

In addition, each tablet contains the following inactive ingredients: Anhydrous lactose, calcium sulfate granular, colloidal silicon dioxide, dibasic calcium phosphate, lactose monohydrate, magnesium stearate, and stearic acid. Film coating and polishing solution contains: D&C yellow no. 10 alminum lake, FD&C blue 1 aluminum lake, hydroxypropyl methylcellulose, polydextrose, polyethylene glycol, titanium dioxide and triacetin. The printing ink contains titanium dioxide.

DONNATAL TABLETS, CAPSULES OR ELIXIR

Each Donnatal tablet, capsule or 5 ml (teaspoonful) of elixir (23% alcohol) contains: Phenobarbital*, 16.2 mg; hyoscyamine sulfate, 0.1037 mg; atropine sulfate, 0.0194 mg; scopolamine hydrobromide, 0.0065 mg.

***Warning:** May be habit forming.

Inactive Ingredients:
Tablets: Dibasic calcium phosphate, magnesium stearate, microcrystalline cellulose, silicon dioxide, sodium starch glycolate, stearic acid, sucrose. May contain corn starch, dextrose, or invert sugar.
Capsules: Corn starch, edible ink, D&C yellow 10 and FD&C green 3 or FD&C blue 1 and FD&C yellow 6, FD&C blue 2 aluminum lake, gelatin, lactose, sucrose. May contain FD&C red 40 and yellow 6 aluminum lakes.
Elixir: D&C yellow 10, FD&C blue 1, FD&C yellow 6, flavors, glucose, saccharin sodium, water.

CLINICAL PHARMACOLOGY

This drug combination provides natural belladonna alkaloids in a specific, fixed ratio combined with phenobarbital to provide peripheral anticholinergic/antispasmodic action and mild sedation.

INDICATIONS AND USAGE

Based on a review of this drug by the National Academy of Sciences — National Research Council and/or other information, FDA has classified the following indications as "possibly" effective:

For use as adjunctive therapy in the treatment of irritable bowel syndrome (irritable colon, spastic colon, mucous colitis) and acute enterocolitis.

May also be useful as adjunctive therapy in the treatment of duodenal ulcer. IT HAS NOT BEEN SHOWN CONCLUSIVELY WHETHER ANTICHOLINERGIC/ANTISPASMODIC DRUGS AID IN THE HEALING OF A DUODENAL ULCER, DECREASE THE RATE OF RECURRENCES OR PREVENT COMPLICATIONS.

CONTRAINDICATIONS

Glaucoma, obstructive uropathy (for example, bladder neck obstruction due to prostatic hypertrophy); obstructive disease of the gastrointestinal tract (as in achalasia, pyloroduodenal stenosis, etc.); paralytic ileus, intestinal atony of the elderly or debilitated patient; unstable cardiovascular status in acute hemorrhage; severe ulcerative colitis especially if complicated by toxic megacolon; myasthenia gravis; hiatal hernia associated with reflux esophagitis.

Donnatal is contraindicated in patients with known hypersensitivity to any of the ingredients. Phenobarbital is contraindicated in acute intermittent porphyria and in those patients in whom phenobarbital produces restlessness and/or excitement.

WARNINGS

In the presence of a high environmental temperature, heat prostration can occur with belladonna alkaloids (fever and heatstroke due to decreased sweating).

Diarrhea may be an early symptom of incomplete intestinal obstruction, especially in patients with ileostomy or colostomy. In this instance treatment with this drug would be inappropriate and possibly harmful.

Donnatal may produce drowsiness or blurred vision. The patient should be warned, should these occur, not to engage in activities requiring mental alertness, such as operating a motor vehicle or other machinery, and not to perform hazardous work.

Phenobarbital may decrease the effect of anticoagulants and necessitate larger doses of the anticoagulant for optimal effect. When phenobarbital is discontinued, the dose of the anticoagulant may have to be decreased.

Phenobarbital may be habit forming and should not be administered to individuals known to be addiction prone or to those with a history of physical and/or psychological dependence upon drugs.

Since barbiturates are metabolized in the liver, they should be used with caution and initial doses should be small in patients with hepatic dysfunction.

PRECAUTIONS

Use with caution in patients with: autonomic neuropathy, hepatic or renal disease, hyperthyroidism, coronary heart disease, congestive heart failure, cardiac arrhythmias, tachycardia, and hypertension.

Belladonna alkaloids may produce a delay in gastric emptying (antral stasis) which would complicate the management of gastric ulcer.

Theoretically, with overdosage, a curare-like action may occur.

CARCINOGENESIS, MUTAGENESIS

Long-term studies in animals have not been performed to evaluate carcinogenic potential.

PREGNANCY CATEGORY C

Animal reproduction studies have not been conducted with Donnatal. It is not known whether Donnatal can cause fetal harm when administered to a pregnant woman or can affect reproduction capacity. Donnatal should be given to a pregnant woman only if clearly needed.

NURSING MOTHERS

It is not known whether this drug is excreted in human milk. Because many drugs are excreted in human milk, caution should be exercised when Donnatal is administered to a nursing mother.

ADVERSE REACTIONS

Adverse reactions may include xerostomia; urinary hesitancy and retention; blurred vision; tachycardia; palpitation; mydriasis; cycloplegia; increased ocular tension; loss of taste sense; headache; nervousness; drowsiness; weakness; dizziness; insomnia; nausea; vomiting; impotence; suppression of lactation; constipation; bloated feeling; musculoskeletal pain; severe allergic reaction or drug idiosyncrasies, including anaphylaxis, urticaria and other dermal manifestations; and decreased sweating. Elderly patients may react with symptoms of excitement, agitation, drowsiness, and other untoward manifestations to even small doses of the drug.

Phenobarbital may produce excitement in some patients, rather than a sedative effect. In patients habituated to barbiturates, abrupt withdrawal may produce delirium or convulsions.

DOSAGE AND ADMINISTRATION

DONNATAL EXTENTABS

The dosage of Donnatal Extentabs should be adjusted to the needs of the individual patient to assure symptomatic control with a minimum of adverse reactions. The usual dose is 1 tablet every 12 hours. If indicated, 1 tablet every 8 hours may be given.

DONNATAL TABLETS, CAPSULES OR ELIXIR

The dosage of Donnatal should be adjusted to the needs of the individual patient to assure symptomatic control with a minimum of adverse effects.

Donnatal Tablets or Capsules

Adults: One or two Donnatal tablets or capsules 3 or 4 times a day according to condition and severity of symptoms.

Donnatal Elixir

Adults: One or two teaspoonfuls of elixir 3 or 4 times a day according to conditions and severity of symptoms.

Children: May be dosed every 4 or 6 hours (see TABLE 1).

TABLE 1

Body Weight	Starting Dosage q4h	Starting Dosage q6h
10 lb (4.5 kg)	0.5 ml	0.75 ml
20 lb (9.1 kg)	1.0 ml	1.5 ml
30 lb (13.6 kg)	1.5 ml	2.0 ml
50 lb (22.7 kg)	½ tsp	¾ tsp
75 lb (34.0 kg)	¾ tsp	1 tsp
100 lb (45.4 kg)	1 tsp	1½ tsp

HOW SUPPLIED

DONNATAL EXTENTABS

Film coated green, round, compressed tablets printed "P421" in black ink.

Storage: Store at controlled room temperature,15-30°C (59-86°F). Protect from light and moisture.

DONNATAL TABLETS, CAPSULES OR ELIXIR

Donnatal Tablets: White, compressed, scored and embossed "R".
Donnatal Capsules: Green and white, monogrammed "AHR" and "4207".
Donnatal Elixir: Green, citrus flavored elixir, containing 23% alcohol.

Storage: Store at controlled room temperature, between 20 and 25°C (68 and 77°F). Dispense in tight, light-resistant container.

PRODUCT LISTING - RATED THERAPEUTICALLY EQUIVALENT

Elixir - Oral - 0.0194 mg;0.1037 mg;16.2 mg;0.0065 mg/5 ml

120 ml	$2.50	GENERIC, Cenci, H.R. Labs Inc	00556-0053-04
120 ml	$5.45	GENERIC, Pharma Pac	52959-0274-03
480 ml	$4.51	GENERIC, Cenci, H.R. Labs Inc	00556-0053-16
3840 ml	$23.20	GENERIC, Cenci, H.R. Labs Inc	00556-0053-28

PRODUCT LISTING - EQUIVALENTS NOT AVAILABLE

Elixir - Oral - 0.0194 mg;0.1037 mg;16.2 mg;0.0065 mg/5 ml

15 ml	$7.50	GENERIC, Marin Pharmaceutical	12539-0315-15
100 ml	$4.25	GENERIC, Cmc-Consolidated Midland Corporation	00223-6419-02
100 ml	$47.50	GENERIC, Cmc-Consolidated Midland Corporation	00223-6419-03
120 ml	$1.82	GENERIC, Allscripts Pharmaceutical Company	54569-3251-00
120 ml	$2.00	GENERIC, Circle Pharmaceuticals Inc	00659-1606-54
120 ml	$2.56	GENERIC, Major Pharmaceuticals Inc	00904-0981-20
120 ml	$3.35	GENERIC, Major Pharmaceuticals Inc	00904-0981-00
120 ml	$3.77	GENERIC, Morton Grove Pharmaceuticals Inc	60432-0009-04
120 ml	$4.13	GENERIC, Pd-Rx Pharmaceuticals	55289-0586-04
120 ml	$5.17	GENERIC, Southwood Pharmaceuticals Inc	58016-0700-24
120 ml	$6.50	GENERIC, Dayton Laboratories Inc	52041-0043-33
120 ml	$7.54	DONNATAL, Southwood Pharmaceuticals Inc	58016-0499-24
120 ml	$7.87	DONNATAL, Esi Lederle Generics	00031-4221-12
120 ml	$8.14	DONNATAL, Allscripts Pharmaceutical Company	54569-0426-00
120 ml	$14.45	DONNATAL, Pbm Pharmaceuticals	66213-0422-04
240 ml	$8.25	GENERIC, Pd-Rx Pharmaceuticals	55289-0586-08
240 ml	$14.96	DONNATAL, Southwood Pharmaceuticals Inc	58016-0499-48
473 ml	$5.25	GENERIC, Seatrace Pharmaceuticals	00551-0195-01
480 ml	$4.66	GENERIC, Geneva Pharmaceuticals	00781-6397-16
480 ml	$7.00	GENERIC, Cypress Pharmaceutical Inc	60258-0822-16
480 ml	$7.35	GENERIC, Mutual/United Research Laboratories	00677-1566-33
480 ml	$7.78	GENERIC, Aligen Independent Laboratories Inc	00405-2350-16
480 ml	$7.97	GENERIC, Alphagen Laboratories Inc	59743-0028-16
480 ml	$8.65	GENERIC, Major Pharmaceuticals Inc	00904-0981-16
480 ml	$9.50	GENERIC, Vita Elixir Company Inc	00181-0626-00
480 ml	$10.70	GENERIC, Physicians Total Care	54868-2087-00
480 ml	$10.74	GENERIC, Ivax Corporation	00182-0686-40
480 ml	$10.85	GENERIC, Moore, H.L. Drug Exchange Inc	00839-5018-69

480 ml	$14.18	GENERIC, Morton Grove Pharmaceuticals Inc	60432-0009-16
480 ml	$14.75	GENERIC, Vintage Pharmaceuticals Inc	00254-9035-58
480 ml	$14.75	GENERIC, Qualitest Products Inc	00603-1030-58
480 ml	$16.61	GENERIC, R.I.D. Inc Distributor	54807-0125-16
480 ml	$27.85	DONNATAL, Esi Lederle Generics	00031-4221-25
480 ml	$51.16	DONNATAL, Pbm Pharmaceuticals	66213-0422-16
1440 ml	$2.45	GENERIC, Cmc-Consolidated Midland Corporation	00223-6419-01
3840 ml	$49.99	GENERIC, Cypress Pharmaceutical Inc	60258-0822-28
3840 ml	$52.00	GENERIC, Vita Elixir Company Inc	00181-0626-01
3840 ml	$59.90	GENERIC, Major Pharmaceuticals Inc	00904-0981-28
3840 ml	$62.59	GENERIC, Ivax Corporation	00182-0686-41
3840 ml	$64.90	GENERIC, Moore, H.L. Drug Exchange Inc	00839-7850-70
3840 ml	$71.77	GENERIC, Morton Grove Pharmaceuticals Inc	60432-0009-28
3840 ml	$174.74	DONNATAL, Esi Lederle Generics	00031-4221-29

Tablet - Oral - 0.0194 mg;0.1037 mg;16.2 mg;0.0065 mg

14's	$3.36	GENERIC, Pd-Rx Pharmaceuticals	55289-0035-14
15's	$0.95	GENERIC, Allscripts Pharmaceutical Company	54569-0427-05
20's	$1.27	GENERIC, Allscripts Pharmaceutical Company	54569-0427-04
20's	$1.70	GENERIC, Pharmaceutical Corporation Of America	51655-0119-52
20's	$1.97	GENERIC, Circle Pharmaceuticals Inc	00659-1607-20
20's	$3.75	GENERIC, Pd-Rx Pharmaceuticals	55289-0035-20
20's	$4.15	GENERIC, Southwood Pharmaceuticals Inc	58016-0709-20
20's	$4.87	GENERIC, Pharma Pac	52959-0023-20
25's	$4.95	GENERIC, Pd-Rx Pharmaceuticals	55289-0035-97
30's	$1.90	GENERIC, Allscripts Pharmaceutical Company	54569-0427-01
30's	$2.18	GENERIC, Physicians Total Care	54868-0031-04
30's	$3.98	GENERIC, Pd-Rx Pharmaceuticals	55289-0035-30
30's	$4.29	GENERIC, Southwood Pharmaceuticals Inc	58016-0709-30
30's	$5.25	GENERIC, Pharma Pac	52959-0023-30
30's	$6.23	GENERIC, St. Mary'S Mpp	60760-0754-30
40's	$2.54	GENERIC, Allscripts Pharmaceutical Company	54569-0427-09
40's	$4.58	GENERIC, Southwood Pharmaceuticals Inc	58016-0709-40
42's	$4.62	GENERIC, Southwood Pharmaceuticals Inc	58016-0709-42
50's	$4.86	GENERIC, Southwood Pharmaceuticals Inc	58016-0709-50
50's	$6.01	GENERIC, Pharma Pac	52959-0023-50
60's	$3.81	GENERIC, Allscripts Pharmaceutical Company	54569-0427-02
60's	$4.43	GENERIC, Pd-Rx Pharmaceuticals	55289-0035-60
60's	$8.85	GENERIC, Pharma Pac	52959-0023-60
100's	$1.29	GENERIC, Global Pharmaceutical Corporation	00115-4652-01
100's	$1.90	GENERIC, Major Pharmaceuticals Inc	00904-3741-60
100's	$2.75	GENERIC, Cmc-Consolidated Midland Corporation	00223-0425-01
100's	$5.30	GENERIC, Moore, H.L. Drug Exchange Inc	00839-5055-06
100's	$5.80	GENERIC, Vintage Pharmaceuticals Inc	00254-2320-28
100's	$5.80	GENERIC, Qualitest Products Inc	00603-2418-21
100's	$5.83	GENERIC, Major Pharmaceuticals Inc	00904-3741-61
100's	$5.83	GENERIC, Southwood Pharmaceuticals Inc	58016-0709-00
100's	$6.30	GENERIC, Pd-Rx Pharmaceuticals	55289-0035-01
100's	$6.35	GENERIC, Allscripts Pharmaceutical Company	54569-0427-08
100's	$11.91	GENERIC, R.I.D. Inc Distributor	54807-0126-01
100's	$20.00	GENERIC, Dayton Laboratories Inc	52041-0044-15
100's	$23.83	CHARDONNA-2, Schwarz Pharma	00091-0202-01
100's	$33.18	DONNATAL, Pbm Pharmaceuticals	66213-0425-10
100's	$55.55	GENERIC, Wallace Laboratories	00037-0301-92

Tablet, Extended Release - Oral - 0.0582 mg;0.0582 mg;48.6 mg;0.0195 mg

100's	$92.96	DONNATAL EXTENTABS, Pbm Pharmaceuticals	66213-0421-10

Auranofin *(000347)*

For complete prescribing information, refer to the CD-ROM included with the book.

Categories: Arthritis, rheumatoid; Pregnancy Category C; FDA Approved 1985 May; Patent Expiration 1992 Jan
Drug Classes: Disease modifying antirheumatic drugs; Gold compounds
Brand Names: Ridaura
Foreign Brand Availability: Aktil (Thailand); Goldar (India); Ridaura Tiltab (Bahrain; Cyprus; Egypt; Hong-Kong; Iran; Iraq; Israel; Jordan; Kuwait; Lebanon; Libya; Malaysia; Oman; Qatar; Republic-of-Yemen; Saudi-Arabia; Syria; United-Arab-Emirates); Ridauran (France)
Cost of Therapy: $170.26 (Rheumatoid Arthritis; Ridaura; 3 mg; 2 capsules/day; 30 day supply)

WARNING

Auranofin contains gold and, like other gold-containing drugs, can cause gold toxicity, signs of which include: fall in hemoglobin, leukopenia below 4000 WBC/cu mm, granulocytes below 1500/cu mm, decrease in platelets below 150,000 cu mm, proteinuria, hematuria, pruritus, rash, stomatitis or persistent diarrhea. Therefore, the results of recommended laboratory work should be reviewed before writing each auranofin prescription. Like other gold preparations, auranofin is only indicated for use in

WARNING — Cont'd

selected patients with active rheumatoid arthritis. Physicians planning to use auranofin should be experienced with chrysotherapy and should thoroughly familiarize themselves with the toxicity and benefits of auranofin.

In addition, the following precautions should be routinely employed:

1. **The possibility of adverse reactions should be explained to patients before starting therapy.**
2. **Patients should be advised to report promptly any symptoms suggesting toxicity.**

DESCRIPTION

Ridaura (auranofin) is available in oral form as capsules containing 3 mg auranofin.

Auranofin is (2,3,4,6-tetra-O-acetyl-1-thio-β-D-glucopyranosato-S-) (triethyl-phosphine) gold.

Auranofin contains 29% gold.

Each Ridaura capsule contains auranofin, 3 mg. Inactive ingredients consist of benzyl alcohol, cellulose, cetylpyridinium chloride, D&C red no. 33, FD&C blue no. 1, FD&C red no. 40, FD&C yellow no. 6, gelatin, lactose, magnesium stearate, povidone, sodium lauryl sulfate, sodium starch glycolate, starch, titanium dioxide and trace amounts of other inactive ingredients.

INDICATIONS AND USAGE

Auranofin is indicated in the management of adults with active classical or definite rheumatoid arthritis (ARA criteria) who have had an insufficient therapeutic response to, or are intolerant of, an adequate trial of full doses of one or more nonsteroidal anti-inflammatory drugs. Auranofin should be added to a comprehensive baseline program, including non-drug therapies.

Unlike anti-inflammatory drugs, auranofin does not produce an immediate response. Therapeutic effects may be seen after 3-4 months of treatment, although improvement has not been seen in some patients before 6 months.

When cartilage and bone damage has already occurred, gold cannot reverse structural damage to joints caused by previous disease. The greatest potential benefit occurs in patients with active synovitis, particularly in its early stage.

In controlled clinical trials comparing auranofin with injectable gold, auranofin was associated with fewer dropouts due to adverse reactions, while injectable gold was associated with fewer dropouts for inadequate or poor therapeutic effect. Physicians should consider these findings when deciding on the use of auranofin in patients who are candidates for chrysotherapy.

CONTRAINDICATIONS

Auranofin is contraindicated in patients with a history of any of the following gold-induced disorders: anaphylactic reactions, necrotizing enterocolitis, pulmonary fibrosis, exfoliative dermatitis, bone marrow aplasia or other severe hematologic disorders.

WARNINGS

Danger signs of possible gold toxicity include fail in hemoglobin, leukopenia below 4000 WBC/cu mm, granulocytes below 1500/cu mm, decrease in platelets below 150,000/cu mm, proteinuria, hematuria, pruritus, rash, stomatitis or persistent diarrhea.

Thrombocytopenia has occurred in 1-3% of patients treated with auranofin, some of whom developed bleeding. The thrombocytopenia usually appears to be peripheral in origin and is usually reversible upon withdrawal of auranofin. Its onset bears no relationship to the duration of auranofin therapy and its course may be rapid. While patients' platelet counts should normally be monitored at least monthly, the occurrence of a precipitous decline in platelets or a platelet count less than 100,000/cu mm or signs and symptoms (*e.g.*, purpura, ecchymoses or petechiae) suggestive of thrombocytopenia indicates a need to immediately withdraw auranofin and other therapies with the potential to cause thrombocytopenia, and to obtain additional platelet counts. No additional auranofin should be given unless the thrombocytopenia resolves and further studies show it was not due to gold therapy.

Proteinuria has developed in 3-9% of patients treated with auranofin. If clinically significant proteinuria or microscopic hematuria is found, auranofin and other therapies with the potential to cause proteinuria or microscopic hematuria should be stopped immediately.

DOSAGE AND ADMINISTRATION

USUAL ADULT DOSAGE

The usual adult dosage of auranofin is 6 mg daily, given either as 3 mg twice daily or 6 mg once daily. Initiation of therapy at dosages exceeding 6 mg daily is not recommended because it is associated with an increased incidence of diarrhea. If response is inadequate after 6 months, an increase to 9 mg (3 mg three times daily) may be tolerated. If response remains inadequate after a 3 month trial of 9 mg daily, auranofin therapy should be discontinued. Safety at dosages exceeding 9 mg daily has not been studied.

TRANSFERRING FROM INJECTABLE GOLD

In controlled clinical studies, patients on injectable gold have been transferred to auranofin by discontinuing the injectable agent and starting oral therapy with auranofin, 6 mg daily. When patients are transferred to auranofin, they should be informed of its adverse reaction profile, in particular the gastrointestinal reactions. At 6 months, control of disease activity of patients transferred to auranofin and those maintained on the injectable agent was not different. Data beyond 6 months are not available.

PRODUCT LISTING - EQUIVALENTS NOT AVAILABLE

Capsule - Oral - 3 mg

60's	$170.26	RIDAURA, Connetics Inc	63032-0011-60
60's	$190.70	RIDAURA, Prometheus Inc	65483-0093-06

A

Aurothioglucose (000348)

For complete prescribing information, refer to the CD-ROM included with the book.

Categories: Arthritis, rheumatoid; Pregnancy Category C; FDA Pre 1938 Drugs
Drug Classes: Disease modifying antirheumatic drugs; Gold compounds
Brand Names: Lomosol; **Solganal**
Foreign Brand Availability: Aureotan (Germany); Auromyose (Netherlands); Gold-50 (Australia); Solganol (Canada)
Cost of Therapy: $61.37 (Rheumatoid Arthritis; Solganal Injection; 50 mg/ml; 1 ml/week; 28 day supply)
HCFA JCODE(S): J2910 up to 50 mg IM

WARNING

Physicians planning to use aurothioglucose suspension should thoroughly familiarize themselves with its toxicity and its benefits. The possibility of toxic reactions should always be explained to the patient before starting therapy. Patients should be warned to report promptly any symptom suggesting toxicity. Before each injection of aurothioglucose suspension, the physician should review the results of laboratory work and see the patient to determine the presence or absence of adverse reactions, since some of these can be severe or even fatal.

DESCRIPTION

Solganal is a sterile suspension, for **intramuscular injection only.** Solganal suspension is an antiarthritic agent which is absorbed gradually following intramuscular injection, producing a therapeutically desired prolonged effect.

Each ml contains 50 mg of aurothioglucose in sterile sesame oil with 2% aluminum monostearate; 1 mg propylparaben is added as preservative. Aurothioglucose contains approximately 50% gold by weight.

The empirical formula for aurothioglucose is $C_6H_{11}AuO_5S$; the molecular weight is 392.18. Chemically it is (1-Thio-D-glucopyranosato) gold.

Aurothioglucose is a nearly odorless, yellow powder which is stable in air. An aqueous solution is unstable on long standing. Aurothioglucose is freely soluble in water but practically insoluble in acetone, in alcohol, in chloroform, and in ether.

INDICATIONS AND USAGE

Aurothioglucose is indicated for the adjunctive treatment of early active rheumatoid arthritis (both of the adult and juvenile types) not adequately controlled by other anti-inflammatory agents and conservative measures. In chronic, advanced cases of rheumatoid arthritis, gold therapy is less valuable.

Antirheumatic measures such as salicylates and other antiinflammatory drugs (both steroidal and non-steroidal) may be continued after initiation of gold therapy. After improvement commences, these measures may be discontinued slowly as symptoms permit.

See DOSAGE AND ADMINISTRATION.

CONTRAINDICATIONS

A history of known hypersensitivity to any component of aurothioglucose contraindicates its use. Gold therapy is contraindicated in patients with uncontrolled diabetes mellitus, severe debilitation, systemic lupus erythematosus, renal disease, hepatic dysfunction, uncontrolled congestive heart failure, marked hypertension, agranulocytosis, other blood dyscrasias, or hemorrhagic diathesis; or if there is a history of infectious hepatitis. Patients who recently have had radiation, and those who have developed severe toxicity from previous exposure to gold or other heavy metals should not receive aurothioglucose.

Urticaria, eczema, and colitis are also contraindications.

Gold therapy is usually contraindicated in pregnancy.

Gold salts should not be used with penicillamine or antimalarials. The safety of coadministration with immunosuppressive agents other than corticosteroids has not been established.

WARNINGS

The following signs should be considered danger signals of gold toxicity, and no additional injection should be given unless further studies reveal some other cause for their presence: rapid reduction of hemoglobin, leukopenia (WBC below 400/cu mm), eosinophilia above 5% platelet count below 100,000/cu mm, albuminuria, hematuria, pruritus, dermatitis, stomatitis, jaundice, and petechiae.

Effects that may occur immediately following an injection, or at any time during gold therapy, include: anaphylactic shock, syncope, bradycardia, thickening of the tongue, difficulty in swallowing and breathing, and angioneurotic edema. If such effects are observed, treatment with aurothioglucose should be discontinued.

Tolerance to gold usually decreases with advancing age. Diabetes mellitus or congestive heart failure should be under control before gold therapy is instituted.

Aurothioglucose should be used with extreme caution in patients with: skin rash, hypersensitivity to other medications, or a history of renal or liver disease.

DOSAGE AND ADMINISTRATION

Adults: The usual dosage schedule for the intramuscular administration of aurothioglucose is as follows: first dose, 10 mg; second and third doses, 25 mg; fourth and subsequent doses, 50 mg. The interval between doses is 1 week. The 50 mg dose is continued at weekly intervals until 0.8-1.0 g aurothioglucose has been given. If the patient has improved and has exhibited no sign of toxicity, the 50 mg dose may be continued many months longer, at 3-4 week intervals. A weekly dose above 50 mg is usually unnecessary and contraindicated; the tendency in gold therapy is toward lower dosage. With this in mind, it may eventually be established that a 25 mg dose is the one of choice. If no improvement has been demonstrated after a total administration of 1.0 g of aurothioglucose, the necessity for gold therapy should be reevaluated.

Children 6-12 Years: One-fourth of the adult dose, governed chiefly by body weight, not to exceed 25 mg per dose.

Aurothioglucose should be injected **intramuscularly** (preferably intragluteally), **never intravenously.** The patient should be lying down and should remain recumbent for approximately 10 minutes after the injection. The vial should be thoroughly shaken in order to suspend all of the active material. Heating the vial to body temperature (by immersion in warm water) will facilitate drawing the suspension into the syringe. An 18-gauge, 1½-inch needle is recommended for depositing the preparation deep into the muscular tissue. For obese patients, an 18-gauge, 2-inch needle may be used. The site usually selected for injection is the upper outer quadrant of the gluteal region.

NOTE: Shake the vial in horizontal position before the dose is withdrawn. Needle and syringe must be dry. The patient should be observed for at least 15 minutes following each injection.

PRODUCT LISTING - EQUIVALENTS NOT AVAILABLE

Suspension - Intramuscular - 50 mg/ml

10 ml	$153.42	SOLGANAL, Allscripts Pharmaceutical Company	54569-2576-00
10 ml	$165.29	SOLGANAL, Physicians Total Care	54868-1133-00
10 ml	$167.70	SOLGANAL, Schering Corporation	00085-0460-03

Azatadine Maleate (000349)

For complete prescribing information, refer to the CD-ROM included with the book.

Categories: Rhinitis, perennial allergic; Rhinitis, seasonal allergic; Urticaria, chronic; Pregnancy Category B; FDA Approved 1977 Mar
Drug Classes: Antihistamines, H1
Brand Names: **Optimine**
Foreign Brand Availability: Idulamine (Colombia; Czech-Republic; Mexico); Idulian (Bulgaria; Italy); Lergocil (Spain); Nalomet (Greece); Verben (Denmark); Zadine (Australia; Hong-Kong; Indonesia; Malaysia; New-Zealand; Taiwan)
Cost of Therapy: $75.60 (Allergic Rhinitis; Optimine; 1 mg; 2 tablets/day; 30 day supply)

DESCRIPTION

Optimine tablets contain azatadine maleate, an antihistamine having the empirical formula, $C_{20}H_{22}N_2 \cdot 2C_4H_4O_4$, the chemical name, 6,11-Dihydro-11-(1-methyl-4-piperidylidene)-*5H*-benzo[5,6] cyclohepta [1,2-b] pyridine maleate (1:2).

The molecular weight of azatadine maleate is 522.55. It is a white to off-white powder and is very soluble in water and soluble in alcohol.

Each Optimine tablet contains 1 mg azatadine maleate. *They Also Contain:* Corn starch, lactose, magnesium stearate, and providone.

INDICATIONS AND USAGE

Azatadine maleate is indicated for the treatment of perennial and seasonal allergic rhinitis and chronic urticaria.

CONTRAINDICATIONS

Antihistamines *should NOT* be used to treat lower respiratory tract symptoms, including asthma.

Antihistamines, including azatadine maleate, are also contraindicated in patients hypersensitive to this medication and to other antihistamines of similar chemical structure, and in patients receiving monoamine oxidase inhibitor therapy.

WARNINGS

Antihistamines should be used with caution in patients with narrow angle glaucoma, stenosing peptic ulcer; pyloroduodenal obstruction; and urinary bladder obstruction due to symptomatic prostatic hypertrophy and narrowing of the bladder neck.

Use with CNS Depressants: Antihistamines have additive effects with alcohol and other CNS depressants (hypnotics, sedatives, tranquilizers, etc.)

Use in Activities Requiring Mental Alertness: Patients should be warned about engaging in activities requiring mental alertness, such as driving a car or operating certain appliances, machinery, etc., until their response to this medication has been determined.

Use in Patients Approximately 60 Years or Older: Antihistamines are more likely to cause dizziness, sedation, and hypotension in patients over 60 years of age.

DOSAGE AND ADMINISTRATION

DOSAGE SHOULD BE INDIVIDUALIZED ACCORDING TO THE NEEDS AND THE RESPONSE OF THE PATIENT.

Azatadine maleate tablets are not recommended for use in children under 12 years of age: The usual adult dosage is 1 or 2 mg, twice a day.

PRODUCT LISTING - EQUIVALENTS NOT AVAILABLE

Tablet - Oral - 1 mg

100's	$126.00	OPTIMINE, Schering Corporation	00085-0282-03

Azathioprine (000351)

Categories: Arthritis, rheumatoid; Rejection, renal transplant, prophylaxis; Pregnancy Category D; FDA Approved 1968 Mar; WHO Formulary
Drug Classes: Disease modifying antirheumatic drugs; Immunosuppressives
Brand Names: Azathioprine Sodium; **Imuran**
Foreign Brand Availability: Azafalk (Germany); Azamedac (Germany); Azamun (Hong-Kong; New-Zealand; Taiwan); Azamune (England); Azanin (Japan); Azapress (South-Africa); Azathiodura (Germany); Azathioprine (Israel); Azatioprina (Peru); Azatrilem (Mexico); Azopi (Israel); Azoran (India); Imuprin (Bahamas; Bahrain; Barbados; Belize; Benin; Bermuda; Burkina-Faso; Curacao; Cyprus; Egypt; Ethiopia; Finland; Gambia; Ghana; Guinea; Guyana; Iran; Iraq; Ivory-Coast; Jamaica; Jordan; Kenya; Kuwait; Lebanon; Liberia; Libya; Malawi; Mali; Mauritania; Mauritius; Morocco; Netherland-Antilles; Niger; Nigeria; Oman; Qatar; Republic-of-Yemen; Saudi-Arabia; Senegal; Seychelles; Sierra-Leone; Sudan; Surinam; Syria; Tanzania; Trinidad; Tunia; Uganda; United-Arab-Emirates; Zambia; Zimbabwe); Imurek (Austria; Germany; Switzerland); Imurel (Denmark; Finland; France; Norway; Spain; Sweden); Thioprine (Australia; New-Zealand); Transimune (India); Zytrim (Germany)
Cost of Therapy: $195.64 (Transplant Rejection; Imuran; 50 mg; 4 tablets/day; 30 day supply)
$157.26 (Transplant Rejection; Generic Tablets; 50 mg; 4 tablets/day; 30 day supply)
HCFA JCODE(S): J7500 50 mg ORAL; J7501 100 mg IV

WARNING

Chronic immunosuppression with this purine antimetabolite increases *risk of neoplasia* in humans. Physicians using this drug should be very familiar with this risk as well as with the mutagenic potential to both men and women and with possible hematologic toxicities (see WARNINGS).

DESCRIPTION

Azathioprine, an immunosuppressive antimetabolite, is available in tablet form for oral administration and 100 mg vials for intravenous injection. Each scored tablet contains 50 mg azathioprine and the inactive ingredients lactose, magnesium stearate, potato starch, povidone, and stearic acid. Each 100 mg vial contains azathioprine, as the sodium salt, equivalent to 100 mg azathioprine sterile lyophilized material and sodium hydroxide to adjust pH.

Azathioprine is chemically 6-[(1-methyl-4-nitro-1*H*-imidazol-5-yl)thio]-1*H*-purine.

It is an imidazolyl derivative of 6-mercaptopurine (Purinethol) and many of its biological effects are similar to those of the parent compound.

Azathioprine is insoluble in water, but may be dissolved with addition of one molar equivalent of alkali. The sodium salt of azathioprine is sufficiently soluble to make a 10 mg/ml water solution which is stable for 24 hours at 15-25°C (59-77°F). Azathioprine is stable in solution at neutral or acid pH but hydrolysis to mercaptopurine occurs in excess sodium hydroxide (0.1N), especially on warming. Conversion to mercaptopurine also occurs in the presence of sulfhydryl compounds such as cysteine, glutathione and hydrogen sulfide.

CLINICAL PHARMACOLOGY

METABOLISM[1]

Azathioprine is well absorbed following oral administration. Maximum serum radioactivity occurs at 1 to 2 hours after oral ^{35}S-azathioprine and decays with a half-life of five hours. This is not an estimate of the half-life of azathioprine itself but is the decay rate for all ^{35}S-containing metabolites of the drug. Because of extensive metabolism, only a fraction of the radioactivity is present as azathioprine. Usual doses produce blood levels of azathioprine, and of mercaptopurine derived from it, which are low (<1 mcg/ml). Blood levels are of little predictive value for therapy since the magnitude and duration of clinical effects correlate with thiopurine nucleotide levels in tissues rather than with plasma drug levels. Azathioprine and mercaptopurine are moderately bound to serum proteins (30%) and are partially dialyzable.

Azathioprine is cleaved *in vivo* to mercaptopurine. Both compounds are rapidly eliminated from blood and are oxidized or methylated in erythrocytes and liver; no azathioprine or mercaptopurine is detectable in urine after 8 hours. Conversion to inactive 6-thiouric acid by xanthine oxidase is an important degradative pathway, and the inhibition of this pathway in patients receiving allopurinol (Zyloprim) is the basis for the azathioprine dosage reduction required in these patients (see DRUG INTERACTIONS). Proportions of metabolites are different in individual patients, and this presumably accounts for variable magnitude and duration of drug effects. Renal clearance is probably not important in predicting biological effectiveness or toxicities, although dose reduction is practiced in patients with poor renal function.

HOMOGRAFT SURVIVAL[1,2]

Summary information from transplant centers and registries indicates relatively universal use of azathioprine with or without other immunosuppressive agents.[3-5] Although the use of azathioprine for inhibition of renal homograft rejection is well established, the mechanism(s) for this action are somewhat obscure. The drug suppresses hypersensitivities of the cell-mediated type and causes variable alterations in antibody production. Suppression of T-cell effects, including ablation of T-cell suppression, is dependent on the temporal relationship to antigenic stimulus or engraftment. This agent has little effect on established graft rejections or secondary responses.

Alterations in specific immune responses or immunologic functions in transplant recipients are difficult to relate specifically to immunosuppression by azathioprine. These patients have subnormal responses to vaccines, low numbers of T-cells, and abnormal phagocytosis by peripheral blood cells, but their mitogenic responses, serum immunoglobulins and secondary antibody responses are usually normal.

IMMUNOINFLAMMATORY RESPONSE

Azathioprine suppresses disease manifestations as well as underlying pathology in animal models of autoimmune disease. For example, the severity of adjuvant arthritis is reduced by azathioprine.

The mechanisms whereby azathioprine affects autoimmune diseases are not known. Azathioprine is immunosuppressive, delayed hypersensitivity and cellular cytotoxicity tests being suppressed to a greater degree than are antibody responses. In the rat model of adjuvant arthritis, azathioprine has been shown to inhibit the lymph node hyperplasia which precedes the onset of the signs of the disease. Both the immunosuppressive and therapeutic effects in animal models are dose-related. Azathioprine is considered a slow-acting drug and effects may persist after the drug has been discontinued.

INDICATIONS AND USAGE

Azathioprine is indicated as an adjunct for the prevention of rejection in renal homotransplantation. It is also indicated for the management of severe, active rheumatoid arthritis unresponsive to rest, aspirin or other nonsteroidal anti-inflammatory drugs, or to agents in the class of which gold is an example.

RENAL HOMOTRANSPLANTATION

Azathioprine is indicated as an adjunct for the prevention of rejection in renal homotransplantation. Experience with over 16,000 transplants shows a 5 year patient survival of 35-55%, but this is dependent on donor, match for HLA antigens, anti-donor or anti B-cell alloantigen antibody and other variables. The effect of azathioprine on these variables has not been tested in controlled trials.

RHEUMATOID ARTHRITIS[6,7]

Azathioprine is indicated only in adult patients meeting criteria for classic or definite rheumatoid arthritis as specified by the American Rheumatism Association.[8] Azathioprine should be restricted to patients with severe, active and erosive disease not responsive to conventional management including rest, aspirin or other nonsteroidal drugs or to agents in the class of which gold is an example. Rest, physiotherapy and salicylates should be continued while azathioprine is given, but it may be possible to reduce the dose of corticosteroids in patients on azathioprine. The combined use of azathioprine with gold, antimalarials or penicillamine has not been studied for either added benefit or unexpected adverse effects. The use of azathioprine with these agents cannot be recommended.

NON-FDA APPROVED INDICATIONS

While not FDA approved indications, azathioprine has also been used in the treatment of systemic lupus erythematosus and other autoimmune diseases as well as some forms of chronic active hepatitis and low-risk gestational trophoblastic disease.

CONTRAINDICATIONS

Azathioprine should not be given to patients who have shown hypersensitivity to the drug.

Azathioprine should not be used for treating rheumatoid arthritis in pregnant women.

Patients with rheumatoid arthritis previously treated with alkylating agents (cyclophosphamide, chlorambucil, melphalan or others) may have a prohibitive risk of neoplasia if treated with azathioprine.[9]

WARNINGS

LEUKOPENIA AND/OR THROMBOCYTOPENIA

Severe leukopenia and/or thrombocytopenia may occur in patients on azathioprine. Macrocytic anemia and severe bone marrow depression may also occur. Hematologic toxicities are dose related and may be more severe in renal transplant patients whose homograft is undergoing rejection. It is suggested that patients on azathioprine have complete blood counts, including platelet counts, weekly during the first month, twice monthly for the second and third months of treatment, then monthly or more frequently if dosage alterations or other therapy changes are necessary. Delayed hematologic suppression may occur. Prompt reduction in dosage or temporary withdrawal of the drug may be necessary if there is a rapid fall in, or persistently low leukocyte count or other evidence of bone marrow depression. Leukopenia does not correlate with therapeutic effect; therefore the dose should not be increased intentionally to lower the white blood cell count.

SERIOUS INFECTIONS

Serious infections are a constant hazard for patients receiving chronic immunosuppression, especially for homograft recipients. Fungal, viral, bacterial and protozoal infections may be fatal and should be treated vigorously. Reduction of azathioprine dosage and/or use of other drugs should be considered.

RISK OF NEOPLASIA

Azathioprine is mutagenic in animals and humans, carcinogenic in animals, and may increase the patient's *risk of neoplasia.* Renal transplant patients are known to have an increased risk of malignancy, predominantly skin cancer and reticulum cell or lymphomatous tumors.[10] The risk of post-transplant lymphomas may be increased in patients who receive aggressive treatment with immunosuppressive drugs.[11] The degree of immunosuppression is determined not only by the immunosuppressive regimen but also by a number of other patient factors. The number of immunosuppressive agents may not necessarily increase the risk of post-transplant lymphomas. However, transplant patients who receive multiple immunosuppressive agents may be at risk for over-immunosuppression; therefore, immunosuppressive drug therapy should be maintained at the lowest effective levels. Information is available on the spontaneous neoplasia risk in rheumatoid arthritis,[12,13] and on neoplasia following immunosuppressive therapy of other autoimmune diseases.[14,15] It has not been possible to define the precise risk of neoplasia due to azathioprine.[16] The data suggest the risk may be elevated in patients with rheumatoid arthritis, though lower than for renal transplant patients.[11,13] However, acute myelogenous leukemia as well as solid tumors have been reported in patients with rheumatoid arthritis who have received azathioprine. Data on neoplasia in patients receiving azathioprine can be found under ADVERSE REACTIONS.

Azathioprine has been reported to cause temporary depression in spermatogenesis and reduction in sperm viability and sperm count in mice at doses 10 times the human therapeutic dose[17]; a reduced percentage of fertile matings occurred when animals received 5 mg/kg.[18]

PREGNANCY CATEGORY D

Azathioprine can cause fetal harm when administered to a pregnant woman. Azathioprine should not be given during pregnancy without careful weighing of risk versus benefit. Whenever possible, use of azathioprine in pregnant patients should be avoided. This drug should not be used for treating rheumatoid arthritis in pregnant women.[19]

Azathioprine is teratogenic in rabbits and mice when given in doses equivalent to the human dose[18] (5 mg/kg daily). Abnormalities included skeletal malformations and visceral anomalies.

Limited immunologic and other abnormalities have occurred in a few infants born of renal allograft recipients on azathioprine. In a detailed case report,[20] documented lymphopenia, diminished IgG and IgM levels, CMV infection, and a decreased thymic shadow were noted in an infant born to a mother receiving 150 mg azathioprine and 30 mg prednisone daily throughout pregnancy. At ten weeks most features were normalized. DeWitte *et al.*[21] reported pancytopenia and severe immune deficiency in a preterm infant whose mother received 125 mg azathioprine and 12.5 mg prednisone daily. There have been two published reports of abnormal physical findings. Williamson and Karp[22] described an infant born with preaxial polydactyly whose mother received azathioprine 200 mg daily and prednisone 20 mg every other day during pregnancy. Tallent et al[23] described an infant with a large myelomeningocele in the upper lumber region, bilateral dislocated hips, and bilateral talipes equinovarus. The father was on long-term azathioprine therapy.

Benefit versus risk must be weighed carefully before use of azathioprine in patients of reproductive potential. There are no adequate and well-controlled studies in pregnant women. If this drug is used during pregnancy or if the patient becomes pregnant while taking this drug, the patient should be apprised of the potential hazard to the fetus. Women of childbearing age should be advised to avoid becoming pregnant.

PRECAUTIONS

GENERAL

A gastrointestinal hypersensitivity reaction characterized by severe nausea and vomiting has been reported.[24-26] These symptoms may also be accompanied by diarrhea, rash, fever, malaise, myalgias, elevations in liver enzymes, and occasionally, hypotension. Symptoms of gastrointestinal toxicity most often develop within the first several weeks of azathioprine therapy and are reversible upon discontinuation of the drug. The reaction can recur within hours after rechallenge with a single dose of azathioprine.

INFORMATION FOR THE PATIENT

Patients being started on azathioprine should be informed of the necessity of periodic blood counts while they are receiving the drug and should be encouraged to report any unusual bleeding or bruising to their physician. They should be informed of the danger of infection while receiving azathioprine and asked to report signs and symptoms of infection to their physician. Careful dosage instructions should be given to the patient, especially when azathioprine is being administered in the presence of impaired renal function or concomitantly with allopurinol (see DOSAGE AND ADMINISTRATION and DRUG INTERACTIONS). Patients should be advised of the potential risks of the use of azathioprine during pregnancy and during the nursing period. The increased risk of neoplasia following azathioprine therapy should be explained to the patient.

LABORATORY TESTS

See WARNINGS and ADVERSE REACTIONS.

CARCINOGENESIS, MUTAGENESIS, AND IMPAIRMENT OF FERTILITY

See WARNINGS.

PREGNANCY, TERATOGENIC EFFECTS, PREGNANCY CATEGORY D

See WARNINGS, Pregnancy Category D.

NURSING MOTHERS

The use of azathioprine in nursing mothers is not recommended. Azathioprine or its metabolites are transferred at low levels, both transplacentally and in breast milk.[29-31] Because of the potential for tumorigenicity shown for azathioprine, a decision should be made whether to discontinue nursing or discontinue the drug, taking into account the importance of the drug to the mother.

PEDIATRIC USE

Safety and efficacy of azathioprine in children have not been established.

DRUG INTERACTIONS

Use with Allopurinol: The principal pathway for detoxification of azathioprine is inhibited by allopurinol. Patients receiving azathioprine and allopurinol concomitantly should have a dose reduction of azathioprine, to approximately 1/3 to 1/4 the usual dose.

Use with Other Agents Effecting Myelopoiesis: Drugs which may affect leukocyte production, including co-trimoxazole, may lead to exaggerated leukopenia, especially in renal transplant recipients. [27]

Use with Angiotensin Converting Enzyme Inhibitors: The use of angiotensin converting enzyme inhibitors to control hypertension in patients on azathioprine has been reported to induce severe leukopenia.[28]

Use with Warfarin: Azathioprine may inhibit the anticoagulant effect of warfarin.

ADVERSE REACTIONS

The principal and potentially serious toxic effects of azathioprine are hematologic and gastrointestinal. The risks of secondary infection and neoplasia are also significant (see WARNINGS). The frequency and severity of adverse reactions depend on the dose and duration of azathioprine as well as on the patient's underlying disease or concomitant therapies. The incidence of hematologic toxicities and neoplasia encountered in groups of renal homograft recipients is significantly higher than that in studies employing azathioprine for rheumatoid arthritis. The relative incidences in clinical studies are summarized in TABLE 1.

TABLE 1

Toxicity	Renal Homograft	Rheumatoid Arthritis
Leukopenia		
Any degree	>50%	28
<2500/mm^3	16%	5.3%
Infections	20%	<1%
Neoplasia		*
Lymphoma	0.5%	
Others	2.8%	

* Data on the rate and risk of neoplasia among persons with rheumatoid arthritis treated with azathioprine are limited. The incidence of lymphoproliferative disease in patients with RA appears to be significantly higher than that in the general population.[12] In one completed study, the rate of lymphoproliferative disease in RA patients receiving higher than recommended doses of azathioprine (5 mg/kg/day) was 1.8 cases per 1000 patient years of follow-up, compared with 0.8 cases per 1000 patient years of follow-up in those not receiving azathioprine.[13] However, the proportion of the increased risk attributable to the azathioprine dosage or to other therapies (*i.e.*, alkylating agents) received by patients treated with azathioprine cannot be determined.

HEMATOLOGIC

Leukopenia and/or thrombocytopenia are dose dependent and may occur late in the course of therapy with azathioprine. Dose reduction or temporary withdrawal allows reversal of these toxicities. Infection may occur as a secondary manifestation of bone marrow suppression or leukopenia, but the incidence of infection in renal homotransplantation is 30-60 times that in rheumatoid arthritis. Macrocytic anemia and/or bleeding have been reported.

There are rare individuals with an inherited deficiency of the enzyme thiopurine methyltransferase (TPMT) who may be unusually sensitive to the myelosuppressive effect of azathioprine and prone to developing rapid bone marrow suppression following the initiation of treatement with azathioprine.

GASTROINTESTINAL

Nausea and vomiting may occur within the first few months of therapy with azathioprine, and occurred in approximately 12% of 676 rheumatoid arthritis patients. The frequency of gastric disturbance often can be reduced by administration of the drug in divided doses and/or after meals. However, in some patients, nausea and vomiting may be severe and may be accompanied by symptoms such as diarrhea, fever, malaise, and myalgias (see PRECAUTIONS). Vomiting with abdominal pain may occur rarely with a hypersensitivity pancreatitis. Hepatotoxicity manifest by elevation of serum alkaline phosphatase, bilirubin and/or serum transaminases is known to occur following azathioprine use, primarily in allograft recipients. Hepatotoxicity has been uncommon (less than 1%) in rheumatoid arthritis patients. Hepatotoxicity following transplantation most often occurs within 6 months of transplantation and is generally reversible after interruption of azathioprine. A rare, but life-threatening hepatic veno-occlusive disease associated with chronic administration of azathioprine has been described in transplant patients and in one patient receiving azathioprine for panuveitis.[32-34] Periodic measurement of serum transaminases, alkaline phosphatase and bilirubin is indicated for early detection of hepatotoxicity. If hepatic veno-occlusive disease is clinically suspected, azathioprine should be permanently withdrawn.

OTHERS

Additional side effects of low frequency have been reported. These include skin rashes, alopecia, fever, arthralgias, diarrhea, steatorrhea and negative nitrogen balance, and reversible interstitial pneumonitis.

DOSAGE AND ADMINISTRATION

RENAL HOMOTRANSPLANTATION

The dose of azathioprine required to prevent rejection and minimize toxicity will vary with individual patients; this necessitates careful management. The initial dose is usually 3-5 mg/kg daily, beginning at the time of transplant. Azathioprine is usually given as a single daily dose on the day of, and in a minority of cases one to three days before, transplantation. Azathioprine is often initiated with the intravenous administration of the sodium salt, with subsequent use of tablets (at the same dose level) after the postoperative period. Intravenous administration of the sodium salt is indicated only in patients unable to tolerate oral medications. Dose reduction to maintenance levels of 1-3 mg/kg daily is usually possible. The dose of azathioprine should not be increased to toxic levels because of threatened rejection. Discontinuation may be necessary for severe hematologic or other toxicity, even if rejection of the homograft may be a consequence of drug withdrawal.

RHEUMATOID ARTHRITIS

Azathioprine is usually given on a daily basis. The initial dose should be approximately 1.0 mg/kg (50-100 mg) given as a single dose or on a twice daily schedule. The dose may be increased, beginning at 6-8 weeks and thereafter by steps at 4 week intervals, if there are no serious toxicities and if initial response is unsatisfactory. Dose increments should be 0.5 mg/kg daily, up to a maximum dose of 2.5 mg/kg/day. Therapeutic response occurs after several weeks of treatment, usually 6-8; an adequate trial should be a minimum of 12 weeks. Patients not improved after 12 weeks can be considered refractory. Azathioprine may be continued long-term in patients with clinical response, but patients should be monitored carefully, and gradual dosage reduction should be attempted to reduce risk of toxicities.

Maintenance therapy should be at the lowest effective dose, and the dose given can be lowered decrementally with changes of 0.5 mg/kg or approximately 25 mg daily every 4 weeks while other therapy is kept constant. The optimum duration of maintenance azathioprine has not been determined. Azathioprine can be discontinued abruptly, but delayed effects are possible.

USE IN RENAL DYSFUNCTION

Relatively oliguric patients, especially those with tubular necrosis in the immediate postcadaveric transplant period, may have delayed clearance of azathioprine or its metabolites, may be particularly sensitive to this drug, and are usually given lower doses.

PARENTERAL ADMINISTRATION

Add 10 ml of sterile water for injection, and swirl until a clear solution results. This solution, equivalent to 100 mg azathioprine, is for intravenous use only; it has a pH of approximately 9.6, and it should be used within 24 hours. Further dilution into sterile saline or dextrose is usually made for infusion; the final volume depends on time for the infusion, usually 30-60 minutes, but as short as 5 minutes and as long as 8 hours for the daily dose.

Parenteral drug products should be inspected visually for particulate matter and discoloration prior to administration, whenever solution and container permit.

Procedures for proper handling and disposal of this immunosuppressive antimetabolite drug should be considered. Several guidelines on this subject have been published.[36-42] There is no general agreement that all of the procedures recommended in the guidelines are necessary or appropriate.

HOW SUPPLIED

50 mg Tablets: Overlapping circle-shaped, yellow to off-white, scored tablets imprinted with "Imuran" and "50" on each tablet.

Store at 15-25°C (59-77°F) in a dry place and protect from light.

20 ml Vial: Each contains the equivalent of 100 mg azathioprine (as the sodium salt).

Store at 15-25°C (59-77°F) and protect from light. The sterile, lyophilized sodium salt is yellow, and should be dissolved in sterile water for injection (see DOSAGE AND ADMINISTRATION, Parenteral Administration).

PRODUCT LISTING - RATED THERAPEUTICALLY EQUIVALENT

Powder For Injection - Intravenous - 100 mg

1's	$85.00	GENERIC, Bedford Laboratories	55390-0600-20
1's	$113.59	IMURAN, Faro Pharmaceuticals Inc	60976-0598-71

Tablet - Oral - 50 mg

50's	$86.84	IMURAN, Physicians Total Care	54868-0921-04
100's	$130.93	GENERIC, Geneva Pharmaceuticals	00781-1059-01
100's	$131.05	GENERIC, Mylan Pharmaceuticals Inc	00378-1005-01
100's	$131.08	GENERIC, Roxane Laboratories Inc	00054-4084-25
100's	$144.18	GENERIC, Roxane Laboratories Inc	00054-8084-25
100's	$163.03	IMURAN, Pharma Pac	52959-0079-00
100's	$231.14	IMURAN, Prometheus Inc	65483-0590-10

PRODUCT LISTING - EQUIVALENTS NOT AVAILABLE

Tablet - Oral - 50 mg

100's	$131.08	GENERIC, Aaipharma	66591-0221-41

Azelaic Acid *(003268)*

Categories: Acne vulgaris; Rosacea; FDA Approved 1995 Sep; Pregnancy Category B
Drug Classes: Anti-infectives, topical; Dermatologics
Brand Names: Azelex; Finacea; Finevin
Foreign Brand Availability: Azalea (Korea); Cutacelan (Mexico; Peru); Skinoderm (Israel); Skinorem (Bahrain; Cyprus; Egypt; Iran; Iraq; Jordan; Kuwait; Lebanon; Libya; Oman; Qatar; Republic-of-Yemen; Saudi-Arabia; Syria; United-Arab-Emirates); Skinoren (Australia; Austria; Belgium; China; Czech-Republic; Denmark; England; Finland; Germany; Greece; Hong-Kong; Indonesia; Ireland; Italy; Malaysia; New-Zealand; Norway; Philippines; Portugal; South-Africa; Spain; Switzerland; Taiwan; Thailand); Zeliris (Indonesia)
Cost of Therapy: $40.19 (Acne; Azelex Cream; 20%; 30 g; 2 applications/day; variable day supply)

DESCRIPTION

AZELAIC ACID CREAM

For Dermatologic Use Only — Not for Ophthalmic Use.

Finevin (azelaic acid cream) 20% contains azelaic acid, a naturally occurring saturated dicarboxylic acid.

The chemical name is 1,7-heptanedicarboxylic acid. The empirical formula is $C_9H_{16}O_4$, and the molecular weight is 188.22.

Active Ingredient: Each gram of Finevin contains azelaic acid 0.2 g (20% w/w).

Inactive Ingredients: Cetearyl octanoate, glycerin, glyceryl stearate, cetearyl alcohol, cetyl palmitate, cocoglycerides, PEG-5 glyceryl stearate, propylene glycol and purified water. Benzoic acid is present as a preservative.

AZELAIC ACID GEL

For Dermatologic Use Only — Not for Ophthalmic, Oral, or Intravaginal Use.

Finacea (azelaic acid) gel, 15%, contains azelaic acid, a naturally occurring saturated dicarboxylic acid. Chemically, azelaic acid is 1,7-heptanedicarboxylic acid, with the molecular formula $C_9H_{16}O_4$, and a molecular weight of 188.22.

Azelaic acid is a white, odorless crystalline solid that is poorly soluble in water at 20°C (0.24%), but freely soluble in boiling water and in ethanol.

Each gram of Finacea gel, 15%, contains 0.15 gm azelaic acid (15% w/w) as the active ingredient in an aqueous gel base containing benzoic acid (as a preservative), disodium-EDTA, lecithin, medium-chain triglycerides, polyacrylic acid, polysorbate 80, propylene glycol, purified water, and sodium hydroxide to adjust pH.

CLINICAL PHARMACOLOGY

AZELAIC ACID CREAM

The exact mechanism of action of azelaic acid is not known. The following *in vitro* data are available, but their clinical significance is unknown. Azelaic acid has been shown to possess antimicrobial activity against *Propionibacterium acnes* and *Staphylococcus epidermidis.* The antimicrobial action may be attributable to inhibition of microbial cellular protein synthesis.

A normalization of keratinization leading to an anticomedonal effect of azelaic acid may also contribute to its clinical activity. Electron microscopic and immunohistochemical evaluation of skin biopsies from human subjects treated with azelaic acid cream 20% demonstrated a reduction in the thickness of the stratum corneum, a reduction in number and size of keratohyalin granules, and a reduction in the amount and distribution of filaggrin (a protein component of keratohyalin) in epidermal layers. This is suggestive of the ability to decrease microcomedo formation.

Pharmacokinetics

Following a single application of azelaic acid cream 20% to human skin *in vitro,* azelaic acid penetrates into the stratum corneum (approximately 3-5% of the applied dose) and other viable skin layers (up to 10% of the dose is found in the epidermis and dermis). Negligible cutaneous metabolism occurs after topical application. Approximately 4% of the topically applied azelaic acid is systemically absorbed. Azelaic acid is mainly excreted unchanged in the urine but undergoes some β-oxidation to shorter chain dicarboxylic acids. The observed half-lives in healthy subjects are approximately 45 minutes after oral dosing and 12 hours after topical dosing, indicating percutaneous absorption rate-limited kinetics.

Azelaic acid is a dietary constituent (whole grain cereals and animal products), and can be formed endogenously from longer-chain dicarboxylic acids, metabolism of oleic acid, and ω-oxidation of monocarboxylic acids. Endogenous plasma concentration (20-80 ng/ml) and daily urinary excretion (4-28 mg) of azelaic acid are highly dependent on dietary intake. After topical treatment with azelaic acid cream 20% in humans, plasma concentration and urinary excretion of azelaic acid are not significantly different from baseline levels.

AZELAIC ACID GEL

The mechanism(s) by which azelaic acid interferes with the pathogenic events in rosacea are unknown.

Pharmacokinetics

The percutaneous absorption of azelaic acid after topical application of azelaic acid gel, 15%, could not be reliably determined. Mean plasma azelaic acid concentrations in rosacea patients treated with azelaic acid gel, 15%, twice daily for at least 8 weeks are in the range of 42-63.1 ng/ml. These values are within the maximum concentration range of 24.0-90.5 ng/ml observed in rosacea patients treated with vehicle only. This indicates that azelaic acid gel, 15%, does not increase plasma azelaic acid concentration beyond the range derived from nutrition and endogenous metabolism.

In vitro and human data suggest negligible cutaneous metabolism of ^{3}H-azelaic acid 20% cream after topical application. Azelaic acid is mainly excreted unchanged in the urine, but undergoes some β-oxidation to shorter chain dicarboxylic acids.

INDICATIONS AND USAGE

AZELAIC ACID CREAM

Azelaic acid cream 20% is indicated for the topical treatment of mild-to-moderate inflammatory acne vulgaris.

AZELAIC ACID GEL

Azelaic acid gel, 15%, is indicated for topical treatment of inflammatory papules and pustules of mild to moderate rosacea. Patients should be instructed to avoid spicy foods, thermally hot foods and drinks, alcoholic beverages and to use only very mild soaps or soapless cleansing lotion for facial cleansing.

NON-FDA APPROVED INDICATIONS

Due to its seemingly selective inhibitory effects on abnormal melanocytes, azelaic acid has also been used to treat cutaneous hyperpigmentary disorders such as melasma and lentigo maligna, the latter with variable success. In addition, results from a preliminary uncontrolled study demonstrated beneficial effects on the primary lesions of malignant melanoma using a regimen of 10-15 g of oral AZA per day with twice daily applications of a 15% cream. However, the use of azelaic acid for conditions other than acne and rosacea is not approved by the FDA, and specifically for lentigo maligna and malignant melanoma, the primary therapy remains surgical excision.

CONTRAINDICATIONS

AZELAIC ACID CREAM

Azelaic acid cream 20% is contraindicated in individuals who have shown hypersensitivity to any of its components.

AZELAIC ACID GEL

Azelaic acid gel, 15%, is contraindicated in individuals with a history of hypersensitivity to propylene glycol or any other component of the formulation.

WARNINGS

AZELAIC ACID CREAM

Azelaic acid cream 20% is for dermatologic use only and not for ophthalmic use.

There have been isolated reports of hypopigmentation after use of azelaic acid. Since azelaic acid has not been well studied in patients with dark complexions, these patients should be monitored for early signs of hypopigmentation.

AZELAIC ACID GEL

Azelaic acid gel, 15%, is for dermatologic use only, and not for ophthalmic, oral or intravaginal use.

There have been isolated reports of hypopigmentation after use of azelaic acid. Since azelaic acid has not been well studied in patients with dark complexion, these patients should be monitored for early signs of hypopigmentation.

PRECAUTIONS

AZELAIC ACID CREAM

General

If sensitivity or severe irritation develop with the use of azelaic acid cream 20%, treatment should be discontinued and appropriate therapy instituted.

Information for the Patient

Patients Should Be Told:

- To use azelaic acid cream 20% for the full prescribed treatment period.
- To avoid the use of occlusive dressings or wrappings.
- To keep azelaic acid cream 20% away from the mouth, eyes, and other mucous membranes. If it does come in contact with the eyes, they should wash their eyes with large amounts of water and consult a physician if eye irritation persists.
- If they have dark complexions, to report abnormal changes in skin color to their physician.
- Due in part to the low pH of azelaic acid, temporary skin irritation (pruritus, burning, or stinging) may occur when azelaic acid cream 20% is applied to broken or inflamed skin, usually at the start of treatment. However, this irritation commonly subsides if treatment is continued. If it continues, azelaic acid cream 20% should be applied only once-a-day, or the treatment should be stopped until these effects have subsided. If troublesome irritation persists, use should be discontinued, and patients should consult their physician. (See ADVERSE REACTIONS, Azelaic Acid Cream.)

Carcinogenesis, Mutagenesis, and Impairment of Fertility

Azelaic acid is a human dietary component of a simple molecular structure that does not suggest carcinogenic potential, and it does not belong to a class of drugs for which there is a concern about carcinogenicity. Therefore, animal studies to evaluate carcinogenic potential with azelaic acid cream 20% were not deemed necessary. In a battery of tests (Ames assay, HGPRT test in Chinese hamster ovary cells, human lymphocyte test, dominant lethal assay in mice), azelaic acid was found to be nonmutagenic. Animal studies have shown no adverse effects on fertility.

Pregnancy, Teratogenic Effects, Pregnancy Category B

Embryotoxic effects were observed in Segment I and Segment II oral studies with rats receiving 2500 mg/kg/day of azelaic acid. Similar effects were observed in Segment II studies in rabbits given 150-500 mg/kg/day and in monkeys given 500 mg/kg/day. The doses at which these effects were noted were all within toxic dose ranges for the dams. No teratogenic effects were observed. There are, however, no adequate and well-controlled studies in pregnant women. Because animal reproduction studies are not always predictive of human response, this drug should be used during pregnancy only if clearly needed.

Nursing Mothers

Equilibrium dialysis was used to assess human milk partitioning *in vitro*. At an azelaic acid concentration of 25 μg/ml, the milk/plasma distribution coefficient was 0.7 and the milk/buffer distribution was 1.0, indicating that passage of drug into maternal milk may occur. Since less than 4% of a topically applied dose is systemically absorbed, the uptake of azelaic acid into maternal milk is not expected to cause a significant change from baseline azelaic acid levels in the milk. However, caution should be exercised when azelaic acid cream 20% is administered to a nursing mother.

Pediatric Use

Safety and effectiveness in pediatric patients under 12 years of age have not been established.

AZELAIC ACID GEL

General

Contact with the eyes should be avoided. If sensitivity or severe irritation develops with the use of azelaic acid gel, 15%, treatment should be discontinued and appropriate therapy instituted. The safety and efficacy of azelaic acid gel, 15%, has not been studied beyond 12 weeks.

Information for the Patient

Patients using azelaic acid gel, 15%, should receive the following information and instructions:

- Azelaic acid gel, 15%, is to be used only as directed by the physician.
- Azelaic acid gel, 15%, is for external use only. It is not to be used orally, intravaginally, or for the eyes.
- Cleanse affected area(s) with a very mild soap or a soapless cleansing lotion and pat dry with a soft towel before applying azelaic acid gel, 15%. Avoid alcoholic cleansers, tinctures and astringents, abrasives and peeling agents.
- Avoid contact of azelaic acid gel, 15%, with the mouth, eyes and other mucous membranes. If it does come in contact with the eyes, wash the eyes with large amounts of water and consult a physician if eye irritation persists.
- The hands should be washed following application of azelaic acid gel, 15%.
- Cosmetics may be applied after azelaic acid gel, 15%, has dried.
- Skin irritation (*e.g.*, pruritus, burning, or stinging) may occur during use of azelaic acid gel, 15%, usually during the first few weeks of treatment. If irritation is excessive or persists, use of azelaic acid gel, 15%, should be discontinued, and patients should consult their physician (see ADVERSE REACTIONS, Azelaic Acid Gel).
- Avoid any foods and beverages that might provoke erythema, flushing, and blushing (including spicy food, alcoholic beverages, and thermally hot drinks, including hot coffee and tea).
- Patients should report abnormal changes in skin color to their physician.
- Avoid the use of occlusive dressings or wrappings.

Carcinogenesis, Mutagenesis, and Impairment of Fertility

Long-term animal studies have not been performed to evaluate the carcinogenic potential of azelaic acid gel, 15%. Azelaic acid was not mutagenic or clastogenic in a battery of *in vitro* (Ames assay, HGPRT in V79 cells [Chinese hamster lung cells], and chromosomal aberration assay in human lymphocytes) and *in vivo* (dominant lethal assay in mice and mouse micronucleus assay) genotoxicity tests.

Oral administration of azelaic acid at dose levels up to 2500 mg/kg/day (162 times the maximum recommended human dose based on body surface area) did not affect fertility or reproductive performance in male or female rats.

Pregnancy, Teratogenic Effects, Pregnancy Category B

There are no adequate and well-controlled studies of topically administered azelaic acid in pregnant women. The experience with azelaic acid gel, 15%, when used by pregnant women is too limited to permit assessment of the safety of its use during pregnancy.

Dermal embryofetal developmental toxicology studies have not been performed with azelaic acid, 15%, gel. Oral embryofetal developmental studies were conducted with azelaic acid in rats, rabbits, and cynomolgus monkeys. Azelaic acid was administered during the period of organogeneisis in all three animal species. Embryotoxicity was observed in rats, rabbits, and monkeys at oral doses of azelaic acid that generated some maternal toxicity. Embryotoxicity was observed in rats given 2500 mg/kg/day (162 times the maximum recommended human dose based on body surface area), rabbits given 150 or 500 mg/kg/day (19 or 65 times the maximum recommended human dose based on body surface area) and cynomolgus monkeys given 500 mg/kg/day (65 times the maximum recommended human dose based on body surface area) azelaic acid. No teratogenic effects were observed in the oral embryofetal developmental studies conducted in rats, rabbits and cynomolgus monkeys.

An oral peri- and postnatal developmental study was conducted in rats. Azelaic acid was administered from gestational Day 15 through Day 21 postpartum up to a dose level of 2500 mg/kg/day. Embryotoxicity was observed in rats at an oral dose that generated some maternal toxicity (2500 mg/kg/day; 162 times the maximum recommended human dose based on body surface area). In addition, slight disturbances in the postnatal development of fetuses was noted in rats at oral doses that generated some maternal toxicity (500 and 2500 mg/kg/day; 32 and 162 times the maximum recommended human dose based on body surface area). No effects on sexual maturation of the fetuses were noted in this study.

Because animal reproduction studies are not always predictive of human response, this drug should be used only if clearly needed during pregnancy.

Nursing Mothers

Equilibrium dialysis was used to assess human milk partitioning *in vitro*. At an azelaic acid concentration of 25 μg/ml, the milk/plasma distribution coefficient was 0.7 and the milk/buffer distribution was 1.0, indicating that passage of drug into maternal milk may occur. Since less than 4% of a topically applied dose of azelaic acid cream, 20%, is systemically absorbed, the uptake of azelaic acid into maternal milk is not expected to cause a significant change from baseline azelaic acid levels in the milk. However, caution should be exercised when azelaic acid gel, 15%, is administered to a nursing mother.

Pediatric Use

Safety and effectiveness of azelaic acid gel, 15%, in pediatric patients have not been established.

Geriatric Use

Clinical studies of azelaic acid gel, 15%, did not include sufficient numbers of subjects aged 65 and over to determine whether they respond differently from younger subjects.

DRUG INTERACTIONS

AZELAIC ACID GEL

There have been no formal studies of the interaction of azelaic acid gel, 15%, with other drugs.

ADVERSE REACTIONS

AZELAIC ACID CREAM

During US clinical trials with azelaic acid cream, 20%, adverse reactions were generally mild and transient in nature. The most common adverse reactions occurring in approximately 1-5% of patients were pruritus, burning, stinging and tingling. Other adverse reactions such as erythema, dryness, rash, peeling, irritation, dermatitis, and contact dermatitis were reported in less than 1% of subjects. There is the potential for experiencing allergic reactions with use of azelaic acid cream, 20%.

In patients using azelaic acid formulations, the following additional adverse experiences have been reported rarely: worsening of asthma, vitiligo depigmentation, small depigmented spots, hypertrichosis, reddening (signs of keratosis pilaris), and exacerbation of recurrent herpes labialis.

AZELAIC ACID GEL

In the two vehicle controlled, identically designed US clinical studies, treatment safety was monitored in 664 patients who used azelaic acid gel, 15%, (n=333), or the gel vehicle (n=331), twice daily for 12 weeks.

Azelaic acid gel, 15%, and its vehicle caused irritant reactions at the application site in human dermal safety studies. Azelaic acid gel, 15%, caused significantly more irritation than its vehicle in a cumulative irritation study. Some improvement in irritation was demonstrated over the course of the clinical studies, but this improvement might be attributed to subject dropouts. No phototoxicity or photoallergenicity were reported in human dermal safety studies.

In patients using azelaic acid formulations, the following additional adverse experiences have been reported rarely: worsening of asthma, vitiligo depigmentation, small depigmented spots, hypertrichosis, reddening (signs of keratosis pilaris), and exacerbation of recurrent herpes labialis.

DOSAGE AND ADMINISTRATION

AZELAIC ACID CREAM

After the skin is thoroughly washed and patted dry, a thin film of azelaic acid cream 20% should be gently but thoroughly massaged into the affected areas twice daily, in the morning and evening. The hands should be washed following application. The duration of use of azelaic acid cream 20% can vary from person to person and depends on the severity of the acne. Improvement of the condition occurs in the majority of patients with inflammatory lesions within 4 weeks.

TABLE 3 *Cutaneous Adverse Events Occurring in ≥1% of Subjects in the Rosacea Trials by Treatment Group and Maximum Intensity**

	Azelaic Acid Gel n=333 (100%)			Vehicle n=331 (100%)		
	Mild n=86 (26%)	Moderate n=44 (13%)	Severe n=20 (6%)	Mild n=49 (15%)	Moderate n=27 (8%)	Severe n=5 (2%)
Burning/stinging/ tingling	66 (20%)	30 (9%)	12 (4%)	8 (2%)	6 (2%)	2 (1%)
Pruritus	24 (7%)	14 (4%)	3 (1%)	9 (3%)	6 (2%)	0 (0%)
Scaling/dry skin/ xerosis	21 (6%)	8 (2%)	4 (1%)	33 (10%)	12 (4%)	1 (0%)
Erythema/irritation	6 (2%)	6 (2%)	1 (0%)	8 (2%)	4 (1%)	2 (1%)
Edema	3 (1%)	2 (1%)	0 (0%)	3 (1%)	0 (0%)	0 (0%)
Contact dermatitis	2 (1%)	2 (1%)	0 (0%)	1 (0%)	0 (0%)	0 (0%)
Acne	2 (1%)	1 (0%)	0 (0%)	1 (0%)	0 (0%)	0 (0%)
Seborrhea	2 (1%)	0 (0%)	0 (0%)	0 (0%)	0 (0%)	0 (0%)
Photosensitivity	1 (0%)	0 (0%)	0 (0%)	3 (1%)	1 (0%)	1 (0%)
Skin disease	1 (0%)	0 (0%)	0 (0%)	1 (0%)	2 (1%)	0 (0%)

* Subjects may have >1 cutaneous adverse event; thus, the sum of the frequencies of preferred terms may exceed the number of subjects with at least 1 cutaneous adverse event.

AZELAIC ACID GEL

A thin layer of azelaic acid gel, 15%, should be gently massaged into the affected areas on the face twice daily, in the morning and evening. Azelaic acid gel, 15%, has only been studied up to 12 weeks in patients with mild to moderate rosacea.

HOW SUPPLIED

AZELAIC ACID CREAM

Finevin Cream

Finevin 20% is supplied in 30 and 50 g collapsible tubes.

Storage: Protect from freezing. Store between 15-30°C (59-86°F).

AZELAIC ACID GEL

Finacea Gel

Finacea gel, 15%, is supplied in 30 g tubes.

Storage: Store at 25°C (77°F); excursions permitted between 15-30°C (59-86°F).

PRODUCT LISTING - EQUIVALENTS NOT AVAILABLE

Cream - Topical - 20%

30 gm	$40.19	AZELEX, Allscripts Pharmaceutical Company	54569-4635-00
30 gm	$40.44	FINEVIN, Berlex Laboratories	50419-0820-01
30 gm	$50.95	AZELEX, Allergan Inc	00023-8694-30
50 gm	$67.38	FINEVIN, Berlex Laboratories	50419-0820-02
50 gm	$84.88	AZELEX, Allergan Inc	00023-8694-50

Gel - Topical - 15%

30 gm	$43.20	FINACEA, Berlex Laboratories	50419-0825-01

Azelastine *(003278)*

Categories: Conjunctivitis, allergic; Rhinitis, seasonal allergic; Rhinitis, vasomotor; FDA Approved 1996 Oct; Pregnancy Category C

Drug Classes: Antihistamines, H1; Antihistamines, inhalation; Antihistamines, ophthalmic; Ophthalmics

Brand Names: **Astelin**

Foreign Brand Availability: Alastine (Korea); Allergodil (Austria; Belgium; Denmark; France; Germany; Hungary; Italy; Netherlands; Portugal; Russia; Switzerland); Amelor (Colombia); Azella (Korea); Azep (Singapore); Azeptin (Japan); Optilast (Israel); Rhinolast (Israel)

Cost of Therapy: $64.35 (Allergic Rhinitis; Optivar; 0.5%; 6ml; 4 drops/day; 14 day supply)
$27.94 (Allergic Rhinitis; Astelin; 137 µg/inh;34 ml; 4 sprays/day; 25 day supply)

INTRANASAL

DESCRIPTION

Astelin (azelastine hydrochloride) nasal spray, 137 µg, is an antihistamine formulated as a metered-spray solution for intranasal administration. Azelastine hydrochloride occurs as a white, almost odorless, crystalline powder with a bitter taste. It has a molecular weight of 418.37. It is sparingly soluble in water, methanol, and propylene glycol and slightly soluble in ethanol, octanol, and glycerine. It has a melting point of about 225°C and the pH of a saturated solution is between 5.0 and 5.4. Its chemical name is (±)-1-(2H)-phthalazinone,4-[(4-chlorophenyl) methyl]-2-(hexahydro-1-methyl-1H-azepin-4-yl)-, monohydrochloride. Its molecular formula is $C_{22}H_{24}ClN_3O{\cdot}HCl$.

Astelin nasal spray contains 0.1% azelastine hydrochloride in an aqueous solution at pH 6.8 ± 0.3. It also contains benzalkonium chloride (125 µg/ml), edetate disodium, hydroxypropyl methyl cellulose, citric acid, dibasic sodium phosphate, sodium chloride, and purified water.

After priming, each metered spray delivers a 0.137 ml mean volume containing 137 µg of azelastine hydrochloride (equivalent to 125 µg of azelastine base). Each bottle can deliver 100 metered sprays.

CLINICAL PHARMACOLOGY

Azelastine hydrochloride, a phthalazinone derivative, exhibits histamine H_1-receptor antagonist activity in isolated tissues, animal models, and humans. Azelastine nasal spray is administered as a racemic mixture with no difference in pharmacologic activity noted between the enantiomers in *in vitro* studies. The major metabolite, desmethylazelastine, also possesses H_1-receptor antagonist activity.

PHARMACOKINETICS AND METABOLISM

After intranasal administration, the systemic bioavailability of azelastine hydrochloride is approximately 40%. Maximum plasma concentrations (C_{max}) are achieved in 2-3 hours. Based on intravenous and oral administration, the elimination half-life, steady-state volume of distribution, and plasma clearance are 22 hours, 14.5 L/kg, and 0.5 L/h/kg, respectively. Approximately 75% of an oral dose of radiolabeled azelastine hydrochloride was excreted in the feces with less than 10% as unchanged azelastine. Azelastine is oxidatively metabolized to the principal active metabolite, desmethylazelastine, by the cytochrome P450 enzyme system. The specific P450 isoforms responsible for the biotransformation of azelastine have not been identified; however, clinical interaction studies with the known CYP3A4 inhibitor erythromycin failed to demonstrate a pharmacokinetic interaction. In a multiple-dose, steady-state drug interaction study in normal volunteers, cimetidine (400 mg twice daily), a nonspecific P450 inhibitor, raised orally administered mean azelastine (4 mg twice daily) concentrations by approximately 65%.

The major active metabolite, desmethylazelastine, was not measurable (below assay limits) after single-dose intranasal administration of azelastine hydrochloride. After intranasal dosing of azelastine hydrochloride to steady-state, plasma concentrations of desmethylazelastine range from 20-50% of azelastine concentrations. When azelastine hydrochloride is administered orally, desmethylazelastine has an elimination half-life of 54 hours. Limited data indicate that the metabolite profile is similar when azelastine hydrochloride is administered via the intranasal or oral route.

In vitro studies with human plasma indicate that the plasma protein binding of azelastine and desmethylazelastine are approximately 88% and 97%, respectively.

Azelastine hydrochloride administered intranasally at doses above 2 sprays per nostril twice daily for 29 days resulted in greater than proportional increases in C_{max} and area under the curve (AUC) for azelastine.

Studies in healthy subjects administered oral doses of azelastine hydrochloride demonstrated linear responses in C_{max} and AUC.

SPECIAL POPULATIONS

Following oral administration, pharmacokinetic parameters were not influenced by age, gender, or hepatic impairment.

Based on oral, single-dose studies, renal insufficiency (creatinine clearance <50 ml/min) resulted in a 70-75% higher C_{max} and AUC compared to normal subjects. Time to maximum concentration was unchanged.

Oral azelastine has been safely administered to over 1400 asthmatic subjects, supporting the safety of administering azelastine nasal spray to allergic rhinitis patients with asthma.

PHARMACODYNAMICS

In a placebo-controlled study (95 subjects with allergic rhinitis), there was no evidence of an effect of azelastine nasal spray (2 sprays per nostril twice daily for 56 days) on cardiac repolarization as represented by the corrected QT interval (QTc) of the electrocardiogram. At higher oral exposures (≥4 mg twice daily), a nonclinically significant mean change on the QTc (3-7 millisecond increase) was observed.

Interaction studies investigating the cardiac repolarization effects of concomitantly administered oral azelastine hydrochloride and erythromycin or ketoconazole were conducted. Oral erythromycin had no effect on azelastine pharmacokinetics or QTc based on analysis of serial electrocardiograms. Ketoconazole interfered with the measurement of azelastine plasma levels; however, no effects on QTc were observed (see DRUG INTERACTIONS).

INDICATIONS AND USAGE

Azelastine nasal spray is indicated for the treatment of the symptoms of seasonal allergic rhinitis such as rhinorrhea, sneezing, and nasal pruritus in adults and children 5 years and older, and for the treatment of the symptoms of vasomotor rhinitis, such as rhinorrhea, nasal congestion and postnasal drip in adults and children 12 years and older.

CONTRAINDICATIONS

Azelastine nasal spray is contraindicated in patients with a known hypersensitivity to azelastine hydrochloride or any of its components.

PRECAUTIONS

ACTIVITIES REQUIRING MENTAL ALERTNESS

In clinical trials, the occurrence of somnolence has been reported in some patients taking azelastine nasal spray; due caution should therefore be exercised when driving a car or operating potentially dangerous machinery. Concurrent use of Azelastine nasal spray with alcohol or other CNS depressants should be avoided because additional reductions in alertness and additional impairment of CNS performance may occur.

INFORMATION FOR THE PATIENT

Patients should be instructed to use azelastine nasal spray only as prescribed. For the proper use of the nasal spray and to attain maximum improvement, the patient should read and follow carefully the accompanying patient instructions. Patients should be instructed to prime the delivery system before initial use and after storage for 3 or more days (see illustrated patient instructions for proper use accompanying each package of azelastine nasal spray.). Patients should also be instructed to store the bottle upright at room temperature with the pump tightly closed and out of the reach of children. In case of accidental ingestion by a young child, seek professional assistance or contact a poison control center immediately.

Patients should be advised against the concurrent use of azelastine nasal spray with other antihistamines without consulting a physician. Patients who are, or may become, pregnant should be told that this product should be used in pregnancy or during lactation only if the potential benefit justifies the potential risks to the fetus or nursing infant. Patients should be advised to assess their individual responses to azelastine nasal spray before engaging in any activity requiring mental alertness, such as driving a car or operating machinery. Patients should be advised that the concurrent use of azelastine nasal spray with alcohol or other

A

CNS depressants may lead to additional reductions in alertness and impairment of CNS performance and should be avoided (see DRUG INTERACTIONS).

CARCINOGENESIS, MUTAGENESIS, AND IMPAIRMENT OF FERTILITY

In 2 year carcinogenicity studies in rats and mice azelastine hydrochloride did not show evidence of carcinogenicity at oral doses up to 30 mg/kg and 25 mg/kg, respectively (approximately 240 and 100 times the maximum recommended daily intranasal dose in adults and children on a mg/m^2 basis).

Azelastine hydrochloride showed no genotoxic effects in the Ames test, DNA repair test, mouse lymphoma forward mutation assay, mouse micronucleus test, or chromosomal aberration test in rat bone marrow.

Reproduction and fertility studies in rats showed no effects on male or female fertility at oral doses up to 30 mg/kg (approximately 240 times the maximum recommended daily intranasal dose in adults on a mg/m^2 basis). At 68.6 mg/kg (approximately 560 times the maximum recommended daily intranasal dose in adults on a mg/m^2 basis), the duration of estrous cycles was prolonged and copulatory activity and the number of pregnancies were decreased. The numbers of corpora lutea and implantations were decreased; however, preimplantation loss was not increased.

PREGNANCY CATEGORY C

Azelastine hydrochloride has been shown to cause developmental toxicity. Treatment of mice with an oral dose of 68.6 mg/kg (approximately 280 times the maximum recommended daily intranasal dose in adults on a mg/m^2 basis) caused embryo-fetal death, malformations (cleft palate; short or absent tail; fused, absent or branched ribs), delayed ossification and decreased fetal weight. This dose also caused maternal toxicity as evidenced by decreased body weight. Neither fetal nor maternal effects occurred at a dose of 3 mg/kg (approximately 10 times the maximum recommended daily intranasal dose in adults on a mg/m^2 basis).

In rats, an oral dose of 30 mg/kg (approximately 240 times the maximum recommended daily intranasal dose in adults on a mg/m^2 basis) caused malformations (oligo-and brachydactylia), delayed ossification and skeletal variations, in the absence of maternal toxicity. At 68.6 mg/kg (approximately 560 times the maximum recommended daily intranasal dose in adults on a mg/m^2 basis) azelastine hydrochloride also caused embryo-fetal death and decreased fetal weight; however, the 68.6 mg/kg dose caused severe maternal toxicity. Neither fetal nor maternal effects occurred at a dose of 3 mg/kg (approximately 25 times the maximum recommended daily intranasal dose in adults on a mg/m^2 basis).

In rabbits, oral doses of 30 mg/kg and greater (approximately 500 times the maximum recommended daily intranasal dose in adults on a mg/m^2 basis) caused abortion, delayed ossification and decreased fetal weight; however, these doses also resulted in severe maternal toxicity. Neither fetal nor maternal effects occurred at a dose of 0.3 mg/kg (approximately 5 times the maximum recommended daily intranasal dose in adults on a mg/m^2 basis).

There are no adequate and well-controlled clinical studies in pregnant women. Azelastine nasal spray should be used during pregnancy only if the potential benefit justifies the potential risk to the fetus.

NURSING MOTHERS

It is not known whether azelastine hydrochloride is excreted in human milk. Because many drugs are excreted in human milk, caution should be exercised when azelastine nasal spray is administered to a nursing woman.

PEDIATRIC USE

The safety and effectiveness of azelastine nasal spray at a dose of 1 spray per nostril twice daily has been established for patients 5-11 years of age for the treatment of symptoms of seasonal allergic rhinitis. The safety of this dosage of azelastine nasal spray was established in well-controlled studies of this dose in 176 patients 5–12 years of age treated for up to 6 weeks. The efficacy of azelastine nasal spray at this dose is based on an extrapolation of the finding of efficacy in adults, on the likelihood that the disease course, pathophysiology and response to treatment are substantially similar in children compared to adults, and on supportive data from controlled clinical trials in patients 5–12 years of age at the dose of 1 spray per nostril twice daily. The safety and effectiveness of azelastine nasal spray in patients below the age of 5 years have not been established.

GERIATRIC USE

Clinical studies of azelastine nasal spray did not include sufficient numbers of subjects aged 65 and over to determine whether they respond differently from younger subjects. Other reported clinical experience has not identified differences in responses between the elderly and younger patients. In general, dose selection for an elderly patient should be cautious, usually starting at the low end of the dosing range, reflecting the greater frequency of decreased hepatic, renal, or cardiac function, and of concomitant disease or other drug therapy.

DRUG INTERACTIONS

Concurrent use of azelastine nasal spray with alcohol or other CNS depressants should be avoided because additional reductions in alertness and additional impairment of CNS performance may occur.

Cimetidine (400 mg twice daily) increased the mean C_{max} and AUC of orally administered azelastine hydrochloride (4 mg twice daily) by approximately 65%. Ranitidine hydrochloride (150 mg twice daily) had no effect on azelastine pharmacokinetics.

Interaction studies investigating the cardiac effects, as measured by the corrected QT interval (QTc), of concomitantly administered oral azelastine hydrochloride and erythromycin or ketoconazole were conducted. Oral erythromycin (500 mg three times daily for 7 days) had no effect on azelastine pharmacokinetics or QTc based on analyses of serial electrocardiograms. Ketoconazole (200 mg twice daily for 7 days) interfered with the measurement of azelastine plasma concentrations; however, no effects on QTc were observed.

No significant pharmacokinetic interaction was observed with the coadministration of an oral 4 mg dose of azelastine hydrochloride twice daily and theophylline 300 or 400 mg twice daily.

ADVERSE REACTIONS

SEASONAL ALLERGIC RHINITIS

Adverse experience information for azelastine nasal spray is derived from six well-controlled, 2 day to 8 week clinical studies which included 391 patients who received azelastine nasal spray at a dose of 2 sprays per nostril twice daily. In placebo-controlled efficacy trials, the incidence of discontinuation due to adverse reactions in patients receiving azelastine nasal spray was not significantly different from vehicle placebo (2.2% vs 2.8%, respectively).

In these clinical studies, adverse events that occurred statistically significantly more often in patients treated with azelastine nasal spray versus vehicle placebo included bitter taste (19.7% vs 0.6%), somnolence (11.5% vs 5.4%), weight increase (2.0% vs 0%), and myalgia (1.5% vs 0%).

The adverse events in TABLE 1 were reported with frequencies ≥2% in the azelastine nasal spray treatment group and more frequently than placebo in short-term (≤2 days) and long-term (2-8 weeks) clinical trials.

TABLE 1

Adverse Reaction	Azelastine Nasal Spray n=391	Vehicle Placebo n=353
Bitter taste	19.7	0.6
Headache	14.8	12.7
Somnolence	11.5	5.4
Nasal burning	4.1	1.7
Pharyngitis	3.8	2.8
Dry mouth	2.8	1.7
Paroxysmal sneezing	3.1	1.1
Nausea	2.8	1.1
Rhinitis	2.3	1.4
Fatigue	2.3	1.4
Dizziness	2.0	1.4
Epistaxis	2.0	1.4
Weight increase	2.0	0.0

P <0.05, Fisher's Exact Test (two-tailed).

A total of 176 patients 5–12 years of age were exposed to azelastine nasal spray at a dose of 1 spray each nostril twice daily in 3 placebo-controlled studies. In these studies, adverse events that occurred more frequently in patients treated with azelastine nasal spray than with placebo, and that were not represented in the adult adverse event table above include rhinitis/cold symptoms (17.0% vs 9.5%), cough (11.4% vs 8.3%), conjunctivitis (5.1% vs 1.8%), and asthma (4.5% vs 4.1%).

The following events were observed infrequently (<2% and exceeding placebo incidence) in patients who received azelastine nasal spray (2 sprays/nostril twice daily) in US clinical trials.

Cardiovascular: Flushing, hypertension, tachycardia.

Dermatologic: Contact dermatitis, eczema, hair and follicle infection, furunculosis.

Digestive: Constipation, gastroenteritis, glossitis, ulcerative stomatitis, vomiting, increased SGPT, aphthous stomatitis.

Metabolic and Nutritional: Increased appetite.

Musculoskeletal: Myalgia, temporomandibular dislocation.

Neurological: Hyperkinesia, hypoesthesia, vertigo.

Psychological: Anxiety, depersonalization, depression, nervousness, sleep disorder, thinking abnormal.

Respiratory: Bronchospasm, coughing, throat burning, laryngitis.

Special Senses: Conjunctivitis, eye abnormality, eye pain, watery eyes, taste loss.

Urogenital: Albuminuria, amenorrhea, breast pain, hematuria, increased urinary frequency.

Whole Body: Allergic reaction, back pain, herpes simplex, viral infection, malaise, pain in extremities, abdominal pain.

VASOMOTOR RHINITIS

Adverse experience information for azelastine nasal spray is derived from two placebo-controlled clinical studies which incuded 216 patients who received azelastine nasal spray at a dose of 2 sprays per nostril twice daily for up to 28 days. The incidence of discontinuation due to adverse reactions in patients receiving azelastine nasal spray was not different from vehicle placebo (2.8% vs 2.9%, respectively).

The adverse events in TABLE 2 were reported with frequencies ≥2% in the azelastine nasal spray treatment group and more frequently than placebo.

TABLE 2

Adverse Reaction	Azelastine Nasal Spray n=216	Vehicle Placebo n=210
Bitter taste	19.4	2.4
Headache	7.9	7.6
Dysesthesia	7.9	3.3
Rhinitis	5.6	2.4
Epistaxis	3.2	2.4
Sinusitis	3.2	1.9
Somnolence	3.2	1.0

Events observed infrequently (<2% and exceeding placebo incidence) in patients who received azelastine nasal spray (2 sprays/nostril twice daily) in US clinical trials in vasomotor rhinitis were similar to those observed in US clinical trials in seasonal allergic rhinitis.

In controlled trials involving nasal and oral azelastine hydrochloride formulations, there were infrequent occurrences of hepatic transaminase elevations. The clinical relevance of these reports has not been established.

A

In addition, the following spontaneous adverse events have been reported during the marketing of azelastine nasal spray and causal relationship with the drug is unknown: Anaphylactoid reaction, application site irritation, chest pain, nasal congestion, confusion, diarrhea, dyspnea, facial edema, involuntary muscle contractions, paresthesia, parosmia, pruritus, rash, tolerance, urinary retention, vision abnormal and xerophthalmia.

DOSAGE AND ADMINISTRATION

SEASONAL ALLERGIC RHINITIS

The recommended dose of azelastine nasal spray in adults and children 12 years and older with seasonal allergic rhinitis is 2 sprays per nostril twice daily. The recommended dose of azelastine nasal spray in children 5–11 years of age is 1 spray per nostril twice daily.

VASOMOTOR RHINITIS

The recommended dose of azelastine nasal spray in adults and children 12 years and older with vasomotor rhinitis is 2 sprays per nostril twice daily.

Before initial use, the screw cap on the bottle should be replaced with the pump unit and the delivery system should be primed with 4 sprays or until a fine mist appears. When 3 or more days have elapsed since the last use, the pump should be reprimed with 2 sprays or until a fine mist appears.

Caution: Avoid spraying in the eyes.

Directions for Use: Illustrated patient instructions for proper use accompany each package of azelastine nasal spray.

HOW SUPPLIED

Astelin nasal spray, 137 μg is supplied as a package containing a total of 200 metered sprays in two high-density polyethylene (HDPE) bottles fitted with screw caps. A separate metered-dose spray pump unit and a leaflet of patient instructions are also provided. The spray pump unit is packaged in a polyethylene wrapper and consists of a nasal spray pump fitted with a blue safety clip and a blue plastic dust cover.

Each Astelin nasal spray, 137 μg, bottle contains 17 mg (1 mg/ml) of azelastine hydrochloride to be used with the supplied metered-dose spray pump unit. Each bottle can deliver 100 metered sprays. Each spray delivers a mean of 0.137 ml solution containing 137 μg of azelastine hydrochloride.

Attention: The imprinted expiration date applies to the product in the bottles with screw caps. After the spray pump is inserted into the first bottle of the dispensing package, both bottles of product should be discarded after 3 months, not to exceed the expiration date imprinted on the label.

Storage: Store at controlled room temperature 20-25°C (68-77°F). Protect from freezing.

OPHTHALMIC

DESCRIPTION

Optivar (azelastine hydrochloride ophthalmic solution) 0.05% is a sterile ophthalmic solution containing azelastine hydrochloride, a relatively selective H_1-receptor antagonist for topical administration to the eyes. Azelastine hydrochloride is a white crystalline powder with a molecular weight of 418.37. Azelastine hydrochloride is sparingly soluble in water, methanol and propylene glycol, and slightly soluble in ethanol, octanol and glycerine. Azelastine hydrochloride is a racemic mixture with a melting point of 225°C. The chemical name for azelastine hydrochloride is (±)-1-(2H)-phthalazinone,4-[(4-chlorophenyl) methyl]-2-(hexahydro-1-methyl-1H-azepin-4-yl)-, monohydrochloride.

Empirical Chemical Structure: $C_{22}H_{24}ClN_3O{\cdot}HCl$.

Each ml of Optivar Contains: *Active:* 0.5 mg azelastine hydrochloride, equivalent to 0.457 mg of azelastine base; *Preservative:* 0.125 mg benzalkonium chloride; *Inactives:* Disodium edetate dihydrate, hydroxypropylmethylcellulose, sorbitol solution, sodium hydroxide and water for injection. It has a pH of approximately 5.0–6.5 and an osmolality of approximately 271–312 mOsmol/L.

CLINICAL PHARMACOLOGY

Azelastine hydrochloride is a relatively selective histamine H_1 antagonist and an inhibitor of the release of histamine and other mediators from cells (*e.g.*, mast cells) involved in the allergic response. Based on *in vitro* studies using human cell lines, inhibition of other mediators involved in allergic reactions (*e.g.*, leukotrienes and PAF) has been demonstrated with azelastine hydrochloride. Decreased chemotaxis and activation of eosinophils has also been demonstrated.

PHARMACOKINETICS AND METABOLISM

Absorption of azelastine following ocular administration was relatively low. A study in symptomatic patients receiving 1 drop azelastine ophthalmic solution in each eye 2–4 times a day (0.06–0.12 mg azelastine hydrochloride) demonstrated plasma concentrations of azelastine hydrochloride to generally be between 0.02 and 0.25 ng/ml after 56 days of treatment. Three (3) of 19 patients had quantifiable amounts of N-desmethylazelastine that ranged from 0.25-0.87 ng/ml at day 56.

Based on intravenous and oral administration, the elimination half-life, steady-state volume of distribution and plasma clearance were 22 hours, 14.5 L/kg and 0.5 L/h/kg, respectively. Approximately 75% of an oral dose of radiolabeled azelastine hydrochloride was excreted in the feces with less than 10% as unchanged azelastine. Azelastine hydrochloride is oxidatively metabolized to the principal metabolite, N-desmethylazelastine, by the cytochrome P450 enzyme system. *In vitro* studies in human plasma indicate that the plasma protein binding of azelastine and N-desmethylazelastine are approximately 88% and 97%, respectively.

INDICATIONS AND USAGE

Azelastine ophthalmic solution is indicated for the treatment of itching of the eye associated with allergic conjunctivitis.

CONTRAINDICATIONS

Azelastine ophthalmic solution is contraindicated in persons with known or suspected hypersensitivity to any of its components.

WARNINGS

Azelastine ophthalmic solution is for ocular use only and not for injection or oral use.

PRECAUTIONS

INFORMATION FOR THE PATIENT

To prevent contaminating the dropper tip and solution, care should be taken not to touch any surface, the eyelids or surrounding areas with the dropper tip of the bottle. Keep bottle tightly closed when not in use. This product is sterile when packaged.

Patients should be advised not to wear a contact lens if their eye is red. Azelastine ophthalmic solution should not be used to treat contact lens related irritation. The preservative in azelastine ophthalmic solution, benzalkonium chloride, may be absorbed by soft contact lenses. Patients who wear soft contact lenses and **whose eyes are not red,** should be instructed to wait at least 10 minutes after instilling azelastine ophthalmic solution before they insert their contact lenses.

CARCINOGENESIS, MUTAGENESIS, AND IMPAIRMENT OF FERTILITY

Azelastine hydrochloride administered orally for 24 months was not carcinogenic in rats and mice at doses up to 30 mg/kg/day and 25 mg/kg/day, respectively. Based on a 30 μl drop size, these doses were approximately 25,000 and 21,000 times higher than the maximum recommended ocular human use level of 0.001 mg/kg/day for a 50 kg adult.

Azelastine hydrochloride showed no genotoxic effects in the Ames test, DNA repair test, mouse lymphoma forward mutation assay, mouse micronucleus test, or chromosomal aberration test in rat bone marrow. Reproduction and fertility studies in rats showed no effects on male or female fertility at oral doses of up to 25,000 times the maximum recommended ocular human use level. At 68.6 mg/kg/day (57,000 times the maximum recommended ocular human use level), the duration of the estrous cycle was prolonged and copulatory activity and the number of pregnancies were decreased. The numbers of corpora lutea and implantations were decreased; however, the implantation ratio was not affected.

PREGNANCY, TERATOGENIC EFFECTS, PREGNANCY CATEGORY C

Azelastine hydrochloride has been shown to be embryotoxic, fetotoxic, and teratogenic (external and skeletal abnormalities) in mice at an oral dose of 68.6 mg/kg/day (57,000 times the recommended ocular human use level). At an oral dose of 30 mg/kg/day (25,000 times the recommended ocular human use level), delayed ossification (undeveloped metacarpus), and the incidence of 14th rib were increased in rats. At 68.6 mg/kg/day (57,000 times the maximum recommended ocular human use level) azelastine hydrochloride caused resorption and fetotoxic effects in rats. The relevance to humans of these skeletal findings noted at only high drug exposure levels is unknown.

There are no adequate and well-controlled studies in pregnant women. Azelastine ophthalmic solution should be used during pregnancy only if the potential benefit justifies the potential risk to the fetus.

NURSING MOTHERS

It is not known whether azelastine hydrochloride is excreted in human milk. Because many drugs are excreted in human milk, caution should be exercised when azelastine ophthalmic solution is administered to a nursing woman.

PEDIATRIC USE

Safety and effectiveness in pediatric patients below the age of 3 have not been established.

GERIATRIC USE

No overall differences in safety or effectiveness have been observed between elderly and younger adult patients.

ADVERSE REACTIONS

In controlled multiple-dose studies where patients were treated for up to 56 days, the most frequently reported adverse reactions were transient eye burning/stinging (approximately 30%), headaches (approximately 15%), and bitter taste (approximately 10%). The occurrence of these events was generally mild.

The following events were reported in 1-10% of patients: Asthma, conjunctivitis, dyspnea, eye pain, fatigue, influenza-like symptoms, pharyngitis, pruritus, rhinitis and temporary blurring. Some of these events were similar to the underlying disease being studied.

DOSAGE AND ADMINISTRATION

The recommended dose is one drop instilled into each affected eye twice a day.

HOW SUPPLIED

Optivar (azelastine hydrochloride ophthalmic solution) 0.05% is supplied as follows: 6 ml solution in a translucent 10 ml HDPE container with a LDPE dropper tip, and a white HDPE screw cap.

Storage: Store UPRIGHT between 2 and 25°C (36 and 77°F).

PRODUCT LISTING - EQUIVALENTS NOT AVAILABLE

Solution - Ophthalmic - 0.05%

3 ml	$46.51	OPTIVAR, Muro Pharmaceuticals Inc	00451-7025-30
6 ml	$64.35	OPTIVAR, Muro Pharmaceuticals Inc	00451-7025-06
6 ml	$68.50	OPTIVAR, Pharma Pac	52959-0710-06
10 ml	$46.64	OPTIVAR, Muro Pharmaceuticals Inc	00451-7025-00

Spray - Nasal - 137 mcg/Inh

34 ml	$47.00	ASTELIN, Almay	54569-4897-00
34 ml	$55.88	ASTELIN, Physicians Total Care	54868-3957-00
34 ml	$59.57	ASTELIN, Wallace Laboratories	00037-0241-10

A

Azithromycin (003066)

For related information, see the comparative table section in Appendix A.

Categories: Bronchitis, chronic, acute exacerbation; Genital ulcer disease; Infection, cervix; Infection, lower respiratory tract; Infection, ear, middle; Infection, skin and skin structures; Infection, upper respiratory tract; Infection, urethra; Mycobacterium avium complex; Pelvic inflammatory disease; Pharyngitis; Pneumonia, community-acquired; Tonsilitis; FDA Approved 1991 Nov; Pregnancy Category B

Drug Classes: Antibiotics, macrolides

Brand Names: Zithromax

Foreign Brand Availability: Aruzilina (Costa-Rica; Dominican-Republic; El-Salvador; Guatemala; Honduras; Nicaragua; Panama); Azadose (France); Azenil (Israel); Azimin (Colombia); Azithral (India); Azitrocin (Italy; Mexico); Azitromax (Norway; Sweden); Aziwok (Benin; Burkina-Faso; Ethiopia; Gambia; Ghana; Guinea; India; Ivory-Coast; Kenya; Liberia; Malawi; Mali; Mauritania; Mauritius; Morocco; Niger; Nigeria; Senegal; Seychelles; Sierra-Leone; Sudan; Tanzania; Tunia; Uganda; Zambia; Zimbabwe); Azomyne (Bahrain; Cyprus; Egypt; Iran; Iraq; Jordan; Kuwait; Lebanon; Libya; Oman; Qatar; Republic-of-Yemen; Saudi-Arabia; Syria; United-Arab-Emirates); Azro (Bahrain; Cyprus; Egypt; Iran; Iraq; Jordan; Kuwait; Lebanon; Libya; Oman; Qatar; Republic-of-Yemen; Saudi-Arabia; Syria; United-Arab-Emirates); Aztrin (Indonesia); Inedol (Peru); Kromicin (Colombia); Macrozit (Peru); Setron (Peru); Sumamed (China); Tobyl (Colombia); Tromix (Colombia); Ultreon (Germany); Zaret (Colombia); Zeto (Israel); Zibramax (Indonesia); Zifin (Indonesia); Zimericina (Colombia); Zistic (Indonesia); Zitrim (Colombia); Zitrim U (Colombia); Zitrobifan (Colombia); Zitromax (Colombia; Ecuador; Italy; Peru; Spain); Zomax (Bahrain; Cyprus; Egypt; Iran; Iraq; Jordan; Kuwait; Lebanon; Libya; Oman; Qatar; Republic-of-Yemen; Saudi-Arabia; Syria; United-Arab-Emirates); Xithrone (Bahrain; Cyprus; Egypt; Iran; Iraq; Jordan; Kuwait; Lebanon; Libya; Oman; Qatar; Republic-of-Yemen; Saudi-Arabia; Syria; United-Arab-Emirates)

Cost of Therapy: $45.48 (Pneumonia; Zithromax Z-Paks; 250 mg; 6 tablets; 5 day supply)
$23.54 (Gonorrhea; Zithromax Suspension; 1 g; 1 g; 1 day supply)

INTRAVENOUS

DESCRIPTION

Note: The trade name has been used throughout this monograph for clarity.
For IV infusion only.

Zithromax contains the active ingredient azithromycin, an azalide, a subclass of macrolide antibiotics, for intravenous (IV) injection. Azithromycin has the chemical name (*2R,3S,4R,5R,8R,10R,11R,12S,13S,14R*)-13-[(2,6-dideoxy-3-*C*-methyl-3-*O*-methyl-α-*L*-*ribo*-hexopyranosyl)oxy]-2-ethyl-3,4,10-trihydroxy-3,5,6,8,10,12,14-hepta-methyl-11-[[3,4,6-trideoxy-3-(dimethylamino)-β-*D*-*xylo*-hexopyranosyl]oxy]-1-oxa-6-azacyclopentadecan-15-one. Azithromycin is derived from erythromycin; however, it differs chemically from erythromycin in that a methyl-substituted nitrogen atom is incorporated into the lactone ring. Its molecular formula is $C_{38}H_{72}N_2O_{12}$, and its molecular weight is 749.00.

Azithromycin, as the dihydrate, is a white crystalline powder with a molecular formula of $C_{38}H_{72}N_2O_{12}{\cdot}2H_2O$ and a molecular weight of 785.0.

Zithromax consists of azithromycin dihydrate and the following inactive ingredients: citric acid and sodium hydroxide. Zithromax is supplied in lyophilized form in a 10 ml vial equivalent to 500 mg of azithromycin for IV administration. Reconstitution, according to label directions, results in approximately 5 ml of Zithromax for IV injection with each ml containing azithromycin dihydrate equivalent to 100 mg of azithromycin.

CLINICAL PHARMACOLOGY

In patients hospitalized with community-acquired pneumonia receiving single daily 1 hour IV infusions for 2-5 days of 500 mg azithromycin at a concentration of 2 mg/ml, the mean C_{max} ±SD achieved was 3.63 ± 1.60 μg/ml, while the 24 hour trough level was 0.20 ± 0.15 μg/ml, and the AUC_{24} was 9.60 ± 4.80 μg·h/ml.

The mean C_{max}, 24 hour trough and AUC_{24} values were 1.14 ± 0.14 μg/ml, 0.18 ± 0.02 μg/ml, and 8.03 ± 0.86 μg·h/ml, respectively, in normal volunteers receiving a 3 hour IV infusion of 500 mg azithromycin at a concentration of 1 mg/ml. Similar pharmacokinetic values were obtained in patients hospitalized with community-acquired pneumonia that received the same 3 hour dosage regimen for 2-5 days.

TABLE 1 *Plasma Concentrations (μg/ml ±SD) After the Last Daily IV Infusion of 500 mg Azithromycin*

Time After Starting the Infusion	Infusion Concentration, Duration: 2 mg/ml, 1 hour*	1 mg/ml, 3 hours†
0.5 hours	2.98 ± 1.12	0.91 ± 0.13
1 hour	3.63 ± 1.73	1.02 ± 0.11
2 hours	0.60 ± 0.31	1.14 ± 0.13
3 hours	0.40 ± 0.23	1.13 ± 0.16
4 hours	0.33 ± 0.16	0.32 ± 0.05
6 hours	0.26 ± 0.14	0.28 ± 0.04
8 hours	0.27 ± 0.15	0.27 ± 0.03
12 hours	0.20 ± 0.12	0.22 ± 0.02
24 hours	0.20 ± 0.15	0.18 ± 0.02

* 500 mg (2 mg/ml) for 2-5 days in Community-acquired pneumonia patients.
† 500 mg (1 mg/ml) for 5 days in healthy subjects.

The average CL_t and V_d values were 10.18 ml/min/kg and 33.3 L/kg, respectively, in 18 normal volunteers receiving 1000-4000 mg doses given as 1 mg/ml over 2 hours.

Comparison of the plasma pharmacokinetic parameters following the 1st and 5th daily doses of 500 mg IV azithromycin showed only an 8% increase in C_{max} but a 61% increase in AUC_{24} reflecting a 3-fold rise in C_{24} trough levels.

Following single oral doses of 500 mg azithromycin to 12 healthy volunteers, C_{max}, trough level, and AUC_{24} were reported to be 0.41 μg/ml, 0.05 μg/ml, and 2.6 μg·h/ml, respectively. These oral values are approximately 38%, 83%, and 52% of the values observed following a single 500 mg IV 3 hour infusion (C_{max}: 1.08 μg/ml, trough: 0.06 μg/ml, AUC_{24}: 5.0 μg·h/ml).

Thus, plasma concentrations are higher following the IV regimen throughout the 24 hour interval. The pharmacokinetic parameters on day 5 of azithromycin 250 mg capsules following a 500 mg oral loading dose to healthy young adults (age 18-40 years old) were as follows: C_{max}: 0.24 μg/ml, AUC_{24}: 2.1 μg·h/ml. Tissue levels have not been obtained following IV infusions of azithromycin. Selected tissue (or fluid) concentration and tissue (or fluid) to plasma/serum concentration ratios following oral administration of azithromycin are shown in TABLE 2.

TABLE 2 *Azithromycin Concentrations Following Two 250 mg (500 mg) Capsules in Adults*

Tissue or Fluid	Time After Dose (hours)	Tissue or Fluid Concentration (μg/g or μg/ml)*	Corresponding Plasma or Serum Level (μg/ml)	Tissue (Fluid) to Plasma (Serum) Ratio*
Skin	72-96	0.4	0.012	35
Lung	72-96	4.0	0.012	>100
Sputum†	2-4	1.0	0.64	2
Sputum‡	10-12	2.9	0.1	30
Tonsil§	9-18	4.5	0.03	>100
Tonsil§	180	0.9	0.006	>100
Cervix¤	19	2.8	0.04	70

* High tissue concentrations should not be interpreted to be quantitatively related to clinical efficacy. The antimicrobial activity of azithromycin is pH related. Azithromycin is concentrated in cell lysosomes which have a low intraorganelle pH, at which the drug's activity is reduced. However, the extensive distribution of drug to tissues may be relevant to clinical activity.
† Sample was obtained 2-4 hours after the first dose.
‡ Sample was obtained 10-12 hours after the first dose.
§ Dosing regimen of 2 doses of 250 mg each, separated by 12 hours.
¤ Sample was obtained 19 hours after a single 500 mg dose.

Tissue levels were determined following a single oral dose of 500 mg azithromycin in 7 gynecological patients. Approximately 17 hours after dosing, azithromycin concentrations were 2.7 μg/g in ovarian tissue, 3.5 μg/g in uterine tissue, and 3.3 μg/g in salpinx. Tissue levels have not been obtained following IV infusion of azithromycin.

In a multiple-dose study in 12 normal volunteers utilizing a 500 mg (1 mg/ml) 1 hour IV-dosage regimen for 5 days, the amount of administered azithromycin dose excreted in urine in 24 hours was about 11% after the 1st dose and 14% after the 5th dose. These values are greater than the reported 6% excreted unchanged in urine after oral administration of azithromycin. Biliary excretion is a major route of elimination for unchanged drug, following oral administration.

The serum protein binding of azithromycin is variable in the concentration range approximating human exposure decreasing from 51% at 0.02 μg/ml to 7% at 2 μg/ml.

MICROBIOLOGY

Azithromycin acts by binding to the 50S ribosomal subunit of susceptible microorganisms and, thus, interfering with microbial protein synthesis. Nucleic acid synthesis is not affected.

Azithromycin concentrates in phagocytes and fibroblasts as demonstrated by *in vitro* incubation techniques. Using such methodology, the ratio of intracellular to extracellular concentration was >30 after 1 hour incubation. *In vivo* studies suggest that concentration in phagocytes may contribute to drug distribution to inflamed tissues.

Azithromycin has been shown to be active against most strains of the following microorganisms, both *in vitro* and in clinical infections as described in INDICATIONS AND USAGE.

Aerobic Gram-Positive Microorganisms:
Staphylococcus aureus and *Streptococcus pneumoniae.*
Note: Azithromycin demonstrates cross-resistance with erythromycin-resistant gram-positive strains. Most strains of *Enterococcus faecalis* and methicillin-resistant staphylococci are resistant to azithromycin.

Aerobic Gram-Negative Microorganisms:
Haemophilus influenzae, Moraxella catarrhalis, and *Neisseria gonorrhoeae.*

"Other" Microorganisms:
Chlamydia pneumoniae, Chlamydia trachomatis, Legionella pneumophila, Mycoplasma hominis, and *Mycoplasma pneumoniae.*

Beta-lactamase production should have no effect on azithromycin activity.

Azithromycin has been shown to be active against most strains of the following microorganisms, both *in vitro* and in clinical infections as described in the INDICATIONS AND USAGE section of the package insert for Zithromax (azithromycin tablets) and Zithromax (azithromycin for oral suspension).

Aerobic Gram-Positive Microorganisms:
Staphylococcus aureus, Streptococcus agalactiae, Streptococcus pneumoniae, and *Streptococcus pyogenes.*

Aerobic Gram-Negative Microorganisms:
Haemophilus ducreyi, Haemophilus influenzae, Moraxella catarrhalis, and *Neisseria gonorrhoeae.*

"Other" Microorganisms:
Chlamydia pneumoniae, Chlamydia trachomatis, and *Mycoplasma pneumoniae.*

The following *in vitro* data are available, **but their clinical significance is unknown.**

Azithromycin exhibits *in vitro* minimum inhibitory concentrations (MICs) of 0.5 μg/ml or less against most (≥90%) strains of streptococci listed below and MICs of 2.0 μg/ml or less against most (≥90%) strains of other listed microorganisms. However, the safety and effectiveness of azithromycin in treating clinical infections due to these microorganisms have not been established in adequate and well-controlled clinical trials.

Aerobic Gram-Positive Microorganisms:
Streptococci (Groups C, F, G), and Viridans group streptococci.

Aerobic Gram-Negative Microorganisms:
Bordetella pertussis.

Anaerobic Microorganisms:
Peptostreptococcus species, and *Prevotella bivia.*

"Other" Microorganisms:
Ureaplasma urealyticum.

Susceptibility Testing
Azithromycin can be solubilized for *in vitro* susceptibility testing using dilution techniques by dissolving in a minimum amount of 95% ethanol and diluting to the working stock concentration with broth.

Dilution Techniques
Quantitative methods are used to determine antimicrobial minimum inhibitory concentrations (MICs). These MICs provide estimates of the susceptibility of bacteria to antimicrobial compounds. The MICs should be determined using a standardized procedure. Standardized procedures are based on a dilution method[1] (broth or agar) or equivalent with standardized inoculum concentrations and standardized concentrations of azithromycin powder. The MIC values should be interpreted according to the following criteria (see TABLES 3-5).

TABLE 3 *For testing aerobic microorganisms other than Haemophilus species, Neisseria gonorrhoeae, and streptococci*

MIC (µg/ml)	Interpretation
≤2	Susceptible (S)
4	Intermediate (I)
≥8	Resistant (R)

TABLE 4 *For testing Haemophilus species**

MIC (µg/ml)	Interpretation
≤4	Susceptible (S)

* This interpretive standard is applicable only to broth microdilution susceptibility testing with *Haemophilus* species using *Haemophilus* Test Medium (HTM).[1]

The current absence of data on resistant strains precludes defining any categories other than "Susceptible". Strains yielding MIC results suggestive of a "nonsusceptible" category should be submitted to a reference laboratory for further testing.

TABLE 5 *For testing streptococci including S. pneumoniae**

MIC (µg/ml)	Interpretation
≤0.5	Susceptible (S)
1	Intermediate (I)
≥2	Resistant (R)

* These interpretive standards are applicable only to broth microdilution susceptibility tests using cation-adjusted Mueller-Hinton broth with 2-5% lysed horse blood.[1]

No interpretive criteria have been established for testing *Neisseria gonorrhoeae.* This species is not usually tested.

A report of "Susceptible" indicates that the pathogen is likely to respond to monotherapy with azithromycin. A report of "Intermediate" indicates that the result should be considered equivocal, and, if the microorganism is not fully susceptible to alternative, clinically feasible drugs, the test should be repeated. This category implies possible clinical applicability in body sites where the drug is physiologically concentrated or in situations where high dosage of drug can be used. This category also provides a buffer zone which prevents small uncontrolled technical factors from causing major discrepancies in interpretation. A report of "Resistant" indicates that achievable drug concentrations are unlikely to be inhibitory; other therapy should be selected.

Standardized susceptibility test procedures require the use of laboratory control microorganisms to control the technical aspects of the laboratory procedures. Standard azithromycin powder should provide the following MIC values (see TABLE 6).

TABLE 6

Microorganism	MIC (µg/ml)
Haemophilus influenzae ATCC 49247*	1.0-4.0
Staphylococcus aureus ATCC 29213	0.5-2.0
Streptococcus pneumoniae ATCC 49619†	0.06-0.25

* This quality control range is applicable to only *H. influenzae* ATCC 49247 tested by a broth microdilution procedure using *Haemophilus* Test Medium (HTM).[1]
† This quality control range is applicable to only *S. pneumoniae* ATCC 49619 tested by a broth microdilution procedure using cation-adjusted Mueller-Hinton broth with 2-5% lysed horse blood.[1]

Diffusion Techniques
Quantitative methods that require measurement of zone diameters also provide reproducible estimates of the susceptibility of bacteria to antimicrobial compounds. One such standardized procedure[2] requires the use of standardized inoculum concentrations. This procedure uses paper disks impregnated with 15 µg azithromycin to test the susceptibility of microorganisms to azithromycin.

Reports from the laboratory providing results of the standard single-disk susceptibility test with a 15 µg azithromycin disk should be interpreted according to the following criteria (see TABLES 7-8).

The current absence of data on resistant strains precludes defining any categories other than "Susceptible". Strains yielding zone diameter results suggestive of a "nonsusceptible" category should be submitted to a reference laboratory for further testing.

TABLE 7 *For testing aerobic microorganisms (including streptococci)* except Haemophilus species and Neisseria gonorrhoeae*

Zone Diameter (mm)	Interpretation
≥18	Susceptible (S)
14-17	Intermediate (I)
≤13	Resistant (R)

* These zone diameter standards for streptococci apply only to tests performed using Mueller-Hinton agar supplemented with 5% sheep blood and incubated in 5% CO_2.[2]

TABLE 8 *For testing Haemophilus species**

Zone Diameter (mm)	Interpretation
≥12	Susceptible (S)

* This zone diameter standard is applicable only to tests with *Haemophilus* species using *Haemophilus* Test Medium (HTM).[2]

No interpretive criteria have been established for testing *Neisseria gonorrhoeae.* This species is not usually tested.

Interpretation should be as stated above for results using dilution techniques. Interpretation involves correlation of the diameter obtained in the disk test with the MIC for azithromycin.

As with standardized dilution techniques, diffusion methods require the use of laboratory control microorganisms that are used to control the technical aspects of the laboratory procedures. For the diffusion technique, the 15 µg azithromycin disk should provide the following zone diameters in these laboratory test quality control strains (see TABLE 9).

TABLE 9

Microorganism	Zone Diameter (mm)
Haemophilus influenzae ATCC 49247*	13-21
Staphylococcus aureus ATCC 25923	21-26
Streptococcus pneumoniae ATCC 49619†	19-25

* These quality control limits are applicable only to tests conducted with *H. influenzae* ATCC 49247 using *Haemophilus* Test Medium (HTM).[2]
† These quality control limits are applicable only to tests conducted with *S. pneumoniae* ATCC 49619 using Mueller-Hinton agar supplemented with 5% sheep blood incubated in 5% CO_2.[2]

INDICATIONS AND USAGE
Zithromax is indicated for the treatment of patients with infections caused by susceptible strains of the designated microorganisms in the conditions listed below. As recommended dosages, durations of therapy, and applicable patient populations vary among these infections, please see DOSAGE AND ADMINISTRATION for dosing recommendations.

Community-acquired pneumonia due to *Chlamydia pneumoniae, Haemophilus influenzae, Legionella pneumophila, Moraxella catarrhalis, Mycoplasma pneumoniae, Staphylococcus aureus,* or *Streptococcus pneumoniae* in patients who require initial IV therapy.

Pelvic inflammatory disease due to *Chlamydia trachomatis, Neisseria gonorrhoeae,* or *Mycoplasma hominis* in patients who require initial IV therapy. If anaerobic microorganisms are suspected of contributing to the infection, an antimicrobial agent with anaerobic activity should be administered in combination with Zithromax.

Zithromax should be followed by Zithromax by the oral route as required. (See DOSAGE AND ADMINISTRATION.)

Appropriate culture and susceptibility tests should be performed before treatment to determine the causative microorganism and its susceptibility to azithromycin. Therapy with Zithromax may be initiated before results of these tests are known; once the results become available, antimicrobial therapy should be adjusted accordingly.

NON-FDA APPROVED INDICATIONS
Azithromycin may also be used to treat Lyme disease, uncomplicated Typhoid Fever, and toxoplasmosis, however, these are not approved indications.

CONTRAINDICATIONS
Zithromax is contraindicated in patients with known hypersensitivity to azithromycin, erythromycin, or any macrolide antibiotic.

WARNINGS
Serious allergic reactions, including angioedema, anaphylaxis, and dermatologic reactions including Stevens Johnson Syndrome and toxic epidermal necrolysis have been reported rarely in patients on azithromycin therapy. Although rare, fatalities have been reported. (See CONTRAINDICATIONS.) Despite initially successful symptomatic treatment of the allergic symptoms, when symptomatic therapy was discontinued, the allergic symptoms **recurred soon thereafter in some patients without further azithromycin exposure.** These patients required prolonged periods of observation and symptomatic treatment. The relationship of these episodes to the long tissue half-life of azithromycin and subsequent prolonged exposure to antigen is unknown at present.

If an allergic reaction occurs, the drug should be discontinued and appropriate therapy should be instituted. Physicians should be aware that reappearance of the allergic symptoms may occur when symptomatic therapy is discontinued.

Pseudomembranous colitis has been reported with nearly all antibacterial agents and may range in severity from mild to life-threatening. Therefore, it is important to consider this diagnosis in patients who present with diarrhea subsequent to the administration of antibacterial agents.

Treatment with antibacterial agents alters the normal flora of the colon and may permit overgrowth of clostridia. Studies indicate that a toxin produced by *Clostridium difficile* is a primary cause of "antibiotic-associated colitis".

After the diagnosis of pseudomembranous colitis has been established, therapeutic measures should be initiated. Mild cases of pseudomembranous colitis usually respond to discontinuation of the drug alone. In moderate to severe cases, consideration should be given to management with fluids and electrolytes, protein supplementation, and treatment with an antibacterial drug clinically effective against *Clostridium difficile* colitis.

PRECAUTIONS

GENERAL

Because azithromycin is principally eliminated via the liver, caution should be exercised when azithromycin is administered to patients with impaired hepatic function. There are no data regarding azithromycin usage in patients with renal impairment; therefore, caution should be exercised when prescribing azithromycin in these patients.

Zithromax should be reconstituted and diluted as directed and administered as an IV infusion over not less than 60 minutes. (See DOSAGE AND ADMINISTRATION.)

Local IV site reactions have been reported with the IV administration of azithromycin. The incidence and severity of these reactions were the same when 500 mg azithromycin were given over 1 hour (2 mg/ml as 250 ml infusion) or over 3 hours (1 mg/ml as 500 ml infusion). (See ADVERSE REACTIONS.) All volunteers who received infusate concentrations above 2.0 mg/ml experienced local IV site reactions and, therefore, higher concentrations should be avoided.

The following adverse events have been reported with macrolide products: ventricular arrhythmias, including ventricular tachycardia, and *torsades de pointes,* in individuals with prolonged QT intervals.

There has been a spontaneous report from the post-marketing experience of a patient with previous history of arrhythmias who experienced *torsades de pointes* and subsequent myocardial infarction following a course of oral azithromycin therapy.

INFORMATION FOR THE PATIENT

Patients should be cautioned not to take aluminum- and magnesium-containing antacids and azithromycin by the oral route simultaneously.

Patients should be directed to discontinue azithromycin and contact a physician if any signs of an allergic reaction occur.

LABORATORY TEST INTERACTIONS

There are no reported laboratory test interactions.

CARCINOGENESIS, MUTAGENESIS, AND IMPAIRMENT OF FERTILITY

Long-term studies in animals have not been performed to evaluate carcinogenic potential. Azithromycin has shown no mutagenic potential in standard laboratory tests: mouse lymphoma assay, human lymphocyte clastogenic assay, and mouse bone marrow clastogenic assay. No evidence of impaired fertility due to azithromycin was found.

PREGNANCY, TERATOGENIC EFFECTS, PREGNANCY CATEGORY B

Reproduction studies have been performed in rats and mice at doses up to moderately maternally toxic dose levels (*i.e.,* 200 mg/kg/day by the oral route). These doses, based on a mg/m^2 basis, are estimated to be 4 and 2 times, respectively, the human daily dose of 500 mg by the oral route. In the animal studies, no evidence of harm to the fetus due to azithromycin was found. There are, however, no adequate and well-controlled studies in pregnant women. Because animal reproduction studies are not always predictive of human response, azithromycin should be used during pregnancy only if clearly needed.

NURSING MOTHERS

It is not known whether azithromycin is excreted in human milk. Because many drugs are excreted in human milk, caution should be exercised when azithromycin is administered to a nursing woman.

PEDIATRIC USE

Safety and effectiveness of azithromycin for injection in children or adolescents under 16 years have not been established. In controlled clinical studies, azithromycin has been administered to pediatric patients (age 6 months to 16 years) by the oral route. For information regarding the use of Zithromax (azithromycin for oral suspension) in the treatment of pediatric patients, refer to the INDICATIONS AND USAGE and DOSAGE AND ADMINISTRATION sections of the prescribing information for Zithromax (azithromycin for oral suspension) 100 mg/5 ml and 200 mg/5 ml bottles.

GERIATRIC USE

Pharmacokinetic studies with IV azithromycin have not been performed in older volunteers. Pharmacokinetics of azithromycin following oral administration in older volunteers (65-85 years old) were similar to those in younger volunteers (18-40 years old) for the 5 day therapeutic regimen.

DRUG INTERACTIONS

Aluminum- and magnesium-containing antacids reduce the peak serum levels (rate) but not the AUC (extent) of orally administered azithromycin.

Administration of cimetidine (800 mg) 2 hours prior to orally administered azithromycin had no effect on azithromycin absorption.

Azithromycin given by the oral route did not affect the plasma levels or pharmacokinetics of theophylline administered as a single IV dose. The effect of azithromycin on the plasma levels or pharmacokinetics of theophylline administered in multiple doses resulting in therapeutic steady-state levels of theophylline is not known. However, concurrent use of macrolides and 12 theophylline has been associated with increases in the serum concentrations of theophylline. Therefore, until further data are available, prudent medical practice dictates careful monitoring of plasma theophylline levels in patients receiving azithromycin and theophylline concomitantly.

Azithromycin given by the oral route did not affect the prothrombin time response to a single dose of warfarin. However, prudent medical practice dictates careful monitoring of prothrombin time in all patients treated with azithromycin and warfarin concomitantly. Concurrent use of macrolides and warfarin in clinical practice has been associated with increased anticoagulant effects.

The following drug interactions have not been reported in clinical trials with azithromycin; however, no specific drug interaction studies have been performed to evaluate potential drug-drug interaction. Nonetheless, they have been observed with macrolide products. Until further data are developed regarding drug interactions when azithromycin and these drugs are used concomitantly, careful monitoring of patients is advised:

- ***Digoxin:*** Elevated digoxin levels.
- ***Ergotamine or dihydroergotamine:*** Acute ergot toxicity characterized by severe peripheral vasospasm and dysesthesia.
- ***Triazolam:*** Increased pharmacologic effect of triazolam by decreasing the clearance of triazolam.
- ***Drugs metabolized by the cytochrome P450 system:*** Elevations of serum carbamazepine, terfenadine, cyclosporine, hexobarbital, and phenytoin levels.

ADVERSE REACTIONS

In clinical trials of IV azithromycin for community-acquired pneumonia, in which 2-5 IV doses were given, most of the reported side effects were mild to moderate in severity and were reversible upon discontinuation of the drug. The majority of patients in these trials had one or more comorbid diseases and were receiving concomitant medications. Approximately 1.2% of the patients discontinued IV Zithromax therapy, and a total of 2.4% discontinued azithromycin therapy by either the IV or oral route because of clinical or laboratory side effects.

In clinical trials conducted in patients with pelvic inflammatory disease, in which 1-2 IV doses were given, 2% of women who received monotherapy with azithromycin and 4% who received azithromycin plus metronidazole discontinued therapy due to clinical side effects.

Clinical side effects leading to discontinuations from these studies were most commonly gastrointestinal (abdominal pain, nausea, vomiting, diarrhea), and rashes; laboratory side effects leading to discontinuation were increases in transaminase levels and/or alkaline phosphatase levels.

CLINICAL

Overall, the most common side effects associated with treatment in adult patients who received IV/PO Zithromax in studies of community-acquired pneumonia were related to the gastrointestinal system with diarrhea/loose stools (4.3%), nausea (3.9%), abdominal pain (2.7%), and vomiting (1.4%) being the most frequently reported. Approximately 12% of patients experienced a side effect related to the IV infusion; most common were pain at the injection site (6.5%) and local inflammation (3.1%).

The most common side effects associated with treatment in adult women who received IV/PO Zithromax in studies of pelvic inflammatory disease were related to the gastrointestinal system. Diarrhea (8.5%) and nausea (6.6%) were most commonly reported, followed by vaginitis (2.8%), abdominal pain (1.9%), anorexia (1.9%), rash and pruritus (1.9%). When azithromycin was co-administered with metronidazole in these studies, a higher proportion of women experienced side effects of nausea (10.3%), abdominal pain (3.7%), vomiting (2.8%), application site reaction, stomatitis, dizziness, or dyspnea (all at 1.9%).

No other side effects occurred in patients on the multiple dose IV/PO regimen of Zithromax in these studies with a frequency greater than 1%.

Side effects that occurred with a frequency of 1% or less included the following:

- ***Gastrointestinal:*** Dyspepsia, flatulence, mucositis, oral moniliasis, and gastritis.
- ***Nervous System:*** Headache, somnolence.
- ***Allergic:*** Bronchospasm.
- ***Special Senses:*** Taste perversion.

POST-MARKETING EXPERIENCE

Adverse events reported with orally administered azithromycin during the post-marketing period in adult and/or pediatric patients for which a causal relationship could not be established include:

- ***Allergic:*** Arthralgia, edema, urticaria, angioedema.
- ***Cardiovascular:*** Arrhythmias, including ventricular tachycardia, hypotension.
- ***Gastrointestinal:*** Anorexia, constipation, dyspepsia, flatulence, vomiting/diarrhea rarely resulting in dehydration, pseudomembranous colitis, pancreatitis, oral candidiasis and rare reports of tongue discoloration.
- ***General:*** Asthenia, paresthesia, fatigue, malaise and anaphylaxis (rarely fatal).
- ***Genitourinary:*** Interstitial nephritis and acute renal failure, vaginitis.
- ***Hematopoietic:*** Thrombocytopenia.
- ***Liver/Biliary:*** Abnormal liver function including hepatitis and cholestatic jaundice, as well as rare cases of hepatic necrosis and hepatic failure, some of which have resulted in death.
- ***Nervous System:*** Convulsions, dizziness/vertigo, headache, somnolence, hyperactivity, nervousness, agitation and syncope.
- ***Psychiatric:*** Aggressive reaction and anxiety.
- ***Skin/Appendages:*** Pruritus, rarely serious skin reactions including erythema multiforme, Stevens Johnson Syndrome, and toxic epidermal necrolysis.
- ***Special Senses:*** Hearing disturbances including hearing loss, deafness, and/or tinnitus, rare reports of taste perversion.

LABORATORY ABNORMALITIES

Significant abnormalities (irrespective of drug relationship) occurring during the clinical trials were reported as follows:

- with an incidence of 4-6%, elevated ALT (SGPT), AST (SGOT), creatinine.
- with an incidence of 1-3%, elevated LDH, bilirubin.
- with an incidence of less than 1%, leukopenia, neutropenia, decreased platelet count, and elevated serum alkaline phosphatase.

When follow-up was provided, changes in laboratory tests appeared to be reversible.

In multiple-dose clinical trials involving more than 750 patients treated with Zithromax (IV/PO), less than 2% of patients discontinued azithromycin therapy because of treatment-related liver enzyme abnormalities.

DOSAGE AND ADMINISTRATION

See INDICATIONS AND USAGE and CLINICAL PHARMACOLOGY.

The recommended dose of Zithromax for the treatment of adult patients with community-acquired pneumonia due to the indicated organisms is: 500 mg as a single daily dose by the IV route for at least 2 days. IV therapy should be followed by azithromycin by the oral route at a single, daily dose of 500 mg, administered as two 250 mg tablets to complete a 7-10 day course of therapy. The timing of the switch to oral therapy should be done at the discretion of the physician and in accordance with clinical response.

The recommended dose of Zithromax for the treatment of adult patients with pelvic inflammatory disease due to the indicated organisms is: 500 mg as a single daily dose by the IV route for 1 or 2 days. IV therapy should be followed by azithromycin by the oral route at a single, daily dose of 250 mg to complete a 7 day course of therapy. The timing of the switch to oral therapy should be done at the discretion of the physician and in accordance with clinical response. If anaerobic microorganisms are suspected of contributing to the infection, an antimicrobial agent with anaerobic activity should be administered in combination with Zithromax.

The infusate concentration and rate of infusion for Zithromax should be either 1 mg/ml over 3 hours or 2 mg/ml over 1 hour.

Preparation of the solution for IV administration is as follows:

RECONSTITUTION

Prepare the initial solution of Zithromax by adding 4.8 ml of sterile water for injection to the 500 mg vial and shaking the vial until all of the drug is dissolved. Since Zithromax is supplied under vacuum, it is recommended that a standard 5 ml (non-automated) syringe be used to ensure that the exact amount of 4.8 ml of sterile water is dispensed. Each ml of reconstituted solution contains 100 mg azithromycin. Reconstituted solution is stable for 24 hours when stored below 30°C or 86°F.

Parenteral drug products should be inspected visually for particulate matter prior to administration. If particulate matter is evident in reconstituted fluids, the drug solution should be discarded.

Dilute this solution further prior to administration as instructed below.

DILUTION

To provide azithromycin over a concentration range of 1.0-2.0 mg/ml, transfer 5 ml of the 100 mg/ml azithromycin solution into the appropriate amount of any of the diluents listed below:

Normal saline (0.9% sodium chloride), 1/2 normal saline (0.45% sodium chloride), 5% dextrose in water, lactated Ringer's solution, 5% dextrose in 1/2 normal saline (0.45% sodium chloride) with 20 mEq KCl, 5% dextrose in lactated Ringer's solution, 5% dextrose in 1/3 normal saline (0.3% sodium chloride), 5% dextrose in 1/2 normal saline (0.45% sodium chloride), Normosol-M in 5% dextrose, Normosol-R in 5% dextrose.

When used with the Vial-Mate drug reconstitution device, please reference the Vial-Mate instructions for assembly and reconstitution.

TABLE 14

Final Infusion Solution Concentration	Amount of Diluent
1.0 mg/ml	500 ml
2.0 mg/ml	250 ml

It is recommended that a 500 mg dose of Zithromax , diluted as above, be infused over a period of not less than 60 minutes.

Zithromax should not be given as a bolus or as an intramuscular injection.

Other IV substances, additives, or medications should not be added to Zithromax , or infused simultaneously through the same IV line.

ANIMAL PHARMACOLOGY

Phospholipidosis (intracellular phospholipid accumulation) has been observed in some tissues of mice, rats, and dogs given multiple doses of azithromycin. It has been demonstrated in numerous organ systems (*e.g.*, eye, dorsal root ganglia, liver, gallbladder, kidney, spleen, and pancreas) in dogs treated with azithromycin at doses which, expressed on a mg/kg basis, are only 2 times greater than the recommended adult human dose and in rats at doses comparable to the recommended adult human dose. This effect has been reversible after cessation of azithromycin treatment. Phospholipidosis has been observed to a similar extent in the tissues of neonatal rats and dogs given daily doses of azithromycin ranging from 10-30 days. Based on the pharmacokinetic data, phospholipidosis has been seen in the rat (30 mg/kg dose) at observed C_{max} value of 1.3 µg/ml (6 times greater than the observed C_{max} of 0.216 µg/ml at the pediatric dose of 10 mg/kg). Similarly, it has been shown in the dog (10 mg/kg dose) at observed C_{max} value of 1.5 µg/ml (7 times greater than the observed same C_{max} and drug dose in the studied pediatric population). On mg/m^2 basis, 30 mg/kg dose in the rat (135 mg/m^2) and 10 mg/kg dose in the dog (79 mg/m^2) are approximately 0.4 and 0.6 times, respectively, the recommended dose in the pediatric patients with an average body weight of 25 kg. This effect, similar to that seen in the adult animals, is reversible after cessation of azithromycin treatment. The significance of these findings for animals and for humans is unknown.

HOW SUPPLIED

Zithromax is supplied in lyophilized form under a vacuum in a 10 ml vial equivalent to 500 mg of azithromycin for IV administration. Each vial also contains sodium hydroxide and 413.6 mg citric acid.

STORAGE

When diluted according to the instructions (1.0-2.0 mg/ml), Zithromax is stable for 24 hours at or below room temperature (30°C or 86°F), or for 7 days if stored under refrigeration (5°C or 41°F).

ORAL

DESCRIPTION

Note: The trade name has been used throughout this monograph for clarity.

ZITHROMAX CAPSULES, 600 MG TABLETS, & ORAL SUSPENSION IN PACKETS

Zithromax contains the active ingredient azithromycin, an azalide, a subclass of macrolide antibiotics, for oral administration. Azithromycin has the chemical name *(2R,3S,4R,5R,8R,10R,11R,12S,13S,14R)*-13-[(2,6-dideoxy-3-*C*-methyl-3-*O*-methyl-α-*L*-*ribo*-hexopyranosyl)oxy]-2-ethyl-3,4,10-trihydroxy-3,5,6,8,10,12,14-heptamethyl-11-[[3,4,6-trideoxy-3-(dimethylamino)-β-*D*-*xylo*-hexopyranosyl]oxy]-1-oxa-6-azacyclopentadecan-15-one. Azithromycin is derived from erythromycin; however, it differs chemically from erythromycin in that a methyl-substituted nitrogen atom is incorporated into the lactone ring. Its molecular formula is $C_{38}H_{72}N_2O_{12}$, and its molecular weight is 749.0.

Azithromycin, as the dihydrate, is a white crystalline powder with a molecular formula of $C_{38}H_{72}N_2O_{12}{\cdot}2H_2O$ and a molecular weight of 785.0.

Zithromax capsules contain azithromycin dihydrate equivalent to 250 mg of azithromycin. The capsules are supplied in red opaque hard-gelatin capsules (containing FD&C red no. 40). They also contain the following inactive ingredients: anhydrous lactose, corn starch, magnesium stearate, and sodium lauryl sulfate.

Zithromax tablets contain azithromycin dihydrate equivalent to 600 mg azithromycin. The tablets are supplied as white, modified oval-shaped, film-coated tablets. They also contain the following inactive ingredients: dibasic calcium phosphate anhydrous, pregelatinized starch, sodium croscarmellose, magnesium stearate, sodium lauryl sulfate and an aqueous film coat consisting of hydroxypropyl methyl cellulose, titanium dioxide, lactose and triacetin.

Zithromax for oral suspension is supplied in a single dose packet containing azithromycin dihydrate equivalent to 1 g azithromycin. It also contains the following inactive ingredients: colloidal silicon dioxide, sodium phosphate tribasic, anhydrous; spray dried artificial banana flavor, spray dried artificial cherry flavor, and sucrose.

ZITHROMAX 250 AND 500 MG TABLETS & ORAL SUSPENSION

Zithromax contains the active ingredient azithromycin, an azalide, a subclass of macrolide antibiotics, for oral administration. Azithromycin has the chemical name *(2R,3S,4R,5R,8R,10R,11R,12S,13S,14R)*-13-[(2,6-dideoxy-3-C-methyl-3-*O*-methyl-α-*L*-*ribo*-hexopyranosyl)oxy]-2-ethyl-3,4,10-trihydroxy-3,5,6,8,10,12,14-heptamethyl-11-[[3,4,6-trideoxy-3-(dimethylamino)-β-*D*-*xylo*-hexopyranosyl]oxy]-1-oxa-6-azacyclopentadecan-15-one. Azithromycin is derived from erythromycin; however, it differs chemically from erythromycin in that a methyl-substituted nitrogen atom is incorporated into the lactone ring. Its molecular formula is $C_{38}H_{72}N_2O_{12}$, and its molecular weight is 749.00.

Azithromycin, as the dihydrate, is a white crystalline powder with a molecular formula of $C_{38}H_{72}N_2O_{12}{\cdot}2H_2O$ and a molecular weight of 785.0.

Zithromax is supplied for oral administration as film-coated, modified capsular shaped tablets containing azithromycin dihydrate equivalent to either 250 or 500 mg azithromycin and the following inactive ingredients: dibasic calcium phosphate anhydrous, pregelatinized starch, sodium croscarmellose, magnesium stearate, sodium lauryl sulfate, hydroxypropyl methylcellulose, lactose, titanium dioxide, triacetin and D&C red no. 30 aluminum lake.

Zithromax for oral suspension is supplied in bottles containing azithromycin dihydrate powder equivalent to 300, 600, 900, or 1200 mg azithromycin per bottle and the following inactive ingredients: sucrose; sodium phosphate, tribasic, anhydrous; hydroxypropyl cellulose; xanthan gum; FD&C red no. 40; and spray dried artificial cherry, creme de vanilla and banana flavors. After constitution, each 5 ml of suspension contains 100 or 200 mg of azithromycin.

CLINICAL PHARMACOLOGY

ZITHROMAX CAPSULES, 600 MG TABLETS, & ORAL SUSPENSION IN PACKETS

Pharmacokinetics

Following oral administration, azithromycin is rapidly absorbed and widely distributed throughout the body. Rapid distribution of azithromycin into tissues and high concentration within cells result in significantly higher azithromycin concentrations in tissues than in plasma or serum. The 1 g single dose packet is bioequivalent to four 250 mg capsules.

The pharmacokinetic parameters of azithromycin in plasma after dosing as per labeled recommendations in healthy young adults and asymptomatic HIV-seropositive adults (age 18-40 years old) are portrayed in TABLE 15A and TABLE 15B.

In these studies (500 mg day 1, 250 mg days 2-5), there was no significant difference in the disposition of azithromycin between male and female subjects. Plasma concentrations of

***TABLE 15A** Mean (CV%) PK Parameter*

Dose/Dosage Form (serum, except as indicated)	Subjects	Day No.	C_{max} (µg/ml)	T_{max} (hours)
500 mg/250 mg capsule	12	Day 1	0.41	2.5
and 250 mg on Days 2-5	12	Day 5	0.24	3.2
1200 mg/600 mg tablets	12	Day 1	0.66	2.5
%CV			(62%)	(79%)
600 mg tablet/day	7	1	0.33	2.0
%CV			25%	(50%)
	7	22	0.55	2.1
%CV			(18%)	(52%)
600 mg tablet/day (leukocytes)	7	22	252	10.9
%CV			(49%)	(28%)

TABLE 15B *Mean (CV%) PK Parameter*

Dose/Dosage Form (serum, except as indicated)	C_{24} (µg/ml)	AUC (µg·h/ml)	T½ (hours)	Urinary Excretion (% of dose)
500 mg/250 mg capsule	0.05	2.6*	—	4.5
and 250 mg on Days 2-5	0.05	2.1*	—	6.5
1200 mg/600 mg tablets	0.074	6.8†	40	—
%CV	(49%)	(64%)	(33%)	
600 mg tablet/day	0.039	2.4*		
%CV	(36%)	(19%)		
	0.14	5.8*	84.5	—
%CV	(26%)	(25%)		—
600 mg tablet/day (leukocytes)	146	4763*	82.8	—
%CV	(33%)	(42%)	—	—

* AUC(0-24).
† 0-last.

azithromycin following single 500 mg oral and IV doses declined in a polyphasic pattern resulting in an average terminal half-life of 68 hours. With a regimen of 500 mg on Day 1 and 250 mg/day on days 2-5, C_{min} and C_{max} remained essentially unchanged from Days 2-5 of therapy. However, without a loading dose, azithromycin C_{min} levels required 5-7 days to reach steady-state.

In asymptomatic HIV-seropositive adult subjects receiving 600 mg Zithromax tablets once daily for 22 days, steady state azithromycin serum levels were achieved by Day 15 of dosing.

When azithromycin capsules were administered with food, the rate of absorption (C_{max}) of azithromycin was reduced by 52% and the extent of absorption (AUC) by 43%.

When the oral suspension of azithromycin was administered with food, the C_{max} increased by 46% and the AUC by 14%.

The absolute bioavailability of two 600 mg tablets was 34% (CV=56%). Administration of two 600 mg tablets with food increased C_{max} by 31% (CV=43%) while the extent of absorption (AUC) was unchanged (mean ratio of AUCs=1.00; CV=55%).

The AUC of azithromycin in 250 mg capsules was unaffected by co-administration of an antacid containing aluminum and magnesium hydroxide with Zithromax; however, the C_{max} was reduced by 24%. Administration of cimetidine (800 mg) 2 hours prior to azithromycin had no effect on azithromycin absorption.

When studied in healthy elderly subjects from age 65-85 years, the pharmacokinetic parameters of azithromycin (500 mg Day 1, 250 mg Days 2-5) in elderly men were similar to those in young adults; however, in elderly women, although higher peak concentrations (increased by 30-50%) were observed, no significant accumulation occurred.

The high values in adults for apparent steady-state volume of distribution (31.1 L/kg) and plasma clearance (630 ml/min) suggest that the prolonged half-life is due to extensive uptake and subsequent release of drug from tissues. Selected tissue (or fluid) concentration and tissue (or fluid) to plasma/serum concentration ratios are shown in TABLE 16.

TABLE 16 *Azithromycin Concentrations Following Two 250 mg (500 mg) Capsules in Adults*

Tissue or Fluid	Time After Dose (hours)	Tissue or Fluid Concentration (µg/g or µg/ml*)	Corresponding Plasma or Serum Level (µg/ml)	Tissue (Fluid) to Plasma (Serum) Ratio*
Skin	72-96	0.4	0.012	35
Lung	72-96	4.0	0.012	>100
Sputum†	2-4	1.0	0.64	2
Sputum‡	10-12	2.9	0.1	30
Tonsil§	9-18	4.5	0.03	>100
Tonsil§	180	0.9	0.006	>100
Cervix¤	19	2.8	0.04	70

* High tissue concentrations should not be interpreted to be quantitatively related to clinical efficacy. The antimicrobial activity of azithromycin is pH related. Azithromycin is concentrated in cell lysosomes which have a low intraorganelle pH, at which the drug's activity is reduced. However, the extensive distribution of drug to tissues may be relevant to clinical activity.
† Sample was obtained 2-4 hours after the first dose.
‡ Sample was obtained 10-12 hours after the first dose.
§ Dosing regimen of 2 doses of 250 mg each, separated by 12 hours.
¤ Sample was obtained 19 hours after a single 500 mg dose.

The extensive tissue distribution was confirmed by examination of additional tissues and fluids (bone, ejaculum, prostate, ovary, uterus, salpinx, stomach, liver, and gallbladder). As there are no data from adequate and well-controlled studies of azithromycin treatment of infections in these additional body sites, the clinical significance of these tissue concentration data is unknown.

Following a regimen of 500 mg on the first day and 250 mg daily for 4 days, only very low concentrations were noted in cerebrospinal fluid (less than 0.01 µg/ml) in the presence of non-inflamed meninges.

Following oral administration of a single 1200 mg dose (two 600 mg tablets), the mean maximum concentration in peripheral leukocytes was 140 µg/ml. Concentrations remained above 32 µg/ml for approximately 60 hours. The mean half-lives for 6 males and 6 females were 34 hours and 57 hours, respectively. Leukocyte to plasma C_{max} ratios for males and females were 258 (±77%) and 175 (±60%), respectively, and the AUC ratios were 804 (±31%) and 541 (±28%), respectively. The clinical relevance of these findings is unknown.

Following oral administration of multiple daily doses of 600 mg (1 tablet/day) to asymptomatic HIV-seropositive adults, mean maximum concentration in peripheral leukocytes was 252 µg/ml (±49%). Trough concentrations in peripheral leukocytes at steady-state averaged 146 µg/ml (±33%). The mean leukocyte to serum C_{max} ratio was 456 (±38%) and the mean leukocyte to serum AUC ratio was 816 (±31%). The clinical relevance of these findings is unknown.

The serum protein binding of azithromycin is variable in the concentration range approximating human exposure, decreasing from 51% at 0.02 µg/ml to 7% at 2 µg/ml. Biliary excretion of azithromycin, predominantly as unchanged drug, is a major route of elimination. Over the course of a week, approximately 6% of the administered dose appears as unchanged drug in urine.

There are no pharmacokinetic data available from studies in hepatically- or renally-impaired individuals.

The effect of azithromycin on the plasma levels or pharmacokinetics of theophylline administered in multiple doses adequate to reach therapeutic steady-state plasma levels is not known. (See PRECAUTIONS.)

Mechanism of Action

Azithromycin acts by binding to the 50S ribosomal subunit of susceptible microorganisms and, thus, interfering with microbial protein synthesis. Nucleic acid synthesis is not affected.

Azithromycin concentrates in phagocytes and fibroblasts as demonstrated by *in vitro* incubation techniques. Using such methodology, the ratio of intracellular to extracellular concentration was >30 after 1 hour incubation. *In vivo* studies suggest that concentration in phagocytes may contribute to drug distribution to inflamed tissues.

Microbiology

Azithromycin has been shown to be active against most strains of the following microorganisms, both *in vitro* and in clinical infections as described in INDICATIONS AND USAGE.

Aerobic Gram-Positive Microorganisms:

Staphylococcus aureus, Streptococcus agalactiae, Streptococcus pneumoniae, and *Streptococcus pyogenes.*

Note: Azithromycin demonstrates cross-resistance with erythromycin-resistant gram-positive strains. Most strains of *Enterococcus faecalis* and methicillin-resistant staphylococci are resistant to azithromycin.

Aerobic Gram-Negative Microorganisms:

Haemophilus influenzae, and *Moraxella catarrhalis.*

"Other" Microorganisms:

Chlamydia trachomatis.

Beta-lactamase production should have no effect on azithromycin activity.

Azithromycin has been shown to be active *in vitro* and in the prevention and treatment of disease caused by the following microorganisms:

Mycobacteria:

Mycobacterium avium complex (MAC) consisting of: Mycobacterium avium, and Mycobacterium intracellulare.

The following in vitro data are available, ***but their clinical significance is unknown.***

Azithromycin exhibits in vitro minimal inhibitory concentrations (MICs) of 2.0 µg/ml or less against most (≥90%) strains of the following microorganisms; however, the safety and effectiveness of azithromycin in treating clinical infections due to these microorganisms have not been established in adequate and well-controlled trials.

Aerobic Gram-Positive Microorganisms:

Streptococci (Groups C, F, G), and Viridans group streptococci.

Aerobic Gram-Negative Microorganisms:

Bordetella pertussis, Campylobacter jejuni, Haemophilus ducreyi, and Legionella pneumophila.

Anaerobic Microorganisms:

Bacteroides bivius, Clostridium perfringens, and Peptostreptococcus species.

"Other" Microorganisms:

Borrelia burgdorferi, Mycoplasma pneumoniae, Treponema pallidum, and Ureaplasma urealyticum.

Susceptibility Testing of Bacteria Excluding Mycobacteria

The *in vitro* potency of azithromycin is markedly affected by the pH of the microbiological growth medium during incubation. Incubation in a 10% CO_2 atmosphere will result in lowering of media pH (7.2 to 6.6) within 18 hours and in an apparent reduction of the *in vitro* potency of azithromycin. Thus, the initial pH of the growth medium should be 7.2-7.4, and the CO_2 content of the incubation atmosphere should be as low as practical.

Azithromycin can be solubilized for *in vitro* susceptibility testing by dissolving in a minimum amount of 95% ethanol and diluting to working concentration with water.

Dilution Techniques

Quantitative methods are used to determine minimal inhibitory concentrations that provide reproducible estimates of the susceptibility of bacteria to antimicrobial compounds. One such standardized procedure uses a standardized dilution method[1] (broth, agar or microdilution) or equivalent with azithromycin powder. The MIC values should be interpreted according to TABLE 17.

TABLE 17

MIC (µg/ml)	Interpretation
≤2	Susceptible (S)
4	Intermediate (I)
≥8	Resistant (R)

A report of "Susceptible" indicates that the pathogen is likely to respond to monotherapy with azithromycin. A report of "Intermediate" indicates that the result should be considered equivocal, and, if the microorganism is not fully susceptible to alternative, clinically feasible drugs, the test should be repeated. This category also provides a buffer zone which prevents small uncontrolled technical factors from causing major discrepancies in interpretation. A report of "Resistant" indicates that usually achievable drug concentrations are unlikely to be inhibitory and that other therapy should be selected.

Measurement of MIC or MBC and achieved antimicrobial compound concentrations may be appropriate to guide therapy in some infections. (See CLINICAL PHARMACOLOGY for further information on drug concentrations achieved in infected body sites and other pharmacokinetic properties of this antimicrobial drug product.)

Standardized susceptibility test procedures require the use of laboratory control microorganisms. Standard azithromycin powder should provide the MIC values shown in TABLE 18.

TABLE 18

Microorganism	MIC (µg/ml)
Escherichia coli ATCC 25922	2.0-8.0
Enterococcus faecalis ATCC 29212	1.0-4.0
Staphylococcus aureus ATCC 29213	0.25-1.0

Diffusion Techniques

Quantitative methods that require measurement of zone diameters also provide reproducible estimates of the susceptibility of bacteria to antimicrobial compounds. One such standardized procedure[2] that has been recommended for use with disks to test the susceptibility of microorganisms to azithromycin uses the 15 µg azithromycin disk. Interpretation involves the correlation of the diameter obtained in the disk test with the minimal inhibitory concentration (MIC) for azithromycin.

Reports from the laboratory providing results of the standard single-disk susceptibility test with a 15 µg azithromycin disk should be interpreted according to the criteria in TABLE 19.

TABLE 19

Zone Diameter (mm)	Interpretation
≥18	(S) Susceptible
14-17	(I) Intermediate
≤13	(R) Resistant

Interpretation should be as stated above for results using dilution techniques.

As with standardized dilution techniques, diffusion methods require the use of laboratory control microorganisms. The 15 µg azithromycin disk should provide the following zone diameters in these laboratory test quality control strains (TABLE 20).

TABLE 20

Microorganism	Zone Diameter (mm)
Staphylococcus aureus ATCC 25923	21-26

In Vitro Activity of Azithromycin Against Mycobacteria

Azithromycin has demonstrated *in vitro* activity against *Mycobacterium avium* complex (MAC) organisms. While gene probe techniques may be used to distinguish between *M. avium* and *M. intracellulare,* many studies only reported results on *M. avium* complex (MAC) isolates. Azithromycin has also been shown to be active against phagocytized *M. avium* complex (MAC) organisms in mouse and human macrophage cell cultures as well as in the beige mouse infection model.

Various *in vitro* methodologies employing broth or solid media at different pHs, with and without oleic acid-albumin dextrose-catalase (OADC), have been used to determine azithromycin MIC values for *Mycobacterium avium* complex strains. In general, azithromycin MIC values decreased 4- to 8-fold as the pH of Middlebrook 7H11 agar media increased from 6.6 to 7.4. At pH 7.4, azithromycin MIC values determined with Mueller-Hinton agar were 4-fold higher than that observed with Middlebrook 7H12 media at the same pH. Utilization of oleic acid-albumin-dextrose-catalase (OADC) in these assays has been shown to further alter MIC values. The relationship between azithromycin and clarithromycin MIC values has not been established. In general, azithromycin MIC values were observed to be 2- to 32-fold higher than clarithromycin independent of the susceptibility method employed.

The ability to correlate MIC values and plasma drug levels is difficult as azithromycin concentrates in macrophages and tissues. (See CLINICAL PHARMACOLOGY.)

Drug Resistance

Complete cross-resistance between azithromycin and clarithromycin has been observed with *Mycobacterium avium* complex (MAC) isolates. In most isolates, a single point mutation at a position that is homologous to the *Escherichia coli* positions 2058 or 2059 on the 23S rRNA gene is the mechanism producing this cross-resistance pattern.[3,4] *Mycobacterium avium* complex (MAC) isolates exhibiting cross-resistance show an increase in azithromycin MICs to ≥128 µg/ml with clarithromycin MICs increasing to ≥32 µg/ml. These MIC values were determined employing the radiometric broth dilution susceptibility testing method with Middlebrook 7H12 medium. The clinical significance of azithromycin and clarithromycin cross-resistance is not fully understood at this time but preclinical data suggest that reduced activity to both agents will occur after *M. avium* complex strains produce the 23S rRNA mutation.

Susceptibility Testing for Mycobacterium avium Complex (MAC)

The disk diffusion techniques and dilution methods for susceptibility testing against gram-positive and gram-negative bacteria should not be used for determining azithromycin MIC values against mycobacteria. *In vitro* susceptibility testing methods and diagnostic products currently available for determining minimal inhibitory concentration (MIC) values against *Mycobacterium avium* complex (MAC) organisms have not been standardized or validated. Azithromycin MIC values will vary depending on the susceptibility testing method employed, composition and pH of media and the utilization of nutritional supplements. Breakpoints to determine whether clinical isolates of *M. avium* or *M. intracellulare* are susceptible or resistant to azithromycin have not been established.

The clinical relevance of azithromycin *in vitro* susceptibility test results for other mycobacterial species, including *Mycobacterium tuberculosis*, using any susceptibility testing method has not been determined.

ZITHROMAX 250 AND 500 MG TABLETS & ORAL SUSPENSION

Pharmacokinetics

Following oral administration of a single 500 mg dose (two 250 mg tablets) to 36 fasted healthy male volunteers, the mean (SD) pharmacokinetic parameters were AUC(0-72) = 4.3 (1.2) mg·h/ml; C_{max} = 0.5 (0.2) µg/ml; T_{max} = 2.2 (0.9) hours.

With a regimen of 500 mg (two 250 mg capsules*) on Day 1, followed by 250 mg daily (one 250 mg capsule) on Days 2-5, the pharmacokinetic parameters of azithromycin in plasma in healthy young adults (18-40 years of age) are portrayed in TABLE 21. C_{min} and C_{max} remained essentially unchanged from Day 2 through Day 5 of therapy.

*Azithromycin 250 mg tablets are equivalent to 250 mg capsules in the fasted state. Azithromycin 250 mg capsules are no longer commercially available.

TABLE 21

Pharmacokinetic Parameters (Mean)	Total n=12 Day 1	Day 5
C_{max} (µg/ml)	0.41	0.24
T_{max} (hours)	2.5	3.2
AUC(0-24) (µg·h/ml)	2.6	2.1
C_{min} (µg/ml)	0.05	0.05
Urinary Excret. (% dose)	4.5	6.5

In a two-way crossover study, 12 adult healthy volunteers (6 males, 6 females) received 1500 mg of azithromycin administered in single daily doses over either 5 days (two 250 mg tablets on Day 1, followed by one 250 mg tablet on Days 2-5) or 3 days (500 mg/day for Days 1-3). Due to limited serum samples on Day 2 (3 day regimen) and Days 2-4 (5 day regimen), the serum concentration-time profile of each subject was fit to a 3-compartment model and the AUC(0-∞) for the fitted concentration profile was comparable between the 5 day and 3 day regimens.

TABLE 22 *Pharmacokinetic Parameter [Mean (SD)]*

	3 Day Regimen		5 Day Regimen	
	Day 1	Day 3	Day 1	Day 5
C_{max} (serum, (µg/ml)	0.44 (0.22)	0.54 (0.25)	0.43 (0.20)	0.24 (0.06)
Serum AUC(0-∞) (µg·h/ml)	17.4 (6.2)*		14.9 (3.1)*	
Serum T½	71.8 hours		68.9 hours	

* Total AUC for the entire 3 day and 5 day regimens.

Median azithromycin exposure [AUC(0-288)] in mononuclear (MN) and polymorphonuclear (PMN) leukocytes following either the 5 day or 3 day regimen was more than a 1000-fold and 800-fold greater than in serum, respectively. Administration of the same total dose with either the 5 day or 3 day regimen may be expected to provide comparable concentrations of azithromycin within MN and PMN leukocytes.

Two azithromycin 250 mg tablets are bioequivalent to a single 500 mg tablet.

Absorption

The absolute bioavailability of azithromycin 250 mg capsules is 38%.

In a two-way crossover study in which 12 healthy subjects received a single 500 mg dose of azithromycin (two 250 mg tablets) with or without a high fat meal, food was shown to increase C_{max} by 23% but had no effect on AUC.

When azithromycin suspension was administered with food to 28 adult healthy male subjects, C_{max} increased by 56% and AUC was unchanged.

The AUC of azithromycin was unaffected by co-administration of an antacid containing aluminum and magnesium hydroxide with azithromycin capsules; however, the C_{max} was reduced by 24%. Administration of cimetidine (800 mg) 2 hours prior to azithromycin had no effect on azithromycin absorption.

Distribution

The serum protein binding of azithromycin is variable in the concentration range approximating human exposure, decreasing from 51% at 0.02 µg/ml to 7% at 2 µg/ml.

Following oral administration, azithromycin is widely distributed throughout the body with an apparent steady-state volume of distribution of 31.1 L/kg. Greater azithromycin concentrations in tissues than in plasma or serum were observed. High tissue concentrations should not be interpreted to be quantitatively related to clinical efficacy. The antimicrobial activity of azithromycin is pH related and appears to be reduced with decreasing pH. However, the extensive distribution of drug to tissues may be relevant to clinical activity.

Selected tissue (or fluid) concentration and tissue (or fluid) to plasma/serum concentration ratios are shown in TABLE 23.

The extensive tissue distribution was confirmed by examination of additional tissues and fluids (bone, ejaculum, prostate, ovary, uterus, salpinx, stomach, liver, and gallbladder). As there are no data from adequate and well-controlled studies of azithromycin treatment of infections in these additional body sites, the clinical importance of these tissue concentration data is unknown.

Following a regimen of 500 mg on the first day and 250 mg daily for 4 days, only very low concentrations were noted in cerebrospinal fluid (less than 0.01 µg/ml) in the presence of non-inflamed meninges.

TABLE 23 *Azithromycin Concentrations Following a 500 mg Dose (Two 250 mg Capsules) in Adults**

Tissue or Fluid	Time After Dose (hours)	Tissue or Fluid Concentration (μg/g or μg/ml)	Corresponding Plasma or Serum Level (μg/ml)	Tissue (Fluid) to Plasma (Serum) Ratio
Skin	72-96	0.4	0.012	35
Lung	72-96	4.0	0.012	>100
Sputum†	2-4	1.0	0.64	2
Sputum‡	10-12	2.9	0.1	30
Tonsil§	9-18	4.5	0.03	>100
Tonsil§	180	0.9	0.006	>100
Cervix¤	19	2.8	0.04	70

* Azithromycin tissue concentrations were originally determined using 250 mg capsules.
† Sample was obtained 2-4 hours after the first dose.
‡ Sample was obtained 10-12 hours after the first dose.
§ Dosing regimen of 2 doses of 250 mg each, separated by 12 hours.
¤ Sample was obtained 19 hours after a single 500 mg dose.

Metabolism

In vitro and *in vivo* studies to assess the metabolism of azithromycin have not been performed.

Elimination

Plasma concentrations of azithromycin following single 500 mg oral and IV doses declined in a polyphasic pattern with a mean apparent plasma clearance of 630 ml/min and terminal elimination half-life of 68 hours. The prolonged terminal half-life is thought to be due to extensive uptake and subsequent release of drug from tissues.

Biliary excretion of azithromycin, predominantly as unchanged drug, is a major route of elimination. Over the course of a week, approximately 6% of the administered dose appears as unchanged drug in urine.

Special Populations

Renal Insufficiency

Azithromycin pharmacokinetics were investigated in 42 adults (21-85 years of age) with varying degrees of renal impairment. Following the oral administration of a single 1000 mg dose of azithromycin, mean C_{max} and AUC(0-120) increased by 5.1% and 4.2%, respectively in subjects with mild to moderate renal impairment (GFR 10-80 ml/min) compared to subjects with normal renal function (GFR >80 ml/min). The mean C_{max} and AUC(0-120) increased 61% and 35%, respectively in subjects with severe renal impairment (GFR <10 ml/min) compared to subjects with normal renal function (GFR >80 ml/min). (See DOSAGE AND ADMINISTRATION.)

Hepatic Insufficiency

The pharmacokinetics of azithromycin in subjects with hepatic impairment have not been established.

Gender

There are no significant differences in the disposition of azithromycin between male and female subjects. No dosage adjustment is recommended based on gender.

Geriatric Patients

When studied in healthy elderly subjects aged 65-85 years, the pharmacokinetic parameters of azithromycin in elderly men were similar to those in young adults; however, in elderly women, although higher peak concentrations (increased by 30-50%) were observed, no significant accumulation occurred.

Pediatric Patients

In two clinical studies, azithromycin for oral suspension was dosed at 10 mg/kg on Day 1, followed by 5 mg/kg on Days 2-5 to two groups of children (aged 1-5 years and 5-15 years, respectively). The mean pharmacokinetic parameters on Day 5 were C_{max} = 0.216 μg/ml, T_{max} = 1.9 hours, and AUC(0-24) = 1.822 μg·h/ml for the 1- to 5-year-old group and were C_{max} = 0.383 μg/ml, T_{max} = 2.4 hours, and AUC(0-24) = 3.109 μg·h/ml for the 5- to 15-year-old group.

Two clinical studies were conducted in 68 children aged 3-16 years to determine the pharmacokinetics and safety of azithromycin for oral suspension in children. Azithromycin was administered following a low-fat breakfast.

The first study consisted of 35 pediatric patients treated with 20 mg/kg/day (maximum daily dose 500 mg) for 3 days of whom 34 patients were evaluated for pharmacokinetics.

In the second study, 33 pediatric patients received doses of 12 mg/kg/day (maximum daily dose 500 mg) for 5 days of whom 31 patients were evaluated for pharmacokinetics.

In both studies, azithromycin concentrations were determined over a 24 hour period following the last daily dose. Patients weighing above 25.0 kg in the 3 day study or 41.7 kg in the 5 day study received the maximum adult daily dose of 500 mg. Eleven (11) patients (weighing 25.0 kg or less) in the first study and 17 patients (weighing 41.7 kg or less) in the second study received a total dose of 60 mg/kg. TABLE 24 shows pharmacokinetic data in the subset of children who received a total dose of 60 mg/kg.

The similarity of the overall exposure [AUC(0-∞)] between the 3 day and 5 day regimens in pediatric patients is unknown.

Single dose pharmacokinetics in children given doses of 30 mg/kg have not been studied. (See DOSAGE AND ADMINISTRATION.)

Drug-Drug Interactions

Drug interaction studies were performed with azithromycin and other drugs likely to be co-administered. The effects of co-administration of azithromycin on the pharmacokinetics

TABLE 24 *Pharmacokinetic Parameter [Mean (SD)]*

	3 Day Regimen (20 mg/kg × 3 days) n=11	5 Day Regimen (12 mg/kg × 5 days) n=17
C_{max} (μg/ml)	1.1 (0.4)	0.5 (0.4)
T_{max} (h)	2.7 (1.9)	2.2 (0.8)
AUC(0-24) (μg·h/ml)	7.9 (2.9)	3.9 (1.9)

of other drugs are shown in TABLE 25 and the effect of other drugs on the pharmacokinetics of azithromycin are shown in TABLE 26.

Co-administration of azithromycin at therapeutic doses had a modest effect on the pharmacokinetics of the drugs listed in TABLE 25. No dosage adjustment of drugs listed in TABLE 25 is recommended when co-administered with azithromycin.

Co-administration of azithromycin with efavirenz or fluconazole had a modest effect on the pharmacokinetics of azithromycin. Nelfinavir significantly increased the C_{max} and AUC of azithromycin. No dosage adjustment of azithromycin is recommended when administered with drugs listed in TABLE 26. (See DRUG INTERACTIONS.)

TABLE 25 *Drug Interactions: Pharmacokinetic Parameters for Co-Administered Drugs in the Presence of Azithromycin*

Co-Administered Drug: Dose of Co-Administered Drug	Dose of Azithromycin	n	Ratio†: Mean C_{max}	Ratio†: Mean AUC
Atorvastatin				
10 mg/day × 8 days	500 mg/day PO on days 6-8	12	0.83 (0.63-1.08)	1.01 (0.81-1.25)
Carbamazepine				
200 mg/day × 2 days, then 200 mg bid × 18 days	500 mg/day PO for days 16-18	7	0.97 (0.88-1.06)	0.96 (0.88-1.06)
Cetirizine				
20 mg/day × 11 days	500 mg PO on day 7, then 250 mg/day on days 8-11	14	1.03 (0.93-1.14)	1.02 (0.92-1.13)
Didanosine				
200 mg PO bid × 21 days	1200 mg/day PO on days 8-21	6	1.44 (0.85-2.43)	1.14 (0.83-1.57)
Efavirenz				
400 mg/day × 7 days	600 mg PO on day 7	14	1.04*	0.95*
Fluconazole				
200 mg PO single dose	1200 mg PO single dose	18	1.04 (0.98-1.11)	1.01 (0.97-1.05)
Indinavir				
800 mg tid × 5 days	1200 mg PO on day 5	18	0.96 (0.86-1.08)	0.90 (0.81-1.00)
Midazolam				
15 mg PO on day 3	500 mg/day PO × 3 days	12	1.27 (0.89-1.81)	1.26 (1.01-1.56)
Nelfinavir				
750 mg tid × 11 days	1200 mg PO on day 9	14	0.90 (0.81-1.01)	0.85 (0.78-0.93)
Rifabutin				
300 mg/day × 10 days	500 mg PO on day 1, then 250 mg/day	6	‡	NA
Sildenafil				
100 mg on days 1 and 4	500 mg/day PO × 3 days	12	1.16 (0.86-1.57)	0.92 (0.75-1.12)
Theophylline				
4 mg/kg IV on days 1, 11, 25	500 mg PO on day 7, 250 mg/day on days 8-11	10	1.19 (1.02-1.40)	1.02 (0.86-1.22)
300 mg PO bid × 15 days	500 mg PO on day 6, then 250 mg/day on days 7-10	8	1.09 (0.92-1.29)	1.08 (0.89-1.31)
Triazolam				
0.125 mg on day 2	500 mg PO on day 1, then 250 mg/day on day 2	12	1.06*	1.02*
Trimethoprim/Sulfamethoxazole				
160 mg/800 mg/day PO × 7 days	1200 mg PO on day 7	12	0.85 (0.75-0.97)/ 0.90 (0.78-1.03)	0.87 (0.80-0.95)/ 0.96 (0.88-1.03)
Zidovudine				
500 mg/day PO × 21 days	600 mg/day PO × 14 days	5	1.12 (0.42-3.02)	0.94 (0.52-1.70)
500 mg/day PO × 21 days	1200 mg/day PO × 14 days	4	1.31 (0.43-3.97)	1.30 (0.69-2.43)

NA Not available.
* 90% confidence interval not reported.
† Ratio (with/without azithromycin) of co-administered drug pharmacokinetic parameters (90% CI); No effect = 1.00.
‡ Mean rifabutin concentrations one-half day after the last dose of rifabutin were 60 ng/ml when co-administered with azithromycin and 71 ng/ml when co-administered with placebo.

Microbiology

Azithromycin acts by binding to the 50S ribosomal subunit of susceptible microorganisms and, thus, interfering with microbial protein synthesis. Nucleic acid synthesis is not affected.

Azithromycin concentrates in phagocytes and fibroblasts as demonstrated by *in vitro* incubation techniques. Using such methodology, the ratio of intracellular to extracellular con-

TABLE 26 *Drug Interactions: Pharmacokinetic Parameters for Azithromycin in the Presence of Co-administered Drugs (see DRUG INTERACTIONS)*

Co-Administered Drug / Dose of Co-Administered Drug	Dose of Azithromycin	n	Ratio† Mean C_{max}	Mean AUC
Efavirenz				
400 mg/day × 7 days	600 mg PO on day 7	14	1.22 (1.04-1.42)	0.92*
Fluconazole				
200 mg PO single dose	1200 mg PO single dose	18	0.82 (0.66-1.02)	1.07 (0.94-1.22)
Nelfinavir				
750 mg tid × 11 days	1200 mg PO on day 9	14	2.36 (1.77-3.15)	2.12 (1.80-2.50)
Rifabutin				
300 mg/day × 10 days	500 mg PO on day 1, then 250 mg/day on days 2-10	6	‡	NA

NA Not available.
* 90% confidence interval not reported.
† Ratio (with/without co-administered drug) of azithromycin pharmacokinetic parameters (90% CI); No effect = 1.00.
‡ Mean azithromycin concentrations 1 day after the last dose were 53 ng/ml when co-administered with 300 mg daily rifabutin and 49 ng/ml when co-administered with placebo.

centration was >30 after 1 hour incubation. *In vivo* studies suggest that concentration in phagocytes may contribute to drug distribution to inflamed tissues.

Azithromycin has been shown to be active against most isolates of the following microorganisms, both *in vitro* and in clinical infections as described in INDICATIONS AND USAGE.

Aerobic and Facultative Gram-Positive Microorganisms:
Staphylococcus aureus, Streptococcus agalactiae, Streptococcus pneumoniae, and *Streptococcus pyogenes.*

Note: Azithromycin demonstrates cross-resistance with erythromycin-resistant gram-positive strains. Most strains of *Enterococcus faecalis* and methicillin-resistant staphylococci are resistant to azithromycin.

Aerobic and Facultative Gram-Negative Microorganisms:
Haemophilus ducreyi, Haemophilus influenzae, Moraxella catarrhalis, and *Neisseria gonorrhoeae.*

"Other" Microorganisms:
Chlamydia pneumoniae, Chlamydia trachomatis, and *Mycoplasma pneumoniae.*

Beta-lactamase production should have no effect on azithromycin activity.

The following *in vitro* data are available, **but their clinical significance is unknown.**

At least 90% of the following microorganisms exhibit an *in vitro* minimum inhibitory concentration (MIC) less than or equal to the susceptible breakpoints for azithromycin. However, the safety and effectiveness of azithromycin in treating clinical infections due to these microorganisms have not been established in adequate and well-controlled trials.

Aerobic and Facultative Gram-Positive Microorganisms:
Streptococci (Groups C, F, G), and Viridans group streptococci.

Aerobic and Facultative Gram-Negative Microorganisms:
Bordetella pertussis, and *Legionella pneumophila.*

Anaerobic Microorganisms:
Peptostreptococcus species, and *Prevotella bivia.*

"Other" Microorganisms:
Ureaplasma urealyticum.

Susceptibility Testing Methods

When available, the results of *in vitro* susceptibility test results for antimicrobial drugs used in resident hospitals should be provided to the physician as periodic reports which describe the susceptibility profile of nosocomial and community-acquired pathogens. These reports may differ from susceptibility data obtained from outpatient use, but could aid the physician in selecting the most effective antimicrobial.

Dilution Techniques

Quantitative methods are used to determine antimicrobial minimum inhibitory concentrations (MICs). These MICs provide estimates of the susceptibility of bacteria to antimicrobial compounds. The MICs should be determined using a standardized procedure. Standardized procedures are based on a dilution method[5,7] (broth or agar) or equivalent with standardized inoculum concentrations and standardized concentrations of azithromycin powder. The MIC values should be interpreted according to criteria provided in TABLE 27.

Diffusion Techniques

Quantitative methods that require measurement of zone diameters also provide reproducible estimates of the susceptibility of bacteria to antimicrobial compounds. One such standardized procedure[6,7] requires the use of standardized inoculum concentrations. This procedure uses paper disks impregnated with 15 mg azithromycin to test the susceptibility of microorganisms to azithromycin. The disk diffusion interpretive criteria are provided in TABLE 27.

No interpretive criteria have been established for testing *Neisseria gonorrhoeae.* This species is not usually tested.

A report of "susceptible" indicates that the pathogen is likely to be inhibited if the antimicrobial compound reaches the concentrations usually achievable. A report of "intermediate" indicates that the result should be considered equivocal, and, if the microorganism is not fully susceptible to alternative, clinically feasible drugs, the test should be repeated. This category implies possible clinical applicability in body sites where the drug is physiologically concentrated or in situations where high dosage of drug can be used. This category also

TABLE 27 *Susceptibility Interpretive Criteria for Azithromycin Susceptibility Test Result Interpretive Criteria*

Pathogen	Minimum Inhibitory Concentrations (µg/ml) S	I	R*	Disk Diffusion (Zone Diameters in mm) S	I	R*
Haemophilus spp.	≤4	—	—	≥12	—	—
Staphylococcus aureus	≤2	4	≥8	≥18	14-17	≤13
Streptococci including *S. pneumoniae*†	≤0.5	1	≥2	≥18	14-17	≤13

* The current absence of data on resistant strains precludes defining any category other than "susceptible". If strains yield MIC results other than susceptible, they should be submitted to a reference laboratory for further testing.
† Susceptibility of streptococci including *S. pneumoniae* to azithromycin and other macrolides can be predicted by testing erythromycin.

provides a buffer zone which prevents small uncontrolled technical factors from causing major discrepancies in interpretation. A report of "resistant" indicates that the pathogen is not likely to be inhibited if the antimicrobial compound reaches the concentrations usually achievable; other therapy should be selected.

Quality Control

Standardized susceptibility test procedures require the use of quality control microorganisms to control the technical aspects of the test procedures. Standard azithromycin powder should provide the following range of values noted in TABLE 28. Quality control microorganisms are specific strains of organisms with intrinsic biological properties. QC strains are very stable trains which will give a standard and repeatable susceptibility pattern. The specific strains used for microbiological quality control are not clinically significant.

TABLE 28 *Acceptable Quality Control Ranges for Azithromycin*

QC Strain	Minimum Inhibitory Concentrations	Disk Diffusion (Zone Diameters)
Haemophilus influenzae ATCC 49247	1.0-4.0 µg/ml	13-21 mm
Staphylococcus aureus ATCC 29213	0.5-2.0 µg/ml	
Staphylococcus aureus ATCC 25923		21-26 mm
Streptococcus pneumoniae ATCC 49619	0.06-0.25 µg/ml	19-25 mm

INDICATIONS AND USAGE

ZITHROMAX CAPSULES, 600 MG TABLETS, & ORAL SUSPENSION IN PACKETS

Zithromax is indicated for the treatment of patients with mild to moderate infections (pneumonia: see WARNINGS) caused by susceptible strains of the designated microorganisms in the specific conditions listed below.

Lower Respiratory Tract

Acute bacterial exacerbations of chronic obstructive pulmonary disease due to *Haemophilus influenzae, Moraxella catarrhalis,* or *Streptococcus pneumoniae.*

Community-acquired pneumonia of mild severity due to *Streptococcus pneumoniae* or *Haemophilus influenzae* in patients appropriate for outpatient oral therapy.

NOTE: Azithromycin should not be used in patients with pneumonia who are judged to be inappropriate for outpatient oral therapy because of moderate to severe illness or risk factors such as any of the following:

- **patients with nosocomially acquired infections,**
- **patients with known or suspected bacteremia,**
- **patients requiring hospitalization,**
- **elderly or debilitated patients, or**
- **patients with significant underlying health problems that may compromise their ability to respond to their illness (including immunodeficiency or functional asplenia).**

Upper Respiratory Tract

Streptococcal pharyngitis/tonsillitis as an alternative to first line therapy of acute pharyngitis/tonsillitis due to *Streptococcus pyogenes* occurring in individuals who cannot use first line therapy.

Note: Penicillin is the usual drug of choice in the treatment of *Streptococcus pyogenes* infection and the prophylaxis of rheumatic fever. Zithromax is often effective in the eradication of susceptible strains of *Streptococcus pyogenes* from the nasopharynx. Data establishing efficacy of azithromycin in subsequent prevention of rheumatic fever are not available.

Skin and Skin Structure

Uncomplicated skin and skin structure infections due to *Staphylococcus aureus, Streptococcus pyogenes,* or *Streptococcus agalactiae.* Abscesses usually require surgical drainage.

Sexually Transmitted Diseases

Non-gonococcal urethritis and cervicitis due to *Chlamydia trachomatis.*

Zithromax, at the recommended dose, should not be relied upon to treat gonorrhea or syphilis. Antimicrobial agents used in high doses for short periods of time to treat non-gonococcal urethritis may mask or delay the symptoms of incubating gonorrhea or syphilis. All patients with sexually-transmitted urethritis or cervicitis should have a serologic test for syphilis and appropriate cultures for gonorrhea performed at the time of diagnosis. Appropriate antimicrobial therapy and follow-up tests for these diseases should be initiated if infection is confirmed.

Appropriate culture and susceptibility tests should be performed before treatment to determine the causative organism and its susceptibility to azithromycin. Therapy with Zithromax may be initiated before results of these tests are known; once the results become available, antimicrobial therapy should be adjusted accordingly.

Mycobacterial Infections

Prophylaxis of Disseminated Mycobacterium avium Complex (MAC) Disease: Zithromax, taken alone or in combination with rifabutin at its approved dose, is indicated for the prevention of disseminated Mycobacterium avium complex (MAC) disease in persons with advanced HIV infection. (See DOSAGE AND ADMINISTRATION.)

Treatment of Disseminated Mycobacterium avium Complex (MAC) Disease: *Zithromax, taken in combination with ethambutol, is indicated for the treatment of disseminated MAC infections in persons with advanced HIV infection. (See DOSAGE AND ADMINISTRATION .)*

ZITHROMAX 250 AND 500 MG TABLETS & ORAL SUSPENSION

Zithromax is indicated for the treatment of patients with mild to moderate infections (pneumonia: see WARNINGS) caused by susceptible strains of the designated microorganisms in the specific conditions listed below. As recommended dosages, durations of therapy and applicable patient populations vary among these infections, please see DOSAGE AND ADMINISTRATION for specific dosing recommendations.

Adults

Acute bacterial exacerbations of chronic obstructive pulmonary disease due to *Haemophilus influenzae, Moraxella catarrhalis* or *Streptococcus pneumoniae.*

Community-acquired pneumonia due to *Chlamydia pneumoniae, Haemophilus influenzae, Mycoplasma pneumoniae* or *Streptococcus pneumoniae* in patients appropriate for oral therapy.

NOTE: Azithromycin should not be used in patients with pneumonia who are judged to be inappropriate for oral therapy because of moderate to severe illness or risk factors such as any of the following:
- **patients with cystic fibrosis,**
- **patients with nosocomially acquired infections,**
- **patients with known or suspected bacteremia,**
- **patients requiring hospitalization,**
- **elderly or debilitated patients, or**
- **patients with significant underlying health problems that may compromise their ability to respond to their illness (including immunodeficiency or functional asplenia).**

Pharyngitis/tonsillitis caused by *Streptococcus pyogenes* as an alternative to first-line therapy in individuals who cannot use first-line therapy.

Note: Penicillin by the intramuscular route is the usual drug of choice in the treatment of *Streptococcus pyogenes* infection and the prophylaxis of rheumatic fever. Zithromax is often effective in the eradication of susceptible strains of *Streptococcus pyogenes* from the nasopharynx. Because some strains are resistant to Zithromax, susceptibility tests should be performed when patients are treated with Zithromax. Data establishing efficacy of azithromycin in subsequent prevention of rheumatic fever are not available.

Uncomplicated skin and skin structure infections due to *Staphylococcus aureus, Streptococcus pyogenes,* or *Streptococcus agalactiae.* Abscesses usually require surgical drainage.

Urethritis and cervicitis due to *Chlamydia trachomatis* or *Neisseria gonorrhoeae.*

Genital ulcer disease in men due to *Haemophilus ducreyi* (chancroid). Due to the small number of women included in clinical trials, the efficacy of azithromycin in the treatment of chancroid in women has not been established.

Zithromax, at the recommended dose, should not be relied upon to treat syphilis. Antimicrobial agents used in high doses for short periods of time to treat nongonococcal urethritis may mask or delay the symptoms of incubating syphilis. All patients with sexually-transmitted urethritis or cervicitis should have a serologic test for syphilis and appropriate cultures for gonorrhea performed at the time of diagnosis. Appropriate antimicrobial therapy and follow-up tests for these diseases should be initiated if infection is confirmed.

Appropriate culture and susceptibility tests should be performed before treatment to determine the causative organism and its susceptibility to azithromycin. Therapy with Zithromax may be initiated before results of these tests are known; once the results become available, antimicrobial therapy should be adjusted accordingly.

Children

See PRECAUTIONS, Pediatric Use.

Acute otitis media caused by *Haemophilus influenzae, Moraxella catarrhalis* or *Streptococcus pneumoniae.* (For specific dosage recommendation, see DOSAGE AND ADMINISTRATION.)

Community-acquired pneumonia due to *Chlamydia pneumoniae, Haemophilus influenzae, Mycoplasma pneumoniae* or *Streptococcus pneumoniae* in patients appropriate for oral therapy. (For specific dosage recommendation, see DOSAGE AND ADMINISTRATION.)

NOTE: Azithromycin should not be used in pediatric patients with pneumonia who are judged to be inappropriate for oral therapy because of moderate to severe illness or risk factors such as any of the following:
- **patients with cystic fibrosis,**
- **patients with nosocomially acquired infections,**
- **patients with known or suspected bacteremia,**
- **patients requiring hospitalization, or**
- **patients with significant underlying health problems that may compromise their ability to respond to their illness (including immunodeficiency or functional asplenia).**

Pharyngitis/tonsillitis caused by *Streptococcus pyogenes* as an alternative to first-line therapy in individuals who cannot use first-line therapy. (For specific dosage recommendation, see DOSAGE AND ADMINISTRATION.)

Note: Penicillin by the intramuscular route is the usual drug of choice in the treatment of *Streptococcus pyogenes* infection and the prophylaxis of rheumatic fever. Zithromax is often effective in the eradication of susceptible strains of *Streptococcus pyogenes* from the nasopharynx. Because some strains are resistant to Zithromax, susceptibility tests should be performed when patients are treated with Zithromax. Data establishing efficacy of azithromycin in subsequent prevention of rheumatic fever are not available.

Appropriate culture and susceptibility tests should be performed before treatment to determine the causative organism and its susceptibility to azithromycin. Therapy with Zithromax may be initiated before results of these tests are known; once the results become available, antimicrobial therapy should be adjusted accordingly.

NON-FDA APPROVED INDICATIONS

Azithromycin may also be used to treat Lyme disease, uncomplicated Typhoid Fever, and toxoplasmosis, however, these are not approved indications.

CONTRAINDICATIONS

ZITHROMAX CAPSULES, 600 MG TABLETS, & ORAL SUSPENSION IN PACKETS

Zithromax is contraindicated in patients with known hypersensitivity to azithromycin, erythromycin, or any macrolide antibiotic.

ZITHROMAX 250 AND 500 MG TABLETS & ORAL SUSPENSION

Zithromax is contraindicated in patients with known hypersensitivity to azithromycin, erythromycin or any macrolide antibiotic.

WARNINGS

ZITHROMAX CAPSULES, 600 MG TABLETS, & ORAL SUSPENSION IN PACKETS

Rare serious allergic reactions, including angioedema and anaphylaxis, have been reported rarely in patients on azithromycin therapy. (See CONTRAINDICATIONS.) Despite initially successful symptomatic treatment of the allergic symptoms, when symptomatic therapy was discontinued, the allergic symptoms **recurred soon thereafter in some patients without further azithromycin exposure.** These patients required prolonged periods of observation and symptomatic treatment. The relationship of these episodes to the long tissue half-life of azithromycin and subsequent prolonged exposure to antigen is unknown at present.

If an allergic reaction occurs, the drug should be discontinued and appropriate therapy should be instituted. Physicians should be aware that reappearance of the allergic symptoms may occur when symptomatic therapy is discontinued.

In the treatment of pneumonia, azithromycin has only been shown to be safe and effective in the treatment of community-acquired pneumonia of mild severity due to *Streptococcus pneumoniae* or *Haemophilus influenzae* in patients appropriate for outpatient oral therapy. Azithromycin should not be used in patients with pneumonia who are judged to be inappropriate for outpatient oral therapy because of moderate to severe illness or risk factors such as any of the following: patients with nosocomially acquired infections, patients with known or suspected bacteremia, patients requiring hospitalization, elderly or debilitated patients, or patients with significant underlying health problems that may compromise their ability to respond to their illness (including immunodeficiency or functional asplenia). Pseudomembranous colitis has been reported with nearly all antibacterial agents and may range in severity from mild to life-threatening. Therefore, it is important to consider this diagnosis in patients who present with diarrhea subsequent to the administration of antibacterial agents.

Treatment with antibacterial agents alters the normal flora of the colon and may permit overgrowth of clostridia. Studies indicate that a toxin produced by *Clostridium difficile* is a primary cause of "antibiotic-associated colitis".

After the diagnosis of pseudomembranous colitis has been established, therapeutic measures should be initiated. Mild cases of pseudomembranous colitis usually respond to discontinuation of the drug alone. In moderate to severe cases, consideration should be given to management with fluids and electrolytes, protein supplementation, and treatment with an antibacterial drug clinically effective against *Clostridium difficile* colitis.

ZITHROMAX 250 AND 500 MG TABLETS & ORAL SUSPENSION

Serious allergic reactions, including angioedema, anaphylaxis, and dermatologic reactions including Stevens Johnson Syndrome and toxic epidermal necrolysis have been reported rarely in patients on azithromycin therapy. Although rare, fatalities have been reported. (See CONTRAINDICATIONS.) Despite initially successful symptomatic treatment of the allergic symptoms, when symptomatic therapy was discontinued, the allergic symptoms **recurred soon thereafter in some patients without further azithromycin exposure.** These patients required prolonged periods of observation and symptomatic treatment. The relationship of these episodes to the long tissue half-life of azithromycin and subsequent prolonged exposure to antigen is unknown at present.

If an allergic reaction occurs, the drug should be discontinued and appropriate therapy should be instituted. Physicians should be aware that reappearance of the allergic symptoms may occur when symptomatic therapy is discontinued.

In the treatment of pneumonia, azithromycin has only been shown to be safe and effective in the treatment of community-acquired pneumonia due to *Chlamydia pneumoniae, Haemophilus influenzae, Mycoplasma pneumoniae* or *Streptococcus pneumoniae* in patients appropriate for oral therapy. Azithromycin should not be used in patients with pneumonia who are judged to be inappropriate for oral therapy because of moderate to severe illness or risk factors such as any of the following: patients with cystic fibrosis, patients with nosocomially acquired infections, patients with known or suspected bacteremia, patients requiring hospitalization, elderly or debilitated patients, or patients with significant underlying health problems that may compromise their ability to respond to their illness (including immunodeficiency or functional asplenia).

Pseudomembranous colitis has been reported with nearly all antibacterial agents and may range in severity from mild to life-threatening. Therefore, it is important to

consider this diagnosis in patients who present with diarrhea subsequent to the administration of antibacterial agents.

Treatment with antibacterial agents alters the normal flora of the colon and may permit overgrowth of clostridia. Studies indicate that a toxin produced by *Clostridium difficile* is a primary cause of "antibiotic-associated colitis".

After the diagnosis of pseudomembranous colitis has been established, therapeutic measures should be initiated. Mild cases of pseudomembranous colitis usually respond to discontinuation of the drug alone. In moderate to severe cases, consideration should be given to management with fluids and electrolytes, protein supplementation, and treatment with an antibacterial drug clinically effective against *Clostridium difficile* colitis.

PRECAUTIONS

ZITHROMAX CAPSULES, 600 MG TABLETS, & ORAL SUSPENSION IN PACKETS

General

Because azithromycin is principally eliminated via the liver, caution should be exercised when azithromycin is administered to patients with impaired hepatic function. There are no data regarding azithromycin usage in patients with renal impairment; thus, caution should be exercised when prescribing azithromycin in these patients.

The following adverse events have been reported with macrolide products: ventricular arrhythmias, including ventricular tachycardia and *torsades de pointes,* in individuals with prolonged QT intervals.

There has been a spontaneous report from the post-marketing experience of a patient with previous history of arrhythmias who experienced *torsades de pointes* and subsequent myocardial infarction following a course of azithromycin therapy.

Information for the Patient

Patients should be cautioned to take azithromycin capsules at least 1 hour prior to a meal or at least 2 hours after a meal. Azithromycin capsules should not be taken with food.

Azithromycin tablets may be taken with or without food. However, increased tolerability has been observed when tablets are taken with food.

Azithromycin for oral suspension in single 1 g packets can be taken with or without food after constitution.

Patients should also be cautioned not to take aluminum- and magnesium-containing antacids and azithromycin simultaneously.

The patient should be directed to discontinue azithromycin immediately and contact a physician if any signs of an allergic reaction occur.

Laboratory Test Interactions

There are no reported laboratory test interactions.

Carcinogenesis, Mutagenesis, and Impairment of Fertility

Long-term studies in animals have not been performed to evaluate carcinogenic potential. Azithromycin has shown no mutagenic potential in standard laboratory tests: mouse lymphoma assay, human lymphocyte clastogenic assay, and mouse bone marrow clastogenic assay.

Pregnancy, Teratogenic Effects, Pregnancy Category B

Reproduction studies have been performed in rats and mice at doses up to moderately maternally toxic dose levels (*i.e.,* 200 mg/kg/day). These doses, based on a mg/m^2 basis, are estimated to be 4 and 2 times, respectively, the human daily dose of 500 mg.

With regard to the MAC treatment dose of 600 mg daily, on a mg/m^2/day basis, the doses in rats and mice are approximately 3.3 and 1.7 times the human dose, respectively.

With regard to the MAC prophylaxis dose of 1200 mg weekly, on a mg/m^2/day basis, the doses in rats and mice are approximately 2 and 1 times the human dose, respectively.

No evidence of impaired fertility or harm to the fetus due to azithromycin was found. There are, however, no adequate and well-controlled studies in pregnant women. Because animal reproduction studies are not always predictive of human response, azithromycin should be used during pregnancy only if clearly needed.

Nursing Mothers

It is not known whether azithromycin is excreted in human milk. Because many drugs are excreted in human milk, caution should be exercised when azithromycin is administered to a nursing woman.

Pediatric Use

In controlled clinical studies, azithromycin has been administered to pediatric patients ranging in age from 6 months to 12 years. For information regarding the use of azithromycin for oral suspension in the treatment of pediatric patients, please refer to the INDICATIONS AND USAGE and DOSAGE AND ADMINISTRATION sections of the prescribing information for azithromycin for oral suspension 100 mg/5 ml and 200 mg/5 ml bottles.

Safety in HIV-Infected Pediatric Patients

Safety and efficacy of azithromycin for the prevention or treatment of MAC in HIV-infected children have not been established. Safety data are available for 72 children 5 months to 18 years of age (mean 7 years) who received azithromycin for treatment of opportunistic infections. The mean duration of therapy was 242 days (range 3-2004 days) at doses of <1 to 52 mg/kg/day (mean 12 mg/kg/day). Adverse events were similar to those observed in the adult population, most of which involved the gastrointestinal tract. Treatment related reversible hearing impairment in children was observed in 4 subjects (5.6%). Two (2.8%) children prematurely discontinued treatment due to side effects: 1 due to back pain and 1 due to abdominal pain, hot and cold flushes, dizziness, headache, and numbness. A third child discontinued due to a laboratory abnormality (eosinophilia). The protocols upon which these data are based specified a daily dose of 10-20 mg/kg/day (oral and/or IV) of azithromycin.

Geriatric Use

Pharmacokinetic parameters in older volunteers (65-85 years old) were similar to those in younger volunteers (18-40 years old) for the 5 day therapeutic regimen. Dosage adjustment does not appear to be necessary for older patients with normal renal and hepatic function receiving treatment with this dosage regimen. (See CLINICAL PHARMACOLOGY.)

Geriatric Patients With Opportunistic Infections, Including Mycobacterium avium Complex (MAC) Disease

Safety data are available for 30 patients (65-94 years old) treated with azithromycin at doses >300 mg/day for a mean of 207 days. These patients were treated for a variety of opportunistic infections, including MAC. The side effect profile was generally similar to that seen in younger patients, except for a higher incidence of side effects relating to the gastrointestinal system and to reversible impairment of hearing. (See DOSAGE AND ADMINISTRATION.)

ZITHROMAX 250 AND 500 MG TABLETS & ORAL SUSPENSION

General

Because azithromycin is principally eliminated via the liver, caution should be exercised when azithromycin is administered to patients with impaired hepatic function. Due to the limited data in subjects with GFR <10 ml/min, caution should be exercised when prescribing azithromycin in these patients. (See CLINICAL PHARMACOLOGY, Special Populations, Renal Insufficiency.)

The following adverse events have been reported with macrolide products: ventricular arrhythmias, including ventricular tachycardia and *torsade de pointes,* in individuals with prolonged QT intervals.

There has been a spontaneous report from the post-marketing experience of a patient with previous history of arrhythmias who experienced *torsade de pointes* and subsequent myocardial infarction following a course of azithromycin therapy.

Information for the Patient

Azithromycin tablets and oral suspension can be taken with or without food.

Patients should also be cautioned not to take aluminum- and magnesium-containing antacids and azithromycin simultaneously.

The patient should be directed to discontinue azithromycin immediately and contact a physician if any signs of an allergic reaction occur.

Laboratory Test Interactions

There are no reported laboratory test interactions.

Carcinogenesis, Mutagenesis, and Impairment of Fertility

Long-term studies in animals have not been performed to evaluate carcinogenic potential. Azithromycin has shown no mutagenic potential in standard laboratory tests: mouse lymphoma assay, human lymphocyte clastogenic assay, and mouse bone marrow clastogenic assay. No evidence of impaired fertility due to azithromycin was found.

Pregnancy, Teratogenic Effects, Pregnancy Category B

Reproduction studies have been performed in rats and mice at doses up to moderately maternally toxic dose concentrations (*i.e.,* 200 mg/kg/day). These doses, based on a mg/m^2 basis, are estimated to be 4 and 2 times, respectively, the human daily dose of 500 mg. In the animal studies, no evidence of harm to the fetus due to azithromycin was found. There are, however, no adequate and well-controlled studies in pregnant women. Because animal reproduction studies are not always predictive of human response, azithromycin should be used during pregnancy only if clearly needed.

Nursing Mothers

It is not known whether azithromycin is excreted in human milk. Because many drugs are excreted in human milk, caution should be exercised when azithromycin is administered to a nursing woman.

Pediatric Use

See CLINICAL PHARMACOLOGY, INDICATIONS AND USAGE, and DOSAGE AND ADMINISTRATION.

Acute Otitis Media (total dosage regimen: 30 mg/kg, see DOSAGE AND ADMINISTRATION): Safety and effectiveness in the treatment of children with otitis media under 6 months of age have not been established.

Community-Acquired Pneumonia (dosage regimen: 10 mg/kg on day 1 followed by 5 mg/kg on days 2-5): Safety and effectiveness in the treatment of children with community-acquired pneumonia under 6 months of age have not been established. Safety and effectiveness for pneumonia due to *Chlamydia pneumoniae* and *Mycoplasma pneumoniae* were documented in pediatric clinical trials. Safety and effectiveness for pneumonia due to *Haemophilus influenzae* and *Streptococcus pneumoniae* were not documented bacteriologically in the pediatric clinical trial due to difficulty in obtaining specimens. Use of azithromycin for these two microorganisms is supported, however, by evidence from adequate and well-controlled studies in adults.

Pharyngitis/Tonsillitis (dosage regimen: 12 mg/kg on days 1-5): Safety and effectiveness in the treatment of children with pharyngitis/tonsillitis under 2 years of age have not been established.

Studies evaluating the use of repeated courses of therapy have not been conducted. (See CLINICAL PHARMACOLOGY and ANIMAL PHARMACOLOGY.)

Geriatric Use

Pharmacokinetic parameters in older volunteers (65-85 years old) were similar to those in younger volunteers (18-40 years old) for the 5 day therapeutic regimen. Dosage adjustment does not appear to be necessary for older patients with normal renal and hepatic function receiving treatment with this dosage regimen. (See CLINICAL PHARMACOLOGY.)

DRUG INTERACTIONS

CAPSULES, 600 MG TABLETS, & ORAL SUSPENSION IN PACKETS

Aluminum- and magnesium-containing antacids reduce the peak serum levels (rate) but not the AUC (extent) of azithromycin (500 mg) absorption.

Administration of cimetidine (800 mg) 2 hours prior to azithromycin had no effect on azithromycin (500 mg) absorption.

A single oral dose of 1200 mg azithromycin (2 × 600 mg azithromycin tablets) did not alter the pharmacokinetics of a single 800 mg oral dose of fluconazole in healthy adult subjects.

Total exposure (AUC) and half-life of azithromycin following the single oral tablet dose of 1200 mg were unchanged and the reduction in C_{max} was not significant (mean decrease of 18%) by co-administration with 800 mg fluconazole.

A single oral dose of 1200 mg azithromycin (2 × 600 mg azithromycin tablets) had no significant effect on the pharmacokinetics of indinavir (800 mg indinavir tid for 5 days) in healthy adult subjects.

Co-administration of a single oral dose of 1200 mg azithromycin (2 × 600 mg azithromycin tablets) with steady-state nelfinavir (750 mg tid) to healthy adult subjects produced a decrease of approximately 15% in mean AUC(0-8) of nelfinavir and its M8 metabolite. Mean C_{max} of nelfinavir and its M8 metabolite were not significantly affected. No dosage adjustment of nelfinavir is required when nelfinavir is co-administered with azithromycin.

Co-administration of nelfinavir (750 mg tid) at steady state with a single oral dose of 1200 mg azithromycin increased the mean AUC(0-∞) of azithromycin by approximately a factor of 2 times (range of up to 4 times) of that when azithromycin was given alone. The mean C_{max} of azithromycin was also increased by approximately a factor of 2 times (range of up to 5 times) of that when azithromycin was given alone. Dose adjustment of azithromycin is not recommended. However, when administered in conjunction with nelfinavir, close monitoring for known side effects of azithromycin, such as liver enzyme abnormalities and hearing impairment, is warranted. (See ADVERSE REACTIONS.)

Following administration of trimethoprim/sulfamethoxazole DS (160 mg/800 mg) for 7 days to healthy adult subjects, co-administration of 1200 mg azithromycin (2 × 600 mg azithromycin tablets) on the 7th day had no significant effects on peak concentrations (C_{max}), total exposure (AUC), and the urinary excretion of either trimethoprim or sulfamethoxazole.

Co-administration of trimethoprim/sulfamethoxazole DS for 7 days had no significant effect on the peak concentration (C_{max}) and total exposure (AUC) of azithromycin following administration of the single 1200 mg tablet dose to healthy adult subjects.

Administration of a 600 mg single oral dose of azithromycin had no effect on the pharmacokinetics of efavirenz given at 400 mg doses for 7 days to healthy adult subjects.

Efavirenz, when administered at a dose of 400 mg for 7 days produced a 22% increase in the C_{max} of azithromycin administered as a 600 mg single oral dose, while the AUC of azithromycin was not affected.

Azithromycin (500 mg Day 1, 250 mg Days 2-5) did not affect the plasma levels or pharmacokinetics of theophylline administered as a single IV dose. The effect of azithromycin on the plasma levels or pharmacokinetics of theophylline administered in multiple doses resulting in therapeutic steady-state levels of theophylline is not known. However, concurrent use of macrolides and theophylline has been associated with increases in the serum concentrations of theophylline. Therefore, until further data are available, prudent medical practice dictates careful monitoring of plasma theophylline levels in patients receiving azithromycin and theophylline concomitantly.

Azithromycin (500 mg Day 1, 250 mg Days 2-5) did not affect the prothrombin time response to a single dose of warfarin. However, prudent medical practice dictates careful monitoring of prothrombin time in all patients treated with azithromycin and warfarin concomitantly. Concurrent use of macrolides and warfarin in clinical practice has been associated with increased anticoagulant effects.

Dose adjustments are not indicated when azithromycin and zidovudine are co-administered. When zidovudine (100 mg q3h × 5) was co-administered with daily azithromycin (600 mg, n=5 or 1200 mg, n=7), mean C_{max}, AUC and CLR increased by 26% (CV 54%), 10% (CV 26%) and 8% (CV 114%), respectively. The mean AUC of phosphorylated zidovudine increased by 75% (CV 95%), while zidovudine glucuronide C_{max} and AUC increased by less than 10%. In another study, addition of 1 g azithromycin/week to a regimen of 10 mg/kg daily zidovudine resulted in 25% (CV 70%) and 13% (CV 37%) increases in zidovudine C_{max} and AUC, respectively. Zidovudine glucuronide mean C_{max} and AUC increased by 16% (CV 61%) and 8.0% (CV 32%), respectively.

Doses of 1200 mg/day azithromycin for 14 days in 6 subjects increased C_{max} of concurrently administered didanosine (200 mg q12h) by 44% (54% CV) and AUC by 14% (23% CV). However, none of these changes were significantly different from those produced in a parallel placebo control group of subjects.

Preliminary data suggest that co-administration of azithromycin and rifabutin did not markedly affect the mean serum concentrations of either drug. Administration of 250 mg azithromycin daily for 10 days (500 mg on the first day) produced mean concentrations of azithromycin 1 day after the last dose of 53 ng/ml when co-administered with 300 mg daily rifabutin and 49 mg/ml when co-administered with placebo. Mean concentrations 5 days after the last dose were 23 and 21 ng/ml in the two groups of subjects. Administration of 300 mg rifabutin for 10 days produced mean concentrations of rifabutin one-half day after the last dose of 60 mg/ml when co-administered with daily 250 mg azithromycin and 71 ng/ml when co-administered with placebo. Mean concentrations 5 days after the last dose were 8.1 ng/ml and 9.2 ng/ml in the two groups of subjects.

The following drug interactions have not been reported in clinical trials with azithromycin; however, no specific drug interaction studies have been performed to evaluate potential drug-drug interaction. Nonetheless, they have been observed with macrolide products. Until further data are developed regarding drug interactions when azithromycin and these drugs are used concomitantly, careful monitoring of patients is advised:

Digoxin: Elevated digoxin levels.

Ergotamine or dihydroergotamine: Acute ergot toxicity characterized by severe peripheral vasospasm and dysesthesia.

Triazolam: Decrease the clearance of triazolam and thus may increase the pharmacologic effect of triazolam.

Drugs metabolized by the cytochrome P 450 system: Elevations of serum carbamazepine, cyclosporine, hexobarbital, and phenytoin levels.

ZITHROMAX 250 AND 500 MG TABLETS & ORAL SUSPENSION

Co-administration of nelfinavir at steady state with a single oral dose of azithromycin resulted in increased azithromycin serum concentrations. Although a dose adjustment of azithromycin is not recommended when administered in combination with nelfinavir, close monitoring for known side effects of azithromycin, such as liver enzyme abnormalities and hearing impairment, is warranted. (See ADVERSE REACTIONS.)

Azithromycin did not affect the prothrombin time response to a single dose of warfarin. However, prudent medical practice dictates careful monitoring of prothrombin time in all patients treated with azithromycin and warfarin concomitantly. Concurrent use of macrolides and warfarin in clinical practice has been associated with increased anticoagulant effects.

Drug interaction studies were performed with azithromycin and other drugs likely to be co-administered. (See CLINICAL PHARMACOLOGY, Drug-Drug Interactions.) When used in therapeutic doses, azithromycin had a modest effect on the pharmacokinetics of atorvastatin, carbamazepine, cetirizine, didanosine, efavirenz, fluconazole, indinavir, midazolam, rifabutin, sildenafil, theophylline (IV and oral), triazolam, trimethoprim/sulfamethoxazole or zidovudine. Co-administration with efavirenz, or fluconazole had a modest effect on the pharmacokinetics of azithromycin. No dosage adjustment of either drug is recommended when azithromycin is co-administered with any of the above agents.

Interactions with the drugs listed below have not been reported in clinical trials with azithromycin; however, no specific drug interaction studies have been performed to evaluate potential drug-drug interaction. Nonetheless, they have been observed with macrolide products. Until further data are developed regarding drug interactions when azithromycin and these drugs are used concomitantly, careful monitoring of patients is advised:

Digoxin: Elevated digoxin concentrations.

Ergotamine or Dihydroergotamine: Acute ergot toxicity characterized by severe peripheral vasospasm and dysesthesia.

Terfenadine, cyclosporine, hexobarbital and phenytoin concentrations.

ADVERSE REACTIONS

ZITHROMAX CAPSULES, 600 MG TABLETS, & ORAL SUSPENSION IN PACKETS

In clinical trials, most of the reported side effects were mild to moderate in severity and were reversible upon discontinuation of the drug. Approximately 0.7% of the patients from the multiple-dose clinical trials discontinued Zithromax therapy because of treatment-related side effects. Most of the side effects leading to discontinuation were related to the gastrointestinal tract, *e.g.*, nausea, vomiting, diarrhea, or abdominal pain. Rarely but potentially serious side effects were angioedema and cholestatic jaundice.

Clinical

Multiple-Dose Regimen

Overall, the most common side effects in adult patients receiving a multiple-dose regimen of azithromycin were related to the gastrointestinal system with diarrhea/loose stools (5%), nausea (3%), and abdominal pain (3%) being the most frequently reported.

No other side effects occurred in patients on the multiple-dose regimen of Zithromax with a frequency greater than 1%. Side effects that occurred with a frequency of 1% or less included the following:

Cardiovascular: Palpitations, chest pain.

Gastrointestinal: Dyspepsia, flatulence, vomiting, melena, and cholestatic jaundice.

Genitourinary: Monilia, vaginitis, and nephritis.

Nervous System: Dizziness, headache, vertigo, and somnolence.

General: Fatigue.

Allergic: Rash, photosensitivity, and angioedema.

Chronic Therapy With 1200 mg Weekly Regimen

The nature of side effects seen with the 1200 mg weekly dosing regimen for the prevention of *Mycobacterium avium* infection in severely immunocompromised HIV-infected patients were similar to those seen with short term dosing regimens.

Chronic Therapy With 600 mg Daily Regimen Combined With Ethambutol

The nature of side effects seen with the 600 mg daily dosing regimen for the treatment of *Mycobacterium avium* complex infection in severely immunocompromised HIV-infected patients were similar to those seen with short term dosing regimens. Five percent (5%) of patients experienced reversible hearing impairment in the pivotal clinical trial for the treatment of disseminated MAC in patients with AIDS. Hearing impairment has been reported with macrolide antibiotics, especially at higher doses. Other treatment related side effects occurring in >5% of subjects and seen at any time during a median of 87.5 days of therapy include: abdominal pain (14%), nausea (14%), vomiting (13%), diarrhea (12%), flatulence (5%), headache (5%) and abnormal vision (5%). Discontinuations from treatment due to laboratory abnormalities or side effects considered related to study drug occurred in 8/88 (9.1%) of subjects.

Single 1 g Dose Regimen

Overall, the most common side effects in patients receiving a single-dose regimen of 1 g of Zithromax were related to the gastrointestinal system and were more frequently reported than in patients receiving the multiple-dose regimen.

Side effects that occurred in patients on the single 1 g dosing regimen of Zithromax with a frequency of 1% or greater included diarrhea/loose stools (7%), nausea (5%), abdominal pain (5%), vomiting (2%), dyspepsia (1%), and vaginitis (1%).

Post-Marketing Experience

Adverse events reported with azithromycin during the post-marketing period in adult and/or pediatric patients for which a causal relationship may not be established include:

Allergic: Arthralgia, edema, urticaria, angioedema.

Cardiovascular: Arrhythmias including ventricular tachycardia, hypotension.

Gastrointestinal: Anorexia, constipation, dyspepsia, flatulence, vomiting/diarrhea rarely resulting in dehydration, pseudomembranous colitis, pancreatitis, oral candidiasis and rare reports of tongue discoloration.
General: Asthenia, paresthesia, fatigue, malaise and anaphylaxis (rarely fatal).
Genitourinary: Interstitial nephritis and acute renal failure, vaginitis.
Hematopoietic: Thrombocytopenia.
Liver/Biliary: Abnormal liver function including hepatitis and cholestatic jaundice, as well as rare cases of hepatic necrosis and hepatic failure, some of which have resulted in death.
Nervous System: Convulsions, dizziness/vertigo, headache, somnolence, hyperactivity, nervousness, agitation and syncope.
Psychiatric: Aggressive reaction and anxiety.
Skin/Appendages: Pruritus, rarely serious skin reactions including erythema multiforme, Stevens Johnson Syndrome, and toxic epidermal necrolysis.
Special Senses: Hearing disturbances including hearing loss, deafness, and/or tinnitus, rare reports of taste perversion.

Laboratory Abnormalities

Significant abnormalities (irrespective of drug relationship) occurring during the clinical trials were reported as follows:

With an incidence of 1-2%, elevated serum creatine phosphokinase, potassium, ALT (SGPT), GGT, and AST (SGOT).

With an incidence of less than 1%, leukopenia, neutropenia, decreased platelet count, elevated serum alkaline phosphatase, bilirubin, BUN, creatinine, blood glucose, LDH, and phosphate.

When follow-up was provided, changes in laboratory tests appeared to be reversible.

In multiple-dose clinical trials involving more than 3000 patients, 3 patients discontinued therapy because of treatment-related liver enzyme abnormalities and 1 because of a renal function abnormality.

In a Phase 1 drug interaction study performed in normal volunteers, 1 of 6 subjects given the combination of azithromycin and rifabutin, 1 of 7 given rifabutin alone and 0 of 6 given azithromycin alone developed a clinically significant neutropenia (<500 cells/mm^3).

Chronic therapy (median duration: 87.5 days, range: 1-229 days) that resulted in laboratory abnormalities in >5% subjects with normal baseline values in the pivotal trial for treatment of disseminated MAC in severely immunocompromised HIV-infected patients treated with azithromycin 600 mg daily in combination with ethambutol include: a reduction in absolute neutrophils to <50% of the lower limit of normal (10/52, 19%) and an increase to 5 times the upper limit of normal in alkaline phosphatase (3/35, 9%). These findings in subjects with normal baseline values are similar when compared to all subjects for analyses of neutrophil reductions (22/75 [29%]) and elevated alkaline phosphatase (16/80 [20%]). Causality of these laboratory abnormalities due to the use of study drug has not been established.

ZITHROMAX 250 AND 500 MG TABLETS & ORAL SUSPENSION

In clinical trials, most of the reported side effects were mild to moderate in severity and were reversible upon discontinuation of the drug. Potentially serious side effects of angioedema and cholestatic jaundice were reported rarely. Approximately 0.7% of the patients (adults and children) from the 5 day multiple-dose clinical trials discontinued Zithromax therapy because of treatment-related side effects. In adults given 500 mg/day for 3 days, the discontinuation rate due to treatment-related side effects was 0.4%. In clinical trials in children given 30 mg/kg, either as a single dose or over 3 days, discontinuation from the trials due to treatment-related side effects was approximately 1%. (See DOSAGE AND ADMINISTRATION.) Most of the side effects leading to discontinuation were related to the gastrointestinal tract, *e.g.*, nausea, vomiting, diarrhea, or abdominal pain.

Clinical

Adults

Multiple-Dose Regimens

Overall, the most common treatment-related side effects in adult patients receiving a multiple-dose regimens of Zithromax were related to the gastrointestinal system with diarrhea/loose stools (4-5%), nausea (3%) and abdominal pain (2-3%) being the most frequently reported.

No other treatment-related side effects occurred in patients on the multiple-dose regimens of Zithromax with a frequency greater than 1%. Side effects that occurred with a frequency of 1% or less included the following:

Cardiovascular: Palpitations, chest pain.
Gastrointestinal: Dyspepsia, flatulence, vomiting, melena and cholestatic jaundice.
Genitourinary: Monilia, vaginitis and nephritis.
Nervous System: Dizziness, headache, vertigo and somnolence.
General: Fatigue.
Allergic: Rash, pruritus, photosensitivity and angioedema.

Single 1 g Dose Regimen

Overall, the most common side effects in patients receiving a single-dose regimen of 1 g of Zithromax were related to the gastrointestinal system and were more frequently reported than in patients receiving the multiple-dose regimen.

Side effects that occurred in patients on the single 1 g dosing regimen of Zithromax with a frequency of 1% or greater included diarrhea/loose stools (7%), nausea (5%), abdominal pain (5%), vomiting (2%), dyspepsia (1%) and vaginitis (1%).

Single 2 g Dose Regimen

Overall, the most common side effects in patients receiving a single 2 g dose of Zithromax were related to the gastrointestinal system. Side effects that occurred in patients in this study with a frequency of 1% or greater included nausea (18%), diarrhea/loose stools (14%), vomiting (7%), abdominal pain (7%), vaginitis (2%), dyspepsia (1%) and dizziness (1%). The majority of these complaints were mild in nature.

Children — Single- and Multiple-Dose Regimens

The types of side effects in children were comparable to those seen in adults, with different incidence rates for the dosage regimens recommended in children.

Acute Otitis Media

For the recommended total dosage regimen of 30 mg/kg, the most frequent side effects (≥1%) attributed to treatment were diarrhea, abdominal pain, vomiting, nausea and rash. (See DOSAGE AND ADMINISTRATION.)

The incidence, based on dosing regimen, is described in TABLE 40.

TABLE 40

	Dosing Regimen		
	1 Day	3 Day	5 Day
Diarrhea	4.3%	2.6%	1.8%
Abdominal pain	1.4%	1.7%	1.2%
Vomiting	4.9%	2.3%	1.1%
Nausea	1.0%	0.4%	0.5%
Rash	1.0%	0.6%	0.4%

Community-Acquired Pneumonia

For the recommended dosage regimen of 10 mg/kg on Day 1 followed by 5 mg/kg on Days 2-5, the most frequent side effects attributed to treatment were diarrhea/loose stools, abdominal pain, vomiting, nausea and rash.

The incidence is described below:

Dosage Regimen (5 day): Diarrhea/loose stools, 5.8%; abdominal pain, 1.9%; vomiting, 1.9%; nausea, 1.9%; rash, 1.6%.

Pharyngitis/Tonsillitis

For the recommended dosage regimen of 12 mg/kg on Days 1-5, the most frequent side effects attributed to treatment were diarrhea, vomiting, abdominal pain, nausea and headache.

The incidence is described below:

Dosage Regimen (5 day): Diarrhea, 5.4%; abdominal pain, 3.4%; vomiting 5.6%; nausea, 1.8%; rash, 0.7%; headache, 1.1%.

With any of the treatment regimens, no other treatment-related side effects occurred in children treated with Zithromax with a frequency greater than 1%. Side effects that occurred with a frequency of 1% or less included the following:

Cardiovascular: Chest pain.
Gastrointestinal: Dyspepsia, constipation, anorexia, enteritis, flatulence, gastritis, jaundice, loose stools and oral moniliasis.
Hematologic and Lymphatic: Anemia and leukopenia.
Nervous System: Headache (otitis media dosage), hyperkinesia, dizziness, agitation, nervousness and insomnia.
General: Fever, face edema, fatigue, fungal infection, malaise and pain.
Allergic: Rash and allergic reaction.
Respiratory: Cough increased, pharyngitis, pleural effusion and rhinitis.
Skin and Appendages: Eczema, fungal dermatitis, pruritus, sweating, urticaria and vesiculobullous rash.
Special Senses: Conjunctivitis.

Post-Marketing Experience

Adverse events reported with azithromycin during the post-marketing period in adult and/or pediatric patients for which a causal relationship may not be established include:

Allergic: Arthralgia, edema, urticaria and angioedema.
Cardiovascular: Arrhythmias including ventricular tachycardia and hypotension.
Gastrointestinal: Anorexia, constipation, dyspepsia, flatulence and vomiting/diarrhea rarely resulting in dehydration, pseudomembranous colitis, pancreatitis, oral candidiasis and rare reports of tongue discoloration.
General: Asthenia, paresthesia, fatigue, malaise and anaphylaxis (rarely fatal).
Genitourinary: Interstitial nephritis and acute renal failure and vaginitis.
Hematopoietic: Thrombocytopenia.
Liver/Biliary: Abnormal liver function including hepatitis and cholestatic jaundice, as well as rare cases of hepatic necrosis and hepatic failure, some of which have resulted in death.
Nervous System: Convulsions, dizziness/vertigo, headache, somnolence, hyperactivity, nervousness, agitation and syncope.
Psychiatric: Aggressive reaction and anxiety.
Skin/Appendages: Pruritus, rarely serious skin reactions including erythema multiforme, Stevens Johnson Syndrome and toxic epidermal necrolysis.
Special Senses: Hearing disturbances including hearing loss, deafness and/or tinnitus and rare reports of taste perversion.

Laboratory Abnormalities

Adults

Clinically significant abnormalities (irrespective of drug relationship) occurring during the clinical trials were reported as follows: With an incidence of greater than 1%: Decreased hemoglobin, hematocrit, lymphocytes and blood glucose; elevated serum creatine phosphokinase, potassium, ALT (SGPT), GGT, and AST (SGOT), BUN, creatinine, blood glucose, platelet count, eosinophils; With an incidence of less than 1%: Leukopenia, neutropenia, decreased platelet count; elevated serum alkaline phosphatase, bilirubin, LDH and phosphate. The majority of subjects with elevated serum creatinine also had abnormal values at baseline.

When follow-up was provided, changes in laboratory tests appeared to be reversible.

In multiple-dose clinical trials involving more than 4500 patients, 3 patients discontinued therapy because of treatment-related liver enzyme abnormalities and 1 because of a renal function abnormality.

Children — 1, 3 and 5 Day Regimens

Laboratory data collected from comparative clinical trials employing two 3 day regimens (30 or 60 mg/kg in divided doses over 3 days), or two 5 day regimens (30 or 60 mg/kg in divided doses over 5 days) were similar for regimens of azithromycin and all comparators combined, with most clinically significant laboratory abnormalities occurring at incidences of 1-5%. Laboratory data for patients receiving 30 mg/kg as a single dose were collected in one single center trial. In that trial, an absolute neutrophil count between 500-1500 cells/mm^3 was observed in 10/64 patients receiving 30 mg/kg as a single dose, 9/62 patients receiving 30 mg/kg given over 3 days, and 8/63 comparator patients. No patient had an absolute neutrophil count <500 cells/mm^3. (See DOSAGE AND ADMINISTRATION.)

In multiple-dose clinical trials involving approximately 4700 pediatric patients, no patients discontinued therapy because of treatment-related laboratory abnormalities.

DOSAGE AND ADMINISTRATION

ZITHROMAX CAPSULES, 600 MG TABLETS, & ORAL SUSPENSION IN PACKETS

See INDICATIONS AND USAGE.

Zithromax capsules should be given at least 1 hour before or 2 hours after a meal. Zithromax capsules should not be mixed with or taken with food.

Zithromax for oral suspension (single dose 1 g packet) can be taken with or without food after constitution. Not for pediatric use. For pediatric suspension, please refer to the INDICATIONS AND USAGE and DOSAGE AND ADMINISTRATION sections of the prescribing information for Zithromax for oral suspension 100 mg/5 ml and 200 mg/5 ml bottles.

Zithromax tablets may be taken without regard to food. However, increased tolerability has been observed when tablets are taken with food.

The recommended dose of Zithromax or the treatment of individuals 16 years of age and older with mild to moderate acute bacterial exacerbations of chronic obstructive pulmonary disease, pneumonia, pharyngitis/tonsillitis (as second line therapy), and uncomplicated skin and skin structure infections due to the indicated organisms is: 500 mg as a single dose on the first day followed by 250 mg once daily on Days 2-5 for a total dose of 1.5 g of Zithromax.

The recommended dose of Zithromax for the treatment of non-gonococcal urethritis and cervicitis due to *C. trachomatis* is: a single 1 g (1000 mg) dose of Zithromax. This dose can be administered as four 250 mg capsules or as 1 single dose packet (1 g).

Prevention of Disseminated MAC Infections: The recommended dose of Zithromax for the prevention of disseminated *Mycobacterium avium* complex (MAC) disease is: 1200 mg taken once weekly. This dose of Zithromax may be combined with the approved dosage regimen of rifabutin.

Treatment of Disseminated MAC Infections: Zithromax should be taken at a daily dose of 600 mg, in combination with ethambutol at the recommended daily dose of 15 mg/kg. Other antimycobacterial drugs that have shown *in vitro* activity against MAC may be added to the regimen of azithromycin plus ethambutol at the discretion of the physician or health care provider.

Directions for Administration of Zithromax for Oral Suspension in the Single Dose Packet (1 g)

The entire contents of the packet should be mixed thoroughly with 2 oz (approximately 60 ml) of water. Drink the entire contents immediately; add an additional 2 oz of water, mix, and drink to assure complete consumption of dosage. **The single dose packet should not be used to administer doses other than 1000 mg of azithromycin. This packet not for pediatric use.**

ZITHROMAX 250 AND 500 MG TABLETS & ORAL SUSPENSION

See INDICATIONS AND USAGE and CLINICAL PHARMACOLOGY.

Adults

The recommended dose of Zithromax for the treatment of community-acquired pneumonia of mild severity, pharyngitis/tonsillitis (as second-line therapy), and uncomplicated skin and skin structure infections due to the indicated organisms is: 500 mg as a single dose on the first day followed by 250 mg once daily on Days 2-5. The recommended dose of Zithromax for the treatment of mild to moderate acute bacterial exacerbations of chronic obstructive pulmonary disease is: either 500 mg/day for 3 days or 500 mg as a single dose on the first day followed by 250 mg once daily on Days 2-5.

Zithromax tablets can be taken with or without food.

The recommended dose of Zithromax for the treatment of genital ulcer disease due to *Haemophilus ducreyi* (chancroid), non-gonococcal urethritis and cervicitis due to *C. trachomatis* is: a single 1 g (1000 mg) dose of Zithromax.

The recommended dose of Zithromax for the treatment of urethritis and cervicitis due to *Neisseria gonorrhoeae* is a single 2 g (2000 mg) dose of Zithromax.

Renal Insufficiency: No dosage adjustment is recommended for subjects with renal impairment (GFR ≤80 ml/min). The mean AUC(0-120) was similar in subjects with GFR 10-80 ml/min compared to subjects with normal renal function, whereas it increased 35% in subjects with GFR <10 ml/min compared to subjects with normal renal function. Caution should be exercised when azithromycin is administered to subjects with severe renal impairment. (See CLINICAL PHARMACOLOGY, Special Populations, Renal Insufficiency.)

Hepatic Insufficiency: The pharmacokinetics of azithromycin in subjects with hepatic impairment have not been established. No dose adjustment recommendations can be made in patients with impaired hepatic function (see CLINICAL PHARMACOLOGY, Special Populations, Hepatic Insufficiency).

No dosage adjustment is recommended based on age or gender (see CLINICAL PHARMACOLOGY, Special Populations).

Children

Zithromax for oral suspension can be taken with or without food.

Acute Otitis Media

The recommended dose of Zithromax for oral suspension for the treatment of children with acute otitis media is 30 mg/kg given as a single dose or 10 mg/kg once daily for 3 days or 10 mg/kg as a single dose on the first day followed by 5 mg/kg/day on Days 2-5. (See TABLES 41-43.)

Community-Acquired Pneumonia

The recommended dose of Zithromax for oral suspension for the treatment of children with community-acquired pneumonia is 10 mg/kg as a single dose on the first day followed by 5 mg/kg on Days 2-5. (See TABLE 41.)

TABLE 41 *Pediatric Dosage Guidelines — Otitis Media and Community-Acquired Pneumonia: 5 Day Regimen (Based on Body Weight)*†‡*

Weight		100 mg/5 ml		200 mg/5 ml		Total per Treatment Course	
kg	lb	Day 1	Days 2-5	Day 1	Days 2-5		
5	11	2.5 ml (½ tsp)	1.25 ml (¼ tsp)			7.5 ml	150 mg
10	22	5 ml (1 tsp)	2.5 ml (½ tsp)			15 ml	300 mg
20	44			5 ml (1 tsp)	2.5 ml (½ tsp)	15 ml	600 mg
30	66			7.5 ml (1½ tsp)	3.75 ml (¾ tsp)	22.5 ml	900 mg
40	88			10 ml (2 tsp)	5 ml (1 tsp)	30 ml	1200 mg
50+	110+			12.5 ml (2½ tsp)	6.25 ml (1¼ tsp)	37.5 ml	1500 mg

* Effectiveness of the 3 day or 1 day regimen in children with community-acquired pneumonia has not been established.
† Dosing calculated on 10 mg/kg/day Day 1 and 5 mg/kg/day Days 2-5.
‡ Age 6 months and above, see PRECAUTIONS, Pediatric Use.

TABLE 42 *Pediatric Dosage Guidelines — Otitis Media: 3 Day Regimen* (Based on Body Weight)†*

Weight		100 mg/5 ml	200 mg/5 ml	Total per Treatment Course	
kg	lb	Day 1-3	Day 1-3		
5	11	2.5 ml (½ tsp)		7.5 ml	150 mg
10	22	5 ml (1 tsp)		15 ml	300 mg
20	44		5 ml (1 tsp)	15 ml	600 mg
30	66		7.5 ml (1½ tsp)	22.5 ml	900 mg
40	88		10 ml (2 tsp)	30 ml	1200 mg
50+	110+		12.5 ml (2½ tsp)	37.5 ml	1500 mg

* Dosing calculated on 10 mg/kg/day.
† Age 6 months and above, see PRECAUTIONS, Pediatric Use.

TABLE 43 *Pediatric Dosage Guidelines — Otitis Media: 1 Day Regimen* (Based on Body Weight)†*

Weight		200 mg/5 ml	Total per Treatment Course	
kg	lb	Day 1		
5	11	3.75 ml (¾ tsp)	7.5 ml	150 mg
10	22	7.5 ml (1½ tsp)	15 ml	300 mg
20	44	15 ml (3 tsp)	15 ml	600 mg
30	66	22.5 ml (4½ tsp)	22.5 ml	900 mg
40	88	30 ml (6 tsp)	30 ml	1200 mg
50+	110+	37.5 ml (7½ tsp)	37.5 ml	1500 mg

* Dosing calculated on 30 mg/kg as a single dose.
† Age 6 months and above, see PRECAUTIONS, Pediatric Use.

The safety of re-dosing azithromycin in children who vomit after receiving 30 mg/kg as a single dose has not been established. In clinical studies involving 487 patients with acute otitis media given a single 30 mg/kg dose of azithromycin, 8 patients who vomited within 30 minutes of dosing were re-dosed at the same total dose.

Pharyngitis/Tonsillitis

The recommended dose of Zithromax for children with pharyngitis/tonsillitis is 12 mg/kg once daily for 5 days. (See TABLE 44.)

TABLE 44 *Pediatric Dosage Guidelines — Pharyngitis/Tonsillitis: 5 Day Regimen (Based on Body Weight)*†*

Weight		200 mg/5 ml	Total per Treatment Course	
kg	lb	Day 1-5		
8	18	2.5 ml (½ tsp)	12.5 ml	500 mg
17	37	5 ml (1 tsp)	25 ml	1000 mg
25	55	7.5 ml (1½ tsp)	37.5 ml	1500 mg
33	73	10 ml (2 tsp)	50 ml	2000 mg
40	88	12.5 ml (2½ tsp)	62.5 ml	2500 mg

* Dosing calculated on 12 mg/kg/day for 5 days.
† Age 2 years and above, see PRECAUTIONS, Pediatric Use.

Following constitution, and for use with the oral syringe, the supplied press in bottle adapter should be inserted into the neck of the bottle then sealed with the original closure. Shake well before each use. Oversized bottle provides shake space. Keep tightly closed.

Use only the dosing device provided to measure the correct amount of suspension. (See HOW SUPPLIED.) The dosing device may need to be filled multiple times to provide the complete dose prescribed. Rinse the device with water after the complete daily dose has been administered.

After mixing, store suspension at 5-30°C (41-86°F) and use within 10 days. Discard after full dosing is completed.

ANIMAL PHARMACOLOGY

ZITHROMAX CAPSULES, 600 MG TABLETS, & ORAL SUSPENSION IN PACKETS

Phospholipidosis (intracellular phospholipid binding) has been observed in some tissues of mice, rats, and dogs given multiple doses of azithromycin. It has been demonstrated in numerous organ systems (*e.g.*, eye, dorsal root ganglia, liver, gallbladder, kidney, spleen, and pancreas) in dogs administered doses which, based on pharmacokinetics, are as low as 2 times greater than the recommended adult human dose and in rats at doses comparable to the recommended adult human dose. This effect has been reversible after cessation of azithromycin treatment. The significance of these findings for humans is unknown.

ZITHROMAX 250 AND 500 MG TABLETS & ORAL SUSPENSION

Phospholipidosis (intracellular phospholipid accumulation) has been observed in some tissues of mice, rats, and dogs given multiple doses of azithromycin. It has been demonstrated in numerous organ systems (*e.g.*, eye, dorsal root ganglia, liver, gallbladder, kidney, spleen, and pancreas) in dogs treated with azithromycin at doses which, expressed on the basis of mg/m^2, are approximately equal to the recommended adult human dose, and in rats treated at doses approximately one-sixth of the recommended adult human dose. This effect has been shown to be reversible after cessation of azithromycin treatment. Phospholipidosis has been observed to a similar extent in the tissues of neonatal rats and dogs given daily doses of azithromycin ranging from 10-30 days. Based on the pharmacokinetic data, phospholipidosis has been seen in the rat (30 mg/kg dose) at observed C_{max} value of 1.3 µg/ml (6 times greater than the observed C_{max} of 0.216 µg/ml at the pediatric dose of 10 mg/kg). Similarly, it has been shown in the dog (10 mg/kg dose) at observed C_{max} value of 1.5 µg/ml (7 times greater than the observed same C_{max} and drug dose in the studied pediatric population). On a mg/m^2 basis, 30 mg/kg dose in the neonatal rat (135 mg/m^2) and 10 mg/kg dose in the neonatal dog (79 mg/m^2) are approximately 0.5 and 0.3 times, respectively, the recommended dose in the pediatric patients with an average body weight of 25 kg. Phospholipidosis similar to that seen in the adult animals, is reversible after cessation of azithromycin treatment. The significance of these findings for animals and for humans is unknown.

HOW SUPPLIED

ZITHROMAX CAPSULES, 600 MG TABLETS, & ORAL SUSPENSION IN PACKETS

Zithromax Capsules

Zithromax capsules (imprinted with "Pfizer 305") are supplied in red opaque hard-gelatin capsules containing azithromycin dihydrate equivalent to 250 mg of azithromycin.
Storage: Store capsules below 30°C.

Zithromax 600 mg Tablets

Zithromax 600 mg tablets (engraved on front with "PFIZER" and on back with "308") are supplied as white, modified oval-shaped, film-coated tablets containing azithromycin dihydrate equivalent to 600 mg azithromycin.
Storage: Tablets should be stored at or below 30°C (86°F).

Zithromax for Oral Suspension in Packets

Zithromax for oral suspension is supplied in single dose packets containing azithromycin dihydrate equivalent to 1 g of azithromycin.
Storage: Store single dose packets between 5 and 30°C (41 and 86°F).

ZITHROMAX 250 AND 500 MG TABLETS & ORAL SUSPENSION

Zithromax Tablets

Zithromax tablets are supplied as film-coated tablets containing azithromycin dihydrate equivalent to 250 or 500 mg of azithromycin.

250 mg: Pink modified capsular shaped, engraved, film-coated tablets engraved with "PFIZER" on one side and "306" on the other.

500 mg: Pink modified capsular shaped, engraved, film-coated tablets engraved with "Pfizer" on one side and "ZTM500" on the other.

Storage: Zithromax tablets should be stored between 15-30°C (59-86°F).

Zithromax for Oral Suspension

Zithromax for oral suspension after constitution contains a flavored suspension. Zithromax for oral suspension is supplied to provide 100 mg/5 ml or 200 mg/5 ml suspension in bottles with accompanying calibrated dosing device.
Storage: Store dry powder below 30°C (86°F). Store constituted suspension between 5-30°C (41-86°F) and discard when full dosing is completed.

PRODUCT LISTING - EQUIVALENTS NOT AVAILABLE

Package	Price	Product	NDC
Capsule - Oral - 250 mg			
6's	$46.38	ZITHROMAX Z-PAK, Physicians Total Care	54868-4183-00
Powder For Injection - Intravenous - 500 mg			
10's	$244.44	ZITHROMAX, Allscripts Pharmaceutical Company	54569-4681-00
10's	$268.93	ZITHROMAX IV, Pfizer U.S. Pharmaceuticals	00069-3150-14
10's	$268.93	ZITHROMAX IV, Pfizer U.S. Pharmaceuticals	00069-3150-83
Powder For Reconstitution - Oral - 1 Gm			
1's	$20.98	ZITHROMAX, Allscripts Pharmaceutical Company	54569-4567-00
3's	$70.63	ZITHROMAX, Pfizer U.S. Pharmaceuticals	00069-3051-75
10's	$235.41	ZITHROMAX, Pfizer U.S. Pharmaceuticals	00069-3051-07
Powder For Reconstitution - Oral - 100 mg/5 ml			
15 ml	$28.60	ZITHROMAX, Allscripts Pharmaceutical Company	54569-4232-00
15 ml	$32.10	ZITHROMAX, Pfizer U.S. Pharmaceuticals	00069-3110-19
15 ml	$32.89	ZITHROMAX, Physicians Total Care	54868-4076-00
Powder For Reconstitution - Oral - 200 mg/5 ml			
15 ml	$28.60	ZITHROMAX, Pharma Pac	54569-4230-00
15 ml	$32.10	ZITHROMAX, Pfizer U.S. Pharmaceuticals	00069-3120-19
15 ml	$32.89	ZITHROMAX, Physicians Total Care	54868-4078-01
15 ml	$38.26	ZITHROMAX, Pharma Pac	52959-0657-03
22.50 ml	$28.60	ZITHROMAX, Pharma Pac	54569-4231-00
22.50 ml	$32.10	ZITHROMAX, Pfizer U.S. Pharmaceuticals	00069-3130-19
22.50 ml	$32.89	ZITHROMAX, Physicians Total Care	54868-4078-00
22.50 ml	$38.26	ZITHROMAX, Pharma Pac	52959-0657-06
30 ml	$28.60	ZITHROMAX, Pharma Pac	54569-4417-00
30 ml	$32.10	ZITHROMAX, Pfizer U.S. Pharmaceuticals	00069-3140-19
30 ml	$32.89	ZITHROMAX, Physicians Total Care	54868-4078-02
Tablet - Oral - 250 mg			
1's	$10.96	ZITHROMAX, Prescript Pharmaceuticals	00247-0280-01
2's	$13.51	ZITHROMAX, Allscripts Pharmaceutical Company	54569-4522-01
2's	$18.58	ZITHROMAX, Prescript Pharmaceuticals	00247-0280-02
3's	$26.19	ZITHROMAX, Prescript Pharmaceuticals	00247-0280-03
4's	$27.03	ZITHROMAX, Allscripts Pharmaceutical Company	54569-4522-00
4's	$33.80	ZITHROMAX, Prescript Pharmaceuticals	00247-0280-04
4's	$37.05	ZITHROMAX, Pd-Rx Pharmaceuticals	55289-0310-04
5's	$41.40	ZITHROMAX, Prescript Pharmaceuticals	00247-0280-05
6 x 3	$136.44	ZITHROMAX Z-PAK, Pfizer U.S. Pharmaceuticals	00069-3060-75
6's	$40.05	ZITHROMAX Z-PAK, Allscripts Pharmaceutical Company	54569-4497-00
6's	$41.00	ZITHROMAX, Southwood Pharmaceuticals Inc	58016-0391-06
6's	$49.01	ZITHROMAX, Prescript Pharmaceuticals	00247-0280-06
6's	$54.23	ZITHROMAX, Pd-Rx Pharmaceuticals	55289-0310-06
6's	$63.78	ZITHROMAX Z-PAK, Pharma Pac	52959-0505-06
6's	$131.85	ZITHROMAX Z-PAK, Southwood Pharmaceuticals Inc	58016-0391-01
10's	$68.33	ZITHROMAX, Southwood Pharmaceuticals Inc	58016-0391-10
10's	$79.46	ZITHROMAX, Prescript Pharmaceuticals	00247-0280-10
11's	$87.07	ZITHROMAX, Prescript Pharmaceuticals	00247-0280-11
14's	$129.71	ZITHROMAX, Pd-Rx Pharmaceuticals	55289-0310-14
15's	$102.50	ZITHROMAX, Southwood Pharmaceuticals Inc	58016-0391-15
18's	$123.00	ZITHROMAX, Southwood Pharmaceuticals Inc	58016-0391-18
20's	$136.67	ZITHROMAX, Southwood Pharmaceuticals Inc	58016-0391-20
28's	$191.33	ZITHROMAX, Southwood Pharmaceuticals Inc	58016-0391-28
30's	$205.00	ZITHROMAX, Southwood Pharmaceuticals Inc	58016-0391-30
30's	$227.39	ZITHROMAX, Pfizer U.S. Pharmaceuticals	00069-3060-30
50's	$378.99	ZITHROMAX, Pfizer U.S. Pharmaceuticals	00069-3060-86
50's	$383.87	ZITHROMAX, Prescript Pharmaceuticals	00247-0280-50
Tablet - Oral - 500 mg			
3 x 3	$136.44	ZITHROMAX TRI-PAK, Pfizer U.S. Pharmaceuticals	00069-3070-75
30's	$454.78	ZITHROMAX, Pfizer U.S. Pharmaceuticals	00069-3070-30
50's	$757.98	ZITHROMAX, Pfizer U.S. Pharmaceuticals	00069-3070-86
Tablet - Oral - 600 mg			
30's	$545.74	ZITHROMAX, Pfizer U.S. Pharmaceuticals	00069-3080-30

Aztreonam *(000354)*

Categories: Cellulitis, pelvic; Endometritis; Infection, gynecologic; Infection, intra-abdominal; Infection, lower respiratory tract; Infection, skin and skin structures; Infection, urinary tract; Peritonitis; Pyelonephritis; Septicemia; Pregnancy Category B; FDA Approved 1986 Dec
Drug Classes: Antibiotics, monobactams
Brand Names: **Azactam**; Primbactam; Urobactam
Foreign Brand Availability: Squibb-Azactam (Colombia)
Cost of Therapy: $226.10 (Infections; Azactam Injection; 1 g; 2 g/day; 7 day supply)

DESCRIPTION

Azactam is a monobactam. It was originally isolated from *Chromobacterium violaceum.* It is a totally synthetic bactericidal antibiotic.

The monobactams, having a unique monocyclic beta-lactam nucleus, are structurally different from other beta-lactam antibiotics (*e.g.*, penicillins, cephalosporins, cephamycins). The sulfonic acid substituent in the 1-position of the ring activates the beta-lactam moiety; an aminothiazolyl oxime side chain in the 3-position and a methyl group in the 4-position confer the specific antibacterial spectrum and beta-lactamase stability.

Aztreonam is designed chemically as (Z)-2-[[[(2-amino-4-thiazolyl)[[(2S,-3S)-2-methyl-4-oxo-1-sulfo-3-azetidinyl]carbamoyl] methylene]amino]oxy]-2-methylpropionic acid.

Azactam for injection is a sterile, nonpyrogenic, sodium-free, white to yellowish-white lyophilized cake containing approximately 780 mg arginine per gram of aztreonam. Following constitution, the product is for intramuscular or intravenous use. Aqueous solutions of the product have a pH in the range of 4.5-7.5.

CLINICAL PHARMACOLOGY

Single 30 minute intravenous infusions of 500 mg, 1 and 2 g doses of aztreonam in healthy subjects produced peak serum levels of 54, 90, and 204 μg/ml, respectively, immediately after administration; at 8 hours, serum levels were 1, 3, and 6 μg/ml, respectively. Single 3 minute intravenous injections of the same doses resulted in serum levels of 58, 125, and 242 μg/ml at 5 minutes following completion of injection.

Maximum serum concentrations of aztreonam in healthy subjects following completion of single intramuscular injections of 500 mg and 1 g doses occur at about 1 hour. After identical single intravenous or intramuscular doses of aztreonam, the serum concentrations of aztreonam are comparable at one hour (1.5 hours from start of intravenous infusion) with similar slopes of serum concentrations thereafter.

The serum levels of aztreonam following single 500 mg or 1 g (intramuscular or intravenous) or 2 g (intravenous) doses of aztreonam exceed the MIC_{90} for *Neisseria* sp., *H. influenzae* and most genera of the *Enterobacteriaceae* for 8 hours (for *Enterobacter* sp., the 8 hour serum levels exceed the MIC for 80% of strains). For *Ps. aeruginosa,* a single 2 g intravenous dose produces serum levels that exceed the MIC_{90} for approximately 4-6 hours. All of the above doses of aztreonam result in average urine levels of aztreonam that exceed the MIC_{90} for the same pathogens for up to 12 hours.

When aztreonam pharmacokinetics were assessed for adult and pediatric patients, they were found to be comparable (down to 9 months old). The serum half-life of aztreonam averaged 1.7 hours (1.5-2.0) in subjects with normal renal function, independent of the dose and route of administration. In healthy subjects, based on a 70 kg person, the serum clearance was 91 ml/min and renal clearance was 56 ml/min; the apparent mean volume of distribution at steady-state averaged 12.6 L, approximately equivalent to extracellular fluid volume.

In a study of healthy elderly male subjects (65-75 years of age), the average elimination half-life of aztreonam was slightly longer than in young healthy males.

In patients with impaired renal function, the serum half-life of aztreonam is prolonged (see DOSAGE AND ADMINISTRATION, Renal Impairment in Adult Patients). The serum half-life of aztreonam is only slightly prolonged in patients with hepatic impairment since the liver is a minor pathway of excretion.

Average urine concentrations of aztreonam were approximately 1100, 3500, and 6600 μg/ml within the first 2 hours following single 500 mg, 1 g, and 2 g intravenous doses of aztreonam (30 minute infusions), respectively. The range of average concentrations for aztreonam in the 8-12 hour urine specimens in these studies was 25-120 μg/ml. After intramuscular injection of single 500 mg and 1 g doses of aztreonam, urinary levels were approximately 500 and 1200 μg/ml, respectively, within the first 2 hours, declining to 180 and 470 μg/ml in the 6-8 hour specimens. In healthy subjects, aztreonam is excreted in the urine about equally by active tubular secretion and glomerular filtration. Approximately 60-70% of an intravenous or intramuscular dose was recovered in the urine by 8 hours. Urinary excretion of a single parenteral dose was essentially complete by 12 hours after injection. About 12% of a single intravenous radiolabeled dose was recovered in the feces. Unchanged aztreonam and the inactive beta-lactam ring hydrolysis product of aztreonam were present in feces and urine.

Intravenous or intramuscular administration of a single 500 mg or 1 g dose of aztreonam every 8 hours for 7 days to healthy subjects produced no apparent accumulation of aztreonam or modification of its disposition characteristics; serum protein binding averaged 56% and was independent of dose. An average of about 6% of a 1 g intramuscular dose was excreted as a microbiologically inactive open beta-lactam ring hydrolysis product (serum half-life approximately 26 hours) of aztreonam in the 0-8 hour urine collection on the last day of multiple dosing.

Renal function was monitored in healthy subjects given aztreonam; standard tests (serum creatinine, creatinine clearance, BUN, urinalysis, and total urinary protein excretion) as well as special tests (excretion of N-acetyl-β-glucosaminidase, alanine aminopeptidase and β_2-microglobulin) were used. No abnormal results were obtained.

Aztreonam achieves measurable concentrations in the body fluids and tissues as shown in TABLE 1.

TABLE 1 *Extravascular Concentrations of Aztreonam After a Single Parenteral Dose**

Fluid or Tissue	Dose (g)	Route	Hours Post injection	Number of Patients	Mean Concentration (μg/ml or μg/g)
Fluids					
Bile	1	IV	2	10	39
Blister fluid	1	IV	1	6	20
Bronchial secretion	2	IV	4	7	5
Cerebrospinal fluid (inflamed meninges)	2	IV	0.9-4.3	16	3
Pericardial fluid	2	IV	1	6	33
Pleural fluid	2	IV	1.1-3.0	3	51
Synovial fluid	2	IV	0.8-1.9	11	83
Tissues					
Atrial appendage	2	IV	0.9-1.6	12	22
Endometrium	2	IV	0.7-1.9	4	9
Fallopian tube	2	IV	0.7-1.9	8	12
Fat	2	IV	1.3-2.0	10	5
Femur	2	IV	1.0-2.1	15	16
Gallbladder	2	IV	0.8-1.3	4	23
Kidney	2	IV	2.4-5.6	5	67
Large intestine	2	IV	0.8-1.9	9	12
Liver	2	IV	0.9-2.0	6	47
Lung	2	IV	1.2-2.1	6	22
Myometrium	2	IV	0.7-1.9	9	11
Ovary	2	IV	0.7-1.9	7	13
Prostate	1	IM	0.8-3.0	8	8
Skeletal muscle	2	IV	0.3-0.7	6	16
Skin	2	IV	0.0-1.0	8	25
Sternum	2	IV	1	6	6

* Tissue penetration is regarded as essential to therapeutic efficacy, but specific tissue levels have not been correlated with specific therapeutic effects.

The concentration of aztreonam in saliva at 30 minutes after a single 1 g intravenous dose (9 patients) was 0.2 μg/ml; in breast milk at 2 hours after a single 1 g intravenous dose (6 patients), 0.2 μg/ml, and at 6 hours after a single 1 g intramuscular dose (6 patients), 0.3 μg/ml; in amniotic fluid at 6-8 hours after a single 1 g intravenous dose (5 patients), 2 μg/ml. The concentration of aztreonam in peritoneal fluid obtained 1-6 hours after multiple 2 g intravenous doses ranged between 12 and 90 μg/ml in 7 of 8 patients studied.

Aztreonam given intravenously rapidly reaches therapeutic concentrations in peritoneal dialysis fluid; conversely, aztreonam given intraperitoneally in dialysis fluid rapidly produces therapeutic serum levels.

DRUG INTERACTIONS

Concomitant administration of probenecid or furosemide and aztreonam causes clinically insignificant increases in the serum levels of aztreonam. Single-dose intravenous pharmacokinetic studies have not shown any significant interaction between aztreonam and concomitantly administered gentamicin, nafcillin sodium, cephradine, clindamycin or metronidazole. No reports of disulfiram-like reactions with alcohol ingestion have been noted; this is not unexpected since aztreonam does not contain a methyl-tetrazole side chain.

MICROBIOLOGY

Aztreonam exhibits potent and specific activity *in vitro* against a wide spectrum of gram-negative aerobic pathogens including *Pseudomonas aeruginosa.* The bactericidal action of aztreonam results from the inhibition of bacterial cell wall synthesis due to a high affinity of aztreonam for penicillin binding protein 3 (PBP3). Aztreonam, unlike the majority of beta-lactam antibiotics, does not induce beta-lactamase activity and its molecular structure confers a high degree of resistance of hydrolysis by beta-lactamases (*i.e.,* penicillinases and cephalosporinases) produced by most gram-negative and gram-positive pathogens; it is therefore usually active against gram-negative aerobic organisms that are resistant to antibiotics hydrolyzed by beta-lactamases. Aztreonam maintains its antimicrobial activity over a pH range of 6-8 *in vitro,* as well as in the presence of human serum and under anaerobic conditions. Aztreonam is active *in vitro* and is effective in laboratory animal models and clinical infections against most strains of the following organisms, including many that are multiply-resistant to other antibiotics (*i.e.,* certain cephalosporins, penicillins, and aminoglycosides):

Escherichia coli.
Enterobacter species.
Klebsiella pneumoniae and *K. oxytoca.*
Proteus mirabilis.
Pseudomonas aeruginosa.
Serratia marcescens.
Haemophilus influenzae (including ampicillin-resistant and other penicillinase-producing strains).
Citrobacter species.

While *in vitro* studies have demonstrated the susceptibility to aztreonam of most strains of the following organisms, clinical efficacy for infections other than those included in INDICATIONS AND USAGE has not been documented:

Neisseria gonorrhoeae (including penicillinase-producing strains).
Proteus vulgaris.
Morganella morganii (formerly *Proteus morganii*).
Providencia species, including *P. stuartii* and *P. rettgeri* (formerly *Proteus rettgeri*).
Pseudomonas species.
Shigella species.
Pasteurella multocida.
Yersinia enterocolitica.
Aeromonas hydrophila.
Neisseria meningitidis.

Aztreonam and aminoglycosides have been shown to be synergistic *in vitro* against most strains of *Ps. aeruginosa,* many strains of *Enterobacteriaceae,* and other gram-negative aerobic bacilli.

Alterations of the anaerobic intestinal flora by broad spectrum antibiotics may decrease colonization resistance, thus permitting overgrowth of potential pathogens (*e.g., Candida* and *Clostridia* species). Aztreonam has little effect on the anaerobic intestinal microflora in *in vitro* studies. *Clostridium difficile* and its cytotoxin were not found in animal models following administration of aztreonam (see ADVERSE REACTIONS, Gastrointestinal).

SUSCEPTIBILITY TESTING

Diffusion Technique

Quantitative procedures that require measurement of zone diameters give precise estimates of microbial susceptibility to antibiotics. One such method, recommended for use with the aztreonam 30 μg disk, is the National Committee of Clinical Laboratory Standards (NCCLS) approved procedure. Only a 30 μg aztreonam disk should be used; there are no suitable surrogate disks.

Results of laboratory tests using 30 μg aztreonam disks should be interpreted using the criteria shown in TABLE 2.

TABLE 2

Zone Diameter (mm)	Interpretation
≥22	(S) Susceptible
16-21	(I) Intermediate (moderate susceptibility)
≤15	(R) Resistant

Dilution Technique

Broth or agar dilution methods may be used to determine the minimal inhibitory concentration (MIC) of aztreonam.

MIC test results should be interpreted according to the concentrations of aztreonam that can be attained in serum, tissues, and body fluids (see TABLE 3).

TABLE 3

MIC (µg/ml)	Interpretation
≤8	(S) Susceptible
16	(I) Intermediate (moderate susceptibility)
≥32	(R) Resistant

For any susceptibility test, a report of "susceptible" indicates that the pathogen is likely to respond to aztreonam therapy; a report of "resistant" indicates that the pathogen is not likely to respond. A report of "intermediate" (moderate susceptibility) indicates that the pathogen is expected to be susceptible to aztreonam if high dosages are used, or if the infection is confined to tissues and fluids (*e.g.*, urine, bile) in which high aztreonam levels are attained.

The quality control cultures should have the assigned daily ranges for aztreonam shown in TABLE 4.

TABLE 4

		Disks	Mode MIC (µg/ml)
E.coli	(ATCC 25922)	28-36 mm	0.06-0.25
Ps. aeruginosa	(ATCC 27853)	23-29 mm	2.0-8.0

INDICATIONS AND USAGE

Before initiating treatment with aztreonam, appropriate specimens should be obtained for isolation of the causative organism(s) and for determination of susceptibility to aztreonam. Treatment with aztreonam may be started empirically before results of the susceptibility testing are available; subsequently, appropriate antibiotic therapy should be continued.

Aztreonam is indicated for the treatment of the following infections caused by susceptible gram-negative microorganisms:

Urinary Tract Infections: (Complicated and uncomplicated), including pyelonephritis and cystitis (initial and recurrent) caused by *Escherichia coli, Klebsiella pneumoniae, Proteus mirabilis, Pseudomonas aeruginosa, Enterobacter cloacae, Klebsiella oxytoca**, *Citrobacter* species* and *Serratia marcescens**.

Lower Respiratory Tract Infections: Including pneumonia and bronchitis caused by *Escherichia coli, Klebsiella pneumoniae, Pseudomonas aeruginosa, Haemophilus influenzae, Proteus mirabilis, Enterobacter* species, and *Serratia marcescens*.*.

Septicemia: Caused by *Escherichia coli, Klebsiella pneumoniae, Pseudomonas aeruginosa, Proteus mirabilis**, *Serratia marcescens** and *Enterobacter* species.

Skin and Skin-structure Infections: Including those associated with postoperative wounds, ulcers, and burns caused by *Escherichia coli, Proteus mirabilis, Serratia marcescens, Enterobacter* species, *Pseudomonas aeruginosa, Klebsiella pneumoniae*, and *Citrobacter* species*.

Intra-Abdominal Infections: Including peritonitis caused by *Escherichia coli, Klebsiella* species including *K. pneumoniae, Enterobacter* species including *E. cloacae**, *Pseudomonas aeruginosa, Citrobacter* species* including *C. freundii** and *Serratia* species* including *S. marcescens**.

Gynecologic Infections: Including endometritis and pelvic cellulitis caused by *Escherichia coli, Klebsiella pneumoniae**, *Enterobacter* species* including *E. cloacae** and *Proteus mirabilis**.

*Efficacy for this organism in this organ system was studied in fewer than ten infections.

Aztreonam is indicated for adjunctive therapy to surgery in the management of infections caused by susceptible organisms, including abscesses, infections complicating hollow viscus perforations, cutaneous infections, and infections of serous surfaces. Aztreonam is effective against most of the commonly encountered gram-negative aerobic pathogens seen in general surgery.

CONCURRENT THERAPY

Concurrent initial therapy with other antimicrobial agents and aztreonam is recommended before the causative organism(s) is known in seriously ill patients who are also at risk of having an infection due to gram-positive aerobic pathogens. If anaerobic organisms are also suspected as etiologic agents, therapy should be initiated using an anti-anaerobic agent concurrently with aztreonam (see DOSAGE AND ADMINISTRATION). Certain antibiotics (*e.g.*, cefoxitin, imipenem) may induce high levels of beta-lactamase *in vitro* in some gram-negative aerobes such as *Enterobacter* and *Pseudomonas* species, resulting in antagonism to many beta-lactam antibiotics including aztreonam. These *in vitro* findings suggest that such beta-lactamase inducing antibiotics not be used concurrently with aztreonam. Following identification and susceptibility testing of the causative organism(s), appropriate antibiotic therapy should be continued.

NON-FDA APPROVED INDICATIONS

Aztreonam has been used for the treatment of uncomplicated nonpharyngeal gonococcal infections; however, it is not approved by the FDA for this purpose.

CONTRAINDICATIONS

This preparation is contraindicated in patients with known hypersensitivity to aztreonam or any other component in the formulation.

WARNINGS

Both animial and human data suggest that aztreonam is rarely cross-reactive with other beta-lactam antibiotics and weakly immunogenic. Treatment with aztreonam can result in hypersensitivity reactions in patients with or without prior exposure. (See CONTRAINDICATIONS.)

Careful inquiry should be made to determine whether the patient has any history of hypersensitivity reactions to any allergens.

While cross-reactivity of aztreonam with other beta-lactam antibiotics is rare, this drug should be administered with caution to any patient with a history of hypersensitivity to beta-lactams (*e.g.*, penicillins, cephalosporins, and/or carbapenems). Treatment with aztreonam can result in hypersensitivity reactions in patients with or without prior exposure to aztreonam. If an allergic reaction to aztreonam occurs, discontinue the drug and institute supportive treatment as appropriate (*e.g.*, maintenance of ventilation, pressor amines, antihistamines, corticosteroids). Serious hypersensitivity reactions may require epinephrine and other emergency measures. (See ADVERSE REACTIONS.)

Pseudomembranous colitis has been reported with nearly all antibacterial agents, including aztreonam, and may range in severity from mild to life-threatening. Therefore, it is important to consider this diagnosis in patients who present with diarrhea subsequent to the administration of antibacterial agents.

Treatment with antibacterial agents alters the normal flora of the colon and may permit overgrowth of *Clostridia*. Studies indicate that a toxin produced by *Clostridium difficile* is one primary cause of "antibiotic-associated colitis".

After the diagnosis of pseudomembranous colitis has been established, therapeutic measures should be initiated. Mild cases of pseudomembranous colitis usually respond to drug discontinuation alone. In moderate to severe cases, consideration should be given to management with fluids and electrolytes, protein supplementation, and treatment with an antibacterial drug clinically effective against *C. difficile* colitis.

Rare cases of toxic epidermal necrolysis have been reported in association with aztreonam in patients undergoing bone marrow transplant with multiple risk factors including sepsis, radiation therapy, and other concomitantly administered drugs associated with toxic epidermal necrolysis.

PRECAUTIONS

GENERAL

In patients with impaired hepatic or renal function, appropriate monitoring is recommended during therapy.

If an aminoglycoside is used concurrently with aztreonam, especially if high dosages of the former are used or if therapy is prolonged, renal function should be monitored because of the potential nephrotoxicity and ototoxicity of aminoglycoside antibiotics.

The use of antibiotics may promote the overgrowth of nonsusceptible organisms, including gram-positive organisms (*Staphylococcus aureus* and *Streptococcus faecalis*) and fungi. Should superinfection occur during therapy, appropriate measures should be taken.

CARCINOGENESIS, MUTAGENESIS, AND IMPAIRMENT OF FERTILITY

Carcinogenicity studies in animals have not been performed.

Genetic toxicology studies performed *in vivo* and *in vitro* with aztreonam in several standard laboratory models revealed no evidence of mutagenic potential at the chromosomal or gene level.

Two-generation reproduction studies in rats at daily doses up to 20 times the maximum recommended human dose, prior to and during gestation and lactation, revealed no evidence of impaired fertility. There was a slightly reduced survival rate during the lactation period in the offspring of rats that received the highest dosage, but not in offspring of rats that received 5 times the maximum recommended human dose.

PREGNANCY CATEGORY B

Aztreonam crosses the placenta and enters the fetal circulation.

Studies in pregnant rats and rabbits, with daily doses up to 15 and 5 times, respectively, the maximum recommended human dose, revealed no evidence of embryo- or fetotoxicity or teratogenicity. No drug induced changes were seen in any of the maternal, fetal, or neonatal parameters that were monitored in rats receiving 15 times the maximum recommended human dose of aztreonam during late gestation and lactation.

There are no adequate and well-controlled studies in pregnant women. Because animal reproduction studies are not always predictive of human response, aztreonam should be used during pregnancy only if clearly needed.

NURSING MOTHERS

Aztreonam is excreted in breast milk in concentrations that are less than 1% of concentrations determined in simultaneously obtained maternal serum; consideration should be given to temporary discontinuation of nursing and use of formula feedings.

PEDIATRIC USE

The safety and effectiveness of intravenous aztreonam have been established in the age groups 9 months to 16 years. Use of aztreonam in these age groups is supported by evidence from adequate and well-controlled studies of aztreonam in adults with additional efficacy, safety, and pharmacokinetic data from non-comparative clinical studies in pediatric patients. Sufficient data are not available for pediatric patients under 9 months of age or for the following treatment indications/pathogens: septicemia and skin and skin-structure infections (where the skin infection is believed or known to be due to *H. influenzae* type b). In pediatric patients with cystic fibrosis, higher doses of aztreonam may be warranted. (See CLINICAL PHARMACOLOGY and DOSAGE AND ADMINISTRATION.)

DRUG INTERACTIONS

See CLINICAL PHARMACOLOGY, Drug Interactions.

ADVERSE REACTIONS

Local reactions such as phlebitis/thrombophlebitis following IV administration, and discomfort/swelling at the injection site following IM administration occurred at rates of approximately 1.9% and 2.4%, respectively.

Systemic reactions (considered to be related to therapy or of uncertain etiology) occurring at an incidence of 1-1.3% include diarrhea, nausea and/or vomiting, and rash. Reactions occurring at an incidence of less than 1% are listed within each body system in order of decreasing severity:

Hypersensitivity: Anaphylaxis, angioedema, bronchospasm.
Hematologic: Pancytopenia, neutropenia, thrombocytopenia, anemia, eosinophilia, leukocytosis, thrombocytosis.
Gastrointestinal: Abdominal cramps; rare cases of *C. difficile*-associated diarrhea, including pseudomembranous colitis, or gastrointestinal bleeding have been reported. Onset of pseudomembranous colitis symptoms may occur during or after antibiotic treatment (see WARNINGS).
Dermatologic: Toxic epidermal necrolysis (see WARNINGS), purpura, erythema multiforme, exfoliative dermatitis, urticaria, petechiae, pruritus, diaphoresis.
Cardiovascular: Hypotension, transient ECG changes (ventricular bigeminy and PVC), flushing.
Respiratory: Wheezing, dyspnea, chest pain.
Hepatobiliary: Hepatitis, jaundice.
Nervous System: Seizure, confusion, vertigo, paresthesia, insomnia, dizziness.
Musculoskeletal: Muscular aches.
Special Senses: Tinnitus, diplopia, mouth ulcer, altered taste, numb tongue, sneezing, nasal congestion, halitosis.
Other: Vaginal candidiasis, vaginitis, breast tenderness.
Body as a Whole: Weakness, headache, fever, malaise.

PEDIATRIC ADVERSE REACTIONS

Of the 612 pediatric patients who were treated with aztreonam in clinical trials, less than 1% required discontinuation of therapy due to adverse events. The following systemic adverse events, regardless of drug relationship, occurred in at least 1% of treated patients in domestic clinical trials: rash (4.3%), diarrhea (1.4%), and fever (1.0%). These adverse events were comparable to those observed in adult clinical trials.

In 343 pediatric patients receiving intravenous therapy, the following local reactions were noted: pain (12%), erythema (2.9%), induration (0.9%), and phlebitis (2.1%). In the US patient population, pain occurred in 1.5% of patients, while each of the remaining three local reactions had an incidence of 0.5%.

The following laboratory adverse events, regardless of drug relationship, occurred in at least 1% of treated patients: increased eosinophils (6.3%), increased platelets (3.6%), neutropenia (3.2%), increased AST (3.8%), increased ALT (6.5%), and increased serum creatinine (5.8%).

In US pediatric clinical trials, neutropenia (absolute neutrophil count less than 1000/mm^3) occurred in 11.3% of patients (8/71) younger than 2 years receiving 30 mg/kg q6h. AST and ALT elevations to greater than 3 times the upper limit of normal were noted in 15-20% of patients aged 2 years or above receiving 50 mg/kg q6h. The increased frequency of these reported laboratory adverse events may be due to either increased severity of illness treated or higher doses of aztreonam administered.

ADVERSE LABORATORY CHANGES

Adverse laboratory changes without regard to drug relationship that were reported during clinical trials were:

Hepatic: Elevations of AST (SGOT), ALT (SGPT), and alkaline phosphatase; signs or symptoms of hepatobiliary dysfunction occurred in less than 1% of recipients (see Hepatobiliary Reactions).
Hematologic: Increases in prothrombin and partial thromboplastin times, positive Coombs test.
Renal: Increases in serum creatinine.

DOSAGE AND ADMINISTRATION

DOSAGE IN ADULT PATIENTS

Aztreonam may be administered intravenously or by intramuscular injection. Dosage and route of administration should be determined by susceptibility of the causative organisms, severity and site of infection, and the condition of the patient (see TABLE 6).

The intravenous route is recommended for patients requiring single doses greater than 1 g or those with bacterial septicemia, localized parenchymal abscess (*e.g.*, intra-abdominal abscess), peritonitis or other severe systemic or life-threatening infections.

The duration of therapy depends on the severity of infection. Generally, aztreonam should be continued for at least 48 hours after the patient becomes asymptomatic or evidence of bacterial eradication has been obtained. Persistent infections may require treatment for several weeks. Doses smaller than those indicated should not be used.

RENAL IMPAIRMENT IN ADULT PATIENTS

Prolonged serum levels of aztreonam may occur in patients with transient or persistent renal insufficiency. Therefore, the dosage of aztreonam should be halved in patients with estimated creatinine clearances between 10 and 30 ml/min/1.73 m^2 after an initial loading dose of 1 or 2 g.

When only the serum creatinine concentration is available, the following formula (based on sex, weight, and age of the patient) may be used to approximate the creatinine clearance (ClCR). The serum creatinine should represent a steady state of renal function.

Males: ClCR = [weight (kg) × (140-age)] ÷ [72 × serum creatinine (mg/dl)]
Females: 0.85 × above value

In patients with severe renal failure (creatinine clearance less than 10 ml/min/1.73 m^2), such as those supported by hemodialysis, the usual dose of 500 mg, 1 g or 2 g should be given initially. The maintenance dose should be ¼ of the usual initial dose given at the usual fixed interval of 6, 8 or 12 hours. For serious or life-threatening infections, in addition to the maintenance doses, one-eighth of the initial dose should be given after each hemodialysis session.

DOSAGE IN THE ELDERLY

Renal status is a major determinant of dosage in the elderly; these patients in particular may have diminished renal function. Serum creatinine may not be an accurate determinant of renal status. Therefore, as with all antibiotics eliminated by the kidneys, estimates of creatinine clearance should be obtained, and appropriate dosage modifications made if necessary.

DOSAGE IN PEDIATRIC PATIENTS

Aztreonam should be administered intravenously to pediatric patients with normal renal function (see TABLE 6). There are insufficient data regarding intramuscular administration to pediatric patients or dosing in pediatric patients with renal impairment. (See PRECAUTIONS, Pediatric Use.)

TABLE 6 *Aztreonam Dosage Guidelines*

Type of Infection	Dose	Frequency
Adults*		
Urinary tract infections	500 mg or 1 g	8 or 12 h
Moderately severe systemic infections	1 or 2 g	8 or 12 h
Severe systemic or life-threatening infections	2 g	6 or 8 h
Pediatric Patients†		
Mild-to-moderate infections	30 mg/kg	8 h
Moderate-to-severe infections	30 mg/kg	6 or 8 h

* Maximum recommended dose is 8 g/day.
† Maximum recommended dose is 120 mg/kg/day.

Because of the serious nature of infections due to *Pseudomonas aeruginosa*, dosage of 2 g every 6 or 8 hours is recommended, at least upon initiation of therapy, in systemic infections caused by this organism in adults.

HOW SUPPLIED

Storage: Store original packages at room temperature; avoid excessive heat.

PRODUCT LISTING - EQUIVALENTS NOT AVAILABLE

Powder For Injection - Injectable - 1 Gm

1's	$16.98	AZACTAM, Bristol-Myers Squibb	00003-2560-20
10's	$161.50	AZACTAM, Bristol-Myers Squibb	00003-2560-10
10's	$188.90	AZACTAM, Dura Pharmaceuticals	51479-0051-10
10's	$188.90	AZACTAM, Dura Pharmaceuticals	51479-0051-15
10's	$216.13	AZACTAM, Elan Pharmaceuticals	51479-0041-15

Powder For Injection - Injectable - 2 Gm

10's	$340.00	AZACTAM, Bristol-Myers Squibb	00003-2570-20
10's	$340.00	AZACTAM, Dura Pharmaceuticals	51479-0052-10
10's	$358.90	AZACTAM, Bristol-Myers Squibb	00003-2570-10
10's	$376.90	AZACTAM, Dura Pharmaceuticals	51479-0052-30
10's	$431.30	AZACTAM, Elan Pharmaceuticals	51479-0042-15

Powder For Injection - Injectable - 500 mg

1's	$8.45	AZACTAM, Dura Pharmaceuticals	00003-2550-10
1's	$9.89	AZACTAM, Dura Pharmaceuticals	51479-0050-05
10's	$116.40	AZACTAM, Elan Pharmaceuticals	51479-0040-05

Solution - Intravenous - 1 Gm/50 ml

50 ml x 24	$451.96	AZACTAM, Bristol-Myers Squibb	00003-2230-51
50 ml x 24	$503.04	AZACTAM, Dura Pharmaceuticals	00003-2231-01

Solution - Intravenous - 2 Gm/50 ml

50 ml x 24	$838.33	AZACTAM, Bristol-Myers Squibb	00003-2240-51
50 ml x 24	$933.12	AZACTAM, Dura Pharmaceuticals	00003-2241-01

Baclofen *(000361)*

Categories: Multiple sclerosis, adjunct; Spasticity; Trauma, spinal cord; FDA Approval Pre 1982; Pregnancy Category C; Orphan Drugs
Drug Classes: Musculoskeletal agents; Relaxants, skeletal muscle
Brand Names: **Lioresal**
Foreign Brand Availability: Alpha-Baclofen (New-Zealand); Backen (Korea); Baclan (Korea); Baclapone (Korea); Baclo (Australia); Baclon (Finland; Taiwan); Baclosal (Israel; Thailand); Bacofen (Korea); Bacron (Korea); Baklofen (Denmark; Norway); Baropan (Korea); Bigafen (Korea); Clofen (Australia); Curofen (Korea); Lebic (Germany); Liotec (Canada); Pacifen (New-Zealand; Taiwan); Spinax (China; Taiwan)
Cost of Therapy: $30.67 (Muscle Spasticity; Generic Tablets; 20 mg; 2 tablets/day; 30 day supply)
HCFA JCODE(S): J0475 10 mg IT

INTRATHECAL

WARNING

Abrupt discontinuation of intrathecal baclofen, regardless of the cause, has resulted in sequelae that include high fever, altered mental status, exaggerated rebound spasticity, and muscle rigidity, that in rare cases has advanced to rhabdomyolysis, multiple organ-system failure and death.

Prevention of abrupt discontinuation of intrathecal baclofen requires careful attention to programming and monitoring of the infusion system, refill scheduling and procedures, and pump alarms. Patients and caregivers should be advised of the importance of keeping scheduled refill visits and should be educated on the early symptoms of baclofen withdrawal. Special attention should be given to patients at apparent risk (*e.g.*, spinal cord injuries at T-6 or above, communication difficulties, history of withdrawal symptoms from oral or intrathecal baclofen). Consult the technical manual of the implantable infusion system for additional postimplant clinician and patient information (see WARNINGS).

DESCRIPTION

Baclofen injection is a muscle relaxant and antispastic. Its chemical name is 4-amino-3-(4 chlorophenyl) butanoic acid.

Baclofen is a white to off-white, odorless or practically odorless crystalline powder, with a molecular weight of 213.66. It is slightly soluble in water, very slightly soluble in methanol, and insoluble in chloroform.

Lioresal Intrathecal is a sterile, pyrogen-free, isotonic solution free of antioxidants, preservatives or other potentially neurotoxic additives indicated only for intrathecal administration. The drug is stable in solution at 37°C and compatible with CSF. Each ml of Lioresal Intrathecal contains baclofen 50, 500 or 2000 μg and sodium chloride 9 mg in water for injection; pH range is 5.0-7.0. Each ampule is intended for SINGLE USE ONLY. Discard any unused portion. **DO NOT AUTOCLAVE.**

CLINICAL PHARMACOLOGY

The precise mechanism of action of baclofen as a muscle relaxant and antispasticity agent is not fully understood. Baclofen inhibits both monosynaptic and polysynaptic reflexes at the spinal level, possibly by decreasing excitatory neurotransmitter release from primary afferent terminals, although actions at supraspinal sites may also occur and contribute to its clinical effect. Baclofen is a structural analog of the inhibitory neurotransmitter gamma-aminobutyric acid (GABA), and may exert its effects by stimulation of the $GABA_B$ receptor subtype.

Baclofen injection when introduced directly into the intrathecal space permits effective CSF concentrations to be achieved with resultant plasma concentrations 100 times less than those occurring with oral administration.

In people, as well as in animals, baclofen has been shown to have general CNS depressant properties as indicated by the production of sedation with tolerance, somnolence, ataxia, and respiratory and cardiovascular depression.

PHARMACODYNAMICS OF BACLOFEN INJECTION

Intrathecal Bolus:

Adult Patients: The onset of action is generally one-half hour to 1 hour after an intrathecal bolus. Peak spasmolytic effect is seen at approximately 4 hours after dosing and effects may last 4-8 hours. Onset, peak response, and duration of action may vary with individual patients depending on the dose and severity of symptoms.

Pediatric Patients: The onset, peak response and duration of action is similar to those seen in adult patients.

Continuous Infusion:

Baclofen injection's antispastic action is first seen at 6-8 hours after initiation of continuous infusion. Maximum activity is observed in 24-48 hours.

No additional information is available for pediatric patients.

PHARMACOKINETICS OF BACLOFEN INJECTION

The pharmacokinetics of CSF clearance of baclofen injection calculated from intrathecal bolus or continuous infusion studies approximates CSF turnover, suggesting elimination is by bulk-low removal of CSF.

Intrathecal Bolus: After a bolus lumbar injection of 50 or 100 μg baclofen injection in 7 patients, the average CSF elimination half-life was 1.51 hours over the first 4 hours and the average CSF clearance was approximately 30 ml/hour.

Continuous Infusion: The mean CSF clearance for baclofen injection was approximately 30 ml/h in a study involving 10 patients on continuous intrathecal infusion.

Concurrent plasma concentrations of baclofen during intrathecal administration are expected to be low (0-5 ng/ml).

Limited pharmacokinetic data suggest that a lumbar-cisternal concentration gradient of about 4:1 is established along the neuroaxis during baclofen infusion. This is based upon simultaneous CSF sampling via cisternal and lumbar tap in 5 patients receiving continuous baclofen infusion at the lumbar level at doses associated with therapeutic efficacy; the interpatient variability was great. The gradient was not altered by position.

Six pediatric patients (age 8-18 years) receiving continuous intrathecal baclofen infusion at doses of 77-400 μg/day had plasma baclofen levels near or below 10 ng/ml.

INDICATIONS AND USAGE

Baclofen injection is indicated for use in the management of severe spasticity. Patients should first respond to a screening dose of intrathecal baclofen prior to consideration for long term infusion via an implantable pump. For spasticity of spinal cord origin, chronic infusion of baclofen injection via an implantable pump should be reserved for patients unresponsive to oral baclofen therapy, or those who experience intolerable CNS side effects at effective doses. Patients with spasticity due to traumatic brain injury should wait at least 1 year after the injury before consideration of long term intrathecal baclofen therapy. Baclofen injection is intended for use by the intrathecal route in single bolus test doses (via spinal catheter or lumbar puncture) and, for chronic use, only in implantable pumps approved by the FDA specifically for the administration of baclofen injection into the intrathecal space.

SPASTICITY OF SPINAL CORD ORIGIN

Evidence supporting the efficacy of baclofen injection was obtained in randomized, controlled investigations that compared the effects of either a single intrathecal dose or a 3 day intrathecal infusion of baclofen injection to placebo in patients with severe spasticity and spasms due to either spinal cord trauma or multiple sclerosis. Baclofen injection was superior to placebo on both principal outcome measures employed: change from baseline in the Ashworth rating of spasticity and the frequency of spasms.

SPASTICITY OF CEREBRAL ORIGIN

The efficacy of baclofen injection was investigated in three controlled clinical trials; two enrolled patients with cerebral palsy and one enrolled patients with spasticity due to previous brain injury. The first study, a randomized controlled cross-over trial of 51 patients with cerebral palsy, provided strong, statistically significant results; baclofen injection was superior to placebo in reducing spasticity as measured by the Ashworth Scale. A second cross-over study was conducted in 11 patients with spasticity arising from brain injury. Despite the small sample size, the study yielded a nearly significant test statistic (p=0.066) and provided directionally favorable results. The last study, however, did not provide data that could be reliably analyzed.

Baclofen injection therapy may be considered an alternative to destructive neurosurgical procedures. Prior to implantation of a device for chronic intrathecal infusion of baclofen injection, patients must show a response to baclofen injection in a screening trial (see DOSAGE AND ADMINISTRATION).

NON-FDA APPROVED INDICATIONS

Baclofen has been used in the treatment of trigeminal neuralgia and intractable hiccups, however these uses are not approved by the FDA. In addition, some investigators have suggested a role for intrathecal baclofen in the treatment of patients with tetanus-induced spasticity.

CONTRAINDICATIONS

Hypersensitivity to baclofen. Baclofen injection is not recommended for intravenous, intramuscular, subcutaneous or epidural administration.

WARNINGS

Baclofen injection is for use in single bolus intrathecal injections (via a catheter placed in the lumbar intrathecal space or injection by lumbar puncture) and in implantable pumps approved by the FDA specifically for the intrathecal administration of baclofen. Because of the possibility of potentially life-threatening CNS depression, cardiovascular collapse, and/or respiratory failure, physicians must be adequately trained and educated in chronic intrathecal infusion therapy.

The pump system should not be implanted until the patient's response to bolus baclofen injection is adequately evaluated. Evaluation (consisting of a screening procedure: see DOSAGE AND ADMINISTRATION) requires that baclofen injection be administered into the intrathecal space via a catheter or lumbar puncture. Because of the risks associated with the screening procedure and the adjustment of dosage following pump implantation, these phases must be conducted in a medically supervised and adequately equipped environment following the instructions outlined in DOSAGE AND ADMINISTRATION.

Resuscitative equipment should be available.

Following surgical implantation of the pump, particularly during the initial phases of pump use, the patient should be monitored closely until it is certain that the patient's response to the infusion is acceptable and reasonably stable.

On each occasion that the dosing rate of the pump and/or the concentration of baclofen injection in the reservoir is adjusted, close medical monitoring is required until it is certain that the patient's response to the infusion is acceptable and reasonably stable.

It is mandatory that the patient, all patient care givers, and the physicians responsible for the patient receive adequate information regarding the risks of this mode of treatment. All medical personnel and care givers should be instructed in (1) the signs and symptoms of overdose, (2) procedures to be followed in the event of overdose and (3) proper home care of the pump and insertion site.

OVERDOSE

Signs of overdose may appear suddenly or insidiously. Acute massive overdose may present as coma. Less sudden and/or less severe forms of overdose may present with signs of drowsiness, lightheadedness, dizziness, somnolence, respiratory depression, seizures, rostral progression of hypotonia and loss of consciousness progressing to coma. Should overdose appear likely, the patient should be taken immediately to a hospital for assessment and emptying of the pump reservoir. In cases reported to date, overdose has generally been related to pump malfunction or dosing error.

Extreme caution must be used when filling an FDA approved implantable pump. Such pumps should only be refilled through the reservoir refill septum. However, some pumps are also equipped with a catheter access port that allows direct access to the intrathecal catheter. Direct injection into this catheter access port may cause a life-threatening overdose.

WITHDRAWAL

Abrupt withdrawal of intrathecal baclofen, regardless of the cause, has resulted in sequelae that included high fever, altered mental status, exaggerated rebound spasticity and muscle rigidity that in rare cases progressed to rhabdomyolysis, multiple organ-system failure, and death. In the first 9 years of post-marketing experience, 27 cases of withdrawal temporally related to the cessation of baclofen therapy were reported; 6 patients died. In most cases, symptoms of withdrawal appeared within hours to a few days following interruption of baclofen therapy. Common reasons for abrupt interruption of intrathecal baclofen therapy included malfunction of the catheter (especially disconnection), low volume in the pump reservoir, and end of pump battery life; human error may have played a causal or contributing role in some cases. Prevention of abrupt discontinuation of intrathecal baclofen requires careful attention to programming and monitoring of the infusion system, refill scheduling and procedures, and pump alarms. Patients and caregivers should be advised of the importance of keeping scheduled refill visits and should be educated on the early symptoms of baclofen withdrawal.

All patients receiving intrathecal baclofen therapy are potentially at risk for withdrawal. Early symptoms of baclofen withdrawal may include return of baseline spasticity, pruritus, hypotension, and paresthesias. Some clinical characteristics of the advanced intrathecal baclofen withdrawal syndrome may resemble autonomic dysreflexia, infection (sepsis), malignant hyperthermia, neuroleptic-malignant syndrome, or other conditions associated with a hypermetabolic state or widespread rhabdomyolysis.

Rapid, accurate diagnosis and treatment in an emergency-room or intensive-care setting are important in order to prevent the potentially life-threatening central nervous system and systemic effects of intrathecal baclofen withdrawal. The suggested treatment for intrathecal baclofen withdrawal is the restoration of intrathecal baclofen at or near the same dosage as before therapy was interrupted. However, if restoration of intrathecal delivery is delayed, treatment with GABA-ergic agonist drugs such as oral or enteral baclofen, or oral, enteral, or intravenous benzodiazepines may prevent potentially fatal sequelae. Oral or enteral baclofen alone should not be relied upon to halt the progression of intrathecal baclofen withdrawal.

Seizures have been reported during overdose and with withdrawal from baclofen injection as well as in patients maintained on therapeutic doses of baclofen injection.

B

FATALITIES

Spasticity of Spinal Cord Origin

There were 16 deaths reported among the 576 US patients treated with baclofen injection in pre- and post-marketing studies evaluated as of December 1992. Because these patients were treated under uncontrolled clinical settings, it is impossible to determine definitively what role, if any, baclofen injection played in their deaths.

As a group, the patients who died were relatively young (mean age was 47 with a range from 25-63), but the majority suffered from severe spasticity of many years duration, were nonambulatory, had various medical complications such as pneumonia, urinary tract infections, and decubiti, and/or had received multiple concomitant medications. A case-by-case review of the clinical course of the 16 patients who died failed to reveal any unique signs, symptoms, or laboratory results that would suggest that treatment with baclofen injection caused their deaths. Two patients, however, did suffer sudden and unexpected death within 2 weeks of pump implantation and 1 patient died unexpectedly after screening.

One patient, a 44-year-old male with MS, died in hospital on the second day following pump implantation. An autopsy demonstrated severe fibrosis of the coronary conduction system. A second patient, a 52-year-old woman with MS and a history of an inferior wall myocardial infarction, was found dead in bed 12 days after pump implantation, 2 hours after having had documented normal vital signs. An autopsy revealed pulmonary congestion and bilateral pleural effusions. It is impossible to determine whether baclofen injection contributed to these deaths. The third patient underwent three baclofen screening trials. His medical history included SCI, aspiration pneumonia, septic shock, disseminated intravascular coagulopathy, severe metabolic acidosis, hepatic toxicity, and status epilepticus. Twelve (12) days after screening (he was not implanted), he again experienced status epilepticus with subsequent significant neurological deterioration. Based upon prior instruction, extraordinary resuscitative measures were not pursued and the patient died.

Spasticity of Cerebral Origin

There were 3 deaths occurring among the 211 patients treated with baclofen injection in pre-marketing studies as of March 1996. These deaths were not attributed to the therapy.

PRECAUTIONS

Children should be of sufficient body mass to accommodate the implantable pump for chronic infusion. Please consult pump manufacturer's manual for specific recommendations.

Safety and effectiveness in pediatric patients below the age of 4 have not been established.

SCREENING

Patients should be infection-free prior to the screening trial with baclofen injection because the presence of a systemic infection may interfere with an assessment of the patient's response to bolus baclofen injection.

PUMP IMPLANTATION

Patients should be infection-free prior to pump implantation because the presence of infection may increase the risk of surgical complications. Moreover, a systemic infection may complicate dosing.

PUMP DOSE ADJUSTMENT AND TITRATION

In most patients, it will be necessary to increase the dose gradually over time to maintain effectiveness; a sudden requirement for substantial dose escalation typically indicates a catheter complication (*i.e.,* catheter kink or dislodgement).

Reservoir refilling must be performed by fully trained and qualified personnel following the directions provided by the pump manufacturer. Refill intervals should be carefully calculated to prevent depletion of the reservoir, as this would result in the return of severe spasticity and possibly symptoms of withdrawal.

Strict aseptic technique in filling is required to avoid bacterial contamination and serious infection. A period of observation appropriate to the clinical situation should follow each refill or manipulation of the drug reservoir.

Extreme caution must be used when filling an FDA approved implantable pump equipped with an injection port that allows direct access to the intrathecal catheter. Direct injection into the catheter through the catheter access port may cause a life-threatening overdose.

Additional Considerations Pertaining to Dosage Adjustment

It may be important to titrate the dose to maintain some degree of muscle tone and allow occasional spasms to: (1) help support circulatory function, (2) possibly prevent the formation of deep vein thrombosis, (3) optimize activities of daily living and ease of care.

Except in overdose related emergencies, the dose of baclofen injection should ordinarily be reduced slowly if the drug is discontinued for any reason.

An attempt should be made to discontinue concomitant oral antispasticity medication to avoid possible overdose or adverse drug interactions, either prior to screening or following implant and initiation of chronic baclofen injection infusion. Reduction and discontinuation of oral antispasmotics should be done slowly and with careful monitoring by the physician. Abrupt reduction or discontinuation of concomitant antispastics should be avoided.

Drowsiness

Drowsiness has been reported in patients on baclofen injection. Patients should be cautioned regarding the operation of automobiles or other dangerous machinery, and activities made hazardous by decreased alertness. Patients should also be cautioned that the central nervous system depressant effects of baclofen injection may be additive to those of alcohol and other CNS depressants.

Precautions in Special Patient Populations

Careful dose titration of baclofen injection is needed when spasticity is necessary to sustain upright posture and balance in locomotion or whenever spasticity is used to obtain optimal function and care.

Patients suffering from psychotic disorders, schizophrenia, or confusional states should be treated cautiously with baclofen injection and kept under careful surveillance, because exacerbations of these conditions have been observed with oral administration.

Baclofen injection should be used with caution in patients with a history of autonomic dysreflexia. The presence of nociceptive stimuli or abrupt withdrawal of baclofen injection may cause an autonomic dysreflexic episode.

Because baclofen injection is primarily excreted unchanged by the kidneys, it should be given with caution in patients with impaired renal function and it may be necessary to reduce the dosage.

LABORATORY TESTS

No specific laboratory tests are deemed essential for the management of patients on baclofen injection.

CARCINOGENESIS, MUTAGENESIS, AND IMPAIRMENT OF FERTILITY

No increase in tumors was seen in rats receiving baclofen orally for 2 years at approximately 30-60 times on a mg/kg basis, or 10-20 times on a mg/m^2 basis, the maximum oral dose recommended for human use. Mutagenicity assays with baclofen have not been performed.

PREGNANCY CATEGORY C

Baclofen given orally has been shown to increase the incidence of omphaloceles (ventral hernias) in fetuses of rats given approximately 13 times on a mg/kg basis, or 3 times on a mg/m^2 basis, the maximum oral dose recommended for human use; this dose also caused reductions in food intake and weight gain in the dams.

This abnormality was not seen in mice or rabbits. There are no adequate and well-controlled studies in pregnant women. Baclofen should be used during pregnancy only if the potential benefit justifies the potential risk to the fetus.

NURSING MOTHERS

In mothers treated with oral baclofen in therapeutic doses, the active substance passes into the breast milk. It is not known whether detectable levels of drug are present in breast milk of nursing mothers receiving baclofen injection. As a general rule, nursing should be undertaken while a patient is receiving baclofen injection only if the potential benefit justifies the potential risks to the infant.

PEDIATRIC USE

Children should be of sufficient body mass to accommodate the implantable pump for chronic infusion. Please consult pump manufacturer's manual for specific recommendations.

Safety and effectiveness in pediatric patients below the age of 4 have not been established.

CONSIDERATIONS BASED ON EXPERIENCE WITH ORAL BACLOFEN

A dose-related increase in incidence of ovarian cysts was observed in female rats treated chronically with oral baclofen. Ovarian cysts have been found by palpation in about 4% of the multiple sclerosis patients who were treated with oral baclofen for up to 1 year. In most cases these cysts disappeared spontaneously while patients continued to receive the drug. Ovarian cysts are estimated to occur spontaneously in approximately 1–5% of the normal female population.

DRUG INTERACTIONS

There is inadequate systematic experience with the use of baclofen injection in combination with other medications to predict specific drug-drug interactions. Interactions attributed to the combined use of baclofen injection and epidural morphine include hypotension and dyspnea.

ADVERSE REACTIONS

SPASTICITY OF SPINAL CORD ORIGIN

Commonly Observed in Patients With Spasticity of Spinal Origin

In pre- and post-marketing clinical trials, the most commonly observed adverse events associated with use of baclofen injection which were not seen at an equivalent incidence among placebo-treated patients were: somnolence, dizziness, nausea, hypotension, headache, convulsions and hypotonia.

Associated With Discontinuation of Treatment

8/474 patients with spasticity of spinal cord origin receiving long term infusion of baclofen injection in pre- and post-marketing clinical studies in the US discontinued treatment due to adverse events. These include: pump pocket infections (3), meningitis (2), wound dehiscence (1), gynecological fibroids (1) and pump overpressurization (1) with unknown, if any, sequela. Eleven (11) patients who developed coma secondary to overdose had their treatment temporarily suspended, but all were subsequently re-started and were not, therefore, considered to be true discontinuations.

Fatalities

See WARNINGS.

Incidence in Controlled Trials

Experience with baclofen injection obtained in parallel, placebo-controlled, randomized studies provides only a limited basis for estimating the incidence of adverse events because the studies were of very brief duration (up to 3 days of infusion) and involved only a total of 63 patients. The following events occurred among the 31 patients receiving baclofen injection in 2 randomized, placebo-controlled trials: hypotension (2), dizziness (2), headache (2), dyspnea (1). No adverse events were reported among the 32 patients receiving placebo in these studies.

Events Observed During the Pre- and Post-Marketing Evaluation of Baclofen Injection

Adverse events associated with the use of baclofen injection reflect experience gained with 576 patients followed prospectively in the US. They received baclofen injection for periods of 1 day (screening) (n=576) to over 8 years (maintenance) (n=10). The usual screening bolus dose administered prior to pump implantation in these studies was typically 50 μg. The maintenance dose ranged from 12-2003 μg/day. Because of the open, uncontrolled nature of the experience, a causal linkage between events observed and the administration of baclofen injection cannot be reliably assessed in many cases and many of the adverse events reported are known to occur in association with the underlying conditions being treated. Nonetheless, many of the more commonly reported reactions — hypotonia, somnolence, dizziness, paresthesia, nausea/vomiting and headache — appear clearly drug-related.

Adverse experiences reported during all US studies (both controlled and uncontrolled) are shown in TABLE 1. Eight (8) of 474 patients who received chronic infusion via implanted pumps had adverse experiences which led to a discontinuation of long term treatment in the pre- and post-marketing studies.

TABLE 1 *Incidence of Most Frequent (≥ 1%) Adverse Events in Patients with Spasticity of Spinal Origin in Prospectively Monitored Clinical Trials*

Adverse Event	Screening* n=576	Titration† n=474	Maintenance‡ n=430
Hypotonia	5.4%	13.5%	25.3%
Somnolence	5.7%	5.9%	20.9%
Dizziness	1.7%	1.9%	7.9%
Paresthesia	2.4%	2.1%	6.7%
Nausea and vomiting	1.6%	2.3%	5.6%
Headache	1.6%	2.5%	5.1%
Constipation	0.2%	1.5%	5.1%
Convulsion	0.5%	1.3%	4.7%
Urinary retention	0.7%	1.7%	1.9%
Dry mouth	0.2%	0.4%	3.3%
Accidental injury	0.0%	0.2%	3.5%
Asthenia	0.7%	1.3%	1.4%
Confusion	0.5%	0.6%	2.3%
Death	0.2%	0.4%	3.0%
Pain	0.0%	0.6%	3.0%
Speech disorder	0.0%	0.2%	3.5%
Hypotension	1.0%	0.2%	1.9%
Ambylopia	0.5%	0.2%	2.3%
Diarrhea	0.0%	0.8%	2.3%
Hypoventilation	0.2%	0.8%	2.1%
Coma	0.0%	1.5%	0.9%
Impotence	0.2%	0.4%	1.6%
Peripheral edema	0.0%	0.0%	2.3%
Urinary incontinence	0.0%	0.8%	1.4%
Insomnia	0.0%	0.4%	1.6%
Anxiety	0.2%	0.4%	0.9%
Depression	0.0%	0.0%	1.6%
Dyspnea	0.3%	0.0%	1.2%
Fever	0.5%	0.2%	0.7%
Pneumonia	0.2%	0.2%	1.2%
Urinary frequency	0.0%	0.6%	0.9%
Urticaria	0.2%	0.2%	1.2%
Anorexia	0.0%	0.4%	0.9%
Diplopia	0.0%	0.4%	0.9%
Dysautonomia	0.2%	0.2%	0.9%
Hallucinations	0.3%	0.4%	0.5%
Hypertension	0.2%	0.6%	0.5%

* Following administration of test bolus.
† Two month period following implant.
‡ Beyond 2 months following implant.
n =Total number of patients entering each period.

In addition to the more common (1% or more) adverse events reported in the prospectively followed 576 domestic patients in pre- and post-marketing studies, experience from an additional 194 patients exposed to baclofen injection from foreign studies has been reported. The following adverse events, not described in TABLE 1, and arranged in decreasing order of frequency, and classified by body system, were reported:

Nervous System: Abnormal gait, thinking abnormal, tremor, amnesia, twitching, vasodilitation, cerebrovascular accident, nystagmus, personality disorder, psychotic depression, cerebral ischemia, emotional lability, euphoria, hypertonia, ileus, drug dependence, incoordination, paranoid reaction and ptosis.

Digestive System: Flatulence, dysphagia, dyspepsia and gastroenteritis.

Cardiovascular: Postural hypotension, bradycardia, palpitations, syncope, arrhythmia ventricular, deep thrombophlebitis, pallor and tachycardia.

Respiratory: Respiratory disorder, aspiration pneumonia, hyperventilation, pulmonary embolus and rhinitis.

Urogenital: Hematuria and kidney failure.

Skin and Appendages: Alopecia and sweating.

Metabolic and Nutritional Disorders: Weight loss, albuminuria, dehydration and hyperglycemia.

Special Senses: Abnormal vision, abnormality of accommodation, photophobia, taste loss and tinnitus.

Body as a Whole: Suicide, lack of drug effect, abdominal pain, hypothermia, neck rigidity, chest pain, chills, face edema, flu syndrome and overdose.

Hemic and Lymphatic System: Anemia.

SPASTICITY OF CEREBRAL ORIGIN

Commonly Observed

In pre-marketing clinical trials, the most commonly observed adverse events associated with use of baclofen injection which were not seen at an equivalent incidence among placebo-treated patients included: agitation, constipation, somnolence, leukocytosis, chills, urinary retention and hypotonia.

Associated With Discontinuation Of Treatment

Nine (9) of 211 patients receiving baclofen injection in pre-marketing clinical studies in the US discontinued long term infusion due to adverse events associated with intrathecal therapy.

The 9 adverse events leading to discontinuation were: Infection (3), CSF leaks (2), meningitis (2), drainage (1), and unmanageable trunk control (1).

Fatalities

Three deaths, none of which were attributed to baclofen injection, were reported in patients in clinical trials involving patients with spasticity of cerebral origin. See WARNINGS on other deaths reported in spinal spasticity patients.

Incidence in Controlled Trials

Experience with baclofen injection obtained in parallel, placebo-controlled, randomized studies provides only a limited basis for estimating the incidence of adverse events because the studies involved a total of 62 patients exposed to a single 50 μg intrathecal bolus. The following events occurred among the 62 patients receiving baclofen injection in two randomized, placebo-controlled trials involving cerebral palsy and head injury patients, respectively: agitation, constipation, somnolence, leukocytosis, nausea, vomiting, nystagmus, chills, urinary retention, and hypotonia.

Events Observed During the Pre-Marketing Evaluation of Baclofen Injection

Adverse events associated with the use of baclofen injection reflect experience gained with a total of 211 US patients with spasticity of cerebral origin, of whom 112 were pediatric patients (under age 16 at enrollment). They received baclofen injection for periods of 1 day (screening) (n=211) to 84 months (maintenance) (n=1). The usual screening bolus dose administered prior to pump implantation in these studies was 50-75 μg. The maintenance dose ranged from 22-1400 μg/day. Doses used in this patient population for long term infusion are generally lower than those required for patients with spasticity of spinal cord origin.

Because of the open, uncontrolled nature of the experience, a causal linkage between events observed and the administration of baclofen injection cannot be reliably assessed in many cases. Nonetheless, many of the more commonly reported reactions — somnolence, dizziness, headache, nausea, hypotension, hypotonia and coma — appear clearly drug-related.

The most frequent (≥1%) adverse events reported during all clinical trials are shown in TABLE 2. Nine patients discontinued long term treatment due to adverse events.

TABLE 2 *Incidence of Most Frequent (≥ 1%) Adverse Events in Patients With Spasticity of Cerebral Origin in Prospectively Monitored Clinical Trials*

Adverse Event	Screening* n=211	Titration† n=153	Maintenance‡ n=150
Hypotonia	2.4%	14.4%	34.7%
Somnolence	7.6%	10.5%	18.7%
Headache	6.6%	7.8%	10.7%
Nausea and vomiting	6.6%	10.5%	4.0%
Vomiting	6.2%	8.5%	4.0%
Urinary retention	0.9%	6.5%	8.0%
Convulsion	0.9%	3.3%	10.0%
Dizziness	2.4%	2.6%	8.0%
Nausea	1.4%	3.3%	7.3%
Hypoventilation	1.4%	1.3%	4.0%
Hypertonia	0.0%	0.7%	6.0%
Paresthesia	1.9%	0.7%	3.3%
Hypotension	1.9%	0.7%	2.0%
Increased salivation	0.0%	2.6%	2.7%
Back pain	0.9%	0.7%	2.0%
Constipation	0.5%	1.3%	2.0%
Pain	0.0%	0.0%	4.0%
Pruritus	0.0%	0.0%	4.0%
Diarrhea	0.5%	0.7%	2.0%
Peripheral edema	0.0%	0.0%	3.3%
Thinking abnormal	0.5%	1.3%	0.7%
Agitation	0.5%	0.0%	1.3%
Asthenia	0.0%	0.0%	2.0%
Chills	0.5%	0.0%	1.3%
Coma	0.5%	0.0%	1.3%
Dry mouth	0.5%	0.0%	1.3%
Pneumonia	0.0%	0.0%	2.0%
Speech disorder	0.5%	0.7%	0.7%
Tremor	0.5%	0.0%	1.3%
Urinary incontinence	0.0%	0.0%	2.0%
Urination impaired	0.0%	0.0%	2.0%

* Following administration of test bolus.
† Two month period following implant.
‡ Beyond 2 months following implant.
n = Total number of patients entering each period. 211 patients received drug; (1 of 212) received placebo only.

The more common (1% or more) adverse events reported in the prospectively followed 211 patients exposed to baclofen injection have been reported. In the total cohort, the following adverse events, not described in TABLE 2, and arranged in decreasing order of frequency, and classified by body system, were reported:

Nervous System: Akathisia, ataxia, confusion, depression, opisthotonos, amnesia, anxiety, hallucinations, hysteria, insomnia, nystagmus, personality disorder, reflexes decreased, and vasodilitation.

Digestive System: Dysphagia, fecal incontinence, gastrointestinal hemorrhage and tongue disorder.

Cardiovascular: Bradycardia.

Respiratory: Apnea, dyspnea and hyperventilation.

Urogenital: Abnormal ejaculation, kidney calculus, oliguria and vaginitis.

Skin and Appendages: Rash, sweating, alopecia, contact dermatitis and skin ulcer.
Special Senses: Abnormality of accommodation.
Body as a Whole: Death, fever, abdominal pain, carcinoma, malaise and hypothermia.
Hemic and Lymphatic System: Leukocytosis and petechial rash.

DOSAGE AND ADMINISTRATION

Refer to the manufacturer's manual for the implantable pump approved for intrathecal infusion for specific instructions and precautions for programming the pump and/or refilling the reservoir.

SCREENING PHASE

Prior to pump implantation and initiation of chronic infusion of baclofen injection, patients must demonstrate a positive clinical response to a baclofen injection bolus dose administered intrathecally in a screening trial. The screening trial employs baclofen injection at a concentration of 50 µg/ml. A 1 ml ampule (50 µg/ml) is available for use in the screening trial. The screening procedure is as follows. An initial bolus containing 50 µg in a volume of 1 ml is administered into the intrathecal space by barbotage over a period of not less than 1 minute. The patient is observed over the ensuing 4-8 hours. A positive response consists of a significant decrease in muscle tone and/or frequency and/or severity of spasms. If the initial response is less than desired, a second bolus injection may be administered 24 hours after the first. The second screening bolus dose consists of 75 µg in 1.5 ml. Again, the patient should be observed for an interval of 4-8 hours. If the response is still inadequate, a final bolus screening dose of 100 µg in 2 ml may be administered 24 hours later.

Pediatric Patients

The starting screening dose for pediatric patients is the same as in adult patients, *i.e.*, 50 µg. However, for very small patients, a screening dose of 25 µg may be tried first.

Patients who do not respond to a 100 µg intrathecal bolus should not be considered candidates for an implanted pump for chronic infusion.

POST-IMPLANT DOSE TITRATION PERIOD

To determine the initial total daily dose of baclofen injection following implant, the screening dose that gave a positive effect should be doubled and administered over a 24 hour period, unless the efficacy of the bolus dose was maintained for more than 8 hours, in which case the starting daily dose should be the screening dose delivered over a 24 hour period. No dose increases should be given in the first 24 hours (*i.e.*, until the steady state is achieved).

Adult patients with spasticity of spinal cord origin: After the first 24 hours, for adult patients, the daily dosage should be increased slowly by 10-30% increments and only once every 24 hours, until the desired clinical effect is achieved.

Adult patients with spasticity of cerebral origin: After the first 24 hours, the daily dose should be increased slowly by 5-15% only once every 24 hours, until the desired clinical effect is achieved.

Pediatric patients: After the first 24 hours, the daily dose should be increased slowly by 5-15% only once every 24 hours, until the desired clinical effect is achieved.

If there is not a substantive clinical response to increases in the daily dose, check for proper pump function and catheter patency.

Patients must be monitored closely in a fully equipped and staffed environment during the screening phase and dose-titration period immediately following implant. Resuscitative equipment should be immediately available for use in case of life-threatening or intolerable side effects.

MAINTENANCE THERAPY

Spasticity of Spinal Cord Origin Patients

The clinical goal is to maintain muscle tone as close to normal as possible, and to minimize the frequency and severity of spasms to the extent possible, without inducing intolerable side effects. Very often, the maintenance dose needs to be adjusted during the first few months of therapy while patients adjust to changes in life style due to the alleviation of spasticity. During periodic refills of the pump, the daily dose may be increased by 10-40%, but no more than 40%, to maintain adequate symptom control. The daily dose may be reduced by 10-20% if patients experience side effects. Most patients require gradual increases in dose over time to maintain optimal response during chronic therapy. A sudden large requirement for dose escalation suggests a catheter complication (*i.e.*, catheter kink or dislodgement).

Maintenance dosage for long term continuous infusion of baclofen injection has ranged from 12-2003 µg/day, with most patients adequately maintained on 300-800 µg/day. There is limited experience with daily doses greater than 1000 µg/day. Determination of the optimal baclofen injection dose requires individual titration. The lowest dose with an optimal response should be used.

Spasticity of Cerebral Origin Patients

The clinical goal is to maintain muscle tone as close to normal as possible and to minimize the frequency and severity of spasms to the extent possible, without inducing intolerable side effects, or to titrate the dose to the desired degree of muscle tone for optimal functions. Very often the maintenance dose needs to be adjusted during the first few months of therapy while patients adjust to changes in life style due to the alleviation of spasticity. During periodic refills of the pump, the daily dose may be increased by 5-20%, but no more than 20%, to maintain adequate symptom control. The daily dose may be reduced by 10-20% if patients experience side effects. Many patients require gradual increases in dose over time to maintain optimal response during chronic therapy. A sudden large requirement for dose escalation suggests a catheter complication (*i.e.*, catheter kink or dislodgement).

Maintenance dosage for long term continuous infusion of baclofen injection has ranged from 22-1400 µg/day, with most patients adequately maintained on 90-703 µg/day. In clinical trials, only 3 of 150 patients required daily doses greater than 1000 µg/day.

Pediatric Patients

Use same dosing recommendations for patients with spasticity of cerebral origin. Pediatric patients under 12 years seemed to require a lower daily dose in clinical trials. Average daily dose for patients under 12 years was 274 µg/day, with a range of 24-1199 µg/day. Dosage requirement for pediatric patients over 12 years does not seem to be different from that of adult patients. Determination of the optimal baclofen injection dose requires individual titration. The lowest dose with an optimal response should be used.

Potential Need for Dose Adjustments in Chronic Use

During long term treatment, approximately 5% (28/627) of patients become refractory to increasing doses. There is not sufficient experience to make firm recommendations for tolerance treatment; however, this "tolerance" has been treated on occasion, in hospital, by a "drug holiday" consisting of the gradual reduction of baclofen injection over a 2-4 week period and switching to alternative methods of spasticity management. After the "drug holiday," baclofen injection may be restarted at the initial continuous infusion dose.

STABILITY

Parenteral drug products should be inspected for particulate matter and discoloration prior to administration, whenever solution and container permit.

DELIVERY SPECIFICATIONS

The specific concentration that should be used depends upon the total daily dose required as well as the delivery rate of the pump. Baclofen injection may require dilution when used with certain implantable pumps. Please consult manufacturer's manual for specific recommendations.

PREPARATION INSTRUCTION

Screening

Use the 1 ml screening ampule only (50 µg/ml) for bolus injection into the subarachnoid space. For a 50 µg bolus dose, use 1 ml of the screening ampule. Use 1.5 ml of 50 µg/ml baclofen injection for a 75 µg bolus dose. For the maximum screening dose of 100 µg, use 2 ml of 50 µg/ml baclofen injection (2 screening ampules).

Maintenance

For patients who require concentrations other than 500 or 2000 µg/ml, baclofen injection must be diluted.

Baclofen injection must be diluted with sterile preservative free sodium chloride for injection.

DELIVERY REGIMEN

Baclofen injection is most often administered in a continuous infusion mode immediately following implant. For those patients implanted with programmable pumps who have achieved relatively satisfactory control on continuous infusion, further benefit may be attained using more complex schedules of baclofen injection delivery. For example, patients who have increased spasms at night may require a 20% increase in their hourly infusion rate. Changes in flow rate should be programmed to start 2 hours before the time of desired clinical effect.

HOW SUPPLIED

Lioresal Intrathecal (baclofen injection) is available in single use ampules of 10 mg/20 ml (500 µg/ml) or 10 mg/5 ml (2000 µg/ml) packaged in a Refill Kit for intrathecal administration.

For screening, Lioresal Intrathecal is available in a single use ampule of 0.05 mg/1 ml.

STORAGE

Does not require refrigeration.

Do not store above 30°C (86°F).

Do not freeze.

Do not heat sterilize.

ORAL

DESCRIPTION

Baclofen is a muscle relaxant and antispastic. Its chemical name is 4-amino-3-(4-chlorophenyl)-butanoic acid.

Baclofen is a white to off-white, odorless or practically odorless crystalline powder, with a molecular weight of 213.66. It is slightly soluble in water, very slightly soluble in methanol, and insoluble in chloroform.

Baclofen tablets are available as 10 and 20 mg tablets for oral administration.

Inactive Ingredients:

Baclofen Tablets: Cellulose compounds, magnesium stearate, povidone, and starch.

CLINICAL PHARMACOLOGY

The precise mechanism of action of baclofen is not fully known. Baclofen is capable of inhibiting both monosynaptic and polysynaptic reflexes at the spinal level, possibly by hyperpolarization of afferent terminals, although actions at supraspinal sites may also occur and contribute to its clinical effect. Although baclofen is an analog of the putative inhibitory neurotransmitter gamma-aminobutyric acid (GABA), there is no conclusive evidence that actions on GABA systems are involved in the production of its clinical effects. In studies with animals, baclofen has been shown to have general CNS depressant properties as indicated by the production of sedation with tolerance, somnolence, ataxia, and respiratory and cardiovascular depression. Baclofen is rapidly and extensively absorbed and eliminated. Absorption may be dose-dependent, being reduced with increasing doses. Baclofen is excreted primarily by the kidney in unchanged form and there is relatively large intersubject variation in absorption and/or elimination.

INDICATIONS AND USAGE

Baclofen is useful for the alleviation of signs and symptoms of spasticity resulting from multiple sclerosis, particularly for the relief of flexor spasms and concomitant pain, clonus, and muscular rigidity. Patients should have reversible spasticity so that baclofen treatment will aid in restoring residual function.

Baclofen may also be of some value in patients with spinal cord injuries and other spinal cord diseases.

Baclofen is not indicated in the treatment of skeletal muscle spasm resulting from rheumatic disorders.

The efficacy of baclofen in stroke, cerebral palsy, and Parkinson's disease has not been established and, therefore, it is not recommended for these conditions.

NON-FDA APPROVED INDICATIONS

Baclofen has been used in the treatment of trigeminal neuralgia and intractable hiccups, however these uses are not approved by the FDA.

CONTRAINDICATIONS

Hypersensitivity to baclofen.

WARNINGS

Abrupt Drug Withdrawal: Hallucinations and seizures have occurred on abrupt withdrawal of baclofen. Therefore, except for serious adverse reactions, the dose should be reduced slowly when the drug is discontinued.

Impaired Renal Function: Because baclofen is primarily excreted unchanged through the kidneys, it should be given with caution, and it may be necessary to reduce the dosage.

Stroke: Baclofen has not significantly benefited patients with stroke. These patients have also shown poor tolerability to the drug.

Pregnancy: Baclofen has been shown to increase the incidence of omphaloceles (ventral hernias) in fetuses of rats given approximately 13 times the maximum dose recommended for human use, at a dose which caused significant reductions in food intake and weight gain in dams. This abnormality was not seen in mice or rabbits. There was also an increased incidence of incomplete sternebral ossification in fetuses of rats given approximately 13 times the maximum recommended human dose, and an increased incidence of unossified phalangeal nuclei of forelimbs and hindlimbs in fetuses of rabbits given approximately 7 times the maximum recommended human dose. In mice, no teratogenic effects were observed, although reductions in mean fetal weight with consequent delays in skeletal ossification were present when dams were given 17 or 34 times the human daily dose. There are no studies in pregnant women. Baclofen should be used during pregnancy only if the benefit clearly justifies the potential risk to the fetus.

PRECAUTIONS

Safe use of baclofen in children under 12 has not been established, and it is, therefore, not recommended for use in children. Because of the possibility of sedation, patients should be cautioned regarding the operation of automobiles or other dangerous machinery, and activities made hazardous by decreased alertness. Patients should also be cautioned that the central nervous system effects of baclofen may be additive to those of alcohol and other CNS depressants.

Baclofen should be used with caution where spasticity is utilized to sustain upright posture and balance in locomotion or whenever spasticity is utilized to obtain increased function.

In patients with epilepsy, the clinical state and electroencephalogram should be monitored at regular intervals, since deterioration in seizure control and EEG have been reported occasionally in patients taking baclofen. It is not known whether this drug is excreted in human milk. As a general rule, nursing should not be undertaken while a patient is on a drug since many drugs are excreted in human milk.

A dose-related increase in incidence of ovarian cysts and a less marked increase in enlarged and/or hemorrhagic adrenal glands was observed in female rats treated chronically with baclofen.

Ovarian cysts have been found by palpation in about 4% of the multiple sclerosis patients that were treated with baclofen for up to 1 year. In most cases these cysts disappeared spontaneously while patients continued to receive the drug. Ovarian cysts are estimated to occur spontaneously in approximately 1%-5% of the normal female population.

PREGNANCY CATEGORY C

Baclofen given orally has been shown to increase the incidence of omphaloceles (ventral hernias) in fetuses of rats given approximately 13 times on a mg/kg basis, or 3 times on a mg/m^2 basis, the maximum oral dose recommended for human use; this dose also caused reductions in food intake and weight gain in the dams.

This abnormality was not seen in mice or rabbits. There are no adequate and well-controlled studies in pregnant women. Baclofen should be used during pregnancy only if the potential benefit justifies the potential risk to the fetus.

NURSING MOTHERS

In mothers treated with oral baclofen in therapeutic doses, the active substance passes into the breast milk.

CONSIDERATIONS BASED ON EXPERIENCE WITH ORAL BACLOFEN

A dose-related increase in incidence of ovarian cysts was observed in female rats treated chronically with oral baclofen. Ovarian cysts have been found by palpation in about 4% of the multiple sclerosis patients who were treated with oral baclofen for up to 1 year. In most cases these cysts disappeared spontaneously while patients continued to receive the drug. Ovarian cysts are estimated to occur spontaneously in approximately 1-5% of the normal female population.

ADVERSE REACTIONS

The most common is transient drowsiness (10-63%). In one controlled study of 175 patients, transient drowsiness was observed in 63% of those receiving baclofen compared to 36% of those in the placebo group. Other common adverse reactions are dizziness (5-15%), weakness (5-15%) and fatigue (2-4%). Others reported:

Neuropsychiatric: Confusion (1-11%), headache (4-8%), insomnia (2-7%); and, rarely, euphoria, excitement, depression, hallucinations, paresthesia, muscle pain, tinnitus, slurred speech, coordination disorder, tremor, rigidity, dystonia, ataxia, blurred vision, nystagmus, strabismus, miosis, mydriasis, diplopia, dysarthria, epileptic seizure.

Cardiovascular: Hypotension (0.9%). Rare instances of dyspnea, palpitation, chest pain, syncope.

Gastrointestinal: Nausea (4-12%), constipation (2-6%); and, rarely, dry mouth, anorexia, taste disorder, abdominal pain, vomiting, diarrhea, and positive test for occult blood in stool.

Genitourinary: Urinary frequency (2-6%); and, rarely, enuresis, urinary retention, dysuria, impotence, inability to ejaculate, nocturia, hematuria.

Other: Instances of rash, pruritus, ankle edema, excessive perspiration, weight gain, nasal congestion.

Some of the CNS and genitourinary symptoms may be related to the underlying disease rather than to the drug therapy.

The following laboratory tests have been found to be abnormal in a few patients receiving baclofen: Increased SGOT, elevated alkaline phosphatase, and elevation of blood sugar.

DOSAGE AND ADMINISTRATION

The determination of optimal dosage requires individual titration. Start therapy at a low dosage and increase gradually until optimum effect is achieved (usually between 40-80 mg daily).

The following dosage schedule is suggested:

5 mg tid for 3 days
10 mg tid for 3 days
15 mg tid for 3 days
20 mg tid for 3 days

Thereafter additional increases may be necessary but the total daily dose should not exceed a maximum of 80 mg daily (20 mg qid).

The lowest dose compatible with an optimal response is recommended. If benefits are not evident after a reasonable trial period, patients should be slowly withdrawn from the drug (see WARNINGS, Abrupt Drug Withdrawal).

HOW SUPPLIED

BACLOFENTABLETS

Dispense in a tight container.

Storage: Do not store above 30°C (86°F).

PRODUCT LISTING - RATED THERAPEUTICALLY EQUIVALENT

Tablet - Oral - 10 mg

25 x 30	$294.38	GENERIC, American Health Packaging	63739-0031-03
30's	$12.56	GENERIC, Heartland Healthcare Services	61392-0706-30
30's	$12.56	GENERIC, Heartland Healthcare Services	61392-0706-39
31 x 10	$127.06	GENERIC, Vangard Labs	00615-3541-53
31 x 10	$127.06	GENERIC, Vangard Labs	00615-3541-63
31's	$12.98	GENERIC, Heartland Healthcare Services	61392-0706-31
32's	$13.40	GENERIC, Heartland Healthcare Services	61392-0706-32
45's	$18.84	GENERIC, Heartland Healthcare Services	61392-0706-45
60's	$25.12	GENERIC, Heartland Healthcare Services	61392-0706-60
60's	$25.12	GENERIC, Heartland Healthcare Services	61392-0706-65
90's	$37.67	GENERIC, Heartland Healthcare Services	61392-0706-90
90's	$37.67	GENERIC, Heartland Healthcare Services	61392-0706-95
100's	$8.99	FEDERAL UPPER LIMIT, H.C.F.A. F F P	99999-0361-01
100's	$18.00	GENERIC, Raway Pharmacal Inc	00686-0668-20
100's	$31.11	GENERIC, Major Pharmaceuticals Inc	00904-3925-61
100's	$31.75	GENERIC, Major Pharmaceuticals Inc	00904-3365-60
100's	$31.75	GENERIC, Major Pharmaceuticals Inc	00904-5216-60
100's	$32.39	GENERIC, Moore, H.L. Drug Exchange Inc	00839-7472-06
100's	$36.20	GENERIC, Aligen Independent Laboratories Inc	00405-4110-01
100's	$36.20	GENERIC, Martec Pharmaceuticals Inc	52555-0513-01
100's	$36.20	GENERIC, Martec Pharmaceuticals Inc	52555-0695-01
100's	$36.28	GENERIC, Watson/Schein Pharmaceuticals Inc	00364-2312-01
100's	$36.28	GENERIC, Watson Laboratories Inc	00591-5730-01
100's	$37.05	GENERIC, Watson Laboratories Inc	52544-0686-01
100's	$39.84	GENERIC, American Health Packaging	62584-0623-01
100's	$40.11	GENERIC, Auro Pharmaceutical	55829-0158-10
100's	$41.00	GENERIC, Ivax Corporation	00182-1295-89
100's	$43.27	GENERIC, Major Pharmaceuticals Inc	00904-3365-61
100's	$43.72	GENERIC, Qualitest Products Inc	00603-2408-21
100's	$54.91	GENERIC, Rosemont Pharmaceutical Corporation	00832-1024-00
100's	$61.01	GENERIC, Ivax Corporation	00172-4096-60
100's	$72.88	LIORESAL, Novartis Pharmaceuticals	00028-0023-01

Tablet - Oral - 20 mg

25 x 30	$540.90	GENERIC, Sky Pharmaceuticals Packaging, Inc	63739-0032-03
30's	$23.77	GENERIC, Heartland Healthcare Services	61392-0707-30
30's	$23.77	GENERIC, Heartland Healthcare Services	61392-0707-39
31 x 10	$227.53	GENERIC, Vangard Labs	00615-3542-53
31 x 10	$227.53	GENERIC, Vangard Labs	00615-3542-63
31's	$24.56	GENERIC, Heartland Healthcare Services	61392-0707-31
32's	$25.36	GENERIC, Heartland Healthcare Services	61392-0707-32
45's	$35.66	GENERIC, Heartland Healthcare Services	61392-0707-45
60's	$47.54	GENERIC, Heartland Healthcare Services	61392-0707-60
60's	$47.54	GENERIC, Heartland Healthcare Services	61392-0707-65
90's	$71.32	GENERIC, Heartland Healthcare Services	61392-0707-90
90's	$71.32	GENERIC, Heartland Healthcare Services	61392-0707-95
100's	$16.88	FEDERAL UPPER LIMIT, H.C.F.A. F F P	99999-0361-05
100's	$31.85	GENERIC, Raway Pharmacal Inc	00686-0669-20

100's	$51.11	GENERIC, Qualitest Products Inc	00603-2409-21
100's	$54.03	GENERIC, Major Pharmaceuticals Inc	00904-3926-01
100's	$54.03	GENERIC, Major Pharmaceuticals Inc	00904-3926-61
100's	$56.69	GENERIC, Moore, H.L. Drug Exchange Inc	00839-7473-06
100's	$56.90	GENERIC, Major Pharmaceuticals Inc	00904-3366-60
100's	$56.90	GENERIC, Major Pharmaceuticals Inc	00904-5222-60
100's	$60.00	GENERIC, Teva Pharmaceuticals Usa	00332-2236-09
100's	$63.90	GENERIC, Aligen Independent Laboratories Inc	00405-4111-01
100's	$64.00	GENERIC, Watson/Schein Pharmaceuticals Inc	00364-2313-01
100's	$64.00	GENERIC, Watson Laboratories Inc	00591-5731-01
100's	$64.08	GENERIC, Watson Laboratories Inc	52544-0687-01
100's	$64.30	GENERIC, Martec Pharmaceuticals Inc	52555-0514-01
100's	$65.84	GENERIC, Auro Pharmaceutical	55829-0159-10
100's	$72.39	GENERIC, American Health Packaging	62584-0624-01
100's	$73.41	GENERIC, Ivax Corporation	00182-1296-89
100's	$98.66	GENERIC, Rosemont Pharmaceutical Corporation	00832-1025-00
100's	$101.39	LIORESAL, Novartis Pharmaceuticals	00028-0033-61
100's	$109.62	GENERIC, Ivax Corporation	00172-4097-60

PRODUCT LISTING - EQUIVALENTS NOT AVAILABLE

Solution - Intrathecal - 0.05 mg/ml			
1 ml	$78.00	LIORESAL INTRATHECAL, Medtronic Neurological	52081-0562-01
1 ml	$84.00	LIORESAL INTRATHECAL, Medtronic Neurological	58281-0562-01
Solution - Intrathecal - 0.5 mg/ml			
20 ml	$208.00	LIORESAL INTRATHECAL, Medtronic Neurological	58281-0560-01
Solution - Intrathecal - 2 mg/ml			
5 ml x 2	$427.00	LIORESAL INTRATHECAL, Medtronic Neurological	58281-0561-02
5 ml x 4	$777.00	LIORESAL INTRATHECAL, Medtronic Neurological	58281-0561-04
Tablet - Oral - 10 mg			
10's	$6.49	GENERIC, Southwood Pharmaceuticals Inc	58016-0486-10
20's	$12.98	GENERIC, Southwood Pharmaceuticals Inc	58016-0486-20
30's	$5.54	GENERIC, Physicians Total Care	54868-3405-00
30's	$19.47	GENERIC, Southwood Pharmaceuticals Inc	58016-0486-30
40's	$25.96	GENERIC, Southwood Pharmaceuticals Inc	58016-0486-40
60's	$22.23	GENERIC, Allscripts Pharmaceutical Company	54569-4330-00
60's	$38.94	GENERIC, Southwood Pharmaceuticals Inc	58016-0486-60
90's	$58.40	GENERIC, Southwood Pharmaceuticals Inc	58016-0486-90
100's	$64.90	GENERIC, Southwood Pharmaceuticals Inc	58016-0486-00
Tablet - Oral - 20 mg			
10's	$11.90	GENERIC, Southwood Pharmaceuticals Inc	58016-0477-10
20's	$12.92	GENERIC, Allscripts Pharmaceutical Company	54569-4171-00
20's	$23.80	GENERIC, Southwood Pharmaceuticals Inc	58016-0477-20
30's	$35.70	GENERIC, Southwood Pharmaceuticals Inc	58016-0477-30
40's	$47.60	GENERIC, Southwood Pharmaceuticals Inc	58016-0477-40
60's	$71.40	GENERIC, Southwood Pharmaceuticals Inc	58016-0477-60
90's	$107.10	GENERIC, Southwood Pharmaceuticals Inc	58016-0477-90
100's	$118.85	GENERIC, Southwood Pharmaceuticals Inc	58016-0477-00

Balsalazide Disodium *(003500)*

Categories: Colitis, ulcerative; FDA Approved 2000 Jul; Pregnancy Category B
Drug Classes: Gastrointestinals; Salicylates
Brand Names: Colazal
Cost of Therapy: $534.24 (Ulcerative Colitis; Colazal; 750 mg; 9 capsules/day; 56 day supply)

DESCRIPTION

Each Colazal capsule contains 750 mg of balsalazide disodium, a prodrug that is enzymatically cleaved in the colon to produce mesalamine (5-aminosalicylic acid), an anti-inflammatory drug. Each daily dose of Colazal (6.75 g) is equivalent to 2.4 g of mesalamine. Balsalazide disodium has the chemical name (E)-5-[[-4-[[(2-carboxyethyl)amino] carbonyl]phenyl]azo]-2-hydroxybenzoic acid, disodium salt, dihydrate.

The molecular weight is 437.32 and the molecular formula is $C_{17}H_{13}N_3O_6Na_2 \cdot 2H_2O$.

Balsalazide disodium is a stable, odorless orange to yellow microcrystalline powder. It is freely soluble in water and isotonic saline, sparingly soluble in methanol and ethanol, and practically insoluble in all other organic solvents.

Inactive ingredients: Each hard gelatin capsule contains colloidal silicon dioxide and magnesium stearate. The sodium content of each capsule is approximately 86 mg.

CLINICAL PHARMACOLOGY

Balsalazide disodium is delivered intact to the colon where it is cleaved by bacterial azoreduction to release equimolar quantities of mesalamine, which is the therapeutically active portion of the molecule, and 4-aminobenzoyl-β-alanine. The recommended dose of 6.75 g/day, for the treatment of active disease, provides 2.4 g of free 5-aminosalicylic acid to the colon.

The 4-aminobenzoyl-β-alanine carrier moiety released when balsalazide disodium is cleaved is only minimally absorbed and largely inert. The mechanism of action of 5-aminosalicylic acid is unknown, but appears to be topical rather than systemic. Mucosal production of arachidonic acid metabolites, both through the cyclooxygenase pathways, *i.e.*, prostanoids, and through the lipoxygenase pathways, *i.e.*, leukotrienes and hydroxyeicosatetraenoic acids, is increased in patients with chronic inflammatory bowel disease, and it is possible that 5-aminosalicylic acid diminishes inflammation by blocking production of arachidonic acid metabolites in the colon.

PHARMACOKINETICS

Colazal capsules contain granules of balsalazide disodium which are insoluble in acid and designed to be delivered to the colon intact. Upon reaching the colon, bacterial azoreductases cleave the compound to release 5-aminosalicylic acid, the therapeutically active portion of the molecule, and 4-aminobenzoyl-β-alanine.

Absorption

In healthy individuals, the systemic absorption of intact balsalazide was very low and variable. The mean C_{max} occurs approximately 1-2 hours after single oral doses of 1.5 or 2.25 g. The absolute bioavailability of this compound was not determined. In a study of ulcerative colitis patients receiving balsalazide, 1.5 g twice daily, for over 1 year, systemic drug exposure, based on mean AUC values, was up to 60 times greater (8-480 ng·h/ml) after equivalent multiple doses of 1.5 g twice daily when compared to healthy subjects who received the same dose. There was a large intersubject variability in the plasma concentration of balsalazide versus time profiles in all studies, thus its half-life could not be determined. The effect of food intake on the absorption of this compound was not studied.

Distribution

The binding of balsalazide to human plasma proteins was ≥99%.

Metabolism

The products of the azoreduction of this compound, 5-aminosalicylic acid and 4-aminobenzoyl-β-alanine, and their N-acetylated metabolites have been identified in plasma, urine and feces.

Elimination

Less than 1% of an oral dose was recovered as parent compound, 5-aminosalicylic acid or 4-aminobenzoyl-β-alanine in the urine of healthy subjects after single and multiple doses of balsalazide disodium, while up to 25% of the dose was recovered as the N-acetylated metabolites. In a study with 10 healthy volunteers, 65% of a single 2.25 g dose of balsalazide disodium was recovered as 5-aminosalicylic acid, 4-aminobenzoyl-β-alanine, and the N-acetylated metabolites in feces, while <1% of the dose was recovered as parent compound.

In a study that examined the disposition of balsalazide in patients who were taking 3-6 g of balsalazide disodium daily for more than 1 year and who were in remission from ulcerative colitis, less than 1% of an oral dose was recovered as intact balsalazide in the urine. Less than 4% of the dose was recovered as 5-aminosalicylic acid, while virtually no 4-aminobenzoyl-β-alanine was detected in urine. The urinary recovery of the N-acetylated metabolites comprised 20-25% of the balsalazide dose. No fecal recovery studies were performed in this population.

SPECIAL POPULATIONS

Geriatric: No information is available for the geriatric population.

Pediatric: The safety and effectiveness of balsalazide in the pediatric population have not been established.

Gender: No adequate and well-controlled studies which examine balsalazide in males versus females are available.

Renal Insufficiency: No adequate and well-controlled studies which examine balsalazide disposition in patients with mild, moderate, and severe renal impairment are available.

Hepatic Insufficiency: No information is available for patients with hepatic impairment.

Race: No information is available which examines balsalazide in different races.

Pharmacodynamic/Pharmacokinetic Relationship: No information is available.

Drug-Drug Interactions: Neither *in vitro* nor *in vivo* drug-drug interaction studies have been performed with balsalazide.

INDICATIONS AND USAGE

Balsalazide disodium is indicated for the treatment of mildly to moderately active ulcerative colitis. Safety and effectiveness of balsalazide disodium beyond 12 weeks has not been established.

CONTRAINDICATIONS

Balsalazide disodium is contraindicated in patients with hypersensitivity to salicylates or to any of the components of balsalazide disodium capsules or balsalazide metabolites.

PRECAUTIONS

Of the 259 patients treated with balsalazide disodium 6.75 g/day in controlled clinical trials of active disease, exacerbation of the symptoms of colitis, possibly related to drug use, has been reported by 3 patients.

GENERAL

Patients with pyloric stenosis may have prolonged gastric retention of balsalazide disodium capsules.

RENAL

At doses up to 2000 mg/kg (approximately 21 times the recommended 6.75 g/day dose on a mg/kg basis for a 70 kg person), balsalazide disodium had no nephrotoxic effects in rats or dogs. Renal toxicity has been observed in animals and patients given other mesalamine products. Therefore, caution should be exercised when administering balsalazide disodium to patients with known renal dysfunction or a history of renal disease.

B

CARCINOGENESIS, MUTAGENESIS, AND IMPAIRMENT OF FERTILITY

In a 24 month rat (Sprague Dawley) carcinogenicity study, oral (dietary) balsalazide disodium at doses up to 2 g/kg/day was not tumorigenic. For a 50 kg person of average height this dose represents 2.4 times the recommended human dose on a body surface area basis.

Balsalazide disodium was not genotoxic in the following *in vitro* or *in vivo* tests: Ames test, human lymphocyte chromosomal aberration test, and mouse lymphoma cell (L5178Y/TK+/-) forward mutation test, or mouse micronucleus test. However, it was genotoxic in the *in vitro* Chinese hamster lung cell (CH V79/HGPRT) forward mutation test.

4-aminobenzoyl-β-alanine, a metabolite of balsalazide disodium, was not genotoxic in the Ames test, and the mouse lymphoma cell (L5178Y/TK+/-) forward mutation test but was positive in the human lymphocyte chromosomal aberration test. N-acetyl-4-aminobenzoyl-β-alanine, a conjugated metabolite of balsalazide disodium, was not genotoxic in the Ames test, the mouse lymphoma cell (L5178Y/TK+/-) forward mutation tests, or the human lymphocyte chromosomal aberration test. Balsalazide disodium at oral doses up to 2 g/kg/day, 2.4 times the recommended human dose based on body surface area, was found to have no effect on fertility and reproductive performance in rats.

PREGNANCY, TERATOGENIC EFFECTS, PREGNANCY CATEGORY B

Reproduction studies were performed in rats and rabbits at oral doses up to 2 g/kg/day, 2.4 and 4.7 times the recommended human dose based on body surface area for the rat and rabbit, respectively, and revealed no evidence of impaired fertility or harm to the fetus due to balsalazide disodium. There are, however, no adequate and well-controlled studies in pregnant women. Because animal reproduction studies are not always predictive of human response, this drug should be used during pregnancy only if clearly needed.

NURSING MOTHERS

It is not known whether balsalazide disodium is excreted in human milk. Because many drugs are excreted in human milk, caution should be exercised when balsalazide disodium is administered to a nursing woman.

PEDIATRIC USE

Safety and effectiveness of balsalazide disodium in pediatric patients have not been established.

DRUG INTERACTIONS

No drug interaction studies have been conducted for balsalazide disodium, however, the use of orally administered antibiotics could, theoretically, interfere with the release of mesalamine in the colon.

ADVERSE REACTIONS

Over 1000 patients received treatment with balsalazide disodium in domestic and foreign clinical trials. In 4 controlled clinical trials patients receiving a balsalazide disodium dose of 6.75 g/day most frequently reported the following events (reporting frequency ≥3%), headache (8%), abdominal pain (6%), diarrhea (5%), nausea (5%), vomiting (4%), and respiratory infection (4%), arthralgia (4%). Withdrawal from therapy due to adverse events was comparable among patients on balsalazide disodium and placebo.

Adverse events reported by 1% or more of patients who participated in the 4 well-controlled, Phase 3 trials are presented by treatment group in TABLE 1.

TABLE 1 *Adverse Events Occurring in at Least 1% of Balsalazide Disodium and Ulcerative Colitis Patients in Controlled Trials*

Adverse Event	Balsalazide Disodium 6.75 g/day (n=259)	Placebo (n=35)
Headache	22 (8%)	3 (9%)
Abdominal pain	16 (6%)	1 (3%)
Nausea	14 (5%)	2 (6%)
Diarrhea	14 (5%)	1 (3%)
Vomiting	11 (4%)	2 (6%)
Respiratory infection	9 (4%)	5 (14%)
Arthralgia	9 (4%)	—
Rhinitis	6 (2%)	—
Insomnia	6 (2%)	—
Fatigue	6 (2%)	—
Rectal bleeding	5 (2%)	1 (3%)
Flatulence	5 (2%)	—
Fever	5 (2%)	—
Dyspepsia	5 (2%)	—
Pharyngitis	4 (2%)	—
Pain	4 (2%)	1 (3%)
Coughing	4 (2%)	—
Back pain	4 (2%)	1 (3%)
Anorexia	4 (2%)	—
Urinary tract infection	3 (1%)	—
Sinusitis	3 (1%)	1 (3%)
Myalgia	3 (1%)	—
Frequent stools	3 (1%)	1 (3%)
Flu-like disorder	3 (1%)	—
Dry mouth	3 (1%)	—
Dizziness	3 (1%)	2 (6%)
Cramps	3 (1%)	—
Constipation	3 (1%)	—

The number of placebo patients is too small for valid comparisons. Some adverse events, such as abdominal pain, fatigue, and nausea were reported more frequently in women subjects than in men. Abdominal pain, rectal bleeding, and anemia can be part of the clinical presentation of ulcerative colitis.

The following adverse events, presented by body system, have also been infrequently reported by patients taking balsalazide disodium during clinical trials (n=513) for the treatment of active acute ulcerative colitis or from foreign post-marketing reports. In most cases no relationship to balsalazide disodium has been established.

Body as a Whole: Abdomen enlarged, asthenia, chest pain, chills, edema, hot flushes, malaise.

Cardiovascular and Vascular: Bradycardia, deep venous thrombosis, hypertension, leg ulcer, palpitations, pericarditis.

Gastrointestinal: Amylase increased, bowel irregularity, ulcerative colitis aggravated, diarrhea with blood, diverticulosis, epigastric pain, eructation, fecal incontinence, feces abnormal, gastroenteritis, giardiasis, glossitis, hemorrhoids, melena, neoplasm benign, pancreatitis, ulcerative stomatitis, stools frequent, tenesmus, tongue discoloration.

Hematologic: Anemia, epistaxis, fibrinogen plasma increase, hemorrhage, prothrombin decrease, prothrombin increase, thrombocythemia.

Liver and Biliary: Bilirubin increase, hepatic function abnormal, SGOT increase, SGPT increase.

Lymphatic: Eosinophilia, granulocytopenia, leukocytosis, leukopenia, lymphadenopathy, lymphoma-like disorder, lymphopenia.

Metabolic and Nutritional: Creatinine phosphokinase increased, hypocalcemia, hypokalemia, hypoproteinemia, LDH increase, weight decrease, weight increase.

Musculoskeletal: Arthritis, arthropathy, stiffness in legs.

Nervous: Aphasia, dysphonia, gait abnormal, hypertonia, hypoesthesia, paresis, spasm generalized, tremor.

Psychiatric: Anxiety, depression, nervousness, somnolence.

Reproductive: Menstrual disorder.

Resistance Mechanism: Abscess, immunoglobulins decrease, infection, moniliasis, viral infection.

Respiratory: Bronchospasm, dyspnea, hemoptysis.

Skin: Alopecia, angioedema, dermatitis, dry skin, erythema nodosum, erythematous rash, pruritus, pruritus ani, psoriasis, skin ulceration.

Special Senses: Conjunctivitis, earache, ear infection, iritis, parosmia, taste perversion, tinnitus, vision abnormal.

Urinary: Hematuria, interstitial nephritis, micturition frequency, polyuria, pyuria.

POST-MARKETING REPORTS

The following events have been identified during post-approval use in clinical practice, of products which contain (or are metabolized to) mesalamine. Because they are reported voluntarily from a population of unknown size estimates of frequency cannot be made. These events have been chosen for inclusion due to a combination of seriousness, frequency of reporting, or potential causal connection to mesalamine.

Gastrointestinal: Reports of hepatotoxicity, including elevated liver function tests (SGOT/AST, SGPT/ALT, GGT, LDH, alkaline phosphatase, bilirubin), jaundice, cholestatic jaundice, cirrhosis, hepatocellular damage including liver necrosis and liver failure. Some of these cases were fatal, however, no fatalities associated with these events were reported in balsalazide disodium clinical trials. One case of Kawasaki-like syndrome which included hepatic function changes was also reported, however, this event was not reported in balsalazide disodium clinical trials.

DOSAGE AND ADMINISTRATION

For treatment of active ulcerative colitis the usual dose in adults is three 750 mg balsalazide disodium capsules to be taken 3 times a day for a total daily dose of 6.75 g for a duration of 8 weeks. Some patients in the clinical trials required treatment for up to 12 weeks.

HOW SUPPLIED

Colazal is available as beige capsules containing 750 mg balsalazide disodium and "CZ" imprinted in black.

Storage: Store at 25°C (77°F); excursions permitted to 15-30°C (59-86°F).

PRODUCT LISTING - EQUIVALENTS NOT AVAILABLE

Capsule - Oral - 750 mg

280's $296.80 COLAZAL, Salix Pharmaceuticals 65649-0101-02

Basiliximab *(003420)*

Categories: Rejection, renal transplant, prophylaxis; FDA Approved 1998 May; Pregnancy Category B; Orphan Drugs
Drug Classes: Immunosuppressives; Monoclonal antibodies
Brand Names: Simulect

WARNING

Only physicians experienced in immunosuppression therapy and management of organ transplantation patients should prescribe basiliximab. The physician responsible for basiliximab administration should have complete information requisite for the follow-up of the patient. Patients receiving the drug should be managed in facilities equipped and staffed with adequate laboratory and supportive medical resources.

DESCRIPTION

Simulect (basiliximab) is a chimeric (murine/human) monoclonal antibody (IgG_{1k}), produced by recombinant DNA technology, that functions as an immunosuppressive agent, specifically binding to and blocking the interleukin-2 receptor α-chain (IL-2Rα, also known as CD25 antigen) on the surface of activated T-lymphocytes. Based on the amino acid sequence, the calculated molecular weight of the protein is 144 kilodaltons. It is a glycoprotein obtained from fermentation of an established mouse myeloma cell line genetically engineered to express plasmids containing the human heavy and light chain constant region genes and mouse heavy and light chain variable region genes encoding the RFT5 antibody that binds selectively to the IL-2Rα.

The active ingredient, basiliximab, is water soluble. The drug product, Simulect, is a sterile lyophilisate which is available in 6 ml colorless glass vials. Each vial contains 20 mg basiliximab, 7.21 mg monobasic potassium phosphate, 0.99 mg disodium hydrogen phosphate (anhydrous), 1.61 mg sodium chloride, 20 mg sucrose, 80 mg mannitol and 40 mg glycine, to be reconstituted in 5 ml of sterile water for injection. No preservatives are added.
Storage: Store lyophilized Simulect under refrigerated conditions 2-8°C (36-46°F). Do not use beyond the expiration date stamped on the vial.

CLINICAL PHARMACOLOGY

GENERAL

Mechanism of Action

Basiliximab functions as an IL-2 receptor antagonist by binding with high affinity (Ka = 1×10^{10} M^{-1}) to the alpha chain of the high affinity IL-2 receptor complex and inhibiting IL-2 binding. Basiliximab is specifically targeted against IL-2Rα, which is selectively expressed on the surface of activated T-lymphocytes. This specific high affinity binding of basiliximab to IL-2Rα competitively inhibits IL-2-mediated activation of lymphocytes, a critical pathway in the cellular immune response involved in allograft rejection.

While in the circulation, basiliximab impairs the response of the immune system to antigenic challenges. Whether the ability to respond to repeated or ongoing challenges with those antigens returns to normal after basiliximab is cleared is unknown. (See PRECAUTIONS.)

PHARMACOKINETICS

Adults

Single-dose and multiple-dose pharmacokinetic studies have been conducted in patients undergoing first kidney transplantation. Cumulative doses ranged from 15 mg up to 150 mg. Peak mean ±SD serum concentration following intravenous infusion of 20 mg over 30 minutes is 7.1 ± 5.1 mg/L. There is a dose-proportional increase in C_{max} and AUC up to the highest tested single dose of 60 mg. The volume of distribution at steady-state is 8.6 ± 4.1 L. The extent and degree of distribution to various body compartments have not been fully studied. The terminal half-life is 7.2 ± 3.2 days. Total body clearance is 41 ± 19 ml/h. No clinically relevant influence of body weight or gender on distribution volume or clearance has been observed in adult patients. Elimination half-life was not influenced by age (20-69 years), gender or race. (See DOSAGE AND ADMINISTRATION.)

Pediatric

The pharmacokinetics of basiliximab were assessed in 12 pediatric renal transplantation patients, children (2-11 years of age, n=8) and adolescents (12-15 years of age, n=4). These data indicate that in children, the volume of distribution at steady-state was 5.2 ± 2.8 L, half-life was 11.5 ± 6.3 days and clearance was 17 ± 6 ml/h. Distribution volume and clearance are reduced by about 50% compared to adult renal transplantation patients. Disposition parameters were not influenced to a clinically relevant extent by age, body weight (9-37 kg) or body surface area (0.44-1.20 m^2) in this age group. In adolescents, the volume of distribution at steady-state was 10.1 ± 7.6 L, half-life was 7.2 ± 3.6 days and clearance was 45 ± 25 ml/h. Disposition in adolescents was similar to that in adult renal transplantation patients. (See DOSAGE AND ADMINISTRATION.)

PHARMACODYNAMICS

Complete and consistent binding to IL-2Rα in adults is maintained as long as serum basiliximab levels exceed 0.2 μg/ml. As concentrations fall below this threshold, the IL-2Rα sites are no longer fully bound and the number of T-cells expressing unbound IL-2Rα returns to pretherapy values within 1-2 weeks. The relationship between serum concentration and receptor saturation was assessed in 2 pediatric patients (2 and 12 years of age) and was similar to that characterized in adult renal transplantation patients. *In vitro* studies using human tissues indicate that basiliximab binds only to lymphocytes.

At the recommended dosing regimen, the mean ±SD duration of basiliximab saturation of IL-2Rα was 36 ± 14 days. (See DOSAGE AND ADMINISTRATION.) The duration of clinically significant IL-2 receptor blockade after the recommended course of basiliximab is not known. No significant changes to circulating lymphocyte numbers or cell phenotypes were observed by flow cytometry.

INDICATIONS AND USAGE

Basiliximab is indicated for the prophylaxis of acute organ rejection in patients receiving renal transplantation when used as part of an immunosuppressive regimen that includes cyclosporine and corticosteroids.

CONTRAINDICATIONS

Basiliximab is contraindicated in patients with known hypersensitivity to basiliximab or any other component of the formulation. See composition of basiliximab in DESCRIPTION.

WARNINGS

See BOXED WARNING.

GENERAL

Basiliximab should be administered under qualified medical supervision. Patients should be informed of the potential benefits of therapy and the risks associated with administration of immunosuppressive therapy.

While neither the incidence of lymphoproliferative disorders nor opportunistic infections was higher in basiliximab-treated patients than in placebo-treated patients, patients on immunosuppressive therapy are at increased risk for developing these complications and should be monitored accordingly.

HYPERSENSITIVITY

Severe acute (onset within 24 hours) hypersensitivity reactions including anaphylaxis have been observed both on initial exposure to basiliximab and/or following re-exposure after several months. These reactions may include hypotension, tachycardia, cardiac failure, dyspnea, wheezing, bronchospasm, pulmonary edema, respiratory failure, urticaria, rash, pruritus, and/or sneezing. If a severe hypersensitivity reaction occurs, therapy with basiliximab should be permanently discontinued. Medications for the treatment of severe hypersensitivity reactions including anaphylaxis should be available for immediate use. Patients previously administered basiliximab should only be re-exposed to a subsequent course of therapy with extreme caution. The potential risks of such readministration, specifically those associated with immunosuppression are not known.

PRECAUTIONS

GENERAL

It is not known whether basiliximab use will have a long-term effect on the ability of the immune system to respond to antigens first encountered during basiliximab-induced immunosuppression.

IMMUNOGENICITY

Of renal transplantation patients treated with basiliximab and tested for anti-idiotype antibodies, 1/246 developed an anti-idiotype antibody response, with no deleterious clinical effect upon the patient. In the US Study, the incidence of human antimurine antibody (HAMA) in renal transplantation patients treated with basiliximab was 2/138 in patients not exposed to muromonab-CD3 and 4/34 in patients who subsequently received muromonab-CD3. The available clinical data on the use of muromonab-CD3 in patients previously treated with basiliximab suggest that subsequent use of muromonab-CD3 or other murine antilymphocytic antibody preparations is not precluded.

CARCINOGENESIS, MUTAGENESIS, AND IMPAIRMENT OF FERTILITY

No mutagenic potential of basiliximab was observed in the *in vitro* assays with *Salmonella* (Ames) and V79 Chinese hamster cells. No long-term or fertility studies in laboratory animals have been performed to evaluate the potential of basiliximab to produce carcinogenicity or fertility impairment, respectively.

PREGNANCY CATEGORY B

There are no adequate and well-controlled studies in pregnant women. No maternal toxicity, embryotoxicity, or teratogenicity was observed in cynomolgus monkeys 100 days post-coitum following dosing with basiliximab during the organogenesis period; blood levels in pregnant monkeys were 13-fold higher than those seen in human patients. Immunotoxicology studies have not been performed in the offspring. Because IgG molecules are known to cross the placental barrier, because the IL-2 receptor may play an important role in development of the immune system, and because animal reproduction studies are not always predictive of human response, basiliximab should only be used in pregnant women when the potential benefit justifies the potential risk to the fetus. Women of childbearing potential should use effective contraception before beginning basiliximab therapy, during therapy, and for 2 months after completion of basiliximab therapy.

NURSING MOTHERS

It is not known whether basiliximab is excreted in human milk. Because many drugs including human antibodies are excreted in human milk, and because of the potential for adverse reactions, a decision should be made to discontinue nursing or to discontinue the drug, taking into account the importance of the drug to the mother.

PEDIATRIC USE

No adequate and well-controlled studies have been completed in pediatric patients. In an ongoing safety and pharmacokinetic study, pediatric patients [2-11 years of age (n=8), 12-15 years of age (n=4), median age 9.5 years] were treated with basiliximab via intravenous bolus injection in addition to standard immunosuppressive agents including cyclosporine, corticosteroids, azathioprine, and mycophenolate mofetil. Preliminary results indicate that 16.7% (2/12) of patients had experienced an acute rejection episode by 3 months post-transplantation. The most frequently reported adverse events were fever and urinary tract infections (41.7% each). Overall, the adverse event profile was consistent with general clinical experience in the pediatric renal transplantation population and with the profile in the controlled adult renal transplantation studies. The available pharmacokinetic data in children and adolescents are described in CLINICAL PHARMACOLOGY and DOSAGE AND ADMINISTRATION.

It is not known whether the immune response to vaccines, infection, and other antigenic stimuli administered or encountered during basiliximab therapy is impaired or whether such response will remain impaired after basiliximab therapy.

GERIATRIC USE

Controlled clinical studies of basiliximab have included a small number of patients 65 years and older (basiliximab 15; placebo 19). From the available data comparing basiliximab- and placebo-treated patients, the adverse event profile in patients ≥65 years of age is not different from patients <65 years of age and no age-related dosing adjustment is required. Caution must be used in giving immunosuppressive drugs to elderly patients.

DRUG INTERACTIONS

No formal drug-drug interaction studies have been conducted. The following medications have been administered in clinical trials with basiliximab with no incremental increase in adverse reactions: ATG/ALG, azathioprine, corticosteroids, cyclosporine, mycophenolate mofetil, and muromonab-CD3.

ADVERSE REACTIONS

The incidence of adverse events for basiliximab was determined in 2 randomized comparative double-blind trials for the prevention of renal allograft rejection. A total of 721 patients received renal allografts, of which 363 received basiliximab and 358 received placebo. All patients received concomitant cyclosporine oral solution and corticosteroids.

Basiliximab did not appear to add to the background of adverse events seen in organ transplantation patients as a consequence of their underlying disease and the concurrent administration of immunosuppressants and other medications. Adverse events were reported by 99% of the patients in the placebo-treated group and 99% of the patients in the basiliximab-treated group. Basiliximab did not increase the incidence of serious adverse events observed compared with placebo. The most frequently reported adverse events were gastrointestinal disorders, reported in 75% of basiliximab-treated patients and 73% of placebo-treated patients.

The incidence and types of adverse events were similar in basiliximab-treated and placebo-treated patients.

The following adverse events occurred in ≥10% of basiliximab-treated patients:

Gastrointestinal System: Constipation, nausea, diarrhea, abdominal pain, vomiting, dyspepsia, moniliasis.

Metabolic and Nutritional: Hyperkalemia, hypokalemia, hyperglycemia, hyperuricemia, hypophosphatemia, hypocalcemia, weight increase, hypercholesterolemia, acidosis.

Central and Peripheral Nervous System: Headache, tremor, dizziness.

Urinary System: Dysuria, increased nonprotein nitrogen, urinary tract infection.

Body as a Whole-General: Pain, peripheral edema, edema, fever, viral infection, leg edema, asthenia.

Cardiovascular Disorders-General: Hypertension.

Respiratory System: Dyspnea, upper respiratory tract infection, coughing, rhinitis, pharyngitis.

Skin and Appendages: Surgical wound complications, acne.

Psychiatric: Insomnia.

Musculoskeletal System: Leg pain, back pain.

Red Blood Cell: Anemia.

The following adverse events, not mentioned above, were reported with an incidence of ≥3% and <10% in patients treated with basiliximab in the two controlled clinical trials:

Body as a Whole: Accidental trauma, chest pain, increased drug level, face edema, fatigue, infection, malaise, generalized edema, rigors, sepsis.

Cardiovascular: Angina pectoris, cardiac failure, chest pain, abnormal heart sounds, aggravated hypertension, hypotension.

Nervous System: Hypoesthesia, neuropathy, paraesthesia.

Endocrine: Increased glucocorticoids.

Gastrointestinal: Enlarged abdomen, flatulence, gastrointestinal disorder, gastroenteritis, GI hemorrhage, gum hyperplasia, melena, esophagitis, ulcerative stomatitis.

Heart Rate and Rhythm: Arrhythmia, atrial fibrillation, tachycardia.

Metabolic and Nutritional: Dehydration, diabetes mellitus, fluid overload, hypercalcemia, hyperlipemia, hypoglycemia, hypoproteinemia, hypomagnesemia.

Musculoskeletal: Arthralgia, arthropathy, bone fracture, cramps, hernia, myalgia.

Nervous System: Paraesthesia, hypoesthesia.

Platelet and Bleeding: Hematoma, hemorrhage, purpura, thrombocytopenia, thrombosis.

Psychiatric: Agitation, anxiety, depression.

Red Blood Cell: Polycythemia.

Reproductive Disorders, Male: Impotence, genital edema.

Respiratory: Bronchitis, bronchospasm, abnormal chest sounds, pneumonia, pulmonary disorder, pulmonary edema, sinusitis.

Skin and Appendages: Cyst, herpes simplex, herpes zoster, hypertrichosis, pruritus, rash, skin disorder, skin ulceration.

Urinary: Albuminuria, bladder disorder, hematuria, frequent micturition, oliguria, abnormal renal function, renal tubular necrosis, surgery, ureteral disorder, urinary retention.

Vascular Disorders: Vascular disorder.

Vision Disorders: Cataract, conjunctivitis, abnormal vision.

INCIDENCE OF MALIGNANCIES

The overall incidence of malignancies among all patients in the two 12 month controlled trials was not significantly different between the basiliximab and placebo treatment groups. Overall, lymphoma/lymphoproliferative disease occurred in 1 patient (0.3%) in the basiliximab group compared with 2 patients (0.6%) in the placebo group. Other malignancies were reported among 5 patients (1.4%) in the basiliximab group compared with 7 patients (1.9%) in patients treated with placebo.

INCIDENCE OF INFECTIOUS EPISODES

Cytomegalovirus infection was reported in 14% of basiliximab-treated patients and 18% of placebo-treated patients. The rates of infections, serious infections, and infectious organisms were similar in the basiliximab and placebo treatment groups.

POSTMARKETING EXPERIENCE

Severe acute hypersensitivity reactions including anaphylaxis characterized by hypotension, tachycardia, cardiac failure, dyspnea, wheezing, bronchospasm, pulmonary edema, respiratory failure, urticaria, rash, pruritus, and/or sneezing, as well as capillary leak syndrome and cytokine release syndrome, have been reported during postmarketing experience with basiliximab.

DOSAGE AND ADMINISTRATION

Basiliximab is used as part of an immunosuppressive regimen that includes cyclosporine and corticosteroids. Basiliximab is for central or peripheral intravenous administration only. Reconstituted basiliximab (20 mg in 5 ml) should be diluted to a volume of 50 ml with normal saline or dextrose 5% and administered as an intravenous infusion over 20-30 minutes.

Basiliximab should only be administered once it has been determined that the patient will receive the graft and concomitant immunosuppression. Patients previously administered basiliximab should only be re-exposed to a subsequent course of therapy with extreme caution.

ADULTS

In adult patients, the recommended regimen is 2 doses of 20 mg each. The first 20 mg dose should be given within 2 hours prior to transplantation surgery. The recommended second 20 mg dose should be given 4 days after transplantation. The second dose should be withheld if complications such as severe hypersensitivity reactions to basiliximab or graft loss occur.

PEDIATRIC

For children and adolescents from 2 up to 15 years of age, the recommended regimen is 2 doses of 12 mg/m^2 each, up to a maximum of 20 mg/dose. The first dose should be given within 2 hours prior to transplantation surgery. The recommended second dose should be given 4 days after transplantation. The second dose should be withheld if complications such as severe hypersensitivity reactions to basiliximab or graft loss occur.

PRODUCT LISTING - EQUIVALENTS NOT AVAILABLE

Powder For Injection - Intravenous - 20 mg

1's $1619.39 SIMULECT, Novartis Pharmaceuticals 00078-0331-84

BCG Live *(003043)*

For complete prescribing information, refer to the CD-ROM included with the book.

Categories: Carcinoma, bladder; Pregnancy Category C; FDA Approved 1991 Dec
Drug Classes: Antineoplastics, biological response modifiers
Brand Names: Theracys
Foreign Brand Availability: Immucyst (Colombia; England; Ireland); PACIS (Canada)
HCFA JCODE(S): J9031 per vial IV

DESCRIPTION

FOR TREATMENT OF CARCINOMA IN-SITU OF THE URINARY BLADDER

BCG Live (Intravesical), TheraCys, is a freeze-dried suspension of an attenuated strain of *Mycobacterium bovis* (Bacillus Calmette and Guerin), which has been grown on Sauton medium (potato and glycerin based medium), used in the non-specific active therapy of carcinoma *in-situ* of the urinary bladder. CAUTION: BCG live is NOT intended to be used as an immunizing agent for the prevention of tuberculosis. BCG live is NOT a vaccine for the prevention of cancer.

TheraCys is formulated to contain 27 mg (dry weight/vial Bacillus of Calmette and Guerin (BCG) and 5% w/v monosodium glutamate. This product contains no preservative. Each vial of TheraCys is ready for use following reconstitution with the accompanying diluent (1.0 ml), which consists of approximately 0.85% sodium chloride, 0.025% Tween 80, 0.06% w/v sodium dihydrogen phosphate and 0.25% disodium hydrogen phosphate. The diluent contains no preservative. One dose consists of three pooled vials of reconstituted material further diluted in sterile, preservative-free saline. The reconstituted product contains $3.4 \pm 3.0 \times 10^8$ colony forming units (CFU) per vial when resuspended in the diluent provided.

To ensure viability of the product through to its labeled expiration date, it is very important that BCG live and diluent be stored continuously between 2 and 8°C (35 and 46°F) until use (see Storage below). It should be used immediately after reconstitution.

STORAGE

BCG live and the accompanying diluent should be kept in a refrigerator at a temperature between 2 and 8°C (35 and 46°F). It should not be used after the expiration date marked on the vial, otherwise it may be inactive. The product should be used immediately after reconstitution; however, it must not be used after 2 hours. Any reconstituted product which exhibits flocculation or clumping that cannot be dispersed with gentle shaking should not be used.

At no time should be freeze-fired or reconstituted BCG live be exposed to sunlight, direct or indirect. Exposure to artificial light should be kept to a minimum.[9]

INDICATIONS AND USAGE

BCG live is indicated for intravesical use in the treatment of primary and relapsed carcinoma *in-situ* of the urinary bladder to eliminate residual tumor cells and to reduce the frequency of tumor recurrence. It is indicated for the treatment of carcinoma *in-situ* with or without associated papillary tumors. BCG live is also indicated for the treatment of papillary tumors occurring alone. BCG live is also indicated as a therapy for patients with carcinoma *in-situ* of the bladder following failure to respond to other treatment regimens. CAUTION: BCG live is NOT a vaccine for the prevention of tuberculosis. BCG live is NOT a vaccine for the prevention of cancer.

CONTRAINDICATIONS

Patients on immunosuppressive therapy or with compromised immune systems should not be receive BCG live due to the risk of overwhelming systemic mycobacterial sepsis.

BCG live should not be administered to patients with fever unless the caused of the fever is determined and evaluated. If the fever is due to an infection, BCG live should be withheld until the patients is afebrile and off all therapy.

Patients with urinary tract infection should not receive BCG live treatment because administration may result in the risk of disseminated BCG infection or in an increased severity of bladder irritation.

BCG live should NOT be administered as an immunizing agent for the prevention of tuberculosis. BCG live is NOT a vaccine for the prevention of cancer.

WARNINGS

BCG live should NOT be administered as an immunizing agent for the prevention of tuberculosis. BCG live is NOT vaccine for the prevention of cancer.

Since administration of intravesical BCG live causes in inflammatory response in the bladder and has been associated with hematuria, urinary frequency, dysuria and bacterial urinary tract infection, careful monitoring of urinary status is required. If there is an increase in the patient's existing symptoms, or if their symptoms persist or if any of these symptoms develop, the patient should be evaluated and managed for urinary tract infection or BCG toxicity.

Since death has occurred due to systemic BCG infection, patients should be closely monitored for symptoms of such an infection. BCG therapy should be withheld upon any suspicion of systemic infection (*e.g.*, granulomatous hepatitis.

Drug combinations containing bone marrow depressants and/or immunosuppressants and/or radiation may impair the response to BCG live or increase the risk of osteomyelitis or disseminated BCG infection.

Patients undergoing antimicrobial therapy for other infections should be evaluated to assess whether the therapy will obviate the effects of BCG live actions.

For patients with small bladder capacity, increased risk of severity of local irritation should be considered in decisions to treat with BCG live.

Intravesical treatment with BCG live may induce a sensitivity to tuberculin which could complicate further interpretations of skin test reactions to tuberculin in the diagnosis of suspected mycobacterial infections. Determination of patient's reactivity to tuberculin prior to administration of BCG live may be desirable in this regard.

In a controlled multi-center clinical trial comparing BCG therapy and doxorubicin HCl for the intravesical treatment of superficial transitional cell carcinoma with and without carcinoma *in-situ* of the bladder, 112 patients received BCG.[4]

In another controlled study using BCG live for the treatment of superficial transitional cell carcinoma, with or without carcinoma *in-situ*, of the bladder, similar adverse reactions were observed.[13] However, 2 deaths were noted in this study which may have been associated with traumatic catheterization.

The incidence of adverse reactions associated with intravesical BCG live therapy is given below. Most local adverse reactions occur following the third intravesical instillation. Symptoms usually begin 2-4 hours after instillation and persist for 24-72 hours. Systemic reactions usually last for 1-3 days after each intravesical instillation.[4,13,14]

TABLE 4 *Local Reactions (n=112)*

Reaction	Total	Severe*
Dysuria	51.8%	3.6%
Frequency	40.2%	1.8%
Hematuria	39.3%	17.0%
Cystitis	29.5%	0.0%
Urgency	17.9%	0.0%
Urinary tract infection	17.9%	1.0%
Urinary incontinence	6.3%	0.0%
Cramps/Pain	6.3%	0.0%
Decreased bladder capacity	5.4%	0.0%
Tissue in urine	0.9%	0.0%
Local infection	0.9%	0.0%

* Severe is defined as grade 3 (severe) or grade 4 (life threatening).

TABLE 5 *Systemic Reactions (n=112)*

Reaction	Total	Severe*
Malaise	40.2%	2.0%
Fever (>30°C)	38.4%	2.6%
Chills	39.9%	2.6%
Anemia	20.5%	0.0%
Nausea/vomiting	16.1%	0.0%
Anorexia	10.7%	0.0%
Myalgia/arthralgia/arthritis	7.1%	1.0%
Diarrhea	6.3%	0.0%
Mild liver involvement	2.7%	0.0%
Mild abdominal pain	2.7%	0.0%
Systemic infection†	2.7%	2.0%
Pulmonary infection†	2.7%	0.0%
Cardiac	2.7%	0.0%
Headache	1.8%	0.0%
Hypersensitivity skin rash	1.8%	0.0%
Constipation	0.9%	0.0%
Dizziness	0.9%	0.0%
Fatigue	0.9%	0.0%
Leukopenia	5.4%	0.0%
Disseminated intravascular coagulation	2.7%	0.0%
Thrombocytopenia	0.9%	0.0%
Renal toxicity	9.8%	2.0%
Genital pain	9.8%	0.0%
Flank pain	0.9%	0.0%

* Severe is defined as grade 3 (severe) or grade 4 (life threatening).
† Includes both BCG and other infections.

No fatalities associated with the use of BCG live were reported in this study. Two fatalities have been reported with the use of BCG live in another study after traumatic catheterization or in the presence of urinary infection.[13]

An increased risk of additional primary malignancies has been reported following radiotherapy and chemotherapy for many types of malignancies. No increase in second primary malignancies after treatment with BCG live was reported in these studies.[4]

Irritative bladder symptoms associated with BCG live administration can be managed symptomatically with phenazopyridine HCl, propantheline bromide, and acetaminophen.[4]

DOSAGE AND ADMINISTRATION

Intravesical treatment and prophylaxis for carcinoma *in-situ* of the urinary bladder should begin between 7-14 days after biopsy or transurethral resection if this procedure is done. A dose of three trials of BCG live is given intravesically under aseptic conditions once weekly for 6 weeks (induction therapy). Each dose (3 reconstituted vials) is further diluted in an additional 50 ml sterile, preservative-free saline for a total of 53 ml. A urethral catheter is inserted into the bladder under aseptic conditions, the bladder drained and then the 53 ml suspension of BCG live is instilled slowly by gravity following which the catheter is withdrawn. During the first hour following instillation, the patient should lie for 15 minutes each in the prone and supine positions and also on each side. The patient is then allowed to be up but retains the suspension for another 60 minutes for a total of 2 hours. All patients may not be able to retain the suspension for the 2 hours and should be instructed to void in less time if necessary. At the end of 2 hours all patients should void in a seated position for safety reasons. Patients should be instructed to maintain adequate hydration.

If the physician believes that the bladder catheterization has been traumatic (*e.g.*, associated with bleeding or possible false passage), then BCG live should not be administered and there must be a treatment delay of at least 1 week. Subsequent treatment should be resumed as if no interruption in the schedule had occurred. That is, all doses of BCG live should be administered even after a temporary halt in administration.

The indication therapy should be followed by one treatment given 3, 6, 12, 18 and 24 months following the initial treatment.

After use, all equipment, materials and containers that may have come in contact with BCG live should be sterilized or disponed of properly as with any other biohazardous waste.

BCG Vaccine *(000375)*

For complete prescribing information, refer to the CD-ROM included with the book.

Categories: Carcinoma, bladder; Immunization, tuberculosis; Pregnancy Category C; FDA Pre 1938 Drugs; WHO Formulary
Drug Classes: Antineoplastics, biological response modifiers; Vaccines
Brand Names: Mycobax; Theracys; **Tice BCG**
Foreign Brand Availability: Immucyst (Australia; Canada; New-Zealand); Immun BCG Pasteur (Germany); OncoTice (Australia; New-Zealand); Oncotice (Austria; Denmark; Finland; Germany; Greece; Netherlands); OncoTICE (Canada; Sweden); Pastimmun (Belgium)

DESCRIPTION

FOR INTRAVESICAL OR PERCUTANEOUS

Tice BCG, a BCG Vaccine for intravesical or percutaneous use, is attenuated, live culture preparation of the Bacillus of Calmette and Guerin (BCG) strain of *Mycobacterium bovis*.[1] The Tice strain was developed at the University of Illinois from a strain originated at the Pasteur Institute.

The medium in which the BCG organism is grown for preparation of the freeze-dried cake is composed of the following ingredients: glycerin, asparagine, citric acid, potassium phosphate, magnesium sulfate, and iron ammonium citrate. The final preparation prior to freeze-drying also contains lactose. The freeze-dried BCG preparation is delivered in a glass-sealed ampules, each containing 1 to 8 $\times$ 10^8 colony forming units (CFU) of Tice BCG which is equivalent to approximately 50 mg net weight.

No preservatives are added.

Storage: Storage of the intact ampules of BCG vaccine should be at refrigerated temperatures of 2-8°C (36-46°F). This agent contains live bacteria and should be protect from light. The product should not be used after the expiration date printed on the label.

INDICATIONS AND USAGE

INTRAVESICAL USE FOR CARCINOMA IN SITU OF THE BLADDER

Intravesical instillation of BCG vaccine is indicated for the treatment of carcinoma *in situ* of the bladder in the following situations: (1) primary treatment in the absence of an associated invasive cancer without papillary tumors or with papillary tumors after TUR, (2) secondary treatment in the absence of an associated invasive cancer, in patients failing to respond to relapsing after intravesical chemotherapy with other agents, (3) primary or secondary treatment in the absence of invasive cancer for patients with medical contraindications to radical surgery. BCG vaccine is not indicated for the treatment of papillary tumors occurring alone.

Percutaneous Use for Immunization Against Tuberculosis: *Exposed tuberculin skin test-negative infants and children:* BCG vaccination is recommended for infants and children with negative skin test who are (1) at high risk of intimate and prolonged exposure to persistently untreated or ineffectively treated patients who cannot be removed from the source of exposure and cannot be placed on long-term preventative therapy, or (2) continuously exposed to persons with tuberculosis who have bacilli resistant to isoniazid and rifampin.[22]

Groups With An Excessive Rate Of New Infections: BCG vaccination is also recommended for tuberculin-negative infants and children in groups in which the rate of new infections exceeds 1% per year and for whom the usual surveillance and treatment programs have been attempted but are not operationally feasible. These groups include persons without regular access to health care, those for whom usual health care is culturally or socially unacceptable, or groups who have demonstrated an inability to effectively use existing accessible care.

The US Immunization Practices Advisory Committee (IPAC) no longer recommends the use of BCG vaccination of health care workers at risk of repeated exposure to tuberculosis but recommends that these individuals be under tuberculin skin testing surveillance and receive isoniazid prophylaxis in case of tuberculin skin test conversion.[22]

For international travelers, the Center for Disease Control (CDC) recommends that BCG vaccination be considered only for travelers with insignificant reaction to tuberculin skin test who will be in a high-risk environment for prolonged periods of time without access to tuberculin skin test surveillance.[22]

CONTRAINDICATIONS

INTRAVESICAL USE FOR CARCINOMA IN SITU OF THE BLADDER

BCG vaccine should not be used in immunosuppressed patients or persons with congenital or acquired immune deficiencies, whether due to concurrent disease (*e.g.*, AIDS, leukemia, lymphoma) or cancer therapy (*e.g.*, cytotoxic drugs, radiation). BCG vaccine should be avoided in asymptomatic carriers with a positive HIV serology and in patients receiving steroids at immunosuppressive therapies because of the possibility of the vaccine establishing a systemic infection.

Treatment should be postponed until a resolution of a concurrent febrile illness, urinary tract infection, or gross hematuria. Seven (7) to 14 days should elapse before BCG is administered following biopsy, TUR, or traumatic catheterization.

A positive Mantoux test is a contraindication only if there is evidence of an active tuberculosis infection.

In the absence of safety data, intravesical BCG vaccine should not be given to pregnant or lactating women.

PERCUTANEOUS USE FOR IMMUNIZATION AGAINST TUBERCULOSIS

BCG vaccine for the prevention of tuberculosis should not be given to persons with impaired immune responses, whether they be congenital, disease produced, drug or therapy induced (*i.e.,* cytotoxic drugs and radiation used in cancer therapy). The concurrent use of steroids requires caution because of the possibility of the vaccine establishing a systemic infection. If necessary, the infection can be treated with anti-tuberculous drugs.

WARNINGS

Intravesical Use for Carcinoma *In Situ* of the Bladder: BCG vaccine is not a vaccine for the prevention of cancer.

There are currently no data on the effectiveness of intravesical instillation of BCG vaccine in the treatment of invasive bladder cancer.

The use of BCG vaccine may cause tuberculin sensitivity. Since this is a valuable aid for the diagnosis of tuberculosis, it may therefore be useful to determine the tuberculin reactivity by PPD skin testing before treatment.

Intravesical instillations should be postponed in the presence of fever, suspected infection, or during treatment with antibiotics, since antimicrobial therapy may interfere with the effectiveness of BCG vaccine.

Instillation of BCG vaccine onto a bleeding mucosa may promote systemic BCG infection.[23] Death has been reported as a result of systemic BCG infection and sepsis. Patients should be monitored for the presence of symptoms and signs of toxicity after each intravesical treatment. Febrile episodes with flu-like symptoms lasting more than 48 hours, fever ≥103°F, systemic manifestations increasing in intensity with repeated instillations, or persistent abnormalities of liver function tests suggest systemic BCG infection and require anti-tuberculous therapy.

Small bladder capacity has been associated with increased risk of severe local reactions and should be considered in deciding to use BCG vaccine therapy.

PERCUTANEOUS USE FOR IMMUNIZATION AGAINST TUBERCULOSIS

Administration should be percutaneous with the multiple puncture disc as described below. DO NOT INJECT INTRAVENOUSLY, SUBCUTANEOUSLY, OR INTRADERMALLY. BCG vaccine Vaccine should not be used in infants, children, or adults with severe immune deficiency syndromes. Children with family history of immune deficiency disease should not be vaccinated. If they are, an infectious disease specialist should be consulted and anti-tuberculous therapy[24] administered if clinically indicated.

DOSAGE AND ADMINISTRATION

INTRAVESICAL USE FOR CARCINOMA IN SITU OF THE BLADDER

The intravesical dose consists of one ampule of BCG vaccine suspended in 50 ml preservative-free saline. *Preparation of Agent:* The preparation of the BCG vaccine suspension should be done using sterile technique. The pharmacist or individual responsible for mixing the agent should wear gloves, mask, and gown to avoid inadvertent exposure of open sores or inhalation of BCG organisms. Draw 1 ml of sterile, preservative-free saline (0.9% sodium chloride injection) at 4-25°C, into a small (*e.g.,* 3 ml) syringe and add to one ampule of BCG vaccine to resuspend. Draw the mixture into the syringe and gently expel back into the ampule 3times to ensure thorough mixing. This mixing minimizes the clumping of the mycobacteria. Dispense the cloudy BCG suspension into the top end of a catheter-tip syringe which contains 49 ml saline diluent bringing the total volume to 50 ml. Gently rotate the syringe. The suspended BCG vaccine should be used immediately after preparation. Discard after 2 hours.

Note: DO NOT filter the contents of the BCG vaccine ampule. Precautions should be taken to avoid exposing the BCG vaccine to light. Bacteriostatic solutions must be avoided. In addition, use only sterile preservative-free saline, 0.9% sodium chloride injection, as diluent and perform all mixing operations in sterile glass or thermosetting plastic containers and syringes.

Treatment and Schedule

Allow 7-14 days to elapse after bladder biopsy or TUR before BCG vaccine is administered. Patients should not drink fluids for 4 hours before treatment and should empty their bladder prior to Tice BC administration. The reconstituted BCG vaccine is instilled into the bladder by gravity flow via the catheter. DO NOT depress the plunger and force the flow of the BCG vaccine. The BCG vaccine is retained in the bladder for 2 hours and then voided. Patients unable to retain the suspension for 2 hours should be allowed to void sooner, if necessary. While the BCG vaccine is retained in the bladder, the patient may be repositioned from left side to right side and also may alternately lie upon the back and the abdomen, changing these positions every 15 minutes to maximize bladder surface exposure to the agent.

A standard treatment schedule consists of one intravesical instillation per week for 6 weeks. This schedule may be repeated once if tumor remission has not been achieved and if the clinical circumstances warrant. Thereafter, intravesical BCG vaccine administration should continue at approximately monthly intervals for at least 6-12 months.

PERCUTANEOUS USE FOR IMMUNIZATION AGAINST TUBERCULOSIS

Preparation of Agent: Using sterile methods, 1 ml of sterile water for injection at 4-25°C, is added to one ampule of vaccine. Draw the mixture into a syringe and expel it back into the ampule 3 times to ensure thorough mixing.

Parenteral drug products should be inspected visually for particulate matter and discoloration prior to administration, whenever solution and container permit. Reconstitution should result in a uniform suspension of the bacilli.

Treatment and Schedule

The vaccine is to be administered after fully explaining the risks and benefits to the vaccinee, parent, or guardian. After the vaccine is prepared, the immunizing dose of 0.2-0.3 ml is dropped on the cleansed surface of the skin, and the vaccine is administered percutaneously utilizing a sterile multiple-puncture disc. The multiple-puncture disc is a thin wafer-like stainless steel plate 7/8″ × 1 1/8″, from which 36 points protrude. The disc is held by a magnet type holder. In this method a drop of vaccine is placed on the arm and spread with the wide edge of disc. The disc is placed gently over the vaccine and the magnet is centered. The arm is grasped firmly from underneath, tensing the skin appreciably. Downward pressure is applied on the magnet so the points of the disc are well buried in skin. With pressure still exerted, the disc is rocked forward and backward and from side to side several times. Pressure underneath the arm is then released and the magnet is slid off the disc. In a successful procedure, the points remain in the skin. If the points are on top of the skin, the procedure must be repeated. Remove the disc after successful puncture and spread vaccine evenly over the puncture area with the wide edge of the disc. Discs should only be used once and discarded after autoclaving. Between individual vaccinations the magnet should be sterilized. Discs may be purchased separately from Organon Teknika Corporation, 115 South Sangamon Street, Chicago, IL 60607; telephone number 800-662-6842. After vaccination the vaccine should flow into the wounds and dry. No dressing is required; however it is recommended that the site be kept dry for 24 hours. The patient should be advised that the vaccine contains live organisms. Although the vaccine will not survive in a dry state, infection of others is possible.

Reconstituted vaccine should be kept refrigerated, protected from exposure to light, and used within 2 hours. Vaccination should be repeated for those who remain tuberculin negative to 5TU of tuberculin after 2-3 months.

Pediatric Dose

In infants less than 1 month old the dosage of vaccine should be reduced by one-half, by using 2 ml of sterile water when reconstituting. If a vaccinated infant remains tuberculin negative to 5TU on skin testing, and if indications for vaccination persist, the infant should receive a full dose after 1 year of age.

PRODUCT LISTING - EQUIVALENTS NOT AVAILABLE

Powder For Injection - Intradermal - Vaccine 50 mg
1's $1475.00 TICE BCG VACCINE, Organon 00052-0601-01

Powder For Injection - Intravesical - 50 mg
1's $183.82 TICE BCG VACCINE, Organon 00052-0602-02

Powder For Injection - Intravesical - 81 mg
1's $175.55 THERACYS INTRAVESICAL, Aventis Pharmaceuticals 49281-0880-01

Becaplermin *(003381)*

Categories: Ulcers, diabetic; FDA Approved 1998 Jan; Pregnancy Category C
Drug Classes: Dermatologics
Brand Names: Regranex
Cost of Therapy: $533.15 (Diabetic Ulcers; Regranex Gel; 0.01%; 15 g; 1 application/day; 15 day supply)

DESCRIPTION

Regranex gel contains becaplermin, a recombinant human platelet-derived growth factor (rhPDGF-BB) for topical administration. Becaplermin is produced by recombinant DNA technology by insertion of the gene for the B chain of platelet-derived growth factor (PDGF) into the yeast, *Saccharomyces cerevisiae.* Becaplermin has a molecular weight of approximately 25 KD and is a homodimer composed of two identical polypeptide chains that are bound together by disulfide bonds. Regranex Gel is a non-sterile, low bioburden, preserved, sodium carboxymethylcellulose-based (CMC) topical gel, containing the active ingredient becaplermin and the following inactive ingredients: sodium chloride, sodium acetate trihydrate, glacial acetic acid, water for injection, and methylparaben, propylparaben, and m-cresol as preservatives and I-lysine hydrochloride as a stabilizer. Each gram of Regranex Gel contains 100 μg of becaplermin.

CLINICAL PHARMACOLOGY

Becaplermin has biological activity similar to that of endogenous platelet-derived growth factor, which includes promoting the chemotactic recruitment and proliferation of cells involved in wound repair and enhancing the formation of granulation tissue.

PHARMACOKINETICS

Ten (10) patients with Stage III or IV (as defined in the International Association of Enterostomal Therapy (IAET) guide to chronic wound staging, *J. Enterostomal Ther* 15:4, 1988 and *Decubitis* 2:24, 1989) lower extremity diabetic ulcers received topical applications of becaplermin gel 0.01% at a dose range of 0.32-2.95 μg/kg (7 μg/cm^2) daily for 14 days. Six (6) patients had non-quantifiable PDGF levels at baseline and throughout the study, 2 patients had PDGF levels at baseline which did not increase substantially, and 2 patients had PDGF levels that increased sporadically above their baseline values during the 14 day study period.

Systemic bioavailability of becaplermin was less than 3% in rats with full thickness wounds receiving single or multiple (5 days) topical applications of 127 μg/kg (20.1 μg/cm^2 of wound area) of becaplermin gel.

INDICATIONS AND USAGE

Becaplermin is indicated for the treatment of lower extremity diabetic neuropathic ulcers that extend into the subcutaneous tissue or beyond and have an adequate blood supply. When used as an adjunct to, and not a substitute for, good ulcer care practices including initial sharp debridement, pressure relief and infection control, becaplermin increases the incidence of complete healing of diabetic ulcers.

The efficacy of becaplermin for the treatment of diabetic neuropathic ulcers that do not extend through the dermis into subcutaneous tissue (Stage I or II, IAET staging classification) or ischemic diabetic ulcers has not been evaluated.

B

CONTRAINDICATIONS

Becaplermin is contraindicated in patients with:

- Known hypersensitivity to any component of this product (*e.g.*, parabens).
- Known neoplasm(s) at the site(s) of application.

WARNINGS

Becaplermin gel is a non-sterile, low bioburden preserved product. Therefore, it should not be used in wounds that close by primary intention.

PRECAUTIONS

For external use only.

If application site reactions occur, the possibility of sensitization or irritation caused by parabens or m-cresol should be considered.

The effects of becaplermin on exposed joints, tendons, ligaments, and bone have not been established in humans. In pre-clinical studies, rats injected at the metatarsals with 3 or 10 μg/site (approximately 60 or 200 μg/kg) of becaplermin every other day for 13 days displayed histological changes indicative of accelerated bone remodeling consisting of periosteal hyperplasia and subperiosteal bone resorption and exostosis. The soft tissue adjacent to the injection site had fibroplasia with accompanying mononuclear cell infiltration reflective of the ability of PDGF to stimulate connective tissue growth.

Information for the Patient:

Patients should be advised that:

- Hands should be washed thoroughly before applying becaplermin.
- The tip of the tube should not come into contact with the ulcer or any other surface; the tube should be recapped tightly after each use.
- A cotton swab, tongue depressor, or other application aid should be used to apply becaplermin.
- Becaplermin should only be applied once a day in a carefully measured quantity (see DOSAGE AND ADMINISTRATION). The measured quantity of gel should be spread evenly over the ulcerated area to yield a thin continuous layer of approximately 1/16 of an inch thickness. The measured length of the gel to be squeezed from the tube should be adjusted according to the size of the ulcer. The amount of becaplermin to be applied daily should be recalculated at weekly or biweekly intervals by the physician or wound care giver.
- After approximately 12 hours, the ulcer should be gently rinsed with saline or water to remove residual gel and covered with a saline-moistened gauze dressing (without becaplermin).
- It is important to use becaplermin together with a good ulcer care program, including a strict non-weight-bearing program.
- Excess application of becaplermin has not been shown to be beneficial.
- Becaplermin should be stored in the refrigerator. Do not freeze becaplermin.
- Becaplermin should not be used after the expiration date on the bottom, crimped end of the tube.

CARCINOGENESIS, MUTAGENESIS, AND IMPAIRMENT OF FERTILITY

Becaplermin was not genotoxic in a battery of *in vitro* assays, (including those for bacterial and mammalian cell point mutation, chromosomal aberration, and DNA damage/repair). Becaplermin was also not mutagenic in an *in vivo* assay for the induction of micronuclei in mouse bone marrow cells.

Carcinogenesis and reproductive toxicity studies have not been conducted with becaplermin.

PREGNANCY CATEGORY C

Animal reproduction studies have not been conducted with becaplermin. It is also not known whether becaplermin can cause fetal harm when administered to a pregnant woman or can affect reproductive capacity. Becaplermin should be given to pregnant women only if clearly needed.

NURSING MOTHERS

It is not known whether becaplermin is excreted in human milk. Because many drugs are secreted in human milk, caution should be exercised when becaplermin is administered to nursing women.

PEDIATRIC USE

Safety and effectiveness of becaplermin in pediatric patients below the age of 16 years have not been established.

DRUG INTERACTIONS

It is not known if becaplermin interacts with other topical medications applied to the ulcer site. The use of becaplermin with other topical drugs has not been studied.

ADVERSE REACTIONS

Patients receiving becaplermin, placebo gel, and good ulcer care alone had a similar incidence of ulcer-related adverse events such as infection, cellulitis, or osteomyelitis. However, erythematous rashes occurred in 2% of patients treated with becaplermin and placebo, and none in patients receiving good ulcer care alone. The incidence of cardiovascular, respiratory, musculoskeletal and central and peripheral nervous system disorders was not different across all treatment groups. Mortality rates were also similar across all treatment groups. Patients treated with becaplermin did not develop neutralizing antibodies against becaplermin.

DOSAGE AND ADMINISTRATION

The amount of becaplermin to be applied will vary depending upon the size of the ulcer area. To calculate the length of gel to apply to the ulcer, measure the greatest length of the ulcer by the greatest width of the ulcer in either inches or centimeters. To calculate the length of gel in inches, use the formula shown in TABLE 2, and to calculate the length of gel in centimeters, use the formula shown in TABLE 3.

TABLE 2 *Formula to Calculate Length of Gel in Inches to be Applied Daily*

Tube Size	Formula
15 gor 7.5 g tube	length × width × 0.6
2 g tube	length × width × 1.3

Using the calculation, each square inch of ulcer surface will require approximately 2/3 inch length of gel squeezed from a 15 g or 7.5 g tube, or approximately 1 1/3 inch length of the gel from a 2 g tube. For example, if the ulcer measures 1 inch by 2 inches, then a 1¼ inch length of gel should be used for 15 g or 7.5 g tubes (1 × 2 × 0.6 = 1¼) and 2¾ inch gel length should be used for 2 g tube (1 × 2 × 1.3 = 2¾).

TABLE 3 *Formula to Calculate Length of Gel in Centimeters to be Applied Daily*

Tube Size	Formula
15 g or 7.5 g tube	(length × width) ÷ 4
2 g tube	(length × width) ÷ 2

Using the calculations for ulcer size in centimeters, each square centimeter of ulcer surface will require approximately a 0.25 centimeter length of gel squeezed from a 15 g or 7.5 g tube, or approximately a 0.5 centimeter length of gel from a 2 g tube. For example, if the ulcer measures 4 cm by 2 cm, then a 2 centimeter length of gel should be used for 15 g or 7.5 g tube [(4 × 2) ÷ 4 = 2] and a 4 centimeter length of gel should be used for 2 g tube [(4 × 2) ÷ 2 = 4].

The amount of becaplermin to be applied should be recalculated by the physician or wound care giver at weekly or biweekly intervals depending on the rate of change in ulcer area. The weight of becaplermin from 7.5 g and 15 g tubes is 0.65g per inch length and 0.25g per centimeter length.

To apply becaplermin, the calculated length of gel should be squeezed on to a clean measuring surface (*e.g.*, wax paper). The measured becaplermin is transferred from the clean measuring surface using an application aid and then spread over the entire ulcer area to yield a thin continuous layer of approximately 1/16 of an inch thickness. The site(s) of application should then be covered by a saline moistened dressing and left in place for approximately 12 hours. The dressing should then be removed and the ulcer rinsed with saline or water to remove residual gel and covered again with a second moist dressing (without becaplermin) for the remainder of the day. Becaplermin should be applied once daily to the ulcer until complete healing has occurred. If the ulcer does not decrease in size by approximately 30% after 10 weeks of treatment or complete healing has not occurred in 20 weeks, continued treatment with becaplermin should be reassessed.

HOW SUPPLIED

Regranex gel, supplied as a clear, colorless to straw-colored preserved gel containing 100 μg of becaplermin per gram of gel.

Becaplermin is for external use only.

Storage: Store refrigerated, 2-8°C (36-46°F). DO NOT FREEZE. DO NOT USE THE GEL AFTER THE EXPIRATION DATE AT THE BOTTOM OF THE TUBE.

PRODUCT LISTING - EQUIVALENTS NOT AVAILABLE

Gel - Topical - 0.01%

15 gm $533.15 REGRANEX, Mcneil Pharmaceutical 00045-0810-15

Beclomethasone Dipropionate *(000376)*

For related information, see the comparative table section in Appendix A.

Categories: Asthma; Polyps, nasal, prevention; Rhinitis, allergic; Rhinitis, vasomotor; FDA Approved 1976 May; Pregnancy Category C; WHO Formulary

Drug Classes: Corticosteroids, inhalation

Brand Names: **Beclovent**; Beconase AQ; Vancenase; Vanceril

Foreign Brand Availability: Aerobec (Germany; Mexico; South-Africa); Alanase (New-Zealand); Aldecin (Belgium; Bulgaria; China; Denmark; Hong-Kong; Malaysia; Netherlands; Switzerland; Taiwan); Aldecin Hayfever Aqueous Nasal Spray (Australia); Aldecina (Costa-Rica; Dominican-Republic; El-Salvador; Guatemala; Honduras; Nicaragua; Panama; Portugal); Anceron (South-Africa); Andion (Denmark); Asmabec Clickhaler (France); Atomase (New-Zealand; Singapore); Beceze (Israel); Beclate (India; South-Africa); Beclazone (Israel; New-Zealand); Beclazone CFC Free (Singapore); Beclo-Asma (Hong-Kong; Singapore); Beclocort Nasel (Poland); Becloforte (Bahrain; Cyprus; Egypt; Hong-Kong; Iran; Iraq; Jordan; Kuwait; Lebanon; Libya; New-Zealand; Oman; Qatar; Republic-of-Yemen; Saudi-Arabia; South-Africa; Syria; United-Arab-Emirates); Beclomet (Bulgaria; Germany; Malaysia; Switzerland; Taiwan); Beclomet Easyhaler (Indonesia; Thailand); Beclomet Nasal (Bahrain; Cyprus; Egypt; Iran; Iraq; Israel; Jordan; Kuwait; Lebanon; Libya; Oman; Qatar; Republic-of-Yemen; Saudi-Arabia; Syria; United-Arab-Emirates); Beclomet Nasal Aqua (Indonesia; Thailand); Beclometasone (France); Beclone (France); Beclo-Rhino (France); Beclorhinol (Germany); Beclo Siozwo Nasenspray (Germany); Becloturmant (Germany); Becodisks (China); Beconase (Australia; Austria; Bahamas; Bahrain; Barbados; Belgium; Belize; Benin; Bermuda; Bulgaria; Burkina-Faso; China; Costa-Rica; Curacao; Cyprus; Dominican-Republic; Ecuador; Egypt; El-Salvador; England; Ethiopia; Finland; France; Gambia; Germany; Ghana; Guatemala; Guinea; Guyana; Honduras; Hong-Kong; Hungary; Indonesia; Iran; Iraq; Israel; Ivory-Coast; Jamaica; Jordan; Kenya; Kuwait; Lebanon; Liberia; Libya; Malawi; Malaysia; Mali; Mauritania; Mauritius; Mexico; Morocco; Netherland-Antilles; Netherlands; Nicaragua; Niger; Nigeria; Oman; Panama; Peru; Philippines; Portugal; Puerto-Rico; Qatar; Republic-of-Yemen; Saudi-Arabia; Senegal; Seychelles; Sierra-Leone; South-Africa; Spain; Sudan; Surinam; Syria; Taiwan; Tanzania; Thailand; Trinidad; Tunia; Uganda; United-Arab-Emirates; Zambia; Zimbabwe); Becotide (Australia; Austria; Bahamas; Bahrain; Barbados; Belgium; Belize; Benin; Bermuda; Bulgaria; Burkina-Faso; Costa-Rica; Curacao; Cyprus; Czech-Republic; Denmark; Dominican-Republic; Ecuador; Egypt; El-Salvador; England; Ethiopia; Finland; France; Gambia; Ghana; Greece; Guatemala; Guinea; Guyana; Honduras; Hong-Kong; Hungary; Indonesia; Iran; Iraq; Israel; Italy; Ivory-Coast; Jamaica; Jordan; Kenya; Kuwait; Lebanon; Liberia; Libya; Malawi; Malaysia; Mali; Mauritania; Mauritius; Mexico; Morocco; Netherland-Antilles; Netherlands; New-Zealand; Nicaragua; Niger; Nigeria; Norway; Oman; Panama; Peru; Philippines; Portugal; Puerto-Rico; Qatar; Republic-of-Yemen; Saudi-Arabia; Senegal; Seychelles; Sierra-Leone; South-Africa; Spain; Sudan; Surinam; Sweden; Switzerland; Syria; Taiwan; Tanzania; Thailand; Trinidad; Tunia; Uganda; United-Arab-Emirates; Zambia; Zimbabwe); Belax (Taiwan); Bemedrex Easyhaler (France); Bronconox (Colombia); Bronconox Forte (Colombia); Clenil (Bahrain; Cyprus; Egypt; Indonesia; Iran; Iraq; Israel; Jordan; Kuwait; Lebanon; Libya; Oman; Philippines; Qatar; Republic-of-Yemen; Saudi-Arabia; Singapore; South-Africa; Syria; Taiwan; United-Arab-Emirates); Clenil Forte (Indonesia; Philippines); Decomit (Singapore); Ecobec (France); Miflasone (France; New-Zealand); Nexxair (France); Nobec (South-Africa); Q Var (New-Zealand; Philippines; Singapore; South-Africa); Qvar Autohaler (Australia; France); Qvar Inhaler (Australia); RatioAllerg (Germany); Respocort (Malaysia; New-Zealand; Philippines); Rhino Clenil (Bahrain; Cyprus; Egypt; Iran; Iraq; Israel; Jordan; Kuwait; Lebanon; Libya; Oman; Qatar; Republic-of-Yemen; Saudi-Arabia; Syria; United-Arab-Emirates); Rhinocort (Israel); Rinaze (South-Africa); Rynconox (Colombia); Viarex (Bahrain; Benin; Burkina-Faso; Cyprus; Egypt; Ethiopia; Gambia; Ghana; Guinea; Iran; Iraq; Israel; Ivory-Coast; Jordan; Kenya; Kuwait; Lebanon; Liberia; Libya; Malawi; Mali; Mauritania; Mauritius; Morocco; Niger; Nigeria; Oman; Qatar; Republic-of-Yemen; Saudi-Arabia; Senegal; Seychelles; Sierra-Leone; South-Africa; Sudan; Syria; Tanzania; Tunia; Uganda; United-Arab-Emirates; Zambia; Zimbabwe); Viarox (Germany; South-Africa); Xiten (Peru)

Cost of Therapy: \$53.33 (Asthma; Vanceril DS Aerosol; 0.084 mg/inh; 12 g; 8 inhalations/day; 15 day supply)
\$55.78 (Allergic Rhinitis; Vancenase AQ DS Nasal Spray; 0.084 mg/spray; 19 g; 2 sprays/day; 60 day supply)

INTRANASAL

DESCRIPTION

Beclomethasone dipropionate, the active component of Beconase inhalation aerosol, is an anti-inflammatory steroid having the chemical name 9-chloro-11β,17,21-trihydroxy-16β-methylpregna-1,4-diene-3,20-dione 17,21-dipropionate.

Beclomethasone dipropionate, monohydrate, the active component of Beconase AQ nasal spray, is an anti-inflammatory steroid having the chemical name 9-chloro-11β,17,21-trihydroxy-16β-methylpregna-1,4-diene-3,20-dione 17,21-dipropionate, monohydrate.

Beclomethasone 17,21-dipropionate is a diester of beclomethasone, a synthetic halogenated corticosteroid. Beclomethasone dipropionate is a white to creamy-white, odorless powder with a molecular weight of 521.25. The molecular weight of beclomethasone dipropionate, monohydrate is 539.06. It is very slightly soluble in water, very soluble in chloroform, and freely soluble in acetone and in alcohol.

BECONASE INHALATION AEROSOL

For Nasal Inhalation Only.

Beconase inhalation aerosol is a metered-dose aerosol unit containing a microcrystalline suspension of beclomethasone dipropionate-trichloromonofluoromethane clathrate in a mixture of propellants (trichloromonofluoromethane and dichlorodifluoromethane) with oleic acid. Each canister contains beclomethasone dipropionate-trichloromonofluoromethane clathrate having a molecular proportion of beclomethasone dipropionate to trichloromonofluoromethane between 3:1 and 3:2. Each actuation delivers from the compact actuator a quantity of clathrate equivalent to 42 μg of beclomethasone dipropionate. The contents of one 6.7 g canister provide at least 80 metered doses, and the contents of one 16.8 g canister provide at least 200 metered doses.

BECONASE AQ NASAL SPRAY

For Intranasal Use Only.

SHAKE WELL BEFORE USE.

Beconase AQ nasal spray is a metered-dose, manual pump spray unit containing a microcrystalline suspension of beclomethasone dipropionate, monohydrate equivalent to 0.042% w/w beclomethasone dipropionate, calculated on the dried basis, in an aqueous medium containing microcrystalline cellulose, carboxymethylcellulose sodium, dextrose, benzalkonium chloride, polysorbate 80, and 0.25% v/w phenylethyl alcohol. Hydrochloric acid may be added to adjust pH. The pH is between 4.5 and 7.0.

After initial priming (3-4 actuations), each actuation of the pump delivers from the nasal adapter 100 mg of suspension containing beclomethasone dipropionate, monohydrate equivalent to 42 μg of beclomethasone dipropionate. Each bottle of Beconase AQ nasal spray will provide at least 200 metered doses.

CLINICAL PHARMACOLOGY

MECHANISM OF ACTION

Following topical administration, beclomethasone dipropionate produces anti-inflammatory and vasoconstrictor effects. The mechanisms responsible for the anti-inflammatory action of beclomethasone dipropionate are unknown. Corticosteroids have been shown to have a wide range of effects on multiple cell types (*e.g.*, mast cells, eosinophils, neutrophils, macrophages, and lymphocytes) and mediators (*e.g.*, histamine, eicosanoids, leukotrienes, and cytokines) involved in inflammation. The direct relationship of these findings to the effects of beclomethasone dipropionate on allergic rhinitis symptoms is not known.

Biopsies of nasal mucosa obtained during clinical studies showed no histopathologic changes when beclomethasone dipropionate was administered intranasally.

Beclomethasone dipropionate is a pro-drug with weak glucocorticoid receptor binding affinity. It is hydrolyzed via esterase enzymes to its active metabolite beclomethasone-17-monopropionate (B-17-MP), which has high topical anti-inflammatory activity.

PHARMACOKINETICS

Absorption

Beclomethasone dipropionate is sparingly soluble in water. When given by nasal inhalation in the form of an aqueous or aerosolized suspension, the drug is deposited primarily in the nasal passages. The majority of the drug is eventually swallowed. Following intranasal administration of aqueous beclomethasone dipropionate, the systemic absorption was assessed by measuring the plasma concentrations of its active metabolite B-17-MP, for which the absolute bioavailability following intranasal administration is 44% (43% of the administered dose came from the swallowed portion and only 1% of the total dose was bioavailable from the nose). The absorption of unchanged beclomethasone dipropionate following oral and intranasal dosing was undetectable (plasma concentrations <50 pg/ml).

Distribution

The tissue distribution at steady-state for beclomethasone dipropionate is moderate (20 L) but more extensive for B-17-MP (424 L). There is no evidence of tissue storage of beclomethasone dipropionate or its metabolites. Plasma protein binding is moderately high (87%).

Metabolism

Beclomethasone dipropionate is cleared very rapidly from the systemic circulation by metabolism mediated via esterase enzymes that are found in most tissues. The main product of metabolism is the active metabolite (B-17-MP). Minor inactive metabolites, beclomethasone-21-monopropionate (B-21-MP) and beclomethasone (BOH), are also formed, but these contribute little to systemic exposure.

Elimination

The elimination of beclomethasone dipropionate and B-17-MP after intravenous administration are characterized by high plasma clearance (150 and 120 L/hour) with corresponding terminal elimination half-lives of 0.5 and 2.7 hours. Following oral administration of tritiated beclomethasone dipropionate, approximately 60% of the dose was excreted in the feces within 96 hours, mainly as free and conjugated polar metabolites. Approximately 12% of the dose was excreted as free and conjugated polar metabolites in the urine. The renal clearance of beclomethasone dipropionate and its metabolites is negligible.

PHARMACODYNAMICS

The effects of beclomethasone dipropionate on hypothalamic-pituitary-adrenal (HPA) function have been evaluated in adult volunteers by other routes of administration. Studies with beclomethasone dipropionate by the intranasal route may demonstrate that there is more or that there is less absorption by this route of administration. There was no suppression of early morning plasma cortisol concentrations when beclomethasone dipropionate was administered in a dose of 1000 μg/day for 1 month as an oral aerosol or for 3 days by intramuscular injection. However, partial suppression of plasma cortisol concentrations was observed when beclomethasone dipropionate was administered in doses of 2000 μg/day either by oral aerosol or intramuscular injection. Immediate suppression of plasma cortisol concentrations was observed after single doses of 4000 μg of beclomethasone dipropionate. Suppression of HPA function (reduction of early morning plasma cortisol levels) has been reported in adult patients who received 1600 μg daily doses of oral beclomethasone dipropionate for 1 month. In clinical studies using beclomethasone dipropionate intranasally, there was no evidence of adrenal insufficiency. The effect of Beconase AQ nasal spray on HPA function was not evaluated but would not be expected to differ from intranasal beclomethasone dipropionate aerosol.

In 1 study in children with asthma, the administration of inhaled beclomethasone at recommended daily doses for at least 1 year was associated with a reduction in nocturnal cortisol secretion. The clinical significance of this finding is not clear. It reinforces other evidence, however, that topical beclomethasone may be absorbed in amounts that can have systemic effects and that physicians should be alert for evidence of systemic effects, especially in chronically treated patients (see PRECAUTIONS).

INDICATIONS AND USAGE

Beconase inhalation aerosol is indicated for the relief of the symptoms of seasonal or perennial rhinitis in those cases poorly responsive to conventional treatment. Beconase AQ nasal spray is indicated for the relief of the symptoms of seasonal or perennial allergic and nonallergic (vasomotor) rhinitis.

Beconase inhalation aerosol and Beconase AQ nasal spray are also indicated for the prevention of recurrence of nasal polyps following surgical removal.

Clinical studies in patients with seasonal or perennial rhinitis have shown that improvement is usually apparent within a few days. However, symptomatic relief may not occur in some patients for as long as 2 weeks. Although systemic effects are minimal at recommended doses, beclomethasone dipropionate should not be continued beyond 3 weeks in the absence of significant symptomatic improvement. Beclomethasone dipropionate should not be used in the presence of untreated localized infection involving the nasal mucosa.

Clinical studies have shown that treatment of the symptoms associated with nasal polyps may have to be continued for several weeks or more before a therapeutic result can be fully assessed. Recurrence of symptoms due to polyps can occur after stopping treatment, depending on the severity of the disease.

CONTRAINDICATIONS

Hypersensitivity to any of the ingredients of this preparation contraindicates its use.

WARNINGS

The replacement of a systemic corticosteroid with beclomethasone dipropionate can be accompanied by signs of adrenal insufficiency.

Careful attention must be given when patients previously treated for prolonged periods with systemic corticosteroids are transferred to beclomethasone dipropionate. This is particularly important in those patients who have associated asthma or other clinical conditions where too rapid a decrease in systemic corticosteroids may cause a severe exacerbation of their symptoms.

Studies have shown that the combined administration of alternate-day prednisone systemic treatment and orally inhaled beclomethasone increases the likelihood of HPA suppression compared to a therapeutic dose of either one alone. Therefore, treatment with beclomethasone dipropionate should be used with caution in patients already on alternate-day prednisone regimens for any disease.

If recommended doses of intranasal beclomethasone are exceeded or if individuals are particularly sensitive or predisposed by virtue of recent systemic steroid therapy, symptoms of hypercorticism may occur, including very rare cases of menstrual irregularities, acneiform lesions, cataracts, and cushingoid features. If such changes occur, beclomethasone dipropionate should be discontinued slowly consistent with accepted procedures for discontinuing oral steroid therapy.

Persons who are on drugs that suppress the immune system are more susceptible to infections than healthy individuals. Chickenpox and measles, for example, can have a more serious or even fatal course in nonimmune children or adults on corticosteroids. In such children or adults who have not had these diseases, particular care should be taken to avoid exposure. How the dose, route, and duration of corticosteroid administration affects the risk of developing a disseminated infection is not known. The contribution of the underlying disease and/or prior corticosteroid treatment to the risk is also not known. If exposed to chickenpox, prophylaxis with varicella zoster immune globulin (VZIG) may be indicated. If exposed to measles, prophylaxis with pooled intramuscular immunoglobulin (IG) may be indicated. (See the respective package inserts for complete VZIG and IG prescribing information.) If chickenpox develops, treatment with antiviral agents may be considered.

PRECAUTIONS

GENERAL

During withdrawal from oral steroids, some patients may experience symptoms of withdrawal, *e.g.*, joint and/or muscular pain, lassitude, and depression.

Rare instances of nasal septum perforation have been spontaneously reported.

Rare instances of wheezing, cataracts, glaucoma, and increased intraocular pressure have been reported following the intranasal use of beclomethasone dipropionate.

In clinical studies with beclomethasone dipropionate administered intranasally, the development of localized infections of the nose and pharynx with *Candida albicans* has occurred only rarely. When such an infection develops, it may require treatment with appropriate local therapy or discontinuation of treatment with beclomethasone dipropionate.

Beclomethasone dipropionate is absorbed into the circulation. Use of excessive doses of beclomethasone dipropionate may suppress HPA function.

Beclomethasone dipropionate should be used with caution, if at all, in patients with active or quiescent tuberculous infections of the respiratory tract; untreated fungal, bacterial, or systemic viral infections; or ocular herpes simplex.

For beclomethasone dipropionate to be effective in the treatment of nasal polyps, the aerosol must be able to enter the nose. Therefore, treatment of nasal polyps with beclomethasone dipropionate should be considered adjunctive therapy to surgical removal and/or the use of other medications that will permit effective penetration of beclomethasone dipropionate into the nose. Nasal polyps may recur after any form of treatment.

As with any long-term treatment, patients using beclomethasone dipropionate over several months or longer should be examined periodically for possible changes in the nasal mucosa.

Because of the inhibitory effect of corticosteroids on wound healing, patients who have experienced recent nasal septum ulcers, nasal surgery, or trauma should not use a nasal corticosteroid until healing has occurred.

Although systemic effects have been minimal with recommended doses, this potential increases with excessive doses. Therefore, larger than recommended doses should be avoided.

If persistent nasopharyngeal irritation occurs, it may be an indication for stopping Beconase AQ nasal spray.

INFORMATION FOR THE PATIENT

Patients being treated with beclomethasone dipropionate should receive the following information and instructions. This information is intended to aid in the safe and effective use of this medication. It is not a disclosure of all possible adverse or intended effects. Patients should use beclomethasone dipropionate at regular intervals since its effectiveness depends on its regular use. The patient should take the medication as directed. It is not acutely effective, and the prescribed dosage should not be increased. Instead, nasal vasoconstrictors or oral antihistamines may be needed until the effects of beclomethasone dipropionate are fully manifested. One (1) to 2 weeks may pass before full relief is obtained. The patient should contact the physician if symptoms do not improve, if the condition worsens, or if sneezing or nasal irritation occurs. For the proper use of this unit and to attain maximum improvement, the patient should read and follow carefully the patient's instructions that are included with the prescription.

Persons who are on immunosuppressant doses of corticosteroids should be warned to avoid exposure to chickenpox or measles. Patients should also be advised that if they are exposed, medical advice should be sought without delay.

CARCINOGENESIS, MUTAGENESIS, AND IMPAIRMENT OF FERTILITY

Treatment of rats for a total of 95 weeks, 13 weeks by inhalation and 82 weeks by the oral route, resulted in no evidence of carcinogenic activity. Mutagenic studies have not been performed.

Impairment of fertility, as evidenced by inhibition of the estrous cycle in dogs, was observed following treatment by the oral route. No inhibition of the estrous cycle in dogs was seen following treatment with beclomethasone dipropionate by the inhalation route.

PREGNANCY CATEGORY C

Teratogenic Effects

Like other corticoids, parenteral (subcutaneous) beclomethasone dipropionate has been shown to be teratogenic and embryocidal in the mouse and rabbit when given in doses approximately 10 times the human dose. In these studies, beclomethasone was found to produce fetal resorption, cleft palate, agnathia, microstomia, absence of tongue, delayed ossification, and agenesis of the thymus. No teratogenic or embryocidal effects have been seen in the rat when beclomethasone dipropionate was administered by inhalation at 10 times the human dose or orally at 1000 times the human dose. There are no adequate and well-controlled studies in pregnant women. Beclomethasone dipropionate should be used during pregnancy only if the potential benefit justifies the potential risk to the fetus.

Nonteratogenic Effects

Hypoadrenalism may occur in infants born of mothers receiving corticosteroids during pregnancy. Such infants should be carefully observed.

NURSING MOTHERS

It is not known whether beclomethasone dipropionate is excreted in human milk. Because other corticosteroids are excreted in human milk, caution should be exercised when beclomethasone dipropionate is administered to a nursing woman.

PEDIATRIC USE

The safety and effectiveness of Beconase inhalation aerosol and Beconase AQ nasal spray have been established in children aged 6 years and above through evidence from extensive clinical use in adult and pediatric patients. The safety and effectiveness of Beconase AQ nasal spray in children below 6 years of age have not been established.

Glucocorticoids have been shown to cause a reduction in growth velocity in children and teenagers with extended use. If a child or teenager on any glucocorticoid appears to have growth suppression, the possibility that they are particularly sensitive to this effect of glucocorticoids should be considered.

GERIATRIC USE

Clinical studies of Beconase AQ nasal spray did not include sufficient numbers of subjects aged 65 and over to determine whether they respond differently from younger subjects. Other reported clinical experience has not identified differences in responses between the elderly and younger patients. In general, dose selection for an elderly patient should be cautious, starting at the low end of the dosing range, reflecting the greater frequency of decreased hepatic, renal, or cardiac function, and of concomitant disease or other drug therapy.

ADVERSE REACTIONS

In general, side effects in clinical studies have been primarily associated with irritation of the nasal mucous membranes. Rare cases of immediate and delayed hypersensitivity reactions, including urticaria, angioedema, rash, and bronchospasm, have been reported following the oral and intranasal inhalation of beclomethasone dipropionate.

Rare cases of ulceration of the nasal mucosa and instances of nasal septum perforation have been spontaneously reported (see PRECAUTIONS).

Reports of dryness and irritation of the nose and throat, and unpleasant taste and smell have been received. There are rare reports of loss of taste and smell.

Rare instances of wheezing, cataracts, glaucoma, and increased intraocular pressure have been reported following the use of intranasal beclomethasone dipropionate (see PRECAUTIONS).

Adverse reactions reported in controlled clinical trials and long-term open studies in patients treated with Beconase inhalation aerosol are described below.

Sensations of irritation and burning in the nose (11/100 patients) following the use of Beconase inhalation aerosol have been reported. Also, occasional sneezing attacks (10/100 adult patients) have occurred immediately following the use of the intranasal inhaler. This symptom may be more common in children. Rhinorrhea may occur occasionally (1/100 patients).

Localized infections of the nose and pharynx with *Candida albicans* have occurred rarely (see PRECAUTIONS).

Transient episodes of epistaxis have been reported in 2/100 patients.

Adverse reactions reported in controlled clinical trials and open studies in patients treated with Beconase AQ nasal spray are described below.

Mild nasopharyngeal irritation following the use of beclomethasone aqueous nasal spray has been reported in up to 24% of patients treated, including occasional sneezing attacks (about 4%) occurring immediately following use of the spray. In patients experiencing these symptoms, none had to discontinue treatment. The incidence of transient irritation and sneezing was approximately the same in the group of patients who received placebo in these studies, implying that these complaints may be related to vehicle components of the formulation.

Fewer than 5/100 patients reported headache, nausea, or lightheadedness following the use of Beconase AQ nasal spray. Fewer than 3/100 patients reported nasal stuffiness, nosebleeds, rhinorrhea, or tearing eyes.

Systemic corticosteroid side effects were not reported during the controlled clinical trials. If recommended doses are exceeded, however, or if individuals are particularly sensitive, symptoms of hypercorticism, *i.e.*, Cushing's syndrome, could occur.

DOSAGE AND ADMINISTRATION

BECONASE INHALATION AEROSOL

Adults and Children 12 Years of Age and Older

The usual dosage is 1 inhalation (42 μg) in each nostril 2-4 times a day (total dose, 168-336 μg/day). Patients can often be maintained on a maximum dose of 1 inhalation in each nostril 3 times a day (252 μg/day).

Children 6-12 Years of Age

The usual dosage is 1 inhalation in each nostril 3 times a day (252 μg/day). Beconase inhalation aerosol is *not* recommended for children below 6 years of age since safety and efficacy studies have not been conducted in this age-group.

BECONASE AQ NASAL SPRAY

Adults and Children 12 Years of Age and Older

The usual dosage is 1 or 2 inhalations (42-84 μg) in each nostril twice a day (total dose, 168-336 μg/day).

Children 6-12 Years of Age

Patients should be started with 1 inhalation in each nostril twice a day; patients not adequately responding to 168 μg or those with more severe symptoms may use 336 μg (2 inhalations in each nostril). Beconase AQ nasal spray is *not* recommended for children below 6 years of age.

In patients who respond to beclomethasone dipropionate, an improvement of the symptoms of seasonal or perennial rhinitis usually becomes apparent within a few days after the start of therapy with beclomethasone dipropionate. However, symptomatic relief may not occur in some patients for as long as 2 weeks. Beclomethasone dipropionate should not be continued beyond 3 weeks in the absence of significant symptomatic improvement.

The therapeutic effects of corticosteroids, unlike those of decongestants, are not immediate. This should be explained to the patient in advance in order to ensure cooperation and continuation of treatment with the prescribed dosage regimen.

In the presence of excessive nasal mucus secretion or edema of the nasal mucosa, the drug may fail to reach the site of intended action. In such cases it is advisable to use a nasal vasoconstrictor during the first 2-3 days of therapy with beclomethasone dipropionate.

HOW SUPPLIED

BECONASE INHALATION AEROSOL

Beconase inhalation aerosol is supplied in a 6.7 g canister containing 80 metered doses and in a 16.8 g canister containing 200 metered doses, each with beige compact actuator and patient's instructions.

Storage: Store between 2 and 30°C (36 and 86°F). As with most inhaled medications in aerosol canisters, the therapeutic effect of this medication may decrease when the canister is cold. Shake well before using.

WARNING: Contains trichloromonofluoromethane and dichlorodifluoromethane, substances that harm public health and environment by destroying ozone in the upper atmosphere.

BECONASE AQ NASAL SPRAY

Beconase AQ nasal spray, 0.042% (calculated on the dried basis) is supplied in an amber glass bottle fitted with a metering atomizing pump and nasal adapter with patient's instructions for use. Each bottle contains 25 g of suspension.

Storage: Store between 15 and 30°C (59 and 86°F).

ORAL

DESCRIPTION

For Oral Inhalation Only.

The active component of Qvar 40 and 80 μg inhalation aerosol is beclomethasone dipropionate, an anti-inflammatory corticosteroid having the chemical name 9-chloro-11β,17,21-trihydroxy-16β-methylpregna-1,4-diene-3,20-dione 17,21-dipropionate. Beclomethasone dipropionate is a diester of beclomethasone, a synthetic corticosteroid chemically related to dexamethasone. Beclomethasone differs from dexamethasone in having a chlorine at the 9-alpha carbon in place of a fluorine, and in having a 16 beta-methyl group instead of a 16 alpha-methyl group. Beclomethasone dipropionate is a white to creamy white, odorless powder with a molecular formula of $C_{28}H_{37}ClO_7$ and a molecular weight of 521.1.

Beclomethasone dipropionate is slightly soluble in water, very soluble in chloroform and freely soluble in acetone and in alcohol.

Qvar is a pressurized, metered-dose aerosol intended for oral inhalation only. Each unit contains a solution of beclomethasone dipropionate in propellant HFA-134a (1,1,1,2 tetrafluoroethane) and ethanol. Qvar 40 μg delivers 40 μg of beclomethasone dipropionate from the actuator and 50 μg from the valve. Qvar 80 μg delivers 80 μg of beclomethasone dipropionate from the actuator and 100 μg from the valve. This product delivers 50 μL (59 mg) of solution formulation from the valve with each actuation. Each canister provides 100 inhalations. Qvar should be "primed" or actuated twice prior to taking the first dose from a new canister, or when the inhaler has not been used for more than 10 days. Avoid spraying in the eyes or face while priming Qvar.

This product does not contain chlorofluorocarbons (CFCs).

CLINICAL PHARMACOLOGY

Airway inflammation is known to be an important component in the pathogenesis of asthma. Inflammation occurs in both large and small airways. Corticosteroids have multiple anti-inflammatory effects, inhibiting both inflammatory cells and release of inflammatory mediators. It is presumed that these anti-inflammatory actions play an important role in the efficacy of beclomethasone dipropionate in controlling symptoms and improving lung function in asthma. Inhaled beclomethasone dipropionate probably acts topically at the site of deposition in the bronchial tree after inhalation.

PHARMACOKINETICS

Bioavailability information on beclomethasone dipropionate (BDP) after inhaled administration is not available in adults. BDP undergoes rapid and extensive conversion to beclomethasone-17-monopropionate (17-BMP) during absorption. The pharmacokinetics of 17-BMP has been studied in asthmatics given single doses.

Absorption

The mean peak plasma concentration (C_{max}) of BDP was 88 pg/ml at 0.5 hours after inhalation of 320 μg using beclomethasone dipropionate inhalation aerosol (4 actuations of the 80 μg/actuation strength). The mean peak plasma concentration of the major and most active metabolite, 17-BMP, was 1419 pg/ml at 0.7 hours after inhalation of 320 μg of beclomethasone dipropionate inhalation aerosol. When the same nominal dose is provided by the two beclomethasone dipropionate inhalation aerosol strengths (40 and 80 μg/actuation), equivalent systemic pharmacokinetics can be expected. The C_{max} of 17-BMP increased dose proportionally in the dose range of 80 and 320 μg.

Metabolism

Three major metabolites are formed via cytochrome P450 3A catalyzed biotransformation — beclomethasone-17-monopropionate (17-BMP), beclomethasone-21-monopropionate (21-BMP) and beclomethasone (BOH). Lung slices metabolize BDP rapidly to 17-BMP and more slowly to BOH. 17-BMP is the most active metabolite.

Distribution

There is no evidence of tissue storage of BDP or its metabolites.

Elimination

The major route of elimination of inhaled BDP appears to be via metabolism. More than 90% of inhaled BDP is found as 17-BMP in the systemic circulation. The mean elimination half-life of 17-BMP is 2.8 hours. Irrespective of the route of administration (injection, oral or inhalation), BDP and its metabolites are mainly excreted in the feces. Less than 10% of the drug and its metabolites are excreted in the urine.

Special Populations

Formal pharmacokinetic studies using beclomethasone dipropionate inhalation aerosol were not conducted in any special populations.

Pediatrics

The pharmacokinetics of 17-BMP, including dose and strength proportionalities, is similar in children and adults, although the exposure is highly variable. In 17 children (mean age 10 years), the C_{max} of 17-BMP was 787 pg/ml at 0.6 hours after inhalation of 160 μg (4 actuations of the 40 μg/actuation strength of HFA beclomethasone dipropionate). The systemic exposure to 17-BMP from 160 μg of HFA-BDP administered without a spacer was comparable to the systemic exposure to 17-BMP from 336 μg CFC-BDP administered with a large volume spacer in 14 children (mean age 12 years).

This implies that approximately twice the systemic exposure to 17-BMP would be expected for comparable mg doses of HFA-BDP without a spacer and CFC-BDP with a large volume spacer.

PHARMACODYNAMICS

Improvement in asthma control following inhalation can occur within 24 hours of beginning treatment in some patients, although maximum benefit may not be achieved for 1-2 weeks, or longer. The effects of beclomethasone dipropionate inhalation aerosol on the hypothalamic-pituitary-adrenal (HPA) axis were studied in 40 corticosteroid naive patients.

Beclomethasone dipropionate inhalation aerosol, at doses of 80, 160 or 320 μg twice daily was compared with placebo and 336 μg twice daily of beclomethasone dipropionate in a CFC propellant based formulation (CFC-BDP). Active treatment groups showed an expected dose-related reduction in 24 hour urinary free cortisol (a sensitive marker of adrenal production of cortisol). Patients treated with the highest recommended dose of beclomethasone dipropionate inhalation aerosol (320 μg twice daily) had a 37.3% reduction in 24 hour urinary free cortisol compared to a reduction of 47.3% produced by treatment with 336 μg twice daily of CFC-BDP. There was a 12.2% reduction in 24 hour urinary free cortisol seen in the group of patients that received 80 μg twice daily of beclomethasone dipropionate inhalation aerosol and a 24.6% reduction in the group of patients that received 160 μg twice daily. An open label study of 354 asthma patients given beclomethasone dipropionate inhalation aerosol at recommended doses for 1 year assessed the effect of beclomethasone dipropionate inhalation aerosol treatment on the HPA axis (as measured by both morning and stimulated plasma cortisol). Less than 1% of patients treated for 1 year with beclomethasone dipropionate inhalation aerosol had an abnormal response (peak less than 18 μg/dl) to short-cosyntropin test.

INDICATIONS AND USAGE

Beclomethasone dipropionate inhalation aerosol is indicated in the maintenance treatment of asthma as prophylactic therapy in patients 5 years of age and older. Beclomethasone dipropionate inhalation aerosol is also indicated for asthma patients who require systemic corticosteroid administration, where adding beclomethasone dipropionate inhalation aerosol may reduce or eliminate the need for the systemic corticosteroids.

Beclomethasone dipropionate is NOT indicated for the relief of acute bronchospasm.

CONTRAINDICATIONS

Beclomethasone dipropionate inhalation aerosol is contraindicated in the primary treatment of status asthmaticus or other acute episodes of asthma where intensive measures are required.

Hypersensitivity to any of the ingredients of this preparation contraindicates its use.

WARNINGS

Particular care is needed in patients who are transferred from systemically active corticosteroids to beclomethasone dipropionate inhalation aerosol because deaths due to adrenal insufficiency have occurred in asthmatic patients during and after transfer from systemic corticosteroids to less systemically available inhaled corticosteroids. After withdrawal from systemic corticosteroids, a number of months are required for recovery of hypothalamic-pituitary-adrenal (HPA) function.

Patients who have been previously maintained on 20 mg or more per day of prednisone (or its equivalent) may be most susceptible, particularly when their systemic corticosteroids have been almost completely withdrawn. During this period of HPA suppression, patients may exhibit signs and symptoms of adrenal insufficiency when exposed to trauma, surgery, or infections (particularly gastroenteritis) or other conditions with severe electrolyte loss. Although beclomethasone dipropionate inhalation aerosol may provide control of asthmatic symptoms during these episodes, in recommended doses it supplies less than normal physiological amounts of glucocorticoid systemically and does NOT provide the mineralocorticoid that is necessary for coping with these emergencies.

During periods of stress or a severe asthmatic attack, patients who have been withdrawn from systemic corticosteroids should be instructed to resume oral corticosteroids (in large doses) immediately and to contact their physician for further instruction. These patients should also be instructed to carry a warning card indicating that they may need supplementary systemic steroids during periods of stress or a severe asthma attack.

Transfer of patients from systemic steroid therapy to beclomethasone dipropionate inhalation aerosol may unmask allergic conditions previously suppressed by the systemic steroid therapy, *e.g.*, rhinitis, conjunctivitis, and eczema.

Persons who are on drugs which suppress the immune system are more susceptible to infections than healthy individuals. Chickenpox and measles, for example, can have a more serious or even fatal course in non-immune children or adults on corticosteroids. In such children or adults who have not had these diseases or been properly immunized, particular care should be taken to avoid exposure. It is not known how the dose, route and duration of corticosteroid administration affects the risk of developing a disseminated infection. Nor is the contribution of the underlying disease and/or prior corticosteroid treatment known. If exposed to chickenpox, prophylaxis with varicella-zoster immune globulin (VZIG) may be indicated. If exposed to measles, prophylaxis with pooled intramuscular immunoglobulin (IG) may be indicated. (See the respective package inserts for complete VZIG and IG prescribing information.) If chickenpox develops, treatment with antiviral agents may be considered.

Beclomethasone dipropionate inhalation aerosol is not a bronchodilator and is not indicated for rapid relief of bronchospasm.

As with other inhaled asthma medications, bronchospasm, with an immediate increase in wheezing, may occur after dosing. If bronchospasm occurs following dosing with beclomethasone dipropionate inhalation aerosol, it should be treated immediately with a short acting inhaled bronchodilator. Treatment with beclomethasone dipropionate inhalation aerosol should be discontinued and alternate therapy instituted. Patients should be instructed to contact their physician immediately when episodes of asthma, which are not responsive to bronchodilators, occur during the course of treatment with beclomethasone dipropionate inhalation aerosol. During such episodes, patients may require therapy with oral corticosteroids.

PRECAUTIONS

GENERAL

During withdrawal from oral corticosteroids, some patients may experience symptoms of systemically active corticosteroid withdrawal, *e.g.*, joint and/or muscular pain, lassitude and depression, despite maintenance or even improvement of respiratory function. Although suppression of HPA function below the clinical normal range did not occur with doses of beclomethasone dipropionate inhalation aerosol up to and including 640 μg/day, a dose dependent reduction of adrenal cortisol production was observed. Since inhaled beclomethasone dipropionate is absorbed into the circulation and can be systemically active, HPA axis suppression by beclomethasone dipropionate inhalation aerosol could occur when recommended doses are exceeded or in particularly sensitive individuals. Since individual sensitivity to effects on cortisol production exist, physicians should consider this information when prescribing beclomethasone dipropionate inhalation aerosol. Because of the possibility of systemic absorption of inhaled corticosteroids, patients treated with these drugs should be observed carefully for any evidence of systemic corticosteroid effect. Particular care should be taken in observing patients postoperatively or during periods of stress for evidence of inadequate adrenal response.

It is possible that systemic corticosteroid effects, such as hypercorticism and adrenal suppression, may appear in a small number of patients, particularly at higher doses. If such changes occur, beclomethasone dipropionate inhalation aerosol should be reduced slowly, consistent with accepted procedures for management of asthma symptoms and for tapering of systemic steroids.

A 12 month randomized controlled clinical trial evaluated the effects of HFA beclomethasone dipropionate without spacer versus CFC beclomethasone dipropionate with large volume spacer on growth in children age 5-11. A total of 520 patients were enrolled, of whom 394 received HFA-BDP (100-400 μg/day ex-valve) and 126 received CFC-BDP (200-800 μg/day ex-valve). Similar control of asthma was noted in each treatment arm. When comparing results at month 12 to baseline, the mean growth velocity in children treated with HFA-BDP was approximately 0.5 cm/year less than that noted with children treated with CFC-BDP via large volume spacer.

A reduction in growth velocity in growing children may occur as a result of inadequate control of chronic diseases such as asthma or from use of corticosteroids for treatment. Physicians should closely follow the growth of all pediatric patients taking corticosteroids by any route and weigh the benefits of corticosteroid therapy and asthma control against the possibility of growth suppression.

The long-term and systemic effects of beclomethasone dipropionate inhalation aerosol in humans are still not fully known. In particular, the effects resulting from chronic use of the agent on developmental or immunologic processes in the mouth, pharynx, trachea, and lung are unknown.

Inhaled corticosteroids should be used with caution, if at all, in patients with active or quiescent tuberculosis infection of the respiratory tract; untreated systemic fungal, bacterial, parasitic or viral infections; or ocular herpes simplex.

Rare instances of glaucoma, increased intraocular pressure, and cataracts have been reported following the inhaled administration of corticosteroids.

INFORMATION FOR THE PATIENT

Patients being treated with beclomethasone dipropionate inhalation aerosol should receive the following information and instructions. This information is intended to aid them in the safe and effective use of this medication. It is not a disclosure of all possible adverse or intended effects.

Persons who are on immunosuppressant doses of corticosteroids should be warned to avoid exposure to chickenpox or measles. Patients should also be advised that if they are exposed to these diseases, medical advice should be sought without delay.

Patients should use beclomethasone dipropionate inhalation aerosol at regular intervals as directed. Results of clinical trials indicated significant improvements may occur within the first 24 hours of treatment in some patients; however, the full benefit may not be achieved until treatment has been administered for 1-2 weeks, or longer. The patient should not increase the prescribed dosage but should contact their physician if symptoms do not improve or if the condition worsens.

Patients should be advised that beclomethasone dipropionate inhalation aerosol is not intended for use in the treatment of acute asthma. The patient should be instructed to contact their physician immediately if there is any deterioration of their asthma.

Patients should be instructed on the proper use of their inhaler. Patients may wish to rinse their mouth after beclomethasone dipropionate inhalation aerosol use. The patient should also be advised that beclomethasone dipropionate inhalation aerosol may have a different taste and inhalation sensation than that of an inhaler containing CFC propellant.

Beclomethasone dipropionate inhalation aerosol use should not be stopped abruptly. The patient should contact their physician immediately if use of beclomethasone dipropionate inhalation aerosol is discontinued.

For the proper use of beclomethasone dipropionate inhalation aerosol, the patient should read and carefully follow the Patient's Instructions that are distributed with the prescription.

CARCINOGENESIS, MUTAGENESIS, AND IMPAIRMENT OF FERTILITY

The carcinogenicity of beclomethasone dipropionate was evaluated in rats which were exposed for a total of 95 weeks, 13 weeks at inhalation doses up to 0.4 mg/kg/day and the remaining 82 weeks at combined oral and inhalation doses up to 2.4 mg/kg/day. There was no evidence of carcinogenicity in this study at the highest dose, which is approximately 30 and 55 times the maximum recommended daily inhalation dose in adults and children, respectively, on a mg/m^2 basis.

Beclomethasone dipropionate did not induce gene mutation in the bacterial cells or mammalian Chinese Hamster ovary (CHO) cells *in vitro.* No significant clastogenic effect was seen in cultured CHO cells *in vitro* or in the mouse micronucleus test *in vivo.*

In rats, beclomethasone dipropionate caused decreased conception rates at an oral dose of 16 mg/kg/day (approximately 200 times the maximum recommended daily inhalation dose in adults on a mg/m^2 basis). Impairment of fertility, as evidence by inhibition of the estrous cycle in dogs, was observed following treatment by the oral route at a dose of 0.5 mg/kg/day (approximately 20 times the maximum recommended daily inhalation dose in adults on a mg/m^2 basis). No inhibition of the estrous cycle in dogs was seen following 12 months of exposure to beclomethasone dipropionate by the inhalation route at an estimated daily dose of 0.33 mg/kg (approximately 15 times the maximum recommended daily inhalation dose in adults on a mg/m^2 basis).

PREGNANCY CATEGORY C

Teratogenic Effects

Like other corticosteroids, parenteral (subcutaneous) beclomethasone dipropionate was teratogenic and embryocidal in the mouse and rabbit when given at a dose of 0.1 mg/kg/day in mice or at a dose of 0.025 mg/kg/day in rabbits. These doses in mice and rabbits were approximately one-half the maximum recommended daily inhalation dose in adults on a mg/m^2 basis. No teratogenicity or embryocidal effects were seen in rats when exposed to an inhalation dose of 15 mg/kg/day (approximately 190 times the maximum recommended daily inhalation dose in adults on a mg/m^2 basis). There are no adequate and well controlled studies in pregnant women. Beclomethasone dipropionate should be used during pregnancy only if the potential benefit justifies the potential risk to the fetus.

Nonteratogenic Effects

Findings of drug-related adrenal toxicity in fetuses following administration of beclomethasone dipropionate to rats suggest that infants born of mothers receiving substantial doses of beclomethasone dipropionate inhalation aerosol during pregnancy should be observed for adrenal suppression.

NURSING MOTHERS

Corticosteroids are secreted in human milk. Because of the potential for serious adverse reactions in nursing infants from beclomethasone dipropionate inhalation aerosol, a decision should be made whether to discontinue nursing or to discontinue the drug, taking into account the importance of the drug to the mother.

PEDIATRIC USE

Eight-hundred and thirty-four (834) children between the ages of 5 and12 were treated with HFA beclomethasone dipropionate (HPA BDP) in clinical trials. The safety and effectiveness of beclomethasone dipropionate inhalation aerosol in children below 5 years of age have not been established. Oral corticosteroids have been shown to cause a reduction in growth velocity in children and teenagers with extended use. If a child or teenager on any corticosteroid appears to have growth suppression, the possibility that they are particularly sensitive to this effect of corticosteroids should be considered (see General).

GERIATRIC USE

Clinical studies of beclomethasone dipropionate inhalation aerosol did not include sufficient numbers of subjects aged 65 and over to determine whether they respond differently from younger subjects. Other reported clinical experience has not identified differences in responses between the elderly and younger patients. In general, dose selection for an elderly patient should be cautious, usually starting at the low end of the dosing range, reflecting the greater frequency of decreased hepatic, renal, or cardiac function, and of concomitant disease or other drug therapy.

ADVERSE REACTIONS

The following reporting rates of common adverse experiences are based upon four clinical trials in which 1196 patients (671 female and 525 male adults previously treated with as-needed bronchodilators and/or inhaled corticosteroids) were treated with beclomethasone dipropionate inhalation aerosol (doses of 40, 80, 160, or 320 µg twice daily) or CFC-BDP (doses of 42, 168, or 336 µg twice daily) or placebo. TABLE 1A and TABLE 1B includes all events reported by patients taking beclomethasone dipropionate inhalation aerosol (whether considered drug related or not) that occurred at a rate over 3% for either beclomethasone dipropionate inhalation aerosol or CFC-BDP. In considering these data, difference in average duration of exposure and clinical trial design should be taken into account.

TABLE 1A *Adverse Events Reported by at Least 3% of the Patients for Beclomethasone Dipropionate Inhalation Aerosol by Treatment and Daily Dose*

			Beclomethasone Dipropionate Inhalation Aerosol		
	Placebo	Total	80-160 µg	320 µg	640 µg
Adverse Event	(n=289)	(n=624)	(n=233)	(n=335)	(n=56)
Headache	9%	12%	15%	8%	25%
Pharyngitis	4%	8%	6%	5%	27%
Upper respiratory tract infection	11%	9%	7%	11%	5%
Rhinitis	9%	6%	8%	3%	7%
Increased asthma symptoms	18%	3%	2%	4%	0%
Oral symptoms — inhalation route	2%	3%	3%	3%	2%
Sinusitis	2%	3%	3%	3%	0%
Pain	<1%	2%	1%	2%	5%
Back pain	1%	1%	2%	<1%	4%
Nausea	0%	1%	<1%	1%	2%
Dysphonia	2%	<1%	1%	0%	4%

TABLE 1B *Adverse Events Reported by at Least 3% of the Patients for CFC—BDP by Treatment and Daily Dose*

		CFC-BDP		
	Total	84 µg	336 µg	672 µg
Adverse Event	(n=283)	(n=59)	(n=55)	(n=169)
Headache	15%	14%	11%	17%
Pharyngitis	10%	12%	9%	10%
Upper respiratory tract infection	12%	3%	9%	17%
Rhinitis	11%	15%	9%	10%
Increased asthma symptoms	8%	14%	5%	7%
Oral symptoms — inhalation route	6%	7%	5%	5%
Sinusitis	4%	7%	2%	4%
Pain	3%	3%	5%	2%
Back pain	4%	2%	4%	4%
Nausea	3%	5%	5%	1%
Dysphonia	4%	0%	0%	6%

Other adverse events that occurred in these clinical trials using beclomethasone dipropionate inhalation aerosol with an incidence of 1-3% and which occurred at a greater incidence than placebo were: Dysphonia, dysmenorrhea and coughing.

No patients treated with beclomethasone dipropionate inhalation aerosol in the clinical development program developed symptomatic oropharyngeal candidiasis. If such an infection develops, treatment with appropriate antifungal therapy or discontinuance of treatment with beclomethasone dipropionate inhalation aerosol may be required.

PEDIATRIC STUDIES

In two 12 week placebo-controlled studies in steroid naïve pediatric patients 5-12 years of age, no clinically relevant differences were found in the pattern, severity, or frequency of adverse events compared with those reported in adults, with the exception of conditions which are more prevalent in a pediatric population generally.

ADVERSE EVENT REPORTS FROM OTHER SOURCES

Rare cases of immediate and delayed hypersensitivity reactions, including urticaria, angioedema, rash, and bronchospasm, have been reported following the oral and intranasal inhalation of beclomethasone dipropionate.

DOSAGE AND ADMINISTRATION

Patients should prime beclomethasone dipropionate inhalation aerosol by actuating into the air twice before using for the first time or if beclomethasone dipropionate inhalation aerosol has not been used for over 10 days. Avoid spraying in the eyes or face when priming beclomethasone dipropionate inhalation aerosol. Beclomethasone dipropionate inhalation aerosol is a solution aerosol, which does not require shaking. Consistent dose delivery is achieved, whether using the 40 or 80 µg strengths, due to proportionality of the 2 products (*i.e.,* 2 actuations of 40 µg strength should provide a dose comparable to 1 actuation of the 80 µg strength).

Beclomethasone dipropionate inhalation aerosol should be administered by the oral inhaled route in patients 5 years of age and older. The onset and degree of symptom relief will vary in individual patients. Improvement in asthma symptoms should be expected within the first or second week of starting treatment, but maximum benefit should not be expected until 3-4 weeks of therapy. For patients who do not respond adequately to the starting dose after 3-4 weeks of therapy, higher doses may provide additional asthma control. The safety and efficacy of beclomethasone dipropionate inhalation aerosol when administered in excess of recommended doses has not been established.

B

TABLE 2 *Recommended Dosage for Beclomethasone Dipropionate Inhalation Aerosol*

Previous Therapy	Recommended Starting Dose	Highest Recommended Dose
Adults and Adolescents:		
Bronchodilators alone	40-80 µg twice daily	320 µg twice daily
Inhaled corticosteroids	40-160 µg twice daily	320 µg twice daily
Children 5-11 Years:		
Bronchodilators alone	40 µg twice daily	80 µg twice daily
Inhaled corticosteroids	40 µg twice daily	80 µg twice daily

The recommended dosage of beclomethasone dipropionate inhalation aerosol relative to CFC-based beclomethasone dipropionate (CFC-BDP) inhalation aerosols is lower due to differences in delivery characteristics between the products. Recognizing that a definitive comparative therapeutic ratio between beclomethasone dipropionate inhalation aerosol and CFC-BDP has not been demonstrated, any patient who is switched from CFC-BDP to beclomethasone dipropionate inhalation aerosol should be dosed appropriately, taking into account the dosing recommendations above, and should be monitored to ensure that the dose of beclomethasone dipropionate inhalation aerosol selected is safe and efficacious. As with any inhaled corticosteroid, physicians are advised to titrate the dose of beclomethasone dipropionate inhalation aerosol downward over time to the lowest level that maintains proper asthma control. This is particularly important in children since a controlled study has shown that beclomethasone dipropionate inhalation aerosol has the potential to affect growth in children.

Patients should be instructed on the proper use of their inhaler. Patients should be advised that beclomethasone dipropionate inhalation aerosol may have a different taste and inhalation sensation than that of an inhaler containing CFC propellant.

PATIENTS NOT RECEIVING SYSTEMIC CORTICOSTEROIDS

Patients who require maintenance therapy of their asthma may benefit from treatment with beclomethasone dipropionate inhalation aerosol at the doses recommended above. In patients who respond to beclomethasone dipropionate inhalation aerosol, improvement in pulmonary function is usually apparent within 1-4 weeks after the start of therapy. Once the desired effect is achieved, consideration should be given to tapering to the lowest effective dose.

PATIENTS MAINTAINED ON SYSTEMIC CORTICOSTEROIDS

Beclomethasone dipropionate inhalation aerosol may be effective in the management of asthmatics maintained on systemic corticosteroids and may permit replacement or significant reduction in the dosage of systemic corticosteroids.

The patient's asthma should be reasonably stable before treatment with beclomethasone dipropionate inhalation aerosol is started. Initially, beclomethasone dipropionate inhalation aerosol should be used concurrently with the patient's usual maintenance dose of systemic corticosteroids. After approximately 1 week, gradual withdrawal of the systemic corticosteroids is started by reducing the daily or alternate daily dose. Reductions may be made after an interval of 1 or 2 weeks, depending on the response of the patient. A slow rate of withdrawal is strongly recommended. Generally these decrements should not exceed 2.5 mg of prednisone or its equivalent. During withdrawal, some patients may experience symptoms of systemic corticosteroid withdrawal, *e.g.,* joint and/or muscular pain, lassitude and depression, despite maintenance or even improvement in pulmonary function. Such patients should be encouraged to continue with the inhaler but should be monitored for objective signs of adrenal insufficiency. If evidence of adrenal insufficiency occurs, the systemic corticosteroid doses should be increased temporarily and thereafter withdrawal should continue more slowly.

During periods of stress or a severe asthma attack, transfer patients may require supplementary treatment with systemic corticosteroids.

HOW SUPPLIED

Qvar is supplied in the following 2 strengths:

40 µg: Supplied in a 7.3 g canister containing 100 actuations with a beige plastic actuator and gray dust cap.

80 µg: Supplied in a 7.3 g canister containing 100 actuations with a dark mauve plastic actuator and gray dust cap.

The correct amount of medication in each inhalation cannot be assured after 100 actuations from the 7.3 g canister even though the canister is not completely empty. The canister should be discarded when the labeled number of actuations have been used.

STORAGE

Store Qvar inhalation aerosol when not being used, so that the product rests on the concave end of the canister with the plastic actuator on top.

Store at 25°C (77°F).

Excursions between 15 and 30°C (59 and 86°F) are permitted. For optimal results, the canister should be at room temperature when used. Qvar inhalation aerosol canister should only be used with the Qvar inhalation aerosol actuator and the actuator should not be used with any other inhalation drug product.

CONTENTS UNDER PRESSURE.

Do not puncture. Do not use or store near heat or open flame. Exposure to temperatures above 49°C (120°F) may cause bursting. Never throw container into fire or incinerator.

PRODUCT LISTING - RATED NOT THERAPEUTICALLY EQUIVALENT

Size	Price	Product, Manufacturer	NDC
Aerosol with Adapter - Inhalation - 0.042 mg/Inh			
6.70 gm	$17.23	BECLOVENT, Southwood Pharmaceuticals Inc	58016-6207-00
6.70 gm	$24.70	BECLOVENT, Glaxo Wellcome	00173-0469-00
6.70 gm	$26.20	BECLOVENT, Allscripts Pharmaceutical Company	55175-4466-01
16.80 gm	$32.78	VANCERIL, Allscripts Pharmaceutical Company	54569-0067-00
16.80 gm	$34.47	VANCERIL, Quality Care Pharmaceuticals Inc	60346-0226-76
16.80 gm	$35.40	VANCERIL, Physicians Total Care	54868-1841-01
16.80 gm	$36.98	BECLOVENT, Allscripts Pharmaceutical Company	54569-1004-00
16.80 gm	$38.13	BECLOVENT, Southwood Pharmaceuticals Inc	58016-6207-01
16.80 gm	$39.31	VANCERIL, Cheshire Drugs	55175-4435-01
16.80 gm	$41.05	BECLOVENT, Physicians Total Care	54868-1269-01
16.80 gm	$43.02	BECLOVENT, Allscripts Pharmaceutical Company	55175-4465-01
16.80 gm	$44.94	BECLOVENT, Glaxo Wellcome	00173-0312-88
16.80 gm	$49.71	VANCERIL, Pharma Pac	52959-0596-01
16.80 gm	$49.91	VANCERIL, Schering Corporation	00085-0736-04
Aerosol with Adapter - Nasal - 0.042 mg/Inh			
6.70 gm	$17.23	BECONASE, Southwood Pharmaceuticals Inc	58016-6092-00
6.70 gm	$47.15	VANCENASE, Schering Corporation	00085-0649-02
7 gm	$40.15	VANCENASE, Pharma Pac	52959-0585-00
7 gm	$45.55	VANCENASE, Allscripts Pharmaceutical Company	54569-3656-00
16.80 gm	$32.78	BECONASE, Allscripts Pharmaceutical Company	54569-0237-00
16.80 gm	$34.47	BECONASE, Quality Care Pharmaceuticals Inc	60346-0338-76
16.80 gm	$35.41	BECONASE, Physicians Total Care	54868-1243-01
16.80 gm	$37.44	BECONASE, Southwood Pharmaceuticals Inc	58016-6092-01
16.80 gm	$39.21	BECONASE, Cheshire Drugs	55175-2570-01
16.80 gm	$45.84	BECONASE, Prescript Pharmaceuticals	00247-0191-88
17 gm	$37.44	VANCENASE, Southwood Pharmaceuticals Inc	58016-6075-01
Spray - Nasal - 0.042 mg/Inh			
25 gm	$32.75	BECONASE AQ, Allscripts Pharmaceutical Company	54569-1729-01
25 gm	$37.55	BECONASE AQ, Quality Care Pharmaceuticals Inc	60346-0308-81
25 gm	$38.10	BECONASE AQ, Physicians Total Care	54868-0175-01
25 gm	$39.71	VANCENASE AQ, Pharma Pac	52959-0586-00
25 gm	$42.22	BECONASE AQ, Cheshire Drugs	55175-1893-01
25 gm	$44.00	BECONASE AQ, Southwood Pharmaceuticals Inc	58016-6451-01
25 gm	$48.00	VANCENASE AQ, Southwood Pharmaceuticals Inc	58016-6204-01
25 gm	$64.06	BECONASE AQ, Glaxosmithkline	00173-0388-79
25 gm	$65.36	BECONASE AQ, Prescript Pharmaceuticals	00247-0192-25
Spray - Nasal - 0.084 mg/Inh			
19 gm	$57.72	VANCENASE AQ DS, Schering Corporation	00085-1049-01

PRODUCT LISTING - EQUIVALENTS NOT AVAILABLE

Size	Price	Product, Manufacturer	NDC
Aerosol with Adapter - Inhalation - 0.084 mg/Inh			
4 gm x 3	$53.34	VANCERIL DS, Schering Corporation	00085-1112-03
5.40 gm x 3	$53.33	VANCERIL DS, Allscripts Pharmaceutical Company	54569-4822-00
12 gm	$53.33	VANCERIL DS, Schering Corporation	00085-1112-01
12.20 gm	$53.33	VANCERIL DS, Allscripts Pharmaceutical Company	54569-4540-00
12.20 gm	$57.52	VANCERIL DS, Pharma Pac	52959-0598-01
Aerosol with Adapter - Inhalation - 40 mcg/Inh			
7.30 gm	$49.70	QVAR, Ivax Corporation	00089-0175-40
7.30 gm	$49.70	QVAR, Ivax Corporation	59310-0175-40
Aerosol with Adapter - Inhalation - 80 mcg/Inh			
7.30 gm	$62.63	QVAR, Ivax Corporation	59310-0177-80
Spray - Nasal - 0.084 mg/Inh			
19 gm	$55.78	VANCENASE AQ DS, Allscripts Pharmaceutical Company	54569-4465-00
19 gm	$60.26	VANCENASE AQ DS, Pharma Pac	52959-0264-01

Benazepril Hydrochloride *(003053)*

For related information, see the comparative table section in Appendix A.

Categories: Hypertension, essential; Pregnancy Category D; FDA Approved 1991 Jun
Drug Classes: Angiotensin converting enzyme inhibitors
Brand Names: **Lotensin**
Foreign Brand Availability: Cibace (South-Africa); Cibacen (Austria; Bahamas; Bahrain; Barbados; Belize; Benin; Bermuda; Burkina-Faso; Curacao; Cyprus; Denmark; Egypt; Ethiopia; Finland; Gambia; Germany; Ghana; Greece; Guinea; Guyana; Indonesia; Iran; Iraq; Israel; Italy; Ivory-Coast; Jamaica; Japan; Jordan; Kenya; Korea; Kuwait; Lebanon; Liberia; Libya; Malawi; Mali; Mauritania; Mauritius; Morocco; Netherland-Antilles; Netherlands; Niger; Nigeria; Oman; Philippines; Portugal; Puerto-Rico; Qatar; Republic-of-Yemen; Saudi-Arabia; Senegal; Seychelles; Sierra-Leone; South-Africa; Spain; Sudan; Surinam; Sweden; Switzerland; Syria; Taiwan; Tanzania; Trinidad; Tunia; Uganda; United-Arab-Emirates; Zambia; Zimbabwe); Cibacen Cor (Germany); Cibacene (France)
Cost of Therapy: $25.99 (Hypertension; Lotensin; 20 mg; 1 tablet/day; 30 day supply)

WARNING

Use in Pregnancy

When used in pregnancy during the second and third trimesters, ACE inhibitors can cause injury and even death to the developing fetus. When pregnancy is detected, benazepril hydrochloride should be discontinued as soon as possible. See WARNINGS, Fetal/Neonatal Morbidity and Mortality.

DESCRIPTION

Benazepril hydrochloride is a white to off-white crystalline powder, soluble (>100 mg/ml) in water, in ethanol, and in methanol. Benazepril's chemical name is 3-[[1-(ethoxycarbonyl)-3-phenyl-(1S)-propyl]amino]-2,3,4,5-tetrahydro-2-oxo-1*H*-1-(3S)-benzazepine-1-acetic acid monohydrochloride. Its empirical formula is $C_{24}H_{28}N_2O_5{\cdot}HCl$, and its molecular weight is 460.96.

Benazeprilat, the active metabolite of benazepril, is a non-sulfhydryl angiotensin-converting enzyme inhibitor. Benazepril is converted to benazeprilat by hepatic cleavage of the ester group.

Lotensin is supplied as tablets containing 5, 10, 20, and 40 mg of benazepril hydrochloride for oral administration. The inactive ingredients are cellulose compounds, colloidal silicon dioxide, crospovidone, hydrogenated castor oil (5, 10, and 20 mg tablets), iron oxides, lactose, magnesium stearate (40 mg tablets), polysorbate 80, propylene glycol (5 and 40 mg tablets), starch, talc, and titanium dioxide.

CLINICAL PHARMACOLOGY

MECHANISM OF ACTION

Benazepril and benazeprilat inhibit angiotensin-converting enzyme (ACE) in human subjects and animals. ACE is a peptidyl dipeptidase that catalyzes the conversion of angiotensin I to the vasoconstrictor substance, angiotensin II. Angiotensin II also stimulates aldosterone secretion by the adrenal cortex.

Inhibition of ACE results in decreased plasma angiotensin II, which leads to decreased vasopressor activity and to decreased aldosterone secretion. The latter decrease may result in a small increase of serum potassium. Hypertensive patients treated with benazepril HCl alone for up to 52 weeks had elevations of serum potassium of up to 0.2 mEq/L. Similar patients treated with benazepril HCl and hydrochlorothiazide for up to 24 weeks had no consistent changes in their serum potassium (see PRECAUTIONS).

Removal of angiotensin II negative feedback on renin secretion leads to increased plasma renin activity. In animal studies, benazepril had no inhibitory effect on the vasopressor response to angiotensin II and did not interfere with the hemodynamic effects of the autonomic neurotransmitters acetylcholine, epinephrine, and norepinephrine.

ACE is identical to kininase, an enzyme that degrades bradykinin. Whether increased levels of bradykinin, a potent vasodepressor peptide, play a role in the therapeutic effects of benazepril HCl remains to be elucidated.

While the mechanism through which benazepril lowers blood pressure is believed to be primarily suppression of the renin-angiotensin-aldosterone system, benazepril has an antihypertensive effect even in patients with low-renin hypertension (see INDICATIONS AND USAGE).

PHARMACOKINETICS AND METABOLISM

Following oral administration of benazepril HCl, peak plasma concentrations of benazepril are reached within 0.5-1.0 hours. The extent of absorption is at least 37% as determined by urinary recovery and is not significantly influenced by the presence of food in the GI tract.

Cleavage of the ester group (primarily in the liver) converts benazepril to its active metabolite, benazeprilat. Peak plasma concentrations of benazeprilat are reached 1-2 hours after drug intake in the fasting state and 2-4 hours after drug intake in the nonfasting state. The serum protein binding of benazepril is about 96.7% and that of benazeprilat about 95.3%, as measured by equilibrium dialysis; on the basis of *in vitro* studies, the degree of protein binding should be unaffected by age, hepatic dysfunction, or concentration (over the concentration range of 0.24-23.6 μmol/L).

Benazepril is almost completely metabolized to benazeprilat, which has much greater ACE inhibitory activity than benazepril, and to the glucuronide conjugates of benazepril and benazeprilat. Only trace amounts of an administered dose of benazepril HCl can be recovered in the urine as unchanged benazepril, while about 20% of the dose is excreted as benazeprilat, 4% as benazepril glucuronide, and 8% as benazeprilat glucuronide.

The kinetics of benazepril are approximately dose-proportional within the dosage range of 10-80 mg.

The effective half-life of accumulation of benazeprilat following multiple dosing of benazepril hydrochloride is 10-11 hours. Thus, steady-state concentrations of benazeprilat should be reached after 2 or 3 doses of benazepril hydrochloride given once daily.

The kinetics did not change, and there was no significant accumulation during chronic administration (28 days) of once-daily doses between 5 mg and 20 mg. Accumulation ratios based on AUC and urinary recovery of benazeprilat were 1.19 and 1.27, respectively.

When dialysis was started 2 hours after ingestion of 10 mg of benazepril, approximately 6% of benazeprilat was removed in 4 hours of dialysis. The parent compound, benazepril, was not detected in the dialysate.

The disposition of benazepril and benazeprilat in patients with mild-to-moderate renal insufficiency (creatinine clearance >30 ml/min) is similar to that in patients with normal renal function. In patients with creatinine clearance ≤30 ml/min, peak benazeprilat levels and the initial (alpha phase) half-life increase, and time to steady state may be delayed (see DOSAGE AND ADMINISTRATION).

Benazepril and benazeprilat are cleared predominantly by renal excretion in healthy subjects with normal renal function. Nonrenal (*i.e.*, biliary) excretion accounts for approximately 11-12% of benazeprilat excretion in healthy subjects. In patients with renal failure, biliary clearance may compensate to an extent for deficient renal clearance.

In patients with hepatic dysfunction due to cirrhosis, levels of benazeprilat are essentially unaltered. The pharmacokinetics of benazepril and benazeprilat do not appear to be influenced by age.

In studies in rats given ^{14}C-benazepril, benazepril and its metabolites crossed the blood-brain barrier only to an extremely low extent. Multiple doses of benazepril did not result in accumulation in any tissue except the lung, where, as with other ACE inhibitors in similar studies, there was a slight increase in concentration due to slow elimination in that organ.

Some placental passage occurred when the drug was administered to pregnant rats.

PHARMACODYNAMICS

Single and multiple doses of 10 mg or more of benazepril HCl cause inhibition of plasma ACE activity by at least 80-90% for at least 24 hours after dosing. Pressor responses to exogenous angiotensin I were inhibited by 60-90% (up to 4 hours post-dose) at the 10 mg dose.

Administration of benazepril HCl to patients with mild-to-moderate hypertension results in a reduction of both supine and standing blood pressure to about the same extent with no compensatory tachycardia. Symptomatic postural hypotension is infrequent, although it can occur in patients who are salt- and/or volume-depleted (see WARNINGS).

In single-dose studies, benazepril HCl lowered blood pressure within 1 hour, with peak reductions achieved 2-4 hours after dosing. The antihypertensive effect of a single dose persisted for 24 hours. In multiple-dose studies, once-daily doses of 20-80 mg decreased seated pressure (systolic/diastolic) 24 hours after dosing by about 6-12/4-7 mm Hg. The trough values represent reductions of about 50% of that seen at peak.

Four dose-response studies using once-daily dosing were conducted in 470 mild-to-moderate hypertensive patients not using diuretics. The minimal effective once-daily dose of benazepril HCl was 10 mg; but further falls in blood pressure, especially at morning trough, were seen with higher doses in the studied dosing range (10-80 mg). In studies comparing the same daily dose of benazepril HCl given as a single morning dose or as a twice-daily dose, blood pressure reductions at the time of morning trough blood levels were greater with the divided regimen.

During chronic therapy, the maximum reduction in blood pressure with any dose is generally achieved after 1-2 weeks. The antihypertensive effects of benazepril HCl have continued during therapy for at least 2 years. Abrupt withdrawal of benazepril HCl has not been associated with a rapid increase in blood pressure.

In patients with mild-to-moderate hypertension, benazepril HCl 10-20 mg was similar in effectiveness to captopril, hydrochlorothiazide, nifedipine SR, and propranolol.

The antihypertensive effects of benazepril HCl were not appreciably different in patients receiving high- or low-sodium diets.

In hemodynamic studies in dogs, blood pressure reduction was accompanied by a reduction in peripheral arterial resistance, with an increase in cardiac output and renal blood flow and little or no change in heart rate. In normal human volunteers, single doses of benazepril caused an increase in renal blood flow but had no effect on glomerular filtration rate.

Use of benazepril HCl in combination with thiazide diuretics gives a blood-pressure-lowering effect greater than that seen with either agent alone. By blocking the renin-angiotensin-aldosterone axis, administration of benazepril HCl tends to reduce the potassium loss associated with the diuretic.

INDICATIONS AND USAGE

Benazepril HCl is indicated for the treatment of hypertension. It may be used alone or in combination with thiazide diuretics.

In using benazepril HCl, consideration should be given to the fact that another angiotensin-converting enzyme inhibitor, captopril, has caused agranulocytosis, particularly in patients with renal impairment or collagen-vascular disease. Available data are insufficient to show that benazepril HCl does not have a similar risk (see WARNINGS).

Black patients receiving ACE-inhibitors have been reported to have a higher incidence of angioedema compared to nonblacks. It should also be noted that in controlled clinical trials ACE inhibitors have an effect on blood pressure that is less in black patients than in non-blacks.

NON-FDA APPROVED INDICATIONS

Data have shown that some ACE inhibitors improve survival and exercise tolerance and reduce the incidence of overt heart failure and associated hospitalization in patients with recent myocardial infarction. Some ACE inhibitors have been shown to reduce the incidence of heart failure in patients with asymptomatic left ventricular dysfunction. ACE inhibitors have been shown to decrease proteinuria and preserve renal function in patients with hypertension and diabetes mellitus better than other antihypertensive agents. ACE inhibitors have also been shown to decrease the progression of nephropathy in normotensive patients with type II diabetes mellitus. Results from at least one study have shown improvement in insulin resistance and glucose tolerance in uremic patients treated with benazepril.

CONTRAINDICATIONS

Benazepril HCl is contraindicated in patients who are hypersensitive to this product or to any other ACE inhibitor.

WARNINGS

ANAPHYLACTOID AND POSSIBLY RELATED REACTIONS

Presumably because angiotensin-converting enzyme inhibitors affect the metabolism of eicosanoids and polypeptides, including endogenous bradykinin, patients receiving ACE inhibitors (including benazepril HCl) may be subject to a variety of adverse reactions, some of them serious.

Angioedema

Angioedema of the face, extremities, lips, tongue, glottis, and larynx has been reported in patients treated with angiotensin-converting enzyme inhibitors. In US clinical trials, symptoms consistent with angioedema were seen in none of the subjects who received placebo and in about 0.5% of the subjects who received benazepril HCl. Angioedema associated with laryngeal edema can be fatal. If laryngeal stridor or angioedema of the face, tongue, or glottis occurs, treatment with benazepril HCl should be discontinued and appropriate therapy instituted immediately. **Where there is involvement of the tongue, glottis, or larynx, likely to cause airway obstruction, appropriate therapy, *e.g.*, subcutaneous epinephrine injection 1:1000 (0.3-0.5 ml) should be promptly administered (see ADVERSE REACTIONS).**

Anaphylactoid Reactions During Desensitization

Two patients undergoing desensitizing treatment with hymenoptera venom while receiving ACE inhibitors sustained life-threatening anaphylactoid reactions. In the same patients, these reactions were avoided when ACE inhibitors were temporarily withheld, but they reappeared upon inadvertent rechallenge.

Anaphylactoid Reactions During Membrane Exposure

Anaphylactoid reactions have been reported in patients dialyzed with high-flux membranes and treated concomitantly with an ACE inhibitor. Anaphylactoid reactions have also been reported in patients undergoing low-density lipoprotein apheresis with dextran sulfate absorption (a procedure dependent upon devices not approved in the US).

HYPOTENSION

Benazepril HCl can cause symptomatic hypotension. Like other ACE inhibitors, benazepril has been only rarely associated with hypotension in uncomplicated hypertensive patients. Symptomatic hypotension is most likely to occur in patients who have been volume- and/or salt-depleted as a result of prolonged diuretic therapy, dietary salt restriction, dialysis, diarrhea, or vomiting. Volume- and/or salt-depletion should be corrected before initiating therapy with benazepril HCl.

In patients with congestive heart failure, with or without associated renal insufficiency, ACE inhibitor therapy may cause excessive hypotension, which may be associated with oliguria or azotemia and, rarely, with acute renal failure and death. In such patients, benazepril HCl therapy should be started under close medical supervision; they should be followed closely for the first 2 weeks of treatment and whenever the dose of benazepril or diuretic is increased.

If hypotension occurs, the patient should be placed in a supine position, and, if necessary, treated with intravenous infusion of physiological saline. Benazepril HCl treatment usually can be continued following restoration of blood pressure and volume.

NEUTROPENIA/AGRANULOCYTOSIS

Another angiotensin-converting enzyme inhibitor, captopril, has been shown to cause agranulocytosis and bone marrow depression, rarely in uncomplicated patients, but more frequently in patients with renal impairment, especially if they also have a collagen-vascular disease such as systemic lupus erythematosus or scleroderma. Available data from clinical trials of benazepril are insufficient to show that benazepril does not cause agranulocytosis at similar rates. Monitoring of white blood cell counts should be considered in patients with collagen-vascular disease, especially if the disease is associated with impaired renal function.

FETAL/NEONATAL MORBIDITY AND MORTALITY

ACE inhibitors can cause fetal and neonatal morbidity and death when administered to pregnant women. Several dozen cases have been reported in the world literature. When pregnancy is detected, ACE inhibitors should be discontinued as soon as possible.

The use of ACE inhibitors during the second and third trimesters of pregnancy has been associated with fetal and neonatal injury, including hypotension, neonatal skull hypoplasia, anuria, reversible or irreversible renal failure, and death. Oligohydramnios has also been reported, presumably resulting from decreased fetal renal function; oligohydramnios in this setting has been associated with fetal limb contractures, craniofacial deformation, and hypoplastic lung development. Prematurity, intrauterine growth retardation, and patent ductus arteriosus have also been reported, although it is not clear whether these occurrences were due to the ACE inhibitor exposure.

These adverse effects do not appear to have resulted from intrauterine ACE inhibitor exposure that has been limited to the first trimester. Mothers whose embryos and fetuses are exposed to ACE inhibitors only during the first trimester should be so informed. Nonetheless, when patients become pregnant, physicians should make every effort to discontinue the use of benazepril as soon as possible.

Rarely (probably less often than once in every thousand pregnancies), no alternative to ACE inhibitors will be found. In these rare cases, the mothers should be apprised of the potential hazards to their fetuses, and serial ultrasound examinations should be performed to assess the intraamniotic environment.

If oligohydramnios is observed, benazepril should be discontinued unless it is considered life-saving for the mother. Contraction stress testing (CST), a nonstress test (NST), or biophysical profiling (BPP) may be appropriate, depending upon the week of pregnancy. Patients and physicians should be aware, however, that oligohydramnios may not appear until after the fetus has sustained irreversible injury.

Infants with histories of *in utero* exposure to ACE inhibitors should be closely observed for hypotension, oliguria, and hyperkalemia. If oliguria occurs, attention should be directed toward support of blood pressure and renal perfusion. Exchange transfusion or dialysis may be required as means of reversing hypotension and/or substituting for disordered renal function. Benazepril, which crosses the placenta, can theoretically be removed from the neonatal circulation by these means; there are occasional reports of benefit from these maneuvers with another ACE inhibitor, but experience is limited.

No teratogenic effects of benazepril HCl were seen in studies of pregnant rats, mice, and rabbits. On a mg/m^2 basis, the doses used in these studies were 60 times (in rats), 9 times (in mice), and more than 0.8 times (in rabbits) the maximum recommended human dose (assuming a 50 kg woman). On a mg/kg basis these multiples are 300 times (in rats), 90 times (in mice), and more than 3 times (in rabbits) the maximum recommended human dose.

HEPATIC FAILURE

Rarely, ACE inhibitors have been associated with a syndrome that starts with cholestatic jaundice and progresses to fulminant hepatic necrosis and (sometimes) death. The mechanism of this syndrome is not understood. Patients receiving ACE inhibitors who develop jaundice or marked elevations of hepatic enzymes should discontinue the ACE inhibitor and receive appropriate medical follow-up.

PRECAUTIONS

GENERAL

Impaired Renal Function

As a consequence of inhibiting the renin-angiotensin-aldosterone system, changes in renal function may be anticipated in susceptible individuals. In patients with severe congestive heart failure whose renal function may depend on the activity of the renin-angiotensin-aldosterone system, treatment with angiotensin-converting enzyme inhibitors, including benazepril HCl, may be associated with oliguria and/or progressive azotemia and (rarely) with acute renal failure and/or death. In a small study of hypertensive patients with renal artery stenosis in a solitary kidney or bilateral renal artery stenosis, treatment with benazepril HCl was associated with increases in blood urea nitrogen and serum creatinine; these increases were reversible upon discontinuation of benazepril HCl or diuretic therapy, or both. When such patients are treated with ACE inhibitors, renal function should be monitored during the first few weeks of therapy. Some hypertensive patients with no apparent preexisting renal vascular disease have developed increases in blood urea nitrogen and serum creatinine, usually minor and transient, especially when benazepril HCl has been given concomitantly with a diuretic. This is more likely to occur in patients with preexisting renal impairment. Dosage reduction of benazepril HCl and/or discontinuation of the diuretic may be required. **Evaluation of the hypertensive patient should always include assessment of renal function (see DOSAGE AND ADMINISTRATION).**

Hyperkalemia

In clinical trials, hyperkalemia (serum potassium at least 0.5 mEq/L greater than the upper limit of normal) occurred in approximately 1% of hypertensive patients receiving benazepril HCl. In most cases, these were isolated values which resolved despite continued therapy. Risk factors for the development of hyperkalemia include renal insufficiency, diabetes mellitus, and the concomitant use of potassium-sparing diuretics, potassium supplements, and/or potassium-containing salt substitutes, which should be used cautiously, if at all, with benazepril HCl (see DRUG INTERACTIONS).

Cough

Presumably due to the inhibition of the degradation of endogenous bradykinin, persistent nonproductive cough has been reported with all ACE inhibitors, always resolving after discontinuation of therapy. ACE inhibitor-induced cough should be considered in the differential diagnosis of cough.

Impaired Liver Function

In patients with hepatic dysfunction due to cirrhosis, levels of benazeprilat are essentially unaltered (see WARNINGS, Hepatic Failure).

Surgery/Anesthesia

In patients undergoing surgery or during anesthesia with agents that produce hypotension, benazepril will block the angiotensin II formation that could otherwise occur secondary to compensatory renin release. Hypotension that occurs as a result of this mechanism can be corrected by volume expansion.

INFORMATION FOR THE PATIENT

Pregnancy

Female patients of childbearing age should be told about the consequences of second- and third-trimester exposure to ACE inhibitors, and they should also be told that these consequences do not appear to have resulted from intrauterine ACE inhibitor exposure that has been limited to the first trimester. These patients should be asked to report pregnancies to their physicians as soon as possible.

Angioedema

Angioedema, including laryngeal edema, can occur at any time with treatment with ACE inhibitors. Patients should be so advised and told to report immediately any signs or symptoms suggesting angioedema (swelling of face, eyes, lips, or tongue, or difficulty in breathing) and to take no more drug until they have consulted with the prescribing physician.

Symptomatic Hypotension

Patients should be cautioned that lightheadedness can occur, especially during the first days of therapy, and it should be reported to the prescribing physician. Patients should be told that if syncope occurs, benazepril HCl should be discontinued until the prescribing physician has been consulted.

All patients should be cautioned that inadequate fluid intake or excessive perspiration, diarrhea, or vomiting can lead to an excessive fall in blood pressure, with the same consequences of lightheadedness and possible syncope.

Hyperkalemia

Patients should be told not to use potassium supplements or salt substitutes containing potassium without consulting the prescribing physician.

Neutropenia

Patients should be told to promptly report any indication of infection (*e.g.*, sore throat, fever), which could be a sign of neutropenia.

CARCINOGENESIS, MUTAGENESIS, AND IMPAIRMENT OF FERTILITY

No evidence of carcinogenicity was found when benazepril was administered to rats and mice for up to 2 years at doses of up to 150 mg/kg/day. When compared on the basis of body weights, this dose is 110 times the maximum recommended human dose. When compared on the basis of body surface areas, this dose is 18 and 9 times (rats and mice, respectively) the maximum recommended human dose (calculations assume a patient weight of 60 kg). No mutagenic activity was detected in the Ames test in bacteria (with or without metabolic activation), in an *in vitro* test for forward mutations in cultured mammalian cells, or in a nucleus anomaly test. In doses of 50-500 mg/kg/day (6-60 times the maximum recommended human dose based on mg/m^2 comparison and 37-375 times the maximum recommended human dose based on a mg/kg comparison), benazepril HCl had no adverse effect on the reproductive performance of male and female rats.

PREGNANCY CATEGORY C (FIRST TRIMESTER) AND D (SECOND AND THIRD TRIMESTERS)

See WARNINGS, Fetal/Neonatal Morbidity and Mortality.

NURSING MOTHERS

Minimal amounts of unchanged benazepril and of benazeprilat are excreted into the breast milk of lactating women treated with benazepril. A newborn child ingesting entirely breast milk would receive less than 0.1% of the mg/kg maternal dose of benazepril and benazeprilat.

GERIATRIC USE

Of the total number of patients who received benazepril in US clinical studies of benazepril HCl, 18% were 65 or older while 2% were 75 or older. No overall differences in effectiveness or safety were observed between these patients and younger patients, and other reported clinical experience has not identified differences in responses between the elderly and younger patients, but greater sensitivity of some older individuals cannot be ruled out.

PEDIATRIC USE

Safety and effectiveness in pediatric patients have not been established.

DRUG INTERACTIONS

DIURETICS

Patients on diuretics, especially those in whom diuretic therapy was recently instituted, may occasionally experience an excessive reduction of blood pressure after initiation of therapy with benazepril HCl. The possibility of hypotensive effects with benazepril HCl can be minimized by either discontinuing the diuretic or increasing the salt intake prior to initiation of treatment with benazepril HCl. If this is not possible, the starting dose should be reduced (see DOSAGE AND ADMINISTRATION).

POTASSIUM SUPPLEMENTS AND POTASSIUM-SPARING DIURETICS

Benazepril HCl can attenuate potassium loss caused by thiazide diuretics. Potassium-sparing diuretics (spironolactone, amiloride, triamterene, and others) or potassium supplements can increase the risk of hyperkalemia. Therefore, if concomitant use of such agents is indicated, they should be given with caution, and the patient's serum potassium should be monitored frequently.

ORAL ANTICOAGULANTS

Interaction studies with warfarin and acenocoumarol failed to identify any clinically important effects on the serum concentrations or clinical effects of these anticoagulants.

LITHIUM

Increased serum lithium levels and symptoms of lithium toxicity have been reported in patients receiving ACE inhibitors during therapy with lithium. These drugs should be coadministered with caution, and frequent monitoring of serum lithium levels is recommended. If a diuretic is also used, the risk of lithium toxicity may be increased.

OTHER

No clinically important pharmacokinetic interactions occurred when benazepril HCl was administered concomitantly with hydrochlorothiazide, chlorthalidone, furosemide, digoxin, propranolol, atenolol, naproxen, or cimetidine.

Benazepril HCl has been used concomitantly with beta-adrenergic-blocking agents, calcium-channel-blocking agents, diuretics, digoxin, and hydralazine, without evidence of clinically important adverse interactions. Benazepril, like other ACE inhibitors, has had less than additive effects with beta-adrenergic blockers, presumably because both drugs lower blood pressure by inhibiting parts of the renin-angiotensin system.

ADVERSE REACTIONS

Benazepril HCl has been evaluated for safety in over 6000 patients with hypertension; over 700 of these patients were treated for at least 1 year. The overall incidence of reported adverse events was comparable in benazepril HCl and placebo patients.

The reported side effects were generally mild and transient, and there was no relation between side effects and age, duration of therapy, or total dosage within the range of 2-80 mg. Discontinuation of therapy because of a side effect was required in approximately 5% of US patients treated with benazepril HCl and in 3% of patients treated with placebo.

The most common reasons for discontinuation were headache (0.6%) and cough (0.5%) (see PRECAUTIONS, General, Cough).

The side effects considered possibly or probably related to study drug that occurred in US placebo-controlled trials in more than 1% of patients treated with benazepril HCl are shown in TABLE 1.

TABLE 1 *Patients in US Placebo-Controlled Studies*

	Benazepril HCl (n=964)		Placebo (n=496)	
	n	%	n	%
Headache	60	6.2%	21	4.2%
Dizziness	35	3.6%	12	2.4%
Fatigue	23	2.4%	11	2.2%
Somnolence	15	1.6%	2	0.4%
Postural dizziness	14	1.5%	1	0.2%
Nausea	13	1.3%	5	1.0%
Cough	12	1.2%	5	1.0%

Other adverse experiences reported in controlled clinical trials (in less than 1% of benazepril patients), and rarer events seen in postmarketing experience, include the following (in some, a causal relationship to drug use is uncertain):

Cardiovascular: Symptomatic hypotension was seen in 0.3% of patients, postural hypotension in 0.4%, and syncope in 0.1%; these reactions led to discontinuation of therapy in 4 patients who had received benazepril monotherapy and in 9 patients who had received benazepril with hydrochlorothiazide (see PRECAUTIONS and WARNINGS). Other reports included angina pectoris, palpitations, and peripheral edema.

Renal: Of hypertensive patients with no apparent preexisting renal disease, about 2% have sustained increases in serum creatinine to at least 150% of their baseline values while receiving benazepril HCl, but most of these increases have disappeared despite continuing treatment. A much smaller fraction of these patients (less than 0.1%) developed simultaneous (usually transient) increases in blood urea nitrogen and serum creatinine.

Fetal/Neonatal Morbidity and Mortality: See WARNINGS, Fetal/Neonatal Morbidity and Mortality.

Angioedema: Angioedema has been reported in patients receiving ACE inhibitors. During clinical trials in hypertensive patients with benazepril, 0.5% of patients experienced edema of the lips or face without other manifestations of angioedema. Angioedema associated with laryngeal edema and/or shock may be fatal. If angioedema of the face, extremities, lips, tongue, or glottis and/or larynx occurs, treatment with benazepril HCl should be discontinued and appropriate therapy instituted immediately (see WARNINGS).

Dermatologic: Stevens-Johnson syndrome, pemphigus, apparent hypersensitivity reactions (manifested by dermatitis, pruritus, or rash), photosensitivity, and flushing.

Gastrointestinal: Pancreatitis, constipation, gastritis, vomiting, and melena.

Hematologic: Thrombocytopenia and hemolytic anemia.

Neurologic and Psychiatric: Anxiety, decreased libido, hypertonia, insomnia, nervousness, and paresthesia.

Other: Asthma, bronchitis, dyspnea, sinusitus, urinary tract infection, infection, arthritis, impotence, alopecia, arthralgia, myalgia, asthenia, and sweating.

Another potentially important adverse experience, eosinophilic pneumonitis, has been attributed to other ACE inhibitors.

DOSAGE AND ADMINISTRATION

The recommended initial dose for patients not receiving a diuretic is 10 mg once-a-day. The usual maintenance dosage range is 20-40 mg/day administered as a single dose or in 2 equally divided doses. A dose of 80 mg gives an increased response, but experience with this dose is limited. The divided regimen was more effective in controlling trough (pre-dosing) blood pressure than the same dose given as a once-daily regimen. Dosage adjustment should be based on measurement of peak (2-6 hours after dosing) and trough responses. If a once-daily regimen does not give adequate trough response, an increase in dosage or divided administration should be considered. If blood pressure is not controlled with benazepril HCl alone, a diuretic can be added.

Total daily doses above 80 mg have not been evaluated.

Concomitant administration of benazepril HCl with potassium supplements, potassium salt substitutes, or potassium-sparing diuretics can lead to increases of serum potassium (see PRECAUTIONS).

In patients who are currently being treated with a diuretic, symptomatic hypotension occasionally can occur following the initial dose of benazepril HCl. To reduce the likelihood of hypotension, the diuretic should, if possible, be discontinued 2-3 days prior to beginning therapy with benazepril HCl (see WARNINGS). Then, if blood pressure is not controlled with benazepril HCl alone, diuretic therapy should be resumed.

If the diuretic cannot be discontinued, an initial dose of 5 mg benazepril HCl should be used to avoid excessive hypotension.

DOSAGE ADJUSTMENT IN RENAL IMPAIRMENT

For patients with a creatinine clearance <30 ml/min/1.73 m^2 (serum creatinine >3 mg/dl), the recommended initial dose is 5 mg benazepril HCl once daily. Dosage may be titrated upward until blood pressure is controlled or to a maximum total daily dose of 40 mg (see WARNINGS).

HOW SUPPLIED

Lotensin is available in tablets in the following strengths:

5 mg: Light yellow tablets imprinted with "LOTENSIN" on one side and "5" on the other.

10 mg: Dark yellow tablets imprinted with "LOTENSIN" on one side and "10" on the other.

20 mg: Pink tablets imprinted with "LOTENSIN" on one side and "20" on the other.

40 mg: Dark rose tablets imprinted with "LOTENSIN" on one side and "40" on the other.

Storage: Do not store above 30°C (86°F). Protect from moisture.

Dispense in tight container.

PRODUCT LISTING - EQUIVALENTS NOT AVAILABLE

Tablet - Oral - 5 mg			
30's	$29.07	LOTENSIN, Physicians Total Care	54868-3690-01
90's	$98.31	LOTENSIN, Novartis Pharmaceuticals	00083-0059-90
100's	$109.25	LOTENSIN, Novartis Pharmaceuticals	00083-0059-30
100's	$109.25	LOTENSIN, Novartis Pharmaceuticals	00083-0059-32
Tablet - Oral - 10 mg			
10's	$8.90	LOTENSIN, Southwood Pharmaceuticals Inc	58016-0420-10
25's	$32.75	LOTENSIN, Pd-Rx Pharmaceuticals	55289-0109-97
30's	$25.99	LOTENSIN, Allscripts Pharmaceutical Company	54569-3423-01
30's	$26.69	LOTENSIN, Southwood Pharmaceuticals Inc	58016-0420-30
30's	$30.75	LOTENSIN, Pd-Rx Pharmaceuticals	55289-0109-30
60's	$53.37	LOTENSIN, Southwood Pharmaceuticals Inc	58016-0420-60
60's	$60.04	LOTENSIN, Physicians Total Care	54868-2350-01
90's	$80.06	LOTENSIN, Southwood Pharmaceuticals Inc	58016-0420-90
90's	$81.00	LOTENSIN, Novartis Pharmaceuticals	00083-0063-90
100's	$86.64	LOTENSIN, Allscripts Pharmaceutical Company	54569-3423-00
100's	$88.95	LOTENSIN, Southwood Pharmaceuticals Inc	58016-0420-00
100's	$98.69	LOTENSIN, Physicians Total Care	54868-2350-02
100's	$109.25	LOTENSIN, Novartis Pharmaceuticals	00083-0063-30
100's	$109.25	LOTENSIN, Novartis Pharmaceuticals	00083-0063-32
Tablet - Oral - 20 mg			
10's	$8.90	LOTENSIN, Southwood Pharmaceuticals Inc	58016-0685-10
25's	$33.75	LOTENSIN, Pd-Rx Pharmaceuticals	55289-0086-97
30's	$24.50	LOTENSIN, Southwood Pharmaceuticals Inc	58016-0685-30
30's	$25.99	LOTENSIN, Allscripts Pharmaceutical Company	54569-3359-00
30's	$30.61	LOTENSIN, Physicians Total Care	54868-2351-00
30's	$33.33	LOTENSIN, Pd-Rx Pharmaceuticals	55289-0086-30
60's	$53.37	LOTENSIN, Southwood Pharmaceuticals Inc	58016-0685-60
90's	$80.06	LOTENSIN, Southwood Pharmaceuticals Inc	58016-0685-90
90's	$81.00	LOTENSIN, Novartis Pharmaceuticals	00083-0079-90
100's	$86.64	LOTENSIN, Allscripts Pharmaceutical Company	54569-3359-01
100's	$88.95	LOTENSIN, Southwood Pharmaceuticals Inc	58016-0685-00
100's	$109.25	LOTENSIN, Novartis Pharmaceuticals	00083-0079-30
100's	$109.25	LOTENSIN, Novartis Pharmaceuticals	00083-0079-32
Tablet - Oral - 40 mg			
10's	$8.90	LOTENSIN, Southwood Pharmaceuticals Inc	58016-0686-10
30's	$25.99	LOTENSIN, Allscripts Pharmaceutical Company	54569-4788-00
30's	$26.69	LOTENSIN, Southwood Pharmaceuticals Inc	58016-0686-30
30's	$29.07	LOTENSIN, Physicians Total Care	54868-2352-00
60's	$53.37	LOTENSIN, Southwood Pharmaceuticals Inc	58016-0686-60
90's	$80.06	LOTENSIN, Southwood Pharmaceuticals Inc	58016-0686-90
90's	$98.31	LOTENSIN, Novartis Pharmaceuticals	00083-0094-90
100's	$88.95	LOTENSIN, Southwood Pharmaceuticals Inc	58016-0686-00
100's	$109.25	LOTENSIN, Novartis Pharmaceuticals	00083-0094-30
100's	$109.25	LOTENSIN, Novartis Pharmaceuticals	00083-0094-32

B

Benazepril Hydrochloride; Hydrochlorothiazide (003124)

For complete prescribing information, refer to the CD-ROM included with the book.

Categories: Hypertension, essential; Pregnancy Category D; FDA Approved 1992 May
Drug Classes: Angiotensin converting enzyme inhibitors; Diuretics, thiazide and derivatives
Brand Names: Lotensin HCT
Foreign Brand Availability: Cibacen HCT (Portugal); Cibadrex (Bahamas; Bahrain; Barbados; Belize; Benin; Bermuda; Burkina-Faso; Curacao; Cyprus; Egypt; Ethiopia; France; Gambia; Germany; Ghana; Guinea; Guyana; Indonesia; Iran; Iraq; Ivory-Coast; Jamaica; Jordan; Kenya; Kuwait; Lebanon; Liberia; Libya; Malawi; Mali; Mauritania; Mauritius; Morocco; Netherland-Antilles; Netherlands; Niger; Nigeria; Oman; Qatar; Republic-of-Yemen; Saudi-Arabia; Senegal; Seychelles; Sierra-Leone; South-Africa; Sudan; Surinam; Switzerland; Syria; Tanzania; Trinidad; Tunia; Uganda; United-Arab-Emirates; Zambia; Zimbabwe)
Cost of Therapy: $32.78 (Hypertension; Lotensin HCT; 20 mg;12.5 mg; 1 tablet/day; 30 day supply)

WARNING

Note: The trade name has been used throughout this monograph for clarity.

USE IN PREGNANCY

When used in pregnancy during the second and third trimesters, ACE inhibitors can cause injury and even death to the developing fetus. When pregnancy is detected, Lotensin HCT should be discontinued as soon as possible. See WARNINGS, Fetal/Neonatal Morbidity and Mortality.

DESCRIPTION

Benazepril hydrochloride is a white to off-white crystalline powder, soluble (>100 mg/ml) in water, in ethanol, and in methanol. Benazepril hydrochloride's chemical name is 3-[[1-(ethoxy-carbonyl)-3-phenyl-(1S)-propyl]amino]-2,3,4,5-tetrahydro-2-oxo-1*H*-1-(3S)-benzazepine-1-acetic acid monohydrochloride.

Its empirical formula is $C_{24}H_{28}N_2O_5$·HCl, and its molecular weight is 460.96.

Benazeprilat, the active metabolite of benazepril, is a nonsulfhydryl angiotensin-converting enzyme inhibitor. Benazepril is converted to benazeprilat by hepatic cleavage of the ester group.

Hydrochlorothiazide is a white, or practically white, practically odorless, crystalline powder. It is slightly soluble in water; freely soluble in sodium hydroxide solution, in n-butylamine, and in dimethylformamide; sparingly soluble in methanol; and insoluble in ether, in chloroform, and in dilute mineral acids. Hydrochlorothiazide's chemical name is 6-chloro-3,4-dihydro-2*H*-1,2,4-benzothiadiazine-7-sulfonamide 1,1-dioxide.

Its empirical formula is $C_7H_8ClN_3O_4S_2$, and its molecular weight is 297.73. Hydrochlorothiazide is a thiazide diuretic.

Lotensin HCT is a combination of benazepril hydrochloride and hydrochlorothiazide. The tablets are formulated for oral administration with a combination of 5, 10, or 20 mg of benazepril hydrochloride and 6.25, 12.5, or 25 mg of hydrochlorothiazide. The inactive ingredients of the tablets are cellulose compounds, crospovidone, hydrogenated castor oil, iron oxides (10/12.5 mg, 20/12.5 mg, and 20/25 mg tablets), lactose, polyethylene glycol, talc, and titanium dioxide.

INDICATIONS AND USAGE

Lotensin HCT is indicated for the treatment of hypertension.

This fixed combination drug is not indicated for the initial therapy of hypertension (see DOSAGE AND ADMINISTRATION).

In using Lotensin HCT, consideration should be given to the fact that another angiotensin-converting enzyme inhibitor, captopril, has caused agranulocytosis, particularly in patients with renal impairment or collagen-vascular disease. Available data are insufficient to show that benazepril does not have a similar risk (see WARNINGS, Neutropenia/Agranulocytosis).

Black patients receiving ACE inhibitors have been reported to have a higher incidence of angioedema compared to nonblacks.

CONTRAINDICATIONS

Lotensin HCT is contraindicated in patients who are anuric.

Lotensin HCT is also contraindicated in patients who are hypersensitive to benazepril, to any other ACE inhibitor, to hydrochlorothiazide, or to other sulfonamide-derived drugs. Hypersensitivity reactions are more likely to occur in patients with a history of allergy or bronchial asthma.

WARNINGS

ANAPHYLACTOID AND POSSIBLY RELATED REACTIONS

Presumably because angiotensin-converting enzyme inhibitors affect the metabolism of eicosanoids and polypeptides, including endogenous bradykinin, patients receiving ACE inhibitors (including Lotensin HCT) may be subject to a variety of adverse reactions, some of them serious.

Angioedema

Angioedema of the face, extremities, lips, tongue, glottis, and larynx has been reported in patients treated with angiotensin-converting enzyme inhibitors. In US clinical trials, symptoms consistent with angioedema were seen in none of the subjects who received placebo and in about 0.5% of the subjects who received benazepril. Angioedema associated with laryngeal edema can be fatal. If laryngeal stridor or angioedema of the face, tongue, or glottis occurs, treatment with Lotensin HCT should be discontinued and appropriate therapy instituted immediately. *When involvement of the tongue, glottis, or larynx appears likely to cause airway obstruction, appropriate therapy, e.g., subcutaneous epinephrine injection 1:1000 (0.3-0.5 ml) should be promptly administered.*

Anaphylactoid Reactions During Desensitization

Two patients undergoing desensitizing treatment with hymenoptera venom while receiving ACE inhibitors sustained life-threatening anaphylactoid reactions. In the same patients, these reactions were avoided when ACE inhibitors were temporarily withheld, but they reappeared upon inadvertent rechallenge.

Anaphylactoid Reactions During Membrane Exposure

Anaphylactoid reactions have been reported in patients dialyzed with high-flux membranes and treated concomitantly with an ACE inhibitor. Anaphylactoid reactions have also been reported in patients undergoing low-density lipoprotein apheresis with dextran sulfate absorption.

HYPOTENSION

Lotensin HCT can cause symptomatic hypotension. Like other ACE inhibitors, benazepril has been only rarely associated with hypotension in uncomplicated hypertensive patients. Symptomatic hypotension is most likely to occur in patients who have been volume and/or salt depleted as a result of prolonged diuretic therapy, dietary salt restriction, dialysis, diarrhea, or vomiting. Volume and/or salt depletion should be corrected before initiating therapy with Lotensin HCT.

Lotensin HCT should be used cautiously in patients receiving concomitant therapy with other antihypertensives. The thiazide component of Lotensin HCT may potentiate the action of other antihypertensive drugs, especially ganglionic or peripheral adrenergic-blocking drugs. The antihypertensive effects of the thiazide component may also be enhanced in the postsympathectomy patient.

In patients with congestive heart failure, with or without associated renal insufficiency, ACE inhibitor therapy may cause excessive hypotension, which may be associated with oliguria, azotemia, and (rarely) with acute renal failure and death. In such patients, Lotensin HCT therapy should be started under close medical supervision; they should be followed closely for the first 2 weeks of treatment and whenever the dose of benazepril or diuretic is increased.

If hypotension occurs, the patient should be placed in a supine position, and, if necessary, treated with intravenous infusion of physiological saline. Lotensin HCT treatment usually can be continued following restoration of blood pressure and volume.

IMPAIRED RENAL FUNCTION

Lotensin HCT should be used with caution in patients with severe renal disease. Thiazides may precipitate azotemia in such patients, and the effects of repeated dosing may be cumulative.

When the renin-angiotensin-aldosterone system is inhibited by benazepril, changes in renal function may be anticipated in susceptible individuals. In patients with **severe congestive heart failure,** whose renal function may depend on the activity of the renin-angiotensin-aldosterone system, treatment with angiotensin-converting enzyme inhibitors (including benazepril) may be associated with oliguria and/or progressive azotemia and (rarely) with acute renal failure and/or death.

In a small study of hypertensive patients with **unilateral or bilateral renal artery stenosis,** treatment with benazepril was associated with increases in blood urea nitrogen and serum creatinine; these increases were reversible upon discontinuation of benazepril therapy, concomitant diuretic therapy, or both. When such patients are treated with Lotensin HCT, renal function should be monitored during the first few weeks of therapy.

Some benazepril-treated hypertensive patients with **no apparent preexisting renal vascular disease** have developed increases in blood urea nitrogen and serum creatinine, usually minor and transient, especially when benazepril has been given concomitantly with a diuretic. Dosage reduction of Lotensin HCT may be required. **Evaluation of the hypertensive patient should always include assessment of renal function (see DOSAGE AND ADMINISTRATION).**

NEUTROPENIA/AGRANULOCYTOSIS

Another angiotensin-converting enzyme inhibitor, captopril, has been shown to cause agranulocytosis and bone marrow depression, rarely in uncomplicated patients (incidence probably less than once per 10,000 exposures) but more frequently (incidence possibly as great as once per 1000 exposures) in patients with renal impairment, especially those who also have collagen-vascular diseases such as systemic lupus erythematosus or scleroderma. Available data from clinical trials of benazepril are insufficient to show that benazepril does not cause agranulocytosis at similar rates. Monitoring of white blood cell counts should be considered in patients with collagen-vascular disease, especially if the disease is associated with impaired renal function.

FETAL/NEONATAL MORBIDITY AND MORTALITY

ACE inhibitors can cause fetal and neonatal morbidity and death when administered to pregnant women. Several dozen cases have been reported in the world literature. When pregnancy is detected, Lotensin HCT should be discontinued as soon as possible.

The use of ACE inhibitors during the second and third trimesters of pregnancy has been associated with fetal and neonatal injury, including hypotension, neonatal skull hypoplasia, anuria, reversible or irreversible renal failure, and death. Oligohydramnios has also been reported, presumably resulting from decreased fetal renal function; oligohydramnios in this setting has been associated with fetal limb contractures, craniofacial deformation, and hypoplastic lung development. Prematurity, intrauterine growth retardation, and patent ductus arteriosus have also been reported, although it is not clear whether these occurrences were due to the ACE-inhibitor exposure.

These adverse effects do not appear to have resulted from intrauterine ACE-inhibitor exposure that has been limited to the first trimester. Mothers whose embryos and fetuses are exposed to ACE inhibitors only during the first trimester should be so informed. Nonetheless, when patients become pregnant, physicians should make every effort to discontinue the use of benazepril as soon as possible.

Rarely (probably less often than once in every thousand pregnancies), no alternative to ACE inhibitors will be found. In these rare cases, the mothers should be apprised of the potential hazards to their fetuses, and serial ultrasound examinations should be performed to assess the intraamniotic environment.

If oligohydramnios is observed, benazepril should be discontinued unless it is considered life-saving for the mother. Contraction stress testing (CST), a nonstress test (NST), or biophysical profiling (BPP) may be appropriate, depending upon the week of pregnancy. Patients and physicians should be aware, however, that oligohydramnios may not appear until after the fetus has sustained irreversible injury.

Infants with histories of *in utero* exposure to ACE inhibitors should be closely observed for hypotension, oliguria, and hyperkalemia. If oliguria occurs, attention should be directed toward support of blood pressure and renal perfusion. Exchange transfusion or peritoneal dialysis may be required as means of reversing hypotension and/or substituting for disordered renal function. Benazepril, which crosses the placenta, can theoretically be removed from the neonatal circulation by these means; there are occasional reports of benefit from these maneuvers, but experience is limited.

Intrauterine exposure to thiazide diuretics is associated with fetal or neonatal jaundice, thrombocytopenia, and possibly other adverse reactions that have occurred in adults.

No teratogenic effects were seen when benazepril and hydrochlorothiazide were administered to pregnant rats at a dose ratio of 4:5. On a mg/kg basis, the doses used were up to 167 times the maximum recommended human dose. Similarly, no teratogenic effects were seen when benazepril and hydrochlorothiazide were administered to pregnant mice at total doses up to 160 mg/kg/day, with benazepril:hydrochlorothiazide ratios of 15:1. When hydrochlorothiazide was orally administered without benazepril to pregnant mice and rats during their respective periods of major organogenesis, at doses up to 3000 and 1000 mg/kg/day respectively, there was no evidence of harm to the fetus. Similarly, no teratogenic effects of benazepril were seen in studies of pregnant rats, mice, and rabbits; on a mg/kg basis, the doses used in these studies were 300 times (in rats), 90 times (in mice), and more than 3 times (in rabbits) the maximum recommended human dose.

HEPATIC FAILURE

Rarely, ACE inhibitors have been associated with a syndrome that starts with cholestatic jaundice and progresses to fulminant hepatic necrosis and (sometimes) death. The mechanism of this syndrome is not understood. Patients receiving ACE inhibitors who develop jaundice or marked elevations of hepatic enzymes should discontinue the ACE inhibitor and receive appropriate medical follow-up.

IMPAIRED HEPATIC FUNCTION

Lotensin HCT should be used with caution in patients with impaired hepatic function or progressive liver disease, since minor alterations of fluid and electrolyte balance may precipitate hepatic coma (see Hepatic Failure). In patients with hepatic dysfunction due to cirrhosis, levels of benazeprilat are essentially unaltered. No formal pharmacokinetic studies have been carried out in hypertensive patients with impaired liver function.

SYSTEMIC LUPUS ERYTHEMATOSUS

Thiazide diuretics have been reported to cause exacerbation or activation of systemic lupus erythematosus.

DOSAGE AND ADMINISTRATION

Benazepril is an effective treatment of hypertension in once-daily doses of 10-80 mg, while hydrochlorothiazide is effective in doses of 12.5-50 mg/day. In clinical trials of benazepril/hydrochlorothiazide combination therapy using benazepril doses of 5-20 mg and hydrochlorothiazide doses of 6.25-25 mg, the antihypertensive effects increased with increasing dose of either component.

The side effects (see WARNINGS) of benazepril are generally rare and apparently independent of dose; those of hydrochlorothiazide are a mixture of dose-dependent phenomena (primarily hypokalemia) and dose-independent phenomena (*e.g.*, pancreatitis), the former much more common than the latter. Therapy with any combination of benazepril and hydrochlorothiazide will be associated with both sets of dose-independent side effects, but regimens in which benazepril is combined with low doses of hydrochlorothiazide produce minimal effects on serum potassium. In clinical trials of Lotensin HCT, the average change in serum potassium was near zero in subjects who received 5/6.25 mg or 20/12.5 mg, but the average subject who received 10/12.5 mg or 20/25 mg experienced a mild reduction in serum potassium, similar to that experienced by the average subject receiving the same dose of hydrochlorothiazide monotherapy.

To minimize dose-independent side effects, it is usually appropriate to begin combination therapy only after a patient has failed to achieve the desired effect with monotherapy.

DOSE TITRATION GUIDED BY CLINICAL EFFECT

A patient whose blood pressure is not adequately controlled with benazepril monotherapy may be switched to Lotensin HCT 10/12.5 or Lotensin HCT 20/12.5. Further increases of either or both components could depend on clinical response. The hydrochlorothiazide dose should generally not be increased until 2-3 weeks have elapsed. Patients whose blood pressures are adequately controlled with 25 mg of daily hydrochlorothiazide, but who experience significant potassium loss with this regimen, may achieve similar blood-pressure control without electrolyte disturbance if they are switched to Lotensin HCT 5/6.25.

REPLACEMENT THERAPY

The combination may be substituted for the titrated individual components.

USE IN RENAL IMPAIRMENT

Regimens of therapy with Lotensin HCT need not take account of renal function as long as the patient's creatinine clearance is >30 ml/min/1.73 m^2 (serum creatinine roughly ≤ 3 mg/dl or 265 μmol/L). In patients with more severe renal impairment, loop diuretics are preferred to thiazides, so Lotensin HCT is not recommended (see WARNINGS).

PRODUCT LISTING - EQUIVALENTS NOT AVAILABLE

Tablet - Oral - 5 mg;6.25 mg

100's $109.25 LOTENSIN HCT, Novartis Pharmaceuticals 00083-0057-30

Tablet - Oral - 10 mg;12.5 mg

100's $109.25 LOTENSIN HCT, Novartis Pharmaceuticals 00083-0072-30

Tablet - Oral - 20 mg;12.5 mg

100's $109.25 LOTENSIN HCT, Novartis Pharmaceuticals 00083-0074-30

Tablet - Oral - 20 mg;25 mg

100's $109.25 LOTENSIN HCT, Novartis Pharmaceuticals 00083-0075-30

B

Benzocaine *(000417)*

Categories: Anesthesia, topical; Pain, secondary to otitis externa; Pain, secondary to otitis media; Pregnancy Category C; FDA Pre 1938 Drugs
Drug Classes: Anesthetics, otic; Anesthetics, topical; Dermatologics; Otics
Brand Names: **Americaine**; Anacaine; Otocain
Foreign Brand Availability: Anaesthesin (Germany); Auralyt (Mexico); Octicaina (Colombia); Solarcaine (Hong-Kong); Topicaine (Australia)

DESCRIPTION

Anesthetic Lubricant: Americaine anesthetic lubricant contains benzocaine 20% with benzethonium chloride 0.1% as a preservative in a water soluble base of polyethylene glycol 300 and 3350.

Topical Anesthetic Ear Drops: Americaine Otic, topical anesthetic ear drops, contains benzocaine 20% (w/w) in a water soluble base of glycerin 1% (w/w) and polyethylene glycol 300 with benzethonium chloride 0.1% as a preservative.

Anesthetic Lubricant and Topical Anesthetic Ear Drops: Benzocaine, a local anesthetic, is chemically ethyl*p*-aminobenzoate, $C_9H_{11}NO_2$, with a molecular weight of 165.19.

CLINICAL PHARMACOLOGY

Anesthetic Lubricant and Topical Anesthetic Ear Drops: Benzocaine reversibly stabilizes the neuronal membrane which decreases its permeability to sodium ions. Depolarization of the neuronal membrane is inhibited thereby blocking the initiation and conduction of nerve impulses.

INDICATIONS AND USAGE

Anesthetic Lubricant: Benzocaine anesthetic lubricant is indicated for general use as a lubricant and topical anesthetic on intratracheal catheters and pharyngeal and nasal airways to obtund the pharyngeal and tracheal reflexes; on nasogastric and endoscopic tubes; urinary catheters; laryngoscopes; proctoscopes; sigmoidoscopes and vaginal specula.

Topical Anesthetic Ear Drops: Benzocaine topical anesthetic ear drops is indicated for relief of pain and pruritus in acute congestive and serous otitis media, acute swimmer's ear, and other forms of otitis externa.

CONTRAINDICATIONS

Anesthetic Lubricant and Topical Anesthetic Ear Drops: Known allergy or hypersensitivity to benzocaine.

Topical Anesthetic Ear Drops: Contraindicated in the presence of a perforated tympanic membrane or ear discharge.

WARNINGS

Topical Anesthetic Ear Drops: Indiscriminate use of anesthetic ear drops may mask symptoms of fulminating infection of the middle ear.

PRECAUTIONS

ANESTHETIC LUBRICANT AND TOPICAL ANESTHETIC EAR DROPS

General: Medication should be discontinued if sensitivity or irritation occurs.

Carcinogenesis, Mutagenesis, and Impairment of Fertility: Long-term studies in animals or humans to evaluate the carcinogenic and mutagenic potential or the effect on fertility have not been conducted.

Pregnancy Category C: Animal reproduction studies have not been conducted with benzocaine. It is also not known whether benzocaine can cause fetal harm when administered to a pregnant woman or can affect reproduction capacity. Benzocaine should be given to a pregnant woman only if clearly needed.

Nursing Mothers: It is not known whether this drug is excreted in human milk. Because many drugs are excreted in human milk, caution should be exercised when benzocaine is administered to a nursing woman.

Pediatric Use: Do not use in infants under 1 year of age.

ADVERSE REACTIONS

Anesthetic Lubricant and Topical Anesthetic Ear Drops: Contact dermatitis and/or hypersensitivity to benzocaine can cause burning, stinging, pruritus, tenderness, erythema, rash, urticaria and edema. Rarely, benzocaine may induce methemoglobinemia causing respiratory distress and cyanosis. Intravenous methylene blue is the specific therapy for this condition.

DOSAGE AND ADMINISTRATION

Anesthetic Lubricant: Apply evenly to exterior of tube or instrument prior to use.

Topical Anesthetic Ear Drops: Instill 4-5 drops of benzocaine topical anesthetic ear drops in the external auditory canal, then insert a cotton pledget into the meatus. Application may be repeated every 1-2 hours if necessary.

HOW SUPPLIED

Anesthetic Lubricant: Store at 15-25°C (59-77°F).

Topical Anesthetic Ear Drops: Keep bottle tightly closed. Store at 15-30°C (59-86°F). Keep out of the reach of children.

PRODUCT LISTING - EQUIVALENTS NOT AVAILABLE

Gel - Topical - 5%

7.10 gm	$4.33	RETRE-GEL, Triton Consumer Products Inc	79511-0400-01

Solution - Otic - 20%

15 ml	$10.80	GENERIC, Andrx Pharmaceuticals	62022-0168-15
15 ml	$12.39	GENERIC, Vintage Pharmaceuticals Inc	00254-9339-43
15 ml	$12.39	GENERIC, Qualitest Products Inc	00603-7238-73
15 ml	$16.93	AMERICAINE OTIC, Allscripts Pharmaceutical Company	54569-0883-00
15 ml	$18.67	AMERICAINE OTIC, Celltech Pharmaceuticals Inc	53014-0377-51
15 ml	$19.37	GENERIC, Jones Pharma Inc	52604-0218-05
15 ml	$24.23	AMERICAINE OTIC, Physicians Total Care	54868-1609-02

Suppository - Rectal - Strength n/a

12's	$37.90	GENERIC, G and W Laboratories Inc	00713-0505-12

Benzocaine; Butamben Picrate; Tetracaine *(000419)*

Categories: Anesthesia, topical; FDA Pre 1938 Drugs
Drug Classes: Anesthetics, topical; Dermatologics
Brand Names: Cetacaine

DESCRIPTION

Active Ingredients: *Benzocaine*, 14.0%; *butyl aminobenzoate*, 2.0%; *tetracaine hydrochloride*, 2.0%.
Contains: *Benzalkonium chloride*, 0.5% and *cetyl dimethyl ethyl ammonium bromide*, 0.005%.
In bland, water-soluble base.

CLINICAL PHARMACOLOGY

Benzocaine; butamben picrate; tetracaine produces anesthesia rapidly in approximately 30 seconds.

INDICATIONS AND USAGE

Benzocaine; butamben picrate; tetracaine is a topical anesthetic indicated for the production of anesthesia of accessible mucous membrane.

Benzocaine; butamben picrate; tetracaine spray is indicated for use to control pain or gagging.

Benzocaine; butamben picrate; tetracaine in all forms is indicated for use to control pain.

CONTRAINDICATIONS

Benzocaine; butamben picrate; tetracaine is not for injection.

Do not use on the eyes.

To avoid excessive systemic absorption, benzocaine; butamben picrate; tetracaine should not be applied to large areas of denuded or inflamed tissue.

Benzocaine; butamben picrate; tetracaine should not be administered to patients who are hypersensitive to any of its ingredients.

Individual dosage of tetracaine HCl in excess of 20 mg is contraindicated. Benzocaine; butamben picrate; tetracaine should not be used under dentures or cotton rolls, as retention of the active ingredients under a denture or cotton roll could possibly cause an escharotic effect.

PRECAUTIONS

Usage in Pregnancy: Safe use of benzocaine; butamben picrate; tetracaine has not been established with respect to possible adverse effects upon fetal development. Therefore benzocaine; butamben picrate; tetracaine should not be used during early pregnancy, unless in the judgement of a physician the potential benefits outweigh the unknown hazards.
Routine precaution for the use of any topical anesthetic should be observed when benzocaine; butamben picrate; tetracaine is used.

ADVERSE REACTIONS

Systemic reactions to benzocaine; butamben picrate; tetracaine have not been reported. Localized allergic reactions may occur after prolonged or repeated use. Dehydration of the epithelium or an escharotic effect may result from prolonged contact. Allergic reactions are known to occur in some patients with preparations containing benzocaine.

DOSAGE AND ADMINISTRATION

Benzocaine; butamben picrate; tetracaine spray should be applied for approximately one second or less for normal anesthesia. Only limited quantity of benzocaine; butamben picrate; tetracaine is required for anesthesia. Spray in excess of 2 seconds is contraindicated. Average expulsion rate of residue from spray, at normal temperatures, is 200 mg/sec.

Tissue need not be dried prior to application of benzocaine; butamben picrate; tetracaine.

Benzocaine; butamben picrate; tetracaine should be applied directly to the site where pain control is required.

Benzocaine; butamben picrate; tetracaine liquid or benzocaine; butamben picrate; tetracaine ointment may be applied with a cotton pledget or directly to tissue. Cotton pledget should not be held in position for extended periods of time, since local reactions to benzoate topical anesthetics are related to the length of time of application.

HOW SUPPLIED

Jetco Spray Cannula: The autoclavable, stainless steel Jetco cannula for Cetacaine spray is specially designed for accessibility and application of Cetacaine, at the required site of pain control.
The Jetco cannula is supplied in various lengths and shapes.

The Jetco cannula is inserted firmly onto the protruding plastic tubing on each bottle of Cetacaine spray.

The Jetco cannula may be removed and reinserted as many times as required for cleansing or sterilization.

PRODUCT LISTING - EQUIVALENTS NOT AVAILABLE

Aerosol - Topical - 14%;2%;2%

56 ml	$52.00	CETACAINE, Cetylite Industries Inc	10223-0201-01
56 ml	$52.00	CETACAINE, Allscripts Pharmaceutical Company	54569-2028-00

Gel - Topical - 14%;2%;2%

29 gm	$7.00	CETACAINE, Cetylite Industries Inc	10223-0215-01

Kit - Topical - 14%;2%;2%

1's	$77.00	CETACAINE, Cetylite Industries Inc	10223-0201-03

Ointment - Topical - 14%;2%;2%

37 gm	$8.00	CETACAINE, Cetylite Industries Inc	10223-0210-01

Solution - Topical - 14%;2%;2%

56 ml	$8.00	CETACAINE, Cetylite Industries Inc	10223-0202-01

Benzonatate *(000446)*

Categories: Cough; Pregnancy Category C; FDA Approved 1958 Feb
Drug Classes: Antitussives
Brand Names: Tessalon Perles
Foreign Brand Availability: Beknol (Mexico); Benzonal (Mexico); Pebegal (Mexico); Tesalon (Mexico); Tessalon (Canada); Tusehli (Mexico)
Cost of Therapy: $23.78 (Cough; Tessalon Perles; 100 mg; 3 capsules/day; 7 day supply)
$11.58 (Cough; Generic Capsules; 100 mg; 3 capsules/day; 7 day supply)

DESCRIPTION

Benzonatate, a non-narcotic antitussive agent, is 2,5,8,11,14,17,20,23,26-nonaoxaoctacosan-28-yl p-(butylamino) benzoate; with a molecular weight of 603.7. Its empirical formula is $C_{30}H_{53}NO_{11}$.
Each Tessalon Perle contains: Benzonatate, 100 mg.
Tessalon Perles also contain: D&C yellow 10, gelatin, glycerin, methylparaben and propylparaben.

CLINICAL PHARMACOLOGY

Benzonatate acts peripherally by anesthetizing the stretch receptors located in the respiratory passages, lungs, and pleura by dampening their activity and thereby reducing the cough reflex at its source. It begins to act within 15-20 minutes and its effect lasts for 3-8 hours. Benzonatate has no inhibitory effect on the respiratory center in recommended dosage.

INDICATIONS AND USAGE

Benzonatate is indicated for the symptomatic relief of cough.

CONTRAINDICATIONS

Hypersensitivity to benzonatate or related compounds.

WARNINGS

Severe hypersensitivity reactions (including bronchospasm, laryngospasm and cardiovascular collapse) have been reported which are possibly related to local anesthesia from sucking or chewing the perle instead of swallowing it. Severe reactions have required intervention with vasopressor agents and supportive measures.

Isolated instances of bizarre behavior, including mental confusion and visual hallucinations, have also been reported in patients taking benzonatate in combination with other prescribed drugs.

PRECAUTIONS

Benzonatate is chemically related to anesthetic agents of the para-amino-benzoic acid class (*e.g.,* procaine; tetracaine) and has been associated with adverse CNS effects possibly related to a prior sensitivity to related agents or interaction with concomitant medication.
Information for the Patient: Release of benzonatate from the perle in the mouth can produce a temporary local anesthesia of the oral mucosa and choking could occur. Therefore, the perles should be swallowed without chewing.
Pregnancy, Pregnancy Category C: Animal reproduction studies have not been conducted with benzonatate. It is also not known whether benzonatate can cause fetal harm when administered to a pregnant woman or can affect reproduction capacity. Benzonatate should be given to a pregnant woman only if clearly needed.
Nursing Mothers: It is not known whether this drug is excreted in human milk. Because many drugs are excreted in human milk caution should be exercised when benzonatate is administered to a nursing woman.
Carcinogenesis, Mutagenesis, and Impairment of Fertility: Carcinogenicity, mutagenicity, and reproduction studies have not been conducted with benzonatate.
Pediatric Use: Safety and effectiveness in children below the age of 10 has not been established.

ADVERSE REACTIONS

Potential adverse reaction to benzonatate may include:

Hypersensitivity reactions including bronchospasm, laryngospasm, cardiovascular collapse possibly related to local anesthesia from chewing or sucking the perle.

CNS: Sedation; headache; dizziness; mental confusion; visual hallucinations.
GI: Constipation; nausea; GI upset.
Dermatologic: Pruritus; skin eruptions.
Other: Nasal congestion; sensation of burning in the eyes; vague "chilly" sensation; numbness of the chest; hypersensitivity.

Rare instances of deliberate or accidental overdose have resulted in death.

DOSAGE AND ADMINISTRATION

Adults and Children over 10: Usual dose is one 100 mg perle tid as required. If necessary, up to 6 perles daily may be given.

Store at controlled room temperature 15-30°C (59-86°F).

PRODUCT LISTING - RATED THERAPEUTICALLY EQUIVALENT

Capsule - Oral - 100 mg

3's	$6.85	TESSALON PERLES, Prescript Pharmaceuticals	00247-0282-03
10's	$15.00	TESSALON PERLES, Prescript Pharmaceuticals	00247-0282-10
15's	$16.98	TESSALON PERLES, Allscripts Pharmaceutical Company	54569-0618-03
15's	$20.82	TESSALON PERLES, Prescript Pharmaceuticals	00247-0282-15
20's	$16.85	GENERIC, Pharma Pac	52959-0411-20
20's	$22.64	TESSALON PERLES, Allscripts Pharmaceutical Company	54569-0618-00
20's	$26.65	TESSALON PERLES, Prescript Pharmaceuticals	00247-0282-20
20's	$27.82	TESSALON PERLES, Physicians Total Care	54868-0714-01
21's	$27.81	TESSALON PERLES, Prescript Pharmaceuticals	00247-0282-21
21's	$38.27	TESSALON PERLES, Pd-Rx Pharmaceuticals	55289-0750-21
30's	$24.05	GENERIC, Pharma Pac	52959-0411-30
30's	$33.97	TESSALON PERLES, Allscripts Pharmaceutical Company	54569-0618-05
30's	$38.29	TESSALON PERLES, Prescript Pharmaceuticals	00247-0282-30
30's	$45.12	TESSALON PERLES, Pd-Rx Pharmaceuticals	55289-0750-30
40's	$45.29	TESSALON PERLES, Allscripts Pharmaceutical Company	54569-0618-01
100's	$29.93	FEDERAL UPPER LIMIT, H.C.F.A. F F P	99999-0446-01
100's	$55.15	GENERIC, Moore, H.L. Drug Exchange	00839-7795-06
100's	$55.15	GENERIC, Moore, H.L. Drug Exchange Inc	00839-7797-06
100's	$55.50	GENERIC, Aligen Independent Laboratories Inc	00405-4115-01
100's	$57.15	GENERIC, Major Pharmaceuticals Inc	00904-7737-60
100's	$69.00	GENERIC, Martec Pharmaceuticals Inc	52555-0484-01
100's	$77.19	GENERIC, Teva Pharmaceuticals Usa	00093-0060-01
100's	$77.19	GENERIC, Ivax Corporation	00182-1080-01
100's	$95.45	GENERIC, Mutual/United Research Laboratories	00677-1472-01
100's	$95.48	GENERIC, Qualitest Products Inc	00603-2426-21
100's	$101.33	GENERIC, Sidmak Laboratories Inc	50111-0851-01
100's	$113.22	TESSALON PERLES, Forest Pharmaceuticals	00456-0688-01

Capsule - Oral - 200 mg

100's	$197.73	GENERIC, Inwood Laboratories Inc	00258-3678-01

PRODUCT LISTING - EQUIVALENTS NOT AVAILABLE

Capsule - Oral - 100 mg

9's	$6.95	GENERIC, Allscripts Pharmaceutical Company	54569-4091-03
9's	$11.40	GENERIC, Pharmaceutical Corporation Of America	51655-0769-05
20's	$9.64	GENERIC, Physicians Total Care	54868-3457-00
20's	$15.44	GENERIC, Allscripts Pharmaceutical Company	54569-4091-00
21's	$13.82	GENERIC, Pd-Rx Pharmaceuticals	55289-0175-21
24's	$18.53	GENERIC, Allscripts Pharmaceutical Company	54569-4091-01
30's	$13.79	GENERIC, Physicians Total Care	54868-3457-01
30's	$21.00	GENERIC, Pd-Rx Pharmaceuticals	55289-0175-30
30's	$23.16	GENERIC, Allscripts Pharmaceutical Company	54569-4091-02
30's	$24.19	GENERIC, Pharmaceutical Corporation Of America	51655-0769-24
30's	$30.72	GENERIC, Heartland Healthcare Services	61392-0094-30
30's	$30.72	GENERIC, Heartland Healthcare Services	61392-0094-39
30's	$32.77	GENERIC, Heartland Healthcare Services	61392-0094-32
31's	$31.74	GENERIC, Heartland Healthcare Services	61392-0094-31
45's	$46.08	GENERIC, Heartland Healthcare Services	61392-0094-45
60's	$61.44	GENERIC, Heartland Healthcare Services	61392-0094-60
90's	$92.16	GENERIC, Heartland Healthcare Services	61392-0094-90
100's	$95.48	GENERIC, Inwood Laboratories Inc	00258-3654-01

Capsule - Oral - 200 mg

100's	$222.17	TESSALON , Forest Pharmaceuticals	00456-0698-01

Benzoyl Peroxide; Clindamycin *(003524)*

Categories: Acne vulgaris; FDA Approved 2000 Dec; Pregnancy Category C
Drug Classes: Antibiotics, lincosamides; Anti-infectives, topical; Dermatologics; Keratolytics
Brand Names: **BenzaClin**
Cost of Therapy: $57.75 (Acne; BenzaClin Gel; 5%; 1%; 25 g; 2 applications/day; variable day supply)

DESCRIPTION

Note: The trade name has been used throughout this monograph for clarity.

For Dermatological Use Only — Not for Ophthalmic Use.

BenzaClin topical gel contains clindamycin phosphate, (7(S)-chloro-7-deoxylincomycin-2-phosphate). Clindamycin phosphate is a water soluble ester of the semi-synthetic antibiotic produced by a 7(S)-chloro-substitution of the 7(R)-hydroxyl group of the parent antibiotic lincomycin.

Chemically, clindamycin phosphate is ($C_{18}H_{34}ClN_2O_8PS$).

Clindamycin phosphate has molecular weight of 504.97 and its chemical name is Methyl 7-chloro-6,7,8-trideoxy-6-(1-methyl-trans-4-propyl-L-2-pyrrolidinecarboxamido)-1-thio-L-threo-alpha-D-galacto-octopyranoside 2-(dihydrogen phosphate).

BenzaClin topical gel also contains benzoyl peroxide, for topical use. Chemically, benzoyl peroxide is ($C_{14}H_{10}O_4$).

Benzoyl peroxide has a molecular weight of 242.23.

Each gram of BenzaClin topical gel contains, as dispensed, 10 mg (1%) clindamycin as phosphate and 50 mg (5%) benzoyl peroxide in a base of carbomer, sodium hydroxide, dioctyl sodium sulfosuccinate, and purified water.

CLINICAL PHARMACOLOGY

An *in vitro* percutaneous penetration study comparing BenzaClin topical gel and topical 1% clindamycin gel alone, demonstrated there was no statistical difference in penetration between the two drugs. Mean systemic bioavailability of topical clindamycin in BenzaClin topical gel is suggested to be less than 1%.

Benzoyl peroxide has been shown to be absorbed by the skin where it is converted to benzoic acid. Less than 2% of the dose enters systemic circulation as benzoic acid. It is suggested that the lipophilic nature of benzoyl peroxide acts to concentrate the compound into the lipid-rich sebaceous follicle.

MICROBIOLOGY

The clindamycin and benzoyl peroxide components individually have been shown to have *in vitro* activity against *Propionibacterium acnes* an organism which has been associated with acne vulgaris; however, the clinical significance of this activity against *P. acnes* was not examined in clinical trials with this product.

INDICATIONS AND USAGE

BenzaClin topical gel is indicated for the topical treatment of acne vulgaris.

CONTRAINDICATIONS

BenzaClin topical gel is contraindicated in those individuals who have shown hypersensitivity to any of its components or to lincomycin. It is also contraindicated in those having a history of regional enteritis, ulcerative colitis, or antibiotic-associated colitis.

WARNINGS

ORALLY AND PARENTERALLY ADMINISTERED CLINDAMYCIN HAS BEEN ASSOCIATED WITH SEVERE COLITIS WHICH MAY RESULT IN PATIENT DEATH. USE OF THE TOPICAL FORMULATION OF CLINDAMYCIN RESULTS IN ABSORPTION OF THE ANTIBIOTIC FROM THE SKIN SURFACE. DIARRHEA, BLOODY DIARRHEA, AND COLITIS (INCLUDING PSEUDOMEMBRANOUS COLITIS) HAVE BEEN REPORTED WITH THE USE OF TOPICAL AND SYSTEMIC CLINDAMYCIN. STUDIES INDICATE A TOXIN(S) PRODUCED BY CLOSTRIDIA IS ONE PRIMARY CAUSE OF ANTIBIOTIC-ASSOCIATED COLITIS. THE COLITIS IS USUALLY CHARACTERIZED BY SEVERE PERSISTENT DIARRHEA AND SEVERE ABDOMINAL CRAMPS AND MAY BE ASSOCIATED WITH THE PASSAGE OF BLOOD AND MUCUS. ENDOSCOPIC EXAMINATION MAY REVEAL PSEUDOMEMBRANOUS COLITIS. STOOL CULTURE FOR *Clostridium difficile* AND STOOL ASSAY FOR *Clostridium difficile* TOXIN MAY BE HELPFUL DIAGNOSTICALLY. WHEN SIGNIFICANT DIARRHEA OCCURS, THE DRUG SHOULD BE DISCONTINUED. LARGE BOWEL ENDOSCOPY SHOULD BE CONSIDERED TO ESTABLISH A DEFINITIVE DIAGNOSIS IN CASES OF SEVERE DIARRHEA. ANTIPERISTALTIC AGENTS SUCH AS OPIATES AND DIPHENOXYLATE WITH ATROPINE MAY PROLONG AND/OR WORSEN THE CONDITION. DIARRHEA, COLITIS, AND PSEUDOMEMBRANOUS COLITIS HAVE BEEN OBSERVED TO BEGIN UP TO SEVERAL WEEKS FOLLOWING CESSATION OF ORAL AND PARENTERAL THERAPY WITH CLINDAMYCIN.

Mild cases of pseudomembranous colitis usually respond to drug discontinuation alone. In moderate to severe cases, consideration should be given to management with fluids and electrolytes, protein supplementation and treatment with an antibacterial drug clinically effective against *Clostridium difficile* colitis.

PRECAUTIONS

GENERAL

For dermatological use only; not for ophthalmic use. Concomitant topical acne therapy should be used with caution because a possible cumulative irritancy effect may occur, especially with the use of peeling, desquamating, or abrasive agents.

The use of antibiotic agents may be associated with the overgrowth of nonsusceptible organisms including fungi. If this occurs, discontinue use of this medication and take appropriate measures.

Avoid contact with eyes and mucous membranes.

Clindamycin and erythromycin containing products should not be used in combination. *In vitro* studies have shown antagonism between these two anti-microbials. The clinical significance of this *in vitro* antagonism is not known.

B

INFORMATION FOR THE PATIENT

Patients using BenzaClin topical gel should receive the following information and instructions:

1. BenzaClin topical gel is to be used as directed by the physician. It is for external use only. Avoid contact with eyes, and inside the nose, mouth, and all mucous membranes, as this product may be irritating.
2. This medication should not be used for any disorder other than that for which it was prescribed.
3. Patients should not use any other topical acne preparation unless otherwise directed by physician.
4. Patients should report any signs of local adverse reactions to their physician.
5. BenzaClin topical gel may bleach hair or colored fabric.
6. Store refrigerated 2-8°C (36-46°F). Do not freeze. Discard any unused product after 2 months.
7. Before applying BenzaClin topical gel to affected areas wash the skin gently, then rinse with warm water and pat dry.

CARCINOGENESIS, MUTAGENESIS, AND IMPAIRMENT OF FERTILITY

Benzoyl peroxide has been shown to be a tumor promoter and progression agent in a number of animal studies. The clinical significance of this is unknown.

Benzoyl peroxide in acetone at doses of 5 and 10 mg administered twice per week induced skin tumors in transgenic Tg.AC mice in a study using 20 weeks of topical treatment.

Genotoxicity studies were not conducted with BenzaClin topical gel. Clindamycin phosphate was not genotoxic in *Salmonella typhimurium* or in a rat micronucleus test. Clindamycin phosphate sulfoxide, an oxidative degradation product of clindamycin phosphate and benzoyl peroxide, was not clastogenic in a mouse micronucleus test. Benzoyl peroxide has been found to cause DNA strand breaks in a variety of mammalian cell types, to be mutagenic in *Salmonella typhimurium* tests by some but not all investigators, and to cause sister chromatid exchanges in Chinese hamster ovary cells. Studies have not been performed with BenzaClin topical gel or benzoyl peroxide to evaluate the effect on fertility. Fertility studies in rats treated orally with up to 300 mg/kg/day of clindamycin (approximately 120 times the amount of clindamycin in the highest recommended adult human dose of 2.5 g BenzaClin topical gel, based on mg/m^2) revealed no effects on fertility or mating ability.

PREGNANCY, TERATOGENIC EFFECTS, PREGNANCY CATEGORY C

Animal reproductive/developmental toxicity studies have not been conducted with BenzaClin topical gel or benzoyl peroxide. Developmental toxicity studies performed in rats and mice using oral doses of clindamycin up to 600 mg/kg/day (240 and 120 times amount of clindamycin in the highest recommended adult human dose based on mg/m^2, respectively) or subcutaneous doses of clindamycin up to 250 mg/kg/day (100 and 50 times the amount of clindamycin in the highest recommended adult human dose based on mg/m^2, respectively) revealed no evidence of teratogenicity.

There are no well-controlled trials in pregnant women treated with BenzaClin topical gel. It also is not known whether BenzaClin topical gel can cause fetal harm when administered to a pregnant woman.

NURSING WOMEN

It is not known whether BenzaClin topical gel is excreted in human milk after topical application. However, orally and parenterally administered clindamycin has been reported to appear in breast milk. Because of the potential for serious adverse reactions in nursing infants, a decision should be made whether to discontinue nursing or to discontinue the drug, taking into account the importance of the drug to the mother.

PEDIATRIC USE

Safety and effectiveness of this product in pediatric patients below the age of 12 have not been established.

ADVERSE REACTIONS

During clinical trials, the most frequently reported adverse event in the BenzaClin treatment group was dry skin (12%). TABLE 2 lists local adverse events reported by at least 1% of patients in the BenzaClin and vehicle groups.

TABLE 2 *Local Adverse Events — All Causalities in ≥ 1% of Patients*

	BenzaClin n=420	Vehicle n=168
Application site reaction	13 (3%)	1 (<1%)
Dry skin	50 (12%)	10 (6%)
Pruritus	8 (2%)	1 (<1%)
Peeling	9 (2%)	—
Erythema	6 (1%)	1 (<1%)
Sunburn	5 (1%)	—

The actual incidence of dry skin might have been greater were it not for the use of a moisturizer in these studies.

DOSAGE AND ADMINISTRATION

BenzaClin topical gel should be applied twice daily, morning and evening, or as directed by a physician, to affected areas after the skin is gently washed, rinsed with warm water and patted dry.

HOW SUPPLIED

BenzaClin topical gel is supplied in 25 g vials containing 19.7 g benzoyl peroxide and 0.3 g clindamycin.

STORAGE

Prior to reconstitution, store at controlled room temperature 20-25°C (68-77°F).

After reconstitution, store refrigerated 2-8°C (36-46°F).

Do not freeze. Keep tightly closed. Keep out of the reach of children.

PRODUCT LISTING - EQUIVALENTS NOT AVAILABLE

Gel - Topical - 5%;1%

25 gm	$57.75	BENZACLIN, Aventis Pharmaceuticals	00066-0494-25
45 gm	$98.75	DUAC , Stiefel Laboratories Inc	00145-2371-05
50 gm	$109.73	BENZACLIN, Aventis Pharmaceuticals	00066-0494-50

Benzoyl Peroxide; Erythromycin *(000448)*

Categories: Acne vulgaris; Pregnancy Category C; FDA Approved 1984 Oct
Drug Classes: Antibiotics, macrolides; Anti-infectives, topical; Dermatologics; Keratolytics
Brand Names: Benzamycin
Foreign Brand Availability: Benzamycine (South-Africa)
Cost of Therapy: $30.57 (Acne; Benzamycin Gel; 5%; 3%; 23.3 g; 2 applications/day; variable day supply)

DESCRIPTION

For Dermatological Use Only — Not for Ophthalmic Use

Benzamycin Pak (benzoyl peroxide) contains erythromycin [(3R*, 4S*, 5S*, 6R*, 7R*, 9R*, 11R*, 12R*, 13S*, 14R*)-4-[(2,6-dideoxy-3-C-methyl-3-O-methyl-a-L-ribo-hexopyranosyl)-oxy]-14-ethyl-7,12,13-trihydroxy-3,5,7,9,11,13-hexa-methyl-6-[[3,4,6-tri-deoxy-3-(dimethylamino)-b-D-xylo-hexopyranosyl]oxy]oxacyclotetradecane-2,10-dione]. Erythromycin is a macrolide antibiotic produced from a strain of *Saccharopolyspora erythraea* (formerly *Streptomyces erythreus*). It is a base and readily forms salts with acids.

Chemically, erythromycin is ($C_{37}H_{67}NO_{13}$).

Benzamycin Pak also contains benzoyl peroxide for topical use. Benzoyl peroxide is an oxidizing agent demonstrating antibacterial activity.

Chemically, benzoyl peroxide is ($C_{14}H_{10}O_4$).

Benzoyl peroxide has the molecular weight of 242.23. It is a white granular powder and is sparingly soluble in water and alcohol and soluble in acetone, chloroform and ether.

Each g of product, as dispensed, contains 30 mg of erythromycin and 50 mg of benzoyl peroxide in a base of SD alcohol 40B, purified water, hydroxypropyl cellulose, carbomer 934, sodium hydroxide, dioctyl sodium sulfosuccinate 75%. Each Benzamycin Pak contains 0.8 g of product.

CLINICAL PHARMACOLOGY

PHARMACOKINETICS

Benzoyl peroxide has been shown to be absorbed by the skin where it is converted to benzoic acid. A single dose pharmacokinetic study, involving the application of either 1 or 3 units of benzoyl peroxide, was performed in 16 adult acne patients to determine systemic absorption of erythromycin. Erythromycin (with a plasma lower limit of quantitation of 2 ng/ml) was not detectable, except in 1 patient who was in the 1 unit application group.

PHARMACODYNAMICS

The exact mechanism by which erythromycin and benzoyl peroxide reduce lesions of acne vulgaris is not fully known.

MICROBIOLOGY

Erythromycin acts by inhibition of protein synthesis in susceptible organisms by reversibly binding to 50 **S** ribosomal subunits, thereby inhibiting translocation of aminoacyl transfer-RNA and inhibiting polypeptide synthesis. Antagonism has been demonstrated *in vitro* between erythromycin, lincomycin, chloramphenicol and clindamycin.

Benzoyl peroxide has been shown to be effective *in vitro* against Propionibacterium acnes, an anaerobe found in sebaceous follicles and comedones. Benzoyl peroxide is believed to act by releasing active oxygen.

INDICATIONS AND USAGE

Benzoyl peroxide is indicated for the topical treatment of acne vulgaris.

CONTRAINDICATIONS

Benzoyl peroxide is contraindicated in those individuals who have shown hypersensitivity to any of its components.

PRECAUTIONS

GENERAL

For topical use only; not for ophthalmic use. Concomitant topical acne therapy should be used with caution because a possible cumulative irritancy effect may occur, especially with the use of peeling, desquamating or abrasive agents. If severe irritation develops, discontinue use and institute appropriate therapy.

The use of antibiotic agents may be associated with the overgrowth of nonsusceptible organisms. If this occurs, discontinue use and take appropriate measures.

Avoid contact with eyes and all mucous membranes.

INFORMATION FOR THE PATIENT

Patients using benzoyl peroxide should receive the following information and instructions:

Patients should be informed that they will need to mix this medication prior to use. The medication will be dispensed in 1 foil pouch which contains medication in 2 separated compartments.

The contents must be mixed thoroughly by the patient (in the palm of the hand), prior to application.

Patients should apply the product immediately after mixing, then the hands should be washed.

Do not mix or apply near an open flame.

Benzoyl peroxide may bleach hair or colored fabric.

Excessive or prolonged exposure to sunlight should be limited. To minimize exposure to sunlight, a hat or other clothing should be worn.

This medication is to be used as directed by the physician. It is for external use only. Avoid contact with the eyes, mouth, and all mucous membranes as this product may be irritating.

Patients should report to their physician any signs of local adverse reactions.

This medication should not be used for any disorder other than that for which it was prescribed.

Patients should not use any other topical acne preparation unless otherwise directed by physician.

Patients should be instructed to review the instructions for use on the product carton.

This medication should be stored at room temperature away from heat and any open flame.

CARCINOGENESIS, MUTAGENESIS, AND IMPAIRMENT OF FERTILITY

The combination of benzoyl peroxide and erythromycin in benzoyl peroxide has not been evaluated for its carcinogenic or mutagenic potential or for its effects on fertility.

Benzoyl peroxide has been shown to be a tumor promoter and progression agent in a number of animal studies. The clinical significance of this is unknown.

Benzoyl peroxide in acetone at doses of 5 and 10 mg administered twice/week induced skin tumors in transgenic Tg.AC mice in a study using 20 weeks of topical treatment.

Benzoyl peroxide has been found to cause DNA strand breaks in a variety of mammalian cell types, to be mutagenic in *Salmonella typhimurium* tests by some but not all investigators, and to cause sister chromatid exchanges in Chinese hamster ovary cells.

No animal studies have been performed to evaluate the carcinogenic potential or effects on fertility of topical erythromycin. However, long-term (2 year) oral studies in rats with erythromycin base and erythromycin ethylsuccinate and in rats and mice with erythromycin stearate did not provide evidence of tumorigenicity.

The genotoxicity of erythromycin stearate has been evaluated in the *Salmonella typhimurium* reverse mutation assay, the mouse L5178Y lymphoma cell assay, and for sister chromatid exchanges and chromosomal aberrations in CHO cells. These studies indicated that erythromycin stearate was not genotoxic.

There was no apparent effect on male or female fertility in rats fed erythromycin base at levels up to 0.25% of diet.

PREGNANCY, TERATOGENIC EFFECTS, PREGNANCY CATEGORY C

Animal reproduction studies have not been conducted with benzoyl peroxide.

There was no evidence of teratogenicity or any other adverse effect on reproduction in female rats fed erythromycin base (up to 0.25% diet) prior to and during mating, during gestation and through weaning of 2 successive litters.

There are no well-controlled trials in pregnant women with benzoyl peroxide. It also is not known whether benzoyl peroxide can cause fetal harm when administered to a pregnant woman or can affect reproductive capacity. Benzoyl peroxide should be given to a pregnant woman only if clearly needed.

NURSING MOTHERS

It is not known whether the ingredients of benzoyl peroxide are excreted in human milk after topical application. However, erythromycin is excreted in human milk following oral and parenteral erythromycin administration. Therefore, caution should be exercised when erythromycin is administered to a nursing woman.

PEDIATRIC USE

Safety and effectiveness of this product in pediatric patients below 12 years of age have not been established.

ADVERSE REACTIONS

During clinical trials, 550 acne patients were studied. Of these patients, 236 were treated with benzoyl peroxide. The most frequently reported adverse event considered at least possibly related was dry skin (7.6%) as compared to vehicle (3.9%). Application site reactions (stinging, burning sensation, tingling, erythema) were reported in 2.5% of patients versus 1.3% for vehicle patients. Blepharitis, pruritus and photosensitivity reactions were reported in <2% of patients who used the dual pouch product.

TABLE 3 *Treatment Group Summaries*

COSTART Term	Benzoyl Peroxide Pak n=236	Benzoyl Peroxide Vehicle n=153	Benzoyl Peroxide Topical Gel n=121	Benzoyl Peroxide Topical Gel Vehicle n=40
Dry skin	18 (7.6%)	6 (3.9%)	6 (5.0%)	0
Application site reaction (stinging, erythema, and burning)	6 (2.5%)	2 (1.3%)	1 (0.8%)	0
Blepharitis	4 (1.7%)	1 (0.7%)	0	1 (2.5%)
Pruritus	4 (1.7%)	2 (1.3%)	3 (2.5%)	0
Photosensitivity reaction (sunburn, stinging with sun exposure)	3 (1.3%)	0	0	0
Peeling	1 (0.5%)	1 (0.7%)	0	0

DOSAGE AND ADMINISTRATION

Benzoyl peroxide requires thorough mixing by the patient immediately prior to each use. The medication should be applied twice daily, morning and evening, or as directed by a physician, to affected areas after the skin is thoroughly washed, rinsed with warm water and gently patted dry.

HOW SUPPLIED

60 pouches/carton

Storage: Store at room temperature 20-25°C (68-77°F).

Keep away from heat and any open flame.

Keep out of the reach of children.

PRODUCT LISTING - EQUIVALENTS NOT AVAILABLE

Gel - Topical - 5%;3%

23.30 gm	$28.00	BENZAMYCIN, Allscripts Pharmaceutical Company	54569-1830-01
23.30 gm	$29.40	BENZAMYCIN, Pharma Pac	52959-1266-01
23.30 gm	$30.57	BENZAMYCIN, Pharma Pac	52959-0259-01
23.30 gm	$58.30	GENERIC, Clay-Park Laboratories Inc	45802-0083-02
23.30 gm	$64.84	BENZAMYCIN, Aventis Pharmaceuticals	00066-0510-23
24 gm	$35.80	BENZAMYCIN, Prescript Pharmaceuticals	00247-0238-24
24 gm	$41.43	BENZAMYCIN, Physicians Total Care	54868-2246-00
46.60 gm	$111.50	GENERIC, Clay-Park Laboratories Inc	45802-0083-86
46.60 gm	$124.05	BENZAMYCIN, Aventis Pharmaceuticals	00066-0510-46
47 gm	$78.54	BENZAMYCIN, Physicians Total Care	54868-2246-01
60 gm	$18.96	BENZAGEL WASH, Aventis Pharmaceuticals	00066-0441-60
60 gm	$79.37	BENZAMYCIN, Aventis Pharmaceuticals	00066-0577-60

Benztropine Mesylate *(000455)*

Categories: Extrapyramidal disorder, drug-induced; Parkinson's disease; FDA Approved 1954 Mar; Pregnancy Category C
Drug Classes: Anticholinergics; Antiparkinson agents
Brand Names: Bensylate; **Cogentin**; Glycopyrrolate
Foreign Brand Availability: Akitan (Finland); Apo-Benzthropine (Canada)
Cost of Therapy: $14.44 (Parkinsonism; Cogentin; 1 mg; 2 tablets/day; 30 day supply)
$3.84 (Parkinsonism; Generic Tablets; 1 mg; 2 tablets/day; 30 day supply)
HCFA JCODE(S): J0515 per 1 mg IM, IV; J0702 3 mg of ea IM

DESCRIPTION

Benztropine mesylate is a synthetic compound containing structural features found in atropine and diphenhydramine.

It is designated chemically as 8-azabicyclo(3.2.1) octane, 3-(diphenylmethoxy)-,*endo*, methanesulfonate. Its empirical formula is $C_{21}H_{25}NO{\cdot}CH_4O_3S$.

Benztropine mesylate is a crystalline white powder, very soluble in water, and has a molecular weight of 403.54.

Benztropine mesylate is supplied as tablets in three strengths (0.5, 1, and 2 mg per tablet), and as a sterile injection for intravenous and intramuscular use.

Tablets contain 0.5, 1 or 2 mg of benztropine mesylate. Each tablet contains the following inactive ingredients: calcium phosphate, cellulose, lactose, magnesium stearate and starch.

Each milliliter of the injection contains:

Benztropine Mesylate: 1 mg
Sodium Chloride: 9 mg
Water for Injection qs: 1 ml

CLINICAL PHARMACOLOGY

Benztropine mesylate possesses both anticholinergic and antihistaminic effects, although only the former have been established as therapeutically significant in the management of parkinsonism.

In the isolated guinea pig ileum, the anticholinergic activity of this drug is about equal to that of atropine; however, when administered orally to unanesthetized cats, it is only about half as active as atropine.

In laboratory animals, its antihistaminic activity and duration of action approach those of pyrilamine maleate.

INDICATIONS AND USAGE

For use as an adjunct in the therapy of all forms of parkinsonism.

Useful also in the control of extrapyramidal disorders (except tardive dyskinesia — see PRECAUTIONS) due to neuroleptic drugs (*e.g.*, phenothiazines).

CONTRAINDICATIONS

Hypersensitivity to benztropine mesylate tablets or to any component of benztropine mesylate injection.

Because of its atropine-like side effects, this drug is contraindicated in children under three years of age, and should be used with caution in older children.

WARNINGS

Safe use in pregnancy has not been established.

Benztropine mesylate may impair mental and/or physical abilities required for performance of hazardous tasks, such as operating machinery or driving a motor vehicle.

When benztropine mesylate is given concomitantly with phenothiazines, haloperidol, or other drugs with anticholinergic or antidopaminergic activity, patients should be advised to report gastrointestinal complaints, fever or heat intolerance promptly. Paralytic ileus, hyperthermia and heat stroke, all of which have sometimes been fatal, have occurred in patients taking anticholinergic-type antiparkinsonism drugs, including benztropine mesylate, in combination with phenothiazines and/or tricyclic antidepressants.

Since benztropine mesylate contains structural features of atropine; it may produce anhidrosis. For this reason, it should be administered with caution during hot weather, especially when given concomitantly with other atropine-like drugs to the chronically ill, the alcoholic, those who have central nervous system disease, and those who do manual labor in a hot environment. Anhidrosis may occur more readily when some disturbance of sweating already exists. If there is evidence of anhidrosis, the possibility of hyperthermia should be considered. Dosage should be decreased at the discretion of the physician so that the ability to maintain body heat equilibrium by perspiration is not impaired. Severe anhidrosis and fatal hyperthermia have occurred.

PRECAUTIONS

GENERAL

Since benztropine mesylate has cumulative action, continued supervision is advisable. Patients with a tendency to tachycardia and patients with prostatic hypertrophy should be observed closely during treatment.

Dysuria may occur, but rarely becomes a problem. Urinary retention has been reported with benztropine mesylate.

The drug may cause complaints of weakness and inability to move particular muscle groups, especially in large doses. For example, if the neck has been rigid and suddenly relaxes, it may feel weak, causing some concern. In this event, dosage adjustment is required.

Mental confusion and excitement may occur with large doses, or in susceptible patients. Visual hallucinations have been reported occasionally. Furthermore, in the treatment of extrapyramidal disorders due to neuroleptic drugs (*e.g.* phenothiazines), in patients with mental disorders, occasionally there may be intensification of mental symptoms. In such cases, antiparkinsonian drugs can precipitate a toxic psychosis. Patients with mental disorders should be kept under careful observation, especially at the beginning of treatment or if dosage is increased.

Tardive dyskinesia may appear in some patients on long-term therapy with phenothiazines and related agents, or may occur after therapy with these drugs has been discontinued. Antiparkinsonism agents do not alleviate the symptoms of tardive dyskinesia, and in some instances may aggravate them. Benztropine mesylate is not recommended for use in patients with tardive dyskinesia.

The physician should be aware of the possible occurrence of glaucoma. Although the drug does not appear to have any adverse effect on simple glaucoma, it probably should not be used in angle-closure glaucoma.

DRUG INTERACTIONS

Antipsychotic drugs such as phenothiazines or haloperidol; tricyclic antidepressants (see WARNINGS).

ADVERSE REACTIONS

The adverse reactions below, most of which are anticholinergic in nature, have been reported and within each category are listed in order of decreasing severity.

Cardiovascular: Tachycardia.

Digestive: Paralytic ileus, constipation, vomiting, nausea, dry mouth.

If dry mouth is so severe that there is difficulty in swallowing or speaking, or loss of appetite and weight, reduce dosage, or discontinue the drug temporarily.

Slight reduction in dosage may control nausea and still give sufficient relief of symptoms. Vomiting may be controlled by temporary discontinuation, followed by resumption at a lower dosage.

Nervous System: Toxic psychosis, including confusion, disorientation, memory impairment, visual hallucinations; exacerbation of pre-existing psychotic symptoms; nervousness; depression; listlessness; numbness of fingers.

Special Senses: Blurred vision, dilated pupils.

Urogenital: Urinary retention, dysuria.

Metabolic/Immune or Skin: Occasionally; an allergic reaction, *e.g.,* skin rash develops. If this can not be controlled by dosage reduction, the medication should be discontinued.

Other: Heat stroke, hyperthermia, fever.

DOSAGE AND ADMINISTRATION

Benztropine mesylate tablets should be used when patients are able to take oral medication.

The injection is especially useful for psychotic patients with acute dystonic reactions or other reaction that make oral medication difficult or impossible. It is recommended also when a more rapid response is desired than can be obtained with the tablets.

Since there is no significant difference in onset of effect after intravenous or intramuscular injection usually there is no need to use the intravenous route. The drug is quickly effective after either route, with improvement sometimes noticeable a few minutes after injection. In emergency situations, when the condition of the patient is alarming, 1-2 ml of the injection normally will provide quick relief. If the parkinsonian effect begins to return, the dose can be repeated.

Because of cumulative action, therapy should be initiated with a low dose which is increased gradually at 5 or 6 day intervals to the smallest amount necessary for optimal relief. Increases should be made in increments of 0.5 mg, to a maximum of 6 mg, or until optimal results are obtained without excessive adverse reactions.

POSTENCEPHALITIC AND IDIOPATHIC PARKINSONISM

The usual daily dose is 1-2 mg, with a range of 0.5 to 6 mg orally or parenterally.

As with any agent used in parkinsonism, dosage must be individualized according to age and weight, and the type of parkinsonism being treated. Generally, older patients, and thin patients cannot tolerate large doses. Most patients with postencephalitic parkinsonism need fairly large doses and tolerate them well. Patients with a poor mental outlook are usually poor candidates for therapy.

In idiopathic parkinsonism, therapy may be initiated with a single daily dose of 0.5 to 1 mg at bedtime. In some patients, this will be adequate; in others 4-6 mg a day may be required.

In postencephalitic parkinsonism, therapy may be initiated in most patients with 2 mg a day in 1 or more doses. In highly sensitive patients, therapy may be initiated with 0.5 mg at bedtime, and increased as necessary.

Some patients experience greatest relief by taking the entire dose at bedtime; others react more favorably to divided doses, 2-4 times a day. Frequently, 1 dose a day is sufficient, and divided doses may be unnecessary or undesirable.

The long duration of action of this drug makes it particularly suitable for bedtime medication when its effects may last throughout the night, enabling patients to turn in bed during the night more easily, and to rise in the morning.

When benztropine mesylate is started, do not terminate therapy with other antiparkinsonian agents abruptly. If the other agents are to be reduced or discontinued, it must be done gradually. Many patients obtain greatest relief with combination therapy.

Benztropine mesylate may be used concomitantly with carbidopa; levodopa (Sinemet, MSD), or with levodopa, in which case periodic dosage adjustment may be required in order to maintain optimum response.

DRUG-INDUCED EXTRAPYRAMIDAL DISORDERS

In treating extrapyramidal disorders due to neuroleptic drugs (*e.g.,* phenothiazines), the recommended dosage is 1-4 mg once or twice a day orally or parenterally. Dosage must be individualized according to the need of the patient. Some patients require more than recommended; others do not need as much.

In acute dystonic reactions, 1-2 ml of the injection usually relieves the condition quickly. After that, the tablets, 1-2 mg twice a day, usually prevent recurrence.

When extrapyramidal disorders develop soon after initiation of treatment with neuroleptic drugs (*e.g.,* phenothiazines), they are likely to be transient. One (1) to 2 mg of benztropine mesylate tablets 2 or 3 times a day usually provides relief within 1 or 2 days. After 1 or 2 weeks, the drug should be withdrawn to determine the continued need for it. If such disorders recur, benztropine mesylate can be reinstituted.

Certain drug-induced extrapyramidal disorders that develop slowly may not respond to benztropine mesylate.

PRODUCT LISTING - RATED THERAPEUTICALLY EQUIVALENT

Tablet - Oral - 0.5 mg			
25 x 30	$137.48	GENERIC, Sky Pharmaceuticals Packaging, Inc	63739-0033-03
25 x 30	$177.56	GENERIC, Sky Pharmaceuticals Packaging, Inc	63739-0033-01
30's	$3.92	GENERIC, Heartland Healthcare Services	61392-0167-30
30's	$3.92	GENERIC, Heartland Healthcare Services	61392-0167-39
31 x 10	$44.24	GENERIC, Vangard Labs	00615-2547-53
31 x 10	$44.24	GENERIC, Vangard Labs	00615-2547-63
60's	$7.84	GENERIC, Heartland Healthcare Services	61392-0167-60
60's	$7.84	GENERIC, Heartland Healthcare Services	61392-0167-65
90's	$11.76	GENERIC, Heartland Healthcare Services	61392-0167-90
90's	$11.76	GENERIC, Heartland Healthcare Services	61392-0167-95
100's	$5.10	GENERIC, Qualitest Products Inc	00603-2430-21
100's	$5.52	GENERIC, Moore, H.L. Drug Exchange Inc	00839-7002-06
100's	$5.70	GENERIC, Invamed Inc	52189-0208-24
100's	$6.51	GENERIC, Geneva Pharmaceuticals	00781-1347-01
100's	$6.53	GENERIC, Apothecon Inc	62269-0208-24
100's	$7.00	GENERIC, Watson/Schein Pharmaceuticals Inc	00364-0834-01
100's	$7.85	GENERIC, Raway Pharmacal Inc	00686-0220-20
100's	$9.60	GENERIC, Ivax Corporation	00182-1299-01
100's	$9.60	GENERIC, Aligen Independent Laboratories Inc	00405-4116-01
100's	$9.60	GENERIC, Martec Pharmaceuticals Inc	52555-0457-01
100's	$9.60	GENERIC, Martec Pharmaceuticals Inc	52555-0676-01
100's	$9.75	GENERIC, Parmed Pharmaceuticals Inc	00349-8941-01
100's	$10.43	GENERIC, Auro Pharmaceutical	55829-0164-10
100's	$11.85	FEDERAL UPPER LIMIT, H.C.F.A. F F P	99999-0455-01
100's	$14.52	GENERIC, Duramed Pharmaceuticals Inc	51285-0827-70
100's	$18.75	GENERIC, Major Pharmaceuticals Inc	00904-1055-60
100's	$18.94	GENERIC, Par Pharmaceutical Inc	49884-0164-01
100's	$19.39	GENERIC, Rosemont Pharmaceutical Corporation	00832-1080-00
100's	$20.83	GENERIC, Major Pharmaceuticals Inc	00904-1055-61
100's	$21.55	GENERIC, Ivax Corporation	00182-1299-89
100's	$22.06	COGENTIN, Merck & Company Inc	00006-0021-68
100's	$26.07	GENERIC, Udl Laboratories Inc	51079-0220-20
200 x 5	$142.71	GENERIC, Vangard Labs	00615-2547-43
Tablet - Oral - 1 mg			
25 x 30	$148.28	GENERIC, Sky Pharmaceuticals Packaging, Inc	63739-0034-03
25's	$3.08	GENERIC, Udl Laboratories Inc	51079-0221-19
30's	$5.24	GENERIC, Heartland Healthcare Services	61392-0170-30
30's	$5.24	GENERIC, Heartland Healthcare Services	61392-0170-39
31 x 10	$60.57	GENERIC, Vangard Labs	00615-2548-53
31 x 10	$60.57	GENERIC, Vangard Labs	00615-2548-63
31's	$5.41	GENERIC, Heartland Healthcare Services	61392-0170-31
32's	$5.59	GENERIC, Heartland Healthcare Services	61392-0170-32
60's	$3.50	GENERIC, Major Pharmaceuticals Inc	00904-1056-52
60's	$4.60	GENERIC, Circle Pharmaceuticals Inc	00659-0705-60

60's	$6.93	GENERIC, Golden State Medical	60429-0027-60
60's	$10.48	GENERIC, Heartland Healthcare Services	61392-0170-60
60's	$10.48	GENERIC, Heartland Healthcare Services	61392-0170-65
90's	$15.71	GENERIC, Heartland Healthcare Services	61392-0170-90
90's	$15.71	GENERIC, Heartland Healthcare Services	61392-0170-95
100's	$5.40	GENERIC, Qualitest Products Inc	00603-2431-21
100's	$6.40	GENERIC, Invamed Inc	52189-0209-24
100's	$6.88	GENERIC, Geneva Pharmaceuticals	00781-1357-01
100's	$7.85	GENERIC, Raway Pharmacal Inc	00686-0221-10
100's	$10.88	GENERIC, Dixon-Shane Inc	17236-0847-01
100's	$10.90	GENERIC, Ivax Corporation	00182-1700-01
100's	$10.90	GENERIC, Aligen Independent Laboratories Inc	00405-4117-01
100's	$10.90	GENERIC, Martec Pharmaceuticals Inc	52555-0458-01
100's	$10.90	GENERIC, Martec Pharmaceuticals Inc	52555-0677-01
100's	$11.05	GENERIC, Moore, H.L. Drug Exchange Inc	00839-6771-06
100's	$11.80	GENERIC, Auro Pharmaceutical	55829-0165-10
100's	$14.03	FEDERAL UPPER LIMIT, H.C.F.A. F F P	99999-0455-03
100's	$14.92	GENERIC, Duramed Pharmaceuticals Inc	51285-0828-70
100's	$16.45	GENERIC, Dixon-Shane Inc	17236-0847-11
100's	$17.75	GENERIC, Major Pharmaceuticals Inc	00904-1056-60
100's	$18.36	GENERIC, Apothecon Inc	62269-0209-24
100's	$19.26	GENERIC, Sidmak Laboratories Inc	50111-0394-01
100's	$19.48	GENERIC, Rosemont Pharmaceutical Corporation	00832-1081-00
100's	$19.60	GENERIC, Ivax Corporation	00182-1700-89
100's	$21.65	GENERIC, Par Pharmaceutical Inc	49884-0165-01
100's	$23.93	GENERIC, Major Pharmaceuticals Inc	00904-1056-61
100's	$25.74	GENERIC, Udl Laboratories Inc	51079-0221-20
Tablet - Oral - 2 mg			
25 x 30	$150.08	GENERIC, Sky Pharmaceuticals Packaging, Inc	63739-0035-03
30's	$4.97	GENERIC, Pd-Rx Pharmaceuticals	55289-0281-30
30's	$5.36	GENERIC, Heartland Healthcare Services	61392-0164-30
30's	$5.36	GENERIC, Heartland Healthcare Services	61392-0164-39
31 x 10	$62.22	GENERIC, Vangard Labs	00615-2549-53
31 x 10	$62.22	GENERIC, Vangard Labs	00615-2549-63
31's	$5.54	GENERIC, Heartland Healthcare Services	61392-0164-31
32's	$5.72	GENERIC, Heartland Healthcare Services	61392-0164-32
60's	$4.10	GENERIC, Major Pharmaceuticals Inc	00904-1057-52
60's	$8.56	GENERIC, Golden State Medical	60429-0028-60
60's	$10.73	GENERIC, Heartland Healthcare Services	61392-0164-60
60's	$10.73	GENERIC, Heartland Healthcare Services	61392-0164-65
90's	$16.09	GENERIC, Heartland Healthcare Services	61392-0164-90
90's	$16.09	GENERIC, Heartland Healthcare Services	61392-0164-95
100's	$6.93	GENERIC, Qualitest Products Inc	00603-2432-21
100's	$7.00	GENERIC, Raway Pharmacal Inc	00686-0222-20
100's	$8.00	GENERIC, Invamed Inc	52189-0210-24
100's	$9.38	GENERIC, Geneva Pharmaceuticals	00781-1367-01
100's	$9.75	GENERIC, Moore, H.L. Drug Exchange Inc	00839-6772-06
100's	$10.58	GENERIC, Parmed Pharmaceuticals Inc	00349-8943-01
100's	$12.64	GENERIC, Mutual Pharmaceutical Co Inc	53489-0184-01
100's	$13.25	GENERIC, Dixon-Shane Inc	17236-0848-01
100's	$13.35	GENERIC, Auro Pharmaceutical	55829-0166-10
100's	$13.75	GENERIC, Ivax Corporation	00182-1701-01
100's	$13.75	GENERIC, Aligen Independent Laboratories Inc	00405-4118-01
100's	$13.75	GENERIC, Martec Pharmaceuticals Inc	52555-0459-01
100's	$13.75	GENERIC, Martec Pharmaceuticals Inc	52555-0678-01
100's	$16.56	GENERIC, Dixon-Shane Inc	17236-0848-11
100's	$17.48	GENERIC, Duramed Pharmaceuticals Inc	51285-0829-70
100's	$17.67	FEDERAL UPPER LIMIT, H.C.F.A. F F P	99999-0455-06
100's	$22.39	GENERIC, Major Pharmaceuticals Inc	00904-1057-60
100's	$23.40	GENERIC, Ivax Corporation	00182-1701-89
100's	$24.29	GENERIC, Sidmak Laboratories Inc	50111-0395-01
100's	$24.71	GENERIC, Rosemont Pharmaceutical Corporation	00832-1082-00
100's	$27.31	GENERIC, Par Pharmaceutical Inc	49884-0166-01
100's	$30.03	GENERIC, Major Pharmaceuticals Inc	00904-1057-61
100's	$30.34	COGENTIN, Merck & Company Inc	00006-0060-68
100's	$32.03	GENERIC, Udl Laboratories Inc	51079-0222-20

PRODUCT LISTING - EQUIVALENTS NOT AVAILABLE

Solution - Injectable - 1 mg/ml			
2 ml x 5	$41.10	COGENTIN, Merck & Company Inc	00006-3275-38
2 ml x 6	$49.32	COGENTIN, Merck & Company Inc	00006-3275-16
Tablet - Oral - 1 mg			
30's	$2.47	GENERIC, Physicians Total Care	54868-2301-02
30's	$5.24	GENERIC, Pharmaceutical Corporation Of America	51655-0233-24
45's	$7.86	GENERIC, Heartland Healthcare Services	61392-0170-45
60's	$7.60	GENERIC, Pharmaceutical Corporation Of America	51655-0233-25
Tablet - Oral - 2 mg			
30's	$2.71	GENERIC, Physicians Total Care	54868-2292-02
30's	$4.02	GENERIC, Pharmaceutical Corporation Of America	51655-0234-24
30's	$4.94	GENERIC, Allscripts Pharmaceutical Company	54569-2862-00
45's	$8.05	GENERIC, Heartland Healthcare Services	61392-0164-45

Bepridil Hydrochloride *(003003)*

For related information, see the comparative table section in Appendix A.

Categories: Angina, chronic stable; Pregnancy Category C; FDA Approved 1990 Dec
Drug Classes: Calcium channel blockers
Brand Names: Vascor
Foreign Brand Availability: Bepricol (Japan); Cordium (Portugal); Cruor (Argentina); Unicordium (France)
Cost of Therapy: $103.45 (Angina; Vascor; 200 mg; 1 tablet/day; 30 day supply)

DESCRIPTION

Bepridil hydrochloride is an anti-anginal agent that inhibits slow calcium as well as fast sodium channels, interferes with calcium binding to calmodulin and blocks both voltage and receptor operated calcium channels. It is not related chemically to other drugs having similar cardioactivity such as diltiazem HCl, nifedipine and verapamil hydrochloride.

Bepridil hydrochloride monohydrate is a white to off-white, crystalline powder with a bitter taste. It is slightly soluble in water, very soluble in ethanol, methanol and chloroform, and freely soluble in acetone. The molecular weight of bepridil hydrochloride monohydrate is 421.02. Its molecular formula is $C_{24}H_{34}N_2O \cdot HCl \cdot H_2O$. Chemically, bepridil hydrochloride is (±)-β[(2-methylpropoxy)methyl)-*N*-phenyl-*N*-(phenylmethyl)-1-pyrrolidineethanamine monohydrochloride monohydrate.

Bepridil HCl is available as film-coated tablets for oral use containing 200, 300, or 400 mg of bepridil hydrochloride monohydrate. Inactive ingredients: hydroxypropyl methylcellulose, lactose, magnesium stearate, microcrystalline cellulose, polyethylene glycol, silicon dioxide, pregelatinized corn starch, corn starch, titanium dioxide, FD&C blue no. 1.
Storage: Store at 15-25°C (59-77°F). Protect from light.

CLINICAL PHARMACOLOGY

Bepridil HCl is a calcium channel blocker anti-anginal agent with Type 1 anti-arrhythmic and minimal anti-hypertensive properties. Bepridil HCl has inhibitory effects on both the slow calcium and fast sodium inward currents in myocardial and vascular smooth muscle.

Bepridil HCl inhibits the transmembrane influx of calcium ions into cardiac and vascular smooth muscle. This has been demonstrated in isolated myocardial and vascular smooth muscle preparations in which both the slope of the calcium dose response curve and the maximum calcium-induced inotropic response were significantly reduced by bepridil HCl. In cardiac myocytes *in vitro,* bepridil HCl was shown to be tightly bound to actin. A negative inotropic effect can be seen in the isolated guinea pig atria.

In *in vitro* studies, bepridil HCl has also been demonstrated to inhibit the sodium inward current. Reductions in the maximal upstroke velocity and the amplitude of the action potential, as well as increases in the duration of the normal action potential, have been observed. Additionally, bepridil HCl has been shown to possess local anesthetic activity in isolated myocardial preparations. It effects electrophysiological changes that are observed with several classes of anti-arrhythmic agents.

MECHANISM OF ACTION

The precise mechanism of action for bepridil HCl as an anti-anginal agent remains to be fully determined, but is believed to include the following mechanisms:

Bepridil HCl regularly reduces heart rate and arterial pressure at rest and at a given level of exercise by dilating peripheral arterioles and reducing total peripheral resistance (afterload) against which the heart works. In exercise tolerance tests in patients with stable angina the heart rate/blood pressure product was reduced with bepridil HCl for a given work load.

HEMODYNAMIC EFFECTS

Bepridil HCl produces dose dependent slowing of the heart, and reflex tachycardia is not seen. The mean decrease in heart rate in US clinical trials was 3 b.p.m. Orally administered bepridil HCl also produces modest decreases (less than 5 mm Hg) in systolic and diastolic blood pressure in normotensive patients and somewhat larger decreases in hypertensive patients.

Intravenous administration of bepridil HCl is associated with a modest reduction in left ventricular contractility (dP/dt), and increased filling pressure, but radionuclide cineangiography studies in angina patients demonstrated improvement in ejection fraction at rest and during exercise following oral bepridil HCl therapy. Patients with impaired cardiac function (overt heart failure) were not included in these studies.

ELECTROPHYSIOLOGICAL EFFECTS

Intravenous administration of bepridil HCl in man prolongs the effective refractory periods of the atria and ventricles, and the functional refractory period of the AV node. There was a tendency for the AV node effective refractory period and A-H interval to be increased as well. Intravenous and oral administration of bepridil HCl slow heart rate, prolong the QT and QTc intervals, and alter the morphology of the T-wave (indentation). In clinical trials with angina patients, the mean percent prolongation of the QTc interval was approximately 8%, and QT of about 10%. The prolongation of QT is dose related, varying from about 0.030 sec at doses of 200 mg once a day to 0.055 sec at 400 mg once a day. Upon cessation of therapy, the ECG gradually normalizes. No instances of greater than first-degree heart block have been observed in US controlled or open clinical studies with bepridil HCl, and first-degree heart block occurred in 0.2% of patients in these studies.

PULMONARY FUNCTION

In healthy subjects and asthmatic patients, intravenous bepridil HCl did not cause bronchoconstriction. Bepridil HCl has been safely used in asthmatic patients and in patients with chronic obstructive lung disease.

PHARMACOKINETICS AND METABOLISM

In studies with healthy volunteers, bepridil HCl is rapidly and completely absorbed after oral administration. The time to peak bepridil plasma concentration is about 2-3 hours. Over a 10 day period, approximately 70% of a single dose of bepridil HCl is excreted in the urine and 22% in the feces, as metabolites of bepridil. Excretion of unmetabolized drug is negligible. In healthy male volunteers, the relationship between dose and steady-state blood levels of bepridil was linear over the range of 200-400 mg/day. Elimination of bepridil is biphasic, with a distribution half-life of about 2 hours. The terminal elimination half-life following the cessation of multiple dosing averaged 42 hours (range 26-64 hours). However, during a given dosing interval, decay from the peak concentration occurs relatively rapidly indicating a dosing interval, decay from the peak concentration occurs relatively rapidly, indicating a dosing interval half-life shorter than 24 hours. Following once-daily dosing with therapeutic doses, steady-state was reached in about 8 days in healthy volunteers. The clearance of bepridil decreases after multiple dosing.

Clearance of bepridil in angina patients was lower than that in healthy volunteers, resulting in higher average plasma bepridil concentrations. At steady state, maximum bepridil concentrations averaged 2332 ng/ml (range 1451-3609) and mean minimum concentrations were 1174 ng/ml (range 226-2639) in angina patients following 300 mg/day doses of bepridil HCl.

Bepridil HCl is more than 99% bound to plasma proteins. Administration of bepridil HCl after a meal resulted in a clinically insignificant delay in time to peak concentration, but neither peak bepridil plasma levels nor the extent of absorption was changed.

Bepridil HCl passes through the placental barrier. Bepridil HCl may cause uterine hypotonia.

INDICATIONS AND USAGE

CHRONIC STABLE ANGINA (CLASSIC EFFORT-ASSOCIATED ANGINA)

Bepridil HCl is indicated for the treatment of chronic stable angina (classic effort-associated). Because bepridil HCl has caused serious ventricular arrhythmias, including torsades de pointes type ventricular tachycardia, and the occurrence of cases of agranulocytosis associated with its use (see WARNINGS), it should be reserved for patients who have failed to respond optimally to, or are intolerant of, other anti-anginal medication.

Bepridil HCl may be used alone or in combination with beta blockers and/or nitrates. Controlled clinical studies have shown an added effect when bepridil HCl is administered to patients already receiving propranolol.

CONTRAINDICATIONS

Bepridil HCl is contraindicated in patients with a known sensitivity to bepridil HCl.

Bepridil HCl is contraindicated in (1) patients with a history of serious ventricular arrhythmias (see WARNINGS, Induction of New Serious Arrhythmias), (2) patients with sick sinus syndrome or patients with second- or third-degree AV block, except in the presence of a functioning ventricular pacemaker, (3) patients with hypotension (less than 90 mm Hg systolic), (4) patients with uncompensated cardiac insufficiency, (5) patients with congenital QT interval prolongation (see WARNINGS), and (6) patients taking other drugs that prolong QT interval (see DRUG INTERACTIONS).

WARNINGS

Induction of New Serious Arrhythmias:

Bepridil HCl has Class 1 anti-arrhythmic properties and, like other such drugs, can induce new arrhythmias, including VT/VF. In addition, because of its ability to prolong the QT interval, bepridil HCl can cause torsades de pointes type ventricular tachycardia. Because of these properties, bepridil HCl should reserved for patients in whom other anti-anginal agents do not offer a satisfactory effect.

In US clinical trials, the QT and QTc intervals were commonly prolonged by bepridil HCl in a dose- related fashion. While the mean prolongation of QTc was 8% and of QT was 10%, QTc increases of 25% or more were not uncommon, 5%; 8.7% QT. Increased QT and QTc may be associated with torsades de pointes type VT, which was seen at least briefly, in about 1.0% of patients in US trials; in many cases, however, patients with marked prolongation of QTc were taken off bepridil HCl therapy. All of the US patients with torsades de pointes had a prolonged QT interval and relatively low serum potassium. French marketing experience has reported over 100 verified cases of torsades de pointes. While this number, based on total use, represents a rate of only 0.01%, the true rate is undoubtedly much higher, as spontaneous reporting systems all suffer from substantial under reporting.

Torsades de pointes is a polymorphic ventricular tachycardia often but not always associated with a prolonged QT interval, and often drug induced. The relation between the degree of QT prolongation and the development of torsades de pointes is not linear and the likelihood of torsades appears to be increased by hypokalemia, use of potassium wasting diuretics, and the presence of antecedent bradycardia. While the safe upper limit of QT is not defined, it is suggested that the interval not be permitted to exceed 0.52 seconds during treatment. If dose reduction does not eliminate the excessive prolongation, bepridil should be stopped.

Because most domestic and foreign cases of torsades have developed in patients with hypokalemia, usually related to diuretic use or significant liver disease, if concomitant diuretics are needed, low doses and addition or primary use of a potassium sparing diuretic should be considered and the serum potassium should be monitored.

Bepridil HCl has been associated with the usual range of pro-arrhythmic effects characteristic of Class 1 anti-arrhythmics (increased premature ventricular contraction rates, new sustained VT, and VT/VF that is more difficult than previously to convert to sinus rhythm). Use in patients with severe arrhythmias (who are most susceptible to certain pro-arrhythmic effects) has been limited, so that risk in these patients is not defined.

In the National Heart, Lung and Blood Institute's Cardiac Arrhythmia Suppression Trial (CAST), a long-term, multi- centered, randomized, double-blind study in patients with asymptomatic non-life-threatening ventricular arrhythmias who had myocardial infarctions more than 6 days but less than 2 years previously, an excess mortality/non-fatal cardiac arrest rate was seen in patients treated with encainide or flecainide (56/730) compared to that seen in patients assigned to matched placebo-treated groups (22/725). The applicability of these results to other populations (*e.g.,* those without recent myocardial infarction) or to other anti-arrhythmic drugs is uncertain, but at present it is prudent to consider any drug documented to provoke new serious arrhythmias or worsening of pre-existing arrhythmias as having a similar risk and to avoid their use in the post-infarction period.

AGRANULOCYTOSIS

In US clinical trials of over 800 patients treated with bepridil HCl for up to 5 years, 2 cases of marked leukopenia and neutropenia were reported. Both patients were diabetic and elderly. One (1) died with overwhelming gram-negative sepsis, itself a possible cause of marked leukopenia. The other patient recovered rapidly when bepridil HCl was stopped.

CONGESTIVE HEART FAILURE

Congestive heart failure has been observed infrequently (about 1%) during US controlled clinical trials, but experience with the use of bepridil HCl in patients with significantly impaired ventricular function is limited. There is little information on the effect of concomitant administration of bepridil HCl and digoxin; therefore, caution should be exercised in treating patients with congestive heart failure.

HEPATIC ENZYME ELEVATION

In US clinical studies with bepridil HCl in about 1000 patients and subjects, clinically significant (at least 2 times the upper limit of normal) transaminase elevations were observed in approximately 1% of the patients. None of these patients became clinically symptomatic or jaundiced and values returned to normal when the drug was stopped.

HYPOKALEMIA

In clinical trials bepridil HCl has not been reported to reduce serum potassium levels. Because hypokalemia has been associated with ventricular arrhythmias, potassium insufficiency should be corrected before bepridil HCl therapy is initiated and normal potassium concentrations should be maintained during bepridil HCl therapy. Serum potassium should be monitored periodically.

PRECAUTIONS

GENERAL

Caution should be exercised when using bepridil HCl in patients with left bundle branch block or sinus bradycardia (less than 50 b.p.m.). Care should also be exercised in patients with serious hepatic or renal disorders because such patients have not been studied and bepridil is highly metabolized, with metabolites excreted primarily in the urine.

RECENT MYOCARDIAL INFARCTION

In US clinical trials with bepridil HCl, patients with myocardial infarctions within 3 months prior to initiation of drug treatment were excluded. The initiation of bepridil HCl therapy in such patients, therefore, cannot be recommended.

INFORMATION FOR THE PATIENT

Since QT prolongation is not associated with defined symptomatology, patients should be instructed on the importance of maintaining any potassium supplementation or potassium sparing diuretic, and the need for routine electrocardiograms and periodic monitoring of serum potassium.

The following patient information is printed on the carton label of each unit of use bottle of 30 tablets:

> As with any medication that you take, you should notify your physician of any changes in your overall condition. Insure that you follow your physician's instructions regarding follow-up visits. Please notify any physician who treats you for a medical condition that you are taking bepridil HCl, as well as any other medications.

CARCINOGENESIS, MUTAGENESIS, AND IMPAIRMENT OF FERTILITY

No evidence of carcinogenicity was revealed in one lifetime study in mice at dosages up to 60 times (for a 60 kg subject) the maximum recommended dosage in man. Unilateral follicular adenomas of the thyroid were observed in a study in rats following lifetime administration of high doses of bepridil HCl, (*i.e.,* ≥100 mg/kg/day) (20 times the usual recommended dose in man). No mutagenic or other genotoxic potential of bepridil HCl was found in the following standard laboratory tests: the Micronucleus Test for Chromosomal Effects, the Liver Microsome Activated Bacterial Assay for Mutagenicity, the Chinese Hamster Ovary Cell Assay for Mutagenicity, and the Sister Chromatid Exchange Assay. No intrinsic effect on fertility by bepridil HCl was demonstrated in rats.

In monkeys, at 200 mg/kg/day, there was a decrease in testicular weight and spermatogenesis. There were no systematic studies in man related to this point. In rats, at doses up to 300 mg/kg/day, there was no observed alteration of mating behavior nor of reproductive performance.

USAGE IN PREGNANCY, PREGNANCY CATEGORY C

Reproductive studies (fertility and peri-postnatal) have been conducted in rats. Reduced litter size at birth and decreased pup survival during lactation were observed at maternal dosages 37 times (on a mg/kg basis) the maximum daily recommended therapeutic dosage.

In teratology studies, no effects were observed in rats or rabbits at these same dosages.

There no well-controlled studies in pregnant women. Use bepridil HCl in pregnant or nursing women only if the potential benefit justifies the potential risk.

NURSING MOTHERS

Bepridil is excreted in human milk. Bepridil concentration in human milk is estimated to reach about one-third the concentration in serum. Because of the potential for serious adverse reactions in nursing infants from bepridil HCl a decision should be made whether to discontinue nursing or to discontinue the drug, taking into account the importance of the drug to the mother.

PEDIATRIC USE

The safety and effectiveness of bepridil HCl in children have not been established.

DRUG INTERACTIONS

NITRATES

The concomitant use of bepridil HCl with long- and short-acting nitrates has been safely tolerated in patients with stable angina pectoris. Sublingual nitroglycerin may be taken if necessary for the control of acute angina attacks during bepridil HCl therapy.

BETA BLOCKING AGENTS

The concomitant use of bepridil HCl and beta-blocking agents has been well tolerated in patients with stable angina. Available data are not sufficient, however, to predict the effects of concomitant medication on patients with impaired ventricular function or cardiac conduction abnormalities (see CLINICAL PHARMACOLOGY and DOSAGE AND ADMINISTRATION).

DIGOXIN

In controlled studies in healthy volunteers, bepridil HCl either had no effect (one study) or was associated with modest increases, about 30% (two studies) in steady-state serum digoxin concentrations. Limited clinical data in angina patients receiving concomitant bepridil HCl and digoxin therapy indicate no discernible changes in serum digoxin levels. Available data are neither sufficient to rule out possible increases in serum digoxin with concomitant treatment in some patients, nor other possible interactions, particularly in patients with cardiac conduction abnormalities (also see WARNINGS, Congestive Heart Failure).

ORAL HYPOGLYCEMICS

Bepridil HCl has been safely used in diabetic patients without significantly lowering their blood glucose levels or altering their need for insulin or oral hypoglycemic agents.

GENERAL INTERACTIONS

Certain drugs could increase the likelihood of potentially serious adverse effects with bepridil HCl. In general, these are drugs that have one or more pharmacologic activities similar to bepridil HCl, including anti-arrhythmic agents such as quinidine and procainamide, cardiac glycosides and tricyclic anti-depressants. Anti-arrhythmics and tricyclic anti-depressants could exaggerate the prolongation of the QT interval observed with bepridil HCl. Cardiac glycosides could exaggerate the depression of AV nodal conduction observed with bepridil HCl.

ADVERSE REACTIONS

Adverse reactions were assessed in placebo and active-drug controlled trials of 4-12 weeks duration and longer-term uncontrolled studies. The most common side effects occurring more frequently than in control groups were upper gastrointestinal complaints (nausea, dyspepsia, or GI distress) in about 22%, diarrhea in about 8%, dizziness in about 15%, asthenia in about 10% and nervousness in about 7%. The adverse reactions seen in at least 2% of bepridil patients in controlled trials are shown in TABLE 1.

TABLE 1 *Adverse Experiences by Body System and Treatment in Greater Than 2% of Bepridil Patients in Controlled Trials*

Adverse Reaction	Bepridil HCl (n=529)	Nifedipine (n=50)	Propanolol (n=88)	Diltiazem (n=41)	Placebo (n=190)
Body as a Whole					
Asthenia	9.83	22.00	22.73	12.20	7.37
Headache	11.34	22.00	13.64	7.32	14.21
Flu syndrome	2.08	8.00	2.27	*	1.05
Cardiovascular/Respiratory					
Palpitations	2.27	6.00	2.27	0.00	1.58
Dyspnea	3.59	4.00	5.68	4.88	2.11
Respiratory Infection	2.84	4.00	3.41	4.88	3.68
Gastrointestinal					
Dyspepsia	6.81	4.00	5.68	4.88	1.58
GI distress	4.35	10.00	6.82	*	2.11
Nausea	12.29	14.00	11.36	2.44	3.68
Dry mouth	3.40	0.00	0.00	2.44	2.63
Anorexia	3.02	0.00	2.27	0.00	1.58
Diarrhea	7.75	2.00	9.09	2.44	2.63
Abdominal pain	3.02	4.00	1.14	*	3.16
Constipation	6.00	1.14	4.88	2.11	2.84
Central Nervous System					
Drowsy	3.78	4.00	4.55	*	3.68
Insomnia	2.65	6.00	3.41	*	1.05
Dizziness	14.74	30.00	10.23	4.88	9.47
Tremor	4.91	4.00	0.00	*	1.05
Tremor of hand	3.02	4.00	0.00	*	0.53
Paresthesia	2.46	2.00	1.14	4.88	3.16
Psychiatric					
Nervous	7.37	16.00	1.14	2.44	3.68

* No data available.

In one 12 week controlled study, daily doses of 200, 300, and 400 mg were compared to placebo. TABLE 2 shows the rates of more common reactions (at least 5% in at least one bepridil group).

Adverse experiences in long-term open studies were generally similar to those seen in controlled trials.

Although adverse experiences were frequent (at least one being reported in 71% of patients participating in controlled clinical trials), most were well-tolerated. About 15% of patients however, left bepridil treatment because of adverse experiences. In controlled clinical trials, these were principally gastrointestinal (1.0%), dizziness (1.0%), ventricular arrhythmias (1.0%), and syncope (0.6%). The major reasons for discontinuation, with comparison to control agents, are shown in TABLE 3

Across all controlled and uncontrolled trials, bepridil HCl was evaluated in over 800 patients with chronic angina. In addition to the adverse reactions noted above, the following were observed in 0.5-2.0% of the bepridil HCl or are rarer, but potentially important events seen in clinical studies or reported in post marketing experience. In most cases it is not possible to determine whether there is a causal relationship to bepridil treatment.

Body as a Whole: Fever, pain, myalgic asthenia, superinfection, flu syndrome.

Cardiovascular/Respiratory: Sinus tachycardia, sinus bradycardia, hypertension vasodilation, edema, ventricular premature contractions, ventricular tachycardia, prolonged QT interval, rhinitis, cough, pharyngitis.

Gastrointestinal: Flatulence, gastritis, appetite increase, dry mouth, constipation.

TABLE 2 *Adverse Experiences by Body System and Treatment in Greater Than 5% of Bepridil Patients in Controlled Trials*

	Bepridil HCl			
Adverse Reaction	200 mg (n=43)	300 mg (n=46)	400 mg (n=44)	Placebo (n=44)
Body as a Whole				
Asthenia	13.95%	6.52%	11.36%	2.27%
Headache	6.88%	8.70%	13.64%	15.91%
Cardiovascular/Respiratory				
Palpitations	0.00%	6.52%	4.55%	0.00%
Dyspnea	2.33%	8.70%	0.00%	2.27%
Gastrointestinal				
GI distress	6.98%	0.00%	4.55%	4.55%
Nausea	6.98%	26.09%	18.18%	2.27%
Anorexia	0.00%	2.17%	6.82%	2.27%
Diarrhea	0.00%	10.87%	6.82%	0.00%
Central Nervous System				
Drowsy	6.98%	6.52%	0.00%	4.55%
Dizziness	11.63%	15.22%	27.27%	6.82%
Tremor	6.98%	0.00%	4.55%	0.00%
Tremor of hand	9.30%	0.00%	4.55%	0.00%
Psychiatric				
Nervous	11.63%	8.70%	11.36%	0.00%
Special Senses				
Tinnitus	0.00%	6.52%	2.27%	2.27%

TABLE 3 *Most Common Events Resulting in Discontinuation*

Bepridil	Placebo	Positive Control	
Adverse Reaction	(n=515)	(n=288)	(n=119)
Dizziness	5 (0.97%)	0 (0.0%)	2 (1.68%)
Gastrointestinal Symptoms	5 (0.97%)	0 (0.0%)	5 (4.20%)
Ventricular Arrhythmia	5 (0.97%)	0 (0.0%)	0 (0.00%)
Syncope	3 (0.58%)	0 (0.0%)	0 (0.00%)

Musculoskeletal: Arthritis.

Central Nervous System: Fainting, vertigo, akathisia, drowsiness, insomnia, tremor.

Psychiatric: Depression, anxiousness, adverse behavior effect.

Skin: Rash, sweating, skin irritation.

Special Senses: Blurred vision, tinnitus, taste change.

Urogenital: Loss of libido, impotence.

Abnormal Lab Values: Abnormal liver function test, SGPT increase.

Certain cardiovascular events, such as acute myocardial infarction (about 3% of patients), worsened heart failure (1.9%), worsened angina (4.5%), severe arrhythmia (about 2.4% VT/VF) and sudden death (1.6%) have occurred in patients receiving bepridil, but have not been included as adverse events because they appear to be, and cannot be distinguished from, manifestations of the patient's underlying cardiac disease. Such events as torsades de pointes arrhythmias, prolonged QT/QTc, bradycardia, first degree heart block, which are probably related to bepridil, are included in the tables.

DOSAGE AND ADMINISTRATION

Therapy with bepridil HCl should be individualized according to each patient's response and the physician's clinical judgement. The usual starting dose of bepridil HCl is 200 mg once daily. After 10 days, dosage may be adjusted upward depending upon the patient's response (*e.g.*, ability to perform activities of daily living, QT interval, heart rate, and frequency and severity of angina). This long interval for dosage adjustment is needed because steady-state blood levels are not achieved until 8 days of therapy. In clinical trials, most patients were maintained at a dose of bepridil HCl of 300 mg once daily. The maximum daily dose of bepridil HCl is 400 mg and the established minimum effective dose is 200 mg daily.

The starting dose for elderly patients does not differ from that for young patients. After therapeutic response is demonstrated, however, elderly patients may require more frequent monitoring.

Food does not interfere with the absorption of bepridil HCl (see CLINICAL PHARMACOLOGY, Pharmacokinetics and Metabolism). If nausea is experienced with bepridil HCl, the drug may be given at meals or at bedtime.

Bepridil HCl has not been studied adequately in patients with impaired hepatic or renal function. It is therefore possible that dosage adjustments may be necessary in these patients.

CONCOMITANT USE WITH OTHER AGENTS

The concomitant use of bepridil hyrdochloride and beta-blocking agents in patients without heart failure is safely tolerated. Physicians wishing to switch patients from beta-blocker therapy to bepridil HCl therapy may initiate bepridil HCl before terminating the beta-blocker in the usual gradual fashion (see CLINICAL PHARMACOLOGY and PRECAUTIONS).

PRODUCT LISTING - RATED THERAPEUTICALLY EQUIVALENT

Tablet - Oral - 200 mg

30's	$76.40	VASCOR, Janssen Pharmaceuticals	00045-0682-30
90's	$359.19	VASCOR, Janssen Pharmaceuticals	00045-0682-33

Tablet - Oral - 300 mg

30's	$93.22	VASCOR, Janssen Pharmaceuticals	00045-0683-30
90's	$438.21	VASCOR, Janssen Pharmaceuticals	00045-0683-33

Tablet - Oral - 400 mg

30's	$105.13	VASCOR, Janssen Pharmaceuticals	00045-0684-30

Betamethasone (000462)

For related information, see the comparative table section in Appendix A.

Categories: Adrenocortical insufficiency; Anemia, acquired hemolytic; Anemia, congenital hypoplastic; Anemia, erythroblastopenia; Ankylosing spondylitis; Arthritis, gouty; Arthritis, osteoarthritis; Arthritis, psoriatic; Arthritis, rheumatoid; Asthma; Berylliosis; Bursitis; Carditis, rheumatic; Chorioretinitis; Choroiditis; Colitis, ulcerative; Conjunctivitis, allergic; Crohn's disease; Dermatitis herpetiformis, bullous; Dermatitis, atopic; Dermatitis, contact; Dermatitis, exfoliative; Dermatitis, seborrheic; Epicondylitis; Erythema multiforme; Herpes zoster ophthalmicus; Hypercalcemia, secondary to neoplasia; Hyperplasia, congenital adrenal; Inflammation, ophthalmic; Inflammatory bowel disease; Iridocyclitis; Iritis; Leukemia; Loffler's syndrome; Lupus erythematosus, systemic; Lymphoma; Meningitis, tuberculous; Mycosis fungoides; Neuritis, optic; Pemphigus; Pneumonitis, aspiration; Psoriasis; Rhinitis, perennial allergic; Rhinitis, seasonal allergic; Sarcoidosis; Serum sickness; Stevens-Johnson syndrome; Synovitis, secondary to osteoarthritis; Tenosynovitis; Thrombocytopenia purpura, idiopathic; Thrombocytopenia, secondary; Thyroiditis, nonsuppurative; Trichinosis; Tuberculosis, disseminated; Tuberculosis, fulminating; Tuberculosis, meningitis; Uveitis; FDA Approved 1961 Apr; Pregnancy Category C; WHO Formulary

Drug Classes: Corticosteroids

Brand Names: Benoson; Betaderm; Betason; **Celestone**; Rinderon; Unicort

Foreign Brand Availability: Benoson (500 mcg) (Indonesia); Betason (500 mcg) (Indonesia); Betnelan (England); Betnelan (500 mcg) (Bahrain; Cyprus; Egypt; India; Iran; Iraq; Jordan; Kuwait; Lebanon; Libya; Netherlands; Oman; Philippines; Qatar; Republic-of-Yemen; Saudi-Arabia; South-Africa; Syria; United-Arab-Emirates); Betnesol (Bulgaria; Greece); Celestamine (Germany); Celestan (Austria); Celestene (France); Celeston (Denmark; Finland; Norway; Sweden); Celestone (500 mcg) (Bahamas; Bahrain; Barbados; Belize; Benin; Bermuda; Burkina-Faso; Canada; CIS; Colombia; Costa-Rica; Curacao; Cyprus; Dominican-Republic; Ecuador; Egypt; El-Salvador; Ethiopia; Gambia; Ghana; Guatemala; Guinea; Guyana; Honduras; Hong-Kong; Iran; Iraq; Ivory-Coast; Jamaica; Jordan; Kenya; Korea; Kuwait; Lebanon; Liberia; Libya; Malawi; Malaysia; Mali; Mauritania; Mauritius; Mexico; Morocco; Netherland-Antilles; Nicaragua; Niger; Nigeria; Oman; Panama; Peru; Philippines; Qatar; Republic-of-Yemen; Saudi-Arabia; Senegal; Seychelles; Sierra-Leone; South-Africa; Sudan; Surinam; Syria; Tanzania; Trinidad; Tunia; Uganda; United-Arab-Emirates; Zambia; Zimbabwe); Walacort (India)

DESCRIPTION

Glucocorticoids are adrenocortical steroids, both naturally occurring and synthetic, that are readily absorbed from the gastrointestinal tract. A derivative of prednisolone, Betamethasone has a 16β-methyl group that enhances the anti-inflammatory action of the molecule and reduces the sodium- and water-retaining properties of the fluorine atom bound at carbon 9.

The formula for betamethasone is $C_{22}H_{29}FO_5$ and has a molecular weight of 329.47. Chemically, it is 9-fluoro-11β,17,21-trihydroxy-16β-methylpregna-1,4-diene-3,20-dione.

Betamethasone is a white to practically white, odorless, crystalline powder. It melts at about 240°C with some decomposition. Betamethasone is sparingly soluble in acetone, alcohol, dioxane, and methanol; very slightly soluble in chloroform and ether; and is insoluble in water.

Each betamethasone tablet contains 0.6 mg betamethasone, betamethasone syrup contains 0.6 mg betamethasone in each 5 ml and less than 1% alcohol.

CLINICAL PHARMACOLOGY

Naturally occurring glucocorticoids (hydrocortisone or cortisone), which also have salt-retaining properties, are used as replacement therapy in adrenocortical deficiency states. Their synthetic analogs are primarily used for their potent anti-inflammatory effects in disorders of many organ systems. Glucocorticoids, such as betamethasone cause profound and varied metabolic effects. In addition, they modify the body's immune responses to diverse stimuli.

INDICATIONS AND USAGE

ENDOCRINE DISORDERS

Primary or secondary adrenocortical insufficiency (hydrocortisone or cortisone is the drug of choice; synthetic analogs may be used in conjunction with mineralocorticoids where applicable; in infancy, mineralocorticoid supplementation is of particular importance).
Congenital adrenal hyperplasia.
Nonsuppurative thyroiditis.
Hypercalcemia associated with cancer.

RHEUMATIC DISORDERS

As adjunctive therapy for short-term administration (to tide the patient over an acute episode or exacerbation) in:

Psoriatic arthritis.
Rheumatoid arthritis, including juvenile rheumatoid arthritis (selected cases may require low-dose maintenance therapy).
Ankylosing spondylitis.
Acute and subacute bursitis.
Acute and nonspecific tenosynovitis.
Acute gouty arthritis.
Post-traumatic osteoarthritis.
Synovitis or osteoarthritis.
Epicondylitis.

COLLAGEN DISEASES

During an exacerbation or as a maintenance therapy in selected cases of:

Systemic lupus erythematosus.
Acute rheumatic carditis.

DERMATOLOGICAL DISEASES

Pemphigus.
Bullous dermatitis herpetiformis.
Severe erythema multiforme (Stevens-Johnson syndrome).
Exfoliative dermatitis.
Mycosis fungoides.
Severe seborrheic dermatitis.
Severe psoriasis.
Systemic lupus erythematosus.
Acute rheumatic carditis.

ALLERGIC STATES

Control of severe or incapacitating allergic conditions intractable to adequate trials of conventional treatment in:

Bronchial asthma.
Contact dermatitis.
Atopic dermatitis.
Serum sickness.
Seasonal or perennial allergic rhinitis.
Drug hypersensitivity.

OPHTHALMIC DISEASES

Severe, acute and chronic allergic and inflammatory processes involving the eye and its adnexa, such as:

Allergic conjunctivitis.
Herpes zoster ophthalmicus.
Iritis, iridocyclitis.
Chorioretinitis.
Anterior segment inflammation.
Diffuse posterior uveitis and chorditis.
Optic neuritis.
Sympathetic ophthalmia.

RESPIRATORY DISEASES

Symptomatic sarcoidosis.
Loftier's syndrome not manageable by any other means.
Berylliosis.
Fulminating or disseminated pulmonary tuberculosis when used concurrently with appropriate antituberculous chemotherapy.
Aspiration pneumonitis.

HEMATOLOGIC DISORDERS

Idiopathic thrombocytopenia purpura in adults (IV and IM administration is contraindicated).
Secondary thrombocytopenia in adults.
Acquired (autoimmune) hemolytic amenia.
Erythroblastopenia (RBC anemia).
Congenital (erythroid) hypoplastic anemia.

NEOPLASTIC DISEASES

For palliative management of:

Leukemias and lymphomas in adults.
Acute leukemia of childhood.

EDEMATOUS STATES

To induce diuresis or remission of proteinuria in the nephrotic syndrome, without uremia, of the idiopathic type or that due to lupus erythematosus.

GASTROINTESTINAL DISEASES

To tide the patient over a critical period of the disease in:

Ulcerative colitis.
Regional enteritis.

MISCELLANEOUS

Tuberculous meningitis with subarachnoid block or impending block when used concurrently with appropriate antituberculosis chemotherapy.
Trichinosis with neurologic or myocardial involvement.

CONTRAINDICATIONS

Betamethasone syrup and tablets contraindicated in systemic fungal infections.

WARNINGS

In patients on corticosteroid therapy subjected to any unusual stress, increased dosage of rapidly acting corticosteroids before, during, and after the stressful situation is indicated.

Corticosteroids may mask some signs of infection, and new infections may appear during their use.

There may be decreased resistance and inability to localize infection when corticosteroids are used.

Prolonged use of corticosteroids may produce posterior subcapsular cataracts, glaucoma with possible damage to the optic nerves, and may enhance the establishment of secondary ocular infections due to fungi or viruses.

Average and large doses of cortisone or hydrocortisone can cause elevation of blood pressure, salt and water retention, and increased excretion of potassium. These effects are less likely to occur with the synthetic derivatives except when used in large doses. Dietary salt restriction and potassium supplementation may be necessary. All corticosteroids increase calcium excretion.

While on corticosteroid therapy patients should not be vaccinated against smallpox. Other immunization procedures should not be undertaken in patients who are on corticosteroids. Especially in high doses, because of the possible hazards of neurological complications and lack of antibody response.

Children who are on immunosuppressant drugs are more susceptible to infections than healthy children. Chickenpox and measles, for example, can have a more serious or even fatal course in children on immunosuppressant corticosteroids. In such children, or in adults who have not had these diseases, particular care should be taken to avoid exposure. If exposed, therapy with varicella zoster immune globulin (VZIG) or pooled intravenous immunoglobulin (IVIG), as appropriate, may be indicated. If chickenpox develops, treatment with antiviral agents may be considered.

The use of betamethasone syrup and tablets in active tuberculosis should be restricted to those cases of fulminating or disseminated tuberculosis in which the corticosteroid is used for the management of the disease in conjunction with appropriate antituberculosis regimen.

If corticosteroids are indicated in patients with latent tuberculosis or tuberculin reactivity, close observation is necessary as reactivation of the disease may occur. During prolonged corticosteroid therapy, these patients should receive chemoprophylaxis.

Because rare instances of anaphylactoid reactions have occurred in patients receiving parenteral corticosteroid therapy, appropriate precautionary measures should be taken prior to administration, especially when the patient has a history of allergy to any drug.

USAGE IN PREGNANCY

Since adequate human reproduction studies have not been done with corticosteroids, the use of these drugs in pregnancy, nursing mothers, or women of childbearing potential requires that the possible benefits of the drug be weighed against the potential hazards to the mother and embryo or fetus. Infants born to mothers who have received substantial doses of corticosteroids during pregnancy should be carefully observed for signs of hypoadrenalism.

PRECAUTIONS

INFORMATION FOR THE PATIENT

Patients who are on immunosuppressant doses of corticosteroids should be warned to avoid exposure to chickenpox or measles and, if exposed, to obtain medical advice.

GENERAL

Drug-induced secondary adrenocortical insufficiency may be minimized by gradual reduction of dosage. This type of relative insufficiency may persist for months after discontinuation of therapy; therefore, in any situation of stress occurring during that period, hormone therapy should be reinstituted. Since mineralocorticoid secretion may be impaired, salt and/or a mineralocorticoid should be administered concurrently.

There is an enhanced effect of corticosteroids in patients with hypothyroidism and in those with cirrhosis.

Corticosteroids should be used cautiously in patients with ocular herpes simplex for fear of corneal perforation.

The lowest possible dose of corticosteroid should be used to control the condition under treatment, and when reduction in dosage is possible, the reduction in dosage is possible, the reduction must be gradual.

Psychic derangements may appear when corticosteroids are used, ranging from euphoria, insomnia, mood swings, personality changes, and severe depression to frank psychotic manifestations. Also, existing emotional instability or psychotic tendencies may be aggravated by corticosteroids.

Aspirin should be used cautiously in conjunction with corticosteroids in hypothrombinemia.

Steroids should be used with caution in nonspecific ulcerative colitis, if there is a probability of impending perforation, abscess or other pyrogenic infection, also in diverticulitis, fresh Intestinal anastomoses, active or latent peptic ulcer, renal insufficiency, hypertension, osteoporosis, and myasthenia gravis. Growth and development or infants and children on prolonged corticosteroid therapy should be carefully followed.

ADVERSE REACTIONS

Fluid and Electrolyte Disturbances: Sodium retention; fluid retention; congestive heart failure in susceptible patients; potassium loss; hypokalemic alkalosis; hypertension.

Musculoskeletal: Muscle weakness; steroid myopathy; loss of muscle mass; osteoporosis, vertebral compression fractures; aseptic necrosis of femoral and humeral heads; pathologic fracture of long bones.

Gastrointestinal: Peptic ulcer with possible subsequent perforation and hemorrhage; pancreatitis; abdominal distention; ulcerative esophagitis.

Dermatological: Impaired wound healing; thin fragile skin; petechiae and ecchymoses; facial erythema; increased sweating; may suppress reactions to skin tests.

Neurological: Convulsions; increased intracranial pressure with papilledema (pseudotumor cerebri) usually after treatment; vertigo; headache.

Endocrine: Menstrual irregularities; development of Cushingoid state; suppression of growth in children; secondary adrenocortical and pituitary unresponsiveness, particularly in times of stress, as in trauma, surgery or illness; decreased carbohydrate tolerance; manifestations of latent diabetes mellitus; increased requirements for insulin or oral hypoglycemic agents in diabetics.

Ophthalmic: Posterior subcapsular cataracts; increased intraocular pressure; glaucoma; exophthalmos.

Metabolic: Negative nitrogen balance due to protein catabolism.

DOSAGE AND ADMINISTRATION

The initial dosage of betamethasone may vary from 0.6-7.2 mg/day depending on the specific disease entity being treated. In situations of less severity lower doses will generally suffice, while in selected patients higher initial doses may be required. The initial dosage should be maintained or adjusted until a satisfactory response is noted. If after a reasonable period of time, there is a lack of satisfactory clinical response, betamethasone should be discontinued and the patient transferred to other therapy. **IT SHOULD BE EMPHASIZED THAT DOSAGE REQUIREMENTS ARE VARIABLE AND MUST BE INDIVIDUALIZED ON THE BASIS OF THE DISEASE UNDER TREATMENT AND RESPONSE OF THE PATIENT**. After a favorable response is noted, the proper maintenance dosage should be determined by decreasing the initial drug dosage in small decrements at appropriate time intervals until the lowest dosage which will maintain an adequate clinical response is reached. It should be kept in mind that constant monitoring is needed in regard to drug dosage. Included in the situations which may make dosage adjustments necessary are changes in clinical status secondary to remissions to exacerbations in the disease process, the patient's individual drug responsiveness, and the effect of patient exposure to stressful situations not directly related to the disease entity under treatment; in this latter situation it may necessary to increase dosage of betamethasone for a period of time consistent with the patient's condition. If after long-term therapy the drug is to be stopped, it is recommended that it be withdrawn gradually rather than abruptly.

Protect syrup from light.

Storage: Store tablets between 2 and 30°C (36 and 86°F). Additionally, protect 21 tablet pack from excessive moisture.

PRODUCT LISTING - EQUIVALENTS NOT AVAILABLE

Syrup - Oral - 0.6 mg/5 ml

120 ml	$41.22	CELESTONE, Schering Corporation	00085-0942-05

Tablet - Oral - 0.6 mg

21's	$41.42	CELESTONE, Schering Corporation	00085-0011-01
100's	$186.54	CELESTONE, Schering Corporation	00085-0011-05

Betamethasone Acetate; Betamethasone Sodium Phosphate *(000463)*

For complete prescribing information, refer to the CD-ROM included with the book.

Categories: Adrenocortical insufficiency; Alopecia areata; Anemia, acquired hemolytic; Anemia, congenital hypoplastic; Anemia, erythroblastopenia; Ankylosing spondylitis; Arthritis, gouty; Arthritis, osteoarthritis; Arthritis, psoriatic; Arthritis, rheumatoid; Asthma; Berylliosis; Bursitis; Carditis, rheumatic; Chorioretinitis; Choroiditis; Colitis, ulcerative; Conjunctivitis, allergic; Crohn's disease; Cyst, aponeurotic; Cyst, ganglionic; Dermatitis herpetiformis, bullous; Dermatitis, atopic; Dermatitis, contact; Dermatitis, exfoliative; Dermatitis, seborrheic; Edema, laryngeal; Epicondylitis; Erythema multiforme; Granuloma annulare; Herpes zoster ophthalmicus; Hypercalcemia, secondary to neoplasia; Hyperplasia, congenital adrenal; Hypersensitivity reactions; Inflammation, ophthalmic; Inflammatory bowel disease; Iridocyclitis; Iritis; Keloid; Keratitis; Leukemia; Lichen planus; Lichen simplex chronicus; Loffler's syndrome; Lupus erythematosus, discoid; Lupus erythematosus, systemic; Lymphoma; Meningitis, tuberculous; Mycosis fungoides; Necrobiosis lipoidica diabeticorum; Neuritis, optic; Pemphigus; Pneumonitis, aspiration; Proteinuria, secondary to lupus erythematosus; Proteinuria, secondary to nephrotic syndrome; Psoriasis; Rhinitis, perennial allergic; Rhinitis, seasonal allergic; Sarcoidosis; Serum sickness; Stevens-Johnson syndrome; Synovitis, secondary to osteoarthritis; Tenosynovitis; Thrombocytopenia purpura, idiopathic; Thrombocytopenia, secondary; Thyroiditis, nonsuppurative; Transfusion reaction; Trichinosis; Tuberculosis, disseminated; Tuberculosis, fulminating; Tuberculosis, meningitis; Ulcer, allergic corneal; Uveitis; FDA Approval Pre 1982; Pregnancy Category C

Drug Classes: Corticosteroids

Brand Names: **Celestone Soluspan**

Foreign Brand Availability: Celestan Biphase (Austria); Celestan Depot (Germany); Celestene Chronodose (France); Celeston (Denmark); Celeston Chronodose (Finland); Celestone Chronodose (Australia; Bahrain; Belgium; Benin; Burkina-Faso; Colombia; Costa-Rica; Cyprus; Dominican-Republic; Egypt; El-Salvador; Ethiopia; Gambia; Ghana; Guatemala; Guinea; Honduras; Hungary; Iran; Iraq; Israel; Italy; Ivory-Coast; Jordan; Kenya; Kuwait; Lebanon; Liberia; Libya; Malawi; Mali; Mauritania; Mauritius; Morocco; Netherlands; New-Zealand; Nicaragua; Niger; Nigeria; Oman; Panama; Qatar; Republic-of-Yemen; Saudi-Arabia; Senegal; Seychelles; Sierra-Leone; Spain; Sudan; Syria; Tanzania; Tunia; Uganda; United-Arab-Emirates; Zambia; Zimbabwe); Celestone Cronodose (Ecuador; Peru); Celestone-Soluspan (South-Africa)

DESCRIPTION

Each ml of Celestone Soluspan suspension contains: 3.0 mg betamethasone as betamethasone sodium phosphate; 3.0 mg betamethasone acetate; 7.1 mg dibasic sodium phosphate; 3.4 mg monobasic sodium phosphate; 0.1 mg edetate disodium; and 0.2 mg benzalkonium chloride. It is a sterile, aqueous suspension with a pH between 6.8 and 7.2. The formula for betamethasone sodium phosphate is $C_{22}H_{28}FNa_2O_8P$ with a molecular weight of 516.41. Chemically it is 9-Fluoro-11β,17,21-trihydroxy-16β-methylpregna-1,4-diene-3,20-dione 21-acetate.

The formula for betamethasone acetate is $C_{24}H_{31}FO_6$ with a molecular weight of 434.50. Chemically it is 9-Fluoro-11β,17,21-trihydroxy-16β-methylpregna-1,4-diene-3,20-dione 21-acetate.

Betamethasone sodium phosphate is a white to practically white, odorless powder, and is hygroscopic. It is freely soluble in water and in methanol, but is practically insoluble in acetone and in chloroform.

Betamethasone acetate is a white to creamy white, odorless powder that sinters and resolidifies at about 165°C, and remelts at about 200-220°C with decomposition. It is practically insoluble in water, but freely soluble in acetone, and is soluble in alcohol and in chloroform.

INDICATIONS AND USAGE

When oral therapy is not feasible and the strength, dosage form, and route of administration of the drug reasonably lend the preparation to the treatment of the condition, this combination drug for intramuscular use is indicated as follows:

Endocrine Disorders: Primary or secondary adrenocortical insufficiency (hydrocortisone or cortisone is the drug of choice; synthetic analogs may be used in conjunction with mineralocorticoids where applicable; in infancy mineralocorticoid supplementation is of particular importance).

Acute adrenocortical insufficiency (hydrocortisone or cortisone is the drug of choice; mineralocorticoid supplementation may be necessary, particularly when synthetic analogs are used). Preoperatively and in the event of serious trauma or illness, in patients with known adrenal insufficiency or when adrenocortical reserve is doubtful. Shock unresponsive ot conventional therapy if adrenocortical insufficiency exists or is suspected. Congenital adrenal hyperplasia. Nonsuppurative thyroiditis. Hypercalcemia associated with cancer.

Rheumatic Disorders: As adjunctive therapy for short-term administration (to tide the patient over an acute episode or exacerbation) in: post-traumatic osteoarthritis, synovitis of osteoarthritis; rheumatoid arthritis, including juvenile rheumatoid arthritis (selected cases may require low-dose maintenance therapy); acute and subacute bursitis; epicondylitis; acute nonspecific tenosynovitis; acute gouty arthritis; psoriatic arthritis; ankylosing spondylitis.

Collagen Diseases: During an exacerbation or as maintenance therapy in selected cases of: systemic lupus erythematosus; acute rheumatic carditis.

B

B

Dermatologic Diseases: Pemphigus; severe erythema multiforme (Stevens-Johnson syndrome); exfoliative dermatitis; bullous dermatitis herpetiformis; severe seborrheic dermatitis; severe psoriasis; mycosis fungoides.
Allergic States: Control of severe or incapacitating allergic conditions intractable to adequate trials of conventional treatment in: bronchial asthma; contact dermatitis; atopic dermatitis; serum sickness; seasonal or perennial allergic rhinitis; drug hypersensitivity reactions; urticarial transfusion reactions; acute noninfectious laryngeal edema (epinephrine is the drug of first choice).
Ophthalmic Diseases: Severe, acute and chronic allergic and inflammatory processes involving the eye, such as: herpes zoster ophthalmicus; iritis, iridocyclitis; chorioretinitis; diffuse posterior uveitis and choroiditis; optic neuritis; sympathetic ophthalmia; anterior segment inflammation; allergic conjunctivitis; allergic corneal marginal ulcers; keratitis.
Gastrointestinal Diseases: To tide the patient over a critical period of disease in: ulcerative colitis-(systemic therapy); regional enteritis-(systemic therapy).
Respiratory Diseases: Symptomatic sarcoidosis; berylliosis; fulminating or disseminated pulmonary tuberculosis when used concurrently with appropriate antituberculous chemotherapy; Loeffler's syndrome not manageable by other means; aspiration pneumonitis.
Hematologic Disorders: Acquired (autoimmune) hemolytic anemia. Secondary thrombocytopenia in adults. Erythroblastopenia (RBC anemia). Congenital (erythroid) hypoplastic anemia.
Neoplastic Diseases: For palliative management of: leukemias and lymphomas in adults; acute leukemia of childhood.
Edematous States: To induce diuresis or remission of proteinuria in the nephrotic syndrome, without uremia, of the idiopathic type or that due to lupus erythematosus.
Miscellaneous: Tuberculosis meningitis with subarachnoid block or impending block when used concurrently with appropriate antituberculous chemotherapy. Trichinosis with neurologic or myocardial involvement.
When the strength and dosage form of the drug lend the preparation to the treatment of the condition, the **intra-articular or soft tissue administration** of this combination drug is indicated as adjunctive therapy for short-term administration (to tide the patient over an acute episode or exacerbation) in: synovitis of osteoarthritis; rheumatoid arthritis; acute and subacute bursitis; acute gouty arthritis; epicondylitis; acute nonspecific tenosynovitis; post-traumatic osteoarthritis.

When the strength and dosage form of the drug lend the preparation to the treatment of the condition, the **intralesional administration** of this combination drug is indicated for: keloids, localized hypertrophic, infiltrated, inflammatory lesions of lichen planus, psoriatic plaques, granuloma annulare, and lichen simplex chronicus (neurodermatitis); discoid lupus erythematosus; necrobiosis lipoidica diabeticorum; alopecia areata.

This combination drug may also be useful in cystic tumors of an aponeurosis or tendon (ganglia).

CONTRAINDICATIONS

This combination drug is contraindicated in systemic fungal infections.

WARNINGS

This combination drug should not be administered intravenously.

In patients on corticosteroid therapy subjected to any unusual stress, increased dosage of rapidly acting corticosteroids before, during, and after the stressful situation is indicated.

Corticosteroids may mask some signs of infection, and new infections may appear during their use. There may be decreased resistance and inability to localize infection when corticosteroids are used.

Prolonged use of corticosteroids may produce posterior subcapsular cataracts, glaucoma with possible damage to the optic nerves, and may enhance the establishment of secondary ocular infections due to fungi or viruses.

This combination drug contains two betamethasone esters one of which, betamethasone sodium phosphate, disappears rapidly from the injection site. The potential for systemic effect produced by the soluble portion of this combination drug should therefore be taken into account by the physician when using the drug.

Average and large doses of cortisone or hydrocortisone can cause elevation of blood pressure, salt and water retention, and increased excretion of potassium. These effects are less likely to occur with the synthetic derivatives except when used in large doses. Dietary salt restriction and potassium supplementation may be necessary. All corticosteroids increase calcium excretion.

While on corticosteroid therapy patients should not be vaccinated against smallpox. Other immunization procedures should not be undertaken in patients who are on corticosteroids, especially in high doses, because of possible hazards of neurological complications and lack of antibody response.

Children who are on immunosuppressant drugs are more susceptible to infections than healthy children. Chickenpox and measles, for example, can have a more serious or even fatal course in children on immunosuppressant corticosteroids. In such children, or in adults who have not had these diseases, particular care should be taken to avoid exposure. If exposed, therapy with varicella zoster immune globulin (VZIG) or pooled intravenous immunoglobulin (IVIG), as appropriate, may be indicated. If chickenpox develops, treatment with antiviral agents may be considered.

The use of this combination drug in active tuberculosis should be restricted ot those cases of fulminating or disseminate tuberculosis in which the corticosteroid is used for the management of the disease in conjunction with appropriate antituberculous regimen.

If corticosteroids are indicated in patients with latent tuberculosis or tuberculin reactivity, close observation is necessary as reactivation of the disease may occur. During prolonged corticosteroid therapy, these patients should receive chemoprophylaxis.

Because rare instances of anaphylactoid reactions have occurred in patients receiving parenteral corticosteroid therapy, appropriate precautionary measures should be taken prior to administration, especially when the patient has a history of allergy to any drug.
Use in Pregnancy: Since adequate human reproduction studies have not been done with corticosteroids, the use of these drugs in pregnancy, nursing mothers, or women of childbearing potential requires that the possible benefits of the drug be weighed against the potential hazards to the mother and embryo or fetus. Infants born of mothers who have received substantial doses of corticosteroids during pregnancy should be carefully observed for signs of hypoadrenalism.

DOSAGE AND ADMINISTRATION

The initial dosage of this combination drug may vary from 0.5 to 9.0 mg/day depending on the specific disease entity being treated. In situations of less severity, lower doses will generally suffice while in selected patients higher initial doses may be required. Usually the parenteral dosage ranges are one-third to one-half the oral dose given every 12 hours. However, in certain overwhelming, acute, life-threatening situations, administration in dosages exceeding the usual dosages may be justified and may be in multiples of the oral dosages.

The initial dosage should be maintained or adjusted until a satisfactory response is noted. If after a reasonable period of time there is a lack of satisfactory clinical response, this combination drug should be discontinued and the patient transferred to other appropriate therapy. *It should be emphasized that dosage requirements are variable and must be individualized on the basis of the disease under treatment and the response of the patient.* After a favorable response is noted, the proper maintenance dosage should be determined by decreasing the initial drug dosage in small decrements at appropriate time intervals until the lowest dosage which will maintain an adequate clinical response is reached. It should be kept in mind that constant monitoring is needed in regard to drug dosage. Included in the situations which may make dosage adjustments necessary are changes in clinical status secondary to remissions or exacerbations in the disease process, the patient's individual drug responsiveness, and the effect of patient exposure to stressful situations not directly related to the disease entity under treatment; in this latter situation it may be necessary to increase the dosage of this combination drug for a period of time consistent with the patient's condition. If after long-term therapy the drug is to be stopped, it is recommended that it be withdrawn gradually rather than abruptly.

If coadministration of a local anesthetic is desired, this combination drug may be mixed with 1 or 2% lidocaine hydrochloride, using the formulations which do not contain parabens. Similar local anesthetics may also be used. Diluents containing methylparaben, propylparaben, phenol, etc. Should be avoided since these compounds may cause flocculation of the steroid. The required dose of this combination drug is first withdrawn from the vial into the syringe. The local anesthetic is then drawn in, and the syringe shaken briefly. **Do not inject local anesthetics into the vial of this combination drug.**
Bursitis, Tenosynovitis, Peritendinitis: In acute subdeltoid, subacromial, olecranon, and prepatellar bursitis, one intrabursal injection of 1.0 ml this combination drug can relieve pain and restore full range of movement. Several intrabursal injections of corticosteroids are usually required in recurrent acute bursitis and in acute exacerbations of chronic bursitis. Partial relief of pain and some increase in mobility can be expected in both conditions after 1 or 2 injections. chronic bursitis may be treated with reduced dosage once the acute condition is controlled. In tenosynovitis and tendinitis, 3 or 4 local injections at intervals of 1-2 weeks between injections are given in most cases. Injections should be made into the affected tendon sheaths rather than into the tendons themselves. In ganglions of joint capsules and tendon sheaths, injection of 0.5 ml directly into the ganglion cysts has produced marked reduction in the size of the lesions.
Rheumatoid Arthritis and Osteoarthritis: Following intra-articular administration of 0.5-2.0 ml of this combination drug, relief of pain, soreness, and stiffness may be experienced. Duration of relief varies widely in both diseases. Intra-articular Injection of this combination drug is well tolerated in joints and periarticular tissues. There is virtually no pain on injection, and the "secondary flare" that sometimes occurs a few hours after intra-articular injection of corticosteroids has not been reported with this combination drug. Using sterile technique, a 20-24 gauge needle on an empty syringe is inserted into the synovial cavity, and a few drops of synovial fluid are withdrawn to confirm that the needle is in the joint. The aspirating syringe is replaced by a syringe containing this combination drug and injection is then made into the joint. See TABLE 1 for recommended doses.

TABLE 1 *Recommended Doses for Intra-articular Injection*

Size of Joint	Location	Dose (ml)
Very large	Hip	1.0-2.0
Large	Knee, ankle, shoulder	1.0
Medium	Elbow, wrist	0.5-1.0
Small		
(Metacarpophalangeal, interphalangeal)	Hand	0.25-0.5
(Sternoclavicular)	Chest	0.25-0.5

A portion of the administered dose of this combination drug is absorbed systemically following intra-articular injection. In patients being treated concomitantly with oral or parenteral corticosteroids, especially those receiving large doses, the systemic absorption of the drug should be considered in determining intra-articular dosage.
Dermatologic Conditions: In intralesional treatment, 0.2 ml/sq cm of this combination drug is injected intradermally (not subcutaneously) using a tuberculin syringe with a 25 gauge, ½ inch needle. Care should be taken to deposit a uniform depot of medication intradermally. A total of no more than 1.0 ml at weekly intervals is recommended.
Disorders of the Foot: A tuberculin syringe with a 25 gauge, ¾ inch needle is suitable for most injections into the foot. The doses shown in TABLE 2 are recommended at intervals of 3 days to a week.

TABLE 2

Diagnosis	Suspension Dose (ml)
Bursitis	
Under heloma durum or heloma molle	0.25-0.5
Under calcaneal spur	0.5
Over hallux rigidus or digiti varus	0.5
Tenosynovitis, periosteitis of cuboid	0.5
Acute gouty arthritis	0.5-1.0

PRODUCT LISTING - RATED THERAPEUTICALLY EQUIVALENT

Suspension - Injectable - acetate;Betamethasone Sodium Phosphate 3 mg;3 mg

5 ml	$14.60	GENERIC, Major Pharmaceuticals Inc	00904-0818-05

PRODUCT LISTING - EQUIVALENTS NOT AVAILABLE

Suspension - Injectable - acetate;Betamethasone Sodium Phosphate 3 mg;3 mg

5 ml	$20.08	CELESTONE SOLUSPAN, Allscripts Pharmaceutical Company	54569-3377-00
5 ml	$25.67	CELESTONE SOLUSPAN, Allscripts Pharmaceutical Company	54569-1630-01
5 ml	$26.18	CELESTONE SOLUSPAN, Southwood Pharmaceuticals Inc	58016-9191-01
5 ml	$28.64	CELESTONE SOLUSPAN, Schering Corporation	00085-0566-05
5 ml	$31.53	CELESTONE SOLUSPAN, Physicians Total Care	54868-0206-00

Betamethasone Dipropionate (000465)

Categories: Dermatosis, corticosteroid-responsive; Pregnancy Category C; FDA Approved 1975 Jan
Drug Classes: Corticosteroids, topical; Dermatologics
Brand Names: Alphatrex; Betanate; Diprolene; Diprolene Af; **Diprosone**; Maxivate
Foreign Brand Availability: Beprosone (Thailand); Betacrem (Peru); Betazone (Hong-Kong); Cleniderm (Bahrain; Cyprus; Egypt; Iran; Iraq; Jordan; Kuwait; Lebanon; Libya; Oman; Qatar; Republic-of-Yemen; Saudi-Arabia; Syria; United-Arab-Emirates); Cortimax (Peru); Cortixyl (Peru); Dicortin (Israel); Diprocel (Hong-Kong; Malaysia; Taiwan); Diproderm (Austria; Denmark; Finland; Spain); Diprolen (Denmark; Finland; Hungary; Switzerland); Diprosone-OV (Australia; Indonesia); Diprotop (Thailand); Mesonta (Indonesia); Metonate (Indonesia); Oviskin (Indonesia); Skizon (Indonesia); Taro-Sone (Canada); Topiderm (Peru); Topilene (Canada); Topilene Glycol (Hong-Kong); Topisone (Canada); Valbet (Thailand)

DESCRIPTION

For Dermatologic Use Only — Not for Ophthalmic Use.

These products contain betamethasone dipropionate, a synthetic adrenocorticosteroid, for dermatologic use. Betamethasone, an analog of prednisolone, has a high degree of corticosteroid activity and a slight degree of mineralocorticoid activity. Betamethasone dipropionate is the 17,21-dipropionate ester of betamethasone.

Chemically, betamethasone dipropionate is 9-fluoro-11β,17,21-trihydroxy-16β-methylpregna-1,4-diene-3,20-dione 17,21-dipropionate, with the empirical formula $C_{28}H_{37}FO_7$, a molecular weight of 504.6.

Betamethasone dipropionate is a white to creamy white, odorless crystalline powder, insoluble in water.

LOTIONS

Each Gram of Diprolene Lotion 0.05% Contains: 0.64 mg betamethasone dipropionate (equivalent to 0.5 mg betamethasone), in a lotion base of isopropyl alcohol (46.8%) and purified water slightly thickened with carbomer 934P; the pH is adjusted to approximately 4.7 with sodium hydroxide.

Each Gram of Diprolene (augmented betamethasone diproprionate) Lotion 0.05% Contains; 0.64 mg betamethasone dipropionate, (equivalent to 0.5 mg betamethasone), in a lotion base of purified water, isopropyl alcohol (30%), hydroxypropylcellulose, propylene glycol, sodium phosphate, phosphoric acid, and sodium hydroxide used to adjust the pH to 4.5.

CREAM

Each Gram of Diprolene AF (augmented betamethasone dipropionate) Cream (0.5%) Contains: 0.64 mg of betamethasone dipropionate (equivalent to 0.5 mg betamethasone), in an emollient cream base consisting of purified water, chlorocresol, propylene glycol, white petrolatum, white wax, cyclomethicone, sorbitol solution, glyceryl monooleate, ceteareth-30, carbomer 940 and sodium hydroxide.

OINTMENT

Each Gram of Diprolene (augmented betamethasone dipropionate) Ointment 0.05% Contains: 0.64 mg betamethasone dipropionate (equivalent to 0.5 mg betamethasone), in ACTIBASE, an optimized vehicle of propylene glycol, propylene glycol, propylene glycol stearate, white wax and white petrolatum.

TOPICAL AEROSOL

Betamethasone Dipropionate Topical Aerosol 0.1% Contains: 6.4 mg betamethasone dipropionate, equivalent to 5.0 mg betamethasone, in a vehicle of mineral oil and caprylic/capric triglyceride; also containing 10% isopropyl alcohol and sufficient inert hydrocarbon (propane and isobutane) propellant to make 85 grams. The aerosol spray deposits betamethasone dipropionate equivalent to approximately 0.1% betamethasone, in a non-volatile, almost invisible film. A 3 second spray delivers betamethasone dipropionate equivalent to approximately 0.06 mg betamethasone.

CLINICAL PHARMACOLOGY

The corticosteroids are a class of compounds comprising steroid hormones secreted by the adrenal cortex and their synthetic analogs. In pharmacologic doses, corticosteroids are used primarily for their anti-inflammatory, and/or immunosuppressive effects.

Topical corticosteroids, such as betamethasone dipropionate, are effective in the treatment of corticosteroid-responsive dermatoses primarily because of their anti-inflammatory, anti-pruritic, and vasoconstrictive actions. However, while the physiologic, pharmacologic, and clinical effects of the corticosteroids are well-known, the exact mechanisms of the their actions in each disease are uncertain. Betamethasone dipropionate, a corticosteroid, has been shown to have topical (dermatologic) and systemic pharmacologic and metabolic effects characteristic of this class of drugs.

PHARMACOKINETICS

The extent of percutaneous absorption of topical corticosteroids is determined by many factors including the vehicle, the integrity of the epidermal barrier, and the use of occlusive dressings (see DOSAGE AND ADMINISTRATION).

Topical corticosteroids can be absorbed through normal intact skin. Inflammation and/or other disease processes in the skin may increase percutaneous absorption. Occlusive dressings substantially increase the percutaneous absorption of topical corticosteroids (see DOSAGE AND ADMINISTRATION).

Once absorbed through the skin, topical corticosteroids enter pharmacokinetic pathways similar to systemically administered corticosteroids. Corticosteroids are bound to plasma proteins in varying degrees. Corticosteroids are metabolized primarily in the liver and excreted by the kidneys. Some of the topical corticosteroids and their metabolites are also excreted into the bile.

AUGMENTED CREAM 0.05%

Augmented betamethasone dipropionate AF cream was applied once daily at 7 g/day for 1 week to diseased skin, in patients with psoriasis or atopic dermatitis, to study its effects on the hypothalamic-pituitary-adrenal (HPA) axis. The results suggested that the drug caused a slight lowering of adrenal corticosteroid secretion, although in no case did plasma cortisol levels go below the lower limit of the normal range.

AUGMENTED OINTMENT 0.05%

At 14 g/day, augmented betamethasone dipropionate ointment was shown to depress the plasma levels of adrenal cortical hormones following repeated application to diseased skin in patients with psoriasis. Adrenal depression in these patients was transient, and rapidly returned to normal upon cessation of treatment. At 7 g/day (3.5 g bid), betamethasone dipropionate ointment was shown to cause minimal inhibition of the hypothalamic-pituitary-adrenal (HPA) axis when applied 2 times daily for 2-3 weeks, in normal patients and in patients with no psoriasis and eczematous disorders.

With 6 or 7 g of betamethasone dipropionate ointment applied once daily for 3 weeks, no significant inhibition of the HPA axis was observed in patients with psoriasis and atopic dermatitis, as measured by plasma cortisol and 24 hour urinary 17-hydroxy-corticosteroid levels.

AUGMENTED LOTION 0.05%

Augmented betamethasone dipropionate lotion was applied once daily at 7 ml/day for 21 days to diseased skin (in patients with scalp psoriasis), to study its effects on the hypothalamic-pituitary-adrenal (HPA) axis. In 2 out of 11 patients, the drug lowered plasma cortisol levels below normal limits. Adrenal depression in these patients was transient, and returned to normal within a week. In 1 of these patients, plasma cortisol levels returned to normal while treatment continued.

INDICATIONS AND USAGE

Betamethasone diproprionate products are indicated for relief of the inflammatory and pruritic manifestations of moderate to severe corticosteroid-responsive dermatoses.

ADDITIONAL INFORMATION FOR AUGMENTED LOTION 0.05%

Treatment beyond 2 weeks is not recommended, and the total dosage should not exceed 50 ml/week because of the potential for the drug to suppress the hypothalamic-pituitary-adrenal axis.

CONTRAINDICATIONS

Betamethasone diproprionate products is contraindicated in patients who are hypersensitive to betamethasone dipropionate, to other corticosteroids, or to any ingredient in these preparations.

PRECAUTIONS

GENERAL

Augmented betamethasone dipropionate lotion is a highly potent topical corticosteroid that has been shown to suppress HPA axis at 7 ml/day.

Systemic absorption of topical corticosteroids has produced reversible HPA axis suppression, manifestations of Cushing's syndrome, hyperglycemia, and glucosuria in some patients.

Conditions which augment systemic absorption include the application of the more potent corticosteroids such as betamethasone diproprionate, use over large surface areas, prolonged use, and the addition of occlusive dressings (see DOSAGE AND ADMINISTRATION).

Therefore, patients receiving large doses of potent topical steroid applied to a large surface area should be evaluated periodically for evidence of HPA axis suppression by using the urinary free cortisol and ACTH stimulation tests. If HPA axis suppression is noted, an attempt should be made to withdraw the drug, to reduce the frequency of application, or to substitute with a less potent steroid.

Recovery of HPA axis function is generally prompt and complete upon discontinuation of the drug. Infrequently, signs and symptoms of steroid withdrawal many occur, requiring supplemental systemic corticosteroids.

Children may absorb proportionally large amounts of topical corticosteroids and thus be more susceptible to systemic toxicity (see Pediatric Use).

If irritation develops, topical corticosteroids should be discontinued and appropriate therapy instituted.

In the presence of dermatological infections, the use of an appropriate antifungal or antibacterial agent should be instituted. If a favorable response does not occur promptly, the corticosteroid should be discontinued until the infection has been adequately controlled.

INFORMATION FOR THE PATIENT

Patients using topical corticosteroids should receive the following information and instructions. This information is intended to aid in the safe and effective use of this medication. It is not a disclosure of all possible adverse or intended effects.

1. This medication is to be used as directed by the physician and should not be used longer than the prescribed time period. It is for external use only. Avoid contact with the eyes.
2. Patients should be advised not to use this medication for any disorder other than that for which it was prescribed.
3. The treated skin areas should be not bandaged or otherwise covered or wrapped so as to be occlusive (see DOSAGE AND ADMINISTRATION).
4. Patients should report any sign of local adverse reactions.
5. Parents of pediatric patients should be advised not to use tight- fitting diapers or plastic pants on a child being treated in the diaper area, as these garments may constitute occlusive dressing (see DOSAGE AND ADMINISTRATION).

LABORATORY TESTS

The following tests may be helpful in evaluating HPA axis suppression:

Urinary free cortisol test
ACTH stimulation test

CARCINOGENESIS, MUTAGENESIS, AND IMPAIRMENT OF FERTILITY

Long-term animal studies have not been performed to evaluate the carcinogenic potential or the effect on fertility of topically applied corticosteroids.

Studies to determine mutagenicity with prednisolone and hydrocortisone have revealed negative results.

PREGNANCY CATEGORY C

Corticosteroids are generally teratogenic in laboratory animal when administered systemically at relatively low dosage levels. The more potent corticosteroids have been shown to be teratogenic after dermal application in laboratory animals. Betamethasone dipropionate has not been tested for teratogenicity by this route; however, it appears to be fairly well-absorbed percutaneously. There are no adequate and well-controlled studies of the teratogenic effects of topically applied corticosteroids in pregnant women. Therefore, topical corticosteroids should be used during pregnancy only if the potential benefit justifies the potential risk to the fetus. Drugs of this class should not be used extensively on pregnant patients, in large amounts, or for prolonged periods of time.

NURSING MOTHERS

It is not known whether topical administration of corticosteroids can result in sufficient systemic absorption to produce detectable quantities in breast milk. Systemically administered corticosteroids are secreted into breast milk in quantities not likely to have deleterious effect on the infant. Nevertheless, a decision should be made whether to discontinue nursing or to discontinue the drug, taking into account the importance of the drug to the mother.

PEDIATRIC USE

The safety and efficacy of betamethasone diproprionate products when used in children 12 years of age have not been established.

Pediatric patients may demonstrate greater susceptibility to topical corticosteroid-induced HPA axis suppression and Cushing's syndrome than mature patients because of a larger skin surface area to body weight ratio.

Hypothalamic-pituitary-adrenal (HPA) axis suppression, Cushing's syndrome, and intracranial hypertension have been reported in children receiving topical corticosteroids. Manifestations of adrenal suppression in children include linear growth retardation, delayed weight gain, low plasma cortisol levels, and absence of response to ACTH stimulation. Manifestations of intracranial hypertension include bulging fontanelles, headaches, and bilateral papilledema.

Administration of topical corticosteroids to children should be limited to the least amount compatible with an effective therapeutic regimen. Chronic corticosteroid therapy may interfere with the growth and development of children.

ADDITIONAL INFORMATION FOR THE TOPICAL AEROSOL

- The spray should be kept away from the eyes or other mucous membranes.
- Avoid freezing tissues by not spraying for more than three seconds, at a distance of not less than six inches between the nozzle and skin.
- Use only as directed; intentional misuse by deliberately concentrating and inhaling the container contents can be harmful or fatal.
- The container contents are under pressure; do not puncture the container.
- The container mixture is flammable; do not use or store the container near heat or an open flame; exposure to temperature above 120°F may cause bursting; never throw container into a fire or incinerator.
- Keep out of reach of children

ADVERSE REACTIONS

The following local adverse reactions are also reported infrequently when betamethasone dipropionate products are used as recommended in DOSAGE AND ADMINISTRATION. These reactions are listed in approximate decreasing order of occurrence: burning; itching; irritation; dryness; folliculitis; hypertrichosis; acneiform eruptions; hypopigmentation; perioral dermatitis; allergic contact dermatitis; maceration of the skin; secondary infection; skin atrophy; striae; miliaria.

Systemic absorption of topical corticosteroids has produced reversible hypothalamic-pituitary-adrenal (HPA) axis suppression, manifestations of Cushing's syndrome, hyperglycemia, and glucosuria in some patients.

AUGMENTED CREAM 0.05%

The only local adverse reaction reported to be possibly or probably related to treatment with betamethasone dipropionate cream during controlled clinical studies was stinging. It occurred in 0.4% of the 242 patients or subjects involved in the studies.

AUGMENTED OINTMENT 0.05%

The local adverse reactions that were reported with betamethasone dipropionate ointment applied either once or twice a day during clinical studies are as follows: Erythema, 3/767 patients, folliculitis, 2/767 patients; pruritus, 2/767 patients; vesiculation, 1/767 patients.

AUGMENTED LOTION 0.05%

The overall incidence of drug-related adverse reactions in the betamethasone dipropionate lotion clinical studies was 5%. The adverse reactions that were reported to be possibly or probably related to treatment with betamethasone dipropionate lotion during controlled clinical studies involving 327 patients or normal volunteers, were as follows: folliculitis occurred in 2%, burning and acneiform papules each occurred in 1%, and hyperesthesia and irritation each occurred in less than 1% of patients.

DOSAGE AND ADMINISTRATION

CREAM

Apply a thin film of betamethasone dipropionate cream 0.05% to the affected areas once daily. In some cases, a twice daily dosage may be necessary.

AUGMENTED CREAM

Apply a thin film of betamethasone dipropionate cream to the affected skin areas once or twice daily. *Treatment with betamethasone dipropionate cream should be limited to 45 g per week.*

Betamethasone dipropionate cream is not to be used with occlusive dressings.

LOTION

Apply a few drops to the affected areas and massage lightly until it disappears. Apply twice daily, in the morning and at night. For the most effective and economical use, apply nozzle very close to affected area and squeeze bottle gently.

AUGMENTED LOTION

Apply a few drops of betamethasone dipropionate lotion to the affected area once or twice daily and massage lightly until the lotion disappears. Treatment must be limited to 14 days, and amounts greater than 50 ml/week should not be used.

Betamethasone dipropionate lotion is not to be used with occlusive dressings.

OINTMENT

Apply a thin film of betamethasone dipropionate ointment to the affected areas once daily. In some cases, a twice daily dosage may be necessary.

AUGMENTED OINTMENT

Apply a thin film of betamethasone dipropionate ointment to the affected skin areas once or twice daily. Treatment with betamethasone dipropionate ointment should be limited to 45 g/week.

Betamethasone dipropionate ointment is not to be used with occlusive dressings.

TOPICAL AEROSOL

Apply sparingly to the affected skin area 3 times a day. The container may be held upright or inverted during use. The spray should be directed onto the affected area from a distance of not more than 6 inches and applied for only 3 seconds. For the most effective and economical use, a 3 second spray is sufficient to cover an area about the size of the hand.

Betamethasone dipropionate products are not to be used with occlusive dressings.

HOW SUPPLIED

Storage: Store all products between 2-30°C (36-86°F).

PRODUCT LISTING - RATED THERAPEUTICALLY EQUIVALENT

Cream - Topical - Dipropionate, augmented 0.05%

Size	Price	Manufacturer	NDC
15 gm	$4.75	GENERIC, Clay-Park Laboratories Inc	45802-0019-35
15 gm	$4.75	GENERIC, Clay-Park Laboratories Inc	45802-0020-35
15 gm	$16.00	GENERIC, Mutual/United Research Laboratories	00677-1569-40
15 gm	$27.81	GENERIC, Alpharma Uspd Makers Of Barre and Nmc	00472-0382-15
45 gm	$9.07	GENERIC, Clay-Park Laboratories Inc	45802-0019-42
45 gm	$9.07	GENERIC, Clay-Park Laboratories Inc	45802-0020-42
45 gm	$29.43	GENERIC, Mutual/United Research Laboratories	00677-1569-49
45 gm	$62.19	GENERIC, Alpharma Uspd Makers Of Barre and Nmc	00472-0382-45

Cream - Topical - Dipropionate 0.05%

Size	Price	Manufacturer	NDC
15 gm	$4.30	GENERIC, Thames Pharmacal Company Inc	49158-0213-20
15 gm	$4.50	GENERIC, Raway Pharmacal Inc	00686-0055-15
15 gm	$5.12	GENERIC, Moore, H.L. Drug Exchange Inc	00839-7049-47
15 gm	$5.31	GENERIC, Qualitest Products Inc	00603-7728-74
15 gm	$5.38	GENERIC, Mason Distributors Inc	11845-0381-01
15 gm	$5.65	GENERIC, Major Pharmaceuticals Inc	00904-0766-36
15 gm	$6.25	GENERIC, Geneva Pharmaceuticals	00781-7009-27
15 gm	$6.90	GENERIC, Ivax Corporation	00182-5010-51
15 gm	$7.02	GENERIC, Taro Pharmaceuticals U.S.A. Inc	51672-1274-01
15 gm	$7.50	GENERIC, Alpharma Uspd Makers Of Barre and Nmc	00472-0380-15
15 gm	$7.80	GENERIC, Fougera	00168-0055-15
15 gm	$23.71	GENERIC, Savage Laboratories	00281-0055-15
15 gm	$24.63	DIPROSONE, Southwood Pharmaceuticals Inc	58016-3023-01

Size	Price	Product	NDC
15 gm	$28.54	DIPROSONE, Schering Corporation	00085-0853-02
45 gm	$8.60	GENERIC, Thames Pharmacal Company Inc	49158-0213-27
45 gm	$8.95	GENERIC, Raway Pharmacal Inc	00686-0055-46
45 gm	$9.17	GENERIC, Moore, H.L. Drug Exchange Inc	00839-7049-52
45 gm	$10.08	GENERIC, Qualitest Products Inc	00603-7728-83
45 gm	$10.57	GENERIC, Major Pharmaceuticals Inc	00904-0766-45
45 gm	$11.50	GENERIC, Watson/Schein Pharmaceuticals Inc	00364-7409-80
45 gm	$11.50	GENERIC, Geneva Pharmaceuticals	00781-7009-19
45 gm	$12.00	GENERIC, Alpharma Uspd Makers Of Barre and Nmc	00472-0380-45
45 gm	$12.00	GENERIC, Alpharma Uspd Makers Of Barre and Nmc	00472-0381-45
45 gm	$12.55	GENERIC, Ivax Corporation	00182-5010-60
45 gm	$13.99	GENERIC, Taro Pharmaceuticals U.S.A. Inc	51672-1274-06
45 gm	$18.17	GENERIC, Fougera	00168-0055-46
45 gm	$20.01	GENERIC, Del Ray Laboratories Inc	00316-0176-45
45 gm	$43.18	GENERIC, Savage Laboratories	00281-0055-46
45 gm	$52.31	DIPROSONE, Schering Corporation	00085-0853-03

Cream - Topical - Valerate 0.1%

Size	Price	Product	NDC
15 gm	$2.30	GENERIC, Thames Pharmacal Company Inc	49158-0184-20
15 gm	$2.48	GENERIC, Clay-Park Laboratories Inc	45802-0069-35
15 gm	$2.59	GENERIC, Clay-Park Laboratories Inc	45802-0015-35
15 gm	$2.78	GENERIC, Genetco Inc	00302-0415-15
15 gm	$3.15	GENERIC, Interstate Drug Exchange Inc	00814-1160-93
15 gm	$3.15	GENERIC, Interstate Drug Exchange Inc	00814-1163-93
15 gm	$3.50	GENERIC, Moore, H.L. Drug Exchange Inc	00839-6371-47
15 gm	$4.23	GENERIC, Qualitest Products Inc	00603-7718-74
15 gm	$4.29	GENERIC, Ivax Corporation	00182-1610-51
15 gm	$4.30	GENERIC, Major Pharmaceuticals Inc	00904-0776-36
15 gm	$4.85	GENERIC, Teva Pharmaceuticals Usa	00093-0673-15
15 gm	$4.95	GENERIC, Alpharma Uspd Makers Of Barre and Nmc	00472-0370-15
15 gm	$5.05	GENERIC, Fougera	00168-0040-15
15 gm	$5.87	GENERIC, Taro Pharmaceuticals U.S.A. Inc	51672-1269-01
15 gm	$9.55	GENERIC, Pharma Pac	52959-0263-00
15 gm	$13.00	GENERIC, Savage Laboratories	00281-3510-44
15 gm	$16.26	VALISONE, Schering Corporation	00085-0136-04
45 gm	$4.70	GENERIC, Thames Pharmacal Company Inc	49158-0184-27
45 gm	$5.08	GENERIC, Clay-Park Laboratories Inc	45802-0069-42
45 gm	$5.29	GENERIC, Clay-Park Laboratories Inc	45802-0015-42
45 gm	$6.30	GENERIC, Interstate Drug Exchange Inc	00814-1160-95
45 gm	$6.30	GENERIC, Interstate Drug Exchange Inc	00814-1163-95
45 gm	$6.55	GENERIC, Moore, H.L. Drug Exchange Inc	00839-6371-52
45 gm	$7.50	GENERIC, Mutual/United Research Laboratories	00677-0842-49
45 gm	$7.51	GENERIC, Qualitest Products Inc	00603-7718-83
45 gm	$7.70	GENERIC, Major Pharmaceuticals Inc	00904-0776-45
45 gm	$8.01	GENERIC, Taro Pharmaceuticals U.S.A. Inc	51672-1269-06
45 gm	$8.03	GENERIC, Teva Pharmaceuticals Usa	00093-0673-95
45 gm	$8.05	GENERIC, Alpharma Uspd Makers Of Barre and Nmc	00472-0370-45
45 gm	$8.14	GENERIC, Fougera	00168-0040-46
45 gm	$14.68	GENERIC, Pharma Pac	52959-0263-01
45 gm	$25.00	GENERIC, Savage Laboratories	00281-3510-50
45 gm	$29.63	VALISONE, Schering Corporation	00085-0136-06
110 gm	$50.88	VALISONE, Schering Corporation	00085-0136-07
430 gm	$171.05	VALISONE, Schering Corporation	00085-0136-08
454 gm	$62.47	GENERIC, Clay-Park Laboratories Inc	45802-0015-05
454 gm	$62.47	GENERIC, Clay-Park Laboratories Inc	45802-0069-05

Cream - Topical - 0.05%

Size	Price	Product	NDC
15 gm	$3.45	FEDERAL UPPER LIMIT, H.C.F.A. F F P	99999-0465-07

Lotion - Topical - Dipropionate 0.05%

Size	Price	Product	NDC
20 ml	$4.30	GENERIC, Thames Pharmacal Company Inc	49158-0245-40
20 ml	$5.64	GENERIC, Alpharma Uspd Makers Of Barre and Nmc	23317-0382-20
20 ml	$10.80	GENERIC, Clay-Park Laboratories Inc	45802-0021-97
20 ml	$31.96	DIPROSONE, Schering Corporation	00085-0028-04
60 ml	$10.52	GENERIC, Moore, H.L. Drug Exchange Inc	00839-7202-53
60 ml	$11.55	GENERIC, Major Pharmaceuticals Inc	00904-0768-03
60 ml	$11.56	GENERIC, Watson/Rugby Laboratories Inc	00536-5038-61
60 ml	$11.85	GENERIC, Clay-Park Laboratories Inc	45802-0021-46
60 ml	$14.23	GENERIC, Alpharma Uspd Makers Of Barre and Nmc	23317-0382-60
60 ml	$15.72	GENERIC, Thames Pharmacal Company Inc	49158-0245-32
60 ml	$16.03	GENERIC, Alpharma Uspd Makers Of Barre and Nmc	00472-1382-02
60 ml	$18.01	GENERIC, Fougera	00168-0057-60
60 ml	$38.85	GENERIC, Teva Pharmaceuticals Usa	00093-0302-39
60 ml	$63.11	GENERIC, Savage Laboratories	00281-0057-60
60 ml	$71.15	DIPROSONE, Schering Corporation	00085-0028-06

Lotion - Topical - Valerate 0.1%

Size	Price	Product	NDC
20 ml	$20.05	VALISONE, Schering Corporation	00085-0002-03
60 ml	$10.10	GENERIC, Major Pharmaceuticals Inc	00904-0778-03
60 ml	$10.50	GENERIC, Watson/Rugby Laboratories Inc	00536-4330-61
60 ml	$10.51	GENERIC, Qualitest Products Inc	00603-7719-49
60 ml	$11.00	GENERIC, Alpharma Uspd Makers Of Barre and Nmc	23317-0372-60
60 ml	$11.07	GENERIC, Moore, H.L. Drug Exchange Inc	00839-7022-64
60 ml	$11.25	GENERIC, Ivax Corporation	00182-1788-68
60 ml	$11.45	GENERIC, Teva Pharmaceuticals Usa	00093-0671-39
60 ml	$12.30	GENERIC, Alpharma Uspd Makers Of Barre and Nmc	00472-0372-02
60 ml	$12.50	GENERIC, Fougera	00168-0041-60
60 ml	$14.55	GENERIC, Pharma Pac	52959-0243-03
60 ml	$39.62	VALISONE, Schering Corporation	00085-0002-05

Lotion - Topical - 0.05%

Size	Price	Product	NDC
60 ml	$8.62	FEDERAL UPPER LIMIT, H.C.F.A. F F P	99999-0465-10

Ointment - Topical - Dipropionate, augmented 0.05%

Size	Price	Product	NDC
15 gm	$20.57	GENERIC, Major Pharmaceuticals Inc	00904-5109-36
15 gm	$21.47	GENERIC, Warrick Pharmaceuticals Corporation	59930-1575-01
15 gm	$29.53	GENERIC, Fougera	00168-0268-15
15 gm	$40.78	DIPROLENE, Schering Corporation	00085-0575-02
50 gm	$51.30	GENERIC, Warrick Pharmaceuticals Corporation	59930-1575-03
50 gm	$66.01	GENERIC, Fougera	00168-0268-50
50 gm	$72.32	DIPROLENE, Allscripts Pharmaceutical Company	54569-4448-00
50 gm	$91.18	DIPROLENE, Schering Corporation	00085-0575-05

Ointment - Topical - Dipropionate 0.05%

Size	Price	Product	NDC
15 gm	$5.00	GENERIC, Major Pharmaceuticals Inc	00904-0767-36
15 gm	$7.50	GENERIC, Alpharma Uspd Makers Of Barre and Nmc	00472-0381-15
15 gm	$9.40	GENERIC, Fougera	00168-0056-15
15 gm	$16.00	GENERIC, Savage Laboratories	00281-0056-15
15 gm	$27.42	DIPROSONE, Schering Corporation	00085-0510-04
45 gm	$9.44	GENERIC, Moore, H.L. Drug Exchange Inc	00839-7110-52
45 gm	$10.00	GENERIC, Major Pharmaceuticals Inc	00904-0767-45
45 gm	$10.65	GENERIC, Pharma Pac	52959-0262-00
45 gm	$12.55	GENERIC, Ivax Corporation	00182-5011-60
45 gm	$20.78	GENERIC, Fougera	00168-0056-46
45 gm	$43.18	GENERIC, Savage Laboratories	00281-0056-46
45 gm	$52.31	DIPROSONE, Schering Corporation	00085-0510-06

Ointment - Topical - Valerate 0.1%

Size	Price	Product	NDC
15 gm	$3.00	GENERIC, Genetco Inc	00302-0416-15
15 gm	$4.29	GENERIC, Ivax Corporation	00182-1735-51
15 gm	$4.55	GENERIC, Major Pharmaceuticals Inc	00904-0777-36
15 gm	$4.71	GENERIC, Moore, H.L. Drug Exchange Inc	00839-6758-47
15 gm	$4.95	GENERIC, Alpharma Uspd Makers Of Barre and Nmc	00472-0371-15
15 gm	$5.26	GENERIC, Fougera	00168-0033-15
15 gm	$13.00	GENERIC, Savage Laboratories	00281-3516-44
15 gm	$16.26	VALISONE, Schering Corporation	00085-0898-04
45 gm	$5.63	GENERIC, Genetco Inc	00302-0416-46
45 gm	$7.29	GENERIC, Moore, H.L. Drug Exchange Inc	00839-6758-52
45 gm	$7.95	GENERIC, Ivax Corporation	00182-1735-60
45 gm	$8.05	GENERIC, Alpharma Uspd Makers Of Barre and Nmc	00472-0371-45
45 gm	$9.10	GENERIC, Major Pharmaceuticals Inc	00904-0777-45
45 gm	$9.24	GENERIC, Fougera	00168-0033-46
45 gm	$25.00	GENERIC, Savage Laboratories	00281-3516-50
45 gm	$29.63	VALISONE, Schering Corporation	00085-0898-06

PRODUCT LISTING - EQUIVALENTS NOT AVAILABLE

Cream - Topical - Benzoate 0.025%

Size	Price	Product	NDC
60 gm	$38.56	UTICORT, Parke-Davis	00071-3027-15

Cream - Topical - Dipropionate, augmented 0.05%

Size	Price	Product	NDC
15 gm	$6.60	GENERIC, Interstate Drug Exchange Inc	00814-1170-93
15 gm	$7.73	GENERIC, Dermol Pharmaceuticals Inc	50744-0108-15
15 gm	$9.62	GENERIC, Del Ray Laboratories Inc	00316-0176-15
15 gm	$32.34	DIPROLENE AF, Allscripts Pharmaceutical Company	54569-2183-00
15 gm	$40.78	DIPROLENE AF, Schering Corporation	00085-0517-01
45 gm	$12.00	GENERIC, Interstate Drug Exchange Inc	00814-1170-95
45 gm	$14.50	GENERIC, Dermol Pharmaceuticals Inc	50744-0108-45
50 gm	$68.74	DIPROLENE AF, Pharma Pac	52959-0575-05
50 gm	$72.32	DIPROLENE AF, Allscripts Pharmaceutical Company	54569-4345-00
50 gm	$91.18	DIPROLENE AF, Schering Corporation	00085-0517-04

Cream - Topical - Dipropionate 0.05%

Size	Price	Product	NDC
15 gm	$4.22	GENERIC, Physicians Total Care	54868-0973-01
15 gm	$4.25	GENERIC, Cmc-Consolidated Midland Corporation	00223-4260-15
15 gm	$4.65	GENERIC, Prescript Pharmaceuticals	00247-0148-15
15 gm	$14.27	GENERIC, Allscripts Pharmaceutical Company	54569-1113-00
15 gm	$19.90	GENERIC, Southwood Pharmaceuticals Inc	58016-6338-01
15 gm	$19.90	GENERIC, Southwood Pharmaceuticals Inc	58016-6338-15
45 gm	$7.25	GENERIC, Prescript Pharmaceuticals	00247-0148-45
45 gm	$7.50	GENERIC, Cmc-Consolidated Midland Corporation	00223-4260-45
45 gm	$7.62	GENERIC, Physicians Total Care	54868-0973-02
45 gm	$27.21	GENERIC, Allscripts Pharmaceutical Company	54569-2556-00
45 gm	$36.30	GENERIC, Bristol-Myers Squibb	00072-9410-45

60 gm	$17.50	GENERIC, Cmc-Consolidated Midland Corporation	00223-4260-60

Cream - Topical - Valerate 0.1%

15 gm	$2.66	GENERIC, Physicians Total Care	54868-0520-01
15 gm	$2.75	GENERIC, Cmc-Consolidated Midland Corporation	00223-4258-15
15 gm	$2.75	GENERIC, Raway Pharmacal Inc	00686-0069-35
15 gm	$4.20	GENERIC, C.O. Truxton Inc	00463-8055-15
15 gm	$4.61	GENERIC, Prescript Pharmaceuticals	00247-0302-15
15 gm	$7.13	GENERIC, Allscripts Pharmaceutical Company	54569-1115-00
15 gm	$10.03	GENERIC, Pharma Pac	52959-1022-00
15 gm	$16.26	GENERIC, Southwood Pharmaceuticals Inc	58016-3097-01
45 gm	$4.67	GENERIC, Physicians Total Care	54868-0520-00
45 gm	$5.50	GENERIC, Raway Pharmacal Inc	00686-0069-42
45 gm	$5.75	GENERIC, Cmc-Consolidated Midland Corporation	00223-4258-45
45 gm	$7.13	GENERIC, Prescript Pharmaceuticals	00247-0302-45
45 gm	$14.43	GENERIC, Allscripts Pharmaceutical Company	54569-1873-01
45 gm	$15.41	GENERIC, Pharma Pac	52959-1022-01
45 gm	$18.65	GENERIC, Southwood Pharmaceuticals Inc	58016-3109-01

Foam - Topical - 0.12%

50 gm	$55.01	LUXIQ, Connetics Inc	63032-0021-50
100 gm	$103.99	LUXIQ, Connetics Inc	63032-0021-00

Gel - Topical - Dipropionate, augmented 0.05%

15 gm	$32.34	DIPROLENE, Allscripts Pharmaceutical Company	54569-2575-00
15 gm	$35.00	DIPROLENE, Schering Corporation	00085-0634-01
45 gm	$51.30	DIPROLENE, Schering Corporation	00085-0634-02
50 gm	$91.18	DIPROLENE, Schering Corporation	00085-0634-03

Lotion - Topical - Dipropionate, augmented 0.05%

30 ml	$46.76	DIPROLENE, Schering Corporation	00085-0962-01
60 ml	$92.18	DIPROLENE, Schering Corporation	00085-0962-02

Lotion - Topical - Dipropionate 0.05%

60 ml	$10.30	GENERIC, Raway Pharmacal Inc	00686-0057-60
60 ml	$13.94	GENERIC, Del Ray Laboratories Inc	00316-0177-02
60 ml	$25.28	GENERIC, Allscripts Pharmaceutical Company	54569-1556-00
60 ml	$53.36	GENERIC, Bristol-Myers Squibb	00072-9490-60

Lotion - Topical - Valerate 0.1%

60 ml	$7.80	GENERIC, Raway Pharmacal Inc	00686-0041-60
60 ml	$12.50	GENERIC, Cmc-Consolidated Midland Corporation	00223-6432-60
60 ml	$18.68	GENERIC, Allscripts Pharmaceutical Company	54569-1874-01

Ointment - Topical - Dipropionate 0.05%

15 gm	$3.75	GENERIC, Cmc-Consolidated Midland Corporation	00223-4261-15
15 gm	$4.50	GENERIC, Raway Pharmacal Inc	00686-0056-15
15 gm	$6.87	GENERIC, Allscripts Pharmaceutical Company	54569-1114-00
45 gm	$7.50	GENERIC, Cmc-Consolidated Midland Corporation	00223-4261-45
45 gm	$8.95	GENERIC, Raway Pharmacal Inc	00686-0056-46
45 gm	$26.46	GENERIC, Allscripts Pharmaceutical Company	54569-2613-00
45 gm	$38.81	GENERIC, Bristol-Myers Squibb	00072-9450-45
1350 gm	$7.23	GENERIC, Physicians Total Care	54868-3280-00

Ointment - Topical - Valerate 0.1%

15 gm	$2.66	GENERIC, Physicians Total Care	54868-2994-01
15 gm	$2.95	GENERIC, Raway Pharmacal Inc	00686-0015-35
15 gm	$4.00	GENERIC, Cmc-Consolidated Midland Corporation	00223-4259-15
15 gm	$7.75	GENERIC, Southwood Pharmaceuticals Inc	58016-3099-01
15 gm	$10.94	GENERIC, Allscripts Pharmaceutical Company	54569-0793-00
45 gm	$4.67	GENERIC, Physicians Total Care	54868-2994-02
45 gm	$5.00	GENERIC, Raway Pharmacal Inc	00686-0015-42
45 gm	$7.95	GENERIC, Cmc-Consolidated Midland Corporation	00223-4259-45
45 gm	$19.79	GENERIC, Allscripts Pharmaceutical Company	54569-2621-00

Spray - Topical - Dipropionate 0.1%

85 ml	$25.97	DIPROSONE, Schering Corporation	00085-0475-06

Betamethasone Dipropionate; Clotrimazole *(000466)*

For complete prescribing information, refer to the CD-ROM included with the book.

Categories: Tinea corporis; Tinea cruris; Tinea pedis; Pregnancy Category C; FDA Approved 1984 Jul
Drug Classes: Antifungals, topical; Corticosteroids, topical; Dermatologics
Brand Names: **Lotrisone**; Sinium
Foreign Brand Availability: Clotrasone (Philippines; Singapore; Taiwan; Thailand); Derzid-c (Thailand); Gynesten-B (Thailand); Lotricomb (Germany); Lotriderm (Bahrain; Belgium; Canada; Colombia; Costa-Rica; Cyprus; Dominican-Republic; Egypt; El-Salvador; England; Guatemala; Honduras; Iran; Iraq; Israel; Jordan; Kuwait; Lebanon; Libya; Nicaragua; Oman; Panama; Qatar; Republic-of-Yemen; Saudi-Arabia; South-Africa; Switzerland; Syria; United-Arab-Emirates)
Cost of Therapy: $23.47 (Tinea pedis; Lotrisone Cream; 0.05%; 1%; 15 g; 2 applications/day; variable day supply)

DESCRIPTION

Note: The trade name has been used throughout this monograph for clarity.

FOR TOPICAL USE ONLY. NOT FOR OPHTHALMIC, ORAL, OR INTRAVAGINAL USE, NOT RECOMMENDED FOR PATIENTS UNDER THE AGE OF 17 YEARS AND NOT RECOMMENDED FOR DIAPER DERMATITIS.

Lotrisone cream and lotion contain combinations of clotrimazole, a synthetic antifungal agent, and betamethasone dipropionate, a synthetic corticosteroid, for dermatologic use.

Chemically, clotrimazole is 1-(*o*-chloro-α,α-diphenylbenzyl)imidazole, with the empirical formula $C_{22}H_{17}ClN_2$ a molecular weight of 344.84.

Clotrimazole is an odorless, white crystalline powder, insoluble in water and soluble in ethanol.

Betamethasone dipropionate has the chemical name 9-fluoro-11β,17,21-trihydroxy-16β-methylpregna-1,4-diene-3,20-dione 17,21-dipropionate, with the empirical formula $C_{28}H_{37}FO_7$, and a molecular weight of 504.59.

Betamethasone dipropionate is a white to creamy white, odorless crystalline powder, insoluble in water.

LOTRISONE CREAM

Each gram of Lotrisone cream contains 10 mg clotrimazole and 0.643 mg betamethasone dipropionate (equivalent to 0.5 mg betamethasone), in a hydrophilic cream consisting of purified water, mineral oil, white petrolatum, cetyl alcohol plus stearyl alcohol, ceteareth-30, propylene glycol, sodium phosphate monobasic monohydrate, and phosphoric acid; benzyl alcohol, as preservative.

Lotrisone cream is smooth, uniform, and white to off-white in color.

LOTRISONE LOTION

Each gram of Lotrisone lotion contains 10 mg clotrimazole and 0.643 mg betamethasone dipropionate (equivalent to 0.5 mg betamethasone), in a hydrophilic base of purified water, mineral oil, white petrolatum, cetyl alcohol plus stearyl alcohol, ceteareth-30, propylene glycol, sodium phosphate monobasic monohydrate, and phosphoric acid, benzyl alcohol as a preservative.

Lotrisone lotion may contain sodium hydroxide. Lotrisone lotion is opaque and white in color.

INDICATIONS AND USAGE

Lotrisone cream and lotion are indicated in patients 17 years and older for the topical treatment of symptomatic inflammatory tinea pedis, tinea cruris and tinea corporis due to *Epidermophyton floccosum, Trichophyton mentagrophytes,* and *Trichophyton rubrum.* Effective treatment without the risks associated with topical corticosteroid use may be obtained using a topical antifungal agent that does not contain a corticosteroid, especially for noninflammatory tinea infections. The efficacy of Lotrisone cream or lotion for the treatment of infections caused by zoophilic dermatophytes (*e.g., Microsporum canis*) has not been established. Several cases of treatment failure of Lotrisone cream in the treatment of infections caused by *Microsporum canis* have been reported.

CONTRAINDICATIONS

Lotrisone cream or lotion is contraindicated in patients who are sensitive to clotrimazole, betamethasone dipropionate, other corticosteroids or imidazoles, or to any ingredient in these preparations.

DOSAGE AND ADMINISTRATION

Gently massage sufficient Lotrisone cream or lotion into the affected skin areas twice a day, in the morning and evening.

Lotrisone cream or lotion should not be used longer than 2 weeks in the treatment of tinea corporis or tinea cruris, and amounts greater than 45 g/week of Lotrisone cream or amounts greater than 45 ml/week of Lotrisone lotion should not be used. If a patient with tinea corporis or tinea cruris shows no clinical improvement after 1 week of treatment with Lotrisone cream or lotion, the diagnosis should be reviewed.

Lotrisone cream or lotion should not be used longer than 4 weeks in the treatment of tinea pedis and amounts greater than 45 g/week of Lotrisone cream or amounts greater than 45 ml/week of Lotrisone lotion should not be used. If a patient with tinea pedis shows no clinical improvement after 2 weeks of treatment with Lotrisone cream or lotion, the diagnosis should be reviewed.

Lotrisone cream or lotion should not be used with occlusive dressings.

PRODUCT LISTING - RATED THERAPEUTICALLY EQUIVALENT

Cream - Topical - 0.05%;1%

15 gm	$22.87	GENERIC, Taro Pharmaceuticals U.S.A. Inc	51672-4048-01
15 gm	$23.57	GENERIC, Fougera	00168-0258-15

45 gm	$49.27	GENERIC, Taro Pharmaceuticals U.S.A. Inc	51672-4048-06
45 gm	$50.75	GENERIC, Fougera	00168-0258-46

PRODUCT LISTING - EQUIVALENTS NOT AVAILABLE

Cream - Topical - 0.05%;1%

15 gm	$23.47	LOTRISONE, Southwood Pharmaceuticals Inc	58016-3046-01
15 gm	$23.47	LOTRISONE, Southwood Pharmaceuticals Inc	58016-3046-15
15 gm	$23.56	GENERIC, Warrick Pharmaceuticals Corporation	59930-1503-01
15 gm	$23.95	GENERIC, Southwood Pharmaceuticals Inc	58016-5612-01
15 gm	$24.37	LOTRISONE, Allscripts Pharmaceutical Company	54569-0772-00
15 gm	$25.56	LOTRISONE, Schering Corporation	00085-0924-01
15 gm	$30.64	LOTRISONE, Physicians Total Care	54868-1062-01
15 gm	$36.58	LOTRISONE, Pharma Pac	52959-0385-00
45 gm	$47.00	LOTRISONE, Southwood Pharmaceuticals Inc	58016-3252-01
45 gm	$50.74	GENERIC, Warrick Pharmaceuticals Corporation	59930-1503-02
45 gm	$52.49	LOTRISONE, Allscripts Pharmaceutical Company	54569-1513-00
45 gm	$55.06	LOTRISONE, Schering Corporation	00085-0924-02
45 gm	$62.33	LOTRISONE, Physicians Total Care	54868-1062-02

Lotion - Topical - 0.05%;1%

30 ml	$54.69	LOTRISONE, Schering Corporation	00085-0809-01

Betamethasone Valerate *(000468)*

Categories: Dermatosis, corticosteroid-responsive; Pregnancy Category C; FDA Approved 1983 Aug

Drug Classes: Corticosteroids, topical; Dermatologics

Brand Names: Beta-Val; Betaderm; Betamethacot; Betatrex; Betnelan-V; Betnesol-V; Betnevate; Celestan-V; Celestone; Dermabet; Ecoval; Luxiq; Metaderm; Muhibeta-V; Nolcot; Rinderon-V; **Valisone**; Valnac

Foreign Brand Availability: Alphacort (Indonesia); Antroquoril (Australia); Beavate (Malaysia); Bemon (Germany); Bennasone (Thailand); Benoson (Indonesia); Besone (Malaysia; Thailand); Bessasone (Thailand); Beta (Philippines; Thailand); Beta cream (New-Zealand); Beta ointment (New-Zealand); Beta Scalp (New-Zealand); Betacort (Bahrain; Cyprus; Egypt; Iran; Iraq; Jordan; Kuwait; Lebanon; Libya; Oman; Qatar; Republic-of-Yemen; Saudi-Arabia; Syria; United-Arab-Emirates); Betacorten (Israel); Betagalen (Germany); Betasone (Hong-Kong; Thailand); Betasone DHA (Malaysia); Betaval (Bahrain; Cyprus; Egypt; Iran; Iraq; Jordan; Kuwait; Lebanon; Libya; Oman; Qatar; Republic-of-Yemen; Saudi-Arabia; Syria; United-Arab-Emirates); Betnelan (Netherlands); Betnelan V (Belgium); Betnesol V (Germany); Betneval (France); Betnovat (Denmark); Betnovate (Australia; Austria; Bahamas; Bahrain; Barbados; Belize; Benin; Bermuda; Bulgaria; Burkina-Faso; Canada; Curacao; Cyprus; Czech-Republic; Ecuador; Egypt; England; Ethiopia; Gambia; Ghana; Guinea; Guyana; Hong-Kong; India; Indonesia; Iran; Iraq; Israel; Ivory-Coast; Jamaica; Jordan; Kenya; Kuwait; Lebanon; Liberia; Libya; Malawi; Malaysia; Mali; Mauritania; Mauritius; Mexico; Morocco; Netherland-Antilles; New-Zealand; Niger; Nigeria; Oman; Peru; Philippines; Portugal; Qatar; Republic-of-Yemen; Saudi-Arabia; Senegal; Seychelles; Sierra-Leone; South-Africa; Spain; Sudan; Surinam; Switzerland; Syria; Tanzania; Thailand; Trinidad; Tunia; Uganda; United-Arab-Emirates; Zambia; Zimbabwe); Betnovate RD (Singapore); Betopic (Indonesia; Taiwan); Betsona (Peru); Bettamousse (Israel); Bipro (Thailand); Celestan V (Germany); Celestoderm (Canada; Colombia; Finland; France; Netherlands); Celestoderm-V (Bahrain; Benin; Burkina-Faso; Cyprus; Egypt; Ethiopia; Gambia; Ghana; Guinea; Hong-Kong; Indonesia; Iran; Iraq; Ivory-Coast; Jordan; Kenya; Kuwait; Lebanon; Liberia; Libya; Malawi; Malaysia; Mali; Mauritania; Mauritius; Morocco; Niger; Nigeria; Oman; Qatar; Republic-of-Yemen; Saudi-Arabia; Senegal; Seychelles; Sierra-Leone; South-Africa; Sudan; Syria; Tanzania; Tunia; Uganda; United-Arab-Emirates; Zambia; Zimbabwe); Celestoderm V (Argentina; Bulgaria; Italy; Mexico; Spain; Switzerland); Celestone-M (Australia); Celestone-V (Australia); Celeston Valerat (Denmark); Corsaderm (Indonesia); Dendri (Korea); Derzid (Hong-Kong; Singapore); Ectosone (Canada; Hong-Kong); Inflacor (Colombia); Lenovate (South-Africa); Medobeta (Taiwan); Repivate (South-Africa); Topivate (South-Africa); Valezone (Philippines); Varol (Korea)

DESCRIPTION

BETAMETHASONE VALERATE CREAM, REDUCED STRENGTH CREAM, OINTMENT, AND LOTION

For Dermatologic Use Only — Not for Ophthalmic Use.

Betamethasone valerate cream, reduced strength cream, ointment and lotion contain betamethasone valerate, a synthetic adrenocorticoid, for dermatologic use. Betamethasone, an analog of prednisolone, has a slight degree of mineralocorticosteroid activity. Betamethasone valerate is the 17-valerate ester of betamethasone.

Chemically, betamethasone valerate is 9-fluoro-11β,17,21-trihydroxy-16β,methylpregna-1, 4-diene-3,20-dione 17-valerate, with the empirical formula $C_{27}H_{37}FO_6$, and a molecular weight of 476.58. Betamethasone valerate is a white to practically white, odorless crystalline powder, and is practically insoluble in water, freely soluble in acetone and in chloroform, soluble in alcohol and slightly soluble in benzene and either.

Each Gram of Valisone Cream 0.1% Contains: 1.2 mg betamethasone valerate (equivalent to 1.0 mg betamethasone), in an aqueous hydrophilic emollient cream consisting of mineral oil, white petrolatum, ceteareth-30, cetearyl alcohol, monobasic sodium phosphate, and phosphoric acid, chlorocresol and propylene glycol as preservatives.

Each Gram of Valisone Ointment 0.1% Contains: 1.2 mg betamethasone valerate (equivalent to 1.0 mg betamethasone), in an ointment base of mineral oil, white petrolatum, and hydrogenated lanolin.

Each Gram of Valisone Lotion 0.1% Contains: 1.2 mg betamethasone valerate (equivalent to 1.0 mg betamethasone), in a lotion base of isopropyl alcohol (47.5%) and water slightly thickened with carbomer 934P, the pH is adjusted to approximately 4.7 with sodium hydroxide.

Each Gram of Valisone Reduced Strength Cream 0.01% Contains: 0.12 mg betamethasone valerate (equivalent to 0.1 mg betamethasone), in an aqueous hydrophilic emollient cream consisting of mineral oil, white petrolatum, cetereth-30, cetearyl alcohol, monobasic sodium phosphate, and phosphoric acid, chlorocresol and propylene glycol as preservatives.

BETAMETHASONE VALERATE FOAM

For Dermatologic Use Only.

Not for Ophthalmic Use.

Luxiq contains betamethasone valerate, a synthetic corticosteroid, for topical dermatologic use. The corticosteroids constitute a class of primarily synthetic steroids used topically as anti-inflammatory agents.

Chemically, betamethasone valerate is 9-fluoro-11β,17,21-trihydroxy-16β-methylpregna-1, 4-diene-3,20-dione 17-valerate, with the empirical formula $C_{27}H_{37}FO_6$, and a molecular weight of 476.58.

Betamethasone valerate is a white to practically white, odorless crystalline powder, and is practically insoluble in water, freely soluble in acetone and in chloroform, soluble in alcohol, and slightly soluble in benzene and in ether.

Each gram of Luxiq contains 1.2 mg betamethasone valerate, in a hydroalcoholic, thermolabile foam. The foam also contains cetyl alcohol, citric acid, ethanol (60.4%), polysorbate 60, potassium citrate, propylene glycol, purified water, and stearyl alcohol, and is dispensed from an aluminum can pressurized with a hydrocarbon propellant (propane/butane).

CLINICAL PHARMACOLOGY

BETAMETHASONE VALERATE CREAM, REDUCED STRENGTH CREAM, OINTMENT, AND LOTION

The corticosteroids are a class of compounds comprising steroid hormones secreted by the adrenal cortex and their synthetic analogs. In pharmacologic doses corticosteroids are used primarily for their anti-inflammatory and/or immunosuppressive effects.

Topical corticosteroids, such as betamethasone valerate, are effective in the treatment of corticosteroid-responsive dermatoses primarily because of their anti-inflammatory, antipruritic, and vasoconstrictive actions. However, while the physiologic, pharmacologic, and clinical effects of the corticosteroids are well-known, the exact mechanisms of their actions in each disease are uncertain. Betamethasone valerate, a corticosteroid, has been shown to have topical (dermatologic) and systemic pharmacologic and metabolic effects characteristic of this class of drugs.

Pharmacokinetics

The extent of percutaneous absorption of topical corticosteroids is determined by many factors including the vehicle, the integrity of the epidermal barrier, and the use of occlusive dressings. Topical corticosteroids can be absorbed from normal intact skin. Inflammation and/or other disease processes in the skin increase percutaneous absorption. Occlusive dressings substantially increase the percutaneous absorption of topical corticosteroids. Thus, occlusive dressings may be a valuable therapeutic adjunct for treatment of resistant dermatoses.

Once absorbed through the skin, topical corticosteroids are handled through pharmacokinetic pathways similar to systemically administered corticosteroids. Corticosteroids are bound to plasma proteins in varying degrees. Corticosteroids are metabolized primarily in the liver and are then excreted by the kidneys. Some of the topical corticosteroids and their metabolites are also excreted into the bile.

BETAMETHASONE VALERATE FOAM

Like other topical corticosteroids, betamethasone valerate foam has anti-inflammatory, antipruritic, and vasoconstrictive properties. The mechanism of the anti-inflammatory activity of the topical steroids, in general, is unclear. However, corticosteroids are thought to act by the induction of phospholipase A_2 inhibitory proteins, collectively called lipocortins. It is postulated that these proteins control the biosynthesis of potent mediators of inflammation such as prostaglandins and leukotrienes by inhibiting the release of their common precursor arachidonic acid. Arachidonic acid is released from membrane phospholipids by phospholipase A_2.

Pharmacokinetics

Topical corticosteroids can be absorbed from intact healthy skin. The extent of percutaneous absorption of topical corticosteroids is determined by many factors, including the vehicle and the integrity of the epidermal barrier. Occlusion, inflammation and/or other disease processes in the skin may also increase percutaneous absorption.

The use of pharmacodynamic endpoints for assessing the systemic exposure of topical corticosteroids is necessary due to the fact that circulating levels are well below the level of detection. Once absorbed through the skin, topical corticosteroids are handled through pharmacokinetic pathways similar to systemically administered corticosteroids. They are metabolized, primarily in the liver, and are then excreted by the kidneys. In addition, some corticosteroids and their metabolites are also excreted in the bile.

INDICATIONS AND USAGE

BETAMETHASONE VALERATE CREAM, REDUCED STRENGTH CREAM, OINTMENT, AND LOTION

Betamethasone valerate cream, reduced strength cream, ointment and lotion indicated for the relief of the inflammatory and pruritic manifestations of corticosteroid-responsive dermatoses.

BETAMETHASONE VALERATE FOAM

Betamethasone valerate foam is a medium potency topical corticosteroid indicated for relief of the inflammatory and pruritic manifestations of corticosteroid-responsive dermatoses of the scalp.

CONTRAINDICATIONS

BETAMETHASONE VALERATE CREAM, REDUCED STRENGTH CREAM, OINTMENT, AND LOTION

Betamethasone valerate cream, reduced strength cream, ointment and lotion contraindicated in those patients who are hypersensitive to betamethasone valerate, to other corticosteroids, or to any ingredient in this preparation.

BETAMETHASONE VALERATE FOAM

Betamethasone valerate foam is contraindicated in patients who are hypersensitive to betamethasone valerate, to other corticosteroids, or to any ingredient in this preparation.

PRECAUTIONS

BETAMETHASONE VALERATE CREAM, REDUCED STRENGTH CREAM, OINTMENT, AND LOTION

General

Systemic absorption of topical corticosteroids has produced reversible hypothalamic-pituitary-adrenal (HPA) axis suppression, manifestations of Cushing's syndrome, hyperglycemia, and glucosuria in some patients.

Conditions which augment systemic absorption include the application of the more potent steroids, use over large surface areas, prolonged use, and the addition of occlusive dressings. Therefore, patients receiving a large dose of a potent topical steroid applied to a large surface area or under an occlusive dressing should be evaluated periodically for evidence of HPA axis suppression by using the urinary free cortisol and ACTH stimulation tests. If HPA axis suppression is noted, an attempt should be made to withdraw the drug, to reduce the frequency of application, or to substitute a less potent steroid.

Recovery of HPA axis function is generally prompt and complete upon discontinuation of the drug. Infrequently, signs and symptoms of steroid withdrawal may occur, requiring supplemental systemic corticosteroids. Children may absorb proportionally larger amounts of topical corticosteroids and thus be more susceptible to systemic toxicity. (See Pediatric Use.)

If irritation develops, topical corticosteroids should be discontinued and appropriate therapy instituted.

In the presence of dermatological infections, the use of an appropriate antifungal or antibacterial agent should be discontinued until the infection has been adequately controlled.

Information for the Patient

Patients using topical corticosteroids should receive the following information and instructions:

- This medication is to be used as directed by the physician. It is for external use only. Avoid contact with the eyes.
- Patients should be advised not to use this medication for any disorder other than for which it was prescribed.
- The treated skin area should not be bandaged or otherwise covered or wrapped as to be occlusive unless directed by the physician.
- Patients should report any signs of local adverse reactions especially under occlusive dressing.
- Parents of pediatric patient should be advised not to use tight-fitting diapers or plastic pants on a child being treated in the diaper area, as these garments may constitute occlusive dressings.

Laboratory Tests

The following tests may be helpful in evaluating the HPA axis suppression:

Urinary free cortisol test
ACTH stimulation test

Carcinogenesis, Mutagenesis, and Impairment of Fertility

Long-term animal studies have not been performed to evaluate the carcinogenic potential or the effect on fertility of topical corticosteroids.

Studies to determine mutagenicity with prednisolone and hydrocortisone have revealed negative results.

Pregnancy Category C

Corticosteroids are generally teratogenic in laboratory animals when administered systemically at relatively low dosage levels. The more potent corticosteroids have been shown to be teratogenic after dermal application in laboratory animals. There are no adequate and well-controlled studies in pregnant women on teratogenic effects from topically applied corticosteroids. Therefore, topical corticosteroids should be used during pregnancy only if the potential benefit justifies the potential risk to the fetus. Drugs of this class should not be used extensively on pregnant patients, in large amounts, or for prolonged periods of time.

Nursing Mothers

It is not know whether topical administration of corticosteroids could result in sufficient systemic absorption to produce detectable quantities in breast milk. Systemically administered corticosteroids are secreted into breast milk in quantities *not* likely to have a deleterious effect on the infant. Nevertheless, caution should be exercised when topical corticosteroids are prescribed to a nursing woman.

Pediatric Use

Pediatric patients may demonstrate greater susceptibility to topical corticosteroid-induced HPA axis suppression and Cushing's syndrome than mature patients because of a larger skin surface area to body weight ratio.

Hypothalamic-pituitary-adrenal (HPA) axis suppression, Cushing's syndrome, and intracranial hypertension have been reported in children receiving topical corticosteroids. Manifestations of adrenal suppression in children include linear growth retardation, delayed weight gain, low plasma cortisol levels, and absence of response to ACTH stimulation. Manifestations of intracranial hypertension include bulging fontanelles, headaches, and bilateral papilledema.

Administration of topical corticosteroids to children should be limited to the least amount compatible with an effective therapeutic regimen. Chronic corticosteroid therapy may interfere with the growth and development of children.

BETAMETHASONE VALERATE FOAM

General

Systemic absorption of topical corticosteroids has caused reversible hypothalamic-pituitary-adrenal (HPA) axis suppression with the potential for glucocorticosteroid insufficiency after withdrawal of treatment. Manifestations of Cushing's syndrome, hyperglycemia, and glucosuria can also be produced in some patients by systemic absorption of topical corticosteroids while on treatment.

Conditions which augment systemic absorption include the application of the more potent steroids, use over large surface areas, prolonged use, and the addition of occlusive dressings.

Therefore, patients applying a topical steroid to a large surface area or to areas under occlusion should be evaluated periodically for evidence of HPA axis suppression. If HPA axis suppression is noted, an attempt should be made to withdraw the drug, to reduce the frequency of application, or to substitute a less potent steroid.

Recovery of HPA axis function is generally prompt upon discontinuation of topical corticosteroids. Infrequently, signs and symptoms of glucocorticosteroid insufficiency may occur requiring supplemental systemic corticosteroids. For information on systemic supplementation, see prescribing information for those products.

Pediatric patients may be more susceptible to systemic toxicity from equivalent doses due to their larger skin surface to body mass ratios. (See Pediatric Use.)

If irritation develops, betamethasone valerate foam should be discontinued and appropriate therapy instituted. Allergic contact dermatitis with corticosteroids is usually diagnosed by observing a failure to heal rather than noting a clinical exacerbation, as with most topical products not containing corticosteroids. Such an observation should be corroborated with appropriate diagnostic patch testing.

In the presence of dermatological infections, the use of an appropriate antifungal or antibacterial agent should be instituted. If a favorable response does not occur promptly, use of betamethasone valerate foam should be discontinued until the infection has been adequately controlled.

Information for the Patient

Patients using topical corticosteroids should receive the following information and instructions:

- This medication is to be used as directed by the physician. It is for external use only. Avoid contact with the eyes.
- This medication should not be used for any disorder other than that for which it was prescribed.
- The treated scalp area should not be bandaged or otherwise covered or wrapped so as to be occlusive unless directed by the physician.
- Patients should report to their physician any signs of local adverse reactions.
- As with other corticosteroids, therapy should be discontinued when control is achieved. If no improvement is seen within 2 weeks, contact the physician.

Laboratory Tests

The following tests may be helpful in evaluating patients for HPA axis suppression:

ACTH stimulation test
AM plasma cortisol test
Urinary free cortisol test

Carcinogenesis, Mutagenesis, and Impairment of Fertility

Long-term animal studies have not been performed to evaluate the carcinogenic potential or the effect on fertility of betamethasone valerate.

Betamethasone was genotoxic in the *in vitro* human peripheral blood lymphocyte chromosome aberration assay with metabolic activation and in the *in vivo* mouse bone marrow micronucleus assay.

Pregnancy Category C

Corticosteroids have been shown to be teratogenic in laboratory animals when administered systemically at relatively low dosage levels. Some corticosteroids have been shown to be teratogenic after dermal application in laboratory animals. There are no adequate and well-controlled studies in pregnant women. Therefore, betamethasone valerate foam should be used during pregnancy only if the potential benefit justifies the potential risk to the fetus.

Drugs of this class should not be used extensively on pregnant patients, in large amounts, or for prolonged periods of time.

Nursing Mothers

Systemically administered corticosteroids appear in human milk and could suppress growth, interfere with endogenous corticosteroid production, or cause other untoward effects. It is not known whether topical administration of corticosteroids could result in sufficient systemic absorption to produce detectable quantities in breast milk. Because many drugs are excreted in human milk, caution should be exercised when betamethasone valerate foam is administered to a nursing woman.

Pediatric Use

Safety and effectiveness in pediatric patients have not been established. Because of a higher ratio of skin surface area to body mass, pediatric patients are at a greater risk than adults of HPA axis suppression and Cushing's syndrome when they are treated with topical corticosteroids. They are therefore also at greater risk of adrenal insufficiency during and/or after withdrawal of treatment. Adverse effects including striae have been reported with inappropriate use of topical corticosteroids in infants and children.

Hypothalamic-pituitary-adrenal (HPA) axis suppression, Cushing's syndrome, linear growth retardation, delayed weight gain, and intracranial hypertension have been reported in children receiving topical corticosteroids. Manifestations of adrenal suppression in children include low plasma cortisol levels and an absence of response to ACTH stimulation. Manifestations of intracranial hypertension include bulging fontanelles, headaches, and bilateral papilledema.

Administration of topical corticosteroids to children should be limited to the least amount compatible with an effective therapeutic regimen. Chronic corticosteroid therapy may interfere with the growth and development of children.

ADVERSE REACTIONS

BETAMETHASONE VALERATE CREAM, REDUCED STRENGTH CREAM, OINTMENT, AND LOTION

The following local adverse reactions are reported infrequently with topical dermatologic corticosteroids, especially under occlusive dressings: burning; itching; irritation; dryness; folliculitis; hypertrichosis; aceneform eruptions; hypopigmentation; periol dermatitis; allergic contact dermatitis; maceration of the skin; secondary infection; skin atrophy; striae; miliaria.

Systemic absorption of topical corticosteroids has produced reversible hypothalamic-pituitary-adrenal (HPA) axis suppression, manifestations of Cushing's syndrome, hyperglycemia, and glucosuria in some patients.

BETAMETHASONE VALERATE FOAM

The most frequent adverse event was burning/itching/stinging at the application site; the incidence and severity of this event were as shown in TABLE 2.

TABLE 2 *Incidence and Severity of Burning/Itching/Stinging*

		Maximum Severity		
Product	Total Incidence	Mild	Moderate	Severe
Betamethasone valerate foam, n=63	34 (54%)	28 (44%)	5 (8%)	1 (2%)
Betamethasone valerate lotion, n=63	33 (52%)	26 (41%)	6 (10%)	1 (2%)
Placebo foam, n=32	24 (75%)	13 (41%)	7 (22%)	4 (12%)
Placebo lotion, n=30	20 (67%)	12 (40%)	5 (17%)	3 (10%)

Other adverse events which were considered to be possibly, probably, or definitely related to betamethasone valerate foam occurred in 1 patient each; these were paresthesia, pruritus, acne, alopecia, and conjunctivitis.

The following additional local adverse reactions have been reported with topical corticosteroids, and they may occur more frequently with the use of occlusive dressings. These reactions are listed in an approximately decreasing order of occurrence: irritation; dryness; folliculitis; acneiform eruptions; hypopigmentation; perioral dermatitis; allergic contact dermatitis; secondary infection; skin atrophy; striae; and miliaria.

Systemic absorption of topical corticosteroids has produced reversible hypothalamic-pituitary-adrenal (HPA) axis suppression, manifestations of Cushing's syndrome, hyperglycemia, and glucosuria in some patients.

DOSAGE AND ADMINISTRATION

BETAMETHASONE VALERATE CREAM, REDUCED STRENGTH CREAM, OINTMENT, AND LOTION

Betamethasone Valerate Cream and Bethamethasone Valerate Ointment: Apply a thin film to the affected skin areas 1-3 times a day. Dosage once or twice daily is often effective.
Betamethasone Valerate Lotion: Apply a few drops of betamethasone valerate 0.1% to the affected area and massage lightly until it disappears. Apply twice daily, in the morning and at night. Dosage may be increased in stubborn cases. Following improvement, apply once daily. For the most effective and economical use, apply nozzle very close to affected area and gently squeeze bottle. **Protect from light. Store in carton until contents are used.**
Betamethasone Valerate Reduced Strength Cream: Apply a thin film of betamethasone valerate reduced strength cream to the affected skin areas 1-3 times daily. Commonly, treatment twice a day is adequate. In some cases, treatment 3 times a day is necessary; in others, once a day suffices.

BETAMETHASONE VALERATE FOAM

Note: For proper dispensing of foam, can must be inverted.
For application to the scalp invert can and dispense a small amount of betamethasone valerate foam onto a saucer or other cool surface. Do not dispense directly onto hands as foam will begin to melt immediately upon contact with warm skin. Pick up small amounts of foam with fingers and gently massage into affected area until foam disappears. Repeat until entire affected scalp area is treated. Apply twice daily, once in the morning and once at night.

As with other corticosteroids, therapy should be discontinued when control is achieved. If no improvement is seen within 2 weeks, reassessment of the diagnosis may be necessary.

Betamethasone valerate foam should not be used with occlusive dressings unless directed by a physician.

HOW SUPPLIED

VALISONE CREAM, REDUCED STRENGTH CREAM, OINTMENT, AND LOTION

Storage: Store between 2-30°C (36-86°F).

LUXIQ FOAM

Luxiq is supplied in 100 and 50 g aluminum cans.
Storage: Store at controlled room temperature 20-25°C (68-77°F).
Warning: FLAMMABLE. AVOID FIRE, FLAME OR SMOKING DURING AND IMMEDIATELY FOLLOWING APPLICATION. Keep out of reach of children. Contents under pressure. Do not puncture or incinerate container. Do not expose to heat or store at temperatures above 49°C (120°F).

PRODUCT LISTING - RATED THERAPEUTICALLY EQUIVALENT

Cream - Topical - 0.1%
45 gm $5.39 FEDERAL UPPER LIMIT, H.C.F.A. F F P 99999-0468-12
Lotion - Topical - 0.1%
60 ml $6.52 FEDERAL UPPER LIMIT, H.C.F.A. F F P 99999-0468-13

Betaxolol Hydrochloride *(000469)*

For related information, see the comparative table section in Appendix A.

Categories: Glaucoma, open-angle; Hypertension, essential; Hypertension, ocular; Pregnancy Category C; FDA Approved 1985 Aug
Drug Classes: Antiadrenergics, beta blocking; Ophthalmics
Brand Names: **Betoptic**; Kerlone
Foreign Brand Availability: Alcon Betoptic (Philippines); Abaxon (Argentina); Betac (Taiwan); Betasel (Argentina); Betoptic S (Australia; Canada; China; Colombia; Hong-Kong; Israel; Mexico; New-Zealand; Philippines; Singapore; South-Africa; Taiwan; Thailand); Betoptima (Germany; Indonesia); Betoquin (Australia); Kerlon (Belgium; Denmark; Finland; Italy; Netherlands; Sweden; Switzerland); Kerlong (Japan); Optipress (India)
Cost of Therapy: $35.16 (Hypertension; Kerlone; 10 mg; 1 tablet/day; 30 day supply)
$26.94 (Glaucoma; Betoptic Ophth. Solution; 0.5%; 5 ml; 2 drops/day; variable day supply)

DESCRIPTION

TABLETS

Kerlone (betaxolol hydrochloride) a β_1-selective (cardioselective) adrenergic receptor blocking agent available as 10 and 20 mg tablets for oral administration. Betaxolol hydrochloride is chemically described as 2-propanol,1-[4-[2-(cyclopropylmethoxy)ethyl] phenoxy]-3-[(1-methylethyl) amino]-, hydrochloride, (±).

Betaxolol hydrochloride is a water-soluble white crystalline powder with a molecular formula of $C_{18}H_{29}NO_3 \cdot HCl$ and a molecular weight of 343.9. It is freely soluble in water, ethanol, chloroform, and methanol, and has a pKa of 9.4.

The inactive ingredients in Kerlone are hydroxypropyl methylcellulose, lactose, magnesium stearate, polyethylene glycol 400, microcrystalline cellulose, colloidal silicon dioxide, sodium starch glycolate, and titanium dioxide.

OPHTHALMIC SOLUTION AND SUSPENSION

This sterile ophthalmic solution and suspension contain betaxolol hydrochloride, a cardioselective beta-adrenergic receptor blocking agent, in a sterile isotonic solution or in a sterile resin suspension formulation. Betaxolol hydrochloride is a white, crystalline powder, soluble in water, with a molecular weight of 343.89.

Its empirical formula is $C_{18}H_{29}NO_3 \cdot HCl$

Its chemical name is (±)-1-[p-[2-(cyclopropylmethoxy)ethyl]phenoxyl]-3-(isopropylamino)-2-propanol HCl.

Each ml of Betopic ophthalmic solution (0.5%) contains: Active: Betaxolol hydrochloride 5.6 mg equivalent to 5 mg betaxolol base. **Preservative:**Benzalkonium chloride 0.01%. **Inactive:**Edetate di sodium, sodium chloride, hydrochloric acid and/or sodium hydroxide (to adjust pH), and purified water.
Each ml of Betopic S ophthalmic suspension contains: Active: Betaxolol hydrochloride 2.8 mg equivalent to 2.5 mg of betaxolol base. **Preservative:**Benzalkonium chloride 0.01%. **Inactive:**Mannitol, Poly(Styrene-Divinyl Benzene) sulfonic acid, Carbomer 934P, edetate disodium, hydrochloric acid or sodium hydroxide (to adjust pH) and purified water.

CLINICAL PHARMACOLOGY

TABLETS

Betaxolol HCl is a β_1-selective (cardioselective) adrenergic receptor blocking agent that has weak membrane-stabilizing activity and no intrinsic sympathomimetic (partial agonist) activity. The preferential effect on β_1 receptors is not absolute, however, and some inhibitory effects on β_2 receptors (found chiefly in the bronchial and vascular musculature) can be expected at higher doses.

Pharmacokinetics and Metabolism

In man, absorption of an oral dose is complete. There is a small and consistent first-pass effect resulting in an absolute bioavailability of 89% ± 5% that is unaffected by the concomitant ingestion of food or alcohol. Mean peak blood concentrations of 21.6 ng/ml (range 16.3-27.9 ng/ml) are reached between 1.5 and 6 (mean about 3) hours after a single oral dose, in healthy volunteers, of 10 mg of betaxolol HCl. Peak concentrations for 20 and 40 mg doses are 2 and 4 times that of a 10 mg dose and have been shown to be linear over the dose range of 5-40 mg. The peak to trough ratio of plasma concentrations over 24 hours is 2.7. The mean elimination half-life in various studies in normal volunteers ranged from about 14-22 hours after single oral doses and is similar in chronic dosing. Steady state plasma concentrations are attained after 5-7 days with once-daily dosing in persons with normal renal function.

Betaxolol HCl is approximately 50% bound to plasma proteins. It is eliminated primarily by liver metabolism and secondarily by renal excretion. Following oral administration, greater than 80% of a dose is recovered in the urine as betaxolol and its metabolites. Approximately 15% of the dose administered is excreted as unchanged drug, the remainder being metabolites whose contribution to the clinical effect is negligible.

Steady state studies in normal volunteers and hypertensive patients found no important differences in kinetics. In patients with hepatic disease, elimination half-life was prolonged by about 33%, but clearance was unchanged, leading to little change in AUC. Dosage reductions have not routinely been necessary in these patients. In patients with chronic renal failure undergoing dialysis, mean elimination half-life was approximately doubled, as was AUC, indicating the need for a lower initial dosage (5 mg) in these patients. The clearance of betaxolol by hemodialysis was 0.015 L/h/kg and by peritoneal dialysis, 0.010 L/h/kg. Patients (n=8) with stable renal failure, not on dialysis, with mean creatinine clearance of 27 ml/min showed slight increases in elimination half-life and AUC, but no change in C_{max}. In a second study of 30 hypertensive patients with mild to severe renal impairment, there was a reduction in clearance of betaxolol with increasing degrees of renal insufficiency. Inulin clearance (ml/min/1.73m^2) ranged from 70-107 in 7 patients with mild impairment, 41-69 in 14 patients with moderate impairment, and 8-37 in 9 patients with severe impairment. Clearance following oral dosing was reduced significantly in patients with moderate and severe renal impairment (26% and 35%, respectively) when compared with those with mildly impaired renal function. In the severely impaired group, the mean C_{max} and the mean elimination half-life tended to increase (28% and 24%, respectively) when compared with the mildly impaired group. A starting dose of 5 mg is recommended in patients with severe renal impairment (see DOSAGE AND ADMINISTRATION).

Studies in elderly patients (n=10) gave inconsistent results but suggested some impairment of elimination, with one small study (n=4) finding a mean half-life of 30 hours. A starting dose of 5 mg is suggested in older patients.

Pharmacodynamics

Clinical pharmacology studies have demonstrated the beta-adrenergic receptor blocking activity of betaxolol HCl (1) reduction in resting and exercise heart rate, cardiac output, and cardiac work load, (2) reduction of systolic and diastolic blood pressure at rest and during exercise, (3) inhibition of isoproterenol-induced tachycardia, and (4) reduction of reflex orthostatic tachycardia.

The β_1 selectivity of betaxolol HCl in man was shown in 3 ways: (1) In normal subjects, 10 and 40 mg oral doses of betaxolol HCl, which reduced resting heart rate at least as much as 40 mg of propranolol, produced less inhibition of isoproterenol-induced increases in forearm blood flow and finger tremor than propranolol. In this study, 10 mg of betaxolol HCl was at least comparable to 50 mg of atenolol. Both doses of betaxolol HCl, and the one dose of atenolol, however, had more effect on the isoproterenol-induced changes than placebo (indicating some β_2 effect at clinical doses) and the higher dose of betaxolol HCl was more inhibitory than the lower. (2) In normal subjects, single intravenous doses of betaxolol and propranolol, which produced equal effects on exercise-induced tachycardia, had differing effects on insulin-induced hypoglycemia, with propranolol, but not betaxolol, prolonging the hypoglycemia compared to placebo. Neither drug affected the maximum extent of the hypoglycemic response. (3) In a single-blind crossover study in asthmatics (n=10), intravenous infusion over 30 minutes of low doses of betaxolol (1.5 mg) and propranolol (2 mg) had similar effects on resting heart rate but had differing effects on FEV_1 and forced vital capacity, with propranolol causing statistically significant (10-20%) reductions from baseline in mean values for both parameters white betaxolol had no effect on mean values. White blood levels were not measured, the dose of betaxolol used in this study would be expected to produce blood concentrations, at the time of the pulmonary function studies, considerably lower than those achieved during antihypertensive therapy with recommended doses of betaxolol HCl. In a randomized double-blind, placebo-controlled crossover (4 × 4 Latin Square) study in 10 asthmatics, betaxolol (about 5 or 10 mg IV) had little effect on isoproterenol-induced increases in FEV_1; in contrast, propranolol (about 7 mg IV) inhibited the response.

Consistent with its negative chronotropic effect, due to beta-blockade of the SA node, and lack of intrinsic sympathomimetic activity, betaxolol HCl increases sinus cycle length and sinus node recovery time. Conduction in the AV node is also prolonged.

Significant reductions in blood pressure and heart rate were observed 24 hours after dosing in double-blind, placebo-controlled trials with doses of 5-40 mg administered once daily. The antihypertensive response to betaxolol was similar at peak blood levels (3-4 hours) and at trough (24 hours). In a large randomized, parallel dose-response study of 5, 10, and 20 mg, the antihypertensive effects of the 5 mg dose were roughly half of the effects of the 20 mg dose (after adjustment for placebo effects) and the 10 mg dose gave more than 80% of the antihypertensive response to the 20 mg dose. The effect of increasing the dose from 10-20 mg was thus small. In this study, while the antihypertensive response to betaxolol showed a dose-response relationship, the heart rate response (reduction in HR) was not dose related. In other trials, there was little evidence of a greater antihypertensive response to 40 mg than to 20 mg. The maximum effect of each dose was achieved within 1 or 2 weeks. In comparative trials against propranolol, atenolol, and chlorthalidone, betaxolol appeared to be at least as effective as the comparative agent.

Betaxolol HCl has been studied in combination with thiazide-type diuretics and the blood pressure effects of the combination appear additive. Betaxolol HCl has also been used concurrently with methyldopa, hydralazine, and prazosin.

The mechanism of the antihypertensive effects of beta-adrenergic receptor blocking agents has not been established. Several possible mechanisms have been proposed, however, including: (1) competitive antagonism of catecholamines at peripheral (especially cardiac) adrenergic-neuronal sites, leading to decreased cardiac output, (2) a central effect leading to reduced sympathetic outflow to the periphery, and (3) suppression of renin activity.

The results from long-term studies have not shown any diminution of the antihypertensive effect of betaxolol HCl with prolonged use.

OPHTHALMIC SOLUTION AND SUSPENSION

Betaxolol HCl, a cardioselective (beta-1-adrenergic) receptor blocking agent, does not have significant membrane-stabilizing (local anesthetic) activity and is devoid of intrinsic sympathomimetic action. Orally administered beta-adrenergic blocking agents reduce cardiac output in healthy subjects and patients with heart disease. In patients with severe impairment of myocardial function beta-adrenergic receptor antagonists may inhibit the sympathetic stimulatory effect necessary to maintain adequate cardiac function.

When instilled in the eye, betaxolol HCl ophthalmic solution and suspension have the action of reducing elevated as well as normal intraocular pressure, whether or not accompanied by glaucoma. Ophthalmic betaxolol has minimal effect on pulmonary and cardiovascular parameters.

Ophthalmic Solution

Ophthalmic betaxolol (1 drop in each eye) was compared to timolol and placebo in a three-way crossover study challenging 9 patients with reactive airway disease who were selected on the basis of having at least a 15% reduction in the forced expiratory volume in 1 second (FEV_1) after administration of ophthalmic timolol. Betaxolol HCl had no significant effect on pulmonary function as measured by FEV_1, Forced Vital Capacity (FVC) and FEV_1/FVC. Additionally, the action of isoproterenol, a beta stimulant, administered at the end of the study was not inhibited by ophthalmic betaxolol. In contrast, ophthalmic timolol significantly decreased these pulmonary functions as shown in TABLE 1.

TABLE 1 *FEV_1-Percent Change from Baseline**

	Means		
	Betaxolol 1.0%†	Timolol 0.5%	Placebo
Baseline	1.6	1.4	1.4
60 Minutes	2.3	-25.7§	5.8
120 Minutes	1.6	-27.4§	7.5
240 Minutes	- 6.4	-26.9§	6.9
Isoproterenol‡	36.1	-12.4§	42.8

* Schoene, R.B., *et al.* Am. J. Ophthal. 97:86, 1984.
† Twice the clinical concentration.
‡ Inhaled at 240 minutes; measurement at 270 minutes.
§ Timolol statistically different from betaxolol and placebo($p<0.05$).

No evidence of cardiovascular beta-adrenergic blockade during exercise was observed with betaxolol in a double masked, three-way crossover study in 24 normal subjects comparing ophthalmic betaxolol, timolol and placebo for effect on blood pressure and heart rate. Mean arterial blood pressure was not affected by any treatment; however, ophthalmic timolol produced a significant decrease in the mean heart rate as shown in TABLE 2.

TABLE 2 *Mean Heart Rates**

	Treatment, Bruce Stress Exercise Test		
Minutes	Betaxolol 1%†	Timolol 0.5%	Placebo
0	79.2	79.3	81.2
2	130.2	126.0	130.4
4	133.4	128.0‡	134.3
6	136.4	129.0‡	137.9
8	139.8	131.8‡	139.4
10	140.8	131.8‡	141.3

* Atkins, J.M., *et al.* Am. J. Oph. 99:173-175, Feb., 1985.
† Twice the clinical concentration.
‡ Mean pulse rate significantly lower for timolol than betaxolol or placebo ($p<0.05$).

Optic nerve head damage and visual field loss are the result of a sustained elevated intraocular pressure and poor ocular perfusion. Betaxolol HCl ophthalmic solution has the action of reducing elevated as well as normal intraocular pressure and the mechanism of ocular hypotensive action appears to be a reduction of aqueous production as demonstrated by tonography and aqueous fluorophotometry. The onset of action with betaxolol HCl ophthalmic solution can generally be noted within 30 minutes and the maximal effect can usually be detected 2 hours after topical administration. A single dose provides a 12 hour reduction in intraocular pressure. Clinical observation of glaucoma patients treated with betaxolol HCl ophthalmic solution for up to 3 years shows that the intraocular pressure lowering effect is well maintained.

Clinical studies show that topical betaxolol HCl ophthalmic solution reduces mean intraocular pressure 25% from baseline. In trials using 22 mm Hg as a generally accepted index of intraocular pressure control, betaxolol HCl ophthalmic solution was effective in more than 94% of the population studied, of which 73% were treated with the beta blocker alone. In controlled, double-masked studies, the magnitude and duration of the ocular hypotensive effect of betaxolol HCl ophthalmic solution and ophthalmic timolol solution were clinically equivalent.

Betaxolol HCl ophthalmic solution has also been used successfully in glaucoma patients who have undergone a laser trabeculoplasty and have needed additional long-term ocular hypotensive therapy.

Betaxolol HCl ophthalmic solution has been well-tolerated in glaucoma patients wearing hard or soft contact lenses and in aphakic patients.

Betaxolol HCl ophthalmic solution does not produce miosis or accommodative spasm which are frequently seen with miotic agents. The blurred vision and night blindness often associated with standard miotic therapy are not associated with betaxolol HCl ophthalmic solution. Thus, patients with central lenticular opacities avoid the visual impairment caused by a constricted pupil.

Ophthalmic Suspension

Elevated IOP presents a major risk factor in glaucomatous field loss. The higher the level of IOP, the greater the likelihood of optic nerve damage and visual field loss. Betaxolol has the action of reducing elevated as well as normal intraocular pressure and the mechanism of ocular hypotensive action appears to be a reduction of aqueous production as demonstrated by tonography and aqueous fluorophotometry. The onset of action with betaxolol can generally be noted within 30 minutes and the maximal effect can usually be detected two hours after topical administration. A single dose provides a 12 hour reduction in intraocular pressure.

In controlled, double-masked studies, the magnitude and duration of the ocular hypotensive effect of betaxolol HCl ophthalmic suspension 0.25% and betaxolol HCl ophthalmic solution 0.5% were clinically equivalent. Betaxolol HCl suspension was significantly more comfortable than betaxolol HCl solution.

Ophthalmic betaxolol solution at 1% (1 drop in each eye) was compared to placebo in a crossover study challenging 9 patients with reactive airway disease. Betaxolol HCl had no significant effect on pulmonary function as measured by FEV_1, Forced Vital Capacity (FVC), FEV_1/FVC and was not significantly different from placebo. The action of isoproterenol, a beta stimulant, administered at the end of the study was not inhibited by ophthalmic betaxolol.

No evidence of cardiovascular beta adrenergic-blockade during exercise was observed with betaxolol in a double-masked, crossover study in 24 normal subjects comparing ophthalmic betaxolol and placebo for effects on blood pressure and heart rate.

INDICATIONS AND USAGE

TABLETS

Betaxolol HCl is indicated in the management of hypertension. It may be used alone or concomitantly with other antihypertensive agents, particularly thiazide-type diuretics.

OPHTHALMIC SOLUTION

Betaxolol HCl ophthalmic solution has been shown to be effective in lowering intraocular pressure and is indicated in the treatment of ocular hypertension and chronic open-angle glaucoma. It may be used alone or in combination with other anti-glaucoma drugs.

In clinical studies betaxolol HCl safely controlled the intraocular pressure of 47 patients with glaucoma and reactive airway disease followed for a mean period of 15 months. However, caution should be used in treating patients with severe reactive airway disease.

OPHTHALMIC SUSPENSION

Betaxolol HCl ophthalmic suspension has been shown to be effective in lowering intraocular pressure and may be used in patients with chronic open-angle glaucoma and ocular hypertension. It may be used alone or in combination with other intraocular pressure lowering medications.

NON-FDA APPROVED INDICATIONS

Limited data have shown that orally administered betaxolol decreases frequency of angina and nitrate consumption and increases time to angina pectoris, time to ST segment changes during exercise, and total exercise time in patients with stable angina pectoris. Use of betaxolol for the treatment or prophylaxis of angina pectoris is not approved by the FDA.

CONTRAINDICATIONS

TABLETS

Betaxolol HCl is contraindicated in patients with known hypersensitivity to the drug.

Betaxolol HCl is contraindicated in patients with sinus bradycardia, heart block greater than first degree, cardiogenic shock, and overt cardiac failure (see WARNINGS).

OPHTHALMIC SOLUTION AND SUSPENSION

Hypersensitivity to any component of this product.

Betaxolol HCl ophthalmic solution and suspension are contraindicated in patients with sinus bradycardia, greater than a first degree atrioventricular block, cardiogenic shock, or patients with overt cardiac failure.

WARNINGS

TABLETS

Cardiac Failure

Sympathetic stimulation may be a vital component supporting circulatory function in congestive heart failure, and beta-adrenergic receptor blockade carries the potential hazard of further depressing myocardial contractility and precipitating more severe heart failure. In hypertensive patients who have congestive heart failure controlled by digitalis and diuretics, beta-blockers should be administered cautiously. Both digitalis and beta-adrenergic receptor blocking agents slow AV conduction.

In Patients Without a History of Cardiac Failure

Continued depression of the myocardium with beta-blocking agents over a period of time can, in some cases, lead to cardiac failure. Therefore, at the first sign or symptom of cardiac failure, discontinuation of betaxolol HCl should be considered. In some cases beta-blocker therapy can be continued while cardiac failure is treated with cardiac glycosides, diuretics, and other agents, as appropriate.

Exacerbation of Angina Pectoris Upon Withdrawal

Abrupt cessation of therapy with certain beta-blocking agents in patients with coronary artery disease has been followed by exacerbations of angina pectoris and, in some cases, myocardial infarction has been reported. Therefore, such patients should be warned against interruption of therapy without the physician's advice. Even in the absence of overt angina pectoris, when discontinuation of betaxolol HCl is planned, the patient should be carefully observed and therapy should be reinstituted, at least temporarily, if withdrawal symptoms occur.

Bronchospastic Diseases

PATIENTS WITH BRONCHOSPASTIC DISEASE SHOULD NOT IN GENERAL RECEIVE BETA-BLOCKERS. Because of its relative β_1 selectively (cardioselectivity), low doses of betaxolol HCl may be used with caution in patients with bronchospastic disease who do not respond to or cannot tolerate alternative treatment. Since β_1 selectivity is not absolute and is inversely related to dose, the lowest possible dose of betaxolol HCl should be used (5-10 mg once daily) and a bronchodilator should be made available. If dosage must be increased, divided dosage should be considered to avoid the higher peak blood levels associated with once-daily dosing.

Anesthesia and Major Surgery

The necessary, or desirability, of withdrawal of a beta-blocking therapy prior to major surgery is controversial. Beta-adrenergic receptor blockade impairs the ability of the heart to respond to beta-adrenergically mediated reflex stimuli. While this might be of benefit in preventing arrhythmic response, the risk of excessive myocardial depression during general anesthesia may be increased and difficulty in restarting and maintaining the heart beat has been reported with beta-blockers. If treatment is continued, particular care should be taken when using anesthetic agents which depress the myocardium, such as ether, cyclopropane, and trichloroethylene, and it is prudent to use the lowest possible dose of betaxolol HCl. Betaxolol HCl, like other beta-blockers, is a competitive inhibitor of beta-receptor agonists and its effect on the heart can be reversed by cautious administration of such agents (*e.g.*, dobutamine or isoproterenol — Manifestations of excessive vagal tone (*e.g.*, profound bradycardia, hypotension) may be corrected with atropine 1-3 mg IV in divided doses.

Diabetes and Hypoglycemia

Beta-blockers should be used with caution in diabetic patients. Beta-blockers may mask tachycardia occurring with hypoglycemia (patients should be warned of this), although other manifestations such as dizziness and sweating may not be significantly affected. Unlike nonselective beta-blockers, betaxolol HCl does not prolong insulin-induced hypoglycemia.

Thyrotoxicosis

Beta-adrenergic blockade may mask certain clinical signs of hyperthyroidism (*e.g.*, tachycardia). Abrupt withdrawal of beta-blockade might precipitate a thyroid storm; therefore, patients known or suspected of being thyrotoxic from whom betaxolol HCl is to be withdrawn should be monitored closely (see DOSAGE AND ADMINISTRATION, Cessation of Therapy).

OPHTHALMIC SOLUTION AND SUSPENSION

Topically applied beta-adrenergic blocking agents may be absorbed systemically. The same adverse reactions found with systemic administration of beta-adrenergic blocking agents may occur with topical administration. For example, severe respiratory reactions and cardiac reactions, including death due to bronchospasm in patients with asthma, and rarely death in association with cardiac failure, have been reported with topical application of beta-adrenergic blocking agents.

Betaxolol HCl ophthalmic solution and suspension have been shown to have a minor effect on heart rate and blood pressure in clinical studies. Caution should be used in treating patients with a history of cardiac failure or heart block. Treatment with betaxolol HCl ophthalmic solution and suspension should be discontinued at the first signs of cardiac failure.

PRECAUTIONS

GENERAL

Tablets

Beta-adrenoceptor blockade can cause reduction of intraocular pressure. Since betaxolol HCl is marketed as an ophthalmic solution for treatment of glaucoma, patients should be told that betaxolol HCl may interfere with the glaucoma-screening test. Withdrawal may lead to a return of increased intraocular pressure. Patients receiving beta-adrenergic blocking agents orally and beta-blocking ophthalmic solutions should be observed for potential additive effects either on the intraocular pressure or on the known systemic effects of beta-blockade.

Impairment Hepatic or Renal Function

Betaxolol HCl is primarily metabolized in the liver to metabolites that are inactive and then excreted by the kidneys; clearance is somewhat reduced in patients with renal failure but little changed in patients with hepatic disease. Dosage reductions have not routinely been necessary when hepatic and/or renal insufficiency is present (see DOSAGE AND ADMINISTRATION) but patients should be observed. Patients with severe renal impairment and those on dialysis require a reduced dose (see DOSAGE AND ADMINISTRATION).

Ophthalmic Solution and Suspension

Diabetes Mellitus

Beta-adrenergic blocking agents should be administered with caution in patients subject to spontaneous hypoglycemia or to diabetic patients (especially those with labile diabetes) who are receiving insulin or oral hypoglycemic agents. Beta-adrenergic receptor blocking agents may mask the signs and symptoms of acute hypoglycemia.

Thyrotoxicosis

Beta-adrenergic blocking agents may mask certain clinical signs (*e.g.*, tachycardia) of hyperthyroidism. Patients suspected of developing thyrotoxicosis should be managed carefully to avoid abrupt withdrawal of beta-adrenergic blocking agents, which might precipitate a thyroid storm.

Muscle Weakness

Beta-adrenergic blockade has been reported to potentiate muscle weakness consistent with certain myasthenic symptoms (*e.g.*, diplopia, ptosis and generalized weakness).

Major Surgery

Consideration should be given to the gradual withdrawal of beta-adrenergic blocking agents prior to general anesthesia because of the reduced ability of the heart to respond to beta-adrenergically medicated sympathetic reflex stimuli.

Pulmonary

Caution should be exercised in the treatment of glaucoma patients with excessive restriction of pulmonary function. There have been reports of asthmatic attacks and pulmonary distress during betaxolol treatment. Although rechallenges of some such patients with ophthalmic betaxolol has not adversely affected pulmonary function test results, the possibility of adverse pulmonary effects in patients sensitive to beta blockers cannot be ruled out.

Ocular

In patients with angle-closure glaucoma, the immediate treatment objective is to reopen the angle by constriction of the pupil with a miotic agent. Betaxolol has little or no effect on the pupil. When betaxolol HCl ophthalmic suspension 0.25% is used to reduce elevated intraocular pressure in angle-closure glaucoma, it should be used with a miotic and not alone.

INFORMATION FOR THE PATIENT

Tablets

Patients, especially those with evidence of coronary artery insufficiency, should be warned against interruption or discontinuation of betaxolol HCl therapy without the physician's advice.

B

Although cardiac failure rarely occurs in appropriately selected patients, patients being treated with beta-adrenergic blocking agents should be advised to consult a physician at the first sign or symptom of failure.

Patients should know how they react to this medicine before they operate automobiles and machinery or engage in other tasks requiring alertness. Patients should contact their physician if any difficulty in breathing occurs, and before surgery of any type. Patients should inform their physicians or dentists that they are taking betaxolol HCl. Patients with diabetes should be warned that beta-blockers may mask tachycardia occurring with hypoglycemia.

Ophthalmic Solution and Suspension

Do not touch dropper tip to any surface, as this may contaminate the contents. Do not use with contact lenses in eyes.

CARCINOGENESIS, MUTAGENESIS, AND IMPAIRMENT OF FERTILITY

Tablets

Lifetime studies with betaxolol HCl in mice at oral dosages of 6, 20, and 60 mg/kg/day (up to 90 × the maximum recommended human dose (MRHD) based on 60 kg body weight) and in rats at 3, 12, or 48 mg/kg/day (up to 72 × MRHD) showed no evidence of a carcinogenic effect. In a variety of *in vitro* and *in vivo* bacterial and mammalian cell assays, betaxolol HCl was nonmutagenic. Betaxolol did not adversely affect fertility or mating performance of male or female rats at doses up to 256 mg/kg/day (380 × MRHD).

Ophthalmic Solution and Suspension

Lifetime studies with betaxolol HCl have been completed in mice at oral doses of 6, 20 or 60 mg/kg/day and in rats at 3, 12 or 48 mg/kg/day; betaxolol HCl demonstrated no carcinogenic effect. Higher dose levels were not tested.

In a variety of *in vitro* and *in vivo* bacterial and mammalian cell assays, betaxolol HCl was nonmutagenic.

PREGNANCY CATEGORY C

Tablets

In a study in which pregnant rats received betaxolol at doses of 4, 40, or 400 mg/kg/day, the highest dose (600 × MRHD) was associated with increased postimplantation loss, reduced litter size and weight, and an increased incidence of skeletal and visceral abnormalities, which may have been a consequence of drug-related maternal toxicity. Other than a possible increased incidence of incomplete descent of testes and sternebral reductions, betaxolol at 4 mg/kg/day and 40 mg/kg/day (6 × MRHD and 60 × MRHD) caused no fetal abnormalities. In a second study with a different strain of rat, 200 mg betaxolol/kg/day (300 × MRHD) was associated with maternal toxicity and an increase in resorptions, but no teratogenicity. In a study in which pregnant rabbits received doses of 1, 4, 12, or 36 mg betaxolol/kg/day (54 × MRHD), a marked increase in postimplantation loss occurred at the highest dose, but no drug-related teratogenicity was observed. The rabbit is more sensitive to betaxolol than other species because of higher bioavailability resulting from saturation on the first-pass effect. In a peri- and postnatal study in rats at doses of 4, 32, and 256 mg betaxolol/kg/day (380 × MRHD), the highest dose was associated with a marked increase in total litter loss within 4 days postpartum. In surviving offspring, growth and development were also affected.

There are no adequate and well-controlled studies in pregnant women. Betaxolol HCl should be used during pregnancy only if the potential benefit justifies the potential risk to the fetus.

Ophthalmic Solution and Suspension

Reproduction, teratology, and perinatal and postnatal studies have been conducted with orally administered betaxolol HCl in rats and rabbits. There was evidence of drug related post-implantation loss in rabbits and rats at dose levels above 12 mg/kg and 128 mg/kg, respectively. Betaxolol HCl was not shown to be teratogenic, however, and there were no other adverse effects on reproduction at subtoxic dose levels. There are, however, no adequate and well-controlled studies in pregnant women. Because animal reproductive studies are not always predictive of human response, this drug should be used during pregnancy only if potential benefit justifies the potential risk to the fetus.

NURSING MOTHERS

Tablets

Since betaxolol HCl is excreted in human milk in sufficient amounts to have pharmacological effects in the infant, caution should be exercised when betaxolol HCl is administered to a nursing mother.

Ophthalmic Solution and Suspension

It is not known whether betaxolol HCl ophthalmic solution and suspension are excreted in human milk. Because many drugs are excreted in human milk, caution should be exercised when betaxolol HCl ophthalmic solution and suspension are administered to nursing women.

PEDIATRIC USE

Safety and efficacy in pediatric patients have not been established.

GERIATRIC USE

Tablets

Betaxolol HCl may produce bradycardia more frequently in elderly patients. In general, patients 65 years of age and older had a higher incidence rate of bradycardia (hear rate <50 BPM) than younger patients in US clinical trials. In a double-blind study in Europe, 19 elderly patients (mean age = 82) received betaxolol 20 mg daily. Dosage reduction to 10 mg or discontinuation was required for 6 patients due to bradycardia (see DOSAGE AND ADMINISTRATION).

DRUG INTERACTIONS

TABLETS

The following drugs have been coadministered with betaxolol HCl and have not altered its pharmacokinetics: cimetidine, nifedipine, chlorthalidone, and hydrochlorothiazide. Concomitant administration of betaxolol HCl with the oral anticoagulant warfarin has been shown not to potentiate the anticoagulant effect of warfarin.

Catecholamine-depleting drugs (*e.g.,* reserpine) may have an additive effect when given with beta-blocking agents. Patients treated with a beta-adrenergic receptor blocking agent plus a catecholamine depletor should therefore be closely observed for evidence of hypotension or marked bradycardia, which may produce vertigo, syncope, or postural hypotension.

Should it be decided to discontinue therapy in patients receiving beta-blockers and clonidine concurrently, the beta-blocker should be discontinued slowly over several days before the gradual withdrawal of clonidine.

Literature reports suggest that oral calcium antagonists may be used in combination with beta-adrenergic blocking agents when heart function is normal, but should be avoided in patients with impaired cardiac function. Hypotension, AV conduction disturbances, and left ventricular failure have been reported in some patients receiving beta-adrenergic blocking agents when an oral calcium antagonist was added to the treatment regimen. Hypotension was more likely to occur if the calcium antagonist were a dihydropyridine derivative, (*e.g.,* nifedipine), while left ventricular failure and AV conduction disturbances, including, complete heart block, were more likely to occur with either verapamil or diltiazem.

Risk of Anaphylactic Reaction: Although it is known that patients on beta-blockers may be refractory to epinephrine in the treatment of anaphylactic shock, beta-blockers can, in addition, interfere with the modulation of allergic reaction and lead to an increased severity and/or frequency of attacks. Severe allergic reactions including anaphylaxis have been reported in patients exposed to a variety of allergens either by repeated challenge, or accidental contact, and with diagnostic or therapeutic agents while receiving beta-blockers. Such patients may be unresponsive to the usual doses of epinephrine used to treat allergic reaction.

OPHTHALMIC SOLUTION AND SUSPENSION

Patients who are receiving a beta-adrenergic blocking agent orally and betaxolol HCl ophthalmic suspension should be observed for a potential additive effect either on the intraocular pressure or on the known systemic effects of beta blockade.

Close observation of the patient is recommended when a beta blocker is administered to patients receiving catecholamine-depleting drugs such as reserpine, because of possible additive effects and the production of hypotension and/or bradycardia.

Betaxolol is an adrenergic blocking agent; therefore, caution should be exercised in patients using concomitant adrenergic psychotropic drugs.

Risk From Anaphylactic Reaction: While taking beta-blockers, patients with a history of atopy or a history of severe anaphylactic reaction to a variety of allergens may be more reactive to repeated accidental, diagnostic, or therapeutic challenge with such allergens. Such patients may be unresponsive to the usual doses of epinephrine used to treat anaphylactic reactions.

ADVERSE REACTIONS

TABLETS

Most adverse reactions have been mild and transient and are typical of beta-adrenergic blocking agents, (*e.g.,* bradycardia, fatigue, dyspnea, and lethargy). Withdrawal of therapy in US and European controlled clinical trials has been necessary in about 3.5% of patients, principally because of bradycardia, fatigue, dizziness, headache, and impotence. Frequency estimates of adverse events were derived from controlled studies in which adverse reactions were volunteered and elicited in US studies and volunteered and/or elicited in European studies.

In the US, the placebo-controlled hypertension studies lasted for 4 weeks, while the active-controlled hypertension studies had a 22-24 week double-blind phase. The following doses were studied: betaxolol-5, 10, 20, and 40 mg once daily; atenolol-25, 50, and 100 mg once daily; and propranolol-40, 80, and 160 mg bid.

Betaxolol HCl, like other beta-blockers, has been associated with the development of antinuclear antibodies (ANA). In controlled clinical studies, conversion of ANA from negative to positive occurred in 5.3% of the patients treated with betaxolol, 6.3% of the patients treated with atenolol, 4.9% of the patients treated with propranolol, and 3.2% of the patients treated with placebo.

Betaxolol adverse events reported with a 2% or greater frequency, and selected events with lower frequency, in US controlled studies are shown in TABLE 3.

Of the adverse reactions associated with the use of betaxolol shown in TABLE 3, only bradycardia was clearly dose related, but there was a suggestion of dose relatedness for fatigue, lethargy, and dyspepsia.

In Europe, the placebo-controlled study lasted for 4 weeks, while the comparative studies had a 4-52 week double-blind phase. The following doses were studied: betaxolol 20 and 40 mg once daily and atenolol 100 mg once daily.

From European controlled clinical trials, the following adverse events reported by 2% or more patients and selected events with lower frequency are presented in TABLE 4.

The only adverse event whose frequency clearly rose with increasing dose was bradycardia. Elderly patients were especially susceptible to bradycardia, which in some cases responded to dose-reduction (see PRECAUTIONS).

The following selected (potentially important) adverse events have been reported at an incidence of less than 2% in US controlled and open, long-term clinical studies, European controlled clinical trials, or in marketing experience. It is not known whether a causal relationship exists between betaxolol and these events; they are listed to alert the physician to a possible relationship:

Autonomic: Flushing, salivation, sweating.

Body as a Whole: Allergy, fever, malaise, pain, rigors.

Cardiovascular: Angina pectoris, arrhythmia, heart failure, hypertension, hypotension, myocardial infarction, thrombosis, syncope.

TABLE 3

Body System/ Adverse Reaction	Betaxolol 5-40 mg qd* (n=509)	Propranolol 40-160 mg bid (n=73)	Atenolol 25-100 mg qd (n=75)	Placebo (n=109)
Cardiovascular				
Bradycardia (heart rate >50 BPM)	8.1%	4.1%	12.0%	0%
Symptomatic bradycardia	0.8%	1.4%	0%	0%
Edema	1.8%	0%	0%	1.8%
Central Nervous System				
Headache	6.5%	4.1%	5.3%	15.6%
Dizziness	4.5%	11.0%	2.7%	5.5%
Fatigue	2.9%	9.6%	4.0%	0%
Lethargy	2.8%	4.1%	2.7%	0.9%
Psychiatric				
Insomnia	1.2%	8.2%	2.7%	0%
Nervousness	0.8%	1.4%	2.7%	0%
Bizarre dreams	1.0%	2.7%	1.3%	0%
Depression	0.8%	2.7%	4.0%	0%
Autonomic				
Impotence	1.2%†	0%	0%	0%
Respiratory				
Dyspnea	2.4%	2.7%	1.3%	0.9%
Pharyngitis	2.0%	0%	4.0%	0.9%
Rhinitis	1.4%	0%	4.0%	0.9%
Upper respiratory infection	2.6%	0%	0%	5.5%
Gastrointestinal				
Dyspepsia	4.7%	6.8%	2.7%	0.9%
Nausea	1.6%	1.4%	4.0%	0%
Diarrhea	2.0%	6.8%	8.0%	0.9%
Musculoskeletal				
Chest pain	2.4%	1.4%	2.7%	0.9%
Arthralgia	3.1%	0%	4.0%	1.8%
Skin				
Rash	1.2%	0%	0%	0%

* Five (5) patients received 80 mg qid.
† n=336 males; impotence is a known possible adverse effect of this pharmacological class.

TABLE 4

Body System/ Adverse Reaction	Betaxolol 20-40 mg gd (n=155)	Atenolol 100 mg qd (n=81)	Placebo (n=60)
Cardiovascular			
Bradycardia (heart rate <50 BPM)	5.8%	5.0%	0%
Symptomatic bradycardia	1.9%	2.5%	0%
Palpitation	1.9%	3.7%	1.7%
Edema	1.3%	1.2%	0%
Cold extremities	1.9%	0%	0%
Central Nervous System			
Headache	14.8%	9.9%	23.3%
Dizziness	14.8%	17.3%	15.0%
Fatigue	9.7%	18.5%	0%
Asthenia	7.1%	0%	16.7%
Insomnia	5.0%	3.7%	3.3%
Paresthesia	1.9%	2.5%	0%
Gastrointestinal			
Nausea	5.8%	1.2%	0%
Dyspepsia	3.9%	7.4%	3.3%
Diarrhea	1.9%	3.7%	0%
Musculoskeletal			
Chest pain	7.1%	6.2%	5.0%
Joint pain	5.2%	4.9%	1.7%
Myalgia	3.2%	3.7%	3.3%

Central and Peripheral Nervous System: Neuropathy, numbness, speech disorder, stupor, tremor, twitching.
Gastrointestinal: anorexia, constipation, dry mouth, increased appetite, mouth ulceration, rectal disorders, vomiting, dysphagia.
Hearing and Vestibular: Earache, labyrinth disorders, tinnitus, deafness.
Hematologic: Leucocytosis, lymphadenopathy, thrombocytopenia.
Liver and Biliary: Increased AST, increased ALT.
Metabolic and Nutritional: Acidosis, diabetes, hypercholesterolemia, hyperglycemia, hyperkalemia, hyperlipemia, hyperuricemia, hypokalemia, weight gain, increased LDH.
Musculoskeletal: Arthropathy, neck pain, muscle cramps tendonitis.
Psychiatric: Abnormal thinking, amnesia, confusion, emotional lability, hallucinations, decreased libido.
Reproductive Disorders: *Female:* Breast pain, breast fibroadenosis, menstrual disorder; *Male:* Peyronie's disease, prostatitis.
Respiratory: Bronchitis, bronchospasm, cough, epistaxis, flu, pneumonia, sinusitis.
Skin: Alopecia, eczema, erythematous rash, hypertrichosis, pruritus, skin disorders.
Special Senses: Abnormal taste, taste loss.
Urinary System: Cystitis, dysuria, proteinuria, abnormal renal function, renal pain.
Vascular: Cerebrovascular disorder, intermittent claudication, leg cramps, peripheral ischemia, thrombophlebitis.
Vision: Abnormal lacrimation, abnormal vision, blepharitis, ocular hemorrhage, conjunctivitis, dry eyes, iritis, cataract, scotoma.

Potential Adverse Effects: Although not reported in clinical studies with betaxolol, a variety of adverse effects have been reported with other beta-adrenergic blocking agents and may be considered potential adverse effects of betaxolol.

Central Nervous System: Reversible mental depression progressing to catatonia, an acute reversible syndrome characterized by disorientation for time and place, short-term memory loss, emotional lability with slightly clouded sensorium, and decreased performance on neuropsychometric tests.
Allergic: Erythematous rash, fever combined with aching and sore throat, laryngospasm, respiratory distress.
Hematologic: Agranulocytosis, thrombocytopenic purpura, and nonthrombocytopenic purpura.
Gastrointestinal: Mesenteric arterial thrombosis, ischemic colitis.
Miscellaneous: Raynaud's phenomena. There have been reports of skin rashes and/or dry eyes associated with the use of beta-adrenergic blocking drugs. The reported incidence is small, and in most cases, the symptoms have cleared when treatment was withdrawn. Discontinuation of the drug should be considered if any such reaction is not otherwise explicable. Patients should be closely monitored following cessation of therapy.

The oculomucocutaneous syndrome associated with the beta-blocker practolol has not been reported with betaxolol HCl during investigational use and extensive foreign experience. However, dry eyes have been reported.

OPHTHALMIC SOLUTION AND SUSPENSION

Ocular

In clinical trials, the most frequent event associated with the use of betaxolol HCl ophthalmic suspension has been transient ocular discomfort. The following other conditions have been reported in small numbers of patients: blurred vision, corneal punctate keratitis, foreign body sensation, photophobia, tearing, itching, dryness of eyes, erythema, inflammation, discharge, ocular pain, decreased visual acuity and crusty lashes.

Additional medical events reported with other formulations of betaxolol include allergic reactions, decreased corneal sensitivity, corneal punctate staining which may appear in dendritic formations, edema and anisocoria.

Systemic

Systemic reactions following administration of betaxolol HCl ophthalmic suspension or betaxolol HCl ophthalmic solution have been rarely reported. These include:

Cardiovascular: Bradycardia, heart block and congestive failure.
Pulmonary: Pulmonary distress characterized by dyspnea, bronchospasm, thickened bronchial secretions, asthma and respiratory failure.
Central Nervous System: Insomnia, dizziness, vertigo, headaches, depression, lethargy, and increase in signs and symptoms of myasthenia gravis.
Other: Hives, toxic epidermal necrolysis, hair loss, and glossitis. Perversions of taste and smell have been reported.

DOSAGE AND ADMINISTRATION

TABLETS

The initial dose of betaxolol HCl in hypertension is ordinarily 10 mg once daily either alone or added to diuretic therapy. The full antihypertensive effect is usually seen within 7-14 days. If the desired response is not achieved the dose can be doubled after 7-14 days. Increasing the dose beyond 20 mg has not been shown to produce a statistically significant additional antihypertensive effect; but the 40 mg dose has been studied and is well tolerated. An increased effect (reduction) on heart rate should be anticipated with increasing dosage. If monotherapy with betaxolol HCl does not produce the desired response, the addition of a diuretic agent or other antihypertensive should be considered (see DRUG INTERACTIONS).

DOSAGE ADJUSTMENT FOR SPECIFIC PATIENTS

Patients With Renal Failure

In patients with renal impairment, clearance of betaxolol declines with decreasing renal function.

In patients with severe renal impairment and those undergoing dialysis, the initial dose of betaxolol HCl is 5 mg once daily. If the desired response in not achieved, dosage may be increased by 5 mg/day increments every 2 weeks to a maximum dose of 20 mg/day.

Patients With Hepatic Disease

Patients with hepatic disease do not have significantly altered clearance. Dosage adjustments are not routinely needed.

Elderly Patients

Consideration should be given to reduction in the starting dose to 5 mg in elderly patients. These patients are especially prone to beta-blocker-induced bradycardia, which appears to be dose related and sometimes responds to reductions in dose.

Cessation of Therapy

If withdrawal of betaxolol HCl therapy is planned, it should be achieved gradually over a period of about 2 weeks. Patients should be carefully observed and advised to limit physical activity to a minimum.

OPHTHALMIC SOLUTION

The usual dose is one drop of betaxolol HCl ophthalmic solution in the affected eye(s) twice daily. In some patients, the intraocular pressure lowering response to betaxolol HCl ophthalmic solution may require a few weeks to stabilize. Clinical follow-up should include a determination of the intraocular pressure during the first month of treatment with betaxolol HCl ophthalmic solution. Thereafter, intraocular pressures should be determined on an individual basis at the judgment of the physician.

When a patient is transferred from a single anti-glaucoma agent, continue the agent already used and add one drop of betaxolol HCl ophthalmic solution in the affected eye(s) twice a day. On the following day, discontinue the previous anti-glaucoma agent completely and continue with betaxolol HCl ophthalmic solution.

Because of diurnal variations of intraocular pressure in individual patients, satisfactory response to twice a day therapy is best determined by measuring intraocular pressure at different times during the day. Intraocular pressures ≤22 mm Hg may not be optimal for control of glaucoma in each patient; therefore, therapy should be individualized.

When a patient is transferred from several concomitantly administered anti-glaucoma agents, individualization is required. Adjustment should involve one agent at a time made at intervals of not less than 1 week. A recommended approach is to continue the agents being used and add 1 drop of betaxolol HCl ophthalmic solution in the affected eye(s) twice a day. On the following day, discontinue one of the other anti-glaucoma agents. The remaining anti-glaucoma agents may be decreased or discontinued according to the patient's response to treatment. The physician may be able to discontinue some or all of the other anti-glaucoma agents.

OPHTHALMIC SUSPENSION

The recommended dose is 1-2 drops of betaxolol HCl ophthalmic suspension in the affected eye(s) twice daily. In some patients, the intraocular pressure lowering responses to betaxolol HCl ophthalmic suspension may require a few weeks to stabilize. As with any new medication, careful monitoring of patients is advised.

OPHTHALMIC SOLUTION AND SUSPENSION

If the intraocular pressure of the patient is not adequately controlled on this regimen, concomitant therapy with pilocarpine and other miotics, and/or epinephrine and/or carbonic anhydrase inhibitors can be instituted.

HOW SUPPLIED

Kerlone 10 mg Tablets: Round, white, film coated, with "KERLONE 10" debossed on one side and scored on the other.

Kerlone 20 mg Tablets: Round, white, film coated, with "KERLONE 20" debossed on one side and β on the other.

STORAGE

Tablets: Store at room temperature, below 30°C (86°F).

Ophthalmic Solution and Suspension: Store upright at room temperature. Shake well before using.

PRODUCT LISTING - RATED THERAPEUTICALLY EQUIVALENT

Size	Price	Product	NDC
Solution - Ophthalmic - 0.5%			
5 ml	$23.03	GENERIC, Falcon Pharmaceuticals, Ltd.	61314-0245-01
5 ml	$26.17	GENERIC, Apotex Usa Inc	60505-0556-02
10 ml	$44.56	GENERIC, Falcon Pharmaceuticals, Ltd.	61314-0245-03
10 ml	$50.64	GENERIC, Apotex Usa Inc	60505-0556-03
15 ml	$57.15	GENERIC, Falcon Pharmaceuticals, Ltd.	61314-0245-02
15 ml	$64.94	GENERIC, Apotex Usa Inc	60505-0556-04
Tablet - Oral - 10 mg			
100's	$95.35	GENERIC, Amide Pharmaceutical Inc	52152-0179-02
Tablet - Oral - 20 mg			
100's	$142.85	GENERIC, Amide Pharmaceutical Inc	52152-0180-02

PRODUCT LISTING - EQUIVALENTS NOT AVAILABLE

Size	Price	Product	NDC
Solution - Ophthalmic - 0.5%			
2.50 ml	$141.72	BETOPTIC, Alcon Laboratories Inc	00065-0245-20
10 ml	$36.56	BETOPTIC, Allscripts Pharmaceutical Company	54569-1180-00
Suspension - Ophthalmic - 0.25%			
2.50 ml	$18.88	BETOPTIC S, Alcon Laboratories Inc	00065-0246-20
5 ml	$26.94	BETOPTIC S, Allscripts Pharmaceutical Company	54569-2854-00
5 ml	$29.32	BETOPTIC S, Physicians Total Care	54868-1639-02
5 ml	$37.56	BETOPTIC S, Alcon Laboratories Inc	00065-0246-05
10 ml	$52.69	BETOPTIC S, Allscripts Pharmaceutical Company	54569-4377-00
10 ml	$54.39	BETOPTIC S, Physicians Total Care	54868-1639-01
10 ml	$70.19	BETOPTIC S, Alcon Laboratories Inc	00065-0246-10
15 ml	$78.63	BETOPTIC S, Allscripts Pharmaceutical Company	54569-3029-00
15 ml	$80.85	BETOPTIC S, Physicians Total Care	54868-1639-03
15 ml	$104.69	BETOPTIC S, Alcon Laboratories Inc	00065-0246-15
Tablet - Oral - 10 mg			
100's	$117.21	KERLONE, Searle	00025-5101-31
Tablet - Oral - 20 mg			
100's	$175.76	KERLONE, Searle	00025-5201-31

Bethanechol Chloride *(000470)*

Categories: Retention, urinary; Pregnancy Category C; FDA Approved 1948 Oct
Drug Classes: Cholinergics
Brand Names: Duvoid; Myocholine; Myotonachol; Myotonine; **Urecholine**
Foreign Brand Availability: Muscaran (Belgium); Myo Hermes (Spain); Myocholine-Glenwood (Austria); Myocholine Glenwood (Switzerland); Myotonine Chloride (England); Ucholine (Thailand); Urotonine (India)
Cost of Therapy: $128.16 (Urinary Retention; Urecholine; 10 mg; 3 tablets/day; 30 day supply)
$3.38 (Urinary Retention; Generic Tablets; 10 mg; 3 tablets/day; 30 day supply)
HCFA JCODE(S): J0520 up to 5 mg SC

DESCRIPTION

Bethanechol chloride, a cholinergic agent, is a synthetic ester which is structurally and pharmacologically related to acetylcholine.

It is designated chemically as 2-((aminocarbonyl) oxy)-*N,N,N*-trimethyl-1-propanaminium chloride. Its empirical formula is $C_7H_{17}ClN_2O_2$.

It is a white, hygroscopic crystalline compound having a slight amine-like odor, freely soluble in water, and has a molecular weight of 196.68.

Bethanechol chloride is supplied as 5, 10, 25, and 50 mg tablets for oral use. Inactive ingredients in the tablets are calcium phosphate, lactose, magnesium stearate, and starch. Bethanechol chloride tablets 10 mg also contain FD&C red 3 and FD&C red 40. Bethanechol chloride tablets 25 and 50 mg also contain D&C yellow 10 and FD&C yellow 6.

Bethanechol chloride is also supplied as a sterile solution **for subcutaneous use only.** The sterile solution is essentially neutral. Each milliliter contains bethanechol chloride, 5 mg, and water for injection, 1 ml. It may be autoclaved at 120°C for 20 minutes without discoloration or loss of potency.

CLINICAL PHARMACOLOGY

Bethanechol chloride acts principally by producing the effects of stimulation of the parasympathetic nervous system. It increases the tone of the detrusor urinae muscle, usually producing a contraction sufficiently strong to initiate micturition and empty the bladder. It stimulates gastric motility, increases gastric tone, and often restores impaired rhythmic peristalsis.

Stimulation of the parasympathetic nervous system releases acetylcholine at the nerve endings. When spontaneous stimulation is reduced and therapeutic intervention is required, acetylcholine can be given, but it is rapidly hydrolyzed by cholinesterase, and its effects are transient. Bethanechol chloride is not destroyed by cholinesterase and its effects are more prolonged than those of acetylcholine.

Effects on the GI and urinary tracts sometimes appear within 30 minutes after oral administration of bethanechol chloride, but more often 60-90 minutes are required to reach maximum effectiveness. Following oral administration, the usual duration of action of bethanechol is one hour, although large doses (300-400 mg) have been reported to produce effects for up to 6 hours. Subcutaneous injection produces a more intense action on bladder muscle than does oral administration of the drug.

Because of the selective action of bethanechol, nicotinic symptoms of cholinergic stimulation are usually absent or minimal when orally or subcutaneously administered in therapeutic doses, while muscarinic effects are prominent. Muscarinic effects usually occur within 5-15 minutes after subcutaneous injection, reach a maximum in 15-30 minutes, and disappear within two hours. Doses that stimulate micturition and defecation and increase peristalsis do not ordinarily stimulate ganglia or voluntary muscles. Therapeutic test doses in normal human subjects have little effect on heart rate, blood pressure, or peripheral circulation.

Bethanechol chloride does not cross the blood-brain barrier because of its charged quaternary amine moiety. The metabolic fate and mode of excretion of the drug have not been elucidated.

A clinical study (Diokno, A.C.; Lapides, J., Urol. 10:23-24, July 1977.) was conducted on the relative effectiveness of oral and subcutaneous doses of bethanechol chloride on the stretch response of bladder muscle in patients with urinary retention. Results showed that 5 mg of the drug given subcutaneously stimulated a response that was more rapid in onset and of larger magnitude than an oral dose of 50, 100, or 200 mg. All the oral doses, however, had a longer duration of effect than the subcutaneous dose. Although the 50 mg oral dose caused little change in intravesical pressure in this study, this dose has been found in other studies to be clinically effective in the rehabilitation of patients with decompensated bladders.

INDICATIONS AND USAGE

For the treatment of acute postoperative and postpartum nonobstructive (functional) urinary retention and for neurogenic atony of the urinary bladder with retention.

CONTRAINDICATIONS

Hypersensitivity to bethanechol chloride tablets or to any component of bethanechol chloride injection, hyperthyroidism, peptic ulcer, latent or active bronchial asthma, pronounced bradycardia or hypotension, vasomotor instability, coronary artery disease, epilepsy, and parkinsonism.

Bethanechol chloride should not be employed when the strength or integrity of the gastrointestinal or bladder wall is in question, or in the presence of mechanical obstruction; when increased muscular activity of the gastrointestinal tract or urinary bladder might prove harmful, as following recent urinary bladder surgery, gastrointestinal resection and anastomosis, or when there is possible gastrointestinal obstruction; in bladder neck obstruction, spastic gastrointestinal disturbances, acute inflammatory lesions of the gastrointestinal tract, or peritonitis; or in marked vagotonia.

WARNINGS

The sterile solution is for subcutaneous use only. It should never be given intramuscularly or intravenously. Violent symptoms of cholinergic over-stimulation, such as circulatory collapse, fall in blood pressure, abdominal cramps, bloody diarrhea, shock, or sudden cardiac arrest are likely to occur if the drug is given by either of these routes. Although rare, these same symptoms have occurred after subcutaneous injection, and may occur in cases of hypersensitivity or overdosage.

PRECAUTIONS

General: In urinary retention, if the sphincter fails to relax as bethanechol chloride contracts the bladder, urine may be forced up the ureter into the kidney pelvis. If there is bacteriuria, this may cause reflux infection.

Information for the Patient: Bethanechol chloride tablets should preferably be taken one hour before or two hours after meals to avoid nausea or vomiting. Dizziness, lightheadedness or fainting may occur, especially when getting up from a lying or sitting position.

Carcinogenesis, Mutagenesis, and Impairment of Fertility: Long-term studies in animals have not been performed to evaluate the effects upon fertility, mutagenic or carcinogenic potential of bethanechol chloride.

Pregnancy Category C: Animal reproduction studies have not been conducted with bethanechol chloride. It is also not known whether bethanechol chloride can cause fetal harm when administered to a pregnant woman or can affect reproduction capacity. Bethanechol chloride should be given to a pregnant woman only if clearly needed.

Nursing Mothers: It is not known whether this drug is secreted in human milk. Because many drugs are secreted in human milk and because of the potential for serious adverse reactions from bethanechol chloride in nursing infants, a decision should be made whether to discontinue nursing or to discontinue the drug, taking into account the importance of the drug to the mother.

Pediatric Use: Safety and effectiveness in children have not been established.

DRUG INTERACTIONS

Special care is required if this drug is given to patients receiving ganglion blocking compounds because a critical fall in blood pressure may occur. Usually, severe abdominal symptoms appear before there is such a fall in the blood pressure.

ADVERSE REACTIONS

Adverse reactions are rare following oral administration of bethanechol, but are more common following subcutaneous injection. Adverse reactions are more likely to occur when dosage is increased.

The following adverse reactions have been observed:

Body as a Whole: Malaise.

Digestive: Abdominal cramps or discomfort, colicky pain, nausea and belching, diarrhea, borborygmi, salivation.

Renal: Urinary urgency.

Nervous System: Headache.

Cardiovascular: A fall in blood pressure with reflex tachycardia, vasomotor response.

Skin: Flushing producing a feeling of warmth, sensation of heat about the face, sweating.

Respiratory: Bronchial constriction, asthmatic attacks.

Special Senses: Lacrimation, miosis.

CAUSAL RELATIONSHIP UNKNOWN

The following adverse reactions have been reported, and a causal relationship to therapy with bethanechol chloride has not been established:

Body as a Whole: Hypothermia.

Nervous System: Seizures.

DOSAGE AND ADMINISTRATION

Dosage and route of administration must be individualized, depending on the type and severity of the condition to be treated.

Preferably give the drug when the stomach is empty. If taken soon after eating, nausea and vomiting may occur.

ORAL

The usual adult dosage is 10-50 mg 3 or 4 times a day. The minimum effective dose is determined by giving 5 or 10 mg initially and repeating the same amount at hourly intervals until satisfactory response occurs or until a maximum of 50 mg has been given. The effects of the drug sometimes appear within 30 minutes and usually within 60-90 minutes. They persist for about an hour.

SUBCUTANEOUS

The usual dose is 1 ml (5 mg), although some patients respond satisfactorily to as little as 0.5 ml (2.5 mg). The minimum effective dose is determined by injecting 0.5 ml (2.5 mg) initially and repeating the same amount at 15-30 minute intervals to a maximum of 4 doses until satisfactory response is obtained, unless disturbing reactions appear. The minimum effective dose may be repeated thereafter 3 or 4 times a day as required.

Rarely, single doses up to 2 ml (10 mg) may be required. Such large doses may cause severe reactions and should be used only after adequate trial of single doses of 0.5 to 1 ml (2.5 to 5 mg) has established that smaller doses are not sufficient.

Bethanechol chloride is usually effective in 5-15 minutes after subcutaneous injection.

If necessary, the effects of the drug can be abolished promptly by atropine.

Parenteral drug products should be inspected visually for particulate matter and discoloration prior to administration, whenever solution and container permit.

STORAGE

Store bethanechol chloride tablets in a tightly-closed container. Avoid storage at temperatures above 40°C (104°F).

Avoid storage of bethanechol chloride injection at temperatures below -20°C (-4°F) and above 40°C (104°F).

PRODUCT LISTING - RATED THERAPEUTICALLY EQUIVALENT

Solution - Subcutaneous - 5 mg/ml

1 ml x 6	$33.72	URECHOLINE, Merck & Company Inc	00006-7786-29

Tablet - Oral - 5 mg

100's	$4.01	GENERIC, Ivax Corporation	00182-0453-01
100's	$4.22	GENERIC, Aligen Independent Laboratories Inc	00405-4123-01
100's	$6.00	GENERIC, Major Pharmaceuticals Inc	00904-0590-60
100's	$7.29	GENERIC, Vangard Labs	00615-2556-01
100's	$13.02	GENERIC, Ivax Corporation	00182-0453-89
100's	$13.47	GENERIC, Major Pharmaceuticals Inc	00904-0590-61
100's	$14.64	GENERIC, Auro Pharmaceutical	55829-0167-10
100's	$29.91	GENERIC, Qualitest Products Inc	00603-2455-21
100's	$45.83	GENERIC, Odyssey Pharmaceutical	65473-0691-01
100's	$75.89	GENERIC, Odyssey Pharmaceutical	65473-0697-01

Tablet - Oral - 10 mg

100's	$3.75	GENERIC, Interstate Drug Exchange Inc	00814-1177-14
100's	$3.75	GENERIC, Major Pharmaceuticals Inc	00904-0591-60
100's	$4.70	GENERIC, Martec Pharmaceuticals Inc	52555-0422-01
100's	$5.05	GENERIC, Geneva Pharmaceuticals	00781-1254-01
100's	$5.27	GENERIC, Aligen Independent Laboratories Inc	00405-4124-01
100's	$5.50	GENERIC, Parmed Pharmaceuticals Inc	00349-2129-01
100's	$6.00	GENERIC, Ivax Corporation	00182-0454-01
100's	$6.34	GENERIC, Moore, H.L. Drug Exchange Inc	00839-6209-06
100's	$16.88	GENERIC, Major Pharmaceuticals Inc	00904-0591-61
100's	$18.20	GENERIC, Ivax Corporation	00182-0454-89
100's	$18.85	GENERIC, Auro Pharmaceutical	55829-0168-10
100's	$41.00	GENERIC, Watson/Schein Pharmaceuticals Inc	00364-0349-01
100's	$43.49	GENERIC, Qualitest Products Inc	00603-2456-21
100's	$51.79	GENERIC, Mutual/United Research Laboratories	00677-0506-01
100's	$80.88	DUVOID, Roberts Pharmaceutical Corporation	54092-0101-01
100's	$142.40	URECHOLINE, Odyssey Pharmaceutical	65473-0703-01
250's	$7.15	GENERIC, Major Pharmaceuticals Inc	00904-0591-70

Tablet - Oral - 25 mg

100's	$4.50	GENERIC, Major Pharmaceuticals Inc	00904-0592-60
100's	$5.39	GENERIC, Us Trading Corporation	56126-0217-11
100's	$5.63	GENERIC, Interstate Drug Exchange Inc	00814-1178-14
100's	$5.90	GENERIC, Parmed Pharmaceuticals Inc	00349-2429-01
100's	$6.30	GENERIC, Martec Pharmaceuticals Inc	52555-0423-01
100's	$6.75	GENERIC, Geneva Pharmaceuticals	00781-1250-01
100's	$6.82	GENERIC, Moore, H.L. Drug Exchange Inc	00839-6210-06
100's	$7.08	GENERIC, Aligen Independent Laboratories Inc	00405-4125-01
100's	$9.40	GENERIC, Ivax Corporation	00182-0455-01
100's	$26.20	GENERIC, Auro Pharmaceutical	55829-0169-10
100's	$32.60	GENERIC, Ivax Corporation	00182-0455-89
100's	$36.82	GENERIC, Major Pharmaceuticals Inc	00904-0592-61
100's	$59.00	GENERIC, Watson/Schein Pharmaceuticals Inc	00364-0410-01
100's	$61.95	GENERIC, Qualitest Products Inc	00603-2457-21
100's	$125.54	DUVOID, Roberts Pharmaceutical Corporation	54092-0102-01
100's	$189.85	URECHOLINE, Odyssey Pharmaceutical	65473-0704-01
250's	$9.00	GENERIC, Major Pharmaceuticals Inc	00904-0592-70

Tablet - Oral - 50 mg

100's	$9.00	GENERIC, Major Pharmaceuticals Inc	00904-0593-60
100's	$9.98	GENERIC, Interstate Drug Exchange Inc	00814-1176-14
100's	$12.06	GENERIC, Aligen Independent Laboratories Inc	00405-4126-01
100's	$15.53	GENERIC, Moore, H.L. Drug Exchange Inc	00839-6537-06
100's	$31.42	GENERIC, Vangard Labs	00615-2559-13
100's	$36.70	GENERIC, Auro Pharmaceutical	55829-0170-10
100's	$42.00	GENERIC, Ivax Corporation	00182-1023-89
100's	$44.69	GENERIC, Major Pharmaceuticals Inc	00904-0593-61
100's	$92.25	GENERIC, Qualitest Products Inc	00603-2458-21
100's	$163.04	URECHOLINE, Merck & Company Inc	00006-0460-68
100's	$194.18	DUVOID, Roberts Pharmaceutical Corporation	54092-0103-01
100's	$303.76	URECHOLINE, Odyssey Pharmaceutical	65473-0700-01

Bexarotene *(003464)*

Categories: Lymphoma, skin manifestations; FDA Approved 1999 Dec; Pregnancy Category X; Orphan Drugs
Drug Classes: Antineoplastics, retinoids; Dermatologics; Retinoids
Foreign Brand Availability: Targretin (Austria; Belgium; Bulgaria; Czech-Republic; Denmark; England; Finland; France; Germany; Greece; Hungary; Ireland; Italy; Netherlands; Norway; Poland; Portugal; Slovenia; Spain; Sweden; Switzerland; Turkey)
Cost of Therapy: $3819.90 (Cutaneous T-cell Lymphoma; Targretin; 75 mg; 7 capsules/day; 30 day supply)
$1177.00 (Cutaneous T-cell Lymphoma; Targretin Gel; 1%; 60 g; 2 applications/day; variable day supply)

ORAL

WARNING

Bexarotene capsules are a member of the retinoid class of drugs that is associated with birth defects in humans. Bexarotene capsules also caused birth defects when administered orally to pregnant rats. Bexarotene capsules must not be administered to a pregnant woman. See CONTRAINDICATIONS.

DESCRIPTION

Bexarotene is a member of a subclass of retinoids that selectively activate retinoid X receptors (RXRs). These retinoid receptors have biologic activity distinct from that of retinoic acid receptors (RARs). Each soft gelatin capsule for oral administration contains 75 mg of bexarotene.

The chemical name is 4-[1-(5,6,7,8-tetrahydro-3,5,5,8,8-pentamethyl-2-naphthalenyl)ethenyl] benzoic acid.

Bexarotene is an off-white to white powder with a molecular weight of 348.48 and a molecular formula of $C_{24}H_{28}O_2$. It is insoluble in water and slightly soluble in vegetable oils and ethanol.

Each Targretin capsule also contains the following inactive ingredients: polyethylene glycol 400, polysorbate 20, povidone, and butylated hydroxyanisole. The capsule shell contains gelatin, sorbitol special-glycerin blend, and titanium dioxide.

B

CLINICAL PHARMACOLOGY

MECHANISM OF ACTION

Bexarotene selectively binds and activates retinoid X receptor subtypes (RXRα, RXRβ,RXRγ). RXRs can form heterodimers with various receptor partners such as retinoic acid receptors (RARs), vitamin D receptor, thyroid receptor, and peroxisome proliferator activator receptors (PPARs). Once activated, these receptors function as transcription factors that regulate the expression of genes that control cellular differentiation and proliferation. Bexarotene inhibits the growth *in vitro* of some tumor cell lines of hematopoietic and squamous cell origin. It also induces tumor regression *in vivo* in some animal models. The exact mechanism of action of bexarotene in the treatment of cutaneous T-cell lymphoma (CTCL) is unknown.

PHARMACOKINETICS

General

After oral administration of bexarotene capsules, bexarotene is absorbed with a T_{max} of about 2 hours. Terminal half-life of bexarotene is about 7 hours. Studies in patients with advanced malignancies show approximate single dose linearity within the therapeutic range and low accumulation with multiple doses. Plasma bexarotene AUC and C_{max} values resulting from a 75-300 mg dose were 35% and 48% higher, respectively, after a fat-containing meal than after a glucose solution (see PRECAUTIONS, Drug-Food Interaction and DOSAGE AND ADMINISTRATION). Bexarotene is highly bound (>99%) to plasma proteins. The plasma proteins to which bexarotene binds have not been elucidated, and the ability of bexarotene to displace drugs bound to plasma proteins and the ability of drugs to displace bexarotene binding have not been studied (see PRECAUTIONS, Protein Binding). The uptake of bexarotene by organs or tissues has not been evaluated.

Metabolism

Four bexarotene metabolites have been identified in plasma: 6- and 7-hydroxy-bexarotene and 6- and 7-oxo-bexarotene. *In vitro* studies suggest that cytochrome P450 3A4 is the major cytochrome P450 responsible for formation of the oxidative metabolites and that the oxidative metabolites may be glucuronidated. The oxidative metabolites are active in *in vitro* assays of retinoid receptor activation, but the relative contribution of the parent and any metabolites to the efficacy and safety of bexarotene capsules is unknown.

Elimination

The renal elimination of bexarotene and its metabolites was examined in patients with Type 2 diabetes mellitus. Neither bexarotene nor its metabolites were excreted in urine in appreciable amounts. Bexarotene is thought to be eliminated primarily through the hepatobiliary system.

Special Populations

Elderly

Bexarotene C_{max} and AUC were similar in advanced cancer patients <60 years old and in patients >60 years old, including a subset of patients >70 years old.

Pediatric

Studies to evaluate bexarotene pharmacokinetics in the pediatric population have not been conducted (see PRECAUTIONS, Pediatric Use).

Gender

The pharmacokinetics of bexarotene were similar in male and female patients with advanced cancer.

Ethnic Origin

The effect of ethnic origin on bexarotene pharmacokinetics is unknown.

Renal Insufficiency

No formal studies have been conducted with bexarotene capsules in patients with renal insufficiency. Urinary elimination of bexarotene and its known metabolites is a minor excretory pathway (<1% of administered dose), but because renal insufficiency can result in significant protein binding changes, pharmacokinetics may be altered in patients with renal insufficiency (see PRECAUTIONS, Renal Insufficiency).

Hepatic Insufficiency

No specific studies have been conducted with bexarotene capsules in patients with hepatic insufficiency. Because less than 1% of the dose is excreted in the urine unchanged and there is *in vitro* evidence of extensive hepatic contribution to bexarotene elimination, hepatic impairment would be expected to lead to greatly decreased clearance (see WARNINGS, Hepatic Insufficiency).

Drug-Drug Interactions

No specific studies to evaluate drug interactions with bexarotene have been conducted. Bexarotene oxidative metabolites appear to be formed by cytochrome P450 3A4.

Because bexarotene is metabolized by cytochrome P450 3A4, ketoconazole, itraconazole, erythromycin, gemfibrozil, grapefruit juice, and other inhibitors of cytochrome P450 3A4 would be expected tolead to an increase in plasma bexarotene concentrations. Furthermore, rifampin, phenytoin, phenobarbital and other inducers of cytochrome P450 3A4 may cause a reduction in plasma bexarotene concentrations.

Concomitant administration of bexarotene capsules and gemfibrozil resulted in substantial increases in plasma concentrations of bexarotene, probably at least partially related to cytochrome P450 3A4 inhibition by gemfibrozil. Under similar conditions, bexarotene concentrations were not affected by concomitant atorvastatin administration. Concomitant administration of gemfibrozil with bexarotene capsules is not recommended (see DRUG INTERACTIONS).

Concomitant administration of bexarotene capsules and tamoxifen in women with breast cancer who were progressing on tamoxifen resulted in a modest decrease in plasma concentrations of tamoxifen, possibly through an induction of cytochrome P450 3A4. Based on this known interaction, bexarotene may theoretically increase the rate of metabolism and reduce plasma concentrations of other substrates metabolized by cytochrome P450 3A4, including hormonal contraceptives (see CONTRAINDICATIONS, Pregnancy, Category X and DRUG INTERACTIONS).

INDICATIONS AND USAGE

Bexarotene capsules are indicated for the treatment of cutaneous manifestations of cutaneous T-cell lymphoma in patients who are refractory to at least one prior systemic therapy.

CONTRAINDICATIONS

Bexarotene capsules are contraindicated in patients with a known hypersensitivity to bexarotene or other components of the product.

PREGNANCY, CATEGORY X

Bexarotene capsules may cause fetal harm when administered to a pregnant woman. Bexarotene capsules must not be given to a pregnant woman or a woman who intends to become pregnant. If a woman becomes pregnant while taking bexarotene capsules, bexarotene capsules must be stopped immediately and the woman given appropriate counseling.

Bexarotene caused malformations when administered orally to pregnant rats during days 7-17 of gestation. Developmental abnormalities included incomplete ossification at 4 mg/kg/day and cleft palate, depressed eye bulge/microphthalmia, and small ears at 16 mg/kg/day. The plasma AUC of bexarotene in rats at 4 mg/kg/day is approximately one-third the AUC in humans at the recommended daily dose. At doses greater than 10 mg/kg/day, bexarotene caused developmental mortality. The no effect dose for fetal effects in rats was 1 mg/kg/day (producing an AUC approximately one-sixth of the AUC at the recommended human daily dose).

Women of child-bearing potential should be advised to avoid becoming pregnant when bexarotene capsules are used. The possibility that a woman of child-bearing potential is pregnant at the time therapy is instituted should be considered. A negative pregnancy test (*e.g.*, serum beta-human chorionic gonadotropin, beta-HCG) with a sensitivity of at least 50 mIU/L should be obtained within 1 week prior to bexarotene capsules therapy, and the pregnancy test must be repeated at monthly intervals while the patient remains on bexarotene capsules. Effective contraception must be used for 1 month prior to the initiation of therapy, during therapy and for at least 1 month following discontinuation of therapy; it is recommended that two reliable forms of contraception be used simultaneously unless abstinence is the chosen method. Bexarotene can potentially induce metabolic enzymes and thereby theoretically reduce the plasma concentrations of hormonal contraceptives (see CLINICAL PHARMACOLOGY, Drug-Drug Interactions and DRUG INTERACTIONS). Thus, if treatment with bexarotene capsules is intended in a woman with child-bearing potential, it is strongly recommended that one of the two reliable forms of contraception should be non-hormonal. Male patients with sexual partners who are pregnant, possibly pregnant, or who could become pregnant must use condoms during sexual intercourse while taking bexarotene capsules and for at least 1 month after the last dose of drug. Bexarotene capsules therapy should be initiated on the second or third day of a normal menstrual period. No more than a 1 month supply of bexarotene capsules should be given to the patient so that the results of pregnancy testing can be assessed and counseling regarding avoidance of pregnancy and birth defects can be reinforced.

WARNINGS

LIPID ABNORMALITIES

Bexarotene capsules induce major lipid abnormalities in most patients. These must be monitored and treated during long-term therapy. About 70% of patients with CTCL who received an initial dose of ≥300 mg/m²/day of bexarotene capsules had fasting triglyceride levels greater than 2.5 times the upper limit of normal. About 55% had values over 800 mg/dl with a median of about 1200 mg/dl in those patients. Cholesterol elevations above 300 mg/dl occurred in approximately 60% and 75% of patients with CTCL who received an initial dose of 300 mg/m²/day or greater than 300 mg/m²/day, respectively. Decreases in high density lipoprotein (HDL) cholesterol to less than 25 mg/dl were seen in about 55% and 90% of patients receiving an initial dose of 300 mg/m²/day or greater than 300 mg/m²/day, respectively, of bexarotene capsules. The effects on triglycerides, HDL cholesterol, and total cholesterol were reversible with cessation of therapy, and could generally be mitigated by dose reduction or concomitant antilipemic therapy.

Fasting blood lipid determinations should be performed before bexarotene capsules therapy is initiated and weekly until the lipid response to bexarotene capsules is established, which usually occurs within 2-4 weeks, and at 8 week intervals thereafter. Fasting triglycerides should be normal or normalized with appropriate intervention prior to initiating bexarotene capsules therapy. Attempts should be made to maintain triglyceride levels below 400 mg/dl to reduce the risk of clinical sequelae (see Pancreatitis). If fasting triglycerides are elevated or become elevated during treatment, antilipemic therapy should be instituted, and if necessary, the dose of bexarotene capsules reduced or suspended. In the 300 mg/m²/day initial dose group, 60% of patients were given lipid lowering drugs. Atorvastatin was used in 48% (73/152) of patients with CTCL. Because of a potential drug-drug interaction (see DRUG INTERACTIONS), gemfibrozil is not recommended for use with bexarotene capsules.

PANCREATITIS

Acute pancreatitis has been reported in 4 patients with CTCL and in 6 patients with non-CTCL cancers treated with bexarotene capsules; the cases were associated with marked elevations of fasting serum triglycerides, the lowest being 770 mg/dl in 1 patient. One (1) patient with advanced non-CTCL cancer died of pancreatitis. Patients with CTCL who have risk factors for pancreatitis (*e.g.*, prior pancreatitis, uncontrolled hyperlipidemia, excessive alcohol consumption, uncontrolled diabetes mellitus, biliary tract disease, and medications known to increase triglyceride levels or to be associated with pancreatic toxicity) should generally not be treated with bexarotene capsules (see Lipids Abnormalities and PRECAUTIONS, Laboratory Tests).

LIVER FUNCTION TEST ABNORMALITIES

For patients with CTCL receiving an initial dose of 300 mg/m^2/day of bexarotene capsules, elevations in liver function tests (LFTs) have been observed in 5% (SGOT/AST), 2% (SGPT/ALT), and 0% (bilirubin). In contrast, with an initial dose greater than 300 mg/m^2/day of bexarotene capsules, the incidence of LFT elevations was higher at 7% (SGOT/AST), 9% (SGPT/ALT), and 6% (bilirubin). Two (2) patients developed cholestasis, including 1 patient who died of liver failure. In clinical trials, elevation of LFTs resolved within 1 month in 80% of patients following a decrease in dose or discontinuation of therapy. Baseline LFTs should be obtained, and LFTs should be carefully monitored after 1, 2 and 4 weeks of treatment initiation, and if stable, at least every 8 weeks thereafter during treatment. Consideration should be given to a suspension or discontinuation of bexarotene capsules if test results reach greater than three times the upper limit of normal values for SGOT/AST, SGPT/ALT, or bilirubin.

HEPATIC INSUFFICIENCY

No specific studies have been conducted with bexarotene capsules in patients with hepatic insufficiency. Because less than 1% of the dose is excreted in the urine unchanged and there is *in vitro* evidence of extensive hepatic contribution to bexarotene elimination, hepatic impairment would be expected to lead to greatly decreased clearance. Bexarotene capsules should be used only with great caution in this population.

THYROID AXIS ALTERATIONS

Bexarotene capsules induce biochemical evidence of or clinical hypothyroidism in about half of all patients treated, causing a reversible reduction in thyroid hormone (total thyroxine [total T4]) and thyroid-stimulating hormone (TSH) levels. The incidence of decreases in TSH and total T4 were about 60% and 45%, respectively, in patients with CTCL receiving an initial dose of 300 mg/m^2/day. Hypothyroidism was reported as an adverse event in 29% of patients. Treatment with thyroid hormone supplements should be considered in patients with laboratory evidence of hypothyroidism. In the 300 mg/m^2/day initial dose group, 37% of patients were treated with thyroid hormone replacement. Baseline thyroid function tests should be obtained and patients monitored during treatment.

LEUKOPENIA

A total of 18% of patients with CTCL receiving an initial dose of 300 mg/m^2/day of bexarotene capsules had reversible leukopenia in the range of 1000 to <3000 WBC/mm^3. Patients receiving an initial dose greater than 300 mg/m^2/day of bexarotene capsules had an incidence of leukopenia of 43%. No patient with CTCL treated with bexarotene capsules developed leukopenia of less than 1000 WBC/mm^3. The time to onset of leukopenia was generally 4-8 weeks. The leukopenia observed in most patients was explained by neutropenia. In the 300 mg/m^2/day initial dose group, the incidence of NCI Grade 3 and Grade 4 neutropenia, respectively, was 12% and 4%. The leukopenia and neutropenia experienced during bexarotene capsules therapy resolved after dose reduction or discontinuation of treatment, on average within 30 days in 93% of the patients with CTCL and 82% of patients with non-CTCL cancers. Leukopenia and neutropenia were rarely associated with severe sequelae or serious adverse events. Determination of WBC with differential should be obtained at baseline and periodically during treatment.

CATARACTS

Posterior subcapsular cataracts were observed in preclinical toxicity studies in rats and dogs administered bexarotene daily for 6 months. In 15 of 79 patients who had serial slit lamp examinations, new cataracts or worsening of previous cataracts were found. Because of the high prevalence and rate of cataract formation in older patient populations, the relationship of bexarotene capsules and cataracts cannot be determined in the absence of an appropriate control group. Patients treated with bexarotene capsules who experience visual difficulties should have an appropriate ophthalmologic evaluation.

PRECAUTIONS

PREGNANCY CATEGORY X

See CONTRAINDICATIONS.

GENERAL

Bexarotene capsules should be used with caution in patients with a known hypersensitivity to retinoids. Clinical instances of cross-reactivity have not been noted.

Vitamin A Supplementation

In clinical studies, patients were advised to limit vitamin A intake to ≤15,000 IU/day. Because of the relationship of bexarotene to vitamin A, patients should be advised to limit vitamin A supplements to avoid potential additive toxic effects.

Patients With Diabetes Mellitus

Caution should be used when administering bexarotene capsules in patients using insulin, agents enhancing insulin secretion (*e.g.,* sulfonylureas), or insulin-sensitizers (*e.g.,* troglitazone). Based on the mechanism of action, bexarotene capsules could enhance the action of these agents, resulting in hypoglycemia. Hypoglycemia has not been associated with the use of bexarotene capsules as monotherapy.

Photosensitivity

Retinoids as a class have been associated with photosensitivity. *In vitro* assays indicate that bexarotene is a potential photosensitizing agent. Mild phototoxicity manifested as sunburn and skin sensitivity to sunlight was observed in patients who were exposed to direct sunlight while receiving bexarotene capsules. Patients should be advised to minimize exposure to sunlight and artificial ultraviolet light while receiving bexarotene capsules.

LABORATORY TESTS

Blood lipid determinations should be performed before bexarotene capsules are given. Fasting triglycerides should be normal or normalized with appropriate intervention prior to therapy. Hyperlipidemia usually occurs within the initial 2-4 weeks. Therefore, weekly lipid determinations are recommended during this interval. Subsequently, in patients not hyperlipidemic, determinations can be performed less frequently (see WARNINGS, Lipid Abnormalities).

A white blood cell count with differential should be obtained at baseline and periodically during treatment. Baseline liver function tests should be obtained and should be carefully monitored after 1, 2 and 4 weeks of treatment initiation, and if stable, periodically thereafter during treatment. Baseline thyroid function tests should be obtained and then monitored during treatment as indicated (see WARNINGS, Leukopenia; Liver Function Test Abnormalities; and Thyroid Axis Alterations).

DRUG-FOOD INTERACTION

In all clinical trials, patients were instructed to take bexarotene capsules with or immediately following a meal. In one clinical study, plasma bexarotene AUC and C_{max} values were substantially higher following a fat-containing meal versus those following the administration of a glucose solution. Because safety and efficacy data are based upon administration with food, it is recommended that bexarotene capsules be administered with food (see CLINICAL PHARMACOLOGY, Pharmacokinetics and DOSAGE AND ADMINISTRATION).

RENAL INSUFFICIENCY

No formal studies have been conducted with bexarotene capsules in patients with renal insufficiency. Urinary elimination of bexarotene and its known metabolites is a minor excretory pathway for bexarotene (<1% of administered dose), but because renal insufficiency can result in significant protein binding changes, and bexarotene is >99% protein bound, pharmacokinetics may be altered in patients with renal insufficiency.

PROTEIN BINDING

Bexarotene is highly bound (>99%) to plasma proteins. The plasma proteins to which bexarotene binds have not been elucidated, and the ability of bexarotene to displace drugs bound to plasma proteins and the ability of drugs to displace bexarotene binding have not been studied.

DRUG/LABORATORY TEST INTERACTIONS

CA125 assay values in patients with ovarian cancer may be increased by bexarotene capsule therapy.

CARCINOGENESIS, MUTAGENESIS, AND IMPAIRMENT OF FERTILITY

Long-term studies in animals to assess the carcinogenic potential of bexarotene have not been conducted. Bexarotene is not mutagenic to bacteria (Ames assay) or mammalian cells (mouse lymphoma assay). Bexarotene was not clastogenic *in vivo* (micronucleus test in mice). No formal fertility studies were conducted with bexarotene. Bexarotene caused testicular degeneration when oral doses of 1.5 mg/kg/day were given to dogs for 91 days (producing an AUC of approximately one-fifth the AUC at the recommended human daily dose).

USE IN NURSING MOTHERS

It is not known whether bexarotene is excreted in human milk. Because many drugs are excreted in human milk and because of the potential for serious adverse reactions in nursing infants from bexarotene, a decision should be made whether to discontinue nursing or to discontinue the drug, taking into account the importance of the drug to the mother.

PEDIATRIC USE

Safety and effectiveness in pediatric patients have not been established.

GERIATRIC USE

Of the total patients with CTCL in clinical studies of bexarotene capsules, 64% were 60 years or older, while 33% were 70 years or older. No overall differences in safety were observed between patients 70 years or older and younger patients, but greater sensitivity of some older individuals to bexarotene capsules cannot be ruled out. Responses to bexarotene capsules were observed across all age group decades, without preference for any individual age group decade.

DRUG INTERACTIONS

No formal studies to evaluate drug interactions with bexarotene have been conducted. Bexarotene oxidative metabolites appear to be formed by cytochrome P450 3A4.

On the basis of the metabolism of bexarotene by cytochrome P450 3A4, ketoconazole, itraconazole, erythromycin, gemfibrozil, grapefruit juice, and other inhibitors of cytochrome P450 3A4 would be expected to lead to an increase in plasma bexarotene concentrations. Furthermore, rifampin, phenytoin, phenobarbital, and other inducers of cytochrome P450 3A4 may cause a reduction in plasma bexarotene concentrations.

Concomitant administration of bexarotene capsules and gemfibrozil resulted in substantial increases in plasma concentrations of bexarotene, probably at least partially related to cytochrome P450 3A4 inhibition by gemfibrozil. Under similar conditions, bexarotene concentrations were not affected by concomitant atorvastatin administration. Concomitant administration of gemfibrozil with bexarotene capsules is not recommended.

Concomitant administration of bexarotene capsules and tamoxifen in women with breast cancer who were progressing on tamoxifen resulted in a modest decrease in plasma concentrations of tamoxifen, possibly through an induction of cytochrome P450 3A4. Based on this known interaction, bexarotene may theoretically increase the rate of metabolism and reduce plasma concentrations of other substrates metabolized by cytochrome P450 3A4, including hormonal contraceptives (see CLINICAL PHARMACOLOGY, Drug-Drug Interactions and CONTRAINDICATIONS, Pregnancy, Category X). Thus, if treatment with bexarotene capsules is intended in a woman with child-bearing potential, it is strongly recommended that two reliable forms of contraception be used concurrently, one of which should be non-hormonal.

B

ADVERSE REACTIONS

The safety of bexarotene capsules has been evaluated in clinical studies of 152 patients with CTCL who received bexarotene capsules for up to 97 weeks and in 352 patients in other studies. The mean duration of therapy for the 152 patients with CTCL was 166 days. The most common adverse events reported with an incidence of at least 10% in patients with CTCL treated at an initial dose of 300 mg/m²/day of bexarotene capsules are shown in TABLE 1. The events at least possibly related to treatment are lipid abnormalities (elevated triglycerides, elevated total and LDL cholesterol and decreased HDL cholesterol), hypothyroidism, headache, asthenia, rash, leukopenia, anemia, nausea, infection, peripheral edema, abdominal pain, and dry skin. Most adverse events occurred at a higher incidence in patients treated at starting doses of greater than 300 mg/m²/day (see TABLE 1).

Adverse events leading to dose reduction or study drug discontinuation in at least 2 patients were hyperlipemia, neutropenia/leukopenia, diarrhea, fatigue/lethargy, hypothyroidism, headache, liver function test abnormalities, rash, pancreatitis, nausea, anemia, allergic reaction, muscle spasm, pneumonia, and confusion.

The moderately severe (NCI Grade 3) and severe (NCI Grade 4) adverse events reported in 2 or more patients with CTCL treated at an initial dose of 300 mg/m²/day of bexarotene capsules (see TABLE 2) were hypertriglyceridemia, pruritus, headache, peripheral edema, leukopenia, rash, and hypercholesteremia. Most of these moderately severe or severe adverse events occurred at a higher rate in patients treated at starting doses of greater than 300 mg/m²/day than in patients treated at a starting dose of 300 mg/m²/day.

As shown in TABLE 3, in patients with CTCL receiving an initial dose of 300 mg/m²/day, the incidence of NCI Grade 3 or 4 elevations in triglycerides and total cholesterol was 28% and 25%, respectively. In contrast, in patients with CTCL receiving greater than 300 mg/m²/day, the incidence of NCI Grade 3 or 4 elevated triglycerides and total cholesterol was 45% and 45%, respectively. Other Grade 3 and 4 laboratory abnormalities are shown in TABLE 3.

In addition to the 152 patients enrolled in the two CTCL studies, 352 patients received bexarotene capsules as monotherapy for various advanced malignancies at doses from 5-1000 mg/m²/day. The common adverse events (incidence greater than 10%) were similar to those seen in patients with CTCL.

In the 504 patients (CTCL and non-CTCL) who received bexarotene capsules as monotherapy, drug-related serious adverse events that were fatal, in one patient each, were acute pancreatitis, subdural hematoma, and liver failure.

In the patients with CTCL receiving an initial dose of 300 mg/m²/day of bexarotene capsules, adverse events reported at an incidence of less than 10% and not included in TABLES 1-3 or discussed in other parts of labeling and possibly related to treatment were as follows:

Body as a Whole: Chills, cellulitis, chest pain, sepsis, and monilia.

Cardiovascular: Hemorrhage, hypertension, angina pectoris, right heart failure, syncope, and tachycardia.

Digestive: Constipation, dry mouth, flatulence, colitis, dyspepsia, cheilitis, gastroenteritis, gingivitis, liver failure, and melena.

Hemic and Lymphatic: Eosinophilia, thrombocythemia, coagulation time increased, lymphocytosis, and thrombocytopenia.

Metabolic and Nutritional: LDH increased, creatinine increased, hypoproteinemia, hyperglycemia, weight decreased, weight increased, and amylase increased.

Musculoskeletal: Arthralgia, myalgia, bone pain, myasthenia, and arthrosis.

Nervous: Depression, agitation, ataxia, cerebrovascular accident, confusion, dizziness, hyperesthesia, hypesthesia, and neuropathy.

Respiratory: Pharyngitis, rhinitis, dyspnea, pleural effusion, bronchitis, cough increased, lung edema, hemoptysis, and hypoxia.

Skin and Appendages: Skin ulcer, acne, alopecia, skin nodule, macular papular rash, pustular rash, serous drainage, and vesicular bullous rash.

Special Senses: Dry eyes, conjunctivitis, ear pain, blepharitis, corneal lesion, keratitis, otitis externa, and visual field defect.

Urogenital: Albuminuria, hematuria, urinary incontinence, urinary tract infection, urinary urgency, dysuria, kidney function abnormal, and breast pain.

TABLE 1 *Adverse Events With Incidence ≥10% in CTCL Trials*

Body System / Adverse Event*†	Initial Assigned Dose Group (mg/m²/day) 300 n=84	>300 n=53
Metabolic and Nutritional Disorders		
Hyperlipemia	66 (78.6%)	42 (79.2%)
Hypercholesteremia	27 (32.1%)	33 (62.3%)
Lactic dehydrogenase increased	6 (7.1%)	7 (13.2%)
Body as a Whole		
Headache	25 (29.8%)	22 (41.5%)
Asthenia	17 (20.2%)	24 (45.3%)
Infection	11 (13.1%)	12 (22.6%)
Abdominal pain	9 (10.7%)	2 (3.8%)
Chills	8 (9.5%)	7 (13.2%)
Fever	4 (4.8%)	9 (17.0%)
Flu syndrome	3 (3.6%)	7 (13.2%)
Back pain	2 (2.4%)	6 (11.3%)
Infection bacterial	1 (1.2%)	7 (13.2%)
Endocrine		
Hypothyroidism	24 (28.6%)	28 (52.8%)
Skin and Appendages		
Rash	14 (16.7%)	12 (22.6%)
Dry skin	9 (10.7%)	5 (9.4%)
Exfoliative dermatitis	8 (9.5%)	15 (28.3%)
Alopecia	3 (3.6%)	6 (11.3%)
Hemic and Lymphatic System		
Leukopenia	14 (16.7%)	25 (47.2%)
Anemia	5 (6.0%)	13 (24.5%)
Hypochromic anemia	3 (3.6%)	7 (13.2%)
Digestive System		
Nausea	13 (15.5%)	4 (7.5%)
Diarrhea	6 (7.1%)	22 (41.5%)
Vomiting	3 (3.6%)	7 (13.2%)
Anorexia	2 (2.4%)	12 (22.6%)
Cardiovascular System		
Peripheral edema	11 (13.1%)	6 (11.3%)
Nervous System		
Insomnia	4 (4.8%)	6 (11.3%)

* Preferred English term coded according to Ligand-modified COSTART 5 Dictionary.
† Patients are counted at most once in each AE category.

TABLE 2 *Incidence of Moderately Severe and Severe Adverse Events Reported in At Least Two Patients (CTCL Trials)*

Body System	Initial Assigned Dose Group (mg/m²/day) 300 (n=84)		>300 (n=53)	
Adverse Event*†	Mod Sev	Severe	Mod Sev	Severe
Body as a Whole				
Asthenia	1 (1.2%)	0 (0.0%)	11 (20.8%)	0 (0.0%)
Headache	3 (3.6%)	0 (0.0%)	5 (9.4%)	1 (1.9%)
Infection bacterial	1 (1.2%)	0 (0.0%)	0 (0.0%)	2 (3.8%)
Cardiovascular System				
Peripheral edema	2 (2.4%)	1 (1.2%)	0 (0.0%)	0 (0.0%)
Digestive System				
Anorexia	0 (0.0%)	0 (0.0%)	3 (5.7%)	0 (0.0%)
Diarrhea	1 (1.2%)	1 (1.2%)	2 (3.8%)	1 (1.9%)
Pancreatitis	1 (1.2%)	0 (0.0%)	3 (5.7%)	0 (0.0%)
Vomiting	0 (0.0%)	0 (0.0%)	2 (3.8%)	0 (0.0%)
Endocrine				
Hypothyroidism	1 (1.2%)	1 (1.2%)	2 (3.8%)	0 (0.0%)
Hemic and Lymphatic System				
Leukopenia	3 (3.6%)	0 (0.0%)	6 (11.3%)	1 (1.9%)
Metabolic and Nutritional Disorders				
Bilirubinemia	0 (0.0%)	1 (1.2%)	2 (3.8%)	0 (0.0%)
Hypercholesteremia	2 (2.4%)	0 (0.0%)	5 (9.4%)	0 (0.0%)
Hyperlipemia	16 (19.0%)	6 (7.1%)	17 (32.1%)	5 (9.4%)
SGOT/AST Increased	0 (0.0%)	0 (0.0%)	2 (3.8%)	0 (0.0%)
SGPT/ALT Increased	0 (0.0%)	0 (0.0%)	2 (3.8%)	0 (0.0%)
Respiratory System				
Pneumonia	0 (0.0%)	0 (0.0%)	2 (3.8%)	2 (3.8%)
Skin and Appendages				
Exfoliative dermatitis	0 (0.0%)	1 (1.2%)	3 (5.7%)	1 (1.9%)
Rash	1 (1.2%)	2 (2.4%)	1 (1.9%)	0 (0.0%)

* Preferred English term coded according to Ligand-modified COSTART 5 Dictionary.
† Patients are counted at most once in each AE category. Patients are classified by the highest severity within each row.

DOSAGE AND ADMINISTRATION

The recommended initial dose of bexarotene capsules is 300 mg/m²/day. (See Table 4.) Bexarotene capsules should be taken as a single oral daily dose with a meal. See CONTRAINDICATIONS, Pregnancy, Category X for precautions to prevent pregnancy and birth defects in women of child-bearing potential.

DOSE MODIFICATION GUIDELINES

The 300 mg/m²/day dose level of bexarotene capsules may be adjusted to 200 mg/m²/day then to 100 mg/m²/day, or temporarily suspended, if necessitated by toxicity. When toxicity is controlled, doses may be carefully readjusted upward. If there is no tumor response after 8 weeks of treatment and if the initial dose of 300 mg/m²/day is well tolerated, the dose may be escalated to 400 mg/m²/day with careful monitoring.

DURATION OF THERAPY

In clinical trials in CTCL, bexarotene capsules were administered for up to 97 weeks.

Bexarotene capsules should be continued as long as the patient is deriving benefit.

HOW SUPPLIED

Targretin capsules are supplied as 75 mg off-white, oblong soft gelatin capsules, imprinted with "Targretin", in high density polyethylene bottles with child-resistant closures.

Storage: Store at 2-25°C (36-77°F). Avoid exposing to high temperatures and humidity after the bottle is opened. Protect from light.

TOPICAL

DESCRIPTION

Targretin gel 1% contains bexarotene and is intended for topical application only. Bexarotene is a member of a subclass of retinoids that selectively activate retinoid X receptors (RXRs). These retinoid receptors have biologic activity distinct from that of retinoic acid receptors (RARs).

The chemical name is 4-[1-(5,6,7,8-tetrahydro-3,5,5,8,8-pentamethyl-2-naphthalenyl)ethenyl] benzoic acid.

Bexarotene is an off-white to white powder with a molecular weight of 348.48 and a molecular formula of $C_{24}H_{28}O_2$. It is insoluble in water and slightly soluble in vegetable oils and ethanol.

Targretin gel is a clear gelled solution containing 1.0% (w/w) bexarotene in a base of dehydrated alcohol, polyethylene glycol 400, hydroxypropyl cellulose, and butylated hydroxytoluene.

CLINICAL PHARMACOLOGY

MECHANISM OF ACTION

Bexarotene selectively binds and activates retinoid X receptor subtypes (RXRα, RXRβ, RXRγ). RXRs can form heterodimers with various receptor partners such as retinoic acid receptors (RARs), vitamin D receptor, thyroid receptor, and peroxisome proliferator acti-

TABLE 3 *Treatment-Emergent Abnormal Laboratory Values in CTCL Trials*

	Initial Assigned Dose Group (mg/m²/day)			
	300 (n=83*)		>300 (n=53*)	
Analyte	Grade 3†	Grade 4†	Grade 3	Grade 4
Triglycerides‡	21.3%	6.7%	31.8%	13.6%
Total cholesterol‡	18.7%	6.7%	15.9%	29.5%
Alkaline phosphatase	1.2%	0.0%	0.0%	1.9%
Hyperglycemia	1.2%	0.0%	5.7%	0.0%
Hypocalcemia	1.2%	0.0%	0.0%	0.0%
Hyponatremia	1.2%	0.0%	9.4%	0.0%
SGPT/ALT	1.2%	0.0%	1.9%	1.9%
Hyperkalemia	0.0%	0.0%	1.9%	0.0%
Hypermatermia	0.0%	1.2%	0.0%	0.0%
SGOT/AST	0.0%	0.0%	1.9%	1.9%
Total bilirubin	0.0%	0.0%	0.0%	1.9%
ANC	12.0%	3.6%	18.9%	7.5%
ALC	7.2%	0.0%	15.1%	0.0%
WBC	3.6%	0.0%	11.3%	0.0%
Hemoglobin	0.0%	0.0%	1.9%	0.0%

* Number of patients with at least one analyte value post-baseline.
† Adapted from NCI Common Toxicity Criteria, Grade 3 and 4, Version 2.0. Patients are considered to have had a Grade 3 or 4 value if either of the following occurred: (a) Value becomes Grade 3 or 4 during the study; (b) Value is abnormal at baseline and worsens to Grade 3 or 4 on study, including all values beyond study drug discontinuation, as defined in data handling conventions.
‡ The denominator used to calculate the incidence rates for fasting Total Cholesterol and Triglycerides were n=75 for the 300 mg/m²/day initial dose group and n=44 for the >300 mg/m²/day initial dose group.

TABLE 4 *Bexarotene Capsule Initial Dose Calculation According to Body Surface Area*

Initial Dose Level (300 mg/m²/day)		
Body Surface Area (m²)	Total Daily Dose (mg/day)	Number of 75 mg Bexarotene Capsules
0.88-1.12	300	4
1.13-1.37	375	5
1.38-1.62	450	6
1.63-1.87	525	7
1.88-2.12	600	8
2.13-2.37	675	9
2.38–2.62	750	10

vator receptors (PPARs). Once activated, these receptors function as transcription factors that regulate the expression of genes that control cellular differentiation and proliferation. Bexarotene inhibits the growth *in vitro* of some tumor cell lines of hematopoietic and squamous cell origin. It also induces tumor regression *in vivo* in some animal models. The exact mechanism of action of bexarotene in the treatment of cutaneous T-cell lymphoma (CTCL) is unknown.

PHARMACOKINETICS

General

Plasma concentrations of bexarotene were determined during clinical studies in patients with CTCL or following repeated single or multiple-daily dose applications of bexarotene gel 1% for up to 132 weeks. Plasma bexarotene concentrations were generally less than 5 ng/ml and did not exceed 55 ng/ml. However, only two patients with very intense dosing regimens (>40% BSA lesions and qid dosing) were sampled. Plasma bexarotene concentrations and the frequency of detecting quantifiable plasma bexarotene concentrations increased with increasing percent body surface area treated and increasing quantity of bexarotene gel applied. The sporadically-observed and generally low plasma bexarotene concentrations indicated that, in patients receiving doses of low to moderate intensity, there is a low potential for significant plasma concentrations following repeated application of bexarotene gel. Bexarotene is highly bound (>99%) to plasma proteins. The plasma proteins to which bexarotene binds have not been elucidated, and the ability of bexarotene to displace drugs bound to plasma proteins and the ability of drugs to displace bexarotene binding have not been studied (see PRECAUTIONS, Protein Binding). The uptake of bexarotene by organs or tissues has not been evaluated.

Metabolism

Four bexarotene metabolites have been identified in plasma following oral administration of bexarotene: 6- and 7-hydroxy-bexarotene and 6- and 7-oxo-bexarotene. *In vitro* studies suggest that cytochrome P450 3A4 is the major cytochrome P450 responsible for formation of the oxidative metabolites and that the oxidative metabolites may be glucuronidated. The oxidative metabolites are active in *in vitro* assays of retinoid receptor activation, but the relative contribution of the parent and any metabolites to the efficacy and safety of bexarotene gel is unknown.

Elimination

The renal elimination of bexarotene and its metabolites was examined in patients with Type 2 diabetes mellitus following oral administration of bexarotene. Neither bexarotene nor its metabolites were excreted in urine in appreciable amounts.

SPECIAL POPULATIONS

Elderly, Gender, Race

Because of a large number of immeasurable plasma concentrations (<1 ng/ml), any potential pharmacokinetic differences between Special Populations could not be assessed.

Pediatric

Studies to evaluate bexarotene pharmacokinetics in the pediatric population have not been conducted (see PRECAUTIONS, Pediatric Use).

Renal Insufficiency

No formal studies have been conducted with bexarotene gel in patients with renal insufficiency. Urinary elimination of bexarotene and its known metabolites is a minor excretory pathway (<1% of an orally administered dose), but because renal insufficiency can result in significant protein binding changes, pharmacokinetics may be altered in patients with renal insufficiency (see PRECAUTIONS, Renal Insufficiency).

Hepatic Insufficiency

No specific studies have been conducted with bexarotene gel in patients with hepatic insufficiency. Because less than 1% of the dose of oral bexarotene is excreted in the urine unchanged and there is *in vitro* evidence of extensive hepatic contribution to bexarotene elimination, hepatic impairment would be expected to lead to greatly decreased clearance (see PRECAUTIONS, Hepatic Insufficiency).

DRUG-DRUG INTERACTIONS

No formal studies to evaluate drug interactions with bexarotene or bexarotene gel have been conducted. Bexarotene oxidative metabolites appear to be formed through cytochrome P450 3A4. Drugs that affect levels or activity of cytochrome P450 3A4 may potentially affect the disposition of bexarotene. Concomitant gemfibrozil was associated with increased bexarotene concentrations following oral administration of bexarotene.

INDICATIONS AND USAGE

Bexarotene gel 1% is indicated for the topical treatment of cutaneous lesions in patients with CTCL (Stage IA and IB) who have refractory or persistent disease after other therapies or who have not tolerated other therapies.

CONTRAINDICATIONS

Bexarotene gel 1% is contraindicated in patients with a known hypersensitivity to bexarotene or other components of the product.

PREGNANCY, CATEGORY X

Bexarotene gel 1% may cause fetal harm when administered to a pregnant woman.

Bexarotene gel must not be given to a pregnant woman or a woman who intends to become pregnant. If a woman becomes pregnant while taking bexarotene gel, bexarotene gel must be stopped immediately and the woman given appropriate counseling.

Bexarotene caused malformations when administered orally to pregnant rats during days 7-17 of gestation. Developmental abnormalities included incomplete ossification at 4 mg/kg/day and cleft palate, depressed eye bulge/microphthalmia, and small ears at 16 mg/kg/day. At doses greater than 10 mg/kg/day, bexarotene caused developmental mortality. The no-effect oral dose in rats was 1 mg/kg/day. Plasma bexarotene concentrations in patients with CTCL applying bexarotene gel 1% were generally less than one-hundredth the C_{max} associated with dysmorphogenesis in rats, although some patients had C_{max} levels that were approximately one-eighth the concentration associated with dysmorphogenesis in rats.

Women of child-bearing potential should be advised to avoid becoming pregnant when bexarotene gel is used. The possibility that a woman of child-bearing potential is pregnant at the time therapy is instituted should be considered. A negative pregnancy test (*e.g.*, serum beta-human chorionic gonadotropin, beta-HCG) with a sensitivity of at least 50 mIU/L should be obtained within 1 week prior to bexarotene gel therapy, and the pregnancy test must be repeated at monthly intervals while the patient remains on bexarotene gel. Effective contraception must be used for 1 month prior to the initiation of therapy, during therapy and for at least 1 month following discontinuation of therapy; it is recommended that two reliable forms of contraception be used simultaneously unless abstinence is the chosen method. Male patients with sexual partners who are pregnant, possibly pregnant, or who could become pregnant must use condoms during sexual intercourse while applying bexarotene gel and for at least 1 month after the last dose of drug. Bexarotene gel therapy should be initiated on the second or third day of a normal menstrual period. No more than a 1 month supply of bexarotene gel should be given to the patient so that the results of pregnancy testing can be assessed and counseling regarding avoidance of pregnancy and birth defects can be reinforced.

PRECAUTIONS

PREGNANCY CATEGORY X

See CONTRAINDICATIONS.

GENERAL

Bexarotene gel should be used with caution in patients with a known hypersensitivity to other retinoids. No clinical instances of cross-reactivity have been noted.

Vitamin A Supplementation

In clinical studies, patients were advised to limit vitamin A intake to ≤15,000 IU/day. Because of the relationship of bexarotene to vitamin A, patients should be advised to limit vitamin A supplements to avoid potential additive toxic effects.

Photosensitivity

Retinoids as a class have been associated with photosensitivity. *In vitro* assays indicate that bexarotene is a potential photosensitizing agent. There were no reports of photosensitivity in patients in the clinical studies. Patients should be advised to minimize exposure to sunlight and artificial ultraviolet light during the use of bexarotene gel.

RENAL INSUFFICIENCY

No formal studies have been conducted with bexarotene gel in patients with renal insufficiency. Urinary elimination of bexarotene and its known metabolites is a minor excretory pathway for bexarotene (<1% of an orally administered dose), but because renal insufficiency can result in significant protein binding changes, and bexarotene is >99% protein bound, pharmacokinetics may be altered in patients with renal insufficiency.

HEPATIC INSUFFICIENCY

No specific studies have been conducted with bexarotene gel in patients with hepatic insufficiency. Because less than 1% of the dose of oral bexarotene is excreted in the urine unchanged and there is *in vitro* evidence of extensive hepatic contribution to bexarotene elimination, hepatic impairment would be expected to lead to greatly decreased clearance.

PROTEIN BINDING

Bexarotene is highly bound (>99%) to plasma proteins. The plasma proteins to which bexarotene binds have not been elucidated, and the ability of bexarotene to displace drugs bound to plasma proteins and the ability of drugs to displace bexarotene binding have not been studied.

CARCINOGENESIS, MUTAGENESIS, AND IMPAIRMENT OF FERTILITY

Long-term studies in animals to assess the carcinogenic potential of bexarotene have not been conducted. Bexarotene was not mutagenic to bacteria (Ames assay) or mammalian cells (mouse lymphoma assay). Bexarotene was not clastogenic *in vivo* (micronucleus test in mice). No formal fertility studies were conducted with bexarotene. Bexarotene caused testicular degeneration when oral doses of 1.5 mg/kg/day were given to dogs for 91 days.

USE IN NURSING MOTHERS

It is not known whether bexarotene is excreted in human milk. Because many drugs are excreted in human milk and because of the potential for serious adverse reactions in nursing infants from bexarotene, a decision should be made whether to discontinue nursing or to discontinue the drug, taking into account the importance of the drug to the mother.

PEDIATRIC USE

Safety and effectiveness in pediatric patients have not been established.

GERIATRIC USE

Of the total patients with CTCL in clinical studies of bexarotene gel, 62% were under 65 years and 38% were 65 years or older. No overall differences in safety were observed between patients 65 years of age or older and younger patients, but greater sensitivity of some older individuals to bexarotene gel cannot be ruled out. Responses to bexarotene gel were observed across all age group decades, without preference for any individual age group decade.

DRUG INTERACTIONS

Patients who are applying bexarotene gel should not concurrently use products that contain DEET (*N,N*-diethyl-*m*-toluamide), a common component of insect repellent products. An animal toxicology study showed increased DEET toxicity when DEET was included as part of the formulation.

No formal studies to evaluate drug interactions with bexarotene have been conducted. Bexarotene oxidative metabolites appear to be formed through cytochrome P450 3A4.

On the basis of the metabolism of bexarotene by cytochrome P450 3A4, concomitant ketoconazole, itraconazole, erythromycin and grapefruit juice could increase bexarotene plasma concentrations. Similarly, based on data that gemfibrozil increases bexarotene concentrations following oral bexarotene administration, concomitant gemfibrozil could increase bexarotene plasma concentrations. However, due to the low systemic exposure to bexarotene after low to moderately intense gel regimens (see CLINICAL PHARMACOLOGY), increases that occur are unlikely to be of sufficient magnitude to result in adverse effects.

No drug interaction data are available on concomitant administration of bexarotene gel and other CTCL therapies.

ADVERSE REACTIONS

The safety of bexarotene gel has been assessed in clinical studies of 117 patients with CTCL who received bexarotene gel for up to 172 weeks. In the multicenter open label study, 50 patients with CTCL received bexarotene gel for up to 98 weeks. The mean duration of therapy for these 50 patients was 199 days. The most common adverse events reported with an incidence at the application site of at least 10% in patients with CTCL were rash, pruritus, skin disorder, and pain.

Adverse events leading to dose reduction or study drug discontinuation in at least two patients were rash, contact dermatitis, and pruritus.

Of the 49 patients (98%) who experienced any adverse event, most experienced events categorized as mild (9 patients, 18%) or moderate (27 patients, 54%). There were 12 patients (24%) who experienced at least one moderately severe adverse event. The most common moderately severe events were rash (7 patients, 14%) and pruritus (3 patients, 6%). Only one patient (2%) experienced a severe adverse event (rash).

In the patients with CTCL receiving bexarotene gel, adverse events reported regardless of relationship to study drug at an incidence of ≥5% are presented in TABLE 5.

A similar safety profile for bexarotene gel was demonstrated in the Phase 1-2 program. For the 67 patients enrolled in the Phase 1-2 program, the mean duration of treatment was 436 days (range: 12-1203 days). As in the multicenter study, the most common adverse events regardless of relationship to study drug in the Phase 1-2 program were rash (78%), pain (40%), and pruritus (40%).

TABLE 5 *Incidence of All Adverse Events* and Application Site Adverse Events With Incidence ≥5% for All Application Frequencies of Bexarotene Gel in the Multicenter CTCL Study*

COSTART 5 Body System/Preferred Term	All Adverse Events n=50	Application Site Adverse Events n=50
Skin and Appendages		
Contact dermatitis†	7 (14%)	4 (8%)
Exfoliative dermatitis	3 (6%)	0
Pruritus‡	18 (36%)	9 (18%)
Rash§	36 (72%)	28 (56%)
Maculopapular rash	3 (6%)	0
Skin disorder (NOS)¤	13 (26%)	9 (18%)
Sweating	3 (6%)	0
Body as a Whole		
Asthenia	3 (6%)	0
Headache	7 (14%)	0
Infection	9 (18%)	0
Pain	15 (30%)	9 (18%)
Cardiovascular		
Edema	5 (10%)	0
Peripheral edema	3 (6%)	0
Hemic and Lymphatic		
Leukopenia	3 (6%)	0
Lymphadenopathy	3 (6%)	0
WBC abnormal	3 (6%)	0
Metabolic and Nutritional		
Hyperlipemia	5 (10%)	0
Nervous		
Paresthesia	3 (6%)	3 (6%)
Respiratory		
Cough increased	3 (6%)	0
Pharyngitis	3 (6%)	0

* Regardless of association with treatment.
Includes Investigator terms such as:
† Contact dermatitis, irritant contact dermatitis, irritant dermatitis.
‡ Pruritus, itching, itching of lesion.
§ Erythema, scaling, irritation, redness, rash, dermatitis.
¤ Skin inflammation, excoriation, sticky or tacky sensation of skin.
NOS = Not Otherwise Specified.

DOSAGE AND ADMINISTRATION

Bexarotene gel should be initially applied once every other day for the first week. The application frequency should be increased at weekly intervals to once daily, then twice daily, then 3 times daily and finally 4 times daily according to individual lesion tolerance. Generally, patients were able to maintain a dosing frequency of 2-4 times per day. Most responses were seen at dosing frequencies of 2 times per day and higher. If application site toxicity occurs, the application frequency can be reduced. Should severe irritation occur, application of drug can be temporarily discontinued for a few days until the symptoms subside. See CONTRAINDICATIONS, Pregnancy, Category X.

Sufficient gel should be applied to cover the lesion with a generous coating. The gel should be allowed to dry before covering with clothing. Because unaffected skin may become irritated, application of the gel to normal skin surrounding the lesions should be avoided. In addition, do not apply the gel near mucosal surfaces of the body.

A response may be seen as soon as 4 weeks after initiation of therapy but most patients require longer application. With continued application, further benefit may be attained. The longest onset time for the first response among the responders was 392 days based on the Composite Assessment of Index Lesion Severity in the multicenter study. In clinical trials, bexarotene gel was applied for up to 172 weeks.

Bexarotene gel should be continued as long as the patient is deriving benefit.

Occlusive dressings should not be used with bexarotene gel.

Bexarotene gel is a topical therapy and is not intended for systemic use. Bexarotene gel has not been studied in combination with other CTCL therapies.

HOW SUPPLIED

Targretin gel is supplied in tubes containing 60 g (600 mg active bexarotene).

Storage: Store at 25°C (77°F); with excursions permitted to 15-30°C (59-86°F). Avoid exposing to high temperatures and humidity after the tube is opened. Protect from light.

PRODUCT LISTING - EQUIVALENTS NOT AVAILABLE

Capsule - Oral - 75 mg

100's $1819.00 TARGRETIN, Ligand Pharmaceuticals 64365-0502-01

Gel - Topical - 1%

60 gm $1177.00 TARGRETIN TOPICAL, Ligand Pharmaceuticals 64365-0504-01

Bicalutamide (003271)

Categories: Carcinoma, prostate; FDA Approved 1995 Oct; Pregnancy Category X
Drug Classes: Antineoplastics, antiandrogens; Hormones/hormone modifiers
Brand Names: Casodex
Foreign Brand Availability: Cosudex (Australia; New-Zealand); Lutamidal (Colombia)
Cost of Therapy: $421.01 (Prostate Cancer; Casodex; 50 mg; 1 tablet/day; 30 day supply)

DESCRIPTION

Casodex tablets for oral administration contain 50 mg of bicalutamide, a nonsteroidal antiandrogen with no other known endocrine activity. The chemical name is propanamide, N-[4-cyano-3-(trifluoromethyl)phenyl]-3-[(4-fluorophenyl)sulfonyl]-2-hydroxy-2-methyl-,(+-). The empirical formula is $C_{18}H_{14}N_2O_4F_4S$.

Bicalutamide has a molecular weight of 430.37. The pKa' is approximately 12. Bicalutamide is a fine white to off-white powder which is practically insoluble in water at 37°C (5 mg per 1000 ml), slightly soluble in chloroform and absolute ethanol, sparingly soluble in methanol, and soluble in acetone and tetrahydrofuran.

Casodex is a racemate with its antiandrogenic activity being almost exclusively exhibited by the R-enantiomer of bicalutamide; the S-enantiomer is essentially inactive.

The inactive ingredients of Casodex tablets are lactose, magnesium stearate, methylhydroxypropylcellulose, polyethylene glycol, polyvidone, sodium starch glycollate, and titanium dioxide.

CLINICAL PHARMACOLOGY

MECHANISM OF ACTION

Bicalutamide is a non-steroidal antiandrogen. It competitively inhibits the action of androgens by binding to cytosol androgen receptors in the target tissue. Prostatic carcinoma is known to be androgen sensitive and responds to treatment that counteracts the effect of androgen and/or removes the source of androgen.

When bicalutamide is combined with luteinizing hormone-releasing hormone (LHRH) analogue therapy, the suppression of serum testosterone induced by the LHRH analogue is not affected. However, in clinical trials with bicalutamide as a single agent for prostate cancer, rises in serum testosterone and estradiol have been noted.

PHARMACOKINETICS

Absorption

Bicalutamide is well-absorbed following oral administration, although the absolute bioavailability is unknown. Coadministration of bicalutamide with food has no clinically significant effect on rate or extent of absorption.

Distribution

Bicalutamide is highly protein-bound (96%). (See Drug-Drug Interactions.)

Metabolism/Elimination

Bicalutamide undergoes stereospecific metabolism. The S (inactive) isomer is metabolized primarily by glucuronidation. The R (active) isomer also undergoes glucuronidation but is predominantly oxidized to an inactive metabolite followed by glucuronidation. Both the parent and metabolite glucuronides are eliminated in the urine and feces. The S-enantiomer is rapidly cleared relative to the R-enantiomer, with the R-enantiomer accounting for about 99% of total steady-state plasma levels.

SPECIAL POPULATIONS

Geriatric

In 2 studies in patients given 50 or 150 mg daily, no significant relationship between age and steady-state levels of total bicalutamide or the active R-enantiomer has been shown.

Hepatic Insufficiency

No clinically significant difference in the pharmacokinetics of either enantiomer of bicalutamide was noted in patients with mild-to-moderate hepatic disease as compared to healthy controls. However, the half-life of the R-enantiomer was increased approximately 76% (5.9 and 10.4 days for normal and impaired patients, respectively) in patients with severe liver disease (n=4).

Renal Insufficiency

Renal impairment (as measured by creatinine clearance) had no significant effect on the elimination of total bicalutamide or the active R-enantiomer.

Women, Pediatrics

Bicalutamide has not been studied in women or pediatric subjects.

Drug-Drug Interactions

Clinical studies have not shown any drug interactions between bicalutamide and LHRH analogues (goserelin or leuprolide). There is no evidence that bicalutamide induces hepatic enzymes. *In vitro* protein-binding studies have shown that bicalutamide can displace coumarin anticoagulants from binding sites. Prothrombin times should be closely monitored in patients already receiving coumarin anticoagulants who are started on bicalutamide.

Pharmacokinetics of the active enantiomer of bicalutamide in normal males and patients with prostate cancer are presented in TABLE 1.

TABLE 1

Parameter	Mean	Standard Deviation
Normal Males (n=30)		
Apparent oral clearance (L/h)	0.320	0.103
Single dose peak concentration (μg/ml)	0.768	0.178
Single dose time to peak concentration (hours)	31.3	14.6
Half-life (days)	5.8	2.29
Patients With Prostate Cancer (n=40)		
Css (μg/ml)	8.939	3.504

Css = Mean Steady-State Concentration.

INDICATIONS AND USAGE

Bicalutamide is indicated for use in combination therapy with a luteinizing hormone-releasing hormone (LHRH) analogue for the treatment of Stage D_2 metastatic carcinoma of the prostate.

CONTRAINDICATIONS

Bicalutamide is contraindicated in any patient who has shown a hypersensitivity reaction to the drug or any of the tablet's components.

Bicalutamide has no indication for women, and should not be used in this population, particularly for non-serious or non-life threatening conditions. Further, bicalutamide should not be used by women who are or may become pregnant. If this drug is used during pregnancy, or if the patient becomes pregnant while taking this drug, the patient should be apprised of the potential hazard to the fetus. Bicalutamide may cause fetal harm when administered to pregnant women. The male offspring of rats receiving doses of 10 mg/kg/day (plasma drug concentrations in rats equal to approximately 2/3 human therapeutic concentrations, based on a maximum dose of 50 mg/day of bicalutamide for an average 70 kg patient) and above were observed to have reduced anogenital distance and hypospadias in reproductive toxicology studies. These pharmacological effects have been observed with other antiandrogens. No other teratogenic effects were observed in rabbits receiving doses up to 200 mg/kg/day (approximately 1/3 human therapeutic concentrations, based on a maximum dose of 50 mg/day of bicalutamide for an average 70 kg patient) or rats receiving doses up to 250 mg/kg/day (approximately 2 times human therapeutic concentrations, based on a maximum dose of 50 mg/day of bicalutamide for an average 70 kg patient).

WARNINGS

HEPATITIS

Rare cases of death or hospitalization due to severe liver injury have been reported post-marketing in association with the use of bicalutamide. Hepatotoxicity in these reports generally occurred within the first 3-4 months of treatment. Hepatitis or marked increases in liver enzymes leading to drug discontinuation occurred in approximately 1% of bicalutamide patients in controlled clinical trials.

Serum transaminase levels should be measured prior to starting treatment with bicalutamide, at regular intervals for the first 4 months of treatment, and periodically thereafter. If clinical symptoms or signs suggestive of liver dysfunction occur (*e.g.,* nausea, vomiting, abdominal pain, fatigue, anorexia, "flu-like" symptoms, dark urine, jaundice, or right upper quadrant tenderness), the serum transaminases, in particular the serum ALT, should be measured immediately. If at any time a patient has jaundice, or their ALT rises above two times the upper limit of normal, bicalutamide should be immediately discontinued with close follow-up of liver function.

PRECAUTIONS

GENERAL

1. Bicalutamide should be used with caution in patients with moderate-to-severe hepatic impairment. Bicalutamide is extensively metabolized by the liver. Limited data in subjects with severe hepatic impairment suggest that excretion of bicalutamide may be delayed and could lead to further accumulation. Periodic liver function tests should be considered for patients on long-term therapy (see WARNINGS.
2. In clinical trials with bicalutamide as a single agent for prostate cancer, gynecomastia and breast pain have been reported in up to 38% and 39% of patients, respectively.
3. Regular assessments of serum Prostate Specific Antigen (PSA) may be helpful in monitoring the patient's response. If PSA levels rise during bicalutamide therapy, the patient should be evaluated for clinical progression. For patients who have objective progression of disease together with an elevated PSA, a treatment-free period of antiandrogen, while continuing the LHRH analogue, may be considered.

INFORMATION FOR THE PATIENT

Patients should be informed that therapy with bicalutamide and the LHRH analogue should be initiated concomitantly, and that they should not interrupt or stop taking these medications without consulting their physician. Treatment with bicalutamide should be started at the same time as treatment with an LHRH analogue.

CARCINOGENESIS, MUTAGENESIS, AND IMPAIRMENT OF FERTILITY

Two year oral carcinogenicity studies were conducted in both male and female rats and mice at doses of 5, 15, or 75 mg/kg/day of bicalutamide. A variety of tumor target organ effects were identified and were attributed to the antiandrogenicity of bicalutamide, namely, testicular benign interstitial (Leydig) cell tumors in male rats at all dose levels (the steady-state plasma concentration with the 5 mg/kg/day dose is approximately 2/3 human therapeutic concentrations, based on a maximum dose of 50 mg/day of bicalutamide for an average 70 kg patient) and uterine adenocarcinoma in female rats at 75 mg/kg/day (approximately 1.5 times the human therapeutic concentrations, based on a maximum dose of 50 mg/day of bicalutamide for an average 70 kg patient). There is no evidence of Leydig cell hyperplasia in patients; uterine tumors are not relevant to the indicated patient population.

A small increase in the incidence of hepatocellular carcinoma in male mice given 75 mg/kg/day of bicalutamide (approximately 4 times human therapeutic concentrations, based on a maximum dose of 50 mg/day of bicalutamide for an average 70 kg patient) and an increased incidence of benign thyroid follicular cell adenomas in rats given 5 mg/kg/day (approximately 2/3 human therapeutic concentrations, based on a maximum dose of 50 mg/day of bicalutamide for an average 70 kg patient) and above were recorded. These neoplastic changes were progressions of non-neoplastic changes related to hepatic enzyme induction observed in animal toxicity studies. Enzyme induction has not been observed following bicalutamide administration in man. There were no tumorigenic effects suggestive of genotoxic carcinogenesis.

A comprehensive battery of both *in vitro* and *in vivo* genotoxicity tests (yeast gene conversion, Ames, *E. coli,* CHO/HGPRT, human lymphocyte cytogenetic, mouse micronucleus, and rat bone marrow cytogenetic tests) has demonstrated that bicalutamide does not have genotoxic activity.

Administration of bicalutamide may lead to inhibition of spermatogenesis. The long-term effects of bicalutamide on male fertility have not been studied.

In male rats dosed at 250 mg/kg/day (approximately 2 times human therapeutic concentrations, based on a maximum dose of 50 mg/day of bicalutamide for an average 70 kg patient), the precoital interval and time to successful mating were increased in the first pairing but no effects on fertility following successful mating were seen. These effects were reversed by 7 weeks after the end of an 11 week period of dosing.

No effects on female rats dosed at 10, 50, and 250 mg/kg/day (approximately 2/3, 1, and 2 times human therapeutic concentrations, respectively, based on a maximum dose of 50 mg/day of bicalutamide for an average 70 kg patient) or their female offspring were observed. Administration of bicalutamide to pregnant females resulted in feminization of the male offspring leading to hypospadias at all dose levels. Affected male offspring were also impotent.

PREGNANCY CATEGORY X

See CONTRAINDICATIONS.

NURSING MOTHERS

Bicalutamide is not indicated for use in women. It is not known whether this drug is excreted in human milk. Because many drugs are excreted in human milk, caution should be exercised when bicalutamide is administered to a nursing woman.

PEDIATRIC USE

Safety and effectiveness of bicalutamide in pediatric patients have not been established.

DRUG INTERACTIONS

In vitro studies have shown bicalutamide can displace coumarin anticoagulants, such as warfarin, from their protein-binding sites. It is recommended that if bicalutamide is started in patients already receiving coumarin anticoagulants, prothrombin times should be closely monitored and adjustment of the anticoagulant dose may be necessary (see CLINICAL PHARMACOLOGY, Special Populations, Drug-Drug Interactions.

ADVERSE REACTIONS

In patients with advanced prostate cancer treated with bicalutamide in combination with an LHRH analogue, the most frequent adverse experience was hot flashes (53%).

In the multicenter, double-blind, controlled clinical trial comparing bicalutamide 50 mg once daily with flutamide 250 mg three times a day, each in combination with an LHRH analogue, the following adverse experiences with an incidence of 5% or greater, regardless of causality, have been reported (see TABLE 2).

TABLE 2 *Incidence of Adverse Events (≥5% In Either Treatment Group) Regardless of Causality*

Body System	Treatment Group: Number of Patients (%)			
	Bicalutamide Plus LHRH Analogue		Flutamide Plus LHRH Analogue	
Adverse Event	(n=401)		(n=407)	
Body as a Whole				
Pain (general)	142	(35%)	127	(31%)
Back pain	102	(25%)	105	(26%)
Asthenia	89	(22%)	87	(21%)
Pelvic pain	85	(21%)	70	(17%)
Infection	71	(18%)	57	(14%)
Abdominal pain	46	(11%)	46	(11%)
Chest pain	34	(8%)	34	(8%)
Headache	29	(7%)	27	(7%)
Flu syndrome	28	(7%)	30	(7%)
Cardiovascular				
Hot flashes	211	(53%)	217	(53%)
Hypertension	34	(8%)	29	(7%)
Digestive				
Constipation	87	(22%)	69	(17%)
Nausea	62	(15%)	58	(14%)
Diarrhea	49	(12%)	107	(26%)
Increased liver enzyme test*	30	(7%)	46	(11%)
Dyspepsia	30	(7%)	23	(6%)
Flatulence	26	(6%)	22	(5%)
Anorexia	25	(6%)	29	(7%)
Vomiting	24	(6%)	32	(8%)
Hemic and Lymphatic				
Anemia†	45	(11%)	53	(13%)
Metabolic and Nutritional				
Peripheral edema	53	(13%)	42	(10%)
Weight loss	30	(7%)	39	(10%)
Hyperglycemia	26	(6%)	27	(7%)
Alkaline phosphatase increased	22	(5%)	24	(6%)
Weight gain	22	(5%)	18	(4%)
Musculoskeletal				
Bone pain	37	(9%)	43	(11%)
Myasthenia	27	(7%)	19	(5%)
Arthritis	21	(5%)	29	(7%)
Pathological fracture	17	(4%)	32	(8%)
Nervous System				
Dizziness	41	(10%)	35	(9%)
Paresthesia	31	(8%)	40	(10%)
Insomnia	27	(7%)	39	(10%)
Anxiety	20	(5%)	9	(2%)
Depression	16	(4%)	33	(8%)
Respiratory System				
Dyspnea	51	(13%)	32	(8%)
Cough increased	33	(8%)	24	(6%)
Pharyngitis	32	(8%)	23	(6%)
Bronchitis	24	(6%)	22	(3%)
Pneumonia	18	(4%)	19	(5%)
Rhinitis	15	(4%)	22	(5%)
Skin and Appendages				
Rash	35	(9%)	30	(7%)
Sweating	25	(6%)	20	(5%)
Urogenital				
Nocturia	49	(12%)	55	(14%)
Hematuria	48	(12%)	26	(6%)
Urinary tract infection	35	(9%)	36	(9%)
Gynecomastia	36	(9%)	30	(7%)
Impotence	27	(7%)	35	(9%)
Breast pain	23	(6%)	15	(4%)
Urinary frequency	23	(6%)	29	(7%)
Urinary retention	20	(5%)	14	(3%)
Urination impaired	19	(5%)	15	(4%)
Urinary incontinence	15	(4%)	32	(8%)

* Increased liver enzyme test includes increases in AST, ALT, or both.
† Anemia includes anemia, hypochromic- and iron-deficiency anemia.

Other adverse experiences (greater than or equal to 2%, but less than 5%) reported in the bicalutamide-LHRH analogue treatment group are listed below by body system and are in order of decreasing frequency within each body system regardless of causality:

Body as a Whole: Neoplasm, neck pain, fever, chills, sepsis, hernia, cyst.

Cardiovascular: Angina pectoris, congestive heart failure, myocardial infarct, heart arrest, coronary artery disorder, syncope.

Digestive: Melena, rectal hemorrhage, dry mouth, dysphagia, gastrointestinal disorder, periodontal abscess, gastrointestinal carcinoma.

Metabolic and Nutritional: Edema, BUN increased, creatinine increased, dehydration, gout, hypercholesteremia.

Musculoskeletal: Myalgia, leg cramps.

Nervous: Hypertonia, confusion, somnolence, libido decreased, neuropathy, nervousness.

Respiratory: Lung disorder, asthma, epistaxis, sinusitis.

Skin and Appendages: Dry skin, alopecia, pruritus, herpes zoster, skin carcinoma, skin disorder.

Special Senses: Cataract specified.

Urogenital: Dysuria, urinary urgency, hydronephrosis, urinary tract disorder.

ABNORMAL LABORATORY TEST VALUES

Laboratory abnormalities including elevated AST, ALT, bilirubin, BUN, and creatinine and decreased hemoglobin and white cell count have been reported in both bicalutamide-LHRH analogue-treated and flutamide-LHRH analogue-treated patients.

POSTMARKETING EXPERIENCE

Rare cases of interstitial pneumonitis and pulmonary fibrosis have been reported with bicalutamide.

DOSAGE AND ADMINISTRATION

The recommended dose for bicalutamide therapy in combination with an LHRH analogue is one 50 mg tablet once daily (morning or evening), with or without food. It is recommended that bicalutamide be taken at the same time each day. Treatment with bicalutamide should be started at the same time as treatment with an LHRH analogue.

DOSAGE ADJUSTMENT IN RENAL IMPAIRMENT

No dosage adjustment is necessary for patients with renal impairment (see CLINICAL PHARMACOLOGY, Special Populations, Renal Insufficiency).

DOSAGE ADJUSTMENT IN HEPATIC IMPAIRMENT

No dosage adjustment is necessary for patients with mild to moderate hepatic impairment. Although there is a 76% (5.9 and 10.4 days for normal and impaired patients, respectively) increase in the half-life of the active enantiomer of bicalutamide in patients with severe liver impairment (n=4), no dosage adjustment is necessary (see CLINICAL PHARMACOLOGY, Special Populations, Hepatic Insufficiency; PRECAUTIONS; and WARNINGS).

HOW SUPPLIED

Casodex 50 mg Tablets: White, film-coated tablets are identified on one side with "CDX50" and on the reverse with the "CASODEX logo".

Storage: Store at controlled room temperature, 20-25°C (68-77°F).

PRODUCT LISTING - EQUIVALENTS NOT AVAILABLE

Tablet - Oral - 50 mg

30's	$421.01	CASODEX, Astra-Zeneca Pharmaceuticals	00310-0705-30
30's	$421.01	CASODEX, Astra-Zeneca Pharmaceuticals	00310-0705-39
100's	$1403.38	CASODEX, Astra-Zeneca Pharmaceuticals	00310-0705-10

Bimatoprost *(003369)*

Categories: Glaucoma, open-angle; Hypertension, ocular; Pregnancy Category C; FDA Approved 2001 Mar
Drug Classes: Ophthalmics; Prostaglandins
Brand Names: Lumigan
Cost of Therapy: $55.79 (Glaucoma; Lumigan Ophth. Solution; 0.3%; 2.5 ml; 1 drop(s)/day; variable day supply day supply)

DESCRIPTION

Lumigan (bimatoprost ophthalmic solution) 0.03% is a synthetic prostamide analog with ocular hypotensive activity. Its chemical name is (Z)-7-[(1R,2R,3R,5S)-3,5-Dihydroxy-2-[1E,3S)-3-hydroxy-5-phenyl-1-pentenyl]cyclopentyl]-5-N-ethylheptenamide, and its molecular weight is 415.58. Its molecular formula is $C_{25}H_{37}NO_4$.

Bimatoprost is a powder, which is very soluble in ethyl alcohol and methyl alcohol and slightly soluble in water. Bimatoprost is a clear, isotonic, colorless, sterile ophthalmic solution with an osmolality of approximately 290 mOsmol/kg.

Each ml contains: *Active:* Bimatoprost 0.3 mg. *Preservative:* Benzalkonium chloride 0.05 mg. *Inactives:* Sodium chloride; sodium phosphate, dibasic; citric acid; and purified water. Sodium hydroxide and/or hydrochloric acid may be added to adjust pH. The pH during its shelf life ranges from 6.8-7.8.

CLINICAL PHARMACOLOGY

MECHANISM OF ACTION

Bimatoprost is a prostamide, a synthetic structural analog of prostaglandin with ocular hypotensive activity. It selectively mimics the effects of naturally occurring substances, prostamides. Bimatoprost is believed to lower intraocular pressure (IOP) in humans by increasing outflow of aqueous humor through both the trabecular meshwork and uveoscleral routes. Elevated IOP presents a major risk factor for glaucomatous field loss. The higher the level of IOP, the greater the likelihood of optic nerve damage and visual field loss.

PHARMACOKINETICS

Absorption

After 1 drop of bimatoprost ophthalmic solution 0.03% was administered once daily to both eyes of 15 healthy subjects for 2 weeks, blood concentrations peaked within 10 minutes after dosing and were below the lower limit of detection (0.025 ng/ml) in most subjects within 1.5 hours after dosing. Mean C_{max} and AUC(0-24h) values were similar on Days 7 and 14 at approximately 0.08 ng/ml and 0.09 ng·h/ml, respectively, indicating that steady state was reached during the first week of ocular dosing. There was no significant systemic drug accumulation over time.

Distribution

Bimatoprost is moderately distributed into body tissues with a steady-state volume of distribution of 0.67 L/kg. In human blood, bimatoprost resides mainly in the plasma. Approximately 12% of bimatoprost remains unbound in human plasma.

Metabolism

Bimatoprost is the major circulating species in the blood once it reaches the systemic circulation following ocular dosing. Bimatoprost then undergoes oxidation, N-deethylation and glucuronidation to form a diverse variety of metabolites.

Elimination

Following an intravenous dose of radiolabeled bimatoprost (3.12 μg/kg) to 6 healthy subjects, the maximum blood concentration of unchanged drug was 12.2 ng/ml and decreased rapidly with an elimination half-life of approximately 45 minutes. The total blood clearance of bimatoprost was 1.5 L/h/kg. Up to 67% of the administered dose was excreted in the urine while 25% of the dose was recovered in the feces.

INDICATIONS AND USAGE

Bimatoprost ophthalmic solution 0.03% is indicated for the reduction of elevated intraocular pressure in patients with open angle glaucoma or ocular hypertension who are intolerant of other intraocular pressure lowering medications or insufficiently responsive (failed to achieve target IOP determined after multiple measurements over time) to another intraocular pressure lowering medication.

CONTRAINDICATIONS

Bimatoprost ophthalmic solution 0.03% is contraindicated in patients with hypersensitivity to bimatoprost or any other ingredient in this product.

WARNINGS

Bimatoprost ophthalmic solution 0.03% has been reported to cause changes to pigmented tissues. These reports include increased pigmentation and growth of eyelashes and increased pigmentation of the iris and periorbital tissue (eyelid). These changes may be permanent.

Bimatoprost ophthalmic solution may gradually change eye color, increasing the amount of brown pigment in the iris by increasing the number of melanosomes (pigment granules) in melanocytes. The long-term effects on the melanocytes and the consequences of potential injury to the melanocytes and/or deposition of pigment granules to other areas of the eye are currently unknown. The change in iris color occurs slowly and may not be noticeable for several months to years. Patients should be informed of the possibility of iris color change.

Eyelid skin darkening has also been reported in association with the use of bimatoprost ophthalmic solution.

Bimatoprost ophthalmic solution may gradually change eyelashes; these changes include increased length, thickness, pigmentation, and number of lashes.

Patients who are expected to receive treatment in only 1 eye should be informed about the potential for increased brown pigmentation of the iris, periorbital tissue, and eyelashes in the treated eye and thus, heterochromia between the eyes. They should also be advised of the potential for a disparity between the eyes in length, thickness, and/or number of eyelashes.

PRECAUTIONS

GENERAL

There have been reports of bacterial keratitis associated with the use of multiple-dose containers of topical ophthalmic products. These containers had been inadvertently contaminated by patients who, in most cases, had a concurrent corneal disease or a disruption of the ocular epithelial surface (see Information for the Patient).

Patients may slowly develop increased brown pigmentation of the iris. This change may not be noticeable for several months to years (see WARNINGS). Typically the brown pigmentation around the pupil is expected to spread concentrically towards the periphery in affected eyes, but the entire iris or parts of it may also become more brownish. Until more information about increased brown pigmentation is available, patients should be examined regularly and, depending on the clinical situation, treatment may be stopped if increased pigmentation ensues. The increase in brown iris pigment is not expected to progress further upon discontinuation of treatment, but the resultant color change may be permanent. Neither nevi nor freckles of the iris are expected to be affected by treatment.

Bimatoprost ophthalmic solution 0.03% should be used with caution in patients with active intraocular inflammation (*e.g.,* uveitis).

Macular edema, including cystoid macular edema, has been reported during treatment with bimatoprost ophthalmic solution. Bimatoprost ophthalmic solution should be used with caution in aphakic patients, in pseudophakic patients with a torn posterior lens capsule, or in patients with known risk factors for macular edema.

Bimatoprost ophthalmic solution has not been evaluated for the treatment of angle closure, inflammatory or neovascular glaucoma.

Bimatoprost ophthalmic solution should not be administered while wearing contact lenses.

INFORMATION FOR THE PATIENT

Patients should be informed that bimatoprost ophthalmic solution has been reported to cause increased growth and darkening of eyelashes and darkening of the skin around the eye in some patients. These changes may be permanent.

Some patients may slowly develop darkening of the iris, which may be permanent.

When only 1 eye is treated, patients should be informed of the potential for a cosmetic difference between the eyes in eyelash length, darkness or thickness, and/or color changes of the eyelid skin or iris.

Patients should be instructed to avoid allowing the tip of the dispensing container to contact the eye, surrounding structures, fingers, or any other surface in order to avoid contamination of the solution by common bacteria known to cause ocular infections. Serious damage to the eye and subsequent loss of vision may result from using contaminated solutions.

Patients should also be advised that if they develop an intercurrent ocular condition (*e.g.,* trauma or infection) or have ocular surgery, they should immediately seek their physician's advice concerning the continued use of the multidose container.

Patients should be advised that if they develop any ocular reactions, particularly conjunctivitis and eyelid reactions, they should immediately seek their physician's advice.

Contact lenses should be removed prior to instillation of bimatoprost ophthalmic solution and may be reinserted 15 minutes following its administration. Patients should be advised that bimatoprost ophthalmic solution contains benzalkonium chloride, which may be absorbed by soft contact lenses.

If more than 1 topical ophthalmic drug is being used, the drugs should be administered at least 5 minutes between applications.

CARCINOGENESIS, MUTAGENESIS, AND IMPAIRMENT OF FERTILITY

Carcinogenicity studies were not performed with bimatoprost.

Bimatoprost was not mutagenic or clastogenic in the Ames test, in the mouse lymphoma test, or in the *in vivo* mouse micronucleus tests.

Bimatoprost did not impair fertility in male or female rats up to doses of 0.6 mg/kg/day (approximately 103 times the recommended human exposure based on blood AUC levels).

PREGNANCY, TERATOGENIC EFFECTS, PREGNANCY CATEGORY C

In embryo/fetal developmental studies in pregnant mice and rats, abortion was observed at oral doses of bimatoprost, which achieved at least 33 or 97 times, respectively, the intended human exposure based on blood AUC levels.

At doses 41 times the intended human exposure based on blood AUC levels, the gestation length was reduced in the dams, the incidence of dead fetuses, late resorptions, peri- and postnatal pup mortality was increased, and pup body weights were reduced.

There are no adequate and well-controlled studies of bimatoprost ophthalmic solution administration in pregnant women. Because animal reproductive studies are not always predictive of human response, bimatoprost ophthalmic solution should be administered during pregnancy only if the potential benefit justifies the potential risk to the fetus.

NURSING MOTHERS

It is not known whether bimatoprost ophthalmic solution is excreted in human milk, although in animal studies, bimatoprost has been shown to be excreted in breast milk. Because many drugs are excreted in human milk, caution should be exercised when bimatoprost ophthalmic solution is administered to a nursing woman.

PEDIATRIC USE

Safety and effectiveness in pediatric patients have not been established.

GERIATRIC USE

No overall clinical differences in safety or effectiveness have been observed between elderly and other adult patients.

ADVERSE REACTIONS

In clinical trials, the most frequent events associated with the use of bimatoprost ophthalmic solution 0.03% occurring in approximately 15-45% of patients, in descending order of incidence, included conjunctival hyperemia, growth of eyelashes, and ocular pruritus. Approximately 3% of patients discontinued therapy due to conjunctival hyperemia.

Ocular adverse events occurring in approximately 3-10% of patients, in descending order of incidence, included ocular dryness, visual disturbance, ocular burning, foreign body sensation, eye pain, pigmentation of the periocular skin, blepharitis, cataract, superficial punctate keratitis, eyelid erythema, ocular irritation, and eyelash darkening. The following ocular adverse events reported in approximately 1-3% of patients, in descending order of incidence, included: eye discharge, tearing, photophobia, allergic conjunctivitis, asthenopia, increases in iris pigmentation, and conjunctival edema. In less than 1% of patients, intraocular inflammation was reported as iritis.

Systemic adverse events reported in approximately 10% of patients were infections (primarily colds and upper respiratory tract infections). The following systemic adverse events reported in approximately 1-5% of patients, in descending order of incidence, included headaches, abnormal liver function tests, asthenia and hirsutism.

DOSAGE AND ADMINISTRATION

The recommended dosage is 1 drop in the affected eye(s) once daily in the evening. The dosage of bimatoprost ophthalmic solution 0.03% should not exceed once daily since it has been shown that more frequent administration may decrease the intraocular pressure lowering effect.

Reduction of the intraocular pressure starts approximately 4 hours after the first administration with maximum effect reached within approximately 8-12 hours.

Bimatoprost ophthalmic solution may be used concomitantly with other topical ophthalmic drug products to lower intraocular pressure. If more than 1 topical ophthalmic drug is being used, the drugs should be administered at 5 minutes apart.

HOW SUPPLIED

Lumigan (bimatoprost ophthalmic solution) 0.03% is supplied sterile in opaque white low density polyethylene ophthalmic dispenser bottles and tips with turquoise polystyrene caps in the following sizes: 2.5 ml fill in 8 ml container, 5 ml fill in 8 ml container, or 7.5 ml fill in 8 ml container.

Storage: Lumigan solution should be stored in the original container at 15-25°C (59-77°F).

PRODUCT LISTING - EQUIVALENTS NOT AVAILABLE

Solution - Ophthalmic - 0.03%

2.50 ml	$55.79	LUMIGAN, Allergan Inc	00023-9187-03
5 ml	$111.56	LUMIGAN, Allergan Inc	00023-9187-05
7.50 ml	$167.35	LUMIGAN, Allergan Inc	00023-9187-07

Biperiden Hydrochloride (000483)

Categories: Extrapyramidal disorder, drug-induced; Parkinson's disease; Pregnancy Category C; FDA Approved 1959 Sep; WHO Formulary

Drug Classes: Anticholinergics; Antiparkinson agents

Brand Names: Akineton

Foreign Brand Availability: Akineton Retard (Austria; Colombia; Costa-Rica; Dominican-Republic; Ecuador; El-Salvador; France; Germany; Guatemala; Honduras; Mexico; Nicaragua; Panama; Peru; Portugal; Spain); Benzum 2 (Peru); Biperen (Taiwan); Biperin (Korea); Bipiden (Taiwan); Desiperiden (Germany); Dyskinon (India); Kinex (Mexico)

Cost of Therapy: $32.57 (Parkinsonism; Akineton; 2 mg; 3 tablets/day; 30 day supply)

HCFA JCODE(S): J0190 per 5 mg IM, IV

DESCRIPTION

Each Akineton tablet for oral administration contains 2 mg biperiden hydrochloride. Other ingredients may include corn syrup, lactose, magnesium stearate, potato starch and talc. Each 1 ml Akineton ampule for intramuscular or intravenous administration contains 5 mg biperiden lactate in an aqueous 1.4% sodium lactate solution. No added preservative.

Biperiden hydrochloride is an anticholinergic agent. Biperiden is α-5-Norbornen-2-yl-α-penyl-1-piperidine-propanol. It is a white, crystalline, odorless powder, slightly soluble in water and alcohol. It is stable in air at normal temperatures.

CLINICAL PHARMACOLOGY

Biperiden HCl is a weak peripheral anticholinergic agent. It has, therefore, some antisecretory, antispasmodic and mydriatic effects. In addition, biperiden HCl possesses nicotinolytic activity. Parkinsonism is thought to result from an imbalance between the excitatory (cholinergic) and inhibitory (dopaminergic) systems in the corpus striatum. The mechanism of action of centrally active anticholinergic drugs such as biperiden HCl is considered to related to competitive antagonism of acetylcholine at cholinergic receptors in the corpus striatum, which then restores the balance.

The parenteral form of biperiden HCl is an effective and reliable agent for the treatment of acute episodes of extrapyramidal disturbances sometimes seen during treatment with neuroleptic agents. Akathisia, akinesia, dyskinetic tremors, rigor, oculogyric crises, spasmodic torticollis, and profuse sweating are markedly reduced or eliminated. With parenteral biperiden HCl, these drug-induced disturbances are rapidly brought under control. Subsequently, this can usually be maintained with oral doses which may be given with tranquilizer therapy in psychotic and other conditions requiring an uninterrupted therapeutic program.

PHARMACOKINETICS AND METABOLISM

Only limited pharmacokinetic studies of biperiden in humans are available. The serum concentration at 1 to 1.5 hours following a single 4 mg oral dose was 4-5 ng/ml. Plasma levels (0.1-0.2 ng/ml) could be determined up to 48 hours after dosing. Six (6) hours after an oral dose of 250 mg/kg in rats, 87% of the drug had been absorbed. The metabolism of biperiden HCl is also incompletely understood, but does involve hydroxylation. In normal volunteers a single 10 mg intravenous dose of biperiden seemed to cause a transient rise in plasma cortisol and prolactin. No change in GH, LH, FSH, or TSH levels were seen. Biperiden lactate (10 mg/ml) was not irritating to the tissue of rabbits when injected intramuscularly (1.0 ml) into the sacrospinalis muscles and intradermally (0.25 ml) and subcutaneously (0.5 ml) into the shaved abdominal skin.

INDICATIONS AND USAGE

- As an adjunct in the therapy of all forms of parkinsonism (idiopathic, post-encephalitic, arteriosclerotic).
- Control of extrapyramidal disorders secondary to neuroleptic drug therapy (*e.g.*, phenothiazines).

CONTRAINDICATIONS

(1) Hypersensitivity to biperiden, (2) Narrow angle glaucoma, (3) Bowel obstruction, (4) Megacolon.

WARNINGS

Isolated instances of mental confusion, euphoria, agitation and disturbed behavior have been reported in susceptible patients. Also, the central anticholinergic syndrome can occur as an adverse reaction to properly prescribed anticholinergic medication, although it is more frequently due to overdosage. It may also result from concomitant administration of an anticholinergic agent and a drug that has secondary anticholinergic actions (see DRUG INTERACTIONS). Caution should be observed in patients with manifest glaucoma, though no prohibitive rise in intraocular pressure has been noted following either oral or parenteral administration. Patients with prostatism, epilepsy or cardiac arrhythmia should be given this drug with caution.

Occasionally, drowsiness may occur, and patients who drive a car or operate any other potentially dangerous machinery should be warned of this possibility. As with other drugs acting on the central nervous system, the consumption of alcohol should be avoided during biperiden HCl therapy.

PRECAUTIONS

Pregnancy Category C: Animal reproduction studies have not been conducted with biperiden HCl. It is also not known whether biperiden HCl can cause fetal harm when administered to a pregnant woman or can affect reproduction capacity. Biperiden HCl should be given to a pregnant woman only if clearly needed.

Nursing Mothers: It is not known whether this drug is excreted in human milk. Because many drugs are excreted in human milk, caution should be exercised when biperiden HCl is administered to a nursing woman.

Pediatric Use: Safety and effectiveness in children have not been established.

DRUG INTERACTIONS

The central anticholinergic syndrome can occur when anticholinergic agents such as Biperiden HCl are administered concomitantly with drugs that have secondary anticholinergic actions, *e.g.*, certain narcotic analgesics such as meperidine, the phenothiazines and other antipsychotics, tricyclic antidepressants, certain antiarrhythmics such as the quinidine salts, and antihistamines.

ADVERSE REACTIONS

Atropine-like side effects such as dry mouth; blurred vision; drowsiness; euphoria or disorientation; urinary retention; postural hypotension; constipation; agitation; disturbed behavior may be seen. There usually are no significant changes in blood pressure or heart rate in patients who have been given the parenteral form of biperiden HCl. Mild transient postural hypotension and bradycardia may occur. These side effects can be minimized or avoided by slow intravenous administration. No local tissue reactions have been reported following intramuscular injection. If gastric irritation occurs following oral administration, it can be avoided by administering the drug during or after meals.

The central anticholinergic syndrome can occur as an adverse reaction to properly prescribed anticholinergic medication.

DOSAGE AND ADMINISTRATION

DRUG INDUCED EXTRAPYRAMIDAL SYMPTOMS

Parenteral: The average adult dose is 2 mg intramuscularly or intravenously. May be repeated every half-hour until there is resolution of symptoms, but not more than four consecutive doses should be given in 24 hour period. *Note:* Parenteral drug product should be inspected visually for particulate matter and discoloration prior to administration, whenever solution and container permit.

Oral: One (1) tablet one to three times daily.

Parkinson's Disease: *Oral:* The usual beginning dose is 1 tablet three or four times daily. This dosage should be individualized with the dose titrated upward to a maximum of 8 tablets (16 mg) per 24 hours.

Storage: All dosage forms of Akineton should be stored at 15- 30°C (59-86°F). Dispense in tight, light-resistant container.

ANIMAL PHARMACOLOGY

Toxicity in Animals: The LD_{50} of biperiden in the white mouse is 545 mg/kg orally, 195 mg/kg subcutaneously, and 56 mg/k intravenously. The acute oral toxicity (LD_{50}) in rats is 750 mg/kg. The intraperitoneal toxicity (LD_{50}) of biperiden lactate in rats was 270 mg/kg and the intravenous toxicity (LD_{50}) in dogs was 222 mg/kg. In dogs under general anesthesia, respiratory arrest occurred at 33 mg/kg (intravenous) and circulatory standstill at 45 mg/kg (intravenous). The oral LD_{50} in dogs is 340 mg/kg. Chronic toxicity studies in both rat and dog have been reported.

PRODUCT LISTING - EQUIVALENTS NOT AVAILABLE

Tablet - Oral - 2 mg

100's	$36.19	AKINETON HCL, Physicians Total Care	54868-2432-00
100's	$46.90	AKINETON HCL, Par Pharmaceutical Inc	49884-0693-01

Bisacodyl (000487)

Categories: Bowel cleansing; Constipation; FDA Pre 1938 Drugs

Drug Classes: Laxatives; Bowel evacuants

Brand Names: Dulcolax

Foreign Brand Availability: Alaxa (Italy); Anulax (Ecuador); Bioyl (Taiwan); Bisalax (Australia); Contalax (France); Correctol (Hong-Kong); Dekalax (Belgium); Dissilax (Bahrain; Cyprus; Egypt; Iran; Iraq; Jordan; Kuwait; Lebanon; Libya; Oman; Qatar; Republic-of-Yemen; Saudi-Arabia; Syria; United-Arab-Emirates); Drix (Germany); Dulcolan (Mexico; Venezuela); Dulco laxo (Spain); Gencolax (Thailand); Kadolax (Thailand); Laxacod (Indonesia); Laxadin (Israel); Laxadyl (Bahrain; Benin; Burkina-Faso; Cyprus; Egypt; Ethiopia; Gambia; Ghana; Guinea; Iran; Iraq; Ivory-Coast; Jordan; Kenya; Kuwait; Lebanon; Liberia; Libya; Malawi; Mali; Mauritania; Mauritius; Morocco; Niger; Nigeria; Oman; Qatar; Republic-of-Yemen; Saudi-Arabia; Senegal; Seychelles; Sierra-Leone; Sudan; Syria; Tanzania; Tunia; Uganda; United-Arab-Emirates; Zambia; Zimbabwe); Laxamex (Indonesia); Laxcodyl (Thailand); Laxitab 5 (Thailand); Mandrolax Bisa (Germany); Melaxan (Indonesia); Stolax (Indonesia); Toilax (Bahrain; Cyprus; Egypt; Finland; Iran; Iraq; Jordan; Kuwait; Lebanon; Libya; Netherlands; Norway; Oman; Qatar; Republic-of-Yemen; Saudi-Arabia; Syria; United-Arab-Emirates); Vacolax (Thailand)

DESCRIPTION

Dulcolax is available as enteric coated tablets of 5 mg each or as suppositories of 10 mg each. Each tablet also contains: acacia, acetylated monoglyceride, carnauba wax, cellulose acetate phthalate, corn starch, D&C red no. 30 aluminum lake, D&C yellow no. 10 aluminum lake, dibutyl phthalate, docusate sodium, gelatin, glycerin, iron oxides, kaolin, lactose, magnesium stearate, methylparaben, pharmaceutical glaze, polyethylene glycol, povidone, propylparaben, sodium benzoate, sorbitan monooleate, sucrose, talc, titanium dioxide, and white wax. Each suppository also contains hydrogenated vegetable oil. Tablets and suppositories contain less than 0.2 mg sodium per dosage unit.

CLINICAL PHARMACOLOGY

Dulcolax is a contact stimulant laxative, administered either orally or rectally, which acts directly on the colonic mucosa to produce normal peristalsis throughout the large intestine. Bisacodyl is a colorless, tasteless compound that is practically insoluble in water or alkaline solution. Its chemical name is: bis(p-acetoxyphenyl)-2-pyridylmethane. Bisacodyl is very poorly absorbed, it at all, in the small intestine following oral administration, or in the large intestine following rectal administration. On contact with the mucosa or submucosal plexi of the large intestine, bisacodyl stimulates sensory nerve endings to produce parasympathetic reflexes resulting in increased peristaltic contractions of the colon. It has also been shown to promote fluid and ion accumulation in the colon, which increases the laxative effect. A bowel movement is usually produced approximately 6 hours after oral administration (8-12 hours if taken at bedtime), and approximately 15 minutes to 1 hour after rectal administration, providing satisfactory cleansing of the bowel which may, under certain circumstances, obviate the need for colonic irrigation.

EXTENT OF DRUG ABSORPTION

In a pharmacokinetic (crossover) study involving 12 patients,[1] plasma levels of bisacodyl were measured following oral administration of a 10 mg reference solution and two 5 mg bisacodyl tablets, and following rectal administration of one 10 mg bisacodyl suppository. With the solution dose, the average C_{max} was 237 ng/ml; with the tablet dose, the average C_{max} was 26 ng/ml (11% of the solution C_{max}); with the suppository dose, in 6 patients the plasma level was below the limit of detection, and in the remaining 6 patients, the average C_{max} was 31 ng/ml (13% of the solution C_{max} in those particular patients). These data demonstrate the low level of systemic absorption of bisacodyl resulting from bisacodyl use.

INDICATIONS AND USAGE

For the relief of occasional constipation and irregularity. For use as part of a bowel cleansing regimen in preparing the patient for surgery or for preparing the colon for x-ray endoscopic examination. Bisacodyl will not replace the colonic irrigations usually given patients before intracolonic surgery, but is useful in the preliminary emptying of the colon prior to those procedures. Bisacodyl may also be used in postoperative care (*i.e.*, restoration of normal bowel hygiene), antepartum care, postpartum care, and in preparation for delivery.

CONTRAINDICATIONS

Stimulant laxatives, such as bisacodyl, are contraindicated for patients with acute surgical abdomen, appendicitis, rectal bleeding, gastroenteritis, or intestinal obstruction.

WARNINGS

Use of bisacodyl is not recommended when abdominal pain, nausea, or vomiting are present. Long term administration of bisacodyl is not recommended in the treatment of chronic constipation. This product should not be used beyond 7 days unless deemed necessary. Rectal bleeding or failure to have a bowel movement after bisacodyl use may indicate a serious condition. If this occurs, the patient should discontinue use of the product and consult a physician.

This and all medication should be kept out of the reach of children.

PRECAUTIONS

PREGNANCY CATEGORY B

Teratology

Reproduction studies of oral doses of bisacodyl have been performed in rats administered up to 70 times the human dose, and have revealed no evidence of impaired fertility or damage to the fetus. At the dose which equated to 70 times the human dose, there was some evidence of lower litter survival at weaning. There are, however, no adequate and well-controlled studies in pregnant women, hence bisacodyl should be used during pregnancy only at the discretion of the physician.

ADVERSE REACTIONS

The process of restoring normal bowel function by use of a laxative may result in some abdominal discomfort.

DOSAGE AND ADMINISTRATION

Tablets:

Adults and children 12 years of age and over: Take 2 or 3 tablets (usually 2) in a single dose once daily.

Children 6 to under 12 years of age: Take 1 tablet once daily. Expect results in 8-12 hours if taken at bedtime, or within 6 hours if taken before breakfast. Do not chew or crush tablets. Do not administer tablets within 1 hour after taking an antacid or milk.

Children under 6 years of age: Oral administration is not recommended due to the requirement to swallow tablets whole.

Suppositories:

Adults and children 12 years of age and over: Use 1 suppository once daily.

Children under 12 years of age: One-half to one 10 mg suppository once daily.

Children under 6 years of age: Consult a physician.

Preparation for X-Ray Endoscopy: For barium enemas, no food should be given following oral administration to prevent reaccumulation of material in the rectum, and a suppository should be administered 1-2 hours prior to examination.

HOW SUPPLIED

Dulcolax is supplied as either light orange enteric coated tablets of 5 mg each, or as suppositories of 10 mg each.

Storage: Store at temperatures below 25°C (77°F). Avoid excessive humidity.

Bisoprolol Fumarate *(003132)*

For related information, see the comparative table section in Appendix A.

Categories: Hypertension, essential; FDA Approved 1992 Jul; Pregnancy Category C
Drug Classes: Antiadrenergics, beta blocking
Brand Names: **Zebeta**
Foreign Brand Availability: Biso (Germany); BisoABZ (Germany); Biso-BASF (Germany); Bisobloc (Netherlands); Bisolol (Israel); Bisomerck (Germany); Cardensiel (France); Cardiloc (Israel); Cardiocor (France); Concor (Austria; China; Colombia; Czech-Republic; Germany; Hong-Kong; India; Indonesia; Israel; Italy; Korea; Malaysia; Portugal; Switzerland; Taiwan; Thailand); Concor COR (Germany); Concore (Philippines); Cordalin (Germany); Detensiel (France); Emconcor (Belgium; Denmark; Finland; Spain; Sweden); Emcor (England; Netherlands); Euradal (Spain); Fondril (Germany); Isoten (Belgium); Maintate (Indonesia; Japan); Monocor (Canada; Denmark; England; Taiwan); Pactens (Greece); Soprol (France)
Cost of Therapy: $40.66 (Hypertension; Zebeta; 5 mg; 1 tablet/day; 30 day supply)

DESCRIPTION

Zebeta (bisoprolol fumarate) is a synthetic, $beta_1$-selective (cardioselective) adrenoreceptor blocking agent. The chemical name for bisoprolol fumarate is (±)-1-[4-[[2-(1-Methylethoxy)ethoxy]methyl]phenoxy]-3-[(1-methylethyl)amino]-2-propanol(*E*)-2-butenedioate (2:1) (salt). It possesses an asymmetric carbon atom in its structure and is provided as a racemic mixture. The S(-) enantiomer is responsible for most of the beta-blocking activity. Its empirical formula is $(C_{18}H_{31}NO_4)_2 \cdot C_4H_4O_4$.

Bisoprolol fumarate has a molecular weight of 766.97. It is a white crystalline powder which is approximately equally hydrophilic and lipophilic, and is readily soluble in water, methanol, ethanol, and chloroform.

Zebeta is available as 5 and 10 mg tablets for oral administration.

Inactive ingredients include colloidal silicon dioxide, corn starch, crospovidone, dibasic calcium phosphate, hypromellose, magnesium stearate, microcrystalline cellulose, polyethylene glycol, polysorbate 80, and titanium dioxide. The 5 mg tablets also contain red and yellow iron oxide.

CLINICAL PHARMACOLOGY

Bisoprolol fumarate is a $beta_1$-selective (cardioselective) adrenoreceptor blocking agent without significant membrane stabilizing activity or intrinsic sympathomimetic activity in its therapeutic dosage range. Cardioselectivity is not absolute, however, and at higher doses (≥20 mg) bisoprolol fumarate also inhibits $beta_2$-adrenoceptors, chiefly located in the bronchial and vascular musculature; to retain selectivity it is therefore important to use the lowest effective dose.

PHARMACOKINETICS AND METABOLISM

The absolute bioavailability after a 10 mg oral dose of bisoprolol fumarate is about 80%. Absorption is not affected by the presence of food. The first pass metabolism of bisoprolol fumarate is about 20%.

Binding to serum proteins is approximately 30%. Peak plasma concentrations occur within 2-4 hours of dosing with 5-20 mg, and mean peak values range from 16 ng/ml at 5 mg to 70 ng/ml at 20 mg. Once daily dosing with bisoprolol fumarate results in less than 2-fold intersubject variation in peak plasma levels. The plasma elimination half-life is 9-12 hours and is slightly longer in elderly patients, in part because of decreased renal function in that population. Steady state is attained within 5 days of once daily dosing. In both young and elderly populations, plasma accumulation is low; the accumulation factor ranges from 1.1-1.3, and is what would be expected from the first order kinetics and once daily dosing. Plasma concentrations are proportional to the administered dose in the range of 5-20 mg. Pharmacokinetic characteristics of the 2 enantiomers are similar.

Bisoprolol fumarate is eliminated equally by renal and non-renal pathways with about 50% of the dose appearing unchanged in the urine and the remainder appearing in the form of inactive metabolites. In humans, the known metabolites are labile or have no known pharmacologic activity. Less than 2% of the dose is excreted in the feces. Bisoprolol fumarate is not metabolized by cytochrome P450 II D6 (debrisoquin hydroxylase).

In subjects with creatinine clearance less than 40 ml/min, the plasma half-life is increased approximately 3-fold compared to healthy subjects.

In patients with cirrhosis of the liver, the elimination of bisoprolol fumarate is more variable in rate and significantly slower than that in healthy subjects, with plasma half-life ranging from 8.3-21.7 hours.

PHARMACODYNAMICS

The most prominent effect of bisoprolol fumarate is the negative chronotropic effect, resulting in a reduction in resting and exercise heart rate. There is a fall in resting and exercise cardiac output with little observed change in stroke volume, and only a small increase in right atrial pressure, or pulmonary capillary wedge pressure at rest or during exercise.

Findings in short-term clinical hemodynamics studies with bisoprolol fumarate are similar to those observed with other beta-blocking agents.

The mechanism of action of its antihypertensive effects has not been completely established. Factors which may be involved include:

Decreased cardiac output,
Inhibition of renin release by the kidneys,
Diminution of tonic sympathetic outflow from the vasomotor centers in the brain.

In normal volunteers, bisoprolol fumarate therapy resulted in a reduction of exercise- and isoproterenol-induced tachycardia. The maximal effect occurred within 1-4 hours post-dosing. Effects persisted for 24 hours at doses equal to or greater than 5 mg.

Electrophysiology studies in man have demonstrated that bisoprolol fumarate significantly decreases heart rate, increases sinus node recovery time, prolongs AV node refractory periods, and, with rapid atrial stimulation, prolongs AV nodal conduction.

$Beta_1$-selectivity of bisoprolol fumarate has been demonstrated in both animal and human studies. No effects at therapeutic doses on $beta_a$-adrenoreceptor density have been observed. Pulmonary function studies have been conducted in healthy volunteers, asthmatics, and patients with chronic obstructive pulmonary disease (COPD). Doses of bisoprolol fumarate ranged from 5-60 mg, atenolol from 50-200 mg, metoprolol from 100-200 mg, and propranolol from 40-80 mg. In some studies, slight, asymptomatic increases in airways resistance (AWR) and decreases in forced expiratory volume (FEV_1) were observed with doses of bisoprolol fumarate 20 mg and higher, similar to the small increases in AWR also noted with the other cardioselective beta-blockers. The changes induced by beta-blockade with all agents were reversed by bronchodilator therapy.

Bisoprolol fumarate had minimal effect on serum lipids during antihypertensive studies. In US placebo-controlled trials, changes in total cholesterol averaged +0.8% for bisoprolol fumarate-treated patients; and +0.7% for placebo. Changes in triglycerides averaged +19% for bisoprolol fumarate-treated patients, and +17% for placebo.

Bisoprolol fumarate has also been given concomitantly with thiazide diuretics. Even very low doses of hydrochlorothiazide (6.25 mg) were found to be additive with bisoprolol fumarate in lowering blood pressure in patients with mild-to-moderate hypertension.

INDICATIONS AND USAGE

Bisoprolol fumarate is indicated in the management of hypertension. It may be used alone or in combination with other antihypertensive agents.

NON-FDA APPROVED INDICATIONS

Bisoprolol is used without approval to treat supraventricular tachycardia, premature ventricular depolarizations, and to prevent angina pectoris. In addition, bisoprolol has been evaluated in the treatment of congestive heart failure, demonstrating a positive effect on the progression of heart failure and frequency of hospitalization in mild-to-moderate heart failure and a decrease in mortality and sudden death in patients with moderate-to-severe heart failure.

CONTRAINDICATIONS

Bisoprolol fumarate is containdicated in patients with cardiogenic shock, overt cardiac failure, second or third degree AV block, and marked sinus bradycardia.

WARNINGS

CARDIAC FAILURE

Sympathetic stimulation is a vital component supporting circulatory function in the setting of congestive heart failure, and beta-blockade may result in further depression of myocardial contractility and precipitate more severe failure. In general, beta-blocking agents should be avoided in patients with overt congestive failure. However, in some patients with compensated cardiac failure it may be necessary to utilize them. In such a situation, they must be used cautiously.

IN PATIENTS WITHOUT A HISTORY OF CARDIAC FAILURE

Continued depression of the myocardium with beta-blockers can, in some patients, precipitate cardiac failure. At the first signs or symptoms of heart failure, discontinuation of bisoprolol fumarate should be considered. In some cases, beta-blocker therapy can be continued while heart failure is treated with other drugs.

ABRUPT CESSATION OF THERAPY

Exacerbation of angina pectoris, and, in some instances, myocardial infarction or ventricular arrhythmia, have been observed in patients with coronary artery disease following abrupt cessation of therapy with beta-blockers. Such patients should, therefore, be cautioned against interruption or discontinuation of therapy without the physician's advice. Even in patients without overt coronary artery disease, it may be advisable to taper therapy with bisoprolol fumarate over approximately 1 week with the patient under careful observation. If withdrawal symptoms occur, bisoprolol fumarate therapy should be reinstituted, at least temporarily.

PERIPHERAL VASCULAR DISEASE

Beta-blockers can precipitate or aggravate symptoms of arterial insufficiency in patients with peripheral vascular disease. Caution should be exercised in such individuals.

BRONCHOSPASTIC DISEASE

PATIENTS WITH BRONCHOSPASTIC DISEASE SHOULD, IN GENERAL, NOT RECEIVE BETA-BLOCKERS. Because of its relative $beta_1$-selectivity, however, bisoprolol fumarate may be used with caution in patients with bronchospastic disease who do not respond to, or who cannot tolerate other antihypertensive treatment. Since $beta_1$-selectivity is not absolute, the lowest possible dose of bisoprolol fumarate should be used, with therapy starting at 2.5 mg. A $beta_2$ agonist (bronchodilator) should be made available.

ANESTHESIA AND MAJOR SURGERY

If bisoprolol fumarate treatment is to be continued perioperatively, particular care should be taken when anesthetic agents which depress myocardial function, such as ether, cyclopropane, and trichloroethylene, are used.

DIABETES AND HYPOGLYCEMIA

Beta-blockers may mask some of the manifestations of hypoglycemia, particularly tachycardia. Nonselective beta-blockers may potentiate insulin-induced hypoglycemia and delay recovery of serum glucose levels. Because of its $beta_1$-selectivity, this is less likely with bisoprolol fumarate. However, patients subject to spontaneous hypoglycemia, or diabetic patients receiving insulin or oral hypoglycemic agents, should be cautioned about these possibilities and bisoprolol fumarate should be used with caution.

THYROTOXICOSIS

Beta-adrenergic blockade may mask clinical signs of hyperthyroidism, such as tachycardia. Abrupt withdrawal of beta-blockade may be followed by an exacerbation of the symptoms of hyperthyroidism or may precipitate thyroid storm.

PRECAUTIONS

IMPAIRED RENAL OR HEPATIC FUNCTION

Use caution in adjusting the dose of bisoprolol fumarate in patients with renal or hepatic impairment (see CLINICAL PHARMACOLOGY and DOSAGE AND ADMINISTRATION).

INFORMATION FOR THE PATIENT

Patients, especially those with coronary artery disease, should be warned about discontinuing use of bisoprolol fumarate without a physician's supervision. Patients should also be advised to consult a physician if any difficulty in breathing occurs, or if they develop signs or symptoms of congestive heart failure or excessive bradycardia.

Patients subject to spontaneous hypoglycemia, or diabetic patients receiving insulin or oral hypoglycemic agents, should be cautioned that beta-blockers may mask some of the manifestations of hypoglycemia, particularly tachycardia, and bisoprolol fumarate should be used with caution.

Patients should know how they react to this medicine before they operate automobiles and machinery or engage in other tasks requiring alertness.

CARCINOGENESIS, MUTAGENESIS, AND IMPAIRMENT OF FERTILITY

Long-term studies were conducted with oral bisoprolol fumarate administered in the feed of mice (20 and 24 months) and rats (26 months). No evidence of carcinogenic potential was seen in mice dosed up to 250 mg/kg/day or rats dosed up to 125 mg/kg/day. On a body weight basis, these doses are 625 and 312 times, respectively, the maximum recommended human dose (MRHD) of 20 mg, (or 0.4 mg/kg/day based on a 50 kg individual); on a body surface area basis, these doses are 59 times (mice) and 64 times (rats) the MRHD. The mutagenic potential of bisoprolol fumarate was evaluated in the microbial mutagenicity (Ames) test, the point mutation and chromosome aberration assays in Chinese hamster V79 cells, the unscheduled DNA synthesis test, the micronucleus test in mice, and the cytogenetics assay in rats. There was no evidence of mutagenic potential in these *in vitro* and *in vivo* assays.

Reproduction studies in rats did not show any impairment of fertility at doses up to 150 mg/kg/day of bisoprolol fumarate, or 375 and 77 times the MRHD on the basis of body weight and body surface area, respectively.

PREGNANCY CATEGORY C

In rats, bisoprolol fumarate was not teratogenic at doses up to 150 mg/kg/day which is 375 and 77 times the MRHD on the basis of body weight and body surface area, respectively. Bisoprolol fumarate was fetotoxic (increased late resorptions) at 50 mg/kg/day and maternotoxic (decreased food intake and body weight gain) at 150 mg/kg/day. The fetotoxicity in rats occurred at 125 times the MRHD on a body weight basis and 26 times the MRHD on the basis of body surface area. The maternotoxicity occurred at 375 times the MRHD on a body weight basis and 77 times the MRHD on the basis of body surface area. In rabbits, bisoprolol fumarate was not teratogenic at doses up to 12.5 mg/kg/day, which is 31 and 12 times the MRHD based on body weight and surface area, respectively, but was embryolethal (increased early resorptions) at 12.5 mg/kg/day.

There are no adequate and well-controlled studies in pregnant women. Bisoprolol fumarate should be used during pregnancy only if the potential benefit justifies the potential risk to the fetus.

NURSING MOTHERS

Small amounts of bisoprolol fumarate (<2% of the dose) have been detected in the milk of lactating rats. It is not known whether this drug is excreted in human milk. Because many drugs are excreted in human milk caution should be exercised when bisoprolol fumarate is administered to nursing women.

PEDIATRIC USE

Safety and effectiveness in pediatric patients have not been established.

GERIATRIC USE

Bisoprolol fumarate has been used in elderly patients with hypertension. Response rate and mean decreases in systolic and diastolic blood pressure were similar to the deceases in younger patients in the US clinical studies. Although no dose response study was conducted in elderly patients, there was a tendency for older patients to be maintained on higher doses of bisoprolol fumarate.

Observed reductions in heart rate were slightly greater in the elderly than in the young and tended to increase with increasing dose. In general, no disparity in adverse experience reports or dropouts for safety reasons was observed between older and younger patients. Dose adjustment based on age is not necessary.

DRUG INTERACTIONS

Bisoprolol fumarate should not be combined with other beta-blocking agents. Patients receiving catecholamine-depleting drugs, such as reserpine or guanethidine, should be closely monitored, because the added beta-adrenergic blocking action of bisoprolol fumarate may produce excessive reduction of sympathetic activity. In patients receiving concurrent therapy with clonidine, if therapy is to be discontinued, it is suggested that bisoprolol fumarate be discontinued for several days before the withdrawal of clonidine.

Bisoprolol fumarate should be used with care when myocardial depressants or inhibitors of AV conduction, such as certain calcium antagonists [particularly of the phenylalkylamine (verapamil) and benzothiazepine (diltiazem) classes], or antiarrhythmic agents, such as disopyramide, are used concurrently.

Concurrent use of rifampin increases the metabolic clearance of bisoprolol fumarate, resulting in a shortened elimination half-life of bisoprolol fumarate. However, initial dose modification is generally not necessary. Pharmacokinetic studies document no clinically relevant interactions with other agents given concomitantly, including thiazide diuretics, digoxin and cimetidine. There was no effect of bisoprolol fumarate on prothrombin time in patients on stable doses of warfarin.

RISK OF ANAPHYLACTIC REACTION

While taking beta-blockers, patients with a history of severe anaphylactic reaction to a variety of allergens may be more reactive to repeated challenge, either accidental, diagnostic, or therapeutic. Such patients may be unresponsive to the usual doses of epinephrine used to treat allergic reactions.

ADVERSE REACTIONS

Safety data are available in more than 30,000 patients or volunteers. Frequency estimates and rates of withdrawal of therapy for adverse events were derived from two US placebo-controlled studies.

In Study A, doses of 5, 10, and 20 mg bisoprolol fumarate were administered for 4 weeks. In Study B, doses of 2.5, 10 and 40 mg of bisoprolol fumarate were administered for 12 weeks. A total of 273 patients were treated with 5-20 mg of bisoprolol fumarate; 132 received placebo.

Withdrawal of therapy for adverse events was 3.3% for patients receiving bisoprolol fumarate and 6.8% for patients on placebo. Withdrawals were less than 1% for either bradycardia or fatigue/lack of energy.

TABLE 2 presents adverse experiences, whether or not considered drug related, reported in at least 1% of patients in these studies, for all patients studied in placebo-controlled clinical trials (2.5-40 mg), as well as for a subgroup that was treated with doses within the recommended dosage range (5-20 mg). Of the adverse events listed in TABLE 2, bradycardia, diarrhea, asthenia, fatigue, and sinusitis appear to be dose related.

TABLE 2

	All Adverse Experiences		
		Bisoprolol Fumarate	
	Placebo	5-20 mg	2.5-40 mg
Body System/Adverse Experience	(n=132)	(n=273)	(n=404)
Skin			
Increased sweating	1.5%	0.7%	1.0%
Musculoskeletal			
Arthralgia	2.3%	2.2%	2.7%
Central Nervous System			
Dizziness	3.8%	2.9%	3.5%
Headache	11.4%	8.8%	10.9%
Hypoaesthesia	0.8%	1.1%	1.5%
Autonomic Nervous System			
Dry mouth	1.5%	0.7%	1.3%
Heart Rate/Rhythm			
Bradycardia	0%	0.4%	0.5%
Psychiatric			
Vivid dreams	0%	0%	0%
Insomnia	2.3%	1.5%	2.5%
Depression	0.8%	0%	0.2%
Gastrointestinal			
Diarrhea	1.5%	2.6%	3.5%
Nausea	1.5%	1.5%	2.2%
Vomiting	0%	1.1%	1.5%
Respiratory			
Bronchospasm	0%	0%	0%
Cough	4.5%	2.6%	2.5%
Dyspnea	0.8%	1.1%	1.5%
Pharyngitis	2.3%	2.2%	2.2%
Rhinitis	3.0%	2.9%	4.0%
Sinusitis	1.5%	2.2%	2.2%
URI	3.8%	4.8%	5.0%
Body as a Whole			
Asthenia	0%	0.4%	1.5%
Chest pain	0.8%	1.1%	1.5%
Fatigue	1.5%	6.6%	8.2%
Edema (peripheral)	3.8%	3.7%	3.0%

The following is a comprehensive list of adverse experiences reported with bisoprolol fumarate in worldwide studies, or in postmarketing experience (in italics):

Central Nervous System: Dizziness, *unsteadiness,* vertigo, *syncope,* headache, paresthesia, hypoaesthesia, hyperesthesia, somnolence, *sleep disturbances,* anxiety/restlessness, decreased, concentration/memory.

Autonomic Nervous System: Dry mouth.

Cardiovascular: Bradycardia; palpitations and other rhythm disturbances, cold extremities, claudication, hypotension, orthostatic hypotension, chest pain, congestive heart failure, dyspnea on exertion.

Psychiatric: Vivid dreams, insomnia, depression.

Gastrointestinal: Gastric/epigastric/abdominal pain, gastritis, dyspepsia, nausea, vomiting, diarrhea, constipation, peptic ulcer.

Musculoskeletal: Muscle/joint pain, *arthralgia,* back/neck pain, muscle cramps, twitching/tremor.

Skin: Rash, acne, eczema, *psoriasis,* skin irritation, pruritus, flushing, sweating, alopecia, *dermatitis, angioedema, exfoliative dermatitis,* cutaneous vasculitis.

Special Senses: Visual disturbances, ocular pain/pressure, abnormal lacrimation, tinnitus, *decreased hearing,* earache, taste abnormalities.

Metabolic: Gout.

Respiratory: Asthma/bronchospasm, bronchitis, coughing, dyspnea, pharyngitis, rhinitis, sinusitis, URI.

Genitourinary: Decreased libido/impotence, *Peyronie's disease,* cystitis, renal colic, polyuria.

Hematologic: Purpura.

General: Fatigue, asthenia, chest pain, malaise, edema, weight gain, angioedema.

In addition, a variety of adverse effects have been reported with other beta-adrenergic blocking agents and should be considered potential adverse effects of bisoprolol fumarate:

Central Nervous System: Reversible mental depression progressing to catatonia, hallucinations, an acute reversible syndrome characterized by disorientation to time and place, emotional lability, slightly clouded sensorium.

Allergic: Fever, combined with aching and sore throat, laryngospasm, respiratory distress.

Hematologic: Agranulocytosis, thrombocytopenia, thrombocytopenic purpura.

Gastrointestinal: Mesenteric arterial thrombosis, ischemic colitis.

Miscellaneous: The oculomucocutaneous syndrome associated with the beta-blocker practolol has not been reported with bisoprolol fumarate during investigational use or extensive foreign marketing experience.

LABORATORY ABNORMALITIES

In clinical trials, the most frequently reported laboratory change was an increase in serum triglycerides, but this was not a consistent finding.

Sporadic liver test abnormalities have been reported. In the US controlled trials experience with bisoprolol fumarate treatment for 4-12 weeks, the incidence of concomitant elevations in SGOT and SGPT from 1-2 times normal was 3.9%, compared to 2.5% for placebo. No patient had concomitant elevations greater than twice normal.

In the long-term, uncontrolled experience with bisoprolol fumarate treatment for 6-18 months, the incidence of 1 or more concomitant elevations in SGOT and SGPT from 1-2 times normal was 6.2%. The incidence of multiple occurrences was 1.9%. For concomitant elevations in SGOT and SGPT of greater than twice normal, the incidence was 1.5%. The incidence of multiple occurrences was 0.3%. In many cases these elevations were attributed to underlying disorders, or resolved during continued treatment with bisprolol fumarate.

Other laboratory changes included small increases in uric acid, creatinine, BUN, serum potassium, glucose, and phosphorus and decreases in WBC and platelets. These were generally not of clinical importance and rarely resulted in discontinuation of bisoprolol fumarate.

As with other beta-blockers, ANA conversions have also been reported on bisoprolol fumarate. About 15% of patients in long-term studies converted to a positive titer, although about one-third of these patients subsequently reconverted to a negative titer while on continued therapy.

DOSAGE AND ADMINISTRATION

The dose of bisoprolol fumarate must be individualized to the needs of the patient. The usual starting dose is 5 mg once daily. In some patients, 2.5 mg may be an appropriate starting dose (see WARNINGS, Bronchospastic Disease). If the antihypertensive effect of 5 mg is inadequate, the dose may be increased to 10 mg and then, if necessary, to 20 mg once daily.

PATIENTS WITH RENAL OR HEPATIC IMPAIRMENT

In patients with hepatic impairment (hepatitis or cirrhosis) or renal dysfunction (creatinine clearance less than 40 ml/min), the initial daily dose should be 2.5 mg and caution should be used in dose-titration. Since limited data suggest that bisoprolol fumarate is not dialyzable, drug replacement is not necessary in patients undergoing dialysis.

GERIATRIC PATIENTS

It is not necessary to adjust the dose in the elderly, unless there is also significant renal or hepatic dysfunction (see DOSAGE AND ADMINISTRATION, Patients with Renal or Hepatic Impairment; PRECAUTIONS, Geriatric Use).

PEDIATRIC PATIENTS

There is no pediatric experience with bisoprolol fumarate.

HOW SUPPLIED

Zebeta is supplied as 5 and 10 mg tablets.

5 mg: Pink, heart-shaped, biconvex, film-coated, and vertically scored in half on both sides, with an engraved "B1" on one side and "LL" on the reverse side.

10 mg: White, heart-shaped, biconvex, film-coated, with an engraved "B3" on one side and "LL" on the reverse side.

Storage: Store at controlled room temperature 20-25°C (68-77°F), protected from moisture.

Dispense in tight containers as defined in the USP.

PRODUCT LISTING - RATED THERAPEUTICALLY EQUIVALENT

Tablet - Oral - 5 mg

30's	$34.24	GENERIC, Esi Lederle Generics	59911-7060-01
30's	$36.58	GENERIC, Mutual/United Research Laboratories	53489-0555-07
30's	$36.59	GENERIC, Eon Labs Manufacturing Inc	00185-0771-30
30's	$40.66	ZEBETA, Lederle Laboratories	00005-3816-38
100's	$121.97	GENERIC, Eon Labs Manufacturing Inc	00185-0771-01
100's	$121.99	GENERIC, Mutual/United Research Laboratories	53489-0555-01

Tablet - Oral - 10 mg

30's	$34.24	GENERIC, Esi Lederle Generics	59911-7061-01
30's	$36.58	GENERIC, United Research Laboratories, Inc.	53489-0556-07
30's	$36.59	GENERIC, Eon Labs Manufacturing Inc	00185-0774-30
30's	$40.66	ZEBETA, Lederle Laboratories	00005-3817-38
100's	$121.97	GENERIC, Eon Labs Manufacturing Inc	00185-0774-01
100's	$121.99	GENERIC, United Research Laboratories, Inc.	53489-0556-01

Bisoprolol Fumarate; Hydrochlorothiazide *(003167)*

B

For complete prescribing information, refer to the CD-ROM included with the book.

Categories: Hypertension, essential; FDA Approved 1993 Mar; Pregnancy Category C
Drug Classes: Antiadrenergics, beta blocking; Diuretics, thiazide and derivatives
Brand Names: Ziac
Foreign Brand Availability: Biconcor (Mexico); Concor Plus (Austria; Switzerland); Concor Plus Forte (Austria); Lodoz (Hong-Kong; Indonesia; Singapore); Wytens (France); Ziak (South-Africa)
Cost of Therapy: $40.98 (Hypertension; Ziac; 2.5 mg; 6.25 mg; 1 tablet/day; 30 day supply)

DESCRIPTION

Ziac (bisoprolol fumarate; hydrochlorothiazide) is indicated for the treatment of hypertension. It combines two antihypertensive agents in a once daily dosage; a synthetic beta$_1$-selective (cardioselective) adrenoceptor blocking agent (bisoprolol fumarate) and a benzothiadiazine diuretic (hydrochlorothiazide).

Bisoprolol fumarate is chemically described as (±)-1-[4-[[2-(1-Methylethoxy) ethoxy]methyl]phenoxy]-3-[(1-methylethyl)amino]-2-propanol(*E*)-2-butenedioate (2:1) (salt). It possesses an asymmetric carbon atom in its structure and is provided as a racemic mixture. The S(-) enantiomer is responsible for most of the beta-blocking activity. Its empirical formula is $(C_{18}H_{31}NO_4)_2 \cdot C_4H_4O_4$ and it has a molecular weight of 766.97.

Bisoprolol fumarate is a white crystalline powder, approximately equally hydrophilic and lipophilic, and readily soluble in water, methanol, ethanol, and chloroform.

Hydrochlorothiazide is 6-Chloro-3,4-dihydro-2*H*-1,2,4-benzothiadiazine-7-sulfonamide 1,1-dioxide. It is a white, or practically white, practically odorless crystalline powder. It is slightly soluble in water, sparingly soluble in dilute sodium hydroxide solution, freely soluble in n-butylamine and dimethylformamide, sparingly soluble in methanol, and insoluble in ether, chloroform, and dilute mineral acids. Its empirical formula is $C_7H_8ClN_3O_4S_2$ and it has a molecular weight of 297.73.

Each bisoprolol fumarate; hydrochlorothiazide 2.5 mg/6.25 mg tablet for oral administration contains bisoprolol fumarate 2.5 mg, hydrochlorothiazide 6.25 mg.

Each bisoprolol fumarate; hydrochlorothiazide 5 mg/6.25 mg tablet for oral administration contains bisoprolol fumarate 5 mg, hydrochlorothiazide 6.25 mg.

Each bisoprolol fumarate; hydrochlorothiazide 10 mg/6.25 mg tablet for oral administration contains bisoprolol fumarate 10 mg, hydrochlorothiazide 6.25 mg.

Inactive ingredients include colloidal silicon dioxide, corn starch, dibasic calcium phosphate, hypromellose, magnesium stearate, microcrystalline cellulose, polyethylene glycol, polysorbate 80, and titanium dioxide. The 5 mg/6.25 mg tablet also contains red and yellow iron oxide. The 2.5 mg/6.25 mg tablet also contains crospovidone, pregelatinized starch and yellow iron oxide.

INDICATIONS AND USAGE

Bisoprolol fumarate; hydrochlorothiazide is indicated in the management of hypertension.

CONTRAINDICATIONS

Bisoprolol fumarate; hydrochlorothiazide is contraindicated in patients in cardiogenic shock, overt cardiac failure (see WARNINGS), second or third degree AV block, marked sinus bradycardia, anuria, and hypersensitivity to either component of this product or to other sulfonamide-derived drugs.

WARNINGS

CARDIAC FAILURE

In general, beta-blocking agents should be avoided in patients with overt congestive failure. However, in some patients with compensated cardiac failure, it may be necessary to utilize these agents. In such situations, they must be used cautiously.

PATIENTS WITHOUT A HISTORY OF CARDIAC FAILURE

Continued depression of the myocardium with beta-blockers can, in some patients, precipitate cardiac failure. At the first signs or symptoms of heart failure, discontinuation of bisoprolol fumarate; hydrochlorothiazide should be considered. In some cases bisoprolol fumarate; hydrochlorothiazide therapy can be continued while heart failure is treated with other drugs.

ABRUPT CESSATION OF THERAPY

Exacerbations of angina pectoris and, in some instances, myocardial infarction or ventricular arrhythmia, have been observed in patients with coronary artery disease following abrupt cessation of therapy with beta-blockers. Such patients should, therefore, be cautioned against interruption or discontinuation of therapy without the physician's advice. Even in patients without overt coronary artery disease, it may be advisable to taper therapy with bisoprolol fumarate; hydrochlorothiazide over approximately 1 week with the patient under careful observation. If withdrawal symptoms occur, beta-blocking agent therapy should be reinstituted, at least temporarily.

PERIPHERAL VASCULAR DISEASE

Beta-blockers can precipitate or aggravate symptoms of arterial insufficiency in patients with peripheral vascular disease. Caution should be exercised in such individuals.

BRONCHOSPASTIC DISEASE

PATIENTS WITH BRONCHOSPASTIC PULMONARY DISEASE SHOULD, IN GENERAL, NOT RECEIVE BETA-BLOCKERS. Because of the relative beta$_1$-selectivity of bisoprolol fumarate, bisoprolol fumarate; hydrochlorothiazide may be used with caution in patients with bronchospastic disease who do not respond to, or who cannot tolerate other antihypertensive treatment. Since beta$_1$-selectivity is not absolute, the lowest possible dose of bisoprolol fumarate; hydrochlorothiazide should be used. A beta$_2$ agonist (bronchodilator) should be made available.

ANESTHESIA AND MAJOR SURGERY

If bisoprolol fumarate; hydrochlorothiazide treatment is to be continued perioperatively, particular care should be taken when anesthetic agents that depress myocardial function, such as ether, cyclopropane, and trichloroethylene, are used.

DIABETES AND HYPOGLYCEMIA

Beta-blockers may mask some of the manifestations of hypoglycemia, particularly tachycardia. Nonselective beta-blockers may potentiate insulin-induced hypoglycemia and delay recovery of serum glucose levels. Because of its beta$_1$-selectivity, this is less likely with bisoprolol fumarate. However, patients subject to spontaneous hypoglycemia, or diabetic patients receiving insulin or oral hypoglycemic agents, should be cautioned about these possibilities. Also, latent diabetes mellitus may become manifest and diabetic patients given thiazides may require adjustment of their insulin dose. Because of the very low dose of hydrochlorothiazide employed, this may be less likely with bisoprolol fumarate; hydrochlorothiazide.

THYROTOXICOSIS

Beta-adrenergic blockade may mask clinical signs of hyperthyroidism, such as tachycardia. Abrupt withdrawal of beta-blockade may be followed by an exacerbation of the symptoms of hyperthyroidism or may precipitate thyroid storm.

RENAL DISEASE

Cumulative effects of the thiazides may develop in patients with impaired renal function. In such patients, thiazides may precipitate azotemia. In subjects with creatinine clearance less than 40 ml/min, the plasma half-life of bisoprolol fumarate is increased up to 3-fold, as compared to healthy subjects. If progressive renal impairment becomes apparent, bisoprolol fumarate; hydrochlorothiazide should be discontinued.

HEPATIC DISEASE

Bisoprolol fumarate; hydrochlorothiazide should be used with caution in patients with impaired hepatic function or progressive liver disease. Thiazides may alter fluid and electrolyte balance, which may precipitate hepatic coma. Also, elimination of bisoprolol fumarate is significantly slower in patients with cirrhosis than in healthy subjects.

DOSAGE AND ADMINISTRATION

Bisoprolol is an effective treatment of hypertension in once daily doses of 2.5 to 40 mg, while hydrochlorothiazide is effective in doses of 12.5 to 50 mg. In clinical trials of bisoprolol; hydrochlorothiazide combination therapy using bisoprolol doses of 2.5 to 20 mg hydrochlorothiazide doses of 6.25 to 25 mg, the antihypertensive effects increased with increasing doses of either component.

The adverse effects (see WARNINGS) of bisoprolol are a mixture of dose-dependent phenomena (primarily bradycardia, diarrhea, asthenia, and fatigue) and dose-independent phenomena (*e.g.*, occasional rash); those of hydrochlorothiazide are a mixture of dose-dependent phenomena (primarily hypokalemia) and dose-independent phenomena (*e.g.*, possibly pancreatitis); the dose-dependent for each being much more common than the dose-independent phenomena. The latter consist of those few that are truly idiosyncratic in nature or those that occur with such low frequency that a dose relationship may be difficult to discern. Therapy with a combination of bisoprolol and hydrochlorothiazide will be associated with both sets of dose-independent adverse effects, and to minimize these, it may be appropriate to begin combination therapy only after a patient has failed to achieve the desired effect with monotherapy. On the other hand, regimens that combine low doses of bisoprolol and hydrochlorothiazide should produce minimal dose-dependent adverse effects, *e.g.*, bradycardia, diarrhea, asthenia and fatigue, and minimal dose-dependent adverse metabolic effects, *i.e.*, decreases in serum potassium.

THERAPY GUIDED BY CLINICAL EFFECT

A patient whose blood pressure is not adequately controlled with 2.5 to 20 mg bisoprolol daily may instead be given bisoprolol fumarate; hydrochlorothiazide. Patients whose blood pressures are adequately controlled with 50 mg of hydrochlorothiazide daily, but who experience significant potassium loss with this regimen, may achieve similar blood pressure control without electrolyte disturbance if they are switched to bisoprolol fumarate; hydrochlorothiazide.

INITIAL THERAPY

Antihypertensive therapy may be initiated with the lowest dose of bisoprolol fumarate; hydrochlorothiazide, one 2.5/6.25 mg tablet once daily. Subsequent titration (14 day intervals) may be carried out with bisoprolol fumarate; hydrochlorothiazide tablets up to the maximum recommended dose 20/12.5 mg (two 10/6.25 mg tablets) once daily, as appropriate.

REPLACEMENT THERAPY

The combination may be substituted for the titrated individual components.

CESSATION OF THERAPY

If withdrawal of bisoprolol fumarate; hydrochlorothiazide therapy is planned, it should be achieved gradually over a period of about 2 weeks. Patients should be carefully observed.

PATIENTS WITH RENAL OR HEPATIC IMPAIRMENT

As noted in WARNINGS, caution must be used in dosing/titrating patients with hepatic impairment or renal dysfunction. Since there is no indication that hydrochlorothiazide is dialyzable, and limited data suggest that bisoprolol is not dialyzable, drug replacement is not necessary in patients undergoing dialysis.

ELDERLY PATIENTS

Dosage adjustment on the basis of age is not usually necessary, unless there is also significant renal or hepatic dysfunction (see DOSAGE AND ADMINISTRATION, WARNINGS).

CHILDREN

There is no pediatric experience with bisoprolol fumarate; hydrochlorothiazide.

PRODUCT LISTING - RATED THERAPEUTICALLY EQUIVALENT

Oral - Tablet - 2.5 mg;6.25 mg			
100's	$82.50	FEDERAL UPPER LIMIT, H.C.F.A. F F P	99999-3167-01
Oral - Tablet - 5 mg;6.25 mg			
100's	$82.50	FEDERAL UPPER LIMIT, H.C.F.A. F F P	99999-3167-02
Oral - Tablet - 10 mg;6.25 mg			
30's	$24.75	FEDERAL UPPER LIMIT, H.C.F.A. F F P	99999-3167-03
Tablet - Oral - 2.5 mg;6.25 mg			
30's	$34.24	GENERIC, Eon Labs Manufacturing Inc	00185-0701-30
30's	$38.05	ZIAC, Allscripts Pharmaceutical Company	54569-4707-00
100's	$113.49	GENERIC, Ivax Corporation	00172-5730-60
100's	$113.50	GENERIC, Watson Laboratories Inc	00591-0841-01
100's	$113.50	GENERIC, Watson Laboratories Inc	52544-0841-01
100's	$114.00	GENERIC, Mylan Pharmaceuticals Inc	00378-0501-01
100's	$114.00	GENERIC, Udl Laboratories Inc	51079-0954-20
100's	$114.02	GENERIC, Geneva Pharmaceuticals	00781-1841-01
100's	$114.14	GENERIC, Purepac Pharmaceutical Company	00228-2650-10
100's	$114.15	GENERIC, Eon Labs Manufacturing Inc	00185-0701-01
100's	$135.60	ZIAC, Lederle Laboratories	00005-3238-23
Tablet - Oral - 5 mg;6.25 mg			
30's	$34.24	GENERIC, Eon Labs Manufacturing Inc	00185-0704-30
30's	$38.05	ZIAC, Allscripts Pharmaceutical Company	54569-4708-00
30's	$41.57	ZIAC, Physicians Total Care	54868-4173-00
100's	$113.49	GENERIC, Ivax Corporation	00172-5731-60
100's	$113.50	GENERIC, Watson Laboratories Inc	00591-0842-01
100's	$113.50	GENERIC, Watson Laboratories Inc	52544-0842-01
100's	$114.00	GENERIC, Mylan Pharmaceuticals Inc	00378-0503-01
100's	$114.00	GENERIC, Udl Laboratories Inc	51079-0955-20
100's	$114.02	GENERIC, Geneva Pharmaceuticals	00781-1824-01
100's	$114.14	GENERIC, Purepac Pharmaceutical Company	00228-2651-10
100's	$114.15	GENERIC, Eon Labs Manufacturing Inc	00185-0704-01
100's	$135.60	ZIAC, Lederle Laboratories	00005-3234-23
Tablet - Oral - 10 mg;6.25 mg			
30's	$34.05	GENERIC, Watson Laboratories Inc	00591-0843-30
30's	$34.05	GENERIC, Watson Laboratories Inc	52544-0843-30
30's	$34.23	GENERIC, Purepac Pharmaceutical Company	00228-2652-03
30's	$34.24	GENERIC, Eon Labs Manufacturing Inc	00185-0707-30
30's	$40.66	ZIAC, Lederle Laboratories	00005-3235-38
30's	$41.55	ZIAC, Physicians Total Care	54868-4179-00
100's	$113.49	GENERIC, Ivax Corporation	00172-5732-60
100's	$114.00	GENERIC, Mylan Pharmaceuticals Inc	00378-0505-01
100's	$114.00	GENERIC, Watson Laboratories Inc	00591-0843-01
100's	$114.00	GENERIC, Udl Laboratories Inc	51079-0956-20
100's	$114.02	GENERIC, Geneva Pharmaceuticals	00781-1833-01
100's	$114.15	GENERIC, Eon Labs Manufacturing Inc	00185-0707-01

PRODUCT LISTING - EQUIVALENTS NOT AVAILABLE

Tablet - Oral - 2.5 mg;6.25 mg			
30's	$34.21	GENERIC, Geneva Pharmaceuticals	00781-1841-31
Tablet - Oral - 5 mg;6.25 mg			
30's	$34.21	GENERIC, Geneva Pharmaceuticals	00781-1824-31
Tablet - Oral - 10 mg;6.25 mg			
30's	$34.21	GENERIC, Geneva Pharmaceuticals	00781-1833-31

Bitolterol Mesylate *(000505)*

For related information, see the comparative table section in Appendix A.

Categories: Asthma; Pregnancy Category C; FDA Approved 1984 Dec
Drug Classes: Adrenergic agonists; Bronchodilators
Brand Names: **Tornalate**
Cost of Therapy: $35.23 (Asthma; Tornalate Aerosol Inhaler; 0.37 mg/inh; 15 ml; 6 inhalations/day; 50 day supply)
HCFA JCODE(S): J7627 per 10 ml INH

DESCRIPTION

Bitolterol mesylate is the di-*p*-toluate ester of the β-adrenergic agonist bronchodilator *N*-t-butylarterenol (colterol). It has a molecular weight of 557.7. Bitolterol mesylate is known chemically as 4-[2-[(1,1-dimethylethyl)amino]-1-hydroxyethyl]-1,2-phenylene 4-methylbenzoate (ester) methanesulfonate (salt).

Tornalate solution for inhalation contains 0.2% bitolterol mesylate in an aqueous vehicle containing alcohol 25% (v/v), citric acid, propylene glycol, and sodium hydroxide. Tornaltate's pH range is 3.0-3.4.

Each ml of Tornalate solution for inhalation, 0.2% contains 0.2% mg of bitolterol mesylate.

Tornalate (bitolterol mesylate) Metered Dose Inhaler is a complete aerosol unit for oral inhalation. It consists of a plastic-coated bottle of ready-to-use aerosol solution and a detachable plastic mouthpiece with built-in-nebulizer. The bottle contains 16.4 g (15 ml) of 0.8% bitolterol mesylate in a vehicle containing 38% alcohol (w/w), inert propellants (dichlorodifluoromethane and dichlorotetrafluoroethane), ascorbic acid, saccharin, and menthol.

Each bottle provides at least 300 actuations. Each actuation delivers a measured dose of 0.37 mg of bitolterol mesylate as a fine, even mist.

CLINICAL PHARMACOLOGY

SOLUTION FOR INHALATION

Bitolteral mesylate is administered as a pro-drug which is hydrolyzed by esterases in tissue and blood to the active moiety colterol. Bitolteral mesylate administered by nebulization has a rapid onset of activity (2-3 minutes) after administration in most patients based on interpolation between baseline and 5 minutes. The duration of action with bitolteral mesylate administered by nebulization is 6 hours or more in most patients and 8 hours in 40% of patients based on 15% or greater increase in forced expiratory volume in one second (FEV_1), as demonstrated in 3 month isoproterenol controlled multicenter trials in non-steroid-dependent patients. Based on mid-maximal expiratory flow (MMEF) measurements, the duration of action is 7.5 to 8 hours in most patients. Median duration of effect in steroid-dependent asthmatic patients ranged from 4.3-7.1 hours based on 15% or greater increase in FEV_1. The mean maximum increase in FEV_1 over baseline in patients during the 3 month studies was 49-55% and occurred by 30-60 minutes in most patients.

In vitro studies and *in vivo* pharmacologic studies have demonstrated that bitolteral mesylate has a preferential effect on beta-2 adrenergic receptors compared with isoproterenol. While it is recognized that beta-2 adrenergic receptors are the prominent receptors in bronchial smooth muscle, recent data indicate that there are between 10-50% beta-2 receptors in the human heart. The precise mechanism of these, however, is not yet established. Bitolteral mesylate has been shown in most controlled clinical trials to have more effect on the respiratory tract, in the form of bronchial smooth muscle relaxation than isoproterenol at comparable doses, while producing fewer cardiovascular effects. Controlled clinical studies and other clinical experience have shown that inhaled bitolteral mesylate, like other beta-adrenergic agonists, can produce a significant cardiovascular effect in some patients, as measured by pulse rate, blood pressure, symptoms and/or ECG changes.

The incidence of cardiovascular side effects such as tachycardia and palpitation was less in patients treated with bitolterol mesylate as compared with patients treated with isoproterenol hydrochloride. The incidence of tachycardia and palpitation was 3.7% and 3.1%, respectively, in patients treated with bitolterol mesylate as compared with an incidence of 12.3% and 12.6% for tachycardia and palpitation for patients treated with isoproterenol.

Blood levels of colterol formed by gradual release from the pro-drug (bitolterol) in the lungs are too low to be measured by currently available assay methods and the bioavailability, pharmacokinetics and metabolism of bitolterol following administration as a solution for inhalation are not known. Data on disposition are available from oral studies in man. Following oral administration of 5.9 mg titrated bitolterol to man, radioactivity measurements indicated mean maximum colterol concentration in blood of approximately 2.1 μg/ml 1 hour after medication. Urinary excretion data indicate that 83% of the radioactivity of this oral dose was excreted within the first 24 hours. By 72 hours, 85.6% of the tritium had been excreted in the urine and 8.1% in the feces. Most of the radioactivity was excreted as conjugated colterol; free colterol accounted for 2.1-3.7% of the total radioactivity excreted in the urine. No intact bitolterol was detected in urine.

The pharmacologic effects of β-adrenergic agonist drugs, including bitolterol mesylate, are at least in part attributable to stimulation through beta-adrenergic receptors to intracellular adenyl cyclase, the enzyme which catalyzes the conversion of adenosine to triphosphate (ATP) to cyclic-3′, 5′-adenosine monophosphate (c-AMP). Increased c-AMP levels are associated with relaxation of bronchial smooth muscle and inhibition of release of mediators of immediate hypersensitivity from cells, especially from mast cells.

In repetitive dosing studies, continued effectiveness was demonstrated throughout the 3 month period of treatment in the majority of patients. In steroid-dependent asthmatics, the median duration of bronchodilator activity as measured by FEV_1 was greater on the first test day as compared with later test days, but patient response remained constant throughout the balance of the three-month period.

Recent studies in laboratory animals (minipigs, rodents, and dogs) recorded the occurrence of cardiac arrhythmias and sudden death (with histologic evidence of myocardial necrosis) when beta-agonists and methylxanthines were administered concurrently. The significance of these findings when applied to humans is currently unknown.

METERED DOSE INHALER

Bitolterol mesylate is administered as a pro-drug which is hydrolyzed by esterases in tissue and blood to the active moiety colterol. Bitolteral mesylate administered as an inhaled aerosol has a rapid (3-4 minutes) onset of bronchodilator activity. The duration of action with bitolteral mesylate is at least 5 hours in most patients and 8 or more hours in 25-35% of patients, based on 15% or greater increase in forced expiratory volume in one second (FEV_1), as demonstrated in 3 month isoproterenol controlled multicenter trials. Based on mean maximal expiratory flow (MMEF) measurements, the duration of action is 6-7 hours. The duration of bronchodilator action with bitolteral mesylate in these trials is longer than that seen with isoproterenol, especially in steroid-dependent patients. Duration of effect was reduced over time in steroid-dependent asthmatic patients where the duration was 3.5 to 5 hours for FEV_1. The mean maximum increase in FEV_1 over baseline in the majority of patients was 39-42% and occurred by 30-60 minutes, similar to that seen in the isoproterenol group.

Bitolteral mesylate is a beta-adrenergic agonist which has been shown by *in vitro* and *in vivo* pharmacological studies in animals to exert a preferential effect on $beta_2$ adrenergic receptors, such as those located in bronchial smooth muscle. However, controlled clinical trials in patients who were administered the drug have not revealed a preferential $beta_2$ adrenergic effect. At doses that produced long duration of bronchodilator activity (up to 8 hours in some patients) with a mean maximum bronchodilating effect of approximately 40% increase in FEV_1 (forced expiratory volume in one second), a less than 10 beat per minute mean maximum increase in heart rate was seen. The effect on the heart rate was transient and similar to the increases seen in the isoproterenol treated patients in these studies.

Although blood levels of colterol formed by gradual release from the pro-drug (bitolterol) in the lungs are too low to be measured by currently available assay methods, data on disposition are available from oral studies in man. Following oral administration of 5.9 mg titrated bitolterol mesylate to man, radioactivity measurements indicated mean maximum colterol concentration in blood of approximately 2.1 μg/ml 1 hour after medication. Urinary excretion data indicate that 83% of the radioactivity of this oral dose was excreted within the first 24 hours. By 72 hours, 85.6% of the tritium had been excreted in the urine and 8.1% in the faces. Most of the radioactivity was excreted as conjugated colterol; free colterol accounted for 2.1-3.7% of the total radioactivity excreted in the urine. No intact bitolterol was detected in urine.

The pharmacologic effects of β-adrenergic drugs including bitolteral mesylate (bitolterol mesylate) are attributable to stimulation of adenyl cyclase, the enzyme which catalyzes the conversion of adenosine triphosphate (ATP) to cyclic-3′, 5′-adenosine monophosphate (c-AMP). Increased c-AMP levels are associated with relaxation of bronchial smooth muscle and with inhibition of release of mediators of immediate hypersensitivity from cells, especially from mast cells.

In a 6 week clinical trial in which 24 asthmatic patients received bitolteral mesylate and theophylline concurrently, improvement in pulmonary function was enhanced over that seen with either drug alone. No potentiation of side effects was observed, and 24 hours ECG recordings (Holter monitoring) indicated no greater degree of cardiac toxicity with bitolteral mesylate alone or in combination with theophylline than that which occurred with theophylline alone.

Bitolteral mesylate did not adversely affect arterial oxygen tension in a blood-gas study in 24 asthmatic patients. However, a decrease in arterial oxygen tension has been reported with other adrenergic bronchodilators and could be anticipated to occur with bitolteral mesylate as well.

In repetitive dosing studies, continued effectiveness was demonstrated throughout the 3 month period of treatment in the majority of patients. However, some overall decrease was observed in steroid-dependent asthmatics.

INDICATIONS AND USAGE

SOLUTION FOR INHALATION

Bitolteral mesylate solution for inhalation, 0.2% is indicated for both prophylaxis and treatment of asthma or other conditions characterized by reversible bronchospasm. It may be used with or without concurrent theophylline and/or steroid therapy.

METERED DOSE INHALER

Bitolterol mesylate is indicated for both prophylactic and therapeutic use as a bronchodilator for bronchial asthma and for reversible bronchospasm. It may be used with or without concurrent theophylline and/or steroid therapy.

CONTRAINDICATIONS

SOLUTION FOR INHALATION AND METERED DOSE INHALER

Bitolteral mesylate is contraindicated in patients who are hypersensitive to bitolterol mesylate or any other ingredients of the formulation.

WARNINGS

SOLUTION FOR INHALATION

As with other β-adrenergic agents, bitolterol mesylate should not be used in excess. Fatalities have been reported in association with excessive use of inhaled sympathomimetic drugs. The exact cause of death is unknown. Use of β-adrenergic drugs may have a deleterious cardiac effect. Paradoxical bronchoconstriction (which can be life-threatening) has been reported with administration of β-adrenergic agents. Immediate hypersensitivity reactions can occur after the administration of sympathomimetic agents. In such instances, the drug should be discontinued immediately and alternative therapy instituted.

In controlled clinical studies, clinically significant increases in pulse rate, increases and decreases in systolic and diastolic blood pressure have been demonstrated in individual patients after administration of bitolteral mesylate. Therefore, caution should be exercised when administering bitolterol mesylate to patients with underlying cardiovascular diseases. Even though the changes may be significant in a small number of patients, these changes occur within a short period of time after administration and have not been shown to be persistent.

If an unusual smell or taste is noted with use of this product, the patient should discontinue use in consultation with his/her physician.

METERED DOSE INHALER

As with other β-adrenergic aerosols, bitolterol mesylate should not be used in excess. Fatalities have been reported in association with excessive use of inhaled sympathomimetic drugs. The exact cause of death is unknown. Use of aerosolized β-adrenergic drugs may have a deleterious cardiac effect. Paradoxical bronchoconstriction (which can be life-threatening) has been reported with administration of β-adrenergic agents. Immediate hypersensitivity (allergic) reactions can occur after the administration of bitolteral mesylate. In such instances, the drug should be discontinued immediately and alternative therapy instituted.

The contents of bitolteral mesylate metered dose inhaler are under pressure. Do not puncture. Do not use or store near heat or open flame. Exposure to temperatures above 120° F may cause bursting. Never throw container into fire or incinerator. Keep out of reach of children.

If an unusual smell or taste is noted with use of this product, the patient should discontinue use in consultation with his/her physician.

PRECAUTIONS

GENERAL

Solution for Inhalation and Metered Dose Inhaler

As with all β-adrenergic stimulating agents, caution should be used when administering bitolterol mesylate to patients with cardiovascular disease such as ischemic heart disease or hypertension. Caution is also advised in patients with hyperthyroidism, diabetes mellitus, cardiac arrhythmias, convulsive disorders or unusual responsiveness to β-adrenergic agonists. Use of any β-adrenergic bronchodilator may produce significant changes in systolic and diastolic blood pressure in some patients. Significant changes in systolic and diastolic blood pressure have been seen in individual patients and could be expected to occur in some patients after use of any β-adrenergic aerosol bronchodilator.

INFORMATION FOR THE PATIENT

Solution for Inhalation

The effects of bitolteral mesylate may last up to eight hours or longer. It should not be used more often than recommended and the patient should not increase the number of treatments or dose without first consulting with the physician. If symptoms of asthma get worse, adverse reactions occur, or the patient does not respond to the usual dose, the patient should be instructed to contact the physician immediately. Drug stability and safety of bitolteral mesylate when mixed with other drugs in a nebulizer have not been established. The patient should be advised as to the proper use of the equipment used for nebulization and to see the Illustrated Patient's Instructions for Use.

Metered Dose Inhaler

The effects of bitolteral mesylate may last up to eight hours or longer. It should not be used more often than recommended and the patient should not increase the number of inhalations or frequency of use without first asking the physician. If symptoms of asthma get worse, adverse reactions occur, or the patient does not respond to the usual dose, the patient should be instructed to contact the physician immediately. The patient should be advised to see the Illustrated Patient's Instructions for Use.

Note: For all illustrations, please see original package insert.

CARCINOGENESIS, MUTAGENESIS, AND IMPAIRMENT OF FERTILITY

Solution for Inhalation

No tumorigenicity (and specifically no increase in leiomyomas) was observed in a 2 year oral study in Sprague-Dawley CD rats at doses of bitolteral mesylate corresponding to 12 or 62 times the maximal total daily human inhalation dose (8.0 mg bitolterol mesylate per day). Bitolteral mesylate was not tumorigenic in an 18 month oral study in Swiss-Webster mice at doses up to 312 times the maximal daily human inhalational dose.

Ames Salmonella and mouse lymphoma mutation assays *in vitro* revealed no mutagenesis due to bitolteral mesylate. Reproductive studies in male and female rats revealed no significant effects on fertility at doses of bitolteral mesylate up to 241 times the maximal daily human inhalational dose.

Metered Dose Inhaler

No tumorigenicity (and specifically no increase in leiomyomas) was observed in a 2 year oral study in Sprague-Dawley CD rats at doses of bitolteral mesylate corresponding to 23 or 114 times the maximal daily human inhalation dose. Bitolteral mesylate was not tumorigenic in an 18 month oral study in Swiss-Webster mice at doses up to 568 times the maximal daily human inhalational dose.

Ames Salmonella and mouse lymphoma mutation assays *in vitro* revealed no mutagenesis due to bitolteral mesylate. Reproductive studies in male and female rats revealed no significant effects on fertility at doses of bitolteral mesylate up to 364 times the maximal daily human inhalational dose.

PREGNANCY, TERATOGENIC EFFECTS, PREGNANCY CATEGORY C

Solution for Inhalation

No teratogenic effects were seen in rats and rabbits after oral doses of bitolteral mesylate up to 361 times the maximal daily human inhalational dose and in mice after oral doses up to 188 times the maximal daily human inhalational dose.

When bitolteral mesylate (as base) was injected subcutaneously into mice in doses of 2, 10, and 20 mg/kg (corresponding to 15, 75, and 151 times the maximal daily human inhalational dose) the incidence of cleft palate was 5.7%, 3.8%, and 3.3%, respectively. Occurrence of cleft palate with isoproterenol (as base) at 10 mg/kg subcutaneously was 10.7%. Since well-controlled studies in pregnant women are not available, bitolteral mesylate should be used during pregnancy only if the potential benefit justifies the potential risk to the fetus.

Metered Dose Inhaler

No teratogenic effects were seen in rats and rabbits after oral doses of bitolteral mesylate up to 557 times the maximal daily human inhalational dose and in mice after oral doses up to 284 times the maximal daily human inhalational dose.

When bitolteral mesylate was injected subcutaneously into mice at doses of 2, 10, and 20 mg/kg (corresponding to 23, 114, and 227 times the maximal daily human inhalational dose) cleft palate incidences of 5.7%, 3.8%, and 3.3% (compared with 0.9% in controls) were found. Cleft palate induction with isoproterenol at 10 mg/kg SC as the positive control was 10.7%. Since no well-controlled studies in pregnant women are available, bitolteral mesylate should be used during pregnancy only if the potential benefit justifies the potential risk to the fetus.

NURSING MOTHERS

Solution for Inhalation and Metered Dose Inhaler

It is not known whether bitolteral mesylate is excreted in human milk. Because many drugs are excreted in human milk, caution should be exercised when bitolteral mesylate is administered to a nursing woman.

PEDIATRIC USE

Solution for Inhalation and Metered Dose Inhaler

Safety and effectiveness of bitolteral mesylate in children 12 years of age or younger has not been established.

DRUG INTERACTIONS

SOLUTION FOR INHALATION

Other sympathomimetic bronchodilators or epinephrine should not be used concomitantly with bitolteral mesylate because they have additive effects.

Bitolteral mesylate should be administered with caution to patients being treated with monoamine oxidase inhibitors or tricyclic antidepressants, since the action of bitolterol on the vascular system may be potentiated.

METERED DOSE INHALER

Other sympathomimetic aerosol bronchodilators should not be used concomitantly with bitolteral mesylate. If additional adrenergic drugs are to be administered by any route, they should be used with caution to avoid deleterious cardiovascular effects.

ADVERSE REACTIONS

SOLUTION FOR INHALATION

The adverse reactions observed with bitolteral mesylate are consistent with those seen with other beta-adrenergic agonists. The frequency of most cardiovascular effects was less after bitolterol mesylate than after isoproterenol in 3 month repetitive dose studies.

Like the findings noted after the administration of other beta-adrenergic agonist drugs, infrequent laboratory abnormalities with undetermined clinical significance were noted after administration of bitolteral mesylate. These include decreases in hemoglobin and hematocrit, decreases in WBC, elevation of liver enzymes, increases in blood sugar, decreases in serum potassium and abnormal urinalysis. In addition, one patient in a bitolteral mesylate controlled clinical trial had increased liver function tests and documented hepatomegaly.

The results of all clinical trials with bitolteral mesylate (323 patients) showed the following side effects:

Central/Peripheral Nervous System: Tremors (26.6%), nervousness (11.1%), headache (8.4%), lightheadedness (6.8%), dizziness (4.0%), paresthesia (1.5%), somnolence (1.2%). In three-month studies, the incidence of tremors decreased from 22% during the first month to 9% during the third month.

Cardiovascular: Tachycardia (3.7%), palpitation (3.1%), irregular pulse (1.2%).

Respiratory: Coughing (2.5%), bronchospasm (1.5%), chest discomfort (1.5%), rhinitis (1.5%).

Oro-Pharyngeal: Throat irritation (2.5%), mouth irritation (1.9%).

Gastrointestinal: Nausea (1.9%).

Other: Fatigue (1.5%).

The incidence of the following adverse reactions was less than 1%:

CNS: Vertigo, insomnia, euphoria, incoordination, hyperkinesia, hypoesthesia, anxiety.

Cardiovascular: Transient ECG changes (ventricular premature contractions, atrial arrhythmia, inverted T waves, junctional rhythm), chest discomfort, increase in blood pressure, chills, heart rate decrease, flushing.

Respiratory: Dyspnea, sputum increase.

Gastrointestinal: Vomiting, hepatomegalia.

Others: Pruritus, urticaria, asthenia, arthralgia, eye irritation, facial discomfort, taste loss.

Clinical relevance or relationship to administration of bitolteral mesylate and rarely reported elevations of SGOT, SGPT, LDH are not known.

METERED DOSE INHALER

The results of all clinical trials with bitolteral mesylate (bitolterol mesylate) in 492 patients showed the following side effects.

CNS: Tremors (14%), nervousness (5%), headache (4%), dizziness (3%), lightheadedness (3%), insomnia (<1%), hyperkinesia (<1%).

Gastrointestinal: Nausea (3%).

Oro-Pharyngeal: Throat irritation (5%).

Cardiovascular: The overall incidence of cardiovascular effects was approximately 5% of patients and these effects included palpitations (approximately 3%), and chest discomfort (approximately 1%). Tachycardia was seen in less than 1%. Premature ventricular contractions and flushing were rarely seen.

Respiratory: Coughing (4%), bronchospasm (<1%), dyspnea (<1%), chest tightness (<1%).

Clinical relevance or relationship to bitolteral mesylate administration of rarely reported elevations of SGOT, decrease in patients, decreases in WBC levels or proteinuria are not known.

In comparing the adverse reactions for bitolterol mesylate treated patients to those of isoproterenol treated patients, during 3 month clinical trails involving approximately 400 patients, the following moderate to severe reactions shown inTABLE 1, as judged by the investigators, were reported for such steroid and non-steroid dependent patients. TABLE 1 does not include mild reactions or those occurring only with the first dose.

TABLE 1 *Percent Incidence of Moderate to Severe Adverse Reactions*

Reaction	Bitolterol n=197	Isoproterenol n=194
Central Nervous System		
Tremors	9.1%	1.5%
Nervousness	1.5%	1.0%
Headache	3.5%	6.1%
Dizziness	1.0%	1.5%
Insomnia	0.5%	0%
Cardiovascular		
Palpitations	1.5%	0%
PVC--transient increase	0.5%	0%
Chest discomfort	0.5%	0%
Respiratory		
Cough	4.1%	1.0%
Bronchospasm	1.0%	0%
Dyspnea	1.0%	0%
Oro-Pharyngeal		
Throat irritation	3.0%	3.1%
Gastrointestinal		
Nausea (dyspepsia)	0.5%	0.5%

NOTE: In most patients, the total isoproterenol dosage was divided into 3 equally dosed inhalations, administered at 3 minute intervals. This procedure may have reduced the incidence of adverse reactions observed with isoproterenol.

DOSAGE AND ADMINISTRATION

SOLUTION FOR INHALATION

Bitolteral mesylate inhalation solution, 0.2% can be administered by nebulization to adults and children over 12 years of age. As with all medications, the physician should begin therapy with the lowest effective dose according to the individual patient's requirements following manufacturer's dosage recommendation. Bitolteral mesylate should be administered during a 10-15 minute period. The treatment period can be adjusted by varying the amount of diluent (normal saline solution) placed in the nebulizer with the medication. The total volume (medication plus diluent) is usually adjusted to 2.0-4.0 ml. Safety of the treatment should be monitored be measuring blood pressure and pulse.

Clinical studies were conducted with 2 types of nebulizer systems.

Intermittent Aerosol Flow (patient-activated nebulizer): This nebulizer is operated by a patient-activated value to permit the release of aerosol mist during inspiration.

Continuous Aerosol Flow Nebulizer: This nebulizer generates a continuous flow of mist while the patient inhales and exhales through the nebulizer resulting in the loss of some medication through an exhaust port.

When using these types of nebulizer systems the dosing regimens in TABLE 2 are recommended.

TABLE 2 *Bitolterol Mesylate for Inhalation, 0.2%*

	Continuous Flow Nebulization		Intermittent Flow Nebulization	
Doses	Volume	Tornalate	Volume	Tornalate
Usual dose	1.25 ml	2.5 mg	0.5 ml	1.0 mg
Decreased dose	0.75 ml	1.5 mg	0.25 ml	0.5 mg
Increased dose	1.75 ml	3.5 mg	0.75 ml	1.5 mg

Up to 1.0 ml of bitolteral mesylate solution for inhalation, 0.2% (2.0 mg bitolteral mesylate), can be administered with the intermittent flow system to severely- obstructed patients.

The usual frequency of treatments is 3 times a day. Treatments may be increased up to 4 times daily, however the interval between treatments should not be less than 4 hours. For some patients 2 treatments a day may be adequate. If a previously effective dosage regimen fails to provide the usual relief, the patient should be advised to seek medical advice immediately as this is often a sign of seriously-worsening asthma that would require reassessment of therapy.

The maximum daily dose should not exceed 8.0 mg bitolteral mesylate with an intermittent flow nebulization system or 14.0 mg bitolteral mesylate with a continuous flow nebulization system.

Bitolteral mesylate solution for inhalation, 0.2% should be added to the nebulizer just prior to use and should not be left in the nebulizer.

Bitolteral mesylate solution for inhalation, 0.2% should not be mixed with other drugs such as cromolyn sodium or acetylcysteine at clinically recommended doses due to chemical and/or physical incompatibles.

METERED DOSE INHALER

The usual dose to relieve bronchospasm for adults and children over 12 years of age is 2 inhalations at an interval of at least 1-3 minutes followed by a third inhalation if needed. For prevention of bronchospasm, the usual dose is 2 inhalations every 8 hours. The dose of bitolteral mesylate (bitolterol mesylate) should never exceed 3 inhalations every 6 hours or 2 inhalations every 4 hours. If a previously effective dosage regimen fails to provide the usual relief, the patient should be advised to seek medical advice immediately as this is often a sign of seriously-worsening asthma that would require reassessment of therapy.

HOW SUPPLIED

SOLUTION FOR INHALATION

Included in each carton is an overwrapped graduated medicine dropper (.75 cc, 1.25 cc , or 1.25 cc) for use with bitolteral mesylate solution for inhalation, 0.2%.

Do not use the solution if it is discolored or contains a precipitate.

Store at controlled room temperature between 15-30°C (59-86°F).

METERED DOSE INHALER

Tornalate (bitolterol mesylate) Metered Dose Inhaler is supplied in 16.4 g (15 ml) self-contained aerosol units. Refill of 16.4 g (15 ml).

Note: The statement below is required by the Federal government's Clean Air Act for all products containing or manufactured with chlorofluorocarbons (CFC's).

WARNING: Contains dichlorodifluoromethane and dichlorotetrafluoroethane, substances which harm public health and environment by destroying ozone in the upper atmosphere.

A notice similar to the above WARNING has been placed in the information for the patient of this product pursuant to EPA regulations.

Store at controlled room temperature between 15°C and 30°C (59°F and 86°F). Use of the product outside this temperature range may result in improper dosing.

PRODUCT LISTING - EQUIVALENTS NOT AVAILABLE

Solution - Inhalation - 0.2%

30 ml	$16.54	TORNALATE, Allscripts Pharmaceutical Company	54569-3959-00

Bivalirudin (003515)

Categories: Angioplasty, adjunct; FDA Approved 2000 Dec; Pregnancy Category B
Drug Classes: Anticoagulants; Thrombin inhibitors
Brand Names: Angiomax

DESCRIPTION

Bivalirudin is a specific and reversible direct thrombin inhibitor. The active substance is a synthetic, 20 amino acid peptide. The chemical name is D-phenylalanyl-L-prolyl-L-arginyl-L-prolyl-glycyl-glycyl-glycyl-glycyl-L-asparagyl-glycyl-L-aspartyl-L-phenylalanyl-L-glutamyl-L-glutamyl-L-isoleucyl-L-prolyl-L-glutamyl-L-glutamyl-L-tyrosyl-L-leucine trifluoroacetate (salt) hydrate. The molecular weight of bivalirudin is 2180 daltons (anhydrous free base peptide). Angiomax is supplied in single-use vials as a white lyophilized cake, which is sterile. Each vial contains 250 mg bivalirudin, 125 mg mannitol, and sodium hydroxide to adjust the pH to 5-6 (equivalent of approximately 12.5 mg sodium). When reconstituted with sterile water for injection the product yields a clear to opalescent, colorless to slightly yellow solution, pH 5-6.

CLINICAL PHARMACOLOGY

GENERAL

Bivalirudin directly inhibits thrombin by specifically binding both to the catalytic site and to the anion-binding exosite of circulating and clot-bound thrombin. Thrombin is a serine proteinase that plays a central role in the thrombotic process, acting to cleave fibrinogen into fibrin monomers and to activate Factor XIII to Factor XIIIa, allowing fibrin to develop a covalently cross-linked framework which stabilizes the thrombus; thrombin also activates Factors V and VIII, promoting further thrombin generation, and activates platelets, stimulating aggregation and granule release. The binding of bivalirudin to thrombin is reversible as thrombin slowly cleaves the bivalirudin-Arg_3-Pro_4 bond, resulting in recovery of thrombin active site functions.

In *in vitro* studies, bivalirudin inhibited both soluble (free) and clot-bound thrombin, was not neutralized by products of the platelet release reaction, and prolonged the activated partial thromboplastin time (aPTT), thrombin time (TT), and prothrombin time (PT) of normal human plasma in a concentration-dependent manner. The clinical relevance of these findings is unknown.

PHARMACOKINETICS

Bivalirudin exhibits linear pharmacokinetics following intravenous (IV) administration to patients undergoing percutaneous transluminal coronary angioplasty (PTCA). In these patients, a mean steady state bivalirudin concentration of 12.3 ± 1.7 μg/ml is achieved following an IV bolus of 1 mg/kg and a 4 hour 2.5 mg/kg/h IV infusion. Bivalirudin is cleared from plasma by a combination of renal mechanisms and proteolytic cleavage, with a half-life in patients with normal renal function of 25 minutes. The disposition of bivalirudin was studied in PTCA patients with mild and moderate renal impairment and in patients with severe renal impairment. Drug elimination was related to glomerular filtration rate (GFR). Total body clearance was similar for patients with normal renal function and with mild renal impairment (60-89 ml/min). Clearance was reduced approximately 20% in patients with moderate and severe renal impairment and was reduced approximately 80% in dialysis-dependent patients. See TABLE 1 for pharmacokinetic parameters and dose reduction recommendations. For patients with renal impairment the activated clotting time (ACT) should be monitored. Bivalirudin is hemodialyzable. Approximately 25% is cleared by hemodialysis.

Bivalirudin does not bind to plasma proteins (other than thrombin) or to red blood cells.

PHARMACODYNAMICS

TABLE 1 *PK Parameters and Dose Adjustments in Renal Impairment**

Renal Function (GFR, ml/min)	Clearance (ml/min/kg)	Half-Life (minutes)	% Reduction in Infusion Dose
Normal renal function (≥90 ml/min)	3.4	25	0
Mild renal impairment (60-89 ml/min)	3.4	22	0
Moderate renal impairment (30-59 ml/min)	2.7	34	20
Severe renal impairment (10-29 ml/min)	2.8	57	60
Dialysis-dependent patients (off dialysis)	1.0	3.5 hours	90

* The ACT should be monitored in renally-impaired patients.

In healthy volunteers and patients (with ≥70% vessel occlusion undergoing routine angioplasty), bivalirudin exhibits linear dose- and concentration-dependent anticoagulant activity as evidenced by prolongation of the ACT, aPTT, PT, and TT. IV administration of bivalirudin produces an immediate anticoagulant effect. Coagulation times return to baseline approximately 1 hour following cessation of bivalirudin administration.

In 291 patients with ≥70% vessel occlusion undergoing routine angioplasty, a positive correlation was observed between the dose of bivalirudin and the proportion of patients achieving ACT values of 300 or 350 seconds. At a bivalirudin dose of 1.0 mg/kg IV bolus plus 2.5 mg/kg/h IV infusion for 4 hours, followed by 0.2 mg/kg/h, all patients reached maximal ACT values >300 seconds.

INDICATIONS AND USAGE

Bivalirudin is indicated for use as an anticoagulant in patients with unstable angina undergoing percutaneous transluminal coronary angioplasty (PTCA). Bivalirudin is intended for use with aspirin and has been studied only in patients receiving concomitant aspirin (see DOSAGE AND ADMINISTRATION).

The safety and effectiveness of bivalirudin have not been established when used in conjunction with platelet inhibitors other than aspirin, such as glycoprotein IIb/IIIa inhibitors (see DRUG INTERACTIONS).

The safety and effectiveness of bivalirudin have not been established in patients with unstable angina who are not undergoing PTCA or in patients with other acute coronary syndromes.

CONTRAINDICATIONS

Bivalirudin is contraindicated in patients with:

Active major bleeding.

Hypersensitivity to bivalirudin or its components.

WARNINGS

Bivalirudin is not intended for intramuscular administration. Although most bleeding associated with the use of bivalirudin in PTCA occurs at the site of arterial puncture, hemorrhage can occur at any site. An unexplained fall in blood pressure or hematocrit, or any unexplained symptom, should lead to serious consideration of a hemorrhagic event and cessation of bivalirudin administration.

There is no known antidote to bivalirudin. Bivalirudin is hemodialyzable (see CLINICAL PHARMACOLOGY, Pharmacokinetics).

PRECAUTIONS

GENERAL

Clinical trials have provided limited information for use of bivalirudin in patients with heparin-induced thrombocytopenia/heparin-induced thrombocytopenia-thrombosis syndrome (HIT/HITTS) undergoing PTCA. The number of HIT/HITTS patients treated is inadequate to reliably assess efficacy and safety in these patients undergoing PTCA. Bivalirudin was administered to a small number of patients with a history of HIT/HITTS or active HIT/HITTS and undergoing PTCA in an uncontrolled, open-label study and in an emergency treatment program and appeared to provide adequate anticoagulation in these patients. In *in vitro* studies, bivalirudin exhibited no platelet aggregation response against sera from patients with a history of HIT/HITTS.

PEDIATRIC USE

The safety and effectiveness of bivalirudin in pediatric patients have not been established.

IMMUNOGENICITY/RE-EXPOSURE

Among 494 subjects who received bivalirudin in clinical trials and were tested for antibodies, 2 subjects had treatment-emergent positive bivalirudin antibody tests. Neither subject demonstrated clinical evidence of allergic or anaphylactic reactions and repeat testing was not performed. Nine additional patients who had initial positive tests were negative on repeat testing.

CARCINOGENESIS, MUTAGENESIS, AND IMPAIRMENT OF FERTILITY

No long-term studies in animals have been performed to evaluate the carcinogenic potential of bivalirudin. Bivalirudin displayed no genotoxic potential in the *in vitro* bacterial cell reverse mutation assay (Ames test), the *in vitro* Chinese hamster ovary cell forward gene mutation test (CHO/HGPRT), the *in vitro* human lymphocyte chromosomal aberration assay, the *in vitro* rat hepatocyte unscheduled DNA synthesis (UDS) assay, and the *in vivo* rat micronucleus assay. Fertility and general reproductive performance in rats were unaffected by subcutaneous doses of bivalirudin up to 150 mg/kg/day, about 1.6 times the dose on a body surface area basis (mg/m^2) of a 50 kg person given the maximum recommended dose of 15 mg/kg/day.

PREGNANCY

Bivalirudin is intended for use with aspirin (see INDICATIONS AND USAGE). Because of possible adverse effects on the neonate and the potential for increased maternal bleeding, particularly during the third trimester, bivalirudin and aspirin should be used together during pregnancy only if clearly needed.

Pregnancy Category B

Teratogenicity studies have been performed in rats at subcutaneous doses up to 150 mg/kg/day, (1.6 times the maximum recommended human dose based on body surface area) and rabbits at subcutaneous doses up to 150 mg/kg/day (3.2 times the maximum recommended human dose based on body surface area). These studies revealed no evidence of impaired fertility or harm to the fetus attributable to bivalirudin. There are, however, no adequate and well-controlled studies in pregnant women. Because animal reproduction studies are not always predictive of human response, this drug should be used during pregnancy only if clearly needed.

NURSING MOTHERS

It is not known whether bivalirudin is excreted in human milk. Because many drugs are excreted in human milk, caution should be exercised when bivalirudin is administered to a nursing woman.

GERIATRIC PATIENTS

Of the total number of patients in clinical studies of bivalirudin undergoing PTCA, 41% were ≥65 years of age, while 11% were >75 years old. A difference of ≥5% between age groups was observed for heparin-treated but not bivalirudin-treated patients with regard to the percentage of patients with major bleeding events. There were no individual bleeding events which were observed with a difference of ≥5% between treatment groups, although puncture site hemorrhage and catheterization site hematoma were each observed in a higher percentage of patients ≥65 years than in patients <65 years. This difference between age groups was more pronounced for heparin-treated than bivalirudin-treated patients.

DRUG INTERACTIONS

Bivalirudin does not exhibit binding to plasma proteins (other than thrombin) or red blood cells.

Drug-drug interaction studies have been conducted with the adenosine diphosphate (ADP) antagonist, ticlopidine, and the glycoprotein IIb/IIIa inhibitor, abciximab, and with low molecular weight heparin. Although data are limited, precluding conclusions regarding efficacy and safety in combination with these agents, the results do not suggest pharmacodynamic interactions. In patients treated with low molecular weight heparin, low molecular weight heparin was discontinued at least 8 hours prior to the procedure and administration of bivalirudin.

The safety and effectiveness of bivalirudin have not been established when used in conjunction with platelet inhibitors other than aspirin, such as glycoprotein IIb/IIIa inhibitors.

In clinical trials in patients undergoing PTCA, coadministration of bivalirudin with heparin, warfarin or thrombolytics was associated with increased risks of major bleeding events compared to patients not receiving these concomitant medications. There is no experience with co-administration of bivalirudin and plasma expanders such as dextran. Bivalirudin should be used with caution in patients with disease states associated with an increased risk of bleeding.

ADVERSE REACTIONS

BLEEDING

In 4312 patients undergoing PTCA for treatment of unstable angina in 2 randomized, double-blind studies comparing bivalirudin to heparin, bivalirudin patients exhibited lower rates of major bleeding and lower requirements for blood transfusions. The incidence of major bleeding is presented in TABLE 3. The incidence of major bleeding was lower in the bivalirudin group than in the heparin group.

TABLE 3 *Major Bleeding and Transfusions — All Patients**

	Bivalirudin n=2161	Heparin n=2151
No. (%) patients with major hemorrhage†	79 (3.7%)	199 (9.3%)
With ≥3 g/dl fall in Hgb	41 (1.9%)	124 (5.8%)
With ≥5 g/dl fall in Hgb	14 (<1%)	47 (2.2%)
Retroperitoneal bleeding	5 (<1%)	15 (<1%)
Intracranial bleeding	1 (<1%)	2 (<1%)
Required transfusion	43 (2.0%)	123 (5.7%)

* No monitoring of ACT (or PTT) was done after a target ACT was achieved.
† Major hemorrhage was defined as the occurrence of any of the following: intracranial bleeding, retroperitoneal bleeding, clinically overt bleeding with a decrease in hemoglobin ≥3 g/dl or leading to a transfusion of ≥2 units of blood. This table includes data from the entire hospitalization period.

OTHER ADVERSE EVENTS

In the 2 randomized double-blind clinical trials of bivalirudin in patients undergoing PTCA, 82% of 2161 bivalirudin-treated patients and 83% of 2151 heparin-treated patients experienced at least 1 treatment-emergent adverse event. The most frequent treatment-emergent events were back pain (42%), pain (15%), nausea (15%), headache (12%), and hypotension (12%) in the bivalirudin-treated group. Treatment-emergent adverse events other than bleeding reported for ≥5% of patients in either treatment group are shown in TABLE 4.

TABLE 4 *Adverse Events Other Than Bleeding Occurring in ≥5% of Patients in Either Treatment Group in Randomized Clinical Trials*

Event	Bivalirudin n=2161	Heparin n=2151
Cardiovascular		
Hypotension	262 (12%)	371 (17%)
Hypertension	135 (6%)	115 (5%)
Bradycardia	118 (5%)	164 (8%)
Gastrointestinal		
Nausea	318 (15%)	347 (16%)
Vomiting	138 (6%)	169 (8%)
Dyspepsia	100 (5%)	111 (5%)
Genitourinary		
Urinary retention	89 (4%)	98 (5%)
Miscellaneous		
Back pain	916 (42%)	944 (44%)
Pain	330 (15%)	358 (17%)
Headache	264 (12%)	225 (10%)
Injection site pain	174 (8%)	274 (13%)
Insomnia	142 (7%)	139 (6%)
Pelvic pain	130 (6%)	169 (8%)
Anxiety	127 (6%)	140 (7%)
Abdominal pain	103 (5%)	104 (5%)
Fever	103 (5%)	108 (5%)
Nervousness	102 (5%)	87 (4%)

Serious, non-bleeding adverse events were experienced in 2% of 2161 bivalirudin-treated patients and 2% of 2151 heparin-treated patients. The following individual serious non-bleeding adverse events were rare (>0.1% to <1%) and similar in incidence between bivalirudin- and heparin-treated patients. These events are listed by body system:

Body as a Whole: Fever, infection, sepsis.
Cardiovascular: Hypotension, syncope, vascular anomaly, ventricular fibrillation.
Nervous: Cerebral ischemia, confusion, facial paralysis.
Respiratory: Lung edema.
Urogenital: Kidney failure, oliguria.

DOSAGE AND ADMINISTRATION

The recommended dosage of bivalirudin is an intravenous (IV) bolus dose of 1.0 mg/kg followed by a 4 hour IV infusion at a rate of 2.5 mg/kg/h. After completion of the initial 4 hour infusion, an additional IV infusion of bivalirudin may be initiated at a rate of 0.2 mg/kg/h for up to 20 hours, if needed. Bivalirudin is intended for use with aspirin (300-325 mg daily) and has been studied only in patients receiving concomitant aspirin. Treatment with bivalirudin should be initiated just prior to PTCA. The dose of bivalirudin may need to be reduced, and anticoagulation status monitored, in patients with renal impairment (see CLINICAL PHARMACOLOGY, Pharmacokinetics).

INSTRUCTIONS FOR ADMINISTRATION

Bivalirudin is intended for IV injection and infusion. To each 250 mg vial add 5 ml of sterile water for injection. Gently swirl until all material is dissolved. Each reconstituted vial should be further diluted in 50 ml of 5% dextrose in water or 0.9% sodium chloride for injection to yield a final concentration of 5 mg/ml (*e.g.,* 1 vial in 50 ml; 2 vials in 100 ml; 5 vials in 250 ml). The dose to be administered is adjusted according to the patient's weight (see TABLE 5).

If the low-rate infusion is used after the initial infusion, a lower concentration bag should be prepared. In order to prepare this bag, reconstitute the 250 mg vial with 5 ml of sterile water for injection. Gently swirl until all material is dissolved. Each reconstituted vial should be further diluted in 500 ml of 5% dextrose in water or 0.9% sodium chloride for injection to yield a final concentration of 0.5 mg/ml. The infusion rate to be administered should be selected from the right-hand column in TABLE 5.

TABLE 5 *Dosing Table*

		Using 5 mg/ml Concentration	Using 0.5 mg/ml Concentration
Weight	Bolus (1 mg/kg)	Initial 4 Hour Infusion (2.5 mg/kg/h)	Subsequent Low-Rate Infusion (0.2 mg/kg/h)
43-47 kg	9 ml	22.5 ml/h	18 ml/h
48-52 kg	10 ml	25 ml/h	20 ml/h
53-57 kg	11 ml	27.5 ml/h	22 ml/h
58-62 kg	12 ml	30 ml/h	24 ml/h
63-67 kg	13 ml	32.5 ml/h	26 ml/h
68-72 kg	14 ml	35 ml/h	28 ml/h
73-77 kg	15 ml	37.5 ml/h	30 ml/h
78-82 kg	16 ml	40 ml/h	32 ml/h
83-87 kg	17 ml	42.5 ml/h	34 ml/h
88-92 kg	18 ml	45 ml/h	36 ml/h
93-97 kg	19 ml	47.5 ml/h	38 ml/h
98-102 kg	20 ml	50 ml/h	40 ml/h
103-107 kg	21 ml	52.5 ml/h	42 ml/h
108-112 kg	22 ml	55 ml/h	44 ml/h
113-117 kg	23 ml	57.5 ml/h	46 ml/h
118-122 kg	24 ml	60 ml/h	48 ml/h
123-127 kg	25 ml	62.5 ml/h	50 ml/h
128-132 kg	26 ml	65 ml/h	52 ml/h
133-137 kg	27 ml	67.5 ml/h	54 ml/h
138-142 kg	28 ml	70 ml/h	56 ml/h
143-147 kg	29 ml	72.5 ml/h	58 ml/h
148-152 kg	30 ml	75 ml/h	60 ml/h

Bivalirudin should be administered via an IV line. No incompatibilities have been observed with glass bottles or polyvinyl chloride bags and administration sets. The following 9 drugs should not be administered in the same IV line with bivalirudin, since they resulted in haze formation, microparticulate formation, or gross precipitation when mixed with bivalirudin: alteplase, amiodarone HCl, amphotericin B, chlorpromazine HCl, diazepam, prochlorperazine edisylate, retaplase, streptokinase, and vancomycin HCl.

Parental drug products should be inspected visually for particulate matter and discoloration prior to administration. Preparations of bivalirudin containing particulate matter should not be used. Reconstituted material will be a clear to slightly opalescent, colorless to slightly yellow solution.

HOW SUPPLIED

Angiomax (bivalirudin) is supplied as a sterile, lyophilized product in single-use, glass vials. After reconstitution, each vial delivers 250 mg of bivalirudin.

Storage: Store Angiomax dosage units at 20-25°C (68-77°F). Excursions to 15-30°C permitted.

Storage after reconstitution: Do not freeze the reconstituted or diluted Angiomax. Reconstituted material may be stored at 2-8°C for up to 24 hours. Diluted Angiomax with a concentration between 0.5 and 5 mg/ml is stable at room temperature for up to 24 hours. Discard any unused portion of reconstituted solution remaining in the vial.

PRODUCT LISTING - EQUIVALENTS NOT AVAILABLE

Powder For Injection - Intravenous - 250 mg

10's $4187.50 ANGIOMAX, The Medicines Company 65293-0001-01

B

Bleomycin Sulfate (000506)

Categories: Carcinoma, cervical; Carcinoma, embryonal cell; Carcinoma, head and neck; Carcinoma, penile; Carcinoma, testicular; Carcinoma, vulvar; Choriocarcinoma; Lymphoma, Hodgkin's; Lymphosarcoma; Pleural effusion, malignant; Sarcoma, reticulum cell; Teratocarcinoma; FDA Approved 1973 Jul; Orphan Drugs; Pregnancy Category D; WHO Formulary
Drug Classes: Antineoplastics, antibiotics; Sclerosing agents
Brand Names: **Blenoxane**
Foreign Brand Availability: Blanoxan (Mexico); Bleocin (Czech-Republic; Greece; Hungary; India; Indonesia; Malaysia; Portugal; Taiwan); Bleolem (Mexico; Thailand); Bleomicina (Italy; Peru; Spain); Bleomycin (Austria; Bulgaria; Denmark; England; Finland; Israel; Netherlands; Norway; Sweden; Switzerland); Bleomycine (Belgium; France); Bleomycinum (Germany)
HCFA JCODE(S): J9040 15 units IM, IV, SC

WARNING

It is recommended that bleomycin sulfate be administered under the supervision of a qualified physician experienced in the use of cancer chemotherapeutic agents. Appropriate management of therapy and complications is possible only when adequate diagnostic and treatment facilities are readily available.

Pulmonary fibrosis is the most severe toxicity associated with bleomycin sulfate. The most frequent presentation is pneumonitis occasionally progressing to pulmonary fibrosis. Its occurrence is higher in elderly patients and in those receiving greater than 400 units total dose, but pulmonary toxicity has been observed in young patients and these treated with low doses.

A severe idiosyncratic reaction consisting of hypotension, mental confusion, fever, chills, and wheezing has been reported in approximately 1% of lymphoma patients treated with bleomycin sulfate.

DESCRIPTION

Blenoxane is a mixture of cytotoxic glycopeptide antibiotics isolated from a strain of *Streptomyces verticillus.* It is freely soluble in water.

Note: A unit of bleomycin is equal to the formerly used milligram activity. The term milligram activity is a misnomer and was changed to units to be more precise.

CLINICAL PHARMACOLOGY

Although the exact mechanism of action of bleomycin sulfate is unknown, available evidence would seem to indicate that the main mode of action is the inhibition of DNA synthesis with some evidence of lesser inhibition of RNA and protein synthesis.

In mice, high concentrations of bleomycin sulfate are found in the skin, lungs, kidneys, peritoneum and lymphatics. Tumor cells of the skin and lungs have been found to have high concentrations of bleomycin sulfate in contrast to the low concentrations found in hematopoietic tissue. The low concentrations of bleomycin sulfate found in bone marrow may be related to high levels of bleomycin sulfate degradative enzymes found in that tissue.

In patients with normal renal function, 60-70% of an administered dose is recovered in the urine as active bleomycin. In patients with a creatinine clearance of >35 ml/min, the serum or plasma terminal elimination half-life of bleomycin is approximately 115 minutes. In patients with a creatinine clearance of <35 ml/min, the plasma or serum terminal elimination half-life increases exponentially as the creatinine clearance decreases. It was reported that patients with moderately severe renal failure excreted less than 20% of the dose in the urine. This result would suggest that severe renal impairment could lead to accumulation of the drug in blood.

Information on the dose proportionality of bleomycin is not available.

When administered intrapluerally for the treatment of malignant pleural effusion, bleomycin acts as a sclerosing agent.

Following intrapleural administration to a limited number of patients (n=4), the resultant bleomycin plasma concentrations suggest a systemic absorbtion of approximately 45%.

The safety and efficacy of bleomycin and tetracycline (1 g) as treatment for malignant pleural effusion were evaluated in a multicenter, randomized trial. Patients were required to have cytologically positive pleural effusion, good performance status (0, 1, 2) lung re-expansion following tube thoracostomy with drainage rates of 100 ml/24 h or less, no prior intrapleural therapy, prior systemic bleomycin therapy, no chest irradiation and no recent change in systemic therapy. Overall survival did not differ between the bleomycin (n=44) and tetracycline (n=41) groups. Of patients evaluated within 30 days of instillation, the recurrence rate was 36% (10/28) with bleomycin and 67% (18/27) with tetracycline (p=0.023). Toxicity was similar between groups.

INDICATIONS AND USAGE

Bleomycin sulfate should be considered a palliative treatment. It has been shown to be useful in the management of the following neoplasms either as a single agent or in proven combinations with other approved chemotherapeutic agents:

Squamous Cell Carcinoma: Head and neck (including mouth, tongue, tonsil, nasopharynx, oropharynx, sinus, palate, lip, buccal mucosa, gingiva, epiglottis, skin, larynx), penis, cervix, and vulva. The response to bleomycin sulfate is poorer in patients with head and neck cancer previously irradiated.

Lymphomas: Hodgkin's, reticulum cell sarcoma, lymphosarcoma.

Testicular Carcinoma: Embryonal cell, choriocarcinoma, and teratocarcinoma.

Bleomycin sulfate has also been shown to be useful in the management of:

Malignant Pleural Effusion: Bleomycin sulfate is effective as a sclerosing agent for the treatment of malignant pleural effusion and prevention of recurrent pleural effusions.

NON-FDA APPROVED INDICATIONS

Bleomycin has been used without FDA approval for treatment of osteosarcoma, melanoma, and certain soft tissue sarcomas including Kaposi's sarcoma.

CONTRAINDICATIONS

Bleomycin sulfate is contraindicated in patients who have demonstrated a hypersensitive or an idiosyncratic reaction to it.

WARNINGS

Patients receiving bleomycin sulfate must be observed carefully and frequently during and after therapy. It should be used with extreme caution in patients with significant impairment of renal function or compromised pulmonary function.

Pulmonary toxicities occur in 10% of treated patients. In approximately 1% the nonspecific pneumonitis induced by bleomycin sulfate progresses to pulmonary fibrosis, and death. Although this is age and dose related, the toxicity is unpredictable. Frequent roentgenograms are recommended.

Idiosyncratic reactions similar to anaphylaxis have been reported in 1% of lymphoma patients treated with bleomycin sulfate. Since these usually occur after the first or second dose, careful monitoring is essential after these doses.

Renal or hepatic toxicity, beginning as a deterioration in renal or liver function tests, have been reported, infrequently. These toxicities may occur, however, at any time after initiation of therapy.

USE IN PREGNANCY

Bleomycin can cause fatal harm when administered to a pregnant woman. It has been shown to be teratogenic in rats. Administration of intraperitoneal doses of 1.5 mg/kg/day to rats (about 1.6 times the recommended human dose on a unit/m^2 basis) on days 5–15 of gestation caused skeletal malformations, shortened innominate artery and hydroureter. Bleomycin is abortifacient but not teratogenic in rabbits, at IV doses of 1.2 mg/kg/day (about 2.4 times the recommended human dose on a unit/m^2 basis) given on gestation days 6–18.

There have been no studies in pregnant women. If bleomycin is used during pregnancy, or if the patient becomes pregnant while receiving this drug, the patient should be apprised of the potential hazard to the fetus. Women of childbearing potential should be advised to avoid becoming pregnant during therapy with bleomycin.

ADVERSE REACTIONS

PULMONARY

This is potentially the most serious side effect, occurring in approximately 10% of treated patients. The most frequent presentation is pneumonitis occasionally progressing to pulmonary fibrosis. Approximately 1% of patients treated have died of pulmonary fibrosis. Pulmonary toxicity is both dose and age-related, being more common in patients over 70 years of age and in those receiving over 400 units total dose. This toxicity, however, is unpredictable and has been seen occasionally in young patients receiving low doses.

Because of lack of specificity of the clinical syndrome, the identification of patients with pulmonary toxicity due to bleomycin sulfate has been extremely difficult. The earliest symptom associated with bleomycin sulfate pulmonary toxicity is dyspnea. The earliest sign is fine rales.

Radiographically, bleomycin sulfate-induced pneumonitis produces nonspecific patchy opacities, usually of the lower lung fields. The most common changes in pulmonary function tests are a decrease in total lung volume and a decrease in vital capacity. However, these changes are not predictive of the development of pulmonary fibrosis.

The microscopic tissue changes due to bleomycin sulfate toxicity include bronchiolar squamous metaplasia, reactive macrophages, atypical alveolar epithelial cells, fibrinous edema, and interstitial fibrosis. The acute stage may involve capillary changes and subsequent fibrinous exudation into alveoli producing a change similar to hyaline membrane formation and progressing to a diffuse interstitial fibrosis resembling the Hamman-Rich syndrome. These microscopic findings are nonspecific, *e.g.,* similar changes are seen in radiation pneumonitis, pneumocystic pneumonitis.

To monitor the onset of pulmonary toxicity, roentgenograms of the chest should be taken every 1-2 weeks. If pulmonary changes are noted, treatment should be discontinued until it can be determined if they are drug related. Recent studies have suggested that sequential measurement of the pulmonary diffusion capacity for carbon monoxide [DL(∞)] during treatment with bleomycin sulfate may be an indicator of subclinical pulmonary toxicity. It is recommended that the DL(∞) be monitored monthly if it is to be employed to detect pulmonary toxicities, and thus the drug should be discontinued when the DL(∞) falls below 30-35% of the pretreatment value.

Because of bleomycin's sensitization of lung tissue, patients who have received bleomycin are at greater risk of developing pulmonary toxicity when oxygen is administered in surgery. While long exposure to very high oxygen concentrations is a known cause of lung damage, after bleomycin administration, lung damage can occur at lower concentrations that are usually considered safe. Suggested preventive measures are:

1. Maintain Fl O_2at concentrations approximating that of room air (25%) during surgery and the postoperative period.
2. Monitor carefully fluid replacement, focusing more on colloid administration than crystalloid.

Sudden onset of an acute chest pain syndrome suggestive of pleuropericarditis has been rarely reported during bleomycin sulfate infusions. Although each patient must be individually evaluated, further courses of bleomycin sulfate do not appear to be contraindicated.

IDIOSYNCRATIC REACTIONS

In approximately 1% of the lymphoma patients treated with bleomycin sulfate, an idiosyncratic reaction, similar to anaphylaxis clinically, has been reported. The reaction may be immediate or delayed for several hours, and usually occurs after the first or second dose. It consists of hypotension, mental confusion, fever, chills, and wheezing. Treatment is symptomatic including volume expansion, pressor agents, antihistamines and corticosteroids.

INTEGUMENT AND MUCOUS MEMBRANES

These are the most frequent side effects, being reported in approximately 50% of treated patients. These consist of erythema, rash, striae, vesiculation, hyperpigmentation, and tenderness of the skin. Hyperkeratosis, nail changes, alopecia, pruritus, and stomatitis have also been reported. It was necessary to discontinue bleomycin sulfate therapy in 2% of treated patients because of these toxicities.

Skin toxicity is a relatively late manifestation usually developing in the 2nd and 3rd week of treatment after 150-200 units of bleomycin sulfate has been administered and appears to be related to the cumulative dose.

OTHER

Vascular toxicities coincident with the use of bleomycin sulfate in combination with other antineoplastic agents have been reported rarely. The events are clinically heterogeneous and may include myocardial infarction, cerebrovascular accident, thrombotic microangiopathy (HUS) or cerebral arteritis. Various mechanisms have been proposed for these vascular complications. There are also reports of Raynaud's phenomenon occurring in patients treated with bleomycin sulfate in combination with vinblastine with or without cisplatin or, in a few cases, with bleomycin sulfate as a single agent. It is currently unknown if the case of Raynaud's phenomenon in these cases is the disease, underlying vascular compromise, bleomycin sulfate, vinblastine, hypomagnesemia, or a combination of any of these factors.

Fever, chills, and vomiting were frequently reported side effects. Anorexia and weight loss are common and may persist long after termination of this medication. Pain at tumor site, phlebitis, and other local reactions were reported infrequently.

DOSAGE AND ADMINISTRATION

DOSAGE

Because of the possibility of an anaphylactoid reaction, lymphoma patients should be treated with 2 units or less for the first 2 doses. If no acute reaction occurs, then the regular dosage schedule may be followed.

The following dose schedule is recommended:

Squamous Cell Carcinoma, Lymphosarcoma, Reticulum Cell Sarcoma, Testicular Carcinoma: 0.25- 0.50 units/kg (10-20 units/m^2) given intravenously, intramuscularly, or subcutaneously weekly or twice weekly.

Hodgkin's Disease: 0.25-0.50 units kg (10-20 units/m^2) given intravenously, intramuscularly, or subcutaneously weekly or twice weekly. After a 50% response, a maintenance dose of 1 units daily or 5 units weekly intravenously or intramuscularly should be given.

Pulmonary toxicity of bleomycin sulfate appears to be dose-related with a striking increase when the total dose is over 400 units. Total doses over 400 units should be given with great caution.

Note: When bleomycin sulfate is used in combination with other antineoplastic agents, pulmonary toxicities may occur at lower doses.

Improvement of Hodgkin's Disease and testicular tumors is prompt and noted within 2 weeks. If no improvement is seen by this time, improvement is unlikely. Squamous cell cancers respond more slowly, sometimes requiring as long as 3 weeks before any improvement is noted.

Malignant Pleural Effusion: 60 units administered as a single dose bolus intrapleural injection.

ADMINISTRATION

Bleomycin sulfate may be given by the intramuscular, intravenous, subcutaneous, intrapleural routes .

Intramuscular or Subcutaneous: The bleomycin 15 units vial should be reconstituted with 1-5 ml of sterile water for injection, sodium chloride for injection, 0.9%, or bacteriostatic water for injection. The bleomycin 30 units vial should be reconstituted with 2-10 ml of the above diluents.

Intravenous: The contents of the 15 or 30 units vial should be dissolved in 5 ml or 10 ml, respectively of sodium chloride for injection, 0.9% and administered slowly over a period of 10 minutes.

Intrapleural: 60 units of bleomycin is dissolved in 50–100 ml sodium chloride injection 0.9%, and administered through a thoracostomy tube following drainage of excess pleural fluid and confirmation of complete lung expansion. The literature suggests that successful pleurodesis is, in part, dependent upon complete drainage of the pleural fluid and reestablishment of negative intrapleural pressure prior to instillation of a sclerosing agent. Therefore, the amount of drainage from the chest tube should be as minimal as possible prior to instillaton of bleomycin. Although there is no conclusive evidence to support this contention, it is generally accepted that chest tube drainage should be less than 100 ml in a 24 hour period prior to sclerosis. However, bleomycin instillation may be appropriate when drainage is between 100–300 ml under clinical conditions that necessitate sclerosis therapy. The thoracostomy tube is clamped after bleomycin instillation. The patient is moved from the supine to the left and right lateral positions several times during the next 4 hours. The clamp is then removed and suction reestablished. The amount of time the chest tube remains in place following sclerosis is dictated by the clinical situation.

The intrapleural injection of topical anesthetics or systemic narcotic analgesia is generally not required. Parental drug products should be inspected visually for particulate matter and discoloration prior to administration, whenever solution and container permit.

STABILITY

The sterile powder is stable under refrigeration 2-8°C (36-46°F) and should not be used after the expiration date is reached.

Bleomycin should not be reconstituted or diluted with D_5W and analyzed by HPLC, bleomycin demonstrates a loss of A^2 and B^2 potency that does not occur when bleomycin is reconstituted in 0.9% sodium chloride.

Bleomycin sulfate is stable for 24 hours at room temperature in sodium chloride.

Procedures for proper handling and disposal of anticancer drugs should be considered. Several guidelines on this subject have been published.[1-7] There is no general agreement that all of the procedures recommended in the guidelines are necessary or appropriate.

PRODUCT LISTING - RATED THERAPEUTICALLY EQUIVALENT

Powder For Injection - Injectable - 15 U

1's	$177.19	GENERIC, Gensia Sicor Pharmaceuticals Inc	00703-3154-01
1's	$292.46	BLENOXANE, Bristol-Myers Squibb	00015-3010-20
1's	$309.00	GENERIC, Faulding Pharmaceutical Company	61703-0332-18

Powder For Injection - Injectable - 30 U

1's	$347.81	GENERIC, Gensia Sicor Pharmaceuticals Inc	00703-3155-01
1's	$584.93	BLENOXANE, Bristol-Myers Squibb	00015-3063-01
1's	$619.00	GENERIC, Faulding Pharmaceutical Company	61703-0323-22

PRODUCT LISTING - EQUIVALENTS NOT AVAILABLE

Powder For Injection - Injectable - 15 U

1's	$268.84	GENERIC, Abbott Pharmaceutical	00074-1616-01
1's	$292.46	BLENOXANE, Bristol-Myers Squibb	00015-3010-26
1's	$304.60	GENERIC, Bedford Laboratories	55390-0005-01

Powder For Injection - Injectable - 30 U

1's	$537.68	GENERIC, Abbott Pharmaceutical	00074-1636-01
1's	$584.93	BLENOXANE, Bristol-Myers Squibb	00015-3063-26

Bortezomib *(003598)*

Categories: Myeloma, multiple; Pregnancy Category D; FDA Approved 2003 May
Drug Classes: Antineoplastics, proteasome inhibitors
Brand Names: Velcade

DESCRIPTION

Velcade (bortezomib) for injection is an antineoplastic agent available for intravenous (IV) injection use only. Each single dose vial contains 3.5 mg of bortezomib as a sterile lyophilized powder. *Inactive ingredient:* 35 mg mannitol.

Bortezomib is a modified dipeptidyl boronic acid. The product is provided as a mannitol boronic ester which, in reconstituted form, consists of the mannitol ester in equilibrium with its hydrolysis product, the monomeric boronic acid. The drug substance exists in its cyclic anhydride form as a trimeric boroxine.

The chemical name for bortezomib, the monomeric boronic acid, is [(1R)-3-methyl-1-[[(2S)-1-oxo-3-phenyl-2-[(pyrazinylcarbonyl)amino]propyl]amino]butyl]boronic acid.

The molecular weight is 384.24. The molecular formula is: $C_{19}H_{25}BN_4O_4$. The solubility of bortezomib, as the monomeric boronic acid, in water is 3.3-3.8 mg/ml in a pH range of 2-6.5.

CLINICAL PHARMACOLOGY

MECHANISM OF ACTION

Bortezomib is a reversible inhibitor of the chymotrypsin-like activity of the 26S proteasome in mammalian cells. The 26S proteasome is a large protein complex that degrades ubiquitinated proteins. The ubiquitin-proteasome pathway plays an essential role in regulating the intracellular concentration of specific proteins, thereby maintaining homeostasis within cells. Inhibition of the 26S proteasome prevents this targeted proteolysis which can affect multiple signaling cascades within the cell. This disruption of normal homeostatic mechanisms can lead to cell death. Experiments have demonstrated that bortezomib is cytotoxic to a variety of cancer cell types *in vitro.* Bortezomib causes a delay in tumor growth *in vivo* in non-clinical tumor models, including multiple myeloma.

PHARMACOKINETICS

Following IV administration of 1.3 mg/m^2 dose, the median estimated maximum plasma concentration of bortezomib was 509 ng/ml (range = 109-1300 ng/ml) in 8 patients with multiple myeloma and creatinine clearance values ranging from 31-169 ml/min. The mean elimination half-life of bortezomib after first dose ranged from 9-15 hours at doses ranging from 1.45-2.00 mg/m^2 in patients with advanced malignancies. The pharmacokinetics of bortezomib as a single agent have not been fully characterized at the recommended dose in multiple myeloma patients.

Distribution

The distribution volume of bortezomib as a single agent was not assessed at the recommended dose in patients with multiple myeloma. The binding of bortezomib to human plasma proteins averaged 83% over the concentration range of 100-1000 ng/ml.

Metabolism

In vitro studies with human liver microsomes and human cDNA-expressed cytochrome P450 isozymes indicate that bortezomib is primarily oxidatively metabolized via cytochrome P450 enzymes, 3A4, 2D6, 2C19, 2C9, and 1A2. The major metabolic pathway is deboronation to form two deboronated metabolites that subsequently undergo hydroxylation to several metabolites. Deboronated-bortezomib metabolites are inactive as 26S proteasome inhibitors. Pooled plasma data from 8 patients at 10 and 30 minutes after dosing indicate that the plasma levels of metabolites are low compared to the parent drug.

Elimination

The pathways of elimination of bortezomib have not been characterized in humans.

SPECIAL POPULATIONS

Age, Gender, and Race: The effects of age, gender, and race on the pharmacokinetics of bortezomib have not been evaluated.

Hepatic Impairment: No pharmacokinetic studies were conducted with bortezomib in patients with hepatic impairment (see PRECAUTIONS).

Renal Impairment: No pharmacokinetic studies were conducted with bortezomib in patients with renal impairment. Clinical studies included patients with creatinine clearances values ranging from 13.8 to 220 ml/min (see PRECAUTIONS).

Pediatric: There are no pharmacokinetic data in pediatric patients.

DRUG INTERACTIONS

No formal drug interaction studies have been conducted with bortezomib.

In vitro studies with human liver microsomes indicate that bortezomib is a substrate of cytochrome P450 3A4, 2D6, 2C19, 2C9, and 1A2 (see PRECAUTIONS).

Bortezomib is a poor inhibitor of human liver microsome cytochrome P450 1A2, 2C9, 2D6, and 3A4, with IC_{50} values of >30 μM (>11.5 μg/ml). Bortezomib may inhibit 2C19 activity (IC_{50} = 18 μM, 6.9 μg/ml) and increase exposure to drugs that are substrates for this enzyme.

Bortezomib did not induce the activities of cytochrome P450 3A4 and 1A2 in primary cultured human hepatocytes.

INDICATIONS AND USAGE

Bortezomib for injection is indicated for the treatment of multiple myeloma patients who have received at least two prior therapies and have demonstrated disease progression on the last therapy.

The effectiveness of bortezomib is based on response rates. There are no controlled trials demonstrating a clinical benefit, such as an improvement in survival.

CONTRAINDICATIONS

Bortezomib is contraindicated in patients with hypersensitivity to bortezomib, boron or mannitol.

WARNINGS

Bortezomib should be administered under the supervision of a physician experienced in the use of antineoplastic therapy.

PREGNANCY CATEGORY D

Women of childbearing potential should avoid becoming pregnant while being treated with bortezomib.

Bortezomib was not teratogenic in nonclinical developmental toxicity studies in rats and rabbits at the highest dose tested (0.075 mg/kg; 0.5 mg/m^2 in the rat and 0.05 mg/kg; 0.6 mg/m^2 in the rabbit) when administered during organogenesis. These dosages are approximately half the clinical dose of 1.3 mg/m^2 based on body surface area.

Pregnant rabbits given bortezomib during organogenesis at a dose of 0.05 mg/kg (0.6 mg/m^2) experienced significant post-implantation loss and decreased number of live fetuses. Live fetuses from these litters also showed significant decreases in fetal weight. The dose is approximately 0.5 times the clinical dose of 1.3 mg/m^2 based on body surface area.

No placental transfer studies have been conducted with bortezomib. There are no adequate and well-controlled studies in pregnant women. If bortezomib is used during pregnancy, or if the patient becomes pregnant while receiving this drug, the patient should be apprised of the potential hazard to the fetus.

PRECAUTIONS

PERIPHERAL NEUROPATHY

Bortezomib treatment causes a peripheral neuropathy that is predominantly sensory, although cases of mixed sensori-motor neuropathy have also been reported. Patients with pre-existing symptoms (numbness, pain or a burning feeling in the feet or hands) and/or signs of peripheral neuropathy may experience worsening during treatment with bortezomib. Patients should be monitored for symptoms of neuropathy, such as a burning sensation, hyperesthesia, hypesthesia, paresthesia, discomfort or neuropathic pain. Patients experiencing new or worsening peripheral neuropathy may require change in the dose and schedule of bortezomib (see DOSAGE AND ADMINISTRATION). Limited follow-up data regarding the outcome of peripheral neuropathy are available. Of the patients who experienced treatment emergent neuropathy more than 70% had previously been treated with neurotoxic agents and more than 80% of these patients had signs or symptoms of peripheral neuropathy at baseline (also see ADVERSE REACTIONS).

HYPOTENSION

Bortezomib treatment can cause orthostatic/postural hypotension in about 12% of patients. These events are observed throughout therapy. Caution should be used when treating patients with a history of syncope, patients receiving medications known to be associated with hypotension, and patients who are dehydrated. Management of orthostatic/postural hypotension may include adjustment of antihypertensive medications, hydration, or administration of mineralocorticoids.

GASTROINTESTINAL ADVERSE EVENTS

Bortezomib treatment can cause nausea, diarrhea, constipation, and vomiting (see ADVERSE REACTIONS) sometimes requiring use of antiemetics and antidiarrheals. Fluid and electrolyte replacement should be administered to prevent dehydration.

THROMBOCYTOPENIA

Thrombocytopenia, which occurred in about 40% of patients throughout therapy, was maximal at Day 11 and usually recovered by the next cycle. Complete blood counts including platelet counts should be frequently monitored throughout treatment. Onset is most common in Cycles 1 and 2 but can continue throughout therapy. There have been reports of gastrointestinal and intracerebral hemorrhage in association with bortezomib induced thrombocytopenia. Bortezomib treatment may be temporarily discontinued if patients experience Grade 4 thrombocytopenia. Bortezomib may be reinitiated at a reduced dose after resolution of thrombocytopenia (see DOSAGE AND ADMINISTRATION and ADVERSE REACTIONS).

PATIENTS WITH HEPATIC IMPAIRMENT

Bortezomib is metabolized by liver enzymes and bortezomib's clearance may decrease in patients with hepatic impairment. These patients should be closely monitored for toxicities when treated with bortezomib. (See CLINICAL PHARMACOLOGY, Special Populations.)

PATIENTS WITH RENAL IMPAIRMENT

No clinical information is available on the use of bortezomib in patients with creatinine clearance values less than 13 ml/min and patients on hemodialysis. These patients should be closely monitored for toxicities when treated with bortezomib (see CLINICAL PHARMACOLOGY, Special Populations).

ANIMAL TOXICITY FINDINGS

Cardiovascular Toxicity

Studies in monkeys showed that administration of dosages approximately twice the recommended clinical dose resulted in heart rate elevations, followed by profound progressive hypotension, bradycardia, and death 12-14 hours post dose. Doses ≥1.2 mg/m^2 induced dose proportional changes in cardiac parameters. Bortezomib has been shown to distribute to most tissues in the body, including the myocardium. In a repeated dosing toxicity study in the monkey, myocardial hemorrhage, inflammation, and necrosis were also observed.

Chronic Administration

In animal studies at a dose and schedule similar to that recommended for patients (twice weekly dosing for 2 weeks followed by 1 week rest) toxicities observed included severe anemia and thrombocytopenia, gastrointestinal, neurological and lymphoid system toxicities. Neurotoxic effects of bortezomib in animal studies included axonal swelling and degeneration in peripheral nerves, dorsal spinal roots, and tracts of the spinal cord. Additionally, multifocal hemorrhage and necrosis in the brain, eye, and heart were observed.

INFORMATION FOR THE PATIENT

Physicians are advised to discuss the following with patients to whom bortezomib will be administered.

Effects on ability to drive or operate machinery or impairment of mental ability: Since bortezomib may be associated with fatigue, dizziness, syncope, orthostatic/postural hypotension, diplopia or blurred vision, patients should be cautious when operating machinery, including automobiles.

Pregnancy/nursing: Patients should be advised to use effective contraceptive measures to prevent pregnancy and to avoid breast feeding during treatment with bortezomib.

Dehydration/hypotension: Since patients receiving bortezomib therapy may experience vomiting and/or diarrhea, patients should be advised regarding appropriate measures to avoid dehydration. Patients should be instructed to seek medical advice if they experience symptoms of dizziness, light headedness or fainting spells.

Concomitant medications: Patients should be cautioned about the use of concomitant medications that may be associated with peripheral neuropathy (such as amiodarone, anti-virals, isoniazid, nitrofurantoin, or statins), or with a decrease in blood pressure.

Peripheral neuropathy: Patients should be instructed to contact their physician if they experience new or worsening symptoms of peripheral neuropathy (see PRECAUTIONS and DOSAGE AND ADMINISTRATION).

DRUG/LABORATORY TEST INTERACTIONS

None known.

CARCINOGENESIS, MUTAGENESIS, AND IMPAIRMENT OF FERTILITY

Carcinogenicity studies have not been conducted with bortezomib.

Bortezomib showed clastogenic activity (structural chromosomal aberrations) in the *in vitro* chromosomal aberration assay using Chinese hamster ovary cells. Bortezomib was not genotoxic when tested in the *in vitro* mutagenicity assay (Ames test) and *in vivo* micronucleus assay in mice.

Fertility studies with bortezomib were not performed but evaluation of reproductive tissues has been performed in the general toxicity studies. In the 6 month rat toxicity study, degenerative effects in the ovary were observed at doses ≥0.3 mg/m^2 (one-fourth of the recommended clinical dose), and degenerative changes in the testes occurred at 1.2 mg/m^2. Bortezomib could have a potential effect on either male or female fertility.

PREGNANCY CATEGORY D

See WARNINGS.

NURSING MOTHERS

It is not known whether bortezomib is excreted in human milk. Because many drugs are excreted in human milk and because of the potential for serious adverse reactions in nursing infants from bortezomib, women should be advised against breast feeding while being treated with bortezomib.

PEDIATRIC USE

The safety and effectiveness of bortezomib in children has not been established.

GERIATRIC USE

Of the 202 patients enrolled, 35% were 65 years of age or older. Nineteen percent (19%) of patients aged 65 years or older experienced responses versus 32% in patients under the age of 65. Across the 256 patients analyzed for safety, the incidence of Grade 3 or 4 events reported was 74%, 80%, and 85% for patients ≤50 years, 51-65 years, and >65 years, respectively.

DRUG INTERACTIONS

No formal drug interaction studies have been conducted with bortezomib.

In vitro studies with human liver microsomes indicate that bortezomib is a substrate for cytochrome P450 3A4, 2D6, 2C19, 2C9, and 1A2. Patients who are concomitantly receiving bortezomib and drugs that are inhibitors or inducers of cytochrome P450 3A4 should be closely monitored for either toxicities or reduced efficacy (see CLINICAL PHARMACOLOGY, Drug Interactions).

During clinical trials, hypoglycemia and hyperglycemia were reported in diabetic patients receiving oral hypoglycemics. Patients on oral antidiabetic agents receiving bortezomib treatment may require close monitoring of their blood glucose levels and adjustment of the dose of their antidiabetic medication.

There have been several SAE reports since filing. These reports were submitted to the IND. If the Agency feels this information is unnecessary, the language can be removed.

ADVERSE REACTIONS

The two studies described evaluated 228 patients with multiple myeloma receiving bortezomib 1.3 mg/m^2/dose twice weekly for 2 weeks followed by a 10 day rest period (21 day treatment cycle length) for a maximum of 8 treatment cycles.

The most commonly reported adverse events were asthenic conditions (including fatigue, malaise and weakness) (65%), nausea (64%), diarrhea (51%), appetite decreased (including anorexia) (43%), constipation (43%), thrombocytopenia (43%), peripheral neuropathy (including peripheral sensory neuropathy and peripheral neuropathy aggravated) (37%), pyrexia (36%), vomiting (36%), and anemia (32%). Fourteen percent (14%) of patients experienced at least 1 episode of Grade 4 toxicity, with the most common toxicity being thrombocytopenia (3%) and neutropenia (3%).

SERIOUS ADVERSE EVENTS (SAES)

Serious Adverse Events are defined as any event, regardless of causality that: Results in death, is life-threatening, requires hospitalization or prolongs a current hospitalization, results in a significant disability or is deemed to be an important medical event. A total of 113 (50%) of the 228 patients experienced SAEs during the studies. The most commonly reported SAEs included pyrexia (7%), pneumonia (7%), diarrhea (6%), vomiting (5%), dehydration (5%), and nausea (4%).

Adverse events thought by the investigator to be drug-related and leading to discontinuation occurred in 18% of patients. The reasons for discontinuation included peripheral neuropathy (5%), thrombocytopenia (4%), diarrhea (2%), and fatigue (2%).

Two deaths were reported and considered by the investigator to be possibly related to study drug: 1 case of cardiopulmonary arrest and 1 case of respiratory failure.

The most common adverse events are shown in TABLE 3. All adverse events occurring at ≥10% are included. In the single arm studies conducted it is often not possible to distinguish adverse events that are drug-caused and those that reflect the patient's underlying disease. See discussion of specific adverse reactions following TABLE 3.

TABLE 3 *Most Commonly Reported (≥10% Overall) Adverse Events (n=228)*

	All Patients (n=228)		
Adverse Event	**All Events**	**Grade 3 Events**	**Grade 4 Events**
Asthenic conditions	149 (65%)	42 (18%)	1 (<1%)
Nausea	145 (64%)	13 (6%)	0
Diarrhea	116 (51%)	16 (7%)	2 (<1%)
Appetite decreased	99 (43%)	6 (3%)	0
Constipation	97 (43%)	5 (2%)	0
Thrombocytopenia	97 (43%)	61 (27%)	7 (3%)
Peripheral neuropathy	84 (37%)	31 (14%)	0
Pyrexia	82 (36%)	9 (4%)	0
Vomiting	82 (36%)	16 (7%)	1 (<1%)
Anemia	74 (32%)	21 (9%)	0
Headache	63 (28%)	8 (4%)	0
Insomnia	62 (27%)	3 (1%)	0
Arthralgia	60 (26%)	11 (5%)	0
Pain in limb	59 (26%)	16 (7%)	0
Edema	58 (35%)	3 (1%)	0
Neutropenia	55 (24%)	30 (13%)	6 (3%)
Paresthesia and dysesthesia	53 (23%)	6 (3%)	0
Dyspnea	50 (22%)	7 (3%)	1 (<1%)
Dizziness (excluding vertigo)	48 (21%)	3 (1%)	0
Rash	47 (21%)	1 (<1%)	0
Dehydration	42 (18%)	15 (7%)	0
Upper respiratory tract infection	41 (18%)	0	0
Cough	39 (17%)	1 (<1%)	0
Bone pain	33 (14%)	5 (2%)	0
Anxiety	32 (14%)	0	0
Myalgia	32 (14%)	5 (2%)	0
Back pain	31 (14%)	9 (4%)	0
Muscle cramps	31 (14%)	1 (<1%)	0
Dyspepsia	30 (13%)	0	0
Abdominal pain	29 (13%)	5 (2%)	0
Dysgeusia	29 (13%)	1 (<1%)	0
Hypotension	27 (12%)	8 (4%)	0
Rigors	27 (12%)	1 (<1%)	0
Herpes zoster	26 (11%)	2 (<1%)	0
Pruritus	26 (11%)	0	0
Vision blurred	25 (11%)	1 (<1%)	0
Pneumonia	23 (10%)	12 (5%)	0

Asthenic Conditions (fatigue, malaise, weakness)

Asthenia was reported in 65% of patients and was predominantly reported as Grade 1 or 2. The first onset of fatigue was most often reported during the 1st and 2nd cycles of therapy. Asthenia was Grade 3 for 18% of patients. Two percent (2%) of patients discontinued treatment due to fatigue.

Gastrointestinal Events

The majority of patients experienced gastrointestinal adverse events during the studies, including nausea, diarrhea, constipation, and vomiting. Grade 3 or 4 gastrointestinal events occurred in 21% of patients and were considered serious in 13% of patients. Vomiting and diarrhea each were of Grade 3 severity in 7% of patients and were Grade 4 in <1%. Five percent (5%) of patients discontinued due to gastrointestinal events. Appetite decreased (anorexia) was reported as an adverse event for 43% of patients. The incidence of Grade 3 decreased appetite was 3%.

Thrombocytopenia

Thrombocytopenia was reported during treatment with bortezomib for 43% of patients. The thrombocytopenia was characterized by a dose related decrease in platelet count during the bortezomib dosing period (Days 1-11) with a return to baseline in platelet count during the rest period (Days 12-21) in each treatment cycle. Thrombocytopenia was Grade 3 or 4 in intensity for 27% and 3% respectively of patients. Four percent (4%) of patients discontinued bortezomib treatment due to thrombocytopenia of any grade.

Peripheral Sensory Neuropathy

Events reported as peripheral neuropathy, peripheral sensory neuropathy, and peripheral neuropathy aggravated occurred in 37% of patients. Peripheral neuropathy was Grade 3 for 14% of patients with no Grade 4 events. New onset or worsening of existing neuropathy was noted throughout the cycles of treatment. Six percent (6%) of patients discontinued bortezomib due to neuropathy. More than 80% of all study patients had signs or symptoms of peripheral neuropathy at baseline evaluation. The incidence of Grade 3 neuropathy was 5% (2 of 41 patients) in patients without baseline neuropathy. Symptoms may improve or return to baseline in some patients upon discontinuation of bortezomib. The complete time-course of this toxicity has not been fully characterized.

Pyrexia

Pyrexia (>38°C) was reported as an adverse event for 36% of patients and was assessed as Grade 3 in 4% of patients.

Neutropenia

Neutropenia occurred in 24% of patients and was Grade 3 in 13% and Grade 4 in 3%. The incidence of febrile neutropenia was <1%.

Hypotension

Hypotension (including reports of orthostatic hypotension) was reported in 12% of patients. Most events were Grade 1 or 2 in severity. Grade 3 hypotension occurred in 4% of patients; no patient experienced Grade 4 hypotension. Patients developing orthostatic hypotension did not have evidence of orthostatic hypotension at study entry; half had pre-existing hypertension and one-third had evidence of peripheral neuropathy. Doses of antihypertensive medications may need to be adjusted in patients receiving bortezomib. Four percent (4%) of patients experienced hypotension, including orthostatic hypotension, and had a concurrent syncopal event.

SERIOUS ADVERSE EVENTS FROM CLINICAL STUDIES

In approximately 580 patients, the following serious adverse events (not described above) were reported, considered at least possibly related to study medication, in at least 1 patient treated with bortezomib administered as monotherapy or in combination with other chemotherapeutics. These studies were conducted in patients with hematological malignancies and in solid tumors.

Blood and Lymphatic System Disorders: Disseminated intravascular coagulation.

Cardiac Disorders: Atrial fibrillation aggravated, atrial flutter, cardiac amyloidosis, cardiac arrest, cardiac failure congestive, myocardial ischemia, myocardial infarction, pericardial effusion, pulmonary edema, ventricular tachycardia.

Gastrointestinal Disorders: Ascites, dysphagia, fecal impaction, gastritis hemorrhagic, gastrointestinal hemorrhage, hematemesis, ileus paralytic, large intestinal obstruction, paralytic intestinal obstruction, small intestinal obstruction, large intestinal perforation, stomatitis, melena, pancreatitis acute.

Hepatobiliary: Hyperbilirubinemia, portal vein thrombosis.

Immune System Disorders: Anaphylactic reaction, drug hypersensitivity, immune complex mediated hypersensitivity.

Infections and Infestations: Bacteremia.

Injury, Poisoning and Procedural Complications: Skeletal fracture, subdural hematoma.

Metabolism and Nutrition Disorders: Hypocalcemia, hyperuricemia, hypokalemia, hyponatremia, tumor lysis syndrome.

Nervous System: Ataxia, coma, dizziness, dysarthria, dysautonomia, cranial palsy, grand mal convulsion, hemorrhagic stroke, motor dysfunction, spinal cord compression, transient ischemic attack.

Psychiatric: Agitation, confusion, psychotic disorder, suicidal ideation.

Renal and Urinary: Calculus renal, bilateral hydronephrosis, bladder spasm, hematuria urinary incontinence, urinary retention, renal failure, acute and chronic, glomerular nephritis proliferative.

Respiratory, Thoracic and Mediastinal: Acute respiratory distress syndrome, atelectasis, chronic obstructive airways disease exacerbated, dysphagia, dyspnea, dyspnea exertional, epistaxis, hemoptysis, hypoxia, lung infiltration, pleural effusion, pneumonitis, respiratory distress, respiratory failure.

Vascular: Cerebrovascular accident, deep venous thrombosis, peripheral embolism, pulmonary embolism.

DOSAGE AND ADMINISTRATION

The recommended dose of bortezomib is 1.3 mg/m^2/dose administered as a bolus IV injection twice weekly for 2 weeks (Days 1, 4, 8, and 11) followed by a 10 day rest period (Days 12-21).

This 3 week period is considered a treatment cycle. At least 72 hours should elapse between consecutive doses of bortezomib.

DOSE MODIFICATION AND REINITIATION OF THERAPY

Bortezomib therapy should be withheld at the onset of any Grade 3 non-hematological or Grade 4 hematological toxicities excluding neuropathy as discussed below (see PRECAUTIONS). Once the symptoms of the toxicity have resolved, bortezomib therapy may be reinitiated at a 25% reduced dose (1.3 mg/m^2/dose reduced to 1.0 mg/m^2/dose; 1.0 mg/m^2/dose reduced to 0.7 mg/m^2/dose). TABLE 4 contains the recommended dose modification for the management of patients who experience bortezomib-related neuropathic pain and/or peripheral sensory neuropathy (TABLE 4). Patients with pre-existing severe neuropathy should be treated with bortezomib only after careful risk/benefit assessment.

ADMINISTRATION PRECAUTIONS

Bortezomib is an antineoplastic. Caution should be used during handling and preparation. Proper aseptic technique should be used. Use of gloves and other protective clothing to

B

TABLE 4 *Recommended Dose Modification for Bortezomib-Related Neuropathic Pain and/or Peripheral Sensory Neuropathy*

Severity of Peripheral Neuropathy Signs and Symptoms	Modification of Dose and Regimen
Grade 1 (paresthesias and/or loss of reflexes) without pain or loss of function	No action
Grade 1 with pain or Grade 2 (interfering with function but not with activities of daily living)	Reduce bortezomib to 1.0 mg/m^2
Grade 2 with pain or Grade 3 (interfering with activities of daily living)	Withhold bortezomib therapy until toxicity resolves. When toxicity resolves reinitiate with a reduced dose of bortezomib at 0.7 mg/m^2 and change treatment schedule to once/week.
Grade 4 (permanent sensory loss that interferes with function)	Discontinue bortezomib

NCI Common Toxicity Criteria website — http://ctep.info.nih.gov/reporting/ctc.html.

prevent skin contact is recommended. In clinical trials, local skin irritation was reported in 5% of patients, but extravasation of bortezomib was not associated with tissue damage.

RECONSTITUTION/PREPARATION FOR IV ADMINISTRATION

Prior to use, the contents of each vial must be reconstituted with 3.5 ml of normal (0.9%) saline, sodium chloride injection. The reconstituted product should be a clear and colorless solution.

Parenteral drug products should be inspected visually for particulate matter and discoloration prior to administration whenever solution and container permit. If any discoloration or particulate matter is observed, the reconstituted product should not be used.

STABILITY

Unopened vials of bortezomib are stable until the date indicated on the package when stored in the original package protected from light.

Bortezomib contains no antimicrobial preservative. When reconstituted as directed, bortezomib may be stored at 25°C (77°F); excursions permitted from 15-30°C (59-86°F). Reconstituted bortezomib should be administered within 8 hours of preparation. The reconstituted material may be stored in the original vial and/or the syringe prior to administration. The product may be stored for up to 3 hours in a syringe, however total storage time for the reconstituted material must not exceed 8 hours when exposed to normal indoor lighting.

HOW SUPPLIED

Velcade (bortezomib) for injection is supplied as individually cartoned 10 ml vials containing 3.5 mg of bortezomib as a white to off-white cake or powder.

Storage: Unopened vials may be stored at controlled room temperature 25°C (77°F); excursions permitted from 15-30°C (59-86°F). Retain in original package to protect from light.

Bosentan *(003537)*

Categories: Hypertension, pulmonary; Pregnancy Category X; FDA Approved 2001 Nov; Orphan Drugs
Drug Classes: Endothelin receptor antagonist
Brand Names: Tracleer
Cost of Therapy: \$2,970.00 (Pulmonary HTN (initial); Tracleer; 62.5 mg; 2 tablets/day; 30 day supply)
\$2,970.00 (Pulmonary HTN (maintenance); Tracleer; 125 mg; 2 tablets/day; 30 day supply)

WARNING

Use of bosentan requires attention to two significant concerns: (1) potential for serious liver injury, and (2) potential damage to a fetus.

WARNING: Potential Liver Injury

Bosentan causes at least 3-fold (upper limit of normal; ULN) elevation of liver aminotransferases (ALT and AST) in about 11% of patients, accompanied by elevated bilirubin in a small number of cases. Because these changes are a marker for potential serious liver injury, serum aminotransferase levels must be measured prior to initiation of treatment and then monthly (see WARNINGS, Potential Liver Injury and DOSAGE AND ADMINISTRATION). To date, in a setting of close monitoring, elevations have been reversible, within a few days to 9 weeks, either spontaneously or after dose reduction or discontinuation, and without sequelae.

Elevations in aminotransferases require close attention (see DOSAGE AND ADMINISTRATION). Bosentan should generally be avoided in patients with elevated aminotransferases (>3 × ULN) at baseline because monitoring liver injury may be more difficult.

If liver aminotransferase elevations are accompanied by clinical symptoms of liver injury (such as nausea, vomiting, fever, abdominal pain, jaundice, or unusual lethargy or fatigue) or increases in bilirubin ≥2 × ULN, treatment should be stopped. There is no experience with the re-introduction of bosentan in these circumstances.

CONTRAINDICATION: Pregnancy

Bosentan is very likely to produce major birth defects if used by pregnant women, as this effect has been seen consistently when it is administered to animals (see CONTRAINDICATIONS). Therefore, pregnancy must be excluded before the start of treatment with bosentan and prevented thereafter by the use of a reliable method of contraception. Hormonal contraceptives, including oral, injectable and implantable contraceptives should not be used as the sole means of contraception because these may not be effective in patients receiving bosentan (see DRUG INTERACTIONS). Monthly pregnancy tests should be obtained.

WARNING — *Cont'd*

Because of potential liver injury and in an effort to make the chance of fetal exposure to bosentan as small as possible, bosentan may be prescribed only through the Tracleer (bosentan) Access Program by calling 1-866-228-3546. Adverse events can also be reported directly via this number.

DESCRIPTION

Bosentan is the first of a new drug class, an endothelin receptor antagonist.

Bosentan belongs to a class of highly substituted pyrimidine derivatives, with no chiral centers. It is designated chemically as 4-tert-butyl-N-[6-(2-hydroxy-ethoxy)-5-(2-methoxy-phenoxy)-[2,2′]-bipyrimidin-4-yl]-benzenesulfonamide monohydrate.

Bosentan has a molecular weight of 569.64 and a molecular formula of $C_{27}H_{29}N_5O_6S{\cdot}H_2O$. Bosentan is a white to yellowish powder. It is poorly soluble in water (1.0 mg/100 ml) and in aqueous solutions at low pH (0.1 mg/100 ml at pH 1.1 and 4.0; 0.2 mg/100 ml at pH 5.0). Solubility increases at higher pH values (43 mg/100 ml at pH 7.5). In the solid state, bosentan is very stable, is not hygroscopic and is not light sensitive.

Bosentan is available as 62.5 and 125 mg film-coated tablets for oral administration, and contains the following excipients: corn starch, pregelatinized starch, sodium starch glycolate, povidone, glyceryl behenate, magnesium stearate, hydroxypropylmethylcellulose, triacetin, talc, titanium dioxide, iron oxide yellow, iron oxide red, and ethylcellulose. Each Tracleer 62.5 mg tablet contains 64.541 mg of bosentan, equivalent to 62.5 mg of anhydrous bosentan. Each Tracleer 125 mg tablet contains 129.082 mg of bosentan, equivalent to 125 mg of anhydrous bosentan.

CLINICAL PHARMACOLOGY

MECHANISM OF ACTION

Endothelin-1 (ET-1) is a neurohormone, the effects of which are mediated by binding to ET_A and ET_B receptors in the endothelium and vascular smooth muscle. ET-1 concentrations are elevated in plasma and lung tissue of patients with pulmonary arterial hypertension, suggesting a pathogenic role for ET-1 in this disease. Bosentan is a specific and competitive antagonist at endothelin receptor types ET_A and ET_B. Bosentan has a slightly higher affinity for ET_A receptors than for ET_B receptors.

PHARMACOKINETICS

General

After oral administration, maximum plasma concentrations of bosentan are attained within 3-5 hours and the terminal elimination half-life ($T_{1/2}$) is about 5 hours. Pharmacokinetics of bosentan was not studied in patients with pulmonary arterial hypertension, but exposure is expected to be greater in such patients because increased (30-40%) bosentan exposure was observed in patients with severe chronic heart failure.

Absorption and Distribution

The absolute bioavailability of bosentan in normal volunteers is about 50% and is unaffected by food. The volume of distribution is about 18 L. Bosentan is highly bound (>98%) to plasma proteins, mainly albumin. Bosentan does not penetrate into erythrocytes.

Metabolism and Elimination

Bosentan has three metabolites, one of which is pharmacologically active and may contribute 10-20% of the effect of bosentan. Bosentan is an inducer of CYP2C9 and CYP3A4 and possibly also of CYP2C19. Total clearance after a single intravenous (IV) dose is about 8 L/h. Upon multiple dosing, plasma concentrations decrease gradually to 50-65% of those seen after single dose administration, probably the effect of auto-induction of the metabolizing liver enzymes. Steady-state is reached within 3-5 days. Bosentan is eliminated by biliary excretion following metabolism in the liver. Less than 3% of an administered oral dose is recovered in urine.

Special Populations

It is not known whether bosentan pharmacokinetics is influenced by gender, body weight, race, or age.

Liver Function Impairment

The influence of liver impairment on the pharmacokinetics of bosentan has not been evaluated, but *in vitro* and *in vivo* evidence showing extensive hepatic metabolism of bosentan suggests that liver impairment would significantly increase exposure of bosentan. Caution should be exercised during the use of bosentan in patients with mildly impaired liver function. Bosentan should generally be avoided in patients with moderate or severe liver abnormalities and/or elevated aminotransferases >3 × ULN (see DOSAGE AND ADMINISTRATION).

Renal Impairment

In patients with severe renal impairment (creatinine clearance 15-30 ml/min), plasma concentrations of bosentan were essentially unchanged and plasma concentrations of the three metabolites were increased about 2-fold compared to people with normal renal function. These differences do not appear to be clinically important (see DOSAGE AND ADMINISTRATION).

INDICATIONS AND USAGE

Bosentan is indicated for the treatment of pulmonary arterial hypertension in patients with WHO Class III or IV symptoms, to improve exercise ability and decrease the rate of clinical worsening.

CONTRAINDICATIONS

See BOXED WARNING for **CONTRAINDICATION** to use in pregnancy.

B

PREGNANCY CATEGORY X

Bosentan is expected to cause fetal harm if administered to pregnant women. Bosentan was teratogenic in rats given oral doses ≥60 mg/kg/day (twice the maximum recommended human oral dose of 125 mg, bid, on a mg/m^2 basis). In an embryo-fetal toxicity study in rats, bosentan showed dose-dependent teratogenic effects, including malformations of the head, mouth, face and large blood vessels. Bosentan increased stillbirths and pup mortality at oral doses of 60 and 300 mg/kg/day (2 and 10 times, respectively, the maximum recommended human dose on a mg/m^2 basis). Although birth defects were not observed in rabbits given oral doses of up to 1500 mg/kg/day, plasma concentrations of bosentan in rabbits were lower than those reached in the rat. The similarity of malformations induced by bosentan and those observed in endothelin-1 knockout mice and in animals treated with other endothelin receptor antagonists indicates that teratogenicity is a class effect of these drugs. There are no data on the use of bosentan in pregnant women.

Pregnancy must be excluded before the start of treatment with bosentan and prevented thereafter by use of reliable contraception. Hormonal contraceptives, including oral, injectable, and implantable contraceptives may not be reliable in the presence of bosentan and should not be used as the sole contraceptive method in patients receiving bosentan (see DRUG INTERACTIONS, Hormonal Contraceptives, Including Oral, Injectable, and Implantable Contraceptives). Input from a gynecologist or similar expert on adequate contraception should be sought as needed.

Bosentan should be started only in patients known not to be pregnant. For female patients of childbearing potential, a prescription for bosentan should not be issued by the prescriber unless the patient assures the prescriber that she is not sexually active or provides negative results from a urine or serum pregnancy test performed during the first 5 days of a normal menstrual period and at least 11 days after the last unprotected act of sexual intercourse.

Follow-up urine or serum pregnancy tests should be obtained monthly in women of childbearing potential taking bosentan. The patient must be advised that if there is any delay in onset of menses or any other reason to suspect pregnancy, she must notify the physician immediately for pregnancy testing. If the pregnancy test is positive, the physician and patient must discuss the risk to the pregnancy and to the fetus.

CYCLOSPORINE A

Co-administration of cyclosporine A and bosentan resulted in markedly increased plasma concentrations of bosentan. Therefore, concomitant use of bosentan and cyclosporine A is contraindicated.

GLYBURIDE

An increased risk of liver enzyme elevations was observed in patients receiving glyburide concomitantly with bosentan. Therefore co-administration of glyburide and bosentan is contraindicated.

HYPERSENSITIVITY

Bosentan is also contraindicated in patients who are hypersensitive to bosentan or any component of the medication.

WARNINGS

POTENTIAL LIVER INJURY

See BOXED WARNING.

Elevations in ALT or AST by more than 3 × ULN were observed in 11% of bosentan-treated patients (n=658) compared to 2% of placebo-treated patients (n=280). Three-fold increases were seen in 12% of 95 PAH patients on 125 mg bid and 14% of 70 PAH patients on 250 mg bid. Eight-fold increases were seen in 2% of PAH patients on 125 mg bid and 7% of PAH patients on 250 mg bid. Bilirubin increases to ≥3 × ULN were associated with aminotransferase increases in 2 of 658 (0.3%) of patients treated with bosentan.

The combination of hepatocellular injury (increases in aminotransferases of >3 × ULN) and increases in total bilirubin (≥3 × ULN) is a marker for potential serious liver injury.[1]

Elevations of AST and/or ALT associated with bosentan are dose-dependent, occur both early and late in treatment, usually progress slowly, are typically asymptomatic, and to date have been reversible after treatment interruption or cessation. These aminotransferase elevations may reverse spontaneously while continuing treatment with bosentan.

Liver aminotransferase levels must be measured prior to initiation of treatment and then monthly. If elevated aminotransferase levels are seen, changes in monitoring and treatment must be initiated (see DOSAGE AND ADMINISTRATION). If liver aminotransferase elevations are accompanied by clinical symptoms of liver injury (such as nausea, vomiting, fever, abdominal pain, jaundice, or unusual lethargy or fatigue) or increases in bilirubin ≥2 × ULN, treatment should be stopped. There is no experience with the re-introduction of bosentan in these circumstances.

PRE-EXISTING LIVER IMPAIRMENT

Liver aminotransferase levels must be measured prior to initiation of treatment and then monthly. Bosentan should generally be avoided in patients with moderate or severe liver impairment (see CLINICAL PHARMACOLOGY and DOSAGE AND ADMINISTRATION). In addition, bosentan should generally be avoided in patients with elevated aminotransferases (>3 × ULN) because monitoring liver injury in these patients may be more difficult (see BOXED WARNING).

PRECAUTIONS

HEMATOLOGIC CHANGES

Treatment with bosentan caused a dose-related decrease in hemoglobin and hematocrit. Hemoglobin levels should be monitored after 1 and 3 months of treatment and then every 3 months. The overall mean decrease in hemoglobin concentration for bosentan-treated patients was 0.9 g/dl (change to end of treatment). Most of this decrease of hemoglobin concentration was detected during the first few weeks of bosentan treatment and hemoglobin levels stabilized by 4-12 weeks of bosentan treatment.

In placebo-controlled studies of all uses of bosentan, marked decreases in hemoglobin (>15% decrease from baseline resulting in values <11 g/dl) were observed in 6% of bosentan-treated patients and 3% of placebo-treated patients. In patients with pulmonary arterial hypertension treated with doses of 125 and 250 mg bid, marked decreases in hemoglobin occurred in 3% compared to 1% in placebo-treated patients.

A decrease in hemoglobin concentration by at least 1 g/dl was observed in 57% of bosentan-treated patients as compared to 29% of placebo-treated patients. In 80% of those patients whose hemoglobin decreased by at least 1 g/dl, the decrease occurred during the first 6 weeks of bosentan treatment.

During the course of treatment the hemoglobin concentration remained within normal limits in 68% of bosentan-treated patients compared to 76% of placebo patients.

The explanation for the change in hemoglobin is not known, but it does not appear to be hemorrhage or hemolysis.

It is recommended that hemoglobin concentrations be checked after 1 and 3 months, and every 3 months thereafter. If a marked decrease in hemoglobin concentration occurs, further evaluation should be undertaken to determine the cause and need for specific treatment.

INFORMATION FOR THE PATIENT

Patients are advised to consult the bosentan medication guide on the safe use of bosentan.

The physician should discuss with the patient the importance of monthly monitoring of serum aminotransferases and urine or serum pregnancy testing and of avoidance of pregnancy. The physician should discuss options for effective contraception and measures to prevent pregnancy with their female patients. Input from a gynecologist or similar expert on adequate contraception should be sought as needed.

CARCINOGENESIS, MUTAGENESIS, AND IMPAIRMENT OF FERTILITY

Two (2) years of dietary administration of bosentan to mice produced an increased incidence of hepatocellular adenomas and carcinomas in males at doses as low as 450 mg/kg/day (about 8 times the maximum recommended human dose [MRHD] of 125 mg bid, on a mg/m^2 basis). In the same study, doses greater than 2000 mg/kg/day (about 32 times the MRHD) were associated with an increased incidence of colon adenomas in both males and females. In rats, dietary administration of bosentan for 2 years was associated with an increased incidence of brain astrocytomas in males at doses as low as 500 mg/kg/day (about 16 times the MRHD). In a comprehensive battery of *in vitro* tests (the microbial mutagenesis assay, the unscheduled DNA synthesis assay, the V-79 mammalian cell mutagenesis assay, and human lymphocyte assay) and an *in vivo* mouse micronucleus assay, there was no evidence for any mutagenic or clastogenic activity of bosentan.

Impairment of Fertility/Testicular Function

Many endothelin receptor antagonists have profound effects on the histology and function of the testes in animals. These drugs have been shown to induce atrophy of the seminiferous tubules of the testes and to reduce sperm counts and male fertility in rats when administered for longer than 10 weeks. Where studied, testicular tubular atrophy and decreases in male fertility observed with endothelin receptor antagonists appear irreversible.

In fertility studies in which male and female rats were treated with bosentan at oral doses of up to 1500 mg/kg/day (50 times the MRHD on a mg/m^2 basis) or IV doses up to 40 mg/kg/day, no effects on sperm count, sperm motility, mating performance or fertility were observed. An increased incidence of testicular tubular atrophy was observed in rats given bosentan orally at doses as low as 125 mg/kg/day (about 4 times the MRHD and the lowest doses tested) for 2 years but not at doses as high as 1500 mg/kg/day (about 50 times the MRHD) for 6 months. Effects on sperm count and motility were evaluated only in the much shorter duration fertility studies in which males had been exposed to the drug for 4-6 weeks. An increased incidence of tubular atrophy was not observed in mice treated for 2 years at doses up to 4500 mg/kg/day (about 75 times the MRHD) or in dogs treated up to 12 months at doses up to 500 mg/kg/day (about 50 times the MRHD).

There are no data on the effects of bosentan or other endothelin receptor antagonists on testicular function in man.

PREGNANCY, TERATOGENIC EFFECTS, PREGNANCY CATEGORY X

See CONTRAINDICATIONS.

NURSING MOTHERS

It is not known whether this drug is excreted in human milk. Because many drugs are excreted in human milk, breastfeeding while taking bosentan is not recommended.

PEDIATRIC USE

Safety and efficacy in pediatric patients have not been established (see DOSAGE AND ADMINISTRATION).

USE IN ELDERLY PATIENTS

Clinical experience with bosentan in subjects aged 65 or older has not included a sufficient number of such subjects to identify a difference in response between elderly and younger patients (see DOSAGE AND ADMINISTRATION).

DRUG INTERACTIONS

Bosentan is metabolized by CYP2C9 and CYP3A4. Inhibition of these isoenzymes may increase the plasma concentration of bosentan (see Ketoconazole). Bosentan is an inducer of CYP3A4 and CYP2C9. Consequently, plasma concentrations of drugs metabolized by these 2 isoenzymes will be decreased when bosentan is co-administered. Bosentan had no relevant inhibitory effect on any CYP isoenzymes tested (CYP1A2, CYP2C9, CYP2C19, CYP2D6, CYP3A4). Consequently, bosentan is not expected to increase the plasma concentrations of drugs metabolized by these enzymes.

HORMONAL CONTRACEPTIVES, INCLUDING ORAL, INJECTABLE, AND IMPLANTABLE CONTRACEPTIVES

Specific interaction studies have not been performed to evaluate the effect of co-administration of bosentan and hormonal contraceptives, including oral, injectable or implantable contraceptives. Since many of these drugs are metabolized by CYP3A4, there is a possibility of failure of contraception when bosentan is co-administered. Women should not rely on hormonal contraception alone when taking bosentan.

Specific interaction studies have demonstrated the following:

Cyclosporine A: During the first day of concomitant administration, trough concentrations of bosentan were increased by about 30-fold. Steady-state bosentan plasma concentrations were 3- to 4-fold higher than in the absence of cyclosporine A. The concomitant administration of bosentan and cyclosporine A is contraindicated (see CONTRAINDICATIONS). Co-administration of bosentan decreased the plasma concentrations of cyclosporine A (a CYP3A4 substrate) by approximately 50%.

Glyburide: An increased risk of elevated liver aminotransferases was observed in patients receiving concomitant therapy with glyburide. Therefore, the concomitant administration of bosentan and glyburide is contraindicated, and alternative hypoglycemic agents should be considered (see CONTRAINDICATIONS).

Co-administration of bosentan decreased the plasma concentrations of glyburide by approximately 40%. The plasma concentrations of bosentan were also decreased by approximately 30%. Bosentan is also expected to reduce plasma concentrations of other oral hypoglycemic agents that are predominantly metabolized by CYP2C9 or CYP3A4. The possibility of worsened glucose control in patients using these agents should be considered.

Ketoconazole: Co-administration of bosentan 125 mg bid and ketoconazole, a potent CYP3A4 inhibitor, increased the plasma concentrations of bosentan by approximately 2-fold. No dose adjustment of bosentan is necessary, but increased effects of bosentan should be considered.

Simvastatin and Other Statins: Co-administration of bosentan decreased the plasma concentrations of simvastatin (a CYP3A4 substrate), and its active β-hydroxy acid metabolite, by approximately 50%. The plasma concentrations of bosentan were not affected. Bosentan is also expected to reduce plasma concentrations of other statins that have significant metabolism by CYP3A4, such as lovastatin and atorvastatin. The possibility of reduced statin efficacy should be considered. Patients using CYP3A4 metabolized statins should have cholesterol levels monitored after bosentan is initiated to see whether the statin dose needs adjustment.

Warfarin: Co-administration of bosentan 500 mg bid for 6 days decreased the plasma concentrations of both S-warfarin (a CYP2C9 substrate) and R-warfarin (a CYP3A4 substrate) by 29 and 38%, respectively. Clinical experience with concomitant administration of bosentan and warfarin in patients with pulmonary arterial hypertension did not show clinically relevant changes in INR or warfarin dose (baseline versus end of the clinical studies), and the need to change the warfarin dose during the trials due to changes in INR or due to adverse events was similar among bosentan- and placebo-treated patients.

Digoxin, Nimodipine and Losartan: Bosentan has been shown to have no pharmacokinetic interactions with digoxin and nimodipine, and losartan has no effect on plasma levels of bosentan.

ADVERSE REACTIONS

See BOXED WARNING for discussion of liver injury and PRECAUTIONS for discussion of hemoglobin and hematocrit abnormalities.

Safety data on bosentan were obtained from 12 clinical studies (8 placebo-controlled and 4 open-label) in 777 patients with pulmonary arterial hypertension, and other diseases. Doses up to 8 times the currently recommended clinical dose (125 mg bid) were administered for a variety of durations. The exposure to bosentan in these trials ranged from 1 day to 4.1 years (n=89 for 1 year; n=61 for 1.5 years and n=39 for more than 2 years). Exposure of pulmonary arterial hypertension patients (n=235) to bosentan ranged from 1 day to 1.7 years (n=126 more than 6 months and n=28 more than 12 months).

Treatment discontinuations due to adverse events other than those related to pulmonary hypertension during the clinical trials in patients with pulmonary arterial hypertension were more frequent on bosentan (5%; 8/165 patients) than on placebo (3%; 2/80 patients). In this database the only cause of discontinuations >1%, and occurring more often on bosentan was abnormal liver function.

The adverse drug reactions that occurred in ≥3% of the bosentan-treated patients and were more common on bosentan in placebo-controlled trials in pulmonary arterial hypertension at doses of 125 or 250 mg bid are shown in TABLE 4.

TABLE 4 *Adverse Events* Occurring in ≥3% of Patients Treated With Bosentan 125-250 mg bid and More Common on Bosentan in Placebo-Controlled Studies in Pulmonary Arterial Hypertension*

Adverse Event	Bosentan (n=165)		Placebo (n=80)	
Headache	36	22%	16	20%
Nasopharyngitis	18	11%	6	8%
Flushing	15	9%	4	5%
Hepatic function abnormal	14	8%	2	3%
Edema, lower limb	13	8%	4	5%
Hypotension	11	7%	3	4%
Palpitations	8	5%	1	1%
Dyspepsia	7	4%	0	0%
Edema	7	4%	2	3%
Fatigue	6	4%	1	1%
Pruritus	6	4%	0	0%

*** Note: Only AEs with onset from start of treatment to 1 calendar day after end of treatment are included. All reported events (at least 3%) are included except those too general to be informative, and those not reasonably associated with the use of the drug because they were associated with the condition being treated or are very common in the treated population.**

In placebo-controlled studies of bosentan in pulmonary arterial hypertension and for other diseases (primarily chronic heart failure), a total of 677 patients were treated with bosentan at daily doses ranging from 100-2000 mg and 288 patients were treated with placebo. The duration of treatment ranged from 4 weeks to 6 months. For the adverse drug reactions that occurred in ≥3% of bosentan-treated patients, the only ones that occurred more frequently on bosentan than on placebo (≥2% difference) were headache (16% vs 13%), flushing (7% vs 2%), abnormal hepatic function (6% vs 2%), leg edema (5% vs 1%), and anemia (3% vs 1%).

LABORATORY ABNORMALITIES

Increased liver aminotransferases (see BOXED WARNING and WARNINGS).

Decreased hemoglobin and hematocrit (see PRECAUTIONS).

DOSAGE AND ADMINISTRATION

GENERAL

Bosentan treatment should be initiated at a dose of 62.5 mg bid for 4 weeks and then increased to the maintenance dose of 125 mg bid. Doses above 125 mg bid did not appear to confer additional benefit sufficient to offset the increased risk of liver injury.

Tablets should be administered morning and evening with or without food.

DOSAGE ADJUSTMENT AND MONITORING IN PATIENTS DEVELOPING AMINOTRANSFERASE ABNORMALITIES

TABLE 5

ALT/AST Levels	Treatment and Monitoring Recommendations
>3 and ≥5 × ULN	Confirm by another aminotransferase test; if confirmed, reduce the daily dose or interrupt treatment, and monitor aminotransferase levels at least every 2 weeks. If the aminotransferase levels return to pre-treatment values, continue or re-introduce the treatment as appropriate (see below).
>5 and ≤8 × ULN	Confirm by another aminotransferase test; if confirmed, stop treatment and monitor aminotransferase levels at least every 2 weeks. Once the aminotransferase levels return to pre-treatment values, consider re-introduction of the treatment (see below).
>8 × ULN	Treatment should be stopped and re-introduction of bosentan should not be considered. There is no experience with re-introduction of bosentan in these circumstances.

If bosentan is re-introduced it should be at the starting dose; aminotransferase levels should be checked within 3 days and thereafter according to the recommendations in TABLE 5.

If liver aminotransferase elevations are accompanied by clinical symptoms of liver injury (such as nausea, vomiting, fever, abdominal pain, jaundice, or unusual lethargy or fatigue) or increases in bilirubin ≥2 × ULN, treatment should be stopped. There is no experience with the re-introduction of bosentan in these circumstances.

USE IN WOMEN OF CHILD-BEARING POTENTIAL

Bosentan treatment should only be initiated in women of child-bearing potential following a negative pregnancy test and only in those who practice adequate contraception that does not rely solely upon hormonal contraceptives, including oral, injectable or implantable contraceptives (see DRUG INTERACTIONS, Hormonal Contraceptives, Including Oral, Injectable and Implantable Contraceptives). Input from a gynecologist or similar expert on adequate contraception should be sought as needed. Urine or serum pregnancy tests should be obtained monthly in women of childbearing potential taking bosentan.

DOSAGE ADJUSTMENT IN RENALLY IMPAIRED PATIENTS

The effect of renal impairment on the pharmacokinetics of bosentan is small and does not require dosing adjustment.

DOSAGE ADJUSTMENT IN GERIATRIC PATIENTS

Clinical studies of bosentan did not include sufficient numbers of subjects aged 65 and older to determine whether they respond differently from younger subjects. Clinical experience has not identified differences in responses between elderly and younger patients. In general, caution should be exercised in dose selection for elderly patients given the greater frequency of decreased hepatic, renal, or cardiac function, and of concomitant disease or other drug therapy in this age group.

DOSAGE ADJUSTMENT IN HEPATICALLY IMPAIRED PATIENTS

The influence of liver impairment on the pharmacokinetics of bosentan has not been evaluated. Because there is *in vivo* and *in vitro* evidence that the main route of excretion of bosentan is biliary, liver impairment would be expected to increase exposure (C_{max}, AUC) to bosentan. There are no specific data to guide dosing in hepatically impaired patients (see WARNINGS); caution should be exercised in patients with mildly impaired liver function. Bosentan should generally be avoided in patients with moderate or severe liver impairment.

DOSAGE ADJUSTMENT IN CHILDREN

Safety and efficacy in pediatric patients have not been established.

DOSAGE ADJUSTMENT IN PATIENTS WITH LOW BODY WEIGHT

In patients with a body weight below 40 kg but who are over 12 years of age the recommended initial and maintenance dose is 62.5 mg bid.

DISCONTINUATION OF TREATMENT

There is limited experience with abrupt discontinuation of bosentan. No evidence for acute rebound has been observed. Nevertheless, to avoid the potential for clinical deterioration, gradual dose reduction (62.5 mg bid for 3-7 days) should be considered.

HOW SUPPLIED

TRACLEER TABLETS

62.5 mg: Film-coated, round, biconvex, orange-white tablets, embossed with identification marking "62,5".

125 mg: Film-coated, oval, biconvex, orange-white tablets, embossed with identification marking "125".

Storage: Store at 20-25°C (68-77°F). Excursions are permitted between 15 and 30°C (59 and 86°F).

PRODUCT LISTING - EQUIVALENTS NOT AVAILABLE

Tablet - Oral - 62.5 mg

60's	$2970.00	TRACLEER, Acetelion Pharmaceuticals Us, Inc	66215-0101-06

Tablet - Oral - 125 mg

60's	$2970.00	TRACLEER, Acetelion Pharmaceuticals Us, Inc	66215-0102-06

Bretylium Tosylate *(000523)*

Categories: Arrhythmia, ventricular; Fibrillation, ventricular; Tachycardia, ventricular; Pregnancy Category C; FDA Approved 1978 Jul
Drug Classes: Antiarrhythmics, class III
Brand Names: **Bretylol**
Foreign Brand Availability: Bretylate (Bahamas; Barbados; Belize; Bermuda; Canada; Curacao; Guyana; Jamaica; Netherland-Antilles; Surinam; Trinidad)

DESCRIPTION

Bretylium tosylate is o-bromobenzyl ethyldimethylammonium p-toluene sulfonate. It is an antifibrillatory and antiarrhythmic agent, intended for intravenous or intramuscular use.

Bretylium tosylate is a white, crystalline powder with an extremely bitter taste. It is freely soluble in water and alcohol. Each ml of sterile, non-pyrogenic solution contains bretylium tosylate 50 mg in water for injection. pH 5.0-7.0; sodium hydroxide and/or hydrochloric acid added, if needed, for pH adjustment. Bretylium tosylate injection contains no preservative.

CLINICAL PHARMACOLOGY

Bretylium is a bromobenzyl quaternary ammonium compound which selectively accumulates in sympathetic ganglia and their postganglionic adrenergic neurons where it inhibits norepinephrine release by depressing adrenergic nerve terminal excitability.

Bretylium also suppresses ventricular fibrillation and ventricular arrhythmias. The mechanisms of the antifibrillatory and antiarrhythmic actions of bretylium are not established. In efforts to define these mechanisms, the following electrophysiologic actions of bretylium have been demonstrated in animal experiments:

1. Increase in ventricular fibrillation threshold.
2. Increase in action potential duration and effective refractory period without changes in heart rate.
3. Little effect on the rate of rise or amplitude of the cardiac action potential (Phase 0) or in resting membrane potential (Phase 4) in normal myocardium. However, when cell injury slows the rate of rise, decreases amplitude, and lowers resting membrane potential, bretylium transiently restores these parameters toward normal.
4. In canine hearts with infarcted areas, bretylium decreases the disparity in action potential duration between normal and infarcted regions.
5. Increase in impulse formation and spontaneous firing rate of pacemaker tissue as well as increased ventricular conduction velocity.

The restoration of injured myocardial cell electrophysiology toward normal, as well as the increase of the action potential duration and effective refractory period without changing their ratio to each other, may be important factors in suppressing re-entry of aberrant impulses and decreasing induced dispersion of local excitable states.

Bretylium induces a chemical sympathectomy-like state which resembles a surgical sympathectomy. Catecholamine stores are not depleted by bretylium, but catecholamine effects on the myocardium and on peripheral vascular resistance are often seen shortly after administration because bretylium causes an early release of norepinephrine from the adrenergic postganglionic nerve terminals. Subsequently, bretylium blocks the release of norepinephrine in response to neuron stimulation. Peripheral adrenergic blockade regularly causes orthostatic hypotension but has less effect on supine blood pressure. The relationship of adrenergic blockade to the antifibrillatory and antiarrhythmic actions of bretylium is not clear. In a study in patients with frequent ventricular premature beats, peak plasma concentration of bretylium and peak hypotensive effects were seen within 1 hour of intramuscular administration, presumably reflecting adrenergic neuronal blockade. However, suppression of premature ventricular beats was not maximal until 6-9 hours after dosing, when mean plasma concentration had declined to less than one-half of peak level. This suggests a slower mechanism, other than neuronal blockade, was involved in suppression of the arrhythmia. On the other hand, antifibrillatory effects can be seen within minutes of an intravenous injection, suggesting that the effect on the myocardium may occur quite rapidly.

Bretylium has a positive inotropic effect on the myocardium, but it is not yet certain whether this effect is direct or is mediated by catecholamine release.

Bretylium is eliminated intact by the kidneys. No metabolites have been identified following administration of bretylium tosylate injection in man and laboratory animals. In man, approximately 70-80% of a ^{14}C-labelled intramuscular dose is excreted in the urine during the first 24 hours, with an additional 10% excreted over the next 3 days.

The terminal half-life in four normal volunteers averaged 7.8 ± 0.6 hours (range 6.9-8.1). In one patient with a creatinine clearance of 21.0 ml/min × 1.73 m^2, the half-life was 16 hours. In one patient with a creatinine clearance of 1.0 ml/min × 1.73 m^2, the half-life was 31.5 hours. During hemodialysis, this patient's arterial and venous bretylium concentrations declined rapidly, resulting in a half-life of 13 hours. During dialysis there was a 2-fold increase in total bretylium clearance.

Effect on Heart Rate: There is sometimes an initial small increase in heart rate when bretylium is administered, but this is an inconsistent and transient occurrence.

Hemodynamic Effects: Following intravenous administration of 5 mg/kg of bretylium tosylate to patients with acute myocardial infarction, there was a mild increase in arterial pressure, followed by a modest decrease, remaining within normal limits throughout. Pulmonary artery pressures, pulmonary capillary wedge pressure, right atrial pressure, cardiac index, stroke volume index and stroke work index were not significantly changed. These hemodynamic effects were not correlated with antiarrhythmic activity.

Onset of Action: Suppression of ventricular fibrillation is rapid, usually occurring within minutes following intravenous administration. Suppression of ventricular tachycardia and other ventricular arrhythmias develops more slowly, usually 20 minutes to 2 hours after parenteral administration.

INDICATIONS AND USAGE

Bretylium tosylate injection is indicated in the prophylaxis and therapy of ventricular fibrillation.

Bretylium tosylate injection is also indicated in the treatment of life-threatening ventricular arrhythmias, such as ventricular tachycardia, that have failed to respond to adequate doses of a first-line antiarrhythmic agent, such as lidocaine.

Use of bretylium tosylate injection should be limited to intensive care units, coronary care units or other facilities where equipment and personnel for constant monitoring of cardiac arrhythmias and blood pressure are available.

Following injection of bretylium tosylate there may be a delay of 20 minutes to 2 hours in the onset of antiarrhythmic action, although it appears to act within minutes in ventricular fibrillation. The delay in effect appears to be longer after intramuscular than after intravenous injection.

CONTRAINDICATIONS

There are no contraindications to use in treatment of ventricular fibrillation or life-threatening refractory ventricular arrhythmias.

WARNINGS

Patients should be kept in the supine position until tolerance to the hypotensive effect of bretylium tosylate injection develops. Tolerance occurs unpredictably but may be present after several days.

HYPOTENSION

Administration of bretylium tosylate injection regularly results in postural hypotension, subjectively recognized by dizziness, lightheadedness, vertigo or faintness. Some degree of hypotension is present in about 50% of patients while they are supine. Hypotension may occur at doses lower than those needed to suppress arrhythmias. Hypotension with supine systolic pressure greater than 75 mm Hg need not be treated unless there are associated symptoms. If supine systolic pressure falls below 75 mm Hg, an infusion of dopamine or norepinephrine may be used to raise blood pressure. When catecholamines are administered, a dilute solution should be employed and blood pressure monitored closely because the pressor effects of the catecholamines are enhanced by bretylium. Volume expansion with blood or plasma and correction of dehydration should be carried out where appropriate.

TRANSIENT HYPERTENSION AND INCREASED FREQUENCY OF ARRHYTHMIAS

Due to the initial release of norepinephrine from adrenergic postganglionic nerve terminals by bretylium, transient hypertension or increased frequency of premature ventricular contractions and other arrhythmias may occur in some patients.

CAUTION DURING USE WITH DIGITALIS GLYCOSIDES

The initial release of norepinephrine caused by bretylium may aggravate digitalis toxicity. When a life-threatening cardiac arrhythmia occurs in a digitalized patient, bretylium tosylate injection should be used only if the etiology of the arrhythmia does not appear to be digitalis toxicity and other antiarrhythmic drugs are not effective. Simultaneous initiation of therapy with digitalis glycosides and bretylium tosylate injection should be avoided.

PATIENTS WITH FIXED CARDIAC OUTPUT

In patients with fixed cardiac output (*i.e.*, severe aortic stenosis or severe pulmonary hypertension) bretylium tosylate injection should be avoided since severe hypotension may result from a fall in peripheral resistance without a compensatory increase in cardiac output. If survival is threatened by the arrhythmia, bretylium tosylate injection may be used but vasoconstrictive catecholamines should be given promptly if severe hypotension occurs.

PRECAUTIONS

GENERAL

Dilution for Intravenous Use: One vial/ampul of bretylium tosylate injection should be diluted with a minimum of 50 ml of dextrose injection 5% or sodium chloride injection prior to intravenous use. Rapid intravenous administration may cause severe nausea and vomiting. Therefore, the diluted solution should be infused over a period greater than 8 minutes. However, in treating existing ventricular fibrillation, bretylium tosylate injection should be given as rapidly as possible and may be given without dilution.

Use Various Sites for Intramuscular Injection: When injected intramuscularly, not more than 5 ml should be given in a site, and injection sites should be varied since repeated intramuscular injection into the same site may cause atrophy and necrosis of muscle tissue, fibrosis, vascular degeneration and inflammatory changes.

Reduce Dosage in Impaired Renal Function: Since bretylium is excreted principally via the kidney, the dosage interval should be increased in patients with impaired renal function. See CLINICAL PHARMACOLOGY for information on the effect of reduced renal function on half-life.

CARCINOGENESIS, MUTAGENESIS, AND IMPAIRMENT OF FERTILITY

No data are available on potential for carcinogenicity, mutagenicity or impairment of fertility in animals or humans.

PREGNANCY CATEGORY C

Animal reproduction studies have not been conducted with bretylium tosylate. It is also not known whether bretylium tosylate can cause harm when administered to a pregnant woman or can affect reproduction capacity. Bretylium tosylate should be given to pregnant women only if clearly needed.

PEDIATRIC USE

The safety and efficacy of this drug in children has not been established. Bretylium tosylate has been administered to a limited number of pediatric patients, but such use has been inadequate to define fully proper dosage and limitations for use.

DRUG INTERACTIONS

1. Digitalis toxicity may be aggravated by the initial release of norepinephrine caused by bretylium.
2. The pressor effects of catecholamines such as dopamine or norepinephrine are enhanced by bretylium. When catecholamines are administered, dilute solutions should be used and blood pressure should be monitored closely (see WARNINGS).
3. Although there is little published information on concomitant administration of lidocaine and bretylium, these drugs are often administered concurrently without any evidence of interactions resulting in adverse effects or diminished efficacy.

ADVERSE REACTIONS

Hypotension and postural hypotension have been the most frequently reported adverse reactions (see WARNINGS). Nausea and vomiting occurred in about 3% of patients, primarily when bretylium tosylate injection was administered rapidly by the intravenous route (see PRECAUTIONS). Vertigo, dizziness, light-headedness and syncope, which sometimes accompanied postural hypotension, were reported in about 7 patients in 1000.

Bradycardia, increased frequency of premature ventricular contractions, transitory hypertension, initial increase in arrhythmias (see WARNINGS), precipitation of anginal attacks, and sensation of substernal pressure have also been reported in a small number of patients, *i.e.,* approximately 1-2 patients in 1000.

Renal dysfunction, diarrhea, abdominal pain, hiccups, erythematous macular rash, flushing, hyperthermia, confusion, paranoid psychosis, emotional lability, lethargy, generalized tenderness, anxiety, shortness of breath, diaphoresis, nasal stuffiness and mild conjunctivitis, have been reported in about 1 patient in 1000. The relationship of bretylium administration to these reactions has not been clearly established.

DOSAGE AND ADMINISTRATION

Bretylium tosylate injection is to be used clinically only for treatment of life-threatening ventricular arrhythmias under constant electrocardiographic monitoring. The clinical use of bretylium tosylate injection is for short-term use only. Patients should either be kept supine during the course of bretylium tosylate therapy or be closely observed for postural hypotension. The optimal dose schedule for parenteral administration of bretylium tosylate injection has not been determined. There is comparatively little experience with dosages greater than 40 mg/kg/day, although such doses have been used without apparent adverse effects. The following schedule is suggested.

FOR IMMEDIATELY LIFE-THREATENING VENTRICULAR ARRHYTHMIAS SUCH AS VENTRICULAR FIBRILLATION OR HEMODYNAMICALLY UNSTABLE VENTRICULAR TACHYCARDIA

Administer undiluted bretylium tosylate injection at a dosage of 5 mg/kg of body weight by rapid intravenous injection. Other usual cardiopulmonary resuscitative procedures, including electrical cardioversion, should be employed prior to and following the injection in accordance with good medical practice. If ventricular fibrillation persists, the dosage may be increased to 10 mg/kg and repeated as necessary.

For continuous suppression, dilute bretylium tosylate injection with dextrose injection or sodium chloride injection using the table below and administer the diluted solution as a constant infusion of 1-2 mg bretylium tosylate per minute. When administering bretylium tosylate injection (or any potent medication) by continuous intravenous infusion, it is advisable to use a precision volume control device. An alternative maintenance schedule is to infuse the diluted solution at a dosage of 5-10 mg bretylium tosylate per kg body weight, over a period greater than 8 minutes, every 6 hours. More rapid infusion may cause nausea and vomiting.

OTHER VENTRICULAR ARRHYTHMIAS

Intravenous Use

Bretylium tosylate injection must be diluted as described above before intravenous use. Administer the diluted solution at a dosage of 5-10 mg bretylium tosylate per kg of body weight by intravenous infusion over a period greater than 8 minutes. More rapid infusion may cause nausea and vomiting. Subsequent doses may be given at 1-2 hour intervals if the arrhythmia persists.

For maintenance therapy, the same dosage may be administered every 6 hours, or a constant infusion of 1-2 mg bretylium tosylate per minute may be given (see TABLE 1).

For Intramuscular Injection

Do not dilute bretylium tosylate injection prior to intramuscular injection. Inject 5-10 mg bretylium tosylate per kg of body weight. Subsequent doses may be given at 1-2 hour intervals if the arrhythmia persists. Thereafter maintain the same dosage every 6-8 hours.

Intramuscular injection should not be made directly into or near a major nerve, and the site of injection should be varied on repeated injections. No more than 5 ml should be injected intramuscularly in one site (see PRECAUTIONS).

As soon as possible, and when indicated, patients should be changed to an oral antiarrhythmic agent for maintenance therapy.

Parenteral drug products should be inspected visually for particulate matter and discoloration prior to administration, whenever solution and container permit.

Storage: Store at controlled room temperature 15-30°C (59-86°F).

***TABLE 1** Suggested Bretylium Tosylate Injection Admixture Dilutions and Administration Rates for Continuous Infusion Maintenance Therapy*

Arranged in descending order of concentration

Preparation			Final Conc. Dose		Administration	
Amount of Bretylium Tosylate Injection	Volume of IV Fluid*	Final Volume	mg/ml	mg/min	Micro-drops/min	ml/h
For Fluid Restricted Patients						
500 mg (10 ml)	50 ml	60 ml	8.3	1	7	7
				1.5	11	11
				2	14	14
2 g (40 ml)	500 ml	540 ml	3.7	1	16	16
1 g (20 ml)	250 ml	270 ml	3.7	1.5	24	24
				2	32	32
1 g (20 ml)	500 ml	520 ml	1.9	1	32	32
500 mg (10 ml)	250 ml	260 ml	1.9	1.5	47	47
				2	63	63

* IV fluid may be either dextrose injection or sodium chloride injection. This table does not consider the overfill volume present in the IV fluid.

PRODUCT LISTING - RATED THERAPEUTICALLY EQUIVALENT

Solution - Injectable - 50 mg/ml

10 ml	$22.44	GENERIC, American Regent Laboratories Inc	00517-8810-01
10 ml x 5	$14.95	GENERIC, Astra-Zeneca Pharmaceuticals	00186-1131-04
10 ml x 10	$23.13	GENERIC, Esi Lederle Generics	00641-2211-41
10 ml x 10	$41.08	GENERIC, Abbott Pharmaceutical	00074-9267-18
10 ml x 10	$41.60	GENERIC, Astra-Zeneca Pharmaceuticals	00186-0663-01
10 ml x 10	$89.50	GENERIC, Abbott Pharmaceutical	00074-1698-10
10 ml x 10	$358.56	GENERIC, Abbott Pharmaceutical	00074-9267-01
10 ml x 25	$50.00	GENERIC, Raway Pharmacal Inc	00686-8810-01

Solution - Intravenous - 200 mg/100 ml;5%

250 ml x 24	$567.60	GENERIC, Abbott Pharmaceutical	00074-7638-62

Solution - Intravenous - 400 mg/100 ml;5%

250 ml x 24	$572.85	GENERIC, Abbott Pharmaceutical	00074-7639-62

PRODUCT LISTING - EQUIVALENTS NOT AVAILABLE

Solution - Injectable - 50 mg/ml

10 ml x 5	$14.96	GENERIC, Allscripts Pharmaceutical Company	54569-2257-00

Brimonidine Tartrate *(003302)*

Categories: Glaucoma, open-angle; Hypertension, ocular; Pregnancy Category B; FDA Approved 1996 Oct
Drug Classes: Adrenergic agonists; Ophthalmics
Brand Names: Alphagan
Cost of Therapy: $30.53 (Glaucoma; Alphagan Ophth. Solution; 0.2%; 5 ml; 3 drops/day; variable day supply)

DESCRIPTION

Note: The trade names have been used throughout this monograph for clarity.

ALPHAGAN 0.2%

Alphagan (brimonidine tartrate ophthalmic solution) 0.2% is a relatively selective alpha-2 adrenergic agonist for ophthalmic use. The chemical name of brimonidine tartrate is 5-bromo-6-(2-imidazolidinylideneamino) quinoxaline L-tartrate. It has a molecular weight of 442.24 as the tartrate salt and is water soluble (34 mg/ml) at pH 6.5. The molecular formula is: $C_{11}H_{10}BrN_5 \cdot C_4H_6O_6$.

In solution, Alphagan 0.2% has a clear, greenish-yellow color. It has an osmolality of 280-330 mOsml/kg and a pH of 5.6-6.6.

Each ml of Alphagan contains: *Active ingredient:* Brimonidine tartrate: 0.2% (2 mg/ml). *Preservative:* Benzalkonium chloride (0.05 mg). *Inactives:* Citric acid; polyvinyl alcohol; sodium chloride; sodium citrate; and purified water. Hydrochloric acid and/or sodium hydroxide may be added to adjust pH.

ALPHAGAN 0.5%

Alphagan (brimonidine tartrate ophthalmic solution) 0.5% is a relatively selective alpha-2 adrenergic agonist for ophthalmic use. The chemical name of brimonidine tartrate is 5-bromo-6-(2-imidazolidinylideneamino) quinoxaline L-tartrate. It has a molecular weight of 442.24 as the tartrate salt and is water soluble (34 mg/ml) pH 6.5.

The molecular formula is $C_{11}H_{10}BrN_5 \cdot C_4H_6O_6$.

In solution, Alphagan 0.5% has a clear, greenish-yellow color. It has a pH of 5.6-6.6.

Each ml of Alphagan contains: *Active ingredient:* Brimonidine tartrate 0.5% (5 mg/ml). *Preservative:* Benzalkonium chloride (0.05 mg). *Inactives:* Citric acid; polyvinyl alcohol; sodium chloride; sodium citrate; and purified water. Hydrochloric acid and/or sodium hydroxide may be added to adjust pH.

ALPHAGAN P

Alphagan P (brimonidine tartrate ophthalmic solution) 0.15% is a relatively selective alpha-2 adrenergic agonist for ophthalmic use. The chemical name of brimonidine tartrate is 5-bromo-6-(2-imidazolidinylideneamino) quinoxaline L-tartrate. It is an off-white to pale yellow powder. It has a molecular weight of 442.24 as the tartrate salt, and is both soluble in water (1.5 mg/ml) and in the product vehicle (3.0 mg/ml) at pH 7.2. The structural formula is: $C_{11}H_{10}BrN_5{\cdot}C_4H_6O_6$.

In solution, Alphagan P 0.15% has a clear, greenish-yellow color. It has an osmolality of 250-350 mOsmol/kg and a pH of 6.6-7.4.

Each ml of Alphagan P contains: *Active ingredient:* Brimonidine tartrate 0.15% (1.5 mg/ml). *Preservative:* Purite 0.005% (0.05mg/ml). *Inactives:* Boric acid; calcium chloride; magnesium chloride; potassium chloride; purified water; sodium borate; sodium carboxymethylcellulose; sodium chloride; with hydrochloric acid and/or sodium hydroxide to adjust pH.

CLINICAL PHARMACOLOGY

ALPHAGAN 0.2%

Mechanism of Action

Alphagan is an alpha adrenergic receptor agonist. It has a peak ocular hypotensive effect occurring at 2 hours post-dosing. Fluorophotometric studies in animals and humans suggest that brimonidine tartrate has a dual mechanism of action by reducing aqueous humor production and increasing uveoscleral outflow.

Pharmacokinetics

After ocular administration of a 0.2% solution, plasma concentrations peaked within 1-4 hours and declined with a systemic half-life of approximately 3 hours. In humans, systemic metabolism of brimonidine is extensive. It is metabolized primarily by the liver. Urinary excretion is the major route of elimination of the drug and its metabolites. Approximately 87% of an orally-administered radioactive dose was eliminated within 120 hours, with 74% found in the urine.

ALPHAGAN 0.5%

Mechanism of Action

Alphagan is an alpha adrenergic receptor agonist. It has a peak ocular hypotensive effect occurring at 2 hours post-dosing.

Fluorophotometric studies in animals and humans suggest that brimonidine tartrate has a dual mechanism of action by reducing aqueous humor production and increasing uveoscleral outflow.

Pharmacokinetics

After ocular administration of a 0.5% solution, plasma concentrations peaked within 1-4 hours and declined with a systemic half-life of approximately 3 hours. In humans, systemic metabolism of brimonidine is extensive. It is metabolized primarily by the liver. Urinary excretion is the major route of elimination of the drug and its metabolites. Approximately 87% of an orally-administered radioactive dose was eliminated within 120 hours, with 74% found in the urine.

ALPHAGAN P

Mechanism of Action

Alphagan P is an alpha adrenergic receptor agonist. It has a peak ocular hypotensive effect occurring at 2 hours post-dosing. Fluorophotometric studies in animals and humans suggest that brimonidine tartrate has a dual mechanism of action by reducing aqueous humor production and increasing uveoscleral outflow.

Pharmacokinetics

After ocular administration of either a 0.1 or 0.2% solution, plasma concentrations peaked within 0.5-2.5 hours and declined with a systemic half-life of approximately 2 hours. In humans, systemic metabolism of brimonidine is extensive. It is metabolized primarily by the liver. Urinary excretion is the major route of elimination of the drug and its metabolites. Approximately 87% of an orally-administered radioactive dose was eliminated within 120 hours, with 74% found in the urine.

INDICATIONS AND USAGE

ALPHAGAN 0.2%

Alphagan is indicated for lowering intraocular pressure in patients with open-angle glaucoma or ocular hypertension. The IOP lowering efficacy of Alphagan ophthalmic solution diminishes over time in some patients. This loss of effect appears with a variable time of onset in each patient and should be closely monitored.

ALPHAGAN 0.5%

Alphagan 0.5% is indicated for the prevention of post-operative IOP elevations in patients undergoing argon laser trabeculoplasty (ALT).

ALPHAGAN P

Alphagan P is indicated for the lowering of intraocular pressure in patients with open-angle glaucoma or ocular hypertension.

CONTRAINDICATIONS

ALPHAGAN 0.2%

Alphagan is contraindicated in patients with hypersensitivity to brimonidine tartrate or any component of this medication. It is also contraindicated in patients receiving monoamine oxidase (MAO) inhibitor therapy.

ALPHAGAN 0.5%

Alphagan is contraindicated in patients with hypersensitivity to brimonidine tartrate or any component of this medication. It is also contraindicated in patients receiving monoamine oxidase (MAO) inhibitor therapy.

ALPHAGAN P

Alphagan P is contraindicated in patients with hypersensitivity to brimonidine tartrate or any component of this medication. It is also contraindicated in patients receiving monoamine oxidase (MAO) inhibitor therapy.

PRECAUTIONS

ALPHAGAN 0.2%

General

Although Alphagan had minimal effect on blood pressure of patients in clinical studies, caution should be exercised in treating patients with severe cardiovascular disease.

Alphagan has not been studied in patients with hepatic or renal impairment; caution should be used in treating such patients.

Alphagan should be used with caution in patients with depression, cerebral or coronary insufficiency, Raynaud's phenomenon, orthostatic hypotension or thromboangiitis obliterans.

During the studies there was a loss of effect in some patients. The IOP-lowering efficacy observed with Alphagan ophthalmic solution during the first month of therapy may not always reflect the long-term level of IOP reduction. Patients prescribed IOP-lowering medication should be routinely monitored for IOP.

Information for the Patient

The preservative in Alphagan, benzalkonium chloride, may be absorbed by soft contact lenses. Patients wearing soft contact lenses should be instructed to wait at least 15 minutes after instilling Alphagan to insert soft contact lenses.

As with other drugs in this class, Alphagan may cause fatigue and/or drowsiness in some patients. Patients who engage in hazardous activities should be cautioned of the potential for a decrease in mental alertness.

Carcinogenesis, Mutagenesis, and Impairment of Fertility

No compound-related carcinogenic effects were observed in either mice or rats following a 21 month and 24 month study, respectively. In these studies, dietary administration of brimonidine tartrate at doses up to 2.5 mg/kg/day in mice and 1.0 mg/kg/day in rats achieved ~77 and 118 times, respectively, the plasma drug concentration estimated in humans treated with 1 drop Alphagan into both eyes 3 times per day.

Brimonidine tartrate was not mutagenic or cytogenic in a series of *in vitro* and *in vivo* studies including the Ames test, chromosomal aberation assay in Chinese Hamster Ovary (CHO) cells, a host-mediated assay and cytogenic studies in mice, and dominant lethal assay.

Reproductive studies performed in rats with oral doses of 0.66 mg base/kg revealed no evidence of harm to the fetus due to Alphagan.

Pregnancy, Teratogenic Effects, Pregnancy Category B

Reproductive studies performed in rats with oral doses of 0.66 mg base/kg revealed no evidence of harm to the fetus due to Alphagan. Dosing at this level produced 100 times the plasma drug concentration level seen in humans following multiple ophthalmic doses.

There are no adequate and well-controlled studies in pregnant women. In animal studies, brimonidine crossed the placenta and entered into the fetal circulation to a limited extent. Alphagan should be used during pregnancy only if the potential benefit to the mother justifies the potential risk to the fetus.

Nursing Mothers

It is not known whether this drug is excreted in human milk; in animal studies brimonidine tartrate was excreted in breast milk. A decision should be made whether to discontinue nursing or to discontinue the drug, taking into account the importance of the drug to the mother.

Pediatric Use

In a well-controlled clinical study conducted in pediatric glaucoma patients (ages 2-7 years) the most commonly observed adverse events with brimonidine tartrate ophthalmic solution 0.2% dosed 3 times daily were somnolence (50-83% in patients ages 2-6 years) and decreased alertness. In pediatric patients 7 years of age or older (>20 kg), somnolence appears to occur less frequently (25%). The most commonly observed adverse event was somnolence. Approximately 16% of patients on brimonidine tartrate ophthalmic solution discontinued from the study due to somnolence.

The safety and effectiveness of Alphagan have not been studied in pediatric patients below the age of 2 years. Alphagan is not recommended for use in pediatric patients under the age of 2 years. (Also refer to ADVERSE REACTIONS.)

Geriatric Use

No overall differences in safety or effectiveness have been observed between elderly and other adult patients.

ALPHAGAN 0.5%

General

Although Alphagan had minimal effect on blood pressure of patients in clinical studies, caution should be exercised in treating patients with severe cardiovascular disease.

Alphagan has not been studied in patients with hepatic or renal impairment; caution should be used in treating such patients.

Alphagan should be used with caution in patients with depression, cerebral or coronary insufficiency, Raynaud's phenomenon, orthostatic hypotension or thromboangiitis obliterans.

Information for the Patient

The preservative in Alphagan, benzalkonium chloride, may be absorbed by soft contact lenses. Patients wearing soft contact lenses should be instructed to wait at least 15 minutes after instilling Alphagan to insert soft contact lenses.

As with other drugs of this class, Alphagan may cause fatigue and/or drowsiness in some patients. On the day of surgery, patients should be cautioned of the potential for a decrease in mental alertness.

Do not touch the tip of the unit-dose container to the eye or any other surface.

B

Carcinogenesis, Mutagenesis, and Impairment of Fertility

No compound-related carcinogenic effects were observed in either mice or rats following a 21 month and 24 month study, respectively. In these studies, dietary administration of brimonidine tartrate at doses up to 2.5 mg/kg/day in mice and 1.0 mg/kg/day in rats achieved ~77 and 118 times, respectively, the plasma drug concentration estimated in humans treated with 1 drop Alphagan into both eyes 3 times per day.

Brimonidine tartrate was not mutagenic or cytogenic in a series of *in vitro* and *in vivo* studies including the Ames test, chromosomal aberation assay in Chinese Hamster Ovary (CHO) cells, a host-mediated assay and cytogenic studies in mice, and dominant lethal assay.

Reproductive studies performed in rats with oral doses of 0.66 mg base/kg revealed no evidence of impaired fertility due to Alphagan.

Pregnancy, Teratogenic Effects, Pregnancy Category B

Reproductive studies performed in rats with oral doses of 0.66 mg base/kg revealed no evidence of harm to the fetus due to Alphagan. Dosing at this level produced 100 times the plasma drug concentration level seen in humans following multiple ophthalmic doses. There are no adequate and well-controlled studies in pregnant women.

In animal studies, brimonidine crossed the placenta and entered into the fetal circulation to a limited extent. Alphagan should be used during pregnancy only if the potential benefit to the mother justifies the potential risk to the fetus.

Nursing Mothers

It is not known whether this drug is excreted in human milk; in animal studies brimonidine tartrate was excreted in breast milk. A decision should be made whether to discontinue nursing or to discontinue the drug, taking into account the importance of the drug to the mother.

Pediatric Use

In a well-controlled clinical study conducted in pediatric glaucoma patients (ages 2-7 years) the most commonly observed adverse events with brimonidine tartrate ophthalmic solution 0.2% dosed 3 times daily were somnolence (50-83% in patients ages 2-6 years) and decreased alertness. In pediatric patients 7 years of age or older (>20 kg), somnolence appears to occur less frequently (25%). Approximately 16% of patients on brimonidine tartrate ophthalmic solution discontinued from the study due to somnolence.

The safety and effectiveness of Alphagan have not been studied in pediatric patients below the age of 2 years. Alphagan is not recommended for use in pediatric patients under the age of 2 years.

Geriatric Use

No overall differences in safety or effectiveness have been observed between elderly and other adult patients.

ALPHAGAN P

General

Although Alphagan P had minimal effect on the blood pressure of patients in clinical studies, caution should be exercised in treating patients with severe cardiovascular disease.

Alphagan P has not been studied in patients with hepatic or renal impairment; caution should be used in treating such patients.

Alphagan P should be used with caution in patients with depression, cerebral or coronary insufficiency, Raynaud's phenomenon, orthostatic hypotension, or thromboangitis obliterans. Patients prescribed IOP-lowering medication should be routinely monitored for IOP.

Information for the Patient

As with other drugs in this class, Alphagan P may cause fatigue and/or drowsiness in some patients. Patients who engage in hazardous activities should be cautioned of the potential for a decrease in mental alertness.

Carcinogenesis, Mutagenesis, and Impairment of Fertility

No compound-related carcinogenic effects were observed in either mice or rats following a 21 month and 24 month study, respectively. In these studies, dietary administration of brimonidine tartrate at doses up to 2.5 mg/kg/day in mice and 1.0 mg/kg/day in rats achieved 86 and 55 times, respectively, the plasma drug concentration estimated in humans treated with 1 drop of Alphagan P into both eyes 3 times per day.

Brimonidine tartrate was not mutagenic or cytogenic in a series of *in vitro* and *in vivo* studies including the Ames test, chromosomal aberration assay in Chinese Hamster Ovary (CHO) cells, a host-mediated assay and cytogenic studies in mice, and dominant lethal assay.

Reproductive studies performed in rats with oral doses of 0.66 mg base/kg revealed no evidence of impaired fertility due to Alphagan P.

Pregnancy, Teratogenic Effects, Pregnancy Category B

Reproductive studies performed in rats with oral doses of 0.66 mg base/kg revealed no evidence of harm to the fetus due to Alphagan P. Dosing at this level produced an exposure that is 189 times higher than the exposure seen in humans following multiple ophthalmic doses.

There are no adequate and well-controlled studies in pregnant women. In animal studies, brimonidine crossed the placenta and entered into the fetal circulation to a limited extent. Alphagan P should be used during pregnancy only if the potential benefit to the mother justifies the potential risk to the fetus.

Nursing Mothers

It is not known whether this drug is excreted in human milk; in animal studies brimonidine tartrate was excreted in breast milk. A decision should be made whether to discontinue nursing or to discontinue the drug, taking into account the importance of the drug to the mother.

Pediatric Use

In a well-controlled clinical study conducted in pediatric glaucoma patients (ages 2-7 years) the most commonly observed adverse events with brimonidine tartrate ophthalmic solution 0.2% dosed 3 times a day were somnolence (50-83% in patients ages 2-6 years) and decreased alertness. In pediatric patients 7 years of age or older (20 kg), somnolence appears to occur less frequently (25%). Approximately 16% of patients on brimonidine tartrate ophthalmic solution discontinued from the study due to somnolence.

The safety and effectiveness of brimonidine tartrate ophthalmic solution have not been studied in pediatric patients below the age of 2 years. Brimonidine tartrate ophthalmic solution is not recommended for use in pediatric patients under the age of 2 years. (Also refer to ADVERSE REACTIONS.)

Geriatric Use

No overall differences in safety or effectiveness have been observed between elderly and other adult patients.

DRUG INTERACTIONS

ALPHAGAN 0.2%

Although specific drug interaction studies have not been conducted with Alphagan, the possibility of an additive or potentiating effect with CNS depressants (alcohol, barbiturates, opiates, sedatives, or anesthetics) should be considered. Alpha-agonists, as a class, may reduce pulse and blood pressure. Caution in using concomitant drugs such as beta-blockers (ophthalmic and systemic), antihypertensives and/or cardiac glycosides is advised.

Tricyclic antidepressants have been reported to blunt the hypotensive effect of systemic clonidine. It is not known whether the concurrent use of these agents with Alphagan in humans can lead to resulting interference with the IOP lowering effect. No data on the level of circulating catecholamines after Alphagan are available. Caution, however, is advised in patients taking tricyclic antidepressants which can affect the metabolism and uptake of circulating amines.

ALPHAGAN 0.5%

Although specific drug interaction studies have not been conducted with Alphagan, the possibility of an additive or potentiating effect with CNS depressants (alcohol, barbiturates, opiates, sedatives, or anesthetics) should be considered. Alpha-agonists, as a class, may reduce pulse and blood pressure. Caution in using concomitant drugs such as beta blockers (ophthalmic and systemic), antihypertensives and/or cardiac glycosides is advised.

Tricyclic antidepressants have been reported to blunt the hypotensive effect of systemic clonidine. It is not known whether the concurrent use of these agents with Alphagan in humans can lead to resulting interference with the IOP lowering effect. No data on the level of circulating catecholamines after Alphagan instillation are available. Caution, however, is advised in patients taking tricyclic antidepressants which can affect the metabolism and uptake of circulating amines.

ALPHAGAN P

Although specific drug interaction studies have not been conducted with Alphagan P, the possibility of an additive or potentiating effect with CNS depressants (alcohol, barbiturates, opiates, sedatives, or anesthetics) should be considered. Alpha-agonists, as a class, may reduce pulse and blood pressure. Caution in using concomitant drugs such as beta-blockers (ophthalmic and systemic), antihypertensives and/or cardiac glycosides is advised.

Tricyclic antidepressants have been reported to blunt the hypotensive effect of systemic clonidine. It is not known whether the concurrent use of these agents with Alphagan P in humans can lead to resulting interference with the IOP lowering effect. No data on the level of circulating catecholamines after Alphagan P administration are available. Caution, however, is advised in patients taking tricyclic antidepressants which can affect the metabolism and uptake of circulating amines.

ADVERSE REACTIONS

ALPHAGAN 0.2%

Adverse events occurring in approximately 10-30% of the subjects, in descending order of incidence, included oral dryness, ocular hyperemia, burning and stinging, headache, blurring, foreign body sensation, fatigue/drowsiness, conjunctival follicles, ocular allergic reactions, and ocular pruritus.

Events occurring in approximately 3-9% of the subjects, in descending order included corneal staining/erosion, photophobia, eyelid erythema, ocular ache/pain, ocular dryness, tearing, upper respiratory symptoms, eyelid edema, conjunctival edema, dizziness, blepharitis, ocular irritation, gastrointestinal symptoms, asthenia, conjunctival blanching, abnormal vision and muscular pain.

The following adverse reactions were reported in less than 3% of the patients: Lid crusting, conjunctival hemorrhage, abnormal taste, insomnia, conjunctival discharge, depression, hypertension, anxiety, palpitations/arrhythmias, nasal dryness and syncope.

The following events have been identified during post-marketing use of Alphagan in clinical practice. Because they are reported voluntarily from a population of unknown size, estimates of frequency cannot be made. The events, which have been chosen for inclusion due to either their seriousness, frequency of reporting, possible causal connection to Alphagan, or a combination of these factors, include: bradycardia; hypotension; iritis; miosis; skin reactions (including erythema, eyelid pruritis, rash, and vasodilation); and tachycardia. Apnea, bradycardia, hypotension, hypothermia, hypotonia, and somnolence have been reported in infants receiving Alphagan.

ALPHAGAN 0.5%

The most common adverse events reported in association with the use of Alphagan 0.5% in conjunction with ALT was transient conjunctival blanching in 50% of patients and upper lid retraction in 30% of patients.

The following adverse reactions were reported in 1-4% of the patients: Corneal edema, dizziness, drowsiness/tiredness, and ocular irritation (encompassing discomfort, foreign body sensation, and ocular pain.

The following were reported in 1% or less of patients: Browache, dry mouth, nausea.

ALPHAGAN P

Adverse events occurring in approximately 10-20% of the subjects included: Allergic conjunctivitis, conjunctival hyperemia, and eye pruritis.

Adverse events occurring in approximately 5-9% of the subjects included: Burning sensation, conjunctival foliculosis, hypertension, oral dryness, and visual disturbance.

Events occurring in approximately 1-4% of subjects included: Allergic reaction, asthenia, blepharitis, bronchitis, conjunctival edema, conjunctival hemorrhage, conjunctivitis, cough, dizziness, dyspepsia, dyspnea, epiphora, eye discharge, eye dryness, eye irritation, eye pain, eyelid edema, eyelid erythema, flu syndrome, follicular conjunctivitis, foreign body sensation, headache, pharyngitis, photophobia, rash, rhinitis, sinus infection, sinusitis, stinging, superficial punctate keratopathy, visual field defect, vitreous floaters, and worsened visual acuity.

The following events were reported in less than 1% of subjects: Corneal erosion, insomnia, nasal dryness, somnolence, and taste perversion.

The following events have been identified during post-marketing use of Alphagan in clinical practice. Because they are reported voluntarily from a population of unknown size, estimates of frequency cannot be made. The events, which have been chosen for inclusion due to either their seriousness, frequency of reporting, possible causal connection to Alphagan, or a combination of these factors, include: bradycardia; hypotension; iritis; miosis; skin reactions (including erythema, eyelid pruritis, rash, and vasodilation); and tachycardia. Apnea, bradycardia, hypotension, hypothermia, hypotonia, and somnolence have been reported in infants receiving Alphagan.

DOSAGE AND ADMINISTRATION

ALPHAGAN 0.2%

The recommended dose is 1 drop of Alphagan in the affected eye(s) 3 times daily, approximately 8 hours apart.

Alphagan may be used concomitantly with other topical ophthalmic drug products to lower intraocular pressure. If more than one topical ophthalmic product is being used, the products should be administered at least 5 minutes apart.

ALPHAGAN 0.5%

Instill 1 drop of Alphagan in the operative eye 30-45 minutes before ALT surgery and immediately following ALT surgery.

ALPHAGAN P

The recommended dose is 1 drop of Alphagan P in the affected eye(s) 3 times daily, approximately 8 hours apart.

Alphagan P may be used concomitantly with other topical ophthalmic drug products to lower intraocular pressure. If more than one topical ophthalmic product is being used, the products should be administered at least 5 minutes apart.

HOW SUPPLIED

ALPHAGAN 0.2%

Alphagan (brimonidine tartrate ophthalmic solution) 0.2% is supplied sterile in white opaque LPDE plastic bottles with tips with purple high impact polystyrene (HIPS) caps in 5, 10, and 15 ml.

Storage: Store between 15-25°C (59-77°F).

ALPHAGAN 0.5%

Alphagan (brimonidine tartrate ophthalmic solution) 0.5% is supplied sterile in unit dose vials of LDPE plastic containing 0.4 ml.

Storage: Store between 15-25°C (59-77°F). Properly dispose of unit-dose vial after each single patient use.

ALPHAGAN P

Alphagan P (brimonidine tartrate ophthalmic solution) 0.15% is supplied sterile in opaque teal LDPE plastic bottles and tips with purple high impact polystyrene (HIPS) caps in 5, 10, and 15 ml.

Storage: Store between 15-25°C (59-77°F).

PRODUCT LISTING - EQUIVALENTS NOT AVAILABLE

Solution - Ophthalmic - 0.15%

5 ml	$38.09	ALPHAGAN-P, Allergan Inc	00023-9177-05
10 ml	$76.11	ALPHAGAN-P, Allergan Inc	00023-9177-10
15 ml	$114.24	ALPHAGAN-P, Allergan Inc	00023-9177-15

Brinzolamide *(003360)*

Categories: Glaucoma, open-angle; Hypertension, ocular; FDA Approved 1998 Apr; Pregnancy Category C
Drug Classes: Carbonic anhydrase inhibitors; Ophthalmics
Brand Names: Azopt
Cost of Therapy: $24.19 (Glaucoma; Azopt Ophth. Suspension; 1%; 5 ml; 3 drops/day; variable day supply)

DESCRIPTION

Azopt (brinzolamide ophthalmic suspension) 1% contains a carbonic anhydrase inhibitor formulated for multidose topical ophthalmic use. Brinzolamide is described chemically as: (R)-(+)-4-Ethylamino-2-(3-methyoxypropyl)-3,4-dihydro-2H-thieno [3,2-e]-1,2-thiazino-6-sulfonamide-1,1-dioxide. Its empirical formula is $C_{12}H_{21}N_3O_5S_3$.

Brinzolamide has a molecular weight of 383.5 and a melting point of about 131°C. It is a white powder, which is insoluble in water, very soluble in methanol and soluble in ethanol.

Azopt 1% is supplied as a sterile, aqueous suspension of brinzolamide which has been formulated to be readily suspended and slow settling, following shaking. It has a pH of approximately 7.5 and an osmolality of 300 mOsm/kg. Each ml of Azopt 1% contains 10 mg brinzolamide. Inactive ingredients are mannitol, carbomer 974P, tyloxapol, edetate disodium, sodium chloride, hydrochloric acid and/or sodium hydroxide (to adjust pH), and purified water. Benzalkonium chloride 0.01 % is added as a preservative.

CLINICAL PHARMACOLOGY

Carbonic anhydrase (CA) is an enzyme found in many tissues of the body including the eye. It catalyzes the reversible reaction including the hydration of carbon dioxide and the dehydration of carbonic acid. In humans, carbonic anhydrase exists as a number of isoenzymes, the most active being carbonic anhydrase II (CA-II), found primarily in red blood cells (RBCs), but also in other tissues. Inhibition of carbonic anhydrase in the cillary processes of the eye decreases aqueous humor secretion, presumably by slowing the formulation of bicarbonate ions with subsequent reduction in sodium and fluid transport. The result is a reduction in intraocular pressure (IOP).

Brinzolamide ophthalmic suspension, an inhibitor of carbonic anhydrase II (CA-II). Following topical ocular administration, brinzolamide inhibits aqueous humor formation and reduces elevated intraocular pressure. Elevated intraocular pressure is a major risk factor in the pathogenesis of optic nerve damage and glaucomatous visual field loss.

Following topical ocular administration, brinzolamide is absorbed into the systemic circulation. Due to its affinity for CA-II, brinzolamide distributes extensively into the RBCs and exhibits a long half-life in whole blood (approximately 111 days). In humans, the metabolite N-desethyl brinzolamide is formed, which also binds to CA and accumulates in RBCs. This metabolite binds mainly to CA-I in the presence of brinzolamide. In plasma, both parent brinzolamide and N-desethyl brinzolamide concentrations are low and generally below assay quantification limits (<10 mg/ml). Binding to plasma proteins is approximately 60%. Brinzolamide is eliminated predominantly in the urine as unchanged drug. N-Desethyl brinzolamide is also found in the urine along with lower concentrations of the N-desmethoxypropyl and O-dosmethyl metabolites.

An oral pharmacokinetic study was conducted in which healthy volunteers received 1 mg capsules of brinzolamide twice per day for up to 32 weeks. This regimen approximates the amount of drug delivered by topical ocular administration of brinzolamide ophthalmic suspension dosed to both eyes three times per day and simulates systemic drug and metabolite concentrations similar to those achieved with long-term topical dosing. RBC CA activity was measured to assess the degree of systemic CA inhibition. Brinzolamide saturation of RBC CA-II was achieved within 4 weeks (RBC concentrations of approximately 20 μM), N-Demsethyl brinzolamide accumulated in RBCs to steady-state within 20-28 weeks reaching concentrations ranging from 6-30 μM. The inhibition of CA-II activity at steady-state was approximately 70-75%, which is below the degree of inhibition expected to have a pharmacological effect on renal function or respiration in healthy subjects.

In two, three-month clinical studies, brinzolamide ophthalmic suspension dosed three times per day (t.i.d.) in patients with elevated intraocular pressure (IOP), produced significant reductions in IOPs (4-5 mmHg). These IOP reductions are equivalent to the reductions observed with dorzolamide hydrochloride ophthalmic solution tid in the same studies.

In two clinical studies in patients with elevated intraocular pressure, brinzolamide ophthalmic suspension was associated with less stinging and burning upon instillation than dorzolamide hydrochloride ophthalmic solution.

INDICATIONS AND USAGE

Brinzolamide ophthalmic suspension is indicated in the treatment of elevated intraocular pressure in patients with ocular hypertension or open-angle glaucoma.

CONTRAINDICATIONS

Brinzolamide ophthalmic suspension is contraindicated in patients who are hypersensitive to any component of this product.

WARNINGS

Brinzolamide ophthalmic suspension is a sulfonamide and although administered topically it is absorbed systemically. Therefore, the same types of adverse reactions that are attributable to sulfonamides may occur with topical administration of brinzolamide ophthalmic suspension. Fatalities have occurred, although rarely, due to severe reactions to sulfonamides including Stevens-Johnson syndrome, toxic epidermal necrolysis, fulminant hepatic necrosis, agranulocytosis, aplastic anemia, and other blood dysorasias. Sensitization may recur when a sulfonamide is re-administered irrespective of the route of administration. If signs of serious reactions or hypersensitivity occur, discontinue the use of this preparation.

PRECAUTIONS

GENERAL

Carbonic anhydrase activity has been observed in both the cytoplasm and around the plasma membranes of the corneal endothelium. The effect of continued administration of brinzolamide ophthalmic suspension on the corneal endothelium has not been fully evaluated. The management of patients with acute angle-closure glaucoma requires therapeutic interventions in addition to ocular hypertensive agents, brinzolamide ophthalmic suspension has not been studied in patients with acute angle-closure glaucoma.

Brinzolamide ophthalmic suspension has not been studied in patients with severe renal impairment (CrCl <30 ml/min). Because brinzolamide ophthalmic suspension and its metabolite are excreted predominantly by the kidney, brinzolamide ophthalmic suspension is not recommended in such patients.

Brinzolamide ophthalmic suspension has not been studied in patients with hepatic impairment and should be used with caution in such patients.

There is a potential for an additive effect on the known systemic effects of carbonic anhydrase inhibition in patients receiving an oral carbonic anhydrase inhibitor and brinzolamide ophthalmic suspension. The concomitant administration of brinzolamide ophthalmic suspension and oral carbonic anhydrase inhibitors is not recommended.

INFORMATION FOR THE PATIENT

Brinzolamide ophthalmic suspension is a sulfonamide and although administered topically, it is absorbed systemically; therefore, the same types of adverse reactions attributable to sulfonamides may occur with topical administration. Patients should be advised that if serious or unusual ocular or systemic reactions or signs of hypersensitivity occur, they should discontinue the use of the product and consult their physician (see WARNINGS).

Vision may be temporarily blurred following dosing with brinzolamide ophthalmic suspension. Care should be exercised in operating machinery or driving a motor vehicle.

Patients should be instructed to avoid allowing the tip of the dispensing container to contact the eye or surrounding structures or other surfaces, since the product can become contaminated by common bacteria known to cause ocular infections. Serious damage to the eye and subsequent loss of vision may result from using contaminated solutions.

Patients should also be advised that if they have ocular surgery or develop an intercurrent ocular condition (*e.g.*, trauma or infection), they should immediately seek their physician's advice concerning the continued use of the present multidose container.

If more than one topical ophthalmic drug is being used, the drugs should be administered at least ten minutes apart. The preservative in brinzolamide ophthalmic suspension, benzalkonium chloride, may be absorbed by soft contact lenses. Contact lenses should be removed during instillation of brinzolamide ophthalmic suspension, but may be reinserted 15 minutes after instillation.

CARCINOGENESIS, MUTAGENESIS, AND IMPAIRMENT OF FERTILITY

Carcinogenicity data on brinzolamide are not available. The following tests for mutagenic potential were negative: (1) *in vivo* mouse micronucleus assay; (2) *in vivo* sister chromatid exchange assay; and (3) Ames *E. coli* test. The *in vitro* mouse lymphoma forward mutation assay was negative in the absence of activation, but positive in the presence of microsomal activation. In reproduction studies of brinzolamide in rats, there were no adverse effects on the fertility or reproductive capacity of males or females at doses up to 18 mg/kg/day (375 times the recommended human ophthalmic dose).

PREGNANCY, TERATOGENIC EFFECTS, PREGNANCY CATEGORY C

Developmental toxicity studies with brinzolamide in rabbits of oral doses at 1, 3, and 6 mg/kg/day (20, 62, and 125 times the recommended human ophthalmic dose) produced maternal toxicity at 6 mg/kg/day and a significant increase in the number of fetal variations, such as accessory skull bones, which was only slightly higher than the historic value at 1 and 6 mg/kg. In rats, statistically decreased body weights of fetuses from dams receiving oral doses of 18 mg/kg/day (375 times the recommended human ophthalmic dose) during gestation were proportional to the reduced maternal weight gain, with no statistically significant effects on organ or tissue development. Increases in unossified sternebrae, reduced ossification of the skull, and unossified hyoid that occurred at 6 and 18 mg/kg were not statistically significant. No treatment-related malformations were seen. Following oral administration of ^{14}C-brinzolamide to pregnant rats, radioactivity was found to cross the placenta and was present in the fetal tissues and blood.

There are no adequate and well-controlled studies in pregnant women. Brinzolamide ophthalmic suspension should be used during pregnancy only if the potential benefit justifies the potential risk to the fetus.

NURSING MOTHERS

In a study of brinzolamide in lactating rats, decreases in body weight gain in offspring at an oral dose of 15 mg/kg/day (312 times the recommended human ophthalmic dose) were seen during lactation. No other effects were observed. However, following oral administration of ^{14}C-brinzolamide to lactating rats, radioactivity was found in milk at concentrations below those in the blood and plasma.

It is not known whether this drug is secreted in human milk. Because many drugs are secreted in human milk and because of the potential for serious adverse reactions in nursing infants from brinzolamide ophthalmic suspension, a decision should be made whether to discontinue nursing or to discontinue the drug, taking into account the importance of the drug to the mother.

PEDIATRIC USE

Safety and effectiveness in pediatric patients have not been established.

DRUG INTERACTIONS

Brinzolamide ophthalmic suspension contains a carbonic anhydrase inhibitor. Acid-base and electrolyte alterations were not reported in the clinical trials with brinzolamide. However, in patients treated with oral carbonic anhydrase inhibitors, rare instances of drug interactions have occurred with high-dose salicylate therapy. Therefore, the potential for such drug interactions should be considered in patients receiving brinzolamide ophthalmic suspension.

ADVERSE REACTIONS

In clinical studies of brinzolamide ophthalmic suspension, the most frequently reported adverse events associated with brinzolamide ophthalmic suspension were blurred vision and bitter, sour or unusual taste. These events occurred in approximately 5-10% of patients. Blepharitis, dermatitis, dry eye, foreign body sensation, headache, hyperemia, ocular discharge, ocular discomfort, ocular keratitis, ocular pain, ocular pruritus and rhinitis were reported at an incidence of 1-5%.

The following adverse reactions were reported at an incidence below 1%: allergic reactions, alopecia, chest pain, conjunctivitis, diarrhea, diplopia, dizziness, dry mouth, dyspnea, dyspepsia, eye fatigue, hypertonia, keratoconjunctivitis, keratopathy, kidney pain, lid margin crusting or sticky sensation, nausea, pharyngitis, tearing and uticaria.

DOSAGE AND ADMINISTRATION

Shake well before use. The recommended dose is 1 drop of brinzolamide ophthalmic suspension in the affected eye(s) three times daily.

Brinzolamide ophthalmic suspension may be used concomitantly with other topical ophthalmic drug products to lower intraocular pressure. If more than one topical ophthalmic drug is being used, the drugs should be administered at least ten minutes apart.

HOW SUPPLIED

Azopt Ophthalmic Suspension 1% is supplied in plastic Drop-Tainer dispensers with a controlled dispensing-tip.

Storage: Store at 4-30°C (38-86°F).

PRODUCT LISTING - EQUIVALENTS NOT AVAILABLE

Suspension - Ophthalmic - 1%

5 ml	$24.19	AZOPT, Allscripts Pharmaceutical Company	54569-4823-00
5 ml	$31.44	AZOPT, Alcon Laboratories Inc	00065-0275-05
10 ml	$62.94	AZOPT, Alcon Laboratories Inc	00065-0275-10
15 ml	$94.38	AZOPT, Alcon Laboratories Inc	00065-0275-15

Bromocriptine Mesylate *(000527)*

Categories: Acromegaly; Adenoma, prolactin-secreting; Hyperprolactinemia; Parkinson's disease; Pregnancy Category B; FDA Approved 1978 Jun

Drug Classes: Antiparkinson agents; Dopaminergics; Ergot alkaloids and derivatives

Brand Names: **Parlodel**

Foreign Brand Availability: Alpha-Bromocriptine (New-Zealand); Antilactin (Korea); Apo-Bromocriptine (New-Zealand); Axialit (Argentina); Barlolin (Taiwan); Brameston (Bahamas; Barbados; Belize; Bermuda; Curacao; Guyana; Jamaica; Netherland-Antilles; Surinam; Trinidad); Bromed (Austria); Bromergon (Denmark); Bromidine (Korea); Bromocorn (Poland); Bromocrel (Germany); Bromohexal (Australia); Bromokin (Finland); Bromo-Kin (France); Bromopar (Denmark); Butin (Singapore); Cryocriptina (Mexico); Demil (Taiwan); Deprolac (Taiwan); Diken (Mexico); Elkrip (Indonesia); Ergolactin (China); Lactismine (Spain); Medocriptine (Hong-Kong); Parilac (Israel); Pravidel (Germany; Sweden); Provasyn (Philippines); Ronalin (Bahrain; Cyprus; Egypt; Iran; Iraq; Jordan; Kuwait; Lebanon; Libya; Oman; Qatar; Republic-of-Yemen; Saudi-Arabia; Syria; United-Arab-Emirates); Serocryptin (Bahrain; China; Cyprus; Egypt; Greece; Hong-Kong; India; Iran; Iraq; Italy; Jordan; Kuwait; Lebanon; Libya; Malaysia; Mexico; Oman; Peru; Qatar; Republic-of-Yemen; Saudi-Arabia; Switzerland; Syria; United-Arab-Emirates); Suplac (Malaysia; Thailand); Umprel (Austria)

Cost of Therapy: $87.57 (Parkinsonism; Parlodel Snap; 2.5 mg; 1 tablet/day; 30 day supply)
$47.31 (Parkinsonism; Generic Tablets; 2.5 mg; 1 tablet/day; 30 day supply)

DESCRIPTION

Parlodel (bromocriptine mesylate) is an ergot derivative with potent dopamine receptor agonist activity. Each Parlodel snap tabs tablet for oral administration contains 2½ mg and each capsule contains 5 mg bromocriptine (as the mesylate). Bromocriptine mesylate is chemically designated as Ergotaman-3′,6′,18-trione,2-bromo-12′-hydroxy-2′-(1-methylethyl)-5′-(2-methylpropyl)-, (5′α) monomethanesulfonate (salt).

2½ mg Snap Tabs: *Active Ingredient:* Bromocriptine mesylate; *Inactive Ingredients:* Colloidal silicon dioxide, lactose, magnesium stearate, povidone, starch, and another ingredient.

5 mg Capsules: *Active Ingredient:* Bromocriptine mesylate; *Inactive Ingredients:* Colloidal silicon dioxide, gelatin, lactose, magnesium stearate, red iron oxide, silicon dioxide, sodium bisulfite, sodium lauryl sulfate, starch, titanium dioxide, yellow iron oxide, and another ingredient.

CLINICAL PHARMACOLOGY

Bromocriptine mesylate is a dopamine receptor agonist, which activates post-synaptic dopamine receptors. The dopaminergic neurons in the tuberoinfundibular process modulate the secretion of prolactin from the anterior pituitary by secreting a prolactin inhibitory factor (thought to be dopamine); in the corpus striatum the dopaminergic neurons are involved in the control of motor function. Clinically, bromocriptine mesylate significantly reduces plasma levels of prolactin in patients with physiologically elevated prolactin as well as in patients with hyperprolactinemia. The inhibition of physiological lactation as well as galactorrhea in pathological hyperprolactinemic states is obtained at dose levels that do not affect secretion of other tropic hormones from the anterior pituitary. Experiments have demonstrated that bromocriptine induces long lasting stereotyped behavior in rodents and turning behavior in rats having unilateral lesions in the substantia nigra. These actions, characteristic of those produced by dopamine, are inhibited by dopamine antagonists and suggest a direct action of bromocriptine on striatal dopamine receptors.

Bromocriptine mesylate is a nonhormonal, nonestrogenic agent that inhibits the secretion of prolactin in humans, with little or no effect on other pituitary hormones, except in patients with acromegaly, where it lowers elevated blood levels of growth hormone in the majority of patients.

In about 75% of cases of amenorrhea and galactorrhea, bromocriptine mesylate therapy suppresses the galactorrhea completely, or almost completely, and reinitiates normal ovulatory menstrual cycles.

Menses are usually reinitiated prior to complete suppression of galactorrhea; the time for this on average is 6-8 weeks. However, some patients respond within a few days, and others may take up to 8 months.

Galactorrhea may take longer to control depending on the degree of stimulation of the mammary tissue prior to therapy. At least a 75% reduction in secretion is usually observed after 8-12 weeks. Some patients may fail to respond even after 12 months of therapy.

In many acromegalic patients, bromocriptine mesylate produces a prompt and sustained reduction in circulating levels of serum growth hormone.

Bromocriptine mesylate produces its therapeutic effect in the treatment of Parkinson's disease, a clinical condition characterized by a progressive deficiency in dopamine synthesis in the substantia nigra, by directly stimulating the dopamine receptors in the corpus striatum. In contrast, levodopa exerts its therapeutic effect only after conversion to dopamine by the neurons of the substantia nigra, which are known to be numerically diminished in this patient population.

PHARMACOKINETICS

The pharmacokinetics and metabolism of bromocriptine in human subjects were studied with the help of radioactively labeled drug. Twenty-eight percent (28%) of an oral dose was absorbed from the gastrointestinal tract. The blood levels following a 2½ mg dose were in the range of 2-3 ng equivalents/ml. Plasma levels were in the range of 4-6 ng equivalents/ml indicating that the red blood cells did not contain appreciable amounts of drug and/or metabolites. *In vitro* experiments showed that the drug was 90-96% bound to serum albumin.

Bromocriptine was completely metabolized prior to excretion. The major route of excretion of absorbed drug was via the bile. Only 2.5-5.5% of the dose was excreted in the urine. Almost all (84.6%) of the administered dose was excreted in the feces in 120 hours.

INDICATIONS AND USAGE

HYPERPROLACTINEMIA-ASSOCIATED DYSFUNCTIONS

Bromocriptine mesylate is indicated for the treatment of dysfunctions associated with **hyperprolactinemia** including **amenorrhea** with or without **galactorrhea, infertility or hypogonadism.** Bromocriptine mesylate treatment is indicated in patients with **prolactin-secreting adenomas,** which may be the basic underlying endocrinopathy contributing to the above clinical presentations. **Reduction** in **tumor size** has been demonstrated in both male and female patients with macroadenomas. In cases where adenectomy is elected, a course of bromocriptine mesylate therapy may be used to reduce the tumor mass prior to surgery.

ACROMEGALY

Bromocriptine mesylate therapy is indicated in the treatment of acromegaly. Bromocriptine mesylate therapy, alone or as adjunctive therapy with pituitary irradiation or surgery, reduces serum growth hormone by 50% or more in approximately ½ of patients treated, although not usually to normal levels.

Since the effects of external pituitary radiation may not become maximal for several years, adjunctive therapy with bromocriptine mesylate offers potential benefit before the effects of irradiation are manifested.

PARKINSON'S DISEASE

Bromocriptine mesylate tablets or capsules are indicated in the treatment of the signs and symptoms of idiopathic or postencephalitic Parkinson's disease. As adjunctive treatment to levodopa (alone or with a peripheral decarboxylase inhibitor), bromocriptine mesylate therapy may provide additional therapeutic benefits in those patients who are currently maintained on optimal dosages of levodopa, those who are beginning to deteriorate (develop tolerance) to levodopa therapy, and those who are experiencing "end of dose failure" on levodopa therapy. Bromocriptine mesylate therapy may permit a reduction of the maintenance dose of levodopa and, thus may ameliorate the occurrence and/or severity of adverse reactions associated with long-term levodopa therapy such as abnormal involuntary movements (*e.g.,* dyskinesias) and the marked swings in motor function ("on-off" phenomenon). Continued efficacy of bromocriptine mesylate therapy during treatment of more than 2 years has not been established.

Data are insufficient to evaluate potential benefit from treating newly diagnosed Parkinson's disease with bromocriptine mesylate. Studies have shown, however, significantly more adverse reactions (notably nausea, hallucinations, confusion and hypotension) in bromocriptine mesylate treated patients than in levodopa/carbidopa treated patients. Patients unresponsive to levodopa are poor candidates for bromocriptine mesylate therapy.

CONTRAINDICATIONS

Uncontrolled hypertension and sensitivity to any ergot alkaloids. In patients being treated for hyperprolactinemia bromocriptine mesylate should be withdrawn when pregnancy is diagnosed (see PRECAUTIONS, Hyperprolactinemic States). In the event that bromocriptine mesylate is reinstituted to control a rapidly expanding macroadenoma (see PRECAUTIONS, Hyperprolactinemic States) and a patient experiences a hypertensive disorder of pregnancy, the benefit of continuing bromocriptine mesylate must be weighted against the possible risk of its use during a hypertensive disorder of pregnancy. When bromocriptine mesylate is being used to treat acromegaly or Parkinson's disease in patients who subsequently become pregnant, a decision should be made as to whether the therapy continues to be medically necessary or can be withdrawn. If it is continued, the drug should be withdrawn in those who may experience hypertensive disorders of pregnancy (including eclampsia, preeclampsia, or pregnancy-induced hypertension) unless withdrawal of bromocriptine mesylate is considered to be medically contraindicated.

WARNINGS

Since hyperprolactinemia with amenorrhea/galactorrhea and infertility has been found in patients with pituitary tumors, a complete evaluation of the pituitary is indicated before treatment with bromocriptine mesylate.

If pregnancy occurs during bromocriptine mesylate administration, careful observation of these patients is mandatory. Prolactin-secreting adenomas may expand and compression of the optic or other cranial nerves may occur, emergency pituitary surgery becoming necessary. In most cases, the compression resolves following delivery. Reinitiation of bromocriptine mesylate treatment has been reported to produce improvement in the visual fields of patients in whom nerve compression has occurred during pregnancy. The safety of bromocriptine mesylate treatment during pregnancy to the mother and fetus has not been established.

Symptomatic hypotension can occur in patients treated with bromocriptine mesylate for any indication. In postpartum studies with bromocriptine mesylate, decreases in supine systolic and diastolic pressures of greater than 20 mm and 10 mm Hg, respectively, have been observed in almost 30% of patients receiving bromocriptine mesylate. On occasion, the drop in supine systolic pressure was as much as 50-59 mm of Hg. **While hypotension during the start of therapy with bromocriptine mesylate occurs in some patients, in postmarketing experience in the US in postpartum patients 89 cases of hypertension have been reported, sometimes at the initiation of therapy, but often developing in the second week of therapy; seizures have been reported in 72 cases (including 4 cases of status epilepticus), both with and without the prior development of hypertension; 30 cases of stroke have been reported mostly in postpartum patients whose prenatal and obstetric courses had been uncomplicated. Many of these patients experiencing seizures and/or strokes reported developing a constant and often progressively severe headache hours to days prior to the acute event. Some cases of strokes and seizures were also preceded by visual disturbances (blurred vision, and transient cortical blindness). Nine cases of acute myocardial infarction have been reported.**

Although a causal relationship between bromocriptine mesylate administration and hypertension, seizures, strokes, and myocardial infarction in postpartum women has not been established, use of the drug for prevention of physiological lactation, or in patients with uncontrolled hypertension is not recommended. In patients being treated for hyperprolactinemia bromocriptine mesylate should be withdrawn when pregnancy is diagnosed (see PRECAUTIONS, Hyperprolactinemic States). In the event that bromocriptine mesylate is reinstituted to control a rapidly expanding macroadenoma (see PRECAUTIONS, Hyperprolactinemic States) **and a patient experiences a hypertensive disorder of pregnancy, the benefit of continuing bromocriptine mesylate must be weighed against the possible risk of its use during a hypertensive disorder of pregnancy. When bromocriptine mesylate is being used to treat acromegaly or Parkinson's disease in patients who have subsequently become pregnant, a decision should be made as to whether the therapy continues to be medically necessary or can be withdrawn. If it is continued, the drug should be withdrawn in those who may experience hypertensive disorders of pregnancy (including eclampsia, preeclampsia, or pregnancy-induced hypertension) unless withdrawal of bromocriptine mesylate is considered to be medically contraindicated. Because of the possibility of an interaction between bromocriptine mesylate and other ergot alkaloids, the concomitant use of these medications is not recommended. Particular attention should be paid to patients who have recently received other drugs that can alter the blood pressure.** Periodic monitoring of the blood pressure, particularly during the first weeks of therapy is prudent. If hypertension, severe, progressive, or unremitting headache (with or without visual disturbance), or evidence of CNS toxicity develops, drug therapy should be discontinued and the patient should be evaluated promptly.

Long-term treatment (6-36 months) with bromocriptine mesylate in doses ranging from 20-100 mg/day has been associated with pulmonary infiltrates, pleural effusion and thickening of the pleura in a few patients. In those instances in which bromocriptine mesylate treatment was terminated, the changes slowly reverted towards normal.

PRECAUTIONS

GENERAL

Safety and efficacy of bromocriptine mesylate have not been established in patients with renal or hepatic disease. Care should be exercised when administering bromocriptine mesylate therapy concomitantly with other medications known to lower blood pressure.

Hyperprolactinemic States: The relative efficacy of bromocriptine mesylate versus surgery in preserving visual fields is not known. Patients with rapidly progressive visual field loss should be evaluated by a neurosurgeon to help decide on the most appropriate therapy. Since pregnancy is often the therapeutic objective in many hyperprolactinemic patients presenting with amenorrhea/galactorrhea and hypogonadism (infertility), a careful assessment of the pituitary is essential to detect the presence of a prolactin-secreting adenoma. Patients not seeking pregnancy, or those harboring large adenomas, should be advised to use contraceptive measures, other than oral contraceptives, during treatment with bromocriptine mesylate. Since pregnancy may occur prior to reinitiation of menses, a pregnancy test is recommended at least every 4 weeks during the amenorrheic period, and, once menses are reinitiated, every time a patient misses a menstrual period. Treatment with bromocriptine mesylate tablets or capsules should be discontinued as soon as pregnancy has been established. Patients must be monitored closely throughout pregnancy for signs and symptoms that may signal the enlargement of a previously undetected or existing prolactin-secreting tumor. Discontinuation of bromocriptine mesylate treatment in patients with known macroadenomas has been associated with rapid regrowth of tumor and increase in serum prolactin in most cases.

Acromegaly: Cold sensitive digital vasospasm has been observed in some acromegalic patients treated with bromocriptine mesylate. The response, should it occur, can be reversed by reducing the dose of bromocriptine mesylate and may be prevented by keeping the fingers warm. Cases of severe gastrointestinal bleeding from peptic ulcers have been reported, some fatal. Although there is no evidence that bromocriptine mesylate increases the incidence of peptic ulcers in acromegalic patients, symptoms suggestive of peptic ulcer should be investigated thoroughly and treated appropriately.

Possible tumor expansion while receiving bromocriptine mesylate therapy has been reported in a few patients. Since the natural history of growth hormone secreting tumors is unknown, all patients should be carefully monitored and, if evidence of tumor expansion develops, discontinuation of treatment and alternative procedures considered.

Parkinson's Disease: Safety during long-term use for more than 2 years at the doses required for parkinsonism has not been established.

As with any chronic therapy, periodic evaluation of hepatic, hematopoietic, cardiovascular, and renal function is recommended. Symptomatic hypotension can occur and, therefore, caution should be exercised when treating patients receiving antihypertensive drugs.

High doses of bromocriptine mesylate may be associated with confusion and mental disturbances. Since parkinsonian patients may manifest mild degrees of dementia, caution should be used when treating such patients.

Bromocriptine mesylate administered alone or concomitantly with levodopa may cause hallucinations (visual or auditory). Hallucinations usually resolve with dosage reduction; occasionally, discontinuation of bromocriptine mesylate is required. Rarely, after high doses, hallucinations have persisted for several weeks following discontinuation of bromocriptine mesylate.

As with levodopa, caution should be exercised when administering bromocriptine mesylate to patients with a history of myocardial infarction who have a residual atrial, nodal, or ventricular arrhythmia.

Retroperitoneal fibrosis has been reported in a few patients receiving long-term therapy (2-10 years) with bromocriptine mesylate in doses ranging from 30-140 mg daily.

INFORMATION FOR THE PATIENT

When initiating therapy, all patients receiving bromocriptine mesylate should be cautioned with regard to engaging in activities requiring rapid and precise responses, such as driving an automobile or operating machinery since dizziness (8%-16%), drowsiness (8%), faintness, fainting (8%), and syncope (less than 1%) have been reported early in the course of therapy. Patients receiving bromocriptine mesylate for hyperprolactinemic states associated with macroadenoma or those who have had previous transsphenoidal surgery, should be told to report any persistent watery nasal discharge to their physician. Patients receiving bromocriptine mesylate for treatment of a macroadenoma should be told that discontinuation of drug may be associated with rapid regrowth of the tumor and recurrence of their original symptoms.

CARCINOGENESIS, MUTAGENESIS, AND IMPAIRMENT OF FERTILITY

A 74 week study was conducted in mice using dietary levels of bromocriptine mesylate equivalent to oral doses of 10 and 50 mg/kg/day. A 100 week study in rats was conducted using dietary levels equivalent to oral doses of 1.7, 9.8, and 44 mg/kg/day. The highest doses tested in mice and rats were approximately 2.5 and 4.4 times, respectively, the maximum human dose administered in controlled clinical trials (100 mg/day) based on body surface area. Malignant uterine tumors, endometrial and myometrial, were found in rats as follows: 0/50 control females, 2/50 females given 1.7 mg/kg daily, 7/49 females given 9.8 mg/kg daily, and 9/50 females given 44 mg/kg daily. The occurrence of these neoplasms is probably attributable to the high estrogen/progesterone ratio which occurs in rats as a result of the prolactin-inhibiting action of bromocriptine mesylate. The endocrine mechanisms believed to be involved in the rats are not present in humans. There is no known correlation between uterine malignancies occurring in bromocriptine-treated rats and human risk. In contrast to the findings in rats, the uteri from mice killed after 74 weeks treatment did not exhibit evidence of drug-related changes.

Bromocriptine mesylate was evaluated for mutagenic potential in the battery of tests that included Ames bacterial mutation assay, mutagenic activity *in vitro* on V79 Chinese hamster fibroblasts, cytogenetic analysis of Chinese hamster bone marrow cells following *in vivo* treatment, and an *in vivo* micronucleus test for mutagenic potential in mice.

No mutagenic effects were obtained in any of these tests.

Fertility and reproductive performance in female rats were not influenced adversely by treatment with bromocriptine beyond the predicted decrease in the weight of pups due to suppression of lactation. In males treated with 50 mg/kg of this drug, mating and fertility were within the normal range. Increased perinatal loss was produced in the subgroups of dams, sacrificed on day 21 postpartum (pp) after mating with males treated with the highest dose (50 mg/kg).

PREGNANCY CATEGORY B

Administration of 10-30 mg/kg of bromocriptine to 2 strains of rats on days 6-15 post coitum (pc) as well as a single dose of 10 mg/kg on day 5 pc interfered with nidation. Three (3) mg/kg given on days 6-15 were without effect on nidation, and did not produce any anomalies. In animals treated from day 8-15 pc, *i.e.,* after implantation, 30 mg/kg produced increased prenatal mortality in the form of increased incidence of embryonic resorption. One anomaly, aplasia of spinal vertebrae and ribs, was found in the group of 262 fetuses derived from the dams treated with 30 mg/kg bromocriptine. No fetotoxic effects were found in offspring of dams treated during the peri- or post-natal period.

Two studies were conducted in rabbits (2 strains) to determine the potential to interfere with nidation. Dose levels of 100 or 300 mg/kg/day from day 1 to day 6 pc did not adversely affect nidation. The high dose was approximately 63 times the maximum human dose administered in controlled clinical trials (100 mg/day), based on body surface area. In New Zealand white rabbits some embryo mortality occurred at 300 mg/kg which was a reflection of overt maternal toxicity. Three studies were conducted in 2 strains of rabbits to determine the teratological potential of bromocriptine at dose levels of 3, 10, 30, 100, and 300 mg/kg given from day 6 to day 18 pc. In 2 studies with the Yellow-silver strain, cleft palate was found in 3 and 2 fetuses at maternally toxic doses of 100 and 300 mg/kg, respectively. One control fetus also exhibited this anomaly. In the third study conducted with New Zealand white rabbits using an identical protocol, no cleft palates were produced.

No teratological or embryo-toxic effects of bromocriptine were produced in any of 6 offspring from 6 monkeys at a dose level of 2 mg/kg.

Information concerning 1276 pregnancies in women taking bromocriptine has been collected. In the majority of cases, bromocriptine was discontinued within 8 weeks into pregnancy (mean 28.7 days), however, 8 patients received the drug continuously throughout pregnancy. The mean daily dose for all patients was 5.8 mg (range 1-40 mg).

Of these 1276 pregnancies, there were 1088 full term deliveries (4 stillborn), 145 spontaneous abortions (11.4%), and 28 induced abortions (2.2%). Moreover, 12 extrauterine gravidities and 3 hydatidiform moles (twice in the same patient) caused early termination of pregnancy. These data compare favorably with the abortion rate (11-25%) cited for pregnancies induced by clomiphene citrate, menopausal gonadotropin, and chorionic gonadotropin.

Although spontaneous abortions often go unreported, especially prior to 20 weeks of gestation, their frequency has been estimated to be 15%.

The incidence of birth defects in the population at large ranges from 2%-4.5%. The incidence in 1109 live births from patients receiving bromocriptine is 3.3%.

There is no suggestion that bromocriptine contributed to the type or incidence of birth defects in this group of infants.

NURSING MOTHERS

Bromocriptine mesylate should not be used during lactation in postpartum women.

PEDIATRIC USE

Safety and efficacy of bromocriptine mesylate have not been established in children under the age of 15.

DRUG INTERACTIONS

Lack or decrease in efficacy may occur in patients receiving bromocriptine mesylate when they are treated concurrently with drugs which have dopamine antagonist activity,*e.g.,* phenothiazines, butyrophenones. This may be a problem particularly for patients treated with bromocriptine mesylate for macroadenomas. Although there is no conclusive evidence demonstrating interactions between bromocriptine mesylate and other ergot derivatives, the concomitant use of these medications is not recommended.

ADVERSE REACTIONS

HYPERPROLACTINEMIC INDICATIONS

The incidence of adverse effects is quite high (69%) but these are generally mild to moderate in degree. Therapy was discontinued in approximately 5% of patients because of adverse effects. These in decreasing order of frequency are: nausea (49%), headache (19%), dizziness (17%), fatigue (7%), lightheadedness (5%), vomiting (5%), abdominal cramps (4%), nasal congestion (3%), constipation (3%), diarrhea (3%) and drowsiness (3%).

A slight hypotensive effect may accompany bromocriptine mesylate treatment. The occurrence of adverse reactions may be lessened by temporarily reducing dosage to ½ tablet 2 or 3 times daily. A few cases of cerebrospinal fluid rhinorrhea have been reported in patients receiving bromocriptine mesylate for treatment of large prolactinomas. This has occurred rarely, usually only in patients who have received previous transsphenoidal surgery, pituitary radiation, or both, and who were receiving bromocriptine mesylate for tumor recurrence. It may also occur in previously untreated patients whose tumor extends into the sphenoid sinus.

ACROMEGALY

The most frequent adverse reactions encountered in acromegalic patients treated with bromocriptine mesylate were: Nausea (18%), constipation (14%), postural/orthostatic hypotension (6%), anorexia (4%), dry mouth/nasal stuffiness (4%), indigestion/dyspepsia (4%), digital vasospasm (3%), drowsiness/tiredness (3%) and vomiting (2%).

Less frequent adverse reactions (less than 2%) were: Gastrointestinal bleeding, dizziness, exacerbation of Raynaud's Syndrome, headache and syncope. Rarely (less than 1%) hair loss, alcohol potentiation, faintness, lightheadedness, arrhythmia, ventricular tachycardia, decreased sleep requirement, visual hallucinations, lassitude, shortness of breath, bradycardia, vertigo, paresthesia, sluggishness, vasovagal attack, delusional psychosis, paranoia, insomnia, heavy headedness, reduced tolerance to cold, tingling of ears, facial pallor and muscle cramps have been reported.

PARKINSON'S DISEASE

In clinical trials in which bromocriptine was administered with concomitant reduction in the dose of levodopa/carbidopa, the most common newly appearing adverse reactions were: Nausea, abnormal involuntary movements, hallucinations, confusion, "on-off" phenomenon, dizziness, drowsiness, faintness/fainting, vomiting, asthenia, abdominal discomfort, visual disturbance, ataxia, insomnia, depression, hypotension, shortness of breath, constipation, and vertigo.

Less common adverse reactions which may be encountered include: Anorexia, blepharospasm, dry mouth, dysphagia, edema of the feet and ankles, erythromelalgia, epileptiform seizure, fatigue, headache, lethargy, mottling of skin, nasal stuffiness, nervousness, nightmares, paresthesia, skin rash, urinary frequency, urinary incontinence, urinary retention, and rarely, signs and symptoms of ergotism such as tingling of fingers, cold feet, numbness, muscle cramps of feet and legs or exacerbation of Raynaud's Syndrome.

Abnormalities in laboratory tests may include elevations in blood urea nitrogen, SGOT, SGPT, GGPT, CPK, alkaline phosphatase and uric acid, which are usually transient and not of clinical significance.

ADVERSE EVENTS OBSERVED IN OTHER CONDITIONS

Postpartum Patients

In postpartum studies with bromocriptine mesylate 23% of postpartum patients treated had at least 1 side effect, but they were generally mild to moderate in degree. Therapy was discontinued in approximately 3% of patients. The most frequently occurring adverse reactions were: headache (10%), dizziness (8%), nausea (7%), vomiting (3%), fatigue (1.0%), syncope (0.7%), diarrhea (0.4%) and cramps (0.4%). Decreases in blood pressure (≥20 mm Hg systolic and ≥10 mm Hg diastolic) occurred in 28% of patients at least once during the first 3 postpartum days; these were usually of a transient nature. Reports of fainting in the puerperium may possibly be related to this effect. In postmarketing experience in the US serious adverse reactions reported include 72 cases of seizures (including 4 cases of status epilepticus), 30 cases of stroke, and 9 cases of myocardial infarction among postpartum patients. Seizure cases were not necessarily accompanied by the development of hypertension. An unremitting and often progressively severe headache, sometimes accompanied by visual disturbance, often preceded by hours to days many cases of seizure and or/stroke. Most patients had shown no evidence of any of the hypertensive disorders of pregnancy including eclampsia, preeclampsia or pregnancy induced hypertension. One stroke case was associated with sagittal sinus thrombosis, and another was associated with cerebral and cerebellar vasculitis. One case of myocardial infarction was associated with unexplained disseminated intravascular coagulation and a second occurred in conjunction with use of another ergot alkaloid. The relationship of these adverse reactions to bromocriptine mesylate administration has not been established.

DOSAGE AND ADMINISTRATION

GENERAL

It is recommended that bromocriptine mesylate be taken with food. Patients should be evaluated frequently during dose escalation to determine the lowest dosage that produces a therapeutic response.

HYPERPROLACTINEMIC INDICATIONS

The initial dosage of bromocriptine mesylate is ½ to one 2½ mg tablet daily. An additional 2½ mg tablet may be added to the treatment regimen as tolerated every 3-7 days until an optimal therapeutic response is achieved. The therapeutic dosage usually is 5-7.5 mg and ranges from 2.5-15 mg/day.

In order to reduce the likelihood of prolonged exposure to bromocriptine mesylate should an unsuspected pregnancy occur, a mechanical contraceptive should be used in conjunction with bromocriptine mesylate therapy until normal ovulatory menstrual cycles have been restored. Contraception may then be discontinued in patients desiring pregnancy.

Thereafter, if menstruation does not occur within 3 days of the expected date, bromocriptine mesylate therapy should be discontinued and a pregnancy test performed.

ACROMEGALY

Virtually all acromegalic patients receiving therapeutic benefit from bromocriptine mesylate also have reductions in circulating levels of growth hormone. Therefore, periodic assessment of circulating levels of growth hormone will, in most cases, serve as a guide in determining the therapeutic potential of bromocriptine mesylate. If, after a brief trial with bromocriptine mesylate therapy, no significant reduction in growth hormone levels has taken place, careful assessment of the clinical features of the disease should be made, and if no change has occurred, dosage adjustment or discontinuation of therapy should be considered.

The initial recommended dosage is ½ to one 2½ mg bromocriptine mesylate tablet on retiring (with food) for 3 days. An additional ½ to 1 tablet should be added to the treatment regimen as tolerated every 3-7 days until the patient obtains optimal therapeutic benefit. Patients should be reevaluated monthly and the dosage adjusted based on reductions of growth hormone or clinical response. The usual optimal therapeutic dosage range of bromocriptine mesylate varies from 20-30 mg/day in most patients. The maximal dosage should not exceed 100 mg/day.

Patients treated with pituitary irradiation should be withdrawn from bromocriptine mesylate therapy on a yearly basis to assess both the clinical effects of radiation on the disease process as well as the effects of bromocriptine mesylate therapy. Usually a 4-8 week withdrawal period is adequate for this purpose. Recurrence of the signs/symptoms or increases in growth hormone indicate the disease process in still active and further courses of bromocriptine mesylate should be considered.

PARKINSON'S DISEASE

The basic principle of bromocriptine mesylate therapy is to initiate treatment at a low dosage and, on an individual basis, increase the daily dosage slowly until a maximum therapeutic response is achieved. The dosage of levodopa during this introductory period should be maintained, if possible. The initial dose of bromocriptine mesylate is ½ of a 2½ mg tablet twice daily with meals. Assessments are advised at 2 week intervals during dosage titration to ensure that the lowest dosage producing an optimal therapeutic response is not exceeded. If necessary, the dosage may be increased every 14-28 days by 2½ mg/day with meals. Should it be advisable to reduce the dosage of levodopa because of adverse reactions, the daily dosage of bromocriptine mesylate, if increased, should be accomplished gradually in small (2½ mg) increments.

The safety of bromocriptine mesylate has not been demonstrated in dosages exceeding 100 mg/day.

HOW SUPPLIED

PARLODEL SNAP TABS

2½ mg Round, white, scored Snap Tabs, each containing 2½ mg bromocriptine (as the mesylate). Engraved "Parlodel 2½" on one side and scored on reverse side.

PARLODEL CAPSULES

5 mg Caramel and white capsules, each containing 5 mg bromocriptine (as the mesylate). Imprinted "Parlodel 5 mg" on one half and "S" on other half.

PRODUCT LISTING - RATED THERAPEUTICALLY EQUIVALENT

Capsule - Oral - 5 mg

100's	$306.06	GENERIC, Geneva Pharmaceuticals	00781-2819-01

Tablet - Oral - 2.5 mg

30's	$50.65	GENERIC, Mylan Pharmaceuticals Inc	00378-0242-93
30's	$54.98	PARLODEL, Southwood Pharmaceuticals Inc	58016-0921-30
30's	$70.18	GENERIC, Lek Pharmaceutical and Chemical Company	66685-5905-03
30's	$87.81	PARLODEL, Novartis Pharmaceuticals	00078-0017-15
100's	$157.70	GENERIC, Mylan Pharmaceuticals Inc	00378-0242-01
100's	$233.31	GENERIC, Lek Pharmaceutical and Chemical Company	66685-5905-00
100's	$291.91	PARLODEL, Novartis Pharmaceuticals	00078-0017-05

PRODUCT LISTING - EQUIVALENTS NOT AVAILABLE

Capsule - Oral - 5 mg

30's	$141.06	PARLODEL, Novartis Pharmaceuticals	00078-0102-15
100's	$445.46	PARLODEL, Novartis Pharmaceuticals	00078-0102-05

Tablet - Oral - 2.5 mg

30's	$60.33	GENERIC, Geneva Pharmaceuticals	00781-1817-31
100's	$200.56	GENERIC, Geneva Pharmaceuticals	00781-1817-01

Budesonide *(003201)*

For related information, see the comparative table section in Appendix A.

Categories: Asthma; Crohn's disease; Inflammatory bowel disease; Rhinitis, allergic; FDA Approved 1994 Feb; Pregnancy Category B, Inhalation; Pregnancy Category C, Oral
Drug Classes: Corticosteroids; Corticosteroids, inhalation
Brand Names: Pulmicort; **Rhinocort**
Foreign Brand Availability: B Cort (Colombia); Budecort (Thailand); Budecort Nasal (Philippines); Budecort NT (Philippines); Budeflam (South-Africa); Budenofalk (Germany; Hong-Kong; Singapore); Budeson 3 (Israel); Budicort Respules (Israel); Butacort (New-Zealand); Clebudan (Colombia; Peru); Desona Nasal (Korea); Duasma (Taiwan); Eltair (New-Zealand; Singapore); Entocort (Bahrain; Canada; Cyprus; Egypt; Iran; Iraq; Jordan; Kuwait; Lebanon; Libya; Mexico; Oman; Qatar; Republic-of-Yemen; Saudi-Arabia; Singapore; Syria; United-Arab-Emirates); Esonide (Singapore); Inflammide (Colombia; Peru; Singapore); Inflanaze (South-Africa); Miflonide (Germany; Israel); Miflonide Inhaler (New-Zealand); Neo-Rinactive (Taiwan); Novopulmon (Bahrain; Cyprus; Egypt; Germany; Iran; Iraq; Israel; Jordan; Kuwait; Lebanon; Libya; Oman; Qatar; Republic-of-Yemen; Saudi-Arabia; Syria; United-Arab-Emirates); Numark (Mexico); Pulmicort Nasal (Taiwan); Pulmicort Nasal Turbohaler (China; Kenya; Korea; Mauritius; Nigeria); Pulmotide (Israel); Rhinocort Aqua (Bahamas; Barbados; Belize; Bermuda; Curacao; Guyana; Jamaica; Netherland-Antilles; Puerto-Rico; Surinam; Trinidad); Rhinocort Aqueous (Australia); Rhinocort Hayfever (Australia)
Cost of Therapy: $50.40 (Allergic Rhinitis; Rhinocort Aqua Nasal Spray; 0.032 mg/inh;5 ml; 2 sprays/day; 30 day supply)
$123.86 (Asthma; Pulmicort Turbuhaler; 200 μg/inh;4 g; 2 inhalations/day; 100 day supply)

INHALATION

DESCRIPTION

Note: The trade names have been used throughout this monograph for clarity.

PULMICORT RESPULES

For inhalation use via compressed air driven jet nebulizers only (not for use with ultrasonic devices). Not for injection. Read patient instructions before using.

Budesonide, the active component of Pulmicort Respules, is a corticosteroid designated chemically as (RS)-11β,16α,17,21-tetrahydroxypregna-1,4-diene-3,20-dione cyclic 16,17-acetal with butyraldehyde. Budesonide is provided as a mixture of two epimers (22R and 22S). The empirical formula of budesonide is $C_{25}H_{34}O_6$ and its molecular weight is 430.5.

Budesonide is a white to off-white, tasteless, odorless powder that is practically insoluble in water and in heptane, sparingly soluble in ethanol, and freely soluble in chloroform. Its partition coefficient between octanol and water at pH 7.4 is 1.6×10^3.

Pulmicort Respules is a sterile suspension for inhalation via jet nebulizer and contains the active ingredient budesonide (micronized), and the inactive ingredients disodium edetate, sodium chloride, sodium citrate, citric acid, polysorbate 80 and water for injection. Two dose strengths are available in single-dose ampules (Respules ampules): 0.25 and 0.5 mg per 2 ml Respule ampule. For Pulmicort Respules, like all other nebulized treatments, the amount delivered to the lungs will depend on patient factors, the jet nebulizer utilized, and compressor performance. Using the Pari-LC-Jet Plus Nebulizer/Pari Master compressor system, under *in vitro* conditions, the mean delivered dose at the mouthpiece (% nominal dose) was approximately 17% at a mean flow rate of 5.5 L/min. The mean nebulization time was 5 minutes or less. Pulmicort Respules should be administered from jet nebulizers at adequate flow rates, via face masks or mouthpieces (see DOSAGE AND ADMINISTRATION, Pulmicort Respules).

PULMICORT TURBUHALER

For Oral Inhalation Only.

Budesonide, the active component of Pulmicort Turbuhaler 200 μg, is a corticosteroid designated chemically as (RS)-11β,16α,17,21-Tetrahydroxypregna-1,4-diene-3,20-dione cyclic 16,17-acetal with butyraldehyde. Budesonide is provided as a mixture of two epimers (22R and 22S). The empirical formula of budesonide is $C_{25}H_{34}O_6$ and its molecular weight is 430.5.

Budesonide is a white to off-white, tasteless, odorless powder that is practically insoluble in water and in heptane, sparingly soluble in ethanol, and freely soluble in chloroform. Its partition coefficient between octanol and water at pH 7.4 is 1.6×10^3.

Pulmicort Turbuhaler is an inhalation-driven multi-dose dry powder inhaler which contains only micronized budesonide. Each actuation of Pulmicort Turbuhaler provides 200 μg budesonide per metered dose, which delivers approximately 160 μg budesonide from the mouthpiece (based on *in vitro* testing at 60 L/min for 2 sec).

In vitro testing has shown that the dose delivery for Pulmicort Turbuhaler is substantially dependent on airflow through the device. Patient factors such as inspiratory flow rates will also affect the dose delivered to the lungs of patients in actual use (see Patient's Instructions for Use that accompany the prescription). In adult patients with asthma (mean FEV_1 2.9 L [0.8-5.1 L]) mean peak inspiratory flow (PIF) through Pulmicort Turbuhaler was 78 (40-111) L/min. Similar results (mean PIF 82 [43-125] L/min) were obtained in asthmatic children (6-15 years, mean FEV_1 2.1 L [0.9-5.4 L]). Patients should be carefully instructed on the use of this drug product to assure optimal dose delivery.

CLINICAL PHARMACOLOGY

PULMICORT RESPULES

Mechanism of Action

Budesonide is an anti-inflammatory corticosteroid that exhibits potent glucocorticoid activity and weak mineralocorticoid activity. In standard *in vitro* and animal models, budesonide has approximately a 200-fold higher affinity for the glucocorticoid receptor and a 1000-fold higher topical anti-inflammatory potency than cortisol (rat croton oil ear edema assay). As a measure of systemic activity, budesonide is 40 times more potent than cortisol when administered subcutaneously and 25 times more potent when administered orally in the rat thymus involution assay.

The precise mechanism of corticosteroid actions on inflammation in asthma is not well known. Corticosteroids have been shown to have a wide range of inhibitory activities against multiple cell types (*e.g.*, mast cells, eosinophils, neutrophils, macrophages and lymphocytes) and mediators (*e.g.*, histamine, eicosanoids, leukotrienes, and cytokines) involved

B

in allergic- and non-allergic-mediated inflammation. The anti-inflammatory actions of corticosteroids may contribute to their efficacy in asthma.

Studies in asthmatic patients have shown a favorable ratio between topical anti-inflammatory activities and systemic corticosteroid effects over a wide dose range of inhaled budesonide in a variety of formulations and delivery systems including Pulmicort Turbuhaler (an inhalation-driven, multi-dose dry powder inhaler) and the inhalation suspension for nebulization. This is explained by a combination of a relatively high local anti-inflammatory effect, extensive first pass hepatic degradation of orally absorbed drug (85-95%) and the low potency of metabolites (see below).

Pharmacokinetics

The activity of Pulmicort Respules is due to the parent drug, budesonide. In glucocorticoid receptor affinity studies, the 22R form was 2 times as active as the 22S epimer. *In vitro* studies indicated that the two forms of budesonide do not interconvert.

Budesonide is primarily cleared by the liver. In asthmatic children 4-6 years of age, the terminal half-life of budesonide after nebulization is 2.3 hours, and the systemic clearance is 0.5 L/min, which is approximately 50% greater than in healthy adults after adjustment for differences in weight.

After a single dose of 1 mg budesonide, a peak plasma concentration of 2.6 nmol/L was obtained approximately 20 minutes after nebulization in asthmatic children 4-6 years of age. The exposure (AUC) of budesonide following administration of a single 1 mg dose of budesonide by nebulization to asthmatic children 4-6 years of age is comparable to healthy adults given a single 2 mg dose by nebulization.

Absorption

In asthmatic children 4-6 years of age, the total absolute bioavailability (*i.e.*, lung + oral) following administration of Pulmicort Respules via jet nebulizer was approximately 6% of the labeled dose.

The peak plasma concentration of budesonide occurred 10-30 minutes after start of nebulization.

Distribution

In asthmatic children 4-6 years of age, the volume of distribution at steady-state of budesonide was 3 L/kg, approximately the same as in healthy adults. Budesonide is 85-90% bound to plasma proteins, the degree of binding being constant over the concentration range (1-100 nmol/L) achieved with, and exceeding, recommended doses. Budesonide showed little or no binding to corticosteroid-binding globulin. Budesonide rapidly equilibrated with red blood cells in a concentration independent manner with a blood/plasma ratio of about 0.8.

Metabolism

In vitro studies with human liver homogenates have shown that budesonide is rapidly and extensively metabolized. Two major metabolites formed via cytochrome P450 (CYP) isoenzyme 3A4 (CYP3A4) catalyzed biotransformation have been isolated and identified as 16α-hydroxyprednisolone and 6β-hydroxybudesonide. The corticosteroid activity of each of these two metabolites is less than 1% of that of the parent compound. No qualitative difference between the *in vitro* and *in vivo* metabolic patterns has been detected. Negligible metabolic inactivation was observed in human lung and serum preparations.

Excretion

Budesonide is excreted in urine and feces in the form of metabolites. In adults, approximately 60% of an IV radiolabeled dose was recovered in the urine. No unchanged budesonide was detected in the urine.

Special Populations

No differences in pharmacokinetics due to race, gender, or age have been identified.

Hepatic Insufficiency

Reduced liver function may affect the elimination of corticosteroids. The pharmacokinetics of budesonide were affected by compromised liver function as evidenced by a doubled systemic availability after oral ingestion. The IV pharmacokinetics of budesonide were, however, similar in cirrhotic patients and in healthy adults.

Pharmacodynamics

The therapeutic effects of conventional doses of orally inhaled budesonide are largely explained by its direct local action on the respiratory tract. To confirm that systemic absorption is not a significant factor in the clinical efficacy of inhaled budesonide, a clinical study in adult patients with asthma was performed comparing 400 μg budesonide administered via a pressurized metered dose inhaler with a tube spacer to 1400 μg of oral budesonide and placebo. The study demonstrated the efficacy of inhaled budesonide but not orally ingested budesonide despite comparable systemic levels.

Improvement in the control of asthma symptoms following inhalation of Pulmicort Respules can occur within 2-8 days of beginning treatment, although maximum benefit may not be achieved for 4-6 weeks.

Budesonide administered via Turbuhaler has been shown in various challenge models (including histamine, methacholine, sodium metabisulfite, and adenosine monophosphate) to decrease bronchial hyperresponsiveness in asthmatic patients. The clinical relevance of these models is not certain.

Pre-treatment with budesonide administered via Turbuhaler 1600 μg daily (800 μg twice daily) for 2 weeks reduced the acute (early-phase reaction) and delayed (late-phase reaction) decrease in FEV_1 following inhaled allergen challenge.

The effects of Pulmicort Respules on the hypothalamic-pituitary-adrenal (HPA) axis were studied in three, 12 week, double-blind, placebo-controlled studies in 293 pediatric patients, 6 months to 8 years of age, with persistent asthma. For most patients, the ability to increase cortisol production in response to stress, as assessed by the short cosyntropin (ACTH) stimulation test, remained intact with Pulmicort Respules treatment at recommended doses. In the subgroup of children age 6 months to 2 years (n=21) receiving a total daily dose of Pulmicort Respules equivalent to 0.25 mg (n=5), 0.5 mg (n=5), 1 mg (n=8), or placebo (n=3), the mean change from baseline in ACTH-stimulated cortisol levels showed a decline in peak stimulated cortisol at 12 weeks compared to an increase in the placebo group. These mean differences were not statistically significant compared to placebo. Another 12 week study in 141 pediatric patients 6–12 months of age with mild to moderate asthma or recurrent/persistent wheezing was conducted. All patients were randomized to receive either 0.5 or 1 mg of Pulmicort Respules or placebo once daily. A total of 28, 17, and 31 patients in the Pulmicort Respules 0.5 mg, 1 mg, and placebo arms respectively, had an evaluation of serum cortisol levels post-ACTH stimulation both at baseline and at the end of the study. The mean change from baseline to Week 12 ACTH-stimulated minus basal plasma cortisol levels did not indicate adrenal suppression in patients treated with Pulmicort Respules versus placebo. However, 7 patients in this study (4 of whom received Pulmicort Respules 0.5 mg, 2 of whom received Pulmicort Respules 1 mg and 1 of whom received placebo) showed a shift from normal baseline stimulated cortisol level (≥500 nmol/L) to a subnormal level (<500 nmol/L) at Week 12. In 4 of these patients receiving Pulmicort Respules, the cortisol values were near the cutoff value of 500 nmol/L.

The effects of Pulmicort Respules at doses of 0.5 mg twice daily, and 1 mg and 2 mg twice daily (2 times and 4 times the highest recommended total daily dose, respectively) on 24 hour urinary cortisol excretion were studied in 18 patients between 6-15 years of age with persistent asthma in a cross-over study design (4 weeks of treatment per dose level). There was a dose-related decrease in urinary cortisol excretion at 2 and 4 times the recommended daily dose. The two higher doses of Pulmicort Respules (1 and 2 mg twice daily) showed statistically significantly reduced (43-52%) urinary cortisol excretion compared to the run-in period. The highest recommended dose of Pulmicort Respules, 1 mg total daily dose, did not show statistically significantly reduced urinary cortisol excretion compared to the run-in period.

Pulmicort Respules, like other inhaled corticosteroid products, may impact the HPA axis, especially in susceptible individuals, in younger children, and in patients given high doses for prolonged periods.

PULMICORT TURBUHALER

Budesonide is an anti-inflammatory corticosteroid that exhibits potent glucocorticoid activity and weak mineralocorticoid activity. In standard *in vitro* and animal models, budesonide has approximately a 200-fold higher affinity for the glucocorticoid receptor and a 1000-fold higher topical anti-inflammatory potency than cortisol (rat croton oil ear edema assay). As a measure of systemic activity, budesonide is 40 times more potent than cortisol when administered subcutaneously and 25 times more potent when administered orally in the rat thymus involution assay.

The precise mechanism of corticosteroid actions on inflammation in asthma is not known. Corticosteroids have been shown to have a wide range of inhibitory activities against multiple cell types (*e.g.*, mast cells, eosinophils, neutrophils, macrophages, and lymphocytes) and mediators (*e.g.*, histamine, eicosanoids, leukotrienes, and cytokines) involved in allergic and non-allergic-mediated inflammation. These anti-inflammatory actions of corticosteroids may contribute to their efficacy in asthma.

Studies in asthmatic patients have shown a favorable ratio between topical anti-inflammatory activity and systemic corticosteroid effects over a wide range of doses from Pulmicort Turbuhaler. This is explained by a combination of a relatively high local anti-inflammatory effect, extensive first pass hepatic degradation of orally absorbed drug (85-95%), and the low potency of formed metabolites (see below).

Pharmacokinetics

The activity of Pulmicort Turbuhaler is due to the parent drug, budesonide. In glucocorticoid receptor affinity studies, the 22R form was 2 times as active as the 22S epimer. *In vitro* studies indicated that the two forms of budesonide do not interconvert. The 22R form was preferentially cleared by the liver with systemic clearance of 1.4 L/min vs 1.0 L/min for the 22S form. The terminal half-life, 2-3 hours, was the same for both epimers and was independent of dose. In asthmatic patients, budesonide showed a linear increase in AUC and C_{max} with increasing dose after both a single dose and repeated dosing from Pulmicort Turbuhaler.

Absorption

After oral administration of budesonide, peak plasma concentration was achieved in about 1-2 hours and the absolute systemic availability was 6-13%. In contrast, most of budesonide delivered to the lungs is systemically absorbed. In healthy subjects, 34% of the metered dose was deposited in the lungs (as assessed by plasma concentration method) with an absolute systemic availability of 39% of the metered dose. Pharmacokinetics of budesonide do not differ significantly in healthy volunteers and asthmatic patients. Peak plasma concentrations of budesonide occurred within 30 minutes of inhalation from Pulmicort Turbuhaler.

Distribution

The volume of distribution of budesonide was approximately 3 L/kg. It was 85-90% bound to plasma proteins. Protein binding was constant over the concentration range (1-100 nmol/L) achieved with, and exceeding, recommended doses of Pulmicort Turbuhaler. Budesonide showed little or no binding to corticosteroid binding globulin. Budesonide rapidly equilibrated with red blood cells in a concentration independent manner with a blood/plasma ratio of about 0.8.

Metabolism

In vitro studies with human liver homogenates have shown that budesonide is rapidly and extensively metabolized. Two major metabolites formed via cytochrome P450 3A catalyzed biotransformation have been isolated and identified as 16α-hydroxyprednisolone and 6β-hydroxybudesonide. The corticosteroid activity of each of these two metabolites is less than 1% of that of the parent compound. No qualitative difference between the *in vitro* and *in vivo* metabolic patterns have been detected. Negligible metabolic inactivation was observed in human lung and serum preparations.

Excretion
Budesonide was excreted in urine and feces in the form of metabolites. Approximately 60% of an IV radiolabelled dose was recovered in the urine. No unchanged budesonide was detected in the urine.

Special Populations
No pharmacokinetic differences have been identified due to race, gender or advanced age.

Pediatric
Following IV dosing in pediatric patients age 10-14 years, plasma half-life was shorter than in adults (1.5 h vs 2.0 h in adults). In the same population following inhalation of budesonide via a pressurized metered-dose inhaler, absolute systemic availability was similar to that in adults.

Hepatic Insufficiency
Reduced liver function may affect the elimination of corticosteroids. The pharmacokinetics of budesonide were affected by compromised liver function as evidenced by a doubled systemic availability after oral ingestion. The IV pharmacokinetics of budesonide were, however, similar in cirrhotic patients and in healthy subjects.

Drug-Drug Interactions
Ketoconazole, a potent inhibitor of cytochrome P450 3A, the main metabolic enzyme for corticosteroids, increased plasma levels of orally ingested budesonide. At recommended doses, cimetidine had a slight but clinically insignificant effect on the pharmacokinetics of oral budesonide.

Pharmacodynamics
To confirm that systemic absorption is not a significant factor in the clinical efficacy of inhaled budesonide, a clinical study in patients with asthma was performed comparing 400 μg budesonide administered via a pressurized metered dose inhaler with a tube spacer to 1400 μg of oral budesonide and placebo. The study demonstrated the efficacy of inhaled budesonide but not orally ingested budesonide despite comparable systemic levels. Thus, the therapeutic effect of conventional doses of orally inhaled budesonide are largely explained by its direct action on the respiratory tract.

Generally, Pulmicort Turbuhaler has a relatively rapid onset of action for an inhaled corticosteroid. Improvement in asthma control following inhalation of Pulmicort Turbuhaler can occur within 24 hours of beginning treatment although maximum benefit may not be achieved for 1-2 weeks, or longer.

Pulmicort Turbuhaler has been shown to decrease airway reactivity to various challenge models, including histamine, methacholine, sodium metabisulfite, and adenosine monophosphate in hyperreactive patients. The clinical relevance of these models is not certain.

Pretreatment with Pulmicort Turbuhaler 1600 μg daily (800 μg twice daily) for 2 weeks reduced the acute (early-phase reaction) and delayed (late-phase reaction) decrease in FEV_1 following inhaled allergen challenge.

The effects of Pulmicort Turbuhaler on the hypothalamic-pituitary-adrenal (HPA) axis were studied in 905 adults and 404 pediatric patients with asthma. For most patients, the ability to increase cortisol production in response to stress, as assessed by cosyntropin (ACTH) stimulation test, remained intact with Pulmicort Turbuhaler treatment at recommended doses. For adult patients treated with 100, 200, 400, or 800 μg twice daily for 12 weeks, 4%, 2%, 6%, and 13% respectively, had an abnormal stimulated cortisol response (peak cortisol <14.5 μg/dl assessed by liquid chromatography following short-cosyntropin test) as compared to 8% of patients treated with placebo. Similar results were obtained in pediatric patients. In another study in adults, doses of 400, 800 and 1600 μg budesonide twice daily via Pulmicort Turbuhaler for 6 weeks were examined; 1600 μg twice daily (twice the maximum recommended dose) resulted in a 27% reduction in stimulated cortisol (6 hour ACTH infusion) while 10 mg prednisone resulted in a 35% reduction. In this study, no patient on Pulmicort Turbuhaler at doses of 400 and 800 μg twice daily met the criterion for an abnormal stimulated cortisol response (peak cortisol <14.5 μg/dl assessed by liquid chromatography) following ACTH infusion. An open-label, long-term follow-up of 1133 patients for up to 52 weeks confirmed the minimal effect on the HPA axis (both basal and stimulated plasma cortisol) of Pulmicort Turbuhaler when administered at recommended doses. In patients who had previously been oral steroid-dependent, use of Pulmicort Turbuhaler in recommended doses was associated with higher stimulated cortisol response compared to baseline following 1 year of therapy.

The administration of budesonide via Pulmicort Turbuhaler in doses up to 800 μg/day (mean daily dose 445 μg/day) or via a pressurized metered-dose inhaler in doses up to 1200 μg/day (mean daily dose 620 μg/day) to 216 pediatric patients (age 3-11 years) for 2-6 years had no significant effect on statural growth compared with non-corticosteroid therapy in 62 matched control patients. However, the long-term effect of Pulmicort Turbuhaler on growth is not fully known.

INDICATIONS AND USAGE

PULMICORT RESPULES
Pulmicort Respules is indicated for the maintenance treatment of asthma and as prophylactic therapy in children 12 months to 8 years of age.

Pulmicort Respules is NOT indicated for the relief of acute bronchospasm.

PULMICORT TURBUHALER
Pulmicort Turbuhaler is indicated for the maintenance treatment of asthma as prophylactic therapy in adult and pediatric patients 6 years of age or older. It is also indicated for patients requiring oral corticosteroid therapy for asthma. Many of those patients may be able to reduce or eliminate their requirement for oral corticosteroids over time.

Pulmicort Turbuhaler is NOT indicated for the relief of acute bronchospasm.

CONTRAINDICATIONS

PULMICORT RESPULES
Pulmicort Respules is contraindicated as the primary treatment of status asthmaticus or other acute episodes of asthma where intensive measures are required.

Hypersensitivity to budesonide or any of the ingredients of this preparation contraindicates the use of Pulmicort Respules.

PULMICORT TURBUHALER
Pulmicort Turbuhaler is contraindicated in the primary treatment of status asthmaticus or other acute episodes of asthma where intensive measures are required.

Hypersensitivity to budesonide contraindicates the use of Pulmicort Turbuhaler.

WARNINGS

PULMICORT RESPULES
Particular care is needed for patients who are transferred from systemically active corticosteroids to inhaled corticosteroids because deaths due to adrenal insufficiency have occurred in asthmatic patients during and after transfer from systemic corticosteroids to less systemically available inhaled corticosteroids. After withdrawal from systemic corticosteroids, a number of months are required for recovery of HPA-axis function.

Patients who have been previously maintained on 20 mg or more per day of prednisone (or its equivalent) may be most susceptible, particularly when their systemic corticosteroids have been almost completely withdrawn.

During this period of HPA-axis suppression, patients may exhibit signs and symptoms of adrenal insufficiency when exposed to trauma, surgery, infection (particularly gastroenteritis) or other conditions associated with severe electrolyte loss. Although Pulmicort Respules may provide control of asthma symptoms during these episodes, in recommended doses it supplies less than normal physiological amounts of corticosteroid systemically and does NOT provide the mineralocorticoid activity that is necessary for coping with these emergencies.

During periods of stress or a severe asthma attack, patients who have been withdrawn from systemic corticosteroids should be instructed to resume oral corticosteroids (in large doses) immediately and to contact their physicians for further instructions. These patients should also be instructed to carry a warning card indicating that they may need supplementary systemic corticosteroids during periods of stress or a severe asthma attack.

Transfer of patients from systemic corticosteroid therapy to Pulmicort Respules may unmask allergic conditions previously suppressed by the systemic corticosteroid therapy, *e.g.*, rhinitis, conjunctivitis, and eczema (see DOSAGE AND ADMINISTRATION, Pulmicort Respules).

Patients who are on drugs which suppress the immune system are more susceptible to infection than healthy individuals. Chicken pox and measles, for example, can have a more serious or even fatal course in susceptible pediatric patients or adults on immunosuppressant doses of corticosteroids. In pediatric or adult patients who have not had these diseases, or who have not been properly vaccinated, particular care should be taken to avoid exposure. How the dose, route, and duration of corticosteroid administration affects the risk of developing a disseminated infection is not known. The contribution of the underlying disease and/or prior corticosteroid treatment to the risk is also not known. If exposed, therapy with varicella zoster immune globulin (VZIG) or pooled IV immunoglobulin (IVIG), as appropriate, may be indicated. If exposed to measles, prophylaxis with pooled intramuscular immunoglobulin (IG) may be indicated. (See the respective package inserts for complete VZIG and IG prescribing information.) If chicken pox develops, treatment with antiviral agents may be considered.

Pulmicort Respules is not a bronchodilator and is not indicated for the rapid relief of acute bronchospasm or other acute episodes of asthma.

As with other inhaled asthma medications, bronchospasm, with an immediate increase in wheezing, may occur after dosing. If acute bronchospasm occurs following dosing with Pulmicort Respules, it should be treated immediately with a fast-acting inhaled bronchodilator. Treatment with Pulmicort Respules should be discontinued and alternate therapy instituted.

Patients should be instructed to contact their physician immediately when episodes of asthma not responsive to their usual doses of bronchodilators occur during treatment with Pulmicort Respules.

PULMICORT TURBUHALER

Particular care is needed for patients who are transferred from systemically active corticosteroids to Pulmicort Turbuhaler because deaths due to adrenal insufficiency have occurred in asthmatic patients during and after transfer from systemic corticosteroids to less systemically available inhaled corticosteroids. After withdrawal from systemic corticosteroids, a number of months are required for recovery of HPA function.

Patients who have been previously maintained on 20 mg or more per day of prednisone (or its equivalent) may be most susceptible, particularly when their systemic corticosteroids have been almost completely withdrawn. During this period of HPA suppression, patients may exhibit signs and symptoms of adrenal insufficiency when exposed to trauma, surgery, or infection (particularly gastroenteritis) or other conditions associated with severe electrolyte loss. Although Pulmicort Turbuhaler may provide control of asthma symptoms during these episodes, in recommended doses it supplies less than normal physiological amounts of glucocorticoid systemically and does NOT provide the mineralocorticoid activity that is necessary for coping with these emergencies.

During periods of stress or a severe asthma attack, patients who have been withdrawn from systemic corticosteroids should be instructed to resume oral corticosteroids (in large doses) immediately and to contact their physicians for further instruction. These patients should also be instructed to carry a medical identification card indicating that they may need supplementary systemic corticosteroids during periods of stress or a severe asthma attack.

Transfer of patients from systemic corticosteroid therapy to Pulmicort Turbuhaler may unmask allergic conditions previously suppressed by the systemic corticosteroid therapy, *e.g.*, rhinitis, conjunctivitis, and eczema (see DOSAGE AND ADMINISTRATION, Pulmicort Turbuhaler).

Patients who are on drugs which suppress the immune system are more susceptible to infection than healthy individuals. Chicken pox and measles, for example, can have a more serious or even fatal course in susceptible pediatric patients or adults on immunosuppressant doses of corticosteroids. In pediatric or adult patients who have not had these diseases, particular care should be taken to avoid exposure. How the dose, route and duration of corticosteroid administration affects the risk of developing a disseminated infection is not known. The contribution of the underlying disease and/or prior corticosteroid treatment to the risk is also not known. If exposed, therapy with varicella zoster immune globulin (VZIG) or pooled IV immunoglobulin (IVIG), as appropriate, may be indicated. If exposed to measles, prophylaxis with pooled intramuscular immunoglobulin (IG) may be indicated. (See the respective package insert for complete VZIG and IG prescribing information.) If chicken pox develops, treatment with antiviral agents may be considered.

Pulmicort Turbuhaler is not a bronchodilator and is not indicated for rapid relief of bronchospasm or other acute episodes of asthma.

As with other inhaled asthma medications, bronchospasm, with an immediate increase in wheezing, may occur after dosing. If bronchospasm occurs following dosing with Pulmicort Turbuhaler, it should be treated immediately with a fast-acting inhaled bronchodilator. Treatment with Pulmicort Turbuhaler should be discontinued and alternate therapy instituted.

Patients should be instructed to contact their physician immediately when episodes of asthma not responsive to their usual doses of bronchodilators occur during treatment with Pulmicort Turbuhaler. During such episodes, patients may require therapy with oral corticosteroids.

PRECAUTIONS

PULMICORT RESPULES

General

Inhaled corticosteroids may cause a reduction in growth velocity when administered to pediatric patients (see Pulmicort Respules, Pediatric Use).

During withdrawal from oral corticosteroids, some patients may experience symptoms of systemically active corticosteroid withdrawal, *e.g.*, joint and/or muscular pain, lassitude, and depression, despite maintenance or even improvement of respiratory function.

Because budesonide is absorbed into the circulation and may be systemically active, particularly at higher doses, suppression of HPA function may be associated when Pulmicort Respules is administered at doses exceeding those recommended (see DOSAGE AND ADMINISTRATION, Pulmicort Respules), or when the dose is not titrated to the lowest effective dose. Since individual sensitivity to effects on cortisol production exists, physicians should consider this information when prescribing Pulmicort Respules.

Because of the possibility of systemic absorption of inhaled corticosteroids, patients treated with these drugs should be observed carefully for any evidence of systemic corticosteroid effects. Particular care should be taken in observing patients post-operatively or during periods of stress for evidence of inadequate adrenal response.

It is possible that systemic corticosteroid effects such as hypercorticism and adrenal suppression may appear in a small number of patients, particularly at higher doses. If such changes occur, Pulmicort Respules should be reduced slowly, consistent with accepted procedures for management of asthma symptoms and for tapering of systemic corticosteroids.

Although patients in clinical trials have received Pulmicort Respules on a continuous basis for periods of up to 1 year, the long-term local and systemic effects of Pulmicort Respules in human subjects are not completely known. In particular, the effects resulting from chronic use of Pulmicort Respules on developmental or immunological processes in the mouth, pharynx, trachea, and lung are unknown.

In clinical trials with Pulmicort Respules, localized infections with *Candida albicans* occurred in the mouth and pharynx in some patients. The incidences of localized infections of *Candida albicans* were similar between the placebo and Pulmicort Respules treatment groups. If symptomatic oropharyngeal candidiasis develops, it should be treated with appropriate local or systemic (*i.e.*, oral) antifungal therapy while still continuing with Pulmicort Respules therapy, but at times therapy with Pulmicort Respules may need to be interrupted under close medical supervision.

Inhaled corticosteroids should be used with caution, if at all, in patients with active or quiescent tuberculosis infection of the respiratory tract, untreated systemic fungal, bacterial, viral, or parasitic infections; or ocular herpes simplex.

Rare instances of glaucoma, increased intraocular pressure, and cataracts have been reported following the inhaled administration of corticosteroids.

Information for the Patient

For instructions on the proper use of Pulmicort Respules and to attain the maximum improvement in asthma symptoms, the patient or the parent/guardian of the patient should receive, read, and follow the accompanying patient information and instructions carefully. In addition, patients being treated with Pulmicort Respules should receive the following information and instructions. This information is intended to aid the patient in the safe and effective use of the medication. It is not a disclosure of all possible adverse or intended effects.

Patients should take Pulmicort Respules at regular intervals once or twice a day as directed, since its effectiveness depends on regular use. The patient should not alter the prescribed dosage unless advised to do so by the physician.

The effects of mixing Pulmicort Respules with other nebulizable medications have not been adequately assessed. Pulmicort Respules should be administered separately in the nebulizer.

Pulmicort Respules is not a bronchodilator, and its use is not intended to treat acute life-threatening episodes of asthma.

Pulmicort Respules should be administered with a jet nebulizer connected to a compressor with an adequate air flow, equipped with a mouthpiece or suitable face mask. The face mask should be properly adjusted to optimize delivery and to avoid exposing the eyes to the nebulized medication (see DOSAGE AND ADMINISTRATION, Pulmicort Respules).

Ultrasonic nebulizers are not suitable for the adequate administration of Pulmicort Respules and, therefore, are not recommended (see DOSAGE AND ADMINISTRATION, Pulmicort Respules).

Rinsing the mouth with water after each treatment may decrease the risk of development of local candidiasis. Corticosteroid effects on the skin can be avoided if the face is washed after the use of a face mask.

Improvement in asthma control following treatment with Pulmicort Respules can occur within 2-8 days of beginning treatment, although maximum benefit may not be achieved for 4-6 weeks after starting treatment. If the asthma symptoms do not improve in that time frame, or if the condition worsens, the patient or the patient's parent/guardian should be instructed to contact the physician.

Care should be taken to avoid exposure to chicken pox and measles. If exposure occurs, and the child has not had chicken pox or been properly vaccinated, a physician should be consulted without delay.

Pulmicort Respules should be stored upright at controlled room temperature 20-25°C (68-77°F) and protected from light. Pulmicort Respules should not be refrigerated or frozen.

When an aluminum foil envelope has been opened, the shelf life of the unused Respules is 2 weeks when protected from light. The date the envelope was opened should be recorded on the back of the envelope in the space provided.

After opening the aluminum foil envelope, the unused Respules ampules should be returned to the envelope to protect them from light. Any individually opened Respules ampules must be used promptly.

For proper usage of Pulmicort Respules and to attain maximum improvement, the accompanying Patient's Instructions for Use should be read and followed.

Carcinogenesis, Mutagenesis, and Impairment of Fertility

In a 2 year study in Sprague-Dawley rats, budesonide caused a statistically significant increase in the incidence of gliomas in male rats at an oral dose of 50 μg/kg (less than the maximum recommended daily inhalation dose in adults and children on a μg/m^2 basis). No tumorigenicity was seen in male and female rats at respective oral doses up to 25 and 50 μg/kg (less than the maximum recommended daily inhalation dose in adults and children on a μg/m^2 basis). In two additional 2 year studies in male Fischer and Sprague-Dawley rats, budesonide caused no gliomas at an oral dose of 50 μg/kg (less than the maximum recommended daily inhalation dose in adults and children on a μg/m^2 basis). However, in the male Sprague-Dawley rats, budesonide caused a statistically significant increase in the incidence of hepatocellular tumors at an oral dose of 50 μg/kg (less than the maximum recommended daily inhalation dose in adults and children on a μg/m^2 basis). The concurrent reference corticosteroids (prednisolone and triamcinolone acetonide) in these two studies showed similar findings.

In a 91 week study in mice, budesonide caused no treatment-related carcinogenicity at oral doses up to 200 μg/kg (less than the maximum recommended daily inhalation dose in adults and children on a μg/m^2 basis).

Budesonide was not mutagenic or clastogenic in six different test systems: Ames *Salmonella*/microsome plate test, mouse micronucleus test, mouse lymphoma test, chromosome aberration test in human lymphocytes, sex-linked recessive lethal test in *Drosophila melanogaster,* and DNA repair analysis in rat hepatocyte culture.

In rats, budesonide had no effect on fertility at SC doses up to 80 μg/kg (less than the maximum recommended daily inhalation dose in adults on a μg/m^2 basis). However, it caused a decrease in prenatal viability and viability in the pups at birth and during lactation, along with a decrease in maternal body-weight gain, at SC doses of 20 μg/kg and above (less than the maximum recommended daily inhalation dose in adults on a μg/m^2 basis). No such effects were noted at 5 μg/kg (less than the maximum recommended daily inhalation dose in adults on a μg/m^2 basis).

Pregnancy

Teratogenic Effects, Pregnancy Category B

As with other corticosteroids, budesonide was teratogenic and embryocidal in rabbits and rats. Budesonide produced fetal loss, decreased pup weights, and skeletal abnormalities at SC doses of 25 μg/kg in rabbits (less than the maximum recommended daily inhalation dose in adults on a μg/m^2 basis) and 500 μg/kg in rats (approximately 4 times the maximum recommended daily inhalation dose in adults on a μg/m^2 basis). In another study in rats, no teratogenic or embryocidal effects were seen at inhalation doses up to 250 μg/kg (approximately 2 times the maximum recommended daily inhalation dose in adults on a μg/m^2 basis).

Experience with oral corticosteroids since their introduction in pharmacologic, as opposed to physiologic, doses suggests that rodents are more prone to teratogenic effects from corticosteroids than humans. In addition, because there is a natural increase in corticosteroid production during pregnancy, most women will require a lower exogenous corticosteroid dose and many will not need corticosteroid treatment during pregnancy.

Studies of pregnant women, however, have not shown that inhaled budesonide increases the risk of abnormalities when administered during pregnancy. The results from a large population-based prospective cohort epidemiological study reviewing data from three Swedish registries covering approximately 99% of the pregnancies from 1995-1997 (*i.e.,* Swedish Medical Birth Registry; Registry of Congenital Malformations; Child Cardiology Registry) indicate no increased risk for congenital malformations from the use of inhaled budesonide during early pregnancy. Congenital malformations were studied in 2014 infants born to mothers reporting the use of inhaled budesonide for asthma in early pregnancy (usually 10-12 weeks after the last menstrual period), the period when most major organ malformations occur. The rate of recorded congenital malformations was similar compared to the general population rate (3.8% vs 3.5%, respectively). In addition, after exposure to inhaled budesonide, the number of infants born with orofacial clefts was similar to the expected number in the normal population (4 children vs 3.3, respectively).

These same data were utilized in a second study bringing the total to 2534 infants whose mothers were exposed to inhaled budesonide. In this study, the rate of congenital malformations among infants whose mothers were exposed to inhaled budesonide during early pregnancy was not different from the rate for all newborn babies during the same period (3.6%).

Despite the animal findings, it would appear that the possibility of fetal harm is remote if the drug is used during pregnancy. Nevertheless, because the studies in humans cannot rule out the possibility of harm, Pulmicort Respules should be used during pregnancy only if clearly needed.

Nonteratogenic Effects

Hypoadrenalism may occur in infants born of mothers receiving corticosteroids during pregnancy. Such infants should be carefully observed.

Nursing Mothers

It is not known whether budesonide is excreted in human milk. Because other corticosteroids are excreted in human milk, caution should be exercised if budesonide is administered to nursing women.

Pediatric Use

Safety in children 6–12 months of age has been evaluated. Safety and effectiveness in children 12 months to 8 years of age have been established (see CLINICAL PHARMACOLOGY, Pulmicort Respules, Pharmacodynamics; and ADVERSE REACTIONS, Pulmicort Respules).

A 12 week study in 141 pediatric patients 6 to 12 months of age with mild to moderate asthma or recurrent/persistent wheezing was conducted. All patients were randomized to receive either 0.5 or 1 mg of Pulmicort Respules or placebo once daily. Adrenal axis function was assessed with an ACTH stimulation test at the beginning and end of the study, and mean changes from baseline in this variable did not indicate adrenal suppression in patients who received Pulmicort Respules versus placebo. However, on an individual basis, 7 patients in this study (6 in the Pulmicort Respules treatment arms and 1 in the placebo arm) experienced a shift from having a normal baseline stimulated cortisol level to having a subnormal level at Week 12 (see CLINICAL PHARMACOLOGY, Pulmicort Respules, Pharmacodynamics). Pneumonia was observed more frequently in patients treated with Pulmicort Respules than in patients treated with placebo, (n=2, 1, and 0) in the Pulmicort Respules 0.5 mg, 1 mg, and placebo groups, respectively.

A dose dependent effect on growth was also noted in this 12 week trial. Infants in the placebo arm experienced an average growth of 3.7 cm over 12 weeks compared with 3.5 cm and 3.1 cm in the Pulmicort Respules 0.5 mg and 1 mg arms respectively. This corresponds to estimated mean (95% CI) reductions in 12 week growth velocity between placebo and Pulmicort Respules 0.5 mg of 0.2 cm (-0.6 to 1.0) and between placebo and Pulmicort Respules 1 mg of 0.6 cm (-0.2 to 1.4). These findings support that the use of Pulmicort Respules in infants 6–12 months of age may result in systemic effects and are consistent with findings of growth suppression in other studies with inhaled corticosteroids.

Controlled clinical studies have shown that inhaled corticosteroids may cause a reduction in growth velocity in pediatric patients. In these studies, the mean reduction in growth velocity was approximately 1 cm/year (range 0.3-1.8 cm/year) and appears to be related to dose and duration of exposure. This effect has been observed in the absence of laboratory evidence of hypothalamic-pituitary-adrenal (HPA)-axis suppression, suggesting that growth velocity is a more sensitive indicator of systemic corticosteroid exposure in pediatric patients than some commonly used tests of HPA-axis function. The long-term effects of this reduction in growth velocity associated with inhaled corticosteroids, including the impact on final adult height, are unknown. The potential for "catch up" growth following discontinuation of treatment with inhaled corticosteroids has not been adequately studied. The growth of pediatric patients receiving inhaled corticosteroids, including Pulmicort Respules, should be monitored routinely (*e.g.*, via stadiometry). The potential growth effects of prolonged treatment should be weighed against clinical benefits obtained and the risks associated with alternative therapies. To minimize the systemic effects of inhaled corticosteroids, including Pulmicort Respules, each patient should be titrated to his/her lowest effective dose.

Geriatric Use

Of the 215 patients in 3 clinical trials of Pulmicort Respules in adult patients, 65 (30%) were 65 years of age or older, while 22 (10%) were 75 years of age or older. No overall differences in safety were observed between these patients and younger patients, and other reported clinical or medical surveillance experience has not identified differences in responses between the elderly and younger patients.

PULMICORT TURBUHALER

General

During withdrawal from oral corticosteroids, some patients may experience symptoms of systemically active corticosteroid withdrawal, *e.g.*, joint and/or muscular pain, lassitude, and depression, despite maintenance or even improvement of respiratory function.

Pulmicort Turbuhaler will often permit control of asthma symptoms with less suppression of HPA function than therapeutically equivalent oral doses of prednisone. Since budesonide is absorbed into the circulation and can be systemically active at higher doses, the full beneficial effects of Pulmicort Turbuhaler in minimizing HPA dysfunction may be expected only when recommended dosages are not exceeded and individual patients are titrated to the lowest effective dose. Since individual sensitivity to effects on cortisol production exists, physicians should consider this information when prescribing Pulmicort Turbuhaler.

Because of the possibility of systemic absorption of inhaled corticosteroids, patients treated with these drugs should be observed carefully for any evidence of systemic corticosteroid effects. Particular care should be taken in observing patients postoperatively or during periods of stress for evidence of inadequate adrenal response.

It is possible that systemic corticosteroid effects such as hypercorticism and adrenal suppression may appear in a small number of patients, particularly at higher doses. If such changes occur, Pulmicort Turbuhaler should be reduced slowly, consistent with accepted procedures for management of asthma symptoms and for tapering of systemic steroids.

A reduction of growth velocity in children or teenagers may occur as a result of inadequate control of chronic diseases such as asthma or from use of corticosteroids for treatment. Physicians should closely follow the growth of all pediatric patients taking corticosteroids by any route and weigh the benefits of corticosteroid therapy and asthma control against the possibility of growth suppression (see Pulmicort Turbuhaler, Pediatric Use).

Although patients in clinical trials have received Pulmicort Turbuhaler on a continuous basis for periods of 1-2 years, the long-term local and systemic effects of Pulmicort Turbuhaler in human subjects are not completely known. In particular, the effects resulting from chronic use of Pulmicort Turbuhaler on developmental or immunological processes in the mouth, pharynx, trachea, and lung are unknown.

In clinical trials with Pulmicort Turbuhaler, localized infections with *Candida albicans* occurred in the mouth and pharynx in some patients. If oropharyngeal candidiasis develops, it should be treated with appropriate local or systemic (*i.e.*, oral) antifungal therapy while still continuing with Pulmicort Turbuhaler therapy, but at times therapy with Pulmicort Turbuhaler may need to be temporarily interrupted under close medical supervision.

Inhaled corticosteroids should be used with caution, if at all, in patients with active or quiescent tuberculosis infection of the respiratory tract, untreated systemic fungal, bacterial, viral or parasitic infections; or ocular herpes simplex.

Rare instances of glaucoma, increased intraocular pressure, and cataracts have been reported following the inhaled administration of corticosteroids.

Information for the Patient

For proper use of Pulmicort Turbuhaler and to attain maximum improvement, the patient should read and follow the accompanying Patient's Instructions for Use carefully. In addition, patients being treated with Pulmicort Turbuhaler should receive the following information and instructions. This information is intended to aid the patient in the safe and effective use of the medication. It is not a disclosure of all possible adverse or intended effects.

- Patients should use Pulmicort Turbuhaler at regular intervals as directed since its effectiveness depends on regular use. The patient should not alter the prescribed dosage unless advised to do so by the physician.
- Pulmicort Turbuhaler is not a bronchodilator and is not intended to treat acute or life-threatening episodes of asthma.
- Pulmicort Turbuhaler must be in the upright position (mouthpiece on top) during loading in order to provide the correct dose. Pulmicort Turbuhaler must be primed when the unit is used for the very first time. To prime the unit, hold the unit in an upright position and turn the brown grip fully to the right, then fully to the left until it clicks. Repeat. The unit is now primed and ready to load the first dose by turning the grip fully to the right and fully to the left until it clicks. On subsequent uses, it is not necessary to prime the unit. However, it must be loaded in the upright position immediately prior to use. Turn the brown grip fully to the right, then fully to the left until it clicks. During inhalation, Pulmicort Turbuhaler must be held in the upright (mouthpiece up) or horizontal position. Do not shake the inhaler. Place the mouthpiece between lips and inhale forcefully and deeply. The powder is then delivered to the lungs.
- Patients should not exhale through Pulmicort Turbuhaler.
- Due to the small volume of powder, the patient may not taste or sense the presence of any medication entering the lungs when inhaling from Turbuhaler. This lack of "sensation" does not indicate that the patient is not receiving benefit from Pulmicort Turbuhaler.
- Rinsing the mouth with water without swallowing after each dosing may decrease the risk of the development of oral candidiasis.
- When there are 20 doses remaining in Pulmicort Turbuhaler, a red mark will appear in the indicator window.
- Pulmicort Turbuhaler should not be used with a spacer.
- The mouthpiece should not be bitten or chewed.
- The cover should be replaced securely after each opening.
- Keep Pulmicort Turbuhaler clean and dry at all times.
- Improvement in asthma control following inhalation of Pulmicort Turbuhaler can occur within 24 hours of beginning treatment although maximum benefit may not be achieved for 1-2 weeks, or longer. If symptoms do not improve in that time frame, or if the condition worsens, the patient should be instructed to contact the physician.
- Patients should be warned to avoid exposure to chicken pox or measles and if they are exposed, to consult their physicians without delay.
- For proper use of Pulmicort Turbuhaler and to attain maximum improvement, the patient should read and follow the accompanying Patient's Instructions for Use.

Carcinogenesis, Mutagenesis, and Impairment of Fertility

Long-term studies were conducted in mice and rats using oral administration to evaluate the carcinogenic potential of budesonide.

There was no evidence of a carcinogenic effect when budesonide was administered orally for 91 weeks to mice at doses up to 200 μg/kg/day (approximately 1/2 the maximum recommended daily inhalation dose in adults and children on a μg/m^2 basis).

In a 104 week oral study in Sprague-Dawley rats, a statistically significant increase in the incidence of gliomas was observed in male rats receiving an oral dose of 50 μg/kg/day (approximately 1/4 the maximum recommended daily inhalation dose on a μg/m^2 basis); no such changes were seen in male rats receiving oral doses of 10 and 25 μg/kg/day (approximately 1/20 and 1/8 the maximum recommended daily inhalation dose on a μg/m^2 basis) or in female rats at oral doses up to 50 μg/kg/day (approximately 1/4 the maximum recommended human daily inhalation dose on a μg/m^2 basis).

Two additional 104 week carcinogenicity studies have been performed with oral budesonide at doses of 50 μg/kg/day (approximately 1/3 the maximum recommended daily inhalation dose in adults and children on a μg/m^2 basis) in male Sprague-Dawley and Fischer rats. These studies did not demonstrate an increased glioma incidence in budesonide-treated animals as compared with concurrent controls or reference corticosteroid-treated groups (prednisolone and triamcinolone acetonide). Compared with concurrent controls, a statistically significant increase in the incidence of hepatocellular tumors was observed in all three steroid groups (budesonide, prednisolone, triamcinolone acetonide) in these studies.

The mutagenic potential of budesonide was evaluated in six different test systems: Ames *Salmonella*/microsome plate test, mouse micronucleus test, mouse lymphoma test, chromosome aberration test in human lymphocytes, sex-linked recessive lethal test in *Drosophila melanogaster,* and DNA repair analysis in rat hepatocyte culture. Budesonide was not mutagenic or clastogenic in any of these tests.

The effect of SC budesonide on fertility and general reproductive performance was studied in rats. At 20 μg/kg/day (approximately 1/8 the maximum recommended daily inhalation dose in adults on a μg/m^2 basis), decreases in maternal body weight gain, prenatal viability, and viability of the young at birth and during lactation were observed. No such effects were noted at 5 μg/kg (approximately 1/32 the maximum recommended daily inhalation dose in adults on a μg/m² basis).

Pregnancy

Teratogenic Effects, Pregnancy Category B

As with other glucocorticoids, budesonide produced fetal loss, decreased pup weight and skeletal abnormalities at SC doses of 25 μg/kg/day in rabbits (approximately 1/3 the maximum recommended daily inhalation dose in adults on a μg/m² basis) and 500 μg/kg/day in rats (approximately 3 times the maximum recommended daily inhalation dose in adults on a μg/m² basis).

No teratogenic or embryocidal effects were observed in rats when budesonide was administered by inhalation at doses up to 250 μg/kg/day (approximately 2 times the maximum recommended daily inhalation dose in adults on a μg/m² basis).

Experience with oral corticosteroids since their introduction in pharmacologic as opposed to physiologic doses suggests that rodents are more prone to teratogenic effects from corticosteroids than humans.

Studies of pregnant women, however, have not shown that Pulmicort Turbuhaler increases the risk of abnormalities when administered during pregnancy. The results from a large population-based prospective cohort epidemiological study reviewing data from three Swedish registries covering approximately 99% of the pregnancies from 1995-1997 (*i.e.*, Swedish Medical Birth Registry; Registry of Congenital Malformations; Child Cardiology Registry) indicate no increased risk for congenital malformations from the use of inhaled budesonide during early pregnancy. Congenital malformations were studied in 2014 infants born to mothers reporting the use of inhaled budesonide for asthma in early pregnancy (usually 10-12 weeks after the last menstrual period), the period when most major organ malformations occur. The rate of recorded congenital malformations was similar compared to the general population rate (3.8% vs 3.5%, respectively). In addition, after exposure to inhaled budesonide, the number of infants born with orofacial clefts was similar to the expected number in the normal population (4 children vs 3.3, respectively).

These same data were utilized in a second study bringing the total to 2534 infants whose mothers were exposed to inhaled budesonide. In this study, the rate of congenital malformations among infants whose mothers were exposed to inhaled budesonide during early pregnancy was not different from the rate for all newborn babies during the same period (3.6%).

Despite the animal findings, it would appear that the possibility of fetal harm is remote if the drug is used during pregnancy. Nevertheless, because the studies in humans cannot rule out the possibility of harm, Pulmicort Turbuhaler should be used during pregnancy only if clearly needed.

Nonteratogenic Effects

Hypoadrenalism may occur in infants born of mothers receiving corticosteroids during pregnancy. Such infants should be carefully observed.

Nursing Mothers

Corticosteroids are secreted in human milk. Because of the potential for adverse reactions in nursing infants from any corticosteroid, a decision should be made whether to discontinue nursing or discontinue the drug, taking into account the importance of the drug to the mother. Actual data for budesonide are lacking.

Pediatric Use

Safety and effectiveness of Pulmicort Turbuhaler in pediatric patients below 6 years of age have not been established.

In pediatric asthma patients the frequency of adverse events observed with Pulmicort Turbuhaler was similar between the 6-12 year age group (n=172) compared with the 13-17 year age group (n=124).

Oral corticosteroids have been shown to cause growth suppression in pediatric and adolescent patients, particularly with higher doses over extended periods. If a pediatric or adolescent patient on any corticosteroid appears to have growth suppression, the possibility that they are particularly sensitive to this effect of corticosteroids should be considered (see PRECAUTIONS, Pulmicort Turbuhaler).

Geriatric Use

One hundred (100) patients 65 years or older were included in the US and non-US controlled clinical trials of Pulmicort Turbuhaler. There were no differences in the safety and efficacy of the drug compared to those seen in younger patients.

DRUG INTERACTIONS

PULMICORT RESPULES

In clinical studies, concurrent administration of budesonide and other drugs commonly used in the treatment of asthma has not resulted in an increased frequency of adverse events. The main route of metabolism of budesonide, as well as other corticosteroids, is via cytochrome P450 (CYP) isoenzyme 3A4 (CYP3A4). After oral administration of ketoconazole, a potent inhibitor of CYP3A4, the mean plasma concentration of orally administered budesonide increased. Concomitant administration of other known inhibitors of CYP3A4 (*e.g.*, itraconazole, clarithromycin, erythromycin, etc.) may inhibit the metabolism of, and increase the systemic exposure to, budesonide. Care should be exercised when budesonide is coadministered with long-term ketoconazole and other known CYP3A4 inhibitors. Omeprazole did not have effects on the pharmacokinetics of oral budesonide, while cimetidine, primarily an inhibitor of CYP1A2, caused a slight decrease in budesonide clearance and a corresponding increase in its oral bioavailability.

PULMICORT TURBUHALER

In clinical studies, concurrent administration of budesonide and other drugs commonly used in the treatment of asthma has not resulted in an increased frequency of adverse events. Ketoconazole, a potent inhibitor of cytochrome P450 3A, may increase plasma levels of budesonide during concomitant dosing. The clinical significance of concomitant administration of ketoconazole with Pulmicort Turbuhaler is not known, but caution may be warranted.

ADVERSE REACTIONS

PULMICORT RESPULES

The following adverse reactions were reported in pediatric patients treated with Pulmicort Respules.

The incidence of common adverse reactions is based on three double-blind, placebo-controlled, US clinical trials in which 945 patients, 12 months to 8 years of age, (98 patients ≥12 months and <2 years of age; 225 patients ≥2 and <4 years of age; and 622 patients ≥4 and ≤8 years of age) were treated with Pulmicort Respules (0.25 to 1 mg total daily dose for 12 weeks) or vehicle placebo. The incidence and nature of adverse events reported for Pulmicort Respules was comparable to that reported for placebo. TABLE 1 shows the incidence of adverse events in US controlled clinical trials, regardless of relationship to treatment, in patients previously receiving bronchodilators and/or inhaled corticosteroids. This population included a total of 605 male and 340 female patients.

TABLE 1 *Adverse Events With ≥3% Incidence Reported by Patients on Pulmicort Respules*

	Vehicle	Pulmicort Respules Total Daily Dose		
	Placebo	0.25 mg	0.5 mg	1 mg
Adverse Event	(n=227)	(n=178)	(n=223)	(n=317)
Respiratory System Disorder				
Respiratory infection	36%	34%	35%	38%
Rhinitis	9%	7%	11%	12%
Coughing	5%	5%	9%	8%
Resistance Mechanism Disorders				
Otitis media	11%	12%	11%	9%
Viral infection	3%	4%	5%	3%
Moniliasis	2%	4%	3%	4%
Gastrointestinal System Disorders				
Gastroenteritis	4%	5%	5%	5%
Vomiting	3%	2%	4%	4%
Diarrhea	2%	4%	4%	2%
Abdominal pain	2%	3%	2%	3%
Hearing and Vestibular Disorders				
Ear infection	4%	2%	4%	5%
Platelet, Bleeding, and Clotting Disorders				
Epistaxis	1%	2%	4%	3%
Vision Disorders				
Conjunctivitis	2%	<1%	4%	2%
Skin and Appendages Disorders				
Rash	3%	<1%	4%	2%

TABLE 1 shows all adverse events with an incidence of 3% or more in at least one active treatment group where the incidence was higher with Pulmicort Respules than with placebo. **The following adverse events occurred with an incidence of 3% or more in at least one Pulmicort Respules group where the incidence was equal to or less than that of the placebo group:** Fever, sinusitis, pain, pharyngitis, bronchospasm, bronchitis, and headache.

Incidence 1 to ≤3% (by body system)

The information below includes all adverse events with an incidence of 1 to ≤3%, in at least one Pulmicort Respules treatment group where the incidence was higher with Pulmicort Respules than with placebo, regardless of relationship to treatment.

Body as a Whole: Allergic reaction, chest pain, fatigue, flu-like disorder.
Respiratory System: Stridor.
Resistance Mechanisms: Herpes simplex, external ear infection, infection.
Central & Peripheral Nervous System: Dysphonia, hyperkinesia.
Skin & Appendages: Eczema, pustular rash, pruritus.
Hearing & Vestibular: Earache.
Vision: Eye infection.
Psychiatric: Anorexia, emotional lability.
Musculoskeletal System: Fracture, myalgia.
Application Site: Contact dermatitis.
Platelet, Bleeding & Clotting: Purpura.
White Cell and Resistance: Cervical lymphadenopathy.

The incidence of reported adverse events was similar between the 447 Pulmicort Respules-treated (mean total daily dose 0.5 to 1 mg) and 223 conventional therapy-treated pediatric asthma patients followed for 1 year in three open-label studies.

Cases of growth suppression have been reported for inhaled corticosteroids including post-marketing reports for Pulmicort Respules (see PRECAUTIONS, Pulmicort Respules, Pediatric Use).

Less frequent adverse events (<1%) reported in the published literature, long-term, open-label clinical trials, or from marketing experience for inhaled budesonide include: immediate and delayed hypersensitivity reactions including rash, contact dermatitis, angioedema, and bronchospasm; symptoms of hypocorticism and hypercorticism; psychiatric symptoms including depression, aggressive reactions, irritability, anxiety, and psychosis; and bone disorders including avascular necrosis of the femoral head and osteoporosis.

PULMICORT TURBUHALER

The following adverse reactions were reported in patients treated with Pulmicort Turbuhaler.

The incidence of common adverse events is based upon double-blind, placebo-controlled US clinical trials in which 1116 adult and pediatric patients age 6-70 years (472 females and 644 males) were treated with Pulmicort Turbuhaler (200-800 μg twice daily for 12-20 weeks) or placebo.

TABLE 2 shows the incidence of adverse events in patients previously receiving bronchodilators and/or inhaled corticosteroids in US controlled clinical trials. This population included 232 male and 62 female pediatric patients (age 6-17 years) and 332 male and 331 female adult patients (age 18 years and greater).

TABLE 2 includes all events (whether considered drug-related or non drug-related by the investigators) that occurred at a rate of ≥3% in any one Pulmicort Turbuhaler group and

TABLE 2 *Adverse Events With ≥3% Incidence Reported by Patients on Pulmicort Turbuhaler*

		Pulmicort Turbuhaler		
	Placebo	200 μg*	400 μg*	800 μg*
Adverse Event	n=284	n=286	n=289	n=98
Respiratory System				
Respiratory infection	17%	20%	24%	19%
Pharyngitis	9%	10%	9%	5%
Sinusitis	7%	11%	7%	2%
Voice alteration	0%	1%	2%	6%
Body as a Whole				
Headache	7%	14%	13%	14%
Flu syndrome	6%	6%	6%	14%
Pain	2%	5%	5%	5%
Back pain	1%	2%	3%	6%
Fever	2%	2%	4%	0%
Digestive System				
Oral candidiasis	2%	2%	4%	4%
Dyspepsia	2%	1%	2%	4%
Gastroenteritis	1%	1%	2%	3%
Nausea	2%	2%	1%	3%
Average duration of exposure (days)	59	79	80	80

* Twice daily.

were more common than in the placebo group. In considering these data, the increased average duration of exposure for Pulmicort Turbuhaler patients should be taken into account.

The following other adverse events occurred in these clinical trials using Pulmicort Turbuhaler with an incidence of 1-3% and were more common on Pulmicort Turbuhaler than on placebo:

Body as a Whole: Neck pain.
Cardiovascular: Syncope.
Digestive: Abdominal pain, dry mouth, vomiting.
Metabolic and Nutritional: Weight gain.
Musculoskeletal: Fracture, myalgia.
Nervous: Hypertonia, migraine.
Platelet, Bleeding and Clotting: Ecchymosis.
Psychiatric: Insomnia.
Resistance Mechanisms: Infection.
Special Senses: Taste perversion.

In a 20 week trial in adult asthmatics who previously required oral corticosteroids, the effects of Pulmicort Turbuhaler 400 μg twice daily (n=53) and 800 μg twice daily (n=53) were compared with placebo (n=53) on the frequency of reported adverse events. Adverse events, whether considered drug-related or non drug-related by the investigators, reported in more than 5 patients in the Pulmicort Turbuhaler group and which occurred more frequently with Pulmicort Turbuhaler than placebo are shown below (% Pulmicort Turbuhaler and % placebo). In considering these data, the increased average duration of exposure for Pulmicort Turbuhaler patients (78 days for Pulmicort Turbuhaler vs 41 days for placebo) should be taken into account.

Body as a whole: Asthenia (9% and 2%), headache (12% and 2%), pain (10% and 2%).
Digestive: Dyspepsia (8% and 0%), nausea (6% and 0%), oral candidiasis (10% and 0%).
Musculoskeletal: Arthralgia (6% and 0%).
Respiratory: Cough increased (6% and 2%), respiratory infection (32% and 13%), rhinitis (6% and 2%), sinusitis (16% and 11%).

Patients Receiving Pulmicort Turbuhaler Once Daily

The adverse event profile of once-daily administration of Pulmicort Turbuhaler 200 and 400 μg, and placebo, was evaluated in 309 adult asthmatic patients in an 18 week study. The study population included both patients previously treated with inhaled corticosteroids, and patients not previously receiving corticosteroid therapy. There was no clinically relevant difference in the pattern of adverse events following once-daily administration of Pulmicort Turbuhaler when compared to twice-daily dosing.

Pediatric Studies

In a 12 week placebo-controlled trial in 404 pediatric patients 6-18 years of age previously maintained on inhaled corticosteroids, the frequency of adverse events for each age category (6-12 years, 13-18 years) was comparable for Pulmicort Turbuhaler (at 100, 200 and 400 μg twice daily) and placebo. There were no clinically relevant differences in the pattern or severity of adverse events in children compared with those reported in adults.

Adverse Event Reports From Other Sources

Rare adverse events reported in the published literature or from marketing experience include: Immediate and delayed hypersensitivity reactions including rash, contact dermatitis, urticaria, angioedema and bronchospasm; symptoms of hypocorticism and hypercorticism; psychiatric symptoms including depression, aggressive reactions, irritability, anxiety and psychosis.

DOSAGE AND ADMINISTRATION

PULMICORT RESPULES

Pulmicort Respules is indicated for use in asthmatic patients 12 months to 8 years of age. Pulmicort Respules should be administered by the inhaled route via jet nebulizer connected to an air compressor. Individual patients will experience a variable onset and degree of symptom relief. Improvement in asthma control following inhaled administration of Pulmicort Respules can occur within 2-8 days of initiation of treatment, although maximum benefit may not be achieved for 4-6 weeks. The safety and efficacy of Pulmicort Respules when administered in excess of recommended doses have not been established. In all patients, it is desirable to downward-titrate to the lowest effective dose once asthma stability is achieved. The recommended starting dose and highest recommended dose of Pulmicort Respules, based on prior asthma therapy, are listed in TABLE 3.

TABLE 3

Previous Therapy	Recommended Starting Dose	Highest Recommended Dose
Bronchodilators alone	0.5 mg total daily dose administered either once or twice daily in divided doses	0.5 mg total daily dose
Inhaled corticosteroids	0.5 mg total daily dose administered either once or twice daily in divided doses	1 mg total daily dose
Oral corticosteroids	1 mg total daily dose administered either as 0.5 mg twice daily or 1 mg once daily	1 mg total daily dose

In symptomatic children not responding to non-steroidal therapy, a starting dose of 0.25 mg once daily of Pulmicort Respules may also be considered.

If once-daily treatment with Pulmicort Respules does not provide adequate control of asthma symptoms, the total daily dose should be increased and/or administered as a divided dose.

Patients Not Receiving Systemic (oral) Corticosteroids

Patients who require maintenance therapy of their asthma may benefit from treatment with Pulmicort Respules at the doses recommended above. Once the desired clinical effect is achieved, consideration should be given to tapering to the lowest effective dose. For the patients who do not respond adequately to the starting dose, consideration should be given to administering the total daily dose as a divided dose, if a once-daily dosing schedule was followed. If necessary, higher doses, up to the maximum recommended doses, may provide additional asthma control.

Patients Maintained on Chronic Oral Corticosteroids

Initially, Pulmicort Respules should be used concurrently with the patient's usual maintenance dose of systemic corticosteroid. After approximately 1 week, gradual withdrawal of the systemic corticosteroid may be initiated by reducing the daily or alternate daily dose. Further incremental reductions may be made after an interval of 1 or 2 weeks, depending on the response of the patient. Generally, these decrements should not exceed 25% of the prednisone dose or its equivalent. A slow rate of withdrawal is strongly recommended. During reduction of oral corticosteroids, patients should be carefully monitored for asthma instability, including objective measures of airway function, and for adrenal insufficiency (see WARNINGS, Pulmicort Respules). During withdrawal, some patients may experience symptoms of systemic corticosteroid withdrawal, *e.g.,* joint and/or muscular pain, lassitude, and depression, despite maintenance or even improvement in pulmonary function. Such patients should be encouraged to continue with Pulmicort Respules but should be monitored for objective signs of adrenal insufficiency. If evidence of adrenal insufficiency occurs, the systemic corticosteroid doses should be increased temporarily and thereafter withdrawal should continue more slowly. During periods of stress or a severe asthma attack, transfer patients may require supplementary treatment with systemic corticosteroids.

A Pari-LC-Jet Plus Nebulizer (with face mask or mouthpiece) connected to a Pari Master compressor was used to deliver Pulmicort Respules to each patient in 3 US controlled clinical studies. The safety and efficacy of Pulmicort Respules delivered by other nebulizers and compressors have not been established.

Pulmicort Respules should be administered via jet nebulizer connected to an air compressor with an adequate air flow, equipped with a mouthpiece or suitable face mask. Ultrasonic nebulizers are not suitable for the adequate administration of Pulmicort Respules and, therefore, are NOT recommended.

The effects of mixing Pulmicort Respules with other nebulizable medications have not been adequately assessed. Pulmicort Respules should be administered separately in the nebulizer (see PRECAUTIONS, Pulmicort Respules, Information for the Patient).

Directions for Use

Illustrated Patient's Instructions for Use accompany each package of Pulmicort Respules.

PULMICORT TURBUHALER

Pulmicort Turbuhaler should be administered by the orally inhaled route in asthmatic patients age 6 years and older. Individual patients will experience a variable onset and degree of symptom relief. Generally, Pulmicort Turbuhaler has a relatively rapid onset of action for an inhaled corticosteroid. Improvement in asthma control following inhaled administration of Pulmicort Turbuhaler can occur within 24 hours of initiation of treatment, although maximum benefit may not be achieved for 1-2 weeks, or longer. The safety and efficacy of Pulmicort Turbuhaler when administered in excess of recommended doses have not been established.

The recommended starting dose and the highest recommended dose of Pulmicort Turbuhaler, based on prior asthma therapy, are listed in TABLE 4.

If the once-daily treatment with Pulmicort Turbuhaler does not provide adequate control of asthma symptoms, the total daily dose should be increased and/or administered as a divided dose.

Patients Maintained on Chronic Oral Corticosteroids

Initially, Pulmicort Turbuhaler should be used concurrently with the patient's usual maintenance dose of systemic corticosteroid. After approximately 1 week, gradual withdrawal of the systemic corticosteroid is started by reducing the daily or alternate daily dose. The next reduction is made after an interval of 1 or 2 weeks, depending on the response of the patient. Generally, these decrements should not exceed 2.5 mg of prednisone or its equivalent. A slow rate of withdrawal is strongly recommended. During reduction of oral corticosteroids, patients should be carefully monitored for asthma instability, including objective measures

B

TABLE 4

Previous Therapy	Recommended Starting Dose	Highest Recommended Dose
Adults		
Bronchodilators alone	200-400 μg twice daily	400 μg twice daily
Inhaled corticosteroids*	200-400 μg twice daily	800 μg twice daily
Oral corticosteroids	400-800 μg twice daily	800 μg twice daily
Children		
Bronchodilators alone	200 μg twice daily	400 μg twice daily
Inhaled corticosteroids*	200 μg twice daily	400 μg twice daily
Oral corticosteroids	The highest recommended dose in children is 400 μg twice daily	

* In patients with mild to moderate asthma who are well controlled on inhaled corticosteroids, dosing with Pulmicort Turbuhaler 200 or 400 μg once daily may be considered. Pulmicort Turbuhaler can be administered once daily either in the morning or in the evening.

of airway function, and for adrenal insufficiency (see WARNINGS, Pulmicort Turbuhaler). During withdrawal, some patients may experience symptoms of systemic corticosteroid withdrawal, *e.g.*, joint and/or muscular pain, lassitude and depression, despite maintenance or even improvement in pulmonary function. Such patients should be encouraged to continue with Pulmicort Turbuhaler but should be monitored for objective signs of adrenal insufficiency. If evidence of adrenal insufficiency occurs, the systemic corticosteroid doses should be increased temporarily and thereafter withdrawal should continue more slowly. During periods of stress or a severe asthma attack, transfer patients may require supplementary treatment with systemic corticosteroids.

Note: In all patients it is desirable to titrate to the lowest effective dose once asthma stability is achieved.

Patients should be instructed to prime Pulmicort Turbuhaler prior to its initial use, and instructed to inhale deeply and forcefully each time the unit is used. Rinsing the mouth after inhalation is also recommended.

Directions for Use

Illustrated Patient's Instructions for Use accompany each package of Pulmicort Turbuhaler.

HOW SUPPLIED

PULMICORT RESPULES

Pulmicort Respules is supplied in sealed aluminum foil envelopes containing one plastic strip of 5 single-dose Respules ampules together with patient instructions for use. There are 30 Respules ampules in a carton. Each single-dose Respule ampule contains 2 ml of sterile liquid suspension.

Pulmicort Respules is available in two strengths 0.25 mg/2 ml and 0.5 mg/2 ml.

Storage

Pulmicort Respules should be stored upright at controlled room temperature 20-25°C (68-77°F), and protected from light. When an envelope has been opened, the shelf life of the unused Respules is 2 weeks when protected. After opening the aluminum foil envelope, the unused Respules ampules should be returned to the aluminum foil envelope to protect them from light. Any opened Respule ampule must be used promptly. Gently shake the Respule ampule using a circular motion before use. Keep out of reach of children. Do not freeze.

PULMICORT TURBUHALER

Pulmicort Turbuhaler consists of a number of assembled plastic details, the main parts being the dosing mechanism, the storage unit for drug substance and the mouthpiece. The inhaler is protected by a white outer tubular cover screwed onto the inhaler. The body of the inhaler is white and the turning grip is brown. The following wording is printed on the grip in raised lettering, "Pulmicort 200 μg". The Turbuhaler cannot be refilled and should be discarded when empty.

Pulmicort Turbuhaler is available as 200 μg/dose, 200 doses and has a target fill weight of 104 mg.

When there are 20 doses remaining in Pulmicort Turbuhaler, a red mark will appear in the indicator window. If the unit is used beyond the point at which the red mark appears at the bottom of the window, the correct amount of medication may not be obtained. The unit should be discarded.

Storage

Store with the cover tightened in a dry place at controlled room temperature 20-25°C (68-77°F).

INTRANASAL

DESCRIPTION

Note: The trade names have been used throughout this monograph for clarity.

For Intranasal Use Only.

Budesonide, the active ingredient of Rhinocort Aqua nasal spray, is an anti-inflammatory synthetic corticosteroid.

It is designated chemically as (RS)-11-β,16-α,17,21-tetrahydroxypregna-1,4-diene-3,20-dione cyclic 16,17-acetal with butyraldehyde.

Budesonide is provided as the mixture of two epimers (22R and 22S).

The empirical formula of budesonide is $C_{25}H_{34}O_6$ and its molecular weight is 430.5.

Budesonide is a white to off-white, odorless powder that is practically insoluble in water and in heptane, sparingly soluble in ethanol, and freely soluble in chloroform.

Its partition coefficient between octanol and water at pH 5 is 1.6×10^3.

Rhinocort Aqua is an unscented, metered-dose, manual-pump spray formulation containing a micronized suspension of budesonide in an aqueous medium. Microcrystalline cellulose and carboxymethyl cellulose sodium, dextrose anhydrous, polysorbate 80, disodium edetate, potassium sorbate and purified water are contained in this medium; hydrochloric acid is added to adjust the pH to a target of 4.5.

Rhinocort Aqua nasal spray delivers 32 μg of budesonide per spray.

Each bottle of Rhinocort Aqua nasal spray 32 μg contains 120 metered sprays after initial priming.

Prior to initial use, the container must be shaken gently and the pump must be primed by actuating 8 times. If used daily, the pump does not need to be reprimed. If not used for 2 consecutive days, reprime with 1 spray or until a fine spray appears. If not used for more than 14 days, rinse the applicator and reprime with 2 sprays or until a fine spray appears.

CLINICAL PHARMACOLOGY

Budesonide is a synthetic corticosteroid having potent glucocorticoid activity and weak mineralocorticoid activity. In standard *in vitro* and animal models, budesonide has approximately a 200-fold higher affinity for the glucocorticoid receptor and a 1000-fold higher topical anti-inflammatory potency than cortisol (rat croton oil ear edema assay). As a measure of systemic activity, budesonide is 40 times more potent than cortisol when administered subcutaneously and 25 times more potent when administered orally in the rat thymus involution assay. In glucocorticoid receptor affinity studies, the 22R form was twice as active as the 22S epimer.

The precise mechanism of corticosteroid actions in seasonal and perennial allergic rhinitis is not known. Corticosteroids have been shown to have a wide range of inhibitory activities against multiple cell types (*e.g.*, mast cells, eosinophils, neutrophils, macrophages, and lymphocytes) and mediators (*e.g.*, histamine, eicosanoids, leukotrienes, and cytokines) involved in allergic mediated inflammation.

Corticosteroids affect the delayed (6 hour) response to an allergen challenge more than the histamine-associated immediate response (20 minute). The clinical significance of these findings is unknown.

PHARMACOKINETICS

The pharmacokinetics of budesonide have been studied following nasal, oral and IV administration. Budesonide is relatively well absorbed after both inhalation and oral administration, and is rapidly metabolized into metabolites with low corticosteroid potency. The clinical activity of Rhinocort Aqua nasal spray is therefore believed to be due to the parent drug, budesonide. *In vitro* studies indicate that the two epimeric forms of budesonide do not interconvert.

Absorption

Following intranasal administration of Rhinocort Aqua, the mean peak plasma concentration occurs at approximately 0.7 hours. Compared to an IV dose, approximately 34% of the delivered intranasal dose reaches the systemic circulation, most of which is absorbed through the nasal mucosa. While budesonide is well absorbed from the GI tract, the oral bioavailability of budesonide is low (~10%) primarily due to extensive first pass metabolism in the liver.

Distribution

Budesonide has a volume of distribution of approximately 2-3 L/kg. The volume of distribution for the 22R epimer is almost twice that of the 22S epimer. Protein binding of budesonide *in vitro* is constant (85-90%) over a concentration range (1-100 nmol/L) which exceeded that achieved after administration of recommended doses. Budesonide shows little to no binding to glucocorticosteroid binding globulin. It rapidly equilibrates with red blood cells in a concentration independent manner with a blood/plasma ratio of about 0.8.

Metabolism

Budesonide is rapidly and extensively metabolized in humans by the liver. Two major metabolites (16α-hydroxyprednisolone and 6β-hydroxybudesonide) are formed via cytochrome P450 3A isoenzyme-catalyzed biotransformation. Known metabolic inhibitors of cytochrome P450 3A (*e.g.*, ketoconazole), or significant hepatic impairment, may increase the systemic exposure of unmetabolized budesonide (see WARNINGS and PRECAUTIONS). *In vitro* studies on the binding of the two primary metabolites to the glucocorticoid receptor indicate that they have less than 1% of the affinity for the receptor as the parent compound budesonide. *In vitro* studies have evaluated sites of metabolism and showed negligible metabolism in skin, lung, and serum. No qualitative difference between the *in vitro* and *in vivo* metabolic patterns could be detected.

Elimination

Budesonide is excreted in the urine and feces in the form of metabolites. After intranasal administration of a radiolabeled dose, 2/3 of the radioactivity was found in the urine and the remainder in the feces. The main metabolites of budesonide in the 0-24 hour urine sample following IV administration are 16α-hydroxyprednisolone (24%) and 6β-hydroxybudesonide (5%). An additional 34% of the radioactivity recovered in the urine was identified as conjugates.

The 22R form was preferentially cleared with clearance value of 1.4 L/min vs 1.0 L/min for the 22S form. The terminal half-life, 2-3 hours, was similar for both epimers and it appeared to be independent of dose.

SPECIAL POPULATIONS

Geriatric

No specific pharmacokinetic study has been undertaken in subjects >65 years of age.

Pediatric

After administration of Rhinocort Aqua nasal spray, the time to reach peak drug concentrations and plasma half-life were similar in children and in adults. Children had plasma concentrations approximately twice those observed in adults due primarily to differences in weight between children and adults.

Gender

No specific pharmacokinetic study has been conducted to evaluate the effect of gender on budesonide pharmacokinetics. However, following administration of 400 μg Rhinocort

Aqua nasal spray to 7 male and 8 female volunteers in a pharmacokinetic study, no major gender differences in the pharmacokinetic parameters were found.

Race

No specific study has been undertaken to evaluate the effect of race on budesonide pharmacokinetics.

Renal Insufficiency

The pharmacokinetics of budesonide have not been investigated in patients with renal insufficiency.

Hepatic Insufficiency

Reduced liver function may affect the elimination of corticosteroids. The pharmacokinetics of orally administered budesonide were affected by compromised liver function as evidenced by a doubled systemic availability. The relevance of this finding to intranasally administered budesonide has not been established.

PHARMACODYNAMICS

A 3 week clinical study in seasonal rhinitis, comparing Rhinocort nasal inhaler, orally ingested budesonide, and placebo in 98 patients with allergic rhinitis due to birch pollen, demonstrated that the therapeutic effect of Rhinocort nasal inhaler can be attributed to the topical effects of budesonide.

The effects of Rhinocort Aqua nasal spray on adrenal function have been evaluated in several clinical trials. In a 4 week clinical trial, 61 adult patients who received 256 µg daily of Rhinocort Aqua nasal spray demonstrated no significant differences from patients receiving placebo in plasma cortisol levels measured before and 60 minutes after 0.25 mg intramuscular cosyntropin. There were no consistent differences in 24 hour urinary cortisol measurements in patients receiving up to 400 µg daily. Similar results were seen in a study of 150 children and adolescents aged 6-17 with perennial rhinitis who were treated with 256 µg daily for up to 12 months.

After treatment with the recommended maximal daily dose of Rhinocort Aqua (256 µg) for 7 days, there was a small, but statistically significant decrease in the area under the plasma cortisol-time curve over 24 hours [AUC(0-24h)] in healthy adult volunteers.

A dose-related suppression of 24 hour urinary cortisol excretion was observed after administration of Rhinocort Aqua doses ranging from 100-800 µg daily for up to 4 days in 78 healthy adult volunteers. The clinical relevance of these results is unknown.

INDICATIONS AND USAGE

Rhinocort Aqua nasal spray is indicated for the management of nasal symptoms of seasonal or perennial allergic rhinitis in adults and children 6 years of age and older.

CONTRAINDICATIONS

Hypersensitivity to any of the ingredients in this preparation contraindicates the use of Rhinocort Aqua nasal spray.

WARNINGS

The replacement of a systemic corticosteroid with a topical corticosteroid can be accompanied by signs of adrenal insufficiency, and in addition some patients may experience symptoms of corticosteroid withdrawal, *e.g.*, joint and/or muscular pain, lassitude, and depression. Patients previously treated for prolonged periods with systemic corticosteroids and transferred to topical corticosteroids should be carefully monitored for acute adrenal insufficiency in response to stress. In those patients who have asthma or other clinical conditions requiring long-term systemic corticosteroid treatment, too rapid a decrease in systemic corticosteroids may cause a severe exacerbation of their symptoms.

Patients who are on drugs which suppress the immune system are more susceptible to infections than healthy individuals. Chicken pox and measles, for example, can have a more serious or even fatal course in non-immune children or adults on immunosuppressant doses of corticosteroids. In such children or adults who have not had these diseases, particular care should be taken to avoid exposure. How the dose, route, and duration of corticosteroid administration affects the risk of developing a disseminated infection is not known. The contribution of the underlying disease and/or prior corticosteroid treatment to the risk is also not known. If exposed to chicken pox, prophylaxis with varicella zoster immune globulin (VZIG) may be indicated. If exposed to measles, prophylaxis with pooled intramuscular immunoglobulin (IG) may be indicated. (See the respective package inserts for complete VZIG and IG prescribing information.) If chicken pox develops, treatment with antiviral agents may be considered.

PRECAUTIONS

GENERAL

Intranasal corticosteroids may cause a reduction in growth velocity when administered to pediatric patients (see Pediatric Use).

Rarely, immediate and/or delayed hypersensitivity reactions may occur after the intranasal administration of budesonide. Rare instances of wheezing, nasal septum perforation, and increased intraocular pressure have been reported following the intranasal application of corticosteroids, including budesonide.

Although systemic effects have been minimal with recommended doses of Rhinocort Aqua nasal spray, any such effect is dose dependent. Therefore, larger than recommended doses of Rhinocort Aqua nasal spray should be avoided and the minimal effective dose for the patient should be used (see DOSAGE AND ADMINISTRATION). When used at larger doses, systemic corticosteroid effects such as hypercorticism and adrenal suppression may appear. If such changes occur, the dosage of Rhinocort Aqua nasal spray should be discontinued slowly, consistent with accepted procedures for discontinuing oral corticosteroid therapy.

In clinical studies with budesonide administered intranasally, the development of localized infections of the nose and pharynx with *Candida albicans* has occurred only rarely. When such an infection develops, it may require treatment with appropriate local or systemic therapy and discontinuation of treatment with Rhinocort Aqua nasal spray. Patients using Rhinocort Aqua nasal spray over several months or longer should be examined periodically for evidence of *Candida* infection or other signs of adverse effects on the nasal mucosa.

Rhinocort Aqua nasal spray should be used with caution, if at all, in patients with active or quiescent tuberculous infection, untreated fungal, bacterial, or systemic viral infections, or ocular herpes simplex.

Because of the inhibitory effect of corticosteroids on wound healing, patients who have experienced recent nasal septal ulcers, nasal surgery, or nasal trauma should not use a nasal corticosteroid until healing has occurred.

Hepatic dysfunction influences the pharmacokinetics of budesonide, similar to the effect on other corticosteroids, with a reduced elimination rate and increased systemic availability (see CLINICAL PHARMACOLOGY,Special Populations).

INFORMATION FOR THE PATIENT

Patients being treated with Rhinocort Aqua nasal spray should receive the following information and instructions. Patients who are on immunosuppressant doses of corticosteroids should be warned to avoid exposure to chicken pox or measles and, if exposed, to obtain medical advice.

Patients should use Rhinocort Aqua nasal spray at regular intervals since its effectiveness depends on its regular use (see DOSAGE AND ADMINISTRATION).

An improvement in nasal symptoms may be noted in patients within 10 hours of first using Rhinocort Aqua nasal spray. This time to onset is supported by an environmental exposure unit study in seasonal allergic rhinitis patients which demonstrated that Rhinocort Aqua nasal spray led to a statistically significant improvement in nasal symptoms compared to placebo by 10 hours. Further support comes from a clinical study of patients with perennial allergic rhinitis which demonstrated a statistically significant improvement in nasal symptoms for both Rhinocort Aqua nasal spray and for the active comparator (mometasone furoate) compared to placebo by 8 hours. Onset was also assessed in this study with peak nasal inspiratory flow rate and this endpoint failed to show efficacy for either active treatment. Although statistically significant improvements in nasal symptoms compared to placebo were noted within 8-10 hours in these studies, about one-half to two-thirds of the ultimate clinical improvement with Rhinocort Aqua nasal spray occurs over the first 1-2 days, and maximum benefit may not be achieved until approximately 2 weeks after initiation of treatment. Initial assessment for response should be made during this time frame and periodically until the patient's symptoms are stabilized.

The patient should take the medication as directed and should not exceed the prescribed dosage. The patient should contact the physician if symptoms do not improve after 2 weeks, or if the condition worsens. Patients who experience recurrent episodes of epistaxis (nosebleeds) or nasal septum discomfort while taking this medication should contact their physician. For proper use of this unit and to attain maximum improvement, the patient should read and follow the accompanying patient instructions carefully.

It is important to shake the bottle well before each use. The Rhinocort Aqua nasal spray 32 µg bottle has been filled with an excess to accommodate the priming activity. The bottle should be discarded after 120 sprays following initial priming, since the amount of budesonide delivered per spray thereafter may be substantially less than the labeled dose. Do not transfer any remaining suspension to another bottle.

CARCINOGENESIS, MUTAGENESIS, AND IMPAIRMENT OF FERTILITY

In a 2 year study in Sprague-Dawley rats, budesonide caused a statistically significant increase in the incidence of gliomas in the male rats receiving an oral dose of 50 µg/kg (approximately twice the maximum recommended daily intranasal dose in adults and children on a µg/m^2 basis). No tumorigenicity was seen in male and female rats at respective oral doses up to 25 and 50 µg/kg (approximately equal to and two times the maximum recommended daily intranasal dose in adults and children on a µg/m^2 basis, respectively). In two additional 2 year studies in male Fischer and Sprague-Dawley rats, budesonide caused no gliomas at an oral dose of 50 µg/kg (approximately twice the maximum recommended daily intranasal dose in adults and children on a µg/m^2 basis). However, in male Sprague-Dawley rats, budesonide caused a statistically significant increase in the incidence of hepatocellular tumors at an oral dose of 50 µg/kg (approximately twice the maximum recommended daily intranasal dose in adults and children on a µg/m^2 basis). The concurrent reference corticosteroids (prednisolone and triamcinolone acetonide) in these two studies showed similar findings.

In a 91 week study in mice, budesonide caused no treatment-related carcinogenicity at oral doses up to 200 µg/kg (approximately 3 times the maximum recommended daily intranasal dose in adults and children on a µg/m^2 basis).

Budesonide was not mutagenic or clastogenic in six different test systems: Ames, *Salmonella*/microsome plate test, mouse micronucleus test, mouse lymphoma test, chromosome aberration test in human lymphocytes, sex-linked recessive lethal test in *Drosophila melanogaster,* and DNA repair analysis in rat hematocyte culture.

In rats, budesonide caused a decrease in prenatal viability and viability of the pups at birth and during lactation, along with a decrease in maternal body-weight gain, at SC doses of 20 µg/kg and above (less than the maximum recommended daily intranasal dose in adults on a µg/m^2 basis). No such effects were noted at 5 µg/kg (less than the maximum recommended daily intranasal dose in adults on a µg/m^2 basis).

PREGNANCY

Teratogenic Effects, Pregnancy Category C

Budesonide was teratogenic and embryocidal in rabbits and rats. Budesonide produced fetal loss, decreased pup weights, and skeletal abnormalities at SC doses of 25 µg/kg in rabbits and 500 µg/kg in rats (approximately 2 and 16 times the maximum recommended daily intranasal dose in adults on a µg/m^2 basis). In another study in rats, no teratogenic or embryocidal effects were seen at inhalation doses up to 250 µg/kg (approximately 8 times the maximum recommended daily intranasal dose in adults on a µg/m^2 basis).

There are no adequate and well-controlled studies in pregnant women. Rhinocort Aqua nasal spray should be used during pregnancy only if the potential benefit justifies the potential risk to the fetus.

Experience with oral corticosteroids since their introduction in pharmacologic, as opposed to physiologic, doses suggests that rodents are more prone to teratogenic effects from corticosteroids than humans. In addition, because there is a natural increase in corticosteroid production during pregnancy, most women will require a lower exogenous corticosteroid dose and many will not need corticosteroid treatment during pregnancy.

Nonteratogenic Effects

Hypoadrenalism may occur in infants born of mothers receiving corticosteroids during pregnancy. Such infants should be carefully observed.

NURSING MOTHERS

It is not known whether budesonide is excreted in human milk. Because other corticosteroids are excreted in human milk, caution should be exercised when Rhinocort Aqua nasal spray is administered to nursing women.

PEDIATRIC USE

Safety and effectiveness in pediatric patients below 6 years of age have not been established.

Controlled clinical studies have shown that intranasal corticosteroids may cause a reduction in growth velocity in pediatric patients. This effect has been observed in the absence of laboratory evidence of hypothalamic-pituitary-adrenal (HPA) axis suppression, suggesting that growth velocity is a more sensitive indicator of systemic corticosteroid exposure in pediatric patients than some commonly used tests of HPA axis function. The long-term effects of this reduction in growth velocity associated with intranasal corticosteroids, including the impact on final adult height, are unknown. The potential for "catch up" growth following discontinuation of treatment with intranasal corticosteroids has not been adequately studied. The growth of pediatric patients receiving intranasal corticosteroids, including Rhinocort Aqua nasal spray, should be monitored routinely (*e.g.*, via stadiometry). The potential growth effects of prolonged treatment should be weighed against clinical benefits obtained and the availability of safe and effective noncorticosteroid treatment alternatives. To minimize the systemic effects of intranasal corticosteroids, including Rhinocort Aqua nasal spray, each patient should be titrated to the lowest dose that effectively controls his/her symptoms.

GERIATRIC USE

Of the 2461 patients in clinical studies of Rhinocort Aqua nasal spray, 5% were 60 years of age and over. No overall differences in safety or effectiveness were observed between these subjects and younger subjects, except for an adverse event reporting frequency of epistaxis which increased with age. Further, other reported clinical experience has not identified any other differences in responses between elderly and younger patients, but greater sensitivity of some older individuals cannot be ruled out.

DRUG INTERACTIONS

The main route of metabolism of budesonide, as well as other corticosteroids, is via cytochrome P450 3A (CYP3A). After oral administration of ketoconazole, a potent inhibitor of cytochrome P450 3A, the mean plasma concentration of orally administered budesonide increased by more than 7-fold. Concomitant administration of other known inhibitors of CYP3A (*e.g.*, itraconazole, clarithromycin, erythromycin, etc.) may inhibit the metabolism of, and increase the systemic exposure to, budesonide (see WARNINGS and PRECAUTIONS, General).

Omeprazole, an inhibitor of cytochrome P450 2C19, did not have effects on the pharmacokinetics of oral budesonide, while cimetidine, primarily an inhibitor of cytochrome P450 1A2, caused a slight decrease in budesonide clearance and corresponding increase in its oral bioavailability.

ADVERSE REACTIONS

The incidence of common adverse reactions is based upon two US and five non-US controlled clinical trials in 1526 patients [110 females and 239 males less than 18 years of age, and 635 females and 542 males 18 years of age and older] treated with Rhinocort Aqua nasal spray at doses up to 400 µg once daily for 3-6 weeks. TABLE 5 describes adverse events occurring at an incidence of 2% or greater and more common among Rhinocort Aqua nasal spray-treated patients than in placebo-treated patients in controlled clinical trials. The overall incidence of adverse events was similar between Rhinocort Aqua and Placebo.

TABLE 5

Adverse Event	Rhinocort Aqua	Placebo Vehicle
Epistaxis	8%	5%
Pharyngitis	4%	3%
Bronchospasm	2%	1%
Coughing	2%	<1%
Nasal irritation	2%	<1%

A similar adverse event profile was observed in the subgroup of pediatric patients 6-12 years of age.

Two to three percent (2-3%) of patients in clinical trials discontinued because of adverse events. Systemic corticosteroid side effects were not reported during controlled clinical studies with Rhinocort Aqua nasal spray.

If recommended doses are exceeded, however, or if individuals are particularly sensitive, symptoms of hypercorticism, *i.e.*, Cushing's Syndrome, could occur.

Rare adverse events reported from post-marketing experience include: Nasal septum perforation, pharynx disorders (throat irritation, throat pain, swollen throat, burning throat, and itchy throat), angioedema, anosmia, and palpitations.

Cases of growth suppression have been reported for intranasal corticosteroids including Rhinocort Aqua nasal spray (see PRECAUTIONS, Pediatric Use).

DOSAGE AND ADMINISTRATION

The recommended starting dose for adults and children 6 years of age and older is 64 µg/day administered as 1 spray per nostril of Rhinocort Aqua nasal spray 32 µg once daily. The maximum recommended dose for adults (12 years of age and older) is 256 µg/day administered as 4 sprays per nostril once daily of Rhinocort Aqua nasal spray 32 µg and the maximum recommended dose for pediatric patients (<12 years of age) is 128 µg/day administered as 2 sprays per nostril once daily of Rhinocort Aqua nasal spray 32 µg (see HOW SUPPLIED).

Prior to initial use, the container must be shaken gently and the pump must be primed by actuating 8 times. If used daily, the pump does not need to be reprimed. If not used for 2 consecutive days, reprime with 1 spray or until a fine spray appears. If not used for more than 14 days, rinse the applicator and reprime with 2 sprays or until a fine spray appears.

INDIVIDUALIZATION OF DOSAGE

It is always desirable to titrate an individual patient to the minimum effective dose to reduce the possibility of side effects. In adults and children 6 years of age and older, the recommended starting dose is 64 µg daily administered as 1 spray per nostril of Rhinocort Aqua nasal spray 32 µg, once daily. Some patients who do not achieve symptom control at the recommended starting dose may benefit from an increased dose. The maximum daily dose is 256 µg for adults and 128 µg for pediatric patients (<12 years of age). When the maximum benefit has been achieved and symptoms have been controlled, reducing the dose may be effective in maintaining control of the allergic rhinitis symptoms in patients who were initially controlled on higher doses.

An improvement in nasal symptoms may be noted in patients within 10 hours of first using Rhinocort Aqua nasal spray. This time to onset is supported by an environmental exposure unit study in seasonal allergic rhinitis patients which demonstrated that Rhinocort Aqua nasal spray led to a statistically significant improvement in nasal symptoms compared to placebo by 10 hours. Further support comes from a clinical study of patients with perennial allergic rhinitis which demonstrated a statistically significant improvement in nasal symptoms for both Rhinocort Aqua nasal spray and for the active comparator (mometasone furoate) compared to placebo by 8 hours. Onset was also assessed in this study with peak nasal inspiratory flow rate and this endpoint failed to show efficacy for either active treatment. Although statistically significant improvements in nasal symptoms compared to placebo were noted within 8-10 hours in these studies, about one-half to two-thirds of the ultimate clinical improvement with Rhinocort Aqua nasal spray occurs over the first 1-2 days, and maximum benefit may not be achieved until approximately 2 weeks after initiation of treatment. Initial assessment for response should be made during this time frame and periodically until the patient's symptoms are stabilized.

DIRECTIONS FOR USE

Illustrated Patient's Instructions for Use accompany each package of Rhinocort Aqua nasal spray 32 µg.

HOW SUPPLIED

Rhinocort Aqua nasal spray 32 µg is available in a green coated glass bottle with a metered-dose pump spray and a green protection cap. Rhinocort Aqua nasal spray 32 µg provides 120 metered sprays after initial priming; net fill weight 8.6 g. The Rhinocort Aqua nasal spray 32 µg bottle has been filled with an excess to accommodate the priming activity. The bottle should be discarded after 120 sprays following initial priming, since the amount of budesonide delivered per spray thereafter may be substantially less than the labeled dose. Each spray delivers 32 µg of budesonide to the patient.

STORAGE

Rhinocort Aqua nasal spray should be stored at controlled room temperature, 20-25°C (68-77°F) with the valve up. Do not freeze. Protect from light. **Shake gently before use.** Do not spray in eyes.

ORAL

DESCRIPTION

Note: The trade names have been used throughout this monograph for clarity.

Budesonide, the active ingredient of Entocort EC capsules, is a synthetic corticosteroid. It is designated chemically as (RS)-11β,16α,17,21-tetrahydroxypregna-1,4-diene-3,20-dione cyclic 16,17-acetal with butyraldehyde. Budesonide is provided as a mixture of two epimers (22R and 22S). The empirical formula of budesonide is $C_{25}H_{34}O_6$ and its molecular weight is 430.5.

Budesonide is a white to off-white, tasteless, odorless powder that is practically insoluble in water and heptane, sparingly soluble in ethanol, and freely soluble in chloroform. Its partition coefficient between octanol and water at pH 5 is 1.6×10^3 ionic strength 0.01.

Each capsule contains 3 mg of micronized budesonide with the following inactive ingredients: Ethylcellulose, acetyltributyl citrate, methacrylic acid copolymer type C, triethyl citrate, antifoam M, polysorbate 80, talc, and sugar spheres. *The capsule shells have the following inactive ingredients:* Gelatin, iron oxide, and titanium dioxide.

CLINICAL PHARMACOLOGY

Budesonide has a high topical glucocorticosteroid (GCS) activity and a substantial first pass elimination. The formulation contains granules which are coated to protect dissolution in gastric juice, but which dissolve at pH >5.5, *i.e.*, normally when the granules reach the duodenum. Thereafter, a matrix of ethylcellulose with budesonide controls the release of the drug into the intestinal lumen in a time-dependent manner.

PHARMACOKINETICS

Absorption

The absorption of Entocort EC seems to be complete, although C_{max} and T_{max} are variable. Time to peak concentration varies in individual patients between 30 and 600 minutes. Following oral administration of 9 mg of budesonide in healthy subjects, a peak plasma concentration of approximately 5 nmol/L is observed and the area under the plasma concentration time curve is approximately 30 nmol·h/L. The systemic availability after a single dose is higher in patients with Crohn's disease compared to healthy volunteers, (21% vs 9%) but approaches that in healthy volunteers after repeated dosing.

Distribution

The mean volume of distribution (Vss) of budesonide varies between 2.2 and 3.9 L/kg in healthy subjects and in patients. Plasma protein binding is estimated to be 85-90% in the concentration range 1-230 nmol/L, independent of gender. The erythrocyte/plasma partition ratio at clinically relevant concentrations is about 0.8.

Metabolism

Following absorption, budesonide is subject to high first pass metabolism (80-90%). *In vitro* experiments in human liver microsomes demonstrate that budesonide is rapidly and extensively biotransformed, mainly by CYP3A4, to its 2 major metabolites, 6β-hydroxy budesonide and 16α-hydroxy prednisolone. The glucocorticoid activity of these metabolites is negligible (<1/100) in relation to that of the parent compound.

In vivo investigations with IV doses in healthy subjects are in agreement with the *in vitro* findings and demonstrate that budesonide has a high plasma clearance, 0.9-1.8 L/min. Similarly, high plasma clearance values have been shown in patients with Crohn's disease. These high plasma clearance values approach the estimated liver blood flow, and, accordingly, suggest that budesonide is a high hepatic clearance drug.

The plasma elimination half-life, $T_{1/2}$, after administration of IV doses ranges between 2.0 and 3.6 hours, and does not differ between healthy adults and patients with Crohn's disease.

Excretion

Budesonide is excreted in urine and feces in the form of metabolites. After oral as well as IV administration of micronized [^{3}H]budesonide, approximately 60% of the recovered radioactivity is found in urine. The major metabolites, including 6β-hydroxy budesonide and 16α-hydroxy prednisolone, are mainly renally excreted, intact or in conjugated forms. No unchanged budesonide is detected in urine.

Special Populations

No significant pharmacokinetic differences have been identified due to sex.

Hepatic Insufficiency

In patients with liver cirrhosis, systemic availability of orally administered budesonide correlates with disease severity and is, on average, 2.5-fold higher compared with healthy controls. Patients with mild liver disease are minimally affected. Patients with severe liver dysfunction were not studied. Absorption parameters are not altered, and for the IV dose, no significant differences in CL or Vss are observed.

Renal Insufficiency

The pharmacokinetics of budesonide in patients with renal impairment has not been studied. Intact budesonide is not renally excreted, but metabolites are to a large extent, and might therefore reach higher levels in patients with impaired renal function. However, these metabolites have negligible corticosteroid activity as compared with budesonide (<1/100). Thus, patients with impaired renal function taking budesonide are not expected to have an increased risk of adverse effects.

DRUG-DRUG INTERACTIONS

Budesonide is metabolized via CYP3A4. Potent inhibitors of CYP3A4 can increase the plasma slevels of budesonide several-fold. Coadministration of ketoconazole results in an 8-fold increase in AUC of budesonide, compared to budesonide alone. Grapefruit juice, an inhibitor of gut mucosal CYP3A, approximately doubles the systemic exposure of oral budesonide. Conversely, induction of CYP3A4 can result in the lowering of budesonide plasma levels. Oral contraceptives containing ethinyl estradiol, which are also metabolized by CYP3A4, do not affect the pharmacokinetics of budesonide. Budesonide does not affect the plasma levels of oral contraceptives (*i.e.*, ethinyl estradiol).

Since the dissolution of the coating of Entocort EC is pH dependent (dissolves at pH >5.5), the release properties and uptake of the compound may be altered after treatment with drugs that change the gastrointestinal pH. However, the gastric acid inhibitory drug omeprazole, 20 mg qd, does not affect the absorption or pharmacokinetics of Entocort EC. When an uncoated oral formulation of budesonide is co-administered with a daily dose of cimetidine 1 g, a slight increase in the budesonide peak plasma concentration and rate of absorption occurs, resulting in significant cortisol suppression.

FOOD EFFECTS

A mean delay in time to peak concentration of 2.5 hours is observed with the intake of a high-fat meal, with no significant differences in AUC.

PHARMACODYNAMICS

Budesonide has a high glucocorticoid effect and a weak mineralocorticoid effect, and the affinity of budesonide to GCS receptors, which reflects the intrinsic potency of the drug, is about 200-fold that of cortisol and 15-fold that of prednisolone.

Treatment with systemically active GCS is associated with a suppression of endogenous cortisol concentrations and an impairment of the hypothalamus-pituitary-adrenal (HPA) axis function. Markers, indirect and direct, of this are cortisol levels in plasma or urine and response to ACTH stimulation.

Plasma cortisol suppression was compared following 5 days' administration of Entocort EC capsules and prednisolone in a crossover study in healthy volunteers. The mean decrease in the integrated 0-24 hour plasma cortisol concentration was greater (78%) with prednisolone 20 mg/day compared to 45% with Entocort EC 9 mg/day.

INDICATIONS AND USAGE

Entocort EC is indicated for the treatment of mild to moderate active Crohn's disease involving the ileum and/or the ascending colon.

CONTRAINDICATIONS

Entocort EC is contraindicated in patients with known hypersensitivity to budesonide.

WARNINGS

Glucocorticosteroids can reduce the response of the hypothalamus-pituitary-adrenal (HPA) axis to stress. In situations where patients are subject to surgery or other stress situations, supplementation with a systemic glucocorticosteroid is recommended. Since Entocort EC is a glucocorticosteroid, general warnings concerning glucocorticoids should be followed.

Care is needed in patients who are transferred from glucocorticosteroid treatment with high systemic effects to corticosteroids with lower systemic availability, since symptoms attributed to withdrawal of steroid therapy, including those of acute adrenal suppression or benign intracranial hypertension, may develop. Adrenocortical function monitoring may be required in these patients and the dose of systemic steroid should be reduced cautiously.

Patients who are on drugs that suppress the immune system are more susceptible to infection than healthy individuals. Chicken pox and measles, for example, can have a more serious or even fatal course in susceptible patients or patients on immunosuppressant doses of glucocorticosteroids. In patients who have not had these diseases, particular care should be taken to avoid exposure. How the dose, route and duration of glucocorticosteroid administration affect the risk of developing a disseminated infection is not known. The contribution of the underlying disease and/or prior glucocorticosteroid treatment to the risk is also not known. If exposed, therapy with varicella zoster immune globulin (VZIG) or pooled IV immunoglobulin (IVIG), as appropriate, may be indicated. If exposed to measles, prophylaxis with pooled intramuscular immunoglobulin (IG) may be indicated. (See the respective package insert for complete VZIG and IG prescribing information.) If chicken pox develops, treatment with antiviral agents may be considered.

PRECAUTIONS

GENERAL

Caution should be taken in patients with tuberculosis, hypertension, diabetes mellitus, osteoporosis, peptic ulcer, glaucoma or cataracts, or with a family history of diabetes or glaucoma, or with any other condition where glucocorticosteroids may have unwanted effects.

Replacement of systemic glucocorticosteroids with Entocort EC capsules may unmask allergies, *e.g.*, rhinitis and eczema, which were previously controlled by the systemic drug.

When Entocort EC capsules are used chronically, systemic glucocorticosteroid effects such as hypercorticism and adrenal suppression may occur.

Reduced liver function affects the elimination of glucocorticosteroids, and increased systemic availability of oral budesonide has been demonstrated in patients with liver cirrhosis.

INFORMATION FOR THE PATIENT

Entocort EC capsules should be swallowed whole and NOT CHEWED OR BROKEN.

Patients should be advised to avoid the consumption of grapefruit juice for the duration of their Entocort EC therapy.

Patients should be given the patient package insert for additional information.

CARCINOGENESIS, MUTAGENESIS, AND IMPAIRMENT OF FERTILITY

Carcinogenicity studies with budesonide were conducted in rats and mice. In a 2 year study in Sprague-Dawley rats, budesonide caused a statistically significant increase in the incidence of gliomas in male rats at an oral dose of 50 μg/kg (approximately 0.05 times the maximum recommended human dose on a body surface area basis). In addition, there were increased incidences of primary hepatocellular tumors in male rats at 25 μg/kg (approximately 0.023 times the maximum recommended human dose on a body surface area basis) and above. No tumorigenicity was seen in female rats at oral doses up to 50 μg/kg (approximately 0.05 times the maximum recommended human dose on a body surface area basis). In an additional 2 year study in male Sprague-Dawley rats, budesonide caused no gliomas at an oral dose of 50 μg/kg (approximately 0.05 times the maximum recommended human dose on a body surface area basis). However, it caused a statistically significant increase in the incidence of hepatocellular tumors at an oral dose of 50 μg/kg (approximately 0.05 times the maximum recommended human dose on a body surface area basis). The concurrent reference corticosteroids (prednisolone and triamcinolone acetonide) showed similar findings. In a 91 week study in mice, budesonide caused no treatment-related carcinogenicity at oral doses up to 200 μg/kg (approximately 0.1 times the maximum recommended human dose on a body surface area basis).

Budesonide was not genotoxic in the Ames test, the mouse lymphoma cell forward gene mutation (TK +/-) test, the human lymphocyte chromosome aberration test, the *Drosophila melanogaster* sex-linked recessive lethality test, the rat hepatocycte UDS test and the mouse micronucleus test. In rats, budesonide had no effect on fertility at SC doses up to 80 μg/kg (approximately 0.07 times the maximum recommended human dose on a body surface area basis). However, it caused a decrease in prenatal viability and viability in pups at birth and during lactation, along with a decrease in maternal body-weight gain, at SC doses of 20 μg/kg (approximately 0.02 times the maximum recommended human dose on a body surface area basis) and above. No such effects were noted at 5 μg/kg (approximately 0.005 times the maximum recommended human dose on a body surface area basis).

PREGNANCY

Teratogenic Effects, Pregnancy Category C

As with other corticosteroids, budesonide was teratogenic and embryocidal in rabbits and rats. Budesonide produced fetal loss, decreased pup weights, and skeletal abnormalities at SC doses of 25 μg/kg in rabbits (approximately 0.05 times the maximum recommended human dose on a body surface area basis) and 500 μg/kg in rats (approximately 0.5 times the maximum recommended human dose on a body surface area basis).

There are no adequate and well-controlled studies in pregnant women. Budesonide should be used during pregnancy only if the potential benefit justifies the potential risk to the fetus.

Nonteratogenic Effects

Hypoadrenalism may occur in infants born of mothers receiving corticosteroids during pregnancy. Such infants should be carefully observed.

NURSING MOTHERS

Glucocorticosteroids are secreted in human milk. Because of the potential for adverse reactions in nursing infants from any corticosteroid, a decision should be made whether to discontinue nursing or discontinue the drug, taking into account the importance of the drug to the mother. The amount of budesonide secreted in breast milk has not been determined.

PEDIATRIC USE

Safety and effectiveness in pediatric patients have not been established.

GERIATRIC USE

Clinical studies of Entocort EC did not include sufficient numbers of subjects aged 65 and over to determine whether they respond differently from younger subjects. Other reported clinical experience has not identified differences in responses between the elderly and younger patients. In general, dose selection for an elderly patient should be cautious, usually starting at the low end of the dosing range, reflecting the greater frequency of decreased hepatic, renal, or cardiac function, and of concomitant disease or other drug therapy.

DRUG INTERACTIONS

Concomitant oral administration of ketoconazole (a known inhibitor of CYP3A4 activity in the liver and in the intestinal mucosa) caused an 8-fold increase of the systemic exposure to oral budesonide. If treatment with inhibitors of CYP3A4 activity (such as ketoconazole, intraconazole, ritonavir, indinavir, saquinavir, erythromycin, etc.) is indicated, reduction of the budesonide dose should be considered. After extensive intake of grapefruit juice (which inhibits CYP3A4 activity predominantly in the intestinal mucosa), the systemic exposure for oral budesonide increased about 2 times. As with other drugs primarily being metabolized through CYP3A4, ingestion of grapefruit or grapefruit juice should be avoided in connection with budesonide administration.

ADVERSE REACTIONS

The safety of Entocort EC was evaluated in 651 patients. They ranged in age from 17-74 (mean 35), 40% were male and 97% were white, 2.6% were ≥65 years of age. Five hundred and twenty (520) patients were treated with Entocort EC 9 mg (total daily dose). In general, Entocort EC was well tolerated in these trials. The most common adverse events reported were headache, respiratory infection, nausea, and symptoms of hypercorticism. Clinical studies have shown that the frequency of glucocorticosteroid-associated adverse events was substantially reduced with Entocort EC capsules compared with prednisolone at therapeutically equivalent doses. Adverse events occurring in ≥5% of the patients are listed in TABLE 7.

TABLE 7 *Adverse Events Occurring in ≥5% of the Patients in any Treated Group*

Adverse Event	Entocort EC 9 mg n=520	Placebo n=107	Prednisolone 40 mg n=145	Comparator* n=88
Headache	107 (21%)	19 (18%)	31 (21%)	11 (13%)
Respiratory infection	55 (11%)	7 (7%)	20 (14%)	5 (6%)
Nausea	57 (11%)	10 (9%)	18 (12%)	7 (8%)
Back pain	36 (7%)	10 (9%)	17 (12%)	5 (6%)
Dyspepsia	31 (6%)	4 (4%)	17 (12%)	3 (3%)
Dizziness	38 (7%)	5 (5%)	18 (12%)	5 (6%)
Abdominal pain	32 (6%)	18 (17%)	6 (4%)	10 (11%)
Flatulence	30 (6%)	6 (6%)	12 (8%)	5 (6%)
Vomiting	29 (6%)	6 (6%)	6 (4%)	6 (7%)
Fatigue	25 (5%)	8 (7%)	11 (8%)	0 (0%)
Pain	24 (5%)	8 (7%)	17 (12%)	2 (2%)

* This drug is not approved for the treatment of Crohn's disease in the US.

Adverse events occurring in 520 patients treated with Entocort EC 9 mg (total daily dose), with an incidence <5% and greater than placebo (n=107), are listed below by body system:

Body as a Whole: Asthenia, C-Reactive protein increased, chest pain, dependent edema, face edema, flu-like disorder, malaise.
Cardiovascular: Hypertension.
Central and Peripheral Nervous System: Hyperkinesia, paresthesia, tremor, vertigo.
Gastrointestinal: Anus disorder, Crohn's disease aggravated, enteritis, epigastric pain, gastrointestinal fistula, glossitis, hemorrhoids, intestinal obstruction, tongue edema, tooth disorder.
Hearing and Vestibular: Ear infection — not otherwise specified.
Heart Rate and Rhythm: Palpitation, tachycardia.
Metabolic and Nutritional: Hypokalemia, weight increase.
Musculoskeletal: Arthritis aggravated, cramps, myalgia.
Psychiatric: Agitation, appetite increased, confusion, insomnia, nervousness, sleep disorder, somnolence.
Resistance Mechanism: Moniliasis.
Reproductive, Female: Intermenstrual bleeding, menstrual disorder.
Respiratory: Bronchitis, dyspnea.
Skin and Appendages: Acne, alopecia, dermatitis, eczema, skin disorder, sweating increased.
Urinary: Dysuria, micturition frequency, nocturia.
Vascular: Flushing.
Vision: Eye abnormality, vision abnormal.
White Blood Cell: Leukocytosis.

GLUCOCORTICOSTEROID ADVERSE REACTIONS

TABLE 8 displays the frequency and incidence of symptoms of hypercorticism by active questioning of patients in clinical trials.

In addition to the symptoms in TABLE 8, 3 cases of benign intracranial hypertension have been reported in patients treated with budesonide from post-marketing surveillance. A cause and effect relationship has not been established.

TABLE 8 *Summary and Incidence of Symptoms of Hypercorticism*

Symptom	Entocort EC 9 mg n=427	Placebo n=107	Prednisolone Taper 40 mg n=145
Acne	63 (15%)	14 (13%)	33 (23%)*
Bruising easily	63 (15%)	12 (11%)	13 (9%)
Moon face	46 (11%)	4 (4%)	53 (37%)*
Swollen ankles	32 (7%)	6 (6%)	13 (9%)
Hirsutism†	22 (5%)	2 (2%)	5 (3%)
Buffalo hump	6 (1%)	2 (2%)	5 (3%)
Skin striae	4 (1%)	2 (2%)	0 (0%)

* Statistically significantly different from Entocort EC 9 mg.
† Adverse event dictionary included term hair growth increased, local and hair growth increased, general.

CLINICAL LABORATORY TEST FINDINGS

The following potentially clinically significant laboratory changes in clinical trials, irrespective of relationship to Entocort EC, were reported in ≥1% of patients: hypokalemia, leukocytosis, anemia, hematuria, pyuria, erythrocyte sedimentation rate increased, alkaline phosphatase increased, atypical neutrophils, C-reactive protein increased, and adrenal insufficiency.

DOSAGE AND ADMINISTRATION

The recommended adult dosage for the treatment of mild to moderate active Crohn's disease involving the ileum and/or the ascending colon is 9 mg taken once daily in the morning for up to 8 weeks. Safety and efficacy of Entocort EC in the treatment of active Crohn's Disease have not been established beyond 8 weeks.

For recurring episodes of active Crohn's Disease, a repeat 8 week course of Entocort EC can be given.

Treatment with Entocort EC capsules can be tapered to 6 mg daily for 2 weeks prior to complete cessation.

Patients with mild to moderate active Crohn's disease involving the ileum and/or ascending colon have been switched from oral prednisolone to Entocort EC with no reported episodes of adrenal insufficiency. Since prednisolone should not be stopped abruptly, tapering should begin concomitantly with initiating Entocort EC treatment.

Hepatic Insufficiency: Patients with moderate to severe liver disease should be monitored for increased signs and/or symptoms of hypercorticism. Reducing the dose of Entocort EC capsules should be considered in these patients.

CYP3A4 Inhibitors: If concomitant administration with ketoconazole, or any other CYP3A4 inhibitor, is indicated, patients should be closely monitored for increased signs and/or symptoms of hypercorticism. Reduction in the dose of Entocort EC capsules should be considered.

Entocort EC capsules should be swallowed whole and not chewed or broken.

HOW SUPPLIED

Entocort EC 3 mg capsules are hard gelatin capsules with an opaque light grey body and an opaque pink cap, coded with "3 mg" on the capsule.

STORAGE

Store at 25°C (77°F); excursions permitted to 15-30°C (59-86°F).

Keep container tightly closed.

PRODUCT LISTING - EQUIVALENTS NOT AVAILABLE

Aerosol with Adapter - Inhalation - 200 mcg/Inh

4 gm	$123.86	PULMICORT TURBUHALER, Allscripts Pharmaceutical Company	54569-4741-00
4 gm	$146.39	PULMICORT TURBUHALER, Astra-Zeneca Pharmaceuticals	00186-0915-42

Aerosol with Adapter - Nasal - 0.032 mg/Inh

7 gm	$39.50	RHINOCORT, Allscripts Pharmaceutical Company	54569-4059-00
7 gm	$43.13	RHINOCORT, Physicians Total Care	54868-3553-00
7 gm	$46.15	RHINOCORT, Astra-Zeneca Pharmaceuticals	00186-1075-09

Capsule, Extended Release - Oral - 3 mg

100's	$233.36	ENTOCORT EC, Astra-Zeneca Pharmaceuticals	00186-0702-10

Spray - Nasal - 0.032 mg/Inh

5 ml	$50.40	RHINOCORT AQUA, Astra-Zeneca Pharmaceuticals	00186-1070-06
9 ml	$67.29	RHINOCORT AQUA, Astra-Zeneca Pharmaceuticals	00186-1070-08

Suspension - Inhalation - 0.25 mg/2 ml

2 ml x 30	$142.50	PULMICORT RESPULES, Astra-Zeneca Pharmaceuticals	00186-1988-04

Suspension - Inhalation - 0.5 mg/2 ml

2 ml x 30	$142.50	PULMICORT RESPULES, Astra-Zeneca Pharmaceuticals	00186-1989-04

Bumetanide *(000544)*

Categories: Edema; Pregnancy Category C; FDA Approved 1983 Feb
Drug Classes: Diuretics, loop
Brand Names: **Bumex**; Pendock; Segurex
Foreign Brand Availability: Budema (Taiwan); Bumedyl (Mexico); Bumet (Dominican-Republic; El-Salvador; Guatemala; Honduras; Panama); Burinax (Brazil); Burinex (Australia; Austria; Bahamas; Barbados; Belgium; Belize; Benin; Bermuda; Burkina-Faso; Canada; Costa-Rica; Curacao; Denmark; Dominican-Republic; El-Salvador; England; Ethiopia; France; Gambia; Germany; Ghana; Greece; Guatemala; Guinea; Guyana; Honduras; Hong-Kong; Ireland; Ivory-Coast; Jamaica; Kenya; Liberia; Malawi; Malaysia; Mali; Mauritania; Mauritius; Morocco; Netherland-Antilles; Netherlands; New-Zealand; Nicaragua; Niger; Nigeria; Norway; Panama; Philippines; Senegal; Seychelles; Sierra-Leone; South-Africa; Sudan; Surinam; Sweden; Switzerland; Taiwan; Tanzania; Thailand; Trinidad; Tunia; Uganda; Zambia; Zimbabwe); Busix (Taiwan); Butinat (Argentina); Butinon (Peru); Cambiex (Argentina); Drenural (Mexico); Farmadiuril (Spain); Fluxil (Brazil); Fontego (Italy); Fordiuran (Spain); Lunetoron (Japan); Miccil (Dominican-Republic; Guatemala; Honduras; Mexico); Primex (Finland)
Cost of Therapy: $12.44 (Edema; Bumex; 0.5 mg; 1 tablet/day; 30 day supply)
$8.15 (Edema; Generic Tablets; 0.5 mg; 1 tablet/day; 30 day supply)

WARNING

Bumetanide is a potent diuretic which, if given in excessive amounts, can lead to a profound diuresis with water and electrolyte depletion. Therefore, careful medical supervision is required, and dose and dosage schedule have to be adjusted to the individual patient's needs. (See DOSAGE AND ADMINISTRATION.)

DESCRIPTION

Bumex is a loop diuretic, available as scored tablets, 0.5 mg (light green), 1 mg (yellow) and 2 mg (peach) for oral administration; each tablet also contains lactose, magnesium stearate, microcrystalline cellulose, corn starch and talc, with the following dye systems: 0.5 mg — D&C yellow no. 10 and FD&C blue no. 1; 1 mg — D&C yellow no. 10; 2 mg — red iron oxide. Also as 2 ml ampuls, 2 ml vials, 4 ml vials and 10 ml vials (0.25 mg/ml) for intravenous or intramuscular injection as a sterile solution, each 2 ml of which contains 0.5 mg (0.25 mg/ml) bumetanide compounded with 0.85% sodium chloride and 0.4% ammonium acetate as buffers; 0.01% edetate disodium; 1% benzyl alcohol as preservative, and pH adjusted to approximately 7 with sodium hydroxide.

Chemically, bumetanide is 3-(butylamino)-4-phenoxy-5-sulfamoylbenzoic acid. It is a practically white powder having a calculated molecular weight of 364.41.

CLINICAL PHARMACOLOGY

Bumetandine is a loop diuretic with a rapid onset and short duration of action. Pharmacological and clinical studies have shown that 1 mg bumetandine has a diuretic potency equivalent to approximately 40 mg furosemide. The major site of bumetandine action is the ascending limb of the loop of Henle.

The mode of action has been determined through various clearance studies in both humans and experimental animals. Bumetandine inhibits sodium reabsorption in the ascending limb of the loop of Henle, as shown by marked reduction of free-water clearance (CH_2O) during hydration and tubular free-water reabsorption (T^cH_2O) during hydropenia. Reabsorption of chloride in the ascending limb is also blocked by bumetandine, and bumetandine is somewhat more chloruretic than natriuretic.

Potassium excretion is also increased by bumetandine, in a dose-related fashion.

Bumetandine may have an additional action in the proximal tubule. Since phosphate reabsorption takes place largely in the proximal tubule, phosphaturia during bumetandine-induced diuresis is indicative of this additional action. This is further supported by the reduction in the renal clearance of bumetandine by probenecid, associated with diminution in the natriuretic response. This proximal tubular activity does not seem to be related to an inhibition of carbonic anhydrase. Bumetandine does not appear to have a noticeable action on the distal tubule.

Bumetandine decreases uric acid excretion and increases serum uric acid. Following oral administration of bumetandine the onset of diuresis occurs in 30-60 minutes. Peak activity is reached between 1 and 2 hours. At usual doses (1-2 mg) diuresis is largely complete within 4 hours; with higher doses, the diuretic action lasts for 4-6 hours. Diuresis starts within minutes following an intravenous injection and reaches maximum levels within 15-30 minutes.

Several pharmacokinetic studies have shown that bumetandine, administered orally or parenterally, is eliminated rapidly in humans, with a half-life of between 1 and 1.5 hours. Plasma protein-binding is in the range of 94-96%.

Oral administration of carbon-14 labeled bumetandine to human volunteers revealed that 81% of the administered radioactivity was excreted in the urine, 45% of it as unchanged drug. Urinary and biliary metabolites identified in this study were formed by oxidation of the N-butyl side chain. Biliary excretion of bumetandine amounted to only 2% of the administered dose.

INDICATIONS AND USAGE

Bumetandine is indicated for the treatment of edema associated with congestive heart failure, hepatic and renal disease, including the nephrotic syndrome.

Almost equal diuretic response occurs after oral and parenteral administration of bumetandine. Therefore, if impaired gastrointestinal absorption is suspected or oral administration is not practical, bumetandine should be given by the intramuscular or intravenous route.

Successful treatment with bumetandine following instances of allergic reactions to furosemide suggests a lack of cross-sensitivity.

CONTRAINDICATIONS

Bumetandine is contraindicated in anuria. Although bumetandine can be used to induce diuresis in renal insufficiency, any marked increase in blood urea nitrogen or creatinine, or the development of oliguria during therapy of patients with progressive renal disease, is an indication for discontinuation of treatment with bumetandine. Bumetandine is also contraindicated in patients in hepatic coma or in states of severe electrolyte depletion until the condition is improved or corrected. Bumetandine is contraindicated in patients hypersensitive to this drug.

WARNINGS

1. ***Volume and electrolyte depletion:*** The dose of bumetandine should be adjusted to the patient's need. Excessive doses or too frequent administration can lead to profound water loss, electrolyte depletion, dehydration, reduction in blood volume and circulatory collapse with the possibility of vascular thrombosis and embolism, particularly in elderly patients.
2. ***Hypokalemia:*** Hypokalemia can occur as a consequence of bumetandine administration. Prevention of hypokalemia requires particular attention in the following conditions: patients receiving digitalis and diuretics for congestive heart failure, hepatic cirrhosis and ascites, states of aldosterone excess with normal renal function, potassium-losing nephropathy, certain diarrheal states, or other states where hypokalemia is thought to represent particular added risks to the patient, *i.e.,* history of ventricular arrhythmias. In patients with hepatic cirrhosis and ascites, sudden alterations of electrolyte balance may precipitate hepatic encephalopathy and coma. Treatment in such patients is best initiated in the hospital with small doses and careful monitoring of the patient's clinical status and electrolyte balance. Supplemental potassium and/or spironolactone may prevent hypokalemia and metabolic alkalosis in these patients.
3. ***Ototoxicity:*** In cats, dogs and guinea pigs, bumetandine has been shown to produce ototoxicity. In these test animals bumetandine was 5-6 times more potent than furosemide and, since the diuretic potency of bumetandine is about 40-60 times furosemide, it is anticipated that blood levels necessary to produce ototoxicity will rarely be achieved. The potential exists, however, and must be considered a risk of intravenous therapy, especially at high doses, repeated frequently in the face of renal excretory function impairment. Potentiation of aminoglycoside ototoxicity has not been tested for bumetandine. Like other members of this class of diuretics, bumetandine probably shares this risk.
4. ***Allergy to sulfonamides:*** Patients allergic to sulfonamides may show hypersensitivity to bumetandine.
5. ***Thrombocytopenia:*** Since there have been rare spontaneous reports of thrombocytopenia from postmarketing experience, patients should be observed regularly for possible occurrence of thrombocytopenia.

PRECAUTIONS

GENERAL

Serum potassium should be measured periodically and potassium supplements or potassium-sparing diuretics added if necessary. Periodic determinations of other electrolytes are advised in patients treated with high doses or for prolonged periods, particularly in those on low salt diets.

Hyperuricemia may occur; it has been asymptomatic in cases reported to date. Reversible elevations of the BUN and creatinine may also occur, especially in association with dehydration and particularly in patients with renal insufficiency. Bumetandine may increase urinary calcium excretion with resultant hypocalcemia.

Diuretics have been shown to increase the urinary excretion of magnesium; this may result in hypomagnesemia.

LABORATORY TESTS

Studies in normal subjects receiving bumetandine revealed no adverse effects on glucose tolerance, plasma insulin, glucagon and growth hormone levels, but the possibility of an effect on glucose metabolism exists. Periodic determinations of blood sugar should be done, particularly in patients with diabetes or suspected latent diabetes.

Patients under treatment should be observed regularly for possible occurrence of blood dyscrasias, liver damage or idiosyncratic reactions, which have been reported occasionally in foreign marketing experience. The relationship of these occurrences to bumetandine use is not certain.

CARCINOGENESIS, MUTAGENESIS, AND IMPAIRMENT OF FERTILITY

Bumetandine was devoid of mutagenic activity in various strains of *Salmonella typhimurium* when tested in the presence or absence of an *in vitro* metabolic activation system. An 18 month study showed an increase in mammary adenomas of questionable significance in female rats receiving oral doses of 60 mg/kg/day (2000 times a 2 mg human dose). A repeat study at the same doses failed to duplicate this finding.

Reproduction studies were performed to evaluate general reproductive performance and fertility in rats at oral dose levels of 10, 30, 60 or 100 mg/kg/day. The pregnancy rate was slightly decreased in the treated animals; however, the differences were small and not statistically significant.

PREGNANCY, TERATOGENIC EFFECTS, PREGNANCY CATEGORY C

Bumetandine is neither teratogenic nor embryocidal in mice when given in doses up to 3400 times the maximum human therapeutic dose.

Bumetandine has been shown to be nonteratogenic, but it has a slight embryocidal effect in rats when given in doses of 3400 times the maximum human therapeutic dose and in rabbits at doses of 3.4 times the maximum human therapeutic dose. In one study, moderate growth retardation and increased incidence of delayed ossification of sternebrae were observed in rats at oral doses of 100 mg/kg/day, 3400 times the maximum human therapeutic dose. These effects were associated with maternal weight reductions noted during dosing. No such adverse effects were observed at 30 mg/kg/day (1000 times the maximum human therapeutic dose). No fetotoxicity was observed at 1000-2000 times the human therapeutic dose.

In rabbits, a dose-related decrease in litter size and an increase in resorption rate were noted at oral doses of 0.1 and 0.3 mg/kg/day (3.4 and 10 times the maximum human therapeutic dose). A slightly increased incidence of delayed ossification of sternebrae occurred at 0.3 mg/kg/day; however, no such adverse effects were observed at the dose of 0.03 mg/kg/day. The sensitivity of the rabbit to bumetandine parallels the marked pharmacologic and toxicologic effects of the drug in this species.

Bumetandine was not teratogenic in the hamster at an oral dose of 0.5 mg/kg/day (17 times the maximum human therapeutic dose). Bumetandine was not teratogenic when given intravenously to mice and rats at doses up to 140 times the maximum human therapeutic dose.

There are no adequate and well-controlled studies in pregnant women. A small investigational experience in the US and marketing experience in other countries to date have not indicated any evidence of adverse effects on the fetus, but these data do not rule out the possibility of harmful effects. Bumetandine should be given to a pregnant woman only if the potential benefit justifies the potential risk to the fetus.

NURSING MOTHERS

It is not known whether this drug is excreted in human milk. As a general rule, nursing should not be undertaken while the patient is on bumetandine since it may be excreted in human milk.

PEDIATRIC USE

Safety and effectiveness in children below the age of 18 have not been established.

DRUG INTERACTIONS

1. ***Drugs With Ototoxic Potential (see WARNINGS):*** Especially in the presence of impaired renal function, the use of parenterally administered bumetandine in patients to whom aminoglycoside antibiotics are also being given should be avoided, except in life-threatening conditions.
2. ***Drugs With Nephrotoxic Potential:*** There has been no experience on the concurrent use of bumetandine with drugs known to have a nephrotoxic potential. Therefore, the simultaneous administration of these drugs should be avoided.
3. ***Lithium:*** Lithium should generally not be given with diuretics (such as bumetandine) because they reduce its renal clearance and add a high risk of lithium toxicity.
4. ***Probenecid:*** Pretreatment with probenecid reduces both the natriuresis and hyperreninemia produced by bumetandine. This antagonistic effect of probenecid on bumetandine natriuresis is not due to a direct action on sodium excretion but is probably secondary to its inhibitory effect on renal tubular secretion of bumetanide. Thus, probenecid should not be administered concurrently with bumetandine.
5. ***Indomethacin:*** Indomethacin blunts the increases in urine volume and sodium excretion seen during bumetandine treatment and inhibits the bumetanide-induced increase in plasma renin activity. Concurrent therapy with bumetandine is thus not recommended.
6. ***Antihypertensives:*** Bumetandine may potentiate the effect of various antihypertensive drugs, necessitating a reduction in the dosage of these drugs.
7. ***Digoxin:*** Interaction studies in humans have shown no effect on digoxin blood levels.
8. ***Anticoagulants:*** Interaction studies in humans have shown bumetandine to have no effect on warfarin metabolism or on plasma prothrombin activity.

ADVERSE REACTIONS

The most frequent clinical adverse reactions considered probably or possibly related to bumetandine are muscle cramps (seen in 1.1% of treated patients), dizziness (1.1%), hypotension (0.8%), headache (0.6%), nausea (0.6%), and encephalopathy (in patients with preexisting liver disease) (0.6%). One or more of these adverse reactions have been reported in approximately 4.1% of bumetandine (bumetandine-treated) patients.

Less frequent clinical adverse reactions to bumetandine are impaired hearing (0.5%), pruritus (0.4%), electrocardiogram changes (0.4%), weakness (0.2%), hives (0.2%), abdominal pain (0.2%), arthritic pain (0.2%), musculoskeletal pain (0.2%), rash (0.2%) and vomiting (0.2%). One or more of these adverse reactions have been reported in approximately 2.9% of bumetandine-treated patients.

Other clinical adverse reactions, which have each occurred in approximately 0.1% of patients, are vertigo, chest pain, ear discomfort, fatigue, dehydration, sweating, hyperventilation, dry mouth, upset stomach, renal failure, asterixis, itching, nipple tenderness, diarrhea, premature ejaculation and difficulty maintaining an erection.

Laboratory abnormalities reported have included hyperuricemia (in 18.4% of patients tested), hypochloremia (14.9%), hypokalemia (14.7%), azotemia (10.6%), hyponatremia (9.2%), increased serum creatinine (7.4%), hyperglycemia (6.6%), and variations in phosphorus (4.5%), CO_2 content (4.3%), bicarbonate (3.1%) and calcium (2.4%). Although manifestations of the pharmacologic action of bumetandine, these conditions may become more pronounced by intensive therapy.

Also reported have been thrombocytopenia (0.2%) and deviations in hemoglobin (0.8%), prothrombin time (0.8%), hematocrit (0.6%), WBC (0.3%) and differential counts (0.1%). There have been rare spontaneous reports of thrombocytopenia from postmarketing experience.

Diuresis induced by bumetandine may also rarely be accompanied by changes in LDH (1.0%), total serum bilirubin (0.8%), serum proteins (0.7%), SGOT (0.6%), SGPT (0.5%), alkaline phosphatase (0.4%), cholesterol (0.4%) and creatinine clearance (0.3%). Increases in urinary glucose (0.7%) and urinary protein (0.3%) have also been seen.

DOSAGE AND ADMINISTRATION

Dosage should be individualized with careful monitoring of patient response.

ORAL ADMINISTRATION

The usual total daily dosage of bumetandine is 0.5 to 2 mg and in most patients is given as a single dose.

If the diuretic response to an initial dose of bumetandine is not adequate, in view of its rapid onset and short duration of action, a second or third dose may be given at 4-5 hour intervals up to a maximum daily dose of 10 mg. An intermittent dose schedule, whereby bumetandine is given on alternate days or for 3-4 days with rest periods of 1-2 days in between, is recommended as the safest and most effective method for the continued control of edema. In patients with hepatic failure, the dosage should be kept to a minimum, and if necessary, dosage increased very carefully.

Because cross-sensitivity with furosemide has rarely been observed, bumetandine can be substituted at approximately a 1:40 ratio of bumetandine to furosemide in patients allergic to furosemide.

PARENTERAL ADMINISTRATION

Bumetandine may be administered parenterally (IV or IM) to patients in whom gastrointestinal absorption may be impaired or in whom oral administration is not practical.

Parenteral treatment should be terminated and oral treatment instituted as soon as possible.

The usual initial dose is 0.5 to 1 mg intravenously or intramuscularly. Intravenous administration should be given over a period of 1-2 minutes. If the response to an initial dose is deemed insufficient, a second or third dose may be given at intervals of 2-3 hours, but should not exceed a daily dosage of 10 mg.

MISCIBILITY AND PARENTERAL SOLUTIONS

The compatibility tests of bumetandine injection (0.25 mg/ml, 2 ml ampuls) with 5% dextrose in water, 0.9% sodium chloride, and lactated Ringer's solution in both glass and plasticized PVC (Viaflex) containers have shown no significant absorption effect with either containers, nor a measurable loss of potency due to degradation of the drug. However, solutions should be freshly prepared and used within 24 hours.

Parenteral drug products should be inspected visually for particulate matter and discoloration prior to administration whenever solution and container permit.

HOW SUPPLIED

Tablets: *0.5 mg:* Light green; *1 mg:* Yellow; *2 mg:* Peach.
Imprint on Tablets: *0.5 mg:* "ROCHE BUMEX 0.5"; *1 mg:* "ROCHE BUMEX 1"; *2 mg:* "ROCHE BUMEX 2".
Ampuls: (0.25 mg/ml), 2 ml.
Vials: (0.25 mg/ml), 2, 4, and 10 ml.
Storage: Store all tablets, vials and ampuls at 59-86°F.

PRODUCT LISTING - RATED THERAPEUTICALLY EQUIVALENT

Solution - Injectable - 0.25 mg/ml			
2 ml x 10	$16.20	GENERIC, Vha Supply	55390-0501-02
2 ml x 10	$16.30	GENERIC, Baxter Pharmaceutical Products, Inc	10019-0506-02
2 ml x 10	$16.90	GENERIC, Bedford Laboratories	55390-0500-02
4 ml x 10	$16.30	GENERIC, Baxter Pharmaceutical Products, Inc	10019-0506-45
4 ml x 10	$17.50	GENERIC, Bedford Laboratories	55390-0500-05
4 ml x 10	$19.00	GENERIC, Abbott Pharmaceutical	00074-1412-14
4 ml x 10	$19.95	GENERIC, Abbott Pharmaceutical	00074-1412-04
4 ml x 10	$28.13	GENERIC, Vha Supply	55390-0501-05
10 ml x 10	$62.50	GENERIC, Bedford Laboratories	55390-0500-10
10 ml x 10	$65.60	GENERIC, Abbott Pharmaceutical	00074-1412-10
10 ml x 10	$76.80	GENERIC, Baxter Pharmaceutical Products, Inc	10019-0506-10
10 ml x 10	$80.00	GENERIC, Vha Supply	55390-0501-10
Tablet - Oral - 0.5 mg			
15's	$8.40	BUMEX, Pd-Rx Pharmaceuticals	55289-0427-15
30's	$8.70	GENERIC, Heartland Healthcare Services	61392-0048-30
30's	$8.70	GENERIC, Heartland Healthcare Services	61392-0048-39
31 x 10	$89.03	GENERIC, Vangard Labs	00615-4541-53
31 x 10	$89.03	GENERIC, Vangard Labs	00615-4541-63
31's	$8.99	GENERIC, Heartland Healthcare Services	61392-0048-31
32's	$9.28	GENERIC, Heartland Healthcare Services	61392-0048-32
45's	$13.05	GENERIC, Heartland Healthcare Services	61392-0048-45
60's	$17.40	GENERIC, Heartland Healthcare Services	61392-0048-60
60's	$17.40	GENERIC, Heartland Healthcare Services	61392-0048-65
90's	$26.10	GENERIC, Heartland Healthcare Services	61392-0048-90
100's	$17.43	FEDERAL UPPER LIMIT, H.C.F.A. F F P	99999-0544-01
100's	$27.18	GENERIC, Qualitest Products Inc	00603-2516-21
100's	$27.18	GENERIC, Major Pharmaceuticals Inc	00904-5102-60
100's	$27.25	GENERIC, Geneva Pharmaceuticals	00781-1821-01
100's	$28.55	GENERIC, Moore, H.L. Drug Exchange Inc	00839-8011-06
100's	$28.55	GENERIC, Dixon-Shane Inc	17236-0870-01
100's	$29.00	GENERIC, Udl Laboratories Inc	51079-0891-20
100's	$37.33	GENERIC, Eon Labs Manufacturing Inc	00185-0128-01
100's	$41.48	BUMEX, Roche Laboratories	00004-0125-01
100's	$47.14	GENERIC, Ivax Corporation	00172-4232-60
Tablet - Oral - 1 mg			
25's	$8.83	GENERIC, Udl Laboratories Inc	51079-0892-19
30's	$11.40	GENERIC, Heartland Healthcare Services	61392-0049-30
30's	$11.70	GENERIC, Heartland Healthcare Services	61392-0049-39
30's	$14.15	BUMEX, Allscripts Pharmaceutical Company	54569-0503-01
30's	$17.78	BUMEX, Physicians Total Care	54868-1293-01
31 x 10	$119.63	GENERIC, Vangard Labs	00615-4536-53
31 x 10	$119.63	GENERIC, Vangard Labs	00615-4536-63
31's	$12.09	GENERIC, Heartland Healthcare Services	61392-0049-31
32's	$12.48	GENERIC, Heartland Healthcare Services	61392-0049-32
45's	$17.55	GENERIC, Heartland Healthcare Services	61392-0049-45
60's	$23.40	GENERIC, Heartland Healthcare Services	61392-0049-60
60's	$23.40	GENERIC, Heartland Healthcare Services	61392-0049-65
60's	$28.30	BUMEX, Allscripts Pharmaceutical Company	54569-0503-03
90's	$35.10	GENERIC, Heartland Healthcare Services	61392-0049-90
90's	$35.10	GENERIC, Heartland Healthcare Services	61392-0049-95
100's	$18.75	FEDERAL UPPER LIMIT, H.C.F.A. F F P	99999-0544-02
100's	$38.15	GENERIC, Major Pharmaceuticals Inc	00904-5103-60
100's	$38.25	GENERIC, Geneva Pharmaceuticals	00781-1822-01
100's	$40.03	GENERIC, Moore, H.L. Drug Exchange Inc	00839-8012-06
100's	$40.03	GENERIC, Dixon-Shane Inc	17236-0871-01
100's	$40.85	GENERIC, Udl Laboratories Inc	51079-0892-20
100's	$47.16	BUMEX, Allscripts Pharmaceutical Company	54569-0503-00

100's	$52.42	GENERIC, Eon Labs Manufacturing Inc	00185-0129-01
100's	$58.24	BUMEX, Roche Laboratories	00004-0121-01
100's	$61.30	GENERIC, Ivax Corporation	00172-4233-60
200 x 5	$385.90	GENERIC, Vangard Labs	00615-4536-43
Tablet - Oral - 2 mg			
30's	$19.50	GENERIC, Heartland Healthcare Services	61392-0050-30
30's	$19.50	GENERIC, Heartland Healthcare Services	61392-0050-39
30's	$22.86	BUMEX, Allscripts Pharmaceutical Company	54569-1988-01
31's	$20.15	GENERIC, Heartland Healthcare Services	61392-0050-31
32's	$20.80	GENERIC, Heartland Healthcare Services	61392-0050-32
45's	$29.25	GENERIC, Heartland Healthcare Services	61392-0050-45
60's	$39.00	GENERIC, Heartland Healthcare Services	61392-0050-60
90's	$58.50	GENERIC, Heartland Healthcare Services	61392-0050-90
100's	$36.75	FEDERAL UPPER LIMIT, H.C.F.A. F F P	99999-0544-03
100's	$64.53	GENERIC, Major Pharmaceuticals Inc	00904-5104-60
100's	$64.65	GENERIC, Geneva Pharmaceuticals	00781-1823-01
100's	$67.76	GENERIC, Moore, H.L. Drug Exchange Inc	00839-8013-06
100's	$67.76	GENERIC, Dixon-Shane Inc	17236-0872-01
100's	$68.90	GENERIC, Udl Laboratories Inc	51079-0893-20
100's	$88.61	GENERIC, Eon Labs Manufacturing Inc	00185-0130-01
100's	$98.45	BUMEX, Roche Laboratories	00004-0162-01
100's	$105.64	GENERIC, Ivax Corporation	00172-4234-60

PRODUCT LISTING - EQUIVALENTS NOT AVAILABLE

Solution - Injectable - 0.25 mg/ml			
2 ml x 10	$18.80	BUMEX, Roche Laboratories	00004-1944-06
2 ml x 10	$21.50	BUMEX, Roche Laboratories	00004-1968-01
4 ml x 10	$31.50	BUMEX, Roche Laboratories	00004-1969-01
10 ml x 10	$101.72	BUMEX, Roche Laboratories	00004-1970-01
Tablet - Oral - 0.5 mg			
100's	$30.20	GENERIC, Mylan Pharmaceuticals Inc	00378-0245-01
Tablet - Oral - 1 mg			
30's	$12.76	GENERIC, Allscripts Pharmaceutical Company	54569-4676-00
100's	$44.52	GENERIC, Mylan Pharmaceuticals Inc	00378-0370-01
Tablet - Oral - 2 mg			
100's	$75.18	GENERIC, Mylan Pharmaceuticals Inc	00378-0417-01

Bupivacaine Hydrochloride *(000545)*

For complete prescribing information, refer to the CD-ROM included with the book.

Categories: Anesthesia, epidural; Anesthesia, local; Anesthesia, regional; Pregnancy Category C; FDA Approved 1972 Oct; WHO Formulary

Drug Classes: Anesthetics, local

Brand Names: Bupivacaine HCl; **Marcaine**; Sensorcaine

Foreign Brand Availability: Bucaine (Bahrain; Cyprus; Egypt; Iran; Iraq; Jordan; Kuwait; Lebanon; Libya; Oman; Qatar; Republic-of-Yemen; Saudi-Arabia; Syria; United-Arab-Emirates); Bupirop (Colombia; Ecuador); Bupirop simple sin preservantes (Peru); Bupivan (Peru); Buvacaina (Mexico); Buvacainas (Colombia); Carbostesin (Austria; Germany; Switzerland); Kamacaine (Israel); Macaine (South-Africa); Marcain (Australia; Denmark; England; Finland; Hungary; India; Indonesia; Ireland; Italy; Malaysia; New-Zealand; Norway; Sweden); Marcaina (El-Salvador; Guatemala); Marcaine Plain (Benin; Burkina-Faso; Ethiopia; Gambia; Ghana; Guinea; Ivory-Coast; Kenya; Liberia; Malawi; Mali; Mauritania; Mauritius; Morocco; Niger; Nigeria; Senegal; Seychelles; Sierra-Leone; Sudan; Tanzania; Tunia; Uganda; Zambia; Zimbabwe); Picain (Finland)

DESCRIPTION

Bupivacaine hydrochloride injections are sterile isotonic solutions that contain a local anesthetic agent with and without epinephrine (as bitartrate) 1:200,000 and are administered parenterally by injection. (See INDICATIONS AND USAGE for specific uses.) Solutions of bupivacaine hydrochloride may be autoclaved if they do not contain epinephrine.

Bupivacaine hydrochloride injections contain bupivacaine hydrochloride which is chemically designated as 2-piperidinecarboxamide,1-butyl-N-(2,6-dimethylphenyl)-, monohydrochloride, monohydrate.

Epinephrine is (-)-3,4-Dihydroxy-α [(methylamino)methyl] benzyl alcohol.

The pK_a of bupivacaine (8.1) is similar to that of lidocaine (7.86). However, bupivacaine possesses a greater degree of lipid solubility and is protein bound to a greater extent than lidocaine.

Bupivacaine is related chemically and pharmacologically to the aminoacyl local anesthetics. It is a homologue of mepivacaine and is chemically related to lidocaine. All three of these anesthetics contain an amide linkage between the aromatic nucleus and the amino or piperidine group. They differ in this respect from the procaine-type local anesthetics, which have an ester linkage.

Dosage forms listed as bupivacaine hydrochloride-MPF indicates single dose solutions that are Methyl Paraben Free (MPF).

Bupivacaine hydrochloride-MPF is a sterile isotonic solution containing sodium chloride. Bupivacaine hydrochloride in multiple dose vials, each ml also contains 1 mg methylparaben as antiseptic preservative. The pH of these solutions is adjusted to between 4.0 and 6.5 with sodium hydroxide and/or hydrochloric acid.

Bupivacaine hydrochloride-MPF with epinephrine 1:200,000 (as bitartrate) is a sterile isotonic solution containing sodium chloride. Each ml contains bupivacaine hydrochloride and 0.005 mg epinephrine, with 0.5 mg sodium metabisulfite as an antioxidant and 0.2 mg citric acid (anhydrous) as stabilizer. Bupivacaine hydrochloride with epinephrine 1:200,000 (as bitartrate) in multiple dose vials, each ml also contains 1 mg methylparaben as antiseptic preservative. The pH of these solutions is adjusted to between 3.3-5.5 with sodium hydroxide and/or hydrochloric acid. Filled under nitrogen.

Note: The user should have an appreciation and awareness of the formulations and their intended uses. (See DOSAGE AND ADMINISTRATION.)

INDICATIONS AND USAGE

Bupivacaine HCl injection is indicated for the production of local or regional anesthesia or analgesia for surgery, for oral surgery procedures, for diagnostic and therapeutic procedures, and for obstetrical procedures. Only the 0.25% and 0.5% concentrations are indicated for obstetrical anesthesia. (See WARNINGS.)

Experience with non-obstetrical surgical procedures in pregnant patients is not sufficient to recommend use of the 0.75% concentration in these patients. Bupivacaine HCl injection is not recommended for intravenous regional anesthesia (Bier Block). (See WARNINGS.)

The routes of administration and indicated bupivacaine HCl concentrations are listed in TABLE 1.

TABLE 1

Type of Block	Concentration
Local infiltration	0.25%
Peripheral nerve block	0.25%, 0.5%
Retrobulbar block	0.75%
Sympathetic block	0.25%
Lumber epidural	0.25%, 0.5% and 0.75% (non-obstetrical)
Caudal	0.25%, 0.5%

(See DOSAGE AND ADMINISTRATION for additional information.) Standard textbooks should be consulted to determine the accepted procedures and techniques for the administration of bupivacaine HCl.

Use only the single dose ampules and single dose vials for caudal or epidural anesthesia, the multiple dose vials contain a preservative and, therefore, should not be used for these procedures.

CONTRAINDICATIONS

Bupivacaine HCl is contraindicated in obstetrical paracervical block anesthesia. Its use by this technique has resulted in fetal bradycardia and death.

Bupivacaine HCl is contraindicated in patients with a known hypersensitivity to it or to any local anesthetic agent of the amide type or to other components of bupivacaine solutions.

WARNINGS

THE 0.75% CONCENTRATION OF BUPIVACAINE HCl INJECTION IS NOT RECOMMENDED FOR OBSTETRICAL ANESTHESIA. THERE HAVE BEEN REPORTS OF CARDIAC ARREST WITH DIFFICULT RESUSCITATION OR DEATH DURING USE OF BUPIVACAINE FOR EPIDURAL ANESTHESIA IN OBSTETRICAL PATIENTS. IN MOST CASES, THIS HAS FOLLOWED USE OF THE 0.75% CONCENTRATION. RESUSCITATION HAS BEEN DIFFICULT OR IMPOSSIBLE DESPITE APPARENTLY ADEQUATE PREPARATION AND APPROPRIATE MANAGEMENT. CARDIAC ARREST HAS OCCURRED AFTER CONVULSIONS RESULTING FROM SYSTEMIC TOXICITY, PRESUMABLY FOLLOWING UNINTENTIONAL INTRAVASCULAR INJECTION. THE 0.75% CONCENTRATION SHOULD BE RESERVED FOR SURGICAL PROCEDURES WHERE A HIGH DEGREE OF MUSCLE RELAXATION AND PROLONGED EFFECT ARE NECESSARY.

LOCAL ANESTHETICS SHOULD ONLY BE EMPLOYED BY CLINICIANS WHO ARE WELL VERSED IN DIAGNOSIS AND MANAGEMENT OF DOSE-RELATED TOXICITY AND OTHER ACUTE EMERGENCIES WHICH MIGHT ARISE FROM THE BLOCK TO BE EMPLOYED, AND THEN ONLY AFTER INSURING THE *IMMEDIATE* AVAILABILITY OF OXYGEN, OTHER RESUSCITATIVE DRUGS, CARDIOPULMONARY RESUSCITATIVE EQUIPMENT, AND THE PERSONNEL RESOURCES NEEDED FOR PROPER MANAGEMENT OF TOXIC REACTIONS AND RELATED EMERGENCIES. DELAY IN PROPER MANAGEMENT OF DOSE-RELATED TOXICITY, UNDERVENTILATION FROM ANY CAUSE AND/OR ALTERED SENSITIVITY MAY LEAD TO THE DEVELOPMENT OF ACIDOSIS, CARDIAC ARREST AND, POSSIBLY, DEATH.

Local anesthetic solutions containing antimicrobial preservatives (*i.e.,* those supplied in multiple dose vials) should not be used for epidural or caudal anesthesia because safety has not been established with regard to intrathecal injection, either intentional or unintentional, of such preservatives.

It is essential that aspiration for blood or cerebrospinal fluid (where applicable) be done prior to injecting any local anesthetic, both the original dose and all subsequent doses, to avoid intravascular or subarachnoid injection. However, a negative aspiration does *not* ensure against an intravascular or subarachnoid injection.

Bupivacaine and epinephrine injection or other vasopressors should not be used concomitantly with ergot-type oxytocic drugs, because a severe persistent hypertension may occur. Likewise, solutions of bupivacaine containing a vasoconstrictor, such as epinephrine, should be used with extreme caution in patients receiving monoamine oxidase (MAO) inhibitors or antidepressants of the triptyline or imipramine types, because severe prolonged hypertension may result.

Until further experience is gained in children younger than 12 years, administration of bupivacaine in this age group is not recommended.

Reports of cardiac arrest and death have occurred with the use of bupivacaine for intravenous regional anesthesia (Bier Block). Information on safe dosages or techniques of administration of this product are lacking; therefore, bupivacaine is not recommended for use by this technique.

Prior use of chloroprocaine may interfere with subsequent use of bupivacaine. Because of this, and because safety of intercurrent use of bupivacaine and chloroprocaine has not been established, such use is not recommended.

Bupivacaine HCl with epinephrine solutions contain sodium metabisulfite, a sulfite that may cause allergic-type reactions including anaphylactic symptoms and life-threatening or less severe asthmatic episodes in certain susceptible people. The overall prevalence of sulfite sensitivity in the general population is unknown and probably low. Sulfite sensitivity is seen more frequently in asthmatic than in nonasthmatic people.

B

DOSAGE AND ADMINISTRATION

The dose of any local anesthetic administered varies with the anesthetic procedure, the area to be anesthetized, the vascularity of the tissues, the number of neuronal segments to be blocked, the depth of anesthesia and degree of muscle relaxation required, the duration of anesthesia desired, individual tolerance, and the physical condition of the patient. The smallest dose and concentration required to produce the desired result should be administered. Dosages of bupivacaine HCl should be reduced for young, elderly and debilitated patients and patients with cardiac and/or liver disease. The rapid injection of a large volume of local anesthetic solution should be avoided and fractional (incremental) doses should be used when feasible.

The specific techniques and procedures, refer to standard textbooks.

In recommended doses, bupivacaine HCl produces complete sensory block, but the effect on motor function differs among the three concentrations.

0.25%: When used for caudal, epidural, or peripheral nerve block, produces incomplete motor block. Should be used for operations in which muscle relaxation is not important, or when another means of providing muscle relaxation is used concurrently. Onset of action may be slower than with the 0.5% or 0.75% solutions.

0.5%: Provides motor blockade for caudal, epidural, or nerve block, but muscle relaxation may be inadequate for operations in which complete muscle relaxation is essential.

0.75%: Produces complete motor block. Most useful for epidural block in abdominal operations requiring complete muscle relaxation, and for retrobulbar anesthesia. Not for obstetrical anesthesia.

The duration of anesthesia with bupivacaine HCl is such that for most indications, a single dose is sufficient.

Maximum dosage limit must be individualized in each case after evaluating the size and physical status of the patient, as well as the usual rate of systemic absorption from a particular injection site. Most experience to date is with single doses of bupivacaine HCl up to 225 mg with epinephrine 1:200,000 and 175 mg without epinephrine; more or less drug may be used depending on individualization of each case.

These doses may be repeated up to once every 3 hours. In clinical studies to date, total daily doses up to 400 mg have been reported. Until further experience is gained, this dose should not be exceeded in 24 hours. The duration of anesthetic effect may be prolonged by the addition of epinephrine.

The dosages in TABLE 2 have generally proved satisfactory and are recommended as a guide for use in the average adult. These dosages should be reduced for young, elderly or debilitated patients. Until further experience is gained bupivacaine HCl is not recommended for children younger than 12 years. Bupivacaine HCl is contraindicated for obstetrical paracervical blocks, and is not recommended for intravenous regional anesthesia (Bier Block).

Use in Epidural Anesthesia: During epidural administration of bupivacaine HCl, 0.5% and 0.75% solutions should be administered in incremental doses of 3-5 ml with sufficient time between doses to detect toxic manifestations of unintentional intravascular or intrathecal injection. In obstetrics, only the 0.5% and 0.25% concentrations should be used; incremental doses of 3-5 ml of the 0.5% solution not exceeding 50-100 mg at any dosing interval are recommended. Repeat doses should be preceded by a test dose containing epinephrine if not contraindicated. Use only the single dose ampules and single dose vials for caudal or epidural anesthesia; the multiple dose vials contain a preservative and therefore should not be used for these procedures.

Unused portions of solutions in single dose containers should be discarded, since this product form contains no preservatives (see TABLE 2).

TABLE 2 *Dosage Recommendations — Bupivacaine HCl Injections*

Type of Block	Conc.	Each Dose (ml)	Each Dose (mg)	Motor Block*
Local infiltration	0.25%§	Up to max	Up to max	—
Epidural	0.75%†§	10-20	75-150	Complete
	0.5%§	10-20	50-100	Moderate to complete
	0.25%§	10-20	25-50	Partial to moderate
Caudal	0.5%§	15-30	75-150	Moderate to complete
	0.25%§	15-30	37.5-75	Moderate
Peripheral nerves	0.5%§	5 to max	25 to max	Moderate to complete
	0.25%§	5 to max	12.5 to max	Moderate to complete
Retrobulbar	0.75%§	2-4	15-30	Complete
Sympathetic	0.25%	20-50	50-125	—
Epidural Test dose	0.5% w/epi	2-3	10-15	—

* With continuous (intermittent) techniques, repeat doses increase the degree of motor block. The first repeat dose of 0.5% may produce complete motor block. Intercostal nerve block with 0.25% may also produce complete motor block for intra-abdominal surgery.

† For single dose use, not for intermittent (catheter) epidural techniques. Not for obstetric anesthesia.

§ Solutions with or without epinephrine.

NOTE: Parenteral drug products should be inspected visually for particulate matter and discoloration prior to administration whenever the solution and container permit. The injection is not to be used if its color is pinkish or darker than slightly yellow or if it contains a precipitate.

PRODUCT LISTING - RATED THERAPEUTICALLY EQUIVALENT

Kit - Injectable - 0.75%

10's	$195.36	GENERIC, Abbott Pharmaceutical	00074-4704-01

Solution - Injectable - 0.25%

2 ml x 10	$27.08	GENERIC, Abbott Pharmaceutical	00074-3613-01
10 ml x 5	$20.65	SENSORCAINE-MPF, Astra-Zeneca Pharmaceuticals	00186-1030-12
10 ml x 10	$32.00	MARCAINE HCL, Abbott Pharmaceutical	00074-1559-10
10 ml x 10	$44.52	MARCAINE HCL, Allscripts Pharmaceutical Company	54569-3952-00
10 ml x 25	$67.69	GENERIC, Abbott Pharmaceutical	00074-1159-01
20 ml x 5	$20.54	GENERIC, Abbott Pharmaceutical	00074-4272-01
30 ml	$5.73	SENSORCAINE-MPF, Astra-Zeneca Pharmaceuticals	00186-1030-01
30 ml x 5	$15.97	GENERIC, Abbott Pharmaceutical	00074-1158-01
30 ml x 5	$28.90	SENSORCAINE-MPF, Astra-Zeneca Pharmaceuticals	00186-1030-02
30 ml x 5	$40.90	SENSORCAINE-MPF, Astra-Zeneca Pharmaceuticals	00186-1030-91
30 ml x 10	$26.40	MARCAINE HCL, Abbott Pharmaceutical	00074-1559-30
30 ml x 25	$87.88	GENERIC, Abbott Pharmaceutical	00074-1159-02
50 ml	$4.07	MARCAINE HCL, Abbott Pharmaceutical	00074-1587-50
50 ml	$7.06	MARCAINE HCL, Allscripts Pharmaceutical Company	54569-3260-00
50 ml	$9.94	SENSORCAINE, Astra-Zeneca Pharmaceuticals	00186-1031-01
50 ml x 5	$47.14	MARCAINE HCL, Abbott Pharmaceutical	00074-1559-50
50 ml x 10	$133.59	GENERIC, Abbott Pharmaceutical	00074-5749-22
50 ml x 25	$112.52	GENERIC, Abbott Pharmaceutical	00074-1158-02
50 ml x 25	$127.75	GENERIC, Abbott Pharmaceutical	00074-1160-01
50 ml x 25	$357.63	GENERIC, Abbott Pharmaceutical	00074-5749-01

Solution - Injectable - 0.5%

10 ml x 5	$22.50	SENSORCAINE-MPF, Astra-Zeneca Pharmaceuticals	00186-1033-12
10 ml x 10	$26.30	MARCAINE HCL, Abbott Pharmaceutical	00074-1560-10
10 ml x 25	$78.08	GENERIC, Abbott Pharmaceutical	00074-1162-01
20 ml x 5	$23.22	GENERIC, Abbott Pharmaceutical	00074-4273-01
30 ml	$6.19	SENSORCAINE-MPF, Astra-Zeneca Pharmaceuticals	00186-1033-01
30 ml x 5	$16.33	GENERIC, Abbott Pharmaceutical	00074-1161-01
30 ml x 5	$25.75	SENSORCAINE-MPF, Astra-Zeneca Pharmaceuticals	00186-1033-02
30 ml x 5	$35.15	MARCAINE HCL, Abbott Pharmaceutical	00074-1560-30
30 ml x 5	$43.95	SENSORCAINE-MPF, Astra-Zeneca Pharmaceuticals	00186-1033-91
30 ml x 10	$59.38	MARCAINE HCL, Abbott Pharmaceutical	00074-1560-29
30 ml x 25	$90.25	GENERIC, Abbott Pharmaceutical	00074-1162-02
30 ml x 25	$124.75	GENERIC, Abbott Pharmaceutical	00074-5748-01
50 ml	$7.77	MARCAINE HCL, Abbott Pharmaceutical	00074-1610-50
50 ml	$8.86	MARCAINE HCL, Southwood Pharmaceuticals Inc	58016-9343-01
50 ml	$11.05	SENSORCAINE, Astra-Zeneca Pharmaceuticals	00186-1035-01
50 ml	$11.18	MARCAINE HCL, Allscripts Pharmaceutical Company	54569-1414-00
50 ml	$12.74	MARCAINE HCL, Prescript Pharmaceuticals	00247-0304-50
50 ml x 25	$112.22	GENERIC, Abbott Pharmaceutical	00074-1163-01
100 ml	$33.61	GENERIC, Allscripts Pharmaceutical Company	54569-2298-00

Solution - Injectable - 0.75%

2 ml x 10	$42.80	SENSORCAINE-MPF, Astra-Zeneca Pharmaceuticals	00186-1026-03
10 ml x 5	$23.45	SENSORCAINE-MPF, Astra-Zeneca Pharmaceuticals	00186-1037-12
10 ml x 10	$37.29	MARCAINE HCL, Abbott Pharmaceutical	00074-1582-10
10 ml x 25	$68.28	GENERIC, Abbott Pharmaceutical	00074-1165-01
20 ml x 5	$26.13	GENERIC, Abbott Pharmaceutical	00074-4274-01
30 ml	$5.93	MARCAINE HCL, Allscripts Pharmaceutical Company	54569-1660-00
30 ml	$6.46	SENSORCAINE-MPF, Astra-Zeneca Pharmaceuticals	00186-1037-01
30 ml x 5	$18.94	GENERIC, Abbott Pharmaceutical	00074-1164-01
30 ml x 5	$20.78	MARCAINE HCL, Abbott Pharmaceutical	00074-1582-30
30 ml x 5	$30.19	SENSORCAINE-MPF, Astra-Zeneca Pharmaceuticals	00186-1037-02
30 ml x 10	$52.30	MARCAINE HCL, Abbott Pharmaceutical	00074-1582-29
30 ml x 25	$108.06	GENERIC, Abbott Pharmaceutical	00074-1165-02

PRODUCT LISTING - EQUIVALENTS NOT AVAILABLE

Kit - Injectable - 0.5%

10's	$579.86	GENERIC, Abbott Pharmaceutical	00074-4038-05

Solution - Intrathecal - 0.75%

2 ml x 10	$46.31	MARCAINE SPINAL, Abbott Pharmaceutical	00074-1761-02

Buprenorphine *(000549)*

For related information, see the comparative table section in Appendix A.

Categories: Opiate dependence; Pain, moderate to severe; Pregnancy Category C; DEA Class CV; FDA Approved 1981 Dec; Orphan Drugs
Drug Classes: Analgesics, narcotic
Brand Names: **Buprenex**
Foreign Brand Availability: Anorfin (Denmark); Buprex (Peru; Portugal; Spain); Buprine (Thailand); Lepetan (Japan); Norphin (India); Pentorel (India); Prefin (Spain); Subutex (Australia; Germany; Hong-Kong; Israel; Singapore); Temgesic (Austria; Bahrain; Belgium; Benin; Brazil; Burkina-Faso; CIS; Costa-Rica; Cyprus; Czech-Republic; Denmark; Dominican-Republic; Egypt; El-Salvador; England; Ethiopia; Finland; France; Gambia; Germany; Ghana; Guatemala; Guinea; Honduras; Hong-Kong; Hungary; Iran; Iraq; Ireland; Italy; Ivory-Coast; Jordan; Kenya; Kuwait; Lebanon; Liberia; Libya; Malawi; Malaysia; Mali; Mauritania; Mauritius; Mexico; Morocco; Netherlands; New-Zealand; Nicaragua; Niger; Nigeria; Norway; Oman; Panama; Peru; Qatar; Republic-of-Yemen; Saudi-Arabia; Senegal; Seychelles; Sierra-Leone; Sudan; Sweden; Switzerland; Syria; Taiwan; Tanzania; Thailand; Tunia; Uganda; United-Arab-Emirates; Venezuela; Zambia; Zimbabwe); Transtec (England; Ireland)

IM-IV

DESCRIPTION

Buprenex (buprenorphine hydrochloride) is a narcotic under the Controlled Substances Act due to its chemical derivation from thebaine. Chemically, it is 17-(cyclopropylmethyl)-α-(1,1-dimethylethyl)-4,5-epoxy-18,19-dihydro-3-hydroxy-6-methoxy-α-methyl-6,14-ethenomorphinan-7-methanol, hydrochloride (5α, 7α(S)). Buprenorphine hydrochloride is a white powder, weakly acidic and with limited solubility in water. Buprenorphine hydrochloride is a clear, sterile, injectable agonist-antagonist analgesic intended for intravenous or intramuscular administration. Each ml of Buprenex contains 0.324 mg buprenorphine hydrochloride (equivalent to 0.3 mg buprenorphine), 50 mg anhydrous dextrose, water for injection and hydrochloride to adjust pH. Buprenorphine hydrochloride has the molecular formula, $C_{29}H_{41}NO_4HCl$. The molecular weight of buprenorphine hydrochloride is 504.09.

CLINICAL PHARMACOLOGY

Buprenorphine HCl is a parenteral opioid analgesic with 0.3 mg buprenorphine HCl being approximately equivalent to 10 mg morphine sulfate in analgesic and respiratory depressant effects in adults. Pharmacological effects occur as soon as 15 minutes after intramuscular injection and persist for 6 hours or longer. Peak pharmacologic effects usually are observed at 1 hour. When used intravenously, the times to onset and peak effect are shortened.

The limits of sensitivity of available analytical methodology precluded demonstration of bioequivalence between intramuscular and intravenous routes of administration. In postoperative adults, pharmacokinetic studies have shown elimination half-lives ranging from 1.2-7.2 hours (mean 2.2 hours) after intravenous administration of 0.3 mg of buprenorphine. A single, 10 patient, pharmacokinetic study of doses of 3 μg/kg in children (age 5-7 years) showed a high inter-patient variability, but suggests that the clearance of the drug may be higher in children than in adults. This is supported by at least one repeat-dose study in postoperative pain that showed an optimal inter-dose interval of 4-5 hours in pediatric patients as opposed to the recommended 6-8 hours in adults.

Buprenorphine, in common with morphine and other phenolic opioid analgesics, is metabolized by the liver and its clearance is related to hepatic blood flow. Studies in patients anesthetized with 0.5% halothane have shown that this anesthetic decreases hepatic blood flow by about 30%.

MECHANISM OF ANALGESIC ACTION

Buprenorphine HCl exerts its analgesic effect via high affinity binding to μ subclass opiate receptors in the central nervous system. Although buprenorphine HCl may be classified as a partial agonist, under the conditions of recommended use it behaves very much like classical μ agonists such as morphine. One unusual property of buprenorphine HCl observed in *in vitro* studies is its very slow rate of dissociation from its receptor. This could account for its longer duration of action than morphine, the unpredictability of its reversal by opioid antagonists, and its low level of manifest physical dependence.

NARCOTIC ANTAGONIST ACTIVITY

Buprenorphine demonstrates narcotic antagonist activity and has been shown to be equipotent with naloxone as an antagonist of morphine in the mouse tail flick test.

CARDIOVASCULAR EFFECTS

Buprenorphine HCl may cause a decrease or, rarely, an increase in pulse rate and blood pressure in some patients.

EFFECTS ON RESPIRATION

Under usual conditions of use in adults, both buprenorphine HCl and morphine show similar dose-related respiratory depressant effects. At adult therapeutic doses, buprenorphine HCl (0.3 mg buprenorphine) can decrease respiratory rate in an equivalent manner to an equianalgesic dose of morphine (10 mg). (See WARNINGS.)

INDICATIONS AND USAGE

Buprenorphine HCl is indicated for the relief of moderate to severe pain.

CONTRAINDICATIONS

Buprenorphine HCl should not be administered to patients who have been shown to be hypertensive to the drug.

WARNINGS

IMPAIRED RESPIRATION

As with other potent opioids, clinically significant respiratory depression may occur within the recommended dose range in patients receiving therapeutic doses of buprenorphine. Buprenorphine HCl should be used with caution in patients with compromised respiratory function (*e.g.*, chronic obstructive pulmonary disease, cor pulmonale, decreased respiratory reserve, hypoxia, hypercapnia, or preexisting respiratory depression). Particular caution is advised if buprenorphine HCl is administered to patients taking or recently receiving drugs with CNS/respiratory depressant effects. In patients with the physical and/or pharmacological risk factors, above, the dose should be reduced by approximately one-half.

NALOXONE MAY NOT BE EFFECTIVE IN REVERSING THE RESPIRATORY DEPRESSION PRODUCED BY BUPRENORPHINE HCl. THEREFORE, AS WITH OTHER POTENT OPIOIDS, THE PRIMARY MANAGEMENT OF OVERDOSE SHOULD BE THE REESTABLISHMENT OF ADEQUATE VENTILATION WITH MECHANICAL ASSISTANCE OF RESPIRATION, IF REQUIRED.

INTERACTION WITH OTHER CENTRAL NERVOUS SYSTEM DEPRESSANTS

Patients receiving buprenorphine HCl in the presence of other narcotic analgesics, general anesthetics, antihistamines, benzodiazepines, phenothiazines, other tranquilizers, sedative/hypnotics or other CNS depressants (including alcohol) may exhibit increased CNS depression. When such combined therapy is contemplated, it is particularly important that the dose of 1 or both agents be reduced.

HEAD INJURY AND INCREASED INTRACRANIAL PRESSURE

Buprenorphine HCl, like other potent analgesics, may itself elevate cerebrospinal fluid pressure and should be used with caution in head injury, intracranial lesions and other circumstances where cerebrospinal pressure may be increased. Buprenorphine HCl can produce miosis and changes in the level of consciousness which may interfere with patient evaluation.

USE IN AMBULATORY PATIENTS

Buprenorphine HCl may impair the mental or physical abilities required for the performance of potentially dangerous tasks such as driving a car or operating machinery. Therefore, buprenorphine HCl should be administered with caution to ambulatory patients who should be warned to avoid such hazards.

USE IN NARCOTIC-DEPENDENT PATIENTS

Because of the narcotic antagonist activity of buprenorphine HCl, use in the physically dependent individual may result in withdrawal effects.

PRECAUTIONS

GENERAL

Buprenorphine HCl should be administered with caution in the elderly, debilitated patients, in children and those with severe impairment of hepatic, pulmonary, or renal function; myxedema or hypothyroidism; adrenal cortical insufficiency (*e.g.*, Addison's disease); CNS depression or coma; toxic psychoses; prostatic hypertrophy or urethral stricture; acute alcoholism; delirium tremens; or kyphoscoliosis.

Because buprenorphine HCl is metabolized by the liver, the activity of buprenorphine HCl may be increased and/or extended in those individuals with impaired hepatic function or those receiving other agents known to decrease hepatic clearance.

Buprenorphine HCl has been shown to increase intracholedochal pressure to a similar degree as other opioid analgesics, and thus should be administered with caution to patients with dysfunction of the biliary tract.

INFORMATION FOR THE PATIENT

The effects of buprenorphine HCl, particularly drowsiness, may be potentiated by other centrally acting agents such as alcohol or benzodiazepines. It is particularly important that in these circumstances patients must not drive or operate machinery. Buprenorphine HCl has some pharmacologic effects similar to morphine which in susceptible patients may lead to self-administration of the drug when pain no longer exists. Patients must not exceed the dosage of buprenorphine HCl prescribed by their physician. Patients should be urged to consult their physician if other prescription medications are currently being used or are prescribed for future use.

CARCINOGENESIS, MUTAGENESIS, AND IMPAIRMENT OF FERTILITY

Carcinogenesis

Carcinogenicity studies were conducted in Sprague-Dawley rats and CD-1 mice. Buprenorphine was administered in the diet at doses of 0.6, 5.5, and 56 mg/kg/day for 27 months in rats. These doses were approximately equivalent to 5.7, 52 and 534 times the recommended human dose (1.2 mg) on a mg/m^2 body surface area basis. Statistically significant dose-related increases in testicular interstitial (Leydig's) cell tumors occurred, according to the trend test adjusted for survival. Pairwise comparison of the high dose against control failed to show statistical significance. In the mouse study, buprenorphine was administered in the diet at doses of 8, 50, and 100 mg/kg/day for 86 weeks.

The high dose was approximately equivalent to 477 times the recommended human dose (1.2 mg) on a mg/m^2 basis. Buprenorphine was not carcinogenic in mice.

Mutagenesis

Buprenorphine was studied in a series of tests. Results were negative in Chinese hamster bone marrow and spermatogonia cells, and negative in mouse lymphoma L5178Y assay. Results were equivocal in the Ames test: negative in studies in two laboratories, but positive in frame shift mutation at high dose (5 mg/plate) in a third study.

Impairment of Fertility

Reproduction studies of buprenorphine in rats demonstrated no evidence of impaired fertility at daily oral doses up to 80 mg/kg (approximately 763 times the recommended human daily dose of 1.2 mg on a mg/m^2 basis) or up to 5 mg/kg IM or SC (approximately 48 times the recommended human daily dose of 1.2 mg on a mg/m^2 basis).

PREGNANCY, TERATOGENIC EFFECTS, PREGNANCY CATEGORY C

Buprenorphine was not teratogenic in rats or rabbits after IM or SC doses up to 5 mg/kg/day (approximately 48 and 95 times the recommended human daily dose of 1.2 mg on a mg/m^2

basis), IV doses up to 0.8 mg/kg/day (approximately 8 times and 15 times the recommended human daily dose of 1.2 mg on a mg/m^2 basis), or oral doses up to 160 mg/kg/day in rats (approximately 1525 times the recommended human daily dose of 1.2 mg on a mg/m^2 basis) and 25 mg/kg/day in rabbits (approximately 475 times the recommended human daily dose of 1.2 mg on a mg/m^2 basis). Significant increases in skeletal abnormalities (*e.g.*, extra thoracic vertebra or thoraco-lumbar ribs) were noted in rats after SC administration of 1 mg/kg/day and up (approximately 9.5 times the recommended human daily dose of 1.2 mg on a mg/m^2 basis) and in rabbits after IM administration of 5 mg/kg/day (approximately 95 times the recommended human daily dose of 1.2 mg on a mg/m^2 basis), but these increases were not statistically significant. Increases in skeletal abnormalities after oral administration were not observed in rats, and increases in rabbits (1-25 mg/kg/day) were not statistically significant.

There are no adequate and well-controlled studies in pregnant women. Buprenorphine HCl should be used during pregnancy only if the potential benefit justifies the potential risk to the fetus.

LABOR AND DELIVERY

The safety of buprenorphine HCl given during labor and delivery has not been established.

NURSING MOTHERS

An apparent lack of milk production during general reproduction studies with buprenorphine HCl in rats caused decreased viability and lactation indices. Use of high doses of sublingual buprenorphine in pregnant women showed that buprenorphine passes into the mother's milk. Breast-feeding is therefore not advised in nursing mothers treated with buprenophine HCl.

PEDIATRIC USE

The safety and effectiveness of buprenorphine HCl have been established for children between 2 and 12 years of age. Use of buprenorphine HCl in children is supported by evidence from adequate and well controlled trials of buprenorphine HCl in adults, with additional data from studies of 960 children ranging in age from 9 months to 18 years of age. Data is available from a pharmacokinetic study, several controlled clinical trials, and several large post-marketing studies and case series. The available information provides reasonable evidence that buprenorphine HCl may be used safely in children ranging from 2-12 years of age, and that it is of similar effectiveness in children as in adults.

DRUG INTERACTIONS

Drug interactions common to other potent opioid analgesics also may occur with buprenorphine HCl. Particular care should be taken when buprenorphine HCl is used in combination with central nervous system depressant drugs (see WARNINGS). Although specific information is not presently available, caution should be exercised when buprenorphine HCl is used in combination with MAO inhibitors. There have been reports of respiratory and cardiovascular collapse in patients who received therapeutic doses of diazepam and buprenorphine HCl. A suspected interaction between buprenorphine HCl and phenprocoumon resulting in purpura has been reported.

CYP3A4 INHIBITORS

Since the metabolism of buprenorphine is mediated by the CYP3A4 isozyme, coadministration of drugs that inhibit CYP3A4 activity may cause decreased clearance of buprenorphine. Thus patients coadministered with inhibitors of CYP3A4 such as macrolide antibiotics (*e.g.*, erythromycin), azole antifungal agents (*e.g.*, ketoconazole), and protease inhibitors (*e.g.*, ritanovir) while receiving buprenophine HCl should be carefully monitored and dosage adjustment made if warranted.

CYP3A4 INDUCERS

Cytochrome P450 inducers, such as rifampin, carbamazepine, and phenytoin, induce metabolism and as such may cause increased clearance of buprenorphine. Caution is advised when administering buprenophine HCl to patients receiving these medications and if necessary dose adjustments should be considered.

ADVERSE REACTIONS

The most frequent side effect in clinical studies involving 1133 patients was sedation which occurred in approximately two-thirds of the patients. Although sedated, these patients could easily be aroused to an alert state.

Other less frequent adverse reactions occurring in 5-10% of the patients were:

Nausea
Dizziness/vertigo

Occurring in 1-5% of the patients:

Sweating
Hypotension
Vomiting
Miosis
Headache
Nausea/vomiting
Hypoventilation

The following adverse reactions were reported to have occurred in less than 1% of the patients:

CNS Effect: Confusion, blurred vision, euphoria, weakness/fatigue, dry mouth, nervousness, depression, slurred speech, paresthesia.
Cardiovascular: Hypertension, tachycardia, bradycardia.
Gastrointestinal: Constipation.
Respiratory: Dyspnea, cyanosis.
Dermatologic: Pruritus.
Ophthalmological: Diplopia, visual abnormalities.
Miscellaneous: Injection site reaction, urinary retention, dreaming, flushing/warmth, chills/cold, tinnitus, conjunctivitis, Wenckebach block, and psychosis.

Other effects observed infrequently include malaise, hallucinations, depersonalization, coma, dyspepsia, flatulence, apnea, rash, amblyopia, tremor and pallor.

The following reactions have been reported to occur rarely: Loss of appetite, dysphoria/agitation, diarrhea, urticaria, and convulsions/lack of muscle coordination.

In the United Kingdom, buprenorphine HCl was made available under monitored release regulation during the first year of sale, and yielded data from 1,736 physicians on 9,123 patients (17,120 administrations). Data on 240 children under the age of 18 years were included in this monitored release program. No important new adverse effects attributable to buprenorphine HCl were observed.

DOSAGE AND ADMINISTRATION

ADULTS

The usual dosage for persons 13 years of age and over is 1 ml of buprenorphine HCl (0.3 mg buprenorphine) given by deep intramuscular or slow (over at least 2 minutes) intravenous injection at up to 6 hour intervals, as needed. Repeat once (up to 0.3 mg) if required, 30-60 minutes after initial dosage, giving consideration to previous dose pharmacokinetics, and thereafter only as needed. In high-risk patients (*e.g.*, elderly, debilitated, presence of respiratory disease, etc.) and/or in patients where other CNS depressants are present, such as in the immediate postoperative period, the dose should be reduced by approximately one-half. Extra caution should be exercised with the intravenous route of administration, particularly with the initial dose.

Occasionally, it may be necessary to administer single doses of up to 0.6 mg to adults depending on the severity of the pain and the response of the patient. This dose should only be given IM and only to adult patients who are not in a high risk category (see WARNINGS and PRECAUTIONS). At this time, there are insufficient data to recommend single doses greater than 0.6 mg for long-term use.

CHILDREN

Buprenorphine HCl has been used in children 2-12 years of age at doses of between 2-6 μg/kg of body weight given every 4-6 hours. There is insufficient experience to recommend a dose in infants below the age of 2 years, single doses greater than 6 μg/kg of body weight, or the use of a repeat or second dose at 30-60 minutes (such as is used in adults). Since there is some evidence that not all children clear buprenorphine faster than adults, fixed interval or "round-the-clock" dosing should not be undertaken until the proper inter-dose interval has been established by clinical observation of the child. Physicians should recognize that, as with adults, some pediatric patients may not need to be remedicated for 6-8 hours.

SAFETY AND HANDLING

Buprenorphine HCl is supplied in sealed ampules and poses no known environmental risk to health care providers. Accidental dermal exposure should be treated by removal of any contaminated clothing and rinsing the affected area with water.

Buprenorphine HCl is a potent narcotic, and like all drugs of this class has been associated with abuse and dependence among health care providers. To control the risk of diversion, it is recommended that measures appropriate to the health care setting be taken to provide rigid accounting, control of wastage, and restriction of access.

Parenteral drug products should be inspected visually for particulate matter and discoloration prior to administration, whenever solution and container permit.

HOW SUPPLIED

Buprenex (buprenorphine hydrochloride) is supplied in clear glass snap-ampules of 1 ml (0.3 mg buprenorphine).

Storage: Avoid excessive heat (over 40°C or 104°F). Protect from prolonged exposure to light.

ORAL

DESCRIPTION

Note: The trade names were used throughout this monograph for clarity.

Under the Drug Addiction Treatment Act of 2000 (DATA) codified at 21 U.S.C. 823(g), prescription use of this product in the treatment of opioid dependence is limited to physicians who meet certain qualifying requirements, and have notified the Secretary of Health and Human Services (HHS) of their intent to prescribe this product for the treatment of opioid dependence.

Suboxone sublingual tablets contain buprenorphine hydrochloride and naloxone hydrochloride dihydrate at a ratio of 4:1 buprenorphine:naloxone (ratio of free bases).

Subutex sublingual tablets contain buprenorphine hydrochloride.

Buprenorphine is a partial agonist at the mu-opioid receptor and an antagonist at the kappa-opioid receptor. Naloxone is an antagonist at the mu-opioid receptor.

Buprenorphine is a Schedule III narcotic under the Controlled Substances Act.

Buprenorphine hydrochloride is a white powder, weakly acidic with limited solubility in water (17 mg/ml). Chemically, buprenorphine is 17-(cyclopropylmethyl)-α-(1,1-dimethylethyl)-4,5-epoxy-18,19-dihydro-3-hydroxy-6-methoxy-α-methyl-6,14-ethenomorphinan-7-methanol, hydrochloride[5α,7α(S)]-. Buprenorphine hydrochloride has the molecular formula $C_{29}H_{41}NO_4HCl$ and the molecular weight is 504.10.

Naloxone hydrochloride is a white to slightly off-white powder and is soluble in water, in dilute acids and in strong alkali. Chemically, naloxone is 17-Allyl-4,5α-epoxy-3,14-dihydroxymorphinan-6-one hydrochloride. Naloxone hydrochloride has the molecular formula $C_{19}H_{21}NO_4HCl{\cdot}2H_2O$ and the molecular weight is 399.87.

Suboxone is an uncoated **hexagonal orange tablet** intended for sublingual administration. It is available in 2 dosage strengths, 2 mg buprenorphine with 0.5 mg naloxone, and 8 mg buprenorphine with 2 mg naloxone free bases. Each tablet also contains lactose, mannitol, cornstarch, povidone K30, citric acid, sodium citrate, FD&C yellow no. 6 color, magnesium stearate, and the tablets also contain Acesulfame K sweetener and a lemon/lime flavor.

Subutex is an uncoated **oval white tablet** intended for sublingual administration. It is available in 2 dosage strengths, 2 mg buprenorphine and 8 mg buprenorphine free base.

Each tablet also contains lactose, mannitol, cornstarch, povidone K30, citric acid, sodium citrate and magnesium stearate.

CLINICAL PHARMACOLOGY

SUBJECTIVE EFFECTS

Comparisons of buprenorphine with full agonists such as methadone and hydromorphone suggest that sublingual buprenorphine produces typical opioid agonist effects which are limited by a ceiling effect.

In non-dependent subjects, acute sublingual doses of Suboxone tablets produced opioid agonist effects, which reached a maximum between doses of 8 and 16 mg of Subutex. The effects of 16 mg Suboxone were similar to those produced by 16 mg Subutex (buprenorphine alone).

Opioid agonist ceiling effects were also observed in a double-blind, parallel group, dose ranging comparison of single doses of buprenorphine sublingual solution (1, 2, 4, 8, 16, or 32 mg), placebo, and a full agonist control at various doses. The treatments were given in ascending dose order at intervals of at least 1 week to 16 opioid-experienced, nondependent subjects. Both drugs produced typical opioid agonist effects. For all the measures for which the drugs produced an effect, buprenorphine produced a dose-related response but, in each case, there was a dose that produced no further effect. In contrast, the highest dose of the full agonist control always produced the greatest effects. Agonist objective rating scores remained elevated for the higher doses of buprenorphine (8-32 mg) longer than for the lower doses and did not return to baseline until 48 hours after drug administrations. The onset of effects appeared more rapidly with buprenorphine than with the full agonist control, with most doses nearing peak effect after 100 minutes for buprenorphine compared to 150 minutes for the full agonist control.

PHYSIOLOGIC EFFECTS

Buprenorphine in intravenous (2, 4, 8, 12 and 16 mg) and sublingual (12 mg) doses has been administered to non-dependent subjects to examine cardiovascular, respiratory and subjective effects at doses comparable to those used for treatment of opioid dependence. Compared with placebo, there were no statistically significant differences among any of the treatment conditions for blood pressure, heart rate, respiratory rate, O_2 saturation or skin temperature across time. Systolic BP was higher in the 8 mg group than placebo (3 hour AUC values). Minimum and maximum effects were similar across all treatments. Subjects remained responsive to low voice and responded to computer prompts. Some subjects showed irritability, but no other changes were observed.

The respiratory effects of sublingual buprenorphine were compared with the effects of methadone in a double-blind, parallel group, dose ranging comparison of single doses of buprenorphine sublingual solution (1, 2, 4, 8, 16, or 32 mg) and oral methadone (15, 30, 45, or 60 mg) in non-dependent, opioid-experienced volunteers. In this study, hypoventilation not requiring medical intervention was reported more frequently after buprenorphine doses of 4 mg and higher than after methadone. Both drugs decreased O_2 saturation to the same degree.

EFFECT OF NALOXONE

Physiologic and subjective effects following acute sublingual administration of Suboxone and Subutex tablets were similar at equivalent dose levels of buprenorphine. Naloxone, in the Suboxone formulation, had no clinically significant effect when administered by the sublingual route, although blood levels of the drug were measurable. Suboxone, when administered sublingually even to an opioid-dependent population, was recognized as an opioid agonist, whereas when administered intramuscularly, combinations of buprenorphine with naloxone produced opioid antagonist actions similar to naloxone. In methadone-maintained patients and heroin-dependent subjects, intravenous administration of buprenorphine/naloxone combinations precipitated opioid withdrawal and was perceived as unpleasant and dysphoric. In morphine-stabilized subjects, intravenously administered combinations of buprenorphine with naloxone produced opioid antagonist and withdrawal effects that were ratio-dependent; the most intense withdrawal effects were produced by 2:1 and 4:1 ratios, less intense by an 8:1 ratio. Suboxone tablets contain buprenorphine with naloxone at a ratio of 4:1.

PHARMACOKINETICS

Absorption

Plasma levels of buprenorphine increased with the sublingual dose of Subutex and Suboxone, and plasma levels of naloxone increased with the sublingual dose of Suboxone (TABLE 1). There was a wide inter-patient variability in the sublingual absorption of buprenorphine and naloxone, but within subjects the variability was low. Both C_{max} and AUC of buprenorphine increased in a linear fashion with the increase in dose (in the range of 4-16 mg), although the increase was not directly dose-proportional.

Naloxone did not affect the pharmacokinetics of buprenorphine and both Subutex and Suboxone deliver similar plasma concentrations of buprenorphine. The levels of naloxone were too low to assess dose-proportionality. At the 3 naloxone doses of 1, 2, and 4 mg, levels above the limit of quantitation (0.05 ng/ml) were not detected beyond 2 hours in 7 of 8 subjects. In 1 individual, at the 4 mg dose, the last measurable concentration was at 8 hours. Within each subject (for most of the subjects), across the doses there was a trend toward an increase in naloxone concentrations with increase in dose. Mean peak naloxone levels ranged from 0.11-0.28 ng/ml in the dose range of 1-4 mg.

TABLE 1 *Pharmacokinetic Parameters of Buprenorphine After the Administration of 4, 8, and 16 mg Suboxone Doses and 16 mg Subutex Dose [Mean (%CV)]*

Pharmacokinetic Parameter	Suboxone 4 mg	Suboxone 8 mg	Suboxone 16 mg	Subutex 16 mg
C_{max}, ng/ml	1.84 (39%)	3.0 (51%)	5.95 (38%)	5.47 (23%)
AUC(0-48), h·ng/ml	12.52 (35%)	20.22 (43%)	34.89 (33%)	32.63 (25%)

Distribution

Buprenorphine is approximately 96% protein bound, primarily to alpha and beta globulin.

Naloxone is approximately 45% protein bound, primarily to albumin.

Metabolism

Buprenorphine undergoes both N-dealkylation to norbuprenorphine and glucuronidation. The N-dealkylation pathway is mediated by cytochrome P-450 3A4 isozyme. Norbuprenorphine, an active metabolite, can further undergo glucuronidation.

Naloxone undergoes direct glucuronidation to naloxone 3-glucuronide as well as N-dealkylation, and reduction of the 6-oxo group.

Elimination

A mass balance study of buprenorphine showed complete recovery of radiolabel in urine (30%) and feces (69%) collected up to 11 days after dosing. Almost all of the dose was accounted for in terms of buprenorphine, norbuprenorphine, and two unidentified buprenorphine metabolites. In urine, most of buprenorphine and norbuprenorphine was conjugated (buprenorphine, 1% free and 9.4% conjugated; norbuprenorphine, 2.7% free and 11% conjugated). In feces, almost all of the buprenorphine and norbuprenorphine were free (buprenorphine, 33% free and 5% conjugated; norbuprenorphine, 21% free and 2% conjugated).

Buprenorphine has a mean elimination half-life from plasma of 37 h.

Naloxone has a mean elimination half-life from plasma of 1.1 h.

SPECIAL POPULATIONS

Hepatic Disease

The effect of hepatic impairment on the pharmacokinetics of buprenorphine and naloxone is unknown. Since both drugs are extensively metabolized, the plasma levels will be expected to be higher in patients with moderate and severe hepatic impairment. However, it is not known whether both drugs are affected to the same degree. Therefore, in patients with hepatic impairment dosage should be adjusted and patients should be observed for symptoms of precipitated opioid withdrawal.

Renal Disease

No differences in buprenorphine pharmacokinetics were observed between 9 dialysis-dependent and 6 normal patients following intravenous administration of 0.3 mg buprenorphine.

The effects of renal failure on naloxone pharmacokinetics are unknown.

DRUG-DRUG INTERACTIONS

CYP 3A4 Inhibitors and Inducers

A pharmacokinetic interaction study of ketoconazole (400 mg/day), a potent inhibitor of CYP 3A4, in 12 patients stabilized on Suboxone [8 mg (n=1) or 12 mg (n=5) or 16 mg (n=6)] resulted in increases in buprenorphine mean C_{max} values (from 4.3-9.8, 6.3-14.4 and 9.0-17.1) and mean AUC values (from 30.9-46.9, 41.9-83.2 and 52.3–120) respectively. Subjects receiving Subutex or Suboxone should be closely monitored and may require dose-reduction if inhibitors of CYP 3A4 such as azole antifungal agents (*e.g.*, ketoconazole), macrolide antibiotics (*e.g.*, erythromycin) and HIV protease inhibitors (*e.g.*, ritonavir, indinavir and saquinavir) are co-administered. The interaction of buprenorphine with CYP 3A4 inducers has not been investigated; therefore it is recommended that patients receiving Subutex or Suboxone should be closely monitored if inducers of CYP 3A4 (*e.g.*, phenobarbital, carbamazepine, phenytoin, rifampicin) are co-administered. (See WARNINGS.)

INDICATIONS AND USAGE

Suboxone and Subutex are indicated for the treatment of opioid dependence.

CONTRAINDICATIONS

Suboxone and Subutex should not be administered to patients who have been shown to be hypersensitive to buprenorphine, and Suboxone should not be administered to patients who have been shown to be hypersensitive to naloxone.

WARNINGS

RESPIRATORY DEPRESSION

Significant respiratory depression has been associated with buprenorphine, particularly by the intravenous route. A number of deaths have occurred when addicts have intravenously misused buprenorphine, usually with benzodiazepines concomitantly. Deaths have also been reported in association with concomitant administration of buprenorphine with other depressants such as alcohol or other opioids. Patients should be warned of the potential danger of the self-administration of benzodiazepines or other depressants while under treatment with Subutex or Suboxone.

IN THE CASE OF OVERDOSE, THE PRIMARY MANAGEMENT SHOULD BE THE REESTABLISHMENT OF ADEQUATE VENTILATION WITH MECHANICAL ASSISTANCE OF RESPIRATION, IF REQUIRED. NALOXONE MAY NOT BE EFFECTIVE IN REVERSING ANY RESPIRATORY DEPRESSION PRODUCED BY BUPRENORPHINE.

Suboxone and Subutex should be used with caution in patients with compromised respiratory function (*e.g.*, chronic obstructive pulmonary disease, cor pulmonale, decreased respiratory reserve, hypoxia, hypercapnia, or pre-existing respiratory depression).

CNS DEPRESSION

Patients receiving buprenorphine in the presence of other narcotic analgesics, general anesthetics, benzodiazepines, phenothiazines, other tranquilizers, sedative/hypnotics or other CNS depressants (including alcohol) may exhibit increased CNS depression. When such combined therapy is contemplated, reduction of the dose of 1 or both agents should be considered.

DEPENDENCE

Buprenorphine is a partial agonist at the mu-opiate receptor and chronic administration produces dependence of the opioid type, characterized by withdrawal upon abrupt discontinuation or rapid taper. The withdrawal syndrome is milder than seen with full agonists, and may be delayed in onset.

B

HEPATITIS, HEPATIC EVENTS

Cases of cytolytic hepatitis and hepatitis with jaundice have been observed in the addict population receiving buprenorphine both in clinical trials and in post-marketing adverse event reports. The spectrum of abnormalities ranges from transient asymptomatic elevations in hepatic transaminases to case reports of hepatic failure, hepatic necrosis, hepatorenal syndrome, and hepatic encephalopathy. In many cases, the presence of pre-existing liver enzyme abnormalities, infection with hepatitis B or hepatitis C virus, concomitant usage of other potentially hepatotoxic drugs, and ongoing injecting drug use may have played a causative or contributory role. In other cases, insufficient data were available to determine the etiology of the abnormality. The possibility exists that buprenorphine had a causative or contributory role in the development of the hepatic abnormality in some cases. Measurements of liver function tests prior to initiation of treatment is recommended to establish a baseline. Periodic monitoring of liver function tests during treatment is also recommended. A biological and etiological evaluation is recommended when a hepatic event is suspected. Depending on the case, the drug should be carefully discontinued to prevent withdrawal symptoms and a return to illicit drug use, and strict monitoring of the patient should be initiated.

ALLERGIC REACTIONS

Cases of acute and chronic hypersensitivity to buprenorphine have been reported both in clinical trials and in the post-marketing experience. The most common signs and symptoms include rashes, hives, and pruritus. Cases of bronchospasm, angioneurotic edema, and anaphylactic shock have been reported. A history of hypersensitivity to buprenorphine is a contraindication to Subutex or Suboxone use. A history of hypersensitivity to naloxone is a contraindication to Suboxone use.

USE IN AMBULATORY PATIENTS

Suboxone and Subutex may impair the mental or physical abilities required for the performance of potentially dangerous tasks such as driving a car or operating machinery, especially during drug induction and dose adjustment. Patients should be cautioned about operating hazardous machinery, including automobiles, until they are reasonably certain that buprenorphine therapy does not adversely affect their ability to engage in such activities. Like other opioids, Suboxone and Subutex may produce orthostatic hypotension in ambulatory patients.

HEAD INJURY AND INCREASED INTRACRANIAL PRESSURE

Suboxone and Subutex, like other potent opioids, may elevate cerebrospinal fluid pressure and should be used with caution in patients with head injury, intracranial lesions and other circumstances where cerebrospinal pressure may be increased. Suboxone and Subutex can produce miosis and changes in the level of consciousness that may interfere with patient evaluation.

OPIOID WITHDRAWAL EFFECTS

Because it contains naloxone, Suboxone is highly likely to produce marked and intense withdrawal symptoms if misused parenterally by individuals dependent on opioid agonists such as heroin, morphine, or methadone. Sublingually, Suboxone may cause opioid withdrawal symptoms in such persons if administered before the agonist effects of the opioid have subsided.

PRECAUTIONS

GENERAL

Suboxone and Subutex should be administered with caution in elderly or debilitated patients and those with severe impairment of hepatic, pulmonary, or renal function; myxedema or hypothyroidism, adrenal cortical insufficiency (*e.g.,* Addison's disease); CNS depression or coma; toxic psychoses; prostatic hypertrophy or urethral stricture; acute alcoholism; delirium tremens; or kyphoscoliosis.

The effect of hepatic impairment on the pharmacokinetics of buprenorphine and naloxone is unknown. Since both drugs are extensively metabolized, the plasma levels will be expected to be higher in patients with moderate and severe hepatic impairment. However, it is not known whether both drugs are affected to the same degree. Therefore, dosage should be adjusted and patients should be watched for symptoms of precipitated opioid withdrawal.

Buprenorphine has been shown to increase intracholedochal pressure, as do other opioids, and thus should be administered with caution to patients with dysfunction of the biliary tract.

As with other mu-opioid receptor agonists, the administration of Suboxone or Subutex may obscure the diagnosis or clinical course of patients with acute abdominal conditions.

INFORMATION FOR THE PATIENT

Patients should inform their family members that, in the event of emergency, the treating physician or emergency room staff should be informed that the patient is physically dependent on narcotics and that the patient is being treated with Suboxone or Subutex.

Patients should be cautioned that a serious overdose and death may occur if benzodiazepines, sedatives, tranquilizers, antidepressants, or alcohol are taken at the same time as Suboxone or Subutex.

Suboxone and Subutex may impair the mental or physical abilities required for the performance of potentially dangerous tasks such as driving a car or operating machinery, especially during drug induction and dose adjustment. Patients should be cautioned about operating hazardous machinery, including automobiles, until they are reasonably certain that buprenorphine therapy does not adversely affect their ability to engage in such activities. Like other opioids, Suboxone and Subutex may produce orthostatic hypotension in ambulatory patients.

Patients should consult their physician if other prescription medications are currently being used or are prescribed for future use.

CARCINOGENESIS, MUTAGENESIS, AND IMPAIRMENT OF FERTILITY

Carcinogenesis

Carcinogenicity data on Suboxone are not available. Carcinogenicity studies of buprenorphine were conducted in Sprague-Dawley rats and CD-1 mice. Buprenorphine was administered in the diet to rats at doses of 0.6, 5.5, and 56 mg/kg/day (estimated exposure was approximately 0.4, 3 and 35 times the recommended human daily sublingual dose of 16 mg on a mg/m^2 basis) for 27 months. Statistically significant dose-related increases in testicular interstitial (Leydig's) cell tumors occurred, according to the trend test adjusted for survival. Pair-wise comparison of the high dose against control failed to show statistical significance. In an 86 week study in CD-1 mice, buprenorphine was not carcinogenic at dietary doses up to 100 mg/kg/day (estimated exposure was approximately 30 times the recommended human daily sublingual dose of 16 mg on a mg/m^2 basis).

Mutagenicity

Suboxone

The 4:1 combination of buprenorphine and naloxone was not mutagenic in a bacterial mutation assay (Ames test) using 4 strains of *S. typhimurium* and 2 strains of *E. coli.* The combination was not clastogenic in an *in vitro* cytogenetic assay in human lymphocytes, or in an intravenous micronucleus test in the rat.

Subutex

Buprenorphine was studied in a series of tests utilizing gene, chromosome, and DNA interactions in both prokaryotic and eukaryotic systems. Results were negative in yeast *(Saccharomyces cerevisiae)* for recombinant, gene convertant, or forward mutations; negative in *Bacillus subtilis* "rec" assay, negative for clastogenicity in CHO cells, Chinese hamster bone marrow and spermatogonia cells, and negative in the mouse lymphoma L5178Y assay. Results were equivocal in the Ames test: negative in studies in two laboratories, but positive for frame shift mutation at a high dose (5 mg/plate) in a third study. Results were positive in the Green-Tweets *(E. coli)* survival test, positive in a DNA synthesis inhibition (DSI) test with testicular tissue from mice, for both *in vivo* and *in vitro* incorporation of [^{3}H]thymidine, and positive in unscheduled DNA synthesis (UDS) test using testicular cells from mice.

Impairment of Fertility

Suboxone

Dietary administration of Suboxone in the rat at dose levels of 500 ppm or greater (equivalent to approximately 47 mg/kg/day or greater; estimated exposure was approximately 28 times the recommended human daily sublingual dose of 16 mg on a mg/m^2 basis) produced a reduction in fertility demonstrated by reduced female conception rates. A dietary dose of 100 ppm (equivalent to approximately 10 mg/kg/day; estimated exposure was approximately 6 times the recommended human daily sublingual dose of 16 mg on a mg/m^2 basis) had no adverse effect on fertility.

Subutex

Reproduction studies of buprenorphine in rats demonstrated no evidence of impaired fertility at daily oral doses up to 80 mg/kg/day (estimated exposure was approximately 50 times the recommended human daily sublingual dose of 16 mg on a mg/m^2 basis) or up to 5 mg/kg/day IM or SC (estimated exposure was approximately 3 times the recommended human daily sublingual dose of 16 mg on a mg/m^2 basis).

PREGNANCY CATEGORY C

Teratogenic Effects

Suboxone

Effects on embryo-fetal development were studied in Sprague-Dawley rats and Russian white rabbits following oral (1:1) and intramuscular (3:2) administration of mixtures of buprenorphine and naloxone. Following oral administration to rats and rabbits, no teratogenic effects were observed at doses up to 250 mg/kg/day and 40 mg/kg/day, respectively (estimated exposure was approximately 150 times and 50 times, respectively, the recommended human daily sublingual dose of 16 mg on a mg/m^2 basis). No definitive drug-related teratogenic effects were observed in rats and rabbits at intramuscular doses up to 30 mg/kg/day (estimated exposure was approximately 20 times and 35 times, respectively, the recommended human daily dose of 16 mg on a mg/m^2 basis). Acephalus was observed in 1 rabbit fetus from the low-dose group and omphacele was observed in 2 rabbit fetuses from the same litter in the mid-dose group; no findings were observed in fetuses from the high-dose group. Following oral administration to the rat, dose-related post-implantation losses, evidenced by increases in the numbers of early resorptions with consequent reductions in the numbers of fetuses, were observed at doses of 10 mg/kg/day or greater (estimated exposure was approximately 6 times the recommended human daily sublingual dose of 16 mg on a mg/m^2 basis). In the rabbit, increased post-implantation losses occurred at an oral dose of 40 mg/kg/day. Following intramuscular administration in the rat and the rabbit, post-implantation losses, as evidenced by decreases in live fetuses and increases in resorptions, occurred at 30 mg/kg/day.

Subutex

Buprenorphine was not teratogenic in rats or rabbits after IM or SC doses up to 5 mg/kg/day (estimated exposure was approximately 3 and 6 times, respectively, the recommended human daily sublingual dose of 16 mg on a mg/m^2 basis), after IV doses up to 0.8 mg/kg/day (estimated exposure was approximately 0.5 times and equal to, respectively, the recommended human daily sublingual dose of 16 mg on a mg/m^2 basis), or after oral doses up to 160 mg/kg/day in rats (estimated exposure was approximately 95 times the recommended human daily sublingual dose of 16 mg on a mg/m^2 basis) and 25 mg/kg/day in rabbits (estimated exposure was approximately 30 times the recommended human daily sublingual dose of 16 mg on a mg/m^2 basis). Significant increases in skeletal abnormalities (*e.g.,* extra thoracic vertebra or thoraco-lumbar ribs) were noted in rats after SC administration of 1 mg/kg/day and up (estimated exposure was approximately 0.6 times the recommended human daily sublingual dose of 16 mg on a mg/m^2 basis), but were not observed at oral doses up to 160 mg/kg/day. Increases in skeletal abnormalities in rabbits after IM administration of 5 mg/kg/day (estimated exposure was approximately 6 times the recommended human daily sublingual dose of 16 mg on a mg/m² basis) or oral administration of 1 mg/kg/day or greater (estimated exposure was approximately equal to the recommended human daily sublingual dose of 16 mg on a mg/m² basis) were not statistically significant.

In rabbits, buprenorphine produced statistically significant pre-implantation losses at oral doses of 1 mg/kg/day or greater and post-implantation losses that were statistically significant at IV doses of 0.2 mg/kg/day or greater (estimated exposure was approximately 0.3 times the recommended human daily sublingual dose of 16 mg on a mg/m² basis).

There are no adequate and well-controlled studies of Suboxone or Subutex in pregnant women. Suboxone or Subutex should only be used during pregnancy if the potential benefit justifies the potential risk to the fetus.

Nonteratogenic Effects

Dystocia was noted in pregnant rats treated IM with buprenorphine 5 mg/kg/day (approximately 3 times the recommended human daily sublingual dose of 16 mg on a mg/m² basis). Both fertility and peri- and postnatal development studies with buprenorphine in rats indicated increases in neonatal mortality after oral doses of 0.8 mg/kg/day and up (approximately 0.5 times the recommended human daily sublingual dose of 16 mg on a mg/m² basis), after IM doses of 0.5 mg/kg/day and up (approximately 0.3 times the recommended human daily sublingual dose of 16 mg on a mg/m² basis), and after SC doses of 0.1 mg/kg/day and up (approximately 0.06 times the recommended human daily sublingual dose of 16 mg on a mg/m² basis). Delays in the occurrence of righting reflex and startle response were noted in rat pups at an oral dose of 80 mg/kg/day (approximately 50 times the recommended human daily sublingual dose of 16 mg on a mg/m² basis).

Neonatal Withdrawal

Neonatal withdrawal has been reported in the infants of women treated with Subutex during pregnancy. From post-marketing reports, the time to onset of neonatal withdrawal symptoms ranged from Day 1-8 of life with most occurring on Day 1. Adverse events associated with neonatal withdrawal syndrome included hypertonia, neonatal tremor, neonatal agitation, and myoclonus. There have been rare reports of convulsions and in 1 case, apnea and bradycardia were also reported.

NURSING MOTHERS

An apparent lack of milk production during general reproduction studies with buprenorphine in rats caused decreased viability and lactation indices. Use of high doses of sublingual buprenorphine in pregnant women showed that buprenorphine passes into the mother's milk. Breast-feeding is therefore not advised in mothers treated with Subutex or Suboxone.

PEDIATRIC USE

Suboxone and Subutex are not recommended for use in pediatric patients. The safety and effectiveness of Suboxone and Subutex in patients below the age of 16 have not been established.

DRUG INTERACTIONS

Buprenorphine is metabolized to norbuprenorphine by cytochrome CYP 3A4. Because CYP 3A4 inhibitors may increase plasma concentrations of buprenorphine, patients already on CYP 3A4 inhibitors such as azole antifungals (*e.g.,* ketoconazole), macrolide antibiotics (*e.g.,* erythromycin), and HIV protease inhibitors (*e.g.,* ritonavir, indinavir and saquinavir) should have their dose of Subutex or Suboxone adjusted.

Based on anecdotal reports, there may be an interaction between buprenorphine and benzodiazepines. There have been a number of reports in the post-marketing experience of coma and death associated with the concomitant intravenous misuse of buprenorphine and benzodiazepines by addicts. In many of these cases, buprenorphine was misused by self-injection of crushed Subutex tablets. Subutex and Suboxone should be prescribed with caution to patients on benzodiazepines or other drugs that act on the central nervous system, regardless of whether these drugs are taken on the advice of a physician or are taken as drugs of abuse. Patients should be warned of the potential danger of the intravenous self-administration of benzodiazepines while under treatment with Suboxone or Subutex.

ADVERSE REACTIONS

The safety of Suboxone has been evaluated in 497 opioid-dependent subjects. The prospective evaluation of Suboxone was supported by clinical trials using Subutex (buprenorphine tablets without naloxone) and other trials using buprenorphine sublingual solutions. In total, safety data are available from 3214 opioid-dependent subjects exposed to buprenorphine at doses in the range used in treatment of opioid addiction.

Few differences in adverse event profile were noted between Suboxone and Subutex or buprenorphine administered as a sublingual solution.

In a comparative study, adverse event profiles were similar for subjects treated with 16 mg Suboxone or 16 mg Subutex. The following adverse events were reported to occur by at least 5% of patients in a 4 week study (TABLE 3).

The adverse event profile of buprenorphine was also characterized in the dose-controlled study of buprenorphine solution, over a range of doses in 4 months of treatment. TABLE 4 shows adverse events reported by at least 5% of subjects in any dose group in the dose-controlled study.

TABLE 3 *Adverse Events (≥5%) by Body System and Treatment Group in a 4 Week Study*

Body System/ Adverse Event (COSTART Terminology)	Suboxone 16 mg/day n=107	Subutex 16 mg/day n=103	Placebo n=107
Body as a Whole			
Asthenia	7 (6.5%)	5 (4.9%)	7 (6.5%)
Chills	8 (7.5%)	8 (7.8%)	8 (7.5%)
Headache	39 (36.4%)	30 (29.1%)	24 (22.4%)
Infection	6 (5.6%)	12 (11.7%)	7 (6.5%)
Pain	24 (22.4%)	19 (18.4%)	20 (18.7%)
Pain abdomen	12 (11.2%)	12 (11.7%)	7 (6.5%)
Pain back	4 (3.7%)	8 (7.8%)	12 (11.2%)
Withdrawal syndrome	27 (25.2%)	19 (18.4%)	40 (37.4%)
Cardiovascular System			
Vasodilation	10 (9.3%)	4 (3.9%)	7 (6.5%)
Digestive System			
Constipation	13 (12.1%)	8 (7.8%)	3 (2.8%)
Diarrhea	4 (3.7%)	5 (4.9%)	16 (15.0%)
Nausea	16 (15.0%)	14 (13.6%)	12 (11.2%)
Vomiting	8 (7.5%)	8 (7.8%)	5 (4.7%)
Nervous System			
Insomnia	15 (14.0%)	22 (21.4%)	17 (15.9%)
Respiratory System			
Rhinitis	5 (4.7%)	10 (9.7%)	14 (13.1%)
Skin and Appendages			
Sweating	15 (14.0%)	13 (12.6%)	11 (10.3%)

TABLE 4 *Adverse Events (≥5%) by Body System and Treatment Group in a 16 Week Study*

Body System/	Buprenorphine Dose*				
Adverse Event (COSTART Terminology)	Very Low* (n=184)	Low* (n=180)	Moderate* (n=186)	High* (n=181)	Total* (n=731)
Body as a Whole					
Abscess	9 (5%)	2 (1%)	3 (2%)	2 (1%)	16 (2%)
Asthenia	26 (14%)	28 (16%)	26 (14%)	24 (13%)	104 (14%)
Chills	11 (6%)	12 (7%)	9 (5%)	10 (6%)	42 (6%)
Fever	7 (4%)	2 (1%)	2 (1%)	10 (6%)	21 (3%)
Flu syndrome	4 (2%)	13 (7%)	19 (10%)	8 (4%)	44 (6%)
Headache	51 (28%)	62 (34%)	54 (29%)	53 (29%)	220 (30%)
Infection	32 (17%)	39 (22%)	38 (20%)	40 (22%)	149 (20%)
Injury accidental	5 (3%)	10 (6%)	5 (3%)	5 (3%)	25 (3%)
Pain	47 (26%)	37 (21%)	49 (26%)	44 (24%)	177 (24%)
Pain back	18 (10%)	29 (16%)	28 (15%)	27 (15%)	102 (14%)
Withdrawal syndrome	45 (24%)	40 (22%)	41 (22%)	36 (20%)	162 (22%)
Digestive System					
Constipation	10 (5%)	23 (13%)	23 (12%)	26 (14%)	82 (11%)
Diarrhea	19 (10%)	8 (4%)	9 (5%)	4 (2%)	40 (5%)
Dyspepsia	6 (3%)	10 (6%)	4 (2%)	4 (2%)	24 (3%)
Nausea	12 (7%)	22 (12%)	23 (12%)	18 (10%)	75 (10%)
Vomiting	8 (4%)	6 (3%)	10 (5%)	14 (8%)	38 (5%)
Nervous System					
Anxiety	22 (12%)	24 (13%)	20 (11%)	25 (14%)	91 (12%)
Depression	24 (13%)	16 (9%)	25 (13%)	18 (10%)	83 (11%)
Dizziness	4 (2%)	9 (5%)	7 (4%)	11 (6%)	31 (4%)
Insomnia	42 (23%)	50 (28%)	43 (23%)	51 (28%)	186 (25%)
Nervousness	12 (7%)	11 (6%)	10 (5%)	13 (7%)	46 (6%)
Somnolence	5 (3%)	13 (7%)	9 (5%)	11 (6%)	38 (5%)
Respiratory System					
Cough increase	5 (3%)	11 (6%)	6 (3%)	4 (2%)	26 (4%)
Pharyngitis	6 (3%)	7 (4%)	6 (3%)	9 (5%)	28 (4%)
Rhinitis	27 (15%)	16 (9%)	15 (8%)	21 (12%)	79 (11%)
Skin and Appendages					
Sweat	23 (13%)	21 (12%)	20 (11%)	23 (13%)	87 (12%)
Special Senses					
Runny eyes	13 (7%)	9 (5%)	6 (3%)	6 (3%)	34 (5%)

* Sublingual solution. Doses in this table cannot necessarily be delivered in tablet form, but for comparison purposes: "Very low" dose (1 mg solution) would be less than a tablet dose of 2 mg, "Low" dose (4 mg solution) approximates a 6 mg tablet dose, "Moderate" dose (8 mg solution) approximates a 12 mg tablet dose, "High" dose (16 mg solution) approximates a 24 mg tablet dose.

DOSAGE AND ADMINISTRATION

Subutex or Suboxone is administered sublingually as a single daily dose in the range of 12-16 mg/day. When taken sublingually, Suboxone and Subutex have similar clinical effects and are interchangeable. There are no adequate and well-controlled studies using Suboxone as initial medication. Subutex contains no naloxone and is preferred for use during induction. Following induction, Suboxone, due to the presence of naloxone, is preferred when clinical use includes unsupervised administration. The use of Subutex for unsupervised administration should be limited to those patients who cannot tolerate Suboxone, for example those patients who have been shown to be hypersensitive to naloxone.

METHOD OF ADMINISTRATION

Suboxone and Subutex tablets should be placed under the tongue until they are dissolved. For doses requiring the use of more than 2 tablets, patients are advised to either place all the tablets at once or alternatively (if they cannot fit in more than 2 tablets comfortably) place 2 tablets at a time under the tongue. Either way, the patients should continue to hold the tablets under the tongue until they dissolve; swallowing the tablets reduces the bioavailability of the drug. To ensure consistency in bioavailability, patients should follow the same manner of dosing with continued use of the product.

INDUCTION

Prior to induction, consideration should be given to the type of opioid dependence (*i.e.,* long- or short-acting opioid), the time since last opioid use, and the degree or level of opioid dependence. To avoid precipitating withdrawal, induction with Subutex should be undertaken when objective and clear signs of withdrawal are evident.

In a 1 month study of Suboxone tablets induction was conducted with Subutex tablets. Patients received 8 mg of Subutex on Day 1 and 16 mg Subutex on Day 2. From Day 3 onward, patients received Suboxone tablets at the same buprenorphine dose as Day 2. Induction in the studies of buprenorphine solution was accomplished over 3-4 days, depending on the target dose. In some studies, gradual induction over several days led to a high rate of drop-out of buprenorphine patients during the induction period. Therefore it is recommended that an adequate maintenance dose, titrated to clinical effectiveness, should be achieved as rapidly as possible to prevent undue opioid withdrawal symptoms.

PATIENTS TAKING HEROIN OR OTHER SHORT-ACTING OPIOIDS

At treatment initiation, the dose of Subutex should be administered at least 4 hours after the patient last used opioids or preferably when early signs of opioid withdrawal appear.

PATIENTS ON METHADONE OR OTHER LONG-ACTING OPIOIDS

There is little controlled experience with the transfer of methadone-maintained patients to buprenorphine. Available evidence suggests that withdrawal symptoms are possible during induction to buprenorphine treatment. Withdrawal appears more likely in patients maintained on higher doses of methadone (>30 mg) and when the first buprenorphine dose is administered shortly after the last methadone dose.

MAINTENANCE

Suboxone is the preferred medication for maintenance treatment due to the presence of naloxone in the formulation.

ADJUSTING THE DOSE UNTIL THE MAINTENANCE DOSE IS ACHIEVED

The recommended target dose of Suboxone is 16 mg/day. Clinical studies have shown that 16 mg of Subutex or Suboxone is a clinically effective dose compared with placebo and indicate that doses as low as 12 mg may be effective in some patients. The dosage of Suboxone should be progressively adjusted in increments/decrements of 2 or 4 mg to a level that holds the patient in treatment and suppresses opioid withdrawal effects. This is likely to be in the range of 4-24 mg/day depending on the individual.

REDUCING DOSAGE AND STOPPING TREATMENT

The decision to discontinue therapy with Suboxone or Subutex after a period of maintenance or brief stabilization should be made as part of a comprehensive treatment plan. Both gradual and abrupt discontinuation have been used, but no controlled trials have been undertaken to determine the best method of dose taper at the end of treatment.

HOW SUPPLIED

SUBOXONE

Suboxone is supplied as sublingual tablets in the following formulations:
- Hexagonal orange tablets containing 2 mg buprenorphine with 0.5 mg naloxone.
- Hexagonal orange tablets containing 8 mg buprenorphine with 2 mg naloxone.

Storage: Store at 25°C (77°F), excursions permitted to 15-30°C (59-86°F).

SUBUTEX

Subutex is supplied as sublingual tablets in the following formulations:
- Oval white tablets containing 2 mg buprenorphine.
- Oval white tablets containing 8 mg buprenorphine.

Storage: Store at 25°C (77°F), excursions permitted to 15-30°C (59-86°F).

PRODUCT LISTING - RATED THERAPEUTICALLY EQUIVALENT

Solution - Injectable - 0.3 mg/ml

1 ml x 10 $29.80 GENERIC, Abbott Pharmaceutical 00074-2012-01

PRODUCT LISTING - EQUIVALENTS NOT AVAILABLE

Solution - Injectable - 0.3 mg/ml

1 ml x 10 $25.46 BUPRENEX, Allscripts Pharmaceutical Company 54569-1416-00

1 ml x 10 $30.60 BUPRENEX, Reckitt and Colman Pharmaceuticals Inc 12496-0757-01

Bupropion Hydrochloride (000550)

For related information, see the comparative table section in Appendix A.

Categories: Depression; Smoking cessation; Pregnancy Category B; FDA Approved 1985 Dec
Drug Classes: Antidepressants, miscellaneous
Brand Names: Wellbutrin; Wellbutrin SR; Zyban
Foreign Brand Availability: Odranal (Colombia); Quomen (Thailand); Well (Korea); Zyban LP (France); Zyban Sustained Release (Australia)
Cost of Therapy: $86.55 (Depression; Wellbutrin; 100 mg; 3 tablets/day; 30 day supply)
$86.45 (Depression; Generic tablets; 100 mg; 3 tablets/day; 30 day supply)
$79.75 (Depression; Wellbutrin SR; 150 mg; 2 tablets/day; 30 day supply)
$91.64 (Smoking Cessation; Zyban SR; 150 mg; 2 tablets/day; 30 day supply)

DESCRIPTION

Note: The trade names have been used thoughout this monograph for clarity.

WELLBUTRIN

Wellbutrin (bupropion hydrochloride), an antidepressant of the aminoketone class, is chemically unrelated to tricyclic, tetracyclic, selective serotonin re-uptake inhibitor, or other known antidepressant agents. Its structure closely resembles that of diethylpropion; it is related to phenylethylamines. It is designated as (±)-1-(3-chlorophenyl)-2-[(1,1-dimethylethyl)amino]-1-propanone hydrochloride. The molecular weight is 276.2. The empirical formula is $C_{13}H_{18}ClNO{\cdot}HCl$. Bupropion hydrochloride powder is white, crystalline, and highly soluble in water. It has a bitter taste and produces the sensation of local anesthesia on the oral mucosa.

Wellbutrin is supplied for oral administration as 75 mg (yellow-gold) and 100 mg (red) film-coated tablets. Each tablet contains the labeled amount of bupropion hydrochloride and the inactive ingredients: *75 mg tablet:* D&C yellow no. 10 lake, FD&C yellow no. 6 lake, hydroxypropyl cellulose, hydroxypropyl methylcellulose, microcrystalline cellulose, polyethylene glycol, talc, and titanium dioxide; *100 mg tablet:* FD&C red no. 40 lake, FD&C yellow no. 6 lake, hydroxypropyl cellulose, hydroxypropyl methylcellulose, microcrystalline cellulose, polyethylene glycol, talc, and titanium dioxide.

WELLBUTRIN SR

Wellbutrin SR (bupropion hydrochloride), an antidepressant of the aminoketone class, is chemically unrelated to tricyclic, tetracyclic, selective serotonin re-uptake inhibitor, or other known antidepressant agents. Its structure closely resembles that of diethylpropion; it is related to phenylethylamines. It is designated as (±)-1-(3-chlorophenyl)-2-[(1,1-dimethylethyl)amino]-1-propanone hydrochloride. The molecular weight is 276.2. The molecular formula is $C_{13}H_{18}ClNO{\cdot}HCl$. Bupropion hydrochloride powder is white, crystalline, and highly soluble in water. It has a bitter taste and produces the sensation of local anesthesia on the oral mucosa.

Wellbutrin SR tablets are supplied for oral administration as 100 mg (blue) 150 mg (purple), and 200 mg (light pink), film-coated, sustained-release tablets. Each tablet contains the labeled amount of bupropion hydrochloride and the inactive ingredients: carnauba wax, cysteine hydrochloride, hydroxypropyl methylcellulose, magnesium stearate, microcrystalline cellulose, polyethylene glycol, polysorbate 80, and titanium dioxide and is printed with edible black ink. In addition, the 100 mg tablet contains FD&C blue no. 1 lake, the 150 mg tablet contains FD&C blue no. 2 lake, and FD&C red no. 40 lake, and the 200 mg tablet contains FD&C red no. 40 lake.

ZYBAN

Zyban (bupropion hydrochloride) sustained-release tablets are a non-nicotine aid to smoking cessation. Zyban is chemically unrelated to nicotine or other agents currently used in the treatment of nicotine addiction. Initially developed and marketed as an antidepressant (Wellbutrin [bupropion hydrochloride] tablets and Wellbutrin SR [bupropion hydrochloride] sustained-release tablets), Zyban is also chemically unrelated to tricyclic, tetracyclic, selective serotonin re-uptake inhibitor, or other known antidepressant agents. Its structure closely resembles that of diethylpropion; it is related to phenylethylamines. It is (±)-1-(3-chlorophenyl)-2-[(1,1-dimethylethyl)amino]-1-propanone hydrochloride. The molecular weight is 276.2. The molecular formula is $C_{13}H_{18}ClNO{\cdot}HCl$. Bupropion hydrochloride powder is white, crystalline, and highly soluble in water. It has a bitter taste and produces the sensation of local anesthesia on the oral mucosa.

Zyban is supplied for oral administration as 150 mg (purple), film-coated, sustained-release tablets. Each tablet contains the labeled amount of bupropion hydrochloride and the inactive ingredients carnauba wax, cysteine hydrochloride, hypromellose, magnesium stearate, microcrystalline cellulose, polyethylene glycol, polysorbate 80 and titanium dioxide and is printed with edible black ink. In addition, the 150 mg tablet contains FD&C blue no. 2 lake and FD&C red no. 40 lake.

CLINICAL PHARMACOLOGY

WELLBUTRIN

Pharmacodynamics

The neurochemical mechanism of the antidepressant effect of bupropion is not known. Bupropion is a relatively weak inhibitor of the neuronal uptake of norepinephrine, serotonin, and dopamine, and does not inhibit monoamine oxidase.

Bupropion produces dose-related central nervous system (CNS) stimulant effects in animals, as evidenced by increased locomotor activity, increased rates of responding in various schedule-controlled operant behavior tasks, and, at high doses, induction of mild stereotyped behavior.

Bupropion causes convulsions in rodents and dogs at doses approximately 10-fold the dose recommended as the human antidepressant dose.

Pharmacokinetics

Bupropion is a racemic mixture. The pharmacological activity and pharmacokinetics of the individual enantiomers have not been studied. In humans, following oral administration of Wellbutrin, peak plasma bupropion concentrations are usually achieved within 2 hours, followed by a biphasic decline. The terminal phase has a mean half-life of 14 hours, with a range of 8-24 hours. The distribution phase has a mean half-life of 3-4 hours. The mean elimination half-life (±SD) of bupropion after chronic dosing is 21 (±9) hours, and steady-state plasma concentrations of bupropion are reached within 8 days. Plasma bupropion concentrations are dose-proportional following single doses of 100-250 mg; however, it is not known if the proportionality between dose and plasma level are maintained in chronic use.

Absorption

The absolute bioavailability of Wellbutrin tablets in humans has not been determined because an intravenous (IV) formulation for human use is not available. However, it appears likely that only a small proportion of any orally administered dose reaches the systemic circulation intact.

Distribution

In vitro tests show that bupropion is 84% bound to human plasma protein at concentrations up to 200 µg/ml. The extent of protein binding of the hydroxybupropion metabolite is similar to that for bupropion, whereas the extent of protein binding of the threohydrobupropion metabolite is about half that seen with bupropion.

Metabolism

Bupropion is extensively metabolized in humans. Three metabolites have been shown to be active: hydroxybupropion, which is formed via hydroxylation of the *tert*-butyl group of bupropion, and the amino-alcohol isomers threohydrobupropion and erythrohydrobupropion, which are formed via reduction of the carbonyl group. *In vitro* findings suggest that cytochrome P450IIB6 (CYP2B6) is the principal isoenzyme involved in the formation of hydroxybupropion, while cytochrome P450 isoenzymes are not involved in the formation of threohydrobupropion. Oxidation of the bupropion side chain results in the formation of a glycine conjugate of metachlorobenzoic acid, which is then excreted as the major urinary metabolite. The potency and toxicity of the metabolites relative to bupropion have not been fully characterized. However, it has been demonstrated in an antidepressant screening test in mice that hydroxybupropion is one half as potent as bupropion, while threohydrobupropion and erythrohydrobupropion are 5-fold less potent than bupropion. This may be of clinical importance because their plasma concentrations are as high or higher than those of bupropion.

Because bupropion is extensively metabolized, there is the potential for drug-drug interactions, particularly with those agents that are metabolized by the cytochrome P450IIB6 (CYP2B6) isoenzyme. Although bupropion is not metabolized by cytochrome P450IID6 (CYP2D6), there is the potential for drug-drug interactions when bupropion is coadministered with drugs metabolized by this isoenzyme (see DRUG INTERACTIONS, Wellbutrin).

Following a single dose in humans, peak plasma concentrations of hydroxybupropion occur approximately 3 hours after administration of Wellbutrin tablets. Peak plasma concentrations of hydroxybupropion are approximately 10 times the peak level of the parent drug at steady-state. The elimination half-life of hydroxybupropion is approximately 20 (±5) hours, and its AUC at steady-state is about 17 times that of bupropion. The times to peak concentrations for the erythrohydrobupropion and threohydrobupropion metabolites are similar to that of the hydroxybupropion metabolite. However, their elimination half-lives are longer, 33 (±10) and 37 (±13) hours, respectively, and steady-state AUCs are 1.5 and 7 times that of bupropion, respectively.

Bupropion and its metabolites exhibit linear kinetics following chronic administration of 300-450 mg/day.

Elimination

Following oral administration of 200 mg of ^{14}C-bupropion in humans, 87% and 10% of the radioactive dose were recovered in the urine and feces, respectively. However, the fraction of the oral dose of Wellbutrin excreted unchanged was only 0.5%, a finding consistent with the extensive metabolism of bupropion.

Populations Subgroups

Factors or conditions altering metabolic capacity (*e.g.,* liver disease, congestive heart failure [CHF], age, concomitant medications, etc.) or elimination may be expected to influence the degree and extent of accumulation of the active metabolites of bupropion. The elimination of the major metabolites of bupropion may be affected by reduced renal or hepatic function because they are moderately polar compounds and are likely to undergo further metabolism or conjugation in the liver prior to urinary excretion.

Hepatic

The effect of hepatic impairment on the pharmacokinetics of bupropion was characterized in 2 single dose studies, one in patients with alcoholic liver disease and one in patients with mild to severe cirrhosis. The first study showed that the half-life of hydroxybupropion was significantly longer in 8 patients with alcoholic liver disease than in 8 healthy volunteers (32 ± 14 hours versus 21 ± 5 hours, respectively). Although not statistically significant, the AUCs for bupropion and hydroxybupropion were more variable and tended to be greater (by 53-57%) in volunteers with alcoholic liver disease. The differences in half-life for bupropion and the other metabolites in the 2 patient groups were minimal.

The second study showed that there were no statistically significant differences in the pharmacokinetics of bupropion and its active metabolites in 9 patients with mild to moderate hepatic cirrhosis compared to 8 healthy volunteers. However, more variability was observed in some of the pharmacokinetic parameters for bupropion (AUC, C_{max}, and T_{max}) and its active metabolites ($T_{1/2}$) in patients with mild to moderate hepatic cirrhosis. In addition, in patients with severe hepatic cirrhosis, the bupropion C_{max} and AUC were substantially increased (mean difference: by approximately 70% and 3-fold, respectively) and more variable when compared to values in healthy volunteers; the mean bupropion half-life was also longer (29 hours in patients with severe hepatic cirrhosis versus 19 hours in healthy subjects). For the metabolite hydroxybupropion, the mean C_{max} was approximately 69% lower. For the combined aminoalcohol isomers threohydrobupropion and erythrohydrobupropion, the mean C_{max} was approximately 31% lower. The mean AUC increased by about 1½-fold for hydroxybupropion and about 2½-fold for threo/erythrohydrobupropion. The median T_{max} was observed 19 hours later for hydroxybupropion and 31 hours later for threo/erythrohydrobupropion. The mean half-lives for hydroxybupropion and threo/erythrohydrobupropion were increased 5- and 2-fold, respectively, in patients with severe hepatic cirrhosis compared to healthy volunteers (see WARNINGS, Wellbutrin; PRECAUTIONS, Wellbutrin; and DOSAGE AND ADMINISTRATION, Wellbutrin).

Renal

The effect of renal disease on the pharmacokinetics of bupropion has not been studied. The elimination of the major metabolites of bupropion may be affected by reduced renal function.

Left Ventricular Dysfunction

During a chronic dosing study in 14 depressed patients with left ventricular dysfunction (history of CHF or an enlarged heart on x-ray), no apparent effect on the pharmacokinetics of bupropion or its metabolites was revealed, compared to healthy volunteers.

Age

The effects of age on the pharmacokinetics of bupropion and its metabolites have not been fully characterized, but an exploration of steady-state bupropion concentrations from several depression efficacy studies involving patients dosed in a range of 300-750 mg/day, on a 3 times daily schedule, revealed no relationship between age (18-83 years) and plasma concentration of bupropion. A single dose pharmacokinetic study demonstrated that the disposition of bupropion and its metabolites in elderly subjects was similar to that of younger subjects. These data suggest there is no prominent effect of age on bupropion concentration; however, another pharmacokinetic study, single and multiple dose, has suggested that the elderly are at increased risk for accumulation of bupropion and its metabolites (see PRECAUTIONS, Wellbutrin, Geriatric Use).

Gender

A single dose study involving 12 healthy male and 12 healthy female volunteers revealed no sex-related differences in the pharmacokinetic parameters of bupropion.

Smokers

The effects of cigarette smoking on the pharmacokinetics of bupropion were studied in 34 healthy male and female volunteers; 17 were chronic cigarette smokers and 17 were nonsmokers. Following oral administration of a single 150 mg dose of bupropion, there were no statistically significant differences in C_{max}, half-life, T_{max}, AUC or clearance of bupropion or its active metabolites between smokers and nonsmokers.

WELLBUTRIN SR

Pharmacodynamics

Bupropion is a relatively weak inhibitor of the neuronal uptake of norepinephrine, serotonin, and dopamine, and does not inhibit monoamine oxidase. While the mechanism of action of bupropion, as with other antidepressants, is unknown, it is presumed that this action is mediated by noradrenergic and/or dopaminergic mechanisms.

Pharmacokinetics

Bupropion is a racemic mixture. The pharmacologic activity and pharmacokinetics of the individual enantiomers have not been studied. The mean elimination half-life (±SD) of bupropion after chronic dosing is 21 (±9) hours, and steady-state plasma concentrations of bupropion are reached within 8 days. In a study comparing chronic dosing with Wellbutrin SR tablets 150 mg twice daily to the immediate-release formulation of bupropion at 100 mg three times daily, peak plasma concentrations of bupropion at steady-state for Wellbutrin SR tablets were approximately 85% of those achieved with the immediate-release formulation. There was equivalence for bupropion AUCs, as well as equivalence for both peak plasma concentration and AUCs for all 3 of the detectable bupropion metabolites. Thus, at steady-state, Wellbutrin SR tablets, given twice daily, and the immediate-release formulation of bupropion, given 3 times daily, are essentially bioequivalent for both bupropion and the 3 quantitatively important metabolites.

Absorption

Following oral administration of Wellbutrin SR tablets to healthy volunteers, peak plasma concentrations of bupropion are achieved within 3 hours. Food increased C_{max} and AUC of bupropion by 11% and 17%, respectively, indicating that there is no clinically significant food effect.

Distribution

In vitro tests show that bupropion is 84% bound to human plasma proteins at concentrations up to 200 µg/ml. The extent of protein binding of the hydroxybupropion metabolite is similar to that for bupropion, whereas the extent of protein binding of the threohydrobupropion metabolite is about half that seen with bupropion.

Metabolism

Bupropion is extensively metabolized in humans. Three metabolites have been shown to be active: hydroxybupropion, which is formed via hydroxylation of the *tert*-butyl group of bupropion, and the amino-alcohol isomers threohydrobupropion and erythrohydrobupropion, which are formed via reduction of the carbonyl group. *In vitro* findings suggest that cytochrome P450IIB6 (CYP2B6) is the principal isoenzyme involved in the formation of hydroxybupropion, while cytochrome P450 isoenzymes are not involved in the formation of threohydrobupropion. Oxidation of the bupropion side chain results in the formation of a glycine conjugate of meta-chlorobenzoic acid, which is then excreted as the major urinary metabolite. The potency and toxicity of the metabolites relative to bupropion have not been fully characterized. However, it has been demonstrated in an antidepressant screening test in mice that hydroxybupropion is one-half as potent as bupropion, while threohydrobupropion and erythrohydrobupropion are 5-fold less potent than bupropion. This may be of clinical importance because the plasma concentrations of the metabolites are as high or higher than those of bupropion.

Because bupropion is extensively metabolized, there is the potential for drug-drug interactions, particularly with those agents that are metabolized by the cytochrome P450IIB6 (CYP2B6) isoenzyme. Although bupropion is not metabolized by cytochrome P450IID6 (CYP2D6), there is the potential for drug-drug interactions when bupropion is coadministered with drugs metabolized by this isoenzyme (see DRUG INTERACTIONS, Wellbutrin SR).

Following a single dose in humans, peak plasma concentrations of hydroxybupropion occur approximately 6 hours after administration of Wellbutrin SR tablets. Peak plasma concentrations of hydroxybupropion are approximately 10 times the peak level of the parent drug at steady-state. The elimination half-life of hydroxybupropion is approximately 20 (±5) hours, and its AUC at steady-state is about 17 times that of bupropion. The times to peak concentrations for the erythrohydrobupropion and threohydrobupropion metabolites are similar to that of the hydroxybupropion metabolite. However, their elimination half-lives are longer, 33 (±10) and 37 (±13) hours, respectively, and steady-state AUCs are 1.5 and 7 times that of bupropion, respectively.

Bupropion and its metabolites exhibit linear kinetics following chronic administration of 300-450 mg/day.

Elimination

Following oral administration of 200 mg of ^{14}C-bupropion in humans, 87% and 10% of the radioactive dose were recovered in the urine and feces, respectively. However, the fraction of the oral dose of bupropion excreted unchanged was only 0.5%, a finding consistent with the extensive metabolism of bupropion.

Population Subgroups

Factors or conditions altering metabolic capacity (*e.g.,* liver disease, congestive heart failure [CHF], age, concomitant medications, etc.) or elimination may be expected to influence the degree and extent of accumulation of the active metabolites of bupropion. The elimination of the major metabolites of bupropion may be affected by reduced renal or hepatic function because they are moderately polar compounds and are likely to undergo further metabolism or conjugation in the liver prior to urinary excretion.

Hepatic

The effect of hepatic impairment on the pharmacokinetics of bupropion was characterized in two single dose studies, one in patients with alcoholic liver disease and one in patients with mild to severe cirrhosis. The first study showed that the half-life of hydroxybupropion was significantly longer in 8 patients with alcoholic liver disease than in 8 healthy volunteers (32 ± 14 hours versus 21 ± 5 hours, respectively). Although not statistically significant, the AUCs for bupropion and hydroxybupropion were more variable and tended to be greater (by 53-57%) in patients with alcoholic liver disease. The differences in half-life for bupropion and the other metabolites in the 2 patient groups were minimal.

The second study showed no statistically significant differences in the pharmacokinetics of bupropion and its active metabolites in 9 patients with mild to moderate hepatic cirrhosis compared to 8 healthy volunteers. However, more variability was observed in some of the pharmacokinetic parameters for bupropion (AUC, C_{max}, and T_{max}) and its active metabolites (T½) in patients with mild to moderate hepatic cirrhosis. In addition, in patients with severe hepatic cirrhosis, the bupropion C_{max} and AUC were substantially increased (mean difference: by approximately 70% and 3-fold, respectively) and more variable when compared to values in healthy volunteers; the mean bupropion half-life was also longer (29 hours in patients with severe hepatic cirrhosis versus 19 hours in healthy subjects). For the metabolite hydroxybupropion, the mean C_{max} was approximately 69% lower. For the combined amino-alcohol isomers threohydrobupropion and erythrohydrobupropion, the mean C_{max} was approximately 31% lower. The mean AUC increased by about 1½-fold for hydroxybupropion and about 2½-fold for threo/erythrohydrobupropion. The median T_{max} was observed 19 hours later for hydroxybupropion and 31 hours later for threo/erythrohydrobupropion. The mean half-lives for hydroxybupropion and threo/erythrohydrobupropion were increased 5- and 2-fold, respectively, in patients with severe hepatic cirrhosis compared to healthy volunteers (see WARNINGS, Wellbutrin SR; PRECAUTIONS, Wellbutrin SR; and DOSAGE AND ADMINISTRATION, Wellbutrin SR).

Renal

The effect of renal disease on the pharmacokinetics of bupropion has not been studied. The elimination of the major metabolites of bupropion may be affected by reduced renal function.

Left Ventricular Dysfunction

During a chronic dosing study with bupropion in 14 depressed patients with left ventricular dysfunction (history of CHF or an enlarged heart on x-ray), no apparent effect on the pharmacokinetics of bupropion or its metabolites was revealed, compared to healthy volunteers.

Age

The effects of age on the pharmacokinetics of bupropion and its metabolites have not been fully characterized, but an exploration of steady-state bupropion concentrations from several depression efficacy studies involving patients dosed in a range of 300-750 mg/day, on a three times daily schedule, revealed no relationship between age (18-83 years) and plasma concentration of bupropion. A single dose pharmacokinetic study demonstrated that the disposition of bupropion and its metabolites in elderly subjects was similar to that of younger subjects. These data suggest there is no prominent effect of age on bupropion concentration; however, another pharmacokinetic study, single and multiple dose, has suggested that the elderly are at increased risk for accumulation of bupropion and its metabolites (see PRECAUTIONS, Wellbutrin SR, Geriatric Use).

Gender

A single dose study involving 12 healthy male and 12 healthy female volunteers revealed no sex-related differences in the pharmacokinetic parameters of bupropion.

Smokers

The effects of cigarette smoking on the pharmacokinetics of bupropion were studied in 34 healthy male and female volunteers; 17 were chronic cigarette smokers and 17 were nonsmokers. Following oral administration of a single 150 mg dose of bupropion, there was no statistically significant difference in C_{max}, half-life, T_{max}, AUC, or clearance of bupropion or its active metabolites between smokers and nonsmokers.

ZYBAN

Pharmacodynamics

Bupropion is a relatively weak inhibitor of the neuronal uptake of norepinephrine, serotonin, and dopamine, and does not inhibit monoamine oxidase. The mechanism by which Zyban enhances the ability of patients to abstain from smoking is unknown. However, it is presumed that this action is mediated by noradrenergic and/or dopaminergic mechanisms.

Pharmacokinetics

Bupropion is a racemic mixture. The pharmacologic activity and pharmacokinetics of the individual enantiomers have not been studied. Bupropion follows biphasic pharmacokinetics best described by a 2-compartment model. The terminal phase has a mean half-life (±% CV) of about 21 hours (±20%), while the distribution phase has a mean half-life of 3-4 hours.

Absorption

Bupropion has not been administered intravenously to humans; therefore, the absolute bioavailability of Zyban sustained-release tablets in humans has not been determined. In rat and dog studies, the bioavailability of bupropion ranged from 5-20%.

Following oral administration of Zyban to healthy volunteers, peak plasma concentrations of bupropion are achieved within 3 hours. The mean peak concentration (C_{max}) values were 91 and 143 ng/ml from two single dose (150 mg) studies. At steady-state, the mean C_{max} following a 150 mg dose every 12 hours is 136 ng/ml.

In a single dose study, food increased the C_{max} of bupropion by 11% and the extent of absorption as defined by area under the plasma concentration-time curve (AUC) by 17%. The mean time to peak concentration (T_{max}) was prolonged by 1 hour. This effect was of no clinical significance.

Distribution

In vitro tests show that bupropion is 84% bound to human plasma proteins at concentrations up to 200 µg/ml. The extent of protein binding of the hydroxybupropion metabolite is similar to that for bupropion, whereas the extent of protein binding of the threohydrobupropion metabolite is about half that seen with bupropion. The volume of distribution (Vss/F) estimated from a single 150 mg dose given to 17 subjects is 1950 L (20% CV).

Metabolism

Bupropion is extensively metabolized in humans. Three metabolites have been shown to be active: hydroxybupropion, which is formed via hydroxylation of the *tert*-butyl group of bupropion, and the amino-alcohol isomers threohydrobupropion and erythrohydrobupropion, which are formed via reduction of the carbonyl group. *In vitro* findings suggest that cytochrome P450IIB6 (CYP2B6) is the principal isoenzyme involved in the formation of hydroxybupropion, while cytochrome P450 isoenzymes are not involved in the formation of threohydrobupropion. Oxidation of the bupropion side chain results in the formation of a glycine conjugate of meta-chlorobenzoic acid, which is then excreted as the major urinary metabolite. The potency and toxicity of the metabolites relative to bupropion have not been fully characterized. However, it has been demonstrated in an antidepressant screening test in mice that hydroxybupropion is one-half as potent as bupropion, while threohydrobupropion and erythrohydrobupropion are 5-fold less potent than bupropion. This may be of clinical importance because the plasma concentrations of the metabolites areas high or higher than those of bupropion.

Because bupropion is extensively metabolized, there is the potential for drug-drug interactions, particularly with those agents that are metabolized by the cytochrome P450IIB6 (CYP2B6) isoenzyme. Although bupropion is not metabolized by cytochrome P450IID6 (CYP2D6), there is the potential for drug-drug interactions when bupropion is coadministered with drugs metabolized by this isoenzyme (see DRUG INTERACTIONS, Zyban).

Following a single dose in humans, peak plasma concentrations of hydroxybupropion occur approximately 6 hours after administration of Zyban tablets. Peak plasma concentrations of hydroxybupropion are approximately 10 times the peak level of the parent drug at steady-state. The elimination half-life of hydroxybupropion is approximately 20 (±5) hours, and its AUC at steady-state is about 17 times that of bupropion. The times to peak concentrations for the erythrohydrobupropion and threohydrobupropion metabolites are similar to that of the hydroxybupropion metabolite; however, their elimination half-lives are longer, 33 (±10) and 37 (±13) hours, respectively, and steady-state AUCs are 1.5 and 7 times that of bupropion, respectively.

Bupropion and its metabolites exhibit linear kinetics following chronic administration of 300-450 mg/day.

Elimination

The mean (±% CV) apparent clearance (Cl/F) estimated from two single dose (150 mg) studies are 135 (±20%) and 209 L/h (±21%). Following chronic dosing of 150 mg of Zyban every 12 hours for 14 days (n=34), the mean Cl/F at steady-state was 160 L/h (±23%). The mean elimination half-life of bupropion estimated from a series of studies is approximately 21 hours. Estimates of the half-lives of the metabolites determined from a multiple dose study were 20 hours (±25%) for hydroxybupropion, 37 hours (±35%) for threohydrobupropion, and 33 hours (±30%) for erythrohydrobupropion. Steady-state plasma concentrations of bupropion and metabolites are reached within 5 and 8 days, respectively.

Following oral administration of 200 mg of ^{14}C-bupropion in humans, 87% and 10% of the radioactive dose were recovered in the urine and feces, respectively. The fraction of the oral dose of bupropion excreted unchanged was only 0.5%.

The effects of cigarette smoking on the pharmacokinetics of bupropion were studied in 34 healthy male and female volunteers; 17 were chronic cigarette smokers and 17 were nonsmokers. Following oral administration of a single 150 mg dose of Zyban, there was no statistically significant difference in C_{max}, half-life, T_{max}, AUC, or clearance of bupropion or its major metabolites between smokers and nonsmokers.

In a study comparing the treatment combination of Zyban and nicotine transdermal system (NTS) versus Zyban alone, no statistically significant differences were observed between the 2 treatment groups of combination Zyban and NTS (n=197) and Zyban alone (n=193) in the plasma concentrations of bupropion or its active metabolites at Weeks 3 and 6.

Population Subgroups

Factors or conditions altering metabolic capacity (*e.g.*, liver disease, congestive heart failure, age, concomitant medications, etc.) or elimination may be expected to influence the degree and extent of accumulation of the active metabolites of bupropion. The elimination of the major metabolites of bupropion may be affected by reduced renal or hepatic function because they are moderately polar compounds and are likely to undergo further metabolism or conjugation in the liver prior to urinary excretion.

Hepatic

The effect of hepatic impairment on the pharmacokinetics of bupropion was characterized in two single dose studies, one in patients with alcoholic liver disease and one in patients with mild to severe cirrhosis.

The first study showed that the half-life of hydroxybupropion was significantly longer in 8 patients with alcoholic liver disease than in 8 healthy volunteers (32 ± 14 hours versus 21 ± 5 hours, respectively). Although not statistically significant, the AUCs for bupropion and hydroxybupropion were more variable and tended to be greater (by 53-57%) in patients with alcoholic liver disease. The differences in half-life for bupropion and the other metabolites in the 2 patient groups were minimal.

The second study showed that there were no statistically significant differences in the pharmacokinetics of bupropion and its active metabolites in 9 patients with mild to moderate hepatic cirrhosis compared to 8 healthy volunteers. However, more variability was observed in some of the pharmacokinetic parameters for bupropion (AUC, C_{max}, and T_{max})

and its active metabolites (T½) in patients with mild to moderate hepatic cirrhosis. In addition, in patients with severe hepatic cirrhosis, the bupropion C_{max} and AUC were substantially increased (mean difference: by approximately 70% and 3-fold, respectively) and more variable when compared to values in healthy volunteers; the mean bupropion half-life was also longer (29 hours in patients with severe hepatic cirrhosis versus 19 hours in healthy subjects). For the metabolite hydroxybupropion, the mean C_{max} was approximately 69% lower.

For the combined amino-alcohol isomers threohydrobupropion and erythrohydrobupropion, the mean C_{max} was approximately 31% lower. The mean AUC increased by 28% for hydroxybupropion and 50% for threo/erythrohydrobupropion.

The median T_{max} was observed 19 hours later for hydroxybupropion and 21 hours later for threo/erythrohydrobupropion. The mean half-lives for hydroxybupropion and threo/erythrohydrobupropion were increased 2- and 4-fold, respectively, in patients with severe hepatic cirrhosis compared to healthy volunteers (see WARNINGS, Zyban; PRECAUTIONS, Zyban; and DOSAGE AND ADMINISTRATION, Zyban).

Renal

The effect of renal disease on the pharmacokinetics of bupropion has not been studied. The elimination of the major metabolites of bupropion may be affected by reduced renal function.

Left Ventricular Dysfunction

During a chronic dosing study with bupropion in 14 depressed patients with left ventricular dysfunction (history of congestive heart failure [CHF] or an enlarged heart on x-ray), no apparent effect on the pharmacokinetics of bupropion or its metabolites, compared to healthy normal volunteers, was revealed.

Age

The effects of age on the pharmacokinetics of bupropion and its metabolites have not been fully characterized, but an exploration of steady-state bupropion concentrations from several depression efficacy studies involving patients dosed in a range of 300-750 mg/day, on a 3 times a day schedule, revealed no relationship between age (18-83 years) and plasma concentration of bupropion. A single dose pharmacokinetic study demonstrated that the disposition of bupropion and its metabolites in elderly subjects was similar to that of younger subjects. These data suggest there is no prominent effect of age on bupropion concentration; however, another pharmacokinetic study, single and multiple dose, has suggested that the elderly are at increased risk for accumulation of bupropion and its metabolites (see PRECAUTIONS, Zyban, Geriatric Use).

Gender

A single dose study involving 12 healthy male and 12 healthy female volunteers revealed no sex-related differences in the pharmacokinetic parameters of bupropion.

INDICATIONS AND USAGE

WELLBUTRIN

Wellbutrin is indicated for the treatment of depression. A physician considering Wellbutrin for the management of a patient's first episode of depression should be aware that the drug may cause generalized seizures in a dose-dependent manner with an approximate incidence of 0.4% (4/1000). This incidence of seizures may exceed that of other marketed antidepressants by as much as 4-fold. This relative risk is only an approximate estimate because no direct comparative studies have been conducted (see WARNINGS, Wellbutrin).

The efficacy of Wellbutrin has been established in three placebo-controlled trials, including two of approximately 3 weeks' duration in depressed inpatients and one of approximately 6 weeks' duration in depressed outpatients. The depressive disorder of the patients studied corresponds most closely to the Major Depression category of the APA Diagnostic and Statistical Manual III.

Major Depression implies a prominent and relatively persistent depressed or dysphoric mood that usually interferes with daily functioning (nearly every day for at least 2 weeks); it should include at least 4 of the following 8 symptoms: change in appetite, change in sleep, psychomotor agitation or retardation, loss of interest in usual activities or decrease in sexual drive, increased fatigability, feelings of guilt or worthlessness, slowed thinking or impaired concentration, and suicidal ideation or attempts.

Effectiveness of Wellbutrin in long-term use, that is, for more than 6 weeks, has not been systematically evaluated in controlled trials. Therefore, the physician who elects to use Wellbutrin for extended periods should periodically reevaluate the long-term usefulness of the drug for the individual patient.

WELLBUTRIN SR

Wellbutrin SR is indicated for the treatment of depression.

The efficacy of bupropion in the treatment of depression was established in two 4 week controlled trials of depressed inpatients and in one 6 week controlled trial of depressed outpatients whose diagnoses corresponded most closely to the Major Depression category of the APA Diagnostic and Statistical Manual (DSM) (see CLINICAL PHARMACOLOGY, Wellbutrin SR).

A major depressive episode (DSM-IV) implies the presence of (1) depressed mood or (2) loss of interest or pleasure; in addition, at least five of the following symptoms have been present during the same 2 week period and represent a change from previous functioning: depressed mood, markedly diminished interest or pleasure in usual activities, significant change in weight and/or appetite, insomnia or hypersomnia, psychomotor agitation or retardation, increased fatigue, feelings of guilt or worthlessness, slowed thinking or impaired concentration, a suicide attempt or suicidal ideation.

The efficacy of Wellbutrin SR in maintaining an antidepressant response for up to 44 weeks following 8 weeks of acute treatment was demonstrated in a placebo-controlled trial (see CLINICAL PHARMACOLOGY, Wellbutrin SR). Nevertheless, the physician who elects to use Wellbutrin SR for extended periods should periodically reevaluate the long-term usefulness of the drug for the individual patient.

ZYBAN

Zyban is indicated as an aid to smoking cessation treatment.

CONTRAINDICATIONS

WELLBUTRIN

Wellbutrin is contraindicated in patients with a seizure disorder.

Wellbutrin is contraindicated in patients treated with Zyban (bupropion hydrochloride) sustained-release tablets, or any other medications that contain bupropion because the incidence of seizure is dose dependent.

Wellbutrin is also contraindicated in patients with a current or prior diagnosis of bulimia or anorexia nervosa because of a higher incidence of seizures noted in such patients treated with Wellbutrin.

Wellbutrin is contraindicated in patients undergoing abrupt discontinuation of alcohol or sedatives (including benzodiazepines).

The concurrent administration of Wellbutrin and a monoamine oxidase (MAO) inhibitor is contraindicated. At least 14 days should elapse between discontinuation of an MAO inhibitor and initiation of treatment with Wellbutrin.

Wellbutrin is contraindicated in patients who have shown an allergic response to bupropion or the other ingredients that make up Wellbutrin tablets.

WELLBUTRIN SR

Wellbutrin SR is contraindicated in patients with a seizure disorder.

Wellbutrin SR is contraindicated in patients treated with Zyban (bupropion hydrochloride) sustained-release tablets, or any other medications that contain bupropion because the incidence of seizure is dose dependent.

Wellbutrin SR is contraindicated in patients with a current or prior diagnosis of bulimia or anorexia nervosa because of a higher incidence of seizures noted in patients treated for bulimia with the immediate-release formulation of bupropion.

Wellbutrin SR is contraindicated in patients undergoing abrupt discontinuation of alcohol or sedatives (including benzodiazepines).

The concurrent administration of Wellbutrin SR tablets and a monoamine oxidase (MAO) inhibitor is contraindicated. At least 14 days should elapse between discontinuation of an MAO inhibitor and initiation of treatment with Wellbutrin SR tablets.

Wellbutrin SR is contraindicated in patients who have shown an allergic response to bupropion or the other ingredients that make up Wellbutrin SR tablets.

ZYBAN

Zyban is contraindicated in patients with a seizure disorder.

Zyban is contraindicated in patients treated with Wellbutrin, Wellbutrin SR, or any other medications that contain bupropion because the incidence of seizure is dose dependent.

Zyban is contraindicated in patients with a current or prior diagnosis of bulimia or anorexia nervosa because of a higher incidence of seizures noted in patients treated for bulimia with the immediate-release formulation of bupropion.

Zyban is contraindicated in patients undergoing abrupt discontinuation of alcohol or sedatives (including benzodiazepines).

The concurrent administration of Zyban and a monoamine oxidase (MAO) inhibitor is contraindicated. At least 14 days should elapse between discontinuation of an MAO inhibitor and initiation of treatment with Zyban.

Zyban is contraindicated in patients who have shown an allergic response to bupropion or the other ingredients that make up Zyban.

WARNINGS

WELLBUTRIN

Patients should be made aware that Wellbutrin contains the same active ingredient found in Zyban, used as an aid to smoking cessation treatment, and that Wellbutrin should not be used in combination with Zyban, or any other medications that contain bupropion.

Seizures

Bupropion is associated with seizures in approximately 0.4% (4/1000) of patients treated at doses up to 450 mg/day. This incidence of seizures may exceed that of other marketed antidepressants by as much as 4-fold. This relative risk is only an approximate estimate because no direct comparative studies have been conducted. The estimated seizure incidence for Wellbutrin increases almost 10-fold between 450 and 600 mg/day, which is twice the usually required daily dose (300 mg) and one and one-third the maximum recommended daily dose (450 mg). Given the wide variability among individuals and their capacity to metabolize and eliminate drugs this disproportionate increase in seizure incidence with dose incrementation calls for caution in dosing.

During the initial development, 25 among approximately 2400 patients treated with Wellbutrin experienced seizures. At the time of seizure, 7 patients were receiving daily doses of 450 mg or below for an incidence of 0.33% (3/1000) within the recommended dose range. Twelve (12) patients experienced seizures at 600 mg/day (2.3% incidence); 6 additional patients had seizures at daily doses between 600 and 900 mg (2.8% incidence).

A separate, prospective study was conducted to determine the incidence of seizure during an 8 week treatment exposure in approximately 3200 additional patients who received daily doses of up to 450 mg. Patients were permitted to continue treatment beyond 8 weeks if clinically indicated. Eight seizures occurred during the initial 8 week treatment period and 5 seizures were reported in patients continuing treatment beyond 8 weeks, resulting in a total seizure incidence of 0.4%.

The risk of seizure appears to be strongly associated with dose. Sudden and large increments in dose may contribute to increased risk. While many seizures occurred early in the course of treatment, some seizures did occur after several weeks at fixed dose. Wellbutrin should be discontinued and not restarted in patients who experience a seizure while on treatment.

The risk of seizure is also related to patient factors, clinical situations, and concomitant medications, which must be considered in selection of patients for therapy with Wellbutrin.

Patient Factors: **Predisposing factors that may increase the risk of seizure with bupropion use include history of head trauma or prior seizure, CNS tumor, the presence of severe hepatic cirrhosis, and concomitant medications that lower seizure threshold.**

Clinical Situations: **Circumstances associated with an increased seizure risk include, among others, excessive use of alcohol or sedatives (including benzodiazepines); addiction to opiates, cocaine, or stimulants; use of over-the-counter stimulants and anorectics; and diabetes treated with oral hypoglycemics or insulin.**

Concomitant Medications: **Many medications (*e.g.,* antipsychotics, antidepressants, theophylline, systemic steroids) are known to lower seizure threshold.**

Recommendations for Reducing the Risk of Seizure

Retrospective analysis of clinical experience gained during the development of Wellbutrin suggests that the risk of seizure may be minimized if:

- **The total daily dose of Wellbutrin does *not* exceed 450 mg,**
- **The daily dose is administered three times daily, with each single dose *not* to exceed 150 mg to avoid high peak concentrations of bupropion and/or its metabolites, and**
- **The rate of incrementation of dose is very gradual.**

Extreme caution should be used when Wellbutrin is administered to patients with a history of seizure, cranial trauma, or other predisposition(s) toward seizure, or prescribed with other agents (*e.g.,* antipsychotics, other antidepressants, theophylline, systemic steroids, etc.) that lower seizure threshold.

Hepatic Impairment

Wellbutrin should be used with extreme caution in patients with severe hepatic cirrhosis. In these patients a reduced dose and/or frequency is required, as peak bupropion levels, as well as AUC, are substantially increased and accumulation is likely to occur in such patients to a greater extent than usual. The dose should not exceed 75 mg once a day in these patients (see CLINICAL PHARMACOLOGY, Wellbutrin; PRECAUTIONS, Wellbutrin; and DOSAGE AND ADMINISTRATION, Wellbutrin).

Potential for Hepatotoxicity

In rats receiving large doses of bupropion chronically, there was an increase in incidence of hepatic hyperplastic nodules and hepatocellular hypertrophy. In dogs receiving large doses of bupropion chronically, various histologic changes were seen in the liver, and laboratory tests suggesting mild hepatocellular injury were noted.

WELLBUTRIN SR

Patients should be made aware that Wellbutrin SR contains the same active ingredient found in Zyban, used as an aid to smoking cessation treatment, and that Wellbutrin SR should not be used in combination with Zyban, or any other medications that contain bupropion.

Seizures

Bupropion is associated with a dose-related risk of seizures. The risk of seizures is also related to patient factors, clinical situations, and concomitant medications, which must be considered in selection of patients for therapy with Wellbutrin SR. Wellbutrin SR should be discontinued and not restarted in patients who experience a seizure while on treatment.

Dose

At doses of Wellbutrin SR up to a dose of 300 mg/day, the incidence of seizure is approximately 0.1% (1/1000) and increases to approximately 0.4% (4/1000) at the maximum recommended dose of 400 mg/day.

Data for the immediate-release formulation of bupropion revealed a seizure incidence of approximately 0.4% (*i.e.,* 13 of 3200 patients followed prospectively) in patients treated at doses in a range of 300-450 mg/day. The 450 mg/day upper limit of this dose range is close to the currently recommended maximum dose of 400 mg/day for Wellbutrin SR tablets. This seizure incidence (0.4%) may exceed that of other marketed antidepressants and Wellbutrin SR tablets up to 300 mg/day by as much as 4-fold. This relative risk is only an approximate estimate because no direct comparative studies have been conducted.

Additional data accumulated for the immediate-release formulation of bupropion suggested that the estimated seizure incidence increases almost 10-fold between 450 and 600 mg/day, which is twice the usual adult dose and one and one-half the maximum recommended daily dose (400 mg) of Wellbutrin SR tablets. This disproportionate increase in seizure incidence with dose incrementation calls for caution in dosing.

Data for Wellbutrin SR tablets revealed a seizure incidence of approximately 0.1% (*i.e.,* 3 of 3100 patients followed prospectively) in patients treated at doses in a range of 100-300 mg/day. It is not possible to know if the lower seizure incidence observed in this study involving the sustained-release formulation of bupropion resulted from the different formulation or the lower dose used. However, as noted above, the immediate-release and sustained-release formulations are bioequivalent with regard to both rate and extent of absorption during steady-state (the most pertinent condition to estimating seizure incidence), since most observed seizures occur under steady-state conditions.

Patient Factors

Predisposing factors that may increase the risk of seizure with bupropion use include history of head trauma or prior seizure, central nervous system (CNS) tumor, the presence of severe hepatic cirrhosis, and concomitant medications that lower seizure threshold.

Clinical Situations

Circumstances associated with an increased seizure risk include, among others, excessive use of alcohol or sedatives (including benzodiazepines); addiction to opiates, cocaine, or stimulants; use of over-the-counter stimulants and anorectics; and diabetes treated with oral hypoglycemics or insulin.

Concomitant Medications

Many medications (*e.g.,* antipsychotics, antidepressants, theophylline, systemic steroids) are known to lower seizure threshold.

Recommendations for Reducing the Risk of Seizure

Retrospective analysis of clinical experience gained during the development of bupropion suggests that the risk of seizure may be minimized if:

The total daily dose of Wellbutrin SR tablets does *not* exceed 400 mg,
The daily dose is administered twice daily, and
The rate of incrementation of dose is gradual.
No single dose should exceed 200 mg to avoid high peak concentrations of bupropion and/or its metabolites.

Wellbutrin SR should be administered with extreme caution to patients with a history of seizure, cranial trauma, or other predisposition(s) toward seizure, or patients treated with other agents (*e.g.,* antipsychotics, other antidepressants, theophylline, systemic steroids, etc.) that lower seizure threshold.

Hepatic Impairment

Wellbutrin SR should be used with extreme caution in patients with severe hepatic cirrhosis. In these patients a reduced frequency and/or dose is required, as peak bupropion levels, as well as AUC, are substantially increased and accumulation is likely to occur in such patients to a greater extent than usual. The dose should not exceed 100 mg every day or 150 mg every other day in these patients (CLINICAL PHARMACOLOGY, Wellbutrin SR; PRECAUTIONS, Wellbutrin SR; and DOSAGE AND ADMINISTRATION, Wellbutrin SR).

Potential for Hepatotoxicity

In rats receiving large doses of bupropion chronically, there was an increase in incidence of hepatic hyperplastic nodules and hepatocellular hypertrophy. In dogs receiving large doses of bupropion chronically, various histologic changes were seen in the liver, and laboratory tests suggesting mild hepatocellular injury were noted.

ZYBAN

Patients should be made aware that Zyban contains the same active ingredient found in Wellbutrin and Wellbutrin SR used to treat depression, and that Zyban should not be used in combination with Wellbutrin, Wellbutrin SR, or any other medications that contain bupropion.

Because the use of bupropion is associated with a dose-dependent risk of seizures, *clinicians should not prescribe doses over 300 mg/day for smoking cessation.* The risk of seizures is also related to patient factors, clinical situation, and concurrent medications, which must be considered in selection of patients for therapy with Zyban. ZYBAN should be discontinued and not restarted in patients who experience a seizure while on treatment.

Dose: For smoking cessation, doses above 300 mg/day should not be used. **The seizure rate associated with doses of sustained-release bupropion up to 300 mg/day is approximately 0.1% (1/1000). This incidence was prospectively determined during an 8 week treatment exposure in approximately 3100 depressed patients. Data for the immediate-release formulation of bupropion revealed a seizure incidence of approximately 0.4% (4/1000) in depressed patients treated at doses in a range of 300-450 mg/day. In addition, the estimated seizure incidence increases almost 10-fold between 450 and 600 mg/day.**

Patient Factors: **Predisposing factors that may increase the risk of seizure with bupropion use include history of head trauma or prior seizure, central nervous system (CNS) tumor, the presence of severe hepatic cirrhosis, and concomitant medications that lower seizure threshold.**

Clinical Situations: **Circumstances associated with an increased seizure risk include, among others, excessive use of alcohol or sedatives (including benzodiazepines); addiction to opiates, cocaine, or stimulants; use of over-the-counter stimulants and anorectics; and diabetes treated with oral hypoglycemics or insulin.**

Concomitant Medications: **Many medications (*e.g.,* antipsychotics, antidepressants, theophylline, systemic steroids) are known to lower seizure threshold.**

Recommendations for Reducing the Risk of Seizure

Retrospective analysis of clinical experience gained during the development of bupropion suggests that the risk of seizure may be minimized if:

- **The total daily dose of Zyban does *not* exceed 300 mg (the maximum recommended dose for smoking cessation), and**
- **The recommended daily dose for most patients (300 mg/day) is administered in divided doses (150 mg twice daily).**
- **No single dose should exceed 150 mg to avoid high peak concentrations of bupropion and/or its metabolites.**

Zyban should be administered with extreme caution to patients with a history of seizure, cranial trauma, or other predisposition(s) toward seizure, or patients treated with other agents (*e.g.,* antipsychotics, antidepressants, theophylline, systemic steroids, etc.) that lower seizure threshold.

Hepatic Impairment

Zyban should be used with extreme caution in patients with severe hepatic cirrhosis. In these patients a reduced frequency of dosing is required, as peak bupropion levels are substantially increased and accumulation is likely to occur in such patients to a greater extent than usual. The dose should not exceed 150 mg every other day in these

patients (see CLINICAL PHARMACOLOGY, Zyban; PRECAUTIONS, Zyban; and DOSAGE AND ADMINISTRATION, Zyban).

Potential for Hepatotoxicity

In rats receiving large doses of bupropion chronically, there was an increase in incidence of hepatic hyperplastic nodules and hepatocellular hypertrophy. In dogs receiving large doses of bupropion chronically, various histologic changes were seen in the liver, and laboratory tests suggesting mild hepatocellular injury were noted.

PRECAUTIONS

WELLBUTRIN

General

Agitation and Insomnia

A substantial proportion of patients treated with Wellbutrin experience some degree of increased restlessness, agitation, anxiety, and insomnia, especially shortly after initiation of treatment. In clinical studies, these symptoms were sometimes of sufficient magnitude to require treatment with sedative/hypnotic drugs. In approximately 2% of patients, symptoms were sufficiently severe to require discontinuation of treatment with Wellbutrin.

Psychosis, Confusion, and Other Neuropsychiatric Phenomena

Patients treated with Wellbutrin have been reported to show a variety of neuropsychiatric signs and symptoms including delusions, hallucinations, psychotic episodes, confusion, and paranoia. Because of the uncontrolled nature of many studies, it is impossible to provide a precise estimate of the extent of risk imposed by treatment with Wellbutrin. In several cases, neuropsychiatric phenomena abated upon dose reduction and/or withdrawal of treatment.

Activation of Psychosis and/or Mania

Antidepressants can precipitate manic episodes in Bipolar Manic Depressive patients during the depressed phase of their illness and may activate latent psychosis in other susceptible patients. Wellbutrin is expected to pose similar risks.

Altered Appetite and Weight

A weight loss of greater than 5 lb occurred in 28% of patients receiving Wellbutrin. This incidence is approximately double that seen in comparable patients treated with tricyclics or placebo. Furthermore, while 34.5% of patients receiving tricyclic antidepressants gained weight, only 9.4% of patients treated with Wellbutrin did. Consequently, if weight loss is a major presenting sign of a patient's depressive illness, the anorectic and/or weight reducing potential of Wellbutrin should be considered.

Suicide

The possibility of a suicide attempt is inherent in depression and may persist until significant remission occurs. Accordingly, prescriptions for Wellbutrin should be written for the smallest number of tablets consistent with good patient management.

Allergic Reactions

Anaphylactoid/anaphylactic reactions characterized by symptoms such as pruritus, urticaria, angioedema, and dyspnea requiring medical treatment have been reported in clinical trials with bupropion. In addition, there have been rare spontaneous post-marketing reports of erythema multiforme, Stevens-Johnson syndrome, and anaphylactic shock associated with bupropion. A patient should stop taking Wellbutrin and consult a doctor if experiencing allergic or anaphylactoid/anaphylactic reactions (*e.g.,* skin rash, pruritus, hives, chest pain, edema, and shortness of breath) during treatment.

Arthralgia, myalgia, and fever with rash and other symptoms suggestive of delayed hypersensitivity have been reported in association with bupropion. These symptoms may resemble serum sickness.

Cardiovascular Effects

In clinical practice, hypertension, in some cases severe, requiring acute treatment, has been reported in patients receiving bupropion alone and in combination with nicotine replacement therapy. These events have been observed in both patients with and without evidence of preexisting hypertension.

Data from a comparative study of the sustained-release formulation of bupropion (Zyban sustained-release tablets), nicotine transdermal system (NTS), the combination of sustained-release bupropion plus NTS, and placebo as an aid to smoking cessation suggest a higher incidence of treatment-emergent hypertension in patients treated with the combination of sustained-release bupropion and NTS. In this study, 6.1% of patients treated with the combination of sustained-release bupropion and NTS had treatment-emergent hypertension compared to 2.5%, 1.6%, and 3.1% of patients treated with sustained-release bupropion, NTS, and placebo, respectively. The majority of these patients had evidence of preexisting hypertension. Three patients (1.2%) treated with the combination of Zyban and NTS and 1 patient (0.4%) treated with NTS had study medication discontinued due to hypertension compared to none of the patients treated with Zyban or placebo. Monitoring of blood pressure is recommended in patients who receive the combination of bupropion and nicotine replacement.

There is no clinical experience establishing the safety of Wellbutrin in patients with a recent history of myocardial infarction or unstable heart disease. Therefore, care should be exercised if it is used in these groups. Bupropion was well tolerated in depressed patients who had previously developed orthostatic hypotension while receiving tricyclic antidepressants and was also generally well tolerated in a group of 36 depressed inpatients with stable congestive heart failure (CHF). However, bupropion was associated with a rise in supine blood pressure in the study of patients with CHF, resulting in discontinuation of treatment in 2 patients for exacerbation of baseline hypertension.

Hepatic Impairment

Wellbutrin should be used with extreme caution in patients with severe hepatic cirrhosis. In these patients, a reduced dose and frequency is required. Wellbutrin should be used with caution in patients with hepatic impairment (including mild to moderate hepatic cirrhosis) and a reduced frequency and/or dose should be considered in patients with mild to moderate hepatic cirrhosis.

All patients with hepatic impairment should be closely monitored for possible adverse effects that could indicate high drug and metabolite levels (see CLINICAL PHARMACOLOGY, Wellbutrin; WARNINGS, Wellbutrin; and DOSAGE AND ADMINISTRATION, Wellbutrin).

Renal Impairment

No studies have been conducted in patients with renal impairment. Bupropion is extensively metabolized in the liver to active metabolites, which are further metabolized and excreted by the kidneys. Wellbutrin should be used with caution in patients with renal impairment and a reduced frequency and/or dose should be considered as bupropion and its metabolites may accumulate in such patients to a greater extent than usual. The patient should be closely monitored for possible adverse effects that could indicate high drug or metabolite levels.

Information for the Patient

See the Patient Instructions that are distributed with the prescription for complete instructions.

Patients should be made aware that Wellbutrin contains the same active ingredient found in Zyban, used as an aid to smoking cessation, and that Wellbutrin should not be used in combination with Zyban or any other medications that contain bupropion hydrochloride.

Physicians are advised to discuss the following issues with patients.

Patients should be instructed to take Wellbutrin in equally divided doses 3 or 4 times a day to minimize the risk of seizure.

Patients should be told that Wellbutrin should be discontinued and not restarted if they experience a seizure while on treatment.

Patients should be told that any CNS-active drug like Wellbutrin may impair their ability to perform tasks requiring judgment or motor and cognitive skills. Consequently, until they are reasonably certain that Wellbutrin does not adversely affect their performance, they should refrain from driving an automobile or operating complex, hazardous machinery.

Patients should be told that the excessive use or abrupt discontinuation of alcohol or sedabives (including benzodiazepines) may alter the seizure threshold. Some patients have reported lower alcohol tolerance during treatment with Wellbutrin. Patients should be advised that the consumption of alcohol should be minimized or avoided.

Patients should be advised to inform their physicians if they are taking or plan to take any prescription or over-the-counter drugs. Concern is warranted because Wellbutrin and other drugs may affect each other's metabolism.

Patients should be advised to notify their physicians if they become pregnant or intend to become pregnant during therapy.

Laboratory Tests

There are no specific laboratory tests recommended.

Carcinogenesis, Mutagenesis, and Impairment of Fertility

Lifetime carcinogenicity studies were performed in rats and mice at doses up to 300 and 150 mg/kg/day, respectively. In the rat study there was an increase in nodular proliferative lesions of the liver at doses of 100-300 mg/kg/day; lower doses were not tested. The question of whether or not such lesions may be precursors of neoplasms of the liver is currently unresolved. Similar liver lesions were not seen in the mouse study, and no increase in malignant tumors of the liver and other organs was seen in either study.

Bupropion produced a borderline positive response (2-3 times control mutation rate) in some strains in the Ames bacterial mutagenicity test, and a high oral dose (300 mg/kg, but not 100 or 200 mg/kg) produced a low incidence of chromosomal aberrations in rats. The relevance of these results in estimating the risk of human exposure to therapeutic doses is unknown.

A fertility study was performed in rats; no evidence of impairment of fertility was encountered at oral doses up to 300 mg/kg/day.

Pregnancy, Teratogenic Effects, Pregnancy Category B

Reproduction studies have been performed in rabbits and rats at doses up to 15-45 times the human daily dose and have revealed no definitive evidence of impaired fertility or harm to the fetus due to bupropion. (In rabbits, a slightly increased incidence of fetal abnormalities was seen in two studies, but there was no increase in any specific abnormality). There are no adequate and well-controlled studies in pregnant women. Because animal reproduction studies are not always predictive of human response, this drug should be used during pregnancy only if clearly needed.

To monitor fetal outcomes of pregnant women exposed to Wellbutrin, GlaxoSmithKline maintains a Bupropion Pregnancy Registry. Health care providers are encouraged to register patients by calling 800-336-2176.

Labor and Delivery

The effect of Wellbutrin on labor and delivery in humans is unknown.

Nursing Mothers

Like many other drugs, bupropion and its metabolites are secreted in human milk. Because of the potential for serious adverse reactions in nursing infants from Wellbutrin, a decision should be made whether to discontinue nursing or to discontinue the drug, taking into account the importance of the drug to the mother.

Pediatric Use

The safety and effectiveness of Wellbutrin in pediatric patients under 18 years old have not been established. The immediate-release formulation of bupropion was studied in 104 pediatric patients (age range, 6-16) in clinical trials of the drug for other indications. Although generally well tolerated, the limited exposure is insufficient to assess the safety of bupropion in pediatric patients.

B

Geriatric Use

Of the approximately 6000 patients who participated in clinical trials with bupropion sustained-release tablets (depression and smoking cessation studies), 275 were 65 and over and 47 were 75 and over. In addition, several hundred patients 65 and over participated in clinical trials using the immediate-release formulation of bupropion (depression studies). No overall differences in safety or effectiveness were observed between these subjects and younger subjects, and other reported clinical experience has not identified differences in responses between the elderly and younger patients, but greater sensitivity of some older individuals cannot be ruled out.

A single dose pharmacokinetic study demonstrated that the disposition of bupropion and its metabolites in elderly subjects was similar to that of younger subjects; however, another pharmacokinetic study, single and multiple dose, has suggested that the elderly are at increased risk for accumulation of bupropion and its metabolites (see CLINICAL PHARMACOLOGY, Wellbutrin).

Bupropion is extensively metabolized in the liver to active metabolites, which are further metabolized and excreted by the kidneys. The risk of toxic reaction to this drug may be greater in patients with impaired renal function. Because elderly patients are more likely to have decreased renal function, care should be taken in dose selection, and it may be useful to monitor renal function (see Renal Impairment and DOSAGE AND ADMINISTRATION, Wellbutrin).

WELLBUTRIN SR

General

Agitation and Insomnia

Patients in placebo-controlled trials with Wellbutrin SR tablets experienced agitation, anxiety, and insomnia as shown in TABLE 4.

TABLE 4 *Incidence of Agitation, Anxiety, and Insomnia in Placebo-Controlled Trials*

	Wellbutrin SR		
	300 mg/day	400 mg/day	Placebo
Adverse Event Term	(n=376)	(n=114)	(n=385)
Agitation	3%	9%	2%
Anxiety	5%	6%	3%
Insomnia	11%	16%	6%

In clinical studies, these symptoms were sometimes of sufficient magnitude to require treatment with sedative/hypnotic drugs.

Symptoms were sufficiently severe to require discontinuation of treatment in 1% and 2.6% of patients treated with 300 and 400 mg/day, respectively, of Wellbutrin SR tablets and 0.8% of patients treated with placebo.

Psychosis, Confusion, and Other Neuropsychiatric Phenomena

Depressed patients treated with an immediate-release formulation of bupropion or with Wellbutrin SR tablets have been reported to show a variety of neuropsychiatric signs and symptoms, including delusions, hallucinations, psychosis, concentration disturbance, paranoia, and confusion. In some cases, these symptoms abated upon dose reduction and/or withdrawal of treatment.

Activation of Psychosis and/or Mania

Antidepressants can precipitate manic episodes in bipolar disorder patients during the depressed phase of their illness and may activate latent psychosis in other susceptible patients. Wellbutrin SR is expected to pose similar risks.

Altered Appetite and Weight

In placebo-controlled studies, patients experienced weight gain or weight loss as shown in TABLE 5.

TABLE 5 *Incidence of Weight Gain and Weight Loss in Placebo-Controlled Trials*

	Wellbutrin SR		
	300 mg/day	400 mg/day	Placebo
Weight Change	(n=339)	(n=112)	(n=347)
Gained >5 lb	3%	2%	4%
Lost >5 lb	14%	19%	6%

In studies conducted with the immediate-release formulation of bupropion, 35% of patients receiving tricyclic antidepressants gained weight, compared to 9% of patients treated with the immediate-release formulation of bupropion. If weight loss is a major presenting sign of a patient's depressive illness, the anorectic and/or weight-reducing potential of Wellbutrin SR tablets should be considered.

Suicide

The possibility of a suicide attempt is inherent in depression and may persist until significant remission occurs. Accordingly, prescriptions for Wellbutrin SR tablets should be written for the smallest number of tablets consistent with good patient management.

Allergic Reactions

Anaphylactoid/anaphylactic reactions characterized by symptoms such as pruritus, urticaria, angioedema, and dyspnea requiring medical treatment have been reported in clinical trials with bupropion. In addition, there have been rare spontaneous post-marketing reports of erythema multiforme, Stevens-Johnson syndrome, and anaphylactic shock associated with bupropion. A patient should stop taking Wellbutrin SR and consult a doctor if experiencing allergic or anaphylactoid/anaphylactic reactions (*e.g.*, skin rash, pruritus, hives, chest pain, edema, and shortness of breath) during treatment.

Arthralgia, myalgia, and fever with rash and other symptoms suggestive of delayed hypersensitivity have been reported in association with bupropion. These symptoms may resemble serum sickness.

Cardiovascular Effects

In clinical practice, hypertension, in some cases severe, requiring acute treatment, has been reported in patients receiving bupropion alone and in combination with nicotine replacement therapy. These events have been observed in both patients with and without evidence of preexisting hypertension.

Data from a comparative study of the sustained-release formulation of bupropion (Zyban sustained-release tablets), nicotine transdermal system (NTS), the combination of sustained-release bupropion plus NTS, and placebo as an aid to smoking cessation suggest a higher incidence of treatment-emergent hypertension in patients treated with the combination of sustained-release bupropion and NTS. In this study, 6.1% of patients treated with the combination of sustained-release bupropion and NTS had treatment-emergent hypertension compared to 2.5%, 1.6%, and 3.1% of patients treated with sustained-release bupropion, NTS, and placebo, respectively. The majority of these patients had evidence of preexisting hypertension. Three patients (1.2%) treated with the combination of Zyban and NTS and one patient (0.4%) treated with NTS had study medication discontinued due to hypertension compared to none of the patients treated with Zyban or placebo. Monitoring of blood pressure is recommended in patients who receive the combination of bupropion and nicotine replacement.

There is no clinical experience establishing the safety of Wellbutrin SR tablets in patients with a recent history of myocardial infarction or unstable heart disease. Therefore, care should be exercised if it is used in these groups. Bupropion was well tolerated in depressed patients who had previously developed orthostatic hypotension while receiving tricyclic antidepressants, and was also generally well tolerated in a group of 36 depressed inpatients with stable congestive heart failure (CHF). However, bupropion was associated with a rise in supine blood pressure in the study of patients with CHF, resulting in discontinuation of treatment in 2 patients for exacerbation of baseline hypertension.

Hepatic Impairment

Wellbutrin SR should be used with extreme caution in patients with severe hepatic cirrhosis. In these patients, a reduced frequency and/or dose is required. Wellbutrin SR should be used with caution in patients with hepatic impairment (including mild to moderate hepatic cirrhosis) and reduced frequency and/or dose should be considered in patients with mild to moderate hepatic cirrhosis.

All patients with hepatic impairment should be closely monitored for possible adverse effects that could indicate high drug and metabolite levels (see CLINICAL PHARMACOLOGY, Wellbutrin SR; WARNINGS, Wellbutrin SR; and DOSAGE AND ADMINISTRATION, Wellbutrin SR).

Renal Impairment

No studies have been conducted in patients with renal impairment. Bupropion is extensively metabolized in the liver to active metabolites, which are further metabolized and subsequently excreted by the kidneys. Wellbutrin SR should be used with caution in patients with renal impairment and a reduced frequency and/or dose should be considered as bupropion and its metabolites may accumulate in such patients to a greater extent than usual. The patient should be closely monitored for possible adverse effects that could indicate high drug or metabolite levels.

Information for the Patient

See the Patient Instructions that are distributed with the prescription for complete instructions.

Patients should be made aware that Wellbutrin SR contains the same active ingredient found in Zyban, used as an aid to smoking cessation treatment, and that Wellbutrin SR should not be used in combination with Zyban or any other medications that contain bupropion hydrochloride.

Physicians are advised to discuss the following issues with patients:

As dose is increased during initial titration to doses above 150 mg/day, patients should be instructed to take Wellbutrin SR tablets in 2 divided doses, preferably with at least 8 hours between successive doses, to minimize the risk of seizures.

Patients should be told that Wellbutrin SR should be discontinued and not restarted if they experience a seizure while on treatment.

Patients should be told that any CNS-active drug like Wellbutrin SR tablets may impair their ability to perform tasks requiring judgment or motor and cognitive skills. Consequently, until they are reasonably certain that Wellbutrin SR tablets do not adversely affect their performance, they should refrain from driving an automobile or operating complex, hazardous machinery.

Patients should be told that the excessive use or abrupt discontinuation of alcohol or sedatives (including benzodiazepines) may alter the seizure threshold. Some patients have reported lower alcohol tolerance during treatment with Wellbutrin SR. Patients should be advised that the consumption of alcohol should be minimized or avoided.

Patients should be advised to inform their physicians if they are taking or plan to take any prescription or over-the-counter drugs. Concern is warranted because Wellbutrin SR tablets and other drugs may affect each other's metabolism.

Patients should be advised to notify their physicians if they become pregnant or intent to become pregnant during therapy.

Patients should be advised to swallow Wellbutrin SR tablets whole so that the release rate is not altered. Do not chew, divide, or crush tablets.

Laboratory Tests

There are no specific laboratory tests recommended.

Carcinogenesis, Mutagenesis, and Impairment of Fertility
Lifetime carcinogenicity studies were performed in rats and mice at doses up to 300 and 150 mg/kg/day, respectively. These doses are approximately 7 and 2 times the maximum recommended human dose (MRHD), respectively, on a mg/m^2 basis. In the rat study there was an increase in nodular proliferative lesions of the liver at doses of 100-300 mg/kg/day (approximately 2-7 times the MRHD on a mg/m^2 basis); lower doses were not tested. The question of whether or not such lesions may be precursors of neoplasms of the liver is currently unresolved. Similar liver lesions were not seen in the mouse study, and no increase in malignant tumors of the liver and other organs was seen in either study.

Bupropion produced a positive response (2-3 times control mutation rate) in 2 of 5 strains in the Ames bacterial mutagenicity test and an increase in chromosomal aberrations in one of three *in vivo* rat bone marrow cytogenetic studies.

A fertility study in rats at doses up to 300 mg/kg revealed no evidence of impaired fertility.

Pregnancy, Teratogenic Effects, Pregnancy Category B
Teratology studies have been performed at doses up to 450 mg/kg in rats, and at doses up to 150 mg/kg in rabbits (approximately 7-11 and 7 times the MRHD, respectively, on a mg/m^2 basis), and have revealed no evidence of harm to the fetus due to bupropion. There are no adequate and well-controlled studies in pregnant women. Because animal reproduction studies are not always predictive of human response, this drug should be used during pregnancy only if clearly needed.

To monitor fetal outcomes of pregnant women exposed to Wellbutrin SR, GlaxoSmithKline maintains a Bupropion Pregnancy Registry. Health care providers are encouraged to register patients by calling 800-336-2176.

Labor and Delivery
The effect of Wellbutrin SR tablets on labor and delivery in humans is unknown.

Nursing Mothers
Like many other drugs, bupropion and its metabolites are secreted in human milk. Because of the potential for serious adverse reactions in nursing infants from Wellbutrin SR tablets, a decision should be made whether to discontinue nursing or to discontinue the drug, taking into account the importance of the drug to the mother.

Pediatric Use
The safety and effectiveness of Wellbutrin SR tablets in pediatric patients below 18 years old have not been established. The immediate-release formulation of bupropion was studied in 104 pediatric patients (age range, 6-16) in clinical trials of the drug for other indications. Although generally well tolerated, the limited exposure is insufficient to assess the safety of bupropion in pediatric patients.

Geriatric Use
Of the approximately 6000 patients who participated in clinical trials with bupropion sustained-release tablets (depression and smoking cessation studies), 275 were 65 and over and 47 were 75 and over. In addition, several hundred patients 65 and over participated in clinical trials using the immediate-release formulation of bupropion (depression studies). No overall differences in safety or effectiveness were observed between these subjects and younger subjects, and other reported clinical experience has not identified differences in responses between the elderly and younger patients, but greater sensitivity of some older individuals cannot be ruled out.

A single dose pharmacokinetic study demonstrated that the disposition of bupropion and its metabolites in elderly subjects was similar to that of younger subjects; however, another pharmacokinetic study, single and multiple dose, has suggested that the elderly are at increased risk for accumulation of bupropion and its metabolites (see CLINICAL PHARMACOLOGY, Wellbutrin SR).

Bupropion is extensively metabolized in the liver to active metabolites, which are further metabolized and excreted by the kidneys. The risk of toxic reaction to this drug may be greater in patients with impaired renal function. Because elderly patients are more likely to have decreased renal function, care should be taken in dose selection, and it may be useful to monitor renal function (see Renal Impairment and DOSAGE AND ADMINISTRATION, Wellbutrin SR).

ZYBAN
General
Allergic Reactions
Anaphylactoid/anaphylactic reactions characterized by symptoms such as pruritus, urticaria, angioedema, and dyspnea requiring medical treatment have been reported at a rate of about 1-3 per thousand in clinical trials of Zyban. In addition, there have been rare spontaneous post-marketing reports of erythema multiforme, Stevens-Johnson syndrome, and anaphylactic shock associated with bupropion. A patient should stop taking Zyban and consult a doctor if experiencing allergic or anaphylactoid/anaphylactic reactions (*e.g.*, skin rash, pruritus, hives, chest pain, edema, and shortness of breath) during treatment.

Arthralgia, myalgia, and fever with rash and other symptoms suggestive of delayed hypersensitivity have been reported in association with bupropion. These symptoms may resemble serum sickness.

Insomnia
In the dose-response smoking cessation trial, 29% of patients treated with 150 mg/day of Zyban and 35% of patients treated with 300 mg/day of Zyban experienced insomnia, compared to 21% of placebo-treated patients. Symptoms were sufficiently severe to require discontinuation of treatment in 0.6% of patients treated with Zyban and none of the patients treated with placebo.

In the comparative trial, 40% of the patients treated with 300 mg/day of Zyban, 28% of the patients treated with 21 mg/day of NTS, and 45% of the patients treated with the combination of Zyban and NTS experienced insomnia compared to 18% of placebo-treated patients. Symptoms were sufficiently severe to require discontinuation of treatment in 0.8% of patients treated with Zyban and none of the patients in the other 3 treatment groups.

Insomnia may be minimized by avoiding bedtime doses and, if necessary, reduction in dose.

Psychosis, Confusion, and Other Neuropsychiatric Phenomena
In clinical trials with Zyban conducted in nondepressed smokers, the incidence of neuropsychiatric side effects was generally comparable to placebo. Depressed patients treated with bupropion in depression trials have been reported to show a variety of neuropsychiatric signs and symptoms including delusions, hallucinations, psychosis, concentration disturbance, paranoia, and confusion. In some cases, these symptoms abated upon dose reduction and/or withdrawal of treatment.

Activation of Psychosis and/or Mania
Antidepressants can precipitate manic episodes in bipolar disorder patients during the depressed phase of their illness and may activate latent psychosis in other susceptible individuals. The sustained-release formulation of bupropion is expected to pose similar risks. There were no reports of activation of psychosis or mania in clinical trials with Zyban conducted in nondepressed smokers.

Cardiovascular Effects
In clinical practice, hypertension, in some cases severe, requiring acute treatment, has been reported in patients receiving bupropion alone and in combination with nicotine replacement therapy. These events have been observed in both patients with and without evidence of preexisting hypertension.

Data from a comparative study of Zyban, nicotine transdermal system (NTS), the combination of sustained-release bupropion plus NTS, and placebo as an aid to smoking cessation suggest a higher incidence of treatment-emergent hypertension in patients treated with the combination of Zyban and NTS. In this study, 6.1% of patients treated with the combination of Zyban and NTS had treatment-emergent hypertension compared to 2.5%, 1.6%, and 3.1% of patients treated with Zyban, NTS, and placebo, respectively. The majority of these patients had evidence of preexisting hypertension. Three patients (1.2%) treated with the combination of Zyban and NTS and 1 patient (0.4%) treated with NTS had study medication discontinued due to hypertension compared to none of the patients treated with Zyban or placebo. Monitoring of blood pressure is recommended in patients who receive the combination of bupropion and nicotine replacement.

There is no clinical experience establishing the safety of Zyban in patients with a recent history of myocardial infarction or unstable heart disease. Therefore, care should be exercised if it is used in these groups. Bupropion was well tolerated in depressed patients who had previously developed orthostatic hypotension while receiving tricyclic antidepressants, and was also generally well tolerated in a group of 36 depressed inpatients with stable congestive heart failure (CHF). However, bupropion was associated with a rise in supine blood pressure in the study of patients with CHF, resulting in discontinuation of treatment in 2 patients for exacerbation of baseline hypertension.

Hepatic Impairment
Zyban should be used with extreme caution in patients with severe hepatic cirrhosis. In these patients, a reduced frequency of dosing is required. Zyban should be used with caution in patients with hepatic impairment (including mild to moderate hepatic cirrhosis) and reduced frequency of dosing should be considered in patients with mild to moderate hepatic cirrhosis.

All patients with hepatic impairment should be closely monitored for possible adverse effects that could indicate high drug and metabolite levels (see CLINICAL PHARMACOLOGY, Zyban; WARNINGS, Zyban; and DOSAGE AND ADMINISTRATION, Zyban).

Renal Impairment
No studies have been conducted in patients with renal impairment. Bupropion is extensively metabolized in the liver to active metabolites, which are further metabolized and excreted by the kidneys. Zyban should be used with caution in patients with renal impairment and a reduced frequency of dosing should be considered as bupropion and its metabolites may accumulate in such patients to a greater extent than usual. The patient should be closely monitored for possible adverse effects that could indicate high drug or metabolite levels.

Information for the Patient
See the Patient Instructions that are distributed with the prescription for complete instructions. Physicians are advised to review the leaflet with their patients and to emphasize that Zyban contains the same active ingredient found in Wellbutrin and Wellbutrin SR used to treat depression and that Zyban should not be used in conjunction with Wellbutrin, Wellbutrin SR, or any other medications that contain bupropion hydrochloride.

Laboratory Tests
There are no specific laboratory tests recommended.

Carcinogenesis, Mutagenesis, and Impairment of Fertility
Lifetime carcinogenicity studies were performed in rats and mice at doses up to 300 and 150 mg/kg/day, respectively. These doses are approximately 10 and 2 times the maximum recommended human dose (MRHD), respectively, on a mg/m^2 basis. In the rat study, there was an increase in nodular proliferative lesions of the liver at doses of 100-300 mg/kg/day (approximately 3-10 times the MRHD on a mg/m^2 basis); lower doses were not tested. The question of whether or not such lesions may be precursors of neoplasms of the liver is currently unresolved. Similar liver lesions were not seen in the mouse study, and no increase in malignant tumors of the liver and other organs was seen in either study.

Bupropion produced a positive response (2-3 times control mutation rate) in 2 of 5 strains in the Ames bacterial mutagenicity test and an increase in chromosomal aberrations in one of three*in vivo* rat bone marrow cytogenic studies.

A fertility study in rats at doses up to 300 mg/kg revealed no evidence of impaired fertility.

Pregnancy, Teratogenic Effects, Pregnancy Category B
Teratology studies have been performed at doses up to 450 mg/kg in rats (approximately 14 times the MRHD on a mg/m^2 basis), and at doses up to 150 mg/kg in rabbits (approximately

10 times the MRHD on a mg/m² basis). There is no evidence of impaired fertility or harm to the fetus due to bupropion. There are no adequate and well-controlled studies in pregnant women. Because animal reproduction studies are not always predictive of human response, this drug should be used during pregnancy only if clearly needed. Pregnant smokers should be encouraged to attempt cessation using educational and behavioral interventions before pharmacological approaches are used.

To monitor fetal outcomes of pregnant women exposed to Zyban, GlaxoSmithKline maintains a Bupropion Pregnancy Registry. Health care providers are encouraged to register patients by calling 800-336-2176.

Labor and Delivery

The effect of Zyban on labor and delivery in humans is unknown.

Nursing Mothers

Bupropion and its metabolites are secreted in human milk. Because of the potential for serious adverse reactions in nursing infants from Zyban, a decision should be made whether to discontinue nursing or to discontinue the drug, taking into account the importance of the drug to the mother.

Pediatric Use

Clinical trials with Zyban did not include individuals under the age of 18. Therefore, the safety and efficacy in a pediatric smoking population have not been established. The immediate-release formulation of bupropion was studied in 104 pediatric patients (age range, 6-16) in clinical trials of the drug for other indications. Although generally well tolerated, the limited exposure is insufficient to assess the safety of bupropion in pediatric patients.

Geriatric Use

Of the approximately 6000 patients who participated in clinical trials with bupropion sustained-release tablets (depression and smoking cessation studies), 275 were 65 and over and 47 were 75 and over. In addition, several hundred patients 65 and over participated in clinical trials using the immediate-release formulation of bupropion (depression studies). No overall differences in safety or effectiveness were observed between these subjects and younger subjects, and other reported clinical experience has not identified differences in responses between the elderly and younger patients, but greater sensitivity of some older individuals cannot be ruled out.

A single dose pharmacokinetic study demonstrated that the disposition of bupropion and its metabolites in elderly subjects was similar to that of younger subjects; however, another pharmacokinetic study, single and multiple dose, has suggested that the elderly are at increased risk for accumulation of bupropion and its metabolites (see CLINICAL PHARMACOLOGY, Zyban).

Bupropion is extensively metabolized in the liver to active metabolites, which are further metabolized and excreted by the kidneys. The risk of toxic reaction to this drug may be greater in patients with impaired renal function. Because elderly patients are more likely to have decreased renal function, care should be taken in dose selection, and it may be useful to monitor renal function (see Renal Impairment and DOSAGE AND ADMINISTRATION, Zyban).

DRUG INTERACTIONS

WELLBUTRIN

Few systemic data have been collected on the metabolism of Wellbutrin following concomitant administration with other drugs or, alternatively, the effect of concomitant administration of Wellbutrin on the metabolism of other drugs.

Because bupropion is extensively metabolized, the coadministration of other drugs may affect its clinical activity. *In vitro* studies indicate that bupropion is primarily metabolized to hydroxybupropion by the CYP2B6 isoenzyme. Therefore, the potential exists for a drug interaction between Wellbutrin and drugs that affect the CYP2B6 isoenzyme (*e.g.*, orphenadrine and cyclophosphamide). The threohydrobupropion metabolite of bupropion does not appear to be produced by the cytochrome P450 isoenzymes. The effects of concomitant administration of cimetidine on the pharmacokinetics of bupropion and its active metabolites were studied in 24 healthy young male volunteers. Following oral administration of two 150 mg sustained-release tablets with and without 800 mg of cimetidine, the pharmacokinetics of bupropion and hydroxybupropion were unaffected. However, there were 16% and 32% increases in the AUC and C_{max}, respectively, of the combined moieties of threohydrobupropion and erythrohydrobupropion.

While not systematically studied, certain drugs may induce the metabolism of bupropion (*e.g.*, carbamazepine, phenobarbital, phenytoin).

Animal data indicated that bupropion may be an inducer of drug-metabolizing enzymes in humans. In one study, following chronic administration of bupropion, 100 mg three times daily to 8 healthy male volunteers for 14 days, there was no evidence of induction of its own metabolism. Nevertheless, there may be the potential for clinically important alterations of blood levels of coadministered drugs.

Drugs Metabolized by Cytochrome P450IID6 (CYP2D6)

Many drugs, including most antidepressants (SSRIs, many tricyclics), beta-blockers, antiarrhythmics, and antipsychotics are metabolized by the CYP2D6 isoenzyme. Although bupropion is not metabolized by this isoenzyme, bupropion and hydroxybupropion are inhibitors of the CYP2D6 isoenzyme *in vitro*. In a study of 15 male subjects (ages 19-35 years) who were extensive metabolizers of the CYP2D6 isoenzyme, daily doses of bupropion given as 150 mg twice daily followed by a single dose of 50 mg desipramine increased the C_{max}, AUC, and $T_{1/2}$ of desipramine by an average of approximately 2-, 5- and 2-fold, respectively. The effect was present for at least 7 days after the last dose of bupropion. Concomitant use of bupropion with other drugs metabolized by CYP2D6 has not been formally studied.

Therefore, coadministration of bupropion with drugs that are metabolized by CYP2D6 isoenzyme including certain antidepressants (*e.g.*, nortriptyline, imipramine, desipramine, paroxetine, fluoxetine, sertraline), antipsychotics (*e.g.*, haloperidol, risperidone, thioridazine), beta-blockers (*e.g.*, metoprolol), and Type 1C antiarrhythmics (*e.g.*, propafenone, flecainide), should be approached with caution and should be initiated at the lower end of the dose range of the concomitant medication. If bupropion is added to the treatment regimen of a patient already receiving a drug metabolized by CYP2D6, the need to decrease the dose of the original medication should be considered, particularly for those concomitant medications with a narrow therapeutic index.

MAO Inhibitors

Studies in animals demonstrate that the acute toxicity of bupropion is enhanced by the MAO inhibitor phenelzine (see CONTRAINDICATIONS, Wellbutrin).

Levodopa and Amantadine

Limited clinical data suggest a higher incidence of adverse experiences in patients receiving bupropion concurrently with either levodopa or amantadine. Administration of Wellbutrin tablets to patients receiving either levodopa or amantadine concurrently should be undertaken with caution, using small initial doses and small gradual dose increases.

Drugs That Lower Seizure Threshold

Concurrent administration of Wellbutrin and agents (*e.g.*, antipsychotics, other antidepressants, theophylline, systemic steroids, etc.) that lower seizure threshold should be undertaken only with extreme caution (see WARNINGS, Wellbutrin). Low initial dosing and small gradual dose increases should be employed.

Nicotine Transdermal System

See PRECAUTIONS, Wellbutrin, General, Cardiovascular Effects.

Alcohol

In post-marketing experience, there have been rare reports of adverse neuropsychiatric events or reduced alcohol tolerance in patients who were drinking alcohol during treatment with Wellbutrin. The consumption of alcohol during treatment with Wellbutrin should be minimized or avoided (also see CONTRAINDICATIONS, Wellbutrin).

WELLBUTRIN SR

Few systemic data have been collected on the metabolism of Wellbutrin SR following concomitant administration with other drugs or, alternatively, the effect of concomitant administration of Wellbutrin SR on the metabolism of other drugs.

Because bupropion is extensively metabolized, the coadministration of other drugs may affect its clinical activity. *In vitro* studies indicate that bupropion is primarily metabolized to hydroxybupropion by the CYP2B6 isoenzyme. Therefore, the potential exists for a drug interaction between Wellbutrin SR and drugs that affect the CYP2B6 isoenzyme (*e.g.*, orphenadrine and cyclophosphamide). The threohydrobupropion metabolite of bupropion does not appear to be produced by the cytochrome P450 isoenzymes. The effects of concomitant administration of cimetidine on the pharmacokinetics of bupropion and its active metabolites were studied in 24 healthy young male volunteers. Following oral administration of two 150 mg Wellbutrin SR tablets with and without 800 mg of cimetidine, the pharmacokinetics of bupropion and hydroxybupropion were unaffected. However, there were 16% and 32% increases in the AUC and C_{max}, respectively, of the combined moieties of threohydrobupropion and erythrohydrobupropion.

While not systematically studied, certain drugs may induce the metabolism of bupropion (*e.g.*, carbamazepine, phenobarbital, phenytoin).

Animal data indicated that bupropion may be an inducer of drug-metabolizing enzymes in humans. In one study, following chronic administration of bupropion, 100 mg three times daily to 8 healthy male volunteers for 14 days, there was no evidence of induction of its own metabolism. Nevertheless, there may be the potential for clinically important alterations of blood levels of coadministered drugs.

Drugs Metabolized by Cytochrome P450IID6 (CYP2D6)

Many drugs, including most antidepressants (SSRIs, many tricyclics), beta-blockers, antiarrhythmics, and antipsychotics are metabolized by the CYP2D6 isoenzyme. Although bupropion is not metabolized by this isoenzyme, bupropion and hydroxybupropion are inhibitors of CYP2D6 isoenzyme *in vitro*. In a study of 15 male subjects (ages 19-35 years) who were extensive metabolizers of the CYP2D6 isoenzyme, daily doses of bupropion given as 150 mg twice daily followed by a single dose of 50 mg desipramine increased the C_{max}, AUC, and $T_{1/2}$ of desipramine by an average of approximately 2-, 5-, and 2-fold, respectively. The effect was present for at least 7 days after the last dose of bupropion. Concomitant use of bupropion with other drugs metabolized by CYP2D6 has not been formally studied.

Therefore, coadministration of bupropion with drugs that are metabolized by CYP2D6 isoenzyme including certain antidepressants (*e.g.*, nortriptyline, imipramine, desipramine, paroxetine, fluoxetine, sertraline), antipsychotics (*e.g.*, haloperidol, risperidone, thioridazine), beta-blockers (*e.g.*, metoprolol), and Type 1C antiarrhythmics (*e.g.*, propafenone, flecainide), should be approached with caution and should be initiated at the lower end of the dose range of the concomitant medication. If bupropion is added to the treatment regimen of a patient already receiving a drug metabolized by CYP2D6, the need to decrease the dose of the original medication should be considered, particularly for those concomitant medications with a narrow therapeutic index.

MAO Inhibitors

Studies in animals demonstrate that the acute toxicity of bupropion is enhanced by the MAO inhibitor phenelzine (see CONTRAINDICATIONS, Wellbutrin SR).

Levodopa and Amantadine

Limited clinical data suggest a higher incidence of adverse experiences in patients receiving bupropion concurrently with either levodopa or amantadine. Administration of Wellbutrin SR tablets to patients receiving either levodopa or amantadine concurrently should be undertaken with caution, using small initial doses and gradual dose increases.

Drugs That Lower Seizure Threshold

Concurrent administration of Wellbutrin SR tablets and agents (*e.g.,* antipsychotics, other antidepressants, theophylline, systemic steroids, etc.) that lower seizure threshold should be undertaken only with extreme caution (see WARNINGS, Wellbutrin SR). Low initial dosing and gradual dose increases should be employed.

Nicotine Transdermal System

See PRECAUTIONS, Wellbutrin SR, General, Cardiovascular Effects.

Alcohol

In post-marketing experience, there have been rare reports of adverse neuropsychiatric events or reduced alcohol tolerance in patients who were drinking alcohol during treatment with Wellbutrin SR. The consumption of alcohol during treatment with Wellbutrin SR should be minimized or avoided (also see CONTRAINDICATIONS, Wellbutrin SR).

ZYBAN

In vitro studies indicate that bupropion is primarily metabolized to hydroxybupropion by the cytochrome P450IIB6 (CYP2B6) isoenzyme. Therefore, the potential exists for a drug interaction between Zyban and drugs that affect the CYP2B6 isoenzyme (*e.g.,* orphenadrine and cyclophosphamide). The threohydrobupropion metabolite of bupropion does not appear to be produced by the cytochrome P450 isoenzymes. Few systemic data have been collected on the metabolism of Zyban following concomitant administration with other drugs or, alternatively, the effect of concomitant administration of Zyban on the metabolism of other drugs.

Animal data indicated that bupropion may be an inducer of drug-metabolizing enzymes in humans. However, following chronic administration of bupropion, 100 mg tid to 8 healthy male volunteers for 14 days, there was no evidence of induction of its own metabolism. Because bupropion is extensively metabolized, the coadministration of other drugs may affect its clinical activity. In particular, certain drugs may induce the metabolism of bupropion (*e.g.,* carbamazepine, phenobarbital, phenytoin), while other drugs may inhibit the metabolism of bupropion (*e.g.,* cimetidine). The effects of concomitant administration of cimetidine on the pharmacokinetics of bupropion and its active metabolites were studied in 24 healthy young male volunteers. Following oral administration of two 150 mg Zyban tablets with and without 800 mg of cimetidine, the pharmacokinetics of bupropion and its hydroxy metabolite were unaffected. However, there were 16% and 32% increases, respectively, in the AUC and C_{max} of the combined moieties of theohydro- and erythrohydrobupropion.

Drugs Metabolized by Cytochrome P450IID6 (CYP2D6)

Many drugs, including most antidepressants (SSRIs, many tricyclics), beta-blockers, antiarrhythmics, and antipsychotics are metabolized by the CYP2D6 isoenzyme. Although bupropion is not metabolized by this isoenzyme, bupropion and hydroxybupropion are inhibitors of the CYP2D6 isoenzyme *in vitro.* In a study of 15 male subjects (ages 19-35 years) who were extensive metabolizers of the CYP2D6 isoenzyme, daily doses of bupropion given as 150 mg twice daily followed by a single dose of 50 mg desipramine increased the C_{max}, AUC, and $T_{½}$ of desipramine by an average of approximately 2-, 5- and 2-fold, respectively. The effect was present for at least 7 days after the last dose of bupropion. Concomitant use of bupropion with other drugs metabolized by CYP2D6 has not been formally studied.

Therefore, coadministration of bupropion with drugs that are metabolized by CYP2D6 isoenzyme including certain antidepressants (*e.g.,* nortriptyline, imipramine, desipramine, paroxetine, fluoxetine, sertraline), antipsychotics (*e.g.,* haloperidol, risperidone, thioridazine), beta-blockers (*e.g.,* metoprolol), and Type 1C antiarrhythmics (*e.g.,* propafenone, flecainide), should be approached with caution and should be initiated at the lower end of the dose range of the concomitant medication. If bupropion is added to the treatment regimen of a patient already receiving a drug metabolized by CYP2D6, the need to decrease the dose of the original medication should be considered, particularly for those concomitant medications with a narrow therapeutic index.

MAO Inhibitors

Studies in animals demonstrate that the acute toxicity of bupropion is enhanced by the MAO inhibitor phenelzine (see CONTRAINDICATIONS, Zyban).

Levodopa and Amantadine

Limited clinical data suggest a higher incidence of adverse experiences in patients receiving bupropion concurrently with either levodopa or amantadine. Administration of Zyban to patients receiving either levodopa or amantadine concurrently should be undertaken with caution, using small initial doses and gradual dose increases.

Drugs That Lower Seizure Threshold

Concurrent administration of Zyban and agents (*e.g.,* antipsychotics, antidepressants, theophylline, systemic steroids, etc.) that lower seizure threshold should be undertaken only with extreme caution (see WARNINGS, Zyban).

Nicotine Transdermal System

See PRECAUTIONS, Zyban, General, Cardiovascular Effects.

Smoking Cessation

Physiological changes resulting from smoking cessation itself, with or without treatment with Zyban, may alter the pharmacokinetics of some concomitant medications, which may require dosage adjustment. Blood concentrations of concomitant medications that are extensively metabolized, such as theophylline and warfarin, may be expected to increase following smoking cessation due to de-induction of hepatic enzymes.

Alcohol

In post-marketing experience, there have been rare reports of adverse neuropsychiatric events or reduced alcohol tolerance in patients who were drinking alcohol during treatment with Zyban. The consumption of alcohol during treatment with Zyban should be minimized or avoided (also see CONTRAINDICATIONS, Zyban).

ADVERSE REACTIONS

WELLBUTRIN

See also WARNINGS, Wellbutrin and PRECAUTIONS, Wellbutrin.

Adverse events commonly encountered in patients treated with Wellbutrin are agitation, dry mouth, insomnia, headache/migraine, nausea/vomiting, constipation, and tremor.

Adverse events were sufficiently troublesome to cause discontinuation of treatment with Wellbutrin in approximately 10% of the 2400 patients and volunteers who participated in clinical trials during the product's initial development. The more common events causing discontinuation include neuropsychiatric disturbances (3.0%), primarily agitation and abnormalities in mental status; gastrointestinal disturbances (2.1%), primarily nausea and vomiting; neurological disturbances (1.7%), primarily seizures, headaches, and sleep disturbances; and dermatologic problems (1.4%), primarily rashes. It is important to note, however, that many of these events occurred at doses that exceed the recommended daily dose.

Accurate estimates of the incidence of adverse events associated with the use of any drug are difficult to obtain. Estimates are influenced by drug dose, detection technique, setting, physician judgments, etc. Consequently, TABLE 6 is presented solely to indicate the relative frequency of adverse events reported in representative controlled clinical studies conducted to evaluate the safety and efficacy of Wellbutrin under relatively similar conditions of daily dosage (300-600 mg), setting, and duration (3-4 weeks). The figures cited cannot be used to predict precisely the incidence of untoward events in the course of usual medical practice where patient characteristics and other factors must differ from those which prevailed in the clinical trials. These incidence figures also cannot be compared with those obtained from other clinical studies involving related drug products as each group of drug trials is conducted under a different set of conditions.

Finally, it is important to emphasize that the tabulation does not reflect the relative severity and/or clinical importance of the events. A better perspective on the serious adverse events associated with the use of Wellbutrin is provided in WARNINGS, Wellbutrin and PRECAUTIONS, Wellbutrin.

Other Events Observed During the Development of Wellbutrin

The conditions and duration of exposure to Wellbutrin varied greatly, and a substantial proportion of the experience was gained in open and uncontrolled clinical settings. During this experience, numerous adverse events were reported; however, without appropriate controls, it is impossible to determine with certainty which events were or were not caused by Wellbutrin. The following enumeration is organized by organ system and describes events in terms of their relative frequency of reporting in the data base. Events of major clinical importance are also described in WARNINGS, Wellbutrin and PRECAUTIONS, Wellbutrin.

The following definitions of frequency are used: *Frequent* adverse events are defined as those occurring in at least 1/100 patients. *Infrequent* adverse events are those occurring in 1/100 to 1/1000 patients, while *rare* events are those occurring in less than 1/1000 patients.

Cardiovascular: *Frequent:* Edema; *Infrequent:* Chest pain, electrocardiogram (ECG) abnormalities (premature beats and nonspecific ST-T changes), and shortness of breath/dyspnea; *Rare:* Flushing, pallor, phlebitis, and myocardial infarction.

Dermatologic: *Frequent:* Nonspecific rashes; *Infrequent:* Alopecia and dry skin; *Rare:* Change in hair color, hirsutism, and acne.

Endocrine: *Infrequent:* Gynecomastia; *Rare:* Glycosuria and hormone level change.

Gastrointestinal: *Infrequent:* Dysphagia, thirst disturbance, and liver damage/jaundice; *Rare:* Rectal complaints, colitis, gastrointestinal bleeding, intestinal perforation, and stomach ulcer.

Genitourinary: *Frequent:* Nocturia; *Infrequent:* Vaginal irritation, testicular swelling, urinary tract infection, painful erection, and retarded ejaculation; *Rare:* Dysuria, enuresis, urinary incontinence, menopause, ovarian disorder, pelvic infection, cystitis, dyspareunia, and painful ejaculation.

Hematologic/Oncologic: *Rare:* Lymphadenopathy, anemia, and pancytopenia.

Musculoskeletal: *Rare:* Musculoskeletal chest pain.

Neurological: (See WARNINGS, Wellbutrin.) *Frequent:* Ataxia/incoordination, seizure, myoclonus, dyskinesia, and dystonia; *Infrequent:* Mydriasis, vertigo, and dysarthria; *Rare:* Electroencephalogram (EEG) abnormality, abnormal neurological exam, impaired attention, sciatica, and aphasia.

Neuropsychiatric: (See PRECAUTIONS, Wellbutrin.) *Frequent:* Mania/hypomania, increased libido, hallucinations, decrease in sexual function, and depression; *Infrequent:* Memory impairment, depersonalization, psychosis, dysphoria, mood instability, paranoia, formal thought disorder, and frigidity; *Rare:* Suicidal ideation.

Oral Complaints: *Frequent:* Stomatitis; *Infrequent:* Toothache, bruxism, gum irritation, and oral edema; *Rare:* Glossitis.

Respiratory: *Infrequent:* Bronchitis and shortness of breath/dyspnea; *Rare:* Epistaxis, rate or rhythm disorder, pneumonia, and pulmonary embolism.

Special Senses: *Infrequent:* Visual disturbance; *Rare:* Diplopia.

Nonspecific: *Frequent:* Flu-like symptoms; *Infrequent:* Nonspecific pain; *Rare:* Body odor, surgically related pain, infection, medication reaction, and overdose.

Postintroduction Reports

Voluntary reports of adverse events temporally associated with bupropion that have been received since market introduction and which may have no causal relationship with the drug include the following:

Body (General): Arthralgia, myalgia, and fever with rash and other symptoms suggestive of delayed hypersensitivity. These symptoms may resemble serum sickness (see PRECAUTIONS, Wellbutrin).

Cardiovascular: Hypertension (in some cases severe, see PRECAUTIONS, Wellbutrin), orthostatic hypotension, third degree heart block.

Endocrine: Syndrome of inappropriate antidiuretic hormone secretion, hyperglycemia, hypoglycemia.

Gastrointestinal: Esophagitis, hepatitis, liver damage.

TABLE 6 *Treatment Emergent Adverse Experience Incidence in Placebo-Controlled Clinical Trials**

Adverse Experience	Wellbutrin (n=323)	Placebo (n=185)
Cardiovascular		
Cardiac arrhythmias	5.3%	4.3%
Dizziness	22.3%	16.2%
Hypertension	4.3%	1.6%
Hypotension	2.5%	2.2%
Palpitations	3.7%	2.2%
Syncope	1.2%	0.5%
Tachycardia	10.8%	8.6%
Dermatologic		
Pruritus	2.2%	0.0%
Rash	8.0%	6.5%
Gastrointestinal		
Anorexia	18.3%	18.4%
Appetite increase	3.7%	2.2%
Constipation	26.0%	17.3%
Diarrhea	6.8%	8.6%
Dyspepsia	3.1%	2.2%
Nausea/vomiting	22.9%	18.9%
Weight gain	13.6%	22.7%
Weight loss	23.2%	23.2%
Genitourinary		
Impotence	3.4%	3.1%
Menstrual complaints	4.7%	1.1%
Urinary frequency	2.5%	2.2%
Urinary retention	1.9%	2.2%
Musculoskeletal		
Arthritis	3.1%	2.7%
Neurological		
Akathisia	1.5%	1.1%
Akinesia/bradykinesia	8.0%	8.6%
Cutaneous temperature disturbance	1.9%	1.6%
Dry mouth	27.6%	18.4%
Excessive sweating	22.3%	14.6%
Headache/migraine	25.7%	22.2%
Impaired sleep quality	4.0%	1.6%
Increased salivary flow	3.4%	3.8%
Insomnia	18.6%	15.7%
Muscle spasms	1.9%	3.2%
Pseudoparkinsonism	1.5%	1.6%
Sedation	19.8%	19.5%
Sensory disturbance	4.0%	3.2%
Tremor	21.1%	7.6%
Neuropsychiatric		
Agitation	31.9%	22.2%
Anxiety	3.1%	1.1%
Confusion	8.4%	4.9%
Decreased libido	3.1%	1.6%
Delusions	1.2%	1.1%
Disturbed concentration	3.1%	1.1%
Euphoria	1.2%	0.5%
Hostility	5.6%	3.8%
Nonspecific		
Fatigue	5.0%	8.6%
Fever/chills	1.2%	0.5%
Respiratory		
Upper respiratory complaints	5.0%	11.4%
Special Senses		
Auditory disturbance	5.3%	3.2%
Blurred vision	14.6%	10.3%
Gustatory disturbance	3.1%	1.1%

* Events reported by at least 1% of patients receiving Wellbutrin are included.

Hemic and Lymphatic: Ecchymosis, leukocytosis, leukopenia, thrombocytopenia. Altered PT and/or INR, infrequently associated with hemorrhagic or thrombotic complications, were observed when bupropion was coadministered with warfarin.

Musculoskeletal: Arthralgia, myalgia, muscle rigidity/fever/rhabdomyolysis, muscle weakness.

Nervous: Coma, delirium, dream abnormalities, paresthesia, unmasking of tardive dyskinesia.

Skin and Appendages: Stevens-Johnson syndrome, angioedema, exfoliative dermatitis, urticaria.

Special Senses: Tinnitus.

WELLBUTRIN SR

See also WARNINGS, Wellbutrin SR and PRECAUTIONS, Wellbutrin SR.

The information included in Incidence in Controlled Trials With Wellbutrin SR is based primarily on data from controlled clinical trials with Wellbutrin SR tablets. Information on additional adverse events associated with the sustained-release formulation of bupropion in smoking cessation trials, as well as the immediate-release formulation of bupropion, is included in a separate section (see Other Events Observed During the Clinical Development and post-marketing Experience of Bupropion).

Incidence in Controlled Trials With Wellbutrin SR

Adverse Events Associated With Discontinuation of Treatment Among Patients Treated With Wellbutrin SR Tablets

In placebo-controlled clinical trials, 9% and 11% of patients treated with 300 and 400 mg/day, respectively, of Wellbutrin SR tablets and 4% of patients treated with placebo discontinued treatment due to adverse events. The specific adverse events in these trials that led to discontinuation in at least 1% of patients treated with either 300 or 400 mg/day of Wellbutrin SR tablets and at a rate at least twice the placebo rate are listed in TABLE 7.

TABLE 7 *Treatment Discontinuations Due to Adverse Events in Placebo-Controlled Trials*

Adverse Event Term	Wellbutrin SR 300 mg/day (n=376)	Wellbutrin SR 400 mg/day (n=114)	Placebo (n=385)
Rash	2.4%	0.9%	0.0%
Nausea	0.8%	1.8%	0.3%
Agitation	0.3%	1.8%	0.3%
Migraine	0.0%	1.8%	0.3%

Adverse Events Occurring at an Incidence of 1% or More Among Patients Treated With Wellbutrin SR Tablets

TABLE 8 enumerates treatment-emergent adverse events that occurred among patients treated with 300 and 400 mg/day of Wellbutrin SR tablets and with placebo in placebo-controlled trials. Events that occurred in either the 300 or 400 mg/day group at an incidence of 1% or more and were more frequent than in the placebo group are included. Reported adverse events were classified using a COSTART-based Dictionary.

Accurate estimates of the incidence of adverse events associated with the use of any drug are difficult to obtain. Estimates are influenced by drug dose, detection technique, setting, physician judgments, etc. The figures cited cannot be used to predict precisely the incidence of untoward events in the course of usual medical practice where patient characteristics and other factors differ from those that prevailed in the clinical trials. These incidence figures also cannot be compared with those obtained from other clinical studies involving related drug products as each group of drug trials is conducted under a different set of conditions.

Finally, it is important to emphasize that the tabulation does not reflect the relative severity and/or clinical importance of the events. A better perspective on the serious adverse events associated with the use of Wellbutrin SR tablets is provided in WARNINGS, Wellbutrin SR and PRECAUTIONS, Wellbutrin SR.

Incidence of Commonly Observed Adverse Events in Controlled Clinical Trials

Adverse events from TABLE 8 occurring in at least 5% of patients treated with Wellbutrin SR tablets and at a rate at least twice the placebo rate are listed below for the 300 and 400 mg/day dose groups.

Wellbutrin SR 300 mg/day: Anorexia, dry mouth, rash, sweating, tinnitus, and tremor.

Wellbutrin SR 400 mg/day: Abdominal pain, agitation, anxiety, dizziness, dry mouth, insomnia, myalgia, nausea, palpitation, pharyngitis, sweating, tinnitus, and urinary frequency.

Other Events Observed During the Clinical Development and Post-Marketing Experience of Bupropion

In addition to the adverse events noted above, the following events have been reported in clinical trials and post-marketing experience with the sustained-release formulation of bupropion in depressed patients and in nondepressed smokers, as well as in clinical trials and post-marketing clinical experience with the immediate-release formulation of bupropion.

Adverse events for which frequencies are provided below occurred in clinical trials with the sustained-release formulation of bupropion. The frequencies represent the proportion of patients who experienced a treatment-emergent adverse event on at least one occasion in placebo-controlled studies for depression (n=987) or smoking cessation (n=1013), or patients who experienced an adverse event requiring discontinuation of treatment in an open-label surveillance study with Wellbutrin SR tablets (n=3100). All treatment-emergent adverse events are included except those listed in TABLE 4, TABLE 5, TABLE 7 and TABLE 8, those events listed in other safety-related sections, those adverse events subsumed under COSTART terms that are either overly general or excessively specific so as to be uninformative, those events not reasonably associated with the use of the drug, and those events that were not serious and occurred in fewer than 2 patients. Events of major clinical importance are described in WARNINGS, Wellbutrin SR and PRECAUTIONS, Wellbutrin SR.

Events are further categorized by body system and listed in order of decreasing frequency according to the following definitions of frequency: *Frequent* adverse events are defined as those occurring in at least 1/100 patients. *Infrequent* adverse events are those occurring in 1/100 to 1/1000 patients, while *rare* events are those occurring in less than 1/1000 patients.

Adverse events for which frequencies are not provided occurred in clinical trials or post-marketing experience with bupropion. Only those adverse events not previously listed for sustained-release bupropion are included. The extent to which these events may be associated with Wellbutrin SR is unknown.

Body (General): *Infrequent:* Chills, facial edema, musculoskeletal chest pain, and photosensitivity. *Rare:* Malaise. Also observed were arthralgia, myalgia, and fever with rash and other symptoms suggestive of delayed hypersensitivity. These symptoms may resemble serum sickness (see PRECAUTIONS, Wellbutrin SR).

Cardiovascular: *Infrequent:* Postural hypotension, stroke, tachycardia, and vasodilation. *Rare:* Syncope. Also observed were complete atrioventricular block, extrasystoles, hypotension, hypertension (in some cases severe, see PRECAUTIONS, Wellbutrin SR), myocardial infarction, phlebitis, and pulmonary embolism.

Digestive: *Infrequent:* Abnormal liver function, bruxism, gastric reflux, gingivitis, glossitis, increased salivation, jaundice, mouth ulcers, stomatitis, and thirst. *Rare:* Edema of tongue. Also observed were colitis, esophagitis, gastrointestinal hemorrhage, gum hemorrhage, hepatitis, intestinal perforation, liver damage, pancreatitis, and stomach ulcer.

Endocrine: Also observed were hyperglycemia, hypoglycemia, and syndrome of inappropriate antidiuretic hormone.

Hemic and Lymphatic: *Infrequent:* Ecchymosis. Also observed were anemia, leukocytosis, leukopenia, lymphadenopathy, pancytopenia, and thrombocytopenia. Altered PT and/or INR, infrequently associated with hemorrhagic or thrombotic complications, were observed when bupropion was coadministered with warfarin.

TABLE 8 *Treatment-Emergent Adverse Events in Placebo-Controlled Trials**

Body System	Wellbutrin SR		
	300 mg/day	400 mg/day	Placebo
Adverse Event	(n=376)	(n=114)	(n=385)
Body (General)			
Headache	26%	25%	23%
Infection	8%	9%	6%
Abdominal pain	3%	9%	2%
Asthenia	2%	4%	2%
Chest pain	3%	4%	1%
Pain	2%	3%	2%
Fever	1%	2%	—
Cardiovascular			
Palpitation	2%	6%	2%
Flushing	1%	4%	—
Migraine	1%	4%	1%
Hot flashes	1%	3%	1%
Digestive			
Dry mouth	17%	24%	7%
Nausea	13%	18%	8%
Constipation	10%	5%	7%
Diarrhea	5%	7%	6%
Anorexia	5%	3%	2%
Vomiting	4%	2%	2%
Dysphagia	0%	2%	0%
Musculoskeletal			
Myalgia	2%	6%	3%
Arthralgia	1%	4%	1%
Arthritis	0%	2%	0%
Twitch	1%	2%	—
Nervous System			
Insomnia	11%	16%	6%
Dizziness	7%	11%	5%
Agitation	3%	9%	2%
Anxiety	5%	6%	3%
Tremor	6%	3%	1%
Nervousness	5%	3%	3%
Somnolence	2%	3%	2%
Irritability	3%	2%	2%
Memory decreased	—	3%	1%
Paresthesia	1%	2%	1%
Central nervous system stimulation	2%	1%	1%
Respiratory			
Pharyngitis	3%	11%	2%
Sinusitis	3%	1%	2%
Increased cough	1%	2%	1%
Skin			
Sweating	6%	5%	2%
Rash	5%	4%	1%
Pruritus	2%	4%	2%
Urticaria	2%	1%	0%
Special Senses			
Tinnitus	6%	6%	2%
Taste perversion	2%	4%	—
Amblyopia	3%	2%	2%
Urogenital			
Urinary frequency	2%	5%	2%
Urinary urgency	—	2%	0%
Vaginal hemorrhage†	0%	2%	—
Urinary tract infection	1%	0%	—

* Adverse events that occurred in at least 1% of patients treated with either 300 or 400 mg/day of Wellbutrin SR tablets, but equally or more frequently in the placebo group, were: abnormal dreams, accidental injury, acne, appetite increased, back pain, bronchitis, dysmenorrhea, dyspepsia, flatulence, flu syndrome, hypertension, neck pain, respiratory disorder, rhinitis, and tooth disorder.
† Incidence based on the number of female patients.
— Denotes adverse events occurring in greater than 0 but less than 0.5% of patients.

Metabolic and Nutritional: *Infrequent:* Edema and peripheral edema. Also observed was glycosuria.

Musculoskeletal: *Infrequent:* Leg cramps. Also observed were muscle rigidity/fever/rhabdomyolysis and muscle weakness.

Nervous System: *Infrequent:* Abnormal coordination, decreased libido, depersonalization, dysphoria, emotional lability, hostility, hyperkinesia, hypertonia, hypesthesia, suicidal ideation, and vertigo. *Rare:* Amnesia, ataxia, derealization, and hypomania. Also observed were abnormal electroencephalogram (EEG), akinesia, aphasia, coma, delirium, dysarthria, dyskinesia, dystonia, euphoria, extrapyramidal syndrome, hallucinations, hypokinesia, increased libido, manic reaction, neuralgia, neuropathy, paranoid reaction, and unmasking tardive dyskinesia.

Respiratory: *Rare:* Bronchospasm. Also observed was pneumonia.

Skin: *Rare:* Maculopapular rash. Also observed were alopecia, angioedema, exfoliative dermatitis, and hirsutism.

Special Senses: *Infrequent:* Accommodation abnormality and dry eye. Also observed were deafness, diplopia, and mydriasis.

Urogenital: *Infrequent:* Impotence, polyuria, and prostate disorder. Also observed were abnormal ejaculation, cystitis, dyspareunia, dysuria, gynecomastia, menopause, painful erection, salpingitis, urinary incontinence, urinary retention, and vaginitis.

ZYBAN

See also WARNINGS, Zyban and PRECAUTIONS, Zyban.

The information included under ADVERSE REACTIONS is based primarily on data from the dose-response trial and the comparative trial that evaluated Zyban for smoking cessation. Information on additional adverse events associated with the sustained-release formulation of bupropion in depression trials, as well as the immediate-release formulation of bupropion, is included in a separate section (see Other Events Observed During the Clinical Development and Post-marketing Experience of Bupropion).

Adverse Events Associated With the Discontinuation of Treatment

Adverse events were sufficiently troublesome to cause discontinuation of treatment in 8% of the 706 patients treated with Zyban and 5% of the 313 patients treated with placebo. The more common events leading to discontinuation of treatment with Zyban included nervous system disturbances (3.4%), primarily tremors, and skin disorders (2.4%), primarily rashes.

Incidence of Commonly Observed Adverse Events

The most commonly observed adverse events consistently associated with the use of Zyban were dry mouth and insomnia. The most commonly observed adverse events were defined as those that consistently occurred at a rate of 5 percentage points greater than that for placebo across clinical studies.

Dose Dependency of Adverse Events

The incidence of dry mouth and insomnia may be related to the dose of Zyban. The occurrence of these adverse events may be minimized by reducing the dose of Zyban. In addition, insomnia may be minimized by avoiding bedtime doses.

Adverse Events Occurring at an Incidence of 1% or More Among Patients Treated With Zyban

TABLE 9 enumerates selected treatment-emergent adverse events from the dose-response trial that occurred at an incidence of 1% or more and were more common in patients treated with Zyban compared to those treated with placebo. TABLE 10 enumerates selected treatment-emergent adverse events from the comparative trial that occurred at an incidence of 1% or more and were more common in patients treated with Zyban, NTS, or the combination of Zyban and NTS compared to those treated with placebo. Reported adverse events were classified using a COSTART-based dictionary.

TABLE 9 *Treatment-Emergent Adverse Event Incidence in the Dose-Response Trial**

Body System	Zyban	
	100-300 mg/day	Placebo
Adverse Experience	(n=461)	(n=150)
Body (General)		
Neck pain	2%	<1%
Allergic reaction	1%	0%
Cardiovascular		
Hot flashes	1%	0%
Hypertension	1%	<1%
Digestive		
Dry mouth	11%	5%
Increased appetite	2%	<1%
Anorexia	1%	<1%
Musculoskeletal		
Arthralgia	4%	3%
Myalgia	2%	1%
Nervous System		
Insomnia	31%	21%
Dizziness	8%	7%
Tremor	2%	1%
Somnolence	2%	1%
Thinking abnormality	1%	0%
Respiratory		
Bronchitis	2%	0%
Skin		
Pruritus	3%	<1%
Rash	3%	<1%
Dry skin	2%	0%
Uriticaria	1%	0%
Special Senses		
Taste perversion	2%	<1%

* Selected adverse events with an incidence of at least 1% of patients treated with Zyban and more frequent than in the placebo group.

Zyban was well-tolerated in the long-term maintenance trial, that evaluated chronic administration of Zyban for up to 1 year and in the COPD trial that evaluated patients with mild to moderate COPD for a 12 week period. Adverse events in both studies were quantitatively and qualitatively similar to those observed in the dose-response and comparative trials.

Other Events Observed During the Clinical Development and Post-Marketing Experience of Bupropion

In addition to the adverse events noted above, the following events have been reported in clinical trials and post-marketing experience with the sustained-release formulation of bupropion in depressed patients and in nondepressed smokers, as well as in clinical trials and post-marketing clinical experience with the immediate-release formulation of bupropion.

Adverse events for which frequencies are provided below occurred in clinical trials with bupropion sustained-release. The frequencies represent the proportion of patients who experienced a treatment-emergent adverse event on at least one occasion in placebo-controlled studies for depression (n=987) or smoking cessation (n=1013), or patients who experienced an adverse event requiring discontinuation of treatment in an open-label surveillance study with bupropion sustained-release tablets (n=3100). All treatment-emergent adverse events are included except those listed in TABLE 9 and TABLE 10, those events listed in other safety-related sections of the insert, those adverse events subsumed under COSTART terms that are either overly general or excessively specified so as to be uninformative, those events not reasonably associated with the use of the drug, and those events that were not serious and occurred in fewer than 2 patients.

TABLE 10 *Treatment-Emergent Adverse Event Incidence in the Comparative Trial**

Adverse Experience (COSTART Term)	Zyban 300 mg/day (n=243)	NTS 21 mg/day (n=243)	Zyban + NTS (n=244)	Placebo (n=159)
Body				
Abdominal pain	3%	4%	1%	1%
Accidental injury	2%	2%	1%	1%
Chest pain	<1%	1%	3%	1%
Neck pain	2%	1%	<1%	0%
Facial edema	<1%	0%	1%	0%
Cardiovascular				
Hypertension	1%	<1%	2%	0%
Palpitations	2%	0%	1%	0%
Digestive				
Nausea	9%	7%	11%	4%
Dry mouth	10%	4%	9%	4%
Constipation	8%	4%	9%	3%
Diarrhea	4%	4%	3%	1%
Anorexia	3%	1%	5%	1%
Mouth ulcer	2%	1%	1%	1%
Thirst	<1%	<1%	2%	0%
Musculoskeletal				
Myalgia	4%	3%	5%	3%
Arthralgia	5%	3%	3%	2%
Nervous System				
Insomnia	40%	28%	45%	18%
Dream abnormality	5%	18%	13%	3%
Anxiety	8%	6%	9%	6%
Disturbed concentration	9%	3%	9%	4%
Dizziness	10%	2%	8%	6%
Nervousness	4%	<1%	2%	2%
Tremor	1%	<1%	2%	0%
Dysphoria	<1%	1%	2%	1%
Respiratory				
Rhinitis	12%	11%	9%	8%
Increased cough	3%	5%	<1%	1%
Pharyngitis	3%	2%	3%	0%
Sinusitis	2%	2%	2%	1%
Dyspnea	1%	0%	2%	1%
Epistaxis	2%	1%	1%	0%
Skin				
Application site reaction†	11%	17%	15%	7%
Rash	4%	3%	3%	2%
Pruritus	3%	1%	5%	1%
Uriticaria	2%	0%	2%	0%
Special Senses				
Taste perversion	3%	1%	3%	2%
Tinnitus	1%	0%	<1%	0%

* Selected adverse events with an incidence of at least 1% of patients treated with either Zyban, NTS, or the combination of Zyban and NTS and more frequent than in the placebo group.
† Patients randomized to Zyban or placebo received placebo patches.

Events are further categorized by body system and listed in order of decreasing frequency according to the following definitions of frequency: *Frequent* adverse events are defined as those occurring in at least 1/100 patients. *Infrequent* adverse events are those occurring in 1/100 to 1/1000 patients, while *rare* events are those occurring in less than 1/1000 patients.

Adverse events for which frequencies are not provided occurred in clinical trials or post-marketing experience with bupropion. Only those adverse events not previously listed for sustained-release bupropion are included. The extent to which these events may be associated with Zyban is unknown.

Body (General): *Frequent:* Asthenia, fever, and headache. *Infrequent:* Back pain, chills, inguinal hernia, musculoskeletal chest pain, pain, and photosensitivity. *Rare:* Malaise. Also observed were arthralgia, myalgia, and fever with rash and other symptoms suggestive of delayed hypersensitivity. These symptoms may resemble serum sickness (see PRECAUTIONS, Zyban).

Cardiovascular: *Infrequent:* Flushing, migraine, postural hypotension, stroke, tachycardia, and vasodilation. *Rare:* Syncope. Also observed were cardiovascular disorder, complete AV block, extrasystoles, hypotension, hypertension (in some cases severe, see PRECAUTIONS, Zyban), myocardial infarction, phlebitis, and pulmonary embolism.

Digestive: *Frequent:* Dyspepsia, flatulence, and vomiting. *Infrequent:* Abnormal liver function, bruxism, dysphagia, gastric reflux, gingivitis, glossitis, jaundice, and stomatitis. *Rare:* Edema of tongue. Also observed were colitis, esophagitis, gastrointestinal hemorrhage, gum hemorrhage, hepatitis, increased salivation, intestinal perforation, liver damage, pancreatitis, stomach ulcer, and stool abnormality.

Endocrine: Also observed were hyperglycemia, hypoglycemia, and syndrome of inappropriate antidiuretic hormone.

Hemic and Lymphatic: *Infrequent:* Ecchymosis. Also observed were anemia, leukocytosis, leukopenia, lymphadenopathy, pancytopenia, and thrombocytopenia. Altered PT and/or INR, infrequently associated with hemorrhagic or thrombotic complications, were observed when bupropion was coadministered with warfarin.

Metabolic and Nutritional: *Infrequent:* Edema, increased weight, and peripheral edema. Also observed was glycosuria.

Musculoskeletal: *Infrequent:* Leg cramps and twitching. Also observed were arthritis and muscle rigidity/fever/rhabdomyolysis, and muscle weakness.

Nervous System: *Frequent:* Agitation, depression, and irritability. *Infrequent:* Abnormal coordination, CNS stimulation, confusion, decreased libido, decreased memory, depersonalization, emotional lability, hostility, hyperkinesia, hypertonia, hypesthesia, paresthesia, suicidal ideation, and vertigo. *Rare:* Amnesia, ataxia, derealization, and hypomania. Also observed were abnormal electroencephalogram (EEG), akinesia, aphasia, coma, delirium, delusions, dysarthria, dyskinesia, dystonia, euphoria, extrapyramidal syndrome, hallucinations, hypokinesia, increased libido, manic reaction, neuralgia, neuropathy, paranoid reaction, and unmasking tardive dyskinesia.

Respiratory: *Rare:* Bronchospasm. Also observed was pneumonia.

Skin: *Frequent:* Sweating. *Infrequent:* Acne and dry skin. *Rare:* Maculopapular rash. Also observed were alopecia, angioedema, exfoliative dermatitis, and hirsutism.

Special Senses: *Frequent:* Amblyopia. *Infrequent:* Accommodation abnormality and dry eye. Also observed were deafness, diplopia, and mydriasis.

Urogenital: *Frequent:* Urinary frequency. *Infrequent:* Impotence, polyuria, and urinary urgency. Also observed were abnormal ejaculation, cystitis, dyspareunia, dysuria, gynecomastia, menopause, painful erection, prostate disorder, salpingitis, urinary incontinence, urinary retention, urinary tract disorder, and vaginitis.

DOSAGE AND ADMINISTRATION

WELLBUTRIN

General Dosing Considerations

It is particularly important to administer Wellbutrin in a manner most likely to minimize the risk of seizure (see WARNINGS, Wellbutrin). Increases in dose should not exceed 100 mg/day in a 3 day period. Gradual escalation in dosage is also important if agitation, motor restlessness, and insomnia, often seen during the initial days of treatment, are to be minimized. If necessary, these effects may be managed by temporary reduction of dose or the short-term administration of an intermediate to long-acting sedative hypnotic. A sedative hypnotic usually is not required beyond the first week of treatment. Insomnia may also be minimized by avoiding bedtime doses. If distressing, untoward effects supervene, dose escalation should be stopped.

No single dose of Wellbutrin should exceed 150 mg. Wellbutrin should be administered 3 times daily, preferably with at least 6 hours between successive doses.

Usual Dosage for Adults

The usual adult dose is 300 mg/day, given 3 times daily. Dosing should begin at 200 mg/day, given as 100 mg twice daily. Based on clinical response, this dose may be increased to 300 mg/day, given as 100 mg three times daily, no sooner than 3 days after beginning therapy (see TABLE 11).

TABLE 11 *Dosing Regimen*

Treatment Day	Total Daily Dose	Number of 100 mg Tablets Morning	Midday	Evening
1	200 mg	1	0	1
4	300 mg	1	1	1

Increasing the Dosage Above 300 mg/Day

As with other antidepressants, the full antidepressant effect of Wellbutrin may not be evident until 4 weeks of treatment or longer. An increase in dosage, up to a maximum of 450 mg/day, given in divided doses of not more than 150 mg each, may be considered for patients in whom no clinical improvement is noted after several weeks of treatment at 300 mg/day. Dosing above 300 mg/day may be accomplished using the 75 or 100 mg tablets. The 100 mg tablet must be administered 4 times daily with at least 4 hours between successive doses, in order not to exceed the limit of 150 mg in a single dose. Wellbutrin should be discontinued in patients who do not demonstrate an adequate response after an appropriate period of treatment at 450 mg/day.

Maintenance

The lowest dose that maintains remission is recommended. Although it is not known how long the patient should remain on Wellbutrin, it is generally recognized that acute episodes of depression require several months or longer of antidepressant drug treatment.

Dosage Adjustment for Patients With Impaired Hepatic Function

Wellbutrin should be used with extreme caution in patients with severe hepatic cirrhosis. The dose should not exceed 75 mg once a day in these patients. Wellbutrin should be used with caution in patients with hepatic impairment (including mild to moderate hepatic cirrhosis) and a reduced frequency and/or dose should be considered in patients with mild to moderate hepatic cirrhosis (see CLINICAL PHARMACOLOGY, Wellbutrin and PRECAUTIONS, Wellbutrin).

Dosage Adjustment for Patients With Impaired Renal Function

Wellbutrin should be used with caution in patients with renal impairment and a reduced frequency and/or dose should be considered (see CLINICAL PHARMACOLOGY, Wellbutrin and PRECAUTIONS, Wellbutrin).

WELLBUTRIN SR

General Dosing Considerations

It is particularly important to administer Wellbutrin SR tablets in a manner most likely to minimize the risk of seizure (see WARNINGS, Wellbutrin SR). Gradual escalation in dosage is also important if agitation, motor restlessness, and insomnia, often seen during the initial days of treatment, are to be minimized. If necessary, these effects may be managed by temporary reduction of dose or the short-term administration of an intermediate to long-acting sedative hypnotic. A sedative hypnotic usually is not required beyond the first week of treatment. Insomnia may also be minimized by avoiding bedtime doses. If distressing, untoward effects supervene, dose escalation should be stopped. Wellbutrin SR should be swallowed whole and not crushed, divided, or chewed.

Initial Treatment

The usual adult target dose for Wellbutrin SR tablets is 300 mg/day, given as 150 mg twice daily. Dosing with Wellbutrin SR tablets should begin at 150 mg/day given as a single daily dose in the morning. If the 150 mg initial dose is adequately tolerated, an increase to the 300 mg/day target dose, given as 150 mg twice daily, may be made as early as day 4 of dosing. There should be an interval of at least 8 hours between successive doses.

Increasing the Dosage Above 300 mg/day

As with other antidepressants, the full antidepressant effect of Wellbutrin SR tablets may not be evident until 4 weeks of treatment or longer. An increase in dosage to the maximum of 400 mg/day, given as 200 mg twice daily, may be considered for patients in whom no clinical improvement is noted after several weeks of treatment at 300 mg/day.

Maintenance Treatment

It is generally agreed that acute episodes of depression require several months or longer of sustained pharmacological therapy beyond response to the acute episode. In a study in which patients with major depressive disorder, recurrent type, who had responded during 8 weeks of acute treatment with Wellbutrin SR were assigned randomly to placebo or to the same dose of Wellbutrin SR (150 mg twice daily) during 44 weeks of maintenance treatment as they had received during the acute stabilization phase, longer-term efficacy was demonstrated. Based on these limited data, it is unknown whether or not the dose of Wellbutrin SR needed for maintenance treatment is identical to the dose needed to achieve an initial response. Patients should be periodically reassessed to determine the need for maintenance treatment and the appropriate dose for such treatment.

Dosage Adjustment for Patients With Impaired Hepatic Function

Wellbutrin SR should be used with extreme caution in patients with severe hepatic cirrhosis. The dose should not exceed 100 mg every day or 150 mg every other day in these patients. Wellbutrin SR should be used with caution in patients with hepatic impairment (including mild to moderate hepatic cirrhosis) and a reduced frequency and/or dose should be considered in patients with mild to moderate hepatic cirrhosis (see CLINICAL PHARMACOLOGY, Wellbutrin SR, WARNINGS, Wellbutrin SR, and PRECAUTIONS, Wellbutrin SR).

Dosage Adjustment for Patients With Impaired Renal Function

Wellbutrin SR should be used with caution in patients with renal impairment and a reduced frequency and/or dose should be considered (see CLINICAL PHARMACOLOGY, Wellbutrin SR and PRECAUTIONS, Wellbutrin SR).

ZYBAN

Usual Dosage for Adults

The recommended and maximum dose of Zyban is 300 mg/day, given as 150 mg twice daily. Dosing should begin at 150 mg/day given every day for the first 3 days, followed by a dose increase for most patients to the recommended usual dose of 300 mg/day. There should be an interval of at least 8 hours between successive doses. Doses above 300 mg/day should not be used (see WARNINGS, Zyban). Zyban should be swallowed whole and not crushed, divided, or chewed. Treatment with Zyban should be initiated **while the patient is still smoking,** since approximately 1 week of treatment is required to achieve steady-state blood levels of bupropion. Patients should set a "target quit date" within the first 2 weeks of treatment with Zyban, generally in the second week. Treatment with Zyban should be continued for 7-12 weeks; longer treatment should be guided by the relative benefits and risks for individual patients. If a patient has not made significant progress towards abstinence by the seventh week of therapy with Zyban, it is unlikely that he or she will quit during that attempt, and treatment should probably be discontinued. Conversely, a patient who successfully quits after 7-12 weeks of treatment should be considered for ongoing therapy with Zyban. Dose tapering of Zyban is not required when discontinuing treatment. It is important that patients continue to receive counseling and support throughout treatment with Zyban, and for a period of time thereafter.

Individualization of Therapy

Patients are more likely to quit smoking and remain abstinent if they are seen frequently and receive support from their physicians or other health care professionals. It is important to ensure that patients read the instructions provided to them and have their questions answered. Physicians should review the patient's overall smoking cessation program that includes treatment with Zyban. Patients should be advised of the importance of participating in the behavioral interventions, counseling, and/or support services to be used in conjunction with Zyban. See the Patient Instructions that are distributed with the prescription for complete instructions.

The goal of therapy with Zyban is complete abstinence. If a patient has not made significant progress towards abstinence by the seventh week of therapy with Zyban, it is unlikely that he or she will quit during that attempt, and treatment should probably be discontinued.

Patients who fail to quit smoking during an attempt may benefit from interventions to improve their chances for success on subsequent attempts. Patients who are unsuccessful should be evaluated to determine why they failed. A new quit attempt should be encouraged when factors that contributed to failure can be eliminated or reduced, and conditions are more favorable.

Maintenance

Nicotine dependence is a chronic condition. Some patients may need continuous treatment. Systematic evaluation of Zyban 300 mg/day for maintenance therapy demonstrated that treatment for up to 6 months was efficacious. Whether to continue treatment with Zyban for periods longer than 12 weeks for smoking cessation must be determined for individual patients.

Combination Treatment With Zyban and a Nicotine Transdermal System (NTS)

Combination treatment with Zyban and NTS may be prescribed for smoking cessation. The prescriber should review the complete prescribing information for both Zyban and NTS before using combination treatment. Monitoring for treatment-emergent hypertension in patients treated with the combination of Zyban and NTS is recommended.

Dosage Adjustment for Patients With Impaired Hepatic Function

Zyban should be used with extreme caution in patients with severe hepatic cirrhosis. The dose should not exceed 150 mg every other day in these patients. Zyban should be used with caution in patients with hepatic impairment (including mild to moderate hepatic cirrhosis) and a reduced frequency of dosing should be considered in patients with mild to moderate hepatic cirrhosis (see CLINICAL PHARMACOLOGY, Zyban, WARNINGS, Zyban, and PRECAUTIONS, Zyban).

Dosage Adjustment for Patients With Impaired Renal Function

Zyban should be used with caution in patients with renal impairment and a reduced frequency of dosing should be considered (see CLINICAL PHARMACOLOGY, Zyban and PRECAUTIONS, Zyban).

HOW SUPPLIED

WELLBUTRIN

Wellbutrin tablets are available in:

75 mg: Yellow-gold, round, biconvex tablets printed with "WELLBUTRIN 75".

100 mg: Red, round, biconvex tablets printed with "WELLBUTRIN 100".

Storage: Store at 15-25°C (59-77°F). Protect from light and moisture.

WELLBUTRIN SR

Wellbutrin SR sustained-release tablets are available in:

100 mg: Blue, round, biconvex, film-coated tablets printed with "WELLBUTRIN SR 100".

150 mg: Purple, round, biconvex, film-coated tablets printed with "WELLBUTRIN SR 150".

200 mg: Light pink, round, biconvex, film-coated tablets printed with "WELLBUTRIN SR 200".

Storage: Store at controlled room temperature, 20-25°C (68-77°F). Dispense in a tight, light-resistant container.

ZYBAN

Zyban sustained-release tablets, 150 mg of bupropion hydrochloride, are purple, round, biconvex, film-coated tablets printed with "ZYBAN 150".

Storage: Store at controlled room temperature, 20-25°C (68-77°F). Dispense in tight, light-resistant containers.

PRODUCT LISTING - RATED THERAPEUTICALLY EQUIVALENT

Tablet - Oral - 75 mg			
7's	$7.61	WELLBUTRIN, Prescript Pharmaceuticals	00247-0676-07
14's	$11.88	WELLBUTRIN, Prescript Pharmaceuticals	00247-0676-14
25's	$20.02	WELLBUTRIN, Allscripts Pharmaceutical Company	54569-3573-04
30's	$21.62	WELLBUTRIN, Prescript Pharmaceuticals	00247-0676-30
60's	$39.88	WELLBUTRIN, Prescript Pharmaceuticals	00247-0676-60
100's	$72.00	GENERIC, Geneva Pharmaceuticals	00781-1053-01
100's	$72.05	GENERIC, Mylan Pharmaceuticals Inc	00378-0433-01
100's	$72.08	GENERIC, Teva Pharmaceuticals Usa	00093-0280-01
100's	$73.00	GENERIC, Udl Laboratories Inc	51079-0943-20
100's	$108.33	WELLBUTRIN, Glaxosmithkline	00173-0177-55
Tablet - Oral - 100 mg			
7's	$10.40	WELLBUTRIN, Prescript Pharmaceuticals	00247-0677-07
14's	$17.44	WELLBUTRIN, Prescript Pharmaceuticals	00247-0677-14
30's	$33.53	WELLBUTRIN, Prescript Pharmaceuticals	00247-0677-30
30's	$36.15	WELLBUTRIN, Southwood Pharmaceuticals Inc	58016-0222-30
50's	$83.37	WELLBUTRIN, Physicians Total Care	54868-1450-00
60's	$63.71	WELLBUTRIN, Prescript Pharmaceuticals	00247-0677-60
60's	$72.30	WELLBUTRIN, Southwood Pharmaceuticals Inc	58016-0222-60
90's	$96.17	WELLBUTRIN, Allscripts Pharmaceutical Company	54569-3190-01
100's	$96.06	GENERIC, Geneva Pharmaceuticals	00781-1064-01
100's	$96.15	GENERIC, Mylan Pharmaceuticals Inc	00378-0435-01
100's	$96.16	GENERIC, Teva Pharmaceuticals Usa	00093-0290-01
100's	$97.00	GENERIC, Udl Laboratories Inc	51079-0944-20
100's	$144.49	WELLBUTRIN, Glaxosmithkline	00173-0178-55

PRODUCT LISTING - EQUIVALENTS NOT AVAILABLE

Tablet - Oral - 75 mg			
60's	$43.20	GENERIC, Southwood Pharmaceuticals Inc	58016-0722-60
Tablet - Oral - 100 mg			
30's	$29.70	GENERIC, Pharma Pac	52959-0655-30
40's	$39.60	GENERIC, Pharma Pac	52959-0655-40
Tablet, Extended Release - Oral - 100 mg			
60's	$112.60	WELLBUTRIN SR, Glaxosmithkline	00173-0947-55
Tablet, Extended Release - Oral - 150 mg			
30's	$49.47	ZYBAN SR, Pharma Pac	52959-0487-30
30's	$54.78	WELLBUTRIN SR, Southwood Pharmaceuticals Inc	58016-0599-30
30's	$70.61	WELLBUTRIN SR, Pharma Pac	52959-0285-30
60's	$91.64	ZYBAN SR, Allscripts Pharmaceutical Company	54569-4496-00
60's	$108.41	ZYBAN SR, Physicians Total Care	54868-4025-00
60's	$108.99	WELLBUTRIN SR, Physicians Total Care	54868-3984-00
60's	$109.55	WELLBUTRIN SR, Southwood Pharmaceuticals Inc	58016-0599-60
60's	$120.69	WELLBUTRIN SR, Glaxosmithkline	00173-0135-55
60's	$120.69	ZYBAN SR, Glaxosmithkline	00173-0556-01
60's	$120.69	ZYBAN SR REFILL, Glaxosmithkline	00173-0556-02
90's	$164.33	WELLBUTRIN SR, Southwood Pharmaceuticals Inc	58016-0599-90
100's	$182.58	WELLBUTRIN SR, Southwood Pharmaceuticals Inc	58016-0599-00
Tablet, Extended Release - Oral - 200 mg			
60's	$224.13	WELLBUTRIN SR, Glaxosmithkline	00173-0722-00

B

Buspirone Hydrochloride (000551)

Categories: Anxiety disorder, generalized; Pregnancy Category B; FDA Approved 1986 Sep
Drug Classes: Anxiolytics
Brand Names: Buspar
Foreign Brand Availability: Ansial (Spain); Ansitec (Brazil); Anxinil (Taiwan); Anxiolan (Thailand); Anxiron (Bahrain; Cyprus; Egypt; Iran; Iraq; Jordan; Kuwait; Lebanon; Libya; Oman; Qatar; Republic-of-Yemen; Saudi-Arabia; Syria; United-Arab-Emirates); Bespar (Germany; Greece); Biron (New-Zealand); Buspin (India); Buspirex (Canada); Buspirone (Greece); Bustab (Canada); Kallmiren (Bahrain; Cyprus; Egypt; Iran; Iraq; Israel; Jordan; Kuwait; Lebanon; Libya; Oman; Qatar; Republic-of-Yemen; Saudi-Arabia; Syria; United-Arab-Emirates); Narol (Spain); Nerbet (Chile); Normaton (Guatemala; Honduras); Pasrin (South-Africa); Paxon (Chile); Relac (Taiwan); Sburol (Korea); Sepirone (Taiwan); Tran-Q (Indonesia); Xiety (Indonesia)
Cost of Therapy: $91.37 (Anxiety; Buspar; 10 mg; 2 tablets/day; 30 day supply)
$80.70 (Anxiety; Generic Tablets; 10 mg; 2 tablets/day; 30 day supply)

DESCRIPTION

Buspirone hydrochloride is an antianxiety agent that is not chemically or pharmacologically related to the benzodiazepines, barbiturates, or other sedative/anxiolytic drugs.

Buspirone hydrochloride is a white crystalline, water soluble compound with a molecular weight of 422.0. Chemically, buspirone hydrochloride is 8-[4-[4-(2-pyrimidinyl)-1-piperazinyl]butyl]-8-azaspiro[4.5]decane-7,9-dione monohydrochloride. The empirical formula is $C_{21}H_{31}N_5O_2$·HCl.

BuSpar is supplied as tablets for oral administration containing 5, 10, 15, or 30 mg of buspirone hydrochloride (equivalent to 4.6, 9.1, 13.7 and 27.4 mg of buspirone free base respectively). The 5 and 10 mg tablets are scored so they can be bisected. Thus, the 5 mg tablet can also provide a 2.5 mg dose, and the 10 mg tablet can provide a 5 mg dose. The 15 and 30 mg tablets are provided in the Dividose tablet design. These tablets are scored so they can be either bisected or trisected. Thus, a single 15 mg tablet can provide the following doses: 15 mg (entire tablet), 10 mg (two-thirds of a tablet), 7.5 mg (one-half of a tablet), or 5 mg (one-third of a tablet). A single 30 mg tablet can provide the following doses: 30 mg (entire tablet), 20 mg (two-thirds of a tablet), 15 mg (one-half of a tablet), or 10 mg (one-third of a tablet). BuSpar tablets contain the following inactive ingredients: Colloidal silicon dioxide, lactose, magnesium stearate, microcrystalline cellulose, and sodium starch glycolate. The 30 mg tablet also contains iron oxide.

CLINICAL PHARMACOLOGY

The mechanism of action of buspirone is unknown. Buspirone differs from typical benzodiazepine anxiolytics in that it does not exert anticonvulsant or muscle relaxant effects. It also lacks the prominent sedative effect that is associated with more typical anxiolytics. *In vitro* preclinical studies have shown that buspirone has a high affinity for serotonin (5-HT_{1A}) receptors. Buspirone has no significant affinity for benzodiazepine receptors and does not affect GABA binding *in vitro* or *in vivo* when tested in preclinical models.

Buspirone has moderate affinity for brain D_2-dopamine receptors. Some studies do suggest that buspirone may have indirect effects on other neurotransmitter systems.

Buspirone HCl is rapidly absorbed in man and undergoes extensive first-pass metabolism. In a radiolabeled study, unchanged buspirone in the plasma accounted for only about 1% of the radioactivity in the plasma. Following oral administration, plasma concentrations of unchanged buspirone are very low and variable between subjects. Peak plasma levels of 1-6 ng/ml have been observed 40-90 minutes after single oral doses of 20 mg. The single-dose bioavailability of unchanged buspirone when taken as a tablet is on the average about 90% of an equivalent dose of solution, but there is large variability.

The effects of food upon the bioavailability of buspirone HCl have been studied in 8 subjects. They were given a 20 mg dose with and without food; the area under the plasma concentration-time curve (AUC) and peak plasma concentration (C_{max}) of unchanged buspirone increased by 84% and 116% respectively, but the total amount of buspirone immunoreactive material did not change. This suggests that food may decrease the extent of presystemic clearance of buspirone (see DOSAGE AND ADMINISTRATION).

A multiple-dose study conducted in 15 subjects suggests that buspirone has nonlinear pharmacokinetics. Thus, dose increases and repeated dosing may lead to somewhat higher blood levels of unchanged buspirone than would be predicted from results of single-dose studies.

An *in vitro* protein binding study indicated that approximately 86% of buspirone is bound to plasma proteins. It was also observed that aspirin increased the plasma levels of free buspirone by 23%, while flurazepam decreased the plasma levels of free buspirone by 20%. However, it is not known whether these drugs cause similar effects on plasma levels of free buspirone *in vivo*, or whether such changes, if they do occur, cause clinically significant differences in treatment outcome. An *in vitro* study indicated that buspirone did not displace highly protein-bound drugs such as phenytoin, warfarin, and propranolol from plasma protein, and that buspirone may displace digoxin.

Buspirone is metabolized primarily by oxidation, which *in vitro* has been shown to be mediated by cytochrome P450 3A4 (CYP3A4). (See DRUG INTERACTIONS.) Several hydroxylated derivatives and a pharmacologically active metabolite, 1-pyrimidinylpiperazine (1-PP), are produced. In animal models predictive of anxiolytic potential, 1-PP has about one-quarter of the activity of buspirone, but is present in up to 20-fold greater amounts. However, this is probably not important in humans: blood samples from humans chronically exposed to buspirone HCl do not exhibit high levels of 1-PP; mean values are approximately 3 ng/ml and the highest human blood level recorded among 108 chronically dosed patients was 17 ng/ml, less than 1/200th of 1-PP levels found in animals given large doses of buspirone without signs of toxicity.

In a single-dose study using ^{14}C-labeled buspirone, 29-63% of the dose was excreted in the urine within 24 hours, primarily as metabolites; fecal excretion accounted for 18-38% of the dose. The average elimination half-life of unchanged buspirone after single doses of 10-40 mg is about 2-3 hours.

SPECIAL POPULATIONS

Age and Gender Effects

After single or multiple doses in adults, no significant differences in buspirone pharmacokinetics (AUC and C_{max}) were observed between elderly and younger subjects or between men and women.

Hepatic Impairment

After multiple-dose administration of buspirone to patients with hepatic impairment, steady-state AUC of buspirone increased 13-fold compared with healthy subjects (see PRECAUTIONS).

Renal Impairment

After multiple-dose administration of buspirone to renally impaired (CLCR = 10-70 ml/min/1.73 m^2) patients, steady-state AUC of buspirone increased 4-fold compared with healthy (CLCR ≥80 ml/min/1.73 m^2) subjects (see PRECAUTIONS).

Race Effects

The effects of race on the pharmacokinetics of buspirone have not been studied.

INDICATIONS AND USAGE

Buspirone HCl is indicated for the management of anxiety disorders or the short-term relief of the symptoms of anxiety. Anxiety or tension associated with the stress of everyday life usually does not require treatment with an anxiolytic.

The efficacy of buspirone HCl has been demonstrated in controlled clinical trials of outpatients whose diagnosis roughly corresponds to Generalized Anxiety Disorder (GAD). Many of the patients enrolled in these studies also had coexisting depressive symptoms and buspirone HCl relieved anxiety in the presence of these coexisting depressive symptoms. The patients evaluated in these studies had experienced symptoms for periods of 1 month to over 1 year prior to the study, with an average symptom duration of 6 months. Generalized Anxiety Disorder (300.02) is described in the American Psychiatric Association's Diagnostic and Statistical Manual, III[1] as follows:

Generalized, persistent anxiety (of at least 1 month continual duration), manifested by symptoms from 3 of the 4 following categories:

- ***Motor Tension:*** Shakiness, jitteriness, jumpiness, trembling, tension, muscle aches, fatigability, inability to relax, eyelid twitch, furrowed brow, strained face, fidgeting, restlessness, easy startle.
- ***Autonomic Hyperactivity:*** Sweating, heart pounding or racing, cold, clammy hands, dry mouth, dizziness, lightheadedness, paresthesias (tingling in hands or feet), upset stomach, hot or cold spells, frequent urination, diarrhea, discomfort in the pit of the stomach, lump in the throat, flushing, pallor, high resting pulse, and respiration rate.
- ***Apprehensive Expectation:*** Anxiety, worry, fear, rumination, and anticipation of misfortune to self or others.
- ***Vigilance and Scanning:*** Hyperattentiveness resulting in distractibility, difficulty in concentrating, insomnia, feeling "on edge", irritability, impatience.

The above symptoms would not be due to another mental disorder, such as a depressive disorder or schizophrenia. However, mild depressive symptoms are common in GAD.

The effectiveness of buspirone HCl in long-term use, that is, for more than 3-4 weeks, has not been demonstrated in controlled trials. There is no body of evidence available that systematically addresses the appropriate duration of treatment for GAD. However, in a study of long-term use, 264 patients were treated with buspirone HCl for 1 year without ill effect. Therefore, the physician who elects to use buspirone HCl for extended periods should periodically reassess the usefulness of the drug for the individual patient.

NON-FDA APPROVED INDICATIONS

Buspirone may also have clinical utility in a number of other disorders including alcohol dependence and cerebellar ataxia. Patients with severe depressive symptoms who are receiving SSRI's may benefit from augmentation with buspirone. Case studies where buspirone has successfully been used in the treatment of Tourette's syndrome and in the treatment of dementia with aggression have been reported. Buspirone has also been shown to have a beneficial effect on smoking abstinence, but only among smokers who were relatively high in anxiety and only for as long as the drug was available. None of these uses have been approved by the FDA.

CONTRAINDICATIONS

Buspirone HCl is contraindicated in patients hypersensitive to buspirone HCl.

WARNINGS

The administration of buspirone HCl to a patient taking a monoamine oxidase inhibitor (MAOI) may pose a hazard. There have been reports of the occurrence of elevated blood pressure when buspirone HCl has been added to a regimen including an MAOI. Therefore, it is recommended that buspirone HCl not be used concomitantly with an MAOI.

Because buspirone HCl has no established antipsychotic activity, it should not be employed in lieu of appropriate antipsychotic treatment.

PRECAUTIONS

GENERAL

Interference With Cognitive and Motor Performance

Studies indicate that buspirone HCl is less sedating than other anxiolytics and that it does not produce significant functional impairment. However, its CNS effects in any individual patient may not be predictable. Therefore, patients should be cautioned about operating an automobile or using complex machinery until they are reasonably certain that buspirone treatment does not affect them adversely.

While formal studies of the interaction of buspirone HCl with alcohol indicate that buspirone does not increase alcohol-induced impairment in motor and mental performance, it is prudent to avoid concomitant use of alcohol and buspirone.

Potential for Withdrawal Reactions in Sedative/Hypnotic/Anxiolytic Drug-Dependent Patients

Because buspirone HCl does not exhibit cross-tolerance with benzodiazepines and other common sedative/hypnotic drugs, it will not block the withdrawal syndrome often seen with cessation of therapy with these drugs. Therefore, before starting therapy with buspirone HCl, it is advisable to withdraw patients gradually, especially patients who have been using a CNS-depressant drug chronically, from their prior treatment. Rebound or withdrawal symptoms may occur over varying time periods, depending in part on the type of drug, and its effective half-life of elimination.

The syndrome of withdrawal from sedative/hypnotic/anxiolytic drugs can appear as any combination of irritability, anxiety, agitation, insomnia, tremor, abdominal cramps, muscle cramps, vomiting, sweating, flu-like symptoms without fever, and occasionally, even as seizures.

Possible Concerns Related to Buspirone's Binding to Dopamine Receptors

Because buspirone can bind to central dopamine receptors, a question has been raised about its potential to cause acute and chronic changes in dopamine-mediated neurological function (*e.g.,* dystonia, pseudo-parkinsonism, akathisia, and tardive dyskinesia). Clinical experience in controlled trials has failed to identify any significant neuroleptic-like activity; however, a syndrome of restlessness, appearing shortly after initiation of treatment, has been reported in some small fraction of buspirone-treated patients. The syndrome may be explained in several ways. For example, buspirone may increase central noradrenergic activity; alternatively, the effect may be attributable to dopaminergic effects (*i.e.,* represent akathisia). Obviously, the question cannot be totally resolved at this point in time. Generally, long-term sequelae of any drug's use can be identified only after several years of marketing.

INFORMATION FOR THE PATIENT

To assure safe and effective use of buspirone HCl, the following information and instructions should be given to patients:

- Inform your physician about any medications, prescription or non-prescription, alcohol, or drugs that you are now taking or plan to take during your treatment with buspirone HCl.
- Inform your physician if you are pregnant, or if you are planning to become pregnant, or if you become pregnant while you are taking buspirone HCl.
- Inform your physician if you are breast-feeding an infant.
- Until you experience how this medication affects you, do not drive a car or operate potentially dangerous machinery.
- You should take buspirone HCl consistently, either always with food or always without food.
- During your treatment with buspirone HCl, avoid drinking large amounts of grapefruit juice.

LABORATORY TESTS

There are no specific laboratory tests recommended.

DRUG/LABORATORY TEST INTERACTIONS

Buspirone is not known to interfere with commonly employed clinical laboratory tests.

CARCINOGENESIS, MUTAGENESIS, AND IMPAIRMENT OF FERTILITY

No evidence of carcinogenic potential was observed in rats during a 24 month study at approximately 133 times the maximum recommended human oral dose; or in mice, during an 18 month study at approximately 167 times the maximum recommended human oral dose.

With or without metabolic activation, buspirone did not induce point mutations in five strains of *Salmonella typhimurium* (Ames Test) or mouse lymphoma L5178YTK+ cell cultures, nor was DNA damage observed with buspirone in Wi-38 human cells. Chromosomal aberrations or abnormalities did not occur in bone marrow cells of mice given 1 or 5 daily doses of buspirone.

PREGNANCY, TERATOGENIC EFFECTS, PREGNANCY CATEGORY B

No fertility impairment or fetal damage was observed in reproduction studies performed in rats and rabbits at buspirone doses of approximately 30 times the maximum recommended human dose. In humans, however, adequate and well-controlled studies during pregnancy have *not* been performed. Because animal reproduction studies are not always predictive of human response, this drug should be used during pregnancy only if clearly needed.

LABOR AND DELIVERY

The effect of buspirone HCl on labor and delivery in women is unknown. No adverse effects were noted in reproduction studies in rats.

NURSING MOTHERS

The extent of the excretion in human milk of buspirone or its metabolites is not known. In rats, however, buspirone and its metabolites are excreted in milk. Buspirone HCl administration to nursing women should be avoided if clinically possible.

PEDIATRIC USE

The safety and effectiveness of buspirone were evaluated in two placebo-controlled 6 week trials involving a total of 559 pediatric patients (ranging from 6-17 years of age) with GAD. Doses studied were 7.5-30 mg bid (15-60 mg/day). There were no significant differences between buspirone and placebo with regard to the symptoms of GAD following doses recommended for the treatment of GAD in adults. Pharmacokinetic studies have shown that, for identical doses, plasma exposure to buspirone and its active metabolite, 1-PP, are equal to or higher in pediatric patients than adults. No unexpected safety findings were associated with buspirone in these trials. There are no long-term safety or efficacy data in this population.

GERIATRIC USE

In one study of 6632 patients who received buspirone for the treatment of anxiety, 605 patients were ≥65 years old and 41 were ≥75 years old; the safety and efficacy profiles for these 605 elderly patients (mean age = 70.8 years) were similar to those in the younger population (mean age = 43.3 years). Review of spontaneously reported adverse clinical events has not identified differences between elderly and younger patients, but greater sensitivity of some older patients cannot be ruled out.

There were no effects of age on the pharmacokinetics of buspirone (see CLINICAL PHARMACOLOGY, Special Populations).

USE IN PATIENTS WITH IMPAIRED HEPATIC OR RENAL FUNCTION

Buspirone is metabolized by the liver and excreted by the kidneys. A pharmacokinetic study in patients with impaired hepatic or renal function demonstrated increased plasma levels and a lengthened half-life of buspirone. Therefore, the administration of buspirone HCl to patients with severe hepatic or renal impairment cannot be recommended (see CLINICAL PHARMACOLOGY).

B

DRUG INTERACTIONS

PSYCHOTROPIC AGENTS

MAO Inhibitors: It is recommended that buspirone HCl *not* be used concomitantly with MAO inhibitors (see WARNINGS).

Amitriptyline: After addition of buspirone to the amitriptyline dose regimen, no statistically significant differences in the steady-state pharmacokinetic parameters (C_{max}, AUC, and C_{min}) of amitriptyline or its metabolite nortriptyline were observed.

Diazepam: After addition of buspirone to the diazepam dose regimen, no statistically significant differences in the steady-state pharmacokinetic parameters (C_{max}, AUC, and C_{min}) were observed for diazepam, but increases of about 15% were seen for nordiazepam, and minor adverse clinical effects (dizziness, headache, and nausea) were observed.

Haloperidol: In a study in normal volunteers, concomitant administration of buspirone HCl and haloperidol resulted in increased serum haloperidol concentrations. The clinical significance of this finding is not clear.

Nefazodone: See Inhibitors and Inducers of Cytochrome P450 3A4 (CYP3A4).

Trazodone: There is one report suggesting that the concomitant use of trazodone HCl and buspirone HCl may have caused 3- to 6-fold elevations on SGPT (ALT) in a few patients. In a similar study attempting to replicate this finding, no interactive effect on hepatic transaminases was identified.

Triazolam/Flurazepam: Coadministration of buspirone with either triazolam or flurazepam did not appear to prolong or intensify the sedative effects of either benzodiazepine.

Other Psychotropics: Because the effects of concomitant administration of buspirone with most other psychotropic drugs have not been studied, the concomitant use of buspirone with other CNS-active drugs should be approached with caution.

INHIBITORS AND INDUCERS OF CYTOCHROME P450 3A4 (CYP3A4)

Buspirone has been shown *in vitro* to be metabolized by CYP3A4. This finding is consistent with the *in vivo* interactions observed between buspirone and the following:

Diltiazem and Verapamil: In a study of 9 healthy volunteers, coadministration of buspirone (10 mg as a single dose) with verapamil (80 mg tid) or diltiazem (60 mg tid) increased plasma buspirone concentrations (verapamil increased AUC and C_{max} of buspirone 3.4-fold while diltiazem increased AUC and C_{max} 5.5-fold and 4-fold, respectively). Adverse events attributable to buspirone may be more likely during concomitant administration with either diltiazem or verapamil. Subsequent dose adjustment may be necessary and should be based on clinical assessment.

Erythromycin: In a study in healthy volunteers, coadministration of buspirone (10 mg as a single dose) with erythromycin (1.5 g/day for 4 days) increased plasma buspirone concentrations (5-fold increase in C_{max} and 6-fold increase in AUC). These pharmacokinetic interactions were accompanied by an increased incidence of side effects attributable to buspirone. If the two drugs are to be used in combination, a low dose of buspirone (*e.g.,* 2.5 mg bid) is recommended. Subsequent dose adjustment of either drug should be based on clinical assessment.

Grapefruit Juice: In a study in healthy volunteers, coadministration of buspirone (10 mg as a single dose) with grapefruit juice (200 ml double-strength tid for 2 days) increased plasma buspirone concentrations (4.3-fold increase in C_{max}; 9.2-fold increase in AUC). Patients receiving buspirone should be advised to avoid drinking such large amounts of grapefruit juice.

Itraconazole: In a study in healthy volunteers, coadministration of buspirone (10 mg as a single dose) with itraconazole (200 mg/day for 4 days) increased plasma buspirone concentrations (13-fold increase in C_{max} and 19-fold increase in AUC). These pharmacokinetic interactions were accompanied by an increased incidence of side effects attributable to buspirone. If the two drugs are to be used in combination, a low dose of buspirone (*e.g.,* 2.5 mg qd) is recommended. Subsequent dose adjustment of either drug should be based on clinical assessment.

Nefazodone: In a study of steady-state pharmacokinetics in healthy volunteers, coadministration of buspirone (2.5 or 5 mg bid) with nefazodone (250 mg bid) resulted in marked increases in plasma buspirone concentrations (increases up to 20-fold in C_{max} and up to 50-fold in AUC) and statistically significant decreases (about 50%) in plasma concentrations of the buspirone metabolite 1-PP. With 5 mg bid doses of buspirone, slight increases in AUC were observed for nefazodone (23%) and its metabolites hydroxynefazodone (HO-NEF) (17%) and meta-chlorophenylpiperazine (9%). Slight increases in C_{max} were observed for nefazodone (8%) and its metabolite HO-NEF (11%). Subjects receiving buspirone 5 mg bid and nefazodone 250 mg bid experienced lightheadedness, asthenia, dizziness, and somnolence, adverse events also observed with either drug alone. If the two drugs are to be used in combination, a low dose of buspirone (*e.g.,* 2.5 mg qd) is recommended. Subsequent dose adjustment of either drug should be based on clinical assessment.

Rifampin: In a study of healthy volunteers, coadministration of buspirone (30 mg as a single dose) with rifampin (600 mg/day for 5 days) decreased the plasma concentrations (83.7% decrease in C_{max}; 89.6% decrease in AUC) and pharmacodynamic effects of buspirone. If the two drugs are to be used in combination, the dosage of buspirone may need adjusting to maintain anxiolytic effect.

Other Inhibitors and Inducers of CYP3A4: Substances that inhibit CYP3A4, such as ketoconazole or ritonavir, may inhibit buspirone metabolism and increase plasma concentrations of buspirone while substances that induce CYP3A4, such as dexamethasone or certain anticonvulsants (phenytoin, phenobarbital, carbamazepine), may increase the rate of buspirone metabolism. If a patient has been titrated to a stable dosage on buspirone, a dose adjustment of buspirone may be necessary to avoid adverse events attributable to buspirone or diminished anxiolytic activity. Consequently, when administered with a potent inhibitor of CYP3A4, a low dose of buspirone used cautiously is recommended. When used in combination with a potent inducer of CYP3A4 the dosage of buspirone may need adjusting to maintain anxiolytic effect.

B

OTHER DRUGS

Cimetidine: Coadministration of buspirone with cimetidine was found to increase C_{max} (40%) and T_{max} (2-fold), but had minimal effects on the AUC of buspirone.

PROTEIN BINDING

In vitro, buspirone does not displace tightly bound drugs like phenytoin, propranolol, and warfarin from serum proteins. However, there has been one report of prolonged prothrombin time when buspirone was added to the regimen of a patient with warfarin. The patient was also chronically receiving phenytoin, phenobarbital, digoxin, and levothyroxine sodium. *In vitro,* buspirone may displace less firmly bound drugs like digoxin. The clinical significance of this property is unknown.

Therapeutic levels of aspirin, desipramine, diazepam, flurazepam, ibuprofen, propranolol, thioridazine, and tolbutamide had only a limited effect on the extent of binding buspirone to plasma proteins (see CLINICAL PHARMACOLOGY).

ADVERSE REACTIONS

See also PRECAUTIONS.

COMMONLY OBSERVED

The more commonly observed untoward events associated with the use of buspirone HCl not seen at an equivalent incidence among placebo-treated patients include dizziness, nausea, headache, nervousness, lightheadedness, and excitement.

ASSOCIATED WITH DISCONTINUATION OF TREATMENT

One guide to the relative clinical importance of adverse events associated with buspirone HCl is provided by the frequency with which they caused drug discontinuation during clinical testing. Approximately 10% of the 2200 anxious patients who participated in the buspirone HCl premarketing clinical efficacy trials in anxiety disorders lasting 3-4 weeks discontinued treatment due to an adverse event. The more common events causing discontinuation included: central nervous system disturbances (3.4%), primarily dizziness, insomnia, nervousness, drowsiness, and lightheaded feeling; gastrointestinal disturbances (1.2%), primarily nausea; and miscellaneous disturbances (1.1%), primarily headache and fatigue. In addition, 3.4% of patients had multiple complaints, none of which could be characterized as primary.

INCIDENCE IN CONTROLLED CLINICAL TRIALS

TABLE 1 enumerates adverse events that occurred at a frequency of 1% or more among buspirone HCl patients who participated in 4 week, controlled trials comparing buspirone HCl with placebo. The frequencies were obtained from pooled data for 17 trials. The prescriber should be aware that these figures cannot be used to predict the incidence of side effects in the course of usual medical practice where patient characteristics and other factors differ from those which prevailed in the clinical trials. Similarly, the cited frequencies cannot be compared with figures obtained from other clinical investigations involving different treatments, uses, and investigators. Comparison of the cited figures, however, does provide the prescribing physician with some basis for estimating the relative contribution of drug and nondrug factors to the side-effect incidence rate in the population studied.

TABLE 1 *Treatment-Emergent Adverse Experience Incidence in Placebo-Controlled Clinical Studies**

Adverse Experience	Buspirone HCl (n=477)	Placebo (n=464)
Cardiovascular		
Tachycardia/palpitations	1%	1%
CNS		
Dizziness	12%	3%
Drowsiness	10%	9%
Nervousness	5%	1%
Insomnia	3%	3%
Lightheadedness	3%	—
Decreased concentration	2%	2%
Excitement	2%	—
Anger/hostility	2%	—
Confusion	2%	—
Depression	2%	2%
EENT		
Blurred vision	2%	—
Gastrointestinal		
Nausea	8%	5%
Dry mouth	3%	4%
Abdominal/gastric distress	2%	2%
Diarrhea	2%	—
Constipation	1%	2%
Vomiting	1%	2%
Musculoskeletal		
Musculoskeletal aches/pains	1%	—
Neurological		
Numbness	2%	—
Paresthesia	1%	—
Incoordination	1%	—
Tremor	1%	—
Skin		
Skin rash	1%	—
Miscellaneous		
Headache	6%	3%
Fatigue	4%	4%
Weakness	2%	—
Sweating/clamminess	1%	—

* Events reported by at least 1% of buspirone HCl patients are included.
— Incidence less than 1%.

OTHER EVENTS OBSERVED DURING THE ENTIRE PREMARKETING EVALUATION OF BUSPIRONE HCl

During its premarketing assessment, buspirone HCl was evaluated in over 3500 subjects. This section reports event frequencies for adverse events occurring in approximately 3000 subjects from this group who took multiple doses of buspirone HCl in the dose range for which buspirone HCl is being recommended (*i.e.,* the modal daily dose of buspirone HCl fell between 10 and 30 mg for 70% of the patients studied) and for whom safety data were systematically collected. The conditions and duration of exposure to buspirone HCl varied greatly, involving well-controlled studies as well as experience in open and uncontrolled clinical settings. As part of the total experience gained in clinical studies, various adverse events were reported. In the absence of appropriate controls in some of the studies, a causal relationship to buspirone HCl treatment cannot be determined. The list includes all undesirable events reasonably associated with the use of the drug.

The following enumeration by organ system describes events in terms of their relative frequency of reporting in this data base. Events of major clinical importance are also described in PRECAUTIONS.

The following definitions of frequency are used: *Frequent* adverse events are defined as those occurring in at least 1/100 patients. *Infrequent* adverse events are those occurring in 1/100 to 1/1000 patients, while *rare* events are those occurring in less than 1/1000 patients.

Cardiovascular: *Frequent:* Nonspecific chest pain; *Infrequent:* Syncope, hypotension, and hypertension; *Rare:* Cerebrovascular accident, congestive heart failure, myocardial infarction, cardiomyopathy, and bradycardia.

Central Nervous System: *Frequent:* Dream disturbances; *Infrequent:* Depersonalization, dysphoria, noise intolerance, euphoria, akathisia, fearfulness, loss of interest, dissociative reaction, hallucinations, involuntary movements, slowed reaction time, suicidal ideation, and seizures; *Rare:* Feelings of claustrophobia, cold intolerance, stupor, and slurred speech and psychosis.

EENT: *Frequent:* Tinnitus, sore throat, and nasal congestion; *Infrequent:* Redness and itching of the eyes, altered taste, altered smell, and conjunctivitis; *Rare:* Inner ear abnormality, eye pain, photophobia, and pressure on eyes.

Endocrine: *Rare:* Galactorrhea and thyroid abnormality.

Gastrointestinal: *Infrequent:* Flatulence, anorexia, increased appetite, salivation, irritable colon, and rectal bleeding; *Rare:* Burning of the tongue.

Genitourinary: *Infrequent:* Urinary frequency, urinary hesitancy, menstrual irregularity and spotting, and dysuria; *Rare:* Amenorrhea, pelvic inflammatory disease, enuresis, and nocturia.

Musculoskeletal: *Infrequent:* Muscle cramps, muscle spasms, rigid/stiff muscles, and arthralgias; *Rare:* Muscle weakness.

Respiratory: *Infrequent:* Hyperventilation, shortness of breath, and chest congestion; *Rare:* Epistaxis.

Sexual Function: *Infrequent:* Decreased or increased libido; *Rare:* Delayed ejaculation and impotence.

Skin: *Infrequent:* Edema, pruritus, flushing, easy bruising, hair loss, dry skin, facial edema, and blisters; *Rare:* Acne and thinning of nails.

Clinical Laboratory: *Infrequent:* Increases in hepatic aminotransferases (SGOT, SGPT); *Rare:* Eosinophilia, leukopenia, and thrombocytopenia.

Miscellaneous: *Infrequent:* Weight gain, fever, roaring sensation in the head, weight loss, and malaise; *Rare:* Alcohol abuse, bleeding disturbance, loss of voice, and hiccoughs.

POSTINTRODUCTION CLINICAL EXPERIENCE

Postmarketing experience has shown an adverse experience profile similar to that given above. Voluntary reports since introduction have included rare occurrences of allergic reactions (including urticaria), angioedema, cogwheel rigidity, dizziness (rarely reported as vertigo), dystonic reactions, ataxias, extrapyramidal symptoms, dyskinesias (acute and tardive), ecchymosis, emotional lability, serotonin syndrome, transient difficulty with recall, urinary retention, and visual changes (including tunnel vision). Because of the uncontrolled nature of these spontaneous reports, a causal relationship to buspirone HCl treatment has not been determined.

DOSAGE AND ADMINISTRATION

The recommended initial dose is 15 mg daily (7.5 mg bid). To achieve an optimal therapeutic response, at intervals of 2-3 days the dosage may be increased 5 mg/day, as needed. The maximum daily dosage should not exceed 60 mg/day. In clinical trials allowing dose titration, divided doses of 20-30 mg/day were commonly employed.

The bioavailability of buspirone is increased when given with food as compared to the fasted state (see CLINICAL PHARMACOLOGY). Consequently, patients should take buspirone in a consistent manner with regard to the timing of dosing; either always with or always without food.

When buspirone is to be given with a potent inhibitor of CYP3A4 the dosage recommendations described in DRUG INTERACTIONS should be followed.

HOW SUPPLIED

BuSpar tablets are available in:

5 mg: White, ovoid-rectangular with score, MJ logo, "5" and "BUSPAR" embossed.

10 mg: White, ovoid-rectangular with score, MJ logo, "10" and "BUSPAR" embossed.

15 mg: White, in the Dividose tablet design imprinted with the MJ logo and scored so that they can be either bisected or trisected with ID number "822" on one side and on the reverse side, the number "5" on each trisect segment.

30 mg: Pink, in the Dividose tablet design imprinted with the MJ logo and scored so that they can be either bisected or trisected with ID number "824" on one side and on the reverse side, the number "10" on each trisect segment.

Storage: Store at room temperature — protect from temperatures greater than 30°C (86°F). Dispense in a tight, light-resistant container.

PRODUCT LISTING - RATED THERAPEUTICALLY EQUIVALENT

Qty	Price	Product	NDC
Tablet - Oral - 5 mg			
8's	$10.35	BUSPAR, Prescript Pharmaceuticals	00247-0959-08
14's	$15.61	BUSPAR, Prescript Pharmaceuticals	00247-0959-14
20's	$18.12	BUSPAR, Southwood Pharmaceuticals Inc	58016-0857-20
20's	$20.86	BUSPAR, Prescript Pharmaceuticals	00247-0959-20
30's	$24.10	BUSPAR, Southwood Pharmaceuticals Inc	58016-0857-30
60's	$39.36	BUSPAR, Southwood Pharmaceuticals Inc	58016-0857-60
60's	$57.19	BUSPAR, Physicians Total Care	54868-1098-02
90's	$73.86	BUSPAR, Allscripts Pharmaceutical Company	54569-0955-03
100's	$77.10	GENERIC, Mylan Pharmaceuticals Inc	00378-1140-01
100's	$77.12	GENERIC, Teva Pharmaceuticals Usa	00093-0053-01
100's	$77.12	GENERIC, Watson Laboratories Inc	00591-0657-01
100's	$77.12	GENERIC, Udl Laboratories Inc	51079-0985-20
100's	$78.05	GENERIC, Ivax Corporation	00172-5663-10
100's	$81.15	GENERIC, Ivax Corporation	00172-5663-60
100's	$81.62	GENERIC, Par Pharmaceutical Inc	49884-0707-01
100's	$90.49	BUSPAR, Bristol-Myers Squibb	00087-0818-43
100's	$90.70	BUSPAR, Bristol-Myers Squibb	00087-0818-41
Tablet - Oral - 10 mg			
20's	$25.65	BUSPAR, Southwood Pharmaceuticals Inc	58016-0160-20
30's	$35.48	BUSPAR, Southwood Pharmaceuticals Inc	58016-0160-30
30's	$42.31	BUSPAR, Prescript Pharmaceuticals	00247-0697-30
30's	$45.68	BUSPAR, Allscripts Pharmaceutical Company	54569-1606-01
30's	$50.02	BUSPAR, Physicians Total Care	54868-1099-00
40's	$70.98	BUSPAR, Pd-Rx Pharmaceuticals	55289-0208-40
60's	$61.96	BUSPAR, Southwood Pharmaceuticals Inc	58016-0160-60
60's	$98.86	BUSPAR, Physicians Total Care	54868-1099-02
90's	$137.05	BUSPAR, Allscripts Pharmaceutical Company	54569-1606-02
100's	$134.50	GENERIC, Teva Pharmaceuticals Usa	00093-0054-01
100's	$134.50	GENERIC, Mylan Pharmaceuticals Inc	00378-1150-01
100's	$134.50	GENERIC, Udl Laboratories Inc	51079-0986-20
100's	$136.25	GENERIC, Ivax Corporation	00172-5664-10
100's	$141.55	GENERIC, Ivax Corporation	00172-5664-60
100's	$142.35	GENERIC, Par Pharmaceutical Inc	49884-0708-01
100's	$152.28	BUSPAR, Allscripts Pharmaceutical Company	54569-1606-00
100's	$154.35	BUSPAR, Physicians Total Care	54868-1099-03
Tablet - Oral - 15 mg			
60's	$121.15	GENERIC, Mylan Pharmaceuticals Inc	00378-1165-91
60's	$126.92	GENERIC, Watson Laboratories Inc	00591-0718-60
60's	$127.61	GENERIC, Par Pharmaceutical Inc	49884-0721-02
100's	$201.90	GENERIC, Udl Laboratories Inc	51079-0960-20
100's	$201.92	GENERIC, Teva Pharmaceuticals Usa	00093-1003-01
100's	$207.36	GENERIC, Par Pharmaceutical Inc	49884-0721-01
100's	$211.45	GENERIC, Ivax Corporation	00172-5665-60
180's	$126.92	GENERIC, Watson Laboratories Inc	00591-0718-18
180's	$358.30	GENERIC, Mylan Pharmaceuticals Inc	00378-1165-80
180's	$369.30	GENERIC, Par Pharmaceutical Inc	49884-0721-13
250's	$521.15	GENERIC, Ivax Corporation	00172-5665-65
Tablet - Oral - 30 mg			
60's	$218.10	GENERIC, Mylan Pharmaceuticals Inc	00378-1175-91

PRODUCT LISTING - EQUIVALENTS NOT AVAILABLE

Qty	Price	Product	NDC
Tablet - Oral - 5 mg			
20's	$17.76	GENERIC, Southwood Pharmaceuticals Inc	58016-0720-20
28's	$24.86	GENERIC, Southwood Pharmaceuticals Inc	58016-0720-28
30's	$26.64	GENERIC, Southwood Pharmaceuticals Inc	58016-0720-30
30's	$48.75	GENERIC, Pharma Pac	52959-0654-30
60's	$53.28	GENERIC, Southwood Pharmaceuticals Inc	58016-0720-60
100's	$68.94	GENERIC, Bristol-Myers Squibb	59772-8818-01
100's	$77.12	BUSPIRONE HYDROCHLORIDE, Watson Laboratories Inc	52544-0657-01
100's	$81.55	GENERIC, Ethex Corporation	58177-0264-04
100's	$81.62	GENERIC, Major Pharmaceuticals Inc	00904-5587-60
100's	$88.80	GENERIC, Southwood Pharmaceuticals Inc	58016-0720-00
Tablet - Oral - 7.5 mg			
100's	$106.32	GENERIC, Par Pharmaceutical Inc	49884-0725-01
Tablet - Oral - 10 mg			
100's	$120.23	GENERIC, Bristol-Myers Squibb	59772-8819-01
100's	$134.50	GENERIC, Watson Laboratories Inc	00591-0658-01
100's	$134.50	GENERIC, Watson Laboratories Inc	52544-0658-01
100's	$142.21	GENERIC, Ethex Corporation	58177-0265-04
100's	$142.35	GENERIC, Major Pharmaceuticals Inc	00904-5588-60
Tablet - Oral - 15 mg			
30's	$107.09	BUSPAR DIVIDOSE, Pd-Rx Pharmaceuticals	55289-0556-30
49's	$110.03	BUSPAR, Bristol-Myers Squibb	00087-0822-34
60's	$141.80	BUSPAR, Bristol-Myers Squibb	00087-0822-32
100's	$176.64	GENERIC, Apothecon Inc	59772-8823-02
100's	$212.49	GENERIC, Ethex Corporation	58177-0309-04
180's	$369.34	GENERIC, Major Pharmaceuticals Inc	00904-5589-93
180's	$419.30	BUSPAR, Bristol-Myers Squibb	00087-0822-33
Tablet - Oral - 30 mg			
60's	$255.27	BUSPAR DIVIDOSE, Bristol-Myers Squibb	00087-0824-81
100's	$363.50	GENERIC, Udl Laboratories Inc	51079-0994-20

Busulfan *(000552)*

Categories: Transplantation, bone marrow; Leukemia, chronic myelogenous; Pregnancy Category D; FDA Approved 1954 Jun; Orphan Drugs
Drug Classes: Antineoplastics, alkylating agents
Brand Names: Busulfex; Citosulfan; Leukosulfan; Misulban; **Myleran**
Foreign Brand Availability: Mablin (Japan)
Cost of Therapy: $68.57 (CML; Myleran; 2 mg; 2 tablets/day; 15 day supply)

INTRAVENOUS

WARNING

CAUTION: MUST BE DILUTED PRIOR TO USE.

Busulfan injection is a potent cytotoxic drug that causes profound myelosuppression at the recommended dosage. It should be administered under the supervision of a qualified physician who is experienced in allogeneic hematopoietic stem cell transplantation, the use of cancer chemotherapeutic drugs and the management of patients with severe pancytopenia. Appropriate management of therapy and complications is only possible when adequate diagnostic and treatment facilities are readily available. SEE WARNINGS FOR INFORMATION REGARDING BUSULFAN-INDUCED PANCYTOPENIA IN HUMANS.

DESCRIPTION

Busulfan is a bifunctional alkylating agent known chemically as 1,4-butanediol, dimethanesulfonate. Busulfan injection is intended for intravenous (IV) administration. It is supplied as a clear, colorless, sterile, solution in 10 ml single use ampoules. Each ampoule of Busulfex contains 60 mg (6 mg/ml) of busulfan, the active ingredient, a white crystalline powder with a molecular formula of $CH_3SO_2O(CH_2)_4OSO_2CH_3$ and a molecular weight of 246 g/mole. Busulfan is dissolved in N,N-dimethylacetamide (DMA) 33% w/w and polyethylene glycol 400, 67% w/w. Busulfan's solubility in water is 0.1 g/L and the pH of a >0.5% solution in 0.9% sodium chloride injection or 5% dextrose injection as recommended for infusion reflects the pH of the diluent used and ranges from 3.4-3.9.

Busulfex is intended for dilution with 0.9% sodium chloride injection or 5% dextrose injection prior to IV infusion.

CLINICAL PHARMACOLOGY

MECHANISM OF ACTION

Busulfan is a bifunctional alkylating agent in which 2 labile methanesulfonate groups are attached to opposite ends of a 4-carbon alkyl chain. In aqueous media, busulfan hydrolyzes to release the methanesulfonate groups. This produces reactive carbonium ions that can alkylate DNA. DNA damage is thought to be responsible for much of the cytotoxicity of busulfan.

PHARMACOKINETICS

The pharmacokinetics of busulfan were studied in 59 patients participating in a prospective trial of a busulfan-cyclophosphamide preparatory regimen prior to allogeneic hematopoietic progenitor stem cell transplantation. Patients received 0.8 mg/kg busulfan every 6 hours, for a total of 16 doses over 4 days. Fifty-five (55) of 59 patients (93%) administered busulfan maintained AUC values below the target value (<1500 μM·min).

TABLE 1 *Steady-State Pharmacokinetic Parameters Following Busulfan Infusion (0.8 mg/kg; n=59)*

	Mean	CV	Range
C_{max} (ng/ml)	1222	18%	496-1684
AUC (μM·min)	1167	20%	556-1673
CL (ml/min/kg)*	2.52	25%	1.49-4.31

* Clearance normalized to actual body weight for all patients.

Busulfan pharmacokinetics showed consistency between dose 9 and dose 13 as demonstrated by reproducibility of steady-state C_{max} and a low coefficient of variation for this parameter.

In a pharmacokinetic study of busulfan in 24 pediatric patients, the population pharmacokinetic (PPK) estimates for busulfan for clearance (CL) and volume of distribution (V) were determined. For actual body weight, PPK estimates of CL and V were 4.04 L/h/20 kg (3.37 ml/min/kg: inter-patient variability 23%); and 12.8 L/20 kg (0.64 l/kg: inter-patient variability 11%).

DISTRIBUTION, METABOLISM, EXCRETION

Studies of distribution, metabolism, and elimination of busulfan have not been done; however, the literature on oral busulfan is relevant. Additionally, for modulating effects on pharmacodynamic parameters, see DRUG INTERACTIONS.

Distribution

Busulfan achieves concentrations in the cerebrospinal fluid approximately equal to those in plasma. Irreversible binding to plasma elements, primarily albumin, has been estimated to be 32.4 ± 2.2% which is consistent with the reactive electrophilic properties of busulfan.

Metabolism

Busulfan is predominantly metabolized by conjugation with glutathione, both spontaneously and by glutathione *S*-transferase (GST) catalysis. This conjugate undergoes further extensive oxidative metabolism in the liver.

B

Excretion

Following administration of ^{14}C-labeled busulfan to humans, approximately 30% of the radioactivity was excreted into the urine over 48 hours; negligible amounts were recovered in feces. The incomplete recovery of radioactivity may be due to the formation of long-lived metabolites or due to nonspecific alkylation of macromolecules.

INDICATIONS AND USAGE

Busulfan injection is indicated for use in combination with cyclophosphamide as a conditioning regimen prior to allogeneic hematopoietic progenitor cell transplantation for chronic myelogenous leukemia.

CONTRAINDICATIONS

Busulfan is contraindicated in patients with a history of hypersensitivity to any of its components.

WARNINGS

Busulfan should be administered under the supervision of a qualified physician experienced in hematopoietic stem cell transplantation. Appropriate management of complications arising from its administration is possible only when adequate diagnostic and treatment facilities are readily available.

The following warnings pertain to different physiologic effects of busulfan in the setting of allogeneic transplantation.

HEMATOLOGIC

The most frequent serious consequence of treatment with busulfan at the recommended dose and schedule is profound myelosuppression, occurring in all patients. Severe granulocytopenia, thrombocytopenia, anemia, or any combination thereof may develop. Frequent complete blood counts, including white blood cell differentials, and quantitative platelet counts should be monitored during treatment and until recovery is achieved. Absolute neutrophil counts dropped below 0.5×10^9/L at a median of 4 days post-transplant in 100% of patients treated in the busulfan clinical trial. The absolute neutrophil count recovered at a median of 13 days following allogeneic transplantation when prophylactic G-CSF was used in the majority of patients. Thrombocytopenia (<25,000/mm^3 or requiring platelet transfusion) occurred at a median of 5-6 days in 98% of patients. Anemia (hemoglobin <8.0 g/dl) occurred in 69% of patients. Antibiotic therapy and platelet and red blood cell support should be used when medically indicated.

NEUROLOGICAL

Seizures have been reported in patients receiving high-dose oral busulfan at doses producing plasma drug levels similar to those achieved following the recommended dosage of busulfan. Despite prophylactic therapy with phenytoin, 1 seizure (1/42 patients) was reported during an autologous transplantation clinical trial of busulfan. This episode occurred during the cyclophosphamide portion of the conditioning regimen, 36 hours after the last busulfan dose. Anti-convulsant prophylactic therapy should be initiated prior to busulfan treatment. Caution should be exercised when administering the recommended dose of busulfan to patients with a history of a seizure disorder or head trauma or who are receiving other potentially epileptogenic drugs.

HEPATIC

Current literature suggests that high busulfan area under the plasma concentration verses time curve (AUC) values (>1500 μM·min) may be associated with an increased risk of developing hepatic veno-occlusive disease (HVOD). Patients who have received prior radiation therapy, greater than or equal to 3 cycles of chemotherapy, or a prior progenitor cell transplant may be at an increased risk of developing HVOD with the recommended busulfan dose and regimen. Based on clinical examination and laboratory findings, HVOD was diagnosed in 8% (5/61) of patients treated with busulfan in the setting of allogeneic transplantation, and was fatal in 2/5 cases (40%), and yielded an overall mortality from HVOD in the entire study population of 2/61 (3%). Three (3) of the 5 patients diagnosed with HVOD were retrospectively found to meet the Jones' criteria. The incidence of HVOD reported in the literature from the randomized, controlled trials was 7.7-12%.

CARDIAC

Cardiac tamponade has been reported in pediatric patients with thalassemia (8/400 or 2% in 1 series) who received high doses of oral busulfan and cyclophosphamide as the preparatory regimen for hematopoietic progenitor cell transplantation. Six (6) of the 8 children died and 2 were saved by rapid pericardiocentesis. Abdominal pain and vomiting preceded the tamponade in most patients. No patients treated in the busulfan clinical trials experienced cardiac tamponade.

PULMONARY

Bronchopulmonary dysplasia with pulmonary fibrosis is a rare but serious complication following chronic busulfan therapy. The average onset of symptoms is 4 years after therapy (range 4 months to 10 years).

CARCINOGENICITY, MUTAGENICITY, AND IMPAIRMENT OF FERTILITY

Busulfan is a mutagen and a clastogen. In *in vitro* tests it caused mutations in *Salmonella typhimurium* and *Drosophila melanogaster.* Chromosomal aberrations induced by busulfan have been reported *in vivo* (rats, mice, hamsters, and humans) and *in vitro* (rodent and human cells). The IV administration of busulfan (48 mg/kg given as biweekly doses of 12 mg/kg, or 30% of the total busulfan dose on a mg/m^2 basis) has been shown to increase the incidence of thymic and ovarian tumors in mice. Four cases of acute leukemia occurred among 19 patients who became pancytopenic in a 243 patient study incorporating busulfan as adjuvant therapy following surgical resection of bronchogenic carcinoma. Clinical appearance of leukemia was observed 5-8 years following oral busulfan treatment. Busulfan is a presumed human carcinogen.

Ovarian suppression and amenorrhea commonly occur in premenopausal women undergoing chronic, low-dose busulfan therapy for chronic myelogenous leukemia. Busulfan depleted oocytes of female rats. Busulfan induced sterility in male rats and hamsters. Sterility, azoospermia, and testicular atrophy have been reported in male patients.

The solvent DMA may also impair fertility. A DMA daily dose of 0.45 g/kg/day given to rats for 9 days (equivalent to 44% of the daily dose of DMA contained in the recommended dose of busulfan on a mg/m^2 basis) significantly decreased spermatogenisis in rats. A single SC dose of 2.2 g/kg (27% of the total DMA dose contained in busulfan on a mg/m^2 basis) 4 days after insemination terminated pregnancy in 100% of tested hamsters.

PREGNANCY

Busulfan may cause fetal harm when administered to a pregnant woman. Busulfan produced teratogenic changes in the offspring of mice, rats, and rabbits when given during gestation. Malformations and anomalies included significant alterations in the musculoskeletal system, body weight gain, and size. In pregnant rats, busulfan produced sterility in both male and female offspring due to the absence of germinal cells in the testes and ovaries. The solvent, DMA, may also cause fetal harm when administered to a pregnant woman. In rats, DMA doses of 400 mg/kg/day (about 40% of the daily dose of DMA in the busulfan dose on a mg/m^2 basis) given during organogenesis caused significant developmental anomalies. The most striking abnormalities included anasarca, cleft palate, vertebral anomalies, rib anomalies, and serious anomalies of the vessels of the heart. There are no adequate and well-controlled studies of either busulfan or DMA in pregnant women. If busulfan is used during pregnancy, or if the patient becomes pregnant while receiving busulfan, the patient should be apprised of the potential hazard to the fetus. Women of childbearing potential should be advised to avoid becoming pregnant.

PRECAUTIONS

HEMATOLOGIC

At the recommended dosage of busulfan, profound myelosuppression is universal, and can manifest as neutropenia, thrombocytopenia, anemia, or a combination thereof. Patients should be monitored for signs of local or systemic infection or bleeding. Their hematologic status should be evaluated frequently.

INFORMATION FOR THE PATIENT

The increased risk of a second malignancy should be explained to the patient.

LABORATORY TESTS

Patients receiving busulfan should be monitored daily with a complete blood count, including differential count and quantitative platelet count, until engraftment has been demonstrated.

To detect hepatotoxicity, which may herald the onset of hepatic veno-occlusive disease, serum transaminases, alkaline phosphatase, and bilirubin should be evaluated daily through BMT Day +28.

PREGNANCY CATEGORY D

See WARNINGS.

NURSING MOTHERS

It is not known whether this drug is excreted in human milk. Because many drugs are excreted in human milk and because of the potential for tumorigenicity shown for busulfan in human and animal studies, a decision should be made whether to discontinue nursing or to discontinue the drug, taking into account the importance of the drug to the mother.

SPECIAL POPULATIONS

Pediatric

The effectiveness of busulfan in the treatment of CML has not been specifically studied in pediatric patients. An open-label, uncontrolled study evaluated the pharmacokinetics of busulfan in 24 pediatric patients receiving busulfan as part of a conditioning regimen administered prior to hematopoietic progenitor cell transplantation for a variety of malignant hematologic (n=15) or non-malignant diseases (n=9). Patients ranged in age from 5 months to 16 years (median 3 years).

Busulfan dosing was targeted to achieve an area under the plasma concentration curve (AUC) of 900-1350 μM·min with an initial dose of 0.8 mg/kg or 1.0 mg/kg (based on ABW) if the patient was >4 or ≤4 years, respectively. The dose was adjusted based on plasma concentration after completion of dose 1.

Patients received busulfan doses every 6 hours as a 2 hour infusion over 4 days for a total of 16 doses, followed by cyclophosphamide 50 mg/kg once daily for 4 days. After 1 rest day, hematopietic progenitor cells well infused. All patients received phenytoin as seizure prophylaxis. The target AUC (900-1350 ± 5% μM·min) for busulfan was achieved at dose 1 in 71% (17/24) of patients. Steady-state pharmacokinetic testing was performed at dose 9 and 13. Busulfan levels were within the target range for 21 of 23 evaluable patients.

All 24 patients experienced neutropenia (absolute neutrophil count $<0.5 \times 10^9$/L) and thrombocytopenia (platelet transfusions or platelet count <20,000/mm^3). Seventy-nine percent (79%) (19/24) of patients experienced lymphopenia (absolute lymphocyte count $<0.1 \times 10^9$). In 23 patients, the ANC recovered to $>0.5 \times 10^9$/L (median time to recovery = BMT Day +13; range = BMT Day +9 to +22). One patient who died on Day +28 had not recovered to an ANC $> 0.5 \times 10^9$/L.

Four (17%) patients died during the study. Two patients died within 28 days of transplant; 1 with pneumonia and capillary leak syndrome, and the other with pneumonia and veno-occlusive disease. Two patients died prior to Day 100; 1 due to progressive disease and 1 due to multi-organ failure.

Adverse events were reported in all 24 patients during the study period (BMT Day —10 through BMT Day +28) or post-study surveillance period (Day +29 through +100). These included vomiting (100%), nausea (83%), stomatitis (79%), hepatic veno-occlusive disease (HVOD) (21%), graft-versus host disease (GVHD) (25%), and pneumonia (21%).

Based on the results of this 24 patient clinical trial, a suggested dosing regimen of busulfan in pediatric patients is shown in the following nomogram. (See TABLE 3.)

TABLE 3 *Busulfan Dosing Nomogram*

Patient's Actual Body Weight (ABW)	Busulfan Dosage
≤12 kg	1.1 (mg/kg)
>12 kg	0.8 (mg/kg)

Simulations based on a pediatric population pharmacokinetic model indicate that approximately 60% of pediatric patients will achieve a target busulfan exposure (AUC) between 900-1350 µM·min with the first dose of busulfan using this dosing nomogram. Therapeutic drug monitoring and dose adjustment following the first dose of busulfan is recommended.

Dose Adjustment Based of Therapeutic Drug Monitoring

Instructions for measuring the AUC of busulfan at dose 1 (see Blood Sample Collection for AUC Determination), and the formula for adjustment of subsequent doses to achieve the desired target AUC (1125 µM·min), are provided below.

Adjusted dose (mg) = Actual dose (mg) × target AUC (µM·min)/actual AUC (µM·min).

For example, if a patient received a dose of 11 mg busulfan and if the corresponding AUC measured was 800 µM·min, for a target AUC of 1125 µM·min, the target mg dose would be:

Mg dose = 11 mg × 1125 µM·min/800 µM·min = 15.5 mg

Busulfan dose adjustment may be made using this formula and instructions below.

Blood Sample Collection for AUC Determination

Calculate the AUC (µM·min) based on blood samples collected at the following time points:

For dose 1: Two hour (end of infusion), 4 and 6 hour (immediately prior to the next scheduled busulfan administration). Actual sampling times should be recorded.

For doses other than dose 1: Pre-infusion (baseline), 2 hour (end of infusion), 4 and 6 hour (immediately prior to the next scheduled busulfan administration).

AUC calculations based on fewer than the 3 specified samples may result in inaccurate AUC determinations.

For each scheduled blood sample, collect 1-3 ml of blood into heparinized (Na or Li heparin) Vacutainer tubes. The blood samples should be placed on wet ice immediately after collection and should be centrifuged (at 4°C) within 1 hour. The plasma, harvested into appropriate cryovial storage tubes, is to be frozen immediately at —20°C. All plasma samples are to be sent in a frozen state (*i.e.,* on dry ice) to the assay laboratory for the determination of plasma busulfan concentrations.

Calculation of AUC

Busulfan AUC calculations may be made using the following instructions and appropriate standard pharmacokinetic formula:

Dose 1 $AUC_{infinity}$ Calculation: $AUC_{infinity}$ = AUC 0-6h + $AUC_{extrapolated}$, where Auc 0-6h is to be estimated using the linear trapezoidal rule and $AUC_{extrapolated}$ can be computed by taking the ratio of the busulfan concentration at Hour 6 and the terminal elimination rate constant, λ^z. The λ^z must be calculated from the terminal elimination phase of the busulfan concentration versus time curve. A "0" pre-dose busulfan concentration should be assumed, and used in the calculation of AUC.

If AUC is assessed subsequent to dose 1, steady-state AUC^{ss} (AUC 0-6h) is to be estimated from the trough, 2, 4 and 6 hour concentrations using the linear trapezoidal rule.

Instructions for Drug Administration and Blood Sample Collection for Therapeutic Drug Monitoring

An administration set with minimal residual hold up (priming) volume (1-3 ml) should be used for drug infusion to ensure accurate delivery of the entire prescribed dose and to ensure accurate collection of blood samples for therapeutic drug monitoring and dose adjustment.

Prime the administration set tubing with drug solution to allow accurate documentation of the start time of busulfan infusion. Collect the blood sample from a peripheral IV line to avoid contamination with infusing drug. If the blood sample is taken directly from the existing central venous catheter (CVC), **DO NOT COLLECT THE BLOOD SAMPLE WHILE THE DRUG IS INFUSING** to ensure that the end of infusion sample is not contaminated with any residual drug. At the end of infusion (2 hour), disconnect the administration tubing and flush the CVC line with 5 cc of normal saline prior to the collection of the end of infusion sample from the CVC port. Collect the blood samples from a different port than that used for the busulfan infusion. When recording the busulfan infusion stop time, do not include the time required to flush the indwelling catheter line. Discard the administration tubing at the end of the 2 hour infusion.

See Preparation for Intravenous Administration for detailed instructions on drug preparation.

Geriatric

Five (5) of 61 patients treated in the busulfan clinical trial were over the age of 55 (range 57-64). All achieved myeloablation and engraftment.

Gender, Race

Adjusting busulfan dosage based on gender or race has not been adequately studied.

Renal Insufficiency

Busulfan has not been studied in patients with renal impairment.

Hepatic Insufficiency

Busulfan has not been administered to patients with hepatic insufficiency.

Other

Busulfan may cause cellular dysplasia in many organs. Cytologic abnormalities characterized by giant, hyperchromatic nuclei have been reported in lymph nodes, pancreas, thyroid, adrenal glands, liver, lungs, and bone marrow. This cytologic dysplasia may be severe enough to cause difficulty in interpretation of exfoliative cytologic examinations of the lungs, bladder, breast, and the uterine cervix.

DRUG INTERACTIONS

Itraconazole decreases busulfan clearance by up to 25%, and may produce AUCs >1500 µM·min in some patients. Fluconazole, and the 5-HT_3 antiemetics odansetron and granisetron have all been used with busulfan.

Phenytoin increases the clearance of busulfan by 15% or more, possibly due to the induction of glutathione-S-transferase. Since the pharmacokinetics of busulfan were studied in patients treated with phenytoin, the clearance of busulfan at the recommended dose may be lower and exposure (AUC) higher in patients not treated with phenytoin. Because busulfan is eliminated from the body via conjugation with glutathione, use of acetaminophen prior to (<72 hours) or concurrent with busulfan may result in reduced busulfan clearance based upon the known property of acetaminophen to decrease glutathione levels in the blood and tissues.

ADVERSE REACTIONS

Dimethylacetamide (DMA), the solvent used in the busulfan formulation, was studied in 1962 as a potential cancer chemotherapy drug. In a Phase 1 trial, the maximum tolerated dose (MTD) was 14.8 g/m²/day for 4 days. The daily recommended dose of busulfan contains DMA equivalent to 42% of the MTD on a mg/m² basis. The dose-limiting toxicities in the Phase 1 study were hepatotoxicity as evidenced by increased liver transaminase (SGOT) levels and neurological symptoms as evidenced by hallucinations. The hallucinations had a pattern of onset at 1 day post completion of DMA administration and were associated with EEG changes. The lowest dose at which hallucinations were recognized was equivalent to 1.9 times that delivered in a conditioning regimen utilizing busulfan 0.8 mg/kg every 6 hours × 16 doses. Other neurological toxicities included somnolence, lethargy, and confusion. The relative contribution of DMA and/or other concomitant medications to neurologic and hepatic toxicities observed with busulfan is difficult to ascertain.

Treatment with busulfan at the recommended dose and schedule will result in profound myelosuppression in 100% of patients, including granulocytopenia, thrombocytopenia, anemia, or a combined loss of formed elements of the blood.

Adverse reaction information is primarily derived from the clinical study (n=61) of busulfan and the data obtained for high-dose oral busulfan conditioning in the setting of randomized, controlled trials identified through a literature review.

BUSULFAN CLINICAL TRIALS

In the busulfan allogeneic stem cell transplantation clinical trial, all patients were treated with busulfan 0.8 mg/kg as a 2 hour infusion every 6 hours for 16 doses over 4 days, combined with cyclophosphamide 60 mg/kg × 2 days. Ninety-three percent (93%) of evaluable patients receiving this dose of busulfan maintained an AUC less than 1500 µM·min for dose 9, which has generally been considered the level that minimizes the risk of HVOD.

The following sections describe clinically significant events occurring in the busulfan clinical trials, regardless of drug attribution. For pediatric information, see Special Populations, Pediatric.

Hematologic: At the indicated dose and schedule, busulfan produced profound myelosuppression in 100% of patients. Following hematopoietic progenitor cell infusion, recovery of neutrophil counts to ≥500 cells/mm³ occurred at median Day 13 when prophylactic G-CSF was administered to the majority of participants on the study. The median number of platelet transfusions/patient on study was 6, and the median number of red blood cell transfusions on study was 4. Prolonged prothrombin time was reported in 1 patient (2%).

Gastrointestinal: Gastrointestinal toxicities were frequent and generally considered to be related to the drug. Few were categorized as serious. Mild or moderate nausea occurred in 92% of patients in the allogeneic clinical trial, and mild or moderate vomiting occurred in 95% through BMT Day +28; nausea was severe in 7%. The incidence of vomiting during busulfan administration (BMT Day -7 to -4) was 43% in the allogeneic clinical trial. Grade 3-4 stomatitis developed in 26% of the participants, and Grade 3 esophagitis developed in 2%. Grade 3-4 diarrhea was reported in 5% of the allogeneic study participants, while mild or moderate diarrhea occurred in 75%. Mild or moderate constipation occurred in 38% of patients; ileus developed in 8% and was severe in 2%. Forty-four percent (44%) of patients reported mild or moderate dyspepsia. Two percent (2%) of patients experienced mild hematemesis. Pancreatitis developed in 2% of patients. Mild or moderate rectal discomfort occurred in 24% of patients. Severe anorexia occurred in 21% of patients and was mild/moderate in 64%.

Hepatic: Hyperbilirubinemia occurred in 49% of patients in the allogeneic BMT trial. Grade 3/4 hyperbilirubinemia occurred in 30% of patients within 28 days of transplantation and was considered life-threatening in 5% of these patients. Hyperbilirubinemia was associated with graft-versus-host disease in 6 patients and with veno-occlusive disease in 5 patients. Grade 3/4 SGPT elevations occurred in 7% of patients. Alkaline phosphatase increases were mild or moderate in 15% of patients. Mild or moderate jaundice developed in 12% of patients, and mild or moderate hepatomegaly developed in 6%.

Hepatic Veno-Occlusive Disease: Hepatic veno-occlusive disease (HVOD) is a recognized potential complication of conditioning therapy prior to transplant. Based on clinical examination and laboratory findings, hepatic veno-occlusive disease was diagnosed in 8% (5/61) of patients treated with busulfan in the setting of allogeneic transplantation, was fatal in 2/5 cases (40%), and yielded an overall mortality from HVOD in the entire study population of 2/61 (3%). Three (3) of the 5 patients diagnosed with HVOD were retrospectively found to meet the Jones' criteria.

Graft-Versus-Host Disease: Graft-versus-host disease developed in 18% of patients (11/61) receiving allogeneic transplants; it was severe in 3%, and mild or moderate in 15%. There were 3 deaths (5%) attributed to GVHD.

Edema: Seventy-nine percent (79%) of patients exhibited some form of edema, hypervolemia, or weight increase; all events were reported as mild or moderate.

Infection/Fever: Fifty-one percent (51%) of patients experienced 1 or more episodes of infection. Pneumonia was fatal in 1 patient (2%) and life-threatening in 3% of pa-

B

TABLE 4 *Summary of the Incidence (≥20%) of Non-Hematologic Adverse Events Through BMT Day +28 in Patients Who Received Busulfan Prior to Allogeneic Hematopoietic Progenitor Cell Transplantation*

Non-Hematological Adverse Events*	% Incidence
Body as a Whole	
Fever	80%
Headache	69%
Asthenia	51%
Chills	46%
Pain	44%
Edema general	28%
Allergic reaction	26%
Chest pain	26%
Inflammation at injection site	25%
Pain back	23%
Cardiovascular System	
Tachycardia	44%
Hypertension	36%
Thrombosis	33%
Vasodilation	25%
Digestive System	
Nausea	98%
Stomatitis (mucositis)	97%
Vomiting	95%
Anorexia	85%
Diarrhea	84%
Abdominal pain	72%
Dyspepsia	44%
Constipation	38%
Dry mouth	26%
Rectal disorder	25%
Abdominal enlargement	23%
Metabolic and Nutritional System	
Hypomagnesemia	77%
Hyperglycemia	66%
Hypokalemia	64%
Hypocalcemia	49%
Hyperbilirubinemia	49%
Edema	36%
SGPT elevation	31%
Creatinine increased	21%
Nervous System	
Insomnia	84%
Anxiety	72%
Dizziness	30%
Depression	23%
Respiratory System	
Rhinitis	44%
Lung disorder	34%
Cough	28%
Epistaxis	25%
Dyspnea	25%
Skin and Appendages	
Rash	57%
Pruritus	28%

* Includes all reported adverse events regardless of severity (toxicity Grades 1-4).

tients. Fever was reported in 80% of patients; it was mild or moderate in 78% and severe in 3%. Forty-six percent (46%) of patients experienced chills.

Cardiovascular: Mild or moderate tachycardia was reported in 44% of patients. In 7 patients (11%) it was first reported during busulfan administration. Other rhythm abnormalities, which were all mild or moderate, included arrhythmia (5%), atrial fibrillation (2%), ventricular extrasystoles (2%), and third degree heart block (2%). Mild or moderate thrombosis occurred in 33% of patients, and all episodes were associated with the central venous catheter. Hypertension was reported in 36% of patients and was Grade 3/4 in 7%. Hypotension occurred in 11% of patients and was Grade 3/4 in 3%. Mild vasodilation (flushing and hot flashes) was reported in 25% of patients. Other cardiovascular events included cardiomegaly (5%), mild ECG abnormality (2%), Grade 3/4 left-sided heart failure in 1 patient (2%), and moderate pericardial effusion (2%). These events were reported primarily in the post-cyclophosphamide phase.

Pulmonary: Mild or moderate dyspnea occurred in 25% of patients and was severe in 2%. One patient (2%) experienced severe hyperventilation; and in 2 (3%) additional patients it was mild or moderate. Mild rhinitis and mild or moderate cough were reported in 44% and 28% of patients, respectively. Mild epistaxis events were reported in 25%. Three patients (5%) on the allogeneic study developed documented alveolar hemorrhage. All required mechanical ventilatory support and all died. Nonspecific interstitial fibrosis was found on wedge biopsies performed with video assisted thoracoscopy in 1 patient on the allogeneic study who subsequently died from respiratory failure on BMT Day +98. Other pulmonary events, reported as mild or moderate, included pharyngitis (18%), hiccup (18%), asthma (8%), atelectasis (2%), pleural effusion (3%), hypoxia (2%), hemoptysis (3%), and sinusitis (3%).

Neurologic: The most commonly reported adverse events of the central nervous system were insomnia (84%), anxiety (75%), dizziness (30%), and depression (23%). Severity was mild or moderate except for 1 patient (1%) who experienced severe insomnia. One patient (1%) developed a life-threatening cerebral hemorrhage and a coma as a terminal event following multi-organ failure after HVOD. Other events considered severe included delirium (2%), agitation (2%), and encephalopathy (2%). The overall incidence of confusion was 11% and 5% of patients were reported to have experienced hallucinations. The patient who developed delirium and hallucination on the allogeneic study had onset of confusion at the completion of busulfan injection. The overall incidence of lethargy in the allogeneic busulfan clinical trial was 7%, and somnolence was reported in 2%. One patient (2%) treated in an autologous transplantation study experienced a seizure while receiving cyclophosphamide, despite prophylactic treatment with phenytoin.

Renal: Creatinine was mildly or moderately elevated in 21% of patients. BUN was increased in 3% of patients and to a Grade 3/4 level in 2%. Seven percent (7%) of patients experienced dysuria, 15% oliguria, and 8% hematuria. There were 4 (7%) Grade 3/4 cases of hemorrhagic cystitis in the allogeneic clinical trial.

Skin: Rash (57%) and pruritus (28%) were reported; both conditions were predominantly mild. Alopecia was mild in 15% of patients and moderate in 2%. Mild vesicular rash was reported in 10% of patients and mild or moderate maculopapular rash in 8%. Vesiculo-bullous rash was reported in 10%, and exfoliative dermatitis in 5%. Erythema nodosum was reported in 2%, acne in 7%, and skin discoloration in 8%.

Metabolic: Hyperglycemia was observed in 67% of patients and Grade 3/4 hyperglycemia was reported in 15%. Hypomagnesemia was mild or moderate in 77% of patients; hypokalemia was mild or moderate in 62% and severe in 2%; hypocalcemia was mild or moderate in 46% and severe in 3%; hypophosphatemia was mild or moderate in 17%; and hyponatremia was reported in 2%.

Other: Other reported events included headache (mild or moderate 64%, severe 5%), abdominal pain (mild or moderate 69%, severe 3%), asthenia (mild or moderate 49%, severe 2%), unspecified pain (mild or moderate 43%, severe 2%), allergic reaction (mild or moderate 24%, severe 2%), injection site inflammation (mild or moderate 25%), injection site pain (mild or moderate 15%), chest pain (mild or moderate 26%), back pain (mild or moderate 23%), myalgia (mild or moderate 16%), arthralgia (mild or moderate 13%), and ear disorder in 3%.

Deaths: There were 2 deaths through BMT Day +28 in the allogeneic transplant setting. There were an additional 6 deaths BMT Day +29 through BMT Day +100 in the allogeneic transplant setting.

ORAL BUSULFAN LITERATURE REVIEW

A literature review identified 4 randomized, controlled trials that evaluated a high-dose oral busulfan-containing conditioning regimen for allogeneic bone marrow transplantation in the setting of CML. The safety outcomes reported in those trials are summarized in TABLE 5 for a mixed population of hematological malignancies (AML, CML, and ALL).

TABLE 5 *Summary of Safety Analyses From the Randomized, Controlled Trials Utilizing a High Dose Oral Busulfan-Containing Conditioning Regimen That Were Identified in a Literature Review*

Clift: CML Chronic Phase	
TRM	
Death ≤100d	4.1% (3/73)
GVHD	
Acute ≥Grade 2	35%
Chronic	41% (30/73)
Pulmonary	1 death from idiopathic interstitial pneumonitis and 1 death from pulmonary fibrosis
Devergie: CML Chronic Phase	
TRM	38%
VOD	7.7% (5/65)
Deaths	4.6% (3/65)
GVHD	
Acute ≥Grade 2	41% (24/59 at risk)
Pulmonary	
Interstitial pneumonitis	16.9% (11/65)
Hemorrhagic Cystitis	10.8% (7/65)
Ringden: CML, AML, ALL	
TRM	28%
VOD	12%
GVHD	
Acute ≥Grade 2	26%
Chronic	45%
Pulmonary	
Interstitial pneumonitis	14%
Hemorrhagic Cystitis	24%
Seizures	6%
Blume: CML, AML, ALL	
VOD	
Deaths	4.9%
GVHD	
Acute ≥Grade 2	22% (13/58 at risk)
Chronic	31% (14/45 at risk)

TRM = Transplantation Related Mortality.
VOD = Veno-Occlusive Disease of the liver.
GVHD = Graft versus Host Disease.

DOSAGE AND ADMINISTRATION

When busulfan is administered as a component of the BuCy conditioning regimen prio to bone marrow or peripheral blood progenitor cell replacement, the recommended doses are as follows:

ADULTS (BUCY2)

The usual adult dose is 0.8 mg/kg of ideal body weight or actual body weight, whichever is lower, administered every 6 hours for 4 days (a total of 16 doses). For obese, or severely obese patients, busulfan should be administered based on adjusted ideal body weight. Ideal body weight (IBW) should be calculated as follows (height in cm, and weight in kg): IBW (kg; men) = 50 + 0.91 × (height in cm —152); IBW (kg; women = 45 + 0.91 × (height in cm —152). Adjusted ideal body weight (AIBW) should be calculated as follows: AIBW = IBW + 0.25 × (actual weight — IBW). Cyclophosphamide is given on each of 2 days as a

1 hour infusion at a dose of 60 mg/kg beginning on BMT Day —3, no sooner than 6 hours following the 16th dose of busulfan.

Busulfan clearance is best predicted when the busulfan dose is administered based on adjusted ideal body weight. Dosing busulfan based on actual body weight, ideal body weight or other factors can produce significant differences in busulfan injection clearance among lean, normal, and obese patients.

Busulfan should be administered intravenously via a central venous catheter as a 2 hour infusion every 6 hours for 4 consecutive days for a total of 16 doses. All patients should be premedicated with phenytoin as busulfan is known to cross the blood brain barrier and induce seizures. Phenytoin reduces busulfan plasma AUC by 15%. Use of other anticonvulsants may result in higher busulfan plasma AUCs, and an increased risk of VOD or seizures. In cases where other anticonvulsants must be used, plasma busulfan exposure should be monitored (see DRUG INTERACTIONS). Antiemetics should be administered prior to the first dose of busulfan and continued on a fixed schedule through administration of busulfan. Where available, pharmacokinetic monitoring may be considered to further optimize therapeutic targeting.

PEDIATRICS

The effectiveness of busulfan in the treatment of CML has not been specifically studied in pediatric patients. For additional information see Special Populations, Pediatrics.

PREPARATION AND ADMINISTRATION PRECAUTIONS

An administration set with minimal residual hold-up volume (2-5 cc) should be used for product administration.

As with other cytotoxic compounds, caution should be exercised in handling and preparing the solution of busulfan. Skin reactions may occur with accidental exposure. The use of gloves is recommended. If busulfan or diluted busulfan solution contacts the skin or mucosa, wash the skin or mucosa thoroughly with water.

Busulfan is a clear, colorless solution. Parenteral drug products should be visually inspected for particulate matter and discoloration prior to administration whenever the solution and container permit. If particulate matter is seen in the busulfan ampoule the drug should not be used.

PREPARATION FOR INTRAVENOUS ADMINISTRATION

Busulfan injection must be diluted prior to use with either 0.9% sodium chloride injection, (normal saline) or 5% dextrose injection, (D_5W). The diluent quantity should be 10 times the volume of busulfan injection, so that the final concentration of busulfan is approximately 0.5 mg/ml.

Calculation of the dose for a 70 kg patient, would be performed as follows:

(70 kg patient) × (0.8 mg/kg) ÷ (6 mg/ml) = 9.3 ml busulfan (56 mg total dose).

To prepare the final solution for infusion, add 9.3 ml of busulfan to 93 ml of diluent (normal saline or D_5W) as calculated below:

(9.3 ml busulfan) × (10) = 93 ml of either diluent plus the 9.3 ml of busulfan to yield a final concentration of busulfan of 0.54 mg/ml (9.3 ml × 6 mg/ml ÷ 102.3 ml = 0.54 mg/ml.

All transfer procedures require strict adherence to aseptic techniques, preferably employing a vertical laminar flow safety hood while wearing gloves and protective clothing. Using sterile transfer techniques, break off the top of the ampoule. Using a syringe fitted with a needle and the 5 micron nylon filter provided with each busulfan from the ampoule. Remove the needle and filter, replace with a new needle and dispense the contents of the syringe into an IV bag (or syringe) which already contains the calculated amount of either normal saline or D^5W, making sure that the drug flows into and through the solution. DO NOT put the busulfan injection into an IV bag that does not contain normal saline or D_5W. Always add the busulfan injection to the diluent, not the diluent to the busulfan injection. Mix thoroughly by inverting several times. USE OF FILTERS OTHER THAN THE SPECIFIC TYPE INCLUDED IN THIS PACKAGE WITH EACH AMPOULE IS NOT RECOMMENDED. DO NOT USE POLYCARBONATE SYRINGES WITH BUSULFAN INJECTION.

Infusion pumps should be used to administer the diluted busulfan solution. Set the flow rate of the pump to deliver the entire prescribed busulfan dose over 2 hours. Prior to and following each infusion, flush the indwelling catheter line with approximately 5 ml of 0.9% sodium chloride injection or 5% dextrose injection. DO NOT infuse concomitantly with another IV solution of unknown compatibility. WARNING: RAPID INFUSION OF BUSULFAN INJECTION HAS NOT BEEN TESTED AND IS NOT RECOMMENDED.

STABILITY

Unopened ampoules of busulfan are stable until the date indicated on the package when stored under refrigeration at 2-8°C (36-46°F).

Busulfan diluted in 0.9% sodium chloride injection or 5% dextrose injection is stable at room temperature (25°C) for up to 8 hours but the infusion must be completed within that time. Busulfan diluted in 0.9% sodium chloride injection is stable at refrigerated conditions (2-8°C) for up to 12 hours but the infusion must be completed within that time.

HOW SUPPLIED

Busulfex is supplied as a sterile solution in 10 ml single-use clear glass ampoules each containing 60 mg of busulfan at a concentration of 6 mg/ml for IV use.

Storage: Unopened ampoules of Busulfex must be stored under refrigerated conditions between 2-8°C (36-46°F).

Handling and Disposal: Procedures for proper handling and disposal of anticancer drugs should be considered. Several guidelines on this subject have been published.[1-6] There is no general agreement that all of the procedures recommended in the guidelines are necessary or appropriate.

ORAL

WARNING

Busulfan is a potent drug. It should not be used unless a diagnosis of chronic myelogenous leukemia has been adequately established and the responsible physician is knowledgeable in assessing response to chemotherapy.

Busulfan can induce severe bone marrow hypoplasia. Reduce or discontinue the dosage immediately at the first sign of any unusual depression of bone marrow function as reflected by an abnormal decrease in any of the formed elements of the blood. A bone marrow examination should be performed if the bone marrow status is uncertain.

SEE WARNINGS FOR INFORMATION REGARDING BUSULFAN-INDUCED LEUKEMOGENESIS IN HUMANS.

DESCRIPTION

Busulfan is a bifunctional alkylating agent. Busulfan is known chemically as 1,4-butanediol dimethanesulfonate and has the structural formula $CH_3SO_2O(CH_2)_4OSO_2CH_3$.

Busulfan is *not* a structural analog of the nitrogen mustards. Myleran is available in tablet form for oral administration. Each scored tablet contains 2 mg busulfan and the inactive ingredients magnesium stearate and sodium chloride.

The activity of busulfan in chronic myelogenous leukemia was first reported by D.A.G. Galton in 1953.

CLINICAL PHARMACOLOGY

No analytical method has been found which permits the quantitation of nonradiolabeled busulfan or its metabolites in biological tissues or plasma. All studies of the pharmacokinetics of busulfan in humans have employed radiolabeled drug using either sulfur-35 (labeling the "carrier" portion of the molecule) or carbon-14 or tritium in the "alkylating" portion of the 4-carbon chain (labels in the alkylating portion of the molecule).

STUDIES WITH ^{35}S-BUSULFAN

Following the intravenous (IV) administration of a single therapeutic dose of ^{35}S-busulfan, there was rapid disappearance of radioactivity from the blood; 90-95% of the ^{35}S-label disappeared within 3-5 minutes after injection. Thereafter, a constant, low level of radioactivity (1-3% of the injected dose) was maintained during the subsequent 48 hour period of observation. Following the oral administration of ^{35}S-busulfan, there was a lag period of ½ to 2 hours prior to the detection of radioactivity in the blood. However, at 4 hours the (low) level of circulating radioactivity was comparable to that obtained following IV administration.

After either oral or IV administration of ^{35}S-busulfan to humans, 45-60% of the radioactivity was recovered in the urine in the 48 hours after administration; the majority of the total urinary excretion occurred in the first 24 hours. In humans, over 95% of the urinary sulfur-35 occurs as ^{35}S-methanesulfonic acid.

The fact that urinary recovery of sulfur-35 was equivalent, irrespective of whether the drug was given intravenously or orally, suggests virtually complete absorption by the oral route.

STUDIES WITH ^{14}C-BUSULFAN

Oral and IV administration of 1,4-^{14}C-busulfan showed the same rapid initial disappearance of plasma radioactivity with a subsequent low-level plateau as observed following the administration of ^{35}S-labeled drug. Cumulative radioactivity in the urine after 48 hours was 25-30% of the administered dose (contrasting with 45-60% for ^{35}S-busulfan) and suggests a slower excretion of the alkylating portion of the molecule and its metabolites than for the sulfonoxymethyl moieties. Regardless of the route of administration, 1,4-^{14}C-busulfan yielded a complex mixture of at least 12 radiolabeled metabolites in urine; the main metabolite being 3-hydroxytetrahydrothiophene-1,1-dioxide.

STUDIES WITH ^{3}H-BUSULFAN

Human pharmacokinetic studies have been conducted employing busulfan labeled with tritium on the tetramethylene chain. These experiments confirmed a rapid initial clearance of the radioactivity from plasma, irrespective of whether the drug was given orally or intravenously, and showed a gradual accumulation of radioactivity in the plasma after repeated doses. Urinary excretion of less than 50% of the total dose given suggested a slow elimination of the metabolic products from the body.

There is 1 report of the impact of hemodialysis on the oral clearance in a patient with chronic renal failure undergoing autologous peripheral stem cell transplantation for non-Hodgkin's lymphoma. A 4 hour hemodialysis session increased the apparent oral clearance of busulfan by about 65%. The factors that favor hemodialysis of busulfan include: (1) low molecular weight, (2) low plasma protein binding, and (3) a blood to plasma partition ratio of close to 1. However, with a 4 hour hemodialysis, the mean daily (24 hours) oral clearance of busulfan was only increased by about 10%.

In patients who receive 16 mg/kg of busulfan over 4 days, the incidence of veno-occlusive disease is higher in patients whose average concentration at steady-state (C_{ss}) area under the concentration time curve [AUC(0-6)] is >900 μg/L or >1500 μmol/L × min (see WARNINGS).

Busulfan clearance may be reduced in the presence of cyclophosphamide. Cyclophosphamide is metabolized to hydroxycyclophosphamide and then to acrolein, which is a hepatotoxin. In addition, acrolein is known to deplete glutathione (the conjugation of which is the main metabolic pathway for the clearance of busulfan), and therefore, could lead to decreased clearance of busulfan.

The concomitant systemic administration of itraconazole to patients receiving high-dose busulfan may result in reduced busulfan clearance, presumably due to possible inhibition of lipoxygenases (by itraconazole), which are important for glutathione conjugation, the primary metabolic pathway for the clearance of busulfan.

No information is available regarding the penetration of busulfan into brain or cerebrospinal fluid.

BIOCHEMICAL PHARMACOLOGY

In aqueous media, busulfan undergoes a wide range of nucleophilic substitution reactions. While this chemical reactivity is relatively non-specific, alkylation of the DNA is felt to be an important biological mechanism for its cytotoxic effect. Coliphage T7 exposed to busulfan was found to have the DNA crosslinked by intrastrand crosslinkages, but no interstrand linkages were found.

The metabolic fate of busulfan has been studied in rats and humans using ^{14}C- and ^{35}S-labeled materials. In humans, as in the rat, almost all of the radioactivity in ^{35}S-labeled busulfan is excreted in the urine in the form of ^{35}S-methanesulfonic acid. No unchanged drug was found in human urine, although a small amount has been reported in rat urine. Roberts and Warwick demonstrated that the formation of methanesulfonic acid *in vivo* in the rat is not due to a simple hydrolysis of busulfan to 1,4-butanediol, since only about 4% of 2,3-^{14}C-busulfan was excreted as carbon dioxide, whereas 2,3-^{14}C-1,4-butanediol was converted almost exclusively to carbon dioxide. The predominant reaction of busulfan in the rat is the alkylation of sulfhydryl groups (particularly cysteine and cysteine-containing compounds) to produce a cyclic sulfonium compound which is the precursor of the major urinary metabolite of the 4-carbon portion of the molecule, 3-hydroxytetrahydrothiophene-1,1-dioxide. This has been termed a "sulfur-stripping" action of busulfan and it may modify the function of certain sulfur-containing amino acids, polypeptides, and proteins; whether this action makes an important contribution to the cytotoxicity of busulfan is unknown.

The biochemical basis for acquired resistance to busulfan is largely a matter of speculation. Although altered transport of busulfan into the cell is 1 possibility, increased intracellular inactivation of the drug before it reaches the DNA is also possible. Experiments with other alkylating agents have shown that resistance to this class of compounds may reflect an acquired ability of the resistant cell to repair alkylation damage more effectively.

INDICATIONS AND USAGE

Busulfan is indicated for the palliative treatment of chronic myelogenous (myeloid, myelocytic, granulocytic) leukemia.

CONTRAINDICATIONS

Busulfan is contraindicated in patients in whom a definitive diagnosis of chronic myelogenous leukemia has not been firmly established.

Busulfan is contraindicated in patients who have previously suffered a hypersensitivity reaction to busulfan or any other component of the preparation.

WARNINGS

The most frequent, serious side effect of treatment with busulfan is the induction of bone marrow failure (which may or may not be anatomically hypoplastic) resulting in severe pancytopenia. The pancytopenia caused by busulfan may be more prolonged than that induced with other alkylating agents. It is generally felt that the usual cause of busulfan-induced pancytopenia is the failure to stop administration of the drug soon enough; individual idiosyncrasy to the drug does not seem to be an important factor. *Busulfan should be used with extreme caution and exceptional vigilance in patients whose bone marrow reserve may have been compromised by prior irradiation or chemotherapy, or whose marrow function is recovering from previous cytotoxic therapy.* Although recovery from busulfan-induced pancytopenia may take from 1 month to 2 years, this complication is potentially reversible, and the patient should be vigorously supported through any period of severe pancytopenia.

A rare, important complication of busulfan therapy is the development of bronchopulmonary dysplasia with pulmonary fibrosis. Symptoms have been reported to occur within 8 months to 10 years after initiation of therapy — the average duration of therapy being 4 years. The histologic findings associated with "busulfan lung" mimic those seen following pulmonary irradiation. Clinically, patients have reported the insidious onset of cough, dyspnea, and low-grade fever. In some cases, however, onset of symptoms may be acute. Pulmonary function studies have revealed diminished diffusion capacity and decreased pulmonary compliance. It is important to exclude more common conditions (such as opportunistic infections or leukemic infiltration of the lungs) with appropriate diagnostic techniques. If measures such as sputum cultures, virologic studies, and exfoliative cytology fail to establish an etiology for the pulmonary infiltrates, lung biopsy may be necessary to establish the diagnosis. Treatment of established busulfan-induced pulmonary fibrosis is unsatisfactory; in most cases the patients have died within 6 months after the diagnosis was established. There is no specific therapy for this complication. Busulfan should be discontinued if this lung toxicity develops. The administration of corticosteroids has been suggested, but the results have not been impressive or uniformly successful.

Busulfan may cause cellular dysplasia in many organs in addition to the lung. Cytologic abnormalities characterized by giant, hyperchromatic nuclei have been reported in lymph nodes, pancreas, thyroid, adrenal glands, liver, and bone marrow. This cytologic dysplasia may be severe enough to cause difficulty in interpretation of exfoliative cytologic examinations from the lung, bladder, breast, and the uterine cervix.

In addition to the widespread epithelial dysplasia that has been observed during busulfan therapy, chromosome aberrations have been reported in cells from patients receiving busulfan.

Busulfan is mutagenic in mice and, possibly, in humans.

Malignant tumors and acute leukemias have been reported in patients who have received busulfan therapy, and this drug may be a human carcinogen. The World Health Organization has concluded that there is a causal relationship between busulfan exposure and the development of secondary malignancies. Four cases of acute leukemia occurred among 243 patients treated with busulfan as adjuvant chemotherapy following surgical resection of bronchogenic carcinoma. All 4 cases were from a subgroup of 19 of these 243 patients who developed pancytopenia while taking busulfan 5-8 years before leukemia became clinically apparent. These findings suggest that busulfan is leukemogenic, although its mode of action is uncertain.

Ovarian suppression and amenorrhea with menopausal symptoms commonly occur during busulfan therapy in premenopausal patients. Busulfan has been associated with ovarian failure including failure to achieve puberty in females. Bulsulfan interferes with spermatogenesis in experimental animals, and there have been clinical reports of sterility, azoospermia, and testicular atrophy in male patients.

Hepatic veno-occlusive disease, which may be life threatening, has been reported in patients receiving busulfan, usually in combination with cyclophosphamide or other chemotherapeutic agents prior to bone marrow transplantation. Possible risk factors for the development of hepatic veno-occlusive disease include: total busulfan dose exceeding 16 mg/kg based on ideal body weight, and concurrent use of multiple alkylating agents (see CLINICAL PHARMACOLOGY and DRUG INTERACTIONS).

A clear cause-and-effect relationship with busulfan has not been demonstrated. Periodic measurement of serum transaminases, alkaline phosphatate, and bilirubin is indicated for early detection of hepatotoxicity. A reduced incidence of hepatic veno-occlusive disease and other regimen-related toxicities have been observed in patients treated with high-dose busulfan and cyclophosphamide when the first dose of cyclophosphamide has been delayed for >24 hours after the last dose of busulphan (see CLINICAL PHARMACOLOGY and DRUG INTERACTIONS).

Cardiac tamponade has been reported in a small number of patients with thalassemia (2% in 1 series) who received busulfan and cyclophosphamide as the preparatory regimen for bone marrow transplantation. In this series, the cardiac tamponade was often fatal. Abdominal pain and vomiting preceded the tamponade in most patients.

PREGNANCY CATEGORY D

Busulfan may cause fetal harm when administered to a pregnant woman. Although there have been a number of cases reported where apparently normal children have been born after busulfan treatment during pregnancy, 1 case has been cited where a malformed baby was delivered by a mother treated with busulfan. During the pregnancy that resulted in the malformed infant, the mother received x-ray therapy early in the first trimester, mercaptopurine until the third month, then busulfan until delivery. In pregnant rats, busulfan produces sterility in both male and female offspring due to the absence of germinal cells in testes and ovaries. Germinal cell aplasia or sterility in offspring of mothers receiving busulfan during pregnancy has not been reported in humans. There are no adequate and well-controlled studies in pregnant women. If this drug is used during pregnancy, or if the patient becomes pregnant while taking this drug, the patient should be apprised of the potential hazard to the fetus. Women of childbearing potential should be advised to avoid becoming pregnant.

PRECAUTIONS

GENERAL

The most consistent, dose-related toxicity is bone marrow suppression. This may be manifest by anemia, leukopenia, thrombocytopenia or any combination of these. It is imperative that patients be instructed to report promptly the development of fever, sore throat, signs of local infection, bleeding from any site, or symptoms suggestive of anemia. Any 1 of these findings may indicate busulfan toxicity; however, they may also indicate transformation of the disease to an acute "blastic" form. Since busulfan may have a delayed effect, it is important to withdraw the medication temporarily at the first sign of an abnormally large or exceptionally rapid fall in any of the formed elements of the blood. *Patients should never be allowed to take the drug without close medical supervision.*

Seizures have been reported in patients receiving busulfan. As with any potentially epileptogenic drug, caution should be exercised when administering busulfan to patients with a history of seizure disorder, head trauma, or receiving other potentially epileptogenic drugs. Some investigators have used prophylactic anticonvulsant therapy in this setting.

INFORMATION FOR THE PATIENT

Patients beginning therapy with busulfan should be informed of the importance of having periodic blood counts and to immediately report any unusual fever or bleeding. Aside from the major toxicity of myelosuppression, patients should be instructed to report any difficulty in breathing, persistent cough, or congestion. They should be told that diffuse pulmonary fibrosis is an infrequent, but serious and potentially life-threatening complication of long-term busulfan therapy. Patients should be alerted to report any signs of abrupt weakness, unusual fatigue, anorexia, weight loss, nausea and vomiting, and melanoderma that could be associated with a syndrome resembling adrenal insufficiency. Patients should never be allowed to take the drug without medical supervision and they should be informed that other encountered toxicities to busulfan include infertility, amenorrhea, skin hyperpigmentation, drug hypersensitivity, dryness of the mucous membranes, and rarely, cataract formation. Women of childbearing potential should be advised to avoid becoming pregnant. The increased risk of a second malignancy should be explained to the patient.

LABORATORY TESTS

It is recommended that evaluation of the hemoglobin or hematocrit, total white blood cell count and differential count, and quantitative platelet count be obtained weekly while the patient is on busulfan therapy. In cases where the cause of fluctuation in the formed elements of the peripheral blood is obscure, bone marrow examination may be useful for evaluation of marrow status. A decision to increase, decrease, continue, or discontinue a given dose of busulfan must be based not only on the absolute hematologic values, but also on the rapidity with which changes are occurring. The dosage of busulfan may need to be reduced if this agent is combined with other drugs whose primary toxicity is myelosuppression. Occasional patients may be unusually sensitive to busulfan administered at standard dosage and suffer neutropenia or thrombocytopenia after a relatively short exposure to the drug. Busulfan should not be used where facilities for complete blood counts, including quantitative platelet counts, are not available at weekly (or more frequent) intervals.

CARCINOGENESIS, MUTAGENESIS, AND IMPAIRMENT OF FERTILITY

See WARNINGS.

The World Health Organization has concluded that there is a causal relationship between busulfan exposure and the development of secondary malignancies.

PREGNANCY CATEGORY D
Teratogenic Effects
See WARNINGS.

Nonteratogenic Effects
There have been reports in the literature of small infants being born after the mothers received busulfan during pregnancy, in particular, during the third trimester. One case was reported where an infant had mild anemia and neutropenia at birth after busulfan was administered to the mother from the eighth week of pregnancy to term.

NURSING MOTHERS
It is not known whether this drug is excreted in human milk. Because of the potential for tumorigenicity shown for busulfan in animal and human studies, a decision should be made whether to discontinue nursing or to discontinue the drug, taking into account the importance of the drug to the mother.

PEDIATRIC USE
See INDICATIONS AND USAGE and DOSAGE AND ADMINISTRATION.

DRUG INTERACTIONS

Busulfan may cause additive myelosuppression when used with other myelosuppressive drugs.

In 1 study, 12 of approximately 330 patients receiving continuous busulfan and thioguanine therapy for treatment of chronic myelogenous leukemia were found to have portal hypertension and esophageal varices associated with abnormal liver function tests. Subsequent liver biopsies were performed in 4 of these patients, all of which showed evidence of nodular regenerative hyperplasia. Duration of combination therapy prior to the appearance of esophageal varices ranged from 6-45 months. With the present analysis of the data, no cases of hepatotoxicity have appeared in the busulfan-alone arm of the study. Long-term continuous therapy with thioguanine and busulfan should be used with caution.

Bulsulfan-induced pulmonary toxicity may be additive to the effects produced by other cytotoxic agents.

The concomitant systemic administration of itraconazole to patients receiving high-dose busulfan may result in reduced busulfan clearance (see CLINICAL PHARMACOLOGY). Patients should be monitored for signs of busulfan toxicity when itraconazole is used concomitantly with busulfan.

Busulfan clearance may be reduced in the presence of cyclophosphamide (see CLINICAL PHARMACOLOGY).

ADVERSE REACTIONS

HEMATOLOGICAL EFFECTS
The most frequent, serious, toxic effect of busulfan is dose-related myelosuppression resulting in leukopenia, thrombocytopenia, and anemia. Myelosuppression is most frequently the result of a failure to discontinue dosage in the face of an undetected decrease in leukocyte or platelet counts.

Aplastic anemia (sometimes irreversible) has been reported rarely, often following long-term conventional doses and also high doses of busulfan.

PULMONARY
Interstitial pulmonary fibrosis has been reported rarely, but it is a clinically significant adverse effect when observed and calls for immediate discontinuation of further administration of the drug. The role of corticosteroids in arresting or reversing the fibrosis has been reported to be beneficial in some cases and without effect in others.

CARDIAC
Cardiac tamponade has been reported in a small number of patients with thalassemia who received busulfan and cyclophosphamide as the preparatory regimen for bone marrow transplantation (see WARNINGS).

One case of endocardial fibrosis has been reported in a 79-year-old woman who received a total dose of 7200 mg of busulfan over a period of 9 years for the management of chronic myelogenous leukemia. At autopsy, she was found to have endocardial fibrosis of the left ventricle in addition to interstitial pulmonary fibrosis.

OCULAR
Busulfan is capable of inducing cataracts in rats and there have been several reports indicating that this is a rare complication in humans.

DERMATOLOGIC
Hyperpigmentation is the most common adverse skin reaction and occurs in 5-10% of patients, particularly those with a dark complexion.

METABOLIC
In a few cases, a clinical syndrome closely resembling adrenal insufficiency and characterized by weakness, severe fatigue, anorexia, weight loss, nausea and vomiting, and melanoderma has developed after prolonged busulfan therapy. The symptoms have sometimes been reversible when busulfan was withdrawn. Adrenal responsiveness to exogenously administered ACTH has usually been normal. However, pituitary function testing with metyrapone revealed a blunted urinary 17-hydroxycorticosteroid excretion in 2 patients. Following the discontinuation of busulfan (which was associated with clinical improvement), rechallenge with metyrapone revealed normal pituitary-adrenal function.

Hyperuricemia and/or hyperuricosuria are not uncommon in patients with chronic myelogenous leukemia. Additional rapid destruction of granulocytes may accompany the initiation of chemotherapy and increase the urate pool. Adverse effects can be minimized by increased hydration, urine alkalinization, and the prophylactic administration of a xanthine oxidase inhibitor such as allopurinol.

HEPATIC EFFECTS
Esophageal varices have been reported in patients receiving continuous busulfan and thioguanine therapy for treatment of chronic myelogenous leukemia (see DRUG INTERACTIONS). Hepatic veno-occlusive disease has been observed in patients receiving busulfan (see WARNINGS).

MISCELLANEOUS
Other reported adverse reactions include: Urticaria, erythema multiforme, erythema nodosum, alopecia, porphyria cutanea tarda, excessive dryness and fragility of the skin with anhidrosis, dryness of the oral mucous membranes and cheilosis, gynecomastia, cholestatic jaundice, and myasthenia gravis. Most of these are single case reports, and in many, a clear cause-and-effect relationship with busulfan has not been demonstrated.
Seizures (see PRECAUTIONS, General) have been observed in patients receiving higher than recommended doses of busulfan.

OBSERVED DURING CLINICAL PRACTICE
The following events have been identified during post-approval use of busulfan. Because they are reported voluntarily from a population of unknown size, estimates of freuqency cannot be made. These events have been chosen for inclusion due to a combination of their seriousness, frequency of reporting, or potential causal connection to busulfan.

Blood and Lymphatic: Aplastic anemia.
Eye: Cataracts, corneal thinning, lens changes.
Hepatobiliary Tract and Pancreas: Centrilobular sinusoidal fibrosis, hepatic veno-occlusive disease, hepatocellular atrophy, hepatocellular necrosis, hyperbilirubinemia (see WARNINGS).
Non-Site Specific: Infection, mucositis, sepsis.
Respiratory: Pneumonia.
Skin: Rash. An increased local cutaneous reaction has been observed in patients receiving radiotherapy soon after busulfan.

DOSAGE AND ADMINISTRATION

Busulfan is administered orally. The usual adult dose range for *remission induction* is 4-8 mg, total dose, daily. Dosing on a weight basis is the same for both pediatric patients and adults, approximately 60 μg/kg of body weight or 1.8 mg/m^2 of body surface, daily. Since the rate of fall of the leukocyte count is dose related, daily doses exceeding 4 mg/day should be reserved for patients with the most compelling symptoms; the greater the total daily dose, the greater is the possibility of inducing bone marrow aplasia.

A decrease in the leukocyte count is not usually seen during the first 10-15 days of treatment; the leukocyte count may actually increase during this period and it should not be interpreted as resistance to the drug, nor should the dose be increased. Since the leukocyte count may continue to fall for more than 1 month after discontinuing the drug, it is important that busulfan be discontinued *prior* to the total leukocyte count falling into the normal range. When the total leukocyte count has declined to approximately 15,000/μl the drug should be withheld.

With a constant dose of busulfan, the total leukocyte count declines exponentially; a weekly plot of the leukocyte count on semi-logarithmic graph paper aids in predicting when therapy should be discontinued. With the recommended dose of busulfan, a normal leukocyte count is usually achieved in 12-20 weeks.

During remission, the patient is examined at monthly intervals and treatment resumed with the induction dosage when the total leukocyte count reaches approximately 50,000/μl. When remission is shorter that 3 months, maintenance therapy of 1-3 mg daily may be advisable in order to keep the hematological status under control and prevent rapid relapse.

Procedures for proper handling and disposal of anticancer drugs should be considered. Several guidelines on this subject have been published.[1-8]

There is no general agreement that all of the procedures recommended in the guidelines are necessary or appropriate.

HOW SUPPLIED

Busulfan is supplied as white, scored tablets containing 2 mg busulfan, imprinted with "MYLERAN" and "K2A" on each tablet.
Storage: Store at 15-25°C (59-77°F) in a dry place.

PRODUCT LISTING - EQUIVALENTS NOT AVAILABLE

Solution - Intravenous - 6 mg/ml

10 ml x 8	$2347.28	BUSULFEX, Orphan Medical	62161-0005-38

Tablet - Oral - 2 mg

25's	$57.14	MYLERAN, Glaxosmithkline	00173-0713-25

Butorphanol Tartrate (000563)

For related information, see the comparative table section in Appendix A.

Categories: Pain; Pain, obstetrical; Preanesthesia; Anesthesia, adjunct; Pregnancy Category C; FDA Approved 1978 Aug; DEA Class CIV
Drug Classes: Analgesics, narcotic agonist-antagonist
Brand Names: Stadol; Stadol NS
Foreign Brand Availability: Bunol (Korea); Busphen (Korea)

DESCRIPTION

Note: The trade names have been used throughout this monograph for clarity.
Butorphanol tartrate is a synthetically derived opioid agonist-antagonist analgesic of the phenanthrene series. The chemical name is (-)-17-(cyclobutylmethyl)morphinan-3, 14-diol [S-(R*,R*)]-2,3-dihydroxybutanedioate (1:1) (salt). The molecular formula is $C_{21}H_{29}NO_2 \cdot C_4H_6O_6$, which corresponds to a molecular weight of 477.55.

Butorphanol tartrate is a white crystalline substance. The dose is expressed as the tartrate salt. One milligram of the salt is equivalent to 0.68 mg of the free base. The n-octanol/aqueous buffer partition coefficient of butorphanol is 180:1 at pH 7.5.

Stadol (butorphanol tartrate) Injection, is a sterile, parenteral, aqueous solution of butorphanol tartrate for intravenous or intramuscular administration. In addition to 1 or 2 mg of butorphanol tartrate, each ml of solution contains 3.3 mg of citric acid, 6.4 mg sodium citrate, and 6.4 mg sodium chloride, and 0.1 mg benzethonium chloride (in multiple dose vial only) as a preservative.

Stadol NS (butorphanol tartrate) Nasal Spray is an aqueous solution of butorphanol tartrate for administration as a metered spray to the nasal mucosa. Each bottle of Stadol NS contains 2.5 ml of a 10 mg/ml solution of butorphanol tartrate with sodium chloride, citric acid, and benzethonium chloride in purified water with sodium hydroxide and/or hydrochloric acid added to adjust the pH to 5.0. The pump reservoir must be fully primed (see the Patient Instructions that are distributed with the prescription) prior to initial use. After initial priming each metered spray delivers an average of 1.0 mg of butorphanol tartrate and the 2.5 ml bottle will deliver an average of 14-15 doses of Stadol NS. If not used for 48 hours or longer, the unit must be reprimed (see the Patient Instructions that are distributed with the prescription). With intermittent use requiring repriming before each dose, the 2.5 ml bottle will deliver an average of 8-10 doses of Stadol NS depending on how much repriming is necessary.

CLINICAL PHARMACOLOGY

GENERAL PHARMACOLOGY AND MECHANISM OF ACTION

Butorphanol is a mixed agonist-antagonist with low intrinsic activity at receptors of the μ-opioid type (morphine-like). It is also an agonist at κ-opioid receptors.

Its interactions with these receptors in the central nervous system apparently mediate most of its pharmacologic effects, including analgesia.

In addition to analgesia, CNS effects include depression of spontaneous respiratory activity and cough, stimulation of the emetic center, miosis, and sedation. Effects possibly mediated by non-CNS mechanisms include alteration in cardiovascular resistance and capacitance, bronchomotor tone, gastrointestinal secretory and motor activity, and bladder sphincter activity.

In an animal model, the dose of butorphanol tartrate required to antagonize morphine analgesia by 50% was similar to that for nalorphine, less than that for pentazocine and more than that for naloxone.

The pharmacological activity of butorphanol metabolites has not been studied in humans; in animal studies, butorphanol metabolites have demonstrated some analgesic activity.

In human studies of butorphanol, sedation is commonly noted at doses of 0.5 mg or more. Narcosis is produced by 10-12 mg doses of butorphanol administered over 10-15 minutes intravenously.

Butorphanol, like other mixed agonist-antagonists with a high affinity for the κ-receptor, may produce unpleasant psychotomimetic effects in some individuals.

Nausea and/or vomiting may be produced by doses of 1 mg or more administered by any route.

In human studies involving individuals without significant respiratory dysfunction, 2 mg of butorphanol IV and 10 mg of morphine sulfate IV depressed respiration to a comparable degree. At higher doses, the magnitude of respiratory depression with butorphanol is not appreciably increased; however, the duration of respiratory depression is longer. Respiratory depression noted after administration of butorphanol to humans by any route is reversed by treatment with naloxone, a specific opioid antagonist.

Butorphanol tartrate demonstrates antitussive effects in animals at doses less than those required for analgesia.

Hemodynamic changes noted during cardiac catheterization in patients receiving single 0.025 mg/kg intravenous doses of butorphanol have included increases in pulmonary artery pressure, wedge pressure and vascular resistance, increases in left ventricular end diastolic pressure, and in systemic arterial pressure.

PHARMACODYNAMICS

The analgesic effect of butorphanol is influenced by the route of administration. Onset of analgesia is within a few minutes for intravenous administration, within 15 minutes for intramuscular injection, and within 15 minutes for the nasal spray doses.

Peak analgesic activity occurs within 30-60 minutes following intravenous and intramuscular administration and within 1-2 hours following the nasal spray administration.

The duration of analgesia varies depending on the pain model as well as the route of administration, but is generally 3-4 hours with IM and IV doses as defined by the time 50% of patients required remedication. In postoperative studies, the duration of analgesia with IV or IM butorphanol was similar to morphine, meperidine, and pentazocine when administered in the same fashion at equipotent doses. Compared to the injectable form and other drugs in this class, Stadol NS has a longer duration of action (4-5 hours).

PHARMACOKINETICS

Stadol Injection is rapidly absorbed after IM injection and peak plasma levels are reached in 20-40 minutes.

After nasal administration, mean peak blood levels of 0.9-1.04 ng/ml occur at 30-60 minutes after a 1 mg dose (see TABLE 1A and TABLE 1B). The absolute bioavailability of Stadol NS is 60-70% and is unchanged in patients with allergic rhinitis. In patients using a nasal vasoconstrictor (oxymetazoline) the fraction of the dose absorbed was unchanged, but the rate of absorption was slowed. The peak plasma concentrations were approximately half those achieved in the absence of the vasoconstrictor.

Serum protein binding is independent of concentration over the range achieved in clinical practice (up to 7 ng/ml) with a bound fraction of approximately 80%.

The volume of distribution of butorphanol varies from 305-901 L and total body clearance from 52-154 L/h (see TABLE 1A and TABLE 1B).

Dose proportionality for Stadol NS has been determined at steady state in doses up to 4 mg at 6 hour intervals. Steady state is achieved within 2 days. The mean peak plasma concentration at steady state was 1.8-fold (maximal 3-fold) following a single dose.

***TABLE 1A** Mean Pharmacokinetic Parameters of Butorphanol in Young and Elderly Subjects* — Intravenous*

Parameters	Young	Elderly
AUC(∞)† (h·ng/ml)	7.24 (1.57) (4.40-9.77)	8.71 (2.02) (4.76-13.03)
Half-life (h)	4.56 (1.67) (2.06-8.70)	5.61 (1.36) (3.25-8.79)
Volume of distribution‡ (L)	487 (155) (305-901)	552 (124) (305-737)
Total body clearance (L/h)	99 (23) (70-154)	82 (21) (52-143)

* Young subjects (n=24) are from 20-40 years old and elderly (n=24) are greater than 65 years of age.
† Area under the plasma concentration-time curve after a 1 mg dose.
‡ Derived from IV data.

***TABLE 1B** Mean Pharmacokinetic Parameters of Butorphanol in Young and Elderly Subjects* — Nasal*

Parameters	Young	Elderly
T_{max}† (h)	0.62 (0.32)¤ (0.15-1.50)¶	1.03 (0.74) (0.25-3.00)
C_{max}‡ (ng/ml)	1.04 (0.40) (0.35-1.97)	0.90 (0.57) (0.10-2.68)
AUC(∞)§ (h·ng/ml)	4.93 (1.24) (2.16-7.27)	5.24 (2.27) (0.30-10.34)
Half-life (h)	4.74 (1.57) (2.89-8.79)	6.56 (1.51) (3.75-9.17)
Absolute bioavailability (%)	69 (16) (44-13)	61 (25) (3-121)

* Young subjects (n=24) are from 20-40 years old and elderly (n=24) are greater than 65 years of age.
† Time to peak plasma concentration.
‡ Peak plasma concentration normalized to 1 mg dose.
§ Area under the plasma concentration-time curve after a 1 mg dose.
¤ Mean (1 SD).
¶ (Range of observed values.)

The drug is transported across the blood brain and placental barriers and into human milk (see PRECAUTIONS: Labor and Delivery and Nursing Mothers).

Butorphanol is extensively metabolized in the liver. Metabolism is qualitatively and quantitatively similar following intravenous, intramuscular, or nasal administration. Oral bioavailability is only 5-17% because of extensive first pass metabolism of butorphanol.

The major metabolite of butorphanol is hydroxybutorphanol, while norbutorphanol is produced in small amounts. Both have been detected in plasma following administration of butorphanol, with norbutorphanol present at trace levels at most time points. The elimination half-life of hydroxybutorphanol is about 18 hours and, as a consequence, considerable accumulation (~5-fold) occurs when butorphanol is dosed to steady state (1 mg transnasally q6h for 5 days).

Elimination occurs by urine and fecal excretion. When ^3H labelled butorphanol is administered to normal subjects, most (70-80%) of the dose is recovered in the urine, while approximately 15% is recovered in the feces.

About 5% of the dose is recovered in the urine as butorphanol. Forty-nine percent (49%) is eliminated in the urine as hydroxybutorphanol. Less than 5% is excreted in the urine as norbutorphanol.

Butorphanol pharmacokinetics in the elderly differ from younger patients (see TABLE 1A and TABLE 1B). The mean absolute bioavailability of Stadol NS in elderly women (48%) was less than that in elderly men (75%), young men (68%), or young women (70%). Elimination half-life is increased in the elderly (6.6 hours as opposed to 4.7 hours in younger subjects).

In renally impaired patients with creatinine clearances <30 ml/min, the elimination half-life was approximately doubled and the total body clearance was approximately one-half (10.5 hours [clearance 150 L/h] compared to 5.8 hours [clearance 260 L/h] in healthy subjects). No effect on C_{max} or T_{max} was observed after a single dose.

After IV administration to patients with hepatic impairment, the elimination half-life of butorphanol was approximately tripled and total body clearance was approximately one-half (half-life 16.8 hours, clearance 92 L/h) compared to healthy subjects (half-life 4.8 hours, clearance 175 L/h). The exposure of hepatically impaired patients to butorphanol was significantly greater (about 2-fold) than that in healthy subjects. Similar results were seen after nasal administration. No effect on C_{max} or T_{max} was observed after a single intranasal dose.

For further recommendations refer to PRECAUTIONS: Hepatic and Renal Disease and Geriatric Use; and DRUG INTERACTIONS.

INDICATIONS AND USAGE

Stadol Injection and Stadol NS Nasal Spray are indicated for the management of pain when the use of an opioid analgesic is appropriate.

Stadol Injection is also indicated as a preoperative or preanesthetic medication, as a supplement to balanced anesthesia, and for the relief of pain during labor.

CONTRAINDICATIONS

Stadol Injection and Stadol NS are contraindicated in patients hypersensitive to butorphanol tartrate or the preservative benzethonium chloride in Stadol NS or Stadol Injection in the multi-dose vial.

WARNINGS

PATIENTS DEPENDENT ON NARCOTICS

Because of its opioid antagonist properties, butorphanol is not recommended for use in patients dependent on narcotics. Such patients should have an adequate period of withdrawal from opioid drugs prior to beginning butorphanol therapy. In patients taking opioid analgesics chronically, butorphanol has precipitated withdrawal symptoms such as anxiety, agitation, mood changes, hallucinations, dysphoria, weakness, and diarrhea.

Because of the difficulty in assessing opioid tolerance in patients who have recently received repeated doses of narcotic analgesic medication, caution should be used in the administration of butorphanol to such patients.

DRUG ABUSE AND DEPENDENCE

Drug abuse: Butorphanol tartrate, by all routes of administration, has been associated with episodes of abuse. Of the cases received, there were more reports of abuse with the nasal spray formulation than with the injectable formulation.

Physical dependence, tolerance, and withdrawal: Prolonged, continuous use of butorphanol tartrate may result in physical dependence or tolerance (a decrease in response to a given dose). Abrupt cessation of use by patients with physical dependence may result in symptoms of withdrawal.

Note: Proper patient selection, dose and prescribing limitations, appropriate directions for use, and frequent monitoring are important to minimize the risk of abuse and physical dependence.

PRECAUTIONS

GENERAL

Hypotension associated with syncope during the first hour of dosing with Stadol NS has been reported rarely, particularly in patients with past history of similar reactions to opioid analgesics. Therefore, patients should be advised to avoid activities with potential risks.

HEAD INJURY AND INCREASED INTRACRANIAL PRESSURE

As with other opioids, the use of butorphanol in patients with head injury may be associated with carbon dioxide retention and secondary elevation of cerebrospinal fluid pressure, drug-induced miosis, and alterations in mental state that would obscure the interpretation of the clinical course of patients with head injuries. In such patients, butorphanol should be used only if the benefits of use outweigh the potential risks.

DISORDERS OF RESPIRATORY FUNCTION OR CONTROL

Butorphanol may produce respiratory depression, especially in patients receiving other CNS active agents, or patients suffering from CNS diseases or respiratory impairment.

HEPATIC AND RENAL DISEASE

In patients with hepatic or renal impairment, the initial dose of Stadol Injection should generally be half the recommended adult dose (0.5 mg IV and 1.0 mg IM). Repeat doses in these patients should be determined by the patient's response rather than at fixed intervals but will generally be no less than 6 hours apart. The initial dose sequence of Stadol NS should be limited to 1 mg followed, if needed, by 1 mg in 90-120 minutes. The repeat dose sequence in these patients should be determined by the patient's response rather than at fixed times but will generally be at intervals of no less than 6 hours (see CLINICAL PHARMACOLOGY, Pharmacokinetics).

CARDIOVASCULAR EFFECTS

Because butorphanol may increase the work of the heart, especially the pulmonary circuit, the use of butorphanol in patients with acute myocardial infarction, ventricular dysfunction, or coronary insufficiency should be limited to those situations where the benefits clearly outweigh the risk (see CLINICAL PHARMACOLOGY).

Severe hypertension has been reported rarely during butorphanol therapy. In such cases, butorphanol should be discontinued and the hypertension treated with antihypertensive drugs. In patients who are not opioid dependent, naloxone has also been reported to be effective.

USE IN AMBULATORY PATIENTS

Opioid analgesics, including butorphanol, impair the mental and physical abilities required for the performance of potentially dangerous tasks such as driving a car or operating machinery. Effects such as drowsiness or dizziness can appear, usually within the first hour after dosing. These effects may persist for varying periods of time after dosing. Patients who have taken butorphanol should not drive or operate dangerous machinery for at least 1 hour and until the effects of the drug are no longer present.

Alcohol should not be consumed while using butorphanol. Concurrent use of butorphanol with drugs that affect the central nervous system (*e.g.*, alcohol, barbiturates, tranquilizers, and antihistamines) may result in increased central nervous system depressant effects such as drowsiness, dizziness, and impaired mental function.

Butorphanol is one of a class of drugs known to be abused and thus should be handled accordingly.

Patients should be instructed on the proper use of Stadol NS (see the Patient Instructions that are distributed with the prescription).

INFORMATION FOR THE PATIENT

See Use in Ambulatory Patients.

CARCINOGENESIS, MUTAGENESIS, AND IMPAIRMENT OF FERTILITY

Two year carcinogenicity studies were conducted in mice and rats given butorphanol tartrate in the diet up to 60 mg/kg/day (180 mg/m^2 for mice and 354 mg/m^2 for rats). There was no evidence of carcinogenicity in either species in these studies.

Butorphanol was not genotoxic in *S. typhimurium* or *E. coli* assays or in unscheduled DNA synthesis and repair assays conducted in cultured human fibroblast cells.

Rats treated orally with 160 mg/kg/day (944 mg/m^2) had a reduced pregnancy rate. However, a similar effect was not observed with a 2.5 mg/kg/day (14.75 mg/m^2) subcutaneous dose.

PREGNANCY CATEGORY C

Reproduction studies in mice, rats, and rabbits during organogenesis did not reveal any teratogenic potential to butorphanol. However, pregnant rats treated subcutaneously with butorphanol at 1 mg/kg (5.9 mg/m^2) had a higher frequency of stillbirths than controls. Butorphanol at 30 mg/kg/oral (360 mg/m^2) and 60 mg/kg/oral (720 mg/m^2) also showed higher incidences of post-implantation loss in rabbits.

There are no adequate and well-controlled studies of Stadol in pregnant women before 37 weeks of gestation. Stadol should be used during pregnancy only if the potential benefit justifies the potential risk to the infant.

LABOR AND DELIVERY

There have been rare reports of infant respiratory distress/apnea following the administration of Stadol Injection during labor. The reports of respiratory distress/apnea have been associated with administration of a dose within 2 hours of delivery, use of multiple doses, use with additional analgesic or sedative drugs, or use in preterm pregnancies.

In a study of 119 patients, the administration of 1 mg of IV Stadol Injection during labor was associated with transient (10-90 minutes) sinusoidal fetal heart rate patterns, but was not associated with adverse neonatal outcomes. In the presence of an abnormal fetal heart rate pattern, Stadol Injection should be used with caution.

Stadol NS is not recommended during labor or delivery because there is no clinical experience with its use in this setting.

NURSING MOTHERS

Butorphanol has been detected in milk following administration of Stadol Injection to nursing mothers. The amount an infant would receive is probably clinically insignificant (estimated 4 μg/L of milk in a mother receiving 2 mg IM four times a day).

Although there is no clinical experience with the use of Stadol NS in nursing mothers, it should be assumed that butorphanol will appear in the milk in similar amounts following the nasal route of administration.

PEDIATRIC USE

Butorphanol is not recommended for use in patients below 18 years of age because safety and efficacy have not been established in this population.

GERIATRIC USE

Of the approximately 1500 patients treated with Stadol Injection in clinical studies, 15% were 61 years of age or older and 1% were 76 years or older. Of the approximately 1700 patients treated with Stadol NS in clinical studies, 8% were 65 years of age or older and 2% were 75 years or older.

Due to changes in clearance, the mean half-life of butorphanol is increased by 25% (to over 6 hours) in patients over the age of 65 years (see CLINICAL PHARMACOLOGY, Pharmacokinetics). Elderly patients may be more sensitive to the side effects of butorphanol. In clinical studies of Stadol NS, elderly patients had an increased frequency of headache, dizziness, drowsiness, vertigo, constipation, nausea and/or vomiting, and nasal congestion compared with younger patients. There are insufficient efficacy data for patients ≥65 years to determine whether they respond differently from younger patients.

The initial dose of Stadol Injection recommended for elderly patients should generally be half the recommended adult dose (0.5 mg IV and 1.0 mg IM). Repeat doses should be determined by the patient's response rather than at fixed intervals, but will generally be no less than 6 hours apart.

Initially a 1 mg dose of Stadol NS should generally be used in geriatric patients and 90-120 minutes should elapse before administering a second 1 mg dose, if needed.

Butorphanol and its metabolites are known to be substantially excreted by the kidney, and the risk of toxic reactions to this drug may be greater in patients with impaired renal function. Because elderly patients are more likely to have decreased renal function, care should be taken in dose selection.

DRUG INTERACTIONS

Concurrent use of butorphanol with central nervous system depressants (*e.g.*, alcohol, barbiturates, tranquilizers, and antihistamines) may result in increased central nervous system depressant effects. When used concurrently with such drugs, the dose of butorphanol should be the smallest effective dose and the frequency of dosing reduced as much as possible when administered concomitantly with drugs that potentiate the action of opioids.

In healthy volunteers, the pharmacokinetics of a 1 mg dose of butorphanol administered as Stadol NS were not affected by the coadministration of a single 6 mg subcutaneous dose of sumatriptan. However, in another study in healthy volunteers, the pharmacokinetics of butorphanol were significantly altered (29% decrease in AUC and 38% decrease in C_{max}) when a 1 mg dose of Stadol NS was administered 1 minute after a 20 mg dose of sumatriptan nasal spray. (The two drugs were administered in opposite nostrils.) When the Stadol NS was administered 30 minutes after the sumatriptan nasal spray, the AUC of butorphanol increased 11% and C_{max} decreased 18%.

In neither case were the pharmacokinetics of sumatriptan affected by coadministration with Stadol NS. These results suggest that the analgesic effect of Stadol NS may be diminished when it is administered shortly after sumatriptan nasal spray, but by 30 minutes any such reduction in effect should be minimal.

The safety of using Stadol NS and Imitrex (sumatriptan) Nasal Spray during the same episode of migraine has not been established. However, it should be noted that both products are capable of producing transient increases in blood pressure.

The pharmacokinetics of a 1 mg dose of butorphanol administered as Stadol NS were not affected by the coadministration of cimetidine (300 mg qid). Conversely, the administration of Stadol NS (1 mg butorphanol qid) did not alter the pharmacokinetics of a 300 mg dose of cimetidine.

It is not known if the effects of butorphanol are altered by other concomitant medications that affect hepatic metabolism of drugs (erythromycin, theophylline, etc.), but physicians should be alert to the possibility that a smaller initial dose and longer intervals between doses may be needed.

The fraction of Stadol NS absorbed is unaffected by the concomitant administration of a nasal vasoconstrictor (oxymetazoline), but the rate of absorption is decreased. Therefore, a slower onset can be anticipated if Stadol NS is administered concomitantly with, or immediately following, a nasal vasoconstrictor.

No information is available about the use of butorphanol concurrently with MAO inhibitors.

ADVERSE REACTIONS

CLINICAL TRIAL EXPERIENCE

A total of 2446 patients were studied in premarketing clinical trials of butorphanol. Approximately half received Stadol Injection with the remainder receiving Stadol NS. In nearly all cases the type and incidence of side effects with butorphanol by any route were those commonly observed with opioid analgesics.

The adverse experiences described below are based on data from short-term and long-term clinical trials in patients receiving butorphanol by any route. There has been no attempt to correct for placebo effect or to subtract the frequencies reported by placebo-treated patients in controlled trials.

The most frequently reported adverse experiences across all clinical trials with Stadol Injection and Stadol NS were somnolence (43%), dizziness (19%), nausea and/or vomiting (13%). In long-term trials with Stadol NS only, nasal congestion (13%) and insomnia (11%) were frequently reported.

The following adverse experiences were reported at a frequency of 1% or greater in clinical trials and were considered to be probably related to the use of butorphanol:

Body as a Whole: Asthenia/lethargy, headache, sensation of heat.

Cardiovascular: Vasodilation, palpitations.

Digestive: Anorexia, constipation, dry mouth, nausea and/or vomiting, stomach pain.

Nervous: Anxiety, confusion, dizziness, euphoria, floating feeling, insomnia, nervousness, paresthesia, somnolence, tremor.

Respiratory: Bronchitis, cough, dyspnea, epistaxis, nasal congestion, nasal irritation, pharyngitis, rhinitis, sinus congestion, sinusitis, upper respiratory infection.

Skin and Appendages: Sweating/clammy, pruritus.

Special Senses: Blurred vision, ear pain, tinnitus, unpleasant taste.

The following adverse experiences were reported with a frequency of less than 1% in clinical trials and were considered to be probably related to the use of butorphanol:

Cardiovascular: Hypotension, syncope.

Nervous: Abnormal dreams, agitation, dysphoria, hallucinations, hostility, withdrawal symptoms.

Skin and Appendages: Rash/hives.

Urogenital: Impaired urination.

The following infrequent additional adverse experiences were reported in a frequency of less than 1% of the patients studied in short-term Stadol NS trials and under circumstances where the association between these events and butorphanol administration is unknown. They are being listed as alerting information for the physician:

Body as a Whole: Edema.

Cardiovascular: Chest pain, hypertension, tachycardia.

Nervous: Depression.

Respiratory: Shallow breathing.

POSTMARKETING EXPERIENCE

Postmarketing experience with Stadol NS and Stadol Injection has shown an adverse event profile similar to that seen during the premarketing evaluation of butorphanol by all routes of administration. Adverse experiences that were associated with the use of Stadol NS or Stadol Injection and that are not listed above have been chosen for inclusion below because of their seriousness, frequency of reporting, or probable relationship to butorphanol. Because they are reported voluntarily from a population of unknown size, estimates of frequency cannot be made. These adverse experiences include apnea, convulsion, delusion, drug dependence, excessive drug effect associated with transient difficulty speaking and/or executing purposeful movements, overdose, and vertigo. Reports of butorphanol overdose with a fatal outcome have usually but not always been associated with ingestion of multiple drugs.

DOSAGE AND ADMINISTRATION

Factors to be considered in determining the dose are age, body weight, physical status, underlying pathological condition, use of other drugs, type of anesthesia to be used, and surgical procedure involved. Use in the elderly, in patients with hepatic or renal disease, or in labor requires extra caution (see PRECAUTIONS). The following doses are for patients who do not have impaired hepatic or renal function and who are not on CNS active agents.

USE FOR PAIN

Stadol Injection

Intravenous: The usual recommended single dose for IV administration is 1 mg repeated every 3-4 hours as necessary. The effective dosage range, depending on the severity of pain, is 0.5 to 2 mg repeated every 3-4 hours.

Intramuscular: The usual recommended single dose for IM administration is 2 mg in patients who will be able to remain recumbent, in the event drowsiness or dizziness occurs. This may be repeated every 3-4 hours, as necessary. The effective dosage range depending on the severity of pain is 1-4 mg repeated every 3-4 hours. There are insufficient clinical data to recommend single doses above 4 mg.

Stadol NS

The usual recommended dose for initial nasal administration is 1 mg (1 spray in **one** nostril). Adherence to this dose reduces the incidence of drowsiness and dizziness. If adequate pain relief is not achieved within 60-90 minutes, an additional 1 mg dose may be given.

The initial dose sequence outlined above may be repeated in 3-4 hours as required after the second dose of the sequence.

Depending on the severity of the pain, an initial dose of 2 mg (1 spray in **each** nostril) may be used in patients who will be able to remain recumbent in the event drowsiness or dizziness occurs. In such patients single additional 2 mg doses should not be given for 3-4 hours.

USE AS PREOPERATIVE/PREANESTHETIC MEDICATION

The preoperative medication dosage of Stadol Injection should be individualized. The usual adult dose is 2 mg IM, administered 60-90 minutes before surgery. This is approximately equivalent in sedative effect to 10 mg morphine or 80 mg meperidine.

USE IN BALANCED ANESTHESIA

The usual dose of Stadol Injection is 2 mg IV shortly before induction and/or 0.5-1.0 mg IV in increments during anesthesia. The increment may be higher, up to 0.06 mg/kg (4 mg/70 kg), depending on previous sedative, analgesic, and hypnotic drugs administered. The total dose of Stadol Injection will vary; however, patients seldom require less than 4 mg or more than 12.5 mg (approximately 0.06-0.18 mg/kg).

The use of Stadol NS is not recommended because it has not been studied in induction or maintenance of anesthesia.

LABOR

In patients at full term in early labor a 1-2 mg dose of Stadol Injection IV or IM may be administered and repeated after 4 hours. Alternative analgesia should be used for pain associated with delivery or if delivery is expected to occur within 4 hours.

If concomitant use of Stadol with drugs that may potentiate its effects is deemed necessary (see DRUG INTERACTIONS), the lowest effective dose should be employed.

The use of Stadol NS is not recommended as it has not been studied in labor.

SAFETY AND HANDLING

Stadol Injection is supplied in sealed delivery systems that have a low risk of accidental exposure to health care workers. Ordinary care should be taken to avoid aerosol generation while preparing a syringe for use. Following skin contact, rinsing with cool water is recommended.

Stadol NS is an open delivery system with increased risk of exposure to health care workers.

In the priming process, a certain amount of butorphanol may be aerosolized; therefore, the pump sprayer should be aimed away from the patient or other people or animals.

The disposal of Schedule IV controlled substances must be consistent with State and Federal Regulations. The unit should be disposed of by unscrewing the cap, rinsing the bottle, and placing the parts in a waste container.

HOW SUPPLIED

STADOL INJECTION

Stadol Injection for IM or IV use is available as 1 mg/ml in a 1 ml vial, and 2 mg/ml in 1 ml vials, 2 ml vials and 10 ml multi-dose vials.

STADOL NS NASAL SPRAY

Stadol NS is supplied as 10 mg/ml in a child-resistant prescription vial containing a metered-dose spray pump with protective clip and dust cover, a bottle of nasal spray solution, and a patient instruction leaflet. On average, one 2.5 ml bottle will deliver 14-15 doses if no repriming is necessary.

STORAGE CONDITIONS

Store at 25°C (77°F) controlled room temperature. Parenteral drug products should be inspected visually for particulate matter and discoloration prior to administration, whenever solution and container permit.

PRODUCT LISTING - RATED THERAPEUTICALLY EQUIVALENT

Solution - Injectable - 1 mg/ml			
1 ml x 10	$46.30	GENERIC, Baxter Pharmaceutical Products, Inc	10019-0461-01
1 ml x 10	$67.50	GENERIC, Bedford Laboratories	55390-0183-01
1 ml x 10	$69.00	GENERIC, Abbott Pharmaceutical	00074-1624-01
1 ml x 10	$80.87	GENERIC, Abbott Pharmaceutical	00074-1623-01
1 ml x 10	$84.20	GENERIC, Vha Supply	00074-1623-49
1 ml x 10	$84.20	GENERIC, Vha Supply	00074-1624-49
1 ml x 10	$87.28	GENERIC, Abbott Pharmaceutical	00074-2301-01
Solution - Injectable - 2 mg/ml			
1 ml	$87.80	STADOL, Geneva Pharmaceuticals	00015-5646-15
1 ml x 10	$80.20	GENERIC, Vha Supply	00074-1626-49
1 ml x 10	$80.20	GENERIC, Vha Supply	00074-1627-49
1 ml x 10	$80.51	GENERIC, Abbott Pharmaceutical	00074-1626-01
1 ml x 10	$266.00	GENERIC, Abbott Pharmaceutical	00074-1627-01
1 ml x 30	$237.60	STADOL, Allscripts Pharmaceutical Company	54569-3799-00
2 ml	$149.60	STADOL, Geneva Pharmaceuticals	00015-5644-15
2 ml x 10	$72.50	GENERIC, Bedford Laboratories	55390-0184-01
2 ml x 10	$84.20	GENERIC, Vha Supply	00074-1626-51
2 ml x 10	$137.51	GENERIC, Abbott Pharmaceutical	00074-1626-02
4 ml x 10	$127.50	GENERIC, Bedford Laboratories	55390-0184-02
10 ml	$52.00	GENERIC, Bedford Laboratories	55390-0185-10
10 ml	$65.00	GENERIC, Apotex Usa Inc	60505-0660-00
10 ml	$76.39	STADOL, Bristol-Myers Squibb	00015-5648-20
10 ml	$79.18	STADOL, Prescript Pharmaceuticals	00247-0335-10
10 ml x 10	$73.33	STADOL, Allscripts Pharmaceutical Company	54569-3109-00
10 ml x 100	$689.16	STADOL, Allscripts Pharmaceutical Company	54569-3109-01
Spray - Nasal - 10 mg/ml			
2.50 ml	$75.25	GENERIC, Mylan Pharmaceuticals Inc	00378-9639-43
2.50 ml	$75.25	GENERIC, Mylan Pharmaceuticals Inc	59911-5944-01
2.50 ml	$79.26	GENERIC, Roxane Laboratories Inc	00054-3090-36

PRODUCT LISTING - EQUIVALENTS NOT AVAILABLE

Solution - Injectable - 1 mg/ml			
1 ml	$84.30	STADOL, Geneva Pharmaceuticals	00015-5645-15
1 ml x 10	$67.50	GENERIC, Apotex Usa Inc	60505-0658-00
1 ml x 10	$242.70	STADOL, Bristol-Myers Squibb	00015-5645-20
30 ml	$252.90	STADOL, Bristol-Myers Squibb	00015-5645-33
Solution - Injectable - 2 mg/ml			
1 ml x 10	$72.50	GENERIC, Apotex Usa Inc	60505-0659-00
1 ml x 30	$252.90	STADOL, Bristol-Myers Squibb	00015-5646-20
1 ml x 30	$263.40	STADOL, Bristol-Myers Squibb	00015-5646-33
2 ml x 10	$127.50	GENERIC, Apotex Usa Inc	60505-0659-01
2 ml x 30	$431.10	STADOL, Bristol-Myers Squibb	00015-5644-20
2 ml x 30	$448.80	STADOL, Bristol-Myers Squibb	00015-5644-33
10 ml x 10	$763.90	STADOL, Bristol-Myers Squibb	00015-5648-97
Spray - Nasal - 10 mg/ml			
2.50 ml	$60.53	STADOL NS, Allscripts Pharmaceutical Company	54569-3681-00
2.50 ml	$66.06	STADOL NS, Cheshire Drugs	55175-4416-01
2.50 ml	$67.52	STADOL NS, Physicians Total Care	54868-3209-00
2.50 ml	$102.65	STADOL NS, Bristol-Myers Squibb	00087-5650-41

Cabergoline *(003323)*

Categories: Galactorrhea; Hyperprolactinemia; FDA Approved 1996 Dec; Pregnancy Category B
Drug Classes: Antiparkinson agents; Dopaminergics; Ergot alkaloids and derivatives; Hormones/hormone modifiers
Brand Names: Dostinex
Foreign Brand Availability: Cabaser (Australia; Israel)
Cost of Therapy: $140.55 (Hyperprolactinemia; Dostinex; 0.5 mg; 1 tablet/day; 28 day supply)

DESCRIPTION

Cabergoline is a dopamine receptor agonist. The chemical name for cabergoline is 1-[(6-allylergolin-8β-yl)-carbonyl]-1-[3-(dimethylamino)propyl]-3-ethylurea. Its empirical formula is $C_{26}H_{37}N_5O_2$, and its molecular weight is 451.62.

Cabergoline is a white powder soluble in ethyl alcohol, chloroform, and N,N-dimethylformamide (DMF); slightly soluble in 0.1 N hydrochloric acid; very slightly soluble in n-hexane; and insoluble in water.

Dostinex tablets, for oral administration, contain 0.5 mg of cabergoline. Inactive ingredients consist of leucine, and lactose.

CLINICAL PHARMACOLOGY

MECHANISM OF ACTION

The secretion of prolactin by the anterior pituitary is mainly under hypothalmic inhibitory control, likely exerted through release of dopamine by tuberoinfundibular neurons. Cabergoline is a long-acting dopamine receptor agonist with a high affinity for D_2 receptors. Results of *in vitro* studies demonstrate that cabergoline exerts a direct inhibitory effect on the secretion of prolactin by rat pituitary lactotrophs. Cabergoline decreased serum prolactin levels in reserpinized rats. Receptor-binding studies indicate that cabergoline has low affinity for dopamine D_1, α_1- and α_2-adrenergic, and 5-HT_1 and 5-HT_2-serotonin receptors.

PHARMACOKINETICS

Absorption

Following single oral doses of 0.5-1.5 mg given to 12 healthy adult volunteers, mean peak plasma levels of 30-70 pg/ml of cabergoline were observed within 2-3 hours. Over the 0.5 to 7 mg dose range, cabergoline plasma levels appeared to be dose-proportional in 12 healthy adult volunteers and 9 adult parkinsonian patients. A repeat-dose study in 12 healthy volunteers suggests that steady-state levels following a once-weekly dosing schedule are expected to be 2- to 3-fold higher than after a single dose. The absolute bioavailability of cabergoline is unknown. A significant fraction of the administered dose undergoes a first-pass effect. The elimination half-life of cabergoline estimated from urinary data of 12 healthy subjects ranged between 63-69 hours. The prolonged prolactin-lowering effect of cabergoline may be related to its slow elimination and long half-life.

Distribution

In animals, based on total radioactivity, cabergoline (and/or its metabolites has shown extensive tissue distribution. Radioactivity in the pituitary exceeded that in plasma by greater than 100-fold and was eliminated with a half-life of approximately 60 hours. This finding is consistent with the long-lasting prolactin-lowering effect of the drug. Whole body autoradiography studies in pregnant rats showed no fetal uptake but high levels in the uterine wall. Significant radioactivity (parent plus metabolites) detected in the milk of lactating rats suggests a potential for exposure to nursing infants. The drug is extensively distributed throughout the body. Cabergoline is moderately bound (40-42%) to human plasma proteins in a concentration-independent manner. Concomitant dosing of highly protein-bound drugs is unlikely to affect its disposition.

Metabolism

In both animals and humans, cabergoline is extensively metabolized, predominantly via hydrolysis of the acylurea bond or the urea moiety. Cytochrome P-450 mediated metabolism appears to be minimal. Cabergoline does not cause enzyme induction and/or inhibition in the rat. Hydrolysis of the acylurea or urea moiety abolishes the prolactin-lowering effect of cabgergoline, and major metabolites identified thus far do not contribute to the therapeutic effect.

Excretion

After oral dosing of radioactive cabergoline to 5 healthy volunteers, approximately 22% and 60% of the dose was excreted within 20 days in the urine and feces, respectively. Less than 4% of the dose was excreted unchanged in the urine. Nonrenal and renal clearances for cabergoline are about 3.2 L/min and 0.08 L/min, respectively. Urinary excretion in hyperprolactinemic patients was similar.

SPECIAL POPULATIONS

Renal Insufficiency

The pharmacokinetics of cabergoline were not altered in 12 patients with moderate-to-severe renal insufficiency as assessed by creatinine clearance.

Hepatic Insufficiency

In 12 patients with mild-to-moderate hepatic dysfunction (Child-Pugh score >10), no effect on mean cabergoline C_{max} or area under the plasma concentrations curve (AUC) was observed. However, patients with severe insufficiency (Child-Pugh score >10) show a substantial increase in the mean cabergoline C_{max} and AUC, and thus necessitate caution.

Elderly

Effect of age on the pharmacokinetics of cabergoline has not been studied.

Food-Drug Interaction

In 12 healthy adult volunteers, food did not alter cabergoline kinetics.

PHARMACODYNAMICS

Dose response with inhibition of plasma prolactin, onset of maximal effect, and duration of effect has been documented following single cabergoline doses to healthy volunteers (0.05 to 1.5 mg) and hyperprolactinemic patients (0.3 to 1 mg). In volunteers, prolactin inhibition was evident at doses >0.2 mg, while doses ≥0.5 mg caused maximal suppression in most subjects. Higher doses produce prolactin suppression in a greater proportion of subjects and with an earlier onset and longer duration of action. In 12 healthy volunteers, 0.5, 1, and 1.5 mg doses resulted in complete prolactin inhibition, with a maximum effect within 3 hours in 92-100% of subjects after the 1 and 1.5 mg doses compared with 50% of subjects after the 0.5 mg dose.

In hyperprolactinemic patients (n=51), the maximal prolactin decrease after a 0.6 mg single dose of cabergoline was comparable to 2.5 mg bromocriptine; however, the duration of effect was markedly longer (14 days vs 24 hours). The time to maximal effect was shorter for bromocriptine than cabergoline (6 hours vs 48 hours).

In 72 healthy volunteers, single or multiple doses (up to 2 mg) of cabergoline resulted in selective inhibition of prolactin with no apparent effect on other anterior pituitary hormones (GH, FSH, LH, ACTH, and TSH) or cortisol.

INDICATIONS AND USAGE

Cabergoline tablets are indicated for the treatment of hyperprolactinemic disorders, either idiopathic or due to pituitary adenomas.

NON-FDA APPROVED INDICATIONS

Cabergoline has been used without FDA approval for the treatment of patients with Parkinson's disease and for the inhibition of physiologic lactation. While use in Parkinson's disease has been approved in some countries in Europe, doses for this indication have been started at 0.5 mg per day (usually along with carbidopa-levodopa) and titrated up to over 10 mg per day. The drug may also have the ability to lower serum growth hormone levels in some dopamine-responsive acromegalic patients. However, further studies are needed.

CONTRAINDICATIONS

Cabergoline tablets are contraindicated in patients with uncontrolled hypertension or known hypersensitivity to ergot derivatives.

WARNINGS

Dopamine agonists in general should not be used in patients with pregnancy-induced hypertension, for example, preclampsia and eclampsia, unless the potential benefit is judged to outweigh the possible risk.

PRECAUTIONS

GENERAL

Initial doses higher than 1.0 mg may produce orthostatic hypotension. Care should be exercised when administering cabergoline with other medications known to lower blood pressure.

Postpartum Lactation Inhibition or Suppression

Cabergoline is not indicated for the inhibition or suppression of physiologic lactation. Use of bromocriptine, another dopamine agonist for this purpose, has been associated with cases of hypertension, stroke, and seizures.

Hepatic Impairment

Since cabergoline is extensively metabolized by the liver, caution should be used, and careful monitoring exercised, when administering cabergoline to patients with hepatic impairment.

INFORMATION FOR THE PATIENT

A patient should be instructed to notify her physician if she suspects she is pregnant, becomes pregnant, or intends to become pregnant during therapy. A pregnancy test should be done if there is any suspicion of pregnancy and continuation of treatment should be discussed with her physician.

CARCINOGENESIS, MUTAGENESIS, AND IMPAIRMENT OF FERTILITY

Carcinogenicity studies were conducted in mice and rats with cabergoline given by gavage at doses up to 0.98 mg/kg/day and 0.32 mg/kg/day, respectively. These doses are 7 times and 4 times the maximum recommended human dose calculated on a body surface area basis using total mg/m^2/week in rodents and mg/m^2/week for a 50 kg human.

There was a slight increase in the incidence of cervical and uterine leiomyomas and uterine leiomyosarcomas in mice. In rats, there was a slight increase in malignant tumors of the cervix and uterus and interstitial cell adenomas. The occurrence of tumors in female rodents may be related to the prolonged suppression of prolactin secretion because prolactin is needed in rodents for the maintenance of the corpus luteum. In the absence of prolactin, the estrogen/progesterone ratio is increased, thereby increasing the risk for uterine tumors. In male rodents, the decrease in serum prolactin levels was associated with an increase in serum luteinizing hormone, which is thought to be a compensatory effect to maintain testicular steroid synthesis. Since these hormonal mechanisms are thought to be species-specific, the relevance of these tumors to humans is not known.

The mutagenic potential of cabergoline was evaluated and found to be negative in a battery of *in vitro* tests. These tests included the bacterial mutation (Ames) test with *Salmonella typhimurium*, the gene mutation assay with *Schizosaccharomyces pombe* P_1 and V79 Chinese hamster cells, DNA damage and repair in *Saccharomyces cerevisiae* D_4, and chromosomal aberrations in human lymphocytes. Cabergoline was also negative in the bone marrow micronucleus test in the mouse.

In female rats, a daily dose of 0.003 mg/kg for 2 weeks prior to mating and throughout the mating period inhibited conception. This dose represents approximately 1/28 the maximum recommended human dose calculated on a body surface area basis using total mg/m^2/week in rats and mg/m^2/week for a 50 kg human.

PREGNANCY, TERATOGENIC EFFECTS, PREGNANCY CATEGORY B

Reproduction studies have been performed with cabergoline in mice, rats, and rabbits administered by gavage.

(Multiples of the maximum recommended human dose in this section are calculated on a body surface area basis using total mg/m^2/week for animals and mg/m^2/week for a 50 kg human.)

There were maternotoxic effects but no teratogenic effects in mice given cabergoline at doses up to 8 mg/kg/day (approximately 55 times the maximum recommended human dose) during the period of organogenesis.)

A dose of 0.012 mg/kg/day (approximately 1/7 the maximum recommended human dose) during the period of organogenesis in rats caused an increase in post-implantation embryofetal loses. These losses could be due to the prolactin inhibitory properties of cabergoline in rats. At daily doses of 0.5 mg/kg/day (approximately 19 times the maximum recommended human dose) during the period of organogenesis in the rabbit, cabergoline caused maternotoxicity characterized by a loss of body weight and decreased food consumption. Doses of 4 mg/kg/day (approximately 150 times the maximum recommended human dose) during the period of organogenesis in the rabbit caused an increased occurrence of various malformations. However, in another study in rabbits, no treatment-related malformations or embryofetotoxicity were observed at doses up to 8 mg/kg/day (approximately 300 times the maximum recommended human dose).

In rats, doses higher than 0.003 mg/kg/day (approximately 1/28 the maximum recommended human dose) from 6 days before parturition and throughout the lactation period inhibited growth and caused death of offspring due to decreased milk secretion.

There are, however, no adequate and well-controlled studies in pregnant women. Because animal reproduction studies are not always predictive of human response, this drug should be used during pregnancy only if clearly needed.

NURSING MOTHERS

It is not known whether this drug is excreted in human milk. Because many drugs are excreted in human milk and because of the potential for serious adverse reactions in nursing infants from cabergoline, a decision should be made whether to discontinue nursing or to discontinue the drug, taking into account the importance of the drug to the mother. Use of cabergoline for the inhibition or suppression of physiologic lactation is not recommended (see PRECAUTIONS).

The prolactin-lowering action of cabergoline suggests that it will interfere with lactation. Due to this interference with lactation, cabergoline should not be given to women postpartum who are breastfeeding or who are planning to breastfeed.

PEDIATRIC USE

Safety and effectiveness of cabergoline in pediatric patients have not been established.

DRUG INTERACTIONS

Cabergoline should not be administered concurrently with D_2-antagonists, such as phenothiazines, butyrophenones, thioxanthines, or metoclopramide.

ADVERSE REACTIONS

The safety of cabergoline tablets has been evaluated in more than 900 patients with hyperprolactinemic disorders. Most adverse events were mild or moderate in severity.

In a 4 week, double-blind, placebo controlled study, treatment consisted of placebo or cabergoline at fixed doses of 0.125, 0.5, 0.75, or 1.0 mg twice weekly. Doses were halved during the first week. Since a possible dose-related effect was observed for nausea only, the four cabergoline treatment groups have been combined. The incidence of the most common adverse events during the placebo-controlled study is presented in TABLE 1.

TABLE 1 *Incidence of Reported Adverse Events During the 4 Week, Double-Blind, Placebo-Controlled Trial*

Adverse Event†	Cabergoline* (n=168)	Placebo (n=20)
Gastrointestinal		
Nausea	45 (27%)	4 (20%)
Constipation	16 (10%)	0
Abdominal pain	9 (5%)	1 (5%)
Dyspepsia	4 (2%)	0
Vomiting	4 (2%)	0
Central and Peripheral Nervous System		
Headache	43 (26%)	5 (25%)
Dizziness	25 (15%)	1 (5%)
Paresthesia	2 (1%)	0
Vertigo	2 (1%)	0
Body as a Whole		
Asthenia	15 (9%)	2 (10%)
Fatigue	12 (7%)	0
Hot flashes	2 (1%)	1 (5%)
Psychiatric		
Somnolence	9 (5%)	1 (5%)
Depression	5 (3%)	1 (5%)
Nervousness	4 (2%)	0
Autonomic Nervous System		
Postural hypotension	6 (4%)	0
Reproductive - Female		
Breast pain	2 (1%)	0
Dysmenorrhea	2 (1%)	0
Vision		
Abnormal vision	2 (1%)	0

* 0.125 to 1 mg two times a week.
† Reported at ≥1% for cabergoline.

In the 8 week, double-blind period of the comparative trial with bromocriptine, cabergoline (at a dose of 0.5 mg twice weekly) was discontinued because of an adverse event in 4 of 221 patients (2%) while bromocriptine (at a dose of 2.5 mg two times a day) was discontinued in 14 of 231 patients (6%). The most common reasons for discontinuation from cabergoline were headache, nausea and vomiting (3, 2 and 2 patients, respectively); the most common reasons for discontinuation from bromocriptine were nausea, vomiting, headache, and dizziness or vertigo (10, 3, 3, and 3 patients respectively). The incidence of the most common adverse events during the double-blind portion of the comparative trial with bromocriptine is presented in TABLE 2.

TABLE 2 *Incidence of Reported Adverse Events During the 8 Week, Double-Blind Period of the Comparative Trial With Bromocriptine*

Adverse Event*	Cabergoline (n=221)	Bromocriptine (n=231)
Gastrointestinal		
Nausea	63 (29%)	100 (43%)
Constipation	15 (7%)	21 (9%)
Abdominal pain	12 (5%)	19 (8%)
Dyspepsia	11 (5%)	16 (7%)
Vomiting	9 (4%)	16 (7%)
Dry mouth	5 (2%)	2 (1%)
Diarrhea	4 (2%)	7 (3%)
Flatulence	4 (2%)	3 (1%)
Throat irritation	2 (1%)	0
Toothache	2 (1%)	0
Central and Peripheral Nervous System		
Headache	58 (26%)	62 (27%)
Dizziness	38 (17%)	42 (18%)
Vertigo	9 (4%)	10 (4%)
Paresthesia	5 (2%)	6 (3%)
Body as a Whole		
Asthenia	13 (6%)	15 (6%)
Fatigue	10 (5%)	18 (8%)
Syncope	3 (1%)	3 (1%)
Influenza-like symptoms	2 (1%)	0
Malaise	2 (1%)	0
Periorbital edema	2 (1%)	2 (1%)
Peripheral edema	2 (1%)	1
Psychiatric		
Depression	7 (3%)	5 (2%)
Somnolence	5 (2%)	5 (2%)
Anorexia	3 (1%)	3 (1%)
Anxiety	3 (1%)	3 (1%)
Insomnia	3 (1%)	2 (1%)
Impaired concentration	2 (1%)	1
Nervousness	2 (1%)	5 (2%)
Cardiovascular		
Hot flashes	6 (3%)	3 (1%)
Hypotension	3 (1%)	4 (2%)
Dependent edema	2 (1%)	1
Palpitation	2 (1%)	5 (2%)
Reproductive - Female		
Breast pain	5 (2%)	8 (3%)
Dysmenorrhea	2 (1%)	1
Skin and Appendages		
Acne	3 (1%)	0
Pruritits	2 (1%)	1
Musculoskeletal		
Pain	4 (2%)	6 (3%)
Arthralgia	2 (1%)	0
Respiratory		
Rhinitis	2 (1%)	9 (4%)
Vision		
Abnormal vision	2 (1%)	2 (1%)

* Reported at ≥1% for cabergoline.

Other adverse events that were reported at an incidence of <1.0% in the overall clinical studies follow:

Body as a Whole: Facial edema, influenza-like symptoms, malaise.

Cardiovascular System: Hypotension, syncope, palpitations.

Digestive System: Dry mouth, flatulence, diarrhea, anorexia.

Metabolic and Nutritional System: Weight loss, weight gain.

Nervous System: Somnolence, nervousness, paresthesia, insomnia, anxiety.

Respiratory System: Nasal stuffiness, epistaxis.

Skin and Appendages: Acne, pruritus.

Special Senses: Abnormal vision.

Urogenital System: Dysmenorrhea, increased libido.

The safety of cabergoline has been evaluated in approximately 1200 patients with Parkinson's disease in controlled and uncontrolled studies at dosages of up to 11.5 mg/day which greatly exceeds the maximum recommended dosage of cabergoline for hyperprolactinemic disorders. In addition to the adverse events that occurred in the patients with hyperprolactinemic disorders, the most common adverse events in patients with Parkinson's disease were dyskinesia, hallucinations, confusion, and peripheral edema. Heart failure, pleural effusion, pulmonary fibrosis, and gastric or duodenal ulcer occurred rarely. One case of constrictive pericarditis has been reported.

DOSAGE AND ADMINISTRATION

The recommended dosage of cabergoline tablets for initiation of therapy is 0.25 mg twice a week. Dosage may be increased by 0.25 mg twice weekly up to a dosage of 1 mg twice a week according to the patient's serum prolactin level.

Dosage increases should not occur more rapidly than every 4 weeks, so that the physician can assess the patient's response to each dosage level. If the patient does not respond adequately, and no additional benefit is observed with higher doses, the lowest dose that achieved maximal response should be used and other therapeutic approaches considered.

After a normal serum prolactin level has been maintained for 6 months, cabergoline may be discontinued, with periodic monitoring of the serum prolactin level to determine whether or when treatment with cabergoline should be reinstituted. The durability of efficacy beyond 24 months of therapy with cabergoline has not been established.

HOW SUPPLIED

Dostinex tablets are white, scored, capsule-shaped tablets containing 0.5 mg cabergoline. Each tablet is scored on one side and has the letter "P" and the letter "U" on either side of the breakline. The other side of the tablet is engraved with the number 700.

Storage: Store at controlled room temperature 20-25°C (68-77°F).

PRODUCT LISTING - EQUIVALENTS NOT AVAILABLE

Tablet - Oral - 0.5 mg

8's $281.10 DOSTINEX, Pharmacia and Upjohn 00013-7001-12

Calcitonin (Salmon) *(000585)*

Categories: Hypercalcemia; Osteoporosis; Paget's disease; Pregnancy Category C; FDA Approval Pre 1982

Drug Classes: Hormones/hormone modifiers

Brand Names: **Calcimar**; Miacalcin; Osteocalcin

Foreign Brand Availability: Biocalcin (Korea); Boncalmon (Korea); Cadens (France); Calcinin (Taiwan); Calco (Singapore; Thailand); Calsynar (Benin; Burkina-Faso; Ethiopia; Gambia; Ghana; Guinea; Ivory-Coast; Kenya; Liberia; Malawi; Mali; Mauritania; Mauritius; Morocco; Niger; Nigeria; Senegal; Seychelles; Sierra-Leone; Sudan; Tanzania; Tunia; Uganda; Zambia; Zimbabwe); Caltine (Canada); Forcaltonin (Austria; Belgium; Bulgaria; Czech-Republic; Denmark; England; Finland; France; Germany; Greece; Hungary; Ireland; Italy; Netherlands; Norway; Poland; Portugal; Slovenia; Spain; Sweden; Switzerland; Turkey); Menocal (Thailand); Miacalcic (Austria; Bahrain; Belgium; Bulgaria; China; Cyprus; Czech-Republic; Denmark; Egypt; England; Finland; France; Germany; Greece; Hong-Kong; Hungary; Iran; Iraq; Ireland; Italy; Jordan; Kuwait; Lebanon; Libya; Mexico; Netherlands; New-Zealand; Norway; Oman; Poland; Portugal; Qatar; Republic-of-Yemen; Saudi-Arabia; Singapore; Slovenia; Spain; Sweden; Switzerland; Syria; Turkey; United-Arab-Emirates); Oseum (Mexico); Tonocalcin (Indonesia; Mexico); Zycalcit (India)

Cost of Therapy: $78.16 (Osteoporosis; Miacalcin Nasal Spray; 200 IU/ml; 4 ml; 200 IU/day; 30 day supply)

HCFA JCODE(S): J0630 up to 400 units SC, IM

DESCRIPTION

Calcitonin is a polypeptide hormone secreted by the parafollicular cells of the thyroid gland in mammals and by the ultimobranchial gland of birds and fish.

Calcitonin (salmon) is a synthetic polypeptide of 32 amino acids in the same linear sequence that is found in calcitonin of salmon origin.

INJECTION

It is provided in sterile solution for subcutaneous or intramuscular injection. Each milliliter contains 200 IU (MRC) of calcitonin (salmon), 5 mg phenol (as preservative), with sodium chloride, sodium acetate, acetic acid, and sodium hydroxide to adjust tonicity and pH.

NASAL SPRAY

It is provided in 2 ml fill glass bottles as a solution for nasal administration. This is sufficient medication for 14 doses. Each milliliter contains calcitonin (salmon) 2200 IU (corresponding to 200 IU/0.09 ml actuation), sodium chloride 8.5 mg, benzalkonium chloride 0.10 mg, nitrogen, hydrochloric acid (added as necessary to adjust pH) and purified water.

The activity of calcitonin (salmon) nasal spray is stated in International Units based on bioassay in comparison with the International Reference Preparation of calcitonin (salmon) for Bioassay, distributed by the National Institute of Biologic Standards and Control, Holly Hill, London.

CLINICAL PHARMACOLOGY

INJECTION

Calcitonin acts primarily on bone, but direct renal effects and actions on the gastrointestinal tract are also recognized. Calcitonin (salmon) appears to have actions essentially identical to calcitonins of mammalian origin, but its potency per mg is greater and it has a longer duration of action. The actions of calcitonin on bone and its role in normal human bone physiology are still incompletely understood.

Bone

Single injections of calcitonin cause a marked transient inhibition of the ongoing bone resorptive process. With prolonged use, there is a persistent, smaller decrease in the rate of bone resorption. Histologically, this is associated with a decreased number of osteoclasts and an apparent decrease in their resorptive activity. Decreased osteocytic resorption may also be involved. There is some evidence that initially bone formation may be augmented by calcitonin through increased osteoblastic activity. However, calcitonin will probably not induce a long-term increase in bone formation.

Animal studies indicate that endogenous calcitonin, primarily through its action on bone, participates with parathyroid hormone in the homeostatic regulation of blood calcium. Thus, high blood calcium levels cause increased secretion of calcitonin which, in turn, inhibits bone resorption. This reduces the transfer of calcium from bone to blood and tends to return blood calcium to the normal level. The importance of this process in humans has not been determined. In normal adults, who have a relatively low rate of bone resorption, the administration of exogenous calcitonin results in only a slight decrease in serum calcium. In normal children and in patients with generalized Paget's disease, bone resorption is more rapid and decreases in serum calcium are more pronounced in response to calcitonin.

Paget's Disease of Bone (osteitis deformans)

Paget's disease is a disorder of uncertain etiology characterized by abnormal and accelerated bone formation and resorption in one or more bones. In most patients only small areas of bone are involved and the disease is not symptomatic. In a small fraction of patients, however, the abnormal bone may lead to bone pain and bone deformity, cranial and spinal nerve entrapment, or spinal cord compression. The increased vascularity of the abnormal bone may lead to high output congestive heart failure.

Active Paget's disease involving a large mass of bone may increase the urinary hydroxyproline excretion (reflecting breakdown of collagen-containing bone matrix) and serum alkaline phosphatase (reflecting increased bone formation).

Calcitonin (salmon), presumably by an initial blocking effect on bone resorption, causes a decreased rate of bone turnover with a resultant fall in the serum alkaline phosphatase and urinary hydroxyproline excretion in approximately ⅔ of patients treated. These biochemical changes appear to correspond to changes toward more normal bone, as evidenced by a small number of documented examples of: (1) radiologic regression of Pagetic lesions, (2) improvement of impaired auditory nerve and other neurologic function, (3) decreases (measured) in abnormally elevated cardiac output. These improvements occur extremely rarely, if ever, spontaneously (elevated cardiac output may disappear over a period of years when the disease slowly enters a sclerotic phase; in the cases treated with calcitonin, however, the decreases were seen in less than 1 year.)

Some patients with Paget's disease who have good biochemical and/or symptomatic responses initially, later relapse. Suggested explanations have included the formation of neutralizing antibodies and the development of secondary hyperparathyroidism, but neither suggestion appears to explain adequately the majority of relapses.

Although the parathyroid hormone levels do appear to rise transiently during each hypocalcemic response to calcitonin, most investigators have been unable to demonstrate persistent hypersecretion of parathyroid hormone in patients treated chronically with calcitonin (salmon).

Circulating antibodies to calcitonin after 2-18 months of treatment have been reported in about half of the patients with Paget's disease in whom antibody studies were done, but calcitonin treatment remained effective in many of these cases. Occasionally, patients with high antibody titers are found. These patients usually will have suffered a biochemical relapse of Paget's disease and are unresponsive to the acute hypocalcemic effects of calcitonin.

Hypercalcemia

In clinical trials, calcitonin (salmon) has been shown to lower the elevated serum calcium of patients with carcinoma (with or without demonstrated metastases), multiple myeloma or primary hyperparathyroidism (lesser response). Patients with higher values for serum calcium tend to show greater reduction during calcitonin therapy. The decrease in calcium occurs about 2 hours after the first injection and lasts for about 6-8 hours. Calcitonin (salmon) given every 12 hours maintained a calcium lowering effect for about 5-8 days, the time period evaluated for most patients during the clinical studies. The average reduction of 8 hour post-injection serum calcium during this period was about 9%.

Kidney

Calcitonin increases the excretion of filtered phosphate, calcium, and sodium by decreasing their tubular reabsorption. In some patients, the inhibition of bone resorption by calcitonin is of such magnitude that the consequent reduction of filtered calcium load more than compensates for the decrease in tubular reabsorption of calcium. The result in these patients is a decrease rather than an increase in urinary calcium.

Transient increases in sodium and water excretion may occur after the initial injection of calcitonin. In most patients, these changes return to pretreatment levels with continued therapy.

Gastrointestinal Tract

Increasing evidence indicates that calcitonin has significant actions on the gastrointestinal tract. Short-term administration results in marked transient decreases in the volume and acidity of gastric juice and in the volume and the trypsin and amylase content of pancreatic juice. Whether these effects continue to be elicited after each injection of calcitonin during chronic therapy has not been investigated.

Metabolism

The metabolism of calcitonin (salmon) has not yet been studied clinically. Information from animal studies with calcitonin (salmon) and from clinical studies with calcitonins of porcine and human origin suggest that calcitonin (salmon) is rapidly metabolized by conversion to smaller inactive fragments, primarily in the kidneys, but also in the blood and peripheral tissues. A small amount of unchanged hormone and its inactive metabolites are excreted in the urine.

It appears that calcitonin (salmon) cannot cross the placental barrier and its passage to the cerebrospinal fluid or to breast milk has not been determined.

NASAL SPRAY

Calcitonin acts primarily on bone, but direct renal effects and actions on the gastrointestinal tract are also recognized. calcitonin (salmon) appears to have actions essentially identical to calcitonins of mammalian origin, but its potency per mg is greater and it has a longer duration of action.

The information below, describing the clinical pharmacology of calcitonin, has been derived from studies with *injectable* calcitonin. The mean bioavailability of calcitonin (salmon) nasal spray is approximately 3% of that of injectable calcitonin in normal subjects and, therefore, the conclusions concerning the clinical pharmacology of this preparation may be different.

The actions of calcitonin on bone and its role in normal human bone physiology are still not completely elucidated, although calcitonin receptors have been discovered in osteoclasts and osteoblasts.

Single injections of calcitonin cause a marked transient inhibition of the ongoing bone resorptive process. With prolonged use, there is a persistent, smaller decrease in the rate of bone resorption. Histologically, this is associated with a decreased number of osteoclasts and an apparent decrease in their resorptive activity. *In vitro* studies have shown that calcitonin (salmon) causes inhibition of osteoclast function with loss of the ruffled osteoclast border responsible for resorption of bone. This activity resumes following removal of calcitonin (salmon) from the test system. There is some evidence from the *in vitro* studies that bone formation may be augmented by calcitonin through increased osteoblastic activity.

Animal studies indicate that endogenous calcitonin, primarily through its action on bone, participates with parathyroid hormone in the homeostatic regulation of blood calcium. Thus, high blood calcium levels cause increased secretion of calcitonin which, in turn, inhibits bone resorption. This reduces the transfer of calcium from bone to blood and tends to return blood calcium towards the normal level. The importance of this process in humans has not been determined. In normal adults, who have a relatively low rate of bone resorption, the administration of exogenous calcitonin results in only a slight decrease in serum calcium in the limits of the normal range. In normal children and in patients with Paget's disease in whom bone resorption is more rapid, decreases in serum calcium are more pronounced in response to calcitonin.

Bone biopsy and radial bone mass studies at baseline and after 26 months of daily injectable calcitonin indicate that calcitonin therapy results in formation of normal bone.

Postmenopausal Osteoporosis

Osteoporosis is a disease characterized by low bone mass and architectural deterioration of bone tissue leading to enhanced bone fragility and a consequent increase in fracture risk as patients approach or fall below a bone mineral density associated with increased frequency of fracture. The most common type of osteoporosis occurs in postmenopausal females. Osteoporosis is a result of a disproportionate rate of bone resorption compared to bone formation which disrupts the structural integrity of bone, rendering it more susceptible to fracture. The most common sites of these fractures are the vertebrae, hip, and distal forearm (Colles' fractures). Vertebral fractures occur with the highest frequency and are associated with back pain, spinal deformity and a loss of height.

Calcitonin, given by the intranasal route, has been shown to increase spinal bone mass in postmenopausal women with established osteoporosis but not in early postmenopausal women.

Calcium Homeostasis

In two clinical studies designed to evaluate the pharmacodynamic response to calcitonin (salmon) nasal spray, administration of 100-1600 IU to healthy volunteers resulted in rapid and sustained small decreases (but still within the normal range) in both total serum calcium and serum ionized calcium. Single doses greater than 400 IU did not produce any further biological response to the drug. The development of hypocalcemia has not been reported in studies in healthy volunteers or postmenopausal females.

Kidney

Studies with injectable calcitonin show increases in the excretion of filtered phosphate, calcium, and sodium by decreasing their tubular reabsorption. Comparable studies have not been carried out with calcitonin (salmon) nasal spray.

Gastrointestinal Tract

Some evidence from studies with injectable preparations suggest that calcitonin may have significant actions on the gastrointestinal tract. Short-term administration of injectable calcitonin results in marked transient decreases in the volume and acidity of gastric juice and in the volume and the trypsin and amylase content of pancreatic juice. Whether these effects continue to be elicited after each injection of calcitonin during chronic therapy has not been investigated. These studies have not been conducted with calcitonin (salmon) nasal spray.

Pharmacokinetics and Metabolism

The data on bioavailability of calcitonin (salmon) nasal spray obtained by various investigators using different methods show great variability. Calcitonin (salmon) nasal spray is absorbed rapidly by the nasal mucosa. Peak plasma concentrations of drug appear 31-39 minutes after nasal administration compared to 16-25 minutes following parenteral dosing. In normal volunteers approximately 3% (range 0.3-30.6%) of a nasally administered dose is bioavailable compared to the same dose administered by intramuscular injection. The half-life of elimination of calcitonin-salmon is calculated to be 43 minutes. There is no accumulation of the drug on repeated nasal administration at 10 hour intervals for up to 15 days. Absorption of nasally administered calcitonin has not been studied in postmenopausal women.

INDICATIONS AND USAGE

PAGET'S DISEASE

Calcitonin (salmon) injection, synthetic is indicated for the treatment of symptomatic Paget's disease of bone, for the treatment of hypercalcemia, and for the treatment of postmenopausal osteoporosis.

Injection

At the present time, effectiveness has been demonstrated principally in patients with moderate to severe disease characterized by polyostotic involvement with elevated serum alkaline phosphatase and urinary hydroxyproline excretion.

In these patients, the biochemical abnormalities were substantially improved (more than 30% reduction) in about ⅔ of patients studied, and bone pain was improved in a similar fraction. A small number of documented instances of reversal of neurologic deficits has occurred, including improvement in the basilar compression syndrome, and improvement of spinal cord and spinal nerve lesions. At present, there is too little experience to predict the likelihood of improvement of any given neurologic lesion. Hearing loss, the most common neurologic lesion of Paget's disease, is improved infrequently (4 of 29 patients studied audiometrically).

Patients with increased cardiac output due to extensive Paget's disease have had measured decreases in cardiac output while receiving calcitonin. The number of treated patients in this category is still too small to predict how likely such a result will be.

The large majority of patients with localized, especially monostotic disease do not develop symptoms and most patients with mild symptoms can be managed with analgesics. There is no evidence that the prophylactic use of calcitonin is beneficial in asymptomatic patients, although treatment may be considered in exceptional circumstances in which there is extensive involvement of the skull or spinal cord with the possibility of irreversible neurologic damage. In these instances, treatment would be based on the demonstrated effect of calcitonin on Pagetic bone, rather than on clinical studies in the patient population in question.

HYPERCALCEMIA

Injection

Calcitonin (salmon) injection, synthetic is indicated for early treatment of hypercalcemic emergencies, along with other appropriate agents, when a rapid decrease in serum calcium is required, until more specific treatment of the underlying disease can be accomplished. It may also be added to existing therapeutic regimens for hypercalcemia such as intravenous fluids and furosemide, oral phosphate or corticosteroids, or other agents.

POSTMENOPAUSAL OSTEOPOROSIS

Injection

Calcitonin (salmon) injection, synthetic is indicated for the treatment of postmenopausal osteoporosis in conjunction with adequate calcium and vitamin D intake to prevent the progressive loss of bone mass. No evidence currently exists to indicate whether or not calcitonin (salmon) decreases the risk of vertebral crush fractures or spinal deformity. A recent controlled study, which was discontinued prior to completion because of questions regarding its design and implementation, failed to demonstrate any benefit of salmon calcitonin on fracture rate. No adequate controlled trials have examined the effect of salmon calcitonin injection on vertebral bone mineral density beyond 1 year of treatment. Two placebo-controlled studies with salmon calcitonin have shown an increase in total body calcium at 1 year, followed by a trend to decreasing total body calcium (still above baseline) at 2 years. The minimum effective dose of calcitonin (salmon) for prevention of vertebral bone mineral density loss has not been established. It has been suggested that those postmenopausal patients having increased rates of bone turnover may be more likely to respond to anti-resorptive agents such as calcitonin (salmon).

Nasal Spray

Calcitonin (salmon) nasal spray is indicated for the treatment of postmenopausal osteoporosis in females greater than 5 years postmenopause with low bone mass relative to healthy premenopausal females. Calcitonin (salmon) nasal spray should be reserved for patients who refuse or cannot tolerate estrogens or in whom estrogens are contraindicated. Use of calcitonin (salmon) nasal spray is recommended in conjunction with an adequate calcium (at least 1000 mg elemental calcium per day) and vitamin D (400 IU/day) intake to retard the progressive loss of bone mass. The evidence of efficacy is based on increases in spinal bone mineral density observed in clinical trials.

Two randomized, placebo controlled trials were conducted in 325 postmenopausal females [227 calcitonin (salmon) nasal spray treated and 98 placebo treated] with spinal, forearm or femoral bone mineral density (BMD) at least one standard deviation below normal for healthy premenopausal females. These studies conducted over 2 years demonstrated that 200 IU daily of calcitonin (salmon) nasal spray increases lumbar vertebral BMD relative to baseline and relative to placebo in osteoporotic females who were greater than 5 years postmenopause. Calcitonin (salmon) nasal spray produced statistically significant increases in lumbar vertebral BMD compared to placebo as early as 6 months after initiation of therapy with persistance of this level for up to 2 years of observation.

No effects of calcitonin (salmon) nasal spray on cortical bone of the forearm or hip were demonstrated. However, in one study, BMD of the hip showed a statistically significant increase compared with placebo in a region composed of predominantly trabecular bone after one year of treatment changing to a trend at 2 years that was no longer statistically significant.

CONTRAINDICATIONS

Clinical allergy to (synthetic) calcitonin (salmon).

WARNINGS

ALLERGIC REACTIONS

Injection

Because calcitonin is protein in nature, the possibility of a systemic allergic reaction exists. **Administration of calcitonin (salmon) has been reported in a few cases to cause serious allergic-type reactions (*e.g.*, bronchospasm, swelling of the tongue or throat, and anaphylactic shock), and in one case, death attributed to anaphylaxis.** The usual provisions should be made for the emergency treatment of such a reaction should it occur. Allergic reactions should be differentiated from generalized flushing and hypotension.

Skin testing should be considered prior to treatment with calcitonin, particularly for patients with suspected sensitivity to calcitonin. The following procedure is suggested: Prepare a dilution at 10 IU/ml by withdrawing 1/20 ml (0.05 ml) in a tuberculin syringe and filling it to 1.0 ml with sodium chloride injection. Mix well, discard 0.9 ml and inject intracutaneously 0.1 ml (approximately 1 IU) on the inner aspect of the forearm. Observe the injection site 15 minutes after injection. The appearance of more than mild erythema or wheal constitutes a positive response.

The incidence of osteogenic sarcoma is known to be increased in Paget's disease. Pagetic lesions, with or without therapy, may appear by x-ray to progress markedly, possibly with some loss of definition of periosteal margins. Such lesions should be evaluated carefully to differentiate these from osteogenic sarcoma.

Nasal Spray

Because calcitonin is a polypeptide, the possibility of a systemic allergic reaction exists. In clinical trials with calcitonin (salmon) nasal spray and foreign marketing experience, no serious allergic-type adverse reactions have been reported. However, with injectable calcitonin (salmon) there have been a few reports of serious allergic-type reactions (*e.g.*, bronchospasm, swelling of the tongue or throat, anaphylactic shock, and in one case death attributed to anaphylaxis). The usual provisions should be made for the emergency treatment of such a reaction should it occur. Allergic reactions should be differentiated from generalized flushing and hypotension.

Skin testing should be considered prior to treatment with nasal calcitonin for patients with suspected sensitivity to calcitonin. The following procedure is suggested: Prepare a dilution at 10 IU/ml by withdrawing 1/20 ml (0.05 ml) of injectable calcitonin (salmon) in a tuberculin syringe and filling it to 1.0 ml with sodium chloride injection. Mix well, discard 0.9 ml and inject intracutaneously 0.1 ml (approximately 1 IU) on the inner aspect of the forearm. Observe the injection site 15 minutes after injection. The appearance of more than mild erythema or wheal constitutes a positive response.

PRECAUTIONS

INJECTION

General

The administration of calcitonin possibly could lead to hypocalcemic tetany under special circumstances although no cases have yet been reported. Provisions for parenteral calcium administration should be available during the first several administrations of calcitonin.

Laboratory Tests

Periodic examinations of urine sediment of patients on chronic therapy are recommended.

Coarse granular casts and casts containing renal tubular epithelial cells were reported in young adult volunteers at bed rest who were given calcitonin (salmon) to study the effect of immobilization on osteoporosis. There was no other evidence of renal abnormality and the urine sediment became normal after calcitonin was stopped. Urine sediment abnormalities have not been reported by other investigators.

Information for the Patient

Careful instruction in sterile injection technique should be given to the patient, and to other persons who may administer calcitonin (salmon) injection, synthetic.

Carcinogenesis, Mutagenesis, and Impairment of Fertility

An increased incidence of pituitary adenomas has been observed in 1 year toxicity studies in Sprague-Dawley rats administered calcitonin (salmon) at dosages of 20 and 80 IU/kg/day and in Fisher 344 rats given 80 IU/kg/day. The relevance of these findings to humans is unknown. Calcitonin (salmon) was not mutagenic in tests using *Salmonella typhimurium, Escherichia coli,* and Chinese Hamster V79 cells.

Pregnancy, Teratogenic Effects, Pregnancy Category C

Calcitonin (salmon) has been shown to cause a decrease in fetal birth weights in rabbits when given in doses 14-56 times the dose recommended for human use. Since calcitonin does not cross the placental barrier, this finding may be due to metabolic effects of calcitonin on the pregnant animal. There are no adequate and well-controlled studies in pregnant women. Calcitonin (salmon) injection, synthetic should be used during pregnancy only if the potential benefit justifies the potential risk to the fetus.

Nursing Mothers

It is not known whether this drug is excreted in human milk. As a general rule, nursing should not be undertaken while a patient is on this drug since many drugs are excreted in human milk. Calcitonin has been shown to inhibit lactation in animals.

Pediatric Use

Disorders of bone in children referred to as juvenile Paget's disease have been reported rarely. The relationship of these disorders to adult Paget's disease has not been established and experience with the use of calcitonin in these disorders is very limited. There are no adequate data to support the use of calcitonin (salmon) injection, synthetic in children.

NASAL SPRAY

Periodic Nasal Examinations

Periodic nasal examinations with visualization of the nasal mucosa, turbinates, septum and mucosal blood vessel status are recommended.

The development of mucosal alterations or transient nasal conditions occurred in up to 9% of patients who received calcitonin (salmon) nasal spray and in up to 12% of patients who received placebo nasal spray in studies in postmenopausal females. The majority of patients (approximately 90%) in whom nasal abnormalities were noted also reported nasally related complaints/symptoms as adverse events. Therefore, a nasal examination should be performed prior to start of treatment with nasal calcitonin and at any time nasal complaints occur.

In all postmenopausal patients treated with calcitonin (salmon) nasal spray, the most commonly reported nasal adverse events included rhinitis (12%), epistaxis (3.5%), and sinusitis (2.3%). Smoking was shown not to have any contributory effect on the occurrence of nasal adverse events. One patient (0.3%) treated with calcitonin (salmon) nasal spray who was receiving 400 IU daily developed a small nasal wound. In clinical trials in another disorder (Paget's Disease), 2.8% of patients developed nasal ulcerations.

If severe ulceration of the nasal mucosa occurs, as indicated by ulcers greater than 1.5 mm in diameter or penetrating below the mucosa, or those associated with heavy bleeding, calcitonin (salmon) nasal spray should be discontinued. Although smaller ulcers often heal without withdrawal of calcitonin (salmon) nasal spray, medication should be discontinued temporarily until healing occurs.

Information for the Patient

Careful instructions on pump assembly, priming of the pump and nasal introduction of calcitonin (salmon) nasal spray should be given to the patient. Although instructions for patients are supplied with individual bottles, procedures for use should be demonstrated to each patient. Patients should notify their physician if they develop significant nasal irritation.

Carcinogenesis, Mutagenesis, and Impairment of Fertility

An increased incidence of non-functioning pituitary adenomas has been observed in one-year toxicity studies in Sprague-Dawley and Fischer 344 Rats administered (subcutaneously) calcitonin (salmon) at dosages of 80 IU/kg/day (16-19 times the recommended human parenteral dose and about 130-160 times the human intranasal dose based on body surface area). The findings suggest that calcitonin (salmon) reduced the latency period for development of pituitary adenomas that do not produce hormones, probably through the perturbation of physiologic processes involved in the evolution of this commonly occurring endocrine lesion in the rat. Although administration of calcitonin (salmon) reduces the latency period of the development of non-functional proliferative lesions in rats, it did not induce the hyperplastic/neoplastic process.

Calcitonin (salmon) was tested for mutagenicity using *Salmonella typhimurium* (5 strains) and *Escherichia coli* (2 strains), with and without rat liver metabolic activation, and found to be non-mutagenic. The drug was also not mutagenic in a chromosome aberration test in mammalian V79 cells of the Chinese Hamster *in vitro.*

Laboratory Tests

Urine sediment abnormalities have not been reported in ambulatory volunteers treated with calcitonin (salmon) nasal spray. Coarse granular casts containing renal tubular epithelial cells were reported in young adult volunteers at bed rest who were given injectable calcitonin (salmon) to study the effect of immobilization on osteoporosis. There was no evidence of renal abnormality and the urine sediment became normal after calcitonin was stopped. Periodic examinations of urine sediment should be considered.

Pregnancy, Teratogenic Effects, Pregnancy Category C

Calcitonin (salmon) has been shown to cause a decrease in fetal birth weights in rabbits when given by injection in doses 8-33 times the parenteral dose and 70-278 times the intranasal dose recommended for human use based on body surface area.

Since calcitonin does not cross the placental barrier, this finding may be due to metabolic effects on the pregnant animal. There are no adequate and well controlled studies in pregnant women with calcitonin (salmon). Calcitonin (salmon) nasal spray is *not* indicated for use in pregnancy.

Nursing Mothers

It is not known whether this drug is excreted in human milk. As a general rule, nursing should not be undertaken while a patient is on this drug since many drugs are excreted in human milk. Calcitonin has been shown to inhibit lactation in animals.

Geriatric Use

Clinical trials using calcitonin (salmon) nasal spray have included post-menopausal patients up to 77 years of age. No unusual adverse events or increased incidence of common adverse events have been noted in patients over 65 years of age.

Pediatric Use

There are no data to support the use of calcitonin (salmon) nasal spray in children. Disorders of bone in children referred to as idiopathic juvenile osteoporosis have been reported rarely. The relationship of these disorders to postmenopausal osteoporosis has not been established and experience with the use of calcitonin in these disorders is very limited.

DRUG INTERACTIONS

NASAL SPRAY

Formal studies designed to evaluate drug interactions with calcitonin (salmon) have not been done. No drug interaction studies have been performed with calcitonin (salmon) nasal spray ingredients.

Currently, no drug interactions with calcitonin (salmon) have been observed. The effects of prior use of diphosphonates in postmenopausal osteoporosis patients have not been assessed; however, in patients with Paget's Disease prior diphosphonate use appears to reduce the anti-resorptive response to calcitonin (salmon) nasal spray.

ADVERSE REACTIONS

GASTROINTESTINAL SYSTEM

Injection

Nausea with or without vomiting has been noted in about 10% of patients treated with calcitonin. It is most evident when treatment is first initiated and tends to decrease or disappear with continued administration.

DERMATOLOGIC/HYPERSENSITIVITY

Injection

Local inflammatory reactions at the site of subcutaneous or intramuscular injection have been reported in about 10% of patients. Flushing of face or hands occurred in about 2%-5% of patients. Skin rashes, nocturia, pruritus of the ear lobes, feverish sensation, pain in the eyes, poor appetite, abdominal pain, edema of feet, and salty taste have been reported in patients treated with calcitonin (salmon). Administration of calcitonin (salmon) has been reported in a few cases to cause serious allergic-type reactions (*e.g.,* bronchospasm, swelling of the tongue or throat, and anaphylactic shock), and in one case, death attributed to anaphylaxis (see WARNINGS).

Nasal Spray

The incidence of adverse reactions reported in studies involving postmenopausal osteoporotic patients chronically exposed to calcitonin (salmon) nasal spray (n=341) and to placebo nasal spray (n=131) and reported in greater than 3% of calcitonin (salmon) nasal spray treated patients are presented below in TABLE 1. Most adverse reactions were mild to moderate in severity. Nasal adverse events were most common with 70% mild, 25% moderate, and 5% severe in nature (placebo rates were 71% mild, 27% moderate, and 2% severe).

In addition, the following adverse events were reported in fewer than 3% of patients during chronic therapy with calcitonin (salmon) nasal spray. Adverse events reported in 1-3% of patients are identified with an asterisk (*). The remainder occurred in less than 1% of patients. Other than flushing, nausea, possible allergic reactions, and possible local irritative effects in the respiratory tract, a relationship to calcitonin (salmon) nasal spray has not been established.

Body as a Whole (general disorders): Influenza-like symptoms*, fatigue*, periorbital edema, fever.

Integumentary: Erythematous rash*, skin ulceration, eczema, alopecia, pruritus, increased sweating.

TABLE 1 Adverse Reactions Occurring in at Least 3% of Postmenopausal Patients Treated Chronically

	Calcitonin (Salmon)	
	Nasal Spray	Placebo
Adverse Reaction	n=341	n=131
Rhinitis	12.0%	6.9%
Symptom of nose*	10.6%	16.0%
Back pain	5.0%	2.3%
Arthralgia	3.8%	5.3%
Epistaxis	3.5%	4.6%
Headache	3.2%	4.6%

* Symptom of nose includes: nasal crusts, dryness, redness or erythema, nasal sores, irritation, itching, thick feeling, soreness, pallor, infection, stenosis, runny/blocked, small wound, bleeding wound, tenderness, uncomfortable feeling and sore across bridge of nose.

Musculoskeletal/Collagen: Arthrosis*, myalgia*, arthritis, polymyalgia rheumatica, stiffness.

Respiratory/Special Senses: Sinusitis*, upper respiratory tract infection*, bronchospasm*, pharyngitis, bronchitis, pneumonia, coughing, dyspnea, taste perversion, parosmia.

Cardiovascular: Hypertension*, angina pectoris*, tachycardia, palpitation, bundle branch block, myocardial infarction.

Gastrointestinal: Dyspepsia*, constipation*, abdominal pain*, nausea*, diarrhea*, vomiting, flatulence, increased appetite, gastritis, dry mouth.

Liver/Metabolic: Cholelithiasis, hepatitis, thirst, weight increase.

Endocrine: Goiter, hyperthyroidism.

Urinary System: Cystitis*, pyelonephritis, hematuria, renal calculus.

Central and Peripheral Nervous System: Dizziness*, paresthesia*, vertigo, migraine, neuralgia, agitation.

Hearing/Vestibular: Tinnitus, hearing loss, earache.

Vision: Abnormal lacrimation*, conjunctivitis*, blurred vision, vitreous floater.

Vascular: Flushing, cerebrovascular accident, thrombophlebitis.

Hematologic/Resistance Mechanisms: Lymphadenopathy*, infection*, anemia.

Psychiatric: Depression*, insomnia, anxiety, anorexia.

Common adverse reactions associated with the use of injectable calcitonin (salmon) occurred less frequently in patients treated with calcitonin (salmon) nasal spray than in those patients treated with injectable calcitonin. Nausea, with or without vomiting, which occurred in 1.8% of patients treated with the nasal spray (and 1.5% of those receiving placebo nasal spray) occurs in about 10% of patients who take injectable calcitonin (salmon). Flushing, which occurred in less than 1% of patients treated with the Nasal Spray, occurs in 2-5% of patients treated with injectable calcitonin (salmon). Although the administered dosages of injectable and nasal spray calcitonin (salmon) are comparable (50-100 units daily of injectable versus 200 units daily of nasal spray), the nasal dosage form has a mean bioavailability of about 3% (range 0.3-30.6%) and therefore provides less drug to the systemic circulation, possibly accounting for the decrease in frequency of adverse reactions.

The collective foreign marketing experience with calcitonin (salmon) nasal spray does not show evidence of any notable difference in the incidence profile of reported adverse reactions when compared with that seen in the clinical trials.

DOSAGE AND ADMINISTRATION

PAGET'S DISEASE

Injection

The recommended starting dose of calcitonin (salmon) in Paget's disease is 100 IU (0.5 ml) per day administered subcutaneously (preferred for outpatient self-administration) or intramuscularly. Drug effect should be monitored by periodic measurement of serum alkaline phosphatase and 24 hour urinary hydroxyproline (if available) and evaluations of symptoms. A decrease toward normal of the biochemical abnormalities is usually seen, if it is going to occur, within the first few months. Bone pain may also decrease during that time. Improvement of neurologic lesions, when it occurs, requires a longer period of treatment, often more than 1 year.

In many patients, doses of 50 IU (0.25 ml) per day or every other day are sufficient to maintain biochemical and clinical improvement. At the present time, however, there are insufficient data to determine whether this reduced dose will have the same effect as the higher dose on forming more normal bone structure. It appears preferable, therefore, to maintain the higher dose in any patient with serious deformity or neurological involvement.

In any patient with a good response initially who later relapses, either clinically or biochemically, the possibility of antibody formation should be explored. The patient may be tested for antibodies by an appropriate specialized test or evaluated for the possibility of antibody formation by critical clinical evaluation.

Patient compliance should also be assessed in the event of relapse.

In patients who relapse, whether because of antibodies or for unexplained reasons, a dosage increase beyond 100 IU/day does not usually appear to elicit an improved response.

HYPERCALCEMIA

Injection

The recommended starting dose of calcitonin (salmon) injection, synthetic in hypercalcemia is 4 IU/kg body weight every 12 hours by subcutaneous or intramuscular injection. If the response to this dose is not satisfactory after 1 or 2 days, the dose may be increased to 8 IU/kg every 12 hours. If the response remains unsatisfactory after 2 more days, the dose may be further increased to a maximum of 8 IU/kg every 6 hours.

POSTMENOPAUSAL OSTEOPOROSIS

Injection

The minimum effective dose of salmon calcitonin for the prevention of vertebral bone mineral density loss has not been established. Data from a single 1 year placebo-controlled study with salmon calcitonin injection suggested that 100 IU (subcutaneously or intramuscularly) every other day might be effective in preserving vertebral bone mineral density. Baseline and interval monitoring of biochemical markers of bone resorption/turnover (*e.g.*, fasting AM, second-voided urine hydroxyproline to creatinine ratio) and of bone mineral density may be useful in achieving the minimum effective dose.

The recommended dose of calcitonin is 100 IU/day administered subcutaneously or intramuscularly. Patients should also receive supplemental calcium such as calcium carbonate 1.5 g daily and an adequate vitamin D intake (400 units daily). An adequate diet is also essential.

If the volume of calcitonin (salmon) injection, synthetic to be injected exceeds 2 ml, intramuscular injection is preferable and multiple sites of injection should be used.

Parenteral drug products should be inspected visually for particulate matter and discoloration prior to administration whenever solution and container permit.

Nasal Spray

The recommended dose of calcitonin (salmon) nasal spray in postmenopausal osteoporotic females is 200 IU/day administered intranasally, alternating nostrils daily.

Drug effect may be monitored by periodic measurements of lumbar vertebral bone mass to document stabilization of bone loss or increases in bone density. Effects of calcitonin (salmon) nasal spray on biochemical markers of bone turnover have not been consistently demonstrated in studies in postmenopausal osteoporosis. Therefore, these parameters should not be solely utilized to determine clinical response to calcitonin (salmon) nasal spray therapy in these patients.

Activation of Pump

Before the first dose, it is necessary to activate the pump. The bottle should be held upright and the 2 white side arms depressed toward the bottle 6 times until a faint spray is emitted. The pump is activated once this first faint spray has been emitted. At this point, the nozzle should be placed firmly into the nostril with the head in the upright position, and the pump depressed toward the bottle. It is not necessary to reactivate the pump before each daily dose.

HOW SUPPLIED

NASAL SPRAY

Available as a metered dose solution in 2 ml fill glass bottles. It is available in a dosage strength of 200 IU per activation (0.09 ml/puff). A screw-on pump is provided. This pump, following activation, will deliver 0.09 ml of solution. Miacalcin Nasal Spray contains 2200 IU/ml calcitonin (salmon). Store unopened in refrigerator between 36-46°F (2-8°C). Protect from freezing.

Once the pump has been activated, the bottle may be maintained at room temperature until the medication has been finished, which is a period of 2 weeks.

INJECTION

Store in Refrigerator: Between 2-8°C (36-46°F).

PRODUCT LISTING - RATED THERAPEUTICALLY EQUIVALENT

Solution - Injectable - 200 IU/ml

2 ml	$42.11	MIACALCIN, Novartis Pharmaceuticals	00078-0149-23

PRODUCT LISTING - EQUIVALENTS NOT AVAILABLE

Solution - Injectable - 200 IU/ml

2 ml	$31.35	GENERIC, Arcola Laboratories	00070-4492-01

Spray - Nasal - 200 IU/Inh

4 ml	$78.16	MIACALCIN NASAL, Novartis Pharmaceuticals	00078-0311-90

Calcium Acetate *(003004)*

Categories: Hyperphosphatemia; Pregnancy Category C; FDA Approved 1990 Dec; Orphan Drugs
Drug Classes: Vitamins/minerals
Brand Names: Calcate; **Phoslo**
Foreign Brand Availability: Calcetat-GRY (Germany); Nephracet 600 (Germany); Phosex (England); Phosphosorb (Germany); Phostrol (Korea); Renacet (Germany); Royen (Dominican-Republic; El-Salvador; Guatemala; Panama)

DESCRIPTION

PHOSLO GELCAPS

Each opaque gelcap with a blue cap and white body is spin printed in blue and white ink with "Phoslo" printed on the cap and "667 mg" printed on the body. Each gelcap contains 667 mg calcium acetate (anhydrous; $Ca(CH_3COO)_2$; MW = 158.17 g) equal to 169 mg (8.45 mEq) calcium, and 10 mg of the inert binder, polyethylene glycol 8000. The gelatin cap and body have the following inactive ingredients: FD&C blue no. 1, D&C red no. 28, titanium dioxide and gelatin.

PHOSLO TABLETS

Each white round tablet (stamped "BRA200") contains 667 mg of calcium acetate (anhydrous; $Ca(CH_3COO)_2$; MW = 158.17 g) equal to 169 mg (8.45 mEq) calcium, and 10 mg of the inert binder, polyethylene glycol 8000.

Calcium acetate is administered orally for the control of hyperphosphatemia in end stage renal failure.

CLINICAL PHARMACOLOGY

Patients with advanced renal insufficiency (creatinine clearance less than 30 ml/min) exhibit phosphate retention and some degree of hyperphosphatemia. The retention of phosphate plays a pivotal role in causing secondary hyperparathyroidism associated with osteodystrophy, and soft-tissue calcification. The mechanism by which phosphate retention leads to hyperparathyroidism is not clearly delineated. Therapeutic efforts directed toward the control of hyperphosphatemia include reduction in the dietary intake of phosphate, inhibition of absorption of phosphate in the intestine with phosphate binders, and removal of phosphate from the body by more efficient methods of dialysis. The rate of removal of phosphate by dietary manipulation or by dialysis is insufficient. Dialysis patients absorb 40-80% of dietary phosphorus. Therefore, the fraction of dietary phosphate absorbed from the diet needs to be reduced by using phosphate binders in most renal failure patients on maintenance dialysis. Calcium acetate when taken with meals, combines with dietary phosphate to form insoluble calcium phosphate which is excreted in the feces. Maintenance of serum phosphorus below 6.0 mg/dl is generally considered as a clinically acceptable outcome of treatment with phosphate binders. Calcium acetate is highly soluble at neutral pH, making the calcium readily available for binding to phosphate in the proximal small intestine.

Orally administered calcium acetate from pharmaceutical dosage forms has been demonstrated to be systemically absorbed up to approximately 40% under fasting conditions and up to approximately 30% under nonfasting conditions. This range represents data from both healthy subjects and renal dialysis patients under various conditions.

INDICATIONS AND USAGE

Calcium acetate is indicated for the control of hyperphosphatemia in end stage renal failure and does not promote aluminum absorption.

CONTRAINDICATIONS

Patients with hypercalcemia.

WARNINGS

Patients with end stage renal failure may develop hypercalcemia when given calcium with meals. No other calcium supplements should be given concurrently with calcium acetate.

Progressive hypercalcemia due to overdose of calcium acetate may be severe as to require emergency measures. Chronic hypercalcemia may lead to vascular calcification, and other soft-tissue calcification. The serum calcium level should be monitored twice weekly during the early dose adjustment period. **The serum calcium times phosphate (CaXP) product should not be allowed to exceed 66.** Radiographic evaluation of suspect anatomical region may be helpful in early detection of soft-tissue calcification.

PRECAUTIONS

GENERAL

Excessive dosage of calcium acetate induces hypercalcemia; therefore, early in the treatment during dosage adjustment serum calcium should be determined twice weekly. Should hypercalcemia develop, the dosage should be reduced or the treatment discontinued immediately depending on the severity of hypercalcemia. Calcium acetate should not be given to patients on digitalis, because hypercalcemia may precipitate cardiac arrhythmias. Calcium acetate therapy should always be started at low dose and should not be increased without careful monitoring of serum calcium. An estimate of daily dietary calcium intake should be made initially and the intake adjusted as needed. Serum phosphorus should also be determined periodically.

INFORMATION FOR THE PATIENT

The patient should be informed about compliance with dosage instructions, adherence to instructions about diet and avoidance of the use of nonprescription antacids. Patients should be informed about the symptoms of hypercalcemia (see ADVERSE REACTIONS).

CARCINOGENESIS, MUTAGENESIS, AND IMPAIRMENT OF FERTILITY

Long-term animal studies have not been performed to evaluate the carcinogenic potential, mutagenicity, or effect on fertility of calcium acetate.

PREGNANCY, TERATOGENIC EFFECTS, PREGNANCY CATEGORY C

Animal reproduction studies have not been conducted with calcium acetate. It is not known whether calcium acetate can cause fetal harm when administered to a pregnant woman or can affect reproduction capacity. Calcium acetate should be given to a pregnant woman only if clearly needed.

PEDIATRIC USE

Safety and effectiveness in pediatric patients have not been established.

GERIATRIC USE

Of the total number of subjects in clinical studies of calcium acetate (n=91), 25% were 65 and over, while 7% were 75 and over. No overall differences in safety or effectiveness were observed between these subjects and younger subjects, and other reported clinical experience has not identified differences in responses between the elderly and younger patients, but greater sensitivity of some older individuals cannot be ruled out.

DRUG INTERACTIONS

Calcium acetate may decrease the bioavailability of tetracyclines.

ADVERSE REACTIONS

In clinical studies, patients have occasionally experienced nausea during calcium acetate therapy. Hypercalcemia may occur during treatment with calcium acetate. Mild hypercalcemia (Ca> 10.5 mg/dl) may be asymptomatic or manifest itself as constipation, anorexia, nausea and vomiting. More severe hypercalcemia (Ca> 12 mg/dl) is associated with confusion, delirium, stupor and coma. Mild hypercalcemia is easily controlled by reducing the calcium acetate dose or temporarily discontinuing therapy. Severe hypercalcemia can be treated by acute hemodialysis and discontinuing calcium acetate therapy. Decreasing dialysate calcium concentration could reduce the incidence and severity of calcium acetate induced hypercalcemia. The long-term effect of calcium acetate on the progression of vascular or soft-tissue calcification has not been determined.

Isolated cases of pruritus have been reported which may represent allergic reactions.

DOSAGE AND ADMINISTRATION

GELCAPS

The recommended initial dose of calcium acetate gelcaps for the adult dialysis patient is 2 gelcaps with each meal. The dosage may be increased gradually to bring the serum phosphate value below 6 mg/dl, as long as hypercalcemia does not develop. Most patients require 3-4 gelcaps with each meal.

TABLETS

The recommended initial dose of calcium acetate tablets for the adult dialysis patient is 2 tablets with each meal. The dosage may be increased gradually to bring the serum phosphate value below 6 mg/dl, as long as hypercalcemia does not develop. Most patients require 3-4 tablets with each meal.

HOW SUPPLIED

PHOSLO GELCAP

White and blue gelcap for oral administration containing 667 mg calcium acetate equal to 169 mg (8.45 mEq) calcium.

Storage: Store at 25°C (77°F); excursions permitted to 15-30°C (59-86°F).

PHOSLO TABLET

White round tablet contains 667 mg of calcium acetate equal to 169 mg (8.45 mEq) calcium, and 10 mg of the inert binder, polyethylene glycol 8000.

Storage: Store at controlled room temperature, 15-30°C.

PRODUCT LISTING - RATED THERAPEUTICALLY EQUIVALENT

Solution - Injectable - 0.5 Meq/ml

10 ml x 25	$22.56	GENERIC, Abbott Pharmaceutical	00074-2553-01
50 ml x 25	$59.97	GENERIC, Abbott Pharmaceutical	00074-2553-02
100 ml x 25	$137.16	GENERIC, Abbott Pharmaceutical	00074-2553-03

Calcium Carbonate *(000593)*

Categories: Gastric hyperacidity; Hyperphosphatemia; Hypertension, pregnancy; Hypocalcemia; Hypoparathyroidism; Osteoporosis; FDA Pre 1938 Drugs

Drug Classes: Vitamins/minerals

Brand Names: Oyster Shell Calcium

Foreign Brand Availability: Apo-Cal (Malaysia); Cal-Sup (Australia); Calcanate (Thailand); Calcefor (Peru); Calci Aid (Philippines); Calcilos (Germany); Calcit (Belgium; France; Italy; Netherlands); Calcitridin (Germany); Calcium (Bulgaria); Calcium Carbonate (France); Calcium Dago (Germany); Calcium Klopfer (Austria); Calcium-Sandoz Forte (Bulgaria); Calcuren (Finland); Caldoral (Colombia); Calsan (Mexico; Philippines); Caltrate (Australia; Bahamas; Bahrain; Barbados; Belize; Bermuda; Colombia; Curacao; Cyprus; Egypt; Guyana; Iran; Iraq; Israel; Jamaica; Jordan; Kuwait; Lebanon; Libya; Malaysia; Mexico; Netherland-Antilles; New-Zealand; Oman; Qatar; Republic-of-Yemen; Saudi-Arabia; South-Africa; Surinam; Syria; Trinidad; United-Arab-Emirates); Caltrate 600 (Canada; Colombia; Costa-Rica; Dominican-Republic; Ecuador; El-Salvador; Guatemala; Honduras; Nicaragua; Panama; Peru); Cantacid (Korea); CC-Nefro 500 (Germany); Chooz Antacid Gum 500 (Bahrain; Cyprus; Egypt; Iran; Iraq; Jordan; Kuwait; Lebanon; Libya; Oman; Qatar; Republic-of-Yemen; Saudi-Arabia; Syria; United-Arab-Emirates); Netra (Israel); Orocal (France); Os-Cal (Canada); Ospur Ca 500 (Germany); Osteocal 500 (France); Osteomin (Mexico); Renacal (Germany); Sandocal (India); Tums (Israel)

CLINICAL PHARMACOLOGY

Neutralizes gastric acidity.

Caution needed for maintenance of nervous, muscular, skeletal, enzyme reactions, normal cardiac contractility, coagulation of blood.

Effects secretory activity of endocrine and exocrine glands.

PHARMACOKINETICS

30% absorbed depending on demand.
Absorption Vitamin D dependent.

INDICATIONS AND USAGE

Calcium carbonate is indicated:

- Hyperphosphatemia
- Hypertension in pregnancy
- Osteoporosis
- Prevention and treatment of hypocalcemia
- Hyperacidity (antacid)
- Hypoparathyroidism

NON-FDA APPROVED INDICATIONS

Calcium carbonate has been used without FDA approval as a phosphate binder for patients with end-stage renal disease.

CONTRAINDICATIONS

Hypercalcemia, hypercalciuria, hyperparathyroidism, bone tumors, digitalis toxicity, ventricular fibrillation, renal calculi, sarcoidosis.

PRECAUTIONS

Elderly, fluid restriction, decreased GI motility, GI obstruction, dehydration.

LABORATORY TEST INTERACTIONS

False Increase: Chloride, green color, benzodiazepine (false positive).
False Decrease: Magnesium, oxylate, lipase.

PREGNANCY

Pregnancy Category C.

NURSING MOTHERS

Calcium carbonate may be excreted in breast milk. Concentrations would not be sufficient to produce an adverse effect in neonates.

C

DRUG INTERACTIONS

Calcium channel blockers: Calcium administration may inhibit calcium channel blocker activity.

Digoxin, digitoxin: Elevated calcium concentrations associated with acute digitalis toxicity.

Doxycycline, tetracycline: Co-therapy with a tetracycline and calcium carbonate can reduce the serum concentrations and efficacy of tetracyclines.

Iron: Some calcium antacids reduce the GI absorption of iron; inhibition of the hematological response to iron has been reported.

Itraconazole, ketoconazole: Antacids containing calcium may reduce antifungal concentrations.

Quinidine: Calcium antacids capable of increasing urine pH may increase serum quinidine concentrations.

Quinolones: Reduced bioavailability of quinolone antibiotics.

Sodium polystyrene sulfonate resin: Combined use with calcium-containing antacid may result in systemic alkalosis.

Thiazides: Large doses of calcium with thiazides may lead to milk-alkali syndrome.

ADVERSE REACTIONS

Cardiovascular: Bradycardia, cardiac arrest, dysrhythmias, heart block, hemorrhage, hypotension, rebound hypertension, shortened QT interval.

Gastrointestinal: Anorexia, constipation, diarrhea, eructation, flatulence, nausea, obstruction, rebound hyperacidity, vomiting.

Genitourinary: Renal dysfunction, renal failure, renal stones.

Metabolic: Hypercalcemia (drowsiness, lethargy, muscle weakness, headache, constipation, coma, anorexia, nausea, vomiting, polyuria, thirst); metabolic alkalosis; milk-alkali syndrome (nausea, vomiting, disorientation, headache).

DOSAGE AND ADMINISTRATION

ADULTS

Hyperphosphatemia: 1-17 g per day in divided doses.

Hypocalcemia (replenish electrolytes): 1.25 g (500 mg Ca^{++}) 4-6 tablets per day, chewed with water.

Antacid: 500 mg to 1 g (250-500 mg Ca^{++}) 1-3 hour after meals and at bedtime as needed.

Hypertension in pregnancy: 500 mg tid during third trimester.

Osteoporosis: 1200 mg per day.

PRODUCT LISTING - EQUIVALENTS NOT AVAILABLE

Tablet, Chewable - Oral - 600 mg

85's	$5.75	MAALOX QUICK DISSOLVE, Novartis Consumer Health	00067-0370-85

Candesartan Cilexetil *(003414)*

For related information, see the comparative table section in Appendix A.

Categories: Hypertension, essential; FDA Approved 1998 Jun; Pregnancy Category C, 1st Trimester; Pregnancy Category D, 2nd & 3rd Trimesters

Drug Classes: Angiotensin II receptor antagonists

Foreign Brand Availability: Amias (England; Ireland); Atacand (Australia; Bahamas; Barbados; Belize; Bermuda; Canada; Colombia; Curacao; France; Germany; Guyana; Israel; Jamaica; Mexico; Netherland-Antilles; New-Zealand; Puerto-Rico; Singapore; South-Africa; Surinam; Sweden; Trinidad); Blopress (Bahrain; Colombia; Cyprus; Egypt; Germany; Hong-Kong; Indonesia; Iran; Iraq; Japan; Jordan; Kuwait; Lebanon; Libya; Mexico; Oman; Philippines; Qatar; Republic-of-Yemen; Saudi-Arabia; Syria; Thailand; United-Arab-Emirates); Candesar (India); Kenzen (France)

Cost of Therapy: $43.41 (Hypertension; Atacand; 16 mg; 1 tablet/day; 30 day supply)

WARNING

Use in Pregnancy

When used in pregnancy during the second and third trimesters, drugs that act directly on the renin-angiotensin system can cause injury and even death to the developing fetus. When pregnancy is detected, candesartan cilexetil should be discontinued as soon as possible. (See WARNINGS, Fetal/Neonatal Morbidity and Mortality.)

DESCRIPTION

Candesartan cilexetil, a prodrug, is hydrolyzed to candesartan during absorption from the gastrointestinal tract. Candesartan is a selective AT_1 subtype angiotensin II receptor antagonist.

Candesartan cilexetil, a nonpeptide, is chemically described as (±)-1-[[(cyclohexyloxy)carbonyl]oxy]ethyl 2-ethoxy-1-[[2′-(1H-tetrazol-5-yl)[1,1′-biphenyl]-4-yl]methyl]-1H-benzimidazole-7-carboxylate.

Its empirical formula is $C_{33}H_{34}N_6O_6$.

Candesartan cilexetil is a white to off-white powder with a molecular weight of 610.67. It is practically insoluble in water and sparingly soluble in methanol. Candesartan cilexetil is a racemic mixture containing one chiral center at the cyclohexyloxycarbonyloxy ethyl ester group. Following oral administration, candesartan cilexetil undergoes hydrolysis at the ester link to form the active drug, candesartan, which is achiral.

Atacand is available for oral use as tablets containing either 4, 8, 16, or 32 mg of candesartan cilexetil and the following inactive ingredients: hydroxypropyl cellulose, polyethylene glycol, lactose, corn starch, carboxymethylcellulose calcium, and magnesium stearate. Ferric oxide (reddish brown) is added to the 8, 16, and 32 mg tablets as a colorant.

CLINICAL PHARMACOLOGY

MECHANISM OF ACTION

Angiotensin II is formed from angiotensin I in a reaction catalyzed by angiotensin-converting enzyme (ACE, kininase II). Angiotensin II is the principal pressor agent of the renin-angiotensin system, with effects that include vasoconstriction, stimulation of synthesis and release of aldosterone, cardiac stimulation, and renal reabsorption of sodium. Candesartan blocks the vasoconstrictor and aldosterone-secreting effects of angiotensin II by selectively blocking the binding of angiotensin II to the AT_1 receptor in many tissues, such as vascular smooth muscle and the adrenal gland. Its action is, therefore, independent of the pathways for angiotensin II synthesis.

There is also an AT_2 receptor found in many tissues, but AT_2 is not known to be associated with cardiovascular homeostasis. Candesartan has much greater affinity (>10,000-fold) for the AT_1 receptor than for the AT_2 receptor.

Blockade of the renin-angiotensin system with ACE inhibitors, which inhibit the biosynthesis of angiotensin II from angiotensin I, is widely used in the treatment of hypertension. ACE inhibitors also inhibit the degradation of bradykinin, a reaction also catalyzed by ACE. Because candesartan does not inhibit ACE (kininase II), it does not affect the response to bradykinin. Whether this difference has clinical relevance is not yet known. Candesartan does not bind to or block other hormone receptors or ion channels known to be important in cardiovascular regulation.

Blockade of the angiotensin II receptor inhibits the negative regulatory feedback of angiotensin II on renin secretion, but the resulting increased plasma renin activity and angiotensin II circulating levels do not overcome the effect of candesartan on blood pressure.

PHARMACOKINETICS

General

Candesartan cilexetil is rapidly and completely bioactivated by ester hydrolysis during absorption from the gastrointestinal tract to candesartan, a selective AT_1 subtype angiotensin II receptor antagonist. Candesartan is mainly excreted unchanged in urine and feces (via bile). It undergoes minor hepatic metabolism by O-deethylation to an inactive metabolite. The elimination half-life of candesartan is approximately 9 hours. After single and repeated administration, the pharmacokinetics of candesartan are linear for oral doses up to 32 mg of candesartan cilexetil. Candesartan and its inactive metabolite do not accumulate in serum upon repeated once-daily dosing.

Following administration of candesartan cilexetil, the absolute bioavailability of candesartan was estimated to be 15%. After tablet ingestion, the peak serum concentration (C_{max}) is reached after 3-4 hours. Food with a high fat content does not affect the bioavailability of candesartan after candesartan cilexetil administration.

Metabolism and Excretion

Total plasma clearance of candesartan is 0.37 ml/min/kg, with a renal clearance of 0.19 ml/min/kg. When candesartan is administered orally, about 26% of the dose is excreted unchanged in urine. Following an oral dose of ^{14}C-labeled candesartan cilexetil, approximately 33% of radioactivity is recovered in urine and approximately 67% in feces. Following an intravenous dose of ^{14}C-labeled candesartan, approximately 59% of radioactivity is recovered in urine and approximately 36% in feces. Biliary excretion contributes to the elimination of candesartan.

Distribution

The volume of distribution of candesartan is 0.13 L/kg. Candesartan is highly bound to plasma proteins (>99%) and does not penetrate red blood cells. The protein binding is constant at candesartan plasma concentrations well above the range achieved with recommended doses. In rats, it has been demonstrated that candesartan crosses the blood-brain barrier poorly, if at all. It has also been demonstrated in rats that candesartan passes across the placental barrier and is distributed in the fetus.

Special Populations

Pediatric

The pharmacokinetics of candesartan cilexetil have not been investigated in patients <18 years of age.

Geriatric and Gender

The pharmacokinetics of candesartan have been studied in the elderly (≥65 years) and in both sexes. The plasma concentration of candesartan was higher in the elderly (C_{max} was approximately 50% higher, and AUC was approximately 80% higher) compared to younger subjects administered the same dose. The pharmacokinetics of candesartan were linear in the elderly, and candesartan and its inactive metabolite did not accumulate in the serum of these subjects upon repeated, once-daily administration. No initial dosage adjustment is necessary. (See DOSAGE AND ADMINISTRATION.) There is no difference in the pharmacokinetics of candesartan between male and female subjects.

Renal Insufficiency

In hypertensive patients with renal insufficiency, serum concentrations of candesartan were elevated. After repeated dosing, the AUC and C_{max} were approximately doubled in patients with severe renal impairment (creatinine clearance <30 ml/min/1.73 m^2) compared to patients with normal kidney function. The pharmacokinetics of candesartan in hypertensive patients undergoing hemodialysis are similar to those in hypertensive patients with severe renal impairment. Candesartan cannot be removed by hemodialysis. No initial dosage adjustment is necessary in patients with renal insufficiency. (See DOSAGE AND ADMINISTRATION.)

Hepatic Insufficiency

The pharmacokinetics of candesartan were compared in patients with mild and moderate hepatic impairment to matched healthy volunteers following a single oral dose of 16 mg candesartan cilexetil. The increase in AUC for candesartan was 30% in patients with mild hepatic impairment (Child-Pugh A) and 145% in patients with moderate hepatic impairment (Child-Pugh B). The increase in C_{max} for candesartan was 56% in patients with mild hepatic impairment and 73% in patients with moderate hepatic impairment. The pharmacokinetics after candesartan cilexetil administration have not been investigated in patients with severe hepatic impairment. No initial dosage adjustment is necessary in patients with mild hepatic impairment. In patients with moderate hepatic impairment, consideration should be given to initiation of candesartan cilexetil at a lower dose. (See DOSAGE AND ADMINISTRATION.)

DRUG INTERACTIONS

See DRUG INTERACTIONS.

PHARMACODYNAMICS

Candesartan inhibits the pressor effects of angiotensin II infusion in a dose-dependent manner. After 1 week of once-daily dosing with 8 mg of candesartan cilexetil, the pressor effect was inhibited by approximately 90% at peak with approximately 50% inhibition persisting for 24 hours.

Plasma concentrations of angiotensin I and angiotensin II, and plasma renin activity (PRA), increased in a dose-dependent manner after single and repeated administration of candesartan cilexetil to healthy subjects and hypertensive patients. ACE activity was not altered in healthy subjects after repeated candesartan cilexetil administration. The once-daily administration of up to 16 mg of candesartan cilexetil to healthy subjects did not influence plasma aldosterone concentrations, but a decrease in the plasma concentration of aldosterone was observed when 32 mg of candesartan cilexetil was administered to hypertensive patients. In spite of the effect of candesartan cilexetil on aldosterone secretion, very little effect on serum potassium was observed.

In multiple-dose studies with hypertensive patients, there were no clinically significant changes in metabolic function, including serum levels of total cholesterol, triglycerides, glucose, or uric acid. In a 12 week study of 161 patients with non-insulin-dependent (Type 2) diabetes mellitus and hypertension, there was no change in the level of HbA_{1c}.

INDICATIONS AND USAGE

Candesartan cilexetil is indicated for the treatment of hypertension. It may be used alone or in combination with other antihypertensive agents.

CONTRAINDICATIONS

Candesartan cilexetil is contraindicated in patients who are hypersensitive to any component of this product.

WARNINGS

FETAL/NEONATAL MORBIDITY AND MORTALITY

Drugs that act directly on the renin-angiotensin system can cause fetal and neonatal morbidity and death when administered to pregnant women. Several dozen cases have been reported in the world literature in patients who were taking angiotensin-converting enzyme inhibitors. When pregnancy is detected, candesartan cilexetil should be discontinued as soon as possible.

The use of drugs that act directly on the renin-angiotensin system during the second and third trimesters of pregnancy has been associated with fetal and neonatal injury, including hypotension, neonatal skull hypoplasia, anuria, reversible or irreversible renal failure, and death. Oligohydramnios has also been reported, presumably resulting from decreased fetal renal function; oligohydramnios in this setting has been associated with fetal limb contractures, craniofacial deformation, and hypoplastic lung development. Prematurity, intrauterine growth retardation, and patent ductus arteriosus have also been reported, although it is not clear whether these occurrences were due to exposure to the drug.

These adverse effects do not appear to have resulted from intrauterine drug exposure that has been limited to the first trimester. Mothers whose embryos and fetuses are exposed to an angiotensin II receptor antagonist only during the first trimester should be so informed. Nonetheless, when patients become pregnant, physicians should have the patient discontinue the use of candesartan cilexetil as soon as possible.

Rarely (probably less often than once in every thousand pregnancies), no alternative to a drug acting on the renin-angiotensin system will be found. In these rare cases, the mothers should be apprised of the potential hazards to their fetuses, and serial ultrasound examinations should be performed to assess the intra-amniotic environment.

If oligohydramnios is observed, candesartan cilexetil should be discontinued unless it is considered life saving for the mother. Contraction stress testing (CST), a nonstress test (NST), or biophysical profiling (BPP) may be appropriate, depending upon the week of pregnancy. Patients and physicians should be aware, however, that oligohydramnios may not appear until after the fetus has sustained irreversible injury.

Infants with histories of *in utero* exposure to an angiotensin II receptor antagonist should be closely observed for hypotension, oliguria, and hyperkalemia. If oliguria occurs, attention should be directed toward support of blood pressure and renal perfusion. Exchange transfusion or dialysis may be required as means of reversing hypotension and/or substituting for disordered renal function.

There is no clinical experience with the use of candesartan cilexetil in pregnant women. Oral doses ≥10 mg candesartan cilexetil/kg/day administered to pregnant rats during late gestation and continued through lactation were associated with reduced survival and an increased incidence of hydronephrosis in the offspring. The 10 mg/kg/day dose in rats is approximately 2.8 times the maximum recommended daily human dose (MRHD) of 32 mg on a mg/m^2 basis (comparison assumes human body weight of 50 kg). Candesartan cilexetil given to pregnant rabbits at an oral dose of 3 mg/kg/day (approximately 1.7 times the MRHD on a mg/m^2 basis) caused maternal toxicity (decreased body weight and death) but, in surviving dams, had no adverse effects on fetal survival, fetal weight, or external, visceral, or skeletal development. No maternal toxicity or adverse effects on fetal development were observed when oral doses up to 1000 mg candesartan cilexetil/kg/day (approximately 138 times the MRHD on a mg/m^2 basis) were administered to pregnant mice.

HYPOTENSION IN VOLUME- AND SALT-DEPLETED PATIENTS

In patients with an activated renin-angiotensin system, such as volume- and/or salt-depleted patients (*e.g.*, those being treated with diuretics), symptomatic hypotension may occur. These conditions should be corrected prior to administration of candesartan cilexetil, or the treatment should start under close medical supervision. (See DOSAGE AND ADMINISTRATION.)

If hypotension occurs, the patients should be placed in the supine position and, if necessary, given an intravenous infusion of normal saline. A transient hypotensive response is not a contraindication to further treatment which usually can be continued without difficulty once the blood pressure has stabilized.

PRECAUTIONS

GENERAL

Impaired Hepatic Function

Based on pharmacokinetic data which demonstrate significant increases in candesartan AUC and C_{max} in patients with moderate hepatic impairment, a lower initiating dose should be considered for patients with moderate hepatic impairment. (See DOSAGE AND ADMINISTRATION and CLINICAL PHARMACOLOGY, Special Populations.)

Impaired Renal Function

As a consequence of inhibiting the renin-angiotensin-aldosterone system, changes in renal function may be anticipated in susceptible individuals treated with candesartan cilexetil. In patients whose renal function may depend upon the activity of the renin-angiotensin-aldosterone system (*e.g.*, patients with severe congestive heart failure), treatment with angiotensin-converting enzyme inhibitors and angiotensin receptor antagonists has been associated with oliguria and/or progressive azotemia and (rarely) with acute renal failure and/or death. Similar results may be anticipated in patients treated with candesartan cilexetil. (See CLINICAL PHARMACOLOGY, Special Populations.)

In studies of ACE inhibitors in patients with unilateral or bilateral renal artery stenosis, increases in serum creatinine or blood urea nitrogen (BUN) have been reported. There has been no long-term use of candesartan cilexetil in patients with unilateral or bilateral renal artery stenosis, but similar results may be expected.

INFORMATION FOR THE PATIENT

Pregnancy

Female patients of childbearing age should be told about the consequences of second- and third-trimester exposure to drugs that act on the renin-angiotensin system, and they should also be told that these consequences do not appear to have resulted from intrauterine drug exposure that has been limited to the first trimester. These patients should be asked to report pregnancies to their physicians as soon as possible.

CARCINOGENESIS, MUTAGENESIS, AND IMPAIRMENT OF FERTILITY

There was no evidence of carcinogenicity when candesartan cilexetil was orally administered to mice and rats for up to 104 weeks at doses up to 100 and 1000 mg/kg/day, respectively. Rats received the drug by gavage, whereas mice received the drug by dietary administration. These (maximally-tolerated) doses of candesartan cilexetil provided systemic exposures to candesartan (AUCs) that were, in mice, approximately 7 times and, in rats, more than 70 times the exposure in man at the maximum recommended daily human dose (32 mg).

Candesartan and its O-deethyl metabolite tested positive for genotoxicity in the *in vitro* Chinese hamster lung (CHL) chromosomal aberration assay. Neither compound tested positive in the Ames microbial mutagenesis assay or the *in vitro* mouse lymphoma cell assay. Candesartan (but not its O-deethyl metabolite) was also evaluated *in vivo*in the mouse micronucleus test and *in vitro* in the Chinese hamster ovary (CHO) gene mutation assay, in both cases with negative results. Candesartan cilexetil was evaluated in the Ames test, the *in vitro* mouse lymphoma cell and rat hepatocyte unscheduled DNA synthesis assays and the *in vivo* mouse micronucleus test, in each case with negative results. Candesartan cilexetil was not evaluated in the CHL chromosomal aberration or CHO gene mutation assay.

Fertility and reproductive performance were not affected in studies with male and female rats given oral doses of up to 300 mg/kg/day (83 times the maximum daily human dose of 32 mg on a body surface area basis).

PREGNANCY CATEGORIES C (FIRST TRIMESTER) AND D (SECOND AND THIRD TRIMESTERS)

See WARNINGS, Fetal/Neonatal Morbidity and Mortality.

NURSING MOTHERS

It is not known whether candesartan is excreted in human milk, but candesartan has been shown to be present in rat milk. Because of the potential for adverse effects on the nursing infant, a decision should be made whether to discontinue nursing or discontinue the drug, taking into account the importance of the drug to the mother.

PEDIATRIC USE

Safety and effectiveness in pediatric patients have not been established.

GERIATRIC USE

Of the total number of subjects in clinical studies of candesartan cilexetil, 21% (683/3260) were 65 and over, while 3% (87/3260) were 75 and over. No overall differences in safety or effectiveness were observed between these subjects and younger subjects, and other reported clinical experience has not identified differences in responses between the elderly and younger patients, but greater sensitivity of some older individuals cannot be ruled out. In a placebo-controlled trial of about 200 elderly hypertensive patients (ages 65-87 years), administration of candesartan cilexetil was well tolerated and lowered blood pressure by about 12/6 mm Hg more than placebo.

DRUG INTERACTIONS

No significant drug interactions have been reported in studies of candesartan cilexetil given with other drugs such as glyburide, nifedipine, digoxin, warfarin, hydrochlorothiazide, and oral contraceptives in healthy volunteers. Because candesartan is not significantly metabolized by the cytochrome P450 system and at therapeutic concentrations has no effects on

C

P450 enzymes, interactions with drugs that inhibit or are metabolized by those enzymes would not be expected.

ADVERSE REACTIONS

Candesartan cilexetil has been evaluated for safety in more than 3600 patients/subjects, including more than 3200 patients treated for hypertension. About 600 of these patients were studied for at least 6 months and about 200 for at least 1 year. In general, treatment with candesartan cilexetil was well tolerated. The overall incidence of adverse events reported with candesartan cilexetil was similar to placebo.

The rate of withdrawals due to adverse events in all trials in patients (7510 total) was 3.3% (*i.e.,* 108 of 3260) of patients treated with candesartan cilexetil as monotherapy and 3.5% (*i.e.,* 39 of 1106) of patients treated with placebo. In placebo-controlled trials, discontinuation of therapy due to clinical adverse events occurred in 2.4% (*i.e.,* 57 of 2350) of patients treated with candesartan cilexetil and 3.4% (*i.e.,* 35 of 1027) of patients treated with placebo.

The most common reasons for discontinuation of therapy with candesartan cilexetil were headache (0.6%) and dizziness (0.3%).

The adverse events that occurred in placebo-controlled clinical trials in at least 1% of patients treated with candesartan cilexetil and at a higher incidence in candesartan cilexetil (n=2350) than placebo (n=1027) patients included back pain (3% vs 2%), dizziness (4% vs 3%), upper respiratory tract infection (6% vs 4%), pharyngitis (2% vs 1%), and rhinitis (2% vs 1%).

The following adverse events occurred in placebo-controlled clinical trials at a more than 1% rate but at about the same or greater incidence in patients receiving placebo compared to candesartan cilexetil: Fatigue, peripheral edema, chest pain, headache, bronchitis, coughing, sinusitis, nausea, abdominal pain, diarrhea, vomiting, arthralgia, albuminuria.

Other potentially important adverse events that have been reported, whether or not attributed to treatment, with an incidence of 0.5% or greater from the 3260 patients worldwide treated in clinical trials with candesartan cilexetil are listed below. It cannot be determined whether these events were causally related to candesartan cilexetil.

Body as a Whole: Asthenia, fever.

Central and Peripheral Nervous System: Paraesthesia, vertigo.

Gastrointestinal System Disorder: Dyspepsia, gastroenteritis.

Heart Rate and Rhythm Disorders: Tachycardia, palpitation.

Metabolic and Nutritional Disorders: Creatine phosphokinase increased, hyperglycemia, hypertriglyceridemia, hyperuricemia.

Musculoskeletal System Disorders: Myalgia.

Platelet/Bleeding-Clotting Disorders: Epistaxis.

Psychiatric Disorders: Anxiety, depression, somnolence.

Respiratory System Disorders: Dyspnea.

Skin and Appendages Disorders: Rash, sweating increased.

Urinary System Disorders: Hematuria.

Other reported events seen less frequently included angina pectoris, myocardial infarction, and angioedema.

Adverse events occurred at about the same rates in men and women, older and younger patients, and black and nonblack patients.

POST-MARKETING EXPERIENCE

The following have been very rarely reported in post-marketing experience:

Digestive: Abnormal hepatic function and hepatitis.

Hematologic: Neutropenia, leukopenia, and agranulocytosis.

Skin and Appendages Disorders: Pruritus and urticaria.

LABORATORY TEST FINDINGS

In controlled clinical trials, clinically important changes in standard laboratory parameters were rarely associated with the administration of candesartan cilexetil.

Creatinine, Blood Urea Nitrogen: Minor increases in blood urea nitrogen (BUN) and serum creatinine were observed infrequently.

Hyperuricemia: Hyperuricemia was rarely found (19 or 0.6% of 3260 patients treated with candesartan cilexetil and 5 or 0.5% of 1106 patients treated with placebo).

Hemoglobin and Hematocrit: Small decreases in hemoglobin and hematocrit (mean decreases of approximately 0.2 g/dl and 0.5 volume percent, respectively) were observed in patients treated with candesartan cilexetil alone but were rarely of clinical importance. Anemia, leukopenia, and thrombocytopenia were associated with withdrawal of 1 patient each from clinical trials.

Potassium: A small increase (mean increase of 0.1 mEq/L) was observed in patients treated with candesartan cilexetil alone but was rarely of clinical importance. One patient from a congestive heart failure trial was withdrawn for hyperkalemia (serum potassium = 7.5 mEq/L). This patient was also receiving spironolactone.

Liver Function Tests: Elevations of liver enzymes and/or serum bilirubin were observed infrequently. Five patients assigned to candesartan cilexetil in clinical trials were withdrawn because of abnormal liver chemistries. All had elevated transaminases. Two had mildly elevated total bilirubin, but 1 of these patients was diagnosed with Hepatitis A.

DOSAGE AND ADMINISTRATION

Dosage must be individualized. Blood pressure response is dose related over the range of 2-32 mg. The usual recommended starting dose of candesartan cilexetil is 16 mg once daily when it is used as monotherapy in patients who are not volume depleted. Candesartan cilexetil can be administered once or twice daily with total daily doses ranging from 8-32 mg. Larger doses do not appear to have a greater effect, and there is relatively little experience with such doses. Most of the antihypertensive effect is present within 2 weeks, and maximal blood pressure reduction is generally obtained within 4-6 weeks of treatment with candesartan cilexetil.

No initial dosage adjustment is necessary for elderly patients, for patients with mildly impaired renal function, or for patients with mildly impaired hepatic function (see CLINICAL PHARMACOLOGY, Special Populations). In patients with moderate hepatic impairment, consideration should be given to initiation of candesartan cilexetil at a lower dose (see CLINICAL PHARMACOLOGY, Special Populations). For patients with possible depletion of intravascular volume (*e.g.,* patients treated with diuretics, particularly those with impaired renal function), candesartan cilexetil should be initiated under close medical supervision and consideration should be given to administration of a lower dose (see WARNINGS, Hypotension in Volume- and Salt-Depleted Patients).

Candesartan cilexetil may be administered with or without food.

If blood pressure is not controlled by candesartan cilexetil alone, a diuretic may be added. Candesartan cilexetil may be administered with other antihypertensive agents.

HOW SUPPLIED

Atacand tablets are available in:

4 mg: White to off-white, circular/biconvex-shaped, non-film-coated tablets, coded "ACF" on one side and "004" on the other.

8 mg: Light pink, circular/biconvex-shaped, non-film-coated tablets, coded "ACG" on one side and "008" on the other.

16 mg: Pink, circular/biconvex-shaped, non-film-coated tablets, coded "ACH" on one side and "016" on the other.

32 mg: Pink, circular/biconvex-shaped, non-film-coated tablets, coded "ACL" on one side and "032" on the other.

Storage: Store at 25°C (77°F); excursions permitted to 15-30°C (59-86°F). Keep container tightly closed.

PRODUCT LISTING - EQUIVALENTS NOT AVAILABLE

Tablet - Oral - 4 mg			
30's	$43.40	ATACAND, Astra-Zeneca Pharmaceuticals	00186-0004-31
Tablet - Oral - 8 mg			
30's	$37.26	ATACAND, Allscripts Pharmaceutical Company	54569-4719-00
30's	$43.40	ATACAND, Astra-Zeneca Pharmaceuticals	00186-0008-31
60's	$74.52	ATACAND, Allscripts Pharmaceutical Company	54569-4719-01
Tablet - Oral - 16 mg			
30's	$38.75	ATACAND, Allscripts Pharmaceutical Company	54569-4714-00
30's	$43.40	ATACAND, Astra-Zeneca Pharmaceuticals	00186-0016-31
90's	$130.23	ATACAND, Astra-Zeneca Pharmaceuticals	00186-0016-54
100's	$134.21	ATACAND, Astra-Zeneca Pharmaceuticals	00186-0016-28
Tablet - Oral - 32 mg			
30's	$58.71	ATACAND, Astra-Zeneca Pharmaceuticals	00186-0032-31
90's	$176.15	ATACAND, Astra-Zeneca Pharmaceuticals	00186-0032-54
100's	$168.00	ATACAND, Astra-Zeneca Pharmaceuticals	00186-0032-28

Candesartan Cilexetil; Hydrochlorothiazide *(003511)*

For complete prescribing information, refer to the CD-ROM included with the book.

Categories: Hypertension, essential; FDA Approved 2000 Sep; Pregnancy Category C
Drug Classes: Angiotensin II receptor antagonists; Diuretics, thiazide and derivatives
Brand Names: Atacand HCT
Foreign Brand Availability: Atacand Plus (Australia; Colombia; Israel; Singapore); Blopress (Germany); Blopress Plus (Thailand); Cokenzen (France); Hytacand (France)
Cost of Therapy: $58.72 (Hypertension; Atacand HCT; 16 mg; 12.5 mg; 1 tablet/day; 30 day supply)

WARNING

Note: The trade names have been used throughout this monograph for clarity.

USE IN PREGNANCY

When used in pregnancy during the second and third trimesters, drugs that act directly on the renin-angiotensin system can cause injury and even death to the developing fetus. When pregnancy is detected, Atacand HCT should be discontinued as soon as possible. See WARNINGS, Fetal/Neonatal Morbidity and Mortality.

DESCRIPTION

Atacand HCT (candesartan cilexetil; hydrochlorothiazide) combines an angiotensin II receptor (type AT_1) antagonist and a diuretic, hydrochlorothiazide.

Candesartan cilexetil, a nonpeptide, is chemically described as (±)-1-[[(cyclohexyloxy)carbonyl]oxy]ethyl 2-ethoxy-1-[[2′-(1H-tetrazol-5-yl)[1,1′-biphenyl]-4-yl]methyl]-1H-benzimidazole-7-carboxylate. Its empirical formula is $C_{33}H_{34}N_6O_6$.

Candesartan cilexetil is a white to off-white powder with a molecular weight of 610.67. It is practically insoluble in water and sparingly soluble in methanol. Candesartan cilexetil is a racemic mixture containing one chiral center at the cyclohexyloxycarbonyloxy ethyl ester group. Following oral administration, candesartan cilexetil undergoes hydrolysis at the ester link to form the active drug, candesartan, which is achiral.

Hydrochlorothiazide is 6-chloro-3,4-dihydro-*2H*-1,2,4-benzothiadiazine-7-sulfonamide 1,1-dioxide. Its empirical formula is $C_7H_8ClN_3O_4S_2$.

Hydrochlorothiazide is a white, or practically white, crystalline powder with a molecular weight of 297.72, which is slightly soluble in water, but freely soluble in sodium hydroxide solution.

Atacand HCT is available for oral administration in two tablet strengths of candesartan cilexetil and hydrochlorothiazide.

Atacand HCT 16-12.5 contains 16 mg of candesartan cilexetil and 12.5 mg of hydrochlorothiazide. Atacand HCT 32-12.5 contains 32 mg of candesartan cilexetil and 12.5 mg of hydrochlorothiazide. The inactive ingredients of the tablets are calcium carboxymethylcellulose, hydroxypropyl cellulose, lactose monohydrate, magnesium stearate, corn starch, polyethylene glycol 8000, and ferric oxide (yellow). Ferric oxide (reddish brown) is also added to the 16-12.5 mg tablet as colorant.

INDICATIONS AND USAGE

Atacand HCT is indicated for the treatment of hypertension. This fixed dose combination is not indicated for initial therapy (see DOSAGE AND ADMINISTRATION).

CONTRAINDICATIONS

Atacand HCT is contraindicated in patients who are hypersensitive to any component of this product.

Because of the hydrochlorothiazide component, this product is contraindicated in patients with anuria or hypersensitivity to other sulfonamide-derived drugs.

WARNINGS

FETAL/NEONATAL MORBIDITY AND MORTALITY

Drugs that act directly on the renin-angiotensin system can cause fetal and neonatal morbidity and death when administered to pregnant women. Several dozen cases have been reported in the world literature in patients who were taking angiotensin-converting enzyme inhibitors. When pregnancy is detected, Atacand HCT should be discontinued as soon as possible.

The use of drugs that act directly on the renin-angiotensin system during the second and third trimesters of pregnancy has been associated with fetal and neonatal injury, including hypotension, neonatal skull hypoplasia, anuria, reversible or irreversible renal failure, and death. Oligohydramnios has also been reported, presumably resulting from decreased fetal renal function; oligohydramnios in this setting has been associated with fetal limb contractures, craniofacial deformation, and hypoplastic lung development. Prematurity, intrauterine growth retardation, and patent ductus arteriosus have also been reported, although it is not clear whether these occurences were due to exposure to the drug.

These adverse effects do not appear to have resulted from intrauterine drug exposure that has been limited to the first trimester. Mothers whose embryos and fetuses are exposed to an angiotensin II receptor antagonist only during the first trimester should be so informed. Nonetheless, when patients become pregnant, physicians should have the patient discontinue the use of Atacand HCT as soon as possible.

Rarely (probably less often than once in every thousand pregnancies), no alternative to a drug acting on the renin-angiotensin system will be found. In these rare cases, the mothers should be apprised of the potential hazards to their fetuses, and serial ultrasound examinations should be performed to assess the intra-amniotic environment.

If oligohydramnios is observed, Atacand HCT should be discontinued unless it is considered life saving for the mother. Contraction stress testing (CST), a nonstress test (NST), or biophysical profiling (BPP) may be appropriate, depending upon the week of pregnancy. Patients and physicians should be aware, however, that oligohydramnios may not appear until after the fetus has sustained irreversible injury.

Infants with histories of *in utero* exposure to an angiotensin II receptor antagonist should be closely observed for hypotension, oliguria, and hyperkalemia. If oliguria occurs, attention should be directed toward support of blood pressure and renal perfusion. Exchange transfusion or dialysis may be required as means of reversing hypotension and/or substituting for disordered renal funtion.

Candesartan Cilexetil; Hydrochlorothiazide

There was no evidence of teratogenicity or other adverse effects on embryo-fetal development when pregnant mice, rats or rabbits were treated orally with candesartan cilexetil alone or in combination with hydrochlorothiazide. For mice, the maximum dose of candesartan cilexetil was 1000 mg/kg/day (about 150 times the maximum recommended daily human dose [MRHD]*). For rats, the maximum dose of candesartan cilexetil was 100 mg/kg/day (about 31 times the MRHD*). For rabbits, the maximum dose of candesartan cilexetil was 1 mg/kg/day (a maternally toxic dose that is about half the MRHD*). In each of these studies, hydrochlorothiazide was tested at the same dose level (10 mg/kg/day, about 4, 8, and 15 times the MRHD* in mouse, rats, and rabbit, respectively). There was no evidence of harm to the rat or mouse fetus or embryo in studies in which hydrochlorothiazide was administered alone to the pregnant rat or mouse at doses of up to 1000 and 3000 mg/kg/day, respectively.

Thiazides cross the placental barrier and appear in cord blood. There is a risk of fetal or neonatal jaundice, thrombocytopenia, and possibly other adverse reactions that have occurred in adults.

* Doses compared on the basis of body surface area. MRHD considered to be 32 mg for candesartan cilexetil and 12.5 mg for hydrochlorothiazide.

HYPOTENSION IN VOLUME- AND SALT-DEPLETED PATIENTS

Based on adverse events reported from all clinical trials of Atacand HCT, excessive reduction of blood pressure was rarely seen in patients with uncomplicated hypertension treated with candesartan cilexetil and hydrochlorothiazide (0.4%). Initiation of antihypertensive therapy may cause symptomatic hypotension in patients with intravascular volume- or sodium-depletion, *e.g.,* in patients treated vigorously with diuretics or in patients on dialysis. These conditions should be corrected prior to administration of Atacand HCT, or the treatment should start under close medical supervision (see DOSAGE AND ADMINISTRATION).

If hypotension occurs, the patients should be placed in the supine position and, if necessary, given an intravenous infusion of normal saline. A transient hypotensive response is not a contraindication to further treatment which usually can be continued without difficulty once the blood pressure has stabilized.

HYDROCHLOROTHIAZIDE

Impaired Hepatic Function

Thiazide diuretics should be used with caution in patients with impaired hepatic function or progressive liver disease, since minor alterations of fluid and electrolyte balance may precipitate hepatic coma.

Hypersensitivity Reaction

Hypersensitivity reactions to hydrochlorothiazide may occur in patients with or without a history of allergy or bronchial asthma, but are more likely in patients with such a history.

Systemic Lupus Erythematosus

Thiazide diuretics have been reported to cause exacerbation or activation of systemic lupus erythematosus.

Lithium Interaction

Lithium generally should not be given with thiazides.

DOSAGE AND ADMINISTRATION

The usual recommended starting dose of candesartan cilexetil is 16 mg once daily when it is used as monotherapy in patients who are not volume depleted. Atacand can be administered once or twice daily with total daily doses ranging from 8 to 32 mg. Patients requiring further reduction in blood pressure should be titrated to 32 mg. Doses larger than 32 mg do not appear to have a greater blood pressure lowering effect.

Hydrochlorothiazide is effective in doses of 12.5 to 50 mg once daily.

To minimize dose-independent side effects, it is usually appropriate to begin combination therapy only after a patient has failed to achieve the desired effect with monotherapy.

The side effects (see WARNINGS) of candesartan cilexetil are generally rare and apparently independent of dose; those of hydrochlorothiazide are a mixture of dose-dependent phenomena (primarily hypokalemia) and dose-independent phenomena (*e.g.,* pancreatitis), the former much more common than the latter.

Therapy with any combination of candesartan cilexetil and hydrochlorothiazide will be associated with both sets of dose-independent side effects.

REPLACEMENT THERAPY

The combination may be substituted for the titrated components.

DOSE TITRATION BY CLINICAL EFFECT

A patient whose blood pressure is not controlled on 25 mg of hydrochlorothiazide once daily can expect an incremental effect from Atacand HCT 16-12.5 mg. A patient whose blood pressure is controlled on 25 mg of hydrochlorothiazide but is experiencing decreases in serum potassium can expect the same or incremental blood pressure effects from Atacand HCT 16-12.5 mg and serum potassium may improve.

A patient whose blood pressure is not controlled on 32 mg of Atacand can expect incremental blood pressure effects from Atacand HCT 32-12.5 mg and then 32-25 mg. The maximal antihypertensive effect of any dose of Atacand HCT can be expected within 4 weeks of initiating that dose.

PATIENTS WITH RENAL IMPAIRMENT

The usual regimens of therapy with Atacand HCT may be followed as long as the patient's creatinine clearance is >30 ml/min. In patients with more severe renal impairment, loop diuretics are preferred to thiazides, so Atacand HCT is not recommended.

PATIENTS WITH HEPATIC IMPAIRMENT

Thiazide diuretics should be used with caution in patients with hepatic impairment; therefore, care should be exercised with dosing of Atacand HCT.

Atacand HCT may be administered with other antihypertensive agents.

Atacand HCT may be administered with or without food.

PRODUCT LISTING - EQUIVALENTS NOT AVAILABLE

Tablet - Oral - 16 mg;12.5 mg

90's	$157.25	ATACAND HCT, Astra-Zeneca Pharmaceuticals	00182-0162-54
90's	$176.15	ATACAND HCT, Merck & Company Inc	00186-0162-54
100's	$195.71	ATACAND HCT, Merck & Company Inc	00186-0162-28

Tablet - Oral - 32 mg;12.5 mg

90's	$160.39	ATACAND HCT, Astra-Zeneca Pharmaceuticals	00182-0322-54
90's	$179.66	ATACAND HCT, Merck & Company Inc	00186-0322-54
100's	$199.63	ATACAND HCT, Merck & Company Inc	00186-0322-28

Capecitabine *(003397)*

Categories: Carcinoma, breast; Carcinoma, colorectal; FDA Approved 1998 Apr; Pregnancy Category D
Drug Classes: Antineoplastics, antimetabolites
Brand Names: Xeloda
Cost of Therapy: $2970.69 (Breast Cancer; Xeloda; 500 mg; 8 tablets/day; 30 day supply)

WARNING

Capecitabine Warfarin Interaction

Patients receiving concomitant capecitabine and oral coumarin-derivative anticoagulant therapy should have their anticoagulant response (INR or prothrombin time) monitored frequently in order to adjust the anticoagulant dose accordingly. A clinically important capecitabine-warfarin drug interaction was demonstrated in a clinical pharmacology trial (see CLINICAL PHARMACOLOGY and PRECAUTIONS). Altered coagulation parameters and/or bleeding, including death, have been reported in patients taking

WARNING — Cont'd

capecitabine concomitantly with coumarin-derivative anticoagulants such as warfarin and phenprocoumon. Postmarketing reports have shown clinically significant increases in prothrombin time (PT) and INR in patients who were stabilized on anticoagulants at the time capecitabine was introduced. These events occurred within several days and up to several months after initiating capecitabine therapy and, in a few cases, within 1 month after stopping capecitabine. These events occurred in patients with and without liver metastases. Age greater than 60 and a diagnosis of cancer independently predispose patients to an increased risk of coagulopathy.

DESCRIPTION

Capecitabine is a fluoropyrimidine carbamate with antineoplastic activity. It is an orally administered systemic prodrug of 5′-deoxy-5-fluorouridine (5′-DFUR) which is converted to 5-fluorouracil.

The chemical name for capecitabine is 5′-deoxy-5-fluoro-N-[(pentyloxy) carbonyl]-cytidine and has a molecular weight of 359.35.

Capecitabine is a white to off-white crystalline powder with an aqueous solubility of 26 mg/ml at 20°C.

Xeloda is supplied as biconvex, oblong film-coated tablets for oral administration. Each light peach-colored tablet contains 150 mg capecitabine and each peach-colored tablet contains 500 mg capecitabine. *The inactive ingredients in Xeloda include:* Anhydrous lactose, croscarmellose sodium, hydroxypropyl methylcellulose, microcrystalline cellulose, magnesium stearate and purified water. The peach or light peach film coating contains hydroxypropyl methylcellulose, talc, titanium dioxide, and synthetic yellow and red iron oxides.

CLINICAL PHARMACOLOGY

Capecitabine is relatively non-cytotoxic *in vitro*. This drug is enzymatically converted to 5-fluorouracil (5-FU) *in vivo*.

BIOACTIVATION

Capecitabine is readily absorbed from the gastrointestinal tract. In the liver, a 60 kDa carboxylesterase hydrolyzes much of the compound to 5′-deoxy-5-fluorocytidine (5′-DFCR). Cytidine deaminase, an enzyme found in most tissues, including tumors, subsequently converts 5′-DFCR to 5′-deoxy-5-fluorouridine (5′-DFUR). The enzyme, thymidine phosphorylase (dThdPase), then hydrolyzes 5′-DFUR to the active drug 5-FU. Many tissues throughout the body express thymidine phosphorylase. Some human carcinomas express this enzyme in higher concentrations than surrounding normal tissues.

MECHANISM OF ACTION

Both normal and tumor cells metabolize 5-FU to 5-fluoro-2′-deoxyuridine monophosphate (FdUMP) and 5-fluorouridine triphosphate (FUTP). These metabolites cause cell injury by two different mechanisms. First, FdUMP and the folate cofactor, N5-10-methylenetetrahydrofolate, bind to thymidylate synthase (TS) to form a covalently bound ternary complex. This binding inhibits the formation of thymidylate from 2′-deoxyuridylate. Thymidylate is the necessary precursor of thymidine triphosphate, which is essential for the synthesis of DNA, so that a deficiency of this compound can inhibit cell division. Second, nuclear transcriptional enzymes can mistakenly incorporate FUTP in place of uridine triphosphate (UTP) during the synthesis of RNA. This metabolic error can interfere with RNA processing and protein synthesis.

PHARMACOKINETICS IN COLORECTAL TUMORS AND ADJACENT HEALTHY TISSUE

Following oral administration of capecitabine 7 days before surgery in patients with colorectal cancer, the median ratio of 5-FU concentration in colorectal tumors to adjacent tissues was 2.9 (range from 0.9-8.0). These ratios have not been evaluated in breast cancer patients or compared to 5-FU infusion.

HUMAN PHARMACOKINETICS

The pharmacokinetics of capecitabine and its metabolites have been evaluated in about 200 cancer patients over a dosage range of 500-3500 mg/m²/day. Over this range, the pharmacokinetics of capecitabine and its metabolite, 5′-DFCR were dose proportional and did not change over time. The increases in the AUCs of 5′-DFUR and 5-FU, however, were greater than proportional to the increase in dose and the AUC of 5-FU was 34% higher on day 14 than on day 1. The elimination half-life of both parent capecitabine and 5-FU was about 3/4 of an hour. The inter-patient variability in the C_{max} and AUC of 5-FU was greater than 85%.

Absorption, Distribution, Metabolism and Excretion

Capecitabine reached peak blood levels in about 1.5 hours (T_{max}) with peak 5-FU levels occurring slightly later, at 2 hours. Food reduced both the rate and extent of absorption of capecitabine with mean C_{max} and AUC(0-∞) decreased by 60% and 35%, respectively. The C_{max} and AUC(0-∞) of 5-FU were also reduced by food by 43% and 21%, respectively. Food delayed T_{max} of both parent and 5-FU by 1.5 hours (see PRECAUTIONS and DOSAGE AND ADMINISTRATION).

Plasma protein binding of capecitabine and its metabolites is less than 60% and is not concentration-dependent. Capecitabine was primarily bound to human albumin (approximately 35%).

Capecitabine is extensively metabolized enzymatically to 5-FU. The enzyme dihydropyrimidine dehydrogenase hydrogenates 5-FU, the product of capecitabine metabolism, to the much less toxic 5-fluoro-5, 6-dihydro-fluorouracil (FUH2). Dihydropyrimidinase cleaves the pyrimidine ring to yield 5-fluoro-ureido-propionic acid (FUPA). Finally, β-ureido-propionase cleaves FUPA to α-fluoro-β-alanine (FBAL) which is cleared in the urine.

Capecitabine and its metabolites are predominantly excreted in urine; 95.5% of administered capecitabine dose is recovered in urine. Fecal excretion is minimal (2.6%). The major metabolite excreted in urine is FBAL which represents 57% of the administered dose. About 3% of the administered dose is excreted in urine as unchanged drug.

A clinical Phase 1 study evaluating the effect of capecitabine on the pharmacokinetics of docetaxel and the effect of docetaxel on the pharmacokinetics of capecitabine was conducted in 26 patients with solid tumors. Capecitabine was found to have no effect on the pharmacokinetics of docetaxel (C_{max} and AUC) and docetaxel has no effect on the pharmacokinetics of capecitabine and the 5-FU precursor 5′-DFUR.

SPECIAL POPULATIONS

A population analysis of pooled data from the two large controlled studies in patients with colorectal cancer (n=505) who were administered capecitabine at 1250 mg/m² twice a day indicated that gender (202 females and 303 males) and race (455 white/Caucasian patients, 22 black patients, and 28 patients of other race) have no influence on the pharmacokinetics of 5′-DFUR, 5-FU and FBAL. Age has no significant influence on the pharmacokinetics of 5′-DFUR and 5-FU over the range of 27-86 years. A 20% increase in age results in a 15% increase in AUC of FBAL (see WARNINGS and DOSAGE AND ADMINISTRATION).

Hepatic Insufficiency

Capecitabine has been evaluated in 13 patients with mild to moderate hepatic dysfunction due to liver metastases defined by a composite score including bilirubin, AST/ALT and alkaline phosphatase following a single 1255 mg/m² dose of capecitabine. Both AUC(0-∞) and C_{max} of capecitabine increased by 60% in patients with hepatic dysfunction compared to patients with normal hepatic function (n=14). The AUC(0-∞) and C_{max} of 5-FU was not affected. In patients with mild to moderate hepatic dysfunction due to liver metastases, caution should be exercised when capecitabine is administered. The effect of severe hepatic dysfunction on capecitabine is not known (see PRECAUTIONS and DOSAGE AND ADMINISTRATION).

Renal Insufficiency

Following oral administration of 1250 mg/m² capecitabine twice a day to cancer patients with varying degrees of renal impairment, patients with moderate (creatinine clearance = 30-50 ml/min) and severe (creatinine clearance <30 ml/min) renal impairment showed 85% and 258% higher systemic exposure to FBAL on day 1 compared to normal renal function patients (creatinine clearance >80 ml/min). Systemic exposure to 5′-DFUR was 42% and 71% greater in moderately and severely renal impaired patients, respectively, than in normal patients. Systemic exposure to capecitabine was about 25% greater in both moderately and severely renal impaired patients (see CONTRAINDICATIONS, WARNINGS, and DOSAGE AND ADMINISTRATION).

DRUG-DRUG INTERACTIONS

Anticoagulants: In 4 patients with cancer, chronic administration of capecitabine (1250 mg/m² bid) with a single 20 mg dose of warfarin increased the mean AUC of S-warfarin by 57% and decreased its clearance by 37%. Baseline corrected AUC of INR in these 4 patients increased by 2.8-fold, and the maximum observed mean INR value was increased by 91% (see BOXED WARNING and DRUG INTERACTIONS).

Drugs Metabolized by Cytochrome P450 Enzymes: *In vitro* enzymatic studies with human liver microsomes indicated that capecitabine and its metabolites (5′-DFUR, 5′-DFCR, 5-FU, and FBAL) had no inhibitory effects on substrates of cytochrome P450 for the major isoenzymes such as 1A2, 2A6, 3A4, 2C9, 2C19, 2D6, and 2E1.

Antacid: When Maalox (20 ml), an aluminum hydroxide- and magnesium hydroxide-containing antacid, was administered immediately after capecitabine (1250 mg/m², n=12 cancer patients), AUC and C_{max} increased by 16% and 35%, respectively, for capecitabine and by 18% and 22%, respectively, for 5′-DFCR. No effect was observed on the other three major metabolites (5′-DFUR, 5-FU, FBAL) of capecitabine.

Capecitabine has a low potential for pharmacokinetic interactions related to plasma protein binding.

INDICATIONS AND USAGE

COLORECTAL CANCER

Capecitabine is indicated as first-line treatment of patients with metastatic colorectal carcinoma when treatment with fluoropyrimidine therapy alone is preferred. Combination chemotherapy has shown a survival benefit compared to 5-FU/LV alone. A survival benefit over 5-FU/LV has not been demonstrated with capecitabine monotherapy. Use of capecitabine instead of 5-FU/LV in combinations has not been adequately studied to assure safety or preservation of the survival advantage.

BREAST CANCER COMBINATION THERAPY

Capecitabine in combination with docetaxel is indicated for the treatment of patients with metastatic breast cancer after failure of prior anthracycline-containing chemotherapy.

BREAST CANCER MONOTHERAPY

Capecitabine monotherapy is also indicated for the treatment of patients with metastatic breast cancer resistant to both paclitaxel and an anthracycline-containing chemotherapy regimen or resistant to paclitaxel and for whom further anthracycline therapy is not indicated, *e.g.*, patients who have received cumulative doses of 400 mg/m² of doxorubicin or doxorubicin equivalents. Resistance is defined as progressive disease while on treatment, with or without an initial response, or relapse within 6 months of completing treatment with an anthracycline-containing adjuvant regimen.

NON-FDA APPROVED INDICATIONS

Capecitabine has been reported to have high activity in preclinical xenograft models of breast, colorectal, gastric, and cervical cancers. However, these uses have not been approved by the FDA.

CONTRAINDICATIONS

Capecitabine is contraindicated in patients who have a known hypersensitivity to 5-fluorouracil. Capecitabine is also contraindicated in patients with severe renal impairment (creatinine clearance below 30 ml/min [Cockroft and Gault]) (see CLINICAL PHARMACOLOGY, Special Populations).

WARNINGS

RENAL INSUFFICIENCY

Patients with moderate renal impairment at baseline require dose reduction (see DOSAGE AND ADMINISTRATION). Patients with mild and moderate renal impairment at baseline should be carefully monitored for adverse events. Prompt interruption of therapy with subsequent dose adjustments is recommended if a patient develops a Grade 2-4 adverse event as outlined in TABLE 13.

COAGULOPATHY

See BOXED WARNING.

DIARRHEA

Capecitabine can induce diarrhea, sometimes severe. Patients with severe diarrhea should be carefully monitored and given fluid and electrolyte replacement if they become dehydrated. In the overall clinical trial safety database of capecitabine monotherapy (n=875), the median time to first occurrence of Grade 2-4 diarrhea was 34 days (range from 1-369 days). The median duration of Grade 3-4 diarrhea was 5 days. National Cancer Institute of Canada (NCIC) Grade 2 diarrhea is defined as an increase of 4-6 stools/day or nocturnal stools, Grade 3 diarrhea as an increase of 7-9 stools/day or incontinence and malabsorption, and Grade 4 diarrhea as an increase of >10 stools/day or grossly bloody diarrhea or the need for parenteral support. If Grade 2, 3 or 4 diarrhea occurs, administration of capecitabine should be immediately interrupted until the diarrhea resolves or decreases in intensity to Grade 1. Following a reoccurrence of Grade 2 diarrhea or occurrence of any Grade 3 or 4 diarrhea, subsequent doses of capecitabine should be decreased (see DOSAGE AND ADMINISTRATION). Standard antidiarrheal treatments (*e.g.,* loperamide) are recommended.

Necrotizing enterocolitis (typhlitis) has been reported.

GERIATRIC PATIENTS

Patients >80 years old may experience a greater incidence of Grade 3 or 4 adverse events (see PRECAUTIONS, Geriatric Use). In the overall clinical trial safety database of capecitabine monotherapy (n=875), 62% of the 21 patients >80 years of age treated with capecitabine experienced a treatment-related Grade 3 or 4 adverse event: diarrhea in 6 (28.6%), nausea in 3 (14.3%), hand-and-foot syndrome in 3 (14.3%), and vomiting in 2 (9.5%) patients. Among the 10 patients 70 years of age and greater (no patients were >80 years of age) treated with capecitabine in combination with docetaxel, 30% (3 out of 10) of patients experienced Grade 3 or 4 diarrhea and stomatitis, and 40% (4 out of 10) experienced Grade 3 hand-and-foot syndrome.

Among the 67 patients >60 years of age receiving capecitabine in combination with docetaxel, the incidence of Grade 3 or 4 treatment-related adverse events, treatment-related serious adverse events, withdrawals due to adverse events, treatment discontinuations due to adverse events and treatment discontinuations within the first two treatment cycles was higher than in the <60 years of age patient group.

PREGNANCY

Capecitabine may cause fetal harm when given to a pregnant woman. Capecitabine at doses of 198 mg/kg/day during organogenesis caused malformations and embryo death in mice. In separate pharmacokinetic studies, this dose in mice produced 5′-DFUR AUC values about 0.2 times the corresponding values in patients administered the recommended daily dose. Malformations in mice included cleft palate, anophthalmia, microphthalmia, oligodactyly, polydactyly, syndactyly, kinky tail and dilation of cerebral ventricles. At doses of 90 mg/kg/day, capecitabine given to pregnant monkeys during organogenesis caused fetal death. This dose produced 5′-DFUR AUC values about 0.6 times the corresponding values in patients administered the recommended daily dose. There are no adequate and well-controlled studies in pregnant women using capecitabine. If the drug is used during pregnancy, or if the patient becomes pregnant while receiving this drug, the patient should be apprised of the potential hazard to the fetus. Women of childbearing potential should be advised to avoid becoming pregnant while receiving treatment with capecitabine.

PRECAUTIONS

GENERAL

Patients receiving therapy with capecitabine should be monitored by a physician experienced in the use of cancer chemotherapeutic agents. Most adverse events are reversible and do not need to result in discontinuation, although doses may need to be withheld or reduced (see DOSAGE AND ADMINISTRATION).

Combination With Other Drugs

Use of capecitabine in combination with irinotecan has not been adequately studied.

Hand-and-Foot Syndrome

Hand-and-foot syndrome (palmar-plantar erythrodysesthesia or chemotherapy-induced acral erythema) is a cutaneous toxicity (median time to onset of 79 days, range from 11-360 days) with a severity range of Grades 1-3. Grade 1 is characterized by any of the following: numbness, dysesthesia/paresthesia, tingling, painless swelling or erythema of the hands and/or feet and/or discomfort which does not disrupt normal activities. Grade 2 hand-and-foot syndrome is defined as painful erythema and swelling of the hands and/or feet and/or discomfort affecting the patients' activities of daily living. Grade 3 hand-and-foot syndrome is defined as moist desquamation, ulceration, blistering or severe pain of the hands and/or feet and/or severe discomfort that causes the patient to be unable to work or perform activities of daily living. If Grade 2 or 3 hand-and-foot syndrome occurs, administration of capecitabine should be interrupted until the event resolves or decreases in intensity to Grade 1. Following Grade 3 hand-and-foot syndrome, subsequent doses of capecitabine should be decreased (see DOSAGE AND ADMINISTRATION).

Cardiotoxicity

The cardiotoxicity observed with capecitabine includes myocardial infarction/ischemia, angina, dysrhythmias, cardiac arrest, cardiac failure, sudden death, electrocardiographic changes, and cardiomyopathy. These adverse events may be more common in patients with a prior history of coronary artery disease.

Hepatic Insufficiency

Patients with mild to moderate hepatic dysfunction due to liver metastases should be carefully monitored when capecitabine is administered. The effect of severe hepatic dysfunction on the disposition of capecitabine is not known (see CLINICAL PHARMACOLOGY and DOSAGE AND ADMINISTRATION).

Hyperbilirubinemia

In the overall clinical trial safety database of capecitabine monotherapy (n=875), Grade 3 (1.5-3 × ULN) hyperbilirubinemia occurred in 15.2% (n=133) and Grade 4 (>3 × ULN) hyperbilirubinemia occurred in 3.9% (n=34) of 875 patients with either metastatic breast or colorectal cancer who received at least 1 dose of capecitabine 1250 mg/m^2 twice daily as monotherapy for 2 weeks followed by a 1 week rest period. Of 566 patients who had hepatic metastases at baseline and 309 patients without hepatic metastases at baseline, Grade 3 or 4 hyperbilirubinemia occurred in 22.8% and 12.3%, respectively. Of the 167 patients with Grade 3 or 4 hyperbilirubinemia, 18.6% (n=31) also had post-baseline elevations (Grades 1-4, without elevations at baseline) in alkaline phosphatase and 27.5% (n=46) had post-baseline elevations in transaminases at any time (not necessarily concurrent). The majority of these patients, 64.5% (n=20) and 71.7% (n=33), had liver metastases at baseline. In addition, 57.5% (n=96) and 35.3% (n=59) of the 167 patients had elevations (Grades 1-4) at both pre-baseline and post-baseline in alkaline phosphatase or transaminases, respectively. Only 7.8% (n=13) and 3.0% (n=5) had Grade 3 or 4 elevations in alkaline phosphatase or transaminases.

In the 596 patients treated with capecitabine as first-line therapy for metastatic colorectal cancer, the incidence of Grade 3 or 4 hyperbilirubinemia was similar to the overall clinical trial safety database of capecitabine monotherapy. The median time to onset for Grade 3 or 4 hyperbilirubinemia in the colorectal cancer population was 64 days and median total bilirubin increased from 8 μm/L at baseline to 13 μm/L during treatment with capecitabine. Of the 136 colorectal cancer patients with Grade 3 or 4 hyperbilirubinemia, 49 patients had Grade 3 or 4 hyperbilirubinemia as their last measured value, of which 46 had liver metastases at baseline.

In 251 patients with metastatic breast cancer who received a combination of capecitabine and docetaxel, Grade 3 (1.5-3 × ULN) hyperbilirubinemia occurred in 7% (n=17) and Grade 4 (>3 × ULN) hyperbilirubinemia occurred in 2% (n=5).

If drug-related Grade 2-4 elevations in bilirubin occur, administration of capecitabine should be immediately interrupted until the hyperbilirubinemia resolves or decreases in intensity to Grade 1. NCIC Grade 2 hyperbilirubinemia is defined as 1.5 times normal, Grade 3 hyperbilirubinemia as 1.5-3 × normal and Grade 4 hyperbilirubinemia as >3 × normal. (See recommended dose modifications under DOSAGE AND ADMINISTRATION.)

Hematologic

In 875 patients with either metastatic breast or colorectal cancer who received a dose of 1250 mg/m^2 administered twice daily as monotherapy for 2 weeks followed by a 1 week rest period, 3.2%, 1.7%, and 2.4% of patients had Grade 3 or 4 neutropenia, thrombocytopenia or decreases in hemoglobin, respectively. In 251 patients with metastatic breast cancer who received a dose of capecitabine in combination with docetaxel, 68% had Grade 3 or 4 neutropenia, 2.8% had Grade 3 or 4 thrombocytopenia, and 9.6% had Grade 3 or 4 anemia.

CARCINOGENESIS, MUTAGENESIS, AND IMPAIRMENT OF FERTILITY

Adequate studies investigating the carcinogenic potential of capecitabine have not been conducted. Capecitabine was not mutagenic *in vitro* to bacteria (Ames test) or mammalian cells (Chinese hamster V79/HPRT gene mutation assay). Capecitabine was clastogenic *in vitro* to human peripheral blood lymphocytes but not clastogenic *in vivo* to mouse bone marrow (micronucleus test). Fluorouracil causes mutations in bacteria and yeast. Fluorouracil also causes chromosomal abnormalities in the mouse micronucleus test *in vivo.*

Impairment of Fertility

In studies of fertility and general reproductive performance in mice, oral capecitabine doses of 760 mg/kg/day disturbed estrus and consequently caused a decrease in fertility. In mice that became pregnant, no fetuses survived this dose. The disturbance in estrus was reversible. In males, this dose caused degenerative changes in the testes, including decreases in the number of spermatocytes and spermatids. In separate pharmacokinetic studies, this dose in mice produced 5′-DFUR AUC values about 0.7 times the corresponding values in patients administered the recommended daily dose.

INFORMATION FOR THE PATIENT

See Patient Package Insert included with prescription.

Patients and patients' caregivers should be informed of the expected adverse effects of capecitabine, particularly nausea, vomiting, diarrhea, and hand-and-foot syndrome, and should be made aware that patient-specific dose adaptations during therapy are expected and necessary (see DOSAGE AND ADMINISTRATION). Patients should be encouraged to recognize the common Grade 2 toxicities associated with capecitabine treatment.

Diarrhea: Patients experiencing Grade 2 diarrhea (an increase of 4-6 stools/day or nocturnal stools) or greater should be instructed to stop taking capecitabine immediately. Standard antidiarrheal treatments (*e.g.,* loperamide) are recommended.

Nausea: Patients experiencing Grade 2 nausea (food intake significantly decreased but able to eat intermittently) or greater should be instructed to stop taking capecitabine immediately. Initiation of symptomatic treatment is recommended.

Vomiting: Patients experiencing Grade 2 vomiting (2-5 episodes in a 24 hour period) or greater should be instructed to stop taking capecitabine immediately. Initiation of symptomatic treatment is recommended.

Hand-and-Foot Syndrome: Patients experiencing Grade 2 hand-and-foot syndrome (painful erythema and swelling of the hands and/or feet and/or discomfort affecting the patients' activities of daily living) or greater should be instructed to stop taking capecitabine immediately.

Stomatitis: Patients experiencing Grade 2 stomatitis (painful erythema, edema or ulcers of the mouth or tongue, but able to eat) or greater should be instructed to stop taking capecitabine immediately. Initiation of symptomatic treatment is recommended (see DOSAGE AND ADMINISTRATION).

Fever and Neutropenia: Patients who develop a fever of 100.5°F or greater or other evidence of potential infection should be instructed to call their physician.

C

DRUG-FOOD INTERACTION

In all clinical trials, patients were instructed to administer capecitabine within 30 minutes after a meal. Since current safety and efficacy data are based upon administration with food, it is recommended that capecitabine be administered with food (see DOSAGE AND ADMINISTRATION).

PREGNANCY, TERATOGENIC EFFECTS, PREGNANCY CATEGORY D

See WARNINGS.

Women of childbearing potential should be advised to avoid becoming pregnant while receiving treatment with capecitabine.

NURSING MOTHERS

Lactating mice given a single oral dose of capecitabine excreted significant amounts of capecitabine metabolites into the milk. Because of the potential for serious adverse reactions in nursing infants from capecitabine, it is recommended that nursing be discontinued when receiving capecitabine therapy.

PEDIATRIC USE

The safety and effectiveness of capecitabine in persons <18 years of age have not been established.

GERIATRIC USE

Physicians should pay particular attention to monitoring the adverse effects of capecitabine in the elderly (see WARNINGS, Geriatric Patients).

DRUG INTERACTIONS

ANTACID

The effect of an aluminum hydroxide- and magnesium hydroxide-containing antacid (Maalox) on the pharmacokinetics of capecitabine was investigated in 12 cancer patients. There was a small increase in plasma concentrations of capecitabine and one metabolite (5′-DFCR); there was no effect on the 3 major metabolites (5′-DFUR, 5-FU and FBAL).

ANTICOAGULANTS

Patients receiving concomitant capecitabine and oral coumarin-derivative anticoagulant therapy should have their anticoagulant response (INR or prothrombin time) monitored closely with great frequency and the anticoagulant dose should be adjusted accordingly (see BOXED WARNING and CLINICAL PHARMACOLOGY). Altered coagulation parameters and/or bleeding have been reported in patients taking capecitabine concomitantly with coumarin-derivative anticoagulants such as warfarin and phenprocoumon. These events occurred within several days and up to several months after initiating capecitabine therapy and, in a few cases, within 1 month after stopping capecitabine. These events occurred in patients with and without liver metastases. In a drug interaction study with single dose warfarin administration, there was a significant increase in the mean AUC of S-warfarin. The maximum observed INR value increased by 91%. This interaction is probably due to an inhibition of cytochrome P450 2C9 by capecitabine and/or its metabolites (see CLINICAL PHARMACOLOGY).

CYP2C9 SUBSTRATES

Other than warfarin, no formal drug-drug interaction studies between capecitabine and other CYP2C9 substrates have been conducted. Care should be exercised when capecitabine is coadministered with CYP2C9 substrates.

PHENYTOIN

The level of phenytoin should be carefully monitored in patients taking capecitabine and phenytoin dose may need to be reduced (see DOSAGE AND ADMINISTRATION, Dose Modification Guidelines). Postmarketing reports indicate that some patients receiving capecitabine and phenytoin had toxicity associated with elevated phenytoin levels. Formal drug-drug interaction studies with phenytoin have not been conducted, but the mechanism of interaction is presumed to be inhibition of the CYP2C9 isoenzyme by capecitabine and/or its metabolites (see Anticoagulants).

LEUCOVORIN

The concentration of 5-fluorouracil is increased and its toxicity may be enhanced by leucovorin. Deaths from severe enterocolitis, diarrhea, and dehydration have been reported in elderly patients receiving weekly leucovorin and fluorouracil.

ADVERSE REACTIONS

COLORECTAL CANCER

TABLE 8 shows the adverse events occurring in >5% of patients from pooling the two Phase 3 trials in colorectal cancer. Rates are rounded to the nearest whole number. A total of 596 patients with metastatic colorectal cancer were treated with 1250 mg/m^2 twice a day of capecitabine administered for 2 weeks followed by a 1 week rest period, and 593 patients were administered 5-FU and leucovorin in the Mayo regimen (20 mg/m^2 leucovorin IV followed by 425 mg/m^2 IV bolus 5-FU, on days 1-5, every 28 days). In the pooled colorectal database the median duration of treatment was 139 days for capecitabine-treated patients and 140 days for 5-FU/LV-treated patients. A total of 78 (13%) and 63 (11%) capecitabine and 5-FU/LV-treated patients, respectively, discontinued treatment because of adverse events/intercurrent illness. A total of 82 deaths due to all causes occurred either on study or within 28 days of receiving study drug: 50 (8.4%) patients randomized to capecitabine and 32 (5.4%) randomized to 5-FU/LV.

***TABLE 8** Pooled Phase 3 Colorectal Trials: Percent Incidence of Adverse Events Related or Unrelated to Treatment in ≥5% of Patients*

	Capecitabine (n=596)			5-FU/LV (n=593)		
		Grade			Grade	
	Total	3	4	Total	3	4
Body System/Adverse Event	n=96*	n=52*	n=9*	n=94*	n=45*	n=9*
GI						
Diarrhea	55%	13%	2%	61%	10%	2%
Nausea	43%	4%	—	51%	3%	<1%
Vomiting	27%	4%	<1%	30%	4%	<1%
Stomatitis	25%	2%	<1%	62%	14%	1%
Abdominal pain	35%	9%	<1%	31%	5%	—
Gastrointestinal motility disorder	10%	<1%	—	7%	<1%	—
Constipation	14%	1%	<1%	17%	1%	—
Oral discomfort	10%	—	—	10%	—	—
Upper GI inflammatory disorders	8%	<1%	—	10%	1%	—
Gastrointestinal hemorrhage	6%	1%	<1%	3%	1%	—
Ileus	6%	4%	1%	5%	2%	1%
Skin and Subcutaneous						
Hand-and-Foot syndrome	54%	17%	NA	6%	1%	NA
Dermatitis	27%	1%	—	26%	1%	—
Skin discoloration	7%	<1%	—	5%	—	—
Alopecia	6%	—	—	21%	<1%	—
General						
Fatigue/weakness	42%	4%	—	46%	4%	—
Pyrexia	18%	1%	—	21%	2%	—
Edema	15%	1%	—	9%	1%	—
Pain	12%	1%	—	10%	1%	—
Chest pain	6%	1%	—	6%	1%	<1%
Neurological						
Peripheral sensory neuropathy	10%	—	—	4%	—	—
Headache	10%	1%	—	7%	—	—
Dizziness†	8%	<1%	—	8%	<1%	—
Insomnia	7%	—	—	7%	—	—
Taste disturbance	6%	1%	—	11%	<1%	1%
Metabolism						
Appetite decreased	26%	3%	<1%	31%	2%	<1%
Dehydration	7%	2%	<1%	8%	3%	1%
Eye						
Eye irritation	13%	—	—	10%	<1%	—
Vision abnormal	5%	—	—	2%	—	—
Respiratory						
Dyspnea	14%	1%	—	10%	<1%	1%
Cough	7%	<1%	1%	8%	—	—
Pharyngeal disorder	5%	—	—	5%	—	—
Epistaxis	3%	<1%	—	6%	—	—
Sore throat	2%	—	—	6%	—	—
Musculoskeletal						
Back pain	10%	2%	—	9%	<1%	—
Arthralgia	8%	1%	—	6%	1%	—
Vascular						
Venous thrombosis	8%	3%	<1%	6%	2%	—
Psychiatric						
Mood alteration	5%	—	—	6%	<1%	—
Depression	5%	—	—	4%	<1%	—
Infections						
Viral	5%	<1%	—	5%	<1%	—
Blood and Lymphatic						
Anemia	80%	2%	<1%	79%	1%	<1%
Neutropenia	13%	1%	2%	46%	8%	13%
Hepatobiliary						
Hyperbilirubinemia	48%	18%	5%	17%	3%	3%

* No. of Patients with >1 Adverse Event.
† Excluding vertigo.
— Not observed.
NA = Not applicable.

BREAST CANCER COMBINATION

The following data are shown for the combination study with capecitabine and docetaxel in patients with metastatic breast cancer in TABLE 9. In the capecitabine and docetaxel combination arm the treatment was capecitabine administered orally 1250 mg/m^2 twice daily as intermittent therapy (2 weeks of treatment followed by 1 week without treatment) for at least 6 weeks and docetaxel administered as a 1 hour IV infusion at a dose of 75 mg/m^2 on the first day of each 3 week cycle for at least 6 weeks. In the monotherapy arm docetaxel was administered as a 1 hour IV infusion at a dose of 100 mg/m^2 on the first day of each 3 week cycle for at least 6 weeks. The mean duration of treatment was 129 days in the combination arm and 98 days in the monotherapy arm. A total of 66 patients (26%) in the combination arm and 49 (19%) in the monotherapy arm withdrew from the study because of adverse events. The percentage of patients requiring dose reductions due to adverse events were 65% in the combination arm and 36% in the monotherapy arm. The percentage of patients requiring treatment interruptions due to adverse events in the combination arm was 79%. Treatment interruptions were part of the dose modification scheme for the combination therapy arm but not for the docetaxel monotherapy-treated patients.

BREAST CANCER CAPECITABINE MONOTHERAPY

The following data are shown for the study in stage IV breast cancer patients who received a dose of 1250 mg/m^2 administered twice daily for 2 weeks followed by a 1 week rest period. The mean duration of treatment was 114 days. A total of 13 out of 162 patients (8%) discontinued treatment because of adverse events/intercurrent illness.

TABLE 9 *Percent Incidence of Adverse Events Considered Related or Unrelated to Treatment in ≥5% of Patients Participating in the Capecitabine and Docetaxel Combination versus Docetaxel Monotherapy Study*

	Capecitabine 1250 mg/m²/bid With Docetaxel 75 mg/m²/3 Weeks (n=255)			Docetaxel 100 mg/m²/3 Weeks (n=255)		
		Grade			Grade	
	Total	3	4	Total	3	4
Body System/Adverse Event	n=99*	n=76.5*	n=29.1*	n=97*	n=57.6*	n=31.8*
GI						
Diarrhea	67%	14%	<1%	48%	5%	<1%
Stomatitis	67%	17%	<1%	43%	5%	—
Nausea	45%	7%	—	36%	2%	—
Vomiting	35%	4%	1%	24%	2%	—
Constipation	20%	2%	—	18%	—	—
Abdominal pain	30%	<3%	<1%	24%	2%	—
Dyspepsia	14%	—	—	8%	1%	—
Dry mouth	6%	<1%	—	5%	—	—
Skin and Subcutaneous						
Hand-and-Foot syndrome	63%	24%	NA	8%	1%	NA
Alopecia	41%	6%	—	42%	7%	—
Nail disorder	14%	2%	—	15%	—	—
Dermatitis	8%	—	—	11%	1%	—
Rash erythematous	9%	<1%	—	5%	—	—
Nail discoloration	6%	—	—	4%	<1%	—
Onycholysis	5%	1%	—	5%	1%	—
Pruritus	4%	—	—	5%	—	—
General						
Pyrexia	28%	2%	—	34%	2%	—
Asthenia	26%	4%	<1%	25%	6%	—
Fatigue	22%	4%	—	27%	6%	—
Weakness	16%	2%	—	11%	2%	—
Pain in limb	13%	<1%	—	13%	2%	—
Lethargy	7%	—	—	6%	2%	—
Pain	7%	<1%	—	5%	1%	—
Chest pain (non-cardiac)	4%	<1%	—	6%	2%	—
Influenza like illness	5%	—	—	5%	—	—
Neurological						
Taste disturbance	16%	<1%	—	14%	<1%	—
Headache	15%	3%	—	15%	2%	—
Paraesthesia	12%	<1%	—	16%	1%	—
Dizziness	12%	—	—	8%	<1%	—
Insomnia	8%	—	—	10%	<1%	—
Peripheral neuropathy	6%	—	—	10%	1%	—
Hypoaesthesia	4%	<1%	—	8%	<1%	—
Metabolism						
Anorexia	13%	1%	—	11%	<1%	—
Appetite decreased	10%	—	—	5%	—	—
Weight decreased	7%	—	—	5%	—	—
Dehydration	10%	2%	—	7%	<1%	<1%
Eye						
Lacrimation increased	12%	—	—	7%	<1%	—
Conjunctivitis	5%	—	—	4%	—	—
Eye irritation	5%	—	—	1%	—	—
Musculoskeletal						
Arthralgia	15%	2%	—	24%	3%	—
Myalgia	15%	2%	—	25%	2%	—
Back pain	12%	<1%	—	11%	3%	—
Bone pain	8%	<1%	—	10%	2%	—
Cardiac						
Edema	33%	<2%	—	34%	<3%	1%
Blood						
Neutropenic fever	16%	3%	13%	21%	5%	16%
Respiratory						
Dyspnea	14%	2%	<1%	16%	2%	—
Cough	13%	1%	—	22%	<1%	—
Sore throat	12%	2%	—	11%	<1%	—
Epistaxis	7%	<1%	—	6%	—	—
Rhinorrhea	5%	—	—	3%	—	—
Pleural effusion	2%	1%	—	7%	4%	—
Infection						
Oral candidiasis	7%	<1%	—	8%	<1%	—
Urinary tract infection	6%	<1%	—	4%	—	—
Upper respiratory tract	4%	—	—	5%	1%	—
Vascular						
Flushing	5%	—	—	5%	—	—
Lymphoedema	3%	<1%	—	5%	1%	—
Psychiatric						
Depression	5%	—	—	5%	1%	—

* No. of patients with at least 1 adverse event.
— Not observed.
NA = Not applicable.

TABLE 10 *Percent of Patients With Laboratory Abnormalities Participating in the Capecitabine and Docetaxel Combination versus Docetaxel Monotherapy Study*

	Capecitabine 1250 mg/m²/bid With Docetaxel 75 mg/m²/3 Weeks (n=251)			Docetaxel 100 mg/m²/3 Weeks (n=255)		
		Grade			Grade	
Body System/Adverse Event	Total	3	4	Total	3	5
Hematologic						
Leukopenia	91%	37%	24%	88%	42%	33%
Neutropenia/granulocytopenia	86%	20%	49%	87%	10%	66%
Thrombocytopenia	41%	2%	1%	23%	1%	2%
Anemia	80%	7%	3%	83%	5%	<1%
Lymphocytopenia	99%	48%	41%	98%	44%	40%
Hepatobiliary						
Hyperbilirubinemia	20%	7%	2%	6%	2%	2%

TABLE 11 *Percent Incidence of Adverse Events Considered Remotely, Possibly or Probably Related to Treatment in ≥5% of Patients Participating in the Single Arm Trial in Stage IV Breast Cancer — Phase 2 Trial in Stage IV Breast Cancer (n=162)*

Body System/Adverse Event	Total	Grade 3	Grade 4
GI			
Diarrhea	57%	12%	3%
Nausea	53%	4%	—
Vomiting	37%	4%	—
Stomatitis	24%	7%	—
Abdominal pain	20%	4%	—
Constipation	15%	1%	—
Dyspepsia	8%	—	—
Skin and Subcutaneous			
Hand-and-Foot syndrome	57%	11%	NA
Dermatitis	37%	1%	—
Nail disorder	7%	—	—
General			
Fatigue	41%	8%	—
Pyrexia	12%	1%	—
Pain in limb	6%	1%	—
Neurological			
Paraesthesia	21%	1%	—
Headache	9%	1%	—
Dizziness	8%	—	—
Insomnia	8%	—	—
Metabolism			
Anorexia	23%	3%	—
Dehydration	7%	4%	1%
Eye			
Eye irritation	15%	—	—
Musculoskeletal			
Myalgia	9%	—	—
Cardiac			
Edema	9%	1%	—
Blood			
Neutropenia	26%	2%	2%
Thrombocytopenia	24%	3%	1%
Anemia	72%	3%	1%
Lymphopenia	94%	44%	15%
Hepatobiliary			
Hyperbilirubinemia	22%	9%	2%

— Not observed.
NA = Not applicable.

OTHER ADVERSE EVENTS

Capecitabine and Docetaxel in Combination

Shown below by body system are the clinically relevant adverse events in <5% of patients in the overall clinical trial safety database of 251 patients (Study Details) reported as related to the administration of capecitabine in combination with docetaxel and that were clinically at least remotely relevant. In parentheses is the incidence of Grade 3 and 4 occurrences of each adverse event.

It is anticipated that the same types of adverse events observed in the capecitabine monotherapy studies may be observed in patients treated with the combination of capecitabine plus docetaxel.

Gastrointestinal: Ileus (0.39), necrotizing enterocolitis (0.39), esophageal ulcer (0.39), hemorrhagic diarrhea (0.80).

Neurological: Ataxia (0.39), syncope (1.20), taste loss (0.80), polyneuropathy (0.39), migraine (0.39).

Cardiac: Supraventricular tachycardia (0.39).

Infection: Neutropenic sepsis (2.39), sepsis (0.39), bronchopneumonia (0.39).

Blood and Lymphatic: Agranulocytosis (0.39), prothrombin decreased (0.39).

Vascular: Hypotension (1.20), venous phlebitis and thrombophlebitis (0.39), postural hypotension (0.80).

Renal: Renal failure (0.39).

Hepatobiliary: Jaundice (0.39), abnormal liver function tests (0.39), hepatic failure (0.39), hepatic coma (0.39), hepatotoxicity (0.39).

Immune System: Hypersensitivity (1.20).

Capecitabine Monotherapy

Shown below by body system are the clinically relevant adverse events in <5% of patients in the overall clinical trial safety database of 875 patients (Phase 3 colorectal studies — 596 patients, Phase 2 colorectal study — 34 patients, Phase 2 breast cancer studies — 245 patients) reported as related to the administration of capecitabine and that were clinically at least remotely relevant. In parentheses is the incidence of Grade 3 or 4 occurrences of each adverse event.

Gastrointestinal: Abdominal distension, dysphagia, proctalgia, ascites (0.1), gastric ulcer (0.1), ileus (0.3), toxic dilation of intestine, gastroenteritis (0.1).
Skin and Subcutaneous: Nail disorder (0.1), sweating increased (0.1), photosensitivity reaction (0.1), skin ulceration, pruritus, radiation recall syndrome (0.2).
General: Chest pain (0.2), influenza-like illness, hot flushes, pain (0.1), hoarseness, irritability, difficulty in walking, thirst, chest mass, collapse, fibrosis (0.1), hemorrhage, edema, sedation.
Neurological: Insomnia, ataxia (0.5), tremor, dysphasia, encephalopathy (0.1), abnormal coordination, dysarthria, loss of consciousness (0.2), impaired balance.
Metabolism: Increased weight, cachexia (0.4), hypertriglyceridemia (0.1), hypokalemia, hypomagnesemia.
Eye: Conjunctivitis.
Respiratory: Cough (0.1), epistaxis (0.1), asthma (0.2), hemoptysis, respiratory distress (0.1), dyspnea.
Cardiac: Tachycardia (0.1), bradycardia, atrial fibrillation, ventricular extrasystoles, extrasystoles, myocarditis (0.1), pericardial effusion.
Infections: Laryngitis (1.0), bronchitis (0.2), pneumonia (0.2), bronchopneumonia (0.2), keratoconjunctivitis, sepsis (0.3), fungal infections (including candidiasis) (0.2).
Musculoskeletal: Myalgia, bone pain (0.1), arthritis (0.1), muscle weakness.
Blood and Lymphatic: Leukopenia (0.2), coagulation disorder (0.1), bone marrow depression (0.1), idiopathic thrombocytopenia purpura (1.0), pancytopenia (0.1).
Vascular: Hypotension (0.2), hypertension (0.1), lymphoedema (0.1), pulmonary embolism (0.2), cerebrovascular accident (0.1).
Psychiatric: Depression, confusion (0.1).
Renal: Renal impairment (0.6).
Ear: Vertigo.
Hepatobiliary: Hepatic fibrosis (0.1), hepatitis (0.1), cholestatic hepatitis (0.1), abnormal liver function tests.
Immune System: Drug hypersensitivity (0.1).
Postmarketing: Hepatic failure.

DOSAGE AND ADMINISTRATION

The recommended dose of capecitabine is 1250 mg/m^2 administered orally twice daily (morning and evening; equivalent to 2500 mg/m^2 total daily dose) for 2 weeks followed by a 1 week rest period given as 3 week cycles. Capecitabine tablets should be swallowed with water within 30 minutes after a meal. TABLE 12 displays the total daily dose by body surface area and the number of tablets to be taken at each dose.

TABLE 12 *Capecitabine Dose Calculation According to Body Surface Area*

Dose Level 1250 mg/m^2 Twice a Day		No. of Tablets to be Taken at Each Dose (morning and evening)	
Surface Area (m^2)	Total Daily* Dose (mg)	150 mg	500 mg
≤1.25	3000	0	3
1.26-1.37	3300	1	3
1.38-1.51	3600	2	3
1.52-1.65	4000	0	4
1.66-1.77	4300	1	4
1.78-1.91	4600	2	4
1.92-2.05	5000	0	5
2.06-2.17	5300	1	5
≥2.18	5600	2	5

* Total daily dose divided by 2 to allow equal morning and evening doses.

DOSE MODIFICATION GUIDELINES

Patients should be carefully monitored for toxicity. Toxicity due to capecitabine administration may be managed by symptomatic treatment, dose interruptions and adjustment of capecitabine dose. Once the dose has been reduced it should not be increased at a later time.

The dose of phenytoin and the dose of a coumarin-derivative anticoagulants may need to be reduced when either drug is administered concomitantly with capecitabine (see DRUG INTERACTIONS).

Dose modification for the use of capecitabine and docetaxel in combination is described in Capecitabine in Combination With Docetaxel Dose Reduction Schedule.

Capecitabine in Combination With Docetaxel Dose Reduction Schedule

Toxicity NCIC Grades* (1st appearance):

Grade 2: Grade 2 occurring during the 14 days of capecitabine treatment: interrupt capecitabine treatment until resolved to Grade 0-1. Treatment may be resumed during the cycle at the same dose of capecitabine. Doses of capecitabine missed during a treatment cycle are not to be replaced. Prophylaxis for toxicities should be implemented where possible.

Grade 2 persisting at the time the next capecitabine/docetaxel treatment is due: delay treatment until resolved to Grade 0-1, then continue at 100% of the original capecitabine and docetaxel dose. Prophylaxis for toxicities should be implemented where possible.

Grade 3: Grade 3 occurring during the 14 days of capecitabine treatment: interrupt the capecitabine treatment until resolved to Grade 0-1. Treatment may be resumed during the cycle at 75% of the capecitabine dose. Doses of capecitabine missed during a treatment cycle are not to be replaced. Prophylaxis for toxicities should be implemented where possible.

Grade 3 persisting at the time the next capecitabine/docetaxel treatment is due: delay treatment until resolved to Grade 0-1.

For patients developing Grade 3 toxicity at any time during the treatment cycle, upon resolution to Grade 0-1, subsequent treatment cycles should be continued at 75% of the original capecitabine dose and at 55 mg/m^2 of docetaxel. Prophylaxis for toxicities should be implemented where possible.

Grade 4: Discontinue treatment unless treating physician considers it to be in the best interest of the patient to continue with capecitabine at 50% of original dose.

* National Cancer Institute of Canada Common Toxicity Criteria were used except for hand-foot syndrome (see PRECAUTIONS).

Toxicity NCIC Grades* (2nd appearance of same toxicity):

Grade 2: Grade 2 occurring during the 14 days of capecitabine treatment: interrupt capecitabine treatment until resolved to Grade 0-1. Treatment may be resumed during the cycle at 75% of original capecitabine dose. Doses of capecitabine missed during a treatment cycle are not to be replaced. Prophylaxis for toxicities should be implemented where possible.

Grade 2 persisting at the time the next capecitabine/docetaxel treatment is due: delay treatment until resolved to Grade 0-1.

For patients developing 2nd occurrence of Grade 2 toxicity at any time during the treatment cycle, upon resolution to Grade 0-1, subsequent treatment cycles should be continued at 75% of the original capecitabine dose and at 55 mg/m^2 of docetaxel. Prophylaxis for toxicities should be implemented where possible.

Grade 3: Grade 3 occurring during the 14 days of capecitabine treatment: interrupt the capecitabine treatment until resolved to Grade 0-1. Treatment may be resumed during the cycle at 50% of the capecitabine dose. Doses of capecitabine missed during a treatment cycle are not to be replaced. Prophylaxis for toxicities should be implemented where possible.

Grade 3 persisting at the time the next capecitabine/docetaxel treatment is due: delay treatment until resolved to Grade 0-1.

For patients developing Grade 3 toxicity at any time during the treatment cycle, upon resolution to Grade 0-1, subsequent treatment cycles should be continued at 50% of the original capecitabine dose and the docetaxel discontinued. Prophylaxis for toxicities should be implemented where possible.

For patients developing Grade 3 toxicity at any time during the treatment cycle, upon resolution to Grade 0-1, subsequent treatment cycles should be continued at 50% of the original capecitabine dose and the docetaxel discontinued. Prophylaxis for toxicities should be implemented where possible.

Grade 4: Discontinue treatment.

* National Cancer Institute of Canada Common Toxicity Criteria were used except for hand-foot syndrome (see PRECAUTIONS).

Toxicity NCIC Grades* (3rd appearance of same toxicity):

Grade 2: Grade 2 occurring during the 14 days of capecitabine treatment: interrupt capecitabine treatment until resolved to Grade 0-1. Treatment may be resumed during the cycle at 50% of the original capecitabine dose. Doses of capecitabine missed during a treatment cycle are not to be replaced. Prophylaxis for toxicities should be implemented where possible.

Grade 2 persisting at the time the next capecitabine/docetaxel treatment is due: delay treatment until resolved to Grade 0-1.

For patients developing 3rd occurrence of Grade 2 toxicity at any time during the treatment cycle, upon resolution to Grade 0-1, subsequent treatment cycles should be continued at 50% of the original capecitabine dose and the docetaxel discontinued. Prophylaxis for toxicities should be implemented where possible.

Grade 3: Discontinue treatment.

* National Cancer Institute of Canada Common Toxicity Criteria were used except for hand-foot syndrome (see PRECAUTIONS).

Toxicity NCIC Grades* (4th appearance of same toxicity):

Grade 2: Discontinue treatment.

* National Cancer Institute of Canada Common Toxicity Criteria were used except for hand-foot syndrome (see PRECAUTIONS).

Dose Modification for the Use of Capecitabine as Monotherapy

Dose modification for the use of capecitabine as monotherapy is shown in TABLE 13.

TABLE 13 *Recommended Dose Modifications*

Toxicity NCIC Grades*	During a Course of Therapy	Dose Adjustment for Next Cycle†
Grade 1	Maintain dose level	Maintain dose level
Grade 2		
1st appearance	Interrupt until resolved to Grade 0-1	100%
2nd appearance	Interrupt until resolved to Grade 0-1	75%
3rd appearance	Interrupt until resolved to Grade 0-1	50%
4th appearance	Discontinue treatment permanently	
Grade 3		
1st appearance	Interrupt until resolved to Grade 0-1	75%
2nd appearance	Interrupt until resolved to Grade 0-1	50%
3rd appearance	Discontinue treatment permanently	
Grade 4		
1st appearance	Discontinue permanently *or* If physician deems it to be in the patient's best interest to continue, interrupt until resolved to Grade 0-1	50%

* National Cancer Institute of Canada Common Toxicity Criteria were used except for the Hand-and-Foot Syndrome (see PRECAUTIONS).
† % of starting dose.

Dosage modifications are not recommended for Grade 1 events. Therapy with capecitabine should be interrupted upon the occurrence of a Grade 2 or 3 adverse experience. Once the adverse event has resolved or decreased in intensity to Grade 1, then capecitabine therapy may be restarted at full dose or as adjusted according to TABLE 13. If a Grade 4 experience occurs, therapy should be discontinued or interrupted until resolved or decreased to Grade 1, and therapy should be restarted at 50% of the original dose. Doses of capecitabine omitted for toxicity are not replaced or restored; instead the patient should resume the planned treatment cycles.

ADJUSTMENT OF STARTING DOSE IN SPECIAL POPULATIONS

Hepatic Impairment

In patients with mild to moderate hepatic dysfunction due to liver metastases, no starting dose adjustment is necessary; however, patients should be carefully monitored. Patients with severe hepatic dysfunction have not been studied.

Renal Impairment

No adjustment to the starting dose of capecitabine is recommended in patients with mild renal impairment (creatinine clearance = 51-80 ml/min [Cockroft and Gault, as shown below]). In patients with moderate renal impairment (baseline creatinine clearance = 30-50 ml/min), a dose reduction to 75% of the capecitabine starting dose when used as monotherapy or in combination with docetaxel (from 1250-950 mg/m^2 twice daily) is recommended (see CLINICAL PHARMACOLOGY, Special Populations). Subsequent dose adjustment is recommended as outlined in TABLE 13 if a patient develops a Grade 2-4 adverse event (see WARNINGS).

Cockroft and Gault equation:

Creatinine clearance for males = (140 - age [years]) (body wt [kg]) ÷ (72) (serum creatinine [mg/dl])

Creatinine clearance for females = 0.85 × male value

Geriatrics

Physicians should exercise caution in monitoring the effects of capecitabine in the elderly. Insufficient data are available to provide a dosage recommendation.

HOW SUPPLIED

Capecitabine is supplied as biconvex, oblong film-coated tablets, available as follows:

150 mg: Color is light peach with the engraving "XELODA" on one side, "150" on the other.

500 mg: Color is peach with the engraving "XELODA" on one side, "500" on the other.

Storage Conditions: Store at 25°C (77°F); excursions permitted to 15-30°C (59-86°F), keep tightly closed.

PRODUCT LISTING - EQUIVALENTS NOT AVAILABLE

Tablet - Oral - 150 mg

120's $445.65 XELODA, Roche Laboratories 00004-1100-51

Tablet - Oral - 500 mg

240's $2970.69 XELODA, Roche Laboratories 00004-1101-16

Captopril *(000642)*

For related information, see the comparative table section in Appendix A.

Categories: Heart failure, congestive; Hypertension, essential; Nephropathy, diabetic; Pregnancy Category C; FDA Approved 1981 Apr; WHO Formulary

Drug Classes: Angiotensin converting enzyme inhibitors

Brand Names: **Capoten**

Foreign Brand Availability: Ace-Bloc (Taiwan); Acenorm (Australia; Germany); Acepress (Indonesia; Italy); Acepril (England); Aceril (Israel); Aceten (India; South-Africa); Adocor (Germany); Alopresin (Spain); Altran (Colombia); Apuzin (Taiwan); Asisten (Argentina); Capace (South-Africa); Capocard (Hong-Kong); Caposan (Peru); Capotena (Mexico); Capotril (Bahrain; Cyprus; Egypt; Iran; Iraq; Jordan; Kuwait; Lebanon; Libya; Oman; Qatar; Republic-of-Yemen; Saudi-Arabia; Syria; United-Arab-Emirates); Capril (Hong-Kong; Korea; Taiwan); Captace (Philippines); Captensin (Indonesia); Capti (Israel); Captoflux (Germany); Captohexal (Australia; New-Zealand); Captolane (France); Captomax (South-Africa); Captopren (Bahrain; Colombia; Cyprus; Egypt; Iran; Iraq; Israel; Jordan; Kuwait; Lebanon; Libya; Oman; Qatar; Republic-of-Yemen; Saudi-Arabia; Syria; United-Arab-Emirates); Captopril (Dominican-Republic); Captoprilan (Dominican-Republic); Captoril (Japan); Captral (Mexico); Cardipril (Mexico); Catona (Mexico); Catoplin (Singapore); Cesplon (Spain); Cryopril (Mexico); Debax (Austria); Dexacap (Hong-Kong; Indonesia); Ecapres (Dominican-Republic); Ecaten (Mexico); Epicordin (Germany); Epsitron (Hong-Kong; Thailand); Farcopril (Bahrain; Cyprus; Egypt; Iran; Iraq; Israel; Jordan; Kuwait; Lebanon; Libya; Oman; Qatar; Republic-of-Yemen; Saudi-Arabia; Syria; United-Arab-Emirates); Farmoten (Indonesia); Hiperil (Portugal); Hypopress (Bahrain; Cyprus; Egypt; Iran; Iraq; Jordan; Kuwait; Lebanon; Libya; Oman; Qatar; Republic-of-Yemen; Saudi-Arabia; Syria; United-Arab-Emirates); Hypotensor (Greece); Inhibace (Israel); Insucar (Colombia); Isopresol (Argentina); Katopil (Slovenia); Ketanine (Singapore); Keyerpril (Mexico); Locap (Indonesia); Lopirin (Austria; Germany; Switzerland); Lopril (Finland; France); Medepres (Argentina); Mereprine (Portugal); Midrat (Mexico); Minitent (Bahrain; Cyprus; Egypt; Iran; Iraq; Israel; Jordan; Kuwait; Lebanon; Libya; Oman; Qatar; Republic-of-Yemen; Saudi-Arabia; Syria; United-Arab-Emirates); Nolectin (Peru); Oltens Ge (France); Petacilon (Singapore); Praten (Indonesia); Primace (Philippines); Rilcapton (Hong-Kong; Singapore; Taiwan); Ropril (Bahrain; Cyprus; Egypt; Hong-Kong; Iran; Iraq; Israel; Jordan; Kuwait; Lebanon; Libya; Oman; Qatar; Republic-of-Yemen; Saudi-Arabia; Syria; United-Arab-Emirates); Smarten (Taiwan); Tenofax (Indonesia); Tensicap (Indonesia); Tensiomen (Bulgaria; Hungary; Thailand); Tensobon (Germany); Tensoprel (Singapore); Tensoril (Philippines); Tenzib (Belgium); Topace (Australia); Toprilem (Mexico); Typril-ACE (Philippines); Vasosta (Philippines); Zapto (South-Africa); Zorkaptil (Slovenia)

Cost of Therapy: $61.37 (Hypertension; Capoten; 25 mg; 2 tablets/day; 30 day supply)
$38.36 (Hypertension; Generic Tablets; 25 mg; 2 tablets/day; 30 day supply)

WARNING

Use in Pregnancy: When used in pregnancy during the second and third trimesters, ACE inhibitors can cause injury and even death to the developing fetus. When pregnancy is detected, captopril should be discontinued as soon as possible. (See WARNINGS, Fetal/Neonatal Morbidity and Mortality.)

DESCRIPTION

Captopril is a specific competitive inhibitor of angiotensin I-converting enzyme (ACE), the enzyme responsible for the conversion of angiotensin I to angiotensin II.

Captopril is designated chemically as 1-[(2S)-3-mercapto-2-methylpropionyl]-L-proline. The molecular weight is 217.28. The empirical formula is $C_9H_{15}NO_3S$.

Captopril is a white to off-white crystalline powder that may have a slight sulfurous odor; it is soluble in water (approx. 160 mg/ml), methanol, and ethanol and sparingly soluble in chloroform and ethyl acetate.

Each tablet for oral administration contains captopril, 12.5, 25, 50, or 100 mg and the following inactive ingredients: corn starch; microcrystalline cellulose; lactose monohydrate, spray dried; and stearic acid.

CLINICAL PHARMACOLOGY

MECHANISM OF ACTION

The mechanism of action of captopril has not yet been fully elucidated. Its beneficial effects in hypertension and heart failure appear to result primarily from suppression of the renin-angiotensin-aldosterone system. However, there is no consistent correlation between renin levels and response to the drug. Renin, an enzyme synthesized by the kidneys, is released into the circulation where it acts on a plasma globulin substrate to produce angiotensin I, a relatively inactive decapeptide. Angiotensin I is then converted by angiotensin converting enzyme (ACE) to angiotensin II, a potent endogenous vasoconstrictor substance. Angiotensin II also stimulates aldosterone secretion from the adrenal cortex, thereby contributing to sodium and fluid retention.

Captopril prevents the conversion of angiotensin I to angiotensin II by inhibition of ACE, a peptidyldipeptide carboxy hydrolase. This inhibition has been demonstrated in both healthy human subjects and in animals by showing that the elevation of blood pressure caused by exogenously administered angiotensin I was attenuated or abolished by captopril. In animal studies, captopril did not alter the pressor responses to a number of other agents, including angiotensin II and norepinephrine, indicating specificity of action.

ACE is identical to "bradykininase," and captopril may also interfere with the degradation of the vasodepressor peptide, bradykinin. Increased concentrations of bradykinin or prostaglandin E_2 may also have a role in the therapeutic effect of captopril.

Inhibition of ACE results in decreased plasma angiotensin II and increased plasma renin activity (PRA), the latter resulting from loss of negative feedback on renin release caused by reduction in angiotensin II. The reduction of angiotensin II leads to decreased aldosterone secretion, and, as a result, small increases in serum potassium may occur along with sodium and fluid loss.

The antihypertensive effects persist for a longer period of time than does demonstrable inhibition of circulating ACE. It is not known whether the ACE present in vascular endothelium is inhibited longer than the ACE in circulating blood.

PHARMACOKINETICS

After oral administration of therapeutic doses of captopril, rapid absorption occurs with peak blood levels at about one hour. The presence of food in the gastrointestinal tract reduces absorption by about 30-40%; captopril therefore should be given 1 hour before meals. Based on carbon-14 labeling, average minimal absorption is approximately 75%. In a 24 hour period, over 95% of the absorbed dose is eliminated in the urine; 40-50% is unchanged drug; most of the remainder is the disulfide dimer of captopril and captopril-cysteine disulfide.

Approximately 25-30% of the circulating drug is bound to plasma proteins. The apparent elimination half-life for total radioactivity in blood is probably less than 3 hours. An accurate determination of half-life of unchanged captopril is not, at present, possible, but it is probably less than 2 hours. In patients with renal impairment, however, retention of captopril occurs (see DOSAGE AND ADMINISTRATION).

PHARMACODYNAMICS

Administration of captopril results in a reduction of peripheral arterial resistance in hypertensive patients with either no change, or an increase, in cardiac output. There is an increase in renal blood flow following administration of captopril and glomerular filtration rate is usually unchanged.

Reductions of blood pressure are usually maximal 60-90 minutes after oral administration of an individual dose of captopril. The duration of effect is dose related. The reduction in blood pressure may be progressive, so to achieve maximal therapeutic effects, several weeks of therapy may be required. The blood pressure lowering effects of captopril and thiazide-type diuretics are additive. In contrast, captopril and beta-blockers have a less than additive effect.

Blood pressure is lowered to about the same extent in both standing and supine positions. Orthostatic effects and tachycardia are infrequent but may occur in volume-depleted patients. Abrupt withdrawal of captopril has not been associated with a rapid increase in blood pressure.

In patients with heart failure, significantly decreased peripheral (systemic vascular) resistance and blood pressure (afterload), reduced pulmonary capillary wedge pressure (preload) and pulmonary vascular resistance, increased cardiac output, and increased exercise tolerance time (ETT) have been demonstrated. These hemodynamic and clinical effects occur after the first dose and appear to persist for the duration of therapy. Placebo controlled studies of 12 weeks duration in patients who did not respond adequately to diuretics and digitalis show no tolerance to beneficial effects on ETT; open studies, with exposure up to 18 months in some cases, also indicate that ETT benefit is maintained. Clinical improvement has been observed in some patients where acute hemodynamic effects were minimal.

The Survival and Ventricular Enlargement (SAVE) study was a multicenter, randomized, double-blind, placebo-controlled trial conducted in 2231 patients (age 21-79 years) who survived the acute phase of a myocardial infarction and did not have active ischemia. Patients had left ventricular dysfunction (LVD), defined as a resting left ventricular ejection fraction ≤40%, but at the time of randomization were not sufficiently symptomatic to require ACE inhibitor therapy for heart failure. About half of the patients had symptoms of heart failure in the past. Patients were given a test dose of 6.25 mg oral captopril and were randomized within 3-16 days post-infarction to receive either captopril or placebo in addition to conventional therapy. Captopril was initiated at 6.25 or 12.5 mg tid and after 2 weeks titrated to a target maintenance dose of 50 mg tid. About 80% of patients were receiving the target dose at the end of the study. Patients were followed for a minimum of 2 years and for up to 5 years, with an average follow-up of 3.5 years.

Baseline blood pressure was 113/70 mm Hg and 112/70 mm Hg for the placebo and captopril groups, respectively. Blood pressure increased slightly in both treatment groups during the study and was somewhat lower in the captopril group (119/74 vs 125/77 mm Hg at 1 yr).

Therapy with captopril improved long-term survival and clinical outcomes compared to placebo. The risk reduction of all cause mortality was 19% (p=0.02) and for cardiovascular death was 21% (p=0.014). Captopril treated subjects had 22% (p=0.034) fewer first hospitalizations for heart failure. Compared to placebo, 22% fewer patients receiving captopril developed symptoms of overt heart failure. There was no significant difference between groups in total hospitalizations for all cause (2056 placebo; 2036 captopril).

Captopril was well tolerated in the presence of other therapies such as aspirin, beta blockers, nitrates, vasodilators, calcium antagonists and diuretics.

In a multicenter, double-blind, placebo controlled trial, 409 patients age 18-49 of either gender, with or without hypertension, with Type 1 (juvenile type, onset below age 30) insulin-dependent diabetes mellitus, retinopathy, proteinuria ≥500 mg/day and serum creatinine ≤2.5 mg/dl, were randomized to placebo or captopril (25 mg tid) and followed for up to 4.8 years (median 3 years). To achieve blood pressure control, additional hypertensive agents (diuretics, beta blockers, centrally acting agents or vasodilators) were added as needed for patients in both groups.

The captopril group had a 51% reduction in risk of doubling of serum creatinine ($p<0.01$) and a 51% reduction in risk for the combined endpoint of end-stage renal disease (dialysis or transplantation) or death ($p<0.01$). Captopril treatment resulted in a 30% reduction in urine protein excretion within the first 3 months ($p<0.05$), which was maintained throughout the trial. The captopril group had somewhat better blood pressure control than the placebo group, but the effects of captopril on renal function were greater than would be expected from the group differences in blood pressure reduction alone. Captopril was well tolerated in this patient population.

In two multicenter, double-blind, placebo controlled studies, a total of 235 normotensive patients with insulin-dependent diabetes mellitus, retinopathy and microalbuminuria (20-200 μg/min) were randomized to placebo or captopril (50 mg bid) and followed for up to 2 years. Captopril delayed the progression to overt nephropathy (proteinuria >500 mg/day) in both studies (risk reduction 67-76%, $p<0.05$). Captopril also reduced the albumin excretion rate. However, the long term clinical benefit of reducing the progression from microalbuminuria to proteinuria has not been established.

Studies in rats and cats indicate that captopril does not cross the blood-brain barrier to any significant extent.

INDICATIONS AND USAGE

HYPERTENSION

Captopril is indicated for the treatment of hypertension.

In using captopril, consideration should be given to the risk of neutropenia/agranulocytosis (see WARNINGS).

Captopril may be used as initial therapy for patients with normal renal function, in whom the risk is relatively low. In patients with impaired renal function, particularly those with collagen vascular disease, captopril should be reserved for hypertensives who have either developed unacceptable side effects on other drugs, or have failed to respond satisfactorily to drug combinations.

Captopril is effective alone and in combination with other antihypertensive agents, especially thiazide-type diuretics. The blood pressure lowering effects of captopril and thiazides are approximately additive.

HEART FAILURE

Captopril is indicated in the treatment of congestive heart failure usually in combination with diuretics and digitalis. The beneficial effect of captopril in heart failure does not require the presence of digitalis, however, most controlled clinical trial experience with captopril has been in patients receiving digitalis; as well as diuretic treatment.

LEFT VENTRICULAR DYSFUNCTION AFTER MYOCARDIAL INFARCTION

Captopril is indicated to improve survival following myocardial infarction in clinically stable patients with left ventricular dysfunction manifested as an ejection fraction ≤40% and to reduce the incidence of overt heart failure and subsequent hospitalizations for congestive heart failure in these patients.

DIABETIC NEPHROPATHY

Captopril is indicated for the treatment of diabetic nephropathy (proteinuria >500 mg/day) in patients with Type 1 insulin-dependent diabetes mellitus and retinopathy. Captopril decreases the rate of progression of renal insufficiency and development of serious adverse clinical outcomes (death or need for renal transplantation or dialysis).

In considering use of captopril tablets, it should be noted that in controlled trials ACE inhibitors have an effect on blood pressure that is less in black patients than in non-blacks. In addition, ACE inhibitors (for which adequate data are available) cause a higher rate of angioedema in black than in non-black patients (see WARNINGS, Angioedema).

CONTRAINDICATIONS

Captopril is contraindicated in patients who are hypersensitive to this product or any other angiotensin-converting enzyme inhibitor (*e.g.*, a patient who has experienced angioedema during therapy with any other ACE inhibitor).

WARNINGS

ANAPHYLACTOID AND POSSIBLY RELATED REACTIONS

Presumably because angiotensin-converting enzyme inhibitors affect the metabolism of eicosanoids and polypeptides, including endogenous bradykinin, patients receiving ACE inhibitors (including captopril) may be subject to a variety of adverse reactions, some of them serious.

ANGIOEDEMA

Angioedema involving the extremities, face, lips, mucous membranes, tongue, glottis or larynx has been seen in patients treated with ACE inhibitors, including captopril. If angioedema involves the tongue, glottis or larynx, airway obstruction may occur and be fatal. Emergency therapy, including but not necessarily limited to, subcutaneous administration of a 1:1000 solution of epinephrine should be promptly instituted.

Swelling confined to the face, mucous membranes of the mouth, lips and extremities has usually resolved with discontinuation of captopril; some cases required medical therapy. (See PRECAUTIONS, Information for the Patient and ADVERSE REACTIONS.)

ANAPHYLACTOID REACTIONS DURING DESENSITIZATION

Two (2) patients undergoing desensitizing treatment with hymenoptera venom while receiving ACE inhibitors sustained life-threatening anaphylactoid reactions. In the same patients, these reactions were avoided when ACE inhibitors were temporarily withheld, but they reappeared upon inadvertent rechallenge.

ANAPHYLACTOID REACTIONS DURING MEMBRANE EXPOSURE

Anaphylactoid reactions should have been reported in patients dialyzed with high-flux membranes and treated concomitantly with an ACE inhibitor. Anaphylactoid reactions have also been reported in patients undergoing low-density lipoprotein apheresis with dextran sulfate absorption.

NEUTROPENIA/AGRANULOCYTOSIS

Neutropenia (<1000/mm^3) with myeloid hypoplasia has resulted from use of captopril. About half of the neutropenic patients developed systemic or oral cavity infections or other features of the syndrome of agranulocytosis.

The risk of neutropenia is dependent on the clinical status of the patient:

In clinical trials in patients with hypertension who have normal renal function (serum creatinine less than 1.6 mg/dl and no collagen vascular disease), neutropenia has been seen in 1 patient out of over 8600 exposed.

In patients with some degree of renal failure (serum creatinine at least 1.6 mg/dl) but no collagen vascular disease, the risk of neutropenia in clinical trials was about 1/500, a frequency over 15 times that for uncomplicated hypertension. Daily doses of captopril were relatively high in these patients, particularly in view of their diminished renal function. In foreign marketing experience in patients with renal failure, use of allopurinol concomitantly with captopril has been associated with neutropenia but this association has not appeared in US reports.

In patients with collagen vascular diseases (*e.g.*, systemic lupus erythematosus, scleroderma) and impaired renal function, neutropenia occurred in 3.7% of patients in clinical trials.

While none of the over 750 patients in formal clinical trials of heart failure developed neutropenia, it has occurred during the subsequent clinical experience. About half of the reported cases had serum creatinine ≥1.6 mg/dl and more than 75% were in patients also receiving procainamide. In heart failure, it appears that the same risk factors for neutropenia are present.

The neutropenia has usually been detected within three months after captopril was started. Bone marrow examinations in patients with neutropenia consistently showed myeloid hypoplasia, frequently accompanied by erythroid hypoplasia and decreased numbers of megakaryocytes (*e.g.*, hypoplastic bone marrow and pancytopenia); anemia and thrombocytopenia were sometimes seen.

In general, neutrophils returned to normal in about 2 weeks after captopril was discontinued, and serious infections were limited to clinically complex patients. About 13% of the cases of neutropenia have ended fatally, but almost all fatalities were in patients with serious illness, having collagen vascular disease, renal failure, heart failure or immunosuppressant therapy, or a combination of these complicating factors.

Evaluation of the hypertensive or heart failure patient should always include assessment of renal function.

If captopril is used in patients with impaired renal function, white blood cell and differential counts should be evaluated prior to starting treatment and at approximately 2 week intervals for about 3 months, then periodically.

In patients with collagen vascular disease or who are exposed to other drugs known to affect the white cells or immune response, particularly when there is impaired renal function, captopril should be used only after an assessment of benefit and risk, and then with caution.

All patients treated with captopril should be told to report any signs of infection (*e.g.*, sore throat, fever). If infection is suspected, white cell counts should be performed without delay.

Since discontinuation of captopril and other drugs has generally led to prompt return of the white count to normal, upon confirmation of neutropenia (neutrophil count <1000/mm^3) the physician should withdraw captopril and closely follow the patient's course.

PROTEINURIA

Total urinary proteins greater than 1 g/day were seen in about 0.7% of patients receiving captopril. About 90% of affected patients had evidence of prior renal disease or received relatively high doses of captopril (in excess of 150 mg/day), or both. The nephrotic syndrome occurred in about one-fifth of proteinuric patients. In most cases, proteinuria subsided or cleared within 6 months whether or not captopril was continued. Parameters of renal function, such as BUN and creatinine, were seldom altered in the patients with proteinuria.

HYPOTENSION

Excessive hypotension was rarely seen in hypertensive patients but is a possible consequence of captopril use in salt/volume depleted persons (such as those treated vigorously with diuretics), patients with heart failure or those patients undergoing renal dialysis. (See DRUG INTERACTIONS.)

In heart failure, where the blood pressure was either normal or low, transient decreases in mean blood pressure greater than 20% were recorded in about half of the patients. This transient hypotension is more likely to occur after any of the first several doses and is usually well tolerated, producing either no symptoms or brief mild lightheadedness, although in rare instances it has been associated with arrhythmia or conduction defects. Hypotension was the reason for discontinuation of drug in 3.6% of patients with heart failure.

BECAUSE OF THE POTENTIAL FALL IN BLOOD PRESSURE IN THESE PATIENTS, THERAPY SHOULD BE STARTED UNDER VERY CLOSE MEDICAL SUPERVISION. A starting dose of 6.25 or 12.5 mg tid may minimize the hypotensive effect. Patients should be followed closely for the first 2 weeks of treatment and whenever the dose of captopril and/or diuretic is increased. In patients with heart failure, reducing the dose of diuretic, if feasible, may minimize the fall in blood pressure.

Hypotension is not *per se* a reason to discontinue captopril. Some decrease of systemic blood pressure is a common and desirable observation upon initiation of captopril treatment in heart failure. The magnitude of the decease is greatest early in the course of treatment; this effect stabilizes within a week or 2, and generally returns to pretreatment levels, without a decrease in therapeutic efficacy, within 2 months.

FETAL/NEONATAL MORBIDITY AND MORTALITY

ACE inhibitors can cause fetal and neonatal morbidity and death when administered to pregnant women. Several dozen cases have been reported in the world literature. When pregnancy is detected, ACE inhibitors should be discontinued as soon as possible.

The use of ACE inhibitors during the second and third trimesters of pregnancy has been associated with fetal and neonatal injury, including hypotension, neonatal skull hypoplasia, anuria, reversible or irreversible renal failure, and death. Oligohydramnios has also been reported, presumably resulting from decreased fetal renal function; oligohydramnios in this setting has been associated with fetal limb contractures, craniofacial deformation, and hypoplastic lung development. Prematurity, intrauterine growth retardation, and patent ductus arteriosus have also been reported, although it is not clear whether these occurrences where due to the ACE-inhibitor exposure.

These adverse effects do not appear to have resulted from intrauterine ACE-inhibitor exposure that has been limited to the first trimester. Mothers whose embryos and fetuses are exposed to ACE inhibitors only during the first trimester should be so informed. Nonetheless, when patients become pregnant, physicians should make every effort to discontinue the use of captopril as soon as possible.

Rarely (probably less often than once in every thousand pregnancies), no alternative to ACE inhibitors will be found. In these rare cases, the mothers should be apprised of the potential hazards to their fetuses, and serial ultrasound examinations should be performed to assess the intraamniotic environment.

If oligohydramnios is observed, captopril should be discontinued unless it is considered life-saving for the mother. Contraction stress testing (CST), a non-stress test (NST), or biophysical profiling (BPP) may be appropriate, depending upon the week of pregnancy. Patients and physicians should be aware, however, that oligohydramnios may not appear until after the fetus has sustained irreversible injury.

Infants with histories of *in utero* exposure to ACE inhibitors should be closely observed for hypotension, oliguria, and hyperkalemia. If oliguria occurs, attention should be directed toward support of blood pressure and renal perfusion. Exchange transfusion or dialysis may be required as a means of reversing hypotension and/or substituting for disordered renal function. While captopril may be removed from the adult circulation by hemodialysis, there is inadequate data concerning the effectiveness of hemodialysis for removing it from the circulation of neonates or children. Peritoneal dialysis is not effective for removing captopril; there is no information concerning exchange transfusion for removing captopril from the general circulation.

When captopril was given to rabbits at doses about 0.8 to 70 times (on a mg/kg basis) the maximum recommended human dose, low incidences of craniofacial malformations were seen. No teratogenic effects of captopril were seen in studies of pregnant rats and hamsters. On a mg/kg basis, the doses used were up to 150 times (in hamsters) and 625 times (in rats) the maximum recommended human dose.

HEPATIC FAILURE

Rarely, ACE inhibitors have been associated with a syndrome that starts with cholestatic jaundice and progresses to fulminant hepatic necrosis and (sometimes) death. The mechanism of this syndrome is not understood. Patients receiving ACE inhibitors who develop jaundice or marked elevations of hepatic enzymes should discontinue the ACE inhibitor and receive appropriate medical follow-up.

PRECAUTIONS

GENERAL

Impaired Renal Function

Hypertension: Some patients with renal disease, particularly those with severe renal artery stenosis, have developed increases in BUN and serum creatinine after reduction of blood pressure with captopril. Captopril dosage reduction and/or discontinuation of diuretic may be required. For some of these patients, it may not be possible to normalize blood pressure and maintain adequate renal perfusion.

Heart Failure: About 20% of patients develop stable elevations of BUN and serum creatinine greater than 20% above normal or baseline upon long-term treatment with captopril. Less than 5% of patients, generally those with severe preexisting renal disease, required discontinuation of treatment due to progressively increasing creatinine; subsequent improvement probably depends upon the severity of the underlying renal disease.

See CLINICAL PHARMACOLOGY; DOSAGE AND ADMINISTRATION; and ADVERSE REACTIONS, Altered Laboratory Findings.

Hyperkalemia

Elevations in serum potassium have been observed in some patients treated with ACE inhibitors, including captopril. When treated with ACE inhibitors, patients at risk for the development of hyperkalemia include those with: renal insufficiency; diabetes mellitus; and those using concomitant potassium-sparing diuretics, potassium supplements or potassium-containing salt substitutes; or other drugs associated with increases in serum potassium. (See PRECAUTIONS, Information for the Patient; DRUG INTERACTIONS; and ADVERSE REACTIONS, Altered Laboratory Findings.)

Cough

Presumably due to the inhibition of the degradation of endogenous bradykinin, persistent nonproductive cough has been reported with all ACE inhibitors, always resolving after discontinuation of therapy. ACE inhibitor-induced cough should be considered in the differential diagnosis of cough.

Valvular Stenosis

There is concern, on theoretical grounds, that patients with aortic stenosis might be at particular risk of decreased coronary perfusion when treated with vasodilators because they do not develop as much afterload reduction as others.

Surgery/Anesthesia

In patients undergoing major surgery or during anesthesia with agents that produce hypotension, captopril will block angiotensin II formation secondary to compensatory renin release. If hypotension occurs and is considered to be due to this mechanism, it can be corrected by volume expansion.

HEMODIALYSIS

Recent clinical observations have shown an association of hypersensitivity-like (anaphylactoid) reactions during hemodialysis with high-flux dialysis membranes (*e.g.,* AN69) in patients receiving ACE inhibitors. In these patients, consideration should be given to using a different type of dialysis membrane or a different class of medication. (See WARNINGS, Anaphylactoid Reactions During Membrane Exposure.)

INFORMATION FOR THE PATIENT

Patients should be advised to immediately report to their physician any signs or symptoms suggesting angioedema (*e.g.,* swelling of face, eyes, lips, tongue, larynx and extremities; difficulty in swallowing or breathing; hoarseness) and to discontinue therapy. (See WARNINGS, Angioedema.)

Patients should be told to report promptly any indication of infection (*e.g.,* sore throat, fever), which may be a sign of neutropenia, or of progressive edema which might be related to proteinuria and nephrotic syndrome.

All patients should be cautioned that excessive perspiration and dehydration may lead to an excessive fall in blood pressure because of reduction in fluid volume. Other causes of volume depletion such as vomiting or diarrhea may also lead to a fall in blood pressure; patients should be advised to consult with the physician.

Patients should be advised not to use potassium-sparing diuretics, potassium supplements or potassium-containing salt substitutes without consulting their physician. (See PRECAUTIONS, General; DRUG INTERACTIONS; and ADVERSE REACTIONS.)

Patients should be warned against interruption or discontinuation of medication unless instructed by the physician.

Heart failure patients on captopril therapy should be cautioned against rapid increases in physical activity.

Patients should be informed that captopril should be taken one hour before meals (see DOSAGE AND ADMINISTRATION).

PREGNANCY CATEGORY C (FIRST TRIMESTER) AND PREGNANCY CATEGORY D (SECOND AND THIRD TRIMESTERS)

(See WARNINGS, Fetal/Neonatal Morbidity and Mortality.) Female patients of childbearing age should be told about the consequences of second- and third-trimester exposure to ACE inhibitors, and they should also be told that these consequences do not appear to have resulted from intrauterine ACE-inhibitor exposure that has been limited to the first trimester. These patients should be asked to report pregnancies to their physicians as soon as possible.

DRUG/LABORATORY TEST INTERACTIONS

Captopril may cause a false-positive urine test for acetone.

CARCINOGENESIS, MUTAGENESIS, AND IMPAIRMENT OF FERTILITY

Two (2) year studies with doses of 50-1350 mg/kg/day in mice and rats failed to show any evidence of carcinogenic potential. The high dose in these studies is 150 times the maximum recommended human dose of 450 mg, assuming a 50 kg subject. On a body-surface-area basis, the high doses for mice and rats are 13 and 26 times the maximum recommended human dose, respectively.

Studies in rats have revealed no impairment of fertility.

NURSING MOTHERS

Concentrations of captopril in human milk are approximately 1% of those in maternal blood. Because of the potential for serious adverse reactions in nursing infants from captopril, a decision should be made whether to discontinue nursing or to discontinue the drug, taking into account the importance of captopril to the mother. (See Pediatric Use.)

PEDIATRIC USE

Safety and effectiveness in pediatric patients have not been established. There is limited experience reported in the literature with the use of captopril in the pediatric population; dosage, on a weight basis, was generally reported to be comparable to or less than that used in adults.

Infants, especially newborns, may be more susceptible to the adverse hemodynamic effects of captopril. Excessive, prolonged and unpredictable decreases in blood pressure and associated complications, including oliguria and seizures, have been reported.

Captopril should be used in pediatric patients only if other measures for controlling blood pressure have not been effective.

C

DRUG INTERACTIONS

HYPOTENSION — PATIENTS ON DIURETIC THERAPY

Patients on diuretics and especially those in whom therapy was recently instituted, as well as those on severe dietary salt restriction or dialysis, may occasionally experience a precipitous reduction of blood pressure usually within the first hour after receiving the initial dose of captopril.

The possibility of hypotensive effects with captopril can be minimized by either discontinuing the diuretic or increasing the salt intake approximately 1 week prior to initiation of treatment with captopril or initiating therapy with small doses (6.25 or 12.5 mg). Alternatively, provide medical supervision for at least 1 hour after the initial dose. If hypotension occurs, the patient should be placed in a supine position and, if necessary, receive an intravenous infusion of normal saline. This transient hypotensive response is not a contraindication to further doses which can be given without difficulty once the blood pressure has increased after volume expansion.

AGENTS HAVING VASODILATOR ACTIVITY

Data on the effect of concomitant use of other vasodilators in patients receiving captopril for heart failure are not available; therefore, nitroglycerin or other nitrates (as used for management of angina) or other drugs having vasodilator activity should, if possible, be discontinued before starting captopril. If resumed during captopril therapy, such agents should be administered cautiously, and perhaps at lower dosage.

AGENTS CAUSING RENIN RELEASE

Captopril's effect will be augmented by antihypertensive agents that cause renin release. For example, diuretics (*e.g.,* thiazides) may activate the renin-angiotensin-aldosterone system.

AGENTS AFFECTING SYMPATHETIC ACTIVITY

The sympathetic nervous system may be especially important in supporting blood pressure in patients receiving captopril alone or with diuretics. Therefore, agents affecting sympathetic activity (*e.g.,* ganglionic blocking agents or adrenergic neuron blocking agents) should be used with caution. Beta-adrenergic blocking drugs add some further antihypertensive effect to captopril, but the overall response is less than additive.

AGENTS INCREASING SERUM POTASSIUM

Since captopril decreases aldosterone production, elevation of serum potassium may occur. Potassium-sparing diuretics such as spironolactone, triamterene, or amiloride, or potassium supplements should be given only for documented hypokalemia, and then with caution, since they may lead to a significant increase of serum potassium. Salt substitutes containing potassium should also be used with caution.

INHIBITORS OF ENDOGENOUS PROSTAGLANDIN SYNTHESIS

It has been reported that indomethacin may reduce the antihypertensive effect of captopril, especially in cases of low renin hypertension. Other nonsteroidal anti-inflammatory agents (*e.g.,* aspirin) may also have this effect.

LITHIUM

Increased serum lithium levels and symptoms of lithium toxicity have been reported in patients receiving concomitant lithium and ACE inhibitor therapy. These drugs should be coadministered with caution and frequent monitoring of serum lithium levels is recommended. If a diuretic is also used, it may increase the risk of lithium toxicity.

ADVERSE REACTIONS

Reported incidences are based on clinical trials involving approximately 7000 patients.

RENAL

About 1 of 100 patients developed proteinuria (see WARNINGS).

Each of the following has been reported in approximately 1-2 of 1000 patients and are of uncertain relationship to drug use: Renal insufficiency, renal failure, nephrotic syndrome, polyuria, oliguria, and urinary frequency.

HEMATOLOGIC

Neutropenia/agranulocytosis has occurred (see WARNINGS). Cases of anemia, thrombocytopenia, and pancytopenia have been reported.

DERMATOLOGIC

Rash, often with pruritus, and sometimes with fever, arthralgia, and eosinophilia, occurred in about 4-7 (depending on renal status and dose) of 100 patients, usually during the first 4 weeks of therapy. It is usually maculopapular and rarely urticarial. The rash is usually mild and disappears within a few days of dosage reduction, short-term treatment with an antihistaminic agent, and/or discontinuing therapy; remission may occur even if captopril is continued. Pruritus, without rash, occurs in about 2 of 100 patients. Between 7 and 10% of patients with skin rash have shown an eosinophilia and/or positive ANA titers. A reversible associated pemphigoid-like lesion, and photosensitivity, have also been reported.

Flushing or pallor has been reported in 2-5 of 1000 patients.

CARDIOVASCULAR

Hypotension may occur; see WARNINGS and DRUG INTERACTIONS for discussion of hypotension with captopril therapy.

Tachycardia, chest pain, and palpitations have each been observed in approximately 1 of 100 patients.

Angina pectoris, myocardial infarction, Raynaud's syndrome, and congestive heart failure have each occurred in 2-3 of 1000 patients.

DYSGEUSIA

Approximately 2-4 (depending on renal status and dose) of 100 patients developed a diminution or loss of taste perception. Taste impairment is reversible and usually self-limited (2-3 months) even with continued drug administration. Weight loss may be associated with the loss of taste.

ANGIOEDEMA

Angioedema involving the extremities, face, lips, mucous membranes, tongue, glottis or larynx has been reported in approximately 1 in 1000 patients. Angioedema involving the upper airways has caused fatal airway obstruction. (See WARNINGS, Angioedema and PRECAUTIONS, Information for the Patient.)

COUGH

Cough has been reported in 0.5-2% of patients treated with captopril in clinical trials. (See PRECAUTIONS, General, Cough.)

The following have been reported in about 0.5 to 2% of patients but did not appear at increased frequency compared to placebo or other treatments used in controlled trials: Gastric irritation, abdominal pain, nausea, vomiting, diarrhea, anorexia, constipation, aphthous ulcers, peptic ulcer, dizziness, headache, malaise, fatigue, insomnia, dry mouth, dyspnea, alopecia, paresthesias.

Other clinical adverse effects reported since the drug was marketed are listed below by body system. In this setting, an incidence or causal relationship cannot be accurately determined.

Body as a Whole: Anaphylactoid reactions (see WARNINGS, Anaphylactoid and Possibly Related Reactions and PRECAUTIONS, Hemodialysis).

General: Asthenia, gynecomastia.

Cardiovascular: Cardiac arrest, cerebrovascular accident/insufficiency, rhythm disturbances, orthostatic hypotension, syncope.

Dermatologic: Bullous pemphigus, erythema multiforme (including Stevens-Johnson syndrome), exfoliative dermatitis.

Gastrointestinal: Pancreatitis, glossitis, dyspepsia.

Hematologic: Anemia, including aplastic and hemolytic.

Hepatobiliary: Jaundice; hepatitis, including rare cases of necrosis; cholestasis.

Metabolic: Symptomatic hyponatremia.

Musculoskeletal: Myalgia, myasthenia.

Nervous/Psychiatric: Ataxia, confusion, depression, nervousness, somnolence.

Respiratory: Bronchospasm, eosinophilic pneumonitis, rhinitis.

Special Senses: Blurred vision.

Urogenital: Impotence.

As with other ACE inhibitors, a syndrome has been reported which may include: Fever, myalgia, arthralgia, interstitial nephritis, vasculitis, rash or other dermatologic manifestations, eosinophilia and an elevated ESR.

FETAL/NEONATAL MORBIDITY AND MORTALITY

See WARNINGS, Fetal/Neonatal Morbidity and Mortality.

ALTERED LABORATORY FINDINGS

Serum Electrolytes: *Hyperkalemia:* Small increases in serum potassium, especially in patients with renal impairment (see PRECAUTIONS).

Hyponatremia: Particularly in patients receiving a low sodium diet or concomitant diuretics.

BUN/Serum Creatinine: Transient elevations of BUN or serum creatinine especially in volume or salt depleted patients or those with renovascular hypertension may occur. Rapid reduction of longstanding or markedly elevated blood pressure can result in decreases in the glomerular filtration rate and, in turn, lead to increases in BUN or serum creatinine.

Hematologic: A positive ANA has been reported.

Liver Function Tests: Elevations of liver transaminases, alkaline phosphatase, and serum bilirubin have occurred.

DOSAGE AND ADMINISTRATION

Captopril should be taken 1 hour before meals. Dosage must be individualized.

HYPERTENSION

Initiation of therapy requires consideration of recent antihypertensive drug treatment, the extent of blood pressure elevation, salt restriction, and other clinical circumstances. If possible, discontinue the patient's previous antihypertensive drug regimen for 1 week before starting captopril.

The initial dose of captopril is 25 mg bid or tid. If satisfactory reduction of blood pressure has not been achieved after 1 or 2 weeks, the dose may be increased to 50 mg bid or tid. Concomitant sodium restriction may be beneficial when captopril is used alone.

The dose of captopril in hypertension usually does not exceed 50 mg tid. Therefore, if the blood pressure has not been satisfactorily controlled after 1-2 weeks at this dose, (and the patient is not already receiving a diuretic), a modest dose of a thiazide-type diuretic (*e.g.,* hydrochlorothiazide, 25 mg daily), should be added. The diuretic dose may be increased at 1-2 week intervals until its highest usual antihypertensive dose is reached.

If captopril is being started in a patient already receiving a diuretic, captopril therapy should be initiated under close medical supervision (see WARNINGS and DRUG INTERACTIONS regarding hypotension), with dosage and titration of captopril as noted above.

If further blood pressure reduction is required, the dose of captopril may be increased to 100 mg bid or tid and then, if necessary, to 150 mg bid or tid (while continuing the diuretic). The usual dose range is 25-150 mg bid or tid. A maximum daily dose of 450 mg captopril should not be exceeded.

For patients with severe hypertension (*e.g.,* accelerated or malignant hypertension), when temporary discontinuation of current antihypertensive therapy is not practical or desirable, or when prompt titration to more normotensive blood pressure levels is indicated, diuretic should be continued but other current antihypertensive medication stopped and captopril dosage promptly initiated at 25 mg bid or tid, under close medical supervision.

When necessitated by the patient's clinical condition, the daily dose of captopril may be increased every 24 hours or less under continuous medical supervision until a satisfactory blood pressure response is obtained or the maximum dose of captopril is reached. In this regimen, addition of a more potent diuretic, *e.g.,* furosemide, may also be indicated.

Beta-blockers may also be used in conjunction with captopril therapy (see DRUG INTERACTIONS), but the effects of the 2 drugs are less than additive.

HEART FAILURE

Initiation of therapy requires consideration of recent diuretic therapy and the possibility of severe salt/volume depletion. In patients with either normal or low blood pressure, who have been vigorously treated with diuretics and who may be hyponatremic and/or hypovolemic, a starting dose of 6.25 or 12.5 mg tid may minimize the magnitude or duration of the hypotensive effect (see WARNINGS, Hypotension); for these patients, titration to the usual daily dosage can then occur within the next several days.

For most patients the usual initial daily dosage is 25 mg tid. After a dose of 50 mg tid is reached, further increases in dosage should be delayed, where possible, for at least 2 weeks to determine if a satisfactory response occurs. Most patients studied have had a satisfactory clinical improvement at 50 or 100 mg tid. A maximum daily dose of 450 mg of captopril should not be exceeded.

Captopril should generally be used in conjunction with a diuretic and digitalis. Captopril therapy must be initiated under very close medical supervision.

LEFT VENTRICULAR DYSFUNCTION AFTER MYOCARDIAL INFARCTION

The recommended dose for long-term use in patients following a myocardial infarction is a target maintenance dose of 50 mg tid.

Therapy may be initiated as early as 3 days following a myocardial infarction. After a single dose of 6.25 mg captopril therapy should be initiated at 12.5 mg tid. Captopril should then be increased to 25 mg tid during the next several days and to a target dose of 50 mg tid over the next several weeks as tolerated (see CLINICAL PHARMACOLOGY).

Captopril may be used in patients treated with other post-myocardial infarction therapies, *e.g.*, thrombolytics, aspirin, beta blockers.

DIABETIC NEPHROPATHY

The recommended dose of captopril for long term use to treat diabetic nephropathy is 25 mg tid.

Other antihypertensives such as diuretics, beta blockers, centrally acting agents or vasodilators may be used in conjunction with captopril if additional therapy is required to further lower blood pressure.

DOSAGE ADJUSTMENT IN RENAL IMPAIRMENT

Because captopril is excreted primarily by the kidneys, excretion rates are reduced in patients with impaired renal function. These patients will take longer to reach steady-state captopril levels and will reach higher steady-state levels for a given daily dose than patients with normal renal function. Therefore, these patients may respond to smaller or less frequent doses.

Accordingly, for patients with significant renal impairment, initial daily dosage of captopril should be reduced, and smaller increments utilized for titration, which should be quite slow (1-2 week intervals). After the desired therapeutic effect has been achieved, the dose should be slowly back-titrated to determine the minimal effective dose. When concomitant diuretic therapy is required, a loop diuretic (*e.g.*, furosemide), rather than a thiazide diuretic, is preferred in patients with severe renal impairment. (See WARNINGS, Anaphylactoid Reactions During Membrane Exposure and PRECAUTIONS, Hemodialysis.)

ANIMAL PHARMACOLOGY

Chronic oral toxicity studies were conducted in rats (2 years), dogs (47 weeks; 1 year), mice (2 years), and monkeys (1 year). Significant drug-related toxicity included effects on hematopoiesis, renal toxicity, erosion/ulceration of the stomach, and variation of retinal blood vessels.

Reductions in hemoglobin and/or hematocrit values were seen in mice, rats, and monkeys at doses 50-150 times the maximum recommended human dose (MRHD) of 450 mg, assuming a 50 kg subject. On a body-surface-area basis, these doses are 5-25 times the maximum recommended human dose (MRHD). Anemia, leukopenia, thrombocytopenia, and bone marrow suppression occurred in dogs at doses 8-30 times MRHD on a body-weight basis (4- 15 times MRHD on a surface-area basis). The reductions in hemoglobin and hematocrit values in rats and mice were only significant at 1 year and returned to normal with continued dosing by the end of the study. Marked anemia was seen at all dose levels (8-30 times MRHD) in dogs, whereas moderate to marked leukopenia was noted only at 15 and 30 times the MRHD and thrombocytopenia at 30 times MRHD. The anemia could be reversed upon discontinuation of dosing. Bone marrow suppression occurred to a varying degree, being associated only with dogs that died or were sacrificed in a moribund condition in the 1 year study. However, in the 47 week study at a dose 30 times MRHD, bone marrow suppression was found to be reversible upon continued drug administration.

Captopril caused hyperplasia of the juxtaglomerular apparatus of the kidneys in mice and rats at doses 7-200 times MRHD on a body-weight basis (0.6 to 35 times MRHD on a surface-area basis); in monkeys at 20-60 times MRHD on a body-weight basis (7-20 times MRHD on a surface-area basis); and in dogs at 30 times MRHD on a body-weight basis (15 times MRHD on a surface-area basis).

Gastric erosions/ulcerations were increased in incidence in male rats at 20-200 times MRHD on a body-weight basis (3.5 and 35 times MRHD on a surface-area basis); in dogs at 30 times MRHD on a body-weight basis (15 times on MRHD on a surface-area basis); and in monkeys at 65 times MRHD on a body-weight basis (20 times MRHD on a surface-area basis). Rabbits developed gastric and intestinal ulcers when given oral doses approximately 30 times MRHD on a body-weight basis (10 times MRHD on a surface-area basis) for only 5-7 days.

In the 2 year rat study, irreversible and progressive variations in the caliber of retinal vessels (focal sacculations and constrictions) occurred at all dose levels (7-200 times MRHD) on a body-weight basis; 1-35 times MRHD on a surface-area basis in a dose-related fashion. The effect was first observed in the 88th week of dosing, with a progressively increased incidence thereafter, even after cessation of dosing.

HOW SUPPLIED

Captopril tablets are supplied as follows:

12.5 mg: White, round, biconvex tablets; one face embossed with "Endo" and partially scored, the other embossed with "721".

25 mg: White, round biconvex tablets; one face embossed with "Endo" and "722", the other plain and quadrisect scored.

50 mg: White, round, biconvex tablets; one face embossed with "Endo" and "724", the other plain and scored.

100 mg: White, round, biconvex tablets; one face embossed with "Endo" and "727", the other plain and scored.

All captopril tablets are white and may exhibit a slight sulfurous odor. Store at controlled room temperature, 15-30°C (59-86°F). Dispense in a tight container (protect from moisture).

PRODUCT LISTING - RATED THERAPEUTICALLY EQUIVALENT

Tablet - Oral - 12.5 mg

Size	Price	Product	NDC
25 x 30	$432.60	GENERIC, Sky Pharmaceuticals Packaging, Inc	63739-0042-03
25's	$19.60	CAPOTEN, Allscripts Pharmaceutical Company	54569-0522-01
30 x 25	$432.60	GENERIC, Sky Pharmaceuticals Packaging, Inc	63739-0042-01
30's	$19.75	CAPOTEN, Pharmaceutical Corporation Of America	51655-0975-24
30's	$33.24	CAPOTEN, Physicians Total Care	54868-1775-01
31 x 10	$199.95	GENERIC, Vangard Labs	00615-4519-53
31 x 10	$199.95	GENERIC, Vangard Labs	00615-4519-63
60's	$47.05	CAPOTEN, Allscripts Pharmaceutical Company	54569-0522-03
90's	$54.79	GENERIC, Golden State Medical	60429-0029-90
90's	$97.36	CAPOTEN, Physicians Total Care	54868-1775-04
100's	$3.98	FEDERAL UPPER LIMIT, H.C.F.A. F F P	99999-0642-01
100's	$58.06	GENERIC, Duramed Pharmaceuticals Inc	51875-0955-02
100's	$59.13	GENERIC, Warrick Pharmaceuticals Corporation	59930-1655-01
100's	$60.30	GENERIC, Eon Labs Manufacturing Inc	00185-0031-01
100's	$60.38	GENERIC, Teva Pharmaceuticals Usa	00093-0091-01
100's	$60.38	GENERIC, Ivax Corporation	00182-2622-01
100's	$60.38	GENERIC, Teva Pharmaceuticals Usa	55953-0132-40
100's	$61.28	GENERIC, Watson Laboratories Inc	52544-0688-01
100's	$63.00	GENERIC, West Ward Pharmaceutical Corporation	00143-1171-01
100's	$63.73	GENERIC, Martec Pharmaceuticals Inc	52555-0637-01
100's	$65.61	GENERIC, West Ward Pharmaceutical Corporation	00143-1171-25
100's	$70.66	GENERIC, Mova Pharmaceutical Corporation	55370-0164-07
100's	$70.67	GENERIC, Mylan Pharmaceuticals Inc	00378-3007-01
100's	$72.79	GENERIC, Udl Laboratories Inc	51079-0863-20
100's	$76.82	GENERIC, Par Pharmaceutical Inc	49884-0619-01
100's	$77.50	GENERIC, Stason Pharmaceuticals Inc	60763-1011-00
100's	$78.41	CAPOTEN, Allscripts Pharmaceutical Company	54569-0522-00
100's	$94.48	CAPOTEN, Bristol-Myers Squibb	00003-0450-51
100's	$118.74	CAPOTEN, Bristol-Myers Squibb	00003-0450-54
100's	$120.94	GENERIC, Duramed Pharmaceuticals Inc	51875-0355-01

Tablet - Oral - 25 mg

Size	Price	Product	NDC
25 x 30	$487.35	GENERIC, Sky Pharmaceuticals Packaging, Inc	63739-0043-03
25's	$6.92	GENERIC, Pd-Rx Pharmaceuticals	55289-0344-97
25's	$36.27	CAPOTEN, Pd-Rx Pharmaceuticals	55289-0506-97
30 x 25	$487.35	GENERIC, Sky Pharmaceuticals Packaging, Inc	63739-0043-01
30's	$4.79	GENERIC, Pd-Rx Pharmaceuticals	55289-0344-30
30's	$35.84	CAPOTEN, Physicians Total Care	54868-0669-02
31 x 10	$203.92	GENERIC, Vangard Labs	00615-4520-53
31 x 10	$203.92	GENERIC, Vangard Labs	00615-4520-63
60's	$39.64	GENERIC, Golden State Medical	60429-0030-60
60's	$61.37	CAPOTEN, Allscripts Pharmaceutical Company	54569-0523-02
60's	$70.49	CAPOTEN, Physicians Total Care	54868-0669-01
90's	$59.20	GENERIC, Golden State Medical	60429-0030-90
90's	$105.15	CAPOTEN, Physicians Total Care	54868-0669-06
100's	$4.42	FEDERAL UPPER LIMIT, H.C.F.A. F F P	99999-0642-02
100's	$63.93	GENERIC, Novopharm Usa Inc	55953-0133-40
100's	$63.93	GENERIC, Warrick Pharmaceuticals Corporation	59930-1656-01
100's	$65.00	GENERIC, Stason Pharmaceuticals Inc	60763-1012-00
100's	$65.00	GENERIC, Boscogen Inc	62033-0101-20
100's	$65.20	GENERIC, Eon Labs Manufacturing Inc	00185-0061-01
100's	$65.27	GENERIC, Teva Pharmaceuticals Usa	00093-0092-01
100's	$65.28	GENERIC, Ivax Corporation	00182-2623-01
100's	$66.25	GENERIC, Royce Laboratories Inc	51875-0348-01
100's	$66.25	GENERIC, Watson Laboratories Inc	52544-0689-01
100's	$68.25	GENERIC, West Ward Pharmaceutical Corporation	00143-1172-01
100's	$68.90	GENERIC, Martec Pharmaceuticals Inc	52555-0638-01
100's	$70.25	GENERIC, West Ward Pharmaceutical Corporation	00143-1172-25
100's	$75.69	GENERIC, Mova Pharmaceutical Corporation	55370-0142-07
100's	$75.71	GENERIC, Mylan Pharmaceuticals Inc	00378-3012-01
100's	$77.98	GENERIC, Udl Laboratories Inc	51079-0864-20
100's	$82.29	GENERIC, Par Pharmaceutical Inc	49884-0620-01

100's	$102.29	CAPOTEN, Allscripts Pharmaceutical Company	54569-0523-00
100's	$110.19	CAPOTEN, Bristol-Myers Squibb	00003-0452-51
100's	$110.29	CAPOTEN, Physicians Total Care	54868-0669-03
100's	$128.37	CAPOTEN, Bristol-Myers Squibb	00003-0452-50
100's	$814.67	GENERIC, Par Pharmaceutical Inc	49884-0620-10
120's	$78.65	GENERIC, Golden State Medical	60429-0030-12
120's	$132.11	CAPOTEN, Physicians Total Care	54868-0669-05
270's	$176.15	GENERIC, Golden State Medical	60429-0030-27
Tablet - Oral - 50 mg			
30's	$4.37	GENERIC, Pd-Rx Pharmaceuticals	55289-0212-30
30's	$33.78	GENERIC, Vangard Labs	00615-4521-65
30's	$340.70	GENERIC, Golden State Medical	60429-0031-30
31 x 10	$349.09	GENERIC, Vangard Labs	00615-4521-63
60's	$67.61	GENERIC, Golden State Medical	60429-0031-60
60's	$120.05	CAPOTEN, Physicians Total Care	54868-1415-01
90's	$1011.60	GENERIC, Golden State Medical	60429-0031-90
100's	$8.92	FEDERAL UPPER LIMIT, H.C.F.A. F F P	99999-0642-03
100's	$100.50	GENERIC, Stason Pharmaceuticals Inc	60763-1013-00
100's	$109.62	GENERIC, Warrick Pharmaceuticals Corporation	59930-1657-01
100's	$111.82	GENERIC, Eon Labs Manufacturing Inc	00185-0471-01
100's	$111.90	GENERIC, Moore, H.L. Drug Exchange Inc	00839-7996-06
100's	$111.93	GENERIC, Teva Pharmaceuticals Usa	00093-0097-01
100's	$111.93	GENERIC, Novopharm Usa Inc	55953-0134-40
100's	$111.94	GENERIC, Ivax Corporation	00182-2624-01
100's	$113.61	GENERIC, Royce Laboratories Inc	51875-0349-01
100's	$113.61	GENERIC, Watson Laboratories Inc	52544-0690-01
100's	$116.50	GENERIC, West Ward Pharmaceutical Corporation	00143-1173-01
100's	$118.15	GENERIC, Martec Pharmaceuticals Inc	52555-0639-01
100's	$119.50	GENERIC, West Ward Pharmaceutical Corporation	00143-1173-25
100's	$131.45	GENERIC, Mova Pharmaceutical Corporation	55370-0144-07
100's	$131.46	GENERIC, Mylan Pharmaceuticals Inc	00378-3017-01
100's	$142.93	GENERIC, Par Pharmaceutical Inc	49884-0621-01
100's	$220.12	CAPOTEN, Bristol-Myers Squibb	00003-0482-50
100's	$226.73	CAPOTEN, Bristol-Myers Squibb	00003-0482-51
100's	$1396.74	GENERIC, Par Pharmaceutical Inc	49884-0621-10
120's	$135.05	GENERIC, Golden State Medical	60429-0031-12
270's	$303.16	GENERIC, Golden State Medical	60429-0031-27
Tablet - Oral - 100 mg			
100's	$18.67	FEDERAL UPPER LIMIT, H.C.F.A. F F P	99999-0642-04
100's	$148.00	GENERIC, West Ward Pharmaceutical Corporation	00143-1174-01
100's	$148.90	GENERIC, Eon Labs Manufacturing Inc	00185-0591-01
100's	$148.97	GENERIC, Moore, H.L. Drug Exchange Inc	00839-8064-06
100's	$149.98	GENERIC, Teva Pharmaceuticals Usa	00093-0098-01
100's	$149.98	GENERIC, Novopharm Usa Inc	55953-0135-40
100's	$149.98	GENERIC, Warrick Pharmaceuticals Corporation	59930-1658-01
100's	$149.99	GENERIC, Ivax Corporation	00182-2625-01
100's	$149.99	GENERIC, Qualitest Products Inc	00603-2558-21
100's	$151.29	GENERIC, Royce Laboratories Inc	51875-0350-01
100's	$151.29	GENERIC, Watson Laboratories Inc	52544-0691-01
100's	$151.50	GENERIC, West Ward Pharmaceutical Corporation	00143-1174-25
100's	$155.02	GENERIC, Geneva Pharmaceuticals	00781-1839-01
100's	$155.82	GENERIC, Martec Pharmaceuticals Inc	52555-0640-01
100's	$159.43	GENERIC, Watson/Rugby Laboratories Inc	00536-3474-01
100's	$172.60	GENERIC, Mova Pharmaceutical Corporation	55370-0145-07
100's	$172.62	GENERIC, Mylan Pharmaceuticals Inc	00378-3022-01
100's	$187.66	GENERIC, Par Pharmaceutical Inc	49884-0622-01
100's	$293.14	CAPOTEN, Bristol-Myers Squibb	00003-0485-50
100's	$293.14	CAPOTEN, Par Pharmaceutical Inc	49884-0796-01

PRODUCT LISTING - EQUIVALENTS NOT AVAILABLE

Tablet - Oral - 12.5 mg			
30's	$2.56	GENERIC, Physicians Total Care	54868-3723-01
60's	$42.40	GENERIC, Allscripts Pharmaceutical Company	54569-4593-01
100's	$54.95	GENERIC, Major Pharmaceuticals Inc	00904-5045-60
100's	$60.29	GENERIC, Vha Supply	59772-7045-07
100's	$60.39	GENERIC, Vha Supply	59772-7045-06
100's	$62.54	GENERIC, Allscripts Pharmaceutical Company	54569-4593-00
100's	$64.57	GENERIC, Watson/Rugby Laboratories Inc	00536-3471-01
100's	$70.00	GENERIC, Apothecon Inc	59772-7045-01
Tablet - Oral - 25 mg			
20's	$15.14	GENERIC, Allscripts Pharmaceutical Company	54569-4246-01
30's	$2.66	GENERIC, Physicians Total Care	54868-3724-01
30's	$22.71	GENERIC, Allscripts Pharmaceutical Company	54569-4246-05
60's	$45.43	GENERIC, Allscripts Pharmaceutical Company	54569-4246-03
90's	$5.32	GENERIC, Physicians Total Care	54868-3724-02
90's	$68.14	GENERIC, Allscripts Pharmaceutical Company	54569-4246-04
100's	$5.76	GENERIC, Physicians Total Care	54868-3724-03
100's	$64.95	GENERIC, Major Pharmaceuticals Inc	00904-5046-60
100's	$65.78	GENERIC, Apothecon Inc	59772-7046-05
100's	$67.80	GENERIC, Allscripts Pharmaceutical Company	54569-4246-00
100's	$75.50	GENERIC, Apothecon Inc	59772-7046-01
Tablet - Oral - 50 mg			
30's	$4.61	GENERIC, Physicians Total Care	54868-3725-02
60's	$78.88	GENERIC, Allscripts Pharmaceutical Company	54569-4247-02
90's	$118.31	GENERIC, Allscripts Pharmaceutical Company	54569-4247-03
100's	$7.67	GENERIC, Physicians Total Care	54868-3725-01
100's	$109.95	GENERIC, Major Pharmaceuticals Inc	00904-5047-60
100's	$116.56	GENERIC, Allscripts Pharmaceutical Company	54569-4247-00
100's	$119.73	GENERIC, Watson/Rugby Laboratories Inc	00536-3473-01
100's	$131.00	GENERIC, Apothecon Inc	59772-7047-01
Tablet - Oral - 100 mg			
100's	$129.95	GENERIC, Major Pharmaceuticals Inc	00904-5048-60
100's	$172.00	GENERIC, Apothecon Inc	59772-7048-01

Captopril; Hydrochlorothiazide *(000643)*

For complete prescribing information, refer to the CD-ROM included with the book.

Categories: Hypertension, essential; Pregnancy Category C; FDA Approved 1984 Oct
Drug Classes: Angiotensin converting enzyme inhibitors; Diuretics, thiazide and derivatives
Brand Names: Aceaide; **Capozide**
Foreign Brand Availability: Acediur (Italy); Acenorm (Germany); Aceplus (Italy; Netherlands); Acezide (England); Adcomp (Germany); Capozid (Denmark); Capozide Forte (Austria); Captea (France); Captoprilan-D (Dominican-Republic); Cesplon Plus (Spain); Ecazide (France); Jutacor Comp (Bahrain; Cyprus; Egypt; Germany; Iran; Iraq; Israel; Jordan; Kuwait; Lebanon; Libya; Oman; Qatar; Republic-of-Yemen; Saudi-Arabia; Syria; United-Arab-Emirates); Lopiretic (Portugal); Zapto-Co (South-Africa)
Cost of Therapy: $80.49 (Hypertension; Capozide 25/15; 25 mg; 15 mg; 2 tablets/day; 30 day supply)
$47.75 (Hypertension; Generic Tablets; 25 mg; 15 mg; 2 tablets/day; 30 day supply)

WARNING

USE IN PREGNANCY:

When used in pregnancy during the second and third semesters, ACE inhibitors can cause injury and even death to the developing fetus. When pregnancy is detected, captopril hydrochlorothiazide should be discontinued as soon as possible. See WARNINGS, Captopril, Fetal/Neonatal Morbidity and Mortality.

DESCRIPTION

Captopril hydrochlorothiazide for oral administration combines two antihypertensive agents: Capoten (captopril) and hydrochlorothiazide. Captopril, the first of a new class of antihypertensive agents, is a specific competitive inhibitor of angiotensin I-converting enzyme (ACE), the enzyme responsible for the conversion of angiotensin I to angiotensin II. Hydrochlorothiazide is a benzothiadiazide (thiazide) diuretic-antihypertensive. Capozide tablets are available in 4 combinations of captopril with hydrochlorothiazide: 25 mg with 15 mg, 25 mg with 25 mg, 50 mg with 15 mg, and 50 mg with 25 mg. *Inactive ingredients:* Microcrystalline cellulose, colorant (FD&C yellow no. 6), lactose, magnesium stearate, pregelatinized starch, and stearic acid.

Captopril is designated chemically a 1-[(2S)-3-mercapto-2-methylpropionyl]-L-proline; hydrochlorothiazide is 6-Chloro-3,4-dihydro-2*H*-1,2,4-benzothiadiazine-7-sulfonamide 1,1-dioxide.

Captopril is a white to off-white crystalline powder that may have a light sulfurous odor; it is soluble in water (approx. 160 mg/ml), methanol, and ethanol and sparingly soluble in chloroform and ethyl acetate.

Hydrochlorothiazide is a white crystalline powder slightly soluble in water but freely soluble in sodium hydroxide solution.

INDICATIONS AND USAGE

Captopril hydrochlorothiazide is indicated for the treatment of hypertension. The blood pressure lowering effects of captopril and thiazides are approximately additive.

This fixed combination drug may be used as initial therapy or substituted for previously titrated doses of the individual components.

When captopril and hydrochlorothiazide are given together it may not be necessary to administer captopril in divided doses to attain blood pressure control at trough (before the next dose). Also, with such a combination, a daily dose of 15 mg of hydrochlorothiazide may be adequate.

Treatment may, therefore, be initiated with captopril hydrochlorothiazide 25 mg/15 mg once daily. Subsequent titration should be with additional doses of the components (captopril, hydrochlorothiazide) as single agents or as captopril hydrochlorothiazide 50 mg/15 mg, 25 mg/25 mg, or 50 mg/25 mg (see DOSAGE AND ADMINISTRATION).

In using captopril hydrochlorothiazide, consideration should be given to the risk of neutropenia/agranulocytosis (see WARNINGS).

Captopril hydrochlorothiazide may be used for patients with normal renal function, in whom the risk is relatively low. In patients with impaired renal function, particularly those with collagen vascular disease, captopril hydrochlorothiazide should be reserved for hypertensives who have either developed unacceptable side effects on other drugs, or have failed to respond satisfactorily to other drug combinations.

NON-FDA APPROVED INDICATIONS

Captopril hydrochlorothiazide is also used without FDA approval for the treatment of congestive heart failure.

CONTRAINDICATIONS

CAPTOPRIL

This product is contraindicated in patients who are hypersensitive to captopril or any other angiotensin-converting enzyme inhibitor (*e.g.*, a patient who has experienced angioedema during therapy with any other ACE inhibitor).

HYDROCHLOROTHIAZIDE

Hydrochlorothiazide is contraindicated in anuria. It is also contraindicated in patients who have previously demonstrated hypersensitivity to hydrochlorothiazide or other sulfonamide-derived drugs.

WARNINGS

CAPTOPRIL

Angioedema

Angioedema involving the extremities, face, lips, mucous membranes, tongue, glottis or larynx has been seen in patients treated with ACE inhibitors, including captopril. If angioedema involves the tongue, glottis or larynx, airway obstruction may occur and be fatal. Emergency therapy, including but not necessarily limited to, subcutaneous administration of a 1:1000 solution of epinephrine should be promptly instituted.

Swelling confined to the face, mucous membranes of the mouth, lips and extremities has usually resolved with discontinuation of treatment; some cases required medical therapy.

Neutropenia/Agranulocytosis

Neutropenia($<1000/mm^3$) with myeloid hypoplasia has resulted from use of captopril. About half of the neutropenic patients developed systemic or oral cavity infections or other features of the syndrome of agranulocytosis.

The risk of neutropenia is dependent on the clinical status of the patient

In clinical trials in patients with hypertension who have normal renal function (serum creatinine less than 1.6 mg/dl and no collagen vascular disease), neutropenia has been seen in one patient out of over 8600 exposed.

In patients with some degree of renal failure (serum creatinine at least 1.6 mg/dl) but no collagen vascular disease, the risk of neutropenia in clinical trials was about 1/500, a frequency over 15 times that for uncomplicated hypertension. Daily doses of captopril were relatively high in these patients, particularly in view of their diminished renal function. In foreign marketing experience in patients with renal failure, use of allopurinol concomitantly with captopril has been associated with neutropenia but this association has not appeared in US reports.

In patients with collagen vascular diseases (*e.g.*, systemic lupus erythematosus, scleroderma) and impaired renal function, neutropenia occurred in 3.7% of patients in clinical trials.

While none of the over 750 patients in formal clinical trials of heart failure developed neutropenia, it has occurred during the subsequent clinical experience. About half of the reported cases had serum creatinine $\geq$1.6 mg/dl and more than 75% were in patients also receiving procainamide. In heart failure, it appears that the same risk factors for neutropenia are present.

The neutropenia has usually been detected within 3 months after captopril was started. Bone marrow examinations in patients with neutropenia consistently showed myeloid hypoplasia, frequently accompanied by erythroid hypoplasia and decreased numbers of megakaryocytes (*e.g.*, hypoplastic bone marrow and pancytopenia); anemia and thrombocytopenia were sometimes seen.

In general, neutrophils returned to normal in about 2 weeks after captopril was discontinued, and serious infections were limited to clinically complex patients. About 13% of the cases of neutropenia have ended fatally, but almost all fatalities were in patients with serious illness, having collagen vascular disease, renal failure, heart failure or immunosuppressant therapy, or a combination of these complicating factors.

Evaluation of the hypertensive or heart failure patient should always include assessment of renal function. If captopril is used in patients with impaired renal function, white blood cell and differential counts should be evaluated prior to starting treatment and at approximately 2 week intervals for about three months, then periodically.

In patients with collagen vascular disease or who are exposed to other drugs known to affect the white cells or immune response, particularly when there is impaired renal function, captopril should be used only after an assessment of benefit and risk, and then with caution.

All patients treated with captopril should be told to report any signs of infection (*e.g.*, sore throat, fever). If infection is suspected, white cell counts should be performed without delay.

Since discontinuation of captopril and other drugs has generally led to prompt return of the white count to normal, upon confirmation of neutropenia (neutrophil count $<1000/mm^3$) the physician should withdraw captopril and closely follow the patient's course.

Proteinuria

Total urinary proteins greater than 1 g/day were seen in about 0.7% of patients receiving captopril. About 90% of affected patients had evidence of prior renal disease or received relatively high doses of captopril (in excess of 150 mg/day), or both. The nephrotic syndrome occurred in about one-fifth of proteinuric patients. In most cases, proteinuria subsided or cleared within 6 months whether or not captopril was continued. Parameters of renal function, such as BUN and creatinine, were seldom altered in the patients with proteinuria.

Since most cases of proteinuria occurred by the eighth month of therapy with captopril, patients with prior renal disease or those receiving captopril at doses greater than 150 mg/day, should have urinary protein estimations (dip-stick on first morning urine) prior to treatment, and periodically thereafter.

Hypotension

Excessive hypotension was rarely seen in hypertensive patients but is a possible consequence of captopril use in salt/volume depleted persons (such as those treated vigorously with diuretics), patients with heart failure or those patients undergoing renal dialysis.

Fetal/Neonatal Morbidity and Mortality

ACE inhibitors can cause fetal and neonatal morbidity and mortality when administered to pregnant women. Several dozen cases have been reported in the world literature. When pregnancy is detected, ACE inhibitors should be discontinued as soon as possible.

The use of ACE inhibitors have been used during the second and third trimesters of pregnancy has been associated with fetal and neonatal injury, including hypotension, neonatal skull hypoplasia, anuria, reversible or irreversible renal failure and death. Oligohydramnios has also been reported, presumably representing decreased renal function; oligohydramnios in this setting has been associated with fetal limb contractures, craniofacial deformation, and hypoplastic lung development. Prematurity, intrauterine growth retardation, and patent ductus arteriosus have also been reported, although it is not clear whether these occurrences were due to the ACE inhibitor exposure.

The adverse effects do not appear to have resulted from intrauterine ACE-inhibitor exposure that has been limited to the first trimester. Mothers whose embryos and fetuses are exposed to ACE inhibitors only during the first trimester should be so informed. Nonetheless, when patients become pregnant, physicians should make every effort to discontinue the use of captopril as soon as possible.

Rarely (probably less often than once in every 1000 pregnancies), no alternative to ACE inhibitors will be found. In these rare cases, the mothers should be apprised of the potential hazards to their fetuses, and serial ultrasound examinations should be performed to assess the intraamniotic environment.

If oligohydramnios is observed, captopril should be discontinued unless it is considered life-saving to the mother. Contraction stress testing (CST), a non-stress test (NST), or biophysical profiling (BPP) may be appropriate, depending upon the week of pregnancy. Patients and physicians should be aware, however, that oligohydramnios may not appear until after the fetus has sustained irreversible injury.

Infants exposed *in utero* to ACE inhibitors should be closely observed for hypotension, oliguria, and hyperkalemia. If oliguria occurs, attention should be directed toward support of blood pressure and renal perfusion. Exchange transfusion or dialysis may be required as a means of reversing hypotension and/or substituting for disordered renal function. While captopril may be removed from the adult circulation by hemodialysis, there is inadequate data concerning the effectiveness of hemodialysis, there is inadequate data concerning the effectiveness of hemodialysis for removing it from the circulation of neonates or children. Peritoneal dialysis is not effective for removing captopril; there is no information concerning exchange transfusion for removing captopril from the general circulation.

When captopril was given to rabbits at doses about 0.8 to 70 times (on a mg/kg basis) the maximum recommended human dose, and low incidence of craniofacial malformations were seen. No teratogenic effect of captopril were seen in studies of pregnant rats and hamsters. On a mg/kg basis, the doses used were up to 150 times (in hamsters) and 625 times (in rats) the maximum recommended human dose.

HYDROCHLOROTHIAZIDE

Thiazides should be used with caution in severe renal disease. In patients with renal disease, thiazides may precipitate azotemia. Cumulative effects of the drug may develop in patients with impaired renal function.

Thiazides should be used with caution in patients with impaired hepatic function or progressive liver disease, since minor alterations of fluid and electrolyte balance may precipitate hepatic coma.

Sensitivity reactions may occur in patients with or without a history of allergy or bronchial asthma.

The possibility of exacerbation or activation of systemic lupus erythematosus has been reported.

In general, lithium should not be given with diuretics.

DOSAGE AND ADMINISTRATION

DOSAGE MUST BE INDIVIDUALIZED ACCORDING TO PATIENT'S RESPONSE.

Captopril hydrochlorothiazide may be substituted for the previously titrated individual components.

Alternatively, therapy may be instituted with a single tablet of captopril hydrochlorothiazide 25 mg/15 mg taken once daily. For patients insufficiently responsive to the initial dose, additional captopril or hydrochlorothiazide may be added as individual components or by using captopril hydrochlorothiazide 50 mg/15 mg, 25 mg/25 mg or 50 mg/25 mg, or divided doses may be used.

Because the full effect of a given dose may not be attained for 6-8 weeks, dosage adjustments should generally be made at 6 week intervals, unless the clinical situation demands more rapid adjustment.

In general, daily doses of captopril should not exceed 150 mg and of hydrochlorothiazide should not exceed 50 mg.

DOSAGE ADJUSTMENT IN RENAL IMPAIRMENT

Because captopril and hydrochlorothiazide are excreted primarily by the kidneys, excretion rates are reduced in patients with impaired renal function. These patients will take longer to reach steady-state captopril levels and will reach higher steady-state levels for a given daily dose than patients with normal renal function. Therefore, these patients may respond to smaller or less frequent doses of captopril hydrochlorothiazide.

After the desired therapeutic effect has been achieved, the dose intervals should be increased or the total daily dose reduced until the minimal effective dose is achieved. When concomitant diuretic therapy is required in patients with severe renal impairment, a loop diuretic (*e.g.*, furosemide), rather than a thiazide diuretic is preferred for use with captopril; therefore, for patients with severe renal dysfunction the captopril-hydrochlorothiazide combination tablet is not usually recommended.

PRODUCT LISTING - RATED THERAPEUTICALLY EQUIVALENT

Tablet - Oral - 25 mg;15 mg

30's	$30.36	CAPOZIDE 25/15, Physicians Total Care	54868-3769-00
100's	$23.59	FEDERAL UPPER LIMIT, H.C.F.A. F F P	99999-0643-01
100's	$71.78	GENERIC, Teva Pharmaceuticals Usa	00093-0176-01

100's	$72.14	GENERIC, Endo Laboratories Llc	60951-0733-70
100's	$77.59	GENERIC, Ivax Corporation	00172-2515-60
100's	$79.59	GENERIC, Mylan Pharmaceuticals Inc	00378-0081-01
100's	$134.15	CAPOZIDE 25/15, Bristol-Myers Squibb	00003-0338-50
Tablet - Oral - 25 mg;25 mg			
100's	$67.69	GENERIC, Endo Laboratories Llc	60951-0741-70
100's	$71.78	GENERIC, Teva Pharmaceuticals Usa	00093-0177-01
100's	$77.59	GENERIC, Ivax Corporation	00172-2525-60
100's	$79.59	GENERIC, Mylan Pharmaceuticals Inc	00378-0083-01
Tablet - Oral - 50 mg;15 mg			
100's	$115.42	GENERIC, Endo Laboratories Llc	60951-0739-70
100's	$123.28	GENERIC, Teva Pharmaceuticals Usa	00093-0181-01
100's	$134.61	GENERIC, Ivax Corporation	00172-5015-60
100's	$136.61	GENERIC, Mylan Pharmaceuticals Inc	00378-0084-01
Tablet - Oral - 50 mg;25 mg			
30's	$47.59	CAPOZIDE 50/25, Physicians Total Care	54868-3891-00
100's	$37.02	FEDERAL UPPER LIMIT, H.C.F.A. F F P	99999-0643-04
100's	$115.42	GENERIC, Endo Laboratories Llc	60951-0731-70
100's	$123.28	GENERIC, Teva Pharmaceuticals Usa	00093-0182-01
100's	$134.61	GENERIC, Ivax Corporation	00172-5025-60
100's	$136.61	GENERIC, Mylan Pharmaceuticals Inc	00378-0086-01
100's	$230.42	CAPOZIDE 50/25, Bristol-Myers Squibb	00003-0390-50

PRODUCT LISTING - EQUIVALENTS NOT AVAILABLE

Tablet - Oral - 25 mg;15 mg			
100's	$79.25	GENERIC, Apothecon Inc	59772-5160-05
Tablet - Oral - 25 mg;25 mg			
100's	$79.25	GENERIC, Apothecon Inc	59772-5161-05
100's	$123.42	CAPOZIDE 25/25, Bristol-Myers Squibb	00003-0349-50
Tablet - Oral - 50 mg;15 mg			
100's	$135.00	GENERIC, Apothecon Inc	59772-5162-05
100's	$196.29	CAPOZIDE 50/15, Bristol-Myers Squibb	00003-0384-50
Tablet - Oral - 50 mg;25 mg			
100's	$135.00	GENERIC, Apothecon Inc	59772-5163-05

Carbamazepine *(000646)*

Categories: Neuralgia, glossopharyngeal; Neuralgia, trigeminal; Seizures, complex partial; Seizures, generalized tonic-clonic; Seizures, mixed pattern; Pregnancy Category C; FDA Approved 1968 Mar; WHO Formulary

Drug Classes: Anticonvulsants

Brand Names: Atretol; Convuline; Epitol; Macrepan; **Tegretol**

Foreign Brand Availability: Apo-Carbamazepine (Canada; Malaysia); Camapine (Taiwan; Thailand); Carbadac (Benin; Burkina-Faso; Ethiopia; Gambia; Ghana; Guinea; Ivory-Coast; Kenya; Liberia; Malawi; Mali; Mauritania; Mauritius; Morocco; Niger; Nigeria; Senegal; Seychelles; Sierra-Leone; South-Africa; Sudan; Tanzania; Tunia; Uganda; Zambia; Zimbabwe); Carbatol (India); Carbazene (Thailand); Carbazep (Mexico); Carbazina (Mexico); Carmaz (India); Carpaz (South-Africa); Carzepin (Malaysia); Carzepine (Thailand); Clostedal (Mexico); Degranol (South-Africa); Epileptol (Korea); Epileptol CR (Korea); Eposal Retard (Colombia); Espa-lepsin (Germany); Foxalepsin (Germany); Foxalepsin Retard (Germany); Hermolepsin (Sweden); Karbamazepin (Sweden); Kodapan (Japan); Lexin (Japan); Mazetol (India; Malaysia); Neugeron (Costa-Rica; Dominican-Republic; Guatemala; Honduras; Mexico; Nicaragua; Panama); Neurotol (Finland); Neurotop (Austria; Hungary; Malaysia); Neurotop Retard (Malaysia); Nordotol (Denmark; Mexico); Panitol (Thailand); Sirtal (Germany); Tardotol (Denmark); Taver (Thailand); Tegol (Taiwan); Tegretal (Germany); Tegretol CR (Australia; Israel; Korea; New-Zealand; South-Africa); Tegretol-S (South-Africa); Telesmin (Japan); Temporol (Bulgaria; South-Africa); Temporal Slow (Bahrain; Cyprus; Egypt; Hungary; Iran; Iraq; Israel; Jordan; Kuwait; Lebanon; Libya; Oman; Qatar; Republic-of-Yemen; Saudi-Arabia; Syria; United-Arab-Emirates); Teril (Australia; Hong-Kong; Israel; New-Zealand; Taiwan); Timonil (Germany; Israel); Timonil Retard (Germany; Israel; Switzerland)

Cost of Therapy: $53.40 (Epilepsy; Tegretol; 200 mg; 4 tablets/day; 30 day supply)
$13.55 (Epilepsy; Generic Tablets; 200 mg; 4 tablets/day; 30 day supply)
$71.83 (Epilepsy; Tegretol XR; 200 mg; 4 tablets/day; 30 day supply)

WARNING

APLASTIC ANEMIA AND AGRANULOCYTOSIS HAVE BEEN REPORTED IN ASSOCIATION WITH THE USE OF CARBAMAZEPINE. DATA FROM A POPULATION-BASED CASE CONTROL STUDY DEMONSTRATE THAT THE RISK OF DEVELOPING THESE REACTIONS IS 5-8 TIMES GREATER THAN IN THE GENERAL POPULATION. HOWEVER, THE OVERALL RISK OF THESE REACTIONS IN THE UNTREATED GENERAL POPULATION IS LOW, APPROXIMATELY SIX PATIENTS PER ONE MILLION POPULATION PER YEAR FOR AGRANULOCYTOSIS AND TWO PATIENTS PER ONE MILLION POPULATION PER YEAR FOR APLASTIC ANEMIA.

ALTHOUGH REPORTS OF TRANSIENT OR PERSISTENT DECREASED PLATELET OR WHITE BLOOD CELL COUNTS ARE NOT UNCOMMON IN ASSOCIATION WITH THE USE OF CARBAMAZEPINE, DATA ARE NOT AVAILABLE TO ESTIMATE ACCURATELY THEIR INCIDENCE OR OUTCOME. HOWEVER, THE VAST MAJORITY OF THE CASES OF LEUKOPENIA HAVE NOT PROGRESSED TO THE MORE SERIOUS CONDITIONS OF APLASTIC ANEMIA OR AGRANULOCYTOSIS.

BECAUSE OF THE VERY LOW INCIDENCE OF AGRANULOCYTOSIS AND APLASTIC ANEMIA, THE VAST MAJORITY OF MINOR HEMATOLOGIC CHANGES OBSERVED IN MONITORING OF PATIENTS ON CARBAMAZEPINE ARE UNLIKELY TO SIGNAL THE OCCURRENCE OF EITHER ABNORMALITY. NONETHELESS, COMPLETE PRETREATMENT HEMATOLOGICAL TESTING SHOULD BE OBTAINED AS BASELINE. IF A PATIENT IN THE COURSE OF TREATMENT EXHIBITS LOW OR DECREASED WHITE BLOOD CELL OR PLATELET COUNTS, THE PATIENT SHOULD BE MONITORED CLOSELY. DISCONTINUATION OF THE DRUG SHOULD BE CONSIDERED IF ANY EVIDENCE OF SIGNIFICANT BONE MARROW DEPRESSION DEVELOPS.

DESCRIPTION

Before prescribing carbamazepine, the physician should be thoroughly familiar with the details of this prescribing information, particularly regarding use with other drugs, especially those which accentuate toxicity potential.

Tegretol, carbamazepine, is an anticonvulsant and specific analgesic for trigeminal neuralgia, available for oral administration as chewable tablets of 100 mg, tablets of 200 mg, extended-release tablets of 100, 200, and 400 mg, and as a suspension of 100 mg/5 ml (teaspoon). Its chemical name is 5*H*-dibenz(*b,f*)azepine-5-carboxamide.

Carbamazepine is a white to off-white powder, practically insoluble in water and soluble in alcohol and in acetone. It molecular weight is 236.27.

Tegretol Inactive Ingredients:

Tegretol Tablets: Colloidal silicon dioxide, D&C red no. 30 aluminum lake (chewable tablets only), FD&C red no. 40 (200 mg tablets only), flavoring (chewable tablets only), gelatin, glycerin, magnesium stearate, sodium starch glycolate (chewable tablets only), starch, stearic acid, and sucrose (chewable tablets only).

Tegretol Suspension: Citric acid, FD&C yellow no. 6, flavoring, polymer, potassium sorbate, propylene glycol, purified water, sorbitol, sucrose, and xanthan gum.

Tegretol XR Tablets: Cellulose compounds, dextrates, iron oxides, magnesium stearate, mannitol, polyethylene glycol, sodium lauryl sulfate, titanium dioxide (200 mg tablets only).

CLINICAL PHARMACOLOGY

In controlled clinical trials, carbamazepine has been shown to be effective in the treatment of psychomotor and grand mal seizures, as well as trigeminal neuralgia.

MECHANISM OF ACTION

Carbamazepine has demonstrated anticonvulsant properties in rats and mice with electrically and chemically induced seizures. It appears to act by reducing polysynaptic responses and blocking the post-tetanic potentiation. Carbamazepine greatly reduces or abolishes pain induced by stimulation of the infraorbital nerve in cats and rats. It depresses thalamic potential and bulbar and polysynaptic reflexes, including the linguomandibular reflex in cats. Carbamazepine is chemically unrelated to other anticonvulsants or other drugs used to control the pain of trigeminal neuralgia. The mechanism of action remains unknown.

The principal metabolite of carbamazepine, carbamazepine-10,11-epoxide, has anticonvulsant activity as demonstrated in several *in vivo* animal models of seizures. Though clinical activity for the epoxide has been postulated, the significance of its activity with respect to the safety and efficacy of carbamazepine has not been established.

PHARMACOKINETICS

In clinical studies carbamazepine suspension, conventional tablets and extended-release tablets delivered equivalent amounts of drug to the systemic circulation. However, the suspension was absorbed somewhat faster, and the extended-release tablet slightly slower, than the conventional tablet. The bioavailability of the extended-release tablet was 89% compared to suspension. Following a bid dosage regimen, the suspension provides higher peak levels and lower trough levels than those obtained from the conventional tablet for the same dosage regimen. On the other hand, following a tid dosage regimen, carbamazepine suspension affords steady-state plasma levels comparable to carbamazepine tablets given bid when administered at the same total mg daily dose. Following a bid regimen, carbamazepine extended-release tablets afford steady-state plasma levels comparable to conventional carbamazepine tablets given qid, when administered at the same total mg daily dose. Carbamazepine in blood is 76% bound to plasma proteins. Plasma levels of carbamazepine are variable and may range from 0.5-25 μg/ml, with no apparent relationship to the daily intake of the drug. Usual adult therapeutic levels are between 4 and 12 μg/ml. In polytherapy, the concentration of carbamazepine and concomitant drugs may be increased or decreased during therapy, and drug effects may be altered (see DRUG INTERACTIONS). Following chronic oral administration of suspension, plasma levels peak at approximately 1.5 hours compared to 4-5 hours after administration of conventional carbamazepine tablets, and 3-12 hours after administration of carbamazepine extended-release tablets. The CSF/serum ratio is 0.22, similar to the 24% unbound carbamazepine in serum. Because carbamazepine may induce its own metabolism, the half-life is also variable. Autoinduction is completed after 3-5 weeks of a fixed dosing regimen. Initial half-life values range from 25-65 hours, decreasing to 12-17 hours on repeated doses. Carbamazepine is metabolized in the liver. Cytochrome P450 3A4 was identified as the major isoform responsible for the formation of carbamazepine-10,11-epoxide from carbamazepine. After oral administration of ^{14}C-carbamazepine, 72% of the administered radioactivity was found in the urine and 28% in the feces. This urinary radioactivity was composed largely of hydroxylated and conjugated metabolites, with only 3% of unchanged carbamazepine.

The pharmacokinetic parameters of carbamazepine disposition are similar in children and in adults. However, there is a poor correlation between plasma concentrations of carbamazepine and carbamazepine dose in children. Carbamazepine is more rapidly metabolized to carbamazepine-10,11-epoxide (a metabolite shown to be equipotent to carbamazepine as an anticonvulsant in animal screens) in the younger age groups than in adults. In children below the age of 15, there is an inverse relationship between CBZ-E/CBZ ratio and increasing age (in one report from 0.44 in children below the age of 1 year to 0.18 in children between 10-15 years of age).

The effects of race and gender on carbamazepine pharmacokinetics have not been systematically evaluated.

INDICATIONS AND USAGE

EPILEPSY

Carbamazepine is indicated for use as an anticonvulsant drug. Evidence supporting efficacy of carbamazepine as an anticonvulsant was derived from active drug-controlled studies that enrolled patients with the following seizure types:

1. Partial seizures with complex symptomatology (psychomotor, temporal lobe). Patients with these seizures appear to show greater improvement than those with other types.
2. Generalized tonic-clonic seizures (grand mal).
3. Mixed seizure patterns which include the above, or other partial or generalized seizures. Absence seizures (petit mal) do not appear to be controlled by carbamazepine (see PRECAUTIONS, General).

TRIGEMINAL NEURALGIA

Carbamazepine is indicated in the treatment of the pain associated with true trigeminal neuralgia.

Beneficial results have also been reported in glossopharyngeal neuralgia.

This drug is not a simple analgesic and should not be used for the relief of trivial aches or pains.

NON-FDA APPROVED INDICATIONS

Carbamazepine has also been used for the treatment of bipolar disorder and diabetic neuropathy, although these uses are not FDA approved.

CONTRAINDICATIONS

Carbamazepine should not be used in patients with a history of previous bone marrow depression, hypersensitivity to the drug, or known sensitivity to any of the tricyclic compounds such as amitriptyline, desipramine, imipramine, protriptyline, nortriptyline, etc. Likewise, on theoretical grounds its use with monoamine oxidase inhibitors is not recommended. Before administration of carbamazepine, MAO inhibitors should be discontinued for a minimum of 14 days, or longer if the clinical situation permits.

WARNINGS

Patients with a history of adverse hematologic reaction to any drug may be particularly at risk.

Severe dermatologic reactions including toxic epidermal necrolysis (Lyell's syndrome) and Stevens-Johnson syndrome, have been reported with carbamazepine. These reactions have been extremely rare. However, a few fatalities have been reported.

Carbamazepine has shown mild anticholinergic activity; therefore, patients with increased intraocular pressure should be closely observed during therapy.

Because of the relationship of the drug to other tricyclic compounds, the possibility of activation of a latent psychosis and, in elderly patients, of confusion or agitation should be borne in mind.

USAGE IN PREGNANCY

Carbamazepine can cause fetal harm when administered to a pregnant woman.

Epidemiological data suggest that there may be an association between the use of carbamazepine during pregnancy and congenital malformations, including spina bifida. In treating or counseling women of childbearing potential, the prescribing physician will wish to weigh the benefits of therapy against the risks. If this drug is used during pregnancy, or if the patient becomes pregnant while taking this drug, the patient should be apprised of the potential hazard to the fetus.

Retrospective case reviews suggest that, compared with monotherapy, there may be a higher prevalence of teratogenic effects associated with the use of anticonvulsants in combination therapy. Therefore, if therapy is to be continued, monotherapy may be preferable for pregnant women.

In humans, transplacental passage of carbamazepine is rapid (30-60 minutes), and the drug is accumulated in the fetal tissues, with higher levels found in liver and kidney than in brain and lung.

Carbamazepine has been shown to have adverse effects in reproduction studies in rats when given orally in dosages 10-25 times the maximum human daily dosage (MHDD) of 1200 mg on a mg/kg basis or 1.5-4 times the MHDD on a mg/m^2 basis. In rat teratology studies, 2 of 135 offspring showed kinked ribs at 250 mg/kg and 4 of 119 offspring at 650 mg/kg showed other anomalies (cleft palate, 1; talipes, 1; anophthalmos, 2). In reproduction studies in rats, nursing offspring demonstrated a lack of weight gain and an unkempt appearance at a maternal dosage level of 200 mg/kg.

Antiepileptic drugs should not be discontinued abruptly in patients in whom the drug is administered to prevent major seizures because of the strong possibility of precipitating status epilepticus with attendant hypoxia and threat to life. In individual cases where the severity and frequency of the seizure disorder are such that removal of medication does not pose a serious threat to the patient, discontinuation of the drug may be considered prior to and during pregnancy, although it cannot be said with any confidence that even minor seizures do not pose some hazard to the developing embryo or fetus.

Tests to detect defects using currently accepted procedures should be considered a part of routine prenatal care in childbearing women receiving carbamazepine.

There have been a few cases of neonatal seizures and/or respiratory depression associated with maternal carbamazepine and other concomitant anticonvulsant drug use. A few cases of neonatal vomiting, diarrhea, and/or decreased feeding have also been reported in association with maternal carbamazepine use. These symptoms may represent a neonatal withdrawal syndrome.

PRECAUTIONS

GENERAL

Before initiating therapy, a detailed history and physical examination should be made.

Carbamazepine should be used with caution in patients with a mixed seizure disorder that includes atypical absence seizures, since in these patients carbamazepine has been associated with increased frequency of generalized convulsions (see INDICATIONS AND USAGE).

Therapy should be prescribed only after critical benefit-to-risk appraisal in patients with a history of cardiac, hepatic or renal damage; adverse hematologic reaction to other drugs including reactions to other anticonvulsants; or interrupted courses of therapy with carbamazepine.

Hepatic effects, ranging from slight elevations in liver enzymes to rare cases of hepatic failure have been reported (see ADVERSE REACTIONS and Laboratory Tests). In some cases, hepatic effects may progress despite discontinuation of the drug.

Multi-organ hypersensitivity reactions occurring days to weeks or months after initiating treatment have been reported in rare cases (see ADVERSE REACTIONS, Other and Information for the Patient).

Discontinuation of carbamazepine should be considered if any evidence of hypersensitivity develops.

Hypersensitivity reactions to carbamazepine have been reported in patients who previously experienced this reaction to anitconvulsants including phenytoin and phenobarbital. A history of hypersensitivity reactions should be obtained for a patient and the immediate family members. If positive, caution should be used in prescribing carbamazepine.

Since a given dose of carbamazepine suspension will produce higher peak levels than the same dose given as the tablet, it is recommended that patients given the suspension be started on lower doses and increased slowly to avoid unwanted side effects (see DOSAGE AND ADMINISTRATION).

INFORMATION FOR THE PATIENT

Patients should be made aware of the early toxic signs and symptoms of a potential hematologic problem, as well as dermatologic, hypersensitivity or hepatic reactions. These symptoms may include, but are not limited to, fever, sore throat, rash, ulcers in the mouth, easy bruising, lymphadenopathy and petechial or purpuric hemorrhage, and in the case of liver reaction, anorexia, nausea/vomiting, or jaundice. The patient should be advised that, because these signs and symptoms may signal a serious reaction, that they must report any occurence immediately to a physician. In addittion, the patient should be advised that these signs and symptoms should be reported even if mild or when occurring after extended use.

Since dizziness and drowsiness may occur, patients should be cautioned about the hazards of operating machinery or automobiles or engaging in other potentially dangerous tasks.

LABORATORY TESTS

Complete pretreatment blood counts, including platelets and possibly reticulocytes and serum iron, should be obtained as a baseline. If a patient in the course of treatment exhibits low or decreased white blood cell or platelet counts, the patient should be monitored closely. Discontinuation of the drug should be considered if any evidence of significant bone marrow depression develops.

Baseline and periodic evaluations of liver function, particularly in patients with a history of liver disease, must be performed during treatment with this drug since liver damage may occur (see PRECAUTIONS, General and ADVERSE REACTIONS). Carbamazepine should be discontinued, based on clinical judgement, if indicated by newly occurring or worsening clinical or laboratory evidence of liver dysfunction or hepatic damage, or in the case of active liver disease.

Baseline and periodic eye examinations, including slit-lamp, funduscopy, and tonometry, are recommended since many phenothiazines and related drugs have been shown to cause eye changes.

Baseline and periodic complete urinalysis and BUN determinations are recommended for patients treated with this agent because of observed renal dysfunction.

Monitoring of blood levels (see CLINICAL PHARMACOLOGY) has increased the efficacy and safety of anticonvulsants. This monitoring may be particularly useful in cases of dramatic increase in seizure frequency and for verification of compliance. In addition, measurement of drug serum levels may aid in determining the cause of toxicity when more than one medication is being used.

Thyroid function tests have been reported to show decreased values with carbamazepine administered alone.

Hyponatremia has been reported in association with carbamazepine use, either alone or in combination with other drugs.

Interference with some pregnancy tests have been reported.

CARCINOGENESIS, MUTAGENESIS, AND IMPAIRMENT OF FERTILITY

Carbamazepine, when administered to Sprague-Dawley rats for 2 years in the diet at doses of 25, 75, and 250 mg/kg/day, resulted in a dose-related increase in the incidence of hepatocellular tumors in females and of benign interstitial cell adenomas in the testes of males.

Carbamazepine must, therefore, be considered to be carcinogenic in Sprague-Dawley rats. Bacterial and mammalian mutagenicity studies using carbamazepine produced negative results. The significance of these findings relative to the use of carbamazepine in humans is, at present, unknown.

PREGNANCY CATEGORY D

See WARNINGS.

LABOR AND DELIVERY

The effect of carbamazepine on human labor and delivery is unknown.

NURSING MOTHERS

Carbamazepine and its epoxide metabolite are transferred to breast milk. The ratio of the concentration in breast milk to that in maternal plasma is about 0.4 for carbamazepine and about 0.5 for the epoxide. The estimated doses given to the newborn during breast feeding are in the range of 2-5 mg daily for carbamazepine and 1-2 mg daily for the epoxide.

Because of the potential of serious adverse reactions in nursing infants from carbamazepine, a decision should be made whether to discontinue nursing or to discontinue the drug, taking into account the importance of the drug to the mother.

PEDIATRIC USE

Substantial evidence of carbamazepine's effectiveness for use in the management of children with epilepsy (see INDICATIONS AND USAGE for specific seizure types) is derived from clinical investigations performed in adults and from studies in several *in vitro* systems which support the conclusion that (1) the pathogenetic mechanisms underlying seizure propagation are essentially identical in adults and children, and (2) the mechanism of action of carbamazepine in treating seizures is essentially identical in adults and children.

Taken as a whole, this information supports a conclusion that the generally accepted therapeutic range of total carbamazepine in plasma (*i.e.,* 4-12 μg/ml) is the same in children and adults.

The evidence assembled was primarily obtained from short-term use of carbamazepine. The safety of carbamazepine in children has been systematically studied up to 6 months. No longer-term data from clinical trials is available.

GERIATRIC USE

No systematic studies in geriatric patients have been conducted.

C

DRUG INTERACTIONS

There has been a report of a patient who passed an orange rubbery precipitate in his stool the day after ingesting carbamazepine suspension immediately followed by chlorpromazine solution. Subsequent testing has shown that mixing carbamazepine suspension and chlorpromazine solution (both generic and brand name) as well as carbamazepine suspension and liquid thioridazine resulted in the occurrence of this precipitate. Because the extent to which this occurs with other liquid medications is not known, carbamazepine suspension should not be administered simultaneously with other liquid medicinal agents or diluents. (See DOSAGE AND ADMINISTRATION.)

Clinically meaningful drug interactions have occurred with concomitant medications and include, but are not limited to, the following:

AGENTS THAT MAY AFFECT CARBAMAZEPINE PLASMA LEVELS

CYP 3A4 inhibitors inhibit carbamazepine metabolism and can thus increase plasma carbamazepine levels. Drugs that have been shown, or would be expected, to increase plasma carbamazepine levels include:

Cimetidine, danazol, diltiazem, macrolides, erythromycin, troleandomycin, clarithromycin, fluoxetine, loratadine, terfenadine, isoniazid, niacinamide, nicotinamide, propoxyphene, ketaconazole, itraconazole, verapamil, valproate*.

CYP 3A4 inducers can increase the rate of carbamazepine metabolism. Drugs that have been shown, or that would be expected, to decrease plasma carbamazepine levels include:

Cisplatin, doxorubicin HCl, felbamate†, rifampin, phenobarbital, phenytoin, primidone, theophylline.

*Increased levels of the active 10,11-epoxide.

†Decreased levels of carbamazepine and increased levels of the 10,11-epoxide.

EFFECT OF CARBAMAZEPINE ON PLASMA LEVELS OF CONCOMITANT AGENTS

Increased Levels: Clomipramine HCl, phenytoin, primidone.

Carbamazepine induces hepatic CYP activity. Carbamazepine causes, or would be expected to cause, decreased levels of the following:

Acetaminophen, alprazolam, clonazepam, clozapine, dicumarol, doxycycline, ethosuximide, haloperidol, lamotrigine, methsuximide, oral contraceptives, phensuximide, phenytoin, theophylline, tiagabine, topiramate, valproate, warfarin.

Concomitant administration of carbamazepine and lithium may increase the risk of neurotoxic side effects.

Alterations of thyroid function have been reported in combination therapy with other anticonvulsant medications.

Breakthrough bleeding has been reported among patients receiving concomitant oral and subdermal implant contraceptives and their reliability may be adversely affected.

ADVERSE REACTIONS

If adverse reactions are of such severity that the drug must be discontinued, the physician must be aware that abrupt discontinuation of any anticonvulsant drug in a responsive epileptic patient may lead to seizures or even status epilepticus with its life-threatening hazards.

The most severe adverse reactions have been observed in the hemopoietic system (see BOXED WARNING), the skin, liver and the cardiovascular system.

The most frequently observed adverse reactions, particularly during the initial phases of therapy, are dizziness, drowsiness, unsteadiness, nausea, and vomiting. To minimize the possibility of such reactions, therapy should be initiated at the low dosage recommended.

The following additional adverse reactions have been reported:

Hemopoietic System: Aplastic anemia, agranulocytosis, pancytopenia, bone marrow depression, thrombocytopenia, leukopenia, leukocytosis, eosinophilia, acute intermittent porphyria.

Skin: Pruritic and erythematous rashes, urticaria, toxic epidermal necrolysis (Lyell's Syndrome) (see WARNINGS), Stevens-Johnson syndrome (see WARNINGS), photosensitivity reactions, alterations in skin pigmentation, exfoliative dermatitis, erythema multiforme and nodosum, purpura, aggravation of disseminated lupus erythematosus, alopecia, and diaphoresis. In certain cases, discontinuation of therapy may be necessary. Isolated cases of hirsutism have been reported, but a causal relationship is not clear.

Cardiovascular System: Congestive heart failure, edema, aggravation of hypertension, hypotension, syncope and collapse, aggravation of coronary artery disease, arrhythmias and AV block, thrombophlebitis, thromboembolism, and adenopathy or lymphadenopathy.

Some of these cardiovascular complications have resulted in fatalities. Myocardial infarction has been associated with other tricyclic compounds.

Liver: Abnormalities in liver function tests, cholestatic and hepatocellular jaundice, hepatitis; very rare cases of hepatic failure.

Pancreatic: Pancreatitis.

Respiratory System: Pulmonary hypersensitivity characterized by fever, dyspnea, pneumonitis or pneumonia.

Genitourinary System: Urinary frequency, acute urinary retention, oliguria with elevated blood pressure, azotemia, renal failure, and impotence. Albuminuria, glycosuria, elevated BUN and microscopic deposits in the urine have also been reported.

Testicular atrophy occurred in rats receiving carbamazepine orally from 4-52 weeks at dosage levels of 50-400 mg/kg/day. Additionally, rats receiving carbamazepine in the diet for 2 years at dosage levels of 25, 75, and 250 mg/kg/day had a dose-related incidence of testicular atrophy and aspermatogenesis. In dogs, it produced a brownish discoloration, presumably a metabolite, in the urinary bladder at dosage levels of 50 mg/kg and higher. Relevance of these findings to humans is unknown.

Nervous System: Dizziness, drowsiness, disturbances of coordination, confusion, headache, fatigue, blurred vision, visual hallucinations, transient diplopia, oculomotor disturbances, nystagmus, speech disturbances, abnormal involuntary movements, peripheral neuritis and paresthesias, depression with agitation, talkativeness, tinnitus, and hyperacusis.

There have been reports of associated paralysis and other symptoms of cerebral arterial insufficiency, but the exact relationship of these reactions to the drug has not been established.

Isolated cases of neuroleptic malignant syndrome have been reported with concomitant use of psychotropic drugs.

Digestive System: Nausea, vomiting, gastric distress and abdominal pain, diarrhea, constipation, anorexia, and dryness of the mouth and pharynx, including glossitis and stomatitis.

Eyes: Scattered punctate cortical lens opacities, as well as conjunctivitis, have been reported. Although a direct causal relationship has not been established, many phenothiazines and related drugs have been shown to cause eye changes.

Musculoskeletal System: Aching joints and muscles, and leg cramps.

Metabolism: Fever and chills. Inappropriate antidiuretic hormone (ADH) secretion syndrome has been reported. Cases of frank water intoxication, with decreased serum sodium (hyponatremia) and confusion, have been reported in association with carbamazepine use (see PRECAUTIONS, Laboratory Tests). Decreased levels of plasma calcium have been reported.

Other: Multi-organ hypersensitivity reactions occurring days to weeks or months after initiating treatment have been reported in rare cases. Signs or symptoms may include, but are not limited to fever, skin rashes, vasculitis, lymphadenopathy, disorders mimicking lymphoma, arthralgia, leukopenia, eosinophilia, hepatosplenomegaly and abnormal liver function tests. These signs and symptoms may occur in various combinations and not necessarily concurrently. Signs and symptoms may initially be mild. Various organs, including but not limited to, liver, skin, immune system, lungs, kidneys, pancreas, myocardium, and colon may be affected (see PRECAUTIONS: General and Information for the Patient).

Isolated cases of lupus erythematosus-like syndrome have been reported. There have been occasional reports of elevated levels of cholesterol, HDL cholesterol and triglycerides in patients taking anticonvulsants.

A case of aseptic meningitis, accompanied by myoclonus and peripheral eosinophilia, has been reported in a patient taking carbamazepine in combination with other medications. The patient was successfully dechallenged, and the meningitis reappeared upon rechallenge with carbamazepine.

DOSAGE AND ADMINISTRATION

See TABLE 1A, TABLE 1B and TABLE 1C.

Carbamazepine suspension in combination with liquid chlorpromazine or thioridazine results in precipitate formation, and, in the case of chlorpromazine, there has been a report of a patient passing an orange rubbery precipitate in the stool following coadministration of the two drugs. (See DRUG INTERACTIONS.) Because the extent to which this occurs with other liquid medications is not known, carbamazepine suspension should not be administered simultaneously with other liquid medications or diluents.

Monitoring of blood levels has increased the efficacy and safety of anticonvulsants (see PRECAUTIONS, Laboratory Tests). Dosage should be adjusted to the needs of the individual patient. A low initial daily dosage with a gradual increase is advised. As soon as adequate control is achieved, the dosage may be reduced very gradually to the minimum effective level. Medication should be taken with meals.

Since a given dose of carbamazepine suspension will produce higher peak levels than the same dose given as the tablet, it is recommended to start with low doses (children 6-12 years: ½ teaspoon qid) and to increase slowly to avoid unwanted side effects.

Conversion of patients from oral carbamazepine tablets to carbamazepine suspension: Patients should be converted by administering the same number of mg/day in smaller, more frequent doses (*i.e.*, bid tablets to tid suspension).

Carbamazepine extended-release is a formulation for twice-a-day administration. When converting patients from carbamazepine conventional tablets to carbamazepine extended-release tablets, the same total daily mg dose of carbamazepine extended-release should be administered. **Carbamazepine extended-release tablets must be swallowed whole and never crushed or chewed.** Carbamazepine extended-release tablets should be inspected for chips or cracks. Damaged tablets, or tablets without a release portal, should not be consumed. Carbamazepine extended-release tablet coating is not absorbed and is excreted in the feces; these coatings may be noticeable in the stool.

EPILEPSY

See INDICATIONS AND USAGE.

Adults and children over 12 years of age:

Initial: Either 200 mg bid for tablets and extended-release tablets or 1 teaspoon qid for suspension (400 mg/day). Increase at weekly intervals by adding up to 200 mg/day using a bid regimen of extended-release or tid or qid regimen of the other formulations until the optimal response is obtained. Dosage generally should not exceed 1000 mg daily in children 12-15 years of age, and 1200 mg daily in patients above 15 years of age. Doses up to 1600 mg daily have been used in adults in rare instances.

Maintenance: Adjust dosage to the minimum effective level, usually 800-1200 mg daily.

Children 6-12 years of age:

Initial: Either 100 mg bid for tablets or extended-release tablets or ½ teaspoon qid for suspension (200 mg/day). Increase at weekly intervals by adding up to 100 mg/day using a bid regimen of carbamazepine extended-release tablets or tid or qid regimen of the other formulations until the optimal response is obtained. Dosage generally should not exceed 1000 mg daily.

Maintenance: Adjust dosage to the minimum effective level, usually 400-800 mg daily.

Children under 6 years of age:

Initial: 10-20 mg/kg/day bid or tid as tablets, or qid as suspension. Increase weekly to achieve optimal clinical response administered tid or qid.

Maintenance: Ordinarily, optimal clinical response is achieved at daily doses below 35 mg/kg. If satisfactory clinical response has not been achieved, plasma levels should be measured to determine whether or not they are in the therapeutic range. No recommendation regarding the safety of carbamazepine for use at doses above 35 mg/kg/24 hours can be made.

Combination Therapy

Carbamazepine may be used alone or with other anticonvulsants. When added to existing anticonvulsant therapy, the drug should be added gradually while the other anticonvulsants are maintained or gradually decreased, except phenytoin, which may have to be increased (see DRUG INTERACTIONS and PRECAUTIONS, Pregnancy Category D).

TRIGEMINAL NEURALGIA

See INDICATIONS AND USAGE.

Initial: On the first day, either 100 mg bid for tablets or extended-release tablets or ½ teaspoon qid for suspension for a total daily dose of 200 mg. This daily dose may be increased by up to 200 mg/day using increments of 100 mg every 12 hours for tablets or extended-release tablets or 50 mg (½ teaspoon) qid for suspension, only as needed to achieve freedom from pain. Do not exceed 1200 mg/daily.

Maintenance: Control of pain can be maintained in most patients with 400-800 mg daily. However, some patients may be maintained on as little as 200 mg daily, while others may require as much as 1200 mg daily. At least once every 3 months throughout the treatment period, attempts should be made to reduce the dose to the minimum effective level or even to discontinue the drug.

TABLE 1A *Dosage Information: Initial Dose*

Indication	Tablet*	Extended-Release Tablet	Suspension
Epilepsy			
Under 6 years	10-20 mg/kg/day bid or tid		10-20 mg/kg/day qid
6-12 years	100 mg bid (200 mg/day)	100 mg bid (200 mg/day)	½ tsp qid (200 mg/day)
Over 12 years	200 mg bid (400 mg/day)	200 mg bid (400 mg/day)	1 tsp qid (400 mg/day)
Trigeminal Neuralgia	100 mg bid (200 mg/day)	100 mg bid (200 mg/day)	½ tsp qid (200 mg/day)

* Tablet = Chewable or conventional tablets.

TABLE 1B *Dosage Information: Subsequent Dose*

	Tablet*	Extended-Release Tablet	Suspension
Epilepsy			
Under 6 years	Increase weekly to achieve optimal clinical response, tid or qid		Increase weekly to achieve optimal clinical response, tid or qid
6-12 years	Add up to 100 mg/day at weekly intervals, tid or qid	Add 100 mg/day at weekly intervals, bid	Add up to 1 tsp (100 mg)/day at weekly intervals, tid or qid
Over 12 years	Add up to 200 mg/day at weekly intervals, tid or qid	Add up to 200 mg/day at weekly intervals, bid	Add up to 2 tsp (200 mg)/day at weekly intervals, tid or qid
Trigeminal Neuralgia	Add up to 200 mg/day in increments of 100 mg every 12 h	Add up to 200 mg/day in increments of 100 mg every 12 h	Add up to 2 tsp (200 mg)/day in increments of 50 mg (½ tsp) qid

* Tablet = Chewable or conventional tablets.

TABLE 1C *Dosage Information: Maximum Daily Dose*

	Tablet*	Extended-Release Tablet	Suspension
Epilepsy			
Under 6 years	35 mg/kg/24 h		35 mg/kg/24 h
6-12 years		1000 mg/24 h	
12-15 years		1000 mg/24 h	
>15 years		1200 mg/24 h	
Adults, in rare instances		1600 mg/24 h	
Trigeminal Neuralgia		1200 mg/24 h	

* Tablets = Chewable or conventional tablets.

HOW SUPPLIED

TEGRETOL CHEWABLE TABLETS

100 mg: Round, red-speckled, pink, single-scored (imprinted "Tegretol" on one side and "52" twice on the scored side).

Storage: Do not store above 30°C (86°F). *Protect from light and moisture. Dispense in tight, light-resistant container.*

TEGRETOL TABLETS

200 mg: Capsule-shaped, pink, single-scored (imprinted "Tegretol" on one side and "27" twice on the partially scored side).

Storage: Do not store above 30°C (86°F). *Protect from moisture. Dispense in tight container.*

TEGRETOL XR TABLETS

100 mg: Round, yellow, coated (imprinted "T" on one side and "100 mg" on the other), release portal on one side.

200 mg: Round, pink, coated (imprinted "T" on one side and "200 mg" on the other), release portal on one side.

400 mg: Round, brown, coated (imprinted "T" on one side and "400 mg" on the other), release portal on one side.

Storage: Store at controlled room temperature 15-30°C (59-86°F). *Protect from moisture. Dispense in tight container.*

SUSPENSION 100 MG/5 ML (TEASPOON)

Suspension is yellow-orange, citrus-vanilla flavored. Shake well before using.

Storage: Do not store above 30°C (86°F). *Dispense in tight, light resistant container.*

PRODUCT LISTING - RATED THERAPEUTICALLY EQUIVALENT

Package	Price	Product, Manufacturer	NDC
Suspension - Oral - 100 mg/5 ml			
450 ml	$29.72	GENERIC, Taro Pharmaceuticals U.S.A. Inc	51672-4047-09
450 ml	$38.55	TEGRETOL, Novartis Pharmaceuticals	00083-0019-76
480 ml	$31.11	GENERIC, Morton Grove Pharmaceuticals Inc	60432-0129-16
Tablet - Oral - 200 mg			
25's	$8.93	GENERIC, Udl Laboratories Inc	51079-0385-19
30 x 25	$263.55	GENERIC, Sky Pharmaceuticals Packaging, Inc	63739-0045-03
30 x 25	$276.68	GENERIC, Sky Pharmaceuticals Packaging, Inc	63739-0045-01
30's	$6.54	GENERIC, Pd-Rx Pharmaceuticals	55289-0210-30
30's	$9.59	GENERIC, Heartland Healthcare Services	61392-0038-30
30's	$9.59	GENERIC, Heartland Healthcare Services	61392-0038-39
31 x 10	$108.34	GENERIC, Vangard Labs	00615-3505-53
31 x 10	$108.34	GENERIC, Vangard Labs	00615-3505-63
31's	$9.90	GENERIC, Heartland Healthcare Services	61392-0038-31
32's	$10.22	GENERIC, Heartland Healthcare Services	61392-0038-32
45's	$14.38	GENERIC, Heartland Healthcare Services	61392-0038-45
60's	$19.17	GENERIC, Heartland Healthcare Services	61392-0038-60
90's	$28.76	GENERIC, Heartland Healthcare Services	61392-0038-90
100's	$10.08	GENERIC, Us Trading Corporation	56126-0352-11
100's	$13.88	FEDERAL UPPER LIMIT, H.C.F.A. F F P	99999-0646-02
100's	$19.95	GENERIC, Raway Pharmacal Inc	00686-0385-20
100's	$23.63	GENERIC, Interstate Drug Exchange Inc	00814-1470-14
100's	$24.91	GENERIC, Moore, H.L. Drug Exchange Inc	00839-7177-06
100's	$25.31	GENERIC, Auro Pharmaceutical	55829-0173-10
100's	$26.80	GENERIC, Elan Pharmaceuticals	59075-0554-10
100's	$27.90	GENERIC, Aligen Independent Laboratories Inc	00405-4131-01
100's	$28.68	GENERIC, Parmed Pharmaceuticals Inc	00349-8977-01
100's	$29.60	GENERIC, Ivax Corporation	00182-1233-01
100's	$29.60	GENERIC, Dixon-Shane Inc	17236-0352-01
100's	$29.85	GENERIC, Purepac Pharmaceutical Company	00228-2143-10
100's	$30.17	GENERIC, Teva Pharmaceuticals Usa	00093-0090-01
100's	$30.17	GENERIC, Teva Pharmaceuticals Usa	00093-0109-01
100's	$31.39	GENERIC, Vangard Labs	00615-3505-13
100's	$35.52	GENERIC, Inwood Laboratories Inc	00258-3587-01
100's	$35.70	GENERIC, Udl Laboratories Inc	51079-0385-20
100's	$41.55	GENERIC, Taro Pharmaceuticals U.S.A. Inc	51672-4005-01
100's	$43.10	GENERIC, Major Pharmaceuticals Inc	00904-3855-60
100's	$44.50	TEGRETOL, Pharma Pac	52959-0174-00
100's	$45.35	GENERIC, Major Pharmaceuticals Inc	00904-3855-61
100's	$45.98	GENERIC, Ivax Corporation	00182-1233-89
100's	$51.74	TEGRETOL, Allscripts Pharmaceutical Company	54569-0163-01
100's	$53.83	TEGRETOL, Physicians Total Care	54868-1975-00
100's	$54.80	TEGRETOL, Novartis Pharmaceuticals	00083-0027-32
100's	$59.86	TEGRETOL, Novartis Pharmaceuticals	00083-0027-30
120's	$38.34	GENERIC, Heartland Healthcare Services	61392-0038-34
Tablet, Chewable - Oral - 100 mg			
8's	$2.28	TEGRETOL, Allscripts Pharmaceutical Company	54569-0165-02
25's	$8.38	GENERIC, Udl Laboratories Inc	51079-0870-19
30's	$5.19	GENERIC, Heartland Healthcare Services	61392-0029-30
30's	$5.19	GENERIC, Heartland Healthcare Services	61392-0029-39
30's	$5.19	GENERIC, Heartland Healthcare Services	61392-0097-30
30's	$5.19	GENERIC, Heartland Healthcare Services	61392-0097-39
30's	$9.56	TEGRETOL, Physicians Total Care	54868-1235-01
31 x 10	$68.13	GENERIC, Vangard Labs	00615-4515-53
31 x 10	$68.13	GENERIC, Vangard Labs	00615-4515-63
31's	$5.36	GENERIC, Heartland Healthcare Services	61392-0029-31
31's	$5.36	GENERIC, Heartland Healthcare Services	61392-0097-31
32's	$5.54	GENERIC, Heartland Healthcare Services	61392-0029-32
32's	$5.54	GENERIC, Heartland Healthcare Services	61392-0097-32
45's	$7.79	GENERIC, Heartland Healthcare Services	61392-0097-45
60's	$10.38	GENERIC, Heartland Healthcare Services	61392-0029-60
60's	$10.38	GENERIC, Heartland Healthcare Services	61392-0097-60
90's	$15.57	GENERIC, Heartland Healthcare Services	61392-0029-90
90's	$15.57	GENERIC, Heartland Healthcare Services	61392-0097-90
100's	$17.40	GENERIC, Moore, H.L. Drug Exchange Inc	00839-7410-06
100's	$18.20	GENERIC, Aligen Independent Laboratories Inc	00405-4130-01
100's	$23.10	GENERIC, Caraco Pharmaceutical Laboratories	57664-0342-88

100's	$23.11	GENERIC, Teva Pharmaceuticals Usa	00093-0778-01
100's	$23.11	GENERIC, Taro Pharmaceuticals U.S.A. Inc	51672-4041-01
100's	$29.13	TEGRETOL, Physicians Total Care	54868-1235-03
100's	$29.48	GENERIC, Udl Laboratories Inc	51079-0870-20
100's	$31.43	TEGRETOL, Novartis Pharmaceuticals	00083-0052-30
100's	$35.30	TEGRETOL, Novartis Pharmaceuticals	00083-0052-32
100's	$35.94	GENERIC, Ivax Corporation	00182-1331-89

PRODUCT LISTING - RATED NOT THERAPEUTICALLY EQUIVALENT

Tablet, Chewable - Oral - 100 mg

100's	$23.99	GENERIC, Major Pharmaceuticals Inc	00904-3854-60

PRODUCT LISTING - EQUIVALENTS NOT AVAILABLE

Capsule, Extended Release - Oral - 200 mg

120's	$60.72	CARBATROL, Shire Richwood Pharmaceutical Company Inc	58521-0177-12
120's	$60.72	CARBATROL, Shire Richwood Pharmaceutical Company Inc	59075-0671-12
120's	$71.03	CARBATROL, Shire Richwood Pharmaceutical Company Inc	58521-0172-12
120's	$73.99	CARBATROL, Shire Richwood Pharmaceutical Company Inc	54092-0172-12

Capsule, Extended Release - Oral - 300 mg

120's	$106.53	CARBATROL, Shire Richwood Pharmaceutical Company Inc	58521-0173-12
120's	$106.53	CARBATROL, Shire Richwood Pharmaceutical Company Inc	59075-0672-12
120's	$110.98	CARBATROL, Shire Richwood Pharmaceutical Company Inc	54092-0173-12

Suspension - Oral - 100 mg/5 ml

10 ml x 50	$112.50	GENERIC, Alpharma Uspd Makers Of Barre and Nmc	50962-0229-60
450 ml	$24.39	TEGRETOL, Basel Pharmaceuticals	58887-0019-76

Tablet - Oral - 200 mg

3's	$3.59	GENERIC, Prescript Pharmaceuticals	00247-0352-03
4's	$3.67	GENERIC, Prescript Pharmaceuticals	00247-0352-04
6's	$3.84	GENERIC, Prescript Pharmaceuticals	00247-0352-06
7's	$3.91	GENERIC, Prescript Pharmaceuticals	00247-0352-07
8's	$3.99	GENERIC, Prescript Pharmaceuticals	00247-0352-08
9's	$4.07	GENERIC, Prescript Pharmaceuticals	00247-0352-09
10's	$4.15	GENERIC, Prescript Pharmaceuticals	00247-0352-10
14's	$4.47	GENERIC, Prescript Pharmaceuticals	00247-0352-14
16's	$4.62	GENERIC, Prescript Pharmaceuticals	00247-0352-16
28's	$8.45	GENERIC, Allscripts Pharmaceutical Company	54569-2655-03
30's	$5.74	GENERIC, Prescript Pharmaceuticals	00247-0352-30
30's	$10.95	GENERIC, Southwood Pharmaceuticals Inc	58016-0968-30
60's	$8.12	GENERIC, Prescript Pharmaceuticals	00247-0352-60
60's	$13.05	GENERIC, Physicians Total Care	54868-0147-05
60's	$18.10	GENERIC, Allscripts Pharmaceutical Company	54569-2655-01
60's	$19.76	GENERIC, St. Mary'S Mpp	60760-0109-60
60's	$21.90	GENERIC, Southwood Pharmaceuticals Inc	58016-0968-60
90's	$10.49	GENERIC, Prescript Pharmaceuticals	00247-0352-90
90's	$32.85	GENERIC, Southwood Pharmaceuticals Inc	58016-0968-90
100's	$11.29	GENERIC, Prescript Pharmaceuticals	00247-0352-00
100's	$20.64	GENERIC, Physicians Total Care	54868-0147-02
100's	$31.32	GENERIC, Allscripts Pharmaceutical Company	54569-2655-00
100's	$36.50	GENERIC, Southwood Pharmaceuticals Inc	58016-0968-00
120's	$43.80	GENERIC, Southwood Pharmaceuticals Inc	58016-0968-02

Tablet, Chewable - Oral - 100 mg

100's	$31.85	GENERIC, Physicians Total Care	54868-2462-01

Tablet, Extended Release - Oral - 100 mg

100's	$27.26	TEGRETOL XR, Physicians Total Care	54868-4067-00
100's	$29.98	TEGRETOL XR, Novartis Pharmaceuticals	00083-0061-30

Tablet, Extended Release - Oral - 200 mg

100's	$59.86	TEGRETOL XR, Novartis Pharmaceuticals	00083-0062-30
120's	$57.60	CARBATROL, Shire Richwood Pharmaceutical Company Inc	59075-6711-20

Tablet, Extended Release - Oral - 400 mg

100's	$98.79	TEGRETOL XR, Physicians Total Care	54868-3862-00
100's	$119.64	TEGRETOL XR, Novartis Pharmaceuticals	00083-0060-30

Carbenicillin Indanyl Sodium (000650)

For related information, see the comparative table section in Appendix A.

Categories: Bacteriuria, asymptomatic; Infection, urinary tract; Prostatitis; Pregnancy Category B; FDA Approved 1972 Oct
Drug Classes: Antibiotics, penicillins
Brand Names: Carbastat; Isopto Carbachol; **Miostat**
Foreign Brand Availability: Carbachol (Poland); Carbamann (Germany); Glaumarin (Japan); Isopto Karbakolin (Sweden); Karbakolin Isopto (Denmark)

DESCRIPTION

Geocillin, a semisynthetic penicillin, is the sodium salt of the indanyl ester of Geopen (carbenicillin disodium). The chemical name is: 1-(5-indanyl)-N-(2-carboxy-3,3-dimethyl-7-oxo-4-thia-1-azabicyclo(3.2.0) hept-6-yl)-2-phenylmalonamate monosodium salt.

The empirical formula is: $C_{26}H_{25}N_2NaO_6S$ and molecular weight is 516.55.

Geocillin tablets are yellow, capsule-shaped and film-coated, made of a white crystalline solid. Carbenicillin is freely soluble in water. Each Geocillin tablet contains 382 mg of carbenicillin, 118 mg of indanyl sodium ester. Each Geocillin tablet contains 23 mg of sodium.

Inert ingredients are glycine; magnesium stearate and sodium lauryl sulfate. *May also include the following:* Hydroxypropyl cellulose; hydroxypropyl methylcellulose; opaspray (which may include blue 2 lake, yellow 6 lake, yellow 10 lake, and other inert ingredients); opadry light yellow (which may contain D&C yellow 10 lake, fd&c yellow 6 lake and other inert ingredients); opadry clear (which may contain other inert ingredients).

CLINICAL PHARMACOLOGY

Free carbenicillin is the predominant pharmacologically active fraction of carbenicillin indanyl sodium. Carbenicillin exerts its antibacterial activity by interference with final cell wall synthesis of susceptible bacteria.

Carbenicillin indanyl sodium is acid stable, and rapidly absorbed from the small intestine following oral administration. It provides relatively low plasma concentrations of antibiotic and is primarily excreted in the urine. After absorption, carbenicillin indanyl sodium is rapidly converted to carbenicillin by hydrolysis of the ester linkage. Following ingestion of a single 500 mg tablet of carbenicillin indanyl sodium, a peak carbenicillin plasma concentration of approximately 6.5 μg/ml is reached in 1 hour. About 30% of this dose is excreted in the urine unchanged within 12 hours, with another 6% excreted over the next 12 hours.

In a multiple dose study utilizing volunteers with normal renal function, the following mean urine and serum levels of carbenicillin were achieved (see TABLE 1).

TABLE 1 *Mean Urine Concentration of Carbenicillin*

	Carbenicillin Indanyl Sodium	
Hours After Initial Dose	**1 tablet q6h**	**2 tablets q6h**
0-3 h	1130 μg/ml	1428μg/ml
3-6 h	352μg/ml	789μg/ml
6-24 h	292μg/ml	809μg/ml

Mean serum concentrations of carbenicillin in this study for these dosages are as listed in TABLE 2.

TABLE 2 *Mean Serum Concentration*

	Carbenicillin Indanyl Sodium	
Hours After Initial Dose	**1 tablet q6h**	**2 tablets q6h**
½ hours	5.1 μg/ml	6.1 μg/ml
1 hours	6.5 μg/ml	9.6 μg/ml
2 hours	3.2 μg/ml	7.9 μg/ml
4 hours	1.9 μg/ml	2.6 μg/ml
6 hours	0.0 μg/ml	0.4 μg/ml
24 hours	0.4 μg/ml	0.8 μg/ml
25 hours	8.8 μg/ml	13.2 μg/ml
26 hours	5.4 μg/ml	12.8 μg/ml
28 hours	0.4 μg/ml	3.8 μg/ml

MICROBIOLOGY

The antibacterial activity of carbenicillin indanyl sodium is due to its rapid conversion to carbenicillin by hydrolysis after absorption. Though carbenicillin indanyl sodium provides substantial *in vitro* activity against a variety of both gram-positive and gram-negative microorganisms, the most important aspect of its profile is in its antipseudomonal and antiproteal activity. Because of the high urine levels obtained following administration, carbenicillin indanyl sodium has demonstrated clinical efficacy in urinary infections due to susceptible strains of:

- *Escherichia coli*
- *Proteus mirabilis*
- *Proteus vulgaris*
- *Morganella morganii* (formerly *Proteus morganii*)
- *Pseudomonas* species
- *Providencia rettgeri* (formerly *Proteus rettgeri*)
- *Enterobacter* species
- Enterococci (*S. faecalis*)

In addition, *in vitro* data, not substantiated by clinical studies, indicate the following pathogens to be usually susceptible to carbenicillin indanyl sodium:

- *Staphylococcus* species (nonpenicillinase producing)
- *Streptococcus* species

RESISTANCE

Most *Klebsiella* species are usually resistant to the action of carbenicillin indanyl sodium. Some strains of *Pseudomonas* species have developed resistance to carbenicillin.

SUSCEPTIBILITY TESTING

Geopen (carbenicillin disodium) Susceptibility Powder or 100 μg Geopen Susceptibility Discs may be used to determine microbial susceptibility to carbenicillin indanyl sodium using one of the following standard methods recommended by the National Committee for Clinical Laboratory Standards:

- M2-A3, "Performance Standards for Antimicrobial Disk Susceptibility Tests"
- M7-A, "Methods for Dilution Antimicrobial Susceptibility Tests for Bacteria that Grow Aerobically"
- M11-A, "Reference Agar Dilution Procedure for Antimicrobial Susceptibility Testing of Anaerobic Bacteria"
- M17-P, "Alternative Methods for Antimicrobial Susceptibility Testing of Anaerobic Bacteria"

Tests should be interpreted by the following criteria (see TABLE 3).

TABLE 3

Disk Diffusion			
		Zone Diameter	
Organisms	**Susceptible**	**Intermediate**	**Resistant**
Enterobacter	≥23 mm	18-22 mm	≤17 mm
Pseudomonas sp.	≥17 mm	14-16 mm	≤13 mm
Dilution			
Organisms	**Susceptible**	**MIC Moderately Susceptible**	**Resistant**
Enterobacter	≤16 µg/ml	32 µg/ml	≥64 µg/ml
Pseudomonas sp.	≤128 µg/ml	—	≥156 µg/ml

Interpretations of susceptible, intermediate, and resistant correlate zone size diameters with MIC values. A laboratory report of "susceptible" indicates that the suspected causative microorganism most likely will respond to therapy with carbenicillin. A laboratory report of "resistant" indicates that the infecting microorganism most likely will not respond to therapy. A laboratory report of "moderately susceptible" indicates that the microorganism is most likely susceptible if a high dosage of carbenicillin is used, or if the infection is such that high levels of carbenicillin may be attained as in urine. A report of "intermediate" using the disk diffusion method may be considered an equivocal result, and dilution tests may be indicated.

INDICATIONS AND USAGE

Carbenicillin indanyl sodium is indicated in the treatment of acute and chronic infections of the upper and lower urinary tract and in asymptomatic bacteriuria due to susceptible strains of the following organisms:

Escherichia coli
Proteus mirabilis
Morganella morganii (formerly *Proteus morganii*)
Providencia rettgeri (formerly *Proteus rettgeri*)
Proteus vulgaris
Pseudomonas
Enterobacter
Enterococci

Carbenicillin indanyl sodium is also indicated in the treatment of prostatitis due to susceptible strains of the following organisms:

Escherichia coli
Enterococcus (S. faecalis)
Proteus mirabilis
Enterobacter sp.

WHEN HIGH AND RAPID BLOOD AND URINE LEVELS OF ANTIBIOTIC ARE INDICATED, THERAPY WITH GEOPEN (CARBENICILLIN DISODIUM) SHOULD BE INITIATED BY PARENTERAL ADMINISTRATION FOLLOWED, AT THE PHYSICIAN'S DISCRETION, BY ORAL THERAPY.

NOTE: Susceptibility testing should be performed prior to and during the course of therapy to detect the possible emergence of resistant organisms which may develop.

CONTRAINDICATIONS

Carbenicillin indanyl sodium is ordinarily contraindicated in patients who have a known penicillin allergy.

WARNINGS

Serious and occasionally fatal hypersensitivity (anaphylactic) reactions have been reported in patients on oral penicillin therapy. Although anaphylaxis is more frequent following parenteral therapy, it has occurred in patients on oral penicillins. These reactions are more apt to occur in individuals with a history of penicillin hypersensitivity and/or a history of sensitivity to multiple allergens.

There have been reports of individuals with a history of penicillin hypersensitivity who have experienced severe hypersensitivity reactions when treated with a cephalosporin, and vice versa. Before initiating therapy with a penicillin, careful inquiry should be made concerning previous hypersensitivity reactions to penicillins, cephalosporins, or other allergens. If an allergic reaction occurs, the drug should be discontinued and the appropriate therapy instituted.

SERIOUS ANAPHYLACTOID REACTIONS REQUIRE IMMEDIATE EMERGENCY TREATMENT WITH EPINEPHRINE. OXYGEN, INTRAVENOUS STEROIDS AND AIRWAY MANAGEMENT, INCLUDING INTUBATION, SHOULD ALSO BE ADMINISTERED AS INDICATED.

PRECAUTIONS

GENERAL

As with any penicillin preparation, an allergic response, including anaphylaxis, may occur particularly in a hypersensitive individual.

Long term use of carbenicillin indanyl sodium may result in the overgrowth of nonsusceptible organisms. If superinfection occurs during therapy, appropriate measures should be taken.

Since carbenicillin is primarily excreted by the kidney, patients with severe renal impairment (creatinine clearance of less than 10 ml/min) will not achieve therapeutic urine levels of carbenicillin.

In patients with creatinine clearance of 10-20 ml/min it may be necessary to adjust dosage to prevent accumulation of drug.

LABORATORY TESTS

As with other penicillins, periodic assessment of organ system function including renal, hepatic, and hematopoietic systems is recommended during prolonged therapy.

CARCINOGENESIS, MUTAGENESIS, AND IMPAIRMENT OF FERTILITY

There are no long-term animal or human studies to evaluate carcinogenic potential. Rats fed 250-1000 mg/kg/day for 18 months developed mild liver pathology (*e.g.*, bile duct hyperplasia) at all dose levels, but there was no evidence of drug-related neoplasia. Carbenicillin indanyl sodium administered at daily doses ranging to 1000 mg/kg had no apparent effect on the fertility or reproductive performance of rats.

PREGNANCY CATEGORY B

Reproduction studies have been performed at dose levels of 1000 or 500 mg/kg in rats, 200 mg/kg in mice, and at 500 mg/kg in monkeys with no harm to fetus due to carbenicillin indanyl sodium. There are, however, no adequate and well controlled studies in pregnant women. Because animal reproduction studies are not always predictive of human response, this drug should be used during pregnancy only if clearly needed.

LABOR AND DELIVERY

It is not known whether the use of carbenicillin indanyl sodium in humans during labor or delivery has immediate or delayed adverse effects on the fetus, prolongs the duration of labor, or increases the likelihood that forceps delivery or other obstetrical intervention or resuscitation of the newborn will be necessary.

NURSING MOTHERS

Carbenicillin class antibiotics are excreted in milk although the amounts excreted are unknown; therefore, caution should be exercised if administered to a nursing woman.

PEDIATRIC USE

Since only limited clinical data is available to date in children, the safety of carbenicillin indanyl sodium administration in this age group has not yet been established.

DRUG INTERACTIONS

Carbenicillin indanyl sodium blood levels may be increased and prolonged by concurrent administration of probenecid.

ADVERSE REACTIONS

The following adverse reactions have been reported as possibly related to carbenicillin indanyl sodium administration in controlled studies which include 344 patients receiving carbenicillin indanyl sodium.

Gastrointestinal: The most frequent adverse reactions associated with carbenicillin indanyl sodium therapy are related to the gastrointestinal tract. Nausea, bad taste, diarrhea, vomiting, flatulence, and glossitis were reported. Abdominal cramps, dry mouth, furry tongue, rectal bleeding, anorexia, and unspecified epigastric distress were rarely reported.

Dermatologic: Hypersensitivity reactions such as skin rash, urticaria, and less frequently pruritus.

Hematologic: As with other penicillins, anemia, thrombocytopenia, leukopenia, neutropenia, and eosinophilia have infrequently been observed. The clinical significance of these abnormalities is not known.

Miscellaneous: Other reactions rarely reported were hyperthermia, headache, itchy eyes, vaginitis, and loose stools.

Abnormalities of Hepatic Function Tests: Mild SGOT elevations have been observed following carbenicillin indanyl sodium administration.

DOSAGE AND ADMINISTRATION

Carbenicillin indanyl sodium is available as a coated tablet to be administered orally. (See TABLE 4.)

TABLE 4 *Usual Adult Dose*

URINARY TRACT INFECTIONS	
Escherichia coli, Proteus species, and *Enterobacter*	1-2 tablets 4 times daily
Pseudomonas and *Enterococcus*	2 tablets 4 times daily
PROSTATITIS	
Escherichia coli, Proteus mirabilis, Enterobacter and *Enterococcus*	2 tablets 4 times daily

PRODUCT LISTING - EQUIVALENTS NOT AVAILABLE

Tablet - Oral - 382 mg

100's	$229.75	GEOCILLIN, Pfizer U.S. Pharmaceuticals	00049-1430-66

Carbidopa; Levodopa (000653)

Categories: Parkinson's disease, adjunct; FDA Approval Pre 1982; Pregnancy Category C; WHO Formulary
Drug Classes: Antiparkinson agents; Dopaminergics
Brand Names: Atamet; Cinetol; Levopa-C; **Sinemet**
Foreign Brand Availability: Carbilev (South-Africa); Cloisone (Mexico); Dopadura (Germany); Dopicar (Israel); Grifoparkin (Peru); Levomed (Hong-Kong); Levomet (Hong-Kong); Menesit (Japan); Neo Dopaston (Japan); Parken (Colombia); Parkin (Korea); Racovel (Mexico); Sindopa (New-Zealand); Sinedopa (Hong-Kong); Sinemet CR (Australia; Bulgaria; Canada; England; Hong-Kong; Hungary; Israel; Italy; Malaysia; Netherlands; New-Zealand; Peru; Portugal; Russia; South-Africa; Switzerland); Sinemet Retard (Spain); Sinemet 25 100 (Hong-Kong; Malaysia; Philippines); Sulconar (Peru); Syndopa (India); Tidomet Forte (India); Tidomet L.S. (India); Tidomet Plus (India); Toniform (Germany); Tremopar (Germany)
Cost of Therapy: $73.61 (Parkinsonism; Sinemet; 25 mg; 100 mg; 3 tablets /day; 30 day supply)
$52.34 (Parkinsonism; Generic tablets ; 25 mg; 100 mg; 3 tablets /day; 30 day supply)
$112.48 (Parkinsonism; Sinemet CR; 50 mg; 200 mg; 2 tablets /day; 30 day supply)
$108.51 (Parkinsonism; Generic CR; 50 mg; 200 mg; 2 tablets /day; 30 day supply)

DESCRIPTION

Note: The trade names have been used throughout this monograph for clarity.

SINEMET

Sinemet is a combination of carbidopa and levodopa for the treatment of Parkinson's disease and syndrome.

Carbidopa, an inhibitor of aromatic amino acid decarboxylation, is a white, crystalline compound, slightly soluble in water, with a molecular weight of 244.3. It is designated chemically as (-)-L-α-hydrazino-α-methyl-β-(3,4-dihydroxybenzene) propanoic acid monohydrate. Its empirical formula is $C_{10}H_{14}N_2O_4 \cdot H_2O$.

Tablet content is expressed in terms of anhydrous carbidopa which has a molecular weight of 226.3.

Levodopa, an aromatic amino acid, is a white, crystalline compound, slightly soluble in water, with a molecular weight of 197.2. It is designated chemically as (-)-L-α-amino-β-(3,4-dihydroxybenzene) propanoic acid. Its empirical formula is $C_9H_{11}NO_4$.

Sinemet is supplied as tablets in three strengths:

Sinemet 25-100, containing 25 mg of carbidopa and 100 mg of levodopa.
Sinemet 10-100, containing 10 mg of carbidopa and 100 mg of levodopa.
Sinemet 25-250, containing 25 mg of carbidopa and 250 mg of levodopa.

Inactive ingredients are cellulose, magnesium stearate, and starch. Sinemet tablets 10-100 and 25-250 also contain FD&C blue 2. Sinemet tablets 25-100 also contain D&C yellow 10 and FD&C yellow 6.

SINEMET CR

Sinemet CR is a sustained-release combination of carbidopa and levodopa for the treatment of Parkinson's disease and syndrome.

Carbidopa, an inhibitor of aromatic amino acid decarboxylation, is a white, crystalline compound, slightly soluble in water, with a molecular weight of 244.3. It is designated chemically as (-)-L-α-hydrazino-α-methyl-β-(3,4-dihydroxybenzene) propanoic acid monohydrate. Its empirical formula is $C_{10}H_{14}N_2O_4 \cdot H_2O$.

Tablet content is expressed in terms of anhydrous carbidopa, which has a molecular weight of 226.3.

Levodopa, an aromatic amino acid, is a white, crystalline compound, slightly soluble in water, with a molecular weight of 197.2. It is designated chemically as (-)-L-α-amino-β-(3,4-dihydroxybenzene) propanoic acid. Its empirical formula is $C_9H_{11}NO_4$.

Sinemet CR is supplied as sustained-release tablets containing either 50 mg of carbidopa and 200 mg of levodopa, or 25 mg of carbidopa and 100 mg of levodopa. Inactive ingredients: hydroxypropyl cellulose, polyvinylacetate-crotonic acid copolymer, magnesium stearate and red ferric oxide. Sinemet CR 50-200 also contains D&C yellow 10.

The 50-200 tablet is supplied as an oval, scored, biconvex, compressed tablet that is peach colored. The 25-100 tablet is supplied as an oval, biconvex, compressed tablet that is pink colored. The Sinemet CR tablet is a polymeric-based drug delivery system that controls the release of carbidopa and levodopa as it slowly erodes. Sinemet CR 25-100 is available to facilitate titration and as an alternative to the half-tablet of Sinemet CR 50-200.

CLINICAL PHARMACOLOGY

SINEMET

Parkinson's disease is a progressive, neurodegenerative disorder of the extrapyramidal nervous system affecting the mobility and control of the skeletal muscular system. Its characteristic features include resting tremor, rigidity, and bradykinetic movements. Symptomatic treatments, such as levodopa therapies, may permit the patient better mobility.

Mechanism of Action

Current evidence indicates that symptoms of Parkinson's disease are related to depletion of dopamine in the corpus striatum. Administration of dopamine is ineffective in the treatment of Parkinson's disease apparently because it does not cross the blood-brain barrier. However, levodopa, the metabolic precursor of dopamine, does cross the blood-brain barrier, and presumably is converted to dopamine in the brain. This is thought to be the mechanism whereby levodopa relieves symptoms of Parkinson's disease.

Pharmacodynamics

When levodopa is administered orally it is rapidly decarboxylated to dopamine in extracerebral tissues so that only a small portion of a given dose is transported unchanged to the central nervous system. For this reason, large doses of levodopa are required for adequate therapeutic effect and these may often be accompanied by nausea and other adverse reactions, some of which are attributable to dopamine formed in extracerebral tissues.

Since levodopa competes with certain amino acids for transport across the gut wall, the absorption of levodopa may be impaired in some patients on a high protein diet.

Carbidopa inhibits decarboxylation of peripheral levodopa. It does not cross the blood-brain barrier and does not affect the metabolism of levodopa within the central nervous system.

The incidence of levodopa-induced nausea and vomiting is less with Sinemet than with levodopa. In many patients, this reduction in nausea and vomiting will permit more rapid dosage titration.

Since its decarboxylase inhibiting activity is limited to extracerebral tissues, administration of carbidopa with levodopa makes more levodopa available for transport to the brain.

Pharmacokinetics

Carbidopa reduces the amount of levodopa required to produce a given response by about 75% and, when administered with levodopa, increases both plasma levels and the plasma half-life of levodopa, and decreases plasma and urinary dopamine and homovanillic acid.

The plasma half-life of levodopa is about 50 minutes, without carbidopa. When carbidopa and levodopa are administered together, the half-life of levodopa is increased to about 1.5 hours. At steady state, the bioavailability of carbidopa from Sinemet tablets is approximately 99% relative to the concomitant administration of carbidopa and levodopa.

In clinical pharmacologic studies, simultaneous administration of carbidopa and levodopa produced greater urinary excretion of levodopa in proportion to the excretion of dopamine than administration of the two drugs at separate times.

Pyridoxine hydrochloride (vitamin B_6), in oral doses of 10-25 mg, may reverse the effects of levodopa by increasing the rate of aromatic amino acid decarboxylation. Carbidopa inhibits this action of pyridoxine; therefore, Sinemet can be given to patients receiving supplemental pyridoxine (vitamin B_6).

SINEMET CR

Mechanism of Action

Parkinson's disease is a progressive, neurodegenerative disorder of the extrapyramidal nervous system affecting the mobility and control of the skeletal muscular system. Its characteristic features include resting tremor, rigidity, and bradykinetic movements. Symptomatic treatments, such as levodopa therapies, may permit the patient better mobility.

Current evidence indicates that symptoms of Parkinson's disease are related to depletion of dopamine in the corpus striatum. Administration of dopamine is ineffective in the treatment of Parkinson's disease apparently because it does not cross the blood-brain barrier. However, levodopa, the metabolic precursor of dopamine, does cross the blood-brain barrier, and presumably is converted to dopamine in the brain. This is thought to be the mechanism whereby levodopa relieves symptoms of Parkinson's disease.

Pharmacodynamics

When levodopa is administered orally it is rapidly decarboxylated to dopamine in extracerebral tissues so that only a small portion of a given dose is transported unchanged to the central nervous system. For this reason, large doses of levodopa are required for adequate therapeutic effect and these may often be accompanied by nausea and other adverse reactions, some of which are attributable to dopamine formed in extracerebral tissues.

Since levodopa competes with certain amino acids for transport across the gut wall, the absorption of levodopa may be impaired in some patients on a high protein diet.

Carbidopa inhibits decarboxylation of peripheral levodopa. It does not cross the blood-brain barrier and does not affect the metabolism of levodopa within the central nervous system.

Since its decarboxylase inhibiting activity is limited to extracerebral tissues, administration of carbidopa with levodopa makes more levodopa available for transport to the brain.

Patients treated with levodopa therapy for Parkinson's disease may develop motor fluctuations characterized by end-of-dose failure, peak dose dyskinesia, and akinesia. The advanced form of motor fluctuations ('on-off' phenomenon) is characterized by unpredictable swings from mobility to immobility. Although the causes of the motor fluctuations are not completely understood, in some patients they may be attenuated by treatment regimens that produce steady plasma levels of levodopa.

Sinemet CR contains either 50 mg of carbidopa and 200 mg of levodopa, or 25 mg of carbidopa and 100 mg of levodopa in a sustained-release dosage form designed to release these ingredients over a 4-6 hour period. With Sinemet CR there is less variation in plasma levodopa levels than with Sinemet, the conventional formulation. *However, Sinemet CR sustained-release is less systemically bioavailable than Sinemet and may require increased daily doses to achieve the same level of symptomatic relief as provided by Sinemet.*

In clinical trials, patients with moderate to severe motor fluctuations who received Sinemet CR *did not experience quantitatively significant reductions* in 'off' time when compared to Sinemet. However, global ratings of improvement as assessed by both patient and physician were better during therapy with Sinemet CR than with Sinemet. In patients without motor fluctuations, Sinemet CR, under controlled conditions, provided the same therapeutic benefit with less frequent dosing when compared to Sinemet.

Pharmacokinetics

Carbidopa reduces the amount of levodopa required to produce a given response by about 75% and, when administered with levodopa, increases both plasma levels and the plasma half-life of levodopa, and decreases plasma and urinary dopamine and homovanillic acid.

Elimination half-life of levodopa in the presence of carbidopa is about 1.5 hours. Following Sinemet CR, the apparent half-life of levodopa may be prolonged because of continuous absorption.

In healthy elderly subjects (56-67 years old) the mean time-to-peak concentration of levodopa after a single dose of Sinemet CR 50-200 was about 2 hours as compared to 0.5 hours after standard Sinemet. The maximum concentration of levodopa after a single dose of Sinemet CR was about 35% of the standard Sinemet (1151 vs 3256 ng/ml). The extent of availability of levodopa from Sinemet CR was about 70-75% relative to intravenous levodopa or standard Sinemet in the elderly. The absolute bioavailability of levodopa from Sinemet CR (relative to IV) in young subjects was shown to be only about 44%. The extent of availability and the peak concentrations of levodopa were comparable in the elderly after a single dose and at steady state after tid administration of Sinemet CR 50-200. In elderly subjects, the average trough levels of levodopa at steady state after the CR tablet were about 2 fold higher than after the standard Sinemet (163 vs 74 ng/ml).

In these studies, using similar total daily doses of levodopa, plasma levodopa concentrations with Sinemet CR fluctuated in a narrower range than with Sinemet. Because the bioavailability of levodopa from Sinemet CR relative to Sinemet is approximately 70-75%, the daily dosage of levodopa necessary to produce a given clinical response with the sustained-release formulation will usually be higher.

The extent of availability and peak concentrations of levodopa after a single dose of Sinemet CR 50-200 increased by about 50% and 25%, respectively, when administered with food.

At steady state, the bioavailability of carbidopa from Sinemet tablets is approximately 99% relative to the concomitant administration of carbidopa and levodopa. At steady state, carbidopa bioavailability from Sinemet CR 50-200 is approximately 58% relative to that from Sinemet.

Pyridoxine hydrochloride (vitamin B_6), in oral doses of 10-25 mg, may reverse the effects of levodopa by increasing the rate of aromatic amino acid decarboxylation. Carbidopa inhibits this action of pyridoxine.

INDICATIONS AND USAGE

SINEMET

Sinemet is indicated in the treatment of the symptoms of idiopathic Parkinson's disease (paralysis agitans), post-encephalitic parkinsonism, and symptomatic parkinsonism which may follow injury to the nervous system by carbon monoxide intoxication and/or manganese intoxication. Sinemet is indicated in these conditions to permit the administration of lower doses of levodopa with reduced nausea and vomiting, with more rapid dosage titration, with a somewhat smoother response, and with supplemental pyridoxine (vitamin B_6).

In some patients a somewhat smoother antiparkinsonian effect results from therapy with Sinemet than with levodopa. However, patients with markedly irregular ("on-off") responses to levodopa have not been shown to benefit from Sinemet.

Although the administration of carbidopa permits control of parkinsonism and Parkinson's disease with much lower doses of levodopa, there is no conclusive evidence at present that this is beneficial other than in reducing nausea and vomiting, permitting more rapid titration, and providing a somewhat smoother response to levodopa.

Certain patients who responded poorly to levodopa have improved when Sinemet was substituted. This is most likely due to decreased peripheral decarboxylation of levodopa which results from administration of carbidopa rather than to a primary effect of carbidopa on the nervous system. Carbidopa has not been shown to enhance the intrinsic efficacy of levodopa in parkinsonian syndromes.

In considering whether to give Sinemet to patients already on levodopa who have nausea and/or vomiting, the practitioner should be aware that, while many patients may be expected to improve, some do not. Since one cannot predict which patients are likely to improve, this can only be determined by a trial of therapy. It should be further noted that in controlled trials comparing Sinemet with levodopa, about half of the patients with nausea and/or vomiting on levodopa improved spontaneously despite being retained on the same dose of levodopa during the controlled portion of the trial.

SINEMET CR

Sinemet CR is indicated in the treatment of the symptoms of idiopathic Parkinson's disease (paralysis agitans), postencephalitic parkinsonism, and symptomatic parkinsonism which may follow injury to the nervous system by carbon monoxide intoxication and/or manganese intoxication.

NON-FDA APPROVED INDICATIONS

Levodopa has also been used for the treatment of a variety of diseases including hepatic coma, bone pain, and herpes zoster. However, none of these uses is approved by the FDA, standard dosage recommendations are not available, and the role of combined levodopa-carbidopa preparations in the treatment of these disorders has not been described.

CONTRAINDICATIONS

SINEMET

Nonselective monoamine oxidase (MAO) inhibitors are contraindicated for use with Sinemet. These inhibitors must be discontinued at least 2 weeks prior to initiating therapy with Sinemet. Sinemet may be administered concomitantly with the manufacturer's recommended dose of an MAO inhibitor with selectivity for MAO type B (*e.g.,* selegiline HCl) (See DRUG INTERACTIONS, Sinemet).

Sinemet is contraindicated in patients with known hypersensitivity to any component of this drug, and in patients with narrow-angle glaucoma.

Because levodopa may activate a malignant melanoma, Sinemet should not be used in patients with suspicious, undiagnosed skin lesions or a history of melanoma.

SINEMET CR

Nonselective MAO inhibitors are contraindicated for use with Sinemet CR. These inhibitors must be discontinued at least 2 weeks prior to initiating therapy with Sinemet CR. Sinemet CR may be administered concomitantly with the manufacturer's recommended dose of an MAO inhibitor with selectivity for MAO type B (*e.g.,* selegiline HCl) (See DRUG INTERACTIONS, Sinemet CR).

Sinemet CR is contraindicated in patients with known hypersensitivity to any component of this drug and in patients with narrow-angle glaucoma.

Because levodopa may activate a malignant melanoma, Sinemet CR should not be used in patients with suspicious, undiagnosed skin lesions or a history of melanoma.

WARNINGS

SINEMET

When Sinemet is to be given to patients who are being treated with levodopa, levodopa must be discontinued at least 12 hours before therapy with Sinemet is started. In order to reduce adverse reactions, it is necessary to individualize therapy. See DOSAGE AND ADMINISTRATION, Sinemet before initiating therapy.

The addition of carbidopa with levodopa in the form of Sinemet reduces the peripheral effects (nausea, vomiting) due to decarboxylation of levodopa; however, carbidopa does not decrease the adverse reactions due to the central effects of levodopa. Because carbidopa permits more levodopa to reach the brain and more dopamine to be formed, certain adverse CNS effects, *e.g.,* dyskinesias (involuntary movements), may occur at lower dosages and sooner with Sinemet than with levodopa alone.

Levodopa alone, as well as Sinemet, is associated with dyskinesias. The occurrence of dyskinesias may require dosage reduction.

As with levodopa, Sinemet may cause mental disturbances. These reactions are thought to be due to increased brain dopamine following administration of levodopa. All patients should be observed carefully for the development of depression with concomitant suicidal tendencies. Patients with past or current psychoses should be treated with caution.

Sinemet should be administered cautiously to patients with severe cardiovascular or pulmonary disease, bronchial asthma, renal, hepatic or endocrine disease.

As with levodopa, care should be exercised in administering Sinemet to patients with a history of myocardial infarction who have residual atrial, nodal, or ventricular arrhythmias. In such patients, cardiac function should be monitored with particular care during the period of initial dosage adjustment, in a facility with provisions for intensive cardiac care.

As with levodopa, treatment with Sinemet may increase the possibility of upper gastrointestinal hemorrhage in patients with a history of peptic ulcer.

Neuroleptic Malignant Syndrome (NMS)

Sporadic cases of a symptom complex resembling NMS have been reported in association with dose reductions or withdrawal of therapy with Sinemet. Therefore, patients should be observed carefully when the dosage of Sinemet is reduced abruptly or discontinued, especially if the patient is receiving neuroleptics.

NMS is an uncommon but life-threatening syndrome characterized by fever or hyperthermia. Neurological findings, including muscle rigidity, involuntary movements, altered consciousness, mental status changes; other disturbances, such as autonomic dysfunction, tachycardia, tachypnea, sweating, hyper- or hypotension; laboratory findings, such as creatine phosphokinase elevation, leukocytosis, myoglobinuria, and increased serum myoglobin have been reported.

The early diagnosis of this condition is important for the appropriate management of these patients. Considering NMS as a possible diagnosis and ruling out other acute illnesses (*e.g.,* pneumonia, systemic infection, etc.) is essential. This may be especially complex if the clinical presentation includes both serious medical illness and untreated or inadequately treated extrapyramidal signs and symptoms (EPS). Other important considerations in the differential diagnosis include central anticholinergic toxicity, heat stroke, drug fever, and primary central nervous system (CNS) pathology.

The management of NMS should include: (1) intensive symptomatic treatment and medical monitoring and (2) treatment of any concomitant serious medical problems for which specific treatments are available. Dopamine agonists, such as bromocriptine, and muscle relaxants, such as dantrolene, are often used in the treatment of NMS, however, their effectiveness has not been demonstrated in controlled studies.

SINEMET CR

When patients are receiving levodopa without a decarboxylase inhibitor, levodopa must be discontinued at least 12 hours before Sinemet CR is started. In order to reduce adverse reactions, it is necessary to individualize therapy. Sinemet CR should be substituted at a dosage that will provide approximately 25% of the previous levodopa dosage (see DOSAGE AND ADMINISTRATION, Sinemet CR).

Carbidopa does not decrease adverse reactions due to central effects of levodopa. By permitting more levodopa to reach the brain, particularly when nausea and vomiting is not a dose-limiting factor, certain adverse CNS effects, e.g., dyskinesias, will occur at lower dosages and sooner during therapy with Sinemet CR sustained-release than with levodopa alone.

Patients receiving Sinemet CR may develop increased dyskinesias compared to Sinemet. Dyskinesias are a common side effect of carbidopa-levodopa treatment. The occurrence of dyskinesias may require dosage reduction.

As with levodopa, Sinemet CR may cause mental disturbances. These reactions are thought to be due to increased brain dopamine following administration of levodopa. All patients should be observed carefully for the development of depression with concomitant suicidal tendencies. Patients with past or current psychoses should be treated with caution.

Sinemet CR should be administered cautiously to patients with severe cardiovascular or pulmonary disease, bronchial asthma, renal, hepatic or endocrine disease.

As with levodopa, care should be exercised in administering Sinemet CR to patients with a history of myocardial infarction who have residual atrial, nodal, or ventricular arrhythmias. In such patients, cardiac function should be monitored with particular care during the period of initial dosage adjustment, in a facility with provisions for intensive cardiac care.

As with levodopa, treatment with Sinemet CR may increase the possibility of upper gastrointestinal hemorrhage in patients with a history of peptic ulcer.

Neuroleptic Malignant Syndrome (NMS)

Sporadic cases of a symptom complex resembling NMS have been reported in association with dose reductions or withdrawal of Sinemet and Sinemet CR.

Therefore, patients should be observed carefully when the dosage of Sinemet CR is reduced abruptly or discontinued, especially if the patient is receiving neuroleptics.

NMS is an uncommon but life-threatening syndrome characterized by fever or hyperthermia. Neurological findings, including muscle rigidity, involuntary movements, altered consciousness, mental status changes; other disturbances, such as autonomic dysfunction, tachycardia, tachypnea, sweating, hyper- or hypotension; laboratory findings, such as creatine phosphokinase elevation, leukocytosis, myoglobinuria, and increased serum myoglobin have been reported.

The early diagnosis of this condition is important for the appropriate management of these patients. Considering NMS as a possible diagnosis and ruling out other acute illnesses (*e.g.,* pneumonia, systemic infection, etc.) is essential. This may be especially complex if the clinical presentation includes both serious medical illness and untreated or inadequately treated extrapyramidal signs and symptoms (EPS). Other important considerations in the differential diagnosis include central anticholinergic toxicity, heat stroke, drug fever, and primary central nervous system (CNS) pathology.

The management of NMS should include: (1) intensive symptomatic treatment and medical monitoring and (2) treatment of any concomitant serious medical problems for which specific treatments are available. Dopamine agonists, such as bromocriptine, and muscle relaxants, such as dantrolene, are often used in the treatment of NMS; however, their effectiveness has not been demonstrated in controlled studies.

PRECAUTIONS

SINEMET

General

As with levodopa, periodic evaluations of hepatic, hematopoietic, cardiovascular, and renal function are recommended during extended therapy.

Patients with chronic wide-angle glaucoma may be treated cautiously with Sinemet provided the intraocular pressure is well controlled and the patient is monitored carefully for changes in intraocular pressure during therapy.

Information for the Patient

The patient should be informed that Sinemet is an immediate-release formulation of carbidopa-levodopa that is designed to begin release of ingredients within 30 minutes. It is important that Sinemet be taken at regular intervals according to the schedule outlined by the physician. The patient should be cautioned not to change the prescribed dosage regimen and not to add any additional antiparkinson medications, including other carbidopa-levodopa preparations, without first consulting the physician.

Patients should be advised that sometimes a 'wearing-off' effect may occur at the end of the dosing interval. The physician should be notified if such response poses a problem to life-style.

Patients should be advised that occasionally, dark color (red, brown, or black) may appear in saliva, urine, or sweat after ingestion of Sinemet. Although the color appears to be clinically insignificant, garments may become discolored.

The patient should be advised that a change in diet to foods that are high in protein may delay the absorption of levodopa and may reduce the amount taken up in the circulation. Excessive acidity also delays stomach emptying, thus delaying the absorption of levodopa. Iron salts (such as in multi-vitamin tablets) may also reduce the amount of levodopa available to the body. The above factors may reduce the clinical effectiveness of the levodopa or carbidopa-levodopa therapy.

Note: The suggested advice to patients being treated with Sinemet is intended to aid in the safe and effective use of this medication. It is not a disclosure of all possible adverse or intended effects.

Laboratory Tests

Abnormalities in laboratory tests may include elevations of liver function tests such as alkaline phosphatase, SGOT (AST), SGPT (ALT), lactic dehydrogenase, and bilirubin. Abnormalities in blood urea nitrogen and positive Coombs test have also been reported. Commonly, levels of blood urea nitrogen, creatinine, and uric acid are lower during administration of Sinemet than with levodopa.

Sinemet may cause a false-positive reaction for urinary ketone bodies when a test tape is used for determination of ketonuria. This reaction will not be altered by boiling the urine specimen. False-negative tests may result with the use of glucose-oxidase methods of testing for glucosuria.

Cases of falsely diagnosed pheochromocytoma in patients on carbidopa-levodopa therapy have been reported very rarely. Caution should be exercised when interpreting the plasma and urine levels of catecholamines and their metabolites in patients on levodopa or carbidopa-levodopa therapy.

Carcinogenesis, Mutagenesis, and Impairment of Fertility

In a 2 year bioassay of Sinemet, no evidence of carcinogenicity was found in rats receiving doses of approximately 2 times the maximum daily human dose of carbidopa and 4 times the maximum daily human dose of levodopa.

In reproduction studies with Sinemet, no effects on fertility were found in rats receiving doses of approximately 2 times the maximum daily human dose of carbidopa and 4 times the maximum daily human dose of levodopa.

Pregnancy Category C

No teratogenic effects were observed in a study in mice receiving up to 20 times the maximum recommended human dose of Sinemet. There was a decrease in the number of live pups delivered by rats receiving approximately 2 times the maximum recommended human dose of carbidopa and approximately 5 times the maximum recommended human dose of levodopa during organogenesis. Sinemet caused both visceral and skeletal malformations in rabbits at all doses and ratios of carbidopa/levodopa tested, which ranged from 10 times/5 times the maximum recommended human dose of carbidopa/levodopa to 20 times/10 times the maximum recommended human dose of carbidopa/levodopa.

There are no adequate or well-controlled studies in pregnant women. It has been reported from individual cases that levodopa crosses the human placental barrier, enters the fetus, and is metabolized. Carbidopa concentrations in fetal tissue appeared to be minimal. Use of Sinemet in women of child-bearing potential requires that the anticipated benefits of the drug be weighed against possible hazards to mother and child.

Nursing Mothers

It is not known whether this drug is excreted in human milk. Because many drugs are excreted in human milk, caution should be exercised when Sinemet is administered to a nursing woman.

Pediatric Use

Safety and effectiveness in pediatric patients have not been established. Use of the drug in patients below the age of 18 is not recommended.

SINEMET CR

General

As with levodopa, periodic evaluations of hepatic, hematopoietic, cardiovascular, and renal function are recommended during extended therapy.

Patients with chronic wide-angle glaucoma may be treated cautiously with Sinemet CR provided the intraocular pressure is well controlled and the patient is monitored carefully for changes in intraocular pressure during therapy.

Information for the Patient

The patient should be informed that Sinemet CR is a sustained-release formulation of carbidopa-levodopa which releases these ingredients over a 4-6 hour period. It is important that Sinemet CR be taken at regular intervals according to the schedule outlined by the physician. The patient should be cautioned not to change the prescribed dosage regimen and not to add any additional antiparkinson medications, including other carbidopa-levodopa preparations, without first consulting the physician.

If abnormal involuntary movements appear or get worse during treatment with Sinemet CR, the physician should be notified, as dosage adjustment may be necessary.

Patients should be advised that sometimes the onset of effect of the first morning dose of Sinemet CR may be delayed for up to 1 hour compared with the response usually obtained from the first morning dose of Sinemet. The physician should be notified if such delayed responses pose a problem in treatment.

Patients should be advised that, occasionally, dark color (red, brown, or black) may appear in saliva, urine, or sweat after ingestion of Sinemet CR. Although the color appears to be clinically insignificant, garments may become discolored.

The patient should be informed that a change in diet to foods that are high in protein may delay the absorption of levodopa and may reduce the amount taken up in the circulation. Excessive acidity also delays stomach emptying, thus delaying the absorption of levodopa. Iron salts (such as in multi-vitamin tablets) may also reduce the amount of levodopa available to the body. The above factors may reduce the clinical effectiveness of the levodopa or carbidopa-levodopa therapy.

Patients must be advised that the whole or half tablet should be swallowed without chewing or crushing.

Note: The suggested advice to patients being treated with Sinemet CR is intended to aid in the safe and effective use of this medication. It is not a disclosure of all possible adverse or intended effects.

Laboratory Tests

Abnormalities in laboratory tests may include elevations of liver function tests such as alkaline phosphatase, SGOT (AST), SGPT (ALT), lactic dehydrogenase, and bilirubin. Abnormalities in blood urea nitrogen and positive Coombs test have also been reported. Commonly, levels of blood urea nitrogen, creatinine, and uric acid are lower during administration of carbidopa-levodopa preparations than with levodopa.

Carbidopa-levodopa preparations, such as Sinemet and Sinemet CR, may cause a false-positive reaction for urinary ketone bodies when a test tape is used for determination of ketonuria. This reaction will not be altered by boiling the urine specimen. False-negative tests may result with the use of glucose-oxidase methods of testing for glucosuria.

Cases of falsely diagnosed pheochromocytoma in patients on carbidopa-levodopa therapy have been reported very rarely. Caution should be exercised when interpreting the plasma and urine levels of catecholamines and their metabolites in patients on levodopa or carbidopa-levodopa therapy.

Carcinogenesis, Mutagenesis, and Impairment of Fertility

In a 2 year bioassay of Sinemet, no evidence of carcinogenicity was found in rats receiving doses of approximately 2 times the maximum daily human dose of carbidopa and 4 times the maximum daily human dose of levodopa (equivalent to 8 Sinemet CR tablets).

In reproduction studies with Sinemet, no effects on fertility were found in rats receiving doses of approximately 2 times the maximum daily human dose of carbidopa and 4 times the maximum daily human dose of levodopa (equivalent to 8 Sinemet CR tablets).

Pregnancy Category C

No teratogenic effects were observed in a study in mice receiving up to 20 times the maximum recommended human dose of Sinemet. There was a decrease in the number of live pups delivered by rats receiving approximately 2 times the maximum recommended human dose of carbidopa and approximately 5 times the maximum recommended human dose of levodopa during organogenesis. Sinemet caused both visceral and skeletal malformations in rabbits at all doses and ratios of carbidopa/levodopa tested, which ranged from 10 times/5 times the maximum recommended human dose of carbidopa/levodopa to 20 times/10 times the maximum recommended human dose of carbidopa/levodopa.

There are no adequate or well-controlled studies in pregnant women. It has been reported from individual cases that levodopa crosses the human placental barrier, enters the fetus, and is metabolized. Carbidopa concentrations in fetal tissue appeared to be minimal. Use of Sinemet CR in women of childbearing potential requires that the anticipated benefits of the drug be weighed against possible hazards to mother and child.

Nursing Mothers

It is not known whether this drug is excreted in human milk. Because many drugs are excreted in human milk, caution should be exercised when Sinemet CR is administered to a nursing woman.

Pediatric Use

Safety and effectiveness in pediatric patients have not been established. Use of the drug in patients below the age of 18 is not recommended.

DRUG INTERACTIONS

SINEMET

Caution should be exercised when the following drugs are administered concomitantly with Sinemet.

Symptomatic postural hypotension has occurred when Sinemet was added to the treatment of a patient receiving antihypertensive drugs. Therefore, when therapy with Sinemet is started, dosage adjustment of the antihypertensive drug may be required.

For patients receiving MAO inhibitors (Type A or B), see CONTRAINDICATIONS, Sinemet. Concomitant therapy with selegiline and carbidopa-levodopa may be associated with severe orthostatic hypotension not attributable to carbidopa-levodopa alone (see CONTRAINDICATIONS, Sinemet).

There have been rare reports of adverse reactions, including hypertension and dyskinesia, resulting from the concomitant use of tricyclic antidepressants and Sinemet.

Dopamine D_2 receptor antagonists (*e.g.*, phenothiazines, butyrophenones, risperidone) and isoniazid may reduce the therapeutic effects of levodopa. In addition, the beneficial effects of levodopa in Parkinson's disease have been reported to be reversed by phenytoin and papaverine. Patients taking these drugs with Sinemet should be carefully observed for loss of therapeutic response.

Iron salts may reduce the bioavailability of levodopa and carbidopa. The clinical relevance is unclear.

Although metoclopramide may increase the bioavailability of levodopa by increasing gastric emptying, metoclopramide may also adversely affect disease control by its dopamine receptor antagonistic properties.

SINEMET CR

Caution should be exercised when the following drugs are administered concomitantly with Sinemet CR sustained-release.

Symptomatic postural hypotension has occurred when carbidopa-levodopa preparations were added to the treatment of patients receiving some antihypertensive drugs. Therefore, when therapy with Sinemet CR is started, dosage adjustment of the antihypertensive drug may be required.

For patients receiving monoamine oxidase (MAO) inhibitors (Type A or B), see CONTRAINDICATIONS, Sinemet CR. Concomitant therapy with selegiline and carbidopa-levodopa may be associated with severe orthostatic hypotension not attributable to carbidopa-levodopa alone (see CONTRAINDICATIONS, Sinemet CR).

There have been rare reports of adverse reactions, including hypertension and dyskinesia, resulting from the concomitant use of tricyclic antidepressants and carbidopa-levodopa preparations.

Dopamine D_2 receptor antagonists (*e.g.*, phenothiazines, butyrophenones, risperidone) and isoniazid may reduce the therapeutic effects of levodopa. In addition, the beneficial effects of levodopa in Parkinson's disease have been reported to be reversed by phenytoin and papaverine. Patients taking these drugs with Sinemet CR should be carefully observed for loss of therapeutic response.

Iron salts may reduce the bioavailability of levodopa and carbidopa. The clinical relevance is unclear.

Although metoclopramide may increase the bioavailability of levodopa by increasing gastric emptying, metoclopramide may also adversely affect disease control by its dopamine receptor antagonistic properties.

ADVERSE REACTIONS

SINEMET

The most common adverse reactions reported with Sinemet have included dyskinesias, such as choreiform, dystonic, and other involuntary movements and nausea.

The following other adverse reactions have been reported with Sinemet:

Body as a Whole: Chest pain, asthenia.

Cardiovascular: Cardiac irregularities, hypotension, orthostatic effects including orthostatic hypotension, hypertension, syncope, phlebitis, palpitation.

Gastrointestinal: Dark saliva, gastrointestinal bleeding, development of duodenal ulcer, anorexia, vomiting, diarrhea, constipation, dyspepsia, dry mouth, taste alterations.

Hematologic: Agranulocytosis, hemolytic and non-hemolytic anemia, thrombocytopenia, leukopenia.

Hypersensitivity: Angioedema, urticaria, pruritus, Henoch-Schonlein purpura, bullous lesions (including pemphigus-like reactions).

Musculoskeletal: Back pain, shoulder pain, muscle cramps.

Nervous System/Psychiatric: Psychotic episodes including delusions, hallucinations, and paranoid ideation, neuroleptic malignant syndrome (see WARNINGS, Sinemet), bradykinetic episodes ("on-off" phenomenon), confusion, agitation, dizziness, somnolence, dream abnormalities including nightmares, insomnia, paresthesia, headache, depression with or without development of suicidal tendencies, dementia, increased libido. Convulsions also have occurred; however, a causal relationship with Sinemet has not been established.

Respiratory: Dyspnea, upper respiratory infection.

Skin: Rash, increased sweating, alopecia, dark sweat.

Urogenital: Urinary tract infection, urinary frequency, dark urine.

Laboratory Tests: Decreased hemoglobin and hematocrit; abnormalities in alkaline phosphatase, SGOT (AST), SGPT (ALT), lactic dehydrogenase, bilirubin, blood urea nitrogen (BUN), Coombs test; elevated serum glucose; white blood cells, bacteria, and blood in the urine.

Other adverse reactions that have been reported with levodopa alone and with various carbidopa-levodopa formulations, and may occur with Sinemet are:

Body as a Whole: Abdominal pain and distress, fatigue.

Cardiovascular: Myocardial infarction.

Gastrointestinal: Gastrointestinal pain, dysphagia, sialorrhea, flatulence, bruxism, burning sensation of the tongue, heartburn, hiccups.

Metabolic: Edema, weight gain, weight loss.

Musculoskeletal: Leg pain.

Nervous System/Psychiatric: Ataxia, extrapyramidal disorder, falling, anxiety, gait abnormalities, nervousness, decreased mental acuity, memory impairment, disorientation, euphoria, blepharospasm (which may be taken as an early sign of excess dosage; consideration of dosage reduction may be made at this time), trismus, increased tremor, numbness, muscle twitching, activation of latent Horner's syndrome, peripheral neuropathy.

Respiratory: Pharyngeal pain, cough.

Skin: Malignant melanoma (see also CONTRAINDICATIONS, Sinemet), flushing.

Special Senses: Oculogyric crises, diplopia, blurred vision, dilated pupils.

Urogenital: Urinary retention, urinary incontinence, priapism.

Miscellaneous: Bizarre breathing patterns, faintness, hoarseness, malaise, hot flashes, sense of stimulation.

Laboratory Tests: Decreased white blood cell count and serum potassium; increased serum creatinine and uric acid; protein and glucose in urine.

SINEMET CR

In controlled clinical trials, patients predominantly with moderate to severe motor fluctuations while on Sinemet were randomized to therapy with either Sinemet or Sinemet CR. The adverse experience frequency profile of Sinemet CR did not differ substantially from that of Sinemet, as shown in TABLE 1.

TABLE 1 *Clinical Adverse Experiences Occurring in 1% or Greater of Patients*

Adverse Experience	Sinemet CR (n=491)	Sinemet (n=524)
Dyskinesia	16.5%	12.2%
Nausea	5.5%	5.7%
Hallucinations	3.9%	3.2%
Confusion	3.7%	2.3%
Dizziness	2.9%	2.3%
Depression	2.2%	1.3%
Urinary tract infection	2.2%	2.3%
Headache	2.0%	1.9%
Dream abnormalities	1.8%	0.8%
Dystonia	1.8%	0.8%
Vomiting	1.8%	1.9%
Upper respiratory infection	1.8%	1.0%
Dyspnea	1.6%	0.4%
"On-Off" phenomena	1.6%	1.1%
Back pain	1.6%	0.6%
Dry mouth	1.4%	1.1%
Anorexia	1.2%	1.1%
Diarrhea	1.2%	0.6%
Insomnia	1.2%	1.0%
Orthostatic hypotension	1.0%	1.1%
Shoulder pain	1.0%	0.6%
Chest pain	1.0%	0.8%
Muscle cramps	0.8%	1.0%
Paresthesia	0.8%	1.1%
Urinary frequency	0.8%	1.1%
Dyspepsia	0.6%	1.1%
Constipation	0.2%	1.5%

Abnormal laboratory findings occurring at a frequency of 1% or greater in approximately 443 patients who received Sinemet CR and 475 who received Sinemet during controlled clinical trials included: Decreased hemoglobin and hematocrit; elevated serum glucose; white blood cells, bacteria and blood in the urine.

The adverse experiences observed in patients in uncontrolled studies were similar to those seen in controlled clinical studies.

Other adverse experiences reported overall in clinical trials in 748 patients treated with Sinemet CR, listed by body system in order of decreasing frequency, include:

Body as a Whole: Asthenia, fatigue, abdominal pain, orthostatic effects.

Cardiovascular: Palpitation, hypertension, hypotension, myocardial infarction.

Gastrointestinal: Gastrointestinal pain, dysphagia, heartburn.

Metabolic: Weight loss.

Musculoskeletal: Leg pain.

Nervous System/Psychiatric: Chorea, somnolence, falling, anxiety, disorientation, decreased mental acuity, gait abnormalities, extrapyramidal disorder, agitation, nervousness, sleep disorders, memory impairment.

Respiratory: Cough, pharyngeal pain, common cold.

Skin: Rash.

Special Senses: Blurred vision.

Urogenital: Urinary incontinence.

Laboratory Tests: Decreased white blood cell count and serum potassium; increased BUN, serum creatinine and serum LDH; protein and glucose in the urine.

The following adverse experiences have been reported in post-marketing experience with Sinemet CR:

Cardiovascular: Cardiac irregularities, syncope.

Gastrointestinal: Taste alterations, dark saliva.

Hypersensitivity: Angioedema, uticaria, pruritus, bullous lesions (including pemphigus-like reactions).

Nervous System/Psychiatric: Neuroleptic malignant syndrome (see WARNINGS, Sinemet CR), increased tremor, peripheral neuropathy, psychotic episodes including delusions and paranoid ideation, increased libido.

Skin: Alopecia, flushing, dark sweat.

Urogenital: Dark urine.

Other adverse reactions that have been reported with levodopa alone and with various carbidopa-levodopa formulations and may occur with Sinemet CR are:

Cardiovascular: Phlebitis.

Gastrointestinal: Gastrointestinal bleeding, development of duodenal ulcer, sialorrhea, bruxism, hiccups, flatulence, burning sensation of tongue.

Hematologic: Hemolytic and nonhemolytic anemia, thrombocytopenia, leukopenia, agranulocytosis.

Hypersensitivity: Henoch-Schonlein purpura.

Metabolic: Weight gain, edema.

Nervous System/Psychiatric: Ataxia, depression with suicidal tendencies, dementia, euphoria, convulsions (however, a causal relationship has not been established);

bradykinetic episodes, numbness, muscle twitching, blepharospasm (which may be taken as an early sign of excess dosage; consideration of dosage reduction may be made at this time), trismus, activation of latent Horner's syndrome, nightmares.

Skin: Malignant melanoma (see also CONTRAINDICATIONS, Sinemet CR), increased sweating.

Special Senses: Oculogyric crises, mydriasis, diplopia.

Urogenital: Urinary retention, priapism.

Miscellaneous: Faintness, hoarseness, malaise, hot flashes, sense of stimulation, bizarre breathing patterns.

Laboratory Tests: Abnormalities in alkaline phosphatase, SGOT (AST), SGPT (ALT), bilirubin, Coombs test, uric acid.

DOSAGE AND ADMINISTRATION

SINEMET

The optimum daily dosage of Sinemet must be determined by careful titration in each patient. Sinemet tablets are available in a 1:4 ratio of carbidopa to levodopa (Sinemet 25-100) as well as 1:10 ratio (Sinemet 25-250 and Sinemet 10-100). Tablets of the two ratios may be given separately or combined as needed to provide the optimum dosage.

Studies show that peripheral dopa decarboxylase is saturated by carbidopa at approximately 70-100 mg a day. Patients receiving less than this amount of carbidopa are more likely to experience nausea and vomiting.

Usual Initial Dosage

Dosage is best initiated with 1 tablet of Sinemet 25-100 three times a day. This dosage schedule provides 75 mg of carbidopa per day. Dosage may be increased by 1 tablet every day or every other day, as necessary, until a dosage of 8 tablets of Sinemet 25-100 a day is reached.

If Sinemet 10-100 is used, dosage may be initiated with 1 tablet 3 or 4 times a day. However, this will not provide an adequate amount of carbidopa for many patients. Dosage may be increased by 1 tablet every day or every other day until a total of 8 tablets (2 tablets qid) is reached.

How to Transfer Patients From Levodopa

Levodopa must be discontinued at least 12 hours before starting Sinemet. A daily dosage of Sinemet should be chosen that will provide approximately 25% of the previous levodopa dosage. Patients who are taking less than 1500 mg of levodopa a day should be started on 1 tablet of Sinemet 25-100 three or four times a day. The suggested starting dosage for most patients taking more than 1500 mg of levodopa is 1 tablet of Sinemet 25-250 three or four times a day.

Maintenance

Therapy should be individualized and adjusted according to the desired therapeutic response. At least 70-100 mg of carbidopa per day should be provided. When a greater proportion of carbidopa is required, 1 tablet of Sinemet 25-100 may be substituted for each tablet of Sinemet 10-100. When more levodopa is required, Sinemet 25-250 should be substituted for Sinemet 25-100 or Sinemet 10-100. If necessary, the dosage of Sinemet 25-250 may be increased by one-half or one tablet every day or every other day to a maximum of 8 tablets a day. Experience with total daily dosages of carbidopa greater than 200 mg is limited.

Because both therapeutic and adverse responses occur more rapidly with Sinemet than with levodopa alone, patients should be monitored closely during the dose adjustment period. Specifically, involuntary movements will occur more rapidly with Sinemet than with levodopa. The occurrence of involuntary movements may require dosage reduction. Blepharospasm may be a useful early sign of excess dosage in some patients.

Addition of Other Antiparkinsonian Medications

Standard drugs for Parkinson's disease, other than levodopa without a decarboxylase inhibitor, may be used concomitantly while Sinemet is being administered, although dosage adjustments may be required.

Interruption of Therapy

Sporadic cases of a symptom complex resembling Neuroleptic Malignant Syndrome (NMS) have been associated with dose reductions and withdrawal of Sinemet. Patients should be observed carefully if abrupt reduction or discontinuation of Sinemet is required, especially if the patient is receiving neuroleptics. (See WARNINGS, Sinemet.)

If general anesthesia is required, Sinemet may be continued as long as the patient is permitted to take fluids and medication by mouth. If therapy is interrupted temporarily, the patient should be observed for symptoms resembling NMS, and the usual daily dosage may be administered as soon as the patient is able to take oral medication.

SINEMET CR

Sinemet CR contains carbidopa and levodopa in a 1:4 ratio as either the 50-200 tablet or the 25-100 tablet. The daily dosage of Sinemet CR must be determined by careful titration. Patients should be monitored closely during the dose adjustment period, particularly with regard to appearance or worsening of involuntary movements, dyskinesias or nausea. Sinemet CR 50-200 may be administered as whole or as half-tablets which should not be chewed or crushed. Sinemet CR 25-100 may be used in combination with Sinemet CR 50-200 to titrate to the optimum dosage, or as an alternative to the 50-200 half-tablet.

Standard drugs for Parkinson's disease, other than levodopa without a decarboxylase inhibitor, may be used concomitantly while Sinemet CR is being administered, although their dosage may have to be adjusted.

Since carbidopa prevents the reversal of levodopa effects caused by pyridoxine, Sinemet CR can be given to patients receiving supplemental pyridoxine (vitamin B_6).

Initial Dosage

Patients Currently Treated With Conventional Carbidopa-Levodopa Preparations

Studies show that peripheral dopa-decarboxylase is saturated by the bioavailable carbidopa at doses of 70 mg a day and greater. Because the bioavailabilities of carbidopa and levodopa in Sinemet and Sinemet CR are different, appropriate adjustments should be made, as shown in TABLE 2.

TABLE 2 Approximate Bioavailabilities at Steady State*

	Sinemet CR 50-200	Sinemet 25-100
Amount of levodopa in each tablet	200 mg	100 mg
Approximate bioavailability	0.70-0.75†	0.99‡
Approximate amount of bioavailable levodopa in each tablet	140-150 mg	99 mg

* This table is only a guide to bioavailabilities since other factors such as food, drugs, and inter-patient variabilities may affect the bioavailability of carbidopa and levodopa.
† The extent of availability of levodopa from Sinemet CR was about 70-75% relative to intravenous levodopa or standard Sinemet in the elderly.
‡ The extent of availability of levodopa from Sinemet was 99% relative to intravenous levodopa in the healthy elderly.

Dosage with Sinemet CR should be substituted at an amount that provides approximately 10% more levodopa per day, although this may need to be increased to a dosage that provides up to 30% more levodopa per day depending on clinical response (see Titration With Sinemet CR). The interval between doses of Sinemet CR should be 4-8 hours during the waking day. (See CLINICAL PHARMACOLOGY, Sinemet CR, Pharmacodynamics.)

A guideline for initiation of Sinemet CR is shown in TABLE 3.

TABLE 3 Guidelines for Initial Conversion from Sinemet to Sinemet CR

Sinemet Total Daily Dose* of Levodopa	Sinemet CR Suggested Dosage Regimen
300-400 mg	200 mg bid
500-600 mg	300 mg bid or 200 mg tid
700-800 mg	A total of 800 mg in 3 or more divided doses (*e.g.*, 300 mg AM, 300 mg early PM, and 200 mg later PM)
900-1000 mg	A total of 1000 mg in 3 or more divided doses (*e.g.*, 400 mg AM, 400 mg early PM, and 200 mg later PM)

* For dosing ranges not shown in the table see Initial Dosage, Patients Currently Treated With Conventional Carbidopa-Levodopa Preparations.

Patients Currently Treated With Levodopa Without a Decarboxylase Inhibitor

Levodopa must be discontinued at least 12 hours before therapy with Sinemet CR is started. Sinemet CR should be substituted at a dosage that will provide approximately 25% of the previous levodopa dosage. In patients with mild to moderate disease, the initial dose is usually 1 tablet of Sinemet CR 50-200 bid.

Patients Not Receiving Levodopa

In patients with mild to moderate disease, the initial recommended dose is 1 tablet of Sinemet CR 50-200 bid. Initial dosage should not be given at intervals of less than 6 hours.

Titration With Sinemet CR

Following initiation of therapy, doses and dosing intervals may be increased or decreased depending upon therapeutic response. Most patients have been adequately treated with doses of Sinemet CR that provide 400-1600 mg of levodopa per day, administered as divided doses at intervals ranging from 4-8 hours during the waking day. Higher doses of Sinemet CR (2400 mg or more of levodopa per day) and shorter intervals (less than 4 hours) have been used, but are not usually recommended.

When doses of Sinemet CR are given at intervals of less than 4 hours, and/or if the divided doses are not equal, it is recommended that the smaller doses be given at the end of the day.

An interval of at least 3 days between dosage adjustments is recommended.

Maintenance

Because Parkinson's disease is progressive, periodic clinical evaluations are recommended; adjustment of the dosage regimen of Sinemet CR may be required.

Addition of Other Antiparkinson Medications

Anticholinergic agents, dopamine agonists, and amantadine can be given with Sinemet CR. Dosage adjustment of Sinemet CR may be necessary when these agents are added.

A dose of Sinemet 25-100 or 10-100 (one-half or a whole tablet) can be added to the dosage regimen of Sinemet CR in selected patients with advanced disease who need additional immediate-release levodopa for a brief time during daytime hours.

Interruption of Therapy

Sporadic cases of a symptom complex resembling Neuroleptic Malignant Syndrome (NMS) have been associated with dose reductions and withdrawal of Sinemet or Sinemet CR.

Patients should be observed carefully if abrupt reduction or discontinuation of Sinemet CR is required, especially if the patient is receiving neuroleptics. (See WARNINGS, Sinemet CR.)

If general anesthesia is required, Sinemet CR may be continued as long as the patient is permitted to take oral medication. If therapy is interrupted temporarily, the patient should be observed for symptoms resembling NMS, and the usual dosage should be administered as soon as the patient is able to take oral medication.

HOW SUPPLIED

SINEMET

Sinemet tablets are available in:

25-100: Yellow, oval, uncoated tablets, that are scored and coded "650" on one side and "SINEMET" on the other side.

10-100: Dark dapple-blue, oval, uncoated tablets, that are scored and coded "647" on one side and "SINEMET" on the other side.

25-250: Light dapple-blue, oval, uncoated tablets, that are scored and coded "654" on one side and "SINEMET" on the other side.

Storage: Sinemet tablets 10-100 and Sinemet tablets 25-250 must be protected from light.

SINEMET CR

Sinemet CR sustained-release tablets are available in:

50-200: Containing 50 mg of carbidopa and 200 mg of levodopa, are peach colored, oval, biconvex, compressed tablets, that are scored and coded "521" on one side and "SINEMET CR" on the other side.

25-100: Containing 25 mg carbidopa and 100 mg of levodopa, are pink colored, oval, biconvex, compressed tablets, that are coded "601" (with bar) on one side and "SINEMET CR" on the other side.

Storage: Avoid temperatures above 30°C (86°F). Store in a tightly closed container.

PRODUCT LISTING - RATED THERAPEUTICALLY EQUIVALENT

Tablet - Oral - 10 mg;100 mg

30 x 25	$859.35	GENERIC, Sky Pharmaceuticals Packaging, Inc	63739-0046-03
30's	$17.69	GENERIC, Heartland Healthcare Services	61392-0177-30
30's	$17.69	GENERIC, Heartland Healthcare Services	61392-0177-39
31 x 10	$203.01	GENERIC, Vangard Labs	00615-3537-53
31 x 10	$203.01	GENERIC, Vangard Labs	00615-3537-63
31's	$18.27	GENERIC, Heartland Healthcare Services	61392-0177-31
32's	$18.86	GENERIC, Heartland Healthcare Services	61392-0177-32
45's	$26.53	GENERIC, Heartland Healthcare Services	61392-0177-45
60's	$35.37	GENERIC, Heartland Healthcare Services	61392-0177-60
90's	$53.06	GENERIC, Heartland Healthcare Services	61392-0177-90
100's	$36.44	FEDERAL UPPER LIMIT, H.C.F.A. F F P	99999-0653-02
100's	$52.10	GENERIC, West Point Pharma	59591-0247-68
100's	$52.60	GENERIC, Qualitest Products Inc	00603-2568-21
100's	$53.95	GENERIC, Major Pharmaceuticals Inc	00904-7718-60
100's	$56.14	GENERIC, Geneva Pharmaceuticals	00781-1626-13
100's	$58.04	GENERIC, Moore, H.L. Drug Exchange Inc	00839-7765-06
100's	$58.05	GENERIC, Geneva Pharmaceuticals	00781-1626-01
100's	$65.50	GENERIC, Ivax Corporation	00182-1948-89
100's	$65.50	GENERIC, Vangard Labs	00615-3537-13
100's	$70.85	GENERIC, Purepac Pharmaceutical Company	00228-2538-10
100's	$70.88	GENERIC, Teva Pharmaceuticals Usa	00093-0292-01
100's	$70.88	GENERIC, Endo Laboratories Llc	60951-0603-68
100's	$72.10	GENERIC, Udl Laboratories Inc	51079-0755-20
100's	$74.60	GENERIC, Major Pharmaceuticals Inc	00904-7718-61
100's	$75.29	SINEMET, Physicians Total Care	54868-1544-01
100's	$82.69	SINEMET, Dupont Pharmaceuticals	00056-0647-68
100's	$90.35	SINEMET, Dupont Pharmaceuticals	00056-0647-28

Tablet - Oral - 25 mg;100 mg

25's	$9.83	GENERIC, Udl Laboratories Inc	51079-0756-19
30 x 25	$573.83	GENERIC, Sky Pharmaceuticals Packaging, Inc	63739-0047-03
30 x 25	$668.25	GENERIC, Sky Pharmaceuticals Packaging, Inc	63739-0048-01
30 x 25	$950.25	GENERIC, Sky Pharmaceuticals Packaging, Inc	63739-0047-01
30's	$18.77	GENERIC, Heartland Healthcare Services	61392-0180-30
30's	$18.77	GENERIC, Heartland Healthcare Services	61392-0180-39
31 x 10	$215.44	GENERIC, Vangard Labs	00615-3561-53
31 x 10	$215.44	GENERIC, Vangard Labs	00615-3561-63
31's	$19.39	GENERIC, Heartland Healthcare Services	61392-0180-31
32's	$20.02	GENERIC, Heartland Healthcare Services	61392-0180-32
45's	$28.15	GENERIC, Heartland Healthcare Services	61392-0180-45
60's	$37.53	GENERIC, Heartland Healthcare Services	61392-0180-60
90's	$56.30	GENERIC, Heartland Healthcare Services	61392-0180-90
100's	$39.15	FEDERAL UPPER LIMIT, H.C.F.A. F F P	99999-0653-05
100's	$58.15	GENERIC, West Point Pharma	59591-0246-68
100's	$58.50	GENERIC, Moore, H.L. Drug Exchange Inc	00839-7766-06
100's	$58.80	GENERIC, Qualitest Products Inc	00603-2569-21
100's	$62.44	GENERIC, Geneva Pharmaceuticals	00781-1627-13
100's	$64.17	GENERIC, Geneva Pharmaceuticals	00781-1627-01
100's	$65.25	GENERIC, Elan Pharmaceuticals	59075-0585-10
100's	$76.92	GENERIC, American Health Packaging	62584-0642-01
100's	$79.80	GENERIC, Udl Laboratories Inc	51079-0756-20
100's	$80.00	GENERIC, Purepac Pharmaceutical Company	00228-2539-10
100's	$80.02	GENERIC, Teva Pharmaceuticals Usa	00093-0293-01
100's	$80.02	GENERIC, Endo Laboratories Llc	60951-0605-68
100's	$84.20	GENERIC, Major Pharmaceuticals Inc	00904-7719-61
100's	$88.91	SINEMET, Physicians Total Care	54868-1270-01
100's	$93.36	SINEMET, Dupont Pharmaceuticals	00056-0650-68
100's	$99.06	SINEMET, Dupont Pharmaceuticals	00056-0650-28
100's	$132.85	GENERIC, Ivax Corporation	00182-1949-89

Tablet - Oral - 25 mg;250 mg

25 x 30	$668.25	GENERIC, Sky Pharmaceuticals Packaging, Inc	63739-0048-03
30's	$24.29	GENERIC, Heartland Healthcare Services	61392-0183-30
30's	$24.29	GENERIC, Heartland Healthcare Services	61392-0183-39
31 x 10	$274.93	GENERIC, Vangard Labs	00615-4504-53
31 x 10	$274.93	GENERIC, Vangard Labs	00615-4504-63
31's	$25.10	GENERIC, Heartland Healthcare Services	61392-0183-31
32's	$25.91	GENERIC, Heartland Healthcare Services	61392-0183-32
45's	$36.44	GENERIC, Heartland Healthcare Services	61392-0183-45
60's	$48.58	GENERIC, Heartland Healthcare Services	61392-0183-60
90's	$72.87	GENERIC, Heartland Healthcare Services	61392-0183-90
100's	$46.57	FEDERAL UPPER LIMIT, H.C.F.A. F F P	99999-0653-09
100's	$71.30	GENERIC, West Point Pharma	59591-0250-68
100's	$73.50	GENERIC, Watson/Schein Pharmaceuticals Inc	00364-2540-01
100's	$75.14	GENERIC, Qualitest Products Inc	00603-2570-21
100's	$75.25	GENERIC, Major Pharmaceuticals Inc	00904-7720-60
100's	$80.22	GENERIC, Geneva Pharmaceuticals	00781-1628-13
100's	$80.31	GENERIC, Moore, H.L. Drug Exchange Inc	00839-7767-06
100's	$81.79	GENERIC, Geneva Pharmaceuticals	00781-1628-01
100's	$83.50	GENERIC, Elan Pharmaceuticals	59075-0587-10
100's	$88.70	GENERIC, Ivax Corporation	00182-1950-89
100's	$89.22	GENERIC, Major Pharmaceuticals Inc	00904-7720-61
100's	$89.55	GENERIC, American Health Packaging	62584-0643-01
100's	$98.20	GENERIC, Udl Laboratories Inc	51079-0783-20
100's	$101.95	GENERIC, Purepac Pharmaceutical Company	00228-2540-10
100's	$101.97	GENERIC, Teva Pharmaceuticals Usa	00093-0294-01
100's	$101.97	GENERIC, Endo Laboratories Llc	60951-0607-68
100's	$118.96	SINEMET, Dupont Pharmaceuticals	00056-0654-68
100's	$125.51	SINEMET, Dupont Pharmaceuticals	00056-0654-28

Tablet, Extended Release - Oral - 25 mg;100 mg

100's	$93.10	GENERIC, Aventis Pharmaceuticals	51079-0978-20
100's	$94.00	GENERIC, Mylan Pharmaceuticals Inc	00378-0088-01

Tablet, Extended Release - Oral - 50 mg;200 mg

25's	$46.16	GENERIC, Udl Laboratories Inc	51079-0923-19
60's	$131.01	SINEMET CR, Physicians Total Care	54868-1882-01
100's	$174.15	GENERIC, Udl Laboratories Inc	51079-0923-20
100's	$180.85	GENERIC, Mylan Pharmaceuticals Inc	00378-0094-01
100's	$187.46	SINEMET CR, Physicians Total Care	54868-1882-00
100's	$201.16	SINEMET CR, Dupont Pharmaceuticals	00056-0521-68
100's	$213.18	SINEMET CR, Dupont Pharmaceuticals	00056-0521-28

PRODUCT LISTING - EQUIVALENTS NOT AVAILABLE

Tablet - Oral - 25 mg;100 mg

30's	$8.75	GENERIC, Physicians Total Care	54868-1334-01
30's	$19.14	GENERIC, Allscripts Pharmaceutical Company	54569-4988-00
100's	$26.05	GENERIC, Physicians Total Care	54868-1334-02

Tablet, Extended Release - Oral - 25 mg;100 mg

100's	$104.59	SINEMET CR, Dupont Pharmaceuticals	00056-0601-68
100's	$110.20	SINEMET CR, Dupont Pharmaceuticals	00056-0601-28

Carbinoxamine Maleate *(003545)*

Categories: Rhinitis, allergic; Pregnancy Category C
Drug Classes: Antihistamines, H1
Brand Names: Histex Pd
Foreign Brand Availability: Allergefon (France); Histin (Thailand); Polistin T-Caps (Germany); Sinumine (Thailand)

DESCRIPTION

Histex Pd is a dye free, alcohol free, and sugar free antihistamine liquid containing 4 mg of carbinoxamine maleate per 5 ml.

The chemical name of carbinoxamine maleate is 2[-*p*-chloro-α-[2-(dimethylamino)ethoxy] benzyl]pyridine maleate. The molecular formula is $C_{16}H_{19}ClN_2O{\cdot}C_4H_4O_4$, and the molecular weight is 406.87.

Inactive ingredients: Sodium saccharin, propylene glycol, sorbitol, glycerin, and gum fruit flavor.

CLINICAL PHARMACOLOGY

Carbinoxamine maleate possesses H_1 antihistaminic activity and mild anticholinergic and sedative effects. Serum halflife for carbinoxamine is estimated to be 10-20 hours. Virtually no intact drug is excreted in the urine.

INDICATIONS AND USAGE

Carbinoxamine maleate is indicated for the relief of nasal and non-nasal symptoms of seasonal and perennial allergic rhinitis.

CONTRAINDICATIONS

Patients with hypersensitivity or idiosyncrasy to any ingredients, patients taking monoamine oxidase (MAO) inhibitors.

PRECAUTIONS

Avoid alcohol and other CNS depressants while taking these products. Patients sensitive to antihistamines may experience moderate to severe drowsiness.

PREGNANCY CATEGORY C

Animal reproduction studies have not been conducted with these products. It is also unknown whether these products can cause fetal harm when administered to a pregnant woman or affect reproduction.

NURSING MOTHERS

Use with caution in nursing mothers.

DRUG INTERACTIONS

Antihistamines may enhance the effects of tricyclic anti-depressants, barbiturates, alcohol, and other CNS depressants, MAO inhibitors prolong and intensify the anticholinergic effects of antihistamines.

ADVERSE REACTIONS

Antihistamines: Sedation, dizziness, diplopia, vomiting, diarrhea, dry mouth, headache, nervousness, nausea, anorexia, heartburn, weakness, polyuria and rarely, excitability in children.

DOSAGE AND ADMINISTRATION

See TABLE 1.

TABLE 1

Age	Dose	Frequency
Adults and children 6 years and over	1 teaspoon	qid
Children 18 months to 6 years	½ teaspoon	qid
Children 9-18 months (titrate dosage individually)	¼-½ teaspoon	qid

HOW SUPPLIED

Histex Pd is bubble gum-flavored and is supplied in plastic bottles of 16 fluid ounces (473 ml).

DISPENSE IN A TIGHT, LIGHT-RESISTANT CONTAINER WITH A CHILD-RESISTANT CLOSURE.

Recommended Storage: Store at controlled room temperature 15-30°C (59-86°F).

Carboplatin *(000660)*

Categories: Carcinoma, ovarian; Pregnancy Category D; FDA Approved 1989 Mar
Drug Classes: Antineoplastics, platinum agents
Brand Names: **Paraplatin**
Foreign Brand Availability: Blastocarb (Mexico); Boplatex (Mexico); Carboplat (Germany; Hungary); Carboplatin (Australia; Denmark; Israel; New-Zealand; Norway); Carboplatin a (Portugal); Carboplatin Abic (Switzerland; Thailand); Carboplatin DBL (Malaysia); Carboplatin dbl (Greece; Portugal); Carboplatin Lederle (Sweden); Carboplatino (Peru); Carbosin (Greece; Norway; South-Africa); Carbosin Lundbeck (Finland); Carbotec (Mexico); Carplan (Korea); Delta West Carboplatin (Indonesia; Philippines); Erbakar (Indonesia); Ercar (Spain); Ifacap (Mexico); Kemocarb (Philippines); Neoplatin (Korea); Oncocarbin (India); Paraplatin-AQ (Canada); Paraplatin RTU (South-Africa); Paraplatine (France)
HCFA JCODE(S): J9045 50 mg IV

WARNING

Carboplatin should be administered under the supervision of a qualified physician experienced in the use of cancer chemotherapeutic agents. Appropriate management of therapy and complications is possible only when adequate treatment facilities are readily available.

Bone marrow suppression is dose-related and may be severe, resulting in infection and/or bleeding. Anemia may be cumulative and may require transfusion support. Vomiting is another frequent drug-related side effect.

Anaphylactic-like reactions to carboplatin have been reported and may occur within minutes of carboplatin administration. Epinephrine, corticosteroids, and antihistamines have been employed to alleviate symptoms.

DESCRIPTION

Paraplatin (carboplatin for injection) is supplied as a sterile, lyophilized white powder available in single-dose vials contains 50, 150, and 450 mg of carboplatin for administration by intravenous infusion. Each vial contains equal parts by weight of carboplatin and mannitol.

Carboplatin is a platinum coordination compound that is used as a cancer chemotherapeutic agent. The chemical name for carboplatin is platinum, diammine [1,1-cyclobutane-dicarboxylato(2-)-0,0']-, (SP-4-2).

Carboplatin is a white crystalline powder with the molecular formula of $C_6H_{12}N_2O_4Pt$ and a molecular weight of 371.25. It is soluble in water at a rate of approximately 14 mg/ml, and the pH of a 1% solution is 5-7. It is virtually insoluble in ethanol, acetone, and dimethylacetamide.

CLINICAL PHARMACOLOGY

Carboplatin, like cisplatin, produces predominantly interstrand DNA cross-links rather than DNA-protein cross-links. This effect is apparently cell-cycle nonspecific. The aquation of carboplatin, which is thought to produce the active species, occurs at a slower rate than in the case of cisplatin. Despite this difference, it appears that both carboplatin and cisplatin induce equal numbers of drug-DNA cross-links, causing equivalent lesions and biological effects. The differences in potencies for carboplatin and cisplatin appear to be directly related to the difference in aquation rates.

In patients with creatinine clearances of about 60 ml/min or greater, plasma levels of intact carboplatin decay in a biphasic manner after a 30 minute intravenous infusion of 300-500 mg/m^2 of carboplatin for injection. The initial plasma half-life (alpha) was found to be 1.1-2.0 hours (n=6), and the postdistribution plasma half-life (beta) was found to be 2.6-5.9 hours (n=6). The total body clearance, apparent volume of distribution, and mean residence time for carboplatin are 4.4 L/h, 16 L, and 3.5 hours, respectively. The C_{max} values and areas under the plasma concentration versus time curves from 0 to infinity (AUC inf) increase linearly with dose, although the increase was slightly more than dose proportional. Carboplatin, therefore, exhibits linear pharmacokinetics over the dosing range studied (300-500 mg/m^2).

Carboplatin is not bound to plasma proteins. No significant quantities of protein-free, ultrafilterable platinum-containing species other than carboplatin are present in plasma. However, platinum from carboplatin becomes irreversibly bound to plasma proteins and is slowly eliminated with a minimum half-life of 5 days.

The major route of elimination of carboplatin is renal excretion. Patients with creatinine clearances of approximately 60 ml/min or greater excrete 65% of the dose in the urine within 12 hours and 71% of the dose within 24 hours. All of the platinum in the 24 hour urine is present as carboplatin. Only 3-5% of the administered platinum is excreted in the urine between 24 and 96 hours. There are insufficient data to determine whether biliary excretion occurs.

In patients with creatinine clearances below 60 ml/min the total body and renal clearances of carboplatin decrease as the creatinine clearance decreases. Carboplatin dosages should therefore be reduced in these patients (see DOSAGE AND ADMINISTRATION).

INDICATIONS AND USAGE

Initial Treatment of Advanced Ovarian Carcinoma: Carboplatin is indicated for the initial treatment of advanced ovarian carcinoma in established combination with other approved chemotherapeutic agents. One established combination regimen consists of carboplatin and cyclophosphamide. Two randomized controlled studies conducted by the NCIC and SWOG with carboplatin vs. cisplatin, both in combination with cyclophosphamide, have demonstrated equivalent overall survival between the 2 groups.

There is limited statistical power to demonstrate equivalence in overall pathologic complete response rates and long-term survival (≥3 years) because of the small number of patients with these outcomes; the small number of patients with residual tumor <2 cm after initial surgery also limits the statistical power to demonstrate equivalence in this subgroup.

Secondary Treatment of Advanced Ovarian Carcinoma: Carboplatin is indicated for the palliative treatment of patients with ovarian carcinoma recurrent after prior chemotherapy, including patients who have been previously treated with cisplatin.

Within the group of patients previously treated with cisplatin, those who have developed progressive disease while receiving cisplatin therapy may have a decreased response rate.

NON-FDA APPROVED INDICATIONS

Studies have reported that Carboplatin may also be useful in the treatment of lung cancer, non-seminomatous testicular cancer, head and neck cancer, and bladder cancer. However, these uses have not been approved by the FDA and further clinical trials are needed.

CONTRAINDICATIONS

Carboplatin is contraindicated in patients with a history of severe allergic reactions to cisplatin or other platinum-containing compounds, or mannitol.

Carboplatin should not be employed in patients with severe bone marrow depression or significant bleeding.

WARNINGS

Bone marrow suppression (leukopenia, neutropenia, and thrombocytopenia) is dose-dependent and is also the dose-limiting toxicity. Peripheral blood counts should be frequently monitored during carboplatin treatment and, when appropriate, until recovery is achieved. Median nadir occurs at day 21 in patients receiving single-agent carboplatin for injection. In general, single intermittent courses of carboplatin should not be repeated until leukocyte, neutrophil, and platelet counts have recovered.

Since anemia is cumulative, transfusions may be needed during treatment with carboplatin for injection, particularly in patients receiving prolonged therapy.

Bone marrow suppression is increased in patients who have received prior therapy, especially regimens including cisplatin. Marrow suppression is also increased in patients with impaired kidney function. Initial carboplatin dosages in these patients should be appropriately reduced (see DOSAGE AND ADMINISTRATION) and blood counts should be carefully monitored between courses. The use of carboplatin in combination with other bone-marrow suppressing therapies must be carefully managed with respect to dosage and timing in order to minimize additive effects.

Carboplatin has limited nephrotoxic potential, but concomitant treatment with aminoglycosides has resulted in increased renal and/or audiologic toxicity, and caution must be exercised when a patient receives both drugs. Clinically significant hearing loss has been reported to occur in pediatric patients when carboplatin was administered at higher than recommended doses in combination with other ototoxic agents.

Carboplatin can induce emesis, which can be more severe in patients previously receiving emetogenic therapy. The incidence and intensity of emesis have been reduced by using premedication with antiemetics. Although no conclusive efficacy data exist with the following schedules of carboplatin for injection, lengthening the duration of single intravenous administration to 24 hours or dividing the total dose over 5 consecutive daily pulse doses has resulted in reduced emesis.

Although peripheral neurotoxicity is infrequent, its incidence is increased in patients older than 65 years and in patients previously treated with cisplatin. Pre-existing cisplatin-induced neurotoxicity does not worsen in about 70% of the patients receiving carboplatin as secondary treatment.

Loss of vision, which can be complete for light and colors, has been reported after the use of carboplatin with doses higher than those recommended in the packaging insert. Vision appears to recover totally or to a significant extent within weeks of stopping these high doses.

As in the case of other platinum coordination compounds, allergic reactions to carboplatin have been reported. These may occur within minutes of administration and should be managed with appropriate supportive therapy. There is increased risk of allergic reactions including anaphylaxis in patients previously exposed to platinum therapy. (See CONTRAINDICATIONS and ADVERSE REACTIONS, Allergic Reactions.)

High dosages of carboplatin (more than 4 times the recommended dose) have resulted in severe abnormalities of liver function tests.

Carboplatin may cause fetal harm when administered to a pregnant woman. Carboplatin has been shown to be embryotoxic and teratogenic in rats. There are no adequate and well-controlled studies in pregnant women. If this drug is used during pregnancy, or if the patient becomes pregnant while receiving this drug, the patient should be apprised of the potential hazard to the fetus. Women of childbearing potential should be advised to avoid becoming pregnant.

PRECAUTIONS

General: Needles or intravenous administration sets containing aluminum parts that may come in contact with carboplatin should not be used for the preparation or administration of the drug. Aluminum can react with carboplatin causing precipitate formation and loss of potency.

Carcinogenesis, Mutagenesis, and Impairment of Fertility: The carcinogenic potential of carboplatin has not been studied, but compounds with similar mechanisms of action and mutagenicity profiles have been reported to be carcinogenic. Carboplatin has been shown to be mutagenic both *in vitro* and *in vivo*. It has also been shown to be embryotoxic and teratogenic in rats receiving the drug during organogenesis. Secondary malignancies have been reported in association with multidrug therapy.

Pregnancy Category D: See WARNINGS.

Nursing Mothers: It is not known whether carboplatin is excreted in human milk. Because there is a possibility of toxicity in nursing infants secondary to carboplatin treatment of the mother, it is recommended that breast-feeding be discontinued if the mother is treated with carboplatin for injection.

Pediatric Use: Safety and effectiveness in pediatric patients have not been established (see WARNINGS).

DRUG INTERACTIONS

The renal effects of nephrotoxic compounds may be potentiated by carboplatin for injection.

ADVERSE REACTIONS

TABLE 4 *Adverse Experiences in Patients With Ovarian Cancer*

		First Line Combination Therapy*	Second Line Single-Agent Therapy†
Bone Marrow			
Thrombocytopenia	$<100,000/mm^3$	66%	62%
	$<50,000/mm^3$	33%	35%
Neutropenia	<2000 cells/mm^3	96%	67%
	<1000 cells/mm^3	82%	21%
Leukopenia	<4000 cells/mm^3	97%	85%
	<2000 cells/mm^3	71%	26%
Anemia	<11 g/dl	90%	90%
	<8 g/dl	14%	21%
Infections		16%	5%
Bleeding		8%	5%
Transfusions		35%	44%
Gastrointestinal			
Nausea and vomiting		93%	92%
Vomiting		83%	81%
Other GI side effects		46%	21%
Neurologic			
Peripheral neuropathies		15%	6%
Ototoxicity		12%	1%
Other sensory side effects		5%	1%
Central neurotoxicity		26%	5%
Renal			
Serum creatinine elevations		6%	10%
Blood urea elevations		17%	22%
Hepatic			
Bilirubin elevations		5%	5%
SGOT elevations		20%	19%
Alkaline phosphatase elevations		29%	37%
Electrolytes Loss			
Sodium		10%	47%
Potassium		16%	28%
Calcium		16%	31%
Magnesium		61%	43%
Other Side Effects			
Pain		44%	23%
Asthenia		41%	11%
Cardiovascular		19%	6%
Respiratory		10%	6%
Allergic		11%	2%
Genitourinary		10%	2%
Alopecia		49%	2%
Mucositis		8%	1%

* **Use with cyclophosphamide for initial treatment of ovarian cancer:** Data are based on the experience of 393 patients with ovarian cancer (regardless of baseline status) who received initial combination therapy with carboplatin and cyclophosphamide in 2 randomized controlled studies conducted by SWOG and NCIC. Combination with cyclophosphamide as well as duration of treatment may be responsible for the differences that can be noted in the adverse experience table.

† **Single-agent use for the secondary treatment of ovarian cancer:** Data are based on the experience of 553 patients with previously treated ovarian carcinoma (regardless of baseline status) who received single-agent carboplatin for injection.

In the narrative section that follows, the incidences of adverse events are based on data from 1893 patients with various types of tumors who received carboplatin as single-agent therapy.

HEMATOLOGIC TOXICITY

Bone marrow suppression is the dose-limiting toxicity of carboplatin for injection. Thrombocytopenia with platelet counts below $50,000/mm^3$ occurs in 25% of the patients (35% of pretreated ovarian cancer patients); neutropenia with granulocyte counts below $1000/mm^3$ occurs in 16% of the patients (21% of pretreated ovarian cancer patients); leukopenia with WBC counts below $2000/mm^3$ occurs in 15% of the patients (26% of pretreated ovarian cancer patients). The nadir usually occurs about day 21 in patients receiving single-agent therapy. By day 28, 90% of patients have platelet counts above $100,000/mm^3$; 74% have neutrophil counts above $2000/mm^3$; 67% have leukocyte counts above $4000/mm^3$.

Marrow suppression is usually more severe in patients with impaired kidney function. Patients with poor performance status have also experienced a higher incidence of severe leukopenia and thrombocytopenia.

The hematologic effects, although usually reversible, have resulted in infectious or hemorrhagic complications in 5% of the patients treated with carboplatin for injection, with drug-related death occurring in less than 1% of the patients. Fever has also been reported in patients with neutropenia.

Anemia with hemoglobin less than 11 g/dl has been observed in 71% of the patients who started therapy with a baseline above that value. The incidence of anemia increases with increasing exposure to carboplatin for injection. Transfusions have been administered to 26% of the patients treated with carboplatin (44% of previously treated ovarian cancer patients).

Bone marrow depression may be more severe when carboplatin is combined with other bone-marrow suppressing drugs or with radiotherapy.

GASTROINTESTINAL TOXICITY

Vomiting occurs in 65% of the patients (81% of previously treated ovarian cancer patients) and in about one-third of these patients it is severe. Carboplatin, as a single-agent or in combination, is significantly less emetogenic than cisplatin; however, patients previously treated with emetogenic agents, especially cisplatin, appear to be more prone to vomiting. Nausea alone occurs in an additional 10-15% of patients. Both nausea and vomiting usually cease within 24 hours of treatment and are often responsive to antiemetic measures. Although no conclusive efficacy data exist with the following schedules, prolonged administration of carboplatin for injection, either by continuous 24-hour infusion or by daily pulse doses given for 5 consecutive days, was associated with less severe vomiting than the single dose intermittent schedule. Emesis was increased when carboplatin was used in combination with other emetogenic compounds. Other gastrointestinal effects observed frequently were pain, in 17% of the patients; diarrhea, in 6%; and constipation, also in 6%.

NEUROLOGIC TOXICITY

Peripheral neuropathies have been observed in 4% of the patients receiving carboplatin (6% of pretreated ovarian cancer patients) with mild paresthesias occurring most frequently. Carboplatin therapy produces significantly fewer and less severe neurologic side effects than does therapy with cisplatin. However, patients older than 65 years and/or previously treated with cisplatin appear to have an increased risk (10%) for peripheral neuropathies. In 70% of the patients with pre-existing cisplatin-induced peripheral neurotoxicity, there was no worsening of symptoms during therapy with carboplatin for injection. Clinical ototoxicity and other sensory abnormalities such as visual disturbances and change in taste have been reported in only 1% of the patients. Central nervous system symptoms have been reported in 5% of the patients and appear to be most often related to the use of antiemetics.

Although the overall incidence of peripheral neurologic side effects induced by carboplatin is low, prolonged treatment, particularly in cisplatin-pretreated patients, may result in cumulative neurotoxicity.

NEPHROTOXICITY

Development of abnormal renal function test results is uncommon, despite the fact that carboplatin, unlike cisplatin, has usually been administered without high-volume fluid hydration and/or forced diuresis. The incidences of abnormal renal function tests reported are 6% for serum creatinine and 14% for blood urea nitrogen (10 and 22%, respectively, in pretreated ovarian cancer patients). Most of these reported abnormalities have been mild and about one half of them were reversible.

Creatinine clearance has proven to be the most sensitive measure of kidney function in patients receiving carboplatin for injection, and it appears to be the most useful test for correlating drug clearance and bone marrow suppression. Twenty-seven percent (27%) of the patients who had a baseline value of 60 ml/min or more demonstrated a reduction below this value during carboplatin therapy.

HEPATIC TOXICITY

The incidences of abnormal liver function tests in patients with normal baseline values were reported as follows: total bilirubin, 5%; SGOT, 15%; and alkaline phosphatase, 24%; (5, 19, and 37%, respectively, in pretreated ovarian cancer patients). These abnormalities have generally been mild and reversible in about one half of the cases, although the rôle of metastatic tumor in the liver may complicate the assessment in many patients. In a limited series of patients receiving very high dosages of carboplatin and autologous bone marrow transplantation, severe abnormalities of liver function tests were reported.

ELECTROLYTE CHANGES

The incidences of abnormally decreased serum electrolyte values reported were as follows: sodium, 29%; potassium, 20%; calcium, 22%: and magnesium, 29%; (47, 28, 31, and 43%, respectively, in pretreated ovarian cancer patients). Electrolyte supplementation was not routinely administered concomitantly with carboplatin for injection, and these electrolyte abnormalities were rarely associated with symptoms.

ALLERGIC REACTIONS

Hypersensitivity to carboplatin has been reported in 2% of the patients. These allergic reactions have been similar in nature and severity to those reported with other platinum-containing compounds, *i.e.*, rash, urticaria, erythema, pruritus, and rarely bronchospasm and hypotension. Anaphylactic reactions have been reported as part of postmarketing surveillance (see WARNINGS). These reactions have been successfully managed with standard epinephrine, corticosteroid, and antihistamine therapy.

OTHER EVENTS

Pain and asthenia were the most frequently reported miscellaneous adverse effects; their relationship to the tumor and to anemia was likely. Alopecia was reported (3%). Cardiovascular, respiratory, genitourinary, and mucosal side effects have occurred in 6% or less of the patients. Cardiovascular events (cardiac failure, embolism, cerebrovascular accidents) were fatal in less than 1% of the patients and did not appear to be related to chemotherapy. Cancer-associated hemolytic uremic syndrome has been reported rarely.

Malaise, anorexia and hypertension have been reported as part of postmarketing surveillance.

DOSAGE AND ADMINISTRATION

NOTE: Aluminum reacts with carboplatin causing precipitate formation and loss of potency, therefore, needles or intravenous sets containing aluminum parts that may come in contact with the drug must not be used for the preparation or administration of carboplatin for injection.

Single-Agent Therapy: Carboplatin for injection, as a single-agent, has been shown to be effective in patients with recurrent ovarian carcinoma at a dosage of 360 mg/m^2 IV on day 1 every 4 weeks (alternatively see Formula Dosing). In general, however, single intermittent courses of carboplatin should not be repeated until the neutrophil count is at least 2000 and the platelet count is at least 100,000.

Combination Therapy With Cyclophosphamide: In the chemotherapy of advanced ovarian cancer, an effective combination for previously untreated patients consists of:

Carboplatin for Injection: 300 mg/m^2 IV on day 1 every 4 weeks for 6 cycles (alternatively see Formula Dosing).

Cyclophosphamide: 600 mg/m^{2}IV on day 1 every 4 weeks for 6 cycles. For directions regarding the use and administration of cyclophosphamide please refer to its package insert.

Intermittent courses of carboplatin in combination with cyclophosphamide should not be repeated until the neutrophil count is at least 2000 and the platelet count is at least 100,000.

Dose Adjustment Recommendations: Pretreatment platelet count and performance status are important prognostic factors for severity of myelosuppression in previously treated patients.

The suggested dose adjustments for single-agent or combination therapy shown in TABLE 5 are modified from controlled trials in previously treated and untreated patients with ovarian carcinoma. Blood counts were done weekly, and the recommendations are based on the lowest post-treatment platelet or neutrophil value.

TABLE 5

Platelets	Neutrophils	Adjusted Dose* (from prior course)
>100,000	>2000	125%
50-100,000	500-2000	No adjustment
<50,000	<500	75%

* Percentages apply to carboplatin as a single-agent or to both carboplatin and cyclophosphamide in combination. In the controlled studies, dosages were also adjusted at a lower level (50-60%) for severe myelosuppression. Escalations above 125% were not recommended for these studies.

Carboplatin is usually administered by an infusion lasting 15 minutes or longer. No pre- or post-treatment hydration or forced diuresis is required.

Patients With Impaired Kidney Function: Patients with creatinine clearance values below 60 ml/min are at increased risk of severe bone marrow suppression. In renally-impaired patients who received single-agent carboplatin therapy, the incidence of severe leukopenia, neutropenia, or thrombocytopenia has been about 25% when the dosage modifications in TABLE 6 have been used.

TABLE 6

Baseline Creatinine Clearance	Recommended Dose on Day 1
41-59 (ml/min)	250 (mg/m^2)
16-40 (ml/min)	200 (mg/m^2)

The data available for patients with severely impaired kidney function (creatinine clearance below 15 ml/min) are too limited to permit a recommendation for treatment.[1,2]

These dosing recommendations apply to the initial course of treatment. Subsequent dosages should be adjusted according to the patient's tolerance based on the degree of bone marrow suppression.

Formula Dosing: Another approach for determining the initial dose of carboplatin is the use of mathematical formulae, which are based on a patient's pre-existing renal function[3-5] or renal function and desired platelet nadir.[6] Renal excretion is the major route of elimination for carboplatin. (See CLINICAL PHARMACOLOGY.) The use of dosing formulae, as compared to empirical dose calculation based on body surface area, allows compensation for patient variations in pretreatment renal function that might otherwise result in either underdosing (in patients with above average renal function) or overdosing (in patients with impaired renal function).

A simple formula for calculating dosage, based upon a patient's glomerular filtration rate (GFR in ml/min) and carboplatin target area under the concentration vs time curve (AUC in mg/ml·min), has been proposed by Calvert.[3-5] In these studies, GFR was measured by ^{51}Cr-EDTA clearance.[7]

TABLE 7

Calvert Formula for Carboplatin Dosing
Total Dose (mg) = (target AUC) × (GFR + 25)
Note: With the Calvert formula, the total dose of carboplatin is calculated in mg, <u>not</u> mg/m^2.

The target of AUC of 4-6 mg/ml·min using single-agent carboplatin appears to provide the most appropriate dose range in previously treated patients.[4] This study also showed a trend between the AUC of single-agent carboplatin administered to previously treated patients and the likelihood of developing toxicity.[1]

TABLE 8

% Actual Toxicity in Previously Treated Patients		
AUC	Gr 3 or Gr 4 Thrombocytopenia	Gr 3 or Gr 4 Leukopenia
4-5 (mg/ml·min)	16%	13%
6-7 (mg/ml·min)	33%	34%

PREPARATION OF INTRAVENOUS SOLUTION

Immediately before use, the content of each vial must be reconstituted with either sterile water for injection, 5% dextrose in water, or 0.9% sodium chloride injection, according to the schedule shown in TABLE 9.

TABLE 9

Vial Strength	Diluent Volume
50 mg	5 ml
150 mg	15 ml
450 mg	45 ml

These dilutions all produce a carboplatin concentration of 10 mg/ml.

Carboplatin can be further diluted to concentrations as low as 0.5 mg/ml with 5% dextrose in water (D_5W) or 0.9% sodium chloride injection.

STABILITY

Unopened vials of carboplatin are stable for the life indicated on the package when stored at controlled room temperature 15-30°C (59-86°F), and protected from light.

When prepared as directed, carboplatin solutions are stable for 8 hours at room temperature (25°C). Since no antibacterial preservative is contained in the formulation, it is recommended that carboplatin solutions be discarded 8 hours after dilution.

Parenteral drug products should be inspected visually for particulate matter and discoloration prior to administration.

HOW SUPPLIED

PARAPLATIN (CARBOPLATIN FOR INJECTION)

50 mg Vial: Yellow flip-off seals.
150 mg Vials: Violet flip-off seals.
450 mg Vials: Blue flip-off seals.

STORAGE

Store the unopened vials at controlled room temperature 15-30°C (59-86°F). Protect unopened vials from light. Solutions for infusion should be discarded 8 hours after preparation.

HANDLING AND DISPOSAL

Procedures for proper handling and disposal of anticancer drugs should be considered. Several guidelines on this subject have been published.[8-14] There is no general agreement that all of the procedures recommended in the guidelines are necessary or appropriate.

PRODUCT LISTING - EQUIVALENTS NOT AVAILABLE

Powder For Injection - Injectable - 50 mg

1's	$96.12	PARAPLATIN, Bristol-Myers Squibb	00015-3213-29
1's	$156.58	PARAPLATIN, Bristol-Myers Squibb	00015-3213-30

Powder For Injection - Injectable - 150 mg

1's	$288.32	PARAPLATIN, Bristol-Myers Squibb	00015-3214-29
1's	$469.69	PARAPLATIN, Bristol-Myers Squibb	00015-3214-30

Powder For Injection - Injectable - 450 mg

1's	$864.97	PARAPLATIN, Bristol-Myers Squibb	00015-3215-29
1's	$1409.09	PARAPLATIN, Bristol-Myers Squibb	00015-3215-30

Carisoprodol *(000664)*

Categories: Pain, musculoskeletal; FDA Approved 1959 Apr
Drug Classes: Musculoskeletal agents; Relaxants, skeletal muscle
Brand Names: Caridolin; Chinchen; Flexartal; Muslax; Neotica; Rela; Rotalin; Scutamil-C; **Soma**
Foreign Brand Availability: Artifar (Greece); Carisoma (England; India); Myolax (Thailand); Somadril (Denmark; Norway; Sweden)
Cost of Therapy: $133.63 (Musculoskeletal Pain; Soma; 350 mg; 4 tablets/day; 10 day supply)
$2.98 (Musculoskeletal Pain; Generic Tablets; 350 mg; 4 tablets/day; 10 day supply)

DESCRIPTION

Carisoprodol is available as 350 mg round, white tablets. Chemically, carisoprodol is 2-methyl-2-propyl-1,3-propanediol carbamate isopropylcarbamate. Carisoprodol is a white, crystalline powder, having a mild, characteristic odor and a bitter taste. It is very slightly soluble in water, freely soluble in alcohol, in chloroform, and in acetone; its solubility is practically independent of pH. Carisoprodol is present as a racemic mixture. The molecular formula is $C_{12}H_{24}N_2O_4$, with a molecular weight of 260.33.

CLINICAL PHARMACOLOGY

Carisoprodol produces muscle relaxation in animals by blocking interneuronal activity in the descending reticular formation and spinal cord. The onset of action is rapid and effects last 4-6 hours.

INDICATIONS AND USAGE

Carisoprodol is indicated as an adjunct to rest, physical therapy, and other measures for the relief of discomfort associated with acute, painful, musculoskeletal conditions. The mode of action of this drug has not been clearly identified, but may be related to its sedative properties. Carisoprodol does not directly relax tense skeletal muscles in man.

CONTRAINDICATIONS

Acute intermittent porphyria as well as allergic or idiosyncratic reactions to carisoprodol or related compounds, such as meprobamate, mebutamate, or tybamate.

WARNINGS

Idiosyncratic Reactions: On very rare occasions, the first dose of carisoprodol has been followed by idiosyncratic symptoms appearing within minutes or hours. *Symptoms Reported Include:* Extreme weakness, transient quadriplegia, dizziness, ataxia, temporary loss of vision, diplopia, mydriasis, dysarthria, agitation, euphoria, confusion, and disorientation. Symptoms usually subside over the course of the next several hours. Supportive and symptomatic therapy, including hospitalization, may be necessary.

Use in Pregnancy and Lactation: Safe usage of this drug in pregnancy or lactation has not been established. Therefore, use of this drug in pregnancy, in nursing mothers, or in women of childbearing potential requires that the potential benefits of the drug be weighed against the potential hazards of the mother and child. Carisoprodol is present in breast milk of lactating mothers at concentrations 2-4 times that of maternal plasma. This factor should be taken into account when use of the drug is contemplated in breastfeeding patients.

Use in Children: Because of limited clinical experience, carisoprodol is not recommended for use in patients under 12 years of age.

Potentially Hazardous Tasks: Patients should be warned that this drug may impair the mental and/or physical abilities required for the performance of potentially hazardous tasks such as driving a motor vehicle or operating machinery.

Additive Effects: Since the effects of carisoprodol and alcohol or carisoprodol and other CNS depressants or psychotropic drugs may be additive, appropriate caution should be exercised with patients who take more than one of these agents simultaneously.

PRECAUTIONS

Carisoprodol is metabolized in the liver and excreted by the kidney; to avoid its excess accumulation, caution should be exercised in administration to patients with compromised liver or kidney function.

ADVERSE REACTIONS

Central Nervous System: Drowsiness and other CNS effects may require dosage reduction. *Also Observed:* Dizziness, vertigo, ataxia, tremor, agitation, irritability, headache, depressive reactions, syncope, and insomnia. (See WARNINGS, Idiosyncratic Reactions.)

Allergic or Idiosyncratic: Allergic or idiosyncratic reactions occasionally develop. They are usually seen within the period of the first to fourth dose in patients having had no previous contact with the drug. Skin rash, erythema multiform, pruritus, eosinophilia, and fixed drug eruption with cross reaction to meprobamate have been reported with carisoprodol. Severe reactions have been manifested by asthmatic episodes, fever, weakness, dizziness, angioneurotic edema, smarting eyes, hypotension, and anaphylactoid shock. (See WARNINGS, Idiosyncratic Reactions.)

In case of allergic or idiosyncratic reactions to carisoprodol, discontinue the drug and initiate appropriate symptomatic therapy, which may include epinephrine, antihistamines, and in severe cases corticosteroids. In evaluating possible allergic reactions, also consider allergy to excipients (information on excipients is available to physicians on request).

Cardiovascular: Tachycardia, postural hypotension, and facial flushing.

Gastrointestinal: Nausea, vomiting, hiccup, and epigastric distress.

Hematologic: Leukopenia, in which other drugs or viral infection may have been responsible, and pancytopenia, attributed to phenylbutazone, have been reported. No serious blood dyscrasias have been attributed to carisoprodol.

DOSAGE AND ADMINISTRATION

The usual adult dosage of carisoprodol is one 350 mg tablet, 3 times daily and at bedtime. Usage in patients under age 12 is not recommended.

HOW SUPPLIED

Carisoprodol tablets are 350 mg white, round, debossed "MP 58".

Storage: Store at controlled room temperature 15-30°C (59-86°F). Dispense in a tight container.

PRODUCT LISTING - RATED THERAPEUTICALLY EQUIVALENT

Tablet - Oral - 350 mg

Qty	Price	Manufacturer	NDC
10's	$18.90	GENERIC, Pd-Rx Pharmaceuticals	55289-0049-10
12's	$8.42	GENERIC, Dhs Inc	55887-0990-12
14's	$9.82	GENERIC, Dhs Inc	55887-0990-14
14's	$22.65	GENERIC, Pd-Rx Pharmaceuticals	55289-0049-14
14's	$41.84	GENERIC, Pharma Pac	52959-0026-14
15's	$23.98	GENERIC, Pd-Rx Pharmaceuticals	55289-0049-15
15's	$25.63	GENERIC, Alpharma Uspd Makers Of Barre and Nmc	63874-0330-15
15's	$44.83	GENERIC, Pharma Pac	52959-0026-15
20's	$12.99	GENERIC, St. Mary'S Mpp	60760-0110-20
20's	$14.03	GENERIC, Dhs Inc	55887-0990-20
20's	$30.63	GENERIC, Pd-Rx Pharmaceuticals	55289-0049-20
20's	$34.22	GENERIC, Alpharma Uspd Makers Of Barre and Nmc	63874-0330-20
20's	$57.22	GENERIC, Pharma Pac	52959-0026-20
20's	$63.27	SOMA, Pd-Rx Pharmaceuticals	55289-0578-20
21's	$31.96	GENERIC, Pd-Rx Pharmaceuticals	55289-0049-21
21's	$58.09	GENERIC, Pharma Pac	52959-0026-21
21's	$61.43	SOMA, Allscripts Pharmaceutical Company	54569-0834-05
24's	$35.95	GENERIC, Pd-Rx Pharmaceuticals	55289-0049-24
25's	$58.39	GENERIC, Pharma Pac	52959-0026-25
28's	$64.89	GENERIC, Pharma Pac	52959-0026-28
30's	$18.44	GENERIC, Mutual/United Research Laboratories	00677-0589-07
30's	$21.05	GENERIC, Dhs Inc	55887-0990-30
30's	$43.93	GENERIC, Pd-Rx Pharmaceuticals	55289-0049-30
30's	$51.32	GENERIC, Alpharma Uspd Makers Of Barre and Nmc	63874-0330-30
30's	$69.46	GENERIC, Pharma Pac	52959-0026-30
32's	$72.20	GENERIC, Pharma Pac	52959-0026-32
40's	$28.02	GENERIC, Dhs Inc	55887-0990-40
40's	$31.14	GENERIC, St. Mary'S Mpp	60760-0110-40
40's	$53.20	GENERIC, Pd-Rx Pharmaceuticals	55289-0049-40
40's	$89.91	GENERIC, Pharma Pac	52959-0026-40
40's	$126.54	SOMA, Pd-Rx Pharmaceuticals	55289-0578-40
50's	$111.98	GENERIC, Pharma Pac	52959-0026-50
52's	$116.18	GENERIC, Pharma Pac	52959-0026-52
56's	$157.25	GENERIC, Pharma Pac	52959-0026-56
60's	$37.26	GENERIC, Mutual/United Research Laboratories	00677-0589-06
60's	$92.23	GENERIC, Pd-Rx Pharmaceuticals	55289-0049-60
60's	$98.89	GENERIC, Pharma Pac	52959-0026-60
90's	$133.39	GENERIC, Pd-Rx Pharmaceuticals	55289-0049-90
100's	$5.94	GENERIC, West Ward Pharmaceutical Corporation	00143-1176-01
100's	$7.45	GENERIC, Vangard Labs	00615-1519-01
100's	$8.75	GENERIC, Cmc-Consolidated Midland Corporation	00223-0657-01
100's	$9.85	GENERIC, Aligen Independent Laboratories Inc	00405-4141-01
100's	$12.22	GENERIC, Moore, H.L. Drug Exchange Inc	00839-6246-06
100's	$12.40	GENERIC, Ivax Corporation	00182-1079-01
100's	$21.01	GENERIC, Major Pharmaceuticals Inc	00904-0355-61
100's	$37.43	FEDERAL UPPER LIMIT, H.C.F.A. F F P	99999-0664-01
100's	$59.61	GENERIC, Qualitest Products Inc	00603-2582-21
100's	$59.62	GENERIC, Geneva Pharmaceuticals	00781-1050-01
100's	$59.63	GENERIC, Watson/Schein Pharmaceuticals Inc	00364-0475-01
100's	$59.63	GENERIC, Watson/Schein Pharmaceuticals Inc	00591-5513-01
100's	$59.63	GENERIC, Major Pharmaceuticals Inc	00904-0355-60
100's	$59.63	GENERIC, Watson Laboratories Inc	52544-0692-01
100's	$59.63	GENERIC, Watson Laboratories Inc	52544-0784-01
100's	$60.03	GENERIC, Udl Laboratories Inc	51079-0055-20
100's	$60.23	GENERIC, Mutual Pharmaceutical Co Inc	53489-0110-01
100's	$60.24	GENERIC, Duramed Pharmaceuticals Inc	51285-0874-02
100's	$61.50	GENERIC, Able Laboratories Inc	53265-0266-10
100's	$83.95	GENERIC, Amide Pharmaceutical Inc	52152-0136-02
100's	$148.23	GENERIC, Pd-Rx Pharmaceuticals	55289-0049-01
100's	$194.64	SOMA, Wallace Laboratories	00037-2001-85
100's	$203.63	GENERIC, Pharma Pac	52959-0026-00
100's	$274.13	GENERIC, Gm Pharmaceuticals	58809-0424-01
100's	$334.07	SOMA, Physicians Total Care	54868-0020-00
100's	$370.81	SOMA, Wallace Laboratories	00037-2001-01
120's	$181.01	GENERIC, Pharma Pac	52959-0026-03
250's	$14.85	GENERIC, Major Pharmaceuticals Inc	00904-0355-70

PRODUCT LISTING - EQUIVALENTS NOT AVAILABLE

Tablet - Oral - 350 mg

Qty	Price	Manufacturer	NDC
2's	$3.48	GENERIC, Prescript Pharmaceuticals	00247-0088-02
4's	$3.62	GENERIC, Prescript Pharmaceuticals	00247-0088-04
7's	$3.81	GENERIC, Prescript Pharmaceuticals	00247-0088-07
7's	$5.21	GENERIC, Allscripts Pharmaceutical Company	54569-3403-01
7's	$19.47	GENERIC, Southwood Pharmaceuticals Inc	58016-0261-07
10's	$4.01	GENERIC, Prescript Pharmaceuticals	00247-0088-10
10's	$9.27	GENERIC, Physicians Total Care	54868-0816-07
10's	$27.82	GENERIC, Southwood Pharmaceuticals Inc	58016-0261-10
10's	$29.88	GENERIC, Pharma Pac	52959-0026-10
12's	$8.93	GENERIC, Allscripts Pharmaceutical Company	54569-3403-04
12's	$33.38	GENERIC, Southwood Pharmaceuticals Inc	58016-0261-12
14's	$4.28	GENERIC, Prescript Pharmaceuticals	00247-0088-14
14's	$11.19	GENERIC, Allscripts Pharmaceutical Company	54569-1709-07
14's	$38.95	GENERIC, Southwood Pharmaceuticals Inc	58016-0261-14
15's	$4.34	GENERIC, Prescript Pharmaceuticals	00247-0088-15
15's	$41.73	GENERIC, Southwood Pharmaceuticals Inc	58016-0261-15
16's	$4.41	GENERIC, Prescript Pharmaceuticals	00247-0088-16
16's	$44.51	GENERIC, Southwood Pharmaceuticals Inc	58016-0261-16
18's	$4.54	GENERIC, Prescript Pharmaceuticals	00247-0088-18
18's	$50.08	GENERIC, Southwood Pharmaceuticals Inc	58016-0261-18
20's	$4.68	GENERIC, Prescript Pharmaceuticals	00247-0088-20
20's	$12.46	GENERIC, Pharmaceutical Corporation Of America	51655-0376-52
20's	$15.99	GENERIC, Allscripts Pharmaceutical Company	54569-1709-03

20's	$16.54	GENERIC, Physicians Total Care	54868-0816-02
20's	$55.64	GENERIC, Southwood Pharmaceuticals Inc	58016-0261-20
21's	$4.74	GENERIC, Prescript Pharmaceuticals	00247-0088-21
21's	$58.42	GENERIC, Southwood Pharmaceuticals Inc	58016-0261-21
24's	$19.19	GENERIC, Allscripts Pharmaceutical Company	54569-1709-05
24's	$19.45	GENERIC, Physicians Total Care	54868-0816-01
24's	$66.77	GENERIC, Southwood Pharmaceuticals Inc	58016-0261-24
25's	$69.55	GENERIC, Southwood Pharmaceuticals Inc	58016-0261-25
28's	$5.21	GENERIC, Prescript Pharmaceuticals	00247-0088-28
28's	$22.39	GENERIC, Allscripts Pharmaceutical Company	54569-3403-00
28's	$77.90	GENERIC, Southwood Pharmaceuticals Inc	58016-0261-28
30's	$5.34	GENERIC, Prescript Pharmaceuticals	00247-0088-30
30's	$5.70	GENERIC, Heartland Healthcare Services	61392-0711-30
30's	$5.70	GENERIC, Heartland Healthcare Services	61392-0711-39
30's	$23.82	GENERIC, Physicians Total Care	54868-0816-03
30's	$23.99	GENERIC, Allscripts Pharmaceutical Company	54569-1709-00
30's	$83.46	GENERIC, Southwood Pharmaceuticals Inc	58016-0261-30
31's	$5.89	GENERIC, Heartland Healthcare Services	61392-0711-31
32's	$6.08	GENERIC, Heartland Healthcare Services	61392-0711-32
40's	$6.00	GENERIC, Prescript Pharmaceuticals	00247-0088-40
40's	$31.98	GENERIC, Allscripts Pharmaceutical Company	54569-1709-02
40's	$111.28	GENERIC, Southwood Pharmaceuticals Inc	58016-0261-40
42's	$116.84	GENERIC, Southwood Pharmaceuticals Inc	58016-0261-42
45's	$8.55	GENERIC, Heartland Healthcare Services	61392-0711-45
45's	$125.19	GENERIC, Southwood Pharmaceuticals Inc	58016-0261-45
50's	$38.36	GENERIC, Physicians Total Care	54868-0816-05
50's	$39.98	GENERIC, Allscripts Pharmaceutical Company	54569-1709-01
50's	$139.10	GENERIC, Southwood Pharmaceuticals Inc	58016-0261-50
56's	$7.06	GENERIC, Prescript Pharmaceuticals	00247-0088-56
56's	$41.75	GENERIC, Allscripts Pharmaceutical Company	54569-3403-06
56's	$155.79	GENERIC, Southwood Pharmaceuticals Inc	58016-0261-56
60's	$7.33	GENERIC, Prescript Pharmaceuticals	00247-0088-60
60's	$11.40	GENERIC, Heartland Healthcare Services	61392-0711-60
60's	$45.63	GENERIC, Physicians Total Care	54868-0816-04
60's	$47.97	GENERIC, Allscripts Pharmaceutical Company	54569-1709-08
60's	$151.50	GENERIC, Southwood Pharmaceuticals Inc	58016-0261-60
80's	$63.96	GENERIC, Allscripts Pharmaceutical Company	54569-3403-07
90's	$17.10	GENERIC, Heartland Healthcare Services	61392-0711-90
90's	$66.97	GENERIC, Allscripts Pharmaceutical Company	54569-3403-05
90's	$250.38	GENERIC, Southwood Pharmaceuticals Inc	58016-0261-90
100's	$9.98	GENERIC, Prescript Pharmaceuticals	00247-0088-00
100's	$74.72	GENERIC, Physicians Total Care	54868-0816-06
100's	$79.75	GENERIC, Allscripts Pharmaceutical Company	54569-1709-04
100's	$278.20	GENERIC, Southwood Pharmaceuticals Inc	58016-0261-00
112's	$311.58	GENERIC, Southwood Pharmaceuticals Inc	58016-0261-92
118's	$11.16	GENERIC, Prescript Pharmaceuticals	00247-0088-52
120's	$333.84	GENERIC, Southwood Pharmaceuticals Inc	58016-0261-02

Carmustine *(000665)*

For complete prescribing information, refer to the CD-ROM included with the book.

Categories: *Astrocytoma; Ependymoma; Glioblastoma; Glioma, brainstem; Lymphoma, Hodgkin's; Lymphoma, non-Hodgkin's; Medulloblastoma; Myeloma, multiple; Pregnancy Category D; FDA Approved 1977 Mar; Orphan Drugs*
Drug Classes: *Antineoplastics, alkylating agents*
Brand Names: *Bicnu*
Foreign Brand Availability: *Bcnu (Hungary; Taiwan); Becenun (Denmark; Finland; Norway; Sweden); BiCNU (Australia; Canada; England; France; Hong-Kong; Ireland; Israel; Korea; Malaysia; Mexico; New-Zealand; Philippines; South-Africa); Carmubris (Germany); Nitrourean (Spain); Nitrumon (Belgium; Germany; Italy)*
HCFA JCODE(S): *J9050 100 mg IV*

IMPLANTATION

DESCRIPTION

Gliadel Wafer (polifeprosan 20 with carmustine implant) is a sterile, off-white to pale yellow wafer approximately 1.45 cm in diameter and 1 mm thick. Each wafer contains 192.3 mg of a biodegradable polyanhydride copolymer and 7.7 mg of carmustine [1,3-bis(2-chloroethyl)-1-nitrosourea, or BCNU]. Carmustine is a nitrosourea oncolytic agent. The copolymer, polifeprosan 20, consists of poly[bis(p-carboxyphenoxy) propane: sebacic acid] in a 20:80 molar ratio and is used to control the local delivery of carmustine. Carmustine is homogeneously distributed in the copolymer matrix.

INDICATIONS AND USAGE

The carmustine implant is indicated in newly-diagnosed high grade malignant glioma patients as an adjunct to surgery and radiation. The carmustine implant is indicated in recurrent glioblastoma multiforme patients as an adjunct to surgery.

CONTRAINDICATIONS

The carmustine implant contains carmustine. The carmustine implant should not be given to individuals who have demonstrated a previous hypersensitivity to carmustine or any of the components of the carmustine implant.

WARNINGS

Patients undergoing craniotomy for malignant glioma and implantation of the carmustine implant should be monitored closely for known complications of craniotomy, including seizures, intracranial infections, abnormal wound healing, and brain edema. Cases of intracerebral mass effect unresponsive to corticosteroids have been described in patients treated with the carmustine implant, including 1 case leading to brain herniation.

PREGNANCY

There are no studies assessing the reproductive toxicity of the carmustine implant. Carmustine, the active component of the carmustine implant, can cause fetal harm when administered to a pregnant woman. Carmustine has been shown to be embryotoxic and teratogenic in rats at intraperitoneal doses of 0.5, 1, 2, 4, or 8 mg/kg/day when given on gestation Days 6-15. Carmustine caused fetal malformations (anophthalmia, micrognathia, omphalocele) at 1.0 mg/kg/day (about 1/6 the recommended human dose (8 wafers of 7.7 mg carmustine/wafer) on a mg/m^2 basis). Carmustine was embryotoxic in rabbits at IV doses of 4.0 mg/kg/day (about 1.2 times the recommended human dose on a mg/m^2 basis). Embryotoxicity was characterized by increased embryo-fetal deaths, reduced numbers of litters, and reduced litter sizes.

There are no studies of the carmustine implant in pregnant women. If the carmustine implant is used during pregnancy, or if the patient becomes pregnant after the carmustine implantation, the patient must be warned of the potential hazard to the fetus.

DOSAGE AND ADMINISTRATION

Each carmustine implant contains 7.7 mg of carmustine, resulting in a dose of 61.6 mg when 8 wafers are implanted. It is recommended that 8 wafers be placed in the resection cavity if the size and shape of it allows. Should the size and shape not accommodate 8 wafers, the maximum number of wafers as allowed should be placed. Since there is no clinical experience, no more than 8 wafers should be used per surgical procedure.

Once the tumor is resected, tumor pathology is confirmed, and hemostasis is obtained, up to 8 carmustine implants may be placed to cover as much of the resection cavity as possible. Slight overlapping of the wafers is acceptable. Wafers broken in half may be used, but wafers broken in more than 2 pieces should be discarded in a biohazard container. Oxidized regenerated cellulose (Surgicel) may be placed over the wafers to secure them against the cavity surface. After placement of the wafers, the resection cavity should be irrigated and the dura closed in a water tight fashion.

Unopened foil pouches may be kept at ambient room temperature for a maximum of 6 hours at a time.

INTRAVENOUS

WARNING

Carmustine should be administered under the supervision of a qualified physician experienced in the use of cancer chemotherapeutic agents.

Bone marrow suppression, notably thrombocytopenia and leukopenia, which may contribute to bleeding and overwhelming infections in an already compromised patient, is the most common and severe of the toxic effects of carmustine (see WARNINGS).

Since the major toxicity is delayed bone marrow suppression, blood counts should be monitored weekly for at least 6 weeks after a dose. At the recommended dosage, courses of carmustine should not be given more frequently than every 6 weeks.

The bone marrow toxicity of carmustine is cumulative and therefore dosage adjustment must be considered on the basis of nadir blood counts from prior dose (see TABLE 4).

Pulmonary toxicity from carmustine appears to be dose related. Patients receiving greater than 1400 mg/m^2 cumulative dose are at significantly higher risk than those receiving less.

Delayed pulmonary toxicity can occur years after treatment, and can result in death, particularly in patients treated in childhood.

DESCRIPTION

Carmustine for injection is one of the nitrosoureas used in the treatment of certain neoplastic diseases. It is 1,3-bis(2-chloroethyl)-1-nitrosourea. It is lyophilized pale yellow flakes or congealed mass with a molecular weight of 214.06. It is highly soluble in alcohol and lipids, and poorly soluble in water. Carmustine is administered by IV infusion after reconstitution as recommended.

Sterile BiCNU is available in 100 mg single dose vials of lyophilized material.

INDICATIONS AND USAGE

Carmustine is indicated as palliative therapy as a single agent or in established combination therapy with other approved chemotherapeutic agents in the following:

Brain Tumors: Glioblastoma, brainstem glioma, medulloblastoma, astrocytoma, ependymoma, and metastatic brain tumors.
Multiple Myeloma: In combination with prednisone.
Hodgkin's Disease: As secondary therapy in combination with other approved drugs in patients who relapse while being treated with primary therapy, or who fail to respond to primary therapy.
Non-Hodgkin's Lymphomas: As secondary therapy in combination with other approved drugs for patients who relapse while being treated with primary therapy, or who fail to respond to primary therapy.

CONTRAINDICATIONS

Carmustine should not be given to individuals who have demonstrated a previous hypersensitivity to it.

WARNINGS

Since the major toxicity is delayed bone marrow suppression, blood counts should be monitored weekly for at least 6 weeks after a dose. At the recommended dosage, courses of carmustine should not be given more frequently than every 6 weeks.

The bone marrow toxicity of carmustine is cumulative and therefore dosage adjustment must be considered on the basis of nadir blood counts from prior dose (see TABLE 4).

Pulmonary toxicity from carmustine appears to be dose related. Patients receiving greater than 1400 mg/m^2 cumulative dose are at a significantly higher risk than those receiving less. Additionally, delayed onset pulmonary fibrosis occurring up to 17 years after treatment has been reported in patients who received carmustine in childhood and early adolescence.

long-term use of nitrosoureas has been reported to be associated with the development of secondary malignancies.

Liver and renal function tests should be monitored periodically.

Carmustine may cause fetal harm when administered to a pregnant woman. Carmustine has been shown to be embryotoxic in rats and rabbits and teratogenic in rats when given in doses equivalent to the human dose. There are no adequate and well-controlled studies in pregnant women. If this drug is used during pregnancy, or if the patient becomes pregnant while taking (receiving) this drug, the patient should be apprised of the potential hazard to the fetus. Women of childbearing potential should be advised to avoid becoming pregnant.

Carmustine has been administered through an intraarterial intracarotid route; this procedure is investigational and has been associated with ocular toxicity.

DOSAGE AND ADMINISTRATION

The recommended dose of carmustine as a single agent in previously untreated patients is 150-200 mg/m^2 intravenously every 6 weeks. This may be given as a single dose or divided into daily injections such as 75-100 mg/m^2 on 2 successive days. When carmustine is used in combination with other myelosuppressive drugs or in patients in whom bone marrow reserve is depleted, the doses should be adjusted accordingly.

Doses subsequent to the initial dose should be adjusted according to the hematologic response of the patient to the preceding dose. The schedule in TABLE 4 is suggested as a guide to dosage adjustment.

TABLE 4

Nadir After Prior Dose		
Leukocytes/mm^3	Platelets/mm^3	Percentage of Prior Dose to Be Given
>4,000	>100,000	100%
3,000-3,999	75,000-99,999	100%
2,000-2,999	25,000-74,999	70%
<2,000	<25,000	50%

A repeat course of carmustine should not be given until circulating blood elements have returned to acceptable levels (platelets above 100,000/mm^3, leukocytes above 4000/mm^3), and this is usually in 6 weeks. Adequate number of neutrophils should be present on a peripheral blood smear. Blood counts should be monitored weekly and repeat courses should not be given before 6 weeks because the hematologic toxicity is delayed and cumulative.

ADMINISTRATION PRECAUTIONS

As with other potentially toxic compounds, caution should be exercised in handling carmustine and preparing the solution of carmustine. Accidental contact of reconstituted carmustine with the skin has caused transient hyperpigmentation of the affected areas. The use of gloves is recommended. If carmustine lyophilized material or solution contacts the skin or mucosa, immediately wash the skin or mucosa thoroughly with soap and water.

The reconstituted solution should be used intravenously only and should be administered by IV drip. Injection of carmustine over shorter periods of time than 1-2 hours may produce intense pain and burning at the site of injection.

PREPARATION OF IV SOLUTIONS

First, dissolve carmustine with 3 ml of the supplied sterile diluent (dehydrated alcohol injection). Second, aseptically add 27 ml sterile water for injection. Each ml of resulting solution contains 3.3 mg of carmustine in 10% ethanol. Such solutions should be protected from light.

Reconstitution as recommended results in a clear, colorless to yellowish solution which may be further diluted with 5% dextrose injection. Parenteral drug products should be inspected visually for particulate matter and discoloration prior to administration, whenever solution and container permit.

Important Note: The lyophilized dosage formulation contains no preservatives and is not intended as a multiple dose vial.

STABILITY

Unopened vials of the dry drug must be stored in a refrigerator (2-8°C, 36-46°F). The recommended storage of unopened vials provides a stable product for 2 years. After reconstitution as recommended, carmustine is stable for 8 hours at room temperature (25°C, 77°F), protected from light.

Vials reconstituted as directed and further diluted to a concentration of 0.2 mg/ml in 5% dextrose injection should be stored at room temperature, protected from light and utilized within 8 hours.

Glass containers were used for the stability data provided in this section. Only use glass containers for carmustine administration.

Important Note: Carmustine has a low melting point (30.5-32.0°C or 86.9-89.6°F). Exposure of the drug to this temperature or above will cause the drug to liquefy and appear as an oil film on the vials. This is a sign of decomposition and vials should be discarded. If there is a question of adequate refrigeration upon receipt of this product, immediately inspect the larger vial in each individual carton. Hold the vial to the bright light for inspection. The carmustine will appear as a very small amount of dry flakes or dry congealed mass. If this is evident, the carmustine is suitable for use and should be refrigerated immediately. Procedures for proper handling and disposal of anticancer drugs should be considered. Several guidelines on this subject have been published.[1-7] There is no general agreement that all of the procedures recommended in the guidelines are necessary or appropriate.

PRODUCT LISTING - EQUIVALENTS NOT AVAILABLE

Device - Implant - 7.7 mg

8's	$13228.80	GLIADEL, Aventis Pharmaceuticals	00075-9995-08
8's	$13731.50	GLIADEL, Guilford Pharmaceuticals	61379-0100-01

Powder For Injection - Injectable - 100 mg

10's	$143.34	BICNU, Bristol-Myers Squibb	00015-3012-38

Carteolol Hydrochloride *(000666)*

For related information, see the comparative table section in Appendix A.

Categories: Glaucoma, open-angle; Hypertension, essential; Hypertension, ocular; Pregnancy Category C; FDA Approved 1988 Dec

Drug Classes: Antiadrenergics, beta blocking; Ophthalmics

Brand Names: Arteoptik; **Cartrol**; Ocupress; Optipress

Foreign Brand Availability: Arteolol (Spain); Arteoptic (Denmark; Germany; Hong-Kong; Portugal; Switzerland; Taiwan; Thailand); Caltamol (Korea); Calte (Korea); Carteol (Belgium; France; Italy); Catelon Eye drop (Korea); Elebloc (Taiwan); Endak (Austria; Germany); Karol (Korea); Karteol (Taiwan); Mikelan (France; Indonesia; Japan; Korea; Philippines; South-Africa; Taiwan); Teoptic (England; South-Africa)

Cost of Therapy: $32.06 (Hypertension; Cartrol; 2.5 mg; 1 tablet/day; 30 day supply)
$32.75 (Glaucoma; Ocupress Ophth. Solution; 1%; 5 ml; 2 drops/day; variable day supply)

DESCRIPTION

TABLETS

Carteolol hydrochloride is a synthetic, nonselective, beta-adrenergic receptor blocking agent with intrinsic sympathomimetic activity. It is chemically described as 5[3-[(1,1-dimethyl-ethyl)amino]- 2-hydroxypropoxy]-3,4-dihydro-2(1H)-quinolinone monohydrochloride.

Carteolol hydrochloride is a stable, white crystalline powder which is soluble in water and slightly soluble in ethanol. The molecular weight is 328.84 and $C_{16}H_{24}N_2O_3 \cdot HCl$ is the empirical formula.

Cartrol (carteolol hydrochloride) is available as tablets containing either 2.5 or 5 mg of carteolol hydrochloride for oral administration.

Cartrol Inactive Ingredients: *2.5 mg Tablet:* Cellulosic polymers, corn starch, iron oxide, lactose, magnesium stearate, microcrystalline cellulose, polyethylene glycol, propylene glycol and titanium dioxide. *5 mg Tablet:* Cellulosic polymers, corn starch, lactose, magnesium stearate, microcrystalline cellulose, polyethylene glycol, propylene glycol and titanium dioxide.

OPHTHALMIC SOLUTION

Carteolol hydrochloride ophthalmic solution, 1% is a nonselective beta-adrenoceptor blocking agent for ophthalmic use.

The chemical name for carteolol hydrochloride is (±)-5-(3-((1,1-dimethylethyl)amino)-2-hydroxypropoxy)-3,4-dihydro-2(1H)- quinolinone monohydrochloride.

Each ml contains 10 mg carteolol hydrochloride and the inactive ingredients sodium chloride, monobasic and dibasic sodium phosphate, and water for injection. Benzalkonium chloride 0.05 mg (0.005%) is added as a preservative. The product has a pH range of 6.2-7.2.

CLINICAL PHARMACOLOGY

Carteolol HCl is a long-acting, nonselective, beta-adrenergic receptor blocking agent with intrinsic sympathomimetic activity (ISA) and without significant membrane stabilizing (local anesthetic) activity.

TABLETS

Pharmacodynamics

Carteolol specifically competes with beta-adrenergic receptor agonists for both beta$_1$-receptors located principally in cardiac muscle and beta$_2$-receptors located in the bronchial and vascular musculature, blocking the chronotropic, inotropic, and vasodilator responses to beta-adrenergic stimulation proportionately. Because of its partial agonist activity, however, carteolol does not reduce resting beta-agonist activity as much as beta-adrenergic blockers lacking this activity. Thus, in clinical trials in man, the decreases in resting pulse rate produced by carteolol (2-5 beats/min in various studies) were less than those produced by beta-blockers (nadolol and propranolol) without ISA (10-12 beats/min). There are also equivocal effects on renin secretion, in contrast to beta-blockers without ISA, which inhibit renin secretion.

In controlled clinical trials carteolol, at doses up to 20 mg as monotherapy or in combination with thiazide type diuretics, produced significantly greater reductions in blood pressure than did placebo, with the full effect seen between two and four weeks. The observed differences from placebo ranged from 3.1-6.7 mm Hg for supine diastolic blood pressure. The antihypertensive effects of carteolol are smaller in black populations but do not seem to be affected by age or sex. Doses of carteolol greater than 10 mg once a day did not produce greater reductions in blood pressure. In fact, doses of 20 mg and above appeared to produce blood pressure reductions less than those produced by 10 mg and below. When carteolol was compared to nadolol and propranolol, although the differences were not statistically significant in relatively small studies, carteolol at doses up to 20 mg produced supine diastolic blood pressure changes consistently 2 mm Hg less than that produced by either nadolol or propranolol.

C

Although the mechanism of the antihypertensive effect of beta-adrenergic blocking agents has not been established, multiple factors are thought to contribute to the lowering of blood pressure, including diminished response to sympathetic nerve outflow from vasomotor centers in the brain, diminished release of renin from the kidneys, and decreased cardiac output. Carteolol does not have a consistent effect on renin and other agents with ISA have been shown to have less effect than other beta-blockers on resting cardiac output (although they cause the usual decrease in exercise cardiac output so that the difference is of uncertain clinical importance), so that the mechanism of its action is particularly uncertain.

Beta-blockade interferes with endogenous adrenergic bronchodilator activity and diminishes the response to exogenous bronchodilators. This is especially important in patients subject to bronchospasm.

Single intravenous doses of carteolol (0.5, 1.0, 2.5 and 5.0 mg) produced statistically, but not clinically, significant increases from baseline in AV node conduction time and RR and PR intervals.

Carteolol HCl induced no significant alteration in total serum cholesterol and triglycerides.

Following discontinuation of carteolol treatment in man, pharmacologic activity (evaluated by blockade of the tachycardia induced by isoproterenol or postural changes) is present for 2-21 days (median 14 days) after the last dose of carteolol. Following administration of recommended doses of carteolol HCl, both beta-blocking and antihypertensive effects persist for at least 24 hours.

Pharmacokinetics and Metabolism

Following oral administration in man, peak plasma concentrations of carteolol usually occur within one to three hours. Carteolol is well absorbed when administered orally as carteolol HCl tablets. The presence of food in the gastrointestinal tract somewhat slows the rate of absorption, but the extent of absorption is not appreciably affected. Compared to intravenous administration, the absolute bioavailability of carteolol from carteolol HCl tablets is approximately 85%.

The plasma half-life carteolol averages approximately 6 hours. Steady-state serum levels are achieved within one to two days after initiating therapeutic doses of carteolol in persons with normal renal function. Since approximately 50-70% of a carteolol dose is eliminated unchanged by the kidneys, the half-life is increased in patients with impaired renal function. Significant reductions in the rate of carteolol elimination (and prolongations of the half-life) occur in patients as creatinine clearance decreases. Therefore, a reduction in maintenance dose and/or prolongation in dosing interval is appropriate (see DOSAGE AND ADMINISTRATION).

Carteolol is 23-30% bound to plasma proteins in humans. The major metabolites of carteolol are 8-hydroxycarteolol and the glucuronic acid conjugates of both carteolol and 8-hydroxycarteolol. In man, 8-hydroxycarteolol is an active metabolite with a half-life of approximately 8-12 hours and represents approximately 5% of the administered dose excreted in the urine.

OPHTHALMIC SOLUTION

Carteolol HCl solution reduces normal and elevated intraocular pressure (IOP) whether or not accompanied by glaucoma. The exact mechanism of the ocular hypotensive effect of beta-blockers has not been definitely demonstrated.

In general, beta-adrenergic blockers reduce cardiac output in patients in good and poor cardiovascular health. In patients with severe impairment of myocardial function, beta-blockers may inhibit the sympathetic stimulation necessary to maintain adequate cardiac function. Beta-adrenergic blockers may also increase airway resistance in the bronchi and bronchioles due to unopposed parasympathetic activity.

Given topically twice daily in controlled clinical trials ranging from 1.5 to 3 months, carteolol HCl solution produced a median percent reduction of IOP 22-25%. No significant effects were noted on corneal sensitivity, tear secretion, or pupil size.

INDICATIONS AND USAGE

TABLETS

Carteolol HCl is indicated in the management of hypertension. It may be used alone or in combination with other antihypertensive agents, especially thiazide diuretics. Preliminary data indicate that carteolol does not have a favorable effect on arrhythmias.

OPHTHALMIC SOLUTION

Carteolol HCl solution, 1%, has been shown to be effective in lowering intraocular pressure and may be used in patients with chronic open-angle glaucoma and intraocular hypertension. It may be used alone or in combination with other intraocular pressure lowering medications.

CONTRAINDICATIONS

TABLETS

Carteolol HCl is contraindicated in patients with: (1) bronchial asthma, (2) severe bradycardia, (3) greater than first degree heart block, (4) cardiogenic shock, and (5) clinically evident congestive heart failure (see WARNINGS).

OPHTHALMIC SOLUTION

Carteolol HCl solution is contraindicated in those individuals with bronchial asthma or with a history of bronchial asthma, or severe chronic obstructive pulmonary disease (see WARNINGS); sinus bradycardia; second- and third-degree atrioventricular block; overt cardiac failure (see WARNINGS); cardiogenic shock; or hypersensitivity to any component of this product.

WARNINGS

OPHTHALMIC SOLUTION

Carteolol HCl solution has not been detected in plasma following ocular instillation. However, as with other topically applied ophthalmic preparations, carteolol HCl solution may be absorbed systemically. The same adverse reactions found with systemic administration of beta-adrenergic blocking agents may occur with topical administration. For example, severe respiratory reactions and cardiac reactions, including death due to bronchospasm in patients with asthma, and rarely death in association with cardiac failure, have been reported with topical application of beta-adrenergic blocking agents (see CONTRAINDICATIONS).

TABLETS AND OPHTHALMIC SOLUTION

Congestive Heart Failure

Sympathetic stimulation may be a vital component supporting circulatory function in patients with congestive heart failure, and impairing that support by beta-blockade may precipitate more severe decompensation.

Although carteolol HCl should be avoided in clinically evident congestive heart failure, it can be used with caution, if necessary, in patients with a history of failure who are well-compensated and are receiving digitalis and diuretics. Beta-adrenergic blocking agents do not abolish the inotropic action of digitalis on heart muscle.

IN PATIENTS WITHOUT A HISTORY OF CONGESTIVE HEART FAILURE, the use of beta-blockers can, in some instances, lead to congestive heart failure. Therefore, at the first sign or symptom of cardiac decompensation, discontinuation of beta-blocker therapy should be considered. The patient should be closely observed and treatment should include a diuretic and/or digitalization as necessary.

Exacerbation of Angina Pectoris Upon Withdrawal

In patients with angina pectoris, exacerbation of angina and, in some cases, myocardial infarction have been reported following abrupt discontinuation of therapy with some beta-blockers. Therefore such patients should be cautioned against interruption of therapy without a physician's advice. The long persistence of beta-adrenergic blockade following abrupt discontinuation of carteolol HCl, however, might be expected to minimize the possibility of this complication. When discontinuation of carteolol HCl is planned, dosage should be tapered gradually as it is with other beta-blockers. If exacerbation of angina occurs when carteolol HCl therapy is interrupted, it is advisable to reinstitute carteolol HCl or other beta-blocker therapy, at least temporarily, and to take other measures appropriate for the management of unstable angina pectoris.

Patients Without Clinically Recognized Angina Pectoris should be carefully monitored after withdrawal of carteolol HCl therapy, since coronary artery disease may be unrecognized.

Nonallergic Bronchospasm (e.g., chronic bronchitis, emphysema)

Patients with bronchospastic disease generally should not receive beta-blocker therapy and carteolol is contraindicated in patients with bronchial asthma. If use of carteolol hydrochloride is essential, it should be administered with caution since it may block bronchodilation produced by endogenous catecholamine stimulation of $beta_2$-receptors or diminish response to therapy with a beta-receptor agonist.

Major Surgery

The necessity, or desirability of withdrawal of beta-blocking therapy prior to major surgery is controversial. Because beta-blockade impairs the ability of the heart to respond to reflex stimuli and may increase risks of general anesthesia and surgical procedures resulting in protracted hypotension or low cardiac output, and difficulty in restarting or maintaining a heartbeat, it has been suggested that beta-blocker therapy should be withdrawn several days prior to surgery. It is also recognized, however, that increased sensitivity to catecholamines of patients recently withdrawn from beta-blocker therapy could increase certain risks. Given the persistence of the beta-blocking activity of carteolol hydrochloride, effective withdrawal would take several weeks and would ordinarily be impractical. When beta-blocker therapy is not discontinued, anesthetic agents that depress the myocardium should be avoided. In one study using intravenous carteolol during surgery, recovery from anesthesia was somewhat delayed in three patients who received carteolol near the end of anesthesia, and respiratory arrest occurred in one of these patients immediately following administration of intravenous carteolol.

In the event that carteolol hydrochloride treatment is not discontinued before surgery, the anesthesiologist should be informed that the patient is receiving carteolol hydrochloride. The effects on the heart of beta-adrenergic blocking agents, such as carteolol HCl, may be reversed by cautious administration of isoproterenol or dobutamine.

Ophthalmic Solution: If necessary during surgery, the effects of beta-adrenergic blocking agents may be reversed by sufficient doses of such agonists as isoproterenol, dopamine, dobutamine or levarterenol.

Diabetes Mellitus and Hypoglycemia

Beta-adrenergic blockade may prevent the appearance of premonitory signs and symptoms (*e.g.*, tachycardia and blood pressure changes) of acute hypoglycemia, and it inhibits glycogenolysis, a normal compensatory mechanism for hypoglycemia. This is especially important for patients with labile diabetes mellitus. Beta-blockade also reduces the release of insulin in response to hyperglycemia; therefore, it may be necessary to adjust the dose of antidiabetic agents used to treat hyperglycemia.

Thyrotoxicosis

Beta-adrenergic blockade may mask certain clinical signs of hyperthyroidism such as tachycardia. Patients suspected of having thyrotoxicosis should be managed carefully to avoid abrupt withdrawal of beta-adrenergic blockade which might precipitate a thyroid storm.

PRECAUTIONS

GENERAL

Tablets

Impaired Renal Function: Carteolol HCl should be used with caution in patients with impaired renal function. Patients with impaired renal function clear carteolol at a reduced rate, and dosage should be reduced accordingly (see DOSAGE AND ADMINISTRATION).

Beta-adrenoreceptor blockade can cause reduction in intraocular pressure. Therefore, carteolol HCl may interfere with glaucoma testing. Withdrawal may lead to a return of increased intraocular pressure.

Ophthalmic Solution

Carteolol HCl solution should be used with caution in patients with known hypersensitivity to other beta-adrenoceptor blocking agents.

Use with caution in patients with known diminished pulmonary function.

In patients with angle-closure glaucoma, the immediate objective of treatment is to reopen the angle. This requires constricting the pupil with a miotic. Carteolol HCl solution has little or no effect on the pupil. When carteolol HCl solution is used to reduce elevated intraocular pressure in angle-closure glaucoma, it should be used with a miotic and not alone.

INFORMATION FOR THE PATIENT

Muscle Weakness

Beta-adrenergic blockade has been reported to potentiate muscle weakness consistent with certain myasthenic symptoms (*e.g.,* diplopia, ptosis and generalized weakness).

Risk from Anaphylactic Reaction

While taking beta-blockers, patients with a history of atopy or a history of severe anaphylactic reaction to a variety of allergens may be more reactive to repeated accidental, diagnostic, or therapeutic challenge with such allergens. Such patients may be unresponsive to the usual doses of epinephrine used to treat anaphylactic reactions.

Tablets

Patients, especially those with evidence of coronary artery insufficiency, should be warned against interruption of discontinuation of carteolol HCl therapy without the physician's advice. Although cardiac failure rarely occurs in properly selected patients, patients being treated with beta-adrenergic blocking agents should be advised to consult the physician at the first sign or symptom of impending failure (*i.e.,* fatigue with exertion, difficulty breathing, cough or unusually fast heartbeat).

Ophthalmic Solution

For topical use only. To prevent contaminating the dropper tip and solution, care should be taken not to touch the eyelids or surrounding areas with the dropper tip of the bottle. Keep bottle tightly closed when not in use. Protect from use.

CARCINOGENESIS, MUTAGENESIS, AND IMPAIRMENT OF FERTILITY

Carteolol HCl did not produce carcinogenic effects at doses 280 times the maximum recommended human dose (10 mg/70 kg/day) in 2 year oral rat and mouse studies.

Tests of mutagenicity, including the Ames Test, recombinant (rec)-assay,*in vivo* cytogenetics and dominant lethal assay demonstrated no evidence for mutagenic potential.

Fertility of male and female rats and male and female mice was unaffected by administration of carteolol hydrochloride at dosages up to 150 mg/kg/day. This dosage is approximately 1052 times the maximum recommended human dose.

PREGNANCY, TERATOGENIC EFFECTS, PREGNANCY CATEGORY C

Carteolol hydrochloride increased resorptions and decreased fetal weights in rabbits and rats at maternally toxic doses approximately 1052 and 5264 times the maximum recommended human dose (10 mg/70 kg/day), respectively. A dose-related increase in wavy ribs was noted in the developing rat fetus when pregnant females received daily doses of approximately 212 times the maximum recommended human dose. No such effects were noted in pregnant mice subjected to up to 1052 times the maximum recommended human dose. There are no adequate and well-controlled studies in pregnant women. Carteolol hydrochloride should be used during pregnancy only if the potential benefit justifies the potential risk to the fetus.

NURSING MOTHERS

Studies have not been conducted in lactating humans and, therefore, it is not known whether carteolol is excreted in human milk. Studies in lactating rats indicate that carteolol hydrochloride is excreted in milk. Because many drugs are excreted in human milk, caution should be exercised when carteolol hydrochloride is administered to a nursing woman.

PEDIATRIC USE

Safety and effectiveness in children have not been established.

DRUG INTERACTIONS

TABLETS

Catecholamine-depending drugs (*e.g.,* reserpine) may have an additive effect when given with beta-blocking agents. Therefore, patients treated with carteolol HCl plus a catecholamine-depleting agent must be observed carefully for evidence of hypotension and/or excessive bradycardia, which may produce syncope or postural hypotension.

Concurrent administration of **general anesthetics** and beta-blocking agents may result in exaggeration of the hypotension induced by general anesthetics (see WARNINGS, Major Surgery).

Blunting of the antihypertensive effect of beta-adrenoreceptor blocking agents by **non-steroidal anti-inflammatory drugs** has been reported. When using these agents concomitantly, patients should be observed carefully to confirm that the desired therapeutic effect has been obtained.

Literature reports suggest that **oral calcium antagonists** may be used in combination with beta-adrenergic blocking agents when heart function is normal, but should be avoided in patients with impaired cardiac function. Hypotension, AV conduction disturbances, and left ventricular failure have been reported in some patients receiving beta-adrenergic blocking agents when an oral calcium antagonist was added to the treatment regimen. Hypotension was more likely to occur if the calcium antagonist were a dihydropyridine derivative *e.g.,* nifedipine, while left ventricular failure and AV conduction disturbances were more likely to occur with either verapamil or diltiazem.

Intravenous calcium antagonists should be used with caution in patients receiving beta-adrenergic blocking agents. The concomitant use of beta-adrenergic blocking agents with digitalis and either diltiazem or verapamil may have additive effects in prolonging AV conduction time.

Concomitant use of oral antidiabetic agents or insulin with beta-blocking agents may be associated with hypoglycemia or possibly hyperglycemia. Dosage of the antidiabetic agent should be adjusted accordingly (see WARNINGS, Diabetes Mellitus and Hypoglycemia).

OPHTHALMIC SOLUTION

Carteolol HCl solution should be used with caution in patients who are receiving a beta-adrenergic blocking agent orally, because of the potential for additive effects on systemic beta-blockade.

Close observation of the patient is recommended when a beta-blocker is administered to patients receiving catecholamine-depleting drugs such as reserpine, because of possible additive effects and the production of hypotension and/or marked bradycardia, which may produce vertigo, syncope, or postural hypotension.

ADVERSE REACTIONS

TABLETS

The prevalence of adverse reactions has been ascertained from clinical studies conducted primarily in the US. All adverse experiences (events) reported during these studies were recorded as adverse reactions. The prevalence rates presented below are based on combined data from nineteen placebo-controlled studies of patients with hypertension, angina or dysrhythmia, using once-daily carteolol at doses up to 60 mg. Table 1 summarizes those adverse experiences reported for patients in these studies where the prevalence in the carteolol group is 1% or greater and exceeds the prevalence in the placebo group. Asthenia and muscle cramps were the only symptoms that were significantly more common in patients receiving carteolol than in patients receiving placebo (TABLE 1). Patients in clinical trials were carefully selected to exclude those, such as patients with asthma or known bronchospasm, or congestive heart failure, who would be at high risk of experiencing beta-adrenergic blocker adverse effect (see WARNINGS and CONTRAINDICATIONS).

TABLE 1 *Adverse Reactions During Placebo-Controlled Studies*

	Placebo (n=448)	Carteolol (n=761)
Body as a Whole		
†Asthenia	4.0%	7.1%*
Abdominal pain	0.4%	1.3%
Back pain	1.6%	2.1%
Chest pain	1.8%	2.2%
Digestive System		
Diarrhea	2.0%	2.1%
Nausea	1.8%	2.1%
Metabolic/Nutritional Disorders		
Abnormal lab test	1.1%	1.2%
Peripheral edema	1.1%	1.7%
Musculoskeletal System		
Arthralgia	1.1%	1.2%
Muscle cramps	0.2%	2.6%*
Lower extremity pain	0.2%	1.2%
Nervous System		
Insomnia	0.7%	1.7%
Paresthesia	1.1%	2.0%
Respiratory System		
Nasal congestion	0.9%	1.1%
Pharyngitis	0.9%	1.1%
Skin and Appendages		
Rash	1.1%	1.3%

† Includes weakness, tiredness, lassitude and fatigue.
* Statistically significant at p = 0.05 level.

The adverse experiences were usually mild or moderate in intensity and transient, but sometimes were serious enough to interrupt treatment. The adverse reactions that were most bothersome, as judged by their being reported as reasons for discontinuation of therapy by at least 0.4% of the carteolol group are shown in TABLE 2.

TABLE 2 *Discontinuations During Placebo-Controlled Studies*

	Placebo (n=448)	Carteolol (n=761)
Body as a Whole		
Asthenia	0.2%	0.5%
Headache	0.7%	0.7%
Chest pain	0.2%	0.4%
Skin and Appendages		
Rash	0.0%	0.4%
Sweating	0.2%	0.4%
Digestive System		
Nausea	0.0%	0.4%
Overall Adverse Reactions	4.2%	3.3%

Additional adverse reactions have been reported, but these are, in general, not distinguishable from symptoms that might have occurred in the absence of exposure to carteolol. The following additional adverse reactions were reported by at least 1% of 1568 patients who received carteolol in controlled or open, short- or long-term clinical studies, or represent less common, but potentially important, reactions reported in clinical studies or marketing experience (these rare reactions are shown in *italics*):

Body as a Whole: Fever, infection, injury, malaise, pain, neck pain, shoulder pain;

Cardiovascular System: Angina pectoris, arrhythmia, *heart failure*, palpitations, *second degree heart block*, vasodilation;

Digestive System: *Acute hepatitis with jaundice*, constipation, dyspepsia, flatulence, gastrointestinal disorder;

Metabolic/Nutritional Disorder: Gout

C

Musculoskeletal System: Pain in extremity, joint disorder, arthritis;
Nervous System: Abnormal dreams, anxiety, depression, dizziness, nervousness, somnolence;
Respiratory System: Bronchitis, *bronchospasm* cold symptoms, cough, dyspnea, flu symptoms, lung disorder, rhinitis, sinusitis, *wheezing;*
Skin and Appendages: Sweating;
Special Senses: Blurred vision, conjunctivitis, eye disorder, tinnitus,
Urogenital: Impotence, urinary frequency, urinary tract infection.

In studies of patients with hypertension or angina pectoris where carteolol and positive reference beta-adrenergic blocking agents (nadolol (n=82) and propranolol (n=50)) have been compared, the differences in prevalence rates between the carteolol group and the reference agent group were statistically significant ($p \leq 0.05$) for the adverse reactions listed in TABLE 3.

TABLE 3 *Adverse Reactions During Positive-Controlled Studies*

	Reference Agents (n=132)	Carteolol (n=135)
Body as a Whole		
Chest pain	5.3%	0.7%
Cardiovascular System		
Bradycardia	4.5%	0.0%
Digestive System		
Diarrhea	11.4%	4.4%
Nervous System		
Somnolence	0.8%	7.4%
Skin and Appendages		
Sweating	5.3%	0.7%

Potential Adverse Reactions

In addition, other adverse reactions not listed above have been reported with other beta-adrenergic blocking agents and should be considered potential adverse reactions of carteolol HCl.

Body as a Whole: Fever combined with aching and sore throat.
Cardiovascular System: Intensification of AV block. (See CONTRAINDICATIONS.)
Digestive System: Mesenteric arterial thrombosis, ischemia colitis.
Hemic/Lymphatic System: Agranulocytosis, thrombocytopenic and nonthrombocytopenic purpura.
Nervous System: Reversible mental depression progressing to catatonia; an acute reversible syndrome characterized by disorientation to time and place, short-term memory loss, emotional lability, slightly clouded sensorium, and decreased performance on neuropsychometric testing.
Respiratory System: Laryngospasm, respiratory distress.
Skin and Appendages: Erythematous rash, reversible alopecia.
Urogenital System: Peyronie's disease.

The oculomucocutaneous syndrome associated with the beta-adrenergic blocking agent practolol has not been reported with carteolol.

OPHTHALMIC SOLUTION

The following adverse reactions have been reported in clinical trials with carteolol HCl solution:

Ocular: Transient eye irritation, burning, tearing, conjunctival hyperemia and edema occurred in about 1 of 4 patients. Ocular symptoms including blurred and cloudy vision, photophobia, decreased night vision, and ptosis and ocular signs including blepharoconjunctivitis, abnormal corneal staining, and corneal sensitivity occurred occasionally.
Systemic: As a characteristic of nonselective adrenergic blocking agents, carteolol HCl solution may cause bradycardia and decreased blood pressure (see WARNINGS).

The following systemic events have occasionally been reported with the use of carteolol HCl solution: Cardiac arrhythmia, heart palpitation, dyspnea, asthenia, headache, dizziness, insomnia, sinusitis, and taste perversion.

The following additional adverse reactions have been reported with ophthalmic use of beta_1 and beta_2 (nonselective) adrenergic receptor blocking agents:

Body As a Whole: Headache
Cardiovascular: Arrhythmia, syncope, heart block, cerebral vascular accident, cerebral ischemia, congestive heart failure, palpitation (see WARNINGS)
Digestive: Nausea
Psychiatric: Depression
Skin: Hypersensitivity, including localized and generalized rash
Respiratory: Bronchospasm (predominantly in patients with pre- existing bronchospastic disease), respiratory failure (see WARNINGS)
Endocrine: Masked symptoms of hypoglycemia in insulin-dependent diabetics (see WARNINGS)
Special Senses: Signs and symptoms of keratitis, blepharoptosis, visual disturbances including refractive changes due to withdrawal of miotic therapy in some cases), diplopia ptosis

Other reactions associated with the oral use of nonselective adrenergic receptor blocking agents should be considered potential effects with ophthalmic use of these agents.

DOSAGE AND ADMINISTRATION

TABLETS

Dosage must be individualized. The initial dose of carteolol HCl is 2.5 mg given as a single daily oral dose either alone or added to diuretic therapy. If an adequate response is not achieved, the dose can be gradually increased to 5 and 10 mg as single daily doses. Increasing the dose above 10 mg/day is unlikely to produce further substantial benefits and, in fact, may decrease the response. The usual maintenance dose of carteolol is 2.5 or 5 mg once daily.

DOSAGE ADJUSTMENT IN RENAL IMPAIRMENT

Carteolol is excreted principally by the kidneys. When administering carteolol HCl to patients with renal impairment, the dosage regimen should be adjusted individually by the physician. Guidelines for dose interval adjustment are shown below (TABLE 4):

TABLE 4

Creatinine Clearance (ml/min)	Dosage Interval (hours)
>60	24
20-60	48
<20	72

OPHTHALMIC SOLUTION

The usual dose is one drop of carteolol HCl solution, 1%, in the affected eye(s) twice a day.

If the patient's IOP is not at a satisfactory level on this regimen, concomitant therapy with pilocarpine and other miotics, and/or epinephrine or dipivefrin, and/or systemically administered carbonic anhydrase inhibitors, such as acetazolamide, can be instituted.

HOW SUPPLIED

TABLETS

Recommended Storage: Avoid exposure to temperatures in excess of 40°C (104°F).

OPHTHALMIC SOLUTION

Storage: Store at 15-25°C (59-77°F) (room temperature) and protect from light.

PRODUCT LISTING - RATED THERAPEUTICALLY EQUIVALENT

Solution - Ophthalmic - 1%

5 ml	$19.44	OCUPRESS, Allscripts Pharmaceutical Company	54569-4304-00
5 ml	$19.64	GENERIC, Akorn Inc	17478-0710-10
5 ml	$19.64	GENERIC, Bausch and Lomb	24208-0367-05
5 ml	$21.28	GENERIC, Falcon Pharmaceuticals, Ltd.	61314-0238-05
5 ml	$32.75	OCUPRESS, Ciba Vision Ophthalmics	58768-0001-01
10 ml	$36.68	FEDERAL UPPER LIMIT, H.C.F.A. F F P	99999-0666-01
10 ml	$37.06	GENERIC, Akorn Inc	17478-0710-11
10 ml	$37.07	GENERIC, Bausch and Lomb	24208-0367-10
10 ml	$40.10	GENERIC, Falcon Pharmaceuticals, Ltd.	61314-0238-10
10 ml	$49.01	OCUPRESS, Allscripts Pharmaceutical Company	54569-4305-00
10 ml	$61.71	OCUPRESS, Ciba Vision Ophthalmics	58768-0001-02
15 ml	$55.59	GENERIC, Akorn Inc	17478-0710-12
15 ml	$55.60	GENERIC, Bausch and Lomb	24208-0367-15
15 ml	$57.25	GENERIC, Falcon Pharmaceuticals, Ltd.	61314-0238-15
15 ml	$92.61	OCUPRESS, Ciba Vision Ophthalmics	58768-0001-04

PRODUCT LISTING - EQUIVALENTS NOT AVAILABLE

Tablet - Oral - 2.5 mg

100's	$106.88	CARTROL, Abbott Pharmaceutical	00074-1664-13

Tablet - Oral - 5 mg

100's	$136.93	CARTROL, Abbott Pharmaceutical	00074-1665-13

Carvedilol (003267)

For related information, see the comparative table section in Appendix A.

Categories: Hypertension, essential; Heart failure, congestive; FDA Approved 1995 Sep; Pregnancy Category C
Drug Classes: Antiadrenergics, beta blocking
Brand Names: Coreg
Foreign Brand Availability: Cardivas (India); Carvedilol (Korea); Carvrol (Korea); Dilbloc (Indonesia); Dilatrend (Australia; Austria; Benin; Burkina-Faso; Colombia; Ecuador; Ethiopia; Gambia; Germany; Ghana; Guinea; Hong-Kong; Italy; Ivory-Coast; Kenya; Korea; Liberia; Malawi; Malaysia; Mali; Mauritania; Mauritius; Mexico; Morocco; New-Zealand; Niger; Nigeria; Norway; Peru; Philippines; Senegal; Seychelles; Sierra-Leone; South-Africa; Sudan; Taiwan; Tanzania; Thailand; Tunia; Uganda; Zambia; Zimbabwe); Eucardic (England; Ireland); Kredex (France); Querto (Germany); V-Bloc (Indonesia)
Cost of Therapy: $95.49 (Congestive Heart Failure; Coreg; 6.25 mg; 2 tablets/day; 30 day supply)

DESCRIPTION

Carvedilol is a nonselective β-adrenergic blocking agent with α_1-blocking activity. It is (±)-1-(carbazol-4-yloxy)-3-[[2-(o-methoxyphenoxy)ethyl]amino]-2-propanol. It is a racemic mixture.

TABLETS FOR ORAL ADMINISTRATION

Coreg is a white, oval, film-coated tablet containing 3.125, 6.25, 12.5 or 25 mg of carvedilol. The 6.25, 12.5 and 25 mg tablets are Tiltab tablets. Inactive ingredients consist of colloidal silicon dioxide, crospovidone, hypromellose, lactose, magnesium stearate, polyethylene glycol, polysorbate 80, povidone, sucrose, and titanium dioxide.

Carvedilol is a white to off-white powder with a molecular weight of 406.5 and a molecular formula of $C_{24}H_{26}N_2O_4$. It is freely soluble in dimethylsulfoxide; soluble in methylene chloride and methanol; sparingly soluble in 95% ethanol and isopropanol; slightly soluble in ethyl ether; and practically insoluble in water, gastric fluid (simulated, TS, pH 1.1) and intestinal fluid (simulated, TS without pancreatin, pH 7.5).

CLINICAL PHARMACOLOGY

Carvedilol is a racemic mixture in which nonselective β-adrenoreceptor blocking activity is present in the S(-) enantiomer and α-adrenergic blocking activity is present in both R(+) and S(-) enantiomers at equal potency. Carvedilol has no intrinsic sympathomimetic activity.

PHARMACOKINETICS

Carvedilol is rapidly and extensively absorbed following oral administration, with absolute bioavailability of approximately 25-35% due to a significant degree of first-pass metabolism. Following oral administration, the apparent mean terminal elimination half-life of carvedilol generally ranges from 7-10 hours. Plasma concentrations achieved are proportional to the oral dose administered. When administered with food, the rate of absorption is slowed, as evidenced by a delay in the time to reach peak plasma levels, with no significant difference in extent of bioavailability. Taking carvedilol with food should minimize the risk of orthostatic hypotension.

Carvedilol is extensively metabolized. Following oral administration of radiolabelled carvedilol to healthy volunteers, carvedilol accounted for only about 7% of the total radioactivity in plasma as measured by area under the curve (AUC). Less than 2% of the dose was excreted unchanged in the urine. Carvedilol is metabolized primarily by aromatic ring oxidation and glucuronidation. The oxidative metabolites are further metabolized by conjugation via glucuronidation and sulfation. The metabolites of carvedilol are excreted primarily via the bile into the feces. Demethylation and hydroxylation at the phenol ring produce three active metabolites with β-receptor blocking activity. Based on preclinical studies, the 4′-hydroxyphenyl metabolite is approximately 13 times more potent than carvedilol for β-blockade.

Compared to carvedilol, the three active metabolites exhibit weak vasodilating activity. Plasma concentrations of the active metabolites are about one-tenth of those observed for carvedilol and have pharmacokinetics similar to the parent.

Carvedilol undergoes stereoselective first-pass metabolism with plasma levels of R(+)-carvedilol approximately 2-3 times higher than S(-)-carvedilol following oral administration in healthy subjects. The mean apparent terminal elimination half-lives for R(+)-carvedilol range from 5-9 hours compared with 7-11 hours for the S(-)-enantiomer.

The primary P450 enzymes responsible for the metabolism of both R(+) and S(-)-carvedilol in human liver microsomes were CYP2D6 and CYP2C9 and to a lesser extent CYP3A4, 2C19, 1A2, and 2E1. CYP2D6 is thought to be the major enzyme in the 4′- and 5′-hydroxylation of carvedilol, with a potential contribution from 3A4. CYP2C9 is thought to be of primary importance in the O-methylation pathway of S(-)-carvedilol.

Carvedilol is subject to the effects of genetic polymorphism with poor metabolizers of debrisoquin (a marker for cytochrome P450 2D6) exhibiting 2- to 3-fold higher plasma concentrations of R(+)-carvedilol compared to extensive metabolizers. In contrast, plasma levels of S(-)-carvedilol are increased only about 20-25% in poor metabolizers, indicating this enantiomer is metabolized to a lesser extent by cytochrome P450 2D6 than R(+)-carvedilol. The pharmacokinetics of carvedilol do not appear to be different in poor metabolizers of S-mephenytoin (patients deficient in cytochrome P450 2C19).

Carvedilol is more than 98% bound to plasma proteins, primarily with albumin. The plasma protein binding is independent of concentration over the therapeutic range. Carvedilol is a basic, lipophilic compound with a steady-state volume of distribution of approximately 115 L, indicating substantial distribution into extravascular tissues. Plasma clearance ranges from 500-700 ml/min.

Congestive Heart Failure

Steady-state plasma concentrations of carvedilol and its enantiomers increased proportionally over the 6.25 to 50 mg dose range in patients with congestive heart failure. Compared to healthy subjects, congestive heart failure patients had increased mean AUC and C_{max} values for carvedilol and its enantiomers, with up to 50-100% higher values observed in 6 patients with NYHA Class IV heart failure. The mean apparent terminal elimination half-life for carvedilol was similar to that observed in healthy subjects.

Pharmacokinetic Drug-Drug Interaction

Since carvedilol undergoes substantial oxidative metabolism, the metabolism and pharmacokinetics of carvedilol may be affected by induction or inhibition of cytochrome P450 enzymes.

Rifampin: In a pharmacokinetic study conducted in 8 healthy male subjects, rifampin (600 mg daily for 12 days) decreased the AUC and C_{max} of carvedilol by about 70%.

Cimetidine: In a pharmacokinetic study conducted in 10 healthy male subjects, cimetidine (1000 mg/day) increased the steady-state AUC of carvedilol by 30% with no change in C_{max}.

Glyburide: In 12 healthy subjects, combined administration of carvedilol (25 mg once daily) and a single dose of glyburide did not result in a clinically relevant pharmacokinetic interaction for either compound.

Hydrochlorothiazide: A single oral dose of carvedilol 25 mg did not alter the pharmacokinetics of a single oral dose of hydrochlorothiazide 25 mg in 12 patients with hypertension. Likewise, hydrochlorothiazide had no effect on the pharmacokinetics of carvedilol.

Digoxin: Following concomitant administration of carvedilol (25 mg once daily) and digoxin (0.25 mg once daily) for 14 days, steady-state AUC and trough concentrations of digoxin were increased by 14% and 16%, respectively, in 12 hypertensive patients.

Torsemide: In a study of 12 healthy subjects, combined oral administration of carvedilol 25 mg once daily and torsemide 5 mg once daily for 5 days did not result in any significant differences in their pharmacokinetics compared with administration of the drugs alone.

Warfarin: Carvedilol (12.5 mg twice daily) did not have an effect on the steady-state prothrombin time ratios and did not alter the pharmacokinetics of R(+)- and S(-)-warfarin following concomitant administration with warfarin in 9 healthy volunteers.

SPECIAL POPULATIONS

Elderly

Plasma levels of carvedilol average about 50% higher in the elderly compared to young subjects.

Hepatic Impairment

Compared to healthy subjects, patients with cirrhotic liver disease exhibit significantly higher concentrations of carvedilol (approximately 4- to 7-fold) following single-dose therapy (see WARNINGS, Hepatic Injury).

Renal Insufficiency

Although carvedilol is metabolized primarily by the liver, plasma concentrations of carvedilol have been reported to be increased in patients with renal impairment. Based on mean AUC data, approximately 40-50% higher plasma concentrations of carvedilol were observed in hypertensive patients with moderate to severe renal impairment compared to a control group of hypertensive patients with normal renal function. However, the ranges of AUC values were similar for both groups. Changes in mean peak plasma levels were less pronounced, approximately 12-26% higher in patients with impaired renal function.

Consistent with its high degree of plasma protein-binding, carvedilol does not appear to be cleared significantly by hemodialysis.

PHARMACODYNAMICS

Congestive Heart Failure

The basis for the beneficial effects of carvedilol in congestive heart failure is not established.

Two placebo-controlled studies compared the acute hemodynamic effects of carvedilol to baseline measurements in 59 and 49 patients with NYHA Class II-IV heart failure receiving diuretics, ACE inhibitors, and digitalis. There were significant reductions in systemic blood pressure, pulmonary artery pressure, pulmonary capillary wedge pressure, and heart rate. Initial effects on cardiac output, stroke volume index, and systemic vascular resistance were small and variable.

These studies measured hemodynamic effects again at 12-14 weeks. Carvedilol significantly reduced systemic blood pressure, pulmonary artery pressure, right atrial pressure, systemic vascular resistance, and heart rate, while stroke volume index was increased.

Among 839 patients with NYHA Class II-III heart failure treated for 26-52 weeks in 4 US placebo-controlled trials, the average left ventricular ejection fraction (EF) measured by radionuclide ventriculography increased by 9 EF units (%) in carvedilol patients and by 2 EF units in placebo patients at a target dose of 25-50 mg bid. The effects of carvedilol on ejection fraction were related to dose. Doses of 6.25 mg bid, 12.5 mg bid and 25 mg bid were associated with placebo-corrected increases in EF of 5 EF units, 6 EF units and 8 EF units, respectively; each of these effects were nominally statistically significant.

Left Ventricular Dysfunction Following Myocardial Infarction

The basis for the beneficial effects of carvedilol in patients with left ventricular dysfunction following an acute myocardial infarction is not established.

Hypertension

The mechanism by which β-blockade produces an antihypertensive effect has not been established.

β-adrenoreceptor blocking activity has been demonstrated in animal and human studies showing that carvedilol (1) reduces cardiac output in normal subjects; (2) reduces exercise-and/or isoproterenol-induced tachycardia and (3) reduces reflex orthostatic tachycardia. Significant β-adrenoreceptor blocking effect is usually seen within 1 hour of drug administration.

α_1-adrenoreceptor blocking activity has been demonstrated in human and animal studies, showing that carvedilol (1) attenuates the pressor effects of phenylephrine; (2) causes vasodilation and (3) reduces peripheral vascular resistance. These effects contribute to the reduction of blood pressure and usually are seen within 30 minutes of drug administration.

Due to the α_1-receptor blocking activity of carvedilol, blood pressure is lowered more in the standing than in the supine position, and symptoms of postural hypotension (1.8%), including rare instances of syncope, can occur. Following oral administration, when postural hypotension has occurred, it has been transient and is uncommon when carvedilol is administered with food at the recommended starting dose and titration increments are closely followed (see DOSAGE AND ADMINISTRATION).

In hypertensive patients with normal renal function, therapeutic doses of carvedilol decreased renal vascular resistance with no change in glomerular filtration rate or renal plasma flow. Changes in excretion of sodium, potassium, uric acid and phosphorus in hypertensive patients with normal renal function were similar after carvedilol and placebo.

Carvedilol has little effect on plasma catecholamines, plasma aldosterone or electrolyte levels, but it does significantly reduce plasma renin activity when given for at least 4 weeks. It also increases levels of atrial natriuretic peptide.

INDICATIONS AND USAGE

CONGESTIVE HEART FAILURE

Carvedilol is indicated for the treatment of mild to severe heart failure of ischemic or cardiomyopathic origin, usually in addition to diuretics, ACE inhibitor, and digitalis, to increase survival and, also, to reduce the risk of hospitalization.

LEFT VENTRICULAR DYSFUNCTION FOLLOWING MYOCARDIAL INFARCTION

Carvedilol is indicated to reduce cardiovascular mortality in clinically stable patients who have survived the acute phase of a myocardial infarction and have a left ventricular ejection fraction of ≤40% (with or without symptomatic heart failure).

HYPERTENSION

Carvedilol is also indicated for the management of essential hypertension. It can be used alone or in combination with other antihypertensive agents, especially thiazide-type diuretics (see DRUG INTERACTIONS).

CONTRAINDICATIONS

Carvedilol is contraindicated in patients with bronchial asthma (two cases of death from status asthmaticus have been reported in patients receiving single doses of carvedilol) or related bronchospastic conditions, second- or third-degree AV block, sick sinus syndrome or severe bradycardia (unless a permanent pacemaker is in place), or in patients with cardiogenic shock or who have decompensated heart failure requiring the use of intravenous inotropic therapy. Such patients should first be weaned from intravenous therapy before initiating carvedilol.

Use of carvedilol in patients with clinically manifest hepatic impairment is not recommended.

Carvedilol is contraindicated in patients with hypersensitivity to any component of the product.

WARNINGS

CESSATION OF THERAPY WITH CARVEDILOL

Patients with coronary artery disease, who are being treated with carvedilol, should be advised against abrupt discontinuation of therapy. Severe exacerbation of angina and the occurrence of myocardial infarction and ventricular arrhythmias have been reported in angina patients following the abrupt discontinuation of therapy with β-blockers. The last two complications may occur with or without preceding exacerbation of the angina pectoris. As with other β-blockers, when discontinuation of carvedilol is planned, the patients should be carefully observed and advised to limit physical activity to a minimum. Carvedilol should be discontinued over 1-2 weeks whenever possible. If the angina worsens or acute coronary insufficiency develops, it is recommended that carvedilol be promptly reinstituted, at least temporarily. Because coronary artery disease is common and may be unrecognized, it may be prudent not to discontinue carvedilol therapy abruptly even in patients treated only for hypertension or heart failure. (See DOSAGE AND ADMINISTRATION.)

HEPATIC INJURY

Mild hepatocellular injury, confirmed by rechallenge, has occurred rarely with carvedilol therapy in the treatment of hypertension. In controlled studies of hypertensive patients, the incidence of liver function abnormalities reported as adverse experiences was 1.1% (13 of 1142 patients) in patients receiving carvedilol and 0.9% (4 of 462 patients) in those receiving placebo. One patient receiving carvedilol in a placebo-controlled trial withdrew for abnormal hepatic function.

In controlled studies of primarily mild-to-moderate congestive heart failure, the incidence of liver function abnormalities reported as adverse experiences was 5.0% (38 of 765 patients) in patients receiving carvedilol and 4.6% (20 of 437 patients) in those receiving placebo. Three patients receiving carvedilol (0.4%) and 2 patients receiving placebo (0.5%) in placebo-controlled trials withdrew for abnormal hepatic function. Similarly, in a long-term, placebo-controlled trial in severe heart failure, there was no difference in the incidence of liver function abnormalities reported as adverse experiences between patients receiving carvedilol and those receiving placebo. No patients receiving carvedilol and 1 patient receiving placebo (0.09%) withdrew for hepatitis. In addition, patients treated with carvedilol had lower values for hepatic transaminases than patients treated with placebo, possibly because carvedilol-induced improvements in cardiac function led to less hepatic congestion and/or improved hepatic blood flow.

In the CAPRICORN study of survivors of an acute myocardial infarction with left ventricular dysfunction the incidence of liver function abnormalities reported as adverse experiences was 2.0% (19 of 969 patients) in patients receiving carvedilol and 1.5% (15 of 980 patients) in those receiving placebo. Of the patients who received carvedilol in the CAPRICORN trial, 1 patient (0.1%) withdrew from the study due to cholestatic jaundice.

Hepatic injury has been reversible and has occurred after short- and/or long-term therapy with minimal clinical symptomatology. No deaths due to liver function abnormalities have been reported in association with the use of carvedilol.

At the first symptom/sign of liver dysfunction (*e.g.*, pruritus, dark urine, persistent anorexia, jaundice, right upper quadrant tenderness or unexplained "flu-like" symptoms), laboratory testing should be performed. If the patient has laboratory evidence of liver injury or jaundice, carvedilol should be stopped and not restarted.

PERIPHERAL VASCULAR DISEASE

β-blockers can precipitate or aggravate symptoms of arterial insufficiency in patients with peripheral vascular disease. Caution should be exercised in such individuals.

ANESTHESIA AND MAJOR SURGERY

If treatment with carvedilol is to be continued perioperatively, particular care should be taken when anesthetic agents which depress myocardial function, such as ether, cyclopropane and trichloroethylene, are used.

DIABETES AND HYPOGLYCEMIA

In general, β-blockers may mask some of the manifestations of hypoglycemia, particularly tachycardia. Nonselective β-blockers may potentiate insulin-induced hypoglycemia and delay recovery of serum glucose levels. Patients subject to spontaneous hypoglycemia, or diabetic patients receiving insulin or oral hypoglycemic agents, should be cautioned about these possibilities. In congestive heart failure patients, there is a risk of worsening hyperglycemia (see PRECAUTIONS).

THYROTOXICOSIS

β-adrenergic blockade may mask clinical signs of hyperthyroidism, such as tachycardia. Abrupt withdrawal of β-blockade may be followed by an exacerbation of the symptoms of hyperthyroidism or may precipitate thyroid storm.

PRECAUTIONS

GENERAL

In clinical trials, carvedilol caused bradycardia in about 2% of hypertensive patients, 9% of congestive heart failure patients, and 6.5% of myocardial infarction patients with left ventricular dysfunction. If pulse rate drops below 55 beats/min, the dosage should be reduced.

In clinical trials of primarily mild-to-moderate heart failure, hypotension and postural hypotension occurred in 9.7% and syncope in 3.4% of patients receiving carvedilol compared to 3.6% and 2.5% of placebo patients, respectively. The risk for these events was highest during the first 30 days of dosing, corresponding to the up-titration period and was a cause for discontinuation of therapy in 0.7% of carvedilol patients, compared to 0.4% of placebo patients. In a long-term, placebo-controlled trial in severe heart failure (COPERNICUS), hypotension and postural hypotension occurred in 15.1% and syncope in 2.9% of heart failure patients receiving carvedilol compared to 8.7% and 2.3% of placebo patients, respectively. These events were a cause for discontinuation of therapy in 1.1% of carvedilol patients, compared to 0.8% of placebo patients.

Postural hypotension occurred in 1.8% and syncope in 0.1% of hypertensive patients, primarily following the initial dose or at the time of dose increase and was a cause for discontinuation of therapy in 1% of patients.

In the CAPRICORN study of survivors of an acute myocardial infarction, hypotension or postural hypotension occurred in 20.2% of patients receiving carvedilol compared to 12.6% of placebo patients. Syncope was reported in 3.9% and 1.9% of patients, respectively. These events were a cause for discontinuation of therapy in 2.5% of patients receiving carvedilol, compared to 0.2% of placebo patients.

To decrease the likelihood of syncope or excessive hypotension, treatment should be initiated with 3.125 mg bid for congestive heart failure patients, and 6.25 mg bid for hypertensive patients and survivors of an acute myocardial infarction with left ventricular dysfunction. Dosage should then be increased slowly, according to recommendations in DOSAGE AND ADMINISTRATION, and the drug should be taken with food. During initiation of therapy, the patient should be cautioned to avoid situations such as driving or hazardous tasks, where injury could result should syncope occur.

Rarely, use of carvedilol in patients with congestive heart failure has resulted in deterioration of renal function. Patients at risk appear to be those with low blood pressure (systolic BP <100 mm Hg), ischemic heart disease and diffuse vascular disease, and/or underlying renal insufficiency. Renal function has returned to baseline when carvedilol was stopped. In patients with these risk factors it is recommended that renal function be monitored during up-titration of carvedilol and the drug discontinued or dosage reduced if worsening of renal function occurs.

Worsening heart failure or fluid retention may occur during up-titration of carvedilol. If such symptoms occur, diuretics should be increased and the carvedilol dose should not be advanced until clinical stability resumes (see DOSAGE AND ADMINISTRATION). Occasionally, it is necessary to lower the carvedilol dose or temporarily discontinue it. Such episodes do not preclude subsequent successful titration of, or a favorable response to, carvedilol. In a placebo-controlled trial of patients with severe heart failure, worsening heart failure during the first 3 months was reported to a similar degree with carvedilol and with placebo. When treatment was maintained beyond 3 months, worsening heart failure was reported less frequently in patients treated with carvedilol than with placebo. Worsening heart failure observed during long-term therapy is more likely to be related to the patients' underlying disease than to treatment with carvedilol.

In patients with pheochromocytoma, an α-blocking agent should be initiated prior to the use of any β-blocking agent. Although carvedilol has both α- and β-blocking pharmacologic activities, there has been no experience with its use in this condition. Therefore, caution should be taken in the administration of carvedilol to patients suspected of having pheochromocytoma.

Agents with non-selective β-blocking activity may provoke chest pain in patients with Prinzmetal's variant angina. There has been no clinical experience with carvedilol in these patients although the α-blocking activity may prevent such symptoms. However, caution should be taken in the administration of carvedilol to patients suspected of having Prinzmetal's variant angina.

In congestive heart failure patients with diabetes, carvedilol therapy may lead to worsening hyperglycemia, which responds to intensification of hypoglycemic therapy. It is recommended that blood glucose be monitored when carvedilol dosing is initiated, adjusted, or discontinued.

RISK OF ANAPHYLACTIC REACTION

While taking β-blockers, patients with a history of severe anaphylactic reaction to a variety of allergens may be more reactive to repeated challenge, either accidental, diagnostic or therapeutic. Such patients may be unresponsive to the usual doses of epinephrine used to treat allergic reaction.

NONALLERGIC BRONCHOSPASM (E.G., CHRONIC BRONCHITIS AND EMPHYSEMA)

Patients with bronchospastic disease should, in general, not receive β-blockers. carvedilol may be used with caution, however, in patients who do not respond to, or cannot tolerate, other antihypertensive agents. It is prudent, if carvedilol is used, to use the smallest effective dose, so that inhibition of endogenous or exogenous β-agonists is minimized.

In clinical trials of patients with congestive heart failure, patients with bronchospastic disease were enrolled if they did not require oral or inhaled medication to treat their bronchospastic disease. In such patients, it is recommended that carvedilol be used with caution. The dosing recommendations should be followed closely and the dose should be lowered if any evidence of bronchospasm is observed during up-titration.

INFORMATION FOR THE PATIENT

Patients taking carvedilol should be advised of the following:

- They should not interrupt or discontinue using carvedilol without a physician's advice.
- Congestive heart failure patients should consult their physician if they experience signs or symptoms of worsening heart failure such as weight gain or increasing shortness of breath.
- They may experience a drop in blood pressure when standing, resulting in dizziness and, rarely, fainting. Patients should sit or lie down when these symptoms of lowered blood pressure occur.
- If patients experience dizziness or fatigue, they should avoid driving or hazardous tasks.
- They should consult a physician if they experience dizziness or faintness, in case the dosage should be adjusted.
- They should take carvedilol with food.
- Diabetic patients should report any changes in blood sugar levels to their physician.
- Contact lens wearers may experience decreased lacrimation.

CARCINOGENESIS, MUTAGENESIS, AND IMPAIRMENT OF FERTILITY

In 2 year studies conducted in rats given carvedilol at doses up to 75 mg/kg/day (12 times the maximum recommended human dose [MRHD] when compared on a mg/m^2 basis) or in mice given up to 200 mg/kg/day (16 times the MRHD on a mg/m^2 basis), carvedilol had no carcinogenic effect.

Carvedilol was negative when tested in a battery of genotoxicity assays, including the Ames and the CHO/HGPRT assays for mutagenicity and the *in vitro* hamster micronucleus and *in vivo* human lymphocyte cell tests for clastogenicity.

At doses ≥200 mg/kg/day (≥32 times the MRHD as mg/m^2) carvedilol was toxic to adult rats (sedation, reduced weight gain) and was associated with a reduced number of successful matings, prolonged mating time, significantly fewer corpora lutea and implants per dam and complete resorption of 18% of the litters. The no-observed-effect dose level for overt toxicity and impairment of fertility was 60 mg/kg/day (10 times the MRHD as mg/m^2).

PREGNANCY, TERATOGENIC EFFECTS, PREGNANCY CATEGORY C

Studies performed in pregnant rats and rabbits given carvedilol revealed increased post-implantation loss in rats at doses of 300 mg/kg/day (50 times the MRHD as mg/m^2) and in rabbits at doses of 75 mg/kg/day (25 times the MRHD as mg/m^2). In the rats, there was also a decrease in fetal body weight at the maternally toxic dose of 300 mg/kg/day (50 times the MRHD as mg/m^2), which was accompanied by an elevation in the frequency of fetuses with delayed skeletal development (missing or stunted 13th rib). In rats the no-observed-effect level for developmental toxicity was 60 mg/kg/day (10 times the MRHD as mg/m^2); in rabbits it was 15 mg/kg/day (5 times the MRHD as mg/m^2). There are no adequate and well-controlled studies in pregnant women. Carvedilol should be used during pregnancy only if the potential benefit justifies the potential risk to the fetus.

NURSING MOTHERS

It is not known whether this drug is excreted in human milk. Studies in rats have shown that carvedilol and/or its metabolites (as well as other β-blockers) cross the placental barrier and are excreted in breast milk. There was increased mortality at 1 week post-partum in neonates from rats treated with 60 mg/kg/day (10 times the MRHD as mg/m^2) and above during the last trimester through Day 22 of lactation. Because many drugs are excreted in human milk and because of the potential for serious adverse reactions in nursing infants from β-blockers, especially bradycardia, a decision should be made whether to discontinue nursing or to discontinue the drug, taking into account the importance of the drug to the mother. The effects of other α- and β-blocking agents have included perinatal and neonatal distress.

PEDIATRIC USE

Safety and efficacy in patients younger than 18 years of age have not been established.

GERIATRIC USE

Of the 765 patients with congestive heart failure randomized to carvedilol in US clinical trials, 31% (235) were 65 years of age or older. Of the 1156 patients randomized to carvedilol in a long-term, placebo-controlled trial in severe heart failure, 47% (547) were 65 years of age or older. Of 3025 patients receiving carvedilol in congestive heart failure trials worldwide, 42% were 65 years of age or older. There were no notable differences in efficacy or the incidence of adverse events between older and younger patients.

Of the 975 myocardial infarction patients randomized to carvedilol in the CAPRICORN trial, 48% (468) were 65 years of age or older, and 11% (111) were 75 years of age or older. There were no notable differences in efficacy or the incidence of adverse events between older and younger patients.

Of the 2065 hypertensive patients in US clinical trials of efficacy or safety who were treated with carvedilol , 21% (436) were 65 years of age or older. Of 3722 patients receiving carvedilol in hypertension clinical trials conducted worldwide, 24% were 65 years of age or older. There were no notable differences in efficacy or the incidence of adverse events between older and younger patients. With the exception of dizziness (incidence 8.8% in the elderly vs 6% in younger patients), there were no events for which the incidence in the elderly exceeded that in the younger population by greater than 2.0%.

Similar results were observed in a postmarketing surveillance study of 3328 carvedilol patients, of whom approximately 20% were 65 years of age or older.

DRUG INTERACTIONS

Also see CLINICAL PHARMACOLOGY, Pharmacokinetics, Pharmacokinetic Drug-Drug Interactions.

Inhibitors of CYP2D6; poor metabolizers of debrisoquin: Interactions of carvedilol with strong inhibitors of CYP2D6 (such as quinidine, fluoxetine, paroxetine, and propafenone) have not been studied, but these drugs would be expected to increase blood levels of the R(+) enantiomer of carvedilol (see CLINICAL PHARMACOLOGY). Retrospective analysis of side effects in clinical trials showed that poor 2D6 metabolizers had a higher rate of dizziness during up-titration, presumably resulting from vasodilating effects of the higher concentrations of the α-blocking R(+) enantiomer.

Catecholamine-depleting agents: Patients taking both agents with β-blocking properties and a drug that can deplete catecholamines (*e.g.*, reserpine and monoamine oxidase inhibitors) should be observed closely for signs of hypotension and/or severe bradycardia.

Clonidine: Concomitant administration of clonidine with agents with β-blocking properties may potentiate blood-pressure- and heart-rate-lowering effects. When concomitant treatment with agents with β-blocking properties and clonidine is to be terminated, the β-blocking agent should be discontinued first. Clonidine therapy can then be discontinued several days later by gradually decreasing the dosage.

Cyclosporin: Modest increases in mean trough cyclosporin concentrations were observed following initiation of carvedilol treatment in 21 renal transplant patients suffering from chronic vascular rejection. In about 30% of patients, the dose of cyclosporin had to be reduced in order to maintain cyclosporin concentrations within the therapeutic range, while in the remainder no adjustment was needed. On the average for the group, the dose of cyclosporin was reduced about 20% in these patients. Due to wide interindividual variability in the dose adjustment required, it is recommended that cyclosporin concentrations be monitored closely after initiation of carvedilol therapy and that the dose of cyclosporin be adjusted as appropriate.

Digoxin: Digoxin concentrations are increased by about 15% when digoxin and carvedilol are administered concomitantly. Both digoxin and carvedilol slow AV conduction. Therefore, increased monitoring of digoxin is recommended when initiating, adjusting or discontinuing carvedilol.

Inducers and inhibitors of hepatic metabolism: Rifampin reduced plasma concentrations of carvedilol by about 70%. Cimetidine increased AUC by about 30% but caused no change in C_{max}.

Calcium channel blockers: Isolated cases of conduction disturbance (rarely with hemodynamic compromise) have been observed when carvedilol is coadministered with diltiazem. As with other agents with β-blocking properties, if carvedilol is to be administered orally with calcium channel blockers of the verapamil or diltiazem type, it is recommended that ECG and blood pressure be monitored.

Insulin or oral hypoglycemics: Agents with β-blocking properties may enhance the blood-sugar-reducing effect of insulin and oral hypoglycemics. Therefore, in patients taking insulin or oral hypoglycemics, regular monitoring of blood glucose is recommended.

C

ADVERSE REACTIONS

CONGESTIVE HEART FAILURE

Carvedilol has been evaluated for safety in congestive heart failure in more than 3000 patients worldwide of whom more than 2100 participated in placebo-controlled clinical trials. Approximately 60% of the total treated population received carvedilol for at least 6 months and 30% received carvedilol for at least 12 months. The adverse experience profile of carvedilol in patients with congestive heart failure was consistent with the pharmacology of the drug and the health status of the patients. Both in US clinical trials in mild-to-moderate heart failure that compared carvedilol in daily doses up to 100 mg (n=765) to placebo (n=437), and in a multinational clinical trial in severe heart failure (COPERNICUS) that compared carvedilol in daily doses up to 50 mg (n=1156) with placebo (n=1133), discontinuation rates for adverse experiences were similar in carvedilol and placebo patients. In these databases, the only cause of discontinuation >1%, and occurring more often on carvedilol was dizziness (1.3% on carvedilol, 0.6% on placebo in the COPERNICUS trial).

TABLE 2 shows adverse events reported in patients with mild-to-moderate heart failure enrolled in US placebo-controlled clinical trials, and with severe heart failure enrolled in the COPERNICUS trial. Shown are adverse events that occurred more frequently in drug-treated patients than placebo-treated patients with an incidence of >3% in patients treated with carvedilol regardless of causality. Median study medication exposure was 6.3 months for both carvedilol and placebo patients in the trials of mild-to-moderate heart failure, and 10.4 months in the trial of severe heart failure patients.

TABLE 2 *Adverse Events Occurring More Frequently With Carvedilol Than With Placebo in Patients With Mild-to-Moderate Heart Failure Enrolled in US Heart Failure Trials or in Patients With Severe Heart Failure in the COPERNICUS Trial (Incidence >3% in Patients Treated With Carvedilol, Regardless of Causality)*

	Mild-to-Moderate HF		Severe Heart Failure	
	Carvedilol (n=765)	Placebo (n=437)	Carvedilol (n=1156)	Placebo (n=1133)
Body as a Whole				
Asthenia	7%	7%	11%	9%
Fatigue	24%	22%	—	—
Pain	9%	8%	1%	1%
Digoxin level increased	5%	4%	2%	1%
Edema generalized	5%	3%	6%	5%
Edema dependent	4%	2%	—	—
Cardiovascular				
Bradycardia	9%	1%	10%	3%
Hypotension	9%	3%	14%	8%
Syncope	3%	3%	8%	5%
Angina pectoris	2%	3%	6%	4%
Central Nervous System				
Dizziness	32%	19%	24%	17%
Headache	8%	7%	5%	3%
Gastrointestinal				
Diarrhea	12%	6%	5%	3%
Nausea	9%	5%	4%	3%
Vomiting	6%	4%	1%	2%
Metabolic				
Hyperglycemia	12%	8%	5%	3%
Weight increase	10%	7%	12%	11%
BUN increased	6%	5%	—	—
NPN increased	6%	5%	—	—
Hypercholesterolemia	4%	3%	1%	1%
Edema peripheral	2%	1%	7%	6%
Musculoskeletal				
Arthralgia	6%	5%	1%	1%
Respiratory				
Sinusitis	5%	4%	2%	1%
Bronchitis	5%	4%	5%	5%
Upper respiratory infection	18%	18%	14%	13%
Cough increased	8%	9%	5%	4%
Rales	4%	4%	4%	2%
Vision				
Vision abnormal	5%	2%	—	—

In addition to the events in TABLE 2, in these trials chest pain, injury, cardiac failure, abdominal pain, gout, insomnia, depression, viral infection, and dyspnea were also reported, but rates were equal or greater in placebo-treated patients. Rates of adverse events were generally similar across demographic subsets (men and women, elderly and non-elderly, blacks and non-blacks).

The following adverse events were reported with a frequency of >1% but ≤3% and more frequently with carvedilol in US placebo-controlled trials in patients with mild-to-moderate heart failure, or in patients with severe heart failure in the COPERNICUS trial.

Incidence >1% to ≤3%:

Body as a Whole: Allergy, malaise, hypovolemia, fever, leg edema, infection, back pain.

Cardiovascular: Fluid overload, postural hypotension, aggravated angina pectoris, AV block, palpitation, hypertension.

Central and Peripheral Nervous System: Hypesthesia, vertigo, paresthesia.

Gastrointestinal: Melena, periodontitis.

Liver and Biliary System: SGPT increased, SGOT increased.

Metabolic and Nutritional: Hyperuricemia, hypoglycemia, hyponatremia, increased alkaline phosphatase, glycosuria, hypervolemia, diabetes mellitus, GGT increased, weight loss, hyperkalemia, creatinine increased.

Musculoskeletal: Muscle cramps.

Platelet, Bleeding and Clotting: Prothrombin decreased, purpura, thrombocytopenia.

Psychiatric: Somnolence.

Resistance Mechanism: Infection.

Reproductive, Male: Impotence.

Special Senses: Blurred vision.

Urinary System: Renal insufficiency, albuminuria, hematuria.

Postmarketing Experience

The following adverse reaction has been reported in postmarketing experience: Reports of aplastic anemia have been rare and received only when carvedilol was administered concomitantly with other medications associated with the event.

LEFT VENTRICULAR DYSFUNCTION FOLLOWING MYOCARDIAL INFARCTION

Carvedilol has been evaluated for safety in survivors of an acute myocardial infarction with left ventricular dysfunction in the CAPRICORN trial which involved 969 patients who received carvedilol and 980 who received placebo. Approximately 75% of the patients received carvedilol for at least 6 months and 53% received carvedilol for at least 12 months. Patients were treated for an average of 12.9 months and 12.8 months with carvedilol and placebo, respectively.

The most common adverse events reported with carvedilol in the CAPRICORN trial were consistent with the profile of the drug in the US heart failure trials and the COPERNICUS trial, as well as the health status of the patients. The only additional adverse events reported in CAPRICORN in >3% of the patients and more commonly on carvedilol were dyspnea, anemia, and lung edema. Hypertension and myocardial infarction were also reported, but rates were equal or greater in placebo-treated patients. The following adverse events were reported with a frequency of >1% but ≤3% and more frequently with carvedilol: flu syndrome, cerebrovascular accident, peripheral vascular disorder, hypotonia, depression, gastrointestinal pain, arthritis, gout and urinary tract infection. The overall rates of discontinuations due to adverse events were similar in both groups of patients. In this database, the only cause of discontinuation >1%, and occurring more often on carvedilol was hypotension (1.5% on carvedilol, 0.2% on placebo).

HYPERTENSION

Carvedilol has been evaluated for safety in hypertension in more than 2193 patients in US clinical trials and in 2976 patients in international clinical trials. Approximately 36% of the total treated population received carvedilol for at least 6 months. In general, carvedilol was well tolerated at doses up to 50 mg daily. Most adverse events reported during carvedilol therapy were of mild to moderate severity. In US controlled clinical trials directly comparing carvedilol monotherapy in doses up to 50 mg (n=1142) to placebo (n=462), 4.9% of carvedilol patients discontinued for adverse events vs 5.2% of placebo patients. Although there was no overall difference in discontinuation rates, discontinuations were more common in the carvedilol group for postural hypotension (1% vs 0). The overall incidence of adverse events in US placebo-controlled trials was found to increase with increasing dose of carvedilol. For individual adverse events this could only be distinguished for dizziness, which increased in frequency from 2-5% as total daily dose increased from 6.25 to 50 mg.

TABLE 3 shows adverse events in US placebo-controlled clinical trials for hypertension that occurred with an incidence of greater than 1% regardless of causality, and that were more frequent in drug-treated patients than placebo-treated patients.

In addition to the events in TABLE 3, abdominal pain, back pain, chest pain, dependent edema, dyspepsia, dyspnea, fatigue, headache, injury, nausea, pain, rhinitis, sinusitis, somnolence, and upper respiratory tract infection were also reported, but rates were equal or greater in placebo-treated patients. Rates of adverse events were generally similar across demographic subsets (men and women, elderly and non-elderly, blacks and non-blacks).

The following adverse events not described above were reported as possibly or probably related to carvedilol in worldwide open or controlled trials with carvedilol in patients with hypertension or congestive heart failure.

Incidence >0.1% to ≤1%:

Cardiovascular: Peripheral ischemia, tachycardia.

Central and Peripheral Nervous System: Hypokinesia.

Gastrointestinal: Bilirubinemia, increased hepatic enzymes (0.2% of hypertension patients and 0.4% of congestive heart failure patients were discontinued from therapy because of increases in hepatic enzymes; see WARNINGS, Hepatic Injury).

Psychiatric: Nervousness, sleep disorder, aggravated depression, impaired concentration, abnormal thinking, paroniria, emotional lability.

Respiratory System: Asthma (see CONTRAINDICATIONS).

Reproductive, Male: Decreased libido.

Skin and Appendages: Pruritus, rash erythematous, rash maculopapular, rash psoriaform, photosensitivity reaction.

Special Senses: Tinnitus.

Urinary System: Micturition frequency increased.

TABLE 3 *Adverse Events in US Placebo-Controlled Hypertension Trials Incidence ≥1%, Regardless of Causality*

	Adverse Reactions	
	Carvedilol (n=1142)	Placebo (n=462)
Cardiovascular		
Bradycardia	2%	—
Postural hypotension	2%	—
Peripheral edema	1%	—
Central Nervous System		
Dizziness	6%	5%
Insomnia	2%	1%
Gastrointestinal		
Diarrhea	2%	1%
Hematologic		
Thrombocytopenia	1%	—
Metabolic		
Hypertriglyceridemia	1%	—
Resistance Mechanism		
Viral infection	2%	1%
Respiratory		
Pharyngitis	2%	1%
Urinary/Renal		
Urinary tract infection	2%	1%

Autonomic Nervous System: Dry mouth, sweating increased.

Metabolic and Nutritional: Hypokalemia, hypertriglyceridemia.

Hematologic: Anemia, leukopenia.

The following events were reported in ≤0.1% of patients and are potentially important: Complete AV block, bundle branch block, myocardial ischemia, cerebrovascular disorder, convulsions, migraine, neuralgia, paresis, anaphylactoid reaction, alopecia, exfoliative dermatitis, amnesia, GI hemorrhage, bronchospasm, pulmonary edema, decreased hearing, respiratory alkalosis, increased BUN, decreased HDL, pancytopenia and atypical lymphocytes.

Other adverse events occurred sporadically in single patients and cannot be distinguished from concurrent disease states or medications.

Carvedilol therapy has not been associated with clinically significant changes in routine laboratory tests in hypertensive patients. No clinically relevant changes were noted in serum potassium, fasting serum glucose, total triglycerides, total cholesterol, HDL cholesterol, uric acid, blood urea nitrogen or creatinine.

DOSAGE AND ADMINISTRATION

CONGESTIVE HEART FAILURE

DOSAGE MUST BE INDIVIDUALIZED AND CLOSELY MONITORED BY A PHYSICIAN DURING UP-TITRATION. Prior to initiation of carvedilol, it is recommended that fluid retention be minimized. The recommended starting dose of carvedilol is 3.125 mg, twice daily for 2 weeks. Patients who tolerate a dose of 3.125 mg twice daily may have their dose increased to 6.25, 12.5 and 25 mg twice daily over successive intervals of at least 2 weeks. Patients should be maintained on lower doses if higher doses are not tolerated. A maximum dose of 50 mg bid has been administered to patients with mild-to-moderate heart failure weighing over 85 kg (187 lb).

Patients should be advised that initiation of treatment and (to a lesser extent) dosage increases may be associated with transient symptoms of dizziness or lightheadedness (and rarely syncope) within the first hour after dosing. Thus during these periods they should avoid situations such as driving or hazardous tasks, where symptoms could result in injury. In addition, carvedilol should be taken with food to slow the rate of absorption. Vasodilatory symptoms often do not require treatment, but it may be useful to separate the time of dosing of carvedilol from that of the ACE inhibitor or to reduce temporarily the dose of the ACE inhibitor. The dose of carvedilol should not be increased until symptoms of worsening heart failure or vasodilation have been stabilized.

Fluid retention (with or without transient worsening heart failure symptoms) should be treated by an increase in the dose of diuretics.

The dose of carvedilol should be reduced if patients experience bradycardia (heart rate <55 beats/min).

Episodes of dizziness or fluid retention during initiation of carvedilol can generally be managed without discontinuation of treatment and do not preclude subsequent successful titration of, or a favorable response to, carvedilol.

LEFT VENTRICULAR DYSFUNCTION FOLLOWING MYOCARDIAL INFARCTION

DOSAGE MUST BE INDIVIDUALIZED AND MONITORED DURING UP-TITRATION. Treatment with carvedilol may be started as an inpatient or outpatient and should be started after the patient is hemodynamically stable and fluid retention has been minimized. It is recommended that carvedilol be started at 6.25 mg twice daily and increased after 3-10 days, based on tolerability to 12.5 mg twice daily, then again to the target dose of 25 mg twice daily. A lower starting dose may be used (3.125 mg twice daily) and/or, the rate of up-titration may be slowed if clinically indicated (*e.g.,* due to low blood pressure or heart rate, or fluid retention). Patients should be maintained on lower doses if higher doses are not tolerated. The recommended dosing regimen need not be altered in patients who received treatment with an IV or oral β-blocker during the acute phase of the myocardial infarction.

HYPERTENSION

DOSAGE MUST BE INDIVIDUALIZED. The recommended starting dose of carvedilol is 6.25 mg twice daily. If this dose is tolerated, using standing systolic pressure measured about 1 hour after dosing as a guide, the dose should be maintained for 7-14 days, and then increased to 12.5 mg twice daily if needed, based on trough blood pressure, again using standing systolic pressure 1 hour after dosing as a guide for tolerance. This dose should also be maintained for 7-14 days and can then be adjusted upward to 25 mg twice daily if tolerated and needed. The full antihypertensive effect of carvedilol is seen within 7-14 days. Total daily dose should not exceed 50 mg. Carvedilol should be taken with food to slow the rate of absorption and reduce the incidence of orthostatic effects.

Addition of a diuretic to carvedilol, or carvedilol to a diuretic can be expected to produce additive effects and exaggerate the orthostatic component of carvedilol action.

USE IN PATIENTS WITH HEPATIC IMPAIRMENT

Carvedilol should not be given to patients with severe hepatic impairment (see CONTRAINDICATIONS).

HOW SUPPLIED

Coreg tablets are available in:

3.125 mg: White, oval, film-coated tablets, engraved with "39" and "SB".
6.25 mg: White, oval, film-coated tablets, engraved with "4140" and "SB".
12.5 mg: White, oval, film-coated tablets, engraved with "4141" and "SB".
25 mg: White, oval, film-coated tablets, engraved with "4142" and "SB".

The 6.25, 12.5 and 25 mg tablets are Tiltab tablets.

Storage: Store below 30°C (86°F). Protect from moisture. Dispense in a tight, light-resistant container.

PRODUCT LISTING - EQUIVALENTS NOT AVAILABLE

Tablet - Oral - 3.125 mg

28's	$48.30	COREG, Glaxosmithkline	00007-4139-55
100's	$179.99	COREG, Glaxosmithkline	00007-4139-20

Tablet - Oral - 6.25 mg

28's	$46.37	COREG, Glaxosmithkline	00007-4140-55
100's	$179.99	COREG, Glaxosmithkline	00007-4140-20

Tablet - Oral - 12.5 mg

28's	$46.37	COREG, Glaxosmithkline	00007-4141-55
100's	$179.99	COREG, Glaxosmithkline	00007-4141-20

Tablet - Oral - 25 mg

28's	$46.37	COREG, Glaxosmithkline	00007-4142-55
100's	$179.99	COREG, Glaxosmithkline	00007-4142-20

Casanthranol; Docusate Sodium *(000670)*

Categories: Constipation; FDA Pre 1938 Drugs; Pregnancy Category C
Drug Classes: Laxatives
Brand Names: Peri-D.S.

DESCRIPTION

Active Ingredients: *Each softgel capsule contains:* Docusate sodium, 100 mg, casanthranol, 30 mg.

Sodium Content: Each capsule contains approximately 5.2 mg of sodium. The maximum daily dose (3) is considered very low sodium.

Inactive Ingredients: Polyethylene glycol 400, gelatin, sorbitol, glycerin, propylene glycol, methylparaben, propylparaben, FD&C blue no. 1, FD&C red no. 40, titanium dioxide.

INDICATIONS AND USAGE

For relief of occasional constipation. This product generally produces a bowel movement in 6-12 hours.

WARNINGS

Do not use when abdominal pain, nausea or vomiting is present, unless directed by a doctor. If you have noticed a sudden change in bowel habits that persists over a period of 2 weeks, consult a doctor before using a laxative. Do not use for a period longer than 1 week, unless directed by a doctor. Rectal bleeding or failure to have a bowel movement after use of a laxative may indicate a serious condition. Discontinue use and consult a doctor. **KEEP THIS AND ALL DRUGS OUT OF THE REACH OF CHILDREN.** In case of accidental overdose, seek professional assistance or contact a Poison Control Center immediately. As with any drug, if you are pregnant or nursing a baby, seek the advice of a health professional before using this product.

DRUG INTERACTIONS

Do not take this product if you are presently taking mineral oil, unless directed by a doctor.

DOSAGE AND ADMINISTRATION

Directions:

Adults and children 12 years of age and over: 1-3 capsules which may be taken as a single daily dose or in divided doses.
Children 2 to under 12 years of age: 1 capsule daily.
Children under 2 years of age: Consult a doctor.

HOW SUPPLIED

Docusate sodium and casanthranol 100 mg/30 mg capsules are supplied as oval, maroon softgel capsule imprinted with **"0057"**.

Storage: Store at controlled room temperature 15-30°C (59-86°). Protect product from moisture.

Caspofungin Acetate *(003518)*

For complete prescribing information, refer to the CD-ROM included with the book.

For related information, see the comparative table section in Appendix A.

Categories: Aspergillosis; Candidemia; Candidiasis; FDA Approved 2001 Jan; Pregnancy Category C
Drug Classes: Antifungals
Brand Names: Cancidas
Cost of Therapy: $5,276.74 (Antifungal; Cancidas; 50 mg; 50 mg/day; 14 day supply)

DESCRIPTION

Cancidas is a sterile, lyophilized product for intravenous (IV) infusion that contains a semi-synthetic lipopeptide (echinocandin) compound synthesized from a fermentation product of *Glarea lozoyensis*. Cancidas is the first of a new class of antifungal drugs (glucan synthesis inhibitors) that inhibit the synthesis of β (1,3)-D-glucan, an integral component of the fungal cell wall.

Caspofungin acetate is 1-[(4*R*,5*S*)-5-[(2-aminoethyl)amino]-N^2-(10,12-dimethyl-1-oxotetradecyl)-4-hydroxy-L-ornithine]-5-[(3*R*)-3-hydroxy-L-ornithine] pneumocandin B_0 diacetate (salt). In addition to the active ingredient caspofungin acetate, Cancidas contains the following inactive ingredients: sucrose, mannitol, acetic acid, and sodium hydroxide. Caspofungin acetate is a hygroscopic, white to off-white powder. It is freely soluble in water and methanol, and slightly soluble in ethanol. The pH of a saturated aqueous solution of caspofungin acetate is approximately 6.6. The empirical formula is $C_{52}H_{88}N_{10}O_{15}\cdot 2C_2H_4O_2$ and the formula weight is 1213.42.

INDICATIONS AND USAGE

Caspofungin acetate is indicated for the treatment of:

Candidemia and the following *Candida* infections: intra-abdominal abscesses, peritonitis and pleural space infections. Caspofungin acetate has not been studied in endocarditis, osteomyelitis, and meningitis due to *Candida*.

Esophageal Candidiasis.

Invasive Aspergillosis in patients who are refractory to or intolerant of other therapies (*i.e.,* amphotericin B, lipid formulations of amphotericin B, and/or itraconazole). Caspofungin acetate has not been studied as initial therapy for invasive aspergillosis.

CONTRAINDICATIONS

Caspofungin acetate is contraindicated in patients with hypersensitivity to any component of this product.

WARNINGS

Concomitant use of caspofungin acetate with cyclosporine is not recommended unless the potential benefit outweighs the potential risk to the patient. In one clinical study, 3 of 4 healthy subjects who received caspofungin acetate 70 mg on Days 1-10, and also received two 3 mg/kg doses of cyclosporine 12 hours apart on Day 10, developed transient elevations of alanine transaminase (ALT) on Day 11 that were 2-3 times the upper limit of normal (ULN). In a separate panel of subjects in the same study, 2 of 8 who received caspofungin acetate 35 mg daily for 3 days and cyclosporine (two 3 mg/kg doses administered 12 hours apart) on Day 1 had small increases in ALT (slightly above the ULN) on Day 2. In both groups, elevations in aspartate transaminase (AST) paralleled ALT elevations, but were of lesser magnitude. Hence, concomitant use of caspofungin acetate with cyclosporine is not recommended until multiple-dose use in patients is studied.

DOSAGE AND ADMINISTRATION

Do not mix or co-infuse caspofungin acetate with other medications, as there are no data available on the compatibility of caspofungin acetate with other IV substances, additives, or medications. DO NOT USE DILUENTS CONTAINING DEXTROSE (α-D-GLUCOSE), as caspofungin acetate is not stable in diluents containing dextrose.

CANDIDEMIA AND OTHER CANDIDA INFECTIONS

A single 70 mg loading dose should be administered on Day 1, followed by 50 mg daily thereafter. Caspofungin acetate should be administered by slow IV infusion over approximately 1 hour. Duration of treatment should be dictated by the patient's clinical and microbiological response. In general, antifungal therapy should continue for at least 14 days after the last positive culture. Patients who remain persistently neutropenic may warrant a longer course of therapy pending resolution of the neutropenia.

ESOPHAGEAL CANDIDIASIS

Fifty (50) mg daily should be administered by slow IV infusion over approximately 1 hour. Because of the risk of relapse of oropharyngeal candidiasis in patients with HIV infections, suppressive oral therapy could be considered. A 70 mg loading dose has not been studied with this indication.

INVASIVE ASPERGILLOSIS

A single 70 mg loading dose should be administered on Day 1, followed by 50 mg daily thereafter. Caspofungin acetate should be administered by slow IV infusion over approximately 1 hour. Duration of treatment should be based upon the severity of the patient's underlying disease, recovery from immunosuppression, and clinical response. The efficacy of a 70 mg dose regimen in patients who are not clinically responding to the 50 mg daily dose is not known. Limited safety data suggests that an increase in dose to 70 mg daily is well tolerated. The safety and efficacy of doses above 70 mg have not been adequately studied.

HEPATIC INSUFFICIENCY

Patients with mild hepatic insufficiency (Child-Pugh score 5-6) do not need a dosage adjustment. For patients with moderate hepatic insufficiency (Child-Pugh score 7-9), caspofungin acetate 35 mg daily is recommended. However, where recommended, a 70 mg loading dose should still be administered on Day 1. There is no clinical experience in patients with severe hepatic insufficiency (Child-Pugh score >9).

CONCOMITANT MEDICATION WITH INDUCERS OF DRUG CLEARANCE

Patients on rifampin should receive 70 mg of caspofungin acetate daily. Patients on nevirapine, efavirenz, carbamazepine, dexamethasone, or phenytoin may require an increase in dose to 70 mg of caspofungin acetate daily.

PREPARATION OF CASPOFUNGIN ACETATE FOR USE

Do not mix or co-infuse caspofungin acetate with other medications, as there are no data available on the compatibility of caspofungin acetate with other IV substances, additives, or medications. DO NOT USE DILUENTS CONTAINING DEXTROSE (α-D-GLUCOSE), as caspofungin acetate is not stable in diluents containing dextrose.

PRODUCT LISTING - EQUIVALENTS NOT AVAILABLE

Powder For Injection - Intravenous - 50 mg
1's $376.91 CANCIDAS, Merck & Company Inc 00006-3822-10
Powder For Injection - Intravenous - 70 mg
1's $485.54 CANCIDAS, Merck & Company Inc 00006-3823-10

Cefaclor (000680)

For related information, see the comparative table section in Appendix A.

Categories: Infection, ear, middle; Infection, lower respiratory tract; Infection, skin and skin structures; Infection, upper respiratory tract; Infection, urinary tract; Pharyngitis; Pyelonephritis; Tonsillitis; Pregnancy Category B; FDA Approved 1979 Apr
Drug Classes: Antibiotics, cephalosporins
Brand Names: **Ceclor**
Foreign Brand Availability: Alfatil (France); Alfatil LP (France); Alphexine (France); Capabiotic (Indonesia); CEC (South-Africa); CEC 500 (Germany); Ceclex (Korea); Ceclor AF (Costa-Rica; Dominican-Republic; El-Salvador; Guatemala; Honduras; Panama; Peru); Ceclor CD (Australia; Philippines); Ceclor MR (Benin; Burkina-Faso; Ethiopia; Gambia; Ghana; Guinea; Hong-Kong; Ivory-Coast; Kenya; Liberia; Malawi; Mali; Mauritania; Mauritius; Morocco; Niger; Nigeria; Senegal; Seychelles; Sierra-Leone; Sudan; Tanzania; Tunia; Uganda; Zambia; Zimbabwe); Ceclor Retard (Colombia; Spain); Cefabac (Bahrain; Cyprus; Egypt; Iran; Iraq; Jordan; Kuwait; Lebanon; Libya; Oman; Qatar; Republic-of-Yemen; Saudi-Arabia; Syria; United-Arab-Emirates); Cefabiocin (Germany); Cefacle (Korea); Cefaclin (Korea); Cefaclostad (Germany); Cefalan (Mexico); Cefaclostad (Germany); Cefkor (Australia); Cefkor CD (Australia); Cefler (Korea); Cefral (Argentina); Celco (Thailand); Cero (Taiwan); Cesid (Korea); Cleancef (China; Korea; Singapore); Cloracef MR (Bahrain; Cyprus; Egypt; Iran; Iraq; Jordan; Kuwait; Lebanon; Libya; Oman; Qatar; Republic-of-Yemen; Saudi-Arabia; Syria; United-Arab-Emirates); Clorotir (New-Zealand); Cyclor (Korea); Distaclor (England; Ireland; Thailand); Distaclor MR (Malaysia); Especlor (Indonesia); hefaclor (Germany); Kefaclor (Tanzania); Keflor (Australia; China; India; Taiwan); Keflor AF (Taiwan); Kefolor (Denmark; Sweden); Kefral (Japan); Kemocin (Korea); Kerfenmycin (Taiwan); Kindoplex (Philippines); Kloclor BD (South-Africa); Mediconcef (Indonesia); Medoclor (Hong-Kong); Miclor (Korea); Newporine (Korea); Panacef (Italy; Peru); Panacef RM (Peru); Panoral (Germany); Panoral Forte (Germany); Pharmaclor (Bahrain; Cyprus; Egypt; Iran; Iraq; Jordan; Kuwait; Lebanon; Libya; Oman; Qatar; Republic-of-Yemen; Saudi-Arabia; Syria; United-Arab-Emirates); Serviclor (Mexico); Sifaclor (Thailand); Sofiklor (Hong-Kong; Singapore); Swiflor (Taiwan); Syntocor (Hong-Kong); Teraclox (Mexico); Vercef (Benin; Burkina-Faso; Ethiopia; Gambia; Ghana; Guinea; Ivory-Coast; Kenya; Liberia; Malawi; Malaysia; Mali; Mauritania; Mauritius; Morocco; Niger; Nigeria; Senegal; Seychelles; Sierra-Leone; South-Africa; Sudan; Tanzania; Tunia; Uganda; Zambia; Zimbabwe); Versef (Philippines); Xelent (Philippines)
Cost of Therapy: $69.95 (Infection; Ceclor Pulvules; 250 mg; 3 capsules/day; 10 day supply)
$136.50 (Infection; Generic Capsules; 250 mg; 3 capsules/day; 10 day supply)

DESCRIPTION

Cefaclor is a semisynthetic cephalosporin antibiotic for oral administration. It is chemically designated as 3-chloro-7-D-(2-phenylglycinamido)-3-cephem-4-carboxylic acid monohydrate. The chemical formula for cefaclor is $C_{15}H_{14}ClN_3O_4S{\cdot}H_2O$ and the molecular weight is 385.82.

Each Pulvule contains cefaclor monohydrate equivalent to 250 mg (0.68 mmol) or 500 mg (1.36 mmol) anhydrous cefaclor. The Pulvules also contain cornstarch, FD&C blue no. 1, FD&C red no. 3, gelatin, magnesium stearate, silicone, titanium dioxide, and other inactive ingredients. The 500 mg Pulvule also contains iron oxide.

After mixing, each 5 ml of Ceclor for oral suspension will contain cefaclor monohydrate equivalent to 125 mg (0.34 mmol), 187 mg (0.51 mmol), 250 mg (0.68 mmol), or 375 mg (1.0 mmol) anhydrous cefaclor. The suspensions also contain cellulose, cornstarch, FD &C red no. 40, flavors, silicone, sodium lauryl sulfate, sucrose, and xanthan gum.

CLINICAL PHARMACOLOGY

Cefaclor is well absorbed after oral administration to fasting subjects. Total absorption is the same whether the drug is given with or without food; however, when it is taken with food, the peak concentration achieved is 50-75% of that observed when the drug is administered to fasting subjects and generally appears from three fourths to 1 hour later. Following administration of 250 mg, 500 mg, and 1 g doses to fasting subjects, average peak serum levels of approximately 7, 13, and 23 μg/ml respectively were obtained within 30-60 minutes. Approximately 60-85% of the drug is excreted unchanged in the urine within 8 hours, the greater portion being excreted within the first 2 hours. During this 8 hour period, peak urine concentrations following the 250 mg, 500 mg, and 1 g doses were approximately 600, 900, and 1900 μg/ml respectively. The serum half-life in normal subjects is 0.6-0.9 hours. In patients with reduced renal function, the serum half-life of cefaclor is slightly prolonged. In those with complete absence of renal function, the biologic half-life of the intact molecule is 2.3-2.8 hours. Excretion pathways in patients with markedly impaired renal function have not been determined. Hemodialysis shortens the half-life by 25-30%.

MICROBIOLOGY

In vitro tests demonstrate that the bactericidal action of the cephalosporins results from inhibition of cell-wall synthesis. Cefaclor is active *in vitro* against most strains of clinical isolates of the following organisms:

Staphylococci, including coagulase-positive, coagulase-negative, and penicillinase-producing strains (when tested by *in vitro* methods), exhibit cross-resistance between cefaclor and methicillin; *Streptococcus pyogenes* (group A β-hemolytic *streptococci*); *Streptococcus pneumoniae; Moraxella (Branhamella) catarrhalis; Haemophilus influenzae,* including β-lactamase-producing ampicillin-resistant strains; *Escherichia coli; Proteus mirabilis; Klebsiella* sp; *Citrobacter diversus; Neisseria gonorrhoeae; Propionibacterium* acnes and *Bacteroides* sp (excluding *Bacteroides fragilis*); *Peptococci; Peptostreptococci.*
Note: *Pseudomonas* sp, *Acinetobacter calcoaceticus* (formerly *Mima* sp and *Herellea* sp), and most strains of *enterococci* (*Enterococcus faecalis* [formerly *Streptococcus faecalis*], group D *streptococci*), *Enterobacter* sp, indole-positive *Proteus,* and *Serratia* sp are resistant to cefaclor. When tested by *in vitro* methods, staphylococci exhibit cross-resistance between cefaclor and methicillin-type antibiotics.

DISK SUSCEPTIBILITY TESTS

Quantitative methods that require measurement of zone diameters give the most precise estimates of antibiotic susceptibility. One such procedure[1] has been recommended for use with disks for testing susceptibility to cephalothin. The currently accepted zone diameter interpretative criteria for the cephalothin disk are appropriate for determining bacterial susceptibility to cefaclor. With this procedure, a report from the laboratory of "resistant" indicates that the infecting organism is not likely to respond to therapy. A report of "intermediate susceptibility" suggests that the organism would be susceptible if the infection is confined to tissues and fluids (*e.g.,* urine) in which high antibiotic levels can be obtained or if high dosage is used.

INDICATIONS AND USAGE

Cefaclor is indicated in the treatment of the following infections when caused by susceptible strains of the designated microorganisms:
Otitis media caused by *S. pneumoniae, H. influenzae, staphylococci,* and *S. pyogenes* (group A β-hemolytic streptococci)
Lower respiratory infections, including pneumonia, caused by *S. pneumoniae, H. influenzae,* and *S. pyogenes* (group A β-hemolytic *streptococci*)
Upper respiratory infections, including pharyngitis and tonsillitis, caused by *S. pyogenes* (group A β-hemolytic *streptococci*).
Note: Penicillin is the usual drug of choice in the treatment and prevention of streptococcal infections, including the prophylaxis of rheumatic fever. Cefaclor is generally effective in the eradication of streptococci from the nasopharynx; however, substantial data establishing the efficacy of cefaclor in the subsequent prevention of rheumatic fever are not available at present.
Urinary tract infections, including pyelonephritis and cystitis, caused by *E. coli, P. mirabilis, Klebsiella* sp, and coagulase-negative staphylococci
Skin and skin structure infections caused by *Staphylococcus aureus* and *S. pyogenes* (group A β-hemolytic streptococci)
Appropriate culture and susceptibility studies should be performed to determine susceptibility of the causative organism to cefaclor.

CONTRAINDICATIONS

Cefaclor is contraindicated in patients with known allergy to the cephalosporin group of antibiotics.

WARNINGS

IN PENICILLIN-SENSITIVE PATIENTS, CEPHALOSPORIN ANTIBIOTICS SHOULD BE ADMINISTERED CAUTIOUSLY. THERE IS CLINICAL AND LABORATORY EVIDENCE OF PARTIAL CROSS-ALLERGENICITY OF THE PENICILLINS AND THE CEPHALOSPORINS AND THERE ARE INSTANCES IN WHICH PATIENTS HAVE HAD REACTIONS, INCLUDING ANAPHYLAXIS, TO BOTH DRUG CLASSES.

Antibiotics, including cefaclor, should be administered cautiously to any patient who has demonstrated some form of allergy, particularly to drugs.

Pseudomembranous colitis has been reported with virtually all broad-spectrum antibiotics (including macrolides, semisynthetic penicillins, and cephalosporins); therefore, it is important to consider its diagnosis in patients who develop diarrhea in association with the use of antibiotics. Such colitis may range in severity from mild to life threatening.

Treatment with broad-spectrum antibiotics alters the normal flora of the colon and may permit overgrowth of clostridia. Studies indicate that a toxin produced by *Clostridium difficile* is a primary cause of antibiotic-associated colitis.

Mild cases of pseudomembranous colitis usually respond to drug discontinuance alone. In moderate to severe cases, management should include sigmoidoscopy, appropriate bacteriologic studies, and fluid, electrolyte, and protein supplementation. When the colitis does not improve after the drug has been discontinued, or when it is severe, oral vancomycin is the drug of choice for antibiotic-associated pseudomembranous colitis produced by *C. difficile.* Other causes of colitis should be ruled out.

PRECAUTIONS

GENERAL

If an allergic reaction to cefaclor occurs, the drug should be discontinued, and, if necessary, the patient should be treated with appropriate agents, *e.g.,* pressor amines, antihistamines, or corticosteroids.

Prolonged use of cefaclor may result in the overgrowth of nonsusceptible organisms. Careful observation of the patient is essential. If superinfection occurs during therapy, appropriate measures should be taken.

Positive direct Coombs' tests have been reported during treatment with the cephalosporin antibiotics. In hematologic studies or in transfusion cross-matching procedures when antiglobulin tests are performed on the minor side or in Coombs' testing of newborns whose mothers have received cephalosporin antibiotics before parturition, it should be recognized that a positive Coombs' test may be due to the drug.

Cefaclor should be administered with caution in the presence of markedly impaired renal function. Since the half-life of cefaclor in anuria is 2.3-2.8 hours, dosage adjustments for patients with moderate or severe renal impairment are usually not required. Clinical experience with cefaclor under such conditions is limited; therefore, careful clinical observation and laboratory studies should be made.

As with other β-lactam antibiotics, the renal excretion of cefaclor is inhibited by probenecid.

As a result of administration of cefaclor, a false-positive reaction for glucose in the urine may occur. This has been observed with Benedict's and Fehling's solutions and also with Clinitest tablets but not with Tes-Tape.

Broad-spectrum antibiotics should be prescribed with caution in individuals with a history of gastrointestinal disease, particularly colitis.

PREGNANCY CATEGORY B

Reproduction studies have been performed in mice and rats at doses up to 12 times the human dose and in ferrets given 3 times the maximum human dose and have revealed no evidence of impaired fertility or harm to the fetus due to cefaclor. There are, however, no adequate and well-controlled studies in pregnant women. Because animal reproduction studies are not always predictive of human response, this drug should be used during pregnancy only if clearly needed.

NURSING MOTHERS

Small amounts of cefaclor have been detected in mother's milk following administration of single 500 mg doses. Average levels were 0.18, 0.20, 0.21, and 0.16 μg/ml at 2, 3, 4, and 5 hours respectively. Trace amounts were detected at 1 hour. The effect on nursing infants is not known. Caution should be exercised when cefaclor is administered to a nursing woman.

PEDIATRIC USE

Safety and effectiveness of this product for use in infants less than 1 month of age have not been established.

ADVERSE REACTIONS

Adverse Effects Considered to be Related to Therapy With Cefaclor are Listed Below:

Hypersensitivity reactions have been reported in about 1.5% of patients and include morbilliform eruptions (1 in 100). Pruritus, urticaria, and positive Coombs' tests each occur in less than 1 in 200 patients.

Cases of **serum-sickness-like** reactions have been reported with the use of cefaclor. These are characterized by findings of erythema multiforme, rashes, and other skin manifestations accompanied by arthritis/arthralgia, with or without fever, and differ from classic serum sickness in that there is infrequently associated lymphadenopathy and proteinuria, no circulating immune complexes, and no evidence to date of sequelae of the reaction. Occasionally, solitary symptoms may occur, but do not represent a **serum-sickness-like** reaction. While further investigation is ongoing, **serum-sickness-like** reactions appear to be due to hypersensitivity and more often occur during or following a second (or subsequent) course of therapy with cefaclor. Such reactions have been reported more frequently in children than in adults with an overall occurrence ranging from 1 in 200 (0.5%) in one focused trial to 2 in 8346 (0.024%) in overall clinical trials (with an incidence in children in clinical trials of 0.055%) to 1 in 38,000 (0.003%) in spontaneous event reports. Signs and symptoms usually occur a few days after initiation of therapy and subside within a few days after cessation of therapy; occasionally these reactions have resulted in hospitalization, usually of short duration (median hospitalization = 2-3 days, based on postmarketing surveillance studies). In those requiring hospitalization, the symptoms have ranged from mild to severe at the time of admission with more of the severe reactions occurring in children. Antihistamines and glucocorticoids appear to enhance resolution of the signs and symptoms. No serious sequelae have been reported.

More severe hypersensitivity reactions, including Stevens-Johnson syndrome, toxic epidermal necrolysis, and anaphylaxis have been reported rarely. Anaphylactoid events may be manifested by solitary symptoms, including angioedema, asthenia, edema (including face and limbs), dyspnea, paresthesias, syncope, or vasodilation. Anaphylaxis may be more common in patients with a history of penicillin allergy.

Rarely, hypersensitivity symptoms may persist for several months.

Gastrointestinal symptoms occur in about 2.5% of patients and include diarrhea (1 in 70).

Symptoms of pseudomembranous colitis may appear either during or after antibiotic treatment. Nausea and vomiting have been reported rarely. As with some penicillins and some other cephalosporins, transient hepatitis and cholestatic jaundice have been reported rarely.

Other effects considered related to therapy included eosinophilia (1 in 50 patients), genital pruritus or vaginitis (less than 1 in 100 patients), and, rarely, thrombocytopenia or reversible interstitial nephritis.

CAUSAL RELATIONSHIP UNCERTAIN

CNS: Rarely, reversible hyperactivity, agitation, nervousness, insomnia, confusion, hypertonia, dizziness, hallucinations, and somnolence have been reported.

Transitory abnormalities in clinical laboratory test results have been reported. Although they were of uncertain etiology, they are listed below to serve as alerting information for the physician.

Hepatic: Slight elevations of AST (SGOT), ALT (SGPT), or alkaline phosphatase values (1 in 40).

Hematopoietic: As has also been reported with other β-lactam antibiotics, transient lymphocytosis, leukopenia, and, rarely, hemolytic anemia and reversible neutropenia of possible clinical significance.

There have been rare reports of increased prothrombin time with or without clinical bleeding in patients receiving cefaclor and warfarin sodium concomitantly.

Renal: Slight elevations in BUN or serum creatinine (less than 1 in 500) or abnormal urinalysis (less than 1 in 200).

DOSAGE AND ADMINISTRATION

Cefaclor is administered orally.

Adults: The usual adult dosage is 250 mg every 8 hours. For more severe infections (such as pneumonia) or those caused by less susceptible organisms, doses may be doubled.

Children: The usual recommended daily dosage for children is 20 mg/kg/day in divided doses every 8 hours. In more serious infections, otitis media, and infections caused by less susceptible organisms, 40 mg/kg/day are recommended, with a maximum dosage of 1 g/day (TABLE 1).

TABLE 1 *Cefaclor Suspension*

Child's Weight	125 mg/5 ml	250 mg/5 ml
20 mg/kg/day		
9 kg	½ tsp tid	
18 kg	1 tsp tid	½ tsp tid
40 mg/kg/day		
9 kg	1 tsp tid	½ tsp tid
18 kg		1 tsp tid

BID Treatment Option: For the treatment of otitis media and pharyngitis, the total daily dosage may be divided and administered every 12 hours (TABLE 2).

TABLE 2 *Cefaclor Suspension*

Child's Weight	187 mg/5 ml	375 mg/5 ml
20 mg/kg/day (pharyngitis)		
9 kg	½ tsp bid	
18 kg	1 tsp bid	½ tsp bid
40 mg/kg/day (otitis media)		
9 kg	1 tsp bid	½ tsp bid
18 kg		1 tsp bid

Cefaclor may be administered in the presence of impaired renal function. Under such a condition, the dosage usually is unchanged (see PRECAUTIONS).

In the treatment of β-hemolytic streptococcal infections, a therapeutic dosage of cefaclor should be administered for at least 10 days.

HOW SUPPLIED

CECLOR

Pulvules:

250 mg, purple and white.

500 mg, purple and gray.

For Oral Suspension:

125 mg/5 ml, strawberry flavor.‡

187 mg/5 ml, strawberry flavor.‡

250 mg/5 ml, strawberry flavor.‡

375 mg/5 ml, strawberry flavor.‡

‡After mixing, store in a refrigerator. Shake well before using. Keep tightly closed. The mixture may be kept for 14 days without significant loss of potency. Discard unused portion after 14 days.

Storage: Store at controlled room temperature, 15-30°C (59-86°F).

PRODUCT LISTING - RATED THERAPEUTICALLY EQUIVALENT

Capsule - Oral - 250 mg

15's	$30.84	GENERIC, Ivax Corporation	00182-2606-28
15's	$30.99	GENERIC, Ivax Corporation	00172-4760-40
15's	$36.77	CECLOR PULVULES, Lilly, Eli and Company	00002-3061-15
15's	$41.72	CECLOR PULVULES, Physicians Total Care	54868-0315-05
15's	$55.07	CECLOR PULVULES, Pd-Rx Pharmaceuticals	55289-0051-15
30's	$44.18	GENERIC, Pd-Rx Pharmaceuticals	55289-0749-30
30's	$82.24	CECLOR PULVULES, Physicians Total Care	54868-0315-01
30's	$106.06	CECLOR PULVULES, Pd-Rx Pharmaceuticals	55289-0051-30
100's	$66.00	FEDERAL UPPER LIMIT, H.C.F.A. F F P	99999-0680-11
100's	$194.94	GENERIC, Moore, H.L. Drug Exchange Inc	00839-7958-06
100's	$195.50	GENERIC, Apothecon Inc	59772-7491-04
100's	$195.60	GENERIC, Ivax Corporation	00182-2606-01
100's	$196.50	GENERIC, Ivax Corporation	00172-4760-60
100's	$198.90	GENERIC, Ivax Corporation	00172-4770-60
100's	$198.93	GENERIC, Mova Pharmaceutical Corporation	55370-0894-07
100's	$198.95	GENERIC, Mylan Pharmaceuticals Inc	00378-7250-01
100's	$198.95	GENERIC, Ranbaxy Laboratories	63304-0658-01
100's	$228.72	CECLOR PULVULES, Lilly, Eli and Company	00002-3061-33
100's	$233.15	CECLOR PULVULES, Lilly, Eli and Company	00002-3061-02

Capsule - Oral - 500 mg

15's	$58.70	GENERIC, Ivax Corporation	00172-4761-40
15's	$58.70	GENERIC, Ivax Corporation	00182-2607-28
15's	$69.77	CECLOR PULVULES, Lilly, Eli and Company	00002-3062-15
30's	$148.02	CECLOR PULVULES, Physicians Total Care	54868-0472-01
100's	$129.00	FEDERAL UPPER LIMIT, H.C.F.A. F F P	99999-0680-12

100's	$372.95	GENERIC, Major Pharmaceuticals Inc	00904-5205-60
100's	$383.00	GENERIC, Apothecon Inc	59772-7494-04
100's	$383.06	GENERIC, Moore, H.L. Drug Exchange Inc	00839-7961-06
100's	$384.07	GENERIC, Ivax Corporation	00182-2607-01
100's	$385.50	GENERIC, Ivax Corporation	00172-4761-60
100's	$389.45	GENERIC, Ivax Corporation	00172-4771-60
100's	$389.48	GENERIC, Mova Pharmaceutical Corporation	55370-0895-07
100's	$389.50	GENERIC, Mylan Pharmaceuticals Inc	00378-7500-01
100's	$389.50	GENERIC, Watson/Rugby Laboratories Inc	00536-1375-01
100's	$389.50	GENERIC, Ranbaxy Laboratories	63304-0659-01

Powder For Reconstitution - Oral - 125 mg/5 ml

75 ml	$13.95	GENERIC, Qualitest Products Inc	00603-6534-62
75 ml	$14.05	GENERIC, Ivax Corporation	00172-4611-22
75 ml	$14.05	GENERIC, Ivax Corporation	00182-7086-69
75 ml	$14.10	GENERIC, Mova Pharmaceutical Corporation	55370-0897-75
75 ml	$14.11	GENERIC, Moore, H.L. Drug Exchange Inc	00839-7956-55
75 ml	$14.12	GENERIC, Mylan Pharmaceuticals Inc	00378-7602-12
75 ml	$14.13	GENERIC, Ivax Corporation	00172-4772-22
75 ml	$14.14	GENERIC, Ranbaxy Laboratories	63304-0954-01
150 ml	$16.61	FEDERAL UPPER LIMIT, H.C.F.A. F F P	99999-0680-13
150 ml	$26.65	GENERIC, Qualitest Products Inc	00603-6534-66
150 ml	$27.95	GENERIC, Ivax Corporation	00172-4611-23
150 ml	$27.95	GENERIC, Ivax Corporation	00182-7086-72
150 ml	$28.00	GENERIC, Moore, H.L. Drug Exchange Inc	00839-7956-75
150 ml	$28.08	GENERIC, Mova Pharmaceutical Corporation	55370-0897-14
150 ml	$28.10	GENERIC, Mylan Pharmaceuticals Inc	00378-7602-06
150 ml	$28.28	GENERIC, Ivax Corporation	00172-4772-23
150 ml	$28.28	GENERIC, Ranbaxy Laboratories	63304-0954-02
150 ml	$31.12	CECLOR, Lilly, Eli and Company	00002-5057-68
150 ml	$37.20	CECLOR, Physicians Total Care	54868-5057-01

Powder For Reconstitution - Oral - 187 mg/5 ml

50 ml	$13.95	GENERIC, Qualitest Products Inc	00603-6535-47
50 ml	$14.05	GENERIC, Ivax Corporation	00172-4613-20
50 ml	$14.05	GENERIC, Ivax Corporation	00182-7087-67
50 ml	$14.11	GENERIC, Moore, H.L. Drug Exchange Inc	00839-7957-59
50 ml	$14.14	GENERIC, Ivax Corporation	00172-4773-20
50 ml	$14.32	GENERIC, Mova Pharmaceutical Corporation	55370-0899-21
50 ml	$14.35	GENERIC, Mylan Pharmaceuticals Inc	00378-7604-09
50 ml	$14.35	GENERIC, Ranbaxy Laboratories	63304-0955-03
100 ml	$16.61	FEDERAL UPPER LIMIT, H.C.F.A. F F P	99999-0680-14
100 ml	$26.65	GENERIC, Qualitest Products Inc	00603-6535-64
100 ml	$27.95	GENERIC, Ivax Corporation	00172-4613-21
100 ml	$27.95	GENERIC, Ivax Corporation	00182-7087-70
100 ml	$28.00	GENERIC, Mylan Pharmaceuticals Inc	00378-7604-02
100 ml	$28.01	GENERIC, Moore, H.L. Drug Exchange Inc	00839-7957-73
100 ml	$28.13	GENERIC, Ranbaxy Laboratories	63304-0955-04
100 ml	$28.26	GENERIC, Mova Pharmaceutical Corporation	55370-0899-13
100 ml	$28.28	GENERIC, Ivax Corporation	00172-4773-21
100 ml	$31.12	CECLOR, Lilly, Eli and Company	00002-5130-48

Powder For Reconstitution - Oral - 250 mg/5 ml

75 ml	$24.85	GENERIC, Qualitest Products Inc	00603-6536-62
75 ml	$26.05	GENERIC, Ivax Corporation	00172-4610-22
75 ml	$26.05	GENERIC, Ivax Corporation	00182-7088-69
75 ml	$26.09	GENERIC, Mova Pharmaceutical Corporation	55370-0839-75
75 ml	$26.12	GENERIC, Moore, H.L. Drug Exchange Inc	00839-7959-55
75 ml	$26.20	GENERIC, Mylan Pharmaceuticals Inc	00378-7610-12
75 ml	$28.22	GENERIC, Mova Pharmaceutical Corporation	55370-0896-75
75 ml	$28.24	GENERIC, Ivax Corporation	00172-4774-22
75 ml	$28.24	GENERIC, Ranbaxy Laboratories	63304-0956-01
75 ml	$29.03	CECLOR, Lilly, Eli and Company	00002-5058-18
150 ml	$44.93	FEDERAL UPPER LIMIT, H.C.F.A. F F P	99999-0680-15
150 ml	$48.27	GENERIC, Qualitest Products Inc	00603-6536-66
150 ml	$50.65	GENERIC, Ivax Corporation	00172-4610-23
150 ml	$50.66	GENERIC, Ivax Corporation	00182-7088-72
150 ml	$50.68	GENERIC, Mova Pharmaceutical Corporation	55370-0839-14
150 ml	$50.74	GENERIC, Moore, H.L. Drug Exchange Inc	00839-7959-75
150 ml	$51.21	GENERIC, Ivax Corporation	00172-4774-23
150 ml	$51.78	GENERIC, Mova Pharmaceutical Corporation	55370-0896-14
150 ml	$51.80	GENERIC, Mylan Pharmaceuticals Inc	00378-7610-06
150 ml	$51.80	GENERIC, Ranbaxy Laboratories	63304-0956-02
150 ml	$56.38	CECLOR, Lilly, Eli and Company	00002-5058-68
150 ml	$56.39	CECLOR, Allscripts Pharmaceutical Company	54569-0103-00
150 ml	$67.50	CECLOR, Pharma Pac	52959-0277-02
150 ml	$68.53	CECLOR, Physicians Total Care	54868-0314-01

Powder For Reconstitution - Oral - 375 mg/5 ml

50 ml	$24.85	GENERIC, Qualitest Products Inc	00603-6537-47
50 ml	$24.85	GENERIC, Qualitest Products Inc	00603-8537-47
50 ml	$26.05	GENERIC, Ivax Corporation	00172-4612-20
50 ml	$26.05	GENERIC, Ivax Corporation	00182-7089-67
50 ml	$26.12	GENERIC, Mylan Pharmaceuticals Inc	00378-7612-09
50 ml	$26.12	GENERIC, Moore, H.L. Drug Exchange Inc	00839-7960-59
50 ml	$26.38	GENERIC, Ranbaxy Laboratories	63304-0957-03
50 ml	$28.23	GENERIC, Mova Pharmaceutical Corporation	55370-0898-21
50 ml	$28.24	GENERIC, Ivax Corporation	00172-4775-20
100 ml	$44.92	FEDERAL UPPER LIMIT, H.C.F.A. F F P	99999-0680-16
100 ml	$48.27	GENERIC, Qualitest Products Inc	00603-6537-64
100 ml	$50.65	GENERIC, Ivax Corporation	00172-4612-21
100 ml	$50.65	GENERIC, Ivax Corporation	00182-7089-70
100 ml	$50.75	GENERIC, Moore, H.L. Drug Exchange Inc	00839-7960-73
100 ml	$51.21	GENERIC, Ivax Corporation	00172-4775-21
100 ml	$51.79	GENERIC, Mova Pharmaceutical Corporation	55370-0898-13
100 ml	$51.80	GENERIC, Mylan Pharmaceuticals Inc	00378-7612-02
100 ml	$51.80	GENERIC, Ranbaxy Laboratories	63304-0957-04
100 ml	$56.38	CECLOR, Lilly, Eli and Company	00002-5132-48

Tablet, Extended Release - Oral - 500 mg

100's	$379.30	GENERIC, Teva Pharmaceuticals Usa	00093-1087-01
100's	$379.30	GENERIC, Ivax Corporation	00172-4194-60

PRODUCT LISTING - EQUIVALENTS NOT AVAILABLE

Capsule - Oral - 250 mg

1's	$3.58	GENERIC, Prescript Pharmaceuticals	00247-0028-01
3's	$4.02	GENERIC, Prescript Pharmaceuticals	00247-0028-03
4's	$4.26	GENERIC, Prescript Pharmaceuticals	00247-0028-04
6's	$4.71	GENERIC, Prescript Pharmaceuticals	00247-0028-06
8's	$5.15	GENERIC, Prescript Pharmaceuticals	00247-0028-08
10's	$8.94	GENERIC, Physicians Total Care	54868-3478-03
12's	$25.99	GENERIC, Southwood Pharmaceuticals Inc	58016-0872-12
14's	$36.05	GENERIC, Pharma Pac	52959-0367-14
15's	$6.73	GENERIC, Prescript Pharmaceuticals	00247-0028-15
15's	$12.75	GENERIC, Physicians Total Care	54868-3478-01
15's	$32.49	GENERIC, Southwood Pharmaceuticals Inc	58016-0872-15
15's	$38.16	GENERIC, Pharma Pac	52959-0367-15
18's	$38.99	GENERIC, Southwood Pharmaceuticals Inc	58016-0872-18
20's	$12.97	GENERIC, Physicians Total Care	54868-3478-02
20's	$43.32	GENERIC, Southwood Pharmaceuticals Inc	58016-0872-20
20's	$51.45	GENERIC, Pharma Pac	52959-0367-20
21's	$8.08	GENERIC, Prescript Pharmaceuticals	00247-0028-21
21's	$41.00	GENERIC, Allscripts Pharmaceutical Company	54569-3901-01
21's	$54.02	GENERIC, Pharma Pac	52959-0367-21
21's	$70.44	GENERIC, Alpharma Uspd Makers Of Barre and Nmc	63874-0119-21
24's	$51.99	GENERIC, Southwood Pharmaceuticals Inc	58016-0872-24
30's	$10.11	GENERIC, Prescript Pharmaceuticals	00247-0028-30
30's	$24.16	GENERIC, Physicians Total Care	54868-3478-00
30's	$58.73	GENERIC, Allscripts Pharmaceutical Company	54569-3901-00
30's	$61.44	GENERIC, Mylan Pharmaceuticals Inc	00378-7250-93
30's	$64.98	GENERIC, Southwood Pharmaceuticals Inc	58016-0872-30
30's	$68.25	GENERIC, Pharma Pac	52959-0367-30
30's	$99.68	GENERIC, Alpharma Uspd Makers Of Barre and Nmc	63874-0119-30
40's	$89.32	GENERIC, Pharma Pac	52959-0367-40
100's	$184.80	GENERIC, Pharma Pac	52959-0367-00
100's	$194.70	GENERIC, Major Pharmaceuticals Inc	00904-7932-60
100's	$218.51	GENERIC, Alpharma Uspd Makers Of Barre and Nmc	63874-0119-01

Capsule - Oral - 500 mg

3's	$7.20	GENERIC, Prescript Pharmaceuticals	00247-0196-03
4's	$8.49	GENERIC, Prescript Pharmaceuticals	00247-0196-04
10's	$12.94	GENERIC, Physicians Total Care	54868-3511-01
10's	$43.05	GENERIC, Pharma Pac	52959-0368-10
12's	$51.07	GENERIC, Southwood Pharmaceuticals Inc	58016-0339-12
14's	$60.27	GENERIC, Pharma Pac	52959-0368-14
15's	$22.61	GENERIC, Prescript Pharmaceuticals	00247-0196-15
15's	$63.85	GENERIC, Southwood Pharmaceuticals Inc	58016-0339-15
18's	$76.62	GENERIC, Southwood Pharmaceuticals Inc	58016-0339-18
20's	$24.54	GENERIC, Physicians Total Care	54868-3511-00
20's	$76.77	GENERIC, Allscripts Pharmaceutical Company	54569-3902-01
20's	$85.13	GENERIC, Southwood Pharmaceuticals Inc	58016-0339-20
20's	$86.10	GENERIC, Pharma Pac	52959-0368-20
20's	$98.37	GENERIC, Alpharma Uspd Makers Of Barre and Nmc	63874-0120-20
24's	$102.16	GENERIC, Southwood Pharmaceuticals Inc	58016-0339-24
30's	$36.15	GENERIC, Physicians Total Care	54868-3511-02
30's	$41.87	GENERIC, Prescript Pharmaceuticals	00247-0196-30
30's	$115.16	GENERIC, Allscripts Pharmaceutical Company	54569-3902-00
30's	$116.64	GENERIC, Mylan Pharmaceuticals Inc	00378-7500-93
30's	$127.55	GENERIC, Southwood Pharmaceuticals Inc	58016-0339-30
30's	$129.15	GENERIC, Pharma Pac	52959-0368-30
30's	$139.40	GENERIC, Alpharma Uspd Makers Of Barre and Nmc	63874-0120-30
100's	$382.65	GENERIC, Major Pharmaceuticals Inc	00904-7933-60
100's	$439.47	GENERIC, Alpharma Uspd Makers Of Barre and Nmc	63874-0120-01

Powder For Reconstitution - Oral - 125 mg/5 ml

75 ml	$14.05	GENERIC, Major Pharmaceuticals Inc	00904-7934-71
75 ml	$18.32	GENERIC, Prescript Pharmaceuticals	00247-0029-75
75 ml	$20.24	GENERIC, Alpharma Uspd Makers Of Barre and Nmc	63874-0151-75

80 ml	$19.32	GENERIC, Prescript Pharmaceuticals	00247-0029-80
150 ml	$14.20	GENERIC, Physicians Total Care	54868-3472-00
150 ml	$27.95	GENERIC, Major Pharmaceuticals Inc	00904-7934-07
150 ml	$28.28	GENERIC, Allscripts Pharmaceutical Company	54569-4241-00
150 ml	$33.29	GENERIC, Prescript Pharmaceuticals	00247-0029-78
150 ml	$34.46	GENERIC, Southwood Pharmaceuticals Inc	58016-4193-05
150 ml	$34.46	GENERIC, Alpharma Uspd Makers Of Barre and Nmc	63874-0151-15
Powder For Reconstitution - Oral - 187 mg/5 ml			
50 ml	$14.08	GENERIC, Major Pharmaceuticals Inc	00904-7935-50
50 ml	$18.14	GENERIC, Prescript Pharmaceuticals	00247-0047-50
50 ml	$21.21	GENERIC, Alpharma Uspd Makers Of Barre and Nmc	63874-0152-50
100 ml	$28.13	GENERIC, Allscripts Pharmaceutical Company	54569-4310-00
100 ml	$32.92	GENERIC, Prescript Pharmaceuticals	00247-0047-00
100 ml	$41.28	GENERIC, Alpharma Uspd Makers Of Barre and Nmc	63874-0152-10
Powder For Reconstitution - Oral - 250 mg/5 ml			
75 ml	$10.60	GENERIC, Prescript Pharmaceuticals	00247-0054-75
75 ml	$26.05	GENERIC, Major Pharmaceuticals Inc	00904-7936-71
75 ml	$35.97	GENERIC, Alpharma Uspd Makers Of Barre and Nmc	63874-0153-75
150 ml	$17.85	GENERIC, Prescript Pharmaceuticals	00247-0054-78
150 ml	$28.50	GENERIC, Physicians Total Care	54868-3473-00
150 ml	$50.66	GENERIC, Major Pharmaceuticals Inc	00904-7936-07
150 ml	$51.35	GENERIC, Allscripts Pharmaceutical Company	54569-3904-00
150 ml	$51.66	GENERIC, Pharma Pac	52959-1399-03
150 ml	$55.93	GENERIC, Southwood Pharmaceuticals Inc	58016-4192-05
150 ml	$67.13	GENERIC, Alpharma Uspd Makers Of Barre and Nmc	63874-0153-15
Powder For Reconstitution - Oral - 375 mg/5 ml			
50 ml	$26.05	GENERIC, Major Pharmaceuticals Inc	00904-7937-50
50 ml	$30.13	GENERIC, Prescript Pharmaceuticals	00247-0055-50
100 ml	$50.74	GENERIC, Major Pharmaceuticals Inc	00904-7937-04
100 ml	$51.37	GENERIC, Allscripts Pharmaceutical Company	54569-4311-00
100 ml	$56.92	GENERIC, Prescript Pharmaceuticals	00247-0055-00
Tablet, Extended Release - Oral - 375 mg			
60's	$264.89	CECLOR CD, Dura Pharmaceuticals	51479-0036-60
100's	$379.30	GENERIC, Teva Pharmaceuticals Usa	00093-1215-01
Tablet, Extended Release - Oral - 500 mg			
14 x 3	$174.84	CECLOR CD, Dura Pharmaceuticals	51479-0035-03
14's	$59.33	CECLOR CD, Allscripts Pharmaceutical Company	54569-4463-01
20's	$69.94	CECLOR CD, Allscripts Pharmaceutical Company	54569-4463-00
60's	$264.89	CECLOR CD, Dura Pharmaceuticals	51479-0035-60

Cefadroxil Monohydrate *(000681)*

For related information, see the comparative table section in Appendix A.

Categories: Infection, skin and skin structures; Infection, upper respiratory tract; Infection, urinary tract; Pharyngitis; Tonsillitis; Pregnancy Category B; FDA Approved 1978 Feb

Drug Classes: Antibiotics, cephalosporins

Brand Names: **Duricef**; Ultracef

Foreign Brand Availability: Alxil (Indonesia); Amben (Hong-Kong); Ancefa (Indonesia); Baxan (England); Bidicef (Indonesia); Biodroxil (Colombia; Hong-Kong; Israel; Peru); Biofaxil (Portugal); Camex (Korea); Cedrox (Bahrain; Cyprus; Egypt; Iran; Iraq; Israel; Jordan; Kuwait; Lebanon; Libya; Oman; Qatar; Republic-of-Yemen; Saudi-Arabia; Syria; United-Arab-Emirates); Cedroxim (Dominican-Republic; El-Salvador; Guatemala; Honduras; Panama); Cefacar (Argentina); Cefacell (Korea); Cefadril (Italy; Thailand); Cefadrol (India); Cefadrox (South-Africa); Cefalom (Greece); Cefamox (Brazil; Mexico; Philippines; Sweden); Cefaroxil (Korea); Cefat (Indonesia); Cefaxil (Taiwan); Ceforal (Portugal); Cefoxil (Korea); Cefra-Om (Portugal); Cefroxil (Spain); Cephos (Italy); Crenodyn (Italy); Curisafe (Bahrain; Cyprus; Egypt; Iran; Iraq; Jordan; Kuwait; Lebanon; Libya; Oman; Qatar; Republic-of-Yemen; Saudi-Arabia; Syria; United-Arab-Emirates); Cyclomycin-K (Greece); Drocef (Korea); Droxicef (Bahrain; Cyprus; Egypt; Iran; Iraq; Jordan; Kuwait; Lebanon; Libya; Oman; Qatar; Republic-of-Yemen; Saudi-Arabia; Syria; United-Arab-Emirates); Droxil (Bahrain; Cyprus; Egypt; Iran; Iraq; Israel; Jordan; Kuwait; Lebanon; Libya; Oman; Qatar; Republic-of-Yemen; Saudi-Arabia; Syria; United-Arab-Emirates); Droxyl (India); Duracef (Austria; Belgium; Benin; Burkina-Faso; Colombia; Costa-Rica; Dominican-Republic; Ecuador; El-Salvador; Ethiopia; Finland; Gambia; Ghana; Guatemala; Guinea; Honduras; Hong-Kong; Israel; Ivory-Coast; Kenya; Liberia; Malawi; Mali; Mauritania; Mauritius; Mexico; Morocco; Nicaragua; Niger; Nigeria; Panama; Peru; Philippines; Senegal; Seychelles; Sierra-Leone; Spain; Sudan; Switzerland; Taiwan; Tanzania; Tunia; Uganda; Zambia; Zimbabwe); Egobiotic (Argentina); Ethicef (Indonesia); Evacef (Korea); Kelfex (Indonesia); Kleotrat (Greece); Lapicef (Indonesia); Lesporina (Colombia); Likodin (Taiwan); Lydroxil (India); Moxacef (Belgium; Greece; Netherlands); Nefalox (Greece); Nor-Dacef (Bahrain; Cyprus; Dominican-Republic; Egypt; El-Salvador; Guatemala; Honduras; Iran; Iraq; Israel; Jordan; Kuwait; Lebanon; Libya; Nicaragua; Oman; Qatar; Republic-of-Yemen; Saudi-Arabia; Syria; United-Arab-Emirates); Odoxil (India); Omnidrox (Slovenia); Oracefal (France); Oradroxil (Italy); QCef (Indonesia); Sedral (Japan; Taiwan); Sofidrox (Singapore); Ucefa (Taiwan); Urocef (Korea); Vepan (India); Versatic (Argentina); Vidcef (Korea)

Cost of Therapy: $81.36 (Infection; Duricef; 500 mg; 2 capsules/day; 10 day supply)
$58.56 (Infection; Generic Capsules; 500 mg; 2 capsules/day; 10 day supply)

DESCRIPTION

Duricef is a semisynthetic cephalosporin antibiotic intended for oral administration. It is a white to yellowish-white crystalline powder. It is soluble in water and it is acid-stable. It is chemically designated as 5-Thia-1-azabicyclo[4.2.0]oct-2-ene-2-carboxylic acid, 7-[[amino(4-hydroxyphenyl)acetyl]amino]-3-methyl-8-oxo-, monohydrate, [6R-[6α,7β(R*)]]-. It has the formula $C_{16}H_{17}N_3O_5S \cdot H_2O$ and the molecular weight of 381.40.

Duricef film-coated tablets, 1 g, contain the following inactive ingredients: microcrystalline cellulose, hydroxypropyl methylcellulose, magnesium stearate, polyethylene glycol, polysorbate 80, simethicone emulsion, and titanium dioxide.

Duricef for Oral Suspension contains the following inactive ingredients: FD&C yellow no. 6, flavors (natural and artificial), polysorbate 80, sodium benzoate, sucrose, and xanthan gum.

Duricef capsules contain the following inactive ingredients: D&C red no. 28, FD&C blue no. 1, FD&C red no. 40, gelatin, magnesium stearate, and titanium dioxide.

CLINICAL PHARMACOLOGY

Cefadroxil is rapidly absorbed after oral administration. Following single doses of 500 mg and 1000 mg, average peak serum concentrations were approximately 16 and 28 μg/ml, respectively. Measurable levels were present 12 hours after administration. Over 90% of the drug is excreted unchanged in the urine within 24 hours. Peak urine concentrations are approximately 1800 μg/ml during the period following a single 500 mg oral dose. Increases in dosage generally produce a proportionate increase in cefadroxil urinary concentration. The urine antibiotic concentration, following a 1 g dose, was maintained well above the MIC of susceptible urinary pathogens for 20-22 hours.

MICROBIOLOGY

In vitro tests demonstrate that the cephalosporins are bactericidal because of their inhibition of cell-wall synthesis. Cefadroxil has been shown to be active against the following organisms both *in vitro* and in clinical infections (see INDICATIONS AND USAGE):

Beta-hemolytic streptococci
Staphylococci, including penicillinase-producing strains
Streptococcus (Diplococcus) pneumoniae
Escherichia coli
Proteus mirabilis
Klebsiella species
Moraxella (Branhamella) catarrhalis

Note: Most strains of *Enterococcus faecalis* (formerly *Streptococcus faecalis*) and *Enterococcus faecium* (formerly *Streptococcus faecium*) are resistant to cefadroxil. It is not active against most strains of *Enterobacter* species, *Morganella morganii* (formerly *Proteus morganii*), and *P. vulgaris*. It has no activity against *Pseudomonas* species and *Acinetobacter calcoaceticus* (formerly *Mima* and *Herellea* species).

SUSCEPTIBILITY TESTS

Diffusion Techniques

The use of antibiotic disk susceptibility test methods which measure zone diameter give an accurate estimation of antibiotic susceptibility. One such standard procedure[1] which has been recommended for use with disks to test susceptibility of organisms to cefadroxil uses the cephalosporin class (cephalothin) disk. Interpretation involves the correlation of the diameters obtained in the disk test with the minimum inhibitory concentration (MIC) for cefadroxil.

Reports from the laboratory giving results of the standard single-disk susceptibility test with a 30 μg cephalothin disk should be interpreted according to the following criteria (see TABLE 1).

TABLE 1

Zone Diameter	Interpretation
≥18 mm	(S) Susceptible
15-17 mm	(I) Intermediate
≤14 mm	(R) Resistant

A report of "Susceptible" indicates that the pathogen is likely to be inhibited by generally achievable blood levels. A report of "Intermediate susceptibility" suggests that the organism would be susceptible if high dosage is used or if the infection is confined to tissue and fluids (*e.g.*, urine) in which high antibiotic levels are attained. A report of "Resistant" indicates that achievable concentrations of the antibiotic are unlikely to be inhibitory and other therapy should be selected.

Standardized procedures require the use of laboratory control organisms. The 30 μg cephalothin disk should give the following zone diameters (see TABLE 2).

TABLE 2

Organism	Zone Diameter
Staphylococcus aureus ATCC 25923	29-37 mm
Escherichia coli ATCC 25922	17-22 mm

Dilution Techniques

When using the NCCLS agar dilution or broth dilution (including microdilution) method[2] or equivalent, a bacterial isolate may be considered susceptible if the MIC (minimum inhibitory concentration) value for cephalothin is 8 μg/ml or less. Organisms are considered resistant if the MIC is 32 μg/ml or greater. Organisms with an MIC value of less than 32 μg/ml but greater than 8 μg/ml are intermediate.

As with standard diffusion methods, dilution procedures require the use of laboratory control organisms. Standard cephalothin powder should give MIC values in the range of 0.12 μg/ml and 0.5 μg/ml for *Staphylococcus aureus* ATCC 29213. For *Escherichia coli* ATCC 25922, the MIC range should be between 4.0 μg/ml and 16.0 μg/ml. For *Streptococcus faecalis* ATCC 29212, the MIC range should be between 8.0 and 32.0 μg/ml.

INDICATIONS AND USAGE

Cefadroxil is indicated for the treatment of patients with infection caused by susceptible strains of the designated organisms in the following diseases:

Urinary tract infections caused by *E. coli, P. mirabilis,* and *Klebsiella* species.
Skin and skin structure infections caused by staphylococci and/or streptococci.
Pharyngitis and/or tonsillitis caused by *Streptococcus pyogenes* (Group A beta-hemolytic streptococci).

Note: Only penicillin by the intramuscular route of administration has been shown to be effective in the prophylaxis of rheumatic fever. Cefadroxil is generally effective in the eradication of streptococci from the oropharynx. However, data establishing the efficacy of cefadroxil for the prophylaxis of subsequent rheumatic fever are not available.
Note: Culture and susceptibility tests should be initiated prior to and during therapy. Renal function studies should be performed when indicated.

CONTRAINDICATIONS

Cefadroxil is contraindicated in patients with known allergy to the cephalosporin group of antibiotics.

WARNINGS

BEFORE THERAPY WITH CEFADROXIL IS INSTITUTED, CAREFUL INQUIRY SHOULD BE MADE TO DETERMINE WHETHER THE PATIENT HAS HAD PREVIOUS HYPERSENSITIVITY REACTIONS TO CEFADROXIL, CEPHALOSPORINS, PENICILLINS, OR OTHER DRUGS. IF THIS PRODUCT IS TO BE GIVEN TO PENICILLIN-SENSITIVE PATIENTS, CAUTION SHOULD BE EXERCISED BECAUSE CROSS-SENSITIVITY AMONG BETA-LACTAM ANTIBIOTICS HAS BEEN CLEARLY DOCUMENTED AND MAY OCCUR IN UP TO 10% OF PATIENTS WITH A HISTORY OF PENICILLIN ALLERGY.

IF AN ALLERGIC REACTION TO CEFADROXIL OCCURS, DISCONTINUE THE DRUG. SERIOUS ACUTE HYPERSENSITIVITY REACTIONS MAY REQUIRE TREATMENT WITH EPINEPHRINE AND OTHER EMERGENCY MEASURES, INCLUDING OXYGEN, INTRAVENOUS FLUIDS, INTRAVENOUS ANTIHISTAMINES, CORTICOSTEROIDS, PRESSOR AMINES, AND AIRWAY MANAGEMENT, AS CLINICALLY INDICATED.

Pseudomembranous colitis has been reported with nearly all antibacterial agents, including cefadroxil, and may range from mild to life-threatening. Therefore, it is important to consider this diagnosis in patients who present with diarrhea subsequent to the administration of antibacterial agents.

Treatment with antibacterial agents alters the normal flora of the colon and may permit overgrowth of clostridia. Studies indicated that a toxin produced by *Clostridium difficile* is a primary cause of "antibiotic-associated colitis".

After the diagnosis of pseudomembranous colitis has been established, therapeutic measures should be initiated. Mild cases of pseudomembranous colitis usually respond to discontinuation of the drug alone. In moderate to severe cases, consideration should be given to management with fluids and electrolytes, protein supplementation and treatment with an antibacterial drug effective against *Clostridium difficile.*

PRECAUTIONS

GENERAL

Cefadroxil should be used with caution in the presence of markedly impaired renal function (creatinine clearance rate of less than 50 ml/min/1.73 m^2). (See DOSAGE AND ADMINISTRATION.) In patients with known or suspected renal impairment, careful clinical observation and appropriate laboratory studies should be made prior to and during therapy.

Prolonged use of cefadroxil may result in the overgrowth of nonsusceptible organisms. Careful observation of the patient is essential. If superinfection occurs during therapy, appropriate measures should be taken.

Cefadroxil should be prescribed with caution in individuals with history of gastrointestinal disease particularly colitis.

DRUG/LABORATORY TEST INTERACTIONS

Positive direct Coombs' tests have been reported during treatment with the cephalosporin antibiotics. In hematologic studies or in transfusion cross-matching procedures when antiglobulin tests are performed on the minor side or in Coombs' testing of newborns whose mothers have received cephalosporin antibiotics before parturition, it should be recognized that a positive Coombs' test may be due to the drug.

CARCINOGENESIS, MUTAGENESIS, AND IMPAIRMENT OF FERTILITY

No long-term studies have been performed to determine carcinogenic potential. No genetic toxicity tests have been performed.

PREGNANCY CATEGORY B

Reproduction studies have been performed in mice and rats at doses up to 11 times the human dose and have revealed no evidence of impaired fertility or harm to the fetus due to cefadroxil monohydrate. There are, however, no adequate and well controlled studies in pregnant women. Because animal reproduction studies are not always predictive of human response, this drug should be used during pregnancy only if clearly needed.

LABOR AND DELIVERY

Cefadroxil has not been studied for use during labor and delivery. Treatment should only be given if clearly needed.

NURSING MOTHERS

Caution should be exercised when cefadroxil monohydrate is administered to a nursing mother.

PEDIATRIC USE

See DOSAGE AND ADMINISTRATION.

GERIATRIC USE

Of approximately 650 patients who received cefadroxil for the treatment of urinary tract infections in three clinical trials, 28% were 60 years and older, while 16% were 70 years and older. Of approximately 1000 patients who received cefadroxil for the treatment of skin and skin structure infection in 14 clinical trials, 12% were 60 years and older while 4% were 70 years and over. No overall differences in safety were observed between the elderly patients in these studies and younger patients. Clinical studies of cefadroxil for the treatment of pharyngitis or tonsillitis did not include sufficient numbers of patients 65 years and older to determine whether they respond differently from younger patients. Other reported clinical experience with cefadroxil has not identified differences in responses between elderly and younger patients, but greater sensitivity of some older individuals cannot be ruled out.

Cefadroxil is substantially excreted by the kidney, and dosage adjustment is indicated for patients with renal impairment (see DOSAGE AND ADMINISTRATION, Renal Impairment). Because elderly patients are more likely to have decreased renal function, care should be taken in dose selection, and it may be useful to monitor renal function.

ADVERSE REACTIONS

GASTROINTESTINAL

Onset of pseudomembranous colitis symptoms may occur during or after antibiotic treatment (see WARNINGS). Dyspepsia, nausea and vomiting have been reported rarely. Diarrhea has also occurred.

HYPERSENSITIVITY

Allergies (in the form of rash, urticaria, angioedema, and pruritus) have been observed. These reactions usually subsided upon discontinuation of the drug. Anaphylaxis has also been reported.

OTHER

Other reactions have included hepatic dysfunction including cholestasis and elevations in serum transaminase, genital pruritus, genital moniliasis, vaginitis, moderate transient neutropenia, fever. Agranulocytosis, thrombocytopenia, idiosyncratic hepatic failure, erythema multiforme, Stevens-Johnson syndrome, serum sickness, and arthralgia have been rarely reported.

In addition to the adverse reactions listed above which have been observed in patients treated with cefadroxil, the following adverse reactions and altered laboratory tests have been reported for cephalosporin-class antibiotics:

Toxic epidermal necrolysis, abdominal pain, superinfection, renal dysfunction, toxic nephropathy, aplastic anemia, hemolytic anemia, hemorrhage, prolonged prothrombin time, positive Coombs' test, increased BUN, increased creatinine, elevated alkaline phosphatase, elevated aspartate aminotransferase (AST), elevated alanine aminotransferase (ALT), elevated bilirubin, elevated LDH, eosinophilia, pancytopenia, neutropenia.

Several cephalosporins have been implicated in triggering seizures, particularly in patients with renal impairment, when the dosage was not reduced (see DOSAGE AND ADMINISTRATION). If seizures associated with drug therapy occur, the drug should be discontinued. Anticonvulsant therapy can be given if clinically indicated.

DOSAGE AND ADMINISTRATION

Cefadroxil is acid-stable and may be administered orally without regard to meals. Administration with food may be helpful in diminishing potential gastrointestinal complaints occasionally associated with oral cephalosporin therapy.

ADULTS

Urinary Tract Infections

For uncomplicated lower urinary tract infections (*i.e.,* cystitis) the usual dosage is 1 or 2 g/day in a single (qd) or divided doses (bid).

For all other urinary tract infections the usual dosage is 2 g/day in divided doses (bid).

Skin and Skin Structure Infections

For skin and skin structure infections the usual dosage is 1 g/day in single (qd) or divided doses (bid).

Pharyngitis and Tonsillitis

Treatment of group A beta-hemolytic streptococcal pharyngitis and tonsillitis — 1 g/day in single (qd) or divided doses (bid) for 10 days.

CHILDREN

For urinary tract infections, the recommended daily dosage for children is 30 mg/kg/day in divided doses every 12 hours. For pharyngitis, tonsillitis, and impetigo, the recommended daily dosage for children is 30 mg/kg/day in a single dose or in equally divided doses every 12 hours. For other skin and skin structure infections, the recommended daily dosage is 30 mg/kg/day in equally divided doses every 12 hours. In the treatment of beta-hemolytic streptococcal infections, a therapeutic dosage of cefadroxil should be administered for at least 10 days.

See TABLE 3 for total daily dosage for children.

TABLE 3 *Daily Dosage of Cefadroxil Suspension*

Child's Weight		125 mg/5 ml	250 mg/5 ml	500 mg/5 ml
10 lb	4.5 kg	1 tsp	—	
20 lb	9.1 kg	2 tsp	1 tsp	
30 lb	13.6 kg	3 tsp	1½ tsp	
40 lb	18.2 kg	4 tsp	2 tsp	1 tsp
50 lb	22.7 kg	5 tsp	2½ tsp	1¼ tsp
60 lb	27.3 kg	6 tsp	3 tsp	1½ tsp
70 lb and above	31.8+ kg	—	—	2 tsp

RENAL IMPAIRMENT

In patients with renal impairment, the dosage of cefadroxil monohydrate should be adjusted according to creatinine clearance rates to prevent drug accumulation. The following schedule is suggested. In adults, the initial dose is 1000 mg of cefadroxil and the maintenance dose (based on the creatinine clearance rate [ml/min/1.73 m^2]) is 500 mg at the time intervals listed in TABLE 4.

Patients with creatinine clearance rates over 50 ml/min may be treated as if they were patients having normal renal function.

TABLE 4

Creatinine Clearances	Dosage Interval
0-10 ml/min	36 hours
10-25 ml/min	24 hours
25-50 ml/min	12 hours

HOW SUPPLIED

DURICEF CAPSULES

Duricef Capsules are Available in:

500 mg: Opaque, maroon and white hard gelatin capsules, imprinted with "PPP" and "784" on one end and with "DURICEF" and "500 mg" on the other end.

Storage: Store at controlled room temperature (15-30°C).

DURICEF TABLETS

Duricef Tablets are Available in:

1 gram: White to off white, top bisected, oval shaped, imprinted with "PPP" on one side of the bisect and "785" on the other side of the bisect.

Storage: Store at controlled room temperature (15-30°C).

DURICEF ORAL SUSPENSION

Duricef for Oral Suspension is orange-pineapple flavored, and is supplied in:

125 mg/5 ml: 50 and 100 ml bottles.

250 mg/5 ml: 50 and 100 ml bottles.

500 mg/5 ml: 50, 75 and 100 ml bottles.

Storage:

Prior to reconstitution: Store at controlled room temperature (15-30°C).

After to reconstitution: Store in refrigerator. Shake well before using. Keep container tightly closed. Discard unused portion after 14 days.

PRODUCT LISTING - RATED THERAPEUTICALLY EQUIVALENT

Capsule - Oral - 500 mg

6's	$35.25	DURICEF, Pd-Rx Pharmaceuticals	55289-0056-06
10's	$37.70	GENERIC, Pd-Rx Pharmaceuticals	55289-0405-10
10's	$46.51	DURICEF, Pharma Pac	52959-0056-10
10's	$58.88	DURICEF, Pd-Rx Pharmaceuticals	55289-0056-10
12's	$54.60	DURICEF, Southwood Pharmaceuticals Inc	58016-0751-12
14's	$45.21	GENERIC, Pd-Rx Pharmaceuticals	55289-0405-14
14's	$45.21	GENERIC, Pd-Rx Pharmaceuticals	55289-0589-14
14's	$65.17	DURICEF, Pharma Pac	52959-0056-14
14's	$82.26	DURICEF, Pd-Rx Pharmaceuticals	55289-0056-14
20's	$85.36	DURICEF, Pharma Pac	52959-0056-20
20's	$143.16	DURICEF, Pd-Rx Pharmaceuticals	55289-0056-20
24's	$73.50	GENERIC, Ivax Corporation	00172-4058-43
25's	$113.75	DURICEF, Southwood Pharmaceuticals Inc	58016-0751-25
40's	$182.00	DURICEF, Southwood Pharmaceuticals Inc	58016-0751-40
50's	$150.10	GENERIC, Major Pharmaceuticals Inc	00904-7878-51
50's	$151.74	GENERIC, Bristol-Myers Squibb	59772-7271-02
50's	$153.95	FEDERAL UPPER LIMIT, H.C.F.A. F F P	99999-0681-03
50's	$168.68	GENERIC, Barr Laboratories Inc	00555-0582-10
50's	$172.75	GENERIC, Ranbaxy Laboratories	63304-0582-50
50's	$188.06	GENERIC, Apothecon Inc	59772-7271-03
50's	$193.42	GENERIC, Ivax Corporation	00172-4058-48
50's	$289.32	DURICEF, Bristol-Myers Squibb	00087-0784-46
60's	$273.00	DURICEF, Southwood Pharmaceuticals Inc	58016-0751-60
90's	$409.50	DURICEF, Southwood Pharmaceuticals Inc	58016-0751-90
100's	$292.78	GENERIC, Apothecon Inc	59772-7271-07
100's	$319.95	GENERIC, Barr Laboratories Inc	00555-0582-02
100's	$327.95	GENERIC, Ranbaxy Laboratories	63304-0582-01
100's	$372.36	GENERIC, Apothecon Inc	59772-7271-04
100's	$414.69	GENERIC, Ivax Corporation	00172-4058-60
100's	$455.00	DURICEF, Southwood Pharmaceuticals Inc	58016-0751-00

Tablet - Oral - 1 Gm

5's	$42.42	DURICEF, Allscripts Pharmaceutical Company	54569-0110-02
5's	$45.99	DURICEF, Pharma Pac	52959-0204-05
7's	$64.36	DURICEF, Pharma Pac	52959-0204-07
10's	$84.83	DURICEF, Allscripts Pharmaceutical Company	54569-0110-04
10's	$91.90	DURICEF, Pharma Pac	52959-0204-10
50's	$357.00	GENERIC, Ranbaxy Laboratories	63304-0512-50
50's	$357.08	GENERIC, Ivax Corporation	00172-4059-48
50's	$544.38	DURICEF, Warner Chilcott Laboratories	00087-0785-43
100's	$695.39	DURICEF, Bristol-Myers Squibb	00087-0785-44
100's	$697.11	DURICEF, Bristol-Myers Squibb	00087-0785-42

PRODUCT LISTING - EQUIVALENTS NOT AVAILABLE

Capsule - Oral - 500 mg

2's	$6.75	GENERIC, Allscripts Pharmaceutical Company	54569-4391-03
2's	$10.29	GENERIC, Prescript Pharmaceuticals	00247-0064-02
3's	$13.75	GENERIC, Prescript Pharmaceuticals	00247-0064-03
4's	$17.22	GENERIC, Prescript Pharmaceuticals	00247-0064-04
7's	$27.62	GENERIC, Prescript Pharmaceuticals	00247-0064-07
10's	$33.76	GENERIC, Allscripts Pharmaceutical Company	54569-4391-00
10's	$36.69	GENERIC, Southwood Pharmaceuticals Inc	58016-0119-10
10's	$38.04	GENERIC, Prescript Pharmaceuticals	00247-0064-10
10's	$53.75	GENERIC, Pharma Pac	52959-0428-10
12's	$44.96	GENERIC, Prescript Pharmaceuticals	00247-0064-12
12's	$54.60	GENERIC, Southwood Pharmaceuticals Inc	58016-0119-12
14's	$35.51	GENERIC, Physicians Total Care	54868-3742-00
14's	$47.26	GENERIC, Allscripts Pharmaceutical Company	54569-4391-01
14's	$51.91	GENERIC, Prescript Pharmaceuticals	00247-0064-14
14's	$63.70	GENERIC, Southwood Pharmaceuticals Inc	58016-0119-14
14's	$68.72	GENERIC, Pharma Pac	52959-0428-14
15's	$55.36	GENERIC, Prescript Pharmaceuticals	00247-0064-15
15's	$68.25	GENERIC, Southwood Pharmaceuticals Inc	58016-0119-15
16's	$78.42	GENERIC, Pharma Pac	52959-0428-16
18's	$88.01	GENERIC, Pharma Pac	52959-0428-18
20's	$50.15	GENERIC, Physicians Total Care	54868-3742-01
20's	$67.52	GENERIC, Allscripts Pharmaceutical Company	54569-4391-02
20's	$72.71	GENERIC, Prescript Pharmaceuticals	00247-0064-20
20's	$91.00	GENERIC, Southwood Pharmaceuticals Inc	58016-0119-20
20's	$97.32	GENERIC, Pharma Pac	52959-0428-20
25's	$113.75	GENERIC, Southwood Pharmaceuticals Inc	58016-0119-25
30's	$107.39	GENERIC, Prescript Pharmaceuticals	00247-0064-30
30's	$136.50	GENERIC, Southwood Pharmaceuticals Inc	58016-0119-30
40's	$182.00	GENERIC, Southwood Pharmaceuticals Inc	58016-0119-40
60's	$273.00	GENERIC, Southwood Pharmaceuticals Inc	58016-0119-60
90's	$409.50	GENERIC, Southwood Pharmaceuticals Inc	58016-0119-90
100's	$350.12	GENERIC, Prescript Pharmaceuticals	00247-0064-00
100's	$455.00	GENERIC, Southwood Pharmaceuticals Inc	58016-0119-00

Powder For Reconstitution - Oral - 125 mg/5 ml

100 ml	$17.11	DURICEF, Allscripts Pharmaceutical Company	54569-2102-00

Powder For Reconstitution - Oral - 250 mg/5 ml

100 ml	$32.14	DURICEF, Allscripts Pharmaceutical Company	54569-0109-00
100 ml	$41.24	DURICEF, Warner Chilcott Laboratories	00087-0782-41

Powder For Reconstitution - Oral - 500 mg/5 ml

75 ml	$42.80	DURICEF, Warner Chilcott Laboratories	00087-0783-05
100 ml	$44.48	DURICEF, Allscripts Pharmaceutical Company	54569-3162-00
100 ml	$57.08	DURICEF, Warner Chilcott Laboratories	00087-0783-41

Cefamandole Nafate *(000682)*

For related information, see the comparative table section in Appendix A.

Categories: Infection, bone; Infection, gynecologic; Infection, intra-abdominal; Infection, joint; Infection, lower respiratory tract; Infection, skin and skin structures; Infection, urinary tract; Pelvic inflammatory disease; Peritonitis; Pneumonia; Prophylaxis, perioperative; Septicemia; Pregnancy Category B; FDA Approved 1978 Sep

Drug Classes: Antibiotics, cephalosporins

Brand Names: **Mandol**

Foreign Brand Availability: Cefadol (Taiwan; Thailand); Dardokef (Indonesia); Dofacef (Indonesia); Kefadol (England; Ireland); Kefdole (Japan; South-Africa); Mancef (Korea); Mandokef (Austria; Bulgaria; Denmark; Finland; Portugal; South-Africa; Spain; Switzerland)

Cost of Therapy: $181.30 (Infection; Mandol Injection; 1 g; 2 g/day; 10 day supply)

DESCRIPTION

Cefamandole nafate for injection is a semisynthetic broad-spectrum cephalosporin antibiotic for parenteral administration. It is 5-Thia-azabicyclo(4.2.0)oct-2-ene-2-carboxylic acid, 7 (((formyloxy)phenylacetyl)amino)-3(((1-methyl-1*H*-tetrazol-5- yl)thio)methyl)-8-oxo-, monosodium salt, (6*R*-(6α, 7β(R*))). Cefamandole has the empirical formula $C_{19}H_{17}N_5NaO_6S_2$ representing a molecular weight of 512.49. Mandol also contains 63 mg sodium carbonate per gram of cefamandole activity. The total sodium content is approximately 77 mg (3.3 mEq sodium ion) per gram of cefamandole activity. After addition of diluent, cefamandole nafate rapidly hydrolyzes to cefamandole and both compounds have microbiologic activity *in vivo*. Solutions of Mandol range from light-yellow to amber, depending on concentration and diluent used. The pH of freshly reconstituted solutions usually ranges from 6.0 to 8.5.

CLINICAL PHARMACOLOGY

After intramuscular administration of a 500 mg dose of cefamandole to normal volunteers, the mean peak serum concentration was 13 μg/ml. After a 1 gram dose, the mean peak concentration was 25 μg/ml. These peaks occurred at 30-120 minutes. Following intravenous doses of 1, 2 and 3 g, serum concentrations were 139, 240, and 533 μg/ml respectively at 10 minutes. These concentrations declined to 0.8, 2.2, and 2.9 μg/ml at 4 hours. Intravenous administration of 4 g doses every 6 hours produced no evidence of accumulation in the serum. The half-life after an intravenous dose is 32 minutes; after intramuscular administration, the half-life is 60 minutes.

Sixty-five percent (65%) to 85% of cefamandole is excreted by the kidneys over an 8 hour period, resulting in high urinary concentrations. Following intramuscular doses of 500 mg and 1 g, urinary concentrations averaged 254 and 1357 μg/ml respectively. Intravenous doses of 1 and 2 gram produced urinary levels averaging 750 and 1380 μg/ml respectively. Probenecid slows tubular excretion and doubles the peak serum level and the duration of measurable serum concentrations.

The antibiotic reaches therapeutic levels in pleural and joint fluids and in bile and bone.

MICROBIOLOGY

The bactericidal action of cefamandole results from inhibition of cell-wall synthesis. Cephalosporins have *in vitro* activity against a wide range of gram-positive and gram-negative organisms. Cefamandole is usually active against the following organisms *in vitro* and in clinical infections:

Gram Positive:

Staphylococcus aureus, including penicillinase and non-penicillinase-producing strains.

Staphylococcus epidermidis.

β-hemolytic and other *streptococci* (Most strains of *enterococci, e.g., Enterococcus faecalis* (formerly *Streptococcus faecalis*), are resistant).

Streptococcus pneumoniae (formerly *Diplococcus pneumoniae*).

Gram Negative:

Escherichia coli.

Klebsiella sp.

*Enterobacter*sp. (Initially susceptible organisms occasionally may become resistant during therapy.)

Haemophilus influenzae.

Proteus mirabilis.

Providencia rettgeri (formerly *Proteus rettgeri*).

Morganella morganii (formerly *Proteus morganii*).

Proteus vulgaris (Some strains of *P. vulgaris* have been shown by *in vitro* tests to be resistant to cefamandole and other cephalosporins).

Anaerobic Organisms:

Gram-positive and gram-negative cocci (including *Peptococcus* and *Peptostreptococcus* sp).

Gram-positive bacilli (including *Clostridium* sp).

Gram-negative bacilli (including *Bacteroides* and *Fusobacterium* sp). Most strains of *Bacteroides fragilis* are resistant.

Pseudomonas, Acinetobacter calcoaceticus (formerly *Mima* and *Herellea* sp), and most *Serratia* strains are resistant to cephalosporins. Cefamandole is resistant to degradation by β-lactamases from certain members of the *Enterobacteriaceae.*

SUSCEPTIBILITY TESTING

Quantitative methods that require measurement of zone diameters give the most precise estimates of antibiotic susceptibility. One such procedure[1] has been recommended for use with disks to test susceptibility to cefamandole. Interpretation involves correlation of the diameters obtained in the disk test with minimum inhibitory concentration (MIC) values for cefamandole.

Reports from the laboratory giving results of the standardized single-disk susceptibility test using a 30 μg cefamandole disk should be interpreted according to the following criteria:

Susceptible organisms produce zones of 18 mm or greater, indicating that the tested organism is likely to respond to therapy.

Organisms of intermediate susceptibility produce zones of 15-17 mm, indicating that the tested organism would be susceptible if high dosage is used or if the infection is confined to tissues and fluids (*e.g.,* urine), in which high antibiotic levels are attained.

Resistant organisms produce zones of 14 mm or less, indicating that other therapy should be selected.

For gram-positive isolates, the test may be performed with either the cephalosporin class disk (30 μg cephalothin) or the cefamandole disk (30 μg cefamandole), and a zone of 18 mm indicative of a cefamandole susceptible organism.

Gram-negative organisms should be tested with the cefamandole disk (using the above criteria), since cefamandole has been shown by *in vitro* tests to have activity against certain strains of *Enterobacteriaceae* found resistant when tested with the cephalosporin-class disk. Gram-negative organisms having zones of less than 18 mm around the cephalothin disk are not necessarily of intermediate susceptibility or resistant to cefamandole.

The cefamandole disk should not be used for testing susceptibility to other cephalosporins.

A bacterial isolate may be considered susceptible if the MIC value for cefamandole[2] is not more than 16 μg/ml. Organisms are considered resistant if the MIC is greater than 32 μg/ml.

INDICATIONS AND USAGE

Cefamandole nafate is indicated for the treatment of serious infections caused by susceptible strains of the designated microorganisms in the diseases listed below:

Lower respiratory infections, including pneumonia caused by *S. pneumoniae, H. influenzae, Klebsiella* sp, *S. aureus* (penicillinase and non-penicillinase-producing), β-hemolytic streptococci, and *P mirabilis.*

Urinary tract infections caused by *E. coli, Proteus* sp (both indole-negative and indole-positive), *Enterobacter* sp, *Klebsiella* sp, group D *streptococci* (*Note:* Most *enterococci, e.g., E. faecalis,* are resistant), and *S. epidermidis.*

Peritonitis caused by *E. coli* and *Enterobacter* sp.

Septicemia caused by *E. coli, S. aureus* (penicillinase and non-penicillinase-producing), *S. pneumoniae, S. pyogenes* (group A β-hemolytic *streptococci*), *H. influenzae,* and *Klebsiella* sp.

Skin and skin-structure infections caused by *S. aureus* (penicillinase and non-penicillinase-producing), *S. pyogenes* (group A β-hemolytic *streptococci*), *H. influenzae, E. coli, Enterobacter* sp, and *P. mirabilis.*

Bone and joint infections caused by *S. aureus* (penicillinase and non-penicillinase-producing).

Clinical microbiologic studies in nongonococcal pelvic inflammatory disease in females, lower respiratory infections, and skin infections frequently reveal the growth of susceptible strains of both aerobic and anaerobic organisms. Cefamandole nafate has been used successfully in these infections in which several organisms have been isolated. Most strains of *B. fragilis* are resistant *in vitro;* however, infections caused by susceptible strains have been treated successfully.

Specimens for bacteriologic cultures should be obtained in order to isolate and identify causative organisms and to determine their susceptibilities to cefamandole. Therapy may be instituted before results of susceptibility studies are known; however, once these results become available, the antibiotic treatment should be adjusted accordingly.

In certain cases of confirmed or suspected gram-positive or gram-negative sepsis or in patients with other serious infections in which the causative organism has not been identified, cefamandole nafate may be used concomitantly with an aminoglycoside (see PRECAUTIONS). The recommended doses of both antibiotics may be given, depending on the security of the infection and the patient's condition. The renal function of the patient should be carefully monitored, especially if higher dosages of the antibiotics are to be administered.

Antibiotic therapy of β-hemolytic streptococcal infections should continue for at least 10 days.

PREVENTIVE THERAPY

The administration of cefamandole nafate preoperatively, intraoperatively, and postoperatively may reduce the incidence of certain postoperative infections in patients undergoing surgical procedures that are classified as contaminated or potentially contaminated (*e.g.,* gastrointestinal surgery, cesarean section, vaginal hysterectomy, or cholecystectomy in high-risk patients such as those with acute cholecystitis, obstructive jaundice, or common-bile-duct stones).

In major surgery in which the risk of postoperative infection is low but serious (cardiovascular surgery, neurosurgery, or prosthetic arthroplasty), cefamandole nafate may be effective in preventing such infections.

The preoperative use of cefamandole nafate should be discontinued after 24 hours; however, in prosthetic arthroplasty, it is recommended that administration be continued for 72 hours. If signs of infection occur, specimens for culture should be obtained for identification of the causative organism so that appropriate antibiotic therapy may be instituted.

CONTRAINDICATIONS

Cefamandole nafate is contraindicated in patients with known allergy to the cephalosporin group of antibiotics.

WARNINGS

BEFORE THERAPY WITH CEFAMANDOLE NAFATE IS INSTITUTED, CAREFUL INQUIRY SHOULD BE MADE TO DETERMINE WHETHER THE PATIENT HAS HAD PREVIOUS HYPERSENSITIVITY REACTIONS TO CEPHALOSPORINS, PENICILLINS, OR OTHER DRUGS. THIS PRODUCT SHOULD BE GIVEN CAUTIOUSLY TO PENICILLIN-SENSITIVE PATIENTS. ANTIBIOTICS SHOULD BE ADMINISTERED WITH CAUTION TO ANY PATIENT WHO HAS DEMONSTRATED SOME FORM OF ALLERGY, PARTICULARLY TO DRUGS. SERIOUS ACUTE HYPERSENSITIVITY REACTIONS MAY REQUIRE EPINEPHRINE AND OTHER EMERGENCY MEASURES.

In newborn infants, accumulation of other cephalosporin-class antibiotics (with resulting prolongation of drug half-life) has been reported.

Pseudomembranous colitis has been reported with virtually all broad-spectrum antibiotics (including macrolides, semisynthetic penicillins, and cephalosporins); therefore, it is important to consider its diagnosis in patients who develop diarrhea in association with the use of antibiotics. Such colitis may range in severity from mild to life-threatening.

Treatment with broad-spectrum antibiotics alters the normal flora of the colon and may permit overgrowth of clostridia. Studies indicate that a toxin produced by *Clostridium difficile* is a primary cause of antibiotic-associated colitis.

Mild cases of pseudomembranous colitis usually respond to drug discontinuance alone. In moderate to severe cases, management should include sigmoidoscopy, appropriate bacteriologic studies, and fluid, electrolyte, and protein supplementation. When the colitis does not improve after the drug has been discontinued, or when it is severe, oral vancomycin is the drug of choice for antibiotic-associated pseudomembranous colitis produced by *C difficile.* Other causes of colitis should be ruled out.

PRECAUTIONS

GENERAL

Although cefamandole nafate rarely produces alteration in kidney function, evaluation of renal status is recommended, especially in seriously ill patients receiving maximum doses.

Prolonged use of cefamandole nafate may result in the overgrowth of nonsusceptible organisms. Careful observation of the patient is essential. If superinfection occurs during therapy, appropriate measures should be taken.

Nephrotoxicity has been reported following concomitant administration of aminoglycoside antibiotics and cephalosporins.

A false-positive reaction for glucose in the urine may occur with Benedict's or Fehling's solution or with Clinitest tablets but not with Tes-Tape (Glucose Enzymatic Test Strip). There may be a false-positive test for proteinuria with acid and denaturization-precipitation tests.

As with other broad-spectrum antibiotics, hypoprothrombinemia, with or without bleeding, has been reported rarely, but it has been promptly reversed by administration of vitamin K. Such episodes usually have occurred in elderly, debilitated, or otherwise compromised patients with deficient stores of vitamin K. Treatment of such individuals with antibiotics possessing significant gram-negative and/or anaerobic activity is thought to alter the number and/or type of intestinal bacterial flora, with consequent reduction in synthesis of vitamin K. Prophylactic administration of vitamin K may be indicated in such patients, especially when intestinal sterilization and surgical procedures are performed.

In a few patients receiving Mandol, nausea, vomiting, and vasomotor instability with hypotension and peripheral vasodilatation occurred following the ingestion of ethanol.

Cefamandole inhibits the enzyme acetaldehyde dehydrogenase in laboratory animals. This causes accumulation of acetaldehyde when ethanol is administered concomitantly.

Broad-spectrum antibiotics should be prescribed with caution in individuals with a history of gastrointestinal disease, particularly colitis.

CARCINOGENESIS, MUTAGENESIS, AND IMPAIRMENT OF FERTILITY

Certain β-lactam antibiotics containing the N-methylthiotetrazole side chain have been reported to cause delayed maturity of the testicular germinal epithelium when given to neonatal rats during initial spermatogenic development (6-36 days of age). In animals that were treated from 6-36 days of age with 1000 mg/kg/day of cefamandole (approximately 5 times the maximum clinical dose), the delayed maturity was pronounced and was associated with decreased testicular weights and a reduced number of germinal cells in the leading waves of spermatogenic development. The effect was slight in rats given 50 or 100 mg/kg/day. Some animals that were given 1000 mg/kg/day during days 6-36 were infertile after becoming sexually mature. No adverse effects have been observed in rats exposed *in utero,* in neonatal rats (4 days of age or younger) treated prior to the initiation of spermatogenesis, or in older rats (more than 36 days of age) after exposure for up to 6 months. The significance to man of these findings in rats is unknown because of differences in the time of initiation of spermatogenesis, rate of spermatogenic development, and duration of puberty.

PREGNANCY CATEGORY B

Reproduction studies have been performed in rats given doses of 500 or 1000 mg/kg/day and have revealed no evidence of impaired fertility or harm to the fetus due to Mandol. There are, however, no adequate and well-controlled studies in pregnant women. Because animal reproduction studies are not always predictive of human response, this drug should be used during pregnancy only if clearly needed.

NURSING MOTHERS

Caution should be exercised when cefamandole nafate is administered to a nursing woman.

USAGE IN INFANCY

Cefamandole nafate has been effectively used in this age group, but all laboratory parameters have not been extensively studied in infants between 1 and 6 months of age; safety of this product has not been established in prematures and infants under 1 month of age. Therefore, if cefamandole nafate is administered to infants, the physician should determine whether the potential benefits outweigh the possible risks involved.

ADVERSE REACTIONS

Gastrointestinal: Symptoms of pseudomembranous colitis may appear either during or after antibiotic treatment. Nausea and vomiting have been reported rarely. As with some penicillins and some other cephalosporins, transient hepatitis and cholestatic jaundice have been reported rarely.

Hypersensitivity: Anaphylaxis, maculopapular rash, urticaria, eosinophilia, and drug fever have been reported. These reactions are more likely to occur in patients with a history of allergy, particularly to penicillin.

Blood: Thrombocytopenia has been reported rarely. Neutropenia has been reported, especially in long courses of treatment. Some individuals have developed positive direct Coombs' tests during treatment with the cephalosporin antibiotics.

Liver: Transient rise in SGOT, SGPT, and alkaline phosphatase levels has been noted.

Kidney: Decreased creatinine clearance has been reported in patients with prior renal impairment. As with some other cephalosporins, transitory elevations of BUN have occasionally been observed with Mandol; their frequency increases in patients over 50 years of age. In some of these cases, there was also a mild increase in serum creatinine.

Local Reactions: Pain on intramuscular injection is infrequent. Thrombophlebitis occurs rarely.

DOSAGE AND ADMINISTRATION

ADULTS

The usual dosage range for cefamandole is 500 mg to 1 g every 4-8 hours.

In infections of skin structures and in uncomplicated pneumonia, a dosage of 500 mg every 6 hours is adequate.

In uncomplicated urinary tract infections, a dosage of 500 mg every 8 hours is sufficient. In more serious urinary tract infections, a dosage of 1 g every 8 hours may be needed.

In severe infections, 1 g doses may be given at 4-6 hour intervals.

In life-threatening infections or infections due to less susceptible organisms, doses up to 2 g every 4 hours (*i.e.,* 12 g/day) may be needed.

INFANTS AND CHILDREN

Administration of 50-100 mg/kg/day in equally divided doses every 4-8 hours has been effective for most infections susceptible to cefamandole nafate. This may be increased to a total daily dose of 150 mg/kg/day (not to exceed the maximum adult dose) for severe infections. (See WARNINGS and PRECAUTIONS, Usage in Infancy for this age group.)

Note: As with antibiotic therapy in general, administration of cefamandole nafate should be continued for a minimum of 48-72 hours after the patient becomes asymptomatic or after evidence of bacterial eradication has been obtained; a minimum of 10 days of treatment is recommended in infections caused by group A β-hemolytic streptococci in order to guard against the risk or rheumatic fever or glomerulonephritis; frequent bacteriologic and clinical appraisal is necessary during therapy of chronic urinary tract infection and may be required for several months after therapy has been completed; persistent infections may require treatment for several weeks; and doses smaller than those indicated above should not be used.

For perioperative use of cefamandole nafate, the following dosages are recommended:

Adults: 1 or 2 g intravenously or intramuscularly one-half to 1 hour prior to the surgical incision followed by 1 or 2 g every 6 hours for 24-48 hours.

Children (3 months of age and older): 50-100 mg/kg/day in equally divided doses by the routes and schedule designated above.

Note: In patients undergoing prosthetic arthroplasty, administration is recommended for as long as 72 hours.

In patients undergoing cesarean section, the initial dose may be administered just prior surgery or immediately after the cord has been clamped.

IMPAIRED RENAL FUNCTION

When renal function is impaired, a reduced dosage must be employed and the serum levels closely monitored. After an initial dose of 1-2 g (depending on the severity of infection), a maintenance dosage schedule should be followed (see TABLE 1). Continued dosage should be determined by degree of renal impairment, severity of infection, and susceptibility of the causative organism.

TABLE 1 *Maintenance Dosage Guide for Patients With Renal Impairment*

Creatinine Clearance (ml/min/1.73 m^2)	Renal Function	Life-Threatening Maximum Dosage	Less Severe Infections
>80	Normal	2 g q4h	1-2 g q6h
80-50	Mild impairment	1.5 g q4h OR 2 g q6h	0.75-1.5 g q6h
50-25	Moderate impairment	1.5 g q6h OR 2 g q8h	0.75-1.5 g q8h
25-10	Severe impairment	1 g q6h OR 1.25 g q8h	0.5 -1 g q8h
10-2	Marked impairment	0.67 g q8h OR 1 g q12h	0.5-0.75 g q12h
<2	None	0.5 g q8h OR 0.75 g q12h	0.25-0.5 g q12h

When only serum creatinine is available, the following formula (based on sex, weight, and age of the patient) may be used to convert this value into creatinine clearance. The serum creatinine should represent a steady state of renal function.

Males: [Weight (kg) × (140 - age)] ÷ [72 × serum creatinine]

Females: 0.9 × above value

MODES OF ADMINISTRATION

Cefamandole nafate may be given intravenously or by deep intramuscular injection into a large muscle mass (such as the gluteus or lateral part of the thigh) to minimize pain.

INTRAMUSCULAR ADMINISTRATION

Each gram of cefamandole nafate should be diluted with 3 ml of one of the following diluents: Sterile water for injection, bacteriostatic water for injection, 0.9% sodium chloride injection, or bacteriostatic sodium chloride injection. Shake well until dissolved.

INTRAVENOUS ADMINISTRATION

The intravenous route may be preferable for patients with bacterial septicemia, localized parenchymal abscesses (such as intra-abdominal abscess), peritonitis, or other severe or life-threatening infections when they may be poor risks because of lowered resistance. In those with normal renal function, the intravenous dosage for such infections is 3-12 g of cefamandole nafate daily. In conditions such as bacterial septicemia, 6-12 g/day may be given initially by the intravenous route for several days, and dosage may then be gradually reduced according to clinical response and laboratory findings.

If combination therapy with cefamandole nafate and an aminoglycoside is indicated, each of these antibiotics should be administered in different sites.*Do not mix an aminoglycoside with cefamandole nafate in the same intravenous fluid container.*

A SOLUTION OF 1 g OF CEFAMANDOLE NAFATE IN 22 ml OF STERILE WATER FOR INJECTION IS ISOTONIC.

The choice of saline, dextrose, or electrolyte solution and the volume to be employed are dictated by fluid and electrolyte management.

For direct intermittent intravenous administration, each gram of cefamandole should be reconstituted with 10 ml of sterile water for injection, 5% dextrose injection, or 0.9% sodium chloride injection. Slowly inject the solution into the vein over a period of 3-5 minutes, or give it through the tubing of an administration set while the patient is also receiving one of the following intravenous fluids:

0.9% Sodium chloride injection; 5% dextrose injection; 10% dextrose injection; 5% dextrose and 0.9% sodium chloride injection; 5% dextrose and 0.45% sodium chloride injection; 5% dextrose and 0.2% sodium chloride injection; or sodium lactate injection (M/6).

Intermittent intravenous infusion with a Y-type administration set or volume control set can also be accomplished while any of the above-mentioned intravenous fluids are being infused. However, during infusion of the solution containing Mandol, it is desirable to discontinue the other solution. When this technique is employed, careful attention should be paid to the volume of the solution containing cefamandole nafate so that the calculated dose will be infused. When a Y-tube hookup is used, 100 ml of the appropriate diluent should be added to the 1 or 2 g piggyback (100 ml) vial. If sterile water for injection is used as the diluent, reconstitute with approximately 20 ml/g to avoid a hypotonic solution.

For continuous intravenous infusion, each gram of cefamandole should be diluted with 10 ml of sterile water for injection. An appropriate quantity of the resulting solution may be added to an IV bottle containing one of the following fluids:

0.9% Sodium chloride injection; 5% dextrose injection; 10% dextrose injection; 5% dextrose and 0.9% sodium chloride injection; 5% dextrose and 0.45% sodium chloride injection; 5% dextrose and 0.2% sodium chloride injection; or sodium lactate injection (M/6).

STABILITY

Reconstituted cefamandole nafate is stable for 24 hours at room temperature (25°C) and for 96 hours if stored under refrigeration (5°C). *During storage at room temperature, carbon dioxide develops inside the vial after reconstitution. This pressure may be dissipated prior to withdrawal of the vial contents, or it may be used to aid withdrawal if the vial is inverted over the syringe needle and the contents are allowed to flow into the syringe.*

Solutions of cefamandole nafate in sterile water for injection, 5% dextrose injection, or 0.9% sodium chloride injection that are frozen immediately after reconstitution in Faspak containers and the conventional vials in which the drugs are supplied are stable for 6 months when stored at -20°C. **If the product is warmed (to a maximum of 37°C), care should be taken to avoid heating it after the thawing is complete. Once thawed, the solution should not be refrozen.**

PRODUCT LISTING - EQUIVALENTS NOT AVAILABLE

Powder For Injection - Injectable - 1 Gm

1's	$9.59	MANDOL, Lilly, Eli and Company	00002-7268-01
10's	$9.06	MANDOL, Lilly, Eli and Company	00002-7061-01
10's	$9.73	MANDOL, Lilly, Eli and Company	00002-7068-01
25's	$226.62	MANDOL, Lilly, Eli and Company	00002-7061-25

25's	$239.70	MANDOL, Lilly, Eli and Company	00002-7068-25
Powder For Injection - Injectable - 2 Gm			
1's	$18.65	MANDOL, Lilly, Eli and Company	00002-7269-01
1's	$18.80	MANDOL, Lilly, Eli and Company	00002-7069-01
10's	$181.30	MANDOL, Lilly, Eli and Company	00002-7064-10
10's	$188.00	MANDOL, Lilly, Eli and Company	00002-7069-10
20's	$18.13	MANDOL, Lilly, Eli and Company	00002-7064-01
Powder For Injection - Injectable - 10 Gm			
1's	$90.65	MANDOL, Lilly, Eli and Company	00002-7072-01

C

Cefazolin Sodium *(000683)*

For related information, see the comparative table section in Appendix A.

Categories: Endocarditis; Epididymitis; Infection, biliary tact; Infection, bone; Infection, genital tract; Infection, joint; Infection, respiratory tract; Infection, skin and skin structures; Infection, urinary tract; Prophylaxis, perioperative; Prostatitis; Septicemia; Pregnancy Category B; FDA Approved 1973 Nov

Drug Classes: Antibiotics, cephalosporins

Brand Names: Ancef; Cefazolin; Kefzol; Zolicef

Foreign Brand Availability: Anzolin (India); Basocef (Germany); Biozolin (Indonesia); Cefa (Taiwan); Cefacidal (Belgium; Ecuador; France; Peru; South-Africa); Cefamezin (Hong-Kong; Indonesia; Israel; Japan; Korea; Portugal; South-Africa; Spain; Thailand); Cefarad (Bahrain; Benin; Burkina-Faso; Cyprus; Egypt; Ethiopia; Gambia; Ghana; Guinea; Iran; Iraq; Ivory-Coast; Jordan; Kenya; Kuwait; Lebanon; Liberia; Libya; Malawi; Mali; Mauritania; Mauritius; Morocco; Niger; Nigeria; Oman; Qatar; Republic-of-Yemen; Saudi-Arabia; Senegal; Seychelles; Sierra-Leone; Sudan; Syria; Tanzania; Tunia; Uganda; United-Arab-Emirates; Zambia; Zimbabwe); Cefazin (Taiwan); Cefazol (Bulgaria; Indonesia; Thailand); Cefazolina (Spain); Cefazoline Panpharma (France); Faxilen (Philippines); Fazolin (Thailand); Fonvicol (Philippines); Gramaxin (Austria); Izacef (South-Africa); Kefarin (Greece); Kefazin (Israel); Kofatol (Taiwan); Lupex (Philippines); Megacef (Philippines); Oricef (Taiwan); Orizolin (Benin; Burkina-Faso; Ethiopia; Gambia; Ghana; Guinea; Ivory-Coast; Kenya; Liberia; Malawi; Mali; Mauritania; Morocco; Niger; Nigeria; Senegal; Seychelles; Sierra-Leone; Sudan; Tanzania; Tunia; Uganda; Zambia; Zimbabwe); Reflin (India); Sanzol (Philippines); Stancef (Philippines); Stazolin (Taiwan); Totacef (Israel); Surzolin (India); Uzolin (Taiwan); Zolecef (Bahrain; Cyprus; Egypt; Iran; Iraq; Jordan; Kuwait; Lebanon; Libya; Oman; Qatar; Republic-of-Yemen; Saudi-Arabia; Syria; United-Arab-Emirates); Zolin (Italy)

Cost of Therapy: $78.75 (Infection; Ancef Injection; 1 g; 3 g/day; 10 day supply)
$49.69 (Infection; Generic Injection; 1 g; 3 g/day; 10 day supply)

HCFA JCODE(S): J0690 up to 500 mg IV, IM

DESCRIPTION

Note: The trade name has been used throughout this monograph for clarity.

Cefazolin sodium is a semi-synthetic cephalosporin for parenteral administration. It is the sodium salt of 3-{[(5-methyl-1,3,4-thiadiazol-2-yl)thio]-methyl}-8-oxo-7-[2-(1H-tetrazol-1-yl)acetamido]-5-thia-1-azabicyclo[4.2.0]oct-2-ene-2-carboxylic acid.

The sodium content is 48 mg per gram of cefazolin.

ANCEF

Ancef in lyophilized form is supplied in vials equivalent to 500 mg or 1 g of cefazolin; in "Piggyback" vials for intravenous admixture equivalent to 1 g of cefazolin; and in pharmacy bulk vials equivalent to 10 g of cefazolin.

Ancef is also supplied as a frozen, sterile, nonpyrogenic solution of cefazolin sodium in an iso-osmotic diluent in plastic containers. After thawing, the solution is intended for intravenous use.

The plastic container is fabricated from a specially designed multilayer plastic, PL 2040. Solutions are in contact with the polyethylene layer of this container and can leach out certain of the chemical components of the plastic in very small amounts within the expiration period. However, the suitability of the plastic has been confirmed in tests in animals according to the USP biological tests for plastic containers as well as by tissue culture toxicity studies.

DUPLEX DRUG DELIVERY SYSTEM

Cefazolin for injection and dextrose injection is a sterile, nonpyrogenic, single use, packaged combination of cefazolin sodium (lyophilized) and sterile iso-osmotic diluent in the Duplex sterile container. The Duplex container is a flexible dual chamber container.

After reconstitution the approximate osmolality for cefazolin for injection and dextrose injection is 290 mOsmol/kg.

The diluent chamber contains dextrose injection, an iso-osmotic diluent using hydrous dextrose in water for injection. Dextrose injection is sterile, nonpyrogenic, and contains no bacteriostatic or antimicrobial agents.

Cefazolin sodium is supplied as a lyophilized form equivalent to either 500 mg or 1 g of cefazolin. Dextrose hydrous has been added to the diluent to adjust osmolality (approximately 2.4 g and 2 g to 500 mg and 1 g dosages, respectively).

After removing the peelable foil strip, activating the seals, and thoroughly mixing, the reconstituted drug product is intended for single intravenous use.

The Duplex dual chamber container is made from a specially formulated material. The product (diluent and drug) contact layer is a mixture of thermoplastic rubber and a polypropylene ethylene copolymer that contains no plasticizers. The safety of the container system is supported by biological evaluation procedures.

CLINICAL PHARMACOLOGY

HUMAN PHARMACOLOGY

After intramuscular administration of Ancef to normal volunteers, the mean serum concentrations were 37 µg/ml at 1 hour and 3 µg/ml at 8 hours following a 500 mg dose, and 64 µg/ml at 1 hour and 7 µg/ml at 8 hours following a 1 g dose.

Studies have shown that following intravenous administration of Ancef to normal volunteers, mean serum concentrations peaked at approximately 185 µg/ml and were approximately 4 µg/ml at 8 hours for a 1 g dose.

The serum half-life for Ancef is approximately 1.8 hours following IV administration and approximately 2.0 hours following IM administration.

In a study (using normal volunteers) of constant intravenous infusion with dosages of 3.5 mg/kg for 1 hour (approximately 250 mg) and 1.5 mg/kg the next 2 hours (approximately 100 mg), Ancef produced a steady serum level at the third hour of approximately 28 µg/ml.

Studies in patients hospitalized with infections indicate that Ancef produces mean peak serum levels approximately equivalent to those seen in normal volunteers.

Bile levels in patients without obstructive biliary disease can reach or exceed serum levels by up to 5 times; however, in patients with obstructive biliary disease, bile levels of Ancef are considerably lower than serum levels (<1.0 µg/ml).

In synovial fluid, the Ancef level becomes comparable to that reached in serum at about 4 hours after drug administration.

Studies of cord blood show prompt transfer of Ancef across the placenta. Ancef is present in very low concentrations in the milk of nursing mothers.

Ancef is excreted unchanged in the urine. In the first 6 hours approximately 60% of the drug is excreted in the urine and this increases to 70-80% within 24 hours. Ancef achieves peak urine concentrations of approximately 2400 µg/ml and 4000 µg/ml respectively following 500 mg and 1 g intramuscular doses.

In patients undergoing peritoneal dialysis (2 L/h), Ancef produced mean serum levels of approximately 10 and 30 µg/ml after 24 hours' instillation of a dialyzing solution containing 50 mg/L and 150 mg/L, respectively. Mean peak levels were 29 µg/ml (range 13-44 µg/ml) with 50 mg/L (3 patients), and 72 µg/ml (range 26-142 µg/ml) with 150 mg/L (6 patients). Intraperitoneal administration of Ancef is usually well tolerated.

Controlled studies on adult normal volunteers, receiving 1 g 4 times a day for 10 days, monitoring CBC, SGOT, SGPT, bilirubin, alkaline phosphatase, BUN, creatinine and urinalysis, indicated no clinically significant changes attributed to Ancef.

MICROBIOLOGY

In vitro tests demonstrate that the bactericidal action of cephalosporins results from inhibition of cell wall synthesis. Ancef is active against the following organisms *in vitro* and in clinical infections:

- *Staphylococcus aureus* (including penicillinase-producing strains)
- *Staphylococcus epidermidis*
- Methicillin-resistant staphylococci are uniformly resistant to cefazolin
- Group A beta-hemolytic streptococci and other strains of streptococci (many strains of enterococci are resistant)
- *Streptococcus pneumoniae*
- *Escherichia coli*
- *Proteus mirabilis*
- *Klebsiella species*
- *Enterobacter aerogenes*
- *Haemophilus influenzae*

Most strains of indole positive Proteus (*Proteus vulgaris*), *Enterobacter cloacae, Morganella morganii* and *Providencia rettgeri* are resistant. *Serratia, Pseudomonas, Mima, Herellea* species are almost uniformly resistant to cefazolin.

DISK SUSCEPTIBILITY TESTS

Disk Diffusion Technique

Quantitative methods that require measurement of zone diameters give the most precise estimates of antibiotic susceptibility. One such procedure[1] has been recommended for use with disks to test susceptibility to cefazolin.

Reports from a laboratory using the standardized single-disk susceptibility test[1] with a 30 µg cefazolin disk should be interpreted according to the following criteria:

Susceptible organisms produce zones of 18 mm or greater, indicating that the tested organism is likely to respond to therapy.

Organisms of intermediate susceptibility produce zones 15-17 mm, indicating that the tested organism would be susceptible if high dosage is used or if the infection is confined to tissues and fluids (*e.g.,* urine), in which high antibiotic levels are attained.

Resistant organisms produce zones of 14 mm or less, indicating that other therapy should be selected.

For gram-positive isolates, a zone of 18 mm is indicative of a cefazolin-susceptible organism when tested with either the cephalosporin-class disk (30 µg cephalothin) or the cefazolin disk (30 µg cefazolin).

Gram-negative organisms should be tested with the cefazolin disk (using the above criteria), since cefazolin has been shown by *in vitro* tests to have activity against certain strains of *Enterobacteriaceae* found resistant when tested with the cephalothin disk. Gram-negative organisms having zones of less than 18 mm around the cephalothin disk may be susceptible to cefazolin.

Standardized procedures require use of control organisms. The 30 µg cefazolin disk should give zone diameter between 23 and 29 mm for *E. coli* ATCC 25922 and between 29 and 35 mm for *S. aureus* ATCC 25923.

The cefazolin disk should not be used for testing susceptibility to other cephalosporins.

Dilution Techniques

A bacterial isolate may be considered susceptible if the minimal inhibitory concentration (MIC) for cefazolin is not more than 16 µg/ml. Organisms are considered resistant if the MIC is equal to or greater than 64 µg/ml.

The range of MIC's for the control strains are as follows:

S. aureus ATCC 25923, 0.25-1.0 µg/ml
E. coli ATCC 25922, 1.0-4.0 µg/ml

INDICATIONS AND USAGE

Ancef is indicated in the treatment of the following serious infections due to susceptible organisms:

RESPIRATORY TRACT INFECTIONS due to *Streptococcus pneumoniae, Klebsiella* species, *Haemophilus influenzae, Staphylococcus aureus* (penicillin-sensitive and penicillin-resistant) and group A beta-hemolytic streptococci.

Injectable benzathine penicillin is considered to be the drug of choice in treatment and prevention of streptococcal infections, including the prophylaxis of rheumatic fever.

Ancef is effective in the eradication of streptococci from the nasopharynx; however, data establishing the efficacy of Ancef in the subsequent prevention of rheumatic fever are not available at present.

URINARY TRACT INFECTIONS due to *Escherichia coli, Proteus mirabilis, Klebsiella* species and some strains of *Enterobacter* and enterococci.

SKIN AND SKIN STRUCTURE INFECTIONS due to *Staphylococcus aureus* (penicillin-sensitive and penicillin-resistant), group A beta-hemolytic streptococci and other strains of streptococci.

BILIARY TRACT INFECTIONS due to *Escherichia coli,* various strains of streptococci, *Proteus mirabilis, Klebsiella* species and *Staphylococcus aureus.*

BONE AND JOINT INFECTIONS due to *Staphylococcus aureus.*

GENITAL INFECTIONS (*i.e.*, prostatitis, epididymitis) due to *Escherichia coli, Proteus mirabilis, Klebsiella* species and some strains of enterococci.

SEPTICEMIA due to *Streptococcus pneumoniae, Staphylococcus aureus* (penicillin-sensitive and penicillin-resistant), *Proteus mirabilis, Escherichia coli* and *Klebsiella* species.

ENDOCARDITIS due to *Staphylococcus aureus* (penicillin-sensitive and penicillin-resistant) and group A beta-hemolytic streptococci.

Appropriate culture and susceptibility studies should be performed to determine susceptibility of the causative organism to Ancef.

PERIOPERATIVE PROPHYLAXIS

The prophylactic administration of Ancef preoperatively, intraoperatively and postoperatively may reduce the incidence of certain postoperative infections in patients undergoing surgical procedures which are classified as contaminated or potentially contaminated (*e.g.,* vaginal hysterectomy, and cholecystectomy in high-risk patients such as those over 70 years of age, with acute cholecystitis, obstructive jaundice or common duct bile stones).

The perioperative use of Ancef may also be effective in surgical patients in whom infection at the operative site would present a serious risk (*e.g.,* during open-heart surgery and prosthetic arthroplasty).

The prophylactic administration of Ancef should usually be discontinued within a 24 hour period after the surgical procedure. In surgery where the occurrence of infection may be particularly devastating (*e.g.,* open-heart surgery and prosthetic arthroplasty), the prophylactic administration of Ancef may be continued for 3-5 days following the completion of surgery.

If there are signs of infection, specimens for cultures should be obtained for the identification of the causative organism so that appropriate therapy may be instituted. (See DOSAGE AND ADMINISTRATION.)

CONTRAINDICATIONS

ANCEF IS CONTRAINDICATED IN PATIENTS WITH KNOWN ALLERGY TO THE CEPHALOSPORIN GROUP OF ANTIBIOTICS.

WARNINGS

BEFORE THERAPY WITH ANCEF IS INSTITUTED, CAREFUL INQUIRY SHOULD BE MADE TO DETERMINE WHETHER THE PATIENT HAS HAD PREVIOUS HYPERSENSITIVITY REACTIONS TO CEFAZOLIN, CEPHALOSPORINS, PENICILLINS, OR OTHER DRUGS. IF THIS PRODUCT IS GIVEN TO PENICILLIN-SENSITIVE PATIENTS, CAUTION SHOULD BE EXERCISED BECAUSE CROSS-HYPERSENSITIVITY AMONG BETA-LACTAM ANTIBIOTICS HAS BEEN CLEARLY DOCUMENTED AND MAY OCCUR IN UP TO 10% OF PATIENTS WITH A HISTORY OF PENICILLIN ALLERGY. IF AN ALLERGIC REACTION TO ANCEF OCCURS, DISCONTINUE TREATMENT WITH THE DRUG. SERIOUS ACUTE HYPERSENSITIVITY REACTIONS MAY REQUIRE TREATMENT WITH EPINEPHRINE AND OTHER EMERGENCY MEASURES, INCLUDING OXYGEN, IV FLUIDS, IV ANTIHISTAMINES, CORTICOSTEROIDS, PRESSOR AMINES AND AIRWAY MANAGEMENT, AS CLINICALLY INDICATED.

Pseudomembranous colitis has been reported with nearly all antibacterial agents, including cefazolin, and may range in severity from mild to life-threatening. Therefore, it is important to consider this diagnosis in patients who present with diarrhea subsequent to the administration of antibacterial agents.

Treatment with antibacterial agents alters the normal flora of the colon and may permit overgrowth of clostridia. Studies indicate that a toxin produced by *Clostridium difficile* is a primary cause of "antibiotic-associated colitis".

After the diagnosis of pseudomembranous colitis has been established, therapeutic measures should be initiated. Mild cases of pseudomembranous colitis usually respond to drug discontinuation alone. In moderate to severe cases, consideration should be given to management with fluids and electrolytes, protein supplementation and treatment with an oral antibacterial drug clinically effective against *C. difficile* colitis.

PRECAUTIONS

GENERAL

Prolonged use of Ancef may result in the overgrowth of nonsusceptible organisms. Careful clinical observation of the patient is essential.

When Ancef is administered to patients with low urinary output because of impaired renal function, lower daily dosage is required (see DOSAGE AND ADMINISTRATION).

As with other beta-lactam antibiotics, seizures may occur if inappropriately high doses are administered to patients with impaired renal function (see DOSAGE AND ADMINISTRATION).

Ancef, as with all cephalosporins, should be prescribed with caution in individuals with a history of gastrointestinal disease, particularly colitis.

DRUG/LABORATORY TEST INTERACTIONS

A false positive reaction for glucose in the urine may occur with Benedict's solution, Fehling's solution or with Clinitest tablets, but not with enzyme-based tests such as Clinistix and Tes-Tape.

Positive direct and indirect antiglobulin (Coombs) tests have occurred; these may also occur in neonates whose mothers received cephalosporins before delivery.

CARCINOGENESIS/MUTAGENESIS

Mutagenicity studies and long-term studies in animals to determine the carcinogenic potential of Ancef have not been performed.

PREGNANCY, TERATOGENIC EFFECTS, PREGNANCY CATEGORY B

Reproduction studies have been performed in rats, mice and rabbits at doses up to 25 times the human dose and have revealed no evidence of impaired fertility or harm to the fetus due to Ancef. There are, however, no adequate and well-controlled studies in pregnant women. Because animal reproduction studies are not always predictive of human response, this drug should be used during pregnancy only if clearly needed.

LABOR AND DELIVERY

When cefazolin has been administered prior to caesarean section, drug levels in cord blood have been approximately one-quarter to one-third of maternal drug levels. The drug appears to have no adverse effect on the fetus.

NURSING MOTHERS

Ancef is present in very low concentrations in the milk of nursing mothers. Caution should be exercised when Ancef is administered to a nursing woman.

PEDIATRIC USE

Safety and effectiveness for use in premature infants and neonates have not been established. See DOSAGE AND ADMINISTRATION for recommended dosage in pediatric patients over 1 month.

The potential for the toxic effect in pediatric patients from chemicals that may leach from the single-dose IV preparation in plastic has not been determined.

DRUG INTERACTIONS

Probenecid may decrease renal tubular secretion of cephalosporins when used concurrently, resulting in increased and more prolonged cephalosporin blood levels.

ADVERSE REACTIONS

The following reactions have been reported:

Gastrointestinal: Diarrhea, oral candidiasis (oral thrush), vomiting, nausea, stomach cramps, anorexia and pseudomembranous colitis. Onset of pseudomembranous colitis symptoms may occur during or after antibiotic treatment (see WARNINGS). Nausea and vomiting have been reported rarely.

Allergic: Anaphylaxis, eosinophilia, itching, drug fever, skin rash, Stevens-Johnson syndrome.

Hematologic: Neutropenia, leukopenia, thrombocytopenia, thrombocythemia.

Hepatic and Renal: Transient rise in SGOT, SGPT, BUN and alkaline phosphatase levels has been observed without clinical evidence of renal or hepatic impairment.

Local Reactions: Rare instances of phlebitis have been reported at site of injection. Pain at the site of injection after intramuscular administration has occurred infrequently. Some induration has occurred.

Other Reactions: Genital and anal pruritus (including vulvar pruritus, genital moniliasis and vaginitis).

DOSAGE AND ADMINISTRATION

ANCEF

Usual Adult Dosage

Moderate to severe infections: 500 mg to 1 g every 6-8 hours.

Mild infections caused by susceptible gram + cocci: 250-500 mg every 8 hours.

Acute, uncomplicated urinary tract infections: 1 g every 12 hours.

Pneumococcal pneumonia: 500 mg every 12 hours.

Severe, life-threatening infections* (e.g., endocarditis, septicemia): 1-1.5 g every 6 hours.

*In rare instances, doses of up to 12 g of Ancef per day have been used.

Perioperative Prophylactic Use

To prevent postoperative infection in contaminated or potentially contaminated surgery, recommended doses are:

- 1 g IV or IM administered ½ to 1 hour prior to the start of surgery.
- For lengthy operative procedures (*e.g.,* 2 hours or more), 500 mg to 1 g IV or IM during surgery (administration modified depending on the duration of the operative procedure).
- 500 mg to 1 g IV or IM every 6-8 hours for 24 hours postoperatively.

It is important that (1) the preoperative dose be given just (½ to 1 hour) prior to the start of surgery so that adequate antibiotic levels are present in the serum and tissues at the time of initial surgical incision; and (2) Ancef be administered, if necessary, at appropriate intervals during surgery to provide sufficient levels of the antibiotic at the anticipated moments of greatest exposure to infective organisms.

In surgery where the occurrence of infection may be particularly devastating (*e.g.,* open-heart surgery and prosthetic arthroplasty), the prophylactic administration of Ancef may be continued for 3-5 days following the completion of surgery.

Dosage Adjustment for Patients With Reduced Renal Function

Ancef may be used in patients with reduced renal function with the following dosage adjustments: Patients with a creatinine clearance of 55 ml/min or greater or a serum creatinine of 1.5 mg % or less can be given full doses. Patients with creatinine clearance rates of 35-54 ml/min or serum creatinine of 1.6-3.0 mg % can also be given full doses but dosage should be restricted to at least 8 hour intervals. Patients with creatinine clearance rates of 11-34 ml/min or serum creatinine of 3.1-4.5 mg % should be given ½ the usual dose every 12 hours. Patients with creatinine clearance rates of 10 ml/min or less or serum creatinine of 4.6 mg % or greater should be given ½ the usual dose every 18-24 hours. All reduced dosage recommendations apply after an initial loading dose appropriate to the severity of the infection. Patients undergoing peritoneal dialysis: See CLINICAL PHARMACOLOGY, Human Pharmacology.

Pediatric Dosage

In pediatric patients, a total daily dosage of 25-50 mg/kg (approximately 10-20 mg/lb) of body weight, divided into 3 or 4 equal doses, is effective for most mild to moderately severe infections. Total daily dosage may be increased to 100 mg/kg (45 mg/lb) of body weight for severe infections. Since safety for use in premature infants and in neonates has not been established, the use of Ancef in these patients is not recommended.

C

TABLE 1 *Pediatric Dosage Guide — 25 mg/kg/day*

Weight		Divided into 3 Doses		Divided into 4 Doses	
lb	kg	App. Single Dose	Vol. needed with dilution of 125 mg/ml	App. Single Dose	Vol. needed with dilution of 125 mg/ml
10	4.5	40 mg	0.35 ml	30 mg	0.25 ml
20	9.0	75 mg	0.60 ml	55 mg	0.45 ml
30	13.6	115 mg	0.90 ml	85 mg	0.70 ml
40	18.1	150 mg	1.20 ml	115 mg	0.90 ml
50	22.7	190 mg	1.50 ml	140 mg	1.10 ml

TABLE 2 *Pediatric Dosage Guide — 50 mg/kg/day*

Weight		Divided into 3 Doses		Divided into 4 Doses	
lb	kg	App. Single Dose	Vol. needed with dilution of 225 mg/ml	App. Single Dose	Vol. needed with dilution of 225 mg/ml
10	4.5	75 mg	0.35 ml	55 mg	0.25 ml
20	9.0	150 mg	0.70 ml	110 mg	0.50 ml
30	13.6	225 mg	1.00 ml	170 mg	0.75 ml
40	18.1	300 mg	1.35 ml	225 mg	1.00 ml
50	22.7	375 mg	1.70 ml	285 mg	1.25 ml

In pediatric patients with mild to moderate renal impairment (creatinine clearance of 70 to 40 ml/min), 60% of the normal daily dose given in equally divided doses every 12 hours should be sufficient. In patients with moderate impairment (creatinine clearance of 40 to 20 ml/min), 25% of the normal daily dose given in equally divided doses every 12 hours should be adequate. Pediatric patients with severe renal impairment (creatinine clearance of 20 to 5 ml/min) may be given 10% of the normal daily dose every 24 hours. All dosage recommendations apply after an initial loading dose.

Reconstitution — Preparation of Parenteral Solution

Parenteral drug products should be SHAKEN WELL when reconstituted, and inspected visually for particulate matter prior to administration. If particulate matter is evident in reconstituted fluids, the drug solutions should be discarded.

When reconstituted or diluted according to the instructions below, Ancef is stable for 24 hours at room temperature or for 10 days if stored under refrigeration (5°C or 41°F). Reconstituted solutions may range in color from pale yellow to yellow without a change in potency.

Administration

Intramuscular Administration

Reconstitute vials with sterile water for injection according to the dilution table. Shake well until dissolved. Ancef should be injected into a large muscle mass. Pain on injection is infrequent with Ancef.

Intravenous Administration

Direct (bolus) injection: Following reconstitution according to the dilution table, further dilute vials with approximately 5 ml sterile water for injection. Inject the solution slowly over 3-5 minutes, directly or through tubing for patients receiving parenteral fluids (see list below).

Intermittent or continuous infusion: Dilute reconstituted Ancef in 50-100 ml of one of the following solutions:

Sodium chloride injection, 5% or 10% dextrose injection, 5% dextrose in lactated Ringer's injection, 5% dextrose and 0.9% sodium chloride injection, 5% dextrose and 0.45% sodium chloride injection, 5% dextrose and 0.2% sodium chloride injection, lactated Ringer's injection, invert sugar 5% or 10% in sterile water for injection, Ringer's injection, 5% sodium bicarbonate injection.

Directions for use of Ancef Galaxy Container

Ancef in Galaxy Container (PL 2040 Plastic) is to be administered either as a continuous or intermittent infusion using sterile equipment.

Storage: Store in a freezer capable of maintaining a temperature of -20°C (-4°F).

Thawing of Plastic Container: Thaw frozen container at 25°C or 77°F or under refrigeration (5°C or 41°F). (DO NOT FORCE THAW BY IMMERSION IN WATER BATHS OR BY MICROWAVE IRRADIATION.)

Check for minute leaks by squeezing container firmly. If leaks are detected, discard solution as sterility may be impaired.

Do not add supplementary medication.

The container should be visually inspected. Components of the solution may precipitate in the frozen state and will dissolve upon reaching room temperature with little or no agitation. Potency is not affected. Agitate after solution has reached room temperature. If after visual inspection the solution remains cloudy or if an insoluble precipitate is noted or if any seals or outlet ports are not intact, the container should be discarded.

The thawed solution is stable for 30 days under refrigeration (5°C or 41°F) and 48 hours at 25°C or 77°F. Do not refreeze thawed antibiotics.

Use sterile equipment. It is recommended that the intravenous administration apparatus be replaced at least once every 48 hours.

CAUTION: Do not use plastic containers in series connections. Such use could result in air embolism due to residual air being drawn from the primary container before administration of the fluid from the secondary container is complete.

Preparation for Administration:

1. Suspend container from eyelet support.
2. Remove plastic protector from outlet port at bottom of container.
3. Attach administration set. Refer to complete directions accompanying set.

ADD-VANTAGE

ADD-Vantage vials of sterile cefazolin sodium are to be reconstituted only with 0.9% sodium chloride injection or 5% dextrose injection in the 50 or 100 ml ADD-Vantage Flexible diluent containers or with 0.45% sodium chloride injection in the 50 ml ADD-Vantage flexible diluent container.

WARNING: Do not use flexible container in series connections.

Compatibility and Stability

Ordinarily ADD-Vantage vials should be reconstituted only when it is certain that the patient is ready to receive the drug. However, sterile cefazolin sodium in ADD-Vantage vials is stable for 24 hours at room temperature when reconstituted as directed.

DUPLEX DRUG DELIVERY SYSTEM

Notes for use:

Protect from light after removal of foil strip.

Note: If foil strip is removed, product must be used within 30 days, but not beyond the labeled expiration date.

Do not use directly after storage by refrigeration, allow the product to equilibrate to room temperature before patient use.

Note: Following reconstitution (activation), product must be used within 24 hours if stored at room temperature or within 7 days if stored under refrigeration.

Precautions:

Do not use in series connection.

Do not introduce additives into the Duplex Container.

Do not freeze.

HOW SUPPLIED

ANCEF

Ancef is supplied in vials equivalent to 500 mg or 1 g of cefazolin; in "Piggyback" vials for intravenous admixture equivalent to 1 g of cefazolin; and in pharmacy bulk vials equivalent to 10 g of cefazolin.

Ancef as a frozen, iso-osmotic, sterile, nonpyrogenic solution in plastic containers - supplied in 50 ml single-dose containers equivalent to 500 mg or 1 g of cefazolin dextrose hydrous, has been added to the above dosages to adjust osmolality (approximately 2.4 g and 2 g, respectively). Store at or below -20°C (-4°F). (See DOSAGE AND ADMINISTRATION, Ancef, Directions for use of Ancef Galaxy Container.)

As with other cephalosporins, Ancef tends to darken depending on storage conditions; within the stated recommendations, however, product potency is not adversely affected.

Storage: Before reconstitution protect from light and store at controlled room temperature 20-25°C (68-77°F).

ADD-VANTAGE

Sterile cefazolin sodium is supplied in ADD-Vantage vials equivalent to 1 g of cefazolin.

Storage: Before reconstitution protect from light and store between 15 and 30°C (59 and 86°F).

DUPLEX DRUG DELIVERY SYSTEM

Cefazolin for injection and dextrose injection in the Duplex drug delivery system is a flexible dual chamber container supplied in two concentrations. After reconstitution, the concentrations are equivalent to 500 mg and 1 g cefazolin. The diluent chamber contains approximately 50 ml of dextrose injection. Dextrose injection has been adjusted to 4.8% and 4.0% for the 500 mg and 1 g doses, respectively, such that the reconstituted solution is iso-osmotic.

Storage: Store the unactivated product at 20-25°C (68-77°F). Excursions permitted to 15-30°C (59-86°F)

PRODUCT LISTING - RATED THERAPEUTICALLY EQUIVALENT

Powder For Injection - Injectable - 1 Gm

1's	$2.83	ANCEF, Glaxosmithkline	00007-3130-01
1's	$3.36	KEFZOL, Lilly, Eli and Company	00002-7266-01
1's	$3.78	ANCEF, Allscripts Pharmaceutical Company	54569-1878-01
1's	$4.13	ANCEF, Abbott Pharmaceutical	00074-3130-01
10's	$19.00	GENERIC, Bristol-Myers Squibb	00015-7339-12
10's	$24.48	GENERIC, Bristol-Myers Squibb	00015-7339-97
10's	$26.64	GENERIC, Bristol-Myers Squibb	00015-7339-31
10's	$33.73	GENERIC, Physicians Total Care	54868-0559-00
10's	$35.00	GENERIC, Bristol-Myers Squibb	00015-7339-99
10's	$39.38	GENERIC, Glaxosmithkline	00007-3137-76
10's	$53.32	ANCEF, Abbott Pharmaceutical	00074-3137-05
10's	$66.54	GENERIC, Geneva Pharmaceuticals	00781-3724-46
10's	$70.00	GENERIC, Ivax Corporation	00182-3048-70
10's	$88.71	GENERIC, American Pharmaceutical Partners	63323-0237-65
10's	$133.25	GENERIC, Faulding Pharmaceutical Company	61703-0329-11
25's	$48.58	GENERIC, Solo Pak Medical Products Inc	39769-0282-10
25's	$68.58	GENERIC, Abbott Pharmaceutical	00074-4732-03
25's	$70.63	ANCEF, Glaxosmithkline	00007-3130-16

25's	$72.00	KEFZOL, Lilly, Eli and Company	00002-1498-25
25's	$84.00	KEFZOL, Lilly, Eli and Company	00002-7266-25
25's	$103.79	GENERIC, Watson/Schein Pharmaceuticals Inc	00364-2465-34
25's	$147.10	GENERIC, Geneva Pharmaceuticals	00781-3157-70
25's	$162.19	GENERIC, American Pharmaceutical Partners	63323-0237-10
Powder For Injection - Injectable - 5 Gm			
10's	$144.38	ANCEF, Glaxosmithkline	00007-3136-05
Powder For Injection - Injectable - 10 Gm			
1's	$10.20	KEFZOL, Lilly, Eli and Company	00002-7014-01
6's	$61.20	KEFZOL, Lilly, Eli and Company	00002-7014-16
10's	$165.63	GENERIC, Bristol-Myers Squibb	00015-7346-39
10's	$172.50	GENERIC, Bristol-Myers Squibb	00015-7346-97
10's	$262.50	ANCEF, Glaxosmithkline	00007-3135-05
10's	$353.20	GENERIC, Geneva Pharmaceuticals	00781-3726-46
10's	$367.13	GENERIC, American Pharmaceutical Partners	63323-0238-61
10's	$375.00	GENERIC, Ivax Corporation	00182-3045-70
10's	$412.40	GENERIC, Faulding Pharmaceutical Company	61703-0330-60
Powder For Injection - Injectable - 20 Gm			
10's	$303.13	GENERIC, American Pharmaceutical Partners	63323-0446-61
Powder For Injection - Injectable - 500 mg			
1's	$11.40	GENERIC, Bristol-Myers Squibb	00015-7338-12
10's	$10.44	GENERIC, Bristol-Myers Squibb	00015-7338-99
10's	$26.52	GENERIC, Marsam Pharmaceuticals Inc	00209-0800-22
10's	$38.00	GENERIC, Solo Pak Medical Products Inc	39769-0281-90
10's	$45.00	GENERIC, Ivax Corporation	00182-3047-70
25's	$32.39	GENERIC, Solo Pak Medical Products Inc	39769-0280-10
25's	$39.38	ANCEF, Glaxosmithkline	00007-3131-76
25's	$47.40	ANCEF, Allscripts Pharmaceutical Company	54569-3067-00
25's	$51.66	ANCEF, Glaxosmithkline	00007-3131-16
25's	$52.23	GENERIC, Watson/Schein Pharmaceuticals Inc	00364-2464-34
25's	$73.68	GENERIC, Geneva Pharmaceuticals	00781-3155-70
25's	$80.94	GENERIC, American Pharmaceutical Partners	63323-0236-10
Solution - Intravenous - 1 Gm/50 ml			
50 ml	$168.00	GENERIC, Baxter Healthcare Corporation	00338-3503-41
Solution - Intravenous - 500 mg/50 ml			
50 ml	$126.00	GENERIC, Baxter Healthcare Corporation	00338-3502-41

PRODUCT LISTING - EQUIVALENTS NOT AVAILABLE

Powder For Injection - Injectable - 1 Gm			
10's	$19.00	GENERIC, Allscripts Pharmaceutical Company	54569-4294-00
10's	$59.89	GENERIC, Vha Supply	00209-1000-92
25's	$103.79	GENERIC, Marsam Pharmaceuticals Inc	00209-0900-24
25's	$103.79	GENERIC, Watson Laboratories Inc	00591-2365-69
Powder For Injection - Injectable - 10 Gm			
10's	$367.88	GENERIC, Vha Supply	00209-1100-92
Powder For Injection - Injectable - 500 mg			
10's	$15.00	GENERIC, Geneva Pharmaceuticals	00781-7338-99
Solution - Intravenous - 1 Gm/50 ml			
50 ml x 24	$136.80	ANCEF, Glaxosmithkline	00007-3143-04
Solution - Intravenous - 500 mg/50 ml			
50 ml x 24	$100.80	ANCEF, Glaxosmithkline	00007-3142-04

Cefdinir *(003366)*

For related information, see the comparative table section in Appendix A.

Categories: Bronchitis, chronic, acute exacerbation; Infection, ear, middle; Infection, lower respiratory tract; Infection, skin and skin structures; Infection, upper respiratory tract; Pharyngitis; Pneumonia, community-acquired; Sinusitis; Tonsillitis; Pregnancy Category B; FDA Approved 1998 Jan

Drug Classes: Antibiotics, cephalosporins

Brand Names: Omnicef

Cost of Therapy: $89.09 (Infection; Omnicef; 300 mg; 2 capsules/day; 10 day supply)

DESCRIPTION

Omnicef capsules and Omnicef for oral suspension contain the active ingredient cefdinir, an extended-spectrum, semisynthetic cehalosporin, for oral administration. Chemically, cefdinir is [6R-[6α,7β(Z)]]-7-[[(2-amino-4-thiazolyl)-(hydroxyimino)acetyl]amino]-3-ethenyl-8-oxo-5-thia-1-azabicy-clo[4.2.0]oct-2-ene-2-carboxylic acid. Cefdinir is a white to slightly brownish-yellow solid. It is slightly soluble in dilute hydrochloric acid and sparingly soluble in 0.1 M pH 7.0 phosphate buffer. The empirical formula is $C_{14}H_{13}N_5O_5S_2$ and the molecular weight is 395.42.

Omnicef capsules contain 300 mg cefdinir and the following inactive ingredients: Carboxymethylcellulose calcium, polyoxyl 40 stearate, magnesium stearate, and silicon dioxide. The capsule shells contain FD&C blue no. 1; FD&C red no. 40; D&C red no. 28; titanium dioxide, gelatin, and sodium lauryl sulfate.

Omnicef oral suspension, after reconstitution, contains 125 mg cefdinir per 5 ml and the following inactive ingredients: Sucrose, citric acid, sodium citrate, sodium benzoate, xanthan gum, guar gum, artificial strawberry and cream flavors; silicon dioxide, and magnesium stearate.

CLINICAL PHARMACOLOGY

PHARMACOKINETICS AND DRUG METABOLISM

Absorption

Oral Bioavailability

Maximal plasma cefdinir concentrations occur 2-4 hours postdose following capsule or suspension administration. Plasma cefdinir concentrations increase with dose, but the increases are less than dose-proportional from 300 mg (7 mg/kg) to 600 mg (14 mg/kg). Following administration of suspension to healthy adults, cefdinir bioavailability is 120% relative to capsules. Estimated bioavailability of cefdinir capsules is 21% following administration of a 300 mg capsule dose, and 16% following administration of a 600 mg capsule dose. Estimated absolute bioavailability of cefdinir suspension is 25%.

Effect of Food

Although the rate (C_{max}) and extent (AUC) of cefdinir absorption from the capsules are reduced by 16% and 10%, respectively, when given with a high-fat meal, the magnitude of these reductions is not likely to be clinically significant. Therefore, cefdinir may be taken without regard to food.

Cefdinir Capsules

Cefdinir plasma concentrations and pharmacokinetic parameter values following administration of single 300 and 600 mg oral doses of cefdinir to adult subjects are presented in TABLE 1.

***TABLE 1** Mean (±SD) Plasma Cefdinir Pharmacokinetic Parameter Values Following Administration of Capsules to Adult Subjects*

Dose	C_{max} (μg/ml)	T_{max} (h)	AUC (μg·h/ml)
300 mg	1.60 (0.55)	2.9 (0.89)	7.05 (2.17)
600 mg	2.87 (1.01)	3.0 (0.66)	11.1 (3.87)

Cefdinir Suspension

Cefdinir plasma concentrations and pharmacokinetic parameter values following administration of single 7 and 14 mg/kg oral doses of cefdinir to pediatric subjects (age 6 months-12 years) are presented in TABLE 2.

***TABLE 2** Mean (±SD) Plasma Cefdinir Pharmacokinetic Parameter Values Following Administration of Suspension to Pediatric Subjects*

Dose	C_{max} (μg/ml)	T_{max} (h)	AUC (μg·h/ml)
7 mg/kg	2.30 (0.65)	2.2 (0.6)	8.31 (2.50)
14 mg/kg	3.86 (0.62)	1.8 (0.4)	13.4 (2.64)

Multiple Dosing

Cefdinir does not accumulate in plasma following once- or twice-daily administration to subjects with normal renal function.

Distribution

The mean volume of distribution (Vd_{area}) of cefdinir in adult subjects is 0.35 L/kg (±0.29); in pediatric subjects (age 6 months-12 years), cefdinir Vd_{area} is 0.67 L/kg (±0.38). Cefdinir is 60% to 70% bound to plasma proteins in both adult and pediatric subjects; binding is independent of concentration.

Skin Blister: In adult subjects, median (range) maximal blister fluid cefdinir concentrations of 0.65 (0.33-1.1) and 1.1 (0.49-1.9) μg/ml were observed 4 to 5 hours following administration of 300 and 600 mg doses, respectively. Mean (±SD) blister C_{max} and AUC(0-∞) values were 48% (±13) and 91% (±18) of corresponding plasma values.

Tonsil Tissue: In adult patients undergoing elective tonsillectomy, respective median tonsil tissue cefdinir concentrations 4 hours after administration of single 300 and 600 mg doses were 0.25 (0.22-0.46) and 0.36 (0.22-0.80) μg/g. Mean tonsil tissue concentrations were 24% (±8) of corresponding plasma concentrations.

Sinus Tissue: In adult patients undergoing elective maxillary and ethmoid sinus surgery, respective median sinus tissue cefdinir concentrations 4 hours after administration of single 300 and 600 mg doses were <0.12 (<0.12 to 0.46) and 0.21 (<0.12 to 2.0) μg/g. Mean sinus tissue concentrations were 16% (±20) of corresponding plasma concentrations.

Lung Tissue: In adult patients undergoing diagnostic bronchoscopy, respective median bronchial mucosa cefdinir concentrations 4 hours after administration of single 300 and 600 mg doses were 0.78 (<0.06 to 1.33) and 1.14 (<0.06 to 1.92) μg/ml, and were 31% (±18) of corresponding plasma concentrations. Respective median epithelial lining fluid concentrations were 0.29 (<0.3 to 4.73) and 0.49 (<0.3 to 0.59) μg/ml, and were 35% (±83) of corresponding plasma concentrations.

Middle Ear Fluid: In 14 pediatric patients with acute bacterial otitis media, respective median middle ear fluid cefdinir concentrations 3 hours after administration of single 7 and 14 mg/kg doses were 0.21 (<0.09 to 0.94) and 0.72 (0.14-1.42) μg/ml. Mean middle ear fluid concentrations were 15% (±15) of corresponding plasma concentrations.

CSF: Data on cefdinir penetration into human cerebrospinal fluid are not available.

Metabolism and Excretion

Cefdinir is not appreciably metabolized. Activity is primarily due to parent drug. Cefdinir is eliminated principally via renal excretion with a mean plasma elimination half-life ($T_{1/2}$) of 1.7 (±0.6) hours. In healthy subjects with normal renal function, renal clearance is 2.0 (±1.0) ml/min/kg, and apparent oral clearance is 11.6 (±6.0) and 15.5 (±5.4) ml/min/kg

C

following doses of 300 and 600 mg, respectively. Mean percent of dose recovered unchanged in the urine following 300 and 600 mg doses is 18.4% (±6.4) and 11.6% (±4.6), respectively. Cefdinir clearance is reduced in patients with renal dysfunction (see Special Populations, Patients With Renal Insufficiency).

Because renal excretion is the predominant pathway of elimination, dosage should be adjusted in patients with markedly compromised renal function or who are undergoing hemodialysis (see DOSAGE AND ADMINISTRATION).

SPECIAL POPULATIONS

Patients With Renal Insufficiency

Cefdinir pharmacokinetics were investigated in 21 adult subjects with varying degrees of renal function. Decreases in cefdinir elimination rate, apparent oral clearance (CL/F), and renal clearance were approximately proportional to the reduction in creatinine clearance (CLCR). As a result, plasma cefdinir concentrations were higher and persisted longer in subjects with renal impairment than in those without renal impairment. In subjects with CLCR between 30 and 60 ml/min, C_{max} and $T_{½}$ increased by approximately 2-fold and AUC by approximately 3-fold. In subjects with CLCR <30 ml/min, C_{max} increased by approximately 2-fold, $T_{½}$ by approximately 5-fold, and AUC by approximately 6-fold. Dosage adjustment is recommended in patients with markedly compromised renal function (creatinine clearance <30 ml/min; see DOSAGE AND ADMINISTRATION).

Hemodialysis

Cefdinir pharmacokinetics were studied in 8 adult subjects undergoing hemodialysis. Dialysis (4 hours duration) removed 63% of cefdinir from the body and reduced apparent elimination $T_{½}$ from 16 (±3.5) to 3.2 (±1.2) hours. Dosage adjustment is recommended in this patient population (see DOSAGE AND ADMINISTRATION).

Hepatic Disease

Because cefdinir is predominantly renally eliminated and not appreciably metabolized, studies in patients with hepatic impairment were not conducted. It is not expected that dosage adjustment will be required in this population.

Geriatric Patients

The effect of age on cefdinir pharmacokinetics after a single 300 mg dose was evaluated in 32 subjects 19 to 91 years of age. Systemic exposure to cefdinir was substantially increased in older subjects (n=16), C_{max} by 44% and AUC by 86%. This increase was due to a reduction in cefdinir clearance. The apparent volume of distribution was also reduced, thus no appreciable alterations in apparent elimination half-life were observed (elderly: 2.2 ± 0.6 hours vs young: 1.8 ± 0.4 hours). Since cefdinir clearance has been shown to be primarily related to changes in renal function rather than age, elderly patients do not require dosage adjustment unless they have markedly compromised renal function (creatinine clearance <30 ml/min, see Patients with Renal Insufficiency).

Gender and Race

The results of a meta-analysis of clinical pharmacokinetics (n=217) indicated no significant impact of either gender or race on cefdinir pharmacokinetics.

MICROBIOLOGY

As with other cephalosporins, bactericidal activity of cefdinir results from inhibition of cell wall synthesis. Cefdinir is stable in the presence of some, but not all, β-lactamase enzymes. As a result, many organisms resistant to penicillins and some cephalosporins are susceptible to cefdinir.

Cefdinir has been shown to be active against most strains of the following microorganisms, both *in vitro* and in clinical infections as described in INDICATIONS AND USAGE.

Aerobic Gram-Positive Microorganisms:

Staphylococcus aureus (including β-lactamase producing strains)
Note: Cefdinir is inactive against methicillin-resistant staphylococci.
Streptococcus pneumoniae (penicillin-susceptible strains only)
Streptococcus pyogenes

Aerobic Gram-Negative Microorganisms:

Haemophilus influenzae (including β-lactamase producing strains)
Haemophilus parainfluenzae (including β-lactamase producing strains)
Moraxella catarrhalis (including β-lactamase producing strains)

The following *in vitro* data are available, **but their clinical significance is unknown.**

Cefdinir exhibits *in vitro* minimum inhibitory concentrations (MICs) of 1 µg/ml or less against (≥90%) strains of the following microorganisms; however, the safety and effectiveness of cefdinir in treating clinical infections due to these microorganisms have not been established in adequate and well-controlled clinical trials.

Aerobic Gram-Positive Microorganisms:

Staphylococcus epidermidis (methicillin-susceptible strains only)
Streptococcus agalactiae
Viridans group *streptococci*
Note: Cefdinir is inactive against *Enterococcus* and methicillin-resistant *Staphylococcus* species.

Aerobic Gram-Negative Microorganisms:

Citrobacter diversus
Escherichia coli
Klebsiella pneumoniae
Proteus mirabilis
Note: Cefdinir is inactive against *Pseudomonas* and *Enterobacter* species.

Susceptibility Tests

Dilution Techniques

Quantitative methods are used to determine antimicrobial minimum inhibitory concentrations (MICs). These MICs provide estimates of the susceptibility of bacteria to antimicrobial compounds. The MICs should be determined using a standardized procedure. Standardized procedures are based on a dilution method[1] (broth or agar) or equivalent with standardized inoculum concentrations and standardized concentrations of cefdinir powder. The MIC values should be interpreted according to the criteria in TABLE 3 and TABLE 4.

For Streptococcus spp.

TABLE 3 *For organisms other than Haemophilus spp. and Streptococcus spp.*

MIC (µg/ml)	Interpretation
≤1	Susceptible (S)
2	Intermediate (I)
≥4	Resistant (R)

TABLE 4 *For Haemophilus spp.**

MIC (µg/ml)	Interpretation†
≤1	Susceptible (S)

* These interpretive standards are applicable only to broth microdilution susceptibility tests with *Haemophilus* spp. using Haemophilus Test Medium (HTM).[1]

† The current absence of data on resistant strains precludes defining any results other than "Susceptible". Strains yielding MIC results suggestive of a "nonsusceptible" category should be submitted to a reference laboratory for further testing.

Streptococcus pneumoniae that are susceptible to penicillin (MIC ≤0.06 µg/ml), or streptococci other than *S. pneumoniae* that are susceptible to penicillin (MIC ≤0.12 µg/ml). can be considered susceptible to cefdinir. Testing of cefdinir against penicillin-intermediate or penicillin-resistant isolates is not recommended. Reliable interpretive criteria for cefdinir are not available.

A report of "Susceptible" indicates that the pathogen is likely to be inhibited if the antimicrobial compound in the blood reaches the concentration usually achievable. A report of "Intermediate" indicates that the result should be considered equivocal, and, if the microorganism is not fully susceptible to alternative, clinically feasible drugs, the test should be repeated. This category implies possible clinical applicability in body sites where the drug is physiologically concentrated or in situations where high dosage of drug can be used. This category also provides a buffer zone which prevents small uncontrolled technical factors from causing major discrepancies in interpretation. A report of "Resistant" indicates that the pathogen is not likely to be inhibited if the antimicrobial compound in the blood reaches the concentrations usually achievable; other therapy should be selected.

Standardized susceptibility test procedures require the use of laboratory control microorganisms to control the technical aspects of laboratory procedures. Standard cefdinir powder should provide the MIC values as shown in TABLE 5.

TABLE 5 *For Streptococcus spp.*

Microorganism	MIC Range (µg/ml)
Escherichia coli ATCC 25922	0.12-0.5
Haemophilus influenzae ATCC 49766	0.12-0.5
Staphylococcus aureus ATCC 29213	0.12-0.5

* This quality control range is applicable only to *H. influenzae* ATCC 49766 tested by a broth microdilution procedure using HTM.

Diffusion Techniques

Quantitative methods that require measurement of zone diameters also provide reproducible estimates of the susceptibility of bacteria to antimicrobial compounds. One such standardized procedure[2] requires the use of standardized inoculum concentrations. This procedure uses paper disks impregnated with 5 µg cefdinir to test the susceptibility of microorganisms to cefdinir.

Reports from the laboratory providing results of the standard single-disk susceptibility test with a 5 µg cefdinir disk should be interpreted according to the criteria in TABLE 6 and TABLE 7.

TABLE 6 *For Organisms Other Than Haemophilus spp. and Streptococcus spp.**

Zone Diameter (mm)	Interpretation
≥20	Susceptible (S)
17-19	Intermediate (I)
≤16	Resistant (R)

* Because certain strains of *Citrobacter, Providencia,* and *Enterobacter* spp. have been reported to give false susceptible results with the cefdinir disk, strains of these genera should not be tested and reported with this disk.

TABLE 7 *For Haemophilus spp.**

Zone Diameter (mm)	Interpretation†
≥20	Susceptible

* These zone diameter standards are applicable only to tests with *Haemophilus* spp. using HTM.[2]

† The current absence of data on resistant strains precludes defining any results other than "Susceptible". Strains yielding MIC results suggestive of a "nonsusceptible" category should be submitted to a reference laboratory for further testing.

For Streptococcus spp.

Isolates of *Streptococcus pneumoniae* should be tested against a 1 µg oxacillin disk. Isolates with oxacillin zone sizes ≥20 mm are susceptible to penicillin and can be considered susceptible to cefdinir. Streptococci other than *S. pneumoniae* should be tested with a 10-unit penicillin disk. Isolates with penicillin zone sizes ≥28 mm are susceptible to penicillin and can be considered susceptible to cefdinir.

Interpretation should be as stated above for results using dilution techniques. Interpretation involves correlation of the diameter obtained in the disk test with the MIC for cefdinir.

As with standardized dilution techniques, diffusion methods require the use of laboratory control microorganisms to control the technical aspects of laboratory procedures. For the diffusion technique, the 5 μg cefdinir disk should provide the following zone diameters in these laboratory quality control strains (see TABLE 8).

TABLE 8 *For Streptococcus spp.*

Organism	Zone Diameter (mm)
Escherichia coli ATCC 25922	24-28
Haemophilus influenzae ATCC 49766*	24-31
Staphylococcus aureus ATCC 25923	25-32

* This quality control range is applicable only to testing of *H. influenzae* ATCC 49766 using HTM.

INDICATIONS AND USAGE

Cefdinir capsules and cefdinir for oral suspension are indicated for the treatment of patients with mild to moderate infections caused by susceptible strains of the designated microorganisms in the conditions listed below.

ADULTS AND ADOLESCENTS

Community-Acquired Pneumonia caused by *Haemophilus influenzae* (including β-lactamase producing strains), *Haemophilus parainfluenzae* (including β-lactamase producing strains), *Streptococcus pneumoniae* (penicillin-susceptible strains only), and *Moraxella catarrhalis* (including β-lactamase producing strains).

Acute Exacerbations of Chronic Bronchitis caused by *Haemophilus influenzae* (including β-lactamase producing strains), *Haemophilus parainfluenzae* (including β-lactamase producing strains), *Streptococcus pneumoniae* (penicillin-susceptible strains only), and *Moraxella catarrhalis* (including β-lactamase producing strains).

Acute Maxillary Sinusitis caused by *Haemophilus influenzae* (including β-lactamase producing strains), *Streptococcus pneumoniae* (penicillin-susceptible strains only), and *Moraxella catarrhalis* (including β-lactamase producing strains).

Note: For information on use in pediatric patients, see PRECAUTIONS, Pediatric Use and DOSAGE AND ADMINISTRATION.

Pharyngitis/Tonsillitis caused by *Streptococcus pyogenes.*

Note: Cefdinir is effective in the eradication of *S. pyogenes* from the oropharynx. Cefdinir has not, however, been studied for the prevention of rheumatic fever following *S. pyogenes* pharyngitis/tonsillitis. Only intramuscular penicillin has been demonstrated to be effective for the prevention of rheumatic fever.

Uncomplicated Skin and Skin Structure Infections caused by *Staphylococcus aureus* (including β-lactamase producing strains) and *Streptococcus pyogenes.*

PEDIATRIC PATIENTS

Acute Bacterial Otitis Media caused by *Haemophilus influenzae* (including β-lactamase producing strains), *Streptococcus pneumoniae* (penicillin-susceptible strains only), and *Moraxella catarrhalis* (including β-lactamase producing strains).

Pharyngitis/Tonsillitis caused by *Streptococcus pyogenes.*

Note: Cefdinir is effective in the eradication of *S. pyogenes* from the oropharynx. Cefdinir has not, however, been studied for the prevention of rheumatic fever following *S. pyogenes* pharyngitis/tonsillitis. Only intramuscular penicillin has been demonstrated to be effective for the prevention of rheumatic fever.

Uncomplicated Skin and Skin Structure Infections caused by *Staphylococcus aureus* (including β-lactamase producing strains) and *Streptococcus pyogenes.*

CONTRAINDICATIONS

Cefdinir is contraindicated in patients with known allergy to the cephalosporin class of antibiotics.

WARNINGS

BEFORE THERAPY WITH CEFDINIR IS INSTITUTED, CAREFUL INQUIRY SHOULD BE MADE TO DETERMINE WHETHER THE PATIENT HAS HAD PREVIOUS HYPERSENSITIVITY REACTIONS TO CEFDINIR, OTHER CEPHALOSPORINS, PENICILLINS, OR OTHER DRUGS. IF CEFDINIR IS TO BE GIVEN TO PENICILLIN-SENSITIVE PATIENTS, CAUTION SHOULD BE EXERCISED BECAUSE CROSS-HYPERSENSITIVITY AMONG β-LACTAM ANTIBIOTICS HAS BEEN CLEARLY DOCUMENTED AND MAY OCCUR IN UP TO 10% OF PATIENTS WITH A HISTORY OF PENICILLIN ALLERGY. IF AN ALLERGIC REACTION TO CEFDINIR OCCURS, THE DRUG SHOULD BE DISCONTINUED. SERIOUS ACUTE HYPERSENSITIVITY REACTIONS MAY REQUIRE TREATMENT WITH EPINEPHRINE AND OTHER EMERGENCY MEASURES, INCLUDING OXYGEN, INTRAVENOUS FLUIDS, INTRAVENOUS ANTIHISTAMINES, CORTICOSTEROIDS, PRESSOR AMINES, AND AIRWAY MANAGEMENT, AS CLINICALLY INDICATED.

Pseudomembranous colitis has been reported with nearly all antibacterial agents, including cefdinir, and may range in severity from mild-to life-threatening. Therefore, it is important to consider this diagnosis in patients who present with diarrhea subsequent to the administration of antibacterial agents.

Treatment with antibacterial agents alters the normal flora of the colon and may permit overgrowth of clostridia. Studies indicate that a toxin produced by *Clostridium difficile* is a primary cause of "antibiotic-associated colitis."

After the diagnosis of pseudomembranous colitis has been established, appropriate therapeutic measures should be initiated. Mild cases of pseudomembranous colitis usually respond to drug discontinuation alone. In moderate to severe cases, consideration should be given to management with fluids and electrolytes, protein supplementation, and treatment with an antibacterial drug clinically effective against *Clostridium difficile.*

PRECAUTIONS

GENERAL

As with other broad-spectrum antibiotics, prolonged treatment may result in the possible emergence and overgrowth of resistant organisms. Careful observation of the patient is essential. If superinfection occurs during therapy, appropriate alternative therapy should be administered.

Cefdinir, as with other broad-spectrum antimicrobials (antibiotics), should be prescribed with caution in individuals with a history of colitis.

In patients with transient or persistent renal insufficiency (creatinine clearance <30 ml/min), the total daily dose of cefdinir should be reduced because high and prolonged plasma concentrations of cefdinir can result following recommended doses (see DOSAGE AND ADMINISTRATION).

INFORMATION FOR THE PATIENT

Antacids containing magnesium or aluminum interfere with the absorption of cefdinir. If this type of antacid is required during cefdinir therapy, cefdinir should be taken at least 2 hours before or after the antacid.

Iron supplements, including multivitamins that contain iron, interfere with the absorption of cefdinir. If iron supplements are required during cefdinir therapy, cefdinir should be taken at least 2 hours before or after the supplement.

Iron-fortified infant formula does not significantly interfere with the absorption of cefdinir. Therefore, cefdinir oral suspension can be administered with iron-fortified infant formula.

If the patient is diabetic, he/she/the guardian should be aware that the oral suspension contains 2.86 g of sucrose per teaspoon.

DRUG/LABORATORY TEST INTERACTIONS

A false-positive reaction for ketones in the urine may occur with tests using nitroprusside, but not with those using nitroferricyanide. The administration of cefdinir may result in a false-positive reaction for glucose in urine using Clinitest, Benedict's solution, or Fehling's solution. It is recommended that glucose tests based on enzymatic glucose oxidase reactions (such as Clinistix or Tes-Tape) be used. Cephalosporins are known to occasionally induce a positive direct Coombs' test.

CARCINOGENESIS, MUTAGENESIS, AND IMPAIRMENT OF FERTILITY

The carcinogenic potential of cefdinir has not been evaluated. No mutagenic effects were seen in the bacterial reverse mutation assay (Ames) or point mutation assay at the hypoxanthine-guanine phosphoribosyltransferase locus (HGPRT) in V79 Chinese hamster lung cells. No clastogenic effects were observed *in vitro* in the structural chromosome aberration assay in V79 Chinese hamster lung cells or *in vivo* in the micronucleus assay in mouse bone marrow. In rats, fertility and reproductive performance were not affected by cefdinir at oral doses up to 1000 mg/kg/day (70 times the human dose based on mg/kg/day, 11 times based on $mg/m^2/day$).

PREGNANCY, TERATOGENIC EFFECTS, PREGNANCY CATEGORY B

Cefdinir was not teratogenic in rats at oral doses up to 1000 mg/kg/day (70 times the human dose based on mg/kg/day, 11 times based on $mg/m^2/day$) or in rabbits at oral doses up to 10 mg/kg/day (0.7 times the human dose based on mg/kg/day, 0.23 times based on $mg/m^2/day$). Maternal toxicity (decreased body weight gain) was observed in rabbits at the maximum tolerated dose of 10 mg/kg/day without adverse effects on offspring. Decreased body weight occurred in rat fetuses at ≥100 mg/kg/day, and in rat offspring at ≥32 mg/kg/day. No effects were observed on maternal reproductive parameters or offspring survival, development, behavior, or reproductive function.

There are, however, no adequate and well-controlled studies in pregnant women. Because animal reproduction studies are not always predictive of human response, this drug should be used during pregnancy only if clearly needed.

LABOR AND DELIVERY

Cefdinir has not been studied for use during labor and delivery.

NURSING MOTHERS

Following administration of single 600 mg doses, cefdinir was not detected in human breast milk.

PEDIATRIC USE

Safety and efficacy in neonates and infants less than 6 months of age have not been established. Use of cefdinir for the treatment of acute maxillary sinusitis in pediatric patients (age 6 months through 12 years) is supported by evidence from adequate and well-controlled studies in adults and adolescents, the similar pathophysiology of acute sinusitis in adult and pediatric patients, and comparative pharmacokinetic data in the pediatric population.

GERIATRIC USE

Efficacy is comparable in geriatric patients and younger adults. While cefdinir has been well-tolerated in all age groups, in clinical trials geriatric patients experienced a lower rate of adverse events, including diarrhea, than younger adults. Dose adjustment in elderly patients is not necessary unless renal function is markedly compromised (see DOSAGE AND ADMINISTRATION).

DRUG INTERACTIONS

ANTACIDS (ALUMINUM- OR MAGNESIUM-CONTAINING)

Concomitant administration of 300 mg cefdinir capsules with 30 ml Maalox TC suspension reduces rate (C_{max}) and extent (AUC) of absorption by approximately 40%. Time to reach C_{max} is also prolonged by 1 hour. There are no significant effects on cefdinir pharmacokinetics if the antacid is administered 2 hours before or 2 hours after cefdinir. If antacids are required during cefdinir therapy, cefdinir should be taken at least 2 hours before or after the antacid.

PROBENECID

As with other β-lactam antibiotics, probenecid inhibits the renal excretion of cefdinir, resulting in an approximate doubling in AUC, a 54% increase in peak cefdinir plasma levels, and a 50% prolongation in the apparent elimination half-life.

C

IRON SUPPLEMENTS AND FOODS FORTIFIED WITH IRON

Concomitant administration of cefdinir with a therapeutic iron supplement containing 60 mg of elemental iron (as $FeSO_4$) or vitamins supplemented with 10 mg of elemental iron reduced extent of absorption by 80% and 31%, respectively. If iron supplements are required during cefdinir therapy, cefdinir should be taken at least 2 hours before or after the supplement.

The effect of foods highly fortified with elemental iron (primarily iron-fortified breakfast cereals) on cefdinir absorption has not been studied.

Concomitantly administered iron-fortified infant formula (2.2 mg elemental iron/6 oz) has no significant effect on cefdinir pharmacokinetics. Therefore, cefdinir oral suspension can be administered with iron-fortified infant formula.

There have been rare reports of reddish stools in patients who have received cefdinir in Japan. The reddish color is due to the formation of a nonabsorbable complex between cefdinir or its breakdown products and iron in the gastrointestinal tract.

ADVERSE REACTIONS

CLINICAL TRIALS

Cefdinir Capsules (Adult and Adolescent Patients)

In clinical trials, 4527 adult and adolescent patients (3275 US and 1252 non-US) were treated with the recommended dose of cefdinir capsules (600 mg/day). Most adverse events were mild and self-limiting in nature. No deaths or permanent disabilities were attributed to cefdinir. One hundred twenty-five of 4527 (3%) patients discontinued medication due to adverse events thought by the investigators to be possibly, probably, or definitely associated with cefdinir therapy. The discontinuations were primarily for gastrointestinal disturbances, usually diarrhea or nausea. Seventeen of 4527 (0.4%) patients were discontinued due to rash thought related to cefdinir administration.

In the US, the following adverse events were thought by the investigators to be possibly, probably, or definitely related to cefdinir capsules in multiple-dose clinical trials (n=3275 cefdinir-treated patients):

Adverse events associated with cefdinir capsules us trials in adult and adolescent patients (n=3275; males=1469, females=1806):

Incidence ≥1%: *Diarrhea:* 16%. *Vaginal moniliasis:* 5% of women. *Nausea:* 3%. *Headache:* 2%. *Abdominal pain:* 1%. *Vaginitis:* 1% of women.

Incidence <1% but >0.1%: *Rash:* 0.9%. *Dyspepsia:* 0.8%. *Flatulence:* 0.6%. *Vomiting:* 0.6%. *Anorexia:* 0.3%. *Constipation:* 0.3%. *Abnormal stools:* 0.2%. *Asthenia:* 0.2%. *Dizziness:* 0.2%. *Insomnia:* 0.2%. *Leukorrhea:* 0.2% of women. *Pruritus:* 0.2%. *Somnolence:* 0.2%.

The following laboratory value changes of possible clinical significance, irrespective of relationship to therapy with cefdinir, were seen during clinical trials conducted in the US:

Laboratory value changes observed with cefdinir capsules US trials in adult and adolescent patients (n=3275):

Incidence ≥1%: *Increased Gamma-Glutamyltransferase:* 1%. *Increased Urine Protein:* 1%. *Increased Urine Red Blood Cells:* 1%.

Incidence <1% but >0.1%: *Increased Glucose, Decreased Glucose:* 0.9%, 0.2%. *Increased Alanine Aminotransferase (ALT):* 0.9%. *Increased Urine Glucose:* 0.9%. *Increased White Blood Cells, Decreased White Blood Cells:* 0.8%, 0.7%. *Decreased Lymphocytes, Increased Lymphocytes:* 0.8%,0.2%. *Increased Urine Specific Gravity:* 0.8%. *Decreased Bicarbonate:* 0.6%. *Increased Eosinophils:* 0.6%. *Increased Phosphorus, Decreased Phosphorus:* 0.6%, 0.3%. *Increased Aspartate Aminotransferase (AST):* 0.4%. *Increased Urine White Blood Cells:* 0.4%. *Decreased Hemoglobin:* 0.3%. *Increased Alkaline Phosphatase:* 0.2%. *Increased Blood Urea Nitrogen (BUN):* 0.2%. *Increased Bilirubin:* 0.2%. *Increased Lactate Dehydrogenase:* 0.2%. *Increased Platelets:* 0.2%. *Decreased Polymorphonuclear Neutrophils (PMNs):* 0.2%. *Increased Potassium:* 0.2%. *Increased Urine pH:* 0.2%.

Cefdinir Oral Suspension (Pediatric Patients)

In clinical trials, 1893 pediatric patients (1387 US and 506 non-US) were treated with the recommended dose of cefdinir suspension (14 mg/kg/day). Most adverse events were mild and self-limiting. No deaths or permanent disabilities were attributed to cefdinir. Thirty-nine of 1893 (2%) patients discontinued medication due to adverse events considered by the investigators to be possibly, probably, or definitely associated with cefdinir therapy. Discontinuations were primarily for gastrointestinal disturbances, usually diarrhea. Five of 1893 (0.3%) patients were discontinued due to rash thought related to cefdinir administration.

In the US, the following adverse events were thought by investigators to be possibly, probably, or definitely related to cefdinir suspension in multiple-dose clinical trials (n=1387 cefdinir-treated patients):

Adverse events associated with cefdinir suspension US trials in pediatric patients (n=1387; males=743, females=644):

Incidence ≥1%: *Diarrhea:* 8%. *Rash:* 3%. *Cutaneous Moniliasis:* 1%. *Vomiting:* 1%.

Incidence <1% but >0.1%: *Abdominal Pain:* 0.9%. *Leukopenia*:* 0.4%. *Nausea:* 0.3%. *Vaginal Moniliasis:* 0.3% of girls. *Vaginitis:* 0.3% of girls. *Dyspepsia:* 0.2%. *Maculopapular Rash:* 0.2%. *Increased AST*:* 0.2%.

*Laboratory changes were occasionally reported as adverse events.

The following laboratory value changes of possible clinical significance, irrespective of relationship to therapy with cefdinir, were seen during clinical trials conducted in the US:

Laboratory value changes observed with cefdinir suspension US trials in pediatric patients (n=1387):

Incidence ≥1%: *Increased Lactate Dehydrogenase:* 2%. *Increased Alkaline Phosphatase:* 1%. *Decreased Bicarbonate:* 1%. *Increased Eosinophils:* 1%. *Increased Urine pH:* 1%.

Incidence <1% but >0.1%: *Increased Lymphocytes, Decreased Lymphocytes:* 0.9%, 0.7%. *Increased Phosphorus, Decreased Phosphorus:* 0.9%, 0.4%. *Decreased White Blood Cells, Increased White Blood Cells:* 0.9%, 0.4%. *Increased Urine Protein:* 0.9%. *Increased PMNs:* 0.8%. *Increased Platelets:* 0.7%. *Decreased Calcium:* 0.5%. *Increased AST:* 0.2%. *Decreased Hemoglobin:* 0.4%. *Increased Potassium:* 0.3%. *Increased ALT:* 0.2%. *Decreased Hematocrit:* 0.2%. *Increased Urine Specific Gravity:* 0.2%. *Increased Urine White Blood Cells:* 0.2.

POSTMARKETING EXPERIENCE

The following adverse experiences and altered laboratory tests, regardless of their relationship to cefdinir, have been reported during extensive postmarketing experience, beginning with approval in Japan in 1991: Stevens-Johnson syndrome, toxic epidermal necrolysis, exfoliative dermatitis, erythema multiforme, erythema nodosum, conjunctivitis, stomatitis, acute hepatitis, cholestasis, fulminant hepatitis, hepatic failure, jaundice, increased amylase, shock, anaphylaxis, facial and laryngeal edema, feeling of suffocation, acute enterocolitis, bloody diarrhea, hemorrhagic colitis, melena, pseudomembranous colitis, pancytopenia, granulocytopenia, leukopenia, thrombocytopenia, idiopathic thrombocytopenic purpura, hemolytic anemia, acute respiratory failure, asthmatic attack, drug-induced pneumonia, eosinophilic pneumonia, idiopathic interstitial pneumonia, fever, acute renal failure, nephropathy, bleeding tendency, coagulation disorder, disseminated intravascular coagulation, upper GI bleed, peptic ulcer, ileus, loss of consciousness, allergic vasculitis, possible cefdinir-diclofenac interaction, cardiac failure, chest pain, myocardial infarction, hypertension, involuntary movements, and rhabdomyolysis.

CEPHALOSPORIN CLASS ADVERSE EVENTS

The following adverse events and altered laboratory tests have been reported for cephalosporin-class antibiotics in general:

Allergic reactions, anaphylaxis, Stevens-Johnson syndrome, erythema multiforme, toxic epidermal necrolysis, renal dysfunction, toxic nephropathy, hepatic dysfunction including cholestasis, aplastic anemia, hemolytic anemia, hemorrhage, false-positive test for urinary glucose, neutropenia, pancytopenia, and agranulocytosis. Pseudomembranous colitis symptoms may begin during or after antibiotic treatment (see WARNINGS).

Several cephalosporins have been implicated in triggering seizures, particularly in patients with renal impairment when the dosage was not reduced (see DOSAGE AND ADMINISTRATION). If seizures associated with drug therapy occur, the drug should be discontinued. Anticonvulsant therapy can be given if clinically indicated.

DOSAGE AND ADMINISTRATION

See INDICATIONS AND USAGE for indicated pathogens.

CAPSULES

The recommended dosage and duration of treatment for infections in adults and adolescents are described in TABLE 13; the total daily dose for all infections is 600 mg. Once-daily dosing for 10 days is as effective as bid dosing. Once-daily dosing has not been studied in pneumonia or skin infections; therefore, cefdinir capsules should be administered twice daily in these infections. Cefdinir capsules may be taken without regard to meals.

TABLE 13 *Adults and Adolescents (Age 13 Years and Older)*

Type of Infection	Dosage	Duration (days)
Community-Acquired Pneumonia	300 mg q12h	10
Acute Exacerbations of Chronic Bronchitis	300 mg q12h or	10
	600 mg q24h	10
Acute Maxillary Sinusitis	300 mg q12h or	10
	600 mg q24h	10
Pharyngitis/Tonsillitis	300 mg q12h or	5-10
	600 mg q24h	10
Uncomplicated Skin and Skin Structure Infections	300 mg q12h	10

POWDER FOR ORAL SUSPENSION

The recommended dosage and duration of treatment for infections in pediatric patients are described in the TABLE 14 and TABLE 15; the total daily dose for all infections is 14 mg/kg, up to a maximum dose of 600 mg/day. Once-daily dosing for 10 days is as effective as bid dosing. Once-daily dosing has not been studied in skin infections; therefore, cefdinir oral suspension should be administered twice daily in this infection. Cefdinir oral suspension may be administered without regard to meals.

TABLE 14 *Pediatric Patients (Age 6 Months Through 12 Years)*

Type of Infection	Dosage	Duration (days)
Acute Bacterial Otitis Media	7 mg/kg q12h or	10
	14 mg/kg q24h	10
Acute Maxillary Sinusitis	7 mg/kg q12h or	10
	14 mg/kg q24h	10
Pharyngitis/Tonsillitis	7 mg/kg q12h or	5-10
	14 mg/kg q24h	10
Uncomplicated Skin and Skin Structure Infections	7 mg/kg q12h	10

PATIENTS WITH RENAL INSUFFICIENCY

For adult patients with creatinine clearance <30 ml/min, the dose of cefdinir should be 300 mg given once daily.

TABLE 15 *Cefdinir Oral Suspension Pediatric Dosage Chart*

Weight	125 mg/5 ml
9 kg/20 lbs	2.5 ml (½ tsp) q12h or 5 ml (1 tsp) q24h
18 kg/40 lbs	5 ml (1 tsp) q12h or 10 ml (2 tsp) q24h
27 kg/60 lbs	7.5 ml (1½ tsp) q12h or 15 ml (3 tsp) q24h
36 kg/80 lbs	10 ml (2 tsp) q12h or 20 ml (4 tsp) q24h
≥43 kg*/95 lbs	12 ml (2½ tsp) q12h or 24 ml (5 tsp) q24h

* Pediatric patients who weigh ≥43 kg should receive the maximum daily dose of 600 mg.

Creatinine clearance is difficult to measure in outpatients. However, the following formula may be used to estimate creatinine clearance (CLCR) in adult patients. For estimates to be valid, serum creatinine levels should reflect steady-state levels of renal function (creatinine clearance is in ml/min, age is in years, weight is in kilograms, and serum creatinine is in mg/dl.[3]).

Males: CLCR = [(weight) × (140-age)] ÷ [(72) × (serum creatinine)]

Females: 0.85 × above value

The following formula may be used to estimate creatinine clearance in pediatric patients (K=0.55 for pediatric patients older than 1 year[4] and 0.45 for infants (up to 1 year)[5]):

CLCR = [K × (body length or height)] ÷ serum creatinine

In the above equation, creatinine clearance is in ml/min/1.73 m^2, body length or height is in centimeters, and serum creatinine is in mg/dl.

For pediatric patients with a creatinine clearance of <30 ml/min/1.73 m^2, the dose of cefdinir should be 7 mg/kg (up to 300 mg) given once daily.

PATIENTS ON HEMODIALYSIS

Hemodialysis removes cefdinir from the body. In patients maintained on chronic hemodialysis, the recommended initial dosage regimen is a 300 mg or 7 mg/kg dose every other day. At the conclusion of each hemodialysis session, 300 mg (or 7 mg/kg) should be given. Subsequent doses (300 mg or 7 mg/kg) are then administered every other day.

After mixing, the suspension can be stored at room temperature (25°C/77°F). The container should be kept tightly closed, and the suspension should be shaken well before each administration. The suspension may be used for 10 days, after which any unused portion must be discarded.

HOW SUPPLIED

Omnicef capsules, containing 300 mg cefdinir, as lavender and turquoise capsules imprinted with the product name.

Omnicef for oral suspension is a cream-colored powder formulation that, when reconstituted as directed, contains 125 mg cefdinir/5 ml. The reconstituted suspension has a cream color and strawberry flavor.

Storage: Store the capsules and unsuspended powder at 25°C (77°F); excursions permitted to 15-30°C (59-86°F). Once reconstituted, the oral suspension can be stored at controlled room temperature for 10 days.

PRODUCT LISTING - EQUIVALENTS NOT AVAILABLE

Capsule - Oral - 300 mg

10 x 3	$133.61	OMNICEF OMNI-PAC, Abbott Pharmaceutical	00074-3769-30
10's	$41.21	OMNICEF OMNI-PAC, Abbott Pharmaceutical	00074-3769-10
60's	$267.26	OMNICEF, Abbott Pharmaceutical	00074-3769-60

Suspension - Oral - 125 mg/5 ml

60 ml	$44.44	OMNICEF, Abbott Pharmaceutical	00074-3771-60
100 ml	$61.57	OMNICEF, Allscripts Pharmaceutical Company	54569-4877-00
100 ml	$70.36	OMNICEF, Abbott Pharmaceutical	00074-3771-13

Cefditoren Pivoxil (003530)

Categories: Bronchitis, chronic, acute exacerbation; Infection, lower respiratory tract; Infection, upper respiratory tract; Infection, skin and skin structures; Pharyngitis; Pneumonia; Tonsillitis; FDA Approved 2001 Aug; Pregnancy Category B
Drug Classes: Antibiotics, cephalosporins
Brand Names: Spectracef
Cost of Therapy: $31.44 (Infection; Spectracef; 200 mg; 2 tablets/day; 10 day supply)

DESCRIPTION

Cefditoren pivoxil tablets contain cefditoren pivoxil, a semi-synthetic cephalosporin antibiotic for oral administration. It is a prodrug which is hydrolyzed by esterases during absorption, and the drug is distributed in the circulating blood as active cefditoren.

Chemically, cefditoren pivoxil is (-)-(6R,7R)-2,2-dimethylpropionyloxymethyl 7-[(Z)-2-(2-aminothiazol-4-yl)-2-methoxyiminoacetamido]-3-[(Z)-2-(4-methylthiazol-5-yl)-ethenyl]-8-oxo-5-thia-1-azabicyclo[4,2,0]oct-2-ene-2-carboxylate. The empirical formula is $C_{25}H_{28}N_6O_7S_3$ and the molecular weight is 620.73.

The amorphous form of cefditoren pivoxil developed for clinical use is a light yellow powder. It is freely soluble in dilute hydrochloric acid and soluble at levels equal to 6.06 mg/ml in ethanol and <0.1 mg/ml in water.

Spectracef tablets contain 200 mg of cefditoren as cefditoren pivoxil and the following inactive ingredients: croscarmellose sodium, sodium caseinate (a milk protein), D-mannitol, magnesium stearate, sodium tripolyphosphate, hydroxypropyl methylcellulose, and hydroxypropyl cellulose. The tablet coating contains hydroxypropyl methylcellulose, titanium dioxide, polyethylene glycol, and carnauba wax. Tablets are printed with ink containing FD&C blue no. 1, D&C red no. 27, shellac, and propylene glycol.

CLINICAL PHARMACOLOGY

PHARMACOKINETICS

Absorption

Oral Bioavailability

Following oral administration, cefditoren pivoxil is absorbed from the gastrointestinal tract and hydrolyzed to cefditoren by esterases. Maximal plasma concentrations (C_{max}) of cefditoren under fasting conditions average 1.8 ± 0.6 µg/ml following a single 200 mg dose and occur 1.5 to 3 hours following dosing. Less than dose-proportional increases in C_{max} and area under the concentration-time curve (AUC) were observed at doses of 400 mg and above. Cefditoren does not accumulate in plasma following twice daily administration to subjects with normal renal function. Under fasting conditions, the estimated absolute bioavailability of cefditoren pivoxil is approximately 14%. The absolute bioavailability of cefditoren pivoxil administered with a low fat meal (693 cal, 14 g fat, 122 g carb, 23 g protein) is 16.1 ± 3.0%.

Food Effect

Administration of cefditoren pivoxil following a high fat meal (858 cal, 64 g fat, 43 g carb, 31 g protein) resulted in a 70% increase in mean AUC and a 50% increase in mean C_{max} compared to administration of cefditoren pivoxil in the fasted state. After a high fat meal, the C_{max} averaged 3.1 ± 1.0 µg/ml following a single 200 mg dose of cefditoren pivoxil and 4.4 ± 0.9 µg/ml following a 400 mg dose. Cefditoren AUC and C_{max} values from studies conducted with a moderate fat meal (648 cal, 27 g fat, 73 g carb, 29 g protein) are similar to those obtained following a high fat meal.

Distribution

The mean volume of distribution at steady state (Vss) of cefditoren is 9.3 ± 1.6 L. Binding of cefditoren to plasma proteins averages 88% from *in vitro* determinations, and is concentration-independent at cefditoren concentrations ranging from 0.05 to 10 µg/ml. Cefditoren is primarily bound to human serum albumin and its binding is decreased when serum albumin concentrations are reduced. Binding to α-1-acid glycoprotein ranges from 3.3-8.1%. Penetration into red blood cells is negligible.

Skin Blister Fluid

Maximal concentrations of cefditoren in suction-induced blister fluid were observed 4-6 hours following administration of a 400 mg dose of cefditoren pivoxil with a mean of 1.1 ± 0.42 µg/ml. Mean blister fluid AUC values were 56 ± 15% of corresponding plasma concentrations.

Tonsil Tissue

In fasted patients undergoing elective tonsillectomy, the mean concentration of cefditoren in tonsil tissue 2-4 hours following administration of a 200 mg dose of cefditoren pivoxil was 0.18 ± 0.07 µg/g. Mean tonsil tissue concentrations of cefditoren were 12 ± 3% of the corresponding serum concentrations.

Cerebrospinal Fluid (CSF)

Data on the penetration of cefditoren into human cerebrospinal fluid are not available.

Metabolism and Excretion

Cefditoren is eliminated from the plasma, with a mean terminal elimination half-life ($T_{½}$) of 1.6 ± 0.4 hours in young healthy adults. Cefditoren is not appreciably metabolized. After absorption, cefditoren is mainly eliminated by excretion into the urine, with a renal clearance of approximately 4-5 L/h. Studies with the renal tubular transport blocking agent probenecid indicate that tubular secretion, along with glomerular filtration is involved in the renal elimination of cefditoren. Cefditoren renal clearance is reduced in patients with renal insufficiency. (See Special Populations, Renal Insufficiency and Hemodialysis.)

Hydrolysis of cefditoren pivoxil to its active component, cefditoren, results in the formation of pivalate. Following multiple doses of cefditoren pivoxil, greater than 70% of the pivalate is absorbed. Pivalate is mainly eliminated (>99%) through renal excretion, nearly exclusively as pivaloylcarnitine. Following a 200 mg bid regimen for 10 days, the mean decrease in plasma concentrations of total carnitine was 18.1 ± 7.2 nmole/ml, representing a 39% decrease in plasma carnitine concentrations. Following a 400 mg bid regimen for 14 days, the mean decrease in plasma concentrations of carnitine was 33.3 ± 9.7 nmole/ml, representing a 63% decrease in plasma carnitine concentrations. Plasma concentrations of carnitine returned to the normal control range within 7-10 days after discontinuation of cefditoren pivoxil. (See PRECAUTIONS, General and CONTRAINDICATIONS.)

Special Populations

Geriatric

The effect of age on the pharmacokinetics of cefditoren was evaluated in 48 male and female subjects aged 25-75 years given 400 mg cefditoren pivoxil bid for 7 days. Physiological changes related to increasing age increased the extent of cefditoren exposure in plasma, as evidenced by a 26% higher C_{max} and a 33% higher AUC for subjects aged ≥65 years compared with younger subjects. The rate of elimination of cefditoren from plasma was lower in subjects aged ≥65 years, with $T_{½}$ values 16-26% longer than for younger subjects. Renal clearance of cefditoren in subjects aged ≥65 years was 20-24% lower than in younger subjects. These changes could be attributed to age-related changes in creatinine clearance. No dose adjustments are necessary for elderly patients with normal (for their age) renal function.

Gender

The effect of gender on the pharmacokinetics of cefditoren was evaluated in 24 male and 24 female subjects given 400 mg cefditoren pivoxil bid for 7 days. The extent of exposure in plasma was greater in females than in males, as evidenced by a 14% higher C_{max} and a 16% higher AUC for females compared to males. Renal clearance of cefditoren in females was 13% lower than in males. These differences could be attributed to gender-related differences in lean body mass. No dose adjustments are necessary for gender.

C

Renal Insufficiency

Cefditoren pharmacokinetics were investigated in 24 adult subjects with varying degrees of renal function following administration of cefditoren pivoxil 400 mg bid for 7 days. Decreased creatinine clearance (CLCR) was associated with an increase in the fraction of unbound cefditoren in plasma and a decrease in the cefditoren elimination rate, resulting in greater systemic exposure in subjects with renal impairment. The unbound C_{max} and AUC were similar in subjects with mild renal impairment (CLCR: 50-80 ml/min/1.73 m^2) compared to subjects with normal renal function (CLCR: >80 ml/min/1.73 m^2). Moderate (CLCR: 30-49 ml/min/1.73 m^2) or severe (CLCR: <30 ml/min/1.73 m^2) renal impairment increased the extent of exposure in plasma, as evidenced by mean unbound C_{max} values 90% and 114% higher and AUC values 232% and 324% higher than that for subjects with normal renal function. The rate of elimination from plasma was lower in subjects with moderate or severe renal impairment, with respective mean T½ values of 2.7 and 4.7 hours. No dose adjustment is necessary for patients with mild renal impairment (CLCR: 50-80 ml/min/1.73 m^2). It is recommended that not more than 200 mg bid be administered to patients with moderate renal impairment (CLCR: 30-49 ml/min/1.73 m^2) and 200 mg qd be administered to patients with severe renal impairment (CLCR: <30 ml/min/1.73 m^2). (See DOSAGE AND ADMINISTRATION.)

Hemodialysis

Cefditoren pharmacokinetics investigated in 6 adult subjects with end-stage renal disease (ESRD) undergoing hemodialysis given a single 400 mg dose of cefditoren pivoxil were highly variable. The mean T½ was 4.7 hours and ranged from 1.5 to 15 hours. Hemodialysis (4 hours duration) removed approximately 30% of cefditoren from systemic circulation but did not change the apparent terminal elimination half-life. The appropriate dose for ESRD patients has not been determined. (See DOSAGE AND ADMINISTRATION.)

Hepatic Disease

Cefditoren pharmacokinetics were evaluated in 6 adult subjects with mild hepatic impairment (Child-Pugh Class A) and 6 with moderate hepatic impairment (Child-Pugh Class B). Following administration of cefditoren pivoxil 400 mg bid for 7 days in these subjects, mean C_{max} and AUC values were slightly (<15%) greater than those observed in normal subjects. No dose adjustments are necessary for patients with mild or moderate hepatic impairment (Child-Pugh Class A or B). The pharmacokinetics of cefditoren in subjects with severe hepatic impairment (Child-Pugh Class C) have not been studied.

MICROBIOLOGY

Cefditoren is a cephalosporin with antibacterial activity against gram-positive and gram-negative pathogens. The bactericidal activity of cefditoren results from the inhibition of cell wall synthesis via affinity for penicillin-binding proteins (PBPs). Cefditoren is stable in the presence of a variety of β-lactamases, including penicillinases and some cephalosporinases.

Cefditoren has been shown to be active against most strains of the following bacteria, both *in vitro* and in clinical infections, as described in INDICATIONS AND USAGE.

Aerobic Gram-Positive Microorganisms:

Staphylococcus aureus (methicillin-susceptible strains, including β-lactamase-producing strains).

Note: Cefditoren is inactive against methicillin-resistant *Staphylococcus aureus.*

Streptococcus pneumoniae (penicillin-susceptible strains only).

Streptococcus pyogenes.

Aerobic Gram-Negative Microorganisms:

Haemophilus influenzae (including β-lactamase-producing strains).

Haemophilus parainfluenzae (including β-lactamase-producing strains).

Moraxella catarrhalis (including β-lactamase-producing strains).

The following *in vitro* data are available, **but their clinical significance is unknown.** Cefditoren exhibits *in vitro* minimum inhibitory concentrations (MICs) of ≤0.125 μg/ml against most (≥90%) strains of the following bacteria; however, the safety and effectiveness of cefditoren in treating clinical infections due to these bacteria have not been established in adequate and well-controlled clinical trials.

Aerobic Gram-Positive Microorganisms:

Streptococcus agalactiae.

Streptococcus Groups C and G.

Streptococcus, viridans group (penicillin-susceptible and -intermediate strains).

SUSCEPTIBILITY TESTING

Dilution Techniques

Quantitative methods that are used to determine MICs provide reproducible estimates of the susceptibility of bacteria to antimicrobial compounds. The MICs should be determined using a standardized procedure. Standardized procedures are based on dilution methods[1] (broth) or equivalent with standardized inoculum concentrations and standardized concentrations of cefditoren powder. The MIC values obtained should be interpreted according to the criteria seen in TABLE 1.

Susceptibility test criteria can not be established for *S. aureus.*

A report of "Susceptible" indicates that the pathogen is likely to be inhibited if the antimicrobial compound in the blood reaches the concentration usually achievable. A report of "Intermediate" indicates that the result should be considered equivocal, and, if the microorganism is not fully susceptible to alternative, clinically feasible drugs, the test should be repeated. This category implies possible clinical applicability in body sites where the drug is physiologically concentrated or in situations where high dosage of drug can be used. This category also provides a buffer zone that prevents small, uncontrolled technical factors from causing major discrepancies in interpretation. A report of "Resistant" indicates that the pathogen is not likely to be inhibited if the antimicrobial compound in the blood reaches the concentration usually achievable and that other therapy should be selected.

Standardized susceptibility test procedures require the use of laboratory control bacterial strains to control the technical aspects of the laboratory procedures. Standard cefditoren powder should provide the following MICs with these quality control strains (see TABLE 2).

TABLE 1 *For Testing Haemophilus spp.* and Streptococcus spp. Including S. pneumoniae†*

Clinical Isolates	MIC	Interpretation
S. pneumoniae	≤0.125 μg/ml 0.250 μg/ml ≥0.50 μg/ml	Susceptible (S) Intermediate (I) Resistant (R)
Haemophilus spp.	≤0.125 μg/ml 0.250 μg/ml ≥0.50 μg/ml	Susceptible (S) Intermediate (I) Resistant (R)
S. pyogenes	≤0.125 μg/ml	Susceptible (S)

* This interpretive standard is applicable only to broth microdilution susceptibility tests with *Haemophilus* spp. using *Haemophilus* Test Medium (HTM).[1]

† These interpretive standards are applicable only to broth microdilution susceptibility tests with *Streptococcus* spp. using cation-adjusted Mueller-Hinton broth with 2-5% lysed horse blood.[1]

TABLE 2

Microorganisms	MIC Ranges
*Streptococcus pneumoniae** ATCC 49619	0.016-0.12 μg/ml
Haemophilus influenzae† ATCC 49766	0.004-0.016 μg/ml
Haemophilus influenzae† ATCC 49247	0.06-0.25 μg/ml

* This quality control range is applicable to only *S. pneumoniae* ATCC 49619 tested by a microdilution procedure using cation-adjusted Mueller-Hinton broth with 2-5% lysed horse blood.[1]

† This quality control range is applicable to only *H. influenzae* ATCC 49247 and ATCC 49766 tested by a microdilution procedure using HTM.[1]

INDICATIONS AND USAGE

Cefditoren pivoxil is indicated for the treatment of mild to moderate infections in adults and adolescents (12 years of age or older) which are caused by susceptible strains of the designated microorganisms in the conditions listed below.

Acute bacterial exacerbation of chronic bronchitis caused by *Haemophilus influenzae* (including β-lactamase-producing strains), *Haemophilus parainfluenzae* (including β-lactamase-producing strains), *Streptococcus pneumoniae* (penicillin susceptible strains only), or *Moraxella catarrhalis* (including β-lactamase-producing strains).

Community-acquired pneumoniacaused by *Haemophilus influenzae* (including β-lactamase-producing strains), *Haemophilus parainfluenzae* (including β-lactamase-producing strains), *Streptococcus pneumoniae* (including β-lactamase-producing strains), or *Moraxella catarrhalis* (including β-lactamase-producing strains).

Pharyngitis/tonsillitis caused by *Streptococcus pyogenes. Note:* Cefditoren pivoxil is effective in the eradication of *Streptococcus pyogenes* from the oropharynx. Cefditoren pivoxil has not been studied for the prevention of rheumatic fever following *Streptococcus pyogenes* pharyngitis/tonsillitis. Only intramuscular penicillin has been demonstrated to be effective for the prevention of rheumatic fever.

Uncomplicated skin and skin-structure infections caused by *Staphylococcus aureus* (including β-lactamase-producing strains) or *Streptococcus pyogenes.*

CONTRAINDICATIONS

Cefditoren pivoxil is contraindicated in patients with known allergy to the cephalosporin class of antibiotics or any of its components.

Cefditoren pivoxil is contraindicated in patients with carnitine deficiency or inborn errors of metabolism that may result in clinically significant carnitine deficiency, because use of cefditoren pivoxil causes renal excretion of carnitine. (See PRECAUTIONS, General.)

Cefditoren pivoxil tablets contain sodium caseinate, a milk protein. Patients with milk protein hypersensitivity (not lactose intolerance) should not be administered cefditoren pivoxil.

WARNINGS

BEFORE THERAPY WITH CEFDITOREN PIVOXIL IS INSTITUTED, CAREFUL INQUIRY SHOULD BE MADE TO DETERMINE WHETHER THE PATIENT HAS HAD PREVIOUS HYPERSENSITIVITY REACTIONS TO CEFDITOREN PIVOXIL, OTHER CEPHALOSPORINS, PENICILLINS, OR OTHER DRUGS. IF CEFDITOREN PIVOXIL IS TO BE GIVEN TO PENICILLIN-SENSITIVE PATIENTS, CAUTION SHOULD BE EXERCISED BECAUSE CROSS-HYPERSENSITIVITY AMONG β-LACTAM ANTIBIOTICS HAS BEEN CLEARLY DOCUMENTED AND MAY OCCUR IN UP TO 10% OF PATIENTS WITH A HISTORY OF PENICILLIN ALLERGY. IF AN ALLERGIC REACTION TO CEFDITOREN PIVOXIL OCCURS, THE DRUG SHOULD BE DISCONTINUED. SERIOUS ACUTE HYPERSENSITIVITY REACTIONS MAY REQUIRE TREATMENT WITH EPINEPHRINE AND OTHER EMERGENCY MEASURES, INCLUDING OXYGEN, INTRAVENOUS (IV) FLUIDS, IV ANTIHISTAMINES, CORTICOSTEROIDS, PRESSOR AMINES, AND AIRWAY MANAGEMENT, AS CLINICALLY INDICATED.

Pseudomembranous colitis has been reported with nearly all antibacterial agents, including cefditoren pivoxil, and may range in severity from mild to life-threatening. Therefore, it is important to consider this diagnosis in patients who present with diarrhea subsequent to the administration of antibacterial agents.

Treatment with antibacterial agents alters normal flora of the colon and may permit overgrowth of clostridia. Studies indicate that a toxin produced by *Clostridium difficile (C. difficile)* is a primary cause of antibiotic-associated colitis.

After the diagnosis of pseudomembranous colitis has been established, appropriate therapeutic measures should be initiated. Mild cases of pseudomembranous colitis usually respond to drug discontinuation alone. In moderate to severe cases, consideration should be given to management with fluids and electrolytes, protein supplementation, and treatment with an antibacterial drug clinically effective against *C. difficile* colitis.

PRECAUTIONS

GENERAL

Cefditoren pivoxil is not recommended when prolonged antibiotic treatment is necessary, since other pivalate-containing compounds have caused clinical manifestations of carnitine deficiency when used over a period of months. No clinical effects of carnitine decrease have been associated with short-term treatment. The effects on carnitine concentrations of repeat short-term courses of cefditoren pivoxil are not known.

In community-acquired pneumonia patients (n=192, mean age 50.3 ± 17.2 years) given a 200 mg bid regimen for 14 days, the mean decrease in serum concentrations of total carnitine while on therapy was 13.8 ± 10.8 nmole/ml, representing a 30% decrease in serum carnitine concentrations. In community-acquired pneumonia patients (n=192, mean age 51.3 ± 17.8 years) given a 400 mg bid regimen for 14 days, the mean decrease in serum concentrations of total carnitine while on therapy was 21.5 ± 13.1 nmole/ml, representing a 46% decrease in serum carnitine concentrations. Plasma concentrations of carnitine returned to the normal control range within 7 days after discontinuation of cefditoren pivoxil. Comparable decreases in carnitine were observed in healthy volunteers (mean age 33.6 ± 7.4 years) following a 200 or 400 mg bid regimen. (See CLINICAL PHARMACOLOGY.) Community-acquired pneumonia clinical trials demonstrated no adverse events attributable to decreases in serum carnitine concentrations.

However, some sub-populations (*e.g.*, patients with renal impairment, patients with decreased muscle mass) may be increased risk for reductions in serum carnitine concentrations during cefditoren pivoxil therapy. Furthermore, the appropriate dose in patients with end-stage renal disease has not been determined. (See DOSAGE AND ADMINISTRATION, Patients with Renal Insufficiency).

As with other antibiotics, prolonged treatment may result in the possible emergence and overgrowth of resistant organisms. Careful observation of the patient is essential. If superinfection occurs during therapy, appropriate alternative therapy should be administered.

Cephalosporins may be associated with a fall in prothrombin activity. Those at risk include patients with renal or hepatic impairment, or poor nutritional state, as well as patients receiving a protracted course of antimicrobial therapy, and patients previously stabilized on anticoagulant therapy. Prothrombin time should be monitored in patients at risk and exogenous vitamin K administered as indicated. In clinical trials, there was no difference between cefditoren and comparator cephalosporins in the incidence of increased prothrombin time.

INFORMATION FOR THE PATIENT

Cefditoren pivoxil should be taken with meals to enhance absorption.

Cefditoren pivoxil may be taken concomitantly with oral contraceptives.

It is not recommended that cefditoren pivoxil be taken concomitantly with antacids or other drugs taken to reduce stomach acids. (See DRUG INTERACTIONS.)

Cefditoren pivoxil tablets contain sodium caseinate, a milk protein. Patients with milk protein hypersensitivity (not lactose intolerance) should not be administered cefditoren pivoxil.

DRUG/LABORATORY TEST INTERACTIONS

Cephalosporins are known to occasionally induce a positive direct Coombs' test. A false-positive reaction for glucose in the urine may occur with copper reduction tests (Benedict's or Fehling's solution or with Clinitest tablets), but not with enzyme-based tests for glycosuria (*e.g.*, Clinistix, Tes-Tape). As a false-negative result may occur in the ferricyanide test, it is recommended that either the glucose oxidase or hexokinase method be used to determine blood/plasma glucose levels in patients receiving cefditoren pivoxil.

CARCINOGENESIS, MUTAGENESIS, AND IMPAIRMENT OF FERTILITY

No long-term animal carcinogenicity studies have been conducted with cefditoren pivoxil. Cefditoren pivoxil was not mutagenic in the Ames bacterial reverse mutation assay, or in the mouse lymphoma mutation assay at the hypoxanthine-guanine phosphoribosyltransferase locus. In Chinese hamster lung cells, chromosomal aberrations were produced by cefditoren pivoxil, but not by cefditoren. Subsequent studies showed that the chromosome aberrations were due to the release of formaldehyde from the pivoxil ester moiety in the *in vitro* assay system. Neither cefditoren nor cefditoren pivoxil produced chromosomal aberrations when tested in an *in vitro* human peripheral blood lymphocyte assay, or in the *in vivo* mouse micronucleus assay. Cefditoren pivoxil did not induce unscheduled DNA synthesis when tested.

In rats, fertility and reproduction were not affected by cefditoren pivoxil at oral doses up to 1000 mg/kg/day, approximately 24 times a human dose of 200 mg bid based on mg/m^2/day.

PREGNANCY, TERATOGENIC EFFECTS, PREGNANCY CATEGORY B

Cefditoren pivoxil was not teratogenic up to the highest doses tested in rats and rabbits. In rats, this dose was 1000 mg/kg/day, which is approximately 24 times a human dose of 200 mg bid based on mg/m^2/day. In rabbits, the highest dose tested was 90 mg/kg/day, which is approximately 4 times a human dose of 200 mg bid based on mg/m^2/day. This dose produced severe maternal toxicity and resulted in fetal toxicity and abortions.

In a postnatal development study in rats, cefditoren pivoxil produced no adverse effects on postnatal survival, physical and behavioral development, learning abilities, and reproductive capability at sexual maturity when tested at doses of up to 750 mg/kg/day, the highest dose tested. This is approximately 18 times a human dose of 200 mg bid based on mg/m^2/day.

There are however, no adequate and well-controlled studies in pregnant women. Because animal reproductive studies are not always predictive of human response, this drug should be used during pregnancy only if clearly needed.

LABOR AND DELIVERY

Cefditoren pivoxil has not been studied for use during labor and delivery.

NURSING MOTHERS

Cefditoren was detected in the breast milk of lactating rats. Because many drugs are excreted in human breast milk, caution should be exercised when cefditoren pivoxil is administered to nursing women.

PEDIATRIC USE

Use of cefditoren pivoxil is not recommended for pediatric patients less than 12 years of age. The safety and efficacy of cefditoren pivoxil tablets in this population, including any effects of altered carnitine concentrations, have not been established. (See PRECAUTIONS, General.)

GERIATRIC USE

Of the 2675 patients in clinical studies who received cefditoren pivoxil 200 mg bid, 308 (12%) were >65 years of age. Of the 2159 patients in clinical studies who received cefditoren pivoxil 400 mg bid, 307 (14%) were >65 years of age. No clinically significant differences in effectiveness or safety were observed between older and younger patients. No dose adjustments are necessary in geriatric patients with normal (for their age) renal function. This drug is known to be substantially excreted by the kidney, and the risk of toxic reactions to this drug may be greater in patients with impaired renal function. Because elderly patients are more likely to have decreased renal function, care should be taken in dose selection, and it may be useful to monitor renal function. (See DOSAGE AND ADMINISTRATION.)

DRUG INTERACTIONS

Oral Contraceptives: Multiple doses of cefditoren pivoxil had no effect on the pharmacokinetics of ethinyl estradiol, the estrogenic component in most oral contraceptives.

Antacids: Coadministration of a single dose of an antacid which contained both magnesium (800 mg) and aluminum (900 mg) hydroxides reduced the oral absorption of a single 400 mg dose of cefditoren pivoxil administered following a meal, as evidenced by a 14% decrease in mean C_{max} and an 11% decrease in mean AUC. Although the clinical significance is not known, it is not recommended that cefditoren pivoxil be taken concomitantly with antacids.

H_2-Receptor Antagonists: Co-administration of a single dose of intravenously administered famotidine (20 mg) reduced the oral absorption of a single 400 mg dose of cefditoren pivoxil administered following a meal, as evidenced by a 27% decrease in mean C_{max} and a 22% decrease in mean AUC. Although the clinical significance is not known, it is not recommended that cefditoren pivoxil be taken concomitantly with H_2 receptor antagonists.

Probenecid: As with other β-lactam antibiotics, co-administration of probenecid with cefditoren pivoxil resulted in an increase in the plasma exposure of cefditoren, with a 49% increase in mean C_{max}, a 122% increase in mean AUC, and a 53% increase in $T_{½}$.

ADVERSE REACTIONS

CLINICAL TRIALS: CEFDITOREN PIVOXIL TABLETS (ADULTS AND ADOLESCENT PATIENTS ≥12 YEARS OF AGE)

In clinical trials, 4834 adult and adolescent patients have been treated with the recommended doses of cefditoren pivoxil tablets (200 or 400 mg bid). Most adverse events were mild and self-limiting. No deaths or permanent disabilities have been attributed to cefditoren.

The following adverse events were thought by the investigators to be possibly, probably, or definitely related to cefditoren tablets in multiple-dose clinical trials (TABLE 3).

TABLE 3 *Treatment-Related Adverse Events in Trials in Adult and Adolescent Patients ≥12 Years*

	Cefditoren Pivoxil		
	200 mg bid	400 mg bid	Comparators*
Incidence ≥1%	(n=2675)	(n=2159)	(n=2648)
Diarrhea	11%	15%	8%
Nausea	4%	6%	5%
Headache	3%	2%	2%
Abdominal pain	2%	2%	1%
Vaginal moniliasis	3%†	6%‡	6%§
Dyspepsia	1%	2%	2%
Vomiting	1%	1%	2%

* Includes amoxicillin/clavulanate, cefadroxil monohydrate, cefuroxime axetil, cefpodoxime proxetil, clarithromycin, and penicillin.
† 1428 females.
‡ 1135 females.
§ 1461 females.

The overall incidence of adverse events, and in particular diarrhea, increased with the higher recommended dose of cefditoren pivoxil.

Treatment related adverse events experienced by <1% but >0.1% of patients who received 200 or 400 mg bid of cefditoren pivoxil were abnormal dreams, allergic reaction, anorexia, asthenia, coagulation time increased, constipation, dizziness, dry mouth, eructation, face edema, fever, flatulence, fungal infection, gastrointestinal disorder, hyperglycemia, increased appetite, insomnia, leukopenia, leukorrhea, liver function test abnormal, myalgia, nervousness, oral moniliasis, pain, peripheral edema, pharyngitis, pseudomembranous colitis, pruritus, rash, rhinitis, sinusitis, somnolence, stomatitis, sweating, taste perversion, thirst, thrombocythemia, urticaria and vaginitis. Pseudomembranous colitis symptoms may begin during or after antibiotic treatment. (See WARNINGS.)

Sixty-one of 2675 (2%) patients who received 200 mg bid and 69 of 2159 (3%) patients who received 400 mg bid of cefditoren pivoxil discontinued medication due to adverse events thought by the investigators to be possibly, probably, or definitely associated with cefditoren therapy. The discontinuations were primarily for gastrointestinal disturbances, usually diarrhea or nausea. Diarrhea was the primary reason for discontinuation in 19 of 2675 (0.7%) patients who received 200 mg bid and in 31 of 2159 (1.4%) patients who received 400 mg bid of cefditoren pivoxil.

Changes in laboratory parameters of possible clinical significance, without regard to drug relationship and which occurred in ≥1% of patients who received cefditoren pivoxil 200 or 400 mg bid, were hematuria (3.0% and 3.1%), increased urine white blood cells (2.3% and 2.3%), decreased hematocrit (2.1% and 2.2%), and increased glucose (1.8% and 1.1%). Those events which occurred in <1% but >0.1% of patients included the following: increased/decreased white blood cells, increased eosinophils, decreased neutrophils, increased lymphocytes, increased platelet count, decreased hemoglobin, decreased sodium, increased potassium, decreased chloride, decreased inorganic phosphorus, decreased calcium, increased SGPT/ALT, increased SGOT/AST, increased cholesterol, decreased albumin, proteinuria, and increased BUN. It is not known if these abnormalities were caused by the drug or the underlying condition being treated.

CEPHALOSPORIN CLASS ADVERSE REACTIONS

In addition to the adverse reactions listed above which have been observed in patients treated with cefditoren pivoxil the following adverse reactions and altered laboratory test results have been reported for cephalosporin class antibiotics:

Adverse Reactions: Allergic reactions, anaphylaxis, drug fever, Stevens-Johnson syndrome, serum sickness-like reaction, erythema multiforme, toxic epidermal necrolysis, colitis, renal dysfunction, toxic nephropathy, reversible hyperactivity, hypertonia, hepatic dysfunction including cholestasis, aplastic anemia, hemolytic anemia, hemorrhage, and superinfection.

Altered Laboratory Findings: Prolonged prothrombin time, positive direct Coombs' test, false-positive test for urinary glucose, elevated alkaline phosphatase, elevated bilirubin, elevated LDH, increased creatinine, pancytopenia, neutropenia, and agranulocytosis.

Several cephalosporins have been implicated in triggering seizures, particularly in patients with renal impairment when the dosage was not reduced. (See DOSAGE AND ADMINISTRATION.) If seizures associated with drug therapy occur, the drug should be discontinued. Anticonvulsant therapy can be given if clinically indicated.

DOSAGE AND ADMINISTRATION

(See INDICATIONS AND USAGE for indicated pathogens.)

TABLE 4 *Cefditoren Pivoxil Dosage and Administration* — Adults and Adolescents (≥12 Years)*

Type of Infection	Dosage	Duration
Community-acquired pneumonia	400 mg bid	14 days
Acute bacterial exacerbation of chronic bronchitis	400 mg bid	10 days
Pharyngitis/tonsillitis	200 mg bid	10 days
Uncomplicated skin and skin structure infections	200 mg bid	10 days

* Should be taken with meals.

PATIENTS WITH RENAL INSUFFICIENCY

No dose adjustment is necessary for patients with mild renal impairment (CLCR: 50-80 ml/min/1.73 m^2). It is recommended that not more than 200 mg bid be administered to patients with moderate renal impairment (CLCR: 30-49 ml/min/1.73 m^2) and 200 mg qd be administered to patients with severe renal impairment (CLCR: <30 ml/min/1.73 m^2). The appropriate dose in patients with end-stage renal disease has not been determined.

PATIENTS WITH HEPATIC DISEASE

No dose adjustments are necessary for patients with mild or moderate hepatic impairment (Child-Pugh Class A or B). The pharmacokinetics of cefditoren have not been studied in patients with severe hepatic impairment (Child-Pugh Class C).

HOW SUPPLIED

Spectracef tablets containing cefditoren pivoxil equivalent to 200 mg of cefditoren are available as white, elliptical, film-coated tablets imprinted with "TAP 200 mg" in blue. These tablets are available in multi-dose tamper-evident containers.

Storage: Store at 52°C (77°F); excursions permitted to 15-30°C (59-86°F). Protect from light and moisture. Dispense in a tight, light resistant container.

PRODUCT LISTING - EQUIVALENTS NOT AVAILABLE

Tablet - Oral - 200 mg

60's $94.32 SPECTRACEF, Tap Pharmaceuticals Inc 00300-7535-60

Cefepime Hydrochloride (003198)

For related information, see the comparative table section in Appendix A.

Categories: Infection, intra-abdominal; Infection, lower respiratory tract; Infection, skin and skin structures; Infection, urinary tract; Neutropenia, febrile; Pneumonia; Pyelonephritis; FDA Approved 1996 Apr; Pregnancy Category B
Drug Classes: Antibiotics, cephalosporins
Brand Names: Maxipime
Foreign Brand Availability: Axepim (France); Cepimax (Philippines); Maxcef (Israel)
Cost of Therapy: $306.00 (Infection; Maxipime Injection; 1 g; 2 g/day; 10 day supply)

DESCRIPTION

For Intravenous or Intramuscular Use.

Cefepime hydrochloride is a semi-synthetic, broad spectrum, cephalosporin antibiotic for parenteral administration. The chemical name is 1-[[(6R,7R)-7-[2-(2-amino-4-thiazolyl)-glyoxylamido]-2-carboxy-8-oxo-5-thia-1-azabicyclo[4.2.0] oct-2-en-3-yl]methyl]-1-methylpyrrolidinium chloride, 7^2-(Z)-(O-methyloxime), monohydrochloride, monohydrate.

Cefepime HCl is a white to pale yellow powder with a molecular formula of $C_{19}H_{25}ClN_6O_5S_2 \cdot HCl \cdot H_2O$ and a molecular weight of 571.5. It is highly soluble in water.

Cefepime HCl for injection is supplied for intramuscular or intravenous administration in strengths equivalent to 500 mg, 1 and 2 g of cefepime. (See DOSAGE AND ADMINISTRATION.) Cefepime HCl is a sterile, dry mixture of cefepime HCl and L-arginine. The L-arginine, at an approximate concentration of 725 mg/g of cefepime, is added to control the pH of the constituted solution at 4.0-6.0. Freshly constituted solutions of cefepime HCl will range in color from colorless to amber.

CLINICAL PHARMACOLOGY

PHARMACOKINETICS

The average plasma concentrations of cefepime observed in healthy adult male volunteers (n=9) at various times following single 30 minute infusions (IV) of cefepime 500 mg, 1 g, and 2 g are summarized in TABLE 1. Elimination of cefepime is principally via renal excretion with an average (±SD) half-life of 2.0 (±0.3) hours and total body clearance of 120.0 (±8.0) ml/min in healthy volunteers. Cefepime pharmacokinetics are linear over the range 250 mg to 2 g. There is no evidence of accumulation in healthy adult male volunteers (n=7) receiving clinically relevant doses for a period of 9 days.

ABSORPTION

The average plasma concentrations of cefepime and its derived pharmacokinetic parameters after IV administration are portrayed in TABLE 1.

TABLE 1 *Average Plasma Concentrations in μg/ml of Cefepime and Derived Pharmacokinetic Parameters (±SD), IV Administration*

	Cefepime HCl		
Parameter	500 mg IV	1 g IV	2 g IV
0.5 h	38.2	78.7	163.1
1.0 h	21.6	44.5	85.8
2.0 h	11.6	24.3	44.8
4.0 h	5.0	10.5	19.2
8.0 h	1.4	2.4	3.9
12.0 h	0.2	0.6	1.1
C_{max}, μg/ml	39.1 (3.5)	81.7 (5.1)	163.9 (25.3)
AUC, h·μg/ml	70.8 (6.7)	148.5 (15.1)	284.8 (30.6)
Number of subjects (male)	9	9	9

Following intramuscular (IM) administration, cefepime is completely absorbed. The average plasma concentrations of cefepime at various times following a single IM injection are summarized in TABLE 2. The pharmacokinetics of cefepime are linear over the range of 500 mg to 2 g IM and do not vary with respect to treatment duration.

TABLE 2 *Average Plasma Concentrations in μg/ml of Cefepime and Derived Pharmacokinetic Parameters (±SD), IM Administration*

	Cefepime HCl		
Parameter	500 mg IM	1 g IM	2 g IM
0.5 h	8.2	14.8	36.1
1.0 h	12.5	25.9	49.9
2.0 h	12.0	26.3	51.3
4.0 h	6.9	16.0	31.5
8.0 h	1.9	4.5	8.7
12.0 h	0.7	1.4	2.3
C_{max}, μg/ml	13.9 (3.4)	29.6 (4.4)	57.5 (9.5)
T_{max}, h	1.4 (0.9)	1.6 (0.4)	1.5 (0.4)
AUC, h·μg/ml	60.0 (8.0)	137.0 (11.0)	262.0 (23.0)
Number of subjects (male)	6	6	12

DISTRIBUTION

The average steady state volume of distribution of cefepime is 18.0 (±2.0) L. The serum protein binding of cefepime is approximately 20% and is independent of its concentration in serum.

Cefepime is excreted in human milk. A nursing infant consuming approximately 1000 ml of human milk per day would receive approximately 0.5 mg of cefepime per day. (See PRECAUTIONS, Nursing Mothers.)

Concentrations of cefepime achieved in specific tissues and body fluids are listed in TABLE 3.

TABLE 3 *Average Concentrations of Cefepime in Specific Body Fluids (μg/ml) or Tissues (μg/g)*

Tissue or Fluid	Dose/Route		Average Time of Sample Post-Dose	Average Concentration
Blister fluid	2 g IV	n=6	1.5 h	81.4 μg/ml
Bronchial mucosa	2 g IV	n=20	4.8 h	24.1 μg/g
Sputum	2 g IV	n=5	4.0 h	7.4 μg/ml
Urine	500 mg IV	n=8	0-4 h	292 μg/ml
	1 g IV	n=12	0-4 h	926 μg/ml
	2 g IV	n=12	0-4 h	3120 μg/ml
Bile	2 g IV	n=26	9.4 h	17.8 μg/ml
Peritoneal fluid	2 g IV	n=19	4.4 h	18.3 μg/ml
Appendix	2 g IV	n=31	5.7 h	5.2 μg/g
Gallbladder	2 g IV	n=38	8.9 h	11.9 μg/g
Prostate	2 g IV	n=5	1.0 h	31.5 μg/g

Data suggest that cefepime does cross the inflamed blood-brain barrier. **The clinical relevance of these data are uncertain at this time.**

METABOLISM AND EXCRETION

Cefepime is metabolized to N-methylpyrrolidine (NMP) which is rapidly converted to the N-oxide (NMP-N-oxide). Urinary recovery of unchanged cefepime accounts for approximately 85% of the administered dose. Less than 1% of the administered dose is recovered from urine as NMP, 6.8% as NMP-N-oxide, and 2.5% as an epimer of cefepime. Because renal excretion is a significant pathway of elimination, patients with renal dysfunction and patients undergoing hemodialysis require dosage adjustment. (See DOSAGE AND ADMINISTRATION.)

SPECIAL POPULATIONS

Pediatric Patients

Cefepime pharmacokinetics have been evaluated in pediatric patients from 2 months to 11 years of age following single and multiple doses on q8h (n=29) and q12h (n=13) schedules. Following a single IV dose, total body clearance and the steady state volume of distribution averaged 3.3 (±1.0) ml/min/kg and 0.3 (±0.1) L/kg, respectively. The urinary recovery of unchanged cefepime was 60.4 (±30.4)% of the administered dose, and the average renal clearance was 2.0 (±1.1) ml/min/kg. There were no significant effects of age or gender (25 male vs 17 female) on total body clearance or volume of distribution, corrected for body weight. No accumulation was seen when cefepime was given at 50 mg/kg q12h (n=13), while C_{max}, AUC, and T½ were increased about 15% at steady state after 50 mg/kg q8h. The exposure to cefepime following a 50 mg/kg IV dose in a pediatric patient is comparable to that in an adult treated with a 2 g IV dose. The absolute bioavailability of cefepime after an IM dose of 50 mg/kg was 82.3 (±15)% in 8 patients.

Geriatric Patients

Cefepime pharmacokinetics have been investigated in elderly (65 years of age and older) men (n=12) and women (n=12) whose mean (SD) creatinine clearance was 74.0 (±15.0) ml/min. There appeared to be a decrease in cefepime total body clearance as a function of creatinine clearance. Therefore, dosage administration of cefepime in the elderly should be adjusted as appropriate if the patient's creatinine clearance is 60 ml/min or less. (See DOSAGE AND ADMINISTRATION.)

Renal Insufficiency

Cefepime pharmacokinetics have been investigated in patients with various degrees of renal insufficiency (n=30). The average half-life in patients requiring hemodialysis was 13.5 (±2.7) hours and in patients requiring continuous peritoneal dialysis was 19.0 (±2.0) hours. Cefepime total body clearance decreased proportionally with creatinine clearance in patients with abnormal renal function, which serves as the basis for dosage adjustment recommendations in this group of patients. (See DOSAGE AND ADMINISTRATION.)

Hepatic Insufficiency

The pharmacokinetics of cefepime were unaltered in patients with impaired hepatic function who received a single 1 g dose (n=11).

MICROBIOLOGY

Cefepime is a bactericidal agent that acts by inhibition of bacterial cell wall synthesis. Cefepime has a broad spectrum of *in vitro* activity that encompasses a wide range of gram-positive and gram-negative bacteria. Cefepime has a low affinity for chromosomally-encoded beta-lactamases. Cefepime is highly resistant to hydrolysis by most beta-lactamases and exhibits rapid penetration into gram-negative bacterial cells. Within bacterial cells, the molecular targets of cefepime are the penicillin binding proteins (PBP).

Cefepime has been shown to be active against most strains of the following microorganisms, both *in vitro* and in clinical infections as described in INDICATIONS AND USAGE.

Aerobic Gram-Negative Microorganisms

Enterobacter, Escherichia coli, Klebsiella pneumoniae, Proteus mirabilis, and *Pseudomonas aeruginosa.*

Aerobic Gram-Positive Microorganisms

Staphylococcus aureus (methicillin-susceptible strains only), *Streptococcus pneumoniae, Streptococcus pyogenes* (Lancefield's Group A streptococci), and Viridans group streptococci.

The following *in vitro* data are available; **but their clinical significance is unknown.** Cefepime has been shown to have *in vitro* activity against most strains of the following microorganisms; however, the safety and effectiveness of cefepime in treating clinical infections due to these microorganisms have not been established in adequate and well-controlled trials.

Aerobic Gram-Positive Microorganisms

Staphylococcus epidermidis (methicillin-susceptible strains only), *Staphylococcus saprophyticus,* and *Streptococcus agalactiae* (Lancefield's Group B streptococci).

Note: Most strains of enterococci, *e.g., Enterococcus faecalis,* and methicillin-resistant staphylococci are resistant to cefepime.

Aerobic Gram-Negative Microorganisms

Acinetobacter calcoaceticus subsp. *lwoffi, Citrobacter diversus, Citrobacter freundii, Enterobacter agglomerans, Haemophilus influenzae* (including beta-lactamase producing strains), *Hafnia alvei, Klebsiella oxytoca, Moraxella catarrhalis* (including beta-lactamase producing strains), *Morganella morganii, Proteus vulgaris, Providencia rettgeri, Providencia stuartii,* and *Serratia marcescens.*

Note: Cefepime is inactive against many strains of *Stenotrophomonas* (formerly *Xanthomonas maltophilia* and *Pseudomonas maltophilia*).

Anaerobic Microorganisms

Note: Cefepime is inactive against most strains of *Clostridium difficile.*

SUSCEPTIBILITY TESTING

Dilution Techniques

Quantitative methods are used to determine antimicrobial minimum inhibitory concentrations (MICs). These MICs provide estimates of the susceptibility of bacteria to antimicrobial compounds. The MICs should be determined using a standardized procedure. Standardized procedures are based on a dilution method[1] (broth or agar) or equivalent with standardized inoculum concentrations and standardized concentrations of cefepime powder. The MIC values should be interpreted according to the criteria in TABLE 4.

TABLE 4

Microorganism	MIC (μg/ml) Susceptible (S)	Intermediate (I)	Resistant (R)z
Microorganisms other than *Haemophilus* spp.* and *S. pneumoniae**	≤8	16	≥32
Haemophilus spp.*	≤2	—*	—*
*Streptococcus pneumoniae**	≤0.5	1	≥2

* **NOTE:** Isolates from these species should be tested for susceptibility using specialized dilution testing methods.[1] Also, strains of *Haemophilus* spp. with MICs greater than 2 μg/ml should be considered equivocal and should be further evaluated.

A report of "Susceptible" indicates that the pathogen is likely to be inhibited if the antimicrobial compound in the blood reaches the concentrations usually achievable. A report of "Intermediate" indicates that the result should be considered equivocal, and, if the microorganism is not fully susceptible to alternative, clinically feasible drugs, the test should be repeated. This category implies possible clinical applicability in body sites where the drug is physiologically concentrated or in situations where high dosage of drug can be used. This category also provides a buffer zone which prevents small uncontrolled technical factors from causing major discrepancies in interpretation. A report of "Resistant" indicates that the pathogen is not likely to be inhibited if the antimicrobial compound in the blood reaches the concentrations usually achievable; other therapy should be selected.

Standardized susceptibility test procedures require the use of laboratory control microorganisms to control the technical aspects of the laboratory procedures. Laboratory control microorganisms are specific strains of microbiological assay organisms with intrinsic biological properties relating to resistance mechanisms and their genetic expression within bacteria; the specific strains are not clinically significant in their current microbiological status. Standard cefepime powder should provide the MIC values in TABLE 5 when tested against the designated quality control strains.

TABLE 5

Microorganism	ATCC	MIC
Escherichia coli	25922	0.016-0.12 μg/ml
Staphylococcus aureus	29213	1-4 μg/ml
Pseudomonas aeruginosa	27853	1-4 μg/ml
Haemophilus influenzae	49247	0.5-2 μg/ml
Streptococcus pneumoniae	49619	0.06-0.25 μg/ml

Diffusion Techniques

Quantitative methods that require measurement of zone diameters also provide reproducible estimates of the susceptibility of bacteria to antimicrobial compounds. One such standardized procedure[2] requires the use of standardized inoculum concentrations. This procedure uses paper disks impregnated with 30 μg of cefepime to test the susceptibility of microorganisms to cefepime. Interpretation is identical to that stated above for results using dilution techniques.

Reports from the laboratory providing results of the standard single-disk susceptibility test with a 30 μg cefepime disk should be interpreted according to the criteria in TABLE 6.

TABLE 6

Microorganism	Zone Diameter (mm) Susceptible (S)	Intermediate (I)	Resistant (R)
Microorganisms other than *Haemophilus* spp.* and *S. pneumoniae**	≥18	15-17	≤14
Haemophilus spp.*	≥26	—*	—*

* **Note:** Isolates from these species should be tested for susceptibility using specialized diffusion testing methods.[2] Isolates of *Haemophilus* spp. with zones smaller than 26 mm should be considered equivocal and should be further evaluated. Isolates of *S. pneumoniae* should be tested against a 1 μg oxacillin disk; isolates with oxacillin zone sizes larger than or equal to 20 mm may be considered susceptible to cefepime.

As with standardized dilution techniques, diffusion methods require the use of laboratory control microorganisms to control the technical aspects of the laboratory procedures. Laboratory control microorganisms are specific strains of microbiological assay organisms with intrinsic biological properties relating to resistance mechanisms and their genetic expression within bacteria; the specific strains are not clinically significant in their current microbiological status. For the diffusion technique, the 30 μg cefepime disk should provide the zone diameters shown in TABLE 7 in these laboratory test quality control strains.

TABLE 7

Microorganism	ATCC	Zone Size Range
Escherichia coli	25922	29-35 mm
Staphylococcus aureus	25923	23-29 mm
Pseudomonas aeruginosa	27853	24-30 mm
Haemophilus influenzae	49247	25-31 mm

INDICATIONS AND USAGE

Cefepime HCl is indicated in the treatment of the following infections caused by susceptible strains of the designated microorganisms (see also PRECAUTIONS, Pediatric Use and DOSAGE AND ADMINISTRATION):

Pneumonia (moderate to severe) caused by *Streptococcus pneumoniae,* including cases associated with concurrent bacteremia, *Pseudomonas aeruginosa, Klebsiella pneumoniae,* or *Enterobacter species.*

Empiric therapy for febrile neutropenic patients. Cefepime as monotherapy is indicated for empiric treatment of febrile neutropenic patients. In patients at high risk for severe infection (including patients with a history of recent bone marrow transplantation, with hypotension at presentation, with an underlying hematologic malignancy, or with severe or prolonged neutropenia), antimicrobial monotherapy may not be appropriate. Insufficient data exist to support the efficacy of cefepime monotherapy in such patients.

Uncomplicated and complicated urinary tract infections (including pyelonephritis) caused by *Escherichia coli* or *Klebsiella pneumoniae,* when the infection is severe, or caused by *Escherichia coli, Klebsiella pneumoniae* or *Proteus mirabilis,* when the infection is mild to moderate, including cases associated with concurrent bacteremia with these microorganisms.

Uncomplicated skin and skin structure infections caused by *Staphylococcus aureus* (methicillin-susceptible strains only) or *Streptococcus pyogenes.*

Complicated intra-abdominal infections (used in combination with metronidazole) caused by *Escherichia coli,* viridans group streptococci, *Pseudomonas aeruginosa, Klebsiella pneumoniae, Enterobacter* species, or *Bacteroides fragilis.*

Culture and susceptibility testing should be performed where appropriate to determine the susceptibility of the causative microorganism(s) to cefepime.

Therapy with cefepime HCl may be instituted before results of susceptibility studies are known; however, once these results become available, the antibiotic treatment should be adjusted accordingly.

CONTRAINDICATIONS

Cefepime HCl is contraindicated in patients who have shown immediate hypersensitivity reactions to cefepime or the cephalosporin class of antibiotics, penicillins or other beta-lactam antibiotics.

WARNINGS

BEFORE THERAPY WITH CEFEPIME HCL FOR INJECTION IS INSTITUTED, CAREFUL INQUIRY SHOULD BE MADE TO DETERMINE WHETHER THE PATIENT HAS HAD PREVIOUS IMMEDIATE HYPERSENSITIVITY REACTIONS TO CEFEPIME, CEPHALOSPORINS, PENICILLINS, OR OTHER DRUGS. IF THIS PRODUCT IS TO BE GIVEN TO PENICILLIN-SENSITIVE PATIENTS, CAUTION SHOULD BE EXERCISED BECAUSE CROSS-HYPERSENSITIVITY AMONG BETA-LACTAM ANTIBIOTICS HAS BEEN CLEARLY DOCUMENTED AND MAY OCCUR IN UP TO 10% OF PATIENTS WITH A HISTORY Of PENICILLIN ALLERGY. IF AN ALLERGIC REACTION TO CEFEPIME HCL OCCURS, DISCONTINUE THE DRUG. SERIOUS ACUTE HYPERSENSITIVITY REACTIONS MAY REQUIRE TREATMENT WITH EPINEPHRINE AND OTHER EMERGENCY MEASURES INCLUDING OXYGEN, CORTICOSTEROIDS, IV FLUIDS, IV ANTIHISTAMINES, PRESSOR AMINES, AND AIRWAY MANAGEMENT, AS CLINICALLY INDICATED.

In patients with impaired renal function (creatinine clearance ≤60 ml/min), the dose of cefepime HCl should be adjusted to compensate for the slower rate of renal elimination. Because high and prolonged serum antibiotic concentrations can occur from usual dosages in patients with renal insufficiency or other conditions that may compromise renal function, the maintenance dosage should be reduced when cefepime is administered to such patients. Continued dosage should be determined by degree of renal impairment, severity of infection, and susceptibility of the causative organisms. (See specific recommendations for dosing adjustment in DOSAGE AND ADMINISTRATION.) During postmarketing surveillance, serious adverse events have been reported including life-threatening or fatal occurrences of the following: encephalopathy (disturbance of consciousness including confusion, hallucinations, stupor, and coma), myoclonus, and seizures (see ADVERSE REACTIONS, Postmarketing Experience). Most cases occurred in patients with renal impairment who received doses of cefepime that exceeded the recommended dosage schedules. However, some cases of encephalopathy occurred in patients receiving a dosage adjustment for their renal function. In the majority of cases, symptoms of neurotoxicity were reversible and resolved after discontinuation of cefepime and/or after hemodialysis.

Pseudomembranous colitis has been reported with nearly all antibacterial agents, including cefepime HCl, and may range in severity from mild to life-threatening. Therefore, it is important to consider this diagnosis in patients who present with diarrhea subsequent to the administration of antibacterial agents.

Treatment with antibacterial agents alters the normal flora of the colon and may permit overgrowth of clostridia. Studies indicate that a toxin produced by *Clostridium difficile* is a primary cause of "antibiotic-associated colitis".

After the diagnosis of pseudomembranous colitis has been established, therapeutic measures should be initiated. Mild cases of pseudomembranous colitis usually respond to drug discontinuation alone. In moderate-to-severe cases, consideration should be given to management with fluids and electrolytes, protein supplementation, and treatment with an antibacterial drug clinically effective against *Clostridium difficile* colitis.

PRECAUTIONS

GENERAL

As with other antimicrobials, prolonged use of cefepime HCl may result in overgrowth of nonsusceptible microorganisms. Repeated evaluation of the patient's condition is essential. Should superinfection occur during therapy, appropriate measures should be taken.

Many cephalosporins, including cefepime, have been associated with a fall in prothrombin activity. Those at risk include patients with renal or hepatic impairment, or poor nutritional state, as well as patients receiving a protracted course of antimicrobial therapy. Prothrombin time should be monitored in patients at risk, and exogenous vitamin K administered as indicated.

Positive direct Coombs' tests have been reported during treatment with cefepime HCl. In hematologic studies or in transfusion cross-matching procedures when antiglobulin tests are performed on the minor side or in Coombs' testing of newborns whose mothers have received cephalosporin antibiotics before parturition, it should be recognized that a positive Coombs' test may be due to the drug.

Cefepime HCl should be prescribed with caution in individuals with a history of gastrointestinal disease, particularly colitis.

Arginine has been shown to alter glucose metabolism and elevate serum potassium transiently when administered at 33 times the amount provided by the maximum recommended human dose of cefepime HCl. The effect of lower doses is not presently known.

DRUG/LABORATORY TEST INTERACTIONS

The administration of cefepime may result in a false-positive reaction for glucose in the urine when using Clinitest tablets. It is recommended that glucose tests based on enzymatic glucose oxidase reactions (such as Clinistix or Tes-Tape) be used.

CARCINOGENESIS, MUTAGENESIS, AND IMPAIRMENT OF FERTILITY

No long-term animal carcinogenicity studies have been conducted with cefepime. A battery of *in vivo* and *in vitro* genetic toxicity tests, including the Ames Salmonella reverse mutation assay, CHO/HGPRT mammalian cell forward gene mutation assay, chromosomal aberration and sister chromatid exchange assays in human lymphocytes, CHO fibroblast clastogenesis assay, and cytogenetic and micronucleus assays in mice were conducted. The overall conclusion of these tests indicated no definitive evidence of genotoxic potential. No untoward effects on fertility or reproduction have been observed in rats, mice, and rabbits when cefepime is administered subcutaneously at 1-4 times the recommended maximum human dose calculated on a mg/m^2 basis.

PREGNANCY, TERATOGENIC EFFECTS, PREGNANCY CATEGORY B

Cefepime was not teratogenic or embryocidal when administered during the period of organogenesis to rats at doses up to 1000 mg/kg/day (4 times the recommended maximum human dose calculated on a mg/m^2 basis) or to mice at doses up to 1200 mg/kg (2 times the recommended maximum human dose calculated on a mg/m^2 basis) or to rabbits at a dose level of 100 mg/kg (approximately equal to the recommended maximum human dose calculated on a mg/m^2 basis).

There are, however, no adequate and well-controlled studies of cefepime use in pregnant women. Because animal reproduction studies are not always predictive of human response, this drug should be used during pregnancy only if clearly needed.

NURSING MOTHERS

Cefepime is excreted in human breast milk in very low concentrations (0.5 μg/ml). Caution should be exercised when cefepime is administered to a nursing woman.

LABOR AND DELIVERY

Cefepime has not been studied for use during labor and delivery. Treatment should only be given if clearly indicated.

PEDIATRIC USE

The safety and effectiveness of cefepime in the treatment of uncomplicated and complicated urinary tract infections (including pyelonephritis), uncomplicated skin and skin structure infections, pneumonia, and as empiric therapy for febrile neutropenic patients have been established in the age groups 2 months up to 16 years. Use of cefepime HCl in these age groups is supported by evidence from adequate and well-controlled studies of cefepime in adults with additional pharmacokinetic and safety data from pediatric trials (see CLINICAL PHARMACOLOGY).

Safety and effectiveness in pediatric patients below the age of 2 months have not been established. There are insufficient clinical data to support the use of cefepime HCl in pediatric patients under 2 months of age or for the treatment of serious infections in the pediatric population where the suspected or proven pathogen is *Haemophilus influenzae* type b.

IN THOSE PATIENTS IN WHOM MENINGEAL SEEDING FROM A DISTANT INFECTION SITE OR IN WHOM MENINGITIS IS SUSPECTED OR DOCUMENTED, AN ALTERNATE AGENT WITH DEMONSTRATED CLINICAL EFFICACY IN THIS SETTING SHOULD BE USED.

GERIATRIC USE

Of the more than 6400 adults treated with cefepime HCl in clinical studies, 35% were 65 years or older while 16% were 75 years or older. When geriatric patients received the usual recommended adult dose, clinical efficacy and safety were comparable to clinical efficacy and safety in nongeriatric adult patients.

Serious adverse events have occurred in geriatric patients with renal insufficiency given unadjusted doses of cefepime, including life-threatening or fatal occurrences of the following: encephalopathy, myoclonus, and seizures. (See WARNINGS and ADVERSE REACTIONS.)

This drug is known to be subtantially excreted by the kidney, and the risk of toxic reactions to this drug may be greater in patients with impaired renal function. Because elderly patients are more likely to have decreased renal function, care should be taken in dose selection, and renal function should be monitored. (See CLINICAL PHARMACOLOGY, Special Populations; WARNINGS; and DOSAGE AND ADMINISTRATION.)

DRUG INTERACTIONS

Renal function should be monitored carefully if high doses of aminoglycosides are to be administered with cefepime HCl because of the increased potential of nephrotoxicity and ototoxicity of aminoglycoside antibiotics. Nephrotoxicity has been reported following concomitant administration of other cephalosporins with potent diuretics such as furosemide.

ADVERSE REACTIONS

CLINICAL TRIALS

In clinical trials using multiple doses of cefepime, 4137 patients were treated with the recommended dosages of cefepime (500 mg to 2 g IV q12h). There were no deaths or permanent disabilities thought related to drug toxicity. Sixty-four (1.5%) patients discontinued medication due to adverse events thought by the investigators to be possibly, probably, or almost certainly related to drug toxicity. Thirty-three (51%) of these 64 patients who discontinued therapy did so because of rash. The percentage of cefepime-treated patients who discontinued study drug because of drug-related adverse events was very similar at daily doses of 500 mg, 1 g and 2 g q12h (0.8%, 1.1%, and 2.0%, respectively). However, the incidence of discontinuation due to rash increased with the higher recommended doses.

The following adverse events were thought to be probably related to cefepime during evaluation of the drug in clinical trials conducted in North America (n=3125 cefepime-treated patients).

TABLE 10 *Adverse Clinical Reactions: Cefepime Multiple-Dose Dosing Regimens Clinical Trials — North America*

Incidence ≥1%	Local reactions (3.0%), including phlebitis (1.3%), pain and/or inflammation (0.6%)*; rash (1.1%)
Incidence <1% but >0.1%	Colitis (including pseudomembranous colitis), diarrhea, fever, headache, nausea, oral moniliasis, pruritus, urticaria, vaginitis, vomiting

* Local reactions, irrespective of relationship to cefepime in those patients who received IV infusion (n=3048).

At the higher dose of 2 g q8h, the incidence of probably-related adverse events was higher among the 795 patients who received this dose of cefepime. They consisted of rash (4%), diarrhea (3%), nausea (2%), vomiting (1%), fever (1%), and headache (1%).

The adverse laboratory changes in TABLE 11, irrespective of relationship to therapy with cefepime, were seen during clinical trials conducted in North America.

TABLE 11 *Adverse Laboratory Changes: Cefepime Multiple-Dose Dosing Regimens Clinical Trials — North America*

Incidence ≥1%	Positive Coombs' test (without hemolysis) (16.2%); decreased phosphorous (2.8%); increased ALT/SGPT (2.8%), AST/SGOT (2.4%), eosinophils (1.7%); abnormal PTT (1.6%), PT (1.4%)
Incidence <1% but >0.1%	Increased alkaline phosphatase, BUN, calcium, creatinine, phosphorous, potassium, total bilirubin; decreased calcium*, hematocrit, neutrophils, platelets, WBC

* Hypocalcemia was more common among elderly patients. Clinical consequences from changes in either calcium or phosphorous were not reported.

A similar safety profile was seen in clinical trials of pediatric patients (see PRECAUTIONS, Pediatric Use).

POSTMARKETING EXPERIENCE

In addition to the events reported during North American clinical trials with cefepime, the following adverse experiences have been reported during worldwide postmarketing experience.

As with some other drugs in this class, encephalopathy (disturbance of consciousness including confusion, hallucinations, stupor, and coma), myoclonus, and seizures have been reported. Although most cases occurred in patients with renal impairment who received doses of cefepime that exceeded the recommended dosage schedules, some cases of encephalopathy occurred in patients receiving a dosage adjustment for their renal function. (See also WARNINGS.) If seizures associated with drug therapy occur, the drug should be discontinued. Anticonvulsant therapy can be given if clinically indicated. Precautions should be taken to adjust daily dosage in patients with renal insufficiency or other conditions that may compromise renal function to reduce antibiotic concentrations that can lead or contribute to these and other serious adverse events, including renal failure.

As with other cephalosporins, anaphylaxis including anaphylactic shock, transient leukopenia, neutropenia, agranulocytosis and thrombocytopenia have been reported.

CEPHALOSPORIN-CLASS ADVERSE REACTIONS

In addition to the adverse reactions listed above that have been observed in patients treated with cefepime, the following adverse reactions and altered laboratory tests have been reported for cephalosporin-class antibiotics: Stevens-Johnson syndrome, erythema multiforme, toxic epidermal necrolysis, renal dysfunction, toxic nephropathy, aplastic anemia, hemolytic anemia, hemorrhage, hepatic dysfunction including cholestasis, and pancytopenia.

DOSAGE AND ADMINISTRATION

The recommended adult and pediatric dosages and routes of administration are outlined in TABLE 12. Cefepime HCl should be administered intravenously over approximately 30 minutes.

TABLE 12 *Recommended Dosage Schedule for Cefepime HCl in Patients With CRCL >60 ml/min*

Site and Type of Infection	Dose	Frequency	Duration
Adults			
Moderate to Severe pneumonia due to *S. pneumoniae**, *P. aeruginosa*, *K. pneumoniae*, or *Enterobacter* species	1-2 g IV	q12h	10 days
Empiric therapy for febrile neutropenic patients†	2 g IV	q8h	7 days‡
Mild to Moderate uncomplicated or complicated urinary tract infections, including pyelonephritis, due to *E. coli*, *K. pneumoniae*, or *P. mirabilis**	0.5-1 g IV/IM§	q12h	7-10 days
Severe uncomplicated or complicated urinary tract infections, including pyelonephritis, due to *E. coli* or *K. pneumoniae**	2 g IV	q12h	10 days
Moderate to Severe uncomplicated skin and skin structure infections due to *S. aureus* or *S. pyogenes*	2 g IV	q12h	10 days
Complicated Intra-abdominal Infections (used in combination with metronidazole) caused by E. coli, viridans group streptococci, *P. aeruginosa*, *K. pneumoniae*, *Enterobacter* species, or *B. fragilis*.	2 g IV	q12h	7-10 days

Pediatric Patients (2 months up to 16 years)
The maximum dose for pediatric patients should not exceed the recommended adult dose. The usual recommended dosage in pediatric patients up to 40 kg in weight for uncomplicated and complicated urinary tract infections (including pyelonephritis), uncomplicated skin and skin structure infections, and pneumonia is 50 mg/kg/dose, administered q12h (50 mg/kg/dose, q8h for febrile neutropenic patients), for durations as given above.

* Including cases associated with concurrent bacteremia.
† See INDICATIONS AND USAGE.
‡ Or until resolution of neutropenia. In patients whose fever resolves but who remain neutropenic for more than 7 days, the need for continued antimicrobial therapy should be re-evaluated frequently.
§ IM route of administration is indicated only for mild to moderate, uncomplicated or complicated UTI's due to *E. coli* when the IM route is considered to be a more appropriate route of drug administration.

IMPAIRED HEPATIC FUNCTION

No adjustment is necessary for patients with impaired hepatic function.

IMPAIRED RENAL FUNCTION

In patients with impaired renal function (creatinine clearance ≤60 ml/min), the dose of cefepime HCl should be adjusted to compensate for the slower rate of renal elimination. The recommended initial dose of cefepime HCl should be the same as in patients with normal renal function except in patients undergoing hemodialysis. The recommended maintenance doses of cefepime HCl in patients with renal insufficiency are presented in TABLE 13.

When only serum creatinine is available, the following formula (Cockcroft and Gault equation)[3] may be used to estimate creatinine clearance. The serum creatinine should represent a steady state of renal function:

Males: Creatinine Clearance (ml/min) = Weight (kg) × (140 - age) ÷ 72 × serum creatinine (mg/dL)

Females: 0.85 × above value

TABLE 13 *Recommended Dosing Schedule for Cefepime HCl in Adult Patients (Normal Renal Function, Renal Insufficiency, and Hemodialysis)*

Creatinine Clearance (ml/min)	Recommended Maintenance Schedule			
>60 Normal recommended dosing schedule	500 mg q12h	1 g q12h	2 g q12h	2 g q8h
30-60	500 mg q24h	1 g q24h	2 g q24h	2 g q12h
11-29	500 mg q24h	500 mg q24h	1 g q24h	2 g q24h
<11	250 mg q24h	250 mg q24h	500 mg q24h	1 g q24h
CAPD	500 mg q48h	1 g q48h	2 g q48h	2 g q48h
Hemodialysis*	1 g on Day 1, then 500 mg q24h thereafter			1 g q24h

* On hemodialysis days, cefepime should be administered following hemodialysis. Whenever possible, cefepime should be administered at the same time each day.

In patients undergoing continuous ambulatory peritoneal dialysis, cefepime HCl may be administered at normally recommended doses at a dosage interval of every 48 hours (see TABLE 13).

In patients undergoing hemodialysis, approximately 68% of the total amount of cefepime present in the body at the start of dialysis will be removed during a 3 hour dialysis period. The dosage of cefepime HCl for hemodialysis patients is 1 g on Day 1 followed by 500 mg q24h for the treatment of all infections except febrile neutropenia, which is 1 g q24h. Cefepime HCl should be administered at the same time each day and following the completion of hemodialysis on hemodialysis days (see TABLE 13).

Data in pediatric patients with impaired renal function are not available; however, since cefepime pharmacokinetics are similar in adults and pediatric patients (see CLINICAL PHARMACOLOGY), changes in the dosing regimen proportional to those in adults (see TABLE 12 and TABLE 13) are recommended for pediatric patients.

ADMINISTRATION

For IV Infusion

Constitute the 1 or 2 g piggyback (100 ml) bottle with 50 or 100 ml of a compatible IV fluid listed in Compatibility and Stability. Alternatively, constitute the 500 mg, 1 g, or 2 g vial, and add an appropriate quantity of the resulting solution to an IV container with one of the compatible IV fluids. **THE RESULTING SOLUTION SHOULD BE ADMINISTERED OVER APPROXIMATELY 30 MINUTES.**

Intermittent IV infusion with a Y-type administration set can be accomplished with compatible solutions. However, during infusion of a solution containing cefepime, it is desirable to discontinue the other solution.

ADD-Vantage vials are to be constituted only with 50 or 100 ml of 5% dextrose injection or 0.9% sodium chloride injection in Abbott ADD-Vantage flexible diluent containers. (See ADD-Vantage Vial Instructions for Use distributed with the ADD-Vantage vial.)

IM Administration

For IM administration, cefepime HCl should be constituted with one of the following diluents: sterile water for injection, 0.9% sodium chloride, 5% dextrose injection, 0.5% or 1.0% lidocaine HCl, or sterile bacteriostatic water for injection with parabens or benzyl alcohol.

COMPATIBILITY AND STABILITY

Intravenous

Cefepime HCl is compatible at concentrations between 1 and 40 mg/ml with the following IV infusion fluids: 0.9% sodium chloride injection, 5% and 10% dextrose injection, M/6 sodium lactate injection, 5% dextrose and 0.9% sodium chloride injection, lactated Ringers and 5% dextrose injection, Normosol-R , and Normosol-M in 5% dextrose injection. These solutions may be stored up to 24 hours at controlled room temperature 20-25°C (68-77°F) or 7 days in a refrigerator 2-8°C (36-46°F). Cefepime HCl in ADD-Vantage vials is stable at concentrations of 10-40 mg/ml in 5% dextrose injection or 0.9% sodium chloride injection for 24 hours at controlled room temperature 20-25°C or 7 days in a refrigerator 2-8°C.

Cefepime HCl admixture compatibility information is summarized in TABLE 14.

TABLE 14 *Cefepime Admixture Stability*

Cefepime HCl Concentration	Admixture and Concentration	IV Infusion Solutions	Stability Time for RT/L (20-25°C)	Refrigeration (2-8°C)
40 mg/ml	Amikacin 6 mg/ml	NS or D5W	24 h	7 days
40 mg/ml	Ampicillin 1 mg/ml	D5W	8 h	8 h
40 mg/ml	Ampicillin 10 mg/ml	D5W	2 h	8 h
40 mg/ml	Ampicillin 1 mg/ml	NS	24 h	48 h
40 mg/ml	Ampicillin 10 mg/ml	NS	8 h	48 h
4 mg/ml	Ampicillin 40 mg/ml	NS	8 h	8 h
4-40 mg/ml	Clindamycin phosphate 0.25-6 mg/ml	NS or D5W	24 h	7 days
4 mg/ml	Heparin 10-50 units/ml	NS or D5W	24 h	7 days
4 mg/ml	Potassium chloride 10-40 mEq/L	NS or D5W	24 h	7 days
4 mg/ml	Theophylline 0.8 mg/ml	D5W	24 h	7 days
1-4 mg/ml	NA	Aminosyn II 4.25% with electrolytes and calcium	8 h	3 days
0.125-0.25 mg/ml	NA	Inpersol with 4.25% dextrose	24 h	7 days

NS = 0.9% sodium chloride injection.
D5W = 5% dextrose injection.
NA = not applicable.
RT/L = Ambient room temperature and light.

Solutions of cefepime HCl, like those of most beta-lactam antibiotics, should not be added to solutions of ampicillin at a concentration greater than 40 mg/ml, and should not be added to metronidazole, vancomycin, gentamicin, tobramycin, netilmicin sulfate or aminophylline because of potential interaction. However, if concurrent therapy with cefepime HCl is indicated, each of these antibiotics can be administered separately.

Intramuscular

Cefepime HCl constituted as directed is stable for 24 hours at controlled room temperature 20-25°C (68-77°F) or for 7 days in a refrigerator 2-8°C (36-46°F) with the following diluents: sterile water for injection, 0.9% sodium chloride injection, 5% dextrose injection, sterile bacteriostatic water for injection with parabens or benzyl alcohol, or 0.5% or 1% lidocaine HCl.

NOTE: PARENTERAL DRUGS SHOULD BE INSPECTED VISUALLY FOR PARTICULATE MATTER BEFORE ADMINISTRATION.

As with other cephalosporins, the color of cefepime HCl powder, as well as its solutions, tend to darken depending on storage conditions; however, when stored as recommended, the product's potency is not adversely affected.

HOW SUPPLIED

Maxipime for injection is supplied as follows:

500 mg*: 15 ml vial.
1 g*: Piggyback bottle 100 ml.
1 g*: ADD-Vantage vial.
1 g*: 15 ml vial.
2 g*: Piggyback bottle 100 ml.
2 g*: ADD-Vantage vial.
2 g*: 20 ml vial.

*Based on cefepime activity.

Storage: MAXIPIME IN THE DRY STATE SHOULD BE STORED BETWEEN 2-25°C (36-77°F) AND PROTECTED FROM LIGHT.

PRODUCT LISTING - EQUIVALENTS NOT AVAILABLE

Powder For Injection - Injectable - 1 Gm

1's	$19.36	MAXIPIME, Elan Pharmaceuticals	51479-0054-10
10's	$153.00	MAXIPIME, Bristol-Myers Squibb	00003-7732-99
10's	$159.00	MAXIPIME, Bristol-Myers Squibb	00003-7732-89
10's	$163.80	MAXIPIME, Bristol-Myers Squibb	00003-7732-95
10's	$180.80	MAXIPIME, Elan Pharmaceuticals	51479-0054-30
10's	$187.90	MAXIPIME, Elan Pharmaceuticals	51479-0054-20

Powder For Injection - Injectable - 2 Gm

1's	$37.14	MAXIPIME, Elan Pharmaceuticals	51479-0055-20
10's	$303.60	MAXIPIME, Bristol-Myers Squibb	00003-7733-99
10's	$314.40	MAXIPIME, Bristol-Myers Squibb	00003-7733-95
10's	$358.60	MAXIPIME, Elan Pharmaceuticals	51479-0055-30
10's	$365.90	MAXIPIME, Elan Pharmaceuticals	51479-0055-10

Powder For Injection - Injectable - 500 mg

10's	$85.60	MAXIPIME, Elan Pharmaceuticals	00003-7731-99

Cefixime *(000684)*

For related information, see the comparative table section in Appendix A.

Categories: Bronchitis, chronic, acute exacerbation; Gonorrhea; Infection, ear, middle; Infection, lower respiratory tract; Infection, sexually transmitted; Infection, upper respiratory tract; Infection, urinary tract; Pharyngitis; Tonsillitis; Pregnancy Category B; FDA Approved 1989 Apr

Drug Classes: Antibiotics, cephalosporins

Brand Names: Suprax

Foreign Brand Availability: Cefix (Bahrain; Cyprus; Egypt; Iran; Iraq; Jordan; Korea; Kuwait; Lebanon; Libya; Oman; Qatar; Republic-of-Yemen; Saudi-Arabia; Syria; United-Arab-Emirates); Cefixmycin (Taiwan); Cefspan (Indonesia; Taiwan; Thailand); Cephoral (Germany; Switzerland); Denvar (Costa-Rica; Dominican-Republic; El-Salvador; Guatemala; Honduras; Mexico; Nicaragua; Panama; Peru; Spain); Devoxim (Colombia); Fixef (Indonesia); Fixim (Netherlands); Fixime (South-Africa); Fixiphar (Indonesia); Fixx (India); Maxpro (Indonesia); Necopen (Spain); Novacef (Mexico); Oroken (France); Pocef (Korea); Sofix (Indonesia); Spancef (Indonesia); Starcef (Indonesia); Sucef (Korea); Supran (Israel); Tergecef (Philippines); Tocef (Indonesia); Tricef (Sweden); Ultraxime (Philippines); Uro-cephoral (Germany); Zefral (Philippines)

Cost of Therapy: $80.08 (Infection; Suprax; 400 mg; 1 tablet/day; 10 day supply)

DESCRIPTION

Cefixime is a semisynthetic, cephalosporin antibiotic for oral administration. Chemically, it is (6*R*,7*R*)-7-[2-(2-Amino-4-thiazolyl) glyoxylamido]-8-oxo-3-vinyl-5-thia-1-azabicyclo[4.2.0]oct-2-ene-2-carboxylic acid, 7^2(*Z*)-[O-(carboxymethyl)oxime]-trihydrate. Molecular weight = 507.50 as the trihydrate.

Suprax is available in scored 200 and 400 mg film coated tablets and in a powder for oral suspension which when reconstituted provides 100 mg/5 ml.

Inactive ingredients contained in the 200 and 400 mg tablets are: Dibasic calcium phosphate, hydroxypropyl methylcellulose 2910, light mineral oil, magnesium stearate, microcrystalline cellulose, pregelatinized starch, sodium lauryl sulfate and titanium dioxide. The powder for oral suspension is strawberry flavored and contains sodium benzoate, sucrose, and xanthan gum.

CLINICAL PHARMACOLOGY

Cefixime, given orally, is about 40-50% absorbed whether administered with or without food; however, time to maximal absorption is increased approximately 0.8 hours when administered with food. A single 200 mg tablet of cefixime produces an average peak serum concentration of approximately 2 µg/ml (range 1-4 µg/ml); a single 400 mg tablet produces an average peak concentration of approximately 3.7 µg/ml (range 1.3-7.7 µg/ml). The oral suspension produces average peak concentrations approximately 25-50% higher than the tablets. Two hundred (200) and 400 mg doses of oral suspension produce average peak concentrations of 3 µg/ml (range 1.0-4.5 µg/ml) and 4.6 µg/ml (range 1.9-7.7 µg/ml), respectively, when tested in normal *adult* volunteers. The area under the time versus concentration curve is greater by approximately 10-25% with the oral suspension than with the tablet after doses of 100-400 mg, when tested in normal *adult* volunteers. This increased absorption should be taken into consideration if the oral suspension is to be substituted for the tablet. Because of the lack of bioequivalence, tablets should not be substituted for oral suspension in the treatment of otitis media. (See DOSAGE AND ADMINISTRATION.) Crossover studies of tablets versus suspension have not been performed in children.

Peak serum concentrations occur between 2 and 6 hours following oral administration of a single 200 or 400 mg tablet, or 400 mg of suspension of cefixime. Peak serum concentrations occur between 2 and 5 hours following a single administration of 200 mg of suspension (see TABLE 1 and TABLE 2).

TABLE 1 *Serum Levels of Cefixime After Administration of Tablets (μg/ml)*

Dose	1 h	2 h	4 h	6 h	8 h	12 h	24 h
100 mg	0.3	0.8	1.0	0.7	0.4	0.2	0.02
200 mg	0.7	1.4	2.0	1.5	1.0	0.4	0.03
400 mg	1.2	2.5	3.5	2.7	1.7	0.6	0.04

TABLE 2 *Serum Levels of Cefixime After Administration of Oral Suspension (μg/ml)*

Dose	1 h	2 h	4 h	6 h	8 h	12 h	24 h
100 mg	0.7	1.1	1.3	0.9	0.6	0.2	0.02
200 mg	1.2	2.1	2.8	2.0	1.3	0.5	0.07
400 mg	1.8	3.3	4.4	3.3	2.2	0.8	0.07

Approximately 50% of the absorbed dose is excreted unchanged in the urine in 24 hours. In animal studies, it was noted that cefixime is also excreted in the bile in excess of 10% of the administered dose. Serum protein binding is concentration independent with a bound fraction of approximately 65%. In a multiple dose study conducted with a research formulation which is less bioavailable than the tablet or suspension, there was little accumulation of drug in serum or urine after dosing for 14 days.

The serum half-life of cefixime in healthy subjects is independent of dosage form and averages 3-4 hours but may range up to 9 hours in some normal volunteers. Average AUCs at steady state in elderly patients are approximately 40% higher than average AUCs in other healthy adults.

In subjects with moderate impairment of renal function (20-40 ml/min creatinine clearance), the average serum half-life of cefixime is prolonged to 6.4 hours. In severe renal impairment (5-20 ml/min creatinine clearance), the half-life increased to an average of 11.5 hours. The drug is not cleared significantly from the blood by hemodialysis or peritoneal dialysis. However, a study indicated that with doses of 400 mg, patients undergoing hemodialysis have similar blood profiles as subjects with creatinine clearances of 21-60 ml/min. There is no evidence of metabolism of cefixime *in vivo*.

Adequate date of CSF levels of cefixime are not available.

MICROBIOLOGY

As with other cephalosporins, bactericidal action of cefixime results from inhibition of cell-wall synthesis. Cefixime is highly stable in the presence of beta-lactamase enzymes. As a result, many organisms resistant to penicillins and some cephalosporins, due to the presence of beta-lactamase, may be susceptible to cefixime. Cefixime has been shown to be active against most strains of the following organisms both *in vitro* and in clinical infections (see INDICATIONS AND USAGE).

Gram-Positive Organisms: *Streptococcus pneumoniae* and *Streptococcus pyogenes.*

Gram-Negative Organisms: *Haemophilus influenzae* (beta-lactamase positive and negative strains), *Moraxella (Branhamella) catarrhalis* (most of which are beta-lactamase positive), *Escherichia coli, Proteus mirabilis,* and *Neisseria gonorrhoeae* (including penicillinase- and non-penicillinase-producing strains).

Cefixime has been shown to be active *in vitro* against most strains of the following organisms; however, clinical efficacy has not been established.

Gram-Positive Organisms: *Streptococcus agalactiae.*

Gram-Negative Organisms: *Haemophilus parainfluenzae* (beta-lactamase positive and negative strains), *Proteus vulgaris, Klebsiella pneumoniae, Klebsiella oxytoca, Pasteurella multocida, Providencia* spp., *Salmonella* spp., *Shigella* spp., *Citrobacter amalonaticus, Citrobacter diversus,* and *Serratia marcescens.*

Note: *Pseudomonas* spp., strains of group D streptococci (including *enterococci*), *Listeria monocytogenes,* most strains of staphylococci (including methicillin-resistant strains) and most strains of *Enterobacter* are resistant to cefixime. In addition, most strains of *Bacteroides fragilis* and *Clostridium* are resistant to cefixime.

SUSCEPTIBILITY TESTING

Diffusion Techniques

Quantitative methods that require measurement of zone diameters give an estimate of antibiotic susceptibility. One such procedure[1-3] has been recommended for use with disks to test susceptibility to cefixime. Interpretation involves correlation of the diameters obtained in the disk test with minimum inhibitory concentration (MIC) for cefixime.

Reports from the laboratory giving results of the standard single-disk susceptibility test with a 5 μg cefixime disk should be interpreted according to TABLE 3.

TABLE 3 *Recommended Susceptibility Ranges — Agar Disk Diffusion*

Organisms	Resistant	Moderately Susceptible	Susceptible
*Neisseria gonorrhoeae**	—	—	≥31 mm
All other organisms	≤15 mm	16-18 mm	≥19 mm

* Using GC agar base with a defined 1% supplement without cysteine.

A report of "Susceptible" indicates that the pathogen is likely to be inhibited by generally achievable blood levels. A report of "Moderately Susceptible" indicates that inhibitory concentrations of the antibiotic may well be achieved if high dosage is used or if the infection is confined to tissues and fluids (*e.g.,* urine) in which high antibiotic levels are attained. A report of "Resistant" indicates that achievable concentrations of the antibiotic are unlikely to be inhibitory and other therapy should be selected.

Standardized procedures require the use of laboratory control organisms. The 5 μg disk should give the following zone diameter (TABLE 4).

TABLE 4

Organism	Zone Diameter (mm)
Escherichia coli ATCC 25922	23-27
Neisseria gonorrhoeae ATCC 49226*	37-45

* Using GC agar base with a defined 1% supplement without cysteine.

The class disk for cephalosporin susceptibility testing (the cephalothin disk) is not appropriate because of spectrum differences with cefixime. The 5 μg cefixime disk should be used for all *in vitro* testing of isolates.

Dilution Techniques

Broth or agar dilution methods can be used to determine the MIC value for susceptibility of bacterial isolates to cefixime. The recommended susceptibility breakpoints are found in TABLE 5.

TABLE 5 *MIC Interpretive Standards (μg/ml)*

Organism	Resistant	Moderately Susceptible	Susceptible
*Neisseria gonorrhoeae**	—	—	≤0.25
All other organisms	≥4	2	≤1

* Using GC agar base with a defined 1% supplement without cysteine.

As with standard diffusion methods, dilution procedures require the use of laboratory control organisms. Standard cefixime powder should give the following MIC ranges in daily testing of quality control organisms (TABLE 6).

TABLE 6

Organism	MIC Range (μg/ml)
Escherichia coli ATCC 25922	0.25-1
Staphylococcus aureus ATCC 29213	8-32
Neisseria gonorrhoeae ATCC 49226*	0.008-0.03

* Using GC agar base with a defined 1% supplement without cysteine.

INDICATIONS AND USAGE

Cefixime is indicated in the treatment of the following infections when caused by susceptible strains of the designated microorganisms:

Uncomplicated Urinary Tract Infections: Caused by *Escherichia coli* and *Proteus mirabilis.*

Otitis Media: Caused by *Haemophilus influenzae* (beta-lactamase positive and negative strains), *Moraxella (Branhamella) catarrhalis* (most of which are beta-lactamase positive) and *Streptococcus pyogenes**.

Note: For information on otitis media caused by *Streptococcus pneumoniae,.*

Pharyngitis and Tonsillitis: Caused by *S. pyogenes.*

Note: Penicillin is the usual drug of choice in the treatment of *S. pyogenes* infections, including the prophylaxis of rheumatic fever. Cefixime is generally effective in the eradication of *S. pyogenes* from the nasopharynx; however, data establishing the efficacy of cefixime in the subsequent prevention of rheumatic fever are not available.

Acute Bronchitis and Acute Exacerbations of Chronic Bronchitis: Caused by *S. pneumoniae* and *H. influenzae* (beta-lactamase positive and negative strains).

Uncomplicated Gonorrhea (Cervical/Urethral): Caused by *Neisseria gonorrhoeae* (penicillinase- and non–penicillinase-producing strains).

Appropriate cultures and susceptibility studies should be performed to determine the causative organism and its susceptibility to cefixime; however, therapy may be started while awaiting the results of these studies. Therapy should be adjusted, if necessary, once these results are known.

*Efficacy for this organism in this organ system was studied in fewer than 10 infections.

CONTRAINDICATIONS

Cefixime is contraindicated in patients with known allergy to the cephalosporin group of antibiotics.

WARNINGS

BEFORE THERAPY WITH CEFIXIME IS INSTITUTED, CAREFUL INQUIRY SHOULD BE MADE TO DETERMINE WHETHER THE PATIENT HAS HAD PREVIOUS HYPERSENSITIVITY REACTIONS TO CEPHALOSPORINS, PENICILLINS, OR OTHER DRUGS. IF THIS PRODUCT IS TO BE GIVEN TO PENICILLIN-SENSITIVE PATIENTS, CAUTION SHOULD BE EXERCISED BECAUSE CROSS HYPERSENSITIVITY AMONG BETA-LACTAM ANTIBIOTICS HAS BEEN CLEARLY DOCUMENTED AND MAY OCCUR IN UP TO 10% OF PATIENTS WITH A HISTORY OF PENICILLIN ALLERGY. IF AN ALLERGIC REACTION TO CEFIXIME OCCURS, DISCONTINUE THE DRUG. SERIOUS ACUTE HYPERSENSITIVITY REACTIONS MAY REQUIRE TREATMENT WITH EPINEPHRINE AND OTHER EMERGENCY MEASURES, INCLUDING OXYGEN, INTRAVENOUS FLUIDS, INTRAVENOUS ANTIHISTAMINES, CORTICOSTEROIDS, PRESSOR AMINES, AND AIRWAY MANAGEMENT, AS CLINICALLY INDICATED.

Antibiotics, including cefixime, should be administered cautiously to any patient who has demonstrated some form of allergy, particularly to drugs.

Treatment with broad, spectrum antibiotics, including cefixime, alters the normal flora of the colon and may permit overgrowth of clostridia. Studies indicate that a toxin produced by *Clostridium difficile* is a primary cause of severe antibiotic-associated diarrhea including pseudomembranous colitis.

Pseudomembranous colitis has been reported with the use of cefixime and other broad-spectrum antibiotics (including macrolides, semisynthetic penicillins, and cephalosporins); therefore, it is important to consider this diagnosis in patients who develop diarrhea in association with the use of antibiotics. Symptoms of pseudomembranous colitis may occur during or after antibiotic treatment and may range in severity from mild to life-threatening. Mild cases of pseudomembranous colitis usually respond to drug discontinuation alone. In moderate to severe cases, management should include fluids, electrolytes, and protein supplementation. If the colitis does not improve after the drug has been discontinued, or if the symptoms are severe, oral vancomycin is the drug of choice for antibiotic-associated pseudomembranous colitis produced by *C. difficile*. Other causes of colitis should be excluded.

PRECAUTIONS

GENERAL

The possibility of the emergence of resistant organisms which might result in overgrowth should be kept in mind, particularly during prolonged treatment. In such use, careful observation of the patient is essential. If superinfection occurs during therapy, appropriate measures should be taken.

The dose of cefixime should be adjusted in patients with renal impairment as well as those undergoing continuous ambulatory peritoneal dialysis (CAPD) and hemodialysis (HD). Patients on dialysis should be monitored carefully. (See DOSAGE AND ADMINISTRATION.)

Cefixime should be prescribed with caution in individuals with a history of gastrointestinal disease, particularly colitis.

DRUG/LABORATORY TEST INTERACTIONS

A false-positive reaction for ketones in the urine may occur with tests using nitroprusside but not with those using nitroferricyanide.

The administration of cefixime may result in a false-positive reaction for glucose in the urine using Clinitest, Benedict's solution, or Fehling's solution. It is recommended that glucose tests based on enzymatic glucose oxidase reactions (such as Clinistix or Tes-Tape) be used.

A false-positive direct Coombs' test has been reported during treatment with other cephalosporin antibiotics; therefore, it should be recognized that a positive Coombs' test may be due to the drug.

CARCINOGENESIS, MUTAGENESIS, AND IMPAIRMENT OF FERTILITY

Lifetime studies in animals to evaluate carcinogenic potential have not been conducted. Cefixime did not cause point mutations in bacteria or mammalian cells, DNA damage, or chromosome damage *in vitro* and did not exhibit clastogenic potential *in vivo* in the mouse micronucleus test. In rats, fertility and reproductive performance were not affected by cefixime at doses up to 125 times the therapeutic dose.

PREGNANCY CATEGORY B

Reproduction studies have been performed in mice and rats at doses up to 400 times the human dose and have revealed no evidence of harm to the fetus due to cefixime. There are no adequate and well-controlled studies in pregnant women. Because animal reproduction studies are not always predictive of human response, this drug should be used during pregnancy only if clearly needed.

LABOR AND DELIVERY

Cefixime has not been studied for use during labor and delivery. Treatment should only be given if clearly needed.

NURSING MOTHERS

It is not known whether cefixime is excreted in human milk. Consideration should be given to discontinuing nursing temporarily during treatment with this drug.

PEDIATRIC USE

Safety and effectiveness of cefixime in children aged less than 6 months old have not been established.

The incidence of gastrointestinal adverse reactions, including diarrhea and loose stools, in the pediatric patients receiving the suspension, was comparable to the incidence seen in adult patients receiving tablets.

DRUG INTERACTIONS

No significant drug interactions have been reported to date.

ADVERSE REACTIONS

Most of adverse reactions observed in clinical trials were of a mild and transient nature. Five percent of patients in the US trials discontinued therapy because of drug-related adverse reactions. The most commonly seen adverse reactions in US trials of the tablet formulation were gastrointestinal events, which were reported in 30% of adult patients on either the bid or the qd regimen. Clinically mild gastrointestinal side effects occurred in 20% of all patients, moderate events occurred in 9% of all patients, and severe adverse reactions occurred in 2% of all patients. Individual event rates included diarrhea 16%, loose or frequent stools 6%, abdominal pain 3%, nausea 7%, dyspepsia 3%, and flatulence 4%. The incidence of gastrointestinal adverse reactions, including diarrhea and loose stools, in pediatric patients receiving the suspension, was comparable to the incidence seen in adult patients receiving tablets.

These symptoms usually responded to symptomatic therapy or ceased when cefixime was discontinued.

Several patients developed severe diarrhea and/or documented pseudomembranous colitis, and a few required hospitalization.

The following adverse reactions have been reported following the use of cefixime. Incidence rated were less than 1 in 50 (less than 2%), except as noted above for gastrointestinal events.

Gastrointestinal: Diarrhea, loose stools, abdominal pain, dyspepsia, nausea, and vomiting. Several cases of documented pseudomembranous colitis were identified during the studies. The onset of pseudomembranous colitis symptoms may occur during or after therapy.

Hypersensitivity Reactions: Skin rashes, urticaria, drug fever, and pruritus. Erythema multiforme, Stevens-Johnson syndrome, and serum sickness-like reactions have been reported.

Hepatic: Transient elevations is SGPT, SGOT, and alkaline phosphatase.

Renal: Transient elevations in BUN or creatinine.

Central Nervous System: Headaches and/or dizziness.

Hemic and Lymphatic Systems: Transient thrombocytopenia, leukopenia, and eosinophilia. Prolongation in prothrombin time was seen rarely.

Other: Genital pruritus, vaginitis, candidiasis.

In addition to the adverse reactions listed above which have been observed in patients treated with cefixime, the following adverse reactions and altered laboratory tests have been reported for cephalosporin class antibiotics:

Adverse Reactions: Allergic reactions including anaphylaxis, toxic epidermal necrolysis, superinfection, renal dysfunction, toxic nephropathy, hepatic dysfunction including cholestasis, aplastic anemia, hemolytic anemia, hemorrhage, and colitis. Several cephalosporins have been implicated in triggering seizures, particularly in patients with renal impairment when the dosage was not reduced (see DOSAGE AND ADMINISTRATION). If seizures associated with drug therapy occur, the drug should be discontinued. Anticonvulsant therapy can be given if clinically indicated.

Abnormal Laboratory Tests: Positive direct Coombs' test, elevated bilirubin, elevated LDH, pancytopenia, neutropenia, agranulocytosis.

DOSAGE AND ADMINISTRATION

ADULTS

The recommended dose of cefixime is 400 mg daily. This may be given as a 400 mg tablet daily or as 200 mg tablet every 12 hours.

For the treatment of uncomplicated cervical/urethral gonococcal infections, a single oral dose of 400 mg is recommended.

CHILDREN

The recommended dose is 8 mg/kg/day of the suspension. This may be administered as a single daily dose or may be given in 2 divided doses, as 4 mg/kg every 12 hours (see TABLE 8).

TABLE 8 *Pediatric Dosage Chart*

Patient Weight	Dose/Day	Dose/Day	Dose/Day (tsp of suspension)
6.25 kg	50 mg	2.5 ml	½
12.5 kg	100 mg	5.0 ml	1
18.75 kg	150 mg	7.5 ml	1½
25.0 kg	200 mg	10.0 ml	2
31.25 kg	250 mg	12.5 ml	2½
37.5 kg	300 mg	15.0 ml	3

Children weighing more than 50 kg or older than 12 years should be treated with the recommended adult dose.

Otitis media should be treated with the suspension. Clinical studies of otitis media were conducted with the suspension, and the suspension results in higher peak blood levels than the tablet when administered at the same dose. Therefore, the tablet should not be substituted for the suspension in the treatment of otitis media (see CLINICAL PHARMACOLOGY).

Efficacy and safety in infants aged less than 6 months have not been established.

In the treatment of infections due to *S. pyogenes*, a therapeutic dosage of cefixime should be administered for at least 10 days.

RENAL IMPAIRMENT

Cefixime may be administered in the presence of impaired renal function. Normal dose and schedule may be employed in patients with creatinine clearances of 60 ml/min or greater. Patients whose clearance is between 21 and 60 ml/min or patients who are on renal hemodialysis may be given 75% of the standard dosage at the standard dosing interval (*i.e.*, 300 mg daily). Patients whose clearance is <20 ml/min, or patients who are on continuous ambulatory peritoneal dialysis may be given half the standard dosage at the standard dosing interval (*i.e.*, 200 mg daily). Neither hemodialysis nor peritoneal dialysis removes significant amounts of drug from the body.

HOW SUPPLIED

200 mg Suprax Tablets: Convex, rectangular, white, film-coated tablets with rounded corners and beveled edges and a divided break line on each side, engraved with "Suprax" across one side and "LL" to the left and "200" to the right on the other side.

400 mg Suprax Tablets: Convex, rectangular, white, film-coated tablets with rounded corners and beveled edges and a divided break line on each side, engraved with "Suprax" across one side and "LL" to the left and "400" to the right on the other side.

Suprax Oral Suspension: The suspension is an off-white to cream-colored powder which when reconstituted as directed contains cefixime 100 mg/5 ml.

STORAGE

Tablets: Store at controlled room temperature 15-30°C (59-86°F).

Oral Suspension: Prior to reconstitution, store at controlled room temperature 15-30°C (59-86°F).

PRODUCT LISTING - EQUIVALENTS NOT AVAILABLE

Powder For Reconstitution - Oral - 100 mg/5 ml

50 ml	$36.51	SUPRAX, Allscripts Pharmaceutical Company	54569-2679-00
50 ml	$39.04	SUPRAX, Lederle Laboratories	00005-3898-40
50 ml	$39.70	SUPRAX, Physicians Total Care	54868-1384-01
75 ml	$62.68	SUPRAX, Lederle Laboratories	00005-3898-42
100 ml	$78.58	SUPRAX, Lederle Laboratories	00005-3898-46
100 ml	$79.34	SUPRAX, Physicians Total Care	54868-1384-02

Tablet - Oral - 400 mg

1's	$7.50	SUPRAX, Allscripts Pharmaceutical Company	54569-2861-02
1's	$13.68	SUPRAX, Pd-Rx Pharmaceuticals	55289-0954-79
5's	$76.25	SUPRAX, Pharma Pac	52959-0664-05
10's	$79.04	SUPRAX, Allscripts Pharmaceutical Company	54569-2861-00
10's	$88.28	SUPRAX, Lederle Laboratories	00005-3897-94
10's	$89.06	SUPRAX, Physicians Total Care	54868-1383-00
10's	$106.80	SUPRAX, Pd-Rx Pharmaceuticals	55289-0954-10
10's	$108.25	SUPRAX, Pharma Pac	52959-0664-10
10's	$128.22	SUPRAX, Pd-Rx Pharmaceuticals	55289-0954-91
50's	$422.50	SUPRAX, Lederle Laboratories	00005-3897-18
100's	$800.81	SUPRAX, Lederle Laboratories	00005-3897-23
100's	$828.04	SUPRAX, Lederle Laboratories	00005-3897-60

Cefonicid Sodium *(000686)*

For related information, see the comparative table section in Appendix A.

Categories: Infection, bone; Infection, joint; Infection, lower respiratory tract; Infection, skin and skin structures; Infection, urinary tract; Prophylaxis, perioperative; Septicemia; Pregnancy Category B; FDA Approved 1984 May
Drug Classes: Antibiotics, cephalosporins
Brand Names: **Monocid**
Foreign Brand Availability: Lisa (Israel); Monocef (Israel)
Cost of Therapy: $271.05 (Infection; Monocid Injection; 1 g; 1 g/day; 10 day supply)
HCFA JCODE(S): J0695 1 g IV

DESCRIPTION

Sterile cefonicid sodium, a sterile, lyophilized, semi-synthetic, broad-spectrum cephalosporin antibiotic for intravenous and intramuscular administration, is 5-Thia-1-azabicyclo [4.2.0] oct-2-ene-2-carboxylic acid, 7-[(hydroxyphenyl-acetyl)-amino]-8-oxo-3-[[[1-(sulfomethyl)-1*H*-te trazol-5-yl]thio]methyl]-disodium salt, [6*R*-[6a, 7β,(*R**)]].

Cefonicid sodium contains 85 mg (3.7 mEq) sodium per gram of cefonicid activity.

CLINICAL PHARMACOLOGY

HUMAN PHARMACOLOGY

TABLE 1 demonstrates the levels and duration of cefoncid sodium in serum following intravenous and intramuscular administration of 1 gram to normal volunteers.

TABLE 1 *Serum Concentrations After 1 g Administration (μg/ml)*

Interval	5 min	15 min	30 min	1 h	2 h	4 h
IV	221.3	176.4	147.6	124.2	88.9	61.4
IM	13.5	45.9	73.1	98.6	97.1	77.8
Interval	**6 h**	**8 h**	**10 h**	**12 h**	**24 h**	
IV	40.0	29.3	20.6	15.2	2.6	
IM	54.9	38.5	28.9	20.6	4.5	

Serum half-life is approximately 4.5 hours with intravenous and intramuscular administration. Cefoncid sodium is highly (greater than 90%) and reversibly protein bound.

Cefoncid sodium is not metabolized; 99% is excreted unchanged in the urine in 24 hours. A 500 mg IM dose provides a high (384 μg/ml) urinary concentration at 6-8 hours. Probenecid, given concurrently with cefoncid sodium, slows renal excretion, produces higher peak serum levels and significantly increases the serum half-life of the drug (8.2 hours).

Cefoncid sodium reaches therapeutic levels in the following tissues and fluids (see TABLE 2).

Note: Although cefoncid sodium reaches therapeutic levels in bile, those levels are lower than those seen with other cephalosporins, and amounts of cefoncid sodium released into the gastrointestinal tract are minute. This small amount of cefoncid sodium in the gastrointestinal tract is thought to be the reason for the low incidence of gastrointestinal reactions following therapy with cefoncid sodium.

No disulfiram-like reactions were reported in a crossover study conducted in healthy volunteers receiving cefoncid sodium and alcohol.

MICROBIOLOGY

The bactericidal action of cefoncid sodium results from inhibition of cell-wall synthesis. Cefoncid sodium is highly resistant to beta-lactamases produced by *Staphylococcus aureus, Hemophilus influenzae, Neisseria gonorrhoeae* and Richmond type I beta-lactamases. Cefoncid sodium is resistant to degradation by beta-lactamases from certain members of *Enterobacteriaceae.* Active against a wide range of gram-positive and gram-negative organisms. Cefoncid sodium is usually active against the following organisms *in vitro* and in clinical situations:

TABLE 2 *Tissue and Body Fluid Levels*

Tissue or Body Fluid	Dosage and Route (No. of Patients Sampled)	Time of Sampling After Dose	Average Tissue or Fluid Levels (μg/g or /ml)
Bone	1 g IM (7)	60-90 min	6.8
	1 g IV (10)	44-99 min	14.0
Gallbladder	1 g IM (10)	60-70 min	15.5
Bile	1 g IM (10)	60-70 min	7.5
Prostate	1 g IM (10)	50-115 min	13.0
Uterine tissue	1 g IM (6)	60-90 min	17.5
Wound fluid	1 g IM (10)	60-75 min	37.7
Purulent wound	1 g IM (9)	60 min	11.5
Adipose tissue	1 g IM (5)	60 min	4.0
Atrial	1 g IM (7)	77-170 min	7.5
Appendage	2 g IM (7)	105-170 min	8.7
	15 mg/kg IV (10)	53-160 min	15.4

Gram-Positive Aerobes: *Staphylococcus aureus* (beta-lactamase producing and non-beta-lactamase producing) and *S. epidermidis* (*Note:* Methicillin-resistant staphylococci are resistant to cephalosporins, including cefonicid.); *Streptococcus pneumoniae, S. pyogenes* (Group A beta-hemolytic *Streptococcus*), and *S. agalactiae* (Group B *Streptococcus*).

Gram-Negative Aerobes: *Escherichia coli; Klebsiella pneumoniae; Providencia rettgeri* (formerly *Proteus rettgeri*); *Proteus vulgaris; Morganella morganii* (formerly *Proteus morganii*); *Proteus mirabilis;* and *Hemophilus influenzae* (ampicillin-sensitive and -resistant).

The following *in vitro* data are available but their clinical significance is unknown. Cefoncid sodium is usually active against the following organisms *in vitro:*

Gram-Negative Aerobes: *Moraxella* (formerly *Branhamella*) *catarrhalis; Klebsiella oxytoca; Enterobacter aerogenes; Neisseria gonorrhoeae* (penicillin-sensitive and -resistant): *Citrobacter freundii* and *C. diversus.*

Gram-Positive Anaerobes: *Clostridium perfringens; Peptostreptococcus anaerobius; Peptococcus magnus; P. prevotii;* and *Propionibacterium acnes.*

Gram-Negative Anaerobes: *Fusobacterium nucleatum.*

Cefoncid sodium is usually inactive *in vitro* against most strains of *Pseudomonas, Serratia, Enterococcus* and *Acinetobacter.* Most strains of *B. fragilis* are resistant.

SUSCEPTIBILITY TESTING

Results from standardized single-disk susceptibility tests using a 30 μg cefoncid sodium disk should be interpreted according to the following criteria:

Zones of 18 mm or greater indicate that the tested organism is susceptible to cefoncid sodium and is likely to respond to therapy.

Zones from 15-17 mm indicate that the tested organism is of intermediate (moderate) susceptibility, and is likely to respond to therapy if a higher dosage is used or if the infection is confined to tissues and fluids in which high antibiotic levels are attained.

Zones of 14 mm or less indicate that the organism is resistant.

Only the cefoncid sodium disk should be used to determine susceptibility, since *in vitro* tests show that cefoncid sodium has activity against certain strains not susceptible to other cephalosporins. The cefoncid sodium disk should not be used for testing susceptibility to other cephalosporins.

A bacterial isolate may be considered susceptible if the MIC value for cefoncid sodium is equal to or less than 8 μg/ml in accordance with the National Committee for Clinical Laboratory Standards (NCCLS) guidelines. Organisms are considered resistant if the MIC is equal to or greater than 32 μg/ml For most organisms the MBC value for cefoncid sodium is the same as the MIC value.

The standardized quality control procedure requires use of control organisms. The 30 μg cefoncid sodium disk should give the zone diameters listed below for the quality control strains.

TABLE 3

Organism	ATCC	Zone Size Range
E. coli	25922	25-29 mm
S. aureus	25923	22-28 mm

INDICATIONS AND USAGE

Due to the long half-life of cefoncid sodium, a 1 g dose results in therapeutic serum levels which provide coverage against susceptible organisms (listed below) for 24 hours.

Studies on specimens obtained prior to therapy should be used to determine the susceptibility of the causative organisms to cefoncid sodium. Therapy with cefoncid sodium may be initiated pending results of the studies; however, treatment should be adjusted according to study findings.

TREATMENT

Cefoncid sodium is indicated in the treatment of infections due to susceptible strains of the microorganisms listed below:

Lower Respiratory Tract Infections: Due to *Streptococcus pneumoniae; Klebsiella pneumoniae**; Escherichia coli;* and *Hemophilus influenzae* (ampicillin-resistant and ampicillin-sensitive).

Urinary Tract Infections: Due to *Escherichia coli; Proteus mirabilis* and *Proteus* spp. (which may include the organisms now called *Proteus vulgaris**, Providencia rettgeri* and *Morganella morganii*); and *Klebsiella pneumoniae**.*

Skin and Skin Structure Infections: Due to *Staphylococcus aureus* and *S. epidermidis; Streptococcus pyogenes* (Group A*Streptococcus*) and *S. agalactiae* (Group B *Streptococcus*).
Septicemia: Due to *Streptococcus pneumoniae* (formerly *D. pneumoniae*) and *Escherichia coli**.
Bone and Joint Infections: Due to *Staphylococcus aureus.*
*Efficacy for this organism on this organ system has been demonstrated in fewer than 10 infections.

C

SURGICAL PROPHYLAXIS

Administration of a single 1 gram dose of cefoncid sodium before surgery may reduce the incidence of postoperative infections in patients undergoing surgical procedures classified as contaminated or potentially contaminated (*e.g.,* colorectal surgery, vaginal hysterectomy, or cholecystectomy in high-risk patients), or in patients in whom infection at the operative site would present a serious risk (*e.g.,* prosthetic arthroplasty, open heart surgery). Although cefonicid has been shown to be as effective as cefazolin in prevention of infection following coronary artery bypass surgery, no placebo-controlled trials have been conducted to evaluate any cephalosporin antibiotic in the prevention of infection following coronary artery bypass surgery or prosthetic heart valve replacement.

In cesarean section, the use of cefoncid sodium (after the umbilical cord has been clamped) may reduce the incidence of certain postoperative infections.

When administered 1 hour prior to surgical procedures for which it is indicated, a single 1 g dose of cefoncid sodium provides protection from most infections due to susceptible organisms throughout the course of the procedure. Intraoperative and/or postoperative administrations of cefoncid sodium are not necessary. Daily doses of cefoncid sodium may be administered for two additional days in patients undergoing prosthetic arthroplasty or open heart surgery.

If there are signs of infection, the causative organisms should be identified and appropriate therapy determined through susceptibility testing.

Before using cefoncid sodium concomitantly with other antibiotics, the prescribing information for those agents should be reviewed for contraindications, warnings, precautions and adverse reactions. Renal function should be carefully monitored.

CONTRAINDICATIONS

Cefoncid sodium is contraindicated in persons who have shown hypersensitivity to cephalosporin antibiotics.

WARNINGS

BEFORE THERAPY WITH STERILE CEFONICID SODIUM IS INSTITUTED, CAREFUL INQUIRY SHOULD BE MADE TO DETERMINE WHETHER THE PATIENT HAS HAD PREVIOUS HYPERSENSITIVITY REACTIONS TO CEPHALOSPORINS, PENICILLINS, OR OTHER DRUGS. THIS PRODUCT SHOULD BE GIVEN CAUTIOUSLY TO PENICILLIN-SENSITIVE PATIENTS. ANTIBIOTICS SHOULD BE ADMINISTERED WITH CAUTION TO ANY PATIENT WHO HAS DEMONSTRATED SOME FORM OF ALLERGY, PARTICULARLY TO DRUGS. SERIOUS ACUTE HYPERSENSITIVITY REACTIONS MAY REQUIRE EPINEPHRINE AND OTHER EMERGENCY MEASURES.

Pseudomembranous colitis has been reported with the use of nearly all antibacterial agents, including cefoncid sodium, and has ranged in severity from mild to life-threatening. Therefore, it is important to consider this diagnosis in patients who present with diarrhea subsequent to the administration of antibacterial agents.

Treatment with antibacterial agents alters the normal flora of the colon and may permit overgrowth of clostridia. Studies indicate that a toxin produced by *Clostridium difficile* is one primary cause of "antibiotic-associated colitis."

Mild cases of pseudomembranous colitis usually respond to drug discontinuation alone. In moderate to severe cases, consideration should be given to management with fluids and electrolytes, protein supplementation and treatment with an antibacterial drug clinically effective against *C. difficile* colitis.

PRECAUTIONS

GENERAL

With any antibiotic, prolonged use may result in overgrowth of nonsusceptible organisms. Careful observation is essential, and appropriate measures should be taken if superinfection occurs.

CARCINOGENESIS, MUTAGENESIS, AND IMPAIRMENT OF FERTILITY

Beta-lactam antibiotics with methyl-thio-tetrazole side chains have been shown to cause testicular atrophy in prepubertal rats, which persisted into adulthood and resulted in decreased spermatogenesis and decreased fertility. Cefonicid, which contains a methylsulfonic-thio-tetrazole moiety, has no adverse effect on the male reproductive system of prepubertal, juvenile or adult rats when given under identical conditions.

Carcinogenicity studies of cefonicid have not been conducted, however, results of mutagenicity studies (*i.e.,* Ames/*Salmonella*/microsome plate assay and the micronucleus test in mice) were negative.

PREGNANCY CATEGORY B

Reproduction studies have been performed in mice, rabbits and rats at doses up to an equivalent of 40 times the usual adult human dose and have revealed no evidence of impaired fertility or harm to the fetus due to cefoncid sodium. There are, however, no adequate and well-controlled studies in pregnant women. Because animal reproduction studies are not always predictive of human response, this drug should be used in pregnancy only if clearly needed.

LABOR AND DELIVERY

In cesarean section, cefoncid sodium should be administered only after the umbilical cord has been clamped.

NURSING MOTHERS

Cefoncid sodium is excreted in human milk in low concentrations. Caution should be exercised when cefoncid sodium is administered to a nursing woman.

PEDIATRIC USE

Safety and effectiveness in children have not been established.

DRUG INTERACTIONS

Nephrotoxicity has been reported following concomitant administration of other cephalosporins and aminoglycosides.

ADVERSE REACTIONS

Cefoncid sodium is generally well tolerated and adverse reactions have occurred infrequently. The most common adverse reaction has been pain on IM injection. On-therapy conditions occurring in greater than 1% of cefoncid sodium-treated patients were:

Injection Site Phenomena: Pain and/or discomfort on injection; less often, burning, phlebitis at IV site.
Increased Platelets: (1.7%).
Increased Eosinophils: (2.9%).
Liver Function Test Alterations: (1.6%): Increased alkaline phosphatase, increased SGOT, increased SGPT, increased GGTP, increased LDH.

Less frequent on-therapy conditions occurring in less than 1% of cefoncid sodium-treated patients were:

Hypersensitivity Reactions: Fever, rash, pruritus, erythema, myalgia and anaphylactoid-type reactions have been reported.
Hematology: Decreased WBC, neutropenia, thrombocytopenia, positive Coombs' test.
Renal: Increased BUN and creatinine levels have occasionally been seen. Rare reports of acute renal failure associated with interstitial nephritis, observed with other beta-lactam antibiotics, have also occurred with Monocid.
Gastrointestinal: Diarrhea and pseudomembranous colitis. Onset of pseudomembranous colitis symptoms may occur during or after antibiotic treatment (see WARNINGS).

DOSAGE AND ADMINISTRATION

GENERAL

The usual adult dosage is 1 g of cefoncid sodium given once every 24 hours, intravenously or by deep intramuscular injection. Doses in excess of 1 g daily are rarely necessary; however, in exceptional cases dosage of up to 2 g given once daily have been well tolerated. When administering 2 g IM doses once daily, ½ the dose should be administered in different large muscle masses.

OUTPATIENT USE

Cefoncid sodium has been used (once daily IM or IV) on an outpatient basis. Individuals responsible for outpatient administration of cefoncid sodium should be instructed thoroughly in appropriate procedures for storage, reconstitution and administration.

SURGICAL PROPHYLAXIS

When administered 1 hour prior to appropriate surgical procedures (see INDICATIONS AND USAGE), a 1 g dose of cefoncid sodium provides protection from most infections due to susceptible organisms throughout the course of the procedure. Intraoperative and/or postoperative administrations of cefoncid sodium are not necessary. Daily doses of cefoncid sodium may be administered for 2 additional days in patients undergoing prosthetic arthroplasty or open heart surgery.

In cesarean section cefoncid sodium should be administered only after the umbilical cord has been clamped.

TABLE 4 *General Guidelines for Dosage of Cefoncid Sodium, IV or IM*

Type of Infection	Daily Dose	Frequency
Uncomplicated Urinary Tract	0.5 g	once every 24 hours
Mild to Moderate	1 g	once every 24 hours
Severe or Life-Threatening	2 g*	once every 24 hours
Surgical Prophylaxis	1 g	1 hour preoperatively

* When administering 2 g IM doses once daily, ½ the dose should be administered in different large muscle masses.

IMPAIRED RENAL FUNCTION

Modification of cefoncid sodium dosage is necessary in patients with impaired renal function. Following an initial loading dosage of 7.5 mg/kg IM or IV, the maintenance dosing schedule shown below should be followed. Further dosing should be determined by severity of the infection and susceptibility of the causative organism.

PREPARATION OF PARENTERAL SOLUTION

Parenteral drug products should be SHAKEN WELL when reconstituted, and inspected visually for particulate matter prior to administration. If particulate matter is evident in reconstituted fluids, the drug solutions should be discarded.

RECONSTITUTION

Single-Dose Vials

For IM injection, IV direct (bolus) injection, or IV infusion, reconstitute with sterile water for injection according to TABLE 6. SHAKE WELL.

These solutions of cefoncid sodium are stable 24 hours at room temperature or 72 hours if refrigerated (5°C). Slight yellowing does not affect potency.

For IV infusion, dilute reconstituted solution in 50-100 ml of the parenteral fluids listed under Administration.

TABLE 5 Dosage of Cefoncid Sodium in Adults With Reduced Renal Function

Monitor renal function and adjust accordingly

Creatinine Clearance (ml/min/ 1.73 M²)	Dosage Regimen Mild to Moderate Infections	Severe Infections
79- 60	10 mg/kg (every 24 hours)	25 mg/kg (every 24 hours)
59-40	8 mg/kg (every 24 hours)	20 mg/kg (every 24 hours)
39-20	4 mg/kg (every 24 hours)	15 mg/kg (every 24 hours)
19-10	4 mg/kg (every 48 hours)	15 mg/kg (every 48 hours)
9-5	4 mg/kg (every 3 to 5 days)	15 mg/kg (every 3 to 5 days)
<5	3 mg/kg (every 3 to 5 days)	4 mg/kg (every 3 to 5 days)

Note: It is not necessary to administer additional dosage following dialysis.

TABLE 6

Vial Size	Diluent to Be Added	Approx. Avail. Volume	Approx. Avg. Concentration
500 mg	2.0 ml	2.2 ml	225 mg/ml
1 g	2.5 ml	3.1 ml	325 mg/ml

Pharmacy Bulk Vials (10 g)

For IM injection, IV direct (bolus) injection or IV infusion, reconstitute with sterile water for injection, bacteriostatic water for injection, or sodium chloride injection according to TABLE 7.

TABLE 7

Amount of Diluent	Approx. Concentration	Approx. Avail. Volume
25 ml	1 g/3 ml	31 ml
45 ml	1 g/5 ml	51 ml

These solutions of cefoncid sodium are stable 24 hours at room temperature or 72 hours if refrigerated (5°C.) Slight yellowing does not affect potency. For IV infusion add to parenteral fluids listed in Administration.

"Piggyback" Vials

Reconstitute with 50-100 ml of sodium chloride injection or other IV solution listed in Administration. Administer with primary IV fluids, as a single dose. These solutions of cefoncid sodium are stable 24 hours at room temperature or 72 hours if refrigerated (5°C). Slight yellowing does not affect potency.

A solution of 1 g of cefoncid sodium in 18 ml of sterile water for injection is isotonic.

ADMINISTRATION

IM Injection: Inject well within the body of a relatively large muscle. Aspiration is necessary to avoid inadvertent injection into a blood vessel. When administering 2 g IM doses once daily, one-half the dose should be given in different large muscle masses.

IV Administration: For direct (bolus) injection, administer reconstituted cefoncid sodium slowly over 3-5 minutes, directly or through tubing for patients receiving parenteral fluids. For infusion, dilute reconstituted cefoncid sodium in 50-100 ml of one of the following solutions: 0.9% sodium chloride injection, 5% dextrose injection, 5% dextrose and 0.9% sodium chloride injection, 5% dextrose and 0.45% sodium chloride injection, 5% dextrose and 0.2% sodium chloride injection, 10% dextrose injection, Ringer's injection, lactated Ringer's injection, 5% dextrose and lactated Ringer's injection, 10% invert sugar in sterile water for injection, 5% dextrose and 0.15% potassium chloride injection, and sodium lactate injection.

In these fluids cefoncid sodium is stable 24 hours at room temperature or 72 hours if refrigerated (5°C). Slight yellowing does not affect potency.

HOW SUPPLIED

Monocid is supplied in vials equivalent to 500 mg and 1 g of cefonicid, in "Piggyback" Vials for IV admixture equivalent to 1 g of cefonicid; and in Pharmacy Bulk Vials equivalent to 10 g of cefonicid.

As with other cephalosporins, cefoncid sodium may darken on storage. However, if stored as recommended, this color change does not affect potency.

Before reconstitution, cefoncid sodium should be protected from light and refrigerated (2-8°C).

Cefoperazone Sodium *(000687)*

For related information, see the comparative table section in Appendix A.

Categories: Endometritis; Infection, gynecologic; Infection, intra-abdominal; Infection, respiratory tract; Infection, skin and skin structures; Infection, urinary tract; Pelvic inflammatory disease; Peritonitis; Septicemia; Pregnancy Category B; FDA Approved 1982 Nov

Drug Classes: Antibiotics, cephalosporins

Brand Names: **Cefobid**

Foreign Brand Availability: Bifotik (Indonesia); CPZ (Taiwan); Cefobactam (Korea); Cefobis (Germany; Philippines; Switzerland); Cefogram (Italy); Cefolatam (Korea); Cefomycin (India); Ceforin (Korea); Cefozone (Singapore; Thailand); Ceperatam (Korea); Dardum (Malaysia; Singapore); Magnamycin (India); Mediper (Italy); Medocef (Thailand); Peratam (Korea); Shinfomycin (Taiwan); Stabixin (India); Tomabef (Italy); Zoncef (Italy)

Cost of Therapy: $351.36 (Infection; Cefobid Injection; 1 g; 2 g/day; 10 day supply)

DESCRIPTION

Cefobid (cefoperazone sodium) is a sterile, semisynthetic, broad-spectrum, parenteral cephalosporin antibiotic for intravenous or intramuscular administration. It is the sodium salt of 7-(D(-)-α-(4-ethyl-2,3-dioxo-1-piperazinecarboxamido)-α-(4-hydroxyphenyl) acetamido)-3-((1-methyl-1H-tetrazol-5-yl)thiomethyl)-3-cephem-4-carboxylic acid. Its chemical formula is $C_{25}H_{26}N_9NaO_8S_2$ with a molecular weight of 667.65.

Cefobid contains 34 mg sodium (1.5 mEq) per gram. Cefobid is a white powder which is freely soluble in water. The pH of a 25% (w/v) freshly reconstituted solution varies between 4.5-6.5 and the solution ranges from colorless to straw yellow depending on the concentration.

Cefobid in crystalline form is supplied in vials equivalent to 1 or 2 g of cefoperazone and in Piggyback Units for intravenous administration equivalent to 1 or 2 g cefoperazone. Cefobid is also supplied premixed as a frozen, sterile, nonpyrogenic, iso-osmotic solution equivalent to 1 or 2 g cefoperazone in plastic containers. After thawing, the solution is intended for intravenous use.

The plastic container is fabricated from specially formulated polyvinyl chloride. Solutions in contact with the plastic container can leach out certain of its chemical components in very small amounts within the expiration period, *e.g.*, di 2-ethylhexyl phthalate (DEHP), up to 5 parts/million. However, the safety of the plastic has been confirmed in tests in animals according to the USP biological tests for plastic containers, as well as by tissue culture toxicity studies.

CLINICAL PHARMACOLOGY

High serum and bile levels of cefoperazone sodium are attained after a single dose of the drug. TABLE 1 demonstrates the serum concentrations of cefoperazone sodium in normal volunteers following either a single 15 minute constant rate intravenous infusion of 1,2,3 or 4 g of the drug, or a single intramuscular injection of 1 or 2 g of the drug (see TABLE 1).

The mean serum half-life of cefoperazone sodium is approximately 2.0 hours, independent of the route of administration.

TABLE 1 Cefoperazone Serum Concentrations

Dose/Route	Mean Serum Concentrations (µg/ml) 0*	0.5 hr	1 hr	2 hr	4 hr	8 hr	12 hr
1 g IV	153	114	73	38	16	4	0.5
2 g IV	252	153	114	70	32	8	2
3 g IV	340	210	142	89	41	9	2
4 g IV	506	325	251	161	71	19	6
1 g IM	32†	52	65	57	33	7	1
2 g IM	40†	69	93	97	58	14	4

* Hours post-administration, with 0 time being the end of the infusion.
† Values obtained 15 minutes post-injection.

In vitro studies with human serum indicate that the degree of cefoperazone sodium reversible protein binding varies with the serum concentration from 93% at 25 µg/ml of cefoperazone sodium to 90% at 250 µg/ml and 82% at 500 µg/ml.

Cefoperazone sodium achieves therapeutic concentrations in the following body tissues and fluids (see TABLE 2).

TABLE 2

Tissue or Fluid	Dose	Concentration
Ascitic Fluid	2 g	64 µg/ml
Cerebrospinal Fluid (in patients with inflamed meninges)	50 mg/k	1.8 µg/ml to 8.0 µg/ml
Urine	2 g	3286 µg/ml
Sputum	3 g	6.0 µg/ml
Endometrium	2 g	74 µg/g
Myometrium	2 g	54 µg/g
Palatine Tonsil	1 g	8 µg/g
Sinus Mucous Membrane	1 g	8 µg/g
Umbilical Cord Blood	1 g	25 µg/ml
Amniotic Fluid	1 g	4.8 µg/ml
Lung	1 g	28 µg/g
Bone	2 g	40 µg/g

Cefoperazone sodium is excreted mainly in the bile. Maximum bile concentrations are generally obtained between 1 and 3 hours following drug administration and exceed concurrent serum concentrations by up to 100 times. Reported biliary concentrations of cefoperazone sodium range from 66 µg/ml at 30 minutes to as high as 6000 µg/ml at 3 hours after an intravenous bolus injection of 2 g.

Following a single intramuscular or intravenous dose, the urinary recovery of cefoperazone sodium over a 12 hour period averages 20-30%. No significant quantity of metabolites has been found in the urine. Urinary concentrations greater than 2200 μg/ml have been obtained following a 15 minute infusion of a 2 g dose. After an IM injection of 2 g, peak urine concentrations of almost 1000 μg/ml have been obtained, and therapeutic levels are maintained for 12 hours.

Repeated administration of cefoperazone sodium at 12 hour intervals does not result in accumulation of the drug in normal subjects. Peak serum concentrations, areas under the curve (AUC's), and serum half-lives in patients with severe renal insufficiency are not significantly different from those in normal volunteers. In patients with hepatic dysfunction, the serum half-life is prolonged and urinary excretion is increased. In patients with combined renal and hepatic insufficiencies, cefoperazone sodium may accumulate in the serum.

Cefoperazone sodium has been used in pediatrics, but the safety and effectiveness in children have not been established. The half-life of cefoperazone sodium in serum is 6-10 hours in low birth-weight neonates.

MICROBIOLOGY

Cefoperazone sodium is active *in vitro* against a wide range of aerobic and anaerobic, gram-positive and gram-negative pathogens. The bactericidal action of cefoperazone sodium results from the inhibition of bacterial cell wall synthesis. Cefoperazone sodium has a high degree of stability in the presence of beta-lactamases produced by most gram-negative pathogens. Cefoperazone sodium is usually active against organisms which are resistant to other beta-lactam antibiotics because of beta-lactamase production. Cefoperazone sodium is usually active against the following organisms *in vitro* and in clinical infections:

Gram-Positive Aerobes: *Staphylococcus aureus,* penicillinase and non-penicillinase-producing strains; *Staphylococcus epidermidis; Streptococcus pneumoniae* (formerly *Diplococcus pneumoniae*); *Streptococcus pyogenes* (Group A beta-hemolytic streptococci); *Streptococcus agalactiae* (Group B beta-hemolytic streptococci); *Enterococcus (Streptococcus faecalis, S. faecium* and *S. durans).*

Gram-Negative Aerobes: *Escherichia coli; Klebsiella* species (including *K. pneumoniae*); *Enterobacter* species; *Citrobacter* species; *Haemophilus influenzae; Proteus mirabilis; Proteus vulgaris; Morganella morganii* (formerly *Proteus morganii*); *Providencia stuartii; Providencia rettgeri* (formerly *Proteus rettgeri*); *Serratia marcescens; Pseudomonas aeruginosa; Pseudomonas* species; some strains of *Acinetobacter calcoaceticu; Neisseria gonorrhoeae.*

Anaerobic Organisms: Gram-positive cocci (including *Peptococcus* and *Peptostreptococcus*); *Clostridium* species; *Bacteroides fragilis;* other *Bacteroides* species.

Cefoperazone sodium is also active *in vitro* against a wide variety of other pathogens although the clinical significance is unknown. These organisms include: *Salmonella* and *Shigella* species, *Serratia liquefaciens, N. meningitidis, Bordetella pertussis, Yersinia enterocolitica, Clostridium difficile, Fusobacterium* species, *Eubacterium* species and beta-lactamase producing strains of *H. influenzae* and *N. gonorrhoeae.*

SUSCEPTIBILITY TESTING

Diffusion Technique

For the disk diffusion method of susceptibility testing, a 75 μg cefoperazone sodium diffusion disk should be used. Organisms should be tested with the cefoperazone sodium 75 μg disk since cefoperazone sodium has been shown *in vitro* to be active against organisms which are found to be resistant to other beta-lactam antibiotics.

Tests should be interpreted by the criteria shown in TABLE 3.

TABLE 3

Zone Diameter	Interpretation
Greater than or equal to 21 mm	Susceptible
16-20 mm	Moderately Susceptible
Less than or equal to 15 mm	Resistant

Quantitative procedures that require measurement of zone diameters give the most precise estimate of susceptibility. One such method which has been recommended for use with the cefoperazone sodium 75 μg disk is the NCCLS approved standard. (Performance Standards for Antimicrobic Disk Susceptibility Tests. Second Information Supplement Vol. 2 No. 2 pp. 49-69. Publisher-National Committee for Clinical Laboratory Standards, Villanova, Pennsylvania.)

A report of "susceptible" indicates that the infecting organism is likely to respond to cefoperazone sodium therapy and a report of "resistant" indicates that the infecting organism is not likely to respond to therapy. A "moderately susceptible" report suggests that the infecting organism will be susceptible to cefoperazone sodium if a higher than usual dosage is used or if the infection is confined to tissues and fluids (*e.g.,* urine or bile) in which high antibiotic levels are attained.

Dilution Techniques

Broth or agar dilution methods may be used to determine the minimal inhibitory concentration (MIC) of cefoperazone sodium. Serial twofold dilutions of cefoperazone sodium should be prepared in either broth or agar. Broth should be inoculated to contain 5×10^5 organisms/ml and agar "spotted" with 10^4organisms.

MIC test results should be interpreted in light of serum, tissue, and body fluid concentrations of cefoperazone sodium. Organisms inhibited by cefoperazone sodium at 16 μg/ml or less are considered susceptible, while organisms with MIC's of 17-63 μg/ml are moderately susceptible. Organisms inhibited at cefoperazone sodium concentrations of greater than or equal to 64 μg/ml are considered resistant, although clinical cures have been obtained in some patients infected by such organisms.

INDICATIONS AND USAGE

Cefoperazone sodium is indicated for the treatment of the following infections when caused by susceptible organisms:

Respiratory Tract Infections: Caused by *S. pneumoniae, H. influenzae, S. aureus* (penicillinase and non-penicillinase producing strains), *S. pyogenes** (Group A beta-hemolytic streptococci), *P. aeruginosa, Klebsiella pneumoniae, E. coli, Proteus mirabilis,* and *Enterobacter* species.

Peritonitis and Other Intra-Abdominal Infections: Caused by *E. coli, P. aeruginosa**, and anaerobic gram-negative bacilli (including *Bacteroides fragilis*).

Bacterial Septicemia: Caused by *S. pneumoniae, S. agalactiae*, S. aureus, Pseudomonas aeruginosa*, E. coli, Klebsiella* spp.*, *Klebsiella pneumoniae*, Proteus* species* (indole-positive and indole-negative), *Clostridium* spp.* and anaerobic gram-positive cocci*.

Infections of the Skin and Skin Structures: Caused by *S. aureus* (penicillinase and non-penicillinase producing strains), *S. pyogenes**, and *P. aeruginosa.*

Pelvic Inflammatory Disease, Endometritis, and Other Infections of the Female Genital Tract: Caused by *N. gonorrhoeae, S. epidermidis*, S. agalactiae, E. coli, Clostridium* spp.*, *Bacteroides* species (including *Bacteroides fragilis*), and anaerobic gram-positive cocci.

Urinary Tract Infections: Caused by *Escherichia coli* and *Pseudomonas aeruginosa.*

Enterococcal Infections: Although cefoperazone has been shown to be clinically effective in the treatment of infections caused by enterococci in cases of **peritonitis and other intra-abdominal infections, infections of the skin and skin structures, pelvic inflammatory disease, endometritis and other infections of the female genital tract, and urinary tract infection***, the majority of clinical isolates of enterococci tested are not susceptible to cefoperazone but fall just at or in the intermediate zone of susceptibility, and are moderately resistant to cefoperazone. However, *in vitro* susceptibility testing may not correlate directly with *in vivo* results. Despite this, cefoperazone therapy has resulted in clinical cures of enterococcal infections, chiefly in polymicrobial infections. Cefoperazone should be used in enterococcal infections with care and at doses that achieve satisfactory serum levels of cefoperazone.

*Efficacy of this organism in this organ system was studied in fewer than 10 infections.

SUSCEPTIBILITY TESTING

Before instituting treatment with cefoperazone sodium, appropriate specimens should be obtained for isolation of the causative organism and for determination of its susceptibility to the drug. Treatment may be started before results of susceptibility testing are available.

COMBINATION THERAPY

Synergy between cefoperazone sodium and aminoglycosides has been demonstrated with many gram-negative bacilli. However, such enhanced activity of these combinations is not predictable. If such therapy is considered, *in vitro* susceptibility tests should be performed to determine the activity of the drugs in combination, and renal function should be monitored carefully. (See PRECAUTIONS, and DOSAGE AND ADMINISTRATION.)

CONTRAINDICATIONS

Cefoperazone sodium is contraindicated in patients with known allergy to the cephalosporin-class of antibiotics.

WARNINGS

BEFORE THERAPY WITH CEFOPERAZONE SODIUM IS INSTITUTED, CAREFUL INQUIRY SHOULD BE MADE TO DETERMINE WHETHER THE PATIENT HAS HAD PREVIOUS HYPERSENSITIVITY REACTIONS TO CEPHALOSPORINS, PENICILLINS OR OTHER DRUGS. THIS PRODUCT SHOULD BE GIVEN CAUTIOUSLY TO PENICILLIN-SENSITIVE PATIENTS. ANTIBIOTICS SHOULD BE ADMINISTERED WITH CAUTION TO ANY PATIENT WHO HAS DEMONSTRATED SOME FORM OF ALLERGY, PARTICULARLY TO DRUGS. SERIOUS ACUTE HYPERSENSITIVITY REACTIONS MAY REQUIRE THE USE OF SUBCUTANEOUS EPINEPHRINE AND OTHER EMERGENCY MEASURES.

PSEUDOMEMBRANOUS COLITIS HAS BEEN REPORTED WITH THE USE OF CEPHALOSPORINS (AND OTHER BROAD-SPECTRUM ANTIBIOTICS); THEREFORE, IT IS IMPORTANT TO CONSIDER ITS DIAGNOSIS IN PATIENTS WHO DEVELOP DIARRHEA IN ASSOCIATION WITH ANTIBIOTIC USE.

Treatment with broad-spectrum antibiotics alters normal flora of the colon and may permit overgrowth of clostridia. Studies indicate a toxin produced by *Clostridium difficile* is one primary cause of antibiotic-associated colitis. Cholestyramine and colestipol resins have been shown to bind the toxin *in vitro.*

Mild cases of colitis may respond to drug discontinuance alone.

Moderate to severe cases should be managed with fluid, electrolyte, and protein supplementation as indicated.

When the colitis is not relieved by drug discontinuance or when it is severe, oral vancomycin is the treatment of choice for antibiotic-associated pseudomembranous colitis produced by *C. difficile*. Other causes of colitis should also be considered.

PRECAUTIONS

GENERAL

Although transient elevations of the BUN and serum creatinine have been observed, cefoperazone sodium alone does not appear to cause significant nephrotoxicity. However, concomitant administration of aminoglycosides and other cephalosporins has caused nephrotoxicity.

Cefoperazone sodium is extensively excreted in bile. The serum half-life of cefoperazone sodium is increased 2- to 4-fold in patients with hepatic disease and/or biliary obstruction. In general, total daily dosage above 4 g should not be necessary in such patients. If higher dosages are used, serum concentrations should be monitored.

Because renal excretion is not the main route of elimination of cefoperazone sodium (see CLINICAL PHARMACOLOGY), patients with renal failure require no adjustment in dosage when usual doses are administered. When high doses of cefoperazone sodium are used, concentrations of drug in the serum should be monitored periodically. If evidence of accumulation exists, dosage should be decreased accordingly.

The half-life of cefoperazone sodium is reduced slightly during hemodialysis. Thus, dosing should be scheduled to follow a dialysis period. In patients with both hepatic dysfunction and significant renal disease, cefoperazone sodium dosage should not exceed 1-2 g daily without close monitoring of serum concentrations.

As with other antibiotics, vitamin K deficiency has occurred rarely in patients treated with cefoperazone sodium. The mechanism is most probably related to the suppression of gut flora which normally synthesize this vitamin. Those at risk include patients with a poor nutritional status, malabsorption states (*e.g.,* cystic fibrosis), alcoholism, and patients on prolonged hyper-alimentation regimens (administered either intravenously or via a naso-gastric tube). Prothrombin time should be monitored in these patients and exogenous vitamin K administered as indicated.

A disulfiram-like reaction characterized by flushing, sweating, headache, and tachycardia has been reported when alcohol (beer, wine) was ingested within 72 hours after cefoperazone sodium administration. Patients should be cautioned about the ingestion of alcoholic beverages following the administration of cefoperazone sodium. A similar reaction has been reported with other cephalosporins.

Prolonged use of cefoperazone sodium may result in the overgrowth of nonsusceptible organisms. Careful observation of the patient is essential. If superinfection occurs during therapy, appropriate measures should be taken.

Cefoperazone sodium should be prescribed with caution in individuals with a history of gastrointestinal disease, particularly colitis.

DRUG/LABORATORY TEST INTERACTIONS

A false-positive reaction for glucose in the urine may occur with Benedict's or Fehling's solution.

CARCINOGENESIS, MUTAGENESIS, AND IMPAIRMENT OF FERTILITY

Long term studies in animals have not been performed to evaluate carcinogenic potential. The maximum duration of cefoperazone sodium animal toxicity studies is six months. In none of the *in vivo* or *in vitro* genetic toxicology studies did cefoperazone sodium show any mutagenic potential at either the chromosomal or subchromosomal level. Cefoperazone sodium produced no impairment of fertility and had no effects on general reproductive performance or fetal development when administered subcutaneously at daily doses up to 500-1000 mg/kg prior to and during mating, and to pregnant female rats during gestation. These doses are 10-20 times the estimated usual single clinical dose. Cefoperazone sodium had adverse effects on the testes of prepubertal rats at all doses tested. Subcutaneous administration of 1000 mg/kg per day (approximately 16 times the average adult human dose) resulted in reduced testicular weight, arrested spermatogenesis, reduced germinal cell population and vacuolation of Sertoli cell cytoplasm. The severity of lesions was dose dependent in the 100-1000 mg/kg per day range; the low dose caused a minor decrease in spermatocytes. This effect has not been observed in adult rats. Histologically the lesions were reversible at all but the highest dosage levels. However, these studies did not evaluate subsequent development of reproductive function in the rats. The relationship of these findings to humans is unknown.

PREGNANCY CATEGORY B

Reproduction studies have been performed in mice, rats, and monkeys at doses up to 10 times the human dose and have revealed no evidence of impaired fertility or harm to the fetus due to cefoperazone sodium. There are, however, no adequate and well controlled studies in pregnant women. Because animal reproduction studies are not always predictive of human response, this drug should be used during pregnancy only if clearly needed.

NURSING MOTHERS

Only low concentrations of cefoperazone sodium are excreted in human milk. Although cefoperazone sodium passes poorly into breast milk of nursing mothers, caution should be exercised when cefoperazone sodium is administered to a nursing woman.

PEDIATRIC USE

Safety and effectiveness in children have not been established. For information concerning testicular changes in prepubertal rats (see Carcinogenesis, Mutagenesis, and Impairment of Fertility).

ADVERSE REACTIONS

In clinical studies the following adverse effects were observed and were considered to be related to cefoperazone sodium therapy or of uncertain etiology:

Hypersensitivity: As with all cephalosporins, hypersensitivity manifested by skin reactions (1 patient in 45), drug fever (1 in 260), or a change in Coombs' test (1 in 60) has been reported. These reactions are more likely to occur in patients with a history of allergies, particularly to penicillin.

Hematology: As with other beta-lactam antibiotics, reversible neutropenia may occur with prolonged administration. Slight decreases in neutrophil count (1 patient in 50) have been reported. Decreased hemoglobins (1 in 20) or hematocrits (1 in 20) have been reported, which is consistent with published literature on other cephalosporins. Transient eosinophilia has occurred in 1 patient in 10.

Hepatic: Of 1285 patients treated with cefoperazone in clinical trials, one patient with a history of liver disease developed significantly elevated liver function enzymes during cefoperazone sodium therapy. Clinical signs and symptoms of nonspecific hepatitis accompanied these increases. After cefoperazone sodium therapy was discontinued, the patient's enzymes returned to pre-treatment levels and the symptomatology resolved. As with other antibiotics that achieve high bile levels, mild transient elevations of liver function enzymes have been observed in 5-10% of the patients receiving cefoperazone sodium therapy. The relevance of these findings, which were not accompanied by overt signs or symptoms of hepatic dysfunction, has not been established.

Gastrointestinal: Diarrhea or loose stools have been reported in 1 in 30 patients. Most of these experiences have been mild or moderate in severity and self-limiting in nature. In all cases, these symptoms responded to symptomatic therapy or ceased when cefoperazone therapy was stopped. Nausea and vomiting have been reported rarely.

Symptoms of pseudomembranous colitis can appear during or for several weeks subsequent to antibiotic therapy (see WARNINGS).

Renal Function Tests: Transient elevations of the BUN (1 in 16) and serum creatinine (1 in 48) have been noted.

Local Reactions: Cefoperazone sodium is well tolerated following intramuscular administration. Occasionally, transient pain (1 in 140) may follow administration by this route. When cefoperazone sodium is administered by intravenous infusion some patients may develop phlebitis (1 in 120) at the infusion site.

DOSAGE AND ADMINISTRATION

C

The usual adult daily dose of cefoperazone sodium is 2-4 g/day administered in equally divided doses every 12 hours.

In severe infections or infections caused by less sensitive organisms, the total daily dose and/or frequency may be increased. Patients have been successfully treated with a total daily dosage of 6-12 g divided into 2, 3 or 4 administrations ranging from 1.5-4 g per dose.

In a pharmacokinetic study, a total daily dose of 16 g was administered to severely immunocompromised patients by constant infusion without complications. Steady state serum concentrations were approximately 150 μg/ml in these patients.

When treating infections caused by *Streptococcus pyogenes,* therapy should be continued for at least 10 days.

Solutions of cefoperazone sodium and aminoglycoside should not be directly mixed, since there is a physical incompatibility between them. If combination therapy with cefoperazone sodium and an aminoglycoside is contemplated (see INDICATIONS AND USAGE) this can be accomplished by sequential intermittent intravenous infusion provided that separate secondary intravenous tubing is used, and that the primary intravenous tubing is adequately irrigated with an approved diluent between doses. It is also suggested that cefoperazone sodium be administered prior to the aminoglycoside. *In vitro* testing of the effectiveness of drug combination(s) is recommended.

RECONSTITUTION

The following solutions may be used for the initial reconstitution of cefoperazone sodium sterile powder:

Vehicles for Initial Reconstitution: 5% dextrose injection, 5% dextrose and 0.9% sodium chloride injection, 5% dextrose and 0.2% sodium chloride injection, 10% dextrose injection bacteriostatic water for injection (benzyl alcohol or parabens)*†, 0.9% sodium chloride injection, normosol M and 5% dextrose injection, normosol R, and sterile water for injection.

*Not to be used as a vehicle for intravenous infusion.

†Preparations containing benzyl alcohol should not be used in neonates.

GENERAL RECONSTITUTION PROCEDURES

Cefoperazone sodium sterile powder for intravenous or intramuscular use may be initially reconstituted with any compatible solution mentioned above in TABLE 1. Solutions should be allowed to stand after reconstitution to allow any foaming to dissipate to permit visual inspection for complete solubilization. Vigorous and prolonged agitation may be necessary to solubilize cefoperazone sodium in higher concentrations (above 333 mg cefoperazone/ml). The maximum solubility of cefoperazone sodium sterile powder is approximately 475 mg cefoperazone/ml of compatible diluent.

PREPARATION FOR INTRAVENOUS USE

General: Cefoperazone sodium concentrations between 2 and 50 mg/ml are recommended for intravenous administration.

Preparation of Vials: Vials of cefoperazone sodium sterile powder may be initially reconstituted with a minimum of 2.8 ml/g of cefoperazone of any compatible reconstituting solution appropriate for intravenous administration listed in TABLE 4. For ease of reconstitution the use of 5 ml of compatible solution per gram of cefoperazone sodium is recommended. The entire quantity of the resulting solution should then be withdrawn for further dilution and administration using any of the following vehicles for intravenous infusion (see TABLE 5).

Vehicles for Intravenous Infusion: 5% dextrose injection, 5% dextrose and lactated Ringer's injection, 5% dextrose and 0.9% sodium chloride injection, 5% dextrose and 0.2% sodium chloride injection, 10% dextrose injection, lactated Ringer's injection, 0.9% sodium chloride injection, normosol M and 5% dextrose injection, and normosol R.

Preparation of Piggy Back Units: Cefoperazone sodium sterile powder in Piggy Back Units for intravenous use may be prepared by adding between 20 and 40 ml of any appropriate diluent listed in TABLE 2 per gram of cefoperazone. If 5% dextrose and lactated ringer's injection or lactated Ringer's injection is the chosen vehicle for administration the cefoperazone sodium sterile powder should initially be reconstituted using 2.8-5 ml/g of any compatible reconstituting solution listed in TABLE 1 prior to the final dilution.

The resulting intravenous solution should be administered in one of the following manners:

Intermittent Infusion: Solutions of cefoperazone sodium should be administered over a 15-30 minute time period.

Continuous Infusion: Cefoperazone sodium can be used for continuous infusion after dilution to a final concentration of between 2 and 25 mg cefoperazone per ml.

PREPARATION FOR INTRAMUSCULAR INJECTION

Any suitable solution listed above may be used to prepare cefoperazone sodium sterile powder for intramuscular injection. When concentrations of 250 mg/ml or more are to be administered, a lidocaine solution should be used. These solutions should be prepared using a combination of sterile water for injection and 2% lidocaine hydrochloride injection that approximates a 0.5% lidocaine hydrochloride solution. A two-step dilution process as follows is recommended: First, add the required amount of sterile water for injection and agitate until cefoperazone sodium powder is completely dissolved. Second, add the required amount of 2% lidocaine and mix (see TABLE 4).

When a diluent other than lidocaine HCl injection is used reconstitute as shown in TABLE 5.

TABLE 4

	Final Cefoperazone Concentration	Step 1 Volume of Sterile Water	Step 2 Volume of 2% Lidocaine	Withdrawable Volume*†
1 g vial	333 mg/ml	2.0 ml	0.6 ml	3 ml
	250 mg/ml	2.8 ml	1.0 ml	4 ml
2 g vial	333 mg/ml	3.8 ml	1.2 ml	6 ml
	250 mg/ml	5.4 ml	1.8 ml	8 ml

* There is sufficient excess present to allow for withdrawal of the stated volume.
† Final lidocaine concentration will approximate that obtained if a 0.5% lidocaine hydrochloride solution is used as diluent.

TABLE 5

	Cefoperazone Concentration	Volume of Diluent to be Added	Withdrawable Volume*
1 g vial	333 mg/ml	2.6 ml	3 ml
	250 mg/ml	3.8 ml	4 ml
2 g vial	333 mg/ml	5.0 ml	6 ml
	250 mg/ml	7.2 ml	8 ml

* There is sufficient excess present to allow for withdrawal of the stated volume.

STORAGE AND STABILITY

Cefoperazone sodium sterile powder is to be stored at or below 25°C (77°F) and protected from light prior to reconstitution. After reconstitution, protection from light is not necessary.

The preceding parenteral diluents and approximate concentrations of cefoperazone sodium provide stable solutions under the following conditions for the indicated time periods (see TABLE 6, TABLE 7, TABLE 8). (After the indicated time periods, unused portions of solutions should be discarded.)

TABLE 6 *Controlled Room Temperature 15-25°C (59-77°F) Approximate*

24 Hours	Concentrations
Bacteriostatic water for injection (benzyl alcohol or parabens)	300 mg/ml
5% Dextrose injection	2 mg to 50 mg/ml
5% Dextrose and lactated Ringer's injection	2 mg to 50 mg/ml
5% Dextrose + 0.9% Sodium chloride injection	2 mg to 50 mg/ml
5% Dextrose + 0.2% sodium chloride injection	2 mg to 50 mg/ml
10% Dextrose injection	2 mg to 50 mg/ml
Lactated Ringer's injection	2 mg/ml
0.5% Lidocaine hydrochloride injection	300 mg/ml
0.9% Sodium chloride injection	2 mg to 300 mg/ml
Normosol M and 5% dextrose injection	2 mg to 50 mg/ml
Normosol	2 mg to 50 mg/ml
Sterile water for injection	300 mg/ml

Reconstituted Cefobid solutions may be stored in glass or plastic syringes, or in glass or flexible plastic parenteral solution containers.

TABLE 7 *Refrigerator Temperature 2-8°C (36-46°F) Approximate*

5 Days	Concentrations
Bacteriostatic water for injection (benzyl alcohol or parabens)	300 mg/ml
5% Dextrose injection	2 mg to 50 mg/ml
5% Dextrose + 0.9% sodium chloride injection	2 mg to 50 mg/ml
5% Dextrose + 0.2% sodium chloride injection	2 mg to 50 mg/ml
Lactated Ringer's injection	2 mg/ml
0.5% Lidocaine hydrochloride injection	300 mg/ml
0.9% Sodium chloride injection	2 mg to 300 mg/ml
Normosol M and 5% dextrose injection	2 mg to 50 mg/ml
Normosol R	2 mg to 50 mg/ml
Sterile water for injection	300 mg/ml

Reconstituted Cefobid solutions may be stored in glass or plastic syringes, or in glass or flexible plastic parenteral solution containers.

TABLE 8 *Freezer Temperature -20 to -10°C (-4 to 14°F) Approximate*

	Concentrations
3 Weeks	
5% Dextrose injection	50 mg/ml
5% Dextrose and 0.9% sodium chloride injection	2 mg/ml
5% Dextrose and 0.2% sodium chloride injection	2 mg/ml
5 Weeks	
0.9% Sodium chloride injection	300 mg/ml
Sterile water for injection	300 mg/ml

Reconstituted Cefobid solutions may be stored in plastic syringes, or in flexible plastic parenteral solution containers.
Frozen samples should be thawed at room temperature before use. After thawing, unused portions should be discarded. Do not refreeze.

PRODUCT LISTING - EQUIVALENTS NOT AVAILABLE

Powder For Injection - Injectable - 1 Gm
10's $179.95 CEFOBID, Pfizer U.S. Pharmaceuticals 00049-1201-83
Powder For Injection - Injectable - 2 Gm
10's $359.89 CEFOBID, Pfizer U.S. Pharmaceuticals 00049-1202-83
Powder For Injection - Injectable - 10 Gm
1's $157.28 CEFOBID, Pfizer U.S. Pharmaceuticals 00049-1219-28

Cefotaxime Sodium *(000689)*

For related information, see the comparative table section in Appendix A.

Categories: Cellulitis, pelvic; Endometritis; Gonorrhea; Infection, bone; Infection, central nervous system; Infection, gynecologic; Infection, intra-abdominal; Infection, joint; Infection, lower respiratory tract; Infection, sexually transmitted; Infection, skin and skin structures; Infection, urinary tract; Meningitis; Pelvic inflammatory disease; Peritonitis; Pneumonia; Prophylaxis, surgical; Septicemia; Ventriculitis; Pregnancy Category B; FDA Approved 1981 Mar
Drug Classes: Antibiotics, cephalosporins
Brand Names: Claforan
Foreign Brand Availability: Baxima (Indonesia); Benaxima (Mexico); Biosint (Mexico); Biotax (India); Biotaxime (Thailand); Cefajet (China); Cefaxim (Mexico); Cefirad (Korea); Cefpiran (Korea); Cefodin (Mexico); Cefomic (China); Cefotax (Bahrain; Cyprus; Egypt; Iran; Iraq; Japan; Jordan; Kuwait; Lebanon; Libya; Oman; Qatar; Republic-of-Yemen; Saudi-Arabia; Syria; Thailand; United-Arab-Emirates); Cetax (Taiwan); Clacef (Indonesia; Singapore); Claforan (Indonesia); Clafoxim (Philippines); Claraxim (Thailand); Clatax (Indonesia); Clavocef (Philippines); Clavox (Taiwan); Efotax (Indonesia); Fotax (Thailand); Fotexina (Colombia; Mexico); Grifotaxima (Peru); Kalfoxim (Indonesia); Lancef (Indonesia); Lyforan (India); Molelant (Greece); Naspor (Peru); Newtaxime (Korea); Omnatax (India); Oritaxim (Benin; Burkina-Faso; Ethiopia; Gambia; Ghana; Guinea; Ivory-Coast; Kenya; Liberia; Malawi; Mali; Mauritania; Mauritius; Morocco; Niger; Nigeria; Senegal; Seychelles; Sierra-Leone; South-Africa; Sudan; Tanzania; Tunia; Uganda; Zambia; Zimbabwe); Oritaxime (Thailand); Primafen (Spain); Ralopar (Portugal); Sepsilem (Mexico); Spirosine (Greece); Stoparen (Greece); Taporin (Mexico); Taxime (Bahrain; Cyprus; Egypt; Iran; Iraq; Jordan; Kuwait; Lebanon; Libya; Oman; Qatar; Republic-of-Yemen; Saudi-Arabia; Syria; United-Arab-Emirates); Tirotax (Mexico); Viken (Mexico); Zariviz (Italy); Zetaxim (India)
Cost of Therapy: $280.96 (Infection; Claforan Injection; 1 g; 2 g/day; 10 day supply)
HCFA JCODE(S): J0698 per 1 g IV, IM

DESCRIPTION

Cefotaxime sodium is a semisynthetic, broad spectrum cephalosporin antibiotic for parenteral administration. It is the sodium salt of 7-[2-(2-amino-4-thiazolyl)glyoxylamido]-3-(hydroxymethyl)-8-oxo-5-thia-1-azabicyclo[4.2.0]oct-2-ene-2-carboxylate 7^2(Z)-(o-methyloxime), acetate (ester). Claforan contains approximately 50.5 mg (2.2 mEq) of sodium/gram of cefotaxime activity. Solutions of Claforan range from very pale yellow to light amber depending on the concentration and the diluent used. The pH of the injectable solutions usually ranges from 5.0-7.5.

Claforan is supplied as a dry powder in conventional and ADD-Vantage System compatible vials, infusion bottles, pharmacy bulk package bottles, and as a frozen, premixed, iso-osmotic injection in a buffered diluent solution in plastic containers. Claforan, equivalent to 1 and 2 g cefotaxime, is supplied as frozen, premixed, iso-osmotic injections in plastic containers. Solutions range from very pale yellow to light amber. Dextrous hydrous has been added to adjust osmolality (approximately 1.7 g and 700 mg to the 1 g and 2 g cefotaxime dosages, respectively). The injections are buffered with sodium citrate hydrous. The pH is adjusted with hydrochloric acid and may be adjusted with sodium hydroxide. The plastic container is fabricated from a specially designed multilayer plastic (PL 2040). Solutions are in contact with the polyethylene layer of this container and can leach out certain chemical components of the plastic in very small amounts within the expiration period. The suitability of the plastic has been confirmed in tests in animals according to the USP biological tests for plastic containers, as well as by tissue culture toxicity studies.

CLINICAL PHARMACOLOGY

Following intramuscular (IM) administration of a single 500 mg or 1 g dose of cefotaxime sodium to normal volunteers, mean peak serum concentrations of 11.7 and 20.5 μg/ml respectively were attained within 30 minutes and declined with an elimination half-life of approximately 1 hour. There was a dose-dependent increase in serum levels after the intravenous (IV) administration of 500 mg, 1 g, and 2 g of cefotaxime sodium (38.9, 101.7, and 214.4 μg/ml respectively) without alteration in the elimination half-life. There is no evidence of accumulation following repetitive IV infusion of 1 g doses every 6 hours for 14 days as there are no alterations of serum or renal clearance. About 60% of the administered dose was recovered from urine during the first 6 hours following the start of the infusion.

Approximately 20-36% of an intravenously administered dose of ^{14}C-cefotaxime is excreted by the kidney as unchanged cefotaxime and 15-25% as the desacetyl derivative, the major metabolite. The desacetyl metabolite has been shown to contribute to the bactericidal activity. Two other urinary metabolites (M_2 and M_3) account for about 20-25%. They lack bactericidal activity.

A single 50 mg/kg dose of cefotaxime sodium was administered as an IV infusion over a 10-15 minute period to 29 newborn infants grouped according to birth weight and age. The mean half-life of cefotaxime in infants with lower birth weights (≤1500 g), regardless of age, was longer (4.6 hours) than the mean half-life (3.4 hours) in infants whose birth weight was greater than 1500 g. Mean serum clearance was also smaller in the lower birth weight infants. Although the differences in mean half-life values are statistically significant for weight, they are not clinically important. Therefore, dosage should be based solely on age. (See DOSAGE AND ADMINISTRATION.)

Additionally, no disulfiram-like reactions were reported in a study conducted in 22 healthy volunteers administered cefotaxime sodium and ethanol.

MICROBIOLOGY

The bactericidal activity of cefotaxime sodium results from inhibition of cell wall synthesis. Cefotaxime sodium has *in vitro* activity against a wide range of gram-positive and gram-negative organisms. Cefotaxime sodium has a high degree of stability in the presence of β-lactamases, both penicillinases and cephalosporinases, of gram-negative and gram-positive bacteria. Cefotaxime sodium has been shown to be active against most strains of the following microorganisms both *in vitro* and in clinical infections as described in INDICATIONS AND USAGE.

Aerobes, Gram-Positive:

Enterococcus spp., *Staphylococcus aureus**, including β-lactamase-positive and negative strains, *Staphylococcus epidermidis, Streptococcus pneumoniae, Streptococcus pyogenes* (Group A beta-hemolytic streptococci), *Streptococcus* spp.

*Staphylococci which are resistant to methicillin/oxacillin must be considered resistant to cefotaxime sodium.

Aerobes, Gram-Negative:

Acinetobacter spp., *Citrobacter* spp., *Enterobacter* spp., *Escherichia coli, Haemophilus influenzae* (including ampicillin-resistant strains), *Haemophilus parainfluenzae, Klebsiella* spp. (including Klebsiella pneumoniae), *Morganella morganii, Neisseria gonorrhoeae* (including β-lactamase-positive and negative strains), *Neisseria meningitidis, Proteus mirabilis, Proteus vulgaris, Providencia rettgeri, Providencia stuartii, Serratia marcescens.*

NOTE: Many strains of the above organisms that are multiply resistant to other antibiotics, *e.g.*, penicillins, cephalosporins, and aminoglycosides, are susceptible to cefotaxime sodium. Cefotaxime sodium is active against some strains of *Pseudomonas aeruginosa*.

Anaerobes:

Bacteroides spp., including some strains of *Bacteroides fragilis, Clostridium* spp. (**Note:** Most strains of *Clostridium difficile* are resistant.) *Fusobacterium* spp. (Including *Fusobacterium nucleatum*). *Peptococcus* spp., *Peptostreptococcus* spp.

Cefotaxime sodium also demonstrates *in vitro* activity against the following microorganisms **but the clinical significance is unknown.**

Cefotaxime sodium exhibits *in vitro* minimal inhibitory concentrations (MIC's) of 8 μg/ml or less against most (≥90%) strains of the following microorganisms; however, the safety and effectiveness of cefotaxime sodium in treating clinical infections due to these microorganisms have not been established in adequate and well controlled clinical trials:

Aerobes, Gram-Negative:

Providencia spp., *Salmonella* spp. (including *Salmonella typhi*) *Shigella* spp.

Cefotaxime sodium is highly stable *in vitro* to 4 of the 5 major classes of 5-lactamases described by Richmond *et al.*[1], including type IIIa (TEM) which is produced by many gram-negative bacteria. The drug is also stable to β-lactamase (penicillinase) produced by staphylococci. In addition, cefotaxime sodium shows high affinity for penicillin-binding proteins in the cell wall, including PBP: Ib and III. Cefotaxime sodium and aminoglycosides have been shown to be synergistic *in vitro* against some strains of *Pseudomonas aeruginosa* but the clinical significance is unknown.

SUSCEPTIBILITY TESTING

Dilution Techniques

Quantitative methods that are used to determine minimum inhibitory concentrations (MIC's) provide reproducible estimates of the susceptibility of bacteria to antimicrobial compounds. One such standardized procedure uses a standardized dilution method[1] (broth or agar) or equivalent with cefotaxime sodium powder. The MIC values obtained should be interpreted according to the criteria (see TABLE 1, TABLE 2, TABLE 3, and TABLE 4).

TABLE 1 *When Testing Organisms* Other Than Haemophilus spp., Neisseria Gonorrhoeae and Streptococcus spp.:*

MIC	Interpretation
≤8 μg/ml	Susceptible (S)
16-32 μg/ml	Intermediate (I)
≥64 μg/ml	Resistant (R)

* Staphylococci exhibiting resistance to methicillin/oxacillin, should be reported as also resistant to cefotaxime despite apparent *in vitro* susceptibility.

TABLE 2 *When Testing Haemophilus spp.*:*

MIC	Interpretation†
≤2 μg/ml	Susceptible (S)

* Interpretive criteria is applicable only to tests performed by broth microdilution method using Haemophilus Test Media.[2]
† The absence of resistant strains precludes defining any interpretations other than susceptible.

TABLE 3 *When Testing Streptococcus*:*

MIC	Interpretation
≤0.5 μg/ml	Susceptible (S)
1 μg/ml	Intermediate (I)
≥2 μg/ml	Resistant (R)

* *Streptococcus pneumoniae* must be tested using cation-adjusted Mueller-Hinton broth with 2-5% lysed horse blood.

TABLE 4 *When Testing Neisseria Gonorrhoeae*:*

MIC	Interpretation†
≤0.5 μg/ml	Susceptible (S)

* Interpretive criteria applicable only to tests performed by agar dilution method using GC agar base with 1% defined growth supplement.[2]
† The absence of resistant strains precludes defining any interpretations other than susceptible.

A report of "Susceptible" indicates that the pathogen is likely to be inhibited if the antimicrobial compound in the blood reaches the concentrations usually achievable. A report of "Intermediate" indicates that the result should be considered equivocal and if the microorganism is not fully susceptible to alternative clinically feasible drugs the test should be repeated. This category implies possible clinical applicability in body sites where the drug is physiologically concentrated or in situations where high dosage of drug can be used. This category also provides a buffer zone that prevents small uncontrolled technical factors from causing major discrepancies in interpretation. A report of "Resistant" indicates that the pathogen is not likely to be inhibited if the antimicrobial compound in the blood reaches the concentrations usually achievable, other therapy should be selected. Standardized susceptibility test procedures require the use of laboratory control microorganisms to control the technical aspects of the laboratory procedure. Standard cefotaxime sodium powder should provide the MIC values as shown in TABLE 5.

TABLE 5

Microorganism	MIC
Escherichia coli ATCC 25922	0.06-0.25 μg/ml
Staphylococcus aureus ATCC 29213	1-4 μg/ml
Pseudomonas aeruginosa ATCC 27853	4-16 μg/ml
*Haemophilus influenzae** ATCC 49247	0.12-0.5 μg/ml
Streptococcus pneumoniae† ATCC 49619	0.06-0.25 μg/ml
Neisseria gonorrhoeae‡ ATCC 49226	0.015-0.06 μg/ml

* Ranges applicable only to tests performed by broth microdilution method using Haemophilus Test Media.[2]
† Ranges applicable only to tests performed by broth microdilution method using cation-adjusted Mueller-Hinton broth with 2-5% lysed horse blood.[2]
‡ Ranges applicable only to tests performed by agar dilution method using GC agar base with 1% defined growth supplement.[2]

Diffusion Techniques

Quantitative methods that require measurements of zone diameters also provide reproducible estimates of the susceptibility of bacteria to antimicrobial compounds. One such standardized procedure[3] requires the use of standardized inoculum concentrations. This procedure uses paper disks impregnated with 30 μg cefotaxime sodium to test the susceptibility of microorganisms to cefotaxime sodium. Reports from the laboratory providing results of the standard single-disk susceptibility test using a 30 μg cefotaxime sodium disk should be interpreted according to the criteria (see TABLE 6, TABLE 7, TABLE 8, and TABLE 9).

TABLE 6 *When Testing Organisms* Other Than Haemophilus spp., Neisseria Gonorrhoeae and Streptococcus spp.:*

MIC	Interpretation
≥23 μg/ml	Susceptible (S)
15-22 μg/ml	Intermediate (I)
≤14 μg/ml	Resistant (R)

* *Staphylococci* exhibiting resistance to methicillin/oxacillin, should be reported as also resistant to cefotaxime despite apparent *in vitro* susceptibility.

TABLE 7 *When Testing Haemophilus spp.*:*

Zone Diameter	Interpretation†
≥26 mm	Susceptible (S)

* Interpretive criteria is applicable only to tests performed by disk diffusion method using Haemophilus Test Media.[3]
† The absence of resistant strains precludes defining any interpretations other than susceptible.

TABLE 8 *When Testing Streptococcus Other Than Streptococcus Pneumoniae:*

Zone Diameter	Interpretation
≥28 mm	Susceptible (S)
26-27 mm	Intermediate (I)
≤25 mm	Resistant (R)

TABLE 9 *When Testing Neisseria Gonorrhoeae*:*

Zone Diameter	Interpretation†
≥31 mm	Susceptible (S)

* Interpretive criteria applicable only to tests performed by disk diffusion method using GC agar base with 1% defined growth supplement.[3]
† The absence of resistant strains precludes defining any interpretations other than susceptible.

Interpretation should be as stated above for results using dilution techniques. Interpretation involves correlation of the diameter obtained in the disk test with the MIC for cefotaxime sodium.

As with standardized dilution techniques, diffusion methods require the use of laboratory control microorganisms that are used to control the technical aspects of the laboratory procedures. For the diffusion technique, the 30 μg cefotaxime sodium disk should provide the following zone diameters in these laboratory test quality control strains (see TABLE 10).

TABLE 10

Microorganism	Zone Diameter
Escherichia coli ATCC 25922	29-35 mm
Staphylococcus aureus ATCC 25923	25-31 mm
Pseudomonas aeruginosa ATCC 27853	18-22 mm
*Haemophilus influenzae** ATCC 49247	31-39 mm
Neisseria gonorrhoeae† ATCC 49226	38-48 mm

* Ranges applicable only to tests performed by disk diffusion method using Haemophilus Test Media.[3]
† Ranges applicable only to tests performed by disk diffusion method using GC agar base with 1% defined growth supplement.[3]

Anaerobic Techniques

For anaerobic bacteria, the susceptibility to cefotaxime sodium as MICs can be determined by standardized test methods.[4] The MIC values obtained should be interpreted according to the criteria (see TABLE 11).

TABLE 11

MIC	Interpretation
≤16 μg/ml	Susceptible (S)
32 μg/ml	Intermediate (I)
≥64 μg/ml	Resistant (R)

Interpretation is identical to that stated above for results using dilution techniques.

As with other susceptibility techniques, the use of laboratory control microorganisms is required to control the technical aspects of the laboratory standardized procedures. Standardized cefotaxime sodium powder should provide the MIC values as shown in TABLE 12.

INDICATIONS AND USAGE

TABLE 12

Microorganism	MIC
*Bacteroides fragilis** ATCC 25285	8-32 μg/ml
Bacteroides thetaiotaomicron ATCC 29741	16-64 μg/ml
Eubacterium lantem ATCC 43055	64-256 μg/ml

* Ranges applicable only to tests performed by agar dilution method.

TREATMENT

Cefotaxime sodium is indicated for the treatment of patients with serious infections caused by susceptible strains of the designated microorganisms in the diseases listed below.

Lower Respiratory Tract Infections: Including pneumonia, caused by *Streptococcus pneumoniae* (formerly *Diplococcus pneumoniae*), *Streptococcus pyogenes** (Group A *streptococci*) and other streptococci (excluding enterococci, *e.g., Streptococcus faecalis*), *Staphylococcus aureus* (penicillinase and non-penicillinase producing), *Escherichia coli, Klebsiella* species, *Haemophilus influenzae* (including ampicillin resistant strains), *Haemophilus parainfluenzae, Proteus mirabilis, Serratia marcescens**, *Enterobacter* species, indole positive *Proteus* and *Pseudomonas* species (including *P. aeruginosa*).

Genitourinary Infections: Urinary tract infections caused by *Enterococcus* species, *Staphylococcus epidermidis, Staphylococcus aureus** (penicillinase and non-penicillinase producing), *Citrobacter* species, *Enterobacter* species, *Escherichia coli, Klebsiella* species, *Proteus mirabilis, Proteus vulgaris**, *Providencia stuartii, Morganella morganii**, *Providencia rettgeri**, *Serratia marcescens* and *Pseudomonas* species (including *P. aeruginosa*). Also, uncomplicated gonorrhea (cervical/urethral and rectal) caused by *Neisseria gonorrhoeae*, including *penicillinase* producing strains.

Gynecologic Infections: Including pelvic inflammatory disease, endometritis and pelvic cellulitis caused by *Staphylococcus epidermidis, Streptococcus* species, *Enterococcus* species, *Enterobacter* species*, *Klebsiella* species*, *Escherichia coli, Proteus mirabilis, Bacteroides* species (including *Bacteroides fragilis**), *Clostridium* species, and anaerobic cocci (including *Peptostreptococcus* species and *Peptococcus* species) and *Fusobacterium* species (including *F. nucleatum**).

Cefotaxime sodium, like other cephalosporins, has no activity against *Chlamydia trachomatis*. Therefore, when cephalosporins are used in the treatment of patients with pelvic inflammatory disease and *C. trachomatis* is one of the suspected pathogens, appropriate anti-chlamydial coverage should be added.

Bacteremia/Septicemia: Caused by *Escherichia coli, Klebsiella* species, and *Serratia marcescens, Staphylococcus aureus*, and *Streptococcus* species (including *S. pneumoniae*).

Skin and Skin Structure Infections: Caused by *Staphylococcus aureus* (penicillinase and non-penicillinase producing), *Staphylococcus epidermidis, Streptococcus pyogenes* (Group A streptococci) and other streptococci, *Enterococcus* species, *Acinetobacter* species*, *Escherichia coli, Citrobacter* species (including *C. freundii**), *Enterobacter* species, *Klebsiella* species, *Proteus mirabilis, Proteus vulgaris**, *Morganella morganii, Providencia rettgeri**, *Pseudomonas* species, *Serratia marcescens, Bacteroides* species, and anaerobic cocci (including *Peptostreptococcus** species and *Peptococcus* species).

Intra-Abdominal Infections: Including peritonitis caused by *Streptococcus*species*, *Escherichia coli, Klebsiella* species, *Bacteroides* species, and anaerobic cocci (including *Peptostreptococcus** species and *Peptococcus** species), *Proteus mirabilis**, and *Clostridium* species*.

Bone and/or Joint Infections: Caused by *Staphylococcus aureus* (penicillinase and non-penicillinase producing strains), *Streptococcus* species (including *S. pyogenes**), *Pseudomonas* species (including *P. aeruginosa**), and *Proteus mirabilis**.

Central Nervous System Infections (e.g., meningitis and ventriculitis): Caused by *Neisseria meningitidis, Haemophilus influenzae, Streptococcus pneumoniae, Klebsiella pneumoniae** and *Escherichia coli**.

*Efficacy for this organism, in this organ system, has been studied in fewer than 10 infections.

Although many strains of enterococci (*e.g., S. faecalis*) and *Pseudomonas* species are resistant to cefotaxime sodium *in vitro*, cefotaxime sodium has been used successfully in treating patients with infections caused by susceptible organisms.

Specimens for bacteriologic culture should be obtained prior to therapy in order to isolate and identify causative organisms and to determine their susceptibilities to cefotaxime sodium. Therapy may be instituted before results of susceptibility studies are known; however, once these results become available, the antibiotic treatment should be adjusted accordingly.

In certain cases of confirmed or suspected gram-positive or gram-negative sepsis or in patients with other serious infections in which the causative organism has not been identified, cefotaxime sodium may be used concomitantly with an aminoglycoside. The dosage recommended in the labeling of both antibiotics may be given and depends on the severity of the infection and the patient's condition. Renal function should be carefully monitored, especially if higher dosages of the aminoglycosides are to be administered or if therapy is prolonged, because of the potential nephrotoxicity and ototoxicity of aminoglycoside antibiotics. It is possible that nephrotoxicity may be potentiated if cefotaxime sodium is used concomitantly with an aminoglycoside.

PREVENTION

The administration of cefotaxime sodium preoperatively reduces the incidence of certain infections in patients undergoing surgical procedures (*e.g.*, abdominal or vaginal hysterectomy, gastrointestinal and genitourinary tract surgery) that may be classified as contaminated or potentially contaminated.

In patients undergoing cesarean section, intraoperative (after clamping the umbilical cord) and postoperative use of cefotaxime sodium may also reduce the incidence of certain post-operative infections. (See DOSAGE AND ADMINISTRATION.)

Effective use for elective surgery depends on the time of administration. To achieve effective tissue levels, cefotaxime sodium should be given ½-1½ hours before surgery. (See DOSAGE AND ADMINISTRATION.)

For patients undergoing gastrointestinal surgery, preoperative bowel preparation by mechanical cleansing as well as with a non-absorbable antibiotic (*e.g.*, neomycin) is recommended.

If there are signs of infection, specimens for culture should be obtained for identification of the causative organism so that appropriate therapy may be instituted.

CONTRAINDICATIONS

Cefotaxime sodium is contraindicated in patients who have shown hypersensitivity to cefotaxime sodium or the cephalosporin group of antibiotics.

WARNINGS

BEFORE THERAPY WITH CEFOTAXIME SODIUM IS INSTITUTED, CAREFUL INQUIRY SHOULD BE MADE TO DETERMINE WHETHER THE PATIENT HAS HAD PREVIOUS HYPERSENSITIVITY REACTIONS TO CEFOTAXIME SODIUM, CEPHALOSPORINS, PENICILLINS, OR OTHER DRUGS. THIS PRODUCT SHOULD BE GIVEN WITH CAUTION TO PATIENTS WITH TYPE I HYPERSENSITIVITY REACTIONS TO PENICILLIN. ANTIBIOTICS SHOULD BE ADMINISTERED WITH CAUTION TO ANY PATIENT WHO HAS DEMONSTRATED SOME FORM OF ALLERGY, PARTICULARLY TO DRUGS. IF AN ALLERGIC REACTION TO CEFOTAXIME SODIUM OCCURS, DISCONTINUE TREATMENT WITH THE DRUG. SERIOUS HYPERSENSITIVITY REACTIONS MAY REQUIRE EPINEPHRINE AND OTHER EMERGENCY MEASURES.

During post-marketing surveillance, a potentially life-threatening arrhythmia was reported in each of 6 patients who received a rapid (less than 60 seconds) bolus injection of cefotaxime through a central venous catheter. Therefore, cefotaxime should only be administered as instructed in DOSAGE AND ADMINISTRATION.

Pseudomembranous colitis has been reported with nearly all antibacterial agents, including cefotaxime, and may range from mild to life threatening. Therefore, it is important to consider its diagnosis in patients with diarrhea subsequent to the administration of antibacterial agents.

Treatment with antibacterial agents alters the normal flora of the colon and may permit overgrowth of Clostridia. Studies indicate that a toxin produced by *Clostridium difficile* is 1 primary cause of antibiotic-associated colitis.

After the diagnosis of pseudomembranous colitis has been established, appropriate therapeutic measures should be initiated. Mild cases of colitis may respond to drug discontinuance alone. In moderate to severe cases, consideration should be given to management with fluids and electrolytes, protein supplementation, and treatment with an antibacterial drug clinically effective against *Clostridium difficile* colitis.

When the colitis is not relieved by drug discontinuance or when it is severe, oral vancomycin is the treatment of choice for antibiotic-associated pseudomembranous colitis produced by *C. difficile*. Other causes of colitis should also be considered.

PRECAUTIONS

GENERAL

Cefotaxime sodium should be prescribed with caution in individuals with a history of gastrointestinal disease, particularly colitis.

Because high and prolonged serum antibiotic concentrations can occur from usual doses in patients with transient or persistent reduction of urinary output because of renal insufficiency, the total daily dosage should be reduced when cefotaxime sodium is administered to such patients. Continued dosage should be determined by degree of renal impairment, severity of infection, and susceptibility of the causative organism. Although there is no clinical evidence supporting the necessity of changing the dosage of cefotaxime sodium in patients with even profound renal dysfunction, it is suggested that, until further data are obtained, the dosage of cefotaxime sodium be halved in patients with estimated creatinine clearances of less than 20 ml/min/1.73 m^2.

When only serum creatinine is available, the following formula[5] (based on sex, weight, and age of the patient) may be used to convert this value into creatinine clearance. The serum creatinine should represent a steady state of renal function.

Males: [Weight (kg) × (140 - age)] ÷ [72 × serum creatinine]

Females: 0.85 × above value

As with other antibiotics, prolonged use of cefotaxime sodium may result in overgrowth of nonsusceptible organisms. Repeated evaluation of the patient's condition is essential. If superinfection occurs during therapy, appropriate measures should be taken.

As with other beta-lactam antibiotics, granulocytopenia and, more rarely, agranulocytosis may develop during treatment with cefotaxime sodium, particularly if given over long periods. For courses of treatment lasting longer than 10 days, blood counts should therefore be monitored.

Cefotaxime sodium, like other parenteral anti-infective drugs, may be locally irritating to tissues. In most cases, perivascular extravasation of cefotaxime sodium responds to changing of the infusion site. In rare instances, extensive perivascular extravasation of cefotaxime sodium may result in tissue damage and require surgical treatment. To minimize the potential for tissue inflammation, infusion sites should be monitored regularly and changed when appropriate.

DRUG/LABORATORY TEST INTERACTIONS

Cephalosporins, including cefotaxime sodium, are known to occasionally induce a positive direct Coombs' test.

CARCINOGENESIS, MUTAGENESIS, AND IMPAIRMENT OF FERTILITY

Lifetime studies in animals to evaluate carcinogenic potential have not been conducted. Cefotaxime sodium was not mutagenic in the mouse micronucleus test or in the Ames' test. Cefotaxime sodium did not impair fertility to rats when administered subcutaneously at doses up to 250 mg/kg/day (0.2 times the maximum recommended human dose based on mg/m^2) or in mice when administered intravenously at doses up to 2000 mg/kg/day (0.7 times the recommended human dose based on mg/m^2.)

PREGNANCY CATEGORY B

Teratogenic Effects

Reproduction studies have been performed in pregnant mice given cefotaxime sodium intravenously at doses up to 1200 mg/kg/day (0.4 times the recommended human dose based on mg/m^2) or in pregnant rats when administered intravenously at doses up to 1200 mg/kg/day (0.8 times the recommended human dose based on mg/m^2). No evidence of embryotoxicity or teratogenicity was seen in these studies. There are no well-controlled studies in pregnant women. Because animal reproductive studies are not always predictive of human response, this drug should be used during pregnancy only if clearly needed.

Nonteratogenic Effects

Use of the drug in women of child-bearing potential requires that the anticipated benefit be weighed against the possible risks.

In perinatal and postnatal studies with rats, the pups in the group given 1200 mg/kg/day of cefotaxime sodium were significantly lighter in weight at birth and remained smaller than pups in the control group during the 21 days of nursing.

NURSING MOTHERS

Cefotaxime sodium is excreted in human milk in low concentrations. Caution should be exercised when cefotaxime sodium is administered to a nursing woman.

PEDIATRIC USE

See PRECAUTIONS regarding perivascular extravasation. The potential for toxic effects in pediatric patients from chemicals that may leach from the plastic in single dose Galaxy containers (premixed Claforan injection) has not been determined.

DRUG INTERACTIONS

Increased nephrotoxicity has been reported following concomitant administration of cephalosporins and aminoglycoside antibiotics.

ADVERSE REACTIONS

Cefotaxime sodium is generally well tolerated. The most common adverse reactions have been local reactions following IM or IV injection. Other adverse reactions have been encountered infrequently.

The most frequent adverse reactions (greater than 1%) are:

Local (4.3%): Injection site inflammation with IV administration. Pain, induration, and tenderness after IM injection.

Hypersensitivity (2.4%): Rash, pruritus, fever, eosinophilia, and less frequently urticaria and anaphylaxis.

Gastrointestinal (1.4%): Colitis, diarrhea, nausea, and vomiting. Symptoms of pseudomembranous colitis can appear during or after antibiotic treatment. Nausea and vomiting have been reported rarely.

Less frequent adverse reactions (less than 1%) are:

Cardiovascular System: Potentially life-threatening arrhymias following rapid (less than 60 seconds) bolus administration via central venous catheter have been observed.

Hematologic System: Neutropenia, transient leukopenia, eosinophilia, thrombocytopenia and agranulocytosis have been reported. Some individuals have developed positive direct Coombs Tests during treatment with cefotaxime sodium and other cephalosporin antibiotics. Rare cases of hemolytic anemia have been reported.

Genitourinary System: Moniliasis, vaginitis.

Central Nervous System: Headache.

Liver: Transient elevations in SGOT, SGPT, serum LDH, and serum alkaline phosphatase levels have been reported.

Kidney: As with some other cephalosporins, interstitial nephritis and transient elevations of BUN and creatinine have been occasionally observed with cefotaxime sodium.

Cutaneous: As with other cephalosporins, isolated cases of erythema multiforme, Stevens-Johnson syndrome, and toxic epidermal necrolysis have been reported.

CEPHALOSPORIN CLASS LABELING

In addition to the adverse reactions listed above which have been observed in patients treated with cefotaxime sodium, the following adverse reactions and altered laboratory tests have been reported for cephalosporin class antibiotics: allergic reactions, hepatic dysfunction including cholestasis, aplastic anemia, hemorrhage, and false-positive test for urinary glucose.

Several cephalosporins have been implicated in triggering seizures, particularly in patients with renal impairment when the dosage was not reduced. See DOSAGE AND ADMINISTRATION. If seizures associated with drug therapy occur, the drug should be discontinued. Anticonvulsant therapy can be given if clinically indicated.

DOSAGE AND ADMINISTRATION

ADULTS

Dosage and route of administration should be determined by susceptibility of the causative organisms, severity of the infection, and the condition of the patient (see TABLE 13) for dosage guideline. Cefotaxime sodium may be administered IM or IV after reconstitution. Premixed cefotaxime sodium injection is intended for IV administration after thawing. The maximum daily dosage should not exceed 12 g.

TABLE 13 *Guidelines for Dosage of Cefotaxime Sodium*

Type of Infection	Daily Dose	Frequency and Route
Gonococcal urethritis/ cervicitis in males and females	0.5 g	0.5 g IM (single dose)
Rectal gonorrhea in females	0.5 g	0.5 g IM (single dose)
Rectal gonorrhea in males	1 g	1 g IM (single dose)
Uncomplicated infections	2 g	1 g every 12 hours IM or IV
Moderate to severe infections	3-6 g	1-2 g every 8 hours IM or IV
Infections commonly needing antibiotics in higher dosage (*e.g.*, septicemia)	6-8 g	2 g every 6-8 hours IV
Life-threatening infections	up to 12 g	2 g every 4 hours IV

If *C. trachomatis* is a suspected pathogen, appropriate anti-chlamydial coverage should be added, because cefotaxime sodium has no activity against this oraganism.

To prevent postoperative infection in contaminated or potentially contaminated surgery, the recommended dose is a single 1 g IM or IV administered 30-90 minutes prior to start of surgery.

CESAREAN SECTION PATIENTS

The first dose of 1 g is administered intravenously as soon as the umbilical cord is clamped. The second and third doses should be given as 1 g intravenously or intramuscularly at 6 and 12 hours after the first dose.

NEONATES, INFANTS, AND CHILDREN

The following dosage schedule is recommended:

Neonates (birth to 1 month):

0-1 week of age: 50 mg/kg/dose every 12 hours IV.

1-4 weeks of age: 50 mg/kg/dose every 8 hours IV.

It is not necessary to differentiate between premature and normal-gestational age infants.

Infants and Children (1 month to 12 years):

For body weights less than 50 kg, the recommended daily dose is 50-180 mg/kg IM or IV body weight divided into 4-6 equal doses. The higher dosages should be used for more severe or serious infections, including meningitis. For body weights 50 kg or more, the usual adult dosage should be used; the maximum daily dosage should not exceed 12 g.

IMPAIRED RENAL FUNCTION

See PRECAUTIONS.

NOTE: As with antibiotic therapy in general, administration of cefotaxime sodium should be continued for a minimum of 48-72 hours after the patient defervesces or after evidence of bacterial eradication has been obtained; a minimum of 10 days of treatment is recommended for infections caused by Group A beta-hemolytic streptococci in order to guard against the risk of rheumatic fever or glomerulonephritis; frequent bacteriologic and clinical appraisal is necessary during therapy of chronic urinary tract infection and may be required for several months after therapy has been completed; persistent infections may require treatment of several weeks and doses smaller than those indicated above should not be used.

PREPARATION OF CEFOTAXIME SODIUM STERILE

Cefotaxime sodium for IM or IV administration should be reconstituted as shown in TABLE 14.

TABLE 14

Strength	Diluent	Withdrawable Volume	Approximate Concentration
500 mg vial* (IM)	2 ml	2.2 ml	230 mg/ml
1 g vial* (IM)	3 ml	3.4 ml	300 mg/ml
2 g vial* (IM)	5 ml	6.0 ml	330 mg/ml
500 mg vial* (IV)	10 ml	10.2 ml	50 mg/ml
1 g vial* (IV)	10 ml	10.4 ml	95 mg/ml
2 g vial* (IV)	10 ml	11.0 ml	180 mg/ml
1 g infusion	50-100 ml	50-100 ml	20-10 mg/ml
2 g infusion	50-100 ml	50-100 ml	40-20 mg/ml

* In conventional vials.

Shake to dissolve; inspect for particulate matter and discoloration prior to use. Solutions of cefotaxime sodium range from very pale yellow to light amber, depending on concentration, diluent used, and length and condition of storage.

For Intramuscular Use: Reconstitute vials with sterile water for injection or bacteriostatic water for injection as described in TABLE 14.

For Intravenous Use: Reconstitute vials with at least 10 ml of sterile water for injection. Reconstitute infusion bottles with 50 or 100 ml of 0.9% sodium chloride injection or 5% dextrose injection. For other diluents, see Compatibility and Stability.
NOTE: Solutions of cefotaxime sodium must not be admixed with aminoglycoside solutions. If cefotaxime sodium and aminoglycosides are to be administered to the same patient, they must be administered separately and not as mixed injection.
A SOLUTION OF 1 G CEFOTAXIME SODIUM IN 14 ML OF STERILE WATER FOR INJECTION IS ISOTONIC.

Intramuscular Administration

As with all IM preparations, cefotaxime sodium should be injected well within the body of a relatively large muscle such as the upper outer quadrant of the buttock (*i.e.,* gluteus maximus); aspiration is necessary to avoid inadvertent injection into a blood vessel. Individual IM doses of 2 g may be given if the dose is divided and is administered in different intramuscular sites.

Intravenous Administration

The IV route is preferable for patients with bacteremia, bacterial septicemia, peritonitis, meningitis, or other severe or life-threatening infections, or for patients who may be poor risks because of lowered resistance resulting from such debilitating conditions as malnutrition, trauma, surgery, diabetes, heart failure, or malignancy, particularly if shock is present or impending.

For intermittent IV administration, a solution containing 1 or 2 g in 10 ml of sterile water for injection can be injected over a period of 3-5 minutes. Cefotaxime should not be administered over a period of less than 3 minutes. (See WARNINGS.) With an infusion system, it may also be given over a longer period of time through the tubing system by which the patient may be receiving other IV solutions. However, during infusion of the solution containing cefotaxime sodium, it is advisable to discontinue temporarily the administration of other solutions at the same site.

For the administration of higher doses by continuous IV infusion, a solution of cefotaxime sodium may be added to IV bottles containing the solutions.

COMPATIBILITY AND STABILITY

Solutions of cefotaxime sodium sterile reconstituted (see Preparation of Cefotaxime Sodium Sterile) remain chemically stable (potency remains above 90%) as shown in TABLE 15 when stored in original containers and disposable plastic syringes.

TABLE 15

Strength	Reconstituted Concentration	Stability at or below 22° C	Stability under Refrigeraton (at or below 5° C): Original Containers	Plastic Syringes
500 mg vial IM	230 mg/ml	12 h	7 days	5 days
1 g vial IM	300 mg/ml	12 h	7 days	5 days
2 g vial IM	330 mg/ml	12 h	7 days	5 days
500 mg vial IV	50 mg/ml	24 h	7 days	5 days
1 g vial IV	95 mg/ml	24 h	7 days	5 days
2 g vial IV	180 mg/ml	12 h	7 days	5 days
1 g infusion bottle	10-20 mg/ml	24 h	10 days	
2 g infusion bottle	20-40 mg/ml	24 h	10 days	

Reconstituted solutions stored in original containers and plastic syringes remain stable for 13 weeks frozen.

Reconstituted solutions may be further diluted up to 1000 ml with the following solutions and maintain satisfactory potency for 24 hours at or below 22°C, and at least 5 days under refrigeration (at or below 5°C): 0.9% sodium chloride injection; 5 or 10% dextrose injection; 5% dextrose and 0.9% sodium chloride injection, 5% dextrose and 0.45% sodium chloride injection; 5% dextrose and 0.2% sodium chloride injection; lactated Ringer's solution; sodium lactate injection (M/6); 10% invert sugar injection, 8.5% travasol (amino acid) injection without electrolytes.

Solutions of cefotaxime sodium sterile reconstituted in 0.9% sodium chloride injection or 5% dextrose injection in Viaflex plastic containers maintain satisfactory potency for 24 hours at or below 22°C, 5 days under refrigeration (at or below 5°C) and 13 weeks frozen. Solutions of cefotaxime sodium sterile reconstituted in 0.9% sodium chloride injection or 5% dextrose injection in the ADD-Vantage flexible containers maintain satisfactory potency for 24 hours at or below 22°C. DO NOT FREEZE.
NOTE: Cefotaxime sodium solutions exhibit maximum stability in the pH 5-7 range. Solutions of cefotaxime sodium should not be prepared with diluents having a pH above 7.5, such as sodium bicarbonate injection.
Parenteral drug products should be inspected visually for particulate matter and discoloration prior to administration, whenever solution and container permit.

HOW SUPPLIED

Sterile Claforan is a dry off-white to pale yellow crystalline powder.
NOTE: Claforan in the dry state should be stored below 30°C. The dry material as well as solutions tend to darken depending on storage conditions and should be protected from elevated temperatures and excessive light.
Premixed Claforan injection is supplied as a frozen, iso-osmotic, sterile, nonpyrogenic solution in 50 ml single dose Galaxy containers (PL 2040 plastic).
NOTE: Store premixed Claforan injection at or below -20°C (-4°F).

PRODUCT LISTING - RATED THERAPEUTICALLY EQUIVALENT

Powder For Injection - Injectable - 1 Gm

25's	$275.00	GENERIC, American Pharmaceutical Partners	63323-0331-15

Powder For Injection - Injectable - 2 Gm

25's	$550.00	GENERIC, American Pharmaceutical Partners	63323-0332-15

Powder For Injection - Injectable - 10 Gm

10's	$886.90	GENERIC, American Pharmaceutical Partners	63323-0333-61

Powder For Injection - Injectable - 500 mg

25's	$181.25	GENERIC, American Pharmaceutical Partners	63323-0335-10

PRODUCT LISTING - EQUIVALENTS NOT AVAILABLE

Powder For Injection - Injectable - 1 Gm

10's	$140.48	CLAFORAN, Aventis Pharmaceuticals	00039-0018-11
10's	$143.93	CLAFORAN, Aventis Pharmaceuticals	00039-0018-10
25's	$339.99	CLAFORAN, Aventis Pharmaceuticals	00039-0018-25
25's	$350.61	CLAFORAN, Aventis Pharmaceuticals	00039-0023-25
50's	$640.66	CLAFORAN, Aventis Pharmaceuticals	00039-0018-50
50's	$663.22	CLAFORAN, Aventis Pharmaceuticals	00039-0023-50

Powder For Injection - Injectable - 2 Gm

10's	$263.86	CLAFORAN, Aventis Pharmaceuticals	00039-0019-11
10's	$266.24	CLAFORAN, Aventis Pharmaceuticals	00039-0019-10
25's	$503.70	CLAFORAN, Abbott Pharmaceutical	00074-0019-25
25's	$628.19	CLAFORAN, Aventis Pharmaceuticals	00039-0019-25
25's	$639.47	CLAFORAN, Aventis Pharmaceuticals	00039-0024-25
50's	$1186.31	CLAFORAN, Aventis Pharmaceuticals	00039-0019-50
50's	$1208.88	CLAFORAN, Aventis Pharmaceuticals	00039-0024-50

Powder For Injection - Injectable - 10 Gm

1's	$118.66	CLAFORAN, Aventis Pharmaceuticals	00039-0020-01

Powder For Injection - Injectable - 500 mg

10's	$86.21	CLAFORAN, Aventis Pharmaceuticals	00039-0017-10

Solution - Intravenous - 1 Gm/50 ml

50 ml x 24	$429.60	CLAFORAN, Aventis Pharmaceuticals	00039-0037-05

Solution - Intravenous - 2 Gm/50 ml

50 ml x 24	$759.00	CLAFORAN, Aventis Pharmaceuticals	00039-0038-05

Cefotetan Disodium *(000690)*

For related information, see the comparative table section in Appendix A.

Categories: Infection, bone; Infection, gynecologic; Infection, intra-abdominal; Infection, joint; Infection, lower respiratory tract; Infection, skin and skin structures; Infection, urinary tract; Prophylaxis, perioperative; Pregnancy Category B; FDA Approved 1985 Dec
Drug Classes: Antibiotics, cephalosporins
Brand Names: Apatef; **Cefotan**
Foreign Brand Availability: Apacef (Belgium; France); Ceftenon (Austria); Cepan (Italy)
Cost of Therapy: $262.40 (Infection; Cefotan Injection; 1 g; 2 g/day; 10 day supply)

DESCRIPTION

Cefotan (cefotetan disodium for injection) and Cefotan (cefotetan injection) in Galaxy plastic container (PL 2040) as cefotetan disodium are sterile, semisynthetic, broad-spectrum, beta-lactamase resistant, cephalosporin (cephamycin) antibiotics for parenteral administration. It is the disodium salt of [6*R*-(6α,7α)]-7-[[[4-(2-amino-1-carboxy-2-oxoethylidene)-1,3-dithietan-2-yl]carbonyl]amino]-7-methoxy-3-[[(1-methyl-1*H*-tetrazol-5-yl)thio]methyl]-8-oxo-5-thia-1-azabicyclo[4.2.0]oct-2-ene-2-carboxylic acid. Its molecular formula is $C_{17}H_{15}N_7Na_2O_8S_4$ with a molecular weight of 619.57.

Cefotan is supplied in vials containing 80 mg (3.5 mEq) of sodium per g of cefotetan activity. It is a white to pale yellow powder which is very soluble in water. Reconstituted solutions of cefotetan disodium for injection are intended for intravenous and intramuscular administration. The solution varies from colorless to yellow depending on the concentration. The pH of freshly reconstituted solutions is usually between 4.5-6.5.

Cefotetan disodium in the ADD-Vantage Vial is intended for intravenous use only after dilution with the appropriate volume of ADD-Vantage diluent solution.

Cefotan is available in 2 vial strengths. Each Cefotan 1 g vial contains cefotetan disodium equivalent to 1 g cefotetan activity. Each Cefotan 2 g vial contains cefotetan disodium equivalent to 2 g cefotetan activity.

Cefotan in the Galaxy plastic container (PL 2040) is a frozen, iso-osmotic, sterile, nonpyrogenic premixed 50 ml solution containing 1 or 2 g cefotetan as cefotetan disodium. Dextrose has been added to adjust the osmolality to 300 mOsmol/kg (approximately 1.9 g and 1.1 g to the 1 g and 2 g dosages, respectively); sodium bicarbonate has been added to convert cefotetan free acid to the sodium salt. The pH has been adjusted between 4 and 6.5 with sodium bicarbonate and may have been adjusted with hydrochloric acid. Cefotan in the Galaxy plastic container (PL 2040) contains 80 mg (3.5 mEq) of sodium per g of cefotetan activity. After thawing to room temperature, the solution is intended for intravenous use only.

This Galaxy container is fabricated from a specially designed multilayer plastic (PL 2040). Solutions are in contact with the polyethylene layer of this container and can leach out certain chemical components of the plastic in very small amounts within the expiration dating period. The suitability of the plastic has been confirmed in tests in animals according to the USP biological tests for plastic containers as well as by tissue culture toxicity.

CLINICAL PHARMACOLOGY

High plasma levels of cefotetan are attained after IV and IM administration of single doses to normal volunteers.

TABLE 1 *Plasma Concentrations After 1 g IV* or IM Dose*

Route	Mean Plasma Concentration (µg/ml)						
	Time After Injection						
	15 min	30 min	1h	2h	4h	8h	12h
IV	92	158	103	72	42	18	9
IM	34	56	71	68	47	20	9

* 30 minute infusion.

TABLE 2 *Plasma Concentrations After 2 g IV* or IM Dose*

Route	Mean Plasma Concentration (µg/ml)						
	Time After Injection						
	5 min	10 min	1h	3h	5h	9h	12h
IV	237	223	135	74	48	22	12†
IM	—	20	75	91	69	33	19

* Injected over 3 minutes.
† Concentrations estimated from regression line.

The plasma elimination half-life of cefotetan is 3 to 4.6 hours after either IV or IM administration.

Repeated administration of cefotetan disodium does not result in accumulation of the drug in normal subjects.

Cefotetan is 88% plasma protein bound.

No active metabolites of cefotetan have been detected; however, small amounts (less than 7%) of cefotetan in plasma and urine may be converted to its tautomer, which has antimicrobial activity similar to the parent drug.

In normal patients, from 51-81% of an administered dose of cefotetan disodium is excreted unchanged by the kidneys over a 24 hour period, which results in high and prolonged urinary concentrations. Following IV doses of 1 and 2 g, urinary concentrations are highest during the first hour and reach concentrations of approximately 1700 and 3500 µg/ml respectively.

In volunteers with reduced renal function, the plasma half-life of cefotetan is prolonged. The mean terminal half-life increases with declining renal function, from approximately 4 hours in volunteers with normal renal function to about 10 hours in those with moderate renal impairment. There is a linear correlation between the systemic clearance of cefotetan and creatinine clearance. When renal function is impaired, a reduced dosing schedule based on creatinine clearance must be used. (See DOSAGE AND ADMINISTRATION).

In pharmacokinetics studies of 8 elderly patients (greater than 65 years) with normal renal function and 6 healthy volunteers (aged 25-28 years), mean (±1 SD) Total Body Clearance [1.8(0.1) L/h vs 1.8 (0.3) L/h] and mean Volume of Distribution [10.4(1.2) L vs 10.3 (1.6)L] were similar following administration of a 1 g IV bolus dose.

Therapeutic levels of cefotetan are achieved in many body tissues and fluids including: skin; muscle; fat; myometrium; endometrium; cervix; ovary; kidney; ureter; bladder; maxillary sinus mucosa; tonsil; bile; peritoneal fluid; umbilical cord serum; amniotic fluid.

MICROBIOLOGY

The bactericidal action of cefotetan results from inhibition of cell wall synthesis. Cefotetan has *in vitro* activity against a wide range of aerobic and anaerobic gram-positive and gram-negative organisms. The methoxy group in the 7-alpha position provides cefotetan with a high degree of stability in the presence of beta-lactamases including both penicillinases and cephalosporinases of gram-negative bacteria.

Cefotetan has been shown to be active against most strains of the following organisms **both *in vitro* and in clinical infections** (see INDICATIONS AND USAGE).

Gram-Negative Aerobes: *Escherichia coli; Haemophilus influenzae* (including ampicillin-resistant strains); *Klebsiella* species (including *K. pneumoniae*); *Morganella morganii; Neisseria gonorrhoeae* (nonpenicillinase-producing strains); *Proteus mirabilis; Proteus vulgaris; Providencia rettgeri; Serratia marcescens.*

NOTE: Approximately one-half of the usually clinically significant strains of *Enterobacter* species (*e.g., E. aerogenes* and *E. cloacae*) are resistant to cefotetan. Most strains of *Pseudomonas aeruginosa* and *Acinetobacter* species are resistant to cefotetan.

Gram-Positive Aerobes: *Staphylococcus aureus* (including penicillinase- and nonpenicillinase-producing strains); *Staphylococcus epidermidis; Streptococcus agalactiae* (Group B beta-hemolytic streptococcus); *Streptococcus pneumoniae; Streptococcus pyogenes.*

NOTE: Methicillin-resistant staphylococci are resistant to cephalosporins. Some strains of *Staphylococcus epidermidis* and most strains of enterococci, *e.g., Enterococcus faecalis* (formerly *Streptococcus faecalis*), are resistant to cefotetan.

Anaerobes: *Prevotella bivia* (formerly *Bacteroides bivius*); *Prevotella disiens* (formerly *Bacteroides disiens*); *Bacteroides fragilis; Prevotella melaninogenica* (formerly *Bacteroides melaninogenicus*); *Bacteroides vulgatus; Fusobacterium* species; Gram-positive bacilli (including *Clostridium* species; see WARNINGS).

NOTE: Many strains of *C. difficile* are resistant (see WARNINGS).

Peptococcus niger; Peptostreptococcus species.

NOTE: Many strains of *B. distasonis, B. ovatus* and *B. thetaiotaomicron* are resistant to cefotetan *in vitro*. However, the therapeutic utility of cefotetan against these organisms cannot be accurately predicted on the basis of *in vitro* susceptibility tests alone.[2]

The following *in vitro* data are available but their clinical significance is unknown. Cefotetan has been shown to be active *in vitro* against most strains of the following organisms:

Gram-Negative Aerobes: *Citrobacter* species (including *C. diversus* and *C. freundii*); *Klebsiella oxytoca; Moraxella (Branhamella) catarrhalis. Neisseria gonorrhoeae* (penicillinase-producing strains); *Salmonella* species; *Serratia* species; *Shigella* species; *Yersinia enterocolitica.*

Anaerobes: *Porphyromonas asaccharolytica* (formerly *Bacteroides asaccharolyticus*); *Prevotella oralis* (formerly *Bacteroides oralis*); *Bacteroides splanchnicus; Clostridium difficile* (see WARNINGS); *Propionibacterium* species; *Veillonella* species.

SUSCEPTIBILITY TESTING

Dilution Techniques

Quantitative methods are used to determine antimicrobial minimum inhibitory concentrations (MICs). These MICs provide estimates of the susceptibility of bacteria to antimicrobial compounds. The MICs should be determined using a standardized procedure. Standardized procedres are based on a dilution method[1] (broth or agar) or equivalent with standardized inoculum concentrations and standardized concentrations of cefotetan powder. The MIC values should be interpreted according to TABLE 3.

TABLE 3

MIC	Interpretation
≤16 µg/ml	Susceptible (S)
32 µg/ml	Intermediate (I)
≥64 µg/ml	Resistant (R)

A report of "Susceptible" indicates that the pathogen is likely to be inhibited if the antimicrobial compound in the blood reaches the concentrations usually achievable. A report of "Intermediate" indicates that the result should be considered equivocal, and if the microorganism is not fully susceptible to alternative, clinically feasible drugs, the test should be repeated. This category implies possible clinical applicability in body sites where the drug is physiologically concentrated or in situations where high dosage of drug can be used. This category also provides a buffer zone which prevents small uncontrolled technical factors from causing major discrepancies in interpretation. A report of "Resistant" indicates that the pathogen is not likely to be inhibited if the antimicrobial compound in the blood reaches the concentrations usually achievable; other therapy should be selected.

Standardized susceptibility text procedures require the use of laboratory control microorganisms to control the technical aspects of the laboratory procedures. Standard cefotetan powder should provide the MIC values in TABLE 4.

TABLE 4

Microorganism	MIC
E. coli ATCC 25922	0.06-0.25 µg/ml
S. aureus ATCC 29213	4-16 µg/ml

Diffusion Techniques

Quantitative methods that require measurement of zone diameters provide reproducible estimates of the susceptibility of bacteria to antimicrobial compounds. One such standardized procedure[2] requires the use of the standardized inoculum concentrations. This procedure uses paper disks impregnated with 30 µg cefotetan to test the susceptibility of microorganisms to cefotetan.

Reports from the laboratory providing results of the standard single-disk susceptibility test with a 30 µg cefotetan disk should be interpreted according to the criteria in TABLE 5.

Interpretation should be as stated above for results using dilution techniques. Interpretation involves correlation of the diameter obtained in the disk test with the MIC for cefotetan.

TABLE 5

Zone Diameter	Interpretation
≥16 mm	Susceptible (S)
13-15 mm	Intermediate (I)
≤12 mm	Resistant (R)

As with standardized dilution techniques, diffusion methods require the use of laboratory control microorganisms that are used to control the technical aspects of the laboratory procedures. For the diffusion technique, the 30 µg cefotetan disk should provide the following zone diameters in these laboratory test quality control strains (see TABLE 6).

TABLE 6

Microorganism	Zone Diameter
E. coli ATCC 25922	28-34 mm
S. aureus ATCC 25923	17-23 mm

Anaerobic Techniques

For anaerobic bacteria, the susceptibility to cefotetan as MICs can be determined by standardized test methods[3]. The MIC values obtained should be interpreted as in TABLE 7.

TABLE 7

MIC	Interpretation
≤16 µg/ml	Susceptible (S)
32 µg/ml	Intermediate (I)
≥64 µg/ml	Resistant (R)

Interpretation is identical to that stated above for results using dilution techniques.

As with other susceptibility techniques, the use of laboratory control microorganisms is required to control the technical aspects of the laboratory standardized procedures. Standard cefotetan powder should provide the following MIC values (see TABLE 8).

TABLE 8

Microorganism	MIC
Bacteroides fragilis ATCC 25285	4-16 µg/ml
Bacteroides thetaiotaomicron ATCC 29741	32-128 µg/ml
Eubacterium lentum ATCC 43055	32-128 µg/ml

C

INDICATIONS AND USAGE

TREATMENT

Cefotetan disodium is indicated for the therapeutic treatment of the following infections when caused by susceptible strains of the designated organisms:

Urinary tract infections: Caused by *E. coli, Klebsiella* spp (including *K. pneumoniae*), *Proteus mirabilis* and *Proteus* spp (which may include the organisms now called *Proteus vulgaris, Providencia rettgeri,* and *Morganella morganii*).

Lower respiratory tract infections: Caused by *Streptococcus pneumoniae, Staphylococcus aureus* (penicillinase- and nonpenicillinase-producing strains), *Haemophilus influenzae* (including ampicillin-resistant strains), *Klebsiella* species (including *K. pneumoniae*), *E. coli, Proteus mirabilis,* and *Serratia marcescens**.

Skin and skin structure infections: Due to *Staphylococcus aureus* (penicillinase- and nonpenicillinase-producing strains), *Staphylococcus epidermidis, Streptococcus pyogenes, Streptococcus* species (excluding *enterococci*), *Escherichia coli, Klebsiella pneumoniae, Peptococcus niger**, *Peptostreptococcus* species.

Gynecologic infections: Caused by *Staphylococcus aureus* (including penicillinase- and nonpenicillinase-producing strains), *Staphylococcus epidermidis, Streptococcus* species (excluding enterococci), *Streptococcus agalactiae, E. coli, Proteus mirabilis, Neisseria gonorrhoeae, Bacteroides* species (excluding *B. distasonis, B. ovatus, B. thetaiotaomicron*), *Fusobacterium* species*, and gram-positive anaerobic cocci (including *Peptococcus* and *Peptostreptococcus* species).

Cefotetan, like other cephalosporins, has no activity against *Chlamydia trachomatis.* Therefore, when cephalosporins are used in the treatment of pelvic inflammatory disease, and *C. trachomatis* is one of the suspected pathogens, appropriate anti-chlamydial coverage should be added.

Intra-abdominal infections: Caused by *E. coli, Klebsiella* species (including *K. pneumoniae*), *Streptococcus* species (excluding enterococci), *Bacteroides* species (excluding *B. distasonis, B. ovatus, B. thetaiotaomicron*) and *Clostridium* species*.

Bone and joint infections: Caused by *Staphylococcus aureus**.

*Efficacy for this organism in this organ system was studied in fewer than ten infections.

Specimens for bacteriological examination should be obtained in order to isolate and identify causative organisms and to determine their susceptibilities to cefotetan. Therapy may be instituted before results of susceptibility studies are known; however, once these results become available, the antibiotic treatment should be adjusted accordingly.

In cases of confirmed or suspected gram-positive or gram-negative sepsis or in patients with other serious infections in which the causative organism has not been identified, it is possible to use cefotetan disodium concomitantly with an aminoglycoside. Cefotetan combinations with aminoglycosides have been shown to be synergistic *in vitro* against many *Enterobacteriaceae* and also some other gram-negative bacteria. The dosage recommended in the labeling of both antibiotics may be given and depends on the severity of the infection and the patient's condition.

NOTE: Increases in serum creatinine have occurred when cefotetan disodium was given alone. If cefotetan disodium and an aminoglycoside are used concomitantly, renal function should be carefully monitored, because nephrotoxicity may be potentiated.

PROPHYLAXIS

The preoperative administration of cefotetan disodium may reduce the incidence of certain postoperative infections in patients undergoing surgical procedures that are classified as clean contaminated or potentially contaminated (*e.g.*, cesarean section, abdominal or vaginal hysterectomy, transurethral surgery, biliary tract surgery, and gastrointestinal surgery).

If there are signs and symptoms of infection, specimens for culture should be obtained for identification of the causative organism so that appropriate therapeutic measures may be initiated.

CONTRAINDICATIONS

Cefotetan disodium is contraindicated in patients with known allergy to the cephalosporin group of antibiotics and in those individuals who have experienced a cephalosporin associated hemolytic anemia.

WARNINGS

BEFORE THERAPY WITH CEFOTETAN DISODIUM IS INSTITUTED, CAREFUL INQUIRY SHOULD BE MADE TO DETERMINE WHETHER THE PATIENT HAS HAD PREVIOUS HYPERSENSITIVITY REACTIONS TO CEFOTETAN DISODIUM, CEPHALOSPORINS, PENICILLINS, OR OTHER DRUGS. IF THIS PRODUCT IS TO BE GIVEN TO PENICILLIN-SENSITIVE PATIENTS, CAUTION SHOULD BE EXERCISED BECAUSE CROSS-HYPERSENSITIVITY AMONG BETA-LACTAM ANTIBIOTICS HAS BEEN CLEARLY DOCUMENTED AND MAY OCCUR IN UP TO 10% OF PATIENTS WITH A HISTORY OF PENICILLIN ALLERGY. IF AN ALLERGIC REACTION TO CEFOTETAN DISODIUM OCCURS, DISCONTINUE THE DRUG. SERIOUS ACUTE HYPERSENSITIVITY REACTIONS MAY REQUIRE TREATMENT WITH EPINEPHRINE AND OTHER EMERGENCY MEASURES, INCLUDING OXYGEN, IV FLUIDS, IV ANTIHISTAMINES, CORTICOSTEROIDS, PRESSOR AMINES, AND AIRWAY MANAGEMENT, AS CLINICALLY INDICATED.

AN IMMUNE MEDIATED HEMOLYTIC ANEMIA HAS BEEN OBSERVED IN PATIENTS RECEIVING CEPHALOSPORIN CLASS ANTIBIOTICS. SEVERE CASES OF HEMOLYTIC ANEMIA, INCLUDING FATALITIES, HAVE BEEN REPORTED IN ASSOCIATION WITH THE ADMINISTRATION OF CEFOTETAN. SUCH REPORTS ARE UNCOMMON. IF A PATIENT DEVELOPS ANEMIA ANYTIME WITHIN 2-3 WEEKS SUBSEQUENT TO THE ADMINISTRATION OF CEFOTETAN, THE DIAGNOSIS OF A CEPHALOSPORIN ASSOCIATED ANEMIA SHOULD BE CONSIDERED AND THE DRUG STOPPED UNTIL THE ETIOLOGY IS DETERMINED WITH CERTAINTY. BLOOD TRANSFUSIONS MAY BE ADMINISTERED AS NEEDED. (SEE CONTRAINDICATIONS).

PATIENTS WHO RECEIVE PROLONGED COURSES OF CEFOTETAN FOR TREATMENT OF INFECTIONS SHOULD HAVE PERIODIC MONITORING FOR SIGNS AND SYMPTOMS OF HEMOLYTIC ANEMIA INCLUDING A MEASUREMENT OF HEMATOLOGICAL PARAMETERS WHERE APPROPRIATE.

Pseudomembranous colitis has been reported with nearly all antibacterial agents, including cefotetan, and may range in severity from mild to life-threatening. Therefore, it is important to consider this diagnosis in patients who present with diarrhea subsequent to the administration of antibacterial agents.

Treatment with antibacterial agents alters the normal flora of the colon and may permit overgrowth of clostridia. Studies indicate that a toxin produced by *Clostridium difficile* is a primary cause of "antibiotic-associated colitis".

After the diagnosis of pseudomembranous colitis has been established, appropriate therapeutic measures should be initiated. Mild cases of pseudomembranous colitis usually respond to drug discontinuation alone. In moderate to severe cases, consideration should be given to management with fluids and electrolytes, protein supplementation, and treatment with an antibacterial drug clinically effective against *Clostridium difficile* colitis. (See ADVERSE REACTIONS.)

In common with many other broad-spectrum antibiotics, cefotetan disodium may be associated with a fall in prothrombin activity and, possibly, subsequent bleeding. Those at increased risk include patients with renal or hepatobiliary impairment or poor nutritional state, the elderly, and patients with cancer. Prothrombin time should be monitored and exogenous vitamin K administered as indicated.

PRECAUTIONS

GENERAL

As with other broad-spectrum antibiotics, prolonged use of cefotetan disodium may result in overgrowth of nonsusceptible organisms. Careful observation of the patient is essential. If superinfection does occur during therapy, appropriate measures should be taken.

Cefotetan disodium should be used with caution in individuals with a history of gastrointestinal disease, particularly colitis.

INFORMATION FOR THE PATIENT

As with some other cephalosporins, a disulfiram-like reaction characterized by flushing, sweating, headache, and tachycardia may occur when alcohol (beer, wine, *etc.*) is ingested within 72 hours after cefotetan disodium administration. Patients should be cautioned about the ingestion of alcoholic beverages following the administration of cefotetan disodium.

DRUG/LABORATORY TEST INTERACTIONS

The administration of cefotetan disodium may result in a false positive reaction for glucose in the urine using Clinitest, Benedict's solution, or Fehling's solution. It is recommended that glucose tests based on enzymatic glucose oxidase be used.

As with other cephalosporins, high concentrations of cefotetan may interfere with measurement of serum and urine creatinine levels by Jaffe' reaction and produce false increases in the levels of creatinine reported.

CARCINOGENESIS, MUTAGENESIS, AND IMPAIRMENT OF FERTILITY

Although long-term studies in animals have not been performed to evaluate carcinogenic potential, no mutagenic potential of cefotetan was found in standard laboratory tests.

Cefotetan has adverse effects on the testes of prepubertal rats. Subcutaneous administration of 500 mg/kg/day (approximately 8-16 times the usual adult human dose) on Days 6-35 of life (thought to be developmentally analogous to late childhood and prepuberty in humans) resulted in reduced testicular weight and seminiferous tubule degeneration in 10 of 10 animals. Affected cells included spermatogonia and spermatocytes; Sertoli and Leydig cells were unaffected. Incidence and severity of lesions were dose-dependent; at 120 mg/kg/day (approximately 2-4 times the usual human dose) only 1 of 10 treated animals was affected, and the degree of degeneration was mild.

Similar lesions have been observed in experiments of comparable design with other methylthiotetrazole-containing antibiotics and impaired fertility has been reported, particularly at high dose levels. No testicular effects were observed in 7 week old rats treated with up to 1000 mg/kg/day SC for 5 weeks, or in infant dogs (3 weeks old) that received up to 300 mg/kg/day IV for 5 weeks. The relevance of these findings to humans is unknown.

PREGNANCY, TERATOGENIC EFFECTS, PREGNANCY CATEGORY B

Reproduction studies have been performed in rats and monkeys at doses up to 20 times the human dose and have revealed no evidence of impaired fertility or harm to the fetus due to cefotetan. There are, however, no adequate and well-controlled studies in pregnant women. Because animal reproductive studies are not always predictive of human response, this drug should be used during pregnancy only if clearly needed.

NURSING MOTHERS

Cefotetan is excreted in human milk in very low concentrations. Caution should be exercised when cefotetan is administered to a nursing woman.

PEDIATRIC USE

Safety and effectiveness in children have not been established.

GERIATRIC USE

Of the 925 subjects who received cefotetan in clinical studies, 492 (53%) were 60 years and older, while 76 (8%) were 80 years and older. No overall differences in safety or effectiveness were observed between these subjects and younger subjects, and the other reported clinical experience has not identified differences in responses between elderly and younger patients, but greater sensitivity of some older individuals cannot be ruled out.

This drug is known to be substantially excreted by the kidney, and the risk of toxic reactions to this drug may be greater in patients with impaired renal function. Because elderly patients are more likely to have decreased renal function, care should be taken in dose selection, and it may be useful to monitor renal function. (See DOSAGE AND ADMINISTRATION, Impaired Renal Function.)

DRUG INTERACTIONS

Increases in serum creatinine have occurred when cefotetan disodium was given alone. If cefotetan disodium and an aminoglycoside are used concomitantly, renal function should be carefully monitored, because nephrotoxicity may be potentiated.

ADVERSE REACTIONS

In clinical studies, the following adverse effects were considered related to cefotetan disodium therapy. Those appearing in italics have been reported during postmarketing experience.

Gastrointestinal: Symptoms occurred in 1.5% of patients, the most frequent were diarrhea (1 in 80) and nausea (1 in 700); *pseudomembranous colitis.* Onset of pseudomembranous colitis symptoms may occur during or after antibiotic treatment or surgical prophylaxis. (See WARNINGS.)

Hematologic: Laboratory abnormalities occurred in 1.4% of patients and included eosinophilia (1 in 200), positive direct Coombs' test (1 in 250), and thrombocytosis (1 in 300); *agranulocytosis, hemolytic anemia, leukopenia, thrombocytopenia,* and *prolonged prothrombin time with or without bleeding.*

Hepatic: Enzyme elevations occurred in 1.2% of patients and included a rise in ALT (SGPT) (1 in 150), AST (SGOT) (1 in 300), alkaline phosphatase (1 in 700), and LDH (1 in 700).

Hypersensitivity: Reactions were reported in 1.2% of patients and included rash (1 in 150) and itching (1 in 700); *anaphylactic reactions and urticaria.*

Local: Effects were reported in less than 1% of patients and included phlebitis at the site of injection (1 in 300), and discomfort (1 in 500).

Renal: *Elevations in BUN and serum creatinine have been reported.*

Urogenital: *Nephrotoxicity has rarely been reported.*

Miscellaneous: *Fever.*

In addition to the adverse reactions listed above which have been observed in patients treated with cefotetan, the following adverse reactions and altered laboratory tests have been reported for cephalosporin-class antibiotics: pruritus, Stevens-Johnson syndrome, erythema multiforme, toxic epidermal necrolysis, vomiting, abdominal pain, colitis, superinfection, vaginitis including vaginal candidiasis, renal dysfunction, toxic nephropathy, hepatic dysfunction including cholestasis, aplastic anemia, hemorrhage, elevated bilirubin, pancytopenia, and neutropenia.

Several cephalosporins have been implicated in triggering seizures, particularly in patients with renal impairment, when the dosage was not reduced. (See DOSAGE AND ADMINISTRATION.) If seizures associated with drug therapy occur, the drug should be discontinued. Anticonvulsant therapy can be given if clinically indicated.

DOSAGE AND ADMINISTRATION

TREATMENT

Cefotetan injection in Galaxy plastic container should not be used for IM administration.

Cefotetan disodium in the ADD-Vantage Vial is intended for IV infusion only, after dilution with the appropriate volume of ADD-Vantage diluent solution.

The usual adult dosage is 1 or 2 g of cefotetan disodium administered intravenously or intramuscularly or cefotetan injection in the Galaxy plastic container (PL 2040) administered intravenously every 12 hours for 5-10 days. Proper dosage and route of administration should be determined by the condition of the patient, severity of the infection, and susceptibility of the causative organism.

TABLE 9 *General Guidelines for Dosage of Cefotetan Disodium*

Type of Infection	Daily Dose	Frequency and Route
Urinary Tract	1-4 g	500 mg q12h IV or IM 1 or 2 g q24h IV or IM 1 or 2 g q12h IV or IM
Skin & Skin Structure		
Mild - Moderate*	2 g	2 g q24h IV 1 g q12h IV or IM
Severe	4 g	2 g q12h IV
Other sites	2-4 g	1 or 2 g q12h IV or IM
Severe	4 g	2 g q12h IV
Life-Threatening	6 g†	3 g q12h IV

* *Klebsiella pneumoniae* skin and skin structure infections should be treated with 1 or 2 g q12h IV or IM.

† Maximum daily dosage should not exceed 6 g.

If *Chlamydia trachomatis* is a suspected pathogen in gynecologic infections, appropriate antichlamydial coverage should be added, since cefotetan has no activity against this organism.

PROPHYLAXIS

To prevent postoperative infection in clean contaminated or potentially contaminated surgery in adults, the recommended dosage is 1 or 2 g of cefotetan disodium administered once, intravenously, 30-60 minutes prior to surgery. In patients undergoing cesarean section, the dose should be administered as soon as the umbilical cord is clamped.

IMPAIRED RENAL FUNCTION

When renal function is impaired, a reduced dosage schedule must be employed. The dosage guidelines in TABLE 10 may be used.

TABLE 10 *Dosage Guidelines for Patients With Impaired Renal Function*

Creatinine Clearance	Dose	Frequency
>30 ml/min	Usual recommended dosage*	q12h
10-30 ml/min	Usual recommended dosage*	q24h
<10 ml/min	Usual recommended dosage*	q48h

* Dose determined by the type and severity of infection, and susceptibility of the causative organism.

Alternatively, the dosing interval may remain constant at 12 hour intervals, but the dose reduced to one-half the usual recommended dose for patients with a creatinine clearance of 10-30 ml/min, and one-quarter the usual recommended dose for patients with a creatinine clearance of less than 10 ml/min. When only serum creatinine levels are available, creatinine clearance may be calculated from the following formula. The serum creatinine level should represent a steady state of renal function.

Males: [Weight (kg) × (140 - age)] ÷ [72 × serum creatinine (mg/100 ml)]

Females: 0.9 × value for males

Cefotetan is dialyzable and it is recommended that for patients undergoing intermittent hemodialysis, one-quarter of the usual recommended dose be given every 24 hours on days between dialysis and one-half the usual recommended dose on the day of dialysis.

HOW SUPPLIED

CEFOTAN FOR IV OR IM INJECTION

Cefotan is a dry, white to pale yellow powder supplied in vials containing cefotetan disodium equivalent to 1 and 2 g cefotetan activity for IV and IM administration. Cefotan is also available as 10 g in a 100 ml vial.

Storage: The vials should not be stored at temperatures above 22°C (72°F) and should be protected from light.

CEFOTAN INJECTION FOR IV USE ONLY

Cefotan is supplied as a frozen, iso-osmotic, premixed solution in single dose Galaxy plastic containers (PL 2040) as 1 and 2 g.

Storage: Store containers at or below -20°C/-4°F.

PRODUCT LISTING - EQUIVALENTS NOT AVAILABLE

Package	Price	Product	NDC
Powder For Injection - Injectable - 1 Gm			
1's	$11.16	CEFOTAN, Astra-Zeneca Pharmaceuticals	00038-0376-10
1's	$11.58	CEFOTAN, Astra-Zeneca Pharmaceuticals	00038-0376-31
1's	$11.72	CEFOTAN, Astra-Zeneca Pharmaceuticals	00038-0376-60
1's	$11.72	CEFOTAN, Astra-Zeneca Pharmaceuticals	00038-0376-61
1's	$11.72	CEFOTAN, Vha Supply	00310-0376-60
1's	$11.72	CEFOTAN, Vha Supply	00310-0376-61
10's	$121.70	CEFOTAN, Astra-Zeneca Pharmaceuticals	00310-0376-11
10's	$126.40	CEFOTAN, Astra-Zeneca Pharmaceuticals	00310-0376-10
10's	$131.88	CEFOTAN, Physicians Total Care	54868-3847-00
25's	$328.00	CEFOTAN, Astra-Zeneca Pharmaceuticals	00310-0376-31
Powder For Injection - Injectable - 2 Gm			
1's	$21.90	CEFOTAN, Astra-Zeneca Pharmaceuticals	00038-0377-20
1's	$22.32	CEFOTAN, Astra-Zeneca Pharmaceuticals	00038-0377-32
1's	$22.32	CEFOTAN, Astra-Zeneca Pharmaceuticals	00038-0377-61
1's	$22.32	CEFOTAN, Astra-Zeneca Pharmaceuticals	00038-0377-62
1's	$22.32	CEFOTAN, Vha Supply	00310-0377-61
1's	$22.32	CEFOTAN, Vha Supply	00310-0377-62
10's	$238.90	CEFOTAN, Astra-Zeneca Pharmaceuticals	00310-0377-21
10's	$243.92	CEFOTAN, Physicians Total Care	54868-3851-00
10's	$263.30	CEFOTAN, Astra-Zeneca Pharmaceuticals	00310-0377-20
25's	$683.25	CEFOTAN, Astra-Zeneca Pharmaceuticals	00310-0377-32
Powder For Injection - Injectable - 10 Gm			
1's	$118.32	CEFOTAN, Astra-Zeneca Pharmaceuticals	00038-0375-61
1's	$118.32	CEFOTAN, Vha Supply	00310-0375-61
6's	$766.68	CEFOTAN, Astra-Zeneca Pharmaceuticals	00310-0375-10
Solution - Intravenous - 1 Gm/50 ml			
50 ml	$376.50	CEFOTAN, Astra-Zeneca Pharmaceuticals	00310-0378-51
Solution - Intravenous - 2 Gm/50 ml			
50 ml	$753.00	CEFOTAN, Astra-Zeneca Pharmaceuticals	00310-0379-51

Cefoxitin Sodium (000691)

For related information, see the comparative table section in Appendix A.

Categories: Abscess, intra-abdominal; Abscess, pulmonary; Cellulitis, pelvic; Endometritis; Gonorrhea; Infection, bone; Infection, gynecologic; Infection, intra-abdominal; Infection, joint; Infection, lower respiratory tract; Infection, sexually transmitted; Infection, skin and skin structures; Infection, urinary tract; Pelvic inflammatory disease; Peritonitis; Pneumonia; Prophylaxis, perioperative; Septicemia; Pregnancy Category B; FDA Approved 1978 Oct
Drug Classes: Antibiotics, cephalosporins
Brand Names: Mefoxin
Foreign Brand Availability: Cefmore (Taiwan); Cefoxin (Thailand); Cefxitin (Thailand); Mefoxil (Greece); Mefoxitin (Austria; Bulgaria; Denmark; Germany; Norway; Spain; Sweden; Switzerland)
Cost of Therapy: $327.00 (Infection; Mefoxin Injection; 1 g; 3 g/day; 10 day supply)
$336.75 (Infection; Generic Injection; 1 g; 3 g/day; 10 day supply)
HCFA JCODE(S): J0694 1 g IV, IM

DESCRIPTION

Cefoxitin is a semi-synthetic, broad-spectrum cepha antibiotic sealed under nitrogen for intravenous administration. It is derived from cephamycin C, which is produced by *Streptomyces lactamdurans*. Its chemical name is (6*R*, 7*S*)-3-(hydroxymethyl)-7-methoxy-8-oxo-7-[2-(2-thienyl)acetamido]-5-thia-1-azabicyclo [4.2.0] oct-2-ene-2-carboxylate carbamate (ester). The empirical formula is $C_{16}H_{16}N_3NaO_7S_2$.

Cefoxin contains approximately 53.8 mg (2.3 milliequivalents) of sodium per gram of cefoxitin activity. Solutions of cefoxitin range from colorless to light amber in color. The pH of freshly constituted solutions usually ranges from 4.2-7.0.

CLINICAL PHARMACOLOGY

Following an intravenous dose of 1 g, serum concentrations were 110 μg/ml at 5 minutes, declining to less than 1 μg/ml at 4 hours. The half-life after an intravenous dose is 41-59 minutes. Approximately 85% of cefoxitin is excreted unchanged by the kidneys over a 6 hour period, resulting in high urinary concentrations. Probenecid slows tubular excretion and produces higher serum levels and increases the duration of measurable serum concentrations.

Cefoxitin passes into pleural and joint fluids and is detectable in antibacterial concentrations in bile.

MICROBIOLOGY

The bactericidal action of cefoxitin results from inhibition of cell wall synthesis. Cefoxitin has *in vitro* activity against a wide range of gram-positive and gram-negative organisms. The methoxy group in the 7α position provides cefoxitin with a high degree of stability in the presence of beta-lactamases, both penicillinases and cephalosporinases, of gram-negative bacteria. While *in vitro* studies have demonstrated the susceptibility of most strains of the following organisms, clinical efficacy for infections other than those included in INDICATIONS AND USAGE is unknown.

Gram-positive:

Staphylococcus aureus, including penicillinase and non-penicillinase producing strains.
Staphylococcus epidermidis.
Beta-hemolytic and other streptococci (most strains of enterococci, *e.g., Enterococcus facalis* [formerly *Streptococcus faecalis*] are resistant).
Streptococcus pneumoniae.

Gram-negative:

Eikenella corrodens (beta-lactamase negative strains).
Escherichia coli..
Klebsiella species (including *K. pneumoniae*).
Hemophilus influenzae.
Neisseria gonorrhoeae, including penicillinase and non-penicillinase producing strains.
Proteus mirabilis..
Morganella morganii.
Proteus vulgaris.
Providencia species, including *Providencia rettgeri.*

Anaerobic Organisms:

Peptococcus niger.
Peptostreptococcus species.
Clostridium species.
Bacteroides species, including the *B. fragilis* group (includes *B. fragilis, B. distasonis, B. ovatus, B. thetaiotaomicron*).

Cefoxitin is inactive *in vitro* against most strains of *Pseudomonas aeruginosa* and enterococci and many strains of *Enterobacter cloacae.*

Methicillin-resistant staphylococci are almost uniformly resistant to cefoxitin.

SUSCEPTIBILITY TESTING

For fast-growing aerobic organisms, quantitative methods that require measurements of zone diameters give the most precise estimates of antibiotic susceptibility. One such procedure* has been recommended for use with discs to test susceptibility to cefoxitin. Interpretation involves correlation of the diameters obtained in the disc test with minimal inhibitory concentration (MIC) values for cefoxitin.

Reports from the laboratory giving results of the standardized single disc susceptibility test* using a 30 μg cefoxitin disc should be interpreted according to the following criteria:

Organisms producing zones of 18 mm or greater are considered susceptible, indicating that the tested organism is likely to respond to therapy.

Organisms of intermediate susceptibility produce zones of 15-17 mm, indicating that the tested organism would be susceptible if high dosage is used or if the infection is confined to tissues and fluids (*e.g.,* urine) in which high antibiotic levels are attained.

Resistant organisms produce zones of 14 mm or less, indicating that other therapy should be selected.

The cefoxitin disc should be used for testing cefoxitin susceptibility.

Cefoxitin has been shown by *in vitro* tests to have activity against certain strains of *Enterobacteriaceae* found resistant when tested with the cephalosporin class disc. For this reason, the cefoxitin disc should not be used for testing susceptibility to cephalosporins, and cephalosporin discs should not be used for testing susceptibility to cefoxitin.

Dilution methods, preferably the agar plate dilution procedure, are most accurate for susceptibility testing of obligate anaerobes.

A bacterial isolate may be considered susceptible if the MIC value for cefoxitin† is not more than 16 μg/ml. Organisms are considered resistant if the MIC is greater than 32 μg/ml.

INDICATIONS AND USAGE

TREATMENT

Cefoxitin is indicated for the treatment of serious infections caused by susceptible strains of the designated microorganisms in the diseases listed below.

(1) ***Lower respiratory tract infections:*** Lower respiratory tract infections, including pneumonia and lung abscess, caused by *Streptococcus pneumoniae,* other streptococci (excluding enterococci, *e.g., Enterococcus facalis* [formerly *Streptococcus faecalis*]), *Staphylococcus aureus* (penicillinase and non-penicillinase producing), *Escherichia coli, Klebsiella* species, *Hemophilus influenzae,* and *Bacteroides* species.

(2) ***Urinary tract infections:*** Urinary tract infections caused by *Escherichia coli, Klebsiella* species, *Proteus mirabilis, Morganella morganii, Proteus vulgaris,* and *Providencia* species (including *Providencia rettgeri*).

(3) ***Intra-abdominal infections:*** Intra-abdominal infections, including peritonitis and intra-abdominal abscess, caused by *Escherichia coli, Klebsiella* species, *Bacteroides* species including the *B. fragilis* group‡, and *Clostridium* species.

(4) ***Gynecological infections:*** Gynecological infections, including endometritis, pelvic cellulitis, and pelvic inflammatory disease caused by *Escherichia coli, Neisseria gonorrhoeae* (penicillinase and non-penicillinase producing), *Bacteroides* species including the *Bacteroides fragilis , Clostridium* species, *Peptococcus niger, Peptostreptococcus* species, and Group B streptococci. Cefoxitin, like cephalosporins, has no activity against *Chlamydia trachomatis.* Therefore, when cefoxitin is used in the treatment of patients with pelvic inflammatory disease and *C. trachomatis* is one of the suspected pathogens, appropriate anti-chlamydial coverage should be added.

(5) ***Septicemia:*** Septicemia caused by *Streptococcus pneumoniae, Staphylococcus aureus* (penicillinase and non-penicillinase producing), *Escherichia coli, Klebsiella* species, and *Bacteroides* species including the *B. fragilis.*

(6) ***Bone and joint infections:*** Bone and joint infections caused by *Staphylococcus aureus* (penicillinase and non-penicillinase producing).

(7) ***Skin and skin structure infections:*** Skin and skin structure infections caused by *Staphylococcus aureus* (penicillinase and non-penicillinase producing), *Staphylococcus epidermidis,* streptococci (excluding enterococci *e.g., Enterococcus facalis* [formerly *Streptococcus faecalis*], *Escherichia coli, Proteus mirabilis, Klebsiella* species, *Bacteroides* species including the *B. fragilis, Clostridium* species, *Peptococcus niger,* and *Peptostreptococcus* species.

Appropriate culture and susceptibility studies should be performed to determine the susceptibility of the causative organisms to cefoxitin. Therapy may be started while awaiting the results of these studies.

In randomized comparative studies, cefoxitin and cephalothin were comparably safe and effective in the management of infections caused by gram-positive cocci and gram-negative rods susceptible to the cephalosporins. Cefoxitin has a high degree of stability in the presence of bacterial beta-lactamases, both penicillinases and cephalosporinases.

Many infections caused by aerobic and anaerobic gram-negative bacteria resistant to some cephalosporins respond to cefoxitin. Similarly, many infections caused by aerobic and anaerobic bacteria resistant to some penicillin antibiotics (ampicillin, carbenicillin, penicillin G) respond to treatment with cefoxitin. Many infections caused by mixtures of susceptible aerobic and anaerobic bacteria respond to treatment with cefoxitin.

* Bauer, A. W.; Kirby, W. M. M.; Sherris, J. C.; Turck, M.: Antibiotic susceptibility testing by a standardized single disc method, Amer. J. Clin. Path. *45*: 493-496, Apr. 1966. Standardized disc susceptibility test, Federal Register *37*: 20527-20529, 1972. National Committee for Clinical Laboratory Standards: Performance Standards for Antimicrobial Disc Susceptibility Tests - Fifth Edition; Approved Standard, NCCLS Document M2-A5, Vol 13, No. 24, NCCLS, Villanova, PA, December 1993.

† Determined by the ICS agar dilution method (Ericsson and Sherris, Acta Path. Microbiol. Scand. (B) Suppl. No 217, 1971) or any other method that has been shown to give equivalent results.

‡*B. fragilis, B. distasonis, B. ovatus, B. thetaiotaomicron, B. vulgatus.*

PREVENTION

Cefoxitin is indicated for the prophylaxis of infection in patients undergoing uncontaminated gastrointestinal surgery, vaginal hysterectomy, abdominal hysterectomy, or cesarean section.

If there are signs of infection, specimens for culture should be obtained for identification of the causative organism so that appropriate treatment may be instituted.

CONTRAINDICATIONS

Cefoxitin is contraindicated in patients who have shown hypersensitivity to cefoxitin and the cephalosporin group of antibiotics.

WARNINGS

BEFORE THERAPY WITH CEFOXITIN IS INSTITUTED, CAREFUL INQUIRY SHOULD BE MADE TO DETERMINE WHETHER THE PATIENT HAS HAD PREVIOUS HYPERSENSITIVITY REACTIONS TO CEFOXITIN, CEPHALOSPORINS, PENICILLINS OR OTHER DRUGS. THIS PRODUCT SHOULD BE GIVEN WITH CAUTION TO PENICILLIN-SENSITIVE PATIENTS. ANTIBIOTICS SHOULD BE ADMINISTERED WITH CAUTION TO ANY PATIENT WHO HAS DEMONSTRATED SOME FORM OF ALLERGY, PARTICULARLY TO DRUGS. IF AN ALLERGIC REACTION TO CEFOXITIN OCCURS, DISCONTINUE THE DRUG. SERIOUS HYPERSEN-

SITIVITY REACTIONS MAY REQUIRE EPINEPHRINE AND OTHER EMERGENCY MEASURES.

Pseudomembranous colitis has been reported with nearly all antibacterial agents, including cefoxitin, and may range in severity from mild to life threatening. Therefore, it is important to consider this diagnosis in patients who present with diarrhea subsequent to the administration of antibacterial agents.

Treatment with antibacterial agents alters the normal flora of the colon and may permit overgrowth of clostridia. Studies indicate a toxin produced by *Clostridium difficile* is one primary cause of "antibiotic-associated colitis".

After the diagnosis of pseudomembranous colitis has been established, appropriate therapeutic measures should be initiated. Mild cases of pseudomembranous colitis usually respond to drug discontinuance alone. In moderate to severe cases, consideration should be given to management with fluids and electrolytes, protein supplementation, and treatment with antibacterial drug clinically effective against *Clostridium difficle* colitis.

PRECAUTIONS

General: The total daily dose should be reduced when cefoxitin is administered to patients with transient or persistent reduction of urinary output due to renal insufficiency (see DOSAGE AND ADMINISTRATION), because high and prolonged serum antibiotic concentrations can occur in such individuals from usual doses.

Antibiotics (including cephalosporins) should be prescribed with caution in individuals with a history of gastrointestinal disease, particularly colitis.

As with other antibiotics, prolonged use of cefoxitin may result in over-growth of non-susceptible organisms. Repeated evaluation of the patient's condition is essential. If superinfection occurs during therapy, appropriate measures should be taken.

Laboratory Tests: As with any potent antibacterial agent, periodic assessment of organ system functions, including renal, hepatic, and hematopoietic, is advisable during prolonged therapy.

Drug/Laboratory Test Interactions: As with cephalothin, high concentrations of cefoxitin (>100 micrograms/ml) may interfere with measurement of serum and urine creatinine levels by the Jaffé reaction, and produce false increases of modest degree in the levels of creatinine reported. Serum samples from patients treated with cefoxitin should not be analyzed for creatinine if withdrawn within 2 hours of drug administration.

High concentrations of cefoxitin in the urine may interfere with measurement of urinary 17-hydroxy-corticosteroids by the Porter-Silber reaction, and produce false increases of modest degree in the levels reported.

A false-positive reaction for glucose in the urine may occur. This has been observed with Clinitest reagent tablets.

Carcinogenesis, Mutagenesis, and Impairment of Fertility: Long-term studies in animals have not been performed with cefoxitin to evaluate carcinogenic or mutagenic potential. Studies in rats treated intravenously with 400 mg/kg of cefoxitin (approximately three times the maximum recommended human dose) revealed no effects on fertility or mating ability.

Pregnancy Category B: Reproduction studies performed in rats and mice at parenteral doses of approximately one to seven and one-half times the maximum recommended human dose did not reveal teratogenic or fetal toxic effects, although a slight decrease in fetal weight was observed.

There are, however, no adequate and well-controlled studies in pregnant women. Because animal reproduction studies are not always predictive of human response, this drug should be used during pregnancy only if clearly needed.

In the rabbit, cefoxitin was associated with a high incidence of abortion and maternal death. This was not considered to be a teratogenic effect but an expected consequence of the rabbit's unusual sensitivity to antibiotic-induced changes in the population of the microflora of the intestine.

Nursing Mothers: Cefoxitin is excreted in human milk in low concentrations. Caution should be exercised when cefoxitin is administered to a nursing woman.

Pediatric Use: Safety and efficacy in pediatric patients from birth to three months of age have not yet been established. In pediatric patients three months of age and older, higher doses of cefoxitin have been associated with an increased incidence of eosinophilia and elevated SGOT.

DRUG INTERACTIONS

Increased nephrotoxicity has been reported following concomitant administration of cephalosporins and aminoglycoside antibiotics.

ADVERSE REACTIONS

Cefoxitin is generally well tolerated. The most common adverse reactions have been local reactions following intravenous injection. Other adverse reactions have been encountered infrequently.

Local Reactions: Thrombophlebitis has occurred with intravenous administration.

Allergic Reactions: Rash (including exfoliative dermatitis and toxic epidermal necrolysis), pruritus, eosinophilia, fever, dyspnea, and other allergic reactions including anaphylaxis, interstitial nephritis and angioedema have been noted.

Cardiovascular: Hypotension.

Gastrointestinal: Diarrhea, including documented pseudomembranous colitis which can appear during or after antibiotic treatment. Nausea and vomiting have been reported rarely.

Neuromuscular: Possible exacerbation of myasthenia gravis.

Blood: Eosinophilia, leukopenia including granulocytopenia, neutropenia, anemia, including hemolytic anemia, thrombocytopenia, and bone marrow depression. A positive direct Coombs test may develop in some individuals, especially those with azotemia.

Liver Function: Transient elevations in SGOT, SGPT, serum LDH, and serum alkaline phosphatase; and jaundice have been reported.

Renal Function: Elevations in serum creatinine and/or blood urea nitrogen levels have been observed. As with the cephalosporins, acute renal failure has been reported rarely. The role of cefoxitin in changes in renal function tests is difficult to assess, since factors predisposing to prerenal azotemia or to impaired renal function usually have been present.

DOSAGE AND ADMINISTRATION

TREATMENT

Adults

The usual adult dosage range is 1 to 2 grams every 6-8 hours. Dosage should be determined by susceptibility of the causative organisms, severity of infection, and the condition of the patient (see TABLE 1 for dosage guidelines).

TABLE 1 *Guidelines for Dosage of Cefoxitin*

Type of Infection	Daily Dosage	Frequency and Route
Uncomplicated forms† of infections such as pneumonia, urinary tract infection, cutaneous infection	3-4 g	1 g every 6-8 hours IV
Moderately severe or severe infections	6-8 g	1 g every 4 hours *or* 2 g every 6-8 hours IV
Infections commonly needing antibiotics in higher dosage (*e.g.*, gas gangrene)	12 g	2 g every 4 hours *or* 3 g every 6 hours IV

† Including patients in whom bacteremia is absent or unlikely.

If *C. trachomatis* is a suspected pathogen, appropriate anti-chlamydial coverage should be added, because cefoxitin has no activity against this organism.

Cefoxitin may be used in patients with reduced renal function with the following dosage adjustments:

In adults with renal insufficiency, an initial loading dose of 1 to 2 g may be given. After a loading dose, the recommendations for *maintenance dosage* (see TABLE 2) may be used as a guide.

TABLE 2 *Maintenance Dosage of Sterile Cefoxitin in Adults With Reduced Renal Function*

Renal Function	Creatinine Clearance (ml/min)	Dose	Frequency
Mild impairment	50-30	1-2 g	every 8-12 hours
Moderate impairment	29-10	1-2 g	every 12-24 hours
Severe impairment	9-5	0.5-1 g	every 12-24 hours
Essentially no function	<5	0.5-1 g	every 24-48 hours

When only the serum creatinine level is available, the following formula (based on sex, weight and age of the patient) may be used to convert this value into creatinine clearance. The serum creatinine should represent a steady state of renal function.

Males: [Weight (kg) × (140 - age)] ÷ [72 × serum creatinine (mg/100 ml)]

Females: 0.85 × above value

In patients undergoing hemodialysis, the loading dose of 1-2 g should be given after each hemodialysis, and the maintenance dose should be given as indicated in TABLE 2.

Antibiotic therapy for group A beta-hemolytic streptococcal infections should be maintained for at least 10 days to guard against the risk of rheumatic fever or glomerulonephritis. In staphylococcal and other infections involving a collection of pus, surgical drainage should be carried out where indicated.

Pediatric Patients

The recommended dosage in pediatric patients three months of age and older is 80-160 mg/kg of body weight per day divided into four to six equal doses. The higher dosages should be used for more severe or serious infections. The total daily dosage should not exceed 12 g.

At this time no recommendation is made for pediatric patients from birth to three months of age (see PRECAUTIONS).

In pediatric patients with renal insufficiency the dosage and frequency of dosage should be modified consistent with the recommendations for adults (see TABLE 2).

PREVENTION

Effective prophylactic use depends on the time of administration. Cefoxitin usually should be given one-half to one hour before the operation, which is sufficient time to acheive effective levels in the wound during the procedure. Prophylactic administraion should usually be stopped within 24 hours since continuing administraion of any antibiotic increases the possibility of adverse reactions but, in the majority of surgical procedures, does not reduce the incidence of subsequent infection.

For prophylactic use in uncontaminated gastrointestinal surgery, vaginal hysterectomy, or abdominal hysterectomy, the following doses are recommended:

Adults: 2 g administered intravenously just prior to surgery (approximately ½ to 1 hour before the initial incision) followed by 2 g every 6 hours after the first dose for no more than 24 hours.

Pediatric Patients (3 months and older): 30-40 mg/kg doses may be given at the times designated above.

Cesarean Section Patients: For patients undergoing cesarean section either a single 2.0 g dose should be administered intravenously as soon as the umbilical cord is clamped OR a 3 dose regimen consisting of 2 g given intravenously as soon as the umbilical cord is clamped followed by 2 grams 4 and 8 hours after the initial dose is recommended.

PREPARATION OF SOLUTION

TABLE 3 is provided for convenience in constituting cefoxitin for intravenous administration.

For Vials: One (1) g should be constituted with at least 10 ml and 2 g with 10 or 20 ml of sterile water for injection, bacteriostatic water for injection, 0.9% sodium chloride injection, or 5% dextrose injection. These primary solutions may be further diluted in 50-1000 ml of the dilutents listed under Compatibility and Stability, Vials and Bulk Packages.

TABLE 3 *Preparation of Solution for Intravenous Administraion*

Strength	Amount of Diluent to be Added (ml)‡	Approximate Withdrawable Volume (ml)	Approximate Average Concentration (mg/ml)
1 g Vial	10	10.5	95
2 g Vial	10 or 20	11.1 or 21.0	180 or 95
1 g Infusion Bottle	50 or 100	50 or 100	20 or 10
2 g Infusion Bottle	50 or 100	50 or 100	40 or 20
10 g Bulk	43 or 93	49 or 98.5	200 or 100

‡ Shake to dissolve and let stand until clear.

For Bulk Packages: The 10 g bulk packages should be constituted with 43 or 93 ml of sterile water for injection, bacteriostatic water for injection, 0.9% sodium chloride injection, or 5% dextrose injection. *CAUTION:* THE 10 g BULK STOCK SOLUTION IS NOT FOR DIRECT INFUSION. These primary solutions may be further diluted in 50-1000 ml of the dilutents listed under Compatibility and Stability, Vials and Bulk Packages.
Benzyl alcohol as a preservative has been associated with toxicity in neonates. While toxicity has not been demonstrated in pediatric patients greater than three months of age, in whom use of cefoxitin may be indicated, small pediatric patients in this age range may also be at risk for benzyl alcohol toxicity. Therefore, diluents containing benzyl alcohol should not be used when cefoxitin is constituted for administration to pediatric patients in this age range.
For Infusion Bottles: One (1) or 2 g of cefoxitin for infusion may be constituted with 50 or 100 ml of 0.9% sodium chloride injection, or 5 or 10% dextrose injection.
For ADD-Vantage vials: See separate INSTRUCTIONS FOR USE OF CEFOXITIN IN ADD-Vantage VIALS included with vial packaging. Cefoxitin in ADD-Vantage vials should be constituted with ADD-Vantage diluent containers containing 50 or 100 ml of either 0.9% sodium chloride injection or 5% dextrose injection. Mefoxin in ADD-Vantage vials is for IV use only.

ADMINISTRATION

Cefoxitin may be administered intravenously after constitution.

Parenteral drug products should be inspected visually for particulate matter and discoloration prior to administration whenever solution and container permit.

Intravenous Administration

The intravenous route is preferable for patients with bacteremia, bacterial septicemia, or other severe or life-threatening infections, or for patients who may be poor risks because of lowered resistance resulting from such debilitating conditions as malnutrition, trauma, surgery, diabetes, heart failure, or malignancy, particularly if shock is present or impending.
For intermittent intravenous administration: A solution containing 1 or 2 g in 10 ml of sterile water for injection can be injected over a period of 3-5 minutes. Using an infusion system, it may also be given over a longer period of time through the tubing system by which the patient may be receiving other intravenous solutions. However, during infusion of the solution containing cefoxitin, it is advisable to temporarily discontinue administration of any other solutions at the same site.
For the administration of higher doses by continuous intravenous infusion: A solution of cefoxitin may be added to an intravenous bottle containing 5% dextrose injection, 0.9% sodium chloride injection, 5% dextrose and 0.9% sodium chloride injection. Butterfly or scalp vein-type needles are preferred for this type of infusion.
Solutions of cefoxitin, like those of most beta-lactam antibiotics, should not be added to aminoglycoside solutions (*e.g.,* gentamicin sulfate, tobramycin sulfate, amikacin sulfate) because of potential interaction. However, cefoxitin and aminoglycosides may be administered separately to the same patient.

COMPATIBILITY AND STABILITY

Vials and Bulk Packages: Mefoxin, as supplied in vials or the bulk package and constituted to 1 g/10 ml with sterile water for injection, bacteriostatic water for injection, (see Preparation of Solution), 0.9% sodium chloride injection, or 5% dextrose injection, maintains satisfactory potency for 6 hours at room temperature or for one week under refrigeration (below 5°C).
These primary solutions may be further diluted in 50-1000 ml of the following solutions and maintain potency for an additional 18 hours at room temperature and an additional 48 hours under refrigeration:

- 0.9% Sodium chloride injection.
- 5% or 10% Dextrose injection.
- 5% Dextrose and 0.9% sodium chloride injection.
- 5% Dextrose injection with 0.2% or 0.45% saline solution.
- Lactated Ringer's injection.
- 5% Dextrose in lactated Ringer's injection.‡
- 10% invert sugar in water.
- 10% invert sugar in saline solution.
- 5% Sodium bicarbonate injection.
- M/6 sodium lactate solution.
- Mannitol 5% and 10%.

Infusion Bottles: Mefoxin, as supplied in infusion bottles and constituted with 50-100 ml of 0.9% sodium chloride injection, or 5 or 10% dextrose injection, maintains satisfactory potency for 24 hours at room temperature for 1 week under refrigeration (below 5°C).

ADD-Vantage Vials: Mefoxin is supplied in single dose ADD-Vantage vials and should be prepared as directed in the accompanying INSTRUCTIONS FOR USE IN ADD-Vantage VIALS using ADD-Vantage diluent containers containing 50 or 100 ml of either 0.9% sodium chloride injection or 5% dextrose injection. When prepared with either of these dilutents cefoxitin maintains satisfactory potency for 24 hours at room temperature.
After the periods mentioned above, any unused solutions should be discarded.

CDC GUIDELINES FOR TREATMENT OF SEXUALLY TRANSMITTED DISEASES
Recommended Treatment Schedules for Gonorrhea and Acute Pelvic Inflammatory Disease (PID):[1,2]

Disseminated Gonococcal Infection: 1 g cefoxitin IV, 4 times/day for at least 7 days for disseminated infections caused by PPNG.
Gonococcal Ophthalmia in Adults: For PPNG, use 1 g cefoxitin IV, 4 times/day.
Acute PID: For hospitalized patients, give 100 mg doxycycline, IV, twice/day plus 2 g cefoxitin, IV, 4 times/day. Continue drugs IV for at least 4 days and at least 48 hours after patient improves. Continue 100 mg oral doxycycline, twice/day after discharge to complete 10-14 days of therapy. For outpatients, give 2 g cefoxitin IM with 1 g oral probenecid, followed by 100 mg oral doxycycline, twice/day for 10-14 days.

HOW SUPPLIED

Sterile cefoxitin is a dry white to off-white powder supplied in vials and infusion bottles.
Special Storage Instructions: Cefoxitin in the dry state should be stored between 2-25°C (36-77°F). Avoid exposure to temperatures above 50°C. The dry material as well as solutions tend to darken depending on storage conditions; product potency, however, is not adversely affected.

PRODUCT LISTING - RATED THERAPEUTICALLY EQUIVALENT

Powder For Injection - Injectable - 1 Gm

10's	$281.25	CEFOXITIN, Esi Lederle Generics	59911-5963-02
25's	$272.50	CEFOXITIN, American Pharmaceutical Partners	63323-0341-20

Powder For Injection - Injectable - 2 Gm

10's	$562.50	CEFOXITIN, Esi Lederle Generics	59911-5964-02
25's	$423.44	CEFOXITIN, American Pharmaceutical Partners	63323-0342-20

Powder For Injection - Injectable - 10 Gm

10's	$1122.50	CEFOXITIN, American Pharmaceutical Partners	63323-0343-61
10's	$1125.00	CEFOXITIN, Esi Lederle Generics	59911-5965-02

PRODUCT LISTING - EQUIVALENTS NOT AVAILABLE

Powder For Injection - Injectable - 1 Gm

25's	$273.73	MEFOXIN, Merck & Company Inc	00006-3548-45
25's	$299.48	MEFOXIN, Merck & Company Inc	00006-3356-45

Powder For Injection - Injectable - 2 Gm

25's	$582.58	MEFOXIN, Merck & Company Inc	00006-3549-53
25's	$596.83	MEFOXIN, Merck & Company Inc	00006-3357-53

Powder For Injection - Injectable - 10 Gm

6's	$716.06	MEFOXIN, Merck & Company Inc	00006-3388-67

Solution - Intravenous - 1 Gm/50 ml

50 ml x 24	$321.36	MEFOXIN, Merck & Company Inc	00006-3545-24

Solution - Intravenous - 2 Gm/50 ml

50 ml x 24	$516.84	MEFOXIN, Merck & Company Inc	00006-3547-25

Cefpodoxime Proxetil *(003126)*

For related information, see the comparative table section in Appendix A.

Categories: Bronchitis, chronic, acute exacerbation; Gonorrhea; Infection, ear, middle; Infection, lower respiratory tract; Infection, sexually transmitted; Infection, skin and skin structures; Infection, upper respiratory tract; Infection, urinary tract; Pharyngitis; Pneumonia, community-acquired; Tonsillitis; FDA Approved 1992 Aug; Pregnancy Category B
Drug Classes: Antibiotics, cephalosporins
Brand Names: Banan; **Vantin**
Foreign Brand Availability: Banan Dry Syrup (Korea); Biocef (Austria); Cefodox (Bahrain; Cyprus; Egypt; Iran; Iraq; Italy; Jordan; Kuwait; Lebanon; Libya; Oman; Qatar; Republic-of-Yemen; Saudi-Arabia; Syria; United-Arab-Emirates); Cepodem (India); Orelox (Bahamas; Barbados; Belize; Bermuda; Costa-Rica; Curacao; Denmark; Dominican-Republic; El-Salvador; England; France; Germany; Guatemala; Guyana; Honduras; Ireland; Italy; Jamaica; Netherland-Antilles; Netherlands; Nicaragua; Panama; Portugal; Puerto-Rico; South-Africa; Spain; Surinam; Sweden; Switzerland; Trinidad); Otreon (Austria; Italy); Podomexef (Germany; Switzerland)
Cost of Therapy: $98.89 (Infection; Vantin ; 200 mg; 2 tablets/day; 10 day supply)

DESCRIPTION

Cefpodoxime proxetil is an orally administered, extended spectrum, semi-synthetic antibiotic of the cephalosporin class. The chemical name is (RS)-1(isopropoxycarbonyloxy)ethyl (+)-(6R,7R)-7-[2-(2-amino-4-thiazolyl)-2-{(Z)-methoxyimino}acetamido]-3-methoxymethyl-8-oxo-5-thia-1-azabicyclo [4.2.0]oct-2-ene-2-carboxylate.

Its empirical formula is $C_{21}H_{27}N_5O_9S_2$.

The molecular weight of cefpodoxime proxetil is 557.6.

Cefpodoxime proxetil is a prodrug; its active metabolite is cefpodoxime. All doses of cefpodoxime proxetil in this product information are expressed in terms of the active cefpodoxime moiety. The drug is supplied both as film-coated tablets and as flavored granules for oral suspension.

Vantin tablets contain cefpodoxime proxetil equivalent to 100 or 200 mg of cefpodoxime activity and the following inactive ingredients: carboxymethylcellulose calcium, carnauba wax, FD&C yellow no. 6, hydroxypropylcellulose, hydroxypropylmethylcellulose, lactose hydrous, magnesium stearate, propylene glycol, sodium lauryl sulfate and titanium dioxide.

In addition, the 100 mg film-coated tablets contain D&C yellow no. 10 and 200 mg film-coated tablets contain FD&C red no. 40.

Each 5 ml of Vantin for oral suspension contains cefpodoxime proxetil equivalent to 50 or 100 mg of cefpodoxime activity after constitution and the following inactive ingredients: artificial flavorings, butylated hydroxy anisole (BHA), carboxymethylcellulose sodium, microcrystalline cellulose, carrageenan, citric acid, colloidal silicon dioxide, croscarmellose sodium, hydroxypropylcellulose, lactose, maltodextrin, natural flavorings, propylene glycol alginate, sodium citrate, sodium benzoate, starch, sucrose, and vegetable oil.

CLINICAL PHARMACOLOGY

ABSORPTION AND EXCRETION

Cefpodoxime proxetil is a prodrug that is absorbed from the gastrointestinal tract and de-esterified to its active metabolite, cefpodoxime. Following oral administration of 100 mg of cefpodoxime proxetil to fasting subjects, approximately 50% of the administered cefpodoxime dose was absorbed systemically. Over the recommended dosing range (100-400 mg), approximately 29-33% of the administered cefpodoxime dose was excreted unchanged in the urine in 12 hours. There is minimal metabolism of cefpodoxime *in vivo*.

Food Effect on Absorption

The extent of absorption (mean AUC) and the mean peak plasma concentration increased when film-coated tablets were administered with food. Following a 200 mg tablet dose taken with food, the AUC was 21-33% higher than under fasting conditions, and the peak plasma concentration averaged 3.1 μg/ml in fed subjects versus 2.6 μg/ml in fasted subjects. Time to peak concentration was not significantly different between fed and fasted subjects.

When a 200 mg dose of the suspension was taken with food, the extent of absorption (mean AUC) and mean peak plasma concentration in fed subjects were not significantly different from fasted subjects, but the rate of absorption was slower with food (48% increase in T_{max}).

PHARMACOKINETICS

Film-Coated Tablets

Over the recommended dosing range (100-400 mg), the rate and extent of cefpodoxime absorption exhibited dose-dependency; dose-normalized C_{max} and AUC decreased by up to 32% with increasing dose. Over the recommended dosing range, the T_{max} was approximately 2-3 hours and the T½ ranged from 2.09-2.84 hours. Mean C_{max} was 1.4 μg/ml for the 100 mg dose, 2.3 μg/ml for the 200 mg dose, and 3.9 μg/ml for the 400 mg dose. In patients with normal renal function, neither accumulation nor significant changes in other pharmacokinetic parameters were noted following multiple oral doses of up to 400 mg q12h (see TABLE 1).

TABLE 1 *Cefpodoxime Plasma Levels (μg/ml) in Fasted Adults After Film-Coated Tablet Administration (single dose)*

	Time After Oral Ingestion (hours)						
Dose*	1	2	3	4	6	8	12
100 mg	0.98	1.4	1.3	1.0	0.59	0.29	0.08
200 mg	1.5	2.2	2.2	1.8	1.2	0.62	0.18
400 mg	2.2	3.7	3.8	3.3	2.3	1.3	0.38

* Cefpodoxime equivalents.

Suspension

In adult subjects, a 100 mg dose of oral suspension produced an average peak cefpodoxime concentration of approximately 1.5 μg/ml (range: 1.1-2.1 μg/ml), which is equivalent to that reported following administration of the 100 mg tablet. Time to peak plasma concentration and area under the plasma concentration-time curve (AUC) for the oral suspension were also equivalent to those produced with film-coated tablets in adults following a 100 mg oral dose.

The pharmacokinetics of cefpodoxime were investigated in 29 patients aged 1-17 years. Each patient received a single, oral, 5 mg/kg dose of cefpodoxime oral suspension. Plasma and urine samples were collected for 12 hours after dosing. The plasma levels reported from this study are as shown in TABLE 2.

TABLE 2 *Cefpodoxime Plasma Levels (μg/ml) in Fasted Patients (1-17 years of age) After Suspension Administration*

	Time After Oral Ingestion (hours)						
Dose*	1	2	3	4	6	8	12
5 mg/kg†	1.4	2.1	2.1	1.7	0.90	0.40	0.090

† Dose did not exceed 200 mg.
* Cefpodoxime equivalents.

Distribution

Protein binding of cefpodoxime ranges from 22-33% in serum and from 21-29% in plasma.

Skin Blister

Following multiple-dose administration every 12 hours for 5 days of 200 or 400 mg cefpodoxime proxetil, the mean maximum cefpodoxime concentration in skin blister fluid averaged 1.6 and 2.8 μg/ml, respectively. Skin blister fluid cefpodoxime levels at 12 hours after dosing averaged 0.2 and 0.4 μg/ml for the 200 and 400 mg multiple-dose regimens, respectively.

Tonsil Tissue

Following a single, oral 100 mg cefpodoxime proxetil film-coated tablet, the mean maximum cefpodoxime concentration in tonsil tissue averaged 0.24 μg/g at 4 hours post-dosing and 0.09 μg/g at 7 hours post-dosing. Equilibrium was achieved between plasma and tonsil tissue within 4 hours of dosing. No detection of cefpodoxime in tonsillar tissue was reported 12 hours after dosing. These results demonstrated that concentrations of cefpodoxime exceeded the MIC_{90} of *S. pyogenes* for at least 7 hours after dosing of 100 mg of cefpodoxime proxetil.

Lung Tissue

Following a single, oral 200 mg cefpodoxime proxetil film-coated tablet, the mean maximum cefpodoxime concentration in lung tissue averaged 0.63 μg/g at 3 hours post-dosing, 0.52 μg/g at 6 hours post-dosing, and 0.19 μg/g at 12 hours post-dosing. The results of this study indicated that cefpodoxime penetrated into lung tissue and produced sustained drug concentrations for at least 12 hours after dosing at levels that exceeded the MIC_{90} for *S. pneumoniae* and *H. influenzae*.

CSF

Adequate data on CSF levels of cefpodoxime are not available.

Effects of Decreased Renal Function

Elimination of cefpodoxime is reduced in patients with moderate to severe renal impairment (<50 ml/min creatinine clearance). (See PRECAUTIONS and DOSAGE AND ADMINISTRATION.) In subjects with mild impairment of renal function (50-80 ml/min creatinine clearance), the average plasma half-life of cefpodoxime was 3.5 hours. In subjects with moderate (30-49 ml/min creatinine clearance) or severe renal impairment (5-29 ml/min creatinine clearance), the half-life increased to 5.9 and 9.8 hours, respectively. Approximately 23% of the administered dose was cleared from the body during a standard 3 hour hemodialysis procedure.

Effect of Hepatic Impairment (cirrhosis)

Absorption was somewhat diminished and elimination unchanged in patients with cirrhosis. The mean cefpodoxime T½ and renal clearance in cirrhotic patients were similar to those derived in studies of healthy subjects. Ascites did not appear to affect values in cirrhotic subjects. No dosage adjustment is recommended in this patient population.

Elderly Subjects

Elderly subjects do not require dosage adjustments unless they have diminished renal function (see PRECAUTIONS). In healthy geriatric subjects, cefpodoxime half-life in plasma averaged 4.2 hours (vs 3.3 in younger subjects) and urinary recovery averaged 21% after a 400 mg dose was administered every 12 hours. Other pharmacokinetic parameters (C_{max}, AUC, and T_{max}) were unchanged relative to those observed in healthy young subjects.

MICROBIOLOGY

Cefpodoxime is active against a wide-spectrum range of gram-positive and gram-negative bacteria. Cefpodoxime is stable in the presence of β-lactamase enzymes. As a result, many organisms resistant to penicillins and some cephalosporins, due to their production of β-lactamase, may be susceptible to cefpodoxime. Cefpodoxime is inactivated by certain extended spectrum β-lactamases.

The bactericidal activity of cefpodoxime results from its inhibition of cell wall synthesis. Cefpodoxime has been shown to be active against most strains of the following microorganisms, *in vitro* and in clinical infections as described in INDICATIONS AND USAGE.

Gram-Positive Aerobes:

Staphylococcus aureus (including penicillinase-producing strains). *Note:* Cefpodoxime is inactive against methicillin-resistant staphylococci.
Staphylococcus saprophyticus.
Streptococcus pneumoniae (excluding penicillin-resistant strains).
Streptococcus pyogenes.

Gram-Negative Aerobes:

Escherichia coli.
Haemophilus influenzae (including β-lactamase-producing strains).
Klebsiella pneumoniae.
Moraxella (Branhamella) catarrhalis.
Neisseria gonorrhoeae (including penicillinase-producing strains).
Proteus mirabilis.

The following *in vitro* data are available, but their clinical significance is unknown. Cefpodoxime exhibits *in vitro* minimum inhibitory concentrations (MICs) of ≤2.0 μg/ml against most (≥90%) of isolates of the following microorganisms. However, the safety and efficacy of cefpodoxime in treating clinical infections due to these microorganisms have not been established in adequate and well controlled trials.

Gram-Positive Aerobes:

Streptococcus agalactiae.
Streptococcus spp. (Groups C, F, G). *Note:* Cefpodoxime is inactive against enterococci.

Gram-Negative Aerobes:

Citrobacter diversus.
Haemophilus parainfluenzae.
Klebsiella oxytoca.
Proteus vulgaris.
Providencia rettgeri. Note: Cefpodoxime is inactive against most strains of *Pseudomonas* and *Enterobacter.*

Gram-Positive Aerobes:

Peptostreptococcus magnus.

SUSCEPTIBILITY TESTING

Dilution Techniques

Quantitative methods are used to determine antimicrobial inhibitory concentrations (MICs). These MICs provide estimates of the susceptibility of microorganisms to antimicrobial compounds. The MICs should be determined using a standardized procedure. Standardized procedures are based on dilution methods[1,2] (broth or agar) or equivalent using standardized inoculum concentrations, and standardized concentrations of cefpodoxime from a powder of unknown potency. The MIC values should be interepreted according to TABLE 3.

TABLE 3 *For Susceptibility Testing of Pathogens*

	Interpretation		
	MIC (μg/ml)		
Pathogen	Susceptible (S)	Intermediate (I)	Resistant (R)
Enterobacteriaceae and *Staphylococcus* spp.	≤2.0	4.0	≥8.0
Haemophilus spp.*	≤2.0	†	†
Neisseria gonorrhoeae‡	≤0.5	†	†
Streptococcus pneumoniae§	≤0.5	1.0	≥2.0

* The interpretive criteria for *Haemophilus* spp. is applicable only to broth microdilution susceptibility testing done with Haemophilus Test Medium (HTM) broth.[2]
† This category has not been determined.
‡ The interpretive value for *N. gonorroheae* is applicable only to agar dilution susceptibility testing done with *Neisseria gonorrhoeae* susceptibility test medium.[2]
§ The interpretive value for *S. pneumoniae* is applicable only to broth microdilution susceptibility testing done with cation-adjusted Mueller-Hinton broth with lysed horse blood (LHB) (2-5% v/v).[2]

For Susceptibility Testing of Streptococcus spp. Other Than Streptococcus pneumoniae
A streptococcal isolate that is susceptible to penicillin (MIC ≤0.12 μg/ml) can be considered susceptible to cefpodoxime for approved indications, and need not be tested against cefpodoxime. The interpretive value for *Streptococcus* spp. is applicable only to broth microdilution susceptibility testing done with cation-adjusted Mueller-Hinton broth with lysed horse blood (LHB) (2-5% v/v).[2]

A report of "Susceptible" indicates that the pathogen is likely to be inhibited if the concentration of the antimicrobial compound in the blood reaches usually achievable levels. A report of "Intermediate" indicates that the results should be considered equivocal, and, if the microorganism is not fully susceptible to alternative, clinically feasible drugs, the test should be repeated. This category implies possible clinical applicability in body sites where the drug is physiologically concentrated or in situations where high dosage of drug can be used. This category also provides a buffer zone which prevents small technical factors from causing major discrepancies in interpretation. A report of "Resistant" indicates that the pathogen is not likely to be inhibited if the antimicrobial compound in the blood reaches the concentrations usually achievable; other therapy should be selected.

Quality Control
A standard susceptibility test procedure requires the use of laboratory control organisms to control the technical aspects of the laboratory procedures. Standard cefpodoxime powder should provide the following MIC values with the indicated quality control strains shown in TABLE 4.

TABLE 4

Microorganism (ATCC *)	MIC Range (μg/ml)
Escherichia coli (25922)	0.25-1.0
Staphylococcus aureus (29213)	1.0-8.0
Haemophilus influenzae (49247)	0.25-1.0†
Neisseria gonorrhoeae (49226)	0.03-0.12‡
Streptococcus pneumoniae (49219)¤	0.03-0.12§

* ATCC is a registered trademark of the American Type Culture Collection.
† These quality control ranges are applicable to tests performed by a broth microdilution procedure using Haemophilus Test Medium (HTM).
‡ These quality control ranges are applicable to tests performed by agar dilution only using GC agar base with 1% defined growth supplement.
§ These quality control ranges are applicable to tests performed by the broth microdilution method only using cation-adjusted Mueller-Hinton broth with 2-5% lysed horse blood.
¤ When susceptibility testing *Streptococcus pneumoniae* or *Streptococcus* spp. this quality control strain should be tested.

Diffusion Techniques
Quannitative methods that require measurement of zone diameters also provide reproducible estimates of the susceptibility of bacteria to antimicrobial compounds. One such standardized procedure3 requires the use of standardized inoculum concentrations. This procedure uses paper disks impregnated with 10 μg cefpodoxime to test the susceptibility of microorganisms to cefpodoxime disk should be interpreted according to the criteria in TABLE 5.

For Susceptibility Testing of Streptococcus Pneumoniae
Isolates of *pneumococci* with oxacillin zone sizes of ≥20 mm are susceptible (MIC ≤0.06 μg/ml) to penicillin and can be considered susceptible to cefpodoxime for approved indications, and cefpodoxime need not be tested.

The zone diameter for *S. pneumoniae* is applicable only to tests performed on Mueller-Hinton agar with 5% sheep blood incubated in 5% CO_2.[2]

For Susceptibility Testing of Streptococcus spp. other than Streptococcus Pneumoniae
A streptococcal isolate that is susceptible to penicillin (zone diameter ≥28 mm) can be considered suspectible to cefpodoxime for approved indications, and cefpodoxime need not be tested.

The zone diameter for *S. pneumoniae* is applicable only to tests performed on Mueller-Hinton agar with 5% sheep blood incubated in 5% CO_2.[2]

TABLE 5

	Interpretation		
	Zone Diameter (mm)		
Pathogen	Susceptible (S)	Intermediate (I)	Resistant (R)
Enterobacteriaceae and *Staphylococcus* spp.	≥21	18-20	≤17
Haemophilus spp.*	≥21	†	†
Neisseria gonorrhoeae‡	≥29	†	†

* The zone diameter of *Haemophilus* spp. is applicable only to tests performed on Haemophilus Test Medium (HTM) agar incubated under 5% CO_2.[2]
† This criteria has not been determined.
‡ The zone diameter for *N. gonorrhoeae* is applicable only to tests perfomed on GC agar base and 1% defined growth supplement incubated under 5% CO_2.[2]

Quality Control
As with standardized dilution techniques, diffusion methods require the use of laboratory control microorganisms that are used to control the technical aspects of the laboratory procedures. For the diffusion technique, the 10 μg cefpodoxime disk should provide the following zone diameters with the quality control strains listed in TABLE 6

TABLE 6

Microorganism (ATCC*)	Zone Diameter Range (mm)
Escherichia coli (25922)	23-28
Staphylococcus aureus (25923)	19-25
Haemophilus influenzae (49247)	25-31†
Neisseria gonorrhoeae (49226)	35-43‡
Streptococcus pneumoniae (49619)§	28-34¤

* ATCC is a registered trademark of the American Type Culture Collection.
† This zone diameter range is only applicable to test performed on Haemophilus Test Medium (HTM) agar incubated in 5% CO_2.
‡ This zone diameter is only applicable to tests performed on GC agar base and 1% defined growth supplement incubated in 5% CD.
§ This zone diameter range is only applicable to tests performed on Mueller-Hinton agar supplemented with 5% defibrinated sheep blood, incubated in 5% CO_2.
¤ This organism is to be used for quality control testing for both *S. pneumoniae* and *Streptococcus* spp.

INDICATIONS AND USAGE

Cefpodoxime proxetil is indicated for the treatment of patients with mild to moderate infections caused by susceptible strains of the designated microorganisms in the conditions listed below. **Recommended dosages, durations of therapy, and applicable patient populations vary among these infections. Please see DOSAGE AND ADMINISTRATION for specific recommendations.**

ACUTE OTITIS MEDIA
Caused by*Streptococcus pneumoniae* (excluding penicillin-resistant strains), *Streptococcus pyogenes, Haemophilus influenzae* (including β-lactamase-producing strains), or *Moraxella (Branhamella) catarrhalis* (including β-lactamase producing strains).

PHARYNGITIS AND/OR TONSILLITIS
Caused by *Streptococcus pyogenes*. *Note:* Only penicillin by the intramuscular route of administration has been shown to be effective in the prophylaxis of rheumatic fever. Cefpodoxime proxetil is generally effective in the eradication of streptococci from the oropharynx. However, data establishing the efficacy of cefpodoxime proxetil for the prophylaxis of subsequent rheumatic fever are not available.

COMMUNITY-ACQUIRED PNEUMONIA
Caused by *S. pneumoniae* or *H. influenzae* (including β-lactamase-producing strains.

ACUTE BACTERIAL EXACERBATION OF CHRONIC BRONCHITIS
Caused by *S. pneumoniae, H. influenzae* (non-β-lactamase-producing strains only), or *M. catarrhalis.* Data are insufficient at this time to establish efficacy in patients with acute bacterial exacerbations of chronic bronchitis caused by β-lactamase-producing strains of *H. influenzae.*

ACUTE, UNCOMPLICATED URETHRAL AND CERVICAL GONORRHEA
Caused by *Neisseria gonorrhoeae* (including penicillinase-producing strains).

ACUTE, UNCOMPLICATED ANO-RECTAL INFECTIONS IN WOMEN
Due to *Neisseria gonorrhoeae* (including penicillinase-producing strains). *Note:* The efficacy of cefpodoxime in treating male patients with rectal infections caused by *N. gonorrhoeae* has not been established. Data do not support the use of cefpodoxime proxetil in the treatment of pharyngeal infections due to *N. gonorrhoeae* in men or women.

UNCOMPLICATED SKIN AND SKIN STRUCTURE INFECTIONS
Caused by *Staphylococcus aureus* (including penicillinase-producing strains) or *Streptococcus pyogenes.* Abscesses should be surgically drained as clinically indicated.*Note:* In clinical trials, successful treatment of uncomplicated skin and skin structure infections was dose-related. The effective therapeutic dose for skin infections was higher than those used in other recommended indications (see DOSAGE AND ADMINISTRATION).

ACUTE MAXILLARY SINUSITIS

Caused by *Haemophilus influenzae* (including β-lactamase producing strains), *Streptococcus pneumoniae*, and *Moraxella catarrhalis.*

UNCOMPLICATED URINARY TRACT INFECTIONS (CYSTITIS)

Caused by *Escherichia coli, Klebsiella pneumoniae, Proteus mirabilis,* or *Staphylococcus saprophyticus. Note:* In considering the use of cefpodoxime proxetil in the treatment of cystitis, cefpodoxime proxetil's lower bacterial eradication rates should be weighed against the increased eradication rates and different safety profiles of some other classes of approved agents.

Appropriate specimens for bacteriological examinations should be obtained in order to isolate and identify causative organisms and to determine their susceptibility to cefpodoxime. Therapy may be instituted while awaiting the results of these studies. Once these results become available, antimicrobial therapy should be adjusted accordingly.

CONTRAINDICATIONS

Cefpodoxime proxetil is contraindicated in patients with a known allergy to cefpodoxime or to the cephalosporin group of antibiotics.

WARNINGS

BEFORE THERAPY WITH CEFPODOXIME PROXETIL IS INSTITUTED, CAREFUL INQUIRY SHOULD BE MADE TO DETERMINE WHETHER THE PATIENT HAS HAD PREVIOUS HYPERSENSITIVITY REACTIONS TO CEFPODOXIME, OTHER CEPHALOSPORINS, PENICILLINS, OR OTHER DRUGS. IF CEFPODOXIME IS TO BE ADMINISTERED TO PENICILLIN-SENSITIVE PATIENTS, CAUTION SHOULD BE EXERCISED BECAUSE CROSS HYPERSENSITIVITY AMONG β-LACTAM ANTIBIOTICS HAS BEEN CLEARLY DOCUMENTED AND MAY OCCUR IN UP TO 10% OF PATIENTS WITH A HISTORY OF PENICILLIN ALLERGY. IF AN ALLERGIC REACTION TO CEFPODOXIME PROXETIL OCCURS, DISCONTINUE THE DRUG. SERIOUS ACUTE HYPERSENSITIVITY REACTIONS MAY REQUIRE TREATMENT WITH EPINEPHRINE AND OTHER EMERGENCY MEASURES, INCLUDING OXYGEN, INTRAVENOUS FLUIDS, INTRAVENOUS ANTIHISTAMINE, AND AIRWAY MANAGEMENT, AS CLINICALLY INDICATED. PSEUDOMEMBRANOUS COLITIS HAS BEEN REPORTED WITH NEARLY ALL ANTIBACTERIAL AGENTS, INCLUDING CEFPODOXIME, AND MAY RANGE IN SEVERITY FROM MILD TO LIFE-THREATENING. THEREFORE, IT IS IMPORTANT TO CONSIDER THIS DIAGNOSIS IN PATIENTS WHO PRESENT WITH DIARRHEA SUBSEQUENT TO THE ADMINISTRATION OF ANTIBACTERIAL AGENTS.

Extreme caution should be observed when using this product in patients at increased risk for antibiotic-induced, pseudomembranous colitis because of exposure to institutional settings, such as nursing homes or hospitals with endemic *C. difficile*.

Treatment with broad-spectrum antibiotics, including cefpodoxime proxetil, alters the normal flora of the colon and may permit overgrowth of clostridia. Studies indicate a toxin produced by *Clostridium difficile* is the primary cause of "antibiotic-associated colitis".

After the diagnosis of pseudomembranous colitis has been established, therapeutic measures should be initiated. Mild cases of pseudomembranous colitis usually respond to drug discontinuation alone. In moderate to severe cases, consideration should be given to management with fluids and electrolytes, protein supplementation, and treatment with an oral antibacterial drug effective against *C. difficile.*

A concerted effort to monitor for *C. difficile* in cefpodoxime-treated patients with diarrhea was undertaken because of an increased incidence of diarrhea associated with *C. difficile* in early trials in normal subjects. *C. difficile* organisms or toxin was reported in 10% of the cefpodoxime-treated adult patients with diarrhea; however, no specific diagnosis of pseudomembranous colitis was made in these patients.

In post-marketing experience outside the US, reports of pseudomembranous colitis associated with the use of cefpodoxime proxetil have been received.

PRECAUTIONS

GENERAL

In patients with transient or persistent reduction in urinary output due to renal insufficiency, the total daily dose of cefpodoxime proxetil should be reduced because high and prolonged serum antibiotic concentrations can occur in such individuals following usual doses. Cefpodoxime, like other cephalosporins, should be administered with caution to patients receiving concurrent treatment with potent diuretics (see DOSAGE AND ADMINISTRATION).

As with other antibiotics, prolonged use of cefpodoxime proxetil may result in overgrowth of non-susceptible organisms. Repeated evaluation of the patient's condition is essential. If superinfection occurs during therapy, appropriate measures should be taken.

DRUG/LABORATORY TEST INTERACTIONS

Cephalosporins, including cefpodoxime proxetil, are known to occasionally induce a positive direct Coombs' test.

CARCINOGENESIS, MUTAGENESIS, AND IMPAIRMENT OF FERTILITY

Long-term animal carcinogenesis studies of cefpodoxime proxetil have not been performed. Mutagenesis studies of cefpodoxime, including the Ames test both with and without metabolic activation, the chromosome aberration test, the unscheduled DNA synthesis assay, mitotic recombination and gene conversion, the forward gene mutation assay and the *in vivo* micronucleus test, were all negative. No untoward effects on fertility or reproduction were noted when 100 mg/kg/day or less (2 times the human dose based on mg/m^2) was administered orally to rats.

PREGNANCY, TERATOGENIC EFFECTS, PREGNANCY CATEGORY B

Cefpodoxime proxetil was neither teratogenic nor embryocidal when administered to rats during organogenesis at doses up to 100 mg/kg/day (2 times the human dose based on mg/m^2) or to rabbits at doses up to 30 mg/kg/day (1-2 times the human dose based on mg/m^2).

There are, however, no adequate and well-controlled studies of cefpodoxime proxetil use in pregnant women. Because animal reproduction studies are not always predictive of human response, this drug should be used during pregnancy only if clearly needed.

LABOR AND DELIVERY

Cefpodoxime proxetil has not been studied for use during labor and delivery. Treatment should only be given if clearly needed.

NURSING MOTHERS

Cefpodoxime is excreted in human milk. In a study of 3 lactating women, levels of cefpodoxime in human milk were 0%, 2% and 6% of concomitant serum levels at 4 hours following a 200 mg oral dose of cefpodoxime proxetil. At 6 hours post-dosing, levels were 0%, 9% and 16% of concomitant serum levels. Because of the potential for serious reactions in nursing infants, a decision should be made whether to discontinue nursing or to discontinue the drug, taking into account the importance of the drug to the mother.

PEDIATRIC USE

Safety and efficacy in infants less than 2 months of age have not been established.

GERIATRIC USE

Of the 3338 patients in multiple-dose clinical studies of cefpodoxime proxetil film-coated tablets, 521 (16%) were 65 and over, while 214 (6%) were 75 and over. No overall differences in effectiveness or safety were observed between the elderly and younger patients. In healthy geriatric subjects with normal renal function, cefpodoxime half-life in plasma averaged 4.2 hours and urinary recovery averaged 21% after a 400 mg dose was given every 12 hours for 15 days. Other pharmacokinetic parameters were unchanged relative to those observed in healthy younger subjects.

Dose adjustment in elderly patients with normal renal function is not necessary.

DRUG INTERACTIONS

Antacids: Concomitant administration of high doses of antacids (sodium bicarbonate and aluminum hydroxide) or H_2 blockers reduces peak plasma levels by 24-42% and the extent of absorption by 27-32%, respectively. The rate of absorption is not altered by these concomitant medications. Oral anti-cholinergics (*e.g.*, propantheline) delay peak plasma levels (47% increase in T_{max}), but do not affect the extent of absorption (AUC).

Probenecid: As with other β-lactam antibiotics, renal excretion of cefpodoxime was inhibited by probenecid and resulted in an approximately 31% increase in AUC and 20% increase in peak cefpodoxime plasma levels.

Nephrotoxic Drugs: Although nephrotoxicity has not been noted when cefpodoxime proxetil was given alone, close monitoring of renal function is advised when cefpodoxime proxetil is administered concomitantly with compounds of known nephrotoxic potential.

ADVERSE REACTIONS

FILM-COATED TABLETS (MULTIPLE DOSE)

In clinical trials using **multiple doses** of cefpodoxime proxetil film-coated tablets, 4696 patients were treated with the recommended dosages of cefpodoxime (100-400 mg q12h). There were no deaths or permanent disabilities thought related to drug toxicity. One-hundred twenty-nine (2.7%) patients discontinued medication due to adverse events thought possibly- or probably-related to drug toxicity. Ninety-three (52%) of the 78 patients who discontinued therapy (whether thought related to drug therapy or not) did so because of gastrointestinal disturbances, nausea, vomiting, or diarrhea. The percentage of cefpodoxime proxetil-treated patients who discontinued study drug because of adverse events was significantly greater at a dose of 800 mg daily than at a dose of 400 mg daily or at a dose of 200 mg daily. Adverse events thought possibly- or probably-related to cefpodoxime in multiple dose clinical trials (n=4696 cefpodoxime-treated patients) were:

Incidence Greater Than 1

Diarrhea: 7.0%. *Diarrhea or loose stools were dose related:* Decreasing from 10.4% of patients receiving 800 mg per day to 5.7% for those receiving 200 mg per day. Of patients with diarrhea, 10% had *C. difficile* organism or toxin in the stool (see WARNINGS).

Nausea: 3.3%.

Vaginal Fungal Infections: 1.0%.

Abdominal Pain: 1.2%.

Vulvovaginal Infections: 1.3%.

Headache: 1.0%.

Incidence Less Than 1% (By Body System in Decreasing Order)

Adverse events thought possibly or probably related to cefpodoxime proxetil that occurred in less than 1% of patients (N=4696).

Body: Fungal infections, abdominal distention, malaise, fatigue, asthenia, fever, chest pain, back pain, chills, generalized pain, abnormal microbiological tests, moniliasis, abscess, allergic reaction, facial edema, bacterial infections, parasitic infections, localized edema, localized pain.

Cardiovascular: Congestive heart failure, migraine, palpitations, vasodilation, hematoma, hypertension, hypotension.

Digestive: Vomiting, dyspepsia, dry mouth, flatulence, decreased appetite, constipation, oral moniliasis, anorexia, eructation, gastritis, mouth ulcers, gastrointestinal disorders, rectal disorders, tongue disorders, tooth disorders, increased thirst, oral lesions, tenesmus, dry throat, toothache.

Hemic and Lymphatic: Anemia.

Metabolic and Nutritional: Dehydration, gout, peripheral edema, weight increase.

Musculoskeletal: Myalgia.

Nervous: Dizziness, insomnia, somnolence, anxiety, shakiness, nervousness, cerebral infarction, change in dreams, impaired concentration, confusion, nightmares, paresthesia, vertigo.

C

Respiratory: Asthma, cough, epistaxis, rhinitis, wheezing, bronchitis, dyspnea, pleural effusion, pneumonia, sinusitis.
Skin: Urticaria, rash, pruritus non-application site, hair loss, vesiculobullous rash, sunburn.
Special Senses: Taste alterations, eye irritation, taste loss, tinnitus.
Urogenital: hematuria, urinary tract infections, metrorrhagia, dysuria, urinary frequency, notcuria, penile infection, proteinuria, vaginal pain.

GRANULES FOR ORAL SUSPENSION (MULTIPLE DOSE)

In clinical trials using **multiple doses** of cefpodoxime proxetil granules for oral suspension, 2128 pediatric patients (93% of whom were less than 12 years of age) were treated with the recommended dosages of cefpodoxime (10 mg/kg/day q24h or divided q12h to a maximum equivalent adult dose). There were no deaths or permanent disabilities in any of the patients in these studies. Twenty-four patients (1.1%) discontinued medication due to adverse events thought possibly- or probably-related to study drug. Primarily, these discontinuations were for gastrointestinal disturbances, usually diarrhea, vomiting, or rashes.

Adverse events thought possibly- or probably-related, or of unknown relationship to cefpodoxime proxetil for oral suspension in multiple dose clinical trials (n=2128 cefpodoxime-treated patients) were:

Incidence Greater Than 1%:
Diarrhea: 6.0%. The incidence of diarrhea in infants and toddlers (age 1 month to 2 years) was 12.8%.
Diaper Rash/Fungal Skin Rash: 2.0% (includes moniliasis). The incidence of diaper rash in infants and toddlers was 8.5%.
Other Skin Rashes: 1.8%.
Vomiting: 2.3%.

Incidence Less Than 1%:
Body: Localized abdominal pain, abdominal cramp, headache, monilia, generalized abdominal pain, asthenia, fever, fungal infection.
Digestive: Nausea, monilia, anorexia, dry mouth, stomatitis, pseudomembranous colitis.
Hemic & Lymphatic: Thrombocythemia, positive direct Coombs' test, eosinophilia, leukocytosis, leukopenia, prolonged partial thromboplastin time, thrombocytopenic purpura.
Metabolic & Nutritional: Increased SGPT.
Musculoskeletal: Myalgia.
Nervous: Hallucination, hyperkinesia, nervousness, somnolence.
Respiratory: Epistaxis, rhinitis.
Skin: Skin moniliasis, urticaria, fungal dermatitis, acne, exfoliative dermatitis, maculopapular rash.
Special Senses: Taste perversion.

FILM-COATED TABLETS (SINGLE DOSE)

In clinical trials using a **single dose** of cefpodoxime proxetil film-coated tablets, 509 patients were treated with the recommended dosage of cefpodoxime (200 mg). There were no deaths or permanent disabilities thought related to drug toxicity in these studies.

Adverse events thought possibly- or probably-related to cefpodoxime in single dose clinical trials conducted in the US were:

Incidence Greater Than 1%:
Nausea: 1.4%.
Diarrhea: 1.2%.

Incidence Less Than 1%:
Central Nervous System: Dizziness, headache, syncope.
Dermatologic: Rash.
Genital: Vaginitis.
Gastrointestinal: Abdominal pain.
Psychiatric: Anxiety.

Laboratory Changes

Significant laboratory changes that have been reported in adult and pediatric patients in clinical trials of cefpodoxime proxetil, without regard to drug relationship, were:
Hepatic: Transient increases in AST (SGOT), ALT (SGPT), GGT, alkaline phosphatase, bilirubin, and LDH.
Hematologic: Eosinophilia, leukocytosis, lymphocytosis, granulocytosis, basophilia, monocytosis, thrombocytosis, decreased hemoglobin, decreased hematocrit, leukopenia, neutropenia, lymphocytopenia, thrombocytopenia, thrombocythemia, positive Coombs' test, and prolonged PT and PTT.
Serum Chemistry: Hyperglycemia, hypoglycemia, hypoalbuminemia, hypoproteinemia, hyperkalemia, and hyponatremia.
Renal: Increases in BUN and creatinine.

Most of these abnormalities were transient and not clinically significant.

Postmarketing Experience

The following serious adverse experiences have been reported: allergic reactions including Stevens-Johnson syndrome, toxic epidermal necrolysis, erythema multiforme and serum sickness-like reactions, pseudomembranous colitis, bloody diarrhea with abdominal pain, ulcerative colitis, rectorrhagia with hypotension, anaphylactic shock, acute liver injury, *in utero* exposure with miscarriage, purpuric nephritis, pulmonary infiltrate with eosinophilia, and eyelid dermatitis.

One death was attributed to pseudomembranous colitis and disseminated intravascular coagulation.

Cephalosporin Class Labeling

In addition to the adverse reactions listed above which have been observed in patients treated with cefpodoxime proxetil, the following adverse reactions and altered laboratory tests have been reported for cephalosporin class antibiotics.

Adverse reactions and abnormal laboratory tests: renal dysfunction, toxic nephropathy, hepatic dysfunction including cholestasis, aplastic anemia, hemolytic anemia, serum sickness-like reaction, hemorrhage, agranulocytosis, and pancytopenia.

Several cephalosporins have been implicated in triggering seizures, particularly in patients with renal impairment when the dosage was not reduced (see DOSAGE AND ADMINISTRATION). If seizures associated with drug therapy occur, the drug should be discontinued. Anticonvulsant therapy can be given if clinically indicated.

DOSAGE AND ADMINISTRATION

See INDICATIONS AND USAGE for indicated pathogens.

FILM-COATED TABLETS

Cefpodoxime proxetil tablets should be administered orally with food to enhance absorption (see CLINICAL PHARMACOLOGY). The recommended dosages, durations of treatment, and applicable patient population are as described in TABLE 9.

TABLE 9 *Adults and Adolescents (age 12 years and older)*

Type of Infection	Total Daily Dose	Dose Frequency	Duration
Pharyngitis and/or tonsillitis	200 mg	100 mg q12h	5-10 days
Acute community-acquired pneumonia	400 mg	200 mg q12h	14 days
Acute bacterial exacerbations of chronic bronchitis	400 mg	200 mg q12h	10 days
Uncomplicated gonorrhea (men and women) and rectal gonococcal infections (women)	200 mg	Single dose	
Skin and skin structure	800 mg	400 mg q12h	7-14 days
Acute maxillary sinusitis	400 mg	200 mg q12h	10 days
Uncomplicated urinary tract infection	200 mg	100 mg q12h	7 days

GRANULES FOR ORAL SUSPENSION

Cefpodoxime proxetil oral suspension may be given without regard to food. The recommended dosages, durations of treatment, and applicable patient populations are as described in TABLE 10A and TABLE 10B.

TABLE 10A *Adults and Adolescents (age 12 years and older)*

Type of Infection	Total Daily Dose	Dose Frequency	Duration
Pharyngitis and/or tonsillitis	200 mg	100 mg q12h	5-10 days
Acute community-acquired pneumonia	400 mg	200 mg q12h	14 days
Uncomplicated gonorrhea (men and women) and rectal gonococcal infections (women)	200 mg	Single dose	
Skin and skin structure	800 mg	400 mg q12h	7-14 days
Acute maxillary sinusitis	400 mg	200 mg q12h	10 days
Uncomplicated urinary tract infection	200 mg	100 mg q12h	7 days

TABLE 10B *Infants and Pediatric Patients (age 2 months through 12 years)*

Type of Infection	Total Daily Dose	Dose Frequency	Duration
Acute otitis media	10 mg/kg/day (max 400 mg/day)	5 mg/kg q12h (max 200 mg/dose)	5 days
Pharyngitis and/or tonsillitis	10 mg/kg/day (max 200 mg/day)	5 mg/kg/dose q12h (max 100 mg/dose)	5-10 days
Acute maxillary sinusitis	10 mg/kg/day (max 400 mg/day)	5 mg/kg q12h (max 200 mg/dose)	10 days

Patients With Renal Dysfunction

For patients with severe renal impairment (<30 ml/min creatinine clearance), the dosing intervals should be increased to q24h. In patients maintained on hemodialysis, the dose frequency should be 3 times/week after hemodialysis.

When only the serum creatinine level is available, the following formula (based on sex, weight, and age of the patient) may be used to estimate creatinine clearance (ml/min). For this estimate to be valid, the serum creatinine level should represent a steady state of renal function.

Males (ml/min): [Weight (kg) × (140 - age)] ÷ [72 × serum creatinine (mg/100 ml)]
Females (ml/min): [0.85 × above value]

Patients With Cirrhosis:

Cefpodoxime pharmacokinetics in cirrhotic patients (with or without ascites) are similar to those in healthy subjects. Dose adjustment is not necessary in this population.

HOW SUPPLIED

VANTIN TABLETS

Vantin tablets are available in the following strengths, colors and sizes:
100 mg: Light orange, elliptical, debossed with "U3617".
200 mg: Coral red, elliptical, debossed with "U3618".

Storage: Store tablets at controlled room temperature 20-25°C (68-77°F). Replace cap securely after each opening. Protect unit dose packs from excessive moisture.

VANTIN FOR ORAL SUSPENSION

Vantin for oral suspension is available in the 50 and 100 mg/5 ml strengths in lemon creme flavor:

Storage: Store unsuspended granules at controlled room temperature 20-25°C (68-77°F).

Directions for mixing are included on the label. After mixing, suspension should be stored in a refrigerator, 2-8°C (36-46°F). Shake well before using. Keep container tightly closed. The mixture may be used for 14 days. Discard unused portion after 14 days.

PRODUCT LISTING - EQUIVALENTS NOT AVAILABLE

Powder For Reconstitution - Oral - 50 mg/5 ml			
50 ml	$22.15	VANTIN, Pharmacia Corporation	00009-3531-03
100 ml	$48.31	VANTIN, Pharmacia and Upjohn	00009-3531-01
Powder For Reconstitution - Oral - 100 mg/5 ml			
50 ml	$48.31	VANTIN, Pharmacia and Upjohn	00009-3615-03
75 ml	$66.39	VANTIN, Pharmacia and Upjohn	00009-3615-02
100 ml	$91.91	VANTIN, Pharmacia and Upjohn	00009-3615-01
Tablet - Oral - 100 mg			
10's	$33.43	VANTIN, Allscripts Pharmaceutical Company	54569-4058-01
20's	$85.70	VANTIN, Pharmacia and Upjohn	00009-3617-01
100's	$355.05	VANTIN, Pharmacia and Upjohn	00009-3617-03
100's	$407.80	VANTIN, Pharmacia and Upjohn	00009-3617-02
Tablet - Oral - 200 mg			
10's	$57.20	VANTIN, Pd-Rx Pharmaceuticals	55289-0390-10
20's	$81.62	VANTIN, Prescript Pharmaceuticals	00247-0339-20
20's	$84.01	VANTIN, Allscripts Pharmaceutical Company	54569-4783-00
20's	$113.24	VANTIN, Pharmacia and Upjohn	00009-3618-01
20's	$117.84	VANTIN, Pd-Rx Pharmaceuticals	55289-0390-20
100's	$430.51	VANTIN, Pharmacia and Upjohn	00009-3618-03
100's	$494.45	VANTIN, Pharmacia and Upjohn	00009-3618-02

Cefprozil *(003102)*

For related information, see the comparative table section in Appendix A.

Categories: Bronchitis, chronic, acute exacerbation; Infection, ear, middle; Infection, lower respiratory tract; Infection, skin and skin structures; Infection, upper respiratory tract; Pharyngitis; Sinusitis; Tonsillitis; FDA Approved 1991 Dec; Pregnancy Category B
Drug Classes: Antibiotics, cephalosporins
Brand Names: Cefzil; Procef
Foreign Brand Availability: Prozef (South-Africa)
Cost of Therapy: $171.45 (Infection; Cefzil; 500 mg; 2 tablets/day; 10 day supply)

DESCRIPTION

Cefprozil is a semi-synthetic broad-spectrum cephalosporin antibiotic.

Cefprozil is a cis and trans isomeric mixture (≥90% cis). The chemical name for the monohydrate is (6R,7R)-7-[(R)-2-amino-2-(p-hydroxyphenyl)acetamido]-8-oxo-3-propenyl-5-thia-1-azabicyclo[4.2.0]oct-2-ene-2-carboxylic acid monohydrate.

Cefprozil is a white to yellowish powder with a molecular formula for the monohydrate of $C_{18}H_{19}N_3O_5S{\cdot}H_2O$ and a molecular weight of 407.45.

Cefprozil tablets and cefprozil for oral suspension are intended for oral administration.

Cefzil tablets contain cefprozil equivalent to 250 or 500 mg of anhydrous cefprozil. In addition, each tablet contains the following inactive ingredients: cellulose, hydroxypropylmethylcellulose, magnesium stearate, methylcellulose, simethicone, sodium starch glycolate, polyethylene glycol, polysorbate 80, sorbic acid and titanium dioxide. The 250 mg tablets also contain FD&C yellow no. 6.

Cefzil for oral suspension contains cefprozil equivalent to 125 or 250 mg anhydrous cefprozil per 5 ml constituted suspension. In addition, the oral suspension contains the following inactive ingredients: aspartame, cellulose, citric acid, colloidal silicone dioxide, FD&C red no. 3, flavors (natural and artificial), glycine, polysorbate 80, simethicone, sodium benzoate, sodium carboxymethylcellulose, sodium chloride, and sucrose.

CLINICAL PHARMACOLOGY

The pharmacokinetic data were derived from the capsule formulation; however, bioequivalence has been demonstrated for the oral solution, capsule, tablet and suspension formulations under fasting conditions.

Following oral administration of cefprozil to fasting subjects, approximately 95% of the dose was absorbed. The average plasma half-life in normal subjects was 1.3 hours, while the steady state volume of distribution was estimated to be 0.23 L/kg. The total body clearance and renal clearance rates were approximately 3 ml/min/kg and 2.3 ml/min/kg, respectively.

Average peak plasma concentrations after administration of 250 mg, 500 mg, or 1 g doses of cefprozil to fasting subjects were approximately 6.1, 10.5, and 18.3 µg/ml, respectively, and were obtained within 1.5 hours after dosing. Urinary recovery accounted for approximately 60% of the administered dose. (See TABLE 1.)

TABLE 1

Dosage	Mean Plasma Cefprozil* Concentrations (µg/ml) Peak appx. 1.5 h	4 h	8 h	8 Hour Urinary Excretion
250 mg	6.1	1.7	0.2	60%
500 mg	10.5	3.2	0.4	62%
1000 mg	18.3	8.4	1.0	54%

* Data represent mean values of 12 healthy volunteers.

During the first 4 hour period after drug administration, the average urine concentrations following 250 mg, 500 mg, and 1 g doses were approximately 700 µg/ml, 1000 µg/ml, and 2900 µg/ml, respectively.

Administration of cefprozil tablet or suspension formulation with food did not affect the extent of absorption (AUC) or the peak plasma concentration (C_{max}) of cefprozil. However, there was an increase of 0.25-0.75 hours in the time to maximum plasma concentration of ceprozil (T_{max}).

The bioavailability of the capsule formulation of cefprozil was not affected when administered 5 minutes following an antacid.

Plasma protein binding is approximately 36% and is independent of concentration in the range of 2-20 µg/ml.

There was no evidence of accumulation of cefprozil in the plasma in individuals with normal renal function following multiple oral doses of up to 1000 mg every 8 hours for 10 days.

In patients with reduced renal function, the plasma half-life may be prolonged up to 5.2 hours depending on the degree of the renal dysfunction. In patients with complete absence of renal function, the plasma half-life of cefprozil has been shown to be as long as 5.9 hours. The half-life is shortened during hemodialysis. Excretion pathways in patients with markedly impaired renal function have not been determined. (See PRECAUTIONS and DOSAGE AND ADMINISTRATION.)

In patients with impaired hepatic function, the half-life increases to approximately 2 hours. The magnitude of the changes does not warrant a dosage adjustment for patients with impaired hepatic function.

Healthy geriatric volunteers (≥65 years old) who received a single 1 g dose of cefprozil had 35-60% higher AUC and 40% lower renal clearance values compared with healthy adult volunteers 20-40 years of age. The average AUC in young and elderly female subjects was approximately 15-20% higher than in young and elderly male subjects.

Adequate data on CSF levels of cefprozil are not available.

Comparable pharmacokinetic parameters of cefprozil are observed between pediatric patients (6 months-12 years) and adults following oral administration of selected matched doses. The maximum concentrations are achieved at 1-2 hours after dosing. The plasma elimination half-life is approximately 1.5 hours. In general, the observed plasma concentrations of cefprozil in pediatric patients at the 7.5, 15, and 30 mg/kg doses are similar to those observed within the same time frame in normal adult subjects at the 250, 500 and 1000 mg doses, respectively. The comparative plasma concentrations of cefprozil in pediatric patients and adult subjects at the equivalent dose level are presented in TABLE 2.

TABLE 2

Population	Dose	Mean (SD) Plasma Cefprozil Concentrations (µg/ml) 1 h	2 h	4 h	6 h	T½ (h)
Children (n=18)	7.5 mg/kg	4.70 (1.57)	3.99 (1.24)	0.91 (0.30)	0.23* (0.13)	0.94 (0.32)
Adults (n=12)	250 mg	4.82 (2.13)	4.92 (1.13)	1.70† (0.53)	0.53 (0.17)	1.28 (0.34)
Children (n=19)	15 mg/kg	10.86 (2.55)	8.47 (2.03)	2.75 (1.07)	0.61‡ (0.27)	1.24 (0.43)
Adults (n=12)	500 mg	8.39 (1.95)	9.42 (0.98)	3.18§ (0.76)	1.00§ (0.24)	1.29 (0.14)
Children (n=10)	30 mg/kg	6.69 (4.26)	17.61 (6.39)	8.66 (2.70)	—	2.06 (0.21)
Adults (n=12)	1000 mg	11.99 (4.67)	16.95 (4.07)	8.36 (4.13)	2.79 (1.77)	1.27 (0.12)

* n=11
† n=5
‡ n=9
§ n=11

MICROBIOLOGY

Cefprozil has *in vitro* activity against a broad range of gram-positive and gram-negative bacteria. The bactericidal action of cefprozil results from inhibition of cell-wall synthesis. Cefprozil has been shown to be active against most strains of the following microorganisms both *in vitro* and in clinical infections as described in INDICATIONS AND USAGE.

Aerobic Gram-Positive Microorganisms:

Staphylococcus aureus (including β-lactamase-producing strains), *Streptococcus pneumoniae, Streptococcus pyogenes.*

NOTE: Cefprozil is inactive against methicillin-resistant *staphylococci.*

Aerobic Gram-Negative Microorganisms:

Haemophilus influenzae (including β-lactamase-producing strains), *Moraxella (Branamella) catarrhalis* (including β-lactamase-producing strains).

The following *in vitro* data are available; however, their clinical significance is unknown. Cefprozil exhibits *in vitro* minimum inhibitory concentrations (MICs) of 8 µg/ml or less against most (≥90%) strains of the following microorganisms; however, the safety and effectiveness of cefprozil in treating clinical infections due to these microorganisms have not been established in adequate and well-controlled clinical trials.

Aerobic Gram-Positive Microorganisms:

Enterococcus durans, Enterococcus faecalis, Listeria monocytogenes, Staphylococcus epidermidis, Staphylococcus saprophyticus, Staphylococcus warneri, Streptococcus agalactiae, Streptococci (Groups C, D, F, and G), Viridans group Streptococci.

NOTE: Cefprozil is inactive against *Enterococcus faecium.*

Aerobic Gram-Negative Microorganisms:

Citrobacter diversus, Eschenchia coli, Kiebsiella pneumoniae, Neissena gonorrhoeae (including β-lactamase-producing strains), *Proteus mirabilis, Salmonella* spp., *Shigella* spp., *Vibrio* spp.

NOTE: Cefprozil is inactive against most strains of *Acinetobacter, Enterobacter, Morganella morganii, Proteus vulgans, Providencia, Pseudomonas,* and *Serratia.*

Anaerobic Microorganisms:

Prevotella (Bacteroides) melaninogenicus, Clostridium difficile, Clostridium perfringens, Fusobacterium spp., *Peptostreptococcus* spp., *Propionibactenum acnes.*

NOTE: Most strains of the *Bacteroides fragilis* group are resistant to cefprozil.

SUSCEPTIBILITY TESTS

Dilution Techniques

Quantitative methods are used to determine antimicrobial minimal inhibitory concentrations (MICs). These MICs provide estimates of the susceptibility of bacteria to antimicrobial compounds. The MICs should be determined using a standardized procedure. Standardized procedures are based on a dilution method[1,2] (broth or agar) or equivalent with standardized inoculum concentrations and standardized concentrations of cefprozil powder. The MIC values should be interpreted according to the criteria found in TABLE 3.

TABLE 3

MIC (µg/ml)	Interpretation
≤8	Susceptible (S)
16	Intermediate (I)
≥32	Resistant (R)

A report of "Susceptible" indicates that the pathogen is likely to be inhibited if the antimicrobial compound in the blood reaches the concentrations usually achievable. A report of "Intermediate" indicates that the result should be considered equivocal, and, if the microorganism is not fully susceptible to alternative, clinically feasible drugs, the test should be repeated. This category implies possible clinical applicability in body sites where the drug is physiologically concentrated or in situations where high dosage of drug can be used. This category also provides a buffer zone which prevents small uncontrolled technical factors from causing major discrepancies in interpretation. A report of "Resistant" indicates that the pathogen is not likely to be inhibited if the antimicrobial compound in the blood reaches the concentrations usually achievable; other therapy should be selected.

Standardized susceptibility test procedures require the use of laboratory control microorganisms to control the technical aspects of the laboratory procedures. Standard cefprozil powder should provide the MIC values found in TABLE 4.

TABLE 4

Microorganism	MIC (µg/ml)
Enterococcus faecalis ATCC 29212	4-16
Escherichia coli ATCC 25922	1-4
Haemophilus influenzae ATCC 49766	1-4
Staphylococcus aureus ATCC 29213	0.25-1
Streptococcus pneumoniae ATCC 49619	0.25-1

Diffusion Techniques

Quantitative methods that require measurement of zone diameters also provide reproducible estimates of the susceptibility of bacteria to antimicrobial compounds. One such standardized procedure[3] requires the use of standardized inoculum concentrations. This procedure uses paper disks impregnated with 30 µg cefprozil to test the susceptibility of microorganisms to cefprozil.

Reports from the laboratory providing results of the standard single-disk susceptibility test with a 30 µg cefprozil disk should be interpreted according to the criteria found in TABLE 5.

TABLE 5

Zone Diameter (mm)	Interpretation
≥18	Susceptible (S)
15-17	Intermediate (I)
≤14	Resistant (R)

Interpretation should be as stated above for results using dilution techniques. Interpretation involves correlation of the diameter obtained in the disk test with the MIC for cefprozil.

As with standardized dilution techniques, diffusion methods require the use of laboratory control microorganisms that are used to control the technical aspects of the laboratory procedures. For the diffusion technique, the 30 µg cefprozil disk should provide the following zone diameters in these laboratory test quality control strains (see TABLE 6).

TABLE 6

Microorganism	Zone Diameter (mm)
Escherichia coli ATCC 25922	21-27
Haemophilus influenzae ATCC 49766	20-27
Staphylococcus aureus ATCC 25923	27-33
Streptococcus pneumoniae ATCC 49619	25-32

INDICATIONS AND USAGE

Cefprozil is indicated for the treatment of patients with mild to moderate infections caused by susceptible strains of the designated microorganisms in the conditions listed below:

Upper Respiratory Tract:

Pharyngitis/Tonsillitis caused by *Streptococcus pyogenes*.

NOTE: The usual drug of choice in the treatment and prevention of streptococcal infections, including the prophylaxis of rheumatic fever, is penicillin given by the intramuscular route. Cefprozil is generally effective in the eradication of *Streptococcus pyogenes* from the nasopharynx; however, substantial data establishing the efficacy of cefprozil in the subsequent prevention of rheumatic fever are not available at present.

Otitis Media caused by *Streptococcus pneumoniae, Haemophilus influenzae* (including β-lactamase-producing strains), and *Moraxella (Branhamella) catarrhalis* (including β-lactamase-producing strains).

NOTE: In the treatment of otitis media due to β-lactamase producing organisms, cefprozil had bacteriologic eradication rates somewhat lower than those observed with a product containing a specific β-lactamase inhibitor. In considering the use of cefprozil, lower overall eradication rates should be balanced against the susceptibility patterns of the common microbes in a given geographic area and the increased potential for toxicity with products containing β-lactamase inhibitors.

Acute Sinusitis caused by *Streptococcus pneumoniae, Haemophilus influenzae* (including β-lactamase-producing strains), and *Moraxella (Branhamella) catarrhalis* (including β-lactamase-producing strains).

Lower Respiratory Tract:

Secondary bacterial infection of acute bronchitis and acute bacterial exacerbation of chronic bronchitis caused by *Streptococcus pneumoniae, Haemophilus influenzae* (including β-lactamase-producing strains), and *Moraxella (Branhamella) catarrhalis,* (including β-lactamase-producing strains).

Skin and Skin Structure:

Uncomplicated skin and skin-structure infections caused by *Staphylococcus aureus* (including penicillinase-producing strains) and *Streptococcus pyogenes.* Abscesses usually require surgical drainage.

Culture and susceptibility testing should be performed when appropriate to determine susceptibility of the causative organism to cefprozil.

CONTRAINDICATIONS

Cefprozil is contraindicated in patients with known allergy to the cephalosporin class of antibiotics.

WARNINGS

BEFORE THERAPY WITH CEFPROZIL IS INSTITUTED, CAREFUL INQUIRY SHOULD BE MADE TO DETERMINE WHETHER THE PATIENT HAS HAD PREVIOUS HYPERSENSITIVITY REACTIONS TO CEFPROZIL, CEPHALOSPORINS, PENICILLINS, OR OTHER DRUGS. IF THIS PRODUCT IS TO BE GIVEN TO PENICILLIN-SENSITIVE PATIENTS, CAUTION SHOULD BE EXERCISED BECAUSE CROSS-SENSITIVITY AMONG β-LACTAM ANTIBIOTICS HAS BEEN CLEARLY DOCUMENTED AND MAY OCCUR IN UP TO 10% OF PATIENTS WITH A HISTORY OF PENICILLIN ALLERGY. IF AN ALLERGIC REACTION TO CEFPROZIL OCCURS, DISCONTINUE THE DRUG. SERIOUS ACUTE HYPERSENSITIVITY REACTIONS MAY REQUIRE TREATMENT WITH EPINEPHRINE AND OTHER EMERGENCY MEASURES, INCLUDING OXYGEN, INTRAVENOUS FLUIDS, INTRAVENOUS ANTIHISTAMINES, CORTICOSTEROIDS, PRESSOR AMINES, AND AIRWAY MANAGEMENT, AS CLINICALLY INDICATED.

Pseudomembranous colitis has been reported with nearly all antibacterial agents, including cefprozil, and may range in severity from mild to life-threatening. Therefore, it is important to consider this diagnosis in patients who present with diarrhea subsequent to the administration of antibacterial agents.

Treatment with antibacterial agents alters the normal flora of the colon and may permit overgrowth of clostridia. Studies indicate that a toxin produced by *Clostridium difficile* is one primary cause of "antibiotic-associated" colitis.

After the diagnosis of pseudomembranous colitis has been established, appropriate therapeutic measures should be initiated. Mild cases of pseudomembranous colitis usually respond to drug discontinuation alone. In moderate to severe cases, consideration should be given to management with fluids and electrolytes, protein supplementation, and treatment with an antibacterial drug clinically effective against *Clostridium difficile* colitis.

PRECAUTIONS

GENERAL

In patients with known or suspected renal impairment (see DOSAGE AND ADMINISTRATION), careful clinical observation and appropriate laboratory studies should be done prior to and during therapy. The total daily dose of cefprozil should be reduced in these patients because high and/or prolonged plasma antibiotic concentrations can occur in such individuals from usual doses. Cephalosporins, including cefprozil, should be given with caution to patients receiving concurrent treatment with potent diuretics since these agents are suspected of adversely affecting renal function.

Prolonged use of cefprozil may result in the overgrowth of nonsusceptible organisms. Careful observation of the patient is essential.

If superinfection occurs during therapy, appropriate measures should be taken.

Cefprozil should be prescribed with caution in individuals with a history of gastrointestinal disease particularly colitis.

Positive direct Coombs' tests have been reported during treatment with cephalosporin antibiotics.

INFORMATION FOR THE PATIENT

Phenylketonurics: Cefprozil for oral suspension contains phenylalanine 28 mg per 5 ml (1 teaspoonful) constituted suspension for both the 125 mg/5 ml and 250 mg/5 ml dosage forms.

DRUG/LABORATORY TEST INTERACTIONS

Cephalosporin antibiotics may produce a false positive reaction for glucose in the urine with copper reduction tests (Benedict's or Fehling's solution or with Clinitest tablets), but not with enzyme-based tests for glycosuria (*e.g.,* Tes-Tape). A false negative reaction may occur in the ferricyanide test for blood glucose. The presence of cefprozil in the blood does not interfere with the assay of plasma or urine creatinine by the alkaline picrate method.

CARCINOGENESIS, MUTAGENESIS, AND IMPAIRMENT OF FERTILITY

Long term *in vivo* studies have not been performed to evaluate the carcinogenic potential of cefprozil.

Cefprozil was not found to be mutagenic in either the Ames *Salmonella* or *E. coli* WP2 urvA reversion assays or the Chinese hamster ovary cell HGPRT forward gene mutation assay and it did not induce chromosomal abnormalities in Chinese hamster ovary cells or unscheduled DNA synthesis in rat hepatocytes *in vitro.* Chromosomal aberrations were not observed in bone marrow cells from rats dosed orally with over 30 times the highest recommended human dose based upon mg/m^2.

Impairment of fertility was not observed in male or female rats given oral doses of cefprozil up to 18.5 times the highest recommended human dose based upon mg/m^2.

PREGNANCY, TERATOGENIC EFFECTS, PREGNANCY CATEGORY B

Reproduction studies have been performed in rabbits, mice, and rats using oral doses of cefprozil of 0.8, 8.5 and 18.5 times the maximum daily human dose (1000 mg) based upon mg/m^2, and have revealed no harm to the fetus. There are, however, no adequate and well-controlled studies in pregnant women. Because animal reproduction studies are not always predictive of human response, this drug should be used during pregnancy only if clearly needed.

LABOR AND DELIVERY

Cefprozil has not been studied for use during labor and delivery. Treatment should only be given if clearly needed.

NURSING MOTHERS

Small amounts of cefprozil (<0.3% of dose) have been detected in human milk following administration of a single 1 g dose to lactating women. The average levels over 24 hours ranged from 0.25-3.3 µg/ml. Caution should be exercised when cefprozil is administered to a nursing woman, since the effect of cefprozil on nursing infants is unknown.

PEDIATRIC USE

See INDICATIONS AND USAGE and DOSAGE AND ADMINISTRATION.

The safety and effectiveness of cefprozil in the treatment of otitis media have been established in the age groups 6 months to 12 years. Use of cefprozil for the treatment of otitis media is supported by evidence from adequate and well-controlled studies of cefprozil in pediatric patients.

The safety and effectiveness of cefprozil in the treatment of pharyngitis/tonsillitis or uncomplicated skin and skin structure infections have been established in the age groups 2-12 years. Use of cefprozil for the treatment of these infections is supported by evidence from adequate and well-controlled studies in pediatric patients.

The safety and effectiveness of cefprozil in the treatment of acute sinusitis have been established in the age groups 6 months to 12 years. Use of cefprozil in these age groups is supported by evidence from adequate and well-controlled studies of cefprozil in adults.

Safety and effectiveness in pediatric patients below the age of 6 months have not been established for the treatment of otitis media or acute sinusitis or below the age of 2 years for the treatment of pharyngitis/tonsillitis or uncomplicated skin and skin structure infections. However, accumulation of other cephalosporin antibiotics in newborn infants (resulting from prolonged drug half-life in this age group) has been reported.

GERIATRIC USE

Of the more than 4500 adults treated with cefprozil in clinical studies, 14% were 65 years and older, while 5% were 75 years and older. When geriatric patients received the usual recommended adult doses, their clinical efficacy and safety were comparable to clinical efficacy and safety in nongeriatric adult patients. Other reported clinical experience has not identified differences in responses between elderly and younger patients, but greater sensitivity of some older individuals to the effects of cefprozil cannot be excluded (see CLINICAL PHARMACOLOGY).

Cefprozil is known to be substantially excreted by the kidney, and the risk of toxic reactions to this drug may be greater in patients with impaired renal function. Because elderly patients are more likely to have decreased renal function, care should be taken in dose selection and it may be useful to monitor renal function. See DOSAGE AND ADMINISTRATION for dosing recommendations for patients with impaired renal function.

DRUG INTERACTIONS

Nephrotoxicity has been reported following concomitant administration of aminoglycoside antibiotics and cephalosporin antibiotics. Concomitant administration of probenecid doubled the AUC for cefprozil.

The bioavailability of the capsule formulation of cefprozil was not affected when administered 5 minutes following an antacid.

ADVERSE REACTIONS

The adverse reactions to cefprozil are similar to those observed with other orally administered cephalosporins. Cefprozil was usually well tolerated in controlled clinical trials. Approximately 2% of patients discontinued cefprozil therapy due to adverse events.

The most common adverse effects observed in patients treated with cefprozil are:

Gastrointestinal: Diarrhea (2.9%), nausea (3.5%), vomiting (1%), and abdominal pain (1%).

Hepatobiliary: Elevations of AST (SGOT) (2%), ALT (SGPT) (2%), alkaline phosphatase (0.2%), and bilirubin values (<0.1%). As with some penicillins and some other cephalosporin antibiotics, cholestatic jaundice has been reported rarely.

Hypersensitivity: Rash (0.9%), urticaria (0.1%). Such reactions have been reported more frequently in children than in adults. Signs and symptoms usually occur a few days after initiation of therapy and subside within a few days after cessation of therapy.

CNS: Dizziness (1%). Hyperactivity, headache, nervousness, insomnia, confusion, and somnolence have been reported rarely (<1%). All were reversible.

Hematopoietic: Decreased leukocyte count (0.2%), eosinophilia (2.3%).

Renal: Elevated BUN (0.1%), serum creatinine (0.1%).

Other: Diaper rash and superinfection (1.5%), genital pruritus and vaginitis (1.6%).

The following adverse events, regardless of established causal relationship to cefprozil have been rarely reported during post-marketing surveillance: Anaphylaxis, angioedema, colitis (including pseudomembranous colitis), erythema multiforme, fever, serum-sickness like reactions, Stevens-Johnson Syndrome, and thrombocytopenia.

CEPHALOSPORIN CLASS PARAGRAPH

In addition to the adverse reactions listed above which have been observed in patients treated with cefprozil, the following adverse reactions and altered laboratory tests have been reported for cephalosporin-class antibiotics:

Aplastic anemia, hemolytic anemia, hemorrhage, renal dysfunction, toxic epidermal necrolysis, toxic nephropathy, prolonged prothrombin time, positive Coombs' test, elevated LDH, pancytopenia, neutropenia, agranulocytosis.

Several cephalosporins have been implicated in triggering seizures, particularly in patients with renal impairment, when the dosage was not reduced. (See DOSAGE AND ADMINISTRATION) If seizures associated with drug therapy occur, the drug should be discontinued. Anticonvulsant therapy can be given if clinically indicated.

DOSAGE AND ADMINISTRATION

Cefprozil is administered orally.

TABLE 10

Population/Infection	Dosage	Duration
Adults (13 years and older)		
Upper Respiratory Tract		
Pharyngitis/tonsillitis	500 mg q24h	10 days*
Acute sinusitis	250 mg q12h or	10 days
(For moderate to severe infections the higher dose should be used)	500 mg q12h	
Lower Respiratory Tract		
Secondary bacterial infection of acute bronchitis and acute bacterial exacerbation of chronic bronchitis	500 mg q12h	10 days
Skin and Skin Structure		
Uncomplicated skin and skin structure infections	250 mg q12h or	10 days
	500 mg q24h or	
	500 mg q12h	
Children (2-12 years)		
Upper Respiratory Tract†		
Pharyngitis/tonsillitis	7.5 mg/kg q12h	10 days*
Skin and Skin Structure†		
Uncomplicated skin and skin structure infections	20 mg/kg q24h	10 days
Infants & Children (6 months-12 years)		
Upper Respiratory Tract†		
Otitis media‡	15 mg/kg q12h	10 days
Acute sinusitis	7.5 mg/kg q12h or	10 days
(For moderate to severe infections, the higher dose should be used)	15 mg/kg q12h	

* In the treatment of infections due to *Streptococcus pyogenes,* cefprozil should be administered for at least 10 days.
† Not to exceed recommended adult doses.
‡ See INDICATIONS AND USAGE.

RENAL IMPAIRMENT

Cefprozil may be administered to patients with impaired renal function. The following dosage schedule should be used (see TABLE 11).

TABLE 11

Creatinine Clearance	Dosage (mg)	Dosing Interval
30-120 ml/min	Standard	Standard
0-29 ml/min*	50% of standard	Standard

* Cefprozil is in part removed by hemodialysis; therefore, cefprozil should be administered after the completion of hemodialysis.

HEPATIC IMPAIRMENT

No dosage adjustment is necessary for patients with impaired hepatic function.

HOW SUPPLIED

CEFZIL TABLETS

250 mg: Each light orange film-coated tablet, imprinted with "7720" on one side and "250" on the other, contains the equivalent of 250 mg anhydrous cefprozil.

500 mg: Each white film-coated tablet, imprinted with "7721" on one side and "500" on the other, contains the equivalent of 500 mg anhydrous cefprozil.

Storage: Store at controlled room temperature, 15-30°C (59-86°F).

CEFZIL FOR ORAL SUSPENSION

125 mg: Each 5 ml of constituted suspension contains the equivalent of 125 mg anhydrous cefprozil.

250 mg: Each 5 ml of constituted suspension contains the equivalent of 250 mg anhydrous cefprozil.

All powder formulations for oral suspension contain cefprozil in a bubble-gum flavored mixture.

Storage: Store at 15-25°C (59-77°F) prior to constitution. After mixing, store in a refrigerator and discard unused portion after 14 days.

PRODUCT LISTING - EQUIVALENTS NOT AVAILABLE

Powder For Reconstitution - Oral - 125 mg/5 ml

50 ml $20.25 CEFZIL, Bristol-Myers Squibb 00087-7718-40

75 ml	$30.23	CEFZIL, Bristol-Myers Squibb	00087-7718-62
100 ml	$32.65	CEFZIL, Allscripts Pharmaceutical Company	54569-3743-00
100 ml	$35.05	CEFZIL, Southwood Pharmaceuticals Inc	58016-4148-01
100 ml	$40.21	CEFZIL, Bristol-Myers Squibb	00087-7718-64
Powder For Reconstitution - Oral - 250 mg/5 ml			
50 ml	$36.46	CEFZIL, Physicians Total Care	54868-2017-01
50 ml	$37.56	CEFZIL, Bristol-Myers Squibb	00087-7719-40
75 ml	$55.20	CEFZIL, Bristol-Myers Squibb	00087-7719-62
100 ml	$59.16	CEFZIL, Allscripts Pharmaceutical Company	54569-3630-00
100 ml	$59.63	CEFZIL, Southwood Pharmaceuticals Inc	58016-4147-01
100 ml	$64.93	CEFZIL, Physicians Total Care	54868-2017-00
100 ml	$72.86	CEFZIL, Bristol-Myers Squibb	00087-7719-64
Tablet - Oral - 250 mg			
10's	$41.38	CEFZIL, Physicians Total Care	54868-3343-00
12's	$50.40	CEFZIL, Southwood Pharmaceuticals Inc	58016-0810-12
15's	$63.00	CEFZIL, Southwood Pharmaceuticals Inc	58016-0810-15
20's	$75.48	CEFZIL, Allscripts Pharmaceutical Company	54569-3652-00
30's	$126.00	CEFZIL, Southwood Pharmaceuticals Inc	58016-0810-30
60's	$232.70	CEFZIL, Southwood Pharmaceuticals Inc	58016-0810-60
100's	$420.00	CEFZIL, Southwood Pharmaceuticals Inc	58016-0810-00
100's	$420.84	CEFZIL, Bristol-Myers Squibb	00087-7720-60
Tablet - Oral - 500 mg			
20's	$127.12	CEFZIL, Pharma Pac	52959-0349-20
20's	$154.01	CEFZIL, Allscripts Pharmaceutical Company	54569-3653-00
50's	$434.55	CEFZIL, Bristol-Myers Squibb	00087-7721-50
100's	$857.23	CEFZIL, Bristol-Myers Squibb	00087-7721-60

Ceftazidime *(003116)*

For related information, see the comparative table section in Appendix A.

Categories: Cellulitis, pelvic; Endometritis; Infection, bone; Infection, central nervous system; Infection, gynecologic; Infection, intra-abdominal; Infection, joint; Infection, lower respiratory tract; Infection, skin and skin structures; Infection, urinary tract; Meningitis; Peritonitis; Pneumonia; Septicemia; Pregnancy Category B; FDA Approved 1990 Sep
Drug Classes: Antibiotics, cephalosporins
Brand Names: **Ceptaz**; Pentacef; Tazicef
Foreign Brand Availability: Ceffotan (Colombia); Cefortam (Portugal); Cefpiran (Peru); Ceftazim (Mexico); Ceftidin (India); Ceftim (Italy; Portugal); Ceftum (Indonesia); Cetazum (Indonesia); Fortam (Spain; Switzerland); Fortum (Australia; Austria; Bahamas; Bahrain; Barbados; Belize; Benin; Bermuda; Bulgaria; Burkina-Faso; China; Costa-Rica; Curacao; Cyprus; Czech-Republic; Denmark; Dominican-Republic; Ecuador; Egypt; El-Salvador; England; Ethiopia; France; Gambia; Germany; Ghana; Guinea; Guyana; Honduras; Hong-Kong; Hungary; India; Indonesia; Iran; Iraq; Ireland; Israel; Ivory-Coast; Jamaica; Jordan; Kenya; Korea; Kuwait; Lebanon; Liberia; Libya; Malawi; Malaysia; Mali; Mauritania; Mauritius; Mexico; Morocco; Netherland-Antilles; Netherlands; New-Zealand; Niger; Nigeria; Norway; Oman; Panama; Peru; Philippines; Qatar; Republic-of-Yemen; Saudi-Arabia; Senegal; Seychelles; Sierra-Leone; South-Africa; Sudan; Surinam; Sweden; Syria; Taiwan; Tanzania; Thailand; Trinidad; Tunia; Uganda; United-Arab-Emirates; Zambia; Zimbabwe); Fortum Pro (Hungary); Fortumset (France); Forzid (Indonesia; Thailand); Fournox (Thailand); Ftazidime (Greece); Izadima (Colombia; Mexico); Kefadim (Belgium; Benin; Burkina-Faso; China; Czech-Republic; Ethiopia; Gambia; Ghana; Guinea; Ivory-Coast; Kenya; Liberia; Malawi; Mali; Mauritania; Mauritius; Morocco; Niger; Nigeria; Senegal; Seychelles; Sierra-Leone; Sudan; Taiwan; Tanzania; Tunia; Uganda; Zambia; Zimbabwe); Kefamin (Spain); Kefazim (Austria); Kefzim (South-Africa); Glazidim (Belgium; Finland; Italy); Modacin (Japan); Panzid (Italy); Pharodime 19 (Indonesia); Potendal (Spain); Solvetan (Greece); Spectrum (Italy); Starcef (Italy); Tagal (Mexico); Tazidime (Canada); Tazime (China; Korea); Thidim (Indonesia); Waytrax (Mexico); Zadolina (Mexico); Zibac (Indonesia); Zytaz (India)
Cost of Therapy: $284.54 (Infection; Fortaz Injection; 1 g; 2 g/day; 10 day supply)
$433.20 (Infection; Tazicef Injection; 1 g; 2 g/day; 10 day supply)

DESCRIPTION

Note: The trade names have been used throughout this monograph for clarity.

For Intravenous or Intramuscular Use.

Ceftazidime is a semisynthetic, broad-spectrum, beta-lactam antibiotic for parenteral administration. It is the pentahydrate of pyridinium, 1-[[7-[[(2-amino-4-thiazolyl)[(1-carboxy-1-methylethoxy)imino]acetyl]amino]-2-carboxy-8-oxo-5-thia-1-azabicyclo[4.2.0]oct-2-en-3-yl]methyl]-, hydroxide, inner salt, [6R-[6α,7β(Z)]].

The empirical formula is $C_{22}H_{32}N_6O_{12}S_2$, representing a molecular weight of 636.6.

CEPTAZ

Ceptaz is a sterile, dry mixture of ceftazidime pentahydrate and L-arginine. The L-arginine is at a concentration of 349 mg/g of ceftazidime activity. Ceptaz dissolves without the evolution of gas. The product contains no sodium ion. Solutions of Ceptaz range in color from light yellow to amber, depending on the diluent and volume used. The pH of freshly constituted solutions usually ranges from 5 to 7.5.

FORTAZ

Fortaz is a sterile, dry powdered mixture of ceftazidime pentahydrate and sodium carbonate. The sodium carbonate at a concentration of 118 mg/g of ceftazidime activity has been admixed to facilitate dissolution. The total sodium content of the mixture is approximately 54 mg (2.3 mEq)/g of ceftazidime activity.

Fortaz in sterile crystalline form is supplied in vials equivalent to 500 mg, 1, 2, or 6 g of anhydrous ceftazidime and in ADD-Vantage vials equivalent to 1 or 2 g of anhydrous ceftazidime. Solutions of Fortaz range in color from light yellow to amber, depending on the diluent and volume used. The pH of freshly constituted solutions usually ranges from 5-8.

Fortaz is available as a frozen, iso-osmotic, sterile, nonpyrogenic solution with 1 or 2 g of ceftazidime as ceftazidime sodium premixed with approximately 2.2 or 1.6 g, respectively, of dextrose hydrous. Dextrose has been added to adjust the osmolality. Sodium hydroxide is used to adjust pH and neutralize ceftazidime pentahydrate free acid to the sodium salt. The pH may have been adjusted with hydrochloric acid. Solutions of premixed Fortaz range in color from light yellow to amber. The solution is intended for intravenous (IV) use after thawing to room temperature. The osmolality of the solution is approximately 300 mOsmol/kg, and the pH of thawed solutions ranges from 5 to 7.5.

The plastic container for the frozen solution is fabricated from a specially designed multilayer plastic, PL 2040. Solutions are in contact with the polyethylene layer of this container and can leach out certain chemical components of the plastic in very small amounts within the expiration period. The suitability of the plastic has been confirmed in tests in animals according to USP biological tests for plastic containers as well as by tissue culture toxicity studies.

CLINICAL PHARMACOLOGY

After IV administration of 500 mg and 1 g doses of ceftazidime over 5 minutes to normal adult male volunteers, mean peak serum concentrations of 45 and 90 μg/ml, respectively, were achieved. After IV infusion of 500 mg, 1 g, and 2 g doses of ceftazidime over 20-30 minutes to normal adult male volunteers, mean peak serum concentrations of 42, 69, and 170 μg/ml, respectively, were achieved. The average serum concentrations following IV infusion of 500 mg, 1 g, and 2 g doses to these volunteers over an 8 hour interval are given in TABLE 1.

TABLE 1 *Average Serum Concentrations of Ceftazidime*

Ceftazidime	Serum Concentrations (μg/ml)				
IV Dose	0.5 h	1 h	2 h	4 h	8 h
500 mg	42	25	12	6	2
1 g	60	39	23	11	3
2 g	129	75	42	13	5

The absorption and elimination of ceftazidime were directly proportional to the size of the dose. The half-life following IV administration was approximately 1.9 hours. Less than 10% of ceftazidime was protein bound. The degree of protein binding was independent of concentration. There was no evidence of accumulation of ceftazidime in the serum in individuals with normal renal function following multiple IV doses of 1 and 2 g every 8 hours for 10 days.

Following intramuscular (IM) administration of 500 mg and 1 g doses of ceftazidime to normal adult volunteers, the main peak serum concentrations were 17 and 39 μg/ml, respectively, at approximately 1 hour. Serum concentrations remained above 4 μg/ml for 6 and 8 hours after the IM administration of 500 mg and 1 g doses, respectively. The half-life of ceftazidime in these volunteers was approximately 2 hours.

The presence of hepatic dysfunction had no effect on the pharmacokinetics of ceftazidime in individuals administered 2 g intravenously every 8 hours for 5 days. Therefore, a dosage adjustment from the normal recommended dosage is not required for patients with hepatic dysfunction, provided renal function is not impaired.

Approximately 80-90% of an IM or IV dose of ceftazidime is excreted unchanged by the kidneys over a 24 hour period. After the IV administration of single 500 mg or 1 g doses, approximately 50% of the dose appeared in the urine in the first 2 hours. An additional 20% was excreted between 2 and 4 hours after dosing, and approximately another 12% of the dose appeared in the urine between 4 and 8 hours later. The elimination of ceftazidime by the kidneys resulted in high therapeutic concentrations in the urine.

The mean renal clearance of ceftazidime was approximately 100 ml/min. The calculated plasma clearance of approximately 115 ml/min indicated nearly complete elimination of ceftazidime by the renal route. Administration of probenecid before dosing had no effect on the elimination kinetics of ceftazidime. This suggested that ceftazidime is eliminated by glomerular filtration and is not actively secreted by renal tubular mechanisms.

Since ceftazidime is eliminated almost solely by the kidneys, its serum half-life is significantly prolonged in patients with impaired renal function. Consequently, dosage adjustments in such patients as described in DOSAGE AND ADMINISTRATION are suggested.

Therapeutic concentrations of ceftazidime achieved in specific body tissues and fluids are depicted in TABLE 2.

TABLE 2 *Ceftazidime Concentrations in Body Tissues and Fluids*

Tissue or Fluid	Dose/Route	No. of Patients	Time of Sample Postdose	Average Tissue or Fluid Level (μg/ml or μg/g)
Urine	500 mg IM	6	0-2 h	2,100.0
	2 g IV	6	0-2 h	12,000.0
Bile	2 g IV	3	90 min	36.4
Synovial fluid	2 g IV	13	2 h	25.6
Peritoneal fluid	2 g IV	8	2 h	48.6
Sputum	1 g IV	8	1 h	9.0
Cerebrospinal fluid	2 g q8h IV	5	120 min	9.8
(Inflamed meninges)	2 g q8h IV	6	180 min	9.4
Aqueous humor	2 g IV	13	1-3 h	11.0
Blister fluid	1 g IV	7	2-3 h	19.7
Lymphatic fluid	1 g IV	7	2-3 h	23.4
Bone	2 g IV	8	0.67 h	31.1
Heart muscle	2 g IV	35	30-280 min	12.7
Skin	2 g IV	22	30-180 min	6.6
Skeletal muscle	2 g IV	35	30-280 min	9.4
Myometrium	2 g IV	31	1-2 h	18.7

MICROBIOLOGY

Ceftazidime is bactericidal in action, exerting its effect by inhibition of enzymes responsible for cell-wall synthesis. A wide range of gram-negative organisms is susceptible to ceftazidime *in vitro,* including strains resistant to gentamicin and other aminoglycosides. In addition, ceftazidime has been shown to be active against gram-positive organisms. It is highly stable to most clinically important beta-lactamases, plasmid or chromosomal, which are produced by both gram-negative and gram-positive organisms and, consequently, is active against many strains resistant to ampicillin and other cephalosporins.

Ceftazidime has been shown to be active against the following organisms both *in vitro* and in clinical infections (see INDICATIONS AND USAGE).

Gram-Negative Aerobes:

Citrobacter spp., including *Citrobacter freundii* and *Citrobacter diversus.*
Enterobacter spp., including *Enterobacter cloacae* and *Enterobacter aerogenes.*
Escherichia coli.
Haemophilus influenzae, including ampicillin-resistant strains.
Klebsiella spp. (including *Klebsiella pneumoniae*).
Neisseria meningitidis.
Proteus mirabilis.
Proteus vulgaris.
Pseudomonas spp. (including *Pseudomonas aeruginosa*).
Serratia spp.

Gram-Positive Aerobes:

Staphylococcus aureus, including penicillinase- and non-penicillinase-producing strains.
Streptococcus agalactiae (group B streptococci).
Streptococcus pneumoniae.
Streptococcus pyogenes (group A beta-hemolytic streptococci).

Anaerobes:

Bacteroides spp. (*Note:* Many strains of *Bacteroides fragilis* are resistant).

Ceftazidime has been shown to be active *in vitro* against most strains of the following organisms; however, the clinical significance of these data is unknown:

Acinetobacter spp.
Clostridium spp. (not including *Clostridium difficile*).
Haemophilus parainfluenzae.
Morganella morganii (formerly *Proteus morganii*).
Neisseria gonorrhoeae.
Peptococcus spp.
Peptostreptococcus spp.
Providencia spp. (including *Providencia rettgeri,* formerly *Proteus rettgeri*).
Salmonella spp.
Shigella spp.
Staphylococcus epidermidis.
Yersinia enterocolitica.

Ceftazidime and the aminoglycosides have been shown to be synergistic *in vitro* against *Pseudomonas aeruginosa* and the enterobacteriaceae. Ceftazidime and carbenicillin have also been shown to be synergistic *in vitro* against *Pseudomonas aeruginosa.*

Ceftazidime is not active *in vitro* against methicillin-resistant staphylococci, *Streptococcus faecalis* and many other enterococci, *Listeria monocytogenes, Campylobacter* spp., or *Clostridium difficile.*

SUSCEPTIBILITY TESTING

Diffusion Techniques

Quantitative methods that require measurement of zone diameters give an estimate of antibiotic susceptibility. One such procedure[1-3] has been recommended for use with disks to test susceptibility to ceftazidime.

Reports from the laboratory giving results of the standard single-disk susceptibility test with a 30 µg ceftazidime disk should be interpreted according to the following criteria:

Susceptible organisms produce zones of 18 mm or greater, indicating that the test organism is likely to respond to therapy.

Organisms that produce zones of 15-17 mm are expected to be susceptible if high dosage is used or if the infection is confined to tissues and fluids (*e.g.,* urine) in which high antibiotic levels are attained.

Resistant organisms produce zones of 14 mm or less, indicating that other therapy should be selected.

Organisms should be tested with the ceftazidime disk since ceftazidime has been shown by *in vitro* tests to be active against certain strains found resistant when other beta-lactam disks are used.

Standardized procedures require the use of laboratory control organisms. The 30 µg ceftazidime disk should give zone diameters between 25 and 32 mm for *Escherichia coli* ATCC 25922. For *Pseudomonas aeruginosa* ATCC 27853, the zone diameters should be between 22 and 29 mm. For *Staphylococcus aureus* ATCC 25923, the zone diameters should be between 16 and 20 mm.

Dilution Techniques

In other susceptibility testing procedures, *e.g.,* ICS agar dilution or the equivalent, a bacterial isolate may be considered susceptible if the minimum inhibitory concentration (MIC) value for ceftazidime is not more than 16 µg/ml. Organisms are considered resistant to ceftazidime if the MIC is ≥64 µg/ml. Organisms having an MIC value of <64 µg/ml but >16 µg/ml are expected to be susceptible if high dosage is used or if the infection is confined to tissues and fluids (*e.g.,* urine) in which high antibiotic levels are attained.

As with standard diffusion methods, dilution procedures require the use of laboratory control organisms. Standard ceftazidime powder should give MIC values in the range of 4-16 µg/ml for *Staphylococcus aureus* ATCC 25923. For *Escherichia coli* ATCC 25922, the MIC range should be between 0.125 and 0.5 µg/ml. For *Pseudomonas aeruginosa* ATCC 27853, the MIC range should be between 0.5 and 2 µg/ml.

INDICATIONS AND USAGE

Ceftazidime is indicated for the treatment of patients with infections caused by susceptible strains of the designated organisms in the following diseases:

Lower Respiratory Tract Infections: Including pneumonia, caused by *Pseudomonas aeruginosa* and other *Pseudomonas* spp.; *Haemophilus influenzae,* including ampicillin-resistant strains; *Klebsiella* spp.; *Enterobacter* spp.; *Proteus mirabilis; Escherichia coli; Serratia* spp.; *Citrobacter* spp.; *Streptococcus pneumoniae;* and *Staphylococcus aureus* (methicillin-susceptible strains).

Skin and Skin-Structure Infections: Caused by *Pseudomonas aeruginosa; Klebsiella* spp.; *Escherichia coli; Proteus* spp., including *Proteus mirabilis* and indole-positive *Proteus; Enterobacter* spp.; *Serratia* spp.; *Staphylococcus aureus* (methicillin-susceptible strains); and *Streptococcus pyogenes* (group A beta-hemolytic streptococci).

Urinary Tract Infections: Both complicated and uncomplicated, caused by *Pseudomonas aeruginosa; Enterobacter* spp.; *Proteus* spp.; including *Proteus mirabilis* and indole-positive *Proteus; Klebsiella* spp.; and *Escherichia coli.*

Bacterial Septicemia: Caused by *Pseudomonas aeruginosa; Klebsiella* spp.; *Haemophilus influenzae; Escherichia coli; Serratia* spp.; *Streptococcus pneumoniae;* and *Staphylococcus aureus* (methicillin-susceptible strains).

Bone and Joint Infections: Caused by *Pseudomonas aeruginosa; Klebsiella* spp.; *Enterobacter* spp.; and *Staphylococcus aureus* (methicillin-susceptible strains).

Gynecologic Infections: Including endometritis, pelvic cellulitis, and other infections of the female genital tract caused by *Escherichia coli.*

Intra-Abdominal Infections: Including peritonitis caused by *Escherichia coli, Klebsiella* spp., and *Staphylococcus aureus* (methicillin-susceptible strains) and polymicrobial infections caused by aerobic and anaerobic organisms and *Bacteroides* spp. (many strains of *Bacteroides fragilis* are resistant).

Central Nervous System Infections: Including meningitis, caused by *Haemophilus influenzae* and *Neisseria meningitidis.* Ceftazidime has also been used successfully in a limited number of cases of meningitis due to *Pseudomonas aeruginosa* and *Streptococcus pneumoniae.*

Specimens for bacterial cultures should be obtained before therapy in order to isolate and identify causative organisms and to determine their susceptibility to ceftazidime. Therapy may be instituted before results of susceptibility studies are known; however, once these results become available, the antibiotic treatment should be adjusted accordingly.

Ceftazidime may be used alone in cases of confirmed or suspected sepsis. Ceftazidime has been used successfully in clinical trials as empiric therapy in cases where various concomitant therapies with other antibiotics have been used.

Ceftazidime may also be used concomitantly with other antibiotics, such as aminoglycosides, vancomycin, and clindamycin; in severe and life-threatening infections; and in the immunocompromised patient (see DOSAGE AND ADMINISTRATION, Compatibility and Stability). When such concomitant treatment is appropriate, prescribing information in the labeling for the other antibiotics should be followed. The dose depends on the severity of the infection and the patient's condition.

CONTRAINDICATIONS

Ceftazidime is contraindicated in patients who have shown hypersensitivity to ceftazidime or the cephalosporin group of antibiotics.

WARNINGS

BEFORE THERAPY WITH CEPTAZIDIME IS INSTITUTED, CAREFUL INQUIRY SHOULD BE MADE TO DETERMINE WHETHER THE PATIENT HAS HAD PREVIOUS HYPERSENSITIVITY REACTIONS TO CEFTAZIDIME, CEPHALOSPORINS, PENICILLINS, OR OTHER DRUGS. IF THIS PRODUCT IS TO BE GIVEN TO PENICILLIN-SENSITIVE PATIENTS, CAUTION SHOULD BE EXERCISED BECAUSE CROSS-HYPERSENSITIVITY AMONG BETA-LACTAM ANTIBIOTICS HAS BEEN CLEARLY DOCUMENTED AND MAY OCCUR IN UP TO 10% OF PATIENTS WITH A HISTORY OF PENICILLIN ALLERGY. IF AN ALLERGIC REACTION TO CEPTAZIDIME OCCURS, DISCONTINUE THE DRUG. SERIOUS ACUTE HYPERSENSITIVITY REACTIONS MAY REQUIRE TREATMENT WITH EPINEPHRINE AND OTHER EMERGENCY MEASURES, INCLUDING OXYGEN, IV FLUIDS, IV ANTIHISTAMINES, CORTICOSTEROIDS, PRESSOR AMINES, AND AIRWAY MANAGEMENT, AS CLINICALLY INDICATED.

Pseudomembranous colitis has been reported with nearly all antibacterial agents, including ceftazidime, and may range in severity from mild to life threatening. Therefore, it is important to consider this diagnosis in patients who present with diarrhea subsequent to the administration of antibacterial agents.

Treatment with antibacterial agents alters the normal flora of the colon and may permit overgrowth of clostridia. Studies indicate that a toxin produced by *Clostridium difficile* is one primary cause of "antibiotic-associated colitis".

After the diagnosis of pseudomembranous colitis has been established, appropriate therapeutic measures should be initiated. Mild cases of pseudomembranous colitis usually respond to drug discontinuation alone. In moderate to severe cases, consideration should be given to management with fluids and electrolytes, protein supplementation, and treatment with an antibacterial drug clinically effective against *Clostridium difficile* colitis.

Elevated levels of ceftazidime in patients with renal insufficiency can lead to seizures, encephalopathy, coma, asterixis, neuromuscular excitability, and myoclonia (see PRECAUTIONS).

PRECAUTIONS

GENERAL

High and prolonged serum ceftazidime concentrations can occur from usual dosages in patients with transient or persistent reduction of urinary output because of renal insufficiency. The total daily dosage should be reduced when ceftazidime is administered to patients with renal insufficiency (see DOSAGE AND ADMINISTRATION). Elevated levels of ceftazidime in these patients can lead to seizures, encephalopathy, coma, asterixis, neuromuscular excitability, and myoclonia. Continued dosage should be determined by degree of renal impairment, severity of infection, and susceptibility of the causative organisms.

As with other antibiotics, prolonged use of ceftazidime may result in overgrowth of nonsusceptible organisms. Repeated evaluation of the patient's condition is essential. If superinfection occurs during therapy, appropriate measures should be taken.

Inducible type I beta-lactamase resistance has been noted with some organisms (*e.g., Enterobacter* spp., *Pseudomonas* spp., and *Serratia* spp.). As with other extended-spectrum beta-lactam antibiotics, resistance can develop during therapy, leading to clinical failure in some cases. When treating infections caused by these organisms, periodic susceptibility testing should be performed when clinically appropriate. If patients fail to respond to monotherapy, an aminoglycoside or similar agent should be considered.

Cephalosporins may be associated with a fall in prothrombin activity. Those at risk include patients with renal or hepatic impairment, or poor nutritional state, as well as patients receiving a protracted course of antimicrobial therapy. Prothrombin time should be monitored in patients at risk and exogenous vitamin K administered as indicated.

Ceftazidime should be prescribed with caution in individuals with a history of gastrointestinal disease, particularly colitis.

Arginine has been shown to alter glucose metabolism and elevate serum potassium transiently when administered at 50 times the recommended dose. The effect of lower dosing is not known.

Distal necrosis can occur after inadvertent intra-arterial administration of ceftazidime.

DRUG/LABORATORY TEST INTERACTIONS

The administration of ceftazidime may result in a false-positive reaction for glucose in the urine when using Clinitest tablets, Benedict's solution, or Fehling's solution. It is recommended that glucose tests based on enzymatic glucose oxidase reactions (such as Clinistix) be used.

CARCINOGENESIS, MUTAGENESIS, AND IMPAIRMENT OF FERTILITY

Long-term studies in animals have not been performed to evaluate carcinogenic potential. However, a mouse micronucleus test and an Ames test were both negative for mutagenic effects.

PREGNANCY, TERATOGENIC EFFECTS, PREGNANCY CATEGORY B

Reproduction studies have been performed in mice and rats at doses up to 40 times the human dose and have revealed no evidence of impaired fertility or harm to the fetus due to ceftazidime. Ceftazidime L-arginine at 23 times the human dose was not teratogenic or embryotoxic in a rat reproduction study. There are, however, no adequate and well-controlled studies in pregnant women. Because animal reproduction studies are not always predictive of human response, this drug should be used during pregnancy only if clearly needed.

NURSING MOTHERS

Ceftazidime is excreted in human milk in low concentrations. It is not known whether the arginine component of Ceptaz is excreted in human milk. Because many drugs are excreted in human milk and because safety of the arginine component of Ceptaz in nursing infants has not been established, a decision should be made whether to discontinue nursing or to discontinue Fortaz or Ceptaz, taking into account the importance of the drug to the mother. Caution should be exercised when Fortaz or Ceptaz is administered to a nursing woman.

PEDIATRIC USE

Safety of the arginine component of Ceptaz in neonates, infants, and children has not been established. This product is for use in patients 12 years and older. If treatment with ceftazidime is indicated for neonates, infants, or children, a sodium carbonate formulation should be used. See DOSAGE AND ADMINISTRATION.

GERIATRIC USE

Clinical studies of Ceptaz (L-arginine formulation of ceftazidime) did not include sufficient numbers of subjects aged 65 and over to determine whether they respond differently from younger subjects. However, of the 2221 subjects who received ceftazidime as Fortaz in 11 clinical studies, 824 (37%) were 65 and over while 391 (18%) were 75 and over. No overall differences in safety or effectiveness were observed between these subjects and younger subjects, and other reported clinical experience has not identified differences in responses between the elderly and younger patients, but greater susceptibility of some older individuals to drug effects cannot be ruled out. This drug is known to be substantially excreted by the kidney, and the risk of toxic reactions to this drug may be greater in patients with impaired renal function. Because elderly patients are more likely to have decreased renal function, care should be taken in dose selection, and it may be useful to monitor renal function (see DOSAGE AND ADMINISTRATION).

DRUG INTERACTIONS

Nephrotoxicity has been reported following concomitant administration of cephalosporins with aminoglycoside antibiotics or potent diuretics such as furosemide. Renal function should be carefully monitored, especially if higher dosages of the aminoglycosides are to be administered or if therapy is prolonged, because of the potential nephrotoxicity and ototoxicity of aminoglycosidic antibiotics. Nephrotoxicity and ototoxicity were not noted when ceftazidime was given alone in clinical trials.

Chloramphenicol has been shown to be antagonistic to beta-lactam antibiotics, including ceftazidime, based on *in vitro* studies and time kill curves with enteric gram-negative bacilli. Due to the possibility of antagonism *in vivo,* particularly when bactericidal activity is desired, this drug combination should be avoided.

ADVERSE REACTIONS

Ceftazidime is generally well tolerated. The incidence of adverse reactions associated with the administration of ceftazidime was low in clinical trials. The most common were local reactions following IV injection and allergic and gastrointestinal reactions. Other adverse reactions were encountered infrequently. No disulfiramlike reactions were reported.

The following adverse effects from clinical trials were considered to be either related to ceftazidime therapy or were of uncertain etiology:

Local Effects: Reported in fewer than 2% of patients, were phlebitis and inflammation at the site of injection (1 in 69 patients).

Hypersensitivity Reactions: Reported in 2% of patients were pruritus, rash, and fever. Immediate reactions, generally manifested by rash and/or pruritus, occurred in 1 in 285 patients. Toxic epidermal necrolysis, Stevens-Johnson syndrome, and erythema multiforme have also been reported with cephalosporin antibiotics, including ceftazidime. Angioedema and anaphylaxis (bronchospasm and/or hypotension) have been reported very rarely.

Gastrointestinal Symptoms: Reported in fewer than 2% of patients, were diarrhea (1 in 78), nausea (1 in 156), vomiting (1 in 500), and abdominal pain (1 in 416). The onset of pseudomembranous colitis symptoms may occur during or after treatment (see WARNINGS).

Central Nervous System Reactions: (Fewer than 1%) included headache, dizziness, and paresthesia. Seizures have been reported with several cephalosporins, including ceftazidime. In addition, encephalopathy, coma, asterixis, neuromuscular excitability, and myoclonia have been reported in renally impaired patients treated with unadjusted dosing regimens of ceftazidime (see PRECAUTIONS, General).

Less Frequent Adverse Events: (Fewer than 1%) were candidiasis (including oral thrush) and vaginitis.

Hematologic: Rare cases of hemolytic anemia have been reported.

LABORATORY TEST CHANGES

Noted during clinical trials with ceftazidime were transient and included: Eosinophilia (1 in 13), positive Coombs test without hemolysis (1 in 23), thrombocytosis (1 in 45), and slight elevations in one or more of the hepatic enzymes, aspartate aminotransferase (AST, SGOT) (1 in 16), alanine aminotransferase (ALT, SGPT) (1 in 15), LDH (1 in 18), GGT (1 in 19), and alkaline phosphatase (1 in 23). As with some other cephalosporins, transient elevations of blood urea, blood urea nitrogen, and/or serum creatinine were observed occasionally. Transient leukopenia, neutropenia, agranulocytosis, thrombocytopenia, and lymphocytosis were seen very rarely.

POSTMARKETING EXPERIENCE WITH CEFTAZIDIME PRODUCTS

In addition to the adverse events reported during clinical trials, the following events have been observed during clinical practice in patients treated with ceftazidime and were reported spontaneously. For some of these events, data are insufficient to allow an estimate of incidence or to establish causation.

General: Anaphylaxis; allergic reactions, which, in rare instances, were severe (*e.g.,* cardiopulmonary arrest); urticaria; pain at injection site.

Hepatobiliary Tract: Hyperbilirubinemia, jaundice.

Renal and Genitourinary: Renal impairment.

CEPHALOSPORIN-CLASS ADVERSE REACTIONS

In addition to the adverse reactions listed above that have been observed in patients treated with ceftazidime, the following adverse reactions and altered laboratory tests have been reported for cephalosporin-class antibiotics:

Adverse Reactions: Colitis, toxic nephropathy, hepatic dysfunction including cholestasis, aplastic anemia, hemorrhage.

Altered Laboratory Tests: Prolonged prothrombin time, false-positive test for urinary glucose, pancytopenia.

DOSAGE AND ADMINISTRATION

DOSAGE

The usual adult dosage is 1 g administered intravenously or intramuscularly every 8-12 hours. The dosage and route should be determined by the susceptibility of the causative organisms, the severity of infection, and the condition and renal function of the patient.

The guidelines for dosage of Ceptaz and Fortaz are listed in TABLE 3. The following dosage schedule is recommended.

TABLE 3 *Recommended Dosage Schedule*

	Dose	Frequency
Ceptaz and Fortaz		
Patients 12 Years and Older		
Usual recommended dosage	**1 g IV or IM**	**q8-12h**
Uncomplicated urinary tract infections	250 mg IV or IM	q12h
Bone and joint infections	2 g IV	q12h
Complicated urinary tract infections	500 mg IV or IM	q8-12h
Uncomplicated pneumonia; mild skin and skin-structure infections	500 mg-1 g IV or IM	q8h
Serious gynecologic and intra-abdominal infections	2 g IV	q8h
Meningitis	2 g IV	q8h
Very severe life-threatening infections, especially in immunocompromised patients	2 g IV	q8h
Lung infections caused by *Pseudomonas* spp. in patients with cystic fibrosis with normal renal function*	30-50 mg/kg IV to a maximum of 6 g/day	q8h
Fortaz Only		
Neonates		
(0-4 weeks)	30 mg/kg IV	q12h
Infants and Children		
(1 month-12 years)	30-50 mg/kg IV to a maximum of 6 g/day†	q8h

* Although clinical improvement has been shown, bacteriologic cures cannot be expected in patients with chronic respiratory disease and cystic fibrosis.

† The higher dose should be reserved for immunocompromised pediatric patients or pediatric patients with cystic fibrosis or meningitis.

Impaired Hepatic Function

No adjustment in dosage is required for patients with hepatic dysfunction.

Impaired Renal Function

Ceftazidime is excreted by the kidneys, almost exclusively by glomerular filtration. Therefore, in patients with impaired renal function (glomerular filtration rate [GFR] <50 ml/min), it is recommended that the dosage of ceftazidime be reduced to compensate for its slower excretion. In patients with suspected renal insufficiency, an initial loading dose of 1 g of ceftazidime may be given. An estimate of GFR should be made to determine the appropriate maintenance dosage. The recommended dosage is presented in TABLE 4.

***TABLE 4** Recommended Maintenance Dosages of Ceftazidime in Renal Insufficiency*

Creatinine Clearance	Recommended Unit Dose of Ceftazidime	Frequency of Dosing
50-31 ml/min	1 g	q12h
30-16 ml/min	1 g	q24h
15-6 ml/min	500 mg	q24h
<5 ml/min	500 mg	q48h

NOTE: IF THE DOSE RECOMMENDED IN TABLE 3 IS LOWER THAN THAT RECOMMENDED FOR PATIENTS WITH RENAL INSUFFICIENCY AS OUTLINED IN TABLE 4, THE LOWER DOSE SHOULD BE USED.

When only serum creatinine is available, the following formula (Cockcroft's equation)[4] may be used to estimate creatinine clearance. The serum creatinine should represent a steady state of renal function:

Males: Creatinine clearance (ml/min) = [Weight (kg) × (140 - age)] ÷ [72 × serum creatinine (mg/dl)]

Females: 0.85 × male value

In patients with severe infections who would normally receive 6 g of ceftazidime daily were it not for renal insufficiency, the unit dose given in TABLE 4 may be increased by 50% or the dosing frequency may be increased appropriately. Further dosing should be determined by therapeutic monitoring, severity of the infection, and susceptibility of the causative organism.

In pediatric patients as for adults, the creatinine clearance should be adjusted for body surface area or lean body mass, and the dosing frequency should be reduced in cases of renal insufficiency.

In patients undergoing hemodialysis, a loading dose of 1 g is recommended, followed by 1 g after each hemodialysis period.

Ceftazidime can also be used in patients undergoing intraperitoneal dialysis and continuous ambulatory peritoneal dialysis. In such patients, a loading dose of 1 g of ceftazidime may be given, followed by 500 mg every 24 hours. In addition to IV use, Fortaz can be incorporated in the dialysis fluid at a concentration of 250 mg for 2 L of dialysis fluid. It is not known whether or not ceftazidime L-arginine can be safely incorporated into dialysis fluid.

Note: Generally ceftazidime should be continued for 2 days after the signs and symptoms of infection have disappeared, but in complicated infections longer therapy may be required.

ADMINISTRATION

Ceftazidime may be given intravenously or by deep IM injection into a large muscle mass such as the upper outer quadrant of the gluteus maximus or lateral part of the thigh. Intra-arterial administration should be avoided (see PRECAUTIONS).

Intramuscular Administration: For IM administration, ceftazidime should be constituted with one of the following diluents: sterile water for injection, bacteriostatic water for injection, or 0.5% or 1% lidocaine HCl injection.

Intravenous Administration: The IV route is preferable for patients with bacterial septicemia, bacterial meningitis, peritonitis, or other severe or life-threatening infections, or for patients who may be poor risks because of lowered resistance resulting from such debilitating conditions as malnutrition, trauma, surgery, diabetes, heart failure, or malignancy, particularly if shock is present or pending.

For direct intermittent IV administration, constitute ceftazidime with sterile water for injection. Slowly inject directly into the vein over a period of 3-5 minutes or give through the tubing of an administration set while the patient is also receiving one of the compatible IV fluids (see Compatibility and Stability).

For IV infusion, constitute the 1 or 2 g infusion pack with 100 ml of sterile water for injection or one of the compatible IV fluids listed under Compatibility and Stability. Alternatively, constitute the 500 mg, 1 g, or 2 g vial and add an appropriate quantity of the resulting solution to an IV container with one of the compatible IV fluids.

Intermittent IV infusion with a Y-type administration set can be accomplished with compatible solutions. However, during infusion of a solution containing ceftazidime, it is desirable to discontinue the other solution.

ADD-Vantage vials are to be constituted only with 50 or 100 ml of 5% dextrose injection, 0.9% sodium chloride injection, or 0.45% sodium chloride injection in Abbott ADD-Vantage flexible diluent containers (see Instructions for Constitution). ADD-Vantage vials that have been joined to Abbott ADD-Vantage diluent containers and activated to dissolve the drug are stable for 24 hours at room temperature or for 7 days under refrigeration. Joined vials that have not been activated may be used within a 14 day period; this period corresponds to that for use of Abbott ADD-Vantage containers following removal of the outer packaging (overwrap).

Freezing solutions of Fortaz in the ADD-Vantage system is not recommended.

All vials of Fortaz as supplied are under reduced pressure. When Fortaz is dissolved, carbon dioxide is released and a positive pressure develops.

Vials of Ceptaz as supplied are under a slightly reduced pressure. This may assist entry of the diluent. No gas-relief needle is required when adding the diluent, except for the infusion pack where it is required during the latter stages of addition (in order to preserve product sterility, a gas-relief needle should not be inserted until an overpressure is produced in the vial). No evolution of gas occurs on constitution. When the vial contents are dissolved, vials other than infusion packs may still be under a reduced pressure. This reduced pressure is particularly noticeable for the 10 g pharmacy bulk package.

Solutions of ceftazidime, like those of most beta-lactam antibiotics, should not be added to solutions of aminoglycoside antibiotics because of potential interaction.

However, if concurrent therapy with ceftazidime and an aminoglycoside is indicated, each of these antibiotics can be administered separately to the same patient.

Directions for Use of Fortaz Frozen in Galaxy Plastic Containers

Fortaz supplied as a frozen, sterile, iso-osmotic, nonpyrogenic solution in plastic containers is to be administered after thawing either as a continuous or intermittent IV infusion. The thawed solution is stable for 24 hours at room temperature or for 7 days if stored under refrigeration. **Do not refreeze.**

Thaw container at room temperature (25°C) or under refrigeration (5°C). Do not force thaw by immersion in water baths or by microwave irradiation. Components of the solution may precipitate in the frozen state and will dissolve upon reaching room temperature with little or no agitation. Potency is not affected. Mix after solution has reached room temperature. Check for minute leaks by squeezing bag firmly. Discard bag if leaks are found as sterility may be impaired. Do not add supplementary medication. Do not use unless solution is clear and seal is intact.

Use sterile equipment.

Caution: Do not use plastic containers in series connections. Such use could result in air embolism due to residual air being drawn from the primary container before administration of the fluid from the secondary container is complete.

COMPATIBILITY AND STABILITY

Fortaz

Intramuscular

Fortaz, when constituted as directed with sterile water for injection, bacteriostatic water for injection, or 0.5% or 1% lidocaine HCl injection, maintains satisfactory potency for 24 hours at room temperature or for 7 days under refrigeration. Solutions in sterile water for injection that are frozen immediately after constitution in the original container are stable for 3 months when stored at -20°C. Once thawed, solutions should not be refrozen. Thawed solutions may be stored for up to 8 hours at room temperature or for 4 days in a refrigerator.

Intravenous

Fortaz, when constituted as directed with sterile water for injection, maintains satisfactory potency for 24 hours at room temperature or for 7 days under refrigeration. Solutions in sterile water for injection in the infusion vial or in 0.9% sodium chloride injection in Viaflex small-volume containers that are frozen immediately after constitution are stable for 6 months when stored at -20°C. Do not force thaw by immersion in water baths or by microwave irradiation. Once thawed, solutions should not be refrozen. Thawed solutions may be stored for up to 24 hours at room temperature or for 7 days in a refrigerator. More concentrated solutions in sterile water for injection in the original container that are frozen immediately after constitution are stable for 3 months when stored at -20°C. Once thawed, solutions should not be refrozen. Thawed solutions may be stored for up to 8 hours at room temperature or for 4 days in a refrigerator.

Ceptaz

Intramuscular

Ceptaz, when constituted as directed with sterile water for injection, bacteriostatic water for injection, or 0.5% or 1% lidocaine HCl injection, maintains satisfactory potency for 18 hours at room temperature or for 7 days under refrigeration. Solutions in sterile water for injection that are frozen immediately after constitution in the original container are stable for 6 months when stored at -20°C. Components of the solution may precipitate in the frozen state and will dissolve on reaching room temperature with little or no agitation. Potency is not affected. Frozen solutions should only be thawed at room temperature. Do not force thaw by immersion in water baths or by microwave irradiation. Once thawed, solutions should not be refrozen. Thawed solutions may be stored for up to 12 hours at room temperature or for 7 days in a refrigerator.

Intravenous

Ceftazidime concentration greater than 100 mg/ml (2 g vial or 10 g pharmacy bulk package): Ceptaz, when constituted as directed with sterile water for injection, 0.9% sodium chloride injection, or 5% dextrose injection, maintains satisfactory potency for 18 hours at room temperature or for 7 days under refrigeration. Solutions of a similar concentration in sterile water for injection that are frozen immediately after constitution in the original container are stable for 6 months when stored at -20°C. Components of the solution may precipitate in the frozen state and will dissolve upon reaching room temperature with little or no agitation. Potency is not affected. Frozen solutions should only be thawed at room temperature. Do not force thaw by immersion in water baths or by microwave irradiation. Once thawed, solutions should not be refrozen. Thawed solutions may be stored for up to 12 hours at room temperature or for 7 days in a refrigerator.

Ceftazidime concentration of 100 mg/ml or less (1 g vial or infusion packs): Ceptaz, when constituted as directed with sterile water for injection, 0.9% sodium chloride injection, or 5% dextrose injection, maintains satisfactory potency for 24 hours at room temperature or for 7 days under refrigeration. Solutions, prepared by a pharmacist, of the approved arginine formulation of ceftazidime of a similar concentration in sterile water for injection, 0.9% sodium chloride injection, or 5% dextrose injection in the original container or in 0.9% sodium chloride injection in Viaflex (PL 146 plastic) small-volume containers that are frozen immediately after constitution by the pharmacist are stable for 6 months when stored at -20°C. Solutions in the PL 146 plastic small-volume containers are in contact with the polyvinyl chloride layer of this container and can leach out certain chemical components of the plastic in very small amounts within the expiration period. The suitability of the plastic has been confirmed in tests in animals according to USP biological tests for plastic containers as well as by tissue culture toxicity studies. Stability of the frozen solution in other containers has not been confirmed. Frozen solutions should only be thawed at room temperature. Do not force thaw by immersion in water baths or by microwave irradiation. For the larger volumes of IV infusion solutions where it may be necessary to warm the frozen product, care should be taken to avoid heating after thawing is complete. Once thawed, solutions should not be refrozen. Thawed solutions may be stored for up to 18 hours at room temperature or for 7 days in a refrigerator.

Components of the solution may precipitate in the frozen state and will dissolve on reaching room temperature with little or no agitation. Potency is not affected. Check for minute leaks in plastic containers by squeezing bag firmly. Discard bag if leaks are found as sterility may be impaired. Do not add supplementary medication to bags. Do not use unless solution is clear and seal is intact.

Use sterile equipment.

Ceptaz and Fortaz

Ceftazidime is compatible with the more commonly used IV infusion fluids. Solutions at concentrations between 1 and 40 mg/ml in 0.9% sodium chloride injection; 1/6 M sodium lactate injection; 5% dextrose injection; 5% dextrose and 0.225% sodium chloride injection; 5% dextrose and 0.45% sodium chloride injection; 5% dextrose and 0.9% sodium chloride injection; 10% dextrose injection; Ringer's injection; lactated Ringer's injection; 10% invert sugar in water for injection; and Normosol-M in 5% dextrose injection may be stored for up to 24 hours at room temperature or for 7 days if refrigerated.

The 1 and 2 g Fortaz ADD-Vantage vials, when diluted in 50 or 100 ml of 5% dextrose injection, 0.9% sodium chloride injection, or 0.45% sodium chloride injection, may be stored for up to 24 hours at room temperature or for 7 days under refrigeration.

Ceftazidime is less stable in sodium bicarbonate injection than in other IV fluids. It is not recommended as a diluent. Solutions of ceftazidime in 5% dextrose injection and 0.9% sodium chloride injection are stable for at least 6 hours at room temperature in plastic tubing, drip chambers, and volume control devices of common IV infusion sets.

Ceftazidime at a concentration of 4 mg/ml has been found compatible for 24 hours at room temperature or for 7 days under refrigeration in 0.9% sodium chloride injection or 5% dextrose injection when admixed with: cefuroxime sodium (Zinacef) 3 mg/ml; heparin 10 or 50 U/ml; or potassium chloride 10 or 40 mEq/L.

Ceftazidime may be constituted at a concentration of 20 mg/ml with metronidazole injection 5 mg/ml, and the resultant solution may be stored for 24 hours at room temperature or for 7 days under refrigeration. Ceftazidime at a concentration of 20 mg/ml has been found compatible for 24 hours at room temperature or for 7 days under refrigeration in 0.9% sodium chloride injection or 5% dextrose injection when admixed with 6 mg/ml clindamycin (as clindamycin phosphate).

Vancomycin solution exhibits a physical incompatibility when mixed with a number of drugs, including ceftazidime. The likelihood of precipitation with ceftazidime is dependent on the concentrations of vancomycin and ceftazidime present. It is therefore recommended, when both drugs are to be administered by intermittent IV infusion, that they be given separately, flushing the IV lines (with 1 of the compatible IV fluids) between the administration of these 2 agents.

Note: Parenteral drug products should be inspected visually for particulate matter before administration whenever solution and container permit.

As with other cephalosporins, ceftazidime powder as well as solutions tend to darken, depending on storage conditions; within the stated recommendations, however, product potency is not adversely affected.

HOW SUPPLIED

FORTAZ

Fortaz in Sterile Crystalline Form

Fortaz in sterile crystalline form is supplied in vials equivalent to 500 mg, 1, 2, or 6 g of anhydrous ceftazidime and in ADD-Vantage vials equivalent to 1 or 2 g of anhydrous ceftazidime.

Storage: Fortaz in the dry state should be stored between 15 and 30°C (59 and 86°F) and protected from light. Fortaz is a dry, white to off-white powder supplied in vials and infusion packs.

Fortaz Frozen as a Premixed Solution

Fortaz is available as a frozen, iso-osmotic, sterile, nonpyrogenic solution with 1 or 2 g of ceftazidime as ceftazidime sodium premixed with approximately 2.2 or 1.6 g, respectively, of dextrose hydrous.

Storage: Fortaz frozen as a premixed solution of ceftazidime sodium should not be stored above -20°C. Fortaz is supplied frozen in 50 ml, single-dose, plastic containers.

CEPTAZ

Ceptaz is a sterile, dry mixture of ceftazidime pentahydrate and L-arginine.

Storage: Ceptaz in the dry state should be stored between 15 and 30°C (59 and 86°F) and protected from light. Ceptaz is a dry, white to off-white powder supplied in vials and infusion packs.

PRODUCT LISTING - RATED THERAPEUTICALLY EQUIVALENT

Powder For Injection - Injectable - 1 Gm

10's	$14.23	TAZIDIME, Lilly, Eli and Company	00002-7231-01
10's	$145.87	FORTAZ, Glaxosmithkline	00173-0380-32
10's	$152.00	GENERIC, Glaxosmithkline	00007-5083-76
24's	$402.00	TAZICEF, Glaxosmithkline	00007-5088-04
25's	$14.71	TAZIDIME, Lilly, Eli and Company	00002-7290-01
25's	$355.67	FORTAZ, Glaxosmithkline	00173-0378-35
25's	$355.68	TAZIDIME, Lilly, Eli and Company	00002-7231-25
25's	$367.68	TAZIDIME, Lilly, Eli and Company	00002-7290-25
25's	$367.68	FORTAZ, Glaxosmithkline	00173-0434-00
25's	$370.50	GENERIC, Glaxosmithkline	00007-5082-76
25's	$400.13	CEPTAZ, Glaxosmithkline	00173-0414-00
25's	$541.50	TAZICEF, Abbott Pharmaceutical	00074-5082-16
25's	$541.50	TAZICEF, Abbott Pharmaceutical	00074-5092-16

Powder For Injection - Injectable - 2 Gm

1's	$28.45	TAZIDIME, Lilly, Eli and Company	00002-7234-01
1's	$28.93	TAZIDIME, Lilly, Eli and Company	00002-7291-01
10's	$284.53	FORTAZ, Glaxosmithkline	00173-0379-34
10's	$284.54	TAZIDIME, Lilly, Eli and Company	00002-7234-10
10's	$288.13	FORTAZ, Glaxosmithkline	00173-0381-32
10's	$289.34	TAZIDIME, Lilly, Eli and Company	00002-7291-10
10's	$289.34	FORTAZ, Glaxosmithkline	00173-0435-00
10's	$300.20	GENERIC, Glaxosmithkline	00007-5085-76
10's	$311.17	CEPTAZ, Glaxosmithkline	00173-0417-00
10's	$311.25	GENERIC, Glaxosmithkline	00007-5084-76
10's	$427.86	TAZICEF, Abbott Pharmaceutical	00074-5084-11
10's	$433.08	TAZICEF, Abbott Pharmaceutical	00074-5093-11
24's	$739.92	TAZICEF, Glaxosmithkline	00007-5089-04
25's	$768.20	CEPTAZ, Glaxosmithkline	00173-0415-00

Powder For Injection - Injectable - 6 Gm

6's	$496.80	FORTAZ, Glaxosmithkline	00173-0382-37
10's	$862.50	TAZICEF, Glaxosmithkline	00007-5086-76
10's	$1244.86	TAZICEF, Abbott Pharmaceutical	00074-5086-11

Powder For Injection - Injectable - 10 Gm

6's	$894.24	CEPTAZ, Glaxosmithkline	00173-0418-00

Powder For Injection - Injectable - 500 mg

25's	$177.84	FORTAZ, Glaxosmithkline	00173-0377-31

Solution - Intravenous - 1 Gm/50 ml

50 ml x 24	$423.16	FORTAZ, Glaxosmithkline	00173-0412-00

Solution - Intravenous - 2 Gm/50 ml

50 ml x 24	$778.83	FORTAZ, Glaxosmithkline	00173-0413-00

PRODUCT LISTING - EQUIVALENTS NOT AVAILABLE

Powder For Injection - Injectable - 6 Gm

1's	$82.80	TAZIDIME, Lilly, Eli and Company	00002-7241-01
6's	$496.82	TAZIDIME, Lilly, Eli and Company	00002-7241-16

Ceftibuten *(003249)*

For related information, see the comparative table section in Appendix A.

Categories: Bronchitis, chronic, acute exacerbation; Infection, ear, middle; Infection, lower respiratory tract; Infection, upper respiratory tract; Pharyngitis; Tonsillitis; Pregnancy Category B
Drug Classes: Antibiotics, cephalosporins
Brand Names: Cedax
Foreign Brand Availability: Ceten (Korea); Keimax (Germany); Seftem (Japan; Korea; Taiwan)
Cost of Therapy: $85.42 (Infection; Cedax; 400 mg; 1 capsule/day; 10 day supply)

DESCRIPTION

Ceftibuten capsules and ceftibuten for oral suspension contain the active ingredient ceftibuten as ceftibuten dihydrate. Ceftibuten dihydrate is a semisynthetic cephalosporin antibiotic for oral administration. Chemically, it is (+)-(6R,7R-7-[(Z)-2-(2-Amino-4-thiazolyl)-4-carboxycrotonamido]-8-oxo-5-thia-1-azabicyclo[4.2.0]oct-2-ene-2-carboxylic acid, dihydrate. Its molecular formula is $C_{15}H_{14}N_4O_6S_2 \cdot 2H_2O$. Its molecular weight is 446.43 as a dihydrate.

Cedax contain ceftibuten dihydrate equivalent to 400 mg of ceftibuten. Inactive ingredients contained in the capsule formulation include: magnesium stearate, microcrystalline cellulose, and sodium startch glycolate. The capsule shell and/or band contains gelatin, sodium lauryl sulfate, titanium dioxide, and polysorbate 80. The capsule shell may also contain benzyl alcohol, sodium propionate, edetate calcium disodium, butylparaben, propylparaben, and methylparaben.

Cedax oral suspension after reconstitution contains ceftibuten dihydrate equivalent to either 90 mg of ceftibuten per ml or 180 mg of ceftibuten per 5 ml. Cedax oral suspension is cherry flavored and contains inactive ingredients: cherry flavoring, polysorbate 80, silicon dioxide, simethicone, sodium benzoate, sucrose (approximately 1 g/5 ml), titanium dioxide, and xanthan gum.

CLINICAL PHARMACOLOGY

PHARMACOKINETICS

Absorption

Capsules

Ceftibuten is rapidly absorbed after oral administration of capsules. The plasma concentrations and pharmacokinetic parameters of ceftibuten after a single 400 mg dose of ceftibuten capsules to 12 healthy adult male volunteers (20-39 years of age) are displayed in the table below. When ceftibuten capsules were administered once daily for 7 days, the average C_{max} was 17.9 µg/ml on day 7. Therefore, ceftibuten accumulation in plasma is about 20% at steady state.

Oral Suspension

Ceftibuten is rapidly absorbed after oral administration of ceftibuten oral suspension. The plasma concentrations and pharmacokinetic parameters of ceftibuten after a single 9 mg/kg dose of ceftibuten oral suspension to 32 fasting pediatric patients (6 months to 12 years of age) are displayed in TABLE 1.

The absolute bioavailability of ceftibuten oral suspension has not been determined. The plasma concentrations of ceftibuten in pediatric patients are dose proportional following single doses of ceftibuten capsules of 200 and 400 mg and of ceftibuten oral suspension between 4.5 and 9 mg/kg.

Distribution

Capsules

The average apparent volume of distribution (V/F) of ceftibuten in 6 adult subjects is 0.21 L/kg (±1 SD = 0.03 L/kg).

Oral Suspension

The average apparent volume of distribution (V/F) of ceftibuten in 32 fasting pediatric patients is 0.5 L/kg (±1 SD = 0.2 L/kg).

TABLE 1

Parameter	Healthy Males Single 400 mg Dose (±1 SD) (n=12)	Pediatric Patients Single 9 mg/kg Dose (±1 SD) (n=32)
Average Plasma Concentration at:		
1.0 hour	6.1 μg/ml (5.1)	9.3 μg/ml (6.3)
1.5 hours	9.9 μg/ml (5.9)	8.6 μg/ml (4.4)
2.0 hours	11.3 μg/ml (5.2)	11.2 μg/ml (4.6)
3.0 hours	13.3 μg/ml (3.0)	9.0 μg/ml (3.4)
4.0 hours	11.2 μg/ml (2.9)	6.6 μg/ml (3.1)
6.0 hours	5.8 μg/ml (1.6)	3.8 μg/ml (2.5)
8.0 hours	3.2 μg/ml (1.0)	1.6 μg/ml (1.3)
12.0 hours	1.1 μg/ml (0.4)	0.5 μg/ml μg/ml (0.4)
C_{max}	15.0 μg/ml (3.3)	13.4 μg/ml (4.9)
T_{max}	2.6 h (0.9)	2.0 h (1.0)
AUC	73.7 μg·h/ml (16.0)	56.0 μg·h/ml (16.9)
$T_{½}$	2.4 h (0.2)	2.0 h (0.6)
Total body clearance (Cl/F)	1.3 ml/min/kg (0.3)	2.9 ml/min/kg (0.7)

Protein Binding

Ceftibuten is 65% bound to plasma proteins. The protein binding is independent of plasma ceftibuten concentration.

Tissue Penetration

Bronchial Secretions

In a study of 15 adults administered a single 400 mg dose of ceftibuten and scheduled to undergo bronchoscopy, the mean concentrations in epithelial lining fluid and bronchial mucosa were 15% and 37%, respectively, of the plasma concentration.

Sputum

Ceftibuten sputum levels average approximately 7% of the concomitant plasma ceftibuten level. In a study of 24 adults administered ceftibuten 200 mg bid or 400 mg qd, the average C_{max} in sputum (1.5 μg/ml) occurred at 2 hours postdose and the average C_{max} in plasma (1.5 μg/ml) occurred at 2 hours postdose.

Middle-Ear Fluid (MEF)

Ceftibuten middle-ear fluid levels average approximately 50% of the concomitant plasma ceftibuten level. In a study of 30 children administered 9 mg/kg of ceftibuten, the average C_{max} in MEF (2.9 ± 0.9 μg/ml) occurred at 4 hours postdose and the average C_{max} in plasma (6.7 ± 1.9 μg/ml) occurred at 2 hours postdose.

Tonsillar Tissue

Data on ceftibuten penetration into tonsillar tissue are not available.

Cerebrospinal Fluid

Data on ceftibuten penetration into cerebrospinal fluid are not available.

Metabolism and Excretion

A study with radiolabeled ceftibuten administered to 6 healthy adult male volunteers demonstrated that *cis*-ceftibuten is the predominant component in both plasma and urine. About 10% of ceftibuten is converted to the *trans*-isomer. The *trans*-isomer is approximately 1/8 as antimicrobially potent as the *cis*-isomer.

Ceftibuten is excreted in the urine; 95% of the administered radioactivity was recovered either in urine or feces. In 6 healthy adult male volunteers, approximately 56% of the administered dose of ceftibuten was recovered from urine and 39% from the feces within 24 hours. Because renal excretion is a significant pathway of elimination, patients with renal dysfunction and patients undergoing hemodialysis require dosage adjustment (see DOSAGE AND ADMINISTRATION).

Food Effect on Absorption

Food affects the bioavailability of ceftibuten from capsules and oral suspension.

The effect of food on the bioavailablility of ceftibuten capsules was evaluated in 26 healthy adult male volunteers who igested 400 mg of ceftibuten capsules after an overnight fast or immediately after a standardized breakfast. Results showed that food delays the time of C_{max} by 1.75 hours, decreases the C_{max} by 18% and decreases the extent of absorption (AUC) by 8%.

The effect of food on the bioavailability of ceftibuten oral suspension was evaluated in 18 healthy adult male volunteers who ingested 400 mg of ceftibuten oral suspension after an overnight fast or immediately after a standardized breakfast. Results obtained demonstrated a decrease in C_{max} of 26% and an AUC of 17% when ceftibuten oral suspension was administered with a high-fat breakfast, and a decrease in C_{max} of 17%and in AUC of 12% when ceftibuten oral suspension was administered with a low-calorie non-fat breakfast (see PRECAUTIONS).

Bioequivalence of Dosage Formulations

A study in 18 healthy adult male volunteers demonstrated that a 400 mg dose of ceftibuten capsules produced equivalent concentrations to a 400 mg dose of ceftibuten oral suspension. Average C_{max} values were 15.6 (3.1) μg/ml for the capsule and 17.0 (3.2) μg/ml for the suspension. Average AUC values were 80.1 (14.4) μg·hr/ml for the capsule and 87.0 (12.2) μg·hr/ml for the suspension.

Special Populations

Geriatric Patients

Ceftibuten pharmacokinetic have been investigated in elderly (65 years of age or older) men (n=8) and women (n=4). Each volunteer received ceftibuten 200 mg capsules twice daily for 3½ days. The average C_{max} was 17.5 (3.7) μg/ml after 3½ days of dosing compared to 12.9 (2.1) μg/ml after the first dose; ceftibuten accumulation in plasma was 40% at steady state. Information regarding the renal function of these volunteers was not available; therefore, the significance of this finding for clinical use of ceftibuten capsules in elderly patients is not clear. Ceftibuten dosage adjustment in elderly patients may be necessary (see DOSAGE AND ADMINISTRATION).

Patients With Renal Insufficiency

Ceftibuten pharmacokinetic have been investigated in adult patients with renal dysfunction. The ceftibuten plasma half-life increased and apparent total clearance (Cl/F) decreased proportionally with increasing degree of renal dysfunction. In 6 patients with moderate renal dysfunction (creatinine clearance 30-49 ml/min), the plasma half-life of ceftibuten increased to 7.1 hours and Cl/F decreased to 30 ml/min. In 6 patients with severe renal dysfunction (creatinine clearance 5-29 ml/min), the half-life increased to 13.4 hours and Cl/F decreased to 16 ml/min. In 6 functionally anephric patients (creatinine clearance <5 ml/min), the half-life increased to 22.3 hours and Cl/F decreased to 11 ml/min (a 7- to 8-fold change compared to healthy volunteers). Hemodialysis removed 65% of the drug from the blood in 2-4 hours. These changes serve as the basis for dosage adjustment recommendations in adult patients with mild to severe renal dysfunction (see DOSAGE AND ADMINISTRATION).

MICROBIOLOGY

Ceftibuten exerts its bactericidal action by binding to essential target proteins of the baterial cell wall. This binding leads to inhibition of cell-wall synthesis.

Ceftibuten is stable in the presence of most plasmid-mediated beta-lactamases, but it is not stable in the presence of chromosomally-mediated cephalosporinases, produced in organisms such as *Bacteroides, Citrobacter, Enterobacter, Morganella,* and *Serratia.* Like other beta-lactam agents, ceftibuten should not be used against strains resistant to beta-lactams due to general mechanisms such as permeability or penicillin binding protein changes like penicillin-resistant *S. pneumoniae.*

Ceftibuten has been shown to be active against most strains of the following organisms both *in vitro* and in clinical infections (see INDICATIONS AND USAGE).

Gram-Positive Aerobes:

Streptococcus pneumoniae (penicillin-suspectible strains only)
Streptococcus pyogenes

Gram-Negative Aerobes:

Haemophilus influenzae (including β-lactamase-producing strains)
Moraxella catarrhalis (including β-lactamase-producing strains)

There are no known organisms which are potential pathogens in the indications approved for ceftibuten for which ceftibuten exhibits *in vitro* activity but for which the safety and efficacy of ceftibuten in treating clinical infections due to these organisms, have not been established in adequate and well-controlled trials.

Note

Ceftibuten is INACTIVE *in vitro* against *Acinetobacter, Bordetella, Campylobacter, Enterobacter, Enterococcus, Flacovacterium, Hafnia, Listeria, Pseudomonas, Staphylococcus,* and *Streptococcus* (except *pneumoniae* and *pyogenes*) species. In addition, it shows little *in vitro* activity against most anaerobes, including most species of *Bacteroides.*

Susceptibility Testing

Dilution Techniques

Quantitative methods are used to determine antimicrobial minimal inhibitory concentrations (MICs). These MICs provide estimates of the susceptibility of bacteria to antimicrobial compounds. The MICs should be determined using a standardized procedure. Standardized procedures are based on a dilution method (broth, agar, or microdilution) or equivalent with standardized inoculum concentrations and standardized concentrations of ceftibuten powder. The MIC values should be interpreted according to the following criteria when testing *Haemophilus* species using Haemophilus Test Media (HTM) (see TABLE 2).

TABLE 2

MIC (μg/ml)	Interpretation
≤2	(S) Susceptible

The current absence of resistant strains precludes defining any categories other than "Susceptible". Strains yielding results suggestive of a "Nonsusceptible" category should be submitted to a reference laboratory for further testing.

A report of a "Susceptible" implies that an infection due to the strain may be appropriately treated with the dosage of antimicrobial agent recommended for that type of infection and infecting species, unless otherwise contraindicated.

Ceftibuten is indicated for penicllin-susceptible only strains of *Streptococcus pneumoniase.* A pneumococcal isolate that is susceptible to penicillin (MIC ≤0.06 μg/ml) can be considered susceptible to ceftibuten for approved indications. Testing of ceftibuten against penicillin-intermediate or penicillin-resistant isolates is not recommended. Reliable interpretive criteria for ceftibuten are not currently available. Physicians should be informed that clinical response rates with ceftibuten may be lower in strains that are not pencillin-susceptible.

Standardized susceptibility test procedures require the use of laboratory control microorganisms to control the technical aspect of laboratory procedures. Standard ceftibuten powder should provide the MIC values listed in TABLE 3.

TABLE 3

Organism	MIC range (μg/ml)
Haemophilus influenzae ATCC 49247	0.25-1.0

Diffusion Techniques

Quantitative methods that require measurement of zone diameters also provide estimates of the susceptibility of bacteria to antimicrobial compounds. One such standardized procedure requires the use of standardized inoculum concentrations. This procedure uses paper disks impregnanted with 30 μg of ceftibuten to test the susceptibility of microorganisms to ceftibuten.

Reports from the laboratory providing results of the standard single-disk susceptibility test with a 30 μg ceftibuten disk should be interpreted according to the criteria listed in TABLE 4 when testing *Haemophilus* species using Haemophilus Test Media (HTM).

TABLE 4

Zone Diameter (mm)	Interpretation
≥28	(S) Susceptible

The current absence of resistant strains precludes defining any categories other than "Susceptible". Strains yielding results suggestive of a "Nonsusceptible" category should be submitted to a reference laboratory for further testing.

Interpretation should be as stated above for the results using dilution techniques.

Ceftibuten is indicated for penicillin-susceptible only strains of *Streptococcus pnemoniae.* Pneumococcal isolates with oxacillin zone sizes of ≥20 mm are susceptible to penicillin and can be considered susceptible for approved indications. Reliable disk diffusion tests for ceftibuten do not yet exist.

As with standard dilution techniques, diffusion methods require the use of laboratory control microorganisms that are used to control the technical aspects of the laboratory procedures. For the diffusion technique, the 30 μg ceftibuten disk should provide the zone diameters listed in TABLE 5 in these laboratory quality control strains.

TABLE 5

Organism	Zone Diameter (mm)
Haemophilus influenzae ATCC 49247	29-35

Cephalosporin-class disks should not be used to test for susceptibility to ceftibuten.

INDICATIONS AND USAGE

Ceftibuten is indicated for the treatment of individuals with mild-to-moderate infections caused by susceptible strains of the designated microorganisms in the specific conditions listed below (see DOSAGE AND ADMINISTRATION).

Acute Bacterial Exacerbations of Chronic Bronchitis: due to *Haemophilus influenzae* (including β-lactamase-producing strains), *Moraxella catarrhalis* (including β-lactamase-producing strains), or *Streptococcus pneumoniae* (penicillin-susceptible strains only). *NOTE:* In acute bacterial exacerbations of chronic bronchitis clinical trials where *Moraxella catarrhalis* was isolated from infected sputum at baseline, ceftibuten clinical efficacy was 22% less than control.

Acute Bacterial Otitis Media: due to *Haemophilus influenzae* (including β-lactamase-producing strains), *Moraxella catarrhalis* (including β-lactamase-producing strains), or *Streptococcus pyogenes. NOTE:* Although ceftibuten used empirically was equivalent to comparators in the treatment of clinically and/or microbiologically documented acute otitis media, the efficacy against *Streptococcus pneumoniae* was 23% less than control. Therefore, ceftibuten should be given empirically only when adequate antimicrobial coverage against *Streptococcus pneumoniae* has been previously administered.

Pharyngitis and Tonsillitis: due to *Streptococcus pyogenes. NOTE:* Only penicillin by the intramuscular route of administration has been shown to be effective in the prophylaxis of rheumatic fever. Ceftibuten is generally effective in the eradication of *Streptococcus pyogenes* from the oropharynx; however, data establishing the efficacy of ceftibuten for the prophylaxis of subsequent rheumatic fever are not available.

NON-FDA APPROVED INDICATIONS

Although not FDA approved uses, ceftibuten has been used in the treatment of sinusitis, urinary tract infections, and gonorrhea.

CONTRAINDICATIONS

Ceftibuten is contraindicated in patients with known allergy to the cephalosporin group of antibiotics.

WARNINGS

BEFORE THERAPY WITH CEFTIBUTIN IS INSTITUTED, CAREFUL INQUIRY SHOULD BE MADE TO DETERMINE WHETHER THE PATIENT HAS HAD PREVIOUS HYPERSENSITIVITY REACTIONS TO CEFTIBUTIN, OTHER CEPHALOSPORINS, PENICILLINS, OR OTHER DRUGS. IF THIS PRODUCT IS TO BE GIVEN TO PENICILLIN-SENSITIVE PATIENTS, CAUTION SHOULD BE EXERCISED BECAUSE CROSS HYPERSENSITIVITY AMONG BETA-LACTAM ANTIBIOTICS HAS BEEN CLEARLY DOCUMENTED AND MAY OCCUR IN UP TO 10% OF PATIENTS WITH A HISTORY OF PENICILLIN ALLERGY. IF AN ALLERGIC REACTION TO CEFTIBUTIN OCCURS, DISCONTINUE THE DRUG. SERIOUS ACUTE HYPERSENSITIVITY REACTIONS MAY REQUIRE TREATMENT WITH EPINEPHRINE AND OTHER EMERGENCY MEASURES, INCLUDING OXYGEN, INTRAVENOUS FLUIDS, INTRAVENOUS ANTIHISTAMINES, CORTICOSTEROIDS, PRESSOR AMINES, AND AIRWAY MANAGEMENT, AS CLINICALLY INDICATED.

Pseudomembranous colitis has been reported with nearly all antibacterial agents, including ceftibuten, and may range in severity from mild to life threatening. Therefore, it is important to consider this diagnosis in patients who present with diarrhea subsequent to the administration of antibacterial agents.

Treatment with antibacterial agents alters normal flora of the colon and may permit overgrowth of clostridia. Studies indicate that a toxin produced by *Clostridium difficile* is one primary cause of "antibiotic-associated colitis".

After the diagnosis of pseudomembranous colitis has been established, appropriate therapeutic measures should be initiated. Mild cases of pseudomembranous colitis usually respond to drug discontinuation alone. In moderate to severe cases, consideration should be given to management with fluids and electrolytes, protein supplementation, and treatment with an antibacterial drug clinically effective against *Clostridium difficile.*

PRECAUTIONS

GENERAL

As with other broad-spectrum antibiotics, prolonged treatment may result in the possible emergence and overgrowth of resistant organisms. Careful observation of the patient is essential. If superinfection occurs during therapy, appropriate measures should be taken.

The dose of ceftibuten may require adjustment in patients with varying degrees of renal insufficiency, particularly in patients with creatinine clearance less than 50 ml/min or undergoing hemodialysis (see DOSAGE AND ADMINISTRATION).

Ceftibuten is readily dialyzable. Dialysis patients should be monitored carefully, and administration of ceftibuten should occur immediately following dialysis.

Ceftibuten should be prescribed with caution to individuals with a history of gastrointestinal disease, particularly colitis.

INFORMATION FOR THE PATIENT

Patients should be informed that:

If the patient is diabetic, he/she should be informed that ceftibuten oral suspension contains 1 g sucrose per teaspoon of suspension.

Ceftibuten oral suspension should be taken at least 2 hours before a meal or at least 1 hour after a meal (see CLINICAL PHARMACOLOGY, Food Effect on Absorption).

DRUG/LABORATORY TEST INTERACTIONS

There have been no chemical or laboratory test interactions with ceftibuten noted to date. False-positive direct Coombs' tests have been reported during treatment with other cephalosporins. Therefore, it should be recognized that a positive Coombs' test could be due to the drug. The results of assays using red cells from healthy subjects to determine whether ceftibuten would cause direct Coombs' reactions *in vitro* showed no positive reaction at ceftibuten concentrations as high as 40 μg/ml.

CARCINOGENESIS, MUTAGENESIS, AND IMPAIRMENT OF FERTILITY

Long-term animal studies have not been performed to evaluate the carcinogenic potential of ceftibuten. No mutagenic effects were seen in the following studies: *in vitro* chromosome assay in human lymphocytes, *in vivo* chromosome assay in mouse bone marrow cells, Chinese Hamster Ovary (CHO) cell point mutation assay at the hypoxanthine-guanine phosphoribosyl transferase (HGPRT) locus, and in a bacterial reversion point mutation test (Ames). No impairment of fertility occurred when rats were administered ceftibuten orally up to 2000 mg/kg/day (approximately 43 times the recommended human dose based on $mg/m^2/day$).

PREGNANCY, TERATOGENIC EFFECTS, PREGNANCY CATEGORY B

Ceftibuten was not teratogenic in the pregnant rat at oral doses up to 400 mg/kg/day (approximately 8.6 times the human dose based on $mg/m^2/day$). Ceftibuten was not teratogenic in the pregnant rabbit at oral doses up to 40 mg/kg/day (approximately 1.5 times the human dose based on $mg/m^2/day$) and has revealed no evidence of harm to the fetus. There are no adequate and well-controlled studies in pregnant women. Because animal reproduction studies are not always predictive of human response, this drug should be used during pregnancy only if clearly needed.

LABOR AND DELIVERY

Ceftibuten has not been studied for use during labor and delivery. Its use during such clinical situations should be weighed in terms of potential risk and benefit to both mother and fetus.

NURSING MOTHERS

It is not known whether ceftibuten (at recommended dosages) is excreted in human milk. Because many drugs are excreted in human milk, caution should be exercised when ceftibuten is administered to a nursing woman.

PEDIATRIC USE

The safety and efficacy of ceftibuten in infants less then 6 months of age have not been established.

GERIATRIC USE

The usual adult dosage recommendation may be followed for patients in this age group. However, these patients should be monitored closely, particularly their renal function, as dosage adjustment may be required.

DRUG INTERACTIONS

THEOPHYLLINE

Twelve healthy male volunteers were administered one 200 mg ceftibuten capsule twice daily for 6 days. With the morning dose of ceftibuten on day 6, each volunteer received a single intravenous infusion of theophylline (4 mg/kg). The pharmacokinetics of theophylline were not altered. The effect of ceftibuten on the pharmacokinetic of theophylline administered orally has not been investigated,

ANTACIDS OR H_2-RECEPTOR ANTAGONISTS

The effect of increases gastric pH on the bioavailability of ceftibuten was evaluated in 18 healthy adult volunteers. Each volunteer was administered one 400 mg ceftibuten capsule.

A single dose of liquid antacid did not affect the C_{max} or AUC of ceftibuten; however, 150 mg of ranitidine q12h for 3 days increased the ceftibuten C_{max} by 23% and ceftibuten AUC by 16%. the clinical relevance of these increases is not known.

ADVERSE REACTIONS

CLINICAL TRIALS

Capsules (Adult Patients)

In clinical trials, 1728 adult patients (1092 US and 636 international) were treated with the recommended dose of ceftibuten capsules (400 mg/day). There were no deaths or permanent disabilities thought due to drug toxicity in any of the patients in these studies. Thirty-six of the 1728 (2%) patients discontinued medication due to adverse events thought by the investigators to be possibly, probably, or almost certainly related to drug toxicity. The discontinuations were primarily for gastrointestinal disturbances, usually diarrhea, vomiting or nausea. Six of 1728 (0.3%) patients were discontinued due to rash or pruritus thought related to ceftibuten administration.

In the US trials, the following adverse events were thought by the investigators to be possibly, probably, or almost certainly related to ceftibuten capsules in multipe-dose clinical trials (n=1092 ceftibuten-treated patients).

TABLE 8 *Adverse Reaction-Ceftibuten Capsules*

US Clinical Studies in Adult Patients (n=1092)

Incidence ≥1%	
Nausea	4%
Headache	3%
Diarrhea	3%
Dyspepsia	2%
Dizziness	1%
Abdominal pain	1%
Vomiting	1%
0.1% < Incidence < 1%	
Anorexia, constipation, dry mouth, dyspnea, dysuria, eructation, fatigue, flatulence, loose stools, moniliasis, nasal congestion, paresthesia, pruritus, rash, somnolence, taste perversion, urticaria, vaginitis.	

TABLE 9 *Laboratory Value Changes* — Ceftibuten Capsules*

US Clinical Studies in Adult Patients

Incidence ≥1%	
Increased BUN	4%
Increased eosinophils	3%
Decreased hemoglobin	2%
Increased ALT (SGPT)	1%
Increased bilirubin	1%
0.1% < Incidence < 1%	
Increased alk phosphatase, increased creatinine, increased platelets, decreased platelets, decreased leukocytes, increased AST (SGOT)	

* Changes in laboratory values with possible clinical significance regardless of whether or not the investigator thought that the change was due to drug toxicity.

Oral Suspension (pediatric patients)

In clinical trials, 1152 pediatric patients (772 US and 380 international), 97% of whom were younger than 12 years of age, were treated with the recommended dose of ceftibuten (9 mg/kg once daily up to a maximum dose of 400 mg/day) for 10 days. There were no deaths, life-threatening adverse events, or permanent disabilities in any of the patients in these studies. Eight of the 1152 (<1%) patients discontinued medication due to adverse events thought by the investigators to be possibly, probably, or almost certainly related to drug toxicty. These discontinuations were primarily (7 out of 8) for gastrointestinal disturbances, usually diarrhea or vomiting. One patient was discontinued due to a cutaneous rash thought possibly related to ceftibuten administration.

In the US trials, the following adverse events were thought by the investigators to be possibly, probably, or almost certainly related to ceftibuten oral suspension in multiple-dose clinical trials (n=772 ceftibuten-treated patients).

Incidence ≥1%:

Diarrhea* 4%
Vomiting 2%
Abdominal pain 2%
Loose stools 2%

0.1% < Incidence < 1%:

Agitation, anorexia, dehydration, diaper dermatitis, dizziness, dyspepsia, fever, headache, hematuria, hyperkinesia, insomnia, irritability, nausea, pruritus, rash, rigors, urticaria

**NOTE:* The incidence of diarrhea in children ≤2 years old was 8% (23/301) compared with 2% (9/471) in children >2 years old.

TABLE 10 *Laboratory Value Changes — Ceftibutin Oral Suspension; US Clinical Studies in Adult Patients*

Incidence ≥ 1%	
Increased eosinophils	3%
Increased BUN	2%
Decreased hemoglobin	1%
Increased platelets	1%
0.1% < Incidence < 1%	
Increased ALT (SGPT), increased AST (SGOT), increased alk phosphatase, increased bilirubin, increased creatinine	

* Changes in laboratory values with possible clinical significance regardless of whether or not the investigator thought that the change was due to drug toxicity.

IN POST-MARKETING EXPERIENCE

In addition to the events reported during clinical trials with ceftibuten, the following adverse experiences have been reported during worldwide post-marketing surveillance:

Capsules: Aphasia, jaundice, psychosis, stridor, toxic epidermal necrolysis.

Oral Suspension: Melena.

CEPHALOSPORIN-CLASS ADVERSE REACTIONS

In addition to the adverse reactions listed above that have been observed in patients treated with ceftibutin capsules, the following adverse events and altered laboratory tests have been reported for cephalosporin-class antibiotics: allergic reactions, anaphylaxis, drug fever, Stevens-Johnson syndrome, renal dysfunction, toxic nephropathy, hepatic cholestasis, aplastic anemia, hemolytic anemia, hemorrhage, false-positive test for urinary glucose, neutropenia, pancytopenia, and agranulocytosis. Pseudomembranous colitis; onset of symptoms may occur during or after antibiotic treatment (see WARNINGS).

Several cephalosporins have been implicated in triggering seizures, particularly in patients with renal impairment when the dosage was not reduced (see DOSAGE AND ADMINISTRATION). If seizures associated with drug therapy occur, the drug should be discontinued. Anticonvulsant therapy can be given if clinically indicated.

DOSAGE AND ADMINISTRATION

The recommended doses of ceftibuten oral suspension are presented in the table below. **Ceftibuten suspension must be administered at least 2 hours before or 1 hour after a meal.**

TABLE 11

Type of Infection*	Daily Maxium Dose	Dose and Frequency	Duration
Adults (12 years of age and older)			
Acute Bacterial Exaberations of Chronic Bronchitis due to:			
H. influenza (including β-lactamase-producing strains)	400 mg	400 mg qd	10 days
M. catarrhalis (including β-lactamas-producing strains)	400 mg	400 mg qd	10 days
Streptococcus pneumoniae (pencillin-susceptible strains only)†	400 mg	400 mg qd	10 days
Pharyngitis and tonsillitis due to:			
S. pyogenes	400 mg	400 mg qd	10 days
Acute Bacterial Otitis Media due to:			
H. influenza (including β-lactamase-producing strains)	400 mg	400 mg qd	10 days
M. catarrhalis (including β-lactamase-producing strains)	400 mg	400 mg qd	10 days
S. pyogenes†	400 mg	400 mg qd	10 days
Children			
Pharyngitis and tonsillitis due to:			
S. pyogenes	400 mg	9 mg/kg qd	10 days
Acute Bacterial Otitis Media due to:			
H. influenza (including β-lactamase-producing strains)	400 mg	9 mg/kg qd	10 days
M. catarrhalis (including β-lactamase-producing strains)	400 mg	9 mg/kg qd	10 days
S. pyogenes†	400 mg	9 mg/kg qd	10 days

* as qualified in INDICATIONS AND USAGE.
† (See INDICATIONS AND USAGE, NOTE.)

TABLE 12 *Ceftibuten Oral Suspension*

Pediatric Dosage Chart

Child's Weight		90 mg/5 ml	180 mg/5 ml
10 kg	22 lb	1 tsp qd	½ tsp qd
20 kg	44 lb	2 tsp qd	1 tsp qd
40 kg	88 lb	4 tsp qd	2 tsp qd

Children weighing more than 45 kg should receive the maximum daily dose of 400 mg.

RENAL IMPAIRMENT

Ceftibuten capsules and oral suspension may be administered at normal doses in the presence of impaired renal function with creatinine clearance of 50 ml/min or greater. The recommendations for dosing in patients with varying degrees of renal insufficiency are presented in TABLE 13.

TABLE 13

Creatinine Clearance	Recommended Dosing Schedules
>50 ml/min	9 mg/kg or 400 mg q24h (normal dosing schedule)
30-49 ml/min	4.5 mg/kg or 200 mg q24h
5-29 ml/min	2.25 mg/kg or 100 mg q24h

HEMODIALYSIS PATIENTS

In patients undergoing hemodialysis 2 or 3 times weekly, a single 400 mg dose of ceftibuten capsules or a single dose of 9 mg/kg (maximum of 400 mg of ceftibuten) oral suspension may be administered at the end of each hemodialysis session.

HOW SUPPLIED

CEDAX CAPSULES

Cedax capsules, containing 400 mg of ceftibuten (as ceftibuten dihydrate) are white, opaque capsules imprinted with the product name and strength.
Storage: Store the capsules between 2-25°C (36-77°F). Replace cap securely after each opening.

CEDAX ORAL SUSPENSION

Cedax oral suspension is an off-white to cream-colored powder that, when reconstituted as directed, contains either ceftibuten equivalent to 90 mg/5 ml or 180 mg/ml.
Storage: Prior to reconsitiution, the powder must be stored between 2-25°C (36-77°F). Once it is reconstituted, the oral suspension is stable for 14 days when stored in a refrigerator between 2-8°C (36-46°F).

PRODUCT LISTING - EQUIVALENTS NOT AVAILABLE

Capsule - Oral - 400 mg			
10's	$78.87	CEDAX, Allscripts Pharmaceutical Company	54569-4551-01
20's	$173.07	CEDAX, Biovail Pharmaceuticals Inc	64455-0691-01
100's	$854.19	CEDAX, Biovail Pharmaceuticals Inc	64455-0691-02
Powder For Reconstitution - Oral - 90 mg/5 ml			
30 ml	$31.74	CEDAX, Biovail Pharmaceuticals Inc	64455-0777-03
60 ml	$43.31	CEDAX, Biovail Pharmaceuticals Inc	64455-0777-01
90 ml	$69.22	CEDAX, Biovail Pharmaceuticals Inc	64455-0777-04
120 ml	$87.34	CEDAX, Biovail Pharmaceuticals Inc	64455-0777-02

Ceftizoxime Sodium *(000693)*

For related information, see the comparative table section in Appendix A.

Categories: Gonorrhea; Infection, bone; Infection, gynecologic; Infection, intra-abdominal; Infection, joint; Infection, lower respiratory tract; Infection, skin and skin structures; Infection, urinary tract; Pelvic inflammatory disease; Septicemia; Pregnancy Category B; FDA Approved 1983 Sep
Drug Classes: Antibiotics, cephalosporins
Brand Names: Cefizox; Cefizox In 5% Dextrose; Cefizox In Dextrose
Foreign Brand Availability: Ceftix (Germany); Epocelin (Finland; Hungary; Japan; Spain; Taiwan); Eposerin (Italy); Tefizox (Israel); Tergecin (Philippines); Ultracef (Mexico)
Cost of Therapy: $21.76 (Infection; Cefizox Injection; 1 g; 2 g/day; 10 day supply)
HCFA JCODE(S): J0715 per 500 mg IV, IM

DESCRIPTION

Ceftizoxime sodium is a sterile, semisynthetic, broad-spectrum, beta-lactamase resistant cephalosporin antibiotic for parenteral (IV, IM) administration. It is the sodium salt of [6R-[6α,7β(Z)]]-7-[[(2,3-dihydro-2-imino-4-thiazolyl) (methoxyimino) acetyl] amino]-8-oxo-5-thia-1-azabicyclo [4.2.0] oct-2-ene-2-carboxylic acid. Its sodium content is approximately 60 mg (2.6 mEq) per gram of ceftizoxime activity.

Its molecular formula is $C_{13}H_{12}N_5NaO_5S_2$ and it has a molecular weight of 405.38.

Sterile ceftizoxime sodium is a white to pale yellow crystalline powder.

Cefizox is supplied in vials equivalent to 500 mg, 1, 2, or 10 g of ceftizoxime, and in "Piggyback" vials for intravenous admixture equivalent to 1 or 2 g of ceftizoxime and in Add-Vantage vials equivalent to 1 and 2 g of ceftizoxime.

Cefizox, equivalent to 1 or 2 g of ceftizoxime, is also supplied as a frozen, iso-osmotic sterile, nonpyrogenic solution of ceftizoxime sodium in an iso-osmotic diluent in plastic containers. After thawing, the solution is intended for intravenous use.

The plastic container is fabricated from specially formulated polyvinyl chloride. Solutions in contact with the plastic container can leach out certain of its chemical components in very small amounts within the expiration period, *e.g.*, di 2-ethylhexyl phthalate (DEHP), up to 5 ppm. However, the suitability of the plastic has been confirmed in tests in animals according to the USP biological tests for plastic containers as well as by tissue culture toxicity studies.

CLINICAL PHARMACOLOGY

TABLE 1 demonstrates the serum levels and duration of ceftizoxime sodium following intramuscular administration of 500 mg and 1 g doses, respectively, to normal volunteers.

Following intravenous administration of 1, 2, and 3 g doses of ceftizoxime sodium to normal volunteers, the serum levels shown in TABLE 2 were obtained.

TABLE 1 *Serum Concentrations After Intramuscular Administration*

Dose	Serum Concentration (µg/ml) ½ h	1 h	2 h	4 h	6 h	8 h
500 mg	13.3	13.7	9.2	4.8	1.9	0.7
1 g	36.0	39.0	31.0	15.0	6.0	3.0

TABLE 2 *Serum Concentrations After Intravenous Administration*

Dose	Serum Concentration (µg/ml) 5 min	10 min	30 min	1 h	2 h	4 h	8 h
1 g	ND	ND	60.5	38.9	21.5	8.4	1.4
2 g	131.8	110.9	77.5	53.6	33.1	12.1	2.0
3 g	221.1	174.0	112.7	83.9	47.4	26.2	4.8

ND=Not Done.

A serum half-life of approximately 1.7 hours was observed after intravenous or intramuscular administration.

Ceftizoxime sodium is 30% protein bound.

Ceftizoxime sodium is not metabolized, and is excreted virtually unchanged by the kidneys in 24 hours. This provides a high urinary concentration. Concentrations greater than 6000 µg/ml have been achieved in the urine by 2 hours after a 1 g dose of ceftizoxime sodium intravenously. Probenecid slows tubular secretion and produces even higher serum levels, increasing the duration of measurable serum concentrations.

Ceftizoxime sodium achieves therapeutic levels in various body fluids, *e.g.*, cerebrospinal fluid (in patients with inflamed meninges), bile, surgical wound fluid, pleural fluid, aqueous humor, ascitic fluid, peritoneal fluid, prostatic fluid and saliva, and in the following body tissues: heart, gallbladder, bone, biliary, peritoneal, prostatic, and uterine.

In clinical experience to date, no disulfiram-like reactions have been reported with ceftizoxime sodium.

MICROBIOLOGY

The bactericidal action of ceftizoxime sodium results from inhibition of cell-wall synthesis. Ceftizoxime sodium is highly resistant to a broad spectrum of beta-lactamases (penicillinase and cephalosporinase), including Richmond types I, II, III, TEM, and IV, produced by both aerobic and anaerobic gram-positive and gram-negative organisms. Ceftizoxime sodium is active against a wide range of gram-positive and gram-negative organisms, and is usually active against the following organisms *in vitro* and in clinical situations. (See INDICATIONS AND USAGE.)

GRAM-POSITIVE AEROBES

Staphylococcus aureus (including penicillinase- and nonpenicillinase-producing strains).

Staphylococcus epidermidis (including penicillinase- and nonpenicillinase-producing strains) *Note:* Methicillin-resistant staphylococci are resistant to cephalosporins, including ceftizoxime.*Streptococcus agalactiae; Streptococcus pneumoniae; Streptococcus pyrogenes Note:* Ceftizoxime is usually inactive against most strains of *Enterococcus faecalis* (formerly *S. faecalis*).

GRAM-NEGATIVE AEROBES

Acinetobacter spp.; *Enterobacter* spp.; *Escherichia coli; Haemophilus influenzae* (including ampicillin-resistant strains); *Klebsiella pneumoniae; Morganella morganii* (formerly *Proteus morganii*); *Neisseria gonorrhoeae; Proteus mirabilis; Proteus vulgaris; Providencia rettgeri* (formerly *Proteus rettgeri*); *Pseudomonas aeruginosa; Serratia marcescens.*

ANAEROBES

Bacteroides spp.; *Peptococcus* spp.; *Peptostreptococcus* spp.

Ceftizoxime is usually active against the following organisms *in vitro,* but the clinical significance of these data is unknown.

GRAM-POSITIVE AEROBES

Corynebacterium diphtheriae.

GRAM-NEGATIVE AEROBES

Aeromonas hydrophilia; Citrobacter spp.; *Moraxella* spp.; *Neisseria meningitidis; Pasteurella multocida; Providence stuartii; Salmonella* spp.; *Shigella* spp.; *Yersinia enterocolitica.*

ANAEROBES

Actinomyces spp.; *Bifidobacterium* spp.; *Clostridium* spp. *NOTE:* Most strains of *Clostridium difficile* are resistant. *Eubacterium* spp.; *Fusobacterium* spp.; *Propionibacterium* spp.; *Veillonella* spp.

SUSCEPTIBILITY TESTING

Diffusion Techniques: Quantitative methods that require measurement of zone diameters give the most precise estimate of the susceptibility of bacteria to antimicrobial agents. One such standard procedure[1] has been recommended for use with disks to test susceptibility of organisms to ceftizoxime. Interpretation involves the correlation of the diameters obtained in the disk test with the minimum inhibitory concentration (MIC) for ceftizoxime.
Organisms should be tested with the ceftizoxime disk, since ceftizoxime has been shown by *in vitro* tests to be active against certain strains found resistant when other beta-lactam disks are used.

Reports from the laboratory giving results of the standard single-disk susceptibility test with a 30 µg ceftizoxime disk should be interpreted according to the criteria in TABLE 3 (with the exception of *Pseudomonas aeruginosa*).

TABLE 3

Zone Diameter (mm)	Interpretation
≥20	(S) Susceptible
15-19	(MS) Moderately Susceptible
≤14	(R) Resistant

A report of "Susceptible" indicates that the pathogen is likely to be inhibited by generally achievable blood levels. A report of "Moderately Susceptible" suggests that the organism would be susceptible if high dosage is used or if the infection is confined to tissue and fluids (*e.g.*, urine) in which high antibiotic levels are attained. A report of "Resistant" indicates that achievable concentrations of the antibiotic are unlikely to be inhibitory and other therapy should be selected.

Standardized procedures require the use of laboratory control organisms. The 30 µg ceftizoxime disk should give the zone diameters shown in TABLE 4.
Pseudomonas in Urinary Tract Infections: Most strains of *Pseudomonas aeruginosa* are moderately susceptible to ceftizoxime. Ceftizoxime achieves high levels in the urine (greater than 6000 µg/ml at 2 hours with 1 g IV) and, therefore, the following zone sizes

TABLE 4

Organism	ATCC	Zone Diameter (mm)
Escherichia coli	25922	30-36
Pseudomonas aeruginosa	27853	12-17
Staphylococcus aureus	25923	27-35

should be used when testing ceftizoxime for treatment of urinary tract infections caused by *Pseudomonas aeruginosa.*
Susceptible organisms produce zones of 20 mm or greater, indicating that the test organism is likely to respond to therapy.

Organisms that produce zones of 11-19 mm are expected to be susceptible when the infection is confined to the urinary tract (in which high antibiotic levels are attained).

Resistant organisms produce zones of 10 mm or less, indicating that other therapy should be selected.

Dilution Techniques: When using the NCCLS agar dilution or broth dilution (including microdilution) method[2] or equivalent, the MIC data shown in TABLE 5 should be used for interpretation.

TABLE 5

MIC (µg/ml)	Interpretation
≤8	(S) Susceptible
16-32	(MS) Moderately Susceptible
≥64	(R) Resistant

As with standard disk diffusion methods, dilution procedures require the use of laboratory control organisms. Standard ceftizoxime powder should give MIC values in the ranges shown in TABLE 6.

TABLE 6

Organism	ATCC	MIC (µg/ml)
Escherichia coli	25922	0.03-0.12
Pseudomonas aeruginosa	27853	16-64
Staphylococcus aureus	29213	2-8

INDICATIONS AND USAGE

Ceftizoxime sodium is indicated in the treatment of infections due to susceptible strains of the microorganisms listed below.

Lower Respiratory Tract Infections: Caused by *Klebsiella* spp.; *Proteus mirabilis; Escherichia coli; Haemophilus influenzae* including ampicillin-resistant strains; *Staphylococcus aureus* (penicillinase- and nonpenicillinase-producing); *Serratia* spp.; *Enterobacter* spp.; *Bacteroides* spp.; and *Streptococcus* spp. including *S. pneumoniae,* but excluding enterococci.

Urinary Tract Infections: Caused by *Staphylococcus aureus* (penicillinase- and nonpenicillinase-producing); *Escherichia coli*; *Pseudomonas* spp. including *P. aeruginosa; Proteus mirabilis; P. vulgaris; Providencia rettgeri* (formerly *Proteus rettgeri*) and *Morganella morganii* (formerly *Proteus morganii*); *Klebsiella* spp.; *Serratia* spp. including *S. marcescens;* and *Enterobacter* spp.

Gonorrhea: Including uncomplicated cervical and urethral gonorrhea caused by *Neisseria gonorrhoeae.*

Pelvic Inflammatory Disease: Caused by *Neisseria gonorrhoeea, Escherichia coli* or *Streptococcus agalactiae. NOTE:* Ceftizoxime, like other cephalosporins, has no activity against *Chlamydia trachomatis.* Therefore, when cephalosporins are used in the treatment of patients with pelvic inflammatory disease and *C. trachomatis* is one of the suspected pathogens, appropriate anti-chlamydial coverage should be added.

Intra-Abdominal Infections: Caused by *Escherichia coli; Staphylococcus epidermidis; Streptococcus* spp. (excluding enterococci); *Enterobacter* spp.; *Klebsiella* spp.; *Bacteroides* spp. including *B. fragilis;* and anaerobic cocci, including *Peptococcus* spp. and *Peptostreptococcus* spp.

Septicemia: Caused by *Streptococcus* spp. including *S. pneumoniae* (but excluding enterococci); *Staphylococcus aureus* (penicillinase- and nonpenicillinase-producing); *Escherichia coli; Bacteroides* spp. including *B. fragilis; Klebsiella* spp.; and *Serratia* spp.

Skin and Skin Structure Infections: Caused by *Staphylococcus aureus* (penicillinase- and nonpenicillinase-producing); *Staphylococcus epidermidis; Escherichia coli; Klebsiella* spp.; *Streptococcus* spp. including *Streptococcus pyogenes* (but excluding enterococci); *Proteus mirabilis; Serratia* spp.; *Enterobacter* spp.; *Bacteroides* spp. including *B. fragilis;* and anaerobic cocci, including *Peptococcus* spp. and *Peptostreptococcus* spp.

Bone and Joint Infections: Caused by *Staphylococcus aureus* (penicillinase- and nonpenicillinase-producing); *Streptococcus* spp. (excluding enterococci); *Proteus mirabilis; Bacteroids* spp.; and *anaerobic cocci,* including *Peptococcus* spp. and *Peptostreptococcus* spp.

Meningitis: Caused by *Haemophilus influenzae.* Ceftizoxime sodium has also been used successfully in the treatment of a limited number of pediatric and adult cases of meningitis caused by *Streptococcus pneumoniae.*

Ceftizoxime sodium has been effective in the treatment of seriously ill, compromised patients, including those who were debilitated, immunosuppressed, or neutropenic.

Infections caused by aerobic gram-negative and by mixtures of organisms resistant to other cephalosporins, aminoglycosides, or penicillins have responded to treatment with ceftizoxime sodium.

Because of the serious nature of some urinary tract infections due to *P. aeruginosa* and because many strains of *Pseudomonas* species are only moderately susceptible to ceftizoxime sodium, higher dosage is recommended. Other therapy should be instituted if the response is not prompt.

Susceptibility studies on specimens obtained prior to therapy should be used to determine the response of causative organisms to ceftizoxime sodium. Therapy with ceftizoxime sodium may be initiated pending results of the studies; however, treatment should be adjusted according to study findings. In serious infections, ceftizoxime sodium has been used concomitantly with aminoglycosides (see PRECAUTIONS). Before using ceftizoxime sodium concomitantly with other antibiotics, the prescribing information for those agents should be reviewed for contraindications, warnings, precautions, and adverse reactions. Renal function should be carefully monitored.

CONTRAINDICATIONS

Ceftizoxime sodium is contraindicated in patients who have known allergy to the drug.

WARNINGS

BEFORE THERAPY WITH CEFTIZOXIME SODIUM IS INSTITUTED, CAREFUL INQUIRY SHOULD BE MADE TO DETERMINE WHETHER THE PATIENT HAS HAD PREVIOUS HYPERSENSITIVITY REACTIONS TO CEFTIZOXIME SODIUM, OTHER CEPHALOSPORINS, PENICILLINS, OR OTHER DRUGS. IF THIS PRODUCT IS TO BE GIVEN TO PENICILLIN-SENSITIVE PATIENTS, CAUTION SHOULD BE EXERCISED BECAUSE CROSS-HYPERSENSITIVITY AMONG BETA-LACTAM ANTIBIOTICS HAS BEEN CLEARLY DOCUMENTED AND MAY OCCUR IN UP TO 10% OF PATIENTS WITH A HISTORY OF PENICILLIN ALLERGY. IF AN ALLERGIC REACTION TO CEFTIZOXIME SODIUM OCCURS, DISCONTINUE THE DRUG, SERIOUS ACUTE HYPERSENSITIVITY REACTIONS MAY REQUIRE TREATMENT WITH EPINEPHRINE AND OTHER EMERGENCY MEASURES, INCLUDING OXYGEN, INTRAVENOUS FLUIDS, INTRAVENOUS ANTIHISTAMINES, CORTICOSTEROIDS, PRESSOR AMINES, AND AIRWAY MANAGEMENT, AS CLINICALLY INDICATED.

Pseudomembranous colitis has been reported with nearly all antibacterial agents, including ceftizoxime, and may range in severity from mild to life threatening. Therefore, it is important to consider this diagnosis in patients who present with diarrhea subsequent to the administration of antibacterial agents.

Treatment with antibacterial agents alters normal flora of the colon and may permit overgrowth of clostridia. Studies indicate that a toxin produced by *Clostridium difficile* is a primary cause of "antibiotic-associated" colitis. After diagnosis of pseudomembranous colitis has been established, appropriate therapeutic measures should be initiated. Mild cases of pseudomembranous colitis usually respond to drug discontinuation alone. In moderate to severe cases, consideration should be given to management with fluids and electrolytes, protein supplementation, and treatment with an antibacterial drug clinically effective against *Clostridium difficile* colitis.

PRECAUTIONS

GENERAL

As with all broad-spectrum antibiotics, ceftizoxime sodium should be prescribed with caution in individuals with a history of gastrointestinal disease, particularly colitis.

Although ceftizoxime sodium has not been shown to produce an alteration in renal function, renal status should be evaluated, especially in seriously ill patients receiving maximum dose therapy. As with any antibiotic, prolonged use may result in overgrowth of nonsusceptible organisms. Careful observation is essential; appropriate measures should be taken if superinfection occurs.

CARCINOGENESIS, MUTAGENESIS, AND IMPAIRMENT OF FERTILITY

Long term studies in animals to evaluate the carcinogenic potential of ceftizoxime have not been conducted. In an *in vitro* bacterial cell assay (*i.e.,* Ames test), there was no evidence of mutagenicity at ceftizoxime concentrations of 0.001-0.5 µg/plate. Ceftizoxime did not produce increases in micronuclei in the *in vivo* mouse micronucleus test when given to animals at doses up to 7500 mg/kg, approximately 6 times greater than the maximum human daily dose on a mg/m^2 basis.

Ceftizoxime had no effect on fertility when administered subcutaneously to rats at daily doses of up to 1000 mg/kg/day, approximately 2 times the maximum human daily dose on a mg/m^2 basis. Ceftizoxime produced no histological changes in the sexual organs of male and female dogs when given intravenously for 13 weeks at a dose of 1000 mg/kg/day, approximately 5 times greater than the maximum human daily dose on a mg/m^2 basis.

PREGNANCY, TERATOGENIC EFFECTS, PREGNANCY CATEGORY B

Reproduction studies performed in rats and rabbits have revealed no evidence of impaired fertility or harm to the fetus due to ceftizoxime sodium. There are, however, no adequate and well-controlled studies in pregnant women. Because animal reproduction studies are not always predictive of human effects, this drug should be used during pregnancy only if clearly needed.

LABOR AND DELIVERY

Safety of ceftizoxime sodium use during labor and delivery has not been established.

NURSING MOTHERS

Ceftizoxime sodium is excreted in human milk in low concentrations. Caution should be exercised when ceftizoxime sodium is administered to a nursing woman.

PEDIATRIC USE

Safety and efficacy in infants from birth to 6 months of age have not been established. In children 6 months of age and older, treatment with ceftizoxime sodium has been associated with transient elevated levels of eosinophils, AST (SGOT), ALT (SGPT), and CPK (creatine phosphokinase). The CPK elevation may be related to IM administration.

The potential for the toxic effect in children from chemicals that may leach from the single-dose IV preparation in plastic has not been determined.

C

DRUG INTERACTIONS

Although the occurrence has not been reported with ceftizoxime sodium, nephrotoxicity has been reported following concomitant administration of other cephalosporins and aminoglycosides.

ADVERSE REACTIONS

Ceftizoxime sodium is generally well tolerated. The *most* frequent adverse reactions (*greater* than 1% but *less* than 5%) are:

Hypersensitivity: Rash, pruritus, fever.

Hepatic: Transient elevation in AST (SGOT), ALT (SGPT), and alkaline phosphatase.

Hematologic: Transient eosinophilia, thrombocytosis. Some individuals have developed a positive Coombs' test.

Local-Injection Site: Burning, cellulitis, phlebitis with IV administration, pain, induration, tenderness, paresthesia.

The *Less* Frequent Adverse Reactions (*less* than 1%) Are:

Hypersensitivity: Numbness and anaphylaxis have been reported rarely.

Hepatic: Elevation of bilirubin has been reported rarely.

Renal: Transient elevations of BUN and creatinine have been occasionally observed with ceftizoxime sodium.

Hematologic: Anemia, including hemolytic anemia with occasional fatal outcome, leukopenia, neutropenia, and thrombocytopenia have been reported rarely.

Urogenital: Vaginitis has occurred rarely.

Gastrointestinal: Diarrhea, nausea and vomiting have been reported occasionally.

Symptoms of pseudomembranous colitis can appear during or after antibiotic treatment (see WARNINGS).

In addition to the adverse reactions listed above which have been observed in patients treated with ceftizoxime, the following adverse reactions and altered laboratory tests have been reported for cephalosporin-class antibiotics:

Stevens-Johnson syndrome, erythema multiforme, toxic epidermal necrolysis, serum-sickness-like reaction, toxic nephropathy, aplastic anemia, hemorrhage, prolonged prothrombin time, elevated LDH, pancytopenia, and agranulocytosis.

Several cephalosporins have been implicated in triggering seizures, particularly in patients with renal impairment, when the dosage was not reduced (see DOSAGE AND ADMINISTRATION). If seizures associated with drug therapy occur, the drug should be discontinued. Anticonvulsant therapy can be given if clinically indicated.

DOSAGE AND ADMINISTRATION

The usual adult dosage is 1 or 2 g of ceftizoxime sodium every 8-12 hours. Proper dosage and route of administration should be determined by the condition of the patient, severity of the infection, and susceptibility of the causative organisms. (See TABLE 7.)

TABLE 7 *General Guidelines for Dosage of Ceftizoxime Sodium*

Type of Infection	Daily Dose	Frequency and Route
Uncomplicated Urinary Tract	1 g	500 mg q12h IM or IV
Other Sites	2-3 g	1 g q8-12h IM or IV
Severe or Refractory	3-6 g	1 g q8h IM or IV 2 g q8-12h IM* or IV
PID†	6 g	2 g q8h IV
Life-Threatening‡	9-12 g	3-4 g q8h IV

* When administering 2 g IM doses, the dose should be divided and given in different large muscle masses.
† If *C. trachomatis* is a suspected pathogen, appropriate anti-chlamydial coverage should be added, because ceftizoxime has no activity against this organism.
‡ In life-threatening infections, dosages up to 2 g every 4 hours have been given.

Because of the serious nature of urinary tract infections due to *P. aeruginosa* and because many strains of *Pseudomonas* species are only moderately susceptible to ceftizoxime sodium, higher dosage is recommended. Other therapy should be instituted if the response is not prompt.

A single, 1 g IM dose is the usual dose for treatment of uncomplicated gonorrhea.

The intravenous route may be preferable for patients with bacterial septicemia, localized parenchymal abscesses (such as intra-abdominal abscess), peritonitis, or other severe or life-threatening infections.

In those with normal renal function, the intravenous dosage for such infections is 2-12 g of ceftizoxime sodium daily. In conditions such as bacterial septicemia, 6-12 g/day may be given initially by the intravenous route for several days, and the dosage may then be gradually reduced according to clinical response and laboratory findings.

For pediatric dosage, see TABLE 8.

TABLE 8 *Pediatric Dosage Schedule*

	Unit Dose	Frequency
Children 6 months and older	50 mg/kg	q6-8h

Dosage may be increased to a total daily dose of 200 mg/kg (not to exceed the maximum adult dose for serious infection).

IMPAIRED RENAL FUNCTION

Modification of ceftizoxime sodium dosage is necessary in patients with impaired renal function. Following an initial loading dose of 500 mg-1 g IM or IV, the maintenance dosing schedule shown in TABLE 9 should be followed. Further dosing should be determined by therapeutic monitoring, severity of the infection, and susceptibility of the causative organisms.

When only the serum creatinine level is available, creatinine clearance may be calculated from the following formula. The serum creatinine level should represent current renal function at the steady state.

Males: Clcr = [Weight (kg) × (140 - age)] ÷ [72 × serum creatinine (mg/100 ml)]
Females: 0.85 of the calculated clearance values for males

In patients undergoing hemodialysis, no additional supplemental dosing is required following hemodialysis; however, dosing should be timed so that the patient receives the dose (according to TABLE 9) at the end of the dialysis.

TABLE 9 *Dosage in Adults With Reduced Renal Function*

Creatinine Clearance	Renal Function	Less Severe Infections	Life-Threatening Infections
79-50 ml/min	Mild Impairment	500 mg q8h	0.75-1.5 g q8h
49-5 ml/min	Moderate to severe impairment	250-500 mg q12h	0.5-1 g q12h
4-0 ml/min	Dialysis patients	500 mg q48h or 250 mg q24h	0.5-1 g q48h or 0.5 g q24h

PREPARATION OF PARENTERAL SOLUTION

Reconstitution

IM Administration: Reconstitute with sterile water for injection. SHAKE WELL. (See TABLE 10.)

TABLE 10

Vial Size	Diluent to Be Added	Approx. Avail. Vol.	Approx. Avg. Concentration
500 mg	1.5 ml	1.8 ml	280 mg/ml
1 g	3.0 ml	3.7 ml	270 mg/ml
2 g*	6.0 ml	7.4 ml	270 mg/ml

* When administering 2 g IM doses, the dose should be divided and given in different large muscle masses.

IV Administration: Reconstitute with sterile water for injection. SHAKE WELL. (See TABLE 11.)

TABLE 11

Vial Size	Diluent to Be Added	Approx. Avail. Vol.	Approx. Avg. Concentration
500 mg	15 ml	5.3 ml	95 mg/ml
1 g	10 ml	10.7 ml	95 mg/ml
2 g	20 ml	21.4 ml	95 mg/ml

These solutions of ceftizoxime sodium are stable 24 hours at room temperature or 96 hours if refrigerated (5°C).

Parenteral drug products should be inspected visually for particulate matter prior to administration. If particulate matter is evident in reconstituted fluids, then the drug solution should be discarded. Reconstituted solutions may range from yellow to amber without changes in potency.

"Piggyback" Vials: Reconstitute with 50-100 ml of sodium chloride injection or any other IV solution listed in IV Administration. SHAKE WELL.

Administer with primary IV fluids, as a single dose. These solutions of ceftizoxime sodium are stable 24 hours at room temperature or 96 hours if refrigerated (5°C).

A solution of 1 g ceftizoxime sodium in 13 ml sterile water for injection is isotonic.

Pharmacy Bulk Vials: For IM or IV direct injection, add sterile water for injection to the 10 g vial according to TABLE 12. SHAKE WELL. For IV intermittent or continuous infusion, add sterile water for injection according to TABLE 12. SHAKE WELL. Add to parenteral fluids listed in IV Administration.

TABLE 12

Vial Size	Diluent to Be Added	Approx. Avail. Vol.	Approx. Avg. Concentration
10 g	30 ml	37 ml	1 g/3.5 ml
	45 ml	51 ml	1 g/5 ml

These reconstituted solutions of ceftizoxime sodium are stable 24 hours at room temperature or 96 hours if refrigerated (5°C).

IM INJECTION

Inject well within the body of a relatively large muscle. Aspiration is necessary to avoid inadvertent injection into a blood vessel. When administering 2 g IM doses, the dose should be divided and given in different large muscle masses.

IV ADMINISTRATION

Direct (bolus) injection, slowly over 3-5 minutes, directly or through tubing for patients receiving parenteral fluids (see list below). Intermittent or continuous infusion, dilute reconstituted ceftizoxime sodium in 50-100 ml of one of the following solutions:

- Sodium chloride injection.
- 5% or 10% dextrose injection.
- 5% dextrose and 0.9%, 0.45%, or 0.2% sodium chloride injection.
- Ringer's injection.
- Lactated Ringer's injection.
- Invert sugar 10% in sterile water for injection.
- 5% sodium bicarbonate in sterile water for injection.
- 5% dextrose in lactated ringer's injection (only when reconstituted with 4% sodium bicarbonate injection).

In these fluids, ceftizoxime sodium is stable 24 hours at room temperature or 96 hours if refrigerated (5°C).

HOW SUPPLIED

Unreconstituted Cefizax should be protected from excessive light, and stored at controlled room temperature 15-30°C (59-86°F) in the original package until used.
Cefizax Injection: Store at or below -20°C (-4°F).

PRODUCT LISTING - EQUIVALENTS NOT AVAILABLE

Powder For Injection - Injectable - 1 Gm

1's	$11.86	CEFIZOX, Fujisawa	00469-7251-01
10's	$128.13	CEFIZOX, Fujisawa	00469-7252-01
10's	$130.00	CEFIZOX, Fujisawa	00469-7271-01

Powder For Injection - Injectable - 2 Gm

1's	$22.03	CEFIZOX, Fujisawa	00469-7253-02
10's	$231.63	CEFIZOX, Fujisawa	00469-7272-02
10's	$240.08	CEFIZOX, Fujisawa	00469-7254-02

Powder For Injection - Injectable - 10 Gm

10's	$1087.96	CEFIZOX, Fujisawa	00469-7255-10

Solution - Intravenous - 1 Gm/50 ml

50 ml	$349.50	CEFIZOX, Fujisawa	00469-7220-01
50 ml x 24	$335.52	CEFIZOX, Fujisawa	00469-7220-50

Solution - Intravenous - 2 Gm/50 ml

50 ml	$569.76	CEFIZOX, Fujisawa	00469-7221-50
50 ml	$593.40	CEFIZOX, Fujisawa	00469-7221-02

Ceftriaxone Sodium *(000694)*

For related information, see the comparative table section in Appendix A.

Categories: Gonorrhea; Infection, bone; Infection, intra-abdominal; Infection, joint; Infection, lower respiratory tract; Infection, ear, middle; Infection, skin and skin structures; Infection, urinary tract; Meningitis; Pelvic inflammatory disease; Prophylaxis, surgical; Septicemia; Pregnancy Category B; FDA Approved 1984 Dec; WHO Formulary

Drug Classes: Antibiotics, cephalosporins

Foreign Brand Availability: Axone (Bahrain; Cyprus; Egypt; Iran; Iraq; Jordan; Kuwait; Lebanon; Libya; Oman; Qatar; Republic-of-Yemen; Saudi-Arabia; Syria; United-Arab-Emirates); Benaxona (Mexico); Biotriax (Indonesia); Broadced (Indonesia); Brospec (Indonesia); Cef-3 (Philippines); Cefalogen (Peru); Cefaxona (Colombia; Mexico); Cefaxone (Korea; Singapore); Cefin (China; Singapore); Cefotal (Peru); Cefriex (Indonesia); Ceftrex (Mexico; Thailand); Ceftrilem (Mexico); Cephin (Thailand); Cerixon (Korea); Chef (Taiwan); Elpicef (Indonesia); Eurocef (Philippines); Ferfacef (Indonesia); Gomcephin (Korea); Grifotriaxona (Peru); Incephin (Indonesia); Keftriaxon (Israel); Keptrix (Philippines); Longacef (Bahrain; Cyprus; Egypt; Iran; Iraq; Jordan; Kuwait; Lebanon; Libya; Oman; Qatar; Republic-of-Yemen; Saudi-Arabia; Syria; United-Arab-Emirates); Lyceft (India); Megion (Mexico); Mesporin IM (Bahamas; Barbados; Belize; Bermuda; Curacao; Guyana; Hong-Kong; Jamaica; Netherland-Antilles; Puerto-Rico; Surinam; Trinidad); Mesporin IV (Bahamas; Barbados; Belize; Bermuda; Curacao; Guyana; Hong-Kong; Jamaica; Netherland-Antilles; Puerto-Rico; Surinam; Trinidad); Monocef (India); Nakaxone (Taiwan); Novosef (Bahrain; Cyprus; Egypt; Iran; Iraq; Jordan; Kuwait; Lebanon; Libya; Oman; Qatar; Republic-of-Yemen; Saudi-Arabia; Syria; United-Arab-Emirates); Oframax (Benin; Burkina-Faso; Ethiopia; Gambia; Ghana; Guinea; India; Ivory-Coast; Kenya; Liberia; Malawi; Mali; Mauritania; Mauritius; Morocco; Niger; Nigeria; Senegal; Seychelles; Sierra-Leone; Singapore; Sudan; Tanzania; Thailand; Tunia; Uganda; Zambia; Zimbabwe); Rocefalin Roche (Spain); Rocefin (Brazil; Colombia; Italy); Rocephalin (Denmark; Finland); Rocephin (Australia; Bahamas; Bahrain; Barbados; Belize; Bermuda; Canada; China; Costa-Rica; Curacao; Cyprus; Dominican-Republic; Ecuador; Egypt; El-Salvador; England; Germany; Ghana; Greece; Guatemala; Guyana; Honduras; Hong-Kong; Hungary; Indonesia; Iran; Iraq; Ireland; Israel; Jamaica; Jordan; Kenya; Korea; Kuwait; Lebanon; Libya; Malaysia; Netherland-Antilles; Netherlands; New-Zealand; Nicaragua; Oman; Panama; Philippines; Portugal; Qatar; Republic-of-Yemen; Saudi-Arabia; Singapore; South-Africa; Surinam; Switzerland; Syria; Taiwan; Tanzania; Thailand; Trinidad; Uganda; United-Arab-Emirates; Zambia); Rocephin "Biochemie" (Austria); Rocephin "Roche" (Austria); Rocephin Roche (Czech-Republic); Rocephine (Belgium; France); Rocephine " Roche" (Bulgaria); Rocidar (Bahrain; Cyprus; Egypt; Iran; Iraq; Jordan; Kuwait; Lebanon; Libya; Oman; Qatar; Republic-of-Yemen; Saudi-Arabia; Syria; United-Arab-Emirates); Rowecef (Costa-Rica; Dominican-Republic; El-Salvador; Guatemala; Honduras; Nicaragua; Panama); Roxcef (Benin; Burkina-Faso; Ethiopia; Gambia; Ghana; Guinea; Ivory-Coast; Kenya; Liberia; Malawi; Mali; Mauritania; Mauritius; Morocco; Niger; Nigeria; Senegal; Seychelles; Sierra-Leone; Sudan; Tanzania; Tunia; Uganda; Zambia; Zimbabwe); Roxon (Philippines); Samixon (Bahrain; Cyprus; Egypt; Iran; Iraq; Jordan; Kuwait; Lebanon; Libya; Oman; Qatar; Republic-of-Yemen; Saudi-Arabia; Syria; United-Arab-Emirates); Sintrex (Taiwan); Sunflow (Taiwan); Tacex (Mexico); Torocef-1 (Republic-Of-Yemen); Trexofin (Singapore); Triaken (Mexico); Triax (Israel); Tricef (Taiwan); Tricefin (Singapore); Tricephin (Thailand); Trijec (Indonesia); Zefaxone (Thailand); Zefone 250 (Benin; Burkina-Faso; Ethiopia; Gambia; Ghana; Guinea; Ivory-Coast; Kenya; Liberia; Malawi; Mali; Mauritania; Mauritius; Morocco; Niger; Nigeria; Senegal; Seychelles; Sierra-Leone; Sudan; Tanzania; Tunia; Uganda; Zambia; Zimbabwe)

Cost of Therapy: $462.89 (Infection; Rocephin Injection; 1 g; 1 g/day; 10 day supply)

HCFA JCODE(S): J0696 per 250 mg IV, IM

DESCRIPTION

Ceftriaxone sodium is a sterile, semisynthetic, broad-spectrum cephalosporin antibiotic for intravenous or intramuscular administration. Ceftriaxone sodium is (6*R*,7*R*)-7-[2-(2-Amino-4-thiazolyl)glyoxylamido]-8-oxo-3-[[(1,2,5,6-tetrahydro-2-methyl-5,6-dioxo-as-triazin-3-yl)thio]methyl]-5-thia-l-azabicyclo[4.2.0]oct-2-ene-2-carboxylic acid, 7^2-(*Z*)-(O-methyloxime), disodium salt, sesquaterhydrate.

The chemical formula of ceftriaxone sodium is $C_{18}H_{16}N_8Na_2O_7S_3 \cdot 3.5H_2O$. It has a calculated molecular weight of 661.59.

Ceftriaxone sodium is a white to yellowish-orange crystalline powder which is readily soluble in water, sparingly soluble in methanol and very slightly soluble in ethanol. The pH of a 1% aqueous solution is approximately 6.7. The color of ceftriazone sodium solutions ranges from light yellow to amber, depending on the length of storage, concentration and diluent used.

Ceftriaxone sodium contains approximately 83 mg (3.6 mEq) of sodium per gram of ceftriaxone activity.

CLINICAL PHARMACOLOGY

Average plasma concentrations of ceftriaxone following a single 30 minute intravenous (IV) infusion of a 0.5, 1 or 2 g dose and intramuscular (IM) administration of a single 0.5 (250 mg/ml or 350 mg/ml concentrations) or 1 g dose in healthy subjects are presented in TABLE 1.

Ceftriaxone was completely absorbed following IM administration with mean maximum plasma concentrations occurring between 2 and 3 hours postdosing. Multiple IV or IM doses ranging from 0.5-2 g at 12-24 hour intervals resulted in 15-36% accumulation of ceftriaxone above single dose values.

TABLE 1 *Ceftriaxone Plasma Concentrations After Single Dose Administration*

	Average Plasma Concentrations (μg/ml)								
Dose/Route	**0.5 h**	**1 h**	**2 h**	**4 h**	**6 h**	**8 h**	**12 h**	**16 h**	**24 h**
0.5 g IV*	82	59	48	37	29	23	15	10	5
0.5 g IM 250 mg/ml	22	33	38	35	30	26	16	ND	5
0.5 g IM 350 mg/ml	20	32	38	34	31	24	16	ND	5
1 g IV*	151	111	88	67	53	43	28	18	9
1 g IM	40	68	76	68	56	44	29	ND	ND
2 g IV*	257	192	154	117	89	74	46	31	15

* IV doses were infused at a constant rate over 30 minutes.
ND = Not determined.

Ceftriaxone concentrations in urine are high, as shown in TABLE 2.

TABLE 2 *Urinary Concentrations of Ceftriaxone After Single Dose Administration*

	Average Urinary Concentrations (μg/ml)					
Dose/Route	**0-2 h**	**2-4 h**	**4-8 h**	**8-12 h**	**12-24 h**	**24-48 h**
0.5 g IV	526	366	142	87	70	15
0.5 g IM	115	425	308	127	96	28
1 g IV	995	855	293	147	132	32
1 g IM	504	628	418	237	ND	ND
2 g IV	2692	1976	757	274	198	40

ND = Not determined.

Thirty three percent (33%) to 67% of a ceftriaxone dose was excreted in the urine as unchanged drug and the remainder was secreted in the bile and ultimately found in the feces as microbiologically inactive compounds. After a 1 g IV dose, average concentrations of ceftriaxone, determined from 1-3 hours after dosing, were 581 μg/ml in the gallbladder bile, 788 μg/ml in the common duct bile, 898 μg/ml in the cystic duct bile, 78.2 μg/g in the gallbladder wall and 62.1 μg/ml in the concurrent plasma.

Over a 0.15-3 g dose range in healthy adult subjects, the values of elimination half-life ranged from 5.8-8.7 hours; apparent volume of distribution from 5.78-13.5 L; plasma clearance from 0.58-1.45 L/h; and renal clearance from 0.32-0.73 L/h. Ceftriaxone is reversibly bound to human plasma proteins, and the binding decreased from a value of 95% bound at plasma concentrations of <25 μg/ml to a value of 85% bound at 300 μg/ml. Ceftriaxone crosses the blood placenta barrier.

The average values of maximum plasma concentration, elimination half-life, plasma clearance and volume of distribution after a 50 mg/kg IV dose and after a 75 mg/kg IV dose in pediatric patients suffering from bacterial meningitis are shown in TABLE 3. Ceftriaxone penetrated the inflamed meninges of infants and pediatric patients; CSF concentrations after a 50 mg/kg IV dose and after a 75 mg/kg IV dose are also shown in TABLE 3.

TABLE 3 *Average Pharmacokinetic Parameters of Ceftriaxone in Pediatric Patients With Meningitis*

	50 mg/kg IV	**75 mg/kg IV**
Maximum plasma concentrations (μg/ml)	216	275
Elimination half-life (h)	4.6	4.3
Plasma clearance (ml/h/kg)	49	60
Volume of distribution (ml/kg)	338	373
CSF concentration — inflamed meninges (μg/ml)	5.6	6.4
Range (μg/ml)	1.3-18.5	1.3-44
Time after dose (h)	3.7 (±1.6)	3.3 (±1.4)

Compared to that in healthy adult subjects, the pharmacokinetics of ceftriaxone were only minimally altered in elderly subjects and in patients with renal impairment or hepatic dysfunction (TABLE 4); therefore, dosage adjustments are not necessary for these patients with ceftriaxone dosages up to 2 g/day. Ceftriaxone was not removed to any significant extent from the plasma by hemodialysis. In 6 of 26 dialysis patients, the elimination rate of ceftriaxone was markedly reduced, suggesting that plasma concentrations of ceftriaxone should be monitored in these patients to determine if dosage adjustments are necessary.

TABLE 4 *Average Pharmacokinetic Parameters of Ceftriaxone in Humans*

Subject Group	**Elimination Half-Life (h)**	**Plasma Clearance (L/h)**	**Volume of Distribution (L)**
Healthy Subjects	5.8-8.7	0.58-1.45	5.8-13.5
Elderly Subjects (mean age, 70.5 y)	8.9	0.83	10.7
Patients With Renal Impairment			
Hemodialysis patients (0-5 ml/min)*	14.7	0.65	13.7
Severe (5-15 ml/min)	15.7	0.56	12.5
Moderate (16-30 ml/min)	11.4	0.72	11.8
Mild (31-60 ml/min)	12.4	0.70	13.3
Patients With Liver Disease	8.8	1.1	13.6

* Creatinine clearance.

PHARMACOKINETICS IN THE MIDDLE EAR FLUID

In one study, total ceftriaxone concentrations (bound and unbound) were measured in middle ear fluid obtained during the insertion of tympanostomy tubes in 42 pediatric patients with otitis media. Sampling times were from 1-50 hours after a single intramuscular injection of 50 mg/kg of ceftriaxone. Mean (±SD) ceftriaxone levels in the middle ear reached a peak of 35 (±12) µg/ml at 24 hours, and remained at 19 (±7) µg/ml at 48 hours. Based on middle ear fluid ceftriaxone concentrations in the 23-25 hour and the 46-50 hour sampling time intervals, a half-life of 25 hours was calculated. Ceftriaxone is highly bound to plasma proteins. The extent of binding to proteins in the middle ear fluid is unknown.

MICROBIOLOGY

The bactericidal activity of ceftriaxone results from inhibition of cell wall synthesis. Ceftriaxone has a high degree of stability in the presence of β-lactamases, both penicillinases and cephalosporinases, of gram-negative and gram-positive bacteria.

Ceftriaxone has been shown to be active against most strains of the following microorganisms, both *in vitro* and in clinical infections described inINDICATIONS AND USAGE.

Aerobic Gram-Negative Microorganisms:

Acinetobacter calcoaceticus
Enterobacter aerogenes
Enterobacter cloacae
Escherichia coli
Haemophilus influenzae (including ampicillin-resistant and β-lactamase producing strains)
Haemophilus parainfluenzae
Klebsiella oxytoca
Klebsiella pneumoniae
Moraxella catarrhalis (including β-lactamase producing strains)
Morganella morganii
Neisseria gonorrhoeae (including penicillinase- and nonpenicillinase-producing strains)
Neisseria meningitidis
Proteus mirabilis
Proteus vulgaris
Serratia marcescens

Ceftriaxone is also active against many strains of *Pseudomonas aeruginosa.*

Note: Many strains of the above organisms that are multiply resistant to other antibiotics, *e.g.,* penicillins, cephalosporins, and aminoglycosides, are susceptible to ceftriaxone.

Aerobic Gram-Positive Microorganisms:

Staphylococcus aureus (including penicillinase-producing strains)
Staphylococcus epidermidis
Streptococcus pneumoniae
Streptococcus pyogenes
Viridans group streptococci

Note: Methicillin-resistant staphylococci are resistant to cephalosporins, including ceftriaxone. Most strains of Group D streptococci and enterococci, *e.g., Enterococcus (Streptococcus) faecalis* are resistant.

Anaerobic Microorganisms:

Bacteroides fragilis
Clostridium species
Peptostreptococcus species

Note: Most strains of *Clostridium difficile* are resistant.

The following *in vitro* data are available, **but their clinical significance is unknown.**

Ceftriaxone exhibits *in vitro* minimal inhibitory concentrations (MICs) of ≤8 µg/ml or less against most strains of the following microorganisms, however, the safety and effectiveness of ceftriaxone in treating clinical infections due to these microorganisms have not been established in adequate and well-controlled clinical trials.

Aerobic Gram-Negative Microorganisms:

Citrobacter diversus
Citrobacter freundii
Providencia species (including *Providencia rettgeri*)
Salmonella species (including *Salmonella typhi*)
Shigella species

Aerobic Gram-Positive Microorganisms:

Streptococcus agalactiae

Anaerobic Microorganisms:

Prevotella (Bacteroides) bivius
Porphyromonas (Bacteroides) melaninogenicus

SUSCEPTIBILITY TESTING

Dilution Techniques

Quantitative methods are used to determine antimicrobial minimal inhibitory concentrations (MICs). These MICs provide estimates of the susceptibility of bacteria to antimicrobial compounds. The MICs should be determined using a standardized procedure.[1] Standardized procedures are based on a dilution method (broth or agar) or equivalent with standardized inoculum concentrations and standardized concentrations of ceftriaxone powder. The MIC values should be interpreted according to the criteria in TABLE 5[2] for aerobic organisms other than *Haemophilus* spp, *Neisseria gonorrhoeae,* and *Streptococcus* spp, including *Streptococcus pneumoniae.*

TABLE 5

MIC (µg/ml)	Interpretation
≤8	(S) Susceptible
16-32	(I) Intermediate
≥64	(R) Resistant

The interpretive criteria in TABLE 6[2] should be used when testing *Haemophilus* species using Haemophilus Test Media (HTM).

TABLE 6

MIC (µg/ml)	Interpretation
≤2	(S) Susceptible

The absence of resistant strains precludes defining any categories other than "Susceptible". Strains yielding results suggestive of a "Nonsusceptible" category should be submitted to a reference laboratory for further testing.

The interpretive criteria in TABLE 7[2] should be used when testing *Neisseria gonorrhoeae* when using GC agar base and 1% defined growth supplement.

TABLE 7

MIC (µg/ml)	Interpretation
≤0.25	(S) Susceptible

The absence of resistant strains precludes defining any categories other than "Susceptible". Strains yielding results suggestive of a "Nonsusceptible" category should be submitted to a reference laboratory for further testing.

The interpretive criteria in TABLE 8[2] should be used when testing *Streptococcus* spp including *Streptococcus pneumoniae* using cation-adjusted Mueller-Hinton broth with 2-5% lysed horse blood.

TABLE 8

MIC (µg/ml)	Interpretation
≤2	(S) Susceptible
1	(I) Intermediate
≥2	(R) Resistant

A report of "Susceptible" indicates that the pathogen is likely to be inhibited if the antimicrobial compound in the blood reaches the concentrations usually achievable. A report of "Intermediate" indicates that the results should be considered equivocal, and if the microorganism is not fully susceptible to alternative, clinically feasible drugs, the test should be repeated. This category implies possible clinical applicability in body sites where the drug is physiologically concentrated or in situations where high dosage of the drug can be used. This category also provides a buffer zone which prevents small uncontrolled technical factors from causing major discrepancies in interpretation. A report of "Resistant" indicates that the pathogen is not likely to be inhibited if the antimicrobial compound in the blood reaches the concentrations usually achievable; other therapy should be selected.

Standardized susceptibility test procedures require the use of laboratory control microorganisms to control the technical aspects of the laboratory procedures. Standardized ceftriaxone powder should provide the MIC values shown in TABLE 9.[2]

TABLE 9

Microorganism	ATCC No.	MIC (µg/ml)
Escherichia coli	25922	0.03-0.12
Staphylococcus aureus	29213	1-8
Pseudomonas aeruginosa	27853	8-32
Haemophilus influenzae	49247	0.006-0.25
Neisseria gonorrhoeae	49226	0.004-0.015
Streptococcus pneumoniae	49619	0.03-0.012

Note: A bimodal distribution of MICs results at the extremes of the acceptable range should be suspect and control validity should be verified with data from other control strains.

Diffusion Techniques

Quantitative methods that require measurement of zone diameters also provide reproducible estimates of the susceptibility of bacteria to antimicrobial compounds. One such standardized procedure[3] requires the use of standardized inoculum concentrations. This procedure uses paper discs impregnated with 30 µg of ceftriaxone to test the susceptibility of microorganisms to ceftriaxone.

Reports from the laboratory providing results of the standard single-disc susceptibility test with a 30 µg ceftriaxone disc should be interpreted according to the criteria in TABLE 10 for aerobic organisms other than *Haemophilus* spp, *Neisseria gonorrhoeae,* and *Streptococcus* spp.

TABLE 10

Zone Diameter (mm)	Interpretation
≥21	(S) Susceptible
14-20	(I) Intermediate
≤13	(R) Resistant

The interpretive criteria in TABLE 11[3] should be used when testing *Haemophilus* species when using Haemophilus Test Media (HTM).

TABLE 11

Zone diameter (mm)	Interpretation
≥26	(S) Susceptible

The absence of resistant strains precludes defining any categories other than "Susceptible". Strains yielding results suggestive of a "Nonsusceptible" category should be submitted to a reference laboratory for further testing.

The interpretive criteria in TABLE 12[3] should be used when testing *Neisseria gonorrhoeae* when using GC agar base and 1% defined growth supplement.

TABLE 12

Zone Diameter (mm)	Interpretation
≥35	(S) Susceptible

The absence of resistant strains precludes defining any categories other than "Susceptible". Strains yielding results suggestive of a "Nonsusceptible" category should be submitted to a reference laboratory for further testing.

The interpretive criteria in TABLE 13[3] should be used when testing *Streptococcus* spp other than *Streptococcus pneumoniae* when using Mueller-Hinton agar supplemented with 5% sheep blood incubated in 5% CO_2.

TABLE 13

Zone Diameter (mm)	Interpretation
≥27	(S) Susceptible
25-26	(I) Intermediate
≤24	(R) Resistant

Interpretation should be as stated above for results using dilution techniques. Interpretation involves correlation of the diameter obtained in the disc test with the MIC for ceftriaxone.

Disc diffusion interpretive criteria for ceftriaxone discs against *Streptococcus pneumoniae* are not available, however, isolates of *pneumococci* with oxacillin zone diameters of >20 mm are susceptible (MIC ≤0.06 μg/ml) to penicillin and can be considered susceptible to ceftriaxone. *Streptococcus pneumoniae* isolates should not be reported as penicillin (ceftriaxone) resistant or intermediate based solely on an oxacillin zone diameter of ≤19 mm. The ceftriaxone MIC should be determined for those isolates with oxacillin zone diameters ≤19 mm.

As with standardized dilution techniques, diffusion methods require the use of laboratory control microorganisms that are used to control the technical aspects of the laboratory procedures. For the diffusion technique, the 30 μg ceftriaxone disc should provide the zone diameters in these laboratory test quality control strains as shown in TABLE 14.[3]

TABLE 14

Microorganism	ATCC No.	Zone Diamter Ranges (mm)
Escherichia coli	25922	29-35
Staphylococcus aureus	25923	22-28
Pseudomonas aeruginosa	27853	17-23
Haemophilus influenzae	49247	31-39
Neisseria gonorrhoeae	49226	39-51
Streptococcus pneumoniae	49619	30-35

Anaerobic Techniques

For anaerobic bacteria, the susceptibility to ceftriaxone as MICs can be determined by standardized test methods.[4] The MIC values obtained should be interpreted according to the criteria shown in TABLE 15.

TABLE 15

MIC (μg/ml)	Interpretation
≤16	(S) Susceptible
32	(I) Intermediate
≥64	(R) Resistant

As with other susceptibility techniques, the use of laboratory control microorganisms is required to control the technical aspects of the laboratory standardized procedures. Standardized ceftriaxone powder should provide the MIC values as shown in TABLE 16 for the indicated standardized anaerobic dilution[4] testing method.

TABLE 16

Method	Microorganism	ATCC No.	MIC (μg/ml)
Agar	*Bacteroides fragilis*	25285	32-128
	Bacteroides thetaiotamicron	29741	64-256
Broth	*Bacteroides thetaiotaomicron*	29741	32-128

INDICATIONS AND USAGE

Ceftriaxone is indicated for the treatment of the following infections when caused by susceptible organisms:

LOWER RESPIRATORY TRACT INFECTIONS

Caused by *Streptococcus pneumoniae, Staphylococcus aureus, Haemophilus influenzae, Haemophilus parainfluenzae, Klebsiella pneumoniae, Escherichia coli, Enterobacter aerogenes, Proteus mirabilis* or *Serratia marcescens.*

ACUTE BACTERIAL OTITIS MEDIA

Caused by *Streptococcus pneumoniae, Haemophilus influenzae* (including β-lactamase producing strains) or *Moraxella catarrhalis* (including β-lactamase producing strains).

Note: In one study lower clinical cure rates were observed with a single dose of ceftrioxone compared to 10 days of oral therapy. In a second study comparable cure rates were observed between single dose ceftrioxone and the comparator. The potentially lower clinical cure rate of ceftrioxone should be balanced against the potential advantages of parenteral therapy.

SKIN AND SKIN STRUCTURE INFECTIONS

Caused by *Staphylococcus aureus, Staphylococcus epidermidis, Streptococcus pyogenes, Viridans* group streptococci, *Escherichia coli, Enterobacter cloacae, Klebsiella oxytoca, Klebsiella pneumoniae, Proteus mirabilis, Morganella morganii,* Pseudomonas aeruginosa, Serratia marcescens, Acinetobacter calcoaceticus, Bacteroides fragilis** or *Peptostreptococcus* species.

C

URINARY TRACT INFECTIONS (COMPLICATED AND UNCOMPLICATED)

Caused by *Escherichia coli, Proteus mirabilis, Proteus vulgaris, Morganella morganii* or *Klebsiella pneumoniae.*

UNCOMPLICATED GONORRHEA (CERVICAL/URETHRAL AND RECTAL)

Caused by *Neisseria gonorrhoeae,* including both penicillinase- and nonpenicillinase-producing strains, and pharyngeal gonorrhea caused by nonpenicillinase-producing strains of *Neisseria gonorrhoeae.*

PELVIC INFLAMMATORY DISEASE

Caused by *Neisseria gonorrhoeae.* Ceftriaxone, like other cephalosporins, has no activity against *Chlamydia trachomatis.* Therefore, when cephalosporins are used in the treatment of patients with pelvic inflammatory disease and *Chlamydia trachomatis* is one of the suspected pathogens, appropriate antichlamydial coverage should be added.

BACTERIAL SEPTICEMIA

Caused by *Staphylococcus aureus, Streptococcus pneumoniae, Escherichia coli, Haemophilus influenzae* or *Klebsiella pneumoniae.*

BONE AND JOINT INFECTIONS

Caused by *Staphylococcus aureus, Streptococcus pneumoniae, Escherichia coli, Proteus mirabilis, Klebsiella pneumoniae* or *Enterobacter* species.

INTRA-ABDOMINAL INFECTIONS

Caused by *Escherichia coli, Klebsiella pneumoniae, Bacteroides fragilis, Clostridium species* (*Note:* most strains of *Clostridium difficile* are resistant) or *Peptostreptococcus* species.

MENINGITIS

Caused by *Haemophilus influenzae, Neisseria meningitidis* or *Streptococcus pneumoniae.* ceftrioxone has also been used successfully in a limited number of cases of meningitis and shunt infection caused by *Staphylococcus epidermidis** and *Escherichia coli.*

*Efficacy for this organism in this organ system was studied in fewer than 10 infections.

SURGICAL PROPHYLAXIS

The preoperative administration of a single 1 g dose of Ceftrioxone may reduce the incidence of postoperative infections in patients undergoing surgical procedures classified as contaminated or potentially contaminated (*e.g.,* vaginal or abdominal hysterectomy or cholecystectomy for chronic calculous cholecystitis in high-risk patients, such as those over 70 years of age, with acute cholecystitis not requiring therapeutic antimicrobials, obstructive jaundice or common duct bile stones) and in surgical patients for whom infection at the operative site would present serious risk (*e.g.,* during coronary artery bypass surgery). Although ceftrioxone has been shown to have been as effective as cefazolin in the prevention of infection following coronary artery bypass surgery, no placebo-controlled trials have been conducted to evaluate any cephalosporin antibiotic in the prevention of infection following coronary artery bypass surgery.

When administered prior to surgical procedures for which it is indicated, a single 1 g dose of ceftrioxone provides protection from most infections due to susceptible organisms throughout the course of the procedure.

Before instituting treatment with ceftrioxone, appropriate specimens should be obtained for isolation of the causative organism and for determination of its susceptibility to the drug. Therapy may be instituted prior to obtaining results of susceptibility testing.

NON-FDA APPROVED INDICATIONS

Ceftriaxone has also been used in the treatment of Lyme's disease, although this use has not been approved by the FDA.

CONTRAINDICATIONS

Ceftrioxone is contraindicated in patients with known allergy to the cephalosporin class of antibiotics.

WARNINGS

BEFORE THERAPY WITH CEFTRIOXONE IS INSTITUTED, CAREFUL INQUIRY SHOULD BE MADE TO DETERMINE WHETHER THE PATIENT HAS HAD PREVIOUS HYPERSENSITIVITY REACTIONS TO CEPHALOSPORINS, PENICILLINS OR OTHER DRUGS. THIS PRODUCT SHOULD BE GIVEN CAUTIOUSLY TO PENICILLIN-SENSITIVE PATIENTS. ANTIBIOTICS SHOULD BE ADMINISTERED WITH CAUTION TO ANY PATIENT WHO HAS DEMONSTRATED SOME FORM OF ALLERGY, PARTICULARLY TO DRUGS. SERIOUS ACUTE HYPERSENSITIVITY REACTIONS MAY REQUIRE THE USE OF SUBCUTANEOUS EPINEPHRINE AND OTHER EMERGENCY MEASURES.

Pseudomembranous colitis has been reported with nearly all antibacterial agents, including ceftriaxone, and may range in severity from mild to life-threatening. Therefore, it is important to consider this diagnosis in patients who present with diarrhea subsequent to the administration of antibacterial agents.

Treatment with antibacterial agents alters the normal flora of the colon and may permit overgrowth of clostridia. Studies indicate that a toxin produced by *Clostridium difficile* is one primary cause of "antibiotic-associated colitis".

After the diagnosis of pseudomembranous colitis has been established, appropriate therapeutic measures should be initiated. Mild cases of pseudomembranous colitis usually respond to drug discontinuation alone. In moderate to severe cases, consideration should be given to management with fluids and electrolytes, protein supplementation and treatment with an antibacterial drug clinically effective against *C. difficile* colitis.

PRECAUTIONS

GENERAL

Although transient elevations of BUN and serum creatinine have been observed, at the recommended dosages, the nephrotoxic potential of ceftriaxone is similar to that of other cephalosporins.

Ceftriaxone is excreted via both biliary and renal excretion (see CLINICAL PHARMACOLOGY). Therefore, patients with renal failure normally require no adjustment in dosage when usual doses of ceftriaxone are administered, but concentrations of drug in the serum should be monitored periodically. If evidence of accumulation exists, dosage should be decreased accordingly.

Dosage adjustments should not be necessary in patients with hepatic dysfunction; however, in patients with both hepatic dysfunction and significant renal disease, ceftriaxone dosage should not exceed 2 g daily without close monitoring of serum concentrations.

Alterations in prothrombin times have occurred rarely in patients treated with ceftriaxone. Patients with impaired vitamin K synthesis or low vitamin K stores (*e.g.*, chronic hepatic disease and malnutrition) may require monitoring of prothrombin time during ceftriaxone treatment. Vitamin K administration (10 mg weekly) may be necessary if the prothrombin time is prolonged before or during therapy.

Prolonged use of ceftriaxone may result in overgrowth of nonsusceptible organisms. Careful observation of the patient is essential. If superinfection occurs during therapy, appropriate measures should be taken.

Ceftriaxone should be prescribed with caution in individuals with a history of gastrointestinal disease, especially colitis.

There have been reports of sonographic abnormalities in the gallbladder of patients treated with ceftriaxone; some of these patients also had symptoms of gallbladder disease. These abnormalities appear on sonography as an echo without acoustical shadowing suggesting sludge or as an echo with acoustical shadowing which may be misinterpreted as gallstones. The chemical nature of the sonographically detected material has been determined to be predominantly a ceftriaxone-calcium salt. **The condition appears to be transient and reversible upon discontinuation of ceftriaxone and institution of conservative management.** Therefore, ceftriaxone should be discontinued in patients who develop signs and symptoms suggestive of gallbladder disease and/or the sonographic findings described above.

CARCINOGENESIS, MUTAGENESIS, AND IMPAIRMENT OF FERTILITY

Carcinogenesis: Considering the maximum duration of treatment and the class of the compound, carcinogenicity studies with ceftriaxone in animals have not been performed. The maximum duration of animal toxicity studies was 6 months.

Mutagenesis: Genetic toxicology tests included the Ames test, a micronucleus test and a test for chromosomal aberrations in human lymphocytes cultured *in vitro* with ceftriaxone. Ceftriaxone showed no potential for mutagenic activity in these studies.

Impairment of Fertility: Ceftriaxone produced no impairment of fertility when given intravenously to rats at daily doses up to 586 mg/kg/day, approximately 20 times the recommended clinical dose of 2 g/day.

PREGNANCY, TERATOGENIC EFFECTS, PREGNANCY CATEGORY B

Reproductive studies have been performed in mice and rats at doses up to 20 times the usual human dose and have no evidence of embryotoxicity, fetotoxicity or teratogenicity. In primates, no embryotoxicity or teratogenicity was demonstrated at a dose approximately 3 times the human dose.

There are, however, no adequate and well-controlled studies in pregnant women. Because animal reproductive studies are not always predictive of human response, this drug should be used during pregnancy only if clearly needed.

Nonteratogenic Effects: In rats, in the Segment I (fertility and general reproduction) and Segment III (perinatal and postnatal) studies with intravenously administered ceftriaxone, no adverse effects were noted on various reproductive parameters during gestation and lactation, including postnatal growth, functional behavior and reproductive ability of the offspring, at doses of 586 mg/kg/day or less.

NURSING MOTHERS

Low concentrations of ceftriaxone are excreted in human milk. Caution should be exercised when ceftriaxone is administered to a nursing woman.

PEDIATRIC USE

Safety and effectiveness of ceftriaxone in neonates, infants and pediatric patients have been established for the dosages described in DOSAGE AND ADMINISTRATION. *In vitro* studies have shown that ceftriaxone, like some other cephalosporins, can displace bilirubin from serum albumin. Ceftriaxone should not be administered to hyperbilirubinemic neonates, especially prematures.

ADVERSE REACTIONS

Ceftriaxone is generally well tolerated. In clinical trials, the following adverse reactions, which were considered to be related to ceftriaxone therapy or of uncertain etiology, were observed:

Local Reactions: Pain, induration and tenderness was 1% overall. Phlebitis was reported in <1% after IV administration. The incidence of warmth, tightness or induration was 17% (3/17) after IM administration of 350 mg/ml and 5% (1/20) after IM administration of 250 mg/ml.

Hypersensitivity: Rash (1.7%). Less frequently reported (<1%) were pruritus, fever or chills.

Hematologic Eosinophilia (6%), thrombocytosis (5.1%) and leukopenia (2.1%). Less frequently reported (<1%) were anemia, hemolytic anemia, neutropenia, lymphopenia, thrombocytopenia and prolongation of the prothrombin time.

Gastrointestinal: Diarrhea (2.7%). Less frequently reported (<1%) were nausea or vomiting, and dysgeusia. The onset of pseudomembranous colitis symptoms may occur during or after antibacterial treatment (see WARNINGS).

Hepatic: Elevations of SGOT (3.1%) or SGPT (3.3%). Less frequently reported (<1%) were elevations of alkaline phosphatase and bilirubin.

Renal: Elevations of the BUN (1.2%). Less frequently reported (<1%) were elevations of creatinine and the presence of casts in the urine.

Central Nervous System: Headache or dizziness were reported occasionally (<1%).

Genitourinary: Moniliasis or vaginitis were reported occasionally (<1%).

Miscellaneous: Diaphoresis and flushing were reported occasionally (<1%).

Other rarely observed adverse reactions (<0.1%) include: Leukocytosis, lymphocytosis, monocytosis, basophilia, a decrease in the prothrombin time, jaundice, gallbladder sludge, glycosuria, hematuria, anaphylaxis, bronchospasm, serum sickness, abdominal pain, colitis, flatulence, dyspepsia, palpitations, epistaxis, biliary lithiasis, agranulocytosis, renal precipitations, and nephrolithiasis.

DOSAGE AND ADMINISTRATION

Ceftriaxone may be administered intravenously or intramuscularly.

ADULTS

The usual adult daily dose is 1-2 g given once a day (or in equally divided doses twice a day) depending on the type and severity of infection. The total daily dose should not exceed 4 g.

If *Chlamydia trachomatis* is a suspected pathogen, appropriate antichlamydial coverage should be added, because ceftriaxone sodium has no activity against this organism.

For the treatment of uncomplicated gonococcal infections, a single intramuscular dose of 250 mg is recommended.

For preoperative use (surgical prophylaxis), a single dose of 1 g administered intravenously ½ to 2 hours before surgery is recommended.

PEDIATRIC PATIENTS

For the treatment of skin and skin structure infections, the recommended total daily dose is 50-75 mg/kg given once a day (or in equally divided doses twice a day). The total daily dose should not exceed 2 g.

For the treatment of acute bacterial otitis media, a single intramuscular dose of 50 mg/kg (not to exceed 1 g) is recommended (see INDICATIONS AND USAGE).

For the treatment of serious miscellaneous infections other than meningitis, the recommended total daily dose is 50-75 mg/kg, given in divided doses every 12 hours. The total daily dose should not exceed 2 g.

In the treatment of meningitis, it is recommended that the initial therapeutic dose be 100 mg/kg (not to exceed 4 g). Thereafter, a total daily dose of 100 mg/kg/day (not to exceed 4 g daily) is recommended. The daily dose may be administered once a day (or in equally divided doses every 12 hours). The usual duration of therapy is 7-14 days.

Generally, ceftriaxone therapy should be continued for at least 2 days after the signs and symptoms of infection have disappeared. The usual duration of therapy is 4-14 days; in complicated infections, longer therapy may be required.

When treating infections caused by *Streptococcus pyogenes,* therapy should be continued for at least 10 days.

No dosage adjustment is necessary for patients with impairment of renal or hepatic function; however, blood levels should be monitored in patients with severe renal impairment (*e.g.*, dialysis patients) and in patients with both renal and hepatic dysfunctions.

COMPATIBILITY AND STABILITY

Ceftriaxone sterile powder should be stored at room temperature [25°C (77°F)] or below and protected from light. After reconstitution, protection from normal light is not necessary. The color of solutions ranges from light yellow to amber, depending on the length of storage, concentration and diluent used.

Ceftriaxone *intramuscular* solutions remain stable (loss of potency less than 10%) for the time periods shown in TABLE 19.

TABLE 19

		Storage	
Diluent	Concentration (mg/ml)	Room Temp. (25°C)	Refrigerated (4°C)
Sterile water for injection	100	3 d	10 d
	250, 350	24 h	3 d
0.9% Sodium chloride solution	100	3 d	10 d
	250, 350	24 h	3 d
5% Dextrose solution	100	3 d	10 d
	250, 350	24 h	3 d
Bacteriostatic water + 0.9% benzyl alcohol	100	24 h	10 d
	250, 350	24 h	3 d
1% Lidocaine solution (without epinephrine)	100	24 h	10 d
	250, 350	24 h	3 d

Ceftriaxone *intravenous* solutions, at concentrations of 10, 20 and 40 mg/ml, remain stable (loss of potency less than 10%) stored in glass or PVC containers for the time periods shown in TABLE 20.

Similarly, ceftriaxone *intravenous* solutions, at concentrations of 100 mg/ml, remain stable in the IV piggyback glass containers for the above specified time periods.

TABLE 20

Diluent	Storage Room Temp. (25°C)	Refrigerated (4°C)
Sterile water for injection	3 d	10 d
0.9% Sodium chloride solution	3 d	10 d
5% Dextrose solution	3 d	10 d
10% Dextrose solution	3 d	10 d
5% Dextrose + 0.9% sodium chloride solution*	3 d	Incompatible
5% Dextrose + 0.45% sodium chloride solution	3 d	Incompatible

* Data available for 10-40 mg/ml concentrations in this diluent in PVC containers only.

The following *intravenous* ceftrioxone solutions are stable at room temperature (25°C) for 24 hours, at concentrations between 10 mg/ml and 40 mg/ml: Sodium lactate (PVC container), 10% invert sugar (glass container), 5% sodium bicarbonate (glass container), Freamine III (glass container), Normosol-M in 5% dextrose (glass and PVC containers), Ionosol-B in 5% dextrose (glass container), 5% mannitol (glass container), 10% mannitol (glass container).

Ceftriaxone has been shown to be compatible with Flagyl IV (metronidazole hydrochloride). The concentration should not exceed 5-7.5 mg/ml metronidazole hydrochloride with ceftriaxone 10 mg/ml as an admixture. The admixture is stable for 24 hours at room temperature only in 0.9% sodium chloride injection or 5% dextrose in water (D5W). No compatibility studies have been conducted with the Flagyl IV RTU (metronidazole) formulation or using other diluents. Metronidazole at concentrations greater than 8 mg/ml will precipitate. Do not refrigerate the admixture as precipitation will occur.

Vancomycin and fluconazole are physically incompatible with ceftriaxone in admixtures. When either of these drugs is to be administered concomitantly with ceftriaxone by intermittent intravenous infusion, it is recommended that they be given sequentially, with thorough flushing of the intravenous lines (with 1 of the compatible fluids) between the administrations.

After the indicated stability time periods, unused portions of solutions should be discarded.

Note: Parenteral drug products should be inspected visually for particulate matter before administration.

Ceftrioxone reconstituted with 5% dextrose or 0.9% sodium chloride solution at concentrations between 10 and 40 mg/ml, and then stored in frozen state (-20°C) in PVC or polyolefin containers, remains stable for 26 weeks.

Frozen solutions should be thawed at room temperature before use. After thawing, unused portions should be discarded. **DO NOT REFREEZE.**

Ceftrioxone solutions should *not* be physically mixed with or piggybacked into solutions containing other antimicrobial drugs or into diluent solutions other than those listed above, due to possible incompatibility.

ANIMAL PHARMACOLOGY

Concretions consisting of the precipitated calcium salt of ceftriaxone have been found in the gallbladder bile of dogs and baboons treated with ceftriaxone.

These appeared as a gritty sediment in dogs that received 100 mg/kg/day for 4 weeks. A similar phenomenon has been observed in baboons but only after a protracted dosing period (6 months) at higher dose levels (335 mg/kg/day or more). The likelihood of this occurrence in humans is considered to be low, since ceftriaxone has a greater plasma half-life in humans, the calcium salt of ceftriaxone is more soluble in human gallbladder bile and the calcium content of human gallbladder bile is relatively low.

HOW SUPPLIED

Rocephin is supplied as a sterile crystalline powder in glass vials and piggyback bottles.

Vials containing 250 mg, 500 mg, 1 g, and 2 g equivalent of ceftriaxone.

Piggyback bottles containing 1 and 2 g equivalent of ceftriaxone.

Bulk pharmacy containers, containing 10 g equivalent of ceftriaxone. NOT FOR DIRECT ADMINISTRATION.

Rochephin is also supplied in an Intramuscular Convenience Kit, available in 2 strengths, consisting of a vial of ceftriaxone sodium as a sterile crystalline powder and a vial of Xylocaine-MPF 1% (lidocaine HCl injection).

Kit containing 1 vial of 500 mg equivalent of ceftriaxone, plus 1 vial of 2.1 ml Xylocaine.

Kit containing 1 vial of 1 g equivalent of ceftriaxone, plus 1 vial of 2.1 ml Xylocaine.

Rocephin is also supplied as a sterile crystalline powder in ADD-Vantage Vials as follows:

ADD-Vantage vials containing 1 and 2 g equivalent of ceftriaxone.

Rocephin is also supplied premixed as a frozen, iso-osmotic, sterile, nonpyrogenic solution of ceftriaxone sodium in 50 ml single dose Galaxy containers. The following strengths are available:

1 g equivalent of ceftriaxone, iso-osmotic with approximately 1.9 g dextrose hydrous, added.

2 g equivalent of ceftriaxone, iso-osmotic with approximately 1.2 g dextrose hydrous, added.

Storage: Store Rocephin in the frozen state at or below -20°C (-4°F).

PRODUCT LISTING - EQUIVALENTS NOT AVAILABLE

Kit - Intramuscular - 1 Gm

1's	$46.48	ROCEPHIN IM CONVENIENCE KIT, Roche Laboratories	00004-2013-92
1's	$47.40	ROCEPHIN IM CONVENIENCE KIT, Allscripts Pharmaceutical Company	54569-4415-00
1's	$50.24	ROCEPHIN IM CONVENIENCE KIT, Roche Laboratories	00004-1964-39

Kit - Intramuscular - 500 mg

1's	$27.09	ROCEPHIN IM CONVENIENCE KIT, Roche Laboratories	00004-2014-92
1's	$29.88	ROCEPHIN IM CONVENIENCE KIT, Roche Laboratories	00004-1963-39

Powder For Injection - Injectable - 1 Gm

1's	$47.40	ROCEPHIN, Allscripts Pharmaceutical Company	54569-3477-00
1's	$48.25	ROCEPHIN, Roche Laboratories	00004-1964-02
1's	$50.24	ROCEPHIN, Southwood Pharmaceuticals Inc	58016-9438-01
1's	$52.34	ROCEPHIN, Roche Laboratories	00004-1964-04
1's	$53.61	ROCEPHIN, Prescript Pharmaceuticals	00247-0331-01
1's	$55.26	ROCEPHIN, Physicians Total Care	54868-2488-01
10's	$462.89	ROCEPHIN, Allscripts Pharmaceutical Company	54569-1802-01
10's	$505.89	ROCEPHIN, Prescript Pharmaceuticals	00247-0331-10
10's	$511.11	ROCEPHIN, Roche Laboratories	00004-1964-01
10's	$527.65	ROCEPHIN, Roche Laboratories	00004-1964-05

Powder For Injection - Injectable - 2 Gm

1's	$100.56	ROCEPHIN, Roche Laboratories	00004-1965-02
10's	$919.82	ROCEPHIN, Allscripts Pharmaceutical Company	54569-3207-00
10's	$1015.65	ROCEPHIN, Roche Laboratories	00004-1965-01
10's	$1042.09	ROCEPHIN, Roche Laboratories	00004-1965-05

Powder For Injection - Injectable - 10 Gm

1's	$498.25	ROCEPHIN, Roche Laboratories	00004-1971-01

Powder For Injection - Injectable - 250 mg

1's	$16.04	ROCEPHIN, Allscripts Pharmaceutical Company	54569-3478-00
1's	$17.73	ROCEPHIN, Roche Laboratories	00004-1962-02
10's	$149.24	ROCEPHIN, Allscripts Pharmaceutical Company	54569-1386-00
10's	$157.00	ROCEPHIN, Southwood Pharmaceuticals Inc	58016-9453-01
10's	$159.96	ROCEPHIN, Physicians Total Care	54868-0934-00
10's	$164.80	ROCEPHIN, Roche Laboratories	00004-1962-01

Powder For Injection - Injectable - 500 mg

1's	$28.19	ROCEPHIN, Allscripts Pharmaceutical Company	54569-3479-00
1's	$31.13	ROCEPHIN, Roche Laboratories	00004-1963-02
1's	$32.45	ROCEPHIN, Physicians Total Care	54868-3221-01
10's	$270.53	ROCEPHIN, Allscripts Pharmaceutical Company	54569-1377-00
10's	$285.00	ROCEPHIN, Southwood Pharmaceuticals Inc	58016-9551-01
10's	$289.49	ROCEPHIN, Physicians Total Care	54868-3221-00
10's	$298.71	ROCEPHIN, Roche Laboratories	00004-1963-01

Solution - Intravenous - 1 Gm/50 ml

50 ml x 24	$980.10	ROCEPHIN, Baxter Healthcare Corporation	00004-2002-78

Solution - Intravenous - 2 Gm/50 ml

50 ml x 24	$1721.10	ROCEPHIN, Baxter Healthcare Corporation	00004-2003-78

Cefuroxime *(000695)*

For related information, see the comparative table section in Appendix A.

Categories: Bronchitis, chronic, acute exacerbation; Gonorrhea; Infection, bone; Infection, central nervous system; Infection, ear, middle; Infection, joint; Infection, lower respiratory tract; Infection, sexually transmitted; Infection, skin and skin structures; Infection, upper respiratory tract; Infection, urinary tract; Meningitis; Pharyngitis; Prophylaxis, perioperative; Septicemia; Tonsillitis; Pregnancy Category B; FDA Approved 1987 Dec

Drug Classes: Antibiotics, cephalosporins

Brand Names: **Ceftin**

Foreign Brand Availability: Axetine (Hong-Kong); Bearcef (Korea); Cefogen (Thailand); Cefuril (India); Cefudura (Germany); Cefuhexal (Germany); Cefuracet (Mexico); Cefurax (Germany); Cefuro-Puren (Germany); Cefurox-wolff (Germany); Cefutil (Bahrain; Cyprus; Egypt; Iran; Iraq; Jordan; Kuwait; Lebanon; Libya; Oman; Qatar; Republic-of-Yemen; Saudi-Arabia; Syria; United-Arab-Emirates); Cepazine (France); Cethixim (Indonesia); Cetoxil (Mexico); Elobact (Germany); Froxime (Bahrain; Cyprus; Egypt; Iran; Iraq; Jordan; Kuwait; Lebanon; Libya; Oman; Qatar; Republic-of-Yemen; Saudi-Arabia; Syria; United-Arab-Emirates); Furoxime (Thailand); Kalcef (Indonesia); Magnaspor (Thailand); Oraxim (Bahrain; Cyprus; Egypt; Iran; Iraq; Jordan; Kuwait; Lebanon; Libya; Oman; Qatar; Republic-of-Yemen; Saudi-Arabia; Syria; United-Arab-Emirates); Sharox-500 (Indonesia); Zinacef (Philippines); Zinat (Switzerland); Zinnat (Australia; Austria; Bahamas; Bahrain; Barbados; Belgium; Belize; Benin; Bermuda; Burkina-Faso; China; Colombia; Costa-Rica; Curacao; Cyprus; Czech-Republic; Denmark; Dominican-Republic; Egypt; El-Salvador; England; Ethiopia; Finland; France; Gambia; Germany; Ghana; Guatemala; Guinea; Guyana; Honduras; Hong-Kong; Indonesia; Iran; Iraq; Ireland; Israel; Italy; Ivory-Coast; Jamaica; Jordan; Kenya; Korea; Kuwait; Lebanon; Liberia; Libya; Malawi; Malaysia; Mali; Mauritania; Mauritius; Mexico; Morocco; Netherland-Antilles; Netherlands; New-Zealand; Niger; Nigeria; Oman; Panama; Philippines; Puerto-Rico; Qatar; Republic-of-Yemen; Saudi-Arabia; Senegal; Seychelles; Sierra-Leone; South-Africa; Spain; Sudan; Surinam; Switzerland; Syria; Taiwan; Tanzania; Thailand; Trinidad; Tunia; Uganda; United-Arab-Emirates; Zambia; Zimbabwe); Zoref (Portugal)

Cost of Therapy: $88.20 (Infection; Ceftin; 250 mg; 2 tablets/day; 10 day supply)

IM-IV

DESCRIPTION

Note: The trade names have been used throughout this monograph for clarity.

Cefuroxime is a semisynthetic, broad-spectrum, cephalosporin antibiotic for parenteral administration. It is the sodium salt of (6R,7R)-3-carbamoyloxymethyl-7-[Z-2-methoxyimino-2-(fur-2-yl)acetamido]ceph-3-em-4-carboxylate.

The empirical formula is $C_{16}H_{15}N_4NaO_8S$, representing a molecular weight of 446.4.

Zinacef contains approximately 54.2 mg (2.4 mEq) of sodium per gram of cefuroxime activity.

Zinacef in sterile crystalline form is supplied in vials equivalent to 750 mg, 1.5 g, or 7.5 g of cefuroxime as cefuroxime sodium and in ADD-Vantage vials equivalent to 750 mg or 1.5 g of cefuroxime as cefuroxime sodium. Solutions of Zinacef range in color from light yellow to amber, depending on the concentration and diluent used. The pH of freshly constituted solutions usually ranges from 6 to 8.5.

Zinacef is available as a frozen, iso-osmotic, sterile, nonpyrogenic solution with 750 mg or 1.5 g of cefuroxime as cefuroxime sodium. Approximately 1.4 g of dextrose hydrous has been added to the 750 mg dose to adjust the osmolality. Sodium citrate hydrous has been added as a buffer (300 mg and 600 mg to the 750 mg and 1.5 g doses, respectively). Zinacef contains approximately 111 mg (4.8 mEq) and 222 mg (9.7 mEq) of sodium in the 750 mg and 1.5 g doses, respectively. The pH has been adjusted with hydrochloric acid and may have been adjusted with sodium hydroxide. Solutions of premixed Zinacef range in color from light yellow to amber. The solution is intended for intravenous (IV) use after thawing to room temperature. The osmolality of the solution is approximately 300 mOsmol/kg, and the pH of thawed solutions ranges from 5 to 7.5.

The plastic container for the frozen solution is fabricated from a specially designed multilayer plastic, PL 2040. Solutions are in contact with the polyethylene layer of this container and can leach out certain chemical components of the plastic in very small amounts within the expiration period. The suitability of the plastic has been confirmed in tests in animals according to USP biological tests for plastic containers as well as by tissue culture toxicity studies.

CLINICAL PHARMACOLOGY

After intramuscular (IM) injection of a 750 mg dose of cefuroxime to normal volunteers, the mean peak serum concentration was 27 μg/ml. The peak occurred at approximately 45 minutes (range, 15-60 minutes). Following IV doses of 750 mg and 1.5 g, serum concentrations were approximately 50 and 100 μg/ml, respectively, at 15 minutes. Therapeutic serum concentrations of approximately 2 μg/ml or more were maintained for 5.3 hours and 8 hours or more, respectively. There was no evidence of accumulation of cefuroxime in the serum following IV administration of 1.5 g doses every 8 hours to normal volunteers. The serum half-life after either IM or IV injections is approximately 80 minutes.

Approximately 89% of a dose of cefuroxime is excreted by the kidneys over an 8 hour period, resulting in high urinary concentrations.

Following the IM administration of a 750 mg single dose, urinary concentrations averaged 1300 μg/ml during the first 8 hours. Intravenous doses of 750 mg and 1.5 g produced urinary levels averaging 1150 and 2500 μg/ml, respectively, during the first 8 hour period.

The concomitant oral administration of probenecid with cefuroxime slows tubular secretion, decreases renal clearance by approximately 40%, increases the peak serum level by approximately 30%, and increases the serum half-life by approximately 30%. Cefuroxime is detectable in therapeutic concentrations in pleural fluid, joint fluid, bile, sputum, bone, and aqueous humor.

Cefuroxime is detectable in therapeutic concentrations in cerebrospinal fluid (CSF) of adults and pediatric patients with meningitis. TABLE 1 shows the concentrations of cefuroxime achieved in cerebrospinal fluid during multiple dosing of patients with meningitis.

Cefuroxime is approximately 50% bound to serum protein.

TABLE 1 *Concentrations of Cefuroxime Achieved in Cerebrospinal Fluid During Multiple Dosing of Patients With Meningitis*

Patients	Dose		Mean (Range)*
Pediatric patients (4 weeks to 6.5 years)	200 mg/kg/day, divided q6h	n=5	6.6 (0.9-17.3)
Pediatric patients (7 months to 9 years)	200-230 mg/kg/day, divided q8h	n=6	8.3 (<2-22.5)
Adults	1.5 g q8h	n=2	5.2 (2.7-8.9)
Adults	1.5 g q6h	n=10	6.0 (1.5-13.5)

* CSF cefuroxime concentrations (μg/ml) achieved within 8 hours post dose.

MICROBIOLOGY

Cefuroxime has *in vitro* activity against a wide range of gram-positive and gram-negative organisms, and it is highly stable in the presence of beta-lactamases of certain gram-negative bacteria. The bactericidal action of cefuroxime results from inhibition of cell-wall synthesis.

Cefuroxime is usually active against the following organisms *in vitro*:

Aerobes, Gram-Positive: *Staphylococcus aureus, Staphylococcus epidermidis, Streptococcus pneumoniae,* and *Streptococcus pyogenes* (and other streptococci).

NOTE: Most strains of enterococci, *e.g., Enterococcus faecalis* (formerly *Streptococcus faecalis*), are resistant to cefuroxime. Methicillin-resistant staphylococci and *Listeria monocytogenes* are resistant to cefuroxime.

Aerobes, Gram-Negative: *Citrobacter* spp., *Enterobacter* spp., *Escherichia coli, Haemophilus influenzae* (including ampicillin-resistant strains), *Haemophilus parainfluenzae, Klebsiella* spp. (including *Klebsiella pneumoniae), Moraxella (Branhamella) catarrhalis* (including ampicillin- and cephalothin-resistant strains), *Morganella morganii* (formerly *Proteus morganii*), *Neisseria gonorrhoeae* (including penicillinase- and non-penicillinase-producing strains), *Neisseria meningitidis, Proteus mirabilis, Providencia rettgeri* (formerly *Proteus rettgeri*), *Salmonella* spp., and *Shigella* spp.

NOTE: Some strains of *Morganella morganii, Enterobacter cloacae,* and *Citrobacter* spp. have been shown by *in vitro* tests to be resistant to cefuroxime and other cephalosporins. *Pseudomonas* and *Campylobacter* spp., *Acinetobacter calcoaceticus,* and most strains of *Serratia* spp. and *Proteus vulgaris* are resistant to most first- and second generation cephalosporins.

Anaerobes: Gram-positive and gram-negative cocci (including *Peptococcus* and *Peptostreptococcus* spp.), gram-positive bacilli (including *Clostridium* spp.), and gram-negative bacilli (including *Bacteroides* and *Fusobacterium* spp.).

NOTE: Clostridium difficile and most strains of *Bacteroides fragilis* are resistant to cefuroxime.

Susceptibility Testing

Diffusion Techniques

Quantitative methods that require measurement of zone diameters give an estimate of antibiotic susceptibility. One such standard procedure[1] that has been recommended for use with disks to test susceptibility of organisms to cefuroxime uses the 30 μg cefuroxime disk. Interpretation involves the correlation of the diameters obtained in the disk test with the minimum inhibitory concentration (MIC) for cefuroxime.

A report of "Susceptible" indicates that the pathogen is likely to be inhibited by generally achievable blood levels. A report of "Moderately Susceptible" suggests that the organism would be susceptible if high dosage is used or if the infection is confined to tissues and fluids in which high antibiotic levels are attained. A report of "Intermediate" suggests an equivocable or indeterminate result. A report of "Resistant" indicates that achievable concentrations of the antibiotic are unlikely to be inhibitory and other therapy should be selected.

Reports from the laboratory giving results of the standard single-disk susceptibility test for organisms other than *Haemophilus* spp. and *Neisseria gonorrhoeae* with a 30 μg cefuroxime disk should be interpreted according to the following criteria (see TABLE 2).

TABLE 2

Zone Diameter	Interpretation
≥18 mm	(S) Susceptible
15-17 mm	(MS) Moderately Susceptible
≤14 mm	(R) Resistant

Results for *Haemophilus* spp. should be interpreted according to the following criteria (see TABLE 3).

TABLE 3

Zone Diameter	Interpretation
≥24 mm	(S) Susceptible
21-23 mm	(I) Intermediate
≤20 mm	(R) Resistant

Results for *Neisseria gonorrhoeae* should be interpreted according to the following criteria (see TABLE 4).

TABLE 4

Zone Diameter	Interpretation
≥31 mm	(S) Susceptible
26-30 mm	(MS) Moderately Susceptible
≤25 mm	(R) Resistant

Organisms should be tested with the cefuroxime disk since cefuroxime has been shown by *in vitro* tests to be active against certain strains found resistant when other beta-lactam disks are used. The cefuroxime disk should not be used for testing susceptibility to other cephalosporins.

Standardized procedures require the use of laboratory control organisms. The 30 μg cefuroxime disk should give the following zone diameters.

Testing for organisms other than *Haemophilus* spp. and *Neisseria gonorrhoeae* (see TABLE 5).

TABLE 5

Organism	Zone Diameter
Staphylococcus aureus ATCC 25923	27-35 mm
Escherichia coli ATCC 25922	20-26 mm

Testing for *Haemophilus* spp. (see TABLE 6).

TABLE 6

Organism	Zone Diameter
Haemophilus influenzae ATCC 49766	28-36 mm

Testing for *Neisseria gonorrhoeae* (see TABLE 7).

TABLE 7

Organism	Zone Diameter
Neisseria gonorrhoeae ATCC 49226	33-41 mm
Staphylococcus aureus ATCC 25923	29-33 mm

Dilution Techniques

Use a standardized dilution method[1] (broth, agar, microdilution) or equivalent with cefuroxime powder. The MIC values obtained for bacterial isolates other than *Haemophilus* spp. and *Neisseria gonorrhoeae* should be interpreted according to the following criteria (see TABLE 8).

MIC values obtained for *Haemophilus* spp. should be interpreted according to the following criteria (see TABLE 9).

MIC values obtained for *Neisseria gonorrhoeae* should be interpreted according to the following criteria (see TABLE 10).

As with standard diffusion techniques, dilution methods require the use of laboratory control organisms. Standard cefuroxime powder should provide the following MIC values.

TABLE 8

MIC	Interpretation
≤8 μg/ml	(S) Susceptible
16 μg/ml	(MS) Moderately Susceptible
≥32 μg/ml	(R) Resistant

TABLE 9

MIC	Interpretation
≤4 μg/ml	(S) Susceptible
8 μg/ml	(I) Intermediate
≥16 μg/ml	(R) Resistant

TABLE 10

MIC	Interpretation
≤1 μg/ml	(S) Susceptible
2 μg/ml	(MS) Moderately Susceptible
≥4 μg/ml	(R) Resistant

For organisms other than *Haemophilus* spp. and *Neisseria gonorrhoeae* (see TABLE 11).
For *Haemophilus* spp. (see TABLE 12).

TABLE 11

Organism	MIC
Staphylococcus aureus ATCC 29213	0.5-2.0 μg/ml
Escherichia coli ATCC 25922	2.0-8.0 μg/ml

TABLE 12

Organism	MIC
Haemophilus influenzae ATCC 49766	0.25-1.0 μg/ml

For *Neisseria gonorrhoeae* (see TABLE 13).

TABLE 13

Organism	MIC
Neisseria gonorrhoeae ATCC 49226	0.25-1.0 μg/ml
Staphylococcus aureus ATCC 29213	0.25-1.0 μg/ml

INDICATIONS AND USAGE

Zinacef is indicated for the treatment of patients with infections caused by susceptible strains of the designated organisms in the following diseases:

Lower respiratory tract infections, including pneumonia, caused by *Streptococcus pneumoniae, Haemophilus influenzae* (including ampicillin-resistant strains), *Klebsiella* spp., *Staphylococcus aureus* (penicillinase- and non-penicillinase-producing strains), *Streptococcus pyogenes,* and *Escherichia coli.*

Urinary tract infections caused by *Escherichia coli* and *Klebsiella* spp.

Skin and skin-structure infections caused by *Staphylococcus aureus* (penicillinase- and non-penicillinase-producing strains), *Streptococcus pyogenes, Escherichia coli, Klebsiella* spp., and *Enterobacter* spp.

Septicemia caused by *Staphylococcus aureus* (penicillinase- and non-penicillinase-producing strains), *Streptococcus pneumoniae, Escherichia coli, Haemophilus influenzae* (including ampicillin-resistant strains), and *Klebsiella* spp.

Meningitis caused by *Streptococcus pneumoniae, Haemophilus influenzae* (including ampicillin-resistant strains), *Neisseria meningitidis,* and *Staphylococcus aureus* (penicillinase and non-penicillinase-producing strains).

Gonorrhea: Uncomplicated and disseminated gonococcal infections due to *Neisseria gonorrhoeae* (penicillinase- and non-penicillinase-producing strains) in both males and females.

Bone and joint infections caused by *Staphylococcus aureus* (penicillinase- and non-penicillinase-producing strains).

Clinical microbiological studies in skin and skin-structure infections frequently reveal the growth of susceptible strains of both aerobic and anaerobic organisms. Zinacef has been used successfully in these mixed infections in which several organisms have been isolated. Appropriate cultures and susceptibility studies should be performed to determine the susceptibility of the causative organisms to Zinacef.

Therapy may be started while awaiting the results of these studies; however, once these results become available, the antibiotic treatment should be adjusted accordingly. In certain cases of confirmed or suspected gram-positive or gram-negative sepsis or in patients with other serious infections in which the causative organism has not been identified, Zinacef may be used concomitantly with an aminoglycoside (see PRECAUTIONS). The recommended doses of both antibiotics may be given depending on the severity of the infection and the patient's condition.

PREVENTION

The preoperative prophylactic administration of Zinacef may prevent the growth of susceptible disease-causing bacteria and thereby may reduce the incidence of certain postoperative infections in patients undergoing surgical procedures (*e.g.,* vaginal hysterectomy) that are classified as clean-contaminated or potentially contaminated procedures. Effective prophylactic use of antibiotics in surgery depends on the time of administration. Zinacef should usually be given ½ to 1 hour before the operation to allow sufficient time to achieve effective antibiotic concentrations in the wound tissues during the procedure. The dose should be repeated intraoperatively if the surgical procedure is lengthy.

Prophylactic administration is usually not required after the surgical procedure ends and should be stopped within 24 hours. In the majority of surgical procedures, continuing prophylactic administration of any antibiotic does not reduce the incidence of subsequent infections but will increase the possibility of adverse reactions and the development of bacterial resistance.

The perioperative use of Zinacef has also been effective during open heart surgery for surgical patients in whom infections at the operative site would present a serious risk. For these patients it is recommended that therapy with Zinacef be continued for at least 48 hours after the surgical procedure ends. If an infection is present, specimens for culture should be obtained for the identification of the causative organism, and appropriate antimicrobial therapy should be instituted.

NON-FDA APPROVED INDICATIONS

Although not approved by the FDA, cefuroxime has also been used for treating sinusitis and pyelonephritis.

CONTRAINDICATIONS

Zinacef is contraindicated in patients with known allergy to the cephalosporin group of antibiotics.

WARNINGS

BEFORE THERAPY WITH ZINACEF IS INSTITUTED, CAREFUL INQUIRY SHOULD BE MADE TO DETERMINE WHETHER THE PATIENT HAS HAD PREVIOUS HYPERSENSITIVITY REACTIONS TO CEPHALOSPORINS, PENICILLINS, OR OTHER DRUGS. THIS PRODUCT SHOULD BE GIVEN CAUTIOUSLY TO PENICILLIN-SENSITIVE PATIENTS. ANTIBIOTICS SHOULD BE ADMINISTERED WITH CAUTION TO ANY PATIENT WHO HAS DEMONSTRATED SOME FORM OF ALLERGY, PARTICULARLY TO DRUGS. IF AN ALLERGIC REACTION TO ZINACEF OCCURS, DISCONTINUE THE DRUG. SERIOUS ACUTE HYPERSENSITIVITY REACTIONS MAY REQUIRE EPINEPHRINE AND OTHER EMERGENCY MEASURES.

Pseudomembranous colitis has been reported with nearly all antibacterial agents, including cefuroxime, and may range in severity from mild to life threatening. Therefore, it is important to consider this diagnosis in patients who present with diarrhea subsequent to the administration of antibacterial agents.

Treatment with antibacterial agents alters the normal flora of the colon and may permit overgrowth of clostridia. Studies indicate that a toxin produced by *Clostridium difficile* is one primary cause of "antibiotic-associated colitis".

After the diagnosis of pseudomembranous colitis has been established, appropriate therapeutic measures should be initiated. Mild cases of pseudomembranous colitis usually respond to drug discontinuation alone. In moderate to severe cases, consideration should be given to management with fluids and electrolytes, protein supplementation, and treatment with an antibacterial drug clinically effective against *Clostridium difficile* colitis.

When the colitis is not relieved by drug discontinuation or when it is severe, oral vancomycin is the treatment of choice for antibiotic-associated pseudomembranous colitis produced by *Clostridium difficile.* Other causes of colitis should also be considered.

PRECAUTIONS

GENERAL

Although Zinacef rarely produces alterations in kidney function, evaluation of renal status during therapy is recommended, especially in seriously ill patients receiving the maximum doses. Cephalosporins should be given with caution to patients receiving concurrent treatment with potent diuretics as these regimens are suspected of adversely affecting renal function.

The total daily dose of Zinacef should be reduced in patients with transient or persistent renal insufficiency (see DOSAGE AND ADMINISTRATION), because high and prolonged serum antibiotic concentrations can occur in such individuals from usual doses.

As with other antibiotics, prolonged use of Zinacef may result in overgrowth of nonsusceptible organisms. Careful observation of the patient is essential. If superinfection occurs during therapy, appropriate measures should be taken.

Broad-spectrum antibiotics should be prescribed with caution in individuals with a history of gastrointestinal disease, particularly colitis.

Nephrotoxicity has been reported following concomitant administration of aminoglycoside antibiotics and cephalosporins.

As with other therapeutic regimens used in the treatment of meningitis, mild-to-moderate hearing loss has been reported in a few pediatric patients treated with cefuroxime. Persistence of positive CSF (cerebrospinal fluid) cultures at 18-36 hours has also been noted with cefuroxime injection, as well as with other antibiotic therapies; however, the clinical relevance of this is unknown.

Cephalosporins may be associated with a fall in prothrombin activity. Those at risk include patients with renal or hepatic impairment, or poor nutritional state, as well as patients receiving a protracted course of antimicrobial therapy, and patients previously stabilized on anticoagulant therapy. Prothrombin time should be monitored in patients at risk and exogenous vitamin K administered as indicated.

DRUG/LABORATORY TEST INTERACTIONS

A false-positive reaction for glucose in the urine may occur with copper reduction tests (Benedict's or Fehling's solution or with CLINITEST tablets) but not with enzyme-based tests for glycosuria. As a false-negative result may occur in the ferricyanide test, it is recommended that either the glucose oxidase or hexokinase method be used to determine blood plasma glucose levels in patients receiving Zinacef.

Cefuroxime does not interfere with the assay of serum and urine creatinine by the alkaline picrate method.

C

CARCINOGENESIS, MUTAGENESIS, AND IMPAIRMENT OF FERTILITY

Although lifetime studies in animals have not been performed to evaluate carcinogenic potential, no mutagenic activity was found for cefuroxime in the mouse lymphoma assay and a battery of bacterial mutation tests. Positive results were obtained in an *in vitro* chromosome aberration assay, however, negative results were found in an *in vivo* micronucleus test at doses up to 10 g/kg. Reproduction studies in mice at doses up to 3200 mg/kg/day (3.1 times the recommended maximum human dose based on mg/m^2) have revealed no impairment of fertility.

Reproductive studies revealed no impairment of fertility in animals.

PREGNANCY, TERATOGENIC EFFECTS, PREGNANCY CATEGORY B

Reproduction studies have been performed in mice at doses up to 6400 mg/kg/day (6.3 times the recommended maximum human dose based on mg/m^2) and rabbits at doses up to 400 mg/kg/day (2.1 times the recommended maximum human dose based on mg/m^2) and have revealed no evidence of impaired fertility or harm to the fetus due to cefuroxime. There are, however, no adequate and well-controlled studies in pregnant women. Because animal reproduction studies are not always predictive of human response, this drug should be used during pregnancy only if clearly needed.

NURSING MOTHERS

Since cefuroxime is excreted in human milk, caution should be exercised when Zinacef is administered to a nursing woman.

PEDIATRIC USE

Safety and effectiveness in pediatric patients below 3 months of age have not been established. Accumulation of other members of the cephalosporin class in newborn infants (with resulting prolongation of drug half-life) has been reported.

GERIATRIC USE

Of the 1914 subjects who received cefuroxime in 24 clinical studies of Zinacef, 901 (47%) were 65 and over while 421 (22%) were 75 and over. No overall differences in safety or effectiveness were observed between these subjects and younger subjects, and other reported clinical experience has not identified differences in responses between the elderly and younger patients, but greater susceptibility of some older individuals to drug effects cannot be ruled out. This drug is known to be substantially excreted by the kidney, and the risk of toxic reactions to this drug may be greater in patients with impaired renal function. Because elderly patients are more likely to have decreased renal function, care should be taken in dose selection, and it may be useful to monitor renal function (see DOSAGE AND ADMINISTRATION).

ADVERSE REACTIONS

Zinacef is generally well tolerated. The most common adverse effects have been local reactions following IV administration. Other adverse reactions have been encountered only rarely.

Local Reactions: Thrombophlebitis has occurred with IV administration in 1 in 60 patients.

Gastrointestinal: Gastrointestinal symptoms occurred in 1 in 150 patients and included diarrhea (1 in 220 patients) and nausea (1 in 440 patients). The onset of pseudomembranous colitis may occur during or after antibacterial treatment (see WARNINGS).

Hypersensitivity Reactions: Hypersensitivity reactions have been reported in fewer than 1% of the patients treated with Zinacef and include rash (1 in 125). Pruritus, urticaria, and positive Coombs' test each occurred in fewer than 1 in 250 patients, and, as with other cephalosporins, rare cases of anaphylaxis, drug fever, erythema multiforme, interstitial nephritis, toxic epidermal necrolysis, and Stevens-Johnson syndrome have occurred.

Blood: A decrease in hemoglobin and hematocrit has been observed in 1 in 10 patients and transient eosinophilia in 1 in 14 patients. Less common reactions seen were transient neutropenia (fewer than 1 in 100 patients) and leukopenia (1 in 750 patients). A similar pattern and incidence were seen with other cephalosporins used in controlled studies. As with other cephalosporins, there have been rare reports of thrombocytopenia.

Hepatic: Transient rise in SGOT and SGPT (1 in 25 patients), alkaline phosphatase (1 in 50 patients), LDH (1 in 75 patients), and bilirubin (1 in 500 patients) levels has been noted.

Kidney: Elevations in serum creatinine and/or blood urea nitrogen and a decreased creatinine clearance have been observed, but their relationship to cefuroxime is unknown.

POSTMARKETING EXPERIENCE WITH ZINACEF PRODUCTS

In addition to the adverse events reported during clinical trials, the following events have been observed during clinical practice in patients treated with Zinacef and were reported spontaneously. Data are generally insufficient to allow an estimate of incidence or to establish causation.

Neurologic: Seizure.

Non-Site Specific: Angioedema.

CEPHALOSPORIN-CLASS ADVERSE REACTIONS

In addition to the adverse reactions listed above that have been observed in patients treated with cefuroxime, the following adverse reactions and altered laboratory tests have been reported for cephalosporin-class antibiotics:

Adverse Reactions: Vomiting, abdominal pain, colitis, vaginitis including vaginal candidiasis, toxic nephropathy, hepatic dysfunction including cholestasis, aplastic anemia, hemolytic anemia, hemorrhage.

Several cephalosporins, including Zinacef, have been implicated in triggering seizures, particularly in patients with renal impairment when the dosage was not reduced (see DOSAGE AND ADMINISTRATION). If seizures associated with drug therapy should occur, the drug should be discontinued. Anticonvulsant therapy can be given if clinically indicated.

Altered Laboratory Tests: Prolonged prothrombin time, pancytopenia, agranulocytosis.

DOSAGE AND ADMINISTRATION

DOSAGE

Adults

The usual adult dosage range for Zinacef is 750 mg to 1.5 g every 8 hours, usually for 5-10 days. In uncomplicated urinary tract infections, skin and skin-structure infections, disseminated gonococcal infections, and uncomplicated pneumonia, a 750 mg dose every 8 hours is recommended. In severe or complicated infections, a 1.5 g dose every 8 hours is recommended.

In bone and joint infections, a 1.5 g dose every 8 hours is recommended. In clinical trials, surgical intervention was performed when indicated as an adjunct to therapy with Zinacef. A course of oral antibiotics was administered when appropriate following the completion of parenteral administration of Zinacef.

In life-threatening infections or infections due to less susceptible organisms, 1.5 g every 6 hours may be required. In bacterial meningitis, the dosage should not exceed 3 g every 8 hours. The recommended dosage for uncomplicated gonococcal infection is 1.5 g given intramuscularly as a single dose at 2 different sites together with 1 g of oral probenecid. For preventive use for clean-contaminated or potentially contaminated surgical procedures, a 1.5 g dose administered intravenously just before surgery (approximately ½ to 1 hour before the initial incision) is recommended. Thereafter, give 750 mg intravenously or intramuscularly every 8 hours when the procedure is prolonged.

For preventive use during open heart surgery, a 1.5 g dose administered intravenously at the induction of anesthesia and every 12 hours thereafter for a total of 6 g is recommended.

Impaired Renal Function

A reduced dosage must be employed when renal function is impaired. Dosage should be determined by the degree of renal impairment and the susceptibility of the causative organism (see TABLE 14).

TABLE 14 *Dosage of Zinacef in Adults With Reduced Renal Function*

Creatinine Clearance	Dose	Frequency
>20 ml/min	750 mg - 1.5 g	q8h
10-20 ml/min	750 mg	q12h
<10 ml/min	750 mg	q24h*

* Since Zinacef is dialyzable, patients on hemodialysis should be given a further dose at the end of the dialysis.

When only serum creatinine is available, the following formula[2] (based on sex, weight, and age of the patient) may be used to convert this value into creatinine clearance. The serum creatinine should represent a steady state of renal function.

Males: Creatinine clearance (ml/min) = [weight (kg) × (140-age)] ÷ [72 × serum creatinine (mg/dl)]

Females: 0.85 × male value

Note: As with antibiotic therapy in general, administration of Zinacef should be continued for a minimum of 48-72 hours after the patient becomes asymptomatic or after evidence of bacterial eradication has been obtained; a minimum of 10 days of treatment is recommended in infections caused by *Streptococcus pyogenes* in order to guard against the risk of rheumatic fever or glomerulonephritis; frequent bacteriologic and clinical appraisal is necessary during therapy of chronic urinary tract infection and may be required for several months after therapy has been completed; persistent infections may require treatment for several weeks; and doses smaller than those indicated above should not be used. In staphylococcal and other infections involving a collection of pus, surgical drainage should be carried out where indicated.

Pediatric Patients Above 3 Months of Age

Administration of 50-100 mg/kg/day in equally divided doses every 6-8 hours has been successful for most infections susceptible to cefuroxime. The higher dosage of 100 mg/kg/day (not to exceed the maximum adult dosage) should be used for the more severe or serious infections.

In bone and joint infections, 150 mg/kg/day (not to exceed the maximum adult dosage) is recommended in equally divided doses every 8 hours. In clinical trials, a course of oral antibiotics was administered to pediatric patients following the completion of parenteral administration of Zinacef.

In cases of bacterial meningitis, a larger dosage of Zinacef is recommended, 200-240 mg/kg/day intravenously in divided doses every 6-8 hours.

In pediatric patients with renal insufficiency, the frequency of dosing should be modified consistent with the recommendations for adults.

PREPARATION OF SOLUTION AND SUSPENSION

The directions for preparing Zinacef for both IV and IM use are summarized in TABLE 15.

Administration

After constitution, Zinacef may be given intravenously or by deep IM injection into a large muscle mass (such as the gluteus or lateral part of the thigh). Before injecting intramuscularly, aspiration is necessary to avoid inadvertent injection into a blood vessel.

Intravenous Administration

The IV route may be preferable for patients with bacterial septicemia or other severe or life-threatening infections or for patients who may be poor risks because of lowered resistance, particularly if shock is present or impending.

TABLE 15 *Preparation of Solution and Suspension*

Strength	Amount of Diluent to be Added	Volume to be Withdrawn	Approx. Cefuroxime Conc.
750 mg vial	3.0 ml (IM)	Total*	200 mg/ml
750 mg vial	8.0 ml (IV)	Total	90 mg/ml
1.5 g vial	16.0 ml (IV)	Total	90 mg/ml
750 mg infusion pack	100 ml (IV)	—	7.5 mg/ml
1.5 g infusion pack	100 ml (IV)	—	15 mg/ml
7.5 g pharmacy bulk package	77 ml (IV)	Amount needed†	95 mg/ml

* Note: Zinacef is a suspension at IM concentrations.
† 8 ml of solution contains 750 mg cefuroxime; 16 ml of solution contains 1.5 g of cefuroxime.

For direct intermittent IV administration, slowly inject the solution into a vein over a period of 3-5 minutes or give it through the tubing system by which the patient is also receiving other IV solutions.

For intermittent IV infusion with a Y-type administration set, dosing can be accomplished through the tubing system by which the patient may be receiving other IV solutions. However, during infusion of the solution containing Zinacef, it is advisable to temporarily discontinue administration of any other solutions at the same site.

ADD-Vantage vials are to be constituted only with 50 or 100 ml of 5% dextrose injection, 0.9% sodium chloride injection, or 0.45% sodium chloride injection in Abbott ADD-Vantage flexible diluent containers. ADD-Vantage vials that have been joined to Abbott ADD-Vantage diluent containers and activated to dissolve the drug are stable for 24 hours room temperature or for 7 days under refrigeration. Joined vials that have not been activated may be used within a 14 day period; this period corresponds to that for use of Abbott ADD-Vantage containers following removal of the outer packaging (overwrap).

Freezing solutions of Zinacef in the ADD-Vantage system is not recommended.

For continuous IV infusion, a solution of Zinacef may be added to an IV infusion pack containing one of the following fluids: 0.9% sodium chloride injection; 5% dextrose injection; 10% dextrose injection; 5% dextrose and 0.9% sodium chloride injection; 5% dextrose and 0.45% sodium chloride injection; or 1/6 M sodium lactate injection.

Solutions of Zinacef, like those of most beta-lactam antibiotics, should not be added to solutions of aminoglycoside antibiotics because of potential interaction.

However, if concurrent therapy with Zinacef and an aminoglycoside is indicated, each of these antibiotics can be administered separately to the same patient.

Directions for Use of Zinacef Frozen in Galaxy Plastic Containers

Zinacef supplied as a frozen, sterile, iso-osmotic, nonpyrogenic solution in plastic containers is to be administered after thawing either as a continuous or intermittent IV infusion. The thawed solution of the premixed product is stable for 28 days if stored under refrigeration (5°C) or for 24 hours if stored at room temperature (25°C). **Do not refreeze.**

Thaw container at room temperature (25°C) or under refrigeration (5°C). Do not force thaw by immersion in water baths or by microwave irradiation. Components of the solution may precipitate in the frozen state and will dissolve upon reaching room temperature with little or no agitation. Potency is not affected. Mix after solution has reached room temperature. Check for minute leaks by squeezing bag firmly. Discard bag if leaks are found as sterility may be impaired. Do not add supplementary medication. Do not use unless solution is clear and seal is intact.

Use sterile equipment.

Caution: Do not use plastic containers in series connections. Such use could result in air embolism due to residual air being drawn from the primary container before administration of the fluid from the secondary container is complete.

COMPATIBILITY AND STABILITY

Intramuscular

When constituted as directed with sterile water for injection, suspensions of Zinacef for IM injection maintain satisfactory potency for 24 hours at room temperature and for 48 hours under refrigeration (5°C).

After the periods mentioned above any unused suspensions should be discarded.

Intravenous

When the 750 mg, 1.5 g, and 7.5 g pharmacy bulk vials are constituted as directed with sterile water for injection, the solutions of Zinacef for IV administration maintain satisfactory potency for 24 hours at room temperature and for 48 hours (750 mg and 1.5 g vials) or for 7 days (7.5 g pharmacy bulk vial) under refrigeration (5°C). More dilute solutions, such as 750 mg or 1.5 g plus 100 ml of sterile water for injection, 5% dextrose injection, or 0.9% sodium chloride injection, also maintain satisfactory potency for 24 hours at room temperature and for 7 days under refrigeration.

These solutions may be further diluted to concentrations of between 1 and 30 mg/ml in the following solutions and will lose not more than 10% activity for 24 hours at room temperature or for at least 7 days under refrigeration: 0.9% sodium chloride injection; 1/6 M sodium lactate injection; Ringer's injection; lactated Ringer's injection; 5% dextrose and 0.9% sodium chloride injection; 5% dextrose injection; 5% dextrose and 0.45% sodium chloride injection; 5% dextrose and 0.225% sodium chloride injection; 10% dextrose injection; and 10% invert sugar in water for injection.

Unused solutions should be discarded after the time periods mentioned above.

Zinacef has also been found compatible for 24 hours at room temperature when admixed in IV infusion with heparin (10 and 50 U/ml) in 0.9% sodium chloride injection and potassium chloride (10 and 40 mEq/L) in 0.9% sodium chloride injection. Sodium bicarbonate injection is not recommended for the dilution of Zinacef.

The 750 mg and 1.5 g Zinacef ADD-Vantage vials, when diluted in 50 or 100 ml of 5% dextrose injection, 0.9% sodium chloride injection, or 0.45% sodium chloride injection, may be stored for up to 24 hours at room temperature or for 7 days under refrigeration.

Frozen Stability

Constitute the 750 mg, 1.5 g, or 7.5 g vial as directed for IV administration in TABLE 15. Immediately withdraw the total contents of the 750 mg or 1.5 g vial or 8 or 16 ml from the 7.5 g bulk vial and add to a Baxter VIAFLEX MINI-BAG containing 50 or 100 ml of 0.9% sodium chloride injection or 5% dextrose injection and freeze. Frozen solutions are stable for 6 months when stored at -20°C. Frozen solutions should be thawed at room temperature and not refrozen. Do not force thaw by immersion in water baths or by microwave irradiation. Thawed solutions may be stored for up to 24 hours at room temperature or for 7 days in a refrigerator.

Note: Parenteral drug products should be inspected visually for particulate matter and discoloration before administration whenever solution and container permit.

As with other cephalosporins, Zinacef powder as well as solutions and suspensions tend to darken, depending on storage conditions, without adversely affecting product potency.

Directions for Dispensing: Pharmacy Bulk Package — Not for Direct Infusion

The pharmacy bulk package is for use in a pharmacy admixture service only under a laminar flow hood. Entry into the vial must be made with a sterile transfer set or other sterile dispensing device, and the contents dispensed in aliquots using aseptic technique. The use of syringe and needle is not recommended as it may cause leakage (see DOSAGE AND ADMINISTRATION). AFTER INITIAL WITHDRAWAL USE ENTIRE CONTENTS OF VIAL PROMPTLY. ANY UNUSED PORTION MUST BE DISCARDED WITHIN 24 HOURS.

HOW SUPPLIED

Zinacef is a dry, white to off-white powder supplied in vials and infusion packs containing either 750 mg or 1.5 g cefuroxime.

Zinacef is supplied frozen in 50 ml, single-dose, plastic containers containing either 750 mg or 1.5 g cefuroxime.

STORAGE

Zinacef in the dry state should be stored between 15 and 30°C (59 and 86°F) and protected from light.

Zinacef frozen as a premixed solution of cefuroxime injection should not be stored above -20°C.

ORAL

DESCRIPTION

Note: The trade names have been used throughout this monograph for clarity.

Ceftin tablets and Ceftin for oral suspension contain cefuroxime as cefuroxime axetil. Ceftin is a semisynthetic, broad-spectrum cephalosporin antibiotic for oral administration.

Chemically, cefuroxime axetil, the 1-(acetyloxy) ethyl ester of cefuroxime, is (*RS*)-1-hydroxyethyl(6*R*,7*R*)-7-[2-(2-furyl)glyoxylamido]-3-(hydroxymethyl)-8-oxo-5-thia-1-azabicyclo[4.2.0]oct-2-ene-2-carboxylate,7^2-(*Z*)-(*O*-methyl-oxime),1-acetate 3-carbamate. Its molecular formula is $C_{20}H_{22}N_4O_{10}S$, and it has a molecular weight of 510.48.

Cefuroxime axetil is in the amorphous form.

Ceftin tablets are film-coated and contain the equivalent of 125, 250, or 500 mg of cefuroxime as cefuroxime axetil. Ceftin tablets contain the inactive ingredients colloidal silicon dioxide, croscarmellose sodium, FD&C blue no. 1 (250 and 500 mg tablets only), hydrogenated vegetable oil, hydroxypropyl methylcellulose, methylparaben, microcrystalline cellulose, propylene glycol, propylparaben, sodium benzoate (125 mg tablets only), sodium lauryl sulfate, and titanium dioxide.

Ceftin for oral suspension, when reconstituted with water, provides the equivalent of 125 or 250 mg of cefuroxime (as cefuroxime axetil) per 5 ml of suspension. Ceftin for oral suspension contains the inactive ingredients povidone K30, stearic acid, sucrose, and tutti-frutti flavoring.

CLINICAL PHARMACOLOGY

ABSORPTION AND METABOLISM

After oral administration, cefuroxime axetil is absorbed from the gastrointestinal tract and rapidly hydrolyzed by nonspecific esterases in the intestinal mucosa and blood to cefuroxime. Cefuroxime is subsequently distributed throughout the extracellular fluids. The axetil moiety is metabolized to acetaldehyde and acetic acid.

PHARMACOKINETICS

Approximately 50% of serum cefuroxime is bound to protein. Serum pharmacokinetic parameters for Ceftin tablets and Ceftin for oral suspension are shown in TABLE 16 and TABLE 17.

TABLE 16 *Postprandial Pharmacokinetics of Cefuroxime Administered as Ceftin Tablets to Adults**

	Dose† (Cefuroxime Equivalent)			
	125 mg	250 mg	500 mg	1000 mg
Peak plasma conc. (µg/ml)	2.1	4.1	7.0	13.6
Time of peak plasma conc. (h)	2.2	2.5	3.0	2.5
Mean elimination half-life (h)	1.2	1.2	1.2	1.3
AUC (µg·h/ml)	6.7	12.9	27.4	50.0

* Mean values of 12 healthy adult volunteers.
† Drug administered immediately after a meal.

COMPARATIVE PHARMACOKINETIC PROPERTIES

A 250 mg/5 ml dose of Ceftin suspension is bioequivalent to 2 times 125 mg/5 ml dose of Ceftin suspension when administered with food (see TABLE 18). **Ceftin for oral suspension was not bioequivalent to Ceftin tablets when tested in healthy adults. The tablet and powder for oral suspension formulations are NOT substitutable on a mg/mg basis.**

TABLE 17 *Postprandial Pharmacokinetics of Cefuroxime Administered as Ceftin for Oral Suspension to Pediatric Patients**

	Dose† (Cefuroxime Equivalent)		
	10 mg/kg	15 mg/kg	20 mg/kg
	n=8	n=12	n=8
Peak plasma conc. (μg/ml)	3.3	5.1	7.0
Time of peak plasma conc. (h)	3.6	2.7	3.1
Mean elimination half-life (h)	1.4	1.9	1.9
AUC (μg·h/ml)	12.4	22.5	32.8

* Mean age = 23 months.
† Drug administered with milk or milk products.

The area under the curve for the suspension averaged 91% of that for the tablet, and the peak plasma concentration for the suspension averaged 71% of the peak plasma concentration of the tablets. Therefore, the safety and effectiveness of both the tablet and oral suspension formulations had to be established in separate clinical trials.

TABLE 18 *Pharmacokinetics of Cefuroxime Administered as 250 mg/5 ml or 2 × 125 mg/5 ml Ceftin for Oral Suspension to Adults* With Food*

	Dose† (Cefuroxime Equivalent)	
	250 mg/5 ml	2 × 125 mg/5 ml
Peak plasma conc. (μg/ml)	2.23	2.37
Time of peak plasma conc. (h)	3	3
Mean elimination half-life (h)	1.40	1.44
AUC (μg·h/ml)	8.92	9.75

* Mean values of 18 healthy adult volunteers.

FOOD EFFECT ON PHARMACOKINETICS

Absorption of the tablet is greater when taken after food (absolute bioavailability of Ceftin tablets increases from 37% to 52%). Despite this difference in absorption, the clinical and bacteriologic responses of patients were independent of food intake at the time of tablet administration in 2 studies where this was assessed.

All pharmacokinetic and clinical effectiveness and safety studies in pediatric patients using the suspension formulation were conducted in the fed state. No data are available on the absorption kinetics of the suspension formulation when administered to fasted pediatric patients.

RENAL EXCRETION

Cefuroxime is excreted unchanged in the urine; in adults, approximately 50% of the administered dose is recovered in the urine within 12 hours. The pharmacokinetics of cefuroxime in the urine of pediatric patients have not been studied at this time. Until further data are available, the renal pharmacokinetic properties of cefuroxime axetil established in adults should not be extrapolated to pediatric patients.

Because cefuroxime is renally excreted, the serum half-life is prolonged in patients with reduced renal function. In a study of 20 elderly patients (mean age = 83.9 years) having a mean creatinine clearance of 34.9 ml/min, the mean serum elimination half-life was 3.5 hours. Despite the lower elimination of cefuroxime in geriatric patients, dosage adjustment based on age is not necessary (see PRECAUTIONS, Geriatric Use).

MICROBIOLOGY

The *in vivo* bactericidal activity of cefuroxime axetil is due to cefuroxime's binding to essential target proteins and the resultant inhibition of cell-wall synthesis.

Cefuroxime has bactericidal activity against a wide range of common pathogens, including many beta-lactamase-producing strains. Cefuroxime is stable to many bacterial beta-lactamases, especially plasmid-mediated enzymes that are commonly found in enterobacteriaceae.

Cefuroxime has been demonstrated to be active against most strains of the following microorganisms both *in vitro* and in clinical infections as described in INDICATIONS AND USAGE.

Aerobic Gram-Positive Microorganisms: *Staphylococcus aureus,* (including beta-lactamase-producing strains) *Streptococcus pneumoniae, Streptococcus pyogenes.*

Aerobic Gram-Negative Microorganisms: *Escherichia coli, Haemophilus influenzae* (including beta-lactamase-producing strains), *Haemophilus parainfluenzae, Klebsiella pneumoniae, Moraxella catarrhalis* (including beta-lactamase-producing strains), *Neisseria gonorrhoeae* (including beta-lactamase-producing strains).

Spirochetes: *Borrelia burgdorferi.*

Cefuroxime has been shown to be active *in vitro* against most strains of the following microorganisms; however, the clinical significance of these findings is unknown.

Cefuroxime exhibits *in vitro* minimum inhibitory concentrations (MICs) of 4.0 μg/ml or less (systemic susceptible breakpoint) against most (≥90%) strains of the following microorganisms; however, the safety and effectiveness of cefuroxime in treating clinical infections due to these microorganisms have not been established in adequate and well-controlled trials.

Aerobic Gram-Positive Microorganisms: *Staphylococcus epidermidis, Staphylococcus saprophyticus, Streptococcus agalactiae.*

NOTE: Certain strains of enterococci, *e.g., Enterococcus faecalis* (formerly *Streptococcus faecalis*), are resistant to cefuroxime. Methicillin-resistant staphylococci are resistant to cefuroxime.

Aerobic Gram-Negative Microorganisms: *Morganella morganii, Proteus inconstans, Proteus mirabilis, Providencia rettgeri.*

NOTE: Pseudomonas spp., *Campylobacter* spp., *Acinetobacter calcoaceticus,* and most strains of *Serratia* spp. and *Proteus vulgaris* are resistant to most first- and second-generation cephalosporins. Some strains of *Morganella morganii, Enterobacter cloacae,* and *Citrobacter* spp. have been shown by *in vitro* tests to be resistant to cefuroxime and other cephalosporins.

Anaerobic Microorganisms: *Peptococcus niger.*

NOTE: Most strains of *Clostridium difficile* and *Bacteroides fragilis* are resistant to cefuroxime.

SUSCEPTIBILITY TESTING

Dilution Techniques

Quantitative methods that are used to determine MICs provide reproducible estimates of the susceptibility of bacteria to antimicrobial compounds. One such standardized procedure uses a standardized dilution method[1] (broth, agar, or microdilution) or equivalent with cefuroxime powder. The MIC values obtained should be interpreted according to the following criteria (see TABLE 19).

TABLE 19

MIC	Interpretation
≤4 μg/ml	(S) Susceptible
8-16 μg/ml	(I) Intermediate
≥32 μg/ml	(R) Resistant

A report of "Susceptible" indicates that the pathogen, if in the blood, is likely to be inhibited by usually achievable concentrations of the antimicrobial compound in blood. A report of "Intermediate" indicates that inhibitory concentrations of the antibiotic may be achieved if high dosage is used or if the infection is confined to tissues or fluids in which high antibiotic concentrations are attained. This category also provides a buffer zone that prevents small, uncontrolled technical factors from causing major discrepancies in interpretation. A report of "Resistant" indicates that usually achievable concentrations of the antimicrobial compound in the blood are unlikely to be inhibitory and that other therapy should be selected.

Standardized susceptibility test procedures require the use of laboratory control microorganisms. Standard cefuroxime powder should give the following MIC values (see TABLE 20).

TABLE 20

Microorganism	MIC
Escherichia coli ATCC 25922	2-8 μg/ml
Staphylococcus aureus ATCC 29213	0.5-2 μg/ml

Diffusion Techniques

Quantitative methods that require measurement of zone diameters provide estimates of the susceptibility of bacteria to antimicrobial compounds. One such standardized procedure[2] that has been recommended (for use with disks) to test the susceptibility of microorganisms to cefuroxime uses the 30 μg cefuroxime disk. Interpretation involves correlation of the diameter obtained in the disk test with the MIC for cefuroxime.

Reports from the laboratory providing results of the standard single-disk susceptibility test with a 30 μg cefuroxime disk should be interpreted according to the following criteria (see TABLE 21).

TABLE 21

Zone Diameter	Interpretation
≥23 mm	(S) Susceptible
15-22 mm	(I) Intermediate
≤14 mm	(R) Resistant

Interpretation should be as stated above for results using dilution techniques.

As with standard dilution techniques, diffusion methods require the use of laboratory control microorganisms. The 30 μg cefuroxime disk provides the following zone diameters in these laboratory test quality control strains (see TABLE 22).

TABLE 22

Microorganism	Zone Diameter
Escherichia coli ATCC 25922	20-26 mm
Staphylococcus aureus ATCC 25923	27-35 mm

INDICATIONS AND USAGE

NOTE: CEFTIN TABLETS AND CEFTIN FOR ORAL SUSPENSION ARE NOT BIOEQUIVALENT AND ARE NOT SUBSTITUTABLE ON A MG/MG BASIS (SEE CLINICAL PHARMACOLOGY).

CEFTIN TABLETS

Ceftin tablets are indicated for the treatment of patients with mild to moderate infections caused by susceptible strains of the designated microorganisms in the conditions listed below:

Pharyngitis/tonsillitis caused by *Streptococcus pyogenes.*

NOTE: The usual drug of choice in the treatment and prevention of streptococcal infections, including the prophylaxis of rheumatic fever, is penicillin given by the intramuscular route. Ceftin tablets are generally effective in the eradication of streptococci from the nasopharynx; however, substantial data establishing the efficacy of cefuroxime in the subsequent prevention of rheumatic fever are not available. Please also note that in all clinical trials, all isolates had to be sensitive to both penicillin and cefuroxime. There are no data from adequate and well-controlled trials to demonstrate the effectiveness of cefuroxime in the treatment of penicillin-resistant strains of *Streptococcus pyogenes.*

Acute bacterial otitis media caused by *Streptococcus pneumoniae, Haemophilus influenzae* (including beta-lactamase-producing strains), *Moraxella catarrhalis* (including beta-lactamase-producing strains), or *Streptococcus pyogenes.*

Acute bacterial maxillary sinusitis caused by *Streptococcus pneumoniae* or *Haemophilus influenzae* (non-beta-lactamase-producing strains only).

NOTE: In view of the insufficient numbers of isolates of beta-lactamase-producing strains of *Haemophilus influenzae* and *Moraxella catarrhalis* that were obtained from clinical trials with Ceftin tablets for patients with acute bacterial maxillary sinusitis, it was not possible to adequately evaluate the effectiveness of Ceftin tablets for sinus infections known, suspected, or considered potentially to be caused by beta-lactamase-producing *Haemophilus influenzae* or *Moraxella catarrhalis.*

Acute bacterial exacerbations of chronic bronchitis and secondary bacterial infections of acute bronchitis caused by *Streptococcus pneumoniae, Haemophilus influenzae* (beta-lactamase negative strains), or *Haemophilus parainfluenzae* (beta-lactamase negative strains). (See DOSAGE AND ADMINISTRATION.)

Uncomplicated skin and skin-structure infections caused by *Staphylococcus aureus* (including beta-lactamase-producing strains) or *Streptococcus pyogenes.*

Uncomplicated urinary tract infections caused by *Escherichia coli* or *Klebsiella pneumoniae.*

Uncomplicated gonorrhea, urethral and endocervical, caused by penicillinase-producing and non-penicillinase-producing strains of *Neisseria gonorrhoeae* and uncomplicated gonorrhea, rectal, in females, caused by non-penicillinase-producing strains of *Neisseria gonorrhoeae.*

Early lyme disease (erythema migrans) caused by *Borrelia burgdorferi.*

CEFTIN FOR ORAL SUSPENSION

Ceftin for oral suspension is indicated for the treatment of pediatric patients 3 months to 12 years of age with mild to moderate infections caused by susceptible strains of the designated microorganisms in the conditions listed below. The safety and effectiveness of Ceftin for oral suspension in the treatment of infections other than those specifically listed below have not been established either by adequate and well-controlled trials or by pharmacokinetic data with which to determine an effective and safe dosing regimen.

Pharyngitis/tonsillitis caused by *Streptococcus pyogenes.*

NOTE: The usual drug of choice in the treatment and prevention of streptococcal infections, including the prophylaxis of rheumatic fever, is penicillin given by the intramuscular route. Ceftin for oral suspension is generally effective in the eradication of streptococci from the nasopharynx; however, substantial data establishing the efficacy of cefuroxime in the subsequent prevention of rheumatic fever are not available. Please also note that in all clinical trials, all isolates had to be sensitive to both penicillin and cefuroxime. There are no data from adequate and well-controlled trials to demonstrate the effectiveness of cefuroxime in the treatment of penicillin-resistant strains of *Streptococcus pyogenes.*

Acute bacterial otitis media caused by *Streptococcus pneumoniae, Haemophilus influenzae* (including beta-lactamase-producing strains), *Moraxella catarrhalis* (including beta-lactamase-producing strains), or *Streptococcus pyogenes.*

Impetigo caused by *Staphylococcus aureus* (including beta-lactamase-producing strains) or *Streptococcus pyogenes.*

Culture and susceptibility testing should be performed when appropriate to determine susceptibility of the causative microorganism(s) to cefuroxime. Therapy may be started while awaiting the results of this testing. Antimicrobial therapy should be appropriately adjusted according to the results of such testing.

NON-FDA APPROVED INDICATIONS

Although not approved by the FDA, cefuroxime has also been used for treating sinusitis and pyelonephritis.

CONTRAINDICATIONS

Ceftin products are contraindicated in patients with known allergy to the cephalosporin group of antibiotics.

WARNINGS

CEFTIN TABLETS AND CEFTIN FOR ORAL SUSPENSION ARE NOT BIOEQUIVALENT AND ARE THEREFORE NOT SUBSTITUTABLE ON A MG/MG BASIS (SEE CLINICAL PHARMACOLOGY).

BEFORE THERAPY WITH CEFTIN PRODUCTS IS INSTITUTED, CAREFUL INQUIRY SHOULD BE MADE TO DETERMINE WHETHER THE PATIENT HAS HAD PREVIOUS HYPERSENSITIVITY REACTIONS TO CEFTIN PRODUCTS, OTHER CEPHALOSPORINS, PENICILLINS, OR OTHER DRUGS. IF THIS PRODUCT IS TO BE GIVEN TO PENICILLIN-SENSITIVE PATIENTS, CAUTION SHOULD BE EXERCISED BECAUSE CROSS-HYPERSENSITIVITY AMONG BETA-LACTAM ANTIBIOTICS HAS BEEN CLEARLY DOCUMENTED AND MAY OCCUR IN UP TO 10% OF PATIENTS WITH A HISTORY OF PENICILLIN ALLERGY. IF A CLINICALLY SIGNIFICANT ALLERGIC REACTION TO CEFTIN PRODUCTS OCCURS, DISCONTINUE THE DRUG AND INSTITUTE APPROPRIATE THERAPY. SERIOUS ACUTE HYPERSENSITIVITY REACTIONS MAY REQUIRE TREATMENT WITH EPINEPHRINE AND OTHER EMERGENCY MEASURES, INCLUDING OXYGEN, INTRAVENOUS FLUIDS, INTRAVENOUS ANTIHISTAMINES, CORTICOSTEROIDS, PRESSOR AMINES, AND AIRWAY MANAGEMENT, AS CLINICALLY INDICATED.

Pseudomembranous colitis has been reported with nearly all antibacterial agents, including cefuroxime, and may range from mild to life threatening. Therefore, it is important to consider this diagnosis in patients who present with diarrhea subsequent to the administration of antibacterial agents.

Treatment with antibacterial agents alters normal flora of the colon and may permit overgrowth of clostridia. Studies indicate that a toxin produced by *Clostridium difficile* is one primary cause of antibiotic-associated colitis.

After the diagnosis of pseudomembranous colitis has been established, appropriate therapeutic measures should be initiated. Mild cases of pseudomembranous colitis usually respond to drug discontinuation alone. In moderate to severe cases, consideration should be given to management with fluids and electrolytes, protein supplementation, and treatment with an antibacterial drug effective against *Clostridium difficile.*

PRECAUTIONS

GENERAL

As with other broad-spectrum antibiotics, prolonged administration of cefuroxime axetil may result in overgrowth of nonsusceptible microorganisms. If superinfection occurs during therapy, appropriate measures should be taken.

Cephalosporins, including cefuroxime axetil, should be given with caution to patients receiving concurrent treatment with potent diuretics because these diuretics are suspected of adversely affecting renal function.

Cefuroxime axetil, as with other broad-spectrum antibiotics, should be prescribed with caution in individuals with a history of colitis. The safety and effectiveness of cefuroxime axetil have not been established in patients with gastrointestinal malabsorption. Patients with gastrointestinal malabsorption were excluded from participating in clinical trials of cefuroxime axetil.

Cephalosporins may be associated with a fall in prothrombin activity. Those at risk include patients with renal or hepatic impairment or poor nutritional state, as well as patients receiving a protracted course of antimicrobial therapy, and patients previously stabilized on anticoagulant therapy. Prothrombin time should be monitored in patients at risk and exogenous vitamin K administered as indicated.

INFORMATION FOR THE PATIENT/CAREGIVERS (PEDIATRIC)

During clinical trials, the tablet was tolerated by pediatric patients old enough to swallow the cefuroxime axetil tablet whole. The crushed tablet has a strong, persistent, bitter taste and should not be administered to pediatric patients in this manner. Pediatric patients who cannot swallow the tablet whole should receive the oral suspension.

Discontinuation of therapy due to taste and/or problems of administering this drug occurred in 1.4% of pediatric patients given the oral suspension. Complaints about taste (which may impair compliance) occurred in 5% of pediatric patients.

DRUG/LABORATORY TEST INTERACTIONS

A false-positive reaction for glucose in the urine may occur with copper reduction tests (Benedict's or Fehling's solution or with Clinitest tablets), but not with enzyme-based tests for glycosuria (*e.g.,* Clinistix). As a false-negative result may occur in the ferricyanide test, it is recommended that either the glucose oxidase or hexokinase method be used to determine blood/plasma glucose levels in patients receiving cefuroxime axetil. The presence of cefuroxime does not interfere with the assay of serum and urine creatinine by the alkaline picrate method.

CARCINOGENESIS, MUTAGENESIS, AND IMPAIRMENT OF FERTILITY

Although lifetime studies in animals have not been performed to evaluate carcinogenic potential, no mutagenic activity was found for cefuroxime axetil in a battery of bacterial mutation tests. Positive results were obtained in an *in vitro* chromosome aberration assay, however, negative results were found in an *in vivo* micronucleus test at doses up to 1.5 g/kg. Reproduction studies in rats at doses up to 1000 mg/kg/day (9 times the recommended maximum human dose based on mg/m^2) have revealed no impairment of fertility.

PREGNANCY, TERATOGENIC EFFECTS, PREGNANCY CATEGORY B

Reproduction studies have been performed in mice at doses up to 3200 mg/kg/day (14 times the recommended maximum human dose based on mg/m^2) and in rats at doses up to 1000 mg/kg/day (9 times the recommended maximum human dose based on mg/m^2) and have revealed no evidence of impaired fertility or harm to the fetus due to cefuroxime axetil. There are, however, no adequate and well-controlled studies in pregnant women. Because animal reproduction studies are not always predictive of human response, this drug should be used during pregnancy only if clearly needed.

LABOR AND DELIVERY

Cefuroxime axetil has not been studied for use during labor and delivery.

NURSING MOTHERS

Because cefuroxime is excreted in human milk, consideration should be given to discontinuing nursing temporarily during treatment with cefuroxime axetil.

PEDIATRIC USE

The safety and effectiveness of Ceftin have been established for pediatric patients aged 3 months to 12 years for acute bacterial maxillary sinusitis based upon its approval in adults. Use of Ceftin in pediatric patients is supported by pharmacokinetic and safety data in adults and pediatric patients, and by clinical and microbiological data from adequate and well-controlled studies of the treatment of acute bacterial maxillary sinusitis in adults and of acute otitis media with effusion in pediatric patients. It is also supported by post-marketing adverse events surveillance (see CLINICAL PHARMACOLOGY, INDICATIONS AND USAGE, ADVERSE REACTIONS, and DOSAGE AND ADMINISTRATION).

GERIATRIC USE

Of the total number of subjects who received cefuroxime axetil in 20 clinical studies of Ceftin, 375 were 65 and over while 151 were 75 and over. No overall differences in safety or effectiveness were observed between these subjects and younger adult subjects. The geriatric patients reported somewhat fewer gastrointestinal events and less frequent vaginal candidiasis compared with patients aged 12–64 years old; however, no clinically significant differences were reported between the elderly and younger adult patients. Other reported clinical experience has not identified differences in responses between the elderly and younger adult patients.

C

DRUG INTERACTIONS

Concomitant administration of probenecid with cefuroxime axetil tablets increases the area under the serum concentration versus time curve by 50%. The peak serum cefuroxime concentration after a 1.5 g single dose is greater when taken with 1 g of probenecid (mean = 14.8 μg/ml) than without probenecid (mean = 12.2 μg/ml).

Drugs that reduce gastric acidity may result in a lower bioavailability of Ceftin compared with that of fasting state and tend to cancel the effect of postprandial absorption.

ADVERSE REACTIONS

CEFTIN TABLETS IN CLINICAL TRIALS

Multiple-Dose Dosing Regimens

7-10 Days Dosing

Using multiple doses of cefuroxime axetil tablets, 912 patients were treated with the recommended dosages of cefuroxime axetil (125-500 mg twice a day). There were no deaths or permanent disabilities thought related to drug toxicity. Twenty (2.2%) patients discontinued medication due to adverse events thought by the investigators to be possibly, probably, or almost certainly related to drug toxicity. Seventeen (85%) of the 20 patients who discontinued therapy did so because of gastrointestinal disturbances, including diarrhea, nausea, vomiting, and abdominal pain. The percentage of cefuroxime axetil tablet-treated patients who discontinued study drug because of adverse events was very similar at daily doses of 1000, 500, and 250 mg (2.3%, 2.1%, and 2.2%, respectively). However, the incidence of gastrointestinal adverse events increased with the higher recommended doses.

The adverse events in TABLE 26 were thought by the investigators to be possibly, probably, or almost certainly related to cefuroxime axetil tablets in multiple-dose clinical trials (n=912 cefuroxime axetil-treated patients).

TABLE 26 *Adverse Reactions: Ceftin Tablets, Multiple-Dose Dosing Regimens — Clinical Trials*

Incidence ≥1%	
Diarrhea/loose stools	3.7%
Nausea/vomiting	3.0%
Transient elevation in AST	2.0%
Transient elevation in ALT	1.6%
Eosinophilia	1.1%
Transient elevation in LDH	1.0%
Incidence <1% but >0.1%	
Abdominal pain, abdominal cramps, flatulence, indigestion, headache, vaginitis, vulvar itch, rash, hives, itch, dysuria, chills, chest pain, shortness of breath, mouth ulcers, swollen tongue, sleepiness, thirst, anorexia, positive Coomb's test	

5 Day Experience

In clinical trials using Ceftin in a dose of 250 mg bid in the treatment of secondary bacterial infections of acute bronchitis, 399 patients were treated for 5 days and 402 patients were treated for 10 days. No difference in the occurrence of adverse events was found between the 2 regimens.

In Clinical Trials for Early Lyme Disease With 20 Days Dosing

Two multicenter trials assessed cefuroxime axetil tablets 500 mg twice a day for 20 days. The most common drug-related adverse experiences were diarrhea (10.6% of patients), Jarisch-Herxheimer reaction (5.6%), and vaginitis (5.4%). Other adverse experiences occurred with frequencies comparable to those reported with 7-10 days dosing.

Single-Dose Regimen for Uncomplicated Gonorrhea

In clinical trials using a single dose of cefuroxime axetil tablets, 1061 patients were treated with the recommended dosage of cefuroxime axetil (1000 mg) for the treatment of uncomplicated gonorrhea. There were no deaths or permanent disabilities thought related to drug toxicity in these studies.

The adverse events in TABLE 27 were thought by the investigators to be possibly, probably, or almost certainly related to cefuroxime axetil in 1000 mg single-dose clinical trials of cefuroxime axetil tablets in the treatment of uncomplicated gonorrhea conducted in the US.

TABLE 27 *Adverse Reactions: Ceftin Tablets, 1 g Single-Dose Regimen for Uncomplicated Gonorrhea — Clinical Trials*

Incidence ≥1%	
Nausea/vomiting	6.8%
Diarrhea	4.2%
Incidence <1% but >0.1%	
Abdominal pain, dyspepsia, erythema, rash, pruritus, vaginal candidiasis, vaginal itch, vaginal discharge, headache, dizziness, somnolence, muscle cramps, muscle stiffness, muscle spasm of neck, tightness/pain in chest, bleeding/pain in urethra, kidney pain, tachycardia, lockjaw-type reaction	

CEFTIN FOR ORAL SUSPENSION IN CLINICAL TRIALS

In clinical trials using multiple doses of cefuroxime axetil powder for oral suspension, pediatric patients (96.7% of whom were younger than 12 years of age) were treated with the recommended dosages of cefuroxime axetil (20-30 mg/kg/day divided twice a day up to a maximum dose of 500 or 1000 mg/day, respectively). There were no deaths or permanent disabilities in any of the patients in these studies. Eleven US patients (1.2%) discontinued medication due to adverse events thought by the investigators to be possibly, probably, or almost certainly related to drug toxicity. The discontinuations were primarily for gastrointestinal disturbances, usually diarrhea or vomiting. During clinical trials, discontinuation of therapy due to the taste and/or problems with administering this drug occurred in 13 (1.4%) pediatric patients enrolled at centers in the US.

The adverse events in TABLE 28 were thought by the investigators to be possibly, probably, or almost certainly related to cefuroxime axetil for oral suspension in multiple-dose clinical trials (n=931 cefuroxime axetil-treated US patients).

TABLE 28 *Adverse Reactions: Ceftin for Oral Suspension, Multiple-Dose Dosing Regimens — Clinical Trials*

Incidence ≥1%	
Diarrhea/loose stools	8.6%
Dislike of taste	5.0%
Diaper rash	3.4%
Nausea/vomiting	2.6%
Incidence <1% but >0.1%	
Abdominal pain, flatulence, gastrointestinal infection, candidiasis, vaginal irritation, rash, hyperactivity, irritable behavior, eosinophilia, positive direct Coomb's test, elevated liver enzymes, viral illness, upper respiratory infection, sinusitis, cough, urinary tract infection, joint swelling, arthralgia, fever, ptyalism	

POSTMARKETING EXPERIENCE WITH CEFTIN PRODUCTS

In addition to adverse events reported during clinical trials, the following events have been identified during clinical practice in patients treated with Ceftin tablets or with Ceftin for oral suspension and were reported spontaneously. Data are generally insufficient to allow an estimate of incidence or to establish causation.

General: The following hypersensitivity reactions have been reported: anaphylaxis, angioedema, pruritus, rash, serum sickness-like reaction, and urticaria.

Gastrointestinal: Pseudomembranous colitis (see WARNINGS).

Hematologic: Hemolytic anemia, leukopenia, pancytopenia, thrombocytopenia, and increased prothrombin time.

Hepatic: Hepatic impairment including hepatitis and cholestasis, jaundice.

Neurologic: Seizure.

Skin: Erythema multiforme, Stevens-Johnson syndrome, toxic epidermal necrolysis.

Urologic: Renal dysfunction.

CEPHALOSPORIN-CLASS ADVERSE REACTIONS

In addition to the adverse reactions listed above that have been observed in patients treated with cefuroxime axetil, the following adverse reactions and altered laboratory tests have been reported for cephalosporin-class antibiotics: toxic nephropathy, aplastic anemia, hemorrhage, increased BUN, increased creatinine, false-positive test for urinary glucose, increased alkaline phosphatase, neutropenia, elevated bilirubin, and agranulocytosis.

Several cephalosporins have been implicated in triggering seizures, particularly in patients with renal impairment when the dosage was not reduced (see DOSAGE AND ADMINISTRATION). If seizures associated with drug therapy occur, the drug should be discontinued. Anticonvulsant therapy can be given if clinically indicated.

DOSAGE AND ADMINISTRATION

NOTE: CEFTIN TABLETS AND CEFTIN FOR ORAL SUSPENSION ARE NOT BIOEQUIVALENT AND ARE NOT SUBSTITUTABLE ON A MG/MG BASIS (SEE CLINICAL PHARMACOLOGY).

CEFTIN TABLETS

See TABLE 29.

TABLE 29 *Ceftin Tablets**

Population/Infection	Dosage	Duration
Adolescents and Adults (13 years and older)		
Pharyngitis/tonsillitis	250 mg bid	10 days
Acute bacterial maxillary sinusitis	250 mg bid	10 days
Acute bacterial exacerbations of chronic bronchitis	250 or 500 mg bid	10† days
Secondary bacterial infections of acute bronchitis	250 or 500 mg bid	5-10 days
Uncomplicated skin and skin-structure infections	250 or 500 mg bid	10 days
Uncomplicated urinary tract infections	125 or 250 mg bid	7-10 days
Uncomplicated gonorrhea	1000 mg once	single dose
Early Lyme disease	500 mg bid	20 days
Pediatric Patients (who can swallow tablets whole)		
Pharyngitis/tonsillitis	125 mg bid	10 days
Acute otitis media	250 mg bid	10 days
Acute bacterial maxillary sinusitis	250 mg bid	10 days

* May be administered without regard to meals.
† The safety and effectiveness of Ceftin administered for less than 10 days in patients with acute exacerbations of chronic bronchitis have not been established.

CEFTIN FOR ORAL SUSPENSION

Ceftin for oral suspension may be administered to pediatric patients ranging in age from 3 months to 12 years, according to dosages in TABLE 30.

TABLE 30 *Ceftin for Oral Suspension**

Population/Infection	Dosage	Daily Maximum Dose	Duration
Pediatric Patients (3 months to 12 years)			
Pharyngitis/tonsillitis	20 mg/kg/day divided bid	500 mg	10 days
Acute otitis media	30 mg/kg/day divided bid	1000 mg	10 days
Acute bacterial maxillary sinusitis	30 mg/kg/day divided bid	1000 mg	10 days
Impetigo	30 mg/kg/day divided bid	1000 mg	10 days

* Must be administered with food. Shake well each time before using.

PATIENTS WITH RENAL FAILURE

The safety and efficacy of cefuroxime axetil in patients with renal failure have not been established. Since cefuroxime is renally eliminated, its half-life will be prolonged in patients with renal failure.

HOW SUPPLIED

CEFTIN TABLETS

Ceftin tablets are available in:

125 mg: White, capsule-shaped, film-coated tablets engraved with "395" on one side and "Glaxo" on the other side.

250 mg: Light blue, capsule-shaped, film-coated tablets engraved with "387" on one side and "Glaxo" on the other side.

500 mg: Dark blue, capsule-shaped, film-coated tablets engraved with "394" on one side and "Glaxo" on the other side.

Storage

Store the tablets between 15 and 30°C (59 and 86°F). Replace cap securely after each opening. Protect unit dose packs from excessive moisture.

CEFTIN FOR ORAL SUSPENSION

Ceftin for oral suspension is provided as dry, white to pale yellow, tutti-frutti-flavored powder. When reconstituted as directed, Ceftin for oral suspension provides the equivalent of 125 or 250 mg of cefuroxime (as cefuroxime axetil) per 5 ml of suspension. It is supplied in amber glass bottles containing 50 or 100 ml of suspension.

NOTE: SHAKE THE ORAL SUSPENSION WELL BEFORE EACH USE. Replace cap securely after each opening.

Storage

Before reconstitution, store dry powder between 2 and 30°C (36 and 86°F).

After reconstitution, store suspension between 2 and 25°C (36 and 77°F), in a refrigerator or at room temperature. DISCARD AFTER 10 DAYS.

PRODUCT LISTING - RATED THERAPEUTICALLY EQUIVALENT

Quantity	Price	Product	NDC
Powder For Injection - Injectable - 1.5 Gm			
1's	$13.46	KEFUROX, Lilly, Eli and Company	00002-7272-01
1's	$13.80	KEFUROX, Lilly, Eli and Company	00002-7274-01
1's	$13.94	KEFUROX, Lilly, Eli and Company	00002-7279-01
1's	$336.45	GENERIC, Faulding Pharmaceutical Company	61703-0334-33
10's	$100.00	GENERIC, American Pharmaceutical Partners	63323-0312-20
10's	$126.36	GENERIC, Geneva Pharmaceuticals	00781-3924-46
10's	$134.01	GENERIC, Geneva Pharmaceuticals	00781-3922-80
10's	$134.58	KEFUROX, Lilly, Eli and Company	00002-5358-10
10's	$134.58	KEFUROX, Lilly, Eli and Company	00002-5363-10
10's	$134.58	KEFUROX, Lilly, Eli and Company	00002-7272-10
10's	$138.04	KEFUROX, Lilly, Eli and Company	00002-7274-10
10's	$138.04	ZINACEF, Glaxosmithkline	00173-0356-32
10's	$139.39	KEFUROX, Lilly, Eli and Company	00002-7279-10
25's	$336.01	GENERIC, Geneva Pharmaceuticals	00781-3922-96
25's	$336.44	ZINACEF, Glaxosmithkline	00173-0354-35
Powder For Injection - Injectable - 7.5 Gm			
1's	$65.94	KEFUROX, Lilly, Eli and Company	00002-7275-01
6's	$292.50	GENERIC, American Pharmaceutical Partners	63323-0313-61
6's	$395.66	ZINACEF, Glaxosmithkline	00173-0400-00
10's	$599.04	GENERIC, Geneva Pharmaceuticals	00781-3926-46
Powder For Injection - Injectable - 750 mg			
1's	$6.76	KEFUROX, Lilly, Eli and Company	00002-7271-01
1's	$7.11	KEFUROX, Lilly, Eli and Company	00002-7273-01
1's	$7.24	KEFUROX, Lilly, Eli and Company	00002-7278-01
1's	$169.00	GENERIC, Faulding Pharmaceutical Company	61703-0333-11
10 x 25	$169.00	GENERIC, Geneva Pharmaceuticals	00781-3918-96
10's	$65.39	GENERIC, Geneva Pharmaceuticals	00781-3920-46
10's	$71.09	KEFUROX, Lilly, Eli and Company	00002-5359-10
10's	$71.09	KEFUROX, Lilly, Eli and Company	00002-7273-10
10's	$71.09	GENERIC, Lilly, Eli and Company	00002-9011-99
10's	$71.09	ZINACEF, Glaxosmithkline	00173-0353-32
10's	$73.80	GENERIC, Geneva Pharmaceuticals	00781-3918-70
25's	$125.00	GENERIC, American Pharmaceutical Partners	63323-0352-10
25's	$169.09	ZINACEF, Glaxosmithkline	00173-0352-31
25's	$169.10	KEFUROX, Lilly, Eli and Company	00002-7271-25
25's	$181.10	KEFUROX, Lilly, Eli and Company	00002-5357-25
25's	$181.10	KEFUROX, Lilly, Eli and Company	00002-5362-25
25's	$181.10	KEFUROX, Lilly, Eli and Company	00002-7278-25
25's	$285.00	GENERIC, Abbott Pharmaceutical	10515-0125-01
25's	$322.50	GENERIC, American Pharmaceutical Partners	63323-0301-10
Solution - Intravenous - 1.5 Gm/50 ml			
50 ml x 24	$403.95	ZINACEF, Glaxosmithkline	00173-0425-00
Solution - Intravenous - 750 mg/50 ml			
50 ml x 24	$236.59	ZINACEF, Glaxosmithkline	00173-0424-00
Tablet - Oral - 250 mg			
2's	$13.28	CEFTIN, Prescript Pharmaceuticals	00247-0262-02
4's	$23.21	CEFTIN, Prescript Pharmaceuticals	00247-0262-04
8's	$43.06	CEFTIN, Prescript Pharmaceuticals	00247-0262-08
10's	$40.30	CEFTIN, Southwood Pharmaceuticals Inc	58016-0114-10
10's	$46.81	CEFTIN, Physicians Total Care	54868-1080-01
10's	$52.99	CEFTIN, Prescript Pharmaceuticals	00247-0262-10
10's	$107.10	CEFTIN, Pd-Rx Pharmaceuticals	55289-0372-10
14's	$56.42	CEFTIN, Southwood Pharmaceuticals Inc	58016-0114-14
14's	$72.84	CEFTIN, Prescript Pharmaceuticals	00247-0262-14
14's	$145.89	CEFTIN, Pd-Rx Pharmaceuticals	55289-0372-14
15's	$46.65	CEFTIN, Southwood Pharmaceuticals Inc	58016-0114-15
15's	$73.13	CEFTIN, Physicians Total Care	54868-1080-00
16's	$82.76	CEFTIN, Prescript Pharmaceuticals	00247-0262-16
20's	$80.55	CEFTIN, Southwood Pharmaceuticals Inc	58016-0114-20
20's	$84.00	CEFTIN, Allscripts Pharmaceutical Company	54569-1792-04
20's	$87.97	GENERIC, Ranbaxy Laboratories	63304-0751-20
20's	$91.88	CEFTIN, Life Cycle Ventures	65939-0387-00
20's	$92.45	CEFTIN, Physicians Total Care	54868-1080-03
20's	$95.33	CEFTIN, Pharma Pac	52959-0029-20
20's	$102.62	CEFTIN, Prescript Pharmaceuticals	00247-0262-20
20's	$107.66	CEFTIN, Glaxosmithkline	00173-0387-00
20's	$130.32	CEFTIN, Pd-Rx Pharmaceuticals	55289-0372-20
24's	$113.76	CEFTIN, Pharma Pac	52959-0029-24
25's	$260.64	CEFTIN, Pd-Rx Pharmaceuticals	55289-0372-97
28's	$117.60	CEFTIN, Allscripts Pharmaceutical Company	54569-1792-03
30's	$120.90	CEFTIN, Southwood Pharmaceuticals Inc	58016-0114-30
60's	$241.80	CEFTIN, Southwood Pharmaceuticals Inc	58016-0114-60
60's	$275.63	CEFTIN, Life Cycle Ventures	65939-0387-42
60's	$322.98	CEFTIN, Glaxosmithkline	00173-0387-42
100's	$441.00	CEFTIN, Life Cycle Ventures	65939-0387-01
100's	$538.30	CEFTIN, Glaxosmithkline	00173-0387-01
Tablet - Oral - 500 mg			
10's	$74.00	CEFTIN, Southwood Pharmaceuticals Inc	58016-0115-10
10's	$109.88	CEFTIN, Pd-Rx Pharmaceuticals	55289-0542-10
14's	$103.60	CEFTIN, Southwood Pharmaceuticals Inc	58016-0115-14
20's	$148.00	CEFTIN, Southwood Pharmaceuticals Inc	58016-0115-20
20's	$160.31	GENERIC, Ranbaxy Laboratories	63304-0752-20
20's	$167.43	CEFTIN, Life Cycle Ventures	65939-0394-00
20's	$196.19	CEFTIN, Glaxosmithkline	00173-0394-00
30's	$222.00	CEFTIN, Southwood Pharmaceuticals Inc	58016-0115-30
50's	$401.82	CEFTIN, Life Cycle Ventures	65939-0394-01
60's	$444.00	CEFTIN, Southwood Pharmaceuticals Inc	58016-0115-60
60's	$482.18	CEFTIN, Life Cycle Ventures	65939-0394-42
60's	$588.56	CEFTIN, Glaxosmithkline	00173-0394-42

PRODUCT LISTING - EQUIVALENTS NOT AVAILABLE

Quantity	Price	Product	NDC
Powder For Injection - Injectable - 1.5 Gm			
10's	$139.38	ZINACEF, Glaxosmithkline	00173-0437-00
Powder For Injection - Injectable - 7.5 Gm			
6's	$395.68	KEFUROX, Lilly, Eli and Company	00002-5361-16
Powder For Injection - Injectable - 750 mg			
25's	$181.09	ZINACEF, Glaxosmithkline	00173-0436-00
Powder For Reconstitution - Oral - 125 mg/5 ml			
100 ml	$37.59	CEFTIN, Life Cycle Ventures	65939-0406-00
100 ml	$44.05	CEFTIN, Glaxo Wellcome	00173-0406-00
Powder For Reconstitution - Oral - 250 mg/5 ml			
50 ml	$30.72	CEFTIN, Life Cycle Ventures	65939-0554-00
50 ml	$34.73	CEFTIN, Glaxosmithkline	00173-0554-00
100 ml	$58.51	CEFTIN, Allscripts Pharmaceutical Company	54569-4737-00
100 ml	$64.00	CEFTIN, Life Cycle Ventures	65939-0555-00
100 ml	$74.99	CEFTIN, Glaxosmithkline	00173-0555-00
Tablet - Oral - 500 mg			
50's	$490.46	CEFTIN, Glaxosmithkline	00173-0394-01

Celecoxib *(003427)*

For related information, see the comparative table section in Appendix A.

Categories: Arthritis, osteoarthritis; Arthritis, rheumatoid; Dysmenorrhea; Familial adenomatous polyposis; Pain, moderate to severe; FDA Approved 1998 Dec; Pregnancy Category C

Drug Classes: Analgesics, non-narcotic; COX-2 inhibitors; Nonsteroidal anti-inflammatory drugs

Foreign Brand Availability: Artroxil (Colombia); Celcox (Israel); Celebra (Israel); Celebrex (Australia; Bahrain; Benin; Burkina-Faso; Canada; Colombia; Cyprus; Egypt; England; Ethiopia; France; Gambia; Germany; Ghana; Guinea; Hong-Kong; Indonesia; Iran; Iraq; Ivory-Coast; Jordan; Kenya; Korea; Kuwait; Lebanon; Liberia; Libya; Malawi; Mali; Mauritania; Mauritius; Mexico; Morocco; New-Zealand; Niger; Nigeria; Oman; Philippines; Qatar; Republic-of-Yemen; Saudi-Arabia; Senegal; Seychelles; Sierra-Leone; Singapore; South-Africa; Sudan; Syria; Taiwan; Tanzania; Thailand; Tunia; Uganda; United-Arab-Emirates; Zambia; Zimbabwe); Celib (India); Coxid (Philippines); Dilox (Colombia); Lexfin (Colombia)

Cost of Therapy: $82.58 (Osteoarthritis; Celebrex; 200 mg; 1 capsule/day; 30 day supply)

DESCRIPTION

Celecoxib is chemically designated as 4-[5-(4-methylphenyl)-3-(trifluoromethyl)-1H-pyrazol-1-yl] benzenesulfonamide and is a diaryl-substituted pyrazole.

The empirical formula for celecoxib is $C_{17}H_{14}F_3N_3O_2S$, and the molecular weight is 381.38.

Celebrex oral capsules contain 100 and 200 mg of celecoxib.

The inactive ingredients in Celebrex capsules include: Croscarmellose sodium, edible inks, gelatin, lactose monohydrate, magnesium stearate, povidone, sodium lauryl sulfate and titanium dioxide.

CLINICAL PHARMACOLOGY

MECHANISM OF ACTION

Celecoxib is a nonsteroidal anti-inflammatory drug that exhibits anti-inflammatory, analgesic, and antipyretic activities in animal models. The mechanism of action of celecoxib is believed to be due to inhibition of prostaglandin synthesis, primarily via inhibition of cyclooxygenase-2 (COX-2), and at therapeutic concentrations in humans, celecoxib does not inhibit the cyclooxygenase-1 (COX-1) isoenzyme. In animal colon tumor models, celecoxib reduced the incidence and multiplicity of tumors.

PHARMACOKINETICS

Absorption

Peak plasma levels of celecoxib occur approximately 3 hours after an oral dose. Under fasting conditions, both peak plasma levels (C_{max}) and area under the curve (AUC) are roughly dose proportional up to 200 mg bid; at higher doses there are less than proportional increases in C_{max} and AUC (see Food Effects). Absolute bioavailability studies have not been conducted. With multiple dosing, steady state conditions are reached on or before day 5.

The pharmacokinetic parameters of celecoxib in a group of healthy subjects are shown in TABLE 1.

TABLE 1 *Summary of Single Dose (200 mg) Disposition Kinetics of Celecoxib in Healthy Subjects**

	Mean (%CV) PK Parameter Values
C_{max} (ng/ml)	705 (38%)
T_{max} (h)	2.8 (37%)
Effective T½ (h)	11.2 (31%)
Vss/F (L)	429 (34%)
CL/F (L/h)	27.7 (28%)

* Subjects under fasting conditions (n=36, 19-52 years).

Food Effects

When celecoxib capsules were taken with a high fat meal, peak plasma levels were delayed for about 1-2 hours with an increase in total absorption (AUC) of 10-20%. Under fasting conditions, at doses above 200 mg, there is less than a proportional increase in C_{max} and AUC, which is thought to be due to the low solubility of the drug in aqueous media. Coadministration of celecoxib with an aluminum- and magnesium-containing antacid resulted in a reduction in plasma celecoxib concentrations with a decrease of 37% in C_{max} and 10% in AUC. Celecoxib, at doses up to 200 mg bid can be administered without regard to timing of meals. Higher doses (400 mg bid) should be administered with food to improve absorption.

Distribution

In healthy subjects, celecoxib is highly protein bound (~97%) within the clinical dose range. *In vitro* studies indicate that celecoxib binds primarily to albumin and, to a lesser extent, α_1-acid glycoprotein. The apparent volume of distribution at steady state (Vss/F) is approximately 400 L, suggesting extensive distribution into the tissues. Celecoxib is not preferentially bound to red blood cells.

Metabolism

Celecoxib metabolism is primarily mediated via cytochrome P450 2C9. Three metabolites, a primary alcohol, the corresponding carboxylic acid, and its glucuronide conjugate, have been identified in human plasma. These metabolites are inactive as COX-1 or COX-2 inhibitors. Patients who are known or suspected to be P450 2C9 poor metabolizers based on a previous history should be administered celecoxib with caution as they may have abnormally high plasma levels due to reduced metabolic clearance.

Excretion

Celecoxib is eliminated predominantly by hepatic metabolism with little (<3%) unchanged drug recovered in the urine and feces. Following a single oral dose of radiolabeled drug, approximately 57% of the dose was excreted in the feces and 27% was excreted into the urine. The primary metabolite in both urine and feces was the carboxylic acid metabolite (73% of dose) with low amounts of the glucuronide also appearing in the urine. It appears that the low solubility of the drug prolongs the absorption process making terminal half-life (T½) determinations more variable. The effective half-life is approximately 11 hours under fasted conditions. The apparent plasma clearance (CL/F) is about 500 ml/min.

SPECIAL POPULATIONS

Geriatric

At steady state, elderly subjects (over 65 years old) had a 40% higher C_{max} and a 50% higher AUC compared to the young subjects. In elderly females, celecoxib C_{max} and AUC are higher than those for elderly males, but these increases are predominantly due to lower body weight in elderly females. Dose adjustment in the elderly is not generally necessary. However, for patients of less than 50 kg in body weight, initiate therapy at the lowest recommended dose.

Pediatric

Celecoxib capsules have not been investigated in pediatric patients below 18 years of age.

Race

Meta-analysis of pharmacokinetic studies has suggested an approximately 40% higher AUC of celecoxib in Blacks compared to Caucasians. The cause and clinical significance of this finding is unknown.

Hepatic Insufficiency

A pharmacokinetic study in subjects with mild (Child-Pugh Class I) and moderate (Child-Pugh Class II) hepatic impairment has shown that steady-state celecoxib AUC is increased about 40% and 180%, respectively, above that seen in healthy control subjects. Therefore, the daily recommended dose of celecoxib capsules should be reduced by approximately 50% in patients with moderate (Child-Pugh Class II) hepatic impairment. Patients with severe hepatic impairment have not been studied. The use of celecoxib in patients with severe hepatic impairment is not recommended.

Renal Insufficiency

In a cross-study comparison, celecoxib AUC was approximately 40% lower in patients with chronic renal insufficiency (GFR 35-60 ml/min) than that seen in subjects with normal renal function. No significant relationship was found between GFR and celecoxib clearance. Patients with severe renal insufficiency have not been studied. Similar to other NSAIDs, celecoxib is not recommended in patients with severe renal insufficiency (see WARNINGS, Advanced Renal Disease.

DRUG INTERACTIONS

Also see DRUG INTERACTIONS.

General

Significant interactions may occur when celecoxib is administered together with drugs that inhibit P450 2C9. *In vitro* studies indicate that celecoxib is not an inhibitor of cytochrome P450 2C9, 2C19 or 3A4.

Clinical studies with celecoxib have identified potentially significant interactions with fluconazole and lithium. Experience with nonsteroidal anti-inflammatory drugs (NSAIDs) suggests the potential for interactions with furosemide and ACE inhibitors. The effects of celecoxib on the pharmacokinetics and/or pharmacodynamics of glyburide, ketoconazole, methotrexate, phenytoin, and tolbutamide have been studied *in vivo* and clinically important interactions have not been found.

INDICATIONS AND USAGE

Celecoxib is Indicated:

For relief of the signs and symptoms of osteoarthritis.

For relief of the signs and symptoms of rheumatoid arthritis in adults.

For the management of acute pain in adults.

For the treatment of primary dysmenorrhea.

To reduce the number of adenomatous colorectal polyps in familial adenomatous polyposis (FAP), as an adjunct to usual care (*e.g.,* endoscopic surveillance, surgery). It is not known whether there is a clinical benefit from a reduction in the number of colorectal polyps in FAP patients. It is also not known whether the effects of celecoxib treatment will persist after celecoxib is discontinued. The efficacy and safety of celecoxib treatment in patients with FAP beyond 6 months have not been studied (see WARNINGS and PRECAUTIONS).

CONTRAINDICATIONS

Celecoxib is contraindicated in patients with known hypersensitivity to celecoxib.

Celecoxib should not be given to patients who have demonstrated allergic-type reactions to sulfonamides.

Celecoxib should not be given to patients who have experienced asthma, urticaria, or allergic-type reactions after taking aspirin or other NSAIDs. Severe, rarely fatal, anaphylactic-like reactions to NSAIDs have been reported in such patients (see WARNINGS, Anaphylactoid Reactions and PRECAUTIONS, Preexisting Asthma).

WARNINGS

GASTROINTESTINAL (GI) EFFECTS — RISK OF GI ULCERATION, BLEEDING, AND PERFORATION

Serious gastrointestinal toxicity such as bleeding, ulceration, and perforation of the stomach, small intestine or large intestine, can occur at any time, with or without warning symptoms, in patients treated with nonsteroidal anti-inflammatory drugs (NSAIDs). Minor upper gastrointestinal problems, such as dyspepsia, are common and may also occur at any time during NSAID therapy. Therefore, physicians and patients should remain alert for ulceration and bleeding, even in the absence of previous GI tract symptoms (see PRECAUTIONS, Hematological Effects). Patients should be informed about the signs and/or symptoms of serious GI toxicity and the steps to take if they occur. The utility of periodic laboratory monitoring has not been demonstrated, nor has it been adequately assessed. Only 1 in 5 patients who develop a serious upper GI adverse event on NSAID therapy is symptomatic. It has been demonstrated that upper GI ulcers, gross bleeding or perforation, caused by NSAIDs, appear to occur in approximately 1% of patients treated for 3-6 months, and in about 2-4% of patients treated for 1 year. These trends continue thus, increasing the likelihood of developing a serious GI event at some time during the course of therapy. However, even short-term therapy is not without risk.

NSAIDs should be prescribed with extreme caution in patients with a prior history of ulcer disease or gastrointestinal bleeding. Most spontaneous reports of fatal GI events are in elderly or debilitated patients and therefore special care should be taken in treating this population. **To minimize the potential risk for an adverse GI event, the lowest effective dose should be used for the shortest possible duration.** For high risk patients, alternate therapies that do not involve NSAIDs should be considered.

Studies have shown that patients with a *prior history of peptic ulcer disease and/or gastrointestinal bleeding* and who use NSAIDs, have a greater than 10-fold higher risk for developing a GI bleed than patients with neither of these risk factors. In addition to a past history of ulcer disease, pharmacoepidemiological studies have identified several other co-therapies or co-morbid conditions that may increase the risk for GI bleeding such as: treatment with oral corticosteroids, treatment with anticoagulants, longer duration of NSAID therapy, smoking, alcoholism, older age, and poor general health status.

CLASS Study

The estimated cumulative rates at 9 months of *complicated and symptomatic ulcers* (an adverse event similar but not identical to the "upper GI ulcers, gross bleeding or perforation" described in the preceding paragraphs) for patients treated with celecoxib 400 mg bid are described in TABLE 5. TABLE 5 also displays results for patients less than or greater than or equal to the age of 65 years. The differences in rates between the celecoxib alone and celecoxib with ASA groups may be due to the higher risk for GI events in ASA users.

In a small number of patients with a history of ulcer disease, the *complicated and symptomatic ulcer* rates in patients taking celecoxib alone or celecoxib with ASA were, respectively, 2.56% (n=243) and 6.85% (n=91) at 48 weeks. These results are to be expected in patients with a prior history of ulcer disease (see WARNINGS, Gastrointestinal (GI) Effects — Risk of GI Ulceration, Bleeding, and Perforation).

TABLE 5 *Complicated and Symptomatic Ulcer Rates in Patients Taking Celecoxib 400 mg bid (Kaplan-Meier rates at 9 months [%]) Based on Risk Factors*

	Complicated and Symptomatic Ulcer Rates
All Patients	
Celecoxib alone (n=3105)	0.78%
Celecoxib with ASA (n=882)	2.19%
Patients <65 years	
Celecoxib alone (n=2025)	0.47%
Celecoxib with ASA (n=403)	1.26%
Patients ≥65 years	
Celecoxib alone (n=1080)	1.40%
Celecoxib with ASA (n=479)	3.06%

ANAPHYLACTOID REACTIONS

As with NSAIDs in general, anaphylactoid reactions have occurred in patients without known prior exposure to celecoxib. In post-marketing experience, rare cases of anaphylactic reactions and angioedema have been reported in patients receiving celecoxib. Celecoxib should not be given to patients with the aspirin triad. This symptom complex typically occurs in asthmatic patients who experience rhinitis with or without nasal polyps, or who exhibit severe, potentially fatal bronchospasm after taking aspirin or other NSAIDs (see CONTRAINDICATIONS and PRECAUTIONS, Preexisting Asthma). Emergency help should be sought in cases where an anaphylactoid reaction occurs.

ADVANCED RENAL DISEASE

No information is available from controlled clinical studies regarding the use of celecoxib in patients with advanced kidney disease. Therefore, treatment with celecoxib is not recommended in these patients with advanced kidney disease. If celecoxib therapy must be initiated, close monitoring of the patient's kidney function is advisable (see PRECAUTIONS, Renal Effects).

PREGNANCY

In late pregnancy celecoxib should be avoided because it may cause premature closure of the ductus arteriosus.

FAMILIAL ADENOMATOUS POLYPOSIS (FAP)

Treatment with celecoxib in FAP has not been shown to reduce the risk of gastrointestinal cancer or the need for prophylactic colectomy or other FAP-related surgeries. Therefore, the usual care of FAP patients should not be altered because of the concurrent administration of celecoxib. In particular, the frequency of routine endoscopic surveillance should not be decreased and prophylactic colectomy or other FAP-related surgeries should not be delayed.

PRECAUTIONS

GENERAL

Celecoxib cannot be expected to substitute for corticosteroids or to treat corticosteroid insufficiency. Abrupt discontinuation of corticosteroids may lead to exacerbation of corticosteroid-responsive illness. Patients on prolonged corticosteroid therapy should have their therapy tapered slowly if a decision is made to discontinue corticosteroids.

The pharmacological activity of celecoxib in reducing inflammation, and possibly fever, may diminish the utility of these diagnostic signs in detecting infectious complications of presumed noninfectious, painful conditions.

HEPATIC EFFECTS

Borderline elevations of 1 or more liver associated enzymes may occur in up to 15% of patients taking NSAIDs, and notable elevations of ALT or AST (approximately 3 or more times the upper limit of normal) have been reported in approximately 1% of patients in clinical trials with NSAIDs. These laboratory abnormalities may progress, may remain unchanged, or may be transient with continuing therapy. Rare cases of severe hepatic reactions, including jaundice and fatal fulminant hepatitis, liver necrosis and hepatic failure (some with fatal outcome) have been reported with NSAIDs, including celecoxib (see ADVERSE REACTIONS). In controlled clinical trials of celecoxib, the incidence of borderline elevations (greater than or equal to 1.2 times and less than 3 times the upper limit of normal) of liver associated enzymes was 6% for celecoxib and 5% for placebo, and approximately 0.2% of patients taking celecoxib and 0.3% of patients taking placebo had notable elevations of ALT and AST.

A patient with symptoms and/or signs suggesting liver dysfunction, or in whom an abnormal liver test has occurred, should be monitored carefully for evidence of the development of a more severe hepatic reaction while on therapy with celecoxib. If clinical signs and symptoms consistent with liver disease develop, or if systemic manifestations occur (*e.g.*, eosinophilia, rash, etc.), celecoxib should be discontinued.

RENAL EFFECTS

Long-term administration of NSAIDs has resulted in renal papillary necrosis and other renal injury. Renal toxicity has also been seen in patients in whom renal prostaglandins have a compensatory role in the maintenance of renal perfusion. In these patients, administration of a nonsteroidal anti-inflammatory drug may cause a dose-dependent reduction in prostaglandin formation and, secondarily, in renal blood flow, which may precipitate overt renal decompensation. Patients at greatest risk of this reaction are those with impaired renal function, heart failure, liver dysfunction, those taking diuretics and ACE inhibitors, and the elderly. Discontinuation of NSAID therapy is usually followed by recovery to the pretreatment state. Clinical trials with celecoxib have shown renal effects similar to those observed with comparator NSAIDs.

Caution should be used when initiating treatment with celecoxib in patients with considerable dehydration. It is advisable to rehydrate patients first and then start therapy with celecoxib. Caution is also recommended in patients with pre-existing kidney disease (see WARNINGS, Advanced Renal Disease).

HEMATOLOGICAL EFFECTS

Anemia is sometimes seen in patients receiving celecoxib. In controlled clinical trials the incidence of anemia was 0.6% with celecoxib and 0.4% with placebo. Patients on long-term treatment with celecoxib should have their hemoglobin or hematocrit checked if they exhibit any signs or symptoms of anemia or blood loss. Celecoxib does not generally affect platelet counts, prothrombin time (PT), or partial thromboplastin time (PTT), and does not appear to inhibit platelet aggregation at indicated dosages.

FLUID RETENTION, EDEMA, AND HYPERTENSION

Fluid retention and edema have been observed in some patients taking celecoxib (see ADVERSE REACTIONS). In the CLASS study, the Kaplan-Meier cumulative rates at 9 months of peripheral edema in patients on celecoxib 400 mg bid (4-fold and 2-fold the recommended OA and RA doses, respectively, and the approved dose for FAP), ibuprofen 800 mg tid and diclofenac 75 mg bid were 4.5%, 6.9% and 4.7%, respectively. The rates of hypertension in the celecoxib, ibuprofen and diclofenac treated patients were 2.4%, 4.2% and 2.5%, respectively. As with other NSAIDs, celecoxib should be used with caution in patients with fluid retention, hypertension, or heart failure.

PREEXISTING ASTHMA

Patients with asthma may have aspirin-sensitive asthma. The use of aspirin in patients with aspirin-sensitive asthma has been associated with severe bronchospasm which can be fatal. Since cross reactivity, including bronchospasm, between aspirin and other nonsteroidal anti-inflammatory drugs has been reported in such aspirin-sensitive patients, celecoxib should not be administered to patients with this form of aspirin sensitivity and should be used with caution in patients with preexisting asthma.

INFORMATION FOR THE PATIENT

Celecoxib can cause discomfort and, rarely, more serious side effects, such as gastrointestinal bleeding, which may result in hospitalization and even fatal outcomes. Although serious GI tract ulcerations and bleeding can occur without warning symptoms, patients should be alert for the signs and symptoms of ulcerations and bleeding, and should ask for medical advice when observing any indicative signs or symptoms. Patients should be apprised of the importance of this follow-up (see WARNINGS, Gastrointestinal (GI) Effects — Risk of GI Ulceration, Bleeding, and Perforation).

Patients should promptly report signs or symptoms of gastrointestinal ulceration or bleeding, skin rash, unexplained weight gain, or edema to their physicians.

Patients should be informed of the warning signs and symptoms of hepatotoxicity (*e.g.*, nausea, fatigue, lethargy, pruritus, jaundice, right upper quadrant tenderness, and "flu-like" symptoms). If these occur, patients should be instructed to stop therapy and seek immediate medical therapy.

Patients should also be instructed to seek immediate emergency help in the case of an anaphylactoid reaction (see WARNINGS).

In late pregnancy celecoxib should be avoided because it may cause premature closure of the ductus arteriosus.

Patients with familial adenomatous polyposis (FAP) should be informed that celecoxib has not been shown to reduce colorectal, duodenal or other FAP-related cancers, or the need for endoscopic surveillance, prophylactic or other FAP-related surgery. Therefore, all patients with FAP should be instructed to continue their usual care while receiving celecoxib.

LABORATORY TESTS

Because serious GI tract ulcerations and bleeding can occur without warning symptoms, physicians should monitor for signs or symptoms of GI bleeding.

In controlled clinical trials, elevated BUN occurred more frequently in patients receiving celecoxib compared with patients on placebo. This laboratory abnormality was also seen in patients who received comparator NSAIDs in these studies. The clinical significance of this abnormality has not been established.

CARCINOGENESIS, MUTAGENESIS, AND IMPAIRMENT OF FERTILITY

Celecoxib was not carcinogenic in rats given oral doses up to 200 mg/kg for males and 10 mg/kg for females [approximately 2- to 4-fold the human exposure as measured by the AUC(0-24) at 200 mg bid] or in mice given oral doses up to 25 mg/kg for males and 50 mg/kg for females [approximately equal to human exposure as measured by the AUC(0-24) at 200 mg bid] for 2 years.

Celecoxib was not mutagenic in an Ames test and a mutation assay in Chinese hamster ovary (CHO) cells, nor clastogenic in a chromosome aberration assay in CHO cells and an *in vivo* micronucleus test in rat bone marrow.

Celecoxib did not impair male and female fertility in rats at oral doses up to 600 mg/kg/day [approximately 11-fold human exposure at 200 mg bid based on the AUC(0-24)].

PREGNANCY CATEGORY C

Teratogenic Effects

Celecoxib at oral doses ≥150 mg/kg/day [approximately 2-fold human exposure at 200 mg bid as measured by AUC(0-24)], caused an increased incidence of ventricular septal defects, a rare event, and fetal alterations, such as ribs fused, sternebrae fused and sternebrae misshapen when rabbits were treated throughout organogenesis. A dose-dependent increase in diaphragmatic hernias was observed when rats were given celecoxib at oral doses ≥30 mg/kg/day [approximately 6-fold human exposure based on the AUC(0-24) at 200 mg bid] throughout organogenesis. There are no studies in pregnant women. Celecoxib should be used during pregnancy only if the potential benefit justifies the potential risk to the fetus.

Nonteratogenic Effects

Celecoxib produced pre-implantation and post-implantation losses and reduced embryo/fetal survival in rats at oral dosages ≥50 mg/kg/day [approximately 6-fold human exposure based on the AUC(0-24) at 200 mg bid]. These changes are expected with inhibition of prostaglandin synthesis and are not the result of permanent alteration of female reproductive function, nor are they expected at clinical exposures. No studies have been conducted to evaluate the effect of celecoxib on the closure of the ductus arteriosus in humans. Therefore, use of celecoxib during the third trimester of pregnancy should be avoided.

LABOR AND DELIVERY

Celecoxib produced no evidence of delayed labor or parturition at oral doses up to 100 mg/kg in rats [approximately 7-fold human exposure as measured by the AUC(0-24) at 200 mg bid]. The effects of celecoxib on labor and delivery in pregnant women are unknown.

NURSING MOTHERS

Celecoxib is excreted in the milk of lactating rats at concentrations similar to those in plasma. It is not known whether this drug is excreted in human milk. Because many drugs are excreted in human milk and because of the potential for serious adverse reactions in nursing infants from celecoxib, a decision should be made whether to discontinue nursing or to discontinue the drug, taking into account the importance of the drug to the mother.

PEDIATRIC USE

Safety and effectiveness in pediatric patients below the age of 18 years have not been evaluated.

GERIATRIC USE

Of the total number of patients who received celecoxib in clinical trials, more than 3300 were 65-74 years of age, while approximately 1300 additional patients were 75 years and over. No substantial differences in effectiveness were observed between these subjects and younger subjects. In clinical studies comparing renal function as measured by the GFR, BUN and creatinine, and platelet function as measured by bleeding time and platelet aggregation, the results were not different between elderly and young volunteers. However, as with other NSAIDs, including those that selectively inhibit COX-2, there have been more spontaneous postmarketing reports of fatal GI events and acute renal failure in the elderly than in younger patients (see WARNINGS, Gastrointestinal (GI) Effects — Risk of GI Ulceration, Bleeding, and Perforation).

DRUG INTERACTIONS

GENERAL

Celecoxib metabolism is predominantly mediated via cytochrome P450 2C9 in the liver. Co-administration of celecoxib with drugs that are known to inhibit 2C9 should be done with caution.

In vitro studies indicate that celecoxib, although not a substrate, is an inhibitor of cytochrome P450 2D6. Therefore, there is a potential for an *in vivo* drug interaction with drugs that are metabolized by P450 2D6.

ACE-Inhibitors: Reports suggest that NSAIDs may diminish the antihypertensive effect of Angiotensin Converting Enzyme (ACE) inhibitors. This interaction should be given consideration in patients taking celecoxib concomitantly with ACE-inhibitors.

Furosemide: Clinical studies, as well as postmarketing observations, have shown that NSAIDs can reduce the natriuretic effect of furosemide and thiazides in some patients. This response has been attributed to inhibition of renal prostaglandin synthesis.

Aspirin: Celecoxib can be used with low-dose aspirin. However, concomitant administration of aspirin with celecoxib increases the rate of GI ulceration or other complications, compared to use of celecoxib alone (see WARNINGS, Gastrointestinal (GI) Effects — Risk of GI Ulceration, Bleeding, and Perforation, CLASS Study).

Because of its lack of platelet effects, celecoxib is not a substitute for aspirin for cardiovascular prophylaxis.

Fluconazole: Concomitant administration of fluconazole at 200 mg qd resulted in a 2-fold increase in celecoxib plasma concentration. This increase is due to the inhibition of celecoxib metabolism via P450 2C9 by fluconazole (see CLINICAL PHARMACOLOGY, Pharmacokinetics, Metabolism). Celecoxib should be introduced at the lowest recommended dose in patients receiving fluconazole.

Lithium: In a study conducted in healthy subjects, mean steady-state lithium plasma levels increased approximately 17% in subjects receiving lithium 450 mg bid with celecoxib 200 mg bid as compared to subjects receiving lithium alone. Patients on lithium treatment should be closely monitored when celecoxib is introduced or withdrawn.

Methotrexate: In an interaction study of rheumatoid arthritis patients taking methotrexate, celecoxib did not have a significant effect on the pharmacokinetics of methotrexate.

Warfarin: Anticoagulant activity should be monitored, particularly in the first few days, after initiating or changing celecoxib therapy in patients receiving warfarin or similar agents, since these patients are at an increased risk of bleeding complications. The effect of celecoxib on the anticoagulant effect of warfarin was studied in a group of healthy subjects receiving daily doses of 2-5 mg of warfarin. In these subjects, celecoxib did not alter the anticoagulant effect of warfarin as determined by prothrombin time. However, in post-marketing experience, bleeding events have been reported, predominantly in the elderly, in association with increases in prothrombin time in patients receiving celecoxib concurrently with warfarin.

ADVERSE REACTIONS

Of the celecoxib treated patients in the premarketing controlled clinical trials, approximately 4250 were patients with OA, approximately 2100 were patients with RA, and approximately 1050 were patients with post-surgical pain. More than 8500 patients have received a total daily dose of celecoxib of 200 mg (100 mg bid or 200 mg qd) or more, including more than 400 treated at 800 mg (400 mg bid). Approximately 3900 patients have received celecoxib at these doses for 6 months or more; approximately 2300 of these have received it for 1 year or more and 124 of these have received it for 2 years or more.

ADVERSE EVENTS FROM CELECOXIB PREMARKETING CONTROLLED ARTHRITIS TRIALS

TABLE 6 lists all adverse events, regardless of causality, occurring in ≥2% of patients receiving celecoxib from 12 controlled studies conducted in patients with OA or RA that included a placebo and/or a positive control group.

TABLE 6 *Adverse Events Occurring in ≥2% of Celecoxib Patients From Celecoxib Premarketing Controlled Arthritis Trials*

	Celecoxib* (n=4146)	Placebo (n=1864)	Naproxen† (n=1366)	Diclofenac‡ (n=387)	Ibuprofen§ (n=345)
Gastrointestinal					
Abdominal pain	4.1%	2.8%	7.7%	9.0%	9.0%
Diarrhea	5.6%	3.8%	5.3%	9.3%	5.8%
Dyspepsia	8.8%	6.2%	12.2%	10.9%	12.8%
Flatulence	2.2%	1.0%	3.6%	4.1%	3.5%
Nausea	3.5%	4.2%	6.0%	3.4%	6.7%
Body as a Whole					
Back pain	2.8%	3.6%	2.2%	2.6%	0.9%
Peripheral edema	2.1%	1.1%	2.1%	1.0%	3.5%
Injury-accidental	2.9%	2.3%	3.0%	2.6%	3.2%
Central and Peripheral Nervous System					
Dizziness	2.0%	1.7%	2.6%	1.3%	2.3%
Headache	15.8%	20.2%	14.5%	15.5%	15.4%
Psychiatric					
Insomnia	2.3%	2.3%	2.9%	1.3%	1.4%
Respiratory					
Pharyngitis	2.3%	1.1%	1.7%	1.6%	2.6%
Rhinitis	2.0%	1.3%	2.4%	2.3%	0.6%
Sinusitis	5.0%	4.3%	4.0%	5.4%	5.8%
Upper respiratory tract infection	8.1%	6.7%	9.9%	9.8%	9.9%
Skin					
Rash	2.2%	2.1%	2.1%	1.3%	1.2%

* 100-200 mg bid or 200 mg qd.
† 500 mg bid.
‡ 75 mg bid.
§ 800 mg tid.

In placebo- or active-controlled clinical trials, the discontinuation rate due to adverse events was 7.1% for patients receiving celecoxib and 6.1% for patients receiving placebo. Among the most common reasons for discontinuation due to adverse events in the celecoxib treatment groups were dyspepsia and abdominal pain (cited as reasons for discontinuation in 0.8% and 0.7% of celecoxib patients, respectively). Among patients receiving placebo, 0.6% discontinued due to dyspepsia and 0.6% withdrew due to abdominal pain.

The following adverse events occurred in 0.1-1.9% of patients regardless of causality with celecoxib doses of 100-200 mg bid or 200 mg qd:

Gastrointestinal: Constipation, diverticulitis, dysphagia, eructation, esophagitis, gastritis, gastroenteritis, gastroesophageal reflux, hemorrhoids, hiatal hernia, melena, dry mouth, stomatitis, tenesmus, tooth disorder, vomiting.

Cardiovascular: Aggravated hypertension, angina pectoris, coronary artery disorder, myocardial infarction.

General: Allergy aggravated, allergic reaction, asthenia, chest pain, cyst NOS, edema generalized, face edema, fatigue, fever, hot flushes, influenza-like symptoms, pain, peripheral pain.

Resistance Mechanism Disorders: Herpes simplex, herpes zoster, infection bacterial, infection fungal, infection soft tissue, infection viral, moniliasis, moniliasis genital, otitis media.

Central, Peripheral Nervous System: Leg cramps, hypertonia, hypoesthesia, migraine, neuralgia, neuropathy, paresthesia, vertigo.

Female Reproductive: Breast fibroadenosis, breast neoplasm, breast pain, dysmenorrhea, menstrual disorder, vaginal hemorrhage, vaginitis.

Male Reproductive: Prostatic disorder.

Hearing and Vestibular: Deafness, ear abnormality, earache, tinnitus.

Heart Rate and Rhythm: Palpitation, tachycardia.

Liver and Biliary System: Hepatic function abnormal, SGOT increased, SGPT increased.

Metabolic and Nutritional: BUN increased, CPK increased, diabetes mellitus, hypercholesterolemia, hyperglycemia, hypokalemia, NPN increase, creatinine increased, alkaline phosphatase increased, weight increase.

Musculoskeletal: Arthralgia, arthrosis, bone disorder, fracture accidental, myalgia, neck stiffness, synovitis, tendinitis.

Platelets (bleeding or clotting): Ecchymosis, epistaxis, thrombocythemia.

Psychiatric: Anorexia, anxiety, appetite increased, depression, nervousness, somnolence.

Hemic: Anemia.

Respiratory: Bronchitis, bronchospasm, bronchospasm aggravated, coughing, dyspnea, laryngitis, pneumonia.

Skin and Appendages: Alopecia, dermatitis, nail disorder, photosensitivity reaction, pruritus, rash erythematous, rash maculopapular, skin disorder, skin dry, sweating increased, urticaria.

Application Site Disorders: Cellulitis, dermatitis contact, injection site reaction, skin nodule.

Special Senses: Taste perversion.

Urinary System: Albuminuria, cystitis, dysuria, hematuria, micturition frequency, renal calculus, urinary incontinence, urinary tract infection.

Vision: Blurred vision, cataract, conjunctivitis, eye pain, glaucoma.

Other serious adverse reactions which occur rarely (estimated <0.1%), regardless of causality: The following serious adverse events have occurred rarely in patients taking celecoxib. Cases reported only in the post-marketing experience are indicated in italics.

Cardiovascular: Syncope, congestive heart failure, ventricular fibrillation, pulmonary embolism, cerebrovascular accident, peripheral gangrene, thrombophlebitis, *vasculitis.*

Gastrointestinal: Intestinal obstruction, intestinal perforation, gastrointestinal bleeding, colitis with bleeding, esophageal perforation, pancreatitis, ileus.

Liver and Biliary System: Cholelithiasis, *hepatitis, jaundice, liver failure.*

Hemic and Lymphatic: Thrombocytopenia, *agranulocytosis, aplastic anemia, pancytopenia, leukopenia.*

Metabolic: *Hypoglycemia, hyponatremia.*

Nervous System: *Aseptic meningitis,* ataxia, suicide.

Renal: Acute renal failure, *interstitial nephritis.*

Skin: *Erythema multiforme, exfoliative dermatitis, Stevens-Johnson syndrome, toxic epidermal necrolysis.*

General: Sepsis, sudden death, *anaphylactoid reaction, angioedema.*

SAFETY DATA FROM CLASS STUDY

Hematological Events

During this study, the incidence of clinically significant decreases in hemoglobin (>2 g/dl) confirmed by repeat testing was lower in patients on celecoxib 400 mg bid (4-fold and 2-fold the recommended OA and RA doses, respectively, and the approved dose for FAP) compared to patients on either diclofenac 75 mg bid or ibuprofen 800 mg tid: 0.5%, 1.3% and 1.9%, respectively. The lower incidence of events with celecoxib was maintained with or without ASA use.

Withdrawals/Serious Adverse Events

Kaplan-Meier cumulative rates at 9 months for withdrawals due to adverse events for celecoxib, diclofenac, and ibuprofen were 24%, 29%, and 26%, respectively. Rates for serious adverse events (*i.e.,* those causing hospitalization or felt to be life threatening or otherwise medically significant) regardless of causality were not different across treatment groups, respectively, 8%, 7%, and 8%.

Based on Kaplan-Meier cumulative rates for investigator-reported serious cardiovascular thromboembolic adverse events*, there were no differences between the celecoxib, diclofenac, or ibuprofen treatment groups. The rates in all patients at 9 months for celecoxib, diclofenac, and ibuprofen were 1.2%, 1.4%, and 1.1%, respectively. The rates for non-ASA users in each of the three treatment groups were less than 1%. The rates for myocardial infarction in each of the three non-ASA treatment groups were less than 0.2%.

*Includes myocardial infarction, pulmonary embolism, deep venous thrombosis, unstable angina, transient ischemic attacks or ischemic cerebrovascular accidents.

ADVERSE EVENTS FROM ANALGESIA AND DYSMENORRHEA STUDIES

Approximately 1700 patients were treated with celecoxib in analgesia and dysmenorrhea studies. All patients in post-oral surgery pain studies recieved a single dose of study medication. Doses up to 600 mg/day of celecoxib were studied in primary dysmenorrhea and post-orthopedic surgery pain studies. The types of adverse events in the analgesia and dysmenorrhea studies were similar to those reported in arthritis studies. The only additional adverse event reported was post-dental extraction alveolar osteitis (dry socket) in the post-oral surgery pain studies.

ADVERSE EVENTS FROM THE CONTROLLED TRIAL IN FAMILIAL ADENOMATOUS POLYPOSIS

The adverse event profile reported for the 83 patients with familial adenomatous polyposis enrolled in the randomized, controlled clinical trial was similar to that reported for patients in the arthritis controlled trials. Intestinal anastomotic ulceration was the only new adverse event reported in the FAP trial, regardless of causality, and was observed in 3 of 58 patients (one at 100 mg bid, and two at 400 mg bid) who had prior intestinal surgery.

DOSAGE AND ADMINISTRATION

For osteoarthritis and rheumatoid arthritis, the lowest dose of celecoxib should be sought for each patient. These doses can be given without regard to timing of meals.

Osteoarthritis: For relief of the signs and symptoms of osteoarthritis the recommended oral dose is 200 mg/day administered as a single dose or as 100 mg twice per day.

Rheumatoid Arthritis: For relief of the signs and symptoms of rheumatoid arthritis the recommended oral dose is 100-200 mg twice per day.

Management of Acute Pain and Treatment of Primary Dysmenorrhea: The recommended dose of celecoxib is 400 mg initially, followed by an additional 200 mg dose if needed on the first day. On subsequent days, the recommended dose is 200 mg twice daily as needed.

Familial Adenomatous Polyposis (FAP): Usual medical care for FAP patients should be continued while on celecoxib. To reduce the number of adenomatous colorectal polyps in patients with FAP, the recommended oral dose is 400 mg (2 × 200 mg capsules) twice per day to be taken with food.

SPECIAL POPULATIONS

Hepatic Insufficiency

The daily recommended dose of celecoxib capsules in patients with moderate hepatic impairment (Child-Pugh Class II) should be reduced by approximately 50% (see CLINICAL PHARMACOLOGY, Special Populations).

HOW SUPPLIED

Celebrex Capsules

100 mg: White, reverse printed white on blue band of body and cap with markings of "7767" on the cap and "100" on the body.

200 mg: White, with reverse printed white on gold band with markings of "7767" on the cap and "200" on the body.

Storage: Store at 25°C (77°F); excursions permitted to 15-30°C (59-86°F).

PRODUCT LISTING - EQUIVALENTS NOT AVAILABLE

Capsule - Oral - 100 mg			
10's	$14.30	CELEBREX, Allscripts Pharmaceutical Company	54569-4671-03
10's	$14.87	CELEBREX, Southwood Pharmaceuticals Inc	58016-0169-10
12's	$17.85	CELEBREX, Southwood Pharmaceuticals Inc	58016-0169-12
14's	$20.82	CELEBREX, Allscripts Pharmaceutical Company	54569-4671-04
14's	$36.74	CELEBREX, Pd-Rx Pharmaceuticals	55289-0451-14
14's	$43.43	CELEBREX, Pharma Pac	52959-0540-14
15's	$46.47	CELEBREX, Pharma Pac	52959-0540-15
20's	$29.75	CELEBREX, Southwood Pharmaceuticals Inc	58016-0169-20
20's	$34.82	CELEBREX, Physicians Total Care	54868-4107-01
20's	$51.33	CELEBREX, Pd-Rx Pharmaceuticals	55289-0451-20
20's	$59.94	CELEBREX, Pharma Pac	52959-0540-20
21's	$31.23	CELEBREX, Southwood Pharmaceuticals Inc	58016-0169-21
21's	$61.97	CELEBREX, Pharma Pac	52959-0540-21
28's	$41.65	CELEBREX, Southwood Pharmaceuticals Inc	58016-0169-28
28's	$82.41	CELEBREX, Pharma Pac	52959-0540-28
30's	$42.90	CELEBREX, Allscripts Pharmaceutical Company	54569-4671-02
30's	$44.62	CELEBREX, Southwood Pharmaceuticals Inc	58016-0169-30
30's	$51.65	CELEBREX, Physicians Total Care	54868-4107-00
30's	$88.20	CELEBREX, Pharma Pac	52959-0540-30
40's	$102.22	CELEBREX, Pharma Pac	52959-0540-40
60's	$89.24	CELEBREX, Southwood Pharmaceuticals Inc	58016-0169-60
60's	$102.12	CELEBREX, Physicians Total Care	54868-4107-02
100's	$148.73	CELEBREX, Southwood Pharmaceuticals Inc	58016-0169-00
100's	$175.56	CELEBREX, Searle	00025-1520-31
100's	$175.56	CELEBREX, Searle	00025-1520-34
Capsule - Oral - 200 mg			
5's	$25.22	CELEBREX, Pharma Pac	52959-0539-05
7's	$35.37	CELEBREX, Pharma Pac	52959-0539-07
10's	$27.53	CELEBREX, Southwood Pharmaceuticals Inc	58016-0223-10
10's	$38.42	CELEBREX, Dhs Inc	55887-0736-10
10's	$40.25	CELEBREX, Pd-Rx Pharmaceuticals	55289-0475-10
10's	$44.84	CELEBREX, Pharma Pac	52959-0539-10
12's	$33.03	CELEBREX, Southwood Pharmaceuticals Inc	58016-0223-12
14's	$38.54	CELEBREX, Southwood Pharmaceuticals Inc	58016-0223-14
14's	$56.18	CELEBREX, Pharma Pac	52959-0539-14
15's	$41.29	CELEBREX, Southwood Pharmaceuticals Inc	58016-0223-15
15's	$43.88	CELEBREX, Physicians Total Care	54868-4101-03
15's	$60.08	CELEBREX, Pharma Pac	52959-0539-15
20's	$50.34	CELEBREX, Allscripts Pharmaceutical Company	54569-4672-05
20's	$55.05	CELEBREX, Southwood Pharmaceuticals Inc	58016-0223-20
20's	$58.12	CELEBREX, Physicians Total Care	54868-4101-02
20's	$74.11	CELEBREX, Dhs Inc	55887-0736-20
20's	$78.55	CELEBREX, Pharma Pac	52959-0539-20
20's	$78.75	CELEBREX, Pd-Rx Pharmaceuticals	55289-0475-20
21's	$57.81	CELEBREX, Southwood Pharmaceuticals Inc	58016-0223-21
21's	$82.52	CELEBREX, Pharma Pac	52959-0539-21
28's	$67.76	CELEBREX, Allscripts Pharmaceutical Company	54569-4672-02
28's	$77.07	CELEBREX, Southwood Pharmaceuticals Inc	58016-0223-28
28's	$98.82	CELEBREX, Pharma Pac	52959-0539-28
28's	$100.32	CELEBREX, Pd-Rx Pharmaceuticals	55289-0475-28
30's	$78.60	CELEBREX, St. Mary'S Mpp	60760-0525-30
30's	$82.58	CELEBREX, Southwood Pharmaceuticals Inc	58016-0223-30
30's	$86.59	CELEBREX, Physicians Total Care	54868-4101-01
30's	$103.62	CELEBREX, Dhs Inc	55887-0736-30
30's	$115.36	CELEBREX, Pharma Pac	52959-0539-30
40's	$177.59	CELEBREX, Pharma Pac	52959-0539-40
45's	$108.90	CELEBREX, Allscripts Pharmaceutical Company	54569-4672-03
45's	$193.13	CELEBREX, Pharma Pac	52959-0539-45
60's	$108.90	CELEBREX, Allscripts Pharmaceutical Company	54569-4672-04
60's	$162.51	CELEBREX, Physicians Total Care	54868-4101-00
60's	$165.16	CELEBREX, Southwood Pharmaceuticals Inc	58016-0223-60
60's	$201.97	CELEBREX, Pharma Pac	52959-0539-60
100's	$275.27	CELEBREX, Southwood Pharmaceuticals Inc	58016-0223-00
100's	$287.95	CELEBREX, Searle	00025-1525-31
100's	$287.95	CELEBREX, Searle	00025-1525-34
Capsule - Oral - 400 mg			
60's	$259.15	CELEBREX, Pharmacia Corporation	00025-1530-02
100's	$438.40	CELEBREX, Pharmacia Corporation	00025-1530-01

Cephalexin (000698)

Categories: Infection, bone; Infection, ear, middle; Infection, skin and skin structures; Infection, upper respiratory tract; Infection, urinary tract; Prostatitis; Pregnancy Category B; FDA Approval Pre 1982

Drug Classes: Antibiotics, cephalosporins

Brand Names: Alsporin; Biocef; Carnosporin; Cefaseptin; Cephin; Ceporexin-E; Check; Ed A-Ceph; Keflet; **Keflex**; Lopilexin; Mamlexin; Syned; Winlex

Foreign Brand Availability: Alexin (India); Anxer (Hong-Kong); Bloflex (Philippines); Cefablan (Colombia); Cefacin-M (Hong-Kong); Cefadal (Benin; Burkina-Faso; Ethiopia; Gambia; Ghana; Guinea; Ivory-Coast; Kenya; Liberia; Malawi; Mali; Mauritania; Mauritius; Morocco; Niger; Nigeria; Senegal; Seychelles; Sierra-Leone; South-Africa; Sudan; Tanzania; Tunia; Uganda; Zambia; Zimbabwe); Cefadin (Ecuador); Cefadina (Spain); Cefadyl (Benin; Burkina-Faso; Ethiopia; Gambia; Ghana; Guinea; Ivory-Coast; Kenya; Liberia; Malawi; Mali; Mauritania; Mauritius; Morocco; Niger; Nigeria; Senegal; Seychelles; Sierra-Leone; South-Africa; Sudan; Tanzania; Tunia; Uganda; Zambia; Zimbabwe); Cefalin (Indonesia; Israel; Philippines); Cefax (Colombia); Ceforal (Israel); Cefovit (Israel); Cefrin (Peru); Celexil (Philippines); Celexin (Thailand); Cepastar (Philippines); Cepexin (Austria); Cephalexyl (Thailand); Cephia (Thailand); Cephanmycin (Singapore); Cepol (Japan); Ceporex (Australia; Bahamas; Bahrain; Barbados; Belgium; Belize; Bermuda; Bulgaria; Curacao; Cyprus; Czech-Republic; Ecuador; Egypt; England; Guyana; Hong-Kong; Iran; Iraq; Ireland; Israel; Italy; Jamaica; Jordan; Kuwait; Lebanon; Libya; Malaysia; Mexico; Netherland-Antilles; Netherlands; New-Zealand; Oman; Philippines; Portugal; Puerto-Rico; Qatar; Republic-of-Yemen; Saudi-Arabia; South-Africa; Spain; Surinam; Switzerland; Syria; Thailand; Trinidad; United-Arab-Emirates); Ceporex Forte (Portugal); Ceporexin (Argentina; Germany); Ceporexine (France); Cerexin (South-Africa); Cromlex (Philippines); Difagen (Philippines); Durantel DS (Japan); Erocetin (Argentina); Falexin (Korea); Farmalex (Thailand); Felexin (Hong-Kong; Malaysia); Fexin (South-Africa); Ibilex (Australia; New-Zealand; Taiwan; Thailand); Inphalex (Indonesia); Kefacin (Korea); Kefalex (Finland); Kefalospes (Greece); Kefaxin (Greece; Ireland); Kefexin (Czech-Republic; Finland; Germany; Ireland); Kefloridina (Spain); Keforal (Argentina; Belgium; France; Italy; Netherlands); Kemolexin (Indonesia); Lenocef (South-Africa); Lexin (Peru); Lonflex (Taiwan); Madlexin (Indonesia); Mamalexin (Japan); Montralex (Philippines); Neokef (Malaysia); Novolexin (Canada); Nufex (India); Oracef (Bulgaria; Czech-Republic; Germany); Oriphex (Benin; Burkina-Faso; Ethiopia; Gambia; Ghana; Guinea; Ivory-Coast; Kenya; Liberia; Malawi; Mali; Mauritania; Mauritius; Morocco; Niger; Nigeria; Senegal; Seychelles; Sierra-Leone; Sudan; Tanzania; Tunia; Uganda; Zambia; Zimbabwe); Ospexin (Austria; Bahrain; Bulgaria; Costa-Rica; Cyprus; Czech-Republic; Dominican-Republic; Egypt; El-Salvador; Guatemala; Honduras; Hong-Kong; Indonesia; Iran; Iraq; Israel; Jordan; Kuwait; Lebanon; Libya; Malaysia; Nicaragua; Oman; Panama; Qatar; Republic-of-Yemen; Saudi-Arabia; Syria; United-Arab-Emirates); Paferxin (Mexico); Palitrex (Ecuador; Indonesia; Peru); Pectril (Philippines); Pharmexin (Bahrain; Cyprus; Egypt; Iran; Iraq; Jordan; Kuwait; Lebanon; Libya; Oman; Qatar; Republic-of-Yemen; Saudi-Arabia; Syria; United-Arab-Emirates); Pondnacef (Thailand); Pyassan (Hungary); Refosporen (Argentina); Relaxin (Philippines); Rofex (India); Sanaxin (Austria); Sefasin (Thailand); Septilisin (Argentina); Sepexin (India); Servicef (Mexico); Servispor (Malaysia); Sialexin (Thailand); Sinlex (Taiwan); Sinthecillin (Greece); Sofilex (Hong-Kong; Singapore); Sporicef (Thailand); Sporidex (India; Philippines); Syncle (Japan); Tepaxin (Indonesia); Tokiolexin (Japan); Uphalexin (Malaysia); Velexin (Thailand); Voxxim (Philippines); Zeplex (Thailand)

Cost of Therapy: $46.12 (Infection; Keflex; 250 mg; 4 capsules/day; 7 day supply)
$10.50 (Infection; Generic Capsules; 250 mg; 4 capsules/day; 7 day supply)

DESCRIPTION

Cephalexin is a semisynthetic cephalosporin antibiotic intended for oral administration. It is 7-(D-α-Amino-α-phenylacetamido)-3-methyl-3-cephem-4-carboxylic acid monohydrate. Cephalexin has the molecular formula $C_{16}H_{17}N_3O_4S{\cdot}H_2O$ and the molecular weight is 365.41.

The nucleus of cephalexin is related to that of other cephalosporin antibiotics. The compound is a zwitterion; *i.e.*, the molecule contains both a basic and an acidic group. The isoelectric point of cephalexin in water is approximately 4.5 to 5.

The crystalline form of cephalexin which is available is a monohydrate. It is a white crystalline solid having a bitter taste. Solubility in water is low at room temperature; 1 or 2 mg/ml may be dissolved readily, but higher concentrations are obtained with increasing difficulty.

The cephalosporins differ from penicillins in the structure of the bicyclic ring system. Cephalexin has a *D*-phenylglycyl group as substituent at the 7-amino position and an unsubstituted methyl group at the 3-position.

Each Pulvule contains cephalexin monohydrate equivalent to 250 mg (720 μmol) or 500 mg (1439 μmol) of cephalexin. The Pulvules also contain cellulose, D&C yellow no. 10, FD&C blue no. 1, F D&C yellow no. 6, gelatin, magnesium stearate, silicone, titanium dioxide, and other inactive ingredients.

Each capsule manufactured by Mylan contains cephalexin monohydrate equivalent to 250 mg (720 μmol) or 500 mg (1439 μmol) of cephalexin. The capsules also contain cellulose, FD&C blue no. 1, gelatin, magnesium stearate, silicone, titanium dioxide, and other inactive ingredients.

After mixing, each 5 ml of Keflex, for oral suspension, will contain cephalexin monohydrate equivalent to 125 mg (360 μmol) or 250 mg (720 μmol) of cephalexin. The suspensions also contain flavors, methylcellulose, silicone, sodium lauryl sulfate, and sucrose. The 125 mg suspension contains FD&C red no. 40, and the 250 mg suspension contains FD&C yellow no. 6.

Each capsule manufactured by Biocraft contains cephalexin monohydrate equivalent to 250 mg (720 μmol) or 500 mg (1439 μmol) of cephalexin. *Inactive Ingredients:* Magnesium stearate, silicone dioxide and may contain talc. Capsule shell and print constituents: black iron oxide, D&C yellow no. 10 aluminium lake, FD&C blue no. 1 aluminium lake, FD&C blue no. 2 aluminium lake, FD&C red no. 40 aluminium lake, gelatin, pharmaceutical glaze modified in SD-45, silcon dioxide or carbomethylcellulose sodium, sodium lauryl sulfate, titanium dioxide and may contian propylene glyceryl. In addition, the 250 mg capsule shell contains yellow iron oxide.

Each tablet manufactured by Biocraft contains cephalexin monohydrate equivalent to 250 mg (720 μmol) or 500 mg (1439 μmol) of cephalexin. Inactive ingredients: hydroxypropyl methylcellulose, magnesium stearate, microcrystalline cellulose, polyethylene glycol, polysorbate 90, sodium starch glycolate and titanium dioxide.

CLINICAL PHARMACOLOGY

HUMAN PHARMACOLOGY

Cephalexin is acid stable and may be given without regard to meals. It is rapidly absorbed after oral administration. Following doses of 250 mg, 500 mg, and 1 g, average peak serum levels of approximately 9, 18, and 32 μg/ml respectively were obtained at 1 hour. Measurable levels were present 6 hours after administration. Cephalexin is excreted in the urine by glomerular filtration and tubular secretion. Studies showed that over 90% of the drug was excreted unchanged in the urine within 8 hours. During this period, peak urine concentrations following the 250 mg, 500 mg, and 1 g doses were approximately 1000, 2200, and 5000 μg/ml respectively.

MICROBIOLOGY

In vitro tests demonstrate that the cephalosporins are bactericidal because of their inhibition of cell-wall synthesis. Cephalexin has been shown to be active against most strains of the following microorganisms both *in vitro* and in clinical infections as described in INDICATIONS AND USAGE.

Aerobes, Gram-positive:

Staphylococcus aureus (including penicillinase-producing strains).
Staphylococcus epidermidis (penicillin-susceptible strains).
Streptococcus pneumoniae.
Streptococcus pyogenes.

Aerobes, Gram-negative:

Escherichia coli.
Haemophilus influenzae.
Klebsiella pneumoniae.
Moraxella (Branhamella) catarrhalis.
Proteus mirabilis.

Note: Methicillin-resistant staphylococci and most strains of enterococci (*Enterococcus faecalis* [formerly *Streptococcus faecalis*]) are resistant to cephalosporins, including cephalexin. It is not active against most strains of *Enterobacter* spp,*Morganella morganii,* and *Proteus vulgaris.* It has no activity against *Pseudomonas* spp or *Acinetobacter calcoaceticus.*

SUSCEPTIBILITY TESTING

Diffusion Techniques: Quantitative methods that require measurement of zone diameters provide reproducible estimates of the susceptibility of bacteria to antimicrobial compounds. One such standard procedure[1] that has been recommended for use with disks to test the susceptibility of microorganisms to cephalexin, uses the 30 μg cephalothin disk. Interpretation involves correlation of the diameter obtained in the disk test with the minimal inhibitory concentration (MIC) for cephalexin.

Reports from the laboratory providing results of the standard single-disk susceptibility test with a 30 μg cephalothin disk should be interpreted according to the criteria found in TABLE 1.

TABLE 1

Zone Diameter (mm)	Interpretation
≥18	(S) Susceptible
15-17	(I) Intermediate
≤14	(R) Resistant

A report of "Susceptible" indicates that the pathogen is likely to be inhibited by usually achievable concentrations of the antimicrobial compound in blood. A report of "Intermediate" indicates that the result should be considered equivocal, and, if the microorganism is not fully susceptible to alternative, clinically feasible drugs, the test should be repeated. This category implies possible clinical applicability in body sites where the drug is physiologically concentrated or in situations where high dosage of drug can be used. This category also provides a buffer zone that prevents small uncontrolled technical factors from causing major discrepancies in interpretation. A report of "Resistant" indicates that usually achievable concentrations of the antimicrobial compound in the blood are unlikely to be inhibitory and that other therapy should be selected.

Measurement of MIC or MBC and achieved antimicrobial compound concentrations may be appropriate to guide therapy in some infections. (See CLINICAL PHARMACOLOGY for information on drug concentrations achieved in infected body sites and other pharmacokinetic properties of this antimicrobial drug product.)

Standardized susceptibility test procedures require the use of laboratory control microorganisms. The 30 μg cephalothin disk should provide the zone diameters in these laboratory test quality control strains (see TABLE 2).

TABLE 2

Microorganism	Zone Diameter (mm)
E. coli ATCC 25922	15-21
S. aureus ATCC 25923	29-37

Dilution Techniques: Quantitative methods that are used to determine MICs provide reproducible estimates of the susceptibility of bacteria to antimicrobial compounds. One such standardized procedure uses a standardized dilution method[2] (broth, agar, microdilution) or equivalent with cephalothin powder. The MIC values obtained should be interpreted according to the criteria found in TABLE 3.

TABLE 3

MIC (μg/ml)	Interpretation
≤8	(S) Susceptible
16	(I) Intermediate
≥32	(R) Resistant

Interpretation should be as stated above for results using diffusion techniques.

As with standard diffusion techniques, dilution methods require the use of laboratory control microorganisms. Standard cephalothin powder should provide the MIC values seen in TABLE 4.

INDICATIONS AND USAGE

Cephalexin is indicated for the treatment of the following infections when caused by susceptible strains of the designated microorganisms:

TABLE 4

Microorganism	MIC (μg/ml)
E. coli ATCC 25922	4-16
S. aureus ATCC 29213	0.12-0.5

Respiratory tract infections caused by *S. pneumoniae* and *S. pyogenes* (Penicillin is the usual drug of choice in the treatment and prevention of streptococcal infections, including the prophylaxis of rheumatic fever. Cephalexin is generally effective in the eradication of streptococci from the nasopharynx; however, substantial data establishing the efficacy of cephalexin in the subsequent prevention of rheumatic fever are not available at present.)

Otitis media due to *S. pneumoniae, H. influenzae, staphylococci, streptococci,* and *M. catarrhalis.*

Skin and skin structure infections caused by *staphylococci* and/or *streptococci.*

Bone infections caused by staphylococci and/or *P. mirabilis.*

Genitourinary tract infections, including acute prostatitis, caused by *E. coli, P. mirabilis,* and *K. pneumoniae.*

Note: Culture and susceptibility tests should be initiated prior to and during therapy. Renal function studies should be performed when indicated.

CONTRAINDICATIONS

Cephalexin is contraindicated in patients with known allergy to the cephalosporin group of antibiotics.

WARNINGS

BEFORE CEPHALEXIN THERAPY IS INSTITUTED, CAREFUL INQUIRY SHOULD BE MADE CONCERNING PREVIOUS HYPERSENSITIVITY REACTIONS TO CEPHALOSPORINS AND PENICILLIN. CEPHALOSPORIN C DERIVATIVES SHOULD BE GIVEN CAUTIOUSLY TO PENICILLIN-SENSITIVE PATIENTS.

SERIOUS ACUTE HYPERSENSITIVITY REACTIONS MAY REQUIRE EPINEPHRINE AND OTHER EMERGENCY MEASURES.

There is some clinical and laboratory evidence of partial cross-allergenicity of the penicillins and the cephalosporins. Patients have been reported to have had severe reactions (including anaphylaxis) to both drugs.

Any patient who has demonstrated some form of allergy, particularly to drugs, should receive antibiotics cautiously. No exception should be made with regard to cephalexin.

Pseudomembranous colitis has been reported with nearly all antibacterial agents, including cephalexin, and may range from mild to life threatening. Therefore, it is important to consider this diagnosis in patients with diarrhea subsequent to the administration of antibacterial agents.

Treatment with antibacterial agents alters the normal flora of the colon and may permit overgrowth of clostridia. Studies indicate that a toxin produced by *Clostridium difficile* is a primary cause of antibiotic-associated colitis.

After the diagnosis of pseudomembranous colitis has been established, appropriate therapeutic measures should be initiated. Mild cases of pseudomembranous colitis usually respond to drug discontinuation alone. In moderate to severe cases, consideration should be given to management with fluids and electrolytes, protein supplementation, and treatment with an antibacterial drug clinically effective against *Clostridium difficile* colitis.

PRECAUTIONS

GENERAL

Patients should be followed carefully so that any side effects or unusual manifestations of drug idiosyncrasy may be detected. If an allergic reaction to cephalexin occurs, the drug should be discontinued and the patient treated with the usual agents (*e.g.,* epinephrine or other pressor amines, antihistamines, or corticosteroids).

Prolonged use of cephalexin may result in the overgrowth of nonsusceptible organisms. Careful observation of the patient is essential. If superinfection occurs during therapy, appropriate measures should be taken.

Positive direct Coombs' tests have been reported during treatment with the cephalosporin antibiotics. In hematologic studies or in transfusion cross-matching procedures when antiglobulin tests are performed on the minor side or in Coombs' testing of newborns whose mothers have received cephalosporin antibiotics before parturition, it should be recognized that a positive Coombs' test may be due to the drug.

Cephalexin should be administered with caution in the presence of markedly impaired renal function. Under such conditions, careful clinical observation and laboratory studies should be made because safe dosage may be lower than that usually recommended.

Indicated surgical procedures should be performed in conjunction with antibiotic therapy.

As a result of administration of cephalexin, a false-positive reaction for glucose in the urine may occur. This has been observed with Benedict's and Fehling's solutions and also with Clinitest tablets.

As with other β-lactams, the renal excretion of cephalexin is inhibited by probenecid.

Broad-spectrum antibiotics should be prescribed with caution in individuals with a history of gastrointestinal disease, particularly colitis.

PREGNANCY CATEGORY B

The daily oral administration of cephalexin to rats in doses of 250 or 500 mg/kg prior to and during pregnancy, or to rats and mice during the period of organogenesis only, had no adverse effect on fertility, fetal viability, fetal weight, or litter size. Note that the safety of cephalexin during pregnancy in humans has not been established.

Cephalexin showed no enhanced toxicity in weanling and newborn rats as compared with adult animals. Nevertheless, because the studies in humans cannot rule out the possibility of harm, cephalexin should be used during pregnancy only if clearly needed.

NURSING MOTHERS

The excretion of cephalexin in the milk increased up to 4 hours after a 500 mg dose; the drug reached a maximum level of 4 μg/ml, then decreased gradually, and had disappeared 8 hours after administration. Caution should be exercised when cephalexin is administered to a nursing woman.

ADVERSE REACTIONS

Gastrointestinal: Symptoms of pseudomembranous colitis may appear either during or after antibiotic treatment. Nausea and vomiting have been reported rarely. The most frequent side effect has been diarrhea. It was very rarely severe enough to warrant cessation of therapy. Dyspepsia, gastritis, and abdominal pain have also occurred. As with some penicillins and some other cephalosporins, transient hepatitis and cholestatic jaundice have been reported rarely.

Hypersensitivity: Allergic reactions in the form of rash, urticaria, angioedema, and, rarely, erythema multiforme, Stevens-Johnson syndrome, or toxic epidermal necrolysis have been observed. These reactions usually subsided upon discontinuation of the drug. In some of these reactions, supportive therapy may be necessary. Anaphylaxis has also been reported. Other reactions have included genital and anal pruritus, genital moniliasis, vaginitis and vaginal discharge, dizziness, fatigue, headache, agitation, confusion, hallucinations, arthralgia, arthritis, and joint disorder. Reversible interstitial nephritis has been reported rarely. Eosinophilia, neutropenia, thrombocytopenia, and slight elevations in AST and ALT have been reported.

DOSAGE AND ADMINISTRATION

Cephalexin is administered orally.

Adults: The adult dosage ranges from 1-4 g daily in divided doses. The usual adult dose is 250 mg every 6 hours. For the following infections, a dosage of 500 mg may be administered every 12 hours: streptococcal pharyngitis, skin and skin structure infections, and uncomplicated cystitis in patients over 15 years of age. Cystitis therapy should be continued for 7-14 days. For more severe infections or those caused by less susceptible organisms, larger doses may be needed. If daily doses of cephalexin greater than 4 g are required, parenteral cephalosporins, in appropriate doses, should be considered.

Pediatric Patients: The usual recommended daily dosage for pediatric patients is 25-50 mg/kg in divided doses. For streptococcal pharyngitis in patients over 1 year of age and for skin and skin structure infections, the total daily dose may be divided and administered every 12 hours (see TABLE 5).

TABLE 5 *Cephalexin Suspension*

Weight	125 mg/5 ml	250 mg/5 ml
10 kg (22 lb)	½-1 tsp qid	¼-½ tsp qid
20 kg (44 lb)	1-2 tsp qid	½-1 tsp qid
40 kg (88 lb)	2-4 tsp qid	1-2 tsp qid
	OR	
10 kg (22 lb)	1-2 tsp bid	½-1 tsp bid
20 kg (44 lb)	2-4 tsp bid	1-2 tsp bid
40 kg (88 lb)	4-8 tsp bid	2-4 tsp bid

In severe infections, the dosage may be doubled.

In the therapy of otitis media, clinical studies have shown that a dosage of 75-100 mg/kg/day in 4 divided doses is required.

In the treatment of β-hemolytic streptococcal infections, a therapeutic dosage of cephalexin should be administered for at least 10 days.

HOW SUPPLIED

Oral Suspension: After mixing, store in refreigerator. May be kept for 14 days without significant loss of potency. Shake well before using. Keep tightly closed.

Pulvules: The 250 mg Pulvules are a white powder filled into size 2 Para0-Posilok Caps (opaque white and opaque light green) that are imprinted with "Dista" and identity code "H69" on the green cap, and Keflex 250 on the white body in edible black ink.

The 500 mg Pulvules are a white powder filled into an elongated, size 0 Para-Posilok Caps (opaque light green and opaque dark green) that are imprinted with "Dista" and identity code "H71" on the light green cap, and Keflex 500 on the dark green body in edible black ink.

Storage: Store at controlled room temperature, 15-30°C (59- 86°F).

PRODUCT LISTING - RATED THERAPEUTICALLY EQUIVALENT

Capsule - Oral - Monohydrate 250 mg

8's	$16.86	KEFLEX, Pd-Rx Pharmaceuticals	55289-0885-08
8's	$23.06	KEFLEX, Quality Care Pharmaceuticals Inc	60346-0649-08
10's	$7.60	GENERIC, Pd-Rx Pharmaceuticals	55289-0057-10
15's	$8.30	GENERIC, Pd-Rx Pharmaceuticals	55289-0057-15
20's	$10.60	GENERIC, Pd-Rx Pharmaceuticals	55289-0057-20
20's	$34.58	KEFLEX, Dista Products Company	00777-0869-20
20's	$57.56	KEFLEX, Pharma Pac	52959-0660-20
21's	$8.26	GENERIC, Dhs Inc	55887-0991-21
24's	$12.00	GENERIC, Pd-Rx Pharmaceuticals	55289-0057-24
24's	$50.64	KEFLEX, Pd-Rx Pharmaceuticals	55289-0885-24
25's	$15.00	GENERIC, Pd-Rx Pharmaceuticals	55289-0057-97
28's	$11.02	GENERIC, Dhs Inc	55887-0991-28
28's	$13.98	GENERIC, Pd-Rx Pharmaceuticals	55289-0057-28
30's	$14.96	GENERIC, Pd-Rx Pharmaceuticals	55289-0057-30
30's	$66.42	KEFLEX, Pd-Rx Pharmaceuticals	55289-0885-30
40's	$6.62	GENERIC, Pd-Rx Pharmaceuticals	55289-0072-40
40's	$17.50	GENERIC, Pd-Rx Pharmaceuticals	55289-0057-40
40's	$18.83	GENERIC, Dhs Inc	55887-0991-40
40's	$37.30	GENERIC, Med-Pro Inc	53978-5020-06
100's	$15.80	GENERIC, Pd-Rx Pharmaceuticals	55289-0072-01
100's	$19.43	GENERIC, Interstate Drug Exchange Inc	00814-1605-14
100's	$20.95	GENERIC, Cmc-Consolidated Midland Corporation	00223-0581-01
100's	$27.00	GENERIC, Pd-Rx Pharmaceuticals	55289-0057-01
100's	$27.00	GENERIC, Pd-Rx Pharmaceuticals	55289-0057-17
100's	$28.00	GENERIC, Raway Pharmacal Inc	00686-0604-20

C

Qty	Price	Product	NDC
100's	$34.95	GENERIC, Major Pharmaceuticals Inc	00904-3800-61
100's	$49.40	GENERIC, Major Pharmaceuticals Inc	00904-3800-60
100's	$50.07	GENERIC, Moore, H.L. Drug Exchange Inc	00839-7311-06
100's	$53.85	GENERIC, Novopharm Usa Inc	55953-0084-40
100's	$54.92	GENERIC, Martec Pharmaceuticals Inc	52555-0970-01
100's	$56.35	GENERIC, Novopharm Usa Inc	55953-0084-01
100's	$56.89	GENERIC, Warner Chilcott Laboratories	00047-0938-24
100's	$62.10	GENERIC, Mutual/United Research Laboratories	00677-1158-01
100's	$62.97	GENERIC, Teva Pharmaceuticals Usa	00686-3145-09
100's	$64.00	GENERIC, Geneva Pharmaceuticals	00781-2531-01
100's	$69.35	GENERIC, Teva Pharmaceuticals Usa	00093-3145-01
100's	$69.35	GENERIC, Mylan Pharmaceuticals Inc	00378-6025-01
100's	$69.93	GENERIC, Mova Pharmaceutical Corporation	55370-0900-07
100's	$73.13	GENERIC, Ivax Corporation	00172-4073-60
100's	$84.20	GENERIC, Udl Laboratories Inc	51079-0604-20
100's	$84.20	GENERIC, Medirex Inc	57480-0468-01
100's	$85.00	GENERIC, Geneva Pharmaceuticals	00781-2531-13
100's	$164.70	KEFLEX, Dista Products Company	00777-0869-02

Capsule - Oral - Monohydrate 500 mg

Qty	Price	Product	NDC
8's	$8.20	GENERIC, Pd-Rx Pharmaceuticals	55289-0058-08
9's	$6.33	GENERIC, Dhs Inc	55887-0958-09
10's	$9.40	GENERIC, Pd-Rx Pharmaceuticals	55289-0058-10
14's	$9.85	GENERIC, Dhs Inc	55887-0958-14
14's	$12.30	GENERIC, Pd-Rx Pharmaceuticals	55289-0058-14
15's	$10.55	GENERIC, Dhs Inc	55887-0958-15
20's	$12.92	GENERIC, Dhs Inc	55887-0958-20
20's	$16.96	GENERIC, Pd-Rx Pharmaceuticals	55289-0058-20
20's	$68.04	KEFLEX, Dista Products Company	00777-0871-20
20's	$68.77	KEFLEX, Pharma Pac	52959-0087-20
20's	$76.21	KEFLEX, Physicians Total Care	54868-0425-01
21's	$13.56	GENERIC, Dhs Inc	55887-0958-21
21's	$17.80	GENERIC, Pd-Rx Pharmaceuticals	55289-0058-21
24's	$18.00	GENERIC, Pd-Rx Pharmaceuticals	55289-0058-24
28's	$14.82	GENERIC, Dhs Inc	55887-0958-28
28's	$19.00	GENERIC, Pd-Rx Pharmaceuticals	55289-0058-28
30's	$15.87	GENERIC, Dhs Inc	55887-0958-30
30's	$20.34	GENERIC, Pd-Rx Pharmaceuticals	55289-0058-30
40's	$27.20	GENERIC, Pd-Rx Pharmaceuticals	55289-0058-40
40's	$47.17	GENERIC, Golden State Medical	60429-0037-40
40's	$62.90	GENERIC, Med-Pro Inc	53978-5021-06
40's	$115.85	KEFLEX, Pharma Pac	52959-0087-40
40's	$118.44	GENERIC, Major Pharmaceuticals Inc	00904-3801-39
40's	$195.60	KEFLEX, Pd-Rx Pharmaceuticals	55289-0582-40
100's	$25.00	GENERIC, Raway Pharmacal Inc	00686-3147-09
100's	$28.00	GENERIC, Raway Pharmacal Inc	00686-0605-20
100's	$38.18	GENERIC, Interstate Drug Exchange Inc	00814-1606-14
100's	$39.84	GENERIC, Pd-Rx Pharmaceuticals	55289-0058-01
100's	$46.50	GENERIC, Cmc-Consolidated Midland Corporation	00223-0582-01
100's	$57.60	GENERIC, Pd-Rx Pharmaceuticals	55289-0058-17
100's	$85.23	GENERIC, Mova Pharmaceutical Corporation	55370-0812-07
100's	$96.38	GENERIC, Moore, H.L. Drug Exchange Inc	00839-7312-06
100's	$98.60	GENERIC, Major Pharmaceuticals Inc	00904-3801-60
100's	$108.75	GENERIC, Martec Pharmaceuticals Inc	52555-0971-01
100's	$110.19	GENERIC, Novopharm Usa Inc	55953-0114-01
100's	$120.65	GENERIC, Mutual/United Research Laboratories	00677-1159-01
100's	$123.76	GENERIC, Aligen Independent Laboratories Inc	00405-4153-01
100's	$125.12	GENERIC, Major Pharmaceuticals Inc	00904-3801-61
100's	$125.95	GENERIC, Novopharm Usa Inc	55953-0114-40
100's	$125.99	GENERIC, Geneva Pharmaceuticals	00781-2532-01
100's	$130.00	GENERIC, International Ethical Laboratories Inc	11584-1034-05
100's	$137.48	GENERIC, Mova Pharmaceutical Corporation	55370-0901-07
100's	$137.50	GENERIC, Mylan Pharmaceuticals Inc	00378-6050-01
100's	$137.60	GENERIC, Teva Pharmaceuticals Usa	00093-3147-01
100's	$137.60	GENERIC, Ranbaxy Laboratories	63304-0657-01
100's	$149.55	GENERIC, Ivax Corporation	00172-4074-60
100's	$173.00	GENERIC, Udl Laboratories Inc	51079-0605-20
100's	$173.00	GENERIC, Medirex Inc	57480-0469-01
100's	$173.25	GENERIC, Geneva Pharmaceuticals	00781-2532-13
100's	$323.71	KEFLEX, Dista Products Company	00777-0871-02
250's	$265.39	GENERIC, Novopharm Usa Inc	55953-0114-58

Capsule - Oral - 250 mg

Qty	Price	Product	NDC
100's	$25.13	FEDERAL UPPER LIMIT, H.C.F.A. F F P	99999-0698-20

Capsule - Oral - 500 mg

Qty	Price	Product	NDC
100's	$44.46	FEDERAL UPPER LIMIT, H.C.F.A. F F P	99999-0698-22

Powder For Reconstitution - Oral - 125 mg/5 ml

Qty	Price	Product	NDC
100 ml	$4.85	GENERIC, Raway Pharmacal Inc	00686-4175-32
100 ml	$6.06	GENERIC, Moore, H.L. Drug Exchange Inc	00839-7313-73
100 ml	$6.40	GENERIC, Geneva Pharmaceuticals	00781-7028-46
100 ml	$7.65	GENERIC, Mova Pharmaceutical Corporation	55370-0903-13
100 ml	$7.76	GENERIC, Aligen Independent Laboratories Inc	00405-2500-60
100 ml	$7.95	GENERIC, Ivax Corporation	00182-7020-70
100 ml	$7.95	GENERIC, Mylan Pharmaceuticals Inc	00378-6030-02
100 ml	$8.93	GENERIC, Teva Pharmaceuticals Usa	00093-4175-73
100 ml	$8.93	GENERIC, Ranbaxy Laboratories	63304-0958-01
100 ml	$9.50	GENERIC, International Ethical Laboratories Inc	11584-1035-01
100 ml	$13.36	GENERIC, Pharma Pac	52959-0200-01
200 ml	$4.65	GENERIC, Raway Pharmacal Inc	00686-4175-36
200 ml	$10.50	GENERIC, Qualitest Products Inc	00603-6541-68
200 ml	$11.00	GENERIC, Moore, H.L. Drug Exchange Inc	00839-7313-78
200 ml	$12.00	GENERIC, Geneva Pharmaceuticals	00781-7028-48
200 ml	$12.80	GENERIC, Mutual/United Research Laboratories	00677-1187-29
200 ml	$13.78	GENERIC, Mova Pharmaceutical Corporation	55370-0903-40
200 ml	$13.83	GENERIC, Allscripts Pharmaceutical Company	54569-1023-00
200 ml	$13.95	GENERIC, Mylan Pharmaceuticals Inc	00378-6030-04
200 ml	$13.96	GENERIC, Ivax Corporation	00182-7020-73
200 ml	$15.75	GENERIC, Teva Pharmaceuticals Usa	00093-4175-74
200 ml	$15.75	GENERIC, Ranbaxy Laboratories	63304-0958-02
200 ml	$18.14	GENERIC, Aligen Independent Laboratories Inc	00405-2500-70
200 ml	$24.12	GENERIC, Pharma Pac	52959-1453-02

Powder For Reconstitution - Oral - 250 mg/5 ml

Qty	Price	Product	NDC
100 ml	$7.95	GENERIC, Raway Pharmacal Inc	00686-4177-32
100 ml	$11.19	GENERIC, Moore, H.L. Drug Exchange Inc	00839-7314-73
100 ml	$11.39	GENERIC, Geneva Pharmaceuticals	00781-7029-46
100 ml	$12.62	GENERIC, Teva Pharmaceuticals Usa	00332-4177-32
100 ml	$14.08	GENERIC, Mova Pharmaceutical Corporation	55370-0902-13
100 ml	$15.20	GENERIC, International Ethical Laboratories Inc	11584-1036-02
100 ml	$18.90	GENERIC, Teva Pharmaceuticals Usa	00093-4177-73
100 ml	$18.90	GENERIC, Ranbaxy Laboratories	63304-0959-01
100 ml	$32.99	GENERIC, Pharma Pac	52959-1029-00
200 ml	$8.95	GENERIC, Raway Pharmacal Inc	00686-4177-36
200 ml	$20.64	GENERIC, Moore, H.L. Drug Exchange Inc	00839-7314-78
200 ml	$22.58	GENERIC, Geneva Pharmaceuticals	00781-7029-48
200 ml	$22.60	GENERIC, Mutual/United Research Laboratories	00677-1188-29
200 ml	$25.23	GENERIC, Mova Pharmaceutical Corporation	55370-0902-40
200 ml	$25.25	GENERIC, Mylan Pharmaceuticals Inc	00378-6035-04
200 ml	$31.50	GENERIC, Teva Pharmaceuticals Usa	00093-4177-74
200 ml	$31.50	GENERIC, Ranbaxy Laboratories	63304-0959-02
200 ml	$47.05	GENERIC, Pharma Pac	52959-1029-01

Tablet - Oral - Monohydrate 250 mg

Qty	Price	Product	NDC
20's	$3.52	GENERIC, Circle Pharmaceuticals Inc	00659-0148-20
40's	$5.79	GENERIC, Circle Pharmaceuticals Inc	00659-0148-40
40's	$24.37	GENERIC, Golden State Medical	60429-0036-40
100's	$32.33	GENERIC, Moore, H.L. Drug Exchange Inc	00839-7461-06
100's	$37.50	GENERIC, Cmc-Consolidated Midland Corporation	00223-0583-01
100's	$49.40	GENERIC, Major Pharmaceuticals Inc	00904-3795-60
100's	$57.00	GENERIC, Ivax Corporation	00182-1886-01
100's	$69.35	GENERIC, Ranbaxy Laboratories	63304-0656-01
100's	$114.50	GENERIC, Teva Pharmaceuticals Usa	00093-2238-01

Tablet - Oral - Monohydrate 500 mg

Qty	Price	Product	NDC
56's	$38.00	GENERIC, Pd-Rx Pharmaceuticals	55289-0058-56
100's	$62.85	GENERIC, Major Pharmaceuticals Inc	00904-3796-60
100's	$64.73	GENERIC, Moore, H.L. Drug Exchange Inc	00839-7462-06
100's	$72.50	GENERIC, Cmc-Consolidated Midland Corporation	00223-0584-01
100's	$89.80	GENERIC, Ivax Corporation	00182-1887-01
100's	$225.02	GENERIC, Teva Pharmaceuticals Usa	00093-2240-01

PRODUCT LISTING - EQUIVALENTS NOT AVAILABLE

Capsule - Oral - Monohydrate 250 mg

Qty	Price	Product	NDC
2's	$3.54	GENERIC, Prescript Pharmaceuticals	00247-0003-02
3's	$3.64	GENERIC, Prescript Pharmaceuticals	00247-0003-03
4's	$2.56	GENERIC, Allscripts Pharmaceutical Company	54569-0304-08
4's	$3.73	GENERIC, Prescript Pharmaceuticals	00247-0003-04
5's	$3.81	GENERIC, Prescript Pharmaceuticals	00247-0003-05
6's	$3.83	GENERIC, Allscripts Pharmaceutical Company	54569-4972-00
6's	$3.91	GENERIC, Prescript Pharmaceuticals	00247-0003-06
8's	$4.09	GENERIC, Prescript Pharmaceuticals	00247-0003-08
8's	$5.12	GENERIC, Allscripts Pharmaceutical Company	54569-0304-06
10's	$4.28	GENERIC, Prescript Pharmaceuticals	00247-0003-10
12's	$4.47	GENERIC, Prescript Pharmaceuticals	00247-0003-12
12's	$18.00	GENERIC, Southwood Pharmaceuticals Inc	58016-0138-12
14's	$4.65	GENERIC, Prescript Pharmaceuticals	00247-0003-14
14's	$21.00	GENERIC, Southwood Pharmaceuticals Inc	58016-0138-14
15's	$4.74	GENERIC, Prescript Pharmaceuticals	00247-0003-15
15's	$22.50	GENERIC, Southwood Pharmaceuticals Inc	58016-0138-15
16's	$4.84	GENERIC, Prescript Pharmaceuticals	00247-0003-16
18's	$5.02	GENERIC, Prescript Pharmaceuticals	00247-0003-18
20's	$4.68	GENERIC, Physicians Total Care	54868-0153-01
20's	$5.21	GENERIC, Prescript Pharmaceuticals	00247-0003-20
20's	$12.78	GENERIC, Allscripts Pharmaceutical Company	54569-0304-02

20's	$14.24	GENERIC, Alpharma Uspd Makers Of Barre and Nmc	63874-0111-20
20's	$30.00	GENERIC, Southwood Pharmaceuticals Inc	58016-0138-20
20's	$31.26	GENERIC, Pharma Pac	52959-0030-20
21's	$5.29	GENERIC, Prescript Pharmaceuticals	00247-0003-21
21's	$31.50	GENERIC, Southwood Pharmaceuticals Inc	58016-0138-21
24's	$33.71	GENERIC, Alpharma Uspd Makers Of Barre and Nmc	63874-0111-24
24's	$36.00	GENERIC, Southwood Pharmaceuticals Inc	58016-0138-24
24's	$36.43	GENERIC, Pharma Pac	52959-0030-24
28's	$5.95	GENERIC, Prescript Pharmaceuticals	00247-0003-28
28's	$17.89	GENERIC, Allscripts Pharmaceutical Company	54569-0304-03
28's	$18.42	GENERIC, Pharmaceutical Corporation Of America	51655-0024-29
28's	$36.51	GENERIC, Alpharma Uspd Makers Of Barre and Nmc	63874-0111-28
28's	$42.00	GENERIC, Southwood Pharmaceuticals Inc	58016-0138-28
28's	$42.41	GENERIC, Pharma Pac	52959-0030-28
30's	$6.13	GENERIC, Prescript Pharmaceuticals	00247-0003-30
30's	$6.18	GENERIC, Physicians Total Care	54868-0153-05
30's	$19.17	GENERIC, Allscripts Pharmaceutical Company	54569-0304-05
30's	$38.95	GENERIC, Alpharma Uspd Makers Of Barre and Nmc	63874-0111-30
30's	$45.00	GENERIC, Southwood Pharmaceuticals Inc	58016-0138-30
30's	$45.99	GENERIC, Pharma Pac	52959-0030-30
32's	$6.32	GENERIC, Prescript Pharmaceuticals	00247-0003-32
40's	$7.06	GENERIC, Prescript Pharmaceuticals	00247-0003-40
40's	$7.69	GENERIC, Physicians Total Care	54868-0153-03
40's	$25.56	GENERIC, Allscripts Pharmaceutical Company	54569-0304-04
40's	$25.88	GENERIC, Pharmaceutical Corporation Of America	51655-0024-51
40's	$51.80	GENERIC, Alpharma Uspd Makers Of Barre and Nmc	63874-0111-40
40's	$59.79	GENERIC, Pharma Pac	52959-0030-40
40's	$60.00	GENERIC, Southwood Pharmaceuticals Inc	58016-0138-40
56's	$84.00	GENERIC, Southwood Pharmaceuticals Inc	58016-0138-56
60's	$8.92	GENERIC, Prescript Pharmaceuticals	00247-0003-60
60's	$90.00	GENERIC, Southwood Pharmaceuticals Inc	58016-0138-60
100's	$12.62	GENERIC, Prescript Pharmaceuticals	00247-0003-00
100's	$16.72	GENERIC, Physicians Total Care	54868-0153-08
100's	$67.96	GENERIC, Mova Pharmaceutical Corporation	64860-0104-07
100's	$85.12	GENERIC, American Health Packaging	62584-0235-01
100's	$150.00	GENERIC, Southwood Pharmaceuticals Inc	58016-0138-00

Capsule - Oral - Monohydrate 500 mg

1's	$3.59	GENERIC, Prescript Pharmaceuticals	00247-0005-01
2's	$3.84	GENERIC, Prescript Pharmaceuticals	00247-0005-02
3's	$4.07	GENERIC, Prescript Pharmaceuticals	00247-0005-03
4's	$2.62	GENERIC, Physicians Total Care	54868-0154-08
4's	$4.31	GENERIC, Prescript Pharmaceuticals	00247-0005-04
4's	$11.84	GENERIC, Southwood Pharmaceuticals Inc	58016-0139-04
4's	$12.54	GENERIC, Pharma Pac	52959-0031-04
5's	$14.80	GENERIC, Southwood Pharmaceuticals Inc	58016-0139-05
6's	$4.79	GENERIC, Prescript Pharmaceuticals	00247-0005-06
6's	$7.56	GENERIC, Allscripts Pharmaceutical Company	54569-3324-03
6's	$17.76	GENERIC, Southwood Pharmaceuticals Inc	58016-0139-06
8's	$5.04	GENERIC, Allscripts Pharmaceutical Company	54569-0305-08
8's	$5.26	GENERIC, Prescript Pharmaceuticals	00247-0005-08
8's	$13.06	GENERIC, Pharma Pac	52959-0031-08
8's	$23.68	GENERIC, Southwood Pharmaceuticals Inc	58016-0139-08
9's	$5.49	GENERIC, Prescript Pharmaceuticals	00247-0005-09
10's	$3.48	GENERIC, Circle Pharmaceuticals Inc	00659-0147-10
10's	$4.06	GENERIC, Physicians Total Care	54868-0154-07
10's	$5.74	GENERIC, Prescript Pharmaceuticals	00247-0005-10
10's	$12.60	GENERIC, Allscripts Pharmaceutical Company	54569-0305-05
10's	$16.19	GENERIC, Pharma Pac	52959-0031-10
10's	$29.60	GENERIC, Southwood Pharmaceuticals Inc	58016-0139-10
12's	$6.21	GENERIC, Prescript Pharmaceuticals	00247-0005-12
12's	$19.18	GENERIC, Pharma Pac	52959-0031-12
12's	$35.52	GENERIC, Southwood Pharmaceuticals Inc	58016-0139-12
14's	$6.69	GENERIC, Prescript Pharmaceuticals	00247-0005-14
14's	$17.63	GENERIC, Allscripts Pharmaceutical Company	54569-0305-03
14's	$22.12	GENERIC, Pharma Pac	52959-0031-14
14's	$23.00	GENERIC, Alpharma Uspd Makers Of Barre and Nmc	63874-0112-14
14's	$41.44	GENERIC, Southwood Pharmaceuticals Inc	58016-0139-14
15's	$6.93	GENERIC, Prescript Pharmaceuticals	00247-0005-15
15's	$23.69	GENERIC, Pharma Pac	52959-0031-15
15's	$44.40	GENERIC, Southwood Pharmaceuticals Inc	58016-0139-15
16's	$7.16	GENERIC, Prescript Pharmaceuticals	00247-0005-16
18's	$53.28	GENERIC, Southwood Pharmaceuticals Inc	58016-0139-18
20's	$6.45	GENERIC, Physicians Total Care	54868-0154-01
20's	$8.12	GENERIC, Prescript Pharmaceuticals	00247-0005-20
20's	$10.11	GENERIC, Circle Pharmaceuticals Inc	00659-0147-20
20's	$25.19	GENERIC, Allscripts Pharmaceutical Company	54569-0305-00
20's	$29.09	GENERIC, Alpharma Uspd Makers Of Barre and Nmc	63874-0112-20
20's	$31.05	GENERIC, Pharma Pac	52959-0031-20
20's	$59.20	GENERIC, Southwood Pharmaceuticals Inc	58016-0139-20
21's	$8.35	GENERIC, Prescript Pharmaceuticals	00247-0005-21
21's	$32.57	GENERIC, Pharma Pac	52959-0031-21
21's	$62.16	GENERIC, Southwood Pharmaceuticals Inc	58016-0139-21
24's	$9.07	GENERIC, Prescript Pharmaceuticals	00247-0005-24
24's	$37.18	GENERIC, Pharma Pac	52959-0031-24
24's	$71.04	GENERIC, Southwood Pharmaceuticals Inc	58016-0139-24
25's	$9.31	GENERIC, Prescript Pharmaceuticals	00247-0005-25
28's	$8.37	GENERIC, Physicians Total Care	54868-0154-03
28's	$10.02	GENERIC, Prescript Pharmaceuticals	00247-0005-28
28's	$35.27	GENERIC, Allscripts Pharmaceutical Company	54569-0305-01
28's	$43.09	GENERIC, Pharma Pac	52959-0031-28
28's	$44.81	GENERIC, Alpharma Uspd Makers Of Barre and Nmc	63874-0112-28
28's	$82.88	GENERIC, Southwood Pharmaceuticals Inc	58016-0139-28
30's	$8.84	GENERIC, Physicians Total Care	54868-0154-02
30's	$10.49	GENERIC, Prescript Pharmaceuticals	00247-0005-30
30's	$37.80	GENERIC, Allscripts Pharmaceutical Company	54569-0305-06
30's	$45.95	GENERIC, Pharma Pac	52959-0031-30
30's	$47.79	GENERIC, Alpharma Uspd Makers Of Barre and Nmc	63874-0112-30
30's	$88.80	GENERIC, Southwood Pharmaceuticals Inc	58016-0139-30
32's	$10.98	GENERIC, Prescript Pharmaceuticals	00247-0005-32
40's	$11.24	GENERIC, Physicians Total Care	54868-0154-04
40's	$12.88	GENERIC, Prescript Pharmaceuticals	00247-0005-40
40's	$41.16	GENERIC, Pharmaceutical Corporation Of America	51655-0025-51
40's	$50.38	GENERIC, Allscripts Pharmaceutical Company	54569-0305-02
40's	$60.00	GENERIC, Pharma Pac	52959-0031-40
40's	$60.69	GENERIC, Alpharma Uspd Makers Of Barre and Nmc	63874-0112-40
40's	$118.40	GENERIC, Southwood Pharmaceuticals Inc	58016-0139-40
50's	$148.00	GENERIC, Southwood Pharmaceuticals Inc	58016-0139-50
56's	$16.69	GENERIC, Prescript Pharmaceuticals	00247-0005-56
56's	$165.76	GENERIC, Southwood Pharmaceuticals Inc	58016-0139-56
60's	$16.02	GENERIC, Physicians Total Care	54868-0154-09
60's	$177.60	GENERIC, Southwood Pharmaceuticals Inc	58016-0139-60
60's	$179.42	GENERIC, Pharma Pac	52959-0031-60
100's	$27.18	GENERIC, Prescript Pharmaceuticals	00247-0005-00
100's	$134.85	GENERIC, Mova Pharmaceutical Corporation	64860-0105-07
100's	$296.00	GENERIC, Southwood Pharmaceuticals Inc	58016-0139-00
120's	$355.20	GENERIC, Southwood Pharmaceuticals Inc	58016-0139-02

Powder For Reconstitution - Oral - 125 mg/5 ml

100 ml	$3.78	GENERIC, Physicians Total Care	54868-0538-02
100 ml	$5.33	GENERIC, Prescript Pharmaceuticals	00247-0393-00
100 ml	$13.37	GENERIC, Alpharma Uspd Makers Of Barre and Nmc	63874-0166-10
100 ml	$15.00	GENERIC, Southwood Pharmaceuticals Inc	58016-1019-01
100 ml	$21.00	GENERIC, Southwood Pharmaceuticals Inc	58016-1021-01
200 ml	$6.14	GENERIC, Physicians Total Care	54868-0538-01
200 ml	$7.31	GENERIC, Prescript Pharmaceuticals	00247-0393-79
200 ml	$29.00	GENERIC, Alpharma Uspd Makers Of Barre and Nmc	63874-0166-20

Powder For Reconstitution - Oral - 250 mg/5 ml

100 ml	$5.69	GENERIC, Physicians Total Care	54868-1385-01
100 ml	$13.04	GENERIC, Allscripts Pharmaceutical Company	54569-1024-00
100 ml	$14.07	GENERIC, Prescript Pharmaceuticals	00247-0004-00
100 ml	$25.92	GENERIC, Alpharma Uspd Makers Of Barre and Nmc	63874-0155-10
200 ml	$7.68	GENERIC, Physicians Total Care	54868-1385-02
200 ml	$21.00	GENERIC, Southwood Pharmaceuticals Inc	58016-1046-01
200 ml	$24.80	GENERIC, Prescript Pharmaceuticals	00247-0004-79
200 ml	$24.95	GENERIC, Southwood Pharmaceuticals Inc	58016-1045-01
200 ml	$25.10	GENERIC, Allscripts Pharmaceutical Company	54569-1025-00
200 ml	$52.89	GENERIC, Alpharma Uspd Makers Of Barre and Nmc	63874-0155-20

Tablet - Oral - Monohydrate 500 mg

20's	$11.69	GENERIC, Physicians Total Care	54868-0155-01

Cephalexin Hydrochloride *(000699)*

For related information, see the comparative table section in Appendix A.

Categories: Infection, bone; Infection, ear, middle; Infection, respiratory tract; Infection, skin and skin structures; Infection, urinary tract; Prostatitis; Pregnancy Category B; FDA Approved 1987 Oct
Drug Classes: Antibiotics, cephalosporins
Brand Names: **Keftab**

DESCRIPTION

Cephalexin hydrochloride is semisynthetic cephalosporin antibiotic intended for oral administration. Chemically, it is designated 7(D-2-amino-2-phenylacetamido)-3-methyl-3-cephem-4-carboxylic acid hydrochloride monohydrate, and the chemical formula is $C_{16}H_{17}N_3O_4S{\cdot}HCl{\cdot}H_2O$. The molecular weight is 401.86.

The nucleus of cephalexin hydrochloride is related to that of other cephalosporin antibiotics. The compound is the hydrochloride salt of cephalexin. The isoelectric point of cephalexin in water is approximately 4.5 to 5.

Cephalexin hydrochloride is in crystalline form and is a monohydrate. It is a white crystalline solid having a bitter taste. Solubility in water is high at room temperature; greater than 10 mg/ml may be dissolved readily.

The cephalosporins differ from penicillins in the structure of the bicyclic ring system. Cephalexin has *D*-phenylglycyl group as substituent at the 7-amino position and an unsubstituted methyl group at the 3-position.

Each Keftab tablet contains cephalexin hydrochloride equivalent to 500 mg (1439 μmol) cephalexin. The tablets also contain D&C yellow no. 10, FD&C blue no. 1, FD&C red no. 40, magnesium stearate, silicon dioxide, stearic acid, sucrose, titanium dioxide, and other inactive ingredients.

CLINICAL PHARMACOLOGY

Human Pharmacology: Cephalexin HCl is acid stable and may be given without regard to meals. It is rapidly absorbed after oral administration. Following doses of 250 and 500 mg, average peak serum levels of approximately 9 and 18 μg/ml respectively were obtained at 1 hour and declined to 1.6 and 3.4 μg/ml respectively at 3 hours. Measurable levels were present 6 hours after administration. Cephalexin is excreted in the urine by glomerular filtration and tubular secretion. Studies showed that approximately 70% of the drug was excreted unchanged in the urine within 12 hours. During the first 6 hours, average urine concentrations following the 250 and 500 mg doses were approximately 200 μg/ml (range, 54 to 663) and 500 μg/ml (range, 137 to 1306) respectively. The average serum half-life is 1.1 hours.

Microbiology: *In vitro* tests demonstrate that the cephalosporins are bactericidal because of their inhibition of cell-wall synthesis. Cephalexin HCl is active against the following organisms *in vitro*.

β-hemolytic *streptococci; Staphylococcus aureus,* including penicillinase-producing strains; *Streptococcus pneumoniae; Escherichia coli; Proteus mirabilis; Klebsiella* sp; *Haemophilus influenzae; Moraxella (Branhamella) catarrhalis.*

Note: Most strains of *enterococci* (*Enterococcus faecalis* [formerly *Streptococcus faecalis*]) and a few strains of staphylococci are resistant to cephalexin HCl. When tested by *in vitro* methods, staphylococci exhibit cross-resistance between cephalexin HCl and methicillin-type antibiotics. Cephalexin HCl is not active against most strains of *Enterobacter* sp, *Morganella morganii* (formerly*Proteus morganii*), *Serratia* sp, and *Proteus vulgaris.* It has no activity against *Pseudomonas* or*Acinetobacter* sp.

Disk Susceptibility Tests: Quantitative methods that require measurement of zone diameters give the most precise estimates of antibiotic susceptibility. One such procedure[1] has been recommended for use with cephalosporin class (cephalothin) disks for testing susceptibility to cephalexin. The currently accepted zone diameter interpretation for the cephalothin disks[1] are appropriate for determining susceptibility to cephalexin. Interpretations correlate zone diameters of the disk test with MIC values for cephalexin. With this procedure, a report from the laboratory of "resistant" indicates a zone diameter of 14 mm or less and suggests that the infecting organism is not likely to respond to therapy. A report of "susceptibility" indicates a zone diameter of 18 mm or greater. A report of "intermediate susceptibility" indicates zone diameters between 15 and 17 mm and suggests that the organism would be susceptible if the infection is confined to the urine, in which high antibiotic levels can be obtained, or if high dosage is used in other types of infection.

Standardized procedures require use of control organisms.[1] The 30 μg cephalothin disk should give zone diameters between 18 and 23 mm and 25 and 37 mm for the reference strains *E. coli* ATCC 25922 and *S. aureus*ATCC 25923 respectively.

INDICATIONS AND USAGE

Cephalexin HCl is indicated for the treatment of the following infections when caused by susceptible strains of the designated microorganisms:

Respiratory tract infections caused by *S. pneumoniae* and group A β-hemolytic streptococci (Penicillin is the usual drug of choice in the treatment and prevention of streptococcal infections, including the prophylaxis of rheumatic fever. Cephalexin HCl is generally effective in the eradication of streptococci from the nasopharynx; however, substantial data establishing the efficacy of cephalexin HCl in the subsequent prevention of rheumatic fever are not available at present.)

Skin and skin structure infections caused by *S. aureus* and/or β-hemolytic *streptococci.*

Bone infections caused by *S. aureus* and/or *P. mirabilis.*

Genitourinary tract infections, including acute prostatitis, caused by *E. coli, P. mirabilis,* and *Klebsiella* sp.

Note: Culture and susceptibility tests should be initiated prior to and during therapy. Renal function studies should be performed when indicated.

CONTRAINDICATIONS

Cephalexin HCl is contraindicated in patients with known allergy to the cephalosporin group of antibiotics.

WARNINGS

BEFORE CEPHALEXIN THERAPY IS INSTITUTED, CAREFUL INQUIRY SHOULD BE MADE CONCERNING PREVIOUS HYPERSENSITIVITY REACTIONS TO CEPHALOSPORINS AND PENICILLIN. CEPHALOSPORIN C DERIVATIVES SHOULD BE GIVEN CAUTIOUSLY TO PENICILLIN-SENSITIVE PATIENTS.

SERIOUS ACUTE HYPERSENSITIVITY REACTIONS MAY REQUIRE EPINEPHRINE AND OTHER EMERGENCY MEASURES.

There is some clinical and laboratory evidence of partial cross-allergenicity of the penicillins and the cephalosporins. Patients have been reported to have had severe reactions (including anaphylaxis) to both drugs.

Any patient who has demonstrated some form of allergy, particularly to drugs, should receive antibiotics cautiously. No exception should be made with regard to cephalexin HCl.

Pseudomembranous colitis has been reported with virtually all broad-spectrum antibiotics (including macrolides, semisynthetic penicillins, and cephalosporins); therefore, it is important to consider its diagnosis in patients who develop diarrhea in association with the use of antibiotics. Such colitis may range in severity from mild to life threatening.

Treatment with broad-spectrum antibiotics alters the normal flora of the colon and may permit overgrowth of clostridia. Studies indicate that a toxin produced by *Clostridium difficile* is a primary cause of antibiotic-associated colitis.

Mild cases of pseudomembranous colitis usually respond to drug discontinuance alone. In moderate to severe cases, management should include sigmoidoscopy, appropriate bacteriologic studies, and fluid, electrolyte, and protein supplementation. When the colitis does not improve after the drug has been discontinued or when it is severe, treatment with an oral antibacterial drug effective against *C. difficile* is recommended. Other causes of colitis should be ruled out.

PRECAUTIONS

GENERAL

Patients should be followed carefully so that any side effects or unusual manifestations of drug idiosyncrasy may be detected. If an allergic reaction to cephalexin HCl occurs, the drug should be discontinued and the patient treated with the usual agents (*e.g.,* epinephrine or other pressor amines, antihistamines, or corticosteroids).

Prolonged use of cephalexin HCl may result in the overgrowth of nonsusceptible organisms. Careful observation of the patient is essential. If superinfection occurs during therapy, appropriate measures should be taken.

Positive direct Coombs' tests have been reported during treatment with the cephalosporin antibiotics. In hematologic studies or in transfusion cross-matching procedures when antiglobulin tests are performed on the minor side or in Coombs' testing of newborns whose mothers have received cephalosporin antibiotics before parturition, it should be recognized that a positive Coombs' test may be due to the drug.

Cephalexin HCl should be administered with caution in the presence of markedly impaired renal function. Under such conditions, careful clinical observation and laboratory studies should be made because safe dosage may be lower than that usually recommended.

As a result of administration of cephalexin HCl, a false-positive reaction for glucose in the urine may occur. This has been observed with Benedict's and Fehling's solutions and also with Clinitest tablets but not with Tes-Tape (Glucose Enzymatic Test Strip).

Broad-spectrum antibiotics should be prescribed with caution in individuals with a history of gastrointestinal disease, particularly colitis.

PREGNANCY CATEGORY B

Reproduction studies have been performed on rats in doses of 250 or 500 mg/kg/day and have revealed no evidence of impaired fertility or harm to the fetus due to cephalexin. There are, however, no adequate and well-controlled studies in pregnant women. Because animal reproduction studies are not always predictive of human response, this drug should be used during pregnancy only if clearly needed.

NURSING MOTHERS:

The excretion of cephalexin in the milk increased up to 4 hours after a 500-mg dose; the drug reached a maximum level of 4 μg/ml, then decreased gradually, and had disappeared 8 hours after administration. A decision should be considered to discontinue nursing temporarily during therapy with cephalexin HCl.

PEDIATRIC USE

Safety and effectiveness in children have not been established.

ADVERSE REACTIONS

Gastrointestinal: Symptoms of pseudomembranous colitis may appear either during or after antibiotic treatment. Nausea and vomiting have been reported rarely. The most frequent side effect has been diarrhea. It was very rarely severe enough to warrant cessation of therapy. Abdominal pain, gastritis, and dyspepsia have also occurred. As with some penicillins and some other cephalosporins, transient hepatitis and cholestatic jaundice have been reported rarely.

Hypersensitivity: Allergic reactions in the form of rash, urticaria, angioedema, and, rarely, erythema multiforme, Stevens-Johnson syndrome, or toxic epidermal necrolysis have been observed. These reactions usually subsided upon discontinuation of the drug. In some of these reactions, supportive therapy may be necessary. Anaphylaxis has also been reported. Other reactions have included genital and anal pruritus, genital moniliasis, vaginitis and vaginal discharge, dizziness, fatigue, headache agitation, confusion, hallucinations, arthralgia, arthritis, and joint disorder. Reversible interstitial nephritis has been reported rarely. Eosinophilia, neutropenia, thrombocytopenia, slight elevations in aspartate aminotransferase (AST, SGOT) and alanine aminotransferase (ALT, SGPT), and elevated creatinine and BUN have been reported.

In addition to the adverse reactions listed above that have been observed in patients treated with cephalexin HCl, the following adverse reactions and altered laboratory tests have been reported for cephalosporin class antibiotics:

Adverse Reactions: Allergic reactions, including fever, colitis, renal dysfunction, toxic nephropathy, and hepatic dysfunction, including cholestasis.

Several cephalosporins have been implicated in triggering seizures, particularly in patients with renal impairment when the dosage was not reduced (see INDICATIONS AND USAGE and PRECAUTIONS, General. If seizures associated with drug therapy should occur, the drug should be discontinued. Anticonvulsant therapy can be given if clinically indicated.

Altered Laboratory Tests: Increased prothrombin time, increased alkaline phosphatase, and leukopenia.

DOSAGE AND ADMINISTRATION

Cephalexin HCl is administered orally.

The adult dosage ranges from 1-4 g daily in divided doses. For the following infections, a dosage of 500 mg may be administered every 12 hours: streptococcal pharyngitis, skin and skin structure infections, and uncomplicated cystitis. Cystitis therapy should be continued for 7-14 days. For other infections, the usual dose is 250 mg every 6 hours. For more severe infections or those caused by less susceptible organisms, larger doses may be needed. If daily doses of cephalexin HCl greater than 4 g are required, parenteral cephalosporins, in appropriate doses, should be considered.

HOW SUPPLIED

Tablets (Elliptical-Shaped): 500 mg* (dark-green).
Storage: Store at controlled room temperature, 15-30°C (59-86°F).

PRODUCT LISTING - EQUIVALENTS NOT AVAILABLE

Tablet - Oral - Hydrochloride 500 mg

4's	$12.98	KEFTAB, Physicians Total Care	54868-1112-01
10's	$30.68	KEFTAB, Physicians Total Care	54868-1112-02
10's	$37.91	KEFTAB, Pd-Rx Pharmaceuticals	55289-0333-10
20's	$68.77	KEFTAB, Pharma Pac	52959-0086-20
20's	$71.91	KEFTAB, Pd-Rx Pharmaceuticals	55289-0333-20
24's	$86.28	KEFTAB, Pd-Rx Pharmaceuticals	55289-0333-24

Cephapirin Sodium *(000701)*

For related information, see the comparative table section in Appendix A.

Categories: Endocarditis; Infection, bone; Infection, respiratory tract; Infection, skin and skin structures; Infection, urinary tract; Prophylaxis, perioperative; Septicemia; Pregnancy Category B; FDA Approval Pre 1982
Drug Classes: Antibiotics, cephalosporins
Brand Names: **Cefadyl**
Foreign Brand Availability: Brisfirina (Portugal; Spain); Cefaloject (France); Cefatrex (Greece; Korea); Cefatrexyl (Bulgaria; Czech-Republic); Lopitrex (Taiwan); Unipirin (Taiwan)
Cost of Therapy: $32.80 (Infection; Cefadyl Injection; 1 g; 2 g/day; 10 day supply)
HCFA JCODE(S): J0710 up to 1 g IV, IM

DESCRIPTION

Cephapirin sodium is a cephalosporin antibiotic intended for intramuscular or intravenous administration only. Each 500 mg contains 1.18 milliequivalents of sodium. Vial headspace contains nitrogen.

Cephapirin is the sodium salt of 7-α-(4-pyridylthio)-acetamido-cephalosporanic acid. The empirical formula is $C_{17}H_{16}N_3NaO_6S_2$ and the molecular weight is 445.44.

CLINICAL PHARMACOLOGY

Human Pharmacology

TABLE 1 *Duration of Blood Levels of Cephapirin in Normal Volunteers (Figures are µg/ml)*

	Time After Injection in Hours		
	½	4	6
Cephapirin 500 mg IM (single dose)	9.0	0.7	0.2
Cephapirin 1 g IM (single dose)	16.4	1.0	0.3

Cephapirin and its metabolites were excreted primarily by the kidneys. Antibiotic activity in the urine was equivalent to 35% of a 500 mg dose 6 hours after IM injection, and to 65% of a 500 mg dose 12 hours after injection. Following an IM dose of 500 mg, peak urine levels averaged 900 µg/ml within the first 6 hours.

TABLE 2 *Duration of Blood Levels of Cephapirin in Normal Volunteers (figures are µg/ml)*

	Time After Injection in Minutes		
	5	30	180
Cephapirin 500 mg rapid IV	35	6.7	0.27
Cephapirin 1 g rapid IV	67	14.0	0.61
Cephapirin 2 g rapid IV	129	31.7	1.11

Seventy percent of the administered dose was recovered in the urine within 6 hours.

Repetitive intravenous administration of 1 g doses over 6 hour periods produced serum levels between 4.5 and 5.5 µg/ml.

At therapeutic drug levels, normal human serum binds cephapirin to the extent of 44-50%. The average serum half-life of cephapirin in patients with normal renal function is approximately 36 minutes.

The major metabolite of cephapirin is desacetyl cephapirin which has been shown to contribute to antibacterial activity.

Controlled studies in normal adult volunteers revealed that cephapirin was well tolerated intramuscularly. In controlled studies of volunteers and of patients receiving IV cephapirin, the incidence of venous irritation was low.

Microbiology: *In vitro* tests demonstrate that the action of cephalosporins results from inhibition of cell-wall synthesis. Cephapirin is active against the following organisms *in vitro:* Beta-hemolytic streptococci and other streptococci. (Many strains of enterococci, *e.g., S. faecalis,* are relatively resistant.)

Staphylococcus aureus (penicillinase- and nonpenicillinase-producing); *Staphylococcus epidermis* (methicillin-susceptible strains); *Streptococcus pneumoniae* (formerly *Diplococcus pneumoniae*); *Proteus mirabilis; Haemophilus influenzae; Escherichia coli; Klebsiella* species.

Most strains of *Enterobacter* and indole-positive *Proteus* (*P. vulgaris, P. morganii, P. rettgeri*) are resistant to cephapirin. Methicillin-resistant staphylococci, *Serratia, Pseudomonas, Mima,* and *Herellea* species are almost uniformly resistant to cephapirin.

Disc Susceptibility Tests: Quantitative methods that require measurement of zone diameters give the most precise estimates of antibiotic susceptibility. One such procedure has been recommended or use with discs for testing susceptibility to cephalosporin class antibiotics. Interpretations correlate diameters of the disc test with MIC values for cephapirin. With this procedure, a report from the laboratory of "susceptible" indicates that the infecting organism is not likely to respond to therapy. A report of "intermediate susceptibility" suggests that the organism would be susceptible if high dosage is used, or if the infection is confined to tissues and fluid (*e.g.,* urine), in which high antibiotic levels are attained.

INDICATIONS AND USAGE

Cephapirin is indicated in the treatment of infections caused by susceptible strains of the designated microorganisms in the diseases listed below. Culture and susceptibility studies should be performed. Therapy may be instituted before results of susceptibility studies are obtained.

Respiratory Tract Infections: Caused by *S. pneumoniae* (formerly *D. pneumoniae*). *Staphylococcus aureus* (penicillinase- and nonpenicillinase-producing), *Klebsiella* species,*H. influenzae* and Group A beta-hemolytic streptococci.

Skin and Skin Structure Infections: Caused by *Staphylococcus aureus* (penicillinase- and nonpenicillinase-producing), *Staphylococcus epidermidis* (methicillin-susceptible strains), *E. coli, P. mirabilis, Klebsiella* species, and Group A beta-hemolytic streptococci.

Urinary Tract Infections: Caused by *Staphylococcus aureus* (penicillinase- and nonpenicillinase-producing), *E. coli, P. mirabilis,* and *Klebsiella* species.

Septicemia: Caused by *Staphylococcus aureus* (penicillinase- and nonpenicillinase-producing), *S. viridans, E. coli, Klebsiella* species and Group A beta-hemolytic streptococci.

Endocarditis: Caused by *Streptococcus viridans* and *Staphylococcus aureus* (penicillinase- and nonpenicillinase-producing).

Osteomyelitis: Caused by *Staphylococcus aureus* (penicillinase- and nonpenicillinase-producing), *Klebsiella* species,*P. mirabilis,* and Group A beta-hemolytic streptococci.

Perioperative Prophylaxis: The prophylactic administration of cephapirin preoperatively and postoperatively may reduce the incidence of certain postoperative infections in patients undergoing surgical procedures which are classified as contaminated or potentially contaminated, *e.g.,* vaginal hysterectomy.

The perioperative use of cephapirin may also be effective in surgical patients in whom infection at the operative site would present a serious risk, *e.g.,* during open-heart surgery and prosthetic arthroplasty.

The prophylactic administration of cephapirin should be discontinued within a 24 hour period after the surgical procedure. In surgery where the occurrence of infection may be particularly devastating, *e.g.,* open-heart surgery and prosthetic arthroplasty, the prophylactic administration of cephapirin may be continued for 3-5 days following completion of surgery. If there are signs of infection, specimens for culture should be obtained for the identification of the causative organism so that appropriate therapy may be instituted. (See DOSAGE AND ADMINISTRATION.)

NOTE: If the susceptibility tests show that the causative organism is resistant to cephapirin, other appropriate therapy should be instituted.

CONTRAINDICATIONS

Cephapirin is contraindicated in persons who have shown hypersensitivity to cephalosporin antibiotics.

WARNINGS

IN PENICILLIN-ALLERGIC PATIENTS, CEPHALOSPORINS SHOULD BE USED WITH GREAT CAUTION. THERE IS CLINICAL AND LABORATORY EVIDENCE OF PARTIAL CROSS-ALLERGENICITY OF THE PENICILLINS AND THE CEPHALOSPORINS, AND THERE ARE INSTANCES OF PATIENTS WHO HAVE HAD REACTIONS TO BOTH DRUGS (INCLUDING ANAPHYLAXIS AFTER PARENTERAL USE).

Any patient who has demonstrated some form of allergy, particularly to drugs, should receive antibiotics cautiously and then only when absolutely necessary. No exceptions should be made with regard to cephapirin.

Pseudomembranous colitis has been reported with the use of cephalosporins; therefore, it is important to consider its diagnosis in patients who develop diarrhea in association with antibiotic use.

SERIOUS ANAPHYLACTOID REACTIONS REQUIRE IMMEDIATE EMERGENCY TREATMENT WITH EPINEPHRINE, OXYGEN, INTRAVENOUS STEROIDS, AND AIRWAY MANAGEMENT, INCLUDING INTUBATION, SHOULD ALSO BE ADMINISTERED AS INDICATED.

PRECAUTIONS

Pregnancy Category B: Reproduction studies have been performed in rats and mice and have revealed no evidence of impaired fertility or harm to the fetus due to cephapirin. There are however no well controlled studies in pregnant women. Because animal studies are not always predictive of human response, this drug should be used during pregnancy only if clearly indicated.

Nursing Mothers: Cephapirin may be present in human milk in small amounts. Caution should be exercised when cephapirin is administered to a nursing woman.

The renal status of the patients should be determined prior to and during cephapirin therapy, since in patients with impaired renal function, a reduced dose may be appropriate (see DOSAGE AND ADMINISTRATION, Adults). When cephapirin was given to patients with marked reduction in renal function and to renal transplant patients, no adverse effects were reported.

Prolonged use of cephapirin may result in the overgrowth of nonsusceptible organisms. Careful observation of the patient is essential. If superinfection occurs during therapy, appropriate measures should be taken.

With high urine concentrations of cephapirin, false-positive glucose reactions may occur if Clinitest, Benedict's Solution, or Fehling's Solution are used. Therefore, it is recommended that glucose tests based on enzymatic glucose oxidase reactions (such as Clinistix or Tes-Tape) be used.

Increased nephrotoxicity has been reported following concomitant administration of cephalosporins and aminoglycoside antibiotics.

C

ADVERSE REACTIONS

Hypersensitivity: Cephalosporins were reported to produce the following reactions: maculopapular rash, urticaria, reactions resembling serum sickness, and anaphylaxis. Eosinophilia and drug fever have been observed to be associated with other allergic reactions. These reactions are most likely to occur in patients with a history of allergy, particularly to penicillin.
Blood: During large scale clinical trials, rare instances of neutropenia, leukopenia, and anemia were reported. Some individuals, particularly those with azotemia, have developed positive direct Coombs' test during therapy with other cephalosporins.
Liver: Elevations in SGPT, or SGOT, alkaline phosphatase, and bilirubin have been reported.
Kidney: Rises in BUN have been observed; their frequency increases in patients over 50 years old.
Gastrointestinal: Symptoms of pseudomembranous colitis can appear during or after antibiotic treatment. (See WARNINGS.)

DOSAGE AND ADMINISTRATION

ADULTS

The usual dose is 500 mg to 1 g every 4-6 hours intramuscularly or intravenously. The lower dose of 500 mg is adequate for certain infections, such as skin and skin structure and most urinary tract infections. However, the higher dose is recommended for more serious infections.

Very serious or life-threatening infections may require doses up to 12 g daily. The intravenous route is preferable when high doses are indicated.

Depending upon the causative organism and the severity of infection, patients with reduced renal function (moderately severe oliguria or serum creatinine above 5.0 mg/100 ml) may be treated adequately with a lower dose, 7.5 to 15 mg/kg of cephapirin every 12 hours. Patients with severely reduced renal function and who are to be dialyzed should receive the same dose just prior to dialysis and every 12 hours thereafter.

PERIOPERATIVE PROPHYLACTIC USE

To prevent postoperative infection in contaminated or potentially contaminated surgery, recommended doses are:

a. 1 to 2 g IM or IV administered ½ to 1 hour prior to the start of surgery.
b. 1 to 2 g during surgery (administration modified depending on the duration of the operative procedure).
c. 1 to 2 grams IV or IM every 6 hours for 24 hours postoperatively.

It is very important (1) the preoperative dose be given just prior to the start of surgery (½-1 hour) so that adequate antibiotic levels are present in the serum and tissues at the time of initial surgical incision, and (2) cephapirin be administered, if necessary, at appropriate intervals during surgery to provide sufficient levels of the antibiotic at the anticipated moments of greatest exposure to infective organisms.

In surgery where the occurrence of infection may be particularly devastating, *e.g.*, open-heart surgery and prosthetic arthroplasty, the prophylactic administration of cephapirin may be continued for 3-5 days following completion of surgery.

CHILDREN

The dosage is in accordance with age, weight, and severity of infection. The recommended total daily dose is 40-80 mg/kg (20-40 mg/lb) administered in 4 equally divided doses.

The drug has not been extensively studied in infants; therefore, in the treatment of children under the age of 3 months the relative benefit/risk should be considered.

Therapy in beta-hemolytic streptococcal infections should continue for at least 10 days.

Where indicated, surgical procedures should be performed in conjunction with antibiotic therapy.

Cephapirin may be administered by the intramuscular or the intravenous routes.

INTRAMUSCULAR INJECTION

The 500 mg and 1 g vials should be reconstituted with 1 or 2 ml of sterile water for injection or bacteriostatic water for injection, respectively. Each 1.2 ml contains 500 mg of cephapirin. All injections should be deep in the muscle mass.

INTRAVENOUS INJECTION

The intravenous route may be preferable for patients with bacteremia, septicemia, or other severe or life-threatening infections who may be poor risks because of lowered resistance resulting from such debilitating conditions as malnutrition, trauma, surgery, diabetes, heart failure, or malignancy, particularly if shock is present or impending. If patient has impaired renal function, a reduced dose may be indicated (see DOSAGE AND ADMINISTRATION, Adults). In conditions such as septicemia, 6-8 g/day may be given intravenously for several days at the beginning of therapy; then, depending on the clinical response and laboratory findings, the dosage may gradually be reduced.

When the infection has been refractory to previous forms of treatment and multiple sites have been involved, daily doses up to 12 g have been used.

Intermittent Intravenous Injection: The contents of the 500 mg, 1 or 2 g vial should be diluted with 10 ml or more of the specified diluent and administered slowly over a 3-5 minute period or may be given with intravenous infusions.

Intermittent Intravenous Infusion with Y-Tube: Intermittent intravenous infusion with a Y-type administration set can also be accomplished while bulk intravenous solutions are being infused. However, during infusion of the solution containing cephapirin it is desirable to discontinue the other solution. When this technique is employed, careful attention should be paid to the volume of the solution containing cephapirin so that the calculated dose will be infused. When a Y-tube hookup is used, the contents of the 4 g vial of cephapirin should be diluted by addition of 40 ml of bacteriostatic water for injection, dextrose injection, or sodium chloride injection.

All of the above solutions can be frozen immediately after reconstitution and stored at -15°C. for 60 days before use. After thawing, at room temperature (25°C), all of the solutions are stable for at least 12 hours at room temperature or 10 days under refrigeration (4°C).

TABLE 3 *Stability Utility Time for Cephapirin Sodium In Various Diluents At Concentrations Ranging From 20-400 mg/ml*

Diluent	Approximate Concentration	Utility Time 25°C	Utility Time 4°C
Water for injection	50-400 mg/ml	12 h	10 days
Bacteriostatic water for injection with benzyl alcohol or parabens	250-400 mg/ml	48 h	10 days
Normal saline	20-100 mg/ml	24 h	10 days
5% Dextrose in water	20-100 mg/ml	24 h	10 days

The pH of the resultant solution ranges from 6.5-8.5. During these storage conditions, no precipitation occurs. A change in solution color during this stage time does not affect the potency.

Compatibility with the Infusion Solution: Cephapirin is stable and compatible for 24 hours at room temperature at concentrations between 2 and 30 mg/ml in the following solutions:

Sodium chloride injection, 5% W/V dextrose in water, sodium lactate injection, 5% dextrose in normal saline, 10% invert sugar in normal saline; 10% invert sugar in water; 5% dextrose + 0.2% sodium chloride injection, lactated Ringer's injection, lactated Ringer's with 5% dextrose; 5% dextrose + 0.45% sodium chloride injection, Ringer's injection, 10% dextrose injection, sterile water for injection, 20% dextrose injection, 5% sodium chloride in water; 5% dextrose in Ringer's injection; Normosol R; Normosol R in 5% dextrose injection; Ionosol D-CM; Ionosol G in 10% dextrose injection.

In addition, cephapirin, at a concentration of 4 mg/ml, is stable and compatible for 10 days under refrigeration (4°C) or 14 days in the frozen state (15°C) followed by 24 hours at room temperature (25°C) in all of the intravenous solutions listed above.

"Piggyback" IV Package: This glass vial contains the labeled quantity of cephapirin and is intended for intravenous administration. The diluent and volume are specified on the label. Parenteral drug products should be inspected visually for particulate matter and discoloration prior to administration, whenever solution and container permit.

HOW SUPPLIED

Storage: Store the dry powder at controlled room temperature, 15-30°C (59-86°F).

Cephradine (000702)

For related information, see the comparative table section in Appendix A.

Categories: Infection, ear, middle; Infection, respiratory tract; Infection, skin and skin structures; Infection, urinary tract; Pharyngitis; Pneumonia; Prostatitis; Tonsillitis; Pregnancy Category B; FDA Approved 1974 Aug
Drug Classes: Antibiotics, cephalosporins
Brand Names: Anspor; Velosef
Foreign Brand Availability: Bactocef (South-Africa); Broadcef (Korea); Cefadin (Taiwan); Cefirex (France); Cefra (Guatemala); Cefradine (China); Cefradur (Dominican-Republic; El-Salvador; Guatemala; Honduras; Panama); Cefrasol (Bahrain; Cyprus; Egypt; Iran; Iraq; Jordan; Kuwait; Lebanon; Libya; Oman; Qatar; Republic-of-Yemen; Saudi-Arabia; Syria; United-Arab-Emirates); Cefril (South-Africa); Cefro (Japan); Celex (Italy); Daicefalin (Japan); Duphratex (Philippines); Dynacef (Indonesia); Eskacef (Benin; Burkina-Faso; Ethiopia; Gambia; Ghana; Guinea; Ivory-Coast; Kenya; Liberia; Malawi; Mali; Mauritania; Mauritius; Morocco; Niger; Nigeria; Senegal; Seychelles; Sierra-Leone; Sudan; Tanzania; Tunia; Uganda; Zambia; Zimbabwe); Lisacef (Taiwan); Lovecef (Indonesia); Maxisporin (Belgium; Netherlands; Portugal); Nakacef-A (Taiwan); Opebrin (Greece); S-60 (Taiwan); Safdin (Korea); Sefril (Austria; Germany; Poland; Switzerland); Sephros (Taiwan); Taicefran (Japan); Tricef (Korea); U-Save (Taiwan); Velocef (Argentina; Peru; Spain); Velosef Viol (Greece); Veracef (Colombia; Costa-Rica; Ecuador; El-Salvador; Guatemala; Honduras; Mexico; Nicaragua; Panama); Zeefra (Hong-Kong); Zolicef (Philippines)
Cost of Therapy: $38.82 (Infection; Velosef; 500 mg; 2 capsules/day; 10 day supply)
$10.40 (Infection; Generic Capsules; 500 mg; 2 capsules/day; 10 day supply)

DESCRIPTION

Cephradine is a semisynthetic cephalosporin antibiotic; oral dosage forms include capsules containing 250 and 500 mg cephradine, and cephradine for oral suspension containing, after constitution, 125 and 250 mg/5 ml dose.

Cephradine is designated chemically as (6R,7R)-7-((R)-2-amino-2-(1,4-cyclohexadien-1-yl) acetamido)-3-methyl-8-oxo-5-thia-1-azabicyclo (4.2.0)oct-2-ene-2-carboxylic acid.

Velosef Inactive Ingredients: *Capsules:* Colorants (D&C red no. 33 and yellow no. 10; FD&C blue no. 1, and, for "250" only, red no. 3), gelatin, lactose, magnesium stearate, talc, and titanium dioxide. *Cephradine for Oral Suspension:* Citric acid, colorants (FD&C red no. 40 for "250" only; FD&C yellow no. 6 for "125" only), flavors, guar gum, methylcellulose, sodium citrate, and sucrose.

CLINICAL PHARMACOLOGY

Cephradine is acid stable. It is rapidly absorbed after oral administration in the fasting state. Following single doses of 250 mg, 500 mg, and 1 g in normal adult volunteers, average peak serum concentrations within 1 hour were approximately 9 μg/ml, 16.5 μg/ml, and 24.2 μg/ml, respectively. *In vitro* studies by an ultracentrifugation technique show that at therapeutic serum antibiotic concentrations, cephradine is minimally bound (8-17%) to normal serum protein. Cephradine does not pass across the blood-brain barrier to any appreciable extent. The presence of food in the gastrointestinal tract delays absorption but does not affect the total amount of cephradine absorbed. Over 90% of the drug is excreted unchanged in the urine within 6 hours. Peak urine concentrations are approximately 1600 μg/ml, 3200 μg/ml, and 4000 μg/ml following single doses of 250 mg, 500 mg, and 1 g, respectively.

MICROBIOLOGY

In vitro tests demonstrate that the cephalosporin are bactericidal because of their inhibition of cell-wall synthesis. Cephradine is active against the following organisms *in vitro:*

Group A beta-hemolytic streptococci.

Staphylococci, including coagulase-positive, coagulase-negative, and penicillinase-producing strains.

Streptococcus pneumoniae (formerly *Diplococcus pneumoniae*).

Escherichia coli.

Proteus mirabilis.

Klebsiella species.

Haemophilus influenzae.

Cephradine is not active against most strains of *Enterobacter* species, *P. morganii,* and *P. vulgaris.* It has no activity against *Pseudomonas* or *Herellea* species. When tested by *in vitro* methods, staphylococci exhibit cross- resistance between cephradine and methicillin-type antibiotics.

Note: Most strains of enterococci *(Streptococcus faecalis)* are resistant to cephradine.

DISC SUSCEPTIBILITY TESTS

Quantitative methods that require measurement of zone diameters give the most precise estimates of antibiotic susceptibility. One recommended procedure (21 CFR 460.1) uses cephalosporin class discs for testing susceptibility; interpretations correlate zone diameters of this disc test with MIC values for cephradine. With this procedure, a report from the laboratory of "resistant" indicates that the infecting organism is not likely to respond to therapy. A report of "intermediate susceptibility" suggests that the organism would be susceptible if the infection is confined to the urinary tract, as high antibiotic levels can be obtained in the urine, or if high dosage is used in other types of infection.

INDICATIONS AND USAGE

Cephradine capsules and cephradine for oral suspension are indicated in the treatment of the following infections when caused by susceptible strains of the designated microorganisms:

Respiratory Tract Infections (*e.g.,* tonsillitis, pharyngitis, and lobar pneumonia): Caused by group A beta-hemolytic streptococci and *S. pneumoniae* (formerly *D. pneumoniae*).

(Penicillin is the usual drug of choice in the treatment and prevention of streptococcal infections, including the prophylaxis of rheumatic fever. Cephradine is generally effective in the eradication of streptococci from the nasopharynx; substantial data establishing the efficacy of cephradine in the subsequent prevention of rheumatic fever are not available at present.)

Otitis Media: Caused by group A beta-hemolytic streptococci, *S. pneumoniae* (formerly *D. pneumoniae*), *H. influenzae,* and *staphylococci.*

Skin and Skin Structures Infections: Caused by staphylococci (penicillin-susceptible and penicillin-resistant) and beta-hemolytic streptococci.

Urinary Tract Infections: Including prostatitis, caused by *E. coli, P. mirabilis, Klebsiella* species, and enterococci *(S. faecalis).* The high concentrations of cephradine achievable in the urinary tract will be effective against many strains of enterococci for which disc susceptibility studies indicate relative resistance. It is to be noted that among beta-lactam antibiotics, ampicillin is the drug of choice for enterococcal urinary tract *(S. faecalis)* infection.

Note: Culture and susceptibility tests should be initiated prior to and during therapy.

Following clinical improvement achieved with parenteral therapy, oral cephradine may be utilized for continuation of treatment of persistent or severe conditions where prolonged therapy is indicated.

CONTRAINDICATIONS

Cephradine is contraindicated in patients with known hypersensitivity to the cephalosporin group of antibiotics.

WARNINGS

In penicillin-sensitive patients, cephalosporin derivatives should be used with great caution. There is clinical and laboratory evidence of partial cross-allergenicity of the penicillins and the cephalosporins, and there are instances of patients who have had reactions to both drug classes (including anaphylaxis after parenteral use).

Any patient who has demonstrated some form of allergy, particularly to drugs, should receive antibiotics, including cephradine, cautiously and then only when absolutely necessary.

Pseudomembranous colitis has been reported with the use of cephalosporins (and other broad spectrum antibiotics); therefore, it is important to consider its diagnosis is patients who develop diarrhea in association with antibiotic use. Treatment with broad spectrum antibiotics alters normal flora of the colon and may permit overgrowth of clostridia. Studies indicate a toxin produced by *Clostridium difficile* is one primary cause of antibiotic-associated colitis. Cholestyramine and colestipol resins have been shown to bind the toxin*in vitro.* Mild cases of colitis may respond to drug discontinuance alone. Moderate to severe cases should be managed with fluid, electrolyte and protein supplementation as indicated. When the colitis is not relieved by drug discontinuance or when it is severe, oral vancomycin is the treatment of choice for antibiotic-associated pseudomembranous colitis produced by *C. difficile.* Other causes of colitis should also be considered.

PRECAUTIONS

GENERAL

Patients should be followed carefully so that any side effects or unusual manifestations of drug idiosyncrasy may be detected. If a hypersensitivity reaction occurs, the drug should be discontinued and the patient treated with the usual agents, *e.g.,* pressor amines, antihistamines, or corticosteroids.

Administer cephradine with caution in the presence of markedly impaired function. In patients with known or suspected renal impairment, careful clinical observation and appropriate laboratory studies should be made prior to and during therapy as cephradine accumulates in the serum and tissues. See DOSAGE AND ADMINISTRATION section for information on treatment of patients with impaired renal function.

Cephradine should be prescribed with caution in individuals with a history of gastrointestinal disease, particularly colitis.

Prolonged use of antibiotics may promote the overgrowth of nonsusceptible organisms. Should superinfection occur during therapy, appropriate measures should be taken.

Indicated surgical procedures should be performed in conjunction with antibiotic therapy.

INFORMATION FOR THE PATIENT

Caution diabetic patients that false results may occur with urine glucose tests (see Drug/Laboratory Test Interactions).

Advise the patient to comply with the full course of therapy even if he begins to feel better and to take a missed dose as soon as possible. Inform the patient that this medication may be taken with food or milk since gastrointestinal upset may be a factor in compliance with the dosage regimen. The patient should report current use of any medicines and should be cautioned not to take other medications unless the physician knows and approves of their use (see DRUG INTERACTIONS).

LABORATORY TESTS

In patients with known or suspected renal impairment, it is advisable to monitor renal function (see DOSAGE AND ADMINISTRATION).

DRUG/LABORATORY TEST INTERACTIONS

After treatment with cephradine, a false-positive reaction for glucose in the urine may occur with Benedict's solution, Fehling's solution, or with Clinitest tablets, but not with enzyme-based tests such as Clinistix and Tes-Tape.

False-positive Coombs test results may occur in newborns whose mothers received a cephalosporin prior to delivery.

Cephalosporins have been reported to cause false-positive reactions in tests for urinary proteins which use sulfosalicylic acid, false elevations of urinary 17-ketosteroid values, and prolonged prothrombin times.

CARCINOGENESIS, MUTAGENESIS

Long-term studies in animals have not been performed to evaluate carcinogenic potential or mutagenesis.

PREGNANCY CATEGORY B

Reproduction studies have been performed in mice and rats at doses up to four times the maximum indicated human dose and have revealed no evidence of impaired fertility or harm to fetus due to cephradine. There are, however, no adequate and well-controlled studies in pregnant women. Because animal reproduction studies are not always predictive of human response, this drug should be used during pregnancy only if clearly needed.

NURSING MOTHERS

Since cephradine is excreted in breast milk during lactation, caution should be exercised when cephradine is administered to a nursing woman.

PEDIATRIC USE

See DOSAGE AND ADMINISTRATION. Adequate information is unavailable on the efficacy of twice daily regimens in children under nine months of age.

DRUG INTERACTIONS

When administered concurrently, the following drugs may interact with cephalosporins.

Other Antibacterial Agents: Bacteriostats may interfere with the bactericidal action of cephalosporins in acute infection; other agents, *e.g.,* aminoglycosides, colistin, polymyxins, vancomycin, may increase the possibility of nephrotoxicity.

Diuretics: (Potent "loop diuretics," *e.g.,* furosemide and ethacrynic acid.) Enhanced possibility for renal toxicity.

Probenecid: Increased and prolonged blood levels of cephalosporins, resulting in increased risk of nephrotoxicity.

ADVERSE REACTIONS

As with other cephalosporins, untoward reactions are limited essentially to gastrointestinal disturbances and, on occasion, to hypersensitivity phenomena. The latter are more likely to occur in individuals who have previously demonstrated hypersensitivity and those with a history of allergy, asthma, hay fever, or urticaria.

The following adverse reactions have been reported following the use of cephradine:

Gastrointestinal: Symptoms of pseudomembranous colitis can appear during antibiotic treatment. Nausea and vomiting have been reported rarely.

Skin and Hypersensitivity Reactions: Mild urticaria or skin rash, pruritus, and joint pains were reported by very few patients.

Hematologic: Mild, transient eosinophilia, leukopenia, and neutropenia have been reported.

Liver: Transient mild rise of SGOT, SGPT, and total bilirubin have been observed with no evidence of hepatocellular damage.

Renal: Transitory rises in BUN have been observed in some patients treated with cephalosporins; their frequency increases in patients over 50 years old. In adults for whom serum creatinine determinations were performed, the rise in BUN was not accompanied by a rise in serum creatinine.

Other adverse reactions have included dizziness and tightness in the chest and candidal vaginitis.

DOSAGE AND ADMINISTRATION

Cephradine may be given without regard to meals.

ADULTS

For respiratory tract infections (other than lobar pneumonia) and skin and skin structures infections, the usual dose is 250 mg every 6 hours or 500 mg every 12 hours.

For lobar pneumonia, the usual dose is 500 mg every 6 hours of 1 g every 12 hours.

For uncomplicated urinary tract infections, the usual dose is 500 mg every 12 hours. In more serious urinary tract infections, including prostatitis, 500 mg every 6 hours or 1 g every 12 hours may be administered.

Larger doses (up to 1 g every 6 hours) may be given for severe or chronic infections.

CHILDREN

No adequate information is available on the efficacy of bid regimens in children under 9 months of age. The usual dose in children over 9 months of age is 25-50 mg/kg/day administered in equally divided doses every 6 or 12 hours. For otitis media due to*H. influenzae,* doses are from 75-100 mg/kg/day administered in equally divided doses every 6 or 12 hours, but should not exceed 4 g/day. Dosage for children should not exceed dosage recommended for adults.

All patients, regardless of age and weight: Larger doses (up to 1 qid) may be given for severe or chronic infections.

As with antibiotic therapy in general, treatment should be continued for a minimum of 48-72 hours after the patient becomes asymptomatic or evidence of bacterial eradication has been obtained. In infections caused by group A beta-hemolytic streptococci, a minimum of 10 days of treatment is recommended to guard against the risk of rheumatic fever or glomerulonephritis. In the treatment of chronic urinary tract infection, frequent bacteriologic and clinical appraisal is necessary during therapy and may be necessary for several months afterwards. Persistent infections may require treatment for several weeks. Prolonged intensive therapy is recommended for prostatitis. Doses smaller than those indicated are not recommended.

PATIENTS WITH IMPAIRED RENAL FUNCTION

Not on Dialysis: The following initial dosage schedule (see TABLE 1), is suggested as a guideline based on creatinine clearance. Further modification in the dosage schedule may be required because of individual variations in absorption.

TABLE 1

Creatinine Clearance	Dose	Time Interval
>20 ml/min	500 mg	6 hours
5-20 ml/min	250 mg	6 hours
<5 ml/min	250 mg	12 hours

On Chronic, Intermittent Hemodialysis:

250 mg Start.

250 mg at 12 hours.

250 mg 36-48 hours (after start).

Children may require dosage modification proportional to their weight and severity of infection.

Capsules: Keep tightly closed. Do not store above 86°F.

Oral Suspension: Prior to constitution, store at room temperature; avoid excessive heat. After constitution, when stored at room temperature, discard unused portion after 14 days. Keep tightly closed.

PRODUCT LISTING - RATED THERAPEUTICALLY EQUIVALENT

Capsule - Oral - 250 mg

Size	Price	Product	NDC
15's	$10.90	GENERIC, Pd-Rx Pharmaceuticals	55289-0608-15
21's	$14.76	GENERIC, Pd-Rx Pharmaceuticals	55289-0608-21
30's	$21.00	GENERIC, Pd-Rx Pharmaceuticals	55289-0608-30
40's	$15.30	GENERIC, Pd-Rx Pharmaceuticals	55289-0074-40
100's	$30.00	GENERIC, Raway Pharmacal Inc	00686-3153-09
100's	$35.00	GENERIC, Cmc-Consolidated Midland Corporation	00223-0611-01
100's	$37.50	GENERIC, Raway Pharmacal Inc	00686-0606-20
100's	$42.25	GENERIC, Ivax Corporation	00182-1253-89
100's	$47.46	GENERIC, Esi Lederle Generics	00005-3406-23
100's	$53.00	GENERIC, Qualitest Products Inc	00603-2619-21
100's	$54.75	GENERIC, Ivax Corporation	00182-1253-01
100's	$55.00	GENERIC, Major Pharmaceuticals Inc	00904-2837-60
100's	$55.05	GENERIC, Geneva Pharmaceuticals	00781-2533-01
100's	$57.90	GENERIC, Moore, H.L. Drug Exchange Inc	00839-7262-06
100's	$59.51	GENERIC, Aligen Independent Laboratories Inc	00405-4158-01
100's	$98.81	VELOSEF, Bristol-Myers Squibb	00003-0113-50

Capsule - Oral - 500 mg

Size	Price	Product	NDC
14's	$15.68	GENERIC, Pd-Rx Pharmaceuticals	55289-0597-14
20's	$21.90	GENERIC, Pd-Rx Pharmaceuticals	55289-0597-20
24's	$18.00	GENERIC, Raway Pharmacal Inc	00686-3155-08
24's	$31.37	GENERIC, Geneva Pharmaceuticals	00781-2534-24
28's	$25.00	GENERIC, Pd-Rx Pharmaceuticals	55289-0597-28
100's	$52.00	GENERIC, Raway Pharmacal Inc	00686-3155-09
100's	$60.00	GENERIC, Raway Pharmacal Inc	00686-0607-20
100's	$65.00	GENERIC, Cmc-Consolidated Midland Corporation	00223-0612-01
100's	$93.71	GENERIC, Esi Lederle Generics	00005-3407-23
100's	$98.00	GENERIC, Qualitest Products Inc	00603-2620-21
100's	$104.70	GENERIC, Major Pharmaceuticals Inc	00904-2838-60
100's	$104.95	GENERIC, Ivax Corporation	00182-1254-01
100's	$105.00	GENERIC, Geneva Pharmaceuticals	00781-2534-01
100's	$105.42	GENERIC, Moore, H.L. Drug Exchange Inc	00839-7263-06
100's	$110.90	GENERIC, Ivax Corporation	00182-1254-89
100's	$114.45	GENERIC, Aligen Independent Laboratories Inc	00405-4159-01
100's	$194.08	VELOSEF, Bristol-Myers Squibb	00003-0114-50

Powder For Reconstitution - Oral - 125 mg/5 ml

Size	Price	Product	NDC
100 ml	$4.25	GENERIC, Raway Pharmacal Inc	00686-4165-32
100 ml	$7.50	GENERIC, Ivax Corporation	00182-7014-70
100 ml	$10.14	VELOSEF, Bristol-Myers Squibb	00003-1193-50
100's	$6.90	GENERIC, Major Pharmaceuticals Inc	00904-2832-04

Powder For Reconstitution - Oral - 250 mg/5 ml

Size	Price	Product	NDC
100 ml	$7.98	GENERIC, Raway Pharmacal Inc	00686-4167-32
100 ml	$12.90	GENERIC, Major Pharmaceuticals Inc	00904-2833-04
100 ml	$13.05	GENERIC, Ivax Corporation	00182-7015-70
100 ml	$13.38	GENERIC, Watson/Schein Pharmaceuticals Inc	00364-2144-61
100 ml	$19.82	GENERIC, Prescript Pharmaceuticals	00247-0779-00
100 ml	$20.33	VELOSEF, Bristol-Myers Squibb	00003-1194-50
200 ml	$37.65	VELOSEF, Bristol-Myers Squibb	00003-1194-80

PRODUCT LISTING - EQUIVALENTS NOT AVAILABLE

Capsule - Oral - 250 mg

Size	Price	Product	NDC
4's	$4.47	GENERIC, Prescript Pharmaceuticals	00247-0344-04
10's	$6.13	GENERIC, Prescript Pharmaceuticals	00247-0344-10
10's	$8.60	GENERIC, Southwood Pharmaceuticals Inc	58016-0154-10
12's	$10.32	GENERIC, Southwood Pharmaceuticals Inc	58016-0154-12
14's	$12.04	GENERIC, Southwood Pharmaceuticals Inc	58016-0154-14
16's	$13.76	GENERIC, Southwood Pharmaceuticals Inc	58016-0154-16
18's	$15.48	GENERIC, Southwood Pharmaceuticals Inc	58016-0154-18
20's	$8.92	GENERIC, Prescript Pharmaceuticals	00247-0344-20
20's	$11.00	GENERIC, Allscripts Pharmaceutical Company	54569-0325-04
20's	$16.00	GENERIC, Pharma Pac	52959-0308-20
20's	$17.20	GENERIC, Southwood Pharmaceuticals Inc	58016-0154-20
20's	$19.09	GENERIC, Alpharma Uspd Makers Of Barre and Nmc	63874-0104-20
21's	$9.19	GENERIC, Prescript Pharmaceuticals	00247-0344-21
24's	$10.02	GENERIC, Prescript Pharmaceuticals	00247-0344-24
24's	$20.64	GENERIC, Southwood Pharmaceuticals Inc	58016-0154-24
28's	$11.14	GENERIC, Prescript Pharmaceuticals	00247-0344-28
28's	$20.09	GENERIC, Alpharma Uspd Makers Of Barre and Nmc	63874-0104-28
30's	$11.69	GENERIC, Prescript Pharmaceuticals	00247-0344-30
30's	$12.19	GENERIC, Physicians Total Care	54868-1997-01
30's	$25.80	GENERIC, Southwood Pharmaceuticals Inc	58016-0154-30
30's	$25.92	GENERIC, Alpharma Uspd Makers Of Barre and Nmc	63874-0104-30
36's	$30.96	GENERIC, Southwood Pharmaceuticals Inc	58016-0154-36
40's	$14.47	GENERIC, Prescript Pharmaceuticals	00247-0344-40
40's	$34.40	GENERIC, Southwood Pharmaceuticals Inc	58016-0154-40
40's	$34.45	GENERIC, Pharma Pac	52959-0308-40
40's	$38.64	GENERIC, Alpharma Uspd Makers Of Barre and Nmc	63874-0104-40
100's	$83.76	GENERIC, Alpharma Uspd Makers Of Barre and Nmc	63874-0104-01
100's	$85.99	GENERIC, Southwood Pharmaceuticals Inc	58016-0154-00

Capsule - Oral - 500 mg

Size	Price	Product	NDC
4's	$5.53	GENERIC, Prescript Pharmaceuticals	00247-0237-04
6's	$6.61	GENERIC, Prescript Pharmaceuticals	00247-0237-06
9's	$8.24	GENERIC, Prescript Pharmaceuticals	00247-0237-09
10's	$8.78	GENERIC, Prescript Pharmaceuticals	00247-0237-10
10's	$10.51	GENERIC, Allscripts Pharmaceutical Company	54569-0326-07
10's	$16.89	GENERIC, Southwood Pharmaceuticals Inc	58016-0155-10
10's	$18.63	GENERIC, Alpharma Uspd Makers Of Barre and Nmc	63874-0238-10
12's	$20.27	GENERIC, Southwood Pharmaceuticals Inc	58016-0155-12
14's	$14.71	GENERIC, Allscripts Pharmaceutical Company	54569-0326-08
14's	$29.35	GENERIC, Pharma Pac	52959-0032-14
15's	$11.49	GENERIC, Prescript Pharmaceuticals	00247-0237-15
15's	$25.33	GENERIC, Southwood Pharmaceuticals Inc	58016-0155-15
16's	$30.08	GENERIC, Southwood Pharmaceuticals Inc	58016-0155-16
18's	$33.84	GENERIC, Southwood Pharmaceuticals Inc	58016-0155-18
20's	$14.21	GENERIC, Prescript Pharmaceuticals	00247-0237-20
20's	$21.01	GENERIC, Allscripts Pharmaceutical Company	54569-0326-04
20's	$37.60	GENERIC, Southwood Pharmaceuticals Inc	58016-0155-20
20's	$38.47	GENERIC, Alpharma Uspd Makers Of Barre and Nmc	63874-0238-20
20's	$41.05	GENERIC, Pharma Pac	52959-0032-20
24's	$45.12	GENERIC, Southwood Pharmaceuticals Inc	58016-0155-24
28's	$18.54	GENERIC, Prescript Pharmaceuticals	00247-0237-28
28's	$47.29	GENERIC, Southwood Pharmaceuticals Inc	58016-0155-28
28's	$52.92	GENERIC, Alpharma Uspd Makers Of Barre and Nmc	63874-0238-28
28's	$56.28	GENERIC, Pharma Pac	52959-0032-28
30's	$19.64	GENERIC, Prescript Pharmaceuticals	00247-0237-30
30's	$23.51	GENERIC, Physicians Total Care	54868-0157-01
30's	$56.40	GENERIC, Southwood Pharmaceuticals Inc	58016-0155-30
36's	$67.68	GENERIC, Southwood Pharmaceuticals Inc	58016-0155-36
40's	$25.06	GENERIC, Prescript Pharmaceuticals	00247-0237-40
40's	$75.20	GENERIC, Southwood Pharmaceuticals Inc	58016-0155-40
40's	$75.45	GENERIC, Pharma Pac	52959-0032-40

40's	$83.34	GENERIC, Alpharma Uspd Makers Of Barre and Nmc	63874-0238-40
42's	$78.96	GENERIC, Pharma Pac	52959-0032-42
100's	$188.00	GENERIC, Southwood Pharmaceuticals Inc	58016-0155-00
100's	$209.05	GENERIC, Alpharma Uspd Makers Of Barre and Nmc	63874-0238-01

Cetirizine Hydrochloride (003162)

For related information, see the comparative table section in Appendix A.

Categories: Rhinitis, allergic; Urticaria, chronic idiopathic; FDA Approved 1995 Dec; Pregnancy Category B
Drug Classes: Antihistamines, H1
Brand Names: **Zyrtec**
Foreign Brand Availability: Acidrine (Colombia); Alercet (Colombia; Peru); Alerid (Bahrain; China; Cyprus; Egypt; Iran; Iraq; Jordan; Kuwait; Lebanon; Libya; Oman; Qatar; Republic-of-Yemen; Saudi-Arabia; Syria; United-Arab-Emirates); Alerviden (Colombia); Alled (Indonesia); Alltec (Taiwan); Alzytec (Singapore); Cerazine (Korea); Cerotec (Korea); Cesta (Korea); Cethis (Thailand); Cetin (Taiwan); Cetirax (Colombia); Cetrimed (Thailand); Cetrine (China; Singapore; Thailand); Cetrizet (Thailand); Cetrizin (Thailand); Cety (Taiwan); Cistamine (Thailand); Falergi (Indonesia); Finallerg (Bahrain; Cyprus; Egypt; Iran; Iraq; Jordan; Kuwait; Lebanon; Libya; Oman; Qatar; Republic-of-Yemen; Saudi-Arabia; Syria; United-Arab-Emirates); Histazine (Israel); Histica (Thailand); Incidal-OD (Indonesia; Thailand); Lergium (Peru); Nosemin (Korea); Nosmin (Korea); Razene (New-Zealand); Reactine (Canada); Rhizin (Singapore); Risima (Indonesia); Ryvel (Indonesia); Ryzen (Indonesia); Sancotec (Korea); Selitex (Korea); Setizin (Taiwan); Sutac (Thailand); Symitec (Taiwan); Terzine (Thailand); Triz (India); Virlix (France; Italy; Mexico; Philippines; Portugal; Spain); Zenriz (Indonesia); Zensil (Thailand); Zeran (Benin; Burkina-Faso; Ethiopia; Gambia; Ghana; Guinea; Ivory-Coast; Kenya; Liberia; Malawi; Mali; Mauritania; Mauritius; Morocco; Niger; Nigeria; Senegal; Seychelles; Sierra-Leone; Sudan; Tanzania; Tunia; Uganda; Zambia; Zimbabwe); Zertine (Thailand); Zinex (Philippines); Zirtin (India); Zyrazine (Thailand); Zyrcon (Thailand); Zyrlex (Sweden)
Cost of Therapy: $63.29 (Allergic Rhinitis; Zyrtec; 10 mg; 1 tablet/day; 30 day supply)

DESCRIPTION

For Oral Use.

Cetirizine hydrochloride is an orally active and selective H_1-receptor antagonist. The chemical name is (±)-[2-[4-[(4-chlorophenyl)phenylmethyl]-1-piperazinyl]ethoxy]acetic acid, dihydrochloride. Cetirizine hydrochloride is a racemic compound with an empirical formula of $C_{21}H_{25}ClN_2O_3 \cdot 2HCl$. The molecular weight is 461.82.

ZYRTEC TABLETS

Cetirizine hydrochloride is a white, crystalline powder and is water soluble. Zyrtec tablets are formulated as white, film-coated, rounded-off rectangular shaped tablets for oral administration and are available in 5 and 10 mg strengths.
Inactive Ingredients: Lactose, magnesium stearate, povidone, titanium dioxide, hydroxypropyl methylcellulose, polyethylene glycol, and corn starch.

ZYRTEC SYRUP

Zyrtec syrup is a colorless to slightly yellow syrup containing cetirizine hydrochloride at a concentration of 1 mg/ml (5 mg/5 ml) for oral administration. The pH is between 4 and 5.
Inactive Ingredients: Banana flavor, glacial acetic acid, glycerin, grape flavor, methylparaben, propylene glycol, propylparaben, sodium acetate, sugar syrup, and water.

CLINICAL PHARMACOLOGY

MECHANISM OF ACTION

Cetirizine, a human metabolite of hydroxyzine, is an antihistamine; its principal effects are mediated via selective inhibition of peripheral H_1 receptors. The antihistaminic activity of cetirizine has been clearly documented in a variety of animal and human models. *In vivo* and *ex vivo* animal models have shown negligible anticholinergic and antiserotonergic activity. In clinical studies, however, dry mouth was more common with cetirizine than with placebo. *In vitro* receptor binding studies have shown no measurable affinity for other than H_1 receptors. Autoradiographic studies with radiolabeled cetirizine in the rat have shown negligible penetration into the brain. *Ex vivo* experiments in the mouse have shown that systemically administered cetirizine does not significantly occupy cerebral H_1 receptors.

PHARMACOKINETICS

Absorption

Cetirizine was rapidly absorbed with a time to maximum concentration (T_{max}) of approximately 1 hour following oral administration of tablets or syrup in adults. Comparable bioavailability was found between the tablet and syrup dosage forms. When healthy volunteers were administered multiple doses of cetirizine (10 mg tablets once daily for 10 days), a mean peak plasma concentration (C_{max}) of 311 ng/ml was observed. No accumulation was observed. Cetirizine pharmacokinetics were linear for oral doses ranging from 5-60 mg. Food had no effect on the extent of cetirizine exposure (AUC) but T_{max} was delayed by 1.7 hours and C_{max} was decreased by 23% in the presence of food.

Distribution

The mean plasma protein binding of cetirizine is 93%, independent of concentration in the range of 25-1000 ng/ml, which includes the therapeutic plasma levels observed.

Metabolism

A mass balance study in 6 healthy male volunteers indicated that 70% of the administered radioactivity was recovered in the urine and 10% in the feces. Approximately 50% of the radioactivity was identified in the urine as unchanged drug. Most of the rapid increase in peak plasma radioactivity was associated with parent drug, suggesting a low degree of first-pass metabolism. Cetirizine is metabolized to a limited extent by oxidative O-dealkylation to a metabolite with negligible antihistaminic activity. The enzyme or enzymes responsible for this metabolism have not been identified.

Elimination

The mean elimination half-life in 146 healthy volunteers across multiple pharmacokinetic studies was 8.3 hours and the apparent total body clearance for cetirizine was approximately 53 ml/min.

INTERACTION STUDIES

Pharmacokinetic interaction studies with cetirizine in adults were conducted with pseudoephedrine, antipyrine, ketoconazole, erythromycin, and azithromycin. No interactions were observed. In a multiple dose study of theophylline (400 mg once daily for 3 days) and cetirizine (20 mg once daily for 3 days), a 16% decrease in the clearance of cetirizine was observed. The disposition of theophylline was not altered by concomitant cetirizine administration.

SPECIAL POPULATIONS

Pediatric Patients

When pediatric patients aged 7-12 years received a single, 5 mg oral cetirizine capsule, the mean C_{max} was 275 ng/ml. Based on cross-study comparisons, the weight-normalized, apparent total body clearance was 33% greater and the elimination half-life was 33% shorter in this pediatric population than in adults. In pediatric patients aged 2-5 years who received 5 mg of cetirizine, the mean C_{max} was 660 ng/ml. Based on cross-study comparisons, the weight-normalized apparent total body clearance was 81-111% greater and the elimination half-life was 33-41% shorter in this pediatric population than in adults. In pediatric patients aged 6-23 months who received a single dose of 0.25 mg/kg cetirizine oral solution (mean dose 2.3 mg), the mean C_{max} was 390 ng/ml. Based on cross-study comparisons, the weight-normalized, apparent total body clearance was 304% greater and the elimination half-life was 63% shorter in this pediatric population compared to adults. The average AUC(0-t) in children 6 months to <2 years of age receiving the maximum dose of cetirizine solution (2.5 mg twice a day) is expected to be 2-fold higher than that observed in adults receiving a dose of 10 mg cetirizine tablets once a day.

Geriatric Patients

Following a single, 10 mg oral dose, the elimination half-life was prolonged by 50% and the apparent total body clearance was 40% lower in 16 geriatric subjects with a mean age of 77 years compared to 14 adult subjects with a mean age of 53 years. The decrease in cetirizine clearance in these elderly volunteers may be related to decreased renal function.

Effect of Gender

The effect of gender on cetirizine pharmacokinetics has not been adequately studied.

Effect of Race

No race-related differences in the kinetics of cetirizine have been observed.

Renal Impairment

The kinetics of cetirizine were studied following multiple, oral, 10 mg daily doses of cetirizine for 7 days in 7 normal volunteers (creatinine clearance 89-128 ml/min), 8 patients with mild renal function impairment (creatinine clearance 42-77 ml/min) and 7 patients with moderate renal function impairment (creatinine clearance 11-31 ml/min). The pharmacokinetics of cetirizine were similar in patients with mild impairment and normal volunteers. Moderately impaired patients had a 3-fold increase in half-life and a 70% decrease in clearance compared to normal volunteers.

Patients on hemodialysis (n=5) given a single, 10 mg dose of cetirizine had a 3-fold increase in half-life and a 70% decrease in clearance compared to normal volunteers. Less than 10% of the administered dose was removed during the single dialysis session.

Dosing adjustment is necessary in patients with moderate or severe renal impairment and in patients on dialysis (see DOSAGE AND ADMINISTRATION).

Hepatic Impairment

Sixteen (16) patients with chronic liver diseases (hepatocellular, cholestatic, and biliary cirrhosis), given 10 or 20 mg of cetirizine as a single, oral dose had a 50% increase in half-life along with a corresponding 40% decrease in clearance compared to 16 healthy subjects.

Dosing adjustment may be necessary in patients with hepatic impairment (see DOSAGE AND ADMINISTRATION).

PHARMACODYNAMICS

Studies in 69 adult normal volunteers (aged 20-61 years) showed that cetirizine HCl at doses of 5 and 10 mg strongly inhibited the skin wheal and flare caused by the intradermal injection of histamine. The onset of this activity after a single 10 mg dose occurred within 20 minutes in 50% of subjects and within 1 hour in 95% of subjects; this activity persisted for at least 24 hours. Cetirizine HCl at doses of 5 and 10 mg also strongly inhibited the wheal and flare caused by intradermal injection of histamine in 19 pediatric volunteers (aged 5-12 years) and the activity persisted for at least 24 hours. In a 35 day study in children aged 5-12, no tolerance to the antihistaminic (suppression of wheal and flare response) effects of cetirizine HCl was found. In 10 infants 7-25 months of age who received 4-9 days of cetirizine in an oral solution (0.25 mg/kg bid), there was a 90% inhibition of histamine-induced (10 mg/ml) cutaneous wheal and 87% inhibition of the flare 12 hours after administration of the last dose. The clinical relevance of this suppression of histamine-induced wheal and flare response on skin testing is unknown.

The effects of intradermal injection of various other mediators or histamine releasers were also inhibited by cetirizine, as was response to a cold challenge in patients with cold-induced urticaria. In mildly asthmatic subjects, cetirizine HCl at 5-20 mg blocked bronchoconstriction due to nebulized histamine, with virtually total blockade after a 20 mg dose. In studies conducted for up to 12 hours following cutaneous antigen challenge, the late phase recruitment of eosinophils, neutrophils and basophils, components of the allergic inflammatory response, was inhibited by cetirizine HCl at a dose of 20 mg.

In four clinical studies in healthy adult males, no clinically significant mean increases in QTc were observed in cetirizine HCl treated subjects. In the first study, a placebo-controlled crossover trial, cetirizine HCl was given at doses up to 60 mg/day, 6 times the maximum clinical dose, for 1 week, and no significant mean QTc prolongation occurred. In the second study, a crossover trial, cetirizine HCl 20 mg and erythromycin (500 mg every 8 hours) were given alone and in combination. There was no significant effect on QTc with the combination or with cetirizine HCl alone. In the third trial, also a crossover study, cetirizine HCl 20 mg and ketoconazole (400 mg/day) were given alone and in combination. Cetirizine HCl caused a mean increase in QTc of 9.1 msec from baseline after 10 days of therapy. Ketoconazole also increased QTc by 8.3 msec. The combination caused an increase of 17.4 msec, equal to the sum of the individual effects. Thus, there was no significant drug interaction on QTc with the combination of cetirizine HCl and ketoconazole. In the fourth study, a placebo-controlled parallel trial, cetirizine HCl 20 mg was given alone or in combination with azithromycin (500 mg as a single dose on the first day followed by 250 mg once daily). There was no significant increase in QTc with cetirizine HCl 20 mg alone or in combination with azithromycin.

In a 4 week clinical trial in pediatric patients aged 6-11 years, results of randomly obtained ECG measurements before treatment and after 2 weeks of treatment showed that cetirizine HCl 5 or 10 mg did not increase QTc versus placebo. In a 1 week clinical trial (n=86) of cetirizine HCl syrup (0.25 mg/kg bid) compared with placebo in pediatric patients 6-11 months of age, ECG measurements taken within 3 hours of the last dose did not show any ECG abnormalities or increases in QTc interval in either group compared to baseline assessments. Data from other studies where cetirizine HCl was administered to patients 6-23 months of age were consistent with the findings in this study.

The effects of cetirizine HCl on the QTc interval at doses higher than the 10 mg dose have not been studied in children less than 12 years of age.

In a 6 week, placebo-controlled study of 186 patients (aged 12-64 years) with allergic rhinitis and mild to moderate asthma, cetirizine HCl 10 mg once daily improved rhinitis symptoms and did not alter pulmonary function. In a 2 week, placebo-controlled clinical trial, a subset analysis of 65 pediatric (aged 6-11 years) allergic rhinitis patients with asthma showed cetirizine HCl did not alter pulmonary function. These studies support the safety of administering cetirizine HCl to pediatric and adult allergic rhinitis patients with mild to moderate asthma.

INDICATIONS AND USAGE

SEASONAL ALLERGIC RHINITIS

Cetirizine HCl is indicated for the relief of symptoms associated with seasonal allergic rhinitis due to allergens such as ragweed, grass and tree pollens in adults and children 2 years of age and older. Symptoms treated effectively include sneezing, rhinorrhea, nasal pruritus, ocular pruritus, tearing, and redness of the eyes.

PERENNIAL ALLERGIC RHINITIS:

Cetirizine HCl is indicated for the relief of symptoms associated with perennial allergic rhinitis due to allergens such as dust mites, animal dander and molds in adults and children 6 months of age and older. Symptoms treated effectively include sneezing, rhinorrhea, post-nasal discharge, nasal pruritus, ocular pruritus, and tearing.

CHRONIC URTICARIA

Cetirizine HCl is indicated for the treatment of the uncomplicated skin manifestations of chronic idiopathic urticaria in adults and children 6 months of age and older. It significantly reduces the occurrence, severity, and duration of hives and significantly reduces pruritus.

CONTRAINDICATIONS

Cetirizine HCl is contraindicated in those patients with a known hypersensitivity to it or any of its ingredients or hydroxyzine.

PRECAUTIONS

ACTIVITIES REQUIRING MENTAL ALERTNESS

In clinical trials, the occurrence of somnolence has been reported in some patients taking cetirizine HCl; due caution should therefore be exercised when driving a car or operating potentially dangerous machinery. Concurrent use of cetirizine HCl with alcohol or other CNS depressants should be avoided because additional reductions in alertness and additional impairment of CNS performance may occur.

CARCINOGENESIS, MUTAGENESIS, AND IMPAIRMENT OF FERTILITY

In a 2 year carcinogenicity study in rats, cetirizine was not carcinogenic at dietary doses up to 20 mg/kg (approximately 15 times the maximum recommended daily oral dose in adults on a mg/m^2 basis, or approximately 7 times the maximum recommended daily oral dose in infants on a mg/m^2 basis). In a 2 year carcinogenicity study in mice, cetirizine caused an increased incidence of benign liver tumors in males at a dietary dose of 16 mg/kg (approximately 6 times the maximum recommended daily oral dose in adults on a mg/m^2 basis, or approximately 3 times the maximum recommended daily oral dose in infants on a mg/m^2 basis). No increase in the incidence of liver tumors was observed in mice at a dietary dose of 4 mg/kg (approximately 2 times the maximum recommended daily oral dose in adults on a mg/m^2 basis, or approximately equivalent to the maximum recommended daily oral dose in infants on a mg/m^2 basis). The clinical significance of these findings during long-term use of cetirizine HCl is not known.

Cetirizine was not mutagenic in the Ames test, and not clastogenic in the human lymphocyte assay, the mouse lymphoma assay, and *in vivo* micronucleus test in rats.

In a fertility and general reproductive performance study in mice, cetirizine did not impair fertility at an oral dose of 64 mg/kg (approximately 25 times the maximum recommended daily oral dose in adults on a mg/m^2 basis).

PREGNANCY CATEGORY B

In mice, rats, and rabbits, cetirizine was not teratogenic at oral doses up to 96, 225, and 135 mg/kg, respectively (approximately 40, 180, and 220 times the maximum recommended daily oral dose in adults on a mg/m^2 basis). There are no adequate and well-controlled studies in pregnant women. Because animal studies are not always predictive of human response, cetirizine HCl should be used in pregnancy only if clearly needed.

NURSING MOTHERS

In mice, cetirizine caused retarded pup weight gain during lactation at an oral dose in dams of 96 mg/kg (approximately 40 times the maximum recommended daily oral dose in adults on a mg/m^2 basis). Studies in beagle dogs indicated that approximately 3% of the dose was excreted in milk. Cetirizine has been reported to be excreted in human breast milk. Because many drugs are excreted in human milk, use of cetirizine HCl in nursing mothers is not recommended.

GERIATRIC USE

Of the total number of patients in clinical studies of cetirizine HCl, 186 patients were 65 years and older, and 39 patients were 75 years and older. No overall differences in safety were observed between these patients and younger patients, but greater sensitivity of some older individuals cannot be ruled out. With regard to efficacy, clinical studies of cetirizine HCl for each approved indication did not include sufficient numbers of patients aged 65 years and older to determine whether they respond differently than younger patients.

Cetirizine HCl is known to be substantially excreted by the kidney, and the risk of toxic reactions to this drug may be greater in patients with impaired renal function. Because elderly patients are more likely to have decreased renal function, care should be taken in dose selection, and it may be useful to monitor renal function. (See CLINICAL PHARMACOLOGY, Special Populations: Geriatric Patients and Renal Impairment.)

PEDIATRIC USE

The safety of cetirizine HCl has been demonstrated in pediatric patients aged 6 months to 11 years. The safety of cetirizine HCl, at daily doses of 5 or 10 mg, has been demonstrated in 376 pediatric patients aged 6-11 years in placebo-controlled trials lasting up to 4 weeks and in 254 patients in a non-placebo-controlled 12 week trial. The safety of cetirizine has been demonstrated in 168 patients aged 2-5 years in placebo-controlled trials of up to 4 weeks duration. On a mg/kg basis, most of the 168 patients received between 0.2 and 0.4 mg/kg of cetirizine HCl. The safety of cetirizine in 399 patients aged 12-24 months has been demonstrated in a placebo-controlled 18 month trial, in which the average dose was 0.25 mg/kg bid, corresponding to a range of 4-11 mg/day. The safety of cetirizine HCl syrup has been demonstrated in 42 patients aged 6-11 months in a placebo-controlled 7 day trial. The prescribed dose was 0.25 mg/kg bid, which corresponded to a mean of 4.5 mg/day, with a range of 3.4-6.2 mg/day.

The effectiveness of cetirizine HCl for the treatment of allergic rhinitis and chronic idiopathic urticaria in pediatric patients aged 6 months to 11 years is based on an extrapolation of the demonstrated efficacy of cetirizine HCl in adults in these conditions and the likelihood that the disease course, pathophysiology and the drug's effect are substantially similar between these two populations. Efficacy is extrapolated down to 6 months of age for perennial allergic rhinitis and down to 2 years of age for seasonal allergic rhinitis became these diseases are thought to occur down to these ages in children. The recommended doses for the pediatric population are based on cross-study comparisons of the pharmacokinetics and pharmacodynamics of cetirizine in adult and pediatric subjects and on the safety profile of cetirizine in both adult and pediatric patients at doses equal to or higher than the recommended doses. The cetirizine AUC and C_{max} in pediatric subjects aged 6-23 months who received a mean of 2.3 mg in a single dose and in subjects aged 2-5 years who received a single dose of 5 mg of cetirizine syrup and in pediatric subjects aged 6-11 years who received a single dose of 10 mg of cetirizine syrup were estimated to be intermediate between that observed in adults who received a single dose of 10 mg of cetirizine tablets and those who received a single dose of 20 mg of cetirizine tablets.

The safety and effectiveness of cetirizine in pediatric patients under the age of 6 months have not been established.

DRUG INTERACTIONS

No clinically significant drug interactions have been found with theophylline at a low dose, azithromycin, pseudoephedrine, ketoconazole, or erythromycin. There was a small decrease in the clearance of cetirizine caused by a 400 mg dose of theophylline; it is possible that larger theophylline doses could have a greater effect.

ADVERSE REACTIONS

Controlled and uncontrolled clinical trials conducted in the US and Canada included more than 6000 patients aged 12 years and older, with more than 3900 receiving cetirizine HCl at doses of 5-20 mg/day. The duration of treatment ranged from 1 week to 6 months, with a mean exposure of 30 days.

Most adverse reactions reported during therapy with cetirizine HCl were mild or moderate. In placebo-controlled trials, the incidence of discontinuations due to adverse reactions in patients receiving cetirizine HCl 5 or 10 mg was not significantly different from placebo (2.9% vs 2.4%, respectively).

The most common adverse reaction in patients aged 12 years and older that occurred more frequently on cetirizine HCl than placebo was somnolence. The incidence of somnolence associated with cetirizine HCl was dose related, 6% in placebo, 11% at 5 mg and 14% at 10 mg. Discontinuations due to somnolence for cetirizine HCl were uncommon (1.0% on cetirizine HCl vs 0.6% on placebo). Fatigue and dry mouth also appeared to be treatment-related adverse reactions. There were no differences by age, race, gender, or by body weight with regard to the incidence of adverse reactions.

TABLE 1 lists adverse experiences in patients aged 12 years and older which were reported for cetirizine HCl 5 and 10 mg in controlled clinical trials in the US and that were more common with cetirizine HCl than placebo.

In addition, headache and nausea occurred in more than 2% of the patients, but were more common in placebo patients.

Pediatric studies were also conducted with cetirizine HCl. More than 1300 pediatric patients aged 6-11 years with more than 900 treated with cetirizine HCl at doses of 1.25-10 mg/day were included in controlled and uncontrolled clinical trials conducted in the US. The duration of treatment ranged from 2-12 weeks. Placebo-controlled trials up to 4 weeks duration included 168 pediatric patients aged 2-5 years who received cetirizine, the majority of whom received single daily doses of 5 mg. A placebo-controlled trial 18 months in duration included 399 patients aged 12-24 months treated with cetirizine (0.25 mg/kg bid), and

TABLE 1 *Adverse Experiences Reported in Patients Aged 12 Years and Older in Placebo-Controlled US Cetirizine HCl Trials (Maximum Dose of 10 mg) at Rates of 2% or Greater (Percent Incidence)*

Adverse Experience	Cetirizine HCl (n=2034)	Placebo (n=1612)
Somnolence	13.7%	6.3%
Fatigue	5.9%	2.6%
Dry mouth	5.0%	2.3%
Pharyngitis	2.0%	1.9%
Dizziness	2.0%	1.2%

another placebo-controlled trial of 7 days duration included 42 patients aged 6-11 months who were treated with cetirizine (0.25 mg/kg bid).

The majority of adverse reactions reported in pediatric patients aged 2-11 years with cetirizine HCl were mild or moderate. In placebo-controlled trials, the incidence of discontinuations due to adverse reactions in pediatric patients receiving up to 10 mg of cetirizine HCl was uncommon (0.4% on cetirizine HCl versus 1.0% on placebo).

TABLE 2 lists adverse experiences which were reported for cetirizine HCl 5 and 10 mg in pediatric patients aged 6-11 years in placebo-controlled clinical trials in the US and were more common with cetirizine HCl than placebo. Of these, abdominal pain was considered treatment-related and somnolence appeared to be dose-related, 1.3% in placebo, 1.9% at 5 mg, and 4.2% at 10 mg. The adverse experiences reported in pediatric patients aged 2-5 years in placebo-controlled trials were qualitatively similar in nature and generally similar in frequency to those reported in trials with children aged 6-11 years.

In the placebo-controlled trials of pediatric patients 6-24 months of age, the incidences of adverse experiences, were similar in the cetirizine and placebo treatment groups in each study. Somnolence occurred with essentially the same frequency in patients who received cetirizine and patients who received placebo. In a study of 1 week duration in children 6-11 months of age, patients who received cetirizine exhibited greater irritability/fussiness than patients on placebo. In a study of 18 months duration in patients 12 months and older, insomnia occurred more frequently in patients who received cetirizine compared to patients who received placebo (9.0% vs 5.3%). In those patients who received 5 mg or more per day of cetirizine as compared to patients who received placebo, fatigue (3.6% vs 1.3%) and malaise (3.6% vs 1.8%) occurred more frequently.

TABLE 2 *Adverse Experiences Reported in Pediatric Patients Aged 6-11 Years in Placebo-Controlled US Cetirizine HCl Trials (5 or 10 mg Dose) Which Occurred at a Frequency of ≥2% in Either the 5 or the 10 mg Cetirizine HCl Group, and More Frequently Than in the Placebo Group*

		Cetirizine HCl	
Adverse Experiences	Placebo (n=309)	5 mg (n=161)	10 mg (n=215)
Headache	12.3%	11.0%	14.0%
Pharyngitis	2.9%	6.2%	2.8%
Abdominal pain	1.9%	4.4%	5.6%
Coughing	3.9%	4.4%	2.8%
Somnolence	1.3%	1.9%	4.2%
Diarrhea	1.3%	3.1%	1.9%
Epistaxis	2.9%	3.7%	1.9%
Bronchospasm	1.9%	3.1%	1.9%
Nausea	1.9%	1.9%	2.8%
Vomiting	1.0%	2.5%	2.3%

The following events were observed infrequently (less than 2%), in either 3982 adults and children 12 years and older or in 659 pediatric patients aged 6-11 years who received cetirizine HCl in US trials, including an open adult study of 6 months duration. A causal relationship of these infrequent events with cetirizine HCl administration has not been established.

Autonomic Nervous System: Anorexia, flushing, increased salivation, urinary retention.

Cardiovascular: Cardiac failure, hypertension, palpitation, tachycardia.

Central and Peripheral Nervous Systems: Abnormal coordination, ataxia, confusion, dysphonia, hyperesthesia, hyperkinesia, hypertonia, hypoesthesia, leg cramps, migraine, myelitis, paralysis, paresthesia, ptosis, syncope, tremor, twitching, vertigo, visual field defect.

Gastrointestinal: Abnormal hepatic function, aggravated tooth caries, constipation, dyspepsia, eructation, flatulence, gastritis, hemorrhoids, increased appetite, melena, rectal hemorrhage, stomatitis including ulcerative stomatitis, tongue discoloration, tongue edema.

Genitourinary: Cystitis, dysuria, hematuria, micturition frequency, polyuria, urinary incontinence, urinary tract infection.

Hearing and Vestibular: Deafness, earache, ototoxicity, tinnitus.

Metabolic/Nutritional: Dehydration, diabetes mellitus, thirst.

Musculoskeletal: Arthralgia, arthritis, arthrosis, muscle weakness, myalgia.

Psychiatric: Abnormal thinking, agitation, amnesia, anxiety, decreased libido, depersonalization, depression, emotional lability, euphoria, impaired concentration, insomnia, nervousness, paroniria, sleep disorder.

Respiratory System: Bronchitis, dyspnea, hyperventilation, increased sputum, pneumonia, respiratory disorder, rhinitis, sinusitis, upper respiratory tract infection.

Reproductive: Dysmenorrhea, female breast pain, intermenstrual bleeding, leukorrhea, menorrhagia, vaginitis.

Reticuloendothelial: Lymphadenopathy.

Skin: Acne, alopecia, angioedema, bullous eruption, dermatitis, dry skin, eczema, erythematous rash, furunculosis, hyperkeratosis, hypertrichosis, increased sweating, maculopapular rash, photosensitivity reaction, photosensitivity toxic reaction, pruritus, purpura, rash, seborrhea, skin disorder, skin nodule, urticaria.

Special Senses: Parosmia, taste loss, taste perversion.

Vision: Blindness, conjunctivitis, eye pain, glaucoma, loss of accommodation, ocular hemorrhage, xerophthalmia.

Body as a Whole: Accidental injury, asthenia, back pain, chest pain, enlarged abdomen, face edema, fever, generalized edema, hot flashes, increased weight, leg edema, malaise, nasal polyp, pain, pallor, periorbital edema, peripheral edema, rigors.

Occasional instances of transient, reversible hepatic transaminase elevations have occurred during cetirizine therapy. Hepatitis with significant transaminase elevation and elevated bilirubin in association with the use of cetirizine HCl has been reported.

In foreign marketing experience the following additional rare, but potentially severe adverse events have been reported: Anaphylaxis, cholestasis, glomerulonephritis, hemolytic anemia, hepatitis, orofacial dyskinesia, severe hypotension, stillbirth, and thrombocytopenia.

DOSAGE AND ADMINISTRATION

ADULTS AND CHILDREN 12 YEARS AND OLDER

The recommended initial dose of cetirizine HCl is 5 or 10 mg/day in adults and children 12 years and older, depending on symptom severity. Most patients in clinical trials started at 10 mg. Cetirizine HCl is given as a single daily dose, with or without food. The time of administration may be varied to suit individual patient needs.

CHILDREN 6-11 YEARS

The recommended initial dose of cetirizine HCl in children aged 6-11 years is 5 or 10 mg (1 or 2 teaspoons) once daily depending on symptom severity. The time of administration may be varied to suit individual patient needs.

CHILDREN 2-5 YEARS

The recommended initial dose of cetirizine HCl syrup in children aged 2-5 years is 2.5 mg (½ teaspoon) once daily. The dosage in this age group can be increased to a maximum dose of 5 mg/day given as 1 teaspoon (5 mg) once daily, or as ½ teaspoon (2.5 mg) given every 12 hours.

CHILDREN 6 MONTHS TO <2 YEARS

The recommended dose of cetirizine HCl syrup in children 6-23 months of age is 2.5 mg (½ teaspoon) once daily. The dose in children 12-23 months of age can be increased to a maximum dose of 5 mg/day, given as ½ teaspoonful (2.5 mg) every 12 hours.

DOSE ADJUSTMENT FOR RENAL AND HEPATIC IMPAIRMENT

In patients 12 years of age and older with decreased renal function (creatinine clearance 11-31 ml/min), patients on hemodialysis (creatinine clearance less than 7 ml/min), and in hepatically impaired patients, a dose of 5 mg once daily is recommended. Similarly, pediatric patients aged 6-11 years with impaired renal or hepatic function should use the lower recommended dose. Because of the difficulty in reliably administering doses of less than 2.5 mg (½ teaspoon) of cetirizine HCl syrup and in the absence of pharmacokinetic and safety information for cetirizine in children below the age of 6 years with impaired renal or hepatic function, its use in this impaired patient population is not recommended.

HOW SUPPLIED

ZYRTEC TABLETS

5 mg: White, film-coated, rounded-off rectangular shaped tablets containing 5 mg cetirizine HCl and engraved with "ZYRTEC" on one side and "5" on the other.

10 mg: White, film-coated, rounded-off rectangular shaped tablets containing 10 mg cetirizine HCl and engraved with "ZYRTEC" on one side and "10" on the other.

Storage: Store at 20-25°C (68-77°F) excursions permitted to 15-30°C (59-86°F).

ZYRTEC SYRUP

Zyrtec syrup is colorless to slightly yellow with a banana-grape flavor. Each teaspoonful (5 ml) contains 5 mg cetirizine HCl.

Storage: Store at 20-25°C (68-77°F) excursions permitted to 15-30°C (36-46°F) or **store refrigerated, 2-8°C (36-46°F).**

PRODUCT LISTING - EQUIVALENTS NOT AVAILABLE

Syrup - Oral - 1 mg/ml

120 ml	$28.03	ZYRTEC, Allscripts Pharmaceutical Company	54569-4509-00
120 ml	$30.83	ZYRTEC, Pfizer U.S. Pharmaceuticals	00069-5530-47
473 ml	$123.30	ZYRTEC, Pfizer U.S. Pharmaceuticals	00069-5530-93

Tablet - Oral - 5 mg

14's	$24.71	ZYRTEC, Allscripts Pharmaceutical Company	54569-4312-00
100's	$210.95	ZYRTEC, Pfizer U.S. Pharmaceuticals	00069-5500-66

Tablet - Oral - 10 mg

5's	$9.59	ZYRTEC, Allscripts Pharmaceutical Company	54569-4290-01
7's	$21.47	ZYRTEC, Pharma Pac	52959-0482-07
7's	$27.05	ZYRTEC, Pd-Rx Pharmaceuticals	55289-0108-07
10's	$20.00	ZYRTEC, Physicians Total Care	54868-3876-02
10's	$29.86	ZYRTEC, Pharma Pac	52959-0482-10
14's	$24.71	ZYRTEC, Allscripts Pharmaceutical Company	54569-4290-00
14's	$39.15	ZYRTEC, Pd-Rx Pharmaceuticals	55289-0108-14
15's	$39.59	ZYRTEC, Pharma Pac	52959-0482-15
20's	$40.76	ZYRTEC, Southwood Pharmaceuticals Inc	58016-0367-20
20's	$41.05	ZYRTEC, Physicians Total Care	54868-3876-01
25's	$62.65	ZYRTEC, Pd-Rx Pharmaceuticals	55289-0108-25
30's	$52.95	ZYRTEC, Allscripts Pharmaceutical Company	54569-4290-02

30's	$57.66	ZYRTEC, Physicians Total Care	54868-3876-00
30's	$61.14	ZYRTEC, Southwood Pharmaceuticals Inc	58016-0367-30
30's	$75.15	ZYRTEC, Pd-Rx Pharmaceuticals	55289-0108-30
30's	$77.15	ZYRTEC, Pharma Pac	52959-0482-30
50's	$109.47	ZYRTEC, Physicians Total Care	54868-3876-04
60's	$114.14	ZYRTEC, Physicians Total Care	54868-3876-03
100's	$210.95	ZYRTEC, Pfizer U.S. Pharmaceuticals	00069-5510-66

C

Cetirizine Hydrochloride; Pseudoephedrine Hydrochloride *(003539)*

For complete prescribing information, refer to the CD-ROM included with the book.

Categories: FDA Approved 2001 Aug; Pregnancy Category C
Brand Names: Zyrtec-D
Foreign Brand Availability: Acidrine-D (Colombia); Alercet-D (Colombia; Peru); Cipan (Korea); Cirrus (Singapore); Cetirax D (Colombia); Lergium Plus (Peru); Zyrtec Decongestant (New-Zealand)
Cost of Therapy: $63.29 (Allergic Rhinitis; Zyrtec-D; 5 mg; 120 mg; 2 tablets/day; 30 day supply)

DESCRIPTION

Note: The trade name has been used throughout this monograph for clarity.

Zyrtec-D 12 Hour (cetirizine hydrochloride 5 mg and pseudoephedrine hydrochloride 120 mg) extended-release tablets for oral administration contain 5 mg of cetirizine hydrochloride for immediate release and 120 mg of pseudoephedrine hydrochloride for extended-release in a bilayer tablet. Tablets also contain as inactive ingredients: colloidal silicon dioxide, croscarmellose sodium, hydroxypropyl methylcellulose, lactose monohydrate, magnesium stearate, microcrystalline cellulose.

Cetirizine hydrochloride, one of the two active components of Zyrtec-D 12 Hour extended-release tablets, is an orally active and selective H_1-receptor antagonist. The chemical name is (+/-)-[2-[4-[(4-chlorophenyl)phenylmethyl]-1-piperazinyl]ethoxy] acetic acid, dihydrochloride. Cetirizine hydrochloride is a racemic compound with an empirical formula of $C_{21}H_{25}ClN_2O_3{\cdot}2HCl$. The molecular weight is 461.82. Cetirizine hydrochloride is a white, crystalline powder and is water-soluble.

Pseudoephedrine hydrochloride, the other active ingredient of Zyrtec-D 12 Hour extended-release tablets, is an adrenergic (vasoconstrictor) agent with the chemical name (1S.2S)-2-methylamino-1-phenyl-1-propanol hydrochloride. The molecular weight is 201.70. The molecular formula is $C_{10}H_{15}NO{\cdot}HCl$. Pseudoephedrine hydrochloride occurs as fine, white to off-white crystals or powder, having a faint characteristic odor. It is very soluble in water, freely soluble in alcohol, and sparingly soluble in chloroform.

INDICATIONS AND USAGE

Zyrtec-D 12 Hour extended-release tablets should be administered when both the antihistaminic properties of cetirizine hydrochloride and the nasal decongestant properties of pseudoephedrine hydrochloride are desired.

Zyrtec-D 12 Hour extended-release tablets are indicated for the relief of nasal and non-nasal symptoms associated with seasonal or perennial allergic rhinitis in adults and children 12 years of age and older.

CONTRAINDICATIONS

Zyrtec-D 12 Hour extended-release tablets are contraindicated in patients with a known hypersensitivity to any of its ingredients or to hydroxyzine.

Due to its pseudoephedrine component, Zyrtec-D 12 Hour extended-release tablets are contraindicated in patients with narrow-angle glaucoma or urinary retention, and in patients receiving monoamine oxidase (MAO) inhibitor therapy or within 14 days of stopping such treatment. It is also contraindicated in patients with severe hypertension, or severe coronary artery disease, and in those who have shown hypersensitivity or idiosyncrasy to its components, to adrenergic agents, or to other drugs of similar 7 chemical structures. Manifestations of patient idiosyncrasy to adrenergic agents include insomnia, dizziness, weakness, tremor, or arrhythmias.

WARNINGS

Sympathomimetic amines should be used judiciously and sparingly in patients with hypertension, diabetes mellitus, ischemic heart disease, increased intraocular pressure, hyperthyroidism, renal impairment, or prostatic hypertrophy (see CONTRAINDICATIONS). Sympathomimetic amines may produce central nervous system stimulation with convulsions or cardiovascular collapse with accompanying hypotension. The elderly are more likely to have adverse reactions to sympathomimetic amines.

DOSAGE AND ADMINISTRATION

ADULTS AND CHILDREN 12 YEARS OF AGE AND OLDER

The recommended dose of Zyrtec-D 12 Hour extended-release tablets is 1 tablet twice daily for adults and children 12 years of age and older. Zyrtec-D 12 Hour extended-release tablets may be given with or without food.

DOSE ADJUSTMENT FOR RENAL AND HEPATIC IMPAIRMENT

In patients with decreased renal function (creatinine clearance 11-31 ml/min), patients on hemodialysis (creatinine clearance less than 7 ml/min), and in hepatically impaired patients, a dose of 1 tablet once daily is recommended.

Zyrtec-D 12 Hour extended-release tablets should be swallowed whole, and should not be broken or chewed.

PRODUCT LISTING - EQUIVALENTS NOT AVAILABLE

Tablet, Extended Release - Oral - 5 mg;120 mg

100's	$105.48	ZYRTEC-D, Pfizer U.S. Pharmaceuticals	00069-1630-66

Cevimeline Hydrochloride *(003469)*

Categories: FDA Approved 2000 Jan; Pregnancy Category C
Drug Classes: Cholinergics
Brand Names: Evoxac
Cost of Therapy: $128.75 (Sjogren's Syndrome; Evoxac; 30 mg; 3 capsules/day; 30 day supply)

DESCRIPTION

Cevimeline is cis-2′-methylspiro[1-azabicyclo [2.2.2] octane - 3,5′-[1,3] oxathiolane] hydrochloride, hydrate (2:1). Its empirical formula is $C_{10}H_{17}NOS{\cdot}HCl{\cdot}½H_2O$.

Cevimeline has a molecular weight of 244.79. It is a white to off white crystalline powder with a melting point range of 201-203°C. It is freely soluble in alcohol and chloroform, very soluble in water, and virtually insoluble in ether. The pH of a 1% solution ranges from 4.6-5.6. Inactive ingredients include lactose monohydrate, hydroxypropyl cellulose, and magnesium stearate.

CLINICAL PHARMACOLOGY

PHARMACODYNAMICS

Cevimeline is a cholinergic agonist which binds to muscarinic receptors. Muscarinic agonists in sufficient dosage can increase secretion of exocrine glands, such as salivary and sweat glands and increase tone of the smooth muscle in the gastrointestinal and urinary tracts.

PHARMACOKINETICS

Absorption

After administration of a single 30 mg capsule, cevimeline was rapidly absorbed with a mean time to peak concentration of 1.5-2 hours. No accumulation of active drug or its metabolites was observed following multiple dose administration. When administered with food, there is a decrease in the rate of absorption, with a fasting T_{max} of 1.53 hours and a T_{max} of 2.86 hours after a meal; the peak concentration is reduced by 17.3%. Single oral doses across the clinical dose range are dose proportional.

Distribution

Cevimeline has a volume of distribution of approximately 6 L/kg and is <20% bound to human plasma proteins. This suggests that cevimeline is extensively bound to tissues; however, the specific binding sites are unknown.

Metabolism

Isozymes CYP2D6 and CYP3A3/4 are responsible for the metabolism of cevimeline. After 24 hours 86.7% of the dose was recovered (16.0% Unchanged, 44.5% as cis and trans-sulfoxide, 22.3% of the dose as glucuronic acid conjugate and 4% of the dose as N-oxide of cevimeline). Approximately 8% of the trans-sulfoxide metabolite is then converted into the corresponding glucuronic acid conjugate and eliminated. Cevimeline did not inhibit cytochrome P450 isozymes 1A2, 2A6, 2C9, 2C19, 2D6, 2E1, and 3A4.

Excretion

The mean half-life of cevimeline is 5 ± 1 hours. After 24 hours, 84% of a 30 mg dose of cevimeline was excreted in urine. After 7 days, 97% of the dose was recovered in the urine and 0.5% was recovered in the feces.

Special Populations

The effects of renal impairment, hepatic impairment, or ethnicity on the pharmacokinetics of cevimeline have not been investigated.

INDICATIONS AND USAGE

Cevimeline is indicated for the treatment of symptoms of dry mouth in patients with Sjögren's Syndrome.

CONTRAINDICATIONS

Cevimeline is contraindicated in patients with uncontrolled asthma, known hypersensitivity to cevimeline, and when miosis is undesirable, *e.g.,* in acute iritis and in narrow-angle (angle-closure) glaucoma.

WARNINGS

CARDIOVASCULAR DISEASE

Cevimeline can potentially alter cardiac conduction and/or heart rate. Patients with significant cardiovascular disease may potentially be unable to compensate for transient changes in hemodynamics or rhythm induced by cevimeline HCl. Cevimeline HCl should be used with caution and under close medical supervision in patients with a history of cardiovascular disease evidenced by angina pectoris or myocardial infarction.

PULMONARY DISEASE

Cevimeline can potentially increase airway resistance, bronchial smooth muscle tone, and bronchial secretions. Cevimeline should be administered with caution and with close medical supervision to patients with controlled asthma, chronic bronchitis, or chronic obstructive pulmonary disease.

OCULAR

Ophthalmic formulations of muscarinic agonists have been reported to cause visual blurring which may result in decreased visual acuity, especially at night and in patients with central lens changes, and to cause impairment of depth perception. Caution should be advised while driving at night or performing hazardous activities in reduced lighting.

PRECAUTIONS

GENERAL

Cevimeline toxicity is characterized by an exaggeration of its parasympathomimetic effects. These may include: headache, visual disturbance, lacrimation, sweating, respiratory distress, gastrointestinal spasm, nausea, vomiting, diarrhea, atrioventricular block, tachycardia, bradycardia, hypotension, hypertension, shock, mental confusion, cardiac arrhythmia, and tremors.

Cevimeline should be administered with caution to patients with a history of nephrolithiasis or cholelithiasis. Contractions of the gallbladder or biliary smooth muscle could precipitate complications such as cholecystitis, cholangitis and biliary obstruction. An increase in the ureteral smooth muscle tone could theoretically precipitate renal colic or ureteral reflux in patients with nephrolithiasis.

INFORMATION FOR THE PATIENT

Patients should be informed that cevimeline may cause visual disturbances, especially at night, that could impair their ability to drive safely.

If a patient sweats excessively while taking cevimeline, dehydration may develop. The patient should drink extra water and consult a health care provider.

CARCINOGENESIS, MUTAGENESIS, AND IMPAIRMENT OF FERTILITY

Lifetime carcinogenicity studies were conducted in CD-1 mice and F-344 rats. A statistically significant increase in the incidence of adenocarcinomas of the uterus was observed in female rats that received cevimeline at a dosage of 100 mg/kg/day (approximately 8 times the maximum human exposure based on comparison of AUC data). No other significant differences in tumor incidence were observed in either mice or rats.

Cevimeline exhibited no evidence of mutagenicity or clastogenicity in a battery of assays that included an Ames test, an *in vitro* chromosomal aberration study in mammalian cells, a mouse lymphoma study in L5178Y cells, or a micronucleus assay conducted *in vivo* in ICR mice.

Cevimeline did not adversely affect the reproductive performance or fertility of male Sprague-Dawley rats when administered for 63 days prior to mating and throughout the period of mating at dosages up to 45 mg/kg/day (approximately 5 times the maximum recommended dose for a 60 kg human following normalization of the data on the basis of body surface area estimates). Females that were treated with cevimeline at dosages up to 45 mg/kg/day from 14 days prior to mating through day 7 of gestation exhibited a statistically significantly smaller number of implantations than did control animals.

PREGNANCY CATEGORY C

Cevimeline was associated with a reduction in the mean number of implantations when given to pregnant Sprague-Dawley rats from 14 days prior to mating through day 7 of gestation at a dosage of 45 mg/kg/day (approximately 5 times the maximum recommended dose for a 60 kg human when compared on the basis of body surface area estimates). This effect may have been secondary to maternal toxicity. There are no adequate and well-controlled studies in pregnant women. Cevimeline should be used during pregnancy only if the potential benefit justifies the potential risk to the fetus.

NURSING MOTHERS

It is not known whether this drug is secreted in human milk. Because many drugs are excreted in human milk, and because of the potential for serious adverse reactions in nursing infants from cevimeline HCl, a decision should be made whether to discontinue nursing or discontinue the drug, taking into account the importance of the drug to the mother.

PEDIATRIC USE

Safety and effectiveness in pediatric patients have not been established.

GERIATRIC USE

Although clinical studies of cevimeline included subjects over the age of 65, the numbers were not sufficient to determine whether they respond differently from younger subjects. Special care should be exercised when cevimeline treatment is initiated in an elderly patient, considering the greater frequency of decreased hepatic, renal, or cardiac function, and of concomitant disease or other drug therapy in the elderly.

DRUG INTERACTIONS

Cevimeline should be administered with caution to patients taking beta adrenergic antagonists, because of the possibility of conduction disturbances. Drugs with parasympathomimetic effects administered concurrently with cevimeline can be expected to have additive effects. Cevimeline might interfere with desirable antimuscarinic effects of drugs used concomitantly.

Drugs which inhibit CYP2D6 and CYP3A3/4 also inhibit the metabolism of cevimeline. Cevimeline should be used with caution in individuals known or suspected to be deficient in CYP2D6 activity, based on previous experience, as they may be at a higher risk of adverse events. In an *in vitro* study cytochrome P450 isozymes 1A2, 2A6, 2C9, 2C19, 2D6, 2E1, and 3A4 were not inhibited by exposure to cevimeline.

ADVERSE REACTIONS

Cevimeline was administered to 1777 patients during clinical trials worldwide, including Sjögren's patients and patients with other conditions. In placebo-controlled studies in the United States, 484 patients received cevimeline doses ranging from 15 mg tid to 60 mg tid, of whom 94% were women and 6% were men. Demographic distribution was 90% Caucasian, 5% Hispanic, 2% Black, and 3% of other origin. In these studies, 11.1% of patients discontinued treatment with cevimeline due to adverse events.

The following adverse events associated with muscarinic agonism were observed in the clinical trials of cevimeline in Sjögren's syndrome patients (see TABLE 1).

In addition, the following adverse events (≥3% incidence) were reported in the Sjögren's clinical trials (see TABLE 2).

TABLE 1

Adverse Event	Cevimeline 30 mg (tid) n=533	Placebo (tid) n=164
Excessive sweating	18.7%	2.4%
Nausea	13.8%	7.9%
Rhinitis	11.2%	5.4%
Diarrhea	10.3%	10.3%
Excessive salivation	2.2%	0.6%
Urinary frequency	0.9%	1.8%
Asthenia	0.5%	0%
Flushing	0.3%	0.6%
Polyuria	0.1%	0.6%

* n is the total number of patients exposed to the dose at any time during the study.

TABLE 2

Adverse Event	Cevimeline 30 mg (tid) n*=533	Placebo (tid) n=164
Headache	14.4%	20.1%
Sinusitis	12.3%	10.9%
Upper respiratory tract infection	11.4%	9.1%
Dyspepsia	7.8%	8.5%
Abdominal pain	7.6%	6.7%
Urinary tract infection	6.1%	3.0%
Coughing	6.1%	3.0%
Pharyngitis	5.2%	5.4%
Vomiting	4.6%	2.4%
Injury	4.5%	2.4%
Back pain	4.5%	4.2%
Rash	4.3%	6.0%
Conjunctivitis	4.3%	3.6%
Dizziness	4.1%	7.3%
Bronchitis	4.1%	1.2%
Arthralgia	3.7%	1.8%
Surgical intervention	3.3%	3.0%
Fatigue	3.3%	1.2%
Pain	3.3%	3.0%
Skeletal pain	2.8%	1.8%
Insomnia	2.4%	1.2%
Hot flushes	2.4%	0%
Rigors	1.3%	1.2%
Anxiety	1.3%	1.2%

* n is the total number of patients exposed to the dose at any time during the study.

The following events were reported in sjögren's patients at incidences of <3% and ≥1%: Constipation, tremor, abnormal vision, hypertonia, peripheral edema, chest pain, myalgia, fever, anorexia, eye pain, ear ache, dry mouth, vertigo, salivary gland pain, pruritus, influenza-like symptoms, eye infection, post-operative pain, vaginitis, skin disorder, depression, hiccup, hyporeflexia, infection, fungal infection, sialoadenitis, otitis media, erythematous rash, pneumonia, edema, salivary gland enlargement, allergy, gastroesophageal reflux, eye abnormality, migraine, tooth disorder, epistaxis, flatulence, tooth ache, ulcerative stomatitis, anemia, hypoesthesia, cystitis, leg cramps, abscess, eructation, moniliasis, palpitation, increased amylase, xerophthalmia, and allergic reaction.

The following events were reported rarely in treated Sjögren's patients (<1%); causal relation is unknown:

Body as a Whole Disorders: Aggravated allergy, precordial chest pain, abnormal crying, hematoma, leg pain, edema, periorbital edema, activated pain trauma, pallor, changed sensation temperature, weight decrease, weight increase, choking, mouth edema, syncope, malaise, face edema, substernal chest pain.

Cardiovascular Disorders: Abnormal ECG, heart disorder, heart murmur, aggravated hypertension, hypotension, arrhythmia, extrasystoles, t wave inversion, tachycardia, supraventricular tachycardia, angina pectoris, myocardial infarction, pericarditis, pulmonary embolism, peripheral ischemia, superficial phlebitis, purpura, deep thrombophlebitis, vascular disorder, vasculitis, hypertension.

Digestive Disorders: Appendicitis, increased appetite, ulcerative colitis, diverticulitis, duodenitis, dysphagia, enterocolitis, gastric ulcer, gastritis, gastroenteritis, gastrointestinal hemorrhage, gingivitis, glossitis, rectum hemorrhage, hemorrhoids, ileus, irritable bowel syndrome, melena, mucositis, esophageal stricture, esophagitis, oral hemorrhage, peptic ulcer, periodontal destruction, rectal disorder, stomatitis, tenesmus, tongue discoloration, tongue disorder, geographic tongue, tongue ulceration, dental caries.

Endocrine Disorders: Increased glucocorticoids, goiter, hypothyroidism.

Hematologic Disorders: Thrombocytopenic purpura, thrombocythemia, thrombocytopenia, hypochromic anemia, eosinophilia, granulocytopenia, leucopenia, leukocytosis, cervical lymphadenopathy, lymphadenopathy.

Liver and Biliary System Disorders: Cholelithiasis, increased gamma-glutamyl transferase, increased hepatic enzymes, abnormal hepatic function, viral hepatitis, increased serum glutamate oxaloacetic transaminase (SGOT) (also called AST—aspartate aminotransferase), increased serum glutamate pyruvate transaminase (SGPT) (also called ALT—alanine aminotransferase).

Metabolic and Nutritional Disorders: Dehydration, diabetes mellitus, hypercalcemia, hypercholesterolemia, hyperglycemia, hyperlipemia, hypertriglyceridemia, hyperuricemia, hypoglycemia, hypokalemia, hyponatremia, thirst.

Musculoskeletal Disorders: Arthritis, aggravated arthritis, arthropathy, femoral head avascular necrosis, bone disorder, bursitis, costochondritis, plantar fasciitis, muscle weakness, osteomyelitis, osteoporosis, synovitis, tendinitis, tenosynovitis.

Neoplasms: Basal cell carcinoma, squamous carcinoma.

C

Nervous Disorders: Carpal tunnel syndrome, coma, abnormal coordination, dysesthesia, dyskinesia, dysphonia, aggravated multiple sclerosis, involuntary muscle contractions, neuralgia, neuropathy, paresthesia, speech disorder, agitation, confusion, depersonalization, aggravated depression, abnormal dreaming, emotional lability, manic reaction, paroniria, somnolence, abnormal thinking, hyperkinesia, hallucination.

Miscellaneous Disorders: Fall, food poisoning, heat stroke, joint dislocation, post-operative hemorrhage.

Resistance Mechanism Disorders: Cellulitis, herpes simplex, herpes zoster, bacterial infection, viral infection, genital moniliasis, sepsis.

Respiratory Disorders: Asthma, bronchospasm, chronic obstructive airway disease, dyspnea, hemoptysis, laryngitis, nasal ulcer, pleural effusion, pleurisy, pulmonary congestion, pulmonary fibrosis, respiratory disorder.

Rheumatologic Disorders: Aggravated rheumatoid arthritis, lupus erythematosus rash, lupus erythematosus syndrome.

Skin and Appendages Disorders: Acne, alopecia, burn, dermatitis, contact dermatitis, lichenoid dermatitis, eczema, furunculosis, hyperkeratosis, lichen planus, nail discoloration, nail disorder, onychia, onychomycosis, paronychia, photosensitivity reaction, rosacea, scleroderma, seborrhea, skin discoloration, dry skin, skin exfoliation, skin hypertrophy, skin ulceration, urticaria, verruca, bullous eruption, cold clammy skin.

Special Senses Disorders: Deafness, decreased hearing, motion sickness, parosmia, taste perversion, blepharitis, cataract, corneal opacity, corneal ulceration, diplopia, glaucoma, anterior chamber eye hemorrhage, keratitis, keratoconjunctivitis, mydriasis, myopia, photopsia, retinal deposits, retinal disorder, scleritis, vitreous detachment, tinnitus.

Urogenital Disorders: Epididymitis, prostatic disorder, abnormal sexual function, amenorrhea, female breast neoplasm, malignant female breast neoplasm, female breast pain, positive cervical smear test, dysmenorrhea, endometrial disorder, intermenstrual bleeding, leukorrhea, menorrhagia, menstrual disorder, ovarian cyst, ovarian disorder, genital pruritus, uterine hemorrhage, vaginal hemorrhage, atrophic vaginitis, albuminuria, bladder discomfort, increased blood urea nitrogen, dysuria, hematuria, micturition disorder, nephrosis, nocturia, increased nonprotein nitrogen, pyelonephritis, renal calculus, abnormal renal function, renal pain, strangury, urethral disorder, abnormal urine, urinary incontinence, decreased urine flow, pyuria.

In one subject with lupus erythematosus receiving concomitant multiple drug therapy, a highly elevated ALT level was noted after the fourth week of cevimeline therapy. In two other subjects receiving cevimeline in the clinical trials, very high AST levels were noted. The significance of these findings is unknown.

Additional adverse events (relationship unknown) which occurred in other clinical studies (patient population different from Sjögren's patients) are as follows: Cholinergic syndrome, blood pressure fluctuation, cardiomegaly, postural hypotension, aphasia, convulsions, abnormal gait, hyperesthesia, paralysis, abnormal sexual function, enlarged abdomen, change in bowel habits, gum hyperplasia, intestinal obstruction, bundle branch block, increased creatine phosphokinase, electrolyte abnormality, glycosuria, gout, hyperkalemia, hyperproteinemia, increased lactic dehydrogenase (LDH), increased alkaline phosphatase, failure to thrive, abnormal platelets, aggressive reaction, amnesia, apathy, delirium, delusion, dementia, illusion, impotence, neurosis, paranoid reaction, personality disorder, hyperhemoglobinemia, apnea, atelectasis, yawning, oliguria, urinary retention, distended vein, lymphocytosis.

DOSAGE AND ADMINISTRATION

The recommended dose of cevimeline is 30 mg taken 3 times a day. There is insufficient safety information to support doses greater than 30 mg tid. There is also insufficient evidence for additional efficacy of cevimeline at doses greater than 30 mg tid.

HOW SUPPLIED

Evoxac is available as white, hard gelatin capsules of cevimeline hydrochloride containing 30 mg of cevimeline.

Storage: Store at 25°C (77°F) excursion permitted to 15-30°C (59-86°F).

PRODUCT LISTING - EQUIVALENTS NOT AVAILABLE

Capsule - Oral - 30 mg

100's $143.06 EVOXAC, Daiichi Pharmaceuticals 63395-0201-13

Chloral Hydrate *(000715)*

Categories: Anesthesia, adjunct; Pain, adjunct; Sedation; Pregnancy Category C; DEA Class CIV; FDA Pre 1938 Drugs; WHO Formulary

Drug Classes: Sedatives/hypnotics

Brand Names: Aquachloral; Chloralhydrat; Chloralix; Dormel; Kloral; Noctec

Foreign Brand Availability: Ansopal (Portugal); Chloraldurat (Austria; Germany; Netherlands; Switzerland); Chloralhydrat 500 (Indonesia); Medianox (Switzerland); Novochlorhydrate (Canada); Pocral (Korea); Somnox (Belgium); Welldorm (England; Ireland)

DESCRIPTION

Chloral hydrate is genotoxic and may be carcinogenic in mice. Chloral hydrate should not be used when less potentially dangerous agents would be effective.

ORAL FORMS

Chloral hydrate capsules and chloral hydrate syrup contain chloral hydrate, an effective sedative and hypnotic agent for oral administration.

Chloral hydrate capsules provide 250 mg (3¾ grains) and 500 mg (7½ grains) chloral hydrate per capsule. *Inactive ingredients:* Colorants (FD&C red no. 3, red no. 40, yellow no. 6), gelatin, glycerin, methylparaben, polyethylene glycol 400, and propylparaben.

Chloral hydrate syrup provides 500 mg (7½ grains) chloral hydrate per 5 ml teaspoonful of clear, pink, aromatic, flavored syrup. *Inactive ingredients:* Citric acid, colorants (FD&C blue no. 2, red no. 40, yellow no. 6), flavors, glycerin, purified water, saccharin sodium, sodium citrate, and sucrose.

Chemically, chloral hydrate (MW 165.40; CAS-302-17-0) is 1,1-0Ethanedial,2,2,2-trichloro-; its graphic formula is: $CCl_3CH(OH)_2$. Chloral hydrate occurs as colorless or white, volatile, hygroscopic crystals very soluble in water and in olive oil and freely soluble in alcohol. It has an aromatic, pungent odor and a slightly bitter, caustic taste.

SUPPOSITORIES

Chloral hydrate suppositories are water soluble rectal suppository dosage forms containing chloral hydrate, color coded as follows:

Green: Chloral hydrate 5 g (325 mg).

Blue: Chloral hydrate 10 g (650 mg).

The Neocera base used to form chloral hydrate suppositories is composed of polyethylene glycol 400, 1450, 8000, and polysorbate 60. FD&C yellow no. 5 (tartrazine) is in the 5 mg suppository.

The active ingredient is represented by: Cl_3CCHOH. The chemical name is 1,1-Ethanedial,2,2,2-trichloro-.

CLINICAL PHARMACOLOGY

ORAL FORMS

The mechanism of action by which the central nervous system is affected is not known. Chloral hydrate is readily absorbed from the gastrointestinal tract following oral administration; however, significant amounts of chloral hydrate have not been detected in the blood after oral administration. It is generally believed that the central depressant effects are due to the principal pharmacologically active metabolite trichloroethanol, which has a plasma half-life of 8-10 hours. A portion of the drug is oxidized to trichloroacetic acid (TCA) in the liver and kidneys; TCA is excreted in the urine and bile along with trichloroethanol in free or conjugated form.

Hypnotic dosage produces mild cerebral depression and quiet, deep sleep with little or no "hangover"; blood pressure and respiration are depressed only slightly more than in normal sleep and reflexes are not significantly depressed, so the patient can be awakened and completely aroused. Chloral hydrate's effect on rapid eye movement (REM) sleep is uncertain.

Chloral hydrate has been detected in cerebrospinal fluid and human milk, and it crosses the placental barrier.

SUPPOSITORIES

Chloral hydrate in the Neocera base is effective when administered rectally as a hypnotic and/or sedative. Irritation has rarely been encountered following correct insertion. Absorption of the drug occurs from the rectum in a short period of time. Somnifacient doses promptly produce drowsiness and/or sedation, followed by quiet sound sleep, generally within an hour. The action of the drug appears to be confined to the cerebral hemispheres. Blood pressures and respiration are depressed only slightly more than in normal REM sleep and reflexes are not greatly depressed so that the patient can be awakened and completely aroused. In contrast to barbiturates and other sedatives, "hangover" and depressant aftereffects are rarely encountered. With the commonly employed therapeutic dosage, the preliminary excitement is rare and tolerance and cumulation are unlikely.

Although the drug is detoxified in the liver and subsequently eliminated by the kidney, moderately impaired function of either organ is not a contraindication for the usual therapeutic doses.

The mechanism of action is not known, but the CNS depressant effects are believed to be due to its active metabolite trichloroethanol.

INDICATIONS AND USAGE

Chloral hydrate is indicated for nocturnal sedation in all types of patients and especially for the ill, the young, and the elderly patient. Older patients usually tolerate chloral hydrate even when they are intolerant of barbiturates. In candidates for surgery, it is a satisfactory preoperative sedative that allays anxiety and induces sleep without depressing respiration or cough reflex. In postoperative care and control of pain, it is a valuable adjunct to opiates and analgesics.

CONTRAINDICATIONS

Chloral hydrate is contraindicated in patients with marked hepatic or renal impairment and in patients with severe cardiac disease. Oral dosage forms of chloral hydrate are contraindicated in the presence of gastritis. Chloral hydrate is also contraindicated in patients who have previously exhibited an idiosyncrasy or hypersensitivity to the drug.

WARNINGS

Chloral hydrate may be habit forming. Tolerance to the drug is also known to occur. Use with caution in patients who are receiving any of the coumarin or coumarin-related anticoagulants as chloral hydrate is known to antagonize the effects of such drugs. When chloral hydrate is added to or subtracted from the therapeutic regimen, or when changes in dosage of chloral hydrate are contemplated, the effect of the sedative on prothrombin time deserves special attention.

Tumorigenicity in mice: Chloral hydrate has shown evidence of carcinogenic activity in studies involving chronic oral administration in mice. Chloral hydrate has also shown mutagenic and clastogenic activity in a number of *in vitro* assay systems and *in vivo* studies in mammals.

PRECAUTIONS

ORAL FORMS

General

Chloral hydrate has been reported to precipitate attacks of acute intermittent porphyria and should be used with caution in susceptible patients.

Continued use of therapeutic doses of chloral hydrate has been shown to be without deleterious effect on the heart. Large doses of chloral hydrate, however, should not be used in patients with *severe* cardiac disease (see CONTRAINDICATIONS).

Information for the Patient

Chloral hydrate may cause gastrointestinal upset. The capsules should be taken with a full glass of water or fruit juice; capsules should be taken whole, and not chewed. The syrup should be diluted in half a glass of water or fruit juice.

Chloral hydrate may cause drowsiness; therefore, patients should be instructed to use caution when driving, operating dangerous machinery, or performing any hazardous task.

Patients should avoid alcohol and other CNS depressants. They should also be informed that chloral hydrate may be habit-forming.

Chloral hydrate and all drugs should be kept out of the reach of children.

Patients should be warned against sudden discontinuation of chloral hydrate except under the advice of the physician; they should also be informed of symptoms that would suggest potential adverse effects.

Drug/Laboratory Test Interactions

Chloral hydrate may interfere with copper sulfate tests for glycosuria (suspected glycosuria should be confirmed by a glucose oxidase test when the patient is receiving chloral hydrate), fluorometric tests for urine catecholamines (it is recommended that the medication not be administered for 48 hours preceding the test), or urinary 17-hydroxycorticosteroid determinations (when using the Reddy, Jenkins, and Thorn procedure).

Carcinogenesis, Mutagenesis, and Impairment of Fertility

Long-term studies in animals have not been performed.

Pregnancy Category C

Animal reproduction studies have not been conducted with chloral hydrate. Chloral hydrate crosses the placental barrier and chronic use during pregnancy may cause withdrawal symptoms in the neonate. It is not known whether chloral hydrate can affect reproduction capacity. Chloral hydrate should be given to a pregnant woman only if clearly needed.

Nursing Mothers

Chloral hydrate is excreted in human milk; use by nursing mothers may cause sedation in the infant. Caution should be exercised when chloral hydrate is administered to a nursing woman

SUPPOSITORIES

General

The concomitant administration of chloral hydrate and alcohol, or other agents which are central nervous system depressants, may significantly potentiate the sedative action of chloral hydrate. Large doses of chloral hydrate should not be used in patients with severe cardiac disease. The 5 g suppository contains FD&C yellow no. 5 (tartrazine) which may cause allergic type reactions (including bronchial asthma) in certain susceptible individuals. Although the overall incidence of FD&C yellow no. 5 (tartrazine) sensitivity in the general population is low, it is frequently seen in patients who also have a hypersensitivity to aspirin.

Pregnancy Category C

Animal reproduction studies have not been conducted with chloral hydrate. Chloral hydrate crosses the placental barrier and chronic use during pregnancy may cause withdrawal symptoms in the neonate. It is not known whether chloral hydrate can affect reproduction capacity. Chloral hydrate should be given to a pregnant woman only if clearly needed.

Nursing Mothers

Chloral hydrate is excreted in human milk; use by nursing mothers may cause sedation in the infant. Caution should be exercised when chloral hydrate is administered to a nursing woman

DRUG INTERACTIONS

Chloral hydrate may cause hypoprothrombinemic effects in patients taking oral anticoagulants (see WARNINGS).

Administration of chloral hydrate followed by intravenous furosemide may result in sweating, hot flashes, and variable blood pressure including hypertension due to a hypermetabolic state caused by displacement of thyroid hormone from its bound state.

Caution is recommended in combining chloral hydrate with other CNS depressants such as alcohol, barbiturates, and tranquilizers. Administration of chloral hydrate should be delayed in patients who have ingested significant amounts of alcohol in the preceding 12-24 hours. CNS depressants are additive in effect and the dosage should be reduced when such combinations are given concurrently.

ADVERSE REACTIONS

Central Nervous System: Occasionally a patient becomes somnambulistic and he may be disoriented and incoherent and show paranoid behavior. Rarely, excitement, tolerance, addiction, delirium, drowsiness, staggering gait, ataxia, lightheadedness, vertigo, dizziness, nightmares, malaise, mental confusion, and hallucinations have been reported.

Hematological: Leukopenia and eosinophilia have occasionally occurred.

Dermatological: Allergic skin rashes including hives, erythema, eczematoid dermatitis, urticaria, and scarlatiniform exanthems have occasionally been reported.

Gastrointestinal: Some patients experience gastric irritation and occasionally nausea and vomiting, flatulence, diarrhea, and unpleasant taste occur.

Miscellaneous: Rarely, headache, hangover, idiosyncratic syndrome, and ketonuria have been reported.

DOSAGE AND ADMINISTRATION

ORAL FORMS

The capsules should be taken with a full glass of liquid. The syrup may be administered in a half glass of water, fruit juice, or ginger ale.

Adults: The usual *hypnotic* dose is 500 mg to 1 g, taken 15-30 minutes before bedtime or ½ hour before surgery. The usual *sedative* dose is 250 mg three times daily after meals. Generally, single doses or daily dosage should not exceed 2 g.

Children: The usual daily *hypnotic* dosage is 50 mg/kg of body weight, with a maximum of 1 g per single dose. Daily dosage may be given in divided doses, if indicated. The *sedative* dosage is half of the hypnotic dosage.

SUPPOSITORIES

Adults: *Hypnotic Use:* 10-20 grains in a single dose on retiring. *Sedative Use:* 5-10 grains three times daily. Total daily dose not to exceed 30 grains.

Children: *Hypnotic Use:* 5 grains per 40 lb body weight. *Sedative Use:* ½ the hypnotic dose. Absorption is dependent on body hydration and not on body temperature. Moisten finger and suppository with water before inserting.

STORAGE

Store chloral hydrate **capsules** and **syrup** at room temperature; avoid excessive heat. Dispense the **syrup** in tight, light-resistant containers.

Store the **suppositories** at room temperature. Do not refrigerate.

PRODUCT LISTING - RATED THERAPEUTICALLY EQUIVALENT

Syrup - Oral - 500 mg/5 ml			
480 ml	$6.00	GENERIC, Cenci, H.R. Labs Inc	00556-0452-16

PRODUCT LISTING - EQUIVALENTS NOT AVAILABLE

Capsule - Oral - 500 mg			
50's	$59.95	GENERIC, Breckenridge Inc	51991-0080-52
50's	$69.95	GENERIC, Breckenridge Inc	51991-0080-51
60's	$8.16	GENERIC, Allscripts Pharmaceutical Company	54569-0897-00
100's	$7.31	GENERIC, Vangard Labs	00615-0413-01
100's	$8.25	GENERIC, Major Pharmaceuticals Inc	00904-3828-60
100's	$8.51	GENERIC, Moore, H.L. Drug Exchange Inc	00839-5005-06
100's	$11.25	GENERIC, Interstate Drug Exchange Inc	00814-1625-14
100's	$12.47	GENERIC, Mutual/United Research Laboratories	00677-0225-01
100's	$13.60	GENERIC, Ivax Corporation	00182-0297-01
100's	$13.60	GENERIC, Ivax Corporation	00182-0324-01
Suppository - Rectal - 325 mg			
12's	$32.31	AQUACHLORAL SUPPRETTES, Polymedica Pharmaceuticals Usa Inc	61451-6005-07
Suppository - Rectal - 500 mg			
100's	$213.50	GENERIC, G and W Laboratories Inc	00713-0122-01
Suppository - Rectal - 650 mg			
12's	$39.75	AQUACHLORAL SUPPRETTES, Polymedica Pharmaceuticals Usa Inc	61451-6010-07
Syrup - Oral - 250 mg/5 ml			
10 ml x 50	$53.95	GENERIC, Pharmaceutical Assoc Inc Div Beach Products	00121-0457-10
Syrup - Oral - 500 mg/5 ml			
5 ml x 100	$39.85	GENERIC, Pharmaceutical Assoc Inc Div Beach Products	00121-0532-05
30 ml	$3.90	GENERIC, Southwood Pharmaceuticals Inc	58016-0852-06
120 ml	$9.75	GENERIC, Southwood Pharmaceuticals Inc	58016-0852-24
480 ml	$3.07	GENERIC, Vangard Labs	00615-1712-16
480 ml	$8.10	GENERIC, Liquipharm Inc	54198-0140-16
480 ml	$9.41	GENERIC, Vintage Pharmaceuticals Inc	00254-9068-58
480 ml	$9.41	GENERIC, Qualitest Products Inc	00603-1088-58
480 ml	$11.28	GENERIC, Aligen Independent Laboratories Inc	00405-2550-16
480 ml	$11.49	GENERIC, Geneva Pharmaceuticals	00781-6605-16
480 ml	$11.66	GENERIC, Ivax Corporation	00182-0364-40
480 ml	$13.43	GENERIC, Major Pharmaceuticals Inc	00904-1300-16
480 ml	$13.79	GENERIC, Morton Grove Pharmaceuticals Inc	60432-0533-16
480 ml	$14.26	GENERIC, Interstate Drug Exchange Inc	00814-1627-82

Chlorambucil *(000716)*

For complete prescribing information, refer to the CD-ROM included with the book.

Categories: Leukemia, chronic lymphocytic; Lymphoma, follicular; Lymphoma, Hodgkin's; Lymphosarcoma; Pregnancy Category D; FDA Approved 1969 Sep; WHO Formulary
Drug Classes: Antineoplastics, alkylating agents
Brand Names: Leukeran
Foreign Brand Availability: Chloraminophene (France)
Cost of Therapy: $178.07 (CLL; Leukeran; 2 mg; 3 tablets/day; 30 day supply)

WARNING

Chlorambucil can severely suppress bone marrow function. Chlorambucil is a carcinogen in humans. Chlorambucil is probably mutagenic and teratogenic in humans. Chlorambucil produces human infertility (see WARNINGS).

C

DESCRIPTION

Chlorambucil was first synthesized by Everett *et al.* It is a bifunctional alkylating agent of the nitrogen mustard type that has been found active against selected human neoplastic diseases. Chlorambucil is known chemically as 4-[bis(2-chlorethyl)amino]benzenebutanoic acid.

Chlorambucil hydrolyzes in water and has a pKa of 5.8.

Leukeran (chlorambucil) is available in tablet form for oral administration. Each film-coated tablet contains 2 mg chlorambucil and the inactive ingredients colloidal silicon dioxide, hypromellose, lactose (anhydrous), macrogol/PEG 400, microcrystalline cellulose, red iron oxide, stearic acid, titanium dioxide, and yellow iron oxide.

INDICATIONS AND USAGE

Chlorambucil is indicated in the treatment of chronic lymphatic (lymphocytic) leukemia, malignant lymphomas including lymphosarcoma, giant follicular lymphoma, and Hodgkin's disease. It is not curative in any of these disorders but may produce clinically useful palliation.

NON-FDA APPROVED INDICATIONS

Chlorambucil has also been reported to be part of a curative combination therapy in the treatment of Hodgkin's disease. This use has not been approved by the FDA.

CONTRAINDICATIONS

Chlorambucil should not be used in patients whose disease has demonstrated a prior resistance to the agent. Patients who have demonstrated hypersensitivity to chlorambucil should not be given the drug. There may be cross-hypersensitivity (skin rash) between chlorambucil and other alkylating agents.

WARNINGS

Because of its carcinogenic properties, chlorambucil should not be given to patients with conditions other than chronic lymphatic leukemia or malignant lymphomas. Convulsions, infertility, leukemia, and secondary malignancies have been observed when chlorambucil was employed in the therapy of malignant and non-malignant diseases.

There are many reports of acute leukemia arising in patients with both malignant and non-malignant diseases following chlorambucil treatment. In many instances, these patients also received other chemotherapeutic agents or some form of radiation therapy. The quantitation of the risk of chlorambucil-induction of leukemia or carcinoma in humans is not possible. Evaluation of published reports of leukemia developing in patients who have received chlorambucil (and other alkylating agents) suggests that the risk of leukemogenesis increases with both chronicity of treatment and large cumulative doses. However, it has proved impossible to define a cumulative dose below which there is no risk of the induction of secondary malignancy. The potential benefits from chlorambucil therapy must be weighed on an individual basis against the possible risk of the induction of a secondary malignancy.

Chlorambucil has been shown to cause chromatid or chromosome damage in humans. Both reversible and permanent sterility have been observed in both sexes receiving chlorambucil.

A high incidence of sterility has been documented when chlorambucil is administered to prepubertal and pubertal males. Prolonged or permanent azoospermia has also been observed in adult males. While most reports of gonadal dysfunction secondary to chlorambucil have related to males, the induction of amenorrhea in females with alkylating agents is well documented and chlorambucil is capable of producing amenorrhea. Autopsy studies of the ovaries from women with malignant lymphoma treated with combination chemotherapy including chlorambucil have shown varying degrees of fibrosis, vasculitis, and depletion of primordial follicles.

Rare instances of skin rash progressing to erythema multiforme, toxic epidermal necrolysis, or Stevens-Johnson syndrome have been reported. Chlorambucil should be discontinued promptly in patients who develop skin reactions.

PREGNANCY CATEGORY D

Chlorambucil can cause fetal harm when administered to a pregnant woman. Unilateral renal agenesis has been observed in 2 offspring whose mothers received chlorambucil during the first trimester. Urogenital malformations, including absence of a kidney, were found in fetuses of rats given chlorambucil. There are no adequate and well-controlled studies in pregnant women. If this drug is used during pregnancy, or if the patient becomes pregnant while taking this drug, the patient should be apprised of the potential hazard to the fetus. Women of childbearing potential should be advised to avoid becoming pregnant.

DOSAGE AND ADMINISTRATION

The usual oral dosage is 0.1-0.2 mg/kg body weight daily for 3-6 weeks as required. This usually amounts to 4-10 mg/day for the average patient. The entire daily dose may be given at one time. These dosages are for initiation of therapy or for short courses of treatment. The dosage must be carefully adjusted according to the response of the patient and must be reduced as soon as there is an abrupt fall in the white blood cell count. Patients with Hodgkin's disease usually require 0.2 mg/kg daily, whereas patients with other lymphomas or chronic lymphocytic leukemia usually require only 0.1 mg/kg daily. When lymphocytic infiltration of the bone marrow is present, or when the bone marrow is hypoplastic, the daily dose should not exceed 0.1 mg/kg (about 6 mg for the average patient).

Alternate schedules for the treatment of chronic lymphocytic leukemia employing intermittent, biweekly, or once-monthly pulse doses of chlorambucil have been reported. Intermittent schedules of chlorambucil begin with an initial single dose of 0.4 mg/kg. Doses are generally increased by 0.1 mg/kg until control of lymphocytosis or toxicity is observed. Subsequent doses are modified to produce mild hematologic toxicity. It is felt that the response rate of chronic lymphocytic leukemia to the biweekly or once-monthly schedule of chlorambucil administration is similar or better to that previously reported with daily administration and that hematologic toxicity was less than or equal to that encountered in studies using daily chlorambucil.

Radiation and cytotoxic drugs render the bone marrow more vulnerable to damage, and chlorambucil should be used with particular caution within 4 weeks of a full course of radiation therapy or chemotherapy. However, small doses of palliative radiation over isolated foci remote from the bone marrow will not usually depress the neutrophil and platelet count. In these cases chlorambucil may be given in the customary dosage.

It is presently felt that short courses of treatment are safer than continuous maintenance therapy, although both methods have been effective. It must be recognized that continuous therapy may give the appearance of "maintenance" in patients who are actually in remission and have no immediate need for further drug. If maintenance dosage is used, it should not exceed 0.1 mg/kg daily and may well be as low as 0.03 mg/kg daily. A typical maintenance dose is 2-4 mg daily, or less, depending on the status of the blood counts. It may, therefore, be desirable to withdraw the drug after maximal control has been achieved, since intermittent therapy reinstituted at time of relapse may be as effective as continuous treatment.

Procedures for proper handling and disposal of anticancer drugs should be considered. Several guidelines on this subject have been published.[1-7]

There is no general agreement that all of the procedures recommended in the guidelines are necessary or appropriate.

PRODUCT LISTING - EQUIVALENTS NOT AVAILABLE

Tablet - Oral - 2 mg

50's	$98.93	LEUKERAN, Glaxosmithkline	00173-0635-35

Chloramphenicol *(000717)*

Categories: Infection, ophthalmic; FDA Approved 1950 Dec; Pregnancy Category C; WHO Formulary

Drug Classes: Antibiotics, chloramphenicol and derivatives; Anti-infectives, ophthalmic; Anti-infectives, otic; Ophthalmics; Otics

Brand Names: Amphicol; Chlorofair; **Chloromycetin**; Chloroptic; Econochlor; I-Chlor; Infa-Chlor; Mychel; Ocu-Chlor; Ophthochlor; Optomycin; Spectro-Chlor

Foreign Brand Availability: Abefen (Colombia); Alchlor (Indonesia); Aquamycetin (Germany); Archifen Eye (Thailand); Aurachlor (Philippines); Biophenicol (Austria); Cadimycetin (Benin; Burkina-Faso; Ethiopia; Gambia; Ghana; Guinea; Ivory-Coast; Kenya; Liberia; Malawi; Mali; Mauritania; Mauritius; Morocco; Niger; Nigeria; Senegal; Seychelles; Sierra-Leone; Sudan; Tanzania; Tunia; Uganda; Zambia; Zimbabwe); Cebenicol (France); Cetina (Mexico); Chemicetina (Italy); Chloment (Hong-Kong); Chlomy (Japan); Chloracil (Thailand); Chloramex (South-Africa); Chloramno (Thailand); Chloramphenicol (Benin; Burkina-Faso; Czech-Republic; Ethiopia; Gambia; Germany; Ghana; Guinea; Israel; Ivory-Coast; Kenya; Liberia; Malawi; Mali; Mauritania; Mauritius; Morocco; Niger; Nigeria; Senegal; Seychelles; Sierra-Leone; Sudan; Tanzania; Tunia; Uganda; Zambia; Zimbabwe); Chloramphenicol "Agepha" Augensalbe (Austria); Chloramphenicol "Agepha" Ohrentropfen (Austria); Chloramphenicol Faure, Ophthadoses (Switzerland); Chloramphenicol PW Ohrentropfen (Germany); Chloramphenicol POS (Germany); Chloramphenicol RIT (Belgium); Chloramsaar N (Germany); Cloranfenicol N.T. (Ecuador); Chlorcol (South-Africa); Chlornicol (South-Africa); Chloromycetin Ear Drops (Australia; New-Zealand); Chloromycetin Eye Drops (New-Zealand); Chloromycetin Eye Ointment (New-Zealand); Chloromycetin Eye Preparations (Australia); Chloromycetine (Belgium); Chlor-Oph (Hong-Kong); Chlorphen (South-Africa); Chlorsig (New-Zealand; Philippines); Chlorsig Eye Preparations (Australia); Clorafen (Mexico); Cloramfeni Ofteno (Mexico); Cloramfeni Ungena (Mexico); Cloromisan (Mexico); Cloroptic (Colombia; Ecuador; Peru); Cogetine (Thailand); Colain (Indonesia); Colircusi Cloramfenicol (Spain); Colsancetine (Indonesia); Diochloram (Canada); Enclor (Malaysia); Enkacetyn (Indonesia); Epiphenicol (Bahrain; Cyprus; Egypt; Iran; Iraq; Jordan; Kuwait; Lebanon; Libya; Oman; Qatar; Republic-of-Yemen; Saudi-Arabia; Syria; United-Arab-Emirates); Fen-Alcon (Philippines); Fenicol (Indonesia); Fenicol oft (Peru); Genercin (Thailand); Gerafen (Philippines); Globenicol (Netherlands); Halomycetin Augensalbe (Austria); Helocetin (Korea); Hinicol (Taiwan); Ikamicetin (Indonesia); Iprobiot (Argentina); Isopto Fenicol (Bahrain; Benin; Burkina-Faso; Cyprus; Egypt; Ethiopia; Gambia; Ghana; Guinea; Iran; Iraq; Ivory-Coast; Jordan; Kenya; Kuwait; Lebanon; Liberia; Libya; Malawi; Mali; Mauritania; Mauritius; Morocco; New-Zealand; Niger; Nigeria; Oman; Qatar; Republic-of-Yemen; Saudi-Arabia; Senegal; Seychelles; Sierra-Leone; Singapore; Spain; Sudan; Sweden; Syria; Tanzania; Tunia; Uganda; United-Arab-Emirates; Zambia; Zimbabwe); Isotic Salmicol (Indonesia); Kemicetin Augensalbe (Austria); Kemicetine (Bahrain; Cyprus; Egypt; Greece; Hong-Kong; India; Indonesia; Iran; Iraq; Jordan; Kuwait; Lebanon; Libya; Oman; Qatar; Republic-of-Yemen; Saudi-Arabia; Syria; Thailand; United-Arab-Emirates); Kemicetine Otologic (Philippines); Kemicetine (Portugal); Keromycin (Taiwan); Kloramfenicol (Denmark; Norway; Sweden); Kloramfenikol (Sweden); Kloramphenicol (Norway); Klorita (Finland); Levomycetin (Thailand); Minims Chloramphenicol (Bahrain; Cyprus; Egypt; Iran; Iraq; Jordan; Kuwait; Lebanon; Libya; Oman; Qatar; Republic-of-Yemen; Saudi-Arabia; Syria; United-Arab-Emirates); Minims Eye Drops (New-Zealand); Miroptic (Colombia); Ocuchloram (Korea); Oftacin (Colombia); Oftan-Akvakol (Finland); Oleomycetin (Germany); Oliphenicol (Philippines); Ophtho-Chloram (Canada); Opticle (Korea); Paraxin (Benin; Burkina-Faso; Ethiopia; Gambia; Germany; Ghana; Guinea; India; Ivory-Coast; Kenya; Liberia; Malawi; Mali; Mauritania; Mauritius; Mexico; Morocco; Niger; Nigeria; Senegal; Seychelles; Sierra-Leone; Sudan; Tanzania; Tunia; Uganda; Zambia; Zimbabwe); Pentamycetin (Canada); Pharmacetin Otic (Thailand); Phenicol (Israel); Quemicitina (Colombia; Mexico); Reclor (India); Scanicol (Philippines); Silmycetin (Thailand); Spersanicol (Hong-Kong; Korea; Malaysia; Philippines); Suismycetin (Bahamas; Barbados; Belize; Bermuda; Curacao; Guyana; Jamaica; Netherland-Antilles; Surinam; Trinidad); Sustachlor (Philippines); Vanafen Otologic (Thailand); Vanafen S (Singapore; Thailand); Vanmycetin (India); Vitamycetin (India); Xepanicol (Hong-Kong; Malaysia); Ximex Avicol (Indonesia)

WARNING

Bone marrow hypoplasia including aplastic anemia and death has been reported following local application of chloramphenicol. Chloramphenicol should not be used when less potentially dangerous agents would be expected to provide effective treatment.

DESCRIPTION

The chemical names for chloramphenicol are:

Acetamide, 2,2-dichloro-*N*-[2-hydroxy-1-(hydroxymethyl)-2-(4-nitrophenyl)ethyl]-, and

D-*threo*-(-)-2,2-dichloro-*N*-[β-hydroxy-α-(hydroxymethyl)-*p*-nitrophenethyl acetamide.

The empirical formula for chloramphenicol is $C_{11}H_{12}Cl_2N_2O_5$. Its molecular weight is 323.13.

Ophthalmic Ointment: Each gram of chloramphenicol ophthalmic ointment, 1%, contains 10 mg chloramphenicol in a special base of liquid petrolatum and polyethylene. It contains no preservatives. Sterile ointment.

Ophthalmic Solution: Each vial of chloramphenicol ophthalmic solution contains 25 mg of chloramphenicol with boric acid-sodium borate buffer. Sodium hydroxide may have been added for adjustment of pH. A 15 ml bottle of sterile distilled water is included in each package of Chloromycetin suitable for ophthalmic use. By varying the quantity of diluent used solutions ranging in strength from 0.16% to 0.5% may be prepared. Both the powder for solution and the diluent contain no preservatives. Sterile powder.

Otic: Each milliliter of chloramphenicol otic contains 5 mg (0.5%) chloramphenicol in propylene glycol. Sterile.

CLINICAL PHARMACOLOGY

Chloramphenicol is a broad-spectrum antibiotic originally isolated from *Streptomyces venezuelae.* It is primarily bacteriostatic and acts by inhibition of protein synthesis by interfering with the transfer of activated amino acids from soluble RNA to ribosomes. Development of resistance to chloramphenicol can be regarded as minimal for staphylococci and many other species of bacteria. *Additional Information for Ophthalmic Forms:* It has been noted that chloramphenicol is found in measurable amounts in the aqueous humor following local application to the eye.

INDICATIONS AND USAGE

OPHTHALMIC SOLUTION AND OINTMENT

Chloramphenicol should be used only in those serious infections for which less potentially dangerous drugs are ineffective or contraindicated. Bacteriological studies should be performed to determine the causative organisms and their sensitivity to chloramphenicol (see BOXED WARNING).

Chloramphenicol ophthalmic solution and ointment are indicated for the treatment of surface ocular infections involving the conjunctiva and/or cornea caused by chloramphenicol-susceptible organisms.

The particular antiinfective drug in these products is active against the following common bacterial eye pathogens:

- *Staphylococcus aureus*
- Streptococci, including *Streptococcus pneumoniae*
- *Escherichia coli*
- *Haemophilus influenzae*
- *Klebsiella/Enterobacter* species
- *Moraxella lacunata* (Morax-Axenfeld bacillus)
- *Neisseria* species

The products do not provide adequate coverage against:

- *Pseudomonas aeruginosa*
- *Serratia marcescens*

OTIC

Chloramphenicol otic is indicated for the treatment of surface infections of the external auditory canal caused by susceptible strains of various gram-positive and gram-negative organisms including: *Staphylococcus aureus, Escherichia coli, Hemophilus influenzae, Pseudomonas aeruginosa, Aerobacter aerogenes, Klebsiella pneumoniae,* and *Proteus* species.

Deeper infections should be treated with appropriate systemic antibiotics.

CONTRAINDICATIONS

This product is contraindicated in persons sensitive to any of its components.

Additional information for otic: Perforated tympanic membrane is considered a contraindication to the use of any medication in the external ear canal.

WARNINGS

See BOXED WARNING.

Ophthalmic Ointment: Ophthalmic ointments may retard corneal wound healing.

Otic: Discontinue promptly if sensitization or irritation occurs.

PRECAUTIONS

The prolonged use of antibiotics may occasionally result in overgrowth of nonsusceptible organisms, including fungi. If new infections appear during medication, the drug should be discontinued and appropriate measures should be taken.

In all seriuos infections the topical use of chloramphenicol should be supplemented by appropriate systemic medication.

Otic: The possibility of the occurrence of ototoxicity must be considered if this product is allowed to enter the middle ear.

ADVERSE REACTIONS

Blood dyscrasias have been reported in association with the use of chloramphenicol (see WARNINGS).

Ophthalmic Ointment: Allergic or inflammatory reactions due to individual hypersensitivity and occasional burning or stinging may occur with the use of chloramphenicol ophthalmic ointment.

Ophthalmic Solution: Transient burning or stinging sensations may occur with use of chloramphenicol ophthalmic solution.

Otic: Signs of local irritation with subjective symptoms of itching or burning, angioneurotic edema, urticaria, vesicular and maculopapular dermatitis have been reported in patients sensitive to chloramphenicol and are causes for discontinuing the medication. Similar sensitivity reactions to other materials in topical preparations may also occur.

DOSAGE AND ADMINISTRATION

OPHTHALMIC SOLUTION

Two drops applied to the affected eye every three hours, or more frequently if deemed advisable by the prescribing physician. Administration should be continued day and night for the first 48 hours, after which the interval between applications may be increased.

Treatment should be continued for at least 48 hours after the eye appears normal.

Solutions remain stable at room temperature for 10 days.

OPHTHALMIC OINTMENT

A small amount of ointment placed in the lower conjunctival sac every 3 hours, or more frequently if deemed advisable by the prescribing physician. Administration should be continued day and night for the first 48 hours, after which the interval between applications may be increased. Treatment should be continued for at least 48 hours after the eye appears normal.

OTIC

Instill 2 or 3 drops into the affected ear 3 times daily.

HOW SUPPLIED

Ophthalmic Solution and Otic: *Storage:* Store below 30°C (86°F).

Ophthalmic Solution Only: *Warning:* Manufactured with CFC-12, a substance which harms public health and environment by destroying ozone in the upper atmosphere.

PRODUCT LISTING - RATED THERAPEUTICALLY EQUIVALENT

Size	Price	Product, Manufacturer	NDC
Ointment - Ophthalmic - 1%			
3.50 gm	$4.57	GENERIC, Akorn Inc	17478-0280-35
3.50 gm	$20.52	CHLOROPTIC S.O.P., Allergan Inc	00023-0301-04
Powder For Injection - Intravenous - 1 Gm			
1's	$6.55	GENERIC, Raway Pharmacal Inc	00686-1100-90
10's	$76.04	GENERIC, Monarch Pharmaceuticals Inc	61570-0405-71
10's	$106.68	GENERIC, King Pharmaceuticals Inc	60793-0405-71
10's	$123.75	GENERIC, Monarch Pharmaceuticals Inc	63323-0011-15
Solution - Ophthalmic - 0.5%			
2.50 ml	$5.31	CHLOROPTIC, Allergan Inc	11980-0109-03
7.50 ml	$3.29	GENERIC, Aligen Independent Laboratories Inc	00405-6030-07
7.50 ml	$3.30	GENERIC, Major Pharmaceuticals Inc	00904-3210-32
7.50 ml	$3.60	GENERIC, Ivax Corporation	00182-1797-83
7.50 ml	$3.90	GENERIC, Interstate Drug Exchange Inc	00814-1632-39
7.50 ml	$5.72	GENERIC, Akorn Inc	17478-0281-09
7.50 ml	$23.26	CHLOROPTIC, Allergan Inc	11980-0109-08
15 ml	$7.60	GENERIC, Akorn Inc	17478-0281-12

PRODUCT LISTING - EQUIVALENTS NOT AVAILABLE

Size	Price	Product, Manufacturer	NDC
Ointment - Ophthalmic - 1%			
3.50 gm	$1.65	OCU-CHLOR, Ocumed Inc	51944-3310-00
3.50 gm	$6.00	GENERIC, Watson/Schein Pharmaceuticals Inc	00364-7373-70
Powder For Reconstitution - Ophthalmic - 25 mg			
1's	$24.40	CHLOROMYCETIN OPHTHALMIC, Monarch Pharmaceuticals Inc	61570-0321-31
Solution - Ophthalmic - 0.5%			
7.50 ml	$2.10	OCU-CHLOR, Ocumed Inc	51944-4425-07
7.50 ml	$3.75	GENERIC, Cmc-Consolidated Midland Corporation	00223-6215-07
15 ml	$2.70	OCU-CHLOR, Ocumed Inc	51944-4425-02
15 ml	$5.25	GENERIC, Cmc-Consolidated Midland Corporation	00223-6225-15

Chloramphenicol Sodium Succinate *(000718)*

Categories: Infection, central nervous system; Infection, rickettsia; Infection, secondary to cystic fibrosis; Meningitis; Septicemia; Typhoid fever; FDA Approved 1959 Feb; WHO Formulary

Drug Classes: Antibiotics, chloramphenicol and derivatives

Brand Names: **Chloromycetin Sodium Succinate**; Mychel-S

Foreign Brand Availability: Acromaxfenicol (Ecuador); Berlicetin (Germany); Biophenicol (Austria); Cetina (Mexico); Chemicetina (Italy); Chloracil (Thailand); Chloram-P (Thailand); Chloramphen (Finland); Chloramphenicol (Czech-Republic; Norway); Chlorocide S (Benin; Burkina-Faso; Ethiopia; Gambia; Ghana; Guinea; Ivory-Coast; Kenya; Liberia; Malawi; Mali; Mauritania; Mauritius; Morocco; Niger; Nigeria; Senegal; Seychelles; Sierra-Leone; Sudan; Tanzania; Tunia; Uganda; Zambia; Zimbabwe); Chloromycetin (Austria; Benin; Burkina-Faso; Canada; England; Ethiopia; Gambia; Ghana; Guinea; Hong-Kong; Ivory-Coast; Kenya; Liberia; Malawi; Mali; Mauritania; Mauritius; Mexico; Morocco; Niger; Nigeria; Peru; Philippines; Portugal; Senegal; Seychelles; Sierra-Leone; South-Africa; Spain; Sudan; Sweden; Switzerland; Tanzania; Tunia; Uganda; Zambia; Zimbabwe); Chloromycetin Injection (Australia); Chloromycetin Succinate Injection (New-Zealand); Chloromycetine (Belgium); Globenicol (Netherlands); Helocetin (Korea); Kemicetin (Austria); Kemicetine (Bahrain; Cyprus; Egypt; England; Hong-Kong; Iran; Iraq; Jordan; Kuwait; Lebanon; Libya; Malaysia; Oman; Philippines; Portugal; Qatar; Republic-of-Yemen; Saudi-Arabia; Syria; United-Arab-Emirates); Kloramfenicol (Sweden); Lyo-Hinicol (Taiwan); Paraxin (Germany); Quemicetina (Mexico); Quemicetina Succinato (Colombia); Solu-Paraxin (Benin; Burkina-Faso; Ethiopia; Gambia; Ghana; Guinea; Ivory-Coast; Kenya; Liberia; Malawi; Mali; Mauritania; Mauritius; Morocco; Niger; Nigeria; Senegal; Seychelles; Sierra-Leone; Sudan; Tanzania; Tunia; Uganda; Zambia; Zimbabwe); Synchlolim (Thailand); Synthomycine Succinate (Israel)

HCFA JCODE(S): J0720 up to 1 g IV

WARNING

Serious and fatal blood dyscrasias (aplastic anemia, hypoplastic anemia, thrombocytopenia, and granulocytopenia) are known to occur after the administration of chloramphenicol. In addition, there have been reports of aplastic anemia attributed to chloramphenicol which later terminated in leukemia. Blood dyscrasias have occurred after both short-term and prolonged therapy with this drug. Chloramphenicol must not be used when less potentially dangerous agents will be effective, as described in INDICATIONS AND USAGE. *It must not be used in the treatment of trivial infections or where it is not indicated, as in colds, influenza, infections of the throat; or as a prophylactic agent to prevent bacterial infections.*

Precautions:

It is essential that adequate blood studies be made during treatment with the drug. While blood studies may detect early peripheral blood changes, such as leukopenia, reticulocytopenia, or granulocytopenia, before they become irreversible, such studies cannot be relied on to detect bone marrow depression prior to development of aplastic anemia. To facilitate appropriate studies and observation during therapy, it is desirable that patients be hospitalized.

C

DESCRIPTION

IMPORTANT CONSIDERATIONS IN PRESCRIBING INJECTABLE CHLORAMPHENICOL SODIUM SUCCINATE: CHLORAMPHENICOL SODIUM SUCCINATE IS INTENDED FOR INTRAVENOUS USE ONLY. IT HAS BEEN DEMONSTRATED TO BE INEFFECTIVE WHEN GIVEN INTRAMUSCULARLY.

Chloramphenicol sodium succinate must be hydrolyzed to its microbiologically active form, and there is a lag in achieving adequate blood levels compared with the base given intravenously.

The oral form of chloramphenicol is readily absorbed, and adequate blood levels are achieved and maintained on the recommended dosage.

Patients started on intravenous chloramphenicol sodium succinate should be changed to the oral form as soon as possible.

Chloramphenicol is an antibiotic that is clinically useful for, *and should be reserved for,* serious infections caused by organisms susceptible to its antimicrobial effects when less potentially hazardous therapeutic agents are ineffective or contraindicated. Sensitivity testing is essential to determine its indicated use, but may be performed concurrently with therapy initiated on clinical impression that one of the indicated conditions exists (see INDICATIONS AND USAGE).

Each gram (10 ml of a 10% solution) of chloramphenicol sodium succinate contains approximately 52 mg (2.25 mEq) of sodium.

CLINICAL PHARMACOLOGY

In vitro chloramphenicol exerts mainly a bacteriostatic effect on a wide range of gram-negative and gram-positive bacteria and is active *in vitro* against rickettsias, the lymphogranuloma-psittacosis group and *Vibrio cholerae.* It is particularly active against *Salmonella typhi* and *Hemophilus influenzae.* The mode of action is through interference or inhibition of protein synthesis in intact cells and in cell-free systems.

Chloramphenicol administered orally is absorbed rapidly from the intestinal tract. In controlled studies in adult volunteers using the recommended dosage of 50 mg/kg/day, a dosage of 1 g every 6 hours for 8 doses was given. Using the microbiological assay method, the average peak serum level was 11.2 µg/ml 1 hour after the first dose. A cumulative effect gave a peak rise to 18.4 µg/ml after the fifth dose of 1 g. Mean serum levels ranged from 8-14 µg/ml over the 48 hour period. Total urinary excretion of chloramphenicol in these studies ranged from a low of 68% to a high of 99% over a 3 day period. From 8-12% of the antibiotic excreted is in the form of free chloramphenicol; the remainder consists of microbiologically inactive metabolites, principally the conjugate with glucuronic acid. Since the glucuronide is excreted rapidly, most chloramphenicol detected in the blood is in the microbiologically active free form. Despite the small proportion of unchanged drug excreted in the urine, the concentration of free chloramphenicol is relatively high, amounting to several hundred µg/ml in patients receiving divided doses of 50 mg/kg/day. Small amounts of active drug are found in bile and feces. Chloramphenicol diffuses rapidly, but its distribution is not uniform. Highest concentrations are found in liver and kidney, and lowest concentrations are found in brain and cerebrospinal fluid. Chloramphenicol enters cerebrospinal fluid even in the absence of meningeal inflammation, appearing in concentrations about half of those found in the blood. Measurable levels are also detected in pleural and in ascitic fluids, saliva, milk and in the aqueous and vitreous humors. Transport across the placental barrier occurs with somewhat lower concentration in cord blood of neonates than in maternal blood.

INDICATIONS AND USAGE

In accord with the concepts in the BOXED WARNING and INDICATIONS AND USAGE, chloramphenicol must be used only in those serious infections for which less potentially dangerous drugs are ineffective or contraindicated. However, chloramphenicol may be chosen to initiate antibiotic therapy on the clinical impression that one of the conditions below is believed to be present; *in vitro* sensitivity tests should be performed concurrently so that the drug may be discontinued as soon as possible if less potentially dangerous agents are indicated by such tests. The decision to continue use of chloramphenicol rather than another antibiotic when both are suggested by *in vitro* studies to be effective against a specific pathogen should be based upon severity of the infection, susceptibility of the pathogen to the various antimicrobial drugs, efficacy of the various drugs in the infection, and the important additional concepts contained in the BOXED WARNING.

Acute infections caused by Salmonella typhi*.

It is not recommended for the routine treatment of the typhoid carrier state.

Serious infections caused by susceptible strains in accordance with the concepts expressed above:

Salmonella species.

H. influenzae, specifically meningeal infections.

Rickettsia.

Lymphogranuloma-psittacosis group.

Various gram-negative bacteria causing bacteremia, meningitis, or other serious gram-negative infections.

Other susceptible organisms which have been demonstrated to be resistant to all other appropriate antimicrobial agents.

Cystic fibrosis regimens.

*In the treatment of typhoid fever some authorities recommend that chloramphenicol be administered at therapeutic levels for 8-10 days after the patient has become afebrile to lessen the possibility of relapse.

CONTRAINDICATIONS

Chloramphenicol is contraindicated in individuals with a history of previous hypersensitivity and/or toxic reaction to it. It must not be used in the treatment of trivial infections or where it is not indicated, as in colds, influenza, infections of the throat; or as a prophylactic agent to prevent bacterial infections.

PRECAUTIONS

Baseline blood studies should be followed by periodic blood studies approximately every 2 days during therapy. The drug should be discontinued upon appearance of reticulocytopenia, leukopenia, thrombocytopenia, anemia, or any other blood study findings attributable to chloramphenicol. However, it should be noted that such studies do not exclude the possible later appearance of the irreversible type of bone marrow depression.

Repeated courses of the drug should be avoided if at all possible. Treatment should not be continued longer than required to produce a cure with little or no risk of relapse of the disease.

Concurrent therapy with other drugs that may cause bone marrow depression should be avoided.

Excessive blood levels may result from administration of the recommended dose to patients with impaired liver or kidney function, including that due to immature metabolic processes in the infant. The dosage should be adjusted accordingly or, preferably, the blood concentration should be determined at appropriate intervals.

There are no studies to establish the safety of this drug in pregnancy.

Since chloramphenicol readily crosses the placental barrier, caution in use of the drug is particularly important during pregnancy at term or during labor because of potential toxic effects on the fetus (gray syndrome).

Precaution should be used in therapy of premature and full-term neonates to avoid "gray syndrome" toxicity. (See ADVERSE REACTIONS, Gray Syndrome.) Serum drug levels should be carefully followed during therapy of the neonate.

Precaution should be used in therapy during lactation because of the possibility of toxic effects on the nursing neonate/infant.

The use of this antibiotic, as with other antibiotics, may result in an overgrowth of nonsusceptible organisms, including fungi. If infections caused by nonsusceptible organisms appear during therapy, appropriate measures should be taken.

ADVERSE REACTIONS

BLOOD DYSCRASIAS

The most serious adverse effect of chloramphenicol is bone marrow depression. Serious and fatal blood dyscrasias (aplastic anemia, hypoplastic anemia, thrombocytopenia, and granulocytopenia) are known to occur after the administration of chloramphenicol. An irreversible type of marrow depression leading to aplastic anemia with a high rate of mortality is characterized by the appearance weeks or months after therapy of bone marrow aplasia or hypoplasia. Peripherally, pancytopenia is most often observed, but in a small number of cases only one or two of the three major cell types (erythrocytes, leukocytes, platelets) may be depressed.

A reversible type of bone marrow depression, which is dose related, may occur. This type of marrow depression is characterized by vacuolization of the erythroid cells, reduction of reticulocytes and leukopenia, and responds promptly to the withdrawal of chloramphenicol.

An exact determination of the risk of serious and fatal blood dyscrasias is not possible because of lack of accurate information regarding (1) the size of the population at risk, (2) the total number of drug-associated dyscrasias, and (3) the total number of non-drug associated dyscrasias.

In a report to the California State Assembly by the California Medical Association and the State Department of Public Health in January 1967, the risk of fatal aplastic anemia was estimated at 1:24,200 to 1:40,500 based on two dosage levels.

There have been reports of aplastic anemia attributed to chloramphenicol which later terminated in leukemia.

Paroxysmal nocturnal hemoglobinuria has also been reported.

GASTROINTESTINAL REACTIONS

Nausea, vomiting, glossitis and stomatitis, diarrhea and enterocolitis may occur in low incidence.

NEUROTOXIC REACTIONS

Headache, mild depression, mental confusion and delirium have been described in patients receiving chloramphenicol. Optic and peripheral neuritis have been reported, usually following long-term therapy. If this occurs, the drug should be promptly withdrawn.

HYPERSENSITIVITY REACTIONS:

Fever, macular and vesicular rashes, angioedema, urticaria and anaphylaxis may occur. Herxheimer reactions have occurred during therapy for typhoid fever.

"GRAY SYNDROME"

Toxic reactions including fatalities have occurred in the premature and neonate; the signs and symptoms associated with these reactions have been referred to as the "gray syndrome". One case of gray syndrome has been reported in a neonate born to a mother having received chloramphenicol during labor. One case has been reported in a 3-month-old infant. The following summarizes the clinical and laboratory studies that have been made on these patients:

In most cases therapy with chloramphenicol had been instituted within the first 48 hours of life.

Symptoms first appeared after 3 to 4 days of continued treatment with high doses of chloramphenicol.

The symptoms appeared in the following order:

1. Abdominal distention with or without emesis.
2. Progressive pallid cyanosis.
3. Vasomotor collapse, frequently accompanied by irregular respiration.
4. Death within a few hours of onset of these symptoms.

The progression of symptoms from onset to exitus was accelerated with higher dose schedules.

Preliminary blood serum level studies revealed unusually high concentrations of chloramphenicol (over 90 µg/ml after repeated doses).

Termination of therapy upon early evidence of the associated symptomatology frequently reversed the process with complete recovery.

DOSAGE AND ADMINISTRATION

ADMINISTRATION

Chloramphenicol, like other potent drugs, should be prescribed at recommended doses known to have therapeutic activity. Administration of 50 mg/kg/day in divided doses will produce blood levels of the magnitude to which the majority of susceptible microorganisms will respond.

As soon as feasible, an oral dosage form of chloramphenicol should be substituted for the intravenous form because adequate blood levels are achieved with chloramphenicol by mouth.

The following method of administration is recommended:

Intravenously as a 10% (100 mg/ml) solution to be injected over at least a 1 minute interval. This is prepared by the addition of 10 ml of an aqueous diluent such as water for injection or 5% dextrose injection.

DOSAGE

Adults

Adults should receive 50 mg/kg/day in divided doses at 6 hour intervals. In exceptional cases, patients with infections due to moderately resistant organisms may require increased dosage up to 100 mg/kg/day to achieve blood levels inhibiting the pathogen, but these high doses should be decreased as soon as possible. Adults with impairment of hepatic or renal function or both may have reduced ability to metabolize and excrete the drug. In instances of impaired metabolic processes, dosages should be adjusted accordingly. (See Neonates.) Precise control of concentration of the drug in the blood should be carefully followed in patients with impaired metabolic processes by the available microtechniques (information available on request).

Pediatric Patients

Dosage of 50 mg/kg/day divided into 4 doses at 6 hour intervals yields blood levels in the range effective against most susceptible organisms. Severe infections (*e.g.,* bacteremia or meningitis), especially when adequate cerebrospinal fluid concentrations are desired, may require dosage up to 100 mg/kg/day; however, it is recommended that dosage be reduced to 50 mg/kg/day as soon as possible. Pediatric patients with impaired liver or kidney function may retain excessive amounts of the drug.

NEONATES

See ADVERSE REACTIONS, Gray Syndrome.

A total of 25 mg/kg/day in 4 equal doses at 6 hour intervals usually produces and maintains concentrations in blood and tissues adequate to control most infections for which the drug is indicated. Increased dosage in these individuals, demanded by severe infections, should be given only to maintain the blood concentration within a therapeutically effective range. After the first 2 weeks of life, full-term neonates ordinarily may receive up to a total of 50 mg/kg/day equally divided into 4 doses at 6 hour intervals. *These dosage recommendations are extremely important because blood concentration in all premature infants and full-term neonates under 2 weeks of age differs from that of other neonates.* This difference is due to variations in the maturity of the metabolic functions of the liver and the kidneys.

When these functions are immature (or seriously impaired in adults), high concentrations of the drug are found which tend to increase with succeeding doses.

PEDIATRIC PATIENTS WITH IMMATURE METABOLIC PROCESSES

In young infants and other pediatric patients in whom immature metabolic functions are suspected, a dose of 25 mg/kg/day will usually produce therapeutic concentrations of the drug in the blood. In this group particularly, the concentration of the drug in the blood should be carefully followed by microtechniques. (Information available on request.)

HOW SUPPLIED

Chloromycetin sodium succinate is freeze-dried in the vial. When reconstituted as directed, each vial contains a sterile solution equivalent to 100 mg of chloramphenical per ml.

Storage: Store between 15-25°C (59-77°F).

Chlordiazepoxide Hydrochloride *(000726)*

Categories: Alcohol withdrawal; Anxiety disorder, generalized; DEA Class CIV; FDA Approved 1961 Jul; Pregnancy Category D

Drug Classes: Anxiolytics; Benzodiazepines

Brand Names: Benzodiapin; Chlordiazachel; Chuichin; Kalbrium; Karmoplex; Libnum; Libritabs; **Librium**; Medilium; Poxi; Reposal; Restocalm; Ripolin; Vapine; Zenecin

Foreign Brand Availability: Apo-Chlordiazepoxide (Canada); Balance (Japan); Benpine (Malaysia; Thailand); Cetabrium (Indonesia); Chlordiazepoxidum (Netherlands); Contol (Japan); Diazebrum (Argentina); Diazepina (Argentina); Disarim (Portugal); Elenium (Bulgaria; Czech-Republic; Hungary; Poland); Epoxide (Thailand); Equilibrium (India); Huberplex (Spain); Klopoxid (Denmark); Lentotran (Portugal); Multum (Germany); Neo-Gnostorid (Greece); Normide (Spain); Nova-Pam (New-Zealand); Novopoxide (Canada); O.C.M. (Argentina); Oasil (Greece); Omnalio (Spain); Paxium (Portugal); Psicofar (Italy); Radepur (Bahrain; Cyprus; Egypt; Germany; Iran; Iraq; Jordan; Kuwait; Lebanon; Libya; Oman; Qatar; Republic-of-Yemen; Saudi-Arabia; Syria; United-Arab-Emirates); Raysedan (Argentina); Reliberan (Italy); Retcol (Japan); Risachief (Japan); Risolid (Denmark; Finland); Seren (Bahrain; Cyprus; Egypt; Iran; Iraq; Israel; Italy; Jordan; Kuwait; Lebanon; Libya; Oman; Qatar; Republic-of-Yemen; Saudi-Arabia; Syria; United-Arab-Emirates); Sintesedan (Argentina); Tensinyl (Indonesia); Tropium (England)

Cost of Therapy: \$59.77 (Anxiety; Librium; 5 mg; 3 capsules/day; 30 day supply)
\$0.85 (Anxiety; Generic Capsules; 5 mg; 3 capsules/day; 30 day supply)

HCFA JCODE(S): J1990 up to 100 mg IM, IV

DESCRIPTION

TABLETS

Chlordiazepoxide, the prototype for the benzodiazepine compounds, was synthesized and developed at Hoffmann-La Roche Inc. It is a versatile therapeutic agent of proven value for the relief of anxiety. Chlordiazepoxide is among the safer of the effective psychopharmacologic compounds available, as demonstrated by extensive clinical evidence.

Chlordiazepoxide is available as tablets containing 5, 10, or 25 mg. Each tablet also contains corn starch, ethylcellulose, hydroxypropyl methylcellulose, lactose, magnesium stearate, microcrystalline cellulose and triacetin; with FD&C blue no. 1, D&C yellow no. 10 and FD&C yellow no. 6 dyes.

Chlordiazepoxide is 7-chloro-2-(methylamino)-5-phenyl-3H-1,4-benzodiazepine 4-oxide. A yellow crystalline substance, it is insoluble in water. The powder must be protected from light. The molecular weight is 299.76.

Note: Chlordiazepoxide tablets are not in the hydrochloride form.

CAPSULES

Chlordiazepoxide hydrochloride is available as capsules containing 5, 10, or 25 mg chlordiazepoxide hydrochloride. Each capsule also contains corn starch, lactose and talc. Gelatin capsules may contain methyl and propyl parabens and potassium sorbate, with the following dye systems: **5 mg capsules** FD&C yellow no. 6 plus D&C yellow no.10 and either FD&C blue no.1 or FD&C green no. 3. **10 mg capsules** FD&C yellow no.6 plus D&C yellow no.10 and either FD&C blue no.1 plus FD&C red no. 3 plus FD&C red no.40. **25 mg capsules** D&C yellow no.10 and either FD&C green no.3 or FD&C blue no.1.

Chlordiazepoxide hydrochloride is 7-chloro-2-(methylamino)-5-phenyl-3H-1,4-benzodiazepine 4-oxide hydrochloride. A white to practically white crystalline substance, it is soluble in water. It is unstable in solution and the powder must be protected from light. The molecular weight is 336.22.

INJECTABLE

Chlordiazepoxide hydrochloride injectable is used for the relief of acute anxiety when rapid action is required

CLINICAL PHARMACOLOGY

Chlordiazepoxide has antianxiety, sedative, appetite-stimulating and weak analgesic actions. The precise mechanism of action is not known. The drug blocks EEG arousal from stimulation of the brain stem reticular formation. It takes several hours for peak blood levels to be reached and the half-life of the drug is between 24 and 48 hours. After the drug is discontinued plasma levels decline slowly over a period of several days. Chlordiazepoxide is excreted in the urine, with 1-2% unchanged and 3-6% as a conjugate.

INDICATIONS AND USAGE

Chlordiazepoxide is indicated for the management of anxiety disorders or for the short-term relief of symptoms of anxiety, withdrawal symptoms of acute alcoholism, and preoperative apprehension and anxiety. Anxiety or tension associated with the stress of everyday life usually does not require treatment with an anxiolytic.

The effectiveness of chlordiazepoxide in long-term use, that is, more than 4 months, has not been assessed by systematic clinical studies. The physician should periodically reassess the usefulness of the drug for the individual patient.

CONTRAINDICATIONS

Chlordiazepoxide is contraindicated in patients with known hypersensitivity to the drug.

WARNINGS

Chlordiazepoxide and chlordiazepoxide hydrochloride may impair the mental and/or physical abilities required for the performance of potentially hazardous tasks such as driving a vehicle or operating machinery. Similarly, it may impair mental alertness in children. The concomitant use of alcohol or other central nervous system depressants may have an additive effect. PATIENTS SHOULD BE WARNED ACCORDINGLY.

Use in Pregnancy: An increased risk of congenital malformations associated with the use of minor tranquilizers (Chlordiazepoxide, diazepam and meprobamate) during the first trimester of pregnancy has been suggested in several studies. Because use of these drugs is rarely a matter of urgency, their use during this period should almost always be avoided. The possibility that a woman of childbearing potential may be pregnant at the time of institution of therapy should be considered. Patients should be advised that if they become pregnant during therapy or intend to become pregnant they should communicate with their physicians about the desirability of discontinuing the drug.

Withdrawal symptoms of the barbiturate type have occurred after the discontinuation of benzodiazepines.

PRECAUTIONS

TABLETS AND CAPSULES

In elderly and debilitated patients, it is recommended that the dosage be limited to the smallest effective amount to preclude the development of ataxia or oversedation (10 mg or less per day initially, to be increased gradually as needed and tolerated). In general, the concomitant administration of chlordiazepoxide and other psychotropic agents is not recommended. If such combination therapy seems indicated, careful consideration should be given to the pharmacology of the agents to be employed - particularly when the known potentiating compounds such as the MAO inhibitors and phenothiazines are to be used. The usual precautions in treating patients with impaired renal or hepatic function should be observed.

Paradoxical reactions, *e.g.,* excitement, stimulation and acute rage, have been reported in psychiatric patients and in hyperactive aggressive children, and should be watched for during chlordiazepoxide therapy. The usual precautions are indicated when chlordiazepoxide is used in the treatment of anxiety states where there is any evidence of impending depression; it should be borne in mind that suicidal tendencies may be present and protective measures may be necessary. Although clinical studies have not established a cause and effect relationship, physicians should be aware that variable effects on blood coagulation have been reported very rarely in patients receiving oral anticoagulants and Chlordiazepoxide. In view of isolated reports associating chlordiazepoxide with exacerbation of porphyria, caution should be exercised in prescribing chlordiazepoxide to patients suffering from this disease.

C

Information for the Patient: To assure the safe and effective use of benzodiazepines, patients should be informed that, since benzodiazepines may produce psychological and physical dependence it is advisable that they consult with their physician before either increasing the dose or abruptly discontinuing this drug.

INJECTABLE

Injectable chlordiazepoxide (intramuscular or intravenous) is indicated primarily in acute states, and patients receiving this form of therapy should be kept under observation, preferably in bed, for a period of up to 3 hours. Ambulatory patients should not be permitted to operate a vehicle following an injection. Injectable chlordiazepoxide should not be given to patients in shock or comatose states. Reduced dosage (usually 25-50 mg) should be used for elderly or debilitated patients, and for children 12 years or older.

ADVERSE REACTIONS

TABLETS AND CAPSULES

The necessity of discontinuing therapy because of undesirable effects has been rare. Drowsiness, ataxia and confusion have been reported in some patients - particularly the elderly and debilitated. While these effects can be avoided in almost all instances by proper dosage adjustment, they have occasionally been observed at the lower dosage ranges. In a few instances syncope has been reported. Other adverse reactions reported during therapy include isolated instances of skin eruptions, edema, minor menstrual irregularities, nausea and constipation, extrapyramidal symptoms, as well as increased and decreased libido. Such side effects have been infrequent and are generally controlled with reduction of dosage. Changes in EEG patterns (low-voltage fast activity) have been observed in patients during and after chlordiazepoxide treatment.

Blood dyscrasias (including agranulocytosis), jaundice and hepatic dysfunction have occasionally been reported during therapy. When chlordiazepoxide treatment is protracted, periodic blood counts and liver function tests are advisable.

Similarly, hypotension associated with spinal anesthesia has occurred. Pain following intramuscular injection has been reported. Changes in EEG patterns (low-voltage fast activity) have been reported in patients during and after treatment.

INJECTABLE

Other adverse reactions reported during therapy include isolated instances of syncope, hypotension, tachycardia, skin eruptions, edema, minor menstrual irregularities, nausea and constipation, extrapyramidal symptoms, blurred vision, as well as increased and decreased libido.

DOSAGE AND ADMINISTRATION

TABLETS AND CAPSULES

Because of the wide range of clinical indications for chlordiazepoxide, the optimum dosage varies with the diagnosis and response of the individual patient. The dosage, therefore, should be individualized for maximum beneficial effects (see TABLE 1 and TABLE 2.

TABLE 1 *Adults — Oral Dosage*

Adults	Usual Daily Dose
Relief of mild and moderate anxiety disorders and symptoms of anxiety	5 or 10 mg, 3 or 4 times daily
Relief of severe anxiety disorders and symptoms of anxiety	20 or 25 mg, 3 or 4 times daily
Geriatric patients, or in the presence of debilitating disease	5 mg, 2 to 4 times daily
Preoperative apprehension and anxiety:	On days preceding surgery, 5-10 mg orally, 3 or 4 times daily. If used as preoperative medication, 50-100 mg IM* 1 hour prior to surgery.

* See TABLE 3.

TABLE 2 *Children — Oral Dosage*

Children	Usual Daily Dose
Because of the varied response of children to CNS-acting drugs, therapy should be initiated with the lowest dose and increased as required.	5 mg, 2 to 4 times daily (may be increased in some children to 10 mg, 2 or 3 times daily)

Since clinical experience in children under 6 years of age is limited, the use of the drug in this age group is not recommended.

For the relief of withdrawal symptoms of acute alcoholism, the parenteral form (see TABLE 3) is usually used initially. If the drug is administered orally, the suggested initial dose is 50-100 mg, to be followed by repeated doses as needed until agitation is controlled - up to 300 mg/day. Dosage should then be reduced to maintenance levels.

INJECTABLE

Preparation And Administration of Solutions: Solutions of chlordiazepoxide HCl for intramuscular or intravenous use should be prepared aseptically. Sterilization by heating should not be attempted.

Intramuscular: Add 2 ml of *Special Intramuscular Diluent* to contents of 5 ml dry-filled amber ampul of chlordiazepoxide HCl sterile powder (100 mg). Avoid excessive pressure in injecting this special diluent into the ampul containing the powder since bubbles will form on the surface of the solution. Agitate gently until completely dissolved. Solution should be prepared immediately before administration. Any unused solution should be discarded. Deep intramuscular injection should be given *slowly* into the upper outer quadrant of the gluteus muscle.

Caution: *Chlordiazepoxide HCl solution made with Special Intramuscular Diluent should not be given intravenously because of the air bubbles which form when the intramuscular diluent is added to the chlordiazepoxide HCl powder. Do not use diluent solution if it is opalescent or hazy.*

Intravenous: In most cases, intramuscular injection is the preferred route of administration of injectable chlordiazepoxide since beneficial effects are usually seen within 15-30 minutes. When, in judgement of the physician, even more rapid action is mandatory, injectable chlordiazepoxide may be administered intravenously. A suitable solution for intravenous administration may be prepared as follows: Add 5 ml or *sterile physiological saline* or *sterile water for injection* to contents of 5 ml dry-filled amber ampul of chlordiazepoxide sterile powder (100 mg). Agitate gently until thoroughly dissolved. Solution should be prepared immediately before administration. Any unused portion should be discarded. *Intravenous solution should be given slowly over a 1 minute period.*

Caution: *Chlordiazepoxide solution made with physiological saline or sterile water for injection should not be given intramuscularly because of pain on injection.*

Dosage: Dosage should be individualized according to the diagnosis and the response of the patient. While 300 mg may be given during a 6 hour period, this dose should not be exceeded in any 24 hour period (TABLE 3).

TABLE 3 *Injectable*

Indication	Adult Dosage*
Withdrawal symptoms of acute alcoholism	50-100 mg IM or IV initially; repeat in 2-4 h, if necessary
Acute or severe anxiety disorders or symptoms of anxiety	50-100 mg IM or IV initially; then 25-50 mg 3 or 4 times daily, if necessary
Preoperative apprehension and anxiety	50-100 IM 1 hour prior to surgery

* Lower doses (usually 25-50 mg) should be used for elderly or debilitated patients and for older children. Since clinical experience in children under 12 years of age is limited, the use of the drug in this age group is not recommended.

In most cases, acute symptoms may be rapidly controlled by parenteral administration so that subsequent treatment, if necessary, may be given orally. See Tablets and Capsules.

Caution: Before preparing solution for intramuscular or intravenous administration, please read instructions for PREPARATION AND ADMINISTRATION OF SOLUTIONS.

ANIMAL PHARMACOLOGY

The drug has been studied extensively in many species of animals and these studies are suggestive of action on the limbic system of the brain, which recent evidence indicates is involved in emotional response.

Hostile monkeys were made tame by oral doses which did not cause sedation. Chlordiazepoxide HCl revealed a "taming" action with the elimination of fear and aggression. The taming effect of chlordiazepoxide hydrochloride was further demonstrated in rats made vicious by lesions in the septal area of the brain. The drug dosage which effectively blocked the vicious reaction was well below the dose which caused sedation in these animals.

The LD_{50} of parenterally administered chlordiazepoxide hydrochloride was determined in mice (72 hours) and rats (5 days), and calculated according to the method of Miller and Tainter, with the following results: mice, IV, 123 ± 12 mg/kg; mice, IM, 366 ± 7 mg/kg; rats, IV, 120 ± 7 mg/kg; rats, IM, >160 mg/kg.

Effects on Reproduction: Reproduction studies in rats fed 10, 20 and 80 mg/kg daily and bred through 1 or 2 matings showed no congenital anomalies, nor were there adverse effects on lactation of the dams or growth of the newborn. However, in another study at 100 mg/kg daily there was noted a significant decrease in the fertilization rate and a marked decrease in the viability and body weight of off-spring which may be attributable to sedative activity, thus resulting in lack of interest in mating and lessened maternal nursing and care of the young. One neonate in each of the first and second matings in the rat reproduction study at the 100 mg/kg dose exhibited major skeletal defects. Further studies are in progress to determine the significance of these findings.

PRODUCT LISTING - RATED THERAPEUTICALLY EQUIVALENT

Capsule - Oral - 5 mg

Size	Price	Product	NDC
100's	$0.94	GENERIC, Global Pharmaceutical Corporation	00115-2758-01
100's	$3.38	GENERIC, Interstate Drug Exchange Inc	00814-1636-14
100's	$5.28	GENERIC, Mutual/United Research Laboratories	00677-0457-01
100's	$5.75	GENERIC, Ivax Corporation	00182-0977-01
100's	$5.84	GENERIC, Aligen Independent Laboratories Inc	00405-0040-01
100's	$6.19	GENERIC, Geneva Pharmaceuticals	00781-2080-01
100's	$6.56	GENERIC, Ivax Corporation	00182-0977-89
100's	$6.56	GENERIC, Auro Pharmaceutical	55829-0844-10
100's	$11.40	FEDERAL UPPER LIMIT, H.C.F.A. F F P	99999-0726-01
100's	$19.20	GENERIC, Udl Laboratories Inc	51079-0374-20
100's	$27.75	GENERIC, Major Pharmaceuticals Inc	00904-0090-60
100's	$27.99	GENERIC, Barr Laboratories Inc	00555-0158-02
100's	$27.99	GENERIC, Watson Laboratories Inc	00591-0785-01
100's	$27.99	GENERIC, Watson Laboratories Inc	52544-0785-01
100's	$39.00	LIBRIUM, Roche Laboratories	00140-0001-50
100's	$39.09	LIBRIUM, Roche Laboratories	00140-0001-49
100's	$66.41	LIBRIUM, Roche Laboratories	00140-0001-01
100's	$66.41	LIBRIUM, Icn Pharmaceuticals Inc	00187-3750-10

Capsule - Oral - 10 mg

Size	Price	Product	NDC
30's	$1.98	GENERIC, Circle Pharmaceuticals Inc	00659-3024-30
100's	$1.11	GENERIC, Global Pharmaceutical Corporation	00115-2760-01
100's	$3.75	GENERIC, Interstate Drug Exchange Inc	00814-1637-14
100's	$4.44	GENERIC, Vangard Labs	00615-0436-01
100's	$5.52	GENERIC, Aligen Independent Laboratories Inc	00405-0041-01

100's	$6.00	GENERIC, Ivax Corporation	00182-0978-01
100's	$6.68	GENERIC, Moore, H.L. Drug Exchange Inc	00839-1131-06
100's	$6.70	GENERIC, Ivax Corporation	00182-0978-89
100's	$7.36	GENERIC, Auro Pharmaceutical	55829-0845-10
100's	$8.77	FEDERAL UPPER LIMIT, H.C.F.A. F F P	99999-0726-04
100's	$19.92	GENERIC, Seneca Pharmaceuticals	47028-0012-01
100's	$22.15	GENERIC, Udl Laboratories Inc	51079-0375-20
100's	$22.15	GENERIC, Udl Laboratories Inc	51079-0375-21
100's	$31.30	GENERIC, Major Pharmaceuticals Inc	00904-0091-60
100's	$31.59	GENERIC, Barr Laboratories Inc	00555-0033-02
100's	$31.59	GENERIC, Watson Laboratories Inc	00591-0786-01
100's	$31.59	GENERIC, Watson Laboratories Inc	52544-0786-01
100's	$48.10	LIBRITABS, Roche Laboratories	00140-0014-01
100's	$55.86	LIBRIUM, Roche Laboratories	00140-0002-49
100's	$56.00	LIBRIUM, Roche Laboratories	00140-0002-50
100's	$96.54	LIBRIUM, Roche Laboratories	00140-0002-01
100's	$96.54	LIBRIUM, Icn Pharmaceuticals Inc	00187-3751-10
Capsule - Oral - 25 mg			
100's	$1.34	GENERIC, Global Pharmaceutical Corporation	00115-2762-01
100's	$4.13	GENERIC, Interstate Drug Exchange Inc	00814-1638-14
100's	$5.18	GENERIC, Vangard Labs	00615-0437-01
100's	$6.24	GENERIC, Aligen Independent Laboratories Inc	00405-0042-01
100's	$6.70	GENERIC, Ivax Corporation	00182-0979-01
100's	$6.95	GENERIC, Moore, H.L. Drug Exchange Inc	00839-1132-06
100's	$7.50	GENERIC, Ivax Corporation	00182-0979-89
100's	$7.50	GENERIC, Mutual/United Research Laboratories	00677-0459-01
100's	$7.60	GENERIC, Geneva Pharmaceuticals	00781-2084-01
100's	$8.35	GENERIC, Auro Pharmaceutical	55829-0846-10
100's	$23.22	GENERIC, Udl Laboratories Inc	51079-0141-20
100's	$33.70	GENERIC, Major Pharmaceuticals Inc	00904-0092-60
100's	$34.02	GENERIC, Barr Laboratories Inc	00555-0159-02
100's	$34.02	GENERIC, Watson Laboratories Inc	00591-0787-01
100's	$34.02	GENERIC, Watson Laboratories Inc	52544-0787-01
100's	$94.19	LIBRIUM, Roche Laboratories	00140-0003-49
100's	$94.76	LIBRIUM, Roche Laboratories	00140-0003-50
100's	$165.56	LIBRIUM, Roche Laboratories	00140-0003-01
100's	$165.56	LIBRIUM, Icn Pharmaceuticals Inc	00187-3758-10

PRODUCT LISTING - EQUIVALENTS NOT AVAILABLE

Capsule - Oral - 5 mg			
12's	$4.29	GENERIC, Southwood Pharmaceuticals Inc	58016-0822-12
15's	$5.37	GENERIC, Southwood Pharmaceuticals Inc	58016-0822-15
20's	$7.16	GENERIC, Southwood Pharmaceuticals Inc	58016-0822-20
30's	$10.73	GENERIC, Southwood Pharmaceuticals Inc	58016-0822-30
100's	$35.78	GENERIC, Southwood Pharmaceuticals Inc	58016-0822-00
Capsule - Oral - 10 mg			
8's	$4.17	GENERIC, Southwood Pharmaceuticals Inc	58016-0821-08
10's	$5.21	GENERIC, Southwood Pharmaceuticals Inc	58016-0821-10
12's	$6.27	GENERIC, Southwood Pharmaceuticals Inc	58016-0821-12
14's	$7.29	GENERIC, Southwood Pharmaceuticals Inc	58016-0821-14
15's	$7.81	GENERIC, Southwood Pharmaceuticals Inc	58016-0821-15
20's	$10.41	GENERIC, Southwood Pharmaceuticals Inc	58016-0821-20
21's	$10.94	GENERIC, Southwood Pharmaceuticals Inc	58016-0821-21
24's	$12.50	GENERIC, Southwood Pharmaceuticals Inc	58016-0821-24
25's	$13.02	GENERIC, Southwood Pharmaceuticals Inc	58016-0821-25
28's	$14.58	GENERIC, Southwood Pharmaceuticals Inc	58016-0821-28
30's	$15.62	GENERIC, Southwood Pharmaceuticals Inc	58016-0821-30
40's	$20.83	GENERIC, Southwood Pharmaceuticals Inc	58016-0821-40
50's	$26.04	GENERIC, Southwood Pharmaceuticals Inc	58016-0821-50
60's	$31.25	GENERIC, Southwood Pharmaceuticals Inc	58016-0821-60
100's	$3.60	GENERIC, Roberts/Hauck Pharmaceutical Corporation	43797-0295-03
100's	$52.08	GENERIC, Southwood Pharmaceuticals Inc	58016-0821-00
Powder For Injection - Injectable - 100 mg			
10's	$263.13	LIBRIUM, Icn Pharmaceuticals Inc	00187-3755-74
Tablet - Oral - 5 mg			
30's	$1.98	GENERIC, Circle Pharmaceuticals Inc	00659-3025-30
100's	$34.73	LIBRITABS, Roche Laboratories	00140-0013-01
Tablet - Oral - 25 mg			
100's	$86.69	LIBRITABS, Roche Laboratories	00140-0015-01

Chlordiazepoxide Hydrochloride; Clidinium Bromide *(000727)*

Categories: Enterocolitis, acute, adjunct; Irritable bowel syndrome; Ulcer, peptic, adjunct; FDA Pre 1938 Drugs
Drug Classes: Anticholinergics; Benzodiazepines; Gastrointestinals
Brand Names: CDP Plus; Chlordinium; Chlorex; Clindex; Clinoxide; Li-Gen; **Librax**; Lidoxide; Lonta; Spazmate; Zebrax
Foreign Brand Availability: Apo-Chlorax (Singapore); Bralix (Bahamas; Bahrain; Barbados; Belize; Bermuda; Curacao; Cyprus; Guyana; Hong-Kong; Jamaica; Jordan; Lebanon; Libya; Netherland-Antilles; Oman; Qatar; Republic-of-Yemen; Saudi-Arabia; Surinam; Syria; Trinidad; United-Arab-Emirates); Braxidin (Indonesia); Chlobax (Singapore); Cliad (Indonesia); Diporax (Taiwan); Epirax (Bahrain; Cyprus; Egypt; Iran; Iraq; Jordan; Kuwait; Lebanon; Libya; Oman; Qatar; Republic-of-Yemen; Saudi-Arabia; Syria; United-Arab-Emirates); Equirex (India); Klidibrax (Indonesia); Lembirax (Ecuador); Libraxin (Ireland); Librocol (Switzerland); Medocalum (Hong-Kong; Singapore); Nirvaxal (Israel); Pehaspas (Indonesia); Poxidium (Bahrain; Cyprus; Egypt; Iran; Iraq; Jordan; Kuwait; Lebanon; Libya; Oman; Qatar; Republic-of-Yemen; Saudi-Arabia; Syria; United-Arab-Emirates); Renagas (Indonesia); Spasmoten (Guatemala; Nicaragua); Zepobrax (Thailand)
Cost of Therapy: $161.99 (Irritable Bowel Syndrome; Librax; 5 mg; 2.5 mg; 3 capsules/day; 30 day supply)
$3.56 (Irritable Bowel Syndrome; Generic Capsules; 5 mg; 2.5 mg; 3 capsules/day; 30 day supply)

DESCRIPTION

To control emotional and somatic factors in gastrointestinal disorders.

This combination of chlordiazepoxide hydrochloride and clidinium bromide will be abbreviated here as chlordiazepoxide w/clidinium.

This drug combines in a single capsule formulation the antianxiety action of chlordiazepoxide hydrochloride and the anticholinergic/spasmolytic effects of clidinium bromide, both exclusive developments of Roche research.

FOR COMPLETE PRESCRIBING INFORMATION, REFER TO THE INDIVIDUAL DRUG MONOGRAPHS (CHLORDIAZEPOXIDE HCL; CLIDINIUM BROMIDE).

INDICATIONS AND USAGE

Based on a review of this drug by the National Academy of Sciences - National Research Council and/or other information, FDA has classified the indications as follows:

"Possibly" effective: as adjunctive therapy in the treatment of peptic ulcer and in the treatment of the irritable bowel syndrome (irritable colon, spastic colon, mucous colitis) and acute enterocolitis.

Final classification of the less-than-effective indications requires further investigation.

DOSAGE AND ADMINISTRATION

Because of the varied individual responses to tranquilizers and anticholinergics, the optimum dosage of chlordiazepoxide w/ clidinium varies with the diagnosis and response of the individual patient. The dosage, therefore, should be individualized for maximum beneficial effects. The usual maintenance dose is 1 or 2 capsules, 3 or 4 times a day administered before meals and at bedtime.

PRODUCT LISTING - RATED THERAPEUTICALLY EQUIVALENT

Capsule - Oral - 5 mg;2.5 mg			
100's	$5.76	GENERIC, Aligen Independent Laboratories Inc	00405-0045-01

PRODUCT LISTING - EQUIVALENTS NOT AVAILABLE

Capsule - Oral - 5 mg;2.5 mg			
6's	$0.29	GENERIC, Allscripts Pharmaceutical Company	54569-0430-01
15's	$4.15	GENERIC, Prescript Pharmaceuticals	00247-0186-15
16's	$4.20	GENERIC, Prescript Pharmaceuticals	00247-0186-16
20's	$4.41	GENERIC, Prescript Pharmaceuticals	00247-0186-20
20's	$13.60	GENERIC, Southwood Pharmaceuticals Inc	58016-0712-20
24's	$4.62	GENERIC, Prescript Pharmaceuticals	00247-0186-24
30's	$2.50	GENERIC, Circle Pharmaceuticals Inc	00659-1609-30
30's	$3.60	GENERIC, Pd-Rx Pharmaceuticals	55289-0062-30
30's	$3.95	GENERIC, Physicians Total Care	54868-0030-05
30's	$4.94	GENERIC, Prescript Pharmaceuticals	00247-0186-30
30's	$5.82	GENERIC, Allscripts Pharmaceutical Company	54569-0430-00
30's	$20.40	GENERIC, Southwood Pharmaceuticals Inc	58016-0712-30
40's	$4.71	GENERIC, Physicians Total Care	54868-0030-00
42's	$2.06	GENERIC, Allscripts Pharmaceutical Company	54569-0430-03
60's	$4.40	GENERIC, Pd-Rx Pharmaceuticals	55289-0062-60
60's	$5.10	GENERIC, Physicians Total Care	54868-0030-04
100's	$3.00	GENERIC, Veratex Corporation	17022-2162-02
100's	$3.96	GENERIC, Vangard Labs	00615-0312-01
100's	$4.17	GENERIC, Moore, H.L. Drug Exchange Inc	00839-6211-06
100's	$5.30	GENERIC, Physicians Total Care	54868-0030-02
100's	$5.95	GENERIC, Eon Labs Manufacturing Inc	00185-0617-01
100's	$5.95	GENERIC, Eon Labs Manufacturing Inc	00185-0968-01
100's	$5.99	GENERIC, Ivax Corporation	00182-1856-01
100's	$5.99	GENERIC, Watson/Rugby Laboratories Inc	52544-0788-01
100's	$6.00	GENERIC, Major Pharmaceuticals Inc	00904-0301-60
100's	$8.12	GENERIC, Pd-Rx Pharmaceuticals	55289-0062-17
100's	$8.87	GENERIC, Us Trading Corporation	56126-0090-11
100's	$9.95	GENERIC, Major Pharmaceuticals Inc	00904-0301-61
100's	$13.45	GENERIC, Major Pharmaceuticals Inc	00904-2503-60
100's	$19.35	GENERIC, Watson/Schein Pharmaceuticals Inc	00364-0559-01
100's	$19.35	GENERIC, Watson/Schein Pharmaceuticals Inc	00591-4007-01
100's	$19.40	GENERIC, Vintage Pharmaceuticals Inc	00254-2732-28
100's	$19.40	GENERIC, Qualitest Products Inc	00603-2714-21

100's	$19.40	GENERIC, Allscripts Pharmaceutical Company	54569-0430-02
100's	$19.60	GENERIC, Amide Pharmaceutical Inc	52152-0018-02
100's	$20.58	GENERIC, Mutual/United Research Laboratories	00677-1247-01
100's	$72.26	LIBRAX, Roche Laboratories	00140-0007-49
100's	$179.99	LIBRAX, Roche Laboratories	00140-0007-01
100's	$206.99	LIBRAX, Icn Pharmaceuticals Inc	00187-4100-10
200's	$16.90	GENERIC, Physicians Total Care	54868-0030-03

Chlorhexidine Gluconate *(000729)*

Categories: Gingivitis; Periodonitis, adjunct; Periodonitis, prevention; Pregnancy Category B, Oral; Pregnancy Category C, Dental; FDA Approved 1986 Aug; WHO Formulary

Drug Classes: Anti-infectives, topical; Dental preparations

Brand Names: **Peridex**; Periogard; Plakicide; Savacol

Foreign Brand Availability: Alcloxidine (Israel); Bactoscrub (Israel); Bactosept Concentrate (Israel); Blend-A-Med (Germany); Chlorhex (Thailand); Chlorhexamed (Belgium; Germany; Switzerland); Chlorhexidine Mouthwash (Australia); Chlorhexidine Obstetric Lotion (Australia); Chlorhexidinium (Poland); Chlorohex gel (Australia); Chlorohex gel Forte (Australia); Chlorohex Mouth Rinse (Australia); Corsodyl (Italy; Portugal; Switzerland); Dosiseptine (France); Exitane (South-Africa); Exoseptoplix (France); Hexadent (Korea); Hexol (Thailand); Hibiclens Solution (New-Zealand); Hibident (Austria; Belgium; Netherlands); Hibidil (South-Africa); Hibigel (Netherlands); Hibiguard (Belgium); Hibiscrub (Belgium; France; Hong-Kong; Indonesia; Netherlands; Spain; Taiwan; Thailand); Hibisol (Bahrain; Benin; Burkina-Faso; Cyprus; Egypt; Ethiopia; Gambia; Ghana; Guinea; Hong-Kong; Indonesia; Iran; Iraq; Ivory-Coast; Jordan; Kenya; Kuwait; Lebanon; Liberia; Libya; Malawi; Mali; Mauritania; Mauritius; Morocco; Niger; Nigeria; Oman; Qatar; Republic-of-Yemen; Saudi-Arabia; Senegal; Seychelles; Sierra-Leone; Sudan; Syria; Tanzania; Tunia; Uganda; United-Arab-Emirates; Zambia; Zimbabwe); Hibitan (Korea); Hibitane (Bahrain; Belgium; Cyprus; Denmark; Egypt; Finland; France; Hong-Kong; Indonesia; Iran; Iraq; Jordan; Kuwait; Lebanon; Libya; Oman; Qatar; Republic-of-Yemen; Saudi-Arabia; South-Africa; Sweden; Syria; United-Arab-Emirates); Hibitane Concentrate (Malaysia; Taiwan; Thailand); Hibitane Cream (Greece); Hibitane Dental (Norway; Sweden); Hibitane Pastillas (Spain); Hibitane Solution (Greece; New-Zealand; Spain); Hidine (Thailand); Improved Phisohex (Philippines); Klorheksidos (Finland); Klorhexidin (Norway); Klorhexol (Finland); Lemocin CX (Germany); Perio Chip (Israel); Periodentix (Israel); Perioxidin (Mexico); Savlon (Spain); Septalone (Israel); Septol (Israel); Trachisan (Germany)

DENTAL

DESCRIPTION

PerioChip is a small, orange-brown, rectangular chip (rounded at 1 end) for insertion into periodontal pockets. Each PerioChip weighs approximately 7.4 mg and contains 2.5 mg of chlorhexidine gluconate in a biodegradable matrix of hydrolyzed gelatin (cross-linked with glutaraldehyde). PerioChip also contains glycerin and purified water.

Chlorhexidine gluconate is an antimicrobial agent. Chemically, it is designated as 1,1'-hexamethylenebis [5-(*p*-chlorophenyl)biguanide] di-D-gluconate, and its molecular formula is $C_{22}H_{30}Cl_2N_{10}{\cdot}2C_6H_{12}O_7$. The molecular weight is 897.8.

CLINICAL PHARMACOLOGY

MICROBIOLOGY

Chlorhexidine gluconate is active against a broad spectrum of microbes. The chlorhexidine molecule, due to its positive charge, reacts with the microbial cell surface, destroys the integrity of the cell membrane, penetrates into the cell, precipitates the cytoplasm, and the cell dies. Studies with chlorhexidine gluconate dental chip showed reductions in the numbers of the putative periodontopathic organisms *Porphyromonas (Bacteriodes) gingivalis, Prevotella (Bacteriodes) intermedia, Bacteriodes forsythus,* and *Campylobacter rectus (Wolinella recta)* after placement of the chip. No overgrowth of opportunistic organisms or other adverse changes in the oral microbial ecosystem were noted. The relationship of the microbial findings to clinical outcome has not been established.

PHARMACOKINETICS

Chlorhexidine gluconate dental chip releases chlorhexidine *in vitro* in a biphasic manner, initially releasing approximately 40% of the chlorhexidine within the first 24 hours and then releasing the remaining chlorhexidine in an almost linear fashion for 7-10 days. This enzymatic release rate assay is an experimental collagenase assay that differs from the Regulatory Specification's Agar Release Rate Assay. This release profile may be explained as an initial burst effect, dependent on diffusion of chlorhexidine from the chip, followed by a further release of chlorhexidine as a result of enzymatic degradation.

In an *in vivo* study of 18 evaluable adult patients, there were no detectable plasma or urine levels of chlorhexidine following the insertion of 4 chlorhexidine gluconate dental chips under clinical conditions. The concentration of chlorhexidine released from the chlorhexidine gluconate dental chip was determined in the gingival crevicular fluid (GCF) of these same subjects. In these subjects, a highly variable biphasic release profile for chlorhexidine was demonstrated, with GCF levels 4 hours after chip insertion (mean: 1444 ± 783 μg/ml), followed by a second peak at 72 hours (mean: 1902 ± 1073 μg/ml). In a second study involving the insertion of 1 chlorhexidine gluconate dental chip under clinical conditions, the mean GCF level of chlorhexidine peaked at 1088 ± 678 μg/ml at 4 hours. The mean GCF levels then declined in a highly erratic fashion to levels of 482 ± 447 μg/ml at 72 hours without producing a true second peak.

The results of these studies confirm a high degree of intersubject variability in chlorhexidine release from the chlorhexidine gluconate dental chip matrix *in vivo* that was not seen *in vitro.* Due to the nature and clinical use of the chlorhexidine gluconate dental chip dosage form, dose proportionality was not and would not be expected to be demonstrated between the two studies.

INDICATIONS AND USAGE

Chlorhexidine gluconate dental chip is indicated as an adjunct to scaling and root planing procedures for reduction of pocket depth in patients with adult periodontitis. Chlorhexidine gluconate dental chip may be used as a part of a periodontal maintenance program, which includes good oral hygiene and scaling and root planing.

CONTRAINDICATIONS

Chlorhexidine gluconate dental chip should not be used in any patient who has a known sensitivity to chlorhexidine.

PRECAUTIONS

GENERAL

The use of chlorhexidine gluconate dental chip in an acutely abscessed periodontal pocket has not been studied and therefore is not recommended. Although rare, infectious events including abscesses and cellulitis, which have been reported after scaling and root planing alone, have also been reported with the adjunctive placement of the chlorhexidine gluconate dental chip post scaling and root planing. Management of patients with periodontal disease should include consideration of potentially contributing medical disorders, such as cancer, diabetes, and immunocompromised status.

INFORMATION FOR THE PATIENT

Patients should avoid dental floss at the site of chlorhexidine gluconate dental chip insertion for 10 days after placement, because flossing might dislodge the chip. All other oral hygiene may be continued as usual. No restrictions regarding dietary habits are needed. Dislodging of the chlorhexidine gluconate dental chip is uncommon; however, patients should be instructed to notify the dentist promptly if the chlorhexidine gluconate dental chip dislodges. Patients should also be advised that, although some mild to moderate sensitivity is normal during the first week after placement of chlorhexidine gluconate dental chip, they should notify the dentist promptly if pain, swelling, or other problems occur.

CARCINOGENESIS, MUTAGENESIS, AND IMPAIRMENT OF FERTILITY

Chlorhexidine gluconate has not been evaluated for carcinogenic potential in connection with the chlorhexidine gluconate dental chip. No evidence that chlorhexidine gluconate has potential to cause genetic toxicity was obtained in a battery of mutagenicity studies, including *(in vitro)* an Ames assay, a chromosome aberration assay in CHO cells, and *(in vitro)* a micronucleus assay conducted in mice.

PREGNANCY, TERATOGENIC EFFECTS, PREGNANCY CATEGORY C

Animal reproduction studies have not been conducted in relation to chlorhexidine gluconate dental chip, because animal models that would permit use of a clinically relevant route of administration are not available. Chlorhexidine gluconate did not induce harm to the fetus when administered to rats by gavage at dosages up to 68.5 mg/kg/day. While chlorhexidine is known to be very poorly absorbed from the GI tract, it may be absorbed following placement within a periodontal pocket. Therefore, it is unclear whether these data are relevant to clinical use of chlorhexidine gluconate dental chip. In clinical studies, placement of 4 chlorhexidine gluconate dental chips within periodontal pockets resulted in plasma concentrations of chlorhexidine that were at or below the limit of detection. However, it is not known whether chlorhexidine gluconate dental chip can cause fetal harm when administered to a pregnant woman or can affect reproductive capacity. Chlorhexidine gluconate dental chip should be used in a pregnant woman only if clearly needed.

PEDIATRIC USE

The safety and effectiveness of chlorhexidine gluconate dental chip in pediatric patients have not been established.

GERIATRIC USE

Although subjects aged 65 years and over were included in clinical studies of chlorhexidine gluconate dental chip, there were not sufficient numbers of these subjects to determine whether they respond differently from younger subjects. Other reported clinical experience has not identified differences in responses between the elderly and younger patients. Overall differences in safety or effectiveness have not been identified between the elderly and younger patients.

ADVERSE REACTIONS

The most frequently observed adverse events in the two pivotal clinical trials were toothache, upper respiratory tract infection, and headache. Toothache was the only adverse reaction that was significantly higher (p=0.042) in the chlorhexidine gluconate dental chip group when compared to placebo. Most oral pain or sensitivity occurred within the first week of the initial chip placement following SRP procedures, was mild to moderate in nature, and spontaneously resolved within days. These reactions were observed less frequently with subsequent chip placement at 3 and 6 months. TABLE 3 lists adverse events, occurring in ≥1% of 225 patients that received chlorhexidine gluconate dental chip, pooled from the two pivotal clinical trials without regard to causality. Gingival bleeding was the only dental adverse event occurring at a rate of ≤1% in both groups.

DOSAGE AND ADMINISTRATION

One chlorhexidine gluconate dental chip is inserted into a periodontal pocket with probing pocket depth (PD) ≥5 mm. Up to 8 chlorhexidine gluconate dental chips may be inserted in a single visit. Treatment is recommended to be administered once every 3 months in pockets with PD remaining ≥5 mm.

The periodontal pocket should be isolated and the surrounding area dried prior to chip insertion. The chlorhexidine gluconate dental chip should be grasped using forceps (such that the rounded end points away from the forceps) and inserted into the periodontal pocket to its maximum depth. If necessary, the chlorhexidine gluconate dental chip can be further maneuvered into position using the tips of the forceps or a flat instrument. The chlorhexidine gluconate dental chip does not need to be removed since it biodegrades completely.

In the unlikely event of chlorhexidine gluconate dental chip dislodgement (in the two pivotal clinical trials, only 8 chips were reported lost), several actions are recommended, depending on the day of chlorhexidine gluconate dental chip loss. If dislodgement occurs 7 days or more after placement, the dentist should consider the subject to have received a full course of treatment. If dislodgement occurs within 48 hours after placement, a new chlorhexidine gluconate dental chip should be inserted. If dislodgement occurs more than 48 hours after placement, the dentist should not replace the chlorhexidine gluconate dental

TABLE 3 *Adverse Events (Frequency ≥1% for the Chlorhexidine Gluconate Dental Chip Group) Reported From 2 Five-Center US Clinical Trials*

	Chlorhexidine Gluconate Dental Chip		Placebo Chip	
	Total n=225		Total n=222	
All patients with adverse events	193	85.8%	189	85.1%
Toothache*	114	50.7%	92	41.4%
Upper resp tract infection	64	28.4%	58	26.1%
Headache	61	27.1%	61	27.5%
Sinusitis	31	13.8%	29	13.1%
Influenza-like symptoms	17	7.6%	21	9.5%
Back pain	15	6.7%	25	11.3%
Tooth disorder†	14	6.2%	15	6.8%
Bronchitis	14	6.2%	7	3.2%
Abscess	13	5.8%	13	5.9%
Pain	11	4.9%	11	5.0%
Allergy	9	4.0%	13	5.9%
Myalgia	9	4.0%	9	4.1%
Gum hyperplasia	8	3.6%	5	2.3%
Pharyngitis	8	3.6%	5	2.3%
Arthralgia	7	3.1%	13	5.9%
Dysmenorrhea	7	3.1%	13	5.9%
Dyspepsia	7	3.1%	6	2.7%
Rhinitis	6	2.7%	11	5.0%
Coughing	6	2.7%	7	3.2%
Arthrosis	6	2.7%	4	1.8%
Hypertension	5	2.2%	6	2.7%
Stomatitis ulcerative	5	2.2%	1	0.5%
Tendinitis	5	2.2%	1	0.5%

* Includes dental, gingival or mouth pain, tenderness, aching, throbbing, soreness, discomfort or sensitivity.
† Includes broken, cracked or fractured teeth, mobile teeth, and lost bridges, crowns, or fillings.

chip, but reevaluate the patient at 3 months and insert a new chlorhexidine gluconate dental chip if the pocket depth has not been reduced to less than 5 mm.

HOW SUPPLIED

PerioChip 2.5 mg is supplied as a small, orange-brown, rectangular chip (rounded at one end).

Storage: Store at controlled room temperature 15-25°C (59-77°F).

ORAL

DESCRIPTION

Peridex is an oral rinse containing 0.12% chlorhexidine gluconate (1, 1′- hexamethylene bis (5-(p-chlorophenyl) biguanide) di-D-gluconate) in a base containing water, 11.6% alcohol, glycerin, PEG-40 sorbitan diisostearate, flavor, sodium saccharin, and FD&C blue no. 1. Peridex is a near-neutral solution (pH range 5-7). Chlorhexidine gluconate is a salt of chlorhexidine and gluconic acid.

CLINICAL PHARMACOLOGY

Chlorhexidine gluconate provides antimicrobial activity during oral rinsing. The clinical significance of chlorhexidine gluconate's antimicrobial activities is not clear. Microbiological sampling of plaque has shown a general reduction of counts of certain assayed bacteria, both aerobic and anaerobic, ranging from 54-97% through 6 months use.

Use of chlorhexidine gluconate in a 6 month clinical study did not result in any significant changes in bacterial resistance, overgrowth of potentially opportunistic organisms or other adverse changes in the oral microbial ecosystem. Three months after chlorhexidine gluconate use was discontinued, the number of bacteria in plaque had returned to baseline levels and resistance of plaque bacteria to chlorhexidine gluconate was equal to that at baseline.

PHARMACOKINETICS

Pharmacokinetic studies with chlorhexidine gluconate indicate approximately 30% of the active ingredient, chlorhexidine gluconate, is retained in the oral cavity following rinsing. This retained drug is slowly released into the oral fluids. Studies conducted on human subjects and animals demonstrate chlorhexidine gluconate is poorly absorbed from the gastrointestinal tract. The mean plasma level of chlorhexidine gluconate reached a peak of 0.206 µg/g in humans 30 minutes after they ingested a 300 mg dose of the drug. Detectable levels of chlorhexidine gluconate were not present in the plasma these subjects 12 hours after the compound was administered. Excretion of chlorhexidine gluconate occurred primarily through the feces (~90%). Less than 1% of the chlorhexidine gluconate ingested by these subjects was excreted in the urine.

INDICATIONS AND USAGE

Chlorhexidine gluconate is indicated for use between dental visits as part of a professional program for the treatment of gingivitis as characterized by redness and swelling of the gingivae, including gingival bleeding upon probing. Chlorhexidine gluconate has not been tested among patients with acute necrotizing ulcerative gingivitis (ANUG). For patients having coexisting gingivitis and periodontitis, see PRECAUTIONS.

NON-FDA APPROVED INDICATIONS

Twice-daily rinsing with chlorhexidine 0.12% has been studied for the prevention of dry socket after extraction of impacted wisdom teeth. This use is not approved by the FDA.

CONTRAINDICATIONS

Chlorhexidine gluconate should not be used by persons who are known to be hypersensitive to chlorhexidine gluconate or other formula ingredients.

WARNINGS

The effect of chlorhexidine gluconate on periodontitis has not been determined. An increase in supragingival calculus was noted in clinical testing in chlorhexidine gluconate users compared with control users. It is not known if chlorhexidine gluconate use results in an increase in subgingival calculus. Calculus deposits should be removed by a dental prophylaxis at intervals not greater than 6 months. Hypersensitivity and generalized allergic reactions have occurred. See CONTRAINDICATIONS.

PRECAUTIONS

GENERAL

For patients having coexisting gingivitis and periodontitis, the presence or absence of gingival inflammation following treatment with chlorhexidine gluconate should not be used as a major indicator of underlying periodontitis.

Chlorhexidine gluconate can cause staining of oral surfaces, such as tooth surfaces, restorations, and the dorsum of the tongue. Not all patients will experience a visually significant increase in toothstaining. In clinical testing, 56% of chlorhexidine gluconate users exhibited a measurable increase in facial anterior stain, compared to 35% of control users after 6 months; 15% of chlorhexidine gluconate users developed what was judged to be heavy stain, compared to 1% of control users after 6 months. Stain will be more pronounced in patients who have heavier accumulations of unremoved plaque.

Stain resulting from use of chlorhexidine gluconate does not adversely affect health of the gingivae of other oral tissues. Stain can be removed from most tooth surfaces by conventional professional prophylactic techniques. Additional time may be required to complete the prophylaxis.

Discretion should be used when prescribing to patients with anterior facial restorations with rough surfaces or margins. If natural stain cannot be removed from these surfaces by a dental prophylaxis, patients should be excluded from chlorhexidine gluconate treatment if permanent discoloration is unacceptable. Stain in these areas may be difficult to remove by dental prophylaxis and on rare occasions may necessitate replacement of these restorations.

Some patients may experience an alteration in taste perception while undergoing treatment with chlorhexidine gluconate. Rare instances of permanent taste alteration following chlorhexidine gluconate use have been reported via post-marketing product surveillance.

PREGNANCY, TERATOGENIC EFFECTS, PREGNANCY CATEGORY B

Reproduction studies have been performed in rats and rabbits at chlorhexidine gluconate doses up to 300 mg/kg/day and 40 mg/kg/day, respectively, and have not revealed evidence of harm to fetus. However, adequate and well-controlled studies in pregnant women have not been done. Because animal reproductions studies are not always predictive of human response, this drug should be used during pregnancy only if clearly needed.

NURSING MOTHERS

It is not known whether this drug is excreted in human milk. Because many drugs are excreted in human milk, caution should be exercised when chlorhexidine gluconate is administered to a nursing woman.

In parturition and lactation studies with rats, no evidence of impaired parturition or of toxic effects to suckling pups was observed when chlorhexidine gluconate was administered to dams at doses that were over 100 times greater than that which would result from a person's ingesting 30 ml (2 capfuls) of chlorhexidine gluconate per day.

PEDIATRIC USE

Clinical effectiveness and safety of chlorhexidine gluconate have been established in children under the age of 18.

CARCINOGENESIS, MUTAGENESIS, AND IMPAIRMENT OF FERTILITY

In a drinking water study in rats, carcinogenic effects were not observed at doses up to 38 mg/kg/day. Mutagenic effects were not observed in two mammalian *in vivo* mutagenesis studies with chlorhexidine gluconate. The highest doses of chlorhexidine used in a mouse dominant-lethal assay and a hamster cytogenetics test were 1000 mg/kg/day and 250 mg/kg/day, respectively. No evidence of impaired fertility was observed in rats at doses up to 100 mg/kg/day.

ADVERSE REACTIONS

The most common side effects associated with chlorhexidine gluconate oral rinses are (1) an increase in staining of teeth and other oral surfaces, (2) an increase in calculus formation, and (3) an alteration in taste perception (see WARNINGS and PRECAUTIONS).

Oral irritation and local allergy-type symptoms have been spontaneously reported as side effects associated with use of chlorhexidine gluconate rinse.

The following oral mucosal side effects were reported during placebo-controlled adult clinical trials: aphthous ulcer, grossly obvious gingivitis, trauma, ulceration, erythema, desquamation, coated tongue, keratinization, geographic tongue, mucocele, and short frenum. Each occurred at a frequency of less that 1.0%.

Among post-marketing reports, the most frequently reported oral mucosal symptoms associated with chlorhexidine gluconate are stomatitis, gingivitis, glossitis, ulcer, dry mouth, hypesthesia, glossal edema, and paresthesia.

Minor irritation and superficial desquamation of the oral mucosa have been noted in patients using chlorhexidine gluconate.

There have been cases of parotid gland swelling and inflammation of the salivary glands (sialadenitis) reported in patients using chlorhexidine gluconate.

DOSAGE AND ADMINISTRATION

Chlorhexidine gluconate therapy should be initiated directly following a dental prophylaxis. Patients using chlorhexidine gluconate should be reevaluated and given a thorough prophylaxis at intervals no longer than 6 months.

Recommended use is twice daily oral rinsing for 30 seconds, morning and evening after toothbrushing. Usual dosage is 15 ml (marked in cap) of undiluted chlorhexidine gluconate. Patients should be instructed to not rinse with water, or other mouthwashes, brush teeth, or eat immediately after using chlorhexidine gluconate. Chlorhexidine gluconate is not intended for ingestion and should be expectorated after rinsing.

HOW SUPPLIED

Peridex is supplied as a blue liquid in 1 pint (473 ml) amber plastic bottles with child-resistant dispensing closures.

Storage: Store above freezing (32°F).

PRODUCT LISTING - RATED THERAPEUTICALLY EQUIVALENT

Liquid - Mucous Membrane - 0.12%

Size	Price	Product	NDC
15 ml x 50	$91.50	GENERIC, Alpharma Uspd Makers Of Barre and Nmc	50962-0800-60
475 ml	$10.40	GENERIC, Apotex Usa Inc	60505-0355-00
480 ml	$7.65	PERIOGARD, Physicians Total Care	54868-3313-00
480 ml	$9.50	GENERIC, Major Pharmaceuticals Inc	00904-5145-16
480 ml	$10.40	GENERIC, Teva Pharmaceuticals Usa	00093-0014-16
480 ml	$10.40	PERIOGARD, Colgate Oral Pharmaceuticals Inc	00126-0271-16
480 ml	$10.41	GENERIC, Moore, H.L. Drug Exchange Inc	00839-8087-69
480 ml	$10.92	GENERIC, Alpharma Uspd Makers Of Barre and Nmc	00472-0036-16
480 ml	$14.50	PERIDEX, Physicians Total Care	54868-2770-00
480 ml x 3	$11.82	PERIDEX, Zila Pharmaceuticals Inc	51284-0620-22

Solution - Dental - 0.12%

Size	Price	Product	NDC
480 ml	$7.01	FEDERAL UPPER LIMIT, H.C.F.A. F F P	99999-0729-01

PRODUCT LISTING - EQUIVALENTS NOT AVAILABLE

Insert - Mucous Membrane - 2.5 mg

Size	Price	Product	NDC
10's	$160.00	PERIOCHIP, Astra-Zeneca Pharmaceuticals	00186-2008-00

Liquid - Mucous Membrane - 0.12%

Size	Price	Product	NDC
473 ml	$8.75	GENERIC, Omnii International	48878-6100-06
480 ml	$9.22	GENERIC, Physicians Total Care	54868-3722-00
480 ml	$10.40	GENERIC, Xttrium Laboratories	00116-2001-16
480 ml	$10.51	GENERIC, Hi-Tech Pharmacal Company Inc	50383-0720-16
480 ml	$17.36	PERIDEX, Southwood Pharmaceuticals Inc	58016-9062-01

Chloroquine *(000736)*

For complete prescribing information, refer to the CD-ROM included with the book.

Categories: Amebiasis, extraintestinal; Malaria; Malaria, prophylaxis; FDA Approved 1946 Aug; Pregnancy Category C; WHO Formulary

Drug Classes: Antiprotozoals

Brand Names: **Aralen**; Aralen Injection; Chlorofoz; Dichinalex; Lariago; Quinalen

Foreign Brand Availability: Anoclor (South-Africa); Avloclor (Benin; Burkina-Faso; England; Ethiopia; Gambia; Ghana; Guinea; Indonesia; Ireland; Israel; Ivory-Coast; Kenya; Liberia; Malawi; Mali; Mauritania; Mauritius; Morocco; Niger; Nigeria; Senegal; Seychelles; Sierra-Leone; Sudan; Tanzania; Tunia; Uganda; Zambia; Zimbabwe); Cadiquin (Benin; Burkina-Faso; Ethiopia; Gambia; Ghana; Guinea; Ivory-Coast; Kenya; Liberia; Malawi; Mali; Mauritania; Mauritius; Morocco; Niger; Nigeria; Senegal; Seychelles; Sierra-Leone; Sudan; Tanzania; Tunia; Uganda; Zambia; Zimbabwe); Chlorquin (Australia); Chloroquini Diphosphas (Netherlands); Cidanchin (Spain); Clo-Kit Junior (India); Delagil (Bahamas; Barbados; Belize; Bermuda; Curacao; Guyana; Jamaica; Netherland-Antilles; Surinam; Trinidad); Diroquine (Thailand); Emquin (India); Genocin (Thailand); Heliopar (Finland); Klorokinfosfat (Denmark); Lagaquin (Bahamas; Barbados; Belize; Benin; Bermuda; Burkina-Faso; Curacao; Ethiopia; Gambia; Ghana; Guinea; Guyana; Ivory-Coast; Jamaica; Kenya; Liberia; Malawi; Mali; Mauritania; Mauritius; Morocco; Netherland-Antilles; Niger; Nigeria; Senegal; Seychelles; Sierra-Leone; Sudan; Surinam; Switzerland; Tanzania; Trinidad; Tunia; Uganda; Zambia; Zimbabwe); Malaquin (Bahrain; Cyprus; Egypt; Iran; Iraq; Jordan; Kuwait; Lebanon; Libya; Oman; Qatar; Republic-of-Yemen; Saudi-Arabia; Syria; United-Arab-Emirates); Malarex (Bahrain; Cyprus; Denmark; Egypt; Indonesia; Iran; Iraq; Jordan; Kuwait; Lebanon; Libya; Malaysia; Oman; Philippines; Qatar; Republic-of-Yemen; Saudi-Arabia; Syria; United-Arab-Emirates); Malaviron (Benin; Burkina-Faso; Ethiopia; Gambia; Ghana; Guinea; Ivory-Coast; Kenya; Liberia; Malawi; Mali; Mauritania; Mauritius; Morocco; Niger; Nigeria; Senegal; Seychelles; Sierra-Leone; Sudan; Tanzania; Tunia; Uganda; Zambia; Zimbabwe); Malarivon (Bahamas; Bahrain; Barbados; Belize; Bermuda; Curacao; Cyprus; Egypt; Guyana; Iran; Iraq; Jamaica; Jordan; Kuwait; Lebanon; Libya; Netherland-Antilles; Oman; Qatar; Republic-of-Yemen; Saudi-Arabia; Surinam; Syria; Trinidad; United-Arab-Emirates); Maquine (Bahrain; Cyprus; Egypt; Iran; Iraq; Jordan; Kuwait; Lebanon; Libya; Oman; Qatar; Republic-of-Yemen; Saudi-Arabia; Syria; United-Arab-Emirates); Melubrin (India); Mexaquin (Indonesia); Mirquin (South-Africa); Nivaquine (Indonesia); Nivaquine DP (Indonesia); P Roquine (Thailand); Repal (Colombia); Resochin (Austria; Bahrain; Benin; Burkina-Faso; Cyprus; Egypt; Ethiopia; Gambia; Germany; Ghana; Guinea; India; Indonesia; Iran; Iraq; Ivory-Coast; Jordan; Kenya; Kuwait; Lebanon; Liberia; Libya; Malawi; Mali; Mauritania; Mauritius; Morocco; Netherlands; Niger; Nigeria; Oman; Qatar; Republic-of-Yemen; Saudi-Arabia; Senegal; Seychelles; Sierra-Leone; Spain; Sudan; Switzerland; Syria; Tanzania; Tunia; Uganda; United-Arab-Emirates; Zambia; Zimbabwe); Resochina (Portugal)

HCFA JCODE(S): J0390 up to 250 mg IM

INTRAMUSCULAR

WARNING

For Malaria and Extraintestinal Amebiasis

PHYSICIANS SHOULD COMPLETELY FAMILIARIZE THEMSELVES WITH THE COMPLETE CONTENTS OF THIS LEAFLET BEFORE PESCRIBING CHLOROQUINE.

DESCRIPTION

Parenteral solution, each ml containing 50 mg of the dihydrochloride salt equivalent to 40 mg of chloroquine base. Chloroquine hydrochloride, a 4-aminoquinoline compound, is chemically 7-(Chloro-4-[[4-diethylamino)-1-methylbutyl]amino]-quinoline dihydrochloride, a white, crystalline substance, freely soluble in water.

INDICATIONS AND USAGE

Chloroquine hydrochloride is indicated for the treatment of extraintestinal amebiasis and for treatment of acute attacks of malaria due to *P. vivax, P. malariae, P. ovale,* and susceptible strains of *P. falciparum* when oral therapy is not feasible.

NON-FDA APPROVED INDICATIONS

Non-FDA approved uses of chloroquine include the treatment of inflammatory and other disorders such as systemic lupus erythematosus, idiopathic pulmonary hemosiderosis, porphyria cutanea tarda, ulcerative colitis, and rheumatoid arthritis.

CONTRAINDICATIONS

Use of this drug is contraindicated in the presence of retinal or visual field changes either attributable to 4-aminoquinoline compounds or to any other etiology, and in patients with known hypersensitivity to 4-aminoquinoline compounds. However, in the treatment of acute attacks of malaria caused by susceptible strains of plasmodia, the physician may elect to use this drug after carefully weighing the possible benefits and risks to the patient.

WARNINGS

Children and infants are extremely susceptible to adverse effects from an overdose of parenteral chloroquine and sudden deaths have been recorded after such administration. In no instance should the single dose of parenteral chloroquine administered to infants or children exceed 5 mg base per kg.

In recent years it has been found that certain strains of *P. falciparum* have become resistant to 4-aminoquinoline compounds (including chloroquine and hydroxychloroquine) as shown by the fact that normally adequate doses have failed to prevent or cure clinical malaria or parasitemia. Treatment with quinine or other specific forms of therapy is therefore advised for patients infected with a resistant strain of parasites.

Use of chloroquine should be avoided in patients with psoriasis, for it may precipitate a severe attack of psoriasis. Some authors consider the use of 4-aminoquinoline compounds contraindicated in patients with porphyria since the condition may be exacerbated.

Irreversible retinal damage has been observed in some patients who had received long-term or high-dosage 4-aminoquinoline therapy. Retinopathy has been reported to be dose related.

If there is any indication (past or present) of abnormality in the visual acuity, visual field, or retinal macular areas (such as pigmentary changes, loss of foveal reflex), or any visual symptoms (such as light flashes and streaks) which are not fully explainable by difficulties of accommodation or corneal opacities, the drug should be discontinued immediately and the patient closely observed for possible progression. Retinal changes (and visual disturbances) may progress even after cessation of therapy.

USAGE IN PREGNANCY

Usage of this drug during pregnancy should be avoided except in the suppression or treatment of malaria when in the judgment of the physician the benefit outweighs the possible hazard. It should be noted that radioactively tagged chloroquine administered intravenously to pregnant pigmented CBA mice passed rapidly across the placenta, accumulated selectively in the melanin structures of the fetal eyes and was retained in the ocular tissues for 5 months after the drug had been eliminated from the rest of the body.[1]

DOSAGE AND ADMINISTRATION

MALARIA

Adult Dose

An initial dose of 4-5 ml (160-200 mg chloroquine base) may be injected intramuscularly and repeated in 6 hours if necessary. The total parenteral dosage in the first 24 hours should not exceed 800 mg chloroquine base. Treatment by mouth should be started as soon as practicable and continued until a course of approximately 1.5 g of base in 3 days is completed.

Pediatric Dose

Infants and children are extremely susceptible to overdosage of parenteral chloroquine. Severe reactions and deaths have occurred. In the pediatric age range, parenteral chloroquine dosage should be calculated in proportion to the adult dose based upon body weight. The recommended single dose in infants and children is 5 mg base per kg. This dose may be repeated in 6 hours; however, the total dose in any 24 hour period should not exceed 10 mg base per kg of body weight. Parenteral administration should be terminated and oral therapy instituted as soon as possible.

EXTRAINTESTINAL AMEBIASIS

In adult patients not able to tolerate oral therapy, from 4-5 ml (160-200 mg chloroquine base) may be injected daily for 10-12 days. Oral administration should be substituted or resumed as soon as possible.

ORAL

WARNING

Note: The trade name has been used throughout this monograph for clarity.

For Malaria and Extraintestinal Amebiasis

PHYSICIANS SHOULD COMPLETELY FAMILIARIZE THEMSELVES WITH THE COMPLETE CONTENTS OF THIS LEAFLET BEFORE PRESCRIBING CHLOROQUINE.

DESCRIPTION

Aralen, chloroquine phosphate, is a 4-aminoquinoline compound for oral administration. It is a white, odorless, bitter tasting, crystalline substance, freely soluble in water. Aralen is an antimalarial and amebicidal drug. Chemically, it is 7-chloro-4-[[4-(diethylamino)-1-methylbutyl]amino]quinoline phosphate (1:2).

Inactive Ingredients: Carnauba wax, colloidal silicon dioxide, dibasic calcium phosphate, hydroxypropyl methylcellulose, magnesium stearate, microcrystalline cellulose, polyethylene glycol, polysorbate 80, pregelatinized starch, sodium starch glycolate, stearic acid, titanium dioxide.

INDICATIONS AND USAGE

Chloroquine phosphate is indicated for the suppressive treatment and for acute attacks of malaria due to *P. vivax, P. malariae, P. ovale,* and susceptible strains of *P. falciparum.* The drug is also indicated for the treatment of extraintestinal amebiasis.

Chloroquine phosphate does not prevent relapses in patients with vivax or malariae malaria because it is not effective against exoerythrocytic forms of the parasite, nor will it prevent vivax or malariae infection when administered as a prophylactic. It is highly effective as a suppressive agent in patients with vivax or malariae malaria, in terminating acute attacks, and significantly lengthening the interval between treatment and relapse. In patients with falciparum malaria it abolishes the acute attack and effects complete cure of the infection, unless due to a resistant strain of *P. falciparum.*

NON-FDA APPROVED INDICATIONS

Non-FDA approved uses of chloroquine include the treatment of inflammatory and other disorders such as systemic lupus erythematosus, idiopathic pulmonary hemosiderosis, porphyria cutanea tarda, ulcerative colitis, and rheumatoid arthritis.

CONTRAINDICATIONS

Use of this drug is contraindicated in the presence of retinal or visual field changes either attributable to 4-aminoquinoline compounds or to any other etiology, and in patients with known hypersensitivity to 4-aminoquinoline compounds. However, in the treatment of acute attacks of malaria caused by susceptible strains of plasmodia, the physician may elect to use this drug after carefully weighing the possible benefits and risks to the patient.

WARNINGS

In recent years it has been found that certain strains of *P. falciparum* have become resistant to 4-aminoquinoline compounds (including chloroquine and hydroxychloroquine) as shown by the fact that normally adequate doses have failed to prevent or cure clinical malaria or parasitemia. Treatment with quinine or other specific forms of therapy is therefore advised for patients infected with a resistant strain of parasites.

Irreversible retinal damage has been observed in some patients who had received long-term or high-dosage 4-aminoquinoline therapy. Retinopathy has been reported to be dose related.

When prolonged therapy with any antimalarial compound is contemplated, initial (base line) and periodic ophthalmologic examinations (including visual acuity, expert slit-lamp, funduscopic, and visual field tests) should be performed.

If there is any indication (past or present) of abnormality in the visual acuity, visual field, or retinal macular areas (such as pigmentary changes, loss of foveal reflex), or any visual symptoms (such as light flashes and streaks) which are not fully explainable by difficulties of accommodation or corneal opacities, the drug should be discontinued immediately and the patient closely observed for possible progression. Retinal changes (and visual disturbances) may progress even after cessation of therapy.

All patients on long-term therapy with this preparation should be questioned and examined periodically, including testing knee and ankle reflexes, to detect any evidence of muscular weakness. If weakness occurs, discontinue the drug.

A number of fatalities have been reported following the accidental ingestion of chloroquine, sometimes in relatively small doses (0.75 g or 1 g chloroquine phosphate in one 3-year-old child). Patients should be strongly warned to keep this drug out of the reach of children because they are especially sensitive to the 4-aminoquinoline compounds.

Use of chloroquine in patients with psoriasis may precipitate a severe attack of psoriasis. When used in patients with porphyria the condition may be exacerbated. The drug should not be used in these conditions unless in the judgment of the physician the benefit to the patient outweighs the possible hazard.

DOSAGE AND ADMINISTRATION

The dosage of chloroquine phosphate is often expressed in terms of equivalent chloroquine base. Each 500 mg tablet of chloroquine contains the equivalent of 300 mg chloroquine base. In infants and children the dosage is preferably calculated by body weight.

MALARIA

Suppression

Adult Dose: 500 mg (= 300 mg base) on exactly the same day of each week.

Pediatric Dose: The weekly suppressive dosage is 5 mg calculated as base, per kg of body weight, but should not exceed the adult dose regardless of weight.

If circumstances permit, suppressive therapy should begin 2 weeks prior to exposure. However, failing this in adults, an initial double (loading) dose of 1 g (= 600 mg base), or in children 10 mg base/kg may be taken in two divided doses, 6 hours apart. The suppressive therapy should be continued for 8 weeks after leaving the endemic area.

For Treatment of Acute Attack

Adults

An initial dose of 1 g (= 600 mg base) followed by an additional 500 mg (= 300 mg base) after 6-8 hours and a single dose of 500 mg (= 300 mg base) on each of 2 consecutive days. This represents a total dose of 2.5 g chloroquine phosphate or 1.5 g base in 3 days.

The dosage for adults may also be calculated on the basis of body weight; this method is preferred for infants and children. A total dose representing 25 mg of base per kg of body weight is administered in 3 days, as follows:

First Dose: 10 mg base per kg (but not exceeding a single dose of 600 mg base).

Second Dose: 5 mg base per kg (but not exceeding a single dose of 300 mg base) 6 hours after first dose.

Third Dose: 5 mg base per kg 18 hours after second dose.

Fourth Dose: 5 mg base per kg 24 hours after third dose.

For radical cure of vivax and malariae malaria concomitant therapy with an 8-aminoquinoline compound is necessary.

EXTRAINTESTINAL AMEBIASIS

Adults, 1 g (600 mg base) daily for 2 days, followed by 500 mg (300 mg base) daily for at least 2-3 weeks. Treatment is usually combined with an effective intestinal amebicide.

PRODUCT LISTING - RATED THERAPEUTICALLY EQUIVALENT

Tablet - Oral - 250 mg

Size	Price	Product	NDC
50's	$124.38	GENERIC, Global Pharmaceutical Corporation	00115-7056-06
100's	$17.50	GENERIC, Cmc-Consolidated Midland Corporation	00223-0691-01
100's	$189.75	GENERIC, Global Pharmaceutical Corporation	00115-7056-01

Tablet - Oral - 500 mg

Size	Price	Product	NDC
6's	$27.02	ARALEN PHOSPHATE, Allscripts Pharmaceutical Company	54569-3777-05
8's	$36.03	ARALEN PHOSPHATE, Allscripts Pharmaceutical Company	54569-3777-02
25's	$125.70	ARALEN PHOSPHATE, Physicians Total Care	54868-3953-00
25's	$145.24	ARALEN PHOSPHATE, Sanofi Winthrop Pharmaceuticals	00024-0084-01

PRODUCT LISTING - EQUIVALENTS NOT AVAILABLE

Solution - Injectable - 50 mg/ml

Size	Price	Product	NDC
5 ml x 5	$103.60	ARALEN HYDROCHLORIDE, Sanofi Winthrop Pharmaceuticals	00024-0074-01

Tablet - Oral - 500 mg

Size	Price	Product	NDC
25's	$101.25	GENERIC, West Ward Pharmaceutical Corporation	00143-2125-22

Chlorothiazide *(000739)*

Categories: Edema; Hypertension, essential; Pregnancy Category B; FDA Approved 1960 Sep
Drug Classes: Diuretics, thiazide and derivatives
Brand Names: Azide; Chlothin; Diurazide; Diuret; **Diuril**; Saluretil
Foreign Brand Availability: Chlotride (Denmark; Japan; Netherlands; Taiwan); Saluric (England)
Cost of Therapy: $8.01 (Edema; Diuril; 500 mg; 1 tablet/day; 30 day supply)
$2.17 (Edema; Generic Tablets; 500 mg; 1 tablet/day; 30 day supply)
HCFA JCODE(S): J1205 per 500 mg IV

DESCRIPTION

Chlorothiazide is a diuretic and antihypertensive. It is 6-chloro- 2*H*-1,2,4-benzothiadiazine-7-sulfonamide 1,1-dioxide. Its empirical formula is $C_7H_6ClN_3O_4S_2$.

It is a white, or practically white, crystalline powder with a molecular weight of 295.72, which is very slightly soluble in water, but readily soluble in dilute aqueous sodium hydroxide. It is soluble in urine to the extent of about 150 mg/100 ml at pH 7.

Tablets: Chlorothiazide is supplied at 250 and 500 mg tablets, for oral use. Each Diuril tablet contains the following inactive ingredients: gelatin, magnesium stearate, starch and talc. The 250 mg tablet also contains lactose.

Oral suspension: Oral suspension chlorothiazide contains 250 mg of chlorothiazide per 5 ml, alcohol 0.5%, with methylparaben 0.12%, propylparaben 0.02%, and benzoic acid 0.1% added as preservatives. The inactive ingredients are D&C yellow 10, flavors, glycerin, purified water, sodium saccharin, sucrose and tragacanth.

Intravenous sodium chlorothiazide is a sterile lyophilized white powder and is supplied in a vial containing: Chlorothiazide sodium equivalent to chlorothiazide, 0.5 g; *Inactive ingredients:* Mannitol, 25 g; sodium hydroxide to adjust pH, with 0.4 mg thimerosal (mercury derivative) added as preservative.

CLINICAL PHARMACOLOGY

The mechanism of the antihypertensive effect of thiazides is unknown. Chlorothiazide does not usually affect normal blood pressure.

Chlorothiazide affects the distal renal tubular mechanism of electrolyte absorption. At maximal therapeutic dosage all thiazides are approximately equal in their diuretic efficacy.

Chlorothiazide increases excretion of sodium and chloride in approximately equivalent amounts. Natriuresis may be accompanied by some loss of potassium and bicarbonate.

After oral use diuresis begins within 2 hours, peaks in about 4 hours and lasts about 6-12 hours. Following intravenous use of sodium chlorothiazide, onset of the diuretic occurs in 15 minutes and the maximal action in 30 minutes.

PHARMACOKINETICS AND METABOLISM

Chlorothiazide is not metabolized but is eliminated rapidly by the kidney. The plasma half-life of chlorothiazide is 45-120 minutes. After oral doses, 10-15% of the dose is excreted unchanged in the urine. Chlorothiazide crosses the placental but not the blood-brain barrier and is excreted in breast milk.

INDICATIONS AND USAGE

Chlorothiazide is indicated as adjunctive therapy in edema associated with congestive heart failure, hepatic cirrhosis, and corticosteroid and estrogen therapy.

Chlorothiazide has also been found useful in edema due to various forms of renal dysfunction such as nephrotic syndrome, acute glomerulonephritis, and chronic renal failure.

Chlorothiazide is indicated in the management of hypertension either as the sole therapeutic agent or to enhance the effectiveness of other antihypertensive drugs in the more severe forms of hypertension.

C

Use in Pregnancy: Routine use of diuretics during normal pregnancy is inappropriate and exposes mother and fetus to unnecessary hazard. Diuretics do not prevent development of toxemia of pregnancy and there is no satisfactory evidence that they are useful in the treatment of toxemia.

Edema during pregnancy may arise from pathologic causes or from the physiologic and mechanical consequences of pregnancy. Thiazides are indicated in pregnancy when edema is due to pathologic causes, just as they are in the absence of pregnancy (see PRECAUTIONS, Pregnancy). Dependent edema in pregnancy, resulting from the restriction of venous return by the gravid uterus, is properly treated through elevation of the lower extremities and use of support stockings. Use of diuretics to lower intravascular volume in this instance is illogical and unnecessary. During normal pregnancy there is hypervolemia which is not harmful to the fetus or the mother in the absence of cardiovascular disease. However, it may be associated with edema, rarely generalized edema. If such edema causes discomfort, increased recumbency will often provide relief. Rarely this edema may cause extreme discomfort which is not relieved by rest In these instances, a short course of diuretic therapy may provide relief and be appropriate.

CONTRAINDICATIONS

Anuria: Hypersensitivity to this product or to other sulfonamide-derived drugs.

WARNINGS

Use with caution in severe renal disease. In patients with renal disease, thiazides may precipitate azotemia. Cumulative effects of the drug may develop in patients with impaired renal function.

Thiazides should be used with caution in patients with impaired hepatic function or progressive liver disease, since minor alterations of fluid and electrolyte balance may precipitate hepatic coma.

Thiazides may add to or potentiate the action of other antihypertensive drugs.

Sensitivity reactions may occur in patients with or without a history of allergy or bronchial asthma.

The possibility of exacerbation or activation of systemic lupus erythematosus has been reported.

Lithium generally should not be given with diuretics (see DRUG INTERACTIONS).

IV ONLY

Intravenous use in infants and children has been limited and is not generally recommended.

PRECAUTIONS

GENERAL

All patients receiving diuretic therapy should be observed for evidence of fluid or electrolyte imbalance: namely, hyponatremia, hypochloremic alkalosis, and hypokalemia. Serum and urine electrolyte determinations are particularly important when the patient is vomiting excessively or receiving parenteral fluids. Warning signs or symptoms of fluid and electrolyte imbalance, irrespective of cause, include dryness of mouth, thirst, weakness, lethargy, drowsiness, restlessness, confusion, seizures, muscle pains or cramps, muscular fatigue, hypotension, oliguria, tachycardia, and gastrointestinal disturbances such as nausea and vomiting.

Hypokalemia may develop, especially with brisk diuresis, when severe cirrhosis is present or after prolonged therapy.

Interference with adequate oral electrolyte intake will also contribute to hypokalemia. Hypokalemia may cause cardiac arrhythmias and may also sensitize or exaggerate the response of the heart to the toxic effects of digitalis (*e.g.*, increased ventricular irritability). Hypokalemia may be avoided or treated by use of potassium sparing diuretics or potassium supplements such as foods with a high potassium content.

Although any chloride deficit is generally mild and usually does not require specific treatment except under extraordinary circumstances (as in liver disease or renal disease), chloride replacement may be required in the treatment of metabolic alkalosis.

Dilutional hyponatremia may occur in edematous patients in hot weather; appropriate therapy is water restriction, rather than administration of salt, except in rare instances when the hyponatremia is life-threatening. In actual salt depletion, appropriate replacement is the therapy of choice.

Hyperuricemia may occur or acute gout may be precipitated in certain patients receiving thiazides.

In diabetic patients dosage adjustments of insulin or oral hypoglycemic agents may be required. Hyperglycemia may occur with thiazide diuretics. Thus latent diabetes mellitus may become manifest during thiazide therapy.

The antihypertensive effects of the drug may be enhanced in the post-sympathectomy patient.

If progressive renal impairment becomes evident, consider withholding or discontinuing diuretic therapy.

Thiazides have been shown to increase the urinary excretion of magnesium; this may result in hypo-magnesemia.

Thiazides may decrease urinary calcium excretion. Thiazides may cause intermittent and slight elevation of serum in the absence of known disorders of calcium metabolism. Marked hyperkalemia may be evidence of a hyperparathyroidism. Thiazides should be discontinued before carrying out tests for parathyroid function.

Increases in cholesterol and triglyceride levels may be associated with thiazide diuretic therapy.

LABORATORY TESTS

Periodic determination of serum electrolytes to detect possible electrolyte imbalance should be done at appropriate intervals.

DRUG/LABORATORY TEST INTERACTIONS

Thiazides should be discontinued before carrying out tests for parathyroid function. (See PRECAUTIONS, General.)

CARCINOGENESIS, MUTAGENESIS, AND IMPAIRMENT OF FERTILITY

Carcinogenicity studies have not been done with chlorothiazide.

Chlorothiazide was not mutagenic *in vitro* in the Ames microbial mutagen test (using a maximum concentration of 5 mg/plate and *Salmonella typhimurium* strains TA98 and TA100) and was not mutagenic and did not induce mitotic nondisjunction in diploid strains of *Aspergillus nidulans.*

Chlorothiazide had no adverse effects on fertility in female rats at doses up to 60 mg/kg/day and no adverse effects on fertility in male rats at doses up to 40 mg/kg/day. These doses are 1.5 and 1.0 times (calculations based on a human body weight of 50 kg) the recommended maximum human dose, respectively, when compared on a body weight basis.

PREGNANCY

Tablets and Oral Suspension Only

Teratogenic Effects — Pregnancy Category C: Although reproduction studies performed with chlorothiazide doses of 50 and 60 mg/kg/day in rats and 500 mg/kg/day in mice revealed no external abnormalities of the fetus or impairment of growth and survival of the fetus due to chlorothiazide, such studies did not include complete examinations for visceral and skeletal abnormalities. It is not known whether chlorothiazide can cause fetal harm when administered to a pregnant woman; however, thiazides cross the placental barrier and appear in cord blood. Chlorothiazide should be used during pregnancy only if clearly needed (see INDICATIONS AND USAGE).

IV Only

Teratogenic Effects — Pregnancy Category C: Although reproduction studies performed with chlorothiazide doses of 50 mg/kg/day in rabbits, 60 mg/kg/day in rats and 500 mg/kg/day in mice revealed no external abnormalities of the fetus or impairment of growth and survival of the fetus due to chlorothiazide, such studies did not include complete examinations for visceral and skeletal abnormalities.It is not known whether chlorothiazide can cause fetal harm when administered to a pregnant woman; however, thiazides cross the placental barrier and appear in cord blood. Chlorothiazide should be used during pregnancy only if clearly needed (see INDICATIONS AND USAGE).

All Forms

Nonteratogenic Effects: These may include fetal or neonatal jaundice, thrombocytopenia, and possibly other adverse reactions which have occurred in the adult.

NURSING MOTHERS

Because of the potential for serious adverse reactions in nursing infants from chlorothiazide, a decision should be made whether to discontinue nursing or to discontinue the drug, taking into account the importance of the drug to the mother.

PEDIATRIC USE

Safety and effectiveness of Intravenous Sodium Chlorothiazide in children has not been established.

DRUG INTERACTIONS

When given concurrently the following drugs may interact with thiazide diuretics.

Alcohol, barbiturates, or narcotics: Potentiation of orthostatic hypotension may occur.

Antidiabetic drugs (oral agents and insulin): Dosage adjustment of the antidiabetic drug may be required.

Other antihypertensive drugs: Addictive effect or potentiation.

Cholestyramine and colestipol resins: Both cholestyramine and colestipol resins have the potential of binding thiazide diuretics and reducing diuretic absorption from the gastrointestinal tract.

Corticosteroids, ACTH: Intensified electrolyte depletion, particularly hypokalemia.

Pressor amines (*e.g.*, norepinephrine): Possible decreased response to pressor amines but not sufficient to preclude their use.

Skeletal muscle relaxants, nondepolarizing (*e.g.*, tubocurarine): Possible increased responsiveness to the muscle relaxant.

Lithium: Generally should not be given with diuretics. Diuretic agents reduce the renal clearance of lithium and add a high risk of lithium toxicity. Refer to the package insert for lithium preparations before use of such preparations with chlorothiazide.

Non-steroidal anti-inflammatory drugs: In some patients, the administration of a non-steroidal anti-inflammatory agent can reduce the diuretic, natriuretic, and antihypertensive effects of loop, potassium-sparing and thiazide diuretics. Therefore, when chlorothiazide and non-steroidal anti-inflammatory agents are used concomitantly, the patient should be observed closely to determine if the desired effect of the diuretic is obtained.

ADVERSE REACTIONS

The following adverse reactions have been reported and, within each category, are listed in order of decreasing severity.

Body as a Whole: Weakness.

Cardiovascular: Hypotension including orthostatic hypotension (may be aggravated by alcohol, barbiturates, narcotics or antihypertensive drugs).

Digestive: Pancreatitis, jaundice (intrahepatic cholestatic jaundice), diarrhea, vomiting, sialadenitis, cramping, constipation, gastric irritation, nausea, anorexia.

Hematologic: Aplastic anemia, agranulocytosis, leukopenia, hemolytic anemia, thrombocytopenia.

Hypersensitivity: Anaphylactic reactions, necrotizing angiitis (vasculitis and cutaneous vasculitis), respiratory distress including pneumonitis and pulmonary edema, photosensitivity, fever, urticaria, rash, purpura.

Metabolic: Electrolyte imbalance (see PRECAUTIONS), hyperglycemia, glycosuria, hyperuricemia.

Musculoskeletal: Muscle spasm.

Nervous System/Psychiatric: Vertigo, paresthesias, dizziness, headache, restlessness.

Renal: Renal failure, renal dysfunction, interstitial nephritis. (See WARNINGS).

Skin: Erythema multiforme including Stevens-Johnson syndrome, exfoliative dermatitis including toxic epidermal necrolysis, alopecia.
Special Senses: Transient blurred vision, xanthopsia.
Urogenital: Impotence.
Whenever adverse reactions are moderate or severe, thiazide dosage should be reduced or therapy withdrawn.

DOSAGE AND ADMINISTRATION

TABLETS AND ORAL SUSPENSION

Therapy should be individualized according to patient response. Use the smallest dosage necessary to achieve the required response.

ADULTS

For Edema: The usual adult dosage is 0.5-1.0 g once or twice a day. Many patients with edema respond to intermittent therapy, *i.e.*, administration on alternate days or on 3-5 days each week. With an intermittent schedule, excessive response and the resulting undesirable electrolyte imbalance are less likely to occur.
For Control of Hypertension: The usual adult dosage is 0.5 or 1.0 g a day as a single or divided dose. Dosage is increased or decreased according to blood pressure response. Rarely some patients may require up to 2.0 g a day in divided doses.

INFANTS AND CHILDREN

For Diuresis and For Control of Hypertension: The usual pediatric dosage is 5-10 mg/lb (10-20 mg/kg) per day in single or 2 divided doses, not to exceed 375 mg/day (2.5-7.5 ml or ½ to 1½ teaspoonfuls of the oral suspension daily) in infants up to 2 years of age or 1 g/day in children 2-12 years of age. In infants less than 6 months of age, doses up to 15 mg/lb (30 mg/kg/day in 2 divided) doses may be required.

STORAGE

Tablets: Keep container tightly closed. Protect from moisture, freezing, 20°C (-4°F) and store at room temperature, 15-30°C (59-86°F).
Oral Suspension: Keep container tightly closed. Protect from freezing, - 20°C (-4°F) and store at room temperature, 15-30°C (59-86°F).

INTRAVENOUS ROUTE

Intravenous sodium chlorothiazide should be reserved for patients unable to take oral medication or for emergency situations.

Therapy should be individualized according to patient response. Use the smallest dosage necessary to achieve the required response.

Intravenous use in infants and children has been limited and is not generally recommended.

When medication can be taken orally, therapy with chlorothiazide tablets or oral suspension may be substituted for intravenous therapy, using the same dosage schedule as for the parenteral route.

Intravenous sodium chlorothiazide may be given slowly by direct intravenous injection or by intravenous infusion.

Add 18 ml of sterile water for injection to the vial to form an isotonic solution for intravenous injection. Never add less than 18 ml. Unused solution may be stored at room temperature for 24 hours, after which it must be discarded. Parenteral drug products should be inspected visually for particulate matter and discoloration prior to use whenever solution and container permit. The solution is compatible with dextrose or sodium chloride solutions for intravenous infusion. Avoid simultaneous administration of solutions of chlorothiazide with whole blood or its derivatives.

EXTRAVASATION MUST BE RIGIDLY AVOIDED. DO NOT GIVE SUBCUTANEOUSLY OR INTRAMUSCULARLY.

The usual adult dosage is 0.5-1.0 g once or twice a day. Many patients with edema respond to intermittent therapy, *i.e.*, administration on alternate days or on 3 or 5 days each week. With an intermittent schedule, excessive response and the resulting undesirable electrolyte imbalance are less likely to occur.

STORAGE

Store reconstituted solution at room temperature and discard unused portion after 24 hours.
Store lyophilized powder between 2-25°C (36-77°F).
Store reconstituted solution at room temperature, 15-30°C (59- 86°F), and discard unused portion after 24 hours.

PRODUCT LISTING - RATED THERAPEUTICALLY EQUIVALENT

Tablet - Oral - 250 mg

100's	$4.00	GENERIC, Cmc-Consolidated Midland Corporation	00223-0654-01
100's	$4.75	GENERIC, Major Pharmaceuticals Inc	00904-0183-60
100's	$5.97	GENERIC, Aligen Independent Laboratories Inc	00405-4179-01
100's	$6.08	GENERIC, Moore, H.L. Drug Exchange Inc	00839-5967-06
100's	$6.31	GENERIC, Qualitest Products Inc	00603-2737-21
100's	$6.60	GENERIC, West Point Pharma	59591-0240-68
100's	$7.19	GENERIC, Major Pharmaceuticals Inc	00904-0183-61
100's	$7.43	GENERIC, Interstate Drug Exchange Inc	00814-1642-14
100's	$7.50	GENERIC, Raway Pharmacal Inc	00686-0060-20
100's	$13.63	GENERIC, West Ward Pharmaceutical Corporation	00143-1209-01
100's	$14.81	GENERIC, Mylan Pharmaceuticals Inc	00378-0150-01
100's	$16.81	DIURIL, Merck & Company Inc	00006-0214-68
100's	$20.25	GENERIC, Udl Laboratories Inc	51079-0060-20
250's	$13.15	GENERIC, Major Pharmaceuticals Inc	00904-0183-70

Tablet - Oral - 500 mg

30's	$6.53	GENERIC, Pd-Rx Pharmaceuticals	55289-0571-30
100's	$7.24	GENERIC, Vita-Rx Corporation	49727-0133-02
100's	$7.95	GENERIC, Cmc-Consolidated Midland Corporation	00223-0655-01
100's	$9.60	GENERIC, West Point Pharma	59591-0245-68
100's	$10.50	GENERIC, Watson/Schein Pharmaceuticals Inc	00364-0390-01
100's	$10.50	GENERIC, Aligen Independent Laboratories Inc	00405-4180-01
100's	$10.79	GENERIC, Moore, H.L. Drug Exchange Inc	00839-7695-06
100's	$11.50	GENERIC, Raway Pharmacal Inc	00686-0061-20
100's	$11.85	GENERIC, Ivax Corporation	00182-0790-01
100's	$12.90	GENERIC, Major Pharmaceuticals Inc	00904-0184-60
100's	$13.65	GENERIC, Interstate Drug Exchange Inc	00814-1643-14
100's	$13.78	GENERIC, Major Pharmaceuticals Inc	00904-0184-61
100's	$25.25	GENERIC, West Ward Pharmaceutical Corporation	00143-1210-01
100's	$25.30	GENERIC, Qualitest Products Inc	00603-2738-21
100's	$25.35	GENERIC, Mylan Pharmaceuticals Inc	00378-0162-01
100's	$25.40	GENERIC, Udl Laboratories Inc	51079-0061-20
100's	$26.69	DIURIL, Merck & Company Inc	00006-0432-68

PRODUCT LISTING - EQUIVALENTS NOT AVAILABLE

Powder For Injection - Intravenous - 0.5 Gm			
1's	$11.04	DIURIL SODIUM, Merck & Company Inc	00006-3619-32
Suspension - Oral - 250 mg/5 ml			
237 ml	$12.26	DIURIL, Merck & Company Inc	00006-3239-66
Tablet - Oral - 250 mg			
100's	$3.32	GENERIC, Vangard Labs	00615-1550-01
Tablet - Oral - 500 mg			
30's	$8.35	GENERIC, Allscripts Pharmaceutical Company	54569-0537-01

Chlorotrianisene *(000742)*

For complete prescribing information, refer to the CD-ROM included with the book.

Categories: Carcinoma, prostate; Hypoestrogenism; Kraurosis vulvae; Menopause; Vaginitis, atrophic; Pregnancy Category X; FDA Approved 1951 Aug
Drug Classes: Antineoplastics, hormones/hormone modifiers; Estrogens; Hormones/hormone modifiers
Brand Names: Tace
Foreign Brand Availability: Estregur (Mexico)
Cost of Therapy: $32.26 (Prostate Cancer; Tace; 12 mg; 1 capsule/day; 30 day supply)

WARNING

ESTROGENS HAVE BEEN REPORTED TO INCREASE THE RISK OF ENDOMETRIAL CARCINOMA IN POST-MENOPAUSAL WOMEN. CLOSE CLINICAL SURVEILLANCE OF ALL WOMEN TAKING ESTROGENS IS IMPORTANT. IN ALL CASES OF UNDIAGNOSED PERSISTENT OR RECURRING ABNORMAL VAGINAL BLEEDING, ADEQUATE DIAGNOSTIC MEASURES INCLUDING ENDOMETRIAL SAMPLING WHEN INDICATED SHOULD BE UNDERTAKEN TO RULE OUT MALIGNANCY. THERE IS CURRENTLY NO EVIDENCE THAT "NATURAL" ESTROGENS ARE MORE OR LESS HAZARDOUS THAN "SYNTHETIC" ESTROGENS AT EQUIESTROGENIC DOSES.

ESTROGENS SHOULD NOT BE USED DURING PREGNANCY. ESTROGEN THERAPY DURING PREGNANCY IS ASSOCIATED WITH AN INCREASED RISK OF CONGENITAL DEFECTS IN THE REPRODUCTIVE ORGANS OF THE MALE AND FEMALE FETUS, AN INCREASED RISK OF VAGINAL ADENOSIS, SQUAMOUS CELL DYSPLASIA OF THE UTERINE CERVIX, AND VAGINAL CANCER IN THE FEMALE LATER IN LIFE. THE 1985 DIETHYLSTILBESTROL (DES) TASK FORCE CONCLUDED THAT WOMEN WHO USED DES DURING THEIR PREGNANCIES MAY SUBSEQUENTLY EXPERIENCE AN INCREASED RISK OF BREAST CANCER. HOWEVER, A CAUSAL RELATIONSHIP IS STILL UNPROVEN, AND THE OBSERVED LEVEL OF RISK IS SIMILAR TO THAT FOR A NUMBER OF OTHER BREAST CANCER RISK FACTORS. THERE IS NO INDICATION FOR ESTROGEN THERAPY DURING PREGNANCY. ESTROGENS ARE INEFFECTIVE FOR THE PREVENTION OR TREATMENT OF THREATENED OR HABITUAL ABORTION.

*** If chlorotrianisene is used during pregnancy, or if the patient becomes pregnant while taking this drug, she should be apprised of the potential risks to the fetus, and the advisability of pregnancy continuation.**

DESCRIPTION

Chlorotrianisene is available in capsule form suitable for oral administration. Each green, soft gelatin capsule contains 12 mg of chlorotrianisene. This capsule also contains inactive ingredients: corn oil (solvent), FD&C blue no. 1, FD&C yellow no. 5 (tartrazine), gelatin, glycerin, methylparaben, propylparaben, titanium dioxide, and water.

Each two-tone green, hard gelatin capsule contains 25 mg of chlorotrianisene. This capsule also contains inactive ingredients: FD&C blue no. 1 or FD&C green no. 3, FD&C Blue No. 2, FD&C red no. 40, FD&C yellow no. 5 (tartrazine), FD&C yellow no. 6, gelatin, iron oxide, magnesium stearate, titanium dioxide, and tristearin (solvent).

Chlorotrianisene is a long-acting, synthetic estrogen with the chemical name 1,1′,1′′-(1-chloro-1-ethenyl-2-ylidene)-tris[4-methoxy]-benzene.

Chlorotrianisene occurs as small, white crystals or as a crystalline powder. It is odorless. It is slightly soluble in alcohol and very slightly soluble in water.

INDICATIONS AND USAGE

Chlorotrianisene is indicated in the treatment of:

Advanced androgen-dependent carcinoma of the prostate (for palliation only).

Moderate to severe vasomotor symptoms associated with the menopause. There is no adequate evidence that estrogens are effective for nervous symptoms or depression which might occur during menopause and they should not be used to treat these conditions.

Atrophic vaginitis.

Kraurosis vulvae.

Hypoestrogenism due to hypogonadism, castration, or primary ovarian failure.

CONTRAINDICATIONS

Chlorotrianisene is contraindicated in patients with a known hypersensitivity to chlorotrianisene or other ingredients of the formulation.

Chlorotrianisene should not be used in women or men with any of the following conditions:

Known or suspected pregnancy. (See BOXED WARNING.) Estrogen may cause fetal harm when administered to a pregnant woman.

Known or suspected cancer of the breast except in appropriately selected patients being treated for metastatic disease.

Known or suspected estrogen-dependent neoplasia.

Undiagnosed abnormal genital bleeding.

Active thrombophlebitis or thromboembolic disorders — Women on estrogen replacement therapy have not been reported to have an increased risk of thrombophlebitis and/or thromboembolic disease. However, there is insufficient information regarding women who have had previous thromboembolic disease.

WARNINGS

INDUCTION OF MALIGNANT NEOPLASMS

Some studies have suggested a possible increased incidence of breast cancer in those women on estrogen therapy taking higher doses for prolonged periods of time. The majority of studies, however, have not shown an association with the usual doses used for estrogen replacement therapy. Women on this therapy should have regular breast examinations and should be instructed in breast self-examination. The reported endometrial cancer risk among estrogen users was about 4-fold or greater than in non-users, and appears dependent on duration of treatment and on estrogen dose. There is no significantly increased risk associated with the use of estrogens for less than 1 year. The greatest risk appears associated with prolonged use — 5 years or more. In one study, persistence of risk was demonstrated for 10 years after cessation of estrogen treatment. In another study, a significant decrease in the incidence of endometrial cancer occurred 6 months after estrogen withdrawal.

Estrogen therapy during pregnancy is associated with an increased risk of fetal congenital reproductive tract disorders. In females, there is an increased risk of vaginal adenosis, squamous cell dysplasia of the cervix, and cancer later in life; in the male, urogenital abnormalities. Although some of these changes are benign, it is not known whether they are precursors of malignancy.

GALLBLADDER DISEASE

The risk of surgically confirmed gallbladder disease has been reported to be 2.5 times higher in women receiving postmenopausal estrogens.

CARDIOVASCULAR DISEASE

Large doses of estrogen (5 mg conjugated estrogens per day), comparable to those used to treat cancer of the prostate and breast, have been shown in a large prospective clinical trial in men to increase the risk of non-fatal myocardial infarction, pulmonary embolism, and thrombophlebitis. It cannot necessarily be extrapolated from men to women. However, to avoid the theoretical cardiovascular risk caused by high estrogen doses, the doses for estrogen replacement therapy should not exceed the recommended dose.

ELEVATED BLOOD PRESSURE

There is no evidence that this may occur with use of estrogens in the menopause. However, blood pressure should be monitored with estrogen use, especially if high doses are used.

HYPERCALCEMIA

Administration of estrogens may lead to severe hypercalcemia in patients with breast cancer and bone metastases. If this occurs, the drug should be stopped and appropriate measures taken to reduce the serum calcium level.

DOSAGE AND ADMINISTRATION

Advanced androgen-dependent carcinoma of the prostate, for palliation only. The usual dosage is 12-25 mg daily (one or two 12 mg capsules or one 25 mg capsule).

For treatment of moderate to severe vasomotor symptoms, atrophic vaginitis, or kraurosis vulvae associated with the menopause. The lowest dose that will control symptoms should be chosen and medication should be discontinued as promptly as possible. Administration should be cyclic (*e.g.,* 3 weeks on and 1 week off).

Attempts to discontinue or taper medication should be made at 3-6 month intervals.

The usual dosage range for vasomotor symptoms, atrophic vaginitis, or kraurosis vulvae associated with the menopause is 12 to 25 mg daily (one or two 12 mg capsules or one 25 mg capsule) for 30 days; one or more courses may be prescribed.

Female hypogonadism; primary ovarian failure.

The usual dosage is 12-25 mg daily (one or two 12 mg capsules or one 25 mg capsule) for 21 days. This course may, if desired, be followed immediately by the intramuscular injection of 100 mg of progesterone; alternatively, an oral progesterone such as medroxyprogesterone may be given during the last 5 days of chlorotrianisene therapy. The next course may begin on the 5th day of the induced uterine bleeding.

Treated patients with an intact uterus should be monitored closely for signs of endometrial cancer, and appropriate diagnostic measures should be taken to rule out malignancy in the event of persistent or recurrent abnormal vaginal bleeding.

PRODUCT LISTING - RATED THERAPEUTICALLY EQUIVALENT

Capsule - Oral - 12 mg

100's	$107.52	TACE, Aventis Pharmaceuticals	00068-0690-61

Capsule - Oral - 25 mg

60's	$113.64	TACE, Aventis Pharmaceuticals	00068-0691-60

Chlorpheniramine Maleate *(000751)*

Categories: Allergy, blood, adjunct; Allergy, plasma, adjunct; Anaphylaxis, adjunct; Angioedema; Conjunctivitis, allergic; Dermographism; Rhinitis, perennial allergic; Rhinitis, seasonal allergic; Rhinitis, vasomotor; Urticaria; Pregnancy Category C; FDA Approved 1972 Dec; WHO Formulary

Drug Classes: Antihistamines, H1

Brand Names: Allerkyn; Chlor-Trimeton; Cloro; Clorten; Comin; Cophene-B; Corometon; Evenin; Histacort; Histex; Kelargine; Methyrit; Polaronil; Reston

Foreign Brand Availability: Ahiston (Israel); Alergical (Peru); Aller (Malaysia); Allerfin (Benin; Burkina-Faso; Ethiopia; Gambia; Ghana; Guinea; Ivory-Coast; Kenya; Liberia; Malawi; Mali; Mauritania; Mauritius; Morocco; Niger; Nigeria; Senegal; Seychelles; Sierra-Leone; Sudan; Tanzania; Tunia; Uganda; Zambia; Zimbabwe); Allergex (South-Africa); Allergin (Japan; Thailand); Allergyl (Benin; Burkina-Faso; Ethiopia; Gambia; Ghana; Guinea; Ivory-Coast; Kenya; Liberia; Malawi; Mali; Mauritania; Mauritius; Morocco; Niger; Nigeria; Senegal; Seychelles; Sierra-Leone; South-Africa; Sudan; Tanzania; Tunia; Uganda; Zambia; Zimbabwe); Allermin (Taiwan); Allerphen (Singapore); Anaphyl (Israel); Antamin (Philippines); Antihistamin (Peru); Apomin (Hong-Kong); Cadistin (Benin; Burkina-Faso; Ethiopia; Gambia; Ghana; Guinea; Ivory-Coast; Kenya; Liberia; Malawi; Mali; Mauritania; Mauritius; Morocco; Niger; Nigeria; Senegal; Seychelles; Sierra-Leone; Sudan; Tanzania; Tunia; Uganda; Zambia; Zimbabwe); Chlometon (Japan); Chlorleate (Thailand); Chlorpheno (Thailand); Chlorpheniramine DHA (Hong-Kong); Chlorphenon (Indonesia); Chlorpyrimine (Hong-Kong; Malaysia; Thailand); Chlor-Tripolon (Canada); Chlortrimeton (South-Africa); Cloroalergan (Peru); Cloro-Trimeton (Costa-Rica; Dominican-Republic; El-Salvador; Guatemala; Honduras; Mexico; Nicaragua; Panama); Cloro Trimeton (Argentina); Clorotrimeton (Colombia; Peru); Cohistan (Indonesia; Thailand); Fenaler (Dominican-Republic; El-Salvador; Guatemala; Honduras; Nicaragua; Panama); Histafen (New-Zealand); Histal (Bahamas; Barbados; Belize; Bermuda; Curacao; Guyana; Jamaica; Netherland-Antilles; Surinam; Trinidad); Histar (Japan); Histat (Bahrain; Cyprus; Egypt; Iran; Iraq; Jordan; Kuwait; Lebanon; Libya; Oman; Qatar; Republic-of-Yemen; Saudi-Arabia; Syria; United-Arab-Emirates); Histatapp (Thailand); Histaton (Peru); Histavil (Bahrain; Cyprus; Egypt; Iran; Iraq; Jordan; Kuwait; Lebanon; Libya; Oman; Qatar; Republic-of-Yemen; Saudi-Arabia; Syria; United-Arab-Emirates); Histin (Bahrain; Cyprus; Egypt; Iran; Iraq; Jordan; Kuwait; Lebanon; Libya; Oman; Qatar; Republic-of-Yemen; Saudi-Arabia; Syria; United-Arab-Emirates); Istamex (Greece); Istaminol (Greece); Kobis (Japan); Losmanin (Greece); Pehachlor (Indonesia); Phenamine (Korea); Piriton (Bahamas; Bahrain; Barbados; Belize; Bermuda; Curacao; Cyprus; Egypt; Guyana; Iran; Iraq; Ireland; Jamaica; Jordan; Kuwait; Lebanon; Libya; Malaysia; Netherland-Antilles; Oman; Qatar; Republic-of-Yemen; Saudi-Arabia; Surinam; Syria; Thailand; Trinidad; United-Arab-Emirates); Polaramine (Bahamas; Bahrain; Barbados; Belize; Benin; Bermuda; Burkina-Faso; Curacao; Cyprus; Egypt; Ethiopia; Gambia; Ghana; Guinea; Guyana; Iran; Iraq; Ivory-Coast; Jamaica; Jordan; Kenya; Kuwait; Lebanon; Liberia; Libya; Malawi; Mali; Mauritania; Mauritius; Morocco; Netherland-Antilles; Niger; Nigeria; Oman; Qatar; Republic-of-Yemen; Saudi-Arabia; Senegal; Seychelles; Sierra-Leone; Sudan; Surinam; Syria; Tanzania; Trinidad; Tunia; Uganda; United-Arab-Emirates; Zambia; Zimbabwe); Prof-N-4 (Argentina); Reston M (Japan); Sprinsol (Hong-Kong); Trimeton (Italy); Trimeton Repetabs (Mexico)

HCFA JCODE(S): J0730 per 10 mg IV, IM, SC

DESCRIPTION

Chlorpheniramine maleate is an antihistaminic agent. It is a white, odorless, crystalline powder, the solutions of which have a pH between 4 and 5.

CLINICAL PHARMACOLOGY

Chlorpheniramine maleate is an antihistaminic drug which possesses anticholinergic and sedative effects.

INDICATIONS AND USAGE

Chlorpheniramine maleate is indicated for the following conditions:

1. Perennial and seasonal allergic rhinitis.
2. Vasomotor rhinitis.
3. Allergic conjunctivitis due to inhalant allergens and foods.
4. Mild, uncomplicated allergic skin manifestations of urticaria and angioedema.
5. Amelioration of allergic reactions to blood or plasma.
6. Dermographism.
7. As therapy for anaphylactic reactions adjunctive to epinephrine and other standard measures after the acute manifestations have been controlled.

CONTRAINDICATIONS

This drug should not be used in newborn or premature infants.

Antihistamines should NOT be used to treat lower respiratory symptoms.

Do Not Use This Drug in Patients With:

Hypersensitivity to preparation
Asthmatic attack
Narrow-angle glaucoma
Prostatic hypertrophy
Stenosing peptic ulcer
Pyloroduodenal obstruction
Bladder neck obstruction
Patients receiving monoamine oxidase inhibitors

WARNINGS

This drug may impair the mental and/or physical abilities required for the performance of potentially hazardous tasks such as driving a vehicle or operating machinery. This drug may impair mental alertness in children. The concomitant use of alcohol or other central nervous system depressants may have an additive effect. Patients should be warned accordingly.

Use in Pregnancy: Although there is no evidence that the use of this drug is detrimental to the mother or fetus, the use of any drug in pregnancy should be carefully deliberated. This product may cause an inhibition of lactation.

Usage In Children: In infants and children particularly, antihistamines in overdosage may produce convulsions and/or death.

PRECAUTIONS

Chlorpheniramine maleate has an atropine-like action and should be used with caution in patients who may have increased intraocular pressure, hyperthyroidism, cardiovascular disease, hypertension or in patients with a history of bronchial asthma.

ADVERSE REACTIONS

The Following Adverse Reactions Have Been Reported: Drowsiness; confusion; nervousness; restlessness; nausea; vomiting; diarrhea; blurring of vision; diplopia; headache; insomnia; urticaria; epigastric distress; nasal stuffiness; difficulty in urination; constipation; tightness of the chest and wheezing; thickening of bronchial secretions; dryness of mouth, nose, and throat; tingling, heaviness, and weakness of hands; vertigo; palpitation; drug rash; hemolytic anemia; hypotension; anaphylaxis.

DOSAGE AND ADMINISTRATION

Adults: The usual adult dose is 4 mg three or four times daily.
Children: For children over 20 lb the usual dose is 2 mg three or four times daily.
Storage: Store at controlled room temperature 15-30°C (59-86°F).

PRODUCT LISTING - RATED THERAPEUTICALLY EQUIVALENT

Solution - Injectable - 10 mg/ml

30 ml	$6.64	GENERIC, Moore, H.L. Drug Exchange Inc	00839-5161-36
30's	$4.50	GENERIC, Cmc-Consolidated Midland Corporation	00223-7310-30

Tablet - Oral - 4 mg

100's	$1.71	FEDERAL UPPER LIMIT, H.C.F.A. F F P	99999-0751-06
100's	$3.50	GENERIC, Major Pharmaceuticals Inc	00904-0012-59

PRODUCT LISTING - EQUIVALENTS NOT AVAILABLE

Solution - Injectable - 10 mg/ml

10's	$4.00	GENERIC, Cmc-Consolidated Midland Corporation	00223-7310-10
30 ml	$7.01	GENERIC, Watson/Schein Pharmaceuticals Inc	00364-6523-56

Chlorpromazine Hydrochloride *(000797)*

Categories: Conduct disorders in children; Bipolar affective disorder; Hiccups, intractable; Mania; Nausea; Porphyria, acute intermittent; Schizophrenia; Vomiting; Tetanus, adjunct; FDA Approved 1954 Mar; Pregnancy Category C; WHO Formulary
Drug Classes: Antiemetics/antivertigo; Antipsychotics; Phenothiazines
Brand Names: **Thorazine**
Foreign Brand Availability: Ampliactil (Argentina); Aspersinal (Argentina); Chlomazine (Japan); Chloractil (England); Chlorazin (Bulgaria; Switzerland); Chlorpromanyl (Canada); Chlorpromed (Thailand); Clonazine (Ireland); Contomin (Japan); Duncan (Thailand); Esmino (Japan); Hibernal (Hungary; Sweden); Klorproman (Czech-Republic; Finland); Klorpromazin (Finland); Laractyl (Philippines); Largactil (Australia; Bahamas; Bahrain; Barbados; Belize; Benin; Bermuda; Burkina-Faso; Canada; Costa-Rica; Curacao; Cyprus; Czech-Republic; Denmark; Dominican-Republic; Ecuador; Egypt; El-Salvador; England; Ethiopia; Finland; France; Gambia; Ghana; Greece; Guatemala; Guinea; Guyana; Honduras; Hong-Kong; Indonesia; Iraq; Italy; Ivory-Coast; Jamaica; Kenya; Kuwait; Lebanon; Liberia; Libya; Malawi; Mali; Mauritania; Mauritius; Morocco; Netherland-Antilles; Netherlands; New-Zealand; Niger; Nigeria; Norway; Oman; Panama; Peru; Portugal; Qatar; Republic-of-Yemen; Saudi-Arabia; Senegal; Seychelles; Sierra-Leone; South-Africa; Spain; Sudan; Surinam; Switzerland; Syria; Tanzania; Trinidad; Tunia; Uganda; United-Arab-Emirates; Zambia; Zimbabwe); Largactil Forte (New-Zealand); Matcine (Malaysia; Thailand); Neomazine (Korea); Plegomazine (Bahamas; Barbados; Belize; Bermuda; Curacao; Guyana; Iraq; Jamaica; Netherland-Antilles; Surinam; Trinidad); Promactil (Indonesia); Promexin (Japan); Propaphenin (Germany); Prozil (Denmark); Prozin (Italy); Psynor (Philippines); Taroctyl (Israel); Winsumin (Taiwan); Wintermin (Japan; Taiwan)
Cost of Therapy: $56.53 (Psychotic Disorders; Thorazine; 25 mg; 3 tablets/day; 30 day supply)
$4.24 (Psychotic Disorders; Generic Tablets; 25 mg; 3 tablets/day; 30 day supply)
$17.00 (Nausea and Vomiting; Thorazine; 10 mg; 4 tablets/day; 10 day supply)
$1.90 (Nausea and Vomiting; Generic Tablets; 10 mg; 4 tablets/day; 10 day supply)
HCFA JCODE(S): J3230 up to 50 mg IM, IV

DESCRIPTION

Chlorpromazine is 10-(3-dimethylaminopropyl)-2-chlorphenothiazine, a dimethylamine derivative of phenothiazine. It is present in oral and injectable forms as the hydrochloride salt, and in the suppositories as the base. It has a chemical formula of $C_{17}H_{19}ClN_2S$.

TABLETS

Thorazine tablets contain 10, 25, 50, 100, or 200 mg of chlorpromazine hydrochloride. Inactive ingredients consist of benzoic acid, croscarmellose sodium, D&C yellow no. 10, FD&C blue no. 2, FD&C yellow no. 6, gelatin, hydroxypropyl methylcellulose, lactose, magnesium stearate, methylparaben, polyethylene glycol, propylparaben, talc, titanium dioxide and trace amounts of other inactive ingredients.

AMPULS

Each milliliter contains, in aqueous solution, chlorpromazine hydrochloride, 25 mg; ascorbic acid, 2 mg; sodium bisulfite, 1 mg; sodium chloride, 6 mg; sodium sulfite, 1 mg.

MULTI-DOSE VIALS

Each milliliter contains, in aqueous solution, chlorpromazine hydrochloride, 25 mg; ascorbic acid, 2 mg; sodium bisulfite, 1 mg; sodium chloride, 1 mg; sodium sulfite, 1 mg; benzyl alcohol, 2%, as a preservative.

SYRUP

Each 5 ml (1 teaspoonful) of clear, orange-custard flavored liquid contains chlorpromazine hydrochloride, 10 mg. Inactive ingredients consist of citric acid, flavors, sodium benzoate, sodium citrate, sucrose, and water.

SUPPOSITORIES

Each suppository contains chlorpromazine, 25 or 100 mg, glycerin, glyceryl monopalmitate, glyceryl monostearate, hydrogenated coconut oil fatty acids and hydrogenated palm kernel oil fatty acids.

CLINICAL PHARMACOLOGY

MECHANISM OF ACTION

The precise mechanism whereby the therapeutic effects of chlorpromazine are produced is not known. The principal pharmacological actions are psychotropic. It also exerts sedative and antiemetic activity. Chlorpromazine has actions at all levels of the central nervous system (CNS) — primarily at subcortical levels — as well as on multiple organ systems. Chlorpromazine has strong antiadrenergic and weaker peripheral anticholinergic activity; ganglionic blocking action is relatively slight. It also possesses slight antihistaminic and antiserotonin activity.

C

INDICATIONS AND USAGE

For the treatment of schizophrenia.
To control nausea and vomiting.
For relief of restlessness and apprehension before surgery.
For acute intermittent porphyria.
As an adjunct in the treatment of tetanus.
To control the manifestations of the manic type of manic-depressive illness.
For relief of intractable hiccups.
For the treatment of severe behavioral problems in children (1-12 years of age) marked by combativeness and/or explosive hyperexcitable behavior (out of proportion to immediate provocations), and in the short-term treatment of hyperactive children who show excessive motor activity with accompanying conduct disorders consisting of some or all of the following symptoms: impulsivity, difficulty sustaining attention, aggressivity, mood lability, and poor frustration tolerance.

NON-FDA APPROVED INDICATIONS

Chlorpromazine has also been used for the treatment of migraine headaches and terminal restlessness, but these uses are not approved by the FDA. In addition, retrobulbar injection of chlorpromazine has been used by some physicians for the relief of pain in patients with irreversible blindness.

CONTRAINDICATIONS

Do not use in patients with known hypersensitivity to phenothiazines.

Do not use in comatose states or in the presence of large amounts of CNS depressants (alcohol, barbiturates, narcotics, etc.).

WARNINGS

The extrapyramidal symptoms which can occur secondary to chlorpromazine may be confused with the CNS signs of an undiagnosed primary disease responsible for the vomiting, *e.g.,* Reye's syndrome or other encephalopathy. The use of chlorpromazine and other potential hepatotoxins should be avoided in children and adolescents whose signs and symptoms suggest Reye's syndrome.

TARDIVE DYSKINESIA

Tardive dyskinesia, a syndrome consisting of potentially irreversible, involuntary, dyskinetic movements, may develop in patients treated with antipsychotic drugs. Although the prevalence of the syndrome appears to be highest among the elderly, especially elderly women, it is impossible to rely upon prevalence estimates to predict, at the inception of antipsychotic treatment, which patients are likely to develop the syndrome. Whether antipsychotic drug products differ in their potential to cause tardive dyskinesia is unknown.

Both the risk of developing the syndrome and the likelihood that it will become irreversible are believed to increase as the duration of treatment and the total cumulative dose of antipsychotic drugs administered to the patient increase. However, the syndrome can develop, although much less commonly, after relatively brief treatment periods at low doses.

There is no known treatment for established cases of tardive dyskinesia, although the syndrome may remit, partially or completely, if antipsychotic treatment is withdrawn. Antipsychotic treatment itself, however, may suppress (or partially suppress) the signs and symptoms of the syndrome and thereby may possibly mask the underlying disease process. The effect that symptomatic suppression has upon the long-term course of the syndrome is unknown.

Given these considerations, antipsychotics should be prescribed in a manner that is most likely to minimize the occurrence of tardive dyskinesia. Chronic antipsychotic treatment should generally be reserved for patients who suffer from a chronic illness that, (1) is known to respond to antipsychotic drugs; and, (2) for whom alternative, equally effective, but potentially less harmful treatments are *not* available or appropriate. In patients who do require chronic treatment, the smallest dose and the shortest duration of treatment producing a satisfactory clinical response should be sought. The need for continued treatment should be reassessed periodically.

If signs and symptoms of tardive dyskinesia appear in a patient on antipsychotics, drug discontinuation should be considered. However, some patients may require treatment despite the presence of the syndrome.

For further information about the description of tardive dyskinesia and its clinical detection, see PRECAUTIONS and ADVERSE REACTIONS.

NEUROLEPTIC MALIGNANT SYNDROME (NMS)

A potentially fatal symptom complex sometimes referred to as Neuroleptic Malignant Syndrome (NMS) has been reported in association with antipsychotic drugs. Clinical manifestations of NMS are hyperpyrexia, muscle rigidity, altered mental status and evidence of autonomic instability (irregular pulse or blood pressure, tachycardia, diaphoresis, and cardiac dysrhythmias).

The diagnostic evaluation of patients with this syndrome is complicated. In arriving at a diagnosis, it is important to identify cases where the clinical presentation includes both serious medical illness (*e.g.,* pneumonia, systemic infection, etc.) and untreated or inadequately treated extrapyramidal signs and symptoms (EPS). Other important considerations in the differential diagnosis include central anticholinergic toxicity, heat stroke, drug fever and primary CNS pathology.

The management of NMS should include (1) immediate discontinuation of antipsychotic drugs and other drugs not essential to concurrent therapy, (2) intensive symptomatic treatment and medical monitoring, and (3) treatment of any concomitant serious medical problems for which specific treatments are available. There is no general agreement about specific pharmacological treatment regimens for uncomplicated NMS.

If a patient requires antipsychotic drug treatment after recovery from NMS, the potential reintroduction of drug therapy should be carefully considered. The patient should be carefully monitored, since recurrences of NMS have been reported.

An encephalopathic syndrome (characterized by weakness, lethargy, fever, tremulousness and confusion, extrapyramidal symptoms, leukocytosis, elevated serum enzymes, BUN and FBS) has occurred in a few patients treated with lithium plus an antipsychotic. In some instances, the syndrome was followed by irreversible brain damage. Because of a possible causal relationship between these events and the concomitant administration if lithium and antipsychotics, patients receiving such combined therapy should be monitored closely for early evidence of neurologic toxicity and treatment discontinued promptly if such signs appear. This encephalopathic syndrome may be similar to or the same as NMS.

Chlorpromazine ampuls and multi-dose vials contain sodium bisulfite and sodium sulfite, sulfites that may cause allergic-type reactions including anaphylactic symptoms and life-threatening or less severe asthmatic episodes in certain susceptible people. The overall prevalence of sulfite sensitivity in the general population is unknown and probably low. Sulfite sensitivity is seen more frequently in asthmatic than in nonasthmatic people.

Patients with bone marrow depression or who have previously demonstrated a hypersensitivity reaction (*e.g.,* blood dyscrasias, jaundice) with a phenothiazine should not receive any phenothiazine, including chlorpromazine, unless in the judgment of the physician the potential benefits of treatment outweigh the possible hazard.

Chlorpromazine may impair mental and/or physical abilities, especially during the first few days of therapy. Therefore, caution patients about activities requiring alertness (*e.g.,* operating vehicles or machinery).

The use of alcohol with this drug should be avoided due to possible additive effects and hypotension.

Chlorpromazine may counteract the antihypertensive effect of guanethidine and related compounds.

USE IN PREGNANCY

Safety for the use of chlorpromazine during pregnancy has not been established. Therefore, it is not recommended that the drug be given to pregnant patients except when, in the judgment of the physician, it is essential. The potential benefits should clearly outweigh possible hazards. There are reported instances of prolonged jaundice, extrapyramidal signs, hyperreflexia or hyporeflexia in newborn infants whose mothers received phenothiazines.

Reproductive studies in rodents have demonstrated potential for embryotoxicity, increased neonatal mortality, and nursing transfer of the drug. Tests in the offspring of the drug-treated rodents demonstrate decreased performance. The possibility of permanent neurological damage cannot be excluded.

NURSING MOTHERS

There is evidence that chlorpromazine is excreted in the breast milk of nursing mothers. Because of the potential for serious adverse reactions in nursing infants from chlorpromazine, a decision should be made whether to discontinue nursing or to discontinue the drug, taking into account the importance of the drug to the mother.

PRECAUTIONS

GENERAL

Given the likelihood that some patients exposed chronically to antipsychotics will develop tardive dyskinesia, it is advised that all patients in whom chronic use is contemplated be given, if possible, full information about this risk. The decision to inform patients and/or their guardians must obviously take into account the clinical circumstances and the competency of the patient to understand the information provided.

Chlorpromazine should be administered cautiously to persons with cardiovascular, liver or renal disease. There is evidence that patients with a history of hepatic encephalopathy due to cirrhosis have increased sensitivity to the CNS effects of chlorpromazine (*i.e.,* impaired cerebration and abnormal slowing of the EEG).

Because of its CNS depressant effect, chlorpromazine should be used with caution in patients with chronic respiratory disorders such as severe asthma, emphysema, and acute respiratory infections, particularly in children (1-12 years of age).

Because chlorpromazine can suppress the cough reflex, aspiration of vomitus is possible.

Chlorpromazine prolongs and intensifies the action of CNS depressants such as anesthetics, barbiturates, and narcotics. When chlorpromazine is administered concomitantly, about ¼-½ the usual dosage of such agents is required. When chlorpromazine is not being administered to reduce requirements of CNS depressants, it is best to stop such depressants before starting chlorpromazine treatment. These agents may subsequently be reinstated at low doses and increased as needed.

Note: Chlorpromazine does not intensify the anticonvulsant action of barbiturates. Therefore, dosage of anticonvulsants, including barbiturates, should not be reduced if chlorpromazine is started. Instead, start chlorpromazine at low doses and increase as needed.

Use with caution in persons who will be exposed to extreme heat, organophosphorus insecticides, and in persons receiving atropine or related drugs.

Antipsychotic drugs elevate prolactin levels; the elevation persists during chronic administration. Tissue culture experiments indicate that approximately 1/3 of human breast cancers are prolactin-dependent *in vitro,* a factor of potential importance if the prescribing of these drugs is contemplated in a patient with a previously detected breast cancer. Although disturbances such as galactorrhea, amenorrhea, gynecomastia and impotence have been reported, the clinical significance of elevated serum prolactin levels is unknown for most patients. An increase in mammary neoplasms has been found in rodents after chronic administration of antipsychotic drugs. Neither clinical nor epidemiologic studies conducted to date, however, have shown an association between chronic administration of these drugs and mammary tumorigenesis; the available evidence is considered too limited to be conclusive at this time.

Chromosomal aberrations in spermatocytes and abnormal sperm have been demonstrated in rodents treated with certain antipsychotics.

As with all drugs which exert an anticholinergic effect, and/or cause mydriasis, chlorpromazine should be used with caution in patients with glaucoma.

Chlorpromazine diminishes the effect of oral anticoagulants.

Phenothiazines can produce alpha-adrenergic blockade.

Chlorpromazine may lower the convulsive threshold; dosage adjustments of anticonvulsants may be necessary. Potentiation of anticonvulsant effects does not occur. However, it has been reported that chlorpromazine may interfere with the metabolism of phenytoin and thus precipitate phenytoin toxicity.

Concomitant administration with propranolol results in increased plasma levels of both drugs.

Thiazide diuretics may accentuate the orthostatic hypotension that may occur with phenothiazines.

The presence of phenothiazines may produce false-positive phenylketonuria (PKU) test results.

Drugs which lower the seizure threshold, including phenothiazine derivatives, should not be used with metrizamide. As with other phenothiazine derivatives, chlorpromazine should be discontinued at least 48 hours before myelography, should not be resumed for at least 24 hours postprocedure, and should not be used for the control of nausea and vomiting occurring either prior to myelography or postprocedure with metrizamide.

Long-Term Therapy

To lessen the likelihood of adverse reactions related to cumulative drug effect, patients with a history of long-term therapy with chlorpromazine and/or other antipsychotics should be evaluated periodically to decide whether the maintenance dosage could be lowered or drug therapy discontinued.

Antiemetic Effect

The antiemetic action of chlorpromazine may mask the signs and symptoms of overdosage of other drugs and may obscure the diagnosis and treatment of other conditions such as intestinal obstruction, brain tumor, and Reye's syndrome. (See WARNINGS.)

When chlorpromazine is used with cancer chemotherapeutic drugs, vomiting as a sign of the toxicity of these agents may be obscured by the antiemetic effect of chlorpromazine.

Abrupt Withdrawal

Like other phenothiazines, chlorpromazine is not known to cause psychic dependence and does not produce tolerance or addiction. There may be, however, following abrupt withdrawal of high-dose therapy, some symptoms resembling those of physical dependence such as gastritis, nausea and vomiting, dizziness, and tremulousness. These symptoms can usually be avoided or reduced by gradual reduction of the dosage or by continuing concomitant anti-parkinsonism agents for several weeks after chlorpromazine is withdrawn.

ADVERSE REACTIONS

Note: Some adverse effects of chlorpromazine may be more likely to occur, or occur with greater intensity, in patients with special medical problems, *e.g.,* patients with mitral insufficiency or pheochromocytoma have experienced severe hypotension following recommended doses.

Drowsiness, usually mild to moderate, may occur, particularly during the first or second week, after which it generally disappears. If troublesome, dosage may be lowered.

Jaundice: Overall incidence has been low, regardless of indication or dosage. Most investigators conclude it is a sensitivity reaction. Most cases occur between the second and fourth weeks of therapy. The clinical picture resembles infectious hepatitis, with laboratory features of obstructive jaundice, rather than those of parenchymal damage. It is usually promptly reversible on withdrawal of the medication; however, chronic jaundice has been reported.

There is no conclusive evidence that preexisting liver disease makes patients more susceptible to jaundice. Alcoholics with cirrhosis have been successfully treated with chlorpromazine without complications. Nevertheless, the medication should be used cautiously in patients with liver disease. Patients who have experienced jaundice with a phenothiazine should not, if possible, be reexposed to chlorpromazine or other phenothiazines.

If fever with grippe-like symptoms occurs, appropriate liver studies should be conducted. If tests indicate an abnormality, stop treatment.

Liver function tests in jaundice induced by the drug may mimic extrahepatic obstruction; withhold exploratory laparotomy until extrahepatic obstruction is confirmed.

Hematological disorders, including agranulocytosis, eosinophilia, leukopenia, hemolytic anemia, aplastic anemia, thrombocytopenic purpura, and pancytopenia have been reported.

Agranulocytosis: Warn patients to report the sudden appearance of sore throat or other signs of infection. If white blood cell and differential counts indicate cellular depression, stop treatment and start antibiotic and other suitable therapy.

Most cases have occurred between the fourth and tenth weeks of therapy; patients should be watched closely during that period.

Moderate suppression of white blood cells is not an indication for stopping treatment unless accompanied by the symptoms described above.

CARDIOVASCULAR

Hypotensive Effects

Postural hypotension, simple tachycardia, momentary fainting, and dizziness may occur after the first injection; occasionally after subsequent injections; rarely, after the first oral dose. Usually recovery is spontaneous and symptoms disappear within ½ to 2 hours. Occasionally, these effects may be more severe and prolonged, producing a shock-like condition.

To minimize hypotension after injection, keep patient lying down and observe for at least ½ hour. To control hypotension, place patient in head-low position with legs raised. If a vasoconstrictor is required, norepinephrine bitartrate and phenylephrine HCl are the most suitable. Other pressor agents, including epinephrine, should not be used as they may cause a paradoxical further lowering of blood pressure.

EKG Changes

Particularly nonspecific, usually reversible Q and T wave distortions, have been observed in some patients receiving phenothiazine antipsychotics, including chlorpromazine.
Note: Sudden death, apparently due to cardiac arrest, has been reported.

CNS REACTIONS

Neuromuscular (extrapyramidal) Reactions

Neuromuscular reactions include dystonias, motor restlessness, pseudo-parkinsonism, and tardive dyskinesia, and appear to be dose-related. They are discussed in the following paragraphs.

Dystonias

Symptoms may include spasm of the neck muscles, sometimes progressing to acute, reversible torticollis; extensor rigidity of back muscles, sometimes progressing to opisthotonos; carpopedal spasm, trismus, swallowing difficulty, oculogyric crisis, and protrusion of the tongue.

These usually subside within a few hours, and almost always within 24-48 hours after the drug has been discontinued.

In mild cases, reassurance or a barbiturate is often sufficient. *In moderate cases,* barbiturates will usually bring rapid relief. *In more severe adult cases,* the administration of an anti-parkinsonism agent, except levodopa (see prescribing information), usually produces rapid reversal of symptoms. *In children (1-12 years of age),* reassurance and barbiturates will usually control symptoms. (Or, parenteral diphenhydramine HCl (see prescribing information) may be useful. See DOSAGE AND ADMINISTRATION, Pediatric Patients (6 months to 12 years of age) for appropriate children's dosage.) If appropriate treatment with anti-parkinsonism agents or diphenhydramine HCl fails to reverse the signs and symptoms, the diagnosis should be reevaluated.

Suitable supportive measures such as maintaining a clear airway and adequate hydration should be employed when needed. If therapy is reinstituted, it should be at a lower dosage. Should these symptoms occur in children or pregnant patients, the drug should not be reinstituted.

Motor Restlessness

Symptoms may include agitation or jitteriness and sometimes insomnia. These symptoms often disappear spontaneously. At times these symptoms may be similar to the original neurotic or psychotic symptoms. Dosage should not be increased until these side effects have subsided.

If these symptoms become too troublesome, they can usually be controlled by a reduction of dosage or change of drug. Treatment with anti-parkinsonian agents, benzodiazepines or propranolol may be helpful.

Pseudo-Parkinsonism

Symptoms may include: Mask-like facies, drooling, tremors, pillrolling motion, cogwheel rigidity, and shuffling gait. In most cases these symptoms are readily controlled when an anti-parkinsonism agent is administered concomitantly. Anti-parkinsonism agents should be used only when required. Generally, therapy of a few weeks to 2 or 3 months will suffice. After this time patients should be evaluated to determine their need for continued treatment. (*Note:* Levodopa has not been found effective in antipsychotic-induced pseudo-parkinsonism.) Occasionally it is necessary to lower the dosage of chlorpromazine or to discontinue the drug.

Tardive Dyskinesia

As with all antipsychotic agents, tardive dyskinesia may appear in some patients on long-term therapy or may appear after drug therapy has been discontinued. The syndrome can also develop, although much less frequently, after relatively brief treatment periods at low doses. This syndrome appears in all age groups. Although its prevalence appears to be highest among elderly patients, especially elderly women, it is impossible to rely upon prevalence estimates to predict at the inception of antipsychotic treatment which patients are likely to develop the syndrome. The symptoms are persistent and in some patients appear to be irreversible. The syndrome is characterized by rhythmical involuntary movements of the tongue, face, mouth or jaw (*e.g.,* protrusion of tongue, puffing of cheeks, puckering of mouth, chewing movements). Sometimes these may be accompanied by involuntary movements of extremities. In rare instances, these involuntary movements of the extremities are the only manifestations of tardive dyskinesia. A variant of tardive dyskinesia, tardive dystonia, has also been described.

There is no known effective treatment for tardive dyskinesia; anti-parkinsonism agents do not alleviate the symptoms of this syndrome. If clinically feasible, it is suggested that all antipsychotic agents be discontinued if these symptoms appear. Should it be necessary to reinstitute treatment, or increase the dosage of the agent, or switch to a different antipsychotic agent, the syndrome may be masked.

It has been reported that fine vermicular movements of the tongue may be an early sign of the syndrome and if the medication is stopped at that time the syndrome may not develop.

Adverse Behavioral Effects

Psychotic symptoms and catatonic-like states have been reported rarely.

Other CNS Effects

NMS has been reported in association with antipsychotic drugs. (See WARNINGS.)

Cerebral edema has been reported.

Convulsive seizures (*petit mal* and *grand mal*) have been reported, particularly in patients with EEG abnormalities or history of such disorders.

Abnormality of the cerebrospinal fluid proteins has also been reported.

Allergic reactions of a mild urticarial type or photosensitivity are seen. Avoid undue exposure to sun. More severe reactions, including exfoliative dermatitis, have been reported occasionally.

Contact dermatitis has been reported in nursing personnel; accordingly, the use of rubber gloves when administering chlorpromazine liquid or injectable is recommended.

In addition, asthma, laryngeal edema, angioneurotic edema, and anaphylactoid reactions have been reported.

ENDOCRINE DISORDERS

Lactation and moderate breast engorgement may occur in females on large doses. If persistent, lower dosage or withdraw drug. False-positive pregnancy tests have been reported, but are less likely to occur when a serum test is used. Amenorrhea and gynecomastia have also been reported. Hyperglycemia, hypoglycemia and glycosuria have been reported.

AUTONOMIC REACTIONS

Occasional dry mouth; nasal congestion; nausea; obstipation; constipation; adynamic ileus; urinary retention; priapism; miosis and mydriasis, atonic colon, ejaculatory disorders/impotence.

SPECIAL CONSIDERATIONS IN LONG-TERM THERAPY

Skin pigmentation and ocular changes have occurred in some patients taking substantial doses of chlorpromazine for prolonged periods.

Skin Pigmentation

Rare instances of skin pigmentation have been observed in hospitalized mental patients, primarily females who have received the drug usually for 3 years or more in dosages ranging from 500-1500 mg daily. The pigmentary changes, restricted to exposed areas of the body, range from an almost imperceptible darkening of the skin to a slate gray color, sometimes with a violet hue. Histological examination reveals a pigment, chiefly in the dermis, which is probably a melanin-like complex. The pigmentation may fade following discontinuance of the drug.

Ocular Changes

Ocular changes have occurred more frequently than skin pigmentation and have been observed both in pigmented and nonpigmented patients receiving chlorpromazine usually for 2 years or more in dosages of 300 mg daily and higher. Eye changes are characterized by deposition of fine particulate matter in the lens and cornea. In more advanced cases, star-shaped opacities have also been observed in the anterior portion of the lens. The nature of the eye deposits has not yet been determined. A small number of patients with more severe ocular changes have had some visual impairment. In addition to these corneal and lenticular changes, epithelial keratopathy and pigmentary retinopathy have been reported. Reports suggest that the eye lesions may regress after withdrawal of the drug.

Since the occurrence of eye changes seems to be related to dosage levels and/or duration of therapy, it is suggested that long-term patients on moderate to high dosage levels have periodic ocular examinations.

Etiology

The etiology of both of these reactions is not clear, but exposure to light, along with dosage/duration of therapy, appears to be the most significant factor. If either of these reactions is observed, the physician should weigh the benefits of continued therapy against the possible risks and, on the merits of the individual case, determine whether or not to continue present therapy, lower the dosage, or withdraw the drug.

OTHER ADVERSE REACTIONS

Mild fever may occur after large IM doses. Hyperpyrexia has been reported. Increases in appetite and weight sometimes occur. Peripheral edema and a systemic lupus erythematosus-like syndrome have been reported.
Note: There have been occasional reports of sudden death in patients receiving phenothiazines. In some cases, the cause appeared to be cardiac arrest or asphyxia due to failure of the cough reflex.

DOSAGE AND ADMINISTRATION

ADULTS

Adjust dosage to individual and the severity of his condition, recognizing that the milligram for milligram potency relationship among all dosage forms has not been precisely established clinically. It is important to increase dosage until symptoms are controlled. Dosage should be increased more gradually in debilitated or emaciated patients. In continued therapy, gradually reduce dosage to the lowest effective maintenance level, after symptoms have been controlled for a reasonable period.

The 100 and 200 mg tablets are for use in severe neuropsychiatric conditions.

Increase parenteral dosage only if hypotension has not occurred. Before using IM, see Important Notes on Injection.

Elderly Patients

In general, dosages in the lower range are sufficient for most elderly patients. Since they appear to be more susceptible to hypotension and neuromuscular reactions, such patients should be observed closely. Dosage should be tailored to the individual, response carefully monitored, and dosage adjusted accordingly. Dosage should be increased more gradually in elderly patients.

Psychotic Disorders

Increase dosage gradually until symptoms are controlled. Maximum improvement may not be seen for weeks or even months. Continue optimum dosage for 2 weeks; then gradually reduce dosage to the lowest effective maintenance level. Daily dosage of 200 mg is not unusual. Some patients require higher dosages (*e.g.,* 800 mg daily is not uncommon in discharged mental patients).

Hospitalized Patients

Acute Schizophrenic or Manic States:

IM: 25 mg (1 ml). If necessary, give additional 25-50 mg injection in 1 hour. Increase subsequent IM doses gradually over several days — up to 400 mg q4-6h in exceptionally severe cases — until patient is controlled. Usually patient becomes quiet and cooperative within 24-48 hours and oral doses may be substituted and increased until the patient is calm. Five-hundred (500) mg a day is generally sufficient. While gradual increases to 2000 mg a day or more may be necessary, there is usually little therapeutic gain to be achieved by exceeding 1000 mg a day for extended periods. In general, dosage levels should be lower in the elderly, the emaciated, and the debilitated.

Less Acutely Disturbed:

Oral: 25 mg tid. Increase gradually until effective dose is reached — usually 400 mg daily.

Outpatients

Oral: 10 mg tid or qid, or 25 mg bid or tid.

More Severe Cases: *Oral:* 25 mg tid. After 1 or 2 days, daily dosage may be increased by 20-50 mg at semiweekly intervals until patient becomes calm and cooperative.

Prompt Control of Severe Symptoms: *IM:* 25 mg (1 ml). If necessary, repeat in 1 hour. Subsequent doses should be oral, 25-50 mg tid.

Nausea and Vomiting

Oral: 10-25 mg q4-6h, prn, increased, if necessary.

IM: 25 mg (1 ml). If no hypotension occurs, give 25-50 mg q3-4h, prn, until vomiting stops. Then switch to oral dosage.

Rectal: One 100 mg suppository q6-8h, prn. In some patients, half this dose will do.

Nausea and Vomiting — During Surgery

IM: 12.5 mg (0.5 ml). Repeat in ½ hour if necessary and if no hypotension occurs.

IV: 2 mg per fractional injection, at 2 minute intervals. Do not exceed 25 mg. Dilute to 1 mg/ml, *i.e.,* 1 ml (25 mg) mixed with 24 ml of saline.

Presurgical Apprehension

Oral: 25-50 mg, 2-3 hours before the operation.

IM: 12.5 to 25 mg (0.5 to 1 ml), 1-2 hours before operation.

Intractable Hiccups

Oral: 25-50 mg tid or qid. If symptoms persist for 2-3 days, give 25-50 mg (1-2 ml) IM. Should symptoms persist, use slow IV infusion with patient flat in bed: 25-50 mg (1-2 ml) in 500-1000 ml of saline. Follow blood pressure closely.

Acute Intermittent Porphyria

Oral: 25-50 mg tid or qid. Can usually be discontinued after several weeks, but maintenance therapy may be necessary for some patients.

IM: 25 mg (1 ml) tid or qid until patient can take oral therapy.

Tetanus

IM: 25-50 mg (1-2 ml) given 3 or 4 times daily, usually in conjunction with barbiturates. Total doses and frequency of administration must be determined by the patient's response, starting with low doses and increasing gradually.

IV: 25-50 mg (1-2 ml). Dilute to at least 1 mg/ml and administer at a rate of 1 mg/min.

PEDIATRIC PATIENTS (6 MONTHS TO 12 YEARS OF AGE)

Chlorpromazine should generally not be used in children under 6 months of age except where potentially lifesaving. It should not be used in conditions for which specific children's dosages have not been established.

Severe Behavioral Problems

Outpatients

Select route of administration according to severity of patient's condition and increase dosage gradually as required.

Oral: ¼ mg/lb body weight q4-6h, prn (*e.g.,* for 40 lb child — 10 mg q4-6h).

Rectal: ½ mg/lb body weight q6-8 h, prn (*e.g.,* for 20-30 lb child — half of a 25 mg suppository q6-8 h).

IM: ¼ mg/lb body weight q6-8 h, prn.

Hospitalized Patients

As with outpatients, start with low doses and increase dosage gradually. In severe behavior disorders, higher dosages (50-100 mg daily, and in older children, 200 mg daily or more) may be necessary. There is little evidence that behavior improvement in severely disturbed mentally retarded patients is further enhanced by doses beyond 500 mg/day.

Maximum IM Dosage: Children up to 5 years (or 50 lb), not over 40 mg/day; 5-12 years (or 50-100 lb), not over 75 mg/day except in unmanageable cases.

Nausea and Vomiting

Dosage and frequency of administration should be adjusted according to the severity of the symptoms and response of the patient. The duration of activity following intramuscular administration may last up to 12 hours. Subsequent doses may be given by the same route if necessary.

Oral: ¼ mg/lb body weight (*e.g.,* 40 lb child — 10 mg q4-6h).

Rectal: ½ mg/lb body weight q6-8h prn (*e.g.,* 20-30 lb child — half of a 25 mg suppository q6-8h).

IM: ¼ mg/lb body weight q6-8h, prn.

Maximum IM Dosage: Pediatric patients 6 months to 5 years (or 50 lbs), not over 40 mg/day; 5-12 years (or 50-100 lbs), not over 75 mg/day except in severe cases.

Nausea and Vomiting — During Surgery

IM: 1/8 mg/lb body weight. Repeat in ½ hour if necessary and if no hypotension occurs.

IV: 1 mg per fractional injection at 2 minute intervals and not exceeding recommended IM dosage. Always dilute to 1 mg/ml, *i.e.,* 1 ml (25 mg) mixed with 24 ml of saline.

Presurgical Apprehension

¼ mg/lb body weight, either:

Orally: 2-3 hours before operation, or

IM: 1-2 hours before.

Tetanus

IM or IV: ¼ mg/lb body weight q6-8h. When given IV, dilute to at least 1 mg/ml and administer at rate of 1 mg/2 minutes. In patients up to 50 lbs, do not exceed 40 mg daily; 50-100 lb, do not exceed 75 mg, except in severe cases.

IMPORTANT NOTES ON INJECTION

Inject slowly, deep into upper outer quadrant of buttock.

Because of possible hypotensive effects, reserve parenteral administration for bedfast patients or for acute ambulatory cases, and keep patient lying down for at least ½ hour after injection. If irritation is a problem, dilute injection with saline or 2% procaine; mixing with other agents in the syringe is not recommended. Subcutaneous injection is not advised. Avoid injecting undiluted chlorpromazine into vein. Intravenous route is only for severe hiccups, surgery, and tetanus.

Because of the possibility of contact dermatitis, avoid getting solution on hands or clothing. This solution should be protected from light. This is a clear, colorless to pale yellow solution; a slight yellowish discoloration will not alter potency. If markedly discolored, solution should be discarded. For information on sulfite sensitivity, see WARNINGS.

NOTE ON CONCENTRATE

When the concentrate is to be used, add the desired dosage of concentrate to 60 ml (2 fl oz) or more of diluent *just prior to administration.* This will insure palatability and stability. *Vehicles suggested for dilution are:* Tomato or fruit juice, milk, simple syrup, orange syrup, carbonated beverages, coffee, tea, or water. Semisolid foods (soups, puddings, etc.) may also be used. The concentrate is light sensitive; it should be protected from light and dispensed in amber glass bottles. *Refrigeration is not required.*

HOW SUPPLIED

THORAZINE TABLETS

Each round, orange, coated tablet contains chlorpromazine HCl as follows:

10 mg: Imprinted "SKF" and "T73".

25 mg: Imprinted "SKF" and "T74".

50 mg: Imprinted "SKF" and "T76".

100 mg: Imprinted "SKF" and "T77".

200 mg: Imprinted "SKF" and "T79".

Storage: Store between 15 and 30°C (59 and 86°F).

THORAZINE AMPULS

Thorazine ampuls are supplied as 1 and 2 ml (25 mg/ml).

Storage: Store between 15 and 30°C (59 and 86°F).

THORAZINE MULTI-DOSE VIALS

Thorazine multi-dose vials are supplied as 10 ml (25 mg/ml).

Storage: Store between 15 and 30°C (59 and 86°F).

THORAZINE SYRUP

Thorazine syrup is supplied as 10 mg/5 ml.

Storage: Store below 25°C (77°F).

THORAZINE SUPPOSITORIES

Thorazine suppositories are supplied as 25 or 100 mg.

Storage: Store between 15 and 30°C (59 and 86°F).

PRODUCT LISTING - RATED THERAPEUTICALLY EQUIVALENT

Concentrate - Oral - 30 mg/ml			
118 ml	$35.55	THORAZINE, Glaxosmithkline	00007-5047-44
120 ml	$5.31	GENERIC, Roxane Laboratories Inc	00054-3144-50
120 ml	$14.95	GENERIC, Major Pharmaceuticals Inc	00904-2159-20
120 ml	$17.66	GENERIC, Geneva Pharmaceuticals	00781-4007-04
Concentrate - Oral - 100 mg/ml			
240 ml	$20.12	GENERIC, Roxane Laboratories Inc	00054-3146-58
240 ml	$20.27	GENERIC, Alpharma Uspd Makers Of Barre and Nmc	00472-0742-98
240 ml	$21.96	GENERIC, Major Pharmaceuticals Inc	00904-2059-09
240 ml	$48.60	GENERIC, Geneva Pharmaceuticals	00781-4009-08
240 ml	$192.20	THORAZINE, Glaxosmithkline	00007-5049-48
Solution - Injectable - 25 mg/ml			
1 ml x 10	$79.65	THORAZINE, Glaxosmithkline	00007-5060-11
1 ml x 10	$83.25	THORAZINE, Allscripts Pharmaceutical Company	54569-2089-00
1 ml x 25	$104.50	GENERIC, Esi Lederle Generics	00641-1397-35
2 ml x 10	$140.10	THORAZINE, Glaxosmithkline	00007-5061-11
2 ml x 25	$115.75	GENERIC, Esi Lederle Generics	00641-1398-35
10 ml	$3.70	GENERIC, Roberts/Hauck Pharmaceutical Corporation	43797-0026-12
10 ml	$9.00	GENERIC, Interstate Drug Exchange Inc	00814-1693-40
10 ml	$12.00	GENERIC, Ivax Corporation	00182-0859-63
10 ml	$52.11	GENERIC, Watson/Schein Pharmaceuticals Inc	00364-6664-54
10 ml	$52.11	GENERIC, Steris Laboratories Inc	00402-0261-10
10 ml	$62.68	THORAZINE, Glaxosmithkline	00007-5062-01
10's	$2.50	GENERIC, Vita-Rx Corporation	49727-0760-10
Syrup - Oral - 10 mg/5 ml			
118 ml	$29.98	THORAZINE, Glaxosmithkline	00007-5072-44
120 ml	$15.95	GENERIC, Geneva Pharmaceuticals	00781-4017-04

Tablet - Oral - 10 mg

100's	$5.95	GENERIC, Major Pharmaceuticals Inc	00904-2075-60

Tablet - Oral - 25 mg

100's	$8.75	GENERIC, Major Pharmaceuticals Inc	00904-2076-60

Tablet - Oral - 50 mg

100's	$10.85	GENERIC, Major Pharmaceuticals Inc	00904-2077-60

Tablet - Oral - 100 mg

100's	$12.50	GENERIC, Major Pharmaceuticals Inc	00904-2078-60

Tablet - Oral - 200 mg

100's	$13.95	GENERIC, Major Pharmaceuticals Inc	00904-2079-60

PRODUCT LISTING - RATED NOT THERAPEUTICALLY EQUIVALENT

Tablet - Oral - 10 mg

30's	$2.15	GENERIC, Heartland Healthcare Services	61392-0039-30
30's	$2.15	GENERIC, Heartland Healthcare Services	61392-0039-39
31's	$2.22	GENERIC, Heartland Healthcare Services	61392-0039-31
32's	$1.98	GENERIC, Vangard Labs	00615-1545-32
32's	$2.29	GENERIC, Heartland Healthcare Services	61392-0039-32
45's	$3.22	GENERIC, Heartland Healthcare Services	61392-0039-45
60's	$4.29	GENERIC, Heartland Healthcare Services	61392-0039-60
90's	$6.44	GENERIC, Heartland Healthcare Services	61392-0039-90
100's	$4.74	GENERIC, Aligen Independent Laboratories Inc	00405-4196-01
100's	$5.12	GENERIC, Moore, H.L. Drug Exchange Inc	00839-1155-06
100's	$5.34	GENERIC, Vangard Labs	00615-1545-01
100's	$6.15	GENERIC, Raway Pharmacal Inc	00686-0518-20
100's	$6.24	GENERIC, Auro Pharmaceutical	55829-0189-10
100's	$6.30	GENERIC, Interstate Drug Exchange Inc	00814-1686-14
100's	$7.76	GENERIC, Major Pharmaceuticals Inc	00904-2161-61
100's	$26.60	GENERIC, Qualitest Products Inc	00603-2808-21
100's	$28.35	GENERIC, Major Pharmaceuticals Inc	00904-2161-60
100's	$29.94	GENERIC, R.I.D. Inc Distributor	54807-0820-01
100's	$31.98	GENERIC, Rosemont Pharmaceutical Corporation	00832-0300-00
100's	$32.00	GENERIC, Geneva Pharmaceuticals	00781-1715-01
100's	$35.10	GENERIC, Udl Laboratories Inc	51079-0518-20
100's	$57.40	GENERIC, Geneva Pharmaceuticals	00781-1715-13

Tablet - Oral - 25 mg

30's	$4.94	GENERIC, Prescript Pharmaceuticals	00247-0816-30
100's	$4.71	GENERIC, Aligen Independent Laboratories Inc	00405-4197-01
100's	$6.53	GENERIC, Auro Pharmaceutical	55829-0190-10
100's	$7.09	GENERIC, Moore, H.L. Drug Exchange Inc	00839-1151-06
100's	$7.60	GENERIC, Raway Pharmacal Inc	00686-0519-20
100's	$8.01	GENERIC, Major Pharmaceuticals Inc	00904-2052-61
100's	$8.40	GENERIC, Interstate Drug Exchange Inc	00814-1688-14
100's	$9.45	GENERIC, Ivax Corporation	00182-0474-01
100's	$28.25	GENERIC, Udl Laboratories Inc	51079-0519-20
100's	$40.50	GENERIC, R.I.D. Inc Distributor	54807-0821-01
100's	$43.25	GENERIC, Major Pharmaceuticals Inc	00904-2052-60
100's	$44.58	GENERIC, Qualitest Products Inc	00603-2809-21
100's	$49.94	GENERIC, Geneva Pharmaceuticals	00781-1716-01
100's	$52.96	GENERIC, Rosemont Pharmaceutical Corporation	00832-0301-00
100's	$53.27	GENERIC, Geneva Pharmaceuticals	00781-1716-13
100's	$62.81	THORAZINE, Glaxosmithkline	00007-5074-20

Tablet - Oral - 50 mg

32's	$2.84	GENERIC, Vangard Labs	00615-1547-32
100's	$7.03	GENERIC, Vangard Labs	00615-1547-01
100's	$7.82	GENERIC, Moore, H.L. Drug Exchange Inc	00839-1158-06
100's	$7.89	GENERIC, Auro Pharmaceutical	55829-0191-10
100's	$8.00	GENERIC, Raway Pharmacal Inc	00686-0130-20
100's	$9.38	GENERIC, Interstate Drug Exchange Inc	00814-1691-14
100's	$9.39	GENERIC, Major Pharmaceuticals Inc	00904-2053-61
100's	$13.27	GENERIC, Ivax Corporation	00182-0475-01
100's	$13.30	GENERIC, Aligen Independent Laboratories Inc	00405-4198-01
100's	$29.60	GENERIC, Udl Laboratories Inc	51079-0130-20
100's	$60.68	GENERIC, R.I.D. Inc Distributor	54807-0822-01
100's	$62.50	GENERIC, Major Pharmaceuticals Inc	00904-2053-60
100's	$64.45	GENERIC, Qualitest Products Inc	00603-2810-21
100's	$70.64	GENERIC, Geneva Pharmaceuticals	00781-1717-01
100's	$72.31	GENERIC, Geneva Pharmaceuticals	00781-1717-13
100's	$75.16	GENERIC, Rosemont Pharmaceutical Corporation	00832-0302-00
100's	$75.40	THORAZINE, Glaxosmithkline	00007-5076-20

Tablet - Oral - 100 mg

100's	$7.00	GENERIC, Cmc-Consolidated Midland Corporation	00223-0673-01
100's	$8.76	GENERIC, Moore, H.L. Drug Exchange Inc	00839-1148-06
100's	$9.00	GENERIC, Raway Pharmacal Inc	00686-0516-20
100's	$9.50	GENERIC, Auro Pharmaceutical	55829-0192-10
100's	$10.52	GENERIC, Major Pharmaceuticals Inc	00904-2191-61
100's	$11.11	GENERIC, Aligen Independent Laboratories Inc	00405-4199-01
100's	$13.35	GENERIC, Interstate Drug Exchange Inc	00814-1692-14
100's	$14.71	GENERIC, Ivax Corporation	00182-0476-01
100's	$14.71	GENERIC, Parmed Pharmaceuticals Inc	00349-2367-01
100's	$40.60	GENERIC, Udl Laboratories Inc	51079-0516-20
100's	$70.15	GENERIC, Major Pharmaceuticals Inc	00904-2191-60
100's	$72.32	GENERIC, Qualitest Products Inc	00603-2811-21
100's	$78.30	GENERIC, R.I.D. Inc Distributor	54807-0823-01
100's	$80.40	GENERIC, Geneva Pharmaceuticals	00781-1718-01
100's	$85.92	GENERIC, Rosemont Pharmaceutical Corporation	00832-0303-00
100's	$92.60	THORAZINE, Glaxosmithkline	00007-5077-20
100's	$93.26	GENERIC, Geneva Pharmaceuticals	00781-1718-13

Tablet - Oral - 200 mg

32's	$4.71	GENERIC, Vangard Labs	00615-1549-32
100's	$10.50	GENERIC, Raway Pharmacal Inc	00686-0517-20
100's	$12.08	GENERIC, Moore, H.L. Drug Exchange Inc	00839-1146-06
100's	$13.68	GENERIC, Aligen Independent Laboratories Inc	00405-4200-01
100's	$13.96	GENERIC, Vangard Labs	00615-1549-01
100's	$15.86	GENERIC, Auro Pharmaceutical	55829-0193-10
100's	$17.10	GENERIC, Interstate Drug Exchange Inc	00814-1694-14
100's	$18.95	GENERIC, Ivax Corporation	00182-0477-01
100's	$18.95	GENERIC, Parmed Pharmaceuticals Inc	00349-2043-01
100's	$20.57	GENERIC, Major Pharmaceuticals Inc	00904-2192-61
100's	$65.27	GENERIC, Udl Laboratories Inc	51079-0517-20
100's	$93.38	GENERIC, Major Pharmaceuticals Inc	00904-2192-60
100's	$96.25	GENERIC, Qualitest Products Inc	00603-2812-21
100's	$99.46	GENERIC, R.I.D. Inc Distributor	54807-0824-01
100's	$100.00	GENERIC, Mutual/United Research Laboratories	00677-0787-01
100's	$104.87	GENERIC, Geneva Pharmaceuticals	00781-1719-01
100's	$114.37	GENERIC, Rosemont Pharmaceutical Corporation	00832-0304-00
100's	$115.77	GENERIC, Geneva Pharmaceuticals	00781-1719-13
100's	$117.65	THORAZINE, Glaxosmithkline	00007-5079-20

C

PRODUCT LISTING - EQUIVALENTS NOT AVAILABLE

Concentrate - Oral - 100 mg/ml

240 ml	$22.50	GENERIC, Cmc-Consolidated Midland Corporation	00223-6246-08

Solution - Injectable - 25 mg/ml

1 ml x 25	$45.00	GENERIC, Cmc-Consolidated Midland Corporation	00223-7326-10
1 ml x 50	$75.00	GENERIC, Raway Pharmacal Inc	00686-1396-35
2 ml	$31.25	GENERIC, Cmc-Consolidated Midland Corporation	00223-7325-02
2 ml x 25	$50.00	GENERIC, Cmc-Consolidated Midland Corporation	00223-7334-01
2 ml x 25	$85.00	GENERIC, Raway Pharmacal Inc	00686-1398-35
10 ml	$4.00	GENERIC, Cmc-Consolidated Midland Corporation	00223-7325-10
10 ml	$4.00	GENERIC, Cmc-Consolidated Midland Corporation	00223-7330-02

Suppository - Rectal - 25 mg

32's	$2.37	GENERIC, Vangard Labs	00615-1546-32
100's	$5.91	GENERIC, Vangard Labs	00615-1546-01

Suppository - Rectal - 100 mg

12's	$59.75	THORAZINE, Glaxosmithkline	00007-5071-03

Tablet - Oral - 25 mg

30's	$2.69	GENERIC, Heartland Healthcare Services	61392-0040-30
30's	$2.69	GENERIC, Heartland Healthcare Services	61392-0040-39
31's	$2.78	GENERIC, Heartland Healthcare Services	61392-0040-31
32's	$2.87	GENERIC, Heartland Healthcare Services	61392-0040-32
45's	$4.03	GENERIC, Heartland Healthcare Services	61392-0040-45
60's	$5.37	GENERIC, Heartland Healthcare Services	61392-0040-60
90's	$8.06	GENERIC, Heartland Healthcare Services	61392-0040-90
100's	$3.00	GENERIC, Cmc-Consolidated Midland Corporation	00223-0671-01

Tablet - Oral - 50 mg

100's	$4.00	GENERIC, Cmc-Consolidated Midland Corporation	00223-0672-01

Tablet - Oral - 200 mg

100's	$10.00	GENERIC, Cmc-Consolidated Midland Corporation	00223-0674-01

Chlorpropamide (000798)

For related information, see the comparative table section in Appendix A.

Categories: Diabetes mellitus; Pregnancy Category C; FDA Approved 1968 Apr
Drug Classes: Antidiabetic agents; Sulfonylureas, first generation
Brand Names: Arodoc; Chlordiabet; Chlorprosil; Diabenil; **Diabinese**; Diamide; Diatanpin; Dibetes; Gliconorm; Glycermin; Glymese; Insilange; Meldian; Mellitos; Milligon; Norgluc; Normoglic; Orodiabin; Promide; Tanpinin
Foreign Brand Availability: Abemide (Japan; Taiwan); Anti-D (Malaysia); Apo-Chlorpropamide (Canada); Arodoc C (Japan); Chlomide (Singapore); Chlormide (Japan); Chlorpropamide Medochemie (Malaysia); Copamide (India); Deavynfar (Mexico); Diabeedol (Thailand); Diabemide (Benin; Burkina-Faso; Ethiopia; Gambia; Ghana; Guinea; Italy; Ivory-Coast; Kenya; Liberia; Malawi; Mali; Mauritania; Mauritius; Morocco; Niger; Nigeria; Senegal; Seychelles; Sierra-Leone; Sudan; Tanzania; Tunia; Uganda; Zambia; Zimbabwe); Diabenese (Argentina; Bahamas; Bahrain; Barbados; Belgium; Belize; Benin; Bermuda; Burkina-Faso; Canada; Colombia; Costa-Rica; Curacao; Ecuador; El-Salvador; England; Ethiopia; Finland; Gambia; Ghana; Greece; Guatemala; Guinea; Guyana; Honduras; Iraq; Ireland; Italy; Ivory-Coast; Jamaica; Jordan; Kenya; Kuwait; Lebanon; Liberia; Libya; Malawi; Mali; Mauritania; Mauritius; Mexico; Morocco; Netherland-Antilles; Nicaragua; Niger; Nigeria; Norway; Oman; Panama; Peru; Portugal; Qatar; Republic-of-Yemen; Saudi-Arabia; Senegal; Seychelles; Sierra-Leone; South-Africa; Spain; Surinam; Switzerland; Syria; Tanzania; Trinidad; Tunia; Uganda; United-Arab-Emirates; Zambia; Zimbabwe); Diabexan (Italy); Diabiclor (Mexico); Diabines (Sweden); Diabitex (Bahamas; Barbados; Belize; Bermuda; Curacao; Guyana; Jamaica; Netherland-Antilles; Puerto-Rico; South-Africa; Surinam; Trinidad); Dibecon (Thailand); Glycemin (Thailand); Hypomide (South-Africa); Insilange C (Japan); Insogen (Mexico); Mellitos C (Japan); Melormin (Finland); Neo-Toltinon (Taiwan); Propamide (Malaysia; Thailand); Tesmel (Indonesia)
Cost of Therapy: \$28.68 (Diabetes; Diabinese; 250 mg; 1 tablet/day; 30 day supply)
\$4.02 (Diabetes; Generic Tablets; 250 mg; 1 tablet/day; 30 day supply)

DESCRIPTION

Chlorpropamide, is an oral blood-glucose-lowering drug of the sulfonylurea class. Chlorpropamide is 1-(p-Chlorophenyl) sulfonyl)-3-propylurea, $C_{10}H_{13}ClN_2O_3S$.

Chlorpropamide is a white crystalline powder, that has a slight odor. It is practically insoluble in water at pH 7.3 (solubility at pH 6 is 2.2 mg/ml). It is soluble in alcohol and moderately soluble in chloroform. The molecular weight of chlorpropamide is 276.74. Chlorpropamide is available as 100 mg and 250 mg tablets.

Inert Ingredient: Alginic acid; blue 1 lake; hydroxypropyl cellulose; magnesium stearate; precipitated calcium carbonate; sodium lauryl sulfate; starch.

CLINICAL PHARMACOLOGY

Chlorpropamide appears to lower the blood glucose acutely by stimulating the release of insulin from the pancreas, an effect dependent upon functioning beta cells in the pancreatic islets. The mechanism by which chlorpropamide lowers blood glucose during long-term administration has not been clearly established. Extra-pancreatic effects may play a part in the mechanism of action of oral sulfonylurea hypoglycemic drugs. While chlorpropamide is a sulfonamide derivative, it is devoid of antibacterial activity.

Chlorpropamide may also prove effective in controlling certain patients who have experienced primary or secondary failure to other sulfonylurea agents.

A method developed which permits easy measurement of the drug in blood is available on request.

Chlorpropamide does not interfere with the usual tests to detect albumin in the urine.

Chlorpropamide is absorbed rapidly from the gastrointestinal tract. Within one hour after a single oral dose, it is readily detectable in the blood, and the level reaches a maximum within 2-4 hours. It undergoes metabolism in humans and it is excreted in the urine as unchanged drug and as hydroxylated or hydrolyzed metabolites. The biological half-life of chlorpropamide averages about 36 hours. Within 96 hours, 80-90% of a single oral dose is excreted in the urine. However, long-term administration of therapeutic doses does not result in undue accumulation in the blood, since absorption and excretion rates become stabilized in about 5-7 days after the initiation of therapy.

Chlorpropamide exerts a hypoglycemic effect in normal humans within one hour, becoming maximal at 3-6 hours and persisting for at least 24 hours. The potency of chlorpropamide is approximately six times that of tolbutamide. Some experimental results suggest that its increased duration of action may be the result of slower excretion and absence of significant deactivation.

INDICATIONS AND USAGE

Chlorpropamide is indicated as an adjunct to diet to lower the blood glucose in patients with non-insulin-dependent diabetes mellitus (Type 2) whose hyperglycemia cannot be controlled by diet alone.

In initiating treatment for non-insulin-dependent diabetes, diet should be emphasized as the primary form of treatment. Caloric restriction and weight loss are essential in the obese diabetic patient. Proper dietary management alone may be effective in controlling the blood glucose and symptoms of hyperglycemia. The importance of regular physical activity should also be stressed, and cardiovascular risk factors should be identified and corrective measures taken where possible.

If this treatment program fails to reduce symptoms and/or blood glucose, the use of an oral sulfonylurea or insulin should be considered. Use of chlorpropamide must be viewed by both the physician and patient as a treatment in addition to diet, and not as a substitute for diet or as a convenient mechanism for avoiding dietary restraint. Furthermore, loss of blood glucose control on diet alone may be transient, thus requiring only short-term administration of chlorpropamide.

During maintenance programs, chlorpropamide should be discontinued if satisfactory lowering of blood glucose is no longer achieved. Judgments should be based on regular clinical and laboratory evaluations.

In considering the use of chlorpropamide in asymptomatic patients, it should be recognized that controlling the blood glucose in non-insulin-dependent diabetes has not been definitely established to be effective in preventing the long-term cardiovascular or neural complications of diabetes.

CONTRAINDICATIONS

Chlorpropamide is contraindicated in patients with:

1. Known hypersensitivity to the drug.
2. Diabetic ketoacidosis, with or without coma. This condition should be treated with insulin.

WARNINGS

SPECIAL WARNING ON INCREASED RISK OF CARDIOVASCULAR MORTALITY

The administration of oral hypoglycemic drugs has been reported to be associated with increased cardiovascular mortality as compared to treatment with diet alone or diet plus insulin. This warning is based on the study conducted by the University Group Diabetes Program (UGDP), a long-term prospective clinical trial designed to evaluate the effectiveness of glucose-lowering drugs in preventing or delaying vascular complications in patients with non-insulin-dependent diabetes. The study involved 823 patients who were randomly assigned to one of four treatment groups (*Diabetes*, 19 (supp. 2): 747-830, 1970.)

UGDP reported that patients treated for 5-8 years with diet plus a fixed dose of tolbutamide (1.5 g/day) had a rate of cardiovascular mortality approximately 2½ times that of patients treated with diet alone. A significant increase in total mortality was not observed, but the use of tolbutamide was discontinued based on the increase in cardiovascular mortality, thus limiting the opportunity for the study to show an increase in overall mortality. Despite controversy regarding the interpretation of these results, the findings of the UGDP study provide an adequate basis for this warning. The patient should be informed of the potential risks and advantages of chlorpropamide and of alternative modes of therapy.

Although only one drug in the sulfonylurea class (tolbutamide) was included in this study, it is prudent from a safety standpoint to consider that this warning may also apply to other oral hypoglycemic drugs in this class, in view of their close similarities in mode of action and chemical structure.

PRECAUTIONS

GENERAL

Hypoglycemia: All sulfonylurea drugs are capable of producing severe hypoglycemia. Proper patient selection, dosage, and instructions are important to avoid hypoglycemic episodes. Renal or hepatic insufficiency may cause elevated blood levels of chlorpropamide and the latter may also diminish gluconeogenic capacity, both of which increase the risk of serious hypoglycemic reactions. Elderly, debilitated or malnourished patients, and those with adrenal or pituitary insufficiency are particularly susceptible to the hypoglycemic action of glucose-lowering drugs. Hypoglycemia may be difficult to recognize in the elderly, and in people who are taking beta-adrenergic blocking drugs. Hypoglycemia is more likely to occur when caloric intake is deficient, after severe or prolonged exercise, when alcohol is ingested, or when more than one glucose-lowering drug is used.

Because of the long half-life of chlorpropamide, patients who become hypoglycemic during therapy require careful supervision of the dose and frequent feedings for at least 3-5 days. Hospitalization and intravenous glucose may be necessary.

Loss Of Control Of Blood Glucose: When a patient stabilized on any diabetic regimen is exposed to stress such as fever, trauma, infection, or surgery, a loss of control may occur. At such times, it may be necessary to discontinue chlorpropamide and administer insulin.

The effectiveness of any oral hypoglycemic drug, including chlorpropamide, in lowering blood glucose to a desired level decreases in many patients over a period of time, which may be due to progression of the severity of the diabetes or to diminished responsiveness to the drug. This phenomenon is known as secondary failure, to distinguish it from primary failure in which the drug is ineffective in an individual patient when first given.

INFORMATION FOR THE PATIENT

Patients should be informed of the potential risks and advantages of chlorpropamide and of alternative modes of therapy. They should also be informed about the importance of adherence to dietary instructions, of a regular exercise program, and of regular testing of urine and/or blood glucose.

The risks of hypoglycemia, its symptoms and treatment, and conditions that predispose to its development should be explained to patients and responsible family members. Primary and secondary failure should also be explained.

Patients should be instructed to contact their physician promptly if they experience symptoms of hypoglycemia or other adverse reactions.

LABORATORY TESTS

Blood and urine glucose should be monitored periodically. Measurement of glycosylated hemoglobin may be useful.

CARCINOGENESIS, MUTAGENESIS, AND IMPAIRMENT OF FERTILITY

Chronic toxicity studies have been carried out in dogs and rats. Dogs treated for 6, 13, or 20 months with doses of chlorpropamide greater than 20 times the human dose, have not shown any gross histological or pathological abnormalities. After treatment with 100 mg/kg of chlorpropamide for 20 months, a dog showed no histopathological liver changes.

Rats treated with continuous chlorpropamide therapy for 6-12 months showed varying degrees of suppression of spermatogenesis at higher dosage levels (up to 125 mg/kg). The extent of suppression seemed to follow that of growth retardation associated with chronic administration of high-dose chlorpropamide in rats.

PREGNANCY, TERATOGENIC EFFECTS, PREGNANCY CATEGORY C

Animal reproductive studies have not been conducted with chlorpropamide. It is also not known whether chlorpropamide can cause fetal harm when administered to a pregnant woman or can affect reproduction capacity. Chlorpropamide should be given to a pregnant woman only if clearly needed.

Because recent information suggests that abnormal blood glucose levels during pregnancy are associated with a higher incidence of congenital abnormalities, many experts recommend that insulin be used during pregnancy to maintain blood glucose levels as close to normal as possible.

Nonteratogenic Effects: Prolonged severe hypoglycemia (4-10 days) has been reported in neonates born to mothers who were receiving a sulfonylurea drug at the time of delivery. This has been reported more frequently with the use of agents with prolonged half-lives. If chlorpropamide is used during pregnancy, it should be discontinued at least one month before the expected delivery date.

NURSING MOTHERS

An analysis of a composite of two samples of human breast milk, each taken five hours after ingestion of 500 mg of chlorpropamide by a patient, revealed a concentration of 5 µg/ml. For reference, the normal peak blood level of chlorpropamide after a single 250 mg dose is 30 µg/ml. Therefore, it is not recommended that a woman breast feed while taking this medication.

PEDIATRIC USE

Safety and effectiveness in children have not been established.

DRUG INTERACTIONS

The hypoglycemic action of sulfonylurea may be potentiated by certain drugs including nonsteroidal anti-inflammatory agents and other drugs that are highly protein bound, salicylates, sulfonamides, chloramphenicol, probenecid, coumarins, monoamine oxidase inhibitors, and beta adrenergic blocking agents. When such drugs are administered to a patient receiving chlorpropamide, the patient should be observed closely for hypoglycemia. When such drugs are withdrawn from a patient receiving chlorpropamide, the patient should be observed closely for loss of control.

Certain drugs tend to produce hyperglycemia and may lead to loss of control. These drugs include the thiazides and other diuretics, corticosteroids, phenothiazines, thyroid products, estrogens, oral contraceptives, phenytoin, nicotinic acid, sympathomimetics, calcium channel blocking drugs, and isoniazid. When such drugs are administered to a patient receiving chlorpropamide, the patient should be closely observed for loss of control. When such drugs are withdrawn from a patient receiving chlorpropamide, the patient should be observed closely for hypoglycemia.

Since animal studies suggest that the action of barbiturates may be prolonged by therapy with chlorpropamide, barbiturates should be employed with caution. In some patients, a disulfiram-like reaction may be produced by the ingestion of alcohol.

A potential interaction between oral miconazole and oral hypoglycemic agents leading to severe hypoglycemia has been reported. Whether this interaction also occurs with the intravenous, topical, or vaginal preparations of miconazole is not known.

ADVERSE REACTIONS

Hypoglycemia: See PRECAUTIONS.

Gastrointestinal Reactions: Cholestatic jaundice may occur rarely; chlorpropamide should be discontinued if this occurs. Gastrointestinal disturbances are the most common reactions; nausea has been reported in less than 5% of patients, and diarrhea, vomiting, anorexia, and hunger in less than 2%. Other gastrointestinal disturbances have occurred in less than 1% of patients including proctocolitis. They tend to be dose related and may disappear when dosage is reduced.

Dermatologic Reactions: Pruritus has been reported in less than 3% of patients. Other allergic skin reactions, e.g., urticaria and maculopapular eruptions have been reported in approximately 1% or less of patients. These may be transient and may disappear despite continued use of chlorpropamide; if skin reactions persist the drug should be discontinued. Porphyria cutanea tarda and photosensitivity reactions have been reported with sulfonylureas.

Skin eruptions rarely progressing to erythema multiforme and exfoliative dermatitis have also been reported.

Hematologic Reactions: Leukopenia, agranulocytosis, thrombocytopenia, hemolytic anemia, aplastic anemia, pancytopenia, and eosinophilia have been reported with sulfonylureas.

Metabolic Reactions: Hepatic porphyria and disulfiram-like reactions have been reported with chlorpropamide. See DRUG INTERACTIONS section.

Endocrine Reactions: On rare occasions, chlorpropamide has caused a reaction identical to the syndrome of inappropriate antidiuretic hormone (ADH) secretion. The features of this syndrome result from excessive water retention and include hyponatremia, low serum osmolality, and high urine osmolality. This reaction has also been reported for other sulfonylureas.

DOSAGE AND ADMINISTRATION

There is no fixed dosage regimen for the management of diabetes mellitus with chlorpropamide or any other hypoglycemic agent. In addition to the usual monitoring of urinary glucose, the patient's blood glucose must also be monitored periodically to determine the minimum effective dose for the patient; to detect primary failure, *i.e.,* inadequate lowering of blood glucose at the maximum recommended dose of medication; and to detect secondary failure, *i.e.,* loss of an adequate blood glucose lowering response after an initial period of effectiveness. Glycosylated hemoglobin levels may also be of value in monitoring the patient's response to therapy.

Short-term administration of chlorpropamide may be sufficient during periods of transient loss of control in patients usually controlled well on diet.

The total daily dosage is generally taken at a single time each morning with breakfast. Occasionally cases of gastrointestinal intolerance may be relieved by dividing the daily dosage. A LOADING OR PRIMING DOSE IS NOT NECESSARY AND SHOULD NOT BE USED.

INITIAL THERAPY

1. The mild to moderately severe, middle-aged, stable, non-insulin-dependent diabetic patient should be started on 250 mg daily. In elderly patients, debilitated or malnourished patients, and patients with impaired renal or hepatic function, the initial and maintenance dosing should be conservative to avoid hypoglycemic reactions (see PRECAUTIONS.) Older patients should be started on smaller amounts of chlorpropamide, in the range of 100-125 mg daily.

2. No transition period is necessary when transferring patients from other oral hypoglycemic agents to chlorpropamide. The other agent may be discontinued abruptly and chlorpropamide started at once. In prescribing chlorpropamide, due consideration must be given to its greater potency.

Many mild to moderately severe, middle-aged, stable non-insulin-dependent diabetic patients receiving insulin can be placed directly on the oral drug and their insulin abruptly discontinued. For patients requiring more than 40 units of insulin daily, therapy with chlorpropamide may be initiated with a 50% reduction in insulin for the first few days, with subsequent further reductions dependent upon the response.

During the initial period of therapy with chlorpropamide, hypoglycemic reactions may occasionally occur, particularly during the transition from insulin to the oral drug. Hypoglycemia within 24 hours after withdrawal of the intermediate or long-acting types of insulin will usually prove to be the result of insulin carry-over and not primarily due to the effect of chlorpropamide.

During the insulin withdrawal period, the patient should test his urine for sugar and ketone bodies at least three times daily and report the results frequently to his physician. If they are abnormal, the physician should be notified immediately. In some cases, it may be advisable to consider hospitalization during the transition period.

Five to seven days after the initial therapy, the blood level of chlorpropamide reaches a plateau. Dosage may subsequently be adjusted upward or downward by increments of not more than 50-125 mg at intervals of 3-5 days to obtain optimal control. More frequent adjustments are usually undesirable.

Maintenance Therapy: Most moderately severe, middle-aged, stable non-insulin-dependent diabetic patients are controlled by approximately 250 mg daily. Many investigators have found that some milder diabetics do well on daily doses of 100 mg or less. Many of the more severe diabetics may require 500 mg daily for adequate control. PATIENTS WHO DO NOT RESPOND COMPLETELY TO 500 mg DAILY WILL USUALLY NOT RESPOND TO HIGHER DOSES. MAINTENANCE DOSES ABOVE 750 mg DAILY SHOULD BE AVOIDED.

Recommended Storage: Store below 30°C (86°F).

PRODUCT LISTING - RATED THERAPEUTICALLY EQUIVALENT

Tablet - Oral - 100 mg

30's	$11.24	GENERIC, Pd-Rx Pharmaceuticals	58864-0100-30
100's	$4.81	GENERIC, Raway Pharmacal Inc	00686-0202-20
100's	$7.97	GENERIC, Geneva Pharmaceuticals	00781-1613-01
100's	$8.00	GENERIC, Ivax Corporation	00182-1851-01
100's	$8.47	GENERIC, Major Pharmaceuticals Inc	00904-0225-61
100's	$16.00	GENERIC, Ivax Corporation	00182-1851-89
100's	$18.37	FEDERAL UPPER LIMIT, H.C.F.A. F F P	99999-0798-01
100's	$27.55	GENERIC, Major Pharmaceuticals Inc	00904-0225-60
100's	$29.05	GENERIC, Qualitest Products Inc	00603-2835-21
100's	$29.06	GENERIC, Sidmak Laboratories Inc	50111-0372-01
100's	$29.90	GENERIC, Martec Pharmaceuticals Inc	52555-0077-01
100's	$33.08	GENERIC, Mylan Pharmaceuticals Inc	00378-0197-01
100's	$34.07	GENERIC, Udl Laboratories Inc	51079-0202-20
100's	$45.24	DIABINESE, Pfizer U.S. Pharmaceuticals	00069-3930-66

Tablet - Oral - 250 mg

25's	$23.46	GENERIC, Pd-Rx Pharmaceuticals	55289-0066-97
90's	$41.27	GENERIC, Pd-Rx Pharmaceuticals	55289-0066-90
100's	$9.70	GENERIC, Major Pharmaceuticals Inc	00904-0226-61
100's	$13.40	GENERIC, Geneva Pharmaceuticals	00781-1623-01
100's	$38.85	FEDERAL UPPER LIMIT, H.C.F.A. F F P	99999-0798-04
100's	$57.95	GENERIC, Major Pharmaceuticals Inc	00904-0226-60
100's	$60.98	GENERIC, Qualitest Products Inc	00603-2836-21
100's	$61.00	GENERIC, Sidmak Laboratories Inc	50111-0373-01
100's	$61.20	GENERIC, Martec Pharmaceuticals Inc	52555-0078-01
100's	$67.31	GENERIC, Mylan Pharmaceuticals Inc	00378-0210-01
100's	$69.33	GENERIC, Udl Laboratories Inc	51079-0203-20
100's	$95.60	DIABINESE, Pfizer U.S. Pharmaceuticals	00069-3940-66

PRODUCT LISTING - EQUIVALENTS NOT AVAILABLE

Tablet - Oral - 100 mg

30's	$8.91	GENERIC, Allscripts Pharmaceutical Company	54569-2017-01
100's	$4.50	GENERIC, Cmc-Consolidated Midland Corporation	00223-0633-01

Tablet - Oral - 250 mg

30's	$18.51	GENERIC, Allscripts Pharmaceutical Company	54569-0203-00
50's	$5.41	GENERIC, Allscripts Pharmaceutical Company	54569-0203-40
100's	$61.81	GENERIC, Allscripts Pharmaceutical Company	54569-0203-01

Chlorthalidone *(000801)*

Categories: Edema; Hypertension, essential; Pregnancy Category B; FDA Approved 1967 Jul
Drug Classes: Diuretics, thiazide and derivatives
Brand Names: Hydro; **Hygroton**; Servidone; Thalidone; Thalitone; Urolin
Foreign Brand Availability: Apo-Chlorthalidone (Canada); Higroton (Ecuador; Mexico); Higrotona (Spain); Hydro-Long (Germany); Hygroton 50 (South-Africa); Hypertol (Finland); Hythalton (India); Igroton (Italy); Urandil (Czech-Republic)
Cost of Therapy: $22.53 (Hypertension; Hygroton; 25 mg; 1 tablet/day; 30 day supply)
$1.65 (Hypertension; Generic Tablets; 25 mg; 1 tablet/day; 30 day supply)

DESCRIPTION

Chlorthalidone is an oral antihypertensive/diuretic. It is a monosulfamyl diuretic that differs chemically from thiazide diuretics in that a double-ring system is incorporated in its structure. It is 2-chloro-5-(1-hydroxy-3-oxo-1-isoindolinyl) benzenesulfonamide.

Chlorthalidone is practically insoluble in water, in ether, and in chloroform: soluble in methanol: slightly soluble in alcohol.

Chlorthalidone tablets also contain colloidal silica, corn starch, gelatin, glycerin, lactose, magnesium stearate, talc, and other ingredients. The 25 mg tablets also contains yellow 6, methylparaben, and propylparaben. The 50 mg tablets also contain FD&C blue no. 1, methylparaben, and propylparaben.

CLINICAL PHARMACOLOGY

Chlorthalidone is an oral diuretic with prolonged action (48-72 hours) and low toxicity. The major portion of the drug is excreted unchanged by the kidneys. The diuretic effect of the drug occurs in approximately 2.6 hours and continues for up to 72 hours. The mean half-life following a 50-200 mg dose is 40 hours. In the first order of absorption, the elimination half-life is 53 hours following a 50 mg dose, and 60 hours following a 100 mg dose. Approximately 75% of the drug is bound to plasma proteins, 58% of the drug being bound to albumin. This is caused by an increased affinity of the drug to erythrocyte carbonic anhydrase. Nonrenal routes of elimination have yet to be clarified. Data are not available regarding percentage of doses as unchanged drug and metabolites, concentration of the drug in body fluids, degree of uptake by a particular organ or in the fetus, or passage across the blood-brain barrier.

The drug produces copious diuresis with greatly increased excretion of sodium and chloride. At maximal therapeutic dosage, chlorthalidone is approximately equal in its diuretic effect to comparable maximal therapeutic doses of benzothiadiazine diuretics. The site of action appears to be the cortical diluting segment of the ascending limb of Henle's loop of the nephron.

INDICATIONS AND USAGE

Diuretics such as chlorthalidone are indicated in the management of hypertension either as the sole therapeutic agent or to enhance the effect of other antihypertensive drugs in the more severe forms of hypertension.

Chlorthalidone is indicated as adjunctive therapy in edema associated with congestive heart failure, hepatic cirrhosis, and corticosteroid and estrogen therapy.

Chlorthalidone has also been found useful in edema due to various forms of renal dysfunction such as nephrotic syndrome, acute glomerulonephritis, and chronic renal failure.

Usage In Pregnancy: The routine use of diuretics in an otherwise healthy woman is inappropriate and exposes mother and fetus to unnecessary hazard. Diuretics do not prevent development of toxemia of pregnancy, and there is no satisfactory evidence that they are useful in the treatment of developed toxemia.

Edema during pregnancy may arise from pathological causes or from the physiologic and mechanical consequences of pregnancy. Chlorthalidone is indicated in pregnancy when edema is due to pathological causes or from the physiologic and mechanical consequences of pregnancy. Chlorthalidone is indicated in pregnancy when edema is due to pathologic causes, just as it is the absence of pregnancy (however, see WARNINGS). Dependent edema in pregnancy, resulting from restriction of venous return by the expanded uterus, is properly treated through elevation of the lower extremities and use of support hose; use of diuretics to lower intravascular volume in this case is illogical and unnecessary. There is hypervolemia during normal pregnancy that is harmful to neither the fetus nor the mother (in the absence of cardiovascular disease), but that is associated with edema, including generalized edema, in the majority of pregnant women. If this edema produces discomfort, increased recumbency will often provide relief. In rare instances, this edema may cause extreme discomfort that is not relieved by rest. In these cases, a short course of diuretics may provide relief and may be appropriate.

NON-FDA APPROVED INDICATIONS

Non FDA-approved uses of thiazide diuretics include treatment of hypercalciuric states, osteoporosis, and diabetes insipidus.

CONTRAINDICATIONS

- Anuria.
- Hypersensitivity to chlorthalidone or other sulfonamide-derived drugs.

WARNINGS

Chlorthalidone should be used with caution in severe renal disease. In patients with renal disease, chlorthalidone or related drugs may precipitate azotemia. Cumulative effects of the drug may develop in patients with impaired renal function.

Chlorthalidone should be used with caution in patients with impaired hepatic function or progressive liver disease, because minor alterations of fluid and electrolyte balance may precipitate hepatic coma.

Sensitivity reactions may occur in patients with a history of allergy or bronchial asthma.

The possibility of exacerbation or activation of systemic lupus erythematosus has been reported with thiazide diuretics, which are structurally related to chlorthalidone. However, systemic lupus erythematosus has not been reported following chlorthalidone administration.

PRECAUTIONS

GENERAL

Hypokalemia may develop with chlorthalidone as with any other potent diuretic, especially with brisk diuresis, when severe cirrhosis is present, or during concomitant use of corticosteroids or ACTH.

Interference with adequate oral electrolyte intake will also contribute to hypokalemia. Digitalis therapy may exaggerate metabolic effects of hypokalemia especially with reference to myocardial activity.

Any chloride deficit is generally mild and usually does not require specific treatment except under extraordinary circumstances (as in liver disease or renal disease). Dilutional hyponatremia may occur in edematous patients in hot weather; appropriate therapy is water restriction, rather than administration of salt except in rare instances when the hyponatremia is life threatening. In actual salt depletion, appropriate replacement is the therapy of choice.

Hyperuricemia may occur or frank gout may be precipitated in certain patients receiving chlorthalidone. Thiazide-like diuretics have been shown to increase the urinary excretion of magnesium; this may result in hypomagnesemia.

The antihypertensive effects of the drug may be enhanced in the postsympathectomy patient.

If progressive renal impairment becomes evident, as indicated by a rising nonprotein nitrogen or blood urea nitrogen, a careful reappraisal of therapy is necessary with consideration given to withholding or discontinuing diuretic therapy.

Calcium excretion is decreased by thiazide-like drugs. Pathological changes in the parathyroid gland with hypercalcemia and hypophosphatemia have been observed in a few patients on thiazide therapy. The common complications of hyperparathyroidism such as renal lithiasis, bone resorption and peptic ulceration have not been seen.

INFORMATION FOR THE PATIENT

Patients should inform their doctor if they have: (1) had an allergic reaction to Hygroton or other diuretics or have asthma (2) kidney disease (3) liver disease (4) gout (5) systemic lupus erythematosus, or (6) been taking other drugs such as cortisone, digitalis, lithium carbonate, or drugs for diabetes.

Patients should be cautioned to contact their physician if they experience any of the following symptoms of potassium loss: excess thirst, tiredness, drowsiness, restlessness, muscle pains or cramps, nausea, vomiting or increased heart rate or pulse.

Patients should also be cautioned that taking alcohol can increase the chance of dizziness occurring.

LABORATORY TESTS

Periodic determination of serum electrolytes to detect possible electrolyte imbalance should be performed at appropriate intervals.

All patients receiving chlorthalidone should be observed for clinical signs of fluid or electrolyte imbalance; namely hyponatremia, hypochloremic alkalosis, and hypokalemia. Serum and urine electrolyte determinations are particularly important when the patient is vomiting excessively or receiving parenteral fluids.

LABORATORY TEST INTERACTIONS

Chlorthalidone and related drugs may decrease serum PBI levels without signs of thyroid disturbance.

CARCINOGENESIS, MUTAGENESIS, AND IMPAIRMENT OF FERTILITY

No information is available.

PREGNANCY, TERATOGENIC EFFECTS, PREGNANCY CATEGORY B

Reproduction studies have been performed in the rat and rabbit at doses up to 420 times the human dose and have revealed no evidence of impaired fertility or harm to the fetus due to chlorthalidone. There are, however, no adequate and well-controlled studies in pregnant women. Because animal reproduction studies are not always predictive of human response, this drug should be used during pregnancy only if clearly needed.

Nonteratogenic Effects: Thiazides cross the placental barrier and appear in cord blood. The use of chlorthalidone and related drugs in pregnant women requires that the anticipated benefits of the drug be weighed against possible hazards to the fetus. These hazards include fetal or neonatal jaundice, thrombocytopenia, and possibly other adverse reactions that have occurred in the adult.

NURSING MOTHERS

Thiazides are excreted in human milk. Because of the potential for serious adverse reactions in nursing infants from chlorthalidone, a decision should be made whether to discontinue the drug, taking into account the importance of the drug to the mother.

PEDIATRIC USE

Safety and effectiveness in children have not been established.

DRUG INTERACTIONS

Chlorthalidone may add to or potentiate the action of other antihypertensive drugs. Potentiation occurs with ganglionic or peripheral adrenergic blocking drugs.

Medication such as digitalis may also influence serum electrolytes. Warning signs, irrespective of cause are: Dryness of mouth, thirst, weakness, lethargy, drowsiness, restlessness, muscle pains or cramps, muscular fatigue, hypotension, oliguria, tachycardia, and gastrointestinal disturbances such as nausea and vomiting.

Insulin requirements in diabetic patients may be increased, decreased, or unchanged. Higher dosage of oral hypoglycemic agents may be required. Latent diabetes mellitus may become manifest during chlorthalidone administration.

Chlorthalidone and related drugs may increase the responsiveness to tubocurarine.

Chlorthalidone and related drugs may decrease arterial responsiveness to norepinephrine. This diminution is not sufficient to preclude effectiveness of the pressor agent for therapeutic use.

ADVERSE REACTIONS

The following adverse reactions have been observed, but there is not enough systematic collection of data to support an estimate of their frequency.

Gastrointestinal System Reactions: Anorexia, gastric irritation, nausea, vomiting, cramping, diarrhea, constipation, jaundice (intrahepatic cholestatic jaundice), pancreatitis.

Central Nervous System Reactions: Dizziness, vertigo, paresthesias, headache, xanthopsia.

Hematologic Reactions: Leukopenia, agranulocytosis, thrombocytopenia, aplastic anemia.

Dermatologic-Hypersensitivity Reactions: Purpura, photosensitivity, rash, urticaria, necrotizing angiitis, (vasculitis), (cutaneous vasculitis), Lyell's syndrome (toxic epidermal necrolysis).

Cardiovascular Reaction: Orthostatic hypotension may occur and may be aggravated by alcohol, barbiturates or narcotics.

Other Adverse Reactions: Hyperglycemia, glycosuria, hyperuricemia, muscle spasm, weakness, restlessness, impotence.

Whenever adverse reactions are moderate or severe, chlorthalidone dosage should be reduced or therapy withdrawn.

DOSAGE AND ADMINISTRATION

Therapy should be initiated with the lowest possible dose. This dose should be titrated according to individual patient response to gain maximal therapeutic benefit while maintaining the minimal dosage possible. A single dose given in the morning with food is recommended, divided doses are unnecessary.

HYPERTENSION

Initiation: Therapy, in most patients should be initiated with a single daily dose of 25 mg. If the response is insufficient after a suitable trial, the dosage may be increased to a single daily dose of 50 mg. If additional control is required, the dosage of chlorthalidone may be increased to 100 mg once daily or a second antihypertensive drug (step-2 therapy) may be added. Dosage above 100 mg daily usually does not increase effectiveness. Increases in serum uric acid and decreases in serum potassium are dose-related over the 25-100 mg day range.

Maintenance: Maintenance doses may be lower than initial doses and should be adjusted according to individual patient response. Effectiveness is well sustained during continued use.

EDEMA

Initiation: Adults, initially 50 to 100 mg daily, or 100 mg on alternate days. Some patients may require 150-200 mg at these intervals, or up to 200 mg daily. Dosages above this level, however, do not usually produce a greater response.

Maintenance: Maintenance doses may often be lower than initial doses and should be adjusted according to the individual patient. Effectiveness is well sustained during continued use.

Store at controlled room temperature, 15-30° C (59-86° F). Avoid excessive heat. Dispense in tight containers as defined in USP.

ANIMAL PHARMACOLOGY

Biochemical studies in animals have suggested reasons for the prolonged effect of chlorthalidone. Absorption from the gastrointestinal tract is slow, due to its slow solubility. After passage to the liver, some of the drug enters the general circulation, while some is excreted in the bile, to be reabsorbed later. In the general circulation, it is distributed widely to the tissues, but is taken up in highest concentrations by the kidneys, where amounts have been found 72 hours after ingestion, long after it has disappeared from other tissues. The drug is excreted unchanged in the urine.

PRODUCT LISTING - RATED THERAPEUTICALLY EQUIVALENT

Tablet - Oral - 25 mg

Qty	Price	Product	NDC
90's	$6.45	GENERIC, Pd-Rx Pharmaceuticals	55289-0067-90
100's	$5.09	FEDERAL UPPER LIMIT, H.C.F.A. F F P	99999-0801-01
100's	$5.50	GENERIC, Major Pharmaceuticals Inc	00904-1349-60
100's	$5.50	GENERIC, Major Pharmaceuticals Inc	00904-7663-60
100's	$5.63	GENERIC, Interstate Drug Exchange Inc	00814-1703-14
100's	$5.78	GENERIC, Warner Chilcott Laboratories	00047-0123-24
100's	$6.75	GENERIC, Cmc-Consolidated Midland Corporation	00223-0629-01
100's	$8.27	GENERIC, Major Pharmaceuticals Inc	00904-1349-61
100's	$8.95	GENERIC, Raway Pharmacal Inc	00686-0528-20
100's	$8.98	GENERIC, Aligen Independent Laboratories Inc	00405-4211-01
100's	$11.95	GENERIC, Moore, H.L. Drug Exchange Inc	00839-6488-06
100's	$11.95	GENERIC, Martec Pharmaceuticals Inc	52555-0372-01
100's	$11.97	GENERIC, Geneva Pharmaceuticals	00781-1726-01
100's	$12.10	GENERIC, Ivax Corporation	00182-1434-01
100's	$13.13	GENERIC, Vangard Labs	00615-1558-13
100's	$15.70	GENERIC, Auro Pharmaceutical	55829-0200-10
100's	$15.94	GENERIC, Qualitest Products Inc	00603-2860-21
100's	$15.95	GENERIC, Sidmak Laboratories Inc	50111-0362-01
100's	$18.07	GENERIC, Udl Laboratories Inc	51079-0058-20
100's	$23.40	GENERIC, Mylan Pharmaceuticals Inc	00378-0222-01
250's	$11.90	GENERIC, Major Pharmaceuticals Inc	00904-1349-70

Tablet - Oral - 50 mg

Qty	Price	Product	NDC
30's	$4.08	GENERIC, Pd-Rx Pharmaceuticals	55289-0068-30
100's	$5.58	FEDERAL UPPER LIMIT, H.C.F.A. F F P	99999-0801-05
100's	$6.45	GENERIC, Major Pharmaceuticals Inc	00904-7665-60
100's	$7.43	GENERIC, Interstate Drug Exchange Inc	00814-1704-14
100's	$7.50	GENERIC, Cmc-Consolidated Midland Corporation	00223-0631-01
100's	$7.70	GENERIC, Warner Chilcott Laboratories	00047-0121-24
100's	$8.55	GENERIC, Major Pharmaceuticals Inc	00904-1350-60
100's	$9.50	GENERIC, Raway Pharmacal Inc	00686-0059-20
100's	$9.58	GENERIC, Aligen Independent Laboratories Inc	00405-4212-01
100's	$10.11	GENERIC, Moore, H.L. Drug Exchange Inc	00839-6369-06
100's	$10.52	GENERIC, Major Pharmaceuticals Inc	00904-1350-61
100's	$12.94	GENERIC, Vangard Labs	00615-1559-01
100's	$12.97	GENERIC, Geneva Pharmaceuticals	00781-1728-01
100's	$13.10	GENERIC, Ivax Corporation	00172-2999-60
100's	$13.10	GENERIC, Ivax Corporation	00182-1435-01
100's	$13.79	GENERIC, Auro Pharmaceutical	55829-0201-10
100's	$14.38	GENERIC, Vangard Labs	00615-1559-13
100's	$17.50	GENERIC, Qualitest Products Inc	00603-2861-21
100's	$17.50	GENERIC, Sidmak Laboratories Inc	50111-0363-01
100's	$18.00	GENERIC, Udl Laboratories Inc	51079-0059-20
100's	$24.55	GENERIC, Mylan Pharmaceuticals Inc	00378-0213-01
250's	$15.90	GENERIC, Major Pharmaceuticals Inc	00904-1350-70

Tablet - Oral - 100 mg

Qty	Price	Product	NDC
100's	$13.65	GENERIC, Martec Pharmaceuticals Inc	52555-0374-01
100's	$13.76	GENERIC, Moore, H.L. Drug Exchange Inc	00839-6370-06
100's	$25.00	GENERIC, Sidmak Laboratories Inc	50111-0364-01
100's	$148.86	HYGROTON, Aventis Pharmaceuticals	00075-0021-00

PRODUCT LISTING - EQUIVALENTS NOT AVAILABLE

Tablet - Oral - 15 mg

Qty	Price	Product	NDC
100's	$84.78	THALITONE, Monarch Pharmaceuticals Inc	61570-0024-01

Tablet - Oral - 25 mg

Qty	Price	Product	NDC
30's	$8.84	GENERIC, Allscripts Pharmaceutical Company	54569-0552-01
100's	$6.75	GENERIC, Cmc-Consolidated Midland Corporation	00223-0630-01
100's	$29.48	GENERIC, Allscripts Pharmaceutical Company	54569-0552-00

Tablet - Oral - 50 mg

Qty	Price	Product	NDC
30's	$5.25	GENERIC, Allscripts Pharmaceutical Company	54569-0554-01

Tablet - Oral - 100 mg

Qty	Price	Product	NDC
100's	$8.45	GENERIC, Cmc-Consolidated Midland Corporation	00223-0632-01
100's	$9.15	GENERIC, Interstate Drug Exchange Inc	00814-1706-14
100's	$9.95	GENERIC, Geneva Pharmaceuticals	00781-1724-01
100's	$10.40	GENERIC, Major Pharmaceuticals Inc	00904-1351-60
100's	$11.90	GENERIC, Eon Labs Manufacturing Inc	00185-0073-01
100's	$13.39	GENERIC, Ivax Corporation	00172-2904-60
100's	$13.39	GENERIC, Ivax Corporation	00182-1194-01
250's	$18.55	GENERIC, Major Pharmaceuticals Inc	00904-1351-70

Chlorthalidone; Clonidine Hydrochloride *(000802)*

Categories: Hypertension, essential; FDA Approval Pre 1982; Pregnancy Category D
Drug Classes: Antiadrenergics, central; Diuretics, thiazide and derivatives
Brand Names: **Combipres**
Foreign Brand Availability: Catapres Diu (India); Clothalton (India); Combipresan (Germany; Italy)
Cost of Therapy: $56.89 (Hypertension; Combipress; 15 mg;0.1 mg; 2 tablets/day; 30 day supply)
$17.73 (Hypertension; Generic Tablets; 15 mg;0.1 mg; 2 tablets/day; 30 day supply)

DESCRIPTION

Each tablet contains: 0.1/15 mg, 0.2/15 mg, 0.3/15 mg of clonidine hydrochloride/chlorthalidone, respectively.

FOR COMPLETE PRESCRIBING INFORMATION REFER TO THE INDIVIDUAL DRUG MONOGRAPHS (CHLORTHALIDONE; CLONIDINE HYDROCHLORIDE).

INDICATIONS AND USAGE

Combipres (clonidine hydrochloride/chlorthalidone) is indicated in the treatment of hypertension. **This fixed combination drug is not indicated for initial therapy of hypertension. Hypertension requires therapy titrated to the individual patient. If the fixed combination represents the dosage so determined, its use may be more convenient in patient management. The treatment of hypertension is not static, but must be reevaluated as conditions in each patient warrant.**

DOSAGE AND ADMINISTRATION

The dosage must be determined by individual titration.

Chlorthalidone is usually initiated at a dose of 25 mg once daily and may be increased to 50 mg if the response is insufficient after a suitable trial.

Clonidine hydrochloride is usually initiated at a dose of 0.1 mg twice daily. Elderly patients may benefit from a lower initial dose. Further increments of 0.1 mg/day may be made if necessary until the desired response is achieved. The therapeutic doses most commonly employed have ranged from 0.2-0.6 mg/day in divided doses.

One Combipres (clonidine hydrochloride/chlorthalidone) tablet administered once or twice daily can be used to administer a minimum of 0.1 mg clonidine hydrochloride and 15 mg chlorthalidone to a maximum of 0.6 mg clonidine hydrochloride and 30 mg chlorthalidone.

PRODUCT LISTING - RATED THERAPEUTICALLY EQUIVALENT

Tablet - Oral - 15 mg;0.1 mg

Qty	Price	Product	NDC
100's	$29.55	GENERIC, Major Pharmaceuticals Inc	00904-1033-60
100's	$31.00	GENERIC, Qualitest Products Inc	00603-2978-21
100's	$36.52	GENERIC, Moore, H.L. Drug Exchange Inc	00839-7285-06
100's	$37.35	GENERIC, Interstate Drug Exchange Inc	00814-1734-14
100's	$37.50	GENERIC, Par Pharmaceutical Inc	49884-0113-01
100's	$39.47	GENERIC, Aligen Independent Laboratories Inc	00405-4248-01
100's	$39.95	GENERIC, Ivax Corporation	00182-1275-01
100's	$63.77	GENERIC, Mylan Pharmaceuticals Inc	00378-0001-01
100's	$91.19	CLORPRES, Bertek Pharmaceuticals Inc	62794-0001-01

Tablet - Oral - 15 mg;0.2 mg

Size	Price	Product	NDC
100's	$39.00	GENERIC, Qualitest Products Inc	00603-2979-21
100's	$39.80	GENERIC, Major Pharmaceuticals Inc	00904-1034-60
100's	$49.50	GENERIC, Par Pharmaceutical Inc	49884-0115-01
100's	$50.29	GENERIC, Moore, H.L. Drug Exchange Inc	00839-7286-06
100's	$52.11	GENERIC, Aligen Independent Laboratories Inc	00405-4249-01
100's	$52.20	GENERIC, Ivax Corporation	00182-1276-01
100's	$85.00	GENERIC, Mylan Pharmaceuticals Inc	00378-0027-01
100's	$121.99	CLORPRES, Bertek Pharmaceuticals Inc	62794-0027-01

Tablet - Oral - 15 mg;0.3 mg

Size	Price	Product	NDC
100's	$41.00	GENERIC, Qualitest Products Inc	00603-2980-21
100's	$47.13	GENERIC, Moore, H.L. Drug Exchange Inc	00839-7287-06
100's	$54.47	GENERIC, Moore, H.L. Drug Exchange Inc	00839-7943-06
100's	$61.50	GENERIC, Par Pharmaceutical Inc	49884-0116-01
100's	$62.00	GENERIC, Ivax Corporation	00182-1277-01
100's	$64.73	GENERIC, Aligen Independent Laboratories Inc	00405-4250-01
100's	$102.88	GENERIC, Mylan Pharmaceuticals Inc	00378-0072-01
100's	$116.57	CLORPRES, Bertek Pharmaceuticals Inc	62794-0072-01

Chlorzoxazone *(000804)*

Categories: Pain, musculoskeletal; FDA Approved 1987 Jun; Pregnancy Category C
Drug Classes: Musculoskeletal agents; Relaxants, skeletal muscle
Brand Names: **Paraflex**; Parafon Forte DSC; Remular-S
Foreign Brand Availability: Escoflex (Switzerland); Klorzoxazon (Denmark); Muscol (Taiwan); Parafon DSC (India); Parafon Forte (Thailand); Prolax (Taiwan); Salalin (Taiwan); Solaxin (Hong-Kong; Indonesia; Malaysia)
Cost of Therapy: $48.54 (Musculoskeletal Pain; Parafon Forte; 500 mg; 3 tablets/day; 10 day supply)
$6.73 (Musculoskeletal Pain; Generic Tablets; 500 mg; 3 tablets/day; 10 day supply)

DESCRIPTION

This monograph contains information on the 250 and 500 mg caplets.

250 MG CAPLET

Each caplet (capsule shaped tablet) contains: Chlorzoxazone* - 250 mg
Inactive ingredients: Docusate sodium, FD&C red no. 40, FD&C yellow no. 6, hydroxypropyl methylcellulose, lactose (hydrous), magnesium stearate, microcrystalline cellulose, polyethylene glycol, polysorbate 80, pregelatinized corn starch, propylene glycol, sodium benzoate, sodium starch glycolate, titanium dioxide.
*5-chlorobenzoxazolinone

500 MG CAPLET

Each caplet (capsule shaped tablet) contains: Chlorzoxazone* - 500 mg
Inactive ingredients: FD&C blue no.1, microcrystalline cellulose, docusate sodium, lactose (hydrous), magnesium stearate, sodium benzoate, sodium starch glycolate, pregelatinized corn starch, D&C yellow no. 10.
*5-chlorobenzoxazolinone.

CLINICAL PHARMACOLOGY

Chlorzoxazone is a centrally-acting agent for painful musculoskeletal conditions. Data available from animal experiments as well as human study indicate that chlorzoxazone acts primarily at the level of the spinal cord and subcortical areas of the brain where it inhibits multisynaptic reflex arcs involved in producing and maintaining skeletal muscle spasm of varied etiology. The clinical result is a reduction of the skeletal muscle spasm with relief of pain and increased mobility of the involved muscles. Blood levels of chlorzoxazone can be detected in people during the first 30 minutes and peak levels may be reached, in the majority of the subjects, in about 1-2 hours after oral administration of chlorzoxazone. Chlorzoxazone is rapidly metabolized and is excreted in the urine, primarily in a conjugated form as the glucuronide. Less than one percent of a dose of chlorzoxazone is excreted unchanged in the urine in 24 hours.

INDICATIONS AND USAGE

Chlorzoxazone is indicated as an adjunct to rest, physical therapy, and other measures for the relief of discomfort associated with acute, painful musculoskeletal conditions. The mode of action of this drug has not been clearly identified, but may be related to its sedative properties. Chlorzoxazone does not directly relax tense skeletal muscles in man.

CONTRAINDICATIONS

Chlorzoxazone is contraindicated in patients with known intolerance to the drug.

WARNINGS

Serious (including fatal) hepatocellular toxicity has been reported rarely in patients receiving chlorzoxazone. The mechanism is unknown but appears to be idiosyncratic and unpredictable. Factors predisposing patients to this reare event are not known. Patients should be instructed to report early signs and/or symptoms of hepatotoxicity such as fever, rash, anorexia, nausea, vomiting, fatigue, right upper quandrant pain, dark urine, or jaundice. Chlorzoxazone should be discontinued immediately and a physician consulted if any of these signs or symptoms develop. Chlorzoxazone use should also be discontinued if a patient develops abnormal liver enzymes (*e.g.*, AST, ALT, alkaline phosphate and bilirubin).

The concomitant use of alcohol or other central nervous system depressants may have an additive effect.

Use in Pregnancy: The safe use of chlorzoxazone has not been established with respect to the possible adverse effects upon fetal development. Therefore, it should be used in women of childbearing potential only when, in the judgment of the physician, the potential benefits outweigh the possible risks.

PRECAUTIONS

Chlorzoxazone should be used with caution in patients with known allergies or with a history of allergic reactions to drugs. If a sensitivity reaction occurs such as urticaria, redness, or itching of the skin, the drug should be stopped.

If any symptoms suggestive of liver dysfunction are observed, the drug should be discontinued.

ADVERSE REACTIONS

After extensive clinical use of chlorzoxazone-containing products, it is apparent that the drug is well tolerated and seldom produces undesirable side effects. Occasional patients may develop gastrointestinal disturbances. It is possible in rare instances that chlorzoxazone may have been associated with gastrointestinal bleeding. Drowsiness, dizziness, lightheadedness, malaise, or overstimulation may be noted by an occasional patient. Rarely, allergic-type skin rashes, petechiae, or ecchymoses may develop during treatment. Angioneurotic edema or anaphylactic reactions are extremely rare. There is no evidence that the drug will cause renal damage. Rarely, a patient may note discoloration of the urine resulting from a phenolic metabolite of chlorzoxazone. This finding is of no known clinical significance.

DOSAGE AND ADMINISTRATION

Usual Adult Dosage: One (1) caplet (250 mg) three or four times daily. Initial dosage for *painful musculoskeletal conditions* should be 2 caplets (500 mg) three or four times daily. If adequate response is not obtained with this dose, it may be increased to 3 caplets (750 mg) three or four times daily. As improvement occurs, dosage can usually be reduced.
Store at room controlled room temperature (15-30°C, 59-86°F).

PRODUCT LISTING - RATED THERAPEUTICALLY EQUIVALENT

Tablet - Oral - 250 mg

Size	Price	Product	NDC
20's	$6.69	GENERIC, Pd-Rx Pharmaceuticals	55289-0376-20
40's	$11.25	GENERIC, Pd-Rx Pharmaceuticals	55289-0376-40
100's	$5.25	GENERIC, Major Pharmaceuticals Inc	00904-0294-60
100's	$6.95	GENERIC, Ivax Corporation	00182-1780-01
100's	$9.50	GENERIC, Par Pharmaceutical Inc	49884-0016-01
100's	$30.00	GENERIC, International Ethical Laboratories Inc	11584-1033-01

Tablet - Oral - 500 mg

Size	Price	Product	NDC
8's	$3.84	GENERIC, Pd-Rx Pharmaceuticals	55289-0633-08
8's	$9.53	GENERIC, Southwood Pharmaceuticals Inc	58016-0291-08
10's	$4.80	GENERIC, Pd-Rx Pharmaceuticals	55289-0633-10
10's	$11.92	GENERIC, Southwood Pharmaceuticals Inc	58016-0291-10
12's	$14.30	GENERIC, Southwood Pharmaceuticals Inc	58016-0291-12
14's	$16.68	GENERIC, Southwood Pharmaceuticals Inc	58016-0291-14
15's	$17.88	GENERIC, Southwood Pharmaceuticals Inc	58016-0291-15
16's	$19.07	GENERIC, Southwood Pharmaceuticals Inc	58016-0291-16
20's	$9.89	GENERIC, Pd-Rx Pharmaceuticals	55289-0633-20
20's	$23.83	GENERIC, Southwood Pharmaceuticals Inc	58016-0291-20
20's	$26.66	PARAFON FORTE DSC, Allscripts Pharmaceutical Company	54569-1506-03
21's	$25.03	GENERIC, Southwood Pharmaceuticals Inc	58016-0291-21
24's	$10.35	GENERIC, Pd-Rx Pharmaceuticals	55289-0633-24
24's	$28.60	GENERIC, Southwood Pharmaceuticals Inc	58016-0291-24
24's	$45.72	PARAFON FORTE DSC, Pd-Rx Pharmaceuticals	55289-0888-24
25's	$14.22	GENERIC, Pd-Rx Pharmaceuticals	55289-0633-97
28's	$10.74	GENERIC, Pd-Rx Pharmaceuticals	55289-0633-28
28's	$33.37	GENERIC, Southwood Pharmaceuticals Inc	58016-0291-28
30's	$8.12	GENERIC, Circle Pharmaceuticals Inc	00659-0433-30
30's	$13.05	GENERIC, Pd-Rx Pharmaceuticals	55289-0633-30
30's	$35.75	GENERIC, Southwood Pharmaceuticals Inc	58016-0291-30
40's	$17.40	GENERIC, Pd-Rx Pharmaceuticals	55289-0633-40
40's	$47.67	GENERIC, Southwood Pharmaceuticals Inc	58016-0291-40
42's	$50.05	GENERIC, Southwood Pharmaceuticals Inc	58016-0291-42
56's	$66.74	GENERIC, Southwood Pharmaceuticals Inc	58016-0291-56
60's	$71.50	GENERIC, Southwood Pharmaceuticals Inc	58016-0291-60
90's	$107.25	GENERIC, Southwood Pharmaceuticals Inc	58016-0291-90
100's	$10.85	FEDERAL UPPER LIMIT, H.C.F.A. F F P	99999-0804-03
100's	$19.00	GENERIC, Raway Pharmacal Inc	00686-0476-20
100's	$22.43	GENERIC, Interstate Drug Exchange Inc	00814-1714-14
100's	$29.95	GENERIC, Seneca Pharmaceuticals	47028-0052-01
100's	$30.41	GENERIC, Pd-Rx Pharmaceuticals	55289-0633-17
100's	$36.13	GENERIC, Bolan Pharmaceutical Inc	44437-0193-01
100's	$44.25	GENERIC, Major Pharmaceuticals Inc	00904-0300-60
100's	$44.32	GENERIC, Aligen Independent Laboratories Inc	00405-4219-01
100's	$44.35	GENERIC, Qualitest Products Inc	00603-2886-21
100's	$46.97	GENERIC, Moore, H.L. Drug Exchange Inc	00839-7445-06
100's	$46.97	GENERIC, Moore, H.L. Drug Exchange Inc	00839-7725-06
100's	$48.90	GENERIC, Martec Pharmaceuticals Inc	52555-0263-01
100's	$48.97	GENERIC, Mutual/United Research Laboratories	00677-1670-01
100's	$48.98	GENERIC, Watson/Rugby Laboratories Inc	00536-3444-01
100's	$48.98	GENERIC, Barr Laboratories Inc	00555-0585-02
100's	$49.48	GENERIC, Udl Laboratories Inc	51079-0476-20
100's	$49.95	GENERIC, Geneva Pharmaceuticals	00781-1304-13
100's	$60.00	GENERIC, International Ethical Laboratories Inc	11584-0411-01
100's	$84.15	GENERIC, Major Pharmaceuticals Inc	00904-0302-60
100's	$84.97	GENERIC, Teva Pharmaceuticals Usa	00093-0542-01
100's	$84.97	GENERIC, Watson Laboratories Inc	52544-0693-01
100's	$96.95	GENERIC, Amide Pharmaceutical Inc	52152-0025-02

100's	$119.17	GENERIC, Southwood Pharmaceuticals Inc	58016-0291-00
100's	$161.81	PARAFON FORTE DSC, Janssen Pharmaceuticals	00045-0325-60

PRODUCT LISTING - EQUIVALENTS NOT AVAILABLE

Tablet - Oral - 250 mg

8's	$7.09	GENERIC, Southwood Pharmaceuticals Inc	58016-0298-08
20's	$3.88	GENERIC, Prescript Pharmaceuticals	00247-0341-20
30's	$4.15	GENERIC, Prescript Pharmaceuticals	00247-0341-30
100's	$16.95	GENERIC, Amide Pharmaceutical Inc	52152-0053-02

Tablet - Oral - 500 mg

3's	$3.64	GENERIC, Prescript Pharmaceuticals	00247-0112-03
4's	$3.73	GENERIC, Prescript Pharmaceuticals	00247-0112-04
8's	$3.61	GENERIC, Physicians Total Care	54868-0735-08
10's	$4.28	GENERIC, Prescript Pharmaceuticals	00247-0112-10
10's	$17.08	GENERIC, Pharma Pac	52959-0035-10
12's	$4.47	GENERIC, Prescript Pharmaceuticals	00247-0112-12
14's	$4.65	GENERIC, Prescript Pharmaceuticals	00247-0112-14
15's	$4.74	GENERIC, Prescript Pharmaceuticals	00247-0112-15
16's	$4.84	GENERIC, Prescript Pharmaceuticals	00247-0112-16
16's	$7.97	GENERIC, Allscripts Pharmaceutical Company	54569-1970-06
20's	$5.21	GENERIC, Prescript Pharmaceuticals	00247-0112-20
20's	$9.98	GENERIC, Allscripts Pharmaceutical Company	54569-1970-01
20's	$20.68	GENERIC, Alpharma Uspd Makers Of Barre and Nmc	63874-0419-20
20's	$27.16	GENERIC, Pharma Pac	52959-0035-20
21's	$20.80	GENERIC, Alpharma Uspd Makers Of Barre and Nmc	63874-0419-21
21's	$28.07	GENERIC, Pharma Pac	52959-0035-21
24's	$4.07	GENERIC, Physicians Total Care	54868-0735-01
24's	$5.58	GENERIC, Prescript Pharmaceuticals	00247-0112-24
25's	$4.17	GENERIC, Physicians Total Care	54868-0735-03
28's	$5.95	GENERIC, Prescript Pharmaceuticals	00247-0112-28
28's	$13.97	GENERIC, Allscripts Pharmaceutical Company	54569-1970-05
28's	$28.08	GENERIC, Alpharma Uspd Makers Of Barre and Nmc	63874-0419-28
28's	$35.71	GENERIC, Pharma Pac	52959-0035-28
30's	$4.75	GENERIC, Physicians Total Care	54868-0735-05
30's	$6.13	GENERIC, Prescript Pharmaceuticals	00247-0112-30
30's	$14.97	GENERIC, Allscripts Pharmaceutical Company	54569-1970-00
30's	$30.16	GENERIC, Alpharma Uspd Makers Of Barre and Nmc	63874-0419-30
30's	$38.03	GENERIC, Pharma Pac	52959-0035-30
40's	$5.89	GENERIC, Physicians Total Care	54868-0735-02
40's	$7.06	GENERIC, Prescript Pharmaceuticals	00247-0112-40
40's	$19.96	GENERIC, Allscripts Pharmaceutical Company	54569-1970-04
40's	$40.56	GENERIC, Alpharma Uspd Makers Of Barre and Nmc	63874-0419-40
40's	$48.59	GENERIC, Pharma Pac	52959-0035-40
50's	$7.03	GENERIC, Physicians Total Care	54868-0735-00
60's	$8.16	GENERIC, Physicians Total Care	54868-0735-04
60's	$64.79	GENERIC, Pharma Pac	52959-0035-60
70's	$71.54	GENERIC, Pharma Pac	52959-0035-70
100's	$102.96	GENERIC, Alpharma Uspd Makers Of Barre and Nmc	63874-0419-01
120's	$143.00	GENERIC, Southwood Pharmaceuticals Inc	58016-0291-02

Cholestyramine (000808)

For related information, see the comparative table section in Appendix A.

Categories: Hypercholesterolemia; Hyperlipoproteinemia; Pruritus, secondary to biliary obstruction; Pregnancy Category C; FDA Approved 1973 Aug
Drug Classes: Antihyperlipidemics; Bile acid sequestrants
Brand Names: Cholybar; Cuemid; **Questran**; Questran Light
Foreign Brand Availability: Chol-Less (Israel); Choles (Taiwan); Colestepril (Colombia); Colestiramina (Colombia); Colestrol (Italy); Lipocol-Merz (Germany); Lismol (Spain); Quantalan (Germany; Portugal; Switzerland); Quantalan Zuckerfrei (Austria); Questran Lite (Australia; Philippines); Questran Loc (Denmark; Sweden); Resincolestiramina (Singapore); Vasosan P-Granulat (Germany); Vasosan S-Granulat (Germany)
Cost of Therapy: $118.84 (Hypercholesterolemia; Questran Light Powder; 4 g/5 g; 8 g/day; 30 day supply)
$82.02 (Hypercholesterolemia; Prevalite; 4 g/5 g; 8 g/day; 30 day supply)
$35.35 (Hypercholesterolemia; Generic Powder; 4 g/5 g; 8 g/day; 30 day supply)

DESCRIPTION

Cholestyramine for oral suspension, the chloride salt of a basic anion exchange resin, a cholesterol lowering agent, is intended for oral administration. Cholestyramine resin is quite hydrophilic, but insoluble in water. Cholestyramine resin is not absorbed from the digestive tract.

Nine (9) g of Questran powder contain 4 g of anhydrous cholestyramine resin. *Inactive Ingredients:* Acacia, citric acid, D&C yellow no. 10, FD&C yellow no. 6, flavor (natural and artificial), polysorbate 80, propylene glycol alginate, and sucrose (421 mg/g powder).

Five (5) g of Questran Light contain 4 g of anhydrous cholestyramine resin.*Inactive Ingredients:* Aspartame, citric acid, D&C yellow no. 10, FD&C red no. 40, flavor (natural and artificial), propylene glycol alginate, colloidal silicon dioxide, sucrose (144 mg/g powder), and xanthan gum.

CLINICAL PHARMACOLOGY

Cholesterol is probably the sole precursor of bile acids. During normal digestion, bile acids are secreted into the intestines. A major portion of the bile acids is absorbed from the intestinal tract and returned to the liver via the enterohepatic circulation. Only very small amounts of bile acids are found in normal serum.

Cholestyramine resin adsorbs and combines with the bile acids in the intestine to form an insoluble complex which is excreted in the feces. This results in a partial removal of bile acids from the enterohepatic circulation by preventing their absorption.

The increased fecal loss of bile acids due to cholestyramine administration leads to an increased oxidation of cholesterol to bile acids, a decrease in beta lipoprotein or low density lipoprotein plasma levels and a decrease in serum cholesterol levels. Although in man, cholestyramine produces an increase in hepatic synthesis of cholesterol, plasma cholesterol levels fall.

In patients with partial biliary obstruction, the reduction of serum bile acid levels by cholestyramine reduces excess bile acids deposited in the dermal tissue with resultant decrease in pruritus.

INDICATIONS AND USAGE

Reduction of Elevated Serum Cholesterol: Cholestyramine is indicated as adjunctive therapy to diet for the reduction of elevated serum cholesterol in patients with primary hypercholesterolemia (elevated low density lipoprotein [LDL] cholesterol) who do not respond adequately to diet. Cholestyramine may be useful to lower LDL cholesterol in patients who also have hypertriglyceridemia, but it is not indicated where hypertriglyceridemia is the abnormality of most concern.
Therapy with lipid-altering agents should be a component of multiple risk factor intervention in those inidividuals at significantly increased risk for atherosclerotic vascular disease due to hypercholesterolemia. Treament should begin and continue with dietary therapy specific for the type of hyperlipoproteinemia determined prior to initiation of drug therapy. Excess body weight may be an important factor and caloric restriction for weight normalization should be addressed prior to drug therapy in the overweight.

Prior to initiating therapy with cholestyramine for oral suspension, secondary causes of hypercholesterolemia (*e.g.*, poorly controlled diabetes mellitus, hypothyroidism, nephrotic syndrome, dysproteinemias, obstructive liver disease, other drug therapy, alcoholism), should be excluded, and a lipid profile performed to assess Total cholesterol, HDL-C, and triglycerides (TG). For individuals with TG less than 400 mg/dl (<4.5 mmol/L), LDL-C can be estimated using the following equation:

LDL-C = Total cholesterol - [(TG/5) + HDL-C]

For TG levels >400 mg/dl, this equation is less accurate and LDL-C concentrations should be determined by ultracentrifugation. In hypertriglyceridemic patients, LDL-C may be low or normal despite elevated Total-C. In such cases cholestyramine may not be indicated.

Serum cholesterol and triglyceride levels should be determined periodically based on NCEP guidelines to confirm inital and adequate long-term response. A favorable trend in cholesterol reduction should occur during the first month of cholestyramine therapy. The therapy should be continued to sustain cholesterol reduction. If adequate cholesterol reduction is not attained, increasing the dosage of cholestyramine or adding other lipid-lowering agents in combination with cholestryramine should be considered.

Since the goal of treatment is to lower LDL-C, the NCEP[4] recommends that LDL-C levels be used to initiate and assess treatment response. If LDL-C levels are not available, then Total-C alone may be used to monitor long-term therapy. A lipoprotein analysis (including LDL-C determination) should be carried out once a year. The NCEP treatment guidelines are summarized in TABLE 1.

TABLE 1

Definite Atherosclerotic Disease*	Two or More Other Risk Factors†	LDL-Cholesterol mg/dl (mmol/L) Initiation Level	Goal
NO	NO	≥190 (≥4.9)	<160 (<4.1)
NO	YES	≥160 (≥4.1)	<130 (<3.4)
YES	YES or NO	≥130 (≥3.4)	≤100 (≤2.6)

* Coronary heart disease or peripheral vascular disease (including symptomatic carotid artery disease).
† Other risk factors for coronary heart disease (CHD) include: age (males: ≥45 years; females: ≥55 years or premature menopause without estrogen replacement therapy); family history of premature CHD; current cigarette smoking; hypertension; confirmed HDL-C <35 mg/dl (<0.91 mmol/L); and diabetes mellitus. Subtract one risk factor if HDL-C is ≥60 mg/dl (≥1.6 mmol/L).

Cholestyramine monotherapy has been demonstrated to retard the rate of progression[2,3] and increase the rate of regression[3] of coronary atherosclerosis.

Relief of Pruritus: Cholestyramine is indicated for the relief of pruritus associated with partial biliary obstruction. Cholestyramine has been shown to have a variable effect on serum cholesterol in these patients. Patients with primary biliary cirrhosis may exhibit an elevated cholesterol as part of their disease.

NON-FDA APPROVED INDICATIONS

Cholestyramine has also been used in the treatment of severe diarrhea. However, this use is not currently FDA approved.

CONTRAINDICATIONS

Cholestyramine is contraindicated in patients with complete biliary obstruction where bile is not secreted into the intestine and in those individuals who have shown hypersensitivity to any of its components.

C

WARNINGS

PHENYLKETONURICS: QUESTRAN LIGHT CONTAINS 16.8 mg PHENYLALANINE PER 5 g DOSE.

PRECAUTIONS

GENERAL

Chronic use of cholestyramine may be associated with increased bleeding tendency due to hypoprothrombinemia associated with vitamin K deficiency. This will usually respond promptly to parenteral vitamin K_1 and recurrences can be prevented by oral administration of vitamin K_1. Reduction of serum or red cell folate has been reported over long term administration of cholestyramine. Supplementation with folic acid should be considered in these cases.

There is a possibility that prolonged use of cholestyramine, since it is a chloride form of anion exchange resin, may produce hyperchloremic acidosis. This would especially be true in younger and smaller patients where the relative dosage may be higher. Caution should also be exercised in patients with renal insufficiency or volume depletion, and in patients receiving concomitant spironolactone.

Cholestyramine may produce or worsen pre-existing constipation. The dosage should be increased gradually in patients to minimize the risk of developing fecal impaction. In patients with pre-existing constipation, the starting dose should be 1 packet or 1 scoop once daily for 5-7 days, increasing to twice daily with monitoring of constipation and of serum lipoproteins, at least twice, 4-6 weeks apart. Increased fluid intake and fiber intake should be encouraged to alleviate constipation and a stool softener may occasionally be indicated. If the inital dose is well tolerated, the dose may be increased as needed by one dose/day (at monthly intervals) with periodic monitoring of serum lipoproteins. If constipation worsens or the desired therapeutic response is not achieved at 1-6 doses/day, combination therapy or alternate therapy should be considered. Particular effort should be made to avoid constipation in patients with sympotmatic coronary artery disease. Constipation associated with cholestyramine may aggravate hemorrhoids.

INFORMATION FOR THE PATIENT

Inform your physician if you are pregnant or plan to become pregnant or are breastfeeding. Drink plenty of fluids and mix each 9 g dose of cholestyramine powder in at least 2-6 ounces of fluid before taking or mix each 5 g dose of cholestyramine light in at least 2-3 ounces of fluid before taking. Sipping or holding the resin suspension in the mouth for prolonged periods may lead to changes in the surface of the teeth resulting in discoloration, erosion of enamel or decay; good oral hygiene should be maintained.

LABORATORY TESTS

Serum cholesterol levels should be determined frequently during the first few months of therapy and periodically thereafter. Serum triglyceride levels should be measured periodically to detect whether significant changes have occurred.

The LRC-CPPT showed a dose-related increase in serum triglycerides of 10.7-17.1% in the cholestyramine-treated group, compared with an increase of 7.9-11.7% in the placebo group. Based on the mean values and adjusting for the placebo group, the cholestyramine-treated group showed an increase of 5% over pre-entry levels the first year of the study and an increase of 4.3% the seventh year.

CARCINOGENESIS, MUTAGENESIS, AND IMPAIRMENT OF FERTILITY

In studies conducted in rats in which cholestyramine resin was used as a tool to investigate the role of various intestinal factors, such as fat, bile salts and microbial flora, in the development of intestinal tumors induced by potent carcinogens, the incidence of such tumors was observed to be greater in cholestyramine resin-treated rats than in control rats.

The relevance of this laboratory observation from studies in rats to the clinical use of cholestyramine is not known. In the LRC-CPPT study referred to above, the total incidence of fatal and nonfatal neoplasms was similar in both treatment groups. When the many different categories of tumors are examined, various alimentary system cancers were somewhat more prevalent in the cholestyramine group. The small numbers and the multiple categories prevent conclusions from being drawn. However, in view of the fact that cholestyramine resin is confined to the GI tract and not absorbed, and in light of the animal experiments referred to above, a 6 year post-trial follow-up of the LRC-CPPT[5] patient population has been completed (a total of 13.4 years of in-trial plus post-trial follow-up) and revealed no significant difference in the incidence of cause-specific mortality or cancer morbidity between cholestyramine and placebo treated patients.

PREGNANCY CATEGORY C

Since cholestyramine is not absorbed systemically, it is not expected to cause fetal harm when administered during pregnancy in recommended dosages. There are, however, no adequate and well controlled studies in pregnant women, and the known interference with absorption of fat soluble vitamins may be detrimental even in the presence of supplementation; accordingly, regular prenatal supplementation may not be adequate (see DRUG INTERACTIONS). The use of cholestyramine in pregnancy or lactation or by women of childbearing age requires that the potential benefits of drug therapy be weighted against the possible hazards to the mother and child.

NURSING MOTHERS

Caution should be exercised when cholestyramine is administered to a nursing mother. The possible lack of proper vitamin absorption may have an effect on nursing infants (see Pregnancy Category C).

PEDIATRIC USE

Although an optimal dosage schedule has not been established, standard texts[6,7] list a usual pediatric dose of 240 mg/kg/day of anhydrous cholestyramine resin in 2-3 divided doses, normally not to exceed 8 g/day with dose titration based on response and tolerance.

In calculating pediatric dosages, 44.4 mg of anhydrous cholestyramine resin are contained in 100 mg of Questran powder and 80 mg of anhydrous cholestyramine resin are contained in 100 mg of Questran Light.

The effects of long-term drug administration, as well as its effect in maintaining lowered cholesterol levels in pediatric patients, are unknown. Also see ADVERSE REACTIONS.

DRUG INTERACTIONS

Cholestyramine may delay or reduce the absorption of concomitant oral medication such as phenylbutazone, warfarin, thiazide diuretics (acidic), or propranolol (basic), as well as tetracycline, penicillin G, phenobarbital, thyroid and thyroxine preparations, estrogens and progestrins, and digitalis. Interference with the absorption of oral phosphate supplements has been observed with another positively-charged bile acid sequestrant. Cholestyramine may interfere with the pharmacokinetics of drugs that undergo enterohepatic circulation. The discontinuance of cholestyramine could pose a hazard to health if a potentially toxic drug such as digitalis has been titrated to a maintenance level while the patient was taking cholestyramine.

Because cholestyramine binds bile acids, cholestyramine may interfere with normal fat digestion and absorption and thus may prevent absorption of fat soluble vitamins such as A, D, E, and K. When cholestyramine is given for long periods of time, concomitant supplementation with water-miscible (or parenteral) forms of fat-soluble vitamins should be considered.

SINCE CHOLESTYRAMINE MAY BIND OTHER DRUGS GIVEN CONCURRENTLY, IT IS RECOMMENDED THAT PATIENTS TAKE OTHER DRUGS AT LEAST ONE HOUR BEFORE OR 4 TO 6 HOURSAFTER CHOLESTYRAMINE (OR AT AS GREAT AN INTERVAL AS POSSIBLE) TO AVOID IMPEDING THEIR ABSORPTION.

ADVERSE REACTIONS

The most common adverse reaction is constipation. When used as a cholesterol-lowering agent predisposing factors for most complaints of constipation are high dose and increased age (more than 60 years old). Most instances of constipation are mild, transient, and controlled with conventional therapy. Some patients require a temporary decrease in dosage or discontinuation of therapy.

Less Frequent Adverse Reactions: Abdominal discomfort and/or pain, flatulence, nausea, vomiting, diarrhea, eructation, anorexia, and steatorrhea, bleeding tendencies due to hypoprothrombinemia (vitamin K deficiency) as well as vitamin A (one case of night blindness reported) and D deficiencies, hyperchloremic acidosis in children, osteoporosis, rash and irritation of the skin, tongue and perianal area. Rare reports of intestinal obstruction, including 2 deaths, have been reported in pediatric patients.

Occasional calcified material has been observed in the biliary tree, including calcification of the gallbladder, in patients to whom cholestyramine resin has been given. However, this may be a manifestation of the liver disease and not drug related.

One patient experienced biliary colic on each of three occasions on which he took cholestyramine. One patient diagnosed as acute abdominal symptom complex was found to have a "pasty mass" in the transverse colon on x-ray.

Other events (not necessarily drug related) reported in patients taking cholestyramine include:

Gastrointestinal: GI-rectal bleeding, black stools, hemorrhoidal bleeding, bleeding from known duodenal ulcer, dysphagia, hiccups, ulcer attack, sour taste, pancreatitis, rectal pain, diverticulitis.

Laboratory Test Changes: Liver function abnormalities.

Hematologic: Prolonged prothrombin time, ecchymosis, anemia.

Hypersensitivity: Urticaria, asthma, wheezing, shortness of breath.

Musculoskeletal: Backache, muscle and joint pains, arthritis.

Neurologic: Headache, anxiety, vertigo, dizziness, fatigue, tinnitus, syncope, drowsiness, femoral nerve pain, paresthesia.

Eye: Uveitis.

Renal: Hematuria, dysuria, burnt odor to urine, diuresis.

Miscellaneous: Weight loss, weight gain, increased libido, swollen glands, edema, dental bleeding, dental caries, erosion of tooth enamel, tooth discoloration.

DOSAGE AND ADMINISTRATION

The recommended starting adult dose for cholestyramine or cholestyramine light is one packet or one level scoopful (9 g of Questran Powder contains 4 g of anhydrous cholestyramine resin) (5 g of Questran Light contains 4 g of anhydrous cholestyramine resin) once or twice a day. The recommended maintenance dose for Questran is 2-4 packets or scoopfuls daily (8-16 g anhydrous cholestyramine resin) divided into 2 doses. It is recommended that increases in dose be gradual with periodic assessment of lipid/lipoprotein levels at intervals of not less than 4 weeks. The maximum recommended daily dose is 6 packets or scoopfuls of Questran (24 g of anhydrous cholestyramine resin). The suggested time of administration is at mealtime but may be modified to avoid interference with absorption of other medications. Although the recommended dosing schedule is twice daily, cholestyramine may be administered in 1-6 doses per day.

Cholestyramine should not be taken in its dry form. Always mix cholestyramine with water or other fluids before ingesting (see Preparation).

Concomitant Therapy: Preliminary evidence suggests that the lipid-lowering effects of cholestyramine on total and LDL-cholesterol are enhanced when combined with a HMG-CoA reductase inhibitor, *e.g.*, pravastatin, lovastatin, simvastatin, and fluvastatin. Additive effects on LDL-cholesterol are also seen with combined nicotinic acid/cholestyramine therapy. See DRUG INTERACTIONS for recommendations on administering concomitant therapy.

Preparation: The color of cholestyramine may vary somewhat from batch to batch but this variation does not affect the performance of the product. Place the contents of one single-dose packet or one level scoopful of cholestyramine in a glass or cup. For Questran Powder, add at least 2-6 ounces of water or the beverage of your choice. For Questran Light, add at least 2-3 ounces of water or the beverage of your choice. Stir to a uniform consistency. Cholestyramine may also be mixed with highly fluid soups or pulpy fruits with a high moisture content such as applesauce or crushed pineapple.

HOW SUPPLIED

Nine (9) g of Questran Powder contain 4 g of anhydrous cholestyramine resin. Five (5) g of Questran Light contain 4 g of anhydrous cholestyramine resin.
Storage: Store at room temperature 15-30°C (59-86°F).

PRODUCT LISTING - RATED THERAPEUTICALLY EQUIVALENT

Size	Price	Product	NDC
Powder - Oral - 4gm Resin/Packet			
60	$73.27	FEDERAL UPPER LIMIT, H.C.F.A. F F P	99999-0808-04
Powder For Reconstitution - Oral - 4 Gm/5 Gm			
4 gm x 42	$36.62	GENERIC, Teva Pharmaceuticals Usa	00093-8111-83
4 gm x 60	$79.49	GENERIC, Watson/Rugby Laboratories Inc	00536-5733-08
4 gm x 60	$82.02	GENERIC, Upsher-Smith Laboratories Inc	00245-0036-60
4 gm x 60	$82.12	GENERIC, Warrick Pharmaceuticals Corporation	59930-1638-01
4 gm x 60	$83.61	GENERIC, Teva Pharmaceuticals Usa	00093-8111-67
4 gm x 60	$83.61	GENERIC, Teva Pharmaceuticals Usa	55953-0111-35
4 gm x 60	$92.50	QUESTRAN LIGHT, Southwood Pharmaceuticals Inc	58016-9111-01
4 gm x 60	$99.00	GENERIC, Major Pharmaceuticals Inc	00904-5235-52
4 gm x 60	$126.65	GENERIC, Bristol-Myers Squibb	59772-5589-01
4 gm x 60	$126.68	GENERIC, Eon Labs Manufacturing Inc	00185-0939-98
4 gm x 60	$168.38	QUESTRAN LIGHT, Bristol-Myers Squibb	00015-9442-14
210 gm	$36.62	GENERIC, Teva Pharmaceuticals Usa	55953-0111-56
210 gm	$46.68	QUESTRAN LIGHT, Southwood Pharmaceuticals Inc	58016-9967-01
210 gm	$51.84	QUESTRAN LIGHT, Allscripts Pharmaceutical Company	54569-3424-00
210 gm	$55.45	GENERIC, Bristol-Myers Squibb	59772-5589-02
231 gm	$35.67	GENERIC, Upsher-Smith Laboratories Inc	00245-0036-23
231 gm	$36.62	GENERIC, Allscripts Pharmaceutical Company	54569-4832-00
231 gm	$37.08	GENERIC, Warrick Pharmaceuticals Corporation	59930-1638-02
239 gm	$37.20	GENERIC, Major Pharmaceuticals Inc	00904-5235-42
239.40 gm	$34.82	GENERIC, Watson/Rugby Laboratories Inc	00536-5733-24
239.40 gm	$55.48	GENERIC, Eon Labs Manufacturing Inc	00185-0939-97
266 gm	$73.76	QUESTRAN LIGHT, Bristol-Myers Squibb	00087-9442-11
Powder For Reconstitution - Oral - 4 Gm/9 Gm			
4 gm x 30	$59.18	QUESTRAN, Allscripts Pharmaceutical Company	54569-1305-02
4 gm x 60	$41.86	GENERIC, Upsher-Smith Laboratories Inc	00245-0036-42
4 gm x 60	$48.68	GENERIC, Ivax Corporation	00182-7091-42
4 gm x 60	$83.61	GENERIC, Teva Pharmaceuticals Usa	00093-8096-67
4 gm x 60	$83.61	GENERIC, Teva Pharmaceuticals Usa	55953-0096-35
4 gm x 60	$99.00	GENERIC, Major Pharmaceuticals Inc	00904-5234-52
4 gm x 60	$118.84	QUESTRAN, Bristol-Myers Squibb	00087-0580-11
4 gm x 60	$126.65	GENERIC, Bristol-Myers Squibb	59772-5585-01
4 gm x 60	$126.68	GENERIC, Eon Labs Manufacturing Inc	00185-0940-98
4 gm x 60	$167.46	QUESTRAN, Bristol-Myers Squibb	00015-0580-11
378 gm	$36.62	GENERIC, Teva Pharmaceuticals Usa	00093-8096-82
378 gm	$36.62	GENERIC, Copley	38245-0266-79
378 gm	$36.62	GENERIC, Teva Pharmaceuticals Usa	55953-0096-65
378 gm	$43.35	GENERIC, Major Pharmaceuticals Inc	00904-5234-42
378 gm	$46.58	QUESTRAN, Southwood Pharmaceuticals Inc	58016-9066-01
378 gm	$55.45	GENERIC, Bristol-Myers Squibb	59772-5585-02
378 gm	$55.48	GENERIC, Eon Labs Manufacturing Inc	00185-0940-97
378 gm	$73.34	QUESTRAN, Bristol-Myers Squibb	00087-0580-05

Ciclopirox *(000817)*

Categories: Candidiasis; Dermatitis, seborrheic ; Onychomycosis; Tinea corporis; Tinea cruris; Tinea pedis; Tinea versicolor; Pregnancy Category B; FDA Approved 1982 Dec
Drug Classes: Antifungals, topical; Dermatologics
Brand Names: **Loprox**
Foreign Brand Availability: Batrafen (Bahamas; Bahrain; Barbados; Belize; Bermuda; Bulgaria; Curacao; Cyprus; Czech-Republic; Ecuador; Egypt; Germany; Greece; Guyana; Hong-Kong; Hungary; India; Indonesia; Iran; Iraq; Ireland; Israel; Italy; Jamaica; Japan; Jordan; Kuwait; Lebanon; Libya; Netherland-Antilles; New-Zealand; Oman; Peru; Qatar; Republic-of-Yemen; Saudi-Arabia; Spain; Surinam; Switzerland; Syria; Trinidad; United-Arab-Emirates); Batrafen Gel (Germany); Batrafen Nail Lacquer (Israel); Brumixol (Italy; Taiwan); Ciclochem (Spain); Cicloderm (Thailand); Fungopirox (Peru); Fungowas (Spain); Loprox Laca (Mexico); Miclast (Italy); Micoxolamina (Italy); Mycoster (France); Nail Batrafen (New-Zealand); Primax (Colombia); Stieprox (Singapore; Thailand); Stiprox (Mexico)
Cost of Therapy: $15.57 (Tinea Pedis; Loprox Cream; 1%;15 g; 2 applications/day; variable day supply)

DESCRIPTION

LOPROX CREAM

FOR DERMATOLOGIC USE ONLY.
NOT FOR USE IN EYES.

Loprox cream 0.77% is for topical use.

Each gram of Loprox cream contains 7.70 mg of ciclopirox (as ciclopirox olamine) in a water miscible vanishing cream base consisting of purified water, octyldodecanol, mineral oil, steryl alcohol, cetyl alcohol, cocamide DEA, Polysorbate 60, myristyl alcohol, sorbitan monostearate, lactic acid, and benzyl alcohol (1%) as preservative.

Loprox cream contains a synthetic, broad-spectrum, antifungal agent ciclopirox (as ciclopirox olamine). The chemical name is 6-cyclohexyl-1-hydroxy-4-methyl-2(*1H*)-pyridone, 2-aminoethanol salt.

Loprox cream has a pH of 7.

LOPROX GEL

FOR DERMATOLOGIC USE ONLY.
NOT FOR USE IN EYES.

Loprox gel 0.77% contains a synthetic antifungal agent, ciclopirox. It is intended for topical dermatologic use only.

Each gram of Loprox gel contains 7.70 mg of ciclopirox in a gel consisting of purified water, isopropyl alcohol, octyldodecanol, dimethicone copolyol 190, carbomer 980, sodium hydroxide, and docusate sodium.

Loprox gel is a white, slightly fluid gel.

The chemical name for ciclopirox is 6-cyclohexyl-1-hydroxy-4-methyl-2(*1H*)-pyridinone, with the empirical formula $C_{12}H_{17}NO_2$ and a molecular weight of 207.27.

LOPROX LOTION

FOR DERMATOLOGIC USE ONLY.
NOT FOR USE IN EYES.

Loprox lotion 0.77% is for topical use. Each gram of Loprox lotion contains 7.70 mg of ciclopirox (as ciclopirox olamine) in a water miscible lotion base consisting of purified water, cocamide DEA, octyldodecanol, mineral oil, stearyl alcohol, cetyl alcohol, polysorbate 60, myristyl alcohol, sorbitan monostearate, lactic acid, and benzyl alcohol (1%) as preservative.

Loprox lotion contains a synthetic, broad-spectrum, antifungal agent ciclopirox (as ciclopirox olamine). The chemical name is 6-cyclohexyl-1-hydroxy-4-methyl-2(*1H*)-pyridone, 2-aminoethanol salt.

Loprox lotion has a pH of 7.

LOPROX SHAMPOO

FOR TOPICAL USE ONLY.
NOT FOR OPHTHALMIC, ORAL, OR INTRAVAGINAL USE.
KEEP OUT OF REACH OF CHILDREN.

Loprox shampoo, 1%, contains the synthetic antifungal agent, ciclopirox.

Each gram (equivalent to 0.96 ml) of Loprox shampoo contains 10 mg ciclopirox in a shampoo base consisting of purified water, sodium laureth sulfate, disodium laureth sulfosuccinate, sodium chloride, and laureth-2.

Loprox shampoo is a colorless, translucent solution. The chemical name for ciclopirox is 6-cyclohexyl-1-hydroxy-4-methyl-2(1H)-pyridone, with the empirical formula $C_{12}H_{17}NO_2$ and a molecular weight of 207.27.

PENLAC NAIL LACQUER TOPICAL SOLUTION

For use on fingernails and toenails and immediately adjacent skin only.
Not for use in eyes.

Penlac nail lacquer topical solution, 8%, contains a synthetic antifungal agent, ciclopirox. It is intended for topical use on fingernails and toenails and immediately adjacent skin.

Each gram of Penlac nail lacquer topical solution, 8%, contains 80 mg ciclopirox in a solution base consisting of ethyl acetate, isopropyl alcohol, and butyl monoester of poly-[methylvinyl ether/maleic acid] in isopropyl alcohol. Ethyl acetate and isopropyl alcohol are solvents that vaporize after application.

Penlac nail lacquer topical solution, 8%, is a clear, colorless to slightly yellowish solution.

The chemical name for ciclopirox is 6-cyclohexyl-1-hydroxy-4-methyl-2(1H)-pyridone, with the empirical formula $C_{12}H_{17}NO_2$ and a molecular weight of 207.27.

CLINICAL PHARMACOLOGY

CICLOPIROX CREAM

Ciclopirox is a broad-spectrum, antifungal agent that inhibits the growth of pathogenic dermatophytes, yeasts, and *Malassezia furfur.* Ciclopirox exhibits fungicidal activity *in vitro* against isolates of *Trichophyton rubrum, Trichophyton mentagrophytes, Epidermophyton floccosum, Microsporum canis,* and *Candida albicans.*

Pharmacokinetic studies in men with tagged ciclopirox solution in polyethylene glycol 400 showed an average of 1.3% absorption of the dose when it was applied topically to 750 cm^2 on the back followed by occlusion for 6 hours. The biological half-life was 1.7 hours and excretion occurred via the kidney. Two days after application only 0.01% of the dose applied could be found in the urine. Fecal excretion was negligible.

Penetration studies in human cadaverous skin from the back, with ciclopirox cream with tagged ciclopirox showed the presence of 0.8-1.6% of the dose in the stratum corneum 1.5-6 hours after application. The levels in the dermis were still 10-15 times above the minimum inhibitory concentrations.

Autoradiographic studies with human cadaverous skin showed that ciclopirox penetrates into the hair and through the epidermis and hair follicles into the sebaceous glands and dermis, while a portion of the drug remains in the stratum corneum.

Draize Human Sensitization Assay, 21-Day Cumulative Irritancy study, Phototoxicity study, and Photo-Draize study conducted in a total of 142 healthy male subjects showed no contact sensitization of the delayed hypersensitivity type, no irritation, no phototoxicity, and no photo-contact sensitization due to ciclopirox cream.

CICLOPIROX GEL

Mechanism of Action

Ciclopirox acts by chelation of polyvalent cations (Fe^{3+} or Al^{3+}) resulting in the inhibition of the metal-dependent enzymes that are responsible for the degradation of peroxides within the fungal cell.

In vitro studies showed that ciclopirox inhibited the formulation of 5-lipoxygenase inflammatory mediators (5-HETE and LTB_4) and also inhibited PGE_2 release in a cell culture model. *In vivo,* ciclopirox inhibited inflammation in an arachidonic acid-induced murine ear edema model. The clinical significance of these findings is unknown.

Pharmacokinetics

A comparative study of the pharmacokinetics of ciclopirox gel and ciclopirox cream 0.77% in 18 healthy males indicated that systemic absorption of ciclopirox from ciclopirox gel was higher than that of ciclopirox cream. A 5 g dose of ciclopirox gel produced a mean (±SD) peak serum concentration of 25.02 (±20.6) ng/ml total ciclopirox and 5 g of ciclopirox cream produced 18.62 (±13.56) ng/ml total ciclopirox. Approximately 3% of the applied ciclopirox was excreted in the urine within 48 hours after application, with a renal elimination half-life of about 5.5 hours.

In a study of ciclopirox gel, 16 men with moderate to severe tinea cruris applied approximately 15 g/day of the gel for 14.5 days. The mean (±SD) dose-normalized values of C_{max} for total ciclopirox in serum were 100 (±42) ng/ml on Day 1 and 238 (±144) ng/ml on Day 15. During the 10 hours after dosing on Day 1, approximately 10% of the administered dose was excreted in the urine.

C

Microbiology

Ciclopirox is a hydroxypyridinone antifungal agent that inhibits the growth of pathogenic dermatophytes. Ciclopirox has been shown to be active against most strains of the following microorganisms both *in vitro* and in clinical infections as described in INDICATIONS AND USAGE, Ciclopirox Gel:

Trichophyton rubrum, Trichophyton mentagrophytes, and *Epidermophyton floccosum.*

CICLOPIROX LOTION

Ciclopirox is a broad-spectrum, antifungal agent that inhibits the growth of pathogenic dermatophytes, yeasts, and *Malassezia furfur.* Ciclopirox exhibits fungicidal activity *in vitro* against isolates of *Trichophyton rubrum, Trichophyton mentagrophytes, Epidermophyton floccosum, Microsporum canis,* and *Candida albicans.*

Pharmacokinetic studies in men with radiolabeled ciclopirox solution in polyethylene glycol 400 showed an average of 1.3% absorption of the dose when it was applied topically to 750 cm^2 on the back followed by occlusion for 6 hours. The biological half-life was 1.7 hours and excretion occurred via the kidney. Two days after application only 0.01% of the dose applied could be found in the urine. Fecal excretion was negligible. Autoradiographic studies with human cadaver skin showed that ciclopirox penetrates into the hair and through the epidermis and hair follicles into the sebaceous glands and dermis, while a portion of the drug remains in the stratum corneum.

In vitro penetration studies in frozen or fresh excised human cadaver and pig skin indicated that the penetration of ciclopirox lotion is equivalent to that of ciclopirox cream (ciclopirox olamine) 0.77%. Therapeutic equivalence of cream and lotion formulations also was indicated by studies of experimentally induced guinea pig and human trichophytosis.

CICLOPIROX SHAMPOO

Mechanism of Action

Ciclopirox is a hydroxypyridone antifungal agent although the relevance of this property for the indication of seborrheic dermatitis is not known. Ciclopirox acts by chelation of polyvalent cations (Fe^{3+} or Al^{3+}), resulting in the inhibition of the metal-dependent enzymes that are responsible for the degradation of peroxides within the fungal cell.

Pharmacokinetics and Pharmacodynamics

In a study in patients with seborrheic dermatitis of the scalp, application of 5 ml ciclopirox shampoo 1% twice weekly for 4 weeks, with an exposure time of 3 minutes per application, resulted in detectable serum concentrations of ciclopirox in 6 out of 18 patients. The serum concentrations measured throughout the dosing interval on Days 1 and 29 ranged from 10.3-13.2 ng/ml. Total urinary excretion of ciclopirox was less than 0.5 % of the administered dose.

Microbiology

Ciclopirox is fungicidal *in vitro* against *Malassezia furfur* (*Pityrosporum* spp.), *P. ovale,* and *P. orbiculare.* Ciclopirox acts by chelation of polyvalent cations (Fe^{3+} or Al^{3+}), resulting in the inhibition of the metal-dependent enzymes that are responsible for the degradation of peroxides within the fungal cell. The clinical significance of antifungal activity in the treatment of seborrheic dermatitis is not known.

CICLOPIROX NAIL LACQUER TOPICAL SOLUTION

Microbiology

Mechanism of Action

The mechanism of action of ciclopirox has been investigated using various *in vitro* and *in vivo* infection models. One *in vitro* study suggested that ciclopirox acts by chelation of polyvalent cations (Fe^{3+} or Al^{3+}) resulting in the inhibition of the metal-dependent enzymes that are responsible for the degradation of peroxides within the fungal cell. The clinical significance of this observation is not known.

Activity In Vitro and Ex Vivo

In vitro methodologies employing various broth or solid media with and without additional nutrients have been utilized to determine ciclopirox minimum inhibitory concentration (MIC) values for the dermatophytic molds.[1-2] As a consequence, a broad range of MIC values, 1-20 μg/ml, were obtained for *Trichophyton rubrum* and *Trichophyton mentagrophytes* species. Correlation between *in vitro* MIC results and clinical outcome has yet to be established for ciclopirox.

One *ex vivo* study was conducted evaluating 8% ciclopirox against new and established *Trichophyton rubrum* and *Trichophyton mentagrophytes* infections in ovine hoof material.[3] After 10 days of treatment the growth of *T. rubrum* and *T. mentagrophytes* in the established infection model was very minimally affected. Elimination of the molds from hoof material was not achieved in either the new or established infection models.

Susceptibility Testing for Trichophyton rubrum Species

In vitro susceptibility testing methods for determining ciclopirox MIC values against the dermatophytic molds, including *Trichophyton rubrum* species, have not been standardized or validated. Ciclopirox MIC values will vary depending on the susceptibility testing method employed, composition and pH of media and the utilization of nutritional supplements. Breakpoints to determine whether clinical isolates of *Trichophyton rubrum* are susceptible or resistant to ciclopirox have not been established.

Resistance

Studies have not been conducted to evaluate drug resistance development in *T. rubrum* species exposed to 8% ciclopirox topical solution. Studies assessing cross-resistance to ciclopirox and other known antifungal agents have not been performed.

Antifungal Drug Interactions

No studies have been conducted to determine whether ciclopirox might reduce the effectiveness of systemic antifungal agents for onychomycosis. Therefore, the concomitant use of 8% ciclopirox topical solution and systemic antifungal agents for onychomycosis is not recommended.

Pharmacokinetics

As demonstrated in pharmacokinetic studies in animals and man, ciclopirox olamine is rapidly absorbed after oral administration and completely eliminated in all species via feces and urine. Most of the compound is excreted either unchanged or as glucuronide. After oral administration of 10 mg of radiolabeled drug (^{14}C-ciclopirox) to healthy volunteers, approximately 96% of the radioactivity was excreted renally within 12 hours of administration. Ninety-four percent (94%) of the renally excreted radioactivity was in the form of glucuronides. Thus, glucuronidation is the main metabolic pathway of this compound.

Systemic absorption of ciclopirox was determined in 5 patients with dermatophytic onychomycoses, after application of ciclopirox nail lacquer topical solution, 8%, to all 20 digits and adjacent 5 mm of skin once daily for 6 months. Random serum concentrations and 24 hour urinary excretion of ciclopirox were determined at 2 weeks and at 1, 2, 4 and 6 months after initiation of treatment and 4 weeks post-treatment. In this study, ciclopirox serum levels ranged from 12-80 ng/ml. Based on urinary data, mean absorption of ciclopirox from the dosage form was <5% of the applied dose. One month after cessation of treatment, serum and urine levels of ciclopirox were below the limit of detection.

In two vehicle-controlled trials, patients applied ciclopirox nail lacquer topical solution, 8%, to all toenails and affected fingernails. Out of a total of 66 randomly selected patients on active treatment, 24 had detectable serum ciclopirox concentrations at some point during the dosing interval (range 10.0-24.6 ng/ml). It should be noted that 11 of these 24 patients took concomitant medication containing ciclopirox as ciclopirox olamine (ciclopirox cream, 0.77%).

The penetration of the ciclopirox nail lacquer topical solution, 8%, was evaluated in an *in vitro* investigation. Radiolabeled ciclopirox applied once to onychomycotic toenails that were avulsed demonstrated penetration up to a depth of approximately 0.4 mm. As expected, nail plate concentrations decreased as a function of nail depth. The clinical significance of these findings in nail plates is unknown. Nail bed concentrations were not determined.

INDICATIONS AND USAGE

CICLOPIROX CREAM

Ciclopirox cream is indicated for the topical treatment of the following dermal infections: tinea pedis, tinea cruris, and tinea corporis due to *Trichophyton rubrum, Trichophyton mentagrophytes, Epidermophyton floccosum,* and *Microsporum canis;* candidiasis (moniliasis) due to *Candida albicans;* and tinea (pityriasis) versicolor due to *Malassezia furfur.*

CICLOPIROX GEL

Superficial Dermatophyte Infections

Ciclopirox gel is indicated for the topical treatment of interdigital tinea pedis and tinea corporis due to *Trichophyton rubrum, Trichophyton mentagrophytes,* or *Epidermophyton floccosum.*

Seborrheic Dermatitis

Ciclopirox gel is indicated for the topical treatment of seborrheic dermatitis of the scalp.

CICLOPIROX LOTION

Ciclopirox lotion is indicated for the topical treatment of the following dermal infections: tinea pedis, tinea cruris and tinea corporis due to *Trichophyton rubrum, Trichophyton mentagrophytes, Epidermophyton floccosum,* and *Microsporum canis;* cutaneous candidiasis (moniliasis) due to *Candida albicans;* and tinea (pityriasis) versicolor due to *Malassezia furfur.*

CICLOPIROX SHAMPOO

Ciclopirox shampoo is indicated for the topical treatment of seborrheic dermatitis of the scalp in adults.

CICLOPIROX NAIL LACQUER TOPICAL SOLUTION

(To understand fully the indication for this product, please read the entire INDICATIONS AND USAGE section of the labeling.)

Ciclopirox nail lacquer topical solution, 8%, as a component of a comprehensive management program, is indicated as topical treatment in immunocompetent patients with mild to moderate onychomycosis of fingernails and toenails without lunula involvement, due to *Trichophyton rubrum.* The comprehensive management program includes removal of the unattached, infected nails as frequently as monthly, by a health care professional who has special competence in the diagnosis and treatment of nail disorders, including minor nail procedures.

- No studies have been conducted to determine whether ciclopirox might reduce the effectiveness of systemic antifungal agents for onychomycosis. Therefore, the concomitant use of 8% ciclopirox topical solution and systemic antifungal agents for onychomycosis, is not recommended.
- Ciclopirox nail lacquer topical solution, 8%, should be used only under medical supervision as described above.
- The effectiveness and safety of ciclopirox nail lacquer topical solution, 8%, in the following populations has not been studied. The clinical trials with use of ciclopirox nail lacquer topical solution, 8%, excluded patients who: were pregnant or nursing, planned to become pregnant, had a history of immunosuppression (*e.g.,* extensive, persistent, or un-

usual distribution of dermatomycoses, extensive seborrheic dermatitis, recent or recurring herpes zoster, or persistent herpes simplex), were HIV seropositive, received organ transplant, required medication to control epilepsy, were insulin dependent diabetics or had diabetic neuropathy. Patients with severe plantar (moccasin) tinea pedis were also excluded.

- The safety and efficacy of using ciclopirox nail lacquer topical solution, 8%, daily for greater than 48 weeks have not been established.

CONTRAINDICATIONS

CICLOPIROX CREAM

Ciclopirox cream is contraindicated in individuals who have shown hypersensitivity to any of its components.

CICLOPIROX GEL

Ciclopirox gel is contraindicated in individuals who have shown hypersensitivity to any of its components.

CICLOPIROX LOTION

Ciclopirox lotion is contraindicated in individuals who have shown hypersensitivity to any of its components.

CICLOPIROX SHAMPOO

Ciclopirox shampoo is contraindicated in individuals who have shown hypersensitivity to any of its components.

CICLOPIROX NAIL LACQUER TOPICAL SOLUTION

Ciclopirox nail lacquer topical solution, 8%, is contraindicated in individuals who have shown hypersensitivity to any of its components.

WARNINGS

CICLOPIROX CREAM

Ciclopirox cream is not for ophthalmic use.

Keep out of reach of children.

CICLOPIROX GEL

Ciclopirox gel is not for ophthalmic, oral, or intravaginal use.

Keep out of reach of children.

CICLOPIROX LOTION

General

Ciclopirox lotion is not for ophthalmic use.

Keep out of reach of children.

CICLOPIROX SHAMPOO

Ciclopirox shampoo is not for ophthalmic, oral, or intravaginal use.

Keep out of reach of children.

CICLOPIROX NAIL LACQUER TOPICAL SOLUTION

Ciclopirox nail lacquer topical solution, 8%, is not for ophthalmic, oral, or intravaginal use. For use on nails and immediately adjacent skin only.

PRECAUTIONS

CICLOPIROX CREAM

If a reaction suggesting sensitivity or chemical irritation should occur with the use of ciclopirox cream, treatment should be discontinued and appropriate therapy instituted.

Information for the Patient

The patient should be told to:

Use the medication for the full treatment time even though symptoms may have improved and notify the physician if there is no improvement after 4 weeks.

Inform the physician if the area of application shows signs of increased irritation (redness, itching, burning, blistering, swelling, or oozing) indicative of possible sensitization.

Avoid the use of occlusive wrappings or dressings.

Carcinogenesis, Mutagenesis, and Impairment of Fertility

A carcinogenicity study in female mice dosed cutaneously twice per week for 50 weeks followed by a 6 month drug-free observation period prior to necropsy revealed no evidence of tumors at the application site.

The following *in vitro* and *in vivo* genotoxicity tests have been conducted with ciclopirox olamine: studies to evaluate gene mutation in the Ames *Salmonella*/Mammalian Microsome Assay (negative) and Yeast Saccharomyces Cerevisiae Assay (negative) and studies to evaluate chromosome aberrations *in vivo* in the Mouse Dominant Lethal Assay and in the Mouse Micronucleus Assay at 500 mg/kg (negative).

The following battery of *in vitro* genotoxicity tests were conducted with ciclopirox: a chromosome aberration assay in V79 Chinese Hamster Cells, with and without metabolic activation (positive); a gene mutation assay in the HGPRT-test with V79 Chinese Hamster Cells (negative); and a primary DNA damage assay (*i.e.*, unscheduled DNA Synthesis Assay in A549 Human Cells (negative). An *in vitro* Cell Transformation Assay in BALB/C3T3 Cells was negative for cell transformation. In an *in vivo* Chinese Hamster Bone Marrow Cytogenetic Assay, ciclopirox was negative for chromosome aberrations at 5000 mg/kg.

Pregnancy Category B

Reproduction studies have been performed in the mouse, rat, rabbit, and monkey (via various routes of administration) at doses 10 times or more the topical human dose and have revealed no significant evidence of impaired fertility or harm to the fetus due to ciclopirox. There are, however, no adequate or well-controlled studies in pregnant woman. Because animal reproduction studies are not always predictive of human response, this drug should be used during pregnancy only if clearly needed.

Nursing Mothers

It is not known whether this drug is excreted in human milk. Because many drugs are excreted in human milk, caution should be exercised when ciclopirox cream is administered to a nursing woman.

Pediatric Use

Safety and effectiveness in pediatric patients below the age of 10 years have not been established.

CICLOPIROX GEL

If a reaction suggesting sensitivity or chemical irritation should occur with the use of ciclopirox gel, treatment should be discontinued and appropriate therapy instituted. A transient burning sensation may occur, especially after application to sensitive areas. Avoid contact with eyes. Efficacy of ciclopirox gel in immunosuppressed individuals has not been studied. Seborrheic dermatitis in association with acne, atopic dermatitis, parkinsonism, psoriasis and rosacea has not been studied with ciclopirox gel. Efficacy in the treatment of plantar and vesicular types of tinea pedis has not been established.

Information for the Patient

The patient should be told the following:

Use ciclopirox gel as directed by the physician. Avoid contact with the eyes and mucous membranes. Ciclopirox gel is for external use only.

Use the medication for fungal infections for the full treatment time even though symptoms may have improved, and notify the physician if there is no improvement after 4 weeks.

A transient burning/stinging sensation may be felt. This may occur in approximately 15-20% of cases, when ciclopirox gel is used to treat seborrheic dermatitis of the scalp.

Inform the physician if the area of application shows signs of increased irritation or possible sensitization (redness with itching, burning, blistering, swelling, and/or oozing).

Avoid the use of occlusive dressings.

Do not use this medication for any disorder other than that for which it is prescribed.

Carcinogenesis, Mutagenesis, and Impairment of Fertility

A carcinogenicity study of ciclopirox (1% and 5% solutions in polyethylene glycol 400) in female mice dose cutaneously twice per week for 50 weeks followed by a 6 month drug-free observation period prior to necropsy revealed no evidence of tumors at the application site.

The following battery of *in vitro* genotoxicity tests was conducted with ciclopirox: evaluation of gene mutation in the Ames *Salmonella* and *E. coli* assays (negative); chromosome aberration assays in V79 Chinese hamster cells, with and without metabolic activation (positive); gene mutation assays in the HGPRT-test with V79 Chinese hamster cells (negative); and a primary DNA damage assay (*i.e.*, unscheduled DNA synthesis assay in A549 human cells) (negative). An *in vitro* cell transformation assay in BALB/c 3T3 cells was negative for cell transformation. In an *in vivo* Chinese hamster bone marrow cytogenetic assay, ciclopirox was negative for chromosome aberrations at 5000 mg/kg.

Pregnancy, Teratogenic Effects, Pregnancy Category B

Reproduction studies of ciclopirox revealed no significant evidence of impaired fertility in rats exposed orally up to 5 mg/kg body weight (approximately 5 times the maximum recommended topical human dose based on surface area). No fetotoxicity was shown due to ciclopirox in the mouse, rat, rabbit, and monkey at oral doses up to 100, 30, 30, and 50 mg/kg body weight, respectively (approximately 37.5, 30, 44, and 77 times the maximum recommended topical human dose based on surface area). By the dermal route of administration, no fetotoxicity was shown due to ciclopirox in the rat and rabbit at doses up to 120 and 100 mg/kg body weight, respectively (approximately 121 and 147 times, respectively, the maximum recommended topical human dose based on surface area).

There are no adequate or well-controlled studies of topically applied ciclopirox in pregnant women. Ciclopirox gel should be used during pregnancy only if the potential benefit justifies the potential risk to the fetus.

Nursing Mothers

It is not known whether this drug is excreted in human milk. Since many drugs are excreted in human milk, caution should be exercised when ciclopirox gel is administered to a nursing woman.

Pediatric Use

The efficacy and safety of ciclopirox gel in pediatric patients below the age of 16 years have not been established.

CICLOPIROX LOTION

If a reaction suggesting sensitivity or chemical irritation should occur with the use of ciclopirox lotion, treatment should be discontinued and appropriate therapy instituted.

Information for the Patient

The patient should be told to:

Use the medication for the full treatment time even though signs/symptoms may have improved and notify the physician if there is no improvement after 4 weeks.

Inform the physician if the area of application shows signs of increased irritation (redness, itching, burning, blistering, swelling, oozing) indicative of possible sensitization.

Avoid the use of occlusive wrappings or dressings.

C

Carcinogenesis, Mutagenesis, and Impairment of Fertility
A carcinogenicity study in female mice dosed cutaneously twice per week for 50 weeks followed by a 6 month drug-free observation period prior to necropsy revealed no evidence of tumors at the application site. The following *in vitro* and *in vivo* genotoxicity tests have been conducted with ciclopirox olamine: studies to evaluate gene mutation in the Ames *Salmonella*/Mammalian Microsome Assay (negative) and Yeast Saccharomyces Cerevisiae Assay (negative) and studies to evaluate chromosome aberrations *in vivo* in the Mouse Dominant Lethal Assay and in the Mouse Micronucleus Assay at 500 mg/kg (negative). The following battery of *in vitro* genotoxicity tests were conducted with ciclopirox: a chromosome aberration assay in V79 Chinese Hamster Cells, with and without metabolic activation (positive); a gene mutation assay in the HGPR -test with V79 Chinese Hamster Cells (negative); and a primary DNA damage assay (*i.e.,* unscheduled DNA Synthesis Assay in A549 Human Cells (negative). An *in vitro* Cell Transformation Assay in BALB/C3T3 Cells was negative for cell transformation. In an *in vivo* Chinese Hamster Bone Marrow Cytogenetic Assay, ciclopirox was negative for chromosome aberrations at 5000 mg/kg.

Pregnancy Category B
Reproduction studies have been performed in the mouse, rat, rabbit, and monkey, via various routes of administration, at doses 10 times or more the topical human dose and have revealed no significant evidence of impaired fertility or harm to the fetus due to ciclopirox. There are, however, no adequate or well-controlled studies in pregnant women. Because animal reproduction studies are not always predictive of human response, this drug should be used during pregnancy only if clearly needed.

Nursing Mothers
It is not known whether this drug is excreted in human milk. Caution should be exercised when ciclopirox lotion is administered to a nursing woman.

Pediatric Use
Safety and effectiveness in pediatric patients below the age of 10 years have not been established.

CICLOPIROX SHAMPOO

General
If a reaction suggesting sensitivity or irritation should occur with the use of ciclopirox shampoo, treatment should be discontinued and appropriate therapy instituted.

Contact of ciclopirox shampoo with the eyes should be avoided. If contact occurs, rinse thoroughly with water.

Seborrheic dermatitis may appear at puberty, however, no clinical studies have been done in patients younger than 16 years.

There is no relevant clinical experience with patients who have a history of immunosuppression (*e.g.,* extensive, persistent, or unusual distribution of dermatomycoses, recent or recurring herpes zoster, or persistent herpes simplex), who are immunocompromised (*e.g.,* HIV-infected patients and transplant patients), or who have a diabetic neuropathy.

Information for the Patient
The patient should be instructed to:

Use ciclopirox shampoo as directed by the physician. Avoid contact with the eyes and mucous membranes. If contact occurs, rinse thoroughly with water. Ciclopirox shampoo is for external use on the scalp only. Do not swallow.

Use the medication for seborrheic dermatitis for the full treatment time even though symptoms may have improved. Notify the physician if there is no improvement after 4 weeks.

Inform the physician if the area of application shows signs of increased irritation (redness, itching, burning, blistering, swelling, or oozing) indicative of possible allergic reaction.

Not use the medication for any disorder other than that for which it is prescribed.

Carcinogenesis, Mutagenesis, and Impairment of Fertility
Long-term animal studies have not been performed to evaluate the carcinogenic potential of ciclopirox shampoo or ciclopirox.

The following *in vitro* genotoxicity tests have been conducted with ciclopirox: evaluation of gene mutation in the Ames *Salmonella* and *E. coli* assays (negative); chromosome aberration assays in V79 Chinese hamster lung fibroblast cells, with and without metabolic activation (positive); chromosome aberration assays in V79 Chinese hamster lung fibroblast cells in the presence of supplemental Fe^{3+}, with and without metabolic activation (negative); gene mutation assays in the HGPRT-test with V79 Chinese hamster lung fibroblast cells (negative); and a primary DNA damage assay (*i.e.,* unscheduled DNA synthesis assay in A549 human cells) (negative). An *in vitro* cell transformation assay in BALB/c 3T3 cells was negative for cell transformation. In an *in vivo* Chinese hamster bone marrow cytogenetic assay, ciclopirox was negative for chromosome aberrations at a dosage of 5000 mg/kg body weight.

A combined oral fertility and embryofetal developmental study was conducted in rats with ciclopirox olamine. No effect on fertility or reproductive performance was noted at the highest dose tested of 3.85 mg/kg/day ciclopirox (approximately 1.3 times the maximum recommended human dose based on body surface area comparisons).

Pregnancy, Teratogenic Effects, Pregnancy Category B
Oral embryofetal developmental studies were conducted in mice, rats, rabbits and monkeys. Ciclopirox or ciclopirox olamine was orally administered during the period of organogenesis. No maternal toxicity, embryotoxicity or teratogenicity were noted at the highest doses of 77, 125, 80 and 38.5 mg/kg/day ciclopirox in mice, rats, rabbits and monkeys, respectively (approximately 13, 42, 54 and 26 times the maximum recommended human dose based on body surface area comparisons, respectively).

Dermal embryofetal developmental studies were conducted in rats and rabbits with ciclopirox olamine dissolved in PEG 400. Ciclopirox olamine was topically administered during the period of organogenesis. No maternal toxicity, embryotoxicity or teratogenicity were noted at the highest doses of 92 mg/kg/day and 77 mg/kg/day ciclopirox in rats and rabbits, respectively (approximately 31 and 54 times the maximum recommended human dose based on body surface area comparisons, respectively).

There are no adequate or well-controlled studies of topically applied ciclopirox in pregnant women. Because animal reproduction studies are not always predictive of human response, ciclopirox shampoo should be used during pregnancy only if clearly needed.

Nursing Mothers
It is not known whether this drug is excreted in human milk. Because many drugs are excreted in human milk, caution should be exercised when ciclopirox shampoo is administered to a nursing woman.

Pediatric Use
Seborrheic dermatitis may appear at puberty, however, no clinical studies have been done in patients younger than 16 years.

Geriatric Use
In clinical studies, the safety and tolerability of ciclopirox shampoo in the population 65 years and older was comparable to that of younger subjects. Results of the efficacy analysis in those patients 65 years and older showed effectiveness in 25 of 85 (29%) patients treated with ciclopirox shampoo, and in 15 of 61 (25%) patients treated with the vehicle; due to the small sample size, a statistically significant difference was not demonstrated. Other reported clinical experience has not identified differences in responses between the elderly and younger subjects, but greater sensitivity to adverse effects in some older individuals cannot be ruled out.

CICLOPIROX NAIL LACQUER TOPICAL SOLUTION

If a reaction suggesting sensitivity or chemical irritation should occur with the use of ciclopirox nail lacquer topical solution, 8%, treatment should be discontinued and appropriate therapy instituted.

So far there is no relevant clinical experience with patients with insulin dependent diabetes or who have diabetic neuropathy. The risk of removal of the unattached, infected nail, by the health care professional and trimming by the patient should be carefully considered before prescribing to patients with a history of insulin dependent diabetes mellitus or diabetic neuropathy.

Information for the Patient
Patients should have detailed instructions regarding the use of ciclopirox nail lacquer topical solution, 8%, as a component of a comprehensive management program for onychomycosis in order to achieve maximum benefit with the use of this product.

The patient should be told to:

Use ciclopirox nail lacquer topical solution, 8%, as directed by a health care professional. Avoid contact with the eyes and mucous membranes. Contact with skin other than skin immediately surrounding the treated nail(s) should be avoided. Ciclopirox nail lacquer topical solution, 8%, is for external use only.

Ciclopirox nail lacquer topical solution, 8%, should be applied evenly over the entire nail plate and 5 mm of surrounding skin. If possible, ciclopirox nail lacquer topical solution, 8%, should be applied to the nail bed, hyponychium, and the under surface of the nail plate when it is free of the nail bed (*e.g.,* onycholysis). Contact with the surrounding skin may produce mild, transient irritation (redness).

Removal of the unattached, infected nail, as frequently as monthly, by a health care professional is needed with use of this medication. Inform a health care professional if they have diabetes for consideraion of the appropriate nail management program.

Inform a health care professional if the area of application shows signs of increased irritation (redness, itching, burning, blistering, swelling, oozing).

Up to 48 weeks of daily applications with ciclopirox nail lacquer topical solution, 8%, and professional removal of the unattached, infected nail, as frequently as monthly, are considered the full treatment needed to achieve a clear or almost clear nail (defined as 10% or less residual nail involvement).

Six months of therapy with professional removal of the unattached, infected nail may be required before initial improvement of symptoms is noticed.

A completely clear nail may not be achieved with use of this medication. In clinical studies less than 12% of patients were able to achieve either a completely clear or almost clear toenail.

Do not use the medication for any disorder other than that for which it is prescribed.

Do not use nail polish or other nail cosmetic products on the treated nails.

Avoid use near heat or open flame, because product is flammable.

Carcinogenesis, Mutagenesis, and Impairment of Fertility
No carcinogenicity study was conducted with ciclopirox nail lacquer topical solution, 8%, formulation. A carcinogenicity study of ciclopirox (1% and 5% solutions in polyethylene glycol 400) in female mice dosed topically twice per week for 50 weeks followed by a 6 month drug-free observation period prior to necropsy revealed no evidence of tumors at the application sites.

In human systemic tolerability studies following daily application ($\sim$340 mg of ciclopirox nail lacquer topical solution, 8%) in subjects with distal subungual onychomycosis, the average maximal serum level of ciclopirox was 31 $\pm$ 28 ng/ml after 2 months of once daily applications. This level was 159 times lower than the lowest toxic dose and 115 times lower than the highest nontoxic dose in rats and dogs fed 7.7 and 23.1 mg ciclopirox (as ciclopirox olamine)/kg/day.

The following *in vitro* genotoxicity tests have been conducted with ciclopirox: evaluation of gene mutation in Ames *Salmonella* and *E. coli* assays (negative); chromosome aberration assays in V79 Chinese hamster lung fibroblasts, with and without metabolic activation (positive); gene mutation assay in the HGPRT-test with V79 Chinese hamster lung fibroblasts (negative); unscheduled DNA synthesis in human A549 cells (negative); and BALB/c3T3 cell transformation assay (negative). In an *in vivo* Chinese hamster bone marrow cytogenetic assay, ciclopirox was negative for chromosome aberrations at 5000 mg/kg.

The following *in vitro* genotoxicity tests were conducted with ciclopirox nail lacquer topical solution, 8%: Ames *Salmonella* test (negative); unscheduled DNA synthesis in the rat hepatocytes (negative); cell transformation assay in BALB/c3T3 cell assay (positive). The positive response of the lacquer formulation in the BALB/c3T3 test was attributed to its butyl monoester of poly[methylvinyl ether/maleic acid] resin component (Gantrez ES-435), which also tested positive in this test. The cell transformation assay may have been confounded because of the film-forming nature of the resin. Gantrez ES-435 tested nonmutagenic in both the *in vitro* mouse lymphoma forward mutation assay with or without activation and unscheduled DNA synthesis assay in rat hepatocytes.

Oral reproduction studies in rats at doses up to 3.85 mg ciclopirox (as ciclopirox olamine)/kg/day [equivalent to approximately 1.4 times the potential exposure at the maximum recommended human topical dose (MRHTD)] did not reveal any specific effects on fertility or other reproductive parameters. MRHTD (mg/m^2) is based on the assumption of 100% systemic absorption of 27.12 mg ciclopirox (~340 mg ciclopirox nail lacquer topical solution, 8%) that will cover all the fingernails and toenails including 5 mm proximal and lateral fold area plus onycholysis to a maximal extent of 50%.

Pregnancy, Teratogenic Effects, Pregnancy Category B

Teratology studies in mice, rats, rabbits, and monkeys at oral doses of up to 77, 23, 23, or 38.5 mg, respectively, of ciclopirox as ciclopirox olamine/kg/day (14, 8, 17, and 28 times MRHTD), or in rats and rabbits receiving topical doses of up to 92.4 and 77 mg/kg/day, respectively (33 and 55 times MRHTD), did not indicate any significant fetal malformations.

There are no adequate or well-controlled studies of topically applied ciclopirox in pregnant women. Ciclopirox nail lacquer topical solution, 8%, should be used during pregnancy only if the potential benefit justifies the potential risk to the fetus.

Nursing Mothers

It is not known whether this drug is excreted in human milk. Since many drugs are excreted in human milk, caution should be exercised when ciclopirox nail lacquer topical solution, 8%, is administered to a nursing woman.

Pediatric Use

Safety and effectiveness in pediatric patients have not been established.

Geriatric Use

Clinical studies of ciclopirox nail lacquer topical solution, 8%, did not include sufficient numbers of subjects aged 65 and over to determine whether they respond differently from younger subjects. Other reported clinical experience has not identified differences in responses between elderly and younger patients.

ADVERSE REACTIONS

CICLOPIROX CREAM

In all controlled clinical studies with 514 patients using ciclopirox cream and in 296 patients using the vehicle cream, the incidence of adverse reactions was low. This included pruritus at the site of application in 1 patient and worsening of the clinical signs and symptoms in another patient using ciclopirox cream and burning in 1 patient and worsening of the clinical signs and symptoms in another patient using the vehicle cream.

CICLOPIROX GEL

In clinical trials, 140 (39%) of 359 subjects treated with ciclopirox gel reported adverse experiences, irrespective of relationship to test materials, which resulted in 8 subjects discontinuing treatment. The most frequent experience reported was skin burning sensation upon application, which occurred in approximately 34% of seborrheic dermatitis patients and 7% of tinea pedis patients. Adverse experiences occurring between 1-5% were contact dermatitis and pruritus. Other reactions that occurred in less than 1% included dry skin, acne, rash, alopecia, pain upon application, eye pain, and facial edema.

CICLOPIROX LOTION

In the controlled clinical trial with 89 patients using ciclopirox lotion and 89 patients using the vehicle, the incidence of adverse reactions was low. Those considered possibly related to treatment or occurring in more than 1 patient were pruritus, which occurred in 2 patients using ciclopirox lotion and 1 patient using the lotion vehicle, and burning, which occurred in 1 patient using ciclopirox lotion.

CICLOPIROX SHAMPOO

In 626 patients treated with ciclopirox shampoo twice weekly in the two pivotal clinical studies, the most frequent adverse events were increased itching in 1% of patients, and application site reactions, such as burning, erythema, and itching, also in 1% of patients. Other adverse events occurred in individual patients only.

Adverse events that led to early study medication termination in clinical trials occurred in 1.5% (26/1738) of patients treated with ciclopirox shampoo and 2.0% (12/661) of patients treated with shampoo vehicle. The most common adverse event leading to termination of study medication in either group was seborrhea. In the ciclopirox shampoo group, other adverse events included rash, pruritus, headache, ventricular tachycardia, and skin disorder. In the shampoo vehicle group, other adverse events included skin disorder and rash.

CICLOPIROX NAIL LACQUER TOPICAL SOLUTION

In the vehicle-controlled clinical trials conducted in the US, 9% (30/327) of patients treated with ciclopirox nail lacquer topical solution, 8%, and 7% (23/328) of patients treated with vehicle reported treatment-emergent adverse events (TEAE) considered by the investigator to be causally related to the test material.

The incidence of these adverse events, within each body system, was similar between the treatment groups except for skin and appendages: 8% (27/327) and 4% (14/328) of subjects in the ciclopirox and vehicle groups reported at least one adverse event, respectively. The most common were rash-related adverse events: periungual erythema and erythema of the proximal nail fold were reported more frequently in patients treated with ciclopirox nail lacquer topical solution, 8%, (5% [16/327]) than in patients treated with vehicle (1% [3/328]). Other TEAEs thought to be causally related included nail disorders such as shape change, irritation, ingrown toenail, and discoloration.

The incidence of nail disorders was similar between the treatment groups (2% [6/327] in the ciclopirox nail lacquer topical solution, 8%, group and 2% [7/328] in the vehicle group). Moreover, application site reactions and/or burning of the skin occurred in 1% of patients treated with ciclopirox nail lacquer topical solution, 8%, (3/327) and vehicle (4/328).

A 21-Day Cumulative Irritancy study was conducted under conditions of semi-occlusion. Mild reactions were seen in 46% of patients with the ciclopirox nail lacquer topical solution, 8%, 32% with the vehicle and 2% with the negative control, but all were reactions of mild transient erythema. There was no evidence of allergic contact sensitization for either the ciclopirox nail lacquer topical solution, 8%, or the vehicle base. In the vehicle-controlled studies, 1 patient treated with ciclopirox nail lacquer topical solution, 8%, discontinued treatment due to a rash, localized to the palm (causal relation to test material undetermined).

Use of ciclopirox nail lacquer topical solution, 8%, for 48 additional weeks was evaluated in an open-label extension study conducted in patients previously treated in the vehicle-controlled studies. Three percent (9/281) of subjects treated with ciclopirox nail lacquer topical solution, 8%, experienced at least one TEAE that the investigator thought was causally related to the test material. Mild rash in the form of periungual erythema (1% [2/281]) and nail disorders (1% [4/281]) were the most frequently reported. Four (4) patients discontinued because of TEAEs. Two (2) of the 4 had events considered to be related to test material: 1 patient's great toenail "broke away" and another had an elevated creatine phosphokinase level on Day 1 (after 48 weeks of treatment with vehicle in the previous vehicle-controlled study).

DOSAGE AND ADMINISTRATION

CICLOPIROX CREAM

Gently massage ciclopirox cream into the affected and surrounding skin areas twice daily, in the morning and evening. Clinical improvement with relief of pruritus and other symptoms usually occurs within the first week of treatment. If a patient shows no clinical improvement after 4 weeks of treatment with ciclopirox cream, the diagnosis should be redetermined. Patients with tinea versicolor usually exhibit clinical and mycological clearing after 2 weeks of treatment.

CICLOPIROX GEL

Superficial Dermatophyte Infections

Gently massage ciclopirox gel into the affected areas and surrounding skin twice daily, in the morning and evening immediately after cleaning or washing the areas to be treated. Interdigital tinea pedis and tinea corporis should be treated for 4 weeks. If a patient shows no clinical improvement after 4 weeks of treatment, the diagnosis should be reviewed.

Seborrheic Dermatitis of the Scalp

Apply ciclopirox gel to affected scalp areas twice daily, in the morning and evening for 4 weeks. Clinical improvement usually occurs within the first week with continuing resolution of signs and symptoms through the fourth week of treatment. If a patient shows no clinical improvement after 4 weeks of treatment, the diagnosis should be reviewed.

CICLOPIROX LOTION

Gently massage ciclopirox lotion into the affected and surrounding skin areas twice daily, in the morning and evening. Clinical improvement with relief of pruritus and other symptoms usually occurs within the first week of treatment. If a patient shows no clinical improvement after 4 weeks of treatment with ciclopirox lotion the diagnosis should be redetermined. Patients with tinea versicolor usually exhibit clinical and mycological clearing after 2 weeks of treatment.

CICLOPIROX SHAMPOO

Wet hair and apply approximately 1 teaspoon (5 ml) of ciclopirox shampoo to the scalp. Up to 2 teaspoons (10 ml) may be used for long hair. Lather and leave on hair and scalp for 3 minutes. A timer may be used. Avoid contact with eyes. Rinse off. Treatment should be repeated twice per week for 4 weeks, with a minimum of 3 days between applications.

If a patient with seborrheic dermatitis shows no clinical improvement after 4 weeks of treatment with ciclopirox shampoo, the diagnosis should be reviewed.

CICLOPIROX NAIL LACQUER TOPICAL SOLUTION

Ciclopirox nail lacquer topical solution, 8%, should be used as a component of a comprehensive management program for onychomycosis. Removal of the unattached, infected nail, as frequently as monthly, by a health care professional, weekly trimming by the patient, and daily application of the medication are all integral parts of this therapy. Careful consideration of the appropriate nail management program should be given to patients with diabetes (see PRECAUTIONS, Ciclopirox Nail Lacquer Topical Solution).

Nail Care by Health Care Professionals

Removal of the unattached, infected nail, as frequently as monthly, trimming of onycholytic nail, and filing of excess horny material should be performed by professionals trained in treatment of nail disorders.

Nail Care by Patient

Patients should file away (with emery board) loose nail material and trim nails, as required, or as directed by the health care professional, every 7 days after ciclopirox nail lacquer topical solution, 8%, is removed with alcohol.

Ciclopirox nail lacquer topical solution, 8%, should be applied once daily (preferably at bedtime or 8 hours before washing) to all affected nails with the applicator brush provided. The ciclopirox nail lacquer topical solution, 8%, should be applied evenly over the entire nail plate.

If possible, ciclopirox nail lacquer topical solution, 8%, should be applied to the nail bed, hyponychium, and the under surface of the nail plate when it is free of the nail bed (*e.g.*, onycholysis).

The ciclopirox nail lacquer topical solution, 8%, should not be removed on a daily basis. Daily applications should be made over the previous coat and removed with alcohol every 7 days. This cycle should be repeated throughout the duration of therapy.

HOW SUPPLIED

LOPROX CREAM

Loprox cream 0.77% is supplied in 15, 30, and 90 g tubes.
Storage: Store at controlled room temperature 15-30°C (59-86°F).

LOPROX GEL

Loprox gel 0.77% is supplied in 30 and 45 g tubes.
Storage: Store at 15-30°C (59-86°F).

LOPROX LOTION

Loprox lotion (ciclopirox) 0.77% is supplied in 30 ml bottles and 60 ml bottles.
Bottle space provided to allow for vigorous shaking before each use.
Storage: Store between 5-25°C (41-77°F).

LOPROX SHAMPOO

Loprox shampoo, 1%, is supplied in 120 ml plastic bottles. Once opened, the shampoo may be used for up to 8 weeks.
Storage: Store between 15 and 30°C (59 and 86°F).

PENLAC NAIL LACQUER TOPICAL SOLUTION

Penlac nail lacquer topical solution, 8%, is supplied in 3.3 and 6.6 ml glass bottles with screw caps which are fitted with brushes.
Protect from light (*e.g.,* store the bottle in the carton after every use).
Storage: Penlac nail lacquer topical solution, 8%, should be stored at room temperature between 59 and 86°F (15 and 30°C).
CAUTION: Flammable. Keep away from heat and flame.

PRODUCT LISTING - EQUIVALENTS NOT AVAILABLE

Size	Price	Product	NDC
Cream - Topical - 0.77%			
15 gm	$15.57	LOPROX, Physicians Total Care	54868-0372-02
15 gm	$22.78	LOPROX, Medicis Dermatologics Inc	99207-0009-15
15 gm	$28.20	LOPROX, Pharma Pac	52959-0381-01
30 gm	$27.35	LOPROX, Physicians Total Care	54868-0372-03
30 gm	$28.33	LOPROX, Allscripts Pharmaceutical Company	54569-4725-00
30 gm	$40.71	LOPROX, Medicis Dermatologics Inc	99207-0009-30
90 gm	$48.97	LOPROX, Physicians Total Care	54868-0372-01
90 gm	$98.50	LOPROX, Medicis Dermatologics Inc	99207-0009-90
Gel - Topical - 0.77%			
30 gm	$40.71	LOPROX, Medicis Dermatologics Inc	99207-0013-30
45 gm	$61.08	LOPROX, Medicis Dermatologics Inc	99207-0013-45
100 gm	$122.31	LOPROX, Medicis Dermatologics Inc	99207-0013-01
Lotion - Topical - 0.77%			
30 ml	$40.18	LOPROX, Medicis Dermatologics Inc	99207-0008-30
30 ml	$40.18	LOPROX TS, Medicis Dermatologics Inc	99207-0022-30
60 ml	$79.56	LOPROX, Medicis Dermatologics Inc	99207-0008-60
60 ml	$79.56	LOPROX TS, Medicis Dermatologics Inc	99207-0022-60
Solution - Topical - 8%			
3.30 ml	$59.94	PENLAC NAIL LACQUER, Allscripts Pharmaceutical Company	54569-4951-00
3.30 ml	$71.60	PENLAC NAIL LACQUER, Aventis Pharmaceuticals	00066-8008-01
6.60 ml	$126.26	PENLAC NAIL LACQUER, Aventis Pharmaceuticals	00066-8008-02

Cilostazol *(003428)*

Categories: Claudication, intermittent; FDA Approved 1999 Jan; Pregnancy Category C
Drug Classes: Platelet inhibitors
Brand Names: **Pletal**
Foreign Brand Availability: Aggravan (Indonesia); Cilosol (Korea); Cilotal (Korea); Lozence (Korea); Pletaal (Thailand); Stazol (Korea)
Cost of Therapy: $106.33 (Intermittent Claudication; Pletal; 100 mg; 2 tablets/day; 30 day supply)

DESCRIPTION

Cilostazol is a quinolinone derivative that inhibits cellular phosphodiesterase (more specific fo phosphodiesterase III). The empirical formula of cilostazol is $C_{20}H_{27}N_5O_2$, and its molecular weight is 369.47. Cilostazol is 6-[4-(1-cyclohexyl-1*H*-tetrazol-5-yl)butoxy]-3,4-dihydro-2(1*H*)-quinolinone.

Cilostazol occurs as white to off-white crystals or as a crystalline powder that is slightly soluble in methanol and ethanol, and is practically insoluble in water, 0.1 N HCl, and 0.1 N NaOH.

Pletal tablets for oral administration are available in 50 mg triangular, and 100 mg round, white debossed tablets. Each tablet, in addition to the active ingredient, contains the following inactive ingredients: carboxymethylcellulose calcium, corn starch, hydroxypropyl methylcellulose 2910, magnesium stearate, and microcrystalline cellulose.

CLINICAL PHARMACOLOGY

MECHANISM OF ACTION

The mechanism of the effects of cilostazol on the symptoms of intermittent claudication is not fully understood. Cilostazol and several of its metabolites are cyclic AMP (cAMP) phosphodiesterase III inhibitors (PDE III inhibitors), inhibiting phosphodiesterase activity and suppressing cAMP degradation with a resultant increase in cAMP in platelets and blood vessels, leading to inhibition of platelet aggregation and vasodilation.

Cilostazol reversibly inhibits platelet aggregation induced by a variety of stimuli, including thrombin, AD collagen, arachidonic acid, epinephrine, and shear stress. Effects on circulating plasma lipids have been examined in patients taking cilostazol. After 12 weeks, as compared to placebo, cilostazol 100 mg bid produced a reduction in triglycerides of 29.3 mg/dl (15%) and an increase in HDL-cholesterol of 4.0 mg/dl (~10%).

Cardiovascular Effects

Cilostazol affects both vascular beds and cardiovascular function. It produces non-homogeneous dilation vascular beds, with greater dilation in femoral beds than in vertebral, carotid or superior mesenteric arteries. Renal arteries were not responsive to the effects of cilostazol.

In dogs or cynomolgous monkeys, cilostazol increased heart rate, myocardial contractile force, and coronary blood flow as well as ventricular automaticity, as would be expected for a PDE III inhibitor. Left ventricular contractility was increased at doses required to inhibit platelet aggregation. AV conduction was accelerated. In humans, heart rate increased in a dose-proportional manner by a mean of 5.1 and 7.4 beats per minute in patients treated with 50 and 100 mg bid, respectively. In 264 patients evaluated with Holt monitors, numerically more cilostazol-treated patients had increases in ventricular premature beats and non-sustained ventricular tachycardia events than did placebo-treated patients; the increases were not dose-related.

PHARMACOKINETICS

Cilostazol is absorbed after oral administration. A high fat meal increases absorption, with an approximate 90% increase in C_{max} and a 25% increase in AUC. Absolute bioavailability is not known. Cilostazol is extensively metabolized by hepatic cytochrome P-450 enzymes, mainly 3A4, with metabolites largely excreted in urine. Two metabolites are active, with one metabolite appearing to account for at least 50% of the pharmacologic (PDE III inhibition) activity after administration of cilostazol. Pharmacokinetics are approximately dose proportional. Cilostazol and its active metabolites have apparent elimination half-live of about 11-13 hours. Cilostazol and its active metabolites accumulate about 2-fold with chronic administration and reach steady state blood levels within a few days. The pharmacokinetics of cilostazol and its two major active metabolites were similar in healthy normal subjects and patients with intermittent claudication due to peripheral arterial disease (PAD).

Distribution

Plasma Protein and Erythrocyte Binding

Cilostazol is 95-98% protein bound, predominantly to albumin. The mean percent binding for 3,4-dehydro-cilostazol is 97.4% and for 4′-trans-hydroxy-cilostazol is 66%. Mild hepatic impairment did not affect protein binding. The free fraction of cilostazol was 27% higher in subjects with renal impairment than in normal volunteers. The displacement of cilostazol from plasma proteins by erythromycin, quinidine warfarin, and omeprazole was not clinically significant.

Metabolism and Excretion

Cilostazol is eliminated predominately by metabolism and subsequent urinary excretion of metabolites. Based on *in vitro* studies, the primary isoenzymes involved in cilostazol's metabolism are CYP3A4 and, a lesser extent, CYP2C19. The enzyme responsible for metabolism of 3,4-dehydro-cilostazol, the most active of the metabolites, is unknown.

Following oral administration of 100 mg radiolabeled cilostazol, 56% of the total analytes in plasma was cilostazol, 15% was 3,4-dehydro-cilostazol (4-7 times as active as cilostazol), and 4% was 4′-trans-hydroxy-cilostazol (one-fifth as active as cilostazol). The primary route of elimination was the urine (74%), with the remainder excreted in the feces (20%). No measurable amount of unchanged cilostazol was excreted in the urine, and less than 2% of the dose was excreted as 3,4-dehydro-cilostazol. About 30% of the dose was excreted in the urine as 4′-trans-hydroxy-cilostazol. The remainder was excreted as other metabolites, none of which exceeded 5%. There was no evidence of induction of hepatic microenzymes.

Special Populations

Age and Gender

The total and unbound oral clearances, adjusted for body weight, of cilostazol and its metabolites were not significantly different with respect to age and/or gender across a 50-80 year-old age range.

Smokers

Population pharmacokinetic analysis suggests that smoking decreased cilostazol exposure by about 20%.

Hepatic Impairment

The pharmacokinetics of cilostazol and its metabolites were similar in subjects with mild hepatic disease compared to healthy subjects.

Patients with moderate or severe hepatic impairment have not been studied.

Renal Impairment

The total pharmacologic activity of cilostazol and its metabolites was similar in subjects with mild to moderate renal impairment and in normal subjects. Severe renal impairment increases metabolite levels and alters protein binding of the parent and metabolites. The expected pharmacologic activity, however, based on plasma concentrations and relative PDE III inhibiting potency of parent drug and metabolites, appeared little changed. Patients on dialysis have not been studied, but, it is unlikely that cilostazol can be removed efficiently by dialysis because of its high protein binding (95-98%).

Pharmacokinetic and Pharmacodynamic Drug-Drug Interactions

Cilostazol could have pharmacodynamic interactions with other inhibitors of platelet function and pharmacokinetic interactions because of effects of other drugs on its metabolism by CYP3A4 or CYP2C19 Cilostazol does not appear to inhibit CYP3A4 (see Lovastatin).

Aspirin: Short-term (≤4 days) coadministration of aspirin with cilostazol showed a 23-35% increase in inhibition of ADP-induced *ex vivo* platelet aggregation compared to aspirin alone; there was no clinically significant impact on PT, aPTT, or bleeding time compared to aspirin alone. There was no additive or synergistic effect on arachidonic acid-induced platelet aggregation. Effects of long-term coadministration in the general population are unknown. In eight randomized, placebo-controlled, double-blind clinical trials, aspirin was coadministered with cilostazol to 201 patients. The most frequent doses and mean durations of aspirin therapy were 75-81 mg daily for 137 days (107 patients) and 325 mg daily for 54 days (85 patients). There was no apparent greater incidence of hemorrhagic adverse effects in patients taking cilostazol and aspirin compared to patients taking placebo and equivalent doses of aspirin.

Warfarin: The cytochrome P-450 isoenzymes involved in the metabolism of R-warfarin are CYP3A4, CYP1A2, and CYP2C19, and in the metabolism of S-warfarin, CYP2C9. Cilostazol did not inhibit either the metabolism or the pharmacologic effects (PT, aPTT, bleeding time, or platelet aggregation) of R- and S-warfarin after single 25 mg dose of warfarin. The effect of concomitant multiple dosing of warfarin and cilostazol on the pharmacokinetics and pharmacodynamics of both drugs is unknown.

Omeprazole: Coadministration of omeprazole did not significantly affect the metabolism of cilostazol, but the systemic exposure to 3,4-dehydro-cilostazol was increased by 69%, probably the result of omeprazole's potent inhibition of CYP2C19 (see DOSAGE AND ADMINISTRATION).

Erythromycin and other macrolide antibiotics: Erythromycin is a moderately strong inhibitor of CYP3A4. Coadministration of erythromycin 500 mg q 8h with a single dose of cilostazol 100 mg increased cilostazol C_{max} by 47% and AUC by 73%. Inhibition of cilostazol metabolism by erythromycin increased the AUC of 4′-trans-hydroxy-cilostazol by 141%. Other macrolide antibiotics would be expected to have similar effect (see DOSAGE AND ADMINISTRATION).

Diltiazem: Diltiazem, a moderate inhibitor of CYP 3A4, has been shown to increase cilostazol plasma concentration by approximately 53% (see DOSAGE AND ADMINISTRATION). This information was obtained from population pharmacokinetic analysis.

Quinidine: Concomitant administration of quinidine with a single dose of cilostazol 100 mg did not alter cilostazol pharmacokinetics.

Strong inhibitors of CYP3A4: Strong inhibitors of CYP3A4, such as ketoconazole, itraconzaole, fluconazole, miconazole, fluvoxamine, fluoxetine, nefazodone, and sertraline have not been studied in combination with cilostazol but would be expected to cause a greater increase in plasma levels of cilostazol and metabolites than erythromycin.

Lovastatin: Coadministration of a single dose of lovastatin 80 mg with cilostazol at steady state did not result in clinically significant increases in lovastatin and its hydroxyacid metabolite plasma concentrations.

INDICATIONS AND USAGE

Cilostazol is indicated for the reduction of symptoms of intermittent claudication, as indicated by an increased walking distance.

NON-FDA APPROVED INDICATIONS

The use of cilostazol is also being studied for prevention of restenosis in patients undergoing coronary angioplasty and stent implantation, and in patients with a history of prior stroke for secondary prevention of cerebral infarction. None of these uses currently has FDA approval.

CONTRAINDICATIONS

Cilostazol and several of its metabolites are inhibitors of phosphodiesterase III. Several drugs with this pharmacologic effect have caused decreased survival compared to placebo in patients with class III-IV congestive heart failure. Cilostazol is contraindicated in patients with congestive heart failure of any severity.

Cilostazol is contraindicated in patients with known or suspected hypersensitivity to any of its components.

PRECAUTIONS

Cilostazol is contraindicated in patients with congestive heart failure. In patients without congestive heart failure, the long-term effects of PDE III inhibitors (including cilostazol) are unknown. Patients in the 3-6 month placebo-controlled trials of cilostazol were relatively stable (no recent myocardial infarction or strokes, no rest pain or other signs of rapidly progressing disease), and only 19 patients died (0.7% in the placebo group and 0.8% in the cilostazol group). The calculated relative risk of death of 1.2 has a wide 95% confidence limit (0.5-3.1). There are no data as to longer-term risk or risk in patients with more severe underlying heart disease.

USE WITH CLOPIDOGREL

There is no information with respect to the efficacy or safety of the concurrent use of cilostazol and clopidogrel, a platelet-aggregation inhibiting drug indicated for use in patients with peripheral arterial disease. Studies of concomitant use of cilostazol and clopidogrel are planned.

INFORMATION FOR THE PATIENT

Patients should be advised:

- To read the patient package insert for cilostazol carefully before starting therapy and to reread it each time therapy is renewed in case the information has changed.
- To take cilostazol at least ½ hour before or 2 hours after food.
- That the beneficial effects of cilostazol on the symptoms of intermittent claudication may not be immediate. Although the patient may experience benefit in 2-4 weeks after initiation of therapy, treatment for up to 12 weeks may be required before a beneficial effect is experienced.
- About the uncertainty concerning cardiovascular risk in long-term use or in patients with severe underlying heart disease, as described in PRECAUTIONS.

HEPATIC IMPAIRMENT

Patients with moderate or severe hepatic impairment have not been studied in clinical trials.

CARDIOVASCULAR TOXICITY

Repeated oral administration of cilostazol to dogs (30 or more mg/kg/day for 52 weeks, 150 or more mg/kg/day for 13 weeks, and 450 mg/kg/day for 2 weeks), produced cardiovascular lesions that included endocardial hemorrhage, hemosiderin deposition and fibrosis in the left ventricle, hemorrhage in the right atrial wall, hemorrhage and necrosis of the smooth muscle in the wall of the coronary artery, intimal thickening of the coronary artery, and coronary arteritis and periarteritis. At the lowest dose associated with cardiovascular lesions in the 52 week study, systemic exposure (AUC) to unbound cilostazol was less than that seen in humans at the maximum recommended human dose (MRHD) of 100 mg bid. Similar lesion have been reported in the dog following the administration of other positive inotropic agents (including PDE III inhibitors) and/or vasodilating agents. No cardiovascular lesions were seen in rats following 5 or 13 weeks of administration of cilostazol at doses up to 1500 mg/kg/day. At this dose, systemic exposures (AUCs) to unbound cilostazol were only about 1.5 and 5 times (male and female rats, respectively) the exposure seen in humans at the MRHD. Cardiovascular lesions were also not seen in rats following 52 weeks of administration of cilostazol at doses up to 150 mg/kg/day. At this dose, systemic exposures (AUCs) to unbound cilostazol were about 0.5 and 5 times (male and female rats, respectively) the exposure in humans at the MRHD. (In female rats, cilostazol AUCs were similar at 150 and 1500 mg/kg/day). Cardiovascular lesions were also not observed in monkeys after oral administration of cilostazol for 13 weeks at doses up to 1800 mg/kg/day. While this dose of cilostazol produced pharmacologic effects in monkeys, plasma cilostazol levels were less than those seen in humans given the MRHD, and those seen dogs given doses associated with cardiovascular lesions.

CARCINOGENESIS, MUTAGENESIS, AND IMPAIRMENT OF FERTILITY

Dietary administration of cilostazol to male and female rats and mice for up to 104 weeks, at doses up to 500 mg/kg/day in rats and 1000 mg/kg/day in mice, revealed no evidence of carcinogenic potential. The maximum doses administered in both rat and mouse studies were, on a systemic exposure basis, less than the human exposure at the MRHD of the drug. Cilostazol tested negative in bacterial gene mutation, bacterial DNA repair, mammalian cell gene mutation, and mouse *in vivo* bone marrow chromosomal aberration assays. It was, however, associated with a significant increase in chromosomal aberrations in the *in vitro* Chinese Hamster Ovary Cell assay.

Cilostazol did not affect fertility or mating performance of male and female rats at doses as high as 1000 mg/kg/day. At this dose, systemic exposures (AUCs) to unbound cilostazol were less than 1.5 times in males, and about 5 times in females, the exposure in humans at the MRHD.

PREGNANCY CATEGORY C

In a rat developmental toxicity study, oral administration of 1000 mg cilostazol/kg/day was associated with decreased fetal weights, and increased incidences of cardiovascular renal, and skeletal anomalies (ventricular septal, aortic arch and subclavian artery abnormalities, renal pelvic dilation, 14th rib and retarded ossification). At this dose, systemic exposure to unbound cilostazol nonpregnant rats was about 5 times the exposure in humans given the MRHD. Increased incidences of ventricular septal defect and retarded ossification were also noted at 150 mg/kg/day (5 times the MRHD on systemic exposure basis). In a rabbit developmental toxicity study, an increased incidence of retardation of ossification of the sternum was seen at doses as low as 150 mg/kg/day. In nonpregnant rabbits given 150 mg/kg/day, exposure to unbound cilostazol was considerably lower than that seen in humans given the MRHD, and exposure to 3,4-dehydro-cilostazol was barely detectable.

When cilostazol was administered to rats during late pregnancy and lactation, an increased incidence of stillborn and decreased birth weights of offspring was seen at doses of 150 mg/kg/day (5 times the MRHD on a systemic exposure basis).

There are no adequate and well-controlled studies in pregnant women.

NURSING MOTHERS

Transfer of cilostazol into milk has been re-ported in experimental animals (rats). Because of the potential risk to nursing infants, a decision should be made to discontinue nursing or to discontinue cilostazol.

PEDIATRIC USE

The safety and effectiveness of cilostazol in pediatric patients have not been established.

GERIATRIC USE

Of the total number of subjects (n=2274) in clinical studies of cilostazol, 56% were 65 years old and over, while 16% were 75 years old and over. No overall differences in safety or effectiveness were observed between these subjects and younger subjects, and other reported clinical experience has not identified differences in responses between the elderly and younger patients, but greater sensitivity of some older individuals cannot be ruled out. Pharmacokinetic studies have not disclosed any age-related effects the absorption, distribution, metabolism, and elimination of cilostazol and its metabolites.

DRUG INTERACTIONS

Since cilostazol is extensively metabolized by cytochrome P-450 isoenzymes, caution should be exercised when cilostazol is coadministered with inhibitors of CYP3A4 such as ketoconazole and erythromycin or inhibitors of CYP2C19 such as omeprazole. Pharmacokinetic studies have demonstrated that omeprazole and erythromycin significantly increased the systemic exposure of cilostazol and/or its major metabolites. Population pharmacokinetic studies showed higher concentrations of cilostazol among patients concurrently treated with diltiazem, an inhibitor of CYP3A4 (see CLINICAL PHARMACOLOGY, Pharmacokinetic and Pharmacodynamic Drug-Drug Interactions). Cilostazol does not, however, appear to cause increased blood levels of drugs metabolized by CYP3A4, as it had no effect on lovastatin, a drug with metabolism very sensitive to CYP3A4 inhibition.

ADVERSE REACTIONS

Adverse events were assessed in eight placebo-controlled clinical trials involving 2274 patients exposed either 50 or 100 mg bid cilostazol (n=1301) or placebo (n=973), with a median treatment duration of 127 days for patients on cilostazol and 134 days for patients on placebo.

The only adverse event resulting in discontinuation of therapy in ≥3% of patients treated with cilostazol 50 or 100 mg bid was headache, which occurred with an incidence of 1.3%, 3.5%, and 0.3% in patients treated with cilostazol 50 mg bid, 100 mg bid, or placebo, respectively. Other frequent causes of discontinuation included palpitation and diarrhea, both 1.1% for cilostazol (all doses) versus 0.1% for placebo.

The most commonly reported adverse events, occurring in ≥2% of patients treated with cilostazol 50 or 100 mg bid, are shown in TABLE 1.

Other events seen with an incidence of ≥2% but occurring in the placebo group, at least as frequently as in the 100 mg bid group were: asthenia, hypertension, vomiting, leg cramps, hyperesthesia, paresthesia, dyspnea, rash, hematuria, urinary tract infection, flu syndrome, angina pectoris, arthritis, and bronchitis.

***TABLE 1** Most Commonly Reported AEs (Incidence ≥2%) in Patients on Cilostazol 50 mg bid or 100 mg bid and Occurring at a Rate in the 100 mg bid Group Higher Than in Patients on Placebo*

Adverse Events (AEs) by Body System	Cilostazol 50 mg bid (n=303)	Cilostazol 100 mg bid (n=998)	Placebo (n=973)
Body as a Whole			
Abdominal pain	4%	5%	3%
Back pain	6%	7%	6%
Headache	27%	34%	14%
Infection	14%	10%	8%
Cardiovascular			
Palpitation	5%	10%	1%
Tachycardia	4%	4%	1%
Digestive			
Abnormal stools	12%	15%	4%
Diarrhea	12%	19%	7%
Dyspepsia	6%	6%	4%
Flatulence	2%	3%	2%
Nausea	6%	7%	6%
Metabolic and Nutritional			
Peripheral edema	9%	7%	4%
Musculo-Skeletal			
Myalgia 2%	3%	2%	
Nervous			
Dizziness	9%	10%	6%
Vertigo 3%	1%	1%	
Respiratory			
Cough increased	3%	4%	3%
Pharyngitis	7%	10%	7%
Rhinitis	12%	7%	5%

Less frequent adverse events (<2%) that were experienced by patients exposed to cilostazol 50 mg bid or 100 mg bid in the eight controlled clinical trials and that occurred at a frequency in the 100 mg bid group than placebo, regardless of suspected drug relationship, are listed below.

Body as a Whole: Chills, face edema, fever, generalized edema, malaise, neck rigidity, pelvic pain, retroperitoneal hemorrhage.

Cardiovascular: Atrial fibrillation, atrial flutter, cerebral infarct, cerebral ischemia, congestive heart failure, heart arrest, hemorrhage, hypotension, myocardial infarction, myocardial ischemia, nodal arrhythmia, postural hypotension, supraventricular tachycardia, syncope, varicose vein, vasodilation, ventricular extrasystoles, ventricular tachycardia.

Digestive: Anorexia, cholelithiasis, colitis, duodenal ulcer, duodenitis, esophageal hemorrhage, esophagitis, GGT increased, gastritis, gastroenteritis, gum hemorrhage, hematemesis, melena, peptic ulcer, periodontal abscess, rectal hemorrhage, stomach ulcer, tongue edema.

Endocrine: Diabetes mellitus.

Hemic and Lymphatic: Anemia, ecchymosis, iron deficiency anemia, polycythemia, purpura.

Metabolic and Nutritional: Creatinine increased, gout, hyperlipemia, hyperuricemia.

Musculoskeletal: Arthralgia, bone pain, bursitis.

Nervous: Anxiety, insomnia, neuralgia.

Respiratory: Asthma, epistaxis, hemoptysis, pneumonia, sinusitis.

Skin and Appendages: Dry skin, furunculosis, skin hypertrophy, urticaria.

Special Senses: Amblyopia, blindness, conjunctivitis, diplopia, ear pain, eye hemorrhage, retinal hemorrhage, tinnitus.

Urogenital: Albuminuria, cystitis, urinary frequency, vaginal hemorrhage, vaginitis.

DOSAGE AND ADMINISTRATION

The recommended dosage of cilostazol is 100 mg bid, taken at least half an hour before or 2 hours after breakfast and dinner. A dose of 50 mg bid should be considered during coadministration of such inhibitors CYP3A4 as ketoconazole, itraconazole, erythromycin and diltiazem, and during coadministration of such inhibitors of CYP2C19 as omeprazole. CYP3A4 is also inhibited by grapefruit juice. Because the magnitude and timing of this interaction have not yet been investigated, patients receiving cilostazol should avoid consuming grapefruit juice.

Patients may respond as early as 2-4 weeks after the initiation of therapy, but treatment for up to 12 weeks may be needed before a beneficial effect is experienced.

DISCONTINUATION OF THERAPY

The available data suggest that the dosage of cilostazol can be reduced or discontinued without rebound (*i.e.*, platelet hyperaggregability).

HOW SUPPLIED

Pletal is supplied as 50 and 100 mg tablets.

50 mg: White, triangular and debossed with "Pletal 50".

100 mg: White, round and debossed with "Pletal 100".

Storage: Store Pletal tablets at 25°C (77°F); excursions permitted to 15-30°C (59-86°F).

PRODUCT LISTING - EQUIVALENTS NOT AVAILABLE

Tablet - Oral - 50 mg

60's $106.33 PLETAL, Pharmacia Corporation 59148-0003-16

Tablet - Oral - 100 mg

60's $106.33 PLETAL, Pharmacia Corporation 59148-0002-16

100's $151.25 PLETAL, Pharmacia Corporation 59148-0002-35

Cimetidine Hydrochloride *(000820)*

For related information, see the comparative table section in Appendix A.

Categories: Adenoma, multiple endocrine; Bleeding, upper gastrointestinal, prophylaxis; Esophagitis, erosive; Gastroesophageal Reflux Disease; Mastocytosis, systemic; Ulcer, duodenal; Ulcer, gastric; Zollinger-Ellison syndrome; Pregnancy Category B; FDA Approved 1986 Apr; WHO Formulary

Drug Classes: Antihistamines, H2; Gastrointestinals

Brand Names: Cimetidine In Sodium Chloride; Procimeti; **Tagamet**

Foreign Brand Availability: Acibilin (Argentina); Acidnor (Bahrain; Cyprus; Egypt; Iran; Iraq; Jordan; Kuwait; Lebanon; Libya; Oman; Qatar; Republic-of-Yemen; Saudi-Arabia; Syria; United-Arab-Emirates); Aciloc (Denmark; Sweden); Aci-Med (South-Africa); Acinil (Denmark; Sweden); Aidar (Thailand); Antag (Philippines); Apo-Cimetidine (Canada; New-Zealand); Asaurex (Mexico); Azucimet (Germany); Biomag (Italy); Brumetidina (Italy); Campanex (Greece); Cemedin 200 (Israel); Cemedin 400 (Israel); Cemedin 800 (Israel); Cementin (Singapore); Ciclem (Philippines); Cidine (Thailand); Cigamet (Thailand); Cignatin (Korea); Ciket M (Philippines); Cimal (Norway); Cimbene (Bahamas; Barbados; Belize; Bermuda; Curacao; Guyana; Jamaica; Netherland-Antilles; Puerto-Rico; Surinam; Trinidad); Cimedine (Bahrain; Cyprus; Egypt; Iran; Iraq; Israel; Jordan; Kuwait; Lebanon; Libya; Oman; Qatar; Republic-of-Yemen; Saudi-Arabia; Syria; United-Arab-Emirates); Cimehexal (Australia; Germany); Cimeldine (Ireland); Cimet (Indonesia; Thailand); Cimlok (South-Africa); Cimetag (Austria; Israel); Cimetalgin (Austria); Cimetase (Mexico); Cimetid (Norway); Cimetidin (Bulgaria; Denmark; Germany; Switzerland); Cimetidina (Spain); Cimetidine (Czech-Republic; Netherlands); Cimetigal (Mexico); Cimetin (Czech-Republic; Ecuador); Cimetum (Argentina); Cimewell (Taiwan); Cimex (Finland); Cimulcer (Malaysia; Thailand); Cinadine (South-Africa); Cinulcus (Spain); Cismetin (Korea); Citidine (Hong-Kong; Singapore); Citius (Bahrain; Cyprus; Egypt; Iran; Iraq; Israel; Jordan; Kuwait; Lebanon; Libya; Oman; Qatar; Republic-of-Yemen; Saudi-Arabia; Syria; United-Arab-Emirates); Corsamet (Indonesia); Cytine (New-Zealand); Defense (Taiwan); Dispamet (Bahrain; Cyprus; Egypt; Iran; Iraq; Israel; Jordan; Kuwait; Lebanon; Libya; Oman; Qatar; Republic-of-Yemen; Saudi-Arabia; Syria; United-Arab-Emirates); Duomet (South-Africa); Dyspamet (England); Erlmetin (Singapore); Eureceptor (Italy); Fremet (Spain); Gastab (Hong-Kong); Gastidine (Hong-Kong); Gastrobitan (Norway); Gastrodin (Taiwan); Gawei (Taiwan); Getidin (Philippines); H-2 (Korea); Haldin (Bahrain; Benin; Burkina-Faso; Cyprus; Egypt; Ethiopia; Gambia; Ghana; Guinea; Iran; Iraq; Israel; Ivory-Coast; Jordan; Kenya; Kuwait; Lebanon; Liberia; Libya; Malawi; Mali; Mauritania; Mauritius; Morocco; Niger; Nigeria; Oman; Qatar; Republic-of-Yemen; Saudi-Arabia; Senegal; Seychelles; Sierra-Leone; South-Africa; Sudan; Syria; Tanzania; Tunia; Uganda; United-Arab-Emirates; Zambia; Zimbabwe); Hexamet (South-Africa); Himetin (Korea); Histodil (Hungary); Inesfay (Mexico); Lenamet (South-Africa); Lenamet OTC (South-Africa); Lock 2 (Benin; Burkina-Faso; Ethiopia; Gambia; Ghana; Guinea; Ivory-Coast; Kenya; Liberia; Malawi; Mali; Mauritania; Mauritius; Morocco; Niger; Nigeria; Senegal; Seychelles; Sierra-Leone; South-Africa; Sudan; Tanzania; Tunia; Uganda; Zambia; Zimbabwe); Magicul (Australia; New-Zealand); Manomet (Thailand); Maritidine (Hong-Kong); Med-Gastramet (Thailand); Meticon (Korea); Neutronorm (Austria); Novocimetine (Canada); Nulcer (Indonesia); Piovalen (Greece); Powegon (Taiwan); Sanmetidin (Indonesia); Secapine (South-Africa); Shintamet (Malaysia; Philippines); Siamidine (Thailand); Sigmetadine (Australia); Simaglen (Hong-Kong); Stogamet (Taiwan); Stomakon (Brazil); Stomedine (France); Stomet (Italy); Tametin (Italy); Timet (Bahrain; Cyprus; Egypt; Iran; Iraq; Israel; Jordan; Kuwait; Lebanon; Libya; Oman; Qatar; Republic-of-Yemen; Saudi-Arabia; Syria; United-Arab-Emirates); Tobymet (Indonesia); Ulcedin (Italy); Ulcedine (Thailand); Ulcemet (Ecuador); Ulcenon (Philippines); Ulcerfen (Argentina); Ulcim (South-Africa); Ulcimet (Argentina; Ecuador; Indonesia; Peru); Ulcodina (Italy); Ulcomedina (Italy); Ulcomet (Hong-Kong); Ulcolind H2 (Germany); Ulcumet (Indonesia); Ulsikur (Indonesia); Weisdin (Taiwan); Xepamet (Malaysia); Zymerol (Mexico)

Cost of Therapy: $89.91 (Duodenal Ulcer; Tagamet; 800 mg; 1 tablet/day; 30 day supply)
$70.95 (Duodenal Ulcer; Generic Tablets; 800 mg; 1 tablet/day; 30 day supply)

DESCRIPTION

Cimetidine hydrochloride is a histamine H_2-receptor antagonist. Chemically it is *N''*-cyano-*N*-methyl-*N'*-[2-[[(5-methyl-1*H*-imidazol-4-yl)methyl]thio]-ethyl]-guanidine.

The empirical formula for cimetidine is $C_{10}H_{16}N_6S$ and for cimetidine hydrochloride, $C_{10}H_{16}N_6SHCl$; these represent molecular weights of 252.34 and 288.80, respectively.

Cimetidine contains an imidazole ring, and is chemically related to histamine.

The liquid and injection dosage forms contain cimetidine as the hydrochloride salt.

Cimetidine hydrochloride has a bitter taste and characteristic odor.

Solubility Characteristics: Cimetidine is soluble in alcohol, slightly soluble in water, very slightly soluble in chloroform and insoluble in ether. Cimetidine hydrochloride is freely soluble in water, soluble in alcohol, very slightly soluble in chloroform, and practically insoluble in ether.

ORAL

Tablets

Each light green, film-coated tablet contains 300, 400, or 800 mg of cimetidine. Inactive ingredients consist of cellulose, D&C yellow no. 10, FD&C blue No. 2, FD&C red no. 40, FD&C yellow no. 6, hydroxypropyl methylcellulose, iron oxides, magnesium stearate, povidone, propylene glycol, sodium lauryl sulfate, sodium starch glycolate, starch, titanium dioxide and trace amounts of other inactive ingredients.

Liquid for Oral Administration

Each 5 ml (1 teaspoonful) of clear, light orange, mint-peach flavored liquid contains cimetidine hydrochloride equivalent to cimetidine, 300 mg; alcohol, 2.8%. Inactive ingredients consist of FD&C yellow no. 6, flavors, methylparaben, polyoxyethylene polyoxypropylene glycol, propylene glycol, propylparaben, saccharin sodium, sodium chloride, sodium phosphate, sorbitol and water.

INJECTION

Single-dose vials for intramuscular or intravenous administration: Each 2 ml contains, in sterile aqueous solution (pH range 3.8 to 6), cimetidine hydrochloride equivalent to cimetidine, 300 mg; phenol, 10 mg.

Multi-dose vials for intramuscular or intravenous administration: *8 ml (300 mg/2 ml):* Each 2 ml contains, in sterile aqueous solution (pH range 3.8 to 6), cimetidine hydrochloride equivalent to cimetidine, 300 mg; phenol, 10 mg.

Single-dose premixed plastic containers for intravenous administration: Each 50 ml of sterile aqueous solution (pH range 5-7) contains cimetidine hydrochloride equivalent to 300 mg cimetidine and 0.45 g sodium chloride.

No preservative has been added.

The plastic container is fabricated from specially formulated polyvinyl chloride. The amount of water that can permeate from inside the container into the overwrap is insufficient to affect the solution significantly. Solutions in contact with the plastic container can leach out certain of its chemical components in very small amounts within the expiration period, *e.g.,* di 2-ethylhexyl phthalate (DEHP), up to 5 parts/million. However, the safety of the plastic has been confirmed in tests in animals according to the USP biological tests for plastic containers as well as by tissue culture toxicity studies.

ADD-Vantage* vials for intravenous administration: Each 2 ml contains, in sterile aqueous solution (pH range 3.8 to 6), cimetidine hydrochloride equivalent to cimetidine, 300 mg; phenol, 10 mg.

All of the above injection formulations are pyrogen free, and sodium hydroxide is used as an ingredient to adjust the pH.

CLINICAL PHARMACOLOGY

Cimetidine competitively inhibits the action of histamine at the histamine H_2 receptors of the parietal cells and thus is a histamine H_2-receptor antagonist.

Cimetidine is not an anticholinergic agent. Studies have shown that cimetidine inhibits both daytime and nocturnal basal gastric acid secretion. Cimetidine also inhibits gastric acid secretion stimulated by food, histamine, pentagastrin, caffeine and insulin.

ANTISECRETORY ACTIVITY

Acid Secretion

Nocturnal

Cimetidine 800 mg orally at bedtime reduces mean hourly H^+ activity by greater than 85% over an 8 hour period in duodenal ulcer patients, with no effect on daytime acid secretion. Cimetidine 1600 mg orally hs produces 100% inhibition of mean hourly H^+ activity over an 8 hour period in duodenal ulcer patients, but also reduces H^+ activity by 35% for an additional 5 hours into the following morning. Cimetidine 400 mg bid and 300 mg qid decrease nocturnal acid secretion in a dose-related manner, *i.e.,* 47-83% over a 6-8 hour period and 54% over a 9 hour period, respectively.

Food Stimulated

During the first hour after a standard experimental meal, oral cimetidine 300 mg inhibited gastric acid secretion in duodenal ulcer patients by at least 50%. During the subsequent 2 hours cimetidine inhibited gastric acid secretion by at least 75%.

The effect of a 300 mg breakfast dose of cimetidine continued for at least 4 hours and there was partial suppression of the rise in gastric acid secretion following the luncheon meal in duodenal ulcer patients. This suppression of gastric acid output was enhanced and could be maintained by another 300 mg dose of cimetidine given with lunch.

In another study, cimetidine 300 mg given with the meal increased gastric pH as compared with placebo.

TABLE 1

	Mean Gastric pH	
	Cimetidine	**Placebo**
1 hour	3.5	2.6
2 hours	3.1	1.6
3 hours	3.8	1.9
4 hours	6.1	2.2

24 Hour Mean H^+ Activity

Cimetidine 800 mg hs, 400 mg bid and 300 mg qid all provide a similar, moderate (less than 60%) level of 24 hour acid suppression. However, the 800 mg hs regimen exerts its entire effect on nocturnal acid, and does not affect daytime gastric physiology.

Chemically Stimulated

Oral cimetidine significantly inhibited gastric acid secretion stimulated by betazole (an isomer of histamine), pentagastrin, caffeine and insulin as shown in TABLE 2.

TABLE 2

Stimulant	Stimulant Dose	Cimetidine HCl	% Inhibition
Betazole	1.5 mg/kg (SC)	300 mg (PO)	85% at 2.5 hours
Pentagastrin	6 μg/kg/h (IV)	100 mg/h (IV)	60% at 1 hour
Caffeine	5 mg/kg/h (IV)	300 mg (PO)	100% at 1 hour
Insulin	0.03 U/kg/h (IV)	100 mg/h (IV)	82% at 1 hour

When food and betazole were used to stimulate secretion, inhibition of hydrogen ion concentration usually ranged from 45-75% and the inhibition of volume ranged from 30-65%.

Injection Only

Parenteral administration also significantly inhibits gastric acid secretion. In a crossover study involving patients with active or healed duodenal or gastric ulcers, either continuous IV infusion of cimetidine 37.5 mg/h (900 mg/day) or intermittent injection of cimetidine 300 mg q6h (1200 mg/day) maintained gastric pH above 4.0 for more than 50% of the time under steady-state conditions.

Pepsin

Oral cimetidine 300 mg reduced total pepsin output as a result of the decrease in volume of gastric juice.

Intrinsic Factor

Intrinsic factor secretion was studied with betazole as a stimulant. Oral cimetidine 300 mg inhibited the rise in intrinsic factor concentration produced by betazole, but some intrinsic factor was secreted at all times.

OTHER

Lower esophageal sphincter pressure and gastric emptying: Cimetidine has no effect on lower esophageal sphincter (LES) pressure or the rate of gastric emptying.

PHARMACOKINETICS

Cimetidine is rapidly absorbed after oral administration and peak levels occur in 45-90 minutes. The half-life of cimetidine is approximately 2 hours. Both oral and parenteral (IV or IM) administration provide comparable periods of therapeutically effective blood levels; blood concentrations remain above that required to provide 80% inhibition of basal gastric acid secretion for 4-5 hours following a dose of 300 mg.

Steady-state blood concentrations of cimetidine with continuous infusion of cimetidine are determined by the infusion rate and clearance of the drug in the individual patient. In a study of peptic ulcer patients with normal renal function, an infusion rate of 37.5 mg/h produced average steady-state plasma cimetidine concentrations of about 0.9 μg/ml. Blood levels with other infusion rates will vary in direct proportion to the infusion rate.

The principal route of excretion of cimetidine is the urine. Following parenteral administration, most of the drug is excreted as the parent compound; following oral administration, the drug is more extensively metabolized, the sulfoxide being the major metabolite. Following a single oral dose, 48% of the drug is recovered from the urine after 24 hours as the parent compound. Following IV or IM administration, approximately 75% of the drug is recovered from the urine after 24 hours as the parent compound.

INDICATIONS AND USAGE

Cimetidine HCl is indicated in:

Short-term treatment of active duodenal ulcer: Most patients heal within 4 weeks and there is rarely reason to use cimetidine at full dosage for longer than 6-8 weeks (see DOSAGE AND ADMINISTRATION, Duodenal Ulcer). Concomitant antacids should be given as needed for relief of pain. However, simultaneous administration of oral cimetidine and antacids is not recommended, since antacids have been reported to interfere with the absorption of oral cimetidine.

Maintenance therapy for duodenal ulcer patients at reduced dosage after healing of active ulcer: Patients have been maintained on continued treatment with cimetidine 400 mg hs for periods of up to 5 years.

Short-term treatment of active benign gastric ulcer: There is no information concerning usefulness of treatment periods of longer than 8 weeks.

Erosive gastroesophageal reflux disease (GERD) (oral solution only): Erosive esophagitis diagnosed by endoscopy. Treatment is indicated for 12 weeks for healing of lesions and control of symptoms. The use of cimetidine beyond 12 weeks has not been established (see DOSAGE AND ADMINISTRATION, Erosive Gastroesophageal Reflux Disease (GERD).

Prevention of upper gastrointestinal bleeding in critically ill patients (injection only).

The treatment of pathological hypersecretory conditions: (*i.e.,* Zollinger-Ellison Syndrome, systemic mastocytosis, multiple endocrine adenomas).

CONTRAINDICATIONS

Cimetidine HCl is contraindicated for patients known to have hypersensitivity to the product.

PRECAUTIONS

GENERAL

Rare instances of cardiac arrhythmias and hypotension have been reported following the rapid administration of cimetidine HCl injection by IV bolus.

Symptomatic response to cimetidine therapy does not preclude the presence of a gastric malignancy. There have been rare reports of transient healing of gastric ulcers despite subsequently documented malignancy.

Reversible confusional states (see ADVERSE REACTIONS) have been observed on occasion, predominantly, but not exclusively, in severely ill patients. Advancing age (50 or more years) and preexisting liver and/or renal disease appear to be contributing factors. In some patients these confusional states have been mild and have not required discontinuation of cimetidine therapy. In cases where discontinuation was judged necessary, the condition usually cleared within 3-4 days of drug withdrawal.

CARCINOGENESIS, MUTAGENESIS, AND IMPAIRMENT OF FERTILITY

In a 24 month toxicity study conducted in rats, at dose levels of 150, 378 and 950 mg/kg/day (approximately 8-48 times the recommended human dose), there was a small increase in the incidence of benign Leydig cell tumors in each dose group; when the combined drug-treated groups and control groups were compared, this increase reached statistical significance. In a subsequent 24 month study, there were no differences between the rats receiving 150 mg/kg/day and the untreated controls. However, a statistically significant increase in benign Leydig cell tumor incidence was seen in the rats that received 378 and 950 mg/kg/day. These tumors were common in control groups as well as treated groups and the difference became apparent only in aged rats.

Cimetidine has demonstrated a weak antiandrogenic effect. In animal studies this was manifested as reduced prostate and seminal vesicle weights. However, there was no impairment of mating performance or fertility, nor any harm to the fetus in these animals at doses 8-48 times the full therapeutic dose of cimetidine, as compared with controls. The cases of gynecomastia seen in patients treated for 1 month or longer may be related to this effect.

In human studies, cimetidine has been shown to have no effect on spermatogenesis, sperm count, motility, morphology or *in vitro* fertilizing capacity.

PREGNANCY, TERATOGENIC EFFECTS, PREGNANCY CATEGORY B

Reproduction studies have been performed in rats, rabbits and mice at doses up to 40 times the normal human dose and have revealed no evidence of impaired fertility or harm to the fetus due to cimetidine. There are, however, no adequate and well-controlled studies in pregnant women. Because animal reproductive studies are not always predictive of human response, this drug should be used during pregnancy only if clearly needed.

NURSING MOTHERS

Cimetidine is secreted in human milk and, as a general rule, nursing should not be undertaken while a patient is on a drug.

PEDIATRIC USE

Clinical experience in children is limited. Therefore, cimetidine therapy cannot be recommended for children under 16, unless, in the judgment of the physician, anticipated benefits outweigh the potential risks. In very limited experience, doses of 20-40 mg/kg/day have been used.

IMMUNOCOMPROMISED PATIENTS

In immunocompromised patients, decreased gastric acidity, including that produced by acid-suppressing agents such as cimetidine, may increase the possibility of a hyperinfection of strongyloidiasis.

DRUG INTERACTIONS

Cimetidine, apparently through an effect on certain microsomal enzyme systems, has been reported to reduce the hepatic metabolism of warfarin-type anticoagulants, phenytoin, propranolol, nifedipine, chlordiazepoxide, diazepam, certain tricyclic antidepressants, lidocaine, theophylline and metronidazole, thereby delaying elimination and increasing blood levels of these drugs.

Clinically significant effects have been reported with the warfarin anticoagulants; therefore, close monitoring of prothrombin time is recommended, and adjustment of the anticoagulant dose may be necessary when cimetidine is administered concomitantly. Interaction with phenytoin, lidocaine and theophylline has also been reported to produce adverse clinical effects.

However, a crossover study in healthy subjects receiving either cimetidine 300 mg qid or 800 mg hs concomitantly with a 300 mg bid dosage of theophylline demonstrated less alteration in steady-state theophylline peak serum levels with the 800 mg hs regimen, particularly in subjects aged 54 years and older. Data beyond 10 days are not available. (*Note:* All patients receiving theophylline should be monitored appropriately, regardless of concomitant drug therapy.)

Dosage of the drugs mentioned above and other similarly metabolized drugs, particularly those of low therapeutic ratio or in patients with renal and/or hepatic impairment, may require adjustment when starting or stopping concomitantly administered cimetidine to maintain optimum therapeutic blood levels.

Alteration of pH may affect absorption of certain drugs (*e.g.,* ketoconazole). If these products are needed, they should be given at least 2 hours before cimetidine administration.

Additional clinical experience may reveal other drugs affected by the concomitant administration of cimetidine.

ADVERSE REACTIONS

Adverse effects reported in patients taking cimetidine are described below by body system. Incidence figures of 1 in 100 and greater are generally derived from controlled clinical studies.

Gastrointestinal: Diarrhea (usually mild) has been reported in approximately 1 in 100 patients.

CNS: Headaches, ranging from mild to severe, have been reported in 3.5% of 924 patients taking 1600 mg/day, 2.1% of 2225 patients taking 800 mg/day and 2.3% of 1897 patients taking placebo. Dizziness and somnolence (usually mild) have been reported in approximately 1 in 100 patients on either 1600 mg/day or 800 mg/day.

Reversible confusional states, *e.g.,* mental confusion, agitation, psychosis, depression, anxiety, hallucinations, disorientation, have been reported predominantly, but not exclusively, in severely ill patients. They have usually developed within 2-3 days of initiation of cimetidine therapy and have cleared within 3-4 days of discontinuation of the drug.

Endocrine: Gynecomastia has been reported in patients treated for 1 month or longer. In patients being treated for pathological hypersecretory states, this occurred in about 4% of cases while in all others the incidence was 0.3 to 1% in various studies. No evidence of induced endocrine dysfunction was found, and the condition remained unchanged or returned toward normal with continuing cimetidine treatment.

Reversible impotence has been reported in patients with pathological hypersecretory disorders (*e.g.,* Zollinger-Ellison Syndrome) receiving cimetidine particularly in high doses, for at least 12 months (range 12-79 months, mean 38 months). However, in large-scale surveillance studies at regular dosage, the incidence has not exceeded that commonly reported in the general population.

Hematologic: Decreased white blood cell counts in cimetidine-treated patients (approximately 1/100,000 patients), including agranulocytosis (approximately 3/million patients), have been reported, including a few reports of recurrence on rechallenge. Most of these reports were in patients who had serious concomitant illnesses and received drugs and/or treatment known to produce neutropenia. Thrombocytopenia (approximately 3/million patients) and, very rarely cases of pancytopenia or aplastic anemia have also been reported. As with some other H_2-receptor antagonists, there have been extremely rare reports of immune hemolytic anemia.

Hepatobiliary: Dose-related increases in serum transaminase have been reported. In most cases they did not progress with continued therapy and returned to normal at the end of therapy. There have been rare reports of cholestatic or mixed cholestatic-hepatocellular effects. These were usually reversible. Because of the predominance of cholestatic features, severe parenchymal injury is considered highly unlikely. However, as in the occasional liver injury with other H_2-receptor antagonists, in exceedingly rare circumstances fatal outcomes have been reported.

There has been reported a single case of biopsy-proven periportal hepatic fibrosis in a patient receiving cimetidine.

Rare cases of pancreatitis, which cleared on withdrawal of the drug, have been reported.

Hypersensitivity: Rare cases of fever and allergic reactions including anaphylaxis and hypersensitivity vasculitis, which cleared on withdrawal of the drug, have been reported.

Renal: Small, possibly dose-related increases in plasma creatinine, presumably due to competition for renal tubular secretion, are not uncommon and do not signify deteriorating renal function. Rare cases of interstitial nephritis and urinary retention, which cleared on withdrawal of the drug, have been reported.

Cardiovascular: Rare cases of bradycardia, tachycardia and A-V heart block have been reported with H_2-receptor antagonists.

Musculoskeletal: There have been rare reports of reversible arthralgia and myalgia; exacerbation of joint symptoms in patients with preexisting arthritis has also been reported. Such symptoms have usually been alleviated by a reduction in cimetidine dosage. Rare cases of polymyositis have been reported, but no causal relationship has been established.

Integumental: Mild rash and, very rarely, cases of severe generalized skin reactions including Stevens-Johnson syndrome, epidermal necrolysis, erythema multiforme, exfoliative dermatitis and generalized exfoliative erythroderma have been reported with H_2-receptor antagonists. Reversible alopecia has been reported very rarely.

Immune Function: There have been extremely rare reports of strongyloidiasis hyperinfection in immunocompromised patients.

DOSAGE AND ADMINISTRATION

DUODENAL ULCER

Active Duodenal Ulcer

Clinical studies have indicated that suppression of nocturnal acid is the most important factor in duodenal ulcer healing (see CLINICAL PHARMACOLOGY, Antisecretory Activity, Acid Secretion). This is supported by recent clinical trials. Therefore, there is no apparent rationale, except for familiarity with use, for treating with anything other than a once-daily at bedtime dosage regimen (hs).

In a US dose-ranging study of 400, 800 and 1600 mg hs, a continuous dose response relationship for ulcer healing was demonstrated.

However, 800 mg hs is the dose of choice for most patients, as it provides a high healing rate (the difference between 800 and 1600 mg hs being small), maximal pain relief, a decreased potential for drug interactions (see DRUG INTERACTIONS) and maximal patient convenience. Patients unhealed at 4 weeks, or those with persistent symptoms, have been shown to benefit from 2-4 weeks of continued therapy.

It has been shown that patients who both have an endoscopically demonstrated ulcer larger than 1.0 cm and are also heavy smokers (*i.e.,* smoke 1 pack of cigarettes or more per day) are more difficult to heal. There is some evidence which suggests that more rapid healing can be achieved in this subpopulation with cimetidine 1600 mg at bedtime. While early pain relief with either 800 or 1600 mg hs is equivalent in all patients, 1600 mg hs provides an appropriate alternative when it is important to ensure healing within 4 weeks for this subpopulation. Alternatively, approximately 94% of all patients will also heal in 8 weeks with cimetidine 800 mg hs.

Other cimetidine oral regimens in the US which have been shown to be effective are: 300 mg 4 times daily, with meals and at bedtime, the original regimen with which US physicians have the most experience, and 400 mg twice daily, in the morning and at bedtime.

Concomitant antacids should be given as needed for relief of pain. However, simultaneous administration of oral cimetidine and antacids is not recommended, since antacids have been reported to interfere with the absorption of cimetidine.

While healing with cimetidine often occurs during the first week or 2, treatment should be continued for 4-6 weeks unless healing has been demonstrated by endoscopic examination.

Maintenance therapy for duodenal ulcer: In those patients requiring maintenance therapy, the recommended adult oral dose is 400 mg at bedtime.

ACTIVE BENIGN GASTRIC ULCER

The recommended adult oral dosage for short-term treatment of active benign gastric ulcer is 800 mg hs, or 300 mg 4 times a day with meals and at bedtime. Controlled clinical studies were limited to 6 weeks of treatment. Eight hundred (800) mg hs is the preferred regimen for most patients based upon convenience and reduced potential for drug interactions. Symptomatic response to cimetidine does not preclude the presence of a gastric malignancy. It is important to follow gastric ulcer patients to assure rapid progress to complete healing.

EROSIVE GASTROESOPHAGEAL REFLUX DISEASE (GERD)

For Oral Solution Only: The recommended adult oral dosage for the treatment of erosive esophagitis that has been diagnosed by endoscopy is 1600 mg daily in divided doses (800 mg bid or 400 mg qid) for 12 weeks. The use of cimetidine beyond 12 weeks has not been established.

PREVENTION OF UPPER GASTROINTESTINAL BLEEDING

For Injection Only: The recommended adult dosing regimen is continuous IV infusion of 50 mg/h. Patients with creatinine clearance less than 30 cc/min should receive half the recommended dose. Treatment beyond 7 days has not been studied.

PATHOLOGICAL HYPERSECRETORY CONDITIONS (SUCH AS ZOLLINGER-ELLISON SYNDROME)

Recommended Adult Oral Dosage: 300 mg 4 times a day with meals and at bedtime. In some patients it may be necessary to administer higher doses more frequently. Doses should be adjusted to individual patient needs, but should not usually exceed 2400 mg/day and should continue as long as clinically indicated.

DOSAGE ADJUSTMENT FOR PATIENTS WITH IMPAIRED RENAL FUNCTION

Patients with severely impaired renal function have been treated with cimetidine. However, such usage has been very limited. On the basis of this experience the recommended dosage is 300 mg every 12 hours orally or by IV injection. Should the patient's condition require, the frequency of dosing may be increased to every 8 hours or even further with caution. In severe renal failure, accumulation may occur and the lowest frequency of dosing compatible with an adequate patient response should be used. When liver impairment is also present, further reductions in dosage may be necessary. Hemodialysis reduces the level of circulating cimetidine. Ideally, the dosage schedule should be adjusted so that the timing of a scheduled dose coincides with the end of hemodialysis.

INJECTION ONLY

Patients with creatinine clearance less than 30 cc/min who are being treated for prevention of upper gastrointestinal bleeding should receive half the recommended dose.

Parenteral Administration

In hospitalized patients with pathological hypersecretory conditions or intractable ulcers, or in patients who are unable to take oral medication, cimetidine may be administered parenterally.

The doses and regimen for parenteral administration in patients with GERD have not been established.

All parenteral drug products should be inspected visually for particulate matter and discoloration prior to administration.

Recommendations for Parenteral Administration

Intramuscular Injection: 300 mg every 6-8 hours (no dilution necessary). Transient pain at the site of injection has been reported.

Intravenous Injection: 300 mg every 6-8 hours. In some patients it may be necessary to increase dosage. When this is necessary, the increases should be made by more frequent administration of a 300 mg dose, but should not exceed 2400 mg/day. Dilute cimetidine HCl injection, 300 mg, in sodium chloride injection (0.9%) or another compatible IV solution (see Stability of Cimetidine Injection) to a total volume of 20 ml and inject over a period of not less than 5 minutes (see PRECAUTIONS).

Intermittent IV Infusion: 300 mg every 6-8 hours, infused over 15-20 minutes. In some patients it may be necessary to increase dosage. When this is necessary, the increases should be made by more frequent administration of a 300 mg dose, but should not exceed 2400 mg/day.

Vials: Dilute cimetidine injection, 300 mg, in at least 50 ml of 5% dextrose injection, or another compatible IV solution (see Stability of Cimetidine Injection).

Plastic Containers: Use premixed cimetidine injection, 300 mg, in 0.9% sodium chloride in 50 ml plastic containers.

ADD-Vantage Vials: Dilute contents of 1 vial in an ADD Vantage diluent container, available in 50 and 100 ml sizes of 0.9% sodium chloride injection, and 5% dextrose injection.

Continuous IV Infusion

37.5 mg/h (900 mg/day): For patients requiring a more rapid elevation of gastric pH, continuous infusion may be preceded by a 150 mg loading dose administered by IV infusion as described above. Dilute 900 mg cimetidine injection in a compatible IV fluid (see Stability of Cimetidine Injection) for constant rate infusion over a 24 hour period. *Note:* Cimetidine may be diluted in 100-1000 ml; however, a volumetric pump is recommended if the volume for 24 hour infusion is less than 250 ml. In one study in patients with pathological hypersecretory states, the mean infused dose of cimetidine was 160 mg/h with a range of 40-600 mg/h.

These doses maintained the intragastric acid secretory rate at 10 mEq/h or less. The infusion rate should be adjusted to individual patient requirements.

Stability of Cimetidine Injection

When added to or diluted with most commonly used IV solutions, *e.g.,* sodium chloride injection (0.9%), dextrose injection (5% or 10%), lactated Ringer's solution, 5% sodium bicarbonate injection, cimetidine HCl injection should not be used after more than 48 hours of storage at room temperature.

Cimetidine injection premixed in plastic containers is stable through the labeled expiration date when stored under the recommended conditions.

HOW SUPPLIED

ORAL

Tablets

Light green, film-coated as follows:

300 mg: Round, debossed with the product name "Tagamet", "SB" and "300".

400 mg: Oval-shaped Tiltab, debossed with the product name "Tagamet", "SB" and "400".

800 mg: Oval-shaped Tiltab, debossed with the product name "Tagamet", "SB" and "800".

Storage: Store between 15-30°C (59-86°F); dispense in a tight light-resistant container.

Liquid

Clear, light orange, mint-peach flavored, as follows: 300 mg/5 ml in 8 fl oz (237 ml).

Storage: Store between 15-30°C (59-86°F); dispense in a tight light-resistant container.

INJECTION AND ORAL SOLUTION

Storage: Store between 15-30°C (59-86°F); do not refrigerate. Dispense in a tight, light resistant container. *Single-Dose Premixed Plastic Containers:* Exposure of the premixed product to excessive heat should be avoided. It is recommended the product be stored at controlled room temperature 15-30°C (59-86°F). Brief exposure up to 40°C does not adversely affect the premixed product.

PRODUCT LISTING - RATED THERAPEUTICALLY EQUIVALENT

Size	Price	Description	NDC
Liquid - Oral - 300 mg/5 ml			
5 ml x 40	$109.80	GENERIC, Roxane Laboratories Inc	00054-8227-16
5 ml x 50	$145.00	GENERIC, Xactdose Inc	50962-0205-05
6.70 ml x 40	$135.31	GENERIC, Roxane Laboratories Inc	00054-8230-16
237 ml	$87.50	GENERIC, Teva Pharmaceuticals Usa	00093-0506-87
237 ml	$89.10	GENERIC, Alpharma Uspd Makers Of Barre and Nmc	00472-0514-08
237 ml	$89.25	GENERIC, Brightstone Pharma	62939-2103-08
237 ml	$89.94	GENERIC, Pharmaceutical Assoc Inc Div Beach Products	00121-0649-08
237 ml	$90.00	GENERIC, Hi-Tech Pharmacal Company Inc	50383-0050-08
240 ml	$86.52	GENERIC, Watson/Rugby Laboratories Inc	00536-2975-59
240 ml	$87.00	GENERIC, Watson/Schein Pharmaceuticals Inc	00364-2602-76
240 ml	$87.24	GENERIC, Ivax Corporation	00182-6164-44
240 ml	$89.00	GENERIC, Morton Grove Pharmaceuticals Inc	60432-0007-08
240 ml	$89.08	GENERIC, Roxane Laboratories Inc	00054-3227-58
240 ml	$89.76	GENERIC, Major Pharmaceuticals Inc	00904-7897-97
240 ml	$89.88	GENERIC, Geneva Pharmaceuticals	00781-6527-08
240 ml	$90.79	GENERIC, Aligen Independent Laboratories Inc	00405-2531-77
240 ml	$91.59	GENERIC, Endo Laboratories Llc	60951-0635-35
250 ml	$91.55	GENERIC, Apotex Usa Inc	60505-0353-02
480 ml	$161.81	GENERIC, Geneva Pharmaceuticals	00781-6527-16
480 ml	$166.90	GENERIC, Alpharma Uspd Makers Of Barre and Nmc	00472-0514-16
480 ml	$170.56	GENERIC, Watson/Rugby Laboratories Inc	00536-2975-85
480 ml	$172.99	GENERIC, Moore, H.L. Drug Exchange Inc	00839-7923-69
Solution - Intravenous - 150 mg/ml			
2 ml x 10	$14.90	GENERIC, Abbott Pharmaceutical	00074-7444-01
2 ml x 10	$33.20	GENERIC, Endo Laboratories Llc	60951-0637-53
2 ml x 25	$84.20	GENERIC, Mova Pharmaceutical Corporation	55370-0202-02
2 ml x 25	$84.50	GENERIC, Endo Laboratories Llc	60951-0637-57
2 ml x 25	$214.25	GENERIC, Abbott Pharmaceutical	00074-7446-02
8 ml x 10	$35.50	GENERIC, Abbott Pharmaceutical	00074-7445-01
8 ml x 10	$102.50	GENERIC, Endo Laboratories Llc	60951-0637-69
8 ml x 25	$260.30	GENERIC, Mova Pharmaceutical Corporation	55370-0202-04
8 ml x 25	$261.60	GENERIC, Endo Laboratories Llc	60951-0637-27
Solution - Intravenous - 300 mg/50 ml;0.9%			
50 ml x 48	$149.91	GENERIC, Abbott Pharmaceutical	00074-7447-16
Solution - Intravenous - 480 mg/100 ml;0.9%			
250 ml x 12	$142.50	GENERIC, Abbott Pharmaceutical	00074-7351-02
Solution - Intravenous - 900 mg;0.9%/250 ml			
250 ml x 12	$108.75	GENERIC, Abbott Pharmaceutical	00074-7350-02
Solution - Oral - 300 mg/5 ml			
240 ml	$27.34	FEDERAL UPPER LIMIT, H.C.F.A. F F P	99999-0820-20
Tablet - Oral - 200 mg			
30's	$21.03	GENERIC, Heartland Healthcare Services	61392-0194-30
30's	$21.03	GENERIC, Heartland Healthcare Services	61392-0194-39
31's	$21.73	GENERIC, Heartland Healthcare Services	61392-0194-31
32's	$22.44	GENERIC, Heartland Healthcare Services	61392-0194-32
45's	$31.55	GENERIC, Heartland Healthcare Services	61392-0194-45
50's	$39.96	GENERIC, Ivax Corporation	00172-7111-48
60's	$42.07	GENERIC, Heartland Healthcare Services	61392-0194-60
90's	$63.10	GENERIC, Heartland Healthcare Services	61392-0194-90
100's	$12.38	FEDERAL UPPER LIMIT, H.C.F.A. F F P	99999-0820-01
100's	$73.40	GENERIC, Dixon-Shane Inc	17236-0445-01
100's	$73.49	GENERIC, West Point Pharma	59591-0259-68
100's	$75.15	GENERIC, Novopharm Usa Inc	55953-0181-01
100's	$75.42	GENERIC, Aligen Independent Laboratories Inc	00405-5370-01
100's	$76.21	GENERIC, Moore, H.L. Drug Exchange Inc	00839-7906-06
100's	$76.30	GENERIC, Martec Pharmaceuticals Inc	52555-0515-01
100's	$78.54	GENERIC, Brightstone Pharma	62939-2111-01
100's	$79.00	GENERIC, Ivax Corporation	00172-7111-60
100's	$79.90	GENERIC, Teva Pharmaceuticals Usa	00093-0111-01
100's	$79.93	GENERIC, Apothecon Inc	62269-0228-24
100's	$80.10	GENERIC, Ivax Corporation	00182-1983-01
100's	$80.35	GENERIC, Endo Laboratories Llc	60951-0630-70
100's	$81.72	GENERIC, Mova Pharmaceutical Corporation	55370-0536-07
100's	$82.15	GENERIC, Apotex Usa Inc	60505-0018-06
100's	$87.00	GENERIC, Mylan Pharmaceuticals Inc	00378-0053-01
120's	$84.13	GENERIC, Heartland Healthcare Services	61392-0194-34
Tablet - Oral - 300 mg			
8's	$6.32	GENERIC, Allscripts Pharmaceutical Company	54569-3837-04
10's	$7.28	GENERIC, Pd-Rx Pharmaceuticals	55289-0799-10
12's	$9.48	GENERIC, Allscripts Pharmaceutical Company	54569-3837-01

Qty	Price	Product	NDC
12's	$12.32	TAGAMET, Allscripts Pharmaceutical Company	54569-0438-05
12's	$13.83	TAGAMET, Pharma Pac	52959-0270-12
12's	$16.53	TAGAMET, Prescript Pharmaceuticals	00247-0189-12
14's	$11.42	GENERIC, Allscripts Pharmaceutical Company	54569-3837-07
21's	$16.59	GENERIC, Allscripts Pharmaceutical Company	54569-3837-02
21's	$26.42	TAGAMET, Prescript Pharmaceuticals	00247-0189-21
25 x 30	$620.18	GENERIC, Sky Pharmaceuticals Packaging, Inc	63739-0056-03
25's	$19.52	GENERIC, Pd-Rx Pharmaceuticals	55289-0799-97
28's	$34.12	TAGAMET, Prescript Pharmaceuticals	00247-0189-28
30's	$23.71	GENERIC, Allscripts Pharmaceutical Company	54569-3837-00
30's	$24.33	GENERIC, Heartland Healthcare Services	61392-0197-30
30's	$24.33	GENERIC, Heartland Healthcare Services	61392-0197-39
30's	$30.81	TAGAMET, Allscripts Pharmaceutical Company	54569-0438-00
30's	$31.81	GENERIC, St. Mary'S Mpp	60760-0192-30
30's	$33.47	TAGAMET, Pharma Pac	52959-0270-30
30's	$36.31	TAGAMET, Prescript Pharmaceuticals	00247-0189-30
30's	$504.00	GENERIC, Medirex Inc	57480-0813-06
31's	$25.14	GENERIC, Heartland Healthcare Services	61392-0197-31
32's	$25.95	GENERIC, Heartland Healthcare Services	61392-0197-32
35's	$38.87	TAGAMET, Pharma Pac	52959-0270-35
40's	$47.29	TAGAMET, Prescript Pharmaceuticals	00247-0189-40
45's	$36.49	GENERIC, Heartland Healthcare Services	61392-0197-45
60's	$27.03	GENERIC, Pd-Rx Pharmaceuticals	55289-0799-60
60's	$48.65	GENERIC, Heartland Healthcare Services	61392-0197-60
60's	$69.27	TAGAMET, Prescript Pharmaceuticals	00247-0189-60
60's	$89.95	TAGAMET, Pd-Rx Pharmaceuticals	55289-0249-60
90's	$72.98	GENERIC, Heartland Healthcare Services	61392-0197-90
90's	$89.43	GENERIC, St. Mary'S Mpp	60760-0192-90
100's	$13.13	FEDERAL UPPER LIMIT, H.C.F.A. F F P	99999-0820-05
100's	$73.40	GENERIC, Mova Pharmaceutical Corporation	55370-0537-07
100's	$76.00	GENERIC, Roxane Laboratories Inc	00054-4224-25
100's	$76.80	GENERIC, Dixon-Shane Inc	17236-0171-01
100's	$76.87	GENERIC, West Point Pharma	59591-0260-68
100's	$77.20	GENERIC, Aligen Independent Laboratories Inc	00405-5371-01
100's	$78.50	GENERIC, Esi Lederle Generics	00005-3416-23
100's	$78.55	GENERIC, Novopharm Usa Inc	55953-0192-01
100's	$79.79	GENERIC, Moore, H.L. Drug Exchange Inc	00839-7907-06
100's	$81.00	GENERIC, Roxane Laboratories Inc	00054-8224-25
100's	$82.90	GENERIC, Vangard Labs	00615-2534-13
100's	$83.55	GENERIC, Brightstone Pharma	62939-2121-01
100's	$83.60	GENERIC, Teva Pharmaceuticals Usa	00093-0112-01
100's	$83.68	GENERIC, Apothecon Inc	62269-0229-24
100's	$84.50	GENERIC, Sidmak Laboratories Inc	50111-0550-01
100's	$88.92	GENERIC, Mova Pharmaceutical Corporation	55370-0135-07
100's	$90.40	GENERIC, Mylan Pharmaceuticals Inc	00378-0317-01
100's	$90.44	GENERIC, Endo Laboratories Llc	60951-0631-70
100's	$90.45	GENERIC, Major Pharmaceuticals Inc	00904-5445-60
100's	$90.75	GENERIC, Ivax Corporation	00172-7117-60
100's	$93.80	GENERIC, Martec Pharmaceuticals Inc	52555-0516-01
100's	$93.89	GENERIC, Par Pharmaceutical Inc	49884-0405-01
100's	$95.20	GENERIC, Major Pharmaceuticals Inc	00904-5445-61
100's	$102.74	GENERIC, Udl Laboratories Inc	51079-0807-20
100's	$113.21	TAGAMET, Prescript Pharmaceuticals	00247-0189-00
100's	$113.63	TAGAMET, Glaxosmithkline	00108-5013-20
120's	$94.82	GENERIC, Allscripts Pharmaceutical Company	54569-3837-03
120's	$97.31	GENERIC, Heartland Healthcare Services	61392-0197-34

Tablet - Oral - 400 mg

Qty	Price	Product	NDC
6's	$8.51	GENERIC, Allscripts Pharmaceutical Company	54569-3838-03
10's	$22.88	TAGAMET, Pd-Rx Pharmaceuticals	55289-0412-10
14's	$19.07	GENERIC, Dhs Inc	55887-0748-14
14's	$19.88	GENERIC, Allscripts Pharmaceutical Company	54569-3838-02
20's	$23.63	GENERIC, Dhs Inc	55887-0748-20
20's	$33.94	TAGAMET, Allscripts Pharmaceutical Company	54569-0439-00
30 x 10	$500.31	GENERIC, Udl Laboratories Inc	51079-0808-24
30 x 25	$1017.83	GENERIC, Sky Pharmaceuticals Packaging, Inc	63739-0057-01
30's	$26.93	GENERIC, Pd-Rx Pharmaceuticals	55289-0581-30
30's	$27.52	GENERIC, Dhs Inc	55887-0748-30
30's	$39.69	GENERIC, Allscripts Pharmaceutical Company	54569-3838-00
30's	$40.20	GENERIC, Heartland Healthcare Services	61392-0200-30
30's	$40.20	GENERIC, Heartland Healthcare Services	61392-0200-39
30's	$59.41	TAGAMET, Physicians Total Care	54868-0319-02
30's	$67.50	TAGAMET, Pd-Rx Pharmaceuticals	55289-0412-30
31's	$41.54	GENERIC, Heartland Healthcare Services	61392-0200-31
32's	$42.88	GENERIC, Heartland Healthcare Services	61392-0200-32
40's	$74.50	TAGAMET, Physicians Total Care	54868-0319-06
45's	$60.30	GENERIC, Heartland Healthcare Services	61392-0200-45
60's	$16.65	GENERIC, Penn Laboratories Inc	58437-0002-18
60's	$32.25	GENERIC, Pd-Rx Pharmaceuticals	55289-0581-60
60's	$38.44	GENERIC, Dhs Inc	55887-0748-60
60's	$71.00	GENERIC, Roxane Laboratories Inc	00054-4225-21
60's	$76.59	GENERIC, Dixon-Shane Inc	17236-0447-60
60's	$78.50	GENERIC, Esi Lederle Generics	00005-3417-32
60's	$80.41	GENERIC, Heartland Healthcare Services	61392-0200-60
60's	$82.00	GENERIC, Sidmak Laboratories Inc	50111-0551-04
60's	$82.00	GENERIC, Apotex Usa Inc	60505-0020-04
60's	$83.40	GENERIC, Teva Pharmaceuticals Usa	00093-0113-06
60's	$88.08	GENERIC, Golden State Medical	60429-0047-60
60's	$97.15	GENERIC, Allscripts Pharmaceutical Company	54569-3838-01
60's	$98.60	GENERIC, Ivax Corporation	00172-7171-49
60's	$113.20	TAGAMET, Glaxosmithkline	00108-5026-18
60's	$117.62	TAGAMET, Physicians Total Care	54868-0319-01
90's	$120.61	GENERIC, Heartland Healthcare Services	61392-0200-90
90's	$138.90	TAGAMET, Allscripts Pharmaceutical Company	54569-8554-01
100's	$15.37	FEDERAL UPPER LIMIT, H.C.F.A. F F P	99999-0820-11
100's	$28.15	GENERIC, Penn Laboratories Inc	58437-0002-21
100's	$86.00	GENERIC, Roxane Laboratories Inc	00054-8225-25
100's	$118.70	GENERIC, Vangard Labs	00615-3566-13
100's	$126.86	GENERIC, West Point Pharma	59591-0261-68
100's	$127.65	GENERIC, Dixon-Shane Inc	17236-0447-01
100's	$127.65	GENERIC, Mova Pharmaceutical Corporation	55370-0539-07
100's	$129.40	GENERIC, Novopharm Usa Inc	55953-0204-01
100's	$132.37	GENERIC, Moore, H.L. Drug Exchange Inc	00839-7908-06
100's	$133.10	GENERIC, Aligen Independent Laboratories Inc	00405-5372-01
100's	$133.23	GENERIC, Moore, H.L. Drug Exchange Inc	00839-7916-06
100's	$138.04	GENERIC, Brightstone Pharma	62939-2131-01
100's	$138.72	GENERIC, Endo Laboratories Llc	60951-0632-75
100's	$138.90	GENERIC, Apothecon Inc	62269-0230-24
100's	$138.95	GENERIC, Teva Pharmaceuticals Usa	00093-0113-01
100's	$138.95	GENERIC, Novopharm Usa Inc	55953-0204-40
100's	$139.20	GENERIC, Martec Pharmaceuticals Inc	52555-0517-01
100's	$140.00	GENERIC, Sidmak Laboratories Inc	50111-0551-01
100's	$146.85	GENERIC, Major Pharmaceuticals Inc	00904-5446-60
100's	$146.85	GENERIC, Apotex Usa Inc	60505-0020-06
100's	$146.88	GENERIC, Endo Laboratories Llc	60951-0632-70
100's	$147.00	GENERIC, Mylan Pharmaceuticals Inc	00378-0372-01
100's	$149.34	GENERIC, Mova Pharmaceutical Corporation	55370-0136-07
100's	$154.55	GENERIC, Major Pharmaceuticals Inc	00904-5446-61
100's	$154.99	GENERIC, Par Pharmaceutical Inc	49884-0406-01
100's	$166.77	GENERIC, Udl Laboratories Inc	51079-0808-20
100's	$167.64	GENERIC, Ivax Corporation	00172-7171-60
180's	$239.98	GENERIC, Allscripts Pharmaceutical Company	54569-8600-00
180's	$252.23	GENERIC, Golden State Medical	60429-0047-18
180's	$277.80	TAGAMET, Allscripts Pharmaceutical Company	54569-8554-00
200 x 5	$1357.10	GENERIC, Vangard Labs	00615-3566-43

Tablet - Oral - 800 mg

Qty	Price	Product	NDC
7's	$14.48	GENERIC, Pd-Rx Pharmaceuticals	55289-0528-07
7's	$19.76	GENERIC, Allscripts Pharmaceutical Company	54569-3839-02
10 x 10	$269.50	GENERIC, Major Pharmaceuticals Inc	00904-5447-61
10's	$34.95	TAGAMET, Pd-Rx Pharmaceuticals	55289-0250-10
15's	$39.56	GENERIC, Allscripts Pharmaceutical Company	54569-3839-01
30's	$9.90	GENERIC, Apotex Usa Inc	60505-0021-02
30's	$14.80	GENERIC, Penn Laboratories Inc	58437-0003-13
30's	$67.93	GENERIC, West Point Pharma	59591-0264-31
30's	$68.90	GENERIC, Roxane Laboratories Inc	00054-4226-13
30's	$69.50	GENERIC, Esi Lederle Generics	00005-3418-38
30's	$70.15	GENERIC, Teva Pharmaceuticals Usa	00093-0122-56
30's	$70.96	GENERIC, Heartland Healthcare Services	61392-0203-30
30's	$70.96	GENERIC, Heartland Healthcare Services	61392-0203-39
30's	$72.00	GENERIC, Sidmak Laboratories Inc	50111-0552-10
30's	$74.71	GENERIC, Major Pharmaceuticals Inc	00904-5447-46
30's	$74.71	GENERIC, Endo Laboratories Llc	60951-0633-30
30's	$74.99	GENERIC, Golden State Medical	60429-0048-30
30's	$78.20	TAGAMET, Glaxosmithkline	00108-5027-76
30's	$79.13	GENERIC, Dixon-Shane Inc	17236-0172-30
30's	$79.13	GENERIC, Allscripts Pharmaceutical Company	54569-3839-00
30's	$85.70	GENERIC, Ivax Corporation	00172-7711-46
31's	$73.32	GENERIC, Heartland Healthcare Services	61392-0203-31
32's	$75.69	GENERIC, Heartland Healthcare Services	61392-0203-32
45's	$106.43	GENERIC, Heartland Healthcare Services	61392-0203-45
60's	$141.91	GENERIC, Heartland Healthcare Services	61392-0203-60
60's	$147.69	GENERIC, Mova Pharmaceutical Corporation	55370-0137-06
60's	$165.45	GENERIC, Par Pharmaceutical Inc	49884-0407-02
90's	$212.87	GENERIC, Heartland Healthcare Services	61392-0203-90
90's	$233.09	GENERIC, Golden State Medical	60429-0048-90
100's	$27.75	FEDERAL UPPER LIMIT, H.C.F.A. F F P	99999-0820-16
100's	$30.86	GENERIC, Apotex Usa Inc	60505-0021-03
100's	$49.65	GENERIC, Penn Laboratories Inc	58437-0003-21
100's	$220.00	GENERIC, Sidmak Laboratories Inc	50111-0552-01
100's	$230.00	GENERIC, Roxane Laboratories Inc	00054-8226-25
100's	$236.26	GENERIC, Geneva Pharmaceuticals	00781-1444-13
100's	$245.10	GENERIC, Novopharm Usa Inc	55953-0235-01
100's	$246.04	GENERIC, Brightstone Pharma	62939-2141-01
100's	$246.15	GENERIC, Mova Pharmaceutical Corporation	55370-0540-07
100's	$250.00	GENERIC, Apothecon Inc	62269-0231-24

100's	$256.05	GENERIC, Major Pharmaceuticals Inc	00904-5447-60
100's	$260.67	GENERIC, Moore, H.L. Drug Exchange Inc	00839-7909-06
100's	$263.75	GENERIC, Teva Pharmaceuticals Usa	00093-0122-01
100's	$263.75	GENERIC, Dixon-Shane Inc	17236-0172-01
100's	$263.75	GENERIC, Teva Pharmaceuticals Usa	55953-0305-40
100's	$264.20	GENERIC, Aligen Independent Laboratories Inc	00405-5373-01
100's	$266.50	GENERIC, Martec Pharmaceuticals Inc	52555-0518-01
100's	$282.35	GENERIC, Mylan Pharmaceuticals Inc	00378-0541-01
100's	$283.80	GENERIC, Ivax Corporation	00172-7711-60
100's	$290.82	GENERIC, Udl Laboratories Inc	51079-0809-20
250's	$323.15	GENERIC, Par Pharmaceutical Inc	49884-0407-04
250's	$649.55	GENERIC, Mova Pharmaceutical Corporation	55370-0137-25

PRODUCT LISTING - EQUIVALENTS NOT AVAILABLE

Liquid - Oral - 300 mg/5 ml			
5 ml x 10	$26.85	TAGAMET, Glaxosmithkline	00108-5014-75
240 ml	$108.84	TAGAMET, Glaxosmithkline	00108-5014-76
Solution - Intravenous - 150 mg/ml			
2 ml x 25	$99.05	TAGAMET, Glaxosmithkline	00108-5017-77
8 ml x 10	$128.61	TAGAMET, Glaxosmithkline	00108-5022-76
200 ml	$306.26	TAGAMET, Glaxosmithkline	00108-5022-75
Solution - Intravenous - 900 mg;0.9%/500 ml			
500 ml x 24	$240.00	GENERIC, Abbott Pharmaceutical	00074-7352-03
Solution - Intravenous - 900 mg;0.9%/1000 ml			
1000 ml x 12	$120.00	GENERIC, Abbott Pharmaceutical	00074-7354-09
Solution - Intravenous - 1200 mg;0.9%/500 ml			
500 ml x 24	$285.00	GENERIC, Abbott Pharmaceutical	00074-7353-03
Solution - Intravenous - 1200 mg;0.9%/1000 ml			
1000 ml x 6	$142.50	GENERIC, Abbott Pharmaceutical	00074-7355-09
Tablet - Oral - 200 mg			
16's	$11.36	GENERIC, Pharma Pac	52959-0374-16
20's	$14.23	GENERIC, Pharma Pac	52959-0374-20
30's	$21.50	GENERIC, Pharma Pac	52959-0374-30
40's	$28.76	GENERIC, Pharma Pac	52959-0374-40
60's	$42.60	GENERIC, Pharma Pac	52959-0374-60
100's	$65.59	GENERIC, Pharma Pac	52959-0374-00
100's	$76.20	GENERIC, Major Pharmaceuticals Inc	00904-7866-60
100's	$96.55	TAGAMET, Glaxosmithkline	00108-5012-20
Tablet - Oral - 300 mg			
12's	$12.12	GENERIC, Southwood Pharmaceuticals Inc	58016-0510-12
12's	$13.05	GENERIC, Pharma Pac	52959-0345-12
20's	$20.20	GENERIC, Southwood Pharmaceuticals Inc	58016-0510-20
21's	$21.21	GENERIC, Southwood Pharmaceuticals Inc	58016-0510-21
30's	$30.31	GENERIC, Southwood Pharmaceuticals Inc	58016-0510-30
30's	$30.36	GENERIC, Pharma Pac	52959-0345-30
35's	$35.37	GENERIC, Pharma Pac	52959-0345-35
40's	$40.40	GENERIC, Southwood Pharmaceuticals Inc	58016-0510-40
40's	$40.42	GENERIC, Pharma Pac	52959-0345-40
50's	$50.50	GENERIC, Southwood Pharmaceuticals Inc	58016-0510-50
60's	$59.59	GENERIC, Pharma Pac	52959-0345-60
60's	$60.62	GENERIC, Southwood Pharmaceuticals Inc	58016-0510-60
90's	$88.19	GENERIC, Pharma Pac	52959-0345-90
100's	$23.50	GENERIC, Raway Pharmacal Inc	00686-0813-01
100's	$79.75	GENERIC, Major Pharmaceuticals Inc	00904-7867-60
100's	$88.92	GENERIC, Stada Pharmaceuticals Inc	67253-0340-10
100's	$101.00	GENERIC, Southwood Pharmaceuticals Inc	58016-0510-00
Tablet - Oral - 400 mg			
6's	$9.40	GENERIC, Pharmaceutical Corporation Of America	51655-0671-87
9's	$15.09	GENERIC, Southwood Pharmaceuticals Inc	58016-0696-09
10's	$16.76	GENERIC, Southwood Pharmaceuticals Inc	58016-0696-10
12's	$17.80	GENERIC, Pharmaceutical Corporation Of America	51655-0671-27
12's	$20.11	GENERIC, Southwood Pharmaceuticals Inc	58016-0696-12
14's	$23.47	GENERIC, Southwood Pharmaceuticals Inc	58016-0696-14
14's	$24.20	GENERIC, Pharma Pac	52959-0375-14
15's	$25.15	GENERIC, Southwood Pharmaceuticals Inc	58016-0696-15
15's	$25.91	GENERIC, Pharma Pac	52959-0375-15
16's	$26.83	GENERIC, Southwood Pharmaceuticals Inc	58016-0696-16
16's	$27.48	GENERIC, Pharma Pac	52959-0375-16
20's	$33.53	GENERIC, Southwood Pharmaceuticals Inc	58016-0696-20
20's	$34.18	GENERIC, Pharma Pac	52959-0375-20
21's	$35.20	GENERIC, Southwood Pharmaceuticals Inc	58016-0696-21
24's	$40.26	GENERIC, Southwood Pharmaceuticals Inc	58016-0696-24
28's	$46.95	GENERIC, Southwood Pharmaceuticals Inc	58016-0696-28
30's	$50.33	GENERIC, Southwood Pharmaceuticals Inc	58016-0696-30
30's	$50.63	GENERIC, Pharma Pac	52959-0375-30
32's	$53.65	GENERIC, Southwood Pharmaceuticals Inc	58016-0696-32
40's	$57.00	GENERIC, Pharmaceutical Corporation Of America	51655-0671-51
40's	$66.91	GENERIC, Pharma Pac	52959-0375-40
40's	$67.06	GENERIC, Southwood Pharmaceuticals Inc	58016-0696-40
60's	$85.00	GENERIC, Pharmaceutical Corporation Of America	51655-0671-25
60's	$100.60	GENERIC, Southwood Pharmaceuticals Inc	58016-0696-60
60's	$100.79	GENERIC, Pharma Pac	52959-0375-60
80's	$134.22	GENERIC, Southwood Pharmaceuticals Inc	58016-0696-80
100's	$36.00	GENERIC, Raway Pharmacal Inc	00686-0814-01
100's	$134.00	GENERIC, Major Pharmaceuticals Inc	00904-7868-60
100's	$149.34	GENERIC, Stada Pharmaceuticals Inc	67253-0341-10
100's	$153.35	GENERIC, Pharma Pac	52959-0375-00
100's	$167.66	GENERIC, Southwood Pharmaceuticals Inc	58016-0696-00
Tablet - Oral - 800 mg			
7's	$20.00	GENERIC, Southwood Pharmaceuticals Inc	58016-0530-07
9's	$25.72	GENERIC, Southwood Pharmaceuticals Inc	58016-0530-09
12's	$34.30	GENERIC, Southwood Pharmaceuticals Inc	58016-0530-12
15's	$42.87	GENERIC, Southwood Pharmaceuticals Inc	58016-0530-15
16's	$47.71	GENERIC, Pharma Pac	52959-0376-16
20's	$57.17	GENERIC, Southwood Pharmaceuticals Inc	58016-0530-20
20's	$57.74	GENERIC, Pharma Pac	52959-0376-20
24's	$68.60	GENERIC, Southwood Pharmaceuticals Inc	58016-0530-24
30's	$85.75	GENERIC, Southwood Pharmaceuticals Inc	58016-0530-30
30's	$86.73	GENERIC, Pharma Pac	52959-0376-30
40's	$110.78	GENERIC, Pharma Pac	52959-0376-40
60's	$149.10	GENERIC, Pharma Pac	52959-0376-60
60's	$159.60	GENERIC, Warner Chilcott Laboratories	00047-0508-20
100's	$236.50	GENERIC, Major Pharmaceuticals Inc	00904-7869-60
100's	$285.83	GENERIC, Southwood Pharmaceuticals Inc	58016-0530-00
100's	$394.43	GENERIC, Pharma Pac	52959-0376-00

Ciprofloxacin Hydrochloride *(000823)*

For related information, see the comparative table section in Appendix A.

Categories: Anthrax; Bronchitis, chronic, acute exacerbation; Conjunctivitis, infectious; Diarrhea, infectious; Gonorrhea; Infection, bone; Infection, genital tract; Infection, intra-abdominal; Infection, joint; Infection, lower respiratory tract; Infection, sexually transmitted; Infection, skin and skin structures; Infection, upper respiratory tract; Infection, urinary tract; Neutropenia, febrile; Pneumonia, nosocomial; Prostatitis; Shigellosis; Typhoid fever; Ulcer, corneal; Pregnancy Category C; FDA Approved 1987 Oct; WHO Formulary

Drug Classes: Antibiotics, quinolones; Anti-infectives, ophthalmic; Ophthalmics

Brand Names: Ciloxan; **Cipro**; Cipro XR

Foreign Brand Availability: Acire (Korea); Alcon Cilox (Colombia; Indonesia); Bacquinor (Indonesia); Bactiflox Lactab (Bahamas; Barbados; Belize; Bermuda; Curacao; Guyana; Jamaica; Netherland-Antilles; Puerto-Rico; Surinam; Trinidad); Baflox (Colombia); Baycip (Spain); Bernoflox (Indonesia); Cetraxal (Guatemala; Honduras; Panama; Spain); C-Flox (Australia); C-Floxacin (Thailand); Ciflox (France; Taiwan); Cifloxin (Thailand); Cifran (Benin; Burkina-Faso; Ethiopia; Gambia; Ghana; Guinea; India; Ivory-Coast; Kenya; Liberia; Malawi; Mali; Mauritania; Mauritius; Morocco; Niger; Nigeria; Senegal; Seychelles; Sierra-Leone; Sudan; Tanzania; Tunia; Uganda; Zambia; Zimbabwe); Cilab (Thailand); Ciloquin (Australia); Cimogal (Mexico); Cinaflox (Peru); Cipide (Hong-Kong); Ciplox (Benin; Burkina-Faso; Ethiopia; Gambia; Ghana; Guinea; India; Israel; Ivory-Coast; Kenya; Liberia; Malawi; Mali; Mauritania; Mauritius; Morocco; Niger; Nigeria; Senegal; Seychelles; Sierra-Leone; South-Africa; Sudan; Tanzania; Tunia; Uganda; Zambia; Zimbabwe); Ciplus (Korea); Ciprecu (Ecuador); Ciprinol (Bulgaria; Hungary); Ciprobac (Mexico); Ciprobay (Bahrain; Bulgaria; China; Cyprus; Czech-Republic; Egypt; Germany; Hungary; Iran; Iraq; Israel; Jordan; Korea; Kuwait; Lebanon; Libya; Malaysia; Oman; Philippines; Qatar; Republic-of-Yemen; Saudi-Arabia; South-Africa; Syria; Thailand; United-Arab-Emirates); Ciprobay Uro (Germany); Ciprobid (Bahrain; Benin; Burkina-Faso; Cyprus; Egypt; Ethiopia; Gambia; Ghana; Guinea; India; Iran; Iraq; Israel; Ivory-Coast; Jordan; Kenya; Kuwait; Lebanon; Liberia; Libya; Malawi; Mali; Mauritania; Mauritius; Morocco; Niger; Nigeria; Oman; Qatar; Republic-of-Yemen; Saudi-Arabia; Senegal; Seychelles; Sierra-Leone; Sudan; Syria; Tanzania; Thailand; Tunia; Uganda; United-Arab-Emirates; Zambia; Zimbabwe); Ciprobiotic (Dominican-Republic); Ciprocan (Korea); Ciprocep (Thailand); Ciprocin (Bahrain; Cyprus; Egypt; Iran; Iraq; Jordan; Kuwait; Lebanon; Libya; Oman; Qatar; Republic-of-Yemen; Saudi-Arabia; Syria; United-Arab-Emirates); Ciprocinol (Bulgaria); Ciprodar (Bahrain; Cyprus; Egypt; Iran; Iraq; Israel; Jordan; Kuwait; Lebanon; Libya; Oman; Qatar; Republic-of-Yemen; Saudi-Arabia; Syria; United-Arab-Emirates); Ciprodex (Israel); Ciproflox (Bulgaria; Mexico; Peru); Ciprogis (Israel); Ciproglen (Thailand); Ciprok (Spain); Ciprolin (Peru); Ciprolon (Bahrain; Cyprus; Egypt; Iran; Iraq; Israel; Jordan; Kuwait; Lebanon; Libya; Oman; Qatar; Republic-of-Yemen; Saudi-Arabia; Syria; United-Arab-Emirates); Cipromycin (Greece); Cipropharm (Bahrain; Cyprus; Egypt; Iran; Iraq; Jordan; Kuwait; Lebanon; Libya; Oman; Qatar; Republic-of-Yemen; Saudi-Arabia; Syria; United-Arab-Emirates); Ciproquin (Bahrain; Cyprus; Egypt; Iran; Iraq; Jordan; Kuwait; Lebanon; Libya; Oman; Qatar; Republic-of-Yemen; Saudi-Arabia; Syria; United-Arab-Emirates); Ciproquinol (Portugal); Ciproxacol (Peru); Ciproxan (Japan; Thailand); Ciproxin (Australia; Austria; Denmark; England; Finland; Greece; Hong-Kong; Indonesia; Ireland; Israel; Italy; Netherlands; New-Zealand; Norway; Sweden; Switzerland; Taiwan); Ciproxina (Bahamas; Barbados; Belize; Bermuda; Costa-Rica; Curacao; Dominican-Republic; Ecuador; El-Salvador; Guatemala; Guyana; Honduras; Jamaica; Mexico; Netherland-Antilles; Nicaragua; Panama; Portugal; Puerto-Rico; Surinam; Trinidad); Ciproxine (Belgium); Ciproxyl (Thailand); Ciprox (Bahrain; Cyprus; Egypt; Iran; Iraq; Jordan; Kuwait; Lebanon; Libya; Oman; Qatar; Republic-of-Yemen; Saudi-Arabia; Syria; United-Arab-Emirates); Ciriax (Peru); Cirokan (Korea); Ciroxin (Singapore); Citopcin (Korea); Cixa (Taiwan); Corsacin (Indonesia); Cosflox (India); Cycin (Korea; Singapore); Cysfec (Korea); Eni (Mexico); Fimoflox (Indonesia); Floroxin (Bahrain; Cyprus; Egypt; Iran; Iraq; Jordan; Kuwait; Lebanon; Libya; Oman; Qatar; Republic-of-Yemen; Saudi-Arabia; Syria; United-Arab-Emirates); Floxager (Mexico); Floxantina (Mexico); Floxbio (Indonesia); Grifociprox (Peru); H-Next (Colombia); Inciflox (Indonesia); Isotic (Indonesia); Jayacin (Indonesia); K-Sacin (Korea); Kenzoflex (Mexico); Lofucin (Korea); Loxan (Colombia; Ecuador); Medociprin (Thailand); Mitroken (Mexico); Neofloxin (Singapore); Nivoflox (Mexico); Opthaflox (Thailand); Otosec (Colombia); Probiox (Peru); Proflaxin (Costa-Rica; Nicaragua); Proflox (Thailand); Proksi 250 (El-Salvador; Guatemala; Honduras); Proksi 500 (El-Salvador; Guatemala; Honduras); Qilaflox (Indonesia); Quinobiotic (Peru); Quinolide (El-Salvador; Guatemala; Honduras); Quintor (Bahrain; India; Republic-Of-Yemen); Qupron (Korea); Rofcin (Korea); Rosacin Eye Drop (Korea); Septicide (Peru); Sifloks (Bahrain; Cyprus; Egypt; Iran; Iraq; Jordan; Kuwait; Lebanon; Libya; Oman; Qatar; Republic-of-Yemen; Saudi-Arabia; Syria; United-Arab-Emirates); Siprogut (Korea); Sophixin Ofteno (Mexico); Spitacin (Korea); Superocin (Taiwan); Unex (Ecuador); Uniflox (France); Uroxin (Singapore); Zipra (Mexico); Zumaflox (Indonesia)

Cost of Therapy: $32.95 (Infection, Ophthalmic; Ciloxan Ophthalmic; 0.3%; 5 ml; 8 drops/day; 7 day supply)
$72.10 (Infection; Cipro; 500 mg; 2 tablets/day; 7 day supply)

ORAL

DESCRIPTION

TABLETS AND ORAL SUSPENSION

Ciprofloxacin hydrochloride tablets and oral suspension are synthetic broad spectrum antimicrobial agents for oral administration. Ciprofloxacin hydrochloride, a fluoroquinolone, is the monohydrochloride monohydrate salt of 1-cyclopropyl-6-fluoro-1, 4-dihydro-4-oxo-7-(1-piperazinyl)-3-quinolinecarboxylic acid. It is a faintly yellowish to light yellow crystalline substance with a molecular weight of 385.8. Its empirical formula is $C_{17}H_{18}FN_3O_3{\cdot}HCl{\cdot}H_2O$.

Ciprofloxacin is 1-cyclopropyl-6-fluoro-1,4-dihydro-4-oxo-7-(1-piperazinyl)-3- quinolinecarboxylic acid. Its empirical formula is $C_{17}H_{18}FN_3O_3$ and its molecular weight is 331.4. It is a faintly yellowish to light yellow crystalline substance.

EXTENDED-RELEASE TABLETS

Ciprofloxacin extended-release tablets contain ciprofloxacin, a synthetic broad-spectrum antimicrobial agent for oral administration. Cipro XR tablets are coated, bilayer tablets consisting of an immediate-release layer and an erosion-matrix type controlled-release layer. The tablets contain a combination of 2 types of ciprofloxacin drug substance, ciprofloxacin hydrochloride and ciprofloxacin betaine (base). Ciprofloxacin hydrochloride is 1-cyclopropyl-6-fluoro-1,4-dihydro-4-oxo-7-(1-piperazinyl)-3-quinolinecarboxylic acid hydrochloride. It is provided as a mixture of the monohydrate and the sesquihydrate. The empirical formula of the monohydrate is $C_{17}H_{18}FN_3O_3 \cdot HCl \cdot H_2O$ and its molecular weight is 385.8. The empirical formula of the sesquihydrate is $C_{17}H_{18}FN_3O3 \cdot HCl \cdot 1.5\ H_2O$ and its molecular weight is 394.8. The drug substance is a faintly yellowish to light yellow crystalline substance.

Ciprofloxacin betaine is 1-cyclopropyl-6-fluoro-1, 4-dihydro-4-oxo-7-(1-piperazinyl)-3-quinolinecarboxylic acid. As a hydrate, its empirical formula is $C_{17}H_{18}FN_3O_3 \cdot 3.5\ H_2O$ and its molecular weight is 394.3. It is a pale yellowish to light yellow crystalline substance.

C

TABLETS

Cipro film-coated tablets are available in 100, 250, 500, and 750 mg (ciprofloxacin equivalent) strengths. Ciprofloxacin tablets are white to slightly yellowish. The inactive ingredients are cornstarch, microcrystalline cellulose, silicon dioxide, crospovidone, magnesium stearate, hydroxypropyl methylcellulose, titanium dioxide, polyethylene glycol and water.

ORAL SUSPENSION

Ciprofloxacin oral suspension is available in 5% (5 g ciprofloxacin in 100 ml) and 10% (10 g ciprofloxacin in 100 ml) strengths. Ciprofloxacin oral suspension is a white to slightly yellowish suspension with strawberry flavor which may contain yellow-orange droplets. It is composed of ciprofloxacin microcapsules and diluent which are mixed prior to dispensing (see instructions for use/handling found in the product packaging).

The components of the suspension have the following compositions:

Microcapsules: Ciprofloxacin, polyvinylpyrrolidone, methacrylic acid copolymer, hydroxypropyl methylcellulose, magnesium stearate, and polysorbate 20.

Diluent: Medium-chain triglycerides, sucrose, lecithin, water, and strawberry flavor.

Does not comply with USP with regards to "loss on drying" and "residue on ignition".

EXTENDED-RELEASE

Cipro XR tablets are available as 500 mg (ciprofloxacin equivalent) tablets strengths. Cipro XR tablets are nearly white to slightly yellowish, film-coated, oblong-shaped tablets. Each Cipro XR 500 mg tablet contains 500 mg of ciprofloxacin as ciprofloxacin HCl (287.5 mg, calculated as ciprofloxacin on the dried basis) and ciprofloxacin* (212.6 mg, calculated on the dried basis). The inactive ingredients are crospovidone, hypromellose, magnesium stearate, polyethylene glycol, silica colloidal anhydrous, succinic acid, and titanium dioxide.

*Does not comply with USP with regards to "loss on drying" and "residue on ignition".

CLINICAL PHARMACOLOGY

ABSORPTION

Ciprofloxacin given as an oral tablet is rapidly and well absorbed from the gastrointestinal tract after oral administration. The absolute bioavailability is approximately 70% with no substantial loss by first pass metabolism. Ciprofloxacin maximum serum concentrations and area under the curve are shown in TABLE 1 for the 250-1000 mg dose range.

TABLE 1

Dose	Maximum Serum Concentration	Area Under Curve (AUC)
250 mg	1.2 μg/ml	4.8 μg·h/ml
500 mg	2.4 μg/ml	11.6 μg·h/ml
750 mg	4.3 μg/ml	20.2 μg·h/ml
1000 mg	5.4 μg/ml	30.8 μg·h/ml

Maximum serum concentrations are attained 1-2 hours after oral dosing. Mean concentrations 12 hours after dosing with 250, 500, or 750 mg are 0.1, 0.2, and 0.4 μg/ml, respectively. The serum elimination half-life in subjects with normal renal function is approximately 4 hours. Serum concentrations increase proportionately with doses up to 1000 mg.

A 500 mg oral dose given every 12 hours has been shown to produce an area under the serum concentration time curve (AUC) equivalent to that produced by an intravenous (IV) infusion of 400 mg ciprofloxacin given over 60 minutes every 12 hours. A 750 mg oral dose given every 12 hours has been shown to produce an AUC at steady-state equivalent to that produced by an IV infusion of 400 mg given over 60 minutes every 8 hours. A 750 mg oral dose results in a C_{max} similar to that observed with a 400 mg IV dose. A 250 mg oral dose given every 12 hours produces an AUC equivalent to that produced by an infusion of 200 mg ciprofloxacin given every 12 hours. See TABLE 2.

TABLE 2 *Steady-State Pharmacokinetic Parameters Following Multiple Oral and IV Doses*

Parameters	500 mg q12h, PO	400 mg q12h, IV	750 mg q12h, PO	400 mg q8h, IV
AUC (μg·h/ml)	13.7*	12.7*	31.6†	32.9‡
C_{max} (μg/ml)	2.97	4.56	3.59	4.07

* AUC(0-12h)
† AUC 24h = AUC(0-12h) × 2
‡ AUC 24h = AUC(0-8h) × 3

Ciprofloxacin extended-release tablets are formulated to release drug at a slower rate compared to immediate-release tablets. Approximately 35% of the dose is contained within an immediate-release component, while the remaining 65% is contained in a slow-release matrix.

Maximum plasma ciprofloxacin concentrations are attained between 1 and 4 hours after dosing with ciprofloxacin extended-release tablets. In comparison to the 250 mg ciprofloxacin immediate-release bid treatment, which is approved for the treatment of uncomplicated urinary tract infections, the C_{max} of ciprofloxacin extended-release tablets 500 mg once daily is higher, while the AUC over 24 hours is equivalent.

TABLE 3 compares the pharmacokinetic parameters obtained at steady state for these 2 treatment regimens (500 mg qd ciprofloxacin extended-release tablets versus 250 mg bid ciprofloxacin immediate-release tablets).

TABLE 3 *Ciprofloxacin Pharmacokinetics (Mean ± SD) Following Ciprofloxacin HCl and Ciprofloxacin XR Administration*

	C_{max} (mg/L)	AUC 0-24h (mg·h/L)	$T_{1/2}$ (hr)	T_{max} (hr)*
Ciprofloxacin XR 500 mg qd	1.59 ± 0.43	7.97 ± 1.87	6.6 ± 1.4	1.5 (1.0-2.5)
Ciprofloxacin 250 mg bid	1.14 ± 0.23	8.25 ± 2.15	4.8 ± 0.6	1.0 (0.5-2.5)

* Median (range).

DISTRIBUTION

The binding of ciprofloxacin to serum proteins is 20-40% which is not likely to be high enough to cause significant protein binding interactions with other drugs.

After oral administration, ciprofloxacin is widely distributed throughout the body. Tissue concentrations often exceed serum concentrations in both men and women, particularly in genital tissue including the prostate. Ciprofloxacin is present in active forem in the saliva, nasal and bronchial secretions, mucosa of the sinuses, sputum, skin blister fluid, lymph, peritoneal fluid, bile, and prostatic secretions. Ciprofloxacin has also been detected in lung, skin, fat, muscle, cartilage, and bone. The drug diffuses into the cerebrospinal fluid (CSF); however, CSF concentrations are generally less than 10% of peak serum concentrations. Low levels of the drug have been detected in the aqueous and vitreous humors of the eye.

Following administration of a single dose of ciprofloxacin XR, ciprofloxacin concentrations in urine collected up to 4 hours after dosing averaged over 300 mg/L; in urine excreted from 12-24 hours after dosing, ciprofloxacin concentration averaged 27 mg/L.

METABOLISM

Four (4) metabolites of ciprofloxacin were identified in human urine. The metabolites have antimicrobial activity, but are less active than unchanged ciprofloxacin. The primary metabolites are oxociprofloxacin (M3) and sulfociprofloxacin (M2), each accounting for roughly 3-8% of the total dose. Other minor metabolites are desethylene ciprofloxacin (M1), and formylciprofloxacin (M4). The relative proportion of drug and metabolite in serum corresponds to the composition found in urine. Excretion of these metabolites was essentially complete by 24 hours after dosing.

EXCRETION

The serum elimination half-life in subjects with normal renal function is approximately 4 hours. Approximately 40-50% of an orally administered dose is excreted in the urine as unchanged drug. After a 250 mg oral dose, urine concentrations of ciprofloxacin usually exceed 200 μg/ml during the first 2 hours and are approximately 30 μg/ml at 8-12 hours after dosing. The urinary excretion of ciprofloxacin is virtually complete within 24 hours after dosing. The renal clearance of ciprofloxacin, which is approximately 300 ml/min, exceeds the normal glomerular filtration rate of 120 ml/min. Thus, active tubular secretion would seem to play a significant role in its elimination. Coadministration of probenecid with ciprofloxacin results in about a 50% reduction in the ciprofloxacin renal clearance and a 50% increase in its concentration in the systemic circulation. Although bile concentrations of ciprofloxacin are several fold higher than serum concentrations after oral dosing, only a small amount of the dose administered is recovered from the bile as unchanged drug. An additional 1-2% of the dose is recovered from the bile in the form of metabolites. Approximately 20-35% of an oral dose is recovered from the feces within 5 days after dosing. This may arise from either biliary clearance or transintestinal elimination.

The elimination kinetics of ciprofloxacin are similar for the immediate-release and the ciprofloxacin XR tablet.

With oral administration, a 500 mg dose, given as 10 ml of the 5% ciprofloxacin oral suspension (containing 250 mg ciprofloxacin/5 ml) is bioequivalent to the 500 mg tablet. A 10 ml volume of the 5% ciprofloxacin oral suspension (containing 250 mg ciprofloxacin/5 ml) is bioequivalent to a 5 ml volume of the 10% ciprofloxacin oral suspension (containing 500 mg ciprofloxacin/5 ml).

DRUG-DRUG INTERACTIONS

When ciprofloxacin HCl tablet is given concomitantly with food, there is a delay in the absorption of the drug, resulting in peak concentrations that occur closer to 2 hours after dosing rather than 1 hour whereas there is no delay observed when ciprofloxacin oral suspension is given with food. The overall absorption of ciprofloxacin HCl tablet or ciprofloxacin oral suspension, however, is not substantially affected. The pharmacokinetics of ciprofloxacin given as the suspension are also not affected by food.

Extended-Release Tablets

Results of the pharmacokinetic studies demonstrate that ciprofloxacin XR may be administered with or without food (*e.g.* high-fat and low-fat meals or under fasted conditions).

Previous studies with immediate-release ciprofloxacin have shown that concomitant administration of ciprofloxacin with theophylline decreases the clearance of theophylline resulting in elevated serum theophylline levels and increased risk of a patient developing CNS or other adverse reactions. Ciprofloxacin also decreases caffeine clearance and inhibits the formation of paraxanthine after caffeine administration. Absorption of ciprofloxacin is significantly reduced by concomitant administration of multivalent cation-containing products such as magnesium/aluminum antacids, sucralfate, Videx (didanosine) chewable/buffered tablets or pediatric powder, or products containing calcium, iron, or zinc (see DRUG INTERACTIONS and PRECAUTIONS, Information for the Patient and DOSAGE AND ADMINISTRATION).

Antacids

Concurrent administration of antacids containing magnesium hydroxide or aluminum hydroxide may reduce the bioavailability of ciprofloxacin by as much as 90%.

When ciprofloxacin XR given as a single 1000 mg dose (twice the recommended daily dose) was administered 2 hours before, or 4 hours after a magnesium/aluminum-containing antacid (900 mg aluminum hydroxide and 600 mg magnesium hydroxide as a single oral dose) to 18 healthy volunteers, there was a 4% and 19% reduction, respectively, in the mean C_{max} of ciprofloxacin. The reduction in the mean AUC was 24% and 26%, respectively. Ciprofloxacin XR should be administered at least 2 hours before or 6 hours after antacids containing magnesium or aluminum, as well as sucralfate, Videx (didanosine) chewable/buffered tablets or pediatric powder, metal cations such as iron, and multivitamin preparations with zinc. Although ciprofloxacin XR may be taken with meals that include milk, concomitant administration with dairy products or with calcium-fortified juices alone should be avoided, since decreased absorption is possible (see DRUG INTERACTIONS and PRECAUTIONS, Information for the Patient and DOSAGE AND ADMINISTRATION).

Omeprazole

When ciprofloxacin XR was administered as a single 1000 mg dose (twice the recommended daily dose) concomitantly with omeprazole (40 mg once daily for 3 days) to 18 healthy volunteers, the mean AUC and C_{max} of ciprofloxacin were reduced by 20% and 23%, respectively (see DRUG INTERACTIONS). These differences are not considered clinically significant.

Metronidazole

The serum concentrations of ciprofloxacin and metronidazole were not altered when these 2 drugs were given concomitantly.

SPECIAL POPULATIONS

Pharmacokinetic studies of the oral (single dose) and IV (single and multiple dose) forms of ciprofloxacin indicate that plasma concentrations of ciprofloxacin are higher in elderly subjects (>65 years) as compared to young adults. Although the C_{max} is increased 16-40%, the increase in mean AUC is approximately 30%, and can be at least partially attributed to decreased renal clearance in the elderly. Elimination half-life is only slightly (~20%) prolonged in the elderly. These differences are not considered clinically significant. (See PRECAUTIONS, Geriatric Use.)

In patients with reduced renal function, the half-life of ciprofloxacin is slightly prolonged. Dosage adjustments may be required. (See DOSAGE AND ADMINISTRATION.)

Extended-Release Tablets

No dose adjustment is required for patients with uncomplicated urinary tract infections receiving 500 mg ciprofloxacin XR. The total drug exposure attained with 500 mg ciprofloxacin XR is similar to or less than that achieved with a single dose of 500 mg immediate-release ciprofloxacin, which is approved for use in patients with severe renal impairment.

In preliminary studies in patients with stable chronic liver cirrhosis, no significant changes in ciprofloxacin pharmacokinetics have been observed. The kinetics of ciprofloxacin in patients with acute hepatic insufficiency, however, have not been fully elucidated.

MICROBIOLOGY

Ciprofloxacin has *in vitro* activity against a wide range of gram-negative and gram-positive microorganisms. The bactericidal action of ciprofloxacin results from inhibition of the enzymes topoisomerase II (DNA gyrase) and topoisomerase IV, which are required for bacterial DNA replication, transcription, repair, and recombination. The mechanism of action of fluoroquinolones, including ciprofloxacin, is different from that of penicillins, cephalosporins, aminoglycosides, macrolides, and tetracyclines; therefore, microorganisms resistant to these classes of drugs may be susceptible to ciprofloxacin and other quinolones. There is no known cross-resistance between ciprofloxacin and other classes of antimicrobials. *In vitro* resistance to ciprofloxacin develops slowly by multiple step mutations.

Resistance to ciprofloxacin due to spontaneous mutations occurs at a general frequency of between $<10^{-9}$ to 1×10^{-6}.

Ciprofloxacin is slightly less active when tested at acidic pH. The inoculum size has little effect when tested *in vitro*. The minimal bactericidal concentration (MBC) generally does not exceed the minimal inhibitory concentration (MIC) by more than a factor of 2.

Ciprofloxacin has been shown to be active against most strains of the following microorganisms, both *in vitro* and in clinical infections as described in INDICATIONS AND USAGE.

Aerobic Gram-Positive Microorganisms

Enterococcus faecalis (many strains are only moderately susceptible), *Staphylococcus aureus* (methicillin—susceptible strains only), *Staphylococcus epidermidis* (methicillin-susceptible strains only), *Staphylococcus saprophyticus, Streptococcus pneumoniae* (penicillin-susceptible strains only), *Streptococcus pyogenes.*

Aerobic Gram-Negative Microorganisms

Campylobacter jejuni, Citrobacter diversus, Citrobacter freundii, Enterobacter cloacae, Escherichia coli, Haemophilus influenzae, Haemophilus parainfluenzae, Klebsiella pneumoniae, Moraxella catarrhalis, Morganella morganii, Neisseria gonorrhoeae, Proteus mirabilis, Proteus vulgaris, Providencia rettgeri, Providencia stuartii, Pseudomonas aeruginosa, Salmonella typhi, Serratia marcescens, Shigella boydii, Shigella dysenteriae, Shigella flexneri, Shigella sonnei.

Ciprofloxacin has been shown to be active against *Bacillus anthracis* both *in vitro* and by use of serum levels as a surrogate marker (see INDICATIONS AND USAGE).

The following *in vitro* data are available, **but their clinical significance is unknown.**

Ciprofloxacin exhibits *in vitro* minimum inhibitory concentrations (MICs) of 1 μg/ml or less against most (≥90%) strains of the following microorganisms; however, the safety and effectiveness of ciprofloxacin in treating clinical infections due to these microorganisms have not been established in adequate and well-controlled clinical trials.

Aerobic Gram-Positive Microorganisms

Staphylococcus haemolyticus, Staphylococcus hominis, Streptococcus pneumoniae (penicillin-resistant strains only).

Aerobic Gram-Negative Microorganisms

Acinetobacter lwoffi, Aeromonas hydrophila, Edwardsiella tarda, Enterobacter aerogenes, Klebsiella oxytoca, Legionella pneumophila, Pasteurella multocida, Salmonella enteritidis, Vibrio cholerae, Vibrio parahaemolyticus, Vibrio vulnificus, Yersinia enterocolitica.

Most strains of *Burkholderia cepacia* and some strains of *Stenotrophomonas maltophilia* are resistant to ciprofloxacin as are most anaerobic bacteria, including *Bacteroides fragilis* and *Clostridium difficile.*

SUSCEPTIBILITY TESTING

Dilution Techniques

Quantitative methods are used to determine antimicrobial minimum inhibitory concentrations (MICs). These MICs provide estimates of the susceptibility of bacteria to antimicrobial compounds. The MICs should be determined using a standardized procedure. Standardized procedures are based on a dilution method[1] (broth or agar) or equivalent with standardized inoculum concentrations and standardized concentrations of ciprofloxacin powder. The MIC values should be interpreted according to the criteria in TABLE 4.

For testing aerobic microorganisms other than *Haemophilus influenzae, Haemophilus parainfluenzae,* and *Neisseria gonorrhoeae**, see TABLE 4.

TABLE 4

MIC	Interpretation
≤1 μg/ml	Susceptible (S)
2 μg/ml	Intermediate (I)
≥4 μg/ml	Resistant (R)

* These interpretive standards are applicable only to broth microdilution susceptibility tests with streptococci using cation-adjusted Mueller-Hinton broth with 2-5% lysed horse blood.

For testing *Haemophilus influenzae* and *Haemophilus parainfluenzae**, see TABLE 5.

TABLE 5

MIC	Interpretation
≤1 μg/ml	Susceptible (S)

* This interpretive standard is applicable only to broth microdilution susceptibility tests with *Haemophilus influenzae* and *Haemophilus parainfluenzae* using *Haemophilus* Test Medium.[1]

The current absence of data on resistant strains precludes defining any results other than "Susceptible". Strains yielding MIC results suggestive of a "nonsusceptible" category should be submitted to a reference laboratory for further testing.

For testing *Neisseria gonorrhoeae**, see TABLE 6.

TABLE 6

MIC	Interpretation
≤0.06 μg/ml	Susceptible (S)
0.12-0.5 μg/ml	Intermediate (I)
≥1 μg/ml	Resistant (R)

* This interpretive standard is applicable only to agar dilution test with GC agar base and 1% defined growth supplement.

A report of "Susceptible" indicates that the pathogen is likely to be inhibited if the antimicrobial compound in the blood reaches the concentrations usually achievable. A report of "Intermediate" indicates that the result should be considered equivocal, and, if the microorganism is not fully susceptible to alternative, clinically feasible drugs, the test should be repeated. This category implies possible clinical applicability in body sites where the drug is physiologically concentrated or in situations where high dosage of drug can be used. This category also provides a buffer zone, which prevents small uncontrolled technical factors from causing major discrepancies in interpretation. A report of "Resistant" indicates that the pathogen is not likely to be inhibited if the antimicrobial compound in the blood reaches the concentrations usually achievable; other therapy should be selected.

Standardized susceptibility test procedures require the use of laboratory control microorganisms to control the technical aspects of the laboratory procedures. Standard ciprofloxacin powder should provide the MIC values in TABLE 7.

TABLE 7

Organism		MIC
E. faecalis	ATCC 29212	0.25-2.0 μg/ml
E. coli	ATCC 25922	0.004-0.015 μg/ml
*H. influenzae**	ATCC 49247	0.004-0.03 μg/ml
N. gonorrhoeae†	ATCC 49226	0.001-0.008 μg/ml
P. aeruginosa	ATCC 27853	0.25-1.0 μg/ml
S. aureus	ATCC 29213	0.12-0.5 μg/ml

* This quality control range is applicable to only *H. influenzae* ATCC 49247 tested by a broth microdilution procedure using *Haemophilus* Test Medium (HTM).[1]

† This quality control range is applicable to only *N. gonorrhoeae* ATCC 49226 tested by an agar dilution procedure using GC agar base and 1% defined growth supplement.

Diffusion Techniques

Quantitative methods that require measurement of zone diameters also provide reproducible estimates of the susceptibility of bacteria to antimicrobial compounds. One such standardized procedure[2] requires the use of standardized inoculum concentrations. This procedure

C

uses paper disks impregnated with 5 µg ciprofloxacin to test the susceptibility of microorganisms to ciprofloxacin.

Reports from the laboratory providing results of the standard single-disk susceptibility test with a 5 µg ciprofloxacin disk should be interpreted according to the following criteria.

For testing aerobic microorganisms other than *Haemophilus influenzae, Haemophilus parainfluenzae*, and *Neisseria gonorrhoeae**, see TABLE 8.

C

TABLE 8

Zone Diameter	Interpretation
≥21 mm	Susceptible (S)
16-20 mm	Intermediate (I)
≤15 mm	Resistant (R)

* These zone diameter standards are applicable only to tests performed for streptococci using Mueller-Hinton agar supplemented with 5% sheep blood incubated in 5% CO_2.

For testing *Haemophilus influenzae* and *Haemophilus parainfluenzae**, see TABLE 9.

TABLE 9

Zone Diameter	Interpretation
≥21 mm	Susceptible (S)

* This zone diameter standard is applicable only to tests with *Haemophilus influenzae* and *Haemophilus parainfluenzae* using *Haemophilus* Test Medium (HTM)[2].

The current absence of data on resistant strains precludes defining any results other than "Susceptible". Strains yielding zone diameter results suggestive of a "nonsusceptible" category should be submitted to a reference laboratory for further testing.

For testing *Neisseria gonorrhoeae**, see TABLE 10.

TABLE 10

Zone Diameter	Interpretation
≥41 mm	Susceptible (S)
28-40 mm	Intermediate (I)
≤27 mm	Resistant (R)

* This zone diameter standard is applicable only to disk diffusion tests with GC agar base and 1% defined growth supplement.

Interpretation should be as stated above for results using dilution techniques. Interpretation involves correlation of the diameter obtained in the disk test with the MIC for ciprofloxacin.

As with standardized dilution techniques, diffusion methods require the use of laboratory control microorganisms that are used to control the technical aspects of the laboratory procedures. For the diffusion technique, the 5 µg ciprofloxacin disk should provide the following zone diameters in these laboratory test quality control strains. (See TABLE 11.)

TABLE 11

Organism		Zone Diameter
E. coli	ATCC 25922	30-40 mm
*H influenzae**	ATCC 49247	34-42 mm
N. gonorrhoeae†	ATCC 49226	48-58 mm
P. aeruginosa	ATCC 27853	25-33 mm
S. aureus	ATCC 25923	22-30 mm

* These quality control limits are applicable to only *H. influenzae* ATCC 49247 testing using *Haemophilus* Test Medium (HTM).[2]

† These quality control limits are applicable only to tests conducted with *N. gonorrhoeae* ATCC 49226 performed by disk diffusion using GC agar base and 1% defined growth supplement.

INDICATIONS AND USAGE

Ciprofloxacin is indicated for the treatment of infections caused by susceptible strains of the designated microorganisms in the conditions listed below. Please see DOSAGE AND ADMINISTRATION for specific recommendations.

Urinary tract infections caused by *Escherichia coli, Klebsiella pneumoniae, Enterobacter cloacae, Serratia marcescens, Proteus mirabilis, Providencia rettgeri, Morganella morganii, Citrobacter diversus, Citrobacter freundii, Pseudomonas aeruginosa, Staphylococcus epidermidis, Staphylococcus saprophyticus*, or *Enterococcus faecalis*.

Acute uncomplicated cystitis in females caused by *Escherichia coli* or *Staphylococcus saprophyticus*. (See DOSAGE AND ADMINISTRATION.)

Chronic bacterial prostatitis caused by *Escherichia coli* or *Proteus mirabilis*.

Lower respiratory tract infections caused by *Escherichia coli, Klebsiella pneumoniae, Enterobacter cloacae, Proteus mirabilis, Pseudomonas aeruginosa, Haemophilus influenzae, Haemophilus parainfluenzae*, or *Streptococcus pneumoniae*. Also, *Moraxella catarrhalis* for the treatment of acute exacerbations of chronic bronchitis.

NOTE: Although effective in clinical trials, ciprofloxacin is not a drug of first choice in the treatment of presumed or confirmed pneumonia secondary to *Streptococcus pneumoniae*.

Acute sinusitis caused by *Haemophilus influenzae, Streptococcus pneumoniae*, or *Moraxella catarrhalis*.

Skin and skin structure infections caused by *Escherichia coli, Klebsiella pneumoniae, Enterobacter cloacae, Proteus mirabilis, Proteus vulgaris, Providencia stuartii, Morganella morganii, Citrobacter freundii, Pseudomonas aeruginosa, Staphylococcus aureus* (methicillin-susceptible), *Staphylococcus epidermidis*, or *Streptococcus pyogenes*.

Bone and joint infections caused by *Enterobacter cloacae, Serratia marcescens*, or *Pseudomonas aeruginosa*.

Complicated intra-abdominal infections (used in combination with metronidazole) caused by *Escherichia coli, Pseudomonas aeruginosa, Proteus mirabilis, Klebsiella pneumoniae*, or *Bacteroides fragilis*. (See DOSAGE AND ADMINISTRATION.)

Infectious diarrhea Caused by *Escherichia coli* (enterotoxigenic strains), *Campylobacter jejuni, Shigella boydii*, Shigella dysenteriae, Shigella flexneri*, or *Shigella sonnei** when antibacterial therapy is indicated.

*Although treatment of infections due to this organism in this organ system demonstrated a clinically significant outcome, efficacy was studied in fewer than 10 patients.

Typhoid fever (enteric fever) caused by *Salmonella typhi*.

NOTE: The efficacy of ciprofloxacin in the eradication of the chronic typhoid carrier state has not been demonstrated.

Uncomplicated cervical and urethral gonorrhea due to *Neisseria gonorrhoeae*.

Inhalational anthrax (post-exposure): To reduce the incidence or progression of disease following exposure to aerosolized *Bacillus anthracis*.

Ciprofloxacin serum concentrations achieved in humans serve as a surrogate endpoint reasonably likely to predict clinical benefit and provide the basis for this indication.[4]

If anaerobic organisms are suspected of contributing to the infection, appropriate therapy should be administered. Appropriate culture and susceptibility tests should be performed before treatment in order to isolate and identify organisms causing infection and to determine their susceptibility to ciprofloxacin. Therapy with ciprofloxacin may be initiated before results of these tests are known; once results become available appropriate therapy should be continued. As with other drugs, some strains of *Pseudomonas aeruginosa* may develop resistance fairly rapidly during treatment with ciprofloxacin. Culture and susceptibility testing performed periodically during therapy will provide information not only on the therapeutic effect of the antimicrobial agent but also on the possible emergence of bacterial resistance.

EXTENDED-RELEASE TABLETS

Ciprofloxacin XR is indicated solely for the treatment of uncomplicated urinary tract infections (acute cystitis) caused by susceptible strains of the designated microorganisms as listed below. Ciprofloxacin XR and ciprofloxacin immediate-release tablets are not interchangeable. Please see DOSAGE AND ADMINISTRATION for specific recommendations.

Uncomplicated urinary tract infections (acute cystitis) caused by *Escherichia coli, Proteus mirabilis, Enterococcus faecalis*, or *Staphylococcus saprophyticus**.

*Treatment of infections due to this organism in this organ system was studied in fewer than 10 patients.

THE SAFETY AND EFFICACY OF CIPROFLOXACIN XR IN TREATING INFECTIONS OTHER THAN UNCOMPLICATED URINARY TRACT INFECTIONS HAVE NOT BEEN DEMONSTRATED.

Appropriate culture and susceptibility tests should be performed before treatment in order to isolate and identify organisms causing infection and to determine their susceptibility to ciprofloxacin. Therapy with ciprofloxacin XR may be initiated before results of these tests are known; once results become available appropriate therapy should be continued. Culture and susceptibility testing performed periodically during therapy will provide information not only on the therapeutic effect of the antimicrobial agent but also on the possible emergence of bacterial resistance.

NON-FDA APPROVED INDICATIONS

Although not approved by the FDA, ciprofloxacin has been used in the treatment of multiple drug resistant tuberculosis, tularemia, and ulcerative colitis.

CONTRAINDICATIONS

Ciprofloxacin HCl is contraindicated in persons with a history of hypersensitivity to ciprofloxacin or any member of the quinolone class of antimicrobial agents.

WARNINGS

THE SAFETY AND EFFECTIVENESS OF CIPROFLOXACIN IN PEDIATRIC PATIENTS AND ADOLESCENTS (LESS THAN 18 YEARS OF AGE), — EXCEPT FOR USE IN INHALATIONAL ANTHRAX (POST-EXPOSURE), PREGNANT WOMEN, AND LACTATING WOMEN HAVE NOT BEEN ESTABLISHED. (See PRECAUTIONS: Pediatric Use, Pregnancy, Teratogenic Effects, Pregnancy Category C, and Nursing Mothers.) The oral administration of ciprofloxacin caused lameness in immature dogs. Histopathological examination of the weight-bearing joints of these dogs revealed permanent lesions of the cartilage. Related quinolone-class drugs also produce erosions of cartilage of weight-bearing joints and other signs of arthropathy in immature animals of various species. (See ANIMAL PHARMACOLOGY.)

Convulsions, increased intracranial pressure, and toxic psychosis have been reported in patients receiving quinolones, including ciprofloxacin. Ciprofloxacin may also cause central nervous system (CNS) events including: dizziness, confusion, tremors, hallucinations, depression, and, rarely, suicidal thoughts or acts. These reactions may occur following the first dose. If these reactions occur in patients receiving ciprofloxacin, the drug should be discontinued and appropriate measures instituted. As with all quinolones, ciprofloxacin should be used with caution in patients with known or suspected CNS disorders that may predispose to seizures or lower the seizure threshold (*e.g.*, severe cerebral arteriosclerosis, epilepsy), or in the presence of other risk factors that may predispose to seizures or lower the seizure threshold (*e.g.*, certain drug therapy, renal dysfunction). (See PRECAUTIONS: General and Information for the Patient; DRUG INTERACTIONS and ADVERSE REACTIONS.)

SERIOUS AND FATAL REACTIONS HAVE BEEN REPORTED IN PATIENTS RECEIVING CONCURRENT ADMINISTRATION OF CIPROFLOXACIN AND THEOPHYLLINE. These reactions have included cardiac arrest, seizure, status epilepticus, and respiratory failure. Although similar serious adverse effects have been reported in patients receiving theophylline alone, the possibility that these reactions may be potentiated by ciprofloxacin cannot be eliminated. If concomitant use cannot be avoided, serum levels of theophylline should be monitored and dosage adjustments made as appropriate.

Serious and occasionally fatal hypersensitivity (anaphylactic) reactions, some following the first dose, have been reported in patients receiving quinolone therapy. Some reactions were accompanied by cardiovascular collapse, loss of consciousness, tingling, pharyngeal or facial edema, dyspnea, urticaria, and itching. Only a few patients had a history of hypersensitivity reactions. Serious anaphylactic reactions require immediate emergency treatment with epinephrine. Oxygen, IV steroids, and airway management, including intubation, should be administered as indicated.

Severe hypersensitivity reactions characterized by rash, fever, eosinophilia, jaundice, and hepatic necrosis with fatal outcome have also been rarely reported in patients receiving ciprofloxacin along with other drugs. The possibility that these reactions were related to ciprofloxacin cannot be excluded. Ciprofloxacin should be discontinued at the first appearance of a skin rash or any other sign of hypersensitivity.

Pseudomembranous colitis has been reported with nearly all antibacterial agents, including ciprofloxacin, and may range in severity from mild to life-threatening. Therefore, it is important to consider this diagnosis in patients who present with diarrhea subsequent to the administration of antibacterial agents.

Treatment with antibacterial agents alters the normal flora of the colon and may permit overgrowth of clostridia. Studies indicate that a toxin produced by *Clostridium difficile* is 1 primary cause of "antibiotic-associated colitis".

After the diagnosis of pseudomembranous colitis has been established, therapeutic measures should be initiated. Mild cases of pseudomembranous colitis usually respond to drug discontinuation alone. In moderate to severe cases, consideration should be given to management with fluids and electrolytes, protein supplementation, and treatment with an antibacterial drug clinically effective against *C. difficile* colitis.

Achilles and other tendon ruptures that required surgical repair or resulted in prolonged disability have been reported with ciprofloxacin and other quinolones. Ciprofloxacin should be discontinued if the patient experiences pain, inflammation, or rupture of a tendon.

Ciprofloxacin has not been shown to be effective in the treatment of syphilis. Antimicrobial agents used in high dose for short periods of time to treat gonorrhea may mask or delay the symptoms of incubating syphilis. All patients with gonorrhea should have a serologic test for syphilis at the time of diagnosis. Patients treated with ciprofloxacin should have a follow-up serologic test for syphilis after 3 months.

PRECAUTIONS

GENERAL

Crystals of ciprofloxacin have been observed rarely in the urine of human subjects but more frequently in the urine of laboratory animals, which is usually alkaline. (See ANIMAL PHARMACOLOGY.) Crystalluria related to ciprofloxacin has been reported only rarely in humans because human urine is usually acidic. Alkalinity of the urine should be avoided in patients receiving ciprofloxacin. Patients should be well hydrated to prevent the formation of highly concentrated urine.

Quinolones, including ciprofloxacin, may also cause CNS events, including: nervousness, agitation, insomnia, anxiety, nightmares or paranoia. (See WARNINGS, PRECAUTIONS, Information for the Patient, and DRUG INTERACTIONS.)

Alteration of the dosage regimen is necessary for patients with impairment of renal function. (See DOSAGE AND ADMINISTRATION.)

Moderate to severe phototoxicity manifested as an exaggerated sunburn reaction has been observed in patients who are exposed to direct sunlight while receiving some members of the quinolone class of drugs. Excessive sunlight should be avoided. Therapy should be discontinued if phototoxicity occurs.

As with any potent drug, periodic assessment of organ system functions, including renal, hepatic, and hematopoietic function, is advisable during prolonged therapy.

INFORMATION FOR THE PATIENT

Patients Should Be Advised:

That ciprofloxacin may be taken with or without meals and to drink fluids liberally. As with other quinolones, concurrent administration of ciprofloxacin with magnesium/aluminum antacids, or sucralfate, didanosine chewable/buffered tablets or pediatric powder, or with other products containing calcium, iron or zinc should be avoided. Ciprofloxacin may be taken 2 hours before or 6 hours after taking these products. Ciprofloxacin should not be taken with dairy products (like milk or yogurt) or calcium-fortified juices alone since absorption of ciprofloxacin may be significantly reduced; however, ciprofloxacin may be taken with a meal that contains these products.

That ciprofloxacin may be associated with hypersensitivity reactions, even following a single dose, and to discontinue the drug at the first sign of a skin rash or other allergic reaction.

To avoid excessive sunlight or artificial ultraviolet light while receiving ciprofloxacin and to discontinue therapy if phototoxicity occurs.

To discontinue treatment; rest and refrain from exercise; and inform their physician if they experience pain, inflammation, or rupture of a tendon.

That ciprofloxacin may cause dizziness and lightheadedness; therefore, patients should know how they react to this drug before they operate an automobile or machinery or engage in activities requiring mental alertness or coordination.

That ciprofloxacin may increase the effects of theophylline and caffeine. There is a possibility of caffeine accumulation when products containing caffeine are consumed while taking quinolones.

That convulsions have been reported in patients receiving quinolones, including ciprofloxacin, and to notify their physician before taking this drug if there is a history of this condition.

If the patient should forget to take ciprofloxacin XR at the usual time, he/she may take the dose later in the day. Do not take more than 1 ciprofloxacin XR tablet/day even if a patient misses a dose. Swallow the ciprofloxacin XR tablet whole. **DO NOT SPLIT, CRUSH, OR CHEW THE TABLET.**

CARCINOGENESIS, MUTAGENESIS, AND IMPAIRMENT OF FERTILITY

Eight *in vitro* mutagenicity tests have been conducted with ciprofloxacin, and the test results are listed below:

- *Salmonella*/Microsome Test (Negative).
- *E. coli* DNA Repair Assay (Negative).
- Mouse Lymphoma Cell Forward Mutation Assay (Positive).
- Chinese Hamster V79 Cell HGPRT Test (Negative).
- Syrian Hamster Embryo Cell Transformation Assay (Negative).
- *Saccharomyces cerevisiae* Point Mutation Assay (Negative).
- *Saccharomyces cerevisiae* Mitotic Crossover and Gene Conversion Assay (Negative).
- Rat Hepatocyte DNA Repair Assay (Positive).

Thus, 2 of the 8 tests were positive, but results of the following 3 *in vivo* test systems gave negative results:

- Rat Hepatocyte DNA Repair Assay.
- Micronucleus Test (Mice).
- Dominant Lethal Test (Mice).

Long-term carcinogenicity studies in mice and rats have been completed. After daily oral doses of 750 mg/kg (mice) and 250 mg/kg (rats) were administered for up to 2 years, there was no evidence that ciprofloxacin had any carcinogenic or tumorigenic effects in these species.

Results from photo co-carcinogenicity testing indicate that ciprofloxacin does not reduce the time to appearance of UV-induced skin tumors as compared to vehicle control. Hairless (Skh-1) mice were exposed to UVA light for 3.5 hours five times every 2 weeks for up to 78 weeks while concurrently being administered ciprofloxacin. The time to development of the first skin tumors was 50 weeks in mice treated concomitantly with UVA and ciprofloxacin (mouse dose approximately equal to maximum recommended human dose based upon mg/m^2), as opposed to 34 weeks when animals were treated with both UVA and vehicle. The times to development of skin tumors ranged from 16-32 weeks in mice treated concomitantly with UVA and other quinolones.[3]

In this model, mice treated with ciprofloxacin alone did not develop skin or systemic tumors. There are no data from similar models using pigmented mice and/or fully haired mice. The clinical significance of these findings to humans is unknown.

Fertility studies performed in rats at oral doses of ciprofloxacin up to 100 mg/kg (1.9 times the highest recommended daily human dose of 500 mg based upon body surface area) revealed no evidence of impairment.

PREGNANCY, TERATOGENIC EFFECTS, PREGNANCY CATEGORY C

There are no adequate and well-controlled studies in pregnant women. An expert review of published data on experiences with ciprofloxacin use during pregnancy by TERIS — the Teratogen Information System — concluded that therapeutic doses during pregnancy are unlikely to pose a substantial teratogenic risk (quantity and quality of data = fair), but the data are insufficient to state that there is no risk.[7]

A controlled prospective observational study followed 200 women exposed to fluoroquinolones (52.5% exposed to ciprofloxacin and 68% first trimester exposures) during gestation.[8] *In utero* exposure to fluoroquinolones during embryogenesis was not associated with increased risk of major malformations. The reported rates of major congenital malformations were 2.2% for the fluoroquinolone group and 2.6% for the control group (background incidence of major malformations is 1-5%). Rates of spontaneous abortions, prematurity and low birth weight did not differ between the groups and there were no clinically significant musculoskelatal dysfunctions up to 1 year of age in the ciprofloxacin exposed children.

Another prospective follow-up study reported on 549 pregnancies with fluoroquinolone exposure (93% first trimetster exposures).[9] There were 70 ciprofloxacin exposures, all within the first trimester. The malformation rates among live-born babies exposed to ciprofloxacin and to fluoroquinolones overall were both within background incidence ranges. No specific patterns of congenital abnormalities were found. The study did not reveal any clear adverse reactions due to *in utero* exposure to ciprofloxacin.

No differences in the rates of prematurity, spontaneous abortions, or birth weight were seen in women exposed to ciprofloxacin during pregnancy.[7,8] However, these small postmarketing epidemiology studies, of which most experience is from short term, first trimester exposure, are insufficient to evaluate the risk for less common defects or to permit reliable and definitive conclusions regarding the safety of ciprofloxacin in pregnant women and their developing fetuses. Ciprofloxacin should not be used during pregnancy unless the potential benefit justifies the potential risk to both fetus and mother (see WARNINGS).

Reproduction studies have been performed in rats and mice using oral doses up to 100 mg/kg (1.4 and 0.7 times the maximum daily human dose of 500 mg based upon body surface area, respectively) and have revealed no evidence of harm to the fetus due to ciprofloxacin. In rabbits, ciprofloxacin (30 and 100 mg/kg orally) produced gastrointestinal disturbances resulting in maternal weight loss and an increased incidence of abortion, but no teratogenicity was observed at either dose. After IV administration of doses up to 20 mg/kg, no maternal toxicity was produced in the rabbit, and no embryotoxicity or teratogenicity was observed. (See WARNINGS.)

NURSING MOTHERS

Ciprofloxacin is excreted in human milk. The amount of ciprofloxacin absorbed by the nursing infant is unknown. Because of the potential for serious adverse reactions in infants nursing from mothers taking ciprofloxacin, a decision should be made whether to discontinue nursing or to discontinue the drug, taking into account the importance of the drug to the mother.

PEDIATRIC USE

Safety and effectiveness in pediatric patients and adolescents less than 18 years of age have not been established, except for use in inhalational anthrax (post-exposure). Ciprofloxacin causes arthropathy in juvenile animals. (See WARNINGS.)

For the indication of inhalational anthrax (post-exposure), the risk-benefit assessment indicates that administration of ciprofloxacin to pediatric patients is appropriate. For information regarding pediatric dosing in inhalational anthrax (post-exposure), see DOSAGE AND ADMINISTRATION.

Short-term safety data from a single trial in pediatric cystic fibrosis patients are available. In a randomized, double-blind clinical trial for the treatment of acute pulmonary exacerbations in cystic fibrosis patients (ages 5-17 years), 67 patients received ciprofloxacin IV 10 mg/kg/dose q8h for 1 week followed by ciprofloxacin tablets 20 mg/kg/dose q12h to complete 10-21 days treatment and 62 patients received the combination of ceftazidime IV 50 mg/kg/dose q8h and tobramycin IV 3 mg/kg/dose q8h for a total of 10-21 days. Patients less than 5 years of age were not studied. Safety monitoring in the study included periodic range of motion examinations and gait assessments by treatment-blinded examiners. Patients were followed for an average of 23 days after completing treatment (range 0-93 days). This study was not designed to determine long term effects and the safety of repeated exposure to ciprofloxacin.

In the study, injection site reactions were more common in the ciprofloxacin group (24%) than in the comparison group (8%). Other adverse events were similar in nature and frequency between treatment arms. Musculoskeletal adverse events were reported in 22% of the patients in the ciprofloxacin group and 21% in the comparison group. Decreased range of motion was reported in 12% of the subjects in the ciprofloxacin group and 16% in the comparison group. Arthralgia was reported in 10% of the patients in the ciprofloxacin group and 11% in the comparison group. One (1) of 67 patients developed arthritis of the knee 9 days after a 10 day course of treatment with ciprofloxacin. Clinical symptoms resolved, but an MRI showed knee effusion without other abnormalities 8 months after treatment. However, the relationship of this event to the patient's course of ciprofloxacin can not be definitively determined, particularly since patients with cystic fibrosis may develop arthralgias/arthritis as part of their underlying disease process.

GERIATRIC USE

In a retrospective analysis of 23 multiple-dose controlled clinical trials of ciprofloxacin encompassing over 3500 ciprofloxacin treated patients, 25% of patients were greater than or equal to 65 years of age and 10% were greater than or equal to 75 years of age. No overall differences in safety or effectiveness were observed between these subjects and younger subjects, and other reported clinical experience has not identified differences in responses between the elderly and younger patients, but greater sensitivity of some older individuals on any drug therapy cannot be ruled out. Ciprofloxacin is known to be substantially excreted by the kidney, and the risk of adverse reactions may be greater in patients with impaired renal function. No alteration of dosage is necessary for patients greater than 65 years of age with normal renal function. However, since some older individuals experience reduced renal function by virtue of their advanced age, care should be taken in dose selection for elderly patients, and renal function monitoring may be useful in these patients. The total drug exposure and maximum serum concentrations attained with ciprofloxacin XR are similar to or less than the corresponding values achieved with 500 mg immediate-release ciprofloxacin, which is approved for use in renally impaired patients. Therefore, no reductions in dosage are required (see CLINICAL PHARMACOLOGY and DOSAGE AND ADMINISTRATION).

DRUG INTERACTIONS

As with some other quinolones, concurrent administration of ciprofloxacin with theophylline may lead to elevated serum concentrations of theophylline and prolongation of its elimination half-life. This may result in increased risk of theophylline-related adverse reactions. (See WARNINGS.) If concomitant use cannot be avoided, serum levels of theophylline should be monitored and dosage adjustments made as appropriate.

Some quinolones, including ciprofloxacin, have also been shown to interfere with the metabolism of caffeine. This may lead to reduced clearance of caffeine and a prolongation of its serum half-life.

Concurrent administration of a quinolone, including ciprofloxacin, with multivalent cation-containing products such as magnesium/aluminum antacids, sucralfate, didanosine chewable/buffered tablets or pediatric powder, or products containing calcium, iron, or zinc may substantially decrease its absorption, resulting in serum and urine levels considerably lower than desired. (See DOSAGE AND ADMINISTRATION for concurrent administration of these agents with ciprofloxacin.)

Histamine H_2-receptor antagonists appear to have no significant effect on the bioavailability of ciprofloxacin.

Altered serum levels of phenytoin (increased and decreased) have been reported in patients receiving concomitant ciprofloxacin.

The concomitant administration of ciprofloxacin with the sulfonylurea glyburide has, on rare occasions, resulted in severe hypoglycemia.

Some quinolones, including ciprofloxacin, have been associated with transient elevations in serum creatinine in patients receiving cyclosporine concomitantly.

Quinolones have been reported to enhance the effects of the oral anticoagulant warfarin or its derivatives. When these products are administered concomitantly, prothrombin time or other suitable coagulation tests should be closely monitored.

Probenecid interferes with renal tubular secretion of ciprofloxacin and produces an increase in the level of ciprofloxacin in the serum. This should be considered if patients are receiving both drugs concomitantly.

EXTENDED-RELEASE TABLETS

Absorption of the ciprofloxacin XR tablet was slightly diminished (20%) when given concomitantly with omeprazole. This difference is not considered clinically significant (see CLINICAL PHARMACOLOGY, Drug-Drug Interactions.)

ADVERSE REACTIONS

During clinical investigation with the tablet, 2799 patients received 2868 courses of the drug. Most of the adverse events reported were described as only mild or moderate in severity, abated soon after the drug was discontinued, and required no treatment. Ciprofloxacin was discontinued because of an adverse event in 3.5% of patients treated.

The most frequently reported events, drug related or not, were nausea (5.2%), diarrhea (2.3%), vomiting (2.0%), abdominal pain/discomfort (1.7%), headache (1.2%), restlessness (1.1%), and rash (1.1%).

Additional events that occurred in less than 1% of ciprofloxacin patients are listed below:

Body as a Whole: Foot pain.

Cardiovascular: Palpitation, atrial flutter, ventricular ectopy, syncope, hypertension, angina pectoris, myocardial infarction, cardiopulmonary arrest, cerebral thrombosis.

Central Nervous System: Dizziness, lightheadedness, insomnia, nightmares, hallucinations, manic reaction, irritability, tremor, ataxia, convulsive seizures, lethargy, drowsiness, weakness, malaise, anorexia, phobia, depersonalization, depression, paresthesia. (See above.) (See PRECAUTIONS.)

Gastrointestinal: Painful oral mucosa, oral candidiasis, dysphagia, intestinal perforation, gastrointestinal bleeding. (See above.) Cholestatic jaundice has been reported.

Hemic/Lymphatic: Lymphadenopathy.

Musculoskeletal: Arthralgia or back pain, joint stiffness, achiness, neck or chest pain, flare up of gout.

Renal/Urogenital: Interstitial nephritis, nephritis, renal failure, polyuria, urinary retention, urethral bleeding, vaginitis, acidosis, breast pain.

Respiratory: Dyspnea, epistaxis, laryngeal or pulmonary edema, hiccough, hemoptysis, bronchospasm, pulmonary embolism.

Skin/Hypersensitivity: Pruritus, urticaria, photosensitivity, flushing, fever, chills, angioedema, edema of the face, neck, lips, conjunctivae or hands, cutaneous candidiasis, hyperpigmentation, erythema nodosum. (See above.) Allergic reactions ranging from urticaria to anaphylactic reactions have been reported. (See WARNINGS.)

Special Senses: Blurred vision, disturbed vision (change in color perception, overbrightness of lights), decreased visual acuity, diplopia, eye pain, tinnitus, hearing loss, bad taste.

In several instances nausea, vomiting, tremor, irritability, or palpitation were judged by investigators to be related to elevated serum levels of theophylline possibly as a result of drug interaction with ciprofloxacin.

In randomized, double-blind controlled clinical trials comparing ciprofloxacin tablets (500 mg bid) to cefuroxime axetil (250-500 mg bid) and to clarithromycin (500 mg bid) in patients with respiratory tract infections, ciprofloxacin demonstrated a CNS adverse event profile comparable to the control drugs.

A clinical trial enrolled 905 ciprofloxacin treated patients, of whom 444 patients received the ciprofloxacin XR 500 mg qd dose and 447 patients received the ciprofloxacin 250 mg bid dose. Most adverse events reported (93.5%) were described as mild to moderate in severity and required no treatment. Ciprofloxacin XR was discontinued due to adverse reactions thought to be drug-related in 0.2% of patients.

Adverse reactions, judged by investigators to be at least possibly drug-related, occurring in greater than or equal to 1% of ciprofloxacin XR treated patients were nausea (3%) and headache (2%).

Additional uncommon events, judged by investigators to be at least possibly drug-related, that occurred in less than 1% of ciprofloxacin XR treated patients were:

Body as a Whole: Abdominal pain, photosensitivity reaction.

Cardiovascular: Migraine.

Digestive: Anorexia, constipation, diarrhea, dyspepsia, flatulence, thirst, vomiting.

Central Nervous System: Depersonalization, dizziness, hypertonia, incoordination, somnolence.

Skin/Appendages: Maculopapular rash, pruritus, rash, skin disorder, vesiculobullous rash.

Special Senses: Taste perversion.

Urogenital: Dysmenorrhea, vaginal candidiasis, vaginitis.

POSTMARKETING ADVERSE EVENTS

The following additional adverse events, in alphabetical order, regardless of incidence or relationship to drug, have been reported during clinical trials and from worldwide postmarketing experience in patients given ciprofloxacin (includes all formulations, all dosages, all drug-therapy durations, and all indications): achiness, acidosis, agitation, agranulocytosis, allergic reactions (ranging from urticaria to anaphylactic reactions), anemia, angina pectoris, angioedema, anosmia, anxiety, arrhythmia, arthralgia, ataxia, atrial flutter, bleeding diathesis, blurred vision, bronchospasm, *C. difficile* associated diarrhea, candidiasis (cutaneous, oral), candiduria, cardiac murmur, cardiopulmonary arrest, cardiovascular collapse, cerebral thrombosis, chills, cholestatic jaundice, confusion, convulsion, delirium, depression, diplopia, drowsiness, dysphagia, dysphasia, dyspnea, edema (conjunctivae, face, hands, laryngeal, lips, lower extremities, neck, pulmonary), epistaxis, erythema multiforme, erythema nodosum, exfoliative dermatitis, fever, flushing, gastrointestinal bleeding, gout (flare up), gynecomastia, hallucinations, hearing loss, hematuria, hemolytic anemia, hemoptysis, hemorrhagic cystitis, hepatic necrosis, hiccup, hyperpigmentation, hypertension, hypotension, ileus, insomnia, interstitial nephritis, intestinal perforation, jaundice, joint stiffness, lethargy, lightheadedness, lymphadenopathy, malaise, manic reaction, mouth dryness, myalgia, myasthenia gravis (possible exacerbation), myocardial infarction, myoclonus, nephritis, nightmares, nystagmus, oral ulceration, pain (arm, back, breast, chest, epigastric, eye, foot, jaw, neck, oral mucosa), palpitation, pancreatitis, paranoia, paresthesia, perspiration (increased), phobia, pleural effusion, polyuria, postural hypotension, pseudomembranous colitis, pulmonary embolism, purpura, renal calculi, renal failure, respiratory arrest, respiratory distress, restlessness, Stevens-Johnson syndrome, syncope, tachycardia, taste loss, tendinitis, tendon rupture, tinnitus, toxic epidermal necrolysis, toxic psychosis, tremor, unresponsiveness, urethral bleeding, urinary retention, urination (frequent), vaginal pruritus, vasculitis, ventricular ectopy, vesicles, visual acuity (decreased), visual disturbances (flashing lights, change in color perception, overbrightness of lights), weakness.

ADVERSE LABORATORY CHANGES

Changes in laboratory parameters listed as adverse events without regard to drug relationship are listed below:

Hepatic: Elevations of ALT (SGPT) (1.9%), AST (SGOT) (1.7%), alkaline phosphatase (0.8%), LDH (0.4%), serum bilirubin (0.3%).

Hematologic: Eosinophilia (0.6%), leukopenia (0.4%), decreased blood platelets (0.1%), elevated blood platelets (0.1%), pancytopenia (0.1%).

For testing *Haemophilus influenzae* and *Haemophilus parainfluenzae**, see TABLE 19.

TABLE 19

MIC	Interpretation
≤1 µg/ml	Susceptible (S)

* This interpretive standard is applicable only to broth microdilution susceptibility tests with *Haemophilus influenzae* and *Haemophilus parainfluenzae* using *Haemophilus* Test Medium.[1]

The current absence of data on resistant strains precludes defining any results other than "Susceptible". Strains yielding MIC results suggestive of a "nonsusceptible" category should be submitted to a reference laboratory for further testing.

A report of "Susceptible" indicates that the pathogen is likely to be inhibited if the antimicrobial compound in the blood reaches the concentrations usually achievable. A report of "Intermediate" indicates that the result should be considered equivocal, and, if the microorganism is not fully susceptible to alternative, clinically feasible drugs, the test should be repeated. This category implies possible clinical applicability in body sites where the drug is physiologically concentrated or in situations where high dosage of drug can be used. This category also provides a buffer zone, which prevents small uncontrolled technical factors from causing major discrepancies in interpretation. A report of "Resistant" indicates that the pathogen is not likely to be inhibited if the antimicrobial compound in the blood reaches the concentrations usually achievable; other therapy should be selected.

Standardized susceptibility test procedures require the use of laboratory control microorganisms to control the technical aspects of the laboratory procedures. Standard ciprofloxacin powder should provide the MIC values found in TABLE 20.

TABLE 20

Organism		MIC
E. faecalis	ATCC 29212	0.25-2.0 µg/ml
E. coli	ATCC 25922	0.004-0.015 µg/ml
*H. influenzae**	ATCC 49247	0.004-0.03 µg/ml
P. aeruginosa	ATCC 27853	0.25-1.0µg/ml
S. aureus	ATCC 29213	0.12-0.5 µg/ml

* This quality control range is applicable to only *H. influenzae* ATCC 49247 tested by a broth microdilution procedure using *Haemophilus* Test Medium (HTM).[1]

Diffusion Techniques

Quantitative methods that require measurement of zone diameters also provide reproducible estimates of the susceptibility of bacteria to antimicrobial compounds. One such standardized procedure[2] requires the use of standardized inoculum concentrations. This procedure uses paper disks impregnated with 5 µg ciprofloxacin to test the susceptibility of microorganisms to ciprofloxacin.

Reports from the laboratory providing results of the standard single-disk susceptibility test with a 5 µg ciprofloxacin disk should be interpreted according to the following criteria.

For testing aerobic microorganisms other than *Haemophilus influenzae* and *Haemophilus parainfluenzae,** see TABLE 21.

TABLE 21

Zone Diameter	Interpretation
≥21 mm	Susceptible (S)
16-20 mm	Intermediate (I)
≤15 mm	Resistant (R)

* These zone diameter standards are applicable only to tests performed for streptococci using Mueller-Hinton agar supplemented with 5% sheep blood incubated in 5% CO_2.

For testing *Haemophilus influenzae* and *Haemophilus parainfluenzae**, see TABLE 22.

TABLE 22

Zone Diameter	Interpretation
≥21 mm	Susceptible (S)

* This zone diameter standard is applicable only to tests with *Haemophilus influenzae* and *Haemophilus parainfluenzae* using *Haemophilus* Test Medium (HTM).[2]

The current absence of data on resistant strains precludes defining any results other than "Susceptible". Strains yielding zone diameter results suggestive of a "nonsusceptible" category should be submitted to a reference laboratory for further testing.

Interpretation should be as stated above for results using dilution techniques. Interpretation involves correlation of the diameter obtained in the disk test with the MIC for ciprofloxacin.

As with standardized dilution techniques, diffusion methods require the use of laboratory control microorganisms that are used to control the technical aspects of the laboratory procedures. For the diffusion technique, the 5 µg ciprofloxacin disk should provide the following zone diameters in these laboratory test quality control strains. (See TABLE 23.)

TABLE 23

Organism		Zone Diameter
E. coli	ATCC 25922	30-40 mm
*H influenzae**	ATCC 49247	34-42 mm
P. aeruginosa	ATCC 27853	25-33 mm
S. aureus	ATCC 25923	22-30 mm

* These quality control limits are applicable to only *H. influenzae* ATCC 49247 testing using *Haemophilus* Test Medium (HTM).[2]

INHALATIONAL ANTHRAX — ADDITIONAL INFORMATION

The mean serum concentrations of ciprofloxacin associated with a statistically significant improvement in survival in the rhesus monkey model of inhalational anthrax are reached or exceeded in adult and pediatric patients receiving oral and IV regimens. (See DOSAGE AND ADMINISTRATION.) Ciprofloxacin pharmacokinetics have been evaluated in various human populations. The mean peak serum concentration achieved at steady-state in human adults receiving 500 mg orally every 12 hours is 2.97 µg/ml, and 4.56 µg/ml following 400 mg intravenously every 12 hours. The mean trough serum concentration at steady-state for both of these regimens is 0.2 µg/ml. In a study of 10 pediatric patients between 6 and 16 years of age, the mean peak plasma concentration achieved is 8.3 µg/ml and trough concentrations range from 0.09-0.26 µg/ml, following two 30 minute IV infusions of 10 mg/kg administered 12 hours apart. After the second IV infusion patients switched to 15 mg/kg orally every 12 hours achieve a mean peak concentration of 3.6 µg/ml after the initial oral dose. Long-term safety data, including effects on cartilage, following the administration of ciprofloxacin to pediatric patients are limited. (For additional information, see PRECAUTIONS, Pediatric Use.) Ciprofloxacin serum concentrations achieved in humans serve as a surrogate endpoint reasonably likely to predict clinical benefit and provide the basis for this indication.[4]

A placebo-controlled animal study in rhesus monkeys exposed to an inhaled mean dose of 11 LD_{50} (~5.5 × 10^5) spores (range 5-30 LD_{50}) of *B. anthracis* was conducted. The minimal inhibitory concentration (MIC) of ciprofloxacin for the anthrax strain used in this study was 0.08 µg/ml. In the animals studied, mean serum concentrations of ciprofloxacin achieved at expected T_{max} (1 hour post-dose) following oral dosing to steady-state ranged from 0.98-1.69 µg/ml. Mean steady-state trough concentrations at 12 hours post-dose ranged from 0.12-0.19 µg/ml.[5] Mortality due to anthrax for animals that received a 30 day regimen of oral ciprofloxacin beginning 24 hours post-exposure was significantly lower (1/9), compared to the placebo group (9/10) [p=0.001]. The 1 ciprofloxacin-treated animal that died of anthrax did so following the 30 day drug administration period.[6]

INDICATIONS AND USAGE

Ciprofloxacin IV is indicated for the treatment of infections caused by susceptible strains of the designated microorganisms in the conditions listed below when the IV administration offers a route of administration advantageous to the patient. Please see DOSAGE AND ADMINISTRATION for specific recommendations.

Urinary tract infections caused by *Escherichia coli* (including cases with secondary bacteremia), *Klebsiella pneumoniae* subspecies *pneumoniae, Enterobacter cloacae, Serratia marcescens, Proteus mirabilis, Providencia rettgeri, Morganella morganii, Citrobacter diversus, Citrobacter freundii, Pseudomonas aeruginosa, Staphylococcus epidermidis, Staphylococcus saprophyticus,* or *Enterococcus faecalis.*

Lower respiratory infections caused by *Escherichia coli, Klebsiella pneumoniae* subspecies *pneumoniae, Enterobacter cloacae, Proteus mirabilis, Pseudomonas aeruginosa, Haemophilus influenzae, Haemophilus parainfluenzae,* or *Streptococcus pneumoniae.* Also, *Moraxella catarrhalis* for the treatment of acute exacerbations of chronic bronchitis.

NOTE: Although effective in clinical trials, ciprofloxacin is not a drug of first choice in the treatment of presumed or confirmed pneumonia secondary to *Streptococcus pneumoniae.*

Nosocomial pneumonia caused by *Haemophilus influenzae* or *Klebsiella pneumoniae.*

Skin and skin structure infections caused by *Escherichia coli, Klebsiella pneumoniae* subspecies *pneumoniae, Enterobacter cloacae, Proteus mirabilis, Proteus vulgaris, Providencia stuartii, Morganella morganii, Citrobacter freundii, Pseudomonas aeruginosa, Staphylococcus aureus* (methicillin susceptible), *Staphylococcus epidermidis,* or *Streptococcus pyogenes.*

Bone and joint infections caused by *Enterobacter cloacae, Serratia marcescens,* or *Pseudomonas aeruginosa.*

Complicated intra-abdominal infections (used in conjunction with metronidazole) caused by *Escherichia coli, Pseudomonas aeruginosa, Proteus mirabilis, Klebsiella pneumoniae,* or *Bacteroides fragilis.*

Acute sinusitis caused by *Haemophilus influenzae, Streptococcus pneumoniae,* or *Moraxella catarrhalis.*

Chronic bacterial prostatitis caused by *Escherichia coli* or *Proteus mirabilis.*

Empirical therapy for febrile neutropenic patients in combination with piperacillin sodium.

Inhalational anthrax (post-exposure): To reduce the incidence or progression of disease following exposure to aerosolized *Bacillus anthracis.*

Ciprofloxacin serum concentrations achieved in humans serve as a surrogate endpoint reasonably likely to predict clinical benefit and provide the basis for this indication.[4] (See also, CLINICAL PHARMACOLOGY, Inhalational Anthrax — Additional Information.)

If anaerobic organisms are suspected of contributing to the infection, appropriate therapy should be administered.

Appropriate culture and susceptibility tests should be performed before treatment in order to isolate and identify organisms causing infection and to determine their susceptibility to ciprofloxacin. Therapy with ciprofloxacin IV may be initiated before results of these tests are known; once results become available, appropriate therapy should be continued.

As with other drugs, some strains of *Pseudomonas aeruginosa* may develop resistance fairly rapidly during treatment with ciprofloxacin. Culture and susceptibility testing performed periodically during therapy will provide information not only on the therapeutic effect of the antimicrobial agent but also on the possible emergence of bacterial resistance.

NON-FDA APPROVED INDICATIONS

Although not approved by the FDA, ciprofloxacin has been used in the treatment of multiple drug resistant tuberculosis, tularemia, and ulcerative colitis.

C

CONTRAINDICATIONS

Ciprofloxacin IV is contraindicated in persons with history of hypersensitivity to ciprofloxacin or any member of the quinolone class of antimicrobial agents.

WARNINGS

THE SAFETY AND EFFECTIVENESS OF CIPROFLOXACIN IN PEDIATRIC PATIENTS AND ADOLESCENTS (LESS THAN 18 YEARS OF AGE), - EXCEPT FOR USE IN INHALATIONAL ANTHRAX (POST-EXPOSURE), PREGNANT WOMEN, AND LACTATING WOMEN HAVE NOT BEEN ESTABLISHED. (See PRECAUTIONS: Pediatric Use;Pregnancy, Teratogenic Effects, Pregnancy Category C; and Nursing Mothers.) Ciprofloxacin causes lameness in immature dogs. Histopathological examination of the weight-bearing joints of these dogs revealed permanent lesions of the cartilage. Related quinolone-class drugs also produce erosions of cartilage of weight-bearing joints and other signs of arthropathy in immature animals of various species. (See ANIMAL PHARMACOLOGY.)

Convulsions, increased intracranial pressure and toxic psychosis have been reported in patients receiving quinolones, including ciprofloxacin. Ciprofloxacin may also cause central nervous system (CNS) events including: dizziness, confusion, tremors, hallucinations, depression, and, rarely, suicidal thoughts or acts. These reactions may occur following the first dose. If these reactions occur in patients receiving ciprofloxacin, the drug should be discontinued and appropriate measures instituted. As with all quinolones, ciprofloxacin should be used with caution in patients with known or suspected CNS disorders that may predispose to seizures or lower the seizure threshold (*e.g.,* severe cerebral arteriosclerosis, epilepsy), or in the presence of other risk factors that may predispose to seizures or lower the seizure threshold (*e.g.,* certain drug therapy, renal dysfunction). (See PRECAUTIONS: General and Information for the Patient; DRUG INTERACTIONS; and ADVERSE REACTIONS.)

SERIOUS AND FATAL REACTIONS HAVE BEEN REPORTED IN PATIENTS RECEIVING CONCURRENT ADMINISTRATION OF IV CIPROFLOXACIN AND THEOPHYLLINE. These reactions have included cardiac arrest, seizure, status epilepticus, and respiratory failure. Although similar serious adverse events have been reported in patients receiving theophylline alone, the possibility that these reactions may be potentiated by ciprofloxacin cannot be eliminated. If concomitant use cannot be avoided, serum levels of theophylline should be monitored and dosage adjustments made as appropriate.

Serious and occasionally fatal hypersensitivity (anaphylactic) reactions, some following the first dose, have been reported in patients receiving quinolone therapy. Some reactions were accompanied by cardiovascular collapse, loss of consciousness, tingling, pharyngeal or facial edema, dyspnea, urticaria, and itching. Only a few patients had a history of hypersensitivity reactions. Serious anaphylactic reactions require immediate emergency treatment with epinephrine and other resuscitation measures, including oxygen, IV fluids, IV antihistamines, corticosteroids, pressor amines, and airway management, as clinically indicated.

Severe hypersensitivity reactions characterized by rash, fever, eosinophilia, jaundice, and hepatic necrosis with fatal outcome have also been reported extremely rarely in patients receiving ciprofloxacin along with other drugs. The possibility that these reactions were related to ciprofloxacin cannot be excluded. Ciprofloxacin should be discontinued at the first appearance of a skin rash or any other sign of hypersensitivity.

Pseudomembranous colitis has been reported with nearly all antibacterial agents, including ciprofloxacin, and may range in severity from mild to life-threatening. Therefore, it is important to consider this diagnosis in patients who present with diarrhea subsequent to the administration of antibacterial agents.

Treatment with antibacterial agents alters the normal flora of the colon and may permit overgrowth of clostridia. Studies indicate that a toxin produced by *Clostridium difficile* is 1 primary cause of "antibiotic-associated colitis".

After the diagnosis of pseudomembranous colitis has been established, therapeutic measures should be initiated. Mild cases of pseudomembranous colitis usually respond to drug discontinuation alone. In moderate to severe cases, consideration should be given to management with fluids and electrolytes, protein supplementation, and treatment with an antibacterial drug clinically effective against *C. difficile* colitis.

Achilles and other tendon ruptures that required surgical repair or resulted in prolonged disability have been reported with ciprofloxacin and other quinolones. Ciprofloxacin should be discontinued if the patient experiences pain, inflammation, or rupture of a tendon.

PRECAUTIONS

GENERAL

INTRAVENOUS CIPROFLOXACIN SHOULD BE ADMINSTERED BY SLOW INFUSION OVER A PERIOD OF 60 MINUTES. Local IV site reactions have been reported with the IV administration of ciprofloxacin. These reactions are more frequent if infusion time is 30 minutes or less or if small veins of the hand are used. (See ADVERSE REACTIONS.)

Quinolones, including ciprofloxacin, may also cause central nervous system (CNS) events, including: nervousness, agitation, insomnia, anxiety, nightmares or paranoia. (See WARNINGS; PRECAUTIONS, Information for the Patient; and DRUG INTERACTIONS.)

Crystals of ciprofloxacin have been observed rarely in the urine of human subjects but more frequently in the urine of laboratory animals, which is usually alkaline. (See ANIMAL PHARMACOLOGY.) Crystalluria related to ciprofloxacin has been reported only rarely in humans because human urine is usually acidic. Alkalinity of the urine should be avoided in patients receiving ciprofloxacin. Patients should be well hydrated to prevent the formation of highly concentrated urine.

Alteration of the dosage regimen is necessary for patients with impairment of renal function. (See DOSAGE AND ADMINISTRATION.)

Moderate to severe phototoxicity manifested as an exaggerated sunburn reaction has been observed in some patients who were exposed to direct sunlight while receiving some members of the quinolone class of drugs. Excessive sunlight should be avoided.

As with any potent drug, periodic assessment of organ system functions, including renal, hepatic, and hematopoietic, is advisable during prolonged therapy.

INFORMATION FOR THE PATIENT

Patients Should Be Advised:

That ciprofloxacin may be associated with hypersensitivity reactions, even following a single dose, and to discontinue the drug at the first sign of a skin rash or other allergic reaction.

That ciprofloxacin may cause dizziness and lightheadedness.

That ciprofloxacin may increase the effects of theophylline and caffeine. There is a possibility of caffeine accumulation when products containing caffeine are consumed while taking ciprofloxacin.

To discontinue treatment; rest and refrain from exercise; and inform their physician if they experience pain, inflammation, or rupture of a tendon.

That convulsions have been reported in patients taking quinolones, including ciprofloxacin, and to notify their physician before taking this drug if there is a history of this condition.

CARCINOGENESIS, MUTAGENESIS, AND IMPAIRMENT OF FERTILITY

Eight *in vitro* mutagenicity tests have been conducted with ciprofloxacin. Test results are listed below:

Salmonella/Microsome Test (Negative).
E. coli DNA Repair Assay (Negative).
Mouse Lymphoma Cell Forward Mutation Assay (Positive).
Chinese Hamster V79 Cell HGPRT Test (Negative).
Syrian Hamster Embryo Cell Transformation Assay (Negative).
Saccharomyces cerevisiae Point Mutation Assay (Negative).
Saccharomyces cerevisiae Mitotic Crossover and Gene Conversion Assay (Negative).
Rat Hepatocyte DNA Repair Assay (Positive).

Thus, 2 of the 8 tests were positive, but results of the following 3 *in vivo* test systems gave negative results:

Rat Hepatocyte DNA Repair Assay.
Micronucleus Test (Mice).
Dominant Lethal Test (Mice).

Long-term carcinogenicity studies in mice and rats have been completed. After daily oral doses of 750 mg/kg (mice) and 250 mg/kg (rats) were administered for up to 2 years, there was no evidence that ciprofloxacin had any carcinogenic or tumorigenic effects in these species.

Results from photo co-carcinogenicity testing indicate that ciprofloxacin does not reduce the time to appearance of UV-induced skin tumors as compared to vehicle control. Hairless (Skh-1) mice were exposed to UVA light for 3.5 hours 5 times every 2 weeks for up to 78 weeks while concurrently being administered ciprofloxacin. The time to development of the first skin tumors was 50 weeks in mice treated concomitantly with UVA and ciprofloxacin (mouse dose approximately equal to maximum recommended human dose based upon mg/m^2), as opposed to 34 weeks when animals were treated with both UVA and vehicle. The times to development of skin tumors ranged from 16-32 weeks in mice treated concomitantly with UVA and other quinolones.[3]

In this model, mice treated with ciprofloxacin alone did not develop skin or systemic tumors. There are no data from similar models using pigmented mice and/or fully haired mice. The clinical significance of these findings to humans is unknown.

Fertility studies performed in rats at oral doses of ciprofloxacin up to 100 mg/kg (0.8 times the highest recommended human dose of 1200 mg based upon body surface area) revealed no evidence of impairment.

PREGNANCY, TERATOGENIC EFFECTS, PREGNANCY CATEGORY C

There are no adequate and well-controlled studies in pregnant women. An expert review of published data on experiences with ciprofloxacin use during pregnancy by TERIS — the Teratogen Information System — concluded that the therapeutic doses during pregnancy are unlikely to pose a substantial teratogenic risk (quantity and quality of data = fair), but the data are insufficient to state that there is no risk.[7]

A controlled prospective observational study followed 200 women exposed to fluoroquinolones (52.5% exposed to ciprofloxacin and 68% first trimester exposures) during gestation.[8] *In utero* exposure to fluoroquinolones during embryogenesis was not associated with increased risk of major malformations. The reported rates of major congenital malformations were 2.2% for the fluoroquinolone group and 2.6% for the control group (background incidence of major malformations is 1-5%.) Rates of spontaneous abortions, prematurity and low birth weight did not differ between the groups and there were no clinically significant musculoskelatal dysfunctions up to 1 year of age in the ciprofloxacin exposed children.

Another prospective follow-up study reported on 549 pregnancies with fluoroquinolone exposure (93% first trimester exposures).[9] There were 70 ciprofloxacin exposures, all within the first trimester. The malformation rates among live-born babies exposed to ciprofloxacin and to fluoroquinolones overall were both within background incidence ranges. No specific patterns of congenital abnormalitites were found. The study did not reveal any clear adverse reactions due to *in utero* exposure to ciprofloxacin.

No differences in the rates of prematurity, spontaneous abortions, or birth weight were seen in women exposed to ciprofloxacin during pregnancy.[7,8] However, these small postmarketing epidemiology studies, of which most experience is from short term, first trimester exposure, are insufficient to evaluate the risk for less common defects or to permit reliable and definitive conclusions regarding the safety of ciprofloxacin in pregnant women and their developing fetuses. Ciprofloxacin should not be used during pregnancy unless the potential benefit justifies the potential risk to both fetus and mother (see WARNINGS).

Reproduction studies have been performed in rats and mice using oral doses up to 100 mg/kg (0.6 and 0.3 times the maximum daily human dose based upon body surface area, respectively) and have revealed no evidence of harm to the fetus due to ciprofloxacin. In rabbits, ciprofloxacin (30 and 100 mg/kg orally) produced gastrointestinal disturbances resulting in maternal weight loss and an increased incidence of abortion, but no teratogenicity was observed at either dose. After IV administration of doses up to 20 mg/kg, no maternal toxicity was produced in the rabbit, and no embryotoxicity or teratogenicity was observed. (See WARNINGS.)

NURSING MOTHERS

Ciprofloxacin is excreted in human milk. The amount of ciprofloxacin absorbed by the nursing infant is unknown. Because of the potential for serious adverse reactions in infants nursing from mothers taking ciprofloxacin, a decision should be made whether to discontinue nursing or to discontinue the drug, taking into account the importance of the drug to the mother.

PEDIATRIC USE

Safety and effectiveness in pediatric patients and adolescents less than 18 years of age have not been established, except for use in inhalational anthrax (post-exposure). Ciprofloxacin causes arthropathy in juvenile animals. (See WARNINGS.)

For the indication of inhalational anthrax (post-exposure), the risk-benefit assessment indicates that administration of ciprofloxacin to pediatric patients is appropriate. For information regarding pediatric dosing in inhalational anthrax (post-exposure), see DOSAGE AND ADMINISTRATION and CLINICAL PHARMACOLOGY, Inhalational Anthrax — Additional Information.

Short-term safety data from a single trial in pediatric cystic fibrosis patients are available. In a randomized, double-blind clinical trial for the treatment of acute pulmonary exacerbations in cystic fibrosis patients (ages 5-17 years), 67 patients received ciprofloxacin IV 10 mg/kg/dose q8h for 1 week followed by ciprofloxacin tablets 20 mg/kg/dose q12h to complete 10-21 days treatment and 62 patients received the combination of ceftazidime IV 50 mg/kg/dose q8h and tobramycin IV 3 mg/kg/dose q8h for a total of 10-21 days. Patients less than 5 years of age were not studied. Safety monitoring in the study included periodic range of motion examinations and gait assessments by treatment-blinded examiners. Patients were followed for an average of 23 days after completing treatment (range 0-93 days). This study was not designed to determine long term effects and the safety of repeated exposure to ciprofloxacin.

In the study, injection site reactions were more common in the ciprofloxacin group (24%) than in the comparison group (8%). Other adverse events were similar in nature and frequency between treatment arms. Musculoskeletal adverse events were reported in 22% of the patients in the ciprofloxacin group and 21% in the comparison group. Decreased range of motion was reported in 12% of the subjects in the ciprofloxacin group and 16% in the comparison group. Arthralgia was reported in 10% of the patients in the ciprofloxacin group and 11% in the comparison group. One (1) of 67 patients developed arthritis of the knee 9 days after a 10 day course of treatment with ciprofloxacin. Clinical symptoms resolved, but an MRI showed knee effusion without other abnormalities 8 months after treatment. However, the relationship of this event to the patient's course of ciprofloxacin can not be definitively determined, particularly since patients with cystic fibrosis may develop arthralgias/arthritis as part of their underlying disease process.

GERIATRIC USE

In a retrospective analysis of 23 multiple-dose controlled clinical trials of ciprofloxacin encompassing over 3500 ciprofloxacin treated patients, 25% of patients were greater than or equal to 65 years of age and 10% were greater than or equal to 75 years of age. No overall differences in safety or effectiveness were observed between these subjects and younger subjects, and other reported clinical experience has not identified differences in responses between the elderly and younger patients, but greater sensitivity of some older individuals on any drug therapy cannot be ruled out. Ciprofloxacin is known to be substantially excreted by the kidney, and the risk of adverse reactions may be greater in patients with impaired renal function. No alteration of dosage is necessary for patients greater than 65 years of age with normal renal function. However, since some older individuals experience reduced renal function by virtue of their advanced age, care should be taken in dose selection for elderly patients, and renal function monitoring may be useful in these patients. (See CLINICAL PHARMACOLOGY and DOSAGE AND ADMINISTRATION.)

DRUG INTERACTIONS

As with some other quinolones, concurrent administration of ciprofloxacin with theophylline may lead to elevated serum concentrations of theophylline and prolongation of its elimination half-life. This may result in increased risk of theophylline-related adverse reactions. (See WARNINGS.) If concomitant use cannot be avoided, serum levels of theophylline should be monitored and dosage adjustments made as appropriate.

Some quinolones, including ciprofloxacin, have also been shown to interfere with the metabolism of caffeine. This may lead to reduced clearance of caffeine and prolongation of its serum half-life.

Some quinolones, including ciprofloxacin, have been associated with transient elevations in serum creatinine in patients receiving cyclosporine concomitantly.

Altered serum levels of phenytoin (increased and decreased) have been reported in patients receiving concomitant ciprofloxacin.

The concomitant administration of ciprofloxacin with the sulfonylurea glyburide has, in some patients, resulted in severe hypoglycemia. Fatalities have been reported.

The serum concentrations of ciprofloxacin and metronidazole were not altered when these 2 drugs were given concomitantly.

Quinolones have been reported to enhance the effects of the oral anticoagulant warfarin or its derivatives. When these products are administered concomitantly, prothrombin time or other suitable coagulation tests should be closely monitored.

Probenecid interferes with renal tubular secretion of ciprofloxacin and produces an increase in the level of ciprofloxacin in the serum. This should be considered if patients are receiving both drugs concomitantly.

Following infusion of 400 mg IV ciprofloxacin every 8 hours in combination with 50 mg/kg IV piperacillin sodium every 4 hours, mean serum ciprofloxacin concentrations were 3.02 μg/ml ½ hour and 1.18 μg/ml between 6-8 hours after the end of infusion.

ADVERSE REACTIONS

The most frequently reported events, without regard to drug relationship, among patients treated with IV ciprofloxacin were nausea, diarrhea, central nervous system disturbance, local IV site reactions, abnormalities of liver associated enzymes (hepatic enzymes), and eosinophilia. Headache, restlessness, and rash were also noted in greater than 1% of patients treated with the most common doses of ciprofloxacin. Many of these events were described as only mild or moderate in severity, abated soon after the drug was discontinued, and required no treatment.

Local IV site reactions have been reported with the IV administration of ciprofloxacin. These reactions are more frequent if the infusion time is 30 minutes or less. These may appear as local skin reactions which resolve rapidly upon completion of the infusion. Subsequent IV administration is not contraindicated unless the reactions recur or worsen.

Additional events, without regard to drug relationship or route of administration, that occurred in 1% or less of ciprofloxacin patients are listed below:

Cardiovascular: Cardiovascular collapse, cardiopulmonary arrest, myocardial infarction, arrhythmia, tachycardia, palpitation, cerebral thrombosis, syncope, cardiac murmur, hypertension, hypotension, angina pectoris.

Central Nervous System: Convulsive seizures, paranoia, toxic psychosis, depression, dysphasia, phobia, depersonalization, manic reaction, unresponsiveness, ataxia, confusion, hallucinations, dizziness, lightheadedness, paresthesia, anxiety, tremor, insomnia, nightmares, weakness, drowsiness, irritability, malaise, lethargy.

Gastrointestinal: Ileus, jaundice, gastrointestinal bleeding, *C. difficile* associated diarrhea, pseudomembranous colitis, pancreatitis, hepatic necrosis, intestinal perforation, dyspepsia, epigastric or abdominal pain, vomiting, constipation, oral ulceration, oral candidiasis, mouth dryness, anorexia, dysphagia, flatulence.

Hemic/Lymphatic: Agranulocytosis, prolongation of prothrombin time.

IV Infusion Site: Thrombophlebitis, burning, pain, pruritus, paresthesia, erythema, swelling.

Musculoskeletal: Arthralgia, jaw, arm or back pain, joint stiffness, neck and chest pain, achiness, flare up of gout, myasthenia gravis.

Renal/Urogenital: Renal failure, interstitial nephritis, hemorrhagic cystitis, renal calculi, frequent urination, acidosis, urethral bleeding, polyuria, urinary retention, gynecomastia, candiduria, vaginitis. Crystalluria, cylindruria, hematuria and albuminuria have also been reported.

Respiratory: Respiratory arrest, pulmonary embolism, dyspnea, pulmonary edema, respiratory distress, pleural effusion, hemoptysis, epistaxis, hiccough.

Skin/Hypersensitivity: Anaphylactic reactions, erythema multiforme/Stevens-Johnson syndrome, exfoliative dermatitis, toxic epidermal necrolysis, vasculitis, angioedema, edema of the lips, face, neck, conjunctivae, hands or lower extremities, purpura, fever, chills, flushing, pruritus, urticaria, cutaneous candidiasis, vesicles, increased perspiration, hyperpigmentation, erythema nodosum, photosensitivity. (See WARNINGS.)

Special Senses: Decreased visual acuity, blurred vision, disturbed vision (flashing lights, change in color perception, overbrightness of lights, diplopia), eye pain, anosmia, hearing loss, tinnitus, nystagmus, a bad taste.

In several instances, nausea, vomiting, tremor, irritability, or palpitation were judged by investigators to be related to elevated serum levels of theophylline possibly as a result of drug interaction with ciprofloxacin.

In randomized, double-blind controlled clinical trials comparing ciprofloxacin (IV and IV PO sequential) with IV β-lactam control antibiotics, the CNS adverse event profile of ciprofloxacin was comparable to that of the control drugs.

POST-MARKETING ADVERSE EVENTS

Additional adverse events, regardless of relationship to drug, reported from worldwide marketing experience with quinolones, including ciprofloxacin, are: change in serum phenytoin, postural hypotension, vasculitis, agitation, delirium, myoclonus, toxic psychosis, hemolytic anemia, methemoglobinemia, elevation of serum triglycerides, cholesterol, blood glucose, and serum potassium, myalgia, tendinitis/tendon rupture, vaginal candidiasis (see PRECAUTIONS).

ADVERSE LABORATORY CHANGES

The most frequently reported changes in laboratory parameters with IV ciprofloxacin therapy, without regard to drug relationship are listed below:

Hepatic: Elevations of AST (SGOT), ALT (SGPT), alkaline phosphatase, LDH, and serum bilirubin.

Hematologic: Elevated eosinophil and platelet counts, decreased platelet counts, hemoglobin and/or hematocrit.

Renal: Elevations of serum creatinine, BUN, and uric acid.

Other: Elevations of serum creatinine phosphokinase, serum theophylline (in patients receiving theophylline concomitantly), blood glucose, and triglycerides.

Other changes occurring infrequently were: decreased leukocyte count, elevated atypical lymphocyte count, immature WBCs, elevated serum calcium, elevation of serum gamma-glutamyl transpeptidase (γ GT), decreased BUN, decreased uric acid, decreased total serum protein, decreased serum albumin, decreased serum potassium, elevated serum potassium, elevated serum cholesterol. Other changes occurring rarely during administration of ciprofloxacin were: elevation of serum amylase, decrease of blood glucose, pancytopenia, leukocytosis, elevated sedimentation rate, change in serum phenytoin, decreased prothrombin time, hemolytic anemia, and bleeding diathesis.

DOSAGE AND ADMINISTRATION

Ciprofloxacin IV should be administered by IV infusion over a period of 60 minutes at dosages described in TABLE 25. Slow infusion of a dilute solution into a larger vein will minimize patient discomfort and reduce the risk of venous irritation. (See Preparation of ciprofloxacin IV for Administration.)

The determination of dosage for any particular patient must take into consideration the severity and nature of the infection, the susceptibility of the causative microorganism, the integrity of the patient's host-defense mechanisms, and the status of renal and hepatic function.

Ciprofloxacin IV should be administered by IV infusion over a period of 60 minutes.

Ciprofloxacin HCl tablets and oral suspension for oral administration are available. Parenteral therapy may be switched to oral ciprofloxacin HCl when the condition warrants, at the discretion of the physician. (See CLINICAL PHARMACOLOGY and TABLE 26 for the equivalent dosing regimens.)

TABLE 25 *Dosage Guidelines: IV*

Infection* Type of Severity	Unit Dose	Frequency	Usual Duration
Urinary Tract			
Mild/moderate	200 mg	q12h	7-14 days
Severe/complicated	400 mg	q12h	7-14 days
Lower Respiratory Tract			
Mild/moderate	400 mg	q12h	7-14 days
Severe/complicated	400 mg	q8h	7-14 days
Nosocomial Pneumonia			
Mild/moderate/severe	400 mg	q8h	10-14 days
Skin and Skin Structure			
Mild/moderate	400 mg	q12h	7-14 days
Severe/complicated	400 mg	q8h	7-14 days
Bone and Joint			
Mild/moderate	400 mg	q12h	≥4-6 weeks
Severe/complicated	400 mg	q8h	≥4-6 weeks
Intra-Abdominal†			
Complicated	400 mg	q12h	7-14 days
Acute Sinusitis			
Mild/moderate	400 mg	q12h	10 days
Chronic Bacterial Prostatitis			
Mild/moderate	400 mg	q12h	28 days
Empirical Therapy in Febrile Neutropenic Patients			
Severe			
Ciprofloxacin +	400 mg	q8h	7-14 days
Piperacillin	50 mg/kg not to exceed 24 g/day	q4h	7-14 days
Inhalational Anthrax (Post-Exposure)‡			
Adult	400 mg	q12h	60 days
Pediatric	10 mg/kg per dose, not to exceed 400 mg per dose	q12h	60 days

* DUE TO THE DESIGNATED PATHOGENS. (See INDICATIONS AND USAGE.)
† Used in conjunction with metronidazole. (See product labeling for prescribing information.)
‡ Drug administration should begin as soon as possible after suspected or confirmed exposure. This indication is based on a surrogate endpoint, ciprofloxacin serum concentrations achieved in humans, reasonably likely to predict clinical benefit.[4] For a discussion of ciprofloxacin serum concentrations in various human populations, see CLINICAL PHARMACOLOGY, Inhalational Anthrax — Additional Information. Total duration of ciprofloxacin administration (IV or oral) for inhalational anthrax (post-exposure) is 60 days.

TABLE 26 *Equivalent AUC Dosing Regimens*

Ciprofloxacin HCl Oral Dosage	Equivalent Ciprofloxacin HCl IV Dosage
250 mg tablet q12h	200 mg IV q12h
500 mg tablet q12h	400 mg IV q12h
750 mg tablet q12h	400 mg IV q8h

Parenteral drug products should be inspected visually for particulate matter and discoloration prior to administration.

IMPAIRED RENAL FUNCTION

TABLE 27 provides dosage guidelines for use in patients with renal impairment; however, monitoring of serum drug levels provides the most reliable basis for dosage adjustment.

TABLE 27 *Recommended Starting and Maintenance Doses for Patients With Impaired Renal Function*

Creatinine Clearance	Dosage
>30 ml/min	See usual dosage
5-29 ml/min	200-400 mg q18-24h

When only the serum creatinine concentration is known, the following formula may be used to estimate creatinine clearance:

Men: Creatinine clearance (ml/min) = [Weight (kg) × (140-age)] ÷ [72 × serum creatinine (mg/dl)]

Women: 0.85 × the value calculated for men.

The serum creatinine should represent a steady state of renal function.

For patients with changing renal function or for patients with renal impairment and hepatic insufficiency, measurement of serum concentrations of ciprofloxacin will provide additional guidance for adjusting dosage.

PREPARATION OF CIPROFLOXACIN IV FOR ADMINISTRATION

Vials (Injection Concentrate)

THIS PREPARATION MUST BE DILUTED BEFORE USE. The IV dose should be prepared by aseptically withdrawing the concentrate from the vial of ciprofloxacin IV. This should be diluted with a suitable IV solution to a final concentration of 1-2 mg/ml. (See Compatibility and Stability.) The resulting solution should be infused over a period of 60 minutes by direct infusion or through a Y-type IV infusion set which may already be in place.

If the Y-type or "piggyback" method of administration is used, it is advisable to discontinue temporarily the administration of any other solutions during the infusion of ciprofloxacin IV. If the concomitant use of ciprofloxacin IV and another drug is necessary each drug should be given separately in accordance with the recommended dosage and route of administration for each drug.

Flexible Containers

Ciprofloxacin IV is also available as a 0.2% premixed solution in 5% dextrose in flexible containers of 100 ml or 200 ml. The solutions in flexible containers do not need to be diluted and may be infused as described above.

COMPATIBILITY AND STABILITY

Ciprofloxacin injection 1% (10 mg/ml), when diluted with the following IV solutions to concentrations of 0.5-2.0 mg/ml, is stable for up to 14 days at refrigerated or room temperature storage.

0.9% Sodium chloride injection
5% Dextrose injection
Sterile water for injection
10% Dextrose for injection
5% Dextrose and 0.225% sodium chloride for injection
5% Dextrose and 0.45% sodium chloride for injection
Lactated Ringer's for injection

ANIMAL PHARMACOLOGY

Ciprofloxacin and other quinolones have been shown to cause arthropathy in immature animals of most species tested. (See WARNINGS.) Damage of weight-bearing joints was observed in juvenile dogs and rats. In young beagles, 100 mg/kg ciprofloxacin given daily for 4 weeks caused degenerative articular changes of the knee joint. At 30 mg/kg, the effect on the joint was minimal. In a subsequent study in beagles, removal of weight-bearing from the joint reduced the lesions but did not totally prevent them.

Crystalluria, sometimes associated with secondary nephropathy, occurs in laboratory animals dosed with ciprofloxacin. This is primarily related to the reduced solubility of ciprofloxacin under alkaline conditions, which predominate in the urine of test animals; in man, crystalluria is rare since human urine is typically acidic. In rhesus monkeys, crystalluria without nephropathy has been noted after IV doses as low as 5 mg/kg. After 6 months of IV dosing at 10 mg/kg/day, no nephropathological changes were noted; however, nephropathy was observed after dosing at 20 mg/kg/day for the same duration.

In dogs, ciprofloxacin administered at 3 and 10 mg/kg by rapid IV injection (15 sec) produces pronounced hypotensive effects. These effects are considered to be related to histamine release because they are partially antagonized by pyrilamine, an antihistamine. In rhesus monkeys, rapid IV injection also produces hypotension, but the effect in this species is inconsistent and less pronounced.

In mice, concomitant administration of nonsteroidal anti-inflammatory drugs, such as phenylbutazone and indomethacin, with quinolones has been reported to enhance the CNS stimulatory effect of quinolones.

Ocular toxicity, seen with some related drugs, has not been observed in ciprofloxacin-treated animals.

HOW SUPPLIED

Cipro IV (ciprofloxacin) is available as a clear, colorless to slightly yellowish solution. Cipro IV is available in 200 and 400 mg strengths. The concentrate is supplied in vials while the premixed solution is supplied in latex-free flexible containers.

STORAGE

Vial: Store between 5-30°C (41-86°F).
Flexible Container: Store between 5-25°C (41-77°F).
Protect from light, avoid excessive heat, protect from freezing.

Cipro IV (ciprofloxacin) is also available as Cipro tablets 100, 250, 500, and 750 mg and Cipro* 5% and 10% oral suspension.

*Does not comply with USP with regards to "loss on drying" and "residue on ignition".

OPHTHALMIC

DESCRIPTION

CIPROFLOXACIN HCl OPHTHALMIC SOLUTION

Ciloxan (ciprofloxacin hydrochloride) ophthalmic solution is a synthetic, sterile, multiple dose, antimicrobial for topical ophthalmic use. Ciprofloxacin is a fluoroquinolone antibacterial active against a broad spectrum of gram-positive and gram-negative ocular pathogens. It is available as the monohydrochloride monohydrate salt of 1-cyclopropyl-6-fluoro-1,4-dihydro-4-oxo-7-(1-piperazinyl)-3-quinoline-carboxylic acid. It is a faint to light yellow crystalline powder with a molecular weight of 385.8. Its empirical formula is $C_{17}H_{18}FN_3O_3HCl \cdot H_2O$.

Ciprofloxacin differs from other quinolones in that it has a fluorine atom at the 6-position, a piperazine moiety at the 7-position, and a cyclopropyl ring at the 1-position.

Each ml of Ciloxan ophthalmic solution contains: *Active:* Ciprofloxacin HCl 3.5 mg equivalent to 3 mg base. *Preservative:* Benzalkonium chloride 0.006%. *Inactive:* Sodium acetate, acetic acid, mannitol 4.6%, edetate disodium 0.05%, hydrochloric acid and/or sodium hydroxide (to adjust pH) and purified water. The pH is approximately 4.5 and the osmolality is approximately 300 mOsm.

CIPROFLOXACIN HCl OPHTHALMIC OINTMENT

Ciloxan (ciprofloxacin hydrochloride ophthalmic ointment) ophthalmic ointment is a synthetic, sterile, multiple dose, antimicrobial for topical use. Ciprofloxacin is a fluoroquinolone antibacterial. It is available as the monohydrochloride monohydrate salt of 1-cyclopropyl-6-fluoro-1,4-dihydro-4-oxo-7-(1-piperazinyl)-3-quinolinecarboxylic acid. Ciprofloxacin is a faint to light yellow crystalline powder with a molecular weight of 385.82. Its empirical formula is $C_{17}H_{18}FN_3O_3HCl \cdot H_2O$.

Ciprofloxacin differs from other quinolones in that it has a fluorine atom at the 6-position, a piperazine moiety at the 7-position, and a cyclopropyl ring at the 1-position.

Each gram of Ciloxan ophthalmic ointment contains: *Active:* Ciprofloxacin HCl 3.33 mg equivalent to 3 mg base. *Inactives:* Mineral oil, white petrolatum.

CLINICAL PHARMACOLOGY

CIPROFLOXACIN HCl OPHTHALMIC SOLUTION

Systemic Absorption

A systemic absorption study was performed in which ciprofloxacin HCl ophthalmic solution was administered in each eye every 2 hours while awake for 2 days followed by every 4 hours while awake for an additional 5 days. The maximum reported plasma concentration of ciprofloxacin was less than 5 ng/ml. The mean concentration was usually less than 2.5 ng/ml.

Microbiology

Ciprofloxacin has *in vitro* activity against a wide range of gram-negative and gram-positive organisms. The bactericidal action of ciprofloxacin results from interference with the enzyme DNA gyrase which is needed for the synthesis of bacterial DNA.

Ciprofloxacin has been shown to be active against most strains of the following organisms both *in vitro* and in clinical infections. (See INDICATIONS AND USAGE, Ciprofloxacin HCl Ophthalmic Solution.)

Gram-Positive

Staphylococcus aureus (including methicillin-susceptible and methicillin-resistant strains), *Staphylococcus epidermidis, Streptococcus pneumoniae, Streptococcus* (Viridans group).

Gram-Negative

Haemophilus influenzae, Pseudomonas aeruginosa, Serratia marcescens.

Ciprofloxacin has been shown to be active *in vitro* against most strains of the following organisms, however, *the clinical significance of these data is unknown:*

Gram-Positive

Enterococcus faecalis (many strains are only moderately susceptible), *Staphylococcus haemolyticus, Staphylococcus hominis, Staphylococcus saprophyticus, Streptococcus pyogenes.*

Gram-Negative

Acinetobacter calcoaceticus subsp. anitratus, Aeromonas caviae, Aeromonas hydrophilia, Brucella melitensis, Campylobacter coli, Campylobacter jejuni, Citrobacter diversus, Citrobacter freundii, Edwardsiella tarda, Enterobacter aerogenes, Enterobacter cloacae, Escherichia coli, Haemophilus ducreyi, Haemophilus parainfluenzae, Klebsiella pneumoniae, Klebsiella oxytoca, Legionella pneumonphila, Moraxella (Branhamella) catarrhalis, Morganella morganii, Neisseria gonorrhoeae, Neisseria meningitidis, Pasteurella multocida, Proteus mirabilis, Proteus vulgaris, Providencia rettgeri, Providencia stuartii, Salmonella enteritidis, Salmonella typhi, Shigella sonneii, Shigella flexneri, Vibrio cholerae, Vibrio parahaeimolyticus, Vibrio vulnificus, Yersinia enterocolitica.

Other Organisms

Chlamydia trachomatis (only moderately susceptible) and *Mycobacterium tuberculosis* (only moderately susceptible).

Most strains of *Pseudomonas cepacia* and some strains of *Pseudomonas maltophilia* are resistant to ciprofloxacin as are most anaerobic bacteria, including *Bacteroides fragilis* and *Clostridium difficile.*

The minimal bactericidal concentration (MBC) generally does not exceed the minimal inhibitory concentration (MIC) by more than a factor of 2. Resistance to ciprofloxacin *in vitro* usually develops slowly (multiple-step mutation).

Ciprofloxacin does not cross-react with other antimicrobial agents such as β-lactams or aminoglycosides; therefore, organisms resistant to these drugs may be susceptible to ciprofloxacin.

CIPROFLOXACIN HCl OPHTHALMIC OINTMENT

Systemic Absorption

Absorption studies in humans with the ciprofloxacin ointment have not been conducted, however, based on studies with ciprofloxacin solution, 0.3%, mean maximal concentrations are expected to be less than 2.5 ng/ml.

Microbiology

Ciprofloxacin has *in vitro* activity against a wide range of gram-negative and gram-positive organisms. The bactericidal action of ciprofloxacin results from interference with the enzyme DNA gyrase which is needed for the synthesis of bacterial DNA.

Ciprofloxacin has been shown to be active against most strains of the following microorganisms both *in vitro* and in clinical infections (see INDICATIONS AND USAGE, Ciprofloxacin HCl Ophthalmic Ointment).

Aerobic Gram-Positive Microorganisms

Staphylococcus aureus (methicillin-susceptible strains), *Staphylococcus epidermidis* (methicillin-susceptible strains), *Streptococcus pneumoniae, Streptococcus* Viridans group.

Aerobic Gram-Negative Microorganisms

Haemophilus influenzae.

The following *in vitro* data are available; **but their clinical significance in ophthalmologic infections is unknown.** The safety and effectiveness of ciprofloxacin in treating conjunctivitis due to these microorganisms have not been established in adequate and well controlled trials. The following organisms are considered susceptible when evaluated using systemic breakpoints. However, a correlation between the *in vitro* systemic breakpoint and ophthalmological efficacy has not been established. Ciprofloxacin exhibits *in vitro* minimal inhibitory concentrations (MIC's) of 1 μg/ml or less (systemic susceptible breakpoint) against most (≥90%) strains of the following ocular pathogens.

Aerobic Gram-Positive Microorganisms

Bacillus species, *Corynebacterium species, Staphylococcus haemolyticus, Staphylococcus hominis.*

Aerobic Gram-Negative Microorganisms

Acinetobacter calcoaceticus, Enterobacter aerogenes, Escherichia coli, Haemophilus parainfluenzae, Klebsielle pneumoniae, Moraxella catarrhalis, Neisseria gonorrhoeae, Proteus mirabilis, Pseudomonas aeruginosa, Serratia marcescens.

Most strains of *Burkholderia cepacia* and some strains of *Stenotrophomonas maltophilia* are resistant to ciprofloxacin as are most anaerobic bacteria, including *Bacteroides fragilis* and *Clostridium difficile.*

The minimal bactericidal concentration (MBC) generally does not exceed the minimal inhibitory concentration (MIC) by more than a factor of 2. Resistance to ciprofloxacin *in vitro* usually develops slowly (multiple-step mutation).

Ciprofloxacin does not cross-react with other antimicrobial agents such as beta-lactams or aminoglycosides; therefore, organisms resistant to these drugs may be susceptible to ciprofloxacin. Organisms resistant to ciprofloxacin may be susceptible to beta-lactams or aminogylcosides.

INDICATIONS AND USAGE

CIPROFLOXACIN HCl OPHTHALMIC SOLUTION

Ciprofloxacin HCl ophthalmic solution is indicated for the treatment of infections caused by susceptible strains of the designated microorganisms in the conditions listed below:

Corneal Ulcers

Pseudomonas aeruginosa, Serratia marcescens, Staphylococcus aureus, Staphylococcus epidermidis, Streptococcus pneumoniae, Streptococcus* (Viridans group)*.

Conjunctivitis

Haemophilus influenzae, Staphylococcus aureus, Staphylococcus epidermidis, Streptococcus pneumoniae.

*Efficacy for this organism was studied in fewer than 10 infections.

CIPROFLOXACIN HCl OPHTHALMIC OINTMENT

Ciprofloxacin HCl ophthalmic ointment is indicated for the treatment of bacterial conjunctivitis caused by susceptible strains of the microorganisms listed below:

Gram-Positive: *Staphylococcus aureus, Staphylococcus epidermidis, Streptococcus pneumoniae, Streptococcus* Viridans group.

Gram-Negative: *Haemophilus influenzae.*

CONTRAINDICATIONS

CIPROFLOXACIN HCl OPHTHALMIC SOLUTION

A history of hypersensitivity to ciprofloxacin or any other component of the medication is a contraindication to its use. A history of hypersensitivity to other quinolones may also contraindicate the use of ciprofloxacin.

CIPROFLOXACIN HCl OPHTHALMIC OINTMENT

A history of hypersensitivity to ciprofloxacin or any other component of the medication is a contraindication to its use. A history of hypersensitivity to other quinolones may also contraindicate the use of ciprofloxacin.

WARNINGS

CIPROFLOXACIN HCl OPHTHALMIC SOLUTION

NOT FOR INJECTION INTO THE EYE.

Serious and occasionally fatal hypersensitivity (anaphylactic) reactions, some following the first dose, have been reported in patients receiving systemic quinolone therapy. Some reactions were accompanied by cardiovascular collapse, loss of consciousness, tingling, pharyngeal or facial edema, dyspnea, urticaria, and itching. Only a few patients had a history of hypersensitivity reactions. Serious anaphylactic reactions require immediate emergency treatment with epinephrine and other resuscitation measures, including oxygen, IV fluids, IV antihistamines, corticosteroids, pressor amines and airway management, as clinically indicated. Remove contact lenses before using.

CIPROFLOXACIN HCl OPHTHALMIC OINTMENT

FOR TOPICAL OPHTHALMIC USE ONLY.

NOT FOR INJECTION INTO THE EYE.

Serious and occasionally fatal hypersensitivity (anaphylactic) reactions, some following the first dose, have been reported in patients receiving systemic quinolone therapy. Some reactions were accompanied by cardiovascular collapse, loss of consciousness, tingling, pharyngeal or facial edema, dyspnea, urticaria, and itching. Only a few patients had a history of hypersensitivity reactions. Serious anaphylactic reactions require immediate emergency treatment with epinephrine and other resuscitation measures, including oxygen, IV fluids, IV antihistamines, corticosteroids, pressor amines and airway management, as clinically indicated.

PRECAUTIONS

CIPROFLOXACIN HCl OPHTHALMIC SOLUTION

General

As with other antibacterial preparations, prolonged use of ciprofloxacin may result in overgrowth of nonsusceptible organisms, including fungi. If superinfection occurs, appropriate therapy should be initiated. Whenever clinical judgment dictates, the patient should be examined with the aid of magnification, such as slit lamp biomicroscopy and, where appropriate, fluorescein staining.

Ciprofloxacin should be discontinued at the first appearance of a skin rash or any other sign of hypersensitivity reaction.

In clinical studies of patients with bacterial corneal ulcer, a white crystalline precipitate located in the superficial portion of the corneal defect was observed in 35 (16.6%) of 210 patients. The onset of the precipitate was within 24 hours to 7 days after starting therapy. In 1 patient, the precipitate was immediately irrigated out upon its appearance. In 17 patients, resolution of the precipitate was seen in 1-8 days (7 within the first 24-72 hours), in 5 patients, resolution was noted in 10-13 days. In 9 patients, exact resolution days were unavailable; however, at follow-up examinations, 18-44 days after onset of the event, complete resolution of the precipitate was noted. In 3 patients, outcome information was unavailable. The precipitate did not preclude continued use of ciprofloxacin, nor did it adversely affect the clinical course of the ulcer or visual outcome. (See ADVERSE REACTIONS.)

C

Information for the Patient
Do not touch dropper tip to any surface, as this may contaminate the solution.

Carcinogenesis, Mutagenesis, and Impairment of Fertility
Eight *in vitro* mutagenicity tests have been conducted with ciprofloxacin and the test results are listed below:

Salmonella/Microsome Test (Negative).
E. coli DNA Repair Assay (Negative).
Mouse Lymphoma Cell Forward Mutation Assay (Positive).
Chinese Hamster V79 Cell HGPRT Test (Negative).
Syrian Hamster Embryo Cell Transformation Assay (Negative).
Saccharomyces cerevisiae Point Mutation Assay (Negative).
Saccharomyces cerevisiae Mitotic Crossover and Gene Conversion Assay (Negative).
Rat Hepatocyte DNA Repair Assay (Positive).

Thus, 2 of the 8 tests were positive, but the results of the following 3 *in vivo* test systems gave negative results:

Rat Hepatocyte DNA Repair Assay.
Micronucleus Test (Mice).
Dominant Lethal Test (Mice).

Long term carcinogenicity studies in mice and rats have been completed. After daily oral dosing for up to 2 years, there is no evidence that ciprofloxacin had any carcinogenic or tumorigenic effects in these species.

Pregnancy Category C
Reproduction studies have been performed in rats and mice at doses up to 6 times the usual daily human oral dose and have revealed no evidence of impaired fertility or harm to the fetus due to ciprofloxacin. In rabbits, as with most antimicrobial agents, ciprofloxacin (30 and 100 mg/kg orally) produced gastrointestinal disturbances resulting in maternal weight loss and an increased incidence of abortion. No teratogenicity was observed at either dose. After IV administration, at doses up to 20 mg/kg, no maternal toxicity was produced and no embryotoxicity or teratogenicity was observed. There are no adequate and well controlled studies in pregnant women. Ciprofloxacin HCl ophthalmic solution should be used during pregnancy only if the potential benefit justifies the potential risk to the fetus.

Nursing Mothers
It is not known whether topically applied ciprofloxacin is excreted in human milk; however, it is known that orally administered ciprofloxacin is excreted in the milk of lactating rats and oral ciprofloxacin has been reported in human breast milk after a single 500 mg dose. Caution should be exercised when ciprofloxacin HCl ophthalmic solution is administered to a nursing mother.

Pediatric Use
Safety and effectiveness in pediatric patients below the age of 1 year have not been established. Although ciprofloxacin and other quinolones cause arthropathy in immature animals after oral administration, topical ocular administration of ciprofloxacin to immature animals did not cause any arthropathy and there is no evidence that the ophthalmic dosage form has any effect on the weight bearing joints.

CIPROFLOXACIN HCl OPHTHALMIC OINTMENT

General
As with other antibacterial preparations, prolonged use of ciprofloxacin may result in overgrowth of nonsusceptible organisms, including fungi. If superinfection occurs, appropriate therapy should be initiated. Whenever clinical judgment dictates, the patient should be examined with the aid of magnification, such as slit lamp biomicroscopy and, where appropriate, fluorescein staining.

Ciprofloxacin should be discontinued at the first appearance of a skin rash or any other sign of hypersensitivity reaction.

Ophthalmic ointments may retard corneal healing and cause visual blurring.

Patients should be advised not to wear contact lenses if they have signs and symptoms of bacterial conjunctivitis.

Information for the Patient
Do not touch tip to any surface as this may contaminate the ointment.

Carcinogenesis, Mutagenesis, and Impairment of Fertility
Eight *in vitro* mutagenicity tests have been conducted with ciprofloxacin and the test results are listed below:

Salmonella/Microsome Test (Negative).
E. coli DNA Repair Assay (Negative).
Mouse Lymphoma Cell Forward Mutation Assay (Positive).
Chinese Hamster V79 Cell HGPRT Test (Negative).
Syrian Hamster Embryo Cell Transformation Assay (Negative).
Saccharomyces cerevisiae Point Mutation Assay (Negative).
Saccharomyces cerevisiae Mitotic Crossover and Gene Conversion Assay (Negative).
Rat Hepatocyte DNA Repair Assay (Positive).

Thus, 2 of the 8 tests were positive, but the results of the following 3 *in vivo* test systems gave negative results:

Rat Hepatocyte DNA Repair Assay.
Micronucleus Test (Mice).
Dominant Lethal Test (Mice).

Long-term carcinogenicity studies in mice and rats have been completed. After daily oral dosing for up to 2 years, there is no evidence that ciprofloxacin had any carcinogenic or tumorigenic effects in these species.

Pregnancy Category C
Reproduction studies have been performed in rats and mice at doses up to 6 times the usual daily human oral dose and have revealed no evidence of impaired fertility or harm to the fetus due to ciprofloxacin. In rabbits, as with most antimicrobial agents, ciprofloxacin (30 and 100 mg/kg orally) produced gastrointestinal disturbances resulting in maternal weight loss and an increased incidence of abortion. No teratogenicity was observed at either dose. After IV administration, at doses up to 20 mg/kg, no maternal toxicity was produced and no embryotoxicity or teratogenicity was observed. There are no adequate and well controlled studies in pregnant women. Ciprofloxacin HCl ophthalmic ointment should be used during pregnancy only if the potential benefit justifies the potential risk to the fetus.

Nursing Mothers
It is not known whether topically applied ciprofloxacin is excreted in human milk. However, it is known that orally administered ciprofloxacin is excreted in the milk of lactating rats and oral ciprofloxacin has been reported in human breast milk after a single 500 mg dose. Caution should be exercised when ciprofloxacin HCl ophthalmic ointment is administered to a nursing mother.

Pediatric Use
Safety and effectiveness of ciprofloxacin HCl ophthalmic ointment 0.3% in pediatric patients below the age of 2 years have not been established. Although ciprofloxacin and other quinolones may cause arthropathy in immature Beagle dogs after oral administration, topical ocular administration of ciprofloxacin to immature animals did not cause any arthropathy and there is no evidence that the ophthalmic dosage form has any effect on the weight bearing joints.

DRUG INTERACTIONS

CIPROFLOXACIN HCl OPHTHALMIC SOLUTION
Specific drug interaction studies have not been conducted with ophthalmic ciprofloxacin. However, the systemic administration of some quinolones has been shown to elevate plasma concentrations of theophylline, interfere with the metabolism of caffeine, enhance the effects of the oral anticoagulant, warfarin, and its derivatives and has been associated with transient elevations in serum creatinine in patients receiving cyclosporine concomitantly.

CIPROFLOXACIN HCl OPHTHALMIC OINTMENT
Specific drug interaction studies have not been conducted with ophthalmic ciprofloxacin. However, the systemic administration of some quinolones has been shown to elevate plasma concentrations of theophylline, interfere with the metabolism of caffeine, enhance the effects of the oral anticoagulant, warfarin, and its derivatives, and has been associated with transient elevations in serum creatinine in patients receiving cyclosporine concomitantly.

ADVERSE REACTIONS

CIPROFLOXACIN HCl OPHTHALMIC SOLUTION
The most frequently reported drug related adverse reaction was local burning or discomfort. In corneal ulcer studies with frequent administration of the drug, white crystalline precipitates were seen in approximately 17% of patients (see PRECAUTIONS). Other reactions occurring in less than 10% of patients included lid margin crusting, crystals/scales, foreign body sensation, itching, conjunctival hyperemia and a bad taste following instillation. Additional events occurring in less than 1% of patients included corneal staining, keratopathy/keratitis, allergic reactions, lid edema, tearing, photophobia, corneal infiltrates, nausea and decreased vision.

CIPROFLOXACIN HCl OPHTHALMIC OINTMENT
The following adverse reactions (incidences) were reported in 2% of the patients in clinical studies for ciprofloxacin HCl ophthalmic ointment: discomfort, keratopathy. Other reactions associated with ciprofloxacin therapy occurring in less than 1% of patients included allergic reactions, blurred vision, corneal staining, decreased visual acuity, dry eye, edema, epitheliopathy, eye pain, foreign body sensation, hyperemia, irritation, keratoconjunctivitis, lid erythema, lid margin hyperemia, photophobia, pruritus, and tearing.

Systemic adverse reactions related to ciprofloxacin therapy occurred at an incidence below 1% and included dermatitis, nausea and taste perversion.

DOSAGE AND ADMINISTRATION

CIPROFLOXACIN HCl OPHTHALMIC SOLUTION
The recommended dosage regimen for the treatment of corneal ulcers is: Two drops into the affected eye every 15 minutes for the first 6 hours and then 2 drops into the affected eye every 30 minutes for the remainder of the first day. On the second day, instill 2 drops in the affected eye hourly. On the third through the fourteenth day, place 2 drops in the affected eye every 4 hours. Treatment may be continued after 14 days if corneal re-epithelialization has not occurred.

The recommended dosage regimen for the treatment of bacterial conjunctivitis is: One (1) or 2 drops instilled into the conjunctival sac(s) every 2 hours while awake for 2 days and 1 or 2 drops every 4 hours while awake for the next 5 days.

CIPROFLOXACIN HCl OPHTHALMIC OINTMENT
Apply a ½" ribbon into the conjunctival sac 3 times a day on the first 2 days, then apply a ½" ribbon 2 times a day for the next 5 days.

ANIMAL PHARMACOLOGY

CIPROFLOXACIN HCl OPHTHALMIC SOLUTION
Ciprofloxacin and related drugs have been shown to cause arthropathy in immature animals of most species tested following oral administration. However, a 1 month topical ocular study using immature Beagle dogs did not demonstrate any articular lesions.

CIPROFLOXACIN HCl OPHTHALMIC OINTMENT
Ciprofloxacin and related drugs have been shown to cause arthropathy in immature animals of most species tested following oral administration. However, a 1 month topical ocular study using immature Beagle dogs did not demonstrate any articular lesions.

HOW SUPPLIED

CILOXAN OPHTHALMIC SOLUTION

As a sterile ophthalmic solution: 2.5 and 5 ml in plastic Drop-Tainer dispensers.
Storage: Store at 2-30°C (36-86°F). Protect from light.

CILOXAN OPHTHALMIC OINTMENT

Sterile ophthalmic ointment: 3.5 g ophthalmic ointment tube.
Storage: Store at 2-25°C (36-77°F).

PRODUCT LISTING - EQUIVALENTS NOT AVAILABLE

Size	Price	Product	NDC
Ointment - Ophthalmic - 0.3%			
3.50 gm	$50.00	CILOXAN, Alcon Laboratories Inc	00065-0654-35
Powder For Reconstitution - Oral - 250 mg/5 ml			
100 ml	$99.96	CIPRO, Bayer	00026-8551-36
Powder For Reconstitution - Oral - 500 mg/5 ml			
100 ml	$117.04	CIPRO, Bayer	00026-8553-36
Solution - Intravenous - 10 mg/ml			
20 ml x 10	$144.10	CIPRO I.V., Bayer	00026-8562-20
40 ml x 10	$288.10	CIPRO I.V., Bayer	00026-8564-64
120 ml x 6	$466.38	CIPRO I.V., Bayer	00026-8566-65
Solution - Intravenous - 200 mg/100 ml			
100 ml x 24	$374.64	CIPRO I.V., Bayer	00026-8527-36
100 ml x 24	$374.64	CIPRO I.V., Bayer	00026-8552-36
Solution - Intravenous - 400 mg/200 ml			
200 ml x 24	$720.24	CIPRO I.V., Bayer	00026-8527-63
200 ml x 24	$720.24	CIPRO I.V., Bayer	00026-8554-63
Solution - Ophthalmic - 0.3%			
2.50 ml	$18.56	CILOXAN, Allscripts Pharmaceutical Company	54569-4103-00
2.50 ml	$23.63	CILOXAN, Alcon Laboratories Inc	00065-0656-25
5 ml	$32.95	CILOXAN, Southwood Pharmaceuticals Inc	58016-6285-01
5 ml	$33.44	CILOXAN, Allscripts Pharmaceutical Company	54569-3296-00
5 ml	$44.63	CILOXAN, Alcon Laboratories Inc	00065-0656-05
5 ml	$53.78	CILOXAN, Pharma Pac	52959-0013-00
10 ml	$89.13	CILOXAN, Alcon Laboratories Inc	00065-0656-10
Tablet - Oral - 100 mg			
6's	$16.83	CIPRO, Allscripts Pharmaceutical Company	54569-4363-00
6's	$21.51	CIPRO, Bayer	00026-8511-06
Tablet - Oral - 250 mg			
1's	$4.59	CIPRO, Quality Care Pharmaceuticals Inc	60346-0433-99
1's	$8.02	CIPRO, Prescript Pharmaceuticals	00247-0197-01
2's	$12.69	CIPRO, Prescript Pharmaceuticals	00247-0197-02
3's	$17.36	CIPRO, Prescript Pharmaceuticals	00247-0197-03
4's	$12.58	CIPRO, Allscripts Pharmaceutical Company	54569-1648-03
4's	$22.05	CIPRO, Prescript Pharmaceuticals	00247-0197-04
4's	$22.93	CIPRO, Quality Care Pharmaceuticals Inc	60346-0433-44
6's	$18.88	CIPRO, Allscripts Pharmaceutical Company	54569-1648-07
6's	$26.98	CIPRO, Pd-Rx Pharmaceuticals	55289-0459-06
6's	$29.15	CIPRO, Quality Care Pharmaceuticals Inc	60346-0433-06
6's	$31.39	CIPRO, Prescript Pharmaceuticals	00247-0197-06
6's	$31.88	CIPRO, Cheshire Drugs	55175-1895-06
6's	$36.15	CIPRO, Pharma Pac	52959-0171-06
10's	$31.46	CIPRO, Allscripts Pharmaceutical Company	54569-1648-05
10's	$44.00	CIPRO, Southwood Pharmaceuticals Inc	58016-0116-10
10's	$44.10	CIPRO, Pd-Rx Pharmaceuticals	55289-0459-10
10's	$46.53	CIPRO, Physicians Total Care	54868-0990-00
10's	$47.06	CIPRO, Cheshire Drugs	55175-1895-01
10's	$47.82	CIPRO, Quality Care Pharmaceuticals Inc	60346-0433-10
10's	$50.07	CIPRO, Prescript Pharmaceuticals	00247-0197-10
10's	$54.46	CIPRO, Pharma Pac	52959-0171-10
12's	$52.80	CIPRO, Southwood Pharmaceuticals Inc	58016-0116-12
12's	$53.77	CIPRO, Pd-Rx Pharmaceuticals	55289-0459-12
12's	$59.42	CIPRO, Prescript Pharmaceuticals	00247-0197-12
14's	$49.02	CIPRO, Physicians Total Care	54868-0990-02
14's	$49.69	CIPRO, Southwood Pharmaceuticals Inc	58016-0116-14
14's	$54.56	CIPRO, Allscripts Pharmaceutical Company	54569-1648-00
14's	$56.06	CIPRO, Cheshire Drugs	55175-1895-04
14's	$57.01	CIPRO, Quality Care Pharmaceuticals Inc	60346-0433-14
14's	$64.88	CIPRO, Pharma Pac	52959-0171-14
14's	$68.76	CIPRO, Prescript Pharmaceuticals	00247-0197-14
14's	$73.50	CIPRO, Pd-Rx Pharmaceuticals	55289-0459-14
15's	$59.29	CIPRO, Quality Care Pharmaceuticals Inc	60346-0433-15
15's	$66.00	CIPRO, Southwood Pharmaceuticals Inc	58016-0116-15
20's	$65.00	CIPRO, Compumed Pharmaceuticals	00403-3027-20
20's	$72.88	CIPRO, Quality Care Pharmaceuticals Inc	60346-0433-20
20's	$72.91	CIPRO, Cheshire Drugs	55175-1895-02
20's	$77.94	CIPRO, Allscripts Pharmaceutical Company	54569-1648-04
20's	$84.39	CIPRO, Pharma Pac	52959-0171-20
20's	$86.82	CIPRO, Physicians Total Care	54868-0990-01
20's	$88.00	CIPRO, Southwood Pharmaceuticals Inc	58016-0116-20
20's	$96.79	CIPRO, Prescript Pharmaceuticals	00247-0197-20
28's	$134.16	CIPRO, Prescript Pharmaceuticals	00247-0197-28
30's	$132.00	CIPRO, Southwood Pharmaceuticals Inc	58016-0116-30
30's	$143.52	CIPRO, Prescript Pharmaceuticals	00247-0197-30
40's	$141.96	CIPRO, Southwood Pharmaceuticals Inc	58016-0116-40
60's	$283.67	CIPRO, Prescript Pharmaceuticals	00247-0197-60
100's	$440.00	CIPRO, Southwood Pharmaceuticals Inc	58016-0116-00
100's	$481.15	CIPRO, Bayer	00026-8512-51
100's	$498.39	CIPRO, Bayer	00026-8512-48
Tablet - Oral - 500 mg			
1's	$3.74	CIPRO, Allscripts Pharmaceutical Company	54569-1723-06
1's	$7.69	CIPRO, Pd-Rx Pharmaceuticals	55289-0371-79
1's	$8.82	CIPRO, Prescript Pharmaceuticals	00247-0167-01
1's	$9.92	CIPRO, Quality Care Pharmaceuticals Inc	60346-0031-99
1's	$17.09	CIPRO, Allscripts Pharmaceutical Company	54569-1723-03
2's	$8.50	CIPRO, Compumed Pharmaceuticals	00403-0601-02
2's	$8.81	CIPRO, Allscripts Pharmaceutical Company	54569-1723-09
2's	$14.28	CIPRO, Prescript Pharmaceuticals	00247-0167-02
2's	$15.60	CIPRO, Cheshire Drugs	55175-1896-01
3's	$19.75	CIPRO, Prescript Pharmaceuticals	00247-0167-03
4's	$16.41	CIPRO, Southwood Pharmaceuticals Inc	58016-0117-04
4's	$17.62	CIPRO, Allscripts Pharmaceutical Company	54569-1723-08
4's	$25.20	CIPRO, Quality Care Pharmaceuticals Inc	60346-0031-44
4's	$25.22	CIPRO, Prescript Pharmaceuticals	00247-0167-04
5's	$22.49	CIPRO, Physicians Total Care	54868-0939-05
6's	$22.47	CIPRO, Allscripts Pharmaceutical Company	54569-1723-05
6's	$28.37	CIPRO, Cheshire Drugs	55175-1896-06
6's	$32.77	CIPRO, Pd-Rx Pharmaceuticals	55289-0371-06
6's	$34.07	CIPRO, Quality Care Pharmaceuticals Inc	60346-0031-06
6's	$36.15	CIPRO, Prescript Pharmaceuticals	00247-0167-06
6's	$40.70	CIPRO, Pharma Pac	52959-0036-06
8's	$31.86	CIPRO, Southwood Pharmaceuticals Inc	58016-0117-08
8's	$47.08	CIPRO, Prescript Pharmaceuticals	00247-0167-08
10's	$36.50	CIPRO, Compumed Pharmaceuticals	00403-0601-10
10's	$37.44	CIPRO, Allscripts Pharmaceutical Company	54569-1723-02
10's	$47.94	CIPRO, Cheshire Drugs	55175-1896-00
10's	$48.06	CIPRO, Quality Care Pharmaceuticals Inc	60346-0031-10
10's	$49.55	CIPRO, St. Mary'S Mpp	60760-0513-10
10's	$51.50	CIPRO, Southwood Pharmaceuticals Inc	58016-0117-10
10's	$55.59	CIPRO, Physicians Total Care	54868-0939-02
10's	$58.01	CIPRO, Prescript Pharmaceuticals	00247-0167-10
10's	$65.85	CIPRO, Pd-Rx Pharmaceuticals	55289-0371-10
10's	$66.54	CIPRO, Pharma Pac	52959-0036-10
12's	$61.80	CIPRO, Southwood Pharmaceuticals Inc	58016-0117-12
12's	$68.95	CIPRO, Prescript Pharmaceuticals	00247-0167-12
14's	$47.00	CIPRO, Compumed Pharmaceuticals	00403-0601-14
14's	$52.42	CIPRO, Allscripts Pharmaceutical Company	54569-1723-00
14's	$62.42	CIPRO, Quality Care Pharmaceuticals Inc	60346-0031-14
14's	$62.96	CIPRO, Cheshire Drugs	55175-1896-04
14's	$72.10	CIPRO, Southwood Pharmaceuticals Inc	58016-0117-14
14's	$74.99	CIPRO, Dhs Inc	55887-0858-14
14's	$77.34	CIPRO, Physicians Total Care	54868-0939-00
14's	$79.88	CIPRO, Prescript Pharmaceuticals	00247-0167-14
14's	$90.99	CIPRO, Pd-Rx Pharmaceuticals	55289-0371-14
14's	$92.60	CIPRO, Pharma Pac	52959-0036-14
15's	$76.20	CIPRO, Pd-Rx Pharmaceuticals	55289-0371-15
15's	$77.25	CIPRO, Southwood Pharmaceuticals Inc	58016-0117-15
15's	$82.78	CIPRO, Physicians Total Care	54868-0939-06
15's	$85.34	CIPRO, Prescript Pharmaceuticals	00247-0167-15
15's	$99.04	CIPRO, Pharma Pac	52959-0036-15
20's	$74.89	CIPRO, Allscripts Pharmaceutical Company	54569-1723-01
20's	$82.22	CIPRO, Cheshire Drugs	55175-1896-02
20's	$88.79	CIPRO, Quality Care Pharmaceuticals Inc	60346-0031-20
20's	$103.00	CIPRO, Southwood Pharmaceuticals Inc	58016-0117-20
20's	$103.93	CIPRO, Physicians Total Care	54868-0939-01
20's	$105.87	CIPRO, Dhs Inc	55887-0858-20
20's	$112.68	CIPRO, Prescript Pharmaceuticals	00247-0167-20
20's	$128.70	CIPRO, Pd-Rx Pharmaceuticals	55289-0371-20
20's	$130.74	CIPRO, Pharma Pac	52959-0036-20
25's	$125.47	CIPRO, Quality Care Pharmaceuticals Inc	60346-0031-25
25's	$153.81	CIPRO, Pd-Rx Pharmaceuticals	55289-0371-97
28's	$123.31	CIPRO, Allscripts Pharmaceutical Company	54569-4820-00
28's	$156.41	CIPRO, Prescript Pharmaceuticals	00247-0167-28
28's	$182.20	CIPRO, Pharma Pac	52959-0036-28
30's	$99.70	CIPRO, Compumed Pharmaceuticals	00403-0601-30
30's	$126.91	CIPRO, Quality Care Pharmaceuticals Inc	60346-0031-30
30's	$132.11	CIPRO, Allscripts Pharmaceutical Company	54569-1723-04
30's	$154.50	CIPRO, Southwood Pharmaceuticals Inc	58016-0117-30
30's	$155.29	CIPRO, Physicians Total Care	54868-0939-03
30's	$167.34	CIPRO, Prescript Pharmaceuticals	00247-0167-30
30's	$191.55	CIPRO, Pd-Rx Pharmaceuticals	55289-0371-30
40's	$258.38	CIPRO, Pd-Rx Pharmaceuticals	55289-0371-40
50's	$198.75	CIPRO, Southwood Pharmaceuticals Inc	58016-0117-50
50's	$316.73	CIPRO, Pd-Rx Pharmaceuticals	55289-0371-50
100's	$515.00	CIPRO, Southwood Pharmaceuticals Inc	58016-0117-00
100's	$549.98	CIPRO, Prescript Pharmaceuticals	00247-0167-00
100's	$563.20	CIPRO, Bayer	00026-8513-51
100's	$581.96	CIPRO, Bayer	00026-8513-48
Tablet - Oral - 750 mg			
4's	$63.71	CIPRO, Allscripts Pharmaceutical Company	54569-2488-01
10's	$53.00	CIPRO, Southwood Pharmaceuticals Inc	58016-0118-10
12's	$63.60	CIPRO, Southwood Pharmaceuticals Inc	58016-0118-12
14's	$74.20	CIPRO, Southwood Pharmaceuticals Inc	58016-0118-14
14's	$75.40	CIPRO, Compumed Pharmaceuticals	00403-3511-14
14's	$95.48	CIPRO, Pharma Pac	52959-0037-14
15's	$79.50	CIPRO, Southwood Pharmaceuticals Inc	58016-0118-15
15's	$94.28	CIPRO, Physicians Total Care	54868-1184-03
20's	$91.01	CIPRO, Allscripts Pharmaceutical Company	54569-2488-00
20's	$106.00	CIPRO, Southwood Pharmaceuticals Inc	58016-0118-20
20's	$107.00	CIPRO, Compumed Pharmaceuticals	00403-3511-20
20's	$125.31	CIPRO, Physicians Total Care	54868-1184-01
20's	$128.99	CIPRO, Pharma Pac	52959-0037-20
20's	$140.10	CIPRO, Cheshire Drugs	55175-1897-02
30's	$159.00	CIPRO, Southwood Pharmaceuticals Inc	58016-0118-30
50's	$265.00	CIPRO, Southwood Pharmaceuticals Inc	58016-0118-50
50's	$292.50	CIPRO, Bayer	00026-8514-50
50's	$311.52	CIPRO, Physicians Total Care	54868-1184-02
100's	$432.70	CIPRO, Southwood Pharmaceuticals Inc	58016-0118-00
100's	$604.45	CIPRO, Bayer	00026-8514-48
Tablet, Extended Release - Oral - 500 mg			
50's	$433.13	CIPRO XR, Bayer	00026-8889-50
100's	$866.25	CIPRO XR, Bayer	00026-8889-51

Ciprofloxacin Hydrochloride; Hydrocortisone (003476)

Categories: Infection, ear, external; FDA Approved 1999 Jan; Pregnancy Category C
Drug Classes: Antibiotics, quinolones; Anti-infectives, otic; Corticosteroids, otic; Otics
Foreign Brand Availability: Cipro HC Otic (Canada; Hong-Kong; Israel); Ciprobay HC (Singapore; South-Africa); Ciproxin (Philippines); Ciproxin HC ear drops (Australia); Otosec HC (Colombia)
Cost of Therapy: $65.63 (Otitis Externa; Cipro HC Otic; 0.2%; 1%; 10 ml; 6 drops/day; 7 day supply)

C

DESCRIPTION

Cipro HC Otic (ciprofloxacin hydrochloride; hydrocortisone otic suspension) contains the synthetic broad spectrum antibacterial agent, ciprofloxacin HCl, combined with the anti-inflammatory corticosteroid, hydrocortisone, in a preserved, nonsterile suspension for otic use. Each ml of Cipro HC Otic contains ciprofloxacin HCl (equivalent to 2 mg ciprofloxacin), 10 mg hydrocortisone, and 9 mg benzyl alcohol as a preservative. The inactive ingredients are polyvinyl alcohol, sodium chloride, sodium acetate, glacial acetic acid, phospholipon 90HB (modified lecithin), polysorbate, and purified water. Sodium hydroxide or hydrochloric acid may be added for adjustment of pH.

Ciprofloxacin, a fluoroquinolone, is available as the monohydrochloride monohydrate salt of 1-cyclopropyl-6-fluoro-1,4-dihydro-4-oxo-7-(1-piperazinyl)-3-quinolinecarboxylic acid. Its empirical formula is $C_{17}H_{18}FN_3O_3 \cdot HCl \cdot H_2O$.

Hydrocortisone, pregn-4-ene-3, 20-dione, 11, 17, 21-trihydroxy-(11b)-, is an anti-inflammatory corticosteroid. Its empirical formula is $C_{21}H_{30}O_5$.

CLINICAL PHARMACOLOGY

The plasma concentrations of ciprofloxacin were not measured following 3 drops of otic suspension administration because the systemic exposure to ciprofloxacin is expected to be below the limit of quantitation of the assay (0.05 mg/ml).

Similarly, the predicted C_{max} of hydrocortisone is within the range of endogenous hydrocortisone concentration (0-150 ng/ml), and therefore can not be differentiated from the endogenous cortisol.

Preclinical studies have shown that ciprofloxacin HCl; hydrocortisone otic suspension was not toxic to the guinea pig cochlea when administered intratympanically twice daily for 30 days and was only weakly irritating to rabbit skin upon repeated exposure.

Hydrocortisone has been added to aid in the resolution of the inflammatory response accompanying bacterial infection.

MICROBIOLOGY

Ciprofloxacin has *in vitro* activity against a wide range of gram-positive and gram-negative microorganisms. The bactericidal action of ciprofloxacin results from interference with the enzyme, DNA gyrase, which is needed for the synthesis of bacterial DNA. Cross-resistance has been observed between ciprofloxacin and other fluoroquinolones. There is generally no cross-resistance between ciprofloxacin and other classes of antibacterial agents such as beta-lactams or aminoglycosides.

Ciprofloxacin has been shown to be active against most strains of the following microorganisms, both *in vitro* and in clinical infections of acute otitis externa as described in the INDICATIONS AND USAGE section:

Aerobic gram-positive microorganism: *Staphylococcus aureus.*
Aerobic gram-negative microorganisms: *Proteus mirabilis, Pseudomonas aeruginosa.*

INDICATIONS AND USAGE

Ciprofloxacin HCl; hydrocortisone otic suspension is indicated for the treatment of acute otitis externa in adult and pediatric patients, 1 year and older, due to susceptible strains of *Pseudomonas aeruginosa, Staphylococcus aureus,* and *Proteus mirabilis.*

CONTRAINDICATIONS

Ciprofloxacin HCl; hydrocortisone otic suspension is contraindicated in persons with a history of hypersensitivity to hydrocortisone, ciprofloxacin or any member of the quinolone class of antimicrobial agents. This nonsterile product should not be used if the tympanic membrane is perforated. Use of this product is contraindicated in viral infections of the external canal including varicella and herpes simplex infections.

WARNINGS

NOT FOR OPHTHALMIC USE. NOT FOR INJECTION.

Ciprofloxacin HCl; hydrocortisone otic suspension should be discontinued at the first appearance of a skin rash or any other sign of hypersensitivity. Serious and occasionally fatal hypersensitivity (anaphylactic) reactions, some following the first dose, have been reported in patients receiving systemic quinolones. Serious acute hypersensitivity reactions may require immediate emergency treatment.

PRECAUTIONS

GENERAL

As with other antibiotic preparations, use of this product may result in overgrowth of non-susceptible organisms, including fungi. If the infection is not improved after 1 week of therapy, cultures should be obtained to guide further treatment.

INFORMATION FOR THE PATIENT

If rash or allergic reaction occurs, discontinue use immediately and contact your physician. Do not use in the eyes. Avoid contaminating the dropper with material from the ear, fingers, or other sources. Protect from light. Shake well immediately before using. Discard unused portion after therapy is completed.

CARCINOGENESIS, MUTAGENESIS, AND IMPAIRMENT OF FERTILITY

Eight *in vitro* mutagenicity tests have been conducted with ciprofloxacin, and the test results are listed below:

- *Salmonella*/Microsome Test (Negative)
- *E. coli* DNA Repair Assay (Negative)
- Mouse Lymphoma Cell Forward Mutation Assay (Positive)
- Chinese Hamster V79 Cell HGPRT Test (Negative)
- Syrian Hamster Embryo Cell Transformation Assay (Negative)
- *Saccharomyces cerevisiae* Point Mutation Assay (Negative)
- *Saccharomyces cerevisiae* Mitotic Crossover and Gene Conversion Assay (Negative)
- Rat Hepatocyte DNA Repair Assay (Positive)

Thus, 2 of the 8 tests were positive, but results of the following three *in vivo* test systems gave negative results:

- Rat Hepatocyte DNA Repair Assay
- Micronucleus Test (Mice)
- Dominant Lethal Test (Mice)

Long-term carcinogenicity studies in mice and rats have been completed for ciprofloxacin. After daily oral doses of 750 mg/kg (mice) and 250 mg/kg (rats) were administered for up to 2 years, there was no evidence that ciprofloxacin had any carcinogenic or tumorigenic effects in these species. No long term studies of ciprofloxacin HCl; hydrocortisone otic suspension have been performed to evaluate carcinogenic potential.

Fertility studies performed in rats at oral doses of ciprofloxacin up to 100 mg/kg/day revealed no evidence of impairment. This would be over 1000 times the maximum recommended clinical dose of ototopical ciprofloxacin based upon body surface area, assuming total absorption of ciprofloxacin from the ear of a patient treated with ciprofloxacin HCl; hydrocortisone otic suspension twice per day.

Long term studies have not been performed to evaluate the carcinogenic potential or the effect on fertility of topical hydrocortisone. Mutagenicity studies with hydrocortisone were negative.

PREGNANCY, TERATOGENIC EFFECTS, PREGNANCY CATEGORY C

Reproduction studies have been performed in rats and mice using oral doses of up to 100 mg/kg and IV doses up to 30 mg/kg and have revealed no evidence of harm to the fetus as a result of ciprofloxacin. In rabbits, ciprofloxacin (30 and 100 mg/kg orally) produced gastrointestinal disturbances resulting in maternal weight loss and an increased incidence of abortion, but no teratogenicity was observed at either dose. After intravenous administration of doses up to 20 mg/kg, no maternal toxicity was produced in the rabbit, and no embryotoxicity or teratogenicity was observed.

Corticosteroids are generally teratogenic in laboratory animals when administered systemically at relatively low dosage levels. The more potent corticosteroids have been shown to be teratogenic after dermal application in laboratory animals.

Animal reproduction studies have not been conducted with ciprofloxacin HCl; hydrocortisone otic suspension. No adequate and well controlled studies have been performed in pregnant women. Caution should be exercised when ciprofloxacin HCl; hydrocortisone otic suspension is used by a pregnant woman.

NURSING MOTHERS

Ciprofloxacin is excreted in human milk with systemic use. It is not known whether ciprofloxacin is excreted in human milk following topical otic administration. Because of the potential for serious adverse reactions in nursing infants, a decision should be made whether to discontinue nursing or to discontinue the drug, taking into account the importance of the drug to the mother.

PEDIATRIC USE

The safety and efficacy of ciprofloxacin HCl; hydrocortisone otic suspension have been established in pediatric patients 2 years and older (131 patients) in adequate and well-controlled clinical trials. Although no data are available on patients less than age 2 years, there are no known safety concerns or differences in the disease process in this population which would preclude use of this product in patients 1 year and older. See DOSAGE AND ADMINISTRATION.

ADVERSE REACTIONS

In Phase 3 clinical trials, a total of 564 patients were treated with ciprofloxacin HCl; hydrocortisone otic suspension. Adverse events with at least remote relationship to treatment included headache (1.2%) and pruritus (0.4%). The following treatment-related adverse events were each reported in a single patient: migraine, hypesthesia, paresthesia, fungal dermatitis, cough, rash, urticaria, and alopecia.

DOSAGE AND ADMINISTRATION

SHAKE WELL IMMEDIATELY BEFORE USING.

For children (age 1 year and older) and adults, 3 drops of the suspension should be instilled into the affected ear twice daily for 7 days. The suspension should be warmed by holding the bottle in the hand for 1-2 minutes to avoid the dizziness which may result from the instillation of a cold solution into the ear canal. The patient should lie with the affected ear upward and then the drops should be instilled. This position should be maintained for 30-60 seconds to facilitate penetration of the drops into the ear. Repeat, if necessary, for the opposite ear. Discard unused portion after therapy is completed.

HOW SUPPLIED

Cipro HC Otic is supplied as a white to off-white opaque suspension.
Storage: Store below 25°C (77°F). Avoid freezing. Protect from light.

PRODUCT LISTING - EQUIVALENTS NOT AVAILABLE

Suspension - Otic - 0.2%;1%

10 ml	$65.63	CIPRO HC, Alcon Laboratories Inc	54569-4723-00
10 ml	$78.75	CIPRO HC, Alcon Laboratories Inc	00065-8531-10

Cisplatin *(000824)*

Categories: Carcinoma, ovarian; Carcinoma, testicular; Carcinoma, bladder; Pregnancy Category D; FDA Approved 1978 Dec; WHO Formulary

Drug Classes: Antineoplastics, platinum agents

Brand Names: **Platinol**

Foreign Brand Availability: Abiplatin (Austria; Israel; South-Africa; Taiwan); Blastolem (Mexico); Briplatin (Japan); Cisplatin (Australia; India; Indonesia; New-Zealand); Cisplatin-Ebewe (Malaysia); Cisplatino (Colombia; Peru); Cisplatinum (Malaysia; Thailand); Cisplatyl (France; Peru); Citoplatino (Italy); Cytoplatin (Bahrain; Cyprus; Egypt; Iran; Iraq; Jordan; Kuwait; Lebanon; Libya; Oman; Qatar; Republic-of-Yemen; Saudi-Arabia; Syria; United-Arab-Emirates); Kemoplat (India); Lederplatin (Sweden); Neoplatin (Spain); Niyaplat (Mexico); Noveldexis (Mexico); Platamine (Bahrain; Bulgaria; Cyprus; Egypt; Greece; Iran; Iraq; Italy; Jordan; Kuwait; Lebanon; Libya; Oman; Philippines; Qatar; Republic-of-Yemen; Saudi-Arabia; South-Africa; Syria; United-Arab-Emirates); Platamine RTU (Indonesia); Platiblastin (Austria; Germany; Switzerland); Platidiam (Bulgaria; Czech-Republic; Hungary); Platinex (Germany; Italy); Platinol-AQ (Canada); Platinoxan (Philippines); Platistil (Portugal; Spain); Platistin (Finland; Norway; Sweden); Platosin (England; Malaysia; Philippines; South-Africa; Taiwan; Thailand); Tecnoplatin (Mexico)

HCFA JCODE(S): J9060 per 10 mg IV; J9062 50 mg IV

WARNING

Cisplatin should be administered under the supervision of a qualified physician experienced in the use of cancer chemotherapeutic agents. Appropriate management of therapy and complications is possible only when adequate diagnostic and treatment facilities are readily available.

Cumulative renal toxicity associated with cisplatin is severe. Other major dose-related toxicities are myelosuppression, nausea, and vomiting.

Ototoxicity, which may be more pronounced in children, and is manifested by tinnitus, and/or loss of high frequency hearing and occasionally deafness, is significant.

Anaphylactic-like reactions to cisplatin have been reported. Facial edema, bronchoconstriction, tachycardia, and hypotension may occur within minutes of cisplatin administration. Epinephrine, corticosteroids, and antihistamines have been effectively employed to alleviate symptoms (see WARNINGS and ADVERSE REACTIONS).

DESCRIPTION

Cisplatin (cis-diamminedichloroplatinum) is a heavy metal complex containing a central atom of platinum surrounded by two chloride atoms and two ammonia molecules in the cis position. It is a white lyophilized powder with the molecular formula $PtCl_2H_6N_2$, and a molecular weight of 300.1. It is soluble in water or saline at 1 mg/ml and in dimethylformamide at 24 mg/ml. It has a melting point of 207°C. Cisplatin-AQ is a sterile aqueous solution, containing 1 mg cisplatin and 9 mg sodium chloride. HCl and/or sodium hydroxide added to adjust pH.

CLINICAL PHARMACOLOGY

Plasma concentrations of the parent compound, cisplatin, decay monoexponentially with a half-life of about 20-30 minutes following bolus administrations of 50 or 100 mg/m^2 doses. Monoexponential decay and plasma half-lives of about 0.5 hour are also seen following two hour or seven hour infusions of 100 mg/m^2. After the latter, the total-body clearances and volumes of distribution at steady-state for cisplatin are about 15-16 L/h/m^2.

Due to its unique chemical structure, the chlorine atoms of cisplatin are more subject to chemical displacement reactions by nucleophiles, such as water or sulfhydryl groups, than to enzyme-catalyzed metabolism. At physiological pH in the presence of 0.1M NaCl, the predominant molecular species are cisplatin and monohydroxymonochloro *cis*-dimmamine platinum (II) in nearly equal concentrations. The latter, combined with the possible direct displacement of the chlorine atoms by sulfhydryl groups of amino acids ot proteins, accounts for the instability of cisplatin in biological matrices. The ratios of cisplatin to total free (ultrafiltrable) platinum in the plasma vary considerably between patients and range from 0.5-1.1 after a dose of 100 mg/m^2.

Cisplatin does not undergo the instantaneous and reversible binding to plasma proteins that is characteristic of normal drug-binding protein. However, the platinum from cisplatin, but not cisplatin itself, becomes bound to several plasma proteins including albumin, transferrin, and gamma globulin. Three (3) hours after a bolus injection and 2 hours after the end of a 3 hour infusion, 90% of the plasma platinum is protein bound. The complexes between albumin and the platinum from cisplatin do not dissociate to a significant extent and are slowly eliminated with a minimum half-life of 5 days or more.

Following cisplatin doses of 20-120 mg/m^2, the concentrations of platinum are highest in liver, prostate, and kidney, and somewhat lower in bladder, muscle, testicle, pancreas, and spleen and lowest in bowel, adrenal, heart, lung, cerebrum, and cerebellum. Platinum is present in tissues for as long as 180 days after the last administration. With the exception of intracerebral tumors, platinum concentrations in tumors are generally somewhat lower than the concentrations in the organ where the tumor is located. Different metastatic sites in the same patient may have different platinum concentrations. Hepatic metastases have the highest platinum concentrations, but these are similar to the platinum concentrations in normal liver. Maximum red blood cell concentrations of platinum are reached within 90-150 minutes after a 100 mg/m^2 dose of cisplatin and decline in a biphasic manner with the terminal half-life of 36 to 47 days.

Over a dose range of 40-140 mg cisplatin/m^2 given as a bolus injection or as infusions varying in length from 1 hour to 24 hours, from 10% to about 40% of the administered platinum is excreted within 24 hours, from 10% to about 40% of the administered platinum is excreted in the urine in 24 hours. Over 5 days following administration of 40-100 mg/m^2 doses given as rapid, 2-3 hour, or 6-8 hour infusions, a mean of 35-51% of the dosed platinum is excreted in the urine. Similar mean urinary recoveries of platinum of about 14-30% of the dose are found following live daily administrations of 20, 30, or 40 mg/m^2/day. Only a small percentage of the administered platinum is excreted beyond 24 hours post-infusion and most of the platinum excreted in the urine in 24 is excreted within the first few hours. Platinum-containing species excreted in the urine are the same as those found following the incubation of cisplatin with urine from healthy subjects, except that the proportions are different.

The parent compound, cisplatin, is excreted in the urine and accounts for 13-17% of the dose excreted within one hour after administration of 50 mg/m^2. The mean renal clearance of cisplatin exceeds creatinine clearance and is 62 and 50 ml/min/m^2 following administration of 100 mg/m^2 as 2 hour or 6-7 hour infusions, respectively.

The renal clearance of free (ultrafiltrable) platinum also exceeds the glomerular filtration rate indicating that cisplatin or other platinum-containing molecules are actively secreted by the kidneys. The renal clearance of free platinum is nonlinear and variable and is dependent on dose, urine flow rate, and individual variability in the extent on of active secretion and possible tubular resorption.

There is a potential for accumulation of ultrafiltrable platinum plasma concentration whenever cisplatin is administered on a daily basis but not when dose on an intermittent basis.

No significant relationships exist between the renal clearance of either free platinum and cisplatin and creatinine clearance.

Although small amounts of platinum are present in the bile and large intestine after administration of cisplatin, the fecal excretion of platinum appears to be insignificant.

INDICATIONS AND USAGE

Cisplatin is indicated as therapy to be employed as follows:

Metastatic Testicular Tumors: In established combination therapy with other approved chemotherapeutic agents in patients with metastatic testicular tumors who have already received appropriate surgical and/or radiotherapeutic procedures.

Metastatic Ovarian Tumors: In established combination therapy with other approved chemotherapeutic agents in patients with metastatic ovarian tumors who have already received appropriate surgical and/or radiotherapeutic procedures. An established combination consists of cisplatin and cyclophosphamide. Cisplatin, as a single agent, is indicated as secondary therapy in patients with metastatic ovarian tumors refractory to standard chemotherapy who have not previously received cisplatin therapy.

Advance Bladder Cancer: Cisplatin is indicated as a single agent for patients with transitional cell bladder cancer which is no longer amenable to local treatments such as surgery and/or radiotherapy.

NON-FDA APPROVED INDICATIONS

Cisplatin has also been used in the treatment of soft tissue sarcomas, mesotheliomas, melanoma, osteosarcoma cancer of unknown primary origin, as salvage treatment of lymphomas, and in bone marrow transplant conditioning regimens. However, these uses have not been approved by the FDA and further clinical trials are needed.

CONTRAINDICATIONS

Cisplatin is contraindicated in patients with preexisting renal impairment. Cisplatin should not be employed in myelosuppressed patients, or patients with hearing impairment.

Cisplatin is contraindicated in patients with a history of allergic reactions to cisplatin or other platinum-containing compounds.

WARNINGS

Cisplatin produces cumulative nephrotoxicity which is potentiated by aminoglycoside antibiotics. The serum creatinine, BUN, creatinine clearance, and magnesium, sodium, potassium, and calcium levels should be measured prior to initiating therapy, and prior to each subsequent course. At the recommended dosage, cisplatin should not be given more frequently than once every 3-4 weeks (see ADVERSE REACTIONS).

There are reports of severe neuropathies in patients in whom regimens are employed using higher doses of cisplatin or greater dose frequencies than those recommended. These neuropathies may be irreversible and are seen as paresthesias in a stocking-glove distribution, areflexia, and loss of proprioception and vibratory sensation.

Loss of motor function has also been reported.

Anaphylactic-like reactions to cisplatin have been reported. These reactions have occurred within minutes of administration to patients with prior exposure to cisplatin, and have been alleviated by administration of epinephrine, corticosteroids, and antihistamines.

Since ototoxicity of cisplatin is cumulative, audiometric testing should be performed prior to initiating therapy and prior to each subsequent dose of drug (see ADVERSE REACTIONS).

Cisplatin can cause fetal harm when administered to a pregnant woman. Cisplatin is mutagenic in bacteria and produces chromosome aberrations in animal cells in tissue culture. In mice cisplatin is teratogenic and embryotoxic. If this drug is used during pregnancy or if the patient becomes pregnant while taking this drug, the patient should be apprised of the potential hazard to the fetus. Patients should be advised to avoid becoming pregnant.

The carcinogenic effect of cisplatin was studied in BD IX rats. Cisplatin was administered i.p. to 50 BD IX rats for 3 weeks, 3 × 1 mg/kg body weight per week. Four hundred and fifty-five (455) days after the first application, 33 animals died, 13 of them related to malignancies: 12 leukemias and 1 renal fibrosarcoma.

The development of acute leukemia coincident with the use of cisplatin has rarely been reported in humans. In these reports, cisplatin was generally given in combination with other leukemogenic agents.

PRECAUTIONS

Peripheral blood counts should be monitored weekly. Liver function should be monitored periodically. Neurologic examination should also be performed regularly (see ADVERSE REACTIONS).

Carcinogenesis, Mutagenesis, and Impairment of Fertility: See WARNINGS.

Pregnancy: See WARNINGS.

DRUG INTERACTIONS

Plasma levels of anticonvulsant agents may become subtherapeutic during cisplatin therapy.

In a randomized trial in advanced ovarian cancer, response duration was adversely affected when pyridoxine was used in combination with altretamine (hexmethylmelamine) and cisplatin.

C

ADVERSE REACTIONS

Nephrotoxicity: Dose-related and cumulative renal insufficiency is the major dose-limiting toxicity of cisplatin. Renal toxicity has been noted in 28-36% of patients treated with a single dose of 50 mg/m^2. It is first noted during the second week after a dose and is manifested by elevations in BUN and creatinine, serum uric acid and/or a decrease in creatinine clearance. **Renal toxicity becomes more prolonged and severe with repeated courses of the drug. Renal function must return to normal before another dose of cisplatin can be given.**

Impairment of renal function has been associated with renal tubular damage. The administration of cisplatin using a 6-8 hour infusion with intravenous hydration, and mannitol has been used to reduce nephrotoxicity. However, renal toxicity still can occur after utilization of these procedures.

Ototoxicity: Ototoxicity has been observed in up to 31% of patients treated with a single dose of cisplatin 50 mg/m^2, and is manifested by tinnitus and/or hearing loss in the high frequency range (4000-8000 Hz). Decreased ability to hear normal conversational tones may occur occasionally. Deafness after the initial dose of cisplatin has been reported rarely. Ototoxic effects may be more severe in children receiving cisplatin. Hearing loss can be unilateral or bilateral and tends to become more frequent and severe with repeated doses. Ototoxicity may be enhanced with prior or simultaneous cranial irradiation. It is unclear whether cisplatin induced ototoxicity is reversible. Careful monitoring of audiometry should be performed prior to initiation of therapy and prior to subsequent doses of cisplatin. Vestibular toxicity has also been reported.

Ototoxicity may become more severe in patients being treated with other drugs with nephrotoxic potential.

Hematologic: Myelosuppression occurs in 25-30% of patients treated with cisplatin. The nadirs in circulating platelets and leukocytes occur between days 18-23 (range 7.5-45) with most patients recovering by day 39 (range 13-62). Leukopenia and thrombocytopenia are more pronounced at higher doses (>50 mg/m^2). Anemia (decrease of 2 g hemoglobin/100 ml) occurs at approximately the same frequency and with the same timing as leukopenia and thrombocytopenia.

In addition to anemia secondary to myelosuppression, a Coombs' positive hemolytic anemia has been reported. in the presence of cisplatin hemolytic anemia, a further course of treatment may be accompanied by increased hemolysis and this risk should be weighed by the treating physician.

The development of acute leukemia coincident with with the use of cisplatin has rarely been reported in humans. In these report, cisplatin was generally given in combination with other leukemogenic agents.

Gastrointestinal: Marked nausea and vomiting occur in almost all patients treated with cisplatin, and are occasionally so severe that the drug must be discontinued. Nausea and vomiting usually begin within 1-4 hours after treatment and last up to 24 hours. Various degrees of nausea and anorexia may persist for up to 1 week after treatment.

Delayed nausea and vomiting (begins or persists 24 hours or more after chemotherapy) has occurred in patients attaining complete emetic control on the day of cisplatin therapy.

Diarrhea has also been reported.

OTHER TOXICITIES

Vascular toxicities coincident with the use of cisplatin in combination with other antineoplastic agents have been reported rarely. The events are clinically heterogeneous and may include myocardial infarction, cerebrovascular accident, thrombotic microangiopathy (HUS), or cerebral arteritis. Various mechanisms have been proposed for these vascular complications. There are also reports of Raynaud's phenomenon occurring in patients treated with the combination of bleomycin, vinblastine with or without cisplatin. It has been suggested that hypomagnesemia developing coincident with the use of cisplatin may be an added, although not essential, factor associated with this event. However, it is currently unknown if the cause of Raynaud's phenomenon in these cases is the disease, underlying vascular compromise, bleomycin, vinblastine, hypomagnesemia, or a combination of any of these factors.

Serum Electrolyte Disturbances: Hypomagnesemia, hypocalcemia, hyponatremia, hypokalemia, and hypophosphatemia have been reported to occur in patients treated with cisplatin and are probably related to renal tubular damage. Tetany has occasionally been reported in those patients with hypocalcemia and hypomagnesemia. Generally, normal serum electrolyte levels are restored by administering supplemental electrolytes and discontinuing cisplatin.

Inappropriate antidiuretic hormone syndrome has also been reported.

Hyperuricemia: Hyperuricemia has been reported to occur at approximately the same frequency as the increases in BUN and serum creatinine.

It is more pronounced after doses greater than 50 mg/m^2, and peak levels of uric acid generally occur between 3-5 days after the dose. Allopurinol therapy for hyperuricemia effectively reduces uric acid levels.

Neurotoxicity: (See WARNINGS.) Neurotoxicity, usually characterized by peripheral neuropathies, has been reported. The neuropathies usually occur after prolonged therapy (4-7 months); however, neurologic symptoms have been reported to occur after a single dose. Cisplatin therapy should be discontinued when the symptoms are first observed. Preliminary evidence suggests peripheral neuropathy may be irreversible in some patients.

Lhermitte's sign and autonomic neuropathy have also been reported.

Loss of taste and seizures have also been reported.

Muscle cramps, defined as localized, painful, involuntary skeletal muscle contractions of sudden onset and short duration, have been reported and were usually associated in patients receiving a relatively high cumulative dose of cisplatin and with a relatively advanced symptomatic stage of peripheral neuropathy.

Ocular Toxicity: Optic neuritis, papilledema, and cerebral blindness have been reported infrequently in patients receiving standard recommended doses of cisplatin. Improvement and/or total recovery usually occurs after discontinuing cisplatin. Steroids with or without mannitol have been used; however, efficacy has not been established.

Blurred vision and altered color perception have been reported after the use of regimens with higher doses of cisplatin or greater dose frequencies than those recommended in the package insert. The altered color perception manifests as a loss of color discrimination, particularly in the blue-yellow axis. The only finding on funduscopic exam is irregular retinal pigmentation of the macular area.

Anaphylactic-like Reactions: Anaphylactic-like reactions have been occasionally reported in patients previously exposed to cisplatin. The reactions consist of facial edema, wheezing, tachycardia, and hypotension within a few minutes of drug administration. Reactions may be controlled by intravenous epinephrine, corticosteroids, or antihistamines. Patients receiving cisplatin should be observed carefully for possible anaphylactic-like reactions and supportive equipment and medication should be available to treat such a complication.

Other Events: Other toxicities reported to occur infrequently are cardiac abnormalities, anorexia, elevated SGOT, and rash. Alopecia has also been reported.

Local soft tissue toxicity has rarely been reported following extravasation of cisplatin. Severity of the local tissue toxicity appears to be related to the concentration of the cisplatin solution. Infusion of solutions with a cisplatin concentration greater than 0.5 mg/ml may result in tissue cellulitis, fibrosis, and necrosis.

DOSAGE AND ADMINISTRATION

Note: Needles or intravenous sets containing aluminum parts that may come in contact with cisplatin should not be used for preparation or administration. Aluminum reacts with cisplatin, causing precipitate formation and a loss of potency.

Metastatic Testicular Tumors: The usual cisplatin dose for the treatment of testicular cancer in combination with other approved chemotherapeutic agents is 20 mg/m^2 IV daily for 5 days.

Metastatic Ovarian Tumors: The usual cisplatin dose for the treatment of metastatic ovarian tumors in combination with Cytoxan is 75-100 mg/m^2 IV once every 4 weeks (DAY 1).[2,3]

The dose of Cytoxan when used in combination with cisplatin is 600 mg/m^2 IV once every 4 weeks (DAY 1). [2,3]

For directions for the administration of Cytoxan, refer to the Cytoxan monograph.

In combination therapy, cisplatin and Cytoxan are administered sequentially.

As a single agent, cisplatin should be administered at a dose of 100 mg/m^2 IV once every 4 weeks.

Advanced Bladder Cancer: Cisplatin should be administered as a single agent at a dose of 50-70 mg/m^2 IV once every 3-4 weeks depending on the extent of prior exposure to radiation therapy and/or prior chemotherapy. For heavily pretreated patients an initial dose of 50 mg/m^2 repeated every 4 weeks is recommended.

Pretreatment hydration with 1-2 L of fluid infused for 8-12 hours prior to a cisplatin dose is recommended. The drug is then diluted in 2 L of 5% dextrose in 1/2 or 1/3 normal saline containing 37.5 g of mannitol, and infused over a 6-8 hour period. If diluted solution is not to be used within 6 hours, protect solution from light. Adequate hydration and urinary output must be maintained during the following 24 hours.

A repeat course of cisplatin should not be given until the serum creatinine is below 1.5 mg/100 ml, and/or the BUN is below 25 mg/100 ml. A repeat course should not be given until circulating blood elements are at an acceptable level (platelets $\geq$100,000/mm^3, WBC $\geq$4000/mm^3). Subsequent doses of cisplatin should not be given until an audiometric analysis indicates that auditory acuity is within normal limits.

As with other potentially toxic compounds, caution should be exercised in handling the powder and preparing the solution of cisplatin. Skin reactions associated with accidental exposure to cisplatin may occur. The use of gloves is recommended. If cisplatin powder or solution contact the skin or mucosae, immediately wash the skin or mucosae thoroughly with soap and water.

The aqueous solution should be used intravenously only and be administered by IV infusion over 6-8 hour period.

STABILITY

Cisplatin is a sterile, multidose vial without preservatives.

Store at 15-25°C. Do not refrigerate. Protect unopened container from light.

The cisplatin remaining in the amber vial following initial entry is stable for 28 days protected from light or for 7 days under fluorescent room light.

Procedures for Proper Handling and Disposal: Anticancer drugs should be considered. Several guidelines on this subject have been published.[4-10] There is no general agreement that all of the procedures recommended in the guidelines are necessary or appropriate.

PRODUCT LISTING - RATED THERAPEUTICALLY EQUIVALENT

Solution - Intravenous - 1 mg/ml

Size	Price	Product	NDC
50 ml	$131.25	GENERIC, Baxter Pharmaceutical Products, Inc	10019-0910-01
50 ml	$222.00	GENERIC, American Pharmaceutical Partners	63323-0103-51
50 ml	$224.98	GENERIC, Bedford Laboratories	55390-0112-50
50 ml	$224.98	GENERIC, Bedford Laboratories	55390-0414-50
50 ml	$231.56	GENERIC, Gensia Sicor Pharmaceuticals Inc	00703-5747-11
50 ml	$240.02	PLATINOL-AQ, Bristol-Myers Squibb	00015-3220-22
100 ml	$256.25	GENERIC, Baxter Pharmaceutical Products, Inc	10019-0910-02
100 ml	$444.00	GENERIC, American Pharmaceutical Partners	63323-0103-65
100 ml	$449.92	GENERIC, Bedford Laboratories	55390-0112-99
100 ml	$449.92	GENERIC, Bedford Laboratories	55390-0414-99
100 ml	$463.13	GENERIC, Gensia Sicor Pharmaceuticals Inc	00703-5748-11
100 ml	$480.00	PLATINOL-AQ, Bristol-Myers Squibb	00015-3221-22
200 ml	$888.00	GENERIC, American Pharmaceutical Partners	63323-0103-64

PRODUCT LISTING - EQUIVALENTS NOT AVAILABLE

Powder For Injection - Intravenous - 10 mg
1's $33.28 PLATINOL, Bristol-Myers Squibb 00015-3070-20
Powder For Injection - Intravenous - 50 mg
1's $122.59 PLATINOL, Bristol-Myers Squibb 00015-3072-20
Solution - Intravenous - 1 mg/ml
50 ml $178.18 PLATINOL-AQ, Bristol-Myers Squibb 00015-3220-26
100 ml $375.94 PLATINOL-AQ, Bristol-Myers Squibb 00015-3221-26

Citalopram Hydrobromide (003408)

For related information, see the comparative table section in Appendix A.

Categories: Depression; FDA Approved 1998 Jul; Pregnancy Category C
Drug Classes: Antidepressants, serotonin specific reuptake inhibitors
Foreign Brand Availability: Celexa (Canada); Cipram (Bahrain; China; Cyprus; Egypt; Hong-Kong; Indonesia; Iran; Iraq; Jordan; Korea; Kuwait; Lebanon; Libya; Oman; Qatar; Republic-of-Yemen; Saudi-Arabia; Singapore; Syria; Taiwan; Thailand; United-Arab-Emirates); Cipramil (Australia; Belgium; Denmark; England; Finland; Germany; Ireland; Israel; Netherlands; New-Zealand; Norway; Peru; South-Africa; Sweden); Citopam (India); Lupram (Philippines); Recital (Israel); Sepram (Germany); Seralgan (Austria); Seropram (Austria; France; Spain; Switzerland); Zentius (Colombia)
Cost of Therapy: $78.49 (Depression; Celexa; 40 mg; 1 tablet/day; 30 day supply)

DESCRIPTION

Citalopram hydrobromide is an orally administered selective serotonin reuptake inhibitor (SSRI) with a chemical structure unrelated to that of other SSRI's or of tricyclic, tetracyclic, or other available antidepressant agents. Citalopram hydrobromide is a racemic bicyclic phthalane derivative designated (±)-1-(3-dimethylaminopropyl)-1-(4-fluorophenyl)-1,3-dihydroisobenzofuran-5-carbonitrile, hydrobromide.

The molecular formula is $C_{20}H_{22}BrFN_2O$ and its molecular weight is 405.35.

Citalopram hydrobromide occurs as a fine white to off-white powder. Citalopram hydrobromide is sparingly soluble in water and soluble in ethanol.

Celexa is available as tablets or as an oral solution.

ORAL SOLUTION

Celexa oral solution contains citalopram hydrobromide equivalent to 2 mg/ml citalopram base. *Inactive Ingredients:* Sorbitol, purified water, propylene glycol, methylparaben, natural peppermint flavor, and propylparaben.

TABLET

Celexa is a film coated, oval, scored tablet containing citalopram hydrobromide in strengths equivalent to 10, 20 or 40 mg citalopram base. *Inactive Ingredients:* Copolyvidone, corn starch, crosscarmellose sodium, glycerin, lactose monohydrate, magnesium stearate, hydroxypropyl methyl cellulose, microcrystalline cellulose, polyethylene glycol and titanium dioxide. Iron oxides are used as coloring agents in the beige (10 mg) and pink (20 mg) tablets.

CLINICAL PHARMACOLOGY

PHARMACODYNAMICS

The mechanism of action of citalopram hydrobromide as an antidepressant is presumed to be linked to potentiation of serotonergic activity in the central nervous system resulting from its inhibition of CNS neuronal reuptake of serotonin (5-HT). *In vitro* and *in vivo* studies in animals suggest that citalopram is a highly selective serotonin reuptake inhibitor (SSRI) with minimal effects on norepinephrine (NE) and dopamine (DA) neuronal reuptake. Tolerance to the inhibition of 5-HT uptake is not induced by long term (14 day) treatment of rats with citalopram. Citalopram is a racemic mixture (50/50), and the inhibition of 5-HT reuptake by citalopram is primarily due to the (S)-enantiomer.

Citalopram has no or very low affinity for 5-HT_{1A}, 5-HT_{2A}, dopamine D_1 and D_2, α_1-, α_2-, and β-adrenergic, histamine H_1, gamma aminobutyric acid (GABA), muscarinic cholinergic, and benzodiazepine receptors. Antagonism of muscarinic, histaminergic and adrenergic receptors has been hypothesized to be associated with various anticholinergic, sedative and cardiovascular effects of other psychotropic drugs.

PHARMACOKINETICS

The single- and multiple-dose pharmacokinetics of citalopram are linear and dose-proportional in a dose range of 10-60 mg/day. Biotransformation of citalopram is mainly hepatic, with a mean terminal half-life of about 35 hours. With once daily dosing, steady state plasma concentrations are achieved within approximately 1 week. At steady state, the extent of accumulation of citalopram in plasma, based on the half-life, is expected to be 2.5 times the plasma concentrations observed after a single dose. The tablet and oral solution dosage forms of citalopram hydrobromide are bioequivalent.

Absorption and Distribution

Following a single oral dose (40 mg tablet) of citalopram, peak blood levels occur at about 4 hours. The absolute bioavailability of citalopram was about 80% relative to an intravenous (IV) dose and absorption is not affected by food. The volume of distribution of citalopram is about 12 L/kg and the binding of citalopram (CT), demethylcitalopram (DCT) and didemethylcitalopram (DDCT) to human plasma proteins is about 80%.

Metabolism andElimination

Following IV administrations of citalopram, the fraction of drug recovered in the urine as citalopram and DCT was about 10% and 5%, respectively. The systemic clearance of citalopram was 330 ml/min, with approximately 20% of that due to renal clearance.

Citalopram is metabolized to demethylcitalopram (DCT), didemethylcitalopram (DDCT), citalopram-N-oxide and a deaminated propionic acid derivative. In humans, unchanged citalopram is the predominant compound in plasma. At steady state, the concentrations of citalopram's metabolites, DCT and DDCT, in plasma are approximately one-half and one-tenth, respectively, that of the parent drug. *In vitro* studies show that citalopram is at least 8 times more potent than its metabolites in the inhibition of serotonin reuptake, suggesting that the metabolites evaluated do not likely contribute significantly to the antidepressant actions of citalopram.

In vitro studies using human liver microsomes indicated that CYP3A4 and CYP2C19 are the primary isozymes involved in the N-demethylation of citalopram.

C

Population Subgroups

Age

Citalopram pharmacokinetics in subjects ≥60 years of age were compared to younger subjects in 2 normal volunteer studies. In a single dose study, citalopram AUC and half-life were increased in the elderly subjects by 30% and 50%, respectively, whereas in a multiple dose study they were increased by 23% and 30% respectively. 20 mg is the recommended dose for most elderly patients (see DOSAGE AND ADMINISTRATION).

Gender

In three pharmacokinetic studies (total n=32), citalopram AUC in women was 1.5-2 times that in men. This difference was not observed in 5 other pharmacokinetic studies (total n=114). In clinical studies, no differences in steady state serum citalopram levels were seen between men (n=237) and women (n=388). There were no gender differences in the pharmacokinetics of DCT and DDCT. No adjustment of dosage on the basis of gender is recommended.

Reduced Hepatic Function

Citalopram oral clearance was reduced by 37% and half-life was doubled in patients with reduced hepatic function compared to normal subjects. 20 mg is the recommended dose for most hepatically impaired patients (see DOSAGE AND ADMINISTRATION).

Reduced Renal Function

In patients with mild to moderate renal function impairment, oral clearance of citalopram was reduced by 17% compared to normal subjects. No adjustment of dosage for such patients is recommended. No information is available about the pharmacokinetics of citalopram in patients with severely reduced renal function (creatinine clearance <20 ml/min).

Drug-Drug Interactions

In vitro enzyme inhibition data did not reveal an inhibitory effect of citalopram on CYP3A4, -2C9, or -2E1, but did suggest that it is a weak inhibitor of CYP-1A2, -2D6, and -2C19. Citalopram would be expected to have little inhibitory effect on *in vivo* metabolism mediated by these cytochromes. However, *in vivo* data to address this question are limited.

Since CYP3A4 and 2C19 are the primary enzymes involved in the metabolism of citalopram, it is expected that potent inhibitors of 3A4, *e.g.,* ketoconazole, itraconazole, and macrolide antibiotics, and potent inhibitors of CYP2C19, *e.g.,* omeprazole, might decrease the clearance of citalopram. However, coadministration of citalopram and the potent 3A4 inhibitor ketaconazole did not significantly affect the pharmacokinetics of citalopram. Because citalopram is metabolized by multiple enzyme systems, inhibition of a single enzyme may not appreciably decrease citalopram clearance. Citalopram steady state levels were not significantly different in poor metabolizers and extensive 2D6 metabolizers after multiple dose administration of citalopram hydrobromide, suggesting that coadministration, with citalopram hydrobromide, of a drug that inhibits CYP2D6, is unlikely to have clinically significant effects on citalopram metabolism. See DRUG INTERACTIONS for more detailed information on available drug interaction data.

INDICATIONS AND USAGE

Citalopram hydrobromide is indicated for the treatment of depression.

The efficacy of citalopram hydrobromide in the treatment of depression was established in 4-6 week controlled trials of outpatients whose diagnosis corresponded most closely to the DSM-III and DSM-III-R category of major depressive disorder (see CLINICAL PHARMACOLOGY).

A major depressive episode (DSM-IV) implies a prominent and relatively persistent (nearly every day for at least 2 weeks) depressed or dysphoric mood that usually interferes with daily functioning, and includes at least 5 of the following 9 symptoms: depressed mood, loss of interest in usual activities, significant change in weight and/or appetite, insomnia or hypersomnia, psychomotor agitation or retardation, increased fatigue, feelings of guilt or worthlessness, slowed thinking or impaired concentration, a suicide attempt or suicidal ideation.

The antidepressant action of citalopram hydrobromide in hospitalized depressed patients has not been adequately studied.

The efficacy of citalopram hydrobromide in maintaining an antidepressant response for up to 24 weeks following 6-8 weeks of acute treatment was demonstrated in two placebo-controlled trials (see CLINICAL PHARMACOLOGY). Nevertheless, the physician who elects to use citalopram hydrobromide for extended periods should periodically re-evaluate the long-term usefulness of the drug for the individual patient.

NON-FDA APPROVED INDICATIONS

Citalopram and other SSRIs may also have clinical utility for the treatment of a number of other conditions including bulimia nervosa, obsessive compulsive disorder, panic disorder, substance abuse, headaches, premenstrual dysphoria, premature ejaculation, post-traumatic stress disorder, seasonal affective disorder and chronic pain, although none of these uses is approved by the FDA for citalopram and comparative efficacy trials for many of these uses have not yet been performed.

CONTRAINDICATIONS

Concomitant use in patients taking monoamine oxidase inhibitors (MAOI's) is contraindicated (see WARNINGS).

Citalopram hydrobromide tablets or oral solution are contraindicated in patients with a hypersensitivity to citalopram or any of the inactive ingredients in either formulation.

WARNINGS

POTENTIAL FOR INTERACTION WITH MONOAMINE OXIDASE INHIBITORS

In patients receiving serotonin reuptake inhibitor drugs in combination with a monoamine oxidase inhibitor (MAOI), there have been reports of serious, sometimes fatal, reactions including hyperthermia, rigidity, myoclonus, autonomic instability with possible rapid fluctuations of vital signs, and mental status changes that include extreme agitation progressing to delirium and coma. These reactions have also been reported in patients who have recently discontinued SSRI treatment and have been started on a MAOI. Some cases presented with features resembling neuroleptic malignant syndrome. Furthermore, limited animal data on the effects of combined use of SSRI's and MAOI's suggest that these drugs may act synergistically to elevate blood pressure and evoke behavioral excitation. Therefore, it is recommended that citalopram hydrobromide should not be used in combination with a MAOI, or within 14 days of discontinuing treatment with a MAOI. Similarly, at least 14 days should be allowed after stopping citalopram hydrobromide before starting a MAOI.

PRECAUTIONS

GENERAL

Hyponatremia

Several cases of hyponatremia and SIADH (syndrome of inappropriate antidiuretic hormone secretion) have been reported in association with citalopram hydrobromide treatment. All patients with these events have recovered with discontinuation of citalopram hydrobromide and/or medical intervention.

Activation of Mania/Hypomania

In placebo-controlled trials of citalopram hydrobromide, some of which included patients with bipolar disorder, activation of mania/hypomania was reported in 0.2% of 1063 patients treated with citalopram hydrobromide and in none of the 446 patients treated with placebo. Activation of mania/hypomania has also been reported in a small proportion of patients with major affective disorders treated with other marketed antidepressants. As with all antidepressants, citalopram hydrobromide should be used cautiously in patients with a history of mania.

Seizures

Although anticonvulsant effects of citalopram have been observed in animal studies, citalopram hydrobromide has not been systematically evaluated in patients with a seizure disorder. These patients were excluded from clinical studies during the product's premarketing testing. In clinical trials of citalopram hydrobromide, seizures occurred in 0.3% of patients treated with citalopram hydrobromide (a rate of 1 patient per 98 years of exposure) and 0.5% of patients treated with placebo (a rate of 1 patient per 50 years of exposure). Like other antidepressants, citalopram hydrobromide should be introduced with care in patients with a history of seizure disorder.

Suicide

The possibility of a suicide attempt is inherent in depression and may persist until significant remission occurs. Close supervision of high risk patients should accompany initial drug therapy. Prescriptions for citalopram hydrobromide should be written for the smallest quantity of tablets consistent with good patient management, in order to reduce the risk of overdose.

Interference With Cognitive and Motor Performance

In studies in normal volunteers, citalopram hydrobromide in doses of 40 mg/day did not produce impairment of intellectual function or psychomotor performance. Because any psychoactive drug may impair judgement, thinking, or motor skills, however, patients should be cautioned about operating hazardous machinery, including automobiles, until they are reasonably certain that citalopram hydrobromide therapy does not affect their ability to engage in such activities.

Use in Patients With Concomitant Illness

Clinical experience with citalopram hydrobromide in patients with certain concomitant systemic illnesses is limited. Caution is advisable in using citalopram hydrobromide in patients with diseases or conditions that produce altered metabolism or hemodynamic responses.

Citalopram hydrobromide has not been systematically evaluated in patients with a recent history of myocardial infarction or unstable heart disease. Patients with these diagnoses were generally excluded from clinical studies during the products premarketing testing. However, the electrocardiograms of 1116 patients who received citalopram hydrobromide in clinical trials were evaluated and the data indicate that citalopram hydrobromide is not associated with the development of clinically significant ECG abnormalities.

In subjects with hepatic impairment, citalopram clearance was decreased and plasma concentrations were increased. The use of citalopram hydrobromide in hepatically impaired patients should be approached with caution and a lower maximum dosage is recommended (see DOSAGE AND ADMINISTRATION).

Because citalopram is extensively metabolized, excretion of unchanged drug in urine is a minor route of elimination. Until adequate numbers of patients with severe renal impairment have been evaluated during chronic treatment with citalopram hydrobromide, however, it should be used with caution in such patients (see DOSAGE AND ADMINISTRATION).

INFORMATION FOR THE PATIENT

Physicians are advised to discuss the following issues with patients for whom they prescribe citalopram hydrobromide:

Although in controlled studies citalopram hydrobromide has not been shown to impair psychomotor performance, any psychoactive drug may impair judgment, thinking or motor skills, and so patients should be cautioned about operating hazardous machinery, including automobiles, until they are reasonably certain that citalopram hydrobromide therapy does not affect their ability to engage in such activities.

Patients should be told that, although citalopram hydrobromide has not been shown in experiments with normal subjects to increase the mental and motor skill impairments caused by alcohol, the concomitant use of citalopram hydrobromide and alcohol in depressed patients is not advised.

Patients should be advised to inform their physician if they are taking, or plan to take, any prescription or over-the-counter drugs, as there is a potential for interactions.

Patients should be advised to notify their physician if they become pregnant or intend to become pregnant during therapy.

Patients should be advised to notify their physician if they are breast feeding an infant.

While patients may notice improvement with citalopram hydrobromide therapy in 1-4 weeks, they should be advised to continue therapy as directed.

LABORATORY TESTS

There are no specific laboratory tests recommended.

CARCINOGENESIS, MUTAGENESIS, AND IMPAIRMENT OF FERTILITY

Carcinogenesis

Citalopram was administered in the diet to NMRI/BOM strain mice and COBS WI strain rats for 18 and 24 months, respectively. There was no evidence for carcinogenicity of citalopram in mice receiving up to 240 mg/kg/day, which is equivalent to 20 times the maximum recommended human daily dose (MRHD) of 60 mg on a surface area (mg/m^2) basis. There was an increased incidence of small intestine carcinoma in rats receiving 8 or 24 mg/kg/day, doses which are approximately 1.3 and 4 times the MRHD, respectively, on a mg/m^2 basis. A no-effect dose for this finding was not established. The relevance of these findings to humans is unknown.

Mutagenesis

Citalopram was mutagenic in the *in vitro* bacterial reverse mutation assay (Ames test) in 2 of 5 bacterial strains (*Salmonella* TA98 and TA1537) in the absence of metabolic activation. It was clastogenic in the *in vitro* Chinese hamster lung cell assay for chromosomal aberrations in the presence and absence of metabolic activation. Citalopram was not mutagenic in the *in vitro* mammalian forward gene mutation assay (HPRT) in mouse lymphoma cells or in a coupled *in vitro/in vivo* unscheduled DNA synthesis (UDS) assay in rat liver. It was not clastogenic in the *in vitro* chromosomal aberration assay in human lymphocytes or in 2 *in vivo* mouse micronucleus assays.

Impairment of Fertility

When citalopram was administered orally to male and female rats prior to and throughout mating and gestation at doses of 16/24 (males/females), 32, 48, and 72 mg/kg/day, mating was decreased at all doses, and fertility was decreased at doses ≥32 mg/kg/day, approximately 5 times the maximum recommended human dose (MRHD) of 60 mg/day on a body surface area (mg/m^2) basis. Gestation duration was increased at 48 mg/kg/day, approximately 8 times the MRHD.

PREGNANCY CATEGORY C

In animal reproduction studies, citalopram has been shown to have adverse effects on embryo/fetal and postnatal development, including teratogenic effects, when administered at doses greater than human therapeutic doses.

In two rat embryo/fetal development studies, oral administration of citalopram (32, 56, or 112 mg/kg/day) to pregnant animals during the period of organogenesis resulted in decreased embryo/fetal growth and survival and an increased incidence of fetal abnormalities (including cardiovascular and skeletal defects) at the high dose, which is approximately 18 times the maximum recommended human dose (MRHD) of 60 mg/day on a body surface area (mg/m^2) basis. This dose was also associated with maternal toxicity (clinical signs, decreased BW gain). The developmental no effect dose of 56 mg/kg/day is approximately 9 times the MRHD on a mg/m^2 basis. In a rabbit study, no adverse effects on embryo/fetal development were observed at doses of up to 16 mg/kg/day, or approximately 5 times the MRHD on a mg/m^2 basis. Thus, teratogenic effects were observed at a maternally toxic dose in the rat and were not observed in the rabbit.

When female rats were treated with citalopram (4.8, 12.8, or 32 mg/kg/day) from late gestation through weaning, increased offspring mortality during the first 4 days after birth and persistent offspring growth retardation were observed at the highest dose, which is approximately 5 times the MRHD on a mg/m^2 basis. The no effect dose of 12.8 mg/kg/day is approximately 2 times the MRHD on a mg/m^2 basis. Similar effects on offspring mortality and growth were seen when dams were treated throughout gestation and early lactation at doses ≥24 mg/kg/day, approximately 4 times the MRHD on a mg/m^2 basis. A no effect dose was not determined in that study.

There are no adequate and well-controlled studies in pregnant women; therefore, citalopram should be used during pregnancy only if the potential benefit justifies the potential risk to the fetus.

LABOR AND DELIVERY

The effect of citalopram hydrobromide on labor and delivery in humans is unknown.

NURSING MOTHERS

As has been found to occur with many other drugs, citalopram is excreted in human breast milk. There have been 2 reports of infants experiencing excessive somnolence, decreased feeding, and weight loss in association with breast feeding from a citalopram-treated mother; in 1 case, the infant was reported to recover completely upon discontinuation of citalopram by its mother, and in the second case, no follow up information was available. The decision whether to continue or discontinue either nursing or citalopram hydrobromide therapy should take into account the risks of citalopram exposure for the infant and the benefits of citalopram hydrobromide treatment for the mother.

PEDIATRIC USE

Safety and effectiveness in pediatric patients have not been established.

GERIATRIC USE

Of 4422 patients in clinical studies of citalopram hydrobromide, 1357 were 60 and over, 1034 were 65 and over, and 457 were 75 and over. No overall differences in safety or effectiveness were observed between these subjects and younger subjects, and other reported clinical experience has not identified differences in responses between the elderly and younger patients, but greater sensitivity of some older individuals cannot be ruled out. Most elderly patients treated with citalopram hydrobromide in clinical trials received daily doses between 20 and 40 mg (see DOSAGE AND ADMINISTRATION).

In two pharmacokinetic studies, citalopram AUC was increased by 23% and 30%, respectively, in elderly subjects as compared to younger subjects, and its half-life was increased by 30% and 50%, respectively (see CLINICAL PHARMACOLOGY). 20 mg/day is the recommended dose for most elderly patients (see DOSAGE AND ADMINISTRATION).

DRUG INTERACTIONS

CNS Drugs: Given the primary CNS effects of citalopram, caution should be used when it is taken in combination with other centrally acting drugs.

Alcohol: Although citalopram did not potentiate the cognitive and motor effects of alcohol in a clinical trial, as with other psychotropic medications, the use of alcohol by depressed patients taking citalopram hydrobromide is not recommended.

Monoamine Oxidase Inhibitors (MAOI's): See CONTRAINDICATIONS and WARNINGS.

Cimetidine: In subjects who had received 21 days of 40 mg/day citalopram hydrobromide, combined administration of 400 mg/day cimetidine for 8 days resulted in an increase in citalopram AUC and C_{max} of 43% and 39%, respectively. The clinical significance of these findings is unknown.

Digoxin: In subjects who had received 21 days of 40 mg/day citalopram hydrobromide, combined administration of citalopram hydrobromide and digoxin (single dose of 1 mg) did not significantly affect the pharmacokinetics of either citalopram or digoxin.

Lithium: Coadministration of citalopram hydrobromide (40 mg/day for 10 days) and lithium (30 mmol/day for 5 days) had no significant effect on the pharmacokinetics of citalopram or lithium. Nevertheless, plasma lithium levels should be monitored with appropriate adjustment to the lithium dose in accordance with standard clinical practice. Because lithium may enhance the serotonergic effects of citalopram, caution should be exercised when citalopram hydrobromide and lithium are coadministered.

Theophylline: Combined administration of citalopram hydrobromide (40 mg/day for 21 days) and the CYP1A2 substrate theophylline (single dose of 300 mg) did not affect the pharmacokinetics of theophylline. The effect of theophylline on the pharmacokinetics of citalopram was not evaluated.

Sumatriptan: There have been rare postmarketing reports describing patients with weakness, hyperreflexia, and incoordination following the use of a selective serotonin reuptake inhibitor (SSRI) and sumatriptan. If concomitant treatment with sumatriptan and an SSRI (*e.g.,* fluoxetine, fluvoxamine, paroxetine, sertraline, citalopram) is clinically warranted, appropriate observation of the patient is advised.

Warfarin: Administration of 40 mg/day citalopram hydrobromide for 21 days did not affect the pharmacokinetics of warfarin, a CYP3A4 substrate. Prothrombin time was increased by 5%, the clinical significance of which is unknown.

Carbamazepine: Combined administration of citalopram hydrobromide (40 mg/day for 14 days) and carbamazepine (titrated to 400 mg/day for 35 days) did not significantly affect the pharmacokinetics of carbamazepine, a CYP3A4 substrate. Although trough citalopram plasma levels were unaffected, given the enzyme inducing properties of carbamazepine, the possibility that carbamazepine might increase the clearance of citalopram should be considered if the 2 drugs are coadministered.

Triazolam: Combined administration of citalopram hydrobromide (titrated to 40 mg/day for 28 days) and the CYP3A4 substrate triazolam (single dose of 0.25 mg) did not significantly affect the pharmacokinetics of either citalopram or triazolam.

Ketoconazole: Combined administration of citalopram hydrobromide (40 mg) and ketoconazole (200 mg) decreased the C_{max} and AUC of ketoconazole by 21% and 10%, respectively, and did not significantly affect the pharmacokinetics of citalopram.

CYP3A4 and 2C19 Inhibitors: *In vitro* studies indicated that CYP3A4 and 2C19 are the primary enzymes involved in the metabolism of citalopram. However, coadministration of citalopram (40 mg) and ketoconazole (200 mg), a potent inhibitor of CYP3A4, did not significantly affect the pharmacokinetics of citalopram. Because citalopram is metabolized by multiple enzyme systems, inhibition of a single enzyme may not appreciably decrease citalopram clearance.

Metoprolol: Administration of 40 mg/day citalopram hydrobromide for 22 days resulted in a 2-fold increase in the plasma levels of the beta-adrenergic blocker metoprolol. Increased metoprolol plasma levels have been associated with decreased cardioselectivity. Coadministration of citalopram hydrobromide and metoprolol had no clinically significant effects on blood pressure or heart rate.

Imipramine and Other Tricyclic Antidepressants (TCAs): *In vitro* studies suggest that citalopram is a relatively weak inhibitor of CYP2D6. Coadministration of citalopram hydrobromide (40 mg/day for 10 days) with the tricyclic antidepressant imipramine (single dose of 100 mg), a substrate for CYP2D6, did not significantly affect the plasma concentrations of imipramine or citalopram. However, the concentration of the imipramine metabolite desipramine was increased by approximately 50%. The clinical significance of the desipramine change is unknown. Nevertheless, caution is indicated in the coadministration of TCA's with citalopram hydrobromide.

Electroconvulsive Therapy (ECT): There are no clinical studies of the combined use of electroconvulsive therapy (ECT) and citalopram hydrobromide.

ADVERSE REACTIONS

The premarketing development program for citalopram hydrobromide included citalopram exposures in patients and/or normal subjects from 3 different groups of studies: 429 normal subjects in clinical pharmacology/pharmacokinetic studies; 4422 exposures from patients in controlled and uncontrolled clinical trials, corresponding to approximately 1370 patient exposure years. There were, in addition, over 19,000 exposures from mostly open-label, European postmarketing studies. The conditions and duration of treatment with citalopram hydrobromide varied greatly and included (in overlapping categories) open-label and double-blind studies, inpatient and outpatient studies, fixed-dose and dose-titration studies, and short-term and long-term exposure. Adverse reactions were assessed by collecting adverse events, results of physical examinations, vital signs, weights, laboratory analyses, ECGs, and results of ophthalmologic examinations.

Adverse events during exposure were obtained primarily by general inquiry and recorded by clinical investigators using terminology of their own choosing. Consequently, it is not possible to provide a meaningful estimate of the proportion of individuals experiencing adverse events without first grouping similar types of events into a smaller number of standardized event categories. In the tables and tabulations that follow, standard World Health Organization (WHO) terminology has been used to classify reported adverse events.

The stated frequencies of adverse events represent the proportion of individuals who experienced, at least once, a treatment-emergent adverse event of the type listed. An event was considered treatment-emergent if it occurred for the first time or worsened while receiving therapy following baseline evaluation.

ADVERSE FINDINGS OBSERVED IN SHORT-TERM, PLACEBO-CONTROLLED TRIALS

Adverse Events Associated With Discontinuation of Treatment

Among 1063 depressed patients who received citalopram hydrobromide at doses ranging from 10-80 mg/day in placebo-controlled trials of up to 6 weeks in duration, 16% discontinued treatment due to an adverse event, as compared to 8% of 446 patients receiving placebo. The adverse events associated with discontinuation and considered drug-related (*i.e.,* associated with discontinuation in at least 1% of citalopram hydrobromide-treated patients at a rate at least twice that of placebo) are shown in TABLE 1. It should be noted that 1 patient can report more than one reason for discontinuation and be counted more than once in this table.

TABLE 1 *Adverse Events Associated With Discontinuation of Treatment in Short-Term, Placebo-Controlled, Depression Trials: Percentage of Patients Discontinuing Due to Adverse Event*

Body System Adverse Event	Citalopram (n=1063)	Placebo (n=446)
General		
Asthenia	1%	<1%
Gastrointestinal Disorders		
Nausea	4%	0%
Dry mouth	1%	<1%
Vomiting	1%	0%
Central and Peripheral Nervous System Disorders		
Dizziness	2%	<1%
Psychiatric Disorders		
Insomnia	3%	1%
Somnolence	2%	1%
Agitation	1%	<1%

Adverse Events Occurring at an Incidence of 2% or More Among Citalopram Hydrobromide-Treated Patients

TABLE 2 enumerates the incidence, rounded to the nearest percent, of treatment emergent adverse events that occurred among 1063 depressed patients who received citalopram hydrobromide at doses ranging from 10-80 mg/day in placebo-controlled trials of up to 6 weeks in duration. Events included are those occurring in 2% or more of patients treated with citalopram hydrobromide and for which the incidence in patients treated with citalopram hydrobromide was greater than the incidence in placebo-treated patients.

The prescriber should be aware that these figures cannot be used to predict the incidence of adverse events in the course of usual medical practice where patient characteristics and other factors differ from those which prevailed in the clinical trials. Similarly, the cited frequencies cannot be compared with figures obtained from other clinical investigations involving different treatments, uses, and investigators. The cited figures, however, do provide the prescribing physician with some basis for estimating the relative contribution of drug and non-drug factors to the adverse event incidence rate in the population studied.

The only commonly observed adverse event that occurred in citalopram hydrobromide patients with an incidence of 5% or greater and at least twice the incidence in placebo patients was ejaculation disorder (primarily ejaculatory delay) in male patients (see TABLE 2).

Dose Dependency of Adverse Events

The potential relationship between the dose of citalopram hydrobromide administered and the incidence of adverse events was examined in a fixed dose study in depressed patients receiving placebo or citalopram hydrobromide 10, 20, 40, and 60 mg. Jonckheere's trend test revealed a positive dose response ($p<0.05$) for the following adverse events: fatigue, impotence, insomnia, sweating increased, somnolence, and yawning.

Male and Female Sexual Dysfunction With SSRIs

Although changes in sexual desire, sexual performance and sexual satisfaction often occur as manifestations of a psychiatric disorder, they may also be a consequence of pharmacologic treatment. In particular, some evidence suggests that selective serotonin reuptake inhibitors (SSRIs) can cause such untoward sexual experiences.

Reliable estimates of the incidence and severity of untoward experiences involving sexual desire, performance and satisfaction are difficult to obtain, however, in part because patients and physicians may be reluctant to discuss them. Accordingly, estimates of the incidence of untoward sexual experience and performance cited in product labeling, are likely to underestimate their actual incidence.

TABLE 3 displays the incidence of sexual side effects reported by at least 2% of patients taking citalopram hydrobromide in a pool of placebo-controlled clinical trials in patients with depression.

In female depressed patients receiving citalopram hydrobromide, the reported incidence of decreased libido and anorgasmia was 1.3% (n=638 females) and 1.1% (n=252 females), respectively.

TABLE 2 *Treatment-Emergent Adverse Events: Incidence in Placebo-Controlled Clinical Trials**

Body System / Adverse Event	Citalopram Hydrobromide (n=1063)	Placebo (n=446)
Autonomic Nervous System Disorders		
Dry mouth	20%	14%
Sweating increased	11%	9%
Central and Peripheral Nervous System Disorders		
Tremor	8%	6%
Gastrointestinal Disorders		
Nausea	21%	14%
Diarrhea	8%	5%
Dyspepsia	5%	4%
Vomiting	4%	3%
Abdominal pain	3%	2%
General		
Fatigue	5%	3%
Fever	2%	<1%
Musculoskeletal System Disorders		
Arthralgia	2%	1%
Myalgia	2%	1%
Psychiatric Disorders		
Somnolence	18%	10%
Insomnia	15%	14%
Anxiety	4%	3%
Anorexia	4%	2%
Agitation	3%	1%
Dysmenorrhea†	3%	2%
Libido decreased	2%	<1%
Yawning	2%	<1%
Respiratory System Disorders		
Upper respiratory tract infection	5%	4%
Rhinitis	5%	3%
Sinusitis	3%	<1%
Urogenital		
Ejaculation disorder‡§	6%	1%
Impotence§	3%	<1%

* Events reported by at least 2% of patients treated with citalopram hydrobromide are reported, except for the following events which had an incidence on placebo ≥ citalopram hydrobromide: headache, asthenia, dizziness, constipation, palpitation, vision abnormal, sleep disorder, nervousness, pharyngitis, micturition disorder, back pain.
† Denominator used was for females only (n=638 citalopram hydrobromide; n=252 placebo).
‡ Primarily ejaculatory delay.
§ Denominator used was for males only (n=425 citalopram hydrobromide; n=194 placebo).

TABLE 3

Treatment	Citalopram Hydrobromide (425 males)	Placebo (194 males)
Abnormal ejaculation*	6.1% (males only)	1% (males only)
Decreased libido	3.8% (males only)	<1% (males only)
Impotence	2.8% (males only)	<1% (males only)

* Mostly ejaculatory delay.

There are no adequately designed studies examining sexual dysfunction with citalopram treatment. Priapism has been reported with all SSRIs.

While it is difficult to know the precise risk of sexual dysfunction associated with the use of SSRIs, physicians should routinely inquire about such possible side effects.

Vital Sign Changes

Citalopram hydrobromide and placebo groups were compared with respect to (1) mean change from baseline in vital signs (pulse, systolic blood pressure, and diastolic blood pressure) and (2) the incidence of patients meeting criteria for potentially clinically significant changes from baseline in these variables. These analyses did not reveal any clinically important changes in vital signs associated with citalopram hydrobromide treatment. In addition, a comparison of supine and standing vital sign measures for citalopram hydrobromide and placebo treatments indicated that citalopram hydrobromide treatment is not associated with orthostatic changes.

Weight Changes

Patients treated with citalopram hydrobromide in controlled trials experienced a weight loss of about 0.5 kg compared to no change for placebo patients.

Laboratory Changes

Citalopram hydrobromide and placebo groups were compared with respect to (1) mean change from baseline in various serum chemistry, hematology, and urinalysis variables and (2) the incidence of patients meeting criteria for potentially clinically significant changes from baseline in these variables. These analyses revealed no clinically important changes in laboratory test parameters associated with citalopram hydrobromide treatment.

ECG Changes

Electrocardiograms from citalopram hydrobromide (n=802) and placebo (n=241) groups were compared with respect to (1) mean change from baseline in various ECG parameters and (2) the incidence of patients meeting criteria for potentially clinically significant changes from baseline in these variables. The only statistically significant drug-placebo difference observed was a decrease in heart rate for citalopram hydrobromide of 1.7 bpm compared to no change in heart rate for placebo. There were no observed differences in QT or other ECG intervals.

OTHER EVENTS OBSERVED DURING THE PREMARKETING EVALUATION OF CITALOPRAM HYDROBROMIDE

Following is a list of WHO terms that reflect treatment-emergent adverse events, as defined in the introduction of ADVERSE REACTIONS, reported by patients treated with citalopram hydrobromide at multiple doses in a range of 10-80 mg/day during any phase of a trial within the premarketing database of 4422 patients. All reported events are included except those already listed in TABLE 2 or elsewhere in labeling, those events for which a drug cause was remote, those event terms which were so general as to be uninformative, and those occurring in only 1 patient. It is important to emphasize that, although the events reported occurred during treatment with citalopram hydrobromide, they were not necessarily caused by it.

Events are further categorized by body system and listed in order of decreasing frequency according to the following definitions: *frequent* adverse events are those occurring on one or more occasions in at least 1/100 patients; *infrequent* adverse events are those occurring in less than 1/100 patients but at least 1/1000 patients; *rare* events are those occurring in fewer than 1/1000 patients.

Cardiovascular: *Frequent:* Tachycardia, postural hypotension, hypotension. *Infrequent:* Hypertension, bradycardia, edema (extremities), angina pectoris, extrasystoles, cardiac failure, flushing, myocardial infarction, cerebrovascular accident, myocardial ischemia. *Rare:* Transient ischemic attack, phlebitis, atrial fibrillation, cardiac arrest, bundle branch block.

Central and Peripheral Nervous System Disorders: *Frequent:* Paresthesia, migraine. *Infrequent:* Hyperkinesia, vertigo, hypertonia, extrapyramidal disorder, leg cramps, involuntary muscle contractions, hypokinesia, neuralgia, dystonia, abnormal gait, hypesthesia, ataxia. *Rare:* Abnormal coordination, hyperesthesia, ptosis, stupor.

Endocrine Disorders: *Rare:* Hypothyroidism, goiter, gynecomastia.

Gastrointestinal Disorders: *Frequent:* Saliva increased, flatulence. *Infrequent:* Gastritis, gastroenteritis, stomatitis, eructation, hemorrhoids, dysphagia, teeth grinding, gingivitis, esophagitis. *Rare:* Colitis, gastric ulcer, cholecystitis, cholelithiasis, duodenal ulcer, gastroesophageal reflux, glossitis, jaundice, diverticulitis, rectal hemorrhage, hiccups.

General: *Infrequent:* Hot flushes, rigors, alcohol intolerance, syncope, influenza-like symptoms. *Rare:* Hayfever.

Hemic and Lymphatic Disorders: *Infrequent:* Purpura, anemia, epistaxis, leukocytosis, leucopenia, lymphadenopathy. *Rare:* Pulmonary embolism, granulocytopenia, lymphocytosis, lymphopenia, hypochromic anemia, coagulation disorder, gingival bleeding.

Metabolic and Nutritional Disorders: *Frequent:* Decreased weight, increased weight. *Infrequent:* Increased hepatic enzymes, thirst, dry eyes, increased alkaline phosphatase, abnormal glucose tolerance. *Rare:* Bilirubinemia, hypokalemia, obesity, hypoglycemia, hepatitis, dehydration.

Musculoskeletal System Disorders: *Infrequent:* Arthritis, muscle weakness, skeletal pain. *Rare:* Bursitis, osteoporosis.

Psychiatric Disorders: *Frequent:* Impaired concentration, amnesia, apathy, depression, increased appetite, aggravated depression, suicide attempt, confusion. *Infrequent:* Increased libido, aggressive reaction, paroniria, drug dependence, depersonalization, hallucination, euphoria, psychotic depression, delusion, paranoid reaction, emotional lability, panic reaction, psychosis. *Rare:* Catatonic reaction, melancholia.

Reproductive Disorders/Female (% Based on Female Subjects Only, 2955): *Frequent:* Amenorrhea. *Infrequent:* Galactorrhea, breast pain, breast enlargement, vaginal hemorrhage.

Respiratory System Disorders: *Frequent:* Coughing. *Infrequent:* Bronchitis, dyspnea, pneumonia. *Rare:* Asthma, laryngitis, bronchospasm, pneumonitis, sputum increased.

Skin and Appendages Disorders: *Frequent:* Rash, pruritus. *Infrequent:* Photosensitivity reaction, urticaria, acne, skin discoloration, eczema, alopecia, dermatitis, skin dry, psoriasis. *Rare:* Hypertrichosis, decreased sweating, melanosis, keratitis, cellulitis, pruritus ani.

Special Senses: *Frequent:* Accommodation abnormal, taste perversion. *Infrequent:* Tinnitus, conjunctivitis, eye pain. *Rare:* Mydriasis, photophobia, diplopia, abnormal lacrimation, cataract, taste loss.

Urinary System Disorders: *Frequent:* Polyuria. *Infrequent:* Micturition frequency, urinary incontinence, urinary retention, dysuria. *Rare:* Facial edema, hematuria, oliguria, pyelonephritis, renal calculus, renal pain.

OTHER EVENTS OBSERVED DURING THE POSTMARKETING EVALUATION OF CITALOPRAM HYDROBROMIDE

It is estimated that over 30 million patients have been treated with citalopram hydrobromide since market introduction. Although no causal relationship to citalopram hydrobromide treatment has been found, the following adverse events have been reported to be temporally associated with citalopram hydrobromide treatment, and have not been described elsewhere in labeling: acute renal failure, akathisia, allergic reaction, anaphylaxis, angioedema, choreoathetosis, chest pain, delirium, dyskinesia, ecchymosis, epidermal necrolysis, erythema multiforme, gastrointestinal hemorrhage, grand mal convulsions, hemolytic anemia, hepatic necrosis, myoclonus, neuroleptic malignant syndrome, nystagmus pancreatitis, priapism, prolactinemia, prothrombin decreased, QT prolonged, rhabdomyolysis, serotonin syndrome, spontaneous abortion, thrombocytopenia, thrombosis, ventricular arrhythmia, Torsades de pointes, and withdrawal syndrome.

DOSAGE AND ADMINISTRATION

INITIAL TREATMENT

Citalopram hydrobromide should be administered at an initial dose of 20 mg once daily, generally with an increase to a dose of 40 mg/day. Dose increases should usually occur in increments of 20 mg at intervals of no less than 1 week. Although certain patients may require a dose of 60 mg/day, the only study pertinent to dose response for effectiveness did not demonstrate an advantage for the 60 mg/day dose over the 40 mg/day dose; doses above 40 mg are therefore not ordinarily recommended.

Citalopram hydrobromide should be administered once daily, in the morning or evening, with or without food.

Special Populations

20 mg/day is the recommended dose for most elderly patients and patients with hepatic impairment, with titration to 40 mg/day only for nonresponding patients.

No dosage adjustment is necessary for patients with mild or moderate renal impairment. Citalopram hydrobromide should be used with caution in patients with severe renal impairment.

MAINTENANCE TREATMENT

It is generally agreed that acute episodes of depression require several months or longer of sustained pharmacologic therapy. Systematic evaluation of citalopram hydrobromide in two studies has shown that its antidepressant efficacy is maintained for periods of up to 24 weeks following 6 or 8 weeks of initial treatment (32 weeks total). In one study, patients were assigned randomly to placebo or to the same dose of citalopram hydrobromide (20-60 mg/day) during maintenance treatment as they had received during the acute stabilization phase, while in the other study, patients were assigned randomly to continuation of citalopram hydrobromide 20 or 40 mg/day, or placebo, for maintenance treatment. In the latter study, the rates of relapse to depression were similar for the 2 dose groups. Based on these limited data, it is not known whether the dose of citalopram needed to maintain euthymia is identical to the dose needed to induce remission. If adverse reactions are bothersome, a decrease in dose to 20 mg/day can be considered.

SWITCHING PATIENTS TO OR FROM A MONOAMINE OXIDASE INHIBITOR

At least 14 days should elapse between discontinuation of an MAOI and initiation of citalopram hydrobromide therapy. Similarly, at least 14 days should be allowed after stopping citalopram hydrobromide before starting a MAOI (see CONTRAINDICATIONS and WARNINGS).

ANIMAL PHARMACOLOGY

RETINAL CHANGES IN RATS

Pathologic changes (degeneration/atrophy) were observed in the retinas of albino rats in the 2 year carcinogenicity study with citalopram. There was an increase in both incidence and severity of retinal pathology in both male and female rats receiving 80 mg/kg/day (13 times the maximum recommended daily human dose of 60 mg on a mg/m^2 basis). Similar findings were not present in rats receiving 24 mg/kg/day for 2 years, in mice treated for 18 months at doses up to 240 mg/kg/day or in dogs treated for 1 year at doses up to 20 mg/kg/day (4, 20 and 10 times, respectively, the maximum recommended daily human dose on a mg/m^2 basis).

Additional studies to investigate the mechanism for this pathology have not been performed, and the potential significance of this effect in humans has not been established.

CARDIOVASCULAR CHANGES IN DOGS

In a 1 year toxicology study, 5 of 10 beagle dogs receiving oral doses of 8 mg/kg/day (4 times the maximum recommended daily human dose of 60 mg on a mg/m^2 basis) died suddenly between weeks 17 and 31 following initiation of treatment. Although appropriate data from that study are not available to directly compare plasma levels of citalopram (CT) and its metabolites, demethylcitalopram (DCT) and didemethylcitalopram (DDCT), to levels that have been achieved in humans, pharmacokinetic data indicate that the relative dog to human exposure was greater for the metabolites than for citalopram. Sudden deaths were not observed in rats at doses up to 120 mg/kg/day, which produced plasma levels of CT, DCT and DDCT similar to those observed in dogs at doses of 8 mg/kg/day. A subsequent IV dosing study demonstrated that in beagle dogs, DDCT caused QT prolongation, a known risk factor for the observed outcome in dogs. This effect occurred in dogs at doses producing peak DDCT plasma levels of 810-3250 nM (39-155 times the mean steady state DDCT plasma level measured at the maximum recommended human daily dose of 60 mg). In dogs, peak DDCT plasma concentrations are approximately equal to peak CT plasma concentrations, whereas in humans, steady state DDCT plasma concentrations are less than 10% of steady state CT plasma concentrations. Assays of DDCT plasma concentrations in 2020 citalopram treated individuals demonstrated that DDCT levels rarely exceeded 70 nM; the highest measured level of DDCT in human overdose was 138 nM. While DDCT is ordinarily present in humans at lower levels than in dogs, it is unknown whether there are individuals who may achieve higher DDCT levels. The possibility that DCT, a principal metabolite in humans, may prolong the QT interval in the dog has not been directly examined because DCT is rapidly converted to DDCT in that species.

HOW SUPPLIED

Celexa Tablets

10 mg: Beige, oval, film coated tablet. They are imprinted on one side with "FP". They are imprinted on the other side with "10 mg".

20 mg: Pink, oval, scored, film coated tablet. They are imprinted on the scored side with "F" on the left side and "P" on the right side. They are imprinted on the non-scored side with "20 mg".

40 mg: White, oval, scored, film coated tablet. They are imprinted on the scored side with "F" on the left side and "P" on the right side. They are imprinted on the non-scored side with "40 mg".

Celexa Oral Solution

The oral solution is a peppermint flavored solution containing 10 mg of citalopram hydrobromide per 5 ml.

Storage: Store Celexa tablets and oral solution at 25°C (77°F); excursions permitted to 15-30°C (59-86°F).

PRODUCT LISTING - EQUIVALENTS NOT AVAILABLE

Solution - Oral - 10 mg/5 ml			
120 ml	$53.60	CELEXA, Forest Pharmaceuticals	00456-4130-04
240 ml	$115.03	CELEXA, Forest Pharmaceuticals	00456-4130-08
Tablet - Oral - 10 mg			
100's	$230.93	CELEXA, Forest Pharmaceuticals	00456-4010-01
Tablet - Oral - 20 mg			
30's	$62.93	CELEXA, Allscripts Pharmaceutical Company	54569-4703-00
30's	$64.82	CELEXA, Southwood Pharmaceuticals Inc	58016-0598-30
30's	$79.30	CELEXA, Physicians Total Care	54868-4159-00
60's	$125.86	CELEXA, Allscripts Pharmaceutical Company	54569-4703-01
60's	$129.64	CELEXA, Southwood Pharmaceuticals Inc	58016-0598-60
90's	$194.46	CELEXA, Southwood Pharmaceuticals Inc	58016-0598-90
100's	$216.07	CELEXA, Southwood Pharmaceuticals Inc	58016-0598-00
100's	$250.73	CELEXA, Forest Pharmaceuticals	00456-4020-01
100's	$255.75	CELEXA, Forest Pharmaceuticals	00456-4020-63
Tablet - Oral - 40 mg			
10's	$28.37	CELEXA, Physicians Total Care	54868-4226-01
30's	$65.67	CELEXA, Allscripts Pharmaceutical Company	54569-4879-00
30's	$82.70	CELEXA, Physicians Total Care	54868-4226-00
100's	$261.64	CELEXA, Forest Pharmaceuticals	00456-4040-01
100's	$266.86	CELEXA, Forest Pharmaceuticals	00456-4040-63

C

Cladribine *(003137)*

For complete prescribing information, refer to the CD-ROM included with the book.

Categories: Leukemia, hairy cell; Pregnancy Category D; FDA Approved 1993 Feb; Orphan Drugs
Drug Classes: Antineoplastics, antimetabolites
Brand Names: CdA; Chlorodeoxyadenosine; **Leustatin**
Foreign Brand Availability: Leustatine (France); Litax (Israel)
Cost of Therapy: $2,984.38 (Hairy Cell Leukemia; Leustatin Injection; 1 mg/ml; 10 ml; 6.3 mg/day; 7 day supply)
HCFA JCODE(S): J9065 per mg IV

WARNING

For intravenous infusion only.

Cladribine injection should be administered under the supervision of a qualified physician experienced in the use of antineoplastic therapy. Suppression of bone marrow function should be anticipated. This is usually reversible and appears to be dose dependent. Serious neurological toxicity (including irreversible paraparesis and quadraparesis) has been reported in patients who received cladribine injection by continuous infusion at high doses (4-9 times the recommended dose for hairy cell leukemia). Neurologic toxicity appears to demonstrate a dose relationship; however, severe neurological toxicity has been reported rarely following treatment with standard cladribine dosing regimens.

Acute nephrotoxicity has been observed with high doses of cladribine (4-9 times the recommended dose for hairy cell leukemia), especially when given concomitantly with other nephrotoxic agents/therapies.

DESCRIPTION

Cladribine injection (also commonly known as 2-chloro-2′-deoxy-β-D-adenosine) is a synthetic antineoplastic agent for continuous intravenous infusion. It is a clear, colorless, sterile, preservative-free, isotonic solution. Leustatin injection is available in single-use vials containing 10 mg (1 mg/ml) of cladribine, a chlorinated purine nucleoside analog. Each milliliter of Leustatin injection contains 1 mg of the active ingredient and 9 mg (0.15 mEq) of sodium chloride as an inactive ingredient. The solution has a pH range of 5.5-8.0. Phosphoric acid and/or dibasic sodium phosphate may have been added to adjust the pH to 6.3 ± 0.3.

The chemical name for cladribine is 2-chloro-6-amino-9-(2-deoxy-β-D-erythropentofuranosyl) purine. Its molecular weight is 285.7.

INDICATIONS AND USAGE

Cladribine injection is indicated for the treatment of active hairy cell leukemia as defined by clinically significant anemia, neutropenia, thrombocytopenia or disease-related symptoms.

NON-FDA APPROVED INDICATIONS

Data have also shown that cladribine has activity in patients with chronic lymphocytic leukemia (CLL), non-Hodgkin's lymphoma, Waldenstom macroglobulinemia, Langerhans cell histiocytosis, cutaneous T-cell lymphoma, and myeloid leukemias. However, these uses have not been approved by the FDA.

CONTRAINDICATIONS

Cladribine is contraindicated in those patients who are hypersensitive to this drug or any of its components.

WARNINGS

Severe bone marrow suppression, including neutropenia, anemia, and thrombocytopenia, has been commonly observed in patients treated with cladribine, especially at high doses. At initiation of treatment, most patients in the clinical studies had hematologic impairment as a manifestation of active hairy cell leukemia. Following treatment with cladribine injection, further hematologic impairment occurred before recovery of peripheral blood counts began. During the first 2 weeks after treatment initiation, mean platelet count, ANC, and hemoglobin concentration declined and subsequently increased with normalization of mean counts by Day 12, Week 5 and Week 8, respectively. The myelosuppressive effects of cladribine were most notable during the first month following treatment. Forty-four percent (44%) of patients received transfusions with RBCs and 14% received transfusions with

C

platelets during Month 1. Careful hematologic monitoring, especially during the first 4-8 weeks after treatment with cladribine injection, is recommended.

Fever (T ≥100°F) was associated with the use of cladribine in approximately two-thirds of patients (131/196) in the first month of therapy. Virtually all of these patients were treated empirically with parenteral antibiotics. Overall, 47% (93/196) of all patients had fever in the setting of neutropenia (ANC ≤1000), including 62 patients (32%) with severe neutropenia (*i.e.,* ANC ≤500).

In a Phase 1 investigational study using cladribine in high doses (4-9 times the recommended dose for hairy cell leukemia) as part of a bone marrow transplant conditioning regimen, which also included high dose cyclophosphamide and total body irradiation, acute nephrotoxicity and delayed onset neurotoxicity were observed. Thirty-one (31) poor-risk patients with drug-resistant acute leukemia in relapse (29 cases) or non-Hodgkins lymphoma (2 cases) received cladribine for 7-14 days prior to bone marrow transplantation. During infusion, 8 patients experienced gastrointestinal symptoms. While the bone marrow was initially cleared of all hematopoietic elements, including tumor cells, leukemia eventually recurred in all treated patients. Within 7-13 days after starting treatment with cladribine, 6 patients (19%) developed manifestations of renal dysfunction (*e.g.,* acidosis, anuria, elevated serum creatinine, etc.) and 5 required dialysis. Several of these patients were also being treated with other medications having known nephrotoxic potential. Renal dysfunction was reversible in 2 of these patients. In the 4 patients whose renal function had not recovered at the time of death, autopsies were performed; in 2 of these, evidence of tubular damage was noted. Eleven patients (35%) experienced delayed onset neurologic toxicity. In the majority, this was characterized by progressive irreversible motor weakness (paraparesis/quadriparesis), of the upper and/or lower extremities, first noted 35-84 days after starting high dose therapy with cladribine. Non-invasive testing (electromyography and nerve conduction studies) was consistent with demyelinating disease. Severe neurologic toxicity has also been noted with high doses of another drug in this class.

Axonal peripheral polyneuropathy was observed in a dose escalation study at the highest dose levels (approximately 4 times the recommended dose for hairy cell leukemia) in patients not receiving cyclophosphamide or total body irradiation. Severe neurological toxicity has been reported rarely following treatment with standard cladribine dosing regimens.

In patients with hairy cell leukemia treated with the recommended treatment regimen (0.09 mg/kg/day for 7 consecutive days), there have been no reports of nephrologic toxicities.

Of the 196 hairy cell leukemia patients entered in the two trials, there were 8 deaths following treatment. Of these, 6 were of infectious etiology , including 3 pneumonias, and 2 occurred in the first month following cladribine therapy. Of the 8 deaths, 6 occurred in previously treated patients who were refractory to α-interferon.

Benzyl alcohol is a constituent of the recommended diluent for the 7 day infusion solution. Benzyl alcohol has been reported to be associated with a fatal "gasping syndrome" in premature infants. (See DOSAGE AND ADMINISTRATION.)

PREGNANCY CATEGORY D

Cladribine injection should not be given during pregnancy.

Cladribine is teratogenic in mice and rabbits and consequently has the potential to cause fetal harm when administered to a pregnant woman. A significant increase in fetal variations was observed in mice receiving 1.5 mg/kg/day (4.5 mg/m^2) and increased resorptions, reduced litter size and increased fetal malformations were observed when mice received 3.0 mg/kg/day (9 mg/m^2). Fetal death and malformations were observed in rabbits that received 3.0 mg/kg/day (33.0 mg/m^2). No fetal effects were seen in mice at 0.5 mg/kg/day (1.5 mg/m^2) or in rabbits at 1.0 mg/kg/day (11.0 mg/m^2).

Although there is no evidence of teratogenicity in humans due to cladribine, other drugs which inhibit DNA synthesis (*e.g.,* methotrexate and aminopterin) have been reported to be teratogenic in humans. Cladribine injection has been shown to be embryotoxic in mice when given at doses equivalent to the recommended dose.

There are no adequate and well controlled studies in pregnant women. If cladribine is used during pregnancy, or if the patient becomes pregnant while taking this drug, the patient should be apprised of the potential hazard to the fetus. Women of childbearing age should be advised to avoid becoming pregnant.

DOSAGE AND ADMINISTRATION

USUAL DOSE

The recommended dose and schedule of cladribine injection for active hairy cell leukemia is as a single course given by continuous infusion for 7 consecutive days at a dose of 0.09 mg/kg/day. Deviations from this dosage regimen are not advised. If the patient does not respond to the initial course of cladribine injection for hairy cell leukemia, it is unlikely they will benefit from additional courses. Physicians should consider delaying or discontinuing the drug if neurotoxicity or renal toxicity occurs (see WARNINGS).

Specific risk factors predisposing to increased toxicity from cladribine have not been defined. In view of the known toxicities of agents of this class, it would be prudent to proceed carefully in patients with known or suspected renal insufficiency or severe bone marrow impairment of any etiology. Patients should be monitored closely for hematologic and non-hematologic toxicity. (See WARNINGS.)

PREPARATION AND ADMINISTRATION OF INTRAVENOUS SOLUTIONS

Cladribine injection must be diluted with the designated diluent prior to administration. Since the drug product does not contain any anti-microbial preservative or bacteriostatic agent, **aseptic technique and proper environmental precautions must be observed in preparation of cladribine injection solutions.**

To Prepare a Single Daily Dose

Add the calculated dose (0.09 mg/kg or 0.09 ml/kg) of cladribine injection to an infusion bag containing 500 ml of 0.9% sodium chloride injection. Infuse continuously over 24 hours. Repeat daily for a total of 7 consecutive days. **The use of 5% dextrose as a diluent is not recommended because of increased degradation of cladribine.** Admixtures of cladribine injection are chemically and physically stable for at least 24 hours at room temperature under normal room fluorescent light in Baxter Viaflex PVC infusion containers. **Since limited compatibility data are available, adherence to the recommended diluents and infusion systems is advised.**

To Prepare a 7 Day Infusion

The 7 day infusion solution should only be prepared with bacteriostatic 0.9% sodium chloride injection (0.9% benzyl alcohol preserved). In order to minimize the risk of microbial contamination, both cladribine injection and the diluent should be passed through a sterile 0.22 μ disposable hydrophilic syringe filter as each solution is being introduced into the infusion reservoir. First add the calculated dose of cladribine injection (7 days × 0.09 mg/kg or ml/kg) to the infusion reservoir through the sterile filter. Then add a calculated amount of bacteriostatic 0.9% sodium chloride injection (0.9% benzyl alcohol preserved) also through the filter to bring the total volume of the solution to 100 ml. After completing solution preparation, clamp off the line, disconnect and discard the filter. Aseptically aspirate air bubbles from the reservoir as necessary using the syringe and a dry second sterile filter or a sterile vent filter assembly. Reclamp the line and discard the syringe and filter assembly. Infuse continuously over 7 days. Solutions prepared with bacteriostatic sodium chloride injection for individuals weighing more than 85 kg may have reduced preservative effectiveness due to greater dilution of the benzyl alcohol preservative. Admixtures for the 7 day infusion have demonstrated acceptable chemical and physical stability for at least 7 days in Sims Deltec Medication Cassettes.

Since limited compatibility data are available, adherence to the recommended diluents and infusion systems is advised. Solutions containing cladribine injection should not be mixed with other intravenous drugs or additives or infused simultaneously via a common intravenous line, since compatibility testing has not been performed. Preparations containing benzyl alcohol should not be used in neonates. (See WARNINGS.)

Care must be taken to assure the sterility of prepared solutions. Once diluted, solutions of cladribine injection should be administered promptly or stored in the refrigerator (2-8°C) for no more than 8 hours prior to start of administration. Vials of cladribine injection are for single-use only. Any unused portion should be discarded in an appropriate manner. (See Handling and Disposal.)

Parenteral drug products should be inspected visually for particulate matter and discoloration prior to administration, whenever solution and container permit. A precipitate may occur during the exposure of cladribine to low temperatures; it may be resolubilized by allowing the solution to warm naturally to room temperature and by shaking vigorously. **DO NOT HEAT OR MICROWAVE.**

CHEMICAL STABILITY OF VIALS

When stored in refrigerated conditions between 2-8°C (36-46°F) protected from light, unopened vials of cladribine injection are stable until the expiration date indicated on the package. Freezing does not adversely affect the solution. If freezing occurs, thaw naturally to room temperature. DO NOT heat or microwave. Once thawed, the vial of cladribine injection is stable until expiry if refrigerated. DO NOT refreeze. Once diluted, solutions containing cladribine injection should be administered promptly or stored in the refrigerator (2-8°C) for no more than 8 hours prior to administration.

HANDLING AND DISPOSAL

The potential hazards associated with cytotoxic agents are well established and proper precautions should be taken when handling, preparing, and administering cladribine injection. The use of disposable gloves and protective garments is recommended. If cladribine injection contacts the skin or mucous membranes, wash the involved surface immediately with copious amounts of water. Several guidelines on this subject have been published.[2-8] There is no general agreement that all of the procedures recommended in the guidelines are necessary or appropriate. Refer to your institution's guidelines and all applicable state/local regulations for disposal of cytotoxic waste.

PRODUCT LISTING - RATED THERAPEUTICALLY EQUIVALENT

Solution - Intravenous - 1 mg/ml

10 ml	$562.00	CLADRIBINE NOVAPLUS, Bedford Laboratories	55390-0115-01
10 ml	$562.50	GENERIC, Bedford Laboratories	55390-0124-01

PRODUCT LISTING - EQUIVALENTS NOT AVAILABLE

Solution - Intravenous - 1 mg/ml

10 ml	$676.73	LEUSTATIN, Ortho Biotech Inc	59676-0201-01

Clarithromycin *(003068)*

For related information, see the comparative table section in Appendix A.

Categories: Bronchitis, chronic, acute exacerbation; Infection, ear, middle; Infection, lower respiratory tract; Infection, sinus; Infection, skin and skin structures; Infection, upper respiratory tract; Mycobacterial avium complex; Pharyngitis; Pneumonia; Tonsillitis; Ulcer, H. pylori associated; Pregnancy Category C; FDA Approved 1991 Oct
Drug Classes: Antibiotics, macrolides
Brand Names: **Biaxin**
Foreign Brand Availability: Abbotic (Indonesia); Adel (Mexico); Bactirel (Colombia); Biaxin HP (Germany); Biclar (Belgium); Bicrolid (Indonesia); Binoklar (Indonesia); Carimycin (Taiwan); Clacine (Indonesia); Clambiotic (Indonesia); Clapharma (Indonesia); Clari (Korea); Claribid (India); Claridar (Bahrain; Cyprus; Egypt; Iran; Iraq; Jordan; Kuwait; Lebanon; Libya; Oman; Qatar; Republic-of-Yemen; Saudi-Arabia; Syria; United-Arab-Emirates); Clarimac (India); Claripen (Singapore); Clarith (Japan); Claritrol (Colombia); Claroma (Korea); Clormicin (Colombia); Crixan (Singapore); Dicupal (Peru); Gervaken (Mexico); Hecobac (Indonesia); Helitic (Indonesia); Klacid (Australia; Austria; Bahrain; China; Cyprus; Denmark; Egypt; Germany; Hong-Kong; Hungary; Iran; Iraq; Ireland; Israel; Italy; Jordan; Kuwait; Lebanon; Libya; Malaysia; Netherlands; New-Zealand; Oman; Portugal; Qatar; Republic-of-Yemen; Saudi-Arabia; South-Africa; Spain; Sweden; Switzerland; Syria; Thailand; United-Arab-Emirates); Klacid XL (Bahrain; Cyprus; Egypt; Iran; Iraq; Jordan; Kuwait; Lebanon; Libya; Oman; Qatar; Republic-of-Yemen; Saudi-Arabia; Syria; United-Arab-Emirates); Klacina (Colombia); Klaribac (Bahrain; Cyprus; Egypt; Iran; Iraq; Jordan; Kuwait; Lebanon; Libya; Oman; Qatar; Republic-of-Yemen; Saudi-Arabia; Syria; United-Arab-Emirates); Klaricid (Bahamas; Barbados; Belize; Bermuda; Colombia; Costa-Rica; Curacao; Dominican-Republic; Ecuador; El-Salvador; England; Greece; Guatemala; Guyana; Honduras; Jamaica; Japan; Korea; Mexico; Netherland-Antilles; Nicaragua; Panama; Peru; Philippines; Surinam; Taiwan; Trinidad); Klaricid H.P. (Mexico); Klaricid O.D. (Mexico); Klaricid Pediatric (Philippines); Klaricid XL (Korea); Klaridex (Israel); Klaridia (Colombia); Klarin (Israel); Klerimed (Bahrain; Cyprus; Egypt; Iran; Iraq; Jordan; Kuwait; Lebanon; Libya; Oman; Qatar; Republic-of-Yemen; Saudi-Arabia; Syria; United-Arab-Emirates); Lagur (Peru); Macladin (Italy); Macrobiol (Mexico); Macrobiol S.R. (Mexico); Mavid (Germany); Naxy (France); Veclam (Italy); Zeclar (France)
Cost of Therapy: $9.10 (Infection; Biaxin; 500 mg; 2 tablets/day; 7 day supply)

DESCRIPTION

Clarithromycin is a semi-synthetic macrolide antibiotic. Chemically, it is 6-*O*-methylerythromycin. The molecular formula is $C_{38}H_{69}NO_{13}$, and the molecular weight is 747.96.

Clarithromycin is a white to off-white crystalline powder. It is soluble in acetone, slightly soluble in methanol, ethanol, and acetonitrile, and practically insoluble in water.

Biaxin is available as immediate-release tablets, extended-release tablets, and granules for oral suspension.

IMMEDIATE-RELEASE TABLETS

Each yellow oval film-coated immediate-release Biaxin tablet contains 250 or 500 mg of clarithromycin and the following inactive ingredients:

250 mg Tablets: Hydroxypropyl methylcellulose, hydroxylpropyl cellulose, croscarmellose sodium, D&C yellow no. 10, FD&C blue no. 1, magnesium stearate, microcrystalline cellulose, povidone, pregelatinized starch, propylene glycol, silicon dioxide, sorbic acid, sorbitan monooleate, stearic acid, talc, titanium dioxide, and vanillin.

500 mg Tablets: Hydroxypropyl methylcellulose, hydroxylpropyl cellulose, collodial silicon dioxide, croscarmellose sodium, D&C yellow no. 10, magnesium stearate, microcrystalline cellulose, povidone, propylene glycol, sorbic acid, sorbitan monooleate, titanium dioxide, and vanillin.

EXTENDED-RELEASE TABLETS

Each yellow oval film-coated Biaxin XL tablet contains 500 mg of clarithromycin and the following inactive ingredients: cellulosic polymers, D&C yellow no. 10, lactose monohydrate, magnesium stearate, propylene glycol, sorbic acid, sorbitan monooleate, talc, titanium dioxide, and vanillin.

GRANULES FOR ORAL SUSPENSION

After constitution, each 5 ml of Biaxin suspension contains 125 or 250 mg of clarithromycin. Each bottle of Biaxin granules contains 1250 mg (50 ml size), 2500 mg (50 and 100 ml sizes), or 5000 mg (100 ml size) of clarithromycin and the following inactive ingredients: carbomer, castor oil, citric acid, hypromellose phthalate, maltodextrin, potassium sorbate, povidone, silicon dioxide, sucrose, xanthan gum, titanium dioxide, and fruit punch flavor.

CLINICAL PHARMACOLOGY

PHARMACOKINETICS

Clarithromycin is rapidly absorbed from the gastrointestinal tract after oral administration. The absolute bioavailability of 250 mg clarithromycin tablets was approximately 50%. For a single 500 mg dose of clarithromycin, food slightly delays both the onset of clarithromycin absorption, increasing the peak time from approximately 2 to 2.5 hours. Food also increases the clarithromycin peak plamsa concentration by about 24%, but does not affect the extent of clarithromycin bioavailability. Food does not affect the onset of formation of the antimicrobially active metabolite, 14-OH clarithromycin or its peak plasma concentration but does slightly decrease the extent of metabolite formation, indicated by an 11% decrease in area under the plasma concentration-time curve (AUC). Therefore, clarithromycin immediate-release tablets may be given without regard to food.

In nonfasting healthy human subjects (males and females), peak plasma concentrations were attained within 2-3 hours after oral dosing. Steady-state peak plasma clarithromycin concentrations were attained within 3 days and were approximately 1-2 μg/ml with a 250 mg dose administered every 12 hours and 3-4 μg/ml with a 500 mg dose administered every 8-12 hours. The elimination half-life of clarithromycin was about 3-4 hours with 250 mg administered every 12 hours but increased to 5-7 hours with 500 mg administered every 8-12 hours. The nonlinearity of clarithromycin pharmacokinetics is slight at the recommended doses of 250 and 500 mg administered every 8-12 hours. With a 250 mg every 12 hours dosing, the principal metabolite, 14-OH clarithromycin, attains a peak steady-state concentration of about 0.6 μg/ml and has an elimination half-life of 5-6 hours. With a 500 mg every 8-12 hours dosing, the peak steady-state concentration of 14-OH clarithromycin is slightly higher (up to 1 μg/ml), and its elimination half-life is about 7-9 hours. With any of these dosing regimens, the steady-state concentration of this metabolite is generally attained within 3-4 days.

After a 250 mg tablet every 12 hours, approximately 20% of the dose is excreted in the urine as clarithromycin, while after a 500 mg tablet every 12 hours, the urinary excretion of clarithromycin is somewhat greater, approximately 30%. In comparison, after an oral dose of 250 mg (125 mg/5 ml) suspension every 12 hours, approximately 40% is excreted in urine as clarithromycin. The renal clearance of clarithromycin is, however, relatively independent of the dose size and approximates the normal glomerular filtration rate. The major metabolite found in urine is 14-OH clarithromycin, which accounts for an additional 10-15% of the dose with either a 250 mg or a 500 mg tablet administered every 12 hours.

Steady-state concentrations of clarithromycin and 14-OH clarithromycin observed following administration of 500 mg doses of clarithromycin every 12 hours to adult patients with HIV infection were similar to those observed in healthy volunteers. In adult HIV-infected patients taking 500 or 1000 mg doses of clarithromycin every 12 hours, steady-state clarithromycin C_{max} values ranged from 2-4 μg/ml and 5-10 μg/ml, respectively.

The steady-state concentrations of clarithromycin in subjects with impaired hepatic function did not differ from those in normal subjects; however, the 14-OH clarithromycin concentrations were lower in the hepatically impaired subjects. The decreased formation of 14-OH clarithromycin was at least partially offset by an increase in renal clearance of clarithromycin in the subjects with impaired hepatic function when compared to healthy subjects.

The pharmacokinetics of clarithromycin was also altered in subjects with impaired renal function. (See PRECAUTIONS and DOSAGE AND ADMINISTRATION.)

Clarithromycin and the 14-OH clarithromycin metabolite distribute readily into body tissues and fluids. There are no data available on cerebrospinal fluid penetration. Because of high intracellular concentrations, tissue concentrations are higher than serum concentrations. Examples of tissue and serum concentrations are presented in TABLE 1.

TABLE 1 *Concentration After 250 mg q12h*

Tissue Type	Tissue	Serum
Tonsil	1.6 μg/g	0.8 μg/ml
Lung	8.8 μg/g	1.7 μg/ml

Clarithromycin extended-release tablets provide extended absorption of clarithromycin from the gastrointestinal tract after oral administration. Relative to an equal total daily dose of immediate-release clarithromycin tablets, clarithromycin extended-release tablets provide lower and later steady-state peak plasma concentrations but equivalent 24 hour AUCs for both clarithromycin and its microbiologically-active metabolite, 14-OH clarithromycin. While the extent of formation of 14-OH clarithromycin following administration of clarithromycin extended-release tablets (2 × 500 mg once daily) is not affected by food, administration under fasting conditions is associated with approximately 30% lower clarithromycin AUC relative to administration with food. Therefore, clarithromycin extended-release tablets should be taken with food.

In healthy human subjects, steady-state peak plasma clarithromycin concentrations of approximately 2-3 μg/ml were achieved about 5-8 hours after oral administration of 2 × 500 mg clarithromycin extended-release tablets once daily; for 14-OH clarithromycin, steady-state peak plasma concentrations of approximately 0.8 μg/ml were attained about 6-9 hours after dosing. Steady-state peak plasma clarithromycin concentrations of approximately 1-2 μg/ml were achieved about 5-6 hours after oral administration of a single 500 mg clarithromycin extended-release tablet once daily; for 14-OH clarithromycin, steady-state peak plasma concentrations of approximately 0.6 μg/ml were attained about 6 hours after dosing.

When 250 mg doses of clarithromycin as clarithromycin suspension were administered to fasting healthy adult subjects, peak plasma concentrations were attained around 3 hours after dosing. Steady-state peak plasma concentrations were attained in 2-3 days and were approximately 2 μg/ml for clarithromycin and 0.7 μg/ml for 14-OH clarithromycin when 250 mg doses of the clarithromycin suspension were administered every 12 hours. Elimination half-life of clarithromycin (3-4 hours) and that of 14-OH clarithromycin (5-7 hours) were similar to those observed at steady state following administration of equivalent doses of clarithromycin tablets.

For adult patients, the bioavailability of 10 ml of the 125 mg/5 ml suspension or 10 ml of the 250 mg/5 ml suspension is similar to a 250 mg or 500 mg tablet, respectively.

In children requiring antibiotic therapy, administration of 7.5 mg/kg q12h doses of clarithromycin as the suspension generally resulted in steady-state peak plasma concentrations of 3-7 μg/ml for clarithromycin and 1-2 μg/ml for 14-OH clarithromycin.

In HIV-infected children taking 15 mg/kg every 12 hours, steady-state clarithromycin peak concentrations generally ranged from 6-15 μg/ml.

Clarithromycin penetrates into the middle ear fluid of children with secretory otitis media. (See TABLE 2.)

TABLE 2 *Concentration After 7.5 mg/kg q12h for 5 doses*

Analyte	Middle Ear Fluid	Serum
Clarithromycin	2.5 μg/ml	1.7 μg/ml
14-OH Clarithromycin	1.3 μg/ml	0.8 μg/ml

In adults given 250 mg clarithromycin as suspension (n=22), food appeared to decrease mean peak plasma clarithromycin concentrations from 1.2 (±0.4) μg/ml to 1.0 (±0.4) μg/ml and the extent of absorption from 7.2 (±2.5) h·μg/ml to 6.5 (±3.7) h·μg/ml.

When children (n=10) were administered a single oral dose of 7.5 mg/kg suspension, food increased mean peak plasma clarithromycin concentrations from 3.6 (±1.5) μg/ml to 4.6 (±2.8) μg/ml and the extent of absorption from 10.0 (±5.5) h·μg/ml to 14.2 (±9.4) h·μg/ml.

Clarithromycin 500 mg every 8 hours was given in combination with omeprazole 40 mg daily to healthy adult males. The plasma levels of clarithromycin and 14-hydroxy-clarithromycin were increased by the concomitant administration of omeprazole. For clarithromycin, the mean C_{max} was 10% greater, the mean C_{min} was 27% greater, and the mean AUC(0-8) was 15% greater when clarithromycin was administered with omeprazole than when clarithromycin was administered alone. Similar results were seen for 14-hydroxy-clarithromycin, the mean C_{max} was 45% greater, the mean C_{min} was 57% greater, and the mean AUC(0-8) was 45% greater. Clarithromycin concentrations in the gastric tissue and mucus were also increased by concomitant administration of omeprazole.

TABLE 3 *Clarithromycin Tissue Concentrations 2 Hours After Dose (μg/ml)/(μg/g)*

Treatment	n	Antrum	Fundus	n	Mucus
Clarithromycin	5	10.48 ± 2.01	20.81 ± 7.64	4	4.15 ± 7.74
Clarithromycin + Omeprazole	5	19.96 ± 4.71	24.25 ± 6.37	4	39.29 ± 32.79

For information about other drugs indicated in combination with clarithromycin, refer to the CLINICAL PHARMACOLOGY section of their prescribing information.

MICROBIOLOGY

Clarithromycin exerts its antibacterial action by binding to the 50S ribosomal subunit of susceptible microorganisms resulting in inhibition of protein synthesis.

Clarithromycin is active *in vitro* against a variety of aerobic and anaerobic gram-positive and gram-negative microorganisms as well as most *Mycobacterium avium* complex (MAC) microorganisms.

Additionally, the 14-OH clarithromycin metabolite also has clinically significant antimicrobial activity. The 14-OH clarithromycin is twice as active against *Haemophilus influenzae* microorganisms as the parent compound. However, for *Mycobacterium avium* complex (MAC) isolates the 14-OH metabolite is 4-7 times less active than clarithromycin. The clinical significance of this activity against *Mycobacterium avium* complex is unknown.

Clarithromycin has been shown to be active against most strains of the following microorganisms both *in vitro* and in clinical infections as described in INDICATIONS AND USAGE.

Aerobic Gram-Positive Microorganisms:
Staphylococcus aureus
Streptococcus pneumoniae
Streptococcus pyogenes
Aerobic Gram-Negative Microorganisms:
Haemophilus influenzae
Haemophilus parainfluenzae
Moraxella catarrhalis
Other Microorganisms:
Mycoplasma pneumoniae
Chlamydia pneumoniae (TWAR)
Mycobacteria:
Mycobacterium avium complex (MAC) consisting of:
Mycobacterium avium
Mycobacterium intracellulare

Beta-lactamase production should have no effect on clarithromycin activity.

Note: Most strains of methicillin-resistant and oxacillin-resistant staphylococci are resistant to clarithromycin.

Omeprazole/clarithromycin dual therapy; ranitidine bismuth citrate/clarithromycin dual therapy; omeprazole/clarithromycin/amoxicillin triple therapy; and lansoprazole/clarithromycin/amoxicillin triple therapy have been shown to be active against most strains of *Helicobacter pylori in vitro* and in clinical infections as described in INDICATIONS AND USAGE.

Helicobacter:
Helicobacter pylori

Pretreatment Resistance

Clarithromycin pretreatment resistance rates were 3.5% (4/113) in the omeprazole/clarithromycin dual-therapy studies (M93-067, M93-100) and 9.3% (41/439) in the omeprazole/clarithromycin/amoxicillin triple-therapy studies (126, 127, M96-446). Clarithromycin pretreatment resistance was 12.6% (44/348) in the ranitidine bismuth citrate/clarithromycin bid versus tid clinical study (H2BA3001). Clarithromycin pretreatment resistance rates were 9.5% (91/960) by E-test and 11.3% (12/106) by agar dilution in the lansoprazole/clarithromycin/amoxicillin triple-therapy clinical trials (M93-125, M93-130, M93-131, M95-392, and M95-399).

Amoxicillin pretreatment susceptible isolates (<0.25 μg/ml) were found in 99.3% (436/439) of the patients in the omeprazole/clarithromycin/amoxicillin clinical studies (126, 127, M96-446). Amoxicillin pretreatment minimum inhibitory concentrations (MICs) >0.25 μg/ml occurred in 0.7% (3/439) of the patients, all of whom were in the clarithromycin/amoxicillin study arm. Amoxicillin pretreatment susceptible isolates (<0.25 μg/ml) occurred in 97.8% (936/957) and 98.0% (98/100) of the patients in the lansoprazole/clarithromycin/amoxicillin triple-therapy clinical trials by E-test and agar dilution, respectively. Twenty-one (21) of the 957 patients (2.2%) by E-test and 2 of 100 patients (2.0%) by agar dilution had amoxicillin pretreatment MICs of >0.25 μg/ml. Two patients had an unconfirmed pretreatment amoxicillin minimum inhibitory concentration (MIC) of >256 μg/ml by E-test.

Patients not eradicated of *H. pylori* following omeprazole/clarithromycin, ranitidine bismuth citrate/clarithromycin, omeprazole/clarithromycin/amoxicillin, or lansoprazole/clarithromycin/amoxicillin therapy would likely have clarithromycin resistant *H. pylori* isolates. Therefore, for patients who fail therapy, clarithromycin susceptibility testing should be done, if possible. Patients with clarithromycin resistant *H. pylori* should not be treated with any of the following: omeprazole/clarithromycin dual therapy; ranitidine bismuth citrate/clarithromycin dual therapy; omeprazole/clarithromycin/amoxicillin triple therapy; lansoprazole/clarithromycin/amoxicillin triple therapy; or other regimens which include clarithromycin as the sole antimicrobial agent.

TABLE 4 *Clarithromycin Susceptibility Test Results and Clinical/Bacteriological Outcomes**

Clarithromycin Pretreatment Results		*H. pylori* Negative — Eradicated	Clarithromycin Post-Treatment Results: *H. pylori* Positive — Not Eradicated, Post-Treatment Susceptibility Results: S†	I†	R†	No MIC
Omeprazole 40 mg qd/clarithromycin 500 mg tid for 14 days followed by omeprazole 20 mg qd for another 14 days (M93-067, M93-100)						
Susceptible†	108	72	1		26	9
Intermediate†	1				1	
Resistant†	4				4	
Ranitidine bismuth citrate 400 mg bid/clarithromycin 500 mg tid for 14 days followed by ranitidine bismuth citrate 400 mg bid for another 14 days (H2BA3001)						
Susceptible†	124	98	4		14	8
Intermediate†	3	2				1
Resistant†	17	1			15	1
Rantidine bismuth citrate 400 mg bid/clarithromycin 500 mg bid for 14 days followed by ranitidine bismuth citrate 400 mg bid for another 14 days (H2BA3001)						
Susceptible†	125	106	1	1	12	5
Intermediate†	2	2				
Resistant†	20	1			19	
Omeprazole 20 mg bid/clarithromycin 500 mg bid/amoxicillin 1 g bid for 10 days (126, 127, M96-446)						
Susceptible†	171	153	7		3	8
Intermediate†						
Resistant†	14	4	1		6	3
Lansoprazole 30 mg bid/clarithromycin 500 mg bid/amoxicillin 1 g bid for 14 days (M95-399, M93-131, M95-392)						
Susceptible†	112	105				7
Intermediate†	3	3				
Resistant†	17	6			7	4
Lansoprazole 30 mg bid/clarithromycin 500 mg bid/amoxicillin 1 g bid for 10 days (M95-399)						
Susceptible†	42	40	1		1	
Intermediate†						
Resistant†	4	1			3	

* Includes only patients with pretreatment clarithromycin susceptibility tests.
† Susceptible (S) MIC <0.25 μg/ml, Intermediate (I) MIC 0.5-1.0 μg/ml, Resistant (R) MIC >2 μg/ml.

Amoxicillin Susceptibility Test Results and Clinical/Bacteriological Outcomes

In the omeprazole/clarithromycin/amoxicillin triple-therapy clinical trials, 84.9% (157/185) of the patients who had pretreatment amoxicillin susceptible MICs (<0.25 μg/ml) were eradicated of *H. pylori* and 15.1% (28/185) failed therapy. Of the 28 patients who failed triple therapy, 11 had no post-treatment susceptibility test results, and 17 had post-treatment *H. pylori* isolates with amoxicillin susceptible MICs. Eleven (11) of the patients who failed triple therapy also had post-treatment *H. pylori* isolates with clarithromycin resistant MICs.

In the lansoprazole/clarithromycin/amoxicillin triple-therapy clinical trials, 82.6% (195/236) of the patients that had pretreatment amoxicillin susceptible MICs (<0.25 μg/ml) were eradicated of *H. pylori.* Of those with pretreatment amoxicillin MICs of >0.25 μg/ml, 3 of 6 had the *H. pylori* eradicated. A total of 12.8% (22/172) of the patients failed the 10 and 14 day triple-therapy regimens. Post-treatment susceptibility results were not obtained on 11 of the patients who failed therapy. Nine (9) of the 11 patients with amoxicillin post-treatment MICs that failed the triple-therapy regimen also had clarithromycin resistant *H. pylori* isolates.

The following *in vitro* data are available, **but their clinical significance is unknown.** Clarithromycin exhibits *in vitro* activity against most strains of the following microorganisms; however, the safety and effectiveness of clarithromycin in treating clinical infections due to these microorganisms have not been established in adequate and well-controlled clinical trials.

Aerobic Gram-Positive Microorganisms:
Streptococcus agalactiae
Streptococci (Groups C, F, G)
Viridans group streptococci
Aerobic Gram-Negative Microorganisms:
Bordetella pertussis
Legionella pneumophila
Pasteurella multocida
Anaerobic Gram-Positive Microorganisms:
Clostridium perfringens
Peptococcus niger
Propionibacterium acnes
Anaerobic Gram-Negative Microorganisms:
Prevotella melaninogenica (formerly *Bacteriodes melaninogenicus*)

SUSCEPTIBILITY TESTING EXCLUDING MYCOBACTERIA AND HELICOBACTER

Dilution Techniques

Quantitative methods are used to determine antimicrobial minimum inhibitory concentrations (MICs). These MICs provide estimates of the susceptibility of bacteria to antimicrobial compounds. The MICs should be determined using a standardized procedure.

Standardized procedures are based on a dilution method[1] (broth or agar) or equivalent with standardized inoculum concentrations and standardized concentrations of clarithromycin powder. The MIC values should be interpreted according to the criteria shown in TABLE 5, TABLE 6 and TABLE 7.

TABLE 5 *For Testing Staphylococcus spp.*

MIC	Interpretation
≤2.0 µg/ml	Susceptible (S)
4.0 µg/ml	Intermediate (I)
≥8.0 µg/ml	Resistant (R)

TABLE 6 *For Testing Streptococcus spp. Including Streptococcus pneumoniaea**

MIC	Interpretation
≤0.25 µg/ml	Susceptible (S)
0.5 µg/ml	Intermediate (I)
≥1.0 µg/ml	Resistant (R)

* These interpretive standards are applicable only to broth microdilution susceptibility tests using cation-adjusted Mueller-Hinton broth with 2-5% lysed horse blood.

TABLE 7 *For Testing Haemophilus spp.**

MIC	Interpretation
≤8.0 µg/ml	Susceptible (S)
16.0 µg/ml	Intermediate (I)
≥32.0 µg/ml	Resistant (R)

* These interpretive standards are applicable only to broth microdilution susceptibility tests with *Haemophilus* spp. using Haemophilus Testing Medium (HTM).[1]

Note: When testing *Streptococcus* spp. including *Streptococcus pneumoniae* susceptibility and resistance to clarithromycin can be predicted using erythromycin.

A report of "Susceptible" indicates that the pathogen is likely to be inhibited if the antimicrobial compound in the blood reaches the concentrations usually achievable. A report of "Intermediate" indicates that the result should be considered equivocal, and, if the microorganism is not fully susceptible to alternative, clinically feasible drugs, the test should be repeated. This category implies possible clinical applicability in body sites where the drug is physiologically concentrated or in situations where high dosage of drug can be used. This category also provides a buffer zone which prevents small uncontrolled technical factors from causing major discrepancies in interpretation. A report of "Resistant" indicates that the pathogen is not likely to be inhibited if the antimicrobial compound in the blood reaches the concentrations usually achievable; other therapy should be selected.

Standardized susceptibility test procedures require the use of laboratory control microorganisms to control the technical aspects of the laboratory procedures. Standard clarithromycin powder should provide the MIC values shown in TABLE 8.

TABLE 8

Microorganism		MIC
S. aureus	ATCC 29213	0.12-0.5 µg/ml
*S. pneumoniae**	ATCC 49619	0.03-0.12 µg/ml
Haemophilus influenzae†	ATCC 49247	4-16 µg/ml

* This quality control range is applicable only to *S. pneumoniae* ATCC 49619 tested by a microdilution procedure using cation-adjusted Mueller-Hinton broth with 2-5% lysed horse blood.
† This quality control range is applicable only to *H. influenzae* ATCC 49247 tested by a microdilution procedure using HTM.[1]

Diffusion Techniques

Quantitative methods that require measurement of zone diameters also provide reproducible estimates of the susceptibility of bacteria to antimicrobial compounds. One such standardized procedure [2] requires the use of standardized inoculum concentrations. This procedure uses paper disks impregnanted with 15 µg clarithromycin to test the susceptibility of microorganisms to clarithromycin.

Reports from the laboratory providing results of the standard single-disk susceptibility test with a 15 µg clarithromycin disk should be interpreted according to the criteria shown in TABLE 9, TABLE 10 and TABLE 11.

TABLE 9 *For Testing Staphylococcus spp.*

Zone Diameter	Interpretation
≥18 mm	Susceptible (S)
14-17 mm	Intermediate (I)
≤13 mm	Resistant (R)

Note: When testing *Streptococcus* spp., including *Streptococcus pneumoniae* susceptibility and resistance to clarithromycin can be predicted by using erythromycin.

Interpretation should be as stated above for results using Dilution Techniques. Interpretation involves correlation of the diameter obtained in the disk test with the MIC for clarithromycin.

As with standardized dilution techniques, diffusion methods require the use of laboratory control microorganisms that are used to control the technical aspects of the laboratory procedures. For the diffusion technique, the 15 µg clarithromycin disk should provide the zone diameters in this laboratory test quality control strain (see TABLE 12).

TABLE 10 *For Testing Streptococcus spp. Including Streptococcus pneumoniaea**

Zone Diameter	Interpretation
≥21 mm	Susceptible (S)
17-20 mm	Intermediate (I)
≤16 mm	Resistant (R)

* These zone diameter standards only apply to tests performed using Mueller-Hinton agar supplemented with 5% sheep blood incubated in 5% CO_2.

TABLE 11 *For Testing Haemophilus spp.**

Zone Diameter	Interpretation
≥13 mm	Susceptible (S)
11-12 mm	Intermediate (I)
≤10 mm	Resistant (R)

* These zone diameter standards are applicable only to tests with *Haemophilus* spp. using HTM.[2]

TABLE 12

Microorganism		Zone Diameter
S. aureus	ATCC 25923	26-32 mm
*S. pneumoniae**	ATCC 49619	25-31 mm
Haemophilus influenzae†	ATCC 49247	11-17 mm

* This quality control range is applicable only to tests performed by disk diffusion using Mueller-Hinton agar supplemented with 5% defibrinated sheep blood.
† This quality control limit applies to tests conducted with *Haemophilus influenzae* ATCC 49247 using HTM.[2]

IN VITRO ACTIVITY OF CLARITHROMYCIN AGAINST MYCOBACTERIA

Clarithromycin has demonstrated *in vitro* activity against *Mycobacterium avium* complex (MAC) microorganisms isolated from both AIDS and non-AIDS patients. While gene probe techniques may be used to distinguish *M. avium* species from *M. intracellulare*, many studies only reported results on *M. avium* complex (MAC) isolates.

Various *in vitro* methodologies employing broth or solid media at different pH's, with and without oleic acid-albumin-dextrose-catalase (OADC), have been used to determine clarithromycin MIC values for mycobacterial species. In general, MIC values decrease more than 16-fold as the pH of Middlebrook 7H12 broth media increases from 5.0-7.4. At pH 7.4, MIC values determined with Mueller-Hinton agar were 4- to 8-fold higher than those observed with Middlebrook 7H12 media. Utilization of oleic acid-albumin-dextrose-catalase (OADC) in these assays has been shown to further alter MIC values.

Clarithromycin activity against 80 MAC isolates from AIDS patients and 211 MAC isolates from non-AIDS patients was evaluated using a microdilution method with Middlebrook 7H9 broth. Results showed an MIC value of ≤4.0 µg/ml in 81% and 89% of the AIDS and non-AIDS MAC isolates, respectively. Twelve percent (12%) of the non-AIDS isolates had an MIC value ≤0.5 µg/ml. Clarithromycin was also shown to be active against phagocytized *M. avium* complex (MAC) in mouse and human macrophage cell cultures as well as in the beige mouse infection model.

Clarithromycin activity was evaluated against *Mycobacterium tuberculosis* microorganisms. In 1 study utilizing the agar dilution method with Middlebrook 7H10 media, 3 of 30 clinical isolates had an MIC of 2.5 µg/ml. Clarithromycin inhibited all isolates at >10.0 µg/ml.

SUSCEPTIBILITY TESTING FOR MYCOBACTERIUM AVIUM COMPLEX (MAC)

The disk diffusion and dilution techniques for susceptibility testing against gram-positive and gram-negative bacteria should not be used for determining clarithromycin MIC values against mycobacteria. *In vitro* susceptibility testing methods and diagnostic products currently available for determining minimum inhibitory concentration (MIC) values against *Mycobacterium avium* complex (MAC) organisms have not been standardized or validated. Clarithromycin MIC values will vary depending on the susceptibility testing method employed, composition and pH of the media, and the utilization of nutritional supplements. Breakpoints to determine whether clinical isolates of *M. avium* or *M. intracellulare* are susceptible or resistant to clarithromycin have not been established.

SUSCEPTIBILITY TESTING FOR HELICOBACTER PYLORI

The reference methodology for susceptibility testing of *H. pylori* is agar dilution MICs.[3] One (1) to 3 ml of an inoculum equivalent to a No. 2 McFarland standard (1×10^7 - 1×10^8 CFU/ml for *H. pylori*) are inoculated directly onto freshly prepared antimicrobial containing Mueller-Hinton agar plates with 5% aged defibrinated sheep blood (>2 weeks old). The agar dilution plates are incubated at 35°C in a microaerobic environment produced by a gas generating system suitable for *Campylobacter* species. After 3 days of incubation, the MICs are recorded as the lowest concentration of antimicrobial agent required to inhibit growth of the organism. The clarithromycin and amoxicillin MIC values should be interpreted according to the criteria shown in TABLE 13.

Standardized susceptibility test procedures require the use of laboratory control microorganisms to control the technical aspects of the laboratory procedures. Standard clarithromycin and amoxicillin powders should provide the MIC values shown in TABLE 14.

INDICATIONS AND USAGE

TABLETS AND GRANULES FOR ORAL SUSPENSION

Clarithromycin tablets and granules for oral suspension are indicated for the treatment of mild to moderate infections caused by susceptible strains of the designated microorganisms in the conditions listed below.

TABLE 13

MIC	Interpretation
Clarithromycin*	
<0.25 μg/ml	Susceptible (S)
0.5-1.0 μg/ml	Intermediate (I)
>2.0 μg/ml	Resistant (R)
Amoxicillin*†	
<0.25 μg/ml	Susceptible (S)

* These are tentative breakpoints for the agar dilution methodology, and they should not be used to interpret results obtained using alternative methods.
† There were not enough organisms with MICs >0.25 μg/ml to determine a resistance breakpoint.

TABLE 14

Microorganisms	Antimicrobial Agent	MIC*
H. pylori ATCC 43504	Clarithromycin	0.015-0.12 μg/ml
H. pylori ATCC 43504	Amoxicillin	0.015-0.12 μg/ml

* These are quality control ranges for the agar dilution methodology and they should not be used to control test results obtained using alternative methods.

Adults

Pharyngitis/tonsillitis due to *Streptococcus pyogenes.* (The usual drug of choice in the treatment and prevention of streptococcal infections and the prophylaxis of rheumatic fever is penicillin administered by either the intramuscular or the oral route. Clarithromycin is generally effective in the eradication of *S. pyogenes* from the nasopharynx; however, data establishing the efficacy of clarithromycin in the subsequent prevention of rheumatic fever are not available at present.)

Acute maxillary sinusitis due to *Haemophilus influenzae, Moraxella catarrhalis,* or *Streptococcus pneumoniae.*

Acute bacterial exacerbation of chronic bronchitis due to *Haemophilus influenzae, Haemophilus parainfluenzae, Moraxella catarrhalis,* or *Streptococcus pneumoniae.*

Community-Acquired pneumonia due to *Haemophilus influenzae, Mycoplasma pneumoniae, Streptococcus pneumoniae,* or *Chlamydia pneumoniae* (TWAR).

Uncomplicated skin and skin structure infections due to *Staphylococcus aureus,* or *Streptococcus pyogenes.* (Abscesses usually require surgical drainage.)

Disseminated mycobacterial infections due to *Mycobacterium avium,* or *Mycobacterium intracellulare.*

Clarithromycin tablets in combination with amoxicillin and lansoprazole or omeprazole delayed-release capsules, as triple therapy, are indicated for the treatment of patients with *H. pylori* infection and duodenal ulcer disease (active or 5 year history of duodenal ulcer) to eradicate *H. pylori.*

Clarithromycin tablets in combination with omeprazole capsules or ranitidine bismuth citrate tablets are also indicated for the treatment of patients with an active duodenal ulcer associated with *H. pylori* infection. However, regimens which contain clarithromycin as the single antimicrobial agent are more likely to be associated with the development of clarithromycin resistance among patients who fail therapy. Clarithromycin-containing regimens should not be used in patients with known or suspected clarithromycin resistant isolates because the efficacy of treatment is reduced in this setting.

In patients who fail therapy, susceptibility testing should be done if possible. If resistance to clarithromycin is demonstrated, a non-clarithromycin-containing therapy is recommended. (For information on development of resistance see CLINICAL PHARMACOLOGY, Microbiology.) The eradication of *H. pylori* has been demonstrated to reduce the risk of duodenal ulcer recurrence.

Children

Pharyngitis/tonsillitis due to *Streptococcus pyogenes.*

Community-Acquired pneumonia due to *Mycoplasma pneumoniae, Streptococcus pneumoniae,* or *Chlamydia pneumoniae* (TWAR).

Acute maxillary sinusitis due to *Haemophilus influenzae, Moraxella catarrhalis,* or *Streptococcus pneumoniae.*

Acute otitis media due to *Haemophilus influenzae, Moraxella catarrhalis,* or *Streptococcus pneumoniae.*

Uncomplicated skin and skin structure infections due to *Staphylococcus aureus,* or *Streptococcus pyogenes.* (Abscesses usually require surgical drainage.)

Disseminated mycobacterial infections due to *Mycobacterium avium,* or *Mycobacterium intracellulare.*

EXTENDED-RELEASE TABLETS

Adults

Clarithromycin extended-release tablets are indicated for the treatment of adults with mild to moderate infection caused by susceptible strains of the designated microorganisms in the conditions listed below:

Acute maxillary sinusitis due to *Haemophilus influenzae, Moraxella catarrhalis,* or *Streptococcus pneumoniae.*

Acute bacterial exacerbation of chronic bronchitis due to *Haemophilus influenzae, Haemophilus parainfluenzae, Moraxella catarrhalis,* or *Streptococcus pneumoniae.*

Community-Acquired Pneumonia due to *Haemophilus influenzae, Haemophilus parainfluenzae, Moraxella catarrhalis, Streptococcus pneumoniae, Chlamydia pneumoniae* (TWAR), or *Mycoplasma pneumoniae.*

THE EFFICACY AND SAFETY OF CLARITHROMYCIN EXTENDED-RELEASE TABLETS IN TREATING OTHER INFECTIONS FOR WHICH OTHER FORMULATIONS OF CLARITHROMYCIN ARE APPROVED HAVE NOT BEEN ESTABLISHED.

PROPHYLAXIS

Clarithromycin tablets and granules for oral suspension are indicated for the prevention of disseminated *Mycobacterium avium* complex (MAC) disease in patients with advanced HIV infection.

CONTRAINDICATIONS

Clarithromycin is contraindicated in patients with a known hypersensitivity to clarithromycin, erythromycin, or any of the macrolide antibiotics.

Concomitant administration of clarithromycin with cisapride, pimozide, astemizole, or terfenadine is contraindicated. There have been post-marketing reports of drug interactions when clarithromycin and/or erythromycin are co-administered with cisapride, pimozide, astemizole, or terfenadine resulting in cardiac arrhythmias (QT prolongation, ventricular tachycardia, ventricular fibrillation, and torsades de pointes) most likely due to inhibition of hepatic metabolism of these drugs by erythromycin and clarithromycin. Fatalities have been reported.

For information about contraindications of other drugs indicated in combination with clarithromycin, refer to the CONTRAINDICATIONS section of their prescribing information.

WARNINGS

CLARITHROMYCIN SHOULD NOT BE USED IN PREGNANT WOMEN EXCEPT IN CLINICAL CIRCUMSTANCES WHERE NO ALTERNATIVE THERAPY IS APPROPRIATE. IF PREGNANCY OCCURS WHILE TAKING THIS DRUG, THE PATIENT SHOULD BE APPRISED OF THE POTENTIAL HAZARD TO THE FETUS. CLARITHROMYCIN HAS DEMONSTRATED ADVERSE EFFECTS OF PREGNANCY OUTCOME AND/OR EMBRYO-FETAL DEVELOPMENT IN MONKEYS, RATS, MICE, AND RABBITS AT DOSES THAT PRODUCED PLASMA LEVELS 2-17 TIMES THE SERUM LEVELS ACHIEVED IN HUMANS TREATED AT THE MAXIMUM RECOMMENDED HUMAN DOSES. (See PRECAUTIONS, Pregnancy, Teratogenic Effects, Pregnancy Category C.)

Pseudomembranous colitis has been reported with nearly all antibacterial agents, including clarithromycin, and may range in severity from mild to life threatening. Therefore, it is important to consider this diagnosis in patients who present with diarrhea subsequent to the administration of antibacterial agents.

Treatment with antibacterial agents alters the normal flora of the colon and may permit overgrowth of clostridia. Studies indicate that a toxin produced by *Clostridium difficile* is a primary cause of "antibiotic-associated colitis".

After the diagnosis of pseudomembranous colitis has been established, therapeutic measures should be initiated. Mild cases of pseudomembranous colitis usually respond to discontinuation of the drug alone. In moderate to severe cases, consideration should be given to management with fluids and electrolytes, protein supplementation, and treatment with an antibacterial drug clinically effective against *Clostridium difficile* colitis.

For information about warnings of other drugs indicated in combination with clarithromycin, refer to the WARNINGS section of their prescribing information.

PRECAUTIONS

GENERAL

Clarithromycin is principally excreted via the liver and kidney. Clarithromycin may be administered without dosage adjustment to patients with hepatic impairment and normal renal function. However, in the presence of severe renal impairment with or without coexisting hepatic impairment, decreased dosage or prolonged dosing intervals may be appropriate.

Clarithromycin in combination with ranitidine bismuth citrate therapy is not recommended in patients with creatinine clearance less than 25 ml/min. (See DOSAGE AND ADMINISTRATION.)

Clarithromycin in combination with ranitidine bismuth citrate should not be used in patients with a history of acute porphyria.

For information about precautions of other drugs indicated in combination with clarithromycin, refer to the PRECAUTIONS section of their prescribing information.

INFORMATION FOR THE PATIENT

Clarithromycin may interact with some drugs; therefore patients should be advised to report to their doctor the use of any other medications.

Clarithromycin tablets and oral suspension can be taken with or without food and can be taken with milk; however, clarithromycin extended-release tablets should be taken with food. Do **NOT** refrigerate the suspension.

CARCINOGENESIS, MUTAGENESIS, AND IMPAIRMENT OF FERTILITY

The following *in vitro* mutagenicity tests have been conducted with clarithromycin:

Salmonella/Mammalian Microsomes Test
Bacterial Induced Mutation Frequency Test
In Vitro Chromosome Aberration Test
Rat Hepatocyte DNA Synthesis Assay
Mouse Lymphoma Assay
Mouse Dominant Lethal Study
Mouse Micronucleus Test

All tests had negative results except the *In Vitro* Chromosome Aberration Test which was weakly positive in 1 test and negative in another.

In addition, a Bacterial Reverse-Mutation Test (Ames Test) has been performed on clarithromycin metabolites with negative results.

Fertility and reproduction studies have shown that daily doses of up to 160 mg/kg/day (1.3 times the recommended maximum human dose based on mg/m^2) to male and female rats caused no adverse effects on the estrous cycle, fertility, parturition, or number and viability of offspring. Plasma levels in rats after 150 mg/kg/day were 2 times the human serum levels.

In the 150 mg/kg/day monkey studies, plasma levels were 3 times the human serum levels. When given orally at 150 mg/kg/day (2.4 times the recommended maximum human dose based on mg/m^2), clarithromycin was shown to produce embryonic loss in monkeys. This effect has been attributed to marked maternal toxicity of the drug at this high dose.

In rabbits, *in utero* fetal loss occurred at an intravenous dose of 33 mg/m^2, which is 17 times less than the maximum proposed human oral daily dose of 618 mg/m^2.

Long-term studies in animals have not been performed to evaluate the carcinogenic potential of clarithromycin.

PREGNANCY, TERATOGENIC EFFECTS, PREGNANCY CATEGORY C

Four teratogenicity studies in rats (3 with oral doses and 1 with IV doses up to 160 mg/kg/day administered during the period of major organogenesis) and 2 in rabbits at oral doses up to 125 mg/kg/day (approximately 2 times the recommended maximum human dose based on mg/m^2) or IV doses of 30 mg/kg/day administered during gestation days 6-18 failed to demonstrate any teratogenicity from clarithromycin. Two additional oral studies in a different rat strain at similar doses and similar conditions demonstrated a low incidence of cardiovascular anomalies at doses of 150 mg/kg/day administered during gestation days 6-15. Plasma levels after 150 mg/kg/day were 2 times the human serum levels. Four studies in mice revealed a variable incidence of cleft palate following oral doses of 1000 mg/kg/day (2 and 4 times the recommended maximum human dose based on mg/m^2, respectively) during gestation days 6-15. Cleft palate was also seen at 500 mg/kg/day. The 1000 mg/kg/day exposure resulted in plasma levels 17 times the human serum levels. In monkeys, an oral dose of 70 mg/kg/day (an approximate equidose of the recommended maximum human dose based on mg/m^2) produced fetal growth retardation at plasma levels that were 2 times the human serum levels.

There are no adequate and well-controlled studies in pregnant women. Clarithromycin should be used during pregnancy only if the potential benefit justifies the potential risk to the fetus. (See WARNINGS.)

NURSING MOTHERS

It is not known whether clarithromycin is excreted in human milk. Because many drugs are excreted in human milk, caution should be exercised when clarithromycin is administered to a nursing woman. It is known that clarithromycin is excreted in the milk of lactating animals and that other drugs of this class are excreted in human milk. Preweaned rats, exposed indirectly via consumption of milk from dams treated with 150 mg/kg/day for 3 weeks, were not adversely affected, despite data indicating higher drug levels in milk than in plasma.

PEDIATRIC USE

Safety and effectiveness of clarithromycin in pediatric patients under 6 months of age have not been established. The safety of clarithromycin has not been studied in MAC patients under the age of 20 months. Neonatal and juvenile animals tolerated clarithromycin in a manner similar to adult animals. Young animals were slightly more intolerant to acute overdosage and to subtle reductions in erythrocytes, platelets and leukocytes but were less sensitive to toxicity in the liver, kidney, thymus, and genitalia.

GERIATRIC USE

In a steady-state study in which healthy elderly subjects (age 65-81 years old) were given 500 mg every 12 hours, the maximum serum concentrations and area under the curves of clarithromycin and 14-OH clarithromycin were increased compared to those achieved in healthy young adults. These changes in pharmacokinetics parallel known age-related decreases in renal function. In clinical trials, elderly patients did not have an increased incidence of adverse events when compared to younger patients. Dosage adjustment should be considered in elderly patients with severe renal impairment.

DRUG INTERACTIONS

Clarithromycin use in patients who are receiving theophylline may be associated with an increase of serum theophylline concentrations. Monitoring of serum theophylline concentrations should be considered for patients receiving high doses of theophylline or with baseline concentrations in the upper therapeutic range. In 2 studies in which theophylline was administered with clarithromycin (a theophylline sustained-release formulation was dosed at either 6.5 or 12 mg/kg together with 250 or 500 mg q12h clarithromycin), the steady-state levels of C_{max}, C_{min}, and the area under the serum concentration time curve (AUC) of theophylline increased about 20%.

Concomitant administration of single doses of clarithromycin and carbamazepine has been shown to result in increased plasma concentrations of carbamazepine. Blood level monitoring of carbamazepine may be considered.

When clarithromycin and terfenadine were coadministered, plasma concentrations of the active acid metabolite of terfenadine were 3-fold higher, on average, than the values observed when terfenadine was administered alone. The pharmacokinetics of clarithromycin and the 14-hydroxy-clarithromycin were not significantly affected by coadministration of terfenadine once clarithromycin reached steady-state conditions. Concomitant administration of clarithromycin with terfenadine is contraindicated. (See CONTRAINDICATIONS.)

Clarithromycin 500 mg every 8 hours was given in combination with omeprazole 40 mg daily to healthy adult subjects. The steady-state plasma concentrations of omeprazole were increased (C_{max}, AUC(0-24), and $T_{1/2}$ increases of 30%, 89%, and 34%, respectively), by the concomitant administration of clarithromycin. The mean 24 hour gastric pH value was 5.2 when omeprazole was administered alone and 5.7 when co-administered with clarithromycin.

Co-administration of clarithromycin with ranitidine bismuth citrate resulted in increased plasma ranitidine concentrations (57%), increased plasma bismuth trough concentrations (48%), and increased 14-hydroxy-clarithromycin plasma concentrations (31%). These effects are clinically insignificant.

Simultaneous oral administration of clarithromycin tablets and zidovudine to HIV-infected adult patients resulted in decreased steady-state zidovudine concentrations. When 500 mg of clarithromycin were administered twice daily, steady-state zidovudine AUC was reduced by a mean of 12% (n=4). Individual values ranged from a decrease of 34% to an increase of 14%. Based on limited data in 24 patients, when clarithromycin tablets were administered 2-4 hours prior to oral zidovudine, the steady-state zidovudine C_{max} was increased by approximately 2-fold, whereas the AUC was unaffected.

Simultaneous administration of clarithromycin tablets and didanosine to 12 HIV-infected adult patients resulted in no statistically significant change in didanosine pharmacokinetics.

Concomitant administration of fluconazole 200 mg daily and clarithromycin 500 mg twice daily to 21 healthy volunteers led to increases in the mean steady-state clarithromycin C_{min} and AUC of 33% and 18%, respectively. Steady-state concentrations of 14-OH clarithromycin were not significantly affected by concomitant administration of fluconazole.

Concomitant administration of clarithromycin and ritonavir (n=22) resulted in a 77% increase in clarithromycin AUC and a 100% decrease in the AUC of 14-OH clarithromycin. Clarithromycin may be administered without dosage adjustment to patients with normal renal function taking ritonavir. However, for patients with renal impairment, the following dosage adjustments should be considered. For patients with CLCR 30-60 ml/min, the dose of clarithromycin should be reduced by 50%. For patients with CLCR <30 ml/min, the dose of clarithromycin should be decreased by 75%.

Spontaneous reports in the post-marketing period suggest that concomitant administration of clarithromycin and oral anticoagulants may potentiate the effects of the oral anticoagulants. Prothrombin times should be carefully monitored while patients are receiving clarithromycin and oral anticoagulants simultaneously.

Elevated digoxin serum concentrations in patients receiving clarithromycin and digoxin concomitantly have also been reported in post-marketing surveillance. Some patients have shown clinical signs consistent with digoxin toxicity, including potentially fatal arrhythmias. Serum digoxin levels should be carefully monitored while patients are receiving digoxin and clarithromycin simultaneously.

Erythromycin and clarithromycin are substrates and inhibitors of the 3A isoform subfamily of the cytochrome P450 enzyme system (CYP3A). Coadministration of erythromycin or clarithromycin and a drug primarily metabolized by CYP3A may be associated with elevations in drug concentrations that could increase or prolong both the therapeutic and adverse effects of the concomitant drug. Dosage adjustments may be considered, and when possible, serum concentrations of drugs primarily metabolized by CYP3A should be monitored closely in patients concurrently receiving clarithromycin or erythromycin.

The following are examples of some clinically significant CYP3A based drug interactions. Interactions with other drugs metabolized by the CYP3A isoform are also possible. Increased serum concentrations of carbamazepine and the active acid metabolite of terfenadine were observed in clinical trials with clarithromycin.

The following CYP3A based drug interactions have been observed with erythromycin products and/or clarithromycin in postmarketing experience:

Antiarrhythmics: There have been postmarketing reports of torsades de pointes occurring with concurrent use of clarithromycin and quinidine or disopyramide. Electrocardiograms should be monitored for QTc prolongation during coadministration of clarithromycin with these drugs. Serum levels of these medications should also be monitored.

Ergotamine/dihydroergotamine: Concurrent use of erythromycin or clarithromycin and ergotamine or dihydroergotamine has been associated in some patients with acute ergot toxicity characterized by severe peripheral vasospasm and dysesthesia.

Triazolobenziodiazepines (such as triazolam and alprazolam) and related benzodiazepines (such as midazolam): Erythromycin has been reported to decrease the clearance of triazolam and midazolam, and thus, may increase the pharmacologic effect of these benzodiazepines. There have been postmarketing reports of drug interactions and CNS effects (*e.g.,* somnolence and confusion) with the concomitant use of clarithromycin and triazolam.

HMG-CoA reductase inhibitors: As with other macrolides, clarithromycin has been reported to increase concentrations of HMG-CoA reductase inhibitors (*e.g.,* lovastatin and simvastatin). Rare reports of rhabdomyolysis have been reported in patients taking these drugs concomitantly.

Sildenafil (Viagra): Erythromycin has been reported to increase the systemic exposure (AUC) of sildenafil. A similar interaction may occur with clarithromycin; reduction of sildenafil dosage should be considered. (See Viagra package insert.)

There have been spontaneous or published reports of CYP3A based interactions of erythromycin and/or clarithromycin with cyclosporine, carbamazepine, tacrolimus, alfentanil, disopyramide, rifabutin, quinidine, methylprednisone, cilostazol, and bromocriptin.

Concomitant administration of clarithromycin with cisapride, pimozide, astemizole, or terfenadine is contraindicated. (See CONTRAINDICATIONS.)

In addition, there have been reports of interactions of erythromycin or clarithromycin with drugs not thought to be metabolized by CYP3A, including hexobarbital, phenytoin, and valproate.

ADVERSE REACTIONS

The majority of side effects observed in clinical trials were of a mild and transient nature. Fewer than 3% of adult patients without mycobacterial infections and fewer than 2% of pediatric patients without mycobacterial infections discontinued therapy because of drug-related side effects. Fewer than 2% of adult patients taking clarithromycin extended-release tablets discontinued therapy because of drug-related side effects.

The most frequently reported events in adults taking clarithromycin tablets were diarrhea (3%), nausea (3%), abnormal taste (3%), dyspepsia (2%), abdominal pain/discomfort (2%), and headache (2%). In pediatric patients, the most frequently reported events were diarrhea (6%), vomiting (6%), abdominal pain (3%), rash (3%), and headache (2%). Most of these events were described as mild or moderate in severity. Of the reported adverse events, only 1% was described as severe.

The most frequently reported events in adults taking clarithromycin extended-release tablets were diarrhea (6%), abnormal taste (7%), and nausea (3%). Most of these events were described as mild or moderate in severity. Of the reported adverse events, less than 1% were described as severe.

In the acute exacerbation of chronic bronchitis and acute maxillary sinusitis studies overall gastrointestinal adverse events were reported by a similar proportion of patients taking either clarithromycin tablets or clarithromycin extended-release tablets; however, patients taking clarithromycin extended-release tablets reported significantly less severe gastrointestinal symptoms compared to patients taking clarithromycin tablets. In addition, patients taking clarithromycin extended-release tablets had significantly fewer premature discontinuations for drug-related gastrointestinal or abnormal taste adverse events compared to clarithromycin tablets.

In community-acquired pneumonia studies conducted in adults comparing clarithromycin to erythromycin base or erythromycin stearate, there were fewer adverse events involving the digestive system in clarithromycin-treated patients compared to erythromycin-treated patients (13% vs 32%; p <0.01). Twenty percent (20%) of erythromycin-treated patients discontinued therapy due to adverse events compared to 4% of clarithromycin-treated patients.

In 2 US studies of acute otitis media comparing clarithromycin to amoxicillin/potassium clavulanate in pediatric patients, there were fewer adverse events involving the digestive system in clarithromycin-treated patients compared to amoxicillin/potassium clavulanate-treated patients (21% vs 40%, p <0.001). One-third as many clarithromycin-treated patients reported diarrhea as did amoxicillin/potassium clavulanate-treated patients.

POST-MARKETING EXPERIENCE

Allergic reactions ranging from urticaria and mild skin eruptions to rare cases of anaphylaxis, Stevens-Johnson syndrome, and toxic epidermal necrolysis have ocurred. Other spontaneously reported adverse events include glossitis, stomatitis, oral moniliasis, anorexia, vomiting, pancreatitis, tongue discoloration, thrombocytopenia, leukopenia, neutropenia, and dizziness. There have been reports of tooth discoloration in patients treated with clarithromycin. Tooth discoloration is usually reversible with professional dental cleaning. There have been isolated reports of hearing loss, which is usually reversible, occurring chiefly in elderly women. Reports of alterations of the sense of smell, usually in conjunction with taste perversion or taste loss have also been reported.

Transient CNS events including anxiety, behavioral changes, confusional states, convulsions, depersonalization, disorientation, hallucinations, insomnia, manic behavior, nightmares, psychosis, tinnitus, tremor, and vertigo have been reported during post-marketing surveillance. Events usually resolve with discontinuation of the drug.

Hepatic dysfunction, including increased liver enzymes, and hepatocellular and/or cholestatic hepatitis, with or without jaundice, has been infrequently reported with clarithromycin. This hepatic dysfunction may be severe and is usually reversible. In very rare instances, hepatic failure with fatal outcome has been reported and generally has been associated with serious underlying diseases and/or concomitant medications.

There have been rare reports of hypoglycemia, some of which have occurred in patients taking oral hypoglycemic agents or insulin.

As with other macrolides, clarithromycin has been associated with QT prolongation and ventricular arrhythmias, including ventricular tachycardia and torsades de pointes.

CHANGES IN LABORATORY VALUES

Changes in laboratory values with possible clinical significance were as follows:

Hepatic: Elevated SGPT (ALT) <1%; SGOT (AST) <1%; GGT <1%; alkaline phosphatase <1%; LDH <1%; total bilirubin <1%.

Hematologic: Decreased WBC <1%; elevated prothrombin time 1%.

Renal: Elevated BUN 4%; elevated serum creatinine <1%.

GGT, alkaline phosphatase, and prothrombin time data are from adult studies only.

DOSAGE AND ADMINISTRATION

Clarithromycin tablets and granules for oral suspension may be given with or without food. Clarithromycin extended-release tablets should be taken with food.

ADULTS

TABLE 31 *Adult Dosage Guidelines — Clarithromycin*

Infection	Tablets Dosage (q12h)	Tablets Duration (days)	Extended-Release Tablets Dosage (q24h)	Extended-Release Tablets Duration (days)
Pharyngitis/tonsillitis due to:				
S. pyogenes	250 mg	10	—	—
Acute maxillary sinusitis due to:				
H. influenzae	500 mg	14	2 × 500 mg	14
M. catarrhalis	500 mg	14	2 × 500 mg	14
S. pneumoniae	500 mg	14	2 × 500 mg	14
Acute exacerbation of chronic bronchitis due to:				
H. influenzae	500 mg	7-14	2 × 500 mg	7
H. parainfluenzae	500 mg	7	2 × 500 mg	7
M. catarrhalis	250 mg	7-14	2 × 500 mg	7
S. pneumoniae	250 mg	7-14	2 × 500 mg	7
Community-Acquired Pneumonia due to:				
H. influenzae	250 mg	7	2 × 500 mg	7
H. parainfluenzae	—	—	2 × 500 mg	7
M. catarrhalis	—	—	2 × 500 mg	7
S. pneumoniae	250 mg	7-14	2 × 500 mg	7
C. pneumoniae	250 mg	7-14	2 × 500 mg	7
M. pneumoniae	250 mg	7-14	2 × 500 mg	7
Uncomplicated skin and skin structure:				
S. aureus	250 mg	7-14	—	—
S. pyogenes	250 mg	7-14	—	—

H. pylori Eradication to Reduce the Risk of Duodenal Ulcer Recurrence

Triple Therapy — Clarithromycin/Lansoprazole/Amoxicillin: The recommended adult dose is 500 mg clarithromycin, 30 mg lansoprazole, and 1 g amoxicillin, all given twice daily (q12h) for 10 or 14 days. (See INDICATIONS AND USAGE.)

Triple Therapy — Clarithromycin/Omeprazole/Amoxicillin: The recommended adult dose is 500 mg clarithromycin, 20 mg omeprazole, and 1 g amoxicillin, all given twice daily (q12h) for 10 days. (See INDICATIONS AND USAGE.) In patients with an ulcer present at the time of initiation of therapy, an additional 18 days of omeprazole 20 mg once daily is recommended for ulcer healing and symptom relief.

Dual Therapy — Clarithromycin/Omeprazole: The recommended adult dose is 500 mg clarithromycin given 3 times daily (q8h) and 40 mg omeprazole given once daily (qAM) for 14 days. (See INDICATIONS AND USAGE.) An additional 14 days of omeprazole 20 mg once daily is recommended for ulcer healing and symptom relief.

Dual Therapy — Clarithromycin/Ranitidine Bismuth Citrate: The recommended adult dose is 500 mg clarithromycin given twice daily (q12h) or 3 times daily (q8h) and 400 mg ranitidine bismuth citrate given twice daily (q12h) for 14 days. An additional 14 days of 400 mg twice daily is recommended for ulcer healing and symptom relief. Clarithromycin and ranitidine bismuth citrate combination therapy is not recommended in patients with creatinine clearance less than 25 ml/min. (See INDICATIONS AND USAGE.)

CHILDREN

The usual recommended daily dosage is 15 mg/kg/day divided q12h for 10 days.

TABLE 32 *Pediatric Dosage Guidelines (based on body weight — dosing calculated on 7.5 mg/kg q12h)*

Weight kg	Weight lb	Dose (q12h)	125 mg/5 ml	250 mg/5 ml
9	20	62.5 mg	2.5 ml q12h	1.25 ml q12h
17	37	125 mg	5 ml q12h	2.5 ml q12h
25	55	187.5 mg	7.5 ml q12h	3.75 ml q12h
33	73	250 mg	10 ml q12h	5 ml q12h

Clarithromycin may be administered without dosage adjustment in the presence of hepatic impairment if there is normal renal function. However, in the presence of severe renal impairment (CLCR <30 ml/min), with or without coexisting hepatic impairment, the dose should be halved or the dosing interval doubled.

MYCOBACTERIAL INFECTIONS

Prophylaxis

The recommended dose of clarithromycin for the prevention of disseminated *Mycobacterium avium* disease is 500 mg bid. In children, the recommended dose is 7.5 mg/kg bid up to 500 mg bid. No studies of clarithromycin for MAC prophylaxis have been performed in pediatric populations and the doses recommended for prophylaxis are derived from MAC treatment studies in children. Dosing recommendations for children are in TABLE 32.

Treatment

Clarithromycin is recommended as the primary agent for the treatment of disseminated infection due to *Mycobacterium avium* complex. Clarithromycin should be used in combination with other antimycobacterial drugs that have shown *in vitro* activity against MAC or clinical benefit in MAC treatment. The recommended dose for mycobacterial infections in adults is 500 mg bid. In children, the recommended dose is 7.5 mg/kg bid up to 500 mg bid. Dosing recommendations for children are in TABLE 32.

Clarithromycin therapy should continue for life if clinical and mycobacterial improvements are observed.

CONSTITUTING INSTRUCTIONS

TABLE 33 indicates the volume of water to be added when constituting.

TABLE 33

Total Volume After Constitution	Clarithromycin Concentration After Constitution	Amount of Water to Be Added*
50ml; 100 ml	125 mg/5 ml; 250 mg/5ml	27 ml; 55 ml

* Add half the volume of water to the bottle and shake vigorously. Add the remainder of water to the bottle and shake.

Shake well before each use. Oversize bottle provides shake space. Keep tightly closed. Do not refrigerate. After mixing, store at 15-30°C (59-86°F) and use within 14 days.

ANIMAL PHARMACOLOGY

Clarithromycin is rapidly and well-absorbed with dose-linear kinetics, low protein binding, and a high volume of distribution. Plasma half-life ranged from 1-6 hours and was species dependent. High tissue concentrations were achieved, but negligible accumulation was observed. Fecal clearance predominated. Hepatotoxicity occurred in all species tested (*i.e.,* in rats and monkeys at doses 2 times greater than and in dogs at doses comparable to the maximum human daily dose, based on mg/m^2). Renal tubular degeneration (calculated on a mg/m^2 basis) occurred in rats at doses 2 times, in monkeys at doses 8 times, and in dogs at doses 12 times greater than the maximum human daily dose. Testicular atrophy (on a mg/m^2 basis) occurred in rats at doses 7 times, in dogs at doses 3 times, and in monkeys at doses 8 times greater than the maximum human daily dose. Corneal opacity (on a mg/m^2 basis) occurred in dogs at doses 12 times and in monkeys at doses 8 times greater than the maximum human daily dose. Lymphoid depletion (on a mg/m^2 basis) occurred in dogs at doses 3 times greater than and in monkeys at doses 2 times greater than the maximum human daily dose. These adverse events were absent during clinical trials.

HOW SUPPLIED

BIAXIN FILMTAB TABLETS

250 mg Tablets

Biaxin filmtabs are supplied as yellow oval film-coated tablets imprinted (on 1 side) in blue with the Abbott logo and a 2 letter Abbo-Code designation, "KT".

Storage: Store Biaxin 250 mg tablets at controlled room temperature 15-30°C (59-86°F) in a well-closed container. Protect from light.

500 mg Tablets

Biaxin Filmtabs are supplied as yellow oval film-coated tablets debossed (on 1 side) in blue with the Abbott logo and a 2 letter Abbo-Code designation, "KL".

Storage: Store Biaxin 500 mg tablets at controlled room temperature 20-25°C (68-77°F) in a well-closed container.

BIAXIN XL EXTENDED-RELEASE TABLETS

Biaxin XL filmtab are supplied as yellow oval film-coated 500 mg tablets debossed (on 1 side) with the Abbott logo and a 2 letter Abbo-Code designation, "KJ".
Storage: Store Biaxin XL tablets at 20-25°C (68-77°F). Excursions permitted to 15-30°C (59-86°F).

BIAXIN GRANULES FOR ORAL SUSPENSION

Biaxin granules for oral suspension are supplied in bottles containing 1250 mg (50 ml size), 2500 mg (50 and 100 ml sizes), or 5000 mg (100 ml size) of clarithromycin.
Storage: Store Biaxin granules for oral suspension at controlled room temperature 15-30°C (59-86°F) in a well-closed container. Do not refrigerate biaxin suspension.

PRODUCT LISTING - EQUIVALENTS NOT AVAILABLE

Size	Price	Product	NDC
Powder For Reconstitution - Oral - 125 mg/5 ml			
50 ml	$15.53	BIAXIN, Allscripts Pharmaceutical Company	54569-4270-00
50 ml	$21.30	BIAXIN, Abbott Pharmaceutical	00074-3163-50
100 ml	$27.85	BIAXIN, Compumed Pharmaceuticals	00403-4621-18
100 ml	$28.71	BIAXIN, Allscripts Pharmaceutical Company	54569-3896-00
100 ml	$39.40	BIAXIN, Abbott Pharmaceutical	00074-3163-13
100 ml	$43.07	BIAXIN, Cheshire Drugs	55175-4427-01
Powder For Reconstitution - Oral - 250 mg/5 ml			
50 ml	$29.55	BIAXIN, Allscripts Pharmaceutical Company	54569-4271-00
50 ml	$40.55	BIAXIN, Abbott Pharmaceutical	00074-3188-50
100 ml	$48.95	BIAXIN, Compumed Pharmaceuticals	00403-4623-18
100 ml	$56.33	BIAXIN, Physicians Total Care	54868-3384-00
100 ml	$65.72	BIAXIN, Allscripts Pharmaceutical Company	54569-3897-00
100 ml	$71.92	BIAXIN, Cheshire Drugs	55175-4428-01
100 ml	$75.10	BIAXIN, Abbott Pharmaceutical	00074-3188-13
Tablet - Oral - 250 mg			
10's	$43.05	BIAXIN, Pd-Rx Pharmaceuticals	55289-0008-10
10's	$48.70	BIAXIN, Pharma Pac	52959-0442-10
14's	$52.96	BIAXIN, Pharma Pac	54569-3556-01
14's	$67.20	BIAXIN, Pharma Pac	52959-0442-14
20's	$75.66	BIAXIN, Pharma Pac	54569-3556-00
20's	$81.50	BIAXIN, Physicians Total Care	54868-3820-00
20's	$94.45	BIAXIN, Pharma Pac	52959-0442-20
20's	$109.47	BIAXIN, Pd-Rx Pharmaceuticals	55289-0008-20
60's	$258.28	BIAXIN, Abbott Pharmaceutical	00074-3368-60
100's	$454.99	BIAXIN, Abbott Pharmaceutical	00074-3368-11
Tablet - Oral - 500 mg			
2's	$7.57	BIAXIN, Allscripts Pharmaceutical Company	54569-3439-04
2's	$12.14	BIAXIN, Prescript Pharmaceuticals	00247-0115-02
3's	$16.53	BIAXIN, Prescript Pharmaceuticals	00247-0115-03
4's	$20.93	BIAXIN, Prescript Pharmaceuticals	00247-0115-04
5's	$22.44	BIAXIN, Physicians Total Care	54868-2338-00
8's	$38.51	BIAXIN, Prescript Pharmaceuticals	00247-0115-08
10's	$32.55	BIAXIN, Southwood Pharmaceuticals Inc	58016-0550-10
10's	$43.70	BIAXIN, Physicians Total Care	54868-2338-06
10's	$47.29	BIAXIN, Prescript Pharmaceuticals	00247-0115-10
10's	$49.22	BIAXIN, Pharma Pac	52959-0230-10
10's	$54.60	BIAXIN, Pd-Rx Pharmaceuticals	55289-0021-10
12's	$39.06	BIAXIN, Southwood Pharmaceuticals Inc	58016-0550-12
14's	$45.57	BIAXIN, Southwood Pharmaceuticals Inc	58016-0550-14
14's	$52.96	BIAXIN, Allscripts Pharmaceutical Company	54569-3439-01
14's	$57.40	BIAXIN, Physicians Total Care	54868-2338-02
14's	$64.87	BIAXIN, Prescript Pharmaceuticals	00247-0115-14
14's	$75.24	BIAXIN, Pd-Rx Pharmaceuticals	55289-0021-14
15's	$48.82	BIAXIN, Southwood Pharmaceuticals Inc	58016-0550-15
20's	$65.10	BIAXIN, Southwood Pharmaceuticals Inc	58016-0550-20
20's	$75.66	BIAXIN, Allscripts Pharmaceutical Company	54569-3439-00
20's	$81.50	BIAXIN, Physicians Total Care	54868-2338-01
20's	$91.24	BIAXIN, Prescript Pharmaceuticals	00247-0115-20
20's	$95.54	BIAXIN, Pharma Pac	52959-0230-20
20's	$106.20	BIAXIN, Pd-Rx Pharmaceuticals	55289-0021-20
28's	$105.92	BIAXIN, Allscripts Pharmaceutical Company	54569-3439-03
28's	$126.39	BIAXIN, Prescript Pharmaceuticals	00247-0115-28
28's	$148.65	BIAXIN, Pd-Rx Pharmaceuticals	55289-0021-28
30's	$97.65	BIAXIN, Southwood Pharmaceuticals Inc	58016-0550-30
40's	$130.20	BIAXIN, Southwood Pharmaceuticals Inc	58016-0550-40
60's	$241.55	BIAXIN, Physicians Total Care	54868-2338-03
60's	$258.28	BIAXIN, Abbott Pharmaceutical	00074-2586-60
100's	$454.99	BIAXIN, Abbott Pharmaceutical	00074-2586-11
Tablet, Extended Release - Oral - 500 mg			
14 x 3	$259.60	BIAXIN XL-PAK, Abbott Pharmaceutical	00074-3165-41
14's	$59.00	BIAXIN XL, Allscripts Pharmaceutical Company	54569-4953-00
14's	$61.90	BIAXIN XL, Abbott Pharmaceutical	00074-3165-14
60's	$280.48	BIAXIN XL, Abbott Pharmaceutical	00074-3165-60
100's	$484.75	BIAXIN XL, Abbott Pharmaceutical	00074-3165-11

Clemastine Fumarate *(000835)*

Categories: Angioedema; Rhinitis, perennial allergic; Rhinitis, seasonal allergic; Urticaria; Pregnancy Category B; FDA Approved 1977 Feb
Drug Classes: Antihistamines, H1
Brand Names: Tavist
Foreign Brand Availability: Aller-Eze (England); Clamist (India); Darvine (Taiwan); Histaverin (Taiwan); Tavegil (Bahamas; Barbados; Belize; Bermuda; Curacao; Germany; Guyana; Ireland; Italy; Jamaica; Netherland-Antilles; Netherlands; Puerto-Rico; Spain; Surinam; Trinidad); Tavegyl (Austria; Belgium; Benin; Bulgaria; Burkina-Faso; Colombia; Czech-Republic; Denmark; Ecuador; Ethiopia; Gambia; Ghana; Guinea; Hungary; Indonesia; Ivory-Coast; Kenya; Liberia; Malawi; Mali; Mauritania; Mauritius; Morocco; Niger; Nigeria; Norway; Philippines; Portugal; Senegal; Seychelles; Sierra-Leone; South-Africa; Sudan; Sweden; Switzerland; Taiwan; Tanzania; Thailand; Tunia; Uganda; Zambia; Zimbabwe)
Cost of Therapy: $87.08 (Allergic Rhinitis; Tavist; 2.68 mg; 2 tablets/day; 30 day supply)
$43.50 (Allergic Rhinitis; Generic Tablets; 2.68 mg; 2 tablets/day; 30 day supply)

DESCRIPTION

TABLETS

Clemastine fumarate belongs to the benzhydryl ether group of antihistaminic compounds. The chemical name is (+)-2-[2]-[(p-chloro-α-methyl-α-phenylbenzyl)oxy]ethyl]-1-methylpyrrolidine* hydrogen fumarate. 1.34 mg and 2.68 tablets. *Inactive Ingredients:* Lactose, povidone, starch, stearic acid and talc.

SYRUP

Each teaspoonful (5 ml) of clemastine fumarate syrup for oral administration contains clemastine 0.5 mg (present as clemastine fumarate 0.67 mg). Other ingredients: alcohol 5.5%, flavors, methylparaben, propylene glycol, propylparaben, purified water, saccharin sodium, sorbitol in a buffered solution. Clemastine fumarate belongs to the benzhydryl ether group of antihistamine compounds. the chemical name is (+)-(2R)-2-[2-[[(R)-p-Chloro-α-methyl-α-phenylbenzyl]-oxy]-ethyl]-1-methylpyrrolidine fumarate*.

Clemastine fumarate occurs as a colorless to faintly yellow, practically odorless, crystalline powder. Clemastine fumarate syrup has an approximate pH of 6.2.

CLINICAL PHARMACOLOGY

TABLETS

Clemastine fumarate is an antihistamine with anticholinergic (drying) and sedative side effects. Antihistamines appear to compete with histamine for cell receptor sites on effector cells. The inherently long duration of antihistaminic effects of clemastine fumarate has been demonstrated in wheal and flare studies. In normal human subjects who received histamine injections over a 24 hour period, the antihistaminic activity of clemastine fumarate reached a peak at 5-7 hours, persisted for 10-12 hours, and, in some cases, for as long as 24 hours. Pharmacokinetic studies in man utilizing ^{3}H and ^{14}C labeled compound demonstrates that: clemastine fumarate is rapidly absorbed from the gastrointestinal tract, peak plasma concentrations are attained in 2-4 hours, and urinary excretion is the major mode of elimination.

SYRUP

Clemastine fumarate is an antihistamine with anticholinergic (drying) and sedative side effects. Antihistamines competitively antagonize various physiological effects of histamine including increased capillary permeability and dilation, the formation of edema, the "flare" and "itch" response, and gastrointestinal and respiratory smooth muscle constriction. Within the vascular tree, H_1-receptor antagonists inhibit both the vasoconstrictor and vasodilator effects of histamine. Depending on the dose, H_1 receptor antagonists can produce CNS stimulation or depression. Most antihistamines exhibit central and/or peripheral anticholinergic activity. Antihistamines act by competitively blocking H_1-receptor sites. Antihistamines do not pharmacologically antagonize or chemically inactivate histamine, nor do they prevent the release of histamine.
Pharmacokinetics: Antihistamines are well-absorbed following oral administration. Chlorpheniramine maleate, clemastine fumarate, and diphenhydramine hydrochloride active peak blood levels within 2-5 hours following oral administration. The absorption of antihistamines is often partially delayed by the use of controlled release dosage forms. In these instances, plasma concentrations from identical doses of the immediate and controlled release dosage forms will not be similar. Tissue distribution of the antihistamines in humans has not been established.
Antihistamines appear to be metabolized in the liver chiefly via mono- and didemethylation and glucuronide conjugation. Antihistamine metabolites and small amounts of unchanged drug excreted in the urine. Small amounts of the drugs may also be excreted in breast milk.

In normal human subjects who received histamine injections over a 24 hour period, the antihistaminic activity of clemastine fumarate reach peak at 5-7 hours, persisted for 10-12 hours and, in some cases, for as long as 24 hours. Pharmacokinetic studies in man utilizing ^{3}H and ^{14}C labeled compound demonstrates that: clemastine fumarate is rapidly absorbed from the gastrointestinal tract, peak plasma concentrations are attained in 2-4 hours, and urinary excretion is the major mode of elimination.

INDICATIONS AND USAGE

TABLETS

Clemastine fumarate tablets, 1.34 mg are indicated for the relief symptoms associated with allergic rhinitis such as sneezing, rhinorrhea, pruritus, and lacrimation.

Clemastine fumarate tablets 2.68 mg are indicated for the relief symptoms associated with allergic rhinitis such as sneezing, rhinorrhea, pruritus, and lacrimation. Clemastine fumarate tablets 2.68 mg are also indicated for the relief of mild, uncomplicated allergic skin manifestations of urticaria and angioedema.

It should be noted that clemastine fumarate is indicated for the dermatologic indications at the 2.68 mg dosage level only.

SYRUP

Clemastine fumarate syrup is indicated for the relief of symptoms associated with allergic rhinitis such as sneezing, rhinorrhea, pruritus and lacrimation. Clemastine fumarate syrup is indicated for use in pediatric populations (age 6 years through 12) and adults (see DOSAGE AND ADMINISTRATION).

It should be noted that clemastine fumarate is indicated for the relief of mild uncomplicated allergic skin manifestations of urticaria and angioedema at the 2 mg dosage level only.

CONTRAINDICATIONS

TABLETS

Use in Nursing Mothers: Because of the higher risk of antihistamines for infants generally and for newborns and prematures in particular antihistamine therapy is contraindicated in nursing mothers.

Use in Lower Respiratory Disease: Antihistamines **should not** be used to treat lower respiratory tract symptoms including asthma.

Antihistamines are also contraindicated in the following conditions:

Hypersensitivity to clemastine fumarate or other antihistamines of similar chemical structure.

Monamine oxidase inhibitor therapy (see DRUG INTERACTIONS).

SYRUP

Antihistamines are contraindicated in patients hypersensitive to the drug or to other antihistamines of similar chemical structure (see DRUG INTERACTIONS.)

Antihistamines **should not** be used **in newborn or premature infants.** Because of the higher risk of antihistamines for infants generally and for newborns and prematures in particular, antihistamine therapy is contraindicated **in nursing mothers** (see CONTRAINDICATIONS, Use in Nursing Mothers).

WARNINGS

TABLETS AND SYRUP

Antihistamines should be used with considerable caution in patients with narrow angle glaucoma, stenosing peptic ulcer, pyloroduodenal obstruction, symptomatic prostatic hypertrophy, and bladder neck obstruction.

SYRUP

Use in Children: Safety and efficacy of clemastine fumarate have not been established in children under the age of 12.

Use in Pregnancy: Experience with this drug in pregnant women is inadequate to determine whether there exists a potential for harm to the developing fetus.

Use with CNS Depressants: Clemastine fumarate has addictive effects with alcohol and other CNS depressants (hypnotics, sedatives, tranquilizers, etc.).

Use in Activities Requiring Mental Alertness: Patients should be warned about engaging in activities requiring mental alertness such as driving a car or operating appliances, machinery, etc.

Use in the Elderly (approximately 60 years or older): Antihistamines are more likely to cause dizziness, sedation, and hypotension in elderly patients.

PRECAUTIONS

TABLETS AND SYRUP

General: Clemastine fumarate should be used with caution in patients with: history of bronchial asthma, increased intraocular pressure, hyperthyroidism, cardiovascular disease, and hypertension.

Information for the Patient: Patients taking antihistamines should receive the following information and instructions:

1. Antihistamines are prescribed to reduce allergic symptoms.
2. Patients should be questioned regarding a history of glaucoma, peptic ulcer, urinary retention or pregnancy before starting antihistamine therapy.
3. Patients should be told not to take alcohol, sleeping pills, sedatives, tranquilizers while taking antihistamines.
4. Antihistamines may cause drowsiness, dizziness, dry mouth, blurred vision, weakness, nausea, headache, or nervousness in some patients.
5. Patients should avoid driving a car or working with hazardous machinery until they assess the effects of this medicine.
6. Patients should be told to store this medicine in a tightly closed container in a dry, cool place away from heat or direct sunlight and out of the reach for children.

DRUG INTERACTIONS

TABLETS

MAO inhibitors prolong and intensify the anticholinergic (drying) effects of antihistamines.

SYRUP

Additive CNS depressions may occur when antihistamines are administered concomitantly with other CNS depressants including barbiturates, tranquilizers, and alcohol. Patients receiving antihistamines should be advised against the concurrent use of other CNS depressant drugs.

Monoamine oxidase (MAO) inhibitors prolong and intensify the anticholinergic effects of antihistamines.

ADVERSE REACTIONS

TABLETS AND SYRUP

Transient drowsiness, the most common adverse reaction associated with clemastine fumarate occurs relatively frequently and may require discontinuation of therapy in some instances.

Antihistaminic Compounds: It should be noted that the following reactions have occurred with one or more antihistamines and, therefore, should be kept in mind when prescribing drugs belonging to this class, including clemastine fumarate. The most frequent adverse reactions are underlined.

1. ***General:*** Urticaria, drug rash, anaphylactic shock, photosensitivity, excessive perspiration, chills, dryness of mouth, nose, and throat.
2. ***Cardiovascular System:*** Hypotension, headache, palpitations, tachycardia, extrasystoles.
3. ***Hematologic System:*** Hemolytic anemia, thrombocytopenia, agranulocytosis.
4. ***Nervous System:*** Sedation, sleepiness, dizziness, disturbedcoordination, fatigue, confusion, restlessness, excitation, nervousness, tremor, irritability, insomnia, euphoria, paresthesia, blurred vision, diplopia, vertigo, tinnitus, acute labyrinthitis, hysteria, neuritis, convulsions.
5. ***GI System:*** Epigastric distress, anorexia, nausea, vomiting, diarrhea, constipation.
6. ***GU System:*** Urinary frequency, difficult urination, urinary retention, early menses.
7. ***Respiratory System:*** Thickening of bronchial secretions, tightness of chest and wheezing, nasal stuffiness.

DOSAGE AND ADMINISTRATION

DOSAGE SHOULD BE INDIVIDUALIZED ACCORDING TO THE NEEDS AND RESPONSE OF THE PATIENT.

TABLETS

Clemastine Fumarate Tablets 1.34 mg: The recommended starting dose is 1 tablet twice daily. Dosage may be increased as required, but not to exceed 6 tablets daily.

Clemastine Fumarate Tablets 2.68 mg: The maximum recommended dosage is 1 tablet three times daily. Many patients respond favorably to a single dose which may be repeated as required, but not to exceed 3 tablets daily.

SYRUP

Pediatric — Children Aged 6-12 Years

For Symptoms of Allergic Rhinitis: The starting dose is 1 teaspoonful (0.5 mg clemastine) twice daily. Since single doses of up to 2.25 mg clemastine were well tolerated by this age group, dosage may be increased as required, but not to exceed 6 teaspoonfuls daily (3 mg clemastine).

For Urticaria and Angioedema: The starting dose is 2 teaspoonfuls (1 mg clemastine) twice daily, not to exceed 6 teaspoonfuls daily (3 mg clemastine).

Adults and Children 12 Years and Over

For Symptoms of Allergic Rhinitis: The starting dose is 2 teaspoonful (1.0 mg clemastine) twice daily. Dosage may be increased as required, but not to exceed 12 teaspoonful daily (6 mg clemastine).

For Urticaria and Angioedema: The starting dose is 4 teaspoonful (2 mg clemastine) twice daily, not to exceed 12 teaspoonful (2 mg clemastine) twice daily, not to exceed 12 teaspoonful daily (6 mg clemastine).

PRODUCT LISTING - RATED THERAPEUTICALLY EQUIVALENT

Syrup - Oral - 0.67 mg/5 ml

120 ml	$16.50	GENERIC, Qualitest Products Inc	00603-1096-54
120 ml	$19.00	GENERIC, Geneva Pharmaceuticals	00781-6128-04
120 ml	$19.50	GENERIC, Silarx Pharmaceuticals Inc	54838-0514-40
120 ml	$19.50	GENERIC, Boca Pharmacal Inc	64376-0401-40
120 ml	$19.95	GENERIC, Geneva Pharmaceuticals	00781-6131-04
120 ml	$20.10	GENERIC, Aligen Independent Laboratories Inc	00405-2529-76
120 ml	$21.35	GENERIC, Teva Pharmaceuticals Usa	00093-0309-12
120 ml	$21.40	GENERIC, Alpharma Uspd Makers Of Barre and Nmc	00472-0857-04
120 ml	$21.40	GENERIC, Apotex Usa Inc	60505-0357-00
120 ml	$22.00	GENERIC, Major Pharmaceuticals Inc	00904-1524-00
120 ml	$22.45	GENERIC, Ivax Corporation	00182-6036-37
120 ml	$22.45	GENERIC, Major Pharmaceuticals Inc	00904-1524-20
120 ml	$29.06	TAVIST, Southwood Pharmaceuticals Inc	58016-4062-01
120 ml	$31.44	TAVIST, Physicians Total Care	54868-1210-01
480 ml	$22.00	GENERIC, Morton Grove Pharmaceuticals Inc	60432-0732-04

Tablet - Oral - 2.68 mg

20's	$29.96	TAVIST, Pd-Rx Pharmaceuticals	55289-0429-20
60's	$87.08	TAVIST, Pd-Rx Pharmaceuticals	55289-0429-60
100's	$72.50	GENERIC, Aligen Independent Laboratories Inc	00405-5356-01
100's	$74.20	GENERIC, Qualitest Products Inc	00603-2900-21
100's	$82.10	GENERIC, Major Pharmaceuticals Inc	00904-7679-60
100's	$83.15	GENERIC, Ivax Corporation	00182-1936-01
100's	$86.05	GENERIC, Geneva Pharmaceuticals	00781-1359-01
100's	$86.08	GENERIC, Teva Pharmaceuticals Usa	00093-0308-01
100's	$128.00	GENERIC, Medirex Inc	57480-0449-01

PRODUCT LISTING - EQUIVALENTS NOT AVAILABLE

Syrup - Oral - 0.67 mg/5 ml

120 ml	$20.41	GENERIC, Moore, H.L. Drug Exchange Inc	00839-7625-65

Tablet - Oral - 2.68 mg

20's	$21.57	GENERIC, Pharma Pac	52959-0501-20
100's	$86.08	GENERIC, Moore, H.L. Drug Exchange Inc	00839-7740-06

Clidinium Bromide (000837)

Categories: Ulcer, peptic, adjunct; FDA Approval Pre 1982; Pregnancy Category D
Drug Classes: Anticholinergics; Gastrointestinals
Brand Names: Quarzan
Cost of Therapy: $18.02 (Peptic Ulcer; Quarzan; 2.5 mg; 3 capsules/day; 30 day supply)

WARNING
NOTE: THIS PRODUCT WAS WITHDRAWN FROM THE MARKET BY THE MANUFACTURER.

DESCRIPTION

Clidinium bromide is 3-hydroxy-1-methyl-quinuclidinium bromide benzilate. A white or nearly white crystalline compound, it is soluble in water and has a calculated molecular weight of 432.36.

Clidinium bromide is a quaternary ammonium compound with anticholinergic and antispasmodic activity. Quarzan is available as green and red opaque capsules each containing 2.5 mg clidinium bromide, and green and grey opaque capsules each containing 5 mg clidinium bromide. Each capsule also contains corn starch, lactose and talc. Gelatin capsule shells contain methyl and propyl parabens and potassium sorbate, with the following dye systems: *2.5 mg Capsules:* FD&C blue no. 1, FD&C green no. 3, FD&C red no. 3, D&C red no. 33 and D&C yellow no. 10. *5 mg Capsules:* FD&C green no. 3, D&C red no. 33, FD&C yellow no. 6 and D&C yellow no. 10.

CLINICAL PHARMACOLOGY

Clidinium bromide inhibits gastrointestinal motility and diminishes gastric acid secretion. Its anticholinergic activity approximates that of atropine sulfate and propantheline bromide.

INDICATIONS AND USAGE

Clidinium bromide is effective as adjunctive therapy in peptic ulcer disease. **Clidinium bromide has not been shown to be effective in contributing to the healing of peptic ulcer, decreasing the rate of recurrence or preventing complications.**

CONTRAINDICATIONS

Known hypersensitivity to clidinium bromide or to other anticholinergic drugs, glaucoma, obstructive uropathy (for example, bladder neck obstruction due to prostatic hypertrophy), obstructive disease of the gastrointestinal tract (for example, pyloroduodenal stenosis), paralytic ileus, intestinal atony of the elderly or debilitated patient, unstable cardiovascular status in acute hemorrhage, severe ulcerative colitis, toxic megacolon complicating ulcerative colitis, myasthenia gravis.

WARNINGS

Clidinium bromide may produce drowsiness or blurred vision. The patient should be cautioned regarding activities requiring mental alertness such as operating a motor vehicle or other machinery or performing hazardous work while taking this drug. In the presence of high environmental temperature, heat prostration (fever and heat stroke) may occur with the use of anticholinergics due to decreased sweating. Diarrhea may be an early symptom of incomplete intestinal obstruction, especially in patients with ileostomy or colostomy. Use of anticholinergics in patients with suspected intestinal obstruction would be inappropriate and possibly harmful. With overdosage, a curare-like action may occur, *i.e.,* neuromuscular blockade leading to muscular weakness and possible paralysis.

Use in Pregnancy: No controlled studies in humans have been performed to establish the safety of the drug in pregnancy. Uncontrolled data derived from clinical usage have failed to show abnormalities attributable to its use. Reproduction studies in rats have failed to show any impaired fertility or abnormality in the fetuses that might be associated with the use of clidinium bromide. Use of any drug in pregnancy or in women of childbearing potential requires that the potential benefit of the drug be weighed against the possible hazards to mother and fetus.

Nursing Mothers: As with all anticholinergic drugs, clidinium bromide may be secreted in human milk and may inhibit lactation. As a general rule, nursing should not be undertaken while a patient is on clidinium bromide, or the drug should not be used by nursing mothers.

Pediatric Use: Since there is no adequate experience in children who have received this drug, safety and efficacy in children have not been established.

PRECAUTIONS

Use clidinium bromide with caution in the elderly and in all patients with autonomic neuropathy, hepatic or renal disease, ulcerative colitis - large doses may suppress intestinal motility to the point of producing a paralytic ileus and for this reason precipitate or aggravate "toxic megacolon," a serious complication of the disease; hyperthyroidism; coronary heart disease; congestive heart failure; cardiac tachy-arrhythmias; tachycardia; hypertension; prostatic hypertrophy; hiatal hernia associated with reflux esophagitis, since anticholinergic drugs may aggravate this condition.

DRUG INTERACTIONS

No specific drug interactions are known.

ADVERSE REACTIONS

As with other anticholinergic drugs, the most frequently reported adverse effects are dryness of mouth, blurring of vision, urinary hesitancy and constipation. Other adverse effects reported with the use of anticholinergic drugs include decreased sweating, urinary retention, tachycardia, palpitations, dilatation of the pupils, cycloplegia, increased ocular tension, loss of taste, headaches, nervousness, mental confusion, drowsiness, weakness, dizziness, insomnia, nausea, vomiting, bloated feeling, impotence, suppression of lactation and severe allergic reactions or drug idiosyncrasies including anaphylaxis, urticaria and other dermal manifestations.

DOSAGE AND ADMINISTRATION

For maximum efficacy, dosage should be individualized according to severity of symptoms and occurrence of side effects. The usual dosage is 2.5 to 5 mg three or four times daily before meals and at bedtime. Dosage in excess of 20 mg daily is usually not required to obtain maximum effectiveness. For the aged or debilitated, one 2.5 mg capsule three times daily before meals is recommended. The desired pharmacological effect of the drug is unlikely to be attained without occasional side effects.

HOW SUPPLIED

Quarzan opaque capsules, 2.5 mg, green and red; 5 mg, green and grey.

PRODUCT LISTING - EQUIVALENTS NOT AVAILABLE

Capsule - Oral - 2.5 mg

100's	$20.02	QUARZAN, Roche Laboratories	00140-0119-01

Capsule - Oral - 5 mg

100's	$27.28	QUARZAN, Roche Laboratories	00140-0120-01

Clindamycin (000838)

Categories: Abscess, intra-abdominal; Abscess, pulmonary; Abscess, tubo-ovarian; Acne vulgaris; Cellulitis, pelvic; Empyema; Endometritis; Infection, bone; Infection, gynecologic; Infection, intra-abdominal; Infection, joint; Infection, lower respiratory tract; Infection, skin and skin structures; Infection, vaginal cuff; Peritonitis; Pneumonia; Pneumonitis, anaerobic; Septicemia; Vaginosis, bacterial; Pregnancy Category B; FDA Approved 1970 May; WHO Formulary
Drug Classes: Antibiotics, lincosamides; Anti-infectives, topical; Dermatologics
Brand Names: Cleocin; Clinda-Derm
Foreign Brand Availability: Aclinda (Germany); Albiotin (Indonesia); BB (Taiwan); Bexon (Colombia); Climadan (Indonesia; Singapore); Clinacin (Bahrain; Cyprus; Egypt; Iran; Iraq; Jordan; Kuwait; Lebanon; Libya; Oman; Qatar; Republic-of-Yemen; Saudi-Arabia; Syria; United-Arab-Emirates); Clinbercin (Indonesia); Clincin (Taiwan); Clinda (Germany); Clindabeta (France); Clindacin (Bahrain; Cyprus; Egypt; Iran; Iraq; Jordan; Kuwait; Lebanon; Libya; Oman; Qatar; Republic-of-Yemen; Saudi-Arabia; Syria; United-Arab-Emirates); Clindal (Philippines); Clindamax (Peru); Clinfol (Peru); Clinimycin (Bahrain; Cyprus; Egypt; Iran; Iraq; Jordan; Kuwait; Lebanon; Libya; Oman; Qatar; Republic-of-Yemen; Saudi-Arabia; Syria; United-Arab-Emirates); Dalacin (Denmark; Finland; India; Japan; Spain; Sweden); Dalacin C (Australia; Austria; Bahrain; Belgium; Benin; Bulgaria; Burkina-Faso; Canada; China; Colombia; Costa-Rica; Cyprus; Czech-Republic; Ecuador; Egypt; El-Salvador; England; Ethiopia; Gambia; Ghana; Guatemala; Guinea; Honduras; Hong-Kong; Hungary; Indonesia; Iran; Iraq; Ireland; Israel; Italy; Ivory-Coast; Jordan; Kenya; Kuwait; Lebanon; Liberia; Libya; Malawi; Malaysia; Mali; Mauritania; Mauritius; Mexico; Morocco; Netherlands; New-Zealand; Nicaragua; Niger; Nigeria; Oman; Panama; Peru; Philippines; Portugal; Qatar; Republic-of-Yemen; Saudi-Arabia; Senegal; Seychelles; Sierra-Leone; South-Africa; Sudan; Switzerland; Syria; Tanzania; Thailand; Tunia; Uganda; United-Arab-Emirates; Zambia; Zimbabwe); Dalacine (France); Dalcap (India); Damicine (Colombia); Euroclin (El-Salvador; Honduras; Panama); Lacin (Thailand); Lanacin (Bahrain; Cyprus; Egypt; Iran; Iraq; Jordan; Kuwait; Lebanon; Libya; Oman; Qatar; Republic-of-Yemen; Saudi-Arabia; Syria; United-Arab-Emirates); Librodan (Indonesia); Lindacin (Taiwan); Lindan (Indonesia); Lisiken (Mexico); Nufaclind (Indonesia); Probiotin (Indonesia); Sobelin (Germany); Tidact (Singapore; Taiwan); Trexen (Mexico)
Cost of Therapy: $100.35 (Infection; Cleocin; 150 mg; 4 capsules/day; 10 day supply)
$23.60 (Infection; Generic Capsules; 150 mg; 4 capsules/day; 10 day supply)

IM-IV

WARNING

Note: The trade names have been used throughout this monograph for clarity.

Sterile Solution is for Intramuscular and Intravenous

Use Cleocin Phosphate in the ADD-Vantage Vial is For Intravenous Use Only

Pseudomembranous colitis has been reported with nearly all antibacterial agents, including clindamycin, and may range in severity from mild to life-threatening. Therefore, it is important to consider this diagnosis in patients who present with diarrhea subsequent to the administration of antibacterial agents.

Because clindamycin therapy has been associated with severe colitis which may end fatally, it should be reserved for serious infections where less toxic antimicrobial agents are inappropriate, as described in INDICATIONS AND USAGE. It should not be used in patients with nonbacterial infections such as most upper respiratory tract infections. Treatment with antibacterial agents alters the normal flora of the colon and may permit overgrowth of clostridia. Studies indicate that a toxin produced by *Clostridium difficile* is one primary cause of "antibiotic-associated colitis".

After the diagnosis of pseudomembranous colitis has been established, therapeutic measures should be initiated. Mild cases of pseudomembranous colitis usually respond to drug discontinuation alone. In moderate to severe cases, consideration should be given to management with fluids and electrolytes, protein supplementation, and treatment with an antibacterial drug clinically effective against *C. difficile* colitis.

Diarrhea, colitis, and pseudomembranous colitis have been observed to begin up to several weeks following cessation of therapy with clindamycin.

DESCRIPTION

Cleocin Phosphate Sterile Solution in vials contains clindamycin phosphate, a water soluble ester of clindamycin and phosphoric acid. Each ml contains the equivalent of 150 mg clindamycin, 0.5 mg disodium edetate and 9.45 mg benzyl alcohol added as preservative in each ml. Clindamycin is a semisynthetic antibiotic produced by a 7(S)-chloro-substitution of the 7(R)-hydroxyl group of the parent compound lincomycin.

The chemical name of clindamycin phosphate is L-*threo*-α-D-*galacto*-Octopyranoside, methyl 7-chloro-6,7,8-trideoxy-6-[[(1-methyl-4-propyl-2-pyrrolidinyl)carbonyl]amino]-1-thio-, 2-(dihydrogen phosphate), (2 *S-trans*)-.

The molecular formula is $C_{18}H_{34}ClN_2O_8PS$ and the molecular weight is 504.96.

Cleocin Phosphate in the ADD-Vantage Vial is intended for intravenous use only after further dilution with appropriate volume of ADD-Vantage diluent base solution.

Cleocin Phosphate IV Solution in the Galaxy plastic container for intravenous use is composed of clindamycin phosphate equivalent to 300, 600 and 900 mg of clindamycin premixed with 5% dextrose as a sterile solution. Disodium edetate has been added at a concentration of 0.04 mg/ml. The pH has been adjusted with sodium hydroxide and/or hydrochloric acid.

The plastic container is fabricated from a specially designed multilayer plastic, PL 2501. Solutions in contact with the plastic container can leach out certain of its chemical components in very small amounts within the expiration period. The suitability of the plastic has been confirmed in tests in animals according to the USP biological tests for plastic containers, as well as by tissue culture toxicity studies.

CLINICAL PHARMACOLOGY

Biologically inactive clindamycin phosphate is rapidly converted to active clindamycin.

By the end of short-term intravenous infusion, peak serum levels of active clindamycin are reached. Biologically inactive clindamycin phosphate disappears rapidly from the serum; the average elimination half-life is 6 minutes; however, the serum elimination half-life of active clindamycin is about 3 hours in adults and 2½ hours in pediatric patients.

After intramuscular injection of clindamycin phosphate, peak levels of active clindamycin are reached within 3 hours in adults and 1 hour in pediatric patients. Serum level curves may be constructed from IV peak serum levels as given in TABLE 1 by application of elimination half-lives listed above.

Serum levels of clindamycin can be maintained above the *in vitro* minimum inhibitory concentrations for most indicated organisms by administration of clindamycin phosphate every 8-12 hours in adults and every 6-8 hours in pediatric patients, or by continuous intravenous infusion. An equilibrium state is reached by the third dose.

The elimination half-life of clindamycin is increased slightly in patients with markedly reduced renal or hepatic function. Hemodialysis and peritoneal dialysis are not effective in removing clindamycin from the serum. Dosage schedules need not be modified in the presence of mild or moderate renal or hepatic disease.

No significant levels of clindamycin are attained in the cerebrospinal fluid even in the presence of inflamed meninges.

Pharmacokinetic studies in elderly volunteers (61-79 years) and younger adults (18-39 years) indicate that age alone does not alter clindamycin pharmacokinetics (clearance, elimination half-life, volume of distribution, and area under the serum concentration-time curve) after IV administration of clindamycin phosphate. After oral administration of clindamycin hydrochloride, elimination half-life is increased to approximately 4.0 hours (range 3.4-5.1 hours) in the elderly compared to 3.2 hours (range 2.1-4.2 hours) in younger adults. The extent of absorption, however, is not different between age groups and no dosage alteration is necessary for the elderly with normal hepatic function and normal (age-adjusted) renal function.[1]

Serum assays for active clindamycin require an inhibitor to prevent *in vitro* hydrolysis of clindamycin phosphate.

TABLE 1 *Average Peak and Trough Serum Concentrations of Active Clindamycin After Dosing With Clindamycin Phosphate*

Dosage Regimen	Peak	Trough
Healthy Adult Males (Post Equilibrium)		
600 mg IV in 30 min q6h	10.9 μg/ml	2.0 μg/ml
600 mg IV in 30 min q8h	10.8 μg/ml	1.1 μg/ml
900 mg IV in 30 min q8h	14.1 μg/ml	1.7 μg/ml
600 mg IM q12h*	9 μg/ml	
Pediatric Patients (first dose)*		
5-7 mg/kg IV in 1 hour	10 μg/ml	
5-7 mg/kg IM	8 μg/ml	
3-5 mg/kg IM	4 μg/ml	

* Data in this group from patients being treated for infection.

MICROBIOLOGY

Although clindamycin phosphate is inactive *in vitro*, rapid *in vivo* hydrolysis converts this compound to the antibacterially active clindamycin.

Clindamycin has been shown to have *in vitro* activity against isolates of the following organisms:

***Aerobic gram positive cocci,* including:**

Staphylococcus aureus

Staphylococcus epidermidis (penicillinase and non-penicillinase producing strains). When tested by *in vitro* methods, some staphylococcal strains originally resistant to erythromycin rapidly develop resistance to clindamycin

Streptococci (except *Enterococcus faecalis*)

Pneumococci

***Anaerobic gram negative bacilli,* including:**

Bacteroides species (including *Bacteroides fragilis* group and *Bacteroides melaninogenicus* group)

Fusobacterium species

***Anaerobic gram positive nonsporeforming bacilli,* including:**

Propionibacterium

Eubacterium

Actinomyces species

***Anaerobic and microaerophilic gram positive cocci,* including:**

Peptococcus species

Peptostreptococcus species

Microaerophilic streptococci

Clostridia:

Clostridia are more resistant than most anaerobes to clindamycin. Most *Clostridium perfringens* are susceptible, but other species, *e.g., Clostridium sporogenes* and *Clostridium tertium* are frequently resistant to clindamycin. Susceptibility testing should be done.

Cross resistance has been demonstrated between clindamycin and lincomycin.

Antagonism has been demonstrated between clindamycin and erythromycin.

In Vitro Susceptibility Testing

Disk Diffusion Technique

Quantitative methods that require measurement of zone diameters give the most precise estimates of antibiotic susceptibility. One such procedure[2] has been recommended for use with disks to test susceptibility to clindamycin.

Reports from a laboratory using the standardized single-disk susceptibility test[1] with a 2 μg clindamycin disk should be interpreted according to the following criteria:

Susceptible organisms produce zones of 17 mm or greater, indicating that the tested organism is likely to respond to therapy.

Organisms of intermediate susceptibility produce zones of 15-16 mm, indicating that the tested organism would be susceptible if a high dosage is used or if the infection is confined to tissues and fluids (*e.g.,* urine), in which high antibiotic levels are attained.

Resistant organisms produce zones of 14 mm or less, indicating that other therapy should be selected.

Standardized procedures require the use of control organisms. The 2 μg clindamycin disk should give a zone diameter between 24 and 30 mm for *S. aureus* ATCC 25923.

Dilution Techniques

A bacterial isolate may be considered susceptible if the minimum inhibitory concentration (MIC) for clindamycin is not more than 1.6 μg/ml. Organisms are considered moderately susceptible if the MIC is greater than 1.6 μg/ml and less than or equal to 4.8 μg/ml. Organisms are considered resistant if the MIC is greater than 4.8 μg/ml.

The range of MICs for the control strains are as follows:

S. aureus ATCC 29213, 0.06 — 0.25 μg/ml.

E. faecalis ATCC 29212, 4.0 — 16 μg/ml.

For anaerobic bacteria the minimum inhibitory concentration (MIC) of clindamycin can be determined by agar dilution and broth dilution (including microdilution) techniques.[3] If MICs are not determined routinely, the disk broth method is recommended for routine use. THE KIRBY-BAUER DISK DIFFUSION METHOD AND ITS INTERPRETIVE STANDARDS ARE NOT RECOMMENDED FOR ANAEROBES.

INDICATIONS AND USAGE

Cleocin Phosphate products are indicated in the treatment of serious infections caused by susceptible anaerobic bacteria.

Cleocin Phosphate products are also indicated in the treatment of serious infections due to susceptible strains of streptococci, pneumococci, and staphylococci. Its use should be reserved for penicillin-allergic patients or other patients for whom, in the judgment of the physician, a penicillin is inappropriate. Because of the risk of antibiotic-associated pseudomembranous colitis, as described in the BOXED WARNING, before selecting clindamycin the physician should consider the nature of the infection and the suitability of less toxic alternatives (*e.g.,* erythromycin).

Bacteriologic studies should be performed to determine the causative organisms and their susceptibility to clindamycin.

Indicated surgical procedures should be performed in conjunction with antibiotic therapy.

Cleocin Phosphate is indicated in the treatment of serious infections caused by susceptible strains of the designated organisms in the conditions listed below:

Lower respiratory tract infections including pneumonia, empyema, and lung abscess caused by anaerobes, *Streptococcus pneumoniae,* other streptococci (except *E. faecalis*), and *Staphylococcus aureus.*

Skin and skin structure infections caused by *Streptococcus pyogenes, Staphylococcus aureus,* and anaerobes.

Gynecological infections including endometritis, nongonococcal tubo-ovarian abscess, pelvic cellulitis, and postsurgical vaginal cuff infection caused by susceptible anaerobes.

Intra-abdominal infections including peritonitis and intra-abdominal abscess caused by susceptible anaerobic organisms.

Septicemia caused by *Staphylococcus aureus,* streptococci (except *Enterococcus faecalis*), and susceptible anaerobes.

Bone and joint infections including acute hematogenous osteomyelitis caused by *Staphylococcus aureus* and as adjunctive therapy in the surgical treatment of chronic bone and joint infections due to susceptible organisms.

NON-FDA APPROVED INDICATIONS

Clindamycin has been investigated for the treatment of periodontitis; however, this use is not approved by the FDA.

CONTRAINDICATIONS

This drug is contraindicated in individuals with a history of hypersensitivity to preparations containing clindamycin or lincomycin.

WARNINGS

See BOXED WARNING.

Pseudomembranous colitis has been reported with nearly all antibacterial agents, including clindamycin, and may range in severity from mild to life-threatening. Therefore, it is important to consider this diagnosis in patients who present with diarrhea subsequent to the administration of antibacterial agents.

Treatment with antibacterial agents alters the normal flora of the colon and may permit overgrowth of clostridia. Studies indicate that a toxin produced by *Clostridium difficile* is one primary cause of "antibiotic-associated colitis".

After the diagnosis of pseudomembranous colitis has been established, therapeutic measures should be initiated. Mild cases of pseudomembranous colitis usually respond to drug discontinuation alone. In moderate to severe cases, consideration should be given to management with fluids and electrolytes, protein supplementation, and treatment with an antibacterial drug clinically effective against *C. difficile* colitis.

A careful inquiry should be made concerning previous sensitivities to drugs and other allergens.

This product contains benzyl alcohol as a preservative. Benzyl alcohol has been associated with a fatal "Gasping Syndrome" in premature infants. (See PRECAUTIONS, Pediatric Use.)

Usage in Meningitis: Since clindamycin does not diffuse adequately into the cerebrospinal fluid, the drug should not be used in the treatment of meningitis.

SERIOUS ANAPHYLACTOID REACTIONS REQUIRE IMMEDIATE EMERGENCY TREATMENT WITH EPINEPHRINE. OXYGEN AND INTRAVENOUS CORTICOSTEROIDS SHOULD ALSO BE ADMINISTERED AS INDICATED.

PRECAUTIONS

GENERAL

Review of experience to date suggests that a subgroup of older patients with associated severe illness may tolerate diarrhea less well. When clindamycin is indicated in these patients, they should be carefully monitored for change in bowel frequency.

Cleocin Phosphate products should be prescribed with caution in individuals with a history of gastrointestinal disease, particularly colitis.

Cleocin Phosphate should be prescribed with caution in atopic individuals.

Certain infections may require incision and drainage or other indicated surgical procedures in addition to antibiotic therapy.

The use of Cleocin Phosphate may result in overgrowth of nonsusceptible organisms — particularly yeasts. Should superinfections occur, appropriate measures should be taken as indicated by the clinical situation.

Cleocin Phosphate should not be injected intravenously undiluted as a bolus, but should be infused over at least 10-60 minutes as directed in DOSAGE AND ADMINISTRATION.

Clindamycin dosage modification may not be necessary in patients with renal disease. In patients with moderate to severe liver disease, prolongation of clindamycin half-life has been found. However, it was postulated from studies that when given every 8 hours, accumulation should rarely occur. Therefore, dosage modification in patients with liver disease may not be necessary. However, periodic liver enzyme determinations should be made when treating patients with severe liver disease.

LABORATORY TESTS

During prolonged therapy periodic liver and kidney function tests and blood counts should be performed.

CARCINOGENESIS, MUTAGENESIS, AND IMPAIRMENT OF FERTILITY

Long term studies in animals have not been performed with clindamycin to evaluate carcinogenic potential. Genotoxicity tests performed included a rat micronucleus test and an Ames *Salmonella* reversion test. Both tests were negative.

Fertility studies in rats treated orally with up to 300 mg/kg/day (approximately 1.1 times the highest recommended adult human dose based on mg/m^2) revealed no effects on fertility or mating ability.

PREGNANCY, TERATOGENIC EFFECTS, PREGNANCY CATEGORY B

Reproduction studies performed in rats and mice using oral doses of clindamycin up to 600 mg/kg/day (2.1 and 1.1 times the highest recommended adult human dose based on mg/m^2, respectively) or subcutaneous doses of clindamycin up to 250 mg/kg/day (0.9 and 0.5 times the highest recommended adult human dose based on mg/m^2, respectively) revealed no evidence of teratogenicity.

There are, however, no adequate and well-controlled studies in pregnant women. Because animal reproduction studies are not always predictive of the human response, this drug should be used during pregnancy only if clearly needed.

NURSING MOTHERS

Clindamycin has been reported to appear in breast milk in the range of 0.7-3.8 μg/ml at dosages of 150 mg orally to 600 mg intravenously. Because of the potential for adverse reactions due to clindamycin in neonates (see Pediatric Use), the decision to discontinue the drug should be made, taking into account the importance of the drug to the mother.

PEDIATRIC USE

When Cleocin Phosphate Sterile Solution is administered to the pediatric population (birth to 16 years) appropriate monitoring of organ system functions is desirable.

USAGE IN NEWBORNS AND INFANTS

This product contains benzyl alcohol as a preservative. Benzyl alcohol has been associated with a fatal "Gasping Syndrome" in premature infants.

The potential for the toxic effect in the pediatric population from chemicals that may leach from the single dose premixed IV preparation in plastic has not been evaluated.

GERIATRIC USE

Clinical studies of clindamycin did not include sufficient numbers of patients age 65 and over to determine whether they respond differently from younger patients. However, other reported clinical experience indicates that antibiotic-associated colitis and diarrhea (due to *Clostridium difficile*) seen in association with most antibiotics occur more frequently in the elderly (>60 years) and may be more severe. These patients should be carefully monitored for the development of diarrhea.

Pharmacokinetic studies with clindamycin have shown no clinically important differences between young and elderly subjects with normal hepatic function and normal (age-adjusted) renal function after oral or intravenous administration.

DRUG INTERACTIONS

Clindamycin has been shown to have neuromuscular blocking properties that may enhance the action of other neuromuscular blocking agents. Therefore, it should be used with caution in patients receiving such agents.

Antagonism has been demonstrated between clindamycin and erythromycin *in vitro*. Because of possible clinical significance, the two drugs should not be administered concurrently.

ADVERSE REACTIONS

The following reactions have been reported with the use of clindamycin:

Gastrointestinal: Antibiotic-associated colitis (see WARNINGS), pseudomembranous colitis, abdominal pain, nausea, and vomiting. The onset of pseudomembranous colitis symptoms may occur during or after antibacterial treatment (see WARNINGS). An unpleasant or metallic taste occasionally has been reported after intravenous administration of the higher doses of clindamycin phosphate.

Hypersensitivity Reactions: Maculopapular rash and urticaria have been observed during drug therapy. Generalized mild to moderate morbilliform-like skin rashes are the most frequently reported of all adverse reactions. Rare instances of erythema multiforme, some resembling Stevens-Johnson syndrome, have been associated with clindamycin. A few cases of anaphylactoid reactions have been reported. If a hypersensitivity reaction occurs, the drug should be discontinued. The usual agents (epinephrine, corticosteroids, antihistamines) should be available for emergency treatment of serious reactions.

Skin and Mucous Membranes: Pruritus, vaginitis, and rare instances of exfoliative dermatitis have been reported (see Hypersensitivity Reactions).

Liver: Jaundice and abnormalities in liver function tests have been observed during clindamycin therapy.

Renal: Although no direct relationship of clindamycin to renal damage has been established, renal dysfunction as evidenced by azotemia, oliguria, and/or proteinuria has been observed in rare instances.

Hematopoietic: Transient neutropenia (leukopenia) and eosinophilia have been reported. Reports of agranulocytosis and thrombocytopenia have been made. No direct etiologic relationship to concurrent clindamycin therapy could be made in any of the foregoing.

Local Reactions: Pain, induration and sterile abscess have been reported after intramuscular injection and thrombophlebitis after intravenous infusion. Reactions can be minimized or avoided by giving deep intramuscular injections and avoiding prolonged use of indwelling intravenous catheters.

Musculoskeletal: Rare instances of polyarthritis have been reported.

Cardiovascular: Rare instances of cardiopulmonary arrest and hypotension have been reported following too rapid intravenous administration. (See DOSAGE AND ADMINISTRATION.)

DOSAGE AND ADMINISTRATION

If diarrhea occurs during therapy, this antibiotic should be discontinued (see BOXED WARNING).

ADULTS

Parenteral (IM or IV Administration): Serious infections due to aerobic gram-positive cocci and the more susceptible anaerobes (NOT generally including *Bacteroides fragilis, Peptococcus* species and *Clostridium* species other than *Clostridium perfringens*):

600-1200 mg/day in 2, 3 or 4 equal doses.

More severe infections, particularly those due to proven or suspected *Bacteroides fragilis, Peptococcus* species, or *Clostridium* species other than *Clostridium perfringens:*

1200-2700 mg/day in 2, 3 or 4 equal doses.

For more serious infections, these doses may have to be increased. In life-threatening situations due to either aerobes or anaerobes these doses may be increased. Doses of as much as 4800 mg daily have been given intravenously to adults. See Dilution and Infusion Rates.

Single intramuscular injections of greater than 600 mg are not recommended.

Alternatively, drug may be administered in the form of a single rapid infusion of the first dose followed by continuous IV infusion as indicated in TABLE 2.

TABLE 2

To Maintain Serum Clindamycin Levels	Rapid Infusion Rate	Maintenance Infusion Rate
Above 4 μg/ml	10 mg/min for 30 min	0.75 mg/min
Above 5 μg/ml	15 mg/min for 30 min	1.00 mg/min
Above 6 μg/ml	20 mg/min for 30 min	1.25 mg/min

NEONATES (LESS THAN 1 MONTH)

15-20 mg/kg/day in 3 to 4 equal doses. The lower dosage may be adequate for small prematures.

PEDIATRIC PATIENTS 1 MONTH OF AGE TO 16 YEARS

Parenteral (IM or IV) administration: 20-40 mg/kg/day in 3 or 4 equal doses. The higher doses would be used for more severe infections. As an alternative to dosing on a body weight basis, pediatric patients may be dosed on the basis of square meters body surface:

350 mg/m^2/day for serious infections and 450 mg/m^2/day for more severe infections.

Parenteral therapy may be changed to oral Cleocin Pediatric Flavored Granules or Cleocin HCl Capsules when the condition warrants and at the discretion of the physician.

In cases of β-hemolytic streptococcal infections, treatment should be continued for at least 10 days.

DILUTION AND INFUSION RATES

Clindamycin phosphate must be diluted prior to IV administration. The concentration of clindamycin in diluent for infusion should not exceed 18 mg/ml. Infusion rates should not exceed 30 mg/min. The usual infusion dilutions and rates are as follows (see TABLE 3).

Administration of more than 1200 mg in a single 1 hour infusion is not recommended.

TABLE 3

Dose	Diluent	Time
300 mg	50 ml	10 min
600 mg	50 ml	20 min
900 mg	50-100 ml	30 min
1200 mg	100 ml	40 min

Parenteral drug products should be inspected visually for particulate matter and discoloration prior to administration, whenever solution and container permit.

DILUTION AND COMPATIBILITY

Physical and biological compatibility studies monitored for 24 hours at room temperature have demonstrated no inactivation or incompatibility with the use of Cleocin Phosphate Sterile Solution in IV solutions containing sodium chloride, glucose, calcium or potassium, and solutions containing vitamin B complex in concentrations usually used clinically. No incompatibility has been demonstrated with the antibiotics cephalothin, kanamycin, gentamicin, penicillin or carbenicillin.

The following drugs are physically incompatible with clindamycin phosphate: ampicillin sodium, phenytoin sodium, barbiturates, aminophylline, calcium gluconate, and magnesium sulfate.

The compatibility and duration of stability of drug admixtures will vary depending on concentration and other conditions. For current information regarding compatibilities of clindamycin phosphate under specific conditions, please contact the Medical and Drug Information Unit, Pharmacia & Upjohn Company.

PHYSICO-CHEMICAL STABILITY OF DILUTED SOLUTIONS OF CLEOCIN PHOSPHATE

Room Temperature

6, 9 and 12 mg/ml (equivalent to clindamycin base) in dextrose injection 5%, sodium chloride injection 0.9%, or lactated Ringer's injection in glass bottles or minibags, demonstrated physical and chemical stability for at least 16 days at 25°C. Also, 18 mg/ml (equivalent to clindamycin base) in dextrose injection 5%, in minibags, demonstrated physical and chemical stability for at least 16 days at 25°C.

Refrigeration

6, 9 and 12 mg/ml (equivalent to clindamycin base) in dextrose injection 5%, sodium chloride injection 0.9%, or lactated Ringer's injection in glass bottles or minibags, demonstrated physical and chemical stability for at least 32 days at 4°C.

IMPORTANT: This chemical stability information in no way indicates that it would be acceptable practice to use this product well after the preparation time. Good professional practice suggests that compounded admixtures should be administered as soon after preparation as is feasible.

Frozen

6, 9 and 12 mg/ml (equivalent to clindamycin base) in dextrose injection 5%, sodium chloride injection 0.9%, or lactated Ringer's injection in minibags demonstrated physical and chemical stability for at least 8 weeks at -10°C.

Frozen solutions should be thawed at room temperature and not refrozen.

DIRECTIONS FOR DISPENSING

Pharmacy Bulk Package — Not for Direct Infusion

The Pharmacy Bulk Package is for use in a Pharmacy Admixture Service only under a laminar flow hood. Entry into the vial should be made with a small diameter sterile transfer set or other small diameter sterile dispensing device, and contents dispensed in aliquots using aseptic technique. Multiple entries with a needle and syringe are not recommended. AFTER ENTRY USE ENTIRE CONTENTS OF VIAL PROMPTLY. ANY UNUSED PORTION MUST BE DISCARDED WITHIN 24 HOURS AFTER INITIAL ENTRY.

DIRECTIONS FOR USE

Cleocin Phosphate IV Solution in Galaxy Plastic Container

Premixed Cleocin Phosphate IV Solution is for intravenous administration using sterile equipment. Check for minute leaks prior to use by squeezing bag firmly. If leaks are found, discard solution as sterility may be impaired. Do not add supplementary medication. Parenteral drug products should be inspected visually for particulate matter and discoloration prior to administration whenever solution and container permit. Do not use unless solution is clear and seal is intact.

Caution: Do not use plastic containers in series connections. Such use could result in air embolism due to residual air being drawn from the primary container before administration of the fluid from the secondary container is complete.

Preparation of Cleocin Phosphate in ADD-Vantage System

For IV Use Only.

Cleocin Phosphate 600 mg and 900 mg may be reconstituted in 50 ml or 100 ml, respectively, of dextrose injection 5% or sodium chloride injection 0.9% in the ADD-diluent container. Refer to separate instructions for ADD-Vantage System.

ANIMAL PHARMACOLOGY

One year oral toxicity studies in Spartan Sprague-Dawley rats and beagle dogs at dose levels up to 300 mg/kg/day (approximately 1.1 and 3.6 times the highest recommended adult human dose based on mg/m^2, respectively) have shown clindamycin to be well tolerated. No appreciable difference in pathological findings has been observed between groups of animals treated with clindamycin and comparable control groups. Rats receiving clindamycin hydrochloride at 600 mg/kg/day (approximately 2.1 times the highest recommended adult human dose based on mg/m^2) for 6 months tolerated the drug well; however, dogs dosed at this level (approximately 7.2 times the highest recommended adult human dose based on mg/m^2) vomited, would not eat, and lost weight.

HOW SUPPLIED

Each ml of Cleocin Phosphate Sterile Solution contains clindamycin phosphate equivalent to 150 mg clindamycin; 0.5 mg disodium edetate; 9.45 mg benzyl alcohol added as preservative. When necessary, pH is adjusted with sodium hydroxide and/or hydrochloric acid. Cleocin Phosphate is available in 2, 4, and 6 ml vials, and a 60 ml Pharmacy Bulk Package.

Cleocin Phosphate is supplied in ADD-Vantage vials containing 4 of clindamycin phosphate per 50 ml diluent (600 mg clindamycin phosphate/vial) or 6 ml of clindamycin phosphate per 100 ml diluent (900 mg clindamycin phosphate/vial).

Storage: Store at controlled room temperature 20-25°C (68-77°F).

Cleocin Phosphate IV Solution in Galaxy plastic containers is a sterile solution of clindamycin phosphate with 5% dextrose. The single dose Galaxy plastic containers are available in 300, 600 or 900 mg/50 ml.

Storage: Exposure of pharmaceutical products to heat should be minimized. It is recommended that Galaxy plastic containers be stored at room temperature (25°C). Avoid temperatures above 30°C.

ORAL

WARNING

Note: The trade names have been used throughout this monograph for clarity.

CLEOCIN HCl CAPSULES

Pseudomembranous colitis has been reported with nearly all antibacterial agents, including clindamycin, and may range in severity from mild to life-threatening. Therefore, it is important to consider this diagnosis in patients who present with diarrhea subsequent to the administration of antibacterial agents.

Because clindamycin therapy has been associated with severe colitis which may end fatally, it should be reserved for serious infections where less toxic antimicrobial agents are inappropriate, as described in INDICATIONS AND USAGE, Cleocin HCl Capsules. It should not be used in patients with nonbacterial infections such as most upper respiratory tract infections. Treatment with antibacterial agents alters the normal flora of the colon and may permit overgrowth of clostridia. Studies indicate that a toxin produced by *Clostridium difficile* is one primary cause of "antibiotic-associated colitis".

After the diagnosis of pseudomembranous colitis has been established, therapeutic measures should be initiated. Mild cases of pseudomembranous colitis usually respond to drug discontinuation alone. In moderate to severe cases, consideration should be given to management with fluids and electrolytes, protein supplementation, and treatment with an antibacterial drug clinically effective against *C. difficile* colitis.

Diarrhea, colitis, and pseudomembranous colitis have been observed to begin up to several weeks following cessation of therapy with clindamycin.

CLEOCIN PEDIATRIC

Pseudomembranous colitis has been reported with nearly all antibacterial agents, including clindamycin, and may range in severity from mild to life-threatening. Therefore, it is important to consider this diagnosis in patients who present with diarrhea subsequent to the administration of antibacterial agents.

Because clindamycin therapy has been associated with severe colitis which may end fatally, it should be reserved for serious infections where less toxic antimicrobial agents are inappropriate, as described in INDICATIONS AND USAGE, Cleocin Pediatric. It should not be used in patients with nonbacterial infections such as most upper respiratory tract infections. Treatment with antibacterial agents alters the normal flora of the colon and may permit overgrowth of clostridia. Studies indicate that a toxin produced by *Clostridium difficile* is one primary cause of "antibiotic-associated colitis".

After the diagnosis of pseudomembranous colitis has been established, therapeutic measures should be initiated. Mild cases of pseudomembranous colitis usually respond to drug discontinuation alone. In moderate to severe cases, consideration should be given to management with fluids and electrolytes, protein supplementation, and treatment with an antibacterial drug clinically effective against *C. difficile* colitis.

Diarrhea, colitis, and pseudomembranous colitis have been observed to begin up to several weeks following cessation of therapy with clindamycin.

DESCRIPTION

CLEOCIN HCl CAPSULES

Clindamycin hydrochloride is the hydrated hydrochloride salt of clindamycin. Clindamycin is a semisynthetic antibiotic produced by a 7(S)-chloro-substitution of the 7(R)-hydroxyl group of the parent compound lincomycin.

Cleocin HCl Capsules contain clindamycin hydrochloride equivalent to 75, 150 or 300 mg of clindamycin.

Inactive ingredients:

75 mg: Corn starch, FD&C blue no. 1, FD&C yellow no. 5, gelatin, lactose, magnesium stearate and talc.

150 mg: Corn starch, FD&C blue no. 1, FD&C yellow no. 5, gelatin, lactose, magnesium stearate, talc and titanium dioxide.

300 mg: Corn starch, FD&C blue no. 1, gelatin, lactose, magnesium stearate, talc and titanium dioxide.

The chemical name for clindamycin hydrochloride is Methyl 7-chloro-6,7,8-trideoxy-6-(1-methyl-*trans*-4-propyl-L-2-pyrrolidinecarboxamido)-1-thio-L-*threo*-α-D-*galacto*-octopyranoside monohydrochloride.

CLEOCIN PEDIATRIC

Not for Injection

Clindamycin palmitate hydrochloride is a water soluble hydrochloride salt of the ester of clindamycin and palmitic acid. Clindamycin is a semisynthetic antibiotic produced by a 7(S)-chloro-substitution of the 7(R)-hydroxyl group of the parent compound lincomycin.

The chemical name for clindamycin palmitate hydrochloride is Methyl 7-chloro-6, 7, 8-trideoxy-6-(1-methyl-*trans*-4-propyl-L-2-pyrrolidinecarboxamido)-1-thio-L-*threo*-α-D-*galacto*-octopyranoside 2-palmitate monohydrochloride.

Cleocin Pediatric Flavored Granules contain clindamycin palmitate hydrochloride for reconstitution. Each 5 ml contains the equivalent of 75 mg clindamycin. Inactive ingredients: artificial cherry flavor, dextrin, ethylparaben, pluronic F68, polymethylsiloxane, sucrose.

CLINICAL PHARMACOLOGY

CLEOCIN HCl CAPSULES

Microbiology

Clindamycin has been shown to have *in vitro* activity against isolates of the following organisms:

***Aerobic gram-positive cocci,* including:**

Staphylococcus aureus

Staphylococcus epidermidis (penicillinase and nonpenicillinase producing strains). When tested by *in vitro* methods some staphylococcal strains originally resistant to erythromycin rapidly develop resistance to clindamycin

Streptococci (except *Streptococcus faecalis*)

Pneumococci

***Anaerobic gram-negative bacilli,* including:**

Bacteroides species (including *Bacteroides fragilis* group and *Bacteroides melaninogenicus* group)

Fusobacterium species

***Anaerobic gram-positive nonsporeforming bacilli,* including:**

Propionibacterium

Eubacterium

Actinomyces species

***Anaerobic and microaerophilic gram-positive cocci,* including:**

Peptococcus species

Peptostreptococcus species

Microaerophilic streptococci

Clostridia:

Clostridia are more resistant than most anaerobes to clindamycin. Most *Clostridium perfringens* are susceptible, but other species, *e.g., Clostridium sporogenes* and *Clostridium tertiumare* frequently resistant to clindamycin. Susceptibility testing should be done.

Cross resistance has been demonstrated between clindamycin and lincomycin.

Antagonism has been demonstrated between clindamycin and erythromycin.

Human Pharmacology

Serum level studies with a 150 mg oral dose of clindamycin hydrochloride in 24 normal adult volunteers showed that clindamycin was rapidly absorbed after oral administration. An average peak serum level of 2.50 µg/ml was reached in 45 minutes; serum levels averaged 1.51 µg/ml at 3 hours and 0.70 µg/ml at 6 hours. Absorption of an oral dose is virtually complete (90%), and the concomitant administration of food does not appreciably modify the serum concentrations; serum levels have been uniform and predictable from person to person and dose to dose. Serum level studies following multiple doses of Cleocin HCl for up to 14 days show no evidence of accumulation or altered metabolism of drug.

Serum half-life of clindamycin is increased slightly in patients with markedly reduced renal function. Hemodialysis and peritoneal dialysis are not effective in removing clindamycin from the serum.

Concentrations of clindamycin in the serum increased linearly with increased dose. Serum levels exceed the MIC (minimum inhibitory concentration) for most indicated organisms for at least 6 hours following administration of the usually recommended doses. Clindamycin is widely distributed in body fluids and tissues (including bones). The average biological half-life is 2.4 hours. Approximately 10% of the bioactivity is excreted in the urine and 3.6% in the feces; the remainder is excreted as bioinactive metabolites.

Doses of up to 2 g of clindamycin per day for 14 days have been well tolerated by healthy volunteers, except that the incidence of gastrointestinal side effects is greater with the higher doses.

No significant levels of clindamycin are attained in the cerebrospinal fluid, even in the presence of inflamed meninges.

Pharmacokinetic studies in elderly volunteers (61-79 years) and younger adults (18-39 years) indicate that age alone does not alter clindamycin pharmacokinetics (clearance, elimination half-life, volume of distribution, and area under the serum concentration-time curve) after IV administration of clindamycin phosphate. After oral administration of clindamycin hydrochloride, elimination half-life is increased to approximately 4.0 hours (range 3.4-5.1 hours) in the elderly compared to 3.2 hours (range 2.1-4.2 hours) in younger adults. The extent of absorption, however, is not different between age groups and no dosage alteration is necessary for the elderly with normal hepatic function and normal (age-adjusted) renal function.[1]

CLEOCIN PEDIATRIC

Microbiology

Although clindamycin palmitate HCl is inactive *in vitro,* rapid *in vivo* hydrolysis converts this compound to the antibacterially active clindamycin.

Clindamycin has been shown to have *in vitro* activity against isolates of the following organisms:

***Aerobic gram positive cocci,* including:**

Staphylococcus aureus

Staphylococcus epidermidis (penicillinase and non-penicillinase producing strains). When tested by *in vitro* methods some staphylococcal strains originally resistant to erythromycin rapidly develop resistance to clindamycin

Streptococci (except *Streptococcus faecalis*)

Pneumococci

***Anaerobic gram negative bacilli,* including:**

Bacteroides species (including *Bacteroides fragilis* group and *Bacteroides melaninogenicus* group)

Fusobacterium species

***Anaerobic gram positive nonsporeforming bacilli,* including:**

Propionibacterium

Eubacterium

Actinomyces species

***Anaerobic and microaerophilic gram positive cocci,* including:**

Peptococcus species

Peptostreptococcus species

Microaerophilic streptococci

Clostridia:

Clostridia are more resistant than most anaerobes to clindamycin. Most *Clostridium perfringensare* susceptible, but other species, *e.g., Clostridium sporogenes* and *Clostridium tertiumare* frequently resistant to clindamycin. Susceptibility testing should be done.

Cross resistance has been demonstrated between clindamycin and lincomycin.

Antagonism has been demonstrated between clindamycin and erythromycin.

Human Pharmacology

Blood level studies comparing clindamycin palmitate HCl with clindamycin hydrochloride show that both drugs reach their peak active serum levels at the same time, indicating a rapid hydrolysis of the palmitate to the clindamycin.

Clindamycin is widely distributed in body fluids and tissues (including bones). Approximately 10% of the biological activity is excreted in the urine. The average serum half-life after doses of Cleocin Pediatric is approximately 2 hours in pediatric patients.

Serum half-life of clindamycin is increased slightly in patients with markedly reduced renal function. Hemodialysis and peritoneal dialysis are not effective in removing clindamycin from the serum.

Serum level studies with clindamycin palmitate HCl in normal pediatric patients weighing 50-100 lb given 2, 3 or 4 mg/kg every 6 hours (8, 12 or 16 mg/kg/day) demonstrated mean peak clindamycin serum levels of 1.24, 2.25 and 2.44 µg/ml respectively, 1 hour after the first dose. By the fifth dose, the 6 hour serum concentration had reached equilibrium. Peak serum concentrations after this time would be about 2.46, 2.98 and 3.79 µg/ml with doses of 8, 12 and 16 mg/kg/day, respectively. Serum levels have been uniform and predictable from person to person and dose to dose. Multiple-dose studies in neonates and infants up to 6 months of age show that the drug does not accumulate in the serum and is excreted rapidly. Serum levels exceed the MICs for most indicated organisms for at least 6 hours following administration of the usually recommended doses of Cleocin Pediatric in adults and pediatric patients.

No significant levels of clindamycin are attained in the cerebrospinal fluid, even in the presence of inflamed meninges.

Pharmacokinetic studies in elderly volunteers (61-79 years) and younger adults (18-39 years) indicate that age alone does not alter clindamycin pharmacokinetics (clearance, elimination half-life, volume of distribution, and area under the serum concentration-time curve) after IV administration of clindamycin phosphate. After oral administration of clindamycin hydrochloride, elimination half-life is increased to approximately 4.0 hours (range 3.4-5.1 hours) in the elderly compared to 3.2 hours (range 2.1-4.2 hours) in younger adults; administration of clindamycin palmitate HCl resulted in a similar elimination half-life value of about 4.5 hours in elderly subjects. However, the extent of absorption is not different between age groups and no dosage alteration is necessary for the elderly with normal hepatic function and normal (age-adjusted) renal function.[1]

INDICATIONS AND USAGE

CLEOCIN HCl CAPSULES

Clindamycin is indicated in the treatment of serious infections caused by susceptible anaerobic bacteria.

Clindamycin is also indicated in the treatment of serious infections due to susceptible strains of streptococci, pneumococci, and staphylococci. Its use should be reserved for penicillin-allergic patients or other patients for whom, in the judgment of the physician, a penicillin is inappropriate. Because of the risk of colitis, as described in the BOXED WARNING, Cleocin HCl Capsules, before selecting clindamycin the physician should consider the nature of the infection and the suitability of less toxic alternatives (*e.g.,* erythromycin).

Anaerobes: Serious respiratory tract infections such as empyema, anaerobic pneumonitis and lung abscess; serious skin and soft tissue infections; septicemia; intra-abdominal infections such as peritonitis and intra-abdominal abscess (typically resulting from anaerobic organisms resident in the normal gastrointestinal tract); infections of the female pelvis and genital tract such as endometritis, nongonococcal tubo-ovarian abscess, pelvic cellulitis and postsurgical vaginal cuff infection.

Streptococci: Serious respiratory tract infections; serious skin and soft tissue infections.

Staphylococci: Serious respiratory tract infections; serious skin and soft tissue infections.

Pneumococci: Serious respiratory tract infections.

Bacteriologic studies should be performed to determine the causative organisms and their susceptibility to clindamycin.

In Vitro Susceptibility Testing

A standardized disk testing procedure* is recommended for determining susceptibility of aerobic bacteria to clindamycin. A description is contained in the Cleocin Susceptibility Disk insert. Using this method, the laboratory can designate isolates as resistant, intermediate, or susceptible. Tube or agar dilution methods may be used for both anaerobic and aerobic bacteria.

When the directions in the Cleocin Susceptibility Powder insert are followed, an MIC of 1.6 µg/ml may be considered susceptible; MICs of 1.6-4.8 µg/ml may be considered intermediate and MICs greater than 4.8 µg/ml may be considered resistant.

*Bauer AW, Kirby WMM, Sherris JC, *et al.*: Antibiotic susceptibility testing by a standardized single disc method. *Am J Clin Pathol* **45**:493-496, 1966. Standardized disc susceptibility test. *Federal Register* **37**:20527-29, 1972.

Cleocin Susceptibility Disks 2 µg. See package insert for use.

Cleocin Susceptibility Powder 20 mg. See package insert for use.

For anaerobic bacteria the minimal inhibitory concentration (MIC) of clindamycin can be determined by agar dilution and broth dilution (including microdilution) techniques.

If MICs are not determined routinely, the disk broth method is recommended for routine use. THE KIRBY-BAUER DISK DIFFUSION METHOD AND ITS INTERPRETIVE STANDARDS ARE NOT RECOMMENDED FOR ANAEROBES.

CLEOCIN PEDIATRIC

Cleocin Pediatric is indicated in the treatment of serious infections caused by susceptible anaerobic bacteria.

Clindamycin is also indicated in the treatment of serious infections due to susceptible strains of streptococci, pneumococci and staphylococci. Its use should be reserved for penicillin-allergic patients or other patients for whom, in the judgment of the physician, a penicillin is inappropriate. Because of the risk of colitis, as described in the BOXED WARNING, Cleocin Pediatric, before selecting clindamycin the physician should consider the nature of the infection and the suitability of less toxic alternatives (*e.g.*, erythromycin).

Anaerobes: Serious respiratory tract infections such as empyema, anaerobic pneumonitis and lung abscess; serious skin and soft tissue infections; septicemia; intra-abdominal infections such as peritonitis and intra-abdominal abscess (typically resulting from anaerobic organisms resident in the normal gastrointestinal tract); infections of the female pelvis and genital tract such as endometritis, nongonococcal tubo-ovarian abscess, pelvic cellulitis and postsurgical vaginal cuff infection.

Streptococci: Serious respiratory tract infections; serious skin and soft tissue infections.

Staphylococci: Serious respiratory tract infections; serious skin and soft tissue infections.

Pneumococci: Serious respiratory tract infections.

Bacteriologic studies should be performed to determine the causative organisms and their susceptibility to clindamycin.

In Vitro Susceptibility Testing

A standardized disk testing procedure[2] is recommended for determining susceptibility of aerobic bacteria to clindamycin. A description is contained in the Cleocin Susceptibility Disk insert. Using this method, the laboratory can designate isolates as resistant, intermediate, or susceptible. Tube or agar dilution methods may be used for both anaerobic and aerobic bacteria. When the directions in the Cleocin Susceptibility Powder insert are followed, an MIC (minimal inhibitory concentration) of 1.6 µg/ml may be considered susceptible; MICs of 1.6-4.8 µg/ml may be considered intermediate and MICs greater than 4.8 µg/ml may be considered resistant.

Cleocin Susceptibility Disks 2 µg. See package insert for use.

Cleocin Susceptibility Powder 20 mg. See package insert for use.

For anaerobic bacteria the minimal inhibitory concentration (MIC) of clindamycin can be determined by agar dilution and broth dilution (including microdilution) techniques. If MICs are not determined routinely, the disk broth method is recommended for routine use. THE KIRBY-BAUER DISK DIFFUSION METHOD AND ITS INTERPRETIVE STANDARDS ARE NOT RECOMMENDED FOR ANAEROBES.

NON-FDA APPROVED INDICATIONS

Clindamycin has been investigated for the treatment of periodontitis; however, this use is not approved by the FDA.

CONTRAINDICATIONS

CLEOCIN HCl CAPSULES

Cleocin HCl is contraindicated in individuals with a history of hypersensitivity to preparations containing clindamycin or lincomycin.

CLEOCIN PEDIATRIC

This drug is contraindicated in individuals with a history of hypersensitivity to preparations containing clindamycin or lincomycin.

WARNINGS

CLEOCIN HCl CAPSULES

See BOXED WARNING, Cleocin HCl Capsules.

Pseudomembranous colitis has been reported with nearly all antibacterial agents, including clindamycin, and may range in severity from mild to life-threatening. Therefore, it is important to consider this diagnosis in patients who present with diarrhea subsequent to the administration of antibacterial agents.

Treatment with antibacterial agents alters the normal flora of the colon and may permit overgrowth of clostridia. Studies indicate that a toxin produced by *Clostridium difficile* is one primary cause of "antibioticassociated colitis".

After the diagnosis of pseudomembranous colitis has been established, therapeutic measures should be initiated.

Mild cases of pseudomembranous colitis usually respond to drug discontinuation alone. In moderate to severe cases, consideration should be given to management with fluids and electrolytes, protein supplementation, and treatment with an antibacterial drug clinically effective against *C. difficile* colitis.

A careful inquiry should be made concerning previous sensitivities to drugs and other allergens.

Usage in Meningitis: Since clindamycin does not diffuse adequately into the cerebrospinal fluid, the drug should not be used in the treatment of meningitis.

CLEOCIN PEDIATRIC

See BOXED WARNING, Cleocin Pediatric.

Pseudomembranous colitis has been reported with nearly all antibacterial agents, including clindamycin, and may range in severity from mild to life-threatening. Therefore, it is important to consider this diagnosis in patients who present with diarrhea subsequent to the administration of antibacterial agents.

Treatment with antibacterial agents alters the normal flora of the colon and may permit overgrowth of clostridia. Studies indicate that a toxin produced by *Clostridium difficile* is one primary cause of "antibiotic-associated colitis".

After the diagnosis of pseudomembranous colitis has been established, therapeutic measures should be initiated. Mild cases of pseudomembranous colitis usually respond to drug discontinuation alone. In moderate to severe cases, consideration should be given to management with fluids and electrolytes, protein supplementation, and treatment with an antibacterial drug clinically effective against *C. difficile* colitis.

A careful inquiry should be made concerning previous sensitivities to drugs and other allergens.

Usage in Meningitis: Since clindamycin does not diffuse adequately into the cerebrospinal fluid, the drug should not be used in the treatment of meningitis.

PRECAUTIONS

CLEOCIN HCl CAPSULES

General

Review of experience to date suggests that a subgroup of older patients with associated severe illness may tolerate diarrhea less well. When clindamycin is indicated in these patients, they should be carefully monitored for change in bowel frequency.

Cleocin HCl should be prescribed with caution in individuals with a history of gastrointestinal disease, particularly colitis.

Cleocin HCl should be prescribed with caution in atopic individuals.

Indicated surgical procedures should be performed in conjunction with antibiotic therapy.

The use of Cleocin HCl occasionally results in overgrowth of nonsusceptible organisms — particularly yeasts. Should superinfections occur, appropriate measures should be taken as indicated by the clinical situation.

Clindamycin dosage modification may not be necessary in patients with renal disease. In patients with moderate to severe liver disease, prolongation of clindamycin half-life has been found. However, it was postulated from studies that when given every 8 hours, accumulation should rarely occur. Therefore, dosage modification in patients with liver disease may not be necessary. However, periodic liver enzyme determinations should be made when treating patients with severe liver disease.

The 75 mg and 150 mg capsules contain FD&C yellow no. 5 (tartrazine) which may cause allergic-type reactions (including bronchial asthma) in certain susceptible individuals. Although the overall incidence of FD&C yellow no. 5 (tartrazine) sensitivity in the general population is low, it is frequently seen in patients who also have aspirin hypersensitivity.

Laboratory Tests

During prolonged therapy, periodic liver and kidney function tests and blood counts should be performed.

Carcinogenesis, Mutagenesis, and Impairment of Fertility

Long term studies in animals have not been performed with clindamycin to evaluate carcinogenic potential. Genotoxicity tests performed included a rat micronucleus test and an Ames *Salmonella* reversion test. Both tests were negative.

Fertility studies in rats treated orally with up to 300 mg/kg/day (approximately 1.6 times the highest recommended adult human dose based on mg/m^2) revealed no effects on fertility or mating ability.

Pregnancy, Teratogenic Effects, Pregnancy Category B

Reproduction studies performed in rats and mice using oral doses of clindamycin up to 600 mg/kg/day (3.2 and 1.6 times the highest recommended adult human dose based on mg/m^2, respectively) or subcutaneous doses of clindamycin up to 250 mg/kg/day (1.3 and 0.7 times the highest recommended adult human dose based on mg/m^2, respectively) revealed no evidence of teratogenicity.

There are, however, no adequate and well-controlled studies in pregnant women. Because animal reproduction studies are not always predictive of the human response, this drug should be used during pregnancy only if clearly needed.

Nursing Mothers

Clindamycin has been reported to appear in breast milk in the range of 0.7-3.8 µg/ml.

Pediatric Use

When Cleocin HCl is administered to the pediatric population (birth to 16 years), appropriate monitoring of organ system functions is desirable.

Geriatric Use

Clinical studies of clindamycin did not include sufficient numbers of patients age 65 and over to determine whether they respond differently from younger patients. However, other reported clinical experience indicates that antibiotic-associated colitis and diarrhea (due to *Clostridium difficile*) seen in association with most antibiotics occur more frequently in the elderly (>60 years) and may be more severe. These patients should be carefully monitored for the development of diarrhea.

Pharmacokinetic studies with clindamycin have shown no clinically important differences between young and elderly subjects with normal hepatic function and normal (age-adjusted) renal function after oral or intravenous administration.

CLEOCIN PEDIATRIC

General

Review of experience to date suggests that a subgroup of older patients with associated severe illness may tolerate diarrhea less well. When clindamycin is indicated in these patients, they should be carefully monitored for change in bowel frequency.

Cleocin Pediatric should be prescribed with caution in individuals with a history of gastrointestinal disease, particularly colitis.

Cleocin Pediatric should be prescribed with caution in atopic individuals.

Indicated surgical procedures should be performed in conjunction with antibiotic therapy.

The use of Cleocin Pediatric occasionally results in overgrowth of nonsusceptible organisms — particularly yeasts. Should superinfections occur, appropriate measures should be taken as indicated by the clinical situation.

Clindamycin dosage modification may not be necessary in patients with renal disease. In patients with moderate to severe liver disease, prolongation of clindamycin half-life has been found. However, it was postulated from studies that when given every 8 hours, accumulation should rarely occur. Therefore, dosage modification in patients with liver disease may not be necessary. However, periodic liver enzyme determinations should be made when treating patients with severe liver disease.

Laboratory Tests

During prolonged therapy, periodic liver and kidney function tests and blood counts should be performed.

Carcinogenesis, Mutagenesis, and Impairment of Fertility

Long term studies in animals have not been performed with clindamycin to evaluate carcinogenic potential. Genotoxicity tests performed included a rat micronucleus test and an Ames *Salmonella* reversion test. Both tests were negative.

Fertility studies in rats treated orally with up to 300 mg/kg/day (approximately 1.6 times the highest recommended adult human oral dose based on mg/m^2) revealed no effects on fertility or mating ability.

Pregnancy, Teratogenic Effects, Pregnancy Category B

Reproduction studies performed in rats and mice using oral doses of clindamycin up to 600 mg/kg/day (3.2 and 1.6 times the highest recommended adult human oral dose based on mg/m^2, respectively) or subcutaneous doses of clindamycin up to 250 mg/kg/day (1.3 and 0.7 times the highest recommended adult human oral dose based on mg/m^2, respectively) revealed no evidence of teratogenicity.

There are, however, no adequate and well-controlled studies in pregnant women. Because animal reproduction studies are not always predictive of the human response, this drug should be used during pregnancy only if clearly needed.

Nursing Mothers

Clindamycin has been reported to appear in breast milk in the range of 0.7-3.8 μg/ml.

Pediatric Use

When Cleocin HCl is administered to the pediatric population (birth to 16 years), appropriate monitoring of organ system functions is desirable.

Geriatric Use

Clinical studies of clindamycin did not include sufficient numbers of patients age 65 and over to determine whether they respond differently from younger patients. However, other reported clinical experience indicates that antibiotic-associated colitis and diarrhea (due to *Clostridium difficile*) seen in association with most antibiotics occur more frequently in the elderly (>60 years) and may be more severe. These patients should be carefully monitored for the development of diarrhea.

Pharmacokinetic studies with clindamycin have shown no clinically important differences between young subjects (18-39 years) and elderly subjects (61-79 years) with normal hepatic function and normal (age-adjusted) renal function after oral or intravenous administration.

DRUG INTERACTIONS

CLEOCIN HCl CAPSULES

Clindamycin has been shown to have neuromuscular blocking properties that may enhance the action of other neuromuscular blocking agents. Therefore, it should be used with caution in patients receiving such agents.

Antagonism has been demonstrated between clindamycin and erythromycin *in vitro*. Because of possible clinical significance, these two drugs should not be administered concurrently.

CLEOCIN PEDIATRIC

Clindamycin has been shown to have neuromuscular blocking properties that may enhance the action of other neuromuscular blocking agents. Therefore, it should be used with caution in patients receiving such agents.

Antagonism has been demonstrated between clindamycin and erythromycin *in vitro*. Because of possible clinical significance, these two drugs should not be administered concurrently.

ADVERSE REACTIONS

CLEOCIN HCl CAPSULES

The following reactions have been reported with the use of clindamycin:

Gastrointestinal: Abdominal pain, pseudomembranous colitis, esophagitis, nausea, vomiting and diarrhea (see BOXED WARNING, Cleocin HCl Capsules). The onset of pseudomembranous colitis symptoms may occur during or after antibacterial treatment (see WARNINGS, Cleocin HCl Capsules).

Hypersensitivity Reactions: Generalized mild to moderate morbilliform-like (maculopapular) skin rashes are the most frequently reported adverse reactions. Vesiculobullous rashes, as well as urticaria, have been observed during drug therapy. Rare instances of erythema multiforme, some resembling Stevens-Johnson syndrome, and a few cases of anaphylactoid reactions have also been reported.

Skin and Mucous Membranes: Pruritus, vaginitis, and rare instances of exfoliative dermatitis have been reported. (See Hypersensitivity Reactions.)

Liver: Jaundice and abnormalities in liver function tests have been observed during clindamycin therapy.

Renal: Although no direct relationship of clindamycin to renal damage has been established, renal dysfunction as evidenced by azotemia, oliguria, and/or proteinuria has been observed in rare instances.

Hematopoietic: Transient neutropenia (leukopenia) and eosinophilia have been reported. Reports of agranulocytosis and thrombocytopenia have been made. No direct etiologic relationship to concurrent clindamycin therapy could be made in any of the foregoing.

Musculoskeletal: Rare instances of polyarthritis have been reported.

CLEOCIN PEDIATRIC

The following reactions have been reported with the use of clindamycin:

Gastrointestinal: Abdominal pain, pseudomembraneous colitis, esophagitis, nausea, vomiting and diarrhea (see BOXED WARNING, Cleocin Pediatric). The onset of pseudomembranous colitis symptoms may occur during or after antibacterial treatment (see WARNINGS, Cleocin Pediatric).

Hypersensitivity Reactions: Generalized mild to moderate morbilliform-like (maculopapular) skin rashes are the most frequently reported adverse reactions. Vesiculobullous rashes, as well as urticaria, have been observed during drug therapy. Rare instances of erythema multiforme, some resembling Stevens-Johnson syndrome, and a few cases of anaphylactoid reactions have also been reported.

Skin and Mucous Membranes: Pruritus, vaginitis, and rare instances of exfoliative dermatitis have been reported. (See Hypersensitivity Reactions.)

Liver: Jaundice and abnormalities in liver function tests have been observed during clindamycin therapy.

Renal: Although no direct relationship of clindamycin to renal damage has been established, renal dysfunction as evidenced by azotemia, oliguria, and/or proteinuria has been observed in rare instances.

Hematopoietic: Transient neutropenia (leukopenia) and eosinophilia have been reported. Reports of agranulocytosis and thrombocytopenia have been made. No direct etiologic relationship to concurrent clindamycin therapy could be made in any of the foregoing.

Musculoskeletal: Rare instances of polyarthritis have been reported.

DOSAGE AND ADMINISTRATION

CLEOCIN HCl CAPSULES

If significant diarrhea occurs during therapy, this antibiotic should be discontinued (see BOXED WARNING, Cleocin HCl Capsules).

Adults:

Serious infections: 150-300 mg every 6 hours.

More severe infections: 300-450 mg every 6 hours.

Pediatric Patients:

Serious infections: 8-16 mg/kg/day (4-8 mg/lb/day) divided into 3 or 4 equal doses.

More severe infections: 16-20 mg/kg/day (8-10 mg/lb/day) divided into 3 or 4 equal doses.

To avoid the possibility of esophageal irritation, Cleocin HCl Capsules should be taken with a full glass of water.

Serious infections due to anaerobic bacteria are usually treated with Cleocin Phosphate Sterile Solution. However, in clinically appropriate circumstances, the physician may elect to initiate treatment or continue treatment with Cleocin HCl Capsules.

In cases of β-hemolytic streptococcal infections, treatment should continue for at least 10 days.

CLEOCIN PEDIATRIC

If significant diarrhea occurs during therapy, this antibiotic should be discontinued (see BOXED WARNING, Cleocin Pediatric).

Concomitant administration of food does not adversely affect the absorption of clindamycin palmitate HCl contained in Cleocin Pediatric Flavored Granules.

Serious Infections: 8-12 mg/kg/day (4-6 mg/lb/day) divided into 3 or 4 equal doses.

Severe Infections: 13-16 mg/kg/day (6.5-8 mg/lb/day) divided into 3 or 4 equal doses.

More Severe Infections: 17-25 mg/kg/day (8.5-12.5 mg/lb/day) divided into 3 or 4 equal doses.

In pediatric patients weighing 10 kg or less, ½ teaspoon (37.5 mg) three times a day should be considered the minimum recommended dose.

Serious infections due to anaerobic bacteria are usually treated with Cleocin Phosphate Sterile Solution. However, in clinically appropriate circumstances, the physician may elect to initiate treatment or continue treatment with Cleocin Pediatric.

NOTE: In cases of β-hemolytic streptococcal infections, treatment should be continued for at least 10 days.

Reconstitution Instructions

When reconstituted with water as follows, each 5 ml (teaspoon) of solution contains clindamycin palmitate HCl equivalent to 75 mg clindamycin.

Reconstitute bottles of 100 ml with **75 ml** of water. Add a large portion of the water and shake vigorously; add the remainder of the water and shake until the solution is uniform.

ANIMAL PHARMACOLOGY

CLEOCIN HCl CAPSULES

One year oral toxicity studies in Spartan Sprague-Dawley rats and beagle dogs at dose levels up to 300 mg/kg/day (approximately 1.6 and 5.4 times the highest recommended adult human dose based on mg/m^2, respectively) have shown clindamycin to be well tolerated. No appreciable difference in pathological findings has been observed between groups of animals treated with clindamycin and comparable control groups. Rats receiving clindamycin hydrochloride at 600 mg/kg/day (approximately 3.2 times the highest recommended adult human dose based on mg/m^2) for 6 months tolerated the drug well; however, dogs dosed at this level (approximately 10.8 times the highest recommended adult human dose based on mg/m^2) vomited, would not eat, and lost weight.

CLEOCIN PEDIATRIC

One year oral toxicity studies in Spartan Sprague-Dawley rats and beagle dogs at dose levels up to 300 mg/kg/day (approximately 1.6 and 5.4 times the highest recommended adult human oral dose based on mg/m^2, respectively) have shown clindamycin to be well tolerated. No appreciable difference in pathological findings has been observed between groups of animals treated with clindamycin and comparable control groups. Rats receiving clindamycin hydrochloride at 600 mg/kg/day (approximately 3.2 times the highest recommended adult human oral dose based on mg/m^2) for 6 months tolerated the drug well; however, dogs dosed at this level (approximately 10.8 times the highest recommended adult human oral dose based on mg/m^2) vomited, would not eat, and lost weight.

HOW SUPPLIED

CLEOCIN HCl CAPSULES

Cleocin HCl Capsules are available in the following strengths and colors: *75 mg:* Green; *150 mg:* Light blue and green; *300 mg:* Light blue.
Storage: Store at controlled room temperature 20-25°C (68-77°F).

CLEOCIN PEDIATRIC

Cleocin Pediatric Flavored Granules for oral solution is available in bottles of 100 ml.

When reconstituted as directed, each bottle yields a solution containing 75 mg of clindamycin per 5 ml.

Storage Conditions

Store at controlled room temperature 20-25°C (68-77°F).

Do **NOT** refrigerate the reconstituted solution; when chilled, the solution may thicken and be difficult to pour. The solution is stable for 2 weeks at room temperature.

TOPICAL

DESCRIPTION

Note: The trade names have been used throughout this monograph for clarity.
For External Use

Cleocin T Topical Solution and Cleocin T Topical Lotion contain clindamycin phosphate, at a concentration equivalent to 10 mg clindamycin per milliliter. Cleocin T Topical Gel contains clindamycin phosphate, at a concentration equivalent to 10 mg clindamycin per gram. Each Cleocin T Topical Solution pledget applicator contains approximately 1 ml of topical solution.

Clindamycin phosphate is a water soluble ester of the semi-synthetic antibiotic produced by a 7(S)-chloro-substitution of the 7(R)-hydroxyl group of the parent antibiotic lincomycin.

The solution contains isopropyl alcohol 50% v/v, propylene glycol, and water.

The gel contains allantoin, carbomer 934P, methylparaben, polyethylene glycol 400, propylene glycol, sodium hydroxide, and purified water.

The lotion contains cetostearyl alcohol (2.5%); glycerin; glyceryl stearate SE (with potassium monostearate); isostearyl alcohol (2.5%); methylparaben (0.3%); sodium lauroyl sarcosinate; stearic acid; and purified water.

The chemical name for clindamycin phosphate is Methyl 7-chloro-6,7,8-trideoxy-6-(1-methyl-*trans*-4-propyl-L-2-pyrrolidinecarboxamido)-1-thio-L-*threo*-α-D-*galacto*-octopyranoside 2-(dihydrogen phosphate).

CLINICAL PHARMACOLOGY

Although clindamycin phosphate is inactive *in vitro*, rapid *in vivo* hydrolysis converts this compound to the antibacterially active clindamycin.

Cross resistance has been demonstrated between clindamycin and lincomycin.

Antagonism has been demonstrated between clindamycin and erythromycin.

Following multiple topical applications of clindamycin phosphate at a concentration equivalent to 10 mg clindamycin per ml in an isopropyl alcohol and water solution, very low levels of clindamycin are present in the serum (0-3 ng/ml) and less than 0.2% of the dose is recovered in urine as clindamycin.

Clindamycin activity has been demonstrated in comedones from acne patients. The mean concentration of antibiotic activity in extracted comedones after application of Cleocin T Topical Solution for 4 weeks was 597 μg/g of comedonal material (range 0-1490). Clindamycin *in vitro* inhibits all *Propionibacterium acnes* cultures tested (MICs 0.4 μg/ml). Free fatty acids on the skin surface have been decreased from approximately 14% to 2% following application of clindamycin.

INDICATIONS AND USAGE

Cleocin T Topical Solution, Cleocin T Topical Gel and Cleocin T Topical Lotion are indicated in the treatment of acne vulgaris. In view of the potential for diarrhea, bloody diarrhea and pseudomembranous colitis, the physician should consider whether other agents are more appropriate. (See CONTRAINDICATIONS, WARNINGS and ADVERSE REACTIONS.)

CONTRAINDICATIONS

Cleocin T Topical Solution, Cleocin T Topical Gel and Cleocin T Topical Lotion are contraindicated in individuals with a history of hypersensitivity to preparations containing clindamycin or lincomycin, a history of regional enteritis or ulcerative colitis, or a history of antibiotic-associated colitis.

WARNINGS

Orally and parenterally administered clindamycin has been associated with severe colitis which may result in patient death. Use of the topical formulation of clindamycin results in absorption of the antibiotic from the skin surface. Diarrhea, bloody diarrhea, and colitis (including pseudomembranous colitis) have been reported with the use of topical and systemic clindamycin.

Studies indicate a toxin(s) produced by clostridia is one primary cause of antibiotic-associated colitis. The colitis is usually characterized by severe persistent diarrhea and severe abdominal cramps and may be associated with the passage of blood and mucus. Endoscopic examination may reveal pseudomembranous colitis. Stool culture for *Clostridium difficile* and stool assay for *C. difficile* toxin may be helpful diagnostically.

When significant diarrhea occurs, the drug should be discontinued. Large bowel endoscopy should be considered to establish a definitive diagnosis in cases of severe diarrhea.

Antiperistaltic agents such as opiates and diphenoxylate with atropine may prolong and/or worsen the condition. Vancomycin has been found to be effective in the treatment of antibiotic-associated pseudomembranous colitis produced by *Clostridium difficile*. The usual adult dosage is 500 mg to 2 g of vancomycin orally per day in three to four divided doses administered for 7-10 days. Cholestyramine or colestipol resins bind vancomycin *in vitro*. If both a resin and vancomycin are to be administered concurrently, it may be advisable to separate the time of administration of each drug.

Diarrhea, colitis, and pseudomembranous colitis have been observed to begin up to several weeks following cessation of oral and parenteral therapy with clindamycin.

PRECAUTIONS

GENERAL

Cleocin T Topical Solution contains an alcohol base which will cause burning and irritation of the eye. In the event of accidental contact with sensitive surfaces (eye, abraded skin, mucous membranes), bathe with copious amounts of cool tap water. The solution has an unpleasant taste and caution should be exercised when applying medication around the mouth.

Cleocin T should be prescribed with caution in atopic individuals.

PREGNANCY, TERATOGENIC EFFECTS, PREGNANCY CATEGORY B

Reproduction studies have been performed in rats and mice using subcutaneous and oral doses of clindamycin ranging from 100-600 mg/kg/day and have revealed no evidence of impaired fertility or harm to the fetus due to clindamycin. There are, however, no adequate and well-controlled studies in pregnant women. Because animal reproduction studies are not always predictive of human response, this drug should be used during pregnancy only if clearly needed.

NURSING MOTHERS

It is not known whether clindamycin is excreted in human milk following use of Cleocin T. However, orally and parenterally administered clindamycin has been reported to appear in breast milk. Because of the potential for serious adverse reactions in nursing infants, a decision should be made whether to discontinue nursing or to discontinue the drug, taking into account the importance of the drug to the mother.

PEDIATRIC USE

Safety and effectiveness in pediatric patients under the age of 12 have not been established.

DRUG INTERACTIONS

Clindamycin has been shown to have neuromuscular blocking properties that may enhance the action of other neuromuscular blocking agents. Therefore it should be used with caution in patients receiving such agents.

ADVERSE REACTIONS

In 18 clinical studies of various formulations of Cleocin T using placebo vehicle and/or active comparator drugs as controls, patients experienced a number of treatment emergent adverse dermatologic events (see TABLE 4).

TABLE 4

Treatment Emergent Adverse Event	Solution n=553	Gel n=148	Lotion n=160
Burning	62 (11%)	15 (10%)	17 (11%)
Itching	36 (7%)	15 (10%)	17 (11%)
Burning/itching	60 (11%)	NR	NR
Dryness	105 (19%)	34 (23%)	29 (18%)
Erythema	86 (16%)	10 (7%)	22 (14%)
Oiliness/oily skin	8 (1%)	26 (18%)	12* (10%)
Peeling	61 (11%)	NR	11 (7%)

NR Not recorded.
* Of 126 subjects.

Orally and parenterally administered clindamycin has been associated with severe colitis which may end fatally.

Cases of diarrhea, bloody diarrhea and colitis (including pseudomembranous colitis) have been reported as adverse reactions in patients treated with oral and parenteral formulations of clindamycin and rarely with topical clindamycin (see WARNINGS).

Abdominal pain and gastrointestinal disturbances as well as gram-negative folliculitis have also been reported in association with the use of topical formulations of clindamycin.

DOSAGE AND ADMINISTRATION

Apply a thin film of Cleocin T Topical Solution, Cleocin T Topical Lotion, Cleocin T Topical Gel, or use a Cleocin T Topical Solution pledget for the application of Cleocin T twice daily to affected area. More than one pledget may be used. Each pledget should be used only once and then be discarded.

Lotion: Shake well immediately before using.

Pledget: Remove pledget from foil just before use. Do not use if the seal is broken. Discard after single use.

Keep all liquid dosage forms in containers tightly closed.

HOW SUPPLIED

Cleocin T Topical Solution containing clindamycin phosphate equivalent to 10 mg clindamycin per milliliter is available in 30 and 60 ml applicator bottles, and a carton of 60 single-use pledget applicators.

Cleocin T Topical Gel containing clindamycin phosphate equivalent to 10 mg clindamycin per gram is available in 30 and 60 g tubes.

Cleocin T Topical Lotion containing clindamycin phosphate equivalent to 10 mg clindamycin per milliliter is available in 60 ml plastic squeeze bottles.

STORAGE

Store at controlled room temperature 20-25°C (68-77°F).

Protect from freezing.

VAGINAL

DESCRIPTION

Note: The trade names have been used throughout this monograph for clarity.

CLEOCIN VAGINAL CREAM

FOR INTRAVAGINAL USE ONLY NOT FOR OPHTHALMIC, DERMAL, OR ORAL USE.

Clindamycin phosphate is a water soluble ester of the semi-synthetic antibiotic produced by a 7(S)-chloro-substitution of the 7(R)-hydroxyl group of the parent antibiotic lincomycin. The chemical name for clindamycin phosphate is methyl 7-chloro-6,7,8-trideoxy-6-(1-methyl-*trans*-4-propyl-L-2-pyrrolidinecarboxamido)-1-thio-L-*threo*-α-D-*galacto*-octopyranoside 2-(dihydrogen phosphate). It has a molecular weight of 504.96, and the molecular formula is $C_{18}H_{34}ClN_2O_8PS$.

Cleocin Vaginal Cream 2%, is a semi-solid, white cream, which contains 2% clindamycin phosphate, at a concentration equivalent to 20 mg clindamycin per gram. The pH of the cream is between 3.0 and 6.0. The cream also contains benzyl alcohol, cetostearyl alcohol, mixed fatty acid esters, mineral oil, polysorbate 60, propylene glycol, purified water, sorbitan monostearate, and stearic acid.

Each applicatorful of 5 g of vaginal cream contains approximately 100 mg of clindamycin phosphate.

CLEOCIN VAGINAL OVULES

FOR INTRAVAGINAL USE ONLY

Clindamycin phosphate is a water-soluble ester of the semisynthetic antibiotic produced by a 7(S)-chloro-substitution of the 7(R)-hydroxyl group of the parent antibiotic lincomycin. The chemical name for clindamycin phosphate is methyl 7-chloro-6,7,8-trideoxy-6-(1-methyl-*trans*-4-propyl-L-2-pyrrolidinecarboxamido)-1-thio-L-*threo*-α-D-*galacto*-octopyranoside 2-(dihydrogen phosphate). The monohydrate form has a molecular weight of 522.98, and the molecular formula is $C_{18}H_{34}ClN_2O_8PS \cdot H_2O$.

Cleocin Vaginal Ovules are semisolid, white to off-white suppositories for intravaginal administration. Each 2.5 g suppository contains clindamycin phosphate equivalent to 100 mg clindamycin in a base consisting of a mixture of glycerides of saturated fatty acids.

CLINICAL PHARMACOLOGY

CLEOCIN VAGINAL CREAM

Following a once a day intravaginal dose of 100 mg of clindamycin phosphate vaginal cream 2%, administered to 6 healthy female volunteers for 7 days, approximately 5% (range 0.6% to 11%) of the administered dose was absorbed systemically. The peak serum clindamycin concentration observed on the first day averaged 18 ng/ml (range 4-47 ng/ml) and on day 7 it averaged 25 ng/ml (range 6-61 ng/ml). These peak concentrations were attained approximately 10 hours post-dosing (range 4-24 hours).

Following a once a day intravaginal dose of 100 mg of clindamycin phosphate vaginal cream 2%, administered for 7 consecutive days to 5 women with bacterial vaginosis, absorption was slower and less variable than that observed in healthy females. Approximately 5% (range 2-8%) of the dose was absorbed systemically. The peak serum clindamycin concentration observed on the first day averaged 13 ng/ml (range 6-34 ng/ml) and on day 7 it averaged 16 ng/ml (range 7-26 ng/ml). These peak concentrations were attained approximately 14 hours post-dosing (range 4-24 hours).

There was little or no systemic accumulation of clindamycin after repeated vaginal dosing of clindamycin phosphate vaginal cream 2%. The systemic half-life was 1.5-2.6 hours.

Microbiology

Clindamycin inhibits bacterial protein synthesis at the level of the bacterial ribosome. The antibiotic binds preferentially to the 50S ribosomal subunit and affects the process of peptide chain initiation. Although clindamycin phosphate is inactive *in vitro,* rapid *in vivo* hydrolysis converts this compound to the antibacterially active clindamycin.

Culture and sensitivity testing of bacteria are not routinely performed to establish the diagnosis of bacterial vaginosis. (See INDICATIONS AND USAGE, Cleocin Vaginal Cream.) Standard methodology for the susceptibility testing of the potential bacterial vaginosis pathogens, *Gardnerella vaginalis, Mobiluncus* spp., or *Mycoplasma hominis,* has not been defined. Nonetheless, clindamycin is an antimicrobial agent active *in vitro* against most strains of the following organisms that have been reported to be associated with bacterial vaginosis:

Bacteroides spp.; *Gardnerella vaginalis; Mobiluncus* spp.; *Mycoplasma hominis; Peptostreptococcus* spp.

CLEOCIN VAGINAL OVULES

Systemic absorption of clindamycin was estimated following a once-a-day intravaginal dose of one clindamycin phosphate vaginal suppository (equivalent to 100 mg clindamycin) administered to 11 healthy female volunteers for 3 days. Approximately 30% (range 6-70%) of the administered dose was absorbed systemically on day 3 of dosing based on area under the concentration-time curve (AUC). Systemic absorption was estimated using a subtherapeutic 100 mg intravenous dose of clindamycin phosphate as a comparator in the same volunteers. The mean AUC following day 3 of dosing with the suppository was 3.2 μg·h/ml (range 0.42 to 11 μg·h/ml). The C_{max} observed on day 3 of dosing with the suppository averaged 0.27 μg/ml (range 0.03-0.67 μg/ml) and was observed about 5 hours after dosing (range 1-10 hours). In contrast, the AUC and C_{max} after the single intravenous dose averaged 11 μg·h/ml (range 5.1 to 26 μg·h/ml) and 3.7 μg/ml (range 2.4-5.0 μg/ml), respectively. The mean apparent elimination half-life after dosing with the suppository was 11 hours (range 4-35 hours) and is considered to be limited by the absorption rate.

The results from this study showed that systemic exposure to clindamycin (based on AUC) from the suppository was, on average, 3-fold lower than that from a single subtherapeutic 100 mg intravenous dose of clindamycin. In addition, the recommended daily and total doses of intravaginal clindamycin suppository are far lower than those typically administered in oral or parenteral clindamycin therapy (100 mg of clindamycin per day for 3 days equivalent to about 30 mg absorbed per day from the ovule relative to 600-2700 mg/day for up to 10 days or more, orally or parenterally). The overall systemic exposure to clindamycin from Cleocin Vaginal Ovules is substantially lower than the systemic exposure from therapeutic doses of oral clindamycin hydrochloride (2- to 20-fold lower) or parenteral clindamycin phosphate (40- to 50-fold lower).

Microbiology

Clindamycin inhibits bacterial protein synthesis at the level of the bacterial ribosome. The antibiotic binds preferentially to the 50S ribosomal subunit and affects the process of peptide chain initiation. Although clindamycin phosphate is inactive *in vitro,* rapid *in vivo* hydrolysis converts this compound to the antibacterially active clindamycin.

Culture and sensitivity testing of bacteria are not routinely performed to establish the diagnosis of bacterial vaginosis. (See INDICATIONS AND USAGE, Cleocin Vaginal Ovules.) Standard methodology for the susceptibility testing of the potential bacterial vaginosis pathogens, *Gardnerella vaginalis, Mobiluncus* spp, or *Mycoplasma hominis,* has not been defined. Nonetheless, clindamycin is an antimicrobial agent active *in vitro* against most strains of the following organisms that have been reported to be associated with bacterial vaginosis:

Bacteroides spp.; *Gardnerella vaginalis; Mobiluncus* spp.; *Mycoplasma hominis; Peptostreptococcus* spp.

INDICATIONS AND USAGE

CLEOCIN VAGINAL CREAM

Cleocin Vaginal Cream 2%, is indicated in the treatment of bacterial vaginosis (formerly referred to as *Haemophilus* vaginitis, *Gardnerella* vaginitis, nonspecific vaginitis, *Corynebacterium* vaginitis, or anaerobic vaginosis). Cleocin Vaginal Cream 2%, can be used to treat non-pregnant women and pregnant women during the second and third trimester.

NOTE: For purposes of this indication, a clinical diagnosis of bacterial vaginosis is usually defined by the presence of a homogeneous vaginal discharge that (a) has a pH of greater than 4.5, (b) emits a "fishy" amine odor when mixed with a 10% KOH solution, and (c) contains clue cells on microscopic examination. Gram's stain results consistent with a diagnosis of bacterial vaginosis include (a) markedly reduced or absent *Lactobacillus* morphology, (b) predominance of *Gardnerella* morphotype, and (c) absent or few white blood cells.

Other pathogens commonly associated with vulvovaginitis, *e.g., Trichomonas vaginalis, Chlamydia trachomatis, N. gonorrhoeae, Candida albicans,* and *Herpes simplex* virus should be ruled out.

CLEOCIN VAGINAL OVULES

Cleocin Vaginal Ovules are indicated for 3 day treatment of bacterial vaginosis in non-pregnant women. There are no adequate and well-controlled studies of Cleocin Vaginal Ovules in pregnant women.

NOTE: For purposes of this indication, a clinical diagnosis of bacterial vaginosis is usually defined by the presence of a homogeneous vaginal discharge that (a) has a pH of greater than 4.5, (b) emits a "fishy" amine odor when mixed with a 10% KOH solution, and (c) contains clue cells on microscopic examination. Gram's stain results consistent with a diagnosis of bacterial vaginosis include (a) markedly reduced or absent *Lactobacillus* morphology, (b) predominance of *Gardnerella* morphotype, and (c) absent or few white blood cells.

Other pathogens commonly associated with vulvovaginitis, *e.g., Trichomonas vaginalis, Chlamydia trachomatis, Neisseria gonorrhoeae, Candida albicans,* and herpes simplex virus, should be ruled out.

CONTRAINDICATIONS

CLEOCIN VAGINAL CREAM

Cleocin Vaginal Cream 2%, is contraindicated in individuals with a history of hypersensitivity to clindamycin, lincomycin, or any of the components of this vaginal cream. Cleocin Vaginal Cream 2%, is also contraindicated in individuals with a history of regional enteritis, ulcerative colitis, or a history of "antibiotic-associated" colitis.

CLEOCIN VAGINAL OVULES

Cleocin Vaginal Ovules are contraindicated in individuals with a history of hypersensitivity to clindamycin, lincomycin, or any of the components of this vaginal suppository. Cleocin Vaginal Ovules are also contraindicated in individuals with a history of regional enteritis, ulcerative colitis, or a history of "antibiotic-associated" colitis.

C

WARNINGS

CLEOCIN VAGINAL CREAM

Pseudomembranous colitis has been reported with nearly all antibacterial agents, including clindamycin, and may range in severity from mild to life-threatening. Orally and parenterally administered clindamycin has been associated with severe colitis which may end fatally. Diarrhea, bloody diarrhea, and colitis (including pseudomembranous colitis) have been reported with the use of orally and parenterally administered clindamycin, as well as with topical (dermal) formulations of clindamycin. Therefore, it is important to consider this diagnosis in patients who present with diarrhea subsequent to the administration of clindamycin, even when administered by the vaginal route, because approximately 5% of the clindamycin dose is systemically absorbed from the vagina.

Treatment with antibacterial agents alters the normal flora of the colon and may permit overgrowth of clostridia. Studies indicate that a toxin produced by *Clostridium difficile* is a primary cause of "antibiotic-associated" colitis.

After the diagnosis of pseudomembranous colitis has been established, therapeutic measures should be initiated. Mild cases of pseudomembranous colitis usually respond to discontinuation of the drug alone. In moderate to severe cases, consideration should be given to management with fluids and electrolytes, protein supplementation, and treatment with an antibacterial drug clinically effective against *Clostridium difficile* colitis.

Onset of pseudomembranous colitis symptoms may occur during or after antimicrobial treatment.

CLEOCIN VAGINAL OVULES

Pseudomembranous colitis has been reported with nearly all antibacterial agents, including clindamycin, and may range in severity from mild to life-threatening. Orally and parenterally administered clindamycin has been associated with severe colitis, which may end fatally. Diarrhea, bloody diarrhea, and colitis (including pseudomembranous colitis) have been reported with the use of orally and parenterally administered clindamycin, as well as with topical (dermal) formulations of clindamycin. Therefore, it is important to consider this diagnosis in patients who present with diarrhea subsequent to the administration of Cleocin Vaginal Ovules, because approximately 30% of the clindamycin dose is systemically absorbed from the vagina.

Treatment with antibacterial agents alters the normal flora of the colon and may permit overgrowth of clostridia. Studies indicate that a toxin produced by *Clostridium difficile* is a primary cause of "antibiotic-associated" colitis.

After the diagnosis of pseudomembranous colitis has been established, therapeutic measures should be initiated. Mild cases of pseudomembranous colitis usually respond to discontinuation of the drug alone. In moderate to severe cases, consideration should be given to management with fluids and electrolytes, protein supplementation, and treatment with an antibacterial drug clinically effective against *Clostridium difficile* colitis.

Onset of pseudomembranous colitis symptoms may occur during or after antimicrobial treatment.

PRECAUTIONS

CLEOCIN VAGINAL CREAM

General

Cleocin Vaginal Cream 2%, contains ingredients that will cause burning and irritation of the eye. In the event of accidental contact with the eye, rinse the eye with copious amounts of cool tap water.

The use of Cleocin Vaginal Cream 2% may result in the overgrowth of nonsusceptible organisms in the vagina. In clinical studies involving 600 non-pregnant women who received treatment for 3 days, *Candida albicans* was detected, either symptomatically or by culture, in 8.8% of patients. In 9% of the patients, vaginitis was recorded. In clinical studies involving 1325 non-pregnant women who received treatment for 7 days, *Candida albicans* was detected, either symptomatically or by culture, in 10.5% of patients. Vaginitis was recorded in 10.7% of the patients.

In 180 pregnant women who received treatment for 7 days, *Candida albicans* was detected, either symptomatically or by culture, in 13.3% of patients. In 7.2% of the patients, vaginitis was recorded. *Candida albicans,* as reported here, includes the terms: vaginal moniliasis and moniliasis (body as a whole). Vaginitis includes the terms: vulvovaginal disorder, vulvovaginitis, vaginal discharge, trichomonal vaginitis, and vaginitis.

Information for the Patient

The patient should be instructed not to engage in vaginal intercourse, or use other vaginal products (such as tampons or douches) during treatment with this product.

The patient should also be advised that this cream contains mineral oil that may weaken latex or rubber products such as condoms or vaginal contraceptive diaphragms. Therefore, use of such products within 72 hours following treatment with Cleocin Vaginal Cream 2%, is not recommended.

Carcinogenesis, Mutagenesis, and Impairment of Fertility

Long term studies in animals have not been performed with clindamycin to evaluate carcinogenic potential. Genotoxicity tests performed included a rat micronucleus test and an Ames test. Both tests were negative. Fertility studies in rats treated orally with up to 300 mg/kg/day (31 times the human exposure based on mg/m^2) revealed no effects on fertility or mating ability.

Pregnancy, Teratogenic Effects, Pregnancy Category B

There are no adequate and well-controlled studies in pregnant women during the first trimester of pregnancy. This drug should be used during the first trimester of pregnancy only if clearly needed.

Cleocin Vaginal Cream 2% has been studied in pregnant women during the second trimester. In women treated for 7 days, abnormal labor was reported in 1.1% of patients who received clindamycin vaginal cream 2% compared with 0.5% of patients who received placebo.

Reproduction studies have been performed in rats and mice using oral and parenteral doses of clindamycin up to 600 mg/kg/day (62 and 25 times, respectively, the maximum human exposure based on mg/m^2) and have revealed no evidence of harm to the fetus due to clindamycin. In one mouse strain, cleft palates were observed in treated fetuses; this outcome was not produced in other mouse strains or in other species and is, therefore, considered to be a strain specific effect.

See INDICATIONS AND USAGE, Cleocin Vaginal Cream; PRECAUTIONS, Cleocin Vaginal Cream, General; and ADVERSE REACTIONS, Cleocin Vaginal Cream.

Nursing Mothers

Clindamycin has been detected in human milk after oral or parenteral administration. It is not known if clindamycin is excreted in human milk following the use of vaginally administered clindamycin phosphate.

Because of the potential for serious adverse reactions in nursing infants from clindamycin phosphate, a decision should be made whether to discontinue nursing or to discontinue the drug, taking into account the importance of the drug to the mother.

Pediatric Use

Safety and effectiveness in pediatric patients have not been established.

CLEOCIN VAGINAL OVULES

General

The use of Cleocin Vaginal Ovules may result in the overgrowth of nonsusceptible organisms in the vagina. In clinical studies using Cleocin Vaginal Ovules, treatment-related moniliasis was reported in 2.7% and vaginitis in 3.6% of 589 nonpregnant women. Moniliasis, as reported here, includes the terms: vaginal or nonvaginal moniliasis and fungal infection. Vaginitis includes the terms: vulvovaginal disorder, vaginal discharge, and vaginitis/vaginal infection.

Information for the Patient

The patient should be instructed not to engage in vaginal intercourse or use other vaginal products (such as tampons or douches) during treatment with this product.

The patient should also be advised that these suppositories use an oleaginous base that may weaken latex or rubber products such as condoms or vaginal contraceptive diaphragms. Therefore, the use of such products within 72 hours following treatment with Cleocin Vaginal Ovules is not recommended.

Carcinogenesis, Mutagenesis, and Impairment of Fertility

Long-term studies in animals have not been performed with clindamycin to evaluate carcinogenic potential. Genotoxicity tests performed included a rat micronucleus test and an Ames test. Both tests were negative. Fertility studies in rats treated orally with up to 300 mg/kg/day (31 times the human exposure based on mg/m^2) revealed no effects on fertility or mating ability.

Pregnancy, Teratogenic Effects, Pregnancy Category B

There are no adequate and well-controlled studies of Cleocin Vaginal Ovules in pregnant women.

Cleocin Vaginal Cream, 2%, has been studied in pregnant women during the second trimester. In women treated for 7 days, abnormal labor was reported more frequently in patients who received Cleocin Vaginal Cream compared to those receiving placebo (1.1% vs 0.5% of patients, respectively).

Reproduction studies have been performed in rats and mice using oral and parenteral doses of clindamycin up to 600 mg/kg/day (62 and 25 times, respectively, the maximum human dose based on mg/m^2) and have revealed no evidence of harm to the fetus due to clindamycin. Cleft palates were observed in fetuses from one mouse strain treated intraperitoneally with clindamycin at 200 mg/kg/day (about 10 times the recommended dose based on body surface area conversions). Since this effect was not observed in other mouse strains or in other species, the effect may be strain specific.

Cleocin Vaginal Ovules should be used during pregnancy only if the potential benefit justifies the potential risk to the fetus.

Nursing Mothers

Clindamycin has been detected in human milk after oral or parenteral administration. It is not known if clindamycin is excreted in human milk following the use of vaginally administered clindamycin phosphate.

Because of the potential for serious adverse reactions in nursing infants from clindamycin phosphate, a decision should be made whether to discontinue nursing or to discontinue the drug, taking into account the importance of the drug to the mother.

Pediatric Use

The safety and efficacy of Cleocin Vaginal Ovules in the treatment of bacterial vaginosis in post-menarchal females have been established on the extrapolation of clinical trial data from adult women. When a post-menarchal adolescent presents to a health professional with bacterial vaginosis symptoms, a careful evaluation for sexually transmitted diseases and other risk factors for bacterial vaginosis should be considered. The safety and efficacy of Cleocin Vaginal Ovules in pre-menarchal females have not been established.

Geriatric Use

Clinical studies of Cleocin Vaginal Ovules did not include sufficient numbers of subjects aged 65 and over to determine whether they respond differently from younger subjects.

DRUG INTERACTIONS

CLEOCIN VAGINAL CREAM

Clindamycin has been shown to have neuromuscular blocking properties that may enhance the action of other neuromuscular blocking agents. Therefore, it should be used with caution in patients receiving such agents.

CLEOCIN VAGINAL OVULES

Clindamycin has been shown to have neuromuscular blocking properties that may enhance the action of other neuromuscular blocking agents. Therefore, it should be used with caution in patients receiving such agents.

ADVERSE REACTIONS

CLEOCIN VAGINAL CREAM

Clinical Trials

Non-Pregnant Women

In clinical trials involving non-pregnant women, 1.8% of 600 patients who received treatment with Cleocin Vaginal Cream 2% for 3 days and 2.7% of 1325 patients who received treatment for 7 days discontinued therapy due to drug-related adverse events. Medical events judged to be related, probably related, possibly related, or of unknown relationship to vaginally administered clindamycin phosphate vaginal cream 2%, were reported for 20.7% of the patients receiving treatment for 3 days and 21.3% of the patients receiving treatment for 7 days. Events occurring in ≥1% of patients receiving clindamycin phosphate vaginal cream 2% are shown in TABLE 6.

TABLE 6 *Events Occurring in ≥1% of Non-Pregnant Patients Receiving Clindamycin Phosphate Vaginal Cream 2%*

	Cleocin Vaginal Cream	
	3 Day	7 Day
Event	n=600	n=1325
Urogenital		
Vaginal moniliasis	7.7%	10.4%
Vulvovaginitis	6.0%	4.4%
Vulvovaginal disorder	3.2%	5.3%
Tichomonal vaginitis	0%	1.3%
Body as a Whole		
Moniliasis (body)	1.3%	0.2%

Other events occurring in <1% of the clindamycin vaginal cream 2% groups include:

Urogenital System: Vaginal discharge, metrorrhagia, urinary tract infection, endometriosis, menstrual disorder, vaginitis/ vaginal infection, and vaginal pain.

Body as a Whole: Localized abdominal pain, generalized abdominal pain, abdominal cramps, halitosis, headache, bacterial infection, inflammatory swelling, allergic reaction, and fungal infection.

Digestive System: Nausea, vomiting, constipation, dyspepsia, flatulence, diarrhea, and gastrointestinal disorder.

Endocrine System: Hyperthyroidism.

Central Nervous System: Dizziness and vertigo.

Respiratory System: Epistaxis.

Skin: Pruritus (non-application site), moniliasis, rash, maculopapular rash, erythema, and urticaria.

Special Senses: Taste perversion.

Pregnant Women

In a clinical trial involving pregnant women during the second trimester, 1.7% of 180 patients who received treatment for 7 days discontinued therapy due to drug-related adverse events. Medical events judged to be related, probably related, possibly related, or of unknown relationship to vaginally administered clindamycin phosphate vaginal cream 2%, were reported for 22.8% of pregnant patients. Events occurring in ≥1% of patients receiving either clindamycin phosphate vaginal cream 2% or placebo are shown in TABLE 7.

TABLE 7 *Events Occurring in ≥1% of Pregnant Patients Receiving Clindamycin Phosphate Vaginal Cream 2% or Placebo*

	Cleocin Vaginal Cream	Placebo
	7 Day	7 Day
Event	n=180	n=184
Urogenital		
Vaginal moniliasis	13.3%	7.1%
Vulvovaginal disorder	6.7%	7.1%
Abnormal labor	1.1%	0.5%
Body as a Whole		
Fungal infection	1.7%	0%
Skin		
Pruritus, non-application site	1.1%	0%

Other events occurring in <1% of the clindamycin vaginal cream 2% group include:

Urogenital System: Dysuria, metrorrhagia, vaginal pain, and trichomonal vaginitis.

Body as a Whole: Upper respiratory infection.

Skin: Pruritus (topical application site) and erythema.

Other Clindamycin Formulations

Clindamycin vaginal cream affords minimal peak serum levels and systemic exposure (AUCs) of clindamycin compared to 100 mg oral clindamycin dosing. Although these lower levels of exposure are less likely to produce the common reactions seen with oral clindamycin, the possibility of these and other reactions cannot be excluded presently. Data from well-controlled trials directly comparing clindamycin administered orally to clindamycin administered vaginally are not available.

The following adverse reactions and altered laboratory tests have been reported with the **oral or parenteral** use of clindamycin:

Gastrointestinal: Abdominal pain, esophagitis, nausea, vomiting, and diarrhea. (See WARNINGS, Cleocin Vaginal Cream.)

Hematopoietic: Transient neutropenia (leukopenia), eosinophilia, agranulocytosis, and thrombocytopenia have been reported. No direct etiologic relationship to concurrent clindamycin therapy could be made in any of these reports.

Hypersensitivity Reactions: Maculopapular rash and urticaria have been observed during drug therapy. Generalized mild to moderate morbilliform-like skin rashes are the most frequently reported of all adverse reactions. Rare instances of erythema multiforme, some resembling Stevens-Johnson syndrome, have been associated with clindamycin. A few cases of anaphylactoid reactions have been reported. If a hypersensitivity reaction occurs, the drug should be discontinued.

Liver: Jaundice and abnormalities in liver function tests have been observed during clindamycin therapy.

Musculoskeletal: Rare instances of polyarthritis have been reported.

Renal: Although no direct relationship of clindamycin to renal damage has been established, renal dysfunction as evidenced by azotemia, oliguria, and/or proteinuria has been observed in rare instances.

CLEOCIN VAGINAL OVULES

Clinical Trials

In clinical trials, 3 (0.5%) of 589 nonpregnant women who received treatment with Cleocin Vaginal Ovules discontinued therapy due to drug-related adverse events. Adverse events judged to have a reasonable possibility of having been caused by clindamycin phosphate vaginal suppositories were reported for 10.5% of patients. Events reported by 1% or more of patients receiving Cleocin Vaginal Ovules were as follows:

Urogenital System: Vulvovaginal disorder (3.4%), vaginal pain (1.9%), and vaginal moniliasis (1.5%).

Body as a Whole: Fungal infection (1.0%).

Other events reported by <1% of patients included:

Urogenital System: Menstrual disorder, dysuria, pyelonephritis, vaginal discharge, and vaginitis/vaginal infection.

Body as a Whole: Abdominal cramps, localized abdominal pain, fever, flank pain, generalized pain, headache, localized edema, and moniliasis.

Digestive System: Diarrhea, nausea, and vomiting.

Skin: Nonapplication-site pruritis, rash, application-site pain, and application-site pruritis.

Other Clindamycin Formulations

The overall systemic exposure to clindamycin from Cleocin Vaginal Ovules is substantially lower than the systemic exposure from therapeutic doses of oral clindamycin hydrochloride (2- to 20-fold lower) or parenteral clindamycin phosphate (40- to 50-fold lower) (see CLINICAL PHARMACOLOGY, Cleocin Vaginal Ovules). Although these lower levels of exposure are less likely to produce the common reactions seen with oral or parenteral clindamycin, the possibility of these and other reactions cannot be excluded.

The following adverse reactions and altered laboratory tests have been reported with the oral or parenteral use of clindamycin and may also occur following administration of Cleocin Vaginal Ovules:

Gastrointestinal: Abdominal pain, esophagitis, nausea, vomiting, and diarrhea. (See WARNINGS, Cleocin Vaginal Ovules.)

Hematopoietic: Transient neutropenia (leukopenia), eosinophilia, agranulocytosis, and thrombocytopenia have been reported. No direct etiologic relationship to concurrent clindamycin therapy could be made in any of these reports.

Hypersensitivity Reactions: Maculopapular rash and urticaria have been observed during drug therapy. Generalized mild to moderate morbilliform-like skin rashes are the most frequently reported of all adverse reactions. Rare instances of erythema multiforme, some resembling Stevens-Johnson syndrome, have been associated with clindamycin. A few cases of anaphylactoid reactions have been reported. If a hypersensitivity reaction occurs, the drug should be discontinued.

Liver: Jaundice and abnormalities in liver function tests have been observed during clindamycin therapy.

Musculoskeletal: Rare instances of polyarthritis have been reported.

Renal: Although no direct relationship of clindamycin to renal damage has been established, renal dysfunction as evidenced by azotemia, oliguria, and/or proteinuria has been observed in rare instances.

DOSAGE AND ADMINISTRATION

CLEOCIN VAGINAL CREAM

The recommended dose is one applicatorful of clindamycin phosphate vaginal cream 2%, (5 g containing approximately 100 mg of clindamycin phosphate) intravaginally, preferably at bedtime, for 3 or 7 consecutive days in non-pregnant patients and for 7 consecutive days in pregnant patients.

CLEOCIN VAGINAL OVULES

The recommended dose is one Cleocin Vaginal Ovule (containing clindamycin phosphate equivalent to 100 mg clindamycin per 2.5 g suppository) intravaginally per day, preferably at bedtime, for 3 consecutive days.

HOW SUPPLIED

CLEOCIN VAGINAL CREAM

Cleocin Vaginal Cream 2%, is supplied in a 40 g tube.

Storage: Store at controlled room temperature 20-25°C (68-77°F). Protect from freezing.

CLEOCIN VAGINAL OVULES

Cleocin Vaginal Ovules are supplied in a carton of 3 suppositories with one applicator.

Important Information: Store at 25°C (77°F); excursions permitted to 15-30°C (59-86°F).

Caution: Avoid heat over 30°C (86°F). Avoid high humidity. See end of carton for the lot number and expiration date.

PRODUCT LISTING - RATED THERAPEUTICALLY EQUIVALENT

Capsule - Oral - 75 mg

Package	Price	Product, Manufacturer	NDC
100's	$114.80	CLEOCIN HCL, Pharmacia and Upjohn	00009-0331-02

Capsule - Oral - 150 mg

Package	Price	Product, Manufacturer	NDC
4's	$4.43	GENERIC, Pd-Rx Pharmaceuticals	55289-0441-04
4's	$4.76	GENERIC, Allscripts Pharmaceutical Company	54569-3456-03
15's	$14.33	GENERIC, Allscripts Pharmaceutical Company	54569-3456-01
16's	$42.69	CLEOCIN HCL, Pharmacia and Upjohn	00009-0225-01
20's	$41.36	CLEOCIN HCL, Allscripts Pharmaceutical Company	54569-0306-00
25's	$16.81	GENERIC, Pd-Rx Pharmaceuticals	55289-0441-97
25's	$28.75	GENERIC, Udl Laboratories Inc	51079-0598-19
28's	$29.48	GENERIC, Pd-Rx Pharmaceuticals	55289-0441-28
30's	$28.66	GENERIC, Allscripts Pharmaceutical Company	54569-3456-00
30's	$33.72	GENERIC, Heartland Healthcare Services	61392-0714-30
30's	$33.72	GENERIC, Heartland Healthcare Services	61392-0714-39
31's	$34.84	GENERIC, Heartland Healthcare Services	61392-0714-31
32's	$35.96	GENERIC, Heartland Healthcare Services	61392-0714-32
36's	$74.45	CLEOCIN HCL, Allscripts Pharmaceutical Company	54569-0306-01
45's	$50.58	GENERIC, Heartland Healthcare Services	61392-0714-45
60's	$67.43	GENERIC, Heartland Healthcare Services	61392-0714-60
80's	$47.64	GENERIC, Pd-Rx Pharmaceuticals	55289-0441-80
80's	$95.29	GENERIC, Allscripts Pharmaceutical Company	54569-3456-02
90's	$101.15	GENERIC, Heartland Healthcare Services	61392-0714-90
100's	$59.00	GENERIC, Raway Pharmacal Inc	00686-3171-09
100's	$73.05	GENERIC, Major Pharmaceuticals Inc	00904-3838-61
100's	$83.76	GENERIC, Us Trading Corporation	56126-0418-11
100's	$90.00	GENERIC, Raway Pharmacal Inc	00686-0598-20
100's	$90.35	GENERIC, Teva Pharmaceuticals Usa	62584-0338-01
100's	$91.80	FEDERAL UPPER LIMIT, H.C.F.A. F F P	99999-0838-03
100's	$96.20	GENERIC, Aligen Independent Laboratories Inc	00405-4233-01
100's	$96.43	GENERIC, Qualitest Products Inc	00603-2909-21
100's	$97.90	GENERIC, Major Pharmaceuticals Inc	00904-3838-60
100's	$99.10	GENERIC, Geneva Pharmaceuticals	00781-2937-01
100's	$104.96	GENERIC, Moore, H.L. Drug Exchange Inc	00839-7534-06
100's	$112.39	GENERIC, Vangard Labs	00615-1310-13
100's	$119.08	GENERIC, Teva Pharmaceuticals Usa	00093-3171-01
100's	$119.11	GENERIC, Allscripts Pharmaceutical Company	54569-3456-04
100's	$119.12	GENERIC, Watson/Schein Pharmaceuticals Inc	00364-2337-01
100's	$119.12	GENERIC, Watson/Schein Pharmaceuticals Inc	00591-5708-01
100's	$119.15	GENERIC, Ranbaxy Laboratories	63304-0692-01
100's	$250.88	CLEOCIN HCL, Pharmacia and Upjohn	00009-0225-02
100's	$258.71	CLEOCIN HCL, Pharmacia and Upjohn	00009-0225-03

Capsule - Oral - 300 mg

Package	Price	Product, Manufacturer	NDC
16's	$64.45	GENERIC, Ranbaxy Laboratories	63304-0693-16
16's	$86.70	CLEOCIN HCL, Pharmacia and Upjohn	00009-0395-13
100's	$371.71	GENERIC, Ranbaxy Laboratories	63304-0693-01
100's	$500.01	CLEOCIN HCL, Pharmacia and Upjohn	00009-0395-14
100's	$519.85	CLEOCIN HCL, Pharmacia and Upjohn	00009-0395-02

Gel - Topical - 1%

Package	Price	Product, Manufacturer	NDC
30 gm	$30.76	CLEOCIN T, Allscripts Pharmaceutical Company	54569-1568-00
30 gm	$32.12	GENERIC, Fougera	00168-0202-30
30 gm	$42.60	CLEOCIN T, Pharmacia and Upjohn	00009-3331-02
60 gm	$57.85	GENERIC, Fougera	00168-0202-60
60 gm	$76.73	CLEOCIN T, Pharmacia and Upjohn	00009-3331-01

Lotion - Topical - 1%

Package	Price	Product, Manufacturer	NDC
60 ml	$44.68	GENERIC, Fougera	00168-0203-60
60 ml	$59.28	CLEOCIN T, Pharmacia and Upjohn	00009-3329-01

Powder For Reconstitution - Oral - 75 mg/5 ml

Package	Price	Product, Manufacturer	NDC
100 ml	$25.26	CLEOCIN PEDIATRIC, Pharmacia and Upjohn	00009-0760-04

Solution - Intravenous - 150 mg/ml

Package	Price	Product, Manufacturer	NDC
2 ml	$7.58	CLEOCIN PHOSPHATE, Pharmacia and Upjohn	00009-0870-21
2 ml x 25	$60.00	GENERIC, Raway Pharmacal Inc	00686-0226-02
2 ml x 25	$93.50	CLEOCIN PHOSPHATE, Pharmacia and Upjohn	00009-0870-26
2 ml x 25	$106.88	GENERIC, Abbott Pharmaceutical	00074-4050-01
2 ml x 25	$121.13	GENERIC, Abbott Pharmaceutical	00074-4053-03
4 ml	$13.86	CLEOCIN PHOSPHATE, Pharmacia and Upjohn	00009-0775-20
4 ml	$14.70	CLEOCIN PHOSPHATE, Pharmacia and Upjohn	00009-3124-01
4 ml x 25	$107.77	GENERIC, Abbott Pharmaceutical	00074-4051-01
4 ml x 25	$120.00	GENERIC, Raway Pharmacal Inc	00686-0226-04
4 ml x 25	$194.75	CLEOCIN PHOSPHATE, Pharmacia and Upjohn	00009-0775-26
4 ml x 25	$211.38	GENERIC, Abbott Pharmaceutical	00074-4054-03
4 ml x 25	$218.00	CLEOCIN PHOSPHATE, Pharmacia and Upjohn	00009-3124-03
6 ml	$19.41	CLEOCIN PHOSPHATE, Pharmacia and Upjohn	00009-3447-01
6 ml x 25	$159.00	GENERIC, Raway Pharmacal Inc	00686-0226-06
6 ml x 25	$212.27	GENERIC, Abbott Pharmaceutical	00074-4052-01
6 ml x 25	$255.25	CLEOCIN PHOSPHATE, Pharmacia and Upjohn	00009-0902-18
6 ml x 25	$260.50	CLEOCIN PHOSPHATE, Pharmacia and Upjohn	00009-3447-03
6 ml x 25	$293.91	GENERIC, Abbott Pharmaceutical	00074-4055-03
6 ml x 25	$462.50	CLEOCIN PHOSPHATE, Pharmacia and Upjohn	00009-0902-11
60 ml	$57.90	GENERIC, Abbott Pharmaceutical	00074-4197-01
60 ml	$181.17	CLEOCIN PHOSPHATE, Pharmacia and Upjohn	00009-0728-05
60 ml	$215.13	GENERIC, Solo Pak Medical Products Inc	39769-0226-60
60 ml x 5	$438.25	CLEOCIN PHOSPHATE, Pharmacia and Upjohn	00009-0728-09

Solution - Intravenous - 300 mg;5%/50 ml

Package	Price	Product, Manufacturer	NDC
50 ml x 12	$78.66	GENERIC, Abbott Pharmaceutical	00074-9621-13
50 ml x 24	$98.76	CLEOCIN PHOSPHATE, Pharmacia and Upjohn	00009-3381-01
50 ml x 24	$163.68	CLEOCIN PHOSPHATE, Pharmacia and Upjohn	00009-3381-02

Solution - Intravenous - 600 mg;5%/50 ml

Package	Price	Product, Manufacturer	NDC
50 ml x 12	$119.70	GENERIC, Abbott Pharmaceutical	00074-9622-13
50 ml x 24	$139.20	CLEOCIN PHOSPHATE, Pharmacia and Upjohn	00009-3375-01
50 ml x 24	$250.56	CLEOCIN PHOSPHATE, Pharmacia and Upjohn	00009-3375-02

Solution - Intravenous - 900 mg;5%/50 ml

Package	Price	Product, Manufacturer	NDC
50 ml x 12	$154.47	GENERIC, Abbott Pharmaceutical	00074-9623-13

Solution - Topical - 1%

Package	Price	Product, Manufacturer	NDC
30 ml	$9.17	GENERIC, Qualitest Products Inc	00603-1098-45
30 ml	$10.50	GENERIC, Morton Grove Pharmaceuticals Inc	60432-0693-30
30 ml	$10.80	GENERIC, Ivax Corporation	00182-6028-66
30 ml	$10.95	GENERIC, Major Pharmaceuticals Inc	00904-7733-30
30 ml	$11.52	GENERIC, Fougera	00168-0201-30
30 ml	$11.65	GENERIC, Alpharma Uspd Makers Of Barre and Nmc	00472-0987-91
30 ml	$17.89	CLEOCIN T, Allscripts Pharmaceutical Company	54569-0750-00
30 ml	$18.04	CLEOCIN T, Southwood Pharmaceuticals Inc	58016-3014-30
30 ml	$24.76	CLEOCIN T, Pharmacia and Upjohn	00009-3116-01
60 ml	$12.36	FEDERAL UPPER LIMIT, H.C.F.A. F F P	99999-0838-04
60 ml	$17.94	GENERIC, Qualitest Products Inc	00603-1098-49
60 ml	$19.85	GENERIC, Moore, H.L. Drug Exchange Inc	00839-7815-64
60 ml	$20.00	GENERIC, Morton Grove Pharmaceuticals Inc	60432-0693-60
60 ml	$21.55	GENERIC, Major Pharmaceuticals Inc	00904-7733-03
60 ml	$23.00	GENERIC, Fougera	00168-0201-60
60 ml	$23.15	GENERIC, Alpharma Uspd Makers Of Barre and Nmc	00472-0987-92
60 ml	$24.10	GENERIC, Paddock Laboratories Inc	00574-0016-02
60 ml	$34.94	CLEOCIN T, Allscripts Pharmaceutical Company	54569-1149-00
60 ml	$48.39	CLEOCIN T, Pharmacia and Upjohn	00009-3116-02

Swab - Topical - 1%

Package	Price	Product, Manufacturer	NDC
60's	$40.56	CLEOCIN T, Allscripts Pharmaceutical Company	54569-4634-00
60's	$42.50	GENERIC, Stiefel Laboratories Inc	00145-2472-60
60's	$46.40	GENERIC, Clay-Park Laboratories Inc	45802-0263-37
60's	$50.25	GENERIC, Glades Pharmaceuticals	59366-2852-06
60's	$56.16	CLEOCIN T, Pharmacia and Upjohn	00009-3116-14
69's	$53.80	GENERIC, Clay-Park Laboratories Inc	45802-0263-93
69's	$65.24	GENERIC, Stiefel Laboratories Inc	00145-2472-80

PRODUCT LISTING - RATED NOT THERAPEUTICALLY EQUIVALENT

Gel - Topical - 1%

Package	Price	Product, Manufacturer	NDC
42 gm	$58.38	CLINDAGEL, Galderma Laboratories Inc	00299-4500-42
77 gm	$95.56	CLINDAGEL, Galderma Laboratories Inc	00299-4500-77

PRODUCT LISTING - EQUIVALENTS NOT AVAILABLE

Capsule - Oral - 150 mg

Package	Price	Product, Manufacturer	NDC
12's	$13.92	GENERIC, Southwood Pharmaceuticals Inc	58016-0453-12
15's	$17.40	GENERIC, Southwood Pharmaceuticals Inc	58016-0453-15
20's	$23.20	GENERIC, Southwood Pharmaceuticals Inc	58016-0453-20
21's	$24.99	GENERIC, Southwood Pharmaceuticals Inc	58016-0453-21
30's	$34.80	GENERIC, Southwood Pharmaceuticals Inc	58016-0453-30
40's	$46.40	GENERIC, Southwood Pharmaceuticals Inc	58016-0453-40
100's	$116.01	GENERIC, Southwood Pharmaceuticals Inc	58016-0453-00
100's	$119.11	GENERIC, Greenstone Limited	59762-3328-01

Capsule - Oral - 300 mg

Package	Price	Product, Manufacturer	NDC
16's	$65.17	GENERIC, Greenstone Limited	59762-5010-01
100's	$375.94	GENERIC, Greenstone Limited	59762-5010-02
100's	$422.40	GENERIC, Southwood Pharmaceuticals Inc	58016-0634-00

Cream - Vaginal - 2%

Package	Price	Product, Manufacturer	NDC
40 gm	$43.16	CLEOCIN VAGINAL, Allscripts Pharmaceutical Company	54569-3723-00
40 gm	$49.78	CLEOCIN VAGINAL, Pharmacia and Upjohn	00009-3448-01

Gel - Topical - 1%

Package	Price	Product, Manufacturer	NDC
30 gm	$32.12	GENERIC, Greenstone Limited	59762-3743-01
60 gm	$57.85	GENERIC, Greenstone Limited	59762-3743-02

Lotion - Topical - 1%

Package	Price	Product, Manufacturer	NDC
60 ml	$45.12	GENERIC, Greenstone Limited	59762-3744-01

Solution - Intravenous - 900 mg;5%/50 ml

50 ml x 24	$306.00	CLEOCIN PHOSPHATE, Pharmacia and Upjohn	00009-3382-02

Solution - Topical - 1%

30 ml	$9.30	GENERIC, Moore, H.L. Drug Exchange Inc	00839-7815-63
30 ml	$11.65	GENERIC, Greenstone Limited	59762-3728-01
60 ml	$20.65	GENERIC, Allscripts Pharmaceutical Company	54569-4349-00
60 ml	$23.15	GENERIC, Greenstone Limited	59762-3728-02

Suppository - Vaginal - 100 mg

3's	$46.54	CLEOCIN OVULES, Pharmacia and Upjohn	00009-7667-01

Clobetasol Propionate *(000839)*

For complete prescribing information, refer to the CD-ROM included with the book.

Categories: Dermatosis, corticosteroid-responsive; Psoriasis; Pregnancy Category C; FDA Approved 1985 Dec
Drug Classes: Corticosteroids, topical; Dermatologics
Brand Names: **Temovate**
Foreign Brand Availability: Betasol (Thailand); Betavate (Korea); Betazol (Colombia); Butavate (Greece); Clobasol (Hong-Kong); Clobasone (Thailand); Clobenate (Peru; Philippines); Clobesol (Italy); Clobeson (Korea); Clobet (Thailand); Cloderm (Bahrain; Cyprus; Egypt; Iran; Iraq; Jordan; Korea; Kuwait; Lebanon; Libya; Oman; Qatar; Republic-of-Yemen; Saudi-Arabia; Syria; United-Arab-Emirates); Clovate (Spain); Crobate (Korea); Decloban (Spain); Delor (Bahrain; Cyprus; Egypt; Iran; Iraq; Jordan; Kuwait; Lebanon; Libya; Oman; Qatar; Republic-of-Yemen; Saudi-Arabia; Syria; United-Arab-Emirates); Dermatovate (Mexico); Dermol (New-Zealand); Dermosol (Korea); Dermotyl (India); Dermoval (France); Dermovat (Denmark; Finland; Norway; Sweden); Dermovate (Austria; Bahamas; Bahrain; Barbados; Belgium; Belize; Benin; Bermuda; Bulgaria; Burkina-Faso; Canada; Colombia; Costa-Rica; Curacao; Cyprus; Czech-Republic; Dominican-Republic; Ecuador; Egypt; El-Salvador; England; Ethiopia; Gambia; Ghana; Guatemala; Guinea; Guyana; Honduras; Hong-Kong; Hungary; Indonesia; Iran; Iraq; Ireland; Israel; Ivory-Coast; Jamaica; Japan; Jordan; Kenya; Kuwait; Lebanon; Liberia; Libya; Malawi; Malaysia; Mali; Mauritania; Mauritius; Morocco; Netherland-Antilles; Netherlands; Nicaragua; Niger; Nigeria; Oman; Panama; Peru; Philippines; Portugal; Qatar; Republic-of-Yemen; Saudi-Arabia; Senegal; Seychelles; Sierra-Leone; South-Africa; Sudan; Surinam; Switzerland; Syria; Taiwan; Tanzania; Thailand; Trinidad; Tunia; Uganda; United-Arab-Emirates; Zambia; Zimbabwe); Dermoxin (Germany); Dhabesol (Korea); Karison Creme (Germany); Karison Salbe (Germany); Kloderma (Indonesia); Lamodex (Indonesia); Lobate (India); Lobesol (Malaysia); Lobevat (Mexico); P-Vate (Thailand); Pentasol (Colombia); Rubocort (Greece); S.Z. (Taiwan); Stivate (Thailand); Tenovate (India); Topifort (India); Uniderm (Hong-Kong; Korea); Univate (Malaysia); Xenovate (South-Africa); Yihfu (Taiwan); Yugofin (Greece)

DESCRIPTION

Cream, Emollient, Gel, Ointment, and Scalp Application: FOR TOPICAL DERMATOLOGIC USE ONLY — NOT FOR OPHTHALMIC, ORAL, OR INTRAVAGINAL USE.

Foam: For dermatologic use only — not for ophthalmic use.

All formulations contain the active compound clobetasol propionate, a synthetic corticosteroid, for topical dermatologic use. Clobetasol, an analog of prednisolone, has a high degree of glucocorticoid activity and a slight degree of mineralocorticoid activity.

Chemically, clobetasol propionate is (11β,16β)-21-chloro-9-fluoro-11-hydroxy-16-methyl-17-(1-oxopropoxy)-pregna-1,4-diene-3,20-dione.

Clobetasol propionate has the empirical formula $C_{25}H_{32}ClFO_5$ and a molecular weight of 467. It is a white to cream-colored crystalline powder insoluble in water.

TEMOVATE CREAM

Temovate cream contains clobetasol propionate 0.5 mg/g in a cream base of propylene glycol, glyceryl monostearate, cetostearyl alcohol, glyceryl stearate, peg 100 stearate, white wax, chlorocresol, sodium citrate, citric acid monohydrate, and purified water.

Storage: Store between 15-30°C (59-86°F). Clobetasol propionate cream should not be refrigerated.

TEMOVATE E EMOLLIENT

Temovate E emollient contains clobetasol propionate 0.5 mg/g in an emollient base of cetostearyl alcohol, isopropyl myristate, propylene glycol, cetomacrogol 1000, dimethicone 360, citric acid, sodium citrate, purified water, and imidurea as a preservative.

Storage: Store between 15-30°C (59-86°F). Clobetasol propionate emollient should not be refrigerated.

OLUX FOAM

Each gram of Olux foam contains 0.5 mg clobetasol propionate in a thermolabile foam which consists of cetyl alcohol, citric acid, ethanol (60%), polysorbate 60, potassium citrate, propylene glycol, purified water, and stearyl alcohol. Olux foam is dispensed from an aluminum can pressurized with a hydrocarbon propellant (propane/butane).

Storage: Store at controlled room temperature 20-25°C (68-77°F).

WARNING: *FLAMMABLE. AVOID FIRE, FLAME OR SMOKING DURING AND IMMEDIATELY FOLLOWING APPLICATION.* Keep out of reach of children. Contents under pressure. Do not puncture or incinerate container. Do not expose to heat or store at temperatures above 49°C (120°F).

TEMOVATE GEL

Temovate gel contains clobetasol propionate 0.5 mg/g in a base of propylene glycol, carbomer 934p, sodium hydroxide, and purified water.

Storage: Store between 2-30°C (36-86°F).

TEMOVATE OINTMENT

Temovate ointment contains clobetasol propionate 0.5 mg/g in a base of propylene glycol, sorbitan sesquioleate, and white petrolatum.

Storage: Store between 15-30°C (59-86°F).

TEMOVATE SCALP APPLICATION

Temovate scalp application contains clobetasol propionate 0.5 mg/g in a base of purified water, isopropyl alcohol (39.3%), carbomer 934p, and sodium hydroxide.

Storage: Store between 4-25°C (39-77°F). Do not use near an open flame.

INDICATIONS AND USAGE

CREAM, EMOLLIENT, GEL, AND OINTMENT

Clobetasol propionate cream, emollient, gel, and ointment are super-high potency corticosteroid formulations indicated for the relief of the inflammatory and pruritic manifestations of corticosteroid-responsive dermatoses. Treatment beyond 2 consecutive weeks is not recommended, and the total dosage should not exceed 50 g/week because of the potential for the drug to suppress the hypothalamic-pituitary-adrenal (HPA) axis. Use in pediatric patients under 12 years of age is not recommended.

Additional information for cream and ointment: As with other highly active corticosteroids, therapy should be discontinued when control has been achieved. If no improvement is seen within 2 weeks, reassessment of the diagnosis may be necessary.

Additional information for emollient: In the treatment of moderate to severe plaque-type psoriasis, clobetasol propionate emollient applied to 5-10% of body surface area can be used up to 4 consecutive weeks. The total dosage should not exceed 50 g/week. When dosing for more than 2 weeks, any additional benefits of extending treatment should be weighed against the risk of HPA suppression. Treatment beyond 4 consecutive weeks is not recommended. Patients should be instructed to use clobetasol propionate emollient for the minimum amount of time necessary to achieve the desired results (see INDICATIONS AND USAGE). Use in pediatric patients under 16 years of age has not been studied.

FOAM

Clobetasol propionate foam is a super-potent topical corticosteroid indicated for short-term topical treatment of the inflammatory and pruritic manifestations of moderate to severe corticosteroid-responsive dermatoses of the scalp, and for short-term topical treatment of mild to moderate plaque-type psoriasis of non-scalp regions excluding the face and intertriginous areas.

Treatment beyond 2 consecutive weeks is not recommended, and the total dosage should not exceed 50 g/week because of the potential for the drug to suppress the hypothalamic-pituitary-adrenal (HPA) axis. In a controlled pharmacokinetic study, some subjects experienced reversible suppression of the adrenals following 14 days of clobetasol propionate foam therapy.

Use in children under 12 years of age is not recommended.

SCALP APPLICATION

Clobetasol propionate scalp application is indicated for short-term topical treatment of inflammatory and pruritic manifestations of moderate to severe corticosteroid-responsive dermatoses of the scalp. Treatment beyond 2 consecutive weeks is not recommended, and the total dosage should not exceed 50 ml/week because of the potential for the drug to suppress the HPA axis.

This product is not recommended for use in pediatric patients under 12 years of age.

CONTRAINDICATIONS

Cream, Emollient, Gel, and Ointment: Clobetasol propionate cream, ointment, emollient, and gel are contraindicated in those patients with a history of hypersensitivity to any of the components of the preparations.

Foam: Clobetasol propionate foam is contraindicated in patients who are hypersensitive to clobetasol propionate, to other corticosteroids, or to any ingredient in this preparation.

Scalp Application: Clobetasol propionate scalp application is contraindicated in patients with primary infections of the scalp, or in patients who are hypersensitive to clobetasol propionate, other corticosteroids, or any ingredient in this preparation.

DOSAGE AND ADMINISTRATION

CREAM, EMOLLIENT, GEL, AND OINTMENT

Apply a thin layer of clobetasol propionate to the affected skin areas twice daily and rub in gently and completely (see INDICATIONS AND USAGE).

Clobetasol propionate is a super-high potency topical corticosteroid; therefore, **treatment should be limited to 2 consecutive weeks, and amounts greater than 50 g/week should not be used.**

Clobetasol propionate should not be used with occlusive dressings.

Additional information for cream, ointment, and gel: As with other highly active corticosteroids, therapy should be discontinued when control has been achieved. If no improvement is seen within 2 weeks, reassessment of diagnosis may be necessary.

Additional information for emollient: In moderate to severe plaque-type psoriasis, clobetasol propionate emollient applied to 5-10% of body surface area can be used up to 4 weeks. The total dosage should not exceed 50 g/week. When dosing for more than 2 weeks, any additional benefits of extending treatment should be weighed against the risk of HPA suppression. As with other highly active corticosteroids, therapy should be discontinued when control has been achieved. If no improvement is seen within 2 weeks, reassessment of diagnosis may be necessary. Treatment beyond 4 consecutive weeks is not recommended. Use in pediatric patients under 16 years of age has not been studied.

Geriatric Use

In studies where geriatric patients (65 years of age or older) have been treated with clobetasol propionate, safety did not differ from that in younger patients; therefore, no dosage adjustment is recommended.

FOAM

Note: For proper dispensing of foam, hold the can upside down and depress the actuator. Clobetasol propionate foam should be applied to the affected area twice daily, once in the morning and once at night. Invert the can and dispense a small amount of clobetasol propionate foam (up to a maximum of a golf-ball-size dollop or 1½ capfuls) into the cap of the can, onto a saucer or other cool surface, or to the lesion, taking care to avoid contact with the eyes. Dispensing directly onto hands is not recommended (unless the hands are the affected area), as the foam will begin to melt immediately upon contact with warm skin. When applying clobetasol propionate foam to a hair-bearing area, move the hair away from the affected area so that the foam can be applied to each affected area. Pick up small amounts with fingertips and gently massage into affected area until the foam disappears. Repeat until entire affected area is treated.

Apply the smallest amount possible that sufficiently covers the affected area(s). No more than one and a half capfuls of foam should be used at each application. Do not apply to face or intertriginous areas.

Clobetasol propionate foam is a super-high-potency topical corticosteroid; therefore, treatment should be limited to 2 consecutive weeks and amounts greater than 50 g/week should not be used. Use in pediatric patients under 12 years of age is not recommended.

Unless directed by a physician, clobetasol propionate foam should not be used with occlusive dressings.

SCALP APPLICATION

Clobetasol propionate should be applied to the affected scalp areas twice daily, once in the morning and once at night.

Clobetasol propionate is potent; therefore, **treatment should be limited to 2 consecutive weeks and amounts greater than 50 ml/week should not be used.**

Clobetasol propionate is not to be used with occlusive dressings.

Geriatric Use

In studies where geriatric patients (65 years of age or older) have been treated with clobetasol propionate scalp application, safety did not differ from that in younger patients; therefore, no dosage adjustment is recommended.

PRODUCT LISTING - RATED THERAPEUTICALLY EQUIVALENT

Cream - Topical - 0.05%

Size	Price	Product	NDC
15 gm	$18.61	GENERIC, Ivax Corporation	00182-5113-51
15 gm	$21.45	GENERIC, Teva Pharmaceuticals Usa	00093-9650-15
15 gm	$23.17	GENERIC, Alpharma Uspd Makers Of Barre and Nmc	00472-0400-15
15 gm	$23.27	GENERIC, Taro Pharmaceuticals U.S.A. Inc	51672-1258-01
15 gm	$23.99	GENERIC, Fougera	00168-0163-15
15 gm	$25.86	TEMOVATE, Dura Pharmaceuticals	51479-0375-73
15 gm	$25.86	TEMOVATE, Allscripts Pharmaceutical Company	54569-1680-01
15 gm	$29.83	TEMOVATE, Physicians Total Care	54868-1807-03
15 gm	$31.34	GENERIC, Watson/Rugby Laboratories Inc	55515-0420-15
30 gm	$24.95	FEDERAL UPPER LIMIT, H.C.F.A. F F P	99999-0839-02
30 gm	$25.75	GENERIC, Ivax Corporation	00182-5113-56
30 gm	$29.65	GENERIC, Teva Pharmaceuticals Usa	00093-9650-30
30 gm	$32.10	GENERIC, Alpharma Uspd Makers Of Barre and Nmc	00472-0400-30
30 gm	$32.19	GENERIC, Taro Pharmaceuticals U.S.A. Inc	51672-1258-02
30 gm	$33.33	GENERIC, Fougera	00168-0163-30
30 gm	$34.94	TEMOVATE, Southwood Pharmaceuticals Inc	58016-1133-01
30 gm	$35.77	TEMOVATE, Dura Pharmaceuticals	51479-0375-72
30 gm	$35.77	TEMOVATE, Allscripts Pharmaceutical Company	54569-3395-00
30 gm	$41.04	TEMOVATE, Physicians Total Care	54868-1807-02
30 gm	$43.37	GENERIC, Watson/Rugby Laboratories Inc	55515-0420-30
45 gm	$43.20	GENERIC, Teva Pharmaceuticals Usa	00093-9650-95
45 gm	$46.70	GENERIC, Alpharma Uspd Makers Of Barre and Nmc	00472-0400-45
45 gm	$46.85	GENERIC, Taro Pharmaceuticals U.S.A. Inc	51672-1258-06
45 gm	$48.75	GENERIC, Fougera	00168-0163-46
45 gm	$52.06	TEMOVATE, Dura Pharmaceuticals	51479-0375-01
45 gm	$52.06	TEMOVATE, Allscripts Pharmaceutical Company	54569-1563-00
45 gm	$59.47	TEMOVATE, Physicians Total Care	54868-1807-01
45 gm	$63.12	GENERIC, Watson/Rugby Laboratories Inc	55515-0420-45
60 gm	$58.47	GENERIC, Taro Pharmaceuticals U.S.A. Inc	51672-1258-03
60 gm	$62.05	GENERIC, Fougera	00168-0163-60
60 gm	$64.97	TEMOVATE, Dura Pharmaceuticals	51479-0375-02

Gel - Topical - 0.05%

Size	Price	Product	NDC
15 gm	$22.80	GENERIC, Taro Pharmaceuticals U.S.A. Inc	51672-1294-01
15 gm	$24.09	GENERIC, Fougera	00168-0293-15
15 gm	$25.86	TEMOVATE, Dura Pharmaceuticals	51479-0455-01
15 gm	$25.86	TEMOVATE, Allscripts Pharmaceutical Company	54569-4069-00
15 gm	$29.16	GENERIC, Glades Pharmaceuticals	59366-2791-01
30 gm	$31.85	GENERIC, Taro Pharmaceuticals U.S.A. Inc	51672-1294-02
30 gm	$33.49	GENERIC, Fougera	00168-0293-30
30 gm	$35.77	TEMOVATE, Dura Pharmaceuticals	51479-0455-02
30 gm	$40.35	GENERIC, Glades Pharmaceuticals	59366-2791-03
60 gm	$57.75	GENERIC, Taro Pharmaceuticals U.S.A. Inc	51672-1294-03
60 gm	$61.12	GENERIC, Fougera	00168-0293-60
60 gm	$64.97	TEMOVATE, Dura Pharmaceuticals	51479-0455-03
60 gm	$73.28	GENERIC, Glades Pharmaceuticals	59366-2791-06

Ointment - Topical - 0.05%

Size	Price	Product	NDC
15 gm	$18.61	GENERIC, Ivax Corporation	00182-5114-51
15 gm	$21.45	GENERIC, Copley	38245-0128-70
15 gm	$23.17	GENERIC, Alpharma Uspd Makers Of Barre and Nmc	00472-0401-15
15 gm	$23.27	GENERIC, Taro Pharmaceuticals U.S.A. Inc	51672-1259-01
15 gm	$23.27	GENERIC, Glades Pharmaceuticals	59366-2796-01
15 gm	$23.99	GENERIC, Fougera	00168-0162-15
15 gm	$25.86	TEMOVATE, Dura Pharmaceuticals	51479-0376-73
15 gm	$25.86	TEMOVATE, Allscripts Pharmaceutical Company	54569-1681-01
15 gm	$28.19	TEMOVATE, Physicians Total Care	54868-1589-01
15 gm	$31.34	GENERIC, Oclassen Pharmaceuticals Inc	55515-0410-15
30 gm	$25.75	GENERIC, Ivax Corporation	00182-5114-56
30 gm	$29.65	GENERIC, Copley	38245-0128-71
30 gm	$31.85	GENERIC, Glades Pharmaceuticals	59366-2796-03
30 gm	$32.10	GENERIC, Alpharma Uspd Makers Of Barre and Nmc	00472-0401-30
30 gm	$32.19	GENERIC, Taro Pharmaceuticals U.S.A. Inc	51672-1259-02
30 gm	$33.33	GENERIC, Fougera	00168-0162-30
30 gm	$35.77	TEMOVATE, Dura Pharmaceuticals	51479-0376-72
30 gm	$41.04	TEMOVATE, Physicians Total Care	54868-1589-02
45 gm	$43.20	GENERIC, Teva Pharmaceuticals Usa	38245-0128-72
45 gm	$46.70	GENERIC, Alpharma Uspd Makers Of Barre and Nmc	00472-0401-45
45 gm	$46.84	GENERIC, Glades Pharmaceuticals	59366-2796-04
45 gm	$46.85	GENERIC, Taro Pharmaceuticals U.S.A. Inc	51672-1259-06
45 gm	$48.75	GENERIC, Fougera	00168-0162-46
45 gm	$52.06	TEMOVATE, Dura Pharmaceuticals	51479-0376-01
45 gm	$63.12	GENERIC, Oclassen Pharmaceuticals Inc	55515-0410-45
50 gm	$42.51	GENERIC, Moore, H.L. Drug Exchange Inc	00839-8063-99
60 gm	$57.95	GENERIC, Glades Pharmaceuticals	59366-2796-06
60 gm	$58.47	GENERIC, Taro Pharmaceuticals U.S.A. Inc	51672-1259-03
60 gm	$62.05	GENERIC, Fougera	00168-0162-60
60 gm	$64.97	TEMOVATE, Dura Pharmaceuticals	51479-0376-02
60 gm	$74.08	TEMOVATE, Physicians Total Care	54868-1589-00

Solution - Topical - 0.05%

Size	Price	Product	NDC
25 ml	$20.55	GENERIC, Morton Grove Pharmaceuticals Inc	60432-0133-25
25 ml	$26.51	GENERIC, Fougera	00168-0269-25
25 ml	$26.60	GENERIC, Alpharma Uspd Makers Of Barre and Nmc	00472-0402-25
25 ml	$26.66	GENERIC, Taro Pharmaceuticals U.S.A. Inc	51672-1293-02
25 ml	$29.62	TEMOVATE, Dura Pharmaceuticals	51479-0432-00
25 ml	$35.43	TEMOVATE, Physicians Total Care	54868-2993-01
50 ml	$39.60	GENERIC, Morton Grove Pharmaceuticals Inc	60432-0133-50
50 ml	$51.26	GENERIC, Taro Pharmaceuticals U.S.A. Inc	51672-1293-03
50 ml	$53.10	GENERIC, Fougera	00168-0269-50
50 ml	$56.96	TEMOVATE, Dura Pharmaceuticals	51479-0432-01

PRODUCT LISTING - RATED NOT THERAPEUTICALLY EQUIVALENT

Cream - Topical - 0.05%

Size	Price	Product	NDC
15 gm	$24.03	GENERIC, Taro Pharmaceuticals U.S.A. Inc	51672-1297-01
15 gm	$26.70	TEMOVATE EMOLLIENT, Dura Pharmaceuticals	51479-0454-01
15 gm	$26.70	TEMOVATE EMOLLIENT, Allscripts Pharmaceutical Company	54569-4173-00
30 gm	$34.79	GENERIC, Taro Pharmaceuticals U.S.A. Inc	51672-1297-02
30 gm	$38.65	TEMOVATE EMOLLIENT, Dura Pharmaceuticals	51479-0454-02
30 gm	$38.65	TEMOVATE EMOLLIENT, Allscripts Pharmaceutical Company	54569-4174-00
30 gm	$40.55	TEMOVATE EMOLLIENT, Physicians Total Care	54868-3734-01
60 gm	$63.19	GENERIC, Taro Pharmaceuticals U.S.A. Inc	51672-1297-03
60 gm	$70.21	TEMOVATE EMOLLIENT, Dura Pharmaceuticals	51479-0454-03
60 gm	$73.18	TEMOVATE EMOLLIENT, Physicians Total Care	54868-3734-00

Solution - Topical - 0.05%

Size	Price	Product	NDC
25 ml	$35.90	GENERIC, Oclassen Pharmaceuticals Inc	55515-0430-25
50 ml	$63.27	GENERIC, Oclassen Pharmaceuticals Inc	55515-0430-50

PRODUCT LISTING - EQUIVALENTS NOT AVAILABLE

Cream - Topical - 0.05%

Size	Price	Product	NDC
15 gm	$21.82	GENERIC, Allscripts Pharmaceutical Company	54569-4200-00
15 gm	$25.46	GENERIC, Fougera	00168-0301-15
15 gm	$27.50	EMBELINE E, Healthpoint	00064-0440-15
30 gm	$31.24	GENERIC, Allscripts Pharmaceutical Company	54569-4550-00
30 gm	$37.87	GENERIC, Fougera	00168-0301-30
30 gm	$42.32	EMBELINE E, Healthpoint	00064-0440-30
60 gm	$62.45	GENERIC, Alpharma Uspd Makers Of Barre and Nmc	00472-0400-60

60 gm	$69.26	GENERIC, Fougera	00168-0301-60
60 gm	$77.35	EMBELINE E, Healthpoint	00064-0440-60
Foam - Topical - 0.05%			
50 gm	$82.68	OLUX, Connetics Inc	63032-0031-50
100 gm	$152.40	OLUX, Connetics Inc	63032-0031-00
Gel - Topical - 0.05%			
45 gm	$107.10	GENERIC, Stiefel Laboratories Inc	00145-2790-04
Ointment - Topical - 0.05%			
15 gm	$21.57	GENERIC, Allscripts Pharmaceutical Company	54569-4649-00
60 gm	$62.45	GENERIC, Alpharma Uspd Makers Of Barre and Nmc	00472-0401-60
Solution - Topical - 0.05%			
25 ml	$27.90	GENERIC, Allscripts Pharmaceutical Company	54569-4656-00

Clocortolone Pivalate *(000840)*

For complete prescribing information, refer to the CD-ROM included with the book.

Categories: Dermatosis, corticosteroid-responsive; Pregnancy Category C; FDA Approved 1977 Aug
Drug Classes: Corticosteroids, topical; Dermatologics
Brand Names: **Cloderm**
Foreign Brand Availability: Kaban (Germany); Lenen (Italy)

DESCRIPTION

Cloderm cream 0.1% contains the medium potency topical corticosteroid, clocortolone pivalate, in a specially formulated water-washable emollient cream base consisting of purified water, white petrolatum, mineral oil, stearyl alcohol, polyoxyl 40 stearate, carbomer 934P, edetate disodium, sodium hydroxide, with methylparaben and propylparaben as preservatives.

The chemical name is 9-chloro-6α-fluoro-11β,21-dihydroxy-16α-methylpregna-1, 4-diene-3,20-dione 21-pivalate.

INDICATIONS AND USAGE

Topical corticosteroids are indicated for the relief of the inflammatory and pruritic manifestations of corticosteroid-responsive dermatoses.

CONTRAINDICATIONS

Topical corticosteroids are contraindicated in those patients with a history of hypersensitivity to any of the components of the preparation.

DOSAGE AND ADMINISTRATION

Apply clocortolone pivalate cream sparingly to the affected areas three times a day and rub in gently.

Occlusive dressings may be used for the management of psoriasis or recalcitrant conditions.

If an infection develops, the use of occlusive dressings should be discontinued and appropriate antimicrobial therapy instituted.

PRODUCT LISTING - EQUIVALENTS NOT AVAILABLE

Cream - Topical - 0.1%			
15 gm	$21.56	GENERIC, Healthpoint	00064-3100-15
45 gm	$43.50	GENERIC, Healthpoint	00064-3100-45

Clofazimine *(000841)*

For complete prescribing information, refer to the CD-ROM included with the book.

Categories: Hansen's disease; Pregnancy Category C; FDA Approved 1986 Dec; WHO Formulary; Orphan Drugs
Drug Classes: Antimycobacterials
Brand Names: **Lamprene**
Foreign Brand Availability: Clofozine (India); Hansepran (India); Lampren (Ireland; Netherlands; Spain; Switzerland); Lapren (Korea)
Cost of Therapy: $12.35 (Hansen's Disease; Lamprene; 50 mg; 2 capsules/day; 30 day supply)

DESCRIPTION

Lamprene, clofazimine, is an antileprosy agent available as capsules for oral administration. Each capsule contains 50 or 100 mg of micronized clofazimine suspended in an oil-wax base. Clofazimine is a substituted iminophenazine bright-red dye. Its chemical name is 3-(*p*-chloroanilino)-10-(*p*-chlorophenyl)-2,10-dihydro-2-isopropyliminophenazine.

Clofazimine is a reddish-brown powder. It is readily soluble in benzene; soluble in chloroform; poorly soluble in acetone and in ethyl acetate; sparingly soluble in methanol and in ethanol; and virtually insoluble in water. Its molecular weight is 473.4.

Inactive Ingredients: Beeswax, butylated hydroxytoluene, citric acid, ethyl vanillin, gelatin, glycerin, iron oxide, lecithin, p-methoxy acetophenone, parabens, plant oils, propylene glycol.

INDICATIONS AND USAGE

Clofazimine is indicated in the treatment of lepromatous leprosy, including dapsone-resistant lepromatous leprosy and lepromatous leprosy complicated by erythema nodosum leprosum. Clofazimine has not been demonstrated to be effective in the treatment of other leprosy-associated inflammatory reactions.

Combination drug therapy has been recommended for initial treatment of multibacillary leprosy to prevent the development of drug resistance.

CONTRAINDICATIONS

There are no known contraindications.

WARNINGS

Severe abdominal symptoms have necessitated exploratory laparotomies in some patients receiving clofazimine. Rare reports have included splenic infarction, bowel obstruction, and gastrointestinal bleeding. There have also been reports of death following severe abdominal symptoms. Autopsies have revealed crystalline deposits of clofazimine in various tissues including the intestinal mucosa, liver, spleen, and mesenteric lymph nodes.

Clofazimine should be used with caution in patients who have gastrointestinal problems such as abdominal pain and diarrhea. Dosages of clofazimine of more than 100 mg daily should be given for as short a period as possible and only under close medical supervision. If a patient complains of colicky or burning pain in the abdomen, nausea, vomiting, or diarrhea, the dose should be reduced, and if necessary, the interval between doses should be increased, or the drug should be discontinued.

DOSAGE AND ADMINISTRATION

Clofazimine should be taken with meals.

Clofazimine should be used preferably in combination with one or more other antileprosy agents to prevent the emergence of drug resistance.

For the treatment of proven dapsone-resistant leprosy, clofazimine should be given at a dosage of 100 mg daily in combination with one or more other antileprosy drugs for 3 years, followed by monotherapy with 100 mg of clofazimine daily. Clinical improvement usually can be detected between the first and third months of treatment and is usually clearly evident by the sixth month.

For dapsone-sensitive multibacillary leprosy, a combination therapy with two other antileprosy drugs is recommended. The triple-drug regimen should be given for at least 2 years and continued, if possible, until negative skin smears are obtained. At this time, monotherapy with an appropriate antileprosy drug can be instituted.

The treatment of erythema nodosum leprosum reactions depends on the severity of symptoms. In general, the basic antileprosy treatment should be continued, and if nerve injury or skin ulceration is threatened, corticosteroids should be given. Where prolonged corticosteroid therapy becomes necessary, clofazimine administered at dosages of 100-200 mg daily for up to 3 months may be useful in eliminating or reducing corticosteroid requirements. Dosages above 200 mg daily are not recommended, and the dosage should be tapered to 100 mg daily as quickly as possible after the reactive episode is controlled. The patient must remain under medical surveillance.

For advice about combination drug regimens, contact the USPHS Gillis W. Long Hansen's Disease Center, Carville, LA (504-642-7771).

Do not store above 86°F. Protect from moisture.

Dispense in tight container.

PRODUCT LISTING - EQUIVALENTS NOT AVAILABLE

Capsule - Oral - 50 mg			
60's	$12.22	LAMPRENE, Physicians Total Care	54868-3417-00
100's	$20.58	LAMPRENE, Novartis Pharmaceuticals	00028-0108-01

Clofibrate *(000842)*

For related information, see the comparative table section in Appendix A.

Categories: Hyperlipidemia; Hyperlipoproteinemia; Hypertriglyceridemia; Pregnancy Category C; FDA Approved 1967 Feb
Drug Classes: Antihyperlipidemics; Fibric acid derivatives
Brand Names: Apoterin; **Atromid-S**; Cartagyl; Clofibral; Clofibrato; Clofipront; Coles
Foreign Brand Availability: Amadol (Japan); Apoterin A (Japan); Arterioflexin (Austria); Arterol (Indonesia); Artes (Finland); Atromid-S 500 (Dominican-Republic; El-Salvador; Guatemala); Atromidin (Belgium; Denmark; Sweden); Cholenal (Taiwan); Clofi ICN (Netherlands); Colebron (Taiwan); Lipilim (Hong-Kong); Miscleron (Bahamas; Barbados; Belize; Bermuda; Curacao; Guyana; Jamaica; Netherland-Antilles; Surinam; Trinidad); Neo Atromid (Spain); Regelan (Austria; Switzerland); Regelan N (Germany); Triglicer (Portugal); Yuclo (Japan)
Cost of Therapy: $138.49 (Hyperlipidemia; Atromid-S; 500 mg; 4 capsules/day; 30 day supply)
$24.00 (Hyperlipidemia; Generic Capsules; 500 mg; 4 capsules/day; 30 day supply)

DESCRIPTION

Clofibrate capsules, ethyl 2-(p-chlorophenoxy)-2-methyl-propionate, an antilipidemic agent.

Its molecular formula is $C_{12}H_{15}O_3Cl$, molecular weight 242.7, and boiling point 148-150°C at 25 mm Hg. It is a stable, colorless to pale-yellow liquid with a faint odor and characteristic taste, soluble in common solvents but not in water. Each clofibrate capsule contains 500 mg clofibrate for oral administration.

Atromid-S capsules contain the following inactive ingredients: D&C red no. 28, D&C red no. 30, D&C yellow no. 10, FD&C blue no. 1, FD&C red no. 3, FD&C yellow no. 6, gelatin.

CLINICAL PHARMACOLOGY

Clofibrate is an antilipidemic agent. It acts to lower elevated serum lipids by reducing the very low-density lipoprotein fraction (S_f 20-400) rich in triglycerides. Serum cholesterol may be decreased, particularly in those patients whose cholesterol elevation is due to the presence of IDL as a result of Type III hyperlipoproteinemia.

The mechanism of action has not been established definitively. Clofibrate may inhibit the hepatic release of lipoproteins (particularly VLDL), potentiate the action of lipoprotein lipase, and increase the fecal excretion of neutral sterols.

Between 95 and 99% of an oral dose of clofibrate is excreted in the urine as free and conjugated clofibric acid; thus, the absorption of clofibrate is virtually complete. The half-life of clofibric acid in normal volunteers averages 18-22 hours (range 14-35 hours) but can vary by up to 7 hours in the same subject at different times. Clofibric acid is highly protein-bound (95-97%). In subjects undergoing continuous clofibrate treatment, 1 g q12h, plasma concentrations of clofibric acid range from 120-125 µg/ml to an approximate peak of 200 µg/ml.

Several investigators have observed in their studies that clofibrate may produce a decrease in cholesterol linoleate but an increase in palmitoleate and oleate, the latter being considered atherogenic in experimental animals. The significance of this finding is unknown at this time.

Reduction of triglycerides in some patients treated with clofibrate or certain of its chemically and clinically similar analogs may be associated with an increase in LDL cholesterol. Increase in LDL cholesterol has been observed in patients whose cholesterol is initially normal.

Animal studies suggest that clofibrate interrupts cholesterol biosynthesis prior to mevalonate formation.

INDICATIONS AND USAGE

The initial treatment of choice for hyperlipidemia is dietary therapy specific for the type of hyperlipidemia.[1]

Excess body weight and alcoholic intake may be important factors in hypertriglyceridemia and should be addressed prior to any drug therapy. Physical exercise can be an important ancillary measure. Estrogen therapy, some beta-blockers, and thiazide diuretics may also be associated with increases in plasma triglycerides. Discontinuation of such products may obviate the need for specific antilipidemic therapy. Contributory diseases such as hypothyroidism or diabetes mellitus should be looked for and adequately treated. The use of drugs should be considered only when reasonable attempts have been made to obtain satisfactory results with non-drug methods. If the decision ultimately is to use drugs, the patient should be instructed that this does not reduce the importance of adhering to diet.

Because clofibrate is associated with certain serious adverse findings reported in two large clinical trials (see WARNINGS), agents other than clofibrate may be more suitable for a particular patient.

Clofibrate is indicated for Primary Dysbetalipoproteinemia (Type III hyperlipidemia) that does not respond adequately to diet.

Clofibrate may be considered for the treatment of adult patients with very high serum-triglyceride levels (Type IV and V hyperlipidemia) who present a risk of abdominal pain and pancreatitis and who do not respond adequately to a determined dietary effort to control them. Patients who present such risk typically have serum triglycerides over 2000 mg/dl and have elevations of VLDL-cholesterol as well as fasting chylomicrons (Type V hyperlipidemia). Subjects who consistently have total serum or plasma triglycerides below 1000 mg/dl are unlikely to present a risk of pancreatitis. Clofibrate therapy may be considered for those subjects with triglyceride elevations between 1000 and 2000 mg/dl who have a history of pancreatitis or of recurrent abdominal pain typical of pancreatitis. It is recognized that some Type IV patients with triglycerides under 1000 mg/dl may, through dietary or alcoholic indiscretion, convert to a Type V pattern with massive triglyceride elevations accompanying fasting chylomicronemia, but the influence of clofibrate therapy on the risk of pancreatitis in such situations has not been adequately studied.

Clofibrate is not useful for the hypertriglyceridemia of Type I hyperlipidemia, where elevations of chylomicrons and plasma triglycerides are accompanied by normal levels of very low-density lipoprotein (VLDL). Inspection of plasma refrigerated for 12-14 hours is helpful in distinguishing Types I, IV, and V hyperlipoproteinemia.[2]

Clofibrate has not been shown to be effective for prevention of coronary heart disease.

The biochemical response to clofibrate is variable, and it is not always possible to predict from the lipoprotein type or other factors which patients will obtain favorable results. LDL cholesterol, as well as triglycerides, should be rechecked during the first several months of therapy in order to detect rises in LDL cholesterol that often accompany fibric-acid-type drug-induced reductions in elevated triglycerides. It is essential that lipid levels be reassessed periodically and that the drug be discontinued in any patient in whom lipids do not show significant improvement.

NON-FDA APPROVED INDICATIONS

Although not FDA approved, clofibrate has been used as adjunct treatment of Fredrickson types IIb and for diabetic hyperlipoproteinemia.

CONTRAINDICATIONS

Clofibrate is contraindicated in pregnant women. While teratogenic studies have not demonstrated any effect attributable to clofibrate, it is known that serum of the rabbit fetus accumulates a higher concentration of clofibrate than that found in maternal serum, and it is possible that the fetus may not have developed the enzyme system required for the excretion of clofibrate.

It is contraindicated in patients with clinically significant hepatic or renal dysfunction. Rhabdomyolysis and severe hyperkalemia have been reported in association with preexisting renal insufficiency.

It is contraindicated in patients with primary biliary cirrhosis, since it may raise the already elevated cholesterol in these cases.

It is contraindicated in patients with a known hypersensitivity to clofibrate.

It is contraindicated in nursing women (see PRECAUTIONS).

WARNINGS

In a large prospective study involving 5000 patients in a clofibrate-treated group and 5000 in a placebo-treated group followed for an average of 5 years on drug or placebo and 1 year beyond (the WHO study), there was a statistically significant 36% higher mortality due to noncardiovascular causes in the clofibrate-treated group than in a comparable placebo group. Half of this difference was due to malignancy; other causes of death included postcholecystectomy complications and pancreatitis.[3] In another prospective study involving 1000 clofibrate and 3000 placebo treated patients followed for an average of 6 years on drug or placebo (the Coronary Drug Project study), the noncardiovascular mortality rate, including that of malignancy, was not significantly

Cont'd

different in the clofibrate and placebo treated groups.[4] This should not be interpreted to mean that clofibrate is not associated with an increased risk of noncardiovascular death, because the patients in the Coronary Drug Project were much older than those in the WHO study and they all had had a previous myocardial infarction, so that the deaths in the Coronary Drug Project were overwhelmingly due to cardiovascular causes, and it would have been very difficult to discern a clofibrate-associated risk of death due to noncardiovascular causes if it existed. Both studies demonstrated that clofibrate users have twice the risk of developing cholelithiasis and cholecystitis requiring surgery as do nonusers.

A potential benefit of clofibrate was, however, reported in the WHO study which involved patients with hypercholesterolemia and no history of myocardial infarction or angina pectoris. In this study, there was a statistically significant 25% decrease in subsequent nonfatal myocardial infarctions in the clofibrate treated group when compared with the placebo group. There was no difference in incidence of fatal myocardial infarction in the two groups. In the Coronary Drug Project study, which involved patients with or without hypercholesterolemia and/or hypertriglyceridemia and with a history of previous myocardial infarction, there was no significant difference in incidence of either nonfatal or fatal myocardial infarction between the clofibrate and placebo treated groups.[3] As a result of these and other studies, the following can be stated:

1. **Clofibrate, in general, causes a relatively modest reduction of serum cholesterol and somewhat greater reduction of serum triglycerides. In Type III hyperlipidemia, however, substantial reductions of both cholesterol and triglycerides can occur with clofibrate use.**
2. **No study to date has shown a convincing reduction in incidence of FATAL myocardial infarction.**
3. **A significantly increased incidence of cholelithiasis has been demonstrated consistently in clofibrate-treated groups, and an increase in morbidity from this complication and mortality from cholecystectomy must be anticipated during clofibrate treatment.**
4. **Several types of other undesirable events have been associated in a statistically significant way with clofibrate administration in the WHO and the Coronary Drug Project studies. There was an increase in incidence of noncardiovascular deaths reported in the WHO study. There was an increase in cardiac arrhythmias, intermittent claudication, and definite or suspected thromboembolic events, and angina reported in the Coronary Drug Project, which was not, however, reported in the WHO study.**
5. **Administration of clofibrate to mice and rats in long-term studies at 8 times the human dose, and to rats at 5 times the human dose, resulted in a higher incidence of benign and malignant liver tumors than in controls. Lower doses were not included in these studies. An increase in benign Leydig-cell tumors in male rats treated at 400 mg/kg (10 times the estimated human dose) was observed in a single study with clofibrate; similar increases were not observed in other studies conducted with clofibrate although they have been observed with other fibric-acid derivatives.**
6. **Administration of clofibrate to male monkeys at dosages of 2-6 times the human dose resulted in increases in mortality of 2- to 5-fold. As in the case of men in the WHO study, no single cause of death was identified. BECAUSE OF THE TUMORIGENICITY OF CLOFIBRATE IN RODENTS AND THE POSSIBLE INCREASED RISK OF MALIGNANCY ASSOCIATED WITH CLOFIBRATE IN THE HUMAN, AS WELL AS THE INCREASED RISK OF CHOLELITHIASIS, AND BECAUSE THERE IS NOT, TO DATE, SUBSTANTIAL EVIDENCE OF A BENEFICIAL EFFECT ON CARDIOVASCULAR MORTALITY FROM CLOFIBRATE, THIS DRUG SHOULD BE UTILIZED ONLY FOR THOSE PATIENTS DESCRIBED IN THE "INDICATIONS AND USAGE" SECTION, AND SHOULD BE DISCONTINUED IF SIGNIFICANT LIPID RESPONSE IS NOT OBTAINED.**

CONCOMITANT ANTICOAGULANTS

CAUTION SHOULD BE EXERCISED WHEN ANTICOAGULANTS ARE GIVEN IN CONJUNCTION WITH CLOFIBRATE. THE DOSAGE OF THE ANTICOAGULANT SHOULD BE REDUCED USUALLY BY ONE-HALF (DEPENDING ON THE INDIVIDUAL CASE) TO MAINTAIN THE PROTHROMBIN TIME AT THE DESIRED LEVEL TO PREVENT BLEEDING COMPLICATIONS. FREQUENT PROTHROMBIN DETERMINATIONS ARE ADVISABLE UNTIL IT HAS BEEN DEFINITELY DETERMINED THAT THE PROTHROMBIN LEVEL HAS BEEN STABILIZED.

SKELETAL MUSCLE

Myalgia, myositis, myopathy, and rhabdomyolysis with or without elevation of CPK have been associated with clofibrate therapy. Consideration should be given to withholding or discontinuing drug therapy in any patient with a risk factor predisposing to the development of renal failure secondary to rhabdomyolysis, including: severe acute infection; hypotension; major surgery; trauma; severe metabolic, endocrine, or electrolyte disorders; and uncontrolled seizures.

Clofibrate therapy should be discontinued if markedly elevated CPK levels occur or myositis is diagnosed.

AVOIDANCE OF PREGNANCY

Strict birth-control procedures must be exercised by women of child-bearing potential. In patients who plan to become pregnant, clofibrate should be withdrawn several months before conception. Because of the possibility of pregnancy occurring despite birth-control precautions in patients taking clofibrate, the possible benefits of the drug to the patient must be weighed against possible hazards to the fetus. (See PRECAUTIONS, Pregnancy, Teratogenic Effects, Pregnancy Category C.)

PRECAUTIONS

GENERAL

Before instituting therapy with clofibrate, attempts should be made to control serum lipids with appropriate dietary regimens, weight loss in obese patients, control of diabetes mellitus, etc.

Because of the long-term administration of a drug of this nature, adequate baseline studies should be performed to determine that the patient has significantly elevated serum-lipid levels. Frequent determinations of serum lipids should be obtained during the first few months of clofibrate administration, and periodic determinations made thereafter. The drug should be withdrawn after 3 months if response is inadequate. However, in the case of xanthoma tuberosum, the drug should be employed for longer periods (even up to 1 year) provided that there is a reduction in the size and/or number of the xanthomata.

Since cholelithiasis is a possible side effect of clofibrate therapy, appropriate diagnostic procedures should be performed if signs and symptoms related to disease of the biliary system should occur.

Clofibrate may produce "flu-like" symptoms (muscular aching, soreness, cramping) associated with increased creatine kinase levels indicative of drug-induced myopathy. The physician should differentiate this from actual viral and/or bacterial disease.

Use with caution in patients with peptic ulcer, since reactivation has been reported. Whether this is drug related is unknown.

Various cardiac arrhythmias have been reported with the use of clofibrate.

LABORATORY TESTS

Subsequent serum lipid determinations should be done to detect a paradoxical rise in serum cholesterol or triglyceride levels. Clofibrate will not alter the seasonal variations of serum cholesterol: peak elevations in midwinter and late summer and decreases in fall and spring. If the drug is discontinued, the patient should be continued on an appropriate hypolipidemic diet, and serum lipids should be monitored until stabilized, as a rise in these values to or above the original baseline may occur.

During clofibrate therapy, frequent serum-transaminase determinations and other liver-function tests should be performed, since the drug may produce abnormalities in these parameters. These effects are usually reversible when the drug is discontinued. Hepatic biopsies are usually within normal limits. If the hepatic-function tests steadily rise or show excessive abnormalities, the drug should be withdrawn. Therefore, use with caution in those patients with a past history of jaundice or hepatic disease.

Complete blood counts should be done periodically since anemia, and more frequently, leukopenia have been reported in patients who have been taking clofibrate.

CARCINOGENESIS, MUTAGENESIS, AND IMPAIRMENT OF FERTILITY

See WARNINGS section for information on carcinogenesis and mutagenesis.

Arrest of spermatogenesis has been seen in both dogs and monkeys at doses approximately 4-6 times the human therapeutic dose.

PREGNANCY, TERATOGENIC EFFECTS, PREGNANCY CATEGORY C

Animal reproduction studies have not been conducted with clofibrate. It is also not known whether clofibrate can cause fetal harm when administered to a pregnant woman or can affect reproductive capacity. However, animal reproduction studies with clofibrate plus androsterone showed increases in neonatal deaths and pup mortality during lactation.

NURSING MOTHERS

Clofibrate is contraindicated in lactating women, since an active metabolite (CPIB) has been measured in breast milk.

PEDIATRIC USE

Safety and efficacy in children have not been established.

DRUG INTERACTIONS

Caution should be exercised when anticoagulants are given in conjunction with clofibrate. Usually, the dosage of the anticoagulant should be reduced by one-half (depending on the individual case) to maintain the prothrombin time at the desired level to prevent bleeding complications. Frequent prothrombin determinations are advisable until it has been determined definitely that the prothrombin level has been stabilized.

Clofibrate may displace acidic drugs such as phenytoin or tolbutamide from their binding sites. Caution should be exercised when treating patients with either of these drugs or other highly protein-bound drugs and clofibrate. The hypoglycemic effect of tolbutamide has been reported to increase when clofibrate is given concurrently.

Fulminant rhabdomyolysis has been seen as early as 3 weeks after initiation of combined therapy with another fibrate and lovastatin but may be seen after several months. For these reasons, it is felt that, in most subjects who have had an unsatisfactory lipid response to either drug alone, the possible benefits of combined therapy with lovastatin and a fibrate do not outweigh the risks of severe myopathy, rhabdomyolysis, and acute renal failure. While it is not known whether this interaction occurs with fibrates other than gemfibrozil, myopathy and rhabdomyolysis have occasionally been associated with the use of fibrates alone, including clofibrate. Therefore, the combined use of lovastatin with fibrates should generally be avoided.

ADVERSE REACTIONS

The most common is nausea. Less frequently encountered gastrointestinal reactions are vomiting, loose stools, dyspepsia, flatulence, and abdominal distress. Reactions reported less often than gastrointestinal ones are headache, dizziness, and fatigue; muscle cramping, aching, and weakness; skin rash, urticaria, and pruritus; dry, brittle hair, and alopecia.

The following reported adverse reactions are listed alphabetically by systems:

Cardiovascular: Increased or decreased angina, cardiac arrhythmias, both swelling and phlebitis at site of xanthomas.

Dermatologic: Allergic reaction including urticaria, skin rash, pruritus, dry skin and dry, brittle hair, alopecia, toxic epidermal necrolysis.

Gastrointestinal: Gallstones, nausea, vomiting, diarrhea, gastrointestinal upset (bloating, flatulence, abdominal distress), hepatomegaly (not associated with hepatotoxicity), stomatitis and gastritis.

Genitourinary: Findings consistent with renal dysfunction as evidenced by dysuria, hematuria, proteinuria, decreased urine output. One patient's renal biopsy suggested "allergic reaction," impotence and decreased libido.

Hematologic: Leukopenia, potentiation of anticoagulant effect, anemia, eosinophilia, agranulocytosis.

Musculoskeletal: Myalgia (muscle cramping, aching, weakness), "flu-like" symptoms, myositis, myopathy, rhabdomyolysis in the setting of preexisting renal insufficiency, aarthralgia.

Neurologic: Fatigue, weakness, drowsiness; dizziness; headache.

Miscellaneous: Weight gain, polyphagia.

Laboratory Findings: Abnormal liver-function tests as evidenced by increased transaminase (SGOT and SGPT), BSP retention, and increased thymol turbidity; proteinuria; increased creatine phosphokinase; hyperkalemia in association with renal insufficiency and continuous ambulatory peritoneal dialysis treatment.

Reported adverse reactions whose direct relationship with the drug has not been established: peptic ulcer, gastrointestinal hemorrhage, rheumatoid arthritis, tremors, increased perspiration, systemic lupus erythematosus, blurred vision, gynecomastia, thrombocytopenic purpura.

DOSAGE AND ADMINISTRATION

Initial: The recommended dosage for adults is 2 g daily in divided doses. Some patients may respond to a lower dosage.

Maintenance: Same as for initial dosage.

HOW SUPPLIED

Store at room temperature (approximately 25° C).
Avoid freezing and excessive heat.

PRODUCT LISTING - RATED THERAPEUTICALLY EQUIVALENT

Capsule - Oral - 500 mg

Qty	Price	Product	NDC
100's	$20.00	GENERIC, Chase Laboratories Inc	54429-3148-01
100's	$23.31	GENERIC, Qualitest Products Inc	00603-2932-21
100's	$24.50	GENERIC, Aligen Independent Laboratories Inc	00405-4236-01
100's	$25.23	GENERIC, Moore, H.L. Drug Exchange Inc	00839-7228-06
100's	$25.75	GENERIC, Watson/Schein Pharmaceuticals Inc	00364-2136-01
100's	$25.81	GENERIC, Caremark Inc	00339-5651-12
100's	$26.08	GENERIC, Geneva Pharmaceuticals	00781-2600-01
100's	$26.40	GENERIC, Major Pharmaceuticals Inc	00904-2916-60
100's	$26.99	GENERIC, Ivax Corporation	00182-1269-01
100's	$28.43	GENERIC, Martec Pharmaceuticals Inc	52555-0111-01
100's	$115.41	ATROMID-S, Wyeth-Ayerst Laboratories	00046-0243-81

Clomipramine Hydrochloride *(000844)*

For related information, see the comparative table section in Appendix A.

Categories: Obsessive compulsive disorder; Pregnancy Category C; FDA Approved 1989 Dec; WHO Formulary
Drug Classes: Antidepressants, tricyclic
Brand Names: **Anafranil**
Foreign Brand Availability: Anafranil 25 (Indonesia); Anafranil Retard (Austria; Denmark; Finland; Netherlands; Sweden; Switzerland); Anafranil SR (Malaysia; Singapore); Clofranil (India); Clopram (Australia); Clopress (New-Zealand); Equinorm (Benin; Burkina-Faso; Ethiopia; Gambia; Ghana; Guinea; Ivory-Coast; Kenya; Liberia; Malawi; Mali; Mauritania; Mauritius; Morocco; Niger; Nigeria; Senegal; Seychelles; Sierra-Leone; Sudan; Tanzania; Tunia; Uganda; Zambia; Zimbabwe); Hydiphen (Germany); Placil (Australia); Zoiral (Hong-Kong)
Cost of Therapy: $79.72 (Obsessive-Compulsive Disorder; Anafranil; 50 mg; 2 capsules/day; 30 day supply)
$60.69 (Obsessive-Compulsive Disorder; Generic Capsules; 50 mg; 2 capsules/day; 30 day supply)

DESCRIPTION

Clomipramine hydrochloride is an antiobsessional drug that belongs to the class (dibenzazepine) of pharmacologic agents known as tricyclic antidepressants. Anafranil is available as capsules of 25, 50, and 75 mg for oral administration.

Clomipramine hydrochloride is 3-chloro-5-[3-(dimethylamino)propyl]-10,11-dihydro-5H-dibenz[b,f]azepine monohydrochloride.

Clomipramine hydrochloride is a white to off-white crystalline powder. It is freely soluble in water, in methanol, and in methylene chloride, and insoluble in ethyl ether and in hexane. Its molecular weight is 351.3.

Anafranil Inactive Ingredients: D&C red no. 33 (25 mg capsules only), D&C yellow no. 10, FD&C blue no. 1 (50 mg capsules only), FD&C yellow no. 6, gelatin, magnesium stearate, methylparaben, propylparaben, silicon dioxide, sodium lauryl sulfate, starch, and titanium dioxide.

CLINICAL PHARMACOLOGY

PHARMACODYNAMICS

Clomipramine (CMI) is presumed to influence obsessive and compulsive behaviors through its effects on serotonergic neuronal transmission. The actual neurochemical mechanism is unknown, but CMI's capacity to inhibit the reuptake of serotonin (5-HT) is thought to be important.

PHARMACOKINETICS

Absorption/Bioavailability

CMI from clomipramine HCl capsules is as bioavailable as CMI from a solution. The bioavailability of CMI from capsules is not significantly affected by food.

In a dose proportionality study involving multiple CMI doses, steady-state plasma concentrations (Css) and area-under-plasma-concentration-time curves (AUC) of CMI and CMI's major active metabolite, desmethylclomipramine (DMI), were not proportional to dose over the ranges evaluated, (*i.e.*, between 25-100 mg/day and between 25-150 mg/day), although Css and AUC are approximately linearly related to dose between 100-150 mg/day. The relationship between dose and CMI/DMI concentrations at higher daily doses has not been systematically assessed, but if there is significant dose dependency at doses above 150 mg/day, there is the potential for dramatically higher Css and AUC even for patients dosed within the recommended range. This may pose a potential risk to some patients (see WARNINGS and DRUG INTERACTIONS).

After a single 50 mg oral dose, maximum plasma concentrations of CMI occur within 2-6 hours (mean, 4.7 hours) and range from 56-154 ng/ml (mean, 92 ng/ml). After multiple daily doses of 150 mg of clomipramine HCl, steady-state maximum plasma concentrations range from 94-339 ng/ml (mean, 218 ng/ml) for CMI and from 134-532 ng/ml (mean, 274 ng/ml) for DMI. No pharmacokinetic information is available for doses ranging from 150-250 mg/day, the maximum recommended daily dose.

Distribution

CMI distributes into cerebrospinal fluid (CSF) and brain and into breast milk. DMI also distributes into CSF, with a mean CSF/plasma ratio of 2.6. The protein binding of CMI is approximately 97%, principally to albumin, and is independent of CMI concentration. The interaction between CMI and other highly protein-bound drugs has not been fully evaluated, but may be important (see DRUG INTERACTIONS).

Metabolism

CMI is extensively biotransformed to DMI and other metabolites and their glucuronide conjugates. DMI is pharmacologically active, but its effects on OCD behaviors are unknown. These metabolites are excreted in urine and feces, following biliary elimination. After a 25 mg radiolabeled dose of CMI in two subjects, 60% and 51%, respectively, of the dose were recovered in the urine and 32% and 24%, respectively, in feces. In the same study, the combined urinary recoveries of CMI and DMI were only about 0.8-1.3% of the dose administered. CMI does not induce drug-metabolizing enzymes, as measured by antipyrine half-life.

Elimination

Evidence that the Css and AUC for CMI and DMI may increase disproportionately with increasing oral doses suggests that the metabolism of CMI and DMI may be capacity limited. This fact must be considered in assessing the estimates of the pharmacokinetic parameters presented below, as these were obtained in individuals exposed to doses of 150 mg. If the pharmacokinetics of CMI and DMI are nonlinear at doses above 150 mg, their elimination half-lives may be considerably lengthened at doses near the upper end of the recommended dosing range (*i.e.,* 200-250 mg/day). Consequently, CMI and DMI may accumulate, and this accumulation may increase the incidence of any dose- or plasma-concentration-dependent adverse reactions, in particular seizures (see WARNINGS).

After a 150 mg dose, the half-life of CMI ranges from 19-37 hours (mean, 32 h) and that of DMI ranges from 54-77 hours (mean, 69 hours). Steady-state levels after multiple dosing are typically reached within 7-14 days for CMI. Plasma concentrations of the metabolite exceed the parent drug on multiple dosing. After multiple dosing with 150 mg/day, the accumulation factor for CMI is approximately 2.5 and for DMI is 4.6. Importantly, it may take 2 weeks or longer to achieve this extent of accumulation at constant dosing because of the relatively long elimination half-lives of CMI and DMI (see DOSAGE AND ADMINISTRATION). The effects of hepatic and renal impairment on the disposition of clomipramine HCl have not been determined.

Interactions

Coadministration of haloperidol with CMI increases plasma concentrations of CMI. Coadministration of CMI with phenobarbital increases plasma concentrations of phenobarbital (see DRUG INTERACTIONS). Younger subjects (18-40 years of age) tolerated CMI better and had significantly lower steady-state plasma concentrations, compared with subjects over 65 years of age. Children under 15 years of age had significantly lower plasma concentration/dose ratios, compared with adults. Plasma concentrations of CMI were significantly lower in smokers than in nonsmokers.

INDICATIONS AND USAGE

Clomipramine HCl is indicated for the treatment of obsessions and compulsions in patients with Obsessive-Compulsive Disorder (OCD). The obsessions or compulsions must cause marked distress, be time-consuming, or significantly interfere with social or occupational functioning, in order to meet the DSM-III-R (circa 1989) diagnosis of OCD.

Obsessions are recurrent, persistent ideas, thoughts, images, or impulses that are ego-dystonic. Compulsions are repetitive, purposeful, and intentional behaviors performed in response to an obsession or in a stereotyped fashion, and are recognized by the person as excessive or unreasonable.

The effectiveness of clomipramine HCl for the treatment of OCD was demonstrated in multicenter, placebo-controlled, parallel-group studies, including two 10 week studies in adults and one 8 week study in children and adolescents 10-17 years of age. Patients in all studies had moderate-to-severe OCD (DSM-III), with mean baseline ratings on the Yale-Brown Obsessive Compulsive Scale (YBOCS) ranging from 26-28 and a mean baseline rating of 10 on the NIMH Clinical Global Obsessive Compulsive Scale (NIMH-OC). Patients taking CMI experienced a mean reduction of approximately 10 on the YBOCS, representing an average improvement on this scale of 35% to 42% among adults and 37% among children and adolescents. CMI treated patients experienced a 3.5 unit decrement on the NIMH-OC. Patients on placebo showed no important clinical response on either scale. The maximum dose was 250 mg/day for most adults and 3 mg/kg/day (up to 200 mg) for all children and adolescents.

The effectiveness of clomipramine HCl for long-term use (*i.e.,* for more than 10 weeks) has not been systematically evaluated in placebo-controlled trials. The physician who elects to use clomipramine HCl for extended periods should periodically reevaluate the long-term usefulness of the drug for the individual patient (see DOSAGE AND ADMINISTRATION).

NON-FDA APPROVED INDICATIONS

Clomipramine has also been used in the treatment of depression and panic disorder, although these uses are not approved by the FDA. Similarly, there has been one case report of clomipramine being effective in treating Tourette's syndrome, another non-FDA approved use.

CONTRAINDICATIONS

Clomipramine HCl is contraindicated in patients with a history of hypersensitivity to clomipramine HCl or other tricyclic antidepressants.

Clomipramine HCl should not be given in combination, or within 14 days before or after treatment, with a monoamine oxidase (MAO) inhibitor. Hyperpyretic crisis, seizures, coma, and death have been reported in patients receiving such combinations.

Clomipramine HCl is contraindicated during the acute recovery period after a myocardial infarction.

WARNINGS

SEIZURES

During premarket evaluation, seizure was identified as the most significant risk of clomipramine HCl use.

The observed cumulative incidence of seizures among patients exposed to clomipramine HCl at doses up to 300 mg/day was 0.64% at 90 days, 1.12% at 180 days, and 1.45% at 365 days. The cumulative rates correct the crude rate of 0.7%, (25 of 3519 patients) for the variable duration of exposure in clinical trials.

Although dose appears to be a predictor of seizure, there is a confounding of dose and duration of exposure, making it difficult to assess independently the effect of either factor alone. The ability to predict the occurrence of seizures in subjects exposed to doses of CMI greater than 250 mg is limited, given that the plasma concentration of CMI may be dose-dependent and may vary among subjects given the same dose. Nevertheless, prescribers are advised to limit the daily dose to a maximum of 250 mg in adults and 3 mg/kg (or 200 mg) in children and adolescents (see DOSAGE AND ADMINISTRATION).

Caution should be used in administering clomipramine HCl to patients with a history of seizures or other predisposing factors (*e.g.,* brain damage of varying etiology, alcoholism, and concomitant use with other drugs that lower the seizure threshold).

Rare reports of fatalities in association with seizures have been reported by foreign postmarketing surveillance, but not in US clinical trials. In some of these cases, clomipramine HCl had been administered with other epileptogenic agents; in others, the patients involved had possibly predisposing medical conditions. Thus a causal association between clomipramine HCl treatment and these fatalities has not been established.

Physicians should discuss with patients the risk of taking clomipramine HCl while engaging in activities in which sudden loss of consciousness could result in serious injury to the patient or others (*e.g.,* the operation of complex machinery, driving, swimming, climbing).

PRECAUTIONS

GENERAL

Suicide

Since depression is a commonly associated feature of OCD, the risk of suicide must be considered. Prescriptions for clomipramine HCl should be written for the smallest quantity of capsules consistent with good patient management, in order to reduce the risk of overdose.

Cardiovascular Effects

Modest orthostatic decreases in blood pressure and modest tachycardia were each seen in approximately 20% of patients taking clomipramine HCl in clinical trials; but patients were frequently asymptomatic. Among approximately 1400 patients treated with CMI in the premarketing experience who had ECGs, 1.5% developed abnormalities during treatment, compared with 3.1% of patients receiving active control drugs and 0.7% of patients receiving placebo. The most common ECG changes were PVCs, ST-T wave changes, and intraventricular conduction abnormalities. These changes were rarely associated with significant clinical symptoms. Nevertheless, caution is necessary in treating patients with known cardiovascular disease, and gradual dose titration is recommended.

Psychosis, Confusion, and Other Neuropsychiatric Phenomena

Patients treated with clomipramine HCl have been reported to show a variety of neuropsychiatric signs and symptoms including delusions, hallucinations, psychotic episodes, confusion, and paranoia. Because of the uncontrolled nature of many of the studies, it is impossible to provide a precise estimate of the extent of risk imposed by treatment with clomipramine HCl. As with tricyclic antidepressants to which it is closely related, clomipramine HCl may precipitate an acute psychotic episode in patients with unrecognized schizophrenia.

Mania/Hypomania

During premarketing testing of clomipramine HCl in patients with affective disorder, hypomania or mania was precipitated in several patients. Activation of mania or hypomania has also been reported in a small proportion of patients with affective disorder treated with marketed tricyclic antidepressants, which are closely related to clomipramine HCl.

Hepatic Changes

During premarketing testing, clomipramine HCl was occasionally associated with elevations in SGOT and SGPT (pooled incidence of approximately 1% and 3% respectively) of potential clinical importance (*i.e.,* values greater than 3 times the upper limit of normal). In the vast majority of instances, these enzyme increases were not associated with other clinical findings suggestive of hepatic injury; none were jaundiced. Rare reports of more severe liver injury, some fatal, have been recorded in foreign postmarketing experience. Caution is indicated in treating patients with known liver disease, and periodic monitoring of hepatic enzyme levels is recommended in such patients.

Hematologic Changes

Although no instances of severe hematologic toxicity were seen in the premarketing experience with clomipramine HCl, there have been postmarketing reports of leukopenia, agranulocytosis, thrombocytopenia, anemia, and pancytopenia in association with clomipramine HCl use. As is the case with tricyclic antidepressants to which clomipramine HCl is closely related, leukocyte and differential blood counts should be obtained in patients who develop fever and sore throat during treatment with clomipramine HCl.

Central Nervous System

More than 30 cases of hyperthermia have been recorded by nondomestic postmarketing surveillance systems. Most cases occurred when clomipramine HCl was used in combination with other drugs. When clomipramine HCl and a neuroleptic were used concomitantly, the cases were sometimes considered to be examples of a neuroleptic malignant syndrome.

Sexual Dysfunction

The rate of sexual dysfunction in male patients with OCD who were treated with clomipramine HCl in the premarketing experience was markedly increased compared with placebo controls (*i.e.*, 42% experienced ejaculatory failure and 20% experienced impotence, compared with 2.0% and 2.6% respectively, in the placebo group). Approximately 85% of males with sexual dysfunction chose to continue treatment.

Weight Changes

In controlled studies of OCD, weight gain was reported in 18% of patients receiving clomipramine HCl, compared with 1% of patients receiving placebo. In these studies, 28% of patients receiving clomipramine HCl had a weight gain of at least 7% of their initial body weight, compared with 4% of patients receiving placebo. Several patients had weight gains in excess of 25% of their initial body weight. Conversely, 5% of patients receiving domipramine HCl and 1% receiving placebo had weight losses of at least 7% of their initial body weight.

Electroconvulsive Therapy

As with closely related tricyclic antidepressants, concurrent administration of clomipramine HCl with electroconvulsive therapy may increase the risks; such treatment should be limited to those patients for whom it is essential, since there is limited clinical experience.

Surgery

Prior to elective surgery with general anesthetics, therapy with clomipramine HCl should be discontinued for as long as is clinically feasible, and the anesthetist should be advised.

Use in Concomitant Illness

As with closely related tricyclic antidepressants, clomipramine HCl should be used with caution in the following:

Hyperthyroid patients or patients receiving thyroid medication, because of the possibility of cardiac toxicity.

Patients with increased intraocular pressure, a history of narrow-angle glaucoma, or urinary retention, because of the anticholinergic properties of the drug.

Patients with tumors of the adrenal medulla (*e.g.*, pheochromocytoma, neuroblastoma) in whom the drug may provoke hypertensive crises.

Patients with significantly impaired renal function.

Withdrawal Symptoms

A variety of withdrawal symptoms have been reported in association with abrupt discontinuation of clomipramine HCl, including dizziness, nausea, vomiting, headache, malaise, sleep disturbance, hyperthermia, and irritability. In addition, such patients may experience a worsening of psychiatric status. While the withdrawal effects of clomipramine HCl have not been systematically evaluated in controlled trials, they are well known with closely related tricyclic antidepressants, and it is recommended that the dosage be tapered gradually and the patient monitored carefully during discontinuation.

INFORMATION FOR THE PATIENT

Physicians are advised to discuss the following issues with patients for whom they prescribe clomipramine HCl:

The risk of seizure (see WARNINGS).

The relatively high incidence of sexual dysfunction among males (see General, Sexual Dysfunction).

Since clomipramine HCl may impair the mental and/or physical abilities required for the performance of complex tasks and since clomipramine HCl is associated with a risk of seizures, patients should be cautioned about the performance of complex and hazardous tasks (see WARNINGS).

Patients should be cautioned about using alcohol, barbiturates, or other CNS depressants concurrently, since clomipramine HCl may exaggerate their response to these drugs.

Patients should notify their physician if they become pregnant or intend to become pregnant during therapy.

Patients should notify their physician if they are breast-feeding.

CARCINOGENESIS, MUTAGENESIS, AND IMPAIRMENT OF FERTILITY

In a 2 year bioassay, no clear evidence of carcinogenicity was found in rats given doses 20 times the maximum daily human dose. Three (3) out of 235 treated rats had a rare tumor (hemangioendothelioma); it is unknown if these neoplasms are compound related.

In reproduction studies, no effects on fertility were found in rats given doses approximately 5 times the maximum daily human dose.

PREGNANCY CATEGORY C

No teratogenic effects were observed in studies performed in rats and mice at doses up to 20 times the maximum daily human dose. Slight nonspecific fetotoxic effects were seen in the offspring of pregnant mice given doses 10 times the maximum daily human dose. Slight nonspecific embryotoxicity was observed in rats given doses 5-10 times the maximum daily human dose.

There are no adequate or well-controlled studies in pregnant women. Withdrawal symptoms, including jitteriness, tremor, and seizures, have been reported in neonates whose mothers had taken clomipramine HCl until delivery. Clomipramine HCl should be used during pregnancy only if the potential benefit justifies the potential risk to the fetus.

NURSING MOTHERS

Clomipramine HCl has been found in human milk. Because of the potential for adverse reactions, a decision should be made whether to discontinue nursing or to discontinue the drug, taking into account the importance of the drug to the mother.

PEDIATRIC USE

In a controlled clinical trial in children and adolescents (10-17 years of age), 46 outpatients received clomipramine HCl for up to 8 weeks. In addition, 150 adolescent patients have received clomipramine HCl in open-label protocols for periods of several months to several years. Of the 196 adolescents studies, 50 were 13 years of age or less and 146 were 14-17 years of age. While the adverse reaction profile in this age group (see ADVERSE REACTIONS) is similar to that in adults, it is unknown what, if any, effects long-term treatment with clomipramine HCl may have on the growth and development of children.

The safety and effectiveness in children below the age of 10 have not been established. Therefore, specific recommendations cannot be made for the use of clomipramine HCl in children under the age of 10.

C

USE IN ELDERLY

Clomipramine HCl has not been systematically studied in older patients; but 152 patients at least 60 years of age participating in US clinical trials received clomipramine HCl for periods of several months to several years. No unusual age-related adverse events have been identified in this elderly population, but these data are insufficient to rule out possible age-related differences, particularly in elderly patients who have concomitant systemic illnesses or who are receiving other drugs concomitantly.

DRUG INTERACTIONS

The risks of using clomipramine HCl in combination with other drugs have not been systematically evaluated. Given the primary CNS effects of clomipramine HCl, caution is advised in using it concomitantly with other CNS-active drugs (see Information for the Patient). Clomipramine HCl should not be used with MAO inhibitors (see CONTRAINDICATIONS.)

Close supervision and careful adjustment of dosage are required when clomipramine HCl is administered with anticholinergic or sympathomimetic drugs.

Several tricyclic antidepressants have been reported to block the pharmacologic effects of guanethidine, clonidine, or similar agents, and such an effect may be anticipated with CMI because of its structural similarity to other tricyclic antidepressants.

The plasma concentration of CMI has been reported to be increased by the concomitant administration of haloperidol; plasma levels of several closely related tricyclic antidepressants have been reported to be increased by the concomitant administration of methylphenidate or hepatic enzyme inhibitors (*e.g.*, cimetidine, fluoxetine) and decreased by the concomitant administration of hepatic enzyme inducers (*e.g.*, barbiturates, phenytoin), and such an effect may be anticipated with CMI as well. Administration of CMI has been reported to increase the plasma levels of phenobarbital, if given concomitantly (see CLINICAL PHARMACOLOGY, Interactions).

DRUGS METABOLIZED BY P450 2D6

The biochemical activity of the drug metabolizing isozyme cytochrome P450 2D6 (debrisoquin hydroxylase) is reduced in a subset of the Caucasian population (about 7-10% of Caucasians are so-called "poor metabolizers"); reliable estimates of the prevalence of reduced P450 2D6 isozyme activity among Asian, African and other populations are not yet available. Poor metabolizers have higher than expected plasma concentrations of tricyclic antidepressants (TCAs) when given usual doses. Depending on the fraction of drug metabolized by P450 2D6, the increase in plasma concentration may be small, or quite large (8-fold increase in plasma AUC of the TCA). In addition, certain drugs inhibit the activity of this isozyme and make normal metabolizers resemble poor metabolizers. An individual who is stable on a given dose of TCA may become abruptly toxic when given one of these inhibiting drugs as concomitant therapy. The drugs that inhibit cytochrome P450 2D6 include some that are not metabolized by the enzyme (quinidine; cimetidine) and many that are substrates for P450 2D6 (many other antidepressants, phenothiazines, and the Type 1C antiarrhythmics propafenone and flecainide). While all the selective serotonin reuptake inhibitors (SSRIs), (*e.g.*, fluoxetine, sertraline, fluvoxamine, and paroxetine) inhibit P450 2D6, they may vary in the extent of inhibition. Fluvoxamine has also been shown to inhibit P450 2D6, an isoform also involved in TCA metabolism. The extent to which SSRI-TCA interactions may pose clinical problems will depend on the degree of inhibition and the pharmacokinetics of the SSRI involved. Nevertheless, caution is indicated in the co-administration of TCAs with any of the SSRIs and also in switching from one class to the other. Of particular importance, sufficient time must elapse before initiating TCA treatment in a patient being withdrawn from fluoxetine, given the long half-life of the parent and active metabolite (at least 5 weeks may be necessary). Concomitant use of agents in the tricyclic antidepressant class (which includes clomipramine HCl) with drugs that can inhibit cytochrome P450 2D6 may require lower doses than usually prescribed for either the tricyclic antidepressant or the other drug. Furthermore, whenever one of these drugs is withdrawn from co-therapy, an increased dose of tricyclic antidepressant agent may be required. It is desirable to monitor TCA plasma levels whenever an agent of the tricyclic antidepressant class (including clomipramine HCl) is going to be co-administered with another drug known to be an inhibitor of P450 2D6 (and/or P450 1A2).

Because clomipramine HCl is highly bound to serum protein, the administration of clomipramine HCl to patients taking other drugs that are highly bound to protein (*e.g.*, warfarin, digoxin) may cause an increase in plasma concentrations of these drugs, potentially resulting in adverse effects. Conversely, adverse effects may result from displacement of protein-bound clomipramine HCl by other highly bound drugs (see CLINICAL PHARMACOLOGY, Pharmacokinetics, Distribution

ADVERSE REACTIONS

COMMONLY OBSERVED

The most commonly observed adverse events associated with the use of clomipramine HCl and not seen at an equivalent incidence among placebo-treated patients were gastrointestinal complaints, including dry mouth, constipation, nausea, dyspepsia, and anorexia; nervous system complaints, including somnolence, tremor, dizziness, nervousness, and myoclonus; genitourinary complaints, including changed libido, ejaculatory failure, impotence, and micturition disorder; and other miscellaneous complaints, including fatigue, sweating, increased appetite, weight gain, and visual changes.

LEADING TO DISCONTINUATION OF TREATMENT

Approximately 20% of 3616 patients who received clomipramine HCl in US premarketing clinical trials discontinued treatment because of an adverse event. Approximately one-half of the patients who discontinued (9% of the total) had multiple complaints, none of which could be classified as primary. Where a primary reason for discontinuation could be identified, most patients discontinued because of nervous system complaints (5.4%), primarily somnolence. The second-most-frequent reason for discontinuation was digestive system complaints (1.3%), primarily vomiting and nausea.

INCIDENCE IN CONTROLLED CLINICAL TRIALS

TABLE 1A and TABLE 1B enumerate adverse events that occurred at an incidence of 1% or greater among patients with OCD who received clomipramine HCl in adult or pediatric placebo-controlled clinical trials. The frequencies were obtained from pooled data of clinical trials involving either adults receiving clomipramine HCl (n=322) or placebo (n=319) or children treated with clomipramine HCl (n=46) or placebo (n=44). The prescriber should be aware that these figures cannot be used to predict the incidence of side effects in the course of usual medical practice, in which patient characteristics and other factors differ from those that prevailed in the clinical trials. Similarly, the cited frequencies cannot be compared with figures obtained from other clinical investigations involving different treatment, uses, and investigators. The cited figures, however, provide the physician with a basis for estimating the relative contribution of drug and nondrug factors to the incidence of side effects in the populations studied.

TABLE 1A *Incidence of Treatment-Emergent Adverse Experience in Placebo-Controlled Clinical Trials*

Body System	Adults		Children and Adolescents	
	CMI	Placebo	CMI	Placebo
Adverse Event*	(n=322)	(n=319)	(n=46)	(n=44)
Nervous System				
Somnolence	54%	16%	46%	11%
Tremor	54%	2%	33%	2%
Dizziness	54%	14%	41%	14%
Headache	52%	41%	28%	34%
Insomnia	25%	15%	11%	7%
Libido change	21%	3%	—	—
Nervousness	18%	2%	4%	2%
Myoclonus	13%	—	2%	—
Increased appetite	11%	2%	—	2%
Paresthesia	9%	3%	2%	2%
Memory impairment	9%	1%	7%	2%
Anxiety	9%	4%	2%	—
Twitching	7%	1%	4%	5%
Impaired concentration	5%	2%	—	—
Depression	5%	1%	—	—
Hypertonia	4%	1%	2%	—
Sleep disorder	4%	—	9%	5%
Psychosomatic disorder	3%	—	—	—
Yawning	3%	—	—	—
Confusion	3%	—	2%	—
Speech disorder	3%	—	—	—
Abnormal dreaming	3%	—	—	2%
Agitation	3%	—	—	—
Migraine	3%	—	—	—
Depersonalization	2%	—	2%	—
Irritability	2%	2%	2%	—
Emotional lability	2%	—	—	2%
Panic reaction	1%	—	2%	—
Aggressive reaction	—	—	2%	—
Paresis	—	—	2%	—
Skin and Appendages				
Increased sweating	29%	3%	9%	—
Rash	8%	1%	4%	2%
Pruritus	6%	—	2%	2%
Dermatitis	2%	—	—	2%
Acne	2%	2%	—	5%
Dry skin	2%	—	—	5%
Urticaria	1%	—	—	—
Abnormal skin odor	—	—	2%	—
Digestive System				
Dry mouth	84%	17%	63%	16%
Constipation	47%	11%	22%	9%
Nausea	33%	14%	9%	11%
Dyspepsia	22%	10%	13%	2%
Diarrhea	13%	9%	7%	5%
Anorexia	12%	—	22%	2%
Abdominal pain	11%	9%	13%	16%
Vomiting	7%	2%	7%	—
Flatulence	6%	3%	—	2%
Tooth disorder	5%	—	—	—
Gastrointestinal disorder	2%	—	—	2%
Dysphagia	2%	—	—	—
Esophagitis	1%	—	—	—
Eructation	—	—	2%	2%
Ulcertative stomatitis	—	—	2%	—
Body as a Whole				
Fatigue	39%	18%	35%	9%
Weight increase	18%	1%	2%	—
Flushing	8%	—	7%	—
Hot flushes	5%	—	2%	—
Chest pain	4%	4%	7%	—
Fever	4%	—	2%	7%
Allergy	3%	3%	7%	5%
Pain	3%	2%	4%	2%
Local edema	2%	4%	—	—
Chills	2%	1%	—	—
Weight decrease	—	—	7%	—
Otitis media	—	—	4%	5%
Asthenia	—	—	2%	—
Halitosis	—	—	2%	—

* Events reported by at least 1% of clomipramine HCl patients are included.

OTHER EVENTS OBSERVED DURING THE PREMARKETING EVALUATION OF CLOMIPRAMINE HCl

During clinical testing in the US, multiple doses of clomipramine HCl were administered to approximately 3600 subjects. Untoward events associated with this exposure were recorded by clinical investigators using terminology of their own choosing. Consequently, it is not possible to provide a meaningful estimate of the proportion of individuals experiencing adverse events without first grouping similar types of untoward events into a smaller number of standardized event categories.

In the tabulations that follow, a modified World Health Organization dictionary of terminology has been used to classify reported adverse events. The frequencies presented, therefore, represent the proportion of the 3525 individuals exposed to clomipramine HCl who experienced an event of the type cited on at least one occasion while receiving clomipramine HCl. All events are included except those already listed in the previous table, those reported in terms so general as to be uninformative, and those in which an association with the drug was remote. It is important to emphasize that although the events reported occurred during treatment with clomipramine HCl, they were not necessarily caused by it.

Events are further categorized by body system and listed in order of decreasing frequency according to the following definitions: *Frequent* adverse events are those occurring on one or more occasions in at least 1/100 patients; *infrequent* adverse events are those occurring in 1/100 to 1/1000 patients; *rare* events are those occurring in less than 1/1000 patients.

Body as a Whole: *Infrequent:* General edema, increased susceptibility to infection, malaise. *Rare:* Dependent edema, withdrawal syndrome.

Cardiovascular System: *Infrequent:* Abnormal ECG, arrhythmia, bradycardia, cardiac arrest, extrasystoles, pallor. *Rare:* Aneurysm, atrial flutter, bundle branch block, cardiac failure, cerebral hemorrhage, heart block, myocardial infarction, myocardial ischemia, peripheral ischemia, thrombophlebitis, vasospasm, ventricular tachycardia.

Digestive System: *Infrequent:* Abnormal hepatic function, blood in stool, colitis, duodenitis, gastric ulcer, gastritis, gastroesophageal reflux, gingivitis, glossitis, hemorrhoids, hepatitis, increased saliva, irritable bowel syndrome, peptic ulcer, rectal hemorrhage, tongue ulceration, tooth caries. *Rare:* Cheilitis, chronic enteritis, discolored feces, gastric dilatation, gingival bleeding, hiccup, intestinal obstruction, oral/pharyngeal edema, paralytic ileus, salivary gland enlargement.

Endocrine System: *Infrequent:* Hypothyroidism. *Rare:* Goiter, gynecomastia, hyperthyroidism.

Hemic and Lymphatic System: *Infrequent:* Lymphadenopathy. *Rare:* Leukemoid reaction, lymphoma-like disorder, marrow depression.

Metabolic and Nutritional Disorder: *Infrequent:* Dehydration, diabetes mellitus, gout, hypercholesterolemia, hyperglycemia, hyperuricemia, hypokalemia. *Rare:* Fat intolerance, glycosuria.

Musculoskeletal System: *Infrequent:* Arthrosis. *Rare:* Dystonia, exostosis, lupus erythematosus rash, bruising, myopathy, myositis, polyarteritis nodosa, torticollis.

Nervous System: *Frequent:* Abnormal thinking, vertigo. *Infrequent:* Abnormal coordination, abnormal EEG, abnormal gait, apathy, ataxia, coma, convulsions, delirium, delusion, dyskinesia, dysphonia, encephalopathy, euphoria, extrapyramidal disorder, hallucination, hostility, hyperkinesia, hypnagogic hallucinations, hypokinesia, leg cramps, manic reaction, neuralgia, paranoia, phobic disorder, psychosis, sensory disturbance, somnambulism, stimulation, suicidal ideation, suicide attempt, teeth-grinding. *Rare:* Anticholinergic syndrome, aphasia, apraxia, catalepsy, cholinergic syndrome, choreoathetosis, generalized spasm, hemiparesis, hyperesthesia, hyperreflexia, hypoesthesia, illusion, impaired impulse control, indecisiveness, mutism, neuropathy, nystagmus, oculogyric crisis, oculomotor nerve paralysis, schizophrenic reaction, stupor, suicide.

Respiratory System: *Infrequent:* Bronchitis, hyperventilation, increased sputum, pneumonia. *Rare:* Cyanosis, hemoptysis, hypoventilation, laryngismus.

Skin and Appendages: *Infrequent:* Alopecia, cellulitis, cyst, eczema, erythematous rash, genital pruritus, maculopapular rash, photosensitivity reaction, psoriasis, pustular rash, skin discoloration. *Rare:* Chloasma, folliculitis, hypertrichosis, piloerection, seborrhea, skin hypertrophy, skin ulceration.

Special Senses: *Infrequent:* Abnormal accommodation, deafness, diplopia, earache, eye pain, foreign body sensation, hyperacusis, parosmia, photophobia, scleritis, taste loss. *Rare:* Blepharitis, chromatopsia, conjunctival hemorrhage, exophthalmos, glaucoma, keratitis, labyrinth disorder, night blindness, retinal disorder, strabismus, visual field defect.

Urogenital System: *Infrequent:* Endometriosis, epididymitis, hematuria, nocturia, oliguria, ovarian cyst, perineal pain, polyuria, prostatic disorder, renal calculus, renal pain, urethral disorder, urinary incontinence, uterine hemorrhage, vaginal hemorrhage. *Rare:* Albuminuria, anorgasmy, breast engorgement, breast fibroadenosis, cervical dysplasia, endometrial hyperplasia, premature ejaculation, pyelonephritis, pyuria, renal cyst, uterine inflammation, vulvar disorder.

DOSAGE AND ADMINISTRATION

The treatment regimens described below are based on those used in controlled clinical trials of clomipramine HCl in 520 adults, and 91 children and adolescents with OCD. During initial titration, clomipramine HCl should be given in divided doses with meals to reduce gastrointestinal side effects. The goal of this initial titration phase is to minimize side effects by permitting tolerance to side effects to develop or allowing the patient time to adapt if tolerance does not develop.

Because both CMI and its active metabolite, DMI, have long elimination half-lives, the prescriber should take into consideration the fact that steady-state plasma levels may not be achieved until 2-3 weeks after dosage change (see CLINICAL PHARMACOLOGY).

TABLE 1B *Incidence of Treatment-Emergent Adverse Experience in Placebo-Controlled Clinical Trials*

Body System	Adults		Children and Adolescents	
	CMI	Placebo	CMI	Placebo
Adverse Event*	(n=322)	(n=319)	(n=46)	(n=44)
Cardiovascular System				
Postural hypotension	6%	—	4%	—
Palpitation	4%	2%	4%	—
Tachycardia	4%	—	2%	—
Syncope	—	—	2%	—
Respiratory System				
Pharyngitis	14%	9%	—	5%
Rhinitis	12%	10%	7%	9%
Sinusitis	6%	4%	2%	5%
Coughing	6%	6%	4%	5%
Bronchospasm	2%	—	7%	2%
Epistaxis	2%	—	—	2%
Dyspnea	—	—	2%	—
Laryngitis	—	1%	2%	—
Urogenital System				
Male and Female Patients Combined				
Micturition disorder	14%	2%	4%	2%
Urinary tract infection	6%	1%	—	—
Micturition frequency	5%	3%	—	—
Urinary retention	2%	—	7%	—
Dysuria	2%	2%	—	—
Cystitis	2%	—	—	—
Female Patients Only	(n=182)	(n=167)	(n=10)	(n=21)
Dysmenorrhea	12%	14%	10%	10%
Lactation (nonpuerperal)	4%	—	—	—
Menstrual disorder	4%	2%	—	—
Vaginitis	2%	—	—	—
Leukorrhea	2%	—	—	—
Breast enlargement	2%	—	—	—
Breast pain	1%	—	—	—
Amenorrhea	1%	—	—	—
Male Patients Only	(n=140)	(n=152)	(n=36)	(n=23)
Ejaculation failure	42%	2%	6%	—
Impotence	20%	3%	—	—
Special Senses				
Abnormal vision	18%	4%	7%	2%
Taste perversion	8%	—	4%	—
Tinnitus	6%	—	4%	—
Abnormal lacrimation	3%	2%	—	—
Mydriasis	2%	—	—	—
Conjunctivitis	1%	—	—	—
Anisocoria	—	—	2%	—
Blepharospasm	—	—	2%	—
Ocular allergy	—	—	2%	—
Vestibular disorder	—	—	2%	2%
Musculoskeletal				
Myalgia	13%	9%	—	—
Back pain	6%	6%	—	—
Arthralgia	3%	5%	—	—
Muscle weakness	1%	—	2%	—
Hemic and Lymphatic				
Purpura	3%	—	—	—
Anemia	—	—	2%	2%
Metabolic and Nutritional				
Thirst	2%	2%	—	2%

* Events reported by at least 1% of clomipramine HCl patients are included

Therefore, after initial titration, it may be appropriate to wait 2-3 weeks between further dosage adjustments.

INITIAL TREATMENT/DOSE ADJUSTMENT

Adults: Treatment with clomipramine HCl should be initiated at a dosage of 25 mg daily and gradually increased, as tolerated, to approximately 100 mg during the first 2 weeks. During initial titration, clomipramine HCl should be given in divided doses with meals to reduce gastrointestinal side effects. Thereafter, the dosage may be increased gradually over the next several weeks, up to a maximum of 250 mg daily. After titration, the total daily dose may be given once daily at bedtime to minimize daytime sedation.

Children and Adolescents: As with adults, the starting dose is 25 mg daily and should be gradually increased (also given in divided doses with meals to reduce gastrointestinal side effects) during the first 2 weeks, as tolerated, up to a daily maximum of 3 mg/kg or 100 mg, whichever is smaller. Thereafter, the dosage may be increased gradually over the next several weeks up to a daily maximum of 3 mg/kg or 200 mg, whichever is smaller (see PRECAUTIONS, Pediatric Use). As with adults, after titration, the total daily dose may be given once daily at bedtime to minimize daytime sedation.

MAINTENANCE/CONTINUATION TREATMENT

While there are no systematic studies that answer the question of how long to continue clomipramine HCl, OCD is a chronic condition and it is reasonable to consider continuation for a responding patient. Although the efficacy of clomipramine HCl after 10 weeks has not been documented in controlled trials, patients have been continued in therapy under double-blind conditions for up to 1 year without loss of benefit. However, dosage adjustments should be made to maintain the patient on the lowest effective dosage, and patients should be periodically reassessed to determine the need for treatment. During maintenance, the total daily dose may be given once daily at bedtime.

ANIMAL PHARMACOLOGY

Testicular and lung changes commonly associated with tricyclic compounds have been observed with clomipramine HCl. In 1 and 2 year studies in rats, changes in the testes (atrophy, aspermatogenesis, and calcification) and drug-induced phospholipidosis in the lungs were observed at doses 4 times the maximum daily human dose. Testicular atrophy was also observed in a 1 year oral toxicity study in dogs at 10 times the maximum daily human dose.

HOW SUPPLIED

Ananfranil capsules are available in:

25 mg: Ivory/melon yellow (imprinted "Anafranil 25 mg").

50 mg: Ivory/aqua blue (imprinted "Anafranil 50 mg").

75 mg: Ivory/yellow (imprinted "Anafranil 75 mg").

Storage: Do not store above 30°C (86°F). Protect from moisture.

Dispense in tight container.

PRODUCT LISTING - RATED THERAPEUTICALLY EQUIVALENT

Capsule - Oral - 25 mg

100's	$33.22	FEDERAL UPPER LIMIT, H.C.F.A. F F P	99999-0844-01
100's	$75.00	GENERIC, Novopharm Usa Inc	55953-0031-40
100's	$75.05	GENERIC, Teva Pharmaceuticals Usa	00093-0956-01
100's	$78.90	GENERIC, Watson Laboratories Inc	52544-0594-01
100's	$78.95	GENERIC, Geneva Pharmaceuticals	00781-2027-01
100's	$82.85	GENERIC, Mylan Pharmaceuticals Inc	00378-3025-01
100's	$83.66	GENERIC, Taro Pharmaceuticals U.S.A. Inc	51672-4011-01

Capsule - Oral - 50 mg

30's	$50.37	ANAFRANIL, Physicians Total Care	54868-1447-00
100's	$51.38	FEDERAL UPPER LIMIT, H.C.F.A. F F P	99999-0844-02
100's	$101.15	GENERIC, Teva Pharmaceuticals Usa	00093-0958-01
100's	$106.30	GENERIC, Watson Laboratories Inc	52544-0595-01
100's	$106.45	GENERIC, Geneva Pharmaceuticals	00781-2037-01
100's	$111.62	GENERIC, Mylan Pharmaceuticals Inc	00378-3050-01
100's	$112.72	GENERIC, Taro Pharmaceuticals U.S.A. Inc	51672-4012-01
100's	$165.14	ANAFRANIL, Novartis Pharmaceuticals	00078-0317-06
100's	$401.85	ANAFRANIL, Novartis Pharmaceuticals	00078-0317-05

Capsule - Oral - 75 mg

100's	$57.72	FEDERAL UPPER LIMIT, H.C.F.A. F F P	99999-0844-03
100's	$133.15	GENERIC, Teva Pharmaceuticals Usa	00093-0960-01
100's	$133.15	GENERIC, Novopharm Usa Inc	55953-0033-40
100's	$139.90	GENERIC, Watson Laboratories Inc	52544-0596-01
100's	$140.14	GENERIC, Geneva Pharmaceuticals	00781-2047-01
100's	$146.90	GENERIC, Mylan Pharmaceuticals Inc	00378-3075-01
100's	$148.35	GENERIC, Taro Pharmaceuticals U.S.A. Inc	51672-4013-01

PRODUCT LISTING - EQUIVALENTS NOT AVAILABLE

Capsule - Oral - 25 mg

100's	$118.13	ANAFRANIL, Novartis Pharmaceuticals	00078-0316-05
100's	$123.10	ANAFRANIL, Novartis Pharmaceuticals	00078-0316-06
100's	$191.69	ANAFRANIL, Mallinckrodt Medical Inc	00406-9906-62
100's	$299.51	ANAFRANIL, Mallinckrodt Medical Inc	00406-9906-01

Capsule - Oral - 50 mg

100's	$401.85	ANAFRANIL, Mallinckrodt Medical Inc	00406-9907-01

Capsule - Oral - 75 mg

100's	$408.00	ANAFRANIL, Novartis Pharmaceuticals	00078-0318-05

Clonazepam *(000845)*

Categories: Lennox-Gastaut syndrome; Panic disorder; Seizures, absence; Seizures, akinetic; Seizures, myoclonic; DEA Class CIV; FDA Approved 1975 Jun; Pregnancy Category D; WHO Formulary

Drug Classes: Anxiolytics; Benzodiazepines

Brand Names: **Klonopin**

Foreign Brand Availability: Amotril (Bahrain; Cyprus; Egypt; Iran; Iraq; Jordan; Kuwait; Lebanon; Libya; Oman; Qatar; Republic-of-Yemen; Saudi-Arabia; Syria; United-Arab-Emirates); Clonex (Israel); Coquan (Colombia); Iktorivil (Sweden); Kenoket (Mexico); Kriadex (Mexico); Landsen (Japan); Lonazep (India); Paxam (Australia); Rivotril (Argentina; Australia; Austria; Bahamas; Bahrain; Barbados; Belgium; Belize; Bermuda; Bolivia; Bulgaria; Canada; CIS; Colombia; Costa-Rica; Curacao; Cyprus; Czech-Republic; Denmark; Dominican-Republic; Ecuador; Egypt; El-Salvador; England; France; Germany; Ghana; Greece; Guatemala; Guyana; Honduras; Hong-Kong; Hungary; Indonesia; Iran; Iraq; Ireland; Israel; Italy; Jamaica; Japan; Jordan; Kenya; Korea; Kuwait; Lebanon; Libya; Malaysia; Mexico; Netherland-Antilles; Netherlands; New-Zealand; Nicaragua; Norway; Oman; Panama; Philippines; Portugal; Puerto-Rico; Qatar; Republic-of-Yemen; Saudi-Arabia; South-Africa; Spain; Surinam; Switzerland; Syria; Taiwan; Tanzania; Thailand; Trinidad; Uganda; United-Arab-Emirates; Zambia; Zimbabwe)

Cost of Therapy: $86.63 (Seizure Disorder; Klonopin; 0.5 mg; 3 tablets/day; 30 day supply)
$63.62 (Seizure Disorder; Generic tablets; 0.5 mg; 3 tablets/day; 30 day supply)

DESCRIPTION

Klonopin, a benzodiazepine, is available as scored tablets with a K-shaped perforation containing 0.5 mg of clonazepam, and unscored tablets with a K-shaped perforation containing 1 or 2 mg of clonazepam. Each tablet also contains lactose, magnesium stearate, microcrystalline cellulose and corn starch, with the following colorants: *0.5 mg:* FD&C yellow no. 6 lake; *1 mg:* FD&C blue no. 1 lake and FD&C blue no. 2 lake.

Chemically, clonazepam is 5-(2-chlorophenyl)-1,3-dihydro-7-nitro-2*H*-1,4-benzodiazepin-2-one. It is a light yellow crystalline powder. It has a molecular weight of 315.72.

CLINICAL PHARMACOLOGY

PHARMACODYNAMICS

The precise mechanism by which clonazepam exerts its antiseizure and antipanic effects is unknown, although it is believed to be related to its ability to enhance the activity of gamma aminobutyric acid (GABA), the major inhibitory neurotransmitter in the central nervous system. Convulsions produced in rodents by pentylenetetrazol or, to a lesser extent, electrical stimulation are antagonized, as are convulsions produced by photic stimulation in susceptible baboons. A taming effect in aggressive primates, muscle weakness and hypnosis are also produced. In humans, clonazepam is capable of suppressing the spike and wave discharge in absence seizures (petit mal) and decreasing the frequency, amplitude, duration and spread of discharge in minor motor seizures.

PHARMACOKINETICS

Clonazepam is rapidly and completely absorbed after oral administration. The absolute bioavailability of clonazepam is about 90%. Maximum plasma concentrations of clonazepam are reached within 1-4 hours after oral administration. Clonazepam is approximately 85% bound to plasma proteins. Clonazepam is highly metabolized, with less than 2% unchanged clonazepam being excreted in the urine. Biotransformation occurs mainly by reduction of the 7-nitro group to the 4-amino derivative. This derivative can be acetylated, hydroxylated and glucuronidated. Cytochrome P-450 including CYP3A, may play an important role in clonazepam reduction and oxidation. The elimination half-life of clonazepam is typically 30-40 hours. Clonazepam pharmacokinetics are dose-independent throughout the dosing range. There is no evidence that clonazepam induces its own metabolism or that of other drugs in humans.

Pharmacokinetics in Demographic Subpopulations and in Disease States

Controlled studies examining the influence of gender and age on clonazepam pharmacokinetics have not been conducted, nor have the effects of renal or liver disease on clonazepam pharmacokinetics been studied. Because clonazepam undergoes hepatic metabolism, it is possible that liver disease will impair clonazepam elimination. Thus, caution should be exercised when administering clonazepam to these patients.

INDICATIONS AND USAGE

SEIZURE DISORDERS

Clonazepam is useful alone or as an adjunct in the treatment of the Lennox-Gastaut syndrome (petit mal variant), akinetic and myoclonic seizures. In patients with absence seizures (petit mal) who have failed to respond to succinimides, clonazepam may be useful.

In some studies, up to 30% of patients have shown a loss of anticonvulsant activity, often within 3 months of administration. In some cases, dosage adjustment may reestablish efficacy.

PANIC DISORDER

Clonazepam is indicated for the treatment of panic disorder, with or without agoraphobia, as defined in DSM-IV. Panic disorder is characterized by the occurrence of unexpected panic attacks and associated concern about having additional attacks, worry about the implications or consequences of the attacks, and/or a significant change in behavior related to the attacks.

The efficacy of clonazepam was established in two 6-9 week trials in panic disorder patients whose diagnoses corresponded to the DSM-IIIR category of panic disorder.

Panic disorder (DSM-IV) is characterized by recurrent unexpected panic attacks, *i.e.*, a discrete period of intense fear or discomfort in which 4 (or more) of the following symptoms develop abruptly and reach a peak within 10 minutes:

1. Palpitations, pounding heart or accelerated heart rate.
2. Sweating.
3. Trembling or shaking.
4. Sensations of shortness of breath or smothering.
5. Feeling of choking.
6. Chest pain or discomfort.
7. Nausea or abdominal distress.
8. Feeling dizzy, unsteady, lightheaded or faint.
9. Derealization (feelings of unreality) or depersonalization (being detached from oneself).
10. Fear of losing control.
11. Fear of dying.
12. Paresthesias (numbness or tingling sensations).
13. Chills or hot flushes.

The effectiveness of clonazepam in long-term use, that is, for more than 9 weeks, has not been systematically studied in controlled clinical trials. The physician who elects to use clonazepam for extended periods should periodically reevaluate the long-term usefulness of the drug for the individual patient (see DOSAGE AND ADMINISTRATION).

NON-FDA APPROVED INDICATIONS

Clonazepam has been used without FDA approval for the treatment of photosensitive epilepsy, partial seizures with complex symptomatology, tonic-clonic seizures, social phobia, anxiety, and bipolar disorder. However, no standard dosage recommendations are available for these conditions. (Please note that clonazepam has been reported to have increased the frequency of tonic-clonic seizures in some patients.)

CONTRAINDICATIONS

Clonazepam should not be used in patients with a history of sensitivity to benzodiazepines, nor in patients with clinical or biochemical evidence of significant liver disease. It may be used in patients with open angle glaucoma who are receiving appropriate therapy but is contraindicated in acute narrow angle glaucoma.

WARNINGS

INTERFERENCE WITH COGNITIVE AND MOTOR PERFORMANCE

Since clonazepam produces CNS depression, patients receiving this drug should be cautioned against engaging in hazardous occupations requiring mental alertness, such as operating machinery or driving a motor vehicle. They should also be warned about the concomitant use of alcohol or other CNS-depressant drugs during clonazepam therapy (see DRUG INTERACTIONS and PRECAUTIONS, Information for the Patient).

PREGNANCY RISKS

Data from several sources raise concerns about the use of clonazepam during pregnancy.

ANIMAL FINDINGS

In three studies in which clonazepam was administered orally to pregnant rabbits at doses of 0.2, 1.0, 5.0, or 10.0 mg/kg/day (low dose approximately 0.2 times the maximum recommended human dose of 20 mg/day for seizure disorders and equivalent to the maximum dose of 4 mg/day for panic disorder, on a mg/m^2 basis) during the period of organogenesis, a similar pattern of malformations (cleft palate, open eyelid, fused sternebrae, and limb defects) was observed in a low, non-dose-related incidence in exposed litters from all dosage groups. Reductions in maternal weight gain occurred at dosages of 5 mg/kg/day or greater and reduction in embryo-fetal growth occurred in one study at a dosage of 10 mg/kg/day. No adverse maternal or embryo-fetal effects were observed in mice and rats following administration during organogenesis of oral doses up to 15 or 40 mg/kg/day, respectively (4 and 20 times the maximum recommended human dose of 20 mg/day for seizure disorders and 20 and 100 times the maximum dose of 4 mg/day for panic disorder, respectively, on a mg/m^2 basis).

GENERAL CONCERNS AND CONSIDERATIONS ABOUT ANTICONVULSANTS

Recent reports suggest an association between the use of anticonvulsant drugs by women with epilepsy and an elevated incidence of birth defects in children born to these women. Data are more extensive with respect to diphenylhydantoin and phenobarbital, but these are also the most commonly prescribed anticonvulsants; less systematic or anecdotal reports suggest a possible similar association with the use of all known anticonvulsant drugs.

In children of women treated with drugs for epilepsy, reports suggesting an elevated incidence of birth defects cannot be regarded as adequate to prove a definite cause and effect relationship. There are intrinsic methodologic problems in obtaining adequate data on drug teratogenicity in humans; the possibility also exists that other factors (*e.g.,* genetic factors or the epileptic condition itself) may be more important than drug therapy in leading to birth defects. The great majority of mothers on anticonvulsant medication deliver normal infants. It is important to note that anticonvulsant drugs should not be discontinued in patients in whom the drug is administered to prevent seizures because of the strong possibility of precipitating status epilepticus with attendant hypoxia and threat to life. In individual cases where the severity and frequency of the seizure disorder are such that the removal of medication does not pose a serious threat to the patient, discontinuation of the drug may be considered prior to and during pregnancy; however, it cannot be said with any confidence that even mild seizures do not pose some hazards to the developing embryo or fetus.

GENERAL CONCERNS ABOUT BENZODIAZEPINES

An increased risk of congenital malformations associated with the use of benzodiazepine drugs has been suggested in several studies.

There may also be non-teratogenic risks associated with the use of benzodiazepines during pregnancy. There have been reports of neonatal flaccidity, respiratory and feeding difficulties, and hypothermia in children born to mothers who have been receiving benzodiazepines late in pregnancy. In addition, children born to mothers receiving benzodiazepines late in pregnancy may be at some risk of experiencing withdrawal symptoms during the postnatal period.

ADVICE REGARDING THE USE OF CLONAZEPAM IN WOMEN OF CHILDBEARING POTENTIAL

In general, the use of clonazepam in women of childbearing potential, and more specifically during known pregnancy, should be considered only when the clinical situation warrants the risk to the fetus.

The specific considerations addressed above regarding the use of anticonvulsants for epilepsy in women of childbearing potential should be weighed in treating or counseling these women.

Because of experience with other members of the benzodiazepine class, clonazepam is assumed to be capable of causing an increased risk of congenital abnormalities when administered to a pregnant woman during the first trimester. Because use of these drugs is rarely a matter of urgency in the treatment of panic disorder, their use during the first trimester should almost always be avoided. The possibility that a woman of childbearing potential may be pregnant at the time of institution of therapy should be considered. If this drug is used during pregnancy, or if the patient becomes pregnant while taking this drug, the patient should be apprised of the potential hazard to the fetus. Patients should also be advised that if they become pregnant during therapy or intend to become pregnant, they should communicate with their physician about the desirability of discontinuing the drug.

WITHDRAWAL SYMPTOMS

Withdrawal symptoms of the barbiturate type have occurred after the discontinuation of benzodiazepines.

PRECAUTIONS

GENERAL

Worsening of Seizures

When used in patients in whom several different types of seizure disorders coexist, clonazepam may increase the incidence or precipitate the onset of generalized tonic-clonic seizures (grand mal). This may require the addition of appropriate anticonvulsants or an increase in their dosages. The concomitant use of valproic acid and clonazepam may produce absence status.

Laboratory Testing During Long-Term Therapy

Periodic blood counts and liver function tests are advisable during long-term therapy with clonazepam.

Risks of Abrupt Withdrawal

The abrupt withdrawal of clonazepam, particularly in those patients on long-term, high-dose therapy, may precipitate status epilepticus. Therefore, when discontinuing clonazepam, gradual withdrawal is essential. While clonazepam is being gradually withdrawn, the simultaneous substitution of another anticonvulsant may be indicated.

Caution in Renally Impaired Patients

Metabolites of clonazepam are excreted by the kidneys; to avoid their excess accumulation, caution should be exercised in the administration of the drug to patients with impaired renal function.

Hypersalivation

Clonazepam may produce an increase in salivation. This should be considered before giving the drug to patients who have difficulty handling secretions. Because of this and the possibility of respiratory depression, clonazepam should be used with caution in patients with chronic respiratory diseases.

INFORMATION FOR THE PATIENT

Physicians are advised to discuss the following issues with patients for whom they prescribe clonazepam:

Dose Changes: To assure the safe and effective use of benzodiazepines, patients should be informed that, since benzodiazepines may produce psychological and physical dependence, it is advisable that they consult with their physician before either increasing the dose or abruptly discontinuing this drug.

Interference With Cognitive and Motor Performance: Because benzodiazepines have the potential to impair judgment, thinking or motor skills, patients should be cautioned about operating hazardous machinery, including automobiles, until they are reasonably certain that clonazepam therapy does not affect them adversely.

Pregnancy: Patients should be advised to notify their physician if they become pregnant or intend to become pregnant during therapy with clonazepam (see WARNINGS).

Nursing: Patients should be advised not to breastfeed an infant if they are taking clonazepam.

Concomitant Medication: Patients should be advised to inform their physicians if they are taking, or plan to take, any prescription or over-the-counter drugs, since there is a potential for interactions.

Alcohol: Patients should be advised to avoid alcohol while taking clonazepam.

CARCINOGENESIS, MUTAGENESIS, AND IMPAIRMENT OF FERTILITY

Carcinogenicity studies have not been conducted with clonazepam.

The data currently available are not sufficient to determine the genotoxic potential of clonazepam.

In a two-generation fertility study in which clonazepam was given orally to rats at 10 and 100 mg/kg/day (low dose approximately 5 and 24 times the maximum recommended human dose of 20 mg/day for seizure disorder and 4 mg/day for panic disorder, respectively, on a mg/m^2 basis), there was a decrease in the number of pregnancies and in the number of offspring surviving until weaning.

PREGNANCY, TERATOGENIC EFFECTS, PREGNANCY CATEGORY D

See WARNINGS.

LABOR AND DELIVERY

The effect of clonazepam on labor and delivery in humans has not been specifically studied; however, perinatal complications have been reported in children born to mothers who have been receiving benzodiazepines late in pregnancy, including findings suggestive of either excess benzodiazepine exposure or of withdrawal phenomena (see WARNINGS, Pregnancy Risks).

NURSING MOTHERS

Mothers receiving clonazepam should not breastfeed their infants.

PEDIATRIC USE

Because of the possibility that adverse effects on physical or mental development could become apparent only after many years, a benefit-risk consideration of the long-term use of clonazepam is important in pediatric patients being treated for seizure disorder (see INDICATIONS AND USAGE and DOSAGE AND ADMINISTRATION).

Safety and effectiveness in pediatric patients with panic disorder below the age of 18 have not been established.

GERIATRIC USE

Clinical studies of clonazepam did not include sufficient numbers of subjects aged 65 and over to determine whether they respond differently from younger subjects. Other reported clinical experience has not identified differences in responses between the elderly and younger patients. In general, dose selection for an elderly patient should be cautious, usually starting at the low end of the dosing range, reflecting the greater frequency of decreased hepatic, renal, or cardiac function, and of concomitant disease or other drug therapy.

Because clonazepam undergoes hepatic metabolism, it is possible that liver disease will impair clonazepam elimination. Metabolites of clonazepam are excreted by kidneys; to avoid their excess accumulation, caution should be exercised in the administration of the drug to patients with impaired renal function. Because elderly patients are more likely to have decreased hepatic and/or renal function, care should be taken in dose selection, and it may be useful to assess hepatic and/or renal functions at the time of dose selection.

Sedating drugs may cause confusion and over-sedation in the elderly; elderly patients generally should be started on low doses of clonazepam and observed closely.

DRUG INTERACTIONS

EFFECT OF CLONAZEPAM ON THE PHARMACOKINETICS OF OTHER DRUGS

Clonazepam does not appear to alter the pharmacokinetics of phenytoin, carbamazepine or phenobarbital. The effect of clonazepam on the metabolism of other drugs has not been investigated.

EFFECT OF OTHER DRUGS ON THE PHARMACOKINETICS OF CLONAZEPAM

Ranitidine and propantheline, agents that decrease stomach acidity, do not greatly alter clonazepam pharmacokinetics. Fluoxetine does not affect the pharmacokinetics of clonazepam. Cytochrome P-450 inducers, such as phenytoin, carbamazepine and phenobarbital, induce clonazepam metabolism, causing an approximately 30% decrease in plasma clonazepam levels. Although clinical studies have not been performed, based on the involvement of the cytochrome P-450 3A family in clonazepam metabolism, inhibitors of this enzyme system, notably oral antifungal agents, should be used cautiously in patients receiving clonazepam.

C

PHARMACODYNAMIC INTERACTIONS

The CNS-depressant action of the benzodiazepine class of drugs may be potentiated by alcohol, narcotics, barbiturates, nonbarbiturate hypnotics, antianxiety agents, the phenothiazines, thioxanthene and butyrophenone classes of antipsychotic agents, monoamine oxidase inhibitors and the tricyclic antidepressants, and by other anticonvulsant drugs.

ADVERSE REACTIONS

The adverse experiences for clonazepam are provided separately for patients with seizure disorders and with panic disorder.

SEIZURE DISORDERS

The most frequently occurring side effects of clonazepam are referable to CNS depression. Experience in treatment of seizures has shown that drowsiness has occurred in approximately 50% of patients and ataxia in approximately 30%. In some cases, these may diminish with time; behavior problems have been noted in approximately 25% of patients.

Others, listed by system, are:

Neurologic: Abnormal eye movements, aphonia, choreiform movements, coma, diplopia, dysarthria, dysdiadochokinesis, ''glassy-eyed'' appearance, headache, hemiparesis, hypotonia, nystagmus, respiratory depression, slurred speech, tremor, vertigo.

Psychiatric: Confusion, depression, amnesia, hallucinations, hysteria, increased libido, insomnia, psychosis, suicidal attempt (the behavior effects are more likely to occur in patients with a history of psychiatric disturbances). *The following paradoxical reactions have been observed:* Excitability, irritability, aggressive behavior, agitation, nervousness, hostility, anxiety, sleep disturbances, nightmares and vivid dreams.

Respiratory: Chest congestion, rhinorrhea, shortness of breath, hypersecretion in upper respiratory passages.

Cardiovascular: Palpitations.

Dermatologic: Hair loss, hirsutism, skin rash, ankle and facial edema.

Gastrointestinal: Anorexia, coated tongue, constipation, diarrhea, dry mouth, encopresis, gastritis, increased appetite, nausea, sore gums.

Genitourinary: Dysuria, enuresis, nocturia, urinary retention.

Musculoskeletal: Muscle weakness, pains.

Miscellaneous: Dehydration, general deterioration, fever, lymphadenopathy, weight loss or gain.

Hematopoietic: Anemia, leukopenia, thrombocytopenia, eosinophilia.

Hepatic: Hepatomegaly, transient elevations of serum trans aminases and alkaline phosphatase.

PANIC DISORDER

Adverse events during exposure to clonazepam were obtained by spontaneous report and recorded by clinical investigators using terminology of their own choosing. Consequently, it is not possible to provide a meaningful estimate of the proportion of individuals experiencing adverse events without first grouping similar types of events into a smaller number of standardized event categories. In the tables and tabulations that follow, CIGY dictionary terminology has been used to classify reported adverse events, except in certain cases in which redundant terms were collapsed into more meaningful terms, as noted below.

The stated frequencies of adverse events represent the proportion of individuals who experienced, at least once, a treatment-emergent adverse event of the type listed. An event was considered treatment-emergent if it occurred for the first time or worsened while receiving therapy following baseline evaluation.

ADVERSE FINDINGS OBSERVED IN SHORT-TERM, PLACEBO-CONTROLLED TRIALS

Adverse Events Associated With Discontinuation of Treatment

Overall, the incidence of discontinuation due to adverse events was 17% in clonazepam compared to 9% for placebo in the combined data of two 6-9 week trials. The most common events (≥1%) associated with discontinuation and a dropout rate twice or greater for clonazepam than that of placebo included those listed in TABLE 1.

TABLE 1

Adverse Event	Clonazepam (n=574)	Placebo (n=294)
Somnolence	7%	1%
Depression	4%	1%
Dizziness	1%	<1%
Nervousness	1%	0%
Ataxia	1%	0%
Intellectual ability reduced	1%	0%

Adverse Events Occurring at an Incidence of 1% or More Among Clonazepam-Treated Patients

TABLE 1 enumerates the incidence, rounded to the nearest percent, of treatment-emergent adverse events that occurred during acute therapy of panic disorder from a pool of two 6-9 week trials. Events reported in 1% or more of patients treated with clonazepam (doses ranging from 0.5-4 mg/day) and for which the incidence was greater than that in placebo-treated patients are included.

The prescriber should be aware that the figures in TABLE 2 cannot be used to predict the incidence of side effects in the course of usual medical practice where patient characteristics and other factors differ from those that prevailed in the clinical trials. Similarly, the cited frequencies cannot be compared with figures obtained from other clinical investigations involving different treatments, uses and investigators. The cited figures, however, do provide the prescribing physician with some basis for estimating the relative contribution of drug and nondrug factors to the side effect incidence in the population studied.

C

TABLE 2 *Treatment-Emergent Adverse Event Incidence in 6-9 Week Placebo-Controlled Clinical Trials**

	Clonazepam Maximum Daily Dose (mg)					
Adverse Event	**<1 (n=96)**	**1 to <2 (n=129)**	**2 to <3 (n=113)**	**≥3 (n=235)**	**All† (n=574)**	**Placebo (n=294)**
Central & Peripheral Nervous System						
Somnolence§	26%	35%	50%	36%	37%	10%
Dizziness	5%	5%	12%	8%	8%	4%
Coordination abnormal§	1%	2%	7%	9%	6%	0%
Ataxia§	2%	1%	8%	8%	5%	0%
Dysarthria§	0%	0%	4%	3%	2%	0%
Psychiatric						
Depression	7%	6%	8%	8%	7%	1%
Memory disturbance	2%	5%	2%	5%	4%	2%
Nervousness	1%	4%	3%	4%	3%	2%
Intellectual ability reduced	0%	2%	4%	3%	2%	0%
Emotional lability	0%	1%	2%	2%	1%	1%
Libido decreased	0%	1%	3%	1%	1%	0%
Confusion	0%	2%	2%	1%	1%	0%
Respiratory System						
Upper respiratory tract infection†	10%	10%	7%	6%	8%	4%
Sinusitis	4%	2%	8%	4%	4%	3%
Rhinitis	3%	2%	4%	2%	2%	1%
Coughing	2%	2%	4%	0%	2%	0%
Pharyngitis	1%	1%	3%	2%	2%	1%
Bronchitis	1%	0%	2%	2%	1%	1%
Gastrointestinal System						
Constipation§	0%	1%	5%	3%	2%	2%
Appetite decreased	1%	1%	0%	3%	1%	1%
Abdominal pain†	2%	2%	2%	0%	1%	1%
Body as a Whole						
Fatigue	9%	6%	7%	7%	7%	4%
Allergic reaction	3%	1%	4%	2%	2%	1%
Musculoskeletal						
Myalgia	2%	1%	4%	0%	1%	1%
Resistance Mechanism Disorder						
Influenza	3%	2%	5%	5%	4%	3%
Urinary System						
Micturition frequency	1%	2%	2%	1%	1%	0%
Urinary tract infection§	0%	0%	2%	2%	1%	0%
Vision Disorders						
Blurred vision	1%	2%	3%	0%	1%	1%
Reproductive Disorders,¤ Female						
Dysmenorrhea	0%	6%	5%	2%	3%	2%
Colpitis	4%	0%	2%	1%	1%	1%
Reproductive Disorders, Male¤						
Ejaculation delayed	0%	0%	2%	2%	1%	0%
Impotence	3%	0%	2%	1%	1%	0%

* Events reported by at least 1% of patients treated with clonazepam and for which the incidence was greater than that for placebo.
† By body system.
‡ All clonazepam groups.
§ Indicates that the p-value for the dose-trend test (Cochran-Mantel-Haenszel) for adverse event incidence was ≤0.10.
¤ Denominators for events in gender-specific systems are: n=240 (clonazepam), 102 (placebo) for male, and 334 (clonazepam), 192 (placebo) for female.

Commonly Observed Adverse Events

TABLE 3 *Incidence of Most Commonly Observed Adverse Events* in Acute Therapy in Pool of 6-9 Week Trials*

Adverse Event (Roche preferred term)	**Clonazepam (n=574)**	**Placebo (n=294)**
Somnolence	37%	10%
Depression	7%	1%
Coordination abnormal	6%	0%
Ataxia	5%	0%

* Treatment-emergent events for which the incidence in the clonazepam patients was ≥5% and at least twice that in the placebo patients.

Treatment-Emergent Depressive Symptoms

In the pool of two short-term placebo-controlled trials, adverse events classified under the preferred term "depression" were reported in 7% of clonazepam-treated patients compared to 1% of placebo-treated patients, without any clear pattern of dose relatedness. In these same trials, adverse events classified under the preferred term "depression" were reported as leading to discontinuation in 4% of clonazepam-treated patients compared to 1% of placebo-treated patients. While these findings are noteworthy, Hamilton Depression Rating Scale (HAM-D) data collected in these trials revealed a larger decline in HAM-D scores in the clonazepam group than the placebo group suggesting that clonazepam-treated patients were not experiencing a worsening or emergence of clinical depression.

Other Adverse Events Observed During the Premarketing Evaluation of Clonazepam in Panic Disorder

Following is a list of modified CIGY terms that reflect treatment-emergent adverse events reported by patients treated with clonazepam at multiple doses during clinical trials. All reported events are included except those already listed in TABLE 1 or elsewhere in labeling, those events for which a drug cause was remote, those event terms which were so general as to be uninformative, and events reported only once and which did not have a substantial probability of being acutely life-threatening. It is important to emphasize that, although the events occurred during treatment with clonazepam, they were not necessarily caused by it.

Events are further categorized by body system and listed in order of decreasing frequency. These adverse events were reported infrequently, which is defined as occurring in 1/100 to 1/1000 patients.

Body as a Whole: Weight increase, accident, weight decrease, wound, edema, fever, shivering, abrasions, ankle edema, edema foot, edema periorbital, injury, malaise, pain, cellulitis, inflammation localized.

Cardiovascular Disorders: Chest pain, hypotension postural.

Central and Peripheral Nervous System Disorders: Migraine, paresthesia, drunkenness, feeling of enuresis, paresis, tremor, burning skin, falling, head fullness, hoarseness, hyperactivity, hypoesthesia, tongue thick, twitching.

Gastrointestinal System Disorders: Abdominal discomfort, gastrointestinal inflammation, stomach upset, toothache, flatulence, pyrosis, saliva increased, tooth disorder, bowel movements frequent, pain pelvic, dyspepsia, hemorrhoids.

Hearing and Vestibular Disorders: Vertigo, otitis, earache, motion sickness.

Heart Rate and Rhythm Disorders: Palpitation.

Metabolic and Nutritional Disorders: Thirst, gout.

Musculoskeletal System Disorders: Back pain, fracture traumatic, sprains and strains, pain leg, pain nape, cramps muscle, cramps leg, pain ankle, pain shoulder, tendinitis, arthralgia, hypertonia, lumbago, pain feet, pain jaw, pain knee, swelling knee.

Platelet, Bleeding and Clotting Disorders: Bleeding dermal.

Psychiatric Disorders: Insomnia, organic disinhibition, anxiety, depersonalization, dreaming excessive, libido loss, appetite increased, libido increased, reactions decreased, aggressive reaction, apathy, attention lack, excitement, feeling mad, hunger abnormal, illusion, nightmares, sleep disorder, suicide ideation, yawning.

Reproductive Disorders, Female: Breast pain, menstrual irregularity.

Reproductive Disorders, Male: Ejaculation decreased.

Resistance Mechanism Disorders: Infection mycotic, infection viral, infection streptococcal, herpes simplex infection, infectious mononucleosis, moniliasis.

Respiratory System Disorders: Sneezing excessive, asthmatic attack, dyspnea, nosebleed, pneumonia, pleurisy.

Skin and Appendages Disorders: Acne flare, alopecia, xeroderma, dermatitis contact, flushing, pruritus, pustular reaction, skin burns, skin disorder.

Special Senses: Taste loss.

Urinary System Disorders: Dysuria, cystitis, polyuria, urinary incontinence, bladder dysfunction, urinary retention, urinary tract bleeding, urine discoloration.

Vascular (extracardiac) Disorders: Thrombophlebitis leg.

Vision Disorders: Eye irritation, visual disturbance, diplopia, eye twitching, styes, visual field defect, xerophthalmia.

DOSAGE AND ADMINISTRATION

SEIZURE DISORDERS

Adults

The initial dose for adults with seizure disorders should not exceed 1.5 mg/day divided into 3 doses. Dosage may be increased in increments of 0.5 to 1 mg every 3 days until seizures are adequately controlled or until side effects preclude any further increase. Maintenance dosage must be individualized for each patient depending upon response. Maximum recommended daily dose is 20 mg.

The use of multiple anticonvulsants may result in an increase of depressant adverse effects. This should be considered before adding clonazepam to an existing anticonvulsant regimen.

Pediatric Patients

Clonazepam is administered orally. In order to minimize drowsiness, the initial dose for infants and children (up to 10 years of age or 30 kg of body weight) should be between 0.01 and 0.03 mg/kg/day but not to exceed 0.05 mg/kg/day given in 2 or 3 divided doses. Dosage should be increased by no more than 0.25-0.5 mg every third day until a daily maintenance dose of 0.1-0.2 mg/kg of body weight has been reached, unless seizures are controlled or side effects preclude further increase. Whenever possible, the daily dose should be divided into 3 equal doses. If doses are not equally divided, the largest dose should be given before retiring.

Geriatric Patients

There is no clinical experience with clonazepam in seizure disorder patients 65 years of age and older. In general, elderly patients should be started on low doses of clonazepam and observed closely (see PRECAUTIONS, Geriatric Use).

PANIC DISORDER

Adults

The initial dose for adults with panic disorder is 0.25 mg bid. An increase to the target dose for most patients of 1 mg/day may be made after 3 days. The recommended dose of 1 mg/day is based on the results from a fixed dose study in which the optimal effect was seen at 1 mg/day. Higher doses of 2, 3 and 4 mg/day in that study were less effective than the 1 mg/day dose and were associated with more adverse effects. Nevertheless, it is possible that some individual patients may benefit from doses of up to a maximum dose of 4 mg/day, and in those instances, the dose may be increased in increments of 0.125-0.25 mg bid every 3 days until panic disorder is controlled or until side effects make further increases undesired. To reduce the inconvenience of somnolence, administration of one dose at bedtime may be desirable.

Treatment should be discontinued gradually, with a decrease of 0.125 mg bid every 3 days, until the drug is completely withdrawn.

There is no body of evidence available to answer the question of how long the patient treated with clonazepam should remain on it. Therefore, the physician who elects to use clonazepam for extended periods should periodically reevaluate the long-term usefulness of the drug for the individual patient.

Pediatric Patients

There is no clinical trial experience with clonazepam in panic disorder patients under 18 years of age.

Geriatric Patients

There is no clinical experience with clonazepam in panic disorder patients 65 years of age and older. In general, elderly patients should be started on low doses of clonazepam and observed closely (see PRECAUTIONS, Geriatric Use).

HOW SUPPLIED

Klonopin is supplied as follows:

0.5 mg: Orange, scored tablets with "1/2 KLONOPIN" on the front side, and "ROCHE" on the scored side of the tablet.

1 mg: Blue, unscored tablets with a K-shaped perforation with "1 KLONOPIN" on the front side, and "ROCHE" on the reverse side.

2 mg: White, unscored tablets with a K-shaped perforation with "2 KLONOPIN" on the front side, and "ROCHE" on the reverse side.

Storage: Store at 15-30°C (59-86°F).

PRODUCT LISTING - RATED THERAPEUTICALLY EQUIVALENT

Package	Price	Product	NDC
Tablet - Oral - 0.5 mg			
20 x 5	$79.79	GENERIC, Udl Laboratories Inc	51079-0881-21
30's	$25.88	GENERIC, Vangard Labs	00615-0456-65
31 x 10	$267.78	GENERIC, Vangard Labs	00615-0456-63
100's	$24.55	FEDERAL UPPER LIMIT, H.C.F.A. F F P	99999-0845-01
100's	$70.69	GENERIC, Vangard Labs	00615-0456-29
100's	$70.76	GENERIC, Par Pharmaceutical Inc	49884-0495-01
100's	$71.24	GENERIC, Apothecon Inc	62269-0353-24
100's	$71.35	GENERIC, Mylan Pharmaceuticals Inc	00378-1910-01
100's	$71.37	GENERIC, Eon Labs Manufacturing Inc	00185-0063-01
100's	$71.37	GENERIC, Andrx Pharmaceuticals	62037-0952-01
100's	$74.90	GENERIC, Teva Pharmaceuticals Usa	00093-0832-01
100's	$74.90	GENERIC, Watson Laboratories Inc	00591-0746-01
100's	$74.90	GENERIC, Watson/Rugby Laboratories Inc	52544-0746-01
100's	$74.90	GENERIC, Novopharm Usa Inc	55953-0027-40
100's	$74.91	GENERIC, Purepac Pharmaceutical Company	00228-3003-11
100's	$79.79	GENERIC, Udl Laboratories Inc	51079-0881-20
100's	$79.79	GENERIC, Novopharm Usa Inc	55953-0027-41
100's	$96.25	KLONOPIN, Roche Laboratories	00004-0068-01
Tablet - Oral - 1 mg			
20 x 5	$90.54	GENERIC, Udl Laboratories Inc	51079-0882-21
31 x 10	$307.64	GENERIC, Vangard Labs	00615-0457-63
100's	$28.52	FEDERAL UPPER LIMIT, H.C.F.A. F F P	99999-0845-02
100's	$81.04	GENERIC, Apothecon Inc	62269-0354-24
100's	$81.40	GENERIC, Mylan Pharmaceuticals Inc	00378-1912-01
100's	$81.41	GENERIC, Eon Labs Manufacturing Inc	00185-0064-01
100's	$81.41	GENERIC, Andrx Pharmaceuticals	62037-0953-01
100's	$85.50	GENERIC, Teva Pharmaceuticals Usa	00093-0833-01
100's	$85.50	GENERIC, Watson Laboratories Inc	00591-0747-01
100's	$85.50	GENERIC, Par Pharmaceutical Inc	49884-0496-01
100's	$85.50	GENERIC, Watson Laboratories Inc	52544-0747-01
100's	$85.50	GENERIC, Novopharm Usa Inc	55953-0028-40
100's	$85.51	GENERIC, Purepac Pharmaceutical Company	00228-3004-11
100's	$90.54	GENERIC, Udl Laboratories Inc	51079-0882-20
100's	$109.78	KLONOPIN, Roche Laboratories	00004-0058-01
Tablet - Oral - 2 mg			
20 x 5	$124.05	GENERIC, Udl Laboratories Inc	51079-0883-21
100's	$39.03	FEDERAL UPPER LIMIT, H.C.F.A. F F P	99999-0845-03
100's	$112.41	GENERIC, Apothecon Inc	62269-0355-24
100's	$112.82	GENERIC, Eon Labs Manufacturing Inc	00185-0065-01
100's	$112.82	GENERIC, Par Pharmaceutical Inc	49884-0497-01
100's	$112.82	GENERIC, Novopharm Usa Inc	55953-0029-40
100's	$112.82	GENERIC, Andrx Pharmaceuticals	62037-0954-01
100's	$118.40	GENERIC, Teva Pharmaceuticals Usa	00093-0834-01
100's	$118.40	GENERIC, Watson Laboratories Inc	00591-0748-01
100's	$118.40	GENERIC, Watson Laboratories Inc	52544-0748-01
100's	$118.40	GENERIC, Caraco Pharmaceutical Laboratories	57664-0275-08
100's	$118.41	GENERIC, Purepac Pharmaceutical Company	00228-3005-11
100's	$118.45	GENERIC, Mylan Pharmaceuticals Inc	00378-1914-01
100's	$124.05	GENERIC, Udl Laboratories Inc	51079-0883-20

PRODUCT LISTING - EQUIVALENTS NOT AVAILABLE

Package	Price	Product	NDC
Tablet - Oral - 0.5 mg			
15's	$10.95	GENERIC, Southwood Pharmaceuticals Inc	58016-0183-15
20's	$14.60	GENERIC, Southwood Pharmaceuticals Inc	58016-0183-20
28's	$20.44	GENERIC, Southwood Pharmaceuticals Inc	58016-0183-28
30's	$21.90	GENERIC, Southwood Pharmaceuticals Inc	58016-0183-30
60's	$43.80	GENERIC, Southwood Pharmaceuticals Inc	58016-0183-60
90's	$65.70	GENERIC, Southwood Pharmaceuticals Inc	58016-0183-90
100's	$73.00	GENERIC, Southwood Pharmaceuticals Inc	58016-0183-00
100's	$77.50	KLONOPIN, Roche Laboratories	00004-0068-50
120's	$87.60	GENERIC, Southwood Pharmaceuticals Inc	58016-0183-02
Tablet - Oral - 1 mg			
15's	$12.83	GENERIC, Southwood Pharmaceuticals Inc	58016-0186-15
20's	$17.10	GENERIC, Southwood Pharmaceuticals Inc	58016-0186-20
28's	$23.94	GENERIC, Southwood Pharmaceuticals Inc	58016-0186-28
30's	$25.65	GENERIC, Southwood Pharmaceuticals Inc	58016-0186-30
60's	$51.30	GENERIC, Southwood Pharmaceuticals Inc	58016-0186-60
90's	$76.95	GENERIC, Southwood Pharmaceuticals Inc	58016-0186-90
100's	$85.50	GENERIC, Southwood Pharmaceuticals Inc	58016-0186-00
100's	$87.94	KLONOPIN, Roche Laboratories	00004-0058-50
120's	$102.60	GENERIC, Southwood Pharmaceuticals Inc	58016-0186-02
Tablet - Oral - 2 mg			
100's	$152.10	KLONOPIN, Roche Laboratories	00004-0098-01

Clonidine Hydrochloride *(000846)*

Categories: Pain, cancer; Hypertension, essential; Pregnancy Category C; FDA Approved 1979 Sep; Orphan Drugs
Drug Classes: Antiadrenergics, central
Brand Names: **Catapres; Catapres-TTS; Duraclon**
Foreign Brand Availability: Arkamin (India); Caprysin (Finland); Catapres (Australia; Bahamas; Bahrain; Barbados; Belize; Benin; Bermuda; Burkina-Faso; Canada; Curacao; Cyprus; Egypt; England; Ethiopia; Gambia; Ghana; Guinea; Guyana; Hong-Kong; India; Indonesia; Iran; Iraq; Ireland; Israel; Ivory-Coast; Jamaica; Japan; Jordan; Kenya; Kuwait; Lebanon; Liberia; Libya; Malawi; Mali; Mauritania; Mauritius; Morocco; Netherland-Antilles; New-Zealand; Niger; Nigeria; Oman; Philippines; Qatar; Republic-of-Yemen; Saudi-Arabia; Senegal; Seychelles; Sierra-Leone; Sudan; Surinam; Syria; Taiwan; Tanzania; Thailand; Trinidad; Tunia; Uganda; United-Arab-Emirates; Zambia; Zimbabwe); Catapres TTS (New-Zealand); Catapresan (Austria; Belgium; Colombia; Denmark; Ecuador; Finland; Germany; Greece; Italy; Netherlands; Norway; Peru; Portugal; Spain; Sweden); Catapresan 100 (Mexico); Catapresan Depot (Czech-Republic; Germany; Switzerland); Catapresan TTS (Italy); Catapressan (Argentina; France); Clonidine (Thailand); Daipres (Japan); Dixarit (Malaysia); Haemiton (Bahrain; Cyprus; Egypt; Germany; Iran; Iraq; Israel; Jordan; Kuwait; Lebanon; Libya; Oman; Qatar; Republic-of-Yemen; Saudi-Arabia; Syria; United-Arab-Emirates); Melzin (Philippines); Normopresan (Israel); Paracefan (Belgium); Sulmidine (Japan); Taitecin (Japan)
Cost of Therapy: $41.42 (Hypertension; Catapres; 0.1 mg; 2 tablets/day; 30 day supply)
$57.35 (Hypertension; Catapres-TTS; 0.1 mg; 1 patch/week; 30 day supply)
$1.80 (Hypertension; Generic Tablets; 0.1 mg; 2 tablets/day; 30 day supply)
HCFA JCODE(S): J0735 1 mg epidural

EPIDURAL

WARNING

The 500 µg/ml strength product should be diluted prior to use in an appropriate solution.

Note: Epidural clonidine is not recommended for obsetrical, post-partum, or peri-operative pain management. The risk of hemodynamic instability, especially hypotension and bradycardia, from epidural clonidine may be unacceptable in these patients. However, in a rare obstetrical, post-partum or peri-operative patient, potential benefits may outweigh the possible risks.

DESCRIPTION

Clonidine hydrochloride injection is a centrally-acting analgesic solution for use in continuous epidural infusion devices.

Clonidine hydrochloride is an imidazoline derivative and exists as a mesomeric compound. The chemical names are benzenamine, 2,6-dichloro-N-2-imidazolidinylidene-monohydrochloride and 2-[(2,6-dichlorophenyl)imino]imidazolidine monohydrochloride. Its molecular formula is $C_9H_9Cl_2N_3 \cdot HCl$, with molecular weight of 266.56.

Clonidine hydrochloride injection is supplied as a clear, colorless, preservative-free, pyrogen-free, aqueous sterile solution (pH 5-7) in a single-dose, 10 ml vial.

100 µg/ml: Each ml of the 100 µg/ml (0.1 mg/ml) concentration contains 100 µg of clonidine hydrochloride and 9 mg sodium chloride in water for injection. Hydrochloric acid and/or sodium hydroxide may have been added for pH adjustment. Each 10 ml vial contains 1 mg (1000 µg) of clonidine HCl.

500 µg/ml: Each ml of the 500 µg/ml (0.5 mg/ml) concentration contains 500 µg of clonidine hydrochloride and 9 mg sodium chloride in water for injection. Hydrochloric acid and/or sodium hydroxide may have been added for pH adjustment. Each 10 ml vial contains 5 mg (5000 µg) of clonidine HCl.

CLINICAL PHARMACOLOGY

MECHANISM OF ACTION

Epidurally administered clonidine produces dose-dependent analgesia not antagonized by opiate antagonists. The analgesia is limited to the body regions innervated by the spinal segments where analgesic concentrations of clonidine are present. Clonidine is thought to produce analgesia at presynaptic and postjunctional alpha-2-adrenoceptors in the spinal cord by preventing pain signal transmission to the brain.

PHARMACOKINETICS

Following a 10 minute intravenous infusion of 300 µg clonidine HCl to 5 male volunteers, plasma clonidine levels showed an initial rapid distribution phase (mean ±SD $T_{½}$ = 11 ± 9 minutes) followed by a slower elimination phase ($T_{½}$ = 9 ± 2 hours) over 24 hours. Clonidine's total body clearance (CL) was 219 ± 92 ml/min.

Following a 700 µg clonidine HCl epidural dose given over 5 minutes to 4 male and 5 female volunteers, peak clonidine plasma levels (4.4 ± 1.4 ng/ml) were obtained in 19 ± 27 minutes. The plasma elimination half-life was determined to be 22 ± 15 hours following sample collection for 24 hours. CL was 190 ± 70 ml/min. In cerebral spinal fluid (CSF), peak clonidine levels (418 ± 255 ng/ml) were achieved in 26 ± 11 minutes. The clonidine CSF elimination half-life was 1.3 ± 0.5 hours when samples were collected for 6 hours. Compared to men, women had a lower mean plasma clearance, longer mean plasma half-life, and higher mean peak level of clonidine in both plasma and CSF.

In cancer patients who received 14 days of clonidine HCl epidural infusion (rate = 30 μg/h) plus morphine by patient-controlled analgesia (PCA), steady state clonidine plasma concentrations of 2.2 ± 1.1 and 2.4 ± 1.4 ng/ml were obtained on dosing days 7 and 14 respectively. CL was 279 ± 184 and 272 ± 163 ml/min on these days. CSF concentrations were not determined in these patients.

C

DISTRIBUTION

Clonidine is highly lipid soluble and readily distributes into extravascular sites including the central nervous system. Clonidine's volume of distribution is 2.1 ± 0.4 L/kg. The binding of clonidine to plasma protein is primarily to albumin and varies between 20 and 40% *in vitro*. Epidurally administered clonidine readily partitions into plasma via the epidural veins and attains systemic concentrations (0.5-2.0 ng/ml) that are associated with a hypotensive effect mediated by the central nervous system.

EXCRETION

Following an intravenous dose of ^{14}C-clonidine, 72% of the administered dose was excreted in urine in 96 hours of which 40-50% was unchanged clonidine. Renal clearance for clonidine was determined to be 133 ± 66 ml/min. In a study where ^{14}C-clonidine was given to subjects with varying degrees of kidney function, elimination half-lives varied (17.5 to 41 hours) as a function of creatinine clearance. In subjects undergoing hemodialysis only 5% of body clonidine stores was removed.

METABOLISM

In humans, clonidine metabolism follows minor pathways with the major metabolite, p-hydroxyclonidine, being present at less than 10% of the concentration of unchanged drug in urine.

SPECIAL POPULATIONS

The pharmacokinetics of epidurally administered clonidine has not been studied in the pediatric population or in patients with renal or hepatic disease.

INDICATIONS AND USAGE

Epidural clonidine HCl is indicated in combination with opiates for the treatment of severe pain in cancer patients that is not adequately relieved by opioid analgesics alone. Epidural clonidine is more likely to be effective in patients with neuropathic pain than somatic or visceral pain.

The safety of this drug product has only been established in a highly selected group of cancer patients, and only after an adequate trial of opioid analgesia. Other use is of unproven safety and is not recommended. In a rare patient, the potential benefits may outweigh the known risks (see WARNINGS).

NON-FDA APPROVED INDICATIONS

Epidural clonidine has been used for obstetrical, postpartum, and perioperative pain management. Injectable clonidine has been investigated for its potential ability to treat postoperative shivering. Intrathecal clonidine has been studied in small doses as an adjunct to anesthesia for knee arthroscopy.

CONTRAINDICATIONS

Clonidine HCl is contraindicated in patients with a history of sensitization or allergic reactions to clonidine. Epidural administration is contraindicated in the presence of an injection site infection, in patients on anticoagulant therapy, and in those with a bleeding diathesis. Administration of epidural clonidine HCl above the C4 dermatome is contraindicated since there are no adequate safety data to support such use (see WARNINGS).

WARNINGS

USE IN POSTOPERATIVE OR OBSTETRICAL ANALGESIA

Epidural clonidine is not recommended for obstetrical, post-partum, or peri-operative pain management. The risk of hemodynamic instability, especially hypotension and bradycardia, from epidural clonidine may be unacceptable in these patients.

HYPOTENSION

Because severe hypotension may follow the administration of clonidine, it should be used with caution in all patients. It is not recommended in most patients with severe cardiovascular disease or in those who are otherwise hemodynamically unstable. The benefit of its administration in these patients should be carefully balanced against the potential risks resulting from hypotension.

Vital signs should be monitored frequently, especially during the first few days of epidural clonidine therapy. When clonidine is infused into the upper thoracic spinal segments, more pronounced decreases in the blood pressure may be seen.

Clonidine decreases sympathetic outflow from the central nervous system resulting in decreases in peripheral resistance, renal vascular resistance, heart rate, and blood pressure. However, in the absence of profound hypotension, renal blood flow and glomerular filtration rate remain essentially unchanged.

In the pivotal double-blind, randomized study of cancer patients, where 38 subjects were administered epidural clonidine HCl at 30 μg/h in addition to epidural morphine, hypertension occurred in 45% of subjects. Most episodes of hypotension occurred within the first 4 days after beginning epidural clonidine. However, hypotensive episodes occurred throughout the duration of the trial. There was a tendency for these episodes to occur more commonly in women, and in those with higher serum clonidine levels. Patients experiencing hypotension also tended to weigh less than those who did not experience hypotension. The hypotension usually responded to intravenous fluids and, if necessary, parenteral ephedrine.

Published reports on the use of epidural clonidine for intraoperative or postoperative analgesia also show a consistent and marked hypotensive response to clonidine. Severe hypotension may occur if intravenous fluid pretreatment is given.

WITHDRAWAL

Sudden cessation of clonidine treatment, regardless of the route of administration, has, in some cases, resulted in symptoms such as nervousness, agitation, headache, and tremor, accompanied or followed by a rapid rise in blood pressure. The likelihood of such reactions appears to be greater after administration of higher doses or with concomitant beta-blocker treatment. Special caution is therefore advised in these situations. Rare instances of hypertensive encephalopathy, cerebrovascular accidents and death have been reported after abrupt clonidine withdrawl. Patients with a history of hypertension and/or other underlying cardiovascular conditions may be at particular risk of the consequences of abrupt discontinuation of clonidine. In the pivotal double-blind, randomized cancer pain study, 4 of 38 subjects receiving 720 μg of clonidine per day experienced rebound hypertension following abrupt withdrawl. One of these patients with rebound hypertension subsequently experienced a cerebrovascular accident.

Careful monitoring of infusion pump function and inspection of catheter tubing for obstruction or dislodgement can help reduce the risk of inadvertent abrupt withdrawl of epidural clonidine. Patients should notify their physician immediately if clonidine administration is inadvertently interrupted for any reason. Patients should also be instructed not to discontinue therapy without consulting their physician.

When discontinuing therapy with epidural clonidine, the physician should reduce the dose gradually over 2-4 days to avoid withdrawl symptoms.

An excessive rise in blood pressure following discontinuation of epidural clonidine can be treated by administration of clonidine or by intravenous phentolamine. If therapy is to be discontinued in patients receiving a beta-blocker and clonidine concurrently, the beta-blocker should be withdrawn several days before the gradual discontinuation of epidural clonidine.

INFECTIONS

Infections related to implantable epidural catheters pose a serious risk. Evaluation of fever in a patient receiving epidural clonidine should include the possibility of catheter-related infection such as meningitis or epidural abscess.

PRECAUTIONS

GENERAL

Cardiac Effects

Epidural clonidine frequently causes decreases in heart rate. Symptomatic bradycardia can be treated with atropine. Rarely, atrioventricular block greater than first degree has been reported. Clonidine does not alter the hemodynamic response to exercise, but may mask the increase in heart rate associated with hypovolemia.

Respiratory Depression and Sedation

Clonidine administration may result in sedation through the activation of alpha-adrenoceptors in the brainstem. High doses of clonidine cause sedation and ventilatory abnormalities that are usually mild. Tolerance to these effects can develop with chronic administration. These effects have been reported with bolus doses that are significantly larger than the infusion rate recommended for treating cancer pain.

Depression

Depression has been seen in a small percentage of patients treated with oral or transdermal clonidine. Depression commonly occurs in cancer patients and may be exacerbated by treatment with clonidine. Patients, especially those with a known history of affective disorders, should be monitored for the signs and symptoms of depression.

Pain of Visceral or Somatic Origin

In the clinical investigations, at doses tested, epidural clonidine HCl was most effective in well-localized, "neuropathic" pain that was characterized as electrical, burning, or shooting in nature, and which was localized to a dermatomal or peripheral nerve distribution. Epidural clonidine HCl may be less effective, or possibly ineffective in the treatment of pain that is diffuse, poorly localized, or visceral in origin.

INFORMATION FOR THE PATIENT

Patients should be instructed about the risks of rebound hypertension and warned not to discontinue clonidine except under the supervision of a physician. Patients should notify their physician immediately if clonidine administration is inadvertently interrupted for any reason. Patients who engage in potentially hazardous activities, such as operating machinery or driving, should be advised of the potential sedative and hypotensive effects of epidural clonidine. They should also be informed that sedative effects may be increased by CNS-depressing drugs such as alcohol and barbiturates, and that hypotensive effects may be increased by opiates.

CARCINOGENESIS, MUTAGENESIS, AND IMPAIRMENT OF FERTILITY

In a 132 week study in rats, clonidine HCl administered as a dietary admixture at 5-8 times (based on body surface area) the 50 μg/kg maximum recommended daily human dose (MRDHD) for hypertension did not show any carcinogenic potential. Clonidine was inactive in the Ames test of mutagenicity. Fertility of male and female rats was unaffected by oral clonidine HCl doses as high as 150 μg/kg, or about 0.5 times the MRDHD. Fertility of female rats did, however, appear to be affected in another experiment at oral dose levels of 500-2000 μg/kg, or 2-7 times the MRDHD.

PREGNANCY, TERATOGENIC EFFECTS, PREGNANCY CATEGORY C

Reproduction studies in rabbits at clonidine HCl doses up to approximately the MRDHD revealed no evidence of teratogenic or embryotoxic potential. In rats, however, doses as low as one-third the MRDHD were associated with increased resorptions in a study in which dams were treated continuously from 2 months prior to mating. Increased resorptions were not associated with treatment with the same or higher doses up to 0.5 times the MRDHD when dams were treated on days 6-15 of gestation. Increased resorptions were observed at higher levels (7 times the MRDHD) in rats and mice treated on days 1-14 of gestation.

Clonidine readily crosses the placenta and its concentrations are equal in maternal and umbilical cord plasma; amniotic fluid concentrations can be 4 times those found in serum. There are no adequate and well-controlled studies in pregnant women during early gestation when organ formation takes place. Studies using epidural clonidine during labor have demonstrated no apparent adverse effects on the infant at the time of delivery. However, these studies did not monitor the infants for hemodynamic effects in the days following delivery. Clonidine HCl injection should be used during pregnancy only if the potential benefits justify the potential risk to the fetus.

LABOR AND DELIVERY

There are no adequate controlled clinical trials evaluating the safety, efficacy, and dosing of epidural clonidine HCl in obstetrical settings. Because maternal perfusion of the placenta is critically dependent on blood pressure, use of epidural clonidine HCl as an analgesic during labor and delivery is not indicated (see WARNINGS).

NURSING MOTHERS

Concentrations of clonidine in human breast milk are approximately twice those found in maternal plasma. Caution should be exercised when clonidine is administered to a nursing woman. Because of the potential for severe adverse reactions in nursing infants, a decision should be made to either discontinue nursing or to discontinue clonidine.

PEDIATRIC USE

The safety and effectiveness of epidural clonidine HCl in this limited indication and clinical population have been established in patients old enough to tolerate placement and management of an epidural catheter, based on evidence from adequate and well controlled studies in adults and experience with the use of clonidine in the pediatric age group for other indications. The use of epidural clonidine HCl should be restricted to pediatric patients with severe intractable pain from malignancy that is unresponsive to epidural or spinal opiates or other more conventional analgesic techniques. The starting dose of epidural clonidine HCl should be selected on per kilogram basis (0.5 μg/kg/h) and cautiously adjusted based on the clinical response.

DRUG INTERACTIONS

Clonidine may potentiate the CNS-depressive effect of alcohol, barbiturates or other sedating drugs. Narcotic analgesics may potentiate the hypotensive effects of clonidine. Tricyclic antidepressants may antagonize the hypotensive effects of clonidine. The effects of tricyclic antidepressants on clonidine's analgesic actions are not known.

Beta-blockers may exacerbate the hypertensive response seen with clonidine withdrawal. Also, due to the potential for additive effects such as bradycardia and AV block, caution is warranted in patients receiving clonidine with agents known to affect sinus node function or AV nodal conduction (*e.g.,* digitalis, calcium channel blockers, and beta-blockers).

There is one reported case of a patient with acute delirium associated with the simultaneous use of fluphenazine and oral clonidine. Symptoms resolved when clonidine was withdrawn and recurred when the patient was rechallenged with clonidine.

Epidural clonidine may prolong the duration of pharmacologic effects of epidural local anesthetics, including both sensory and motor blockade.

ADVERSE REACTIONS

Adverse reactions seen during continuous epidural clonidine infusion are dose-dependent and typical for a compound of this pharmacologic class. The adverse events most frequently reported in the pivotal controlled clinical trial of continuous epidural clonidine administration consisted of hypotension, postural hypotension, decreased heart rate, rebound hypertension, dry mouth, nausea, confusion, dizziness, somnolence, and fever. Hypotension is the adverse event that most frequently requires treatment. The hypotension is usually responsive to intravenous fluids and, if necessary, parenterally-administered ephedrine. Hypotension was observed more frequently in women and in lower weight patients, but no dose-related response was established.

Implantable epidural catheters are associated with a risk of catheter-related infections, including meningitis and/or epidural abscess. The risk depends on the clinical situation and the type of catheter used, but catheter related infections occur in 5-20% of patients, depending on the kind of catheter used, catheter placement technique, quality of catheter care, and length of catheter placement.

The inadvertent intrathecal administration of clonidine has not been associated with a significantly increased risk of adverse events, but there are inadequate safety and efficacy data to support the use of intrathecal clonidine.

Epidural clonidine was compared to placebo in a 2 week double-blind study of 85 terminal cancer patients with intractable pain receiving epidural morphine. The adverse events in TABLE 1 were reported in 2 or more patients and may be related to administration of either epidural clonidine HCl or morphine.

An open label long-term extension of the trial was performed. Thirty-two (32) subjects received epidural clonidine and morphine for up to 94 weeks with a median dosing period of 10 weeks. The following adverse events (and percent incidence) were reported: hypotension/postural hypotension (47%); nausea (13%); anxiety/confusion (38%); somnolence (25%); urinary tract infection (22%); constipation, dyspnea, fever, infection (6% each); asthenia, hyperaesthesia, pain, skin ulcer, and vomiting (5% each). Eighteen percent (18%) of subjects discontinued this study as a result of catheter-related problems (infections, accidental dislodging, etc.), and 1 subject developed meningitis, possibly as a result of a catheter-related infection. In this study, rebound hypertension was not assessed, and ECG and laboratory data were not systemically sought.

The following adverse reactions have also been reported with the use of any dosage form of clonidine. In many cases patients were receiving concomitant medication and a causal relationship has not been established:

Body as a Whole: Weakness, 10%; fatigue, 4%; headache and withdrawl syndrome, each 1%. Also reported were pallor, a weakly positive Coomb's test, and increased sensitivity to alcohol.

TABLE 1 *Incidence of Adverse Events in the 2 week Trial*

Adverse Events	Clonidine (n=38)	Placebo (n=47)
Total number of patients who experienced at least one adverse event.	37 (97.4%)	38 (80.5%)
Hypotension	17 (44.8%)	5 (10.6%)
Postural hypotension	12 (31.6%)	0 (0%)
Dry mouth	5 (13.2%)	4 (8.5%)
Nausea	5 (13.2%)	10 (21.3%)
Somnolence	5 (13.2%)	10 (21.3%)
Dizziness	5 (13.2%)	2 (4.3%)
Confusion	5 (13.2%)	5 (10.6%)
Vomiting	4 (10.5%)	7 (14.9%)
Nausea/vomiting	3 (7.9%)	1 (2.1%)
Sweating	2 (5.3%)	0 (0%)
Chest pain	2 (5.3%)	0 (0%)
Hallucination	2 (5.3%)	1 (2.1%)
Tinnitus	2 (5.3%)	0 (0%)
Constipation	1 (2.6%)	2 (4.3%)
Tachycardia	1 (2.6%)	2 (4.3%)
Hypoventilation	1 (2.6%)	2 (4.3%)

Cardiovascular: Palpitations and tachycardia, and bradycardia, each 0.5%. Syncope, Raynaud's phenomenon, congestive heart failure, and electrocardiographic abnormalities (*i.e.,* sinus node arrest, functional bradycardia, high degree AV block) have been reported rarely. Rare case of sinus bradycardia and atrioventricular block have been reported, both with and without the use of concomitant digitalis.

Central Nervous System: Nervousness and agitation, 3%; mental depression, 1%; insomnia, 0.5%. Cerebrovascular accidents, other behavioral changes, vivid dreams or nightmares, restlessness, and delirium have been reported rarely.

Dermatological: Rash, 1%; pruritus, 0.7%; hives, angioneurotic edema and urticaria, 0.5%; alopecia, 0.2%.

Gastrointestinal: Anorexia and malaise, each 1%; mild transient abnormalities in liver function tests, 1%; hepatitis, parotitis, ileus and pseudo obstruction, and abdominal pain, rarely.

Genitourinary: Decreased sexual activity, impotence, and libido, 3%; nocturia, about 1%; difficulty in micturition, about 0.2%; urinary retention, about 0.1%.

Hematologic: Theombocytopenia, rarely.

Metabolic: Weight gain, 0.1%; gynecomastia, 1%; transient elevation of glucose or serum phosphatase, rarely.

Musculoskeletal: Muscle or joint pain, about 0.6%; leg cramps, 0.3%.

Oro-Otolaryngeal: Dryness of the nasal mucosa was rarely reported.

Ophthalmological: Dryness of the eyes, burning of the eyes and blurred vision were rarely reported.

DOSAGE AND ADMINISTRATION

The recommended starting dose of epidural clonidine HCl for continuous epidural infusion is 30 μg/h. Although dosage may be titrated up or down depending on pain relief and occurrence of adverse events, experience with dosage rates above 40 μg/h is limited.

Familiarization with the continuous epidural infusion device is essential. Patients receiving epidural clonidine from a continuous infusion device should be closely monitored for the first few days to assess their response.

The 500 μg/ml (0.5 mg/ml) strength product must be diluted prior to use in 0.9% sodium chloride for injection, to a final concentration of 100 μg/ml.

Renal Impairment: Dosage should be adjusted according to the degree of renal impairment, and patients should be carefully monitored. Since only a minimal amount of clonidine is removed during routine hemodialysis, there is no need to give supplemental clonidine following dialysis.

Epidural clonidine HCl must *not* be used with a preservative.

Parenteral drug products should be inspected visually for particulate matter and discoloration prior to administration, whenever solution and container permit.

HOW SUPPLIED

Duraclon is supplied in 100 μg/ml (0.1 mg/ml) and 500 μg/ml (0.5 mg/ml) strengths in 10 ml vials.

Storage: Store at 25°C controlled room temperature. **Preservative Free.** Discard unused portion.

ORAL

DESCRIPTION

Catapres (clonidine hydrochloride) is a centrally acting antihypertensive agent available as tablets for oral administration in three dosage strengths: 0.1, 0.2, and 0.3 mg. The 0.1 mg tablet is equivalent to 0.087 mg of the free base.

The inactive ingredients in Catapres are colloidal silicon dioxide, corn starch, dibasic calcium phosphate, FD&C yellow no. 6, gelatin, glycerin, lactose, magnesium stearate, methylparaben, propylparaben. The Catapres 0.1 mg tablet also contains FD&C blue no. 1 and FD&C red no. 3.

Clonidine hydrochloride is an imidazoline derivative and exists as a mesomeric compound. The chemical name is 2-(2,6-dichlorophenylamino)-2-imidazoline hydrochloride. It has the following molecular formula $C_9H_9Cl_2N_3 \cdot HCl$, with molecular weight of 266.56.

Clonidine hydrochloride is an odorless, bitter, white, crystalline substance soluble in water and alcohol.

CLINICAL PHARMACOLOGY

Clonidine HCl acts relatively rapidly. The patient's blood pressure declines within 30-60 minutes after an oral dose, the maximum decrease occurring within 2-4 hours. The plasma level of clonidine HCl peaks in approximately 3-5 hours and the plasma half-life ranges from 12-16 hours. The half-life increases up to 41 hours in patients with severe impairment of renal function. Following oral administration about 40-60% of the absorbed dose is recovered in the urine as unchanged drug in 24 hours. About 50% of the absorbed dose is metabolized in the liver.

Clonidine stimulates alpha-adrenoreceptors in the brain stem, resulting in reduced sympathetic outflow from the central nervous system and a decrease in peripheral resistance: at a 45° tilt there is a smaller reduction in cardiac output and a decrease of peripheral resistance. During long-term therapy, cardiac output tends to return to control values, while peripheral resistance remains decreased. Slowing of the pulse rate has been observed in most patients given clonidine, but the drug does not alter normal hemodynamic response to exercise.

Other studies in patients have provided evidence of a reduction in plasma renin activity and in the excretion of aldosterone and catecholamines, but the exact relationship of these pharmacologic actions to the antihypertensive effect has not been fully elucidated.

Clonidine acutely stimulates growth hormone release in both children and adults, but does not produce a chronic elevation of growth hormone with long-term use.

Tolerance may develop in some patients, necessitating a reevaluation of therapy.

INDICATIONS AND USAGE

Clonidine HCl is indicated in the treatment of hypertension. Clonidine HCl may be employed alone or concomitantly with other antihypertensive agents.

NON-FDA APPROVED INDICATIONS

Unlabeled and investigational uses of Clonidine have included analgesia potentiation, anxiety, atrial fibrillation, attention deficit disorder, bipolar disorder, chronic stable angina, congestive heart failure, diagnosis of depression, diagnosis of pheochromocytoma, diarrhea, dysmenorrhea, growth hormone stimulation test, malignant hypertension, menopausal vasomotor symptoms, migraine prophylaxis, neurogenic bladder, neuroleptic-induced akathisia, obstructive sleep apnea, opiate withdrawal symptoms, panic disorder, paroxysmal hyperhidrosis, perioperative myocardial ischemia, portal hypertension, post-traumatic stress disorder, premenstrual syndrome, preoperative sedation and anxiolysis, prevention of cyclosporine-induced nephrotoxicity, prevention of postoperative nausea and vomiting, proctalgia fugax, Raynaud's disease, reduction of anesthetic requirements, reflex sympathetic dystrophy, restless leg syndrome, sialorrhea, smoking cessation, social phobia, tardive dyskinesia, Tourette's syndrome, and transmural and/or lateral wall myocardial infarction.

CONTRAINDICATIONS

None known.

PRECAUTIONS

GENERAL

In patients who have developed localized contact sensitization to clonidine film, substitution of oral clonidine HCl therapy may be associated with the development of a generalized skin rash.

In patients who develop an allergic reaction from clonidine film that extends beyond the local patch site (such as generalized skin rash, urticaria, or angioedema), oral clonidine HCl substitution may elicit a similar reaction.

As with all antihypertensive therapy, clonidine HCl should be used with caution in patients with severe coronary insufficiency, recent myocardial infarction, cerebrovascular disease or chronic renal failure.

WITHDRAWAL

Patients should be instructed not to discontinue therapy without consulting their physician. Sudden cessation of clonidine treatment has resulted in subjective symptoms such as nervousness, agitation and headache, accompanied or followed by a rapid rise in blood pressure and elevated catecholamine concentrations in the plasma, but such occurrences have usually been associated with previous administration of high oral doses (exceeding 1.2 mg/day) and/or with continuation of concomitant beta-blocker therapy. Rare instances of hypertensive encephalopathy and death have been reported. When discontinuing therapy with clonidine HCl, the physician should reduce the dose gradually over 2-4 days withdrawal symptomatology.

An excessive rise in blood pressure following clonidine HCl discontinuance can be reversed by administration of oral clonidine or by intravenous phentolamine. If therapy is to be discontinued in patients receiving beta-blockers and clonidine concurrently, beta-blockers should be discontinued several days before the gradual withdrawal of clonidine HCl.

PERIOPERATIVE USE

Administration of clonidine HCl should be continued to within 4 hours of surgery and resumed as soon as possible thereafter. The blood pressure should be carefully monitored and appropriate measures instituted to control it as necessary.

INFORMATION FOR THE PATIENT

Patients who engage in potentially hazardous activities, such as operating machinery or driving, should be advised of a potential sedative effect of clonidine. Patients should be cautioned against interruption of clonidine HCl therapy without a physician's advice.

CARCINOGENESIS, MUTAGENESIS, AND IMPAIRMENT OF FERTILITY

In a 132 week (fixed concentration) dietary administration study in rats, clonidine HCl administered at 32-46 times the maximum recommended daily human dose was unassociated with evidence of carcinogenic potential.

Fertility of male or female rats was unaffected by clonidine HCl doses as high as 150 μg/kg or about 3 times the maximum recommended daily human dose (MRDHD). Fertility of female rats did, however, appear to be affected (in another experiment) at dose levels of 500-2000 μg/kg or 10-40 times the MRDHD.

PREGNANCY, TERATOGENIC EFFECTS, PREGNANCY CATEGORY C

Reproduction studies performed in rabbits at doses up to approximately 3 times the maximum recommended daily human dose (MRDHD) of clonidine HCl have revealed no evidence of teratogenic or embryotoxic potential in rabbits. In rats, however, doses as low as 1/3 the MRDHD were associated with increased resorptions in a study in which dams were treated continuously from 2 months prior to mating. Increased resorptions were not associated with treatment at the same or at higher dose levels (up to 3 times the MRDHD) when dams were treated days 6-15 of gestation. Increased resorptions were observed at much higher levels (40 times the MRDHD) in rats and mice treated days 1-14 of gestation (lowest dose employed in that study was 500 μg/kg). There are, however, no adequate and well-controlled studies in pregnant women. Because animal reproduction studies are not always predictive of human response, this drug should be used during pregnancy only if clearly needed.

NURSING MOTHERS

As clonidine HCl is excreted in human milk, caution should be exercised when clonidine HCl is administered to a nursing woman.

PEDIATRIC USE

Safety and effectiveness in children have not been established.

DRUG INTERACTIONS

If a patient receiving clonidine HCl is also taking tricyclic antidepressants, the effect of clonidine may be reduced, thus necessitating an increase in dosage. Clonidine HCl may enhance the CNS-depressive effects of alcohol, barbiturates or other sedatives. Amitriptyline in combination with clonidine enhances the manifestation of corneal lesions in rats (see ANIMAL PHARMACOLOGY).

ADVERSE REACTIONS

Most adverse effects are mild and tend to diminish with continued therapy. The most frequent (which appear to be dose-related) are dry mouth, occurring in about 40 in 100 patients; drowsiness, about 33 in 100; dizziness, about 16 in 100; constipation and sedation, each about 10 in 100.

The following less frequent adverse experiences have also been reported in patients receiving clonidine HCl, but in many cases patients were receiving concomitant medication and a causal relationship has not been established.

Gastrointestinal: Nausea and vomiting, about 5 in 100 patients; anorexia and malaise, each about 1 in 100; mild transient abnormalities in liver function tests, about 1 in 100; rare reports of hepatitis; parotitis, rarely.

Metabolic: Weight gain, about 1 in 100 patients; gynecomastia, about 1 in 1000; transient elevation of blood glucose or serum creatine phosphokinase, rarely.

Central Nervous System: Nervousness and agitation, about 3 in 100 patients; mental depression, about 1 in 100; headache, about 1 in 100; insomnia, about 5 in 1000. Vivid dreams or nightmares, other behavioral changes, restlessness, anxiety, visual and auditory hallucinations and delirium have been reported.

Cardiovascular: Orthostatic symptoms, about 3 in 100 patients; palpitations and tachycardia, and bradycardia, each about 5 in 1000. Raynaud's phenomenon, congestive heart failure, and electrocardiographic abnormalities (*i.e.*, conduction disturbances and arrhythmias) have been reported rarely. Rare cases of sinus bradycardia and atrioventricular block have been reported, both with and without the use of concomitant digitalis.

Dermatological: Rash, about 1 in 100 patients; pruritus, about 7 in 1000; hives, angioneurotic edema and urticaria, about 5 in 1000; alopecia, about 2 in 1000.

Genitourinary: Decreased sexual activity, impotence and loss of libido, about 3 in 100 patients; nocturia, about 1 in 100; difficulty in micturition, about 2 in 1000; urinary retention, about 1 in 1000.

Other: Weakness, about 10 in 100 patients; fatigue, about 4 in 100; discontinuation syndrome, about 1 in 100; muscle or joint pain, about 6 in 1000 and cramps of the lower limbs, about 3 in 1000. Dryness, burning of the eyes, blurred vision, dryness of the nasal mucosa, pallor, weakly positive Coombs' test, increased sensitivity to alcohol and fever have been reported.

DOSAGE AND ADMINISTRATION

ADULTS

The dose of clonidine HCl must be adjusted according to the patient's individual blood pressure response. The following is a general guide to its administration.

Initial Dose: 0.1 mg tablet twice daily (morning and bedtime). Elderly patients may benefit from a lower initial dose.

Maintenance Dose: Further increments of 0.1 mg/day may be made if necessary until the desired response is achieved. Taking the larger portion of the oral daily dose at bedtime may minimize transient adjustment effects of dry mouth and drowsiness. The therapeutic doses most commonly employed have ranged from 0.2-0.6 mg/day given in divided doses. Studies have indicated that 2.4 mg is the maximum effective daily dose, but doses as high as this have rarely been employed.

RENAL IMPAIRMENT

Dosage must be adjusted according to the degree of impairment, and patients should be carefully monitored. Since only a minimal amount of clonidine is removed during routine hemodialysis, there is no need to give supplemental clonidine following dialysis.

ANIMAL PHARMACOLOGY

In several studies, oral clonidine HCl produced a dose-dependent increase in the incidence and severity of spontaneously occurring retinal degeneration in albino rats treated for 6 months or longer. Tissue distribution studies in dogs and monkeys revealed that clonidine HCl was concentrated in the choroid of the eye. In view of the retinal degeneration observed in rats, eye examinations were performed in 908 patients prior to the start of clonidine HCl therapy, who were then examined periodically thereafter. In 353 of these 908 patients, examinations were performed for periods of 24 months or longer. Except for some dryness of the eyes, no drug-related abnormal ophthalmologic findings were recorded and clonidine HCl did not alter retinal function as shown by specialized tests such as the electroretinogram and macular dazzle. In rats, clonidine HCl in combination with amitriptyline produced corneal lesions within 5 days.

HOW SUPPLIED

Catapres is supplied in tablets containing 0.1, 0.2, and 0.3 mg of clonidine HCl.

0.1 mg: Tan, oval shaped and single scored with the marking "BI 6".

0.2 mg: Orange, oval shaped and single scored with the marking "BI 7".

0.3 mg: Peach, oval shaped and single scored with the marking "BI 11".

Storage: Store below 30°C (86°F). Dispense in tight, light-resistant container.

TRANSDERMAL

DESCRIPTION

TRANSDERMAL THERAPEUTIC SYSTEM

Programmed delivery *in vivo* of 0.1, 0.2, or 0.3 mg clonidine per day, for 1 week.

Catapres-TTS (clonidine) is a transdermal system providing continuous systemic delivery of clonidine for 7 days at an approximately constant rate. Clonidine is a centrally acting alpha-agonist and is an antihypertensive agent. It is an imidazoline derivative whose chemical name is 2,6-dichloro-N-2-imidazolidinylidenebenzenamine.

System Structure and Components

Catapres-TTS is a multilayered film, 0.2 mm thick, containing clonidine as the active agent. System area is 3.5, 7.0, or 10.5 cm^2 and the amount of drug released is directly proportional to area. (See Release Rate Concept.) The composition per unit area of all three dosages is identical.

Proceeding from the visible surface towards the surface attached to the skin, are four layers (1) a backing layer of pigmented polyester film; (2) a drug reservoir of clonidine, mineral oil, polyisobutylene, and colloidal silicon dioxide; (3) a microporous polypropylene membrane that controls the rate of delivery of clonidine from the system to the skin surface; (4) an adhesive formulation of clonidine, mineral oil, polyisobutylene, and colloidal silicon dioxide. Prior to use, a protective peel strip of polyester that covers layer 4 is removed.

Release Rate Concept

Clonidine film is programmed to release clonidine at an approximately constant rate for 7 days. The energy source for drug release derives from the concentration gradient existing between a saturated solution of drug in the system and the much lower concentration prevailing in the skin. Clonidine flows in the direction of the lower concentration at a constant rate, limited by the rate-controlling membrane, so long as a saturated solution is maintained in the drug reservoir.

Following system application to intact skin, clonidine in the adhesive layer saturates the skin sites below the system. Clonidine from the drug reservoir then begins to flow through the rate-controlling membrane and the adhesive layer of the system into the systemic circulation via the capillaries beneath the skin. Therapeutic plasma clonidine levels are achieved 2-3 days after initial application of clonidine film.

The 3.5, 7.0, and 10.5 cm^2 systems respectively deliver 0.1, 0.2, and 0.3 mg clonidine per day. To ensure constant release of drug over 7 days, the total drug content of the system is greater than the total amount of drug delivered. Application of a new system to a fresh skin site at weekly intervals continuously maintains therapeutic plasma concentrations of clonidine. If the clonidine film is removed and not replaced with a new system, therapeutic plasma clonidine levels will persist for about 8 hours and than decline slowly over several days. Over this time period, blood plasma returns gradually to pretreatment levels. If the patient experiences localized skin irritation before completing 7 days of use, the system may be removed and replaced with a new one applied on a fresh skin site.

CLINICAL PHARMACOLOGY

Clonidine stimulates alpha-adrenoreceptors in the brain stem, resulting in reduced sympathetic outflow from the central nervous system and a decrease in peripheral resistance, renal vascular resistance, heart rate, and blood pressure. Renal blood flow and glomerular filtration rate remain essentially unchanged. Normal postural reflexes are intact, and therefore orthostatic symptoms are mild and infrequent.

Acute studies with clonidine HCl in human have demonstrated a moderate reduction (15-20%) of cardiac output in the supine position with no change in the peripheral resistance; at a 45° tilt there is a smaller reduction in cardiac output and a decrease of peripheral resistance. During long-term therapy, cardiac output tends to return to control values, while peripheral resistance remains decreased. Slowing of the pulse rate has been observed in most patients given clonidine, but the drug does not alter normal hemodynamic response to exercise.

Other studies in patients have provided evidence of a reduction in plasma renin activity and in the excretion of aldosterone and catecholamines, but the exact relationship of these pharmacologic actions to the antihypertensive effect has not been fully elucidated.

Clonidine acutely stimulates growth hormone release in both children and adults, but does not produce a chronic elevation of growth hormone with long-term use.

Tolerance may develop in some patients, necessitating a reevaluation of therapy.

The plasma half-life of clonidine is 12.7 ± 7 hours. Following oral administration about 40-60% of the absorbed dose is recovered in the urine as unchanged drug in 24 hours. About 50% of the absorbed dose is metabolized in the liver.

INDICATIONS AND USAGE

Clonidine film is indicated in the treatment of hypertension. It may be employed alone or concomitantly with other antihypertensive agents.

CONTRAINDICATIONS

Clonidine film should not be used in patients with known hypersensitivity to clonidine or to any other component of the adhesive layer of the therapeutic system.

PRECAUTIONS

GENERAL

In patients who have developed localized contact sensitization to clonidine film, substitution of oral clonidine HCl therapy may be associated with development of a generalized skin rash.

In patients who develop an allergic reaction to clonidine film that extends beyond the local patch site (such as generalized skin rash, urticaria, or angioedema) oral clonidine HCl substitution may elicit a similar reaction.

As with all antihypertensive therapy, clonidine film should be used with caution in patients with severe coronary insufficiency, recent myocardial infarction, cerebrovascular disease, or chronic renal failure.

Transdermal clonidine systems should be removed before attempting defibrillation or cardioversion because of the potential for altered electrical conductivity which may enhance the possibility of arcing, a phenomenon associated with the use of defibrillators.

WITHDRAWAL

Patients should be instructed not to discontinue therapy without consulting their physician. Sudden cessation of clonidine treatment has resulted in subjective symptoms such as nervousness, agitation and headache, accompanied or followed by a rapid rise in blood pressure and elevated catecholamine concentrations in the plasma, but such occurrences have usually been associated with previous administration of high oral doses (exceeding 1.2 mg/day) and/or with continuation of concomitant beta-blocker therapy. Rare instances of hypertensive encephalopathy and death have been reported.

An excessive rise in blood pressure following clonidine film discontinuance can be reversed by administration of oral clonidine or by intravenous phentolamine. If therapy is to be discontinued in patients receiving beta-blockers and clonidine concurrently, beta-blockers should be discontinued several days before cessation of clonidine film administration.

PERIOPERATIVE USE

As with oral clonidine therapy, clonidine film therapy should not be interrupted during the surgical period. Blood pressure should be carefully monitored during surgery and additional measures to control blood pressure should be available if required. Physicians considering starting clonidine film therapy during the perioperative period must be aware that therapeutic plasma clonidine levels are not achieved until 2-3 days after initial application of clonidine film (see DOSAGE AND ADMINISTRATION).

INFORMATION FOR THE PATIENT

Patients who engage in potentially hazardous activities, such as operating machinery or driving, should be advised of a potential sedative effect of clonidine. Patients should be cautioned against interruption of clonidine film therapy without a physician's advice. Patients should be advised that if the system begins to loosen from the skin after application, the adhesive overlay should be applied directly over the system to ensure good adhesion over its 7 day lifetime. Instructions for using the system are provided. Patients who develop moderate or severe erythema and/or localized vesicle formation at the site of application, or a generalized skin rash, should consult their physician promptly about the possible need to remove the patch.

CARCINOGENESIS, MUTAGENESIS, AND IMPAIRMENT OF FERTILITY

In a 132 week (fixed concentration) dietary administration study in rats, clonidine HCl administered at 32-46 times the oral maximum recommended daily human dose (MRDHD) was unassociated with evidence of carcinogenic potential. Results from the Ames test with clonidine HCl reveled no evidence of mutagenesis. Fertility of male or female rats was unaffected by clonidine doses as high as 150 μg/kg or about 3 times the oral MRDHD. Fertility of female rats did, however, appear to be affected (in another experiment) at the dose levels of 500-2000 μg/kg or 10-40 times the oral MRDHD.

PREGNANCY, TERATOGENIC EFFECTS, PREGNANCY CATEGORY C

Reproduction studies performed in rabbits at doses up to approximately 3 times the oral maximum recommended daily human dose (MRDHD) of clonidine HCl tablets have revealed no evidence of teratogenic or embryotoxic potential in rabbits. In rats, however, doses as low as 1/3 the MRDHD of clonidine were associated with increased resorptions in a study in which dams were treated continuously from 2 months prior to mating. Increased resorptions were not associated with treatment at the same or at higher dose levels (up to 3 times the oral MRDHD) when dams were treated days 6-15 of gestation. Increased resorptions were observed at much higher levels (40 times the MRDHD) in rats and mice treated days 1-14 of gestation (lowest dose employed in the study was 500 μg/kg). There are, however, no adequate and well-controlled studies in pregnant women. Because animal reproduction studies are not always predictive of human response, this drug should be used during pregnancy only if clearly needed.

NURSING MOTHERS

As clonidine is excreted in human milk, caution should be exercised when clonidine film is administered to a nursing woman.

PEDIATRIC USE

Safety and effectiveness in children below the age of 12 have not been established.

DRUG INTERACTIONS

If a patient receiving clonidine is also taking tricyclic antidepressants, the effect of clonidine may be reduced, thus necessitating an increase in dosage. Clonidine may enhance the CNS-depressive effects of alcohol, barbiturates or other sedatives. Amitriptyline in combination with clonidine enhances the manifestation of corneal lesions in rats (see ANIMAL PHARMACOLOGY).

ADVERSE REACTIONS

Most systemic adverse effects during therapy with clonidine film have been mild and have tended to diminish with continued therapy. In a 3 month, multiclinic trial of clonidine film in 101 hypertensive patients, the most frequent systemic reactions were dry mouth (25 patients) and drowsiness (12 patients).

Transient localized skin reactions, primarily localized pruritus, occurred in 51 patients. Twenty-six (26) patients experienced localized erythema. This erythema and pruritus were more common in patients utilizing an adhesive overlay for the entire 7 day treatment period. Allergic contact sensitization to clonidine film was observed in 5 patients.

In additional clinical experience contact dermatitis resulting in treatment discontinuation was observed in 128 of 673 patients (about 19 in 100) after a mean duration of treatment of 37 weeks. The incidence in white females was about 34 in 100; in white males about 18 in 100; in black females about 14 in 100; and in black males about 8 in 100.

The following less frequent adverse experiences were also reported in patients involved in the multiclinic trial with clonidine film:

Gastrointestinal: Constipation (1 patient); nausea (1); and change in taste (1).

Central Nervous System: Fatigue (6 patients); headache (5); lethargy (3); sedation (3); insomnia (2); dizziness (2); and nervousness (1).

Genitourinary: Impotence/sexual dysfunction (2 patients).

Dermatological: Localized vesiculation (7 patients); hyperpigmentation (5); edema (3); excoriation (3); burning (3); papules (1); throbbing (1); blanching (1); and generalized macular rash (1). In additional clinical experience involving 3539 patients, less common dermatological reactions have occurred, where a causal relationship to clonidine film was not established: maculopapular skin rash (10 cases); urticaria (2 cases); angioedema involving the face (2 cases), 1 of which also involved the tongue.

Oro-Otolaryngeal: Dry throat (2 patients). In long experience with oral Catapres, the most common adverse reactions have been dry mouth (about 40%), drowsiness (about 35%) and sedation (about 8%).

In addition, the following adverse reactions have been reported less frequently:

Gastrointestinal: Nausea and vomiting, about 5 in 100 patients; anorexia and malaise, each about 1 in 100; mild transient abnormalities in liver function tests, about 1 in 100; rare reports of hepatitis; parotitis, rarely.

Metabolic: Weight gain, about 1 in 100 patients; gynecomastia, about 1 in 1000; transient elevation of blood glucose or serum creatine phosphokinase, rarely.

Central Nervous System: Nervousness and agitation, about 3 in 100 patients; mental depression, about 1 in 100 and insomnia, about 5 in 1000. Vivid dreams or nightmares, other behavioral changes, restlessness, anxiety, visual and auditory hallucinations and delirium have been reported.

Cardiovascular: Orthostatic symptoms, about 3 in 100 patients; palpitations and tachycardia, and bradycardia, each about 5 in 1000. Raynaud's phenomenon, congestive heart failure, and electrocardiographic abnormalities (*i.e.,* conduction disturbances and arrhythmias) have been reported rarely. Rare cases of sinus bradycardia and atrioventricular block have been reported, both with and without the use of concomitant digitalis.

Dermatological: Rash, about 1 in 100 patients; pruritus, about 7 in 1000; hives, angioneurotic edema and urticaria, about 5 in 100; alopecia, about 2 in 1000.

Genitourinary: Decreased sexual activity, impotence and loss of libido, about 3 in 100 patients; nocturia, about 1 in 100; difficulty in micturition, about 2 in 1000; urinary retention, about 1 in 1000.

Other: Weakness, about 10 in 100 patients; fatigue, about 4 in 100; headache, and discontinuation syndrome, each about 1 in 100; muscle or joint pain, about 6 in 1000 and cramps of the lower limbs, about 3 in 1000. Dryness, burning of the eyes, blurred vision, dryness of the nasal mucosa, pallor, weakly positive Coombs' test, increased sensitivity to alcohol and fever have been reported.

DOSAGE AND ADMINISTRATION

Apply clonidine film to a hairless area of intact skin on the upper arm or torso, once every 7 days. Each new application of clonidine film should be on a different skin site from the previous location. If the system loosens during 7 day wearing, the adhesive overlay should be applied directly over the system to ensure good adhesion.

To initiate therapy, clonidine film dosage should be titrated according to individual therapeutic requirements, starting with clonidine film 0.1 mg. If after 1 or 2 weeks the desired reduction in blood pressure is not achieved, increase the dosage by adding an additional clonidine film 0.1 mg or changing to a larger system. An increase in dosage above the two clonidine film 0.3 mg is usually not associated with additional efficacy.

When substituting clonidine film in patients on prior antihypertensive therapy, physicians should be aware that the antihypertensive effect of clonidine film may not commence until 2-3 days after initial application. Therefore, gradual reduction of prior drug dosage is advised. Some or all previous antihypertensive treatment may have to be continued, particularly in patients with more severe forms of hypertension.

ANIMAL PHARMACOLOGY

In several studies, oral clonidine HCl produced a dose-dependent increase in the incidence and severity of spontaneously occurring retinal degeneration in albino rats treated for 6 months or longer. Tissue distribution studies in dogs and monkeys revealed that clonidine HCl was concentrated in the choroid of the eye. In view of the retinal degeneration observed in rats, eye examinations were performed in 908 patients prior to the start of clonidine HCl therapy, who were then examined periodically thereafter. In 353 of these 908 patients, examinations were performed for periods of 24 months or longer. Except for some dryness of the eyes, no drug-related abnormal ophthalmologic findings were recorded and clonidine HCl did not alter retinal function as shown by specialized tests such as the electroretinogram and macular dazzle.

In rats, clonidine HCl in combination with amitriptyline produced corneal lesions within 5 days.

HOW SUPPLIED

Catapres-TTS-1, Catapres-TTS-2 and Catapres-TTS-3 are supplied as 4 pouched systems and 4 adhesive overlays per carton. (See TABLE 2.)

TABLE 2

	Catapres-TTS 1	Catapres-TTS 2	Catapres-TTS 3
Programmed delivery of clonidine *in vivo* per day over 1 week	0.1 mg	0.2 mg	0.3 mg
Clonidine content	2.5 mg	5.0 mg	7.5 mg
Size (cm^2)	3.5	7.0	10.5
Code	BI-31	BI-32	BI-33

Storage: Store below 30°C (86°F).

PRODUCT LISTING - RATED THERAPEUTICALLY EQUIVALENT

Size	Price	Product	NDC
Solution - Intrathecal - 100 mcg/ml			
10 ml	$58.06	DURACLON, Roxane Laboratories Inc	00054-8233-01
Solution - Intrathecal - 500 mcg/ml			
10 ml	$290.32	DURACLON, Roxane Laboratories Inc	00054-8234-01
Tablet - Oral - 0.1 mg			
8's	$6.22	GENERIC, Pd-Rx Pharmaceuticals	55289-0073-08
25's	$2.53	GENERIC, Udl Laboratories Inc	51079-0299-19
25's	$2.58	GENERIC, Udl Laboratories Inc	51079-0300-19
25's	$5.40	GENERIC, Pd-Rx Pharmaceuticals	55289-0073-97
30's	$4.12	GENERIC, Pd-Rx Pharmaceuticals	58864-0110-30
30's	$7.02	GENERIC, Heartland Healthcare Services	61392-0513-30
30's	$7.02	GENERIC, Heartland Healthcare Services	61392-0513-39
30's	$7.98	GENERIC, Pd-Rx Pharmaceuticals	55289-0073-30
30's	$26.63	CATAPRES, Physicians Total Care	54868-0535-00
31 x 10	$82.94	GENERIC, Vangard Labs	00615-2572-53
31 x 10	$82.94	GENERIC, Vangard Labs	00615-2572-63
31's	$7.25	GENERIC, Heartland Healthcare Services	61392-0513-31
32's	$7.49	GENERIC, Heartland Healthcare Services	61392-0513-32
45's	$10.53	GENERIC, Heartland Healthcare Services	61392-0513-45
60's	$6.90	GENERIC, Golden State Medical	60429-0050-60
60's	$9.00	GENERIC, Pd-Rx Pharmaceuticals	58864-0110-60
60's	$10.24	GENERIC, Pd-Rx Pharmaceuticals	55289-0073-60
60's	$14.04	GENERIC, Heartland Healthcare Services	61392-0513-60
90's	$10.39	GENERIC, Golden State Medical	60429-0050-90
90's	$12.36	GENERIC, Pd-Rx Pharmaceuticals	58864-0110-90
90's	$21.06	GENERIC, Heartland Healthcare Services	61392-0513-90
100's	$3.00	GENERIC, Interstate Drug Exchange Inc	00814-1730-14
100's	$3.25	GENERIC, Cmc-Consolidated Midland Corporation	00223-0660-01
100's	$3.41	GENERIC, Us Trading Corporation	56126-0110-11
100's	$5.25	GENERIC, Interpharm Inc	53746-0045-01
100's	$5.50	GENERIC, Raway Pharmacal Inc	00686-0299-20
100's	$6.45	GENERIC, Major Pharmaceuticals Inc	00904-1025-60
100's	$9.00	FEDERAL UPPER LIMIT, H.C.F.A. F F P	99999-0846-01
100's	$10.38	GENERIC, Qualitest Products Inc	00603-2954-21
100's	$10.40	GENERIC, Moore, H.L. Drug Exchange Inc	00839-7182-06
100's	$11.19	GENERIC, Major Pharmaceuticals Inc	00904-1025-61
100's	$11.52	GENERIC, Aligen Independent Laboratories Inc	00405-4241-01
100's	$14.00	GENERIC, Pd-Rx Pharmaceuticals	55289-0073-01
100's	$15.00	GENERIC, Watson/Schein Pharmaceuticals Inc	00364-0820-90
100's	$18.00	GENERIC, Parmed Pharmaceuticals Inc	00349-8921-01
100's	$18.10	GENERIC, Esi Lederle Generics	00005-3180-23
100's	$18.10	GENERIC, Ivax Corporation	00182-1250-01
100's	$21.32	GENERIC, Mylan Pharmaceuticals Inc	00378-0152-01
100's	$23.15	GENERIC, Purepac Pharmaceutical Company	00228-2127-10
100's	$23.62	GENERIC, Udl Laboratories Inc	51079-0299-20
100's	$26.00	GENERIC, Ivax Corporation	00182-1250-89
100's	$42.69	GENERIC, Auro Pharmaceutical	55829-0211-10
100's	$90.83	CATAPRES, Boehringer-Ingelheim	00597-0006-01
180's	$20.72	GENERIC, Golden State Medical	60429-0050-18
270's	$31.08	GENERIC, Golden State Medical	60429-0050-27
Tablet - Oral - 0.2 mg			
30's	$9.23	GENERIC, Heartland Healthcare Services	61392-0516-30
30's	$9.23	GENERIC, Heartland Healthcare Services	61392-0516-39
30's	$10.24	GENERIC, Pd-Rx Pharmaceuticals	58864-0111-30
30's	$21.90	GENERIC, Pd-Rx Pharmaceuticals	55289-0074-30
30's	$40.11	CATAPRES, Physicians Total Care	54868-0931-00
31 x 10	$106.02	GENERIC, Vangard Labs	00615-2573-53
31 x 10	$106.02	GENERIC, Vangard Labs	00615-2573-63
31's	$9.54	GENERIC, Heartland Healthcare Services	61392-0516-31
32's	$4.20	GENERIC, Vangard Labs	00615-2573-32
32's	$9.85	GENERIC, Heartland Healthcare Services	61392-0516-32
45's	$13.85	GENERIC, Heartland Healthcare Services	61392-0516-45
60's	$9.25	GENERIC, Golden State Medical	60429-0051-60
60's	$13.18	GENERIC, Pd-Rx Pharmaceuticals	55289-0074-60
60's	$16.48	GENERIC, Pd-Rx Pharmaceuticals	58864-0111-60
60's	$18.47	GENERIC, Heartland Healthcare Services	61392-0516-60
90's	$13.88	GENERIC, Golden State Medical	60429-0051-90
90's	$27.70	GENERIC, Heartland Healthcare Services	61392-0516-90
100's	$3.38	GENERIC, Interstate Drug Exchange Inc	00814-1731-14
100's	$3.57	GENERIC, Us Trading Corporation	56126-0111-11
100's	$4.25	GENERIC, Cmc-Consolidated Midland Corporation	00223-0661-01
100's	$5.85	GENERIC, Interpharm Inc	53746-0046-01

100's	$6.55	GENERIC, Raway Pharmacal Inc	00686-0300-20
100's	$7.45	GENERIC, Ivax Corporation	00182-1768-01
100's	$9.95	GENERIC, Major Pharmaceuticals Inc	00904-1026-60
100's	$10.92	GENERIC, Moore, H.L. Drug Exchange Inc	00839-7183-06
100's	$11.48	GENERIC, Qualitest Products Inc	00603-2955-21
100's	$12.16	GENERIC, Auro Pharmaceutical	55829-0212-10
100's	$12.75	FEDERAL UPPER LIMIT, H.C.F.A. F F P	99999-0846-04
100's	$12.85	GENERIC, Major Pharmaceuticals Inc	00904-1026-61
100's	$15.86	GENERIC, Aligen Independent Laboratories Inc	00405-4242-01
100's	$18.75	GENERIC, Ivax Corporation	00182-1768-89
100's	$20.00	GENERIC, Watson/Schein Pharmaceuticals Inc	00364-0821-90
100's	$24.50	GENERIC, Ivax Corporation	00182-1251-01
100's	$26.95	GENERIC, Esi Lederle Generics	00005-3181-23
100's	$31.50	GENERIC, Mylan Pharmaceuticals Inc	00378-0186-01
100's	$32.45	GENERIC, Udl Laboratories Inc	51079-0300-20
100's	$33.85	GENERIC, Purepac Pharmaceutical Company	00228-2128-10
100's	$34.20	GENERIC, Ivax Corporation	00182-1251-89
100's	$138.95	CATAPRES, Boehringer-Ingelheim	00597-0007-01
180's	$27.75	GENERIC, Golden State Medical	60429-0051-18
Tablet - Oral - 0.3 mg			
30's	$10.34	GENERIC, Heartland Healthcare Services	61392-0519-30
30's	$10.34	GENERIC, Heartland Healthcare Services	61392-0519-39
31's	$10.69	GENERIC, Heartland Healthcare Services	61392-0519-31
32's	$11.03	GENERIC, Heartland Healthcare Services	61392-0519-32
45's	$15.51	GENERIC, Heartland Healthcare Services	61392-0519-45
60's	$20.68	GENERIC, Heartland Healthcare Services	61392-0519-60
90's	$31.02	GENERIC, Heartland Healthcare Services	61392-0519-90
100's	$4.20	GENERIC, Interstate Drug Exchange Inc	00814-1732-14
100's	$4.75	GENERIC, Cmc-Consolidated Midland Corporation	00223-0662-01
100's	$6.00	GENERIC, Us Trading Corporation	56126-0112-11
100's	$7.92	GENERIC, Interpharm Inc	53746-0047-01
100's	$9.50	GENERIC, Raway Pharmacal Inc	00686-0301-20
100's	$11.68	GENERIC, Qualitest Products Inc	00603-2956-21
100's	$11.73	GENERIC, Moore, H.L. Drug Exchange Inc	00839-7184-06
100's	$12.40	GENERIC, Major Pharmaceuticals Inc	00904-1027-60
100's	$16.50	FEDERAL UPPER LIMIT, H.C.F.A. F F P	99999-0846-07
100's	$18.49	GENERIC, Major Pharmaceuticals Inc	00904-1027-61
100's	$18.64	GENERIC, Auro Pharmaceutical	55829-0213-10
100's	$20.01	GENERIC, Aligen Independent Laboratories Inc	00405-4243-01
100's	$22.50	GENERIC, Ivax Corporation	00182-1769-89
100's	$36.00	GENERIC, Watson/Schein Pharmaceuticals Inc	00364-0824-90
100's	$39.64	GENERIC, Ivax Corporation	00182-1252-01
100's	$39.75	GENERIC, Esi Lederle Generics	00005-3182-23
100's	$45.30	GENERIC, Ivax Corporation	00182-1252-89
100's	$46.31	GENERIC, Mylan Pharmaceuticals Inc	00378-0199-01
100's	$47.70	GENERIC, Udl Laboratories Inc	51079-0301-20
100's	$49.55	GENERIC, Purepac Pharmaceutical Company	00228-2129-10
100's	$174.36	CATAPRES, Boehringer-Ingelheim	00597-0011-01

PRODUCT LISTING - EQUIVALENTS NOT AVAILABLE

Film, Extended Release - Transdermal - 0.1 mg/24 Hr			
4 x 3	$160.59	CATAPRES-TTS-1, Boehringer-Ingelheim	00597-0031-12
4's	$39.68	CATAPRES-TTS-1, Allscripts Pharmaceutical Company	54569-1437-00
4's	$45.09	CATAPRES-TTS-1, Physicians Total Care	54868-0537-01
Film, Extended Release - Transdermal - 0.2 mg/24 Hr			
4 x 3	$270.30	CATAPRES-TTS-2, Boehringer-Ingelheim	00597-0032-12
4's	$71.34	CATAPRES-TTS-2, Physicians Total Care	54868-0532-01
Film, Extended Release - Transdermal - 0.3 mg/24 Hr			
4's	$125.00	CATAPRES-TTS-3, Boehringer-Ingelheim	00597-0033-34
Tablet - Oral - 0.1 mg			
8's	$4.48	GENERIC, Southwood Pharmaceuticals Inc	58016-0517-08
10's	$3.44	GENERIC, Pharmaceutical Corporation Of America	51655-0353-53
30's	$6.48	GENERIC, Allscripts Pharmaceutical Company	54569-0478-00
30's	$16.80	GENERIC, Southwood Pharmaceuticals Inc	58016-0517-30
60's	$12.96	GENERIC, Allscripts Pharmaceutical Company	54569-0478-01
60's	$33.70	GENERIC, Southwood Pharmaceuticals Inc	58016-0517-60
100's	$21.60	GENERIC, Allscripts Pharmaceutical Company	54569-0478-02
100's	$56.16	GENERIC, Southwood Pharmaceuticals Inc	58016-0517-00
Tablet - Oral - 0.2 mg			
10's	$8.58	GENERIC, Southwood Pharmaceuticals Inc	58016-0518-10
12's	$10.29	GENERIC, Southwood Pharmaceuticals Inc	58016-0518-12
14's	$12.01	GENERIC, Southwood Pharmaceuticals Inc	58016-0518-14
20's	$17.15	GENERIC, Southwood Pharmaceuticals Inc	58016-0518-20
21's	$18.01	GENERIC, Southwood Pharmaceuticals Inc	58016-0518-21
24's	$20.58	GENERIC, Southwood Pharmaceuticals Inc	58016-0518-24
28's	$24.01	GENERIC, Southwood Pharmaceuticals Inc	58016-0518-28
30's	$9.53	GENERIC, Allscripts Pharmaceutical Company	54569-1853-00
30's	$25.73	GENERIC, Southwood Pharmaceuticals Inc	58016-0518-30
40's	$34.30	GENERIC, Southwood Pharmaceuticals Inc	58016-0518-40
60's	$16.48	GENERIC, Pharmaceutical Corporation Of America	51655-0362-25
60's	$19.05	GENERIC, Allscripts Pharmaceutical Company	54569-1853-01
60's	$51.46	GENERIC, Southwood Pharmaceuticals Inc	58016-0518-60
100's	$85.79	GENERIC, Southwood Pharmaceuticals Inc	58016-0518-00
Tablet - Oral - 0.3 mg			
12's	$12.93	GENERIC, Southwood Pharmaceuticals Inc	58016-0605-12
15's	$16.16	GENERIC, Southwood Pharmaceuticals Inc	58016-0605-15
20's	$21.55	GENERIC, Southwood Pharmaceuticals Inc	58016-0605-20
30's	$32.33	GENERIC, Southwood Pharmaceuticals Inc	58016-0605-30
60's	$64.66	GENERIC, Southwood Pharmaceuticals Inc	58016-0605-60
100's	$46.56	GENERIC, Allscripts Pharmaceutical Company	54569-2801-00
100's	$107.76	GENERIC, Southwood Pharmaceuticals Inc	58016-0605-00

Clopidogrel Bisulfate *(003380)*

Categories: Myocardial infarction, prophylaxis; Stroke, prophylaxis; Pregnancy Category B; FDA Approved 1997 Nov
Drug Classes: Platelet inhibitors
Brand Names: Plavix
Foreign Brand Availability: Clopilet (India); Iscover (Australia; Austria; Belgium; Bulgaria; Colombia; Czech-Republic; Denmark; England; Finland; France; Germany; Greece; Hungary; Ireland; Italy; Mexico; Netherlands; Norway; Poland; Portugal; Slovenia; Spain; Sweden; Switzerland; Turkey)
Cost of Therapy: $86.75 (Atherosclerosis Events; Plavix; 75 mg; 1 tablet/day; 30 day supply)

DESCRIPTION

Plavix (clopidogrel bisulfate) is an inhibitor of ADP-induced platelet aggregation acting by direct inhibition of adenosine diphosphate (ADP) binding to its receptor and of the subsequent ADP-mediated activation of the glycoprotein GPIIb/IIIa complex. Chemically it is methyl (+)-(*S*)-α-(2-chlorophenyl)-6,7-dihydrothieno[3,2-c]pyridine-5(4*H*)-acetate sulfate (1:1). The empirical formula of clopidogrel bisulfate is $C_{16}H_{16}ClNO_2S{\cdot}H_2SO_4$ and its molecular weight is 419.9.

Clopidogrel bisulfate is a white to off-white powder. It is practically insoluble in water at neutral pH but freely soluble at pH 1. It also dissolves freely in methanol, dissolves sparingly in methylene chloride, and is practically insoluble in ethyl ether. It has a specific optical rotation of about +56°.

Plavix for oral administration is provided as pink, round, biconvex, debossed film-coated tablets containing 97.875 mg of clopidogrel bisulfate which is the molar equivalent of 75 mg of clopidogrel base.

Each tablet contains hydrogenated castor oil, hydroxypropylcellulose, mannitol, microcrystalline cellulose and polyethylene glycol 6000 as inactive ingredients. The pink film coating contains ferric oxide, hydroxypropyl methylcellulose 2910, lactose monohydrate, titanium dioxide and triacetin. The tablets are polished with Carnauba wax.

CLINICAL PHARMACOLOGY

MECHANISM OF ACTION

Clopidogrel is an inhibitor of platelet aggregation. A variety of drugs that inhibit platelet function have been shown to decrease morbid events in people with established atherosclerotic disease as evidenced by stroke or transient ischemic attacks, myocardial infarction, unstable angina or the need for vascular bypass or angioplasty. This indicates that platelets participate in the initiation and/or evolution of these events and that inhibiting them can reduce the event rate.

PHARMACODYNAMIC PROPERTIES

Clopidogrel selectively inhibits the binding of adenosine diphosphate (ADP) to its platelet receptor and the subsequent ADP-mediated activation of the glycoprotein GPIIb/IIIa complex, thereby inhibiting platelet aggregation. Biotransformation of clopidogrel is necessary to produce inhibition of platelet aggregation, but an active metabolite responsible for the activity of the drug has not been isolated. Clopidogrel also inhibits platelet aggregation induced by agonists other than ADP by blocking the amplification of platelet activation by released ADP. Clopidogrel does not inhibit phosphodiesterase activity.

Clopidogrel acts by irreversibly modifying the platelet ADP receptor. Consequently, platelets exposed to clopidogrel are affected for the remainder of their lifespan.

Dose dependent inhibition of platelet aggregation can be seen 2 hours after single oral doses of clopidogrel bisulfate. Repeated doses of 75 mg clopidogrel bisulfate per day inhibit ADP-induced platelet aggregation on the first day, and inhibition reaches steady state between Day 3 and Day 7. At steady state, the average inhibition level observed with a dose of 75 mg clopidogrel bisulfate per day was between 40% and 60%. Platelet aggregation and bleeding time gradually return to baseline values after treatment is discontinued, generally in about 5 days.

Pharmacokinetics and Metabolism

After repeated 75 mg oral doses of clopidogrel (base), plasma concentrations of the parent compound, which has no platelet inhibiting effect, are very low and are generally below the quantification limit (0.00025 mg/L) beyond 2 hours after dosing. Clopidogrel is extensively metabolized by the liver. The main circulating metabolite is the carboxylic acid derivative, and it too has no effect on platelet aggregation. It represents about 85% of the circulating drug-related compounds in plasma.

Following an oral dose of ^{14}C-labeled clopidogrel in humans, approximately 50% was excreted in the urine and approximately 46% in the feces in the 5 days after dosing. The elimination half-life of the main circulating metabolite was 8 hours after single and repeated administration. Covalent binding to platelets accounted for 2% of radiolabel with a half-life of 11 days.

Effect of Food

Administration of clopidogrel bisulfate with meals did not significantly modify the bioavailability of clopidogrel as assessed by the pharmacokinetics of the main circulating metabolite.

Absorption and Distribution

Clopidogrel is rapidly absorbed after oral administration of repeated doses of 75 mg clopidogrel (base), with peak plasma levels (~3 mg/L) of the main circulating metabolite occurring approximately 1 hour after dosing. The pharmacokinetics of the main circulating metabolite are linear (plasma concentrations increased in proportion to dose) in the dose range of 50-150 mg of clopidogrel. Absorption is at least 50% based on urinary excretion of clopidogrel-related metabolites.

Clopidogrel and the main circulating metabolite bind reversibly *in vitro* to human plasma proteins (98% and 94%, respectively). The binding is nonsaturable *in vitro* up to a concentration of 100 μg/ml.

Metabolism and Elimination

In vitro and *in vivo*, clopidogrel undergoes rapid hydrolysis into its carboxylic acid derivative. In plasma and urine, the glucuronide of the carboxylic acid derivative is also observed.

SPECIAL POPULATIONS

Geriatric Patients

Plasma concentrations of the main circulating metabolite are significantly higher in elderly (≥75 years) compared to young healthy volunteers but these higher plasma levels were not associated with differences in platelet aggregation and bleeding time. No dosage adjustment is needed for the elderly.

Renally Impaired Patients

After repeated doses of 75 mg clopidogrel bisulfate per day, plasma levels of the main circulating metabolite were lower in patients with severe renal impairment (creatinine clearance from 5-15 ml/min) compared to subjects with moderate renal impairment (creatinine clearance 30-60 ml/min) or healthy subjects. Although inhibition of ADP-induced platelet aggregation was lower (25%) than that observed in healthy volunteers, the prolongation of bleeding time was similar to healthy volunteers receiving 75 mg of clopidogrel bisulfate per day. No dosage adjustment is needed in renally impaired patients.

Gender

No significant difference was observed in the plasma levels of the main circulating metabolite between males and females. In a small study comparing men and women, less inhibition of ADP-induced platelet aggregation was observed in women, but there was no difference in prolongation of bleeding time. In the large, controlled clinical study (Clopidogrel vs Aspirin in Patients at Risk of Ischemic Events; CAPRIE), the incidence of clinical outcome events, other adverse clinical events, and abnormal clinical laboratory parameters was similar in men and women.

Race

Pharmacokinetic differences due to race have not been studied.

INDICATIONS AND USAGE

Clopidogrel bisulfate is indicated for the reduction of atherosclerotic events as follows:

Recent MI, Recent Stroke or Established Peripheral Arterial Disease: For patients with a history of recent myocardial infarction (MI), recent stroke, or established peripheral arterial disease, clopidogrel bisulfate has been shown to reduce the rate of a combined endpoint of new ischemic stroke (fatal or not), new MI (fatal or not), and other vascular death.

Acute Coronary Syndrome: For patients with acute coronary syndrome (unstable angina/non-Q-wave MI), including patients who are to be managed medically and those who are to be managed with percutaneous coronary intervention (with or without stent) or CABG, clopidogrel bisulfate has been shown to decrease the rate of a combined endpoint of cardiovascular death, MI, or stroke as well as the rate of a combined endpoint of cardiovascular death, MI, stroke, or refractory ischemia.

NON-FDA APPROVED INDICATIONS

Although not currently approved by the FDA, clopidogrel has been used successfully in combination with aspirin alone or aspirin and a glycoprotein IIb/IIIa inhibitor (abciximab or tirofiban) to prevent thrombotic complications and adverse cardiovascular events in patients undergoing coronary artery stenting. In addition, results from a study in patients with acute coronary syndromes receiving clopidogrel in combination with aspirin therapy found the risk of heart attack, stroke and cardiovascular death was reduced by 20%. A second study of similar design resulted in nearly identical results and the benefit of clopidogrel therapy was maintained throughout a 12 month follow-up period.

CONTRAINDICATIONS

The use of clopidogrel bisulfate is contraindicated in the following conditions:

Hypersensitivity to the drug substance or any component of the product.

Active pathological bleeding such as peptic ulcer or intracranial hemorrhage.

WARNINGS

THROMBOTIC THROMBOCYTOPENIC PURPURA (TTP)

TTP has been reported rarely following use of clopidogrel bisulfate, sometimes after a short exposure (<2 weeks). TTP is a serious condition requiring prompt treatment. It is characterized by thrombocytopenia, microangiopathic hemolytic anemia (schistocytes [fragmented RBCs] seen on peripheral smear), neurological findings, renal dysfunction, and fever. TTP was not seen during clopidogrel's clinical trials, which included over 17,500 clopidogrel-treated patients. In worldwide postmarketing experience, however, TTP has been reported at a rate of about 4 cases per million patients exposed, or about 11 cases per million patient-years. The background rate is thought to be about 4 cases per million person-years.

PRECAUTIONS

GENERAL

As with other antiplatelet agents, clopidogrel bisulfate should be used with caution in patients who may be at risk of increased bleeding from trauma, surgery, or other pathological conditions. If a patient is to undergo elective surgery and an antiplatelet effect is not desired, clopidogrel bisulfate should be discontinued 5 days prior to surgery.

GI Bleeding

Clopidogrel bisulfate prolongs the bleeding time. In CAPRIE, clopidogrel bisulfate was associated with a rate of gastrointestinal bleeding of 2.0%, vs 2.7% on aspirin. In CURE, the incidence of major gastrointestinal bleeding was 1.3% vs 0.7% (clopidogrel bisulfate + aspirin vs placebo + aspirin, respectively). Clopidogrel bisulfate should be used with caution in patients who have lesions with a propensity to bleed (such as ulcers). Drugs that might induce such lesions should be used with caution in patients taking clopidogrel bisulfate.

Use in Hepatically Impaired Patients

Experience is limited in patients with severe hepatic disease, who may have bleeding diatheses. Clopidogrel bisulfate should be used with caution in this population.

INFORMATION FOR THE PATIENT

Patients should be told that it may take them longer than usual to stop bleeding when they take clopidogrel bisulfate, and that they should report any unusual bleeding to their physician. Patients should inform physicians and dentists that they are taking clopidogrel bisulfate before any surgery is scheduled and before any new drug is taken.

DRUG/LABORATORY TEST INTERACTIONS

None known.

CARCINOGENESIS, MUTAGENESIS, AND IMPAIRMENT OF FERTILITY

There was no evidence of tumorigenicity when clopidogrel was administered for 78 weeks to mice and 104 weeks to rats at dosages up to 77 mg/kg/day, which afforded plasma exposures >25 times that in humans at the recommended daily dose of 75 mg.

Clopidogrel was not genotoxic in four *in vitro* tests (Ames test, DNA-repair test in rat hepatocytes, gene mutation assay in Chinese hamster fibroblasts, and metaphase chromosome analysis of human lymphocytes) and in one *in vivo* test (micronucleus test by oral route in mice).

Clopidogrel was found to have no effect on fertility of male and female rats at oral doses up to 400 mg/kg/day (52 times the recommended human dose on a mg/m^2 basis).

PREGNANCY CATEGORY B

Reproduction studies performed in rats and rabbits at doses up to 500 and 300 mg/kg/day (respectively, 65 and 78 times the recommended daily human dose on a mg/m^2 basis), revealed no evidence of impaired fertility or fetotoxicity due to clopidogrel. There are, however, no adequate and well-controlled studies in pregnant women. Because animal reproduction studies are not always predictive of a human response, clopidogrel bisulfate should be used during pregnancy only if clearly needed.

NURSING MOTHERS

Studies in rats have shown that clopidogrel and/or its metabolites are excreted in the milk. It is not known whether this drug is excreted in human milk. Because many drugs are excreted in human milk and because of the potential for serious adverse reactions in nursing infants, a decision should be made whether to discontinue nursing or to discontinue the drug, taking into account the importance of the drug to the nursing woman.

PEDIATRIC USE

Safety and effectiveness in the pediatric population have not been established.

DRUG INTERACTIONS

Study of specific drug interactions yielded the following results:

Aspirin: Aspirin did not modify the clopidogrel-mediated inhibition of ADP-induced platelet aggregation. Concomitant administration of 500 mg of aspirin twice a day for 1 day did not significantly increase the prolongation of bleeding time induced by clopidogrel bisulfate. Clopidogrel bisulfate potentiated the effect of aspirin on collagen-induced platelet aggregation. Clopidogrel bisulfate and aspirin have been administered together for up to 1 year.

Heparin: In a study in healthy volunteers, clopidogrel bisulfate did not necessitate modification of the heparin dose or alter the effect of heparin on coagulation. Coadministration of heparin had no effect on inhibition of platelet aggregation induced by clopidogrel bisulfate.

Nonsteroidal Anti-Inflammatory Drugs (NSAIDs): In healthy volunteers receiving naproxen, concomitant administration of clopidogrel bisulfate was associated with increased occult gastrointestinal blood loss. NSAIDs and clopidogrel bisulfate should be coadministered with caution.

Warfarin: The safety of the coadministration of clopidogrel bisulfate with warfarin has not been established. Consequently, concomitant administration of these two agents should be undertaken with caution. (See PRECAUTIONS, General.)

Other Concomitant Therapy: No clinically significant pharmacodynamic interactions were observed when clopidogrel bisulfate was coadministered with **atenolol, nifedipine,** or both atenolol and nifedipine. The pharmacodynamic activity of clopidogrel bisulfate was also not significantly influenced by the coadministration of **phenobarbital, cimetidine** or **estrogen.**

The pharmacokinetics of **digoxin** or **theophylline** were not modified by the coadministration of clopidogrel bisulfate.

At high concentrations *in vitro,* clopidogrel inhibits P450 (2C9). Accordingly, clopidogrel bisulfate may interfere with the metabolism of **phenytoin, tamoxifen, tolbutamide, warfarin, torsemide, fluvastatin,** and many **non-steroidal anti-inflammatory agents,** but there are no data with which to predict the magnitude of these interactions. Caution should be used when any of these drugs is coadministered with clopidogrel bisulfate.

In addition to the above specific interaction studies, patients entered into clinical trials with clopidogrel bisulfate received a variety of concomitant medications including **diuretics, beta-blocking agents, angiotensin converting enzyme inhibitors, calcium antagonists, cholesterol lowering agents, coronary vasodilators, antidiabetic agents** (including **insulin**), **antiepileptic agents, hormone replacement therapy, heparins** (unfractionated and LMWH) and **GPIIb/IIIa antagonists** without evidence of clinically significant adverse interactions. The use of oral anticoagulants, non-study anti-platelet drug and chronic NSAIDS was not allowed in CURE and there are no data on their concomitant use with clopidogrel.

ADVERSE REACTIONS

Clopidogrel bisulfate has been evaluated for safety in more than 17,500 patients, including over 9,000 patients treated for 1 year or more. The overall tolerability of clopidogrel bisulfate in CAPRIE was similar to that of aspirin regardless of age, gender and race, with an approximately equal incidence (13%) of patients withdrawing from treatment because of adverse reactions. The clinically important adverse events observed in CAPRIE and CURE are discussed below.

HEMORRHAGIC

In CAPRIE patients receiving clopidogrel bisulfate, gastrointestinal hemorrhage occurred at a rate of 2.0%, and required hospitalization in 0.7%. In patients receiving aspirin, the corresponding rates were 2.7% and 1.1%, respectively. The incidence of intracranial hemorrhage was 0.4% for clopidogrel bisulfate compared to 0.5% for aspirin.

In CURE, clopidogrel bisulfate use with aspirin was associated with an increase in bleeding compared to placebo with aspirin (see TABLE 4). There was an excess in major bleeding in patients receiving clopidogrel bisulfate plus aspirin compared with placebo plus aspirin, primarily gastrointestinal and at puncture sites. The incidence of intracranial hemorrhage (0.1%), and fatal bleeding (0.2%), was the same in both groups.

In patients receiving both clopidogrel bisulfate and aspirin in CURE, the incidence of bleeding is described in TABLE 4.

TABLE 4 *CURE Incidence of Bleeding Complications*

	Clopidogrel Bisulfate (+ aspirin)* (n=6259)	Placebo (+ aspirin)* (n=6303)	P-value
Major Bleeding†	3.7%‡	2.7%§	0.001
Life-Threatening Bleeding	2.2%	1.8%	0.13
Fatal	0.2%	0.2%	
5 g/dl hemoglobin drop	0.9%	0.9%	
Requiring surgical intervention	0.7%	0.7%	
Hemorrhagic strokes	0.1%	0.1%	
Requiring inotropes	0.5%	0.5%	
Requiring transfusion (≥4 units)	1.2%	1.0%	
Other Major Bleeding	1.6%	1.0%	0.005
Significantly disabling	0.4%	0.3%	
Intraocular bleeding with significant loss of vision	0.05%	0.03%	
Requiring 2-3 units of blood	1.3%	0.9%	
Minor Bleeding¶	5.1%	2.4%	<0.001

* Other standard therapies were used as appropriate.
† Life threatening and other major bleeding.
‡ Major bleeding event rate for clopidogrel bisulfate + aspirin was dose-dependent on aspirin: <100 g=2.6%; 100-200 g=3.5%; >200 g=4.9%.
§ Major bleeding event rate for placebo + aspirin was dose-dependent on aspirin: <100 mg=2.0%; 100-200 mg=2.3%; >200 mg=4.0%.
¶ Led to interruption of study medication.

Ninety-two percent (92%) of the patients in the CURE study received heparin/LMWH, and the rate of bleeding in these patients was similar to the overall results.

There was no excess in major bleeds within 7 days after coronary bypass graft surgery in patients who stopped therapy more than 5 days prior to surgery (event rate 4.4% clopidogrel bisulfate + aspirin; 5.3% placebo + aspirin). In patients who remained on therapy within 5 days of bypass graft surgery, the event rate was 9.6% for clopidogrel bisulfate + aspirin, and 6.3% for placebo + aspirin.

NEUTROPENIA/AGRANULOCYTOSIS

Ticlopidine, a drug chemically similar to clopidogrel bisulfate, is associated with a 0.8% rate of severe neutropenia (less than 450 neutrophils/µl). In CAPRIE severe neutropenia was observed in 6 patients, 4 on clopidogrel bisulfate and 2 on aspirin. Two (2) of the 9599 patients who received clopidogrel bisulfate and none (0) of the 9586 patients who received aspirin had neutrophil counts of zero. One (1) of the 4 clopidogrel bisulfate patients in CAPRIE was receiving cytotoxic chemotherapy, and another recovered and returned to the trial after only temporarily interrupting treatment with clopidogrel bisulfate. In CURE, the numbers of patients with thrombocytopenia (19 clopidogrel bisulfate + aspirin vs 24 placebo + aspirin) or neutropenia (3 vs 3) were similar.

Although the risk of myelotoxicity with clopidogrel bisulfate thus appears to be quite low, this possibility should be considered when a patient receiving clopidogrel bisulfate demonstrates fever or other sign of infection.

GASTROINTESTINAL

Overall, the incidence of gastrointestinal events (*e.g.,* abdominal pain, dyspepsia, gastritis and constipation) in patients receiving clopidogrel bisulfate was 27.1%, compared to 29.8% in those receiving aspirin in the CAPRIE trial. In the CURE trial the incidence of these gastrointestinal events for patients receiving clopidogrel bisulfate + aspirin was 11.7% compared to 12.5% for those receiving placebo + aspirin.

In the CAPRIE trial, the incidence of peptic, gastric or duodenal ulcers was 0.7% for clopidogrel bisulfate and 1.2% for aspirin. In the CURE trial the incidence of peptic, gastric or duodenal ulcers was 0.4% for clopidogrel bisulfate + aspirin and 0.3% for placebo + aspirin.

Cases of diarrhea were reported in the CAPRIE trial in 4.5% of patients in the clopidogrel bisulfate group compared to 3.4% in the aspirin group. However, these were rarely severe (clopidogrel bisulfate=0.2% and aspirin=0.1%). In the CURE trial, the incidence of diarrhea for patients receiving clopidogrel bisulfate + aspirin was 2.1% compared to 2.2% for those receiving placebo + aspirin.

In the CAPRIE trial, the incidence of patients withdrawing from treatment because of gastrointestinal adverse reactions was 3.2% for clopidogrel bisulfate and 4.0% for aspirin. In the CURE trial, the incidence of patients withdrawing from treatment because of gastrointestinal adverse reactions was 0.9% for clopidogrel bisulfate + aspirin compared with 0.8% for placebo + aspirin.

RASH AND OTHER SKIN DISORDERS

In the CAPRIE trial, the incidence of skin and appendage disorders in patients receiving clopidogrel bisulfate was 15.8% (0.7% serious); the corresponding rate in aspirin patients was 13.1% (0.5% serious). In the CURE trial the incidence of rash or other skin disorders in patients receiving clopidogrel bisulfate + aspirin was 4.0% compared to 3.5% for those receiving placebo + aspirin.

In the CAPRIE trial, the overall incidence of patients withdrawing from treatment because of skin and appendage disorders adverse reactions was 1.5% for clopidogrel bisulfate and 0.8% for aspirin. In the CURE trial, the incidence of patients withdrawing because of skin and appendage disorders adverse reactions was 0.7% for clopidogrel bisulfate + aspirin compared with 0.3% for placebo + aspirin.

Adverse events occurring in ≥2.5% of patients on clopidogrel bisulfate in the CAPRIE controlled clinical trial are shown below regardless of relationship to clopidogrel bisulfate. The median duration of therapy was 20 months, with a maximum of 3 years.

TABLE 5 *Adverse Events Occurring in ≥2.5% of Clopidogrel Bisulfate Patients in CAPRIE*

Body System Event	% Incidence (% Discontinuation) Clopidogrel Bisulfate (n=9599)	 Aspirin (n=9586)
Body as Whole — General Disorders		
Chest pain	8.3% (0.2%)	8.3% (0.3%)
Accidental/inflicted injury	7.9% (0.1%)	7.3% (0.1%)
Influenza-like symptoms	7.5% (<0.1%)	7.0% (<0.1%)
Pain	6.4% (0.1%)	6.3% (0.1%)
Fatigue	3.3% (0.1%)	3.4% (0.1%)
Cardiovascular Disorders, General		
Edema	4.1% (<0.1%)	4.5% (<0.1%)
Hypertension	4.3% (<0.1%)	5.1% (<0.1%)
Central and Peripheral Nervous System Disorders		
Headache	7.6% (0.3%)	7.2% (0.2%)
Dizziness	6.2% (0.2%)	6.7% (0.3%)
Gastrointestinal System Disorders		
Abdominal pain	5.6% (0.7%)	7.1% (1.0%)
Dyspepsia	5.2% (0.6%)	6.1% (0.7%)
Diarrhea	4.5% (0.4%)	3.4% (0.3%)
Nausea	3.4% (0.5%)	3.8% (0.4%)
Metabolic and Nutritional Disorders		
Hypercholesterolemia	4.0% (0%)	4.4% (<0.1%)
Musculo-Skeletal System Disorders		
Arthralgia	6.3% (0.1%)	6.2% (0.1%)
Back pain	5.8% (0.1%)	5.3% (<0.1%)
Platelet, Bleeding and Clotting Disorders		
Purpura/bruise	5.3% (0.3%)	3.7% (0.1%)
Epistaxis	2.9% (0.2%)	2.5% (0.1%)
Psychiatric Disorders		
Depression	3.6% (0.1%)	3.9% (0.2%)
Respiratory System Disorders		
Upper resp tract infection	8.7% (<0.1%)	8.3% (<0.1%)
Dyspnea	4.5% (0.1%)	4.7% (0.1%)
Rhinitis	4.2% (0.1%)	4.2% (<0.1%)
Bronchitis	3.7% (0.1%)	3.7% (0%)
Coughing	3.1% (<0.1%)	2.7% (<0.1%)
Skin and Appendage Disorders		
Rash	4.2% (0.5%)	3.5% (0.2%)
Pruritus	3.3% (0.3%)	1.6% (0.1%)
Urinary System Disorders		
Urinary tract infection	3.1% (0%)	3.5% (0.1%)

Incidence of discontinuation, regardless of relationship to therapy, is shown in parentheses.

Adverse events occurring in ≥2.0% of patients on clopidogrel bisulfate in the CURE controlled clinical trial are shown below regardless of relationship to clopidogrel bisulfate.

Other adverse experiences of potential importance occurring in 1% to 2.5% of patients receiving clopidogrel bisulfate in the CAPRIE or CURE controlled clinical trials are listed below regardless of relationship to clopidogrel bisulfate. In general, the incidence of these events was similar to that in patients receiving aspirin (in CAPRIE) or placebo + aspirin (in CURE):

Autonomic nervous system disorders: Syncope, palpitation.
Body as a whole-general disorders: Asthenia, fever, hernia.
Cardiovascular disorders: Cardiac failure.

C

TABLE 6 *Adverse Events Occurring in ≥2.0% of Clopidogrel Bisulfate Patients in CURE*

	% Incidence (% Discontinuation)	
Body System	Clopidogrel Bisulfate (+ aspirin)*	Aspirin (+ aspirin)*
Event	(n=6259)	(n=6303)
Body as a Whole — General Disorders		
Chest pain	2.7% (<0.1%)	2.8% (0.0%)
Central and Peripheral Nervous System Disorders		
Headache	3.1% (0.1%)	3.2% (0.1%)
Dizziness	2.4% (0.1%)	2.0% (<0.1%)
Gastrointestinal System Disorders		
Abdominal pain	2.3% (0.3%)	2.8% (0.3%)
Dyspepsia	2.0% (0.1%)	1.9% (<0.1%)
Diarrhea	2.1% (0.1%)	2.2% (0.1%)

* Other standard therapies were used as appropriate.

Central and peripheral nervous system disorders: Cramps legs, hypoaesthesia, neuralgia, paraesthesia, vertigo.
Gastrointestinal system disorders: Constipation, vomiting.
Heart rate and rhythm disorders: Fibrillation atrial.
Liver and biliary system disorders: Hepatic enzymes increased.
Metabolic and nutritional disorders: Gout, hyperuricemia, non-protein nitrogen (NPN) increased.
Musculo-skeletal system disorders: Arthritis, arthrosis.
Platelet, bleeding and clotting disorders: GI hemorrhage, hematoma, platelets decreased.
Psychiatric disorders: Anxiety, insomnia.
Red blood cell disorders: Anemia.
Respiratory system disorders: Pneumonia, sinusitis.
Skin and appendage disorders: Eczema, skin ulceration.
Urinary system disorders: Cystitis.
Vision disorders: Cataract, conjunctivitis.

Other potentially serious adverse events which may be of clinical interest but were rarely reported (<1%) in patients who received clopidogrel bisulfate in the CAPRIE or CURE controlled clinical trials are listed below regardless of relationship to clopidogrel bisulfate. In general, the incidence of these events was similar to that in patients receiving aspirin (in CAPRIE) or placebo + aspirin (in CURE):

Body as a whole: Allergic reaction, necrosis ischemic.
Cardiovascular disorders: Edema generalized.
Gastrointestinal system disorders: Gastric ulcer perforated, gastritis hemorrhagic, upper GI ulcer hemorrhagic.
Liver and biliary system disorders: Bilirubinemia, hepatitis infectious, liver fatty.
Platelet, bleeding and clotting disorders: Hemarthrosis, hematuria, hemoptysis, hemorrhage intracranial, hemorrhage retroperitoneal, hemorrhage of operative wound, ocular hemorrhage, pulmonary hemorrhage, purpura allergic, thrombocytopenia.
Red blood cell disorders: Anemia aplastic, anemia hypochromic.
Reproductive disorders, female: Menorrhagia.
Respiratory system disorders: Hemothorax.
Skin and appendage disorders: Bullous eruption, rash erythematous, rash maculopapular, urticaria.
Urinary system disorders: Abnormal renal function, acute renal failure.
White cell and reticuloendothelial system disorders: Agranulocytosis, granulocytopenia, leukemia, leukopenia, neutrophils decreased.

POSTMARKETING EXPERIENCE

The following events have been reported spontaneously from worldwide postmarketing experience: fever, very rare cases of hypersensitivity reactions including angioedema, bronchospasms, and anaphylactoid reactions. Suspected thrombotic thrombocytopenic purpura (TTP) has been reported as part of the world-wide postmarketing experience, see WARNINGS.

DOSAGE AND ADMINISTRATION

RECENT MI, RECENT STROKE OR ESTABLISHED PERIPHERAL ARTERIAL DISEASE

The recommended daily dose of clopidogrel bisulfate is 75 mg once daily.

ACUTE CORONARY SYNDROME

For patients with acute coronary syndrome (unstable angina/non-Q-wave MI), clopidogrel bisulfate should be initiated with a single 300 mg loading dose and then continued at 75 mg once daily. Aspirin (75-325 mg once daily) should be initiated and continued in combination with clopidogrel bisulfate. In CURE, most patients with Acute Coronary Syndrome also received heparin acutely.

Clopidogrel bisulfate can be administered with or without food.

No dosage adjustment is necessary for elderly patients or patients with renal disease. (See CLINICAL PHARMACOLOGY, Special Populations.)

HOW SUPPLIED

Plavix (clopidogrel bisulfate) is available as a pink, round, biconvex, film-coated tablet debossed with "75" on one side and "1171" on the other.

Storage: Store at 25°C (77°F); excursions permitted to 15-30°C (59-86°F).

PRODUCT LISTING - EQUIVALENTS NOT AVAILABLE

Tablet - Oral - 75 mg

30's	$96.46	PLAVIX, Allscripts Pharmaceutical Company	54569-4700-00
30's	$126.49	PLAVIX, Bristol-Myers Squibb	63653-1171-06
90's	$260.28	PLAVIX, Bristol-Myers Squibb	63653-1171-10
90's	$379.50	PLAVIX, Bristol-Myers Squibb	63653-1171-01
100's	$289.15	PLAVIX, Bristol-Myers Squibb	63653-1171-30
100's	$421.65	PLAVIX, Bristol-Myers Squibb	63653-1171-03

Clorazepate Dipotassium *(000847)*

Categories: Alcohol withdrawal; Anxiety disorder, generalized; Seizures, partial; DEA Class CIV; FDA Approved 1975 Mar
Drug Classes: Anxiolytics; Benzodiazepines
Brand Names: Gen-Xene; **Tranxene**
Foreign Brand Availability: Ansiospaz (Peru); Anxidin (Finland); Anxielax (Thailand); Audilex (Greece); Covengar (Argentina); Cloramed (Thailand); Clozene (Taiwan); Dipot (Thailand); Disposef (Thailand); Enadine (Argentina); Flulium (Thailand); Justum (Argentina); Manotran (Thailand); Moderane (Argentina); Nansius (Dominican-Republic; Spain); Novo-Clopate (Canada); Sanor (Malaysia); Serene (Thailand); Tencilan (Argentina); Trancon (Thailand); Transene (Italy); Tranxal (Israel); Tranxen (Denmark); Tranxilen (Norway; Sweden); Tranxilium (Argentina; Austria; Germany; Spain; Switzerland; Taiwan); Travex (Slovenia); Zetran-5 (Thailand)
Cost of Therapy: $226.64 (Anxiety; Tranxene; 15 mg; 2 tablets/day; 30 day supply)
$24.28 (Anxiety; Generic Tablets; 15 mg; 2 tablets/day; 30 day supply)

DESCRIPTION

Clorazepate dipotassium is a benzodiazepine. The molecular formula is $C_{16}H_{11}ClK_2N_2O_4$; the molecular weight is 408.92.

It is a fine, light yellow, practically odorless compound insoluble in the common organic solvents, but very soluble in water. Aqueous solutions are unstable, clear, light yellow, and alkaline.

It is available for oral administration as 3.75, 7.5, 11.25, 15, and 22.5 mg tablets.

The inactive ingredients include lactose anhydrous, magnesium stearate, microcrystalline cellulose, polacrilin potassium, silicon dioxide colloidal and talc.

In addition, the following coloring agents are used: *3.75 mg Tablets:* FD&C blue no. 2; *7.5 mg Tablets:* FD&C yellow no. 6; *15 mg Tablets:* FD&C red no. 3.

CLINICAL PHARMACOLOGY

Pharmacologically, clorazepate dipotassium has the characteristics of benzodiazepines. It has depressant effects on the central nervous system (CNS). The primary metabolite, nordiazepam, quickly appears in the blood stream. The serum half-life is about 2 days. The drug is metabolized in the liver and excreted primarily in the urine.

(See also ANIMAL PHARMACOLOGY.)

Studies in healthy men have shown that clorazepate has depressant effects on the central nervous system. Prolonged administration of single daily doses as high as 120 mg was without toxic effects. Abrupt cessation of high doses was followed in some patients by nervousness, insomnia, irritability, diarrhea, muscle aches, or memory impairment.

Absorption — Excretion: After oral administration of clorazepate dipotassium, there is essentially no circulating parent drug. Nordiazepam, its primary metabolite, quickly appears in the blood stream. In 2 volunteers given 15 mg of (50 microcuries) of ^{14}C-clorazepate dipotassium, about 80% was recovered in the urine and feces within 10 days. Excretion was primarily in the urine with about 1% excreted per day on day 10.

INDICATIONS AND USAGE

Clorazepate dipotassium is indicated for the management of anxiety disorders or for the short-term relief of the symptoms of anxiety. Anxiety or tension associated with the stress of everyday life usually does not require treatment with an anxiolytic.

Clorazepate dipotassium is indicated as adjunctive therapy in the management of partial seizures.

The effectiveness of clorazepate in the long-term management of anxiety, that is, for more than 4 months, has not been assessed by systematic clinical studies. Long-term studies in epileptic patients, however, have shown continued therapeutic activity. The physician should reassess periodically the usefulness of the drug for the individual patient.

Clorazepate dipotassium is indicated for the symptomatic relief of acute alcohol withdrawal.

CONTRAINDICATIONS

Clorazepate dipotassium is contraindicated in patients with a known hypersensitivity to the drug, and in those with acute narrow angle glaucoma.

WARNINGS

Clorazepate is not recommended for use in depressive neuroses or in psychotic reactions.

Patients on clorazepate dipotassium should be cautioned against engaging in hazardous occupations requiring mental alertness, such as operating dangerous machinery, including motor vehicles.

Since clorazepate has a CNS depressant effect, patients should be advised against the simultaneous use of other CNS-depressant drugs, and cautioned that the effects of alcohol may be increased.

Because of the lack of sufficient clinical experience, clorazepate dipotassium is not recommended for use in patients less than 9 years of age.

USE IN PREGNANCY

An increased risk of congenital malformations associated with the use of minor tranquilizers (chlordiazepoxide, diazepam, and meprobamate) during the first trimester of pregnancy has been suggested in several studies. Clorazepate, a benzodiazepine derivative, has not been studied adequately to determine whether it, too, may be associated with an increased risk of fetal abnormality. Because use of these drugs is rarely a

matter of urgency, their use during this period should almost always be avoided. The possibility that a woman of childbearing potential may be pregnant at the time of institution of therapy should be considered. Patients should be advised that if they become pregnant during therapy or intend to become pregnant they should communicate with their physician about the desirability of discontinuing the drug.

USAGE DURING LACTATION

Clorazepate dipotassium should not be given to nursing mothers since it has been reported that nordiazepam is excreted in human breast milk.

PRECAUTIONS

In those patients in which a degree of depression accompanies the anxiety, suicidal tendencies may be present and protective measures may be required. The least amount of drug that is feasible should be available to the patients.

Patients on clorazepate for prolonged periods should have blood counts and liver function tests periodically. The usual precautions in treating patients with impaired renal or hepatic function should also be observed.

In elderly or debilitated patients, initial dose should be small, and increments should be made gradually, in accordance with the response of the patient, to preclude ataxia or excessive sedation.

DRUG INTERACTIONS

If clorazepate dipotassium is to be combined with other drugs acting on the CNS, careful consideration should be given to the pharmacology of the agents to be employed. Animal experience indicates that clorazepate prolongs the sleeping time after hexobarbital or after ethyl alcohol, increases the inhibitory effects of chlorpromazine, but does not exhibit monoamine oxidase inhibition. Clinical studies have shown increased sedation with concurrent hypnotic medications. The actions of the benzodiazepines may be potentiated by barbiturates, narcotics, phenothiazines, monoamine oxidase inhibitors or other antidepressants.

If clorazepate dipotassium is used to treat anxiety associated with somatic disease states, careful attention must be paid to possible drug interaction with concomitant medication.

In bioavailability studies with normal subjects, the concurrent administration of antacids at therapeutic levels did not significantly influence the bioavailability of clorazepate.

ADVERSE REACTIONS

The side effect most frequently reported was drowsiness. Less commonly reported (in descending order of occurrence) were: dizziness, various gastrointestinal complaints, nervousness, blurred vision, dry mouth, headache, and mental confusion. Other side effects included insomnia, transient skin rashes, fatigue, ataxia, genitourinary complaints, irritability, diplopia, depression and slurred speech.

There have been reports of abnormal liver and kidney function tests and decrease in hematocrit.

Decrease in systolic blood pressure has been observed.

DOSAGE AND ADMINISTRATION

FOR THE SYMPTOMATIC RELIEF OF ANXIETY

Clorazepate dipotassium T-Tabs tablets are administered orally in divided doses. The usual daily dose is 30 mg. The dose should be adjusted gradually within the range of 15-60 mg daily in accordance with the response of the patient. In elderly or debilitated patients, it is advisable to initiate treatment at a daily dose of 7.5-15 mg.

Clorazepate dipotassium tablets may also be administered in a single dose daily at bedtime; the recommended initial dose is 15 mg. After the initial dose, the response of the patient may require adjustment of subsequent dosage. Lower doses may be indicated in the elderly patient. Drowsiness may occur at the initiation of treatment and with dosage increment.

Clorazepate dipotassium-SD (22.5 mg tablet) may be administered as a single dose every 24 hours. The tablet is intended as an alternative form for the convenience of patients stabilized on a dose of 7.5 mg tablets 3 times a day. Clorazepate dipotassium-SD should not be used to initiate therapy.

Clorazepate dipotassium-SD half strength (11.25 mg tablet) may be administered as a single dose every 24 hours. This tablet is intended as an alternate dosage form for the convenience of patients stabilized on a dose of 3.75 mg tablets 3 times a day. Clorazepate dipotassium-SD half strength should not be used to initiate therapy.

FOR THE SYMPTOMATIC RELIEF OF ACUTE ALCOHOL WITHDRAWAL

The following dosage schedule is recommended (see TABLE 1).

TABLE 1

	Dosage
1st 24 hours (Day 1)	30 mg Clorazepate dipotassium initially; followed by 30-60 mg in divided doses
2nd 24 hours (Day 2)	45-90 mg in divided doses
3rd 24 hours (Day 3)	22.5-45 mg in divided doses
Day 4	15-30 mg in divided doses

Thereafter, gradually reduce the daily dose to 7.5-15 mg. Discontinue drug therapy as soon as patient's condition is stable.

The maximum recommended total daily dose is 90 mg. Avoid excessive reductions in the total amount of drug administered on successive days.

AS AN ADJUNCT TO ANTIEPILEPTIC DRUGS

In order to minimize drowsiness, the recommended initial dosages and dosage increments should not be exceeded.

Adults: The maximum recommended initial dose in patients over 12 years old is 7.5 mg three times a day. Dosage should be increased by no more than 7.5 mg every week and should not exceed 90 mg/day.

Children (9-12 years): The maximum recommended initial dose is 7.5 mg two times a day. Dosage should be increased by no more than 7.5 mg every week and should not exceed 60 mg/day.

ANIMAL PHARMACOLOGY

Studies in rats and monkeys have shown a substantial difference between doses producing tranquilizing, sedative and toxic effects. In rats, conditioned avoidance response was inhibited at an oral dose of 10 mg/kg; sedation was induced at 32 mg/kg; the LD_{50} was 1320 mg/kg. In monkeys, aggressive behavior was reduced at an oral dose of 0.25 mg/kg; sedation (ataxia) was induced at 7.5 mg/kg; the LD_{50} could not be determined because of the emetic effect of large doses, but the LD_{50} exceeds 1600 mg/kg.

Twenty-four (24) dogs were given clorazepate dipotassium orally in a 22 month toxicity study; doses up to 75 mg/kg were given. Drug-related changes occurred in the liver; weight was increased and cholestasis with minimal hepatocellular damage was found, but lobular architecture remained well preserved.

Eighteen (18) rhesus monkeys were given oral doses of clorazepate dipotassium from 3-36 mg/kg daily for 52 weeks. All treated animals remained similar to control animals. Although total leukocyte count remained within normal limits it tended to fall in the female animals on the highest doses.

Examination of all organs revealed no alterations attributable to clorazepate. There was no damage to liver function or structure.

Reproduction Studies: Standard fertility, reproduction, and teratology studies were conducted in rats and rabbits. Oral doses in rats up to 150 mg/kg and in rabbits up to 15 mg/kg produced no abnormalities in the fetuses. Clorazepate dipotassium did not alter the fertility indices or reproductive capacity of adult animals. As expected, the sedative effect of high doses interfered with care of the young by their mothers (see WARNINGS, Use in Pregnancy).

HOW SUPPLIED

Recommended Storage: Store below 25°C (77°F)

PRODUCT LISTING - RATED THERAPEUTICALLY EQUIVALENT

Tablet - Oral - 3.75 mg

7's	$5.02	GENERIC, Prescript Pharmaceuticals	00247-0790-07
14's	$6.69	GENERIC, Prescript Pharmaceuticals	00247-0790-14
30's	$10.49	GENERIC, Prescript Pharmaceuticals	00247-0790-30
50's	$15.27	GENERIC, Prescript Pharmaceuticals	00247-0790-50
100's	$6.38	GENERIC, Interstate Drug Exchange Inc	00814-1620-14
100's	$22.31	GENERIC, Purepac Pharmaceutical Company	00228-2078-10
100's	$23.50	GENERIC, Major Pharmaceuticals Inc	00904-3970-60
100's	$25.18	GENERIC, Moore, H.L. Drug Exchange Inc	00839-7335-06
100's	$26.97	GENERIC, Geneva Pharmaceuticals	00781-1865-01
100's	$30.27	GENERIC, Ivax Corporation	00182-0009-01
100's	$31.95	GENERIC, Martec Pharmaceuticals Inc	52555-0986-01
100's	$38.49	GENERIC, Major Pharmaceuticals Inc	00904-3970-61
100's	$58.85	GENERIC, Alpharma Uspd Makers Of Barre and Nmc	00472-0047-10
100's	$78.47	GENERIC, Aligen Independent Laboratories Inc	00405-0050-01
100's	$83.50	FEDERAL UPPER LIMIT, H.C.F.A. F F P	99999-0847-02
100's	$103.00	GENERIC, Watson Laboratories Inc	52544-0363-01
100's	$118.42	GENERIC, Watson/Rugby Laboratories Inc	52544-0835-01
100's	$128.41	GENERIC, Qualitest Products Inc	00603-3004-21
100's	$128.41	GENERIC, Taro Pharmaceuticals U.S.A. Inc	51672-4042-01
100's	$128.42	GENERIC, Mylan Pharmaceuticals Inc	00378-0030-01
100's	$128.45	GENERIC, Able Laboratories Inc	53265-0048-10
100's	$223.79	TRANXENE T-TAB, Abbott Pharmaceutical	00074-4389-13

Tablet - Oral - 7.5 mg

7's	$5.39	GENERIC, Prescript Pharmaceuticals	00247-0791-07
14's	$7.44	GENERIC, Prescript Pharmaceuticals	00247-0791-14
30's	$12.09	GENERIC, Prescript Pharmaceuticals	00247-0791-30
100's	$7.13	GENERIC, Interstate Drug Exchange Inc	00814-1621-14
100's	$28.03	GENERIC, Purepac Pharmaceutical Company	00228-2081-10
100's	$31.45	GENERIC, Major Pharmaceuticals Inc	00904-3971-60
100's	$31.45	GENERIC, Major Pharmaceuticals Inc	00904-5160-60
100's	$31.95	GENERIC, Watson Laboratories Inc	52544-0364-01
100's	$31.98	GENERIC, Moore, H.L. Drug Exchange Inc	00839-7336-06
100's	$32.47	GENERIC, Prescript Pharmaceuticals	00247-0791-00
100's	$34.27	GENERIC, Geneva Pharmaceuticals	00781-1866-01
100's	$34.95	GENERIC, Ivax Corporation	00182-0010-01
100's	$39.95	GENERIC, Martec Pharmaceuticals Inc	52555-0987-01
100's	$47.52	GENERIC, Major Pharmaceuticals Inc	00904-3971-61
100's	$73.20	GENERIC, Alpharma Uspd Makers Of Barre and Nmc	00472-0049-10
100's	$97.61	GENERIC, Aligen Independent Laboratories Inc	00405-0051-01
100's	$103.88	FEDERAL UPPER LIMIT, H.C.F.A. F F P	99999-0847-05
100's	$159.70	GENERIC, Taro Pharmaceuticals U.S.A. Inc	51672-4043-01
100's	$159.70	GENERIC, Able Laboratories Inc	53265-0049-10
100's	$159.71	GENERIC, Mylan Pharmaceuticals Inc	00378-0040-01
100's	$159.71	GENERIC, Qualitest Products Inc	00603-3005-21
100's	$159.71	GENERIC, Watson Laboratories Inc	52544-0836-01

100's	$278.43	TRANXENE T-TAB, Abbott Pharmaceutical	00074-4390-13
Tablet - Oral - 15 mg			
2's	$4.28	GENERIC, Prescript Pharmaceuticals	00247-0792-02
7's	$6.60	GENERIC, Prescript Pharmaceuticals	00247-0792-07
14's	$9.84	GENERIC, Prescript Pharmaceuticals	00247-0792-14
30's	$17.25	GENERIC, Prescript Pharmaceuticals	00247-0792-30
100's	$40.46	GENERIC, Purepac Pharmaceutical Company	00228-2083-10
100's	$45.35	GENERIC, Moore, H.L. Drug Exchange Inc	00839-7337-06
100's	$45.75	GENERIC, Major Pharmaceuticals Inc	00904-3973-60
100's	$45.75	GENERIC, Major Pharmaceuticals Inc	00904-5159-60
100's	$49.85	GENERIC, Ivax Corporation	00182-0014-01
100's	$49.87	GENERIC, Geneva Pharmaceuticals	00781-1867-01
100's	$59.55	GENERIC, Martec Pharmaceuticals Inc	52555-0988-01
100's	$69.90	GENERIC, Major Pharmaceuticals Inc	00904-3973-61
100's	$99.33	GENERIC, Alpharma Uspd Makers Of Barre and Nmc	00472-0051-10
100's	$132.44	GENERIC, Aligen Independent Laboratories Inc	00405-0052-01
100's	$140.94	FEDERAL UPPER LIMIT, H.C.F.A. F F P	99999-0847-08
100's	$175.00	GENERIC, Watson Laboratories Inc	52544-0365-01
100's	$217.24	GENERIC, Qualitest Products Inc	00603-3006-21
100's	$217.24	GENERIC, Taro Pharmaceuticals U.S.A. Inc	51672-4044-01
100's	$217.25	GENERIC, Mylan Pharmaceuticals Inc	00378-0070-01
100's	$217.25	GENERIC, Watson Laboratories Inc	52544-0837-01
100's	$217.25	GENERIC, Able Laboratories Inc	53265-0050-10
100's	$377.73	TRANXENE T-TAB, Abbott Pharmaceutical	00074-4391-13

PRODUCT LISTING - EQUIVALENTS NOT AVAILABLE

Tablet - Oral - 11.25 mg			
100's	$592.18	TRANXENE SD, Abbott Pharmaceutical	00074-2699-13
Tablet - Oral - 22.5 mg			
100's	$758.41	TRANXENE SD, Abbott Pharmaceutical	00074-2997-13

Clotrimazole *(000848)*

Categories: Candidiasis; Tinea corporis; Tinea cruris; Tinea pedis; Tinea versicolor; Pregnancy Category B; FDA Approved 1975 Feb

Drug Classes: Antifungals, topical; Dermatologics

Brand Names: Gyne-Lotrimin; **Lotrimin**; Mycelex; Mycelex-G

Foreign Brand Availability: Agisten (Israel); Apocanda (Germany); Baby Agisten (Israel); Caginal (Thailand); Canazol (Thailand); Candazole (Singapore); Candespor (South-Africa); Candid (Benin; Burkina-Faso; Ethiopia; Gambia; Ghana; Guinea; Ivory-Coast; Kenya; Liberia; Malawi; Malaysia; Mali; Mauritania; Mauritius; Morocco; Niger; Nigeria; Senegal; Seychelles; Sierra-Leone; Sudan; Tanzania; Tunia; Uganda; Zambia; Zimbabwe); Candid-V3 (Thailand); Candimon (Mexico); Candinox (Thailand); Candizole (South-Africa); Canesten (Australia; Austria; Bahamas; Bahrain; Barbados; Belize; Benin; Bermuda; Bolivia; Bulgaria; Burkina-Faso; Canada; CIS; Colombia; Costa-Rica; Curacao; Cyprus; Czech-Republic; Denmark; Dominican-Republic; Ecuador; Egypt; El-Salvador; England; Ethiopia; Finland; Gambia; Germany; Ghana; Greece; Guatemala; Guinea; Guyana; Honduras; Hong-Kong; Hungary; Indonesia; Iran; Iraq; Ireland; Italy; Ivory-Coast; Jamaica; Jordan; Kenya; Korea; Kuwait; Lebanon; Liberia; Libya; Malawi; Malaysia; Mali; Mauritania; Mauritius; Mexico; Morocco; Netherland-Antilles; Netherlands; New-Zealand; Nicaragua; Niger; Nigeria; Norway; Oman; Panama; Philippines; Portugal; Qatar; Republic-of-Yemen; Saudi-Arabia; Senegal; Seychelles; Sierra-Leone; South-Africa; Spain; Sudan; Surinam; Sweden; Switzerland; Syria; Taiwan; Tanzania; Thailand; Trinidad; Tunia; Uganda; United-Arab-Emirates; Zambia; Zimbabwe); Canesten 1 (China); Canestene (Belgium); Canifug (Germany); Catima (Korea); Chingazol (Thailand); Cinabel (Mexico); Clocreme (New-Zealand); Cloderm (Germany); Clogesten (Philippines); Clomacinvag (Peru); Clomaderm (South-Africa); Clomizol (Dominican-Republic); Clonea (Australia); Clonitia (Indonesia); Clostrin (Japan); Clotrihexal (New-Zealand); Clotrimaderm (Canada; Israel; New-Zealand); Cloxy (Philippines); Clozol (Peru); Clozole (Hong-Kong); Cotren (Malaysia; Thailand); Covospor (South-Africa); Dermasten (Mexico); Dermatin (Bahrain; Cyprus; Egypt; Iran; Iraq; Jordan; Kuwait; Lebanon; Libya; Oman; Qatar; Republic-of-Yemen; Saudi-Arabia; Syria; United-Arab-Emirates); Durafungol (Germany); Elcid (Japan); Empecid (Argentina; Japan); Epicort (Colombia); Esporex (Peru); Factodin (Greece); Fungicip (Bahrain; Cyprus; Egypt; Iran; Iraq; Jordan; Kuwait; Lebanon; Libya; Oman; Qatar; Republic-of-Yemen; Saudi-Arabia; Syria; United-Arab-Emirates); Fungicon (Thailand); Fungiderm (Indonesia); Fungistin (Philippines); Fungizid (New-Zealand); Gino-Lotrimin (Colombia); Gyne-Lotremin (Australia; Hong-Kong); Gyne Lotremin (Indonesia; Malaysia); Gynesol (Philippines); Gyno Canesten (Italy); Gyno-Canestene (Belgium); Holfungin (Germany); Imazol (Germany); Jenamazol (Germany); Kanezin (Taiwan); Krema-Rosa (Bahrain; Cyprus; Egypt; Iran; Iraq; Jordan; Kuwait; Lebanon; Libya; Oman; Qatar; Republic-of-Yemen; Saudi-Arabia; Syria; United-Arab-Emirates); Lotramina (Peru); Lotremin (Malaysia; Singapore); Medizol (Colombia); Micoter (Malaysia); Myco-Hermal (Israel; Singapore; Taiwan); Mycoban (South-Africa); Mycocid (India); Mycoril (Singapore; Taiwan); Mycoril Spray (Hong-Kong); Mycozole (Thailand); Nalbix (Portugal); Oralten Troche (Israel); Pan-Fungex (Portugal); Sastid Anti-Fungal (Singapore); Sinium (India); Panmicol (Argentina); Taon (Japan); Taraten (Thailand); Tinaderm Extra (Australia); Tricloderm (Hong-Kong); Trimadan (Indonesia); Trimaze (South-Africa); Vanesten (Singapore; Thailand); Warimazol (Hong-Kong); Xeraspor V (South-Africa)

Cost of Therapy: $14.83 (Candidiasis; Lotrimin Cream; 1%;15 g; 2 applications/day; variable day supply)
$11.16 (Candidiasis; Mycelex Cream; 1%;15 g; 2 applications/day; variable day supply)
$4.49 (Candidiasis; Generic Cream; 1%;15 g; 2 applications/day; variable day supply)

ORAL

DESCRIPTION

FOR TOPICAL ORAL ADMINISTRATION.

Each Mycelex troche contains 10 mg clotrimazole [1-(o-chloro-α,α-diphenylbenzyl)imidazole], a synthetic antifungal agent, for topical use in the mouth.

The chemical formula is $C_{22}H_{17}ClN_2$.

The troche dosage form is a large, slowly dissolving tablet (lozenge) containing 10 mg of clotrimazole dispersed in dextrose, microcrystalline cellulose, povidone, and magnesium stearate.

CLINICAL PHARMACOLOGY

Clotrimazole is a broad-spectrum antifungal agent that inhibits the growth of pathogenic yeasts by altering the permeability of cell membranes. The action of clotrimazole is fungistatic at concentrations of drug up to 20 µg/ml and may be fungicidal *in vitro* against *Candida albicans* and other species of the genus *Candida* at higher concentrations. No single-step or multiple-step resistance to clotrimazole has developed during successive passages of *Candida albicans* in the laboratory; however, individual organism tolerance has been observed during successive passages in the laboratory. Such *in vitro* tolerance has resolved once the organism has been removed from the antifungal environment.

After oral administration of a 10 mg clotrimazole troche to healthy volunteers, concentrations sufficient to inhibit most species of *Candida* persist in saliva for up to 3 hours following the approximately 30 minutes needed for a troche to dissolve. The long term persistence of drug in saliva appears to be related to the slow release of clotrimazole from the oral mucosa to which the drug is apparently bound. Repetitive dosing at 3 hour intervals maintains salivary levels above the minimum inhibitory concentrations of most strains of *Candida;* however, the relationship between *in vitro* susceptibility of pathogenic fungi to clotrimazole and prophylaxis or cure of infections in humans has not been established.

In another study, the mean serum concentrations were 4.98 ± 3.7 and 3.23 ± 1.4 ng/ml of clotrimazole at 30 and 60 minutes, respectively, after administration as a troche.

INDICATIONS AND USAGE

Clotrimazole troches are indicated for the local treatment of oropharyngeal candidiasis. The diagnosis should be confirmed by a KOH smear and/or culture prior to treatment.

Clotrimazole troches are also indicated prophylactically to reduce the incidence of oropharyngeal candidiasis in patients immunocompromised by conditions that include chemotherapy, radiotherapy, or steroid therapy utilized in the treatment of leukemia, solid tumors, or renal transplantation. There are no data from adequate and well-controlled trials to establish the safety and efficacy of this product for prophylactic use in patients immunocompromised by etiologies other than those listed in the previous sentence. (See DOSAGE AND ADMINISTRATION.)

CONTRAINDICATIONS

Clotrimazole troches are contraindicated in patients who are hypersensitive to any of its components.

WARNINGS

Clotrimazole troches are not indicated for the treatment of systemic mycoses including systemic candidiasis.

PRECAUTIONS

Abnormal liver function tests have been reported in patients treated with clotrimazole troches; elevated SGOT levels were reported in about 15% of patients in the clinical trials. In most cases the elevations were minimal and it was often impossible to distinguish effects of clotrimazole from those of other therapy and the underlying disease (malignancy in most cases). Periodic assessment of hepatic function is advisable particularly in patients with pre-existing hepatic impairment.

Since patients must be instructed to allow each troche to dissolve slowly in the mouth in order to achieve maximum effect of the medication, they must be of such an age and physical and/or mental condition to comprehend such instructions.

CARCINOGENESIS

An 18 month dosing study with clotrimazole in rats has not revealed any carcinogenic effect.

PREGNANCY CATEGORY C

Clotrimazole has been shown to be embryotoxic in rats and mice when given in doses 100 times the adult human dose (in mg/kg), possibly secondary to maternal toxicity. The drug was not teratogenic in mice, rabbits, and rats when given in doses up to 200, 180, and 100 times the human dose.

Clotrimazole given orally to mice from 9 weeks before mating through weaning at a dose 120 times the human dose was associated with impairment of mating, decreased number of viable young, and decreased survival to weaning. No effects were observed at 60 times the human dose. When the drug was given to rats during a similar time period at 50 times the human dose, there was a slight decrease in the number of pups per litter and decreased pup viability.

There are no adequate and well controlled studies in pregnant women. Clotrimazole troches should be used during pregnancy only if the potential benefit justifies the potential risk to the fetus.

PEDIATRIC USE

Safety and effectiveness of clotrimazole in children below the age of 3 years have not been established; therefore, its use in such patients is not recommended.

The safety and efficacy of the prophylactic use of clotrimazole troches in children have not been established.

GERIATRIC USE

Clinical studies of clotrimazole did not include sufficient numbers of subjects aged 65 and over to determine whether they respond differently from younger subjects. Other reported clinical experience has not identified differences in responses between the elderly and younger patients.

ADVERSE REACTIONS

Abnormal liver function tests have been reported in patients treated with clotrimazole troches; elevated SGOT levels were reported in about 15% of patients in the clinical trials (see PRECAUTIONS).

Nausea, vomiting, unpleasant mouth sensations and pruritus have also been reported with the use of the troche.

DOSAGE AND ADMINISTRATION

Clotrimazole troches are administered only as a lozenge that must be slowly dissolved in the mouth. The recommended dose is 1 troche five times a day for 14 consecutive days. Only limited data are available on the safety and effectiveness of the clotrimazole troche after prolonged administration; therefore, therapy should be limited to short term use, if possible.

For prophylaxis to reduce the incidence of oropharyngeal candidiasis in patients immunocompromised by conditions that include chemotherapy, radiotherapy, or steroid therapy utilized in the treatment of leukemia, solid tumors, or renal transplantation, the recommended dose is 1 troche three times daily for the duration of chemotherapy or until steroids are reduced to maintenance levels.

HOW SUPPLIED

MYCELEX TROCHES

Mycelex troches are white discoid, uncoated tablets identified with "Mycelex 10".
Storage: Store below 30°C (86°F). Avoid freezing.

TOPICAL

DESCRIPTION

For Dermatologic Use Only. Not For Ophthalmic Use.

These preparations are also available without a prescription.

Clotrimazole products contain clotrimazole, a synthetic antifungal agent having the chemical name [1-(*o*-Chloro-α,α-diphenylbenzyl)imidazole]; the empirical formula, $C_{22}H_{17}ClN_2$; and a molecular weight of 344.84.

Clotrimazole is an odorless, white crystalline substance. It is practically insoluble in water, sparingly soluble in ether, and very soluble in polyethylene glycol 400, ethanol, and chloroform.

CREAM

Each gram of clotrimazole cream contains 10 mg clotrimazole in vanishing cream base of benzyl alcohol, cetearyl alcohol, cetyl esters wax, octyldodecanol, polysorbate, sorbitan monostearate, and water.
Storage: Store between 2-30°C (36-86°F).

LOTION

Each gram of clotrimazole lotion contains 10 mg clotrimazole dispersed in an emulsion vehicle composed of benzyl alcohol, cetearyl alcohol, cetyl esters wax, octyldodecanol, polysorbate, sodium phosphate, sorbitan monostearate, and water.
Lotion: Store between 2-25°C (36-77°F).

TOPICAL SOLUTION

Each milliliter of clotrimazole topical solution contains 10 mg clotrimazole in a nonaqueous vehicle of PEG.
Storage: Store between 2-30°C (36-86°F).

CLINICAL PHARMACOLOGY

Clotrimazole is a broad-spectrum antifungal agent that is used for the treatment of dermal infections caused by various species of pathogenic dermatophytes, yeasts, and *Malassezia furfur.* The primary action of clotrimazole is against dividing and growing organisms.

In vitro, clotrimazole exhibits fungistatic and fungicidal activity against isolates of *Trichophyton rubrum, Trichophyton mentagrophytes, Epidermophyton floccosum, Microsporum canis,* and *Candida* species, including *Candida albicans.* In general, the *in vitro* activity of clotrimazole corresponds to that of tolnaftate and griseofulvin against the mycelia of dermatophytes *(Trichophyton, Microsporum,* and *Epidermophyton),* and to that of the polyenes (amphotericin B and nystatin) against budding fungi *(Candida).* Using an *in vitro* (mouse) and an *in vitro* (mouse kidney homogenate) testing system, clotrimazole and miconazole were equally effective in preventing the growth of the pseudomycelia and mycelia of *Candida albicans.*

Strains of fungi having a natural resistance to clotrimazole are rare. Only a single isolate of *Candida guilliermondi* has been reported to have primary resistance to clotrimazole.

No single-step or multiple-step resistance to clotrimazole has developed during successive passages of *Candida albicans* and *Trichophyton mentagrophytes.* No appreciable change in sensitivity was detected after successive passages of isolates of *C. albicans, C. krusei,* or *C. pseudotropicalis* in liquid or solid media containing clotrimazole. Also, resistance could not be developed in chemically induced mutant strains of polyene-resistant isolates of *C. albicans.* Slight, reversible resistance was noted in three isolates of *C. albicans* tested by 1 investigator. There is a single report that records the clinical emergence of a *C. albicans* strain with considerable resistance of flucytosine and miconazole, and with cross-resistance to clotrimazole; the strain remained sensitive to nystatin and amphotericin B.

In studies of the mechanism of action, the minimum fungicidal concentration of clotrimazole caused leakage of intracellular phosphorus compounds into the ambient medium with concomitant breakdown of cellular nucleic acids and accelerated potassium efflux. Both these events began rapidly and extensively after addition of the drug.

Clotrimazole appears to be well absorbed in humans following oral administration and is eliminated mainly as inactive metabolites. Following topical and vaginal administration, however, clotrimazole appears to be minimally absorbed.

Six hours after the application of radioactive clotrimazole 1% cream and 1% solution onto intact and acutely inflamed skin, the concentration of clotrimazole varied from 100 μg/cm^3 in the stratum corneum to 0.5-1 μg/cm^3 in the stratum reticulare and 0.1 μg/cm^3 in the subcutis. No measurable amount of radioactivity (≤0.001 μg/ml) was found in the serum within 48 hours after application under occlusive dressing of 0.5 ml of the solution or 0.8 g of the cream. Only 0.5% or less of the applied radioactivity was excreted in the urine.

Following intravaginal administration of 100 mg ^{14}C-clotrimazole vaginal tablets to 9 adult females, an average peak serum level, corresponding to only 0.03 μg equivalents/ml of clotrimazole, was reached 1-2 days after application. After intravaginal administration of 5 g of 1% ^{14}C-clotrimazole vaginal cream containing 50 mg active drug to 5 subjects (1 with candidal colpitis), serum levels corresponding to approximately 0.01 μg equivalents/ml were reached between 8 and 24 hours after application.

INDICATIONS AND USAGE

Prescription clotrimazole cream, lotion and solution 1% products are indicated for the topical treatment of candidiasis due to *Candida albicans* and tinea versicolor due to *Malassezia furfur.*

These formulations are also available as the clotrimazole (cream, lotion, and solution 1%) line of nonprescription products which are indicated for the topical treatment of the following dermal infections: tinea pedis, tinea cruris, and tinea corporis due to *Trichophyton rubrum, Trichophyton mentagrophytes, Epidermophyton floccosum,* and *Microsporum canis.*

CONTRAINDICATIONS

Clotrimazole products are contraindicated in individuals who have shown hypersensitivity to any of their components.

WARNINGS

Clotrimazole products are not for ophthalmic use.

PRECAUTIONS

GENERAL

If irritation or sensitivity develops with the use of clotrimazole, treatment should be discontinued and appropriate therapy instituted.

INFORMATION FOR THE PATIENT

This information is intended to aid in the safe and effective use of this medication. It is not a disclosure of all possible adverse or intended effects.

The Patient Should be Advised To:

- Use the medication for the full treatment time even though the symptoms may have improved. Notify the physician if there is no improvement after 4 weeks of treatment.
- Inform the physician if the area of application shows signs of increased irritation (redness, itching, burning, blistering, oozing) indicative of possible sensitization.
- Avoid sources of infection or reinfection.

LABORATORY TESTS

If there is lack of response to clotrimazole, appropriate microbiological studies should be repeated to confirm the diagnosis and rule out other pathogens before instituting another course of antimycotic therapy.

CARCINOGENESIS, MUTAGENESIS, AND IMPAIRMENT OF FERTILITY

An 18 month oral dosing study with clotrimazole in rats has not revealed any carcinogenic effect.

In tests for mutagenesis, chromosomes of the spermatophores of Chinese hamsters which had been exposed to clotrimazole were examined for structural changes during the metaphase. Prior to testing, the hamsters had received 5 oral clotrimazole doses of 100 mg/kg body weight. The results of this study showed that clotrimazole had no mutagenic effect.

PREGNANCY CATEGORY B

The disposition of ^{14}C-clotrimazole has been studied in humans and animals. Clotrimazole is very poorly absorbed following dermal application or intravaginal administration to humans. (See CLINICAL PHARMACOLOGY.)

In clinical trials, use of vaginally applied clotrimazole in pregnant women in their second and third trimesters has not been associated with ill effects. There are, however, no adequate and well-controlled studies in pregnant women during the first trimester of pregnancy.

Studies in pregnant rats with **intravaginal** doses up to 100 mg/kg have revealed no evidence of harm to the fetus due to clotrimazole.

High **oral** doses of clotrimazole in rats and mice ranging from 50-120 mg/kg resulted in embryotoxicity (possible secondary to maternal toxicity) impairment of mating, decreased litter size and number of viable young and decreased pup survival to weaning. However, clotrimazole was **not** teratogenic in mice, rabbits and rats at oral doses up to 200, 180 and 100 mg/kg, respectively. Oral absorption in the rat amounts to approximately 90% of the administered dose.

Because animal reproduction studies are not always predictive of human response, this drug should be used only if clearly indicated during the first trimester of pregnancy.

NURSING MOTHERS

It is not known whether this drug is excreted in human milk. Because many drugs are excreted in human milk, caution should be exercised when clotrimazole is used by a nursing woman.

PEDIATRIC USE

Safety and effectiveness in children have been established for clotrimazole when used as indicated and in the recommended dosage.

DRUG INTERACTIONS

Synergism or antagonism between clotrimazole and nystatin, or amphotericin B, or flucytosine against strains of *C. albicans* has not been reported.

ADVERSE REACTIONS

The following adverse reactions have been reported in connection with the use of clotrimazole: erythema, stinging, blistering, peeling, edema, pruritus, urticaria, burning, and general irritation of the skin.

DOSAGE AND ADMINISTRATION

Gently massage sufficient clotrimazole into the affected and surrounding skin areas twice a day, in the morning and evening.

Clinical improvement, with relief of pruritus, usually occurs within the first week of treatment with clotrimazole. If the patient shows no clinical improvement after 4 weeks of treatment with clotrimazole, the diagnosis should be reviewed.

Shake well before using.

PRODUCT LISTING - RATED THERAPEUTICALLY EQUIVALENT

Cream - Topical - 1%

Size	Price	Product	NDC
15 gm	$7.85	GENERIC, Qualitest Products Inc	00603-7730-74
15 gm	$7.85	GENERIC, Warrick Pharmaceuticals Corporation	59930-1570-01
15 gm	$8.85	GENERIC, Major Pharmaceuticals Inc	00904-7794-36
15 gm	$9.44	GENERIC, Moore, H.L. Drug Exchange Inc	00839-7836-47
15 gm	$9.93	GENERIC, Taro Pharmaceuticals U.S.A. Inc	51672-1275-01
15 gm	$13.20	GENERIC, Ivax Corporation	00182-5094-51
15 gm	$14.78	LOTRIMIN, Southwood Pharmaceuticals Inc	58016-3045-01
15 gm	$16.21	LOTRIMIN, Schering Corporation	00085-0613-02
15 gm	$18.04	LOTRIMIN, Physicians Total Care	54868-0613-01
30 gm	$13.40	GENERIC, Qualitest Products Inc	00603-7730-78
30 gm	$13.40	GENERIC, Warrick Pharmaceuticals Corporation	59930-1570-02
30 gm	$15.05	GENERIC, Major Pharmaceuticals Inc	00904-7794-31
30 gm	$16.05	GENERIC, Moore, H.L. Drug Exchange Inc	00839-7836-49
30 gm	$17.32	GENERIC, Taro Pharmaceuticals U.S.A. Inc	51672-1275-02
30 gm	$23.69	LOTRIMIN, Southwood Pharmaceuticals Inc	58016-3105-01
30 gm	$27.53	LOTRIMIN, Schering Corporation	00085-0613-05
30 gm	$29.21	LOTRIMIN, Physicians Total Care	54868-0613-02
45 gm	$16.25	GENERIC, Ivax Corporation	00182-5094-60
45 gm	$16.25	GENERIC, Warrick Pharmaceuticals Corporation	59930-1570-03
45 gm	$16.75	GENERIC, Qualitest Products Inc	00603-7730-83
45 gm	$18.75	GENERIC, Major Pharmaceuticals Inc	00904-7794-45
45 gm	$22.33	GENERIC, Taro Pharmaceuticals U.S.A. Inc	51672-1275-06
45 gm	$33.37	LOTRIMIN, Schering Corporation	00085-0613-04
45 gm x 2	$22.25	GENERIC, Warrick Pharmaceuticals Corporation	59930-1570-09
45 gm x 2	$28.38	GENERIC, Taro Pharmaceuticals U.S.A. Inc	51672-1275-07
90 gm	$36.28	LOTRIMIN, Schering Corporation	00085-0613-03

Kit - Vaginal - 100 mg;1%

Size	Price	Product	NDC
1's	$17.51	MYCELEX TWIN PAK, Bayer	00026-3098-22

Solution - Topical - 1%

Size	Price	Product	NDC
10 ml	$1.43	LOTRIMIN, Schering Corporation	00085-0182-02
10 ml	$6.00	GENERIC, Teva Pharmaceuticals Usa	51672-0203-71
10 ml	$7.40	GENERIC, Teva Pharmaceuticals Usa	00093-0248-43
10 ml	$9.48	MYCELEX, Bayer	00026-3092-10
10 ml	$15.52	GENERIC, Taro Pharmaceuticals U.S.A. Inc	51672-1260-03
30 ml	$2.97	LOTRIMIN, Schering Corporation	00085-0182-04
30 ml	$15.52	GENERIC, Teva Pharmaceuticals Usa	00093-0248-31
30 ml	$19.86	MYCELEX, Bayer	00026-3092-30

PRODUCT LISTING - RATED NOT THERAPEUTICALLY EQUIVALENT

Cream - Topical - 1%

Size	Price	Product	NDC
15 gm	$11.16	MYCELEX, Bayer	00026-3091-61
15 gm	$13.50	MYCELEX, Southwood Pharmaceuticals Inc	58016-3192-01
30 gm	$20.28	MYCELEX, Bayer	00026-3091-59
90 gm	$30.66	MYCELEX, Bayer	00026-3091-67

PRODUCT LISTING - EQUIVALENTS NOT AVAILABLE

Cream - Topical - 1%

Size	Price	Product	NDC
15 gm	$5.29	GENERIC, Major Pharmaceuticals Inc	00904-7822-36
15 gm	$5.39	GENERIC, Bergen Brunswig Drug Company	24385-0205-01
15 gm	$5.79	GENERIC, Mckesson Drug Company	49348-0827-69
15 gm	$11.08	GENERIC, Southwood Pharmaceuticals Inc	58016-3503-01
15 gm	$12.00	GENERIC, Pharma Pac	52959-0112-03
15 gm	$12.60	GENERIC, Pharma Pac	52959-0493-15
30 gm	$5.44	GENERIC, Leader Brand Products	37205-0160-10
30 gm	$8.25	GENERIC, Major Pharmaceuticals Inc	00904-7822-31
30 gm	$16.95	GENERIC, Pharma Pac	52959-0112-05
30 gm	$17.80	GENERIC, Pharma Pac	52959-0493-30
45 gm	$16.00	FUNGOID (CLOTRIMAZOLE), Pedinol Pharmacal Inc	00884-2495-45
45 gm	$26.64	GENERIC, Pharma Pac	52959-0493-45

Lotion - Topical - 1%

Size	Price	Product	NDC
30 ml	$31.06	LOTRIMIN, Schering Corporation	00085-0707-02

Lozenge - Oral - 10 mg

Size	Price	Product	NDC
70 x 2	$202.54	MYCELEX TROCHE, Alza	17314-9400-03
70's	$73.26	MYCELEX TROCHE, Bayer	00026-3095-55
70's	$78.26	MYCELEX TROCHE, Bayer	00026-3095-38
70's	$86.78	MYCELEX TROCHE, Physicians Total Care	54868-2498-01
70's	$111.50	MYCELEX TROCHE, Alza	17314-9400-01
70's	$119.14	MYCELEX TROCHE, Alza	17314-9400-02
140's	$133.04	MYCELEX TROCHE, Bayer	00026-3095-56
140's	$157.12	MYCELEX TROCHE, Physicians Total Care	54868-2498-02

Solution - Topical - 1%

Size	Price	Product	NDC
30 ml	$18.00	GENERIC, Pedinol Pharmacal Inc	00884-3197-01

Tablet - Vaginal - 500 mg

Size	Price	Product	NDC
1's	$13.88	MYCELEX-G, Allscripts Pharmaceutical Company	54569-1246-00
1's	$15.38	MYCELEX-G, Physicians Total Care	54868-3047-00
1's	$15.40	MYCELEX-G, Bayer	00026-3097-01

Clozapine *(000851)*

Categories: Schizophrenia; Pregnancy Category B; FDA Approved 1989 Sep
Drug Classes: Antipsychotics
Brand Names: **Clozaril**
Foreign Brand Availability: Clopine (Australia; New-Zealand; Taiwan); Clopsine (Mexico); Elcrit (Germany); Leponex (Austria; Bahrain; Bulgaria; Colombia; Cyprus; Czech-Republic; Denmark; Egypt; Finland; France; Germany; Greece; Hungary; Iran; Iraq; Israel; Jordan; Kuwait; Lebanon; Libya; Mexico; Netherlands; Norway; Oman; Peru; Philippines; Portugal; Qatar; Republic-of-Yemen; Saudi-Arabia; South-Africa; Spain; Sweden; Switzerland; Syria; Turkey; United-Arab-Emirates); Lozapin (India); Lozapine (Israel); Sizopin (India); Zapen (Colombia)
Cost of Therapy: $342.24 (Schizophrenia; Clozaril; 100 mg; 3 tablets/day; 30 day supply)
$285.26 (Schizophrenia; Generic Tablets; 100 mg; 3 tablets/day; 30 day supply)

WARNING

Before prescribing clozapine, the physician should be thoroughly familiar with the details of this prescribing information.

AGRANULOCYTOSIS

BECAUSE OF A SIGNIFICANT RISK OF AGRANULOCYTOSIS, A POTENTIALLY LIFE-THREATENING ADVERSE EVENT, CLOZAPINE SHOULD BE RESERVED FOR USE IN THE TREATMENT OF SEVERELY ILL SCHIZOPHRENIC PATIENTS WHO FAIL TO SHOW AN ACCEPTABLE RESPONSE TO ADEQUATE COURSES OF STANDARD ANTIPSYCHOTIC DRUG TREATMENT.

PATIENTS BEING TREATED WITH CLOZAPINE MUST HAVE A BASELINE WHITE BLOOD CELL (WBC) AND DIFFERENTIAL COUNT BEFORE INITIATION OF TREATMENT AS WELL AS REGULAR WBC COUNTS DURING TREATMENT AND FOR 4 WEEKS AFTER DISCONTINUATION OF TREATMENT.

CLOZAPINE IS AVAILABLE ONLY THROUGH A DISTRIBUTION SYSTEM THAT ENSURES MONITORING OF WBC COUNTS ACCORDING TO THE SCHEDULE DESCRIBED BELOW PRIOR TO DELIVERY OF THE NEXT SUPPLY OF MEDICATION. (SEE WARNINGS.)

SEIZURES

SEIZURES HAVE BEEN ASSOCIATED WITH THE USE OF CLOZAPINE. DOSE APPEARS TO BE AN IMPORTANT PREDICTOR OF SEIZURE, WITH A GREATER LIKELIHOOD AT HIGHER CLOZAPINE DOSES. CAUTION SHOULD BE USED WHEN ADMINISTERING CLOZAPINE TO PATIENTS HAVING A HISTORY OF SEIZURES OR OTHER PREDISPOSING FACTORS. PATIENTS SHOULD BE ADVISED NOT TO ENGAGE IN ANY ACTIVITY WHERE SUDDEN LOSS OF CONSCIOUSNESS COULD CAUSE SERIOUS RISK TO THEMSELVES OR OTHERS. (SEE WARNINGS.)

MYOCARDITIS

ANALYSES OF POSTMARKETING SAFETY DATABASES SUGGEST THAT CLOZAPINE IS ASSOCIATED WITH AN INCREASED RISK OF FATAL MYOCARDITIS, ESPECIALLY DURING, BUT NOT LIMITED TO, THE FIRST MONTH OF THERAPY. IN PATIENTS IN WHOM MYOCARDITIS IS SUSPECTED, CLOZAPINE TREATMENT SHOULD BE PROMPTLY DISCONTINUED. (SEE WARNINGS.)

OTHER ADVERSE CARDIOVASCULAR AND RESPIRATORY EFFECTS

ORTHOSTATIC HYPOTENSION, WITH OR WITHOUT SYNCOPE, CAN OCCUR WITH CLOZAPINE TREATMENT. RARELY, COLLAPSE CAN BE PROFOUND AND BE ACCOMPANIED BY RESPIRATORY AND/OR CARDIAC ARREST. ORTHOSTATIC HYPOTENSION IS MORE LIKELY TO OCCUR DURING INITIAL TITRATION IN ASSOCIATION WITH RAPID DOSE ESCALATION. IN PATIENTS WHO HAVE HAD EVEN A BRIEF INTERVAL OFF CLOZAPINE, *i.e.*, 2 OR MORE DAYS SINCE THE LAST DOSE, TREATMENT SHOULD BE STARTED WITH 12.5 MG ONCE OR TWICE DAILY. (SEE WARNINGS and DOSAGE AND ADMINISTRATION.)

SINCE COLLAPSE, RESPIRATORY ARREST AND CARDIAC ARREST DURING INITIAL TREATMENT HAS OCCURRED IN PATIENTS WHO WERE BEING ADMINISTERED BENZODIAZEPINES OR OTHER PSYCHOTROPIC DRUGS, CAUTION IS ADVISED WHEN CLOZAPINE IS INITIATED IN PATIENTS TAKING A BENZODIAZEPINE OR ANY OTHER PSYCHOTROPIC DRUG. (SEE WARNINGS.)

DESCRIPTION

Clozaril (clozapine), an atypical antipsychotic drug, is a tricyclic dibenzodiazepine derivative, 8-chloro-11-(4-methyl-1-piperazinyl)-5*H*-dibenzo [*b,e*] [1,4] diazepine.

The molecular formula is $C_{18}H_{19}ClN_4$, and the molecular weight is 326.83.

Clozaril is available in pale yellow tablets of 25 and 100 mg for oral administration.

Clozaril 25 and 100 mg tablets:

Active Ingredient: Clozapine is a yellow, crystalline powder, very slightly soluble in water.

Inactive Ingredients: Colloidal silicon dioxide, lactose, magnesium stearate, povidone, starch (corn), and talc.

CLINICAL PHARMACOLOGY

PHARMACODYNAMICS

Clozapine is classified as an 'atypical' antipsychotic drug because its profile of binding to dopamine receptors and its effects on various dopamine mediated behaviors differ from those exhibited by more typical antipsychotic drug products. In particular, although clozapine does interfere with the binding of dopamine at D_1, D_2, D_3 and D_5 receptors, and has a high affinity for the D_4 receptor, it does not induce catalepsy nor inhibit apomorphine-induced stereotypy. This evidence, consistent with the view that clozapine is preferentially more active at limbic than at striatal dopamine receptors, may explain the relative freedom of clozapine from extrapyramidal side effects.

Clozapine also acts as an antagonist at adrenergic, cholinergic, histaminergic and serotonergic receptors.

ABSORPTION, DISTRIBUTION, METABOLISM AND EXCRETION

In man, clozapine tablets (25 and 100 mg) are equally bioavailable relative to a clozapine solution. Following a dosage of 100 mg bid, the average steady state peak plasma concentration was 319 ng/ml (range: 102-771 ng/ml), occurring at the average of 2.5 hours (range: 1-6 hours) after dosing. The average minimum concentration at steady state was 122 ng/ml (range: 41-343 ng/ml), after 100 mg bid dosing. Food does not appear to affect the systemic bioavailability of clozapine. Thus, clozapine may be administered with or without food.

Clozapine is approximately 97% bound to serum proteins. The interaction between clozapine and other highly protein-bound drugs has not been fully evaluated but may be important. (See PRECAUTIONS.)

Clozapine is almost completely metabolized prior to excretion and only trace amounts of unchanged drug are detected in the urine and feces. Approximately 50% of the administered dose is excreted in the urine and 30% in the feces. The demethylated, hydroxylated and N-oxide derivatives are components in both urine and feces. Pharmacological testing has shown the desmethyl metabolite to have only limited activity, while the hydroxylated and N-oxide derivatives were inactive.

The mean elimination half-life of clozapine after a single 75 mg dose was 8 hours (range: 4-12 hours), compared to a mean elimination half-life, after achieving steady state with 100 mg bid dosing, of 12 hours (range: 4-66 hours). A comparison of single-dose and multiple-dose administration of clozapine showed that the elimination half-life increased significantly after multiple dosing relative to that after single-dose administration, suggesting the possibility of concentration dependent pharmacokinetics. However, at steady state, linearly dose-proportional changes with respect to AUC (area under the curve), peak and minimum clozapine plasma concentrations were observed after administration of 37.5, 75, and 150 mg bid.

HUMAN PHARMACOLOGY

In contrast to more typical antipsychotic drugs, clozapine therapy produces little or no prolactin elevation.

As is true of more typical antipsychotic drugs, clinical EEG studies have shown that clozapine increases delta and theta activity and slows dominant alpha frequencies. Enhanced synchronization occurs, and sharp wave activity and spike and wave complexes may also develop. Patients, on rare occasions, may report an intensification of dream activity during clozapine therapy. REM sleep was found to be increased to 85% of the total sleep time. In these patients, the onset of REM sleep occurred almost immediately after falling asleep.

INDICATIONS AND USAGE

Clozapine is indicated for the management of severely ill schizophrenic patients who fail to respond adequately to standard drug treatment for schizophrenia. Because of the significant risk of agranulocytosis and seizure associated with its use, clozapine should be used only in patients who have failed to respond adequately to treatment with appropriate courses of standard drug treatments for schizophrenia, either because of insufficient effectiveness or the inability to achieve an effective dose due to intolerable adverse effects from those drugs. (See WARNINGS.)

The effectiveness of clozapine in a treatment resistant schizophrenic population was demonstrated in a 6 week study comparing clozapine and chlorpromazine. Patients meeting DSM-III criteria for schizophrenia and having a mean BPRS total score of 61 were demonstrated to be treatment resistant by history and by open, prospective treatment with haloperidol before entering into the double-blind phase of the study. The superiority of clozapine to chlorpromazine was documented in statistical analyses employing both categorical and continuous measures of treatment effect.

Because of the significant risk of agranulocytosis and seizure, events which both present a continuing risk over time, the extended treatment of patients failing to show an acceptable level of clinical response should ordinarily be avoided. In addition, the need for continuing treatment in patients exhibiting beneficial clinical responses should be periodically re-evaluated.

NON-FDA APPROVED INDICATIONS

Some investigators have suggested that clozapine may be effective in the treatment of tremor associated with Parkinson's Disease. However this use is not approved by the FDA.

CONTRAINDICATIONS

Clozapine is contraindicated in patients with a previous hypersensitivity to clozapine or any other component of this drug, in patients with myeloproliferative disorders, uncontrolled epilepsy, or a history of clozapine induced agranulocytosis or severe granulocytopenia. As with more typical antipsychotic drugs, clozapine is contraindicated in severe central nervous system depression or comatose states from any cause.

Clozapine should not be used simultaneously with other agents having a well-known potential to cause agranulocytosis or otherwise suppress bone marrow function. The mechanism of clozapine induced agranulocytosis is unknown; nonetheless, it is possible that causative factors may interact synergistically to increase the risk and/or severity of bone marrow suppression.

WARNINGS

GENERAL

BECAUSE OF THE SIGNIFICANT RISK OF AGRANULOCYTOSIS, A POTENTIALLY LIFE-THREATENING ADVERSE EVENT (SEE FOLLOWING), CLOZAPINE SHOULD BE RESERVED FOR USE IN THE TREATMENT OF SEVERELY ILL SCHIZOPHRENIC PATIENTS WHO FAIL TO SHOW AN ACCEPTABLE RESPONSE TO ADEQUATE COURSES OF STANDARD DRUG TREATMENT FOR SCHIZOPHRENIA, EITHER BECAUSE OF INSUFFICIENT EFFECTIVENESS OR THE INABILITY TO ACHIEVE AN EFFECTIVE DOSE DUE TO INTOLERABLE ADVERSE EFFECTS FROM THOSE DRUGS. CONSEQUENTLY, BEFORE INITIATING TREATMENT WITH CLOZAPINE, IT IS STRONGLY RECOMMENDED THAT A PATIENT BE GIVEN AT LEAST 2 TRIALS, EACH WITH A DIFFERENT STANDARD DRUG PRODUCT FOR SCHIZOPHRENIA, AT AN ADEQUATE DOSE, AND FOR AN ADEQUATE DURATION.

PATIENTS WHO ARE BEING TREATED WITH CLOZAPINE MUST HAVE A BASELINE WHITE BLOOD CELL (WBC) AND DIFFERENTIAL COUNT BEFORE INITIATION OF TREATMENT, AND A WBC COUNT EVERY WEEK FOR THE FIRST 6 MONTHS. THEREAFTER, IF ACCEPTABLE WBC COUNTS (WBC greater than or equal to 3000/mm^3, ANC ≥1500/mm^3) HAVE BEEN MAINTAINED DURING THE FIRST 6 MONTHS OF CONTINUOUS THERAPY, WBC COUNTS CAN BE MONITORED EVERY OTHER WEEK. WBC COUNTS MUST BE MONITORED WEEKLY FOR AT LEAST 4 WEEKS AFTER THE DISCONTINUATION OF CLOZAPINE.

CLOZAPINE IS AVAILABLE ONLY THROUGH A DISTRIBUTION SYSTEM THAT ENSURES MONITORING OF WBC COUNTS ACCORDING TO THE SCHEDULE DESCRIBED BELOW PRIOR TO DELIVERY OF THE NEXT SUPPLY OF MEDICATION.

AGRANULOCYTOSIS

Agranulocytosis, defined as an absolute neutrophil count (ANC) of less than 500/mm^3, has been estimated to occur in association with clozapine use at a cumulative incidence at 1 year of approximately 1.3%, based on the occurrence of 15 US cases out of 1743 patients exposed to clozapine during its clinical testing prior to domestic marketing. All of these cases occurred at a time when the need for close monitoring of WBC counts was already recognized. This reaction could prove fatal if not detected early and therapy interrupted. Of the 149 cases of agranulocytosis reported worldwide in association with clozapine use as of December 31, 1989, 32% were fatal. However, few of these deaths occurred since 1977, at which time the knowledge of clozapine induced agranulocytosis became more widespread, and close monitoring of WBC counts more widely practiced. Nevertheless, it is unknown at present what the case fatality rate will be for clozapine induced agranulocytosis, despite strict adherence to the required frequency of monitoring. In the US, under a weekly WBC monitoring system with clozapine, there have been 585 cases of agranulocytosis as of August 21, 1997; 19 were fatal. During this period 150,409 patients received clozapine. A hematologic risk analysis was conducted based upon the available information in the Clozaril National Registry (CNR) for US patients. Based upon a cut-off date of April 30, 1995, the incidence rates of agranulocytosis based upon a weekly monitoring schedule, rose steeply during the first 2 months of therapy, peaking in the third month. Among clozapine patients who continued the drug beyond the third month, the weekly incidence of agranulocytosis fell to a substantial degree, so that by the sixth month the weekly incidence of agranulocytosis was reduced to 3/1000 person-years. After 6 months, the weekly incidence of agranulocytosis declines still further, however, never reaches 0. It should be noted that any type of reduction in the frequency of monitoring WBC counts may result in an increase incidence of agranulocytosis.

Because of the substantial risk for developing agranulocytosis in association with clozapine use, which may persist over an extended period of time, patients must have a blood sample drawn for a WBC count before initiation of treatment with clozapine, and must have subsequent WBC counts done at least weekly for the first 6 months of continuous treatment. If WBC counts remain acceptable (WBC greater than or equal to 3000/mm^3, ANC ≥1500/mm^3) during this period, WBC counts may be monitored every other week thereafter. After the discontinuation of clozapine, weekly WBC counts should be continued for an additional 4 weeks.

If a patient is on clozapine therapy for less than 6 months with no abnormal blood events and there is a break on therapy which is less than or equal to 1 month, then patients can continue where they left off with weekly WBC testing for 6 months. When this 6 month period has been completed, the frequency of WBC count monitoring can be reduced to every other week. If a patient is on clozapine therapy for less than 6 months with no abnormal blood events and there is a break on therapy which is greater than 1 month, then patients should be tested weekly for an additional 6 month period before biweekly testing is initiated. If a patient is on clozapine therapy for less than 6 months and experiences an abnormal blood event as described below but remains a rechallengeable patient [patients cannot be reinitiated on clozapine therapy if WBC counts fall below 2000/mm^3 or the ANC falls below 1000/mm^3 during clozapine therapy], the patient must restart the 6 month period of weekly WBC monitoring at day 0.

If a patient is on clozapine therapy for 6 months or longer with no abnormal blood events and there is a break on therapy which is 1 year or less, then the patient can continue WBC count monitoring every other week if clozapine therapy is reinitiated. If a patient is on clozapine therapy for 6 months or longer with no abnormal blood events and there is a break on therapy which is greater than 1 year, then, if clozapine therapy is reinitiated, the patient must have WBC counts monitored weekly for an additional 6 months. If a patient is on clozapine therapy for 6 months or longer and subsequently has an abnormal blood event, but remains a rechallengeable patient, then the patient must restart weekly WBC count monitoring until an additional 6 months of clozapine therapy has been received. The distribution of clozapine is contingent upon performance of the required blood tests.

Treatment should not be initiated if the WBC count is less than 3500/mm^3, or if the patient has a history of a myeloproliferative disorder, or previous clozapine induced agranulocytosis or granulocytopenia. Patients should be advised to report immediately the appearance of lethargy, weakness, fever, sore throat or any other signs of infection. If, after the initiation of treatment, the total WBC count has dropped below 3500/mm^3 or it has dropped by a substantial amount from baseline, even if the count is above 3500/mm^3, or if immature forms are present, a repeat WBC count and a differential count should be done. A substantial drop is defined as a single drop of 3000 or more in the WBC count or a cumulative drop of 3000 or more within 3 weeks. If subsequent

WBC counts and the differential count reveal a total WBC count between 3000 and 3500/mm³ and an ANC above 1500/mm³, twice weekly WBC counts and differential counts should be performed.

If the total WBC count falls below 3000/mm³ or the ANC below 1500/mm³, clozapine therapy should be interrupted, WBC count and differential should be performed daily, and patients should be carefully monitored for flu-like symptoms or other symptoms suggestive of infection. Clozapine therapy may be resumed if no symptoms of infection develop, and if the total WBC count returns to levels above 3000/mm³ and the ANC returns to levels above 1500/mm³. However, in this event, twice weekly WBC counts and differential counts should continue until total WBC counts return to levels above 3500/mm³.

If the total WBC count falls below 2000/mm³ or the ANC falls below 1000/mm³, bone marrow aspiration should be considered to ascertain granulopoietic status. Protective isolation with close observation may be indicated if granulopoiesis is determined to be deficient. Should evidence of infection develop, the patient should have appropriate cultures performed and an appropriate antibiotic regimen instituted.

Patients whose total WBC counts fall below 2000/mm³, or ANCs below 1000/mm³ during clozapine therapy should have daily WBC count and differential. These patients should not be rechallenged with clozapine. Patients discontinued from clozapine therapy due to significant WBC suppression have been found to develop agranulocytosis upon rechallenge, often with a shorter latency on re-exposure. To reduce the chances of rechallenge occurring in patients who have experienced significant bone marrow suppression during clozapine therapy, a single, national master file will be maintained confidentially.

Except for evidence of significant bone marrow suppression during initial clozapine therapy, there are no established risk factors, based on world-wide experience, for the development of agranulocytosis in association with clozapine use. However, a disproportionate number of the US cases of agranulocytosis occurred in patients of Jewish background compared to the overall proportion of such patients exposed during domestic development of clozapine. Most of the US cases occurred within 4-10 weeks of exposure, but neither dose nor duration is a reliable predictor of this problem. No patient characteristics have been clearly linked to the development of agranulocytosis in association with clozapine use, but agranulocytosis associated with other antipsychotic drugs has been reported to occur with a greater frequency in women, the elderly and in patients who are cachectic or have serious underlying medical illness; such patients may also be at particular risk with clozapine.

To reduce the risk of agranulocytosis developing undetected, clozapine is available only through a distribution system that ensures monitoring of WBC counts according to the schedule described above prior to delivery of the next supply of medication.

EOSINOPHILIA

In clinical trials, 1% of patients developed eosinophilia, which, in rare cases, can be substantial. If a differential count reveals a total eosinophil count above 4000/mm³, clozapine therapy should be interrupted until the eosinophil count falls below 3000/mm³.

SEIZURES

Seizure has been estimated to occur in association with clozapine use at a cumulative incidence at 1 year of approximately 5%, based on the occurrence of 1 or more seizures in 61 of 1743 patients exposed to clozapine during its clinical testing prior to domestic marketing (*i.e.,* a crude rate of 3.5%). Dose appears to be an important predictor of seizure, with a greater likelihood of seizure at the higher clozapine doses used.

Caution should be used in administering clozapine to patients having a history of seizures or other predisposing factors. Because of the substantial risk of seizure associated with clozapine use, patients should be advised not to engage in any activity where sudden loss of consciousness could cause serious risk to themselves or others, *e.g.,* the operation of complex machinery, driving an automobile, swimming, climbing, etc.

MYOCARDITIS

Post-marketing surveillance data from 4 countries that employ hematological monitoring of clozapine-treated patients revealed: 30 reports of myocarditis with 17 fatalities in 205,493 US patients (August 2001); 7 reports of myocarditis with 1 fatality in 15,600 Canadian patients (April 2001); 30 reports of myocarditis with 8 fatalities in 24,108 UK patients (August 2001); 15 reports of myocarditis with 5 fatalities in 8,000 Australian patients (March 1999). These reports represent an incidence of 5.0, 16.3, 43.2, and 96.6 cases per 100,000 patient years, respectively. The number of fatalities represent an incidence of 2.8, 2.3, 11.5, and 32.2 cases per 100,000 patient years, respectively.

The overall incidence rate of myocarditis in patients with schizophrenia treated with antipsychotic agents is unknown. However, for the established market economies (WHO), the incidence of myocarditis is 0.3 cases per 100,000 patient years and the fatality rate is 0.2 cases per 100,000 patient years. Therefore, the rate of myocarditis in clozapine-treated patients appears to be 17-322 times greater than the general population and is associated with an increased risk of fatal myocarditis that is 14-161 times greater than the general population.

The total reports of myocarditis for these 4 countries was 82 of which 51 (62%) occurred within the first month of clozapine treatment, 25 (31%) occurred after the first month of therapy and 6 (7%) were unknown. The median duration of treatment was 3 weeks. Of 5 patients rechallenged with clozapine, 3 had a recurrence of myocarditis. Of the 82 reports, 31 (38%) were fatal and 25 patients who died had evidence of myocarditis at autopsy. These data also suggest that the incidence of fatal myocarditis may be highest during the first month of therapy.

Therefore, the possibility of myocarditis should be considered in patients receiving clozapine who present with unexplained fatigue, dyspnea, tachypnea, fever, chest pain, palpitations, other signs or symptoms of heart failure, or electrocardiographic findings such as ST-T wave abnormalities or arrhythmias. It is not known whether eosinophilia is a reliable predictor of myocarditis. Tachycardia, which has been associated with clozapine treatment, has also been noted as a presenting sign in patients with myocarditis. Therefore, tachycardia during the first month of therapy warrants close monitoring for other signs of myocarditis.

Prompt discontinuation of clozapine treatment is warranted upon suspicion of myocarditis. Patients with clozapine-related myocarditis should not be rechallenged with clozapine.

OTHER ADVERSE CARDIOVASCULAR AND RESPIRATORY EFFECTS

Orthostatic hypotension with or without syncope can occur with clozapine treatment and may represent a continuing risk in some patients. Rarely (approximately 1 case per 3000 patients), collapse can be profound and be accompanied by respiratory and/or cardiac arrest. Orthostatic hypotension is more likely to occur during initial titration in association with rapid dose escalation and may even occur on first dose. In 1 report, initial doses as low as 12.5 mg were associated with collapse and respiratory arrest. When restarting patients who have had even a brief interval off clozapine, *i.e.,* 2 days or more since the last dose, it is recommended that treatment be reinitiated with one-half of a 25 mg tablet (12.5 mg) once or twice daily. (See DOSAGE AND ADMINISTRATION.)

Some of the cases of collapse/respiratory arrest/cardiac arrest during initial treatment occurred in patients who were being administered benzodiazepines; similar events have been reported in patients taking other psychotropic drugs or even clozapine by itself. Although it has not been established that there is an interaction between clozapine and benzodiazepines or other psychotropics, caution is advised when clozapine is initiated in patients taking a benzodiazepine or any other psychotropic drug.

Tachycardia, which may be sustained, has also been observed in approximately 25% of patients taking clozapine, with patients having an average increase in pulse rate of 10-15 bpm. The sustained tachycardia is not simply a reflex response to hypotension, and is present in all positions monitored. Either tachycardia or hypotension may pose a serious risk for an individual with compromised cardiovascular function.

A minority of clozapine treated patients experience ECG repolarization changes similar to those seen with other antipsychotic drugs, including S-T segment depression and flattening or inversion of T waves, which all normalize after discontinuation of clozapine. The clinical significance of these changes is unclear. However, in clinical trials with clozapine, several patients experienced significant cardiac events, including ischemic changes, myocardial infarction, arrhythmias and sudden death. In addition there have been postmarketing reports of congestive heart failure, pericarditis, and pericardial effusions. Causality assessment was difficult in many of these cases because of serious preexisting cardiac disease and plausible alternative causes. Rare instances of sudden death have been reported in psychiatric patients, with or without associated antipsychotic drug treatment, and the relationship of these events to antipsychotic drug use is unknown.

Clozapine should be used with caution in patients with known cardiovascular and/or pulmonary disease, and the recommendation for gradual titration of dose should be carefully observed.

NEUROLEPTIC MALIGNANT SYNDROME (NMS)

A potentially fatal symptom complex sometimes referred to as Neuroleptic Malignant Syndrome (NMS) has been reported in association with antipsychotic drugs. Clinical manifestations of NMS are hyperpyrexia, muscle rigidity, altered mental status and evidence of autonomic instability (irregular pulse or blood pressure, tachycardia, diaphoresis, and cardiac dysrhythmias).

The diagnostic evaluation of patients with this syndrome is complicated. In arriving at a diagnosis, it is important to identify cases where the clinical presentation includes both serious medical illness (*e.g.,* pneumonia, systemic infection, etc.) and untreated or inadequately treated extrapyramidal signs and symptoms (EPS). Other important considerations in the differential diagnosis include central anticholinergic toxicity, heat stroke, drug fever and primary central nervous system (CNS) pathology.

The management of NMS should include (1) immediate discontinuation of antipsychotic drugs and other drugs not essential to concurrent therapy, (2) intensive symptomatic treatment and medical monitoring, and (3) treatment of any concomitant serious medical problems for which specific treatments are available. There is no general agreement about specific pharmacological treatment regimens for uncomplicated NMS.

If a patient requires antipsychotic drug treatment after recovery from NMS, the potential reintroduction of drug therapy should be carefully considered. The patient should be carefully monitored, since recurrences of NMS have been reported.

There have been several reported cases of NMS in patients receiving clozapine alone or in combination with lithium or other CNS-active agents.

TARDIVE DYSKINESIA

A syndrome consisting of potentially irreversible, involuntary, dyskinetic movements may develop in patients treated with antipsychotic drugs. Although the prevalence of the syndrome appears to be highest among the elderly, especially elderly women, it is impossible to rely upon prevalence estimates to predict, at the inception of treatment, which patients are likely to develop the syndrome.

There are several reasons for predicting that clozapine may be different from other antipsychotic drugs in its potential for inducing tardive dyskinesia, including the preclinical finding that it has a relatively weak dopamine-blocking effect and the clinical finding of a virtual absence of certain acute extrapyramidal symptoms, *e.g.,* dystonia. A few cases of tardive dyskinesia have been reported in patients on clozapine who had been previously treated with other antipsychotic agents, so that a causal relationship cannot be established. There have been no reports of tardive dyskinesia directly attributable to clozapine alone. Nevertheless, it cannot be concluded, without more extended experience, that clozapine is incapable of inducing this syndrome.

Both the risk of developing the syndrome and the likelihood that it will become irreversible are believed to increase as the duration of treatment and the total cumulative dose of antipsychotic drugs administered to the patient increase. However, the syndrome can develop, although much less commonly, after relatively brief treatment periods at low doses. There is no known treatment for established cases of tardive dyskinesia, although the syndrome may remit, partially or completely, if antipsychotic drug treatment is withdrawn. Antipsychotic drug treatment, itself, however, may suppress (or partially suppress) the signs and symptoms of the syndrome and thereby may possibly mask the underlying process. The effect that symptom suppression has upon the long-term course of the syndrome is unknown.

Given these considerations, clozapine should be prescribed in a manner that is most likely to minimize the occurrence of tardive dyskinesia. As with any antipsychotic drug, chronic clozapine use should be reserved for patients who appear to be obtaining substantial benefit from the drug. In such patients, the smallest dose and the shortest duration of treatment should be sought. The need for continued treatment should be reassessed periodically.

If signs and symptoms of tardive dyskinesia appear in a patient on clozapine, drug discontinuation should be considered. However, some patients may require treatment with clozapine despite the presence of the syndrome.

PRECAUTIONS

GENERAL

Because of the significant risk of agranulocytosis and seizure, both of which present a continuing risk over time, the extended treatment of patients failing to show an acceptable level of clinical response should ordinarily be avoided. In addition, the need for continuing treatment in patients exhibiting beneficial clinical responses should be periodically re-evaluated. Although it is not known whether the risk would be increased, it is prudent either to avoid clozapine or use it cautiously in patients with a previous history of agranulocytosis induced by other drugs.

CARDIOMYOPATHY

Cases of cardiomyopathy have been reported in patients treated with clozapine. The reporting rate for cardiomyopathy in clozapine-treated patients in the US (8.9/100,000 person-years) was similar to an estimate of the cardiomyopathy incidence in the US general population derived from the 1999 National Hospital Discharge Survey data (9.7/100,000 person-years). Approximately 80% of clozapine-treated patients in whom cardiomyopathy was reported were less than 50 years of age; the duration of treatment with clozapine prior to cardiomyopathy diagnosis varied, but was >6 months in 65% of the reports. Dilated cardiomyopathy was most frequently reported, although a large percentage of reports did not specify the type of cardiomyopathy. Signs and symptoms suggestive of cardiomyopathy, particularly exertional dyspnea, fatigue, orthopnea, paroxysmal nocturnal dyspnea, and peripheral edema should alert the clinician to perform further investigations. If the diagnosis of cardiomyopathy is confirmed, the prescriber should discontinue clozapine unless the benefit to the patients clearly outweighs the risk.

FEVER

During clozapine therapy, patients may experience transient temperature elevations above 38°C (100.4°F), with the peak incidence within the first 3 weeks of treatment. While this fever is generally benign and self limiting, it may necessitate discontinuing patients from treatment. On occasion, there may be an associated increase or decrease in WBC count. Patients with fever should be carefully evaluated to rule out the possibility of an underlying infectious process or the development of agranulocytosis. In the presence of high fever, the possibility of Neuroleptic Malignant Syndrome (NMS) must be considered. There have been several reports of NMS in patients receiving clozapine, usually in combination with lithium or other CNS-active drugs. [See WARNINGS, Neuroleptic Malignant Syndrome (NMS).]

PULMONARY EMBOLISM

The possibility of pulmonary embolism should be considered in patients receiving clozapine who present with deep vein thrombosis, acute dyspnea, chest pain or with other respiratory signs and symptoms. As of December 31, 1993 there were 18 cases of fatal pulmonary embolism in association with clozapine therapy in users 10-54 years of age. Based upon the extent of use observed in the Clozaril National Registry, the mortality rate associated with pulmonary embolus was 1 death per 3450 person-years of use. This rate was about 27.5 times higher than that in the general population of a similar age and gender (95% Confidence Interval; 17.1, 42.2). Deep vein thrombosis has also been observed in association with clozapine therapy. Whether pulmonary embolus can be attributed to clozapine or some characteristic(s) of its users is not clear, but the occurrence of deep vein thrombosis or respiratory symptomatology should suggest its presence.

HYPERGLYCEMIA

Severe hyperglycemia, sometimes leading to ketoacidosis, has been reported during clozapine treatment in patients with no prior history of hyperglycemia. While a causal relationship to clozapine use has not been definitively established, glucose levels normalized in most patients after discontinuation of clozapine, and a rechallenge in 1 patient produced a recurrence of hyperglycemia. The effect of clozapine on glucose metabolism in patients with diabetes mellitus has not been studied. The possibility of impaired glucose tolerance should be considered in patients receiving clozapine who develop symptoms of hyperglycemia, such as polydipsia, polyuria, polyphagia, and weakness. In patients with significant treatment-emergent hyperglycemia, the discontinuation of clozapine should be considered.

HEPATITIS

Caution is advised in patients using clozapine who have concurrent hepatic disease. Hepatitis has been reported in both patients with normal and pre-existing liver function abnormalities. In patients who develop nausea, vomiting, and/or anorexia during clozapine treatment, liver function tests should be performed immediately. If the elevation of these values is clinically relevant or if symptoms of jaundice occur, treatment with clozapine should be discontinued.

ANTICHOLINERGIC TOXICITY

Eye

Clozapine has potent anticholinergic effects and care should be exercised in using this drug in the presence of narrow angle glaucoma.

Gastrointestinal

Clozapine use has been associated with varying degrees of impairment of intestinal peristalsis, ranging from constipation to intestinal obstruction, fecal impaction and paralytic ileus (see ADVERSE REACTIONS). On rare occasions, these cases have been fatal. Constipation should be initially treated by ensuring adequate hydration, and use of ancillary therapy such as bulk laxatives. Consultation with a gastroenterologist is advisable in more serious cases.

Prostate

Clozapine has potent anticholinergic effects and care should be exercised in using this drug in the presence of prostatic enlargement.

INTERFERENCE WITH COGNITIVE AND MOTOR PERFORMANCE

Because of initial sedation, clozapine may impair mental and/or physical abilities, especially during the first few days of therapy. The recommendations for gradual dose escalation should be carefully adhered to, and patients cautioned about activities requiring alertness.

USE IN PATIENTS WITH CONCOMITANT ILLNESS

Clinical experience with clozapine in patients with concomitant systemic diseases is limited. Nevertheless, caution is advisable in using clozapine in patients with renal or cardiac disease.

USE IN PATIENTS UNDERGOING GENERAL ANESTHESIA

Caution is advised in patients being administered general anesthesia because of the CNS effects of clozapine. Check with the anesthesiologist regarding continuation of clozapine therapy in a patient scheduled for surgery.

INFORMATION FOR THE PATIENT

Physicians are advised to discuss the following issues with patients for whom they prescribe clozapine:

Patients who are to receive clozapine should be warned about the significant risk of developing agranulocytosis. They should be informed that weekly blood tests are required for the first 6 months, if acceptable WBC counts (WBC greater than or equal to 3000/mm^3, ANC $\geq$1500/mm^3) have been maintained during the first 6 months of continuous therapy, then WBC counts can be monitored every other week in order to monitor for the occurrence of agranulocytosis, and that clozapine tablets will be made available only through a special program designed to ensure the required blood monitoring. Patients should be advised to report immediately the appearance of lethargy, weakness, fever, sore throat, malaise, mucous membrane ulceration or other possible signs of infection. Particular attention should be paid to any flu-like complaints or other symptoms that might suggest infection.

Patients should be informed of the significant risk of seizure during clozapine treatment, and they should be advised to avoid driving and any other potentially hazardous activity while taking clozapine.

Patients should be advised of the risk of orthostatic hypotension, especially during the period of initial dose titration.

Patients should be informed that if they stop taking clozapine for more than 2 days, they should not restart their medication at the same dosage, but should contact their physician for dosing instructions.

Patients should notify their physician if they are taking, or plan to take, any prescription or over-the-counter drugs or alcohol.

Patients should notify their physician if they become pregnant or intend to become pregnant during therapy.

Patients should not breast feed an infant if they are taking clozapine.

CARCINOGENESIS, MUTAGENESIS, AND IMPAIRMENT OF FERTILITY

No carcinogenic potential was demonstrated in long-term studies in mice and rats at doses approximately 7 times the typical human dose on a mg/kg basis. Fertility in male and female rats was not adversely affected by clozapine. Clozapine did not produce genotoxic or mutagenic effects when assayed in appropriate bacterial and mammalian tests.

PREGNANCY CATEGORY B

Reproduction studies have been performed in rats and rabbits at doses of approximately 2-4 times the human dose and have revealed no evidence of impaired fertility or harm to the fetus due to clozapine. There are, however, no adequate and well-controlled studies in pregnant women. Because animal reproduction studies are not always predictive of human response, and in view of the desirability of keeping the administration of all drugs to a minimum during pregnancy, this drug should be used only if clearly needed.

NURSING MOTHERS

Animal studies suggest that clozapine may be excreted in breast milk and have an effect on the nursing infant. Therefore, women receiving clozapine should not breast feed.

PEDIATRIC USE

Safety and effectiveness in pediatric patients have not been established.

GERIATRIC USE

Clinical studies of clozapine did not include sufficient numbers of subjects age 65 and over to determine whether they respond differently from younger subjects.

Orthostatic hypotension can occur with clozapine treatment and tachycardia, which may be sustained, has been observed in about 25% of patients taking clozapine (see WARNINGS, Other Adverse Cardiovascular and Respiratory Effects). Elderly patients, particularly those with compromised cardiovascular functioning, may be more susceptible to these effects.

Also, elderly patients may be particularly susceptible to the anticholinergic effects of clozapine, such as urinary retention and constipation. (See Anticholinergic Toxicity.)

Dose selection for an elderly patient should be cautious, reflecting the greater frequency of decreased hepatic, renal, or cardiac function, and of concomitant disease or other drug therapy. Other reported clinical experience does suggest that the prevalence of tardive dyskinesia appears to be highest among the elderly, especially elderly women. (See WARNINGS, Tardive Dyskinesia.)

DRUG INTERACTIONS

The risks of using clozapine in combination with other drugs have not been systematically evaluated.

C

PHARMACODYNAMIC-RELATED INTERACTIONS

The mechanism of clozapine induced agranulocytosis is unknown; nonetheless, the possibility that causative factors may interact synergistically to increase the risk and/or severity of bone marrow suppression warrants consideration. Therefore, clozapine should not be used with other agents having a well-known potential to suppress bone marrow function.

Given the primary CNS effects of clozapine, caution is advised in using it concomitantly with other CNS-active drugs or alcohol.

Orthostatic hypotension in patients taking clozapine can, in rare cases (approximately 1 case per 3000 patients), be accompanied by profound collapse and respiratory and/or cardiac arrest. Some of the cases of collapse/respiratory arrest/cardiac arrest during initial treatment occurred in patients who were being administered benzodiazepines; similar events have been reported in patients taking other psychotropic drugs or even clozapine by itself. Although it has not been established that there is an interaction between clozapine and benzodiazepines or other psychotropics, caution is advised when clozapine is initiated in patients taking a benzodiazepine or any other psychotropic drug.

Clozapine may potentiate the hypotensive effects of antihypertensive drugs and the anticholinergic effects of atropine-type drugs. The administration of epinephrine should be avoided in the treatment of drug induced hypotension because of a possible reverse epinephrine effect.

PHARMACOKINETIC-RELATED INTERACTIONS

Clozapine is a substrate for many CYP 450 isozymes, in particular 1A2, 2D6, and 3A4. The risk of metabolic interactions caused by an effect on an individual isoform is therefore minimized. Nevertheless, caution should be used in patients receiving concomitant treatment with other drugs which are either inhibitors or inducers of these enzymes.

Concomitant administration of drugs known to induce cytochrome P450 enzymes may decrease the plasma levels of clozapine. Phenytoin, nicotine, and rifampin may decrease clozapine plasma levels, resulting in a decrease in effectiveness of a previously effective clozapine dose.

Concomitant administration of drugs known to inhibit the activity of cytochrome P450 isozymes may increase the plasma levels of clozapine. Cimetidine, caffeine, and erythromycin may increase plasma levels of clozapine, potentially resulting in adverse effects. Although concomitant use of clozapine and carbamazepine is not recommended, it should be noted that discontinuation of concomitant carbamazepine administration may result in an increase in clozapine plasma levels.

In a study of schizophrenic patients who received clozapine under steady state conditions, fluvoxamine or paroxetine was added in 16 and 14 patients, respectively. After 14 days of co-administration, mean trough concentrations of clozapine and its metabolites, *N*-desmethylclozapine and clozapine *N*-oxide, were elevated with fluvoxamine by about 3-fold compared to baseline concentrations. Paroxetine produced only minor changes in the levels of clozapine and its metabolites. However, other published reports describe modest elevations (less than 2-fold) of clozapine and metabolite concentrations when clozapine was taken with paroxetine, fluoxetine, and sertraline. Therefore, such combined treatment should be approached with caution and patients should be monitored closely when clozapine is combined with these drugs, particularly with fluvoxamine. A reduced clozapine dose should be considered.

A subset (3-10%) of the population has reduced activity of certain drug metabolizing enzymes such as the cytochrome P450 isozyme P450 2D6. Such individuals are referred to as "poor metabolizers" of drugs such as debrisoquin, dextromethorphan, the tricyclic antidepressants, and clozapine. These individuals may develop higher than expected plasma concentrations of clozapine when given usual doses. In addition, certain drugs that are metabolized by this isozyme, including many antidepressants (clozapine, selective serotonin reuptake inhibitors, and others), may inhibit the activity of this isozyme, and thus may make normal metabolizers resemble poor metabolizers with regard to concomitant therapy with other drugs metabolized by this enzyme system, leading to drug interaction.

Concomitant use of clozapine with other drugs metabolized by cytochrome P450 2D6 may require lower doses than usually prescribed for either clozapine or the other drug. Therefore, co-administration of clozapine with other drugs that are metabolized by this isozyme, including antidepressants, phenothiazines, carbamazepine, and Type 1C antiarrhythmics (*e.g.*, propafenone, flecainide and encainide), or that inhibit this enzyme (*e.g.*, quinidine), should be approached with caution.

ADVERSE REACTIONS

ASSOCIATED WITH DISCONTINUATION OF TREATMENT

Sixteen percent (16%) of 1080 patients who received clozapine in premarketing clinical trials discontinued treatment due to an adverse event, including both those that could be reasonably attributed to clozapine treatment and those that might more appropriately be considered intercurrent illness. The more common events considered to be causes of discontinuation included: CNS, primarily drowsiness/sedation, seizures, dizziness/syncope; cardiovascular, primarily tachycardia, hypotension and ECG changes; gastrointestinal, primarily nausea/vomiting; hematologic, primarily leukopenia/granulocytopenia/agranulocytosis; and fever. None of the events enumerated accounts for more than 1.7% of all discontinuations attributed to adverse clinical events.

COMMONLY OBSERVED

Adverse events observed in association with the use of clozapine in clinical trials at an incidence of greater than 5% were: central nervous system complaints, including drowsiness/sedation, dizziness/vertigo, headache and tremor; autonomic nervous system complaints, including salivation, sweating, dry mouth and visual disturbances; cardiovascular findings, including tachycardia, hypotension and syncope; and gastrointestinal complaints, including constipation and nausea; and fever. Complaints of drowsiness/sedation tend to subside with continued therapy or dose reduction. Salivation may be profuse, especially during sleep, but may be diminished with dose reduction.

INCIDENCE IN CLINICAL TRIALS

TABLE 1 enumerates adverse events that occurred at a frequency of 1% or greater among clozapine patients who participated in clinical trials. These rates are not adjusted for duration of exposure.

TABLE 1 *Treatment-Emergent Adverse Experience Incidence Among Patients Taking Clozapine in Clinical Trials (n=842)*

Body System/Adverse Event*	Percent
Central Nervous System	
Drowsiness/sedation	39%
Dizziness/vertigo	19%
Headache	7%
Tremor	6%
Syncope	6%
Disturbed sleep/nightmares	4%
Restlessness	4%
Hypokinesia/akinesia	4%
Agitation	4%
Seizures (convulsions)	3%†
Rigidity	3%
Akathisia	3%
Confusion	3%
Fatigue	2%
Insomnia	2%
Hyperkinesia	1%
Weakness	1%
Lethargy	1%
Ataxia	1%
Slurred speech	1%
Depression	1%
Epileptiform movements/myoclonic jerks	1%
Anxiety	1%
Cardiovascular	
Tachycardia	25%†
Hypotension	9%
Hypertension	4%
Chest pain/angina	1%
ECG change/cardiac abnormality	1%
Gastrointestinal	
Constipation	14%
Nausea	5%
Abdominal discomfort/heartburn	4%
Nausea/vomiting	3%
Vomiting	3%
Diarrhea	2%
Liver test abnormality	1%
Anorexia	1%
Urogenital	
Urinary abnormalities	2%
Incontinence	1%
Abnormal ejaculation	1%
Urinary urgency/frequency	1%
Urinary retention	1%
Autonomic Nervous System	
Salivation	31%
Sweating	6%
Dry mouth	6%
Visual disturbances	5%
Integumentary (skin)	
Rash	2%
Musculoskeletal	
Muscle weakness	1%
Pain (back, neck, legs)	1%
Muscle spasm	1%
Muscle pain, ache	1%
Respiratory	
Throat discomfort	1%
Dyspnea, shortness of breath	1%
Nasal congestion	1%
Hemic/Lymphatic	
Leukopenia/decreased WBC/neutropenia	3%
Agranulocytosis	1%†
Eosinophilia	1%
Miscellaneous	
Fever	5%
Weight gain	4%
Tongue numb/sore	1%

* Events reported by at least 1% of clozapine patients are included.
† Rate based on population of approximately 1700 exposed during premarket clinical evaluation of clozapine.

OTHER EVENTS OBSERVED DURING THE PREMARKETING EVALUATION OF CLOZAPINE

This section reports additional, less frequent adverse events which occurred among the patients taking clozapine in clinical trials. Various adverse events were reported as part of the total experience in these clinical studies; a causal relationship to clozapine treatment cannot be determined in the absence of appropriate controls in some of the studies. TABLE 1 enumerates adverse events that occurred at a frequency of at least 1% of patients treated with clozapine. The list below includes all additional adverse experiences reported as being temporally associated with the use of the drug which occurred at a frequency less than 1%, enumerated by organ system.

Central Nervous System: Loss of speech, amentia, tics, poor coordination, delusions/hallucinations, involuntary movement, stuttering, dysarthria, amnesia/memory loss, histrionic movements, libido increase or decrease, paranoia, shakiness, Parkinsonism, and irritability.

Cardiovascular System: Edema, palpitations, phlebitis/thrombophlebitis, cyanosis, premature ventricular contraction, bradycardia, and nose bleed.

Gastrointestinal System: Abdominal distention, gastroenteritis, rectal bleeding, nervous stomach, abnormal stools, hematemesis, gastric ulcer, bitter taste, and eructation.

Urogenital System: Dysmenorrhea, impotence, breast pain/discomfort, and vaginal itch/infection.

Autonomic Nervous System: Numbness, polydypsia, hot flashes, dry throat, and mydriasis.

Integumentary (skin): Pruritus, pallor, eczema, erythema, bruise, dermatitis, petechiae, and urticaria.

Musculoskeletal System: Twitching and joint pain.

Respiratory System: Coughing, pneumonia/pneumonia-like symptoms, rhinorrhea, hyperventilation, wheezing, bronchitis, laryngitis, and sneezing.

Hemic and Lymphatic System: Anemia and leukocytosis.

Miscellaneous: Chills/chills with fever, malaise, appetite increase, ear disorder, hypothermia, eyelid disorder, bloodshot eyes, and nystagmus.

POSTMARKETING CLINICAL EXPERIENCE

Postmarketing experience has shown an adverse experience profile similar to that presented above. Voluntary reports of adverse events temporally associated with clozapine not mentioned above that have been received since market introduction and that may have no causal relationship with the drug include the following:

Central Nervous System: Delirium; EEG abnormal; exacerbation of psychosis; myoclonus; overdose; paresthesia; possible mild cataplexy; and status epilepticus.

Cardiovascular System: Atrial or ventricular fibrillation and periorbital edema.

Gastrointestinal System: Acute pancreatitis; dysphagia; fecal impaction; intestinal obstruction/paralytic ileus; and salivary gland swelling.

Hepatobiliary System: Cholestasis; hepatitis; jaundice.

Hepatic System: Cholestasis.

Urogenital System: Acute interstitial nephritis and priapism.

Integumentary (skin): Hypersensitivity reactions: Photosensitivity, vasculitis, erythema multiforme, and Stevens-Johnson syndrome.

Musculoskeletal System: Myasthenic syndrome and rhabdomyolysis.

Respiratory System: Aspiration and pleural effusion.

Hemic and Lymphatic System: Deep vein thrombosis; elevated hemoglobin/hematocrit; ESR increased; pulmonary embolism; sepsis; thrombocytosis; and thrombocytopenia.

Vision Disorders: Narrow angle glaucoma.

Miscellaneous: CPK elevation; hyperglycemia; hyperuricemia; hyponatremia; and weight loss.

DOSAGE AND ADMINISTRATION

Upon initiation of clozapine therapy, up to a 1 week supply of additional clozapine tablets may be provided to the patient to be held for emergencies (*e.g.*, weather, holidays).

INITIAL TREATMENT

It is recommended that treatment with clozapine begin with one-half of a 25 mg tablet (12.5 mg) once or twice daily and then be continued with daily dosage increments of 25-50 mg/day, if well-tolerated, to achieve a target dose of 300-450 mg/day by the end of 2 weeks. Subsequent dosage increments should be made no more than once or twice weekly, in increments not to exceed 100 mg. Cautious titration and a divided dosage schedule are necessary to minimize the risks of hypotension, seizure, and sedation.

In the multicenter study that provides primary support for the effectiveness of clozapine in patients resistant to standard drug treatment for schizophrenia, patients were titrated during the first 2 weeks up to a maximum dose of 500 mg/day, on a tid basis, and were then dosed in a total daily dose range of 100-900 mg/day, on a tid basis thereafter, with clinical response and adverse effects as guides to correct dosing.

THERAPEUTIC DOSE ADJUSTMENT

Daily dosing should continue on a divided basis as an effective and tolerable dose level is sought. While many patients may respond adequately at doses between 300-600 mg/day, it may be necessary to raise the dose to the 600-900 mg/day range to obtain an acceptable response. [Note: In the multicenter study providing the primary support for the superiority of clozapine in treatment resistant patients, the mean and median clozapine doses were both approximately 600 mg/day.]

Because of the possibility of increased adverse reactions at higher doses, particularly seizures, patients should ordinarily be given adequate time to respond to a given dose level before escalation to a higher dose is contemplated. Clozapine can cause EEG changes, including the occurrence of spike and wave complexes. It lowers the seizures threshold in a dose-dependent manner and may induce myoclonic jerks or generalized seizures. These symptoms may be likely to occur with rapid dose increase and in patients with pre-existing epilepsy. In this case, the dose should be reduced and, if necessary, anticonvulsant treatment initiated.

Dosing should not exceed 900 mg/day.

Because of the significant risk of agranulocytosis and seizure, events which both present a continuing risk over time, the extended treatment of patients failing to show an acceptable level of clinical response should ordinarily be avoided.

MAINTENANCE TREATMENT

While the maintenance effectiveness of clozapine in schizophrenia is still under study, the effectiveness of maintenance treatment is well established for many other drugs used to treat schizophrenia. It is recommended that responding patients be continued on clozapine, but at the lowest level needed to maintain remission. Because of the significant risk associated with the use of clozapine, patients should be periodically reassessed to determine the need for maintenance treatment.

DISCONTINUATION OF TREATMENT

In the event of planned termination of clozapine therapy, gradual reduction in dose is recommended over a 1-2 week period. However, should a patient's medical condition require abrupt discontinuation (*e.g.*, leukopenia), the patient should be carefully observed for the recurrence of psychotic symptoms and symptoms related to cholinergic rebound such as headache, nausea, vomiting, and diarrhea.

REINITIATION OF TREATMENT IN PATIENTS PREVIOUSLY DISCONTINUED

When restarting patients who have had even a brief interval off clozapine, *i.e.*, 2 days or more since the last dose, it is recommended that treatment be reinitiated with one-half of a 25 mg tablet (12.5 mg) once or twice daily (see WARNINGS). If that dose is well tolerated, it may be feasible to titrate patients back to a therapeutic dose more quickly than is recommended for initial treatment. However, any patient who has previously experienced respiratory or cardiac arrest with initial dosing, but was then able to be successfully titrated to a therapeutic dose, should be re-titrated with extreme caution after even 24 hours of discontinuation.

Certain additional precautions seem prudent when reinitiating treatment. The mechanisms underlying clozapine induced adverse reactions are unknown. It is conceivable, however, that re-exposure of a patient might enhance the risk of an untoward event's occurrence and increase its severity. Such phenomena, for example, occur when immune mediated mechanisms are responsible. Consequently, during the reinitiation of treatment, additional caution is advised. Patients discontinued for WBC counts below 2000/mm^3 or an ANC below 1000/mm^3 must *not* be restarted on clozapine. (See WARNINGS.)

HOW SUPPLIED

Clozaril is available as 25 and 100 mg round, pale-yellow, uncoated tablets with a facilitated score on 1 side.

25 mg tablets: Engraved with "CLOZARIL" once on the periphery of 1 side. Engraved with a facilitated score and "25" once on the other side.

100 mg tablets: Engraved with "CLOZARIL" once on the periphery of 1 side. Engraved with a facilitated score and "100" once on the other side.

STORE AND DISPENSE

Storage temperature should not exceed 30°C (86°F). Drug dispensing should not ordinarily exceed a weekly supply. If a patient is eligible for WBC testing every other week, then a 2 week supply of clozaril can be dispensed. Dispensing should be contingent upon the results of a WBC count.

PRODUCT LISTING - RATED THERAPEUTICALLY EQUIVALENT

Tablet - Oral - 25 mg			
100's	$122.35	GENERIC, Ivax Corporation	00172-4359-10
100's	$122.35	GENERIC, Mylan Pharmaceuticals Inc	00378-0825-01
100's	$132.32	GENERIC, Udl Laboratories Inc	51079-0921-20
100's	$135.96	CLOZARIL, Novartis Pharmaceuticals	00078-0126-06
100's	$146.77	CLOZARIL, Novartis Pharmaceuticals	00078-0126-05
Tablet - Oral - 100 mg			
100's	$316.95	GENERIC, Mylan Pharmaceuticals Inc	00378-0860-01
100's	$342.78	GENERIC, Ivax Corporation	00172-4360-10
100's	$342.78	GENERIC, Udl Laboratories Inc	51079-0922-20
100's	$352.26	CLOZARIL, Novartis Pharmaceuticals	00078-0127-06
100's	$380.27	CLOZARIL, Novartis Pharmaceuticals	00078-0127-05

Codeine Phosphate (000870)

For related information, see the comparative table section in Appendix A.

Categories: Pain, mild to moderate; DEA Class CII; FDA Pre 1938 Drugs; Pregnancy Category C; WHO Formulary
Drug Classes: Analgesics, narcotic; Antitussives
Brand Names: Codate; **Codeine Phosphate Injection**; Codephos; Melrosum
Foreign Brand Availability: Actacode (Australia); Codein Knoll (Switzerland); Codein Kwizda (Austria); Codein Phosphate (Czech-Republic); Codein Slovakofarma (Czech-Republic); Codeine Linctus (Australia); Codeine Phosphate (Australia; Czech-Republic; India; New-Zealand); Codeinum Phosphorcum (Poland); Codeisan (Portugal; Spain); Codenfan (France); Codicompren Retard (Germany); Codiforton (Germany); Codipront N (Philippines); Pulmocodeina (Ecuador); Solcodein (Spain); Tricodein (Benin; Burkina-Faso; Gambia; Germany; Ghana; Guinea; Ivory-Coast; Liberia; Malawi; Mali; Mauritania; Mauritius; Morocco; Niger; Senegal; Seychelles; Sierra-Leone; Sudan; Tanzania; Tunia; Uganda; Zambia; Zimbabwe); Tricodein Solco (Austria; Switzerland)
Cost of Therapy: $12.49 (Pain; Generic Tablets; 30 mg; 4 tablets/day; 7 day supply)
HCFA JCODE(S): J0745 per 30 mg IM, IV, SC

DESCRIPTION

WARNING: MAY BE HABIT FORMING.

Codeine is an alkaloid obtained from opium or prepared from morphine by methylation and occurs as white crystals. Codeine effloresces slowly in dry air and is effected by light.

The chemical name of codeine phosphate is 7,8-didehydro-4,5α-epoxy-3-methoxy-17-methylmorphinan-6α-ol phosphate (1:1)(salt) hemihydrate and has the empirical formula of $C_{18}H_{21}NO_3 \cdot H_3PO_4 \cdot \frac{1}{2}H_2O$. Its molecular weight is 406.4.

Each soluble tablet contains 30 mg (0.074 mmol) or 60 mg (0.15 mmol) of codeine phosphate. These tablets also contain lactose and sucrose.

Soluble tablets of codeine phosphate are freely soluble in water. They are intended for the preparation of solutions for parenteral administration. These tablets are not sterile. Codeine phosphate is an analgesic.

CLINICAL PHARMACOLOGY

Codeine phosphate is a centrally active analgesic. When administered parenterally, 120 mg of codeine phosphate produces an analgesic response equivalent to that from 10 mg of morphine. Other actions include respiratory depression; depression of the cough center; release of antidiuretic hormone; activation of the vomiting center; pupillary constriction; a decrease in gastric, pancreatic, and biliary secretion; a reduction in intestinal motility; an increase in biliary tract pressure; and an increased amplitude of ureteral contractions.

Onset of analgesia following intramuscular or subcutaneous administration occurs within 10-30 minutes. The effect persists for 4-6 hours.

Most of a dose of codeine is excreted within 24 hours, 5-15% as unchanged codeine and the remainder as a product of glucuronide conjugates of codeine and its metabolites.

INDICATIONS AND USAGE

Codeine phosphate is an analgesic indicated for the relief of mild to moderate pain.

CONTRAINDICATIONS

Hypersensitivity to codeine.

PRECAUTIONS

GENERAL

Head Injury and Increased Intracranial Pressure

The respiratory depressant effects of narcotics and their capacity to elevate cerebrospinal-fluid pressure may be markedly exaggerated in the presence of head injury, other intracranial lesions, or a pre-existing increase in intracranial pressure. Furthermore, narcotics produce adverse reactions that may obscure the clinical course in patients with head injuries.

Acute Abdominal Conditions

The administration of codeine or other narcotics may obscure the diagnosis or clinical course in patients with acute abdominal conditions.

Special-Risk Patients

Codeine should be given with caution to certain patients, such as the elderly or debilitated and those with severe impairment of hepatic or renal function, hypothyroidism, Addison's disease, and prostatic hypertrophy or urethral stricture.

Kidney or Liver Dysfunction

Codeine phosphate may have a prolonged cumulative effect in patients with kidney or liver dysfunction.

INFORMATION FOR THE PATIENT

Codeine may impair the mental and/or physical abilities required for the performance of potentially hazardous tasks, such as driving a car or operating machinery. Codeine in combination with other narcotic analgesics, phenothiazines, sedative hypnotics, and alcohol has additive depressant effects.

PREGNANCY CATEGORY C

Animal reproduction studies have not been conducted with codeine phosphate. It is also not known whether codeine phosphate can cause fetal harm when administered to a pregnant woman or can affect reproduction capacity. On the basis of the historical use of codeine phosphate during all stages of pregnancy, there is no known risk of fetal abnormality. Codeine phosphate should be given to a pregnant woman only if clearly needed.

LABOR AND DELIVERY

The use of codeine phosphate in obstetrics may prolong labor. It passes the placental barrier and may produce depression of respiration in the newborn. Resuscitation and, in severe depression, the administration of naloxone may be required.

NURSING MOTHERS

Codeine appears in the milk of nursing mothers. Caution should be exercised when it is administered to a nursing woman.

DRUG INTERACTIONS

Codeine in combination with other narcotic analgesics, general anesthetics, phenothiazines, tranquilizers, sedative-hypnotics, or other CNS depressants (including alcohol) has additive depressant effects. When such combination therapy is contemplated, the dosage of one or both agents should be reduced.

ADVERSE REACTIONS

The most frequent adverse reactions include lightheadedness, dizziness, sedation, nausea, and vomiting. These effects seem to be more prominent in ambulatory than in nonambulatory patients, and some of these adverse reactions may be alleviated if the patient lies down.

Other adverse reactions include euphoria, dysphoria, constipation, and pruritus.

DOSAGE AND ADMINISTRATION

FOR ANALGESIA

Dosage should be adjusted according to the severity of the pain and the response of the patient.

Adults: 15-60 mg every 4-6 hours (usual adult dose, 30 mg).

Children: *1 Year of Age and Older:* 0.5 mg/kg of body weight or 15 mg/m^2 of body surface every 4-6 hours.

Soluble tablets codeine phosphate are administered subcutaneously or intramuscularly.

Solutions for injection should be prepared with sterile water and filtered through a 0.22 μ membrane filter.

Note: Do not use the solution if it is more than slightly discolored or contains a precipitate.

PRODUCT LISTING - RATED THERAPEUTICALLY EQUIVALENT

Solution - Injectable - 15 mg/ml

2 ml x 10	$9.30	GENERIC, Abbott Pharmaceutical	00074-1097-32

Solution - Injectable - 30 mg/ml

2 ml x 10	$9.90	GENERIC, Abbott Pharmaceutical	00074-1102-32

PRODUCT LISTING - EQUIVALENTS NOT AVAILABLE

Solution - Injectable - 15 mg/ml

2 ml x 10	$8.55	GENERIC, Abbott Pharmaceutical	00074-1097-02

Solution - Injectable - 30 mg/ml

1 ml x 10	$11.80	GENERIC, Esi Lederle Generics	00008-0728-01
2 ml x 10	$9.38	GENERIC, Abbott Pharmaceutical	00074-1102-02

Solution - Injectable - 60 mg/ml

1 ml x 10	$12.60	GENERIC, Wyeth-Ayerst Laboratories	00008-0729-01

Solution - Oral - 15 mg/5 ml

5 ml x 40	$59.20	GENERIC, Roxane Laboratories Inc	00054-8160-16
500 ml	$35.78	GENERIC, Roxane Laboratories Inc	00054-3161-63

Tablet - Oral - Phosphate 30 mg

100's	$58.94	GENERIC, Lilly, Eli and Company	00002-2557-02
100's	$80.50	GENERIC, Ranbaxy Laboratories	63304-0748-01

Tablet - Oral - Phosphate 60 mg

100's	$112.62	GENERIC, Lilly, Eli and Company	00002-2558-02
100's	$148.93	GENERIC, Ddn/Obergfel	63304-0749-01

Tablet - Oral - Sulfate 15 mg

100's	$37.41	GENERIC, Roxane Laboratories Inc	00054-8155-24

Tablet - Oral - Sulfate 30 mg

100's	$40.27	GENERIC, Roxane Laboratories Inc	00054-4156-25
100's	$44.59	GENERIC, Roxane Laboratories Inc	00054-8156-24

Tablet - Oral - Sulfate 60 mg

100's	$73.77	GENERIC, Roxane Laboratories Inc	00054-4157-25
100's	$80.97	GENERIC, Roxane Laboratories Inc	00054-8157-24

Codeine Phosphate; Phenylephrine Hydrochloride; Promethazine Hydrochloride *(000875)*

Categories: Congestion, nasal; Cough; Pregnancy Category C; DEA Class CV; FDA Approved 1984 Apr

Drug Classes: Antiemetics/antivertigo; Antihistamines, H1; Antitussives; Decongestants, nasal; Phenothiazines

Brand Names: M-Phen; **Phenergan Vc W/Codeine**; Promethazine Vc W/Codeine

DESCRIPTION

FOR COMPLETE PRESCRIBING INFORMATION, REFER TO CODEINE PHOSPHATE; PHENYLEPHRINE HCL; AND PROMETHAZINE HCL .

INDICATIONS AND USAGE

Promethazine/phenylephrine with codeine is indicated for the temporary relief of coughs and upper respiratory symptoms, including nasal congestion, associated with allergy or the common cold.

DOSAGE AND ADMINISTRATION

The average effective dose is given in TABLE 1.

TABLE 1

	Dosage
Adults	1 teaspoon (5 ml) q4-6h, not to exceed 30.0 ml in 24 h
Children 6 years to under 12 years	½-1 teaspoon (2.5-5 ml) q4-6h, not to exceed 30.0 ml in 24 h
Children under 6 years (weight: 18 kg or 40 lb)	¼-½ teaspoon (1.25-2.5 ml) q4-6h, not to exceed 9.0 ml in 24 h
Children under 6 years (weight: 16 kg or 35 lb)	¼-½ teaspoon (1.25-2.5 ml) q4-6h, not to exceed 8.0 ml in 24 h
Children under 6 years (weight: 14 kg or 30 lb)	¼-½ teaspoon (1.25-2.5 ml) q4-6h, not to exceed 7.0 ml in 24 h
Children under 6 years (weight: 12 kg or 25 lb)	¼-½ teaspoon (1.25-2.5 ml) q4-6h, not to exceed 6.0 ml in 24 h

Promethazine/phenylephrine with codeine is not recommended for children under 2 years of age.

HOW SUPPLIED

Storage: Store at room temperature, between 15-25°C (59-77°F).

PRODUCT LISTING - RATED THERAPEUTICALLY EQUIVALENT

Syrup - Oral - 10 mg;5 mg;6.25 mg/5 ml

120 ml	$2.86	GENERIC, Major Pharmaceuticals Inc	00904-1514-20
120 ml	$2.90	GENERIC, Cenci, H.R. Labs Inc	00556-0345-04
120 ml	$3.85	GENERIC, Moore, H.L. Drug Exchange Inc	00839-7061-65
120 ml	$4.10	GENERIC, Major Pharmaceuticals Inc	00904-1514-00
120 ml	$4.38	GENERIC, Qualitest Products Inc	00603-1581-54
120 ml	$4.66	GENERIC, Halsey Drug Company Inc	00879-0515-04
120 ml	$5.68	GENERIC, Morton Grove Pharmaceuticals Inc	60432-0607-04
120 ml	$13.30	GENERIC, Alpharma Uspd Makers Of Barre and Nmc	00472-1629-04
480 ml	$8.74	GENERIC, Aligen Independent Laboratories Inc	00405-0170-16
480 ml	$10.90	GENERIC, Major Pharmaceuticals Inc	00904-1514-16
480 ml	$11.80	GENERIC, Qualitest Products Inc	00603-1581-58
480 ml	$12.24	GENERIC, Halsey Drug Company Inc	00879-0515-16
480 ml	$13.97	GENERIC, Moore, H.L. Drug Exchange Inc	00839-7061-69

480 ml	$16.36	GENERIC, Morton Grove Pharmaceuticals Inc	60432-0607-16
480 ml	$17.70	GENERIC, Geneva Pharmaceuticals	00781-6950-16
480 ml	$47.85	GENERIC, Alpharma Uspd Makers Of Barre and Nmc	00472-1629-16
480 ml	$61.44	GENERIC, Ivax Corporation	00182-1713-41
3840 ml	$59.20	GENERIC, Cenci, H.R. Labs Inc	00556-0345-28
3840 ml	$63.36	GENERIC, Halsey Drug Company Inc	00879-0515-28
3840 ml	$65.66	GENERIC, Moore, H.L. Drug Exchange Inc	00839-7061-70
3840 ml	$70.27	GENERIC, Major Pharmaceuticals Inc	00904-1514-28

PRODUCT LISTING - EQUIVALENTS NOT AVAILABLE

Syrup - Oral - 10 mg;5 mg;6.25 mg/5 ml

120 ml	$7.39	GENERIC, Southwood Pharmaceuticals Inc	58016-0491-24
240 ml	$10.88	GENERIC, Southwood Pharmaceuticals Inc	58016-0491-48

Codeine Phosphate; Promethazine Hydrochloride *(000876)*

Categories: Common cold; Cough; DEA Class CV; Pregnancy Category C; FDA Approved 1984 Apr
Drug Classes: Antiemetics/antivertigo; Antihistamines, H1; Antitussives; Phenothiazines
Foreign Brand Availability: Phensedyl (Malaysia)

DESCRIPTION

FOR COMPLETE PRESCRIBING INFORMATION, REFER TO CODEINE PHOSPHATE; PROMETHAZINE HCl.

INDICATIONS AND USAGE

Codeine phosphate; promethazine HCl is indicated for the temporary relief of coughs and upper respiratory symptoms associated with allergy or the common cold.

DOSAGE AND ADMINISTRATION

The average effective dose is given in TABLE 1.

TABLE 1

Adults	1 teaspoon (5 ml) q4-6h, not to exceed 30.0 ml in 24 h
Children 6 years to under 12 years	½-1 teaspoon (2.5-5 ml) q4-6h, not to exceed 30.0 ml in 24 h
Children under 6 years (weight: 18 kg or 40 lb)	¼-½ teaspoon (1.25-2.5 ml) q4-6h, not to exceed 9.0 ml in 24 h
Children under 6 years (weight: 16 kg or 35 lb)	¼-½ teaspoon (1.25-2.5 ml) q4-6h, not to exceed 8.0 ml in 24 h
Children under 6 years (weight: 14 kg or 30 lb)	¼- ½ teaspoon (1.25-2.5 ml) q4-6h, not to exceed 7.0 ml in 24 h
Children under 6 years (weight: 12 kg or 25 lb)	¼- ½ teaspoon (1.25-2.5 ml) q4-6h, not to exceed 6.0 ml in 24 h

Codeine phosphate; promethazine HCl is not recommended for children under 2 years of age.

HOW SUPPLIED

Storage: Keep bottles tightly closed—store at room temperature, between 15-25°C (59-77°F).

Protect from light.

Dispense in light-resistant, glass, tight containers.

PRODUCT LISTING - RATED THERAPEUTICALLY EQUIVALENT

Syrup - Oral - 10 mg/5 ml;6.25 mg/5 ml

480 ml	$11.95	FEDERAL UPPER LIMIT, H.C.F.A. F F P	99999-0876-05

Syrup - Oral - 10 mg;6.25 mg/5 ml

5 ml x 100	$80.45	GENERIC, Pharmaceutical Assoc Inc Div Beach Products	00121-0547-05
120 ml	$2.50	GENERIC, Cenci, H.R. Labs Inc	00556-0343-04
120 ml	$2.80	GENERIC, Ivax Corporation	00182-0346-37
120 ml	$2.80	GENERIC, Ivax Corporation	00182-1712-37
120 ml	$3.83	GENERIC, Major Pharmaceuticals Inc	00904-1510-00
120 ml	$4.45	GENERIC, Halsey Drug Company Inc	00879-0513-04
120 ml	$6.04	GENERIC, Geneva Pharmaceuticals	00781-6930-04
120 ml	$9.05	GENERIC, Alpharma Uspd Makers Of Barre and Nmc	00472-1627-04
120 ml	$9.62	GENERIC, Morton Grove Pharmaceuticals Inc	60432-0606-04
120 ml x 24	$341.54	PHENERGAN WITH CODEINE, Wyeth-Ayerst Laboratories	00008-0550-02
480 ml	$5.62	GENERIC, Esi Lederle Generics	59911-5819-03
480 ml	$7.30	GENERIC, Aligen Independent Laboratories Inc	00405-0166-16
480 ml	$7.44	GENERIC, Cenci, H.R. Labs Inc	00556-0343-16
480 ml	$9.36	GENERIC, Moore, H.L. Drug Exchange Inc	00839-7059-69
480 ml	$9.75	GENERIC, Major Pharmaceuticals Inc	00904-1510-16
480 ml	$10.94	GENERIC, Halsey Drug Company Inc	00879-0513-16
480 ml	$14.83	GENERIC, Watson/Rugby Laboratories Inc	00536-1805-85
480 ml	$14.83	GENERIC, Geneva Pharmaceuticals	00781-6930-16
480 ml	$16.35	GENERIC, Mutual/United Research Laboratories	00677-1733-33
480 ml	$22.92	GENERIC, Mutual/United Research Laboratories	00677-1735-33
480 ml	$22.92	GENERIC, Mutual/United Research Laboratories	00677-1828-33
480 ml	$32.55	GENERIC, Alpharma Uspd Makers Of Barre and Nmc	00472-1627-16
480 ml	$32.70	GENERIC, Morton Grove Pharmaceuticals Inc	60432-0606-16
480 ml	$32.75	GENERIC, Hi-Tech Pharmacal Company Inc	50383-0804-16
480 ml	$51.32	PHENERGAN WITH CODEINE, Wyeth-Ayerst Laboratories	00008-0550-03
3840 ml	$49.60	GENERIC, Cenci, H.R. Labs Inc	00556-0343-28
3840 ml	$52.49	GENERIC, Ivax Corporation	00182-1712-41
3840 ml	$53.38	GENERIC, Moore, H.L. Drug Exchange Inc	00839-7059-70
3840 ml	$53.38	GENERIC, Halsey Drug Company Inc	00879-0513-28
3840 ml	$55.30	GENERIC, Geneva Pharmaceuticals	00781-6930-28
3840 ml	$58.37	GENERIC, Major Pharmaceuticals Inc	00904-1510-28
3840 ml	$234.36	GENERIC, Alpharma Uspd Makers Of Barre and Nmc	00472-1627-28

PRODUCT LISTING - EQUIVALENTS NOT AVAILABLE

Syrup - Oral - 10 mg;6.25 mg/5 ml

4 ml	$3.46	GENERIC, Prescript Pharmaceuticals	00247-0081-04
30 ml	$4.14	GENERIC, Prescript Pharmaceuticals	00247-0081-30
60 ml	$4.93	GENERIC, Prescript Pharmaceuticals	00247-0081-60
89 ml	$5.68	GENERIC, Prescript Pharmaceuticals	00247-0081-89
118 ml	$6.45	GENERIC, Prescript Pharmaceuticals	00247-0081-52
120 ml	$5.75	GENERIC, Southwood Pharmaceuticals Inc	58016-0674-24
120 ml	$6.49	GENERIC, Prescript Pharmaceuticals	00247-0081-77
120 ml	$14.23	GENERIC, Southwood Pharmaceuticals Inc	58016-0390-01
180 ml	$8.07	GENERIC, Prescript Pharmaceuticals	00247-0081-59

Colchicine *(000890)*

Categories: Arthritis, gouty; Pregnancy Category D; FDA Pre 1938 Drugs; WHO Formulary
Drug Classes: Antigout agents
Brand Names: Colsalide Improved
Foreign Brand Availability: Artrichine (Ecuador); Colchicin (Bulgaria); Colchicine (Israel; New-Zealand); Colchicine capsules (Netherlands); Colchicine Houde (South-Africa); Colchicum-Dispert (Hungary); Colchily (Thailand); Colchimedio (Colombia; Dominican-Republic; El-Salvador; Guatemala; Honduras; Panama); Colchiquim (Mexico); Colchisol (Peru); Colcine (Thailand); Colgout (Australia; Hong-Kong); Conicine (Taiwan); Goutichine (Thailand); Goutnil (India); Kolkicin (Denmark); Tolchicine (Thailand)
Cost of Therapy: $7.11 (Gout; Generic tablets; 0.6 mg; 6 tablets/day; 30 day supply)
HCFA JCODE(S): J0760 per 1 mg IV

DESCRIPTION

A phenanthrene derivative, colchicine is the active alkaloidal principle derived from various species of *Colchicum;* it appears as pale-yellow amorphous scales or powder that darkens on exposure to light. For the injection, 1 g dissolves in 25 ml of water and in 220 ml of ether. Colchicine is soluble in water, freely soluble in alcohol and chloroform and slightly soluble in ether.

Chemically it is Acetamide, *N*-(5,6,7,9-tetrahydro-1,2,3,10-tetramethoxy-9-oxobenzo(α)heptalen-7-yl)-,(*S*)-. The molecular weight is 399.44, the empirical formula is $C_{22}H_{25}NO_6$.

Colchicine, an acetyltrimethylcolchicinic acid, is hydrolyzed in the presence of dilute acids or alkalies, with cleavage of a methyl group as methanol and formation of *colchiceine,* which has very little therapeutic activity. On hydrolysis with strong acids, colchicine is converted to trimethylcolchicinic acid.

For Tablets Only: Each tablet contains colchicine 0.6 mg. *Inactive Ingredients:* Hydrogenated vegetable oil, lactose, povidone, sodium starch glycolate, starch, syloid.

For Injection Only: Colchicine injection provides a sterile aqueous solution of colchicine for intravenous use. Each ampoule contains 1 mg (2.5 μmol) of colchicine in 2 ml of solution. Sodium hydroxide may have been added during manufacture to adjust the pH.

CLINICAL PHARMACOLOGY

The mechanism of the relief afforded by colchicine in acute attacks of gouty arthritis is not completely known, but studies on the processes involved in precipitation of an acute attack have helped elucidate how this drug may exert its effects. The drug is not an analgesic, does not relieve other types of pain or inflammation, and is of no value in other types of arthritis. It is not a diuretic and does not influence the renal excretion of uric acid or its level in the blood or the magnitude of the "miscible pool" of uric acid. It also does not alter the solubility of urate in the plasma.

Colchicine is not a uricosuric agent. An acute attack of gout apparently occurs as a result of an inflammatory reaction to crystals of monosodium urate that are deposited in the joint tissue from hyperuric body fluids; the reaction is aggravated as more urate crystals accumulate. The initial inflammatory response involves local infiltration of granulocytes that phagocytize the urate crystals. Interference with these processes will prevent the development of an acute attack. Colchicine apparently exerts its effect by reducing the inflammatory response to the deposited crystals and also by diminishing phagocytosis. The deposition of uric acid is favored by an acid pH. In synovial tissues and in leukocytes associated with inflammatory processes, lactic acid production is high; this favors a local decrease in pH that enhances uric acid deposition. Colchicine diminishes lactic acid production by leukocytes both directly and by diminishing phagocytosis, and thereby interrupts the cycle of urate crystal deposition and inflammatory response that sustains the acute attack. The oxidation of glucose in phagocytizing as well as in nonphagocytizing leukocytes *in vitro* is suppressed by colchicine; this suppression may explain the diminished lactic acid production. The precise biochemical step that is affected by colchicine is not yet known. The antimitotic activity of colchicine is unrelated to its effectiveness in the treatment of acute gout, as indicated by the fact that trimethylcolchicinic acid, an analog of colchicine, has no antimitotic activity except in extremely high doses.

INDICATIONS AND USAGE

Colchicine is indicated for the treatment of gout. It is effective in relieving the pain of acute attacks, especially if therapy is begun early in the attack and in adequate dosage. Many therapists use colchicine as interval therapy to prevent acute attacks of gout. It has no effect on nongouty arthritis or on uric acid metabolism.

The intravenous use of colchicine is advantageous when a rapid response is desired or when gastrointestinal side effects interfere with oral administration of the medication. Occasionally, intravenous colchicine is effective when the oral preparation is not. After the acute attack has subsided, the patient can usually be given colchicine tablets by mouth.

NON-FDA APPROVED INDICATIONS

Colchicine has also been used to prevent amyloidosis in patients with familial Mediterranean fever, to treat pseudogout, prostate cancer (with estramustine), relapsing polychondritis, sarcoid arthropathy, hepatic cirrhosis and fibrosis, biliary cirrhosis, Behcet's disease, fibromatosis, palmar and plantar pustulosis, chronic cutaneous leukocytoclastic vasculitis, psoriasis, dermatitis herpetiformis, splenectomy-resistant idiopathic thrombocytopenic purpura, scleroderma, pyoderma gangrenosum and recurrent pericarditis.

CONTRAINDICATIONS

Colchicine is contraindicated in patients with gout who also have serious gastrointestinal, renal, hepatic, or cardiac disorders. Colchicine should not be given in the presence of combined renal and hepatic disease.

WARNINGS

Colchicine can cause fetal harm when administered to a pregnant woman. If this drug is used during pregnancy, or if the patient becomes pregnant while taking it, the woman should be apprised of the potential hazard to the fetus.

Mortality Related to Overdosage: Cumulative intravenous doses of colchicine above 4 mg have resulted in irreversible multiple organ failure and death (see DOSAGE AND ADMINISTRATION).

PRECAUTIONS

General: Reduction in dosage is indicated if weakness, anorexia, nausea, vomiting or diarrhea occurs. Rarely, thrombophlebitis occurs at the site of injection. Colchicine should be administered with great caution to aged and debilitated patients, especially those with renal, hepatic, gastrointestinal, or heart disease.

Pregnancy Category D: See WARNINGS.

Nursing Mothers: It is not known whether this drug is excreted in human milk. Because many drugs are excreted in human milk, caution should be exercised when colchicine is administered to a nursing woman.

Pediatric Use: Safety and effectiveness in children have not been established.

DRUG INTERACTIONS

Colchicine has been shown to induce reversible malabsorption of vitamin B_{12}, apparently by altering the function of ileal mucosa. The possibility that colchicine may increase response to central nervous system (CNS) depressants and to sympathomimetic agents is suggested by the results of experiments on animals.

ADVERSE REACTIONS

FOR INJECTION

These are usually gastrointestinal in nature and consist of abdominal pain, nausea, vomiting, and diarrhea. The diarrhea may be severe. The gastrointestinal symptoms may occur even though the drug is given intravenously; however, such symptoms are unusual unless the recommended dose is exceeded.

Prolonged administration may cause bone marrow depression, with agranulocytosis, thrombocytopenia, and aplastic anemia. Peripheral neuritis and epilation have also been reported.

Myopathy may occur in patients on usual maintenance doses, especially in the presence of renal impairment.

FOR TABLETS

Adverse reactions to colchicine appear to be a function of dosage. The possibility of increased colchicine toxicity in the presence of hepatic dysfunction should be considered. The appearance of any of the following symptoms may require reduction of dosage or discontinuation of the drug.

Central Nervous System: Peripheral neuritis.

Musculoskeletal: Muscular weakness.

Gastrointestinal: Nausea, vomiting, abdominal pain or diarrhea may be particularly troublesome in the presence of peptic ulcer or spastic colon.

Hypersensitivity: Urticaria.

Hematologic: Aplastic anemia, agranulocytosis, or thrombocytopenia.

Integumentary: Dermatitis, purpura, alopecia.

At toxic doses, colchicine may cause severe diarrhea, generalized vascular damage, and renal damage with hematuria oliguria.

DOSAGE AND ADMINISTRATION

FOR TABLETS ONLY

Colchicine should be started at the first warning of an acute attack; a delay of a few hours impairs its effectiveness. The usual adult dose is 1 or 2 tablets initially, followed by 1 tablet every 1-2 hours until pain is relieved or nausea, vomiting, or diarrhea develops. Some physicians use 2 tablets every 2 hours. Since the number of doses required may range from 6-16, the total dose is variable. As interval treatment, 1 tablet may be taken 1-4 times a week for the mild or moderate case, once or twice daily for the severe case.

FOR INJECTION ONLY

Colchicine injection is for intravenous use only. Severe local irritation occurs if it is administered subcutaneously or intramuscularly.

It is extremely important that the needle be properly positioned in the vein before colchicine is injected. If leakage into surrounding tissue or outside the vein along its course should occur during intravenous administration, considerable irritation and possible tissue damage may follow. There is no specific antidote for the prevention of this irritation. Local application of heat or cold, as well as the administration of analgesics, may afford relief.

The injection should take 2-5 minutes for completion. To minimize the risk of extravasation, it is recommended that the injection be made into an established intravenous line into a large vein using normal saline as the intravenous fluid. Colchicine injection should not be diluted with 5% dextrose in water. If a decrease in concentration of colchicine in solution is required, 0.9% sodium chloride injection, which does not contain a bacteriostatic agent, should be used. Solutions that become turbid should not be used.

In the treatment of acute gouty arthritis, the average initial dose of colchicine injection is 2 mg (4 ml). This may be followed by 0.5 (1 ml) every 6 hours until a satisfactory response is achieved. In general, a total dosage for the first 24 hour period should be achieved. In general, the total dosage for the first 24 hour period should not exceed 4 mg (8 ml). Cumulative doses of colchicine above 4 mg have resulted in irreversible multiple organ failure and death. The total dosage for a single course of treatment should not exceed 4 mg. Some clinicians recommend a single intravenous dose of 3 mg, whereas others recommend an initial dose of not more than 1 mg of colchicine intravenously, followed by 0.5 mg once or twice daily if needed.

If pain recurs, it may be necessary to administer a daily dose of 1-2 mg (2-4 ml) for several days; however, **no more colchicine should be given by any route for at least 7 days after a full course of IV therapy (4 mg).**[1,2] Many patients can be transferred to oral colchicine at a dosage similar to that being given intravenously.

In the prophylactic or maintenance therapy of recurrent or chronic gouty arthritis, a dosage of 0.5-1 mg (1-2 ml) once or twice daily may be used. However, in these cases, oral administration of colchicine is preferable, usually taken in conjunction with a uricosuric agent. If an acute attack of gout occurs while the patient is taking colchicine as maintenance therapy, an alternative drug should be instituted in preference to increasing the dose of colchicine.

Parenteral drug products should be inspected visually for particulate matter and discoloration prior to administration, whenever solution and container permit.

HOW SUPPLIED

TABLETS

Colchicine tablets, 0.6 mg, are available as round, white tablets imprinted with "T 024" logo on one side and no imprint on the opposite side.

Storage: Store at controlled room temperature, 15-30°C (59-86°F) in a dry place. Dispense in a tight, light-resistant container.

INJECTION

Storage: Store at controlled room temperature, 15-30°C (59-86°F).

PRODUCT LISTING - RATED THERAPEUTICALLY EQUIVALENT

Tablet - Oral - 0.6 mg

100's	$5.78	GENERIC, Us Trading Corporation	56126-0472-11

PRODUCT LISTING - RATED NOT THERAPEUTICALLY EQUIVALENT

Tablet - Oral - 0.6 mg

100's	$25.98	GENERIC, Qualitest Products Inc	00603-3052-21

PRODUCT LISTING - EQUIVALENTS NOT AVAILABLE

Solution - Intravenous - 0.5 mg/ml			
2 ml	$50.40	GENERIC, Bedford Laboratories	55390-0605-02
Tablet - Oral - 0.5 mg			
30's	$16.92	GENERIC, Pd-Rx Pharmaceuticals	55289-0724-30
100's	$39.64	GENERIC, Abbott Pharmaceutical	00074-0074-02
Tablet - Oral - 0.6 mg			
10's	$2.84	GENERIC, Pharmaceutical Corporation Of America	51655-0424-53
20's	$1.20	GENERIC, Allscripts Pharmaceutical Company	54569-0236-02
25's	$6.14	GENERIC, Pd-Rx Pharmaceuticals	55289-0156-97
30's	$1.80	GENERIC, Allscripts Pharmaceutical Company	54569-0236-06
30's	$3.50	GENERIC, Pd-Rx Pharmaceuticals	58864-0119-30
30's	$4.20	GENERIC, Heartland Healthcare Services	61392-0715-30
30's	$4.20	GENERIC, Heartland Healthcare Services	61392-0715-39
31's	$4.34	GENERIC, Heartland Healthcare Services	61392-0715-31
32's	$4.48	GENERIC, Heartland Healthcare Services	61392-0715-32
45's	$6.30	GENERIC, Heartland Healthcare Services	61392-0715-45
60's	$3.61	GENERIC, Allscripts Pharmaceutical Company	54569-0236-03
60's	$8.40	GENERIC, Heartland Healthcare Services	61392-0715-60
90's	$12.60	GENERIC, Heartland Healthcare Services	61392-0715-90
100's	$3.95	GENERIC, Cmc-Consolidated Midland Corporation	00223-0703-01
100's	$4.30	GENERIC, Major Pharmaceuticals Inc	00904-2147-60
100's	$5.00	GENERIC, Shire Richwood Pharmaceutical Company Inc	58521-0187-01

100's	$6.01	GENERIC, Moore, H.L. Drug Exchange Inc	00839-5152-06
100's	$6.01	GENERIC, Allscripts Pharmaceutical Company	54569-0236-05
100's	$18.99	GENERIC, Major Pharmaceuticals Inc	00904-2047-60
100's	$19.30	GENERIC, Watson/Schein Pharmaceuticals Inc	00364-0074-01
100's	$19.30	GENERIC, Watson/Schein Pharmaceuticals Inc	00591-0944-01
100's	$19.49	GENERIC, Integrity Pharmaceutical Corporation	64731-0187-01
100's	$19.85	GENERIC, West Ward Pharmaceutical Corporation	00143-1201-01
100's	$25.99	GENERIC, Mutual/United Research Laboratories	00677-1683-01
100's	$31.54	GENERIC, Abbott Pharmaceutical	00074-3781-01
100's	$33.25	GENERIC, West Ward Pharmaceutical Corporation	00143-1201-25
250's	$7.45	GENERIC, Major Pharmaceuticals Inc	00904-2047-70

Colesevelam Hydrochloride *(003493)*

For related information, see the comparative table section in Appendix A.

Categories: Hypercholesterolemia; FDA Approved 2000 Jun; Pregnancy Category B
Drug Classes: Antihyperlipidemics; Bile acid sequestrants
Brand Names: **Welchol**
Cost of Therapy: $147.65 (Hypercholesterolemia; Welchol; 625 mg; 6 tablets/day; 30 day supply)

DESCRIPTION

Welchol contains colesevelam hydrochloride (hereafter referred to as colesevelam), a non-absorbed, polymeric, lipid-lowering agent intended for oral administration. Colesevelam is a high capacity bile acid binding molecule. Colesevelam is poly(allylamine hydrochloride) cross-linked with epichlorohydrin and alkylated with 1-bromodecane and (6-bromohexyl)-trimethylammonium bromide. Colesevelam is hydrophilic and insoluble in water.

Welchol is an off-white, film-coated, solid tablet containing 625 mg colesevelam. In addition, each tablet contains the following inactive ingredients: magnesium stearate, microcrystalline cellulose, and silicon dioxide. The tablets are imprinted using a water-soluble black ink.

CLINICAL PHARMACOLOGY

MECHANISM OF ACTION

The mechanism of action for the lipid-lowering activity of colesevelam, the active pharmaceutical ingredient in colesevelam HCl , has been evaluated in various *in vitro* and *in vivo* studies. These studies have demonstrated that colesevelam binds bile acids, including glycocholic acid, the major bile acid in humans.

Cholesterol is the sole precursor of bile acids. During normal digestion, bile acids are secreted into the intestine. A major portion of bile acids are then absorbed from the intestinal tract and returned to the liver via the enterohepatic circulation.

Colesevelam is a nonabsorbed, lipid-lowering polymer that binds bile acids in the intestine, impeding their reabsorption. As the bile acid pool becomes depleted, the hepatic enzyme, cholesterol 7-α-hydroxylase, is upregulated, which increases the conversion of cholesterol to bile acids. This causes an increased demand for cholesterol in the liver cells, resulting in the dual effect of increasing transcription and activity of the cholesterol biosynthetic enzyme, hydroxymethyl-glutaryl-coenzyme A (HMG-CoA) reductase, and increasing the number of hepatic low-density lipoprotein (LDL) receptors. These compensatory effects result in increased clearance of LDL cholesterol (LDL-C) from the blood, resulting in decreased serum LDL-C levels.[1,2]

Clinical studies have demonstrated that elevated levels of total cholesterol (total-C), LDL-C, and apolipoprotein B (Apo B, a protein associated with LDL-C) are associated with an increased risk of atherosclerosis in humans. Similarly, decreased levels of high-density lipoprotein cholesterol (HDL-C) are associated with the development of atherosclerosis.[1] Epidemiological investigations have established that cardiovascular morbidity and mortality vary directly with the levels of total-C and LDL-C, and inversely with the level of HDL-C.

The combination of colesevelam and an HMG-CoA reductase inhibitor is effective in further lowering serum total-C and LDL-C levels beyond that achieved by either agent alone. The effects of colesevelam either alone or with an HMG-CoA reductase inhibitor on cardiovascular morbidity and mortality have not been determined.

PHARMACOKINETICS

Colesevelam is a hydrophilic, water-insoluble polymer that is not hydrolyzed by digestive enzymes and is not absorbed. In 16 healthy volunteers, an average of 0.05% of a single ^{14}C-labeled colesevelam dose was excreted in the urine when given following 28 days of chronic dosing of 1.9 g of colesevelam twice per day.

INDICATIONS AND USAGE

Colesevelam HCl , administered alone or in combination with an HMG-CoA reductase inhibitor, is indicated as adjunctive therapy to diet and exercise for the reduction of elevated LDL cholesterol in patients with primary hypercholesterolemia (Fredrickson Type IIa).

Therapy with lipid-lowering agents should be a component of multiple risk-factor intervention in patients at significant increased risk for atherosclerotic vascular disease due to hypercholesterolemia. Lipid-altering agents should be used in addition to a diet restricted in saturated fat and cholesterol and when the response to diet and other nonpharmacological means has been inadequate.

Prior to initiating therapy with colesevelam HCl, secondary causes of hypercholesterolemia (*i.e.,* poorly controlled diabetes mellitus, hypothyroidism, nephrotic syndrome, dysproteinemias, obstructive liver disease, other drug therapy, alcoholism) should be excluded, and a lipid profile obtained to assess total-C, HDL-C, and TG. For individuals with TG less than 400 mg/dl, LDL-C can be estimated using the following equation.[3]

LDL-C = Total-C - [(TG/5) + HDL-C]

Periodic determination of serum cholesterol levels in patients as outlined in the National Cholesterol Education Program (NCEP) guidelines should be done to confirm a favorable initial and long-term response. The NCEP treatment guidelines are presented in TABLE 3.

Other risk factors for CHD include the following: age (males >45 years, females >55 years or premature menopause without estrogen replacement therapy); family history of premature CHD; current cigarette smoking; hypertension; confirmed HDL-C, <35 mg/dl (<0.01 mmol/L); and diabetes mellitus. Subtract risk factor if HDL-C >60 mg/dl (>1.6 mmol/L).

TABLE 3 *NCEP Guideline*

Patient Assessment Criteria	LDL-C Initiation Level	LDL-C Minimum Goal
Without CHD* and with fewer than 2 risk factors	≥190 mg/dl	<160 mg/dl
Without CHD and with 2 or more risk factors	≥160 mg/dl	<130 mg/dl
With CHD	≥130 mg/dl	≤100 mg/dl

* CHD = Coronary Heart Disease.

In CHD patients with LDL-C levels of 100-129 mg/dl, the physician should exercise clinical judgment in deciding whether to initiate drug treatment.

CONTRAINDICATIONS

Colesevelam HCl is contraindicated in individuals with bowel obstruction and in individuals who have shown hypersensitivity to any of the components of colesevelam HCl.

PRECAUTIONS

GENERAL

Patients with TG levels greater than 300 mg/dl were excluded from colesevelam HCl clinical trials. Caution should be exercised when treating patients with TG levels greater than 300 mg/dl.

In nonclinical safety studies, rats administered colesevelam at doses greater than 30-fold the projected human clinical dose experienced hemorrhage from vitamin K deficiency. Colesevelam HCl did not induce any clinically significant reduction in the absorption of vitamins A, D, E, or K during clinical trials of up to 1 year. However, caution should be exercised when treating patients with a susceptibility to vitamin K or fat soluble vitamin deficiencies.

The safety and efficacy of colesevelam HCl in patients with dysphagia, swallowing disorders, severe gastrointestinal motility disorders, or major gastrointestinal tract surgery have not been established. Consequently, caution should be exercised when colesevelam HCl is used in patients with these gastrointestinal disorders.

INFORMATION FOR THE PATIENT

Colesevelam HCl may be taken once per day with a meal, or taken twice per day in divided doses with meals. Patients should be directed to take colesevelam HCl with a liquid and a meal, and to adhere to their NCEP-recommended diet. Patients should tell their physicians if they are pregnant, are intending to become pregnant, or are breast-feeding.

LABORATORY TESTS

Serum total-C, LDL-C and TG levels should be determined periodically based on NCEP guidelines to confirm favorable initial and adequate long-term responses.

CARCINOGENESIS, MUTAGENESIS, AND IMPAIRMENT OF FERTILITY

A 104 week carcinogenicity study with colesevelam was conducted in CD-1 mice, at oral dietary doses up to 3 g/kg/day. This dose was approximately 50 times the maximum recommended human dose of 4.5 g/day, based on body weight, mg/kg. There were no significant drug-induced tumor findings in male or female mice. In a 104 week carcinogenicity study with colesevelam in Harlan Sprague-Dawley rats, a statistically significant increase in the incidence of pancreatic acinar cell adenoma was seen in male rats at doses >1.2 g/kg/day (approximately 20 times the maximum human dose, based on body weight, mg/kg) (trend test only). A statistically significant increase in thyroid C-cell adenoma was seen in female rats at 2.4 g/kg/day (approximately 40 times the maximum human dose, based on body weight, mg/kg).

Colesevelam and 4 degradants present in the drug substance have been evaluated for mutagenicity in the Ames test and a mammalian chromosomal aberration test. The 4 degradants and an extract of the parent compound did not exhibit genetic toxicity in an *in vitro* bacterial mutagenesis assay in *S. typhimurium* and *E. coli* (Ames assay) with or without rat liver metabolic activation. An extract of the parent compound was positive in the Chinese Hamster Ovary (CHO) cell chromosomal aberration assay in the presence of metabolic activation and negative in the absence of metabolic activation. The results of the CHO cell chromosomal aberration assay with 2 of the 4 degradants, decylamine HCl and aminohexyltrimethyl ammonium chloride HCl, were equivocal in the absence of metabolic activation and negative in the presence of metabolic activation. The other two degradants, didecylamine HCl and 6-decylamino-hexyltrimethyl ammonium chloride HCl, were negative in the presence and absence of metabolic activation.

Colesevelam did not impair fertility in rats at doses of up to 3 g/kg/day (approximately 50 times the maximum human dose, based on body weight, mg/kg).

PREGNANCY CATEGORY B

Reproduction studies have been performed in rats and rabbits at doses up to 3 g/kg/day and 1 g/kg/day, respectively (approximately 50 and 17 times the maximum human dose, based on body weight, mg/kg) and have revealed no evidence of harm to the fetus due to colesevelam. There are, however, no adequate and well-controlled studies in pregnant women. Because animal reproduction studies are not always predictive of human response, this drug should be used during pregnancy only if clearly needed.

Requirements for vitamins and other nutrients are increased in pregnancy. The effect of colesevelam HCl on the absorption of vitamins has not been studied in pregnant women.

PEDIATRIC USE

The safety and efficacy of colesevelam HCl have not been established in pediatric patients.

GERIATRIC USE

There is no evidence for special considerations when colesevelam HCl is administered to elderly patients.

DRUG INTERACTIONS

Colesevelam HCl has been studied in several human drug interaction studies in which it was administered with a meal and the test drug. Colesevelam HCl was found to have no significant effect on the bioavailability of digoxin, lovastatin, metoprolol, quinidine, valproic acid, and warfarin. Colesevelam HCl decreased the C_{max} and AUC of sustained-release verapamil by approximately 31% and 11%, respectively. Since there is a high degree of variability in the bioavailability of verapamil, the clinical significance of this finding is unclear. In clinical studies, coadministration of colesevelam HCl with atorvastatin, lovastatin, or simvastatin did not interfere with the lipid-lowering activity of the HMG-CoA reductase inhibitor. Other drugs have not been studied. When administering other drugs for which alterations in blood levels could have a clinically significant effect on safety or efficacy, physicians should consider monitoring drug levels or effects.

ADVERSE REACTIONS

Colesevelam HCl treatment-emergent adverse events that occurred in greater than 2% of patients in an integrated safety analysis are presented in TABLE 4.

TABLE 4 *Frequent (>2%) Treatment-Emergent Adverse Events by Treatment Category*

Body System / Adverse Event	Placebo (n=258)	Colesevelam HCl (n=807)
Body as a Whole		
Infection	13%	10%
Headache	8%	6%
Pain	7%	5%
Back pain	6%	3%
Abdominal pain	5%	5%
Flu syndrome	3%	3%
Accidental injury	3%	4%
Asthenia	2%	4%
Digestive System		
Flatulence	14%	12%
Constipation	7%	11%
Diarrhea	7%	5%
Nausea	4%	4%
Dyspepsia	3%	8%
Respiratory System		
Sinusitis	4%	2%
Rhinitis	3%	3%
Cough increased	2%	2%
Pharyngitis	2%	3%
Musculoskeletal System		
Myalgia	0%	2%

DOSAGE AND ADMINISTRATION

MONOTHERAPY

The recommended starting dose of colesevelam HCl is 3 tablets taken twice per day with meals or 6 tablets once per day with a meal. The colesevelam HCl dose can be increased to 7 tablets, depending upon the desired therapeutic effect. Colesevelam HCl should be taken with a liquid.

COMBINATION THERAPY

Colesevelam HCl , at doses of 4-6 tablets per day, has been shown to be safe and effective when dosed at the same time (*i.e.,* coadministered) as an HMG-CoA reductase inhibitor or when the 2 drugs are dosed apart. Colesevelam HCl should be taken with a liquid. For maximal therapeutic effect in combination with an HMG-CoA reductase inhibitor, the recommended dose of colesevelam HCl is 3 tablets taken twice per day with meals or 6 tablets taken once per day with a meal.

HOW SUPPLIED

Wechol is supplied as an off-white, solid tablet imprinted with the word "Sankyo" over "C01", containing 625 mg colesevelam, magnesium stearate, microcrystalline cellulose, silicon dioxide, HPMC (hydroxypropyl methylcellulose), and acetylated monoglyceride.

Storage: Store at room temperature (25°C). Brief exposure to 40°C does not adversely affect the product. Protect from moisture.

PRODUCT LISTING - EQUIVALENTS NOT AVAILABLE

Tablet - Oral - 625 mg

180's $147.65 WELCHOL, Sankyo Parke Davis 65597-0701-18

Colestipol Hydrochloride (000892)

For related information, see the comparative table section in Appendix A.

Categories: Hypercholesterolemia; Hyperlipidemia; Hyperlipoproteinemia; FDA Approved 1977 Apr
Drug Classes: Antihyperlipidemics; Bile acid sequestrants
Brand Names: Colestid
Foreign Brand Availability: Cholestabyl (Germany); Lestid (Denmark; Finland; Norway; Sweden)
Cost of Therapy: $99.79 (Hypercholesterolemia; Colestid Granules; 5 g; 10 g/day; 30 day supply)
$69.09 (Hypercholesterolemia; Colestid; 1 g; 4 tablets/day; 30 day supply)

DESCRIPTION

The active ingredient in Colestid is micronized colestipol hydrochloride, which is a lipid-lowering agent for oral use. Colestipol is an insoluble, high molecular weight basic anion-exchange copolymer of diethylenetriamine and 1-chloro-2, 3-epoxypropane, with approximately 1 out of 5 amine nitrogens protonated (chloride form). It is a light yellow water-insoluble resin which is hygroscopic and swells when suspended in water or aqueous fluids.

Colestid Tablets: Colestid tablets are light yellow in color and are tasteless and odorless. Each Colestid tablet contains 1 g of micronized colestipol hydrochloride. *Inactive Ingredients:* Cellulose acetate phthalate, glyceryl triacetate, carnauba wax, hydroxypropyl methylcellulose, magnesium stearate, povidone, silicon dioxide. Colestid tablets contain no calories.

Colestid Oral Suspension: Colestid is tasteless and odorless. One dose (1 packet or 1 level teaspoon) of Colestid contains 5 g of colestipol hydrochloride. Flavored Colestid is orange flavored and light orange in color. One dose (1 packet or 1 level scoopful) of Flavored Colestid is approximately 7.5 g which contains 5 g of colestipol hydrochloride. *Inactive Ingredients:* Silicon dioxide, aspartame, beta carotene, citric acid, flavor (natural and artificial), glycerine, maltol, mannitol, and methylcellulose.

CLINICAL PHARMACOLOGY

Cholesterol is the major, and probably the sole precursor of bile acids. During normal digestion, bile acids are secreted via the bile from the liver and gall bladder into the intestines. Bile acids emulsify the fat and lipid materials present in food, thus facilitating absorption. A major portion of the bile acids secreted is reabsorbed from the intestines and returned via the portal circulation to the liver, thus completing the enterohepatic cycle. Only very small amounts of bile acids are found in normal serum.

Colestipol HCl binds bile acids in the intestine forming a complex that is excreted in the feces. This nonsystemic action results in a partial removal of the bile acids from the enterohepatic circulation, preventing their reabsorption. Since colestipol HCl is an anion exchange resin, the chloride anions of the resin can be replaced by other anions, usually those with a greater affinity for the resin than the chloride ion.

Colestipol HCl is hydrophilic, but it is virtually water insoluble (99.75%) and it is not hydrolyzed by digestive enzymes. The high molecular weight polymer in colestipol HCl apparently is not absorbed. In humans, less than 0.17% of a single ^{14}C-labeled colestipol HCl dose is excreted in the urine when given following 60 days of dosing of 20 g of colestipol HCl per day.

The increased fecal loss of bile acids due to colestipol HCl administration leads to an increased oxidation of cholesterol to bile acids. This results in an increase in the number of low-density lipoprotein (LDL) receptors, increased hepatic uptake of LDL and a decrease in beta lipoprotein or LDL serum levels, and a decrease in serum cholesterol levels. Although colestipol HCl produces an increase in the hepatic synthesis of cholesterol in man, serum cholesterol levels fall.

There is evidence to show that this fall in cholesterol is secondary to an increased rate of clearance of cholesterol-rich lipoproteins (beta or low-density lipoproteins) from the plasma. Serum triglyceride levels may increase or remain unchanged in colestipol HCl treated patients.

The decline in serum cholesterol levels with colestipol HCl treatment is usually evident by 1 month. When colestipol HCl is discontinued, serum cholesterol levels usually return to baseline levels within 1 month. Periodic determinations of serum cholesterol levels as outlined in the National Cholesterol Education Program (NCEP) guidelines, should be done to confirm a favorable initial and long-term response.[1]

In a large, placebo-controlled, multiclinic study, the LRC-CPPT[2], hypercholesterolemic subjects treated with cholestyramine, a bile-acid sequestrant with a mechanism of action and an effect on serum cholesterol similar to that of colestipol HCl, had reductions in total and LDL-C. Over the 7 year study period the cholestyramine group experienced a 19% reduction (relative to the incidence in the placebo group) in the combined rate of coronary heart disease (CHD) death plus nonfatal myocardial infarction (cumulative incidences of 7% cholestyramine and 8.6% placebo). The subjects included in the study were middle-aged men (aged 35-59) with serum cholesterol levels above 265 mg/dl, LDL-C above 175 mg/dl on a moderate cholesterol-lowering diet, and no history of heart disease. It is not clear to what extent these findings can be extrapolated to other segments of the hypercholesterolemic population not studied.

Treatment with colestipol results in a significant increase in lipoprotein LpAI. Lipoprotein LpAI is one of the two major lipoprotein particles within the high-density lipoprotein (HDL) density range[3], and has been shown in cell culture to promote cholesterol efflux or removal from cells.[4] Although the significance of this finding has not been established in clinical studies, the elevation of the lipoprotein LpAI particle within the HDL fraction is consistent with an antiatherogenic effect of colestipol HCl, even though little change is observed in HDL cholesterol (HDL-C).

In patients with heterozygous familial hypercholesterolemia who have not obtained an optimal response to colestipol HCl alone in maximal doses, the combination of colestipol HCl and nicotinic acid has been shown to further lower serum cholesterol, triglyceride, and LDL-cholesterol (LDL-C) values. Simultaneously, HDL-C values increased significantly. In many such patients it is possible to normalize serum lipid values.[5-7]

Preliminary evidence suggests that the cholesterol-lowering effects of lovastatin and the bile acid sequestrant, colestipol HCl, are additive.

The effect of intensive lipid-lowering therapy on coronary atherosclerosis has been assessed by arteriography in hyperlipidemic patients. In these randomized, controlled clinical trials, patients were treated for 2-4 years by either conventional measures (diet, placebo, or in some cases low-dose resin), or with intensive combination therapy using diet and colestipol HCl granules plus either nicotinic acid or lovastatin. When compared to conventional measures, intensive lipid-lowering combination therapy significantly reduced the frequency of progression and increased the frequency of regression of coronary atherosclerotic lesions in patients with or at risk for coronary artery disease.[8-11]

INDICATIONS AND USAGE

Since no drug is innocuous, strict attention should be paid to the indications and contraindications, particularly when selecting drugs for chronic long-term use.

Colestipol HCl is indicated as adjunctive therapy to diet for the reduction of elevated serum total and LDL-C in patients with primary hypercholesterolemia (elevated LDL-C) who do not respond adequately to diet. Generally, colestipol HCl has no clinically significant effect on serum triglycerides, but with its use, triglyceride levels may be raised in some patients.

Therapy with lipid-altering agents should be a component of multiple risk factor intervention in those individuals at significantly increased risk for atherosclerotic vascular disease due to hypercholesterolemia. Treatment should begin and continue with dietary therapy (see NCEP guidelines; TABLE 1). A minimum of 6 months of intensive dietary therapy and counseling should be carried out prior to initiation of drug therapy. Shorter periods may be considered in patients with severe elevations of LDL-C or with definite CHD.

According to the NCEP guidelines, the goal of treatment is to lower LDL-C, and LDL-C is to be used to initiate and assess treatment response. Only if LDL-C levels are not available, should the total-C be used to monitor therapy. The NCEP treatment guidelines are shown in TABLE 1.

TABLE 1

Definite Atherosclerotic Disease*	Two or More Other Risk Factors†	LDL-Cholesterol mg/dl (mmol/L) Initiation Level	Goal
No	No	≥190 (≥4.9)	<160 (<4.1)
No	Yes	≥160 (≥4.1)	<130 (<3.4)
Yes	Yes or No	≥130 (≥3.4)	≤100 (≤2.6)

* Coronary heart disease or peripheral vascular disease (including symptomatic carotid artery disease).

† Other risk factors for coronary heart disease (CHD) include: age (males: ≥45 years; female: ≥55 years or premature menopause without estrogen replacement therapy); family history of premature CHD; current cigarette smoking; hypertension; confirmed HDL-C <35 mg/dl (0.91 mmol/L); and diabetes mellitus. Subtract one risk factor if HDL-C is ≥60 mg/dl (1.6 mmol/L).

CONTRAINDICATIONS

Colestipol HCl tablets and granules for oral suspension are contraindicated in those individuals who have shown hypersensitivity to any of their components.

WARNINGS

Oral Suspension: TO AVOID ACCIDENTAL INHALATION OR ESOPHAGEAL DISTRESS, COLESTIPOL HCl SHOULD NOT BE TAKEN IN ITS DRY FORM. ALWAYS MIX COLESTIPOL HCl WITH WATER OR OTHER FLUIDS BEFORE INGESTING. *PHENYLKETONURICS:* **COLESTIPOL HCl CONTAINS 18.2 mg PHENYLALANINE PER 7.5 g DOSE.**

PRECAUTIONS

Prior to initiating therapy with colestipol HCl, secondary causes of hypercholesterolemia (*e.g.,* poorly controlled diabetes mellitus, hypothyroidism, nephrotic syndrome, dysproteinemias, obstructive liver disease, other drug therapy, alcoholism), should be excluded, and a lipid profile performed to assess total cholesterol, HDL-C, and triglycerides (TG). For individuals with TG less than 400 mg/dl (<4.5 mmol/L), LDL-C can be estimated using the following equation:

LDL-C = Total cholesterol − [(Triglycerides/5) + HDL-C]

For TG levels >400 mg/dl, this equation is less accurate and LDL-C concentrations should be determined by ultracentrifugation. In hypertriglyceridemic patients, LDL-C may be low or normal despite elevated Total-C. In such cases colestipol HCl may not be indicated.

Because it sequesters bile acids, colestipol HCl may interfere with normal fat absorption and, thus, may reduce absorption of folic acid and fat soluble vitamins such as A, D, and K.

Chronic use of colestipol HCl may be associated with an increased bleeding tendency due to hypoprothrombinemia from vitamin K deficiency. This will usually respond promptly to parenteral vitamin K_1 and recurrences can be prevented by oral administration of vitamin K_1.

Serum cholesterol and triglyceride levels should be determined periodically based on NCEP guidelines to confirm a favorable initial and adequate long-term response.

Colestipol HCl may produce or severely worsen pre-existing constipation. The dosage should be increased gradually in patients to minimize the risk of developing fecal impaction.

TABLETS

In patients with pre-existing constipation, the starting dose should be 2 g once or twice a day. Increased fluid and fiber intake should be encouraged to alleviate constipation and a stool softener may occasionally be indicated. If the initial dose is well tolerated, the dose may be increased as needed by a further 2-4 g/day (at monthly intervals) with periodic monitoring of serum lipoproteins. If constipation worsens or the desired therapeutic response is not achieved at 2-16 g/day, combination therapy or alternate therapy should be considered.

ORAL SUSPENSION

In patients with pre-existing constipation, the starting dose should be 1 packet or 1 scoop once daily for 5-7 days, increasing to twice daily with monitoring of constipation and of serum lipoproteins, at least twice, 4-6 weeks apart. Increased fluid and fiber intake should be encouraged to alleviate constipation and a stool softener may occasionally be indicated. If the initial dose is well tolerated, the dose may be increased as needed by one dose/day (at monthly intervals) with periodic monitoring of serum lipoproteins. If constipation worsens or the desired therapeutic response is not achieved at 1-6 doses/day, combination therapy or alternate therapy should be considered.

TABLETS AND ORAL SUSPENSION

Particular effort should be made to avoid constipation in patients with symptomatic coronary artery disease. Constipation associated with colestipol HCl may aggravate hemorrhoids.

While there have been no reports of hypothyroidism induced in individuals with normal thyroid function, the theoretical possibility exists, particularly in patients with limited thyroid reserve.

Since colestipol HCl is a chloride form of an anion exchange resin, there is a possibility that prolonged use may lead to the development of hyperchloremia acidosis.

CARCINOGENESIS, MUTAGENESIS, AND IMPAIRMENT OF FERTILITY

In studies conducted in rats in which cholestyramine resin (a bile acid sequestering agent similar to colestipol HCl) was used as a tool to investigate the role of various intestinal factors, such as fat, bile salts, and microbial flora, in the development of intestinal tumors induced by potent carcinogens, the incidence of such tumors was observed to be greater in cholestyramine resin treated rats than in control rats.

The relevance of this laboratory observation from studies in rats with cholestyramine resin to the clinical use of colestipol HCl is not known. In the LRC-CPPT study referred to above, the total incidence of fatal and nonfatal neoplasms was similar in both treatment groups. When the many different categories of tumors are examined, various alimentary system cancers were somewhat more prevalent in the cholestyramine group. The small numbers and the multiple categories prevent conclusions from being drawn. Further follow-up of the LRC-CPPT participants by the sponsors of that study is planned for cause-specific mortality and cancer morbidity. When colestipol HCl was administered in the diet to rats for 18 months, there was no evidence of any drug related intestinal tumor formation. In the Ames assay, colestipol HCl was not mutagenic.

PREGNANCY

Since colestipol HCl is essentially not absorbed systemically (less than 0.17% of the dose), it is not expected to cause fetal harm when administered during pregnancy in recommended dosages. There are no adequate and well-controlled studies in pregnant women, and the known interference with absorption of fat-soluble vitamins may be detrimental even in the presence of supplementation.

Additional Information for Oral Suspension

The use of colestipol HCl oral suspension in pregnancy or by women of childbearing potential requires that the potential benefits of drug therapy be weighed against possible hazards to the mother or child.

NURSING MOTHERS

Caution should be exercised when colestipol HCl is administered to a nursing mother. The possible lack of proper vitamin absorption described in Pregnancy may have an effect on nursing infants.

PEDIATRIC USE

Safety and effectiveness in the pediatric population have not been established.

INFORMATION FOR THE PATIENT

Colestipol HCl Tablets Only

Colestipol HCl tablets may be larger than pills you have taken before. If you have had swallowing problems or choking with food, liquids or other tablets or capsules in the past, you should discuss this with your doctor before taking colestipol HCl tablets.

It is important that you take colestipol HCl tablets correctly:

1. Always take 1 tablet at a time and swallow promptly.
2. Swallow each tablet whole. Do not cut, crush, or chew the tablets.
3. Colestipol HCl tablets must be taken with water or another liquid that you prefer. Swallowing the tablets will be easier if you drink plenty of liquid as you swallow each tablet.

Difficulty swallowing and temporary obstruction of the esophagus (the tube between your mouth and stomach) have been rarely reported in patients taking colestipol HCl tablets. If a tablet does get stuck after you swallow it, you may notice pressure or discomfort. If this happens to you, you should contact your doctor. Do not take colestipol HCl tablets again without your doctor's advice.

If you are taking other medications, you should take them at least 1 hour before or 4 hours after taking colestipol HCl tablets.

DRUG INTERACTIONS

Since colestipol HCl is an anion exchange resin, it may have a strong affinity for anions other than the bile acids. *In vitro* studies have indicated that colestipol HCl binds a number of drugs. Therefore, colestipol HCl may delay or reduce the absorption of concomitant oral medication. The interval between the administration of colestipol HCl and any other medication should be as long as possible. Patients should take other drugs at least 1 hour before or 4 hours after colestipol HCl to avoid impeding their absorption.

Repeated doses of colestipol HCl given prior to a single dose of propranolol in human trials have been reported to decrease propranolol absorption. However, in a follow-up study in normal subjects, single-dose administration of colestipol HCl and propranolol and twice-a-day administration for 5 days of both agents did not affect the extent of propranolol absorption, but had a small yet statistically significant effect on its rate of absorption; the time to reach maximum concentration was delayed approximately 30 minutes. Effects on the absorption of other beta-blockers have not been determined. Therefore, patients on propranolol should be observed when colestipol HCl is either added or deleted from a therapeutic regimen.

Studies in humans show that the absorption of chlorothiazide as reflected in urinary excretion is markedly decreased even when administered 1 hour before colestipol HCl. The absorption of tetracycline, furosemide, penicillin G, hydrochlorothiazide, and gemfibrozil was significantly decreased when given simultaneously with colestipol HCl; these drugs were not tested to determine the effect of administration 1 hour before colestipol HCl.

No depressant effect on blood levels in humans was noted when colestipol HCl was administered with any of the following drugs: aspirin, clindamycin, clofibrate, methyldopa, nicotinic acid (niacin), tolbutamide, phenytoin or warfarin. Particular caution should be observed with digitalis preparations since there are conflicting results for the effect of colestipol HCl on the availability of digoxin and digitoxin. The potential for binding of these drugs if given concomitantly is present. Discontinuing colestipol HCl could pose a hazard to health if a potentially toxic drug that is significantly bound to the resin has been titrated to a maintenance level while the patient was taking colestipol HCl.

Bile acid binding resins may also interfere with the absorption of oral phosphate supplements and hydrocortisone.

ADVERSE REACTIONS

GASTROINTESTINAL

The most common adverse reactions are confined to the gastrointestinal tract. To achieve minimal GI disturbance with an optimal LDL-C lowering effect, a gradual increase of dosage starting with 2 g, once or twice daily is recommended for the tablets, and one dose/day for the oral suspension. Constipation is the major single complaint and at times is severe. Most instances of constipation are mild, transient, and controlled with standard treatment. Increased fluid intake and inclusion of additional dietary fiber should be the first step; a stool softener may be added if needed. Some patients require decreased dosage or discontinuation of therapy. Hemorrhoids may be aggravated.

Other, less frequent gastrointestinal complaints consist of abdominal discomfort (abdominal pain and cramping), intestinal gas (bloating and flatulence), indigestion and heartburn, diarrhea and loose stools, and nausea and vomiting. Bleeding hemorrhoids and blood in the stool have been infrequently reported. Peptic ulceration, cholecystitis, and cholelithiasis have been rarely reported in patients receiving colestipol HCl granules, and are not necessarily drug related.

Difficulty swallowing and transient esophageal obstruction have been rarely reported in patients taking colestipol HCl tablets.

Transient and modest elevations of aspartate aminotransferase (AST, SGOT), alanine aminotransferase (ALT, SGPT) and alkaline phosphatase were observed on one or more occasions in various patients treated with colestipol HCl.

The following nongastrointestinal adverse reactions have been reported with generally equal frequency in patients receiving colestipol HCl tablets, colestipol granules, flavored colestipol granules, or placebo in clinical studies:

Cardiovascular: Chest pain, angina, and tachycardia have been infrequently reported.

Hypersensitivity: Rash has been infrequently reported. Urticaria and dermatitis have been rarely noted in patients receiving colestipol HCl granules.

Musculoskeletal: Musculoskeletal pain, aches and pains in the extremities, joint pain and arthritis, and backache have been reported.

Neurologic: Headache, migraine headache, and sinus headache have been reported. Other infrequently reported complaints include dizziness, lightheadedness, and insomnia.

Miscellaneous: Anorexia, fatigue, weakness, shortness of breath, and swelling of the hands or feet, have been infrequently reported.

DOSAGE AND ADMINISTRATION

TABLETS

For adults, colestipol HCl tablets are recommended in doses of 2-16 g/day given once or in divided doses. The starting dose should be 2 g once or twice daily. Dosage increases of 2 g, once or twice daily should occur at 1 or 2 month intervals. Appropriate use of lipid profiles as per NCEP guidelines including LDL-C and triglycerides, is advised so that optimal but not excessive doses are used to obtain the desired therapeutic effect on LDL-C level. If the desired therapeutic effect is not obtained at a dose of 2-16 g/day with good compliance and acceptable side effects, combined therapy or alternate treatment should be considered.

Colestipol HCl tablets must be taken one at a time and be promptly swallowed whole, using plenty of water or other appropriate liquid. Do not cut, crush, or chew the tablets. Patients should take other drugs at least 1 hour before or 4 hours after colestipol HCl tablets to minimize possible interference with their absorption. (See DRUG INTERACTIONS.)

ORAL SUSPENSION

One dose (1 packet or 1 level teaspoon) contains 5 g of colestipol HCl. One dose (1 packet or 1 level scoopful) of flavored colestipol HCl is approximately 7.5 g which contains 5 g of colestipol HCl. The recommended daily adult dose is 1-6 packets or level scoopfuls given once or in divided doses. Treatment should be started with 1 dose once or twice daily with an increment of 1 dose/day at 1 or 2 month intervals. Appropriate use of lipid profiles as per NCEP guidelines including LDL-cholesterol and trigylcerides is advised so that optimal, but not excessive doses are used to obtain the desired therapeutic effect on LDL-cholesterol level. If the desired therapeutic effect is not obtained at 1-6 doses/day with good compliance and acceptable side effects, combined therapy or alternate treatment should be considered.

To avoid accidental inhalation or esophageal distress, colestipol HCl and flavored colestipol HCl should not be taken in its dry form. Colestipol HCl and flavored colestipol HCl should always be mixed with water or other fluids before ingesting. Patients should take other drugs at least 1 hour before or 4 hours after colestipol HCl or flavored colestipol HCl to minimize possible interference with their absorption. (See DRUG INTERACTIONS.)

Mixing and Administration Guide

Colestipol HCl and flavored colestipol HCl should always be mixed in a liquid such as water or the beverage of your choice. It may also be taken in soups or with cereals or pulpy fruits. Colestipol HCl or flavored colestipol HCl *should never be taken in its dry form.*

Flavored colestipol HCl is an orange-flavored product. Although it may be mixed with a variety of liquids or foods, the selection should be based on patient preference.

With Beverages:

1. Add the prescribed amount of colestipol HCl or flavored colestipol HCl to a glassful (3 oz or more) of water or the beverage of your choice. A heavy or pulpy juice may minimize complaints relative to consistency.
2. Stir the mixture until the medication is completely mixed. (Colestipol HCl and flavored colestipol HCl will not dissolve in the liquid.) Colestipol HCl and flavored colestipol HCl may also be mixed with carbonated beverages, slowly stirred in a large glass; however, this mixture may be associated with GI complaints.

Rinse the glass with a small amount of additional beverage to make sure all the medication is taken.

With Cereals, Soups, and Fruits: Colestipol HCl and flavored colestipol HCl may be taken mixed with milk in hot or regular breakfast cereals, or even mixed in soups that have a high fluid content. It may also be added to fruits that are pulpy such as crushed pineapple, pears, peaches, or fruit cocktail.

TABLETS AND ORAL SUSPENSION

Before Administration of Colestipol HCl:

1. Define the type of hyperlipoproteinemia, as described in NCEP guidelines.
2. Institute a trial of diet and weight reduction.
3. Establish baseline serum total and LDL-C and triglyceride levels.

During Administration of Colestipol HCl:

1. The patient should be carefully monitored clinically, including serum cholesterol and triglyceride levels. Periodic determinations of serum cholesterol levels as outlined in the NCEP guidelines should be done to confirm a favorable initial and long-term response.
2. Failure of total or LDL-C to fall within the desired range should lead one to first examine dietary and drug compliance. If these are deemed acceptable, combined therapy or alternate treatment should be considered.
3. Significant rise in triglyceride level should be considered as indication for dose reduction, drug discontinuation, or combined or alternate therapy.

HOW SUPPLIED

COLESTID TABLETS

Colestid tablets are yellow, elliptical, imprinted "U".

Each tablet contains 1 g of colestipol HCl.

Storage: *Flavored Colestid, Tablets, and Oral Suspension:* Store at controlled room temperature 20-25°C (68-77°F).

PRODUCT LISTING - EQUIVALENTS NOT AVAILABLE

Granule For Reconstitution - Oral - 5 Gm

5 gm x 30	$56.57	COLESTID, Pharmacia and Upjohn	00009-0260-01
5 gm x 90	$166.32	COLESTID, Pharmacia and Upjohn	00009-0260-04
300 gm	$67.39	COLESTID, Pharmacia and Upjohn	00009-0260-17
500 gm	$112.33	COLESTID, Pharmacia and Upjohn	00009-0260-02

Granule For Reconstitution - Oral - 5 Gm/7.5 Gm

7.50 gm x 60	$132.85	COLESTID FLAVORED, Pharmacia and Upjohn	00009-0370-03
450 gm	$88.76	COLESTID FLAVORED, Pharmacia and Upjohn	00009-0370-05

Tablet - Oral - 1 Gm

120's	$69.09	COLESTID, Pharmacia and Upjohn	00009-0450-03

Cortisone Acetate *(000907)*

For related information, see the comparative table section in Appendix A.

Categories: Adrenocortical insufficiency; Anemia, acquired hemolytic; Anemia, congenital hypoplastic; Anemia, erythroblastopenia; Ankylosing spondylitis; Arthritis, gouty; Arthritis, post-traumatic; Arthritis, psoriatic; Arthritis, rheumatoid; Asthma; Berylliosis; Bursitis; Carditis, rheumatic; Chorioretinitis; Choroiditis; Colitis, ulcerative; Conjunctivitis, allergic; Crohn's disease; Dermatitis herpetiformis, bullous; Dermatitis, atopic; Dermatitis, contact; Dermatitis, exfoliative; Dermatitis, seborrheic; Dermatomyositis, systemic; Epicondylitis; Erythema multiforme; Herpes zoster ophthalmicus; Hypercalcemia, secondary to neoplasia; Hypersensitivity reactions; Inflammation, anterior segment, ophthalmic; Inflammation, ophthalmic; Inflammatory bowel disease; Iridocyclitis; Iritis; Keratitis; Leukemia; Loffler's syndrome; Lupus erythematosus, systemic; Lymphoma; Meningitis, tuberculous; Multiple sclerosis; Mycosis fungoides; Nephrotic syndrome; Neuritis, optic; Ophthalmia, sympathetic; Pemphigus; Pneumonitis, aspiration; Polymyositis; Psoriasis; Rhinitis, perennial allergic; Rhinitis, seasonal allergic; Sarcoidosis; Serum sickness; Stevens-Johnson syndrome; Synovitis, secondary to osteoarthritis; Tenosynovitis; Thrombocytopenia, secondary; Thyroiditis, nonsuppurative; Trichinosis; Tuberculosis, disseminated; Tuberculosis, fulminating; Tuberculosis, meningitis; Ulcer, allergic corneal marginal; Uveitis; FDA Approved 1951 Nov; Pregnancy Category D

Drug Classes: Corticosteroids

Brand Names: **Cortone**

Foreign Brand Availability: Adreson (Hungary; Netherlands); Altesona (Spain); Cortate (Australia; Hong-Kong; Malaysia); Cortison Ciba (Germany; Switzerland); Cortison Nycomed (Norway); Cortisone (France); Cortisone Acetate (Israel; New-Zealand); Cortisoni Acetas (Netherlands); Cortogen (South-Africa); Cortone Acetato (Italy); Cortone-Azetat (Austria); Scheroson (Japan)

Cost of Therapy: $1.00 (Asthma; Generic Tablet; 25 mg; 1 tablet/day; 30 day supply)

HCFA JCODE(S): J0810 up to 50 mg IM

DESCRIPTION

Cortisone acetate is a white to practically white, odorless, crystalline powder. It is insoluble in water; freely soluble in chloroform; soluble in dioxane; sparingly soluble in acetone; slightly soluble in alcohol.

The chemical name for cortisone acetate is pregn-4-ene-3,11,20-trione, 21-(acetyloxy)-17-hydroxy and the molecular weight is 402.49. The empirical formula is $C_{23}H_{30}O_6$.

TABLETS

Cortisone acetate is a glucocorticoid. Glucocorticoids are adrenocortical steroids, both naturally occurring and synthetic, which are readily absorbed from the gastrointestinal tract.

Cortone tablets contain 25 mg of cortisone acetate in each tablet. *Inactive Ingredients:* Lactose, magnesium stearate, and starch.

IM INJECTION

Cortone sterile suspension is a sterile suspension containing 50 mg/ml of cortisone acetate in an aqueous medium (pH 5.0-7.0). *Inactive Ingredients per ml:* Sodium chloride, 9 mg; polysorbate 80, 4 mg; sodium carboxymethylcellulose, 5 mg; water for injection qs 1 ml; benzyl alcohol, 9 mg, added as preservative.

No attempt should be made to alter cortone acetate sterile suspension. Diluting it or mixing it with other substances may affect the state of suspension or change the rate of absorption and reduce its effectiveness.

CLINICAL PHARMACOLOGY

Naturally occurring glucocorticoids (hydrocortisone and cortisone), which also have salt-retaining properties, are used as replacement therapy in adrenocortical deficiency states. Their synthetic analogs are primarily used for their potent anti-inflammatory effects in disorders of many organ systems.

Glucocorticoids cause profound and varied metabolic effects. In addition, they modify the body's immune responses to diverse stimuli.

IM Injection: Cortisone acetate sterile suspension has a slow onset but long duration of action when compared with more soluble preparations. When daily corticosteroid therapy is required and oral therapy is not feasible, the required daily dosage may be given in a single intramuscular (IM) injection of this preparation.

INDICATIONS AND USAGE

Cortisone Acetate is Indicated in the Following Conditions:

Endocrine Disorders: Primary or secondary adrenocortical insufficiency (hydrocortisone or cortisone is the first choice; synthetic analogs may be used in conjunction with mineralocorticoids where applicable; in infancy mineralocorticoid supplementation is of particular importance); congenital adrenal hyperplasia; hypercalcemia associated with cancer; nonsuppurative thyroiditis. *IM Injection Only:* Acute adrenocortical insufficiency (hydrocortisone or cortisone is the drug of choice; mineralocorticoid supplementation may be necessary, particularly when synthetic analogs are used).

Rheumatic Disorders: As adjunctive therapy for short-term administration (to tide the patient over an acute episode or exacerbation) in:

Psoriatic arthritis, rheumatoid arthritis, including juvenile rheumatoid arthritis (selected cases may require low-dose maintenance therapy), ankylosing spondylitis, post-traumatic osteoarthritis, acute and subacute bursitis, synovitis of osteoarthritis, acute nonspecific tenosynovitis, epicondylitis, acute gouty arthritis.

Collagen Diseases: During an exacerbation or as maintenance therapy in selected cases of:

Systemic lupus erythematosus, acute rheumatic carditis, systemic dermatomyositis (polymyositis).

Dermatologic Diseases: Pemphigus, exfoliative dermatitis, bullous dermatitis herpetiformis, mycosis fungoides, severe erythema multiforme (Stevens-Johnson syndrome), severe psoriasis, severe seborrheic dermatitis.

Allergic States: Control of severe or incapacitating allergic conditions intractable to adequate trials of conventional treatment:

Seasonal or perennial allergic rhinitis, contact dermatitis, atopic dermatitis, serum sickness, drug hypersensitivity reactions, bronchial asthma. *IM Injection Only:* Urticarial transfusion reactions.

Ophthalmic Diseases: Severe acute and chronic allergic and inflammatory processes involving the eye and its adnexa such as:

Allergic conjunctivitis, anterior segment inflammation, keratitis, allergic corneal marginal ulcers, diffuse posterior uveitis and choroiditis, herpes zoster ophthalmicus, iritis and iridocyclitis, optic neuritis, chorioretinitis, sympathetic ophthalmia.

Respiratory Diseases: Symptomatic sarcoidosis, Loeffler's syndrome not manageable by other means, fulminating or disseminated pulmonary tuberculosis when used concurrently with appropriate antituberculous chemotherapy, berylliosis, aspiration pneumonitis.

Hematologic Disorders: Acquired (autoimmune) hemolytic anemia, erythroblastopenia (RBC anemia), congenital (erythroid) hypoplastic anemia. *Tablets Only:* Idiopathic thrombocytopenic purpura in adults, secondary thrombocytopenia in adults.

Neoplastic Diseases: For palliative management of:

Leukemias and lymphomas in adults, acute leukemia of childhood.

Edematous States: To induce a diuresis or remission of proteinuria in the nephrotic syndrome, without uremia, of the idiopathic type or that due to lupus erythematosus.

Gastrointestinal Diseases: To tide the patient over a critical period of the disease in:

Ulcerative colitis, regional enteritis.

Miscellaneous: Tuberculous meningitis with subarachnoid block or impending block when used concurrently with appropriate antituberculous chemotherapy; trichinosis with neurologic or myocardial involvement.

IM Injection Only:

- Preoperatively, and in the event of serious trauma or illness, in patients with known adrenal insufficiency or when adrenocortical reserve is doubtful.
- Shock unresponsive to conventional therapy if adrenocortical insufficiency exists or is suspected.
- Acute noninfectious laryngeal edema (epinephrine is the drug of first choice).

CONTRAINDICATIONS

Systemic fungal infections and known hypersensitivity to components.

WARNINGS

In patients on corticosteroid therapy subjected to unusual stress, increased dosage of rapidly acting corticosteroids before, during, and after the stressful situation is indicated.

Corticosteroids may mask some signs of infection, and new infections may appear during their use. Infections with any pathogen including viral, bacterial, fungal, protozoan or helminthic infections, in any location of the body, may be associated with the use of corticosteroids alone or in combination with other immunosuppressive agents that affect cellular immunity, humoral immunity, or neutrophil function.[1]

These infections may be mild, but can be severe and at times fatal. With increasing doses of corticosteroids, the rate of occurrence of infectious complications increases.[2] There may be decreased resistance and inability to localize infection when corticosteroids are used.

Prolonged use of corticosteroids may produce posterior subcapsular cataracts, glaucoma with possible damage to the optic nerves, and may enhance the establishment of secondary ocular infections due to fungi or viruses.

USE IN PREGNANCY

Since adequate human reproduction studies have not been done with corticosteroids, use of these drugs in pregnancy, nursing mothers, or in women of childbearing potential requires that the possible benefits of the drug be weighed against the potential hazards to the mother and embryo or fetus. Infants born of mothers who have received substantial doses of corticosteroids during pregnancy should be carefully observed for signs of hypoadrenalism.

Average and large doses of hydrocortisone or cortisone can cause elevation of blood pressure, salt and water retention, and increased excretion of potassium. These effects are less likely to occur with the synthetic derivatives except when used in large doses. Dietary salt restriction and potassium supplementation may be necessary. All corticosteroids increase calcium excretion.

Administration of live or live, attenuated vaccines is contraindicated in patients receiving immunosuppressive doses of corticosteroids. Killed or inactivated vaccines may be administered to patients receiving immunosuppressive doses of corticosteroids; however, the response to such vaccines may be diminished. Indicated immunization procedures may be undertaken in patients receiving nonimmunosuppressive doses of corticosteroids.

The use of cortisone acetate tablets or sterile suspension in active tuberculosis should be restricted to those cases of fulminating or disseminated tuberculosis in which the corticosteroid is used for the management of the disease in conjunction with an appropriate anti-tuberculosis regimen.

If corticosteroids are indicated in patients with latent tuberculosis or tuberculin reactivity, close observation is necessary as reactivation of the disease may occur. During prolonged corticosteroid therapy, these patients should receive chemoprophylaxis.

Persons who are on drugs which suppress the immune system are more susceptible to infections than healthy individuals. Chicken pox and measles, for example, can have a more serious or even fatal course in nonimmune children or adults on corticosteroids. In such children or adults who have not had these diseases, particular care should be taken to avoid exposure. How the dose, route, and duration of corticosteroid administration affects the risk of developing a disseminated infection is not known. The contribution of the underlying disease and/or prior corticosteroid treatment to the risk is also not known. If exposed to chicken pox, prophylaxis with varicella zoster immune globulin (VZIG) may be indicated. If exposed to measles, prophylaxis with pooled intramuscular immunoglobulin (IG) may be indicated. (See the respective prescribing information for VZIG and IG.) If chicken pox develops, treatment with antiviral agents may be considered. Similarly, corticosteroids should be used with great care in patients with known or suspected *Strongyloides* (threadworm) infestation. In such patients, corticosteroid-induced immunosuppression may lead to *Strongyloides* hyperinfection and dissemination with widespread larval migration, often accompanied by severe enterocolitis and potentially fatal gram-negative septicemia.

IM INJECTION ONLY

Because rare instances of anaphylactoid reactions have occurred in patients receiving parenteral corticosteroid therapy, appropriate precautionary measures should be taken prior to administration, especially when the patient has a history of allergy to any drug. Anaphylactoid and hypersensitivity reactions have been reported for sterile suspension cortisone acetate (see ADVERSE REACTIONS).

PRECAUTIONS

Drug-induced secondary adrenocortical insufficiency may be minimized by gradual reduction of dosage. This type of relative insufficiency may persist for months after discontinuation of therapy; therefore, in any situation of stress occurring during that period, hormone therapy should be reinstituted. Since mineralocorticoid secretion may be impaired, salt and/or a mineralocorticoid should be administered concurrently.

There is an enhanced effect of corticosteroids on patients with hypothyroidism and in those with cirrhosis.

Corticosteroids should be used cautiously in patients with ocular herpes simplex because of possible corneal perforation.

The lowest possible dose of corticosteroid should be used to control the condition under treatment, and when reduction in dosage is possible, the reduction should be gradual.

Psychic derangements may appear when corticosteroids are used, ranging from euphoria, insomnia, mood swings, personality changes, and severe depression, to frank psychotic manifestations. Also, existing emotional instability or psychotic tendencies may be aggravated by corticosteroids.

Steroids should be used with caution in nonspecific ulcerative colitis, if there is a probability of impending perforation, abscess or other pyogenic infection, diverticulitis, fresh intestinal anastomoses, active or latent peptic ulcer, renal insufficiency, hypertension, osteoporosis, and myasthenia gravis.

Growth and development of infants and children on prolonged corticosteroid therapy should be carefully observed.

Kaposi's sarcoma has been reported to occur in patients receiving corticosteroid therapy. Discontinuation of corticosteroids may result in clinical remission.

Information for the Patient: Persons who are on immunosuppressant doses of corticosteroids should be warned to avoid exposure to chicken pox or measles. Patients should also be advised that if they are exposed, medical advice should be sought without delay.
IM Injection Only: Cortisone acetate sterile suspension, like many other steroid formulations, is sensitive to heat. Therefore, it should not be autoclaved when it is desirable to sterilize the exterior of the vial.

DRUG INTERACTIONS

The pharmacokinetic interactions listed below are potentially clinically important. Drugs that induce hepatic enzymes such as phenobarbital, phenytoin, and rifampin may increase the clearance of corticosteroids and may require increases in corticosteroid dose to achieve the desired response. Drugs such as troleandomycin and ketoconazole may inhibit the metabolism of corticosteroids and thus decrease their clearance. Therefore, the dose of corticosteroid should be titrated to avoid steroid toxicity. Corticosteroids may increase the clearance of chronic high dose aspirin. This could lead to decreased salicylate serum levels or increase the risk of salicylate toxicity when corticosteroid is withdrawn. Aspirin should be used cautiously in conjunction with corticosteroids in patients suffering from hypoprothrombinemia. The effect of corticosteroids on oral anticoagulants is variable. There are reports of enhanced as well as diminished effects of anticoagulants when given concurrently with corticosteroids. Therefore, coagulation indices should be monitored to maintain the desired anticoagulant effect.

ADVERSE REACTIONS

Fluid and Electrolyte Disturbances: Sodium retention, potassium loss, fluid retention, hypokalemic alkalosis, congestive heart failure in susceptible patients, hypertension.
Musculoskeletal: Muscle weakness, vertebral compression fractures, steroid myopathy, aseptic necrosis of femoral and humeral heads, loss of muscle mass, osteoporosis, tendon rupture (particularly of the Achilles tendon), pathologic fracture of long bones.
Gastrointestinal: Peptic ulcer with possible perforation and hemorrhage, abdominal distention, ulcerative esophagitis, pancreatitis, increases in alanine transaminase (ALT, SGPT), aspartate transaminase (AST, SGOT) and alkaline phosphatase have been observed following corticosteroid treatment. These changes are usually small, not associated with any clinical syndrome and are reversible upon discontinuation.
Dermatologic: Impaired wound healing, facial erythema, thin fragile skin, increased sweating, petechiae and ecchymosis, may suppress reactions to skin tests.
Neurological: Increased intracranial pressure with papilledema (pseudotumor cerebri) usually after treatment, convulsions, vertigo, headache.
Endocrine: Menstrual irregularities, suppression of growth in children, development of cushingoid state, decreased carbohydrate tolerance, secondary adrenocortical and pituitary unresponsiveness, particularly in times of stress, as in trauma, surgery or illness, manifestations of latent diabetes mellitus, increased requirements for insulin or oral hypoglycemic agents in diabetics.
Ophthalmic: Posterior subcapsular cataracts, glaucoma, increased intraocular pressure, exophthalmos.
Metabolic: Negative nitrogen balance due to protein catabolism.
Cardiovascular: IM Injection Only: Myocardial rupture following recent myocardial infarction (see WARNINGS).
Other: IM Injection Only: Hypersensitivity, thromboembolism, weight gain, increased appetite, nausea.

DOSAGE AND ADMINISTRATION

Tablets: For oral administration.
IM Injection: For IM injection only. NOT FOR INTRAVENOUS USE.
The initial dosage of cortisone acetate may vary from 25-300 mg/day depending on the specific disease entity being treated. In situations of less severity, lower doses will generally suffice; while in selected patients higher initial doses may be required. The initial dosage should be maintained or adjusted until a satisfactory response is noted. If after a reasonable period of time there is a lack of satisfactory clinical response, cortisone acetate should be discontinued and the patient transferred to other appropriate therapy. **IT SHOULD BE EMPHASIZED THAT DOSAGE REQUIREMENTS ARE VARIABLE AND MUST BE INDIVIDUALIZED ON THE BASIS OF THE DISEASE UNDER TREATMENT AND THE RESPONSE OF THE PATIENT.** After a favorable response is noted, the proper maintenance dosage should be determined by decreasing the initial drug dosage in small decrements at appropriate time intervals until the lowest dosage which will maintain an adequate clinical response is reached. It should be kept in mind that constant monitoring is needed in regard to drug dosage. Included in the situations which may make dosage adjustments necessary are changes in clinical status secondary to remissions or exacerbations in the disease process, the patient's individual drug responsiveness, and the effect of patient exposure to stressful situations not directly related to the disease entity under treatment; in this latter situation it may be necessary to increase the dosage of cortisone acetate for a period of time consistent with the patient's condition. If after long-term therapy the drug is to be stopped, it is recommended that it be withdrawn gradually rather than abruptly.

HOW SUPPLIED

Storage: The tablets should be stored at controlled room temperature 20-25°C (68-77°F).

PRODUCT LISTING - RATED NOT THERAPEUTICALLY EQUIVALENT

Tablet - Oral - 25 mg

Qty	Price	Manufacturer	NDC
100's	$3.34	GENERIC, Global Pharmaceutical Corporation	00115-2920-01
100's	$37.50	GENERIC, Moore, H.L. Drug Exchange Inc	00839-5084-06
100's	$41.00	GENERIC, Raway Pharmacal Inc	00686-1202-01
100's	$42.50	GENERIC, Cmc-Consolidated Midland Corporation	00223-0704-01
100's	$43.48	GENERIC, Qualitest Products Inc	00603-3062-21
100's	$43.50	GENERIC, Major Pharmaceuticals Inc	00904-2043-60
100's	$45.75	GENERIC, West Ward Pharmaceutical Corporation	00143-1202-01
100's	$48.00	GENERIC, Ivax Corporation	00182-1648-01
100's	$50.48	GENERIC, Watson Laboratories Inc	52544-0798-01

PRODUCT LISTING - EQUIVALENTS NOT AVAILABLE

Qty	Price	Manufacturer	NDC
Suspension - Injectable - 50 mg/ml			
10 ml	$9.50	GENERIC, Hyrex Pharmaceuticals	00314-0620-70
Tablet - Oral - 25 mg			
100's	$7.07	GENERIC, Vita-Rx Corporation	49727-0092-02

Cromolyn Sodium *(000916)*

For related information, see the comparative table section in Appendix A.

Categories: Asthma; Bronchospasm, exercise-induced; Conjunctivitis, vernal; Keratitis, vernal; Keratoconjunctivitis, vernal; Mastocytosis, systemic; Pregnancy Category B; FDA Approved 1973 Jun; WHO Formulary; Orphan Drugs

Drug Classes: Mast cell stabilizers; Ophthalmics

Brand Names: Cromoglicic Acid; Gastrocrom; **Intal**; Nasalcrom; Opticrom

Foreign Brand Availability: Alerbul Nasal (Colombia); Alerbul Oftalmico (Colombia); Alerg (Germany); Allergo-comod (Germany); Allergocrom (Korea; Taiwan); Clesin (Korea); Cromabak (Hong-Kong; Singapore); Cromadoses (France); Cromal-5 Inhaler (South-Africa); Cromo-Asma (Spain); Cromogen (Israel); Cromolyn (Bahrain; Cyprus; Egypt; Iran; Iraq; Jordan; Kuwait; Lebanon; Libya; Oman; Qatar; Republic-of-Yemen; Saudi-Arabia; Syria; United-Arab-Emirates); Crom-Ophtal (Indonesia); Cromoptic (France); Cronase (Israel); Cusicrom (Taiwan); Dadcrome (Bahrain; Cyprus; Egypt; Iran; Iraq; Jordan; Kuwait; Lebanon; Libya; Oman; Qatar; Republic-of-Yemen; Saudi-Arabia; Syria; United-Arab-Emirates); DNCG Trom (Taiwan); Epicrom (Bahrain; Cyprus; Egypt; Iran; Iraq; Jordan; Kuwait; Lebanon; Libya; Oman; Qatar; Republic-of-Yemen; Saudi-Arabia; Syria; United-Arab-Emirates); Fintal (India); Frenal (Italy); Ifiral (India; Thailand); Lomudal (Belgium; Benin; Burkina-Faso; Denmark; Ethiopia; Finland; France; Gambia; Ghana; Greece; Guinea; Italy; Ivory-Coast; Kenya; Liberia; Malawi; Mali; Mauritania; Mauritius; Morocco; Netherlands; Niger; Nigeria; Norway; Peru; Senegal; Seychelles; Sierra-Leone; South-Africa; Sudan; Sweden; Switzerland; Tanzania; Tunia; Uganda; Zambia; Zimbabwe); Lomudal Gastrointestinum (Finland); Lomudal Nasal (Finland; Sweden); Lomudal Nesespray (Norway); Lomupren-Nasenspray (Austria); Lomusol (Austria; Belgium; France); Lomusol Forte (Netherlands); Lomusol Nasenspray (Austria); Multicrom (France); Nalcrom (Canada; England; Hong-Kong; Italy; Netherlands; New-Zealand; South-Africa); Nasotal (Bahrain; Cyprus; Egypt; Iran; Iraq; Jordan; Kuwait; Lebanon; Libya; Oman; Qatar; Republic-of-Yemen; Saudi-Arabia; Syria; United-Arab-Emirates); Nazotral (Colombia); Noaler (Colombia); Noaler Nasal (Colombia); Opticron (France); Optrex (New-Zealand); Rynacrom (Australia; Bahamas; Bahrain; Barbados; Belize; Benin; Bermuda; Burkina-Faso; Costa-Rica; Curacao; Cyprus; Dominican-Republic; Egypt; El-Salvador; Ethiopia; Finland; Gambia; Ghana; Guatemala; Guinea; Guyana; Honduras; Hong-Kong; Iran; Iraq; Ivory-Coast; Jamaica; Jordan; Kenya; Korea; Kuwait; Lebanon; Liberia; Libya; Malawi; Malaysia; Mali; Mauritania; Mauritius; Mexico; Morocco; Netherland-Antilles; New-Zealand; Nicaragua; Niger; Nigeria; Oman; Panama; Portugal; Qatar; Republic-of-Yemen; Saudi-Arabia; Senegal; Seychelles; Sierra-Leone; Singapore; South-Africa; Sudan; Surinam; Syria; Tanzania; Trinidad; Tunia; Uganda; United-Arab-Emirates; Zambia; Zimbabwe); Rynacrom M (Bahamas; Barbados; Belize; Bermuda; Curacao; Guyana; Hong-Kong; Jamaica; Netherland-Antilles; Singapore; Surinam; Thailand; Trinidad); Sificrom (Singapore); Vicrom (New-Zealand); Vipront (Indonesia); Vistacrom (Costa-Rica; Dominican-Republic; El-Salvador; Guatemala; Honduras; Nicaragua; Panama; South-Africa); Vividrin (Malaysia; Philippines; Thailand)

HCFA JCODE(S): J7630 per 20 mg INH

INHALATION

DESCRIPTION

Note: The trade names have been used throughout this monograph for clarity.

INTAL INHALER

For Oral Inhalation Only.

The active ingredient of Intal Inhaler is cromolyn sodium. It is an inhaled anti-inflammatory agent for the preventive management of asthma. Cromolyn sodium is disodium 5,5′-[(2-hydroxytrimethylene)dioxy]bis[4-oxo-4*H*-1-benzopyran-2-carboxylate]. The empirical formula is $C_{23}H_{14}Na_2O_{11}$; the molecular weight is 512.34. Cromolyn sodium is a water soluble, odorless, white, hydrated crystalline powder. It is tasteless at first, but leaves a slightly bitter aftertaste.

Intal Inhaler is a metered dose aerosol unit for oral inhalation containing micronized cromolyn sodium, sorbitan trioleate with dichlorotetrafluoroethane and dichlorodifluoromethane as propellants. Each actuation delivers approximately 1 mg cromolyn sodium from the valve and 800 μg cromolyn sodium through the mouthpiece to the patient. Each 8.1 g canister delivers at least 112 metered inhalations (56 doses); each 14.2 g canister delivers at least 200 metered inhalations (100 doses).

INTAL NEBULIZER SOLUTION

For Inhalation Use Only — Not for Injection.

The active ingredient of Intal Nebulizer Solution is cromolyn sodium. It is an inhaled anti-inflammatory agent for the preventive management of asthma. Cromolyn sodium is disodium 5,5′-[(2-hydroxytrimethylene)dioxy]bis[4-oxo-4*H*-1-benzopyran-2-carboxylate]. The empirical formula is $C_{23}H_{14}Na_2O_{11}$; the molecular weight is 512.34. Cromolyn sodium is a water soluble, odorless, white, hydrated crystalline powder. It is tasteless at first, but leaves a slightly bitter aftertaste. Intal Nebulizer Solution is clear, colorless, sterile, and has a target pH of 5.5.

Each 2 ml ampule of Intal Nebulizer Solution contains 20 mg cromolyn sodium in purified water.

CLINICAL PHARMACOLOGY

INTAL INHALER

In vitro and *in vivo* animal studies have shown that cromolyn sodium inhibits sensitized mast cell degranulation which occurs after exposure to specific antigens. Cromolyn sodium acts by inhibiting the release of mediators from mast cells. Studies show that cromolyn sodium indirectly blocks calcium ions from entering the mast cell, thereby preventing mediator release.

Cromolyn sodium inhibits both the immediate and non-immediate bronchoconstrictive reactions to inhaled antigen. Cromolyn sodium also attenuates bronchospasm caused by exercise, toluene diisocyanate, aspirin, cold air, sulfur dioxide, and environmental pollutants, at least in some patients.

Cromolyn sodium has no intrinsic bronchodilator or antihistamine activity.

After administration of cromolyn sodium capsules by inhalation, approximately 8% of the total dose administered is absorbed and rapidly excreted unchanged, approximately equally divided between urine and bile. The remainder of the dose is either exhaled or deposited in the oropharynx, swallowed, and excreted via the alimentary tract.

INTAL NEBULIZER SOLUTION

In vitro and *in vivo* animal studies have shown that cromolyn sodium inhibits sensitized mast cell degranulation which occurs after exposure to specific antigens. Cromolyn sodium acts by inhibiting the release of mediators from mast cells. Studies show that cromolyn sodium indirectly blocks calcium ions from entering the mast cell, thereby preventing mediator release.

Cromolyn sodium inhibits both the immediate and non-immediate bronchoconstrictive reactions to inhaled antigen. Cromolyn sodium also attenuates bronchospasm caused by exercise, toluene diisocyanate, aspirin, cold air, sulfur dioxide, and environmental pollutants.

Cromolyn sodium has no intrinsic bronchodilator or antihistamine activity.

After administration by inhalation, approximately 8% of the total cromolyn sodium dose administered is absorbed and rapidly excreted unchanged, approximately equally divided between urine and bile. The remainder of the dose is either exhaled or deposited in the oropharynx, swallowed, and excreted via the alimentary tract.

INDICATIONS AND USAGE

INTAL INHALER

Intal Inhaler is a prophylactic agent indicated in the management of patients with bronchial asthma.

In patients whose symptoms are sufficiently frequent to require a continuous program of medication, Intal Inhaler is given by inhalation on a regular daily basis (see DOSAGE AND ADMINISTRATION). The effect of Intal Inhaler is usually evident after several weeks of treatment, although some patients show an almost immediate response.

If improvement occurs, it will ordinarily occur within the first 4 weeks of administration as manifested by a decrease in the severity of clinical symptoms of asthma, or in the need for concomitant therapy, or both.

In patients who develop acute bronchoconstriction in response to exposure to exercise, toluene diisocyanate, environmental pollutants, known antigens, etc., Intal Inhaler should be used shortly before exposure to the precipitating factor, *i.e.,* within 10-15 minutes but not more than 60 minutes (see DOSAGE AND ADMINISTRATION). Intal Inhaler may be effective in relieving bronchospasm in some, but not all, patients with exercise induced bronchospasm.

INTAL NEBULIZER SOLUTION

Intal Nebulizer Solution is a prophylactic agent indicated in the management of patients with bronchial asthma.

In patients whose symptoms are sufficiently frequent to require a continuous program of medication, Intal is given by inhalation on a regular daily basis (see DOSAGE AND ADMINISTRATION). The effect of Intal is usually evident after several weeks of treatment, although some patients show an almost immediate response.

In patients who develop acute bronchoconstriction in response to exposure to exercise, toluene diisocyanate, environmental pollutants, etc., Intal Nebulizer Solution should be used shortly before exposure to the precipitating factor (see DOSAGE AND ADMINISTRATION).

CONTRAINDICATIONS

INTAL INHALER

Intal Inhaler is contraindicated in those patients who have shown hypersensitivity to cromolyn sodium or other ingredients in this preparation.

INTAL NEBULIZER SOLUTION

Intal is contraindicated in those patients who have shown hypersensitivity to cromolyn sodium or other ingredients in this preparation.

WARNINGS

INTAL INHALER

Intal Inhaler has no role in the treatment of an acute attack of asthma, especially status asthmaticus. Severe anaphylactic reactions can occur after cromolyn sodium administration. The recommended dosage should be decreased in patients with decreased renal or hepatic function. Intal Inhaler should be discontinued if the patient develops eosinophilic pneumonia (or pulmonary infiltrates with eosinophilia). Because of the propellants in this preparation, it should be used with caution in patients with coronary artery disease or a history of cardiac arrhythmias.

INTAL NEBULIZER SOLUTION

Intal has no role in the treatment of status asthmaticus.

Anaphylactic reactions with cromolyn sodium administration have been reported rarely.

PRECAUTIONS

INTAL INHALER

General

In view of the biliary and renal routes of excretion for cromolyn sodium, consideration should be given to decreasing the dosage or discontinuing the administration of the drug in patients with impaired renal or hepatic function.

Occasionally, patients may experience cough and/or bronchospasm following cromolyn sodium inhalation. At times, patients who develop bronchospasm may not be able to continue administration despite prior bronchodilator administration. Rarely, very severe bronchospasm has been encountered.

Carcinogenesis, Mutagenesis, and Impairment of Fertility

Long term studies of cromolyn sodium in mice (12 months intraperitoneal administration at doses up to 150 mg/kg three days per week), hamsters (intraperitoneal administration at doses up to 53 mg/kg three days per week for 15 weeks followed by 17.5 mg/kg three days per week for 37 weeks), and rats (18 months subcutaneous administration at doses up to 75 mg/kg six days per week) showed no neoplastic effects. These doses in mice, hamsters, and rats correspond to approximately 40, 10, and 80 times, respectively the maximum recommended daily inhalation dose in adults on a mg/m^2 basis, or approximately 20, 5, and 40 times, respectively the maximum recommended daily inhalation dose in children on a mg/m^2 basis.

Cromolyn sodium showed no mutagenic potential in Ames *Salmonella*/microsome plate assays, mitotic gene conversion in *Saccharomyces cerevisiae* and in an *in vitro* cytogenic study in human peripheral lymphocytes.

No evidence of impaired fertility was shown in laboratory reproduction studies conducted subcutaneously in rats at the highest doses tested 175 mg/kg/day in males and 100 mg/kg/day in females. These doses are approximately 220 and 130 times, respectively, the maximum recommended daily inhalation dose in adults on a mg/m^2 basis.

Pregnancy Category B

Reproduction studies with cromolyn sodium administered subcutaneously to pregnant mice and rats at maximum daily doses of 540 mg/kg/day and 160 mg/kg/day, respectively and intravenously to rabbits at a maximum daily dose of 485 mg/kg/day produced no evidence of fetal malformations. These doses represent approximately 340, 210, and 1200 times, respectively, the maximum recommended daily inhalation dose in adults on a mg/m^2 basis. Adverse fetal effects (increased resorption and decreased fetal weight) were noted only at the very high parenteral doses that produced maternal toxicity. There are, however, no adequate and well-controlled studies in pregnant women.

Because animal reproduction studies are not always predictive of human response, Intal Inhaler should be used during pregnancy only if clearly needed.

Drug Interaction During Pregnancy

Cromolyn sodium and isoproterenol were studied following subcutaneous injections in pregnant mice. Cromolyn sodium alone in doses up to 540 mg/kg/day (approximately 340 times the maximum recommended daily inhalation dose in adults on a mg/m^2 basis) did not cause significant increases in resorptions or major malformations. Isoproternol alone at a dose of 2.7 mg/kg/day (approximately 7 times the maximum recommended daily inhalation dose in adults on a mg/m^2 basis) increased both resorptions and malformations. The addition of 540 mg/kg/day of cromolyn sodium (approximately 340 times the maximum recommended daily inhalation dose in adults on a mg/m^2 basis) to 2.7 mg/kg/day isoproterenol (approximately 7 times the maximum recommended daily inhalation dose in adults on a mg/m^2 basis) appears to have increased the incidence of both resorptions and malformations.

Nursing Mothers

It is not known whether this drug is excreted in human milk, therefore, caution should be exercised when Intal Inhaler is administered to a nursing woman and the attending physician must make a benefit/risk assessment in regard to its use in this situation.

Pediatric Use

Safety and effectiveness in pediatric patients below the age of 5 years have not been established. For young pediatric patients unable to utilize the Inhaler, Intal Nebulizer Solution is recommended. Because of the possibility that adverse effects of this drug could become apparent only after many years, a benefit/risk consideration of the long-term use of Intal Inhaler is particularly important in pediatric patients.

INTAL NEBULIZER SOLUTION

General

Occasionally, patients may experience cough and/or bronchospasm following Intal inhalation. At times, pati^nts who develop bronchospasm may not be able to continue administration despite prior bronchodilator administration. Rarely, very severe bronchospasm has been encountered.

Symptoms of asthma may recur if Intal is reduced below the recommended dosage or discontinued.

Information for the Patient

Intal is to be taken as directed by the physician. Because it is preventative medication, it may take up to 4 weeks before the patient experiences maximum benefit.

Intal Nebulizer Solution should be used in a power-driven nebulizer with an adequate airflow rate equipped with a suitable face mask or mouthpiece.

Drug stability and safety of Intal Nebulizer Solution when mixed with other drugs in a nebulizer have not been established.

Carcinogenesis, Mutagenesis, and Impairment of Fertility

Long term studies of cromolyn sodium in mice (12 months intraperitoneal administration at doses up to 150 mg/kg three days per week), hamsters (intraperitoneal administration at doses up to 52.6 mg/kg three days per week for 15 weeks followed by 17.5 mg/kg three days per week for 37 weeks), and rats (18 months subcutaneous administration at doses up to 75 mg/kg six days per week) showed no neoplastic effects. The average daily maximum dose levels administered in these studies were 192.9 mg/m^2 for mice, 47.2 mg/m^2 for hamsters and 385.8 mg/m^2 for rats. These doses correspond to approximately 330%, 80%, and 650% of the maximum daily human dose of 59.2 mg/m^2.

Cromolyn sodium showed no mutagenic potential in Ames *Salmonella*/microsome plate assays, mitotic gene conversion in *Saccharomyces cerevisiae* and in an *in vitro* cytogenetic study in human peripheal lymphocytes.

No evidence of impaired fertility was shown in laboratory reproductive studies conducted subcutaneously in rats in the highest doses tested, 175 mg/kg/day (1050 mg/m^2) in males and 100 mg/kg/day (600 mg/m^2) in females. These doses are approximately 18 and 10 times the maximum daily human dose, respectively, based on mg/m^2.

Pregnancy Category B

Reproduction studies with cromolyn sodium administered subcutaneously to pregnant mice and rats at maximum daily doses of 540 mg/kg (1620 mg/m^2) and 164 mg/kg (984 mg/m^2), respectively, and intravenously to rabbits at a maximum daily dose of 485 mg/kg (5820 mg/m^2) produced no evidence of fetal malformations. These doses represent approximately 27, 16, and 98 times the maximum daily human dose, respectively, on a mg/m^2 basis. Adverse fetal effects (increased resorptions and decreased fetal weight) were noted only at the very high parenteral doses that produced maternal toxicity. There are, however, no adequate and well-controlled studies in pregnant women.

C

Because animal reproduction studies are not always predictive of human response, Intal Nebulizer Solution should be used during pregnancy only if clearly needed.

Drug Interaction During Pregnancy

Cromolyn sodium and isoproterenol were studied following subcutaneous injections in pregnant mice. Cromolyn sodium alone in doses of 60-540 mg/kg/day (38-338 times the human dose) did not cause significant increases in resorptions or major malformations. Isoproternol alone at a dose of 2.7 mg/kg/day (90 times the human dose) increased both resorptions and malformations. The addition of cromolyn sodium (338 times the human dose) to isoproterenol (90 times the human dose) appears to have increased the incidence of both resorptions and malformations.

Nursing Mothers

It is not known whether this drug is excreted in human milk. Because many drugs are excreted in human milk, caution should be exercised when Intal Nebulizer Solution is administered to a nursing woman.

Pediatric Use

Safety and effectiveness in pediatric patients below the age of 2 years have not been established.

ADVERSE REACTIONS

INTAL INHALER

In controlled clinical studies of Intal Inhaler, the most frequently reported adverse reactions attributed to cromolyn sodium treatment were: Throat irritation or dryness, bad taste, cough, wheeze, nausea.

The most frequently reported adverse reactions attributed to other forms of cromolyn sodium (on the basis of reoccurrence following readministration) involve the respiratory tract and are: Bronchospasm [sometimes severe, associated with a precipitous fall in pulmonary function (FEV_1)], cough, laryngeal edema (rare), nasal congestion (sometimes severe), pharyngeal irritation, and wheezing.

Adverse reactions which occur infrequently and are associated with administration of the drug are: Anaphylaxis, angioedema, dizziness, dysuria and urinary frequency, joint swelling and pain, lacrimation, nausea and headache, rash, swollen parotid gland, urticaria, pulmonary infiltrates with eosinophilia, substernal burning, and myopathy.

The following adverse reactions have been reported as rare events and it is unclear whether they are attributable to the drug: Anemia, exfoliative dermatitis, hemoptysis, hoarseness, myalgia, nephrosis, periarteritic vasculitis, pericarditis, peripheral neuritis, photodermatitis, sneezing, drowsiness, nasal itching, nasal bleeding, nasal burning, serum sickness, stomachache, polymyositis, vertigo, and liver disease.

INTAL NEBULIZER SOLUTION

Clinical experience with the use of Intal suggests that adverse reactions are rare events. The following adverse reactions have been associated with Intal Nebulizer Solution: cough, nasal congestion, nausea, sneezing, and wheezing.

Other reactions have been reported in clinical trials; however, a causal relationship could not be established: drowsiness, nasal itching, nose bleed, nose burning, serum sickness, and stomachache.

In addition, adverse reactions have been reported with Intal Inhaler. The most common side effects are associated with inhalation of the powder and include transient cough (1 in 5 patients) and mild wheezing (1 in 25 patients). These effects rarely require treatment or discontinuation of the drug.

Information on the incidence of adverse reactions to Intal Inhaler have been derived from US postmarketing surveillance experience. The following adverse reactions attributed to Intal Inhaler, based upon recurrence following readministration, have been reported in less than 1 in 10,000 patients: laryngeal edema, swollen parotid gland, angioedema, bronchospasm, joint swelling and pain, dizziness, dysuria and urinary frequency, nausea, cough, wheezing, headache, nasal congestion, rash, urticaria, and lacrimation.

Other adverse reactions have been reported in less than 1 in 100,000 patients, and it is unclear whether these are attributable to the drug: anaphylaxis, nephrosis, periarteritic vasculitis, pericarditis, peripheral neuritis, pulmonary infiltrates with eosinophilia, polymyositis, exfoliative dermatitis, hemoptysis, anemia, myalgia, hoarseness, photodermatitis, and vertigo.

DOSAGE AND ADMINISTRATION

INTAL INHALER

For management of bronchial asthma in adults and pediatric patients (5 years of age and over) who are able to use the Inhaler, the usual starting dosage is two metered inhalations 4 times daily at regular intervals. This dose should not be exceeded. Not all patients will respond to the recommended dose and there is evidence to suggest, at least in younger patients, that a lower dose may provide efficacy.

Patients with chronic asthma should be advised that the effect of Intal Inhaler therapy is dependent upon its administration at regular intervals, as directed. Intal Inhaler should be introduced into the patient's therapeutic regimen when the acute episode has been controlled, the airway has been cleared, and the patient is able to inhale adequately.

For the prevention of acute bronchospasm which follows exercise, exposure to cold, dry air, or environmental agents, the usual dose is two metered inhalations shortly before exposure to the precipitating factor, *i.e.*, 10-15 minutes but not more than 60 minutes.

Intal Inhaler Therapy in Relation to Other Treatments for Asthma

Non-Steroidal Agents

Intal Inhaler should be *added* to the patient's existing treatment regimen (*e.g.*, bronchodilators). When a clinical response to Intal Inhaler is evident, usually within 2-4 weeks, and if the asthma is under good control, an attempt may be made to decrease concomitant medication usage gradually.

If concomitant medications are eliminated or required on no more than a prn basis, the frequency of administration of Intal Inhaler may be titrated downward to the lowest level consistent with the desired effect. The usual decrease is from two metered inhalations 4 times daily to 3 times daily to twice daily. It is important that the dosage be reduced gradually to avoid exacerbation of asthma. It is emphasized that in patients whose dosage has been titrated to fewer than 4 inhalations per day, an increase in the dosage of Intal Inhaler and the introduction of, or increase in, symptomatic medications may be needed if the patient's clinical condition deteriorates.

Corticosteroids

In patients chronically receiving corticosteroids for the management of bronchial asthma, the dosage should be maintained following the introduction of Intal Inhaler. If the patient improves, an attempt to decrease corticosteroids should be made. Even if the corticosteroid-dependent patient fails to show symptomatic improvement following Intal Inhaler administration, the potential to reduce corticosteroids may nonetheless be present. Thus, gradual tapering of corticosteroid dosage may be attempted. It is important that the dose be reduced slowly, maintaining close supervision of the patient to avoid an exacerbation of asthma.

It should be borne in mind that prolonged corticosteroid therapy frequently causes an impairment in the activity of the hypothalamic-pituitary-adrenal axis and a reduction in the size of the adrenal cortex. A potentially critical degree of impairment or insufficiency may persist asymptomatically for some time even after gradual discontinuation of adrenocortical steroids. Therefore, if a patient is subjected to significant stress, such as a severe asthmatic attack, surgery, trauma, or severe illness while being treated or within 1 year (occasionally up to 2 years) after corticosteroid treatment has been terminated, consideration should be given to reinstituting corticosteroid therapy. When respiratory function is impaired, as may occur in severe exacerbation of asthma, a temporary increase in the amount of corticosteroids may be required to regain control of the patient's asthma.

It is particularly important that great care be exercised if for any reason cromolyn sodium is withdrawn in cases where its use has permitted a reduction in the maintenance dose of corticosteroids. In such cases, continued close supervision of the patient is essential since there may be sudden reappearance of severe manifestations of asthma which will require immediate therapy and possible reintroduction of corticosteroids.

For best results, the canister should be at room temperature before use.

INTAL NEBULIZER SOLUTION

For management of bronchial asthma in adults and pediatric patients (2 years of age and over), the usual starting dosage 1 ampule administered by nebulization 4 times a day at regular intervals.

Drug stability and safety of Intal Nebulizer Solution when mixed with other drugs in a nebulizer have not been established.

Patients with chronic asthma should be advised that the effect of Intal therapy is dependent upon its administration at regular intervals, as directed. Intal should be introduced into the patient's therapeutic regimen when the acute episode has been controlled, the airway has been cleared, and the patient is able to inhale adequately.

For the prevention of acute bronchospasm which follows exercise, exposure to cold dry air, environmental agents (*e.g.*, animal dander, toluene diisocyanate, pollutants), etc., the usual dose is the contents of 1 ampule administered by nebulization shortly before exposure to the precipitating factor.

It should be emphasized to the patient that the drug is poorly absorbed when swallowed and is not effective by this route of administration.

Intal Therapy in Relation to Other Treatments for Asthma

Non-Steroidal Agents

Intal Nebulizer Solution should be *added* to the patient's existing treatment regimen (*e.g.*, bronchodilators). When a clinical response to Intal is evident, usually within 2-4 weeks, and if the asthma is under good control, an attempt may be made to decrease concomitant medication usage gradually.

If concomitant medications are eliminated or required on no more than a prn basis, the frequency of administration of Intal Nebulizer Solution may be titrated downward to the lowest level consistent with the desired effect. The usual decrease is from 4 to 3 ampules per day. It is important that the dosage be reduced gradually to avoid exacerbation of asthma. It is emphasized that in patients whose dosage has been titrated to fewer than 4 ampules per day, an increase in the dosage of Intal and the introduction of, or increase in, symptomatic medications may be needed if the patient's clinical condition deteriorates.

Corticosteroids

In patients chronically receiving corticosteroids for the management of bronchial asthma, the dosage should be maintained following the introduction of Intal. If the patient improves, an attempt to decrease corticosteroids should be made. Even if the corticosteroid-dependent patient fails to show symptomatic improvement following Intal administration, the potential to reduce corticosteroids may nonetheless be present. Thus, gradual tapering of corticosteroid dosage may be attempted. It is important that the dose be reduced slowly, maintaining close supervision of the patient to avoid an exacerbation of asthma.

It should be borne in mind that prolonged corticosteroid therapy frequently causes an impairment in the activity of the hypothalamic-pituitary-adrenal axis and a reduction in the size of the adrenal cortex. A potentially critical degree of impairment or insufficiency may persist asymptomatically for some time even after gradual discontinuation of adrenocortical steroids. Therefore, if a patient is subjected to significant stress, such as a severe asthmatic attack, surgery, trauma, or severe illness while being treated or within 1 year (occasionally up to 2 years) after corticosteroid treatment has been terminated, consideration should be given to reinstituting corticosteroid therapy. When respiratory function is impaired, as may occur in severe exacerbation of asthma, a temporary increase in the amount of corticosteroids may be required to regain control of the patient's asthma.

It is particularly important that great care be exercised if for any reason Intal is withdrawn in cases where its use has permitted a reduction in the maintenance dose of corticosteroids. In such cases, continued close supervision of the patient is essential since there may be sudden reappearance of severe manifestations of asthma which will require immediate therapy and possible reintroduction of corticosteroids.

HOW SUPPLIED

INTAL INHALER

Intal Inhaler is supplied as an aerosol canister which provides 112 metered dose actuations from the 8.1 g canister or 200 metered dose actuations from the 14.2 g canister. The correct amount of medication in each inhalation cannot be assured after 112 actuations from the 8.1 g canister or 200 actuations from the 14.2 g canister even though the canister may not feel empty. The canister should be discarded when the labeled number of actuations have been used.

Each actuation delivers 1 mg cromolyn sodium from the valve and 800 µg cromolyn sodium through the mouthpiece to the patient. The Intal Inhaler canister and accompanying mouthpiece are designed to be used together. The Intal Inhaler canister should not be used with other mouthpieces and the supplied mouthpiece should not be used with other products' canisters. Intal Inhaler is supplied with a white plastic mouthpiece with blue dust cap and patient instructions.

Storage: Store between 15-30°C (59-86°F). Contents under pressure. Do not puncture, incinerate, or place near sources of heat. Exposure to temperatures above 120°F may cause bursting. **Avoid spraying in eyes. Keep out of the reach of children.**

Note: The indented statement below is required by the Federal government's Clean Air Act for all products containing or manufactured with chlorofluorocarbons (CFCs).

> ***WARNING:*** Contains CFC-12 (dichlorodifluoromethane) and CFC-114 (dichlorotetrafluoroethane), substances which harm public health and the environment by destroying ozone in the upper atmosphere.

A notice similar to the above WARNING has been placed in the "Information For The Patient" package insert under the Environmental Protection Agency's (EPA's) regulations. The patient's warning states that the patient should consult his or her physician if there are questions about alternatives.

INTAL NEBULIZER SOLUTION

Intal Nebulizer Solution is a colorless solution supplied in a low density polyethylene plastic unit dose ampule with 12 ampules per foil pouch. Each 2 ml ampule contains 20 mg cromolyn sodium in purified water.

Storage

Store at controlled room temperature 20-25°C (68-77°F). Protect from light. Do not use if it contains a precipitate or becomes discolored. Keep out of the reach of children.

Store ampules in foil pouch until ready for use.

OPHTHALMIC

DESCRIPTION

Note: The trade name has been used throughout this monograph for clarity.

Opticrom (cromolyn sodium ophthalmic solution) 4% is a clear, colorless, sterile solution intended for topical ophthalmic use.

Cromolyn sodium has a molecular weight of 512.34. Its chemical name is disodium 5-5′-[(2-hydroxytrimethylene)dioxy]bis[4-oxo-4H-1-benzopyran-2-carboxylate].

The empirical formula is $C_{23}H_{14}Na_2O_{11}$; the molecular weight is 512.34.

Each ml of Opticrom contains:

Active: Cromolyn sodium 40 mg (4%)

Preservative: Benzalkonium chloride 0.01%

Inactives: Edetate disodium 0.1% and purified water. It has a pH of 4.0-7.0.

CLINICAL PHARMACOLOGY

In vitro and *in vivo* animal studies have shown that cromolyn sodium inhibits the degranulation of sensitized mast cells which occurs after exposure to specific antigens. Cromolyn sodium acts by inhibiting the release of histamine and SRS-A (slow-reacting substance of anaphylaxis) from the mast cell.

Another activity demonstrated *in vitro* is the capacity of cromolyn sodium to inhibit the degranulation of non-sensitized rat mast cells by phospholipase A and the subsequent release of chemical mediators. Another study showed that cromolyn sodium did not inhibit the enzymatic activity of released phospholipase A on its specific substrate.

Cromolyn sodium has no intrinsic vasoconstrictor, antihistamine, or anti-inflammatory activity.

Cromolyn sodium is poorly absorbed. When multiple doses of cromolyn sodium ophthalmic solution are instilled into normal rabbit eyes, less than 0.07% of the administered dose of cromolyn sodium is absorbed into the systemic circulation (presumably by way of the eye, nasal passages, buccal cavity, and gastrointestinal tract). Trace amounts (less than 0.01%) of the cromolyn sodium dose penetrate into the aqueous humor and clearance from this chamber is virtually complete within 24 hours after treatment is stopped.

In normal volunteers, analysis of drug excretion indicates that approximately 0.03% of cromolyn sodium is absorbed following administration to the eye.

INDICATIONS AND USAGE

Opticrom is indicated in the treatment of vernal keratoconjunctivitis, vernal conjunctivitis, and vernal keratitis.

CONTRAINDICATIONS

Opticrom is contraindicated in those patients who have shown hypersensitivity to cromolyn sodium or to any of the other ingredients.

PRECAUTIONS

GENERAL

Patients may experience a transient stinging or burning sensation following application of Opticrom.

The recommended frequency of administration should not be exceeded (see DOSAGE AND ADMINISTRATION).

INFORMATION FOR THE PATIENT

Patients should be advised to follow the patient instructions listed on the Information for Patients sheet.

Users of contact lenses should refrain from wearing lenses while exhibiting the signs and symptoms of vernal keratoconjunctivitis, vernal conjunctivitis, or vernal keratitis. Do not wear contact lenses during treatment with Opticrom.

CARCINOGENESIS, MUTAGENESIS, AND IMPAIRMENT OF FERTILITY

Long term studies of cromolyn sodium in mice (12 months intraperitoneal administration at doses up to 150 mg/kg three days per week), hamsters (intraperitoneal administration at doses up to 52.6 mg/kg three days per week for 15 weeks followed by 17.5 mg/kg three days per week for 37 weeks), and rats (18 months subcutaneous administration at doses up to 75 mg/kg six days per week) showed no neoplastic effects. The average daily maximum dose levels administered in these studies were 192.9 mg/m^2 for mice, 47.2 mg/m^2 for hamsters and 385.8 mg/m^2 for rats. These doses correspond to approximately 6.8, 1.7, and 14 times the maximum daily human dose of 28 mg/m^2.

Cromolyn sodium showed no mutagenic potential in the Ames *Salmonella*/microsome plate assays, mitotic gene conversion in *Saccharomyes cerevisiae* and in an *in vitro* cytogenetic study in human peripheral lymphocytes.

No evidence of impaired fertility was shown in laboratory reproduction studies conducted subcutaneously in rats at the highest doses tested, 175 mg/kg/day (1050 mg/m^2) in males and 100 mg/kg/day (600 mg/m^2) in females. These doses are approximately 37 and 21 times the maximum daily human dose, respectively, based on mg/m^2.

PREGNANCY, TERATOGENIC EFFECTS, PREGNANCY CATEGORY B

Reproduction studies with cromolyn sodium administered subcutaneously to pregnant mice and rats at maximum daily doses of 540 mg/kg (1620 mg/m^2) and 164 mg/kg (984 mg/m^2), respectively, and intravenously to rabbits at a maximum daily dose of 485 mg/kg (5820 mg/m^2) produced no evidence of fetal malformation. These doses represent approximately 57, 35, and 205 times the maximum daily human dose, respectively, on a mg/m^2 basis. Adverse fetal effects (increased resorption and decreased fetal weight) were noted only at the very high parenteral doses that produced maternal toxicity. There are, however, no adequate and well-controlled studies in pregnant women. Because animal reproduction studies are not always predictive of human response, this drug should be used during pregnancy only if clearly needed.

NURSING MOTHERS

It is not known whether this drug is excreted in human milk. Because many drugs are excreted in human milk, caution should be exercised when Opticrom is administered to a nursing woman.

PEDIATRIC USE

Safety and effectiveness in children below the age of 4 years have not been established.

GERIATRIC USE

No overall differences in safety or effectiveness have been observed between elderly and younger patients.

ADVERSE REACTIONS

The most frequently reported adverse reaction attributed to the use of Opticrom on the basis of reoccurrence following readministration, is transient ocular stinging or burning upon instillation.

The following adverse reactions have been reported as infrequent events. It is unclear whether they are attributed to the drug: Conjunctival injection; watery eyes; itchy eyes; dryness around the eye; puffy eyes; eye irritation; and styes.

Immediate hypersensitivity reactions have been reported rarely and include dyspnea, edema, and rash.

DOSAGE AND ADMINISTRATION

The dose is 1-2 drops in each eye 4-6 times a day at regular intervals. One drop contains approximately 1.6 mg cromolyn sodium.

Patients should be advised that the effect of Opticrom therapy is dependent upon its administration at regular intervals, as directed.

Symptomatic response to therapy (decreased itching, tearing, redness, and discharge) is usually evident within a few days, but longer treatment for up to 6 weeks is sometimes required. Once symptomatic improvement has been established, therapy should be continued for as long as needed to sustain improvement.

If required, corticosteroids may be used concomitantly with Opticrom.

HOW SUPPLIED

Opticrom (cromolyn sodium ophthalmic solution) 4% is supplied as 10 ml of solution in an opaque polyethylene eye drop bottle.

STORAGE

Store at controlled room temperature 20-25°C (68-77°F).

Protect from light — store in original carton. Keep tightly closed and out of the reach of children.

ORAL

DESCRIPTION

Note: The trade name has been used throughout this monograph for clarity.

For Oral Use Only — Not for Inhalation or Injection.

Each 5 ml ampule of Gastrocrom contains 100 mg cromolyn sodium, in purified water. Cromolyn sodium is a hygroscopic, white powder having little odor. It may leave a slightly bitter aftertaste. Gastrocrom oral concentrate is clear, colorless, and sterile. It is intended for oral use.

C

Chemically, cromolyn sodium is disodium 5,5′-[(2-hydroxytrimethylene)dioxy]bis[4-oxo-4*H*-1-benzopyran-2-carboxylate]. The empirical formula is $C_{23}H_{14}Na_2O_{11}$ and the molecular weight is 512.34.

CLINICAL PHARMACOLOGY

In vitro and *in vivo* animal studies have shown that cromolyn sodium inhibits the release of mediators from sensitized mast cells. Cromolyn sodium acts by inhibiting the release of histamine and leukotrienes (SRS-A) from the mast cell.

Cromolyn sodium has no intrinsic vasoconstrictor, antihistamine, or glucocorticoid activity.

Cromolyn sodium is poorly absorbed from the gastrointestinal tract. No more than 1% of an administered dose is absorbed by humans after oral administration, the remainder being excreted in the feces. Very little absorption of cromolyn sodium was seen after oral administration of 500 mg by mouth to each of 12 volunteers. From 0.28-0.50% of the administered dose was recovered in the first 24 hours of urinary excretion in 3 subjects. The mean urinary excretion of an administered dose over 24 hours in the remaining 9 subjects was 0.45%.

INDICATIONS AND USAGE

Gastrocrom is indicated in the management of patients with mastocytosis. Use of this product has been associated with improvement in diarrhea, flushing, headaches, vomiting, urticaria, abdominal pain, nausea, and itching in some patients.

CONTRAINDICATIONS

Gastrocrom is contraindicated in those patients who have shown hypersensitivity to cromolyn sodium.

WARNINGS

The recommended dosage should be decreased in patients with decreased renal or hepatic function. Severe anaphylactic reactions may occur rarely in association with cromolyn sodium administration.

PRECAUTIONS

In view of the biliary and renal routes of excretion of Gastrocrom, consideration should be given to decreasing the dosage of the drug in patients with impaired renal or hepatic function.

CARCINOGENESIS, MUTAGENESIS, AND IMPAIRMENT OF FERTILITY

In carcinogenicity studies in mice, hamsters, and rats, cromolyn sodium had no neoplastic effects at intraperitoneal doses up to 150 mg/kg three days per week for 12 months in mice, at intraperitoneal doses up to 53 mg/kg three days per week to 15 weeks followed by 17.5 mg/kg three days per week for 37 weeks in hamsters, and at subcutaneous doses up to 75 mg/kg six days per week for 18 months in rats. These doses in mice, hamsters, and rats are less than the maximum recommended daily oral dose in adults and children on a mg/m^2 basis.

Cromolyn sodium showed no mutagenic potential in Ames *Salmonella*/microsome plate assays, mitotic gene conversion in *Saccharomyes cerevisiae* and in an *in vitro* cytogenetic study in human peripheral lymphocytes.

In rats, cromolyn sodium showed no evidence of impaired fertility at subcutaneous doses up to 175 mg/kg in males (approximately equal to the maximum recommended daily oral dose in adults on a mg/m^2 basis) and 100 mg/kg in females (less than the maximum recommended daily oral dose in adults on a mg/m^2 basis).

PREGNANCY CATEGORY B

In reproductive studies in pregnant mice, rats, and rabbits, cromolyn sodium produced no evidence of fetal malformations at subcutaneous doses up to 540 mg/kg in mice (approximately equal to the maximum recommended daily oral dose in adults on a mg/m^2 basis) and 164 mg/kg in rats (less than the maximum recommended daily oral dose in adults on a mg/m^2 basis) or at intravenous doses up to 485 mg/kg in rabbits (approximately 4 times the maximum recommended daily oral dose in adults on a mg/m^2 basis). There are, however, no adequate and well controlled studies in pregnant women.

Because animal reproduction studies are not always predictive of human response, this drug should be used during pregnancy only if clearly needed.

DRUG INTERACTION DURING PREGNANCY

In pregnant mice, cromolyn sodium alone did not cause significant increases in resorptions or major malformations at subcutaneous doses up to 540 mg/kg (approximately equal to the maximum recommended daily oral dose in adults on a mg/m^2 basis). Isoproterenol alone increased both resorptions and major malformations (primarily cleft palate) at a subcutaneous dose of 2.7 mg/kg (approximately 7 times the maximum recommended daily inhalation dose in adults on a mg/m^2 basis). The incidence of major malformations increased further when cromolyn sodium at a subcutaneous dose of 540 mg/kg was added to isoproterenol at a subcutaneous dose of 2.7 mg/kg. No such interaction was observed in rats or rabbits.

NURSING MOTHERS

It is not known whether this drug is excreted in human milk. Because many drugs are excreted in human milk, caution should be exercised when Gastrocrom is administered to a nursing woman.

PEDIATRIC USE

In adult rats no adverse effects of cromolyn sodium were observed at oral doses up to 6144 mg/kg (approximately 25 times the maximum recommended daily oral dose in adults on a mg/m^2 basis). In neonatal rats, cromolyn sodium increased mortality at oral doses of 1000 mg/kg or greater (approximately 9 times the maximum recommended daily oral dose in infants on a mg/m^2 basis) but not at doses of 300 mg/kg or less (approximately 3 times the maximum recommended daily oral dose in infants on a mg/m^2 basis). Plasma and kidney concentrations of cromolyn after oral administration to neonatal rats were up to 20 times greater than those in older rats. In term infants up to 6 months of age, available clinical data suggest that the dose should not exceed 20 mg/kg/day. The use of this product in pediatric patients less than 2 years of age should be reserved for patients with severe disease in which the potential benefits clearly outweigh the risks.

ADVERSE REACTIONS

Most of the adverse events reported in mastocytosis patients have been transient and could represent symptoms of the disease. The most frequently reported adverse events in mastocytosis patients who have received Gastrocrom during clinical studies were headache and diarrhea, each of which occurred in 4 of the 87 patients. Pruritus, nausea, and myalgia were each reported in 3 patients and abdominal pain, rash, and irritability in 2 patients each. One report of malaise was also recorded.

OTHER ADVERSE EVENTS

Additional adverse events have been reported during studies in other clinical conditions and from worldwide postmarketing experience. In most cases the available information is incomplete and attribution to the drug cannot be determined. The majority of these reports involve the gastrointestinal system and include: diarrhea, nausea, abdominal pain, constipation, dyspepsia, flatulence, glossitis, stomatitis, vomiting, dysphagia, esophagospasm.

Other less commonly reported events (the majority representing only a single report) include the following:

Skin: Pruritus, rash, urticaria/angioedema, erythema/burning, photosensitivity.

Musculoskeletal: Arthralgia, myalgia, stiffness/weakness of legs.

Neurologic: Headache, dizziness, hypoesthesia, paresthesia, migraine, convulsions, flushing.

Psychiatric: Psychosis, anxiety, depression, hallucinations, behavior change, insomnia, nervousness.

Heart Rate: Tachycardia, premature ventricular contractions (PVCs), palpitations.

Respiratory: Pharyngitis, dyspnea.

Miscellaneous: Fatigue, edema, unpleasant taste, chest pain, postprandial lightheadedness and lethargy, dysuria, urinary frequency, purpura, hepatic function test abnormal, polycythemia, neutropenia, pancytopenia, tinnitus, lupus erythematosus (LE) syndrome.

DOSAGE AND ADMINISTRATION

NOT FOR INHALATION OR INJECTION. SEE DIRECTIONS FOR USE.

The usual starting dose is as follows:

Adults and adolescents (13 years and older): Two ampules 4 times daily, taken one-half hour before meals and at bedtime.

Children 2-12 years: One ampule 4 times daily, taken one-half hour before meals and at bedtime.

Pediatric patients under 2 years: Not recommended.

If satisfactory control of symptoms is not achieved within 2-3 weeks, the dosage may be increased but should not exceed 40 mg/kg/day.

Patients should be advised that the effect of Gastrocrom therapy is dependent upon its administration at regular intervals, as directed.

Maintenance Dose:

Once a therapeutic response has been achieved, the dose may be reduced to the minimum required to maintain the patient with a lower degree of symptomatology. To prevent relapses, the dosage should be maintained.

HOW SUPPLIED

Gastrocrom oral concentrate is an unpreserved, colorless solution supplied in a low density polyethylene plastic unit dose ampule with 8 ampules per foil pouch. Each 5 ml ampule contains 100 mg cromolyn sodium in purified water.

STORAGE

Gastrocrom oral concentrate should be stored between 15-30°C (59-86°F) and protected from light. Do not use if it contains a precipitate or becomes discolored. Keep out of the reach of children.

Store ampules in foil pouch until ready for use.

PRODUCT LISTING - RATED THERAPEUTICALLY EQUIVALENT

Solution - Inhalation - 10 mg/ml

2 ml x 60	$42.00	GENERIC, Dey Laboratories	49502-0689-02
2 ml x 60	$42.00	GENERIC, Warrick Pharmaceuticals Corporation	59930-1509-01
2 ml x 60	$42.00	GENERIC, Morton Grove Pharmaceuticals Inc	60432-0157-06
2 ml x 60	$49.20	GENERIC, Roxane Laboratories Inc	00054-8167-21
2 ml x 60	$49.20	GENERIC, Ivax Corporation	00172-6406-49
2 ml x 60	$49.20	GENERIC, Bausch and Lomb	24208-0373-60
2 ml x 60	$49.80	GENERIC, Alpharma Uspd Makers Of Barre and Nmc	00472-0750-60
2 ml x 60	$73.80	INTAL, Aventis Pharmaceuticals	00585-0673-02
2 ml x 120	$61.58	INTAL, Allscripts Pharmaceutical Company	54569-0048-00
2 ml x 120	$84.00	GENERIC, Dey Laboratories	49502-0689-12
2 ml x 120	$84.00	GENERIC, Warrick Pharmaceuticals Corporation	59930-1509-02

2 ml x 120	$84.00	GENERIC, Morton Grove Pharmaceuticals Inc	60432-0157-21
2 ml x 120	$92.40	GENERIC, Roxane Laboratories Inc	00054-8167-23
2 ml x 120	$92.40	GENERIC, Ivax Corporation	00172-6406-59
2 ml x 120	$92.40	GENERIC, Alpharma Uspd Makers Of Barre and Nmc	00472-0750-21
2 ml x 120	$92.40	GENERIC, Bausch and Lomb	24208-0373-62
2 ml x 120	$136.80	INTAL, Aventis Pharmaceuticals	00585-0673-03
Solution - Ophthalmic - 4%			
10 ml	$33.75	FEDERAL UPPER LIMIT, H.C.F.A. F F P	99999-0916-01
10 ml	$37.15	GENERIC, Pacific Pharma	60758-0458-10
10 ml	$37.20	GENERIC, Falcon Pharmaceuticals, Ltd.	61314-0237-10
10 ml	$37.25	GENERIC, Akorn Inc	17478-0291-11
10 ml	$37.25	GENERIC, Apotex Usa Inc	60505-0811-02
10 ml	$44.56	CROLOM, Bausch and Lomb	24208-0300-10
10 ml	$44.56	CROLOM, Allscripts Pharmaceutical Company	54569-4060-00
10 ml	$54.08	OPTICROM, Allergan Inc	00023-6422-10

PRODUCT LISTING - RATED NOT THERAPEUTICALLY EQUIVALENT

Solution - Inhalation - 10 mg/ml			
2 ml x 60	$42.06	GENERIC, Allscripts Pharmaceutical Company	54569-4549-00
2 ml x 120	$88.20	GENERIC, Allscripts Pharmaceutical Company	54569-4772-00

PRODUCT LISTING - EQUIVALENTS NOT AVAILABLE

Aerosol with Adapter - Inhalation - 0.8 mg/Inh			
8.10 gm	$49.00	INTAL INHALER, Allscripts Pharmaceutical Company	54569-0049-00
8.10 gm	$58.24	INTAL INHALER, Physicians Total Care	54868-1894-02
8.10 gm	$58.41	INTAL INHALER, Aventis Pharmaceuticals	00585-0675-02
14.20 gm	$77.95	INTAL INHALER, Allscripts Pharmaceutical Company	54569-1012-00
14.20 gm	$92.94	INTAL INHALER, Aventis Pharmaceuticals	00585-0675-01
Solution - Ophthalmic - 4%			
10 ml	$36.47	GENERIC, Teva Pharmaceuticals Usa	00093-1389-43
Solution - Oral - 20 mg/ml			
5 ml x 96	$218.88	GASTROCROM, Celltech Pharmacueticals Inc	53014-0678-70
Spray - Nasal - 5.2 mg/Inh			
13 ml	$8.39	NASALCROM, Pharmacia and Upjohn	00009-7709-01
13 ml	$8.74	NASALCROM CHILD, Pharmacia and Upjohn	00009-5003-01
26 ml	$13.91	NASALCROM CHILD, Pharmacia and Upjohn	00009-5003-02
26 ml	$13.91	NASALCROM, Pharmacia and Upjohn	00009-7709-02

Cyanocobalamin *(000922)*

Categories: Anemia, pernicious; Deficiency, vitamin B12; Pregnancy Category C; FDA Approved 1951 Nov
Drug Classes: Hematinics; Vitamins/minerals
Brand Names: Antipernicin; B-12-1000; Berubigen; Betalin 12; Betlovex; Blu-12; Cobal; Cobalparen; Cobavite; Cobex; Cobolin-M; Compensal; Corubeen; Corubin; Cpc-Carpenters; Crystamine; Crysti-12; Cyano-Plex; Cyanocob; Cyanoject; Cyomin; Cytacon; Cytaman; Depinar; Depo-Cobolin; Docemine; Dodecamin; La-12; Lifaton; Nascobal; Neurin-12; Neurodex; Neuroforte-R; Norivite; Ottovit; Pan B-12; Primabalt; Rubesol-1000; Rubisol; Rubivite; Rubramin Pc; Ruvite; Shovite; Sytobex; Vibal; Vibisone; Vita Liver; Vita-Plus B-12; Vitabee 12; **Vitamin B-12**; Yobramin
Foreign Brand Availability: Arcored (Indonesia); Bedoc (Greece); Bedodeka (Israel); Behepan (Denmark; Sweden); Betolvex (Denmark; Finland; Norway; Sweden; Switzerland); Bevitex (Israel); Cobalin (Bahrain; Cyprus; Egypt; Iran; Iraq; Jordan; Kuwait; Lebanon; Libya; Oman; Qatar; Republic-of-Yemen; Saudi-Arabia; Syria; United-Arab-Emirates); Cobalmed (South-Africa); Cobamin Ophth Soln (Hong-Kong); Compensal 25,000 (Mexico); Creliverol-12 (Peru); Cytamen (Argentina; Australia; England; Ireland; Turkey); Dobetin (Italy); Hematolamin (Japan); Lagavit B12 (Bahamas; Bahrain; Barbados; Belize; Bermuda; Curacao; Cyprus; Egypt; Guyana; Iran; Iraq; Jamaica; Jordan; Kuwait; Lebanon; Libya; Netherland-Antilles; Oman; Qatar; Republic-of-Yemen; Saudi-Arabia; Surinam; Syria; Trinidad; United-Arab-Emirates); Lifaton B12 (Spain); Nascobal Intranasal Gel (Israel); Norivite-12 (South-Africa); Redisol (Japan; Thailand); Rojamin (Ecuador); Rubramin (Philippines); Rubranova (Mexico); Vicapan N (Germany); Vitamina B12-Ecar (Colombia); Vitarubin (Switzerland)
HCFA JCODE(S): J3420 up to 1,000 µg IM, SC

DESCRIPTION

Cyanocobalamin injection is a sterile solution of cyanocobalamin. Each ml contains 100 or 1000 µg cyanocobalamin. The vials also contain sodium chloride, 0.25%. Benzyl alcohol, 2% is present as a preservative. Sodium hydroxide and/or hydrochloric acid may have been added during manufacture to adjust the pH.

Cyanocobalamin occurs as dark-red crystals or orthorhombic needles or crystalline red powder. It is very hygroscopic in the anhydrous form and sparingly soluble in water (1:80). Its pharmacological activity is destroyed by heavy metals (iron) and strong oxidizing or reducing agents (vitamin C), but not by autoclaving for short periods of time (15-20 minutes) at 121°C. The vitamin B_{12} coenzymes are very unstable in light.

The chemical name is 5, 6-dimethyl-benzimidazolyl cyanocobalamine; the empirical formula is $C_{63}H_{88}CoN_{14}O_{14}P$. The cobalt content is 4.35%. The molecular weight is 1355.38. **Gel for Intranasal Administration:** Cyanocobalamin gel for intranasal administration is a solution of cyanocobalamin (vitamin B_{12}) for administration as a metered gel to the nasal mucosa. Each bottle of Nascobal contains 5 ml of a 500 µg/ 0. 1 ml gel solution of cyanocobalamin with methylcellulose, sodium citrate, citric acid, glycerin, benzalkonium chloride in purified water. The gel solution has a pH between 4.5 and 5.5. The gel pump unit must be fully primed (see HOW SUPPLIED) prior to initial use. After initial priming, each metered gel delivers an average of 500 µg of cyanocobalamin and the 5 ml bottle will deliver 8 doses of Nascobal. If not used for 48 hours or longer, the unit must be reprimed (see HOW SUPPLIED).

CLINICAL PHARMACOLOGY

INJECTION

Vitamin B_{12} is essential to growth, cell reproduction, hematopoiesis, and nucleoprotein and myelin synthesis. Cyanocobalamin is quantitatively and rapidly absorbed from intramuscular (IM) and subcutaneous sites of injection; the plasma level of the compound reaches its peak within 1 hour after IM injection. Absorbed vitamin B_{12} is transported via specific B_{12}-binding proteins, transcobalamin I and II, to the various tissues. The liver is the main organ for vitamin B_{12} storage.

Within 48 hours after injection of 100 or 1000 µg of vitamin B_{12}, 50-98% of the injected dose may appear in the urine. The major portion is excreted within the first 8 hours. Intravenous administration results in even more rapid excretion with little opportunity for liver storage. Gastrointestinal absorption of vitamin B_{12} depends on the presence of sufficient intrinsic factor and calcium ions. Intrinsic factor deficiency causes pernicious anemia, which may be associated with subacute combined degeneration of the spinal cord. Prompt parenteral administration of vitamin B_{12} prevents progression of neurologic damage.

The average diet supplies about 5-15 µg/day of vitamin B_{12} in a protein-bound form that is available for absorption after normal digestion. Vitamin B_{12} is not present in foods of plant origin but is abundant in foods of animal origin. In people with normal absorption, deficiencies have been reported only in strict vegetarians who consume no products of animal origin (including no milk products or eggs).

Vitamin B_{12} is bound to intrinsic factor during transit through the stomach; separation occurs in the terminal ileum in the presence of calcium, and vitamin B_{12} enters the mucosal cell for absorption. It is then transported by the transcobalamin-binding proteins. A small amount (approximately 1% of the total amount ingested) is absorbed by simple diffusion, but this mechanism is adequate only with very large doses. Oral absorption is considered too undependable to rely on in patients with pernicious anemia or other conditions resulting in malabsorption of vitamin B_{12}.

Cyanocobalamin is the most widely used form of vitamin B_{12} and has hematopoietic activity apparently identical to that of the antianemia factor in purified liver extract. Hydroxycobalamin is equally as effective as cyanocobalamin, and they share the cobalamin molecular structure.

Colchicine, para-aminosalicylic acid, and heavy alcohol intake for longer than 2 weeks may produce malabsorption of vitamin B_{12}.

GEL FOR INTRANASAL ADMINISTRATION

Cells characterized by rapid division (*e.g.*, epithelial cells, bone marrow, myeloid cells) appear to have the greatest requirement for vitamin B_{12}. Vitamin B_{12} can be converted to coenzyme B_{12} in tissues, and as such is essential for conversion of methylmalonate to succinate and synthesis of methionine from homocysteine, a reaction which also requires folate. In the absence of coenzyme B_{12}, tetrahydrofolate cannot be regenerated from its inactive storage form, 5-methyl tetrahydrofolate, and a functional folate deficiency occurs. Vitamin B_{12} also may be involved in maintaining sulfhydryl (SH) groups in the reduced form required by many SH-activated enzyme systems. Through these reactions, vitamin B_{12} is associated with fat and carbohydrate metabolism and protein synthesis. Vitamin B_{12} deficiency results in megaloblastic anemia, GI lesions, and neurologic damage that begins with an inability to produce myelin and is followed by gradual degeneration of the axon and nerve head.

Cyanocobalamin is the most stable and widely used form of vitamin B_{12}, and has hematopoietic activity apparently identical to that of the antianemia factor in purified liver extract. The information below, describing the clinical pharmacology of cyanocobalamin, has been derived from studies with injectable vitamin B_{12}.

Vitamin B_{12} is quantitatively and rapidly absorbed from IM and subcutaneous sites of injection. It is bound to plasma proteins and stored in the liver. Vitamin B_{12} is excreted in the bile and undergoes some enterohepatic recycling. Absorbed vitamin B_{12} is transported via specific B_{12} binding proteins, transcobalamin I and II, to the various tissues. The liver is the main organ for vitamin B_{12} storage.

Parenteral (intramuscular) administration of vitamin B_{12} completely reverses the megaloblastic anemia and GI symptoms of vitamin B_{12} deficiency; the degree of improvement in neurologic symptoms depends on the duration and severity of the lesions, although progression of the lesions is immediately arrested.

Gastrointestinal absorption of vitamin B_{12} depends on the presence of sufficient intrinsic factor and calcium ions. Intrinsic factor deficiency causes pernicious anemia, which may be associated with subacute combined degeneration of the spinal cord. Prompt parenteral administration of vitamin B_{12} prevents progression of neurologic damage.

PHARMACOKINETICS

Absorption

In a bioavailability study in 23 pernicious anemia patients comparing B_{12} nasal gel to intramuscular B_{12}, peak concentrations of B_{12} after intranasal administration were reached in 1-2 hours. The average peak concentration of B_{12} after intranasal administration was 1414 ± 1003 pg/ml. The bioavailability of the nasal gel relative to an IM injection was found to be 8.9% (90% confidence intervals 7.1-11.2%).

In pernicious anemia patients, once weekly intranasal dosing with 500 µg B_{12} resulted in a consistent increase in predose serum B_{12} levels during 1 month of treatment ($p<0.003$) above that seen 1 month after 100 µg IM dose.

Distribution

In the blood, B_{12} is bound to transcobalamin II, a specific B-globulin carrier protein, and is distributed and stored primarily in the liver and bone marrow.

Elimination

About 3-8 µg of B_{12} is secreted into the GI tract daily via the bile; in normal subjects with sufficient intrinsic factor, all but about 1 µg is reabsorbed. When B_{12} is administered in doses which saturate the binding capacity of plasma proteins and the liver, the unbound B_{12} is rapidly eliminated in the urine. Retention of B_{12} in the body is dose-dependent. About 80-90% of an IM dose up to 50 μg is retained in the body; this percentage drops to 55% for a 100 μg dose, and decreases to 15% when a 1000 μg dose is given.

INDICATIONS AND USAGE

INJECTION AND GEL FOR INTRANASAL ADMINISTRATION

Cyanocobalamin gel for intranasal administration is indicated for the maintenance of the hematologic status of patients who are in remission following IM vitamin B_{12} therapy for the following conditions:

1. Pernicious anemia. Indicated only in patients who are in hematologic remission with no nervous system involvement.
2. Dietary deficiency of vitamin B_{12} occurring in strict vegetarians. (Isolated vitamin B_{12} deficiency is very rare.)
3. Malabsorption of vitamin B_{12} resulting from structural or functional damage to the stomach, where intrinsic factor is secreted or to the ileum, where intrinsic factor facilitates vitamin B_{12} absorption. These conditions include tropical sprue, and nontropical sprue (idiopathic steatorrhea, gluten-induced enteropathy). Folate deficiency in these patients is usually more severe than vitamin B_{12} deficiency.
4. Inadequate secretion of intrinsic factor, resulting from lesions that destroy the gastric mucosa (ingestion of corrosives, extensive neoplasia), and a number of conditions associated with a variable degree of gastric atrophy (such as multiple sclerosis, certain endocrine disorders, iron deficiency, and subtotal gastrectomy). Total gastrectomy always produces vitamin B_{12} deficiency. Structural lesions leading to vitamin B_{12} deficiency include regional ileitis, ileal resections, malignancies, etc.
5. Competition for vitamin B_{12} by intestinal parasites or bacteria. The fish tapeworm *(Diphyllobothrium latum)* absorbs huge quantities of vitamin B_{12} and infested patients often have associated gastric atrophy. The blind-loop syndrome may produce deficiency of vitamin B_{12} or folate.
6. Inadequate utilization of vitamin B_{12}. This may occur if antimetabolites for the vitamin are employed in the treatment of neoplasia.
7. Malignancy of pancreas or bowel folic acid deficiency.

It may be possible to treat the underlying disease by surgical correction of anatomic lesions leading to small bowel bacterial overgrowth, expulsion of fish tapeworm, discontinuation of drugs leading to vitamin malabsorption (see PRECAUTIONS, Drug/Laboratory Test Interactions), use of a gluten-free diet in nontropical sprue, or administration of antibiotics in tropical sprue. Such measures remove the need for long-term administration of vitamin B_{12}.

Requirements of vitamin B_{12} in excess of normal (due to pregnancy, thyrotoxicosis, hemolytic anemia, hemorrhage, malignancy, hepatic and renal disease) can usually be met with intranasal or oral supplementation.

Injection Only

Cyanocobalamin injection is suitable for the vitamin B_{12} absorption test (Schilling Test).

Gel for Intranasal Administration Only

Cyanocobalamin gel for intranasal administration has only been tested in patients with vitamin B_{12} malabsorption who have received prior IM cyanocobalamin treatment and are in hematologic remission.

Cyanocobalamin gel for intranasal administration is not suitable for the vitamin B_{12} absorption test (Schilling Test).

NON-FDA APPROVED INDICATIONS

Although not approved by the FDA, cyanocobalamin has been used for the prevention and treatment of cyanide toxicity associated with sodium nitroprusside. Addidtional unapproved uses of cyanocobalamin include the treatment of trigeminal neuralgia, multiple sclerosis and other neuropathies, various psychiatric disorders, poor growth or nutrition, and as a "tonic" for patients with easy fatigability. There is no evidence that cyanocobalamin is a valid treatment in any of these conditions.

CONTRAINDICATIONS

Sensitivity to cobalt and/or vitamin B_{12}, or any component of the medication is a contraindication.

WARNINGS

Patients with early Leber's disease (hereditary optic nerve atrophy) who were treated with cyanocobalamin suffered severe and swift optic atrophy.

Hypokalemia and sudden death may occur in severe megaloblastic anemia which is treated intensively with vitamin B_{12}. Folic acid is not a substitute for vitamin B_{12} although it may improve vitamin B_{12} deficient megaloblastic anemia. Exclusive use of folic acid in treating vitamin B_{12}-deficient megaloblastic anemia could result in progressive and irreversible neurologic damage.

Anaphylactic shock and death have been reported after parenteral vitamin B_{12} administration. No such reactions have been reported in clinical trials with cyanocobalamin gel for intranasal administration.

Blunted or impeded therapeutic response to vitamin B_{12} may be due to such conditions as infection, uremia, drugs having bone marrow suppressant properties such as chloramphenicol, and concurrent iron or folic acid deficiency.

PRECAUTIONS

GENERAL

Vitamin B_{12} deficiency that is allowed to progress for longer than 3 months may produce permanent degenerative lesions of the spinal cord. Doses of folic acid greater than 0.1 mg/day may result in hematologic remission in patients with vitamin B_{12} deficiency. Neurologic manifestations will not be prevented with folic acid, and if they are not treated with vitamin B_{12}, irreversible damage will result. Doses of cyanocobalamin exceeding 10 μg daily may produce hematologic response in patients with folate deficiency. Indiscriminate administration may mask the true diagnosis.

Gel for Intranasal Administration

An intradermal test dose of parenteral vitamin B_{12} is recommended before cyanocobalamin gel for intranasal administration is administered to patients suspected of cyanocobalamin sensitivity. Vitamin B_{12} deficiency that is allowed to progress for longer than 3 months may produce permanent degenerative lesions of the spinal cord. Doses of folic acid greater than 0.1 mg/day may result in hematologic remission in patients with vitamin B_{12} deficiency. Neurologic manifestations will not be prevented with folic acid, and if not treated with vitamin B_{12}, irreversible damage will result.

Doses of vitamin B_{12} exceeding 10 μg daily may produce hematologic response in patients with folate deficiency. Indiscriminate administration may mask the true diagnosis.

The validity of diagnostic vitamin B_{12} or folic acid blood assays could be compromised by medications, and this should be considered before relying on such tests for therapy.

Vitamin B_{12} is not a substitute for folic acid and since it might improve folic acid deficient megaloblastic anemia, indiscriminate use of vitamin B_{12} could mask the true diagnosis.

Hypokalemia and thrombocytosis could occur upon conversion of severe megaloblastic to normal erythropoiesis with vitamin B_{12} therapy. Therefore, serum potassium levels and the platelet count should be monitored carefully during therapy.

Vitamin B_{12} deficiency may suppress the signs of polycythemia vera. Treatment with vitamin B_{12} may unmask this condition.

If a patient is not properly maintained with cyanocobalamin gel for intranasal administration, intramuscular vitamin B_{12} is necessary for adequate treatment of the patient. No single regimen fits all cases, and the status of the patient observed in follow-up is the final criterion for adequacy of therapy.

The effectiveness of cyanocobalamin gel for intranasal administration in patients with nasal congestion, allergic rhinitis and upper respiratory infections has not been determined. Therefore, treatment with cyanocobalamin gel for intranasal administration should be deferred until symptoms have subsided.

INFORMATION FOR THE PATIENT

Patients with pernicious anemia should be informed that they will require monthly injections of vitamin B_{12} (or weekly intranasal administration of cyanocobalamin gel for intranasal administration) for the remainder of their lives. Failure to do so will result in return of the anemia and in development of incapacitating and irreversible damage to the nerves of the spinal chord. Also, patients should be warned about the danger of taking folic acid in place of vitamin B_{12}, because the former may prevent anemia but allow progression of subacute combined degeneration.

A vegetarian diet which contains no animal products (including milk products or eggs) does not supply any vitamin B_{12}. Patients following such a diet should be advised to take oral vitamin B_{12} regularly, or cyanocobalamin gel for intranasal administration, weekly. The need for vitamin B_{12} is increased by pregnancy and lactation. Deficiency has been recognized in infants of vegetarian mothers who were breast fed, even though the mothers had no symptoms of deficiency at the time.

Gel for Intranasal Administration

Hot foods may cause nasal secretions and a resulting loss of medication; therefore, patients should be told to administer cyanocobalamin gel for intranasal administration at least 1 hour before or 1 hour after ingestion of hot foods or liquids.

The patient should also understand the importance of returning for follow-up blood tests every 3-6 months to confirm adequacy of the therapy. Careful instructions on the actuator assembly, priming of the actuator and nasal administration of cyanocobalamin gel for intranasal administration should be given to the patient. Although instructions for patients are supplied with individual bottles, procedures for use should be demonstrated to each patient.

LABORATORY TESTS

During the initial treatment of patients with pernicious anemia, serum potassium must be observed closely during the first 48 hours and potassium should be replaced, if necessary.

Hematocrit, reticulocyte count, and vitamin B_{12}, folate, and iron levels should be obtained prior to treatment. Hematocrit and reticulocyte counts should be repeated daily from the fifth to seventh days of therapy and then frequently until the hematocrit is normal. If folate levels are low, folic acid should also be administered. If reticulocytes have not increased after treatment or if reticulocyte counts do not continue at least twice the normal level (as long as the hematocrit is less than 35%), diagnosis or treatment should be re-evaluated. Repeat determinations of iron and folic acid may reveal a complicating illness that might inhibit the response of the marrow. Since patients with pernicious anemia have about 3 times the incidence of carcinoma of the stomach as the general population, appropriate tests for this condition should be carried out when indicated.

All hematologic parameters should be normal when beginning treatment with cyanocobalamin gel for intranasal administration.

Vitamin B_{12} blood levels and peripheral blood counts must be monitored initially at 1 month after the start of treatment with cyanocobalamin gel for intranasal administration, and then at intervals of 3-6 months.

A decline in the serum levels of B_{12} after 1 month after treatment with B_{12} nasal gel may indicate that the dose may need to be adjusted upward. Patients should be seen 1 month after each dose adjustment, continued low levels of serum B_{12} may indicate that the patient is not a candidate for this mode of administration.

Patients with pernicious anemia have about 3 times the incidence of carcinoma of the stomach as in the general population, so appropriate tests for this condition should be carried out when indicated.

DRUG/LABORATORY TEST INTERACTIONS

Persons taking most antibiotics, methotrexate, and pyrimethamine invalidate folic acid and vitamin B_{12} diagnostic blood assays. *Gel for Intranasal Administration:* Colchicine, para-aminosalicylic acid and heavy alcohol intake for longer than 2 weeks may produce malabsorption of vitamin B_{12}.

CARCINOGENESIS, MUTAGENESIS, AND IMPAIRMENT OF FERTILITY

Long-term studies in animals to evaluate carcinogenic potential have not been done. There is no evidence from long-term use in patients with pernicious anemia that cyanocobalamin is carcinogenic. Pernicious anemia is associated with an increased incidence of carcinoma of the stomach, but this is believed to be related to the underlying pathology and not to treatment with cyanocobalamin.

PREGNANCY CATEGORY C

Animal reproduction studies have not been conducted with vitamin B_{12}. It is also not known whether vitamin B_{12} can cause fetal harm when administered to a pregnant woman or can affect reproduction capacity. Adequate and well-controlled studies have not been done in pregnant women. However, vitamin B_{12} is an essential vitamin, and requirements are increased during pregnancy. Amounts of vitamin B_{12} that are recommended by the Food and Nutrition Board, National Academy of Science-National Research Council, for pregnant women (4 µg daily) should be consumed during pregnancy.

NURSING MOTHERS

Vitamin B_{12} appears in the milk of nursing mothers in concentrations which approximate the mother's level of vitamin B_{12} in the blood. Amounts of vitamin B_{12} that are recommended by the Food and Nutrition Board, National Academy of Science-National Research Council, for lactating women (4 µg daily) should be consumed during lactation.

PEDIATRIC USE

Intake for children should be the amount (0.5-3 µg daily) recommended by the Food and Nutrition Board, National Academy of Science-National Research Council.

ADVERSE REACTIONS

The incidence of adverse experiences described in TABLE 1 are based on data from a short-term clinical trial in vitamin B_{12} deficient patients in hematologic remission receiving cyanocobalamin gel for intranasal administration (n=24) and IM vitamin B_{12} (n=25).

TABLE 1 *Adverse Experiences by Body System, Number of Patients and Number of Occurrences by Treatment Following Intramuscular and Intranasal Administration of Cyanocobalamin*

Body System/ Adverse Experience	Number of Patients (occurrences): Vitamin B_{12} Nasal Gel, 500 µg (n=24)	IM Vitamin B_{12} 100 µg (n=25)
Body as a Whole		
Asthenia	1 (1)	4 (4)
Back pain	0 (0)	1 (1)
Generalized pain	0 (0)	2 (3)
Headache	1 (2)*	5 (11)
Infection†	3 (4)	3 (3)
Cardiovascular System		
Peripheral vascular disorder	0 (0)	1 (1)
Digestive System		
Dyspepsia	0 (0)	1 (2)
Glossitis	1 (1)	0 (0)
Nausea	1 (1)*	1 (1)
Nausea & vomiting	0 (0)	1 (1)
Vomiting	0 (0)	1 (1)
Musculoskeletal System		
Arthritis	0 (0)	2 (2)
Myalgia	0 (0)	1 (1)
Nervous System		
Abnormal gait	0 (0)	1 (1)
Anxiety	0 (0)	1 (1)*
Dizziness	0 (0)	3 (3)
Hypesthesia	0 (0)	1 (1)
Incoordination	0 (0)	1 (2)*
Nervousness	0 (0)	1 (3)*
Paresthesia	1 (1)	1 (1)
Respiratory System		
Dyspnea	0 (0)	1 (1)
Rhinitis	1 (1)*	2 (2)

* There may be a possible relationship between these adverse experiences and the study drugs. These adverse experiences could also have been produced by the patient's clinical state or other concomitant therapy.
† Sore throat, common cold.

The intensity of the reported adverse experiences following the administration of cyanocobalamin gel for intranasal administration and IM vitamin B_{12} were generally mild. One patient reported severe headache following IM dosing. Similarly, a few adverse experiences of moderate intensity were reported following IM dosing (2 headaches and rhinitis; 1 dyspepsia, arthritis, and dizziness), and dosing with cyanocobalamin gel for intranasal administration (1 headache, infection, and paresthesia).

The majority of the reported adverse experiences following dosing with cyanocobalamin gel for intranasal administration and IM vitamin B_{12} were judged to be intercurrent events. For the other reported adverse experiences, the relationship to study drug was judged as "possible" or "remote". Of the adverse experiences judged to be of "possible" relationship to the study drug, anxiety, incoordination, and nervousness were reported following IM vitamin B_{12} and headache, nausea, and rhinitis were reported following dosing with cyanocobalamin gel for intranasal administration.

The following adverse reactions have been reported with *parenteral* vitamin B_{12}:

Generalized: Anaphylactic shock and death. (See WARNINGS and PRECAUTIONS.)
Cardiovascular: Pulmonary edema and congestive heart failure early in treatment; peripheral vascular thrombosis.
Hematologic: Polycythemia vera.
Gastrointestinal: Mild transient diarrhea.
Dermatologic: Itching; transitory exanthema.
Miscellaneous: Feeling of swelling of entire body.

DOSAGE AND ADMINISTRATION

ORAL AND INJECTABLE FORMS

Avoid using the intravenous route. Use of this product intravenously will result in almost all of the vitamin being lost in the urine. *Pernicious Anemia:* Parenteral vitamin B_{12} is the recommended treatment and will be required for the remainder of the patient's life. The oral form is not dependable. A dose of 100 µg daily for 6 or 7 days should be administered by IM or deep subcutaneous injection.

If there is clinical improvement and if a reticulocyte response is observed, the same amount may be given on alternate days for 7 doses, then every 3-4 days for another 2-3 weeks. By this time, hematologic values should have become normal. This regimen should be followed by 100 µg monthly for life. Folic acid should be administered concomitantly, if needed.

Patients With Normal Intestinal Absorption

When the oral route is not deemed adequate, initial treatment similar to that for patients with pernicious anemia may be indicated, depending on the severity of the deficiency. Chronic treatment should be with an oral B_{12} preparation.

If other vitamin deficiencies are present, they should be treated.

Other Indications In Patients With Inadequate Intestinal Absorption

Doses similar to those for pernicious anemia are generally appropriate.

The individual patient and specific condition must be assessed to help guide needs and dosage.

Schilling Test

The flushing dose is 1000 µg.

GEL FOR INTRANASAL ADMINISTRATION

The recommended initial dose of cyanocobalamin gel for intranasal administration in patients with vitamin B_{12} malabsorption who are in remission following injectable vitamin B_{12} therapy is 500 µg administered intranasally once weekly. Patients should be in hematologic remission before treatment with cyanocobalamin gel for intranasal administration. See PRECAUTIONS, Laboratory Tests, for monitoring B_{12} levels and adjustment of dosage.

HOW SUPPLIED

INJECTION

Parenteral drug products should be inspected visually for particulate matter and discoloration prior to administration, whenever solution and container permit.

Cyanocobalamin Injection should be protected from light. Vials should be stored at controlled room temperature, 15-30°C (59-86°F).

GEL FOR INTRANASAL ADMINISTRATION

Nascobal (cyanocobalamin) gel for intranasal administration is available as a metered dose gel in 5 ml glass bottles. It is available in a dosage strength of 500 µg per actuation (0.1 ml/actuation). A screw-on actuator is provided. This actuator, following priming, will deliver 0.1 ml of the gel. Nascobal (cyanocobalamin) gel for intranasal administration is provided in a sealed prescription vial containing a metered dose nasal gel actuator with dust cover, a bottle of nasal gel solution, and a patient instruction leaflet. One bottle will deliver 8 doses.

Storage: Protect from light. Keep covered in prescription vial until ready to use. Store at room temperature 15-30°C (59-86°F). Protect from freezing.

PRODUCT LISTING - RATED THERAPEUTICALLY EQUIVALENT

Solution - Injectable - 100 mcg/ml

Size	Price	Manufacturer	NDC
30 ml	$1.85	GENERIC, C.O. Truxton Inc	00463-1021-30
30 ml	$3.00	GENERIC, Interstate Drug Exchange Inc	00814-8448-46
30 ml	$3.85	GENERIC, Ivax Corporation	00182-0693-66

Solution - Injectable - 1000 mcg/ml

Size	Price	Manufacturer	NDC
1 ml x 25	$16.00	GENERIC, American Regent Laboratories Inc	00517-0031-25
1 ml x 25	$20.25	GENERIC, Esi Lederle Generics	00641-0370-25
1 ml x 25	$45.00	GENERIC, American Pharmaceutical Partners	63323-0044-01
10 ml	$1.00	GENERIC, Dunhall Pharmaceuticals Inc	00217-8806-08
10 ml	$2.05	GENERIC, Geneva Pharmaceuticals	00781-3020-70
10 ml	$2.25	GENERIC, Roberts/Hauck Pharmaceutical Corporation	43797-0004-12
10 ml	$2.30	GENERIC, Major Pharmaceuticals Inc	00904-0889-10
10 ml	$2.31	GENERIC, Pasadena Research Laboratories Inc	00418-0151-41
10 ml	$2.40	GENERIC, Hyrex Pharmaceuticals	00314-0622-70
10 ml	$10.00	GENERIC, International Ethical Laboratories Inc	11584-1025-01
10 ml x 25	$36.00	GENERIC, American Regent Laboratories Inc	00517-0032-25
30 ml	$1.56	GENERIC, American Regent Laboratories Inc	00517-0130-01
30 ml	$1.69	GENERIC, Mcguff Company	49072-0145-30
30 ml	$1.95	GENERIC, C.O. Truxton Inc	00463-1015-30
30 ml	$2.25	GENERIC, Geneva Pharmaceuticals	00781-3021-90
30 ml	$2.50	GENERIC, Dunhall Pharmaceuticals Inc	00217-8806-10
30 ml	$3.25	GENERIC, Major Pharmaceuticals Inc	00904-0889-30
30 ml	$3.25	GENERIC, Roberts/Hauck Pharmaceutical Corporation	43797-0004-13
30 ml	$3.30	GENERIC, Merit Pharmaceuticals	30727-0314-80
30 ml	$3.95	GENERIC, Jones Pharma Inc	52604-0091-08

30 ml	$4.50	GENERIC, Hyrex Pharmaceuticals	00314-0622-30
30 ml	$4.50	GENERIC, Forest Pharmaceuticals	00456-1015-30
30 ml	$6.25	GENERIC, Esi Lederle Generics	00641-2270-41
30 ml	$10.90	GENERIC, Hyrex Pharmaceuticals	00314-0678-30

PRODUCT LISTING - RATED NOT THERAPEUTICALLY EQUIVALENT

Solution - Injectable - 100 mcg/ml

30 ml	$4.00	GENERIC, Consolidated Midland Corporation	00223-8871-30

PRODUCT LISTING - EQUIVALENTS NOT AVAILABLE

Gel - Nasal - 500 mcg/0.1 ml			
2.30 ml	$60.00	NASCOBAL, Schwarz Pharma	00091-7033-13
2.30 ml	$62.40	NASCOBAL, Nastech Pharmaceutical Company Inc	57459-1002-01
Injection - Intramuscular - 2 mcg/ml			
30 ml	$10.99	GENERIC, Hauser, A.F. Inc	52637-2020-30
30 ml	$35.99	GENERIC, Merit Pharmaceuticals	30727-0335-80
30 ml	$126.00	GENERIC, Pro Metic Pharma	62174-0493-72
Solution - Injectable - 100 mcg/ml			
30 ml	$2.60	GENERIC, Steris Laboratories Inc	00402-0090-30
30 ml	$2.69	GENERIC, Moore, H.L. Drug Exchange Inc	00839-5660-36
Solution - Injectable - 1000 mcg/ml			
1 ml x 10	$0.96	GENERIC, Vangard Labs	00615-0006-11
1 ml x 10	$3.90	GENERIC, Cmc-Consolidated Midland Corporation	00223-8859-10
1 ml x 25	$31.25	GENERIC, Cmc-Consolidated Midland Corporation	00223-8861-01
10 ml	$0.95	GENERIC, Carpenter Pharmaceuticals	55726-0091-10
10 ml	$1.14	GENERIC, Hauser, A.F. Inc	52637-0282-10
10 ml	$1.50	GENERIC, Vita-Rx Corporation	49727-0722-10
10 ml	$1.89	GENERIC, Moore, H.L. Drug Exchange Inc	00839-5661-30
10 ml	$2.30	GENERIC, Forest Pharmaceuticals	00785-8010-10
10 ml	$2.63	GENERIC, Interstate Drug Exchange Inc	00814-8449-40
10 ml	$2.75	GENERIC, Cmc-Consolidated Midland Corporation	00223-8870-00
10 ml	$2.90	GENERIC, Primedics Laboratories	00684-0123-10
10 ml	$4.50	GENERIC, Clint Pharmaceutical Inc	55553-0091-10
30 ml	$1.20	GENERIC, Hauser, A.F. Inc	52637-0312-30
30 ml	$1.65	GENERIC, Pegasus Laboratories Inc	10974-0092-30
30 ml	$1.94	GENERIC, Vangard Labs	00615-0006-13
30 ml	$2.00	GENERIC, Vita-Rx Corporation	49727-0722-30
30 ml	$2.77	GENERIC, Forest Pharmaceuticals	00785-8010-30
30 ml	$2.93	GENERIC, Interstate Drug Exchange Inc	00814-8449-46
30 ml	$3.00	GENERIC, Med Tek Pharmaceuticals Inc	52349-0113-30
30 ml	$3.50	GENERIC, Pasadena Research Laboratories Inc	00418-0151-61
30 ml	$4.75	GENERIC, Primedics Laboratories	00684-0153-30
30 ml	$5.50	GENERIC, Cmc-Consolidated Midland Corporation	00223-8870-30
30 ml	$5.95	GENERIC, Clint Pharmaceutical Inc	55553-0091-30
30 ml	$6.08	GENERIC, Physicians Total Care	54868-0762-00
30 ml	$6.95	COBOLIN-M, Legere Pharmaceuticals	25332-0004-30
30 ml	$17.95	DEPO-COBOLIN, Legere Pharmaceuticals	25332-0078-10
30 ml	$27.55	GENERIC, Steris Laboratories Inc	00402-0208-30
30 ml x 10	$2.28	GENERIC, Moore, H.L. Drug Exchange Inc	00839-5661-36

Cyclobenzaprine Hydrochloride *(000926)*

Categories: Muscle spasm; Pain, musculoskeletal; Pregnancy Category B; FDA Approved 1977 Aug
Drug Classes: Musculoskeletal agents; Relaxants, skeletal muscle
Brand Names: Flexeril
Foreign Brand Availability: Cyben (Korea); Flexiban (Italy; Portugal); Tensodox (Peru); Yurelax (Spain)
Cost of Therapy: $36.04 (Musculoskeletal Pain; Flexeril; 10 mg; 3 tablets/day; 10 day supply)
$2.20 (Musculoskeletal Pain; Generic tablets; 10 mg; 3 tablets/day; 10 day supply)

DESCRIPTION

Cyclobenzaprine hydrochloride is a white, crystalline tricyclic amine salt with the empirical formula $C_{20}H_{21}N{\cdot}HCl$ and a molecular weight of 311.9. It has a melting point of 217°C, and a pK_a of 8.47 at 25°C. It is freely soluble in water and alcohol, sparingly soluble in isopropanol, and insoluble in hydrocarbon solvents. If aqueous solutions are made alkaline, the free base separates. Cyclobenzaprine hydrochloride is designated chemically as 3-(5*H*-dibenzo[*a,d*]cyclohepten-5-ylidene)-*N*, *N*-dimethyl-1-propanamine hydrochloride.

Cyclobenzaprine hydrochloride is supplied as 10 mg tablets for oral administration. *Inactive Ingredients:* Hydroxypropyl cellulose, hydroxypropyl methylcellulose, iron oxide, lactose, magnesium stearate, starch, and titanium dioxide.

CLINICAL PHARMACOLOGY

Cyclobenzaprine HCl relieves skeletal muscle spasm of local origin without interfering with muscle function. It is ineffective in muscle spasm due to central nervous system disease (CNS).

Cyclobenzaprine reduced or abolished skeletal muscle hyperactivity in several animal models. Animal studies indicate that cyclobenzaprine does not act at the neuromuscular junction or directly on skeletal muscle. Such studies show that cyclobenzaprine acts primarily within the CNS at brain stem as opposed to spinal cord levels, although its action on the latter may contribute to its overall skeletal muscle relaxant activity. Evidence suggests that the net effect of cyclobenzaprine is a reduction of tonic somatic motor activity, influencing both gamma (γ) and alpha (α) motor systems.

Pharmacological studies in animals showed a similarity between the effects of cyclobenzaprine and the structurally related tricyclic antidepressants, including reserpine antagonism, norepinephrine potentiation, potent peripheral and central anticholinergic effects, and sedation. Cyclobenzaprine caused slight to moderate increase in heart rate in animals.

Cyclobenzaprine is well absorbed after oral administration, but there is a large intersubject variation in plasma levels. Cyclobenzaprine is eliminated quite slowly with a half-life as long as 1-3 days. It is highly bound to plasma proteins, is extensively metabolized primarily to glucuronide-like conjugates, and is excreted primarily via the kidneys.

No significant effect on plasma levels or bioavailability of cyclobenzaprine HCl or aspirin was noted when single or multiple doses of the 2 drugs were administered concomitantly. Concomitant administration of cyclobenzaprine HCl and aspirin is usually well tolerated and no unexpected or serious clinical or laboratory adverse effects have been observed. No studies have been performed to indicate whether cyclobenzaprine HCl enhances the clinical effect of aspirin or other analgesics, or whether analgesics enhance the clinical effect of cyclobenzaprine HCl in acute musculoskeletal conditions.

INDICATIONS AND USAGE

Cyclobenzaprine HCl is indicated as an adjunct to rest and physical therapy for relief of muscle spasm associated with acute, painful musculoskeletal conditions.

Improvement is manifested by relief of muscle spasm and its associated signs and symptoms, namely, pain, tenderness, limitation of motion, and restriction in activities of daily living.

Cyclobenzaprine HCl should be used only for short periods (up to 2 or 3 weeks) because adequate evidence of effectiveness for more prolonged use is not available and because muscle spasm associated with acute, painful musculoskeletal conditions is generally of short duration and specific therapy for longer periods is seldom warranted.

Cyclobenzaprine HCl has not been found effective in the treatment of spasticity associated with cerebral or spinal cord disease, or in children with cerebral palsy.

CONTRAINDICATIONS

- Hypersensitivity to the drug.
- Concomitant use of monoamine oxidase inhibitors or within 14 days after their discontinuation.
- Acute recovery phase of myocardial infarction, and patients with arrhythmias, heart block or conduction disturbances, or congestive heart failure.
- Hyperthyroidism.

WARNINGS

Cyclobenzaprine is closely related to the tricyclic antidepressants, *e.g.*, amitriptyline and imipramine. In short-term studies for indications other than muscle spasm associated with acute musculoskeletal conditions, and usually at doses somewhat greater than those recommended for skeletal muscle spasm, some of the more serious CNS reactions noted with the tricyclic antidepressants have occurred (see ADVERSE REACTIONS).

Cyclobenzaprine HCl may interact with monoamine oxidase (MAO) inhibitors. Hyperpyretic crisis, severe convulsions, and deaths have occurred in patients receiving tricyclic antidepressants and MAO inhibitor drugs.

Tricyclic antidepressants have been reported to produce arrhythmias, sinus tachycardia, prolongation of the conduction time leading to myocardial infarction, and stroke.

Cyclobenzaprine HCl may enhance the effects of alcohol, barbiturates, and other CNS depressants.

PRECAUTIONS

GENERAL

Because of its atropine-like action, cyclobenzaprine HCl should be used with caution in patients with a history of urinary retention, angle-closure glaucoma, increased intraocular pressure, and in patients taking anticholinergic medication.

INFORMATION FOR THE PATIENT

Cyclobenzaprine HCl may impair mental and/or physical abilities required for performance of hazardous tasks, such as operating machinery or driving a motor vehicle.

CARCINOGENESIS, MUTAGENESIS, AND IMPAIRMENT OF FERTILITY

In rats treated with cyclobenzaprine HCl for up to 67 weeks at doses of approximately 5-40 times the maximum recommended human dose, pale, sometimes enlarged, livers were noted and there was a dose-related hepatocyte vacuolation with lipidosis. In the higher dose groups this microscopic change was seen after 26 weeks and even earlier in rats which died prior to 26 weeks; at lower doses, the change was not seen until after 26 weeks.

Cyclobenzaprine did not affect the onset, incidence or distribution of neoplasia in an 81-week study in the mouse or in a 105 week study in the rat.

At oral doses of up to 10 times the human dose, cyclobenzaprine did not adversely affect the reproductive performance or fertility of male or female rats. Cyclobenzaprine did not demonstrate mutagenic activity in the male mouse at dose levels of up to 20 times the human dose.

PREGNANCY CATEGORY B

Reproduction studies have been performed in rats, mice, and rabbits at doses up to 20 times the human dose, and have revealed no evidence of impaired fertility or harm to the fetus due to cyclobenzaprine HCl. There are, however, no adequate and well-controlled studies in pregnant women. Because animal reproduction studies are not always predictive of human response, this drug should be used during pregnancy only if clearly needed.

NURSING MOTHERS

It is not known whether this drug is excreted in human milk. Because cyclobenzaprine is closely related to the tricyclic antidepressants, some of which are known to be excreted in human milk, caution should be exercised when cyclobenzaprine HCl is administered to a nursing woman.

PEDIATRIC USE

Safety and effectiveness of cyclobenzaprine HCl in pediatric patients below 15 years of age have not been established.

DRUG INTERACTIONS

Cyclobenzaprine HCl may enhance the effects of alcohol, barbiturates, and other CNS depressants.

Tricyclic antidepressants may block the antihypertensive action of guanethidine and similarly acting compounds.

ADVERSE REACTIONS

The following list of adverse reactions is based on the experience in 473 patients treated with cyclobenzaprine HCl in controlled clinical studies, 7607 patients in the postmarketing surveillance program, and reports received since the drug was marketed. The overall incidence of adverse reactions among patients in the surveillance program was less than the incidence in the controlled clinical studies.

The adverse reactions reported most frequently with cyclobenzaprine HCl were drowsiness, dry mouth, and dizziness. The incidence of these common adverse reactions was lower in the surveillance program than in the controlled clinical studies (see TABLE 1).

TABLE 1

	Clinical Studies	Surveillance Program
Drowsiness	39%	16%
Dry mouth	27%	7%
Dizziness	11%	3%

Among the less frequent adverse reactions, there was no appreciable difference in incidence in controlled clinical studies or in the surveillance program. Adverse reactions which were reported in 1-3% of the patients were: fatigue/tiredness, asthenia, nausea, constipation, dyspepsia, unpleasant taste, blurred vision, headache, nervousness, and confusion.

The following adverse reactions have been reported at an incidence of less than 1 in 100:

Body as a Whole: Syncope, malaise.

Cardiovascular: Tachycardia, arrhythmia, vasodilatation, palpitation, hypotension.

Digestive: Vomiting, anorexia, diarrhea, gastrointestinal pain, gastritis, thirst, flatulence, edema of the tongue, abnormal liver function and rare reports of hepatitis, jaundice, and cholestasis.

Hypersensitivity: Anaphylaxis, angioedema, pruritus, facial edema, urticaria, rash.

Musculoskeletal: Local weakness.

Nervous System and Psychiatric: Ataxia, vertigo, dysarthria, tremors, hypertonia, convulsions, muscle twitching, disorientation, insomnia, depressed mood, abnormal sensations, anxiety, agitation, abnormal thinking and dreaming, hallucinations, excitement, paresthesia, diplopia.

Skin: Sweating.

Special Senses: Ageusia, tinnitus.

Urogenital: Urinary frequency and/or retention.

Other reactions, reported rarely for cyclobenzaprine HCl under circumstances where a causal relationship could not be established or reported for other tricyclic drugs, are listed to serve as alerting information to physicians:

Body as a Whole: Chest pain, edema.

Cardiovascular: Hypertension, myocardial infarction, heart block, stroke.

Digestive: Paralytic ileus, tongue discoloration, stomatitis, parotid swelling.

Endocrine: Inappropriate ADH syndrome.

Hematic and Lymphatic: Purpura, bone marrow depression, leukopenia, eosinophilia, thrombocytopenia.

Metabolic, Nutritional, and Immune: Elevation and lowering of blood sugar levels, weight gain or loss.

Musculoskeletal: Myalgia.

Nervous System and Psychiatric: Decreased or increased libido, abnormal gait, delusions, peripheral neuropathy, Bell's palsy, alteration in EEG patterns, extrapyramidal symptoms.

Respiratory: Dyspnea.

Skin: Photosensitization, alopecia.

Urogenital: Impaired urination, dilatation of urinary tract, impotence, testicular swelling, gynecomastia, breast enlargement, galactorrhea.

DOSAGE AND ADMINISTRATION

The usual dosage of cyclobenzaprine HCl is 10 mg 3 times a day, with a range of 20-40 mg a day in divided doses. Dosage should not exceed 60 mg a day. Use of cyclobenzaprine HCl for periods longer than 2 or 3 weeks is not recommended (see INDICATIONS AND USAGE).

HOW SUPPLIED

Cyclobenzaprine HCl tablets are D-shaped, film coated tablets. *10 mg Tablets:* Butterscotch yellow colored, with code "156" one side and "WPPh" on the other.

PRODUCT LISTING - RATED THERAPEUTICALLY EQUIVALENT

Tablet - Oral - 10 mg

Size	Price	Product	NDC
7's	$8.39	FLEXERIL, Allscripts Pharmaceutical Company	54569-4008-01
7's	$10.48	FLEXERIL, Prescript Pharmaceuticals	00247-0391-07
10's	$8.93	GENERIC, Heartland Healthcare Services	55289-0567-10
10's	$19.16	FLEXERIL, Pharma Pac	52959-0069-10
12's	$5.76	GENERIC, Heartland Healthcare Services	55289-0567-12
12's	$14.38	FLEXERIL, Allscripts Pharmaceutical Company	54569-0835-08
14's	$6.72	GENERIC, Heartland Healthcare Services	55289-0567-14
14's	$16.78	FLEXERIL, Allscripts Pharmaceutical Company	54569-4008-00
15's	$7.20	GENERIC, Heartland Healthcare Services	55289-0567-15
15's	$17.98	FLEXERIL, Allscripts Pharmaceutical Company	54569-0835-00
15's	$18.64	FLEXERIL, Prescript Pharmaceuticals	00247-0391-15
15's	$25.95	FLEXERIL, Pd-Rx Pharmaceuticals	55289-0115-15
15's	$27.05	FLEXERIL, Pharma Pac	52959-0069-15
18's	$8.91	GENERIC, Heartland Healthcare Services	55289-0567-18
20's	$9.90	GENERIC, Heartland Healthcare Services	55289-0567-20
20's	$20.85	GENERIC, St. Mary'S Mpp	60760-0418-20
20's	$23.74	FLEXERIL, Prescript Pharmaceuticals	00247-0391-20
20's	$34.60	FLEXERIL, Pharma Pac	52959-0069-20
21's	$10.43	GENERIC, Heartland Healthcare Services	55289-0567-21
21's	$32.91	FLEXERIL, Pd-Rx Pharmaceuticals	55289-0115-21
21's	$35.66	FLEXERIL, Pharma Pac	52959-0069-21
25 x 30	$717.23	GENERIC, Sky Pharmaceuticals Packaging, Inc	63739-0066-03
25's	$5.08	GENERIC, Udl Laboratories Inc	51079-0644-19
30's	$4.70	GENERIC, Heartland Healthcare Services	55289-0128-30
30's	$13.95	GENERIC, Heartland Healthcare Services	55289-0567-30
30's	$23.75	GENERIC, St. Mary'S Mpp	60760-0418-30
30's	$27.98	GENERIC, Golden State Medical	60429-0052-30
30's	$30.10	GENERIC, Heartland Healthcare Services	61392-0716-30
30's	$30.10	GENERIC, Heartland Healthcare Services	61392-0716-39
30's	$33.93	FLEXERIL, Prescript Pharmaceuticals	00247-0391-30
30's	$35.96	FLEXERIL, Allscripts Pharmaceutical Company	54569-0835-02
30's	$45.26	FLEXERIL, Pd-Rx Pharmaceuticals	55289-0115-30
30's	$50.11	FLEXERIL, Pharma Pac	52959-0069-30
31 x 10	$297.56	GENERIC, Vangard Labs	00615-3520-53
31 x 10	$297.56	GENERIC, Vangard Labs	00615-3520-63
31's	$31.11	GENERIC, Heartland Healthcare Services	61392-0716-31
32's	$32.11	GENERIC, Heartland Healthcare Services	61392-0716-32
40's	$44.12	FLEXERIL, Prescript Pharmaceuticals	00247-0391-40
40's	$65.39	FLEXERIL, Pharma Pac	52959-0069-40
42's	$22.53	GENERIC, Heartland Healthcare Services	55289-0567-42
45's	$45.16	GENERIC, Heartland Healthcare Services	61392-0716-45
45's	$58.13	GENERIC, Udl Laboratories Inc	51079-0644-97
60's	$48.50	GENERIC, St. Mary'S Mpp	60760-0418-60
60's	$52.50	GENERIC, Heartland Healthcare Services	55289-0567-60
60's	$60.21	GENERIC, Heartland Healthcare Services	61392-0716-60
90's	$75.60	GENERIC, Heartland Healthcare Services	55289-0567-90
90's	$90.31	GENERIC, Heartland Healthcare Services	61392-0716-90
100's	$7.40	GENERIC, Heartland Healthcare Services	55289-0128-01
100's	$8.58	FEDERAL UPPER LIMIT, H.C.F.A. F F P	99999-0926-02
100's	$34.00	GENERIC, Raway Pharmacal Inc	00686-0644-20
100's	$40.65	GENERIC, Ivax Corporation	00182-1919-89
100's	$63.90	GENERIC, Heartland Healthcare Services	55289-0567-17
100's	$70.66	GENERIC, Qualitest Products Inc	00603-3077-21
100's	$73.00	GENERIC, Duramed Pharmaceuticals Inc	51285-0873-02
100's	$73.00	GENERIC, Invamed Inc	52189-0252-24
100's	$75.90	GENERIC, West Point Pharma	59591-0156-68
100's	$78.20	GENERIC, Aligen Independent Laboratories Inc	00405-4290-01
100's	$79.25	GENERIC, Major Pharmaceuticals Inc	00904-2221-60
100's	$79.25	GENERIC, Major Pharmaceuticals Inc	00904-7586-60
100's	$79.95	GENERIC, Moore, H.L. Drug Exchange Inc	00839-7711-06
100's	$81.68	GENERIC, Royce Laboratories Inc	51875-0257-01
100's	$84.00	GENERIC, Sidmak Laboratories Inc	50111-0563-01
100's	$84.50	GENERIC, Creighton Products Corporation	50752-0285-05
100's	$85.75	GENERIC, Martec Pharmaceuticals Inc	52555-0441-01
100's	$86.73	GENERIC, Endo Laboratories Llc	60951-0767-70
100's	$88.42	GENERIC, Major Pharmaceuticals Inc	00904-7586-61
100's	$92.07	GENERIC, Major Pharmaceuticals Inc	00904-2221-61
100's	$95.66	GENERIC, Mylan Pharmaceuticals Inc	00378-0751-01
100's	$96.90	GENERIC, Udl Laboratories Inc	51079-0644-20
100's	$99.81	GENERIC, American Health Packaging	62584-0354-01
100's	$100.60	GENERIC, Major Pharmaceuticals Inc	00904-7809-60
100's	$101.60	GENERIC, Watson/Schein Pharmaceuticals Inc	00364-2348-01
100's	$101.60	GENERIC, Watson Laboratories Inc	00591-5658-01
100's	$101.60	GENERIC, Watson Laboratories Inc	52544-0418-01
100's	$104.18	FLEXERIL, Merck & Company Inc	00006-0931-28
100's	$105.90	GENERIC, Major Pharmaceuticals Inc	00904-7809-61
100's	$120.13	FLEXERIL, Merck & Company Inc	00006-0931-68
100's	$127.63	FLEXERIL, Alza	17314-8700-01
100's	$137.81	FLEXERIL, Mcneil Consumer Healthcare	50580-0874-11
200 x 5	$959.87	GENERIC, Vangard Labs	00615-3520-43

PRODUCT LISTING - EQUIVALENTS NOT AVAILABLE

Tablet - Oral - 10 mg

Size	Price	Product	NDC
1's	$3.39	GENERIC, Prescript Pharmaceuticals	00247-0059-01
2's	$1.91	GENERIC, Allscripts Pharmaceutical Company	54569-3193-07
2's	$3.44	GENERIC, Prescript Pharmaceuticals	00247-0059-02
3's	$2.87	GENERIC, Allscripts Pharmaceutical Company	54569-3193-00
3's	$3.47	GENERIC, Prescript Pharmaceuticals	00247-0059-03
4's	$3.52	GENERIC, Prescript Pharmaceuticals	00247-0059-04
4's	$12.00	GENERIC, Pharma Pac	52959-0042-04
5's	$3.55	GENERIC, Prescript Pharmaceuticals	00247-0059-05
6's	$3.59	GENERIC, Prescript Pharmaceuticals	00247-0059-06
6's	$5.04	GENERIC, Allscripts Pharmaceutical Company	54569-3193-08

7's	$3.64	GENERIC, Prescript Pharmaceuticals	00247-0059-07
7's	$6.04	GENERIC, Allscripts Pharmaceutical Company	54569-2573-06
7's	$8.40	GENERIC, Southwood Pharmaceuticals Inc	58016-0234-07
7's	$15.00	GENERIC, Pharma Pac	52959-0042-07
8's	$3.67	GENERIC, Prescript Pharmaceuticals	00247-0059-08
9's	$3.71	GENERIC, Prescript Pharmaceuticals	00247-0059-09
9's	$7.56	GENERIC, Allscripts Pharmaceutical Company	54569-3193-09
9's	$8.30	GENERIC, Pharmaceutical Corporation Of America	51655-0440-85
10's	$3.75	GENERIC, Prescript Pharmaceuticals	00247-0059-10
10's	$8.63	GENERIC, Allscripts Pharmaceutical Company	54569-2573-09
10's	$12.00	GENERIC, Southwood Pharmaceuticals Inc	58016-0234-10
10's	$18.25	GENERIC, Pharma Pac	52959-0042-10
12's	$3.84	GENERIC, Prescript Pharmaceuticals	00247-0059-12
12's	$10.36	GENERIC, Allscripts Pharmaceutical Company	54569-3193-01
12's	$14.39	GENERIC, Southwood Pharmaceuticals Inc	58016-0234-12
12's	$20.50	GENERIC, Pharma Pac	52959-0042-12
14's	$3.91	GENERIC, Prescript Pharmaceuticals	00247-0059-14
14's	$12.08	GENERIC, Allscripts Pharmaceutical Company	54569-2573-07
14's	$16.79	GENERIC, Southwood Pharmaceuticals Inc	58016-0234-14
14's	$23.75	GENERIC, Pharma Pac	52959-0042-14
15's	$3.95	GENERIC, Prescript Pharmaceuticals	00247-0059-15
15's	$13.17	GENERIC, Pharmaceutical Corporation Of America	51655-0440-54
15's	$14.35	GENERIC, Allscripts Pharmaceutical Company	54569-2573-00
15's	$14.56	GENERIC, Alpharma Uspd Makers Of Barre and Nmc	63874-0315-15
15's	$17.99	GENERIC, Southwood Pharmaceuticals Inc	58016-0234-15
15's	$25.02	GENERIC, Pharma Pac	52959-0042-15
18's	$4.07	GENERIC, Prescript Pharmaceuticals	00247-0059-18
18's	$21.59	GENERIC, Southwood Pharmaceuticals Inc	58016-0234-18
20's	$4.15	GENERIC, Prescript Pharmaceuticals	00247-0059-20
20's	$17.26	GENERIC, Allscripts Pharmaceutical Company	54569-2573-01
20's	$19.76	GENERIC, Alpharma Uspd Makers Of Barre and Nmc	63874-0315-20
20's	$23.99	GENERIC, Southwood Pharmaceuticals Inc	58016-0234-20
20's	$28.98	GENERIC, Pharma Pac	52959-0042-20
21's	$4.19	GENERIC, Prescript Pharmaceuticals	00247-0059-21
21's	$18.12	GENERIC, Allscripts Pharmaceutical Company	54569-2573-08
21's	$25.19	GENERIC, Southwood Pharmaceuticals Inc	58016-0234-21
21's	$30.07	GENERIC, Pharma Pac	52959-0042-21
24's	$28.79	GENERIC, Southwood Pharmaceuticals Inc	58016-0234-24
25's	$35.50	GENERIC, Pharma Pac	52959-0042-25
28's	$4.47	GENERIC, Prescript Pharmaceuticals	00247-0059-28
28's	$33.59	GENERIC, Southwood Pharmaceuticals Inc	58016-0234-28
28's	$39.50	GENERIC, Pharma Pac	52959-0042-28
30's	$4.54	GENERIC, Prescript Pharmaceuticals	00247-0059-30
30's	$25.33	GENERIC, Pharmaceutical Corporation Of America	51655-0440-24
30's	$25.89	GENERIC, Allscripts Pharmaceutical Company	54569-2573-02
30's	$29.12	GENERIC, Alpharma Uspd Makers Of Barre and Nmc	63874-0315-30
30's	$35.99	GENERIC, Southwood Pharmaceuticals Inc	58016-0234-30
30's	$42.25	GENERIC, Pharma Pac	52959-0042-30
40's	$4.94	GENERIC, Prescript Pharmaceuticals	00247-0059-40
40's	$47.98	GENERIC, Southwood Pharmaceuticals Inc	58016-0234-40
40's	$50.50	GENERIC, Pharma Pac	52959-0042-40
42's	$5.02	GENERIC, Prescript Pharmaceuticals	00247-0059-42
45's	$37.40	GENERIC, Allscripts Pharmaceutical Company	54569-3193-05
45's	$53.98	GENERIC, Southwood Pharmaceuticals Inc	58016-0234-45
45's	$55.75	GENERIC, Pharma Pac	52959-0042-45
50's	$59.98	GENERIC, Southwood Pharmaceuticals Inc	58016-0234-50
56's	$67.17	GENERIC, Southwood Pharmaceuticals Inc	58016-0234-56
60's	$5.74	GENERIC, Prescript Pharmaceuticals	00247-0059-60
60's	$49.66	GENERIC, Pharmaceutical Corporation Of America	51655-0440-25
60's	$51.78	GENERIC, Allscripts Pharmaceutical Company	54569-2573-03
60's	$71.50	GENERIC, Pharma Pac	52959-0042-60
60's	$71.97	GENERIC, Southwood Pharmaceuticals Inc	58016-0234-60
90's	$6.93	GENERIC, Prescript Pharmaceuticals	00247-0059-90
90's	$107.96	GENERIC, Southwood Pharmaceuticals Inc	58016-0234-90
100's	$7.33	GENERIC, Prescript Pharmaceuticals	00247-0059-00
100's	$86.30	GENERIC, Allscripts Pharmaceutical Company	54569-2573-04
100's	$98.80	GENERIC, Alpharma Uspd Makers Of Barre and Nmc	63874-0315-01
100's	$119.55	GENERIC, Southwood Pharmaceuticals Inc	58016-0234-00
120's	$143.95	GENERIC, Southwood Pharmaceuticals Inc	58016-0234-02

Cyclophosphamide *(000930)*

Categories: Carcinoma, breast; Carcinoma, ovarian; Leukemia, acute lymphoblastic; Leukemia, acute myelogenous; Leukemia, chronic granulocytic; Leukemia, chronic lymphocytic; Leukemia, monocytic; Lymphoma, Burkitt's; Lymphoma, Hodgkin's; Lymphoma, lymphocytic; Myeloma, multiple; Mycosis fungoides; Nephrotic syndrome; Neuroblastoma; Retinoblastoma; Pregnancy Category D; FDA Approved 1959 Nov; WHO Formulary

Drug Classes: Antineoplastics, alkylating agents; Disease modifying antirheumatic drugs

Brand Names: Cytokan; **Cytoxan**; Endoxon; Neosar; Neosar For Injection

Foreign Brand Availability: Alkyroxan (Korea); Carloxan (Denmark); Ciclofosfamida (Colombia; Peru); Ciclolen (Mexico); Cicloxal (Spain); Cycloblastin (Australia; New-Zealand; South-Africa); Cycloblastine (Belgium; Netherlands); Cyclo-Cell (Germany); Cyclophar (Philippines); Cyclostin (Germany); Cyclostin N (Germany); Cytophosphan (Israel); Endoxan (Austria; Belgium; Bulgaria; China; Germany; Greece; Hungary; Israel; Japan; New-Zealand; Portugal; Russia; South-Africa; Turkey); Endoxan Asta (Philippines); Endoxan-Asta (Argentina; Australia; Bahrain; Costa-Rica; Cyprus; Dominican-Republic; Egypt; El-Salvador; France; Guatemala; Honduras; Hong-Kong; India; Indonesia; Iran; Iraq; Italy; Jordan; Kuwait; Lebanon; Libya; Malaysia; Netherlands; Nicaragua; Oman; Panama; Philippines; Qatar; Republic-of-Yemen; Saudi-Arabia; Switzerland; Syria; Taiwan; Thailand; United-Arab-Emirates); Endoxana (England; Ireland); Endoxon-Asta (Australia); Enduxan (Brazil); Genoxal (Mexico; Spain); Ledoxan (Philippines); Ledoxina (Mexico); Lyophilisate (Indonesia); Procytox (Canada); Sendoxan (Denmark; Finland; Norway; Sweden); Syklofosfamid (Finland; Taiwan; Turkey)

Cost of Therapy: $203.26 (Malignancies; Cytoxan; 25 mg; 3 tablets/day; 30 day supply)
$182.90 (Malignancies; Generic Tablets; 25 mg; 3 tablets/day; 30 day supply)

HCFA JCODE(S): J9070 100 mg IV; J9080 200 mg IV; J9090 500 mg IV; J9091 1 g IV; J9092 2 g IV; J9093 100 mg IV; J9094 200 mg IV; J9095 500 mg IV; J9096 1 g IV; J9097 2 g IV; J8530 25 mg ORAL

DESCRIPTION

Cytoxan (cyclophosphamide for injection) is a sterile white lyophilized cake, or partially broken cake, containing 75 mg mannitol per 100 mg cyclophosphamide (anhydrous). Cytoxan (cyclophosphamide) tablets are for oral use and contain 25 or 50 mg cyclophosphamide (anhydrous). *Inactive ingredients in Cytoxan tablets are:* Acacia, FD&C blue no. 1, D&C yellow no. 10 aluminum lake, lactose, magnesium stearate, starch, stearic acid and talc. Cyclophosphamide is a synthetic antineoplastic drug chemically related to the nitrogen mustards. Cyclophosphamide is a white crystalline powder with the molecular formula $C_7H_{15}Cl_2N_2O_2P{\cdot}H_2O$ and a molecular weight of 279.1. The chemical name for cyclophosphamide is 2-[bis(2-chloroethyl)amino] tetrahydro-2H-1,3,2-oxazaphosphorine 2-oxide monohydrate. Cyclophosphamide is soluble in water, saline, or ethanol.

CLINICAL PHARMACOLOGY

Cyclophosphamide is biotransformed principally in the liver to active alkylating metabolites by a mixed function microsomal oxidase system. These metabolites interfere with the growth of susceptible rapidly proliferating malignant cells. The mechanism of action is thought to involve cross-linking of tumor cell DNA.

Cyclophosphamide is well absorbed after oral administration with a bioavailability greater than 75%. The unchanged drug has an elimination half-life of 3-12 hours. It is eliminated primarily in the form of metabolites, but from 5-25% of the dose is excreted in urine as unchanged drug. Several cytotoxic and noncytotoxic metabolites have been identified in urine and in plasma. Concentrations of metabolites reach a maximum in plasma 2-3 hours after an intravenous dose. Plasma protein binding of unchanged drug is low but some metabolites are bound to an extent greater than 60%. It has not been demonstrated that any single metabolite is responsible for either the therapeutic or toxic effects of cyclophosphamide. Although elevated levels of metabolites of cyclophosphamide have been observed in patients with renal failure, increased clinical toxicity in such patients has not been demonstrated.

INDICATIONS AND USAGE

MALIGNANT DISEASES

Cyclophosphamide, although effective alone in susceptible malignancies, is more frequently used concurrently or sequentially with other antineoplastic drugs.

The following malignancies are often susceptible to cyclophosphamide treatment:

1. Malignant lymphomas (Stages III and IV of the Ann Arbor staging system), Hodgkin's disease, lymphocytic lymphoma (nodular or diffuse), mixed-cell type lymphoma, histiocytic lymphoma, Burkitt's lymphoma.
2. Multiple myeloma.
3. ***Leukemias:*** Chronic lymphocytic leukemia, chronic granulocytic leukemia (it is usually ineffective in acute blastic crisis), acute myelogenous and monocytic leukemia, acute lymphoblastic (stem cell) leukemia in children (cyclophosphamide given during remission is effective in prolonging its duration).
4. Mycosis fungoides (advanced disease).
5. Neuroblastoma (disseminated disease).
6. Adenocarcinoma of the ovary.
7. Retinoblastoma.
8. Carcinoma of the breast.

NONMALIGNANT DISEASES

Biopsy Proven "Minimal Change" Nephrotic Syndrome in Children

Cyclophosphamide is useful in carefully selected cases of biopsy proven "minimal change" nephrotic syndrome in children but should not be used as primary therapy. In children whose disease fails to respond adequately to appropriate adrenocorticosteroid therapy or in whom the adrenocorticosteroid therapy produces or threatens to produce intolerable side effects, cyclophosphamide may induce a remission. Cyclophosphamide is not indicated for the nephrotic syndrome in adults or for any other renal disease.

NON-FDA APPROVED INDICATIONS

Cyclophosphamide is used without FDA approval for the treatment of breast, ovarian, cervical, bladder, head and neck, prostrate, and lung cancers (usually small cell lung cancer), Ewing's sarcoma, retinoblastoma and neuroblastoma. Cyclophosphamide is also used without FDA approval to treat transplant rejection, pure red cell aplasia, idiopathic thrombocytopenia (ITP),Wegener's granulomatosis (drug of first choice), polyarteritis nodosa (with glucocorticoids), lupus nephritis, severe refractory rheumatoid arthritis, systemic lupus erythematosus, and it is used in bone marrow transplant conditioning regimens.

CONTRAINDICATIONS

Continued use of cyclophosphamide is contraindicated in patients with severely depressed bone marrow function. Cyclophosphamide is contraindicated in patients who have demonstrated a previous hypersensitivity to it (see WARNINGS and PRECAUTIONS).

WARNINGS

CARCINOGENESIS, MUTAGENESIS, IMPAIRMENT OF FERTILITY

Second malignancies have developed in some patients treated with cyclophosphamide used alone or in association with other antineoplastic drugs and/or modalities. Most frequently, they have been urinary bladder, myeloproliferative, or lymphoproliferative malignancies. Second malignancies most frequently were detected in patients treated for primary myeloproliferative or lymphoproliferative malignancies or nonmalignant disease in which immune processes are believed to be involved pathologically.

In some cases, the second malignancy developed several years after cyclophosphamide treatment had been discontinued. In a single breast cancer trial utilizing 2-4 times the standard dose of cyclophosphamide in conjunction with doxorubicin a small number of cases of secondary acute myeloid leukemia occurred within 2 years of treatment initiation. Urinary bladder malignancies generally have occurred in patients who previously had hemorrhagic cystitis. In patients treated with cyclophosphamide-containing regimens for a variety of solid tumors, isolated case reports of secondary malignancies have been published. One case of carcinoma of the renal pelvis was reported in a patient receiving long-term cyclophosphamide therapy for cerebral vasculitis. The possibility of cyclophosphamide-induced malignancy should be considered in any benefit-to-risk assessment for use of the drug.

Cyclophosphamide can cause fetal harm when administered to a pregnant woman and such abnormalities have been reported following cyclophosphamide therapy in pregnant women. Abnormalities were found in 2 infants and a 6-month-old fetus born to women treated with cyclophosphamide. Ectrodactylia was found in 2 of the 3 cases. Normal infants have also been born to women treated with cyclophosphamide during pregnancy, including the first trimester. If this drug is used during pregnancy, or if the patient becomes pregnant while taking (receiving) this drug, the patient should be apprised of the potential hazard to the fetus. Women of childbearing potential should be advised to avoid becoming pregnant.

Cyclophosphamide interferes with oogenesis and spermatogenesis. It may cause sterility in both sexes. Development of sterility appears to depend on the dose of cyclophosphamide, duration of therapy, and the state of gonadal function at the time of treatment. Cyclophosphamide-induced sterility may be irreversible in some patients.

Amenorrhea associated with decreased estrogen and increased gonadotropin secretion develops in a significant proportion of women treated with cyclophosphamide. Affected patients generally resume regular menses within a few months after cessation of therapy. Girls treated with cyclophosphamide during prepubescence generally develop secondary sexual characteristics normally and have regular menses. Ovarian fibrosis with apparently complete loss of germ cells after prolonged cyclophosphamide treatment in late prepubescence has been reported. Girls treated with cyclophosphamide during prepubescence subsequently have conceived.

Men treated with cyclophosphamide may develop oligospermia or azoospermia associated with increased gonadotropin but normal testosterone secretion. Sexual potency and libido are unimpaired in these patients. Boys treated with cyclophosphamide during prepubescence develop secondary sexual characteristics normally, but may have oligospermia or azoospermia and increased gonadotropin secretion. Some degree of testicular atrophy may occur. Cyclophosphamide-induced azoospermia is reversible in some patients, though the reversibility may not occur for several years after cessation of therapy. Men temporarily rendered sterile by cyclophosphamide have subsequently fathered normal children.

URINARY SYSTEM

Hemorrhagic cystitis may develop in patients treated with cyclophosphamide. Rarely, this condition can be severe and even fatal. Fibrosis of the urinary bladder, sometimes extensive, also may develop with or without accompanying cystitis. Atypical urinary bladder epithelial cells may appear in the urine. These adverse effects appear to depend on the dose of cyclophosphamide and the duration of therapy. Such bladder injury is thought to be due to cyclophosphamide metabolites excreted in the urine. Forced fluid intake helps to assure an ample output of urine, necessitates frequent voiding, and reduces the time the drug remains in the bladder. This helps to prevent cystitis. Hematuria usually resolves in a few days after cyclophosphamide treatment is stopped, but it may persist. Medical and/or surgical supportive treatment may be required, rarely, to treat protracted cases of severe hemorrhagic cystitis. It is usually necessary to discontinue cyclophosphamide therapy in instances of severe hemorrhagic cystitis.

CARDIAC TOXICITY

Although a few instances of cardiac dysfunction have been reported following use of recommended doses of cyclophosphamide, no causal relationship has been established. Acute cardiac toxicity has been reported with doses as low as 2.4 g/m^2 to as high as 26 g/m^2, usually as a portion of an intensive antineoplastic multidrug regimen or in conjunction with transplantation procedures. In a few instances with high doses of cyclophosphamide, severe, and sometimes fatal, congestive heart failure has occurred after the first cyclophosphamide dose. Histopathologic examination has primarily shown hemorrhagic myocarditis. Hemopericardium has occurred secondary to hemorrhagic myocarditis and myocardial necrosis. Pericarditis has been reported independent of any hemopericardium.

No residual cardiac abnormalities, as evidenced by electrocardiogram or echocardiogram appear to be present in patients surviving episodes of apparent cardiac toxicity associated with high doses of cyclophosphamide.

Cyclophosphamide has been reported to potentiate doxorubicin-induced cardiotoxicity.

INFECTIONS

Treatment with cyclophosphamide may cause significant suppression of immune responses. Serious, sometimes fatal, infections may develop in severely immunosuppressed patients. Cyclophosphamide treatment may not be indicated or should be interrupted or the dose reduced in patients who have or who develop viral, bacterial, fungal, protozoan, or helminthic infections.

OTHER

Anaphylactic reactions have been reported; death has also been reported in association with this event. Possible cross-sensitivity with other alkylating agents has been reported.

PRECAUTIONS

GENERAL

Special attention to the possible development of toxicity should be exercised in patients being treated with cyclophosphamide if any of the following conditions are present:

1. Leukopenia.
2. Thrombocytopenia.
3. Tumor cell infiltration of bone marrow.
4. Previous X-ray therapy.
5. Previous therapy with other cytotoxic agents.
6. Impaired hepatic function.
7. Impaired renal function.

LABORATORY TESTS

During treatment, the patient's hematologic profile (particularly neutrophils and platelets) should be monitored regularly to determine the degree of hematopoietic suppression. Urine should also be examined regularly for red cells which may precede hemorrhagic cystitis.

ADRENALECTOMY

Since cyclophosphamide has been reported to be more toxic in adrenalectomized dogs, adjustment of the doses of both replacement steroids and cyclophosphamide may be necessary for the adrenalectomized patient.

WOUND HEALING

Cyclophosphamide may interfere with normal wound healing.

CARCINOGENESIS, MUTAGENESIS, AND IMPAIRMENT OF FERTILITY

See WARNINGS for information on carcinogenesis, mutagenesis, and impairment of fertility.

PREGNANCY CATEGORY D

See WARNINGS.

NURSING MOTHERS

Cyclophosphamide is excreted in breast milk. Because of the potential for serious adverse reactions and the potential for tumorigenicity shown for cyclophosphamide in humans, a decision should be made whether to discontinue nursing or to discontinue the drug, taking into account the importance of the drug to the mother.

DRUG INTERACTIONS

The rate of metabolism and the leukopenic activity of cyclophosphamide reportedly are increased by chronic administration of high doses of phenobarbital.

The physician should be alert for possible combined drug actions, desirable or undesirable, involving cyclophosphamide even though cyclophosphamide has been used successfully concurrently with other drugs, including other cytotoxic drugs.

Cyclophosphamide treatment, which causes a marked and persistent inhibition of cholinesterase activity, potentiates the effect of succinylcholine chloride.

If a patient has been treated with cyclophosphamide within 10 days of general anesthesia, the anesthesiologist should be alerted.

ADVERSE REACTIONS

Information on adverse reactions associated with the use of cyclophosphamide is arranged according to body system affected or type of reaction. The adverse reactions are listed in order of decreasing incidence. The most serious adverse reactions are described in WARNINGS.

Reproductive System: See WARNINGS for information on impairment of fertility.

Digestive System: Nausea and vomiting commonly occur with cyclophosphamide therapy. Anorexia and, less frequently, abdominal discomfort or pain and diarrhea may occur. There are isolated reports of hemorrhagic colitis, oral mucosal ulceration and jaundice occurring during therapy. These adverse drug effects generally remit when cyclophosphamide treatment is stopped.

Skin and Its Structures: Alopecia occurs commonly in patients treated with cyclophosphamide. The hair can be expected to grow back after treatment with the drug or even during continued drug treatment, though it may be different in texture or color. Skin rash occurs occasionally in patients receiving the drug. Pigmentation of the skin and changes in nails can occur. Very rare reports of Stevens-Johnson syndrome and toxic epidermal necrolysis have been received during postmarketing surveillance; due to the nature of spontaneous adverse event reporting, a definitive causal relationship to cyclophosphamide has not been established.

Hematopoietic System: Leukopenia occurs in patients treated with cyclophosphamide, is related to the dose of drug, and can be used as a dosage guide. Leukopenia of less than 2000 cells/mm^3 develops commonly in patients treated with an initial loading dose of the drug, and less frequently in patients maintained on smaller doses. The degree of neutropenia is particularly important because it correlates with a reduction in resistance to infections. Fever without documented infection has been reported in neutropenic patients.

Thrombocytopenia or anemia develop occasionally in patients treated with cyclophosphamide. These hematologic effects usually can be reversed by reducing the drug dose or by interrupting treatment. Recovery from leukopenia usually begins in 7-10 days after cessation of therapy.

Urinary System: See WARNINGS for information on cystitis and urinary bladder fibrosis.

C

Hemorrhagic ureteritis and renal tubular necrosis have been reported to occur in patients treated with cyclophosphamide. Such lesions usually resolve following cessation of therapy.

Infections: See WARNINGS for information on reduced host resistance to infections.

Carcinogenesis: See WARNINGS for information on carcinogenesis.

Respiratory System: Interstitial pneumonitis has been reported as part of the postmarketing experience. Interstitial pulmonary fibrosis has been reported in patients receiving high doses of cyclophosphamide over a prolonged period.

Other: Anaphylactic reactions have been reported; death has also been reported in association with this event. Possible cross-sensitivity with other alkylating agents has been reported. SIADH (syndrome of inappropriate ADH secretion) has been reported with the use of cyclophosphamide. Malaise and asthenia have been reported as part of the postmarketing experience.

DOSAGE AND ADMINISTRATION

TREATMENT OF MALIGNANT DISEASES

Adults and Children

When used as the only oncolytic drug therapy, the initial course of cyclophosphamide for patients with no hematologic deficiency usually consists of 40-50 mg/kg given intravenously in divided doses over a period of 2-5 days. Other intravenous regimens include 10-15 mg/kg given every 7-10 days or 3-5 mg/kg twice weekly.

Oral cyclophosphamide dosing is usually in the range of 1-5 mg/kg/day for both initial and maintenance dosing.

Many other regimens of intravenous and oral cyclophosphamide have been reported. Dosages must be adjusted in accord with evidence of antitumor activity and/or leukopenia. The total leukocyte count is a good, objective guide for regulating dosage. Transient decreases in the total white blood cell count to 2000 cells/mm^3 (following short courses) or more persistent reduction to 3000 cells/mm^3 (with continuing therapy) are tolerated without serious risk of infection if there is no marked granulocytopenia.

When cyclophosphamide is included in combined cytotoxic regimens, it may be necessary to reduce the dose of cyclophosphamide as well as that of the other drugs.

Cyclophosphamide and its metabolites are dialyzable although there are probably quantitative differences depending upon the dialysis system being used. Patients with compromised renal function may show some measurable changes in pharmacokinetic parameters of cyclophosphamide metabolism, but there is no consistent evidence indicating a need for cyclophosphamide dosage modification in patients with renal function impairment.

TREATMENT OF NONMALIGNANT DISEASES

Biopsy Proven "Minimal Change" Nephrotic Syndrome in Children

An oral dose of 2.5-3 mg/kg daily for a period of 60-90 days is recommended. In males, the incidence of oligospermia and azoospermia increases if the duration of cyclophosphamide treatment exceeds 60 days. Treatment beyond 90 days increases the probability of sterility. Adrenocorticosteroid therapy may be tapered and discontinued during the course of cyclophosphamide therapy. See PRECAUTIONS concerning hematologic monitoring.

HOW SUPPLIED

Lyophilized Cytoxan for injection contains 75 mg of mannitol per 100 mg of cyclophosphamide (anhydrous) and is supplied in vials for single-dose use.

Cytoxan tablets, 25 and 50 mg, are white tablets with blue flecks containing 25 and 50 mg cyclophosphamide (anhydrous), respectively.

Storage: Storage at or below 25°C (77°F) is recommended; this product will withstand brief exposure to temperatures up to 30°C (86°F) but should be protected from temperatures above 30°C (86°F).

Procedures for proper handling and disposal of anticancer drugs should be considered. Several guidelines on this subject have been published.[1-7] There is no general agreement that all of the procedures recommended in the guidelines are necessary or appropriate.

PRODUCT LISTING - RATED THERAPEUTICALLY EQUIVALENT

Powder For Injection - Intravenous - Lyophilized 1 Gm
6's $296.28 CYTOXAN LYOPHILIZED, Bristol-Myers Squibb 00015-0548-41

Powder For Injection - Intravenous - Lyophilized 2 Gm
6's $592.74 CYTOXAN LYOPHILIZED, Bristol-Myers Squibb 00015-0549-41

Powder For Injection - Intravenous - Lyophilized 100 mg
12's $74.28 CYTOXAN LYOPHILIZED, Bristol-Myers Squibb 00015-0539-41

Powder For Injection - Intravenous - Lyophilized 200 mg
12's $141.12 CYTOXAN LYOPHILIZED, Bristol-Myers Squibb 00015-0546-41

Powder For Injection - Intravenous - Lyophilized 500 mg
12's $296.28 CYTOXAN LYOPHILIZED, Bristol-Myers Squibb 00015-0547-41

Powder For Injection - Intravenous - 1 Gm
6's $300.90 NEOSAR, Pharmacia and Upjohn 00013-5636-70

Powder For Injection - Intravenous - 2 Gm
1's $86.00 NEOSAR, Pharmacia and Upjohn 00013-5646-70
6's $489.60 CYTOXAN, Bristol-Myers Squibb 00015-0506-41

Powder For Injection - Intravenous - 100 mg
6's $68.52 NEOSAR, Pharmacia and Upjohn 00013-5606-93

Powder For Injection - Intravenous - 200 mg
1's $10.24 NEOSAR, Pharmacia and Upjohn 00013-5616-93

Powder For Injection - Intravenous - 500 mg
6's $300.72 NEOSAR, Pharmacia and Upjohn 00013-5626-93

Tablet - Oral - 25 mg
100's $203.22 GENERIC, Roxane Laboratories Inc 00054-4129-25
100's $213.38 GENERIC, Roxane Laboratories Inc 00054-8089-25
100's $225.84 CYTOXAN, Bristol-Myers Squibb 00015-0504-01

Tablet - Oral - 50 mg
100's $341.68 CYTOXAN, Bristol-Myers Squibb 00015-0503-03
100's $372.96 GENERIC, Roxane Laboratories Inc 00054-4130-25
100's $391.61 GENERIC, Roxane Laboratories Inc 00054-8130-25
100's $414.47 CYTOXAN, Bristol-Myers Squibb 00015-0503-01

PRODUCT LISTING - EQUIVALENTS NOT AVAILABLE

Powder For Injection - Intravenous - Lyophilized 1 Gm
6's $308.55 CYTOXAN LYOPHILIZED, Bristol-Myers Squibb 00015-0548-12

Powder For Injection - Intravenous - Lyophilized 2 Gm
6's $617.33 CYTOXAN LYOPHILIZED, Bristol-Myers Squibb 00015-0549-12

Powder For Injection - Intravenous - Lyophilized 500 mg
12's $308.55 CYTOXAN LYOPHILIZED, Bristol-Myers Squibb 00015-0547-12

Powder For Injection - Intravenous - 1 Gm
6's $132.15 NEOSAR, Pharmacia and Upjohn 00013-5636-01

Cyclosporine *(000932)*

Categories: Arthritis, rheumatoid; Keratoconjunctivitis sicca; Psoriasis; Rejection, heart transplant, prophylaxis; Rejection, liver transplant, prophylaxis; Rejection, renal transplant, prophylaxis; Pregnancy Category C; FDA Approved 1983 Nov; WHO Formulary

Drug Classes: Immunosuppressives

Brand Names: Cidosporin; Neoral; **Sandimmune**

Foreign Brand Availability: Cipol (Korea); Cipol-N (Korea); Consupren (Bahrain; Cyprus; Egypt; Iran; Iraq; Jordan; Kuwait; Lebanon; Libya; Oman; Qatar; Republic-of-Yemen; Saudi-Arabia; Syria; Thailand; United-Arab-Emirates); Deximune (Israel); Gengraf (Hong-Kong); Implanta (China; Korea); Imusporin (Colombia; India); Sandimmun (Australia; Austria; Belgium; Benin; Burkina-Faso; Canada; Czech-Republic; Denmark; Ecuador; England; Ethiopia; Finland; France; Gambia; Germany; Ghana; Greece; Guinea; Hong-Kong; Hungary; Indonesia; Ireland; Israel; Italy; Ivory-Coast; Japan; Kenya; Korea; Liberia; Malawi; Malaysia; Mali; Mauritania; Mauritius; Mexico; Morocco; New-Zealand; Niger; Nigeria; Norway; Peru; Philippines; Portugal; Senegal; Seychelles; Sierra-Leone; Spain; Sudan; Sweden; Switzerland; Tanzania; Thailand; Tunia; Turkey; Uganda; Zambia; Zimbabwe); Sandimmun Neoral (Australia; Austria; Bahrain; Canada; China; Colombia; Cyprus; Czech-Republic; Denmark; Egypt; England; Finland; Greece; Hong-Kong; Indonesia; Iran; Iraq; Israel; Jordan; Korea; Kuwait; Lebanon; Libya; Mexico; Norway; Oman; Peru; Philippines; Qatar; Republic-of-Yemen; Saudi-Arabia; South-Africa; Sweden; Switzerland; Syria; Thailand; Turkey; United-Arab-Emirates); Sangcya (Israel)

Cost of Therapy: $740.64 (Transplant Rejection; Sandimmune; 100 mg; 4 capsules/day; 30 day supply)
$732.84 (Transplant Rejection; Neoral; 100 mg; 4 capsules/day; 30 day supply)

HCFA JCODE(S): J7503 50 mg IV

WARNING

Note: Trade names have been used throughout this monograph for clarity.

NEORAL

Only physicians experienced in management of systemic immunosuppressive therapy for the indicated disease should prescribe Neoral. At doses used in solid organ transplantation, only physicians experienced in immunosuppressive therapy and management of organ transplant recipients should prescribe Neoral. Patients receiving the drug should be managed in facilities equipped and staffed with adequate laboratory and supportive medical resources. The physician responsible for maintenance therapy should have complete information requisite for the follow-up of the patient.

Neoral, a systemic immunosuppressant, may increase the susceptibility to infection and the development of neoplasia. In kidney, liver, and heart transplant patients Neoral may be administered with other immunosuppressive agents. Increased susceptibility to infection and the possible development of lymphoma and other neoplasms may result from the increase in the degree of immunosuppression in transplant patients.

Neoral soft gelatin capsules MODIFIED and Neoral oral solution MODIFIED have increased bioavailability in comparison to Sandimmune soft gelatin capsules and Sandimmune oral solution. Neoral and Sandimmune are not bioequivalent and cannot be used interchangeably without physician supervision. For a given trough concentration, cyclosporine exposure will be greater with Neoral than with Sandimmune. If a patient who is receiving exceptionally high doses of Sandimmune is converted to Neoral, particular caution should be exercised. Cyclosporine blood concentrations should be monitored in transplant and rheumatoid arthritis patients taking Neoral to avoid toxicity due to high concentrations. Dose adjustments should be made in transplant patients to minimize possible organ rejection due to low concentrations. Comparison of blood concentrations in the published literature with blood concentrations obtained using current assays must be done with detailed knowledge of the assay methods employed.

For Psoriasis Patients

See also BOXED WARNING, Neoral.

Psoriasis patients previously treated with PUVA and to a lesser extent, methotrexate or other immunosuppressive agents, UVB, coal tar, or radiation therapy, are at an increased risk of developing skin malignancies when taking Neoral.

Cyclosporine, the active ingredient in Neoral, in recommended dosages, can cause systemic hypertension and nephrotoxicity. The risk increases with increasing dose and duration of cyclosporine therapy. Renal dysfunction, including structural kidney damage, is a potential consequence of cyclosporine, and therefore, renal function must be monitored during therapy.

SANDIMMUNE

Only physicians experienced in immunosuppressive therapy and management of organ transplant patients should prescribe Sandimmune. Patients receiving the drug should be managed in facilities equipped and staffed with adequate laboratory and supportive medical resources. The physician responsible for maintenance therapy should have complete information requisite for the follow-up of the patient.

WARNING — Cont'd

Sandimmune should be administered with adrenal corticosteroids but not with other immunosuppressive agents. Increased susceptibility to infection and the possible development of lymphoma may result from immunosuppression.

Sandimmune soft gelatin capsules and Sandimmune oral solution have decreased bioavailability in comparison to Neoral soft gelatin capsules MODIFIED and Neoral oral solution MODIFIED.

Sandimmune and Neoral are not bioequivalent and cannot be used interchangeably without physician supervision.

The absorption of cyclosporine during chronic administration of Sandimmune soft gelatin capsules and oral solution was found to be erratic. It is recommended that patients taking the soft gelatin capsules or oral solution over a period of time be monitored at repeated intervals for cyclosporine blood levels and subsequent dose adjustments be made in order to avoid toxicity due to high levels and possible organ rejection due to low absorption of cyclosporine. This is of special importance in liver transplants. Numerous assays are being developed to measure blood levels of cyclosporine. Comparison of levels in published literature to patient levels using current assays must be done with detailed knowledge of the assay methods employed. (See DOSAGE AND ADMINISTRATION, Sandimmune, Blood Level Monitoring.)

DESCRIPTION

NEORAL

Neoral is an oral formulation of cyclosporine that immediately forms a microemulsion in an aqueous environment.

Cyclosporine, the active principle in Neoral, is a cyclic polypeptide immunosuppressant agent consisting of 11 amino acids. It is produced as a metabolite by the fungus species *Beauveria nivea.*

Chemically, cyclosporine is designated as [*R*-[*R**,*R**-(*E*)]]-cyclic-(L-alanyl-D-alanyl-*N*-methyl-L-leucyl-*N*-methyl-L-leucyl-*N*-methyl-L-valyl-3-hydroxy-*N*,4-dimethyl-L-2-amino-6-octenoyl-L-α-amino-butyryl-*N*-methylglycyl-*N*-methyl-L-leucyl-L-valyl-*N*-methyl-L-leucyl).

Neoral Soft Gelatin Capsules

Neoral soft gelatin capsules (cyclosporine capsules) MODIFIED are available in 25 and 100 mg strengths.

Each 25 mg capsule contains: Cyclosporine 25 mg; alcohol, dehydrated 11.9% v/v (9.5% wt/vol).

Each 100 mg capsule contains: Cyclosporine 100 mg; alcohol, dehydrated 11.9% v/v (9.5% wt/vol).

Inactive ingredients: Corn oil-mono-di-triglycerides, polyoxyl 40 hydrogenated castor oil, DL-α-tocopherol, gelatin, glycerol, iron oxide black, propylene glycol, titanium dioxide, carmine, and other ingredients.

Neoral Oral Solution

Neoral oral solution (cyclosporine oral solution) MODIFIED is available in 50 ml bottles.

Each ml contains: Cyclosporine 100 mg/ml; alcohol, dehydrated 11.9% v/v (9.5% wt/vol).

Inactive ingredients: Corn oil-mono-di-triglycerides, polyoxyl 40 hydrogenated castor oil, DL-α-tocopherol, propylene glycol.

SANDIMMUNE

Cyclosporine, the active principle in Sandimmune (cyclosporine), is a cyclic polypeptide immunosuppressant agent consisting of 11 amino acids. It is produced as a metabolite by the fungus species *Beauveria nivea.*

Chemically, cyclosporine is designated as [*R*-[*R**,*R**-(*E*)]]-cyclic-(L-alanyl-D-alanyl-*N*-methyl-L-leucyl-*N*-methyl-L-leucyl-*N*-methyl-L-valyl-3-hydroxy-*N*,4-dimethyl-L-2-amino-6-octenoyl-L-α-amino-butyryl-*N*-methylglycyl-*N*-methyl-L-leucyl-L-valyl-*N*-methyl-L-leucyl).

Sandimmune Soft Gelatin Capsules

Sandimmune soft gelatin capsules (cyclosporin capsules) are available in 25 and 100 mg strengths.

Each 25 mg capsule contains: Cyclosporine 25 mg; alcohol, dehydrated max 12.7% by volume.

Each 100 mg capsule contains: Cyclosporine 100 mg; alcohol, dehydrated max 12.7% by volume.

Inactive ingredients: Corn oil, gelatin, glycerol, Labrafil M 2125 CS (polyoxyethylated glycolysed glycerides), red iron oxide (25 and 100 mg capsule only), sorbitol, titanium dioxide, and other ingredients.

Sandimmune Oral Solution

Sandimmune oral solution (cyclosporine oral solution) is available in 50 ml bottles.

Each ml contains: Cyclosporine 100 mg; and alcohol, Ph. Helv. 12.5% by volume dissolved in an olive oil, Ph. Helv./Labrafil M 1944 CS (polyoxyethylated oleic glycerides) vehicle which must be further diluted with milk, chocolate milk, or orange juice before oral administration.

Sandimmune Injection

Sandimmune injection (cyclosporine injection) is available in a 5 ml sterile ampul for IV administration.

Each ml contains: Cyclosporine 50 mg; Cremophor EL (polyoxyethylated castor oil) 650 mg; alcohol, Ph. Helv. 32.9% by volume, and nitrogen qs which must be diluted further with 0.9% sodium chloride injection or 5% dextrose injection before use.

RESTASIS

Restasis Ophthalmic Emulsion

Restasis (cyclosporine ophthalmic emulsion) 0.05% contains a topical immunomodulator with anti-inflammatory effects. Cyclosporine's chemical name is Cyclo[[(*E*)-(2*S*,3*R*,4*R*)-3-hydroxy-4-methyl-2-(methylamino)-6-octen125yl]-L-2-aminobutyryl-*N*-methylglycyl-*N*-methyl-L-leucyl-L-valyl-*N*-methyl-L-leucyl-L-alanyl-D-alanyl-*N*-methyl-L-leucyl-*N*-methyl-L-leucyl-*N*-methyl-L-valyl].

Its empirical formula is $C_{62}H_{111}N_{11}O_{12}$ and molecular weight is 1202.6.

Cyclosporine is a fine white powder. Restasis appears as a white opaque to slightly translucent homogeneous emulsion. It has an osmolality of 230-320 mOsmol/kg and a pH of 6.5-8.0.

Each ml of Restasis ophthalmic emulsion contains: *Active:* Cyclosporine 0.05%. *Inactives:* Glycerin; castor oil; polysorbate 80; carbomer 1342; purified water, and sodium hydroxide to adjust the pH.

CLINICAL PHARMACOLOGY

NEORAL

Cyclosporine is a potent immunosuppressive agent that in animals prolongs survival of allogeneic transplants involving skin, kidney, liver, heart, pancreas, bone marrow, small intestine, and lung. Cyclosporine has been demonstrated to suppress some humoral immunity and to a greater extent, cell-mediated immune reactions such as allograft rejection, delayed hypersensitivity, experimental allergic encephalomyelitis, Freund's adjuvant arthritis, and graft versus host disease in many animal species for a variety of organs.

The effectiveness of cyclosporine results from specific and reversible inhibition of immunocompetent lymphocytes in the G_0- and G_1-phase of the cell cycle. T-lymphocytes are preferentially inhibited. The T-helper cell is the main target, although the T-suppressor cell may also be suppressed. Cyclosporine also inhibits lymphokine production and release including interleukin-2.

No effects on phagocytic function (changes in enzyme secretions, chemotactic migration of granulocytes, macrophage migration, carbon clearance *in vivo*) have been detected in animals. Cyclosporine does not cause bone marrow suppression in animal models or man.

Pharmacokinetics

The immunosuppressive activity of cyclosporine is primarily due to parent drug. Following oral administration, absorption of cyclosporine is incomplete. The extent of absorption of cyclosporine is dependent on the individual patient, the patient population, and the formulation. Elimination of cyclosporine is primarily biliary with only 6% of the dose (parent drug and metabolites) excreted in urine. The disposition of cyclosporine from blood is generally biphasic, with a terminal half-life of approximately 8.4 hours (range 5-18 hours). Following intravenous (IV) administration, the blood clearance of cyclosporine (assay: HPLC) is approximately 5-7 ml/min/kg in adult recipients of renal or liver allografts. Blood cyclosporine clearance appears to be slightly slower in cardiac transplant patients.

The Neoral soft gelatin capsules MODIFIED and Neoral oral solution MODIFIED are bioequivalent. Neoral oral solution diluted with orange juice or with apple juice is bioequivalent to Neoral oral solution diluted with water. The effect of milk on the bioavailability of cyclosporine when administered as Neoral oral solution has not been evaluted.

The relationship between administered dose and exposure (area under the concentration versus time curve, AUC) is linear within the therapeutic dose range. The intersubject variability (total, %CV) of cyclosporine exposure (AUC) when Neoral or Sandimmune is administered ranges from approximately 20-50% in renal transplant patients. This intersubject variability contributes to the need for individualization of the dosing regimen for optimal therapy (see DOSAGE AND ADMINISTRATION, Neoral). Intrasubject variability of AUC in renal transplant recipients (%CV) was 9-21% for Neoral and 19-26% for Sandimmune. In the same studies, intrasubject variability of trough concentrations (%CV) was 17-30% for Neoral and 16-38% for Sandimmune.

Absorption

Neoral has increased bioavailability compared to Sandimmune. The absolute bioavailability of cyclosporine administered as Sandimmune is dependent on the patient population, estimated to be less than 10% in liver transplant patients and as great as 89% in some renal transplant patients. The absolute bioavailability of cyclosporine administered as Neoral has not been determined in adults. In studies of renal transplant, rheumatoid arthritis and psoriasis patients, the mean cyclosporine AUC was approximately 20-50% greater and the peak blood cyclosporine concentration (C_{max}) was approximately 40-106% greater following administration of Neoral compared to following administration of Sandimmune. The dose normalized AUC in *de novo* liver transplant patients administered Neoral 28 days after transplantation was 50% greater and C_{max} was 90% greater than in those patients administered Sandimmune. AUC and C_{max} are also increased (Neoral relative to Sandimmune) in heart transplant patients, but data are very limited. Although the AUC and C_{max} values are higher on Neoral relative to Sandimmune, the pre-dose trough concentrations (dose-normalized) are similar for the 2 formulations.

Following oral administration of Neoral, the time to peak blood cyclosporine concentrations (T_{max}) ranged from 1.5-2.0 hours. The administration of food with Neoral decreases the cyclosporine AUC and C_{max}. A high fat meal (669 kcal, 45 g fat) consumed within one-half hour before Neoral administration decreased the AUC by 13% and C_{max} by 33%. The effects of a low fat meal (667 kcal, 15 g fat) were similar.

The effect of T-tube diversion of bile on the absorption of cyclosporine from Neoral was investigated in 11 *de novo* liver transplant patients. When the patients were administered Neoral with and without T-tube diversion of bile, very little difference in absorption was observed, as measured by the change in maximal cyclosporine blood concentrations from pre-dose values with the T-tube closed relative to when it was open: 6.9 ± 41% (range -55% to 68%).

Distribution

Cyclosporine is distributed largely outside the blood volume. The steady state volume of distribution during IV dosing has been reported as 3-5 L/kg in solid organ transplant recipients. In blood, the distribution is concentration dependent. Approximately 33-47% is in

C

TABLE 1A *Pharmacokinetic Parameters (mean ± SD)*

Patient Population	Dose/Day* (mg/day)	Dose/Weight (mg/kg/day)	AUC† (ng·h/ml)
De novo renal transplant‡ Week 4 (n=37)	597 ± 174	7.95 ± 2.81	8772 ± 2089
Stable renal transplant‡(n=55)	344 ± 122	4.10 ± 1.58	6035 ± 2194
De novo liver transplant§ Week 4 (n=18)	458 ± 190	6.89 ± 3.68	7187 ± 2816
De novo rheumatoid arthritis¤ (n=23)	182 ± 55.6	2.37 ± 0.36	2641 ± 877
De novo psoriasis¤ Week 4 (n=18)	189 ± 69.8	2.48 ± 0.65	2324 ± 1048

* Total daily dose was divided into 2 doses administered every 12 hours.
† AUC was measured over 1 dosing interval.
‡ Assay: TDx specific monoclonal fluorescence polarization immunoassay.
§ Assay: Cyclo-trac specific monoclonal radioimmunoassay.
¤ Assay: INCSTAR specific monoclonal radioimmunoassay.

TABLE 1B *Pharmacokinetic Parameters (mean ± SD)*

Patient Population	C_{max} (ng/ml)	Trough* (ng/ml)	CL/F (ml/min)	CL/F (ml/min/kg)
De novo renal transplant† Week 4 (n=37)	1802 ± 428	361 ± 129	593 ± 204	7.8 ± 2.9
Stable renal transplant†(n=55)	1333 ± 469	251 ± 116	492 ± 140	5.9 ± 2.1
De novo liver transplant‡ Week 4 (n=18)	1555 ± 740	268 ± 101	577 ± 309	8.6 ± 5.7
De novo rheumatoid arthritis§ (n=23)	728 ± 263	96.4 ± 37.7	613 ± 196	8.3 ± 2.8
De novo psoriasis§ Week 4 (n=18)	655 ± 186	74.9 ± 46.7	723 ± 186	10.2 ± 3.9

* Trough concentration was measured just prior to the morning Neoral dose, approximately 12 hours after the previous dose.
† Assay: TDx specific monoclonal fluorescence polarization immunoassay.
‡ Assay: Cyclo-trac specific monoclonal radioimmunoassay.
§ Assay: INCSTAR specific monoclonal radioimmunoassay.

plasma, 4-9% in lymphocytes, 5-12% in granulocytes, and 41-58% in erythrocytes. At high concentrations, the binding capacity of leukocytes and erythrocytes becomes saturated. In plasma, approximately 90% is bound to proteins, primarily lipoproteins. Cyclosporine is excreted in human milk. (See PRECAUTIONS, Neoral, Nursing Mothers.)

Metabolism

Cyclosporine is extensively metabolized by the cytochrome P-450 3A enzyme system in the liver, and to a lesser degree in the gastrointestinal tract, and the kidney. The metabolism of cyclosporine can be altered by the coadministration of a variety of agents. (See DRUG INTERACTIONS, Neoral.) At least 25 metabolites have been identified from human bile, feces, blood, and urine. The biological activity of the metabolites and their contributions to toxicity are considerably less than those of the parent compound. The major metabolites (M1, M9, and M4N) result from oxidation at the 1-beta, 9-gamma, and 4-N-demethylated positions, respectively. At steady state following the oral administration of Sandimmune, the mean AUCs for blood concentrations of M1, M9, and M4N are about 70%, 21%, and 7.5% of the AUC for blood cyclosporine concentrations, respectively. Based on blood concentration data from stable renal transplant patients (13 patients administered Neoral and Sandimmune in a crossover study), and bile concentration data from *de novo* liver transplant patients (4 administered Neoral, 3 administered Sandimmune), the percentage of dose present as M1, M9, and M4N metabolites is similar when either Neoral or Sandimmune is administered.

Excretion

Only 0.1% of a cyclosporine dose is excreted unchanged in the urine. Elimination is primarily biliary with only 6% of the dose (parent drug and metabolites) excreted in the urine. Neither dialysis nor renal failure alter cyclosporine clearance significantly.

Drug Interactions

See DRUG INTERACTIONS, Neoral.

When diclofenac or methotrexate was co-administered with cyclosporine in rheumatoid arthritis patients, the AUC of diclofenac and methotrexate, each was significantly increased (see DRUG INTERACTIONS, Neoral). No clinically significant pharmacokinetic interactions occurred between cyclosporine and aspirin, ketoprofen, piroxicam, or indomethacin.

Special Populations

Pediatric Population

Pharmacokinetic data from pediatric patients administered Neoral or Sandimmune are very limited. In 15 renal transplant patients aged 3-16 years, cyclosporine whole blood clearance after IV administration of Sandimmune was 10.6 ± 3.7 ml/min/kg (assay: Cyclo-trac specific RIA). In a study of 7 renal transplant patients aged 2-16, the cyclosporine clearance ranged from 9.8-15.5 ml/min/kg. In 9 liver transplant patients aged 0.6-5.6 years, clearance was 9.3 ± 5.4 ml/min/kg (assay: HPLC).

In the pediatric population, Neoral also demonstrates an increased bioavailability as compared to Sandimmune. In 7 liver *de novo* transplant patients aged 1.4-10 years, the absolute bioavailability of Neoral was 43% (range 30-68%) and for Sandimmune in the same individuals absolute bioavailability was 28% (range 17-42%).

TABLE 2A *Pediatric Pharmacokinetic Parameters (mean ± SD)*

Patient Population	Dose/Day (mg/day)	Dose/Weight (mg/kg/day)	AUC* (ng·h/ml)
Stable Liver Transplant†			
Age 2-8, dosed tid (n=9)	101 ± 25	5.95 ± 1.32	2163 ± 801
Age 8-15, dosed bid (n=8)	188 ± 55	4.96 ± 2.09	4272 ± 1462
Stable Liver Transplant‡			
Age 3, dosed bid (n=1)	120	8.33	5832
Age 8-15, dosed bid (n=5)	158 ± 55	5.51 ± 1.91	4452 ± 2475
Stable Renal Transplant‡			
Age 7-15, dosed bid (n=5)	328 ± 83	7.37 ± 4.11	6922 ± 1988

* AUC was measured over one dosing interval.
† Assay: Cyclo-trac specific monoclonal radioimmunoassay.
‡ Assay: TDx specific monoclonal fluorescence polarization immunoassay.

TABLE 2B *Pediatric Pharmacokinetic Parameters (mean ± SD)*

Patient Population	C_{max} (ng/ml)	CL/F (ml/min)	CL/F (ml/min/kg)
Stable Liver Transplant*			
Age 2-8, dosed tid (n=9)	629 ± 219	285 ± 94	16.6 ± 4.3
Age 8-15, dosed bid (n=8)	975 ± 281	378 ± 80	10.2 ± 4.0
Stable Liver Transplant†			
Age 3, dosed bid (n=1)	1050	171	11.9
Age 8-15, dosed bid (n=5)	1013 ± 635	328 ± 121	11.0 ± 1.9
Stable Renal Transplant†			
Age 7-15, dosed bid (n=5)	1827 ± 487	418 ± 143	8.7 ± 2.9

* Assay: Cyclo-trac specific monoclonal radioimmunoassay.
† Assay: TDx specific monoclonal fluorescence polarization immunoassay.

Geriatric Population

Comparison of single dose data from both normal elderly volunteers (n=18, mean age 69 years) and elderly rheumatoid arthritis patients (n=16, mean age 68 years) to single dose data in young adult volunteers (n=16, mean age 26 years) showed no significant difference in the pharmacokinetic parameters.

SANDIMMUNE

Sandimmune is a potent immunosuppressive agent which in animals prolongs survival of allogeneic transplants involving skin, heart, kidney, pancreas, bone marrow, small intestine, and lung. Sandimmune has been demonstrated to suppress some humoral immunity and to a greater extent, cell-mediated reactions such as allograft rejection, delayed hypersensitivity, experimental allergic encephalomyelitis, Freund's adjuvant arthritis, and graft-versus-host disease in many animal species for a variety of organs.

Successful kidney, liver, and heart allogeneic transplants have been performed in man using Sandimmune.

The exact mechanism of action of Sandimmune is not known. Experimental evidence suggests that the effectiveness of cyclosporine is due to specific and reversible inhibition of immunocompetent lymphocytes in the G_0- or G_1-phase of the cell cycle. T-lymphocytes are preferentially inhibited. The T-helper cell is the main target, although the T-suppressor cell may also be suppressed. Sandimmune also inhibits lymphokine production and release including interleukin-2 or T-cell growth factor (TCGF).

No functional effects on phagocytic (changes in enzyme secretions not altered, chemotactic migration of granulocytes, macrophage migration, carbon clearance *in vivo*) or tumor cells (growth rate, metastasis) can be detected in animals. Sandimmune does not cause bone marrow suppression in animal models or man.

The absorption of cyclosporine from the gastrointestinal tract is incomplete and variable. Peak concentrations (C_{max}) in blood and plasma are achieved at about 3.5 hours. C_{max} and area under the plasma or blood concentration/time curve (AUC) increase with the administered dose; for blood the relationship is curvilinear (parabolic) between 0 and 1400 mg. As determined by a specific assay, C_{max} is approximately 1.0 ng/ml/mg of dose for plasma and 2.7-1.4 ng/ml/mg of dose for blood (for low to high doses). Compared to an intravenous (IV) infusion, the absolute bioavailability of the oral solution is approximately 30% based upon the results in 2 patients. The bioavailability of Sandimmune soft gelatin capsules is equivalent to Sandimmune oral solution.

Cyclosporine is distributed largely outside the blood volume. In blood the distribution is concentration dependent. Approximately 33-47% is in plasma, 4-9% in lymphocytes, 5-12% in granulocytes, and 41-58% in erythrocytes. At high concentrations, the uptake by leukocytes and erythrocytes becomes saturated. In plasma, approximately 90% is bound to proteins, primarily lipoproteins.

The disposition of cyclosporine from blood is biphasic with a terminal half-life of approximately 19 hours (range: 10-27 hours). Elimination is primarily biliary with only 6% of the dose excreted in the urine.

Cyclosporine is extensively metabolized but there is no major metabolic pathway. Only 0.1% of the dose is excreted in the urine as unchanged drug. Of 15 metabolites characterized in human urine, 9 have been assigned structures. The major pathways consist of hydroxylation of the Cγ-carbon of 2 of the leucine residues, Cη-carbon hydroxylation, and cyclic ether formation (with oxidation of the double bond) in the side chain of the amino acid 3-hydroxyl-*N*,4-dimethyl-L-2-amino-6-octenoic acid and *N*-demethylation of *N*-methyl leucine residues. Hydrolysis of the cyclic peptide chain or conjugation of the aforementioned metabolites do not appear to be important biotransformation pathways.

RESTASIS

Restasis Ophthalmic Emulsion

Mechanism of Action

Cyclosporine is an immunosuppressive agent when administered systemically.

In patients whose tear production is presumed to be suppressed due to ocular inflammation associated with keratoconjunctivitis sicca, cyclosporine emulsion is thought to act as a partial immunomodulator. The exact mechanism of action is not known.

Pharmacokinetics

Blood cyclosporin A concentrations were measured using a specific high pressure liquid chromatographymass spectrometry assay. Blood concentrations of cyclosporine, in all the samples collected, after topical administration of Restasis 0.05%, bid, in humans for up to 12 months, were below the quantitation limit of 0.1 ng/ml. There was no detectable drug accumulation in blood during 12 months of treatment with Restasis ophthalmic emulsion.

INDICATIONS AND USAGE

NEORAL

Kidney, Liver, and Heart Transplantation

Neoral is indicated for the prophylaxis of organ rejection in kidney, liver, and heart allogeneic transplants. Neoral has been used in combination with azathioprine and corticosteroids.

Rheumatoid Arthritis

Neoral is indicated for the treatment of patients with severe active, rheumatoid arthritis where the disease has not adequately responded to methotrexate. Neoral can be used in combination with methotrexate in rheumatoid arthritis patients who do not respond adequately to methotrexate alone.

Psoriasis

Neoral is indicated for the treatment of *adult, nonimmunocompromised* patients with severe (*i.e.,* extensive and/or disabling), recalcitrant, plaque psoriasis who have failed to respond to at least 1 systemic therapy (*e.g.,* PUVA, retinoids, or methotrexate) or in patients for whom other systemic therapies are contraindicated, or cannot be tolerated.

While rebound rarely occurs, most patients will experience relapse with Neoral as with other therapies upon cessation of treatment.

SANDIMMUNE

Sandimmune is indicated for the prophylaxis of organ rejection in kidney, liver, and heart allogeneic transplants. It is always to be used with adrenal corticosteroids. The drug may also be used in the treatment of chronic rejection in patients previously treated with other immunosuppressive agents.

Because of the risk of anaphylaxis, Sandimmune injection should be reserved for patients who are unable to take the soft gelatin capsules or oral solution.

RESTASIS

Restasis Ophthalmic Emulsion

Restasis ophthalmic emulsion is indicated to increase tear production in patients whose tear production is presumed to be suppressed due to ocular inflammation associated with keratoconjunctivitis sicca. Increased tear production was not seen in patients currently taking topical anti-inflammatory drugs or using punctal plugs.

Non-FDA Approved Indications

While not well established, cyclosporine has also been used in bone marrow, pancreatic, and corneal transplantation as well as in the treatment of other immunologic based diseases. Studies are conflicting over the use of cyclosporine for Crohn's disease and ulcerative colitis. The use of cyclosporine for these indications has not been approved by the FDA and further clinical trials are needed.

CONTRAINDICATIONS

NEORAL

General

Neoral is contraindicated in patients with a hypersensitivity to cyclosporine or to any of the ingredients of the formulation.

Rheumatoid Arthritis

Rheumatoid arthritis patients with abnormal renal function, uncontrolled hypertension, or malignancies should not receive Neoral.

Psoriasis

Psoriasis patients who are treated with Neoral should not receive concomitant PUVA or UVB therapy, methotrexate or other immunosuppressive agents, coal tar or radiation therapy. Psoriasis patients with abnormal renal function, uncontrolled hypertension, or malignancies should not receive Neoral.

SANDIMMUNE

Sandimmune injection is contraindicated in patients with a hypersensitivity to Sandimmune and/or Cremophor EL (polyoxyethylated castor oil).

RESTASIS

Restasis Ophthalmic Emulsion

Restasis is contraindicated in patients with active ocular infections and in patients with known or suspected hypersensitivity to any of the ingredients in the formulation.

WARNINGS

NEORAL

See also BOXED WARNING, Neoral.

All Patients

Cyclosporine, the active ingredient of Neoral, can cause nephrotoxicity and hepatotoxicity. The risk increases with increasing doses of cyclosporine. Renal dysfunction including structural kidney damage is a potential consequence of Neoral and therefore renal function must be monitored during therapy. **Care should be taken in using cyclosporine with nephrotoxic drugs. (See PRECAUTIONS, Neoral.)**

Patients receiving Neoral require frequent monitoring of serum creatinine. (See Special Monitoring under DOSAGE AND ADMINISTRATION, Neoral.) Elderly patients should be monitored with particular care, since decreases in renal function also occur with age. If patients are not properly monitored and doses are not properly adjusted, cyclosporine therapy can be associated with the occurrence of structural kidney damage and persistent renal dysfunction.

An increase in serum creatinine and BUN may occur during Neoral therapy and reflect a reduction in the glomerular filtration rate. Impaired renal function at any time requires close monitoring, and frequent dosage adjustment may be indicated. The frequency and severity of serum creatinine elevations increase with dose and duration of cyclosporine therapy. These elevations are likely to become more pronounced without dose reduction or discontinuation.

Because Neoral is not bioequivalent to Sandimmune, conversion from Neoral to Sandimmune using a 1:1 ratio (mg/kg/day) may result in lower cyclosporine blood concentrations. Conversion from Neoral to Sandimmune should be made with increased monitoring to avoid the potential of underdosing.

Kidney, Liver, and Heart Transplant

Cyclosporine, the active ingredient of Neoral, can cause nephrotoxicity and hepatotoxicity when used in high doses. It is not unusual for serum creatinine and BUN levels to be elevated during cyclosporine therapy. These elevations in renal transplant patients do not necessarily indicate rejection, and each patient must be fully evaluated before dosage adjustment is initiated.

Based on the historical Sandimmune experience with oral solution, nephrotoxicity associated with cyclosporine had been noted in 25% of cases of renal transplantation, 38% of cases of cardiac transplantation, and 37% of cases of liver transplantation. Mild nephrotoxicity was generally noted 2-3 months after renal transplant and consisted of an arrest in the fall of the pre-operative elevations of BUN and creatinine at a range of 35-45 mg/dl and 2.0-2.5 mg/dl respectively. These elevations were often responsive to cyclosporine dosage reduction.

More overt nephrotoxicity was seen early after transplantation and was characterized by a rapidly rising BUN and creatinine. Since these events are similar to renal rejection episodes, care must be taken to differentiate between them. This form of nephrotoxicity is usually responsive to cyclosporine dosage reduction.

Although specific diagnostic criteria which reliably differentiate renal graft rejection from drug toxicity have not been found, a number of parameters have been significantly associated with one or the other. It should be noted however, that up to 20% of patients may have simultaneous nephrotoxicity and rejection.

Nephrotoxicity Versus Rejection

History

Nephrotoxicity:

Donor >50 years old or hypotensive.
Prolonged kidney preservation.
Prolonged anastomosis time.
Concomitant nephrotoxic drugs.

Rejection:

Anti-donor immune response.
Retransplant patient.

Clinical

Nephrotoxicity:

Often >6 weeks postop*.
Prolonged initial nonfunction (acute tubular necrosis).

Rejection:

Often <4 weeks postop*.
Fever >37.5°C.
Weight gain >0.5 kg.
Graft swelling and tenderness.
Decrease in daily urine volume >500 ml (or 50%).

Laboratory

Nephrotoxicity:

CyA serum trough level >200 ng/ml.
Gradual rise in Cr (<0.15 mg/dl/day)†.
Cr plateau <25% above baseline.
BUN/Cr ≥20.

Rejection:

CyA serum trough level <150 ng/ml.
Rapid rise in Cr (>0.3 mg/dl/day)†.
Cr >25% above baseline.
BUN/Cr <20.

Biopsy

Nephrotoxicity:

Arteriolopathy (medial hypertrophy†, hyalinosis, nodular deposits, intimal thickening, endothelial vacuolization, progressive scarring).
Tubular atrophy, isometric vacuolization, isolated calcifications.

Minimal edema.
Mild focal infiltrates‡.
Diffuse interstitial fibrosis, often striped form.
Rejection:
Endovasculitis‡ (proliferation†, intimal arteritis*, necrosis, sclerosis).
Tubulitis with RBC* and WBC* casts, some irregular vacuolization.
Interstitial edema‡ and hemorrhage*.
Diffuse moderate to severe mononuclear infiltrates§.
Glomerulitis (mononuclear cells)‡.

Aspiration Cytology
Nephrotoxicity:
CyA deposits in tubular and endothelial cells.
Fine isometric vacuolization of tubular cells.
Rejection:
Inflammatory infiltrate with mononuclear phagocytes, macrophages, lymphoblastoid cells, and activated T-cells.
These strongly express HLA-DR antigens.

Urine Cytology
Nephrotoxicity:
Tubular cells with vacuolization and granularization.
Rejection:
Degenerative tubular cells, plasma cells, and lymphocyturia >20% of sediment.

Manometry
Nephrotoxicity:
Intracapsular pressure <40 mm Hg*.
Rejection:
Intracapsular pressure <40 mm Hg*.

Ultrasonography
Nephrotoxicity:
Unchanged graft cross sectional area.
Rejection:
Increase in graft cross sectional area.
AP diameter ≥ Transverse diameter.

Magnetic Resonance Imagery
Nephrotoxicity:
Normal appearance.
Rejection:
Loss of distinct corticomedullary junction, swelling image intensity of parachyma approaching that of psoas, loss of hilar fat.

Radionuclide Scan
Nephrotoxicity:
Normal or generally decreased perfusion.
Decrease in tubular function.
(^{131}I-hippuran) > decrease in perfusion (^{99m}Tc DTPA).
Rejection:
Patchy arterial flow.
Decrease in perfusion > decrease in tubular function.
Increased uptake of Indium 111 labeled platelets or Tc-99m in colloid.

Therapy
Nephrotoxicity:
Responds to decreased cyclosporine.
Rejection:
Responds to increased steroids or antilymphocyte globulin.

* p <0.05.
† p <0.01.
‡ p <0.001.
§ p <0.0001.

A form of a cyclosporine-associated nephropathy is characterized by serial deterioration in renal function and morphologic changes in the kidneys. From 5-15% of transplant recipients who have received cyclosporine will fail to show a reduction in rising serum creatinine despite a decrease or discontinuation of cyclosporine therapy. Renal biopsies from these patients will demonstrate 1 or several of the following alterations: tubular vacuolization, tubular microcalcifications, peritubular capillary congestion, arteriolopathy, and a striped form of interstitial fibrosis with tubular atrophy. Though none of these morphologic changes is entirely specific, a diagnosis of cyclosporine-associated structural nephrotoxicity requires evidence of these findings.

When considering the development of cyclosporine-associated nephropathy, it is noteworthy that several authors have reported an association between the appearance of interstitial fibrosis and higher cumulative doses or persistently high circulating trough levels of cyclosporine. This is particularly true during the first 6 post-transplant months when the dosage tends to be highest and when, in kidney recipients, the organ appears to be most vulnerable to the toxic effects of cyclosporine. Among other contributing factors to the development of interstitial fibrosis in these patients are prolonged perfusion time, warm ischemia time, as well as episodes of acute toxicity, and acute and chronic rejection. The reversibility of interstitial fibrosis and its correlation to renal function have not yet been determined. Reversibility of arteriolopathy has been reported after stopping cyclosporine or lowering the dosage.

Impaired renal function at any time requires close monitoring, and frequent dosage adjustment may be indicated.

In the event of severe and unremitting rejection, when rescue therapy with pulse steroids and monoclonal antibodies fail to reverse the rejection episode, it may be preferable to switch to alternative immunosuppressive therapy rather than increase the Neoral dose to excessive levels.

Occasionally patients have developed a syndrome of thrombocytopenia and microangiopathic hemolytic anemia which may result in graft failure. The vasculopathy can occur in the absence of rejection and is accompanied by avid platelet consumption within the graft as demonstrated by Indium 111 labeled platelet studies. Neither the pathogenesis nor the management of this syndrome is clear. Though resolution has occurred after reduction or discontinuation of cyclosporine and (1) administration of streptokinase and heparin or (2) plasmapheresis, this appears to depend upon early detection with Indium 111 labeled platelet scans. (See ADVERSE REACTIONS, Neoral.)

Significant hyperkalemia (sometimes associated with hyperchloremic metabolic acidosis) and hyperuricemia have been seen occasionally in individual patients.

Hepatotoxicity associated with cyclosporine use had been noted in 4% of cases of renal transplantation, 7% of cases of cardiac transplantation, and 4% of cases of liver transplantation. This was usually noted during the first month of therapy when high doses of cyclosporine were used and consisted of elevations of hepatic enzymes and bilirubin. The chemistry elevations usually decreased with a reduction in dosage.

As in patients receiving other immunosuppressants, those patients receiving cyclosporine are at increased risk for development of lymphomas and other malignancies, particularly those of the skin. The increased risk appears related to the intensity and duration of immunosuppression rather than to the use of specific agents. Because of the danger of oversuppression of the immune system resulting in increased risk of infection or malignancy, a treatment regimen containing multiple immunosuppressants should be used with caution.

There have been reports of convulsions in adult and pediatric patients receiving cyclosporine, particularly in combination with high dose methylprednisolone.

Encephalopathy has been described both in post-marketing reports and in the literature. Manifestations include impaired consciousness, convulsions, visual disturbances (including blindness), loss of motor function, movement disorders and psychiatric disturbances. In many cases, changes in the white matter have been detected using imaging techniques and pathologic specimens. Predisposing factors such as hypertension, hypomagnesemia, hypocholesterolemia, high-dose corticosteroids, high cyclosporine blood concentrations, and graft-versus-host disease have been noted in many but not all of the reported cases. The changes in most cases have been reversible upon discontinuation of cyclosporine, and in some cases improvement was noted after reduction of dose. It appears that patients receiving liver transplant are more susceptible to encephalopathy than those receiving kidney transplant.

Care should be taken in using cyclosporine with nephrotoxic drugs. (See PRECAUTIONS, Neoral.)

Rheumatoid Arthritis

Cyclosporine nephropathy was detected in renal biopsies of 6 out of 60 (10%) rheumatoid arthritis patients after the average treatment duration of 19 months. Only 1 patient, out of these 6 patients, was treated with a dose ≤4 mg/kg/day. Serum creatinine improved in all but 1 patient after discontinuation of cyclosporine. The "maximal creatinine increase" appears to be a factor in predicting cyclosporine nephropathy.

There is a potential, as with other immunosuppressive agents, for an increase in the occurrence of malignant lymphomas with cyclosporine. It is not clear whether the risk with cyclosporine is greater than that in rheumatoid arthritis patients or in rheumatoid arthritis patients on cytotoxic treatment for this indication. Five cases of lymphoma were detected: 4 in a survey of approximately 2300 patients treated with cyclosporine for rheumatoid arthritis, and another case of lymphoma was reported in a clinical trial. Although other tumors (12 skin cancers, 24 solid tumors of diverse types, and 1 multiple myeloma) were also reported in this survey, epidemiologic analyses did not support a relationship to cyclosporine other than for malignant lymphomas.

Patients should be thoroughly evaluated before and during Neoral treatment for the development of malignancies. Moreover, use of Neoral therapy with other immunosuppressive agents may induce an excessive immunosuppression which is known to increase the risk of malignancy.

Psoriasis

See also BOXED WARNING, Neoral, For Psoriasis Patients. Since cyclosporine is a potent immunosuppressive agent with a number of potentially serious side effects, the risks and benefits of using Neoral should be considered before treatment of patients with psoriasis. Cyclosporine, the active ingredient in Neoral, can cause nephrotoxicity and hypertension (see PRECAUTIONS, Neoral) and the risk increases with increasing dose and duration of therapy. Patients who may be at increased risk such as those with abnormal renal function, uncontrolled hypertension or malignancies, should not receive Neoral.

Renal dysfunction is a potential consequence of Neoral therefore renal function must be monitored during therapy.

Patients receiving Neoral require frequent monitoring of serum creatinine. (See Special Monitoring under DOSAGE AND ADMINISTRATION, Neoral.) Elderly patients should be monitored with particular care, since decreases in renal function also occur with age. If patients are not properly monitored and doses are not properly adjusted, cyclosporine therapy can cause structural kidney damage and persistent renal dysfunction.

An increase in serum creatinine and BUN may occur during Neoral therapy and reflects a reduction in the glomerular filtration rate.

Kidney biopsies from 86 psoriasis patients treated for a mean duration of 23 months with 1.2-7.6 mg/kg/day of cyclosporine showed evidence of cyclosporine nephropathy in 18/86 (21%) of the patients. The pathology consisted of renal tubular atrophy and interstitial fibrosis. On repeat biopsy of 13 of these patients maintained on various dosages of cyclosporine for a mean of 2 additional years, the number with cyclosporine induced nephropathy rose to 26/86 (30%). The majority of patients (19/26) were on a dose of ≥5.0 mg/kg/day (the highest recommended dose is 4 mg/kg/day). The patients were also on cyclosporine for greater than 15 months (18/26) and/or had a clinically significant increase in serum creatinine for greater than 1 month (21/26). Creatinine levels returned to normal range in 7 of 11 patients in whom cyclosporine therapy was discontinued.

There is an increased risk for the development of skin and lymphoproliferative malignancies in cyclosporine-treated psoriasis patients. The relative risk of malignancies is comparable to that observed in psoriasis patients treated with other immunosuppressive agents.

Tumors were reported in 32 (2.2%) of 1439 psoriasis patients treated with cyclosporine worldwide from clinical trials. Additional tumors have been reported in 7 patients in cyclosporine postmarketing experience. Skin malignancies were reported in 16 (1.1%) of these patients; all but 2 of them had previously received PUVA therapy. Methotrexate was received by 7 patients. UVB and coal tar had been used by 2 and 3 patients, respectively. Seven patients had either a history of previous skin cancer or a potentially predisposing lesion was present prior to cyclosporine exposure. Of the 16 patients with skin cancer, 11 patients had 18 squamous cell carcinomas and 7 patients had 10 basal cell carcinomas.

There were 2 lymphoproliferative malignancies; 1 case of non-Hodgkin's lymphoma which required chemotherapy, and 1 case of mycosis fungoides which regressed spontaneously upon discontinuation of cyclosporine. There were 4 cases of benign lymphocytic infiltration: 3 regressed spontaneously upon discontinuation of cyclosporine, while the fourth regressed despite continuation of the drug. The remainder of the malignancies, 13 cases (0.9%), involved various organs.

Patients should not be treated concurrently with cyclosporine and PUVA or UVB, other radiation therapy, or other immunosuppressive agents, because of the possibility of excessive immunosuppression and the subsequent risk of malignancies. (See CONTRAINDICATIONS, Neoral.) Patients should also be warned to protect themselves appropriately when in the sun, and to avoid excessive sun exposure. Patients should be thoroughly evaluated before and during treatment for the presence of malignancies remembering that malignant lesions may be hidden by psoriatic plaques. Skin lesions not typical of psoriasis should be biopsied before starting treatment. Patients should be treated with Neoral only after complete resolution of suspicious lesions, and only if there are no other treatment options. (See PRECAUTIONS, Neoral, General, Special Monitoring for Psoriasis Patients.)

SANDIMMUNE

See BOXED WARNING, Sandimmune.

Sandimmune, when used in high doses, can cause hepatotoxicity and nephrotoxicity.

It is not unusual for serum creatinine and BUN levels to be elevated during Sandimmune therapy. These elevations in renal transplant patients do not necessarily indicate rejection, and each patient must be fully evaluated before dosage adjustment is initiated.

Nephrotoxicity has been noted in 25% of cases of renal transplantation, 38% of cases of cardiac transplantation, and 37% of cases of liver transplantation. Mild nephrotoxicity was generally noted 2-3 months after transplant and consisted of an arrest in the fall of the preoperative elevations of BUN and creatinine at a range of 35-45 mg/dl and 2.0-2.5 mg/dl, respectively. These elevations were often responsive to dosage reduction.

More overt nephrotoxicity was seen early after transplantation and was characterized by a rapidly rising BUN and creatinine. Since these events are similar to rejection episodes care must be taken to differentiate between them. This form of nephrotoxicity is usually responsive to Sandimmune dosage reduction.

Although specific diagnostic criteria which reliably differentiate renal graft rejection from drug toxicity have not been found, a number of parameters have been significantly associated to one or the other. It should be noted however, that up to 20% of patients may have simultaneous nephrotoxicity and rejection.

Nephrotoxicity Versus Rejection

History

Nephrotoxicity:

Donor >50 years old or hypotensive.
Prolonged kidney preservation.
Prolonged anastomosis time.
Concomitant nephrotoxic drugs.

Rejection:

Anti-donor immune response.
Retransplant patient.

Clinical

Nephrotoxicity:

Often >6 weeks postop*.
Prolonged initial nonfunction (acute tubular necrosis).

Rejection:

Often <4 weeks postop*.
Fever >37.5°C.
Weight gain >0.5 kg.
Graft swelling and tenderness.
Decrease in daily urine volume >500 ml (or 50%).

Laboratory

Nephrotoxicity:

CyA serum trough level >200 ng/ml.
Gradual rise in Cr (<0.15 mg/dl/day)†.
Cr plateau <25% above baseline.
BUN/Cr ≥20.

Rejection:

CyA serum trough level <150 ng/ml.
Rapid rise in Cr (>0.3 mg/dl/day)†.
Cr >25% above baseline.
BUN/Cr <20.

Biopsy

Nephrotoxicity:

Arteriolopathy (medial hypertrophy†, hyalinosis, nodular deposits, intimal thickening, endothelial vacuolization, progressive scarring).
Tubular atrophy, isometric vacuolization, isolated calcifications.
Minimal edema.
Mild focal infiltrates‡.
Diffuse interstitial fibrosis, often striped form.

Rejection:

Endovasculitis‡ (proliferation†, intimal arteritis*, necrosis, sclerosis).
Tubulitis with RBC* and WBC* casts, some irregular vacuolization.
Interstitial edema‡ and hemorrhage*.
Diffuse moderate to severe mononuclear infiltrates§.
Glomerulitis (mononuclear cells)‡.

Aspiration Cytology

Nephrotoxicity:

CyA deposits in tubular and endothelial cells.
Fine isometric vacuolization of tubular cells.

Rejection:

Inflammatory infiltrate with mononuclear phagocytes, macrophages, lymphoblastoid cells, and activated T-cells.
These strongly express HLA-DR antigens.

Urine Cytology

Nephrotoxicity:

Tubular cells with vacuolization and granularization.

Rejection:

Degenerative tubular cells, plasma cells, and hocyturia >20% of sediment.

Manometry

Nephrotoxicity:

Intracapsular pressure <40 mm Hg*.

Rejection:

Intracapsular pressure >40 mm Hg*.

Ultrasonography

Nephrotoxicity:

Unchanged graft cross-sectional area.

Rejection:

Increase in graft cross-sectional area.
AP diameter ≥ transverse diameter.

Magnetic Resonance Imagery

Nephrotoxicity:

Normal appearance.

Rejection:

Loss of distinct corticomedullary junction, swelling, image intensity of parachyma approaching that of psoas, loss of hilar fat.

Radionuclide Scan

Nephrotoxicity:

Normal or generally decreased perfusion.
Decrease in tubular function.
(^{131}I-hippuran) > decrease in perfusion (^{99m}Tc DTPA).

Rejection:

Patchy arterial flow.
Decrease in perfusion > decrease in tubular function.
Increased uptake of Indium 111 labeled platelets or Tc-99m in colloid.

Therapy

Nephrotoxicity:

Responds to decreased Sandimmune.

Rejection:

Responds to increased steroids or antilymphocyte globulin.

* p <0.01.
† p <0.05.
‡ p <0.001.
§ p <0.0001.

A form of chronic progressive cyclosporine-associated nephrotoxicity is characterized by serial deterioration in renal function and morphologic changes in the kidneys. From 5-15% of transplant recipients will fail to show a reduction in a rising serum creatinine despite a decrease or discontinuation of cyclosporine therapy. Renal biopsies from these patients will demonstrate an interstitial fibrosis with tubular atrophy. In addition, toxic tubulopathy, peritubular capillary congestion, arteriolopathy, and a striped form of interstitial fibrosis with tubular atrophy may be present. Though none of these morphologic changes is entirely specific, a histologic diagnosis of chronic progressive cyclosporine-associated nephrotoxicity requires evidence of these.

When considering the development of chronic nephrotoxicity it is noteworthy that several authors have reported an association between the appearance of interstitial fibrosis and higher cumulative doses or persistently high circulating trough levels of cyclosporine. This is particularly true during the first 6 posttransplant months when the dosage tends to be highest and when, in kidney recipients, the organ appears to be most vulnerable to the toxic effects of cyclosporine. Among other contributing factors to the development of interstitial fibrosis in these patients must be included, prolonged perfusion time, warm ischemia time, as well as episodes of acute toxicity, and acute and chronic rejection. The reversibility of interstitial fibrosis and its correlation to renal function have not yet been determined.

Impaired renal function at any time requires close monitoring, and frequent dosage adjustment may be indicated. In patients with persistent high elevations of BUN and creatinine who are unresponsive to dosage adjustments, consideration should be given to switching to other immunosuppressive therapy. In the event of severe and unremitting rejection, it is preferable to allow the kidney transplant to be rejected and removed rather than increase the Sandimmune dosage to a very high level in an attempt to reverse the rejection.

C

Occasionally patients have developed a syndrome of thrombocytopenia and microangiopathic hemolytic anemia which may result in graft failure. The vasculopathy can occur in the absence of rejection and is accompanied by avid platelet consumption within the graft as demonstrated by Indium 111 labeled platelet studies. Neither the pathogenesis nor the management of this syndrome is clear. Though resolution has occurred after reduction or discontinuation of Sandimmune and (1) administration of streptokinase and heparin or (2) plasmapheresis, this appears to depend upon early detection with Indium 111 labeled platelet scans. (See ADVERSE REACTIONS, Sandimmune.)

Significant hyperkalemia (sometimes associated with hyperchloremic metabolic acidosis) and hyperuricemia have been seen occasionally in individual patients.

Hepatotoxicity has been noted in 4% of cases of renal transplantation, 7% of cases of cardiac transplantation, and 4% of cases of liver transplantation. This was usually noted during the first month of therapy when high doses of Sandimmune were used and consisted of elevations of hepatic enzymes and bilirubin. The chemistry elevations usually decreased with a reduction in dosage.

As in patients receiving other immunosuppressants, those patients receiving Sandimmune are at increased risk for development of lymphomas and other malignancies, particularly those of the skin. The increased risk appears related to the intensity and duration of immunosuppression rather than to the use of specific agents. Because of the danger of oversuppression of the immune system, which can also increase susceptibility to infection, Sandimmune should not be administered with other immunosuppressive agents except adrenal corticosteroids. The efficacy and safety of cyclosporine in combination with other immunosuppressive agents have not been determined.

There have been reports of convulsions in adult and pediatric patients receiving cyclosporine, particularly in combination with high dose methylprednisolone.

Encephalopathy has been described both in post-marketing reports and in the literature. Manifestations include impaired consciousness, convulsions, visual disturbances (including blindness) loss of motor function, movement disorders and psychiatric disturbances. In many cases, changes in the white matter have been detected using imaging techniques and pathologic specimens. Predisposing factors such as hypertension, hypomagnesemia, hypocholesterolemia, high-dose corticosteroids, high cyclosporine blood concentrations, and graft-versus-host disease have been noted in many but not all of the reported cases. The changes in most cases have been reversible upon discontinuation of cyclosporine and in some cases improvement was noted after reduction of dose. It appears that patients receiving liver transplant are more susceptible to encephalopathy than those patients receiving kidney transplant.

Rarely (approximately 1 in 1000), patients receiving Sandimmune injection have experienced anaphylactic reactions. Although the exact cause of these reactions is unknown, it is believed to be due to the Cremophor EL (polyoxyethylated castor oil) used as the vehicle for the IV formulation. These reactions have consisted of flushing of the face and upper thorax, acute respiratory distress with dyspnea and wheezing, blood pressure changes, and tachycardia. One (1) patient died after respiratory arrest and aspiration pneumonia. In some cases, the reaction subsided after the infusion was stopped.

Patients receiving Sandimmune injection should be under continuous observation for at least the first 30 minutes following the start of the infusion and at frequent intervals thereafter. If anaphylaxis occurs, the infusion should be stopped. An aqueous solution of epinephrine 1:1000 should be available at the bedside as well as a source of oxygen.

Anaphylactic reactions have not been reported with the soft gelatin capsules or oral solution which lack Cremophor EL (polyoxyethylated castor oil). In fact, patients experiencing anaphylactic reactions have been treated subsequently with the soft gelatin capsules or oral solution without incident.

Care should be taken in using Sandimmune with nephrotoxic drugs. (See PRECAUTIONS, Sandimmune.)

Because Sandimmune is not bioequivalent to Neoral, conversion from Neoral to Sandimmune using a 1:1 ratio (mg/kg/day) may result in a lower cyclosporine blood concentration. Conversion from Neoral to Sandimmune should be made with increased blood concentration monitoring to avoid the potential of underdosing.

RESTASIS

Restasis ophthalmic emulsion has not been studied in patients with a history of herpes keratitis.

PRECAUTIONS

NEORAL

General

Hypertension

Cyclosporine is the active ingredient of Neoral. Hypertension is a common side effect of cyclosporine therapy which may persist. (See ADVERSE REACTIONS, Neoral, and DOSAGE AND ADMINISTRATION, Neoral, for monitoring recommendations.) Mild or moderate hypertension is encountered more frequently than severe hypertension and the incidence decreases over time. In recipients of kidney, liver, and heart allografts treated with cyclosporine, antihypertensive therapy may be required. (See Special Monitoring of Rheumatoid Arthritis Patients and Special Monitoring for Psoriasis Patients.) However, since cyclosporine may cause hyperkalemia, potassium-sparing diuretics should not be used. While calcium antagonists can be effective agents in treating cyclosporine-associated hypertension, they can interfere with cyclosporine metabolism. (See DRUG INTERACTIONS, Neoral.)

Vaccination

During treatment with cyclosporine, vaccination may be less effective; and the use of live attenuated vaccines should be avoided.

Special Monitoring of Rheumatoid Arthritis Patients

Before initiating treatment, a careful physical examination, including blood pressure measurements (on at least 2 occasions) and two creatinine levels to estimate baseline should be performed. Blood pressure and serum creatinine should be evaluated every 2 weeks during the initial 3 months and then monthly if the patient is stable. It is advisable to monitor serum creatinine and blood pressure always after an increase of the dose of nonsteroidal anti-inflammatory drugs and after initiation of new nonsteroidal anti-inflammatory drug therapy during Neoral treatment. If coadministered with methotrexate, CBC and liver function tests are recommended to be monitored monthly. (See also Hypertension.)

In patients who are receiving cyclosporine, the dose of Neoral should be decreased by 25-50% if hypertension occurs. If hypertension persists, the dose of Neoral should be further reduced or blood pressure should be controlled with antihypertensive agents. In most cases, blood pressure has returned to baseline when cyclosporine was discontinued.

In placebo-controlled trials of rheumatoid arthritis patients, systolic hypertension (defined as an occurrence of 2 systolic blood pressure readings >140 mm Hg) and diastolic hypertension (defined as 2 diastolic blood pressure readings >90 mm Hg) occurred in 33% and 19% of patients treated with cyclosporine, respectively. The corresponding placebo rates were 22% and 8%.

Special Monitoring for Psoriasis Patients

Before initiating treatment, a careful dermatological and physical examination, including blood pressure measurements (on at least 2 occasions) should be performed. Since Neoral is an immunosuppressive agent, patients should be evaluated for the presence of occult infection on their first physical examination and for the presence of tumors initially, and throughout treatment with Neoral. Skin lesions not typical for psoriasis should be biopsied before starting Neoral. Patients with malignant or premalignant changes of the skin should be treated with Neoral only after appropriate treatment of such lesions and if no other treatment option exists.

Baseline laboratories should include serum creatinine (on 2 occasions), BUN, CBC, serum magnesium, potassium, uric acid, and lipids.

The risk of cyclosporine nephropathy is reduced when the starting dose is low (2.5 mg/kg/day), the maximum dose does not exceed 4.0 mg/kg/day, serum creatinine is monitored regularly while cyclosporine is administered, and the dose of Neoral is decreased when the rise in creatinine is greater than or equal to 25% above the patients pretreatment level. The increase in creatinine is generally reversible upon timely decrease of the dose of Neoral or its discontinuation.

Serum creatinine and BUN should be evaluated every 2 weeks during the initial 3 months of therapy and then monthly if the patient is stable. If the serum creatinine is greater than or equal to 25% above the patient's pretreatment level, serum creatinine should be repeated within 2 weeks. If the change in serum creatinine remains greater than or equal to 25% above baseline, Neoral should be reduced by 25-50%. If at **any time** the serum creatinine increases by greater than or equal to 50% above pretreatment level, Neoral should be reduced by 25-50%. Neoral should be discontinued if reversibility (within 25% of baseline) of serum creatinine is not achievable after 2 dosage modifications. It is advisable to monitor serum creatinine after an increase of the dose of nonsteroidal anti-inflammatory drug and after initiation of new nonsteroidal anti-inflammatory therapy during Neoral treatment.

Blood pressure should be evaluated every 2 weeks during the initial 3 months of therapy and then monthly if the patient is stable, or more frequently when dosage adjustments are made. Patients without a history of previous hypertension before initiation of treatment with Neoral, should have the drug reduced by 25-50% if found to have sustained hypertension. If the patient continues to be hypertensive despite multiple reductions of Neoral, then Neoral should be discontinued. For patients with treated hypertension, before the initiation of Neoral therapy, their medication should be adjusted to control hypertension while on Neoral. Neoral should be discontinued if a change in hypertension management is not effective or tolerable.

CBC, uric acid, potassium, lipids, and magnesium should also be monitored every 2 weeks for the first 3 months of therapy, and then monthly if the patient is stable or more frequently when dosage adjustments are made. Neoral dosage should be reduced by 25-50% for any abnormality of clinical concern.

In controlled trials of cyclosporine in psoriasis patients, cyclosporine blood concentrations did not correlate well with either improvement or with side effects such as renal dysfunction.

Information for the Patient

Patients should be advised that any change of cyclosporine formulation should be made cautiously and only under physician supervision because it may result in the need for a change in dosage.

Patients should be informed of the necessity of repeated laboratory tests while they are receiving cyclosporine. Patients should be advised of the potential risks during pregnancy and informed of the increased risk of neoplasia. Patients should also be informed of the risk of hypertension and renal dysfunction.

Patients should be advised that during treatment with cyclosporine, vaccination may be less effective and the use of live attenuated vaccines should be avoided.

Patients should be given careful dosage instructions. Neoral oral solution MODIFIED should be diluted, preferably with orange or apple juice that is at room temperature. The combination of Neoral oral solution MODIFIED with milk can be unpalatable.

Patients should be advised to take Neoral on a consistent schedule with regard to time of day and relation to meals. Grapefruit and grapefruit juice affect metabolism, increasing blood concentration of cyclosporine, thus should be avoided.

Laboratory Tests

In all patients treated with cyclosporine, renal and liver functions should be assessed repeatedly by measurement of serum creatinine, BUN, serum bilirubin, and liver enzymes. Serum lipids, magnesium, and potassium should also be monitored. Cyclosporine blood concentrations should be routinely monitored in transplant patients (see DOSAGE AND ADMINISTRATION, Neoral, Blood Concentration Monitoring in Transplant Patients), and periodically monitored in rheumatoid arthritis patients.

Carcinogenesis, Mutagenesis, and Impairment of Fertility

Carcinogenicity studies were carried out in male and female rats and mice. In the 78 week mouse study, evidence of a statistically significant trend was found for lymphocytic lymphomas in females, and the incidence of hepatocellular carcinomas in mid-dose males significantly exceeded the control value. In the 24 month rat study, pancreatic islet cell adenomas significantly exceeded the control rate in the low dose level. Doses used in the mouse and rat studies were 0.01-0.16 times the clinical maintenance dose (6 mg/kg). The hepatocellular carcinomas and pancreatic islet cell adenomas were not dose related. Published reports indicate that co-treatment of hairless mice with UV irradiation and cyclosporine or other immunosuppressive agents shorten the time to skin tumor formation compared to UV irradiation alone.

Cyclosporine was not mutagenic in appropriate test systems. Cyclosporine has not been found to be mutagenic/genotoxic in the Ames Test, the V79-HGPRT Test, the micronucleus test in mice and Chinese hamsters, the chromosome-aberration tests in Chinese hamster bone-marrow, the mouse dominant lethal assay, and the DNA-repair test in sperm from treated mice. A recent study analyzing sister chromatid exchange (SCE) induction by cyclosporine using human lymphocytes *in vitro* gave indication of a positive effect (*i.e.,* induction of SCE), at high concentrations in this system.

No impairment in fertility was demonstrated in studies in male and female rats.

Widely distributed papillomatosis of the skin was observed after chronic treatment of dogs with cyclosporine at 9 times the human initial psoriasis treatment dose of 2.5 mg/kg, where doses are expressed on a body surface area basis. This papillomatosis showed a spontaneous regression upon discontinuation of cyclosporine.

An increased incidence of malignancy is a recognized complication of immunosuppression in recipients of organ transplants and patients with rheumatoid arthritis and psoriasis. The most common forms of neoplasms are non-Hodgkin's lymphoma and carcinomas of the skin. The risk of malignancies in cyclosporine recipients is higher than in the normal, healthy population but similar to that in patients receiving other immunosuppressive therapies. Reduction or discontinuance of immunosuppression may cause the lesions to regress.

In psoriasis patients on cyclosporine, development of malignancies, especially those of the skin has been reported. (See WARNINGS, Neoral.) Skin lesions not typical for psoriasis should be biopsied before starting cyclosporine treatment. Patients with malignant or premalignant changes of the skin should be treated with cyclosporine only after appropriate treatment of such lesions and if no other treatment option exists.

Pregnancy Category C

Cyclosporine was not teratogenic in appropriate test systems. Only at dose levels toxic to dams, were adverse effects seen in reproduction studies in rats. Cyclosporine has been shown to be embryo- and fetotoxic in rats and rabbits following oral administration at maternally toxic doses. Fetal toxicity was noted in rats at 0.8 and rabbits at 5.4 times the transplant doses in humans of 6.0 mg/kg, where dose corrections are based on body surface area. Cyclosporine was embryo- and fetotoxic as indicated by increased pre- and postnatal mortality and reduced fetal weight together with related skeletal retardation.

There are no adequate and well-controlled studies in pregnant women. Neoral should be used during pregnancy only if the potential benefit justifies the potential risk to the fetus.

The following data represent the reported outcomes of 116 pregnancies in women receiving cyclosporine during pregnancy, 90% of whom were transplant patients, and most of whom received cyclosporine throughout the entire gestational period. The only consistent patterns of abnormality were premature birth (gestational period of 28-36 weeks) and low birth weight for gestational age. Sixteen (16) fetal losses occurred. Most of the pregnancies (85 of 100) were complicated by disorders; including, pre-eclampsia, eclampsia, premature labor, abruptio placentae, oligohydramnios, Rh incompatibility, and fetoplacental dysfunction. Pre-term delivery occurred in 47%. Seven malformations were reported in 5 viable infants and in 2 cases of fetal loss. Twenty-eight percent (28%) of the infants were small for gestational age. Neonatal complications occurred in 27%. Therefore, the risks and benefits of using Neoral during pregnancy should be carefully weighed.

Because of the possible disruption of maternal-fetal interaction, the risk/benefit ratio of using Neoral in psoriasis patients during pregnancy should carefully be weighed with serious consideration for discontinuation of Neoral.

Nursing Mothers

Since cyclosporine is excreted in human milk, breast-feeding should be avoided.

Pediatric Use

Although no adequate and well-controlled studies have been completed in children, transplant recipients as young as 1 year of age have received Neoral with no unusual adverse effects. The safety and efficacy of Neoral treatment in children with juvenile rheumatoid arthritis or psoriasis below the age of 18 have not been established.

Geriatric Use

In rheumatoid arthritis clinical trials with cyclosporine, 17.5% of patients were age 65 or older. These patients were more likely to develop systolic hypertension on therapy, and more likely to show serum creatinine rises ≥50% above the baseline after 3-4 months of therapy.

SANDIMMUNE

General

Patients with malabsorption may have difficulty in achieving therapeutic levels with Sandimmune soft gelatin capsules or oral solution.

Hypertension is a common side effect of Sandimmune therapy. (See ADVERSE REACTIONS, Sandimmune.) Mild or moderate hypertension is more frequently encountered than severe hypertension and the incidence decreases over time. Antihypertensive therapy may be required. Control of blood pressure can be accomplished with any of the common antihypertensive agents. However, since cyclosporine may cause hyperkalemia, potassium-sparing diuretics should not be used. While calcium antagonists can be effective agents in treating cyclosporine-associated hypertension, care should be taken since interference with cyclosporine metabolism may require a dosage adjustment. (See DRUG INTERACTIONS, Sandimmune.)

During treatment with Sandimmune, vaccination may be less effective; and the use of live attenuated vaccines should be avoided.

Information for the Patient

Patients should be advised that any change of cyclosporine formulation should be made cautiously and only under physician supervision because it may result in the need for a change in dosage.

Patients should be informed of the necessity of repeated laboratory tests while they are receiving the drug. They should be given careful dosage instructions, advised of the potential risks during pregnancy, and informed of the increased risk of neoplasia.

Patients using cyclosporine oral solution with its accompanying syringe for dosage measurement should be cautioned not to rinse the syringe either before or after use. Introduction of water into the product by any means will cause variation in dose.

Laboratory Tests

Renal and liver functions should be assessed repeatedly by measurement of BUN, serum creatinine, serum bilirubin, and liver enzymes.

Carcinogenesis, Mutagenesis, and Impairment of Fertility

Cyclosporine gave no evidence of mutagenic or teratogenic effects in appropriate test systems. Only at dose levels toxic to dams, were adverse effects seen in reproduction studies in rats. (See Pregnancy Category C.)

Carcinogenicity studies were carried out in male and female rats and mice. In the 78 week mouse study, at doses of 1, 4, and 16 mg/kg/day, evidence of a statistically significant trend was found for lymphocytic lymphomas in females, and the incidence of hepatocellular carcinomas in mid-dose males significantly exceeded the control value. In the 24 month rat study, conducted at 0.5, 2, and 8 mg/kg/day, pancreatic islet cell adenomas significantly exceeded the control rate in the low dose level. The hepatocellular carcinomas and pancreatic islet cell adenomas were not dose related.

No impairment in fertility was demonstrated in studies in male and female rats.

Cyclosporine has not been found mutagenic/genotoxic in the Ames Test, the V79-HGPRT test, the micronucleus test in mice and Chinese hamsters, the chromosome-aberration tests in Chinese hamster bone-marrow, the mouse dominant lethal assay, and the DNA-repair test in sperm from treated mice. A recent study analyzing sister chromatid exchange (SCE) induction by cyclosporine using human lymphocytes *in vitro* gave indication of a positive effect (*i.e.,* induction of SCE), at high concentrations in this system.

An increased incidence of malignancy is a recognized complication of immunosuppression in recipients of organ transplants. The most common forms of neoplasms are non-Hodgkin's lymphoma and carcinomas of the skin. The risk of malignancies in cyclosporine recipients is higher than in the normal, healthy population but similar to that in patients receiving other immunosuppressive therapies. It has been reported that reduction or discontinuance of immunosuppression may cause the lesions to regress.

Pregnancy Category C

Sandimmune oral solution has been shown to be embryo- and fetotoxic in rats and rabbits when given in doses 2-5 times the human dose. At toxic doses (rats at 30 mg/kg/day and rabbits at 100 mg/kg/day), Sandimmune oral solution was embryo- and fetotoxic as indicated by increased pre- and postnatal mortality and reduced fetal weight together with related skeletal retardations. In the well-tolerated dose range (rats at up to 17 mg/kg/day and rabbits at up to 30 mg/kg/day), Sandimmune oral solution proved to be without any embryolethal or teratogenic effects.

There are no adequate and well-controlled studies in pregnant women. Sandimmune should be used during pregnancy only if the potential benefit justifies the potential risk to the fetus.

The following data represent the reported outcomes of 116 pregnancies in women receiving Sandimmune during pregnancy, 90% of whom were transplant patients, and most of whom received Sandimmune throughout the entire gestational period. Since most of the patients were not prospectively identified, the results are likely to be biased toward negative outcomes. The only consistent patterns of abnormality were premature birth (gestational period of 28-36 weeks) and low birth weight for gestational age. It is not possible to separate the effects of Sandimmune on these pregnancies from the effects of the other immunosuppressants, the underlying maternal disorders, or other aspects of the transplantation milieu. Sixteen (16) fetal losses occurred. Most of the pregnancies (85 of 100) were complicated by disorders; including, pre-eclampsia, eclampsia, premature labor, abruptio placentae, oligohydramnios, Rh incompatibility and fetoplacental dysfunction. Preterm delivery occurred in 47%. Seven (7) malformations were reported in 5 viable infants and in 2 cases of fetal loss. Twenty-eight percent (28%) of the infants were small for gestational age. Neonatal complications occurred in 27%. In a report of 23 children followed up to 4 years, postnatal development was said to be normal. More information on cyclosporine use in pregnancy is available from Novartis Pharmaceuticals Corporation.

Nursing Mothers

Since Sandimmune is excreted in human milk, nursing should be avoided.

Pediatric Use

Although no adequate and well-controlled studies have been conducted in children, patients as young as 6 months of age have received the drug with no unusual adverse effects.

RESTASIS

General

For ophthalmic use only.

Information for the Patient

The emulsion from 1 individual single-use vial is to be used immediately after opening for administration to 1 or both eyes, and the remaining contents should be discarded immediately after administration.

Do not allow the tip of the vial to touch the eye or any surface, as this may contaminate the emulsion.

Restasis should not be administered while wearing contact lenses. Patients with decreased tear production typically should not wear contact lenses. If contact lenses are worn, they should be removed prior to the administration of the emulsion. Lenses may be reinserted 15 minutes following administration of Restasis ophthalmic emulsion.

Carcinogenesis, Mutagenesis, and Impairment of Fertility

Systemic carcinogenicity studies were carried out in male and female mice and rats. In the 78 week oral (diet) mouse study, at doses of 1, 4, and 16 mg/kg/day, evidence of a statistically significant trend was found for lymphocytic lymphomas in females, and the incidence of hepatocellular carcinomas in mid-dose males significantly exceeded the control value.

C

In the 24 month oral (diet) rat study, conducted at 0.5, 2, and 8 mg/kg/day, pancreatic islet cell adenomas significantly exceeded the control rate in the low dose level. The hepatocellular carcinomas and pancreatic islet cell adenomas were not dose related. The low doses in mice and rats are approximately 1000 and 500 times greater, respectively, than the daily human dose of 1 drop (28 µl) of 0.05% Restasis bid into each eye of a 60 kg person (0.001 mg/kg/day), assuming that the entire dose is absorbed.

Cyclosporine has not been found mutagenic/genotoxic in the Ames Test, the V79-HGPRT Test, the micronucleus test in mice and Chinese hamsters, the chromosome-aberration tests in Chinese hamster bone-marrow, the mouse dominant lethal assay, and the DNA-repair test in sperm from treated mice. A study analyzing sister chromatid exchange (SCE) induction by cyclosporine using human lymphocytes *in vitro* gave indication of a positive effect (*i.e.*, induction of SCE).

No impairment in fertility was demonstrated in studies in male and female rats receiving oral doses of cyclosporine up to 15 mg/kg/day (approximately 15,000 times the human daily dose of 0.001 mg/kg/day) for 9 weeks (male) and 2 weeks (female) prior to mating.

Pregnancy, Teratogenic Effects

Pregnancy Category C

Teratogenic Effects

No evidence of teratogenicity was observed in rats or rabbits receiving oral doses of cyclosporine up to 300 mg/kg/day during organogenesis. These doses in rats and rabbits are approximately 300,000 times greater than the daily human dose of 1 drop (28 µl) 0.05% Restasis bid into each eye of a 60 kg person (0.001 mg/kg/day), assuming that the entire dose is absorbed.

Nonteratogenic Effects

Adverse effects were seen in reproduction studies in rats and rabbits only at dose levels toxic to dams. At toxic doses (rats at 30 mg/kg/day and rabbits at 100 mg/kg/day), cyclosporine oral solution was embryo- and fetotoxic as indicated by increased pre- and postnatal mortality and reduced fetal weight together with related skeletal retardations. These doses are 30,000 and 100,000 times greater, respectively than the daily human dose of 1 drop (28 µl) of 0.05% Restasis bid into each eye of a 60 kg person (0.001 mg/kg/day), assuming that the entire dose is absorbed. No evidence of embryofetal toxicity was observed in rats or rabbits receiving cyclosporine at oral doses up to 17/mg/kg/day or 30 mg/kg/day, respectively, during organogenesis. These doses in rats and rabbits are approximately 17,000 and 30,000 times greater, respectively, than the daily human dose.

Offspring of rats receiving a 45 mg/kg/day oral dose of cyclosporine from Day 15 of pregnancy until Day 21 post partum, a maternally toxic level, exhibited an increase in postnatal mortality; this dose is 45,000 times greater than the daily human topical dose, 0.001 mg/kg/day, assuming that the entire dose is absorbed. No adverse events were observed at oral doses up to 15 mg/kg/day (15,000 times greater than the daily human dose).

There are no adequate and well-controlled studies of Restasis in pregnant women. Restasis should be administered to a pregnant woman only if clearly needed.

Nursing Mothers

Cyclosporine is known to be excreted in human milk following systemic administration but excretion in human milk after topical treatment has not been investigated. Although blood concentrations are undetectable after topical administration of Restasis ophthalmic emulsion, caution should be exercised when Restasis is administered to a nursing woman.

Pediatric Use

The safety and efficacy of Restasis ophthalmic emulsion have not been established in pediatric patients below the age of 16.

Geriatric Use

No overall difference in safety or effectiveness has been observed between elderly and younger patients.

DRUG INTERACTIONS

NEORAL

All of the individual drugs cited below are well substantiated to interact with cyclosporine. In addition, concomitant non-steroidal anti-inflammatory drugs, particularly in the setting of dehydration, may potentiate renal dysfunction.

Drugs That May Potentiate Renal Dysfunction

Antibiotics: Gentamicin, tobramycin, vancomycin, trimethoprim with sulfamethoxazole.
Antineoplastics: Melphalan.
Antifungals: Amphotericin B, ketoconazole.
Anti-Inflammatory Drugs: Azapropazon, diclofenac, naproxen, sulindac, colchicine.
Gastrointestinal Agents: Cimetidine, ranitidine.
Immunosuppressives: Tacrolimus.

Drugs That Alter Cyclosporine Concentrations

Compounds that decrease cyclosporine absorption such as orlistat should be avoided. Cyclosporine is extensively metabolized cytochrome P-450 3A. Substances that inhibit this enzyme could decrease metabolism and increase cyclosporine concentrations. Substances that are inducers of cytochrome P-450 activity could increase metabolism and decrease cyclosporine concentrations. Monitoring of circulating cyclosporine concentrations and appropriate Neoral dosage adjustment are essential when these drugs are used concomitantly. (See DOSAGE AND ADMINISTRATION, Neoral, Blood Concentration Monitoring in Transplant Patients.)

Drugs That Increase Cyclosporine Concentrations

Calcium Channel Blockers: Diltiazem, nicardipine, verapamil.
Antifungals: Fluconazole, itraconazole, ketoconazole.
Antibiotics: Clarithromycin, erythromycin, quinupristin/daldopristin.
Glucocorticoids: Methylprednisolone.
Other Drugs: Allopurinol, bromocriptine, danazol, metoclopramide, colchicine, amiodarone.

The HIV protease inhibitors (*e.g.*, indinavir, nelfinavir, ritonavir, and saquinavir) are known to inhibit cytochrome P-450 3A and thus could potentially increase the concentrations of cyclosporine, however no formal studies of the interaction are available. Care should be exercised when these drugs are administered concomitantly.

Grapefruit and grapefruit juice affect metabolism, increasing blood concentrations of cyclosporine, thus should be avoided.

Drugs/Dietary Supplements That Decrease Cyclosporine Concentrations

Antibiotics: Nafcillin, rifampin.
Anticonvulsants: Carbamazepine, phenobarbital, phenytoin.
Other Drugs: Octreotide, ticlopidine, orlistat, St. John's Wort.

There have been reports of a serious drug interaction between cyclosporine and the herbal dietary supplement, St. John's Wort. This interaction has been reported to produce a marked reduction in the blood concentrations of cyclosporine, resulting in subtherapeutic levels, rejection of transplanted organs, and graft loss.

Rifabutin is known to increase the metabolism of other drugs metabolized by the cytochrome P-450 system. The interaction between rifabutin and cyclosporine has not been studied. Care should be exercised when these 2 drugs are administered concomitantly.

Nonsteroidal Anti-Inflammatory Drug (NSAID) Interactions

Clinical status and serum creatinine should be closely monitored when cyclosporine is used with nonsteroidal anti-inflammatory agents in rheumatoid arthritis patients. (See WARNINGS, Neoral.)

Pharmacodynamic interactions have been reported to occur between cyclosporine and both naproxen and sulindac, in that concomitant use is associated with additive decreases in renal function, as determined by 99 mTc-diethylenetriaminepentaacetic acid (DTPA) and (p-aminohippuric acid) PAH clearances. Although concomitant administration of diclofenac does not affect blood levels of cyclosporine, it has been associated with approximate doubling of diclofenac blood levels and occasional reports of reversible decreases in renal function. Consequently, the dose of diclofenac should be in the lower end of the therapeutic range.

Methotrexate Interaction

Preliminary data indicate that when methotrexate and cyclosporine were coadministered to rheumatoid arthritis patients (n=20), methotrexate concentrations (AUCs) were increased approximately 30% and the concentrations (AUCs) of its metabolite, 7-hydroxy methotrexate, were decreased by approximately 80%. The clinical significance of this interaction is not known. Cyclosporine concentrations do not appear to have been altered (n=6).

Other Drug Interactions

Reduced clearance of prednisolone, digoxin, and lovastatin has been observed when these drugs are administered with cyclosporine. In addition, a decrease in the apparent volume of distribution of digoxin has been reported after cyclosporine administration. Severe digitalis toxicity has been seen within days of starting cyclosporine in several patients taking digoxin. Cyclosporine should not be used with potassium-sparing diuretics because hyperkalemia can occur.

During treatment with cyclosporine, vaccination may be less effective. The use of live vaccines should be avoided. Myositis has occurred with concomitant lovastatin, frequent gingival hyperplasia with nifedipine, and convulsions with high dose methylprednisolone.

Psoriasis patients receiving other immunosuppressive agents or radiation therapy (including PUVA and UVB) should not receive concurrent cyclosporine because of the possibility of excessive immunosuppression.

For additional information on Cyclosporine Drug Interactions please contact Novartis Medical Affairs Department at 888-NOW-NOVA (888-669-6682).

SANDIMMUNE

All of the individual drugs cited below are well substantiated to interact with cyclosporine. In addition, concomitant non-steroidal anti-inflammatory drugs, particularly in the setting of dehydration, may potentiate renal dysfunction.

Drugs That May Potentiate Renal Dysfunction:

Antibiotics: Gentamicin, tobramycin, vancomycin, trimethoprim with sulfamethoxazole.
Antineoplastic: Melphalan.
Antifungals: Amphotericin B, ketoconazole.
Anti-Inflammatory Drugs: Azapropazon, diclofenac, naproxen, sulindac, colchicine.
Gastrointestinal Agents: Cimetidine, ranitidine.
Immunosuppressives: Tacrolimus.

Careful monitoring of renal function should be practiced when Sandimmune is used with nephrotoxic drugs.

Drugs That Alter Cyclosporine Concentrations

Compounds that decrease cyclosporine absorption such as orlistat should be avoided. Cyclosporine is extensively metabolized by cytochrome P-450 3A. Substances that inhibit this enzyme could decrease metabolism and increase cyclosporine concentrations. Substances that are inducers of cytochrome P-450 activity could increase metabolism and decrease cyclosporine concentrations. Monitoring of circulating cyclosporine concentrations and appropriate Sandimmune dosage adjustment are essential when these drugs are used concomitantly. (See DOSAGE AND ADMINISTRATION, Blood Level Monitoring.)

Drugs That Increase Cyclosporine Concentrations:

Calcium Channel Blockers: Diltiazem, nicardipine, verapamil.

Antifungals: Fluconazole, itraconazole, ketoconazole.

Antibiotics: Clarithromycin, erythromycin, quinupristin/dalfopristin.

Glucorticoids: Methylprednisolone.

Other Drugs: Allopurinol, bromocriptine, danazol, metoclopromide, colchicine, amiodarone.

The HIV protease inhibitors (*e.g.,* indinavir, nelfinavir, ritonavir, and saquinavir) are known to inhibit cytochrome P-450 3A and thus could potentially increase the concentrations of cyclosporine, however no formal studies of the interaction are available. Care should be exercised when these drugs are administered concomitantly.

Grapefruit and grapefruit juice affect metabolism, increasing blood concentrations of cyclosporine, thus should be avoided.

Drugs/Dietary Supplements That Decrease Cyclosporine Concentrations:

Antibiotics: Nafcillin, rifampin.

Anticonvulsants: Carbamazepine, phenobarbital, phenytoin.

Other Drugs/Dietary Supplements: Octreotide, ticlopidine, orlistat, St. John's Wort.

There have been reports of a serious drug interaction between cyclosporine and the herbal dietary supplement, St. John's Wort. This interaction has been reported to produce a marked reduction in the blood concentrations of cyclosporine, resulting in subtherapeutic levels, rejection of transplanted organs, and graft loss.

Rifabutin is known to increase the metabolism of other drugs metabolized by the cytochrome P-450 system. The interaction between rifabutin and cyclosporine has not been studied. Care should be exercised when these 2 drugs are administered concomitantly.

Nonsteroidal Anti-Inflammatory Drug (NSAID) Interactions

Clinical status and serum creatinine should be closely monitored when cyclosporine is used with nonsteroidal anti-inflammatory agents in rheumatoid arthritis patients. (See WARNINGS, Sandimmune.)

Pharmacodynamic interactions have been reported to occur between cyclosporine and both naproxen and sulindac, in that concomitant use is associated with additive decreases in renal function, as determined by ^{99m}Tc-diethylenetriaminepentaacetic acid (DTPA) and (*p*-aminohippuric acid) PAH clearances. Although concomitant administration of diclofenac does not affect blood levels of cyclosporine, it has been associated with approximate doubling of diclofenac blood levels and occasional reports of reversible decreases in renal function. Consequently, the dose of diclofenac should be in the lower end of the therapeutic range.

Methotrexate Interaction

Preliminary data indicate that when methotrexate and cyclosporine were coadministered to rheumatoid arthritis patients (n=20), methotrexate concentrations (AUCs) were increased approximately 30% and the concentrations (AUCs) of its metabolite, 7-hydroxy methotrexate, were decreased by approximately 80%. The clinical significance of this interaction is not known. Cyclosporine concentrations do not appear to have been altered (n=6).

Other Drug Interactions

Reduced clearance of prednisolone, digoxin, and lovastatin has been observed when these drugs are administered with cyclosporine. In addition, a decrease in the apparent volume of distribution of digoxin has been reported after cyclosporine administration. Severe digitalis toxicity has been seen within days of starting cyclosporine in several patients taking digoxin. Cyclosporine should not be used with potassium-sparing diuretics because hyperkalemia can occur.

During treatment with cyclosporine, vaccination may be less effective. The use of live vaccines should be avoided. Myositis has occurred with concomitant lovastatin, frequent gingival hyperplasia with nifedipine, and convulsions with high dose methylprednisolone.

Psoriasis patients receiving other immunosuppressive agents or radiation therapy (including PUVA and UVB) should not receive concurrent cyclosporine because of the possibility of excessive immunosuppression.

For additional information on Cyclosporine Drug Interactions please contact Novartis Medical Affairs Department at 888-NOW-NOVA (888-669-6682).

ADVERSE REACTIONS

NEORAL

Kidney, Liver, and Heart Transplantation

The principal adverse reactions of cyclosporine therapy are renal dysfunction, tremor, hirsutism, hypertension, and gum hyperplasia.

Hypertension, which is usually mild to moderate, may occur in approximately 50% of patients following renal transplantation and in most cardiac transplant patients.

Glomerular capillary thrombosis has been found in patients treated with cyclosporine and may progress to graft failure. The pathologic changes resembled those seen in the hemolytic-uremic syndrome and included thrombosis of the renal microvasculature, with platelet-fibrin thrombi occluding glomerular capillaries and afferent arterioles, microangiopathic hemolytic anemia, thrombocytopenia, and decreased renal function. Similar findings have been observed when other immunosuppressives have been employed post-transplantation.

Hypomagnesemia has been reported in some, but not all, patients exhibiting convulsions while on cyclosporine therapy. Although magnesium-depletion studies in normal subjects suggest that hypomagnesemia is associated with neurologic disorders, multiple factors, including hypertension, high dose methylprednisolone, hypocholesterolemia, and nephrotoxicity associated with high plasma concentrations of cyclosporine appear to be related to the neurological manifestations of cyclosporine toxicity.

In controlled studies, the nature, severity, and incidence of the adverse events that were observed in 493 transplanted patients treated with Neoral were comparable with those observed in 208 transplanted patients who received Sandimmune in these same studies when the dosage of the 2 drugs was adjusted to achieve the same cyclosporine blood trough concentrations.

Based on the historical experience with Sandimmune, the following reactions occurred in 3% or greater of 892 patients involved in clinical trials of kidney, heart, and liver transplants.

TABLE 3

Body System/Adverse Reactions	Randomized Kidney Patients		Cyclosporine Patients*		
	Sandimmune (n=277)	Azathioprine (n=228)	Kidney (n=705)	Heart (n=112)	Liver (n=75)
Genitourinary					
Renal dysfunction	32%	6%	25%	38%	37%
Cardiovascular					
Hypertension	26%	18%	13%	53%	27%
Cramps	4%	<1%	2%	<1%	0%
Skin					
Hirsutism	2%	<1%	21%	28%	45%
Acne	6%	8%	2%	2%	1%
Central Nervous System					
Tremor	12%	0%	21%	31%	55%
Convulsions	3%	1%	1%	4%	5%
Headache	2%	<1%	2%	15%	4%
Gastrointestinal					
Gum hyperplasia	4%	0%	9%	5%	16%
Diarrhea	3%	<1%	3%	4%	8%
Nausea/vomiting	2%	<1%	4%	10%	4%
Hepatotoxicity	<1%	<1%	4%	7%	4%
Abdominal discomfort	<1%	0%	<1%	7%	0%
Autonomic Nervous System					
Paresthesia	3%	0%	1%	2%	1%
Flushing	<1%	0%	4%	0%	4%
Hematopoietic					
Leukopenia	2%	19	<1%	6%	0%
Lymphoma	<1%	0%	1%	6%	1%
Respiratory					
Sinusitis	<1%	0%	4%	3%	7%
Miscellaneous					
Gynecomastia	<1%	0%	<1%	4%	3%

* Sandimmune.

Among 705 kidney transplant patients treated with Sandimmune in clinical trials, the reason for treatment discontinuation was renal toxicity in 5.4%, infection in 0.9%, lack of efficacy in 1.4%, acute tubular necrosis in 1.0%, lymphoproliferative disorders in 0.3%, hypertension in 0.3%, and other reasons in 0.7% of the patients.

The following reactions occurred in 2% or less of Sandimmune-treated patients: Allergic reactions, anemia, anorexia, confusion, conjunctivitis, edema, fever, brittle fingernails, gastritis, hearing loss, hiccups, hyperglycemia, muscle pain, peptic ulcer, thrombocytopenia, tinnitus.

The following reactions occurred rarely: Anxiety, chest pain, constipation, depression, hair breaking, hematuria, joint pain, lethargy, mouth sores, myocardial infarction, night sweats, pancreatitis, pruritus, swallowing difficulty, tingling, upper GI bleeding, visual disturbance, weakness, weight loss.

TABLE 4 *Infectious Complications in Historical Randomized Studies in Renal Transplant Patients Using Sandimmune*

Complication	Cyclosporine Treatment (n=227)	Azathioprine with Steroids* (n=228)
Septicemia	5.3%	4.8%
Abscesses	4.4%	5.3%
Systemic fungal infection	2.2%	3.9%
Local fungal infection	7.5%	9.6%
Cytomegalovirus	4.8%	12.3%
Other viral infections	15.9%	18.4%
Urinary tract infections	21.1%	20.2%
Wound and skin infections	7.0%	10.1%
Pneumonia	6.2%	9.2%

* Some patients also received ALG.

Rheumatoid Arthritis

The principal adverse reactions associated with the use of cyclosporine in rheumatoid arthritis are renal dysfunction (see WARNINGS, Neoral), hypertension (see PRECAUTIONS, Neoral), headache, gastrointestinal disturbances, and hirsutism/hypertrichosis.

In rheumatoid arthritis patients treated in clinical trials within the recommended dose range, cyclosporine therapy was discontinued in 5.3% of the patients because of hypertension and in 7% of the patients because of increased creatinine. These changes are usually reversible with timely dose decrease or drug discontinuation. The frequency and severity of serum creatinine elevations increase with dose and duration of cyclosporine therapy. These elevations are likely to become more pronounced without dose reduction or discontinuation.

The adverse events listed in TABLE 5A and TABLE 5B occurred in controlled clinical trials.

In addition, the following adverse events have been reported in 1% to <3% of the rheumatoid arthritis patients in the cyclosporine treatment group in controlled clinical trials:

Autonomic Nervous System: Dry mouth, increased sweating.

C

TABLE 5A *Neoral/Sandimmune Rheumatoid Arthritis — Percentage of Patients With Adverse Events ≥3% in any Cyclosporine Treated Group*

	Sandimmune		Methotrexate & Sandimmune
Body System/Preferred Term	**(n=269)*†**	**(n=155)‡**	**(n=74)§**
Autonomic Nervous System Disorders			
Flushing	2%	2%	3%
Body as a Whole — General Disorders			
Accidental trauma	0%	1%	10%
Edema NOS¤	5%	14%	12%
Fatigue	6%	3%	8%
Fever	2%	3%	0%
Influenza-like symptoms	<1%	6%	1%
Pain	6%	9%	10%
Rigors	1%	1%	4%
Cardiovascular Disorders			
Arrhythmia	2%	5%	5%
Chest pain	4%	5%	1%
Hypertension	8%	26%	16%
Central and Peripheral Nervous System Disorders			
Dizziness	8%	6%	7%
Headache	17%	23%	22%
Migraine	2%	3%	0%
Paresthesia	8%	7%	8%
Tremor	8%	7%	7%
Gastrointestinal System Disorders			
Abdominal pain	15%	15%	15%
Anorexia	3%	3%	1%
Diarrhea	12%	12%	18%
Dyspepsia	12%	12%	10%
Flatulence	5%	5%	5%
Gastrointestinal disorder NOS¤	0%	2%	1%
Gingivitis	4%	3%	0%
Gum hyperplasia	2%	4%	1%
Nausea	23%	14%	24%
Rectal hemorrhage	0%	3%	0%
Stomatitis	7%	5%	16%
Vomiting	9%	8%	14%
Hearing and Vestibular Disorders			
Ear disorder NOS¤	0%	5%	0%
Metabolic and Nutritional Disorders			
Hypomagnesemia	0%	4%	0%
Musculoskeletal System Disorders			
Arthropathy	0%	5%	0%
Leg cramps/involuntary muscle contractions	2%	11%	11%
Psychiatric Disorders			
Depression	3%	6%	3%
Insomnia	4%	1%	1%
Renal			
Creatinine elevations ≥30%	43%	39%	55%
Creatinine elevations ≥50%	24%	18%	26%
Reproductive Disorders, Female			
Leukorrhea	1%	0%	4%
Menstrual disorder	3%	2%	1%
Respiratory System Disorders			
Bronchitis	1%	3%	1%
Coughing	5%	3%	5%
Dyspnea	5%	1%	3%
Infection NOS¤	9%	5%	0%
Pharyngitis	3%	5%	5%
Pneumonia	1%	0%	4%
Rhinitis	0%	3%	11%
Sinusitis	4%	4%	8%
Upper respiratory tract	0%	14%	23%
Skin and Appendages Disorders			
Alopecia	3%	0%	1%
Bullous eruption	1%	0%	4%
Hypertrichosis	19%	17%	12%
Rash	7%	12%	10%
Skin ulceration	1%	1%	3%
Urinary System Disorders			
Dysuria	0%	0%	11%
Micturition frequency	2%	4%	3%
NPN, increased	0%	19%	12%
Urinary tract infection	0%	3%	5%
Vascular (extracardiac) Disorders			
Purpura	3%	4%	1%

* Includes patients in 2.5 mg/kg/day dose group only.
† Studies 651 + 652 + 2008.
‡ Study 302.
§ Study 654.
¤ NOS = Not Otherwise Specified.

Body as a Whole: Allergy, asthenia, hot flushes, malaise, overdose, procedure NOS*, tumor NOS*, weight decrease, weight increase.

Cardiovascular: Abnormal heart sounds, cardiac failure, myocardial infarction, peripheral ischemia.

Central and Peripheral Nervous System: Hypoesthesia, neuropathy, vertigo.

Endocrine: Goiter.

Gastrointestinal: Constipation, dysphagia, enanthema, eructation, esophagitis, gastric ulcer, gastritis, gastroenteritis, gingival bleeding, glossitis, peptic ulcer, salivary gland enlargement, tongue disorder, tooth disorder.

Infection: Abscess, bacterial infection, cellulitis, folliculitis, fungal infection, herpes simplex, herpes zoster, renal abscess, moniliasis, tonsillitis, viral infection.

Hematologic: Anemia, epistaxis, leukopenia, lymphadenopathy.

Liver and Biliary System: Bilirubinemia.

TABLE 5B *Neoral/Sandimmune Rheumatoid Arthritis — Percentage of Patients With Adverse Events ≥3% in any Cyclosporine Treated Group*

Body System/Preferred Term	Methotrexate & Placebo (n=73)*	Neoral (n=143)†	Placebo (n=201)‡
Autonomic Nervous System Disorders			
Flushing	0%	5%	2%
Body as a Whole — General Disorders			
Accidental trauma	4%	4%	0%
Edema NOS§	4%	10%	<1%
Fatigue	12%	3%	7%
Fever	0%	2%	4%
Influenza-like symptoms	0%	3%	2%
Pain	15%	13%	4%
Rigors	0%	3%	1%
Cardiovascular Disorders			
Arrhythmia	6%	2%	1%
Chest pain	1%	6%	1%
Hypertension	12%	25%	2%
Central and Peripheral Nervous System Disorders			
Dizziness	3%	8%	3%
Headache	11%	25%	9%
Migraine	0%	3%	1%
Paresthesia	4%	11%	1%
Tremor	3%	13%	4%
Gastrointestinal System Disorders			
Abdominal pain	7%	15%	10%
Anorexia	0%	3%	3%
Diarrhea	15%	13%	8%
Dyspepsia	8%	8%	4%
Flatulence	4%	4%	1%
Gastrointestinal disorder NOS§	4%	4%	0%
Gingivitis	0%	0%	1%
Gum hyperplasia	3%	4%	1%
Nausea	15%	18%	14%
Rectal hemorrhage	0%	1%	1%
Stomatitis	12%	6%	8%
Vomiting	7%	6%	5%
Hearing and Vestibular Disorders			
Ear disorder NOS§	0%	1%	0%
Metabolic and Nutritional Disorders			
Hypomagnesemia	0%	6%	0%
Musculoskeletal System Disorders			
Arthropathy	1%	4%	0%
Leg cramps/involuntary muscle contractions	3%	12%	1%
Psychiatric Disorders			
Depression	1%	1%	2%
Insomnia	0%	3%	2%
Renal			
Creatinine elevations ≥30%	19%	48%	13%
Creatinine elevations ≥50%	8%	18%	3%
Reproductive Disorders, Female			
Leukorrhea	0%	1%	0%
Menstrual disorder	0%	1%	1%
Respiratory System Disorders			
Bronchitis	0%	1%	3%
Coughing	7%	4%	4%
Dyspnea	3%	1%	2%
Infection NOS§	7%	3%	10%
Pharyngitis	6%	4%	4%
Pneumonia	0%	1%	1%
Rhinitis	10%	1%	0%
Sinusitis	4%	3%	3%
Upper respiratory tract	15%	13%	0%
Skin and Appendages Disorders			
Alopecia	1%	4%	4%
Bullous eruption	1%	1%	1%
Hypertrichosis	0%	15%	3%
Rash	7%	8%	10%
Skin ulceration	4%	0%	2%
Urinary System Disorders			
Dysuria	3%	1%	2%
Micturition frequency	1%	2%	2%
NPN, increased	0%	18%	0%
Urinary tract infection	4%	3%	0%
Vascular (extracardiac) Disorders			
Purpura	1%	2%	0%

* Study 654.
† Study 302.
‡ Studies 651 + 652 + 2008.
§ NOS = Not Otherwise Specified.

Metabolic and Nutritional: Diabetes mellitus, hyperkalemia, hyperuricemia, hypoglycemia.

Musculoskeletal System: Arthralgia, bone fracture, bursitis, joint dislocation, myalgia, stiffness, synovial cyst, tendon disorder.

Neoplasms: Breast fibroadenosis, carcinoma.

Psychiatric: Anxiety, confusion, decreased libido, emotional lability, impaired concentration, increased libido, nervousness, paroniria, somnolence.

Reproductive (female): Breast pain, uterine hemorrhage.

Respiratory System: Abnormal chest sounds, bronchospasm.

Skin and Appendages: Abnormal pigmentation, angioedema, dermatitis, dry skin, eczema, nail disorder, pruritus, skin disorder, urticaria.

Special Senses: Abnormal vision, cataract, conjunctivitis, deafness, eye pain, taste perversion, tinnitus, vestibular disorder.

Urinary System: Abnormal urine, hematuria, increased BUN, micturition urgency, nocturia, polyuria, pyelonephritis, urinary incontinence.

*NOS = Not Otherwise Specified.

Psoriasis

The principal adverse reactions associated with the use of cyclosporine in patients with psoriasis are renal dysfunction, headache, hypertension, hypertriglyceridemia, hirsutism/hypertrichosis, paresthesia or hyperesthesia, influenza-like symptoms, nausea/vomiting, diarrhea, abdominal discomfort, lethargy, and musculoskeletal or joint pain.

In psoriasis patients treated in US controlled clinical studies within the recommended dose range, cyclosporine therapy was discontinued in 1.0% of the patients because of hypertension and in 5.4% of the patients because of increased creatinine. In the majority of cases, these changes were reversible after dose reduction or discontinuation of cyclosporine.

There has been 1 reported death associated with the use of cyclosporine in psoriasis. A 27-year-old male developed renal deterioration and was continued on cyclosporine. He had progressive renal failure leading to death.

Frequency and severity of serum creatinine increases with dose and duration of cyclosporine therapy. These elevations are likely to become more pronounced and may result in irreversible renal damage without dose reduction or discontinuation.

TABLE 6 *Adverse Events Occurring in 3% or More of Psoriasis Patients in Controlled Clinical Trials*

Body System*/Preferred Term	Neoral (n=182)	Sandimmune (n=185)
Infection or Potential Infection	24.7%	24.3%
Influenza-like symptoms	9.9%	8.1%
Upper respiratory tract infections	7.7%	11.3%
Cardiovascular System	28.0%	25.4%
Hypertension†	27.5%	25.4%
Urinary System	24.2%	16.2%
Increased creatinine	19.8%	15.7%
Central and Peripheral Nervous System	26.4%	20.5%
Headache	15.9%	14.0%
Paresthesia	7.1%	4.8%
Musculoskeletal System	13.2%	8.7%
Arthralgia	6.0%	1.1%
Body as a Whole — General	29.1%	22.2%
Pain	4.4%	3.2%
Metabolic and Nutritional	9.3%	9.7%
Reproductive, Female	8.5% (4 of 47 females)	11.5% (6 of 52 females)
Resistance Mechanism	18.7%	21.1%
Skin and Appendages	17.6%	15.1%
Hypertrichosis	6.6%	5.4%
Respiratory System	5.0%	6.5%
Bronchospasm, coughing, dyspnea, rhinitis	5.0%	4.9%
Psychiatric	5.0%	3.8%
Gastrointestinal System	19.8%	28.7%
Abdominal pain	2.7%	6.0%
Diarrhea	5.0%	5.9%
Dyspepsia	2.2%	3.2%
Gum hyperplasia	3.8%	6.0%
Nausea	5.5%	5.9%
White Cell and RES	4.4%	2.7%

* Total % of events within the system.
† Newly occurring hypertension = SBP ≥160 mm Hg and/or DBP ≥90 mm Hg.

The following events occurred in 1% to less than 3% of psoriasis patients treated with cyclosporine:

Body as a Whole: Fever, flushes, hot flushes.

Cardiovascular: Chest pain.

Central and Peripheral Nervous System: Appetite increased, insomnia, dizziness, nervousness, vertigo.

Gastrointestinal: Abdominal distention, constipation, gingival bleeding.

Liver and Biliary System: Hyperbilirubinemia.

Neoplasms: Skin malignancies [squamous cell (0.9%) and basal cell (0.4%) carcinomas].

Reticuloendothelial: Platelet, bleeding, and clotting disorders, red blood cell disorder.

Respiratory: Infection, viral and other infection.

Skin and Appendages: Acne, folliculitis, keratosis, pruritus, rash, dry skin.

Urinary System: Micturition frequency.

Vision: Abnormal vision.

Mild hypomagnesemia and hyperkalemia may occur but are asymptomatic. Increases in uric acid may occur and attacks of gout have been rarely reported. A minor and dose related hyperbilirubinemia has been observed in the absence of hepatocellular damage. Cyclosporine therapy may be associated with a modest increase of serum triglycerides or cholesterol. Elevations of triglycerides (>750 mg/dl) occur in about 15% of psoriasis patients; elevations of cholesterol (>300 mg/dl) are observed in less than 3% of psoriasis patients. Generally these laboratory abnormalities are reversible upon dose reduction or discontinuation of cyclosporine.

SANDIMMUNE

The principal adverse reactions of Sandimmune therapy are renal dysfunction, tremor, hirsutism, hypertension, and gum hyperplasia.

Hypertension, which is usually mild to moderate, may occur in approximately 50% of patients following renal transplantation and in most cardiac transplant patients.

Glomerular capillary thrombosis has been found in patients treated with cyclosporine and may progress to graft failure. The pathologic changes resemble those seen in the hemolytic-uremic syndrome and include thrombosis of the renal microvasculature, with platelet-fibrin thrombi occluding glomerular capillaries and afferent arterioles, microangiopathic hemolytic anemia, thrombocytopenia, and decreased renal function. Similar findings have been observed when other immunosuppressives have been employed posttransplantation.

Hypomagnesemia has been reported in some, but not all, patients exhibiting convulsions while on cyclosporine therapy. Although magnesium-depletion studies in normal subjects suggest that hypomagnesemia is associated with neurologic disorders, multiple factors, including hypertension, high dose methylprednisolone, hypocholesterolemia, and nephrotoxicity associated with high plasma concentrations of cyclosporine appear to be related to the neurological manifestations of cyclosporine toxicity.

The reactions shown in TABLE 7 occurred in 3% or greater of 892 patients involved in clinical trials of kidney, heart, and liver transplants.

TABLE 7

Body System/ Adverse Reactions	Randomized Kidney Patients: Sandimmune (n=227)	Randomized Kidney Patients: Azathioprine (n=228)	All Sandimmune Patients: Kidney (n=705)	All Sandimmune Patients: Heart (n=112)	All Sandimmune Patients: Liver (n=75)
Genitourinary					
Renal dysfunction	32%	6%	25%	38%	37%
Cardiovascular					
Hypertension	26%	18%	13%	53%	27%
Cramps	4%	<1%	2%	<1%	0%
Skin					
Hirsutism	21%	<1%	21%	28%	45%
Acne	6%	8%	2%	2%	1%
Central Nervous System					
Tremor	12%	0%	21%	31%	55%
Convulsions	3%	1%	1%	4%	5%
Headache	2%	<1%	2%	15%	4%
Gastrointestinal					
Gum hyperplasia	4%	0%	9%	5%	16%
Diarrhea	3%	<1%	3%	4%	8%
Nausea/vomiting	2%	<1%	4%	10%	4%
Hepatotoxicity	<1%	<1%	4%	7%	4%
Abdominal discomfort	<1%	0%	<1%	7%	0%
Autonomic Nervous System					
Paresthesia	3%	0%	1%	2%	1%
Flushing	<1%	0%	4%	0%	4%
Hematopoietic					
Leukopenia	2%	19%	<1%	6%	0%
Lymphoma	<1%	0%	1%	6%	1%
Respiratory					
Sinusitis	<1%	0%	4%	3%	7%
Miscellaneous					
Gynecomastia	<1%	0%	<1%	4%	3%

The following reactions occurred in 2% or less of patients: Allergic reactions, anemia, anorexia, confusion, conjunctivitis, edema, fever, brittle fingernails, gastritis, hearing loss, hiccups, hyperglycemia, muscle pain, peptic ulcer, thrombocytopenia, tinnitus.

The following reactions occurred rarely: Anxiety, chest pain, constipation, depression, hair breaking, hematuria, joint pain, lethargy, mouth sores, myocardial infarction, night sweats, pancreatitis, pruritus, swallowing difficulty, tingling, upper GI bleeding, visual disturbance, weakness, weight loss.

TABLE 8 *Renal Transplant Patients in Whom Therapy Was Discontinued*

Reason for Discontinuation	Randomized Patients: Sandimmune (n=227)	Randomized Patients: Azathioprine (n=228)	All Sandimmune Patients (n=705)
Renal toxicity	5.7%	0%	5.4%
Infection	0%	0.4%	0.9%
Lack of efficacy	2.6%	0.9%	1.4%
Acute tubular necrosis	2.6%	0%	1.0%
Lymphoma/lymphoproliferative disease	0.4%	0%	0.3%
Hypertension	0%	0%	0.3%
Hematological abnormalities	0%	0.4%	0%
Other	0%	0%	0.7%

Sandimmune was discontinued on a temporary basis and then restarted in 18 additional patients.

TABLE 9 *Infectious Complications in the Randomized Renal Transplant Patients*

Complication	Sandimmune Treatment (n=227)	Standard Treatment* (n=228)
Septicemia	5.3%	4.8%
Abscesses	4.4%	5.3%
Systemic fungal infection	2.2%	3.9%
Local fungal infection	7.5%	9.6%
Cytomegalovirus	4.8%	12.3%
Other viral infections	15.9%	18.4%
Urinary tract infections	21.1%	20.2%
Wound and skin infections	7.0%	10.1%
Pneumonia	6.2%	9.2%

* Some patients also received ALG.

Cremophor EL (polyoxyethylated castor oil) is known to cause hyperlipemia and electrophoretic abnormalities of lipoproteins. These effects are reversible upon discontinuation of treatment but are usually not a reason to stop treatment.

RESTASIS

Restasis Ophthalmic Emulsion

The most common adverse event following the use of Restasis was ocular burning (17%).

Other events reported in 1- 5% of patients included conjunctival hyperemia, discharge, epiphora, eye pain, foreign body sensation, pruritus, stinging, and visual disturbance (most often blurring).

DOSAGE AND ADMINISTRATION

NEORAL

Neoral Soft Gelatin Capsules MODIFIED and Neoral Oral Solution MODIFIED

Neoral has increased bioavailability in comparison to Sandimmune. Neoral and Sandimmune are not bioequivalent and cannot be used interchangeably without physician supervision.

The daily dose of Neoral should always be given in 2 divided doses (bid). It is recommended that Neoral be administered on a consistent schedule with regard to time of day and relation to meals. Grapefruit and grapefruit juice affect metabolism, increasing blood concentration of cyclosporine, thus should be avoided.

Newly Transplanted Patients

The initial oral dose of Neoral can be given 4-12 hours prior to transplantation or be given postoperatively. The initial dose of Neoral varies depending on the transplanted organ and the other immunosuppressive agents included in the immunosuppressive protocol. In newly transplanted patients, the initial oral dose of Neoral is the same as the initial oral dose of Sandimmune. Suggested initial doses are available from the results of a 1994 survey of the use of Sandimmune in US transplant centers. The mean ±SD initial doses were 9 ± 3 mg/kg/day for renal transplant patients (75 centers), 8 ± 4 mg/kg/day for liver transplant patients (30 centers), and 7 ± 3 mg/kg/day for heart transplant patients (24 centers). Total daily doses were divided into 2 equal daily doses. The Neoral dose is subsequently adjusted to achieve a pre-defined cyclosporine blood concentration. (See Blood Concentration Monitoring in Transplant Patients.) If cyclosporine trough blood concentrations are used, the target range is the same for Neoral as for Sandimmune. Using the same trough concentration target range for Neoral as for Sandimmune results in greater cyclosporine exposure when Neoral is administered. (See CLINICAL PHARMACOLOGY, Neoral, Pharmacokinetics, Absorption.) Dosing should be titrated based on clinical assessments of rejection and tolerability. Lower Neoral doses may be sufficient as maintenance therapy.

Adjunct therapy with adrenal corticosteroids is recommended initially. Different tapering dosage schedules of prednisone appear to achieve similar results. A representative dosage schedule based on the patient's weight started with 2.0 mg/kg/day for the first 4 days tapered to 1.0 mg/kg/day by 1 week, 0.6 mg/kg/day by 2 weeks, 0.3 mg/kg/day by 1 month, and 0.15 mg/kg/day by 2 months and thereafter as a maintenance dose. Steroid doses may be further tapered on an individualized basis depending on status of patient and function of graft. Adjustments in dosage of prednisone must be made according to the clinical situation.

Conversion From Sandimmune to Neoral in Transplant Patients

In transplanted patients who are considered for conversion to Neoral from Sandimmune, Neoral should be started with the same daily dose as was previously used with Sandimmune (1:1 dose conversion). The Neoral dose should subsequently be adjusted to attain the pre-conversion cyclosporine blood trough concentration. Using the same trough concentration target range for Neoral as for Sandimmune results in greater cyclosporine exposure when Neoral is administered. (See CLINICAL PHARMACOLOGY, Neoral, Pharmacokinetics, Absorption.) Patients with suspected poor absorption of Sandimmune require different dosing strategies. (See Transplant Patients With Poor Absorption of Sandimmune.) In some patients, the increase in blood trough concentration is more pronounced and may be of clinical significance.

Until the blood trough concentration attains the pre-conversion value, it is strongly recommended that the cyclosporine blood trough concentration be monitored every 4-7 days after conversion to Neoral. In addition, clinical safety parameters such as serum creatinine and blood pressure should be monitored every 2 weeks during the first 2 months after conversion. If the blood trough concentrations are outside the desired range and/or if the clinical safety parameters worsen, the dosage of Neoral must be adjusted accordingly.

Transplant Patients With Poor Absorption of Sandimmune

Patients with lower than expected cyclosporine blood trough concentrations in relation to the oral dose of Sandimmune may have poor or inconsistent absorption of cyclosporine from Sandimmune. After conversion to Neoral, patients tend to have higher cyclosporine concentrations. **Due to the increase in bioavailability of cyclosporine following conversion to Neoral, the cyclosporine blood trough concentration may exceed the target range. Particular caution should be exercised when converting patients to Neoral at doses greater than 10 mg/kg/day.** The dose of Neoral should be titrated individually based on cyclosporine trough concentrations, tolerability, and clinical response. In this population the cyclosporine blood trough concentration should be measured more frequently, at least twice a week (daily, if initial dose exceeds 10 mg/kg/day) until the concentration stabilizes within the desired range.

Rheumatoid Arthritis

The initial dose of Neoral is 2.5 mg/kg/day, taken twice daily as a divided (bid) oral dose. Salicylates, nonsteroidal anti-inflammatory agents, and oral corticosteroids may be continued. (See WARNINGS, Neoral and DRUG INTERACTIONS, Neoral.) Onset of action generally occurs between 4 and 8 weeks. If insufficient clinical benefit is seen and tolerability is good (including serum creatinine less than 30% above baseline), the dose may be increased by 0.5-0.75 mg/kg/day after 8 weeks and again after 12 weeks to a maximum of 4 mg/kg/day. If no benefit is seen by 16 weeks of therapy, Neoral therapy should be discontinued.

Dose decreases by 25-50% should be made at any time to control adverse events, *e.g.*, hypertension elevations in serum creatinine (30% above patient's pretreatment level) or clinically significant laboratory abnormalities. (See WARNINGS, Neoral, and PRECAUTIONS, Neoral.)

If dose reduction is not effective in controlling abnormalities or if the adverse event or abnormality is severe, Neoral should be discontinued. The same initial dose and dosage range should be used if Neoral is combined with the recommended dose of methotrexate. Most patients can be treated with Neoral doses of 3 mg/kg/day or below when combined with methotrexate doses of up to 15 mg/week.

There is limited long-term treatment data. Recurrence of rheumatoid arthritis disease activity is generally apparent within 4 weeks after stopping cyclosporine.

Psoriasis

The initial dose of Neoral should be 2.5 mg/kg/day. Neoral should be taken twice daily, as a divided (1.25 mg/kg bid) oral dose. Patients should be kept at that dose for at least 4 weeks, barring adverse events. If significant clinical improvement has not occurred in patients by that time, the patient's dosage should be increased at 2 week intervals. Based on patient response, dose increases of approximately 0.5 mg/kg/day should be made to a maximum of 4.0 mg/kg/day.

Dose decreases by 25-50% should be made at any time to control adverse events, *e.g.*, hypertension, elevations in serum creatinine (≥25% above the patient's pretreatment level), or clinically significant laboratory abnormalities. If dose reduction is not effective in controlling abnormalities, or if the adverse event or abnormality is severe, Neoral should be discontinued. (See PRECAUTIONS, Neoral, General, Special Monitoring for Psoriasis Patients.)

Patients generally show some improvement in the clinical manifestations of psoriasis in 2 weeks. Satisfactory control and stabilization of the disease may take 12-16 weeks to achieve. Results of a dose-titration clinical trial with Neoral indicate that an improvement of psoriasis by 75% or more (based on PASI) was achieved in 51% of the patients after 8 weeks and in 79% of the patients after 16 weeks. Treatment should be discontinued if satisfactory response cannot be achieved after 6 weeks at 4 mg/kg/day or the patient's maximum tolerated dose. Once a patient is adequately controlled and appears stable the dose of Neoral should be lowered, and the patient treated with the lowest dose that maintains an adequate response (this should not necessarily be total clearing of the patient). In clinical trials, cyclosporine doses at the lower end of the recommended dosage range were effective in maintaining a satisfactory response in 60% of the patients. Doses below 2.5 mg/kg/day may also be equally effective.

Upon stopping treatment with cyclosporine, relapse will occur in approximately 6 weeks (50% of the patients) to 16 weeks (75% of the patients). In the majority of patients rebound does not occur after cessation of treatment with cyclosporine. Thirteen (13) cases of transformation of chronic plaque psoriasis to more severe forms of psoriasis have been reported. There were 9 cases of pustular and 4 cases of erythrodermic psoriasis. Long term experience with Neoral in psoriasis patients is limited and continuous treatment for extended periods greater than 1 year is not recommended. Alternation with other forms of treatment should be considered in the long term management of patients with this life long disease.

Neoral Oral Solution MODIFIED — Recommendations for Administration

To make Neoral oral solution MODIFIED more palatable, it should be diluted with orange or apple juice that is at room temperature. Patients should avoid switching diluents frequently. Grapefruit juice affects metabolism of cyclosporine and should be avoided. The combination of Neoral solution with milk can be unpalatable. The effect of milk on the bioavailability of cyclosporine when admininstered as Neoral oral solution has not been evaluated.

Take the prescribed amount of Neoral oral solution MODIFIED from the container using the dosing syringe supplied, after removal of the protective cover, and transfer the solution to a glass of orange or apple juice. Stir well and drink at once. Do not allow diluted oral solution to stand before drinking. Use a glass container (not plastic). Rinse the glass with more diluent to ensure that the total dose is consumed. After use, dry the outside of the dosing syringe with a clean towel and replace the protective cover. Do not rinse the dosing syringe with water or other cleaning agents. If the syringe requires cleaning, it must be completely dry before resuming use.

Blood Concentration Monitoring in Transplant Patients

Transplant centers have found blood concentration monitoring of cyclosporine to be an essential component of patient management. Of importance to blood concentration analysis are the type of assay used, the transplanted organ, and other immunosuppressant agents being administered. While no fixed relationship has been established, blood concentration monitoring may assist in the clinical evaluation of rejection and toxicity, dose adjustments, and the assessment of compliance.

Various assays have been used to measure blood concentrations of cyclosporine. Older studies using a nonspecific assay often cited concentrations that were roughly twice those of the specific assays. Therefore, comparison between concentrations in the published literature and an individual patient concentration using current assays must be made with detailed knowledge of the assay methods employed. Current assay results are also not interchangeable and their use should be guided by their approved labeling. A discussion of the different assay methods is contained in *Annals of Clinical Biochemistry* 1994;31:420-446. While several assays and assay matrices are available, there is a consensus that parent-compound-specific assays correlate best with clinical events. Of these, HPLC is the standard reference, but the monoclonal antibody RIAs and the monoclonal antibody FPIA offer sensitivity, reproducibility, and convenience. Most clinicians base their monitoring on trough cyclosporine concentrations. *Applied Pharmacokinetics, Principles of Therapeutic Drug Monitoring* (1992) contains a broad discussion of cyclosporine pharmacokinetics and drug monitoring techniques. Blood concentration monitoring is not a replacement for renal function monitoring or tissue biopsies.

SANDIMMUNE

Sandimmune Soft Gelatin Capsules and Oral Solution

Sandimmune soft gelatin capsules and Sandimmune oral solution have decreased bioavailability in comparison to Neoral soft gelatin capsules MODIFIED and Neoral oral solution MODIFIED. Sandimmune and Neoral are not bioequivalent and cannot be used interchangeably without physician supervision.

The initial oral dose of Sandimmune should be given 4-12 hours prior to transplantation as a single dose of 15 mg/kg. Although a daily single dose of 14-18 mg/kg was used in most clinical trials, few centers continue to use the highest dose, most favoring the lower end of the scale. There is a trend towards use of even lower initial doses for renal transplantation in the ranges of 10-14 mg/kg/day. The initial single daily dose is continued postoperatively for 1-2 weeks and then tapered by 5% per week to a maintenance dose of 5-10 mg/kg/day. Some centers have successfully tapered the maintenance dose to as low as 3 mg/kg/day in selected *renal* transplant patients without an apparent rise in rejection rate.

See Blood Level Monitoring.

In pediatric usage, the same dose and dosing regimen may be used as in adults although in several studies children have required and tolerated higher doses than those used in adults.

Adjunct therapy with adrenal corticosteroids is recommended. Different tapering dosage schedules of prednisone appear to achieve similar results. A dosage schedule based on the patient's weight started with 2.0 mg/kg/day for the first 4 days tapered to 1.0 mg/kg/day by 1 week, 0.6 mg/kg/day by 2 weeks, 0.3 mg/kg/day by 1 month, and 0.15 mg/kg/day by 2 months and thereafter as a maintenance dose. Another center started with an initial dose of 200 mg tapered by 40 mg/day until reaching 20 mg/day. After 2 months at this dose, a further reduction to 10 mg/day was made. Adjustments in dosage of prednisone must be made according to the clinical situation.

To make Sandimmune oral solution more palatable, the oral solution may be diluted with milk, chocolate milk, or orange juice preferably at room temperature. Patients should avoid switching diluents frequently. Sandimmune soft gelatin capsules and oral solution should be administered on a consistent schedule with regard to time of day and relation to meals.

Take the prescribed amount of Sandimmune from the container using the dosage syringe supplied after removal of the protective cover, and transfer the solution to a glass of milk, chocolate milk, or orange juice. Stir well and drink at once. Do not allow to stand before drinking. It is best to use a glass container and rinse it with more diluent to ensure that the total dose is taken. After use, replace the dosage syringe in the protective cover. Do not rinse the dosage syringe with water or other cleaning agents either before or after use. If the dosage syringe requires cleaning, it must be completely dry before resuming use. Introduction of water into the product by any means will cause variation in dose.

Sandimmune Injection FOR INFUSION ONLY

Note: Anaphylactic reactions have occurred with Sandimmune injection. (See WARNINGS, Sandimmune.)

Patients unable to take Sandimmune soft gelatin capsules or oral solution pre- or postoperatively may be treated with the IV concentrate. **Sandimmune injection is administered at 1/3 the oral dose.** The initial dose of Sandimmune injection should be given 4-12 hours prior to transplantation as a single IV dose of 5-6 mg/kg/day. This daily single dose is continued postoperatively until the patient can tolerate the soft gelatin capsules or oral solution. Patients should be switched to Sandimmune soft gelatin capsules or oral solution as soon as possible after surgery. In pediatric usage, the same dose and dosing regimen may be used, although higher doses may be required.

Adjunct steroid therapy is to be used. (See aforementioned.)

Immediately before use, the IV concentrate should be diluted 1 ml Sandimmune injection in 20-100 ml 0.9% sodium chloride injection or 5% dextrose injection and given in a slow IV infusion over approximately 2-6 hours.

Diluted infusion solutions should be discarded after 24 hours.

The Cremophor EL (polyoxyethylated castor oil) contained in the concentrate for IV infusion can cause phthalate stripping from PVC.

Parenteral drug products should be inspected visually for particulate matter and discoloration prior to administration, whenever solution and container permit.

Blood Level Monitoring

Several study centers have found blood level monitoring of cyclosporine useful in patient management. While no fixed relationships have yet been established, in one series of 375 consecutive cadaveric renal transplant recipients, dosage was adjusted to achieve specific whole blood 24 hour trough levels of 100-200 ng/ml as determined by high-pressure liquid chromatography (HPLC).

Of major importance to blood level analysis is the type of assay used. The above levels are specific to the parent cyclosporine molecule and correlate directly to the new monoclonal specific radioimmunoassays (mRIA-sp). Nonspecific assays are also available which detect the parent compound molecule and various of its metabolites. Older studies often cited levels using a nonspecific assay which were roughly twice those of specific assays. Assay results are not interchangeable and their use should be guided by their approved labeling. If plasma specimens are employed, levels will vary with the temperature at the time of separation from whole blood. Plasma levels may range from 1/2-1/5 of whole blood levels. Refer to individual assay labeling for complete instructions. In addition, *Transplantation Proceedings* (June 1990) contains position papers and a broad consensus generated at the Cyclosporine-Therapeutic Drug Monitoring conference that year. Blood level monitoring is not a replacement for renal function monitoring or tissue biopsies.

RESTASIS

Restasis Ophthalmic Emulsion

Invert the unit dose vial a few times to obtain a uniform, white, opaque emulsion before using. Instill 1 drop of Restasis ophthalmic emulsion twice a day in each eye approximately 12 hours apart. Restasis can be used concomitantly with artificial tears, allowing a 15 minute interval between products. Discard vial immediately after use.

HOW SUPPLIED

NEORAL

Neoral Soft Gelatin Capsules (cyclosporine capsules) MODIFIED

25 mg: Oval, blue-gray imprinted in red, "Neoral" over "25 mg".

100 mg: Oblong, blue-gray imprinted in red, "NEORAL" over "100 mg".

Store and Dispense: In the original unit-dose container at controlled room temperature 20-25°C (68-77°F).

Neoral Oral Solution (cyclosporine oral solution) MODIFIED

A clear, yellow liquid supplied in 50 ml bottles containing 100 mg/ml.

Store and Dispense: In the original container at controlled room temperature 20-25°C (68-77°F). Do not store in the refrigerator. Once opened, the contents must be used within 2 months. At temperatures below 20°C (68°F) the solution may gel; light flocculation or the formation of a light sediment may also occur. There is no impact on product performance or dosing using the syringe provided. Allow to warm to room temperature 25°C (77°F) to reverse these changes.

SANDIMMUNE

Sandimmune Soft Gelatin Capsules (cyclosporine capsules)

25 mg: Oblong, pink, branded with the Sandoz logo and "78/240".

100 mg: Oblong, dusty rose, branded with the Sandoz logo and "78/241".

Store and Dispense: Store at 25°C (77°F); excursions permitted to 15-30°C (59-86°F). An odor may be detected upon opening the unit dose container, which will dissipate shortly thereafter. This odor does not affect the quality of the product.

Sandimmune Oral Solution (cyclosporine oral solution)

Supplied in 50 ml bottles containing 100 mg of cyclosporine per ml. A dosage syringe is provided for dispensing.

Store and Dispense: In the original container at temperatures below 30°C (86°F). Do not store in the refrigerator. Protect from freezing. Once opened, the contents must be used within 2 months.

Sandimmune Injection (cyclosporine injection) FOR INTRAVENOUS INFUSION

Supplied as a 5 ml sterile ampul containing 50 mg of cyclosporine per ml.

Store and Dispense: At temperatures below 30°C (86°F) and protected from light.

RESTASIS

Restasis Ophthalmic Emulsion (cyclosporine ophthalmic emulsion) 0.05%

Restasis ophthalmic emulsion is packaged in single use vials. Each vial contains 0.4 ml fill in a 0.9 ml LDPE vial; 32 vials are packaged in a polypropylene tray with an aluminum peelable lid.

Storage: Store Restasis ophthalmic emulsion at 15-25°C (59-77°F).

KEEP OUT OF THE REACH OF CHILDREN.

PRODUCT LISTING - RATED THERAPEUTICALLY EQUIVALENT

Size	Price	Product	NDC
Capsule - Oral - 25 mg			
30's	$41.25	GENERIC, Eon Labs Manufacturing Inc	00185-0932-30
30's	$41.26	GENERIC, Eon Labs Manufacturing Inc	50111-0909-43
30's	$46.82	GENERIC, Apotex Usa Inc	60505-0133-00
Capsule - Oral - 100 mg			
30's	$164.88	GENERIC, Eon Labs Manufacturing Inc	50111-0920-43
30's	$164.89	GENERIC, Eon Labs Manufacturing Inc	00185-0933-30
30's	$186.97	GENERIC, Apotex Usa Inc	60505-0134-00
Liquid - Oral - Microemulsion 100 mg/ml			
50 ml	$332.83	NEORAL, Novartis Pharmaceuticals	00078-0274-22
Solution - Injectable - 50 mg/ml			
5 ml x 10	$275.00	GENERIC, Bedford Laboratories	55390-0122-10
5 ml x 10	$291.60	SANDIMMUNE, Novartis Pharmaceuticals	00078-0109-01

PRODUCT LISTING - RATED NOT THERAPEUTICALLY EQUIVALENT

Size	Price	Product	NDC
Capsule - Oral - Microemulsion 25 mg			
30's	$45.85	NEORAL, Novartis Pharmaceuticals	00078-0246-15
Capsule - Oral - Microemulsion 100 mg			
30's	$183.21	NEORAL, Novartis Pharmaceuticals	00078-0248-15
Capsule - Oral - 25 mg			
30's	$52.09	SANDIMMUNE, Novartis Pharmaceuticals	00078-0240-15
Capsule - Oral - 100 mg			
30's	$185.16	SANDIMMUNE, Allscripts Pharmaceutical Company	54569-2872-00
30's	$207.98	SANDIMMUNE, Novartis Pharmaceuticals	00078-0241-15
Solution - Oral - 100 mg/ml			
50 ml	$299.53	GENERIC, Sidmak Laboratories Inc	50111-0885-42
50 ml	$308.40	SANDIMMUNE, Allscripts Pharmaceutical Company	54569-2563-00
50 ml	$336.64	SANDIMMUNE, Novartis Pharmaceuticals	00078-0110-22

PRODUCT LISTING - EQUIVALENTS NOT AVAILABLE

Size	Price	Product	NDC
Capsule - Oral - 25 mg			
30's	$41.28	GENERIC, Eon Labs Manufacturing Inc	00074-6463-32
Capsule - Oral - 100 mg			
30's	$164.88	GENERIC, Sangstat Medical Corporation	00074-6479-32
Emulsion - Ophthalmic - 0.05%			
0.40 ml x 32	$93.75	RESTASIS, Allergan Inc	00023-9163-32
Solution - Oral - 100 mg/ml			
50 ml	$311.34	GENERIC, Sangstat Medical Corporation	00074-7269-50

Cyproheptadine Hydrochloride *(000934)*

For complete prescribing information, refer to the CD-ROM included with the book.

Categories: Anaphylaxis, adjunct; Angioedema; Conjunctivitis, allergic, secondary to inhalant allergens; Dermatographism; Rhinitis, perennial allergic; Rhinitis, seasonal allergic; Rhinitis, vasomotor; Transfusion reaction; Urticaria; Urticaria, secondary to cold; Pregnancy Category B; FDA Approved 1961 Aug
Drug Classes: Antihistamines, H1
Brand Names: Periactin
Foreign Brand Availability: Adekin (Greece); Antisemin (Taiwan); Apeton 4 (Indonesia); Ciplactin (India); Ciproral (Germany); Ciprovit-A (Peru); Cyheptine (Thailand); Cylat (Indonesia); Cypro H (Taiwan); Cyproatin (Japan); Cyprogin (Hong-Kong; Thailand); Cypromin (Japan); Cyprono (Thailand); Cyprosian (Thailand); Cytadine (Taiwan); Ennamax (Indonesia); Glocyp (Indonesia); Heptasan (Indonesia); Ifrasal (Japan); Istam-Far (Greece); Klarivitina (Spain); Kulinet (Greece); Periactine (France); Peritol (Bahamas; Barbados; Belize; Bermuda; Curacao; Guyana; India; Jamaica; Netherland-Antilles; Surinam; Trinidad); Petina (Malaysia); Pilian (Malaysia); Pronicy (Indonesia); Sinapdin (Indonesia); Trimetabol (Colombia)
Cost of Therapy: $45.80 (Allergic Rhinitis; Periactin; 4 mg; 3 tablets/day; 30 day supply)
$2.64 (Allergic Rhinitis; Generic Tablets; 4 mg; 3 tablets/day; 30 day supply)

DESCRIPTION

Cyproheptadine hydrochloride is an antihistaminic and antiserotonergic agent.

Cyproheptadine hydrochloride is a white to slightly yellowish, crystalline solid, with a molecular weight of 350.89, which is soluble in water, freely soluble in methanol, sparingly soluble in ethanol, soluble in chloroform, and practically insoluble in ether. It is the sesquihydrate of 4-(5*H*-dibenzo(*a,d*)cyclohepten-5-ylidene)-1-methylpiperidine hydrochloride. The empirical formula of the anhydrous salt is $C_{21}H_{21}N{\cdot}HCl$.

Cyproheptadine hydrochloride is available in tablets, containing 4 mg of cyproheptadine HCl, and as a syrup in which 5 ml contains 2 mg of cyproheptadine hydrochloride, with a pH range of 3.5-4.5.

The tablets also contain the following inactive ingredients: calcium phosphate, lactose, magnesium stearate, and starch. The syrup contains the following inactive ingredients: D&C yellow 10, artificial flavors, glycerin, purified water, sodium saccharin, and sucrose, with sorbic acid 0.1% added as preservative.

STORAGE

Store cyproheptadine HCl tablets in a well-closed container. Avoid storage at temperatures above 40°C (104°F).

Store cyproheptadine HCl syrup in a container which is kept tightly closed. Avoid storage at temperatures below -20°C (-4°F) and above 40°C (104°F).

INDICATIONS AND USAGE

- Perennial and seasonal allergic rhinitis.
- Vasomotor rhinitis.
- Allergic conjunctivitis due to inhalant allergens and foods.
- Mild, uncomplicated allergic skin manifestations of urticaria and angioedema.
- Amelioration of allergic reactions to blood or plasma.
- Cold urticaria.
- Dermatographism.
- As therapy for anaphylactic reactions *adjunctive* to epinephrine and other standard measures after the acute manifestations have been controlled.

NON-FDA APPROVED INDICATIONS

Cyproheptadine has also been used for the treatment of Cushing's syndrome secondary to pituitary disorders, and anorexia nervosa because of its effect on appetite and weight gain. In addition, there have been isolated preliminary reports of efficacy in treating the serotonin syndrome, neuroleptic-induced akathisia, and the galactorrhea-amenorrhea syndrome. However, these indications are not approved by the FDA.

CONTRAINDICATIONS

NEWBORN OR PREMATURE INFANTS

This drug should not be used in newborn or premature infants.

NURSING MOTHERS

Because of the higher risk of antihistamines for infants generally and for newborns and prematures in particular, antihistamine therapy is contraindicated in nursing mothers.

OTHER CONDITIONS

Hypersensitivity to cyproheptadine and other drugs of similar chemical structure:
Monoamine oxidase inhibitor therapy.
Angle-closure glaucoma.
Stenosing peptic ulcer.
Symptomatic prostatic hypertrophy.
Bladder neck obstruction.
Pyloroduodenal obstruction.
Elderly, debilitated patients.

WARNINGS

CHILDREN

Overdosage: Of antihistamines, particularly in infants and children, may produce hallucinations, central nervous system depression, convulsions, and death.

Antihistamines may diminish mental alertness; conversely, particularly, in the young child, they may occasionally produce excitation.

CNS DEPRESSANTS

Antihistamines may have additive effects with alcohol and other CNS depressants, *e.g.*, hypnotics, sedatives, tranquilizers, antianxiety agents.

ACTIVITIES REQUIRING MENTAL ALERTNESS

Patients should be warned about engaging in activities requiring mental alertness and motor coordination, such as driving a car or operating machinery.

Antihistamines are more likely to cause dizziness, sedation, and hypotension in elderly patients.

DOSAGE AND ADMINISTRATION

DOSAGE SHOULD BE INDIVIDUALIZED ACCORDING TO THE NEEDS AND THE RESPONSE OF THE PATIENT.

Each cyproheptadine HCl tablet contains 4 mg of cyproheptadine HCl. Each 5 ml of cyproheptadine HCl syrup contains 2 mg of cyproheptadine HCl.

Although intended primarily for administration to children, the syrup is also useful for administration to adults who cannot swallow tablets.

CHILDREN

The total daily dosage for children may be calculated on the basis of body weight or body area using approximately 0.25 mg/kg/day (0.11 mg/lb/day) or 8 mg/m^2. In small children for whom the calculation of dosage based upon body size is most important, it may be necessary to use cyproheptadine HCl syrup to permit accurate dosage.

Age 2-6 Years: The usual dose is 2 mg (½ tablet or 1 teaspoon) 2 or 3 times a day, adjusted as necessary to the size and response of the patient. The dose is not to exceed 12 mg a day.

Age 7-14 Years: The usual dose is 4 mg (1 tablet or 2 teaspoons) 2 or 3 times a day, adjusted as necessary to the size and response of the patient. The dose is not to exceed 16 mg a day.

ADULTS

The total daily dose for adults should not exceed 0.5 mg/kg/day (0.23 mg/lb/day).

The therapeutic range is 4-20 mg a day, with the majority of patients requiring 12-16 mg a day. An occasional patient may require as much as 32 mg a day for adequate relief. It is suggested that dosage be initiated with 4 mg (1 tablet or 2 teaspoons) three times a day and adjusted according to the size and response of the patient.

PRODUCT LISTING - RATED THERAPEUTICALLY EQUIVALENT

Syrup - Oral - 2 mg/5 ml			
100 ml	$57.50	GENERIC, Cmc-Consolidated Midland Corporation	00223-6489-02
120 ml	$2.60	GENERIC, Circle Pharmaceuticals Inc	00659-0724-54
480 ml	$10.43	GENERIC, Major Pharmaceuticals Inc	00904-1146-16
480 ml	$10.49	GENERIC, Qualitest Products Inc	00603-1117-58
480 ml	$10.50	GENERIC, Ivax Corporation	00182-1355-40
480 ml	$10.75	GENERIC, Watson/Rugby Laboratories Inc	00536-1930-85
480 ml	$10.75	GENERIC, Halsey Drug Company Inc	00879-0473-16
480 ml	$12.67	GENERIC, Aligen Independent Laboratories Inc	00405-2600-16
480 ml	$37.93	GENERIC, Alpharma Uspd Makers Of Barre and Nmc	00472-0755-16
3840 ml	$58.37	GENERIC, Major Pharmaceuticals Inc	00904-1146-28
3840 ml	$62.16	GENERIC, Halsey Drug Company Inc	00879-0473-28
Tablet - Oral - 4 mg			
20's	$2.25	GENERIC, Circle Pharmaceuticals Inc	00659-0717-20
20's	$4.88	GENERIC, Pd-Rx Pharmaceuticals	55289-0089-20
30's	$4.98	GENERIC, Heartland Healthcare Services	61392-0209-30
60's	$9.96	GENERIC, Heartland Healthcare Services	61392-0209-60
90's	$14.94	GENERIC, Heartland Healthcare Services	61392-0209-90
100's	$2.93	GENERIC, Interstate Drug Exchange Inc	00814-2090-14
100's	$3.55	GENERIC, Camall Company	00147-0236-10
100's	$3.90	GENERIC, Geneva Pharmaceuticals	00781-1125-01
100's	$4.25	GENERIC, Balan, J.J. Inc	00304-1145-60
100's	$4.71	GENERIC, Moore, H.L. Drug Exchange Inc	00839-6300-06
100's	$4.71	GENERIC, Moore, H.L. Drug Exchange Inc	00839-7866-06
100's	$5.55	GENERIC, Raway Pharmacal Inc	00686-0159-20
100's	$5.75	GENERIC, Cmc-Consolidated Midland Corporation	00223-0709-01
100's	$6.55	GENERIC, Aligen Independent Laboratories Inc	00405-4295-01
100's	$6.55	GENERIC, Martec Pharmaceuticals Inc	52555-0043-01
100's	$7.18	GENERIC, Qualitest Products Inc	00603-3098-21
100's	$8.50	GENERIC, Cmc-Consolidated Midland Corporation	00223-6489-01
100's	$11.40	GENERIC, Auro Pharmaceutical	55829-0220-10
100's	$19.45	GENERIC, Vangard Labs	00615-1536-13
100's	$38.50	GENERIC, Ivax Corporation	00182-1132-89
100's	$38.61	GENERIC, Major Pharmaceuticals Inc	00904-1145-60
100's	$42.69	GENERIC, Ivax Corporation	00172-2929-60
100's	$42.69	GENERIC, Par Pharmaceutical Inc	49884-0043-01
100's	$42.69	GENERIC, Sidmak Laboratories Inc	50111-0314-01
100's	$42.90	GENERIC, Major Pharmaceuticals Inc	00904-1145-61
100's	$50.89	PERIACTIN, Merck & Company Inc	00006-0062-68
250's	$7.70	GENERIC, Major Pharmaceuticals Inc	00904-1145-70

PRODUCT LISTING - EQUIVALENTS NOT AVAILABLE

Syrup - Oral - 2 mg/5 ml			
120 ml	$7.47	GENERIC, Allscripts Pharmaceutical Company	54569-2984-01
480 ml	$9.00	GENERIC, Cmc-Consolidated Midland Corporation	00223-6248-01
Tablet - Oral - 4 mg			
30's	$11.70	GENERIC, Allscripts Pharmaceutical Company	54569-0411-01

Cytarabine *(000935)*

Categories: Leukemia, acute lymphoblastic; Leukemia, chronic myelogenous; Leukemia, meningeal; Pregnancy Category D; FDA Approved 1969 Jun; WHO Formulary
Drug Classes: Antineoplastics, antimetabolites
Brand Names: ***Cytosar-U;*** Tarabine Pfs
Foreign Brand Availability: Alexan (Austria; Belgium; Bulgaria; China; Czech-Republic; Denmark; England; Germany; Hong-Kong; Hungary; Indonesia; Ireland; Italy; Malaysia; Mexico; Philippines; Portugal; South-Africa; Sweden; Switzerland; Thailand; Turkey); Arabitin (Japan); Aracytin (Colombia; Greece; Italy); Aracytine (France); Citarabina (Peru); Cytarabine (Australia); Cytarabine Injection (Australia; New-Zealand); Cytarine (India; Thailand); Cytonal (Turkey); Cytosa U (Korea); Cytosar (Austria; Bahrain; Belgium; Bulgaria; Canada; China; Cyprus; Czech-Republic; Denmark; Egypt; England; Finland; Ghana; Hong-Kong; Hungary; Iran; Iraq; Israel; Jordan; Kenya; Kuwait; Lebanon; Libya; Netherlands; Norway; Oman; Philippines; Portugal; Qatar; Republic-of-Yemen; Saudi-Arabia; South-Africa; Sweden; Switzerland; Syria; Tanzania; Uganda; United-Arab-Emirates; Zambia); Cytosar U (New-Zealand); Iretin (Japan); Laracit (Mexico); Novumtrax (Mexico); Udicil (Germany); Udicil CS (Germany)
HCFA JCODE(S): J9100 100 mg SC, IV; J9110 500 mg SC, IV

WARNING

Only physicians experienced in cancer chemotherapy should use cytarabine.

For induction therapy patients should be treated in a facility with laboratory and supportive resources sufficient to monitor drug tolerance and protect and maintain a patient compromised by drug toxicity. The main toxic effect of cytarabine is bone marrow suppression with leukopenia, thrombocytopenia and anemia. Less serious toxicity includes nausea, vomiting, diarrhea and abdominal pain, oral ulceration, and hepatic dysfunction.

The physician must judge possible benefit to the patient against known toxic effects of this drug in considering the advisability of therapy with cytarabine. Before making this judgment or beginning treatment, the physician should be familiar with the following text.

DESCRIPTION

Cytosar-U sterile powder, commonly known as ara-C, an antineoplastic, is a sterile lyophilized material for reconstitution and intravenous, intrathecal or subcutaneous administration. It is available in multi-dose vials containing 100 mg, 500 mg, 1 g or 2 g sterile cytarabine. The pH of cytarabine was adjusted, when necessary, with hydrochloric acid and/or sodium hydroxide.

Cytarabine is chemically 4-amino-1-β-D-arabinofuranosyl-2 (IH)-pyrimidinone.

Cytosar-U is an odorless, white to off-white, crystalline powder which is freely soluble in water and slightly soluble in alcohol and in chloroform.

Storage: Store Cytosar-U at controlled room temperature 20-25°C (68-77°F).

CLINICAL PHARMACOLOGY

CELL CULTURE STUDIES

Cytarabine is cytotoxic to a wide variety of proliferating mammalian cells in culture. It exhibits cell phase specificity, primarily killing cells undergoing DNA synthesis (S-phase) and under certain conditions blocking the progression of cells from the G_1 phase to the S-phase. Although the mechanism of action is not completely understood, it appears that cytarabine acts through the inhibition of DNA polymerase. A limited, but significant, incorporation of cytarabine into both DNA and RNA has also been reported. Extensive chromosomal damage, including chromatoid breaks, have been produced by cytarabine and malignant transformation of rodent cells in culture has been reported. Deoxycytidine prevents or delays (but does not reverse) the cytotoxic activity.

Cell culture studies have shown an antiviral effect.[1] However, efficacy against herpes zoster or smallpox could not be demonstrated in controlled clinical trials.[2-4]

CELLULAR RESISTANCE AND SENSITIVITY

Cytarabine is metabolized by deoxycytidine kinase and other nucleotide kinases to the nucleotide triphosphate, an effective inhibitor of DNA polymerase; it is inactivated by a pyrimidine nucleoside deaminase which converts it to the nontoxic uracil derivative. It appears that the balance of kinase and deaminase levels may be an important factor in determining sensitivity or resistance of the cell to cytarabine.

ANIMAL STUDIES

In experimental studies with mouse tumors, cytarabine was most effective in those tumors with a high growth fraction. The effect was dependent on the treatment schedule; optimal effects were achieved when the schedule (multiple closely spaced doses or constant infusion) ensured contact of the drug with the tumor cells when the maximum number of cells were in the susceptible S-phase. The best results were obtained when courses of therapy were separated by intervals sufficient to permit adequate host recovery.

HUMAN PHARMACOLOGY

Cytarabine is rapidly metabolized and is not effective orally; less than 20% of the orally administered dose is absorbed from the gastrointestinal tract.

Following rapid intravenous injection of cytarabine labeled with tritium, the disappearance from plasma is biphasic. There is an initial distributive phase with a half-life of about 10 minutes, followed by a second elimination phase with a half-life of about 1-3 hours. After the distributive phase, more than 80% of plasma radioactivity can be accounted for by the inactive metabolite 1-β-D-arabinofuranosyluracil (ara-U). Within 24 hours about 80% of the administered radioactivity can be recovered in the urine, approximately 90% of which is excreted as ara-U.

Relatively constant plasma levels can be achieved by continuous intravenous infusion.

After subcutaneous or intramuscular administration of cytarabine labeled with tritium, peak-plasma levels of radioactivity are achieved about 20-60 minutes after injection and are considerably lower than those after intravenous administration.

Cerebrospinal fluid levels of cytarabine are low in comparison to plasma levels after single intravenous injection. However, in 1 patient in whom cerebrospinal levels were examined after 2 hours of constant intravenous infusion, levels approached 40% of the steady state plasma level. With intrathecal administration, levels of cytarabine in the cerebrospinal fluid declined with a first order half-life of about 2 hours. Because cerebrospinal fluid levels of deaminase are low, little conversion to ara-U was observed.

IMMUNOSUPPRESSIVE ACTION

Cytarabine is capable of obliterating immune responses in man during administration with little or no accompanying toxicity.[5,6] Suppression of antibody responses to *E. coli*-VI antigen and tetanus toxoid have been demonstrated. This suppression was obtained during both primary and secondary antibody responses.

Cytarabine also suppressed the development of cell-mediated immune responses such as delayed hypersensitivity skin reaction to dinitrochlorobenzene. However, it had no effect on already established delayed hypersensitivity reactions.

Following 5 day courses of intensive therapy with cytarabine the immune response was suppressed, as indicated by the following parameters: macrophage ingress into skin windows; circulating antibody response following primary antigenic stimulation; lymphocyte blastogenesis with phytohemagglutinin. A few days after termination of therapy there was a rapid return to normal.[7]

INDICATIONS AND USAGE

Cytarabine in combination with other approved anticancer drugs is indicated for remission induction in acute non-lymphocytic leukemia of adults and pediatric patients. It has also been found useful in the treatment of acute lymphocytic leukemia and the blast phase of chronic myelocytic leukemia. Intrathecal administration of cytarabine is indicated in the prophylaxis and treatment of meningeal leukemia.

CONTRAINDICATIONS

Cytarabine is contraindicated in those patients who are hypersensitive to the drug.

WARNINGS

See BOXED WARNING.

Cytarabine is a potent bone marrow suppressant. Therapy should be started cautiously in patients with pre-existing drug-induced bone marrow suppression. Patients receiving this drug must be under close medical supervision and, during induction therapy, should have leukocyte and platelet counts performed daily. Bone marrow examinations should be performed frequently after blasts have disappeared from the peripheral blood. Facilities should be available for management of complications, possibly fatal, of bone marrow suppression (infection resulting from granulocytopenia and other impaired body defenses, and hemorrhage secondary to thrombocytopenia). One case of anaphylaxis that resulted in acute cardiopulmonary arrest and required resuscitation has been reported. This occurred immediately after the intravenous administration of cytarabine.

Severe and at times fatal CNS, GI and pulmonary toxicity (different from that seen with conventional therapy regimens of cytarabine) has been reported following some experimental dose schedules for cytarabine.[8-11] These reactions include reversible corneal toxicity, and hemorrhagic conjunctivitis, which may be prevented or diminished by prophylaxis with a local corticosteroid eye drop; cerebral and cerebellar dysfunction, including personality changes, somnolence and coma, usually reversible; severe gastrointestinal ulceration, including pneumatosis cystoides intestinalis leading to peritonitis; sepsis and liver abscess; pulmonary edema, liver damage with increased hyperbilirubinemia; bowel necrosis; and necrotizing colitis. Rarely, severe skin rash, leading to desquamation has been reported. Complete alopecia is more commonly seen with experimental high dose therapy than with standard treatment programs using cytarabine. If experimental high dose therapy is used, do not use a diluent containing benzyl alcohol.

Cases of cardiomyopathy with subsequent death has been reported following experimental high dose therapy with cytarabine in combination with cyclophosphamide when used for bone marrow transplant preparation.[12]

A syndrome of sudden respiratory distress, rapidly progressing to pulmonary edema and radiographically pronounced cardiomegaly has been reported following experimental high dose therapy with cytarabine used for the treatment of relapsed leukemia from one institution in 16/72 patients. The outcome of this syndrome can be fatal.[13]

Benzyl alcohol is contained in the diluent for this product. Benzyl alcohol has been reported to be associated with a fatal "Gasping Syndrome" in premature infants.

Two patients with childhood acute myelogenous leukemia who received intrathecal and intravenous cytarabine at conventional doses (in addition to a number of other concomitantly administered drugs) developed delayed progressive ascending paralysis resulting in death in 1 of the 2 patients.[14]

PREGNANCY CATEGORY D

Cytarabine can cause fetal harm when administered to a pregnant woman. (See ANIMAL PHARMACOLOGY.) There are no adequate and well-controlled studies in pregnant women. If cytarabine is used during pregnancy, or if the patient becomes pregnant while taking cytarabine, the patient should be apprised of the potential hazard to the fetus. Women of childbearing potential should be advised to avoid becoming pregnant.

A review of the literature has shown 32 reported cases where cytarabine was given during pregnancy, either alone or in combination with other cytotoxic agents.

Eighteen (18) normal infants were delivered. Four (4) of these had first trimester exposure. Five (5) infants were premature or of low birth weight. Twelve (12) of the 18 normal infants were followed up at ages ranging from 6 weeks to 7 years, and showed no abnormalities. One apparently normal infant died at 90 days of gastroenteritis.

Two cases of congenital abnormalities have been reported, 1 with upper and lower distal limb defects,[16] and the other with extremity and ear deformities.[17] Both of these cases had first trimester exposure.

There were 7 infants with various problems in the neonatal period, including pancytopenia; transient depression of WBC, hematocrit or platelets; electrolyte abnormalities; transient eosinophilia; and 1 case of increased IgM levels and hyperpyrexia possibly due to sepsis. Six (6) of the 7 infants were also premature. The child with pancytopenia died at 21 days of sepsis.

Therapeutic abortions were done in 5 cases. Four (4) fetuses were grossly normal, but 1 had an enlarged spleen and another showed Trisomy C chromosome abnormality in the chorionic tissue.

Because of the potential for abnormalities with cytotoxic therapy, particularly during the first trimester, a patient who is or who may become pregnant while on cytarabine should be apprised of the potential risk to the fetus and the advisability of pregnancy continuation. There is a definite, but considerably reduced risk if therapy is initiated during the second or third trimester. Although normal infants have been delivered to patients treated in all three trimesters of pregnancy, follow-up of such infants would be advisable.

PRECAUTIONS

GENERAL

Patients receiving cytarabine must be monitored closely. Frequent platelet and leukocyte counts and bone marrow examinations are mandatory. Consider suspending or modifying therapy when drug-induced marrow depression has resulted in a platelet count under 50,000 or a polymorphonuclear granulocyte count under $1000/mm^3$. Counts of formed elements in the peripheral blood may continue to fall after the drug is stopped and reach lowest values after drug-free intervals of 12-24 days. When indicated, restart therapy when definite signs of marrow recovery appear (on successive bone marrow studies). Patients whose drug is withheld until "normal" peripheral blood values are attained may escape from control.

When large intravenous doses are given quickly, patients are frequently nauseated and may vomit for several hours postinjection. This problem tends to be less severe when the drug is infused.

The human liver apparently detoxifies a substantial fraction of an administered dose. In particular, patients with renal or hepatic function impairment may have a higher likelihood of CNS toxicity after high-dose cytarabine treatment.[46,47,49] Use the drug with caution and possibly at reduced dose in patients whose liver or kidney function is poor.

Periodic checks of bone marrow, liver and kidney functions should be performed in patients receiving cytarabine.

Like other cytotoxic drugs, cytarabine may induce hyperuricemia secondary to rapid lysis of neoplastic cells. The clinician should monitor the patients's blood uric acid level and be prepared to use such supportive and pharmacologic measures as might be necessary to control this problem.

Acute pancreatitis has been reported to occur in patients being treated with cytarabine who have had prior treatment with L-asparaginase.[15] There is evidence that this may be schedule dependent.[50]

INFORMATION FOR THE PATIENT

Not applicable.

LABORATORY TESTS

See General.

CARCINOGENESIS, MUTAGENESIS, AND IMPAIRMENT OF FERTILITY

Extensive chromosomal damage, including chromatoid breaks have been produced by cytarabine and malignant transformation of rodent cells in culture has been reported.

PREGNANCY CATEGORY D

See WARNINGS.

LABOR AND DELIVERY

Not applicable.

NURSING MOTHERS

It is not known whether this drug is excreted in human milk. Because many drugs are excreted in human milk and because of the potential for serious adverse reactions in nursing infants from cytarabine, a decision should be made whether to discontinue nursing or to discontinue the drug, taking into account the importance of the drug to the mother.

PEDIATRIC USE

See INDICATIONS AND USAGE.

DRUG INTERACTIONS

Reversible decreases in steady-state plasma digoxin concentrations and renal glycoside excretion were observed in patients receiving beta-acetyldigoxin and chemotherapy regimens containing cyclophosphamide, vincristine and prednisone with or without cytarabine or procarbazine.[39] Steady-state plasma digitoxin concentrations did not appear to change. Therefore, monitoring of plasma digoxin levels may be indicated in patients receiving similar combination chemotherapy regimens. The utilization of digitoxin for such patients may be considered as an alternative.

An *in vitro* interaction study between gentamicin and cytarabine showed a cytarabine related antagonism for the susceptibility of *K. pneumoniae* strains. This study suggests that in patients on cytarabine being treated with gentamicin for a *K. pneumoniae* infection, the lack of a prompt therapeutic response may indicate the need for reevaluation of antibacterial therapy.[40]

Clinical evidence in 1 patient showed possible inhibition of fluorocytosine efficacy during therapy with cytarabine.[41] This may be due to potential competitive inhibition of its uptake.[42]

ADVERSE REACTIONS

EXPECTED REACTIONS

Because cytarabine is a bone marrow suppressant, anemia, leukopenia, thrombocytopenia, megaloblastosis and reduced reticulocytes can be expected as a result of administration with cytarabine. The severity of these reactions are dose and schedule dependent.[18] Cellular changes in the morphology of bone marrow and peripheral smears can be expected.[19]

Following 5 day constant infusions or acute injections of 50-600 mg/m^2, white cell depression follows a biphasic course. Regardless of initial count, dosage level, or schedule, there is an initial fall starting the first 24 hours with a nadir at days 7-9. This is followed by a brief rise which peaks around the twelfth day. A second and deeper fall reaches nadir at days 15-24. Then there is rapid rise to above baseline in the next 10 days. Platelet depression is noticeable at 5 days with a peak depression occurring between days 12-15. Thereupon, a rapid rise to above baseline occurs in the next 10 days.[20]

INFECTIOUS COMPLICATIONS

Infection: Viral, bacterial, fungal, parasitic, or saprophytic infections, in any location in the body may be associated with the use of cytarabine alone or in combination with other immunosuppressive agents following immunosuppressant doses that affect cellular or humoral immunity. These infections may be mild, but can be severe and at times fatal.

THE CYTARABINE (ARA-C) SYNDROME

A cytarabine syndrome has been described by Castleberry.[21] It is characterized by fever, myalgia, bone pain, occasionally chest pain, maculopapular rash, conjunctivitis and malaise. It usually occurs 6-12 hours following drug administration. Corticosteroids have been shown to be beneficial in treating or preventing this syndrome. If the symptoms of the syndrome are deemed treatable, corticosteroids should be contemplated as well as continuation of therapy with cytarabine.

Most frequent adverse reactions: Anorexia, nausea, vomiting, diarrhea, oral and anal inflammation or ulceration, hepatic dysfunction, fever, rash, thrombophlebitis, bleeding (all sites).

Nausea and vomiting are most frequent following rapid intravenous injection.

Less frequent adverse reactions: Sepsis, pneumonia, cellulitis at injection site, skin ulceration, urinary retention, renal dysfunction, neuritis, neural toxicity, sore throat, esophageal ulceration, esophagitis, chest pain, pericarditis, bowel necrosis, abdominal pain, pancreatitis, freckling, jaundice, conjunctivitis (may occur with rash), dizziness, alopecia, anaphylaxis (See WARNINGS), allergic edema, pruritus, shortness of breath, urticaria, headache.

EXPERIMENTAL DOSES

Severe and at times fatal CNS, GI and pulmonary toxicity (different from that seen with conventional therapy regimens of cytarabine) has been reported following some experimental dose schedules of cytarabine.[8-11] These reactions include reversible corneal toxicity and hemorrhagic conjunctivitis, which may be prevented or diminished by prophylaxis with a local corticosteroid eye drop; cerebral and cerebellar dysfunction, including personality changes, somnolence and coma, usually reversible; severe gastrointestinal ulceration, including pneumatosis cystoides intestinalis leading to peritonitis; sepsis and liver abscess; pulmonary edema, liver damage with increased hyperbilirubinemia; bowel necrosis; and necrotizing colitis. Rarely, severe skin rash, leading to desquamation has been reported. Complete alopecia is more commonly seen with experimental high dose therapy than with standard treatment programs using cytarabine. If experimental high dose therapy is used, do not use a diluent containing benzyl alcohol.

Cases of cardiomyopathy with subsequent death has been reported following experimental high dose therapy with cytarabine in combination with cyclophosphamide when used for bone marrow transplant preparation.[12] **This cardiac toxicity may be schedule dependent.**[45]

A syndrome of sudden respiratory distress, rapidly progressing to pulmonary edema and radiographically pronounced cardiomegaly has been reported following experimental high dose therapy with cytarabine used for the treatment of relapsed leukemia from one institution in 16/72 patients. The outcome of this syndrome can be fatal.[13]

Two (2) patients with adult acute nonlymphocytic leukemia developed peripheral motor and sensory neuropathies after consolidation with high-dose cytarabine, daunorubicin, and asparaginase. Patients treated with high-dose cytarabine should be observed for neuropathy since dose schedule alterations may be needed to avoid irreversible neurologic disorders.[22]

Ten (10) patients treated with experimental intermediate doses of cytarabine (1 g/m^2) with and without other chemotherapeutic agents (meta-AMSA, daunorubicin, etoposide) at various dose regimes developed a diffuse interstitial pneumonitis without clear cause that may have been related to the cytarabine.[43]

Two (2) cases of pancreatitis have been reported following experimental doses of cytarabine and numerous other drugs. Cytarabine could have been the causative agent.[44]

DOSAGE AND ADMINISTRATION

Cytarabine is not active orally. The schedule and method of administration varies with the program of therapy to be used. Cytarabine may be given by intravenous infusion or injection, subcutaneously, or intrathecally. Thrombophlebitis has occurred at the site of drug injection or infusion in some patients, and rarely patients have noted pain and inflammation at subcutaneous injection sites. In most instances, however, the drug has been well tolerated.

Patients can tolerate higher total doses when they receive the drug by rapid intravenous injection as compared with slow infusion. This phenomenon is related to the drug's rapid inactivation and brief exposure of susceptible normal and neoplastic cells to significant levels after rapid injection. Normal and neoplastic cells seem to respond in somewhat parallel fashion to these different modes of administration and no clear-cut clinical advantage has been demonstrated for either.

In the induction therapy of acute nonlymphocytic leukemia, the usual cytarabine dose in combination with other anti-cancer drugs is 100 mg/m^2/day by continuous IV infusion (Days 1-7) or 100 mg/m^2 IV every 12 hours (Days 1-7).

The literature should be consulted for the current recommendations for use in acute lymphocytic leukemia.

INTRATHECAL USE IN MENINGEAL LEUKEMIA

Cytarabine has been used intrathecally in acute leukemia in doses ranging from 5-75 mg/m^2 of body surface area. The frequency of administration varied from once a day for 4 days to once every 4 days. The most frequently used dose was 30 mg/m^2 every 4 days until cerebrospinal fluid findings were normal, followed by one additional treatment.[24-28] The dosage schedule is usually governed by the type and severity of central nervous system manifestations and the response to previous therapy.

If used intrathecally, do not use a diluent containing benzyl alcohol. Many clinicians reconstitute with autologous spinal fluid or preservative-free 0.9% sodium chloride for injection and use immediately.

Cytarabine given intrathecally may cause systemic toxicity and careful monitoring of the hemopoietic system is indicated. Modification of other anti-leukemia therapy may be necessary. Major toxicity is rare. The most frequently reported reactions after intrathecal administration were nausea, vomiting and fever; these reactions are mild and self-limiting. Paraplegia has been reported.[29] Necrotizing leukoencephalopathy occurred in 5 children; these patients had also been treated with intrathecal methotrexate and hydrocortisone, as well as by central nervous system radiation.[30] Isolated neurotoxicity has been reported.[31] Blindness occurred in 2 patients in remission whose treatment had consisted of combination systemic chemotherapy, prophylactic central nervous system radiation and intrathecal cytarabine.[32]

When cytarabine is administered both intrathecally and intravenously within a few days, there is an increased risk of spinal cord toxicity, however, in serious life-threatening disease, concurrent use of intravenous and intrathecal cytarabine is left to the discretion of the treating physician.[48]

Focal leukemic involvement of the central nervous system may not respond to intrathecal cytarabine and may better be treated with radiotherapy.

The 100 mg vial may be reconstituted with 5 ml of bacteriostatic water for injection with benzyl alcohol 0.945% w/v added as preservative. The resulting solution contains 20 mg of cytarabine per ml. (Do not use bacteriostatic water for injection with benzyl alcohol 0.945% w/v as a diluent for intrathecal use. See WARNINGS.)

The 500 mg vial may be reconstituted with 10 ml bacteriostatic water for injection with benzyl alcohol 0.945% w/v added as preservative. The resulting solution contains 50 mg of cytarabine per ml. (Do not use bacteriostatic water for injection with benzyl alcohol 0.945% w/v as a diluent for intrathecal use. See WARNINGS.)

The 1 g vial may be reconstituted with 10 ml of bacteriostatic water for injection with benzyl alcohol 0.945% w/v added as preservative. The resulting solution contains 100 mg of cytarabine per ml. (Do not use bacteriostatic water for injection with benzyl alcohol 0.945% w/v as a diluent for intrathecal use. See WARNINGS.)

The 2 g vial may be reconstituted with 20 ml of bacteriostatic water for injection with benzyl alcohol 0.945% w/v added as preservative. The resulting solution contains 100 mg of cytarabine per ml. (Do not use bacteriostatic water for injection with benzyl alcohol 0.945% w/v as a diluent for intrathecal use. See WARNINGS.)

If used intrathecally many clinicians reconstitute with preservative-free 0.9% sodium chloride for injection and use immediately.

The pH of the reconstituted solutions is about 5. Solutions reconstituted with bacteriostatic water for injection with benzyl alcohol 0.945% w/v may be stored at controlled room temperature, 20-25°C (68-77°F) for 48 hours. Discard any solutions in which a slight haze develops.

Solutions reconstituted without a preservative should be used immediately.

CHEMICAL STABILITY OF INFUSION SOLUTIONS

Chemical stability studies were performed by ultraviolet assay on cytarabine in infusion solutions. These studies showed that when reconstituted cytarabine was added to water for injection, 5% dextrose in water or sodium chloride injection, 94-96% of the cytarabine was present after 192 hours storage at room temperature.

Parenteral drugs should be inspected visually for particulate matter and discoloration, prior to administration, whenever solution and container permit.

Procedures for proper handling and disposal of anticancer drugs should be considered. Several guidelines on this subject have been published.[33-38] There is no general agreement that all of the procedures recommended in the guidelines are necessary or appropriate.

ANIMAL PHARMACOLOGY

Toxicity of cytarabine in experimental animals, as well as activity, is markedly influenced by the schedule of administration. For example, in mice, the LD_{10} for single intraperitoneal administration is greater than 6000 mg/m^2. However, when administered as 8 doses, each separated by 3 hours, the LD_{10} is less than 750 mg/m^2 total dose. Similarly, although a total dose of 1920 mg/m^2 administered as 12 injections at 6 hour intervals was lethal to beagle dogs (severe bone marrow hypoplasia with evidence of liver and kidney damage), dogs receiving the same total dose administered in 8 injections (again at 6 hour intervals) over a 48 hour period survived with minimal signs of toxicity. The most consistent observation in surviving dogs was elevated transaminase levels. In all experimental species the primary limiting toxic effect is marrow suppression with leukopenia. In addition, cytarabine causes abnormal cerebellar development in the neonatal hamster and is teratogenic to the rat fetus.

PRODUCT LISTING - RATED THERAPEUTICALLY EQUIVALENT

Powder For Injection - Injectable - 1 Gm

1's	$25.00	GENERIC, Bedford Laboratories	55390-0133-01
1's	$49.46	GENERIC, Abbott Pharmaceutical	00703-5194-01
1's	$50.00	GENERIC, Vha Supply	55390-0808-01
1's	$67.73	CYTOSAR-U, Pharmacia and Upjohn	00009-3295-01

Powder For Injection - Injectable - 2 Gm

1's	$50.00	GENERIC, Bedford Laboratories	55390-0134-01
1's	$98.90	GENERIC, Bedford Laboratories	55390-0809-01
1's	$98.92	GENERIC, Abbott Pharmaceutical	00703-5195-01
1's	$100.00	GENERIC, Faulding Pharmaceutical Company	61703-0319-22
1's	$132.58	CYTOSAR-U, Pharmacia and Upjohn	00009-3296-01

Powder For Injection - Injectable - 100 mg

1's	$8.98	CYTOSAR-U, Pharmacia and Upjohn	00009-0373-01
10's	$37.50	GENERIC, Bedford Laboratories	55390-0131-10
10's	$62.24	GENERIC, Abbott Pharmaceutical	00703-5182-03
10's	$62.50	GENERIC, Vha Supply	55390-0806-10

Powder For Injection - Injectable - 500 mg

1's	$35.64	CYTOSAR-U, Pharmacia and Upjohn	00009-0473-01
5's	$130.15	GENERIC, Abbott Pharmaceutical	00703-5193-02
10's	$106.25	GENERIC, Bedford Laboratories	55390-0132-10
10's	$250.00	GENERIC, Vha Supply	55390-0807-10

Solution - Injectable - 20 mg/ml

5 ml	$69.40	GENERIC, Faulding Pharmaceutical Company	61703-0305-09
25 ml x 5	$143.65	GENERIC, Faulding Pharmaceutical Company	61703-0304-25
50 ml	$268.95	GENERIC, Faulding Pharmaceutical Company	61703-0303-50

PRODUCT LISTING - EQUIVALENTS NOT AVAILABLE

Solution - Injectable - 20 mg/ml

5 ml	$6.58	GENERIC, Fujisawa	00469-1030-05
50 ml	$51.87	GENERIC, Fujisawa	00469-1030-50

Cytarabine Liposome (003434)

Categories: FDA Approved 1999 April; Pregnancy Category D; Orphan Drugs
Drug Classes: Antineoplastics, antimetabolites
Brand Names: **DepoCyt**

WARNING

Cytarabine liposome should be administered only under the supervision of a qualified physician experienced in the use of intrathecal cancer chemotherapeutic agents. Appropriate management of complications is possible only when adequate diagnostic and treatment facilities are readily available. In all clinical studies, chemical arachnoiditis, a syndrome manifested primarily by nausea, vomiting, headache, and fever was a common adverse event. If left untreated, chemical arachnoiditis may be fatal. The incidence and severity of chemical arachnoiditis can be reduced by coadministration of dexamethasone (see WARNINGS). Patients receiving cytarabine liposome should be treated concurrently with dexamethasone to mitigate the symptoms of chemical arachnoiditis (see DOSAGE AND ADMINISTRATION).

DESCRIPTION

DepoCyt is a sterile, injectable suspension of the antimetabolite cytarabine, encapsulated into multivesicular lipid-based particles. Chemically, cytarabine is 4-amino-1-β-D-arabinofuranosyl-2(1H)-pyrimidinone, also known as cytosine arabinoside ($C_9H_{13}N_3O_5$, molecular weight 243.22).

DepoCyt is available in 5 ml, ready-to-use, single-use vials containing 50 mg of cytarabine. DepoCyt is formulated as a sterile, non-pyrogenic, white to off-white suspension of cytarabine in sodium chloride 0.9% w/v in water for injection. DepoCyt is preservative-free. Cytarabine, the active ingredient, is present at a concentration of 10 mg/ml, and is encapsulated in the particles. Inactive ingredients at their respective approximate concentrations are cholesterol 4.1 mg/ml, triolein 1.2 mg/ml, dioleoylphosphatidylcholine (DOPC) 5.7 mg/ml, and dipalmitoylphosphatidylglycerol (DPPG) 1.0 mg/ml. The pH of the product falls within the range from 5.5-8.5.

CLINICAL PHARMACOLOGY

MECHANISM OF ACTION

Cytarabine liposome is a sustained-release formulation of the active ingredient cytarabine designed for direct administration into the cerebrospinal fluid (CSF). Cytarabine is a cell cycle phase-specific antineoplastic agent, affecting cells only during the S-phase of cell division. Intracellularly, cytarabine is converted into cytarabine-5′-triphosphate (ara-CTP), which is the active metabolite. The mechanism of action is not completely understood, but it appears that ara-CTP acts primarily through inhibition of DNA polymerase. Incorporation into DNA and RNA may also contribute to cytarabine cytotoxicity. Cytarabine is cytotoxic to a wide variety of proliferating mammalian cells in culture.

PHARMACOKINETICS

The pharmacokinetics of cytarabine liposome administered intrathecally to patients at a 50 mg dose every 2 weeks is currently under investigation. However, preliminary analysis of the pharmacokinetic data show that following cytarabine liposome intrathecal administration in patients, in either the lumbar sac or by intraventricular reservoir, peak levels of free cytarabine were observed within 5 hours in both the ventricle and lumbar sac. These peak levels were followed by a biphasic elimination profile with a terminal phase half-life of 100-263 hours over a dose range of 12.5 to 75 mg. In contrast, intrathecal administration of 30 mg of free cytarabine showed a biphasic CSF concentration profile with a terminal phase half-life of 3.4 hours. Since the transfer rate of cytarabine from the CSF to plasma is slow and the conversion of cytarabine to ara-U in the plasma is fast, systemic exposure to cytarabine was negligible following intrathecal administration of cytarabine liposome, 50 or 75 mg.

Metabolism and Elimination

The primary route of elimination of cytarabine is metabolism to the inactive compound ara-U (1-β-D-arabinofuranosyluracil or uracilarabinoside), followed by urinary excretion of ara-U. In contrast to systemically administered cytarabine, which is rapidly metabolized to ara-U, conversion to ara-U in the CSF is negligible after intrathecal administration because of the significantly lower cytidine deaminase activity in the CNS tissues and CSF. The CSF clearance rate of cytarabine is similar to the CSF bulk flow rate of 0.24 ml/min.

Drug Interactions

No formal assessments of pharmacokinetic drug-drug interactions between cytarabine liposome and other agents have been conducted.

Special Populations
The effects of gender or race on the pharmacokinetics of cytarabine liposome have not been studied, nor has the effect of renal or hepatic impairment.

INDICATIONS AND USAGE

Cytarabine liposome is indicated for the intrathecal treatment of lymphomatous meningitis. This indication is based on demonstration of increased complete response rate compared to unencapsulated cytarabine. There are no controlled trials that demonstrate a clinical benefit resulting from this treatment, such as improvement in disease-related symptoms, or increased time to disease progression, or increased survival.

CONTRAINDICATIONS

Cytarabine liposome is contraindicated in patients who are hypersensitive to cytarabine or any component of the formulation, and in patients with active meningeal infection.

WARNINGS

See BOXED WARNING.

Cytarabine liposome should be administered only under the supervision of a qualified physician experienced in the use of cancer chemotherapeutic agents. Appropriate management of complications is possible only when adequate diagnostic and treatment facilities are readily available. Chemical arachnoiditis, a syndrome manifested primarily by nausea, vomiting, headache, and fever, has been a common adverse event in all studies. If left untreated, chemical arachnoiditis may be fatal. The incidence and severity of chemical arachnoiditis can be reduced by coadministration of dexamethasone. Patients receiving cytarabine liposome should be treated concurrently with dexamethasone to mitigate the symptoms of chemical arachnoiditis (see DOSAGE AND ADMINISTRATION).

During the clinical studies, 2 deaths related to cytarabine liposome were reported. One patient died after developing encephalopathy 36 hours after an intraventricular dose of cytarabine liposome, 125 mg. This patient was receiving concurrent whole-brain irradiation and had previously received systemic chemotherapy with cyclophosphamide, doxorubicin, and fluorouracil, as well as intraventricular methotrexate. The other patient received cytarabine liposome 50 mg by the intraventricular route and developed focal seizures progressing to status epilepticus. This patient died approximately 8 weeks after the last dose of study medication. The death of 1 additional patient was considered "possibly" related to cytarabine liposome. He was a 63-year-old with extensive lymphoma involving the nasopharynx, brain, and meninges with multiple neurologic deficits who died of apparent disease progression 4 days after his second dose of cytarabine liposome.

After intrathecal administration of free cytarabine the most frequently reported reactions are nausea, vomiting and fever. Intrathecal administration of free cytarabine may cause myelopathy and other neurologic toxicity and can rarely lead to a permanent neurologic deficit. Administration of intrathecal cytarabine in combination with other chemotherapeutic agents or with cranial/spinal irradiation may increase this risk of neurotoxicity.

Blockage to CSF flow may result in increased free cytarabine concentrations in the CSF and an increased risk of neurotoxicity.

PREGNANCY CATEGORY D

There are no studies assessing the reproductive toxicity of cytarabine liposome. Cytarabine, the active component of cytarabine liposome, can cause fetal harm if a pregnant woman is exposed to the drug systemically. Three anecdotal cases of major limb malformations have been reported in infants after their mothers received intravenous cytarabine, alone or in combination with other agents, during the first trimester. The concern for fetal harm following intrathecal cytarabine liposome administration is low, however, because systemic exposure to cytarabine is negligible. Cytarabine was teratogenic in mice (cleft palate, phocomelia, deformed appendages, skeletal abnormalities) when doses ≥2 mg/kg/day were administered IP during the period of organogenesis (about 0.2 times the recommended human dose on mg/m^2 basis), and in rats (deformed appendages) when 20 mg/kg was administered as a single IP dose on day 12 of gestation (about 4 times the recommended human dose on mg/m^2 basis). Single IP doses of 50 mg/kg in rats (about 10 times the recommended human dose on mg/m^2 basis) on day 14 of gestation also cause reduced prenatal and postnatal brain size and permanent impairment of learning ability. Cytarabine was embryotoxic in mice when administered during the period of organogenesis. Embryotoxicity was characterized by decreased fetal weight at 0.5 mg/kg/day (about 0.05 times the recommended human dose on mg/m^2 basis), and increased early and late resorptions and decreased live litter sizes at 8 mg/kg/day (approximately equal to the recommended human dose on mg/m^2 basis). There are no adequate and well controlled studies in pregnant women. If this drug is used during pregnancy or if the patient becomes pregnant while taking this drug, the patient should be apprised of the potential harm to the fetus. Despite the low apparent risk for fetal harm, women of childbearing potential should be advised to avoid becoming pregnant.

PRECAUTIONS

GENERAL

Cytarabine liposome has the potential of producing serious toxicity (see BOXED WARNING). All patients receiving cytarabine liposome should be treated concurrently with dexamethasone to mitigate the symptoms of chemical arachnoiditis (see DOSAGE AND ADMINISTRATION). Toxic effects may be related to a single dose or to cumulative administration. Because toxic effects can occur at any time during therapy (although they are most likely within 5 days of drug administration), patients receiving intrathecal therapy with cytarabine liposome should be monitored continuously for the development of neurotoxicity. If patients develop neurotoxicity, subsequent doses of cytarabine liposome should be reduced, and cytarabine liposome should be discontinued if toxicity persists.

Some patients with neoplastic meningitis receiving treatment with cytarabine liposome may require concurrent radiation or systemic therapy with other chemotherapeutic agents; this may increase the rate of adverse events.

Anaphylactic reactions following intravenous administration of free cytarabine have been reported.

Although significant systemic exposure to free cytarabine following intrathecal treatment is not expected, some effect on bone marrow function cannot be excluded. Systemic toxicity due to intravenous administration of cytarabine consists primarily of bone marrow suppression with leukopenia, thrombocytopenia, and anemia. Accordingly, careful monitoring of the hematopoietic system is advised.

Transient elevations in CSF protein and white blood cells have been observed in patients following cytarabine liposome administration and have also been noted after intrathecal treatment with methotrexate or cytarabine.

INFORMATION FOR THE PATIENT

Patients should be informed about the expected adverse events of headache, nausea, vomiting, and fever, and about the early signs and symptoms of neurotoxicity. The importance of concurrent dexamethasone administration should be emphasized at the initiation of each cycle of cytarabine liposome treatment. Patients should be instructed to seek medical attention if signs or symptoms of neurotoxicity develop, or if oral dexamethasone is not well tolerated (see DOSAGE AND ADMINISTRATION).

LABORATORY TEST INTERACTIONS

Since cytarabine liposome particles are similar in size and appearance to white blood cells, care must be taken in interpreting CSF examinations following cytarabine liposome administration.

CARCINOGENESIS, MUTAGENESIS, AND IMPAIRMENT OF FERTILITY

No carcinogenicity, mutagenicity or impairment of fertility studies have been conducted with cytarabine liposome. The active ingredient of cytarabine liposome, cytarabine, was mutagenic in *in vitro* tests and was clastogenic *in vitro* (chromosome aberrations and SCE in human leukocytes) and *in vivo* (chromosome aberrations and SCE assay in rodent bone marrow, mouse micronucleus assay). Cytarabine caused the transformation of hamster embryo cells and rat H43 cells *in vitro*. Cytarabine was clastogenic to meiotic cells; a dose-dependent increase in sperm-head abnormalities and chromosomal aberrations occurred in mice given IP cytarabine.

Impairment of Fertility

No studies assessing the impact of cytarabine on fertility are available in the literature. Because the systemic exposure to free cytarabine following intrathecal treatment with cytarabine liposome was negligible, the risk of impaired fertility after intrathecal cytarabine liposome is likely to be low.

PREGNANCY CATEGORY D

See WARNINGS, Pregnancy Category D.

NURSING MOTHERS

It is not known whether cytarabine is excreted in human milk following intrathecal cytarabine liposome administration. The systemic exposure to free cytarabine following intrathecal treatment with cytarabine liposome was negligible. Despite the low apparent risk, because many drugs are excreted in human milk and because of the potential for serious adverse reactions in nursing infants, the use of cytarabine liposome is not recommended in nursing women.

PEDIATRIC USE

The safety and efficacy of cytarabine liposome in pediatric patients has not been established.

DRUG INTERACTIONS

No formal drug interaction studies of cytarabine liposome and other drugs were conducted. Concomitant administration of cytarabine liposome with other antineoplastic agents administered by the intrathecal route has not been studied. With intrathecal cytarabine and other cytotoxic agents administered intrathecally, enhanced neurotoxicity has been associated with co-administration of drugs.

ADVERSE REACTIONS

The toxicity database consists of the observations made during an early uncontrolled study and the controlled multi-arm study described above. In the early study, patients received cytarabine liposome at doses ranging from 12.5 to 125 mg. In the randomized multi-arm study cytarabine liposome was administered at a dose of 50 mg every 2 weeks and was compared to standard intrathecal chemotherapy (cytarabine or methotrexate) in patients with lymphoma, leukemia and solid tumors; 28 lymphoma patients, 5 leukemia patients and 59 solid tumor patients received study drug.

Arachnoiditis is an expected and well-documented side effect of both neoplastic meningitis and of intrathecal chemotherapy. For clinical studies of cytarabine liposome, chemical arachnoiditis was defined as the occurrence of any one of the symptoms of neck rigidity, neck pain, meningism, or any two of the symptoms of nausea, vomiting, headache, fever, back pain, or CSF pleocytosis; the grade assigned to an episode of chemical arachnoiditis was the highest severity grade of its component symptoms. Since most of the adverse events reported in the trials were transient episodes associated with drug exposure, the incidence of these events is best expressed by drug cycle. A cycle of treatment for all treatment groups was defined as the 14 day period between cytarabine liposome doses. The duration of reported symptoms was from 1-5 days. Although it was sometimes difficult to distinguish between drug-related chemical arachnoiditis, infectious meningitis, or disease progression, >90% of the chemical arachnoiditis cases reported occurred within 48 hours of the administration of intrathecal drug, indicating a drug etiology.

In the early study, chemical arachnoiditis was observed in 100% of cycles without dexamethasone prophylaxis; with concurrent administration of dexamethasone, chemical arachnoiditis was observed in 33% of cycles. Patients receiving cytarabine liposome should be treated concurrently with dexamethasone to mitigate the symptoms of chemical arachnoiditis (see DOSAGE AND ADMINISTRATION).

TABLE 2 shows the rate of all adverse events occurring in ≥10% of patients, as a rate per cycle, in the lymphoma randomized study.

TABLE 2 *Comparison of Adverse Events Occurring in ≥10% of Patients, by Cycle*

Patients with lymphomatous meningitis receiving cytarabine liposome or cytarabine (ara-C) in the randomized study

Body System	All Adverse Events		Grade 3 or 4	
	CL	Ara-C	CL	Ara-C
Adverse Event	n=74	n=45	n=74	n=45
Body as a Whole	53%	60%	18%	22%
Headache*	28%	9%	5%	2%
Asthenia	19%	33%	5%	9%
Fever*	11%	24%	4%	0%
Back pain*	7%	11%	0%	2%
Pain	11%	20%	3%	0%
Nervous System	45%	53%	18%	18%
Confusion	14%	7%	4%	2%
Somnolence	12%	11%	4%	2%
Abnormal gait	4%	11%	1%	2%
Digestive System	27%	44%	7%	9%
Nausea*	11%	16%	0%	4%
Vomiting*	12%	18%	3%	2%
Constipation	7%	11%	0%	0%
Metabolic and Nutritional Disorders	16%	24%	0%	0%
Peripheral Edema	7%	11%	0%	0%
Hematologic	19%	22%	11%	13%
Neutropenia	9%	11%	8%	11%
Thrombocytopenia	8%	16%	5%	11%
Anemia	1%	13%	1%	4%
Urogenital System	11%	20%	3%	2%
Urinary incontinence	3%	11%	0%	0%
Special Senses	16%	18%	1%	2%

* Components of Chemical Arachnoiditis.
CL Cytarabine liposome.
Ara-C Cytarabine.

DOSAGE AND ADMINISTRATION

PREPARATION OF CYTARABINE LIPOSOME

Cytarabine liposome is a cytotoxic anticancer drug and, as with other potentially toxic compounds, caution should be used in handling cytarabine liposome. The use of gloves is recommended. If cytarabine liposome suspension contacts the skin, wash immediately with soap and water. If it contacts mucous membranes, flush thoroughly with water (see Handling and Disposal). Cytarabine liposome particles are more dense than the diluent and have a tendency to settle with time. Vials of cytarabine liposome should be allowed to warm to room temperature and gently agitated or inverted to re-suspend the particles immediately prior to withdrawal from the vial. Avoid aggressive agitation. No further reconstitution or dilution is required.

CYTARABINE LIPOSOME ADMINISTRATION

Cytarabine liposome should be withdrawn from the vial immediately before administration. Cytarabine liposome is a single-use vial and does not contain any preservative; cytarabine liposome should be used within 4 hours of withdrawal from the vial. Unused portions of each vial should be discarded properly (see Handling and Disposal). Do not save any unused portions for later administration. Do not mix cytarabine liposome with any other medications.

In-line filters must not be used when administering cytarabine liposome. Cytarabine liposome is administered directly into the CSF via an intraventricular reservoir or by direct injection into the lumbar sac. Cytarabine liposome should be injected slowly over a period of 1-5 minutes. Following drug administration by lumbar puncture, the patient should be instructed to lie flat for 1 hour. Patients should be observed by the physician for immediate toxic reactions.

Patients should be started on dexamethasone 4 mg bid either PO or IV for 5 days beginning on the day of cytarabine liposome injection.

Cytarabine liposome must only be administered by the intrathecal route.

Further dilution of cytarabine liposome is not recommended.

DOSING REGIMEN

For the treatment of lymphomatous meningitis, cytarabine liposome 50 mg (1 vial of cytarabine liposome) is recommended to be given according to the following schedule:

Induction Therapy: Cytarabine liposome, 50 mg, administered intrathecally (intraventricular or lumbar puncture) every 14 days for 2 doses (weeks 1 and 3).

Consolidation Therapy: Cytarabine liposome, 50 mg, administered intrathecally (intraventricular or lumbar puncture) every 14 days for 3 doses (weeks 5, 7 and 9) followed by 1 additional dose at week 13.

Maintenance: Cytarabine liposome, 50 mg, administered intrathecally (intraventricular or lumbar puncture) every 28 days for 4 doses (weeks 17, 21, 25 and 29).

If drug related neurotoxicity develops, the dose should be reduced to 25 mg. If it persists, treatment with cytarabine liposome should be discontinued.

HANDLING AND DISPOSAL

Procedures for proper handling and disposal of anticancer drugs should be considered. Several guidelines on this subject have been published.[1-7] There is no general agreement that all of the procedures recommended in the guidelines are necessary or appropriate.

HOW SUPPLIED

DepoCyt is available in 5 ml, ready-to-use, single-use vials containing 50 mg of cytarabine. DepoCyt is formulated as a sterile, non-pyrogenic, white to off-white suspension of cytarabine in sodium chloride 0.9% w/v in water for injection.

STORAGE

Refrigerate at 2-8°C. Protect from freezing and avoid aggressive agitation.

Do not use beyond expiration date printed on the label.

PRODUCT LISTING - EQUIVALENTS NOT AVAILABLE

Suspension - Intrathecal - 10 mg/ml

5 ml $1955.00 DEPOCYT, Chiron Therapeutics 53905-0331-01

Dacarbazine (000938)

D

Categories: Lymphoma, Hodgkin's; Melanoma, malignant; Pregnancy Category C; FDA Approved 1975 May; WHO Formulary
Drug Classes: Antineoplastics, alkylating agents
Brand Names: Dtic-Dome
Foreign Brand Availability: Dacarbazin (Czech-Republic); Dacarbazine DBL (Malaysia); Dacarbazine Dome (Denmark); Dacarbazine For Injection (Australia); Dacatic (Finland); D.T.I.C. (Australia); D.T.I.C.-Dome (South-Africa); DTI (Korea); DTIC (Austria; Canada; Germany; Japan; Sweden); DTIC Dome (Ireland); DTIC-Dome (Belgium; England; Korea; New-Zealand; Spain; Switzerland; Taiwan); DTIC-VHB (India); Deticene (Czech-Republic; France; Greece; Hong-Kong; Israel; Italy; Malaysia; Mexico; Netherlands; Portugal; Russia; Switzerland; Turkey); Detimedac (Germany)
Cost of Therapy: $277.27 (Malignant Melanoma; Dtic-Dome Injection; 200 mg; 200 mg/day; 10 day supply)
HCFA JCODE(S): J9130 100 mg IV; J9140 200 mg IV

WARNING

It is recommended that dacarbazine be administered under the supervision of a qualified physician experienced in the use of cancer chemotherapeutic agents.

Hemopoietic depression is the most common toxicity with dacarbazine (see WARNINGS).

Hepatic necrosis has been reported (see WARNINGS).

Studies have demonstrated this agent to have a carcinogenic and teratogenic effect when used in animals.

In treatment of each patient, the physician must weigh carefully the possibility of achieving therapeutic benefit against the risk of toxicity.

DESCRIPTION

Dacarbazine is a colorless to an ivory colored solid which is light sensitive. Each vial contains 100 or 200 mg of dacarbazine (the active ingredient), anhydrous citric acid and mannitol. Dacarbazine is reconstituted and administered intravenously (pH 3-4). Dacarbazine is an anticancer agent. Chemically, dacarbazine is 5-(3,3-dimethyl-l-triazeno)-imidazole-4-carboxamide (DTIC).

CLINICAL PHARMACOLOGY

After IV administration of dacarbazine, the volume of distribution exceeds total body water content in some body tissue, probably the liver. Its disappearance from the plasma is biphasic with initial half- life of 19 minutes and a terminal half-life of 5 hours.[1] In a patient with renal and hepatic dysfunctions, the half-lives were lengthened to 55 minutes and 7.2 hours.[1] The average cumulative excretion of unchanged dacarbazine in the urine is 40% of the injected dose in 6 hours.[1] Dacarbazine is subject to renal tubular secretion rather than glomerular filtration. At therapeutic concentrations, dacarbazine is not appreciably bound to plasma proteins.

In man, dacarbazine is extensively degraded. Besides unchanged dacarbazine, 5-aminoimidazole-4 carboxamide (AIC) is a major metabolite of dacarbazine excreted in the urine. AIC is a major metabolite of dacarbazine excreted on the urine. AIC is not derived endogenously but from the injected dacarbazine, because the administration of radioactive dacarbazine labeled with ^{14}C in the imidazole portion of the molecule (dacarbazine-2-^{14}) gives rise to AIC-2-^{14}C.[1]

Although the exact mechanism of action of dacarbazine is not known, three hypotheses have been offered:

Inhibition of DNA-synthesis by acting as a purine analog.
Action as an alkylating agent.
Interaction with SH groups.

INDICATIONS AND USAGE

Dacarbazine is indicated in the treatment of metastatic malignant melanoma. In addition, dacarbazine is also indicated for Hodgkin's disease as a second-line therapy when used in combination with other effective agents.

NON-FDA APPROVED INDICATIONS

Dacarbazine has been used without FDA approval in the treatment of soft tissue sarcomas.

CONTRAINDICATIONS

Dacarbazine is contraindicated in patients who have demonstrated a hypersensitivity to it in the past.

WARNINGS

Hemopoietic depression is the most common toxicity with dacarbazine and involves primarily the leukocytes and platelets, although anemia may sometimes occur. Leukopenia and thrombocytopenia may be severe enough to cause death. The possible bone marrow depression requires careful monitoring of white blood cells, red blood cells, and platelet levels. Hemopoietic toxicity may warrant temporary suspension or cessation of therapy with dacarbazine.

Hepatic toxicity, accompanied by hepatic vein thrombosis and hepatocellular necrosis resulting in death, has been reported. The incidence of such reactions has been low; approximately 0.01% of patients treated. This toxicity has been observed mostly when dacarbazine has been administered concomitantly with other anti-neoplastic drugs; however, it has also been reported in some patients treated with dacarbazine alone.

Anaphylaxis can occur following the administration of dacarbazine.

PRECAUTIONS

Hospitalization is not always necessary but adequate laboratory study capability must be available. Extravasation of the drug subcutaneously during IV administration may result in tissue damage and severe pain. Local pain, burning sensation, and irritation at the site of injection may be relieved by locally applied hot packs.

Carcinogenicity of dacarbazine was studied in rats and mice. Proliferative endocardial lesions, including fibrocarcinomas and sarcomas, were induced by dacarbazine in rats. In mice, administration of dacarbazine resulted in the induction of angiosarcomas of the spleen.

D

PREGNANCY CATEGORY C

Dacarbazine has been shown to be teratogenic in rats when given in doses 20 times the human daily dose on day 12 of gestation. Dacarbazine when administered in 10 times the human dose female rats mated to male rats (twice weekly for 9 weeks) did not affect the male libido, although female rats mated to male rats had higher incidence of resorptions than controls. In rabbits, dacarbazine daily dose 7 times the human daily dose given on days 6-15 of gestation resulted in fetal skeletal abnormalities. There are no adequate and well controlled studies in pregnant women. Dacarbazine should be used during pregnancy only if the potential benefit justifies the potential risk to the fetus. It is not known whether this drug is excreted in human milk. Because many drugs are excreted in human milk and because the potential for tumorigenicity shown for dacarbazine in animal studies, a decision should be made whether to continue nursing or to discontinue the drug, taking into account the importance of the drug to the mother.

ADVERSE REACTIONS

Symptoms of anorexia, nausea, and vomiting are the most frequently noted of all toxic reactions. Over 90% of the patients are affected with the initial few doses. The vomiting lasts 1-12 hours and is incompletely and unpredictably palliated with phenobarbital and/or prochlorperazine. Rarely, intractable nausea and vomiting have necessitated discontinuance of therapy with dacarbazine. Rarely, dacarbazine has caused diarrhea. Some helpful suggestions include restricting the patient's oral intake of food for 4-6 hours prior to treatment. The rapid toleration of these symptoms suggests that a central nervous system mechanism may be involved, and usually these symptoms subside after the first 1 or 2 days.

There are a number of minor toxicities that are infrequently noted. Patients have experienced an influenzae-like syndrome of fever to 39°C, myalgias and malaise. These symptoms occur usually after large single doses, may last for several days, and then may occur with successive treatments.

Alopecia has been noted as has facial flushing and facial paresthesia. There have been few reports of significant liver or renal function test abnormalities in man. However, these abnormalities have been observed more frequently in animal studies.

Erythematous and urticarial rashes have been observed infrequently after administration of dacarbazine. Rarely, photosensitivity reactions may occur.

DOSAGE AND ADMINISTRATION

Malignant Melanoma: The recommended dosage is 2-4.5 mg/kg/day for 10 days. Treatment may be repeated at 4 week intervals.[2]

An alternativee recommended dosage is 250 mg/square meter body surface/day IV for 5 days. Treatment may be repeated every 3 weeks.[3,4]

Hodgkin's Disease: The recommended dosage of dacarbazine in the treatment of Hodgkin's disease is 150 mg/square meter body surface for 5 days, in combination with other effective drugs. Treatment may be repeated every 4 weeks.[5] An alternative recommended dosage is 375 mg/kg square meter body surface on day 1, in combination with other effective drugs, to be repeated every 15 days.[6]

Dacarbazine 100 and 200 mg/vial are reconstituted with 9.9 ml and 19.7 ml, respectively, of sterile water for injection. The resulting solution contains 10 mg/ml of dacarbazine having a pH of 3.0-4.0. The calculated dose of the resulting solution is drawn into a syringe and administered *only* intravenously.

The reconstituted solution may be further diluted with 5% dextrose injection or sodium chloride injection and administered as an IV infusion.

After reconstitution and prior to use, the solution in the vial may be stored at 4°C for up to 72 hours or at normal room conditions (temperature and light) for up to 8 hours. If the reconstituted solution is further diluted in 5% dextrose injection or sodium chloride injection the resulting solution may be stored at 4°C for up to 24 hours or at normal room conditions for up to 8 hours.

Procedures for proper handling and disposal of anticancer drugs should be considered. Several guidelines on this subject have been published.[7-12] There is no general agreement that all of the procedures recommended in the guidelines are necessary or appropriate.

PRODUCT LISTING - RATED THERAPEUTICALLY EQUIVALENT

Powder For Injection - Intravenous - 100 mg

10's	$13.35	GENERIC, American Pharmaceutical Partners	63323-0127-10
12's	$165.92	DTIC-DOME, Bayer	00026-8151-10

Powder For Injection - Intravenous - 200 mg

1's	$25.27	GENERIC, Gensia Sicor Pharmaceuticals Inc	00703-5075-01
1's	$26.65	GENERIC, American Pharmaceutical Partners	63323-0128-20
10's	$236.25	GENERIC, Bedford Laboratories	55390-0090-10
10's	$252.70	GENERIC, Gensia Sicor Pharmaceuticals Inc	00703-5075-03
12's	$332.72	DTIC-DOME, Bayer	00026-8151-20

Powder For Injection - Intravenous - 500 mg

1's	$59.38	GENERIC, Abbott Pharmaceutical	00703-4658-01

PRODUCT LISTING - EQUIVALENTS NOT AVAILABLE

Powder For Injection - Intravenous - 200 mg

1's	$23.00	GENERIC, Faulding Pharmaceutical Company	61703-0327-22

Daclizumab *(003376)*

Categories: Rejection, renal transplant, prophylaxis; FDA Approved 1997 Dec; Pregnancy Category C; Orphan Drugs
Drug Classes: Immunosuppressives; Monoclonal antibodies
Brand Names: Zenapax
HCFA JCODE(S): J7513 25 mg IV

> **WARNING**
>
> **Only physicians experienced in immunosuppressive therapy and management of organ transplant patients should prescribe daclizumab. The physician responsible for daclizumab administration should have complete information requisite for the follow-up of the patient. Patients receiving the drug should be managed in facilities equipped and staffed with adequate laboratory and supportive medical resources.**

DESCRIPTION

Daclizumab is an immunosuppressive, humanized IgG1 monoclonal antibody produced by recombinant DNA technology that binds specifically to the alpha subunit (p55 alpha, CD25, or Tac subunit) of the human high-affinity interleukin-2 (IL-2) receptor that is expressed on the surface of activated lymphocytes.

Daclizumab is a composite of human (90%) and murine (10%) antibody sequences. The human sequences were derived from the constant domains of human IgG1 and the variable framework regions of the Eu myeloma antibody. The murine sequences were derived from the complementarity-determining regions of a murine anti-Tac antibody. The molecular weight predicted from DNA sequencing is 144 kilodaltons.

Zenapax 25 mg/5ml is supplied as a clear, sterile, colorless concentrate for further dilution and intravenous administration. Each milliliter of Zenapax contains 5 mg of daclizumab and 3.6 mg sodium phosphate monobasic monohydrate, 11 mg sodium phosphate dibasic heptahydrate, 4.6 mg sodium chloride, 0.2 mg polysorbate 80 and may contain hydrochloric acid or sodium hydroxide to adjust the pH to 6.9. No preservatives are added.

CLINICAL PHARMACOLOGY

MECHANISM OF ACTION

Daclizumab functions as an IL-2 receptor antagonist that binds with high-affinity to the Tac subunit of the high-affinity IL-2 receptor complex and inhibits IL-2 binding. Daclizumab binding is highly specific for Tac, which is expressed on activated but not resting lymphocytes. Administration of daclizumab inhibits IL-2-mediated activation of lymphocytes, a critical pathway in the cellular immune response involved in allograft rejection.

While in the circulation, daclizumab impairs the response of the immune system to antigenic challenges. Whether the ability to respond to repeated or ongoing challenges with those antigens returns to normal after daclizumab is cleared is unknown (see PRECAUTIONS).

PHARMACOKINETICS

In clinical trials involving renal allograft patients treated with a 1 mg/kg IV dose of daclizumab every 14 days for a total of five doses, peak serum concentration (mean ± SD) rose between the first dose (21 ± 14 μg/ml) and fifth dose (32 ± 22 μg/ml). The mean trough serum concentration before the fifth dose was 7.6 ± 4.0 μg/ml. *In vitro* and *in vivo* data suggest that serum levels of 5 to 10 μg/ml are necessary for saturation of the Tac subunit of the IL-2 receptors to block the responses of activated T lymphocytes.

Population pharmacokinetic analysis of the data using a two-compartment open model gave the following values for a reference patient (45-year-old male Caucasian patient with a body weight of 80 kg and no proteinuria): systemic clearance = 15 ml/hour, volume of central compartment = 2.5 liter, volume of peripheral compartment = 3.4 liter. The estimated terminal elimination half-life for the reference patient was 20 days (480 hours), which is similar to the terminal elimination half-life for human IgG (18-23 days). Bayesian estimates of terminal elimination half-life ranged from 11-38 days for the 123 patients included in the population analysis.

The influence of body weight on systemic clearance supports the dosing of daclizumab on a milligram per kilogram (mg/kg) basis. For patients studied, this dosing maintained drug exposure within 30% of the reference exposure. Covariate analyses showed that no dosage adjustments based on age, race, gender or degree of proteinuria, are required for renal allograft patients. The estimated interpatient variability (percent coefficient of variation) in systemic clearance and central volume of distribution were 15% and 27%, respectively.

PHARMACODYNAMICS

At the recommended dosage regimen, daclizumab saturates the Tac subunit of the IL-2 receptor for approximately 120 days post-transplant. The duration of clinically significant IL-2 receptor blockade after the recommended course of daclizumab is not known. No significant changes to circulating lymphocyte numbers or cell phenotypes were observed by flow cytometry. Cytokine release syndrome has not been observed after daclizumab administration.

INDICATIONS AND USAGE

Daclizumab is indicated for the prophylaxis of acute organ rejection in patients receiving renal transplants. It is used as part of an immunosuppressive regimen that includes cyclosporine and corticosteroids.

NON-FDA APPROVED INDICATIONS

Daclizumab may also have potential in the management of various T cell derived cancers including leukemia and several autoimmune T cell mediated disorders including uveitis, rheumatoid arthritis, and systemic lupus erythematosus. However, these uses have not been approved by the FDA and further clinical trials are needed.

CONTRAINDICATIONS

Daclizumab is contraindicated in patients with known hypersensitivity to daclizumab or to any components of this product.

WARNINGS

See BOXED WARNING.

Daclizumab should be administered under qualified medical supervision. Patients should be informed of the potential benefits of therapy and the risks associated with administration of immunosuppressive therapy.

While the incidence of lymphoproliferative disorders and opportunistic infections, in the limited clinical trial experience, was no higher in daclizumab-treated patients compared with placebo-treated patients, patients on immunosuppressive therapy are at increased risk for developing lymphoproliferative disorders and opportunistic infections and should be monitored accordingly.

Anaphylactoid reactions following the administration of daclizumab have not been observed but can occur following the administration of proteins. Medications for the treatment of severe hypersensitivity reactions should, therefore, be available for immediate use.

PRECAUTIONS

GENERAL

It is not known whether daclizumab use will have a long-term effect on the ability of the immune system to respond to antigens first encountered during daclizumab-induced immunosuppression.

Re-administration of daclizumab after an initial course of therapy has not been studied in humans. The potential risks of such re-administration, specifically those associated with immunosuppression and/or the occurrence of anaphylaxis/anaphylactoid reactions, are not known.

IMMUNOGENICITY

Low titers of anti-idiotype antibodies to daclizumab were detected in the daclizumab-treated patients with an overall incidence of 8.4%. No antibodies that affected efficacy, safety, serum daclizumab levels or any other clinically relevant parameter examined were detected.

CARCINOGENESIS, MUTAGENESIS, AND IMPAIRMENT OF FERTILITY

Long-term studies to evaluate the carcinogenic potential of daclizumab have not been performed. Daclizumab was not genotoxic in the Ames or the V79 chromosomal aberration assays, with or without metabolic activation. The effect of daclizumab on fertility is not known, because animal reproduction studies have not been conducted with daclizumab (see WARNINGS and ADVERSE REACTIONS).

PREGNANCY CATEGORY C

Animal reproduction studies have not been conducted with daclizumab. Therefore, it is not known whether daclizumab can cause fetal harm when administered to pregnant women or can affect reproductive capacity. In general, IgG molecules are known to cross the placental barrier. Daclizumab should not be used in pregnant women unless the potential benefit justifies the potential risk to the fetus. Women of childbearing potential should use effective contraception before beginning daclizumab therapy, during therapy, and for 4 months after completion of daclizumab therapy.

NURSING MOTHERS

It is not known whether daclizumab is excreted in human milk. Because many drugs are excreted in human milk, including human antibodies, and because of the potential for adverse reactions, a decision should be made to discontinue nursing or to discontinue the drug, taking into account the importance of the drug to the mother.

PEDIATRIC USE

No adequate and well-controlled studies have been completed in pediatric patients. The preliminary results of an ongoing safety and pharmacokinetic study (n=25) in pediatric patients (median age: 12 years of age, range: 11 months to 17 years of age; 11 months to 5 years = 7 patients; 6 years to 12 years = 6 patients; 13 years to 17 years = 12 patients) treated with daclizumab in addition to standard immunosuppressive agents including mycophenolate mofetil, cyclosporine, tacrolimus, azathioprine, and corticosteroids indicate that the most frequently reported adverse events were hypertension (48%), post-operative (post-traumatic) pain (44%), diarrhea (36%), and vomiting (32%). The reported rates of hypertension and dehydration were higher for pediatric patients than for adult patients. It is not known whether the immune response to vaccines, infection, and other antigenic stimuli administered or encountered during daclizumab therapy is impaired or whether such response will remain impaired after daclizumab therapy.

The preliminary pharmacokinetic results from this ongoing study in pediatric patients indicate daclizumab serum levels (n=6) appear to be somewhat lower in pediatric renal transplant patients than in adult transplant patients administered the same dosing regimen. However, daclizumab levels in these pediatric patients were sufficient to saturate the Tac subunit of the IL-2 receptor on lymphocytes as measured by flow cytometry (n=24). The Tac subunit of the IL-2 receptor was saturated immediately after the first dose of 1.0 mg/kg of daclizumab and remained saturated for at least the first 3 months post-transplant. Saturation of the Tac subunit of the IL-2 receptor was similar to that observed in adult patients receiving the same dose regimen.

GERIATRIC USE

Clinical studies of daclizumab did not include sufficient numbers of subjects age 65 and older to determine whether they respond differently from younger subjects. Caution must be used in giving immunosuppressive drugs to elderly patients.

DRUG INTERACTIONS

The following medications have been administered in clinical trials with daclizumab with no incremental increase in adverse reactions: cyclosporine, mycophenolate mofetil, ganciclovir, acyclovir, azathioprine, and corticosteroids. Very limited experience exists with the use of daclizumab concomitantly with tacrolimus, muromonab-CD3, antithymocyte globulin, and antilymphocyte globulin.

In renal allograft recipients treated with daclizumab and mycophenolate mofetil, no pharmacokinetic interaction between daclizumab and mycophenolic acid, the active metabolite of mycophenolate mofetil, was observed.

ADVERSE REACTIONS

The safety of daclizumab was determined in four clinical studies, three of which were randomized controlled clinical trials, in 629 patients receiving renal allografts of whom 336 received daclizumab and 293 received placebo. All patients received concomitant cyclosporine and corticosteroids.

Daclizumab did not appear to alter the pattern, frequency or severity of known major toxicities associated with the use of immunosuppressive drugs.

Adverse events were reported by 95% of the patients in the placebo-treated group and 96% of the patients in the daclizumab-treated group. The proportion of patients prematurely withdrawn from the combined studies because of adverse events was 8.5% in the placebo-treated group and 8.6% in the daclizumab-treated group.

Daclizumab did not increase the number of serious adverse events observed compared with placebo. The most frequently reported adverse events were gastrointestinal disorders, which were reported with equal frequency in daclizumab- (67%) and placebo-treated (68%) patient groups.

The incidence and types of adverse events were similar in both placebo-treated and daclizumab-treated patients. The following adverse events occurred in ≥5% of daclizumab-treated patients. These events included:

Gastrointestinal System: Constipation, nausea, diarrhea, vomiting, abdominal pain, pyrosis, dyspepsia, abdominal distention, epigastric pain not food-related.
Metabolic and Nutritional: Edema extremities, edema.
Central and Peripheral Nervous System: Tremor, headache, dizziness.
Urinary System: Oliguria, dysuria, renal tubular necrosis.
Body as a Whole — General: Post-traumatic pain, chest pain, fever, pain, fatigue.
Autonomic Nervous System: Hypertension, hypotension, aggravated hypertension.
Respiratory System: Dyspnea, pulmonary edema, coughing.
Skin and Appendages: Impaired wound healing without infection, acne.
Psychiatric: Insomnia.
Musculoskeletal System: Musculoskeletal pain, back pain.
Heart Rate and Rhythm: Tachycardia.
Vascular Extracardiac: Thrombosis.
Platelet, Bleeding and Clotting Disorders: Bleeding.
Hemic and Lymphatic: Lymphocele.

The following adverse events occurred in <5% and ≥2% of daclizumab-treated patients. These included:

Gastrointestinal System: Flatulence, gastritis, hemorrhoids.
Metabolic and Nutritional: Fluid overload, diabetes mellitus, dehydration.
Urinary System: Renal damage, hydronephrosis, urinary tract bleeding, urinary tract disorder, renal insufficiency.
Body as a Whole — General: Shivering, generalized weakness.
Central and Peripheral Nervous System: Urinary retention, leg cramps, prickly sensation.
Respiratory System: Atelectasis, congestion, pharyngitis, rhinitis, hypoxia, rales, abnormal breath sounds, pleural effusion.
Skin and Appendages: Pruritus, hirsutism, rash, night sweats, increased sweating.
Psychiatric: Depression, anxiety.
Musculoskeletal System: Arthralgia, myalgia.
Vision: Vision blurred.
Application Site: Application site reaction.

INCIDENCE OF MALIGNANCIES

One year after treatment, the incidence of malignancies was 2.7% in the placebo group compared with 1.5% in the daclizumab group. Addition of daclizumab did not increase the number of post-transplant lymphomas, which occurred with a frequency of <1% in both placebo-treated and daclizumab-treated groups.

HYPERGLYCEMIA

No differences in abnormal hematologic or chemical laboratory test results were seen between placebo-treated and daclizumab-treated groups with the exception of fasting blood glucose. Fasting blood glucose was measured in a small number of placebo- and daclizumab-treated patients. A total of 16% (10 of 64 patients) of placebo-treated and 32% (28 of 88 patients) of daclizumab-treated patients had high fasting blood glucose values. Most of these high values occurred either on the first day post-transplant when patients received high doses of corticosteroids or in patients with diabetes.

INCIDENCE OF INFECTIOUS EPISODES

The overall incidence of infectious episodes, including viral infections, fungal infections, bacteremia and septicemia, and pneumonia, was not higher in daclizumab-treated patients than in placebo-treated patients. The types of infections reported were similar in both the daclizumab-treated and the placebo-treated groups. Cytomegalovirus infection was reported in 16% of the patients in the placebo group and 13% of the patients in the daclizumab group. One exception was cellulitis and wound infections, which occurred in 4.1% of placebo-treated and 8.4% of daclizumab-treated patients. At 1 year post-transplant, 7 placebo patients and only 1 daclizumab-treated patient had died of an infection.

DOSAGE AND ADMINISTRATION

Daclizumab is used as part of an immunosuppressive regimen that includes cyclosporine and corticosteroids. The recommended dose for daclizumab is 1.0 mg/kg. The calculated volume of daclizumab should be mixed with 50 ml of sterile 0.9% sodium chloride solution and administered via a peripheral or central vein over a 15 minute period.

Based on the clinical trials, the standard course of daclizumab therapy is five doses. The first dose should be given no more than 24 hours before transplantation. The four remaining doses should be given at intervals of 14 days.

No dosage adjustment is necessary for patients with severe renal impairment. No dosage adjustments based on other identified covariates (age, gender, proteinuria, race) are required for renal allograft patients. No data are available for administration in patients with severe hepatic impairment.

D

INSTRUCTIONS FOR ADMINISTRATION

- DACLIZUMAB IS NOT FOR DIRECT INJECTION. The calculated volume should be diluted in 50 ml of sterile 0.9% sodium chloride solution before intravenous administration to patients. When mixing the solution, gently invert the bag in order to avoid foaming; DO NOT SHAKE.
- Parenteral drug products should be inspected visually for particulate matter and discoloration before administration. If particulate matter is present or the solution colored, do not use.
- Care must be taken to assure sterility of the prepared solution, since the drug product does not contain any antimicrobial preservative or bacteriostatic agents.
- Daclizumab is a colorless solution provided as a single-use vial; any unused portion of the drug should be discarded.
- Once the infusion is prepared, it should be administered intravenously within 4 hours. If it must be held longer, it should be refrigerated between 2-8°C (36-46°F) for up to 24 hours. After 24 hours, the prepared solution should be discarded.
- No incompatibility between daclizumab and polyvinyl chloride or polyethylene bags or infusion sets has been observed. No data are available concerning the incompatibility of daclizumab with other drug substances. However, other drug substances should not be added or infused simultaneously through the same intravenous line.

HOW SUPPLIED

Each vial of Zenapax contains 25 mg of daclizumab in 5 ml of solution. Vials should be stored between the temperatures of 2-8°C (36-46°F); do not shake or freeze. Protect undiluted solution against direct light. Diluted medication is stable for 24 hours at 4°C or for 4 hours at room temperature.

PRODUCT LISTING - EQUIVALENTS NOT AVAILABLE

Solution - Intravenous - 5 mg/ml

5 ml $466.13 ZENAPAX, Roche Laboratories 00004-0501-09

Dactinomycin *(000939)*

Categories: Carcinoma, testicular; Carcinoma, uterine; Rhabdomyosarcoma; Sarcoma, Ewing's; Wilms' tumor; Pregnancy Category C; FDA Approved 1964 Dec; WHO Formulary
Drug Classes: Antineoplastics, antibiotics
Brand Names: Cosmegen
Foreign Brand Availability: Ac-De (Mexico); Cosmegen, Lyovac (England); Cosmogen Lyovac (Hong-Kong; Malaysia); Dacmozen (India); Lyovac (England)
HCFA JCODE(S): J9120 0.5 mg IV

WARNING

Dactinomycin for injection should be administered only under the supervision of a physician who is experienced in the use of cancer chemotherapeutic agents.

This drug is HIGHLY TOXIC and both powder and solution must be handled and administered with care. Inhalation of dust or vapors and contact with skin or mucous membranes, especially those of the eyes, must be avoided. Due to the toxic properties of dactinomycin (*e.g.,* corrosivity, carcinogenicity, mutagenicity, teratogenicity), special handling procedures should be reviewed prior to handling and followed diligently. Dactinomycin is extremely corrosive to soft tissue. If extravasation occurs during intravenous use, severe damage to soft tissues will occur. In at least one instance, this has led to contracture of the arms.

DESCRIPTION

Dactinomycin is one of the actinomycins, a group of antibiotics produced by various species of *Streptomyces.* Dactinomycin is the principal component of the mixture of actinomycins produced by *Streptomyces parvullus.* Unlike other species of *Streptomyces,* this organism yields an essentially pure substance that contains only traces of similar compounds differing in the amino acid content of the peptide side chains. The empirical formula is $C_{62}H_{86}N_{12}O_{16}$.

Cosmegen is a sterile, yellow to orange lyophilized powder for injection by the intravenous route or by regional perfusion after reconstitution. Each vial contains 0.5 mg (500 µg) of dactinomycin and 20.0 mg of mannitol.

CLINICAL PHARMACOLOGY

ACTION

Generally, the actinomycins exert an inhibitory effect on gram-positive and gram-negative bacteria and on some fungi. However, the toxic properties of the actinomycins (including dactinomycin) in relation to antibacterial activity are such as to preclude their use as antibiotics in the treatment of infectious diseases.

Because the actinomycins are cytotoxic, they have an antineoplastic effect which has been demonstrated in experimental animals with various types of tumor implants. This cytotoxic action is the basis for their use in the treatment of certain types of cancer. Dactinomycin is believed to produce its cytotoxic effects by binding DNA and inhibiting RNA synthesis.

PHARMACOKINETICS AND METABOLISM

Results of a study in patients with malignant melanoma indicate that dactinomycin (^3H actinomycin D) is minimally metabolized, is concentrated in nucleated cells, and does not penetrate the blood-brain barrier. Approximately 30% of the dose was recovered in urine and feces in 1 week. The terminal plasma half-life for radioactivity was approximately 36 hours.

INDICATIONS AND USAGE

Dactinomycin, as part of a combination chemotherapy and/or multi-modality treatment regimen, is indicated for the treatment of Wilms' tumor, childhood rhabdomyosarcoma, Ewing's sarcoma and metastatic, nonseminomatous testicular cancer.

Dactinomycin is indicated as a single agent, or as part of a combination chemotherapy regimen, for the treatment of gestational trophoblastic neoplasia.

Dactinomycin, as a component of regional perfusion, is indicated for the palliative and/or adjunctive treatment of locally recurrent or locoregional solid malignancies.

CONTRAINDICATIONS

Dactinomycin should not be given at or about the time of infection with chickenpox or herpes zoster because of the risk of severe generalized disease which may result in death.

WARNINGS

Reports indicate an increased incidence of second primary tumors (including leukemia) following treatment with radiation and antineoplastic agents, such as dactinomycin. Multimodal therapy creates the need for careful, long-term observation of cancer survivors.

PREGNANCY CATEGORY D

Dactinomycin may cause fetal harm when administered to a pregnant woman. Dactinomycin has been shown to cause malformations and embryotoxicity in rat, rabbit, and hamster when given in doses of 50-100 µg/kg (approximately 0.5-2 times the maximum recommended daily human dose on a body surface area basis). If this drug is used during pregnancy, or if the patient becomes pregnant while receiving this drug, the patient should be apprised of the potential hazard to the fetus. Women of childbearing potential must be warned to avoid becoming pregnant.

PRECAUTIONS

GENERAL

This drug is **HIGHLY TOXIC** and both powder and solution must be handled and administered with care (see BOXED WARNING; and HOW SUPPLIED, Special Handling). Since dactinomycin is extremely corrosive to soft tissues, it is intended for intravenous use. Inhalation of dust or vapors and contact with skin or mucous membranes, especially those of the eyes, must be avoided. Appropriate protective equipment should be worn when handling dactinomycin. Should accidental eye contact occur, copious irrigation for at least 15 minutes with water, normal saline or a balanced salt ophthalmic irrigating solution should be instituted immediately, followed by prompt ophthalmologic consultation. Should accidental skin contact occur, the affected part must be irrigated immediately with copious amounts of water for at least 15 minutes while removing contaminated clothing and shoes. Medical attention should be sought immediately. Contaminated clothing should be destroyed and shoes cleaned thoroughly before reuse (see HOW SUPPLIED, Special Handling).

As with all antineoplastic agents, dactinomycin is a toxic drug and very careful and frequent observation of the patient for adverse reactions is necessary. These reactions may involve any tissue of the body, most commonly the hematopoietic system resulting in myelosuppression. The possibility of an anaphylactoid reaction should be borne in mind.

It is extremely important to observe the patient daily for toxic side effects when combination chemotherapy is employed, since a full course of therapy occasionally is not tolerated. If stomatitis, diarrhea, or severe hematopoietic depression appear during therapy, these drugs should be discontinued until the patient has recovered.

DACTINOMYCIN AND RADIATION THERAPY

An increased incidence of gastrointestinal toxicity and marrow suppression has been reported with combined therapy incorporating dactinomycin and radiation. Moreover, the normal skin, as well as the buccal and pharyngeal mucosa, may show early erythema. A smaller than usual radiation dose administered in combination with dactinomycin causes erythema and vesiculation, which progress more rapidly through the stages of tanning and desquamation. Healing may occur in 4-6 weeks rather than 2-3 months. Erythema from previous radiation therapy may be reactivated by dactinomycin alone, even when radiotherapy was administered many months earlier, and especially when the interval between the two forms of therapy is brief. This potentiation of radiation effect represents a special problem when the radiotherapy involves the mucous membrane. When irradiation is directed toward the nasopharynx, the combination may produce severe oropharyngeal mucositis. *Severe reactions may ensue if high doses of both dactinomycin and radiation therapy are used or if the patient is particularly sensitive to such combined therapy.*

Particular caution is necessary when administering dactinomycin within 2 months of irradiation for the treatment of right-sided Wilms' tumor, since hepatomegaly and elevated AST levels have been noted. In general, dactinomycin should not be concomitantly administered with radiotherapy in the treatment of Wilms' tumor unless the benefit outweighs the risk.

DACTINOMYCIN AND REGIONAL PERFUSION THERAPY

Complications of the perfusion technique are related mainly to the amount of drug that escapes into the systemic circulation and may consist of hematopoietic depression, absorption of toxic products from massive destruction of neoplastic tissue, increased susceptibility to infection, impaired wound healing, and superficial ulceration of the gastric mucosa. Other side effects may include edema of the extremity involved, damage to soft tissues of the perfused area, and (potentially) venous thrombosis.

LABORATORY TESTS

Many abnormalities of renal, hepatic, and bone marrow function have been reported in patients with neoplastic diseases receiving dactinomycin. Renal, hepatic, and bone marrow functions should be assessed frequently.

DRUG/LABORATORY TEST INTERACTIONS

Dactinomycin may interfere with bioassay procedures for the determination of antibacterial drug levels.

CARCINOGENESIS, MUTAGENESIS, AND IMPAIRMENT OF FERTILITY

Reports indicate an increased incidence of second primary tumors (including leukemia) following treatment with radiation and antineoplastic agents, such as dactinomycin. Multi-modal therapy creates the need for careful, long-term observation of cancer survivors.

The International Agency on Research on Cancer has judged that dactinomycin is a positive carcinogen in animals. Local sarcomas were produced in mice and rats after repeated subcutaneous or intraperitoneal injection. Mesenchymal tumors occurred in male F344 rats given intraperitoneal injections of 50 μg/kg, 2-5 times per week for 18 weeks. The first tumor appeared at 23 weeks.

Dactinomycin has been shown to be mutagenic in a number of test systems *in vitro* and *in vivo* including human fibroblasts and leukocytes, and HeLa cells. DNA damage and cytogenetic effects have been demonstrated in the mouse and the rat.

Adequate fertility studies have not been reported, although, reports suggest an increased incidence of infertility following treatment with other antineoplastic agents.

PREGNANCY CATEGORY D

See WARNINGS.

NURSING MOTHERS

It is not known whether this drug is excreted in human milk. Because many drugs are excreted in human milk and because of the potential for serious adverse reactions in nursing infants from dactinomycin, a decision should be made as to discontinuation of nursing and/or drug, taking into account the importance of the drug to the mother.

PEDIATRIC USE

The greater frequency of toxic effects of dactinomycin in infants suggest that this drug should be administered to infants only over the age of 6-12 months.

ADVERSE REACTIONS

Toxic effects (excepting nausea and vomiting) usually do not become apparent until 2-4 days after a course of therapy is stopped, and may not peak until 1-2 weeks have elapsed. Deaths have been reported. However, adverse reactions are usually reversible on discontinuance of therapy. They include the following:

Miscellaneous: Malaise, fatigue, lethargy, fever, myalgia, proctitis, hypocalcemia, growth retardation, infection.

Oral: Cheilitis, dysphagia, esophagitis, ulcerative stomatitis, pharyngitis.

Lung: Pneumonitis.

Gastrointestinal: Anorexia, nausea, vomiting, abdominal pain, diarrhea, gastrointestinal ulceration, liver toxicity including ascites, hepatomegaly, hepatic veno-occlusive disease, hepatitis, and liver function test abnormalities. Nausea and vomiting, which occur early during the first few hours after administration, may be alleviated by the administration of anti-emetics.

Hematologic: Anemia, even to the point of aplastic anemia, agranulocytosis, leukopenia, thrombocytopenia, pancytopenia, reticulocytopenia. Platelet and white cell counts should be performed *frequently* to detect severe hematopoietic depression. If either count markedly decreases, the drug should be withheld to allow marrow recovery. This often takes up to 3 weeks.

Dermatologic: Alopecia, skin eruptions, acne, flare-up of erythema or increased pigmentation of previously irradiated skin.

Soft Tissues: Dactinomycin is extremely corrosive. If extravasation occurs during intravenous use, severe damage to soft tissues will occur. In at least one instance, this has led to contracture of the arms. Epidermolysis, erythema, and edema, at times severe, have been reported with regional limb perfusion.

LABORATORY TESTS

Many abnormalities of renal, hepatic, and bone marrow function have been reported in patients with neoplastic diseases receiving dactinomycin. Renal, hepatic, and bone marrow functions should be assessed frequently.

DOSAGE AND ADMINISTRATION

Toxic reactions due to dactinomycin are frequent and may be severe (see ADVERSE REACTIONS), thus limiting in many instances the amount that may be administered. However, the severity of toxicity varies markedly and is only partly dependent on the dose employed.

INTRAVENOUS USE

The dosage of dactinomycin varies depending on the tolerance of the patient, the size and location of the neoplasm, and the use of other forms of therapy. It may be necessary to decrease the usual dosages suggested below when additional chemotherapy or radiation therapy is used concomitantly or has been used previously.

The dosage for dactinomycin is calculated in micrograms (μg). The dose intensity per 2 week cycle for adults or children should not exceed 15 μg/kg/day or 400-600 μg/m²/day intravenously for 5 days. Calculation of the dosage for obese or edematous patients should be performed on the basis of surface area in an effort to more closely relate dosage to lean body mass.

A wide variety of single agent and combination chemotherapy regimens with dactinomycin may be employed. Because chemotherapeutic regimens are constantly changing, dosing and administration should be performed under the direct supervision of physicians familiar with current oncologic practices and new advances in therapy. The following suggested regimens are based upon a review of current literature concerning therapy with dactinomycin and are on a per cycle basis.

D

WILMS' TUMOR, CHILDHOOD RHABDOMYOSARCOMA AND EWING'S SARCOMA

Regimens of 15 μg/kg intravenously daily for 5 days administered in various combinations and schedules with other chemotherapeutic agents have been utilized in the treatment of Wilms' tumor[1], rhabdomyosarcoma[2] and Ewing's sarcoma.[5,6]

METASTATIC NONSEMINOMATOUS TESTICULAR CANCER

1000 μg/m² intravenously on Day 1 as part of a combination regimen with cyclophosphamide, bleomycin, vinblastine, and cisplatin.[3]

GESTATIONAL TROPHOBLASTIC NEOPLASIA

12 μg/kg intravenously daily for 5 days as a single agent.[7]

500 μg intravenously on Days 1 and 2 as part of a combination regimen with etoposide, methotrexate, folinic acid, vincristine, cyclophosphamide and cisplatin.[8]

REGIONAL PERFUSION IN LOCALLY RECURRENT AND LOCOREGIONAL SOLID MALIGNANCIES

The dosage schedules and the technique itself vary from one investigator to another; the published literature, therefore, should be consulted for details. In general, the following doses are suggested:

50 μg (0.05 mg)/kg of body weight for lower extremity or pelvis.

35 μg (0.035 mg)/kg of body weight for upper extremity.

It may be advisable to use lower doses in obese patients, or when previous chemotherapy or radiation therapy has been employed.

MANAGEMENT OF EXTRAVASATION

Care in the administration of dactinomycin will reduce the chance of perivenous infiltration (see BOXED WARNING and ADVERSE REACTIONS). It may also decrease the chance of local reactions such as urticaria and erythematous streaking. On intravenous administration of dactinomycin, extravasation may occur with or without an accompanying burning or stinging sensation, even if blood returns well on aspiration of the infusion needle. If any signs or symptoms of extravasation have occurred, the injection or infusion should be immediately terminated and restarted in another vein. If extravasation is suspected, intermittent application of ice to the site for 15 minutes qid for 3 days may be useful. The benefit of local administration of drugs has not been clearly established. Because of the progressive nature of extravasation reactions, close observation and plastic surgery consultation is recommended. Blistering, ulceration and/or persistent pain are indications for wide excision surgery, followed by split-thickness skin grafting.[9]

HOW SUPPLIED

Cosmegen for injection is a lyophilized powder. In the dry form the compound is an amorphous yellow to orange powder. The solution is clear and gold-colored. Cosmegen for injection is supplied in vials containing 0.5 mg (500 μg) of dactinomycin and 20.0 mg of mannitol.

Storage: Store at 25°C (77°F); excursions permitted to 15-30°C (59-86°F). Protect from light and humidity.

SPECIAL HANDLING

Animal studies have shown dactinomycin to be corrosive to skin, irritating to the eyes and mucous membranes of the respiratory tract and highly toxic by the oral route. It has also been shown to be carcinogenic, mutagenic, embryotoxic and teratogenic. Due to the drug's toxic properties, appropriate precautions including the use of appropriate safety equipment are recommended for the preparation of dactinomycin for parenteral administration. Inhalation of dust or vapors and contact with skin or mucous membranes, especially those of the eyes, must be avoided. The National Institutes of Health presently recommends that the preparation of injectable antineoplastic drugs should be performed in a Class II laminar flow biological safety cabinet.[10] Personnel preparing drugs of this class should wear chemical resistant, impervious gloves, safety goggles, outer garments and shoe covers. Additional body garments should be used based upon the task being performed (*e.g.,* sleevelets, apron, gauntlets, disposable suits) to avoid exposed skin surfaces and inhalation of vapors and dust. Appropriate techniques should be used to remove potentially contaminated clothing.

Several other guidelines for proper handling and disposal of antineoplastic drugs have been published and should be considered.[11-16]

ACCIDENTAL CONTACT MEASURES

Should accidental eye contact occur, copious irrigation for at least 15 minutes with water, normal saline or a balanced salt ophthalmic irrigating solution should be instituted immediately, followed by prompt ophthalmologic consultation. Should accidental skin contact occur, the affected part must be irrigated immediately with copious amounts of water for at least 15 minutes while removing contaminated clothing and shoes. Medical attention should be sought immediately. Contaminated clothing should be destroyed and shoes cleaned thoroughly before reuse (see PRECAUTIONS, General; and DOSAGE AND ADMINISTRATION).

PRODUCT LISTING - EQUIVALENTS NOT AVAILABLE

Solution - Intravenous - 0.5 mg
1's $14.60 COSMEGEN, Merck & Company Inc 00006-3298-22

Dalfopristin; Quinupristin (003447)

Categories: Infection, skin and skin structures; Pregnancy Category B
Drug Classes: Antibiotics, streptogramins
Brand Names: Synercid
Cost of Therapy: $2368.72 (Infection; Synercid; 150 mg; 350 mg; 1575 mg/day; 7 day supply)

D

WARNING

One of dalfopristin; quinupristin's approved indications is for the treatment of patients with serious or life-threatening infections associated with vancomycin-resistant *Enterococcus faecium* (VREF) bacteremia. Dalfopristin; quinupristin has been approved for marketing in the United States for this indication under FDA's accelerated approval regulations that allow marketing of products for use in life-threatening conditions when other therapies are not available. Approval of drugs for marketing under these regulations is based upon a demonstrated effect on a surrogate endpoint that is likely to predict clinical benefit.

Approval of this indication is based upon dalfopristin; quinupristin's ability to clear VREF from the bloodstream, with clearance of bacteremia considered to be a surrogate endpoint. There are no results from well-controlled clinical studies that confirm the validity of this surrogate marker. However, a study to verify the clinical benefit of therapy with dalfopristin; quinupristin on traditional clinical endpoints (such as cure of the underlying infection) is presently underway.

DESCRIPTION

Synercid IV, a streptogramin antibacterial agent for intravenous administration, is a sterile lyophilized formulation of two semisynthetic pristinamycin derivatives, quinupristin (derived from pristinamycin I) and dalfopristin (derived from pristinamycin IIA) in the ratio of 30:70 (w/w).

Quinupristin is a white to very slightly yellow, hygroscopic powder. It is a combination of three peptide macrolactones. The main component of quinupristin (>88.0%) has the following chemical name: N-[(6*R*,9*S*,10*R*,13*S*,15a*S*,18*R*,22*S*,24a*S*)-22-[*p*-(dimethylamino) benzyl]-6-ethyldocosahydro-10,23-dimethyl-5,8,12,15,17,21,24-heptaoxo-13-phenyl-18-[[(3*S*)-3-quinuclidinylthio]methyl]-12*H*-pyrido[2,1-*f*]pyrrolo-[2,1-*l*][1,4,7,10,13,16] oxapentaazacyclononadecin-9-yl]-3-hydroxypicolinamide.

The main component of quinupristin has an empirical formula of $C_{53}H_{67}N_9O_{10}S$ and a molecular weight of 1022.24.

Dalfopristin is a slightly yellow to yellow, hygroscopic, powder. The chemical name for dalfopristin is: (3*R*,4*R*,5*E*,10*E*,12*E*,14*S*,26*R*,26a*S*)-26-[[2-(diethylamino)ethyl]sulfonyl]-8,9,14,15,24,25,26,26a-octahydro-14-hydroxy-3-isopropyl-4,12-dimethyl-3*H*-21,18-nitrilo-1*H*,22*H*-pyrrolo[2,1-*c*][1,8,4,19]-dioxadiazacyclotetracosine-1,7,16,22(4*H*,17*H*)-tetrone.

Dalfopristin has an empirical formula of $C_{34}H_{50}N_4O_9S$ and a molecular weight of 690.85.

CLINICAL PHARMACOLOGY

PHARMACOKINETICS

Dalfopristin and quinupristin are the main active components circulating in plasma in human subjects. Dalfopristin and quinupristin are converted to several active major metabolites: two conjugated metabolites for quinupristin (one with glutathione and one with cysteine) and one non-conjugated metabolite for dalfopristin (formed by drug hydrolysis).

Pharmacokinetic profiles of dalfopristin and quinupristin in combination with their metabolites were determined using a bioassay following multiple 60 minute infusions of dalfopristin; quinupristin in two groups of healthy young adult male volunteers. Each group received 7.5 mg/kg of dalfopristin; quinupristin intravenously q12h or q8h for a total of 9 or 10 doses, respectively. The pharmacokinetic parameters were proportional with q12h and q8h dosing; those of the q8h regimen are shown in TABLE 1.

TABLE 1 *Mean Steady-State Pharmacokinetic Parameters of Quinupristin and Dalfopristin in Combination With Their Metabolites (±SD) (Dose = 7.5 mg/kg q8h; n=10)*

	C_{max} (µg/ml)	AUC (µg·h/ml)	T½ (h)
Quinupristin and metabolites	3.20 ± 0.67	7.20 ± 1.24	3.07 ± 0.51
Dalfopristin and metabolite	7.96 ± 1.30	10.57 ± 2.24	1.04 ± 0.20

SD = Standard Deviation.
C_{max} = Maximum drug plasma concentration.
AUC = Area under the drug plasma concentration-time curve.
T½ = Half-life.

The clearances of unchanged dalfopristin and quinupristin are similar (0.72 L/h/kg), and the steady-state volume of distribution for quinupristin is 0.45 L/kg and for dalfopristin is 0.24 L/kg. The elimination half-life of dalfopristin and quinupristin is approximately 0.85 and 0.70 hours, respectively.

The protein binding of dalfopristin; quinupristin is moderate.

Penetration of unchanged dalfopristin and quinupristin in noninflammatory blister fluid corresponds to about 19% and 11% of that estimated in plasma, respectively. The penetration into blister fluid of dalfopristin and quinupristin in combination with their major metabolites was in total approximately 40% compared to that in plasma.

In vitro, the transformation of the parent drugs into their major active metabolites occurs by non-enzymatic reactions and is not dependent on cytochrome-P450 or glutathione-transferase enzyme activities.

Dalfopristin; quinupristin has been shown to be a major inhibitor (*in vitro* inhibits 70% cyclosporin A biotransformation at 10 µg/ml of dalfopristin; quinupristin) of the activity of cytochrome P450 3A4 isoenzyme. (See WARNINGS.)

Dalfopristin; quinupristin can interfere with the metabolism of other drug products that are associated with QTc prolongation. However, electrophysiologic studies confirm that dalfopristin; quinupristin does not itself induce QTc prolongation. (See WARNINGS.)

Fecal excretion constitutes the main elimination route for both parent drugs and their metabolites (75-77% of dose). Urinary excretion accounts for approximately 15% of the quinupristin and 19% of the dalfopristin dose. Preclinical data in rats have demonstrated that approximately 80% of the dose is excreted in the bile and suggest that in man, biliary excretion is probably the principal route for fecal elimination.

SPECIAL POPULATIONS

Elderly

The pharmacokinetics of dalfopristin and quinupristin were studied in a population of elderly individuals (range 69-74 years). The pharmacokinetics of the drug products were not modified in these subjects.

Gender

The pharmacokinetics of dalfopristin and quinupristin are not modified by gender.

Renal Insufficiency

In patients with creatinine clearance 6-28 ml/min, the AUC of dalfopristin and quinupristin in combination with their major metabolites increased about 40% and 30%, respectively.

In patients undergoing Continuous Ambulatory Peritoneal Dialysis, dialysis clearance for dalfopristin, quinupristin, and their metabolites is negligible. The plasma AUC of unchanged dalfopristin and quinupristin increased about 20% and 30%, respectively. The high molecular weight of both components of dalfopristin; quinupristin suggests that it is unlikely to be removed by hemodialysis.

Hepatic Insufficiency

In patients with hepatic dysfunction (Child-Pugh scores A and B), the terminal half-life of dalfopristin and quinupristin was not modified. However, the AUC of dalfopristin and quinupristin in combination with their major metabolites increased about 180% and 50%, respectively. (See DOSAGE AND ADMINISTRATION and PRECAUTIONS.)

Obesity (Body Mass Index ≥30)

In obese patients the C_{max} and AUC of quinupristin increased about 30% and those of dalfopristin about 40%.

Pediatric Patients

The pharmacokinetics of dalfopristin; quinupristin in patients less than 16 years of age have not been studied.

MICROBIOLOGY

The streptogramin components of dalfopristin; quinupristin, dalfopristin, quinupristin, are present in a ratio of 70 parts dalfopristin to 30 parts quinupristin. These two components act synergistically so that dalfopristin; quinupristin's microbiologic *in vitro* activity is greater than that of the components individually. Dalfopristin and quinupristin's metabolites also contribute to the antimicrobial activity of dalfopristin; quinupristin. *In vitro* synergism of the major metabolites with the complementary parent compound has been demonstrated.

Dalfopristin; quinupristin is bacteriostatic against *Enterococcus faecium* and bactericidal against strains of methicillin-susceptible and methicillin-resistant staphylococci.

The site of action of dalfopristin and quinupristin is the bacterial ribosome. Dalfopristin has been shown to inhibit the early phase of protein synthesis while quinupristin inhibits the late phase of protein synthesis.

In vitro combination testing of dalfopristin; quinupristin with aztreonam, cefotaxime, ciprofloxacin, and gentamicin against Enterobacteriaceae and *Pseudomonas aeruginosa* did not show antagonism.

In vitro combination testing of dalfopristin; quinupristin with prototype drugs of the following classes: aminoglycosides (gentamicin), β-lactams (cefepime, ampicillin, and amoxicillin), glycopeptides (vancomycin), quinolones (ciprofloxacin), tetracyclines (doxycycline), and also chloramphenicol against enterococci and staphylococci did not show antagonism.

The mode of action differs from that of other classes of antibacterial agents such as β-lactams, aminoglycosides, glycopeptides, quinolones, macrolides, lincosamides, and tetracyclines. There is no cross resistance between dalfopristin; quinupristin and these agents when tested by the minimum inhibitory concentration (MIC) method.

In non-comparative studies, emerging resistance to dalfopristin; quinupristin during treatment of VREF infections occurred. Resistance to dalfopristin; quinupristin is associated with resistance to both components (*i.e.,* dalfopristin and quinupristin).

Dalfopristin; quinupristin has been shown to be active against most strains of the following microorganisms, both *in vitro* and in clinical infections, as described in INDICATIONS AND USAGE.

AEROBIC GRAM-POSITIVE MICROORGANISMS

Enterococcus faecium **(Vancomycin-resistant and multi-drug resistant strains only).**
Staphylococcus aureus (methicillin-susceptible strains only).
Streptococcus pyogenes.

NOTE: Dalfopristin; quinupristin is **not active** against *Enterococcus faecalis.* Differentiation of enterococcal species is important to avoid misidentification of *Enterococcus faecalis* as *Enterococcus faecium.*

The following *in vitro* data are available, **but their clinical significance is unknown.**

The combination of dalfopristin and quinupristin exhibits *in vitro* minimum inhibitory concentrations (MICs) of ≤1.0 µg/ml against most (≥90%) isolates of the following microorganisms; however, the safety and effectiveness of dalfopristin; quinupristin in treating clinical infections due to these microorganisms have not been established in adequate and well-controlled clinical trials.

AEROBIC GRAM-POSITIVE MICROORGANISMS

Corynebacterium jeikeium.
Staphylococcus aureus (methicillin-resistant strains).
Staphylococcus epidermidis (including methicillin-resistant strains).
Streptococcus agalactiae.

SUSCEPTIBILITY TESTING

Dilution Techniques

Quantitative methods are used to determine antimicrobial minimum inhibitory concentrations (MICs). These MICs provide estimates of the susceptibility of microorganisms to antimicrobial compounds. The MICs should be determined using a standardized procedure. Standardized procedures are based on a dilution[1] method (broth or agar) or equivalent using standardized inoculum concentrations, and standardized concentrations of quinupristin/dalfopristin in a 30:70 ratio made from powder of known potency. The MIC values should be interpreted according to the criteria shown in TABLE 2.

TABLE 2 *For Susceptibility Testing of Enterococcus Faecium, Staphylococcus Spp., and Streptococcus Spp. (Excluding Streptococcus Pneumoniae)**

MIC (µg/ml)	Interpretation
≤1.0	Susceptible (S)
2.0	Intermediate (I)
≥4.0	Resistant (R)

* The interpretive values for *Streptococcus* spp. are applicable only to broth microdilution susceptibility testing using cation-adjusted Mueller-Hinton broth with 2-5% lysed horse blood.

A report of "Susceptible" indicates that the pathogen is likely to be inhibited if the concentration of the antimicrobial compound in the blood reaches usually achievable levels. A report of "Intermediate" indicates that the result should be considered equivocal, and if the microorganism is not fully susceptible to alternative, clinically feasible drugs, the test should be repeated. This category implies possible clinical applicability in body sites where the drug is physiologically concentrated or in situations where high dosage of drug can be used. This category provides a buffer zone which prevents small uncontrolled technical factors from causing major discrepancies in interpretation. A report of "Resistant" indicates that the pathogen is not likely to be inhibited if the antimicrobial compound in the blood reaches the concentrations usually achievable; other therapy should be selected.

Quality Control

A standardized susceptibility test procedure requires the use of laboratory control organisms to control the technical aspects of the laboratory procedures. Standard quinupristin/dalfopristin powder in a 30:70 ratio should provide the following MIC values with the indicated quality control strains as shown in TABLE 3.

TABLE 3

Microorganism (ATCC#)	MIC (µg/ml)
Enterococcus faecalis (29212)	2.0-8.0
Staphylococcus aureus (29213)	0.25-1.0

Diffusion Techniques

Quantitative methods that require measurement of zone diameters also provide reproducible estimates of the susceptibility of bacteria to antimicrobial compounds. One such standardized procedure[2] requires the use of standardized inoculum concentrations. This procedure uses paper disks impregnated with 15 µg quinupristin/dalfopristin in a ratio of 30:70 to test the susceptibility of microorganisms to dalfopristin; quinupristin. Reports from the laboratory providing results of the standard single-disk susceptibility test with a 15 µg dalfopristin; quinupristin disk should be interpreted according to the criteria shown in TABLE 4.

TABLE 4 *For Susceptibility Testing of Enterococcus Faecium, Staphylococcus Spp., and Streptococcus Spp. (Excluding Streptococcus Pneumoniae)**

Zone Diameter (mm)	Interpretation
≥19	Susceptible (S)
16-18	Intermediate (I)
≤15	Resistant (R)

* The zone diameter for *Streptococcus* spp. are applicable only to tests performed using Mueller-Hinton agar supplemented with 5% sheep blood when incubated in 5% CO_2.

These zone diameters are applicable only to tests performed using Mueller-Hinton agar supplemented with 5% sheep blood when incubated in 5% CO_2.

Interpretation should be as stated above for results using dilution techniques. Interpretation involves correlation of the diameter obtained in the disk test with the MIC for dalfopristin; quinupristin.

Quality Control

As with standardized dilution techniques, diffusion methods require the use of laboratory control microorganisms that are used to control the technical aspects of the laboratory procedures. For the diffusion technique, the 15 µg quinupristin/dalfopristin (30:70 ratio) disk should provide the following zone diameter with the quality control strain listed in TABLE 5.

TABLE 5

Microorganism (ATCC #)	Zone Diameter Range (mm)
Staphylococcus aureus (25923)	23-29

ATCC is a registered trademark of the American Type Culture Collection.

INDICATIONS AND USAGE

Dalfopristin; quinupristin is indicated in adults for the treatment of the following infections when caused by susceptible strains of the designated microorganisms.

VANCOMYCIN-RESISTANT ENTEROCOCCUS FAECIUM (VREF)

Dalfopristin; quinupristin is indicated for the treatment of patients with serious or life-threatening infections associated with vancomycin-resistant *Enterococcus faecium* (VREF) bacteremia.

One of dalfopristin; quinupristin's approved indications is for the treatment of patients with serious or life-threatening infections associated with vancomycin-resistant *Enterococcus faecium* (VREF) bacteremia. Dalfopristin; quinupristin has been approved for marketing in the United States for this indication under FDA's accelerated approval regulations that allow marketing of products for use in life-threatening conditions when other therapies are not available. Approval of drugs for marketing under these regulations is based upon a demonstrated effect on a surrogate endpoint that is likely to predict clinical benefit.

Approval of this indication is based upon dalfopristin; quinupristin's ability to clear VREF from the bloodstream, with clearance of bacteremia considered to be a surrogate endpoint. There are no results from well-controlled clinical studies that confirm the validity of this surrogate marker. However, a study to verify the clinical benefit of therapy with dalfopristin; quinupristin on traditional clinical endpoints (such as cure of the underlying infection) is presently underway.

Complicated skin and skin structure infections caused by *Staphylococcus aureus* (methicillin susceptible) or *Streptococcus pyogenes.*

NON-FDA APPROVED INDICATIONS

Individual case reports have described intrathecal administration of low doses (1-2 mg/day) of dalfopristin-quinupristin to treat vancomycin-resistant *Enterococcus faecium* shunt infections; however, this route is not approved by the FDA.

CONTRAINDICATIONS

Dalfopristin; quinupristin is contraindicated in patients with known hypersensitivity to dalfopristin; quinupristin, or with prior hypersensitivity to other streptogramins (*e.g.*, pristinamycin or virginiamycin).

WARNINGS

DRUG INTERACTIONS

In vitro drug interaction studies have demonstrated that dalfopristin; quinupristin significantly inhibits cytochrome P450 3A4 metabolism of cyclosporin A, midazolam, nifedipine, and terfenadine. In addition, 24 subjects given dalfopristin; quinupristin 7.5 mg/kg q8hr for 2 days and 300 mg of cyclosporine on day 3 showed an increase of 63% in the AUC of cyclosporine, an increase of 30% in the C_{max} of cyclosporine, a 77% increase in the $T_{1/2}$ of cyclosporine, and, a decrease of 34% in the clearance of cyclosporine. **Therapeutic level monitoring of cyclosporine should be performed when cyclosporine must be used concomitantly with dalfopristin; quinupristin.**

It is reasonable to expect that the concomitant administration of dalfopristin; quinupristin and other drugs primarily metabolized by the cytochrome P450 3A4 enzyme system may likely result in increased plasma concentrations of these drugs that could increase or prolong their therapeutic effect and/or increase adverse reactions. (See Selected Drugs That Are Predicted to Have Plasma Concentrations Increased by Dalfopristin; Quinupristin.) Therefore, coadministration of dalfopristin; quinupristin with drugs which are cytochrome P450 3A4 substrates and possess a narrow therapeutic window requires caution and monitoring of these drugs (*e.g.*, cyclosporine), whenever possible. Concomitant medications metabolized by the cytochrome P450 3A4 enzyme system that may prolong the QTc interval should be avoided.

Concomitant administration of dalfopristin; quinupristin and nifedipine (repeated oral doses) and midazolam (intravenous bolus dose) in healthy volunteers led to elevated plasma concentrations of these drugs. The C_{max} increased by 18% and 14% (median values) and the AUC increased by 44% and 33% for nifedipine and midazolam, respectively.

*Selected Drugs That Are Predicted to Have Plasma Concentrations Increased by Dalfopristin; Quinupristin**

Antihistamines: Astemizole, terfenadine.
Anti-HIV (NNRTIs and Protease Inhibitors: Delavirdine, nevirapine, indinavir, ritonavir.
Antineoplastic Agents: Vinca alkaloids (*e.g.*, vinblastine), docetaxel, paclitaxel.
Benzodiazepines: Midazolam, diazepame.
Calcium Channel Blockers: Dihydropyridines (*e.g.*, nifedipine), verapamil, diltiazem.
Cholesterol-lowering Agents: HMG-CoA reductase inhibitors (*e.g.*, lovastatin).
GI Motility Agents: Cisapride.
Immunosuppressive Agents: Cyclosporine, tacrolimus.
Steroids: Methylprednisolone.
Other: Carbamazepine, quinidine, lidocaine, disopyramide.

*This list of drugs is not all inclusive.

Pseudomembranous colitis has been reported with nearly all antibacterial agents, including dalfopristin; quinupristin, and may range in severity from mild to life-threatening. Therefore, it is important to consider this diagnosis in patients who present with diarrhea subsequent to the administration of antibacterial agents.

Treatment with antibacterial agents alters the normal flora of the colon and may permit overgrowth of clostridia. Studies indicate that a toxin produced by *Clostridium difficile* is one primary cause of "antibiotic-associated colitis".

After the diagnosis of pseudomembranous colitis has been established, therapeutic measures should be initiated. Mild cases usually respond to drug discontinuation alone. In moderate to severe cases, consideration should be given to management with fluids and electrolytes, protein supplementation, and treatment with an antibacterial drug clinically effective against *C. difficile* colitis.

PRECAUTIONS

GENERAL

Venous Irritation

Following completion of a peripheral infusion, the vein should be flushed with 5% dextrose in water solution to minimize venous irritation. **DO NOT FLUSH** with saline or heparin **after** dalfopristin; quinupristin administration because of incompatibility concerns.

If moderate to severe venous irritation occurs following peripheral administration of dalfopristin; quinupristin diluted in 250 ml of dextrose 5% in water, consideration should be given to increasing the infusion volume to 500 or 750 ml, changing the infusion site, or infusing by a peripherally inserted central catheter (PICC) or a central venous catheter. In clinical trials, concomitant administration of hydrocortisone or diphenhydramine did not appear to alleviate venous pain or inflammation.

Rate of Infusion

In animal studies toxicity was higher when dalfopristin; quinupristin was administered as a bolus compared to slow infusion. However, the safety of an intravenous bolus of dalfopristin; quinupristin has not been studied in humans. Clinical trial experience has been exclusively with an intravenous duration of 60 minutes and, thus, other infusion rates cannot be recommended.

Arthralgias/Myalgias

Episodes of arthralgia and myalgia, some severe, have been reported in patients treated with dalfopristin; quinupristin. In some patients, improvement has been noted with a reduction in dose frequency to q12 hours. In those patients available for follow-up, treatment discontinuation has been followed by resolution of symptoms. The etiology of these myalgias and arthralgias is under investigation.

Superinfections

The use of antibiotics may promote the overgrowth of nonsusceptible organisms. Should superinfection occur during therapy, appropriate measures should be taken.

Hyperbilirubinemia

Elevations of total biliburin greater than 5 times the upper limit of normal were noted in approximately 25% of patients in the non-comparative studies. In some patients, isolated hyperbilirubinemia (primarily conjugated) can occur during treatment, possibly resulting from competition between dalfopristin; quinupristin and biliburin for excretion. Of note, in the comparative trials, elevations in ALT and AST occurred at a similar frequency in both the dalfopristin; quinupristin and comparator groups.

CARCINOGENESIS, MUTAGENESIS, AND IMPAIRMENT OF FERTILITY

Long-term carcinogenicity studies in animals have not been conducted with dalfopristin; quinupristin. Five genetic toxicity tests were performed. Dalfopristin; quinupristin, dalfopristin, and quinupristin were tested in the bacterial reverse mutation assay, the Chinese hamster ovary cell HGPRT gene mutation assay, the unscheduled DNA synthesis assay in rat hepatocytes, the Chinese hamster ovary cell chromosome aberration assay, and the mouse micronucleus assay in bone marrow. Dalfopristin was associated with the production of structural chromosome aberrations when tested in the Chinese hamster ovary cell chromosome aberration assay. Dalfopristin; quinupristin and quinupristin were negative in this assay. Dalfopristin; quinupristin, dalfopristin, and quinupristin were all negative in the other four genetic toxicity assays.

No impairment of fertility or perinatal/postnatal development was observed in rats at doses up to 12-18 mg/kg (approximately 0.3-0.4 times the human dose based on body-surface area).

PREGNANCY, TERATOGENIC EFFECTS, PREGNANCY CATEGORY B

Reproductive studies have been performed in mice at doses up to 40 mg/kg/day (approximately half the human dose based on body-surface area), in rats at doses up to 120 mg/kg/day (approximately 2.5 times the human dose based on body-surface area), and in rabbits at doses up to 12 mg/kg/day (approximately half the human dose based on body-surface area) and have revealed no evidence of impaired fertility or harm to the fetus due to dalfopristin; quinupristin.

There are, however, no adequate and well-controlled studies with dalfopristin; quinupristin in pregnant women. Because animal reproduction studies are not always predictive of the human response, this drug should be used during pregnancy only if clearly needed.

NURSING MOTHERS

In lactating rats, dalfopristin; quinupristin was excreted in milk. It is not known whether dalfopristin; quinupristin is excreted in human breast milk. Because many drugs are excreted in human milk, caution should be exercised when dalfopristin; quinupristin is administered to a nursing woman.

HEPATIC INSUFFICIENCY

Following a single 1-hour infusion of dalfopristin; quinupristin (7.5 mg/kg) to patients with hepatic insufficiency, plasma concentrations were significantly increased. (See CLINICAL PHARMACOLOGY, Special Populations.) However, the effect of dose reduction or increase in dosing interval on the pharmacokinetics of dalfopristin; quinupristin in these patients has not been studied. Therefore, no recommendations can be made at this time regarding the appropriate dose modification.

PEDIATRIC USE

Dalfopristin; quinupristin has been used in a limited number of pediatric patients under emergency-use conditions at a dose of 7.5 mg/kg q8h or q12h. However, the safety and effectiveness of dalfopristin; quinupristin in patients under 16 years of age have not been established.

GERIATRIC USE

In phase 3 comparative trials of dalfopristin; quinupristin, 37% of patients (n=404) were ≥65 years of age, of which 145 were ≥75 years of age. In the Phase 3 non-comparative trials, 29% of patients (n=346) were ≥65 years of age, of which 112 were ≥75 years of age. There were no apparent differences in the frequency, type, or severity of related adverse reactions including cardiovascular events between elderly and younger individuals.

DRUG INTERACTIONS

In vitro drug interaction studies have shown that dalfopristin; quinupristin significantly inhibits cytochrome P450 3A4. (See WARNINGS.)

Dalfopristin; quinupristin does not significantly inhibit human cytochrome P450 1A2, 2A6, 2C9, 2C19, 2D6, or 2E1. Therefore, clinical interactions with drugs metabolized by these cytochrome P450 isoenzymes are not expected.

A drug interaction between dalfopristin; quinupristin and digoxin cannot be excluded but is unlikely to occur via CYP3A4 enzyme inhibition. Dalfopristin; quinupristin has shown *in vitro* activity (MICs of 0.25 µg/ml when tested on two strains) against *Eubacterium lentum.* Digoxin is metabolized in part by bacteria in the gut and as such, a drug interaction based on dalfopristin; quinupristin's inhibition of digoxin's gut metabolism (by *Eubacterium lentum*) may be possible.

In vitro combination testing of dalfopristin; quinupristin with aztreonam, cefotaxime, ciprofloxacin, and gentamicin, against *Enterobacteriaceae* and *Pseudomonas aeruginosa* did not show antagonism.

In vitro combination testing of dalfopristin; quinupristin with prototype drugs of the following classes: aminoglycosides (gentamicin), β-lactams (cefepime, ampicillin, and amoxicillin), glycopeptides (vancomycin), quinolones (ciprofloxacin), tetracyclines (doxycycline), and also chloramphenicol against enterococci and staphyococci did not show antagonism.

ADVERSE REACTIONS

The safety of dalfopristin; quinupristin was evaluated in 1099 patients enrolled in 5 comparative clinical trials. Additionally, 4 non-comparative clinical trials (3 prospective and 1 retrospective in design) were conducted in which 1199 patients received dalfopristin; quinupristin for infections due to gram-positive pathogens for which no other treatment option was available. In non-comparative trials, the patients were severely ill, often with multiple co-morbidities or physiological impairments, and may have been intolerant to or failed other antibacterial therapies.

COMPARATIVE TRIALS

Adverse Reaction Summary—All Comparative Studies

Safety data are available from five comparative clinical studies (n=1099 dalfopristin; quinupristin, n=1095 comparator). One of the deaths in the comparative studies was assessed as possibly related to dalfopristin; quinupristin. The most frequent reasons for discontinuation due to drug-related adverse reactions were as shown in TABLE 7.

TABLE 7 *Percent of Patients Discontinuing Therapy by Reaction Type*

Type	Dalfopristin; Quinupristin	Comparator
Venous	9.2%	2.0%
Non-Venous	9.6%	4.3%
Rash	1.0%	0.5%
Nausea	0.9%	0.6%
Vomiting	0.5%	0.5%
Pain	0.5%	0.0%
Pruritus	0.5%	0.3%

Clinical Reactions — All Comparative Studies

Adverse reactions with an incidence of ≥1% and possibly or probably related to dalfopristin; quinupristin administration include those shown in TABLE 8.

TABLE 8 *Percent of Patients With Adverse Reactions*

Adverse Reactions	Dalfopristin; Quinupristin	Comparator
Inflammation at infusion site	42.0%	25.0%
Pain at infusion site	40.0%	23.7%
Edema at infusion site	17.3%	9.5%
Infusion site reaction	13.4%	10.1%
Nausea	4.6%	7.2%
Thrombophlebitis	2.4%	0.3%
Diarrhea	2.7%	3.2%
Vomiting	2.7%	3.8%
Rash	2.5%	1.4%
Headache	1.6%	0.9%
Pruritus	1.5%	1.1%
Pain	1.5%	0.1%

Additional adverse reactions that were possibly or probably related to dalfopristin; quinupristin with an incidence less than 1% within each body system are listed below.

Body as a Whole: Abdominal pain, worsening of underlying illness, allergic reaction, chest pain, fever, infection.

Cardiovascular: Palpitation, phlebitis.

Digestive: Constipation, dyspepsia, oral moniliasis, pancreatitis, pseudomembranous enterocolitis, stomatitis.

Metabolic: Gout, peripheral edema.

Musculoskeletal: Arthralgia, myalgia, myasthenia.
Nervous: Anxiety, confusion, dizziness, hypertonia, insomnia, leg cramps, paresthesia, vasodilation.
Respiratory: Dyspnea, pleural effusion.
Skin and Appendages: Maculopapular rash, sweating, urticaria.
Urogenital: Hematuria, vaginitis.

Clinical Reactions — Skin And Skin Structure Studies

In two of the five comparative clinical trials dalfopristin; quinupristin (n=450) and comparator regimens (*e.g.*, oxacillin/vancomycin or cefazolin/vancomycin; n=443) were studied for safety and efficacy in the treatment of complicated skin and skin structure infections. The adverse event profile seen in the dalfopristin; quinupristin patients in these two studies differed significantly from that seen in the other comparative studies. What follows is safety data from these two studies.

Discontinuation of therapy was most frequently due to the drug related events shown in TABLE 9.

TABLE 9 *Percent of Patients Discontinuing Therapy by Reaction Type*

Type	Dalfopristin; Quinupristin	Comparator
Venous	12.0%	2.0%
Non-Venous	11.8%	4.0%
Rash	2.0%	0.9%
Nausea	1.1%	0.0%
Vomiting	0.9%	0.0%
Pain	0.9%	0.0%
Pruritus	0.9%	0.5%

Venous adverse events were seen predominately in patients who had peripheral infusions. The most frequently reported venous and non-venous adverse reactions possibly or probably related to study drug were as shown in TABLE 10.

TABLE 10 *Percent of Patients With Adverse Reactions*

	Dalfopristin; Quinupristin	Comparator
Venous	68.0%	32.7%
Pain at infusion site	44.7%	17.8%
Inflammation at infusion site	38.2%	14.7%
Edema at infusion site	18.0%	7.2%
Infusion site reaction	11.6%	3.6%
Non-Venous	24.7%	13.1%
Nausea	4.0%	2.0%
Vomiting	3.7%	1.0%
Rash	3.1%	1.3%
Pain	3.1%	0.2%

There were eight (1.7%) episodes of thrombus or thrombophlebitis in the dalfopristin; quinupristin arms and none in the comparator arms.

Laboratory Events—All Comparative Studies

TABLE 11 shows the number (%) of patients exhibiting laboratory values above or below the clinically relevant "critical" values during treatment phase (with an incidence of 0.1% or greater in either treatment group).

TABLE 11

		Critically High or Low	
Parameter	**Critically High or Low Value**	**Dalfopristin; Quinupristin**	**Comparator**
AST	>10 × ULN	9 (0.9%)	2 (0.2%)
ALT	>10 × ULN	4 (0.4%)	4 (0.4%)
Total bilirubin	>5 × ULN	9 (0.9%)	2 (0.2%)
Conjugated bilirubin	>5 × ULN	29 (3.1%)	12 (1.3%)
LDH	>5 × ULN	10 (2.6%)	8 (2.1%)
Alk. phosphatase	>5 × ULN	3 (0.3%)	7 (0.7%)
Gamma-GT	>10 × ULN	19 (1.9%)	10 (1.0%)
CPK	>10 × ULN	6 (1.6%)	5 (1.4%)
Creatinine	≥440 μmol/L	1 (0.1%)	1 (0.1%)
BUN	≥35.5 mmol/L	2 (0.3%)	9 (1.2%)
Blood glucose	>22.2 mmol/L	11 (1.3%)	11 (1.3%)
	<2.2 mmol/L	1 (0.1%)	1 (0.1%)
Bicarbonates	>40 mmol/L	2 (0.3%)	3 (0.5%)
	< 10 mmol/L	3 (0.5%)	3 (0.5%)
CO_2	>50 mmol/L	0 (0.0%)	0 (0.0%)
	<15 mmol/L	1 (0.2%)	0 (0.0%)
Sodium	>160 mmol/L	0 (0.0%)	0 (0.0%)
	<120 mmol/L	5 (0.5%)	3 (0.3%)
Potassium	>6.0 mmol/L	3 (0.3%)	6 (0.6%)
	<2.0 mmol/L	0 (0.0%)	1 (0.1%)
Hemoglobin	<8 g/dl	25 (2.6%)	16 (1.6%)
Hematocrit	>60%	2 (0.2%)	0 (0.0%)
Platelets	>1,000,000/mm^3	2 (0.2%)	2 (0.2%)
	<50,000/mm^3	6 (0.6%)	7 (0.7%)

NON-COMPARATIVE TRIALS

Clinical Adverse Reactions

Approximately one-third of patients discontinued therapy in these trials due to adverse events. However, the discontinuation rate due to adverse reactions assessed by the investigator as possibly or probably related to dalfopristin; quinupristin therapy was approximately 5.0%.

There were three prospectively designed non-comparative clinical trials in patients (n=972) treated with dalfopristin; quinupristin. One of these studies (301), had more complete documentation than the other two (398 and 398B). The most common events probably or possibly related to therapy were as shown in TABLE 12.

TABLE 12

Adverse Reactions	Study 301	Study 398A	Study 398B
Arthralgia	7.8%	5.2%	4.3%
Myalgia	5.1%	0.95%	3.1%
Arthralgia and myalgia	7.4%	3.3%	6.8%
Nausea	3.8%	2.8%	4.9%

The percentage of patients who experienced severe related arthralgia and myalgia was 3.3% and 3.1%, respectively. The percentage of patients who discontinued treatment due to related arthralgia and myalgia was 2.3% and 1.8%, respectively.

LABORATORY EVENTS

The most frequently observed abnormalities in laboratory studies were in total and conjugated bilirubin, with increases greater than 5 times upper limit of normal, irrespective of relationship to dalfopristin; quinupristin, reported in 25.0% and 34.6% of patients, respectively. The percentage of patients who discontinued treatment due to increased total and conjugated bilirubin was 2.7% and 2.3%, respectively. Of note, 46.5% and 59.0% of patients had high baseline total and conjugated bilirubin levels before study entry.

OTHER

Serious adverse reactions in clinical trials, including non-comparative studies, considered possibly or probably related to dalfopristin; quinupristin administration with an incidence <0.1% include: acidosis, anaphylactoid reaction, apnea, arrhythmia, bone pain, cerebral hemorrhage, cerebrovascular accident, coagulation disorder, convulsion, dysautonomia, encephalopathy, grand mal convulsion, hemolysis, hemolytic anemia, heart arrest, hepatitis, hypoglycemia, hyponatremia, hypoplastic anemia, hypoventilation, hypovolemia, hypoxia, jaundice, mesenteric arterial occlusion, neck rigidity, neuropathy, pancytopenia, paraplegia, pericardial effusion, pericarditis, respiratory distress syndrome, shock, skin ulcer, supraventricular tachycardia, syncope, tremor, ventricular extrasystoles, and ventricular fibrillation. Cases of hypotension and gastrointestinal hemorrhage were reported in less than 0.2% of patients.

DOSAGE AND ADMINISTRATION

Dalfopristin; quinupristin should be administered by intravenous infusion in 5% dextrose in water solution over a 60 minute period. (See WARNINGS.) The recommended dosage for the treatment of infections is described in TABLE 13. An infusion pump or device may be used to control the rate of infusion. If necessary, central venous access (*e.g.*, PICC) can be used to administer dalfopristin; quinupristin to decrease the incidence of venous irritation.

TABLE 13

	Dose
Vancomycin-Resistant *Enterococcus faecium*	7.5 mg/kg q8h
Complicated Skin and Skin Structure Infection	7.5 mg/kg q12h

The minimum recommended treatment duration for Complicated Skin and Skin Structure Infections is 7 days. For Vancomycin-Resistant *Enterococcus faecium* infection, the treatment duration should be determined based on the site and severity of the infection.

SPECIAL POPULATIONS

Elderly

No dosage adjustment of dalfopristin; quinupristin is required for use in the elderly. (See CLINICAL PHARMACOLOGY, Pharmacokinetics and PRECAUTIONS, Geriatric Use.)

Renal Insufficiency

No dosage adjustment of dalfopristin; quinupristin is required for use in patients with renal impairment or patients undergoing peritoneal dialysis. (See CLINICAL PHARMACOLOGY, Pharmacokinetics.)

Hepatic Insufficiency

Data from clinical trials of dalfopristin; quinupristin suggest that the incidence of adverse effects in patients with chronic liver insufficiency or cirrhosis was comparable to that in patients with normal hepatic function. Pharmacokinetic data in patients with hepatic cirrhosis (Child Pugh A or B) suggest that dosage reduction may be necessary but exact recommendations cannot be made at this time. (See CLINICAL PHARMACOLOGY, Special Populations and PRECAUTIONS, Hepatic Insufficiency.)

Pediatric Patients (less than 16 years of age)

Based on a limited number of pediatric patients treated under emergency-use conditions, no dosage adjustment of dalfopristin; quinupristin is required. (See PRECAUTIONS, Pediatric Use.)

COMPATIBILITY

Note: As for other parenteral drug products, dalfopristin; quinupristin should be inspected visually for particulate matter prior to administration.

DO NOT DILUTE WITH SALINE SOLUTIONS BECAUSE DALFOPRISTIN; QUINUPRISTIN IS NOT COMPATIBLE WITH THESE AGENTS. Dalfopristin; quinupristin should not be mixed with, or physically added to, other drugs except for the following drugs where compatibility by Y-site injection has been established. (See TABLE 14.)

If dalfopristin; quinupristin is to be given concomitantly with another drug, each drug should be given separately in accordance with the recommended dosage and route of administration for each drug.

TABLE 14 *Y-Site Injection Compatibility of Dalfopristin; Quinupristin at 2 mg/ml Concentration*

Admixture and Concentration	IV Infusion Solutions for Admixture
Aztreonam 20 mg/ml	D5W
Ciprofloxacin 1 mg/ml	D5W
Fluconazole 2 mg/ml	Used as the undiluted solution
Haloperidol 0.2 mg/ml	D5W
Metoclopramide 5 mg/ml	D5W
Potassium Chloride 40 mEq/L	D5W

D5W = 5% dextrose injection.

With intermittent infusion of dalfopristin; quinupristin and other drugs through a common intravenous line, the line should be flushed before and after administration with 5% dextrose in water solution.

HOW SUPPLIED

Each 10 ml vial contains sufficient dalfopristin; quinupristin to deliver 500 mg (150 mg of quinupristin and 350 mg of dalfopristin) for intravenous administration.

STABILITY AND STORAGE

Before Reconstitution: The unopened vials should be stored in a refrigerator at 2-8°C (36-46°F).

Reconstituted and Infusions Solutions: Because dalfopristin; quinupristin contains no antibacterial preservative, it should be reconstituted under strict aseptic conditions (*e.g.*, Laminar Air Flow Hood). The reconstituted solution should be diluted within 30 minutes. Vials are for single use. The storage time of the diluted solution should be as short as possible to minimize the risk of microbial contamination. Stability of the diluted solution prior to the infusion is established as 5 hours at room temperature or 54 hours if stored under refrigeration 2-8°C (36-46°F). The solution should not be frozen.

PRODUCT LISTING - EQUIVALENTS NOT AVAILABLE

Powder For Injection - Intravenous - 150 mg;350 mg

10's $1074.25	SYNERCID, Allscripts Pharmaceutical Company	54569-4838-00
10's $1206.06	SYNERCID, Aventis Pharmaceuticals	00075-9051-10

Dalteparin Sodium *(003197)*

For related information, see the comparative table section in Appendix A.

Categories: Embolism, pulmonary, prophylaxis; Ischemia, myocardial, prophylaxis; Thrombosis, deep vein, prophylaxis; FDA Approved 1994 Dec; Pregnancy Category B
Drug Classes: Anticoagulants
Brand Names: **Fragmin**
Foreign Brand Availability: Fragmin P Forte (Austria; Belgium; Bulgaria; Czech-Republic; Denmark; England; Finland; France; Germany; Greece; Hungary; Ireland; Italy; Netherlands; Norway; Poland; Portugal; Slovenia; Spain; Sweden; Switzerland; Turkey); Fragmine (France)
Cost of Therapy: $84.00 (Deep Vein Thrombosis; Fragmin Injection; 1000 units/ml; 2500 units/day; 7 day supply)
HCFA JCODE(S): J1645 per 2500 IU SC

WARNING

SPINAL/EPIDURAL HEMATOMAS

When neuraxial anesthesia (epidural/spinal anesthesia) or spinal puncture is employed, patients anticoagulated or scheduled to be anticoagulated with low molecular weight heparins or heparinoids for prevention of thromboembolic complications are at risk of developing an epidural or spinal hematoma which can result in long-term or permanent paralysis.

The risk of these events is increased by the use of indwelling epidural catheters for administration of analgesia or by the concomitant use of drugs affecting hemostasis such as nonsteroidal anti-inflammatory drugs (NSAIDs), platelet inhibitors, or other anticoagulants. The risk also appears to be increased by traumatic or repeated epidural or spinal puncture.

Patients should be frequently monitored for signs and symptoms of neurological impairment. If neurological compromise is noted, urgent treatment is necessary.

The physician should consider the potential benefit versus risk before neuraxial intervention in patients anticoagulated or to be anticoagulated for thromboprophylaxis (also see WARNINGS, Hemorrhage and DRUG INTERACTIONS).

DESCRIPTION

Dalteparin sodium injection is a sterile, low molecular weight heparin. It is available in single-dose, prefilled syringes preassembled with a needle guard device, and a multiple-dose vial. With reference to the WHO First International Low Molecular Weight Heparin Reference Standard, each syringe contains either 2500, 5000, 7500, or 10,000 anti-Factor Xa international units (IU), equivalent to 16, 32, 48, or 64 mg dalteparin sodium, respectively. Each vial contains 10,000 or 25,000 anti-Factor Xa IU/1 ml (equivalent to 64 or 160 mg dalteparin sodium, respectively), for a total of 95,000 anti-Factor Xa IU/vial.

Each prefilled syringe also contains water for injection and sodium chloride, when required, to maintain physiologic ionic strength. The prefilled syringes are preservtive free. Each mulitple-dose vial also contains water for injection and 14 mg of benzyl alcohol per ml as a preservative. The pH of both formulations is 5.0-7.5.

Dalteparin sodium is produced through controlled nitrous acid depolymerization of sodium heparin from porcine intestinal mucosa followed by a chromatographic purification process. It is composed of strongly acidic sulphated polysaccharide chains (oligosaccharide, containing 2,5-anhydro-D-mannitol residues as end groups) with an average molecular weight of 5000 and about 90% of the material within the range 2000-9000.

The molecular weight distribution is:

<3000 daltons: 3.0-15.0%
3000-8000 daltons: 65.0-78.0%
>8000 daltons: 14.0-26.0%

CLINICAL PHARMACOLOGY

Dalteparin sodium is a low molecular weight heparin with antithrombotic properties. It acts by enhancing the inhibition of Factor Xa and thrombin by antithrombin. In man, dalteparin potentiates preferentially the inhibition of coagulation Factor Xa, while only slightly affecting clotting time, *e.g.*, activated partial thromboplastin time (APTT).

PHARMACODYNAMICS

Doses of dalteparin sodium injection of up to 10,000 anti-Factor Xa IU administered subcutaneously as a single dose or two 5000 IU doses 12 hours apart to healthy subjects do not produce a significant change in platelet aggregation, fibrinolysis, or global clotting tests such as prothrombin time (PT), thrombin time (TT) or APTT. Subcutaneous (SC) administration of doses of 5000 IU bid of dalteparin sodium for 7 consecutive days to patients undergoing abdominal surgery did not markedly affect APTT, Platelet Factor 4 (PF4), or lipoprotein lipase.

PHARMACOKINETICS

Mean peak levels of plasma anti-Factor Xa activity following single SC doses of 2,500, 5,000 and 10,000 IU were 0.19 ± 0.04, 0.41 ± 0.07 and 0.82 ± 0.10 IU/ml, respectively, and were attained in about 4 hours in most subjects. Absolute bioavailability in healthy volunteers, measured as the anti-Factor Xa activity, was 87 ± 6%. Increasing the dose from 2,500 to 10,000 IU resulted in an overall increase in anti-Factor Xa AUC that was greater than proportional by about one-third.

Peak anti-Factor Xa activity increased more or less linearly with dose over the same dose range. There appeared to be no appreciable accumulation of anti-Factor Xa activity with twice-daily dosing of 100 IU/kg SC for up to 7 days.

The volume of distribution for dalteparin anti-Factor Xa activity was 40-60 ml/kg. The mean plasma clearances of dalteparin anti-Factor Xa activity in normal volunteers following single intravenous (IV) bolus doses of 30 and 120 anti-Factor Xa IU/kg were 24.6 ± 5.4 and 15.6 ± 2.4 ml/h/kg, respectively. The corresponding mean disposition half-lives are 1.47 ± 0.3 and 2.5 ± 0.3 hours.

Following IV doses of 40 and 60 IU/kg, mean terminal half-lives were 2.1 ± 0.3 and 2.3 ± 0.4 hours, respectively. Longer apparent terminal half-lives (3-5 hours) are observed following SC dosing, possibly due to delayed absorption. In patients with chronic renal insufficiency requiring hemodialysis, the mean terminal half-life of anti-Factor Xa activity following a single IV dose of 5000 IU dalteparin sodium was 5.7 ± 2.0 hours, *i.e.*, considerably longer than values observed in healthy volunteers, therefore, greater accumulation can be expected in these patients.

INDICATIONS AND USAGE

Dalteparin sodium injection is indicated for the prophylaxis of ischemic complications in unstable angina and non-Q-wave myocardial infarction, when concurrently administered with aspirin therapy.

Dalteparin sodium is also indicated for the prophylaxis of deep vein thrombosis (DVT), which may lead to pulmonary embolism (PE):

- In patients undergoing hip replacement surgery.
- In patients undergoing abdominal surgery who are at risk for thromboembolic complications.

NON-FDA APPROVED INDICATIONS

Although not approved by the FDA, additional uses of dalteparin have included the prophylaxis of deep vein thrombosis (DVT) following general surgery, treatment of acute DVT, PE, or stroke, outpatient perioperative anticoagulation, long-term DVT prophylaxis in warfarin-failure cancer patients, and anticoagulation during hemodialysis.

CONTRAINDICATIONS

Dalteparin sodium injection is contraindicated in patients with known hypersensitivity to the drug, active major bleeding, or thrombocytopenia associated with positive *in vitro* tests for antiplatelet antibody in the presence of dalteparin sodium.

Patients undergoing regional anesthesia should not receive dalteparin sodium for unstable angina or non-Q-wave myocardial infarction due to an increased risk of bleeding associated with the dosage of dalteparin sodium recommended for unstable angina and non-Q-wave myocardial infarction.

Patients with known hypersensitivity to heparin or pork products should not be treated with dalteparin sodium.

WARNINGS

Dalteparin sodium injection is not intended for intramuscular administration.

Dalteparin sodium cannot be used interchangeably (unit for unit) with unfractionated heparin or other low molecular weight heparins.

Dalteparin sodium should be used with extreme caution in patients with history of heparin-induced thrombocytopenia.

HEMORRHAGE

Dalteparin sodium, like other anticoagulants, should be used with extreme caution in patients who have an increased risk of hemorrhage, such as those with severe uncontrolled hypertension, bacterial endocarditis, congenital or acquired bleeding disorders, active ulceration and angiodysplastic gastrointestinal disease, hemorrhagic stroke, or shortly after brain, spinal or ophthalmological surgery.

Spinal or epidural hematomas can occur with the associated use of low molecular weight heparins or heparinoids and neuraxial (spinal/epidural) anesthesia or spinal puncture, which can result in long-term or permanent paralysis. The risk of these events is higher with the use of indwelling epidural catheters or concomitant use of additional drugs affecting hemostasis such as NSAIDs (see BOXED WARNING and ADVERSE REACTIONS, Other, Ongoing Safety Surveillance).

As with other anticoagulants, bleeding can occur at any site during therapy with dalteparin sodium. An unexpected drop in hematocrit or blood pressure should lead to a search for a bleeding site.

THROMBOCYTOPENIA

In clinical trials, thrombocytopenia with platelet counts of <100,000/mm^3 and <50,000/mm^3 occurred in <1% and <1%, respectively. In clinical practice, rare cases of thrombocytopenia with thrombosis have also been observed.

Thrombocytopenia of any degree should be monitored closely. Heparin-induced thrombocytopenia can occur with the administration of dalteparin sodium. The incidence of this complication is unknown at present.

MISCELLANEOUS

The multiple-dose vial of dalteparin sodium contains benzyl alcohol as a preservative. Benzyl alcohol has been reported to be associated with a fatal "Gasping Syndrome" in premature infants. Because benzyl alcohol may cross the placenta, dalteparin sodium preserved with benzyl alcohol should not be used in pregnant women. (See PRECAUTIONS, Pregnancy Category B, Nonteratogenic Effects.)

PRECAUTIONS

GENERAL

Dalteparin sodium should not be mixed with other injections or infusions unless specific compatability data are available that support such mixing.

Dalteparin sodium injection should be used with caution in patients with bleeding diathesis, thrombocytopenia or platelet defects, severe liver or kidney insufficiency, hypertensive or diabetic retinopathy, and recent gastrointestinal bleeding.

If a thromboembolic event should occur despite dalteparin sodium prophylaxis, dalteparin sodium should be discontinued and appropriate therapy initiated.

LABORATORY TESTS

Periodic routine complete blood counts, including platelet count, and stool occult blood tests are recommended during the course of treatment with dalteparin sodium. No special monitoring of blood clotting times (*e.g.*, APTT) is needed.

When administered at recommended prophylaxis doses, routine coagulation tests such as Prothrombin Time (PT) and Activated Partial Thromboplastin Time (APTT) are relatively insensitive measures of dalteparin sodium activity and, therefore, unsuitable for monitoring.

DRUG/LABORATORY TEST INTERACTIONS

Elevations of Serum Transaminases

Asymptomatic increases in transaminase levels (SGOT/AST and SGPT/ALT) greater than 3 times the upper limit of normal of the laboratory reference range have been reported in 1.7 and 4.3%, respectively, of patients during treatment with dalteparin sodium. Similar significant increases in transaminase levels have also been observed in patients treated with heparin and other low molecular weight heparins. Such elevations are fully reversible and are rarely associated with increases in bilirubin. Since transaminase determinations are important in the differential diagnosis of myocardial infarction, liver disease and pulmonary emboli, elevations that might be caused by drugs like dalteparin sodium should be interpreted with caution.

CARCINOGENESIS, MUTAGENESIS, AND IMPAIRMENT OF FERTILITY

Dalteparin sodium has not been tested for its carcinogenic potential in long-term animal studies. It was not mutagenic in the *in vitro* Ames test, mouse lymphoma cell forward mutation test and human lymphocyte chromosomal aberration test and in the *in vivo* mouse micronucleus test. Dalteparin sodium at SC doses up to 1200 IU/kg (7080 IU/m^2) did not affect the fertility of reproductive performance of male and female rats.

PREGNANCY CATEGORY B

Teratogenic Effects

Reproduction studies with dalteparin sodium at IV doses up to 2400 IU/kg (14,160 IU/m^2) in pregnant rats and 4800 IU/kg (40,800 IU/m^2) in pregnant rabbits did not produce any evidence of impaired fertility or harm to the fetuses. There are, however, no adequate and well-controlled studies in pregnant women. Because animal reproduction studies are not always predictive of human response, this drug should be used during pregnancy only if clearly needed.

Nonteratogenic Effects

Cases of "Gasping Syndrome" have occurred when large amounts of benzyl alcohol have been administered (99-404 mg/kg/day). The 9.5 ml multiple-dose vial of dalteparin sodium contains 14 mg/ml of benzyl alcohol.

NURSING MOTHERS

It is not known whether dalteparin sodium is excreted in human milk. Because many drugs are excreted in human milk, caution should be exercised when dalteparin sodium is administered to a nursing mother.

PEDIATRIC USE

Safety and effectiveness in pediatric patients have not been established.

DRUG INTERACTIONS

Dalteparin sodium should be used with care in patients receiving oral anticoagulants, platelet inhibitors, and thrombolytic agents because of increased risk of bleeding (see PRECAUTIONS, Laboratory Tests). Aspirin, unless contraindicated, is recommended in patients treated for unstable angina or non-Q-wave myocardial infarction (see DOSAGE AND ADMINISTRATION).

ADVERSE REACTIONS

HEMORRHAGE

The incidence of hemorrhagic complications during treatment with dalteparin sodium injection has been low. The most commonly reported side effect is hematoma at the injection site. The incidence of bleeding may increase with higher doses; however, in abdominal surgery patients with malignancy, no significant increase in bleeding was observed when comparing dalteparin sodium 5000 IU to either dalteparin sodium 2500 IU or low dose heparin.

In a trial comparing dalteparin sodium 5000 IU once daily to dalteparin sodium 2500 IU once daily in patients undergoing surgery for malignancy, the incidence of bleeding events was 4.6% and 3.6%, respectively (n.s.). In a trial comparing dalteparin sodium 5000 IU once daily to heparin 5000 U twice daily, the incidence of bleeding events was 3.2% and 2.7%, respectively (n.s.) in the malignancy subroup.

Unstable Angina and Non-Q-Wave Myocardial Infarction

TABLE 6 summarizes major bleeding events that occurred with dalteparin sodium, heparin, and placebo in clinical trials of unstable angina and non-Q-wave myocardial infarction.

TABLE 6 *Major Bleeding Events in Unstable Angina and Non-Q-Wave Myocardial Infarction*

Indication	Dosing Regimen: Dalteparin Sodium	Dosing Regimen: Heparin	Dosing Regimen: Placebo
Unstable Angina and Non-Q-Wave MI	120 IU/kg/12h SC*	IV and SC†	q12h SC
Major bleeding events‡§	15/1497 (1.0%)	7/731 (1.0%)	4/760 (0.5%)

* Treatment was administered for 5-8 days.
† Heparin IV infusion for at least 48 hours, APPT 1.5 to 2 times control, then 12,500 U SC every 12 hours for 5-8 days.
‡ Aspirin (75-165 mg/day) and beta blocker therapies were administered concurrently.
§ Bleeding events were considered major if: (1) accompanied by a decrease in hemoglobin of ≥2 g/dl in connection with clinical symptoms; (2) a transfusion was required; (3) bleeding led to interruption of treatment or death; or (4) intracranial bleeding.

Hip Replacement Surgery

TABLE 7 summarizes: (1) all major bleeding events and, (2) other bleeding events possibly or probably related to treatment with dalteparin sodium (preoperative dosing regimen), warfarin sodium, or heparin in 2 hip replacement surgery clinical trials.

TABLE 7 *Bleeding Events Following Hip Replacement Surgery*

	Dalteparin Sodium vs Warfarin Sodium		Dalteparin Sodium vs Heparin	
	Dosing Regimen		Dosing Regimen	
	Dalteparin Sodium	Warfarin Sodium†	Dalteparin Sodium	Heparin
Indication	5000 IU qd SC	Oral	5000 IU qd SC	5000 U tid SC
Hip Replacement Surgery	(n=274*)	(n=279)	(n=69‡)	(n=69)
Major Bleeding Events§	7/274 (2.6%)	1/279 (0.4%)	0	3/69 (4.3%)
Other Bleeding Events¤				
Hematuria	8/274 (2.9%)	5/279 (1.8%)	0	0
Wound hematoma	6/274 (2.2%)	0	0	0
Injection site hematoma	3/274 (1.1%)	NA	2/69 (2.9%)	7/69 (10.1%)

* Includes 3 treated patients who did not undergo a surgical procedure.
† Warfarin sodium dosage was adjusted to maintain a prothrombin time index of 1.4-1.5, corresponding to an International Normalized Ratio (INR) of approximately 2.5.
‡ Includes 2 treated patients who did not undergo a surgical procedure.
§ A bleeding event was considered major if: (1) hemorrhage caused a significant clinical event, (2) it was associated with a hemoglobin decrease of ≥2 g/dl or transfusion of 2 or more units of blood products, (3) it resulted in reoperation due to bleeding, or (4) it involved retroperitoneal or intracranial hemorrhage.
¤ Occurred at a rate of at least 2% in the group treated with dalteparin sodium 5000 IU once daily.

Six of the patients treated with dalteparin sodium experienced 7 major bleeding events. Two (2) of the events were wound hematoma (1 requiring reoperation), 3 were bleeding from the operative site, 1 was intraoperative bleeding due to vessel damage, and 1 was gastrointestinal bleeding. None of the patients experienced retroperitoneal or intracranial hemorrhage nor died of bleeding complications.

In the third hip replacement surgery clinical trial, the incidence of major bleeding events was similar in all 3 treatment groups: 3.6% (18/496) for patients who started dalteparin sodium before surgery; 2.5% (12/487) for patients who started dalteparin sodium after surgery; and 3.1% (15/489) for patients treated with warfarin sodium.

Abdominal Surgery

TABLE 8A and TABLE 8B summarizes bleeding events that occurred in clinical trials which studied dalteparin sodium 2500 and 5000 IU administered once daily to abdominal surgery patients.

TABLE 8A *Bleeding Events Following Abdominal Surgery — Dalteparin Sodium Versus Heparin*

Indication	Dalteparin Sodium	Heparin	Dalteparin Sodium	Heparin
	Dosing Regimen			
Abdominal Surgery	2500 IU qd SC	5000 U bid SC	5000 IU qd SC	5000 U bid SC
Postoperative transfusions	26/459 (5.7%)	36/454 (7.9%)	81/508 (15.9%)	63/498 (12.7%)
Wound hematoma	16/467 (3.4%)	18/467 (3.9%)	12/508 (2.4%)	6/498 (1.2%)
Reoperation due to bleeding	2/392 (0.5%)	3/392 (0.8%)	4/508 (0.8%)	2/498 (0.4%)
Injection site hematoma	1/466 (0.2%)	5/464 (1.1%)	36/506 (7.1%)	47/493 (9.5%)

TABLE 8B *Bleeding Events Following Abdominal Surgery*

Indication	Dalteparin Sodium vs Placebo		Dalteparin Sodium vs Dalteparin Sodium	
	Dosing Regimen			
	Dalteparin Sodium	Placebo	Dalteparin Sodium	Dalteparin Sodium
Abdominal Surgery	2500 IU qd SC	qd SC	2500 IU qd SC	5000 IU qd SC
Postoperative transfusions	14/182 (7.7%)	13/182 (7.1%)	89/1025 (8.7%)	125/1033 (12.1%)
Wound hematoma	2/79 (2.5%)	2/77 (2.6%)	1/1030 (0.1%)	4/1039 (0.4%)
Reoperation due to bleeding	1/79 (1.3%)	1/78 (1.3%)	2/1030 (0.2%)	13/1038 (1.3%)
Injection site hematoma	8/172 (4.7%)	2/174 (1.1%)	36/1026 (3.5%)	57/1035 (5.5%)

THROMBOCYTOPENIA

See WARNINGS, Thrombocytopenia.

OTHER

Allergic Reactions

Allergic reactions (*i.e.*, pruritus, rash, fever, injection site reaction, bulleous eruption) and skin necrosis have occurred rarely. A few cases of anaphylactoid reactions have been reported.

Local Reactions

Pain at the injection site, the only non-bleeding event determined to be possibly or probably related to treatment with dalteparin sodium and reported at a rate of at least 2% in the group treated with dalteparin sodium, was reported in 4.5% of patients treated with dalteparin sodium 5000 IU qd vs 11.8% of patients treated with heparin 5000 U bid in the abdominal surgery trials. In the hip replacement trials, pain at injection site was reported in 12% of patients treated with dalteparin sodium 5000 IU qd vs 13% of patients treated with heparin 5000 U tid.

Ongoing Safety Surveillance

Since first international market introduction in 1985, there have been 6 reports of epidural or spinal hematoma formation with concurrent use of dalteparin sodium and spinal/epidural anesthesia or spinal puncture. Five (5) of the 6 patients had post-operative indwelling epidural catheters placed for analgesia or received additional drugs affecting hemostasis. The hematomas caused long-term or permanent paralysis (partial or complete) in 4 of these cases. The sixth patient experienced temporary paraplegia but made a full recovery. Because these events were reported voluntarily from a population of unknown size, estimates of frequency cannot be made.

DOSAGE AND ADMINISTRATION

UNSTABLE ANGINA AND NON-Q-WAVE MYOCARDIAL INFARCTION

In patients with unstable angina or non-Q-wave myocardial infarction, the recommended dose of dalteparin sodium injection is 120 IU/kg of body weight, but not more than 10,000 IU, SC every 12 hours with concurrent oral aspirin (75-165 mg once daily) therapy. Treatment should be continued until the patient is clinically stabilized. The usual duration of administration is 5-8 days. Concurrent aspirin therapy is recommended except when contraindicated.

TABLE 9 lists the volume of dalteparin sodium to be administered for a range of patient weights.

TABLE 9 *Volume of Dalteparin Sodium to Be Administered by Patient Weight*

Patient Weight		Volume of Dalteparin Sodium*
<110 lb	<50 kg	0.55 ml
110-131 lb	50-59 kg	0.65 ml
132-153 lb	60-69 kg	0.75 ml
154-175 lb	70-79 kg	0.90 ml
176-197 lb	80-89 kg	1.00 ml
≥198 lb	≥90 kg	1.00 ml

* Calculated volume based on the 9.5 ml multiple-dose vial (10,000 anti-Factor Xa IU/ml).

HIP REPLACEMENT SURGERY

TABLE 10 presents the dosing options for patients undergoing hip replacement surgery. The usual duration of administration is 5-10 days after surgery; up to 14 days of treatment with dalteparin sodium have been well tolerated in clinical trials.

TABLE 10 *Dosing Options for Patients Undergoing Hip Replacement Surgery*

Timing of First Dose of Dalteparin Sodium	Dose of Dalteparin Sodium to Be Given SC			
	10-14 h Before Surgery	Within 2 h Before Surgery	4-8 h After Surgery*	Postoperative Period†
Postoperative start	—	—	2500 IU‡	5000 IU qd
Preoperative start — day of surgery	—	2500 IU	2500 IU‡	5000 IU qd
Preoperative start — evening before surgery§	5000 IU	—	5000 IU	5000 IU qd

* Or later, if hemostasis has not been achieved.
† Up to 14 days of treatment was well tolerated in controlled clinical trials, where the usual duration of treatment was 5-10 days postoperatively.
‡ Allow a minimum of 6 hours between this dose and the dose to be given on Postoperative Day 1. Adjust the timing of the dose on Postoperative Day 1 accordingly.
§ Allow approximately 24 hours between doses.

ABDOMINAL SURGERY

In patients undergoing abdominal surgery with a risk of thromboembolic complications, the recommended dose of dalteparin sodium is 2500 IU administered by SC injection once daily, starting 1-2 hours prior to surgery and repeated once daily postoperatively. The usual duration of administration is 5-10 days.

In patients undergoing abdominal surgery associated with a high risk of thromboembolic complications, such as malignant disorder, the recommended dose of dalteparin sodium is 5000 IU SC the evening before surgery, then once daily postoperatively. The usual duration of administration is 5-10 days. Alternatively, in patients with malignancy, 2500 IU of dalteparin sodium can be administered SC 1-2 hours before surgery followed by 2500 IU SC 12 hours later, and then 5000 IU once daily postoperatively. The usual duration of administration is 5-10 days.

Dosage adjustment and routine monitoring of coagulation parameters are not required if the dosage and administration recommendations specified above are followed.

ADMINISTRATION

Dalteparin sodium is administered by SC injection. It must not be administered by IM injection.

Subcutaneous Injection Technique

Patients should be sitting or lying down and dalteparin sodium administered by deep SC injection. Dalteparin sodium may be injected in a U-shape area around the navel, the upper outer side of the thigh or the upper outer quadrangle of the buttock. The injection site should be varied daily. When the area around the navel or the thigh is used, using the thumb and forefinger, you **must** lift up a fold of skin while giving the injection. The entire length of the needle should be inserted at a 45-90 degree angle.

Parenteral drug products should be inspected visually for particulate matter and discoloration prior to administration, whenever solution and container permit.

After first penetration of the rubber stopper, store the multiple-dose vials at room temperature for up to 2 weeks. Discard any unused solution after 2 weeks.

Instructions for Using the Prefilled Single-dose Syringes Preassembled With Needle Guard Devices

Hold the syringe assembly by the open sides of the device. Remove the needle shield. Insert the needle into the injection area as instructed above. Depress the plunger of the syringe while holding the finger flange **until the entire dose has been given.** The needle guard will **not** be activated unless the **entire** dose has been given. Remove needle from the patient. Let go of the plunger and allow syringe to move up inside the device until the entire needle is guarded. Discard the syringe assembly in approved containers.

HOW SUPPLIED

Fragmin injection is available in 0.2 and 0.3 ml single-dose prefilled syringes, a 1.0 ml single-dose graduated syringe, and 3.5 or 9.5 ml multiple-dose vial.
Storage: Store at controlled room temperature 20-25°C (68-77°F).

PRODUCT LISTING - RATED THERAPEUTICALLY EQUIVALENT

Solution - Subcutaneous - 2500 IU/0.2 ml
0.20 ml x 10 $172.09 FRAGMIN, Pharmacia and Upjohn 00013-2406-91

PRODUCT LISTING - EQUIVALENTS NOT AVAILABLE

Solution - Subcutaneous - 5000 U/0.2 ml
0.20 ml x 10 $279.24 FRAGMIN, Pharmacia and Upjohn 00013-2426-91
0.30 ml x 10 $418.85 FRAGMIN, Pharmacia and Upjohn 00013-2426-01
3.80 ml $479.99 FRAGMIN, Pharmacia and Upjohn 00013-5191-01
Solution - Subcutaneous - 10000 U/ml
1 ml x 10 $558.46 FRAGMIN, Pharmacia and Upjohn 00013-5190-01
10 ml $479.99 FRAGMIN, Pharmacia and Upjohn 00013-2436-06

Danazol (000940)

Categories: Angioedema; Endometriosis; Fibrocystic breast disease; Pregnancy Category X; FDA Approved 1976 Jun
Drug Classes: Hormones/hormone modifiers
Brand Names: Danocrine
Foreign Brand Availability: Anargil (Hong-Kong; Thailand); Azol (Australia; Malaysia; Taiwan); Bonzol (Japan); Cyclomen (Canada); D-Zol (New-Zealand); Danasin (Turkey); Danatrol (Belgium; France; Greece; Italy; Netherlands; Portugal; Spain; Switzerland); Danazol (Korea; Poland); Danazol-Ratiopharm (Germany); Danazol Jean Marie (Hong-Kong); Danokrin (Austria); Danodiol (Bahamas; Bahrain; Barbados; Belize; Bermuda; Curacao; Cyprus; Egypt; Ghana; Guyana; Israel; Jamaica; Jordan; Kenya; Lebanon; Libya; Mauritius; Netherland-Antilles; Oman; Qatar; Republic-of-Yemen; Saudi-Arabia; Surinam; Syria; Tanzania; Trinidad; United-Arab-Emirates); Danogen (India; Russia); Danol (Bahrain; Cyprus; Czech-Republic; Egypt; England; Hungary; Iran; Iraq; Ireland; Jordan; Kuwait; Lebanon; Libya; Oman; Qatar; Republic-of-Yemen; Saudi-Arabia; Syria; United-Arab-Emirates); Danoval (Bulgaria; Hungary); Dorink (Taiwan); Ectopal (Taiwan; Thailand); Gonablok (India); Kendazol (Mexico); Ladazol (South-Africa); Ladogal (CIS; Colombia; Costa-Rica; Dominican-Republic; Ecuador; El-Salvador; Guatemala; Honduras; Malaysia; Mexico; Nicaragua; Panama; Peru; Philippines; Taiwan; Thailand); Nazol (Malaysia); Norciden (Mexico); Vabon (Thailand); Winobanin (Germany); Zendol (India); Zoldan-A (Mexico)
Cost of Therapy: $275.38 (Endometriosis; Danocrine; 200 mg; 2 capsules/day; 30 day supply)
$171.60 (Endometriosis; Generic capsules; 200 mg; 2 capsules/day; 30 day supply)

WARNING

Use of danazol in pregnancy is contraindicated. A sensitive test (*e.g.,* beta subunit test if available) capable of determining early pregnancy is recommended immediately prior to start of therapy. Additionally a non-hormonal method of contraception should be used during therapy. If a patient becomes pregnant while taking danazol administration of the drug should be discontinued and the patient should be apprised of the potential risk to the fetus. Exposure to danazol in utero may result in androgenic effects on the female fetus; reports of clitoral hypertrophy, labial fusion, urogenital sinus defect, vaginal atresia, and ambiguous genitalia have been received. (See PRECAUTIONS, Pregnancy, Teratogenic Effects, Pregnancy Category X.)

Thromboembolism, thrombotic and thrombophlebitic events including sagittal sinus thrombosis and life-threatening or fetal strokes have been reported.

Experience with long-term therapy with danazol is limited. Peliosis hepatis and benign hepatic adenoma have been observed with long-term use. Peliosis hepatis and benign hepatic adenoma may be silent until complicated by acute, potentially life-threatening intraabdominal hemorrhage. The physician therefore should be alert to this possibility. Attempts should be made to determine the lowest dose that will provide adequate protection. If the drug was begun at a time of exacerbation of hereditary angioneurotic edema due to trauma, stress or other cause, periodic attempts to decrease or withdraw therapy should be considered.

Danazol has been associated with several cases of benign intracranial hypertension also known as pseudotumor cerebri. Early signs and symptoms of benign intracranial hypertension include papilledema headache, nausea and vomiting, and visual disturbances. Patients with these symptoms should be screened for papilledema and, if present, the patients should be advised to discontinue danazol immediately and be referred to a neurologist for further diagnosis and care.

DESCRIPTION

Danazol, is a synthetic steroid derived from ethisterone. Chemically, danazol is 17α-pregna-2,4-dien-20-yno[2,3-*dl*-isoxazol-17-ol

Danocrine Inactive Ingredients: benzyl alcohol, gelatin, lactose, magnesium stearate, parabens, sodium propionate, starch, talc. Capsules 50 and 200 mg contain D&C yellow no. 10, FD&C red no. 3. Capsules 100 mg contains D&C yellow no. 10, FD&C yellow no. 6.

CLINICAL PHARMACOLOGY

Danazol suppresses the pituitary-ovarian axis. This suppression is probably a combination of depressed hypothalamic-pituitary response to lowered estrogen production, the alteration of sex steroid metabolism, and interaction of danazol with sex hormone receptors. The only other demonstrable hormonal effect is weak androgenic activity. Danazol depresses the output of both follicle-stimulating hormone (FSH) and luteinizing hormone (LH).

Recent evidence suggests a direct inhibitory effect at gonadal sites and a binding of danazol to receptors of gonadal steroids at target organs. In addition, danazol has been shown to significantly decrease IgG, IgM, and IgA levels, as well as phospholipid and IgG isotope autoantibodies in patients with endometriosis and associated elevations of autoantibodies, suggesting this could be another mechanism by which it facilitates regression of the disease.

Bioavailability studies indicate that blood levels do not increase proportionally with increases in the administered dose. When the dose of danazol is doubled the increase in plasma levels is only about 35-40%.

Separate single dosing of 100 and 200 mg capsules of danazol to female volunteers showed that both the extent of availability and the maximum plasma concentration increased by 3- to 4-fold, respectively, following a meal (>30 g of fat), when compared to the fasted state. Further, food also delayed mean time to peak concentration of danazol by about 30 minutes.

In the treatment of endometriosis, danazol alters the normal and ectopic endometrial tissue so that it becomes inactive and atrophic. Complete resolution of endometrial lesions occurs in the majority of cases.

Changes in vaginal cytology and cervical mucus reflect the suppressive effect of danazol on the pituitary-ovarian axis.

In the treatment of fibrocystic breast disease, danazol usually produces partial to complete disappearance of nodularity and complete relief of pain and tenderness. Changes in the menstrual pattern may occur.

Generally, the pituitary-suppressive action of danazol is reversible. Ovulation and cyclic bleeding usually return within 60-90 days when therapy with danazol is discontinued.

In the treatment of hereditary angioedema, danazol at effective doses prevents attacks of the disease characterized by episodic edema of the abdominal viscera, extremities, face, and airway which may be disabling and, if the airway is involved, fatal. In addition, danazol corrects partially or completely the primary biochemical abnormality of hereditary angioedema by increasing the levels of the deficient C1 esterase inhibitor (C1EI). As a result of this action the serum levels of the C4 component of the complement system are also increased.

INDICATIONS AND USAGE

ENDOMETRIOSIS

Danazol is indicated for the treatment of endometriosis amenable to hormonal management.

FIBROCYSTIC BREAST DISEASE

Most cases of symptomatic fibrocystic breast disease may be treated by simple measures (*e.g.,* padded brassieres and analgesics).

In infrequent patients, symptoms of pain and tenderness may be severe enough to warrant treatment by suppression of ovarian function. Danazol is usually effective in decreasing nodularity, pain, and tenderness. It should be stressed to the patient that this treatment is not innocuous in that it involves considerable alterations of hormone levels and that recurrence of symptoms is very common after cessation of therapy.

HEREDITARY ANGIOEDEMA

Danazol is indicated for the prevention of attacks of angioedema of all types (cutaneous, abdominal, laryngeal) in males and females.

NON-FDA APPROVED INDICATIONS

Danazol has been used in treatment of gynecomastia, menorrhagia, and precocious puberty. It has also been used in female or male contraception, breast cancer, certain anemias (red cell aplasia and other deficient red cell production anemias) to enhance red cell production, as treatment in select coagulopathies (Antithrombin III deficiency or fibrinogen excess), in inflammatory responses (autoimmune hemolytic anemia, asthma, SLE) and to modulate growth failure (primary or secondary) or short stature associated with Turner's syndrome.

CONTRAINDICATIONS

Danazol should not be administered to patients with:

Undiagnosed abnormal genital bleeding.
Markedly impaired hepatic, renal, or cardiac function.
Pregnancy. (See WARNINGS.)
Breast feeding.
Porphyria-danazol can induce ALA synthetase activity and hence porphyrin metabolism.

WARNINGS

A temporary alteration of lipoproteins in the form of decreased high density lipoproteins and possibly increased low density lipoproteins has been reported during danazol therapy. These alterations may be marked, and prescribers should consider the potential impact on the risk of atherosclerosis and coronary artery disease in accordance with the potential benefit of the therapy to the patient.

Before initiating therapy of fibrocystic breast disease with danazol, carcinoma of the breast should be excluded. However, nodularity, pain, tenderness due to fibrocystic breast disease may prevent recognition of underlying carcinoma before treatment is begun. Therefore, if any nodule persists or enlarges during treatment, carcinoma should be considered and ruled out.

Patients should be watched closely for signs of androgenic effects some of which may not be reversible even when drug administration is stopped.

PRECAUTIONS

Because danazol may cause some degree of fluid retention, conditions that might be influenced by this factor, such as epilepsy, migraine, or cardiac or renal dysfunction, require careful observation.

Since hepatic dysfunction manifested by modest increases in serum transaminase levels has been reported in patients treated with danazol, periodic liver function tests should be performed (see WARNINGS and ADVERSE REACTIONS).

Administration of danazol has been reported to cause exacerbation of the manifestations of acute intermittent porphyria. (see CONTRAINDICATIONS.)

LABORATORY TESTS

Danazol treatment may interfere with laboratory determinations of testosterone, androstenedione and dehydroepiandrosterone.

CARCINOGENESIS, MUTAGENESIS, AND IMPAIRMENT OF FERTILITY

No valid studies have been performed to assess the carcinogenicity of danazol.

PREGNANCY, TERATOGENIC EFFECTS, PREGNANCY CATEGORY X

See CONTRAINDICATIONS.

Danazol administered orally to pregnant rats from the 6th through the 15th day of gestation at doses up to 250 mg/kg/day (7-15 times the human dose) did not result in drug-induced embryotoxicity or teratogenicity, nor difference in litter size, viability or weight of offspring compared to controls. In rabbits, the administration of danazol on days 6-18 of gestation at doses of 60 mg/kg/day and above (2-4 times the human dose) resulted in inhibition of fetal development.

NURSING MOTHERS

See CONTRAINDICATIONS.

PEDIATRIC USE

Safety and effectiveness in children have not been established.

DRUG INTERACTIONS

Prolongation of prothrombin time occurs in patients stabilized on warfarin. Therapy with danazol may cause an increase in carbamazepine in patients taking both drugs.

ADVERSE REACTIONS

The following events have been reported in association with the use of danazol:

Androgen like effects include weight gain, acne and seborrhea. Mild hirsutism, edema, hair loss, voice change, which may take the form of hoarseness, sore throat or of instability or deepening of pitch, may occur and may persist after cessation of therapy. Hypertrophy of the clitoris is rare.

Other possible endocrine effects include menstrual disturbances in the form of spotting, alteration of the timing of the cycle and amenorrhea. Although cyclical bleeding and ovulation usually return within 60-90 days after discontinuation of therapy with danazol, persistent amenorrhea has occasionally been reported.

Flushing, sweating, vaginal dryness and irritation and reduction in breast size, may reflect lowering of estrogen. Nervousness and emotional liability have been reported. In the male a modest reduction in spermatogenesis may be evident during treatment. Abnormalities in semen volume, viscosity, sperm count, and motility may occur in patients receiving long-term therapy.

Hepatic dysfunction, as evidenced by reversible elevated serum enzymes and/or jaundice, has been reported in patients receiving a daily dosage of danazol of 400 mg or more. It is recommended that patients receiving danazol be monitored for hepatic dysfunction by laboratory tests and clinical observation. Serious hepatic toxicity including cholestatic jaundice, peliosis hepatis, and hepatic adenoma have been reported. (See WARNINGS and PRECAUTIONS.)

Abnormalities is laboratory tests may occur during therapy with danazol including CPK, glucose tolerance, glucagon, thyroid binding globulin, sex hormone binding globulin, other plasma proteins, lipids and lipoproteins.

The following reactions have been reported, a causal relationship to the administration of danazol has neither been confirmed nor refuted:

Allergic: Urticaria, pruritus and rarely, nasal congestion.

CNS Effects: Headache, nervousness and emotional lability, dizziness and fainting, depression, fatigue, sleep disorders, tremor, paresthesias, weakness, visual disturbances, and rarely, benign intracranial hypertension, anxiety, changes in appetite, chills, and rarely convulsions Guillain-Barre syndrome.

Gastrointestinal: Gastroenteritis, nausea, vomiting, constipation, and rarely, pancreatitis.

Musculoskeletal: Muscle cramps or spasms, or pains, joint pain, joint lockup, joint swelling, pain in back, neck, or extremities, and rarely, carpal tunnel syndrome which may be secondary to fluid retention.

Genitourinary: Hematuria, prolonged posttherapy amenorrhea,

Hematologic: Increase in red cell and platelet count. Reversible erythrocytosis, leukocytosis or polycythemia may be provoked. Eosinophilia, leukopenia and thrombocytopenia have also been noted.

Skin: Rashes (maculopapular, vesicular, papular, purpuric, petechial), and rarely, sun sensitivity, Stevens-Johnson syndrome.

Other: Increased insulin requirements in diabetic patients, change in libido, elevation in blood pressure, and rarely, cataracts, bleeding gums, fever, pelvic pain, nipple discharge.

Malignant liver tumors have been reported in rare instances, after long-term use.

DOSAGE AND ADMINISTRATION

ENDOMETRIOSIS

In moderate to severe disease, or in patients infertile due to endometriosis, a starting dose of 800 mg given in two divided doses is recommended. Amenorrhea and rapid response to painful symptoms is best achieved at this dosage level. Gradual downward titration to a dose sufficient to maintain amenorrhea may be considered depending upon patient response. For mild cases, an initial daily dose of 200-400 mg given in two divided doses is recommended and may be adjusted depending on patient response. **Therapy should begin during menstruation. Otherwise, appropriate tests should be performed to ensure that the patient is not pregnant while on therapy with danazol.** (See CONTRAINDICATIONS and WARNINGS.) **It is essential that therapy continue uninterrupted for 3-6 months but may be extended to 9 months if necessary.** After termination of therapy, if symptoms recur, treatment can be reinstituted.

FIBROCYSTIC BREAST DISEASE

The total daily dosage of danazol for fibrocystic breast disease ranges from 100-400 mg given in two divided doses depending upon patient response. **Therapy should begin during menstruation. Otherwise, appropriate tests should be performed to ensure that the patient is not pregnant while on therapy with danazol.** A nonhormonal method of contraception is recommended when danazol is administered at this dose, since ovulation may not be suppressed.

In most instances breast pain and tenderness are significantly relieved by the first month and eliminated in 2-3 months. Usually elimination of nodularity requires 4-6 months of uninterrupted therapy. Regular menstrual patterns, irregular menstrual patterns, and amenorrhea each occur in approximately one-third of patients treated with 100 mg of danazol. Irregular menstrual patterns and amenorrhea are observed more frequently with higher doses. Clinical studies have demonstrated that 50% of patients may show evidence of recurrence of symptoms within 1 year. In this event, treatment may be reinstated.

HEREDITARY ANGIOEDEMA

The dosage requirements of continuous treatment of hereditary angioedema with danazol should be individualized on the basis of the clinical response of the patient. It is recommended that the patient be started on 200 mg, two or three times a day. After a favorable initial response is obtained in terms of prevention of episodes of edematous attacks, the proper continuing dosage should be determined by decreasing the dosage by 50% or less at intervals of one to three or longer if frequency of attacks prior to treatment dictates. If an attack occurs, the daily dosage may be increased by up to 200 mg. During the dose adjusting phase, close monitoring of the patient's response is indicated, particularly if the patient has a history of airway involvement.

PRODUCT LISTING - RATED THERAPEUTICALLY EQUIVALENT

Capsule - Oral - 50 mg

100's	$158.60	GENERIC, Barr Laboratories Inc	00555-0633-02
100's	$159.86	DANOCRINE, Sanofi Winthrop Pharmaceuticals	00024-0303-06

Capsule - Oral - 100 mg

100's	$237.96	GENERIC, Barr Laboratories Inc	00555-0634-02
100's	$275.44	DANOCRINE, Sanofi Winthrop Pharmaceuticals	00024-0304-06

Capsule - Oral - 200 mg

60's	$242.14	DANOCRINE, Sanofi Winthrop Pharmaceuticals	00024-0305-60
60's	$269.81	GENERIC, Barr Laboratories Inc	00555-0635-09
100's	$286.00	GENERIC, Warner Chilcott Laboratories	00047-0360-24
100's	$396.50	GENERIC, Barr Laboratories Inc	00555-0635-02
100's	$458.96	DANOCRINE, Sanofi Winthrop Pharmaceuticals	00024-0305-06

Dantrolene Sodium *(000944)*

For complete prescribing information, refer to the CD-ROM included with the book.

Categories: Hyperthermia, malignant; Spasticity; Pregnancy Category C; FDA Approved 1974 Jan
Drug Classes: Musculoskeletal agents; Relaxants, skeletal muscle
Brand Names: **Dantrium**
Foreign Brand Availability: Anorex (Korea); Dantamacrin (Austria; Bulgaria; Switzerland); Dantrolen (Austria; Bulgaria; Czech-Republic; Russia)
Cost of Therapy: $241.43 (Spasticity; Dantrium; 100 mg; 4 capsules/day; 30 day supply)

INTRAVENOUS

DESCRIPTION

Note: The trade names have been used throughout this monograph for clarity.

Dantrium intravenous is a sterile, non-pyrogenic, lyophilized formulation of dantrolene sodium for injection. Dantrium intravenous is supplied in 70 ml vials containing 20 mg dantrolene sodium, 3000 mg mannitol, and sufficient sodium hydroxide to yield a pH of approximately 9.5 when reconstituted with 60 ml sterile water for injection (without a bacteriostatic agent).

Dantrium is classified as a direct-acting skeletal muscle relaxant. Chemically, Dantrium is hydrated 1-[[[5-(4-nitrophenyl)-2-furanyl]methylene]amino]-2,4-imidazolidinedione sodium salt.

The hydrated salt contains approximately 15% water (3½ moles) and has a molecular weight of 399. The anhydrous salt (dantrolene) has a molecular weight of 336.

INDICATIONS AND USAGE

Dantrium IV is indicated, along with appropriate supportive measures, for the management of the fulminant hypermetabolism of skeletal muscle characteristic of malignant hyperthermia crises in patients of all ages. Dantrium IV should be administered by continuous rapid IV push as soon as the malignant hyperthermia reaction is recognized (*i.e.,* tachycardia, tachypnea, central venous desaturation, hypercarbia, metabolic acidosis, skeletal muscle rigidity, increased utilization of anesthesia circuit carbon dioxide absorber, cyanosis and mottling of the skin, and, in many cases, fever).

Dantrium IV is also indicated preoperatively, and sometimes postoperatively, to prevent or attenuate the development of clinical and laboratory signs of malignant hyperthermia in individuals judged to be malignant hyperthermia susceptible.

NON-FDA APPROVED INDICATIONS

Dantrolene has also been used for hyperthermia and/or spasticity associated with other disorders including neuroleptic malignant syndrome, heat stroke, tetanus, Black Widow spider bites, lethal catatonia, phenelzine overdose, ecstacy overdose, and other myopathic conditions in which standard agents are poorly tolerated or ineffective.

CONTRAINDICATIONS

None.

WARNINGS

The use of Dantrium IV *in the management of malignant hyperthermia crisis is not a substitute for previously known supportive measures. These measures must be individualized, but it will usually be necessary to discontinue the suspect triggering agents, attend to increased oxygen requirements, manage the metabolic acidosis, institute cooling when necessary, monitor urinary output, and monitor for electrolyte imbalance.*

Since the effect of disease state and other drugs on Dantrium related skeletal muscle weakness, including possible respiratory depression, cannot be predicted, patients who receive IV Dantrium preoperatively should have vital signs monitored.

If patients judged malignant hyperthermia susceptible are administered IV or oral Dantrium preoperatively, anesthetic preparation must still follow a standard malignant hyperthermia susceptible regimen, including the avoidance of known triggering agents.

Monitoring for early clinical and metabolic signs of malignant hyperthermia is indicated because attenuation of malignant hyperthermia, rather than prevention, is possible. These signs usually call for the administration of additional IV dantrolene.

DOSAGE AND ADMINISTRATION

As soon as the malignant hyperthermia reaction is recognized, all anesthetic agents should be discontinued; the administration of 100% oxygen is recommended. Dantrium IV should be administered by continuous rapid IV push beginning at a minimum dose of 1 mg/kg, and continuing until symptoms subside or the maximum cumulative dose of 10 mg/kg has been reached.

If the physiologic and metabolic abnormalities reappear, the regimen may be repeated. It is important to note that administration of Dantrium IV should be continuous until symptoms subside. The effective dose to reverse the crisis is directly dependent upon the individual's degree of susceptibility to malignant hyperthermia, the amount and time of exposure to the triggering agent, and the time elapsed between onset of the crisis and initiation of treatment.

PEDIATRIC DOSE

Experience to date indicates that the dose of Dantrium IV for pediatric patients is the same as for adults.

PREOPERATIVELY

Dantrium IV and/or Dantrium capsules may be administered preoperatively to patients judged malignant hyperthermia susceptible as part of the overall patient management to prevent or attenuate the development of clinical and laboratory signs of malignant hyperthermia.

Dantrium IV

The recommended prophylactic dose of Dantrium IV is 2.5 mg/kg, starting approximately 1¼ hours before anticipated anesthesia and infused over approximately 1 hour. This dose should prevent or attenuate the development of clinical and laboratory signs of malignant hyperthermia provided that the usual precautions, such as avoidance of established malignant hyperthermia triggering agents, are followed.

Additional Dantrium IV may be indicated during anesthesia and surgery because of the appearance of early clinical and/or blood gas signs of malignant hyperthermia or because of prolonged surgery (see also WARNINGS). Additional doses must be individualized.

Oral Administration of Dantrium Capsules

Administer 4-8 mg/kg/day of oral Dantrium in 3 or 4 divided doses for 1 or 2 days prior to surgery, with the last dose being given with a minimum of water approximately 3-4 hours before scheduled surgery. Adjustment can usually be made within the recommended dosage range to avoid incapacitation (weakness, drowsiness, etc.) or excessive gastrointestinal irritation (nausea and/or vomiting). See also the package insert for Dantrium capsules.

POST CRISIS FOLLOW-UP

Dantrium capsules, 4-8 mg/kg/day, in 4 divided doses should be administered for 1-3 days following a malignant hyperthermia crisis to prevent recurrence of the manifestations of malignant hyperthermia.

Intravenous Dantrium may be used postoperatively to prevent or attenuate the recurrence of signs of malignant hyperthermia when oral Dantrium administration is not practical. The IV dose of Dantrium in the postoperative period must be individualized, starting with 1 mg/kg or more as the clinical situation dictates.

PREPARATION

Each vial of Dantrium IV should be reconstituted by adding 60 ml of sterile water for injection (without a bacteriostatic agent), and the vial shaken until the solution is clear. 5% dextrose injection, 0.9% sodium chloride injection, and other acidic solutions are not compatible with Dantrium IV and should not be used. The contents of the vial must be protected from direct light and used within 6 hours after reconstitution. Store reconstituted solutions at controlled room temperature (15-30°C or 59-86°F).

Reconstituted Dantrium IV should not be transferred to large glass bottles for prophylactic infusion due to precipitate formation observed with the use of some glass bottles as reservoirs.

For prophylactic infusion, the required number of individual vials of Dantrium IV should be reconstituted as outlined above. The contents of individual vials are then transferred to a larger volume sterile intravenous plastic bag. Stability data on file at Procter & Gamble Pharmaceuticals indicate commercially available sterile plastic bags are acceptable drug delivery devices. However, it is recommended that the prepared infusion be inspected carefully for cloudiness and/or precipitation prior to dispensing and administration. Such solutions should not be used. While stable for 6 hours, it is recommended that the infusion be prepared immediately prior to the anticipated dosage administration time.

Parenteral drug products should be inspected visually for particulate matter and discoloration prior to administration.

ORAL

WARNING

Note: The trade names have been used throughout this monograph for clarity.

Dantrium has a potential for hepatotoxicity, and should not be used in conditions other than those recommended. Symptomatic hepatitis (fatal and non-fatal) has been reported at various dose levels of the drug. The incidence reported in patients taking up to 400 mg/day is much lower than in those taking doses of 800 mg or more per day. Even sporadic short courses of these higher dose levels within a treatment regimen markedly increased the risk of serious hepatic injury. Liver dysfunction as evidenced by blood chemical abnormalities alone (liver enzyme elevations) has been observed in patients exposed to Dantrium for varying periods of time. Overt hepatitis has occurred at varying intervals after initiation of therapy, but has been most frequently observed between the third and twelfth month of therapy. The risk of hepatic injury appears to be greater in females, in patients over 35 years of age, and in patients taking other medication(s) in addition to Dantrium. Dantrium should be used only in conjunction with appropriate monitoring of hepatic function including frequent determination of SGOT or SGPT. If no observable benefit is derived from the administration of Dantrium after a total of 45 days,

WARNING — *Cont'd*

therapy should be discontinued. The lowest possible effective dose for the individual patient should be prescribed.

DESCRIPTION

The chemical formula of Dantrium is hydrated 1-[[[5-(4-nitrophenyl)-2-furanyl]methylene]amino]-2,4-imidazolidinedione sodium salt. It is an orange powder, slightly soluble in water, but due to its slightly acidic nature the solubility increases somewhat in alkaline solution. The anhydrous salt has a molecular weight of 336. The hydrated salt contains approximately 15% water (3½ moles) and has a molecular weight of 399.

Dantrium is supplied in capsules of 25, 50, and 100 mg.

Inactive Ingredients: Each capsule contains edible black ink, FD&C yellow no. 6, gelatin, lactose, magnesium stearate, starch, synthetic iron oxide red, synthetic iron oxide yellow, talc, and titanium dioxide.

INDICATIONS AND USAGE

IN CHRONIC SPASTICITY

Dantrium is indicated in controlling the manifestations of clinical spasticity resulting from upper motor neuron disorders (*e.g.*, spinal cord injury, stroke, cerebral palsy, or multiple sclerosis). It is of particular benefit to the patient whose functional rehabilitation has been retarded by the sequelae of spasticity. Such patients must have presumably reversible spasticity where relief of spasticity will aid in restoring residual function. Dantrium is not indicated in the treatment of skeletal muscle spasm resulting from rheumatic disorders.

If improvement occurs, it will ordinarily occur within the dosage titration (see DOSAGE AND ADMINISTRATION), and will be manifested by a decrease in the severity of spasticity and the ability to resume a daily function not quite attainable without Dantrium.

Occasionally, subtle but meaningful improvement in spasticity may occur with Dantrium therapy. In such instances, information regarding improvement should be solicited from the patient and those who are in constant daily contact and attendance with him. Brief withdrawal of Dantrium for a period of 2-4 days will frequently demonstrate exacerbation of the manifestations of spasticity and may serve to confirm a clinical impression.

A decision to continue the administration of Dantrium on a long-term basis is justified if introduction of the drug into the patient's regimen:

Produces a significant reduction in painful and/or disabling spasticity such as clonus, or
Permits a significant reduction in the intensity and/or degree of nursing care required, or
Rids the patient of any annoying manifestation of spasticity considered important by the patient himself.

IN MALIGNANT HYPERTHERMIA

Oral Dantrium is also indicated preoperatively to prevent or attenuate the development of signs of malignant hyperthermia in known, or strongly suspect, malignant hyperthermia susceptible patients who require anesthesia and/or surgery. Currently accepted clinical practices in the management of such patients must still be adhered to (careful monitoring for early signs of malignant hyperthermia, minimizing exposure to triggering mechanisms and prompt use of IV dantrolene sodium and indicated supportive measures should signs of malignant hyperthermia appear); see also the package insert for Dantrium IV.

Oral Dantrium should be administered following a malignant hyperthermic crisis to prevent recurrence of the signs of malignant hyperthermia.

NON-FDA APPROVED INDICATIONS

Dantrolene has also been used for hyperthermia and/or spasticity associated with other disorders including neuroleptic malignant syndrome, heat stroke, tetanus, Black Widow spider bites, lethal catatonia, phenelzine overdose, ecstacy overdose, and other myopathic conditions in which standard agents are poorly tolerated or ineffective.

CONTRAINDICATIONS

Active hepatic disease, such as hepatitis and cirrhosis, is a contraindication for use of Dantrium. Dantrium is contraindicated where spasticity is utilized to sustain upright posture and balance in locomotion or whenever spasticity is utilized to obtain or maintain increased function.

WARNINGS

It is important to recognize that fatal and non-fatal liver disorders of an idiosyncratic or hypersensitivity type may occur with Dantrium therapy.

At the start of Dantrium therapy, it is desirable to do liver function studies (SGOT, SGPT, alkaline phosphatase, total bilirubin) for a baseline or to establish whether there is preexisting liver disease. If baseline liver abnormalities exist and are confirmed, there is a clear possibility that the potential for Dantrium hepatotoxicity could be enhanced, although such a possibility has not yet been established.

Liver function studies (*e.g.*, SGOT or SGPT) should be performed at appropriate intervals during Dantrium therapy. If such studies reveal abnormal values, therapy should generally be discontinued. Only where benefits of the drug have been of major importance to the patient, should reinitiation or continuation of therapy be considered. Some patients have revealed a return to normal laboratory values in the face of continued therapy while others have not.

If symptoms compatible with hepatitis, accompanied by abnormalities in liver function tests or jaundice appear, Dantrium should be discontinued. If caused by Dantrium and detected early, the abnormalities in liver function characteristically have reverted to normal when the drug was discontinued. Dantrium therapy has been reinstituted in a few patients who have developed clinical and/or laboratory evidence of hepatocellular injury. If such reinstitution of therapy is done, it should be attempted only in patients who clearly need Dantrium and only after previous symptoms and laboratory abnormalities have cleared. The patient should be hospitalized and the drug should be restarted in very small and gradually increasing doses. Laboratory monitoring should be frequent and the drug should be withdrawn immediately if there is any indication of recurrent liver involvement. Some patients have reacted with unmistakable signs of liver abnormality upon administration of a challenge dose, while others have not.

Dantrium should be used with particular caution in females and in patients over 35 years of age in view of apparent greater likelihood of drug-induced, potentially fatal, hepatocellular disease in these groups.

Long-term safety of Dantrium in humans has not been established. Chronic studies in rats, dogs, and monkeys at dosages greater than 30 mg/kg/day showed growth or weight depression and signs of hepatopathy and possible occlusion nephropathy, all of which were reversible upon cessation of treatment. Sprague-Dawley female rats fed dantrolene sodium for 18 months at dosage levels of 15, 30, and 60 mg/kg/day showed an increased incidence of benign and malignant mammary tumors compared with concurrent controls. At the highest dose level, there was an increase in the incidence of benign hepatic lymphatic neoplasms. In a 30 month study at the same dose levels also in Sprague-Dawley rats, dantrolene sodium produced a decrease in the time of onset of mammary neoplasms. Female rats at the highest dose level showed an increased incidence of hepatic lymphangiomas and hepatic angiosarcomas.

The only drug-related effect seen in a 30 month study in Fischer-344 rats was a dose-related reduction in the time of onset of mammary and testicular tumors. A 24 month study in HaM/ICR mice revealed no evidence of carcinogenic activity. Carcinogenicity in humans cannot be fully excluded, so that this possible risk of chronic administration must be weighed against the benefits of the drug (*i.e.*, after a brief trial) for the individual patient.

USAGE IN PREGNANCY

The safety of Dantrium for use in women who are or who may become pregnant has not been established. Dantrium should not be used in nursing mothers.

USAGE IN PEDIATRIC PATIENTS

The long-term safety of Dantrium in pediatric patients under the age of 5 years has not been established. Because of the possibility that adverse effects of the drug could become apparent only after many years, a benefit-risk consideration of the long-term use of Dantrium is particularly important in pediatric patients.

DOSAGE AND ADMINISTRATION

FOR USE IN CHRONIC SPASTICITY

Prior to the administration of Dantrium, consideration should be given to the potential response to treatment. A decrease in spasticity sufficient to allow a daily function not otherwise attainable should be the therapeutic goal of treatment with Dantrium. Refer to INDICATIONS AND USAGE for description of response to be anticipated.

It is important to establish a therapeutic goal (regain and maintain a specific function such as therapeutic exercise program, utilization of braces, transfer maneuvers, etc.) before beginning Dantrium therapy. Dosage should be increased until the maximum performance compatible with the dysfunction due to underlying disease is achieved. No further increase in dosage is then indicated.

Usual Dosage

It is important that the dosage be titrated and individualized for maximum effect. The lowest dose compatible with optimal response is recommended.

In view of the potential for liver damage in long-term Dantrium use, therapy should be stopped if benefits are not evident within 45 days.

Adults

The following gradual titration schedule is suggested. Some patients will not respond until higher daily dosage is achieved. Each dosage level should be maintained for 7 days to determine the patient's response. If no further benefit is observed at the next higher dose, dosage should be decreased to the previous lower dose.

25 mg once daily for 7 days, then
25 mg tid for 7 days
50 mg tid for 7 days
100 mg tid

Therapy with a dose 4 times daily may be necessary for some individuals. Doses higher than 100 mg four times daily should not be used. (See BOXED WARNING.)

Pediatric Patients

The following gradual titration schedule is suggested. Some patients will not respond until higher daily dosage is achieved. Each dosage level should be maintained for 7 days to determine the patient's response. If no further benefit is observed at the next higher dose, dosage should be decreased to the previous lower dose.

0.5 mg/kg once daily for 7 days, then
0.5 mg/kg tid for 7 days
1 mg/kg tid for 7 days
2 mg/kg tid

Therapy with a dose 4 times daily may be necessary for some individuals. Doses higher than 100 mg four times daily should not be used. (See BOXED WARNING.)

FOR MALIGNANT HYPERTHERMIA

Preoperatively

Administer 4-8 mg/kg/day of oral Dantrium in 3 or 4 divided doses for 1 or 2 days prior to surgery, with the last dose being given approximately 3-4 hours before scheduled surgery with a minimum of water.

This dosage will usually be associated with skeletal muscle weakness and sedation (sleepiness or drowsiness); adjustment can usually be made within the recommended dosage range to avoid incapacitation or excessive gastrointestinal irritation (including nausea and/or vomiting).

Post Crisis Follow-Up

Oral Dantrium should also be administered following a malignant hyperthermia crisis, in doses of 4-8 mg/kg/day in four divided doses, for a 1-3 day period to prevent recurrence of the manifestations of malignant hyperthermia.

PRODUCT LISTING - EQUIVALENTS NOT AVAILABLE

Capsule - Oral - 25 mg

100's	$102.23	DANTRIUM, Procter and Gamble Pharmaceuticals	00149-0030-77
100's	$107.98	DANTRIUM, Procter and Gamble Pharmaceuticals	00149-0030-05

Capsule - Oral - 50 mg

100's	$161.75	DANTRIUM, Procter and Gamble Pharmaceuticals	00149-0031-05

Capsule - Oral - 100 mg

100's	$201.19	DANTRIUM, Procter and Gamble Pharmaceuticals	00149-0033-05

Powder For Injection - Intravenous - 20 mg

1's	$71.10	DANTRIUM INTRAVENOUS, Procter and Gamble Pharmaceuticals	00149-0734-02

Dapsone *(000945)*

For complete prescribing information, refer to the CD-ROM included with the book.

Categories: Dermatitis herpetiformis; Hansen's disease; Pregnancy Category C; FDA Approved 1979 Jul; WHO Formulary
Drug Classes: Antimycobacterials
Foreign Brand Availability: Avlosulfon (Canada); Dapsoderm-X (Mexico); Dapson (Denmark; Norway; Sweden); Dapson-Fatol (Germany); Dapsone (Australia); Diaphenylsulfon (Hungary; Netherlands); Dopsan (Thailand); Novasulfon (Mexico); Protogen (Japan); Servidapsone (Thailand); Sulfona (Portugal; Spain)
Cost of Therapy: $5.93 (Leprosy; Generic tablets; 100 mg; 1 tablet/day; 30 day supply)

DESCRIPTION

Dapsone, 4,4'-diaminodiphenylsulfone (DDS), is a primary treatment for Dermatitis herpetiformis. It is an antibacterial drug for susceptible cases of leprosy. It is a white, odorless crystalline powder, practically insoluble in water and insoluble in fixed and vegetable oils.

Dapsone is issued on prescription in tablets of 25 and 100 mg for oral use.

Jacobus Dapsone Inactive Ingredients: Colloidal silicone dioxide, magnesium stearate, microcrystalline cellulose and corn starch.

INDICATIONS AND USAGE

Dermatitis Herpetiformis: (D.H.)
Leprosy: All forms of leprosy except for cases of proven dapsone resistance.

CONTRAINDICATIONS

Hypersensitivity to dapsone and/or its derivatives.

WARNINGS

The patient should be warned to respond to the presence of clinical signs such as sore throat, fever, pallor, purpura or jaundice. Deaths associated with the administration of dapsone have been reported from agranulocytosis, aplastic anemia and other blood dyscrasias. Complete blood counts should be done frequently in patients receiving dapsone.

The FDA Dermatology Advisory Committee recommended that, when feasible, counts should be done weekly for the first month, monthly for 6 months and semi-annually thereafter. If a significant reduction in leucocytes, platelets or hemopoiesis is noted, dapsone should be discontinued and the patient followed intensively. Folic acid antagonists have similar effects and may increase the incidence of hematologic reactions; if co- administered with dapsone the patient should be monitored more frequently. Patients on weekly pyrimethamine and dapsone have developed agranulocytosis during the second and third month of therapy.

Severe anemia should be treated prior to initiation of therapy and hemoglobin monitored. Hemolysis and methemoglobin may be poorly tolerated by patients with severe cardiopulmonary disease.

Carcinogenesis, Mutagenesis: Dapsone has been found carcinogenic (sarcomagenic) for male rats and female mice causing mesenchymal tumors in the spleen and peritoneum, and thyroid carcinoma in female rats. Dapsone is not mutagenic with or without microsomal activation in *S. typhimurium* tester strains 1535, 1537, 1538, 98 or 100.

Cutaneous reactions, especially bullous, include exfoliative dermatitis and are probably one of the most serious, though rare, complications of sulfone therapy. They are directly due to drug sensitization. Such reactions include toxic erythema, erythema multiforme, toxic epidermal necrolysis, morbilliform and scarlatiniform reactions, urticaria and erythema nodosum. If new or toxic dermatologic reactions occur, sulfone therapy must be promptly discontinued and appropriate therapy instituted.

Leprosy reactional states, including cutaneous, are not hypersensitivity reactions to dapsone and do not require discontinuation. See special section.

DOSAGE AND ADMINISTRATION

DERMATITIS HERPETIFORMIS

The dosage should be individually titrated starting in adults with 50 mg daily and correspondingly smaller doses in children. If full control is not achieved within the range of 50-300 mg daily, higher doses may be tried. Dosage should be reduced to a minimum maintenance level as soon as possible. In responsive patients there is a prompt reduction in pruritus followed by clearance of skin lesions. There is no effect on the gastrointestinal component of the disease.

Dapsone levels are influenced by acetylation rates. Patients with high acetylation rates, or who are receiving treatment affecting acetylation may require an adjustment in dosage.

A strict gluten free diet is an option for the patient to elect, permitting many to reduce or eliminate the need for dapsone; the average time for dosage reduction is 8 months with a range of 4 months to 2½ years and for dosage elimination 29 months with a range of 6 months to 9 years.

LEPROSY

In order to reduce secondary dapsone resistance, the WHO Expert Committee on Leprosy and the USPHS at Carville, LA, recommend that dapsone should be commenced in combination with one or more anti- leprosy drugs. In the multidrug program. Dapsone should be maintained at the full dosage of 100 mg daily without interruption (with corresponding smaller doses for children) and provided to all patients who have sensitive organisms with new or recrudescent disease or who have not yet completed a 2 year course of dapsone monotherapy. For advice and other drugs, the USPHS at Carville, LA (800-642-2477) should be contacted. Before using other drugs, consult appropriate product labeling.

In bacteriologically negative tuberculoid and indeterminate disease, the recommendation is the coadministration of dapsone 100 mg daily with 6 months of Rifampin 600 mg daily. Under WHO, daily Rifampin may be replaced 600 mg Rifampin monthly, if supervised. The dapsone is continued until all signs of clinical activity are controlled-usually after an additional 6 months. Then dapsone should be continued for an additional 3 years for tuberculoid and indeterminate patients and for 5 years for borderline tuberculoid patients.

In lepromatous and borderline lepromatous patients, the recommendation is the coadministration of dapsone 100 mg daily with 2 years of Rifampin 600 mg daily. Under WHO daily Rifampin may be replaced by 600 mg Rifampin monthly, if supervised. One may elect the concurrent administration of a third anti-leprosy drug, usually either Clofazamine 50-100 mg daily or Ethionamide 250-500 mg daily. Dapsone 100 mg daily is continued 3-10 years until all signs of clinical activity are controlled with skin scrapings and biopsies negative for 1 year. Dapsone should then be continued for an additional 10 years for borderline patients and for life for lepromatous patients.

Secondary dapsone resistance should be suspected whenever a lepromatous or borderline lepromatous patient receiving dapsone treatment relapses clinically and bacteriologically, solid staining bacilli being found in the smears taken from the new active lesions. If such cases show no response to regular and supervised dapsone therapy within 3-6 months or good compliance for the past 3-6 months can be assured, dapsone resistance should be considered confirmed clinically. Determination of drug sensitivity using the mouse footpad method is recommended and, after prior arrangement, is available without charge from the USPHS, Carville, LA. Patients with proven dapsone resistance should be treated with other drugs.

LEPROSY REACTIONAL STATES

Abrupt changes in clinical activity occur in leprosy with any effective treatment and are known as reactional states. The majority can be classified into two groups.

The "Reversal" reaction (Type 1) may occur in borderline or tuberculoid leprosy patients often soon after chemotherapy is started. The mechanism is presumed to result from a reduction in the antigenic load: the patient is able to mount an enhanced delayed hypersensitivity response to residual infection leading to swelling ("Reversal") of existing skin and nerve lesions. If severe, or if neuritis is present, large doses of steroids should always be used. If severe, the patient should be hospitalized. In general, anti-leprosy treatment is continued and therapy to suppress the reaction is indicated such as analgesics, steroids, or surgical decompression of swollen nerve trunks. USPHS, at Carville, LA should be contacted for advice in management.

Erythema nodosum leprosum (ENL) (lepromatous reaction) (Type 2 reaction) occurs mainly in lepromatous patients and small numbers of borderline patients. Approximately 50% of treated patients show this reaction in the first year. The principal clinical features are fever and tender erythematous skin nodules sometimes associated with malaise, neuritis, orchitis, albuminuria, joint swelling, iritis, epistaxis or depression. Skin lesions can become pustular and/or ulcerate. Histologically there is a vasculitis with an intense polymorphonuclear infiltrate. Elevated circulating immune complexes are considered to be mechanism of reaction. If severe, patients should be hospitalized. In general, anti-leprosy treatment is continued. Analgesics, steroids, and other agents available from USPHS, Carville, LA, are used to suppress the reaction.

PRODUCT LISTING - EQUIVALENTS NOT AVAILABLE

Tablet - Oral - 25 mg			
40's	$11.40	GENERIC, Pd-Rx Pharmaceuticals	55289-1088-40
40's	$13.99	GENERIC, Physicians Total Care	54868-2817-02
100's	$18.90	GENERIC, Jacobus Pharmaceutical Company	49938-0102-01
120's	$30.36	GENERIC, Physicians Total Care	54868-2817-01
Tablet - Oral - 100 mg			
14's	$2.52	GENERIC, Allscripts Pharmaceutical Company	54569-2015-02
30's	$10.73	GENERIC, Cheshire Drugs	55175-1590-03
100's	$19.75	GENERIC, Jacobus Pharmaceutical Company	49938-0101-01

Darbepoetin alfa *(003531)*

Categories: Anemia, secondary to renal failure; FDA Approved 2001 Sep; Pregnancy Category C
Drug Classes: Hematopoietic agents; Hormones/hormone modifiers
Brand Names: Aranesp
Cost of Therapy: $498.76 (Anemia; Aranesp Injection; 25 μg/ml; 1 ml; 1 injection/week; 28 day supply)

DESCRIPTION

Aranesp is an erythropoiesis stimulating protein closely related to erythropoietin that is produced in Chinese hamster ovary (CHO) cells by recombinant DNA technology. Aranesp is a 165-amino acid protein that differs from recombinant human erythropoietin in containing 5 N-linked oligosaccharide chains, whereas recombinant human erythropoietin contains 3.1 The 2 additional N-glycosylation sites result from amino acid substitutions in the erythropoietin peptide backbone. The additional carbohydrate chains increase the approximate molecular weight of the glycoprotein from 30,000-37,000 daltons. Aranesp is formulated as a sterile, colorless, preservative-free protein solution for intravenous (IV) or subcutaneous (SC) administration.

Single-dose vials are available containing either 25, 40, 60, 100, or 200 μg of Aranesp. Two formulations contain excipients as follows:

Polysorbate solution contains 0.05 mg polysorbate 80, 2.12 mg sodium phosphate monobasic monohydrate, 0.66 mg sodium phosphate dibasic anhydrous, and 8.18 mg sodium chloride in water for injection (per 1 ml) at pH 6.2 ± 0.2.

Albumin solution contains 2.5 mg albumin (human), 2.23 mg sodium phosphate monobasic monohydrate, 0.53 mg sodium phosphate dibasic anhydrous, and 8.18 mg sodium chloride in water for injection (per 1 ml) at pH 6.0 ± 0.3.

D

CLINICAL PHARMACOLOGY

MECHANISM OF ACTION

Darbepoetin alfa stimulates erythropoiesis by the same mechanism as endogenous erythropoietin. A primary growth factor for erythroid development, erythropoietin is produced in the kidney and released into the bloodstream in response to hypoxia. In responding to hypoxia, erythropoietin interacts with progenitor stem cells to increase red cell production. Production of endogenous erythropoietin is impaired in patients with chronic renal failure (CRF), and erythropoietin deficiency is the primary cause of their anemia. Increased hemoglobin levels are not generally observed until 2-6 weeks after initiating treatment with darbepoetin alfa.

PHARMACOKINETICS

Darbepoetin alfa has an approximately 3-fold longer terminal half-life than Epoetin alfa when administered by either the IV or SC route.

Following IV administration to adult CRF patients, darbepoetin alfa serum concentration-time profiles are biphasic, with a distribution half-life of approximately 1.4 hours and mean terminal half-life of approximately 21 hours.

Following SC administration, the absorption is slow and rate-limiting, and the terminal half-life is 49 hours (range: 27-89 hours), which reflects the absorption half-life. The peak concentration occurs at 34 hours (range: 24-72 hours) post-SC administration in adult CRF patients, and bioavailability is approximately 37% (range: 30-50%).

The distribution of darbepoetin alfa in adult CRF patients is predominantly confined to the vascular space (approximately 60 ml/kg). The pharmacokinetic parameters indicate dose-linearity over the therapeutic dose range. With once weekly dosing, steady-state serum levels are achieved within 4 weeks with <2-fold increase in peak concentration when compared to the initial dose. Accumulation was negligible following both IV and SC dosing over 1 year of treatment.

INDICATIONS AND USAGE

Darbepoetin alfa is indicated for the treatment of anemia associated with chronic renal failure, including patients on dialysis and patients not on dialysis.

CONTRAINDICATIONS

Darbepoetin alfa is contraindicated in patients with:

- Uncontrolled hypertension.
- Known hypersensitivity to the active substance or any of the excipients.

WARNINGS

CARDIOVASCULAR EVENTS, HEMOGLOBIN, AND RATE OF RISE OF HEMOGLOBIN

Darbepoetin alfa and other erythropoietic therapies may increase the risk of cardiovascular events, including death, in patients with CRF. The higher risk of cardiovascular events may be associated with higher hemoglobin and/or higher rates of rise of hemoglobin.

In a clinical trial of Epoetin alfa treatment in hemodialysis patients with clinically evident cardiac disease, patients were randomized to a target hemoglobin of either 14 ± 1 g/dl or 10 ± 1 g/dl.2 Higher mortality (35% vs 29%) was observed in the 634 patients randomized to a target hemoglobin of 14 g/dl than in the 631 patients assigned a target hemoglobin of 10 g/dl. The reason for the increased mortality observed in this study is unknown; however, the incidence of nonfatal myocardial infarction, vascular access thrombosis, and other thrombotic events was also higher in the group randomized to a target hemoglobin of 14 g/dl.

In CRF patients the hemoglobin should be managed carefully, not to exceed a target of 12 g/dl.

In patients treated with darbepoetin alfa or other recombinant erythropoietins in darbepoetin alfa clinical trials, increases in hemoglobin greater than approximately 1.0 g/dl during any 2 week period were associated with increased incidence of cardiac arrest, neurologic events (including seizures and stroke), exacerbations of hypertension, congestive heart failure, vascular thrombosis/ischemia/infarction, acute myocardial infarction, and fluid overload/edema. It is recommended that the dose of darbepoetin alfa be decreased if the hemoglobin increase exceeds 1.0 g/dl in any 2 week period, because of the association of excessive rate of rise of hemoglobin with these events.

HYPERTENSION

Patients with uncontrolled hypertension should not be treated with darbepoetin alfa; blood pressure should be controlled adequately before initiation of therapy. Blood pressure may rise during treatment of anemia with darbepoetin alfa or Epoetin alfa. In darbepoetin alfa clinical trials, approximately 40% of patients required initiation or intensification of antihypertensive therapy during the early phase of treatment when the hemoglobin was increasing. Hypertensive encephalopathy and seizures have been observed in patients with CRF treated with darbepoetin alfa or Epoetin alfa.

Special care should be taken to closely monitor and control blood pressure in patients treated with darbepoetin alfa. During darbepoetin alfa therapy, patients should be advised of the importance of compliance with antihypertensive therapy and dietary restrictions. If blood pressure is difficult to control by pharmacologic or dietary measures, the dose of darbepoetin alfa should be reduced or withheld (see DOSAGE AND ADMINISTRATION,

Dose Adjustment). A clinically significant decrease in hemoglobin may not be observed for several weeks.

SEIZURES

Seizures have occurred in patients with CRF participating in clinical trials of darbepoetin alfa and Epoetin alfa. During the first several months of therapy, blood pressure and the presence of premonitory neurologic symptoms should be monitored closely. While the relationship between seizures and the rate of rise of hemoglobin is uncertain, it is recommended that the dose of darbepoetin alfa be decreased if the hemoglobin increase exceeds 1.0 g/dl in any 2 week period.

ALBUMIN (HUMAN)

Darbepoetin alfa is supplied in 2 formulations with different excipients, one containing polysorbate 80 and another containing albumin (human), a derivative of human blood (see DESCRIPTION). Based on effective donor screening and product manufacturing processes, darbepoetin alfa formulated with albumin carries an extremely remote risk for transmission of viral diseases. A theoretical risk for transmission of Creutzfeldt-Jakob disease (CJD) also is considered extremely remote. No cases of transmission of viral diseases or CJD have ever been identified for albumin.

PRECAUTIONS

GENERAL

A lack of response or failure to maintain a hemoglobin response with darbepoetin alfa doses within the recommended dosing range should prompt a search for causative factors. Deficiencies of folic acid or vitamin B_{12} should be excluded or corrected. Intercurrent infections, inflammatory or malignant processes, osteofibrosis cystica, occult blood loss, hemolysis, severe aluminum toxicity, and bone marrow fibrosis may compromise an erythropoietic response.

The safety and efficacy of darbepoetin alfa therapy have not been established in patients with underlying hematologic diseases (*e.g.*, hemolytic anemia, sickle cell anemia, thalassemia, porphyria).

HEMATOLOGY

Sufficient time should be allowed to determine a patient's responsiveness to a dosage of darbepoetin alfa before adjusting the dose. Because of the time required for erythropoiesis and the red cell half-life, an interval of 2-6 weeks may occur between the time of a dose adjustment (initiation, increase, decrease, or discontinuation) and a significant change in hemoglobin.

In order to prevent the hemoglobin from exceeding the recommended target (12 g/dl) or rising too rapidly (greater than 1.0 g/dl in 2 weeks), the guidelines for dose and frequency of dose adjustments should be followed (see DOSAGE AND ADMINISTRATION, Dose Adjustment).

PATIENTS WITH CRF NOT REQUIRING DIALYSIS

Patients with CRF not yet requiring dialysis may require lower maintenance doses of darbepoetin alfa than patients receiving dialysis. Though predialysis patients generally receive less frequent monitoring of blood pressure and laboratory parameters than dialysis patients, predialysis patients may be more responsive to the effects of darbepoetin alfa, and require judicious monitoring of blood pressure and hemoglobin. Renal function and fluid and electrolyte balance should also be closely monitored.

DIALYSIS MANAGEMENT

Therapy with darbepoetin alfa results in an increase in red blood cells and a decrease in plasma volume, which could reduce dialysis efficiency; patients who are marginally dialyzed may require adjustments in their dialysis prescription.

LABORATORY TESTS

After initiation of darbepoetin alfa therapy, the hemoglobin should be determined weekly until it has stabilized and the maintenance dose has been established (see DOSAGE AND ADMINISTRATION). After a dose adjustment, the hemoglobin should be determined weekly for at least 4 weeks until it has been determined that the hemoglobin has stabilized in response to the dose change. The hemoglobin should then be monitored at regular intervals.

In order to ensure effective erythropoiesis, iron status should be evaluated for all patients before and during treatment, as the majority of patients will eventually require supplemental iron therapy. Supplemental iron therapy is recommended for all patients whose serum ferritin is below 100 µg/L or whose serum transferrin saturation is below 20%.

INFORMATION FOR THE PATIENT

Patients should be informed of the possible side effects of darbepoetin alfa and be instructed to report them to the prescribing physician. Patients should be informed of the signs and symptoms of allergic drug reactions and be advised of appropriate actions. Patients should be counseled on the importance of compliance with their darbepoetin alfa treatment, dietary and dialysis prescriptions, and the importance of judicious monitoring of blood pressure and hemoglobin concentration should be stressed.

If it is determined that a patient can safely and effectively administer darbepoetin alfa at home, appropriate instruction on the proper use of darbepoetin alfa should be provided for patients and their caregivers, including careful review of the "Information for Patients and Caregivers" leaflet.

Patients and caregivers should also be cautioned against the reuse of needles, syringes, or drug product, and be thoroughly instructed in their proper disposal. A puncture-resistant container for the disposal of used syringes and needles should be made available to the patient.

CARCINOGENESIS, MUTAGENESIS, AND IMPAIRMENT OF FERTILITY

Carcinogenesis

The carcinogenic potential of darbepoetin alfa has not been evaluated in long-term animal studies. Darbepoetin alfa did not alter the proliferative response of nonhematological cells *in vitro* or *in vivo*. In toxicity studies of approximately 6 months duration in rats and dogs, no tumorigenic or unexpected mitogenic responses were observed in any tissue type. Using a panel of human tissues, the *in vitro* tissue binding profile of darbepoetin alfa was identical to Epoetin alfa. Neither molecule bound to human tissues other than those expressing the erythropoietin receptor.

Mutagenicity

Darbepoetin alfa was negative in the *in vitro* bacterial and CHO cell assays to detect mutagenicity and in the *in vivo* mouse micronucleus assay to detect clastogenicity.

Impairment of Fertility

When administered intravenously to male and female rats prior to and during mating, reproductive performance, fertility, and sperm assessment parameters were not affected at any doses evaluated (up to 10 µg/kg/dose, administered 3 times weekly). An increase in postimplantation fetal loss was seen at doses equal to or greater than 0.5 µg/kg/dose, administered 3 times weekly (3-fold higher than the recommended weekly starting human dose).

PREGNANCY CATEGORY C

When darbepoetin alfa was administered intravenously to rats and rabbits during gestation, no evidence of a direct embryotoxic, fetotoxic, or teratogenic outcome was observed at doses up to 20 µg/kg/day (40-fold higher than the recommended weekly starting human dose). The only adverse effect observed was a slight reduction in fetal weight, which occurred at doses causing exaggerated pharmacological effects in the dams (1 µg/kg/day and higher). No deleterious effects on uterine implantation were seen in either species. No significant placental transfer of darbepoetin alfa was observed in rats. An increase in postimplantation fetal loss was observed in studies assessing fertility (see Impairment of Fertility).

Intravenous injection of darbepoetin alfa to female rats every other day from day 6 of gestation through day 23 of lactation at doses of 2.5 µg/kg/dose and higher resulted in offspring (F1 generation) with decreased body weights, which correlated with a low incidence of deaths, as well as delayed eye opening and delayed preputial separation. No adverse effects were seen in the F2 offspring.

There are no adequate and well controlled studies in pregnant women. Darbepoetin alfa should be used during pregnancy only if the potential benefit justifies the potential risk to the fetus.

NURSING MOTHERS

It is not known whether darbepoetin alfa is excreted in human milk. Because many drugs are excreted in human milk, caution should be exercised when darbepoetin alfa is administered to a nursing woman.

PEDIATRIC USE

The safety and efficacy of darbepoetin alfa in pediatric patients have not been established.

GERIATRIC USE

Of the 1598 CRF patients in clinical studies of darbepoetin alfa, 42% were age 65 and over, while 15% were 75 and over. No overall differences in safety or efficacy were observed between these patients and younger patients, but greater sensitivity of some older individuals cannot be ruled out.

DRUG INTERACTIONS

No formal drug interaction studies of darbepoetin alfa with other medications commonly used in CRF patients have been performed.

ADVERSE REACTIONS

In all studies, the most frequently reported serious adverse reactions with darbepoetin alfa were vascular access thrombosis, congestive heart failure, sepsis, and cardiac arrhythmia. The most commonly reported adverse reactions were infection, hypertension, hypotension, myalgia, headache, and diarrhea (see WARNINGS: Cardiovascular Events, Hemoglobin, and Rate of Rise of Hemoglobin; and Hypertension). The most frequently reported adverse reactions resulting in clinical intervention (*e.g.*, discontinuation of darbepoetin alfa, adjustment in dosage, or the need for concomitant medication to treat an adverse reaction symptom) were hypotension, hypertension, fever, myalgia, nausea, and chest pain.

Because clinical trials are conducted under widely varying conditions, adverse reaction rates observed in the clinical trials of darbepoetin alfa cannot be directly compared to rates in the clinical trials of other drugs and may not reflect the rates observed in practice.

The data described below reflect exposure to darbepoetin alfa in 1598 CRF patients, including 675 exposed for at least 6 months, of whom 185 were exposed for greater than 1 year. Darbepoetin alfa was evaluated in active-controlled (n=823) and uncontrolled studies (n=775).

The rates of adverse events and association with darbepoetin alfa are best assessed in the results from studies in which darbepoetin alfa was used to stimulate erythropoiesis in patients anemic at study baseline (n=348), and, in particular, the subset of these patients in randomized controlled trials (n=276). Because there were no substantive differences in the rates of adverse reactions between these subpopulations, or between these subpopulations and the entire population of patients treated with darbepoetin alfa, data from all 1598 patients were pooled.

The population encompassed an age range from 18-91 years. Fifty-seven percent (57%) of the patients were male. The percentages of Caucasian, Black, Asian, and Hispanic patients were 83%, 11%, 3%, and 1%, respectively. The median weekly dose of darbepoetin alfa was 0.45 µg/kg (25th, 75th percentiles: 0.29, 0.66 µg/kg).

Some of the adverse events reported are typically associated with CRF, or recognized complications of dialysis, and may not necessarily be attributable to darbepoetin alfa therapy. No important differences in adverse event rates between treatment groups were observed in controlled studies in which patients received darbepoetin alfa or other recombinant erythropoietins.

The data in TABLE 1 reflect those adverse events occurring in at least 5% of patients treated with darbepoetin alfa.

The incidence rates for other clinically significant events are shown in TABLE 2.

TABLE 1 *Adverse Events Occurring in ≥5% of Patients*

Event	Darbepoetin alfa (n=1598)
Application Site	
Injection site pain	7%
Body as a Whole	
Peripheral edema	11%
Fatigue	9%
Fever	9%
Death	7%
Chest pain, unspecified	6%
Fluid overload	6%
Access infection	6%
Influenza-like symptoms	6%
Access hemorrhage	6%
Asthenia	5%
Cardiovascular	
Hypertension	23%
Hypotension	22%
Cardiac arrhythmias/cardiac arrest	10%
Angina pectoris/cardiac chest pain	8%
Thrombosis vascular access	8%
Congestive heart failure	6%
CNS/PNS	
Headache	16%
Dizziness	8%
Gastrointestinal	
Diarrhea	16%
Vomiting	15%
Nausea	14%
Abdominal pain	12%
Constipation	5%
Musculoskeletal	
Myalgia	21%
Arthralgia	11%
Limb pain	10%
Back pain	8%
Resistance Mechanism	
Infection*	27%
Respiratory	
Upper respiratory infection	14%
Dyspnea	12%
Cough	10%
Bronchitis	6%
Skin and Appendages	
Pruritus	8%

* Infection includes sepsis, bacteremia, pneumonia, peritonitis, and abscess.

TABLE 2 *Percent Incidence of Other Clinically Significant Events*

Event	Darbepoetin alfa (n=1598)
Acute myocardial infarction	2%
Seizure	1%
Stroke	1%
Transient ischemic attack	1%

THROMBOTIC EVENTS

Vascular access thrombosis in hemodialysis patients occurred in clinical trials at an annualized rate of 0.22 events per patient year of darbepoetin alfa therapy. Rates of thrombotic events (*e.g.*, vascular access thrombosis, venous thrombosis, and pulmonary emboli) with darbepoetin alfa therapy were similar to those observed with other recombinant erythropoietins in these trials.

IMMUNOGENICITY

As with all therapeutic proteins, there is a potential for immunogenicity. The incidence of antibody development in patients receiving darbepoetin alfa has not been adequately determined. Radioimmunoprecipitation and neutralizing antibody assays were performed on sera from 1534 patients treated with darbepoetin alfa. High-titer antibodies were not detected, but assay sensitivity may be inadequate to reliably detect lower titers. Since the incidence of antibody formation is highly dependent on the sensitivity and specificity of the assay, and the observed incidence of antibody positivity in an assay may additionally be influenced by several factors including sample handling, concomitant medications, and underlying disease, comparison of the incidence of antibodies to darbepoetin alfa with the incidence of antibodies to other products may be misleading.

Erythrocyte aplasia, in association with antibodies to erythropoietin, has been reported on rare occasions in patients treated with other recombinant erythropoietins. Due to the close relationship of darbepoetin alfa to endogenous erythropoietin, such a response is a theoretical possibility with darbepoetin alfa treatment, but has not been observed to date.

There have been rare reports of potentially serious allergic reactions including skin rash and urticaria associated with darbepoetin alfa. Symptoms have recurred with rechallenge, suggesting a causal relationship exists in some instances. If an anaphylactic reaction occurs, darbepoetin alfa should be immediately discontinued and appropriate therapy should be administered.

DOSAGE AND ADMINISTRATION

GENERAL

Darbepoetin alfa is administered either IV or SC as a single weekly injection. The dose should be started and slowly adjusted as described below based on hemoglobin levels. If a patient fails to respond or maintain a response, other etiologies should be considered and evaluated (see PRECAUTIONS: General and Laboratory Tests). When darbepoetin alfa therapy is initiated or adjusted, the hemoglobin should be followed weekly until stabilized and monitored at least monthly thereafter.

For patients who respond to darbepoetin alfa with a rapid increase in hemoglobin (*e.g.*, more than 1.0 g/dl in any 2 week period), the dose of darbepoetin alfa should be reduced (see Adults) because of the association of excessive rate of rise of hemoglobin with adverse events (see WARNINGS, Cardiovascular Events, Hemoglobin, and Rate of Rise of Hemoglobin).

The dose should be adjusted for each patient to achieve and maintain a target hemoglobin level not to exceed 12 g/dl.

STARTING DOSE

Correction of Anemia

The recommended starting dose of darbepoetin alfa for the correction of anemia in CRF patients is 0.45 μg/kg body weight, administered as a single IV or SC injection once weekly. Because of individual variability, doses should be titrated to not exceed a target hemoglobin concentration of 12 g/dl (see Dose Adjustment). For many patients, the appropriate maintenance dose will be lower than this starting dose. Predialysis patients, in particular, may require lower maintenance doses. Also, some patients have been treated successfully with a SC dose of darbepoetin alfa administered once every 2 weeks.

Conversion From Epoetin alfa to Darbepoetin alfa

The starting weekly dose of darbepoetin alfa should be estimated on the basis of the weekly Epoetin alfa dose at the time of substitution (see TABLE 3). Because of individual variability, doses should then be titrated to maintain the target hemoglobin. Due to the longer serum half-life, darbepoetin alfa should be administered less frequently than Epoetin alfa. Darbepoetin alfa should be administered once a week if a patient was receiving Epoetin alfa 2-3 times weekly. Darbepoetin alfa should be administered once every 2 weeks if a patient was receiving Epoetin alfa once per week. The route of administration (IV or SC) should be maintained.

TABLE 3 *Estimated Darbepoetin alfa Starting Doses (μg/week) Based on Previous Epoetin alfa Dose (Units/week)*

Previous Weekly Epoetin alfa Dose	Weekly Darbepoetin alfa Dose
<2,500 units/week	6.25 μg/week
2,500-4,999 units/week	12.5 μg/week
5,000-10,999 units/week	25 μg/week
11,000-17,999 units/week	40 μg/week
18,000-33,999 units/week	60 μg/week
34,000-89,999 units/week	100 μg/week
≥90,000 units/week	200 μg/week

DOSE ADJUSTMENT

The dose should be adjusted for each patient to achieve and maintain a target hemoglobin not to exceed 12 g/dl.

Increases in dose should not be made more frequently than once a month. If the hemoglobin is increasing and approaching 12 g/dl, the dose should be reduced by approximately 25%. If the hemoglobin continues to increase, doses should be temporarily withheld until the hemoglobin begins to decrease, at which point therapy should be reinitiated at a dose approximately 25% below the previous dose. If the hemoglobin increases by more than 1.0 g/dl in a 2 week period, the dose should be decreased by approximately 25%.

If the increase in hemoglobin is less than 1 g/dl over 4 weeks and iron stores are adequate (see PRECAUTIONS, Laboratory Tests), the dose of darbepoetin alfa may be increased by approximately 25% of the previous dose. Further increases may be made at 4 week intervals until the specified hemoglobin is obtained.

MAINTENANCE DOSE

Darbepoetin alfa dosage should be adjusted to maintain a target hemoglobin not to exceed 12 g/dl. If the hemoglobin exceeds 12 g/dl, the dose may be adjusted as described above. Doses must be individualized to ensure that hemoglobin is maintained at an appropriate level for each patient.

Preparation and Administration of Darbepoetin alfa:

1. Do not shake darbepoetin alfa. Vigorous shaking may denature darbepoetin alfa, rendering it biologically inactive.
2. Parenteral drug products should be inspected visually for particulate matter and discoloration prior to administration. Do not use any vials exhibiting particulate matter or discoloration.
3. Do not dilute darbepoetin alfa.
4. Do not administer darbepoetin alfa in conjunction with other drug solutions.
5. Darbepoetin alfa is packaged in single-use vials and contains no preservative. Discard any unused portion. Do not pool unused portions.
6. See the "Information for Patients and Caregivers" leaflet for complete instructions on the preparation and administration of darbepoetin alfa.

HOW SUPPLIED

Aranesp is available in 2 solutions, an albumin solution and a polysorbate solution. The words "Albumin Free" appear on the polysorbate container labels and the package main panels as well as other panels as space permits. Aranesp is available in the following packages:

1 ml Single-dose Vial, Polysorbate Solution: 25, 40, 60, 100, and 200 μg/1 ml.

1 ml Single-dose Vial, Albumin Solution: 25, 40, 60, 100, and 200 μg/1 ml.

Storage: Store at 2-8°C (36-46°F). Do not freeze or shake. Protect from light.

PRODUCT LISTING - EQUIVALENTS NOT AVAILABLE

Solution - Injectable - 25 mcg/ml

1 ml	$124.69	ARANESP, Amgen	55513-0010-01
1 ml x 4	$498.76	ARANESP, Amgen	55513-0010-04

Solution - Injectable - 40 mcg/ml

1 ml	$199.50	ARANESP, Amgen	55513-0011-01
1 ml x 4	$798.00	ARANESP, Amgen	55513-0011-04

Solution - Injectable - 60 mcg/ml

1 ml $299.25	ARANESP, Amgen	55513-0012-01
1 ml x 4 $1197.00	ARANESP, Amgen	55513-0012-04

Solution - Injectable - 100 mcg/ml

1 ml x 4 $1995.00	ARANESP, Amgen	55513-0013-04

Solution - Injectable - 200 mcg/ml

0.75 ml x 4 $2992.52	ARANESP, Amgen	55513-0054-04
1 ml $997.50	ARANESP, Amgen	55513-0014-01

Solution - Injectable - 300 mcg/ml

1 ml x 4 $1496.25	ARANESP, Amgen	55513-0015-01

D

Daunorubicin Citrate Liposome *(003285)*

Categories: Sarcoma, Kaposi's; Pregnancy Category D; Orphan Drugs
Drug Classes: Antineoplastics, antibiotics
Brand Names: DaunoXome
Foreign Brand Availability: Daunoxome (Sweden)
HCFA JCODE(S): J9151 10 mg IV

WARNING

1. **Cardiac function should be monitored regularly in patients receiving daunorubicin because of the potential risk for cardiac toxicity and congestive heart failure. Cardiac monitoring is advised especially in those patients who have received prior anthracyclines or who have pre-existing cardiac disease.**
2. **Severe myelosuppression may occur.**
3. **Daunorubicin should be administered only under the supervision of a physician who is experienced in the use of cancer chemotherapeutic agents.**
4. **Dosage should be reduced in patients with impaired hepatic function (see DOSAGE AND ADMINISTRATION).**
5. **A triad of back pain, flushing, and chest tightness has been reported in 13.8% of the patients (16/116) treated with daunorubicin in the Phase 3 clinical trial, and in 2.7% of treatment cycles (27/994). This triad generally occurs during the first 5 minutes of the infusion, subsides with interruption of the infusion, and generally does not recur if the infusion is then resumed at a slower rate.**

DESCRIPTION

Daunoxome (daunorubicin) is a sterile, pyrogen-free, preservative-free product in a single use vial for intravenous (IV) infusion.

Daunoxome contains an aqueous solution of the citrate salt of daunorubicin encapsulated within lipid vesicles (liposomes) composed of a lipid bilayer of distearoylphosphatidylcholine and cholesterol (2:1 molar ratio), with a mean diameter of about 45 nm. The lipid to drug weight ratio is 18.7:1 (total lipid:daunorubicin base), equivalent to a 10:5:1 molar ratio of distearoylphosphatidylcholine: cholesterol: daunorubicin. Daunoxome is an anthracycline antibiotic with antineoplastic activity, originally obtained from *Streptomyces peucetius*. Daunoxome has a 4-ring anthracycline moiety linked by a glycosidic bond to daunosamine, an amino sugar. Daunoxome may also be isolated from *Streptomyces coeruleorubidus* and has the following chemical name: (8S-*cis*)-8-acetyl-10-[(3-amino-2,3,6-trideoxy-α-L-*lyxo*-hexopyranosyl)oxy]-7,8,9,10-tetrahydro-6,8,11-trihydroxy-1-methoxy-5,12-naphthacenedione hydrochloride.

The diameter of the liposomes in Daunoxome is between 35 and 65 nm.

Note: Liposomal encapsulation can substantially affect a drug's functional properties relative to those of the unencapsulated drug.

In addition, different liposomal drug products may vary from one another in the chemical composition and physical form of the liposomes. Such differences can substantially affect the functional properties of liposomal drug products.

Each vial of Daunoxome contains daunorubicin citrate equivalent to 50 mg of daunorubicin base, encapsulated in liposomes consisting of 701 mg distearoylphosphatidylcholine and 171 mg cholesterol. The liposomes encapsulating daunorubicin are dispersed in an aqueous medium containing 2125 mg sucrose, 94 mg glycine, and 7 mg calcium chloride dihydrate in a total volume of 25 ml/vial. The pH of the dispersion is between 4.9 and 6.0. The liposome dispersion should appear red and translucent.

CLINICAL PHARMACOLOGY

MECHANISM OF ACTION

Daunorubicin is a liposomal preparation formulated to maximize the selectivity of daunorubicin for solid tumors *in situ*. While in the circulation, the daunorubicin citrate liposome formulation helps to protect the entrapped daunorubicin from chemical and enzymatic degradation, minimizes protein binding, and generally decreases uptake by normal (non-reticuloendothelial system) tissues. The specific mechanism by which daunorubicin citrate liposome is able to deliver daunorubicin to solid tumors *in situ* is not known. However, it is believed to be a function of increased permeability of the tumor neovasculature to some particles in the size range of daunorubicin citrate liposome. In animal studies, daunorubicin has been shown to accumulate in tumors to a greater extent when administered as daunorubicin citrate liposome than when administered as daunorubicin. Once within the tumor environment, daunorubicin is released over time enabling it to exert its antineoplastic activity.

PHARMACOKINETICS

Following IV injection of daunorubicin citrate liposome, plasma clearance of daunorubicin shows monoexponential decline. The pharmacokinetic parameter values for total daunorubicin following a single 40 mg/m^2 dose of daunorubicin citrate liposome administered over a 30-60 minute period to patients with AIDS-related Kaposi's sarcoma and following a single rapid IV, 80 mg/m^2 dose of conventional daunorubicin to patients with disseminated solid malignancies are shown in TABLE 1.

***TABLE 1** Pharmacokinetic Parameters of Daunorubicin Citrate Liposome in AIDS Patients With Kaposi's Sarcoma and Reported Parameters for Conventional Daunorubicin*

Parameter (units)	Daunorubicin Citrate Liposome*	Conventional Daunorubicin†
Plasma clearance (ml/min)	17.3 ± 6.1	236 ± 181‡
Volume of distribution	6.4 ± 1.5	1006 ± 622
Distribution of half-life (h)	4.41 ± 2.33	0.77 ± 0.3
Elimination half-life (h)	-	55.4 ± 13.7

* n=30.
† n=4.
c Calculated.

The plasma pharmacokinetics of daunorubicin citrate liposome differ significantly from the results reported for conventional daunorubicin hydrochloride. Daunorubicin citrate liposome has a small steady-state volume of distribution 6.4 L, (probably because it is confined to vascular fluid volume), and clearance of 17 ml/min. These differences in the volume of distribution and clearance result in a higher daunorubicin exposure (in terms of plasma AUC) from daunorubicin citrate liposome than with conventional daunorubicin hydrochloride. The apparent elimination half-life of daunorubicin citrate liposome is 4.4 hours, far shorter than that of daunorubicin, and probably represents a distribution half-life. Although preclinical biodistribution data in animals suggest that daunorubicin citrate liposome crosses the normal blood-brain barrier, it is unknown whether daunorubicin citrate liposome crosses the blood-brain barrier in humans.

METABOLISM

Daunorubicinol, the major active metabolite of daunorubicin, was detected at low levels in the plasma following IV administration of daunorubicin citrate liposome.

No formal assessments of pharmacokinetic drug-drug interactions between daunorubicin citrate liposome and other agents have been conducted.

SPECIAL POPULATIONS

The pharmacokinetics of daunorubicin citrate liposome have not been evaluated in women, in different ethnic groups, or in subjects with renal and hepatic insufficiency.

INDICATIONS AND USAGE

Daunorubicin citrate liposome is indicated as a first line cytotoxic therapy for advanced HIV-associated Kaposi's sarcoma. Daunorubicin citrate liposome is not recommended in patients with less than advanced HIV-related Kaposi's sarcoma.

NON-FDA APPROVED INDICATIONS

Daunorubicin liposomal has been investigated for the treatment of acute leukemia, multiple myeloma, metastatic colon cancer, and as an adjunct in lymphoma; however, none of these uses has been approved by the FDA.

CONTRAINDICATIONS

Therapy with daunorubicin citrate liposome is contraindicated in patients who have experienced a serious hypersensitivity reaction to previous doses of daunorubicin citrate liposome or to any of its constituents.

WARNINGS

Daunorubicin citrate liposome is intended for administration under the supervision of a physician who is experienced in the use of cancer chemotherapeutic agents.

The primary toxicity of daunorubicin citrate liposome is myelosuppression, especially of the granulocytic series, which may be severe, with much less marked effects on the platelets and erythroid series. Careful hematologic monitoring is required and since patients with HIV infection are immunocompromised, patients must be observed carefully for evidence of intercurrent or opportunistic infections.

Special attention must be given to the potential cardiac toxicity of daunorubicin citrate liposome, particularly in patients who have received prior anthracyclines or who have pre-existing cardiac disease. Although there is no reliable means of predicting congestive heart failure, cardiomyopathy induced by anthracyclines is usually associated with a decrease of the left ventricular ejection fraction (LVEF). Cardiac function should be evaluated in each patient by means of a history and physical examination before each course of daunorubicin citrate liposome and determination of LVEF should be performed at total cumulative doses of daunorubicin citrate liposome of 320 mg/m^2, 480 mg/m^2 and every 240 mg/m^2 thereafter.

A triad of back pain, flushing, and chest tightness has been reported in 13.8% of the patients (16/116) treated with daunorubicin citrate liposome in the randomized clinical trial and in 2.7% of treatment cycles (27/994). This triad generally occurs during the first 5 minutes of the infusion, subsides with interruption of the infusion, and generally does not recur if the infusion is then resumed at a slower rate. This combination of symptoms appears to be related to the lipid component of daunorubicin citrate liposome, as a similar set of signs and symptoms has been observed with other liposomal products not containing daunorubicin.

Daunorubicin has been associated with local tissue necrosis at the site of drug extravasation. Although no such local tissue necrosis has been observed with daunorubicin citrate liposome, care should be taken to ensure that there is no extravasation of drug when daunorubicin citrate liposome is administered.

Dosage should be reduced in patients with impaired hepatic function (see DOSAGE AND ADMINISTRATION).

PREGNANCY CATEGORY D

Daunorubicin citrate liposome can cause fetal harm when administered to a pregnant woman. Daunorubicin citrate liposome was administered to rats on gestation days 6-15 at 0.3, 1.0, or 2.0 mg/kg/day, (about 1/20, 1/6, or 1/3 the recommended human dose on a mg/m^2 basis). Daunorubicin citrate liposome produced severe maternal toxicity and embryolethality at 2.0 mg/kg/day and was embryotoxic and caused fetal malformations (anophthalmia, microphthalmia, incomplete ossification) at 0.3 mg/kg/day. Embryotoxicity was characterized by increased embryo-fetal deaths, reduced numbers of litters, and reduced litter sizes.

There are no studies of daunorubicin citrate liposome in pregnant women. If daunorubicin citrate liposome is used during pregnancy, or if the patient becomes pregnant while taking daunorubicin citrate liposome, the patient must be warned of the potential hazard to the fetus. Patients should be advised to avoid becoming pregnant while taking daunorubicin citrate liposome.

PRECAUTIONS

CARCINOGENESIS, MUTAGENESIS, AND IMPAIRMENT OF FERTILITY

No carcinogenesis, mutagenesis, or impairment of fertility studies were conducted with daunorubicin citrate liposome.

Carcinogenesis

Carcinogenicity and mutagenicity studies have been conducted with daunorubicin, the active component of daunorubicin citrate liposome. A high incidence of mammary tumors was observed about 120 days after a single IV dose of 12.5 mg/kg daunorubicin in rats (about 2 times the human dose on a mg/m^2 basis).

Mutagenesis

Daunorubicin was mutagenic *in vitro* tests (Ames assay, V79 hamster cell assay), and clastogenic *in vitro* (CCRF-CEM human lymphoblasts) and *in vivo* (SCE assay in mouse bone marrow) tests.

Impairment of Fertility

Daunorubicin IV doses of 0.25 mg/kg/day (about 8 times the human dose on a mg/m^2 basis) in male dogs caused testicular atrophy and total aplasia of spermatocytes in the seminiferous tubules.

PREGNANCY CATEGORY D

See WARNINGS.

PEDIATRIC USE

Safety and effectiveness in pediatric patients have not been established.

GERIATRIC USE

Safety and effectiveness in the elderly have not been established. Special populations safety has not been established in patients with pre-existing hepatic or renal dysfunction.

DRUG INTERACTIONS

In the patient population studied, daunorubicin citrate liposome has been administered to patients receiving a variety of concomitant medications (*e.g.,* antiretroviral agents, antiviral agents, anti-infective agents). Although interactions of daunorubicin citrate liposome with other drugs have not been observed, no systematic studies of interactions have been conducted.

ADVERSE REACTIONS

Daunorubicin citrate liposome contains daunorubicin, encapsulated within a liposome. Conventional daunorubicin has acute myelosuppression as its dose limiting side effect, with the greatest effect on the granulocytic series. In addition, daunorubicin causes alopecia, and nausea and vomiting in a significant number of patients treated. Extravasation of conventional daunorubicin can cause severe local tissue necrosis. Chronic therapy at total doses above 300 mg/m^2 causes a cumulative-dose-related cardiomyopathy with congestive heart failure.

Administered as daunorubicin citrate liposome, daunorubicin has substantially altered pharmacokinetics and some differences in toxicity. The most important acute toxicity of daunorubicin citrate liposome remains myelosuppression, principally of the granulocytic series, with much less marked effects on the platelets and erythroid series.

In an open-label, randomized, controlled clinical trial conducted in 13 centers in the US and Canada in advanced HIV-related Kaposi's sarcoma, two treatment regimens were compared as first line cytotoxic therapy: daunorubicin citrate liposome and ABV (doxorubicin [adriamycin], bleomycin, and vincristine). All drugs were administered intravenously every 2 weeks. The safety data presented below include ail reported or observed adverse experiences, including those not considered to be drug related. Patients with advanced HIV-associated Kaposi's sarcoma are seriously ill due to their underlying infection and are receiving several concomitant medications including potentially toxic antiviral and antiretroviral agents. The contribution of the study drugs to the adverse experience profile is therefore difficult to establish.

TABLE 3 summarizes the important safety data.

A triad of back pain, flushing and chest tightness was reported in 13.8% of the patients (16/116) treated with daunorubicin citrate liposome in the Phase 3 clinical trial and in 2.7% of treatment cycles (27/994). Most of the episodes were mild to moderate in severity (12% of patients and 2.5% of treatment cycles).

Mild alopecia was reported in 6% of patients treated with daunorubicin citrate liposome and moderate alopecia in 2% of patients. Mild nausea was reported in 35% of daunorubicin citrate liposome patients, moderate nausea in 16% of patients and severe nausea in 3% of patients. For patients treated with daunorubicin citrate liposome, mild vomiting was reported in 10%, moderate in 10%, and severe in 3% of patients. Although Grade 3-4 injection site inflammation was reported in 2 patients treated with daunorubicin citrate liposome, no instances of local tissue necrosis were observed with extravasation.

***TABLE 3** Summary of Important Safety Data*

	Daunorubicin Citrate Liposome* (n=116)	ABV* (n=111)
Neutropenia (<1000 cells/mm^3)	36%	35%
Neutropenia (<500 cells/mm^3)	15%	5%
Opportunistic infections/illnesses, % of patients	40%	27%
Median time to first opportunistic infections/illnesses	214 days	412 days‡
Number of cases with absolute reduction in ejection fraction of 20-25%†	3	1
Number of cases removed from therapy due to cardiac causes†	2	0
Alopecia All grades % of patients	8%	36%§
Neuropathy all grades % of patients	13%	41%§

* % of patients.
† The denominator is uncertain since there were several instances of missing repeat cardiac evaluations.
‡ p=0.21.
§ p <0.001.

TABLE 4 is a listing of all the mild-moderate and severe adverse events reported on both treatment arms in Protocol 103-09 in 5% of daunorubicin citrate liposome patients.

***TABLE 4** Adverse Experiences: Protocol 103-09*

	Daunorubicin Citrate Liposome (n=116)		ABV (n=111)	
Adverse Event	Mild Moderate	Severe	Mile Moderate	Severe
Nausea	51%	3%	45%	5%
Fatigue	43%	6%	44%	7%
Fever	42%	5%	49%	5%
Diarrhea	34%	4%	29%	6%
Cough	26%	2%	19%	0%
Dyspnea	23%	3%	17%	3%
Headache	22%	3%	23%	2%
Allergic reactions	21%	3%	19%	2%
Abdominal pain	20%	3%	23%	4%
Anorexia	21%	2%	26%	2%
Vomiting	20%	3%	26%	2%
Rigors	19%	0%	23%	0%
Back pain	16%	0%	8%	0%
Increased sweating	12%	2%	12%	0%
Neuropathy	12%	1%	38%	3%
Rhinitis	12%	0%	6%	0%
Edema	9%	2%	8%	1%
Chest pain	9%	1%	7%	0%
Depression	7%	3%	6%	0%
Malaise	9%	1%	11%	0%
Stomatitis	9%	1%	8%	0%
Alopecia	8%	0%	36%	0%
Dizziness	8%	0%	9%	0%
Sinusitis	8%	0%	5%	1%
Arthraigia	7%	0%	6%	0%
Constipation	7%	0%	18%	0%
Myalgia	7%	0%	12%	0%
Pruritus	7%	0%	14%	0%
Insomnia	6%	0%	14%	0%
Influena-like symptoms	5%	0%	5%	0%
Tenesmus	4%	1%	1%	0%
Abnormal vision	3%	2%	3%	0%

The following adverse events were reported in 5% of patients treated with daunorubicin citrate liposome, tabulated by body system:

Body as a Whole: Infection site inflammation.

Cardiovascular: Hot flushes, hypertension, palpitation, syncope, tachycardia.

Digestive: Increased appetite, dysphagia, GI hemorrhage, gastritis, gingival bleeding, hemorrhoids, hepatomegaly, melena, dry mouth, tooth caries.

Hemic and Lymphatic: Lymphadenopathy, splenomegaly.

Metabolic and Nutritional: Dehydration, thirst.

Nervous: Amnesia, anxiety, ataxia, confusion, convulsions, emotional lability, abnormal gait, hallucination, hyperkinesia, hypertonia, meningitis, somnolence, abnormal thinking, tremor.

Respiratory: Hemoptysis, hiccups, pulmonary infiltration, increased sputum.

Skin: Folliculitis, seborrhea, dry skin.

Special Senses: Conjunctivitis, deafness, earache, eye pain, taste perversion, tinnitus.

Urogenital: Dysuria, nocturia, polyuria.

DOSAGE AND ADMINISTRATION

Daunorubicin citrate liposome should be administered intravenously over a 60 minute period at a dose of 40 mg/m^2, with doses repeated every 2 weeks. Blood counts should be repeated prior to each dose, and therapy withheld if the absolute granulocyte count is less than 750 cells/mm^3. Treatment should be continued until there is evidence of progressive disease (*e.g.,* based on best response achieved: new visceral sites of involvement, or progression of visceral disease; development of 10 or more new, cutaneous lesions or a 25% increase in the number of lesions compared to baseline; a change in the character of 25% or more of all previously counted flat lesions to raised; increase in surface area of the indicator lesions), or until other intercurrent complications of HIV disease preclude continuation of therapy.

PATIENTS WITH IMPAIRED HEPATIC AND RENAL FUNCTION

Limited clinical experience exists in treating hepatically and renally impaired patients with daunorubicin citrate liposome.

Therefore, based on experience with daunorubicin HCl, it is recommended that the dosage of daunorubicin citrate liposome be reduced if the bilirubin or creatinine is elevated as follows: Serum bilirubin 1.2 to 3 mg/dl, give 3/4 the normal dose; serum bilirubin or creatinine >3 mg/dl, give ½ the normal dose.

Do not mix daunorubicin citrate liposome with other drugs.

HOW SUPPLIED

Daunoxome is a translucent, red, liposomal dispersion supplied in single use vials, each sealed with a synthetic rubber stopper and aluminum sealing ring with a plastic cap. Daunoxome provides daunorubicin citrate equivalent to 50 mg of daunorubicin base, at a concentration of 2 mg/ml.

Storage: Store Daunoxome in a refrigerator, 2-8°C (36-46°F). Do not freeze. Protect from light.

PRODUCT LISTING - EQUIVALENTS NOT AVAILABLE

Dispersion - Intravenous - 2 mg/ml

25 ml $340.00 DAUNOXOME, Gilead Sciences 61958-0301-01

Daunorubicin Hydrochloride *(000946)*

Categories: Leukemia, acute erythroid; Leukemia, acute lymphoblastic; Leukemia, acute monocytic; Leukemia, acute myelogenous; Pregnancy Category D; FDA Approved 1995 Feb; WHO Formulary

Drug Classes: Antineoplastics, antibiotics

Brand Names: Cerubidine

Foreign Brand Availability: Cerubidin (Bahrain; Cyprus; Denmark; Egypt; England; Hong-Kong; Hungary; Iraq; Ireland; Kuwait; Lebanon; Libya; Malaysia; Norway; Oman; Qatar; Republic-of-Yemen; Saudi-Arabia; South-Africa; Sweden; Syria; United-Arab-Emirates); Daunoblastin (Austria; Germany); Daunoblastina (Bahrain; Cyprus; Czech-Republic; Egypt; Greece; Indonesia; Iran; Iraq; Italy; Jordan; Korea; Kuwait; Lebanon; Libya; Malaysia; Oman; Portugal; Qatar; Republic-of-Yemen; Saudi-Arabia; Spain; Syria; United-Arab-Emirates); Daunomycin (Japan); Daunorubicin Injection (Australia); Rubilem (Mexico); Trixilem (Mexico)

HCFA JCODE(S): J9150 10 mg IV

WARNING

- **Daunorubicin HCl must be given into a rapidly flowing intravenous infusion. It must NEVER be given by the intramuscular or subcutaneous route. Severe local tissue necrosis will occur if there is extravasation during administration.**
- **Myocardial toxicity manifested in its most severe form by potentially fatal congestive heart failure may be encountered when total cumulative dosage exceeds 550 mg/square m in adults, 300 mg/square m in children more than 2 years of age, or 10 mg/kg in children less than 2 years of age. This may occur either during therapy or several months after termination of therapy.**
- **Severe myelosuppression occurs when used in therapeutic doses.**
- **It is recommended that daunorubicin HCl be administered only by physicians who are experienced in leukemia chemotherapy and in facilities with laboratory and supportive resources adequate to monitor drug tolerance and protect and maintain a patient compromised by drug toxicity. The physician and institution must be capable of responding rapidly and completely to severe hemorrhagic conditions and/or overwhelming infection.**
- **Dosage should be reduced in patients with impaired hepatic or renal function.**

DESCRIPTION

Daunorubicin hydrochloride is the hydrochloride salt of an anthracycline cytotoxic antibiotic produced by a strain of*Streptomyces coeruleorubidus*. It is provided as a sterile reddish lyophilized powder in vials for intravenous administration only. Each vial contains 20 mg of base activity (21.4 mg as the hydrochloride salt) and 100 mg of mannitol. It is soluble in water when adequately agitated and produces a reddish solution. It has the following structural formula which may be described with the chemical name of 7-(3-amino-2,3,6-trideoxy-L-lyxohexosyioxy)-9-acetyl-7,8,9,10-tetrahydro-6,9,11-trihydroxy-4-methoxy-5,12-naphthacenequinone hydrochloride. Its empirical formula is $C_{27}H_{29}NO_{10}HCl$ with a molecular weight of 563.99. It is a hygroscopic crystalline powder. The pH of a 5 mg/ml aqueous solution is 4.5-6.5.

Storage: Store at 15-25°C.

CLINICAL PHARMACOLOGY

Daunorubicin HCl inhibits the synthesis of nucleic acids; its effect on deoxyribonucleic acid is particularly rapid and marked. Daunorubicin HCl has antimitotic and cytotoxic activity although the precise mode of action is unknown. daunorubicin HCl displays an immunosuppressive effect. It has been shown to inhibit the production of heterohemagglutinins in mice. *In vitro,* it inhibits blast-cell transformation of canine lymphocytes at 0.01 mcg/ml.

Daunorubicin HCl possesses a potent antitumor effect against a wide spectrum of animal tumors either grafted or spontaneous.

Following intravenous injection of daunorubicin HCl, plasma levels of daunorubicin decline rapidly, indicating rapid tissue uptake and concentration. Thereafter, plasma levels decline slowly with a half-life of 18.5 hours. By 1 hour after drug administration, the predominant plasma species is daunorubicinol, an active metabolite, which disappears with a half-life of 26.7 hours. Further metabolism via reduction cleavage of the glycosidic bond, 4-0 demethylation, and conjugation with both sulfate and glucuronide have been demonstrated. Simple glycosidic cleavage of daunorubicin or daunorubicinol is not a significant metabolic pathway in man. Twenty-five percent (25%) of an administered dose of daunorubicin HCl is eliminated in an active form by urinary excretion and an estimated 40% by biliary excretion.

There is no evidence that daunorubicin HCl crosses the blood-brain barrier.

In the treatment of adult acute nonlymphocytic leukemia, daunorubicin HCl, used as a single agent, has produced complete remission rates of 40-50%, and in combination with cytarabine, has produced complete remission rates of 53-65%.

The addition of daunorubicin HCl to the two-drug induction regimen of vincristine-prednisone in the treatment of childhood acute lymphocytic leukemia does not increase the rate of complete remission. In children receiving identical CNS prophylaxis and maintenance therapy (without consolidation), there is prolongation of complete remission duration (statistically significant, $p < 0.02$) in those children induced with the three-drug (daunorubicin HCl-vincristine-prednisone) regimen as compared to two drugs. There is no evidence of any impact of daunorubicin HCl on the duration of complete remission when a consolidation (intensification) phase is employed as part of a total treatment program.

In adult acute lymphocytic leukemia, in contrast to childhood acute lymphocytic leukemia, daunorubicin HCl during induction significantly increases the rate of complete remission, but not remission duration, compared to that obtained with vincristine, prednisone, and L-asparaginase alone. The use of daunorubicin HCl in combination with vincristine, prednisone, and L-asparaginase has produced complete remission rates of 83% in contrast to a 47% remission in patients not receiving daunorubicin HCl.

INDICATIONS AND USAGE

Daunorubicin HCl in combination with other approved anticancer drugs is indicated for remission induction in acute nonlymphocytic leukemia (myelogenous, monocytic, erythroid) of adults and for remission induction in acute lymphocytic leukemia of children and adults.

WARNINGS

BONE MARROW

Daunorubicin HCl is a potent bone-marrow suppressant. Suppression will occur in all patients given a therapeutic dose of this drug. Therapy with daunorubicin HCl should not be started in patients with preexisting drug-induced bone-marrow suppression unless the benefit from such treatment warrants the risk.

CARDIAC EFFECTS

Special attention must be given to the potential cardiac toxicity of daunorubicin HCl, particularly in infants and children. Preexisting heart disease and previous therapy with doxorubicin are co-factors of increased risk of daunorubicin HCl-induced cardiac toxicity and the benefit-to-risk ratio of daunorubicin HCl therapy in such patients should be weighed before starting daunorubicin HCl. In adults, at total cumulative doses less than 550 mg/m^2, acute congestive heart failure is seldom encountered. However, rare instances of pericarditis-myocarditis, not dose-related, have been reported.

In adults, at cumulative doses exceeding 550 mg/m^2, there is an increased incidence of drug-induced congestive heart failure. Based on prior clinical experience with doxorubicin, this limit appears lower, namely 400 mg/m^2, in patients who received radiation therapy that encompassed the heart.[1]

In infants and children, there appears to be a greater susceptibility to anthracycline-induced cardiotoxicity compared to that in adults, which is more clearly dose-related. However, there is very little risk for children over 2 years of age in developing daunorubicin HCl-related cardiotoxicity below a cumulative dose of 300 mg/m^2 [2-4] or in children less than 2 years of age (or <0.5 m^2 body-surface area) below a cumulative dose of 10 mg/kg. In both children and adults, the total dose of daunorubicin HCl administered should also take into account any previous or concomitant therapy with other potentially cardiotoxic agents or related compounds such as doxorubicin.

There is no absolutely reliable method of predicting the patients in whom acute congestive heart failure will develop as a result of the cardiac toxic effect of daunorubicin HCl. However, certain changes in the electrocardiogram and a decrease in the systolic ejection fraction from pretreatment baseline may help to recognize those patients at greatest risk to develop congestive heart failure. On the basis of the electrocardiogram, a decrease equal to or greater than 30% in limb lead QRS voltage has been associated with a significant risk of drug-induced cardiomyopathy. Therefore, an electrocardiogram and/or determination of systolic ejection fraction should be performed before each course of daunorubicin HCl. In the event that one or the other of these predictive parameters should occur, the benefit of continued therapy must be weighed against the risk of producing cardiac damage.

Early clinical diagnosis of drug-induced congestive heart failure appears to be essential for successful treatment with digitalis, diuretics, sodium restriction, and bed rest.

EVALUATION OF HEPATIC AND RENAL FUNCTION

Significant hepatic or renal impairment can enhance the toxicity of the recommended doses of daunorubicin HCl; therefore, prior to administration, evaluation of hepatic function and renal function using conventional clinical laboratory tests is recommended (see DOSAGE AND ADMINISTRATION).

PREGNANCY

Daunorubicin HCl may cause fetal harm when administered to a pregnant woman because of its teratogenic potential. An increased incidence of fetal abnormalities (parietooccipital cranioschisis, umbilical hernias, or rachischisis) and abortions was reported in rabbits. Decreases in fetal birth weight and postdelivery growth rate were observed in mice. There are no adequate and well-controlled studies in pregnant women. If this drug is used during pregnancy, or if the patient becomes pregnant while taking this drug, the patient should be apprised of the potential hazard to the fetus. Women of childbearing potential should be advised to avoid becoming pregnant.

EXTRAVASATION AT INJECTION SITE

Extravasation of daunorubicin HCl at the site of intravenous administration can cause severe local tissue necrosis.

PRECAUTIONS

Therapy with daunorubicin HCl requires close patient observation and frequent complete blood-count determinations. Cardiac, renal, and hepatic function should be evaluated prior to each course of treatment.

Daunorubicin HCl may induce hyperuricemia secondary to rapid lysis of leukemic cells. As a precaution, allopurinol administration is usually begun prior to initiating antileukemic therapy. Blood uric acid levels should be monitored and appropriate therapy initiated in the event that hyperuricemia develops.

Appropriate measures must be taken to control any systemic infection before beginning therapy with daunorubicin HCl.

Daunorubicin HCl may transiently impart a red coloration to the urine after administration, and patients should be advised to expect this.

CARCINOGENESIS, MUTAGENESIS, AND IMPAIRMENT OF FERTILITY

Daunorubicin HCl, when injected subcutaneously into mice, causes fibrosarcomas to develop at the injection site. When administered to mice orally or intraperitoneally, no carcinogenic effect was noted after 22 months of observation.

In male dogs at a daily dose of 0.25 mg/kg administered intravenously, testicular atrophy was noted at autopsy. Histologic examination revealed total aplasia of the spermatocyte series in the seminiferous tubules with complete aspermatogenesis.

PREGNANCY CATEGORY D

See WARNINGS.

ADVERSE REACTIONS

Dose-limiting toxicity includes myelosuppression and cardiotoxicity (see WARNINGS). Other reactions include:

Cutaneous: Reversible alopecia occurs in most patients.

Gastrointestinal: Acute nausea and vomiting occur but are usually mild. Antiemetic therapy may be of some help. Mucositis may occur 3-7 days after administration. Diarrhea has occasionally been reported.

Local: If extravasation occurs during administration, tissue necrosis can result at the site.

Acute Reactions: Rarely, anaphylactoid reaction, fever, chills, and skin rash can occur.

DOSAGE AND ADMINISTRATION

Parenteral drug products should be inspected visually for particulate matter and discoloration prior to administration, whenever solution and container permit.

PRINCIPLES

In order to eradicate the leukemic cells and induce a complete remission, a profound suppression of the bone marrow is usually required. Evaluation of both the peripheral blood and bone marrow are mandatory in the formulation of appropriate treatment plans.

It is recommended that the dosage of daunorubicin HCl be reduced in instances of hepatic or renal impairment. For example, using serum bilirubin and serum creatinine as indicators of liver and kidney function, the following dose modifications are recommended (TABLE 1).

TABLE 1

Serum Bilirubin	Serum Creatinine	Recommended Dose
1.2-3.0 mg%		3/4 normal dose
> 3 mg%	>3 mg%	½ normal dose

REPRESENTATIVE DOSE SCHEDULES AND COMBINATION FOR THE APPROVED INDICATION OF REMISSION INDUCTION IN ADULT ACUTE NONLYMPHOCYTIC LEUKEMIA

In Combination[6,7]: For patients under age 60, daunorubicin HCl 45 mg/m^2/day IV on days 1, 2, 3 of the first course and on days 1, 2 of subsequent courses AND cytosine arabinoside 100 mg/m^2/day IV infusion daily for 7 days for the first course and for 5 days for subsequent courses.

For patients 60 years of age and above, daunorubicin HCl 30 mg/m^2/day IV on days 1, 2, 3, of the first course and on days 1, 2 of subsequent courses AND cytosine arabinoside 100 mg/m^2/day IV infusion daily for 7 days for the first course and for 5 days for subsequent courses.[7] This daunorubicin HCl dose-reduction is based on a single study and may not be appropriate if optimal supportive care is available.

The attainment of a normal-appearing bone marrow may require up to three courses of induction therapy. Evaluation of the bone marrow following recovery from the previous course of induction therapy determines whether a further course of induction treatment is required.

REPRESENTATIVE DOSE SCHEDULE AND COMBINATION FOR THE APPROVED INDICATION OF REMISSION INDUCTION IN PEDIATRIC ACUTE LYMPHOCYTIC LEUKEMIA

In Combination: Daunorubicin HCl 25 mg/m^2 IV on day 1 every week, vincristine 1.5 mg/m^2 IV on day 1 every week, prednisone 40 mg/m^2 PO daily. Generally, a complete remission will be obtained within four such courses of therapy; however, if after four courses the patient is in partial remission, an additional one or, if necessary, two courses may be given in an effort to obtain a complete remission.

In children less than 2 years of age or below 0.5 m^2 body-surface area, it has been recommended that the daunorubicin HCl dosage calculation should be based on weight (1.0 mg/kg) instead of body-surface area.[15]

REPRESENTATIVE DOSE SCHEDULE AND COMBINATION FOR THE APPROVED INDICATION OF REMISSION INDUCTION IN ADULT ACUTE LYMPHOCYTIC LEUKEMIA

In Combination[8]: Daunorubicin HCl 45 mg/m^2/day IV on days 1,2, and 3 AND vincristine 2 mg IV on days 1,8, and 15; prednisone 40 mg/m^2/day PO on days 1-22, then tapered between days 22-29; L-asparaginase 500 IU/kg/day × 10 days IV on days 22-32.

The contents of a vial should be reconstituted with 4 ml of sterile water for injection and agitated gently until the material has completely dissolved. The withdrawable vial contents provide 20 mg of daunorubicin activity, with 5 mg of daunorubicin activity per ml. The desired dose is withdrawn into a syringe containing 10-15 ml of normal saline and then injected into the tubing or sidearm of a rapidly flowing IV infusion of 5% glucose or normal saline solution. Daunorubicin HCl should not be administered mixed with other drugs or heparin. The reconstituted solution is stable for 24 hours at room temperature and 48 hours under refrigeration. It should be protected from exposure to sunlight.

Procedures for proper handling and disposal of anticancer drugs should be considered. Several guidelines on this subject have been published.[9-14] There is no general agreement that all of the procedures recommended in the guidelines are necessary or appropriate.

PRODUCT LISTING - RATED THERAPEUTICALLY EQUIVALENT

Powder For Injection - Intravenous - 20 mg

10's	$1685.00	GENERIC, Vha Supply	55390-0805-10
10's	$1698.00	GENERIC, Gensia Sicor Pharmaceuticals Inc	00703-5032-03
10's	$1768.75	CERUBIDINE, Bedford Laboratories	55390-0281-10
10's	$1768.80	GENERIC, Bedford Laboratories	55390-0108-10
10's	$1768.80	GENERIC, Bedford Laboratories	55390-0142-10

PRODUCT LISTING - EQUIVALENTS NOT AVAILABLE

Powder For Injection - Intravenous - 20 mg

1's	$169.75	GENERIC, American Pharmaceutical Partners	63323-0119-08

Delavirdine Mesylate *(003335)*

For related information, see the comparative table section in Appendix A.

Categories: Infection, human immunodeficiency virus; Pregnancy Category C; FDA Approved 1997 Mar
Drug Classes: Antivirals; Non-nucleoside reverse transcriptase inhibitors
Brand Names: Rescriptor
Cost of Therapy: $282.96 (HIV; Rescriptor; 100 mg; 12 tablets/day; 7 day supply)

DESCRIPTION

Rescriptor tablets contain delavirdine mesylate, a synthetic non-nucleoside reverse transcriptase inhibitor of the human immunodeficiency virus Type 1 (HIV-1). The chemical name of delavirdine mesylate is piperazine, 1-[3-[(1-methyl-ethyl)amino]-2-pyridinyl]-4-[[5-[(methylsulfonyl)amino]-1H-indol-2-yl]carbonyl]-, monomethanesulfonate. Its molecular formula is $C_{22}H_{28}N_6O_3S{\cdot}CH_4O_3S$, and its molecular weight is 552.68.

Delavirdine mesylate is an odorless white-to-tan crystalline powder. The aqueous solubility of delavirdine free base at 23°C is 2942 μg/ml at pH 1.0, 295 μg/ml at pH 2.0, and 0.81 μg/ml at pH 7.4.

Each Rescriptor tablet, for oral administration, contains 100 or 200 mg of delavirdine mesylate (henceforth referred to as delavirdine). Inactive ingredients consist of lactose, microcrystalline cellulose, croscarmellose sodium, magnesium stearate, colloidal silicon dioxide, and carnauba wax. In addition, the 100 mg tablet contains Opadry white YS-1-7000-E and the 200 mg tablet contains hydroxypropyl methylcellulose, Opadry white YS-1-18202-A, and pharmaceutical ink black.

CLINICAL PHARMACOLOGY

MICROBIOLOGY

Mechanism of Action

Delavirdine is a non-nucleoside reverse transcriptase inhibitor (NNRTI) of HIV-1. Delavirdine binds directly to reverse transcriptase (RT) and blocks RNA-dependent and DNA-dependent DNA polymerase activities. Delavirdine does not compete with template: primer or deoxynucleoside triphosphates. HIV-2 RT and human cellular DNA polymerases α, γ, or δ are not inhibited by delavirdine. In addition, HIV-1 group O, a group of highly divergent strains that are uncommon in North America, may not be inhibited by delavirdine.

In vitro HIV-1 Susceptibility

In vitro anti-HIV-1 activity of delavirdine was assessed by infecting cell lines of lymphoblastic and monocytic origin and peripheral blood lymphocytes with laboratory and clinical isolates of HIV-1. IC_{50} and IC_{90} values (50 and 90% inhibitory concentrations) for laboratory isolates (n=5) ranged from 0.005-0.030 μM and 0.04-0.10 μM, respectively. Mean IC_{50} of clinical isolates (n=74) was 0.038 μM (range 0.001-0.69 μM); 73 of 74 clinical isolates had an IC_{50} ≤0.18 μM. The IC_{90} of 24 of these clinical isolates ranged from 0.05-0.10 μM. In drug combination studies of delavirdine with zidovudine, didanosine, zalcitabine, lamivudine, interferon-α, and protease inhibitors, additive to synergistic anti-HIV-1 activity was observed in cell culture. The relationship between the *in vitro* susceptibility of HIV-1 RT inhibitors and the inhibition of HIV replication in humans has not been established.

Drug Resistance

Phenotypic analyses of isolates from patients treated with delavirdine as monotherapy showed a 50- to 500-fold reduced susceptibility in 14 of 15 patients by week 8 of therapy. Genotypic analysis of HIV-1 isolates from patients receiving delavirdine plus zidovudine combination therapy (n=79) showed resistance conferring mutations in all isolates by week

D

24 of therapy. In delavirdine treated patients the mutations in RT occurred predominantly at amino acid positions 103 and less frequently at positions 181 and 236. In a separate study, an average of 86-fold increase in the zidovudine susceptibility of patient isolates (n=24) was observed after 24 weeks of delavirdine and zidovudine combination therapy. The clinical relevance of the phenotypic and the genotypic changes associated with delavirdine therapy has not been established.

Cross-Resistance

Delavirdine may confer cross-resistance to other non-nucleoside RT inhibitors when used alone or in combination. Mutations at positions 103 and/or 181 have been found in resistant virus during treatment with delavirdine and other non-nucleoside RT inhibitors. These mutations have been associated with cross-resistance among non-nucleoside RT inhibitors *in vitro.*

PHARMACOKINETICS

Absorption and Bioavailability

Delavirdine is rapidly absorbed following oral administration, with peak plasma concentrations occurring at approximately 1 hour. Following administration of delavirdine 400 mg tid (n=67, HIV-1-infected patients), the mean ±SD steady-state peak plasma concentration (C_{max}) was 35 ± 20 μM (range 2-100 μM), systemic exposure (AUC) was 180 ± 100 μM·h (range 5-515 μM·h) and trough concentration (C_{min}) was 15 ± 10 μM (range 0.1 to 45 μM). The single-dose bioavailability of delavirdine tablets relative to an oral solution was 85 ± 25% (n=16, non-HIV-infected subjects). The single-dose bioavailability of delavirdine tablets (100 mg strength) was increased by approximately 20% when a slurry of drug was prepared by allowing delavirdine tablets to disintegrate in water before administration (n=16, non-HIV-infected subjects). The bioavailability of the 200 mg strength delavirdine tablets has not been evaluated when administered as a slurry, because they are not readily dispersed in water (see DOSAGE AND ADMINISTRATION).

Delavirdine may be administered with or without food. In a multiple-dose crossover study, delavirdine was administered every 8 hours with food or every 8 hours, 1 hour before or 2 hours after a meal (n=13, HIV-1-infected patients). Patients remained on their typical diet throughout the study; meal content was not standardized. When multiple doses of delavirdine were administered with food, geometric mean C_{max} was reduced by 22% but AUC and C_{min} were not altered.

Distribution

Delavirdine is extensively bound (approximately 98%) to plasma proteins, primarily albumin. The percentage of delavirdine that is protein bound is constant over a delavirdine concentration range of 0.5 to 196 μM. In 5 HIV-1-infected patients whose total daily dose of delavirdine ranged from 600-1200 mg, cerebrospinal fluid concentrations of delavirdine averaged 0.4 ± 0.07% of the corresponding plasma delavirdine concentrations; this represents about 20% of the fraction not bound to plasma proteins. Steady-state delavirdine concentrations in saliva (n=5, HIV-1-infected patients who received delavirdine 400 mg tid) and semen (n=5 healthy volunteers who received delavirdine 300 mg tid) were about 6% and 2%, respectively, of the corresponding plasma delavirdine concentrations collected at the end of a dosing interval.

Metabolism and Elimination

Delavirdine is extensively converted to several inactive metabolites. Delavirdine is primarily metabolized by cytochrome P450 3A (CYP3A), but *in vitro* data suggest that delavirdine may also be metabolized by CYP2D6. The major metabolic pathways for delavirdine are N-desalkylation and pyridine hydroxylation. Delavirdine exhibits nonlinear steady-state elimination pharmacokinetics, with apparent oral clearance decreasing by about 22-fold as the total daily dose of delavirdine increases from 60-1200 mg/day. In a study of ^{14}C-delavirdine in 6 healthy volunteers who received multiple doses of delavirdine tablets 300 mg tid, approximately 44% of the radiolabeled dose was recovered in feces, and approximately 51% of the dose was excreted in urine. Less than 5% of the dose was recovered unchanged in urine. The parent plasma half-life of delavirdine increases with dose; mean half-life following 400 mg tid is 5.8 hours, with a range of 2-11 hours.

In vitro and *in vivo* studies have shown that delavirdine reduces CYP3A activity and inhibits its own metabolism. *In vitro* studies have also shown that delavirdine reduces CYP2C9, CYP2D6, and CYP2C19 activity. Inhibition of hepatic CYP3A activity by delavirdine is reversible within 1 week after discontinuation of drug.

SPECIAL POPULATIONS

Hepatic or Renal Impairment

The pharmacokinetics of delavirdine in patients with hepatic or renal impairment have not been investigated (see PRECAUTIONS).

Age

The pharmacokinetics of delavirdine have not been adequately studied in patients <16 years or >65 years of age.

Gender

Data from population pharmacokinetics suggest that the plasma concentrations of delavirdine tend to be higher in females than in males. However, this difference is not considered to be clinically significant.

Race

No significant differences in the mean trough delavirdine concentrations were observed between different racial or ethnic groups.

DRUG INTERACTIONS

See also DRUG INTERACTIONS.

Specific drug interaction studies were performed with delavirdine and a number of drugs. TABLE 1 summarizes the effects of delavirdine on the geometric mean AUC, C_{max} and C_{min} of coadministered drugs. TABLE 2 shows the effects of coadministered drugs on the geometric mean AUC, C_{max} and C_{min} of delavirdine.

For information regarding clinical recommendations, see CONTRAINDICATIONS, WARNINGS, and DRUG INTERACTIONS.

***TABLE 1** Pharmacokinetic Parameters for Coadministered Drugs in the Presence of Delavirdine*

Coadminstered Drug	Dose of Coadministered Drug	Dose of Delavirdine	n	% Change in Pharmacokinetic Parameters of Coadministered Drug (90% DI) C_{max}	AUC	C_{min}
HIV-Protease Inhibitors						
Indinavir	400 mg tid × 7 days	400 mg tid × 7 days	28	D 36* (D 52-D 14)	NC	I 118* (I 16-I 312)
	600 mg tid × 7 days	400 mg tid × 7 days	28	NC	I 53* (I 7-I 120)	I 298* (I 104-I 678)
Nelfinavir†	750 mg tid × 14 days	400 mg tid × 7 days	12	I 88 (I 66-I 113)	I 107 (I 83-I 135)	I 136 (I 103-I 175)
Saquinavir	Soft gel capsule 1000 mg tid × 28 days	400 mg tid × 28 days	20	I 98‡ (I 4-I 277	I 121‡ (I 14-I 340)	I 199‡ (I 37-I 553)
Nucleoside Reverse Transcriptase Inhibitors						
Didanosine (buffered tablets)	125 or 250 mg bid × 28 days	400 mg tid × 28 days	9	D 20§ (D 44-I 15)	D 21§ (D 40-I 5)	—
Zidovudine	200 mg tid for >38 days	100 mg qid to 400 mg tid for 8-10 days	34	NC	NC	—
Anti-Infective Agents						
Clarithromycin	500 mg bid × 15 days	300 mg tid × 30 days	6	—	I 100	—
Rifabutin	300 mg qd for 15-99 days	400-1000 mg for 45-129 days	5	I 128 (I 71-I 203)	I 230 (I 119-I 396)	I 452 (I 246-I 781)

I Indicates increase.
D Indicates decrease.
NC Indicates no significant change.
* Relative to indinavir 800 mg tid without delavirdine.
† Plasma concentrations of the nelfinavir active metabolite (nelfinavir hydroxy-t-butylamide) were significantly reduced by delavirdine, which is more than compensated for by increased nelfinavir concentration.
‡ Saquinavir soft gel capsule 1000 mg tid plus delavirdine 400 mg tid relative to saquinavir soft gel capsule 1200 mg tid without delavirdine.
§ Delavirdine taken with didanosine (buffered tablets) relative to doses of delavirdine and didanosine (buffered tablets) separated by at least 1 hour.
— No data available.

INDICATIONS AND USAGE

Delavirdine tablets are indicated for the treatment of HIV-1 infection in combination with at least 2 other active antiretroviral agents when therapy is warranted.

The following should be considered before initiating therapy with delavirdine in treatment-naïve patients. There are insufficient data directly comparing delavirdine containing antiretroviral regimens with currently preferred 3 drug regimens for initial treatment of HIV. In studies comparing regimens consisting of 2 NRTIs (currently considered suboptimal) to delavirdine plus 2 NRTIs, the proportion of patients receiving the delavirdine regimen who achieved and sustained an HIV-1 RNA level <400 copies/ml over 1 year of therapy was relatively low.

Resistant virus emerges rapidly when delavirdine is administered as monotherapy. Therefore, delavirdine should always be administered in combination with other antiretroviral agents.

CONTRAINDICATIONS

Delavirdine tablets are contraindicated in patients with known hypersensitivity to any of its ingredients. Coadministration of delavirdine is contraindicated with drugs that are highly dependent on CYP3A for clearance and for which elevated plasma concentrations are associated with serious and/or life-threatening events. These drugs are listed in TABLE 5. **(Also, see TABLE 6.)**

WARNINGS

ALERT: Find out about medicines that should NOT be taken with delavirdine. This statement is included on the product's bottle label.

DRUG INTERACTIONS

Because delavirdine may inhibit the metabolism of many different drugs (*e.g.,* antiarrhythmics, calcium channel blockers, sedative hypnotics and others), **serious and/or life threatening drug interactions could result from inappropriate coadministration of some drugs with delavirdine.** In addition, some drugs may markedly reduce delavirdine plasma concentrations, resulting in suboptimal antiviral activity and subsequent emergence of drug resistance. All prescribers should become familiar with the following tables in this package insert: **TABLE 5, TABLE 6, and TABLE 7.** Additional details on drug interactions can be found in TABLE 1 and TABLE 2.

Concomitant use of lovastatin or simvastatin with delavirdine is not recommended. Caution should be exercised if delavirdine is used concurrently with other HMG-CoA reductase inhibitors that are also metabolized by the CYP3A4 pathway (*e.g.,* atorvastatin or cerivastatin). The risk of myopathy including rhabdomyolysis may be increased when delavirdine is used in combination with these drugs.

Particular caution should be used when prescribing sildenafil in patients receiving delavirdine. Coadministration of sildenafil with delavirdine is expected to substantially increase

TABLE 2 *Pharmacokinetic Parameters for Delavirdine in the Presence of Coadministered Drugs*

Coadminstered Drug	Dose of Coadministered Drug	Dose of Delavirdine	n	% Change in Delavirdine Pharmacokinetic Parameters (90% CI) C_{max}	AUC	C_{min}
HIV-Protease Inhibitors						
Indinavir	400 or 600 mg tid × 7 days	400 mg tid × 7 days	81	No apparent changes based on a comparison to historical data		
Nelfinavir	750 mg tid × 7 days	400 mg tid × 14 days	7	D 27 (D 49-I 4)	D 31 (D 57-I 10)	D 33 (D 70-I 49)
Saquinavir	Soft gel capsule 1000 mg tid × 28 days	400 mg tid for 7-28 days	23	No apparent changes based on a comparison to historical data		
Nucleoside Reverse Transcriptase Inhibitors						
Didanosine (buffered tablets)	125 or 200 mg bid × 28 days	400 mg tid × 28 days	9	D 32* (D 48-D 11)	D 19* (D 37-I 6)	NC*
Zidovudine	200 mg tid for ≥7 days	400 mg tid for 7-14 days	42	No apparent changes based on a comparison to historical data		
Anti-Infective Agents						
Clarithromycin	500 mg bid × 15 days	300 mg tid × 30 days	6	NC	NC	NC
Fluconazole	400 mg qd × 15 days	300 mg tid × 30 days	8	NC	NC	NC
Ketoconazole	Various	200-400 mg tid	26	—	—	I 50†
Rifabutin	300 mg qd × 14 days	400 mg tid × 28 days	7	D 72 (D 61-D 80)	D 82 (D 74-D 88)	D 94 (D 90-D 96)
Rifampin	600 mg qd × 15 days	400 mg tid × 30 days	7	D 90 (D 94-D 83)	D 97 (D 98-D 95)	D 100
Sulfamethoxazole or trimethoprim & sulfamethoxazole	Various	200-400 mg tid	311	—	—	NC†
Other						
Antacid	20 ml	300 mg single-dose	12	D 52 (D 68-D 29)	D 44 (D 58-D 27)	—
Fluoxetine	Various	200-400 mg tid	36	—	—	I 50†
Phenytoin, phenobarbital, carbamazepine	Various	300-400 mg tid	8	—	—	D 90†

I Indicates increase.
D Indicates decrease.
NC Indicates no significant change.
* Delavirdine taken with didanosine (buffered tablets) relative to doses of delavirdine and didanosine (buffered tablets) separated by at least 1 hour.
† Population pharmacokinetic data from efficacy studies.
— No data available.

TABLE 5 *Drugs That Are Contraindicated With Delavirdine*

Drug Class	Drugs Within Class That Are Contraindicated With Delavirdine
Antihistamines	Astemizole, terfenadine
Ergot derivatives	Dihydroergotamine, ergonovine, ergotamine, methylergonovine
GI motility agent	Cisapride
Neuroleptic	Pimozide
Sedative/hypnotics	Alprazolam, midazolam, triazolam

sildenafil concentrations and may result in an increase in sildenafil-associated adverse events, including hypotension, visual changes, and priapism (see DRUG INTERACTIONS and PRECAUTIONS, Information for the Patient, and the complete prescribing information for sildenafil).

Concomitant use of St. John's wort (hypericum perforatum) or St. John's wort containing products and delavirdine is not recommended. Coadministration of St. John's wort with non-nucleoside reverse transcriptase inhibitors (NNRTIs), including delavirdine, is expected to substantially decrease NNRTI concentrations and may result in sub-optimal levels of delavirdine and lead to loss of virologic response and possible resistance to delavirdine or to the class of NNRTIs.

PRECAUTIONS

GENERAL

Delavirdine is metabolized primarily by the liver. Therefore, caution should be exercised when administering delavirdine tablets to patients with impaired hepatic function.

RESISTANCE/CROSS-RESISTANCE

Non-nucleoside reverse transcriptase inhibitors, when used alone or in combination, may confer cross-resistance to other non-nucleoside reverse transcriptase inhibitors.

FAT REDISTRIBUTION

Redistribution/accumulation of body fat including central obesity, dorsocervical fat enlargement (buffalo hump), peripheral wasting, facial wasting, breast enlargement, and "cushingoid appearance" have been observed in patients receiving antiretroviral therapy. The mechanism and long-term consequences of these events are currently unknown. A causal relationship has not been established.

SKIN RASH

Severe rash, including rare cases of erythema multiforme and Stevens-Johnson syndrome, has been reported in patients receiving delavirdine. Erythema multiforme and Stevens-Johnson syndrome were rarely seen in clinical trials and resolved after withdrawal of delavirdine. Any patient experiencing severe rash or rash accompanied by symptoms such as fever, blistering, oral lesions, conjunctivitis, swelling, and muscle or joint aches should discontinue delavirdine and consult a physician. Two cases of Stevens-Johnson syndrome have been reported through postmarketing surveillance out of a total of 339 surveillance reports.

In studies 21 Part II and 13C, rash (including maculopapular rash) was reported in more patients who were treated with delavirdine 400 mg tid (35% and 32%, respectively) than in those who were not treated with delavirdine (21% and 16%, respectively). The highest intensity of rash reported in these studies was severe (grade 3), which was observed in approximately 4% of patients treated with delavirdine in each study and in none of the patients who were not treated with delavirdine. Also in studies 21 Part II and 13C, discontinuations due to rash were reported in more patients who received delavirdine 400 mg tid (3% and 4%, respectively) than in those who did not receive delavirdine (0% and 1%, respectively).

In most cases, the duration of the rash was less than 2 weeks and did not require dose reduction or discontinuation of delavirdine. Most patients were able to resume therapy after rechallenge with delavirdine following a treatment interruption due to rash. The distribution of the rash was mainly on the upper body and proximal arms, with decreasing intensity of the lesions on the neck and face, and progressively less on the rest of the trunk and limbs. Occurrence of a delavirdine-associated rash after 1 month is uncommon. Symptomatic relief has been obtained using diphenhydramine HCl, hydroxyzine HCl, and/or topical corticosteroids.

INFORMATION FOR THE PATIENT

A statement to patients and health care providers is included on the product's bottle label: **ALERT: Find out about medicines that should NOT be taken with delavirdine.** A patient package insert (PPI) for delavirdine is available for patient information.

Patients should be informed that delavirdine is not a cure for HIV-1 infection and that they may continue to acquire illnesses associated with HIV-1 infection, including opportunistic infections. Treatment with delavirdine has not been shown to reduce the incidence or frequency of such illnesses, and patients should be advised to remain under the care of a physician when using delavirdine.

Patients should be advised that the use of delavirdine has not been shown to reduce the risk of transmission of HIV-1.

Patients should be instructed that the major toxicity of delavirdine is rash and should be advised to promptly notify their physician should rash occur. The majority of rashes associated with delavirdine occur within 1-3 weeks after initiating treatment with delavirdine. The rash normally resolves in 3-14 days and may be treated symptomatically while therapy with delavirdine is continued. Any patient experiencing severe rash or rash accompanied by symptoms such as fever, blistering, oral lesions, conjunctivitis, swelling, muscle or joint aches should discontinue medication and consult a physician.

Patients should be informed that redistribution or accumulation of body fat may occur in patients receiving antiretroviral therapy and that the cause and long-term health effects of these conditions are not known at this time.

Patients should be informed to take delavirdine every day as prescribed. Patients should not alter the dose of delavirdine without consulting their doctor. If a dose is missed, patients should take the next dose as soon as possible. However, if a dose is skipped, the patient should not double the next dose.

Patients with achlorhydria should take delavirdine with an acidic beverage (*e.g.,* orange or cranberry juice). However, the effect of an acidic beverage on the absorption of delavirdine in patients with achlorhydria has not been investigated.

Patients taking both delavirdine and antacids should be advised to take them at least 1 hour apart.

Because delavirdine may interact with certain drugs, patients should be advised to report to their doctor the use of any prescription, nonprescription medication or herbal products, particularly St. John's wort.

Patients receiving sildenafil and delavirdine should be advised that they may be at an increased risk of sildenafil-associated adverse events, including hypotension, visual changes, and prolonged penile erection, and should promptly report any symptoms to their doctor.

CARCINOGENESIS, MUTAGENESIS, AND IMPAIRMENT OF FERTILITY

Delavirdine was negative in a battery of genetic toxicology tests which included an Ames assay, an *in vitro* rat hepatocyte unscheduled DNA synthesis assay, an *in vitro* chromosome aberration assay in human peripheral lymphocytes, an *in vitro* mutation assay in Chinese hamster ovary cells, and an *in vivo* micronucleus test in mice.

Lifetime carcinogenicity studies were conducted in rats at doses of 10, 32 and 100 mg/kg/day and in mice at doses of 62.5, 250 and 500 mg/kg/day for males and 62.5, 125 and 250 mg/kg/day for females. In rats, delavirdine was noncarcinogenic at maximally tolerated doses that produced exposures (AUC) up to 12 (male rats) and 9 (female rats) times human exposure at the recommended clinical dose. In mice, delavirdine produced significant increases in the incidence of hepatocellular adenoma/adenocarcinoma in both males and females, hepatocellular adenoma in females, and mesenchymal urinary bladder tumors in males. The systemic drug exposures (AUC) in female mice were 0.5- to 3-fold and in male mice 0.2- to 4-fold of those in humans at the recommended clinical dose. Given the lack of genotoxic activity of delavirdine, the relevance of urinary bladder and hepatocellular neoplasm in delavirdine-treated mice to humans is not known.

Delavirdine at doses of 20, 100, and 200 mg/kg/day did not cause impairment of fertility in rats when males were treated for 70 days and females were treated for 14 days prior to mating.

PREGNANCY CATEGORY C

Delavirdine has been shown to be teratogenic in rats. Delavirdine caused ventricular septal defects in rats at doses of 50, 100, and 200 mg/kg/day when administered during the period of organogenesis. The lowest dose of delavirdine that caused malformations produced systemic exposures in pregnant rats equal to or lower than the expected human exposure to delavirdine (C_{min} = 15 μM) at the recommended dose. Exposure in rats approximately 5-fold higher than the expected human exposure resulted in marked maternal toxicity, embryotoxicity, fetal developmental delay, and reduced pup survival. Additionally, reduced pup survival on postpartum day 0 occurred at an exposure (mean C_{min}) approximately equal to the expected human exposure. Delavirdine was excreted in the milk of lactating rats at a concentration 3-5 times that of rat plasma.

Delavirdine at doses of 200 and 400 mg/kg/day administered during the period of organogenesis caused maternal toxicity, embryotoxicity, and abortions in rabbits. The lowest dose of delavirdine that resulted in these toxic effects produced systemic exposures in pregnant rabbits approximately 6-fold higher than the expected human exposure to delavirdine (C_{min} = 15 μM) at the recommended dose. The no-observed-adverse-effect dose in the pregnant rabbit was 100 mg/kg/day. Various malformations were observed at this dose, but the incidence of such malformations was not statistically significantly different from those observed in the control group. Systemic exposures in pregnant rabbits at a dose of 100 mg/kg/day were lower than those expected in humans at the recommended clinical dose. Malformations were not apparent at 200 and 400 mg/kg/day; however, only a limited number of fetuses were available for examination as a result of maternal and embryo death.

No adequate and well-controlled studies in pregnant women have been conducted. Delavirdine should be used during pregnancy only if the potential benefit justifies the potential risk to the fetus. Of 9 pregnancies reported in premarketing clinical studies and postmarketing experience, a total of 10 infants were born (including 1 set of twins). Eight of the infants were born healthy. One infant was born HIV-positive but was otherwise healthy and with no congenital abnormalities detected, and 1 infant was born prematurely (34-35 weeks) with a small muscular ventricular septal defect that spontaneously resolved. The patient received approximately 6 weeks of treatment with delavirdine and zidovudine early in the course of the pregnancy.

Antiretroviral Pregnancy Registry: To monitor maternal-fetal outcomes of pregnant women exposed to delavirdine and other antiretroviral agents, an Antiretroviral Pregnancy Registry has been established. Physicians are encouraged to register patients by calling 800-258-4263.

NURSING MOTHERS

The Centers for Disease Control and Prevention recommend that HIV-infected mothers not breast-feed their infants to avoid risking postnatal transmission of HIV. Because of both the potential for HIV transmission and any possible adverse reactions in nursing infants, **mothers should be instructed not to breast-feed if they are receiving delavirdine.**

PEDIATRIC USE

Safety and effectiveness of delavirdine in combination with other antiretroviral agents have not been established in HIV-1-infected individuals younger than 16 years of age.

GERIATRIC USE

Clinical studies of delavirdine did not include sufficient numbers of subjects aged 65 and over to determine whether they respond differently from younger subjects. In general, caution should be taken when dosing delavirdine in elderly patients due to the greater frequency of decreased hepatic, renal or cardiac function and of concomitant disease or other drug therapy.

DRUG INTERACTIONS

See also CONTRAINDICATIONS; WARNINGS; andCLINICAL PHARMACOLOGY, Drug Interactions.

Delavirdine is an inhibitor of CYP3A isoform and other CYP isoforms to a lesser extent, including CYP2C9, CYP2D6, and CYP2C19. Coadministration of delavirdine and drugs primarily metabolized by CYP3A (*e.g.*, HMG-CoA reductase inhibitors and sildenafil) may result in increased plasma concentrations of the coadministered drug that could increase or prolong both its therapeutic or adverse effects.

Delavirdine is metabolized primarily by CYP3A, but *in vitro* data suggest that delavirdine may also be metabolized by CYP2D6. Coadministration of delavirdine and drugs that induce CYP3A, such as rifampin, may decrease delavirdine plasma concentrations and reduce its therapeutic effect. Coadministration of delavirdine and drugs that inhibit CYP3A may increase delavirdine plasma concentrations. **See TABLE 6 and TABLE 7.**

ADVERSE REACTIONS

The safety of delavirdine tablets alone and in combination with other therapies has been studied in approximately 6000 patients receiving delavirdine. The majority of adverse events were of mild or moderate (*i.e.*, ACTG Grade 1 or 2) intensity. The most frequently reported drug-related adverse event (*i.e.*, events considered by the investigator to be related to the blinded study medication, or events with an unknown or missing causal relationship to the blinded medication) among patients receiving delavirdine was skin rash **(see TABLE 8 and PRECAUTIONS, Skin Rash).**

Adverse events of moderate to severe intensity reported by at least 5% of evaluable patients in any treatment group in the pivotal trials, which includes patients receiving delavirdine in combination with zidovudine and/or lamivudine in Study 21 Part II for up to 98 weeks and in combination with zidovudine and either lamivudine, didanosine, or zalcitabine in Study 13C for up to 72 weeks are summarized in TABLE 9A and TABLE 9B.

Other adverse events that occurred in patients receiving delavirdine (in combination treatment) in all Phase 2 and 3 studies, and considered possibly related to treatment, and of at least ACTG Grade 2 in intensity are listed below by body system.

Body as a Whole: Abdominal cramps, abdominal distention, abdominal pain (localized), abscess, allergic reaction, chills, edema (generalized or localized), epidermal cyst, fever, infection, infection viral, lip edema, malaise, *Mycobacterium tuberculosis* infection, neck rigidity, sebaceous cyst, and redistribution/accumulation of body fat (see PRECAUTIONS, Fat Redistribution).

Cardiovascular System: Abnormal cardiac rate and rhythm, cardiac insufficiency, cardiomyopathy, hypertension, migraine, pallor, peripheral vascular disorder, and postural hypotension.

Digestive System: Anorexia, bloody stool, colitis, constipation, decreased appetite, diarrhea *(Clostridium difficile)*, diverticulitis, dry mouth, dyspepsia, dysphagia, enteritis at all levels, eructation, fecal incontinence, flatulence, gagging, gastroenteritis, gastroesophageal reflux, gastrointestinal bleeding, gastrointestinal disorder, gingivitis, gum hemorrhage, hepatomegaly, increased appetite, increased saliva, increased thirst, jaundice, mouth or tongue inflammation or ulcers, nonspecific hepatitis, oral/enteric moniliasis, pancreatitis, rectal disorder, sialadenitis, tooth abscess, and toothache.

Hemic and Lymphatic System: Adenopathy, bruising, eosinophilia, granulocytosis, leukopenia, pancytopenia, purpura, spleen disorder, thrombocytopenia, and prolonged prothrombin time.

Metabolic and Nutritional Disorders: Alcohol intolerance, amylase increased, bilirubinemia, hyperglycemia, hyperkalemia, hypertriglyceridemia, hyperuricemia, hypocalcemia, hyponatremia, hypophosphatemia, increased AST (SGOT), increased gamma glutamyl transpeptidase, increased lipase, increased serum alkaline phosphatase, increased serum creatinine, and weight increase or decrease.

Musculoskeletal System: Arthralgia or arthritis of single and multiple joints, bone disorder, bone pain, myalgia, tendon disorder, tenosynovitis, tetany, and vertigo.

TABLE 6 *Drugs That Should Not Be Coadministered With Delavirdine*

Drug Class: Drug Name	Clinical Comment
Anticonvulsant Agents: phenytoin, phenobarbital, carbamazepine	May lead to loss of virologic response and possible resistance to delavirdine or to the class of non-nucleoside reverse transcriptase inhibitors.
Antihistamines: astemizole, terfenadine	CONTRAINDICATED due to potential for serious and/or life-threatening reactions such as cardiac arrhythmias.
Antimycobacterials: rifabutin*, rifampin*	May lead to loss of virologic response and possible resistance to delavirdine or to the class of non-nucleoside reverse transcriptase inhibitors or other co-administered antiviral agents.
Ergot Derivatives: dihydroergotamine, ergonovine, ergotamine, methylergonovine	CONTRAINDICATED due to potential for serious and/or life threatening reactions such as acute ergot toxicity characterized by peripheral vasospasm and ischemia of the extremities and other tissues.
GI Motility Agent: cisapride	CONTRAINDICATED due to potential for serious and/or life-threatening reactions such as cardiac arrhythmias.
Herbal Products: St. John's wort (hypericum perforatum)	May lead to loss of virologic response and possible resistance to delavirdine or to the class of non-nucleoside reverse transcriptase inhibitors.
HMG-CoA Reductase Inhibitors: lovastatin, simvastatin	Potential for serious reactions such as risk of myopathy including rhabdomyolysis.
Neuroleptic: pimozide	CONTRAINDICATED due to potential for serious and/or life-threatening reactions such as cardiac arrhythmias.
Sedative/Hypnotics: alprazolam, midazolam, triazolam	CONTRAINDICATED due to potential for serious and/or life-threatening reactions such as prolonged or increased sedation or respiratory depression.

* See TABLE 1 and TABLE 2 for magnitude of interaction.

TABLE 7 *Established and Other Potentially Significant Drug Interactions: Alteration in Dose or Regimen May Be Recommended Based on Drug Interaction Studies or Predicted Interaction**

	Clinical Comment
HIV-Antiviral Agents	
Amprenavir	
Increases amprenavir concentration.	Appropriate doses of this combination, with respect to safety, efficacy and pharmacokinetics, have not been established.
Didanosine*	
Decreases delavirdine and didanosine concentraion.	Administration of didanosine (buffered tablets) and delavirdine should be separated by at least 1 hour.
Indinavir*	
Increases indinavir concentration.	A dose reduction of indinavir to 600 mg tid should be considered when delavirdine and indinavir are coadministered.
Lopinavir/Ritonavir	
Increases lopinavir and ritonavir concentration.	Appropriate doses of this combination, with respect to safety, efficacy and pharmacokinetics, have not been established.
Nelfinavir*	
Increases nelfinavir concentration and decreases delavirdine concentration.	Appropriate doses of this combination, with respect to safety, efficacy and pharmacokinetics, have not been established.*
Ritonavir	
Increases ritonavir concentration.	Appropriate doses of this combination, with respect to safety, efficacy and pharmacokinetics, have not been established.
Saquinavir	
Increases saquinavir concentration.	A dose reduction of saquinavir (soft gelatin capsules) may be considered when delavirdine and saquinavir are coadministered.† Appropriate doses with respect to safety, efficacy and pharmacokinetics, have not been established.

(Table continued in next column)

TABLE 7 (cont.) *Established and Other Potentially Significant Drug Interactions: Alteration in Dose or Regimen May Be Recommended Based on Drug Interaction Studies or Predicted Interaction**

	Clinical Comment
Other Agents	
Acid Blockers: Antacids*	
Decreases delavirdine concentration.	Doses of an antacid and delavirdine should be separated by at least 1 hour, because the absorption of delavirdine is reduced when coadministered with antacids.
Acid Blockers: H_2 Receptor Antagonists: cimetidine, famotidine, nizatidine, ranitidine; Proton Pump Inhibitors: omeprazole, lansoprazole	
Decreases delavirdine concentration.	These agents increase gastric pH and may reduce the absorption of delavirdine. Although the effect of these drugs on delavirdine absorption has not been evaluated, chronic use of these drugs with delavirdine is not recommended.
Amphetamines	
Increases amphetamines concentration.	Use with caution.
Antiarrhythmics: Bepridil	
Increases antiarrhythmics concentration.	Use with caution. Increased bepridil exposure may be associated with life-threatening reactions such as cardiac arrhythmias.
Antiarrhythmics: Amiodarone, lidocaine (systemic), quinidine, flecainide, propafenone	
Increases antiarrhythmics concentration.	Caution is warranted and therapeutic concentration monitoring is recommended, if available, for antiarrhythmics when coadministered with delavirdine.
Anticoagulant: Warfarin	
Increases warfarin concentration	It is recommended that INR (international normalized ratio) be monitored.
Anti-Infective: Clarithromycin*	
Increases clarithromycin concentration.	When coadministered with delavirdine, clarithromycin should be adjusted in patients with impaired renal function: For patients with CLCR 30-60 ml/min the dose of clarithromycin should be reduced by 50%. For patients with CLCR <30 ml/min the dose of clarithromycin should be reduced by 75%.
Dihydropyridine: Calcium Channel Blockers Amlodipine, diltiazem, felodipine, isradipine, nifedipine, nicardipine, nimodipine, nisoldipine, verapamil	
Increases dihydropyridine calcium channel blockers concentration.	Caution is warranted and clinical monitoring of patients is recommended.
Corticosteroid: Dexamethasone	
Decreases delavirdine concentration.	Use with caution. Delavirdine may be less effective due to decreased delavirdine plasma concentrations in patients taking these agents concomitantly.
Erectile Dysfunction Agent: Sildenafil	
Increases sildenafil concentration.	Sildenafil should not exceed a maximum single dose of 25 mg in a 48 hour period.
HMG-CoA Reductase Inhibitors: Atorvastatin, cerivastatin, fluvastatin	
Increases atorvastatin, cerivastatin, and fluvastatin concentrations.	Use lowest possible dose of atorvastatin or cerivastatin, or fluvastatin with careful monitoring, or consider other HMG-CoA reductase inhibitors such as pravastatin in combination with delavirdine.
Immunosuppressants: Cyclosporine, tacrolimus, rapamycin	
Increases immunosuppressants concentration.	Therapeutic concentration monitoring is recommended for immunosuppressant agents when coadministered with delavirdine.
Narcotic Analgesic: Methadone	
Increases methadone concentration.	Dosage of methadone may need to be decreased when coadministered with delavirdine.
Oral Contraceptives: Ethinyl estradiol	
Inreases ethinyl estradiol concentration.	Concentrations of ethinyl estradiol may increase. However, the clinical significance is unknown.

* See TABLE 1 and TABLE 2 for magnitude of interaction.
† See TABLE 1.

Nervous System: Abnormal coordination, agitation, amnesia, change in dreams, cognitive impairment, confusion, decreased libido, disorientation, dizziness, emotional lability, euphoria, hallucination, hyperesthesia, hyperreflexia, hypertonia, hypesthesia, impaired concentration, manic symptoms, muscle cramp, nervousness, neuropathy, nystagmus, paralysis, paranoid symptoms, restlessness, sleep cycle disorder, somnolence, tingling, tremor, vertigo, and weakness.

Respiratory System: Chest congestion, dyspnea, epistaxis, hiccups, laryngismus, pneumonia, and rhinitis.

Skin and Appendages: Angioedema, dermal leukocytoclastic vasculitis, dermatitis, desquamation, diaphoresis, discolored skin, dry skin, erythema, erythema multiforme, folliculitis, fungal dermatitis, hair loss, herpes zoster or simplex, nail disorder, petechiae, non-application site pruritus, seborrhea, skin hypertrophy, skin disorder, skin nodule, Stevens-Johnson syndrome, urticaria, vesiculobullous rash, and wart.

Special Senses: Blepharitis, blurred vision, conjunctivitis, diplopia, dry eyes, ear pain, parosmia, otitis media, photophobia, taste perversion, tinnitus.

Urogenital System: Amenorrhea, breast enlargement, calculi of the kidney, chromaturia, epididymitis, hematuria, hemospermia, impaired urination, impotence, kidney pain, metrorrhagia, nocturia, polyuria, proteinuria, testicular pain, urinary tract infection, and vaginal moniliasis.

TABLE 8 *Percent of Patients With Treatment-Emergent Rash in Pivotal Trials: Studies 21 Part II and 13C**

	Description of Rash Grade†	Delavirdine 400 mg tid n=412	Control Group Patients n=295
Grade 1 rash	Erythema, pruritis	69 (16.7%)	35 (11.9%)
Grade 2 rash	Diffuse maculopapular rash, dry desquamation	59 (14.3%)	17 (5.8%)
Grade 3 rash	Vesiculation, moist desquamation, ulceration	18 (4.4%)	0 (0.0%)
Grade 4 rash	Erythema multiforme, Stevens-Johnson syndrome, toxic epideral necrolysis, necrosis requiring surgery, exfoliative dermatitis	0 (0.0%)	0 (0.0%)
Rash of any Grade		146 (35.4%)	52 (17.6%)
Treatment discontinuation as a result of rash		13 (3.2%)	1 (0.3%)

* Includes events reported regardless of causality.
† ACTG Toxicity Grading System; includes events reported as "rash", "maculopapular rash", and "urticaria".

TABLE 9A *Treatment-Emergent Events, Regardless of Causality, of Moderate-to-Severe or Life- Threatening Intensity Reported by at Least 5% of Evaluable* Patients in any Treatment Group: Study 21 Part II*

	% of Patients (n)		
Adverse Events	ZDV + 3TC (n=123)	400 mg tid Delavirdine + ZDV (n=123)	400 mg tid Delavirdine + ZDV + 3TC (n=119)
Body as a Whole			
Abdominal pain, generalized	2.4% (3)	3.3% (4)	5.0% (6)
Asthenia/fatigue	16.3% (20)	15.4% (19)	16.0% (19)
Fever	2.4% (3)	1.6% (2)	3.4% (4)
Flu syndrome	4.9% (6)	7.3% (9)	5.0% (6)
Headache	14.6% (18)	12.2% (15)	16.8% (20)
Localized pain	4.9% (6)	5.7% (7)	5.0% (6)
Digestive			
Diarrhea	8.1% (10)	2.4% (3)	4.2% (5)
Nausea	17.1% (21)	20.3% (25)	16.8% (20)
Vomiting	8.9% (11)	4.9% (6)	2.5% (3)
Nervous			
Anxiety	1.6% (2)	2.4% (3)	6.7% (8)
Depressive symptoms	6.5% (8)	4.9% (6)	12.6% (15)
Insomnia	4.9% (6)	4.9% (6)	5.0% (6)
Respiratory			
Bronchitis	4.1% (5)	6.5% (8)	6.7% (8)
Cough	9.8% (12)	4.1% (5)	5.0% (6)
Pharyngitis	6.5% (8)	1.6% (2)	5.0% (6)
Sinusitis	8.9% (11)	7.3% (9)	5.0% (6)
Upper respiratory infection	11.4% (14)	6.5% (8)	7.6% (9)
Skin			
Rashes	3.3% (4)	19.5% (24)	13.4% (16)

* Evaluble patients in Study 21 Part II were those who received at least 1 dose of study medication and returned for at least 1 clinic study visit.

POSTMARKETING EXPERIENCE

Adverse event terms reported from postmarking surveillance that were not reported in the Phase 2 and 3 trials are presented below.

Digestive System: Hepatic failure.
Hemic and Lymphatic System: Hemolytic anemia.
Musculoskeletal System: Rhabdomyolysis.
Urogenital System: Acute kidney failure.

LABORATORY ABNORMALITIES

Marked laboratory abnormalities observed in at least 2% of patients during Studies 21 Part II and 13C are summarized in TABLE 10A and TABLE 10B. Marked laboratory abnormalities are defined as any Grade 3 or 4 abnormality found in patients at any time during study.

DOSAGE AND ADMINISTRATION

The recommended dosage for delavirdine tablets is 400 mg (four 100 or two 200 mg tablets) 3 times daily. Delavirdine should be used in combination with other antiretroviral therapy. The complete prescribing information for other antiretroviral agents should be consulted for information on dosage and administration.

The 100 mg delavirdine tablets may be dispersed in water prior to consumption. To prepare a dispersion, add four 100 mg delavirdine tablets to at least 3 oz of water, allow to stand for a few minutes, and then stir until a uniform dispersion occurs (see CLINICAL PHARMACOLOGY, Pharmacokinetics, Absorption and Bioavailability). The dispersion should be consumed promptly. The glass should be rinsed with water and the rinse swallowed to insure the entire dose is consumed. **The 200 mg tablets should be taken as intact tablets, because they are not readily dispersed in water.** *Note:* The 200 mg tablets are approximately one-third smaller in size than the 100 mg tablets.

TABLE 9B *Treatment-Emergent Events, Regardless of Causality, of Moderate-to-Severe or Life-Threatening Intensity Reported by at Least 5% of Evaluable* Patients in Any Treatment Group: Study 13C*

	% of Patients (n)	
	ZDV + ddI, ddC or 3TC	400 mg tid Delavirdine + ZDV + ddl, ddC or 3TC
Adverse Events	(n=172)	(n=170)
Body as a Whole		
Abdominal pain, generalized	1.7% (3)	2.4% (4)
Asthenia/fatigue	8.1% (14)	5.3% (9)
Fever	6.4% (11)	7.1% (12)
Flu syndrome	5.2% (9)	2.4% (4)
Headache	12.8% (22)	11.2% (19)
Localized pain	2.9% (5)	1.8% (3)
Digestive		
Diarrhea	8.1% (14)	5.9% (10)
Nausea	9.3% (16)	14.7% (25)
Vomiting	4.1% (7)	6.5% (11)
Nervous		
Anxiety	4.1% (7)	3.5% (6)
Depressive symptoms	3.5% (6)	5.9% (10)
Insomnia	2.9% (5)	1.2% (2)
Respiratory		
Bronchitis	3.5% (6)	3.5% (6)
Cough	5.2% (9)	3.5% (6)
Pharyngitis	4.1% (7)	3.5% (6)
Sinusitis	2.3% (4)	1.2% (2)
Upper respiratory infection	8.7% (15)	4.7% (8)
Skin		
Rashes	7.6% (13)	18.8% (32)

* Evaluble patients in Study 13C were those who received at least 1 dose of study medication.

TABLE 10A *Marked Laboratory Abnormalities Reported by ≥2% of Patients: Study 21 Part II*

Adverse Events	Toxicity Limit	ZDV + 3TC	400 mg tid Delavirdine + ZDV	400 mg tid Delavirdine + ZDV + 3TC
		n=123	n=123	n=119
Hematology				
Hemoglobin	<7 mg/dl	4.1%	2.5%	0.9%
Neutrophils	<750/mm^3	5.7%	4.9%	3.4%
Prothrombin time (PT)	>1.5 × ULN	0%	0%	1.7%
Activated partial thromboplastin (APTT)	>2.33 × ULN	0%	0.8%	0%
Chemistry				
Alananine aminotransferase (ALT/SGPT)	>5 × ULN	2.5%	4.1%	5.1%
Amylase	>2 × ULN	0.8%	2.5%	2.6%
Aspartate aminotransferase (AST/SGOT)	>5 × ULN	1.6%	2.5%	3.4%
Bilirubin	>2.5 × ULN	0.8%	2.5%	1.7%
Gamma glutamyl transferase (GGT)	>5 × ULN	N/A	N/A	N/A
Glucose (hypo-/ hyperglycemia)	<40 mg/dl >250 mg/dl	4.1%	0.8%	1.7%

N/C Not applicable because no predose values were obtained for patients.

TABLE 10B *Marked Laboratory Abnormalities Reported by ≥2% of Patients: Study 13C*

Adverse Events	Toxicity Limit	ZDV + ddl, ddC or 3TC	400 mg tid Delavirdine + ZDV + ddl, ddC or 3TC
		n=172	n=170
Hematology			
Hemoglobin	<7 mg/dl	1.7%	2.9%
Neutrophils	<750/mm^3	10.4%	7.6%
Prothrombin time (PT)	>1.5 × ULN	2.9%	2.4%
Activated partial thromboplastin (APTT)	>2.33 × ULN	5.8%	2.4%
Chemistry			
Alananine aminotransferase (ALT/SGPT)	>5 × ULN	3.5%	4.1%
Amylase	>2 × ULN	3.5%	2.9%
Aspartate aminotransferase (AST/SGOT)	>5 × ULN	3.5%	2.3%
Bilirubin	>2.5 × ULN	1.2%	0%
Gamma glutamyl transferase (GGT)	>5 × ULN	4.1%	1.8%
Glucose (hypo-/ hyperglycemia)	<40 mg/dl >250 mg/dl	1.2%	0.0%

Delavirdine tablets may be administered with or without food (see CLINICAL PHARMACOLOGY, Pharmacokinetics, Absorption and Bioavailability). Patients with achlorhydria should take delavirdine with an acidic beverage (*e.g.,* orange or cranberry juice). However, the effect of an acidic beverage on the absorption of delavirdine in patients with achlorhydria has not been investigated.

Patients taking both delavirdine and antacids should be advised to take them at least 1 hour apart.

ANIMAL PHARMACOLOGY

Toxicities among various organs and organ systems in rats, mice, rabbits, dogs, and monkeys were observed following the administration of delavirdine. Necrotizing vasculitis was the most significant toxicity that occurred in dogs when mean nadir serum concentrations of delavirdine were at least 7-fold higher than the expected human exposure to delavirdine (C_{min} 15 μM) at the recommended dose. Vasculitis in dogs was not reversible during a 2.5 month recovery period; however, partial resolution of the vascular lesion characterized by reduced inflammation, diminished necrosis, and intimal thickening occurred during this period. Other major target organs included the gastrointestinal tract, endocrine organs, liver, kidneys, bone marrow, lymphoid tissue, lung, and reproductive organs.

HOW SUPPLIED

RESCRIPTOR TABLETS

Rescriptor tablets are available as follows:

100 mg: White, capsule-shaped tablets marked with "U 3761".

200 mg: White, capsule-shaped tablets marked with "RESCRIPTOR 200 mg".

Storage: Store at controlled room temperature 20-25°C (68-77°F). Keep container tightly closed. Protect from high humidity.

PRODUCT LISTING - EQUIVALENTS NOT AVAILABLE

Tablet - Oral - 200 mg

180's	$292.02	RESCRIPTOR, Pharmacia and Upjohn	00009-7576-01
180's	$316.35	RESCRIPTOR, Pfizer U.S. Pharmaceuticals	63010-0021-18

Demeclocycline Hydrochloride *(000956)*

Categories: Amebiasis, intestinal; Chancroid; Conjunctivitis, inclusion; Gonorrhea; Granuloma inguinale; Infection, sexually transmitted; Infection, skin and skin structures; Infection, upper respiratory tract; Lymphogranuloma venereum; Psittacosis; Q fever; Relapsing fever; Rickettsialpox; Rocky mountain spotted fever; Syphilis; Tick fever; Trachoma; Typhus fever; Vincent's infection; Yaws; Pregnancy Category D; FDA Approved 1960 Jan

Drug Classes: Antibiotics, tetracyclines

Brand Names: **Declomycin**

Foreign Brand Availability: Ledermicina (Italy; Peru); Ledermycin (Australia; Austria; Belgium; England; India; Japan; Korea; Netherlands)

Cost of Therapy: $192.36 (Infection; Declomycin; 300 mg; 2 tablets/day; 10 day supply)

DESCRIPTION

Demeclocycline hydrochloride is an antibiotic isolated from a mutant strain of *Streptomyces aureofaciens.* Chemically it is (4S-(4α,4aα,5aα,6β,12aα))-7-Chloro-4-dimethylamino)-1,4,4a,5,5a,6,11,12a-octahydro-3,6,10,12,12a-pentahydroxy-1,11-dioxo-2-naphthacenecarboxamide monohydrochloride.

Declomycin contains the following inactive ingredients:

Declomycin Capsules: Benzoin gum, blue 1, colloidal silicon dioxide, corn starch, FD&C yellow no. 6, ethyl vanillin, gelatin, glycerin, methylparaben, propenyl guaethol, propylene glycol, propylparaben, red 33, red 40, terpene resin, titanium dioxide, and other ingredients.

Declomycin Tablets: Alginic acid, corn starch, ethylcellulose, hydroxypropyl methylcellulose, magnesium stearate, red 7, sorbitol, titanium dioxide, yellow 10 and other ingredients. may also contain sodium lauryl sulfate.

Storage: Store at controlled room temperature 15-30°C (59-86°F).

CLINICAL PHARMACOLOGY

The tetracyclines are primarily bacteriostatic and are thought to exert their antimicrobial effect by the inhibition of protein synthesis. Tetracyclines are active against a wide range of gram-negative and gram-positive organisms. The drugs in the tetracycline class have closely similar antimicrobial spectra, and cross-resistance among them is common. Microorganisms may be considered susceptible if the MIC (minimum inhibitory concentration) is not more than 4 μg/ml and intermediate if the MIC is 4-12.5 μg/ml.

Susceptibility plate testing: A tetracycline disc may be used to determine microbial susceptibility to drugs in the tetracycline class. If the Kirby-Bauer method of disc susceptibility testing is used, a 30 μg tetracycline disc should give a zone of at least 19 mm when tested against a tetracycline-susceptible bacterial strain.

Tetracyclines are readily absorbed and are bound to plasma proteins in varying degrees. They are concentrated by the liver in the bile and excreted in the urine and feces at high concentrations and in a biologically active form.

INDICATIONS AND USAGE

Demeclocycline HCl is indicated in infections caused by the following microorganisms:

Rickettsiae: (Rocky Mountain spotted fever, typhus fever and the typhus group, Q fever, rickettsialpox, tick fevers).

Mycoplasma pneumoniae (PPLO, Eaton agent).

Agents of psittacosis and ornithosis.

Agents of lymphogranuloma venereum and granuloma inguinale.

The spirochetal agent of relapsing fever (*Borrelia recurrentis*).

The following gram-negative microorganisms:

Haemophilus ducreyi (chancroid), *Yersinia pestis and Francisella tularensis,* formerly *Pasteurella pestis* and *Pasteurella tularensis, Bartonella bacilliformis, Bacteroides*

species, *Vibrio comma* and *Vibrio fetus, Brucella* species (in conjunction with streptomycin).

Because many strains of the following groups of microorganisms have been shown to be resistant to tetracyclines, culture and susceptibility testing are recommended.

Demeclocycline is indicated for treatment of infections caused by the following gram-negative microorganisms, when bacteriologic testing indicates appropriate susceptibility to the drug:

Escherichia coli, Enterobacter aerogenes (formerly *Aerobacter aerogenes*), *Shigella* species, *Mima* species and *Herellea* species, *Haemophilus influenzae* (respiratory infections), *Klebsiella* species (respiratory and urinary infections).

Declomycin is indicated for treatment of infections caused by the following gram-positive microorganisms when bacteriologic testing indicates appropriate susceptibility to the drug:

***Streptococcus* species:**

Up to 44% of strains of *Streptococcus pyogenes* and 74% of *Streptococcus faecalis* have been found to be resistant to tetracycline drugs. Therefore, tetracyclines should not be used for streptococcal disease unless the organism has been demonstrated to be sensitive.

For upper respiratory infections due to Group A beta-hemolytic streptococci, penicillin is the usual drug of choice, including prophylaxis of rheumatic fever.

Streptococcus pneumoniae.

Staphylococcus aureus, skin and soft tissue infections.

Tetracyclines are not the drugs of choice in the treatment of any type of Staphylococcal infection.

When penicillin is contraindicated, tetracyclines are alternative drugs in the treatment of infections due to:

Neisseria gonorrhoeae, Treponema pallidum and *Treponema pertenue* (syphilis and yaws), *Listeria monocytogenes, Clostridium* species, *Bacillus anthracis, Fusobacterium fusiforme* (Vincent's infection), *Actinomyces* species.

In acute intestinal amebiasis, the tetracyclines may be a useful adjunct to amebicides.

Demeclocycline HCl is indicated in the treatment of trachoma, although the infectious agent is not always eliminated, as judged by immunofluorescence.

Inclusion conjunctivitis may be treated with oral tetracyclines or with a combination of oral and topical agents.

CONTRAINDICATIONS

This drug is contraindicated in persons who have shown hypersensitivity to any of the tetracyclines.

WARNINGS

THE USE OF DRUGS OF THE TETRACYCLINE CLASS DURING TOOTH DEVELOPMENT (LAST HALF OF PREGNANCY, INFANCY AND CHILDHOOD TO THE AGE OF 8 YEARS) MAY CAUSE PERMANENT DISCOLORATION OF THE TEETH (YELLOW-GRAY-BROWN). This adverse reaction is more common during long-term use of the drugs but has been observed following repeated short-term courses. Enamel hypoplasia has also been reported. TETRACYCLINE DRUGS, THEREFORE, SHOULD NOT BE USED IN THIS AGE GROUP UNLESS OTHER DRUGS ARE NOT LIKELY TO BE EFFECTIVE OR ARE CONTRAINDICATED. If renal impairment exists, even usual oral or parenteral doses may lead to excessive systemic accumulation of the drug and possible liver toxicity. Under such conditions, lower than usual total doses are indicated and, if therapy is prolonged, serum level determinations of the drug may be advisable.

Phototoxic reactions can occur in individuals taking demeclocycline, and are characterized by severe burn of exposed surfaces resulting from direct exposure of patients to sunlight during therapy with moderate or large doses of demeclocycline. Patients apt to be exposed to direct sunlight or ultraviolet light should be advised that this reaction can occur, and treatment should be discontinued at the first evidence of skin erythema.

The anti-anabolic action of the tetracyclines may cause in increase in BUN. While this is not a problem in those with normal renal function, in patients with significantly impaired function, higher serum levels of tetracycline may lead to azotemia, hyperphosphatemia, and acidosis.

Administration of demeclocycline HCl has resulted in appearance of the diabetes insipidus syndrome (polyuria, polydipsia and weakness) in some patients on long-term therapy. The syndrome has been shown to be nephrogenic, dose-dependent and reversible on discontinuance of therapy.

PREGNANCY CATEGORY D

See WARNINGS about use during tooth development. Results of animal studies indicate that tetracyclines cross the placets, are found in fetal tissues and can have toxic effects on the developing fetus (often related to retardation of skeletal development). Evidence of embryotoxicity has also been noted in animals treated early in pregnancy.

USAGE IN NEWBORNS, INFANTS, AND CHILDREN

See WARNINGS about use during tooth development.

All tetracyclines form stable calcium complex in bone forming tissue. A decrease in the fibula growth rate has been observed in prematures given oral tetracycline in doses of 25 mg/kg every 6 hours. This reaction was shown to be reversible when the drug was discontinued.

Tetracyclines are present in the milk of lactating women who are taking a drug in this class.

PRECAUTIONS

GENERAL

Pseudotumor cerebri (benign intracranial hypertension) in adults has been associated with the use of tetracyclines. The usual clinical manifestations are headache and blurred vision. Bulging fontanels have been associated with the use of tetracyclines in infants. While both of these conditions and related symptoms usually resolve soon after discontinuation of the tetracyclines, the possibility for permanent sequelae exists.

As with other antibiotic preparations, use of this drug may result in overgrowth of nonsusceptible organisms, including fungi. If superinfection occurs, the antibiotic should be discontinued and appropriate therapy should be instituted. In venereal diseases when coexistent syphilis is suspected, darkfield examination should be done before treatment is started and the blood serology repeated monthly for at least 4 months.

In long-term therapy, periodic laboratory evaluation of organ systems, including hematopoietic, renal and hepatic studies should be performed.

All infections due to Group A beta-hemolytic streptococci should be treated for at least 10 days.

Interpretation of Bacteriologic Studies: Following a course of therapy, persistence for several days in both urine and blood of bacterio-suppressive levels of demeclocycline may interfere with culture studies. These levels should not be considered therapeutic.

DRUG INTERACTIONS

Because the tetracyclines have been shown to depress plasma prothrombin activity, patients who are on anticoagulant therapy may require downward adjustment of their anticoagulant dosage.

Since bacteriostatic drugs, such as the tetracycline class of antibiotics, may interfere with the bactericidal action of penicillins, it is not advisable to administer these drugs concomitantly.

Concurrent use of tetracyclines with oral contraceptives may render oral contraceptives less effective. Breakthrough bleeding has been reported.

ADVERSE REACTIONS

Gastrointestinal: Anorexia, nausea, vomiting, diarrhea, glossitis, dysphagia, enterocolitis, pancreatitis, and inflammatory lesions (with monilial overgrowth) in the anogenital region, increases in liver enzymes, and hepatic toxicity has been reported rarely. Rare instances of esophagitis and esophageal ulcerations have been reported in patients taking the tetracycline-class antibiotics in capsule and tablet form. Most of these patients took the medication immediately before going to bed (see DOSAGE AND ADMINISTRATION).

Skin: Maculopapular and erythematous rashes. Exfoliative dermatitis has been reported but is uncommon. Photosensitivity is discussed above. (See WARNINGS).

Renal Toxicity: Rise in BUN has been reported and is apparently dose related. Nephrogenic diabetes insipidus. (See WARNINGS).

Hypersensitivity Reactions: Urticaria, angioneurotic edema, anaphylaxis, anaphylactoid purpura, pericarditis and exacerbation of systemic lupus erythematosus.

Blood: Hemolytic anemia, thrombocytopenia, neutropenia and eosinophilia have been reported.

CNS: Pseudotumor cerebri (benign intracranial hypertension) in adults and bulging fontanels in infants (see PRECAUTIONS, General). Dizziness, tinnitus, and visual disturbances have been reported. Myasthenic syndrome has been reported rarely.

Other: When given over prolonged periods, tetracyclines have been reported to produce brown-black microscopic discoloration of thyroid glands. No abnormalities of thyroid function studies are known to occur.

DOSAGE AND ADMINISTRATION

Therapy should be continued for at least 24-48 hours after symptoms and fever have subsided.

Concomitant Therapy: Antacids containing aluminum, calcium, or magnesium impair absorption and should not be given to patients taking oral tetracycline. Foods and some diary products also interfere with absorption. Oral forms of tetracycline should be given 1 hour before or 2 hours after meals.

In Patients With Renal Impairment: (See WARNINGS). Total dosage should be decreased by reduction recommended individual doses and/or by extending time intervals between doses.

In the treatment of streptococcal infections, a therapeutic dose of demeclocycline should be administered for at least 10 days.

Adults: *Usual Daily Dose:* Four divided doses of 150 mg each or two divided doses of 300 mg each.

For Children Above 8 Years of Age: *Usual Daily Dose:* 3-6 mg per pound body weight per day, depending upon the severity of the disease, divided into 2-4 doses.

Gonorrhea patients sensitive to penicillin may be treated with demeclocycline administered as an initial oral dose of 600 mg followed by 300 mg every 12 hours for 4 days to a total of 3 grams.

PRODUCT LISTING - EQUIVALENTS NOT AVAILABLE

Tablet - Oral - 150 mg

100's	$528.56	DECLOMYCIN, Lederle Laboratories	00005-9218-23

Tablet - Oral - 300 mg

48's	$461.66	DECLOMYCIN, Lederle Laboratories	00005-9270-29

Denileukin Diftitox (003474)

For complete prescribing information, refer to the CD-ROM included with the book.

Categories: Lymphoma, T-cell, cutaneous; FDA Approved 1999 Feb; Pregnancy Category C; Orphan Drugs
Drug Classes: Antineoplastics, biological response modifiers
Brand Names: **Ontak**

WARNING

Only physicians experienced in the use of antineoplastic therapy and management of patients with cancer should use denileukin diftitox. Patients treated with denileukin diftitox must be managed in a

> **WARNING — Cont'd**
> **facility equipped and staffed for cardiopulmonary resuscitation and where the patient can be closely monitored for an appropriate period based on his or her health status.**

DESCRIPTION

Ontak (denileukin diftitox), a recombinant DNA-derived cytotoxic protein composed of the amino acid sequences for diphtheria toxin fragments A and B (Met1-Thr_{387})-His followed by the sequences for interleukin-2 (IL-2; Ala1-Thr_{133}), is produced in an *E. coli* expression system. Ontak has a molecular weight of 58 kD. Neomycin is used in the fermentation process but is undetectable in the final product. The product is purified using reverse phase chromatography followed by a multistep diafiltration process.

D

Ontak is supplied in single use vials as a sterile, frozen solution intended for intravenous (IV) administration. Each 2 ml vial of Ontak contains 300 μg of recombinant denileukin diftitox in a sterile solution of citric acid (20 mM), EDTA (0.05 mM) and polysorbate 20 (<1%) in water for injection. The solution has a pH of 6.9-7.2.

INDICATIONS AND USAGE

Denileukin diftitox is indicated for the treatment of patients with persistent or recurrent cutaneous T-cell lymphoma whose malignant cells express the CD25 component of the IL-2 receptor. The safety and efficacy of denileukin diftitox in patients with CTCL whose malignant cells do not express the CD25 component of the IL-2 receptor have not been examined.

NON-FDA APPROVED INDICATIONS

The drug has also been reported to have efficacy in the treatment of severe psoriasis. However, this use has not been approved by the FDA.

CONTRAINDICATIONS

Denileukin diftitox is contraindicated for use in patients with a known hypersensitivity to denileukin diftitox or any of its components: diphtheria toxin, interleukin-2, or excipients.

WARNINGS

ACUTE HYPERSENSITIVITY-TYPE REACTIONS

Acute hypersensitivity reactions were reported in 98 of 143 patients (69%) during or within 24 hours of denileukin diftitox infusion; approximately half of the events occurred on the first day of dosing regardless of the treatment cycle. The constellation of symptoms included one or more of the following, defined as the incidence (%) in these 98 patients: hypotension (50%), back pain (30%), dyspnea (28%), vasodilation (28%), rash (25%), chest pain or tightness (24%), tachycardia (12%), dysphagia or laryngismus (5%), syncope (3%), allergic reaction (1%) or anaphylaxis (1%). These events were severe in 2% of patients. Management consists of interruption or a decrease in the rate of infusion (depending on the severity of the reaction); 3% of infusions were terminated prematurely and reduction in rate occurred in 4% of the infusions during the clinical trials. The administration of IV antihistamines, corticosteroids, and epinephrine may also be required; 2 subjects received epinephrine and 18 (13%) received systemic corticosteroids in the clinical studies. These drugs and resuscitative equipment should be readily available during denileukin diftitox administration.

VASCULAR LEAK SYNDROME

This syndrome, characterized by 2 or more of the following 3 symptoms (hypotension, edema, hypoalbuminemia) was reported in 27% (38/143) of patients in the clinical studies. Six percent (8/143) of patients were hospitalized for the management of these symptoms. The onset of symptoms in patients with vascular leak syndrome was delayed, usually occurring within the first 2 weeks of infusion and may persist or worsen after the cessation of denileukin diftitox. Special caution should be taken in patients with preexisting cardiovascular disease.

Weight, edema, blood pressure and serum albumin levels should be carefully monitored on an outpatient basis. This syndrome is usually self-limited and treatment should be used only if clinically indicated. The type of treatment will depend on whether edema or hypotension is the primary clinical problem. Pre-existing low serum albumin levels appear to predict and may predispose patients to the syndrome.

DOSAGE AND ADMINISTRATION

Denileukin diftitox is for intravenous (IV) use only. The recommended treatment regimen (1 treatment cycle) is 9 or 18 μg/kg/day administered intravenously for 5 consecutive days every 21 days. Denileukin diftitox should be infused over at least 15 minutes. If infusional adverse reactions occur, the infusion should be discontinued or the rate should be reduced depending on the severity of the reaction. There is no clinical experience with prolonged infusion times (>80 minutes).

The optimal duration of therapy has not been determined; however, only 2% (1/50) of patients who did not demonstrate at least a 25% decrease in tumor burden prior to the fourth course of treatment subsequently responded.

Special Handling

- Denileukin diftitox must be brought to room temperature, up to 2°C (77°F), before preparing the dose. The vials may be thawed in the refrigerator at 2-8°C (36- 46°F) for not more than 24 hours or at room temperature for 1-2 hours. **DENILEUKIN DIFTITOX MUST NOT BE HEATED.**
- The solution in the vial may be mixed by gentle swirling; **DO NOT VIGOROUSLY SHAKE DENILEUKIN DIFTITOX SOLUTION.**
- After thawing, a haze may be visible. This haze should clear when the solution is at room temperature.
- Denileukin diftitox solution must not be used unless the solution is clear, colorless and without visible particulate matter.
- **DENILEUKIN DIFTITOX MUST NOT BE REFROZEN.**

Preparation and Administration

- USE APPROPRIATE ASEPTIC TECHNIQUE IN DILUTION AND ADMINISTRATION OF DENILEUKIN DIFTITOX.
- Prepare and hold diluted denileukin diftitox in plastic syringes or soft plastic IV bags. **Do not use a glass container** because adsorption to glass may occur in the dilute state.
- The concentration of denileukin diftitox must be at least 15 μg/ml during all steps in the preparation of the solution for IV infusion. This is best accomplished by withdrawing the calculated dose from the vial(s) and injecting it into an empty IV infusion bag. **FOR EACH 1 ML OF DENILEUKIN DIFTITOX FROM THE VIAL(S), NO MORE THAN 9 ML OF STERILE SALINE WITHOUT PRESERVATIVE SHOULD THEN BE ADDED TO THE IV BAG.**
- The denileukin diftitox dose should be infused over at least 15 minutes.
- **DENILEUKIN DIFTITOX SHOULD NOT BE ADMINISTERED AS A BOLUS INJECTION.**
- Do not physically mix denileukin diftitox with other drugs.
- **DO NOT ADMINISTER DENILEUKIN DIFTITOX THROUGH AN IN-LINE FILTER.**
- Prepared solutions of denileukin diftitox should be administered within 6 hours, using a syringe pump or IV infusion bag.
- Unused portions of denileukin diftitox should be discarded immediately.

PRODUCT LISTING - EQUIVALENTS NOT AVAILABLE

Solution - Intravenous - 150 mcg/ml

2 ml x 6 $1273.75 ONTAK, Ligand Pharmaceuticals 64365-0503-01

Desipramine Hydrochloride *(000964)*

For related information, see the comparative table section in Appendix A.

Categories: Depression; FDA Approved 1967 Jan; Pregnancy Category C
Drug Classes: Antidepressants, tricyclic
Brand Names: Norpramin
Foreign Brand Availability: Deprexan (Israel); Nebril (Argentina); Nortimil (Italy); Pertofran (Austria; Belgium; England; France; Netherlands; New-Zealand); Petylyl (Bulgaria; Czech-Republic; Russia)
Cost of Therapy: $80.70 (Depression; Norpramin; 100 mg; 1 tablet/day; 30 day supply)
$33.03 (Depression; Generic Tablets; 100 mg; 1 tablet/day; 30 day supply)

DESCRIPTION

Desipramine hydrochloride is an antidepressant drug of the tricyclic type, and is chemically: 5*H*-Dibenz[*bf*]azepine-5-propanamine,10,11-dihydro-*N*-methyl-, monohydrochloride

The following inactive ingredients are contained in all Norpramin tablet dosage strengths: acacia, calcium carbonate, corn starch, D&C red no. 30 and D&C yellow no. 10 (except 10 and 150 mg), FD&C blue no. 1 (except 50, 75, and 100 mg), hydrogenated soy oil, iron oxide, light mineral oil, magnesium stearate, mannitol, polyethylene glycol 8000, pregelatinized corn starch, sodium benzoate (except 150 mg), sucrose, talc, titanium dioxide, and other ingredients.

Desipramine hydrochloride capsule form, is a metabolite of imipramine HCl. It is a dibenzazepine derivative, representing the dimethyl analog of imipramine hydrochloride. Chemically it is 10,11-dihydro-5-(3-(methylamino) propyl)-5H-dibenz (bf) azepine monohydrochloride, and differs from the parent substance by having only one methyl group on the side chain of nitrogen.

CLINICAL PHARMACOLOGY

MECHANISM OF ACTION

Available evidence suggests that many depressions have a biochemical basis in the form of a relative deficiency of neurotransmitters such as norepinephrine and serotonin. Norepinephrine deficiency may be associated with relatively low urinary 3-methoxy-4-hydroxyphenyl glycol (MHPG) levels, while serotonin deficiencies may be associated with low spinal fluid levels of 5-hydroxyindoleacetic acid.

While the precise mechanism of action of the tricyclic antidepressants is unknown, a leading theory suggests that they restore normal levels of neurotransmitters by blocking the re-uptake of these substances from the synapse in the central nervous system. Evidence indicates that the secondary amine tricyclic antidepressants, including desipramine HCl, may have greater activity in blocking the re-uptake of norepinephrine. Tertiary amine tricyclic antidepressants, such as amitriptyline, may have greater effect on serotonin re-uptake.

Desipramine HCl is not a monoamine oxidase (MAO) inhibitor and does not act primarily as a central nervous system stimulant. It has been found in some studies to have a more rapid onset of action than imipramine. Earliest therapeutic effects may occasionally be seen in 2-5 days, but full treatment benefit usually requires 2-3 weeks to obtain.

METABOLISM

Tricyclic antidepressants, such as desipramine HCl, are rapidly absorbed from the gastrointestinal tract. Tricyclic antidepressants or their metabolites are to some extent excreted through the gastric mucosa and reabsorbed from the gastrointestinal tract. Desipramine is metabolized in the liver and approximately 70% is excreted in the urine.

The rate of metabolism of tricyclic antidepressants varies widely from individual to individual, chiefly on a genetically determined basis. Up to a 36-fold difference in plasma level may be noted among individuals taking the same oral dose of desipramine. In general, the elderly metabolize tricyclic antidepressants more slowly than do younger adults.

Certain drugs, particularly the psychostimulants and the phenothiazines, increase plasma levels of concomitantly administered tricyclic antidepressants through competition for the same metabolic enzyme systems. Concurrent administration of cimetidine and tricyclic antidepressants can produce clinically significant increases in the plasma concentrations of the tricyclic antidepressants. Conversely, decreases in plasma levels of the tricyclic antidepressants have been reported upon discontinuation of cimetidine which may result in the loss of the therapeutic efficacy of the tricyclic antidepressant. Other substances, particularly barbiturates and alcohol, induce liver enzyme activity and thereby reduce tricyclic antidepressant plasma levels. Similar effects have been reported with tobacco smoke.

Research on the relationship of plasma level to therapeutic response with the tricyclic antidepressants has produced conflicting results. While some studies report no correlation, many studies cite therapeutic levels for most tricyclics in the range of 50-300 ng/ml. The therapeutic range is different for each tricyclic antidepressant. For desipramine, an optimal range of therapeutic plasma levels has not been established.

INDICATIONS AND USAGE

Desipramine HCl is indicated for the treatment of depression.

NON-FDA APPROVED INDICATIONS

Desipramine has also been used in the treatment of neuropathic pain, bulimia, and stimulant abuse (particularly cocaine abuse), although these uses are not explicitly approved by the FDA.

CONTRAINDICATIONS

Desipramine HCl should not be given in conjunction with, or within 2 weeks of, treatment with an MAO inhibitor drug; hyperpyretic crises, severe convulsions, and death have occurred in patients taking MAO inhibitors and tricyclic antidepressants. When despiramine HCl is substituted for an MAO inhibitor, at least 2 weeks should elapse between treatments. Desipramine HCl should then be started cautiously and should be increased gradually.

The drug is contraindicated in the acute recovery period following myocardial infarction. It should not be used in those who have shown prior hypersensitivity to the drug. Cross-sensitivity between this and other dibenzazepines is a possibility.

WARNINGS

Extreme caution should be used when this drug is given in the following situations:

In patients with cardiovascular disease, because of the possibility of conduction defects, arrhythmias, tachycardias, strokes, and acute myocardial infarction.

In patients with a history of urinary retention or glaucoma, because of the anticholinergic properties of the drug.

In patients with thyroid disease or those taking thyroid medication, because of the possibility of cardiovascular toxicity, including arrhythmias.

In patients with a history of seizure disorder, because this drug has been shown to lower the seizure threshold.

This drug is capable of blocking the antihypertensive effect of guanethidine and similarly acting compounds.

The patient should be cautioned that this drug may impair the mental and/or physical abilities required for the performance of potentially hazardous tasks such as driving a car or operating machinery.

In patients who may use alcohol excessively, it should be borne in mind that the potentiation may increase the danger inherent in any suicide attempt or overdosage.

USE IN PREGNANCY

Safe use of despiramine HCl during pregnancy and lactation has not been established; therefore, if it is to be given to pregnant patients, nursing mothers, or women of childbearing potential, the possible benefits must be weighed against the possible hazards to mother and child. Animal reproductive studies have been inconclusive.

USE IN CHILDREN

Desipramine HCl is not recommended for use in children since safety and effectiveness in the pediatric age group have not been established. (See ADVERSE REACTIONS, Cardiovascular.)

PRECAUTIONS

It is important that this drug be dispensed in the least possible quantities to depressed outpatients, since suicide has been accomplished with this class of drug. Ordinary prudence requires that children not have access to this drug or to potent drugs of any kind; if possible, this drug should be dispensed in containers with child-resistant safety closures. Storage of this drug in the home must be supervised responsibly.

If serious adverse effects occur, dosage should be reduced or treatment should be altered.

Desipramine HCl therapy in patients with manic-depressive illness may induce a hypomanic state after the depressive phase terminates.

The drug may cause exacerbation of psychosis in schizophrenic patients.

Close supervision and careful adjustment of dosage are required when this drug is given concomitantly with anticholinergic or sympathomimetic drugs.

Patients should be warned that while taking this drug their response to alcoholic beverages may be exaggerated.

Clinical experience in the concurrent administration of ECT and antidepressant drugs is limited. Thus, if such treatment is essential, the possibility of increased risk relative to benefits should be considered.

If despiramine HCl is to be combined with other psychotropic agents such as tranquilizers or sedative/hypnotics, careful consideration should be given to the pharmacology of the agents employed since the sedative effects of despiramine HCl and benzodiazepines (*e.g.,* chlordiazepoxide or diazepam) are additive. Both the sedative and anticholinergic effects of the major tranquilizers are also additive to those of despiramine HCl.

There have been greater than 2-fold increases of previously stable plasma levels of tricyclic antidepressants when fluoxetine has been administered in combination with these agents.

This drug should be discontinued as soon as possible prior to elective surgery because of the possible cardiovascular effects. Hypertensive episodes have been observed during surgery in patients taking desipramine HCl.

Both elevation and lowering of blood sugar levels have been reported.

Leukocyte and differential counts should be performed in any patient who develops fever and sore throat during therapy; the drug should be discontinued if there is evidence of pathologic neutrophil depression.

DRUG INTERACTIONS

DRUGS METABOLIZED BY P450 2D6

The biochemical activity of the drug metabolizing isozyme cytochrome P450 2D6 (debrisoquin hydroxylase) is reduced in a subset of the Caucasian population (about 7-10% of Caucasians are so called "poor metabolizers"); reliable estimates of the prevalence of reduced P450 2D6 isozyme activity among Asian, African and other populations are not yet available. Poor metabolizers have higher than expected plasma concentrations of tricyclic antidepressants (TCAs) when given usual doses. Depending on the fraction of drug metabolized by P450 2D6, the increase in plasma concentration may be small, or quite large (8-fold increase in plasma AUC of the TCA).

In addition, certain drugs inhibit the activity of the isozyme and make normal metabolizers resemble poor metabolizers. An individual who is stable on a given dose of TCA may become abruptly toxic when given one of these inhibiting drugs as concomitant therapy. The drugs that inhibit cytochrome P450 2D6 include some that are not metabolized by the enzyme (quinidine; cimetidine) and many that are substrates for P450 2D6 (many other antidepressants, phenothiazines, and the Type 1C antiarrhythmic propafenone and flecainide). While all the selective serotonin reuptake inhibitors (SSRIs) *e.g.,* fluoxetine, sertraline, paroxetine, inhibit P450 2D6, they may vary in the extent of inhibition. The extent to which SSRTI TCA interactions may pose clinical problems will depend on the degree of inhibition and the pharmacokinetics of the SSRI involved. Nevertheless, caution is indicated in the co-administration of TCAs with any of the SSRIs and also in switching from one class to the other. Of particular importance, sufficient time must elapse before initiating TCA treatment in a patient being withdrawn from fluoxetine, given the long half-life of the parent and active metabolite (at least 5 weeks may be necessary).

Concomitant use of tricyclic antidepressants with drugs that can inhibit cytochrome P450 2D6 may require lower doses than usually prescribed for either the tricyclic antidepressant or the other drug. Furthermore, whenever one to these other drugs is withdrawn from co-therapy, an increased dose of tricyclic antidepressant may be required. It is desirable to monitor TCA plasma levels whenever a TCA is going to be coadministered with another drug known to be an inhibitor of P450 2D6.

Close supervision and careful adjustment of dosage are required when this drug is given concomitantly with anticholinergic or sympathomimetic drugs.

Patients should be warned that while taking this drug their response to alcoholic beverages may be exaggerated.

If desipramine HCl is to be combined with other psychotropic agents such as tranquilizers or sedative/hypnotics, careful consideration should be given to the pharmacology of the agents employed since the sedative effects of desipramine HCl and benzodiazepines (*e.g.,*chlorodiazepoxide or diazepam) are additive. Both the sedative and anticholinergic effects of the major tranquilizers are also additive to those of desipramine HCl.

ADVERSE REACTIONS

Included in the following listing are a few adverse reactions that have not been reported with this specific drug. However, the pharmacologic similarities among the tricyclic antidepressant drugs require that each of the reactions be considered when desipramine HCl is given.

Cardiovascular: Hypotension, hypertension, palpitations, heart block, myocardial infarction, stroke, arrhythmias, premature ventricular contractions, tachycardia, ventricular tachycardia, ventricular fibrillation, sudden death.

There has been a report of an "acute collapse" and "sudden death" in an 8-year-old (18 kg) male, treated for 2 years for hyperactivity. There have been additional reports of sudden death in children (see WARNINGS, Use in Children).

Psychiatric: Confusional states (especially in the elderly) with hallucinations, disorientation, delusions; anxiety, restlessness, agitation; insomnia and nightmares; hypomania; exacerbation of psychosis.

Neurologic: Numbness, tingling, paresthesia of extremities; incoordination, ataxia, tremors; peripheral neuropathy; extrapyramidal symptoms; seizures; alteration in EEG patterns; tinnitus. Symptoms attributed to Neuroleptic Malignant Syndrome have been reported during desipramine use with and without concomitant neuroleptic therapy.

Anticholinergic: Dry mouth, and rarely associated sublingual adenitis; blurred vision, disturbance of accommodation, mydriasis, increased intraocular pressure; constipation, paralytic ileus; urinary retention, delayed micturition, dilatation of urinary tract.

Allergic: Skin rash, petechiae, urticaria, itching, photosensitization (avoid excessive exposure to sunlight), edema (of face and tongue or general), drug fever, cross sensitivity with other tricyclic drugs.

Hematologic: Bone marrow depressions including agranulocytosis, eosinophilia, purpura, thrombocytopenia.

Endocrine: Gynecomastia in the male, breast enlargement and galactorrhea in the female; increased or decreased libido, impotence, painful ejaculation, testicular swelling; elevation or depression of blood sugar levels; syndrome of inappropriate antidiuretic hormone secretion (SIADH).

Other: Weight gain or loss; perspiration, flushing; urinary frequency, nocturia; parotid swelling; drowsiness, dizziness, weakness and fatigue, headache; fever; alopecia; elevated alkaline phosphatase.

Withdrawal Symptoms: Though not indicative of addiction, abrupt cessation of treatment after prolonged therapy may produce nausea, headache, and malaise.

DOSAGE AND ADMINISTRATION

Tablets: Not recommended for use in children (see WARNINGS).

Lower dosages are recommended for elderly patients and adolescents. Lower dosages are also recommended for outpatients compared to hospitalized patients, who are closely supervised. Dosage should be initiated at a low level and increased according to clinical response and any evidence of intolerance. Following remission, maintenance medication may be required for a period of time and should be at the lowest dose that will maintain remission.

USUAL ADULT DOSE

The usual adult dose is 100-200 mg/day. In more severely ill patients, dosage may be further increased gradually to 300 mg/day if necessary. Dosages above 300 mg/day are not recommended. Dosage should be initiated at a lower level and increased according to tolerance and clinical response.

Treatment of patients requiring as much as 300 mg should generally be initiated in hospitals, where regular visits by the physician, skilled nursing care, and frequent electrocardiograms (ECGs) are available.

The best available evidence of impending toxicity from very high doses of desipramine HCl is prolongation of the QRS or QT intervals on the ECG. Prolongation of the PR interval is also significant, but less closely correlated with plasma levels. Clinical symptoms of intolerance, especially drowsiness, dizziness, and postural hypotension, should also alert the physician to the need for reduction in dosage. Plasma desipramine measurement would constitute the optimal guide to dosage monitoring.

Initial therapy may be administered in divided doses or a single daily dose.

Maintenance therapy may be given on a once-daily schedule for patient convenience and compliance.

ADOLESCENT AND GERIATRIC DOSE

The usual adolescent and geriatric dose is 25-100 mg daily.

Dosage should be initiated at a lower level and increased according to tolerance and clinical response to a usual maximum of 100 mg daily. In more severely ill patients, dosage may be further increased to 150 mg/day. Doses above 150 mg/day are not recommended in these age groups.

Initial therapy may be administered in divided doses or a single daily dose.

Maintenance therapy may be given on a once-daily schedule for patient convenience and compliance.

HOW SUPPLIED

Norpramin is available in:

10 mg: Blue coated tablets imprinted "68-7".
25 mg: Yellow coated tablets imprinted "NORPRAMIN 25".
50 mg: Green coated tablets imprinted "NORPRAMIN 50".
75 mg: Orange coated tablets imprinted "NORPRAMIN 75".
100 mg: Peach coated tablets imprinted "NORPRAMIN 100".
150 mg: White coated tablets imprinted "NORPRAMIN 150".

Storage: Desipramine HCl tablets should be stored at room temperature, preferably below 30°C (86°F). Protect from excessive heat.

PRODUCT LISTING - RATED THERAPEUTICALLY EQUIVALENT

Tablet - Oral - 10 mg

30's	$18.76	NORPRAMIN, Allscripts Pharmaceutical Company	54569-2006-00
100's	$12.24	FEDERAL UPPER LIMIT, H.C.F.A. F F P	99999-0964-02
100's	$15.90	GENERIC, Ivax Corporation	00182-2652-01
100's	$39.76	GENERIC, Geneva Pharmaceuticals	00781-1971-01
100's	$39.78	GENERIC, Eon Labs Manufacturing Inc	00185-0029-01
100's	$71.11	NORPRAMIN, Aventis Pharmaceuticals	00068-0007-01

Tablet - Oral - 25 mg

100's	$6.75	FEDERAL UPPER LIMIT, H.C.F.A. F F P	99999-0964-01
100's	$12.63	GENERIC, Us Trading Corporation	56126-0376-11
100's	$12.75	GENERIC, Raway Pharmacal Inc	00686-0489-20
100's	$16.80	GENERIC, Interstate Drug Exchange Inc	00814-2300-14
100's	$23.48	GENERIC, Qualitest Products Inc	00603-3166-21
100's	$23.90	GENERIC, Major Pharmaceuticals Inc	00904-1570-60
100's	$26.72	GENERIC, Moore, H.L. Drug Exchange Inc	00839-7551-06
100's	$27.00	GENERIC, Watson/Rugby Laboratories Inc	00536-4881-01
100's	$27.90	GENERIC, Mutual/United Research Laboratories	00677-1198-01
100's	$27.95	GENERIC, Watson/Rugby Laboratories Inc	52544-0808-01
100's	$28.00	GENERIC, Martec Pharmaceuticals Inc	52555-0286-01
100's	$46.35	GENERIC, Ivax Corporation	00182-1332-89
100's	$46.36	GENERIC, Geneva Pharmaceuticals	00781-1972-13
100's	$47.78	GENERIC, Geneva Pharmaceuticals	00781-1972-01
100's	$48.76	GENERIC, Eon Labs Manufacturing Inc	00185-0019-01
100's	$85.44	NORPRAMIN, Aventis Pharmaceuticals	00068-0011-01

Tablet - Oral - 50 mg

30's	$8.12	GENERIC, Prescript Pharmaceuticals	00247-0815-30
100's	$8.25	FEDERAL UPPER LIMIT, H.C.F.A. F F P	99999-0964-04
100's	$16.95	GENERIC, Raway Pharmacal Inc	00686-0490-20
100's	$17.19	GENERIC, Us Trading Corporation	56126-0377-11
100's	$19.24	GENERIC, Prescript Pharmaceuticals	00247-0815-00
100's	$25.28	GENERIC, Interstate Drug Exchange Inc	00814-2301-14
100's	$43.19	GENERIC, Major Pharmaceuticals Inc	00904-1582-61
100's	$45.15	GENERIC, Major Pharmaceuticals Inc	00904-1582-60
100's	$47.50	GENERIC, Major Pharmaceuticals Inc	00904-1571-60
100's	$52.36	GENERIC, Mutual/United Research Laboratories	00677-1199-01
100's	$52.72	GENERIC, Moore, H.L. Drug Exchange Inc	00839-7552-06
100's	$59.29	GENERIC, Sidmak Laboratories Inc	50111-0437-01
100's	$59.35	GENERIC, Watson/Rugby Laboratories Inc	00536-4882-01
100's	$59.35	GENERIC, Watson Laboratories Inc	00591-0809-01
100's	$62.12	GENERIC, Geneva Pharmaceuticals	00781-1973-13
100's	$66.15	GENERIC, Ivax Corporation	00182-1333-89
100's	$89.95	GENERIC, Geneva Pharmaceuticals	00781-1973-01
100's	$91.79	GENERIC, Eon Labs Manufacturing Inc	00185-0721-01
100's	$160.84	NORPRAMIN, Aventis Pharmaceuticals	00068-0015-01

Tablet - Oral - 75 mg

100's	$9.00	FEDERAL UPPER LIMIT, H.C.F.A. F F P	99999-0964-07
100's	$25.00	GENERIC, Raway Pharmacal Inc	00686-0491-20
100's	$53.15	GENERIC, Major Pharmaceuticals Inc	00904-1583-60
100's	$56.35	GENERIC, Watson/Schein Pharmaceuticals Inc	00364-2243-01
100's	$59.85	GENERIC, Martec Pharmaceuticals Inc	52555-0288-01
100's	$59.90	GENERIC, Major Pharmaceuticals Inc	00904-1572-60
100's	$62.84	GENERIC, Moore, H.L. Drug Exchange Inc	00839-7553-06
100's	$65.00	GENERIC, Medirex Inc	57480-0320-01
100's	$65.55	GENERIC, Vangard Labs	00615-3526-13
100's	$66.15	GENERIC, Martec Pharmaceuticals Inc	52555-0566-01
100's	$72.09	GENERIC, Sidmak Laboratories Inc	50111-0438-01
100's	$72.10	GENERIC, Watson/Rugby Laboratories Inc	00536-4883-01
100's	$114.48	GENERIC, Geneva Pharmaceuticals	00781-1974-01
100's	$114.50	GENERIC, Eon Labs Manufacturing Inc	00185-0722-01
100's	$190.80	NORPRAMIN, Aventis Pharmaceuticals	00068-0019-01

Tablet - Oral - 100 mg

100's	$38.97	FEDERAL UPPER LIMIT, H.C.F.A. F F P	99999-0964-10
100's	$110.10	GENERIC, Watson Laboratories Inc	00591-0545-01
100's	$110.10	GENERIC, Major Pharmaceuticals Inc	00904-1573-60
100's	$150.43	GENERIC, Geneva Pharmaceuticals	00781-1975-01
100's	$150.45	GENERIC, Eon Labs Manufacturing Inc	00185-0736-01
100's	$269.00	NORPRAMIN, Aventis Pharmaceuticals	00068-0020-01

Tablet - Oral - 150 mg

50's	$108.98	GENERIC, Geneva Pharmaceuticals	00781-1976-50
50's	$109.00	GENERIC, Eon Labs Manufacturing Inc	00185-0760-53
50's	$194.89	NORPRAMIN, Aventis Pharmaceuticals	00068-0021-50

PRODUCT LISTING - EQUIVALENTS NOT AVAILABLE

Tablet - Oral - 10 mg

15's	$18.00	GENERIC, Southwood Pharmaceuticals Inc	58016-0502-15
28's	$33.60	GENERIC, Southwood Pharmaceuticals Inc	58016-0502-28
30's	$7.90	GENERIC, Pharma Pac	52959-0128-30
30's	$36.00	GENERIC, Southwood Pharmaceuticals Inc	58016-0502-30
50's	$60.00	GENERIC, Southwood Pharmaceuticals Inc	58016-0502-50
60's	$72.00	GENERIC, Southwood Pharmaceuticals Inc	58016-0502-60
100's	$120.00	GENERIC, Southwood Pharmaceuticals Inc	58016-0502-00

Tablet - Oral - 25 mg

7's	$4.00	GENERIC, Prescript Pharmaceuticals	00247-0038-07
14's	$4.65	GENERIC, Prescript Pharmaceuticals	00247-0038-14
14's	$9.00	GENERIC, Southwood Pharmaceuticals Inc	58016-0853-14
14's	$9.86	GENERIC, Pharma Pac	52959-0458-14
15's	$4.74	GENERIC, Prescript Pharmaceuticals	00247-0038-15
15's	$11.27	GENERIC, Southwood Pharmaceuticals Inc	58016-0191-15
20's	$5.21	GENERIC, Prescript Pharmaceuticals	00247-0038-20
20's	$12.85	GENERIC, Southwood Pharmaceuticals Inc	58016-0853-20
20's	$13.73	GENERIC, Pharma Pac	52959-0458-20
25's	$5.67	GENERIC, Prescript Pharmaceuticals	00247-0038-25
28's	$18.00	GENERIC, Southwood Pharmaceuticals Inc	58016-0853-28
28's	$21.03	GENERIC, Southwood Pharmaceuticals Inc	58016-0191-28
30's	$6.13	GENERIC, Prescript Pharmaceuticals	00247-0038-30
30's	$8.39	GENERIC, Allscripts Pharmaceutical Company	54569-0404-01
30's	$19.28	GENERIC, Southwood Pharmaceuticals Inc	58016-0853-30
30's	$22.53	GENERIC, Southwood Pharmaceuticals Inc	58016-0191-30
40's	$7.06	GENERIC, Prescript Pharmaceuticals	00247-0038-40
50's	$37.55	GENERIC, Southwood Pharmaceuticals Inc	58016-0191-50
60's	$8.92	GENERIC, Prescript Pharmaceuticals	00247-0038-60
60's	$38.55	GENERIC, Southwood Pharmaceuticals Inc	58016-0853-60
60's	$45.06	GENERIC, Southwood Pharmaceuticals Inc	58016-0191-60
90's	$11.69	GENERIC, Prescript Pharmaceuticals	00247-0038-90
100's	$27.95	GENERIC, Allscripts Pharmaceutical Company	54569-0404-00
100's	$64.25	GENERIC, Southwood Pharmaceuticals Inc	58016-0853-00
100's	$75.10	GENERIC, Southwood Pharmaceuticals Inc	58016-0191-00

Tablet - Oral - 50 mg

12's	$9.83	GENERIC, Pharma Pac	52959-0464-12
14's	$15.22	GENERIC, Pharma Pac	52959-0464-14
20's	$15.22	GENERIC, Pharma Pac	52959-0464-20
30's	$17.79	GENERIC, Allscripts Pharmaceutical Company	54569-1701-02

Desirudin *(003597)*

Categories: Thrombosis, deep vein, prophylaxis; Pregnancy Category C; FDA Approved 2003 Apr
Drug Classes: Anticoagulants; Thrombin inhibitors
Brand Names: **Iprivask**

WARNING

Spinal/Epidural Hematomas

When neuraxial anesthesia (epidural/spinal anesthesia) or spinal puncture is employed, patients anticoagulated or scheduled to be anticoagulated with selective inhibitors of thrombin such as desirudin may be at risk of developing an epidural or spinal hematoma which can result in long-term or permanent paralysis.

The risk of these events may be increased by the use of indwelling spinal catheters for administration of analgesia or by the concomitant use of drugs affecting hemostasis such as non-steroidal anti-inflammatory drugs (NSAIDs), platelet inhibitors, or other anticoagulants. Likewise with such agents, the risk appears to be increased by traumatic or repeated epidural or spinal puncture.

WARNING — Cont'd

Patients should be frequently monitored for signs and symptoms of neurological impairment. If neurological compromise is noted, urgent treatment is necessary.

The physician should consider the potential benefit versus risk before neuraxial intervention, in patients anticoagulated or to be anticoagulated for thromboprophylaxis (see also WARNINGS).

DESCRIPTION

Iprivask (desirudin for injection) is a specific inhibitor of human thrombin. It has a protein structure that is similar to that of hirudin, the naturally occurring anticoagulant present in the peripharyngeal glands in the medicinal leech, *Hirudo medicinalis.* Hirudin is a single polypeptide chain of 65 amino acids residues and contains three disulfide bridges. Desirudin has a chemical formula of $C_{287}H_{440}N_{80}O_{110}S_6$ with a molecular weight of 6963.52. Desirudin, which is expressed in yeast (*Saccharomyces cerevisiae,* strain TR 1456) by recombinant DNA technology differs from the natural hirudin by lack of a sulfate group on Tyr-63. The biological activity of desirudin is determined through a chromogenic assay which measures the ability of desirudin to inhibit the hydrolysis of a chromogenic peptidic substrate by thrombin in comparison to a desirudin standard. One vial of desirudin contains 15.75 mg desirudin corresponding to approximately 315,000 antithrombin units (ATU) or 20,000 ATU/mg of desirudin with reference to the WHO International Standard (prepared 1991) for alphathrombin.

Iprivask 15 mg is supplied as a sterile, white, freeze dried powder for injection. Each **vial** contains 15.75 mg desirudin and the following inactive ingredients: 1.31 mg anhydrous magnesium chloride, sodium hydroxide for injection. Each **ampule** of diluent for Iprivask contains 0.6 ml sterile mannitol (3%) in water for injection and is preservative free. Iprivask 15 mg is administered by subcutaneous (SC) injection, preferably at an abdominal or thigh site.

To prepare the reconstituted aqueous solution, 0.5 ml of the mannitol diluent is added under aseptic conditions to the vial containing the sterile powder. Shaking gently rapidly disperses the drug. The reconstituted solution has a pH of 7.4.

CLINICAL PHARMACOLOGY

MECHANISM OF ACTION

Desirudin is a selective inhibitor of free circulating and clot-bound thrombin. The anticoagulant properties of desirudin are demonstrated by its ability to prolong the clotting time of human plasma. One molecule of desirudin binds to one molecule of thrombin and thereby blocks the thrombogenic activity of thrombin. As a result, all thrombin-dependent coagulation assays are affected. Activated partial thromboplastin time (aPTT) is a measure of the anticoagulant activity of desirudin and increases in a dose-dependent fashion. The pharmacodynamic effect of desirudin on proteolytic activity of thrombin was assessed as an increase in aPTT. A mean peak aPTT prolongation of about 1.38 times baseline value (range 0.58-3.41) was observed following SC bid injections of 15 mg desirudin. Thrombin time (TT) frequently exceeds 200 seconds even at low plasma concentrations of desirudin, which renders this test unsuitable for routine monitoring of desirudin therapy. At therapeutic serum concentrations, desirudin has no effect on other enzymes of the hemostatic system such as factors IXa, Xa, kallikrein, plasmin, tissue plasminogen activator, or activated protein C. In addition, it does not display any effect on other serine proteases, such as the digestive enzymes trypsin, chymotrypsin, or on complement activation by the classical or alternative pathways.

PHARMACOKINETIC PROPERTIES

Pharmacokinetic parameters were calculated based on plasma concentration data obtained by a non-specific ELISA method that does not discriminate between native desirudin and its metabolites. It is not known if the metabolites are pharmacologically active.

Absorption

The absorption of desirudin is complete when subcutaneously administered at doses of 0.3 or 0.5 mg/kg. Following SC administration of single doses of 0.1-0.75 mg/kg, plasma concentrations of desirudin increased to a maximum level (C_{max}) between 1 and 3 hours. Both C_{max} and area-under-the-curve (AUC) values are dose proportional.

Distribution

The pharmacokinetic properties of desirudin following intravenous (IV) administration are well described by a two- or three-compartment disposition model. Desirudin is distributed in the extracellular space with a volume of distribution at steady state of 0.25 L/kg, independent of the dose. Desirudin binds specifically and directly to thrombin, forming an extremely tight, non-covalent complex with an inhibition constant of approximately 2.6×10^{-13} M. Thus, free or protein bound desirudin immediately binds circulating thrombin. The pharmacological effect of desirudin is not modified when coadministered with highly protein bound drugs (>99%).

Metabolism

Human and animal data suggest that desirudin is primarily eliminated and metabolized by the kidney. The total urinary excretion of unchanged desirudin amounts to 40-50% of the administered dose. Metabolites lacking one or two C-terminal amino acids constitute a minor proportion of the material recovered from urine (<7%). There is no evidence for the presence of other metabolites. This indicates that desirudin is metabolized by stepwise degradation from the C-terminus probably catalyzed by carboxypeptidase(s) such as carboxypeptidase A, originating from the pancreas. Total clearance of desirudin is approximately 1.5-2.7 ml/min/kg following either SC or IV administration and is independent of dose. This clearance value is close to the glomerular filtration rate.

Elimination

The elimination of desirudin from plasma is rapid after IV administration, with approximately 90% of the dose disappearing from the plasma within 2 hours of the injection. Plasma concentrations of desirudin then decline with a mean terminal elimination half-life of 2-3 hours. After SC administration, the mean terminal elimination half-life is also approximately 2 hours.

Special Populations

Renal Insufficiency

In a pharmacokinetic study of renally impaired subjects, subjects with mild [creatinine clearance (CC) between 61 and 90 ml/min/1.73 m² body surface area], moderate (CC between 31 and 60 ml/min/1.73 m² body surface area), and severe (CC below 31 ml/min/1.73 m² body surface area) renal insufficiency, were administered a single IV dose of 0.5, 0.25, or 0.125 mg/kg desirudin, respectively. This resulted in mean dose-normalized AUC(effect) [AUC(0-60th) for aPTT prolongation] increases of approximately 3- and 9-fold for the moderate and severe renally impaired subjects, respectively, compared with healthy individuals. In subjects with mild renal impairment, there was no increase in AUC(effect) compared with healthy individuals. In subjects with severe renal insufficiency, terminal elimination half-lives were prolonged up to 12 hours compared with 2-4 hours in normal volunteers or subjects with mild to moderate renal insufficiency (see WARNINGS). Dose adjustments are recommended in certain circumstances in relation to the degree of impairment or degree of aPTT abnormality (see WARNINGS, Renal Insufficiency; PRECAUTIONS, Laboratory Tests; and TABLE 4).

D

Hepatic Insufficiency

No pharmacokinetic studies have been conducted to investigate the effects of desirudin in hepatic insufficiency (see PRECAUTIONS, Hepatic Insufficiency/Liver Injury and DOSAGE AND ADMINISTRATION).

Age/Gender

The mean plasma clearance of desirudin in patients ≥65 years of age (n=12; 110 ml/min) is approximately 28% lower than in patients <65 years of age (n=8; 153 ml/min). Population pharmacokinetics conducted in 301 patients undergoing elective total hip replacement indicate that age or gender do not affect the systemic clearance of desirudin when renal creatinine clearance is considered. This drug is substantially excreted by the kidney, and the risk of adverse events due to it may be greater in patients with impaired renal function. Because elderly patients are more likely to have decreased renal function, care should be taken in dose selection, and it may be useful to monitor renal function. Dosage adjustment in the case of moderate and severe renal impairment is necessary. (See Renal Insufficiency and DOSAGE AND ADMINISTRATION, Initial Dosage, Use in Renal Insufficiency.)

INDICATIONS AND USAGE

Desirudin is indicated for the prophylaxis of deep vein thrombosis, which may lead to pulmonary embolism, in patients undergoing elective hip replacement surgery.

CONTRAINDICATIONS

Desirudin is contraindicated in patients with known hypersensitivity to natural or recombinant hirudins, and in patients with active bleeding and/or irreversible coagulation disorders.

WARNINGS

RENAL INSUFFICIENCY

Desirudin must be used with caution in patients with renal impairment, particularly in those with moderate and severe renal impairment (creatinine clearance ≤60 ml/min/1.73 m² body surface area) (see CLINICAL PHARMACOLOGY, Pharmacokinetics, Special Populations, Renal Insufficiency). Dose reductions by factors of 3 and 9 are recommended for patients with moderate and severe renal impairment respectively (see DOSAGE AND ADMINISTRATION). In addition, daily aPTT and serum creatinine monitoring are recommended for patients with moderate or severe renal impairment (see PRECAUTIONS, Laboratory Tests).

HEMORRHAGIC EVENTS

Desirudin is not intended for intramuscular injection as local hematoma formation may result.

Desirudin, like other anticoagulants, should be used with caution in patients with increased risks of hemorrhage such as those with recent major surgery, organ biopsy or puncture of a non-compressible vessel within the last month; a history of hemorrhagic stroke, intracranial or intraocular bleeding including diabetic (hemorrhagic) retinopathy; recent ischemic stroke, severe uncontrolled hypertension, bacterial endocarditis, a known hemostatic disorder (congenital or acquired, *e.g.,* hemophilia, liver disease) or a history of gastrointestinal or pulmonary bleeding within the past 3 months.

Bleeding can occur at any site during therapy with desirudin. An unexplained fall in hematocrit or blood pressure should lead to a search for a bleeding site.

SPINAL/EPIDURAL ANESTHESIA

As with other anticoagulants, there is a risk of neuraxial hematoma formation with the concurrent use of desirudin and spinal/epidural anesthesia, which has the potential to result in long term or permanent paralysis. The risk may be greater with the use of post-operative indwelling catheters or the concomitant use of additional drugs affecting hemostasis such as NSAIDs (Non-Steroidal Anti-Inflammatory Drugs), platelet inhibitors or other anticoagulants (see BOXED WARNING and DRUG INTERACTIONS). The risk may also be increased by traumatic or repeated neuraxial puncture.

To reduce the potential risk of bleeding associated with the concurrent use of desirudin and epidural or spinal anesthesia/analgesia, the pharmacokinetic profile of the drug should be considered (see CLINICAL PHARMACOLOGY, Pharmacokinetic Properties) when scheduling or using epidural or spinal anesthesia in proximity to desirudin administration. The physician should consider placement of the catheter prior to initiating desirudin and removal of the catheter when the anticoagulant effect of desirudin is low (see DOSAGE AND ADMINISTRATION).

Should the physician decide to administer anticoagulation in the context of epidural/spinal anesthesia, extreme vigilance and frequent monitoring must be exercised to detect any signs and symptoms of neurological impairment such as midline back pain, sensory and motor deficits (numbness or weakness in lower limbs), bowel and/or bladder dysfunction. Patients should be instructed to inform their physician immediately if they experience any of the above signs or symptoms. If signs or symptoms of spinal hematoma are suspected, urgent diagnosis and treatment including spinal cord decompression should be initiated.

The physician should consider the potential benefit versus risk before neuraxial intervention in patients anticoagulated or to be anticoagulated for thromboprophylaxis (see also Hemorrhage and DRUG INTERACTIONS).

Desirudin cannot be used interchangeably with other hirudins as they differ in manufacturing process and specific biological activity (ATUs). Each of these medicines has its own instructions for use.

PRECAUTIONS

ANTIBODIES/RE-EXPOSURE

Antibodies have been reported in patients treated with hirudins. Potential for cross-sensitivity to hirudin products cannot be excluded. Irritative skin reactions were observed in 9/322 volunteers exposed to desirudin by SC injection or IV bolus or infusion in single or multiple administrations of the drug. Allergic events were reported in <2% of patients who were administered desirudin in Phase 3 clinical trials. Allergic events were reported in 1% of patients receiving unfractionated heparin and 1% of patients receiving enoxaparin. Hirudin-specific IgE evaluations may not be indicative of sensitivity to desirudin as this test was not always positive in the presence of symptoms. Very rarely, anti-hirudin antibodies have been detected upon re-exposure to desirudin. (See ADVERSE REACTIONS, Non-Hemorrhagic Events, Allergic Reactions.) Fatal anaphylactoid reactions have been reported during hirudin therapy.

HEPATIC INSUFFICIENCY/LIVER INJURY

No information is available about the use of desirudin in patients with hepatic insufficiency/liver injury. Although desirudin is not significantly metabolized by the liver, hepatic impairment or serious liver injury (*e.g.*, liver cirrhosis) may alter the anticoagulant effect of desirudin due to coagulation defects secondary to reduced generation of vitamin K-dependent coagulation factors. Desirudin should be used with caution in these patients.

LABORATORY TESTS

Activated partial thromboplastin time (aPTT) should be monitored daily in patients with increased risk of bleeding and/or renal impairment. Serum creatinine should be monitored daily in patients with renal impairment. Peak aPTT should not exceed 2 times control. Should peak aPTT exceed this level, dose reduction is advised based on the degree of aPTT abnormality (see DOSAGE AND ADMINISTRATION, Initial Dosage, Use in Renal Insufficiency). If necessary, therapy with desirudin should be interrupted until aPTT falls to less than 2 times control, at which time treatment with desirudin can be resumed at a reduced dose. (See DRUG INTERACTIONS for information on use of desirudin in conjunction with other drugs affecting coagulation.) Thrombin time (TT) is not a suitable test for routine monitoring of desirudin therapy (see CLINICAL PHARMACOLOGY, Mechanism of Action). Dose adjustments based on serum creatinine may be necessary (see DOSAGE AND ADMINISTRATION, Initial Dosage, Use in Renal Insufficiency).

ANIMAL PHARMACOLOGY AND TOXICOLOGY

General Toxicity

Desirudin produced bleeding, local inflammation, and granulation at injection sites in rat and dog toxicity studies. In a 28 day study in Rhesus monkeys, there was also evidence of SC bleeding and local inflammation at the injection sites. In addition, desirudin was immunogenic in dogs and formed antibody complexes resulting in prolonged half-life and accumulation. Desirudin showed sensitization potential in guinea pig immediate and delayed hypersensitivity models.

CARCINOGENESIS, MUTAGENESIS, AND IMPAIRMENT OF FERTILITY

No long-term studies in animals have been performed to evaluate the carcinogenic potential of desirudin.

Desirudin was not genotoxic in the Ames test, the Chinese hamster lung cell (V79/HGPRT) forward mutation test or the rat micronucleus test. It was, however, equivocal in its genotoxic effect in Chinese hamster ovarian cell (CCL 61) chromosome aberration tests.

Desirudin at SC doses up to 10 mg/kg/day (about 2.7 times the recommended human dose based on body surface area) was found to have no effect on fertility and reproductive performance of male and female rats.

PREGNANCY, TERATOGENIC EFFECTS, PREGNANCY CATEGORY C

Teratology studies have been performed in rats at SC doses in a range of 1-15 mg/kg/day (about 0.3 to 4 times the recommended human dose based on body surface area) and in rabbits at IV doses in a range of 0.6 to 6 mg/kg/day (about 0.3 to 3 times the recommended human dose based on body surface area) and have revealed desirudin to be teratogenic. Observed teratogenic findings were: omphalocele, asymmetric and fused sternebrae, edema, shortened hind limbs, etc. in rats; and spina bifida, malrotated hind limb, hydrocephaly, gastroschisis, etc. in rabbits. There are no adequate and well controlled studies in pregnant women. Desirudin should be used during pregnancy only if the potential benefit justifies the potential risk to the fetus.

NURSING MOTHERS

It is not known whether desirudin is excreted in human milk. Because many drugs are excreted in human milk, caution should be exercised when desirudin is administered to a nursing woman.

PEDIATRIC USE

Safety and effectiveness in pediatric patients have not been established.

GERIATRIC USE

In three clinical studies of desirudin, the percentage of patients greater than 65 years of age treated with 15 mg of desirudin subcutaneously every 12 hours was 58.5%, while 20.8% were 75 years of age or older. Elderly patients treated with desirudin had a reduction in the incidence of VTE similar to that observed in the younger patients, and a slightly lower incidence of VTE compared to those patients treated with heparin or enoxaparin.

Regarding safety, in the clinical studies the incidence of hemorrhage (major or otherwise) in patients 65 years of age or older was similar to that in patients less than 65 years of age. In addition, the elderly had a similar incidence of total, treatment-related, or serious adverse events compared to those patients less than 65 years of age. Serious adverse events occurred more frequently in patients 75 years of age or older as compared to those less than 65 years of age. In general, 15 mg desirudin every 12 hours can be used safely in the geriatric population as in the population of patients less than 65 years of age so long as renal function is adequate (see CLINICAL PHARMACOLOGY, Pharmacokinetics, Special Populations, Renal Insufficiency and DOSAGE AND ADMINISTRATION, Initial Dosage, Use in Renal Insufficiency).

DRUG INTERACTIONS

Any agent which may enhance the risk of hemorrhage should be discontinued prior to initiation of desirudin therapy. These agents include medications such as Dextran 40, systemic glucocorticoids, thrombolytics, and anticoagulants. If coadministration cannot be avoided, close clinical and laboratory monitoring should be conducted. During prophylaxis of venous thromboembolism, concomitant treatment with heparins (unfractionated and low-molecular weight heparins) or dextrans is not recommended. The effects of desirudin and unfractionated heparins on prolongation of aPTT are additive.

As with other anticoagulants, desirudin should be used with caution in conjunction with drugs which affect platelet function. These medications include systemic salicylates, NSAIDS including ketorolac, acetylsalicylic acid, ticlopidine, dipyridamole, sulfinpyrazone, clopidogrel, abciximab and other glycoprotein IIb/IIIa antagonists (see PRECAUTIONS, Laboratory Tests).

USE IN PATIENTS SWITCHING FROM ORAL ANTICOAGULANTS TO DESIRUDIN OR FROM DESIRUDIN TO ORAL ANTICOAGULANTS

The concomitant administration of warfarin did not significantly affect the pharmacokinetic effects of desirudin. When warfarin and desirudin were coadministered, greater inhibition of hemostasis measured by activated partial thromboplastin time (aPTT), prothrombin time (PT), and international normalized ratio (INR) was observed. If a patient is switched from oral anticoagulants to desirudin therapy or from desirudin to oral anticoagulants, the anticoagulant activity should continue to be closely monitored with appropriate methods. That activity should be taken into account in the evaluation of the overall coagulation status of the patient during the switch.

ADVERSE REACTIONS

In the Phase 2 and 3 clinical studies, desirudin was administered to 2159 patients undergoing elective hip replacement surgery to determine the safety and efficacy of desirudin in preventing VTE in this population. Below is the safety profile of the desirudin 15 mg (q12h) regimen from these 5 multicenter clinical trials.

HEMORRHAGIC EVENTS

TABLE 2 shows the rates of hemorrhagic events that have been reported during clinical trials.

TABLE 2 *Hemorrhage in Patients Undergoing Hip Replacement Surgery*

	Dosing Regimen		
	Desirudin 15 mg q12h SC	Heparin 5000 IU q8h SC	Enoxaparin 40 mg qd SC
	n=1561	n=501	n=1036
Patients with any hemorrhage*	464 (30%)	111 (22%)	341 (33%)
Patients with serious hemorrhage†	41 (3%)	15 (3%)	21 (2%)
Patients with major hemorrhage‡	13 (<1%)	0 (0%)	2 (<1%)

* Includes hematomas which occurred at an incidence of 6% in the desirudin and enoxaparin treatment groups and 5% in the heparin treatment group.

† Bleeding complications were considered *serious* if perioperative transfusion requirements exceeded 5 units of whole blood or packed red cells, or if total transfusion requirements up to postoperative Day 6 inclusive exceeded 7 units of whole blood or packed red cells, or total blood loss up to postoperative Day 6 inclusive exceeded 3500 ml.

‡ Bleeding complications were considered *major* if the hemorrhage was: (1) overt and it produced a fall in hemoglobin of ≥2 g/dl or if it lead to a transfusion of 2 or more units of whole or packed cells outside the perioperative period (the time from start of surgery until up to 12 hours after); (2) Retroperitoneal, intracranial, intraocular, intraspinal, or occurred in a major prosthetic joint.

NON-HEMORRHAGIC EVENTS

Non-hemorrhagic adverse events occurring at ≥2% incidence in patients treated with desirudin 15 mg (q12h) during elective hip replacement surgery *and* considered to be remotely, possibly, or probably related to desirudin are provided in TABLE 3.

Related adverse events with a frequency of <2% and >0.2% (in decreasing order of frequency): Thrombosis, hypotension, leg edema, fever, decreased hemoglobin, hematuria, dizziness, epistaxis, vomiting, impaired healing, cerebrovascular disorder, leg pain, hematemesis.

Allergic reactions: In clinical studies, allergic events were reported <2% overall and in 2% of patients who were administered 15 mg desirudin. (See PRECAUTIONS, Antibodies/Re-Exposure.)

TABLE 3 *Adverse Events Occurring at ≥2% in Desirudin Treated Patients Undergoing Hip Replacement Surgery*†*

Body System (Preferred Term)	Desirudin 15 mg q12h SC n=1561	Heparin 5000 IU q8h SC n=501	Enoxaparin 40 mg qd SC n=1036
Injection site mass	56 (4%)	32 (6%)	7 (<1%)
Wound secretion	59 (4%)	23 (5%)	34 (3%)
Anemia	51 (3%)	11 (2%)	37 (4%)
Deep thrombophlebitis	24 (2%)	41 (8%)	22 (2%)
Nausea	24 (2%)	5 (<1%)	10 (<1%)

* Represents events reported while on treatment, excluding unrelated adverse events.
† All hemorrhages that occurred are included in Hemorrhagic Events.

POST MARKETING

In addition to adverse events reported from clinical trials the following adverse events have been identified during post approval use of desirudin. These events were reported voluntarily from a population of unknown size and the frequency of occurrence cannot be determined precisely: rare reports of major hemorrhages, some of which were fatal, and anaphylactic/anaphylactoid reactions.

DOSAGE AND ADMINISTRATION

All patients should be evaluated for bleeding disorder risk before prophylactic administration of desirudin (see DRUG INTERACTIONS).

INITIAL DOSAGE

In patients undergoing hip replacement surgery, the recommended dose of desirudin is **15 mg every 12 hours** administered by SC injection with the initial dose given up to 5-15 minutes prior to surgery, but *after* induction of regional block anesthesia, if used (see WARNINGS, Spinal/Epidural Anesthesia). Up to 12 days administration (average duration 9-12 days) of desirudin has been well tolerated in controlled clinical trials.

Use in Renal Insufficiency

TABLE 4

Degree of Renal Insufficiency	Creatinine Clearance [ml/min/1.73 m^2 body surface area]	aPTT Monitoring & Dosing Instructions
Moderate	≥31 to 60	Initiate therapy at 5 mg every 12 hours by SC injection. Monitor aPTT and serum creatinine at least daily. *If* aPTT exceeds 2 times control: 1. Interrupt therapy until the value returns to less than 2 times control; 2. Resume therapy at a reduced dose guided by the initial degree of aPTT abnormality.
Severe*	<31	Initiate therapy at 1.7 mg every 12 hours. Monitor aPTT and serum creatinine at least daily. *If* aPTT exceeds 2 times control: 1. Interrupt therapy until the value returns to less than 2 times control; 2. Consider further dose reductions guided by the initial degree of aPTT abnormality.

* See CLINICAL PHARMACOLOGY, Pharmacokinetics, Special Populations, Renal Insufficiency and WARNINGS, Renal Insufficiency.

Use in Hepatic Insufficiency

In the absence of clinical studies in this population, dosing recommendations cannot be made at this time (see CLINICAL PHARMACOLOGY: Metabolism and Pharmacokinetics, Special Populations, Hepatic Insufficiency; and PRECAUTIONS, Hepatic Insufficiency/Liver Injury).

HOW SUPPLIED

Iprivask (desirudin for injection) is supplied as a single dose (15.75 mg) lyophilized powder with an accompanying sterile, non-pyrogenic diluent [0.6 ml of mannitol (3%) in water for injection].

Storage: Protect from light.

Unopened vials or ampules: Store at 25°C (77°F); excursions permitted to 15-30°C (59-86°F).

Keep this and all medicines out of the reach of children.

Desloratadine *(003543)*

For related information, see the comparative table section in Appendix A.

Categories: Rhinitis, allergic; Urticaria, chronic idiopathic; FDA Approved 2001 Dec; Pregnancy Category C
Drug Classes: Antihistamines, H1
Brand Names: **Clarinex**; Clarinex RediTabs
Foreign Brand Availability: Aerius (Austria; Belgium; Bulgaria; Colombia; Czech-Republic; Denmark; England; Finland; France; Germany; Greece; Hong-Kong; Hungary; Ireland; Israel; Italy; Netherlands; Norway; Poland; Portugal; Slovenia; Spain; Sweden; Switzerland; Turkey); Allex (Austria; Belgium; Bulgaria; Czech-Republic; Denmark; England; Finland; France; Germany; Greece; Hungary; Ireland; Italy; Netherlands; Norway; Poland; Portugal; Slovenia; Spain; Sweden; Switzerland; Turkey); Azomyr (Austria; Belgium; Bulgaria; Czech-Republic; Denmark; England; Finland; France; Germany; Greece; Hungary; Ireland; Italy; Netherlands; Norway; Poland; Portugal; Slovenia; Spain; Sweden; Switzerland; Turkey); Claramax (New-Zealand); Desalex (Colombia); Deslor (India); Neoclarityn (Austria; Belgium; Bulgaria; Czech-Republic; Denmark; England; Finland; France; Germany; Greece; Hungary; Ireland; Italy; Netherlands; Norway; Poland; Portugal; Slovenia; Spain; Sweden; Switzerland; Turkey); Opulis (Austria; Belgium; Bulgaria; Czech-Republic; Denmark; England; Finland; France; Germany; Greece; Hungary; Ireland; Italy; Netherlands; Norway; Poland; Portugal; Slovenia; Spain; Sweden; Switzerland; Turkey)
Cost of Therapy: $70.55 (Allergic Rhinitis; Clarinex; 5 mg; 1 tablet/day; 30 day supply)

DESCRIPTION

Clarinex (desloratadine) tablets are light blue, round, film coated tablets containing 5 mg desloratadine, an antihistamine, to be administered orally. It also contains the following excipients: dibasic calcium phosphate dihydrate, microcrystalline cellulose, corn starch, talc, carnauba wax, white wax, coating material consisting of lactose monohydrate, hydroxypropyl methylcellulose, titanium dioxide, polyethylene glycol, and FD&C blue no. 2 aluminum lake.

The Clarinex RediTabs brand of desloratadine orally-disintegrating tablets is a pink colored round tablet shaped unit with a "C" debossed on one side. Each RediTabs unit contains 5 mg of desloratadine. It also contains the following inactive ingredients: gelatin Type B, mannitol, aspartame, polarcrillin potassium, citric acid, red dye and tutti frutti flavoring.

Desloratadine is a white to off-white powder that is slightly soluble in water, but very soluble in ethanol and propylene glycol. It has an empirical formula: $C_{19}H_{19}ClN_2$ and a molecular weight of 310.8. The chemical name is 8-chloro-6,11-dihydro-11-(4-piperdinylidene)-5*H*-benzo[5,6]cyclohepta[1,2-*b*]pyridine.

CLINICAL PHARMACOLOGY

MECHANISM OF ACTION

Desloratadine is a long-acting tricyclic histamine antagonist with selective H_1-receptor histamine antagonist activity. Receptor binding data indicates that at a concentration of 2-3 ng/ml (7 nmol), desloratadine shows significant interaction with the human histamine H_1 receptor. Desloratadine inhibited histamine release from human mast cells *in vitro*.

Results of a radiolabeled tissue distribution study in rats and a radioligand H_1-receptor binding study in guinea pigs showed that desloratadine does not readily cross the blood brain barrier.

PHARMACOKINETICS

Absorption

Following oral administration of desloratadine 5 mg once daily for 10 days to normal healthy volunteers, the mean time to maximum plasma concentrations (T_{max}) occurred at approximately 3 hours post dose and mean steady state peak plasma concentrations (C_{max}) and area under the concentration-time curve (AUC) of 4 ng/ml and 56.9 ng·h/ml were observed, respectively. Neither food nor grapefruit juice had an effect on the bioavailability (C_{max} and AUC) of desloratadine.

The pharmacokinetic profile of desloratadine orally-disintegrating tablets was evaluated in a three way crossover study in 30 adult volunteers. A single desloratadine orally-disintegrating tablet containing 5 mg of desloratadine was bioequivalent to a single 5 mg desloratadine tablet and was bioequivalent to 10 ml of desloratadine syrup containing 5 mg of desloratadine for both desloratadine and 3-hydroxydesloratadine. In a separate study with 30 adult volunteers, food or water had no effect on the bioavailability (AUC and C_{max}) of desloratadine orally-disintegrating tablets, however, food shifted the desloratadine median T_{max} value from 2.5 to 4 hours.

Distribution

Desloratadine and 3-hydroxydesloratadine are approximately 82-87% and 85-89%, bound to plasma proteins, respectively. Protein binding of desloratadine and 3-hydroxydesloratadine was unaltered in subjects with impaired renal function.

Metabolism

Desloratadine (a major metabolite of loratadine) is extensively metabolized to 3-hydroxydesloratadine, an active metabolite, which is subsequently glucuronidated. The enzyme(s) responsible for the formation of 3-hydroxydesloratadine have not been identified. Data from clinical trials indicate that a subset of the general patient population has a decreased ability to form 3-hydroxydesloratadine, and are slow metabolizers of desloratadine. In pharmacokinetic studies (n=1087), approximately 7% of subjects were slow metabolizers of desloratadine (defined as a subject with an AUC ratio of 3-hydroxydesloratadine to desloratadine less than 0.1, or a subject with a desloratadine half-life exceeding 50 hours). The frequency of slow metabolizers is higher in Blacks (approximately 20% of Blacks were slow metabolizers in pharmacokinetic studies, n=276). The median exposure (AUC) to desloratadine in the slow metabolizers was approximately 6-fold greater than the subjects who are not slow metabolizers. Subjects who are slow metabolizers of desloratadine cannot be prospectively identified and will be exposed to higher levels of desloratadine following dosing with the recommended dose of desloratadine. Although not seen in these pharmacokinetic studies, patients who are slow metabolizers may be more susceptible to dose-related adverse events.

Elimination

The mean elimination half-life of desloratadine was 27 hours. C_{max} and AUC values increased in a dose proportional manner following single oral doses between 5 and 20 mg. The degree of accumulation after 14 days of dosing was consistent with the half-life and dosing frequency. A human mass balance study documented a recovery of approximately 87% of the ^{14}C-desloratadine dose, which was equally distributed in urine and feces as metabolic products. Analysis of plasma 3-hydroxydesloratadine showed similar T_{max} and half-life values compared to desloratadine.

SPECIAL POPULATIONS

Geriatric

D

In older subjects (≥65 years old; n=17) following multiple-dose administration of desloratadine tablets, the mean C_{max} and AUC values for desloratadine were 20% greater than in younger subjects (<65 years old). The oral total body clearance (CL/F) when normalized for body weight was similar between the two age groups. The mean plasma elimination half-life of desloratadine was 33.7 hours in subjects ≥65 years old. The pharmacokinetics for 3-hydroxydesloratadine appeared unchanged in older versus younger subjects. These age-related differences are unlikely to be clinically relevant and no dosage adjustment is recommended in elderly subjects.

Renally Impaired

Desloratadine pharmacokinetics following a single dose of 7.5 mg were characterized in patients with mild (n=7; creatinine clearance 51-69 ml/min/1.73 m^2), moderate (n=6; creatinine clearance 34-43 ml/min/1.73 m^2), and severe (n=6; creatinine clearance 5-29 ml/min/1.73 m^2) renal impairment or hemodialysis dependent (n=6) patients. In patients with mild and moderate renal impairment, median C_{max} and AUC values increased by approximately 1.2- and 1.9-fold, respectively, relative to subjects with normal renal function. In patients with severe renal impairment or who were hemodialysis dependent, C_{max} and AUC values increased by approximately 1.7- and 2.5-fold, respectively. Minimal changes in 3-hydroxydesloratadine concentrations were observed. Desloratadine and 3-hydroxydesloratadine were poorly removed by hemodialysis. Plasma protein binding of desloratadine and 3-hydroxydesloratadine was unaltered by renal impairment. Dosage adjustment for patients with renal impairment is recommended (see DOSAGE AND ADMINISTRATION).

Hepatically Impaired

Desloratadine pharmacokinetics were characterized following a single oral dose in patients with mild (n=4), moderate (n=4), and severe (n=4) hepatic impairment as defined by the Child-Pugh classification of hepatic function and 8 subjects with normal hepatic function. Patients with hepatic impairment, regardless of severity, had approximately a 2.4-fold increase in AUC as compared with normal subjects. The apparent oral clearance of desloratadine in patients with mild, moderate, and severe hepatic impairment was 37%, 36%, and 28% of that in normal subjects, respectively. An increase in the mean elimination half-life of desloratadine in patients with hepatic impairment was observed. For 3-hydroxydesloratadine, the mean C_{max} and AUC values for patients with hepatic impairment were not statistically significantly different from subjects with normal hepatic function. Dosage adjustment for patients with hepatic impairment is recommended (see DOSAGE AND ADMINISTRATION).

Gender

Female subjects treated for 14 days with desloratadine tablets had 10% and 3% higher desloratadine C_{max} and AUC values, respectively, compared with male subjects. The 3-hydroxydesloratadine C_{max} and AUC values were also increased by 45% and 48%, respectively, in females compared with males. However, these apparent differences are not likely to be clinically relevant and therefore no dosage adjustment is recommended.

Race

Following 14 days of treatment with desloratadine tablets, the C_{max} and AUC values for desloratadine were 18% and 32% higher, respectively, in Blacks compared with Caucasians. For 3-hydroxydesloratadine there was a corresponding 10% reduction in C_{max} and AUC values in Blacks compared to Caucasians. These differences are not likely to be clinically relevant and therefore no dose adjustment is recommended.

DRUG INTERACTIONS

In two controlled crossover clinical pharmacology studies in healthy male (n=12 in each study) and female (n=12 in each study) volunteers, desloratadine 7.5 mg (1.5 times the daily dose) once daily was coadministered with erythromycin 500 mg every 8 hours or ketoconazole 200 mg every 12 hours for 10 days. In 3 separate controlled, parallel group clinical pharmacology studies, desloratadine at the clinical dose of 5 mg has been coadministered with azithromycin 500 mg followed by 250 mg once daily for 4 days (n=18) or with fluoxetine 20 mg once daily for 7 days after a 23 day pretreatment period with fluoxetine (n=18) or with cimetidine 600 mg every 12 hours for 14 days (n=18) under steady state conditions to normal healthy male and female volunteers. Although increased plasma concentrations [C_{max} and AUC(0-24h)] of desloratadine and 3-hydroxydesloratadine were observed (see TABLE 1), there were no clinically relevant changes in the safety profile of desloratadine, as assessed by electrocardiographic parameters (including the corrected QT interval), clinical laboratory tests, vital signs, and adverse events.

PHARMACODYNAMICS

Wheal and Flare

Human histamine skin wheal studies following single and repeated 5 mg doses of desloratadine have shown that the drug exhibits an antihistaminic effect by 1 hour; this activity may persist for as long as 24 hours. There was no evidence of histamine-induced skin wheal tachyphylaxis within the desloratadine 5 mg group over the 28 day treatment period. The clinical relevance of histamine wheal skin testing is unknown.

TABLE 1 *Changes in Desloratadine and 3-Hydroxydesloratadine Pharmacokinetics in Healthy Male and Female Volunteers*

	Desloratadine		3-Hydroxydesloratadine	
	C_{max}	AUC(0-24h)	C_{max}	AUC(0-24h)
Erythromycin (500 mg q8h)	+24%	+14%	+43%	+40%
Ketoconazole (200 mg q12h)	+45%	+39%	+43%	+72%
Azithromycin (500 mg day 1, 250 mg qd × 4 days)	+15%	+5%	+15%	+4%
Fluoxetine (20 mg qd)	+15%	+0%	+17%	+13%
Cimetidine (600 mg q12h)	+12%	+19%	-11%	-3%

Effects on QTc

Single dose administration of desloratadine did not alter the corrected QT interval (QTc) in rats (up to 12 mg/kg, oral), or guinea pigs (25 mg/kg, intravenous). Repeated oral administration at doses up to 24 mg/kg for durations up to 3 months in monkeys did not alter the QTc at an estimated desloratadine exposure (AUC) that was approximately 955 times the mean AUC in humans at the recommended daily oral dose.

INDICATIONS AND USAGE

ALLERGIC RHINITIS

Desloratadine tablets 5 mg are indicated for the relief of the nasal and non-nasal symptoms of allergic rhinitis (seasonal and perennial) in patients 12 years of age and older.

CHRONIC IDIOPATHIC URTICARIA

Desloratadine tablets are indicated for the symptomatic relief of pruritus, reduction in the number of hives, and size of hives, in patients with chronic idiopathic urticaria 12 years of age and older.

CONTRAINDICATIONS

Desloratadine tablets 5 mg are contraindicated in patients who are hypersensitive to this medication or to any of its ingredients, or to loratadine.

PRECAUTIONS

CARCINOGENESIS, MUTAGENESIS, AND IMPAIRMENT OF FERTILITY

The carcinogenic potential of desloratadine was assessed using loratadine studies. In an 18 month study in mice and a 2 year study in rats, loratadine was administered in the diet at doses up to 40 mg/kg/day in mice (estimated desloratadine and desloratadine metabolite exposures were approximately 3 times the AUC in humans at the recommended daily oral dose) and 25 mg/kg/day in rats (estimated desloratadine and desloratadine metabolite exposures were approximately 30 times the AUC in humans at the recommended daily oral dose). Male mice given 40 mg/kg/day loratadine had a significantly higher incidence of hepatocellular tumors (combined adenomas and carcinomas) than concurrent controls. In rats, a significantly higher incidence of hepatocellular tumors (combined adenomas and carcinomas) was observed in males given 10 mg/kg/day and in males and females given 25 mg/kg/day. The estimated desloratadine and desloratadine metabolite exposures of rats given 10 mg/kg of loratadine were approximately 7 times the AUC in humans at the recommended daily oral dose. The clinical significance of these findings during long-term use of desloratadine is not known.

In genotoxicity studies with desloratadine, there was no evidence of genotoxic potential in a reverse mutation assay (*Salmonella/E. coli* mammalian microsome bacterial mutagenicity assay) or in two assays for chromosomal aberrations (human peripheral blood lymphocyte clastogenicity assay and mouse bone marrow micronucleus assay).

There was no effect on female fertility in rats at desloratadine doses up to 24 mg/kg/day (estimated desloratadine and desloratadine metabolite exposures were approximately 130 times the AUC in humans at the recommended daily oral dose). A male specific decrease in fertility, demonstrated by reduced female conception rates, decreased sperm numbers and motility, and histopathologic testicular changes, occurred at an oral desloratadine dose of 12 mg/kg in rats (estimated desloratadine exposures were approximately 45 times the AUC in humans at the recommended daily oral dose). Desloratadine had no effect on fertility in rats at an oral dose of 3 mg/kg/day (estimated desloratadine and desloratadine metabolite exposures were approximately 8 times the AUC in humans at the recommended daily oral dose).

PREGNANCY CATEGORY C

Desloratadine was not teratogenic in rats at doses up to 48 mg/kg/day (estimated desloratadine and desloratadine metabolite exposures were approximately 210 times the AUC in humans at the recommended daily oral dose) or in rabbits at doses up to 60 mg/kg/day (estimated desloratadine exposures were approximately 230 times the AUC in humans at the recommended daily oral dose). In a separate study, an increase in pre-implantation loss and a decreased number of implantations and fetuses were noted in female rats at 24 mg/kg (estimated desloratadine and desloratadine metabolite exposures were approximately 120 times the AUC in humans at the recommended daily oral dose). Reduced body weight and slow righting reflex were reported in pups at doses of 9 mg/kg/day or greater (estimated desloratadine and desloratadine metabolite exposures were approximately 50 times or greater than the AUC in humans at the recommended daily oral dose). Desloratadine had no effect on pup development at an oral dose of 3 mg/kg/day (estimated desloratadine and desloratadine metabolite exposures were approximately 7 times the AUC in humans at the recommended daily oral dose). There are, however, no adequate and well-controlled studies in pregnant women. Because animal reproduction studies are not always predictive of human response, desloratadine should be used during pregnancy only if clearly needed.

NURSING MOTHERS

Desloratadine passes into breast milk, therefore a decision should be made whether to discontinue nursing or to discontinue desloratadine, taking into account the importance of the drug to the mother.

PEDIATRIC USE

The safety and effectiveness of desloratadine tablets in pediatric patients under 12 years of age have not been established.

GERIATRIC USE

Clinical studies of desloratadine did not include sufficient numbers of subjects aged 65 and over to determine whether they respond differently from younger subjects. Other reported clinical experience has not identified differences between the elderly and younger patients. In general, dose selection for an elderly patient should be cautious, reflecting the greater frequency of decreased hepatic, renal, or cardiac function, and of concomitant disease or other drug therapy. (See CLINICAL PHARMACOLOGY, Special Populations.)

INFORMATION FOR THE PATIENT

Patients should be instructed to use desloratadine tablets as directed. As there are no food effects on bioavailability, patients can be instructed that desloratadine tablets may be taken without regard to meals. Patients should be advised not to increase the dose or dosing frequency as studies have not demonstrated increased effectiveness at higher doses and somnolence may occur.

Phenylketonurics: Desloratadine orally-disintegrating tablets contain phenylalanine 1.75 mg per tablet.

ADVERSE REACTIONS

ALLERGIC RHINITIS

In multiple-dose placebo-controlled trials, 2834 patients received desloratadine tablets at doses of 2.5 to 20 mg daily, of whom 1655 patients received the recommended daily dose of 5 mg. In patients receiving 5 mg daily, the rate of adverse events was similar between desloratadine and placebo-treated patients. The percent of patients who withdrew prematurely due to adverse events was 2.4% in the desloratadine group and 2.6% in the placebo group. There were no serious adverse events in these trials in patients receiving desloratadine. All adverse events that were reported by greater than or equal to 2% of patients who received the recommended daily dose of desloratadine tablets (5.0 mg once-daily), and that were more common with desloratadine tablet than placebo, are listed in TABLE 5.

***TABLE 5** Incidence of Adverse Events Reported by ≥2% of Allergic Rhinitis Patients in Placebo-Controlled, Multiple-Dose Clinical Trials*

Adverse Experience	Desloratadine 5 mg (n=1655)	Placebo (n=1652)
Pharyngitis	4.1%	2.0%
Dry mouth	3.0%	1.9%
Myalgia	2.1%	1.8%
Fatigue	2.1%	1.2%
Somnolence	2.1%	1.8%
Dysmenorrhea	2.1%	1.6%

The frequency and magnitude of laboratory and electrocardiographic abnormalities were similar in desloratadine and placebo-treated patients.

There were no differences in adverse events for subgroups of patients as defined by gender, age, or race.

CHRONIC IDIOPATHIC URTICARIA

In multiple-dose, placebo-controlled trials of chronic idiopathic urticaria, 211 patients received desloratadine tablets and 205 received placebo. Adverse events that were reported by greater than or equal to 2% of patients who received desloratadine tablets and that were more common with desloratadine than placebo were (rates for desloratadine and placebo, respectively): headache (14%, 13%), nausea (5%, 2%), fatigue (5%, 1%), dizziness (4%, 3%), pharyngitis (3%, 2%), dyspepsia (3%, 1%), and myalgia (3%, 1%).

The following spontaneous adverse events have been reported during the marketing of desloratadine: Tachycardia, and rarely hypersensitivity reactions (such as rash, pruritus, urticaria, edema, dyspnea, and anaphylaxis), and elevated liver enzymes including bilirubin.

DOSAGE AND ADMINISTRATION

In adults and children 12 years of age and over; the recommended dose of desloratadine tablets is 5 mg once daily. In patients with liver or renal impairment, a starting dose of one 5 mg tablet every other day is recommended based on pharmacokinetic data.

Administration of desloratadine orally-disintegrating tablets: Place desloratadine orally-disintegrating tablets on the tongue. Tablet disintegration occurs rapidly. Administer with or without water. Take tablet immediately after opening the blister.

HOW SUPPLIED

CLARINEX TABLETS

5 mg: Embossed "C5", light blue film coated tablets.

Storage

Protect Unit-of-Use packaging and Unit Dose-Hospital Pack from excessive moisture. Store between 2 and 25°C (36 and 77°F).

Heat sensitive. Avoid exposure at or above 30°C (86°F).

CLARINEX REDITABS

5 mg: "C" debossed, pink tablets in foil/foil blisters.

Storage: Store RediTabs Tablets at 25°C (77°F); excursions permitted between 15-30°C (59-86°F).

PRODUCT LISTING - EQUIVALENTS NOT AVAILABLE

Tablet - Oral - 5 mg

30's	$70.54	CLARINEX, Schering Corporation	00085-1264-04
100's	$235.15	CLARINEX, Schering Corporation	00085-1264-01
100's	$235.15	CLARINEX, Schering Corporation	00085-1264-03

Desmopressin Acetate *(000966)*

For complete prescribing information, refer to the CD-ROM included with the book.

Categories: Diabetes insipidus; Enuresis, primary nocturnal; Hemophilia A; Von Willebrand's disease; Pregnancy Category B; FDA Approved 1978 Feb; Orphan Drugs; WHO Formulary

Drug Classes: Antidiuretics; Hormones/hormone modifiers

Brand Names: Concentraid; **DDAVP**; Stimate

Foreign Brand Availability: DDAVP Desmopressin (Portugal); Defirin (Greece); Desmopressin Nasal Solution (Japan); Desmospray (England; Ireland); Minirin (Australia; Austria; Denmark; Finland; France; Germany; Israel; Korea; Malaysia; Mexico; New-Zealand; Norway; Sweden; Switzerland; Taiwan; Turkey); Minirin DDAVP (Bahrain; Cyprus; Egypt; Greece; Iran; Iraq; Italy; Jordan; Kuwait; Lebanon; Libya; Oman; Qatar; Republic-of-Yemen; Saudi-Arabia; Syria; United-Arab-Emirates); Minirin DDAVP (Hong-Kong; Thailand); Minirin Nasal Spray (Australia; New-Zealand); Minrin (Belgium; Netherlands); Minurin (Spain); Nucotil nasenspray (Germany); Octim (France); Octostim (Bahrain; Cyprus; Egypt; Finland; Hong-Kong; Iran; Iraq; Israel; Jordan; Korea; Kuwait; Lebanon; Libya; Netherlands; New-Zealand; Norway; Oman; Qatar; Republic-of-Yemen; Saudi-Arabia; Sweden; Switzerland; Syria; United-Arab-Emirates)

HCFA JCODE(S): J2597 4mcg IV, SC

DESCRIPTION

Desmopressin acetate nasal spray, rhinal tube, and injection) is an antidiuretic hormone affecting renal water conservation and a synthetic analogue of 8-arginine vasopressin. It is chemically defined as follows:

Empirical formula: $C_{48}H_{74}N_{14}O_{17}S_2$

SCH_2CH_2CO-Tyr-Phe-Gln-Asn-Cys-Pro-D-Arg-Gly-$NH_2 \cdot C_2H_4O_2 \cdot 3H_2O$ 1-(3-mercaptopropionic acid)-8-D-arginine vasopressin monoacetate (salt) trihydrate.

The molecular weight is 1183.2

NASAL SPRAY/RHINAL TUBE

Desmopressin is provided as a sterile, aqueous solution for intranasal use. Each ml contains:

Desmopressin acetate: 0.1 mg
Chlorobutanol: 5.0 mg
Sodium chloride: 9.0 mg
Hydrochloric acid to adjust pH to approximately 4.0

The desmopressin nasal spray compression pump delivers 0.1 ml (10 µg) of desmopressin per spray.

Nasal Spray Storage: Keep refrigerated at 2-8°C (36-46°F). When traveling, product will maintain stability for up to 3 weeks when stored at room temperature, 22°C (72°F).

Rhinal Tube Storage: KEEP REFRIGERATED AT ABOUT 4°C (39°F). When traveling — controlled room temperature 22°C (72°F) closed sterile bottles will maintain stability for 3 weeks.

INJECTION

Desmopressin is provided as a sterile, aqueous solution for injection. Each ml contains:

Desmopressin acetate: 4.0 µg
Sodium chloride: 9.0 mg
Hydrochloric acid to adjust pH to 4.0

The 10 ml vial contains chlorobutanol as a preservative (5.0 mg/ml).

INDICATIONS AND USAGE

PRIMARY NOCTURNAL ENURESIS

Nasal Spray/Rhinal Tube

Desmopressin is indicated for the management of primary nocturnal enuresis. It may be used alone or adjunctive to behavioral conditioning or other non-pharmacological intervention. It has been shown to be effective in some cases that are refractory to conventional therapies.

CENTRAL CRANIAL DIABETES INSIPIDUS

Nasal Spray/Rhinal Tube/Injection

Desmopressin is indicated as antidiuretic replacement therapy in the management of central cranial diabetes insipidus and for management of the temporary polyuria and polydipsia following head trauma or surgery in the pituitary region. It is ineffective for the treatment of nephrogenic diabetes insipidus.

The use of desmopressin in patients with an established diagnosis will result in a reduction in urinary output with increase in urine osmolality and a decrease in plasma osmolality. This will allow the resumption of a more normal life-style with a decrease in urinary frequency and nocturia.

There are reports of an occasional change in response with time, usually greater than 6 months. Some patients may show a decreased responsiveness, others a shortened duration of effect. There is no evidence this effect is due to the development of binding antibodies but may be due to a local inactivation of the peptide.

Patients are selected for therapy by establishing the diagnosis by means of the water deprivation test, the hypertonic saline infusion test, and/or the response to antidiuretic hormone. Continued response to desmopressin can be monitored by urine volume and osmolality.

Desmopressin is also available as a solution for injection when the intranasal route may be compromised. These situations include nasal congestion and blockage, nasal discharge, atrophy of nasal mucosa, and severe atrophic rhinitis. Intranasal delivery may also be inappropriate where there is an impaired level of consciousness. In addition, cranial surgical procedures, such as transsphenoidal hypophysectomy create situations where an alternative route of administration is needed as in cases of nasal packing or recovery from surgery.

HEMOPHILIA A
Injection
Desmopressin injection is indicated for patients with hemophilia A with factor VIII coagulant activity levels greater than 5%.

Desmopressin will often maintain hemostasis in patients with hemophilia A during surgical procedures and postoperatively when administered 30 minutes prior to scheduled procedure.

Desmopressin will also stop bleeding in hemophilia A patients with episodes of spontaneous or trauma-induced injuries such as hemarthroses, intramuscular hematoses or mucosal bleeding.

Desmopressin is not indicated for the treatment of hemophilia A with factor VII coagulant activity levels equal to or less than 5%, or for the treatment of hemophilia B, or in patients who should have factor VIII antibodies.

In certain clinical situations, it may be justified to try desmopressin in patients with factor VIII levels between 2%-5%; however, these patients should be carefully monitored.

VON WILLEBRAND'S DISEASE (TYPE I)
Injection
Desmopressin injection is indicated for patients with mild to moderate classic von Willebrand's disease (Type I) with factor VIII levels greater than 5%. Desmopressin will often maintain hemostasis in patients with mild to moderate von Willebrand's disease during surgical procedure and postoperatively when administered 30 minutes prior to the scheduled procedure.

Desmopressin will usually stop bleeding in mild to moderate von Willebrand's patients with episodes of spontaneous or trauma-induced injuries such as hemarthroses, intramuscular hematoses or mucosal bleeding.

Those von Willebrand's disease patients who are least likely to respond are those with severe homozygous von Willebrand's disease with factor VIII coagulant activity and factor VIII von Willebrand's factor antigen levels less than 1%. Other patients may respond in a variable fashion depending on the type of molecular defect they have. Bleeding time and factor VIII coagulant activity, ristocetin cofactor activity, and von Willebrand's factor antigen should be checked during administration of desmopressin to ensure that adequate levels are being achieved.

Desmopressin is not indicated for the treatment of severe classic von Willebrand's disease (Type I) and when there is evidence of an abnormal molecular form of factor VIII antigen. (See WARNINGS.)

DIABETES INSIPIDUS
Injection
Desmopressin injection is indicated as antidiuretic replacement therapy in the management of central (cranial) diabetes insipidus and for the management of the temporary polyuria and polydipsia following head trauma or surgery in the pituitary region. Desmopressin is ineffective for the treatment of nephrogenic diabetes insipidus.

Desmopressin is also available as an intranasal preparation. However, this means of delivery can be compromised by a variety of factors that can make nasal insufflation ineffective or inappropriate. These include poor intranasal absorption, nasal congestion and blockage, nasal discharge, atrophy of nasal mucosa, and severe atrophic rhinitis. Intranasal delivery may be inappropriate where there is an impaired level of consciousness. In addition, cranial surgical procedures, such as transsphenoidal hypophysectomy, create situations where an alternative route of administration is needed as in cases of nasal packing or recovery from surgery.

NON-FDA APPROVED INDICATIONS
Unapproved uses of desmopressin include treatment of chronic autonomic failure, assessment of renal concentrating capacity, nocturia, and bleeding disorders in patients with uremia or liver cirrhosis.

CONTRAINDICATIONS

Known hypersensitivity to desmopressin.

WARNINGS

NASAL SPRAY/RHINAL TUBE

For intranasal use only.

In very young and elderly patients in particular, fluid intake should be adjusted in order to decrease the potential occurrence of water intoxication and hyponatremia. Particular attention should be paid to the possibility of the rare occurrence of an extreme decrease in plasma osmolality that may result in seizures which could lead to coma.

INJECTION
Patients who do not have need of antidiuretic hormone and for its diuretic effect, in particularly those who are young or elderly, should be cautioned to ingest only enough fluid to satisfy thirst, in order to decrease the potential occurrence of water intoxication and hyponatremia.

Fluid intake should be adjusted, particularly in very young and elderly patients, in order to decrease the potential occurrence of water intoxication and hyponatremia. Particular attention should be paid to the possibility of the rare occurrence of an extreme decrease in plasma molality that may result in seizures which could lead to coma.

Desmopressin should not be used to treat patients with type IIB von Willebrand's disease since platelet aggregation may be induced.

DOSAGE AND ADMINISTRATION

NASAL SPRAY/RHINAL SPRAY
Primary Nocturnal Enuresis
Dosage should be adjusted according to the individual. The recommended initial dose for those 6 years of age and older is 20 μg or 0.2 ml solution intranasally at bedtime. Adjustment up to 40 μg is suggested if the patient does not respond. Some patients may respond to 10 μg and adjustment to that lower dose may be done if the patient has shown a response to 20 μg. It is recommended that one-half of the dose be administered per nostril. Adequately controlled studies with desmopressin Nasal Spray in primary nocturnal enuresis have not been conducted beyond 4-8 weeks.

RHINAL SPRAY
Central Cranial Diabetes Insipidus
This drug is administered into the nose through a soft, flexible plastic rhinal tube which has four graduation marks on it that measures 0.2, 0.15, 0.1 and 0.5 ml. Desmopressin rhinal tube dosage must be determined for each individual patient and adjusted according to the diurnal pattern of response. Response should be estimated by two parameters: adequate duration of sleep and adequate, not excessive, water turnover. Patients with nasal congestion and blockage have often responded well to desmopressin Rhinal tube. The usual dosage range in adults is 0.1 to 0.4 nl daily, either as a single dose or divided doses into 2 or 3 doses. Most adults require 0.2 ml daily in two divided doses. The morning and evening doses should be separately adjusted for an adequate diurnal rhythm of water turnover. For children aged 3 months to 12 years, the usual dived dosage range is 0.05 to 0.3 ml daily, either as single dose or divided into two doses.

About 1/4 to 1/3 of patients can be controlled by a single dose.

INJECTION
Hemophilia A and von Willebrand's Disease (Type I)
DDAVP injection is administered as an IV infusion at a dose of 0.3 μg desmopressin/kg body weight diluted in sterile physiological saline and infused slowly over 15-30 minutes. In adults and children weighing more than 10 kg, 50 ml of diluent is used; in children weighing 10 kg or less, 10 ml of diluent is used. Blood pressure and pulse should be monitored during infusion. If desmopressin injection is used preoperatively, it should be administered 30 minutes prior to the scheduled procedure.

The necessity for repeat administration of desmopressin or use of any blood products for hemostasis should be determined by laboratory response as well as the clinical condition of the patient. The tendency toward tachyphylaxis (lessening of response) with repeated administration given more frequently than every 48 hours should be considered in treating each patient.

Diabetes Insipidus
The formulation is administered subcutaneously by direct IV injection. Desmopressin injection dosage must be administered for each patient and adjusted according to the pattern of response. response should be estimated by two parameters: adequate duration of sleep and adequate, not excessive, water turnover.

The usual dosage range in adults is 0.5 ml (2.0 μg) to 1 ml (4.0 μg) daily, administered intravenously or subcutaneously, usually in two divided doses. The morning and evening doses should be separately adjusted for an adequate diurnal rhythm of water turnover. For patients who have been controlled on intranasal desmopressin and who must be switched to the injection form, wither because of poor intranasal absorption or because of the need for surgery, the comparable antidiuretic dose of the injection is about one-tenth the intranasal dose.

Parenteral drug products should be inspected visually for particulate matter and discoloration prior to administration whenever solution and container permit.

PRODUCT LISTING - RATED THERAPEUTICALLY EQUIVALENT

Solution - Intravenous - 4 mcg/ml

1 ml x 10	$83.36	GENERIC, Abbott Pharmaceutical	00074-2265-01
10 ml	$145.20	GENERIC, Gensia Sicor Pharmaceuticals Inc	00703-5051-03
10 ml	$145.20	GENERIC, Gensia Sicor Pharmaceuticals Inc	00703-5054-01
Spray - Nasal - 10 mcg/Inh			
5 ml	$121.26	DDAVP NASAL, Aventis Pharmaceuticals	00075-2450-02
5 ml	$143.34	GENERIC, Bausch and Lomb	24208-0342-05
5 ml	$151.95	DDAVP NASAL, Allscripts Pharmaceutical Company	54569-4818-00
5 ml	$165.90	DDAVP NASAL, Aventis Pharmaceuticals	00075-2452-01

PRODUCT LISTING - EQUIVALENTS NOT AVAILABLE

Solution - Intravenous - 4 mcg/ml

1 ml x 10	$228.90	GENERIC, Ferring Pharmaceuticals Inc	55566-5030-01
1 ml x 10	$274.80	DDAVP, Aventis Pharmaceuticals	00075-2451-01
10 ml	$228.86	GENERIC, Ferring Pharmaceuticals Inc	55566-5040-01
10 ml	$278.10	DDAVP, Aventis Pharmaceuticals	00075-2451-53
Solution - Nasal - 0.01%			
2 ml	$87.61	DDAVP RHINAL TUBE, Aventis Pharmaceuticals	00075-2450-01
2.50 ml	$77.77	GENERIC, Ferring Pharmaceuticals Inc	55566-5020-01
30 ml	$618.00	GENERIC, Ferring Pharmaceuticals Inc	55566-5020-02
Spray - Nasal - 0.15 mg/Inh			
2 ml	$600.00	STIMATE NASAL SPRAY, Centeon	00053-2453-00
Tablet - Oral - 0.1 mg			
100's	$253.90	DDAVP, Aventis Pharmaceuticals	00075-0016-00
Tablet - Oral - 0.2 mg			
100's	$335.50	DDAVP, Aventis Pharmaceuticals	00075-0026-00

Desogestrel; Ethinyl Estradiol *(003143)*

Categories: Contraception; Pregnancy Category X; FDA Approved 1992 Dec
Drug Classes: Contraceptives; Estrogens; Hormones/hormone modifiers; Progestins
Brand Names: **Desogen**; Ortho-Cept
Foreign Brand Availability: Desmin (Germany); Desolett (Turkey); Gracial 28 (Bahrain; Cyprus; Egypt; Indonesia; Iran; Iraq; Jordan; Kuwait; Lebanon; Libya; Oman; Peru; Philippines; Qatar; Republic-of-Yemen; Saudi-Arabia; Syria; United-Arab-Emirates); Lamuna (Germany); Lovina (Germany); Marvelon (Austria; Bahrain; Belgium; Benin; Bulgaria; Burkina-Faso; Canada; China; Colombia; Costa-Rica; Cyprus; Czech-Republic; Denmark; Ecuador; Egypt; England; Ethiopia; Finland; Gambia; Germany; Ghana; Greece; Guatemala; Guinea; Honduras; Hong-Kong; Hungary; Iran; Iraq; Ireland; Israel; Ivory-Coast; Jordan; Kenya; Kuwait; Lebanon; Liberia; Libya; Malawi; Malaysia; Mali; Mauritania; Mauritius; Mexico; Morocco; Netherlands; Niger; Nigeria; Norway; Oman; Peru; Portugal; Qatar; Republic-of-Yemen; Russia; Saudi-Arabia; Senegal; Seychelles; Sierra-Leone; South-Africa; Sudan; Switzerland; Syria; Tanzania; Tunia; Uganda; United-Arab-Emirates; Zambia; Zimbabwe); Marvelon 21 (New-Zealand; Taiwan; Thailand); Marvelon 28 (Australia; Denmark; Indonesia; New-Zealand; Philippines; Thailand); Mercilon (France; Philippines); Mircodiol (Israel; Spain); Miravelle (Colombia); Miravelle Suave (Colombia); Novelon (India); Novynette (Bahamas; Barbados; Belize; Bermuda; Curacao; Guyana; Jamaica; Netherland-Antilles; Puerto-Rico; Surinam; Trinidad); Varnoline (France; Switzerland)
Cost of Therapy: $26.12 (Contraceptive; Desogen; 0.15 mg;0.03 mg; 1 tablet/day; 28 day supply)
$31.45 (Contraceptive; Ortho-Cept; 0.15 mg;0.03 mg; 1 tablet/day; 28 day supply)

DESCRIPTION

Note: The trade name has been used throughout this monograph for clarity.

Patients should be counseled that this product does not protect against HIV infection (AIDS) and other sexually transmitted diseases.

Desogen (desogestrel and ethinyl estradiol) tablets provide an oral contraceptive regimen of 21 white round tablets each containing 0.15 mg desogestrel (13-ethyl-11-methylene-18,19-dinor-17α-pregn-4-en-20-yn-17-ol) and 0.03 mg ethinyl estradiol (19-nor-17α-pregna-1,3,5(10)-trien-20-yne-3,17-diol). Inactive ingredients include vitamin E, corn starch, povidone, stearic acid, colloidal silicon dioxide, lactose, hydroxypropyl methylcellulose, polyethylene glycol, titanium dioxide, and talc. Desogen also contains 7 green round tablets containing the following inactive ingredients: lactose, corn starch, magnesium stearate, FD&C blue no. 2 aluminum lake, ferric oxide, hydroxypropyl methylcellulose, polyethylene glycol, titanium dioxide, and talc. The molecular weights for desogestrel and ethinyl estradiol are 310.48 and 296.41, respectively. The molecular formulas for desogestrel and ethinyl estradiol are $C_{22}H_{30}O$ and $C_{20}H_{24}O_2$, respectively.

CLINICAL PHARMACOLOGY

PHARMACODYNAMICS

Combination oral contraceptives act by suppression of gonadotropins. Although the primary mechanism of this action is inhibition of ovulation, other alterations include changes in the cervical mucus (which increase the difficulty of sperm entry into the uterus) and the endometrium (which reduce the likelihood of implantation).

Receptor binding studies, as well as studies in animals, have shown that etonogestrel, the biologically active metabolite of desogestrel, combines high progestational activity with minimal intrinsic androgenicity.[91,92] The relevance of this latter finding in humans is unknown. Desogestrel, in combination with ethinyl estradiol, does not counteract the estrogen induced increase in SHBG, resulting in lower serum levels of free testosterone.[96-99]

PHARMACOKINETICS

Desogestrel is rapidly and almost completely absorbed and converted into etonogestrel, its biologically active metabolite. Following oral administration, the relative bioavailability of desogestrel, as measured by serum levels of etonogestrel, is approximately 84%.

In the third cycle of use after a single dose of Desogen tablets, maximum concentrations of etonogestrel of 2805 ± 1203 pg/ml (mean ±SD) are reached at 1.4 ± 0.8 hours. The area under the curve AUC(0-∞) is 33,858 ± 11,043 pg/ml·h after a single dose. At steady state, attained from at least day 19 onwards, maximum concentrations of 5840 ± 1667 pg/ml are reached at 1.4 ± 0.9 hours. The minimum plasma levels of etonogestrel at steady state are 1400 ± 560 pg/ml. The AUC(0-24) at steady state is 52,299 ± 17,878 pg/ml·h. The mean AUC(0-∞) for etonogestrel at single dose is significantly lower than the mean AUC(0-24) at steady state. This indicates that the kinetics of etonogestrel are non-linear due to an increase in binding of etonogestrel to sex hormone-binding globulin in the cycle, attributed to increased sex hormone-binding globulin levels which are induced by the daily administration of ethinyl estradiol. Sex hormone-binding globulin levels increased significantly in the third treatment cycle from day 1 (150 ± 64 nmol/L) to day 21 (230 ± 59 nmol/L).

The elimination half-life of etonogestrel is approximately 38 ± 20 hours at steady state. In addition to etonogestrel, other phase I metabolites are 3α-OH-desogestrel, 3β-OH-desogestrel, and 3α-OH-5α-H-desogestrel. These other metabolites are not known to have any pharmacologic effects, and are further converted in part by conjugation (phase II metabolism) into polar metabolites, mainly sulfates and glucuronides.

Ethinyl estradiol is rapidly and almost completely absorbed. In the third cycle of use after a single dose of Desogen, the relative bioavailability is approximately 83%.

In the third cycle of use after a single dose of Desogen, maximum concentrations of ethinyl estradiol of 95 ± 34 pg/ml are reached at 1.5 ± 0.8 hours. The AUC(0-∞) is 1471 ± 268 pg/ml·h after a single dose. At steady state, attained from at least day 19 onwards, maximum ethinyl estradiol concentrations of 141 ± 48 pg/ml are reached at about 1.4 ± 0.7 hours. The minimum serum levels of ethinyl estradiol at steady state are 24 ± 8.3 pg/ml. The AUC(0-24), at steady state is 1117 ± 302 pg/ml·h. The mean AUC(0-∞) for ethinyl estradiol following a single dose during treatment cycle 3 does not significantly differ from the mean AUC(0-24) at steady state. This finding indicates linear kinetics for ethinyl estradiol.

The elimination half-life is 26 ± 6.8 hours at steady state. Ethinyl estradiol is subject to a significant degree of presystemic conjugation (phase II metabolism). Ethinyl estradiol escaping gut wall conjugation undergoes phase I metabolism and hepatic conjugation (phase II metabolism). Major phase I metabolites are 2-OH-ethinyl estradiol and 2-methoxy-ethinyl estradiol. Sulfate and glucuronide conjugates of both ethinyl estradiol and phase I metabolites, which are excreted in bile, can undergo enterohepatic circulation.

NON-CONTRACEPTIVE HEALTH BENEFITS

The following non-contraceptive health benefits related to the use of oral contraceptives are supported by epidemiological studies which largely utilized oral contraceptive formulations containing estrogen doses exceeding 0.035 mg of ethinyl estradiol or 0.05 mg of mestranol.[73-78]

Effects on menses:

- Increased menstrual cycle regularity.
- Decreased blood loss and decreased incidence of iron deficiency anemia.
- Decreased incidence of dysmenorrhea.

Effects related to inhibition of ovulation:

- Decreased incidence of functional ovarian cysts.
- Decreased incidence of ectopic pregnancies.

Effects from long-term use:

- Decreased incidence of fibroadenomas and fibrocystic disease of the breast.
- Decreased incidence of acute pelvic inflammatory disease.
- Decreased incidence of endometrial cancer.
- Decreased incidence of ovarian cancer.

INDICATIONS AND USAGE

Desogen tablets are indicated for the prevention of pregnancy in women who elect to use this product as a method of contraception.

Oral contraceptives are highly effective. TABLE 1 lists the typical accidental pregnancy rates for users of combination oral contraceptives and other methods of contraception. The efficacy of these contraceptive methods, except sterilization, depends upon the reliability with which they are used. Correct and consistent use of these methods can result in lower failure rates.

TABLE 1 *Percentage of Women Experiencing an Unintended Pregnancy During the First Year of Typical Use and the First Year of Perfect Use of Contraception and the Percentage Continuing Use at the End of the First Year, United States*

	% of Women Experiencing an Unintended Pregnancy Within the First Year of Use		% of Women Continuing Use
Method	Typical Use*	Perfect Use†	at 1 Year‡
(1)	(2)	(3)	(4)
Chance§	85%	85%	
Spermicides¤	26%	6%	40%
Periodic abstinence	25%		63%
Calendar		9%	
Ovulation method		3%	
Sympto-thermal¶		2%	
Post-ovulation		1%	
Withdrawal	19%	4%	
Cap**			
Parous women	40%	26%	42%
Nulliparous women	20%	9%	56%
Sponge			
Parous women	40%	20%	42%
Nulliparous women	20%	9%	56%
Diaphragm**	20%	6%	56%
Condom††			
Female (Reality)	21%	5%	56%
Male	14%	3%	61%
Pill	5%		71%
Progestin only		0.5%	
Combined		0.1%	
IUD			
Progesterone T	2.0%	1.6%	81%
Copper T 380A	0.8%	0.6%	78%
LNg 20	0.1%	0.1%	81%
Depo-Provera	0.3%	0.3%	70%
Norplant and Norplant-2	0.05%	0.05%	88%
Female sterilization	0.5%	0.5%	100%
Male sterilization	0.15%	0.10%	100%

Adapted from Hatcher *et al.*, 1998.[1]

* Among typical couples who initiate use of a method (not necessarily for the first time), the percentage who experience an accidental pregnancy during the first year if they do not stop use for any other reason.

† Among couples who initiate use of a method (not necessarily for the first time) and who use it *perfectly* (both consistently and correctly), the percentage who experience an accidental pregnancy during the first year if they do not stop use for any other reason.

‡ Among couples attempting to avoid pregnancy, the percentage who continue to use a method for 1 year.

§ The percents becoming pregnant in columns (2) and (3) are based on data from populations where contraception is not used and from women who cease using contraception in order to become pregnant. Among such populations, about 89% become pregnant within 1 year. This estimate was lowered slightly (to 85%) to represent the percent who would become pregnant within 1 year among women now relying on reversible methods of contraception if they abandoned contraception altogether.

¤ Foams, creams, gels, vaginal suppositories, and vaginal film.

¶ Cervical mucus (ovulation) method supplemented by calendar in the pre-ovulatory and basal body temperature in the post-ovulatory phases.

** With spermicidal cream or jelly.

†† Without spermicides.

CONTRAINDICATIONS

Oral contraceptives should not be used in women who currently have the following conditions:

- Thrombophlebitis or thromboembolic disorders.
- A past history of deep vein thrombophlebitis or thromboembolic disorders.
- Cerebral vascular or coronary artery disease.
- Known or suspected carcinoma of the breast.

Carcinoma of the endometrium or other known or suspected estrogen-dependent neoplasia.
Undiagnosed abnormal genital bleeding.
Cholestatic jaundice of pregnancy or jaundice with prior pill use.
Hepatic adenomas or carcinomas.
Known or suspected pregnancy.

WARNINGS

Cigarette smoking increases the risk of serious cardiovascular side effects from oral contraceptive use. This risk increases with age and with heavy smoking (15 or more cigarettes per day) and is quite marked in women over 35 years of age. Women who use oral contraceptives should be strongly advised not to smoke.

The use of oral contraceptives is associated with increased risks of several serious conditions including myocardial infarction, thromboembolism, stroke, hepatic neoplasia, and gallbladder disease, although the risk of serious morbidity or mortality is very small in healthy women without underlying risk factors. The risk of morbidity and mortality increases significantly in the presence of other underlying risk factors such as hypertension, hyperlipidemias, obesity, and diabetes.

Practitioners prescribing oral contraceptives should be familiar with the following information relating to these risks.

The information contained in this package insert is principally based on studies carried out in patients who used oral contraceptives with formulations of higher doses of estrogens and progestogens than those in common use today. The effect of long-term use of the oral contraceptives with formulations of lower doses of both estrogens and progestogens remains to be determined.

Throughout this labeling, epidemiologic studies reported are of two types: retrospective or case control studies and prospective or cohort studies. Case control studies provide a measure of the relative risk of a disease, namely, a ratio of the incidence of a disease among oral contraceptive users to that among non-users. The relative risk does not provide information on the actual clinical occurrence of a disease. Cohort studies provide a measure of attributable risk, which is the difference in the incidence of disease between oral contraceptive users and non-users. The attributable risk does provide information about the actual occurrence of a disease in the population (Adapted from refs. 2 and 3 with the authors' permission). For further information, the reader is referred to a text on epidemiologic methods.

THROMBOEMBOLIC DISORDERS AND OTHER VASCULAR PROBLEMS

Thromboembolism

An increased risk of thromboembolic and thrombotic disease associated with the use of oral contraceptives is well established. Case control studies have found the relative risk of users compared to non-users to be 3 for the first episode of superficial venous thrombosis, 4 to 11 for deep vein thrombosis or pulmonary embolism, and 1.5 to 6 for women with predisposing conditions for venous thromboembolic disease.[2,3,19-24] Cohort studies have shown the relative risk to be somewhat lower, about 3 for new cases and about 4.5 for new cases requiring hospitalization.[25] The risk of thromboembolic disease associated with oral contraceptives is not related to length of use and disappears after pill use is stopped.[2]

Several epidemiologic studies indicate that third generation oral contraceptives, including those containing desogestrel, are associated with a higher risk of venous thromboembolism than certain second generation oral contraceptives.[100-102] In general, these studies indicate an approximate 2-fold increased risk, which corresponds to an additional 1-2 cases of venous thromboembolism per 10,000 women-years of use. However, data from additional studies have not shown this 2-fold increase in risk.

A 2- to 4-fold increase in relative risk of post-operative thromboembolic complications has been reported with the use of oral contraceptives.[9,26] The relative risk of venous thrombosis in women who have predisposing conditions is twice that of women without such medical conditions.[9,26] If feasible, oral contraceptives should be discontinued at least 4 weeks prior to and for 2 weeks after elective surgery of a type associated with an increase in risk of thromboembolism and during and following prolonged immobilization. Since the immediate postpartum period is associated with an increased risk of thromboembolism, oral contraceptives should be started no earlier than 4 weeks after delivery in women who elect not to breast feed.

Myocardial Infarction

An increased risk of myocardial infarction has been attributed to oral contraceptive use. This risk is primarily in smokers or women with other underlying risk factors for coronary artery disease such as hypertension, hypercholesterolemia, morbid obesity, and diabetes. The relative risk of heart attack for current oral contraceptive users has been estimated to be two to six.[4-10] The risk is very low in women under the age of 30.

Smoking in combination with oral contraceptive use has been shown to contribute substantially to the incidence of myocardial infarction in women in their mid-thirties or older with smoking accounting for the majority of excess cases.[11] Mortality rates associated with circulatory disease have been shown to increase substantially in smokers over the age of 35 and non-smokers over the age of 40 (TABLE 2) among women who use oral contraceptives.

Oral contraceptives may compound the effects of well-known risk factors, such as hypertension, diabetes, hyperlipidemias, age, and obesity.[13] In particular, some progestogens are known to decrease HDL cholesterol and cause glucose intolerance, while estrogens may create a state of hyperinsulinism.[14-18] Oral contraceptives have been shown to increase blood pressure among users (see Elevated Blood Pressure). Similar effects on risk factors have been associated with an increased risk of heart disease. Oral contraceptives must be used with caution in women with cardiovascular disease risk factors.

Cerebrovascular Diseases

Oral contraceptives have been shown to increase both the relative and attributable risks of cerebrovascular events (thrombotic and hemorrhagic strokes), although, in general, the risk is greatest among older (>35 years), hypertensive women who also smoke. Hypertension was found to be a risk factor for both users and nonusers, for both types of strokes, while smoking interacted to increase the risk of hemorrhagic stroke.[27-29]

In a large study, the relative risk of thrombotic strokes has been shown to range from 3 for normotensive users to 14 for users with severe hypertension.[30] The relative risk of hemorrhagic stroke is reported to be 1.2 for non-smokers who used oral contraceptives, 2.6 for smokers who did not use oral contraceptives, 7.6 for smokers who used oral contraceptives, 1.8 for normotensive users, and 25.7 for users with severe hypertension.[30] The attributable risk is also greater in older women.[3]

Dose-Related Risk of Vascular Disease From Oral Contraceptives

A positive association has been observed between the amount of estrogen and progestogen in oral contraceptives and the risk of vascular disease.[31-33] A decline in serum high-density lipoproteins (HDL) has been reported with many progestational agents.[14-16] A decline in serum high-density lipoproteins has been associated with an increased incidence of ischemic heart disease. Because estrogens increase HDL cholesterol, the net effect of an oral contraceptive depends on a balance achieved between doses of estrogen and progestogen and the nature and absolute amount of progestogens used in the contraceptives. The amount of both hormones should be considered in the choice of an oral contraceptive.

Minimizing exposure to estrogen and progestogen is in keeping with good principles of therapeutics. For any particular estrogen/progestogen combination, the dosage regimen prescribed should be one which contains the least amount of estrogen and progestogen that is compatible with a low failure rate and the needs of the individual patient. New acceptors of oral contraceptive agents should be started on preparations containing 0.035 mg or less of estrogen.

Persistence of Risk of Vascular Disease

There are two studies which have shown persistence of risk of vascular disease for ever-users of oral contraceptives. In a study in the US, the risk of developing myocardial infarction after discontinuing oral contraceptives persists for at least 9 years for women 40-49 years old who had used oral contraceptives for 5 or more years, but this increased risk was not demonstrated in other age groups.[8] In another study in Great Britain, the risk of developing cerebrovascular disease persisted for at least 6 years after discontinuation of oral contraceptives, although excess risk was very small.[34] However, both studies were performed with oral contraceptive formulations containing 0.05 mg or higher of estrogens.

ESTIMATES OF MORTALITY FROM CONTRACEPTIVE USE

One study gathered data from a variety of sources which have estimated the mortality rate associated with different methods of contraception at different ages (TABLE 2).

These estimates include the combined risk of death associated with contraceptive methods plus the risk attributable to pregnancy in the event of method failure. Each method of contraception has its specific benefits and risks. The study concluded that with the exception of oral contraceptive users 35 and older who smoke and 40 and older who do not smoke, mortality associated with all methods of birth control is low and below that associated with childbirth.

The observation of a possible increase in risk of mortality with age for oral contraceptive users is based on data gathered in the 1970s — but not reported until 1983.[35] However, current clinical practice involves the use of lower estrogen formulations combined with careful consideration of risk factors.

Because of these changes in practice and, also, because of some limited new data which suggest that the risk of cardiovascular disease with the use of oral contraceptives may now be less than previously observed,[103-104] the Fertility and Maternal Health Drugs Advisory Committee was asked to review the topic in 1989. The Committee concluded that although cardiovascular disease risks may be increased with oral contraceptive use after age 40 in healthy non-smoking women (even with the newer low-dose formulations), there are also greater potential health risks associated with pregnancy in older women and with the alternative surgical and medical procedures which may be necessary if such women do not have access to effective and acceptable means of contraception.

Therefore, the Committee recommended that the benefits of low-dose oral contraceptive use by healthy non-smoking women over 40 may outweigh the possible risks. Of course, older women, as all women who take oral contraceptives, should take the lowest possible dose formulation that is effective.

TABLE 2 *Annual Number of Birth-Related or Method-Related Deaths Associated With Control of Fertility Per 100,000 Nonsterile Women, by Fertility Control Method According to Age*

Method of Control and Outcome	15-19	20-24	25-29	30-34	35-39	40-44
No fertility control methods*	7.0	7.4	9.1	14.8	25.7	28.2
Oral contraceptives non-smoker†	0.3	0.5	0.9	1.9	13.8	31.6
Oral contraceptives smoker†	2.2	3.4	6.6	13.5	51.1	117.2
IUD†	0.8	0.8	1.0	1.0	1.4	1.4
Condom*	1.1	1.6	0.7	0.2	0.3	0.4
Diaphragm/spermicide*	1.9	1.2	1.2	1.3	2.2	2.8
Periodic abstinence*	2.5	1.6	1.6	1.7	2.9	3.6

* Deaths are birth-related.
† Deaths are method-related.
Adapted from H.W. Ory.[35]

CARCINOMA OF THE REPRODUCTIVE ORGANS AND BREASTS

Numerous epidemiologic studies have been performed on the incidence of breast, endometrial, ovarian, and cervical cancer in women using oral contraceptives. While there are conflicting reports, most studies suggest that the use of oral contraceptives is not associated with an overall increase in the risk of developing breast cancer. Some studies have reported an increased relative risk of developing breast cancer, particularly at a younger age. This increased relative risk appears to be related to duration of use.[36-43,79-89]

Some studies suggest that oral contraceptive use has been associated with an increase in the risk of cervical intra-epithelial neoplasia in some populations of women.[45-48] However, there continues to be controversy about the extent to which such findings may be due to differences in sexual behavior and other factors.

HEPATIC NEOPLASIA

Benign hepatic adenomas are associated with oral contraceptive use, although the incidence of benign tumors is rare in the US. Indirect calculations have estimated the attributable risk to be in the range of 3.3 cases/100,000 for users, a risk that increases after 4 or more years of use especially with oral contraceptives of higher dose.[49] Rupture of rare, benign, hepatic adenomas may cause death through intraabdominal hemorrhage.[50,51]

Studies from Britain have shown an increased risk of developing hepatocellular carcinoma[52-54] in long-term (>8 years) oral contraceptive users. However, these cancers are extremely rare in the US and the attributable risk (the excess incidence) of liver cancers in oral contraceptive users approaches less than one per million users.

OCULAR LESIONS

There have been clinical case reports of retinal thrombosis associated with the use of oral contraceptives. Oral contraceptives should be discontinued if there is unexplained partial or complete loss of vision; onset of proptosis or diplopia; papilledema; or retinal vascular lesions. Appropriate diagnostic and therapeutic measures should be undertaken immediately.

ORAL CONTRACEPTIVE USE BEFORE OR DURING EARLY PREGNANCY

Extensive epidemiologic studies have revealed no increased risk of birth defects in women who have used oral contraceptives prior to pregnancy.[55-57] Studies also do not suggest a teratogenic effect, particularly in so far as cardiac anomalies and limb reduction defects are concerned,[55-56,58-59] when oral contraceptives are taken inadvertently during early pregnancy.

The administration of oral contraceptives to induce withdrawal bleeding should not be used as a test for pregnancy. Oral contraceptives should not be used during pregnancy to treat threatened or habitual abortion. It is recommended that for any patient who has missed two consecutive periods, pregnancy should be ruled out before continuing oral contraceptive use. If the patient has not adhered to the prescribed schedule, the possibility of pregnancy should be considered at the first missed period. Oral contraceptive use should be discontinued until pregnancy is ruled out.

GALLBLADDER DISEASE

Earlier studies have reported an increased lifetime relative risk of gallbladder surgery in users of oral contraceptives and estrogens.[60,61] More recent studies, however, have shown that the relative risk of developing gallbladder disease among oral contraceptive users may be minimal.[62-64] The recent findings of minimal risk may be related to the use of oral contraceptive formulations containing lower hormonal doses of estrogens and progestogens.

CARBOHYDRATE AND LIPID METABOLIC EFFECTS

Oral contraceptives have been shown to cause a decrease in glucose tolerance in a significant percentage of users.[17] Oral contraceptives containing greater than 75 µg of estrogen cause hyperinsulinism, while lower doses of estrogen cause less glucose intolerance.[65] Progestogens increase insulin secretion and create insulin resistance, this effect varying with different progestational agents.[17,66] However, in the non-diabetic woman, oral contraceptives appear to have no effect on fasting blood glucose.[67] Because of these demonstrated effects, prediabetic and diabetic women should be carefully monitored while taking oral contraceptives.

A small proportion of women will have persistent hypertriglyceridemia while on the pill. As discussed earlier (see WARNINGS), changes in serum triglycerides and lipoprotein levels have been reported in oral contraceptive users.

ELEVATED BLOOD PRESSURE

An increase in blood pressure has been reported in women taking oral contraceptives[68] and this increase is more likely in older oral contraceptive users.[69] and with continued use.[61] Data from the Royal College of General Practitioners[12] and subsequent randomized trials have shown that the incidence of hypertension increases with increasing quantities of progestogens.

Women with a history of hypertension or hypertension-related diseases, or renal disease[70] should be encouraged to use another method of contraception. If women elect to use oral contraceptives, they should be monitored closely and if significant elevation of blood pressure occurs, oral contraceptives should be discontinued. For most women, elevated blood pressure will return to normal after stopping oral contraceptives,[69] and there is no difference in the occurrence of hypertension between ever and never-users.[68,70,71]

HEADACHE

The onset or exacerbation of migraine or development of headache with a new pattern which is recurrent, persistent, or severe requires discontinuation of oral contraceptives and evaluation of the cause.

BLEEDING IRREGULARITIES

Breakthrough bleeding and spotting are sometimes encountered in patients on oral contraceptives, especially during the first 3 months of use. Non-hormonal causes should be considered and adequate diagnostic measures taken to rule out malignancy or pregnancy in the event of breakthrough bleeding, as in the case of any abnormal vaginal bleeding. If pathology has been excluded, time or a change to another formulation may solve the problem. In the event of amenorrhea, pregnancy should be ruled out.

Some women may encounter post-pill amenorrhea or oligomenorrhea, especially when such a condition was pre-existent.

ECTOPIC PREGNANCY

Ectopic as well as intrauterine pregnancy may occur in contraceptive failures.

PRECAUTIONS

GENERAL

Patients should be counseled that this product does not protect against HIV infection (AIDS) and other sexually transmitted diseases.

PHYSICAL EXAMINATION AND FOLLOW UP

It is good medical practice for all women to have annual history and physical examinations, including women using oral contraceptives. The physical examination, however, may be deferred until after initiation of oral contraceptives if requested by the woman and judged appropriate by the clinician. The physical examination should include special reference to blood pressure, breasts, abdomen and pelvic organs, including cervical cytology, and relevant laboratory tests. In case of undiagnosed, persistent or recurrent abnormal vaginal bleeding, appropriate measures should be conducted to rule out malignancy. Women with a strong family history of breast cancer or who have breast nodules should be monitored with particular care.

LIPID DISORDERS

Women who are being treated for hyperlipidemias should be followed closely if they elect to use oral contraceptives. Some progestogens may elevate LDL levels and may render the control of hyperlipidemias more difficult.

LIVER FUNCTION

If jaundice develops in any woman receiving such drugs, the medication should be discontinued. Steroid hormones may be poorly metabolized in patients with impaired liver function.

FLUID RETENTION

Oral contraceptives may cause some degree of fluid retention. They should be prescribed with caution, and only with careful monitoring, in patients with conditions which might be aggravated by fluid retention.

EMOTIONAL DISORDERS

Women with a history of depression should be carefully observed and the drug discontinued if depression recurs to a serious degree.

CONTACT LENSES

Contact lens wearers who develop visual changes or changes in lens tolerance should be assessed by an ophthalmologist.

INTERACTIONS WITH LABORATORY TESTS

Certain endocrine and liver function tests and blood components may be affected by oral contraceptives:

- Increased prothrombin and factors VII, VIII, IX and X; decreased antithrombin 3; increased norepinephrine-induced platelet aggregability.
- Increased thyroid binding globulin (TBG) leading to increased circulating total thyroid hormone, as measured by protein-bound iodine (PBI), T4 by column or by radioimmunoassay. Free T3 resin uptake is decreased, reflecting the elevated TBG; free T4 concentration is unaltered.
- Other binding proteins may be elevated in serum.
- Sex hormone-binding globulins are increased and result in elevated levels of total circulating sex steroids; however, free or biologically active levels either decrease or remain unchanged.
- High-density lipoprotein cholesterol (HDL-C) and triglycerides may be increased, while low-density lipoprotein cholesterol (LDL-C) and total cholesterol (Total-C) may be decreased or unchanged.
- Glucose tolerance may be decreased.
- Serum folate levels may be depressed by oral contraceptive therapy. This may be of clinical significance if a woman becomes pregnant shortly after discontinuing oral contraceptives.

CARCINOGENESIS

See WARNINGS.

PREGNANCY CATEGORY X

See CONTRAINDICATIONS and WARNINGS.

NURSING MOTHERS

Small amounts of oral contraceptive steroids have been identified in the milk of nursing mothers and a few adverse effects on the child have been reported, including jaundice and breast enlargement. In addition, oral contraceptives given in the postpartum period may interfere with lactation by decreasing the quantity and quality of breast milk. If possible, the nursing mother should be advised not to use oral contraceptives but to use other forms of contraception until she has completely weaned her child.

PEDIATRIC USE

Safety and efficacy of Desogen tablets have been established in women of reproductive age. Safety and efficacy are expected to be the same for postpubertal adolescents under the age of 16 and for users 16 years and older. Use of this product before menarche is not indicated.

INFORMATION FOR THE PATIENT

See Patient Labeling available with the prescription.

DRUG INTERACTIONS

Reduced efficacy and increased incidence of breakthrough bleeding and menstrual irregularities have been associated with concomitant use of rifampin. A similar association, though less marked, has been suggested with barbiturates, phenylbutazone, phenytoin sodium, carbamazepine and possibly with griseofulvin, ampicillin, and tetracyclines.[72]

D

ADVERSE REACTIONS

An increased risk of the following serious adverse reactions has been associated with the use of oral contraceptives (see WARNINGS): Thrombophlebitis and venous thrombosis with or without embolism, arterial thromboembolism, pulmonary embolism, myocardial infarction, cerebral hemorrhage, cerebral thrombosis, hypertension, gallbladder disease, hepatic adenomas or benign liver tumors.

There is evidence of an association between the following conditions and the use of oral contraceptives: Mesenteric thrombosis, retinal thrombosis.

The following adverse reactions have been reported in patients receiving oral contraceptives and are believed to be drug-related: Nausea; vomiting; gastrointestinal symptoms (such as abdominal cramps and bloating); breakthrough bleeding; spotting; change in menstrual flow; amenorrhea; temporary infertility after discontinuation of treatment; edema; melasma which may persist; breast changes: tenderness, enlargement, secretion; change in weight (increase or decrease); change in cervical erosion and secretion; diminution in lactation when given immediately postpartum; cholestatic jaundice; migraine; rash (allergic); mental depression; reduced tolerance to carbohydrates; vaginal candidiasis; change in corneal curvature (steepening); intolerance to contact lenses.

The following adverse reactions have been reported in users of oral contraceptives and the association has been neither confirmed nor refuted: Pre-menstrual syndrome, cataracts, changes in appetite, cystitis-like syndrome, headache, nervousness, dizziness, hirsutism, loss of scalp hair, erythema multiforme, erythema nodosum, hemorrhagic eruption, vaginitis, porphyria, impaired renal function, hemolytic uremic syndrome, acne, changes in libido, colitis, Budd-Chiari syndrome.

DOSAGE AND ADMINISTRATION

To achieve maximum contraceptive effectiveness, Desogen tablets must be taken exactly as directed and at intervals not exceeding 24 hours. Desogen may be initiated using either a Sunday start or a Day 1 start.

NOTE: Each cycle pack dispenser is preprinted with the days of the week, starting with Sunday, to facilitate a Sunday start regimen. Six different "day label strips" are provided with each cycle pack dispenser in order to accommodate a Day 1 start regimen. In this case, the patient should place the self-adhesive "day label strip" that corresponds to her starting day over the preprinted days.

IMPORTANT: The possibility of ovulation and conception prior to initiation of use of Desogen should be considered.

The use of Desogen for contraception may be initiated 4 weeks postpartum in women who elect not to breast feed. When the tablets are administered during the postpartum period, the increased risk of thromboembolic disease associated with the postpartum period must be considered see CONTRAINDICATIONS and WARNINGS concerning thromboembolic disease. See also PRECAUTIONS, Nursing Mothers.

If the patient starts on Desogen postpartum, and has not yet had a period, she should be instructed to use another method of contraception until a white tablet has been taken daily for 7 days.

SUNDAY START

When initiating a Sunday start regimen, another method of contraception should be used until after the first 7 consecutive days of administration.

Using a Sunday start, tablets are taken daily without interruption as follows: The first white tablet should be taken on the first Sunday after menstruation begins (if menstruation begins on Sunday, the first white tablet is taken on that day). One white tablet is taken daily for 21 days, followed by 1 green (inert) tablet daily for 7 days. For all subsequent cycles, the patient then begins a new 28 tablet regimen on the next day (Sunday) after taking the last green tablet. [If switching from a Sunday Start oral contraceptive, the first Desogen (desogestrel and ethinyl estradiol) tablet should be taken on the second Sunday after the last tablet of a 21 day regimen or should be taken on the first Sunday after the last inactive tablet of a 28 day regimen.] If a patient misses 1 white tablet, she should take the missed tablet as soon as she remembers.

If the patient misses 2 consecutive white tablets in Week 1 or Week 2, the patient should take 2 tablets the day she remembers and 2 tablets the next day; thereafter, the patient should resume taking 1 tablet daily until she finishes the cycle pack. The patient should be instructed to use a back-up method of birth control if she has intercourse in the 7 days after missing pills. If the patient misses 2 consecutive white tablets in the third week or misses 3 or more white tablets in a row at any time during the cycle, the patient should keep taking 1 white tablet daily until the next Sunday. On Sunday the patient should throw out the rest of that cycle pack and start a new cycle pack that same day. The patient should be instructed to use a back-up method of birth control if she has intercourse in the 7 days after missing pills.

DAY 1 START

Counting the first day of menstruation as "Day 1", tablets are taken without interruption as follows: One white tablet daily for 21 days, then one green (inert) tablet daily for 7 days. For all subsequent cycles, the patient then begins a new 28 tablet regimen on the next day after taking the last green tablet. [If switching directly from another oral contraceptive, the first white tablet should be taken on the first day of menstruation which begins after the last ACTIVE tablet of the previous product.] If a patient misses 1 white tablet, she should take the missed tablet as soon as she remembers.

If the patient misses 2 consecutive white tablets in Week 1 or Week 2, the patient should take 2 tablets the day she remembers and 2 tablets the next day; thereafter, the patient should resume taking 1 tablet daily until she finishes the cycle pack. The patient should be instructed to use a back-up method of birth control if she has intercourse in the 7 days after missing pills. If the patient misses 2 consecutive white tablets in the third week or misses 3 or more white tablets in a row at any time during the cycle, the patient should throw out the rest of that cycle pack and start a new cycle pack that same day. The patient should be instructed to use a back-up method of birth control if she has intercourse in the 7 days after missing pills.

ALL ORAL CONTRACEPTIVES

Breakthrough bleeding, spotting, and amenorrhea are frequent reasons for patients discontinuing oral contraceptives. In breakthrough bleeding, as in all cases of irregular bleeding from the vagina, non-functional causes should be borne in mind. In undiagnosed persistent or recurrent abnormal bleeding from the vagina, adequate diagnostic measures are indicated to rule out pregnancy or malignancy. If both pregnancy and pathology have been excluded, time or a change to another preparation may solve the problem. Changing to an oral contraceptive with a higher estrogen content, while potentially useful in minimizing menstrual irregularity, should be done only if necessary since this may increase the risk of thromboembolic disease.

Use of oral contraceptives in the event of a missed menstrual period:

If the patient has not adhered to the prescribed schedule, the possibility of pregnancy should be considered at the time of the first missed period and oral contraceptive use should be discontinued until pregnancy is ruled out.

If the patient has adhered to the prescribed regimen and misses two consecutive periods, pregnancy should be ruled out before continuing oral contraceptive use.

HOW SUPPLIED

Desogen tablets contain 21 round white tablets and 7 round green tablets in a blister card within a recyclable plastic dispenser. Each white tablet (debossed with "T5R" on one side and "Organon" on the other side) contains 0.15 mg desogestrel and 0.03 mg ethinyl estradiol. Each green tablet (debossed with "K2H" on one side and "Organon" on the other side) contains inert ingredients.

Storage: Store below 30°C (86°F).

PRODUCT LISTING - RATED THERAPEUTICALLY EQUIVALENT

Tablet - Oral - Biphasic

28 x 6	$177.66	GENERIC, Barr Laboratories Inc	00555-9050-58

Tablet - Oral - 0.15 mg;0.03 mg

28 x 6	$24.62	APRI, Allscripts Pharmaceutical Company	54569-4878-00
28 x 6	$26.13	DESOGEN, Allscripts Pharmaceutical Company	54569-4222-01
28 x 6	$141.84	APRI, Allscripts Pharmaceutical Company	54569-4878-01
28 x 6	$156.75	DESOGEN, Allscripts Pharmaceutical Company	54569-4222-00
28 x 6	$162.90	APRI, Duramed Pharmaceuticals Inc	51285-0576-28
28 x 6	$175.20	APRI, Barr Laboratories Inc	00555-9043-58
28 x 6	$194.70	DESOGEN, Organon	00052-0261-06

PRODUCT LISTING - EQUIVALENTS NOT AVAILABLE

Tablet - Oral - Biphasic

28 x 6	$214.86	MIRCETTE, Organon	00052-0281-06
28's	$26.13	MIRCETTE, Allscripts Pharmaceutical Company	54569-4890-00

Tablet - Oral - Triphasic

28 x 6	$205.68	CYCLESSA, Organon	00052-0283-06

Tablet - Oral - 0.15 mg;0.03 mg

28 x 6	$227.58	ORTHO-CEPT, Janssen Pharmaceuticals	00062-1796-15

Desonide *(000967)*

Categories: Dermatosis, corticosteroid-responsive; Pregnancy Category C; FDA Approved 1972 Jan
Drug Classes: Corticosteroids, topical; Dermatologics
Brand Names: **Desowen**; Locapred; Tridesilon
Foreign Brand Availability: Apolar (Indonesia); Desocort (Canada); Desonida (Colombia); Prenacid (Peru); Sterax (Ecuador); Tresilen (Colombia)

DESCRIPTION

Desonide cream 0.05%, ointment 0.05%, and lotion 0.05% contain desonide (pregna-1,4-diene-3,20-dione,11,21-dihydroxy-16,17-[(1-methylethylidene)bis(oxy)]-,(11β,16α-) a synthetic nonfluorinated corticosteroid for topical dermatologic use. The corticosteroids constitute a class of primarily synthetic steroids used topically as anti-inflammatory and antipruritic agents.

Chemically, desonide is $C_{24}H_{32}O_6$.

Desonide has the molecular weight of 416.51. It is a white to off white odorless powder which is soluble in methanol and practically insoluble in water.

Each gram of desonide cream contains 0.5 mg of desonide in a compatible vehicle buffered to the pH range of normal skin. It contains dehydag wax, beeswax, white petrolatum, mineral oil, aluminum acetate basic, glycerin, and purified water. It is preserved with methylparaben.

Each gram of desonide ointment contains 0.5 mg of desonide in an ointment base consisting of white petrolatum and mineral oil. It is a smooth, uniform petrolatum-type ointment.

Each gram of desonide lotion contains 0.5 mg of desonide in a lotion vehicle consisting of sodium lauryl sulfate, light mineral oil, cetyl alcohol, stearyl paraben, sorbitan monostearate, glyceryl stearate SE, edetate sodium and purified water. May contain citric acid and/or sodium hydroxide for pH adjustment.

Storage: Store between 2-30°C (36-86°F). Avoid freezing.

CLINICAL PHARMACOLOGY

Like other topical corticosteroids, desonide has anti-inflammatory, antipruritic, and vasoconstrictive properties. The mechanism of the anti-inflammatory activity of the topical corticosteroids, in general, is unclear. However corticosteroids are thought to act by the induction of phospholipase A_2 inhibitory proteins, collectively called lipcortins. It is postulated that these proteins control the biosynthesis of potent mediators of inflammation such as prostaglandins and leukotrienes by inhibiting the release of their common precursor arachidonic acid. Arachidonic acid is released from membrane phospholipids by phospholipase A_2.

PHARMACOKINETICS

The extent of percutaneous absorption of topical corticosteroids is determined by many factors including the vehicle and the integrity of the epidermal barrier. Occlusive dressings with hydrocortisone for up to 24 hours have not been demonstrated to increase penetration; however, occlusion of hydrocortisone for 96 hours markedly enhances penetration. Topical corticosteroids can be absorbed from normal intact skin. Inflammation and/or other disease processes in the skin increase percutaneous absorption.

INDICATIONS AND USAGE

Desonide is a low to medium potency corticosteroid indicated for the relief of the inflammatory and pruritic manifestations of corticosteroid responsive dermatoses.

CONTRAINDICATIONS

Desonide is contraindicated in those patients with a history of hypersensitivity to any of the components of the preparations.

PRECAUTIONS

GENERAL

Systemic absorption of topical corticosteroids can produce reversible hypothalamic-pituitary-adrenal (HPA) axis suppression with the potential for glucocorticosteroid insufficiency after withdrawal of treatment. Manifestations of Cushing's syndrome, hyperglycemia, and glucosuria can also be produced in some patients by systemic absorption of topical corticosteroids while on treatment.

Patients applying a topical steroid to a large surface area or to areas under occlusion should be evaluated periodically for evidence of HPA axis suppression. This may be done by using the ACTH stimulation, AM plasma cortisol, and urinary free cortisol tests. Patients receiving superpotent corticosteroids should not be treated for more than 2 weeks at a time and only small areas should be treated at any one time due to the increased risk of HPA axis suppression.

If HPA axis suppression is noted, an attempt should be made to withdraw the drug, to reduce the frequency of application, or to substitute a less potent corticosteroid. Recovery of HPA axis function is generally prompt and complete upon discontinuation of topical corticosteroids. Infrequently, signs and symptoms of glucocorticosteroid insufficiency may occur requiring supplemental systemic corticosteroids. For information on systemic supplementation, see product information for those products.

Pediatric patients may be more susceptible to systemic toxicity from equivalent doses due to their larger skin surface to body mass ratios (see Pediatric Use).

If irritation develops, desonide should be discontinued and appropriate therapy instituted. Allergic contact dermatitis with corticosteroids is usually diagnosed by observing *failure to heal* rather than noting a clinical exacerbation as with most topical products not containing corticosteroids. Such an observation should be corroborated with appropriate diagnostic patch testing.

If concomitant skin infections are present or develop, an appropriate antifungal or antibacterial agent should be used. If a favorable response does not occur promptly, use of desonide should be discontinued until the infection has been adequately controlled.

INFORMATION FOR THE PATIENT

Patients using topical corticosteroids should receive the following information and instructions:

This medication is to be used as directed by the physician. It is for external use only. Avoid contact with the eyes.

This medication should not be used for any disorder other than that for which it was prescribed.

The treated skin area should not be bandaged or otherwise covered or wrapped so as to be occlusive unless directed by the physician.

Patients should report to their physician any signs of local adverse reactions.

LABORATORY TESTS

The following tests may be helpful in evaluating patients for HPA axis suppression:

ACTH stimulation test.
A.M. plasma cortisol test.
Urinary free cortisol test.

CARCINOGENESIS, MUTAGENESIS, AND IMPAIRMENT OF FERTILITY

Long-term animal studies have not been performed to evaluate the carcinogenic potential or the effect on reproduction with the use of desonide.

PREGNANCY, TERATOGENIC EFFECTS, PREGNANCY CATEGORY C

Corticosteroids have been shown to be teratogenic in laboratory animals when administered systemically at relatively low dosage levels. Some corticosteroids have been shown to be teratogenic after dermal application in laboratory animals. Animal reproduction studies have not been conducted with desonide. It is also not known whether desonide can cause fetal harm when administered to a pregnant woman or can affect reproduction capacity. Desonide should be given to a pregnant woman only if clearly needed.

NURSING MOTHERS

Systemically administered corticosteroids appear in human milk and could suppress growth, interfere with endogenous corticosteroid production, or cause other untoward effects. It is not known whether topical administration of corticosteroids could result in sufficient systemic absorption to produce detectable quantities in human milk. Because many drugs are excreted in human milk, caution should be exercised when desonide is administered to a nursing woman.

PEDIATRIC USE

Safety and effectiveness in pediatric patients have not been established. Because of a higher ratio of skin surface area to body mass, pediatric patients are at a greater risk than adults of HPA axis suppression when they are treated with topical corticosteroids. They are therefore also at greater risk of glucocorticosteroid insufficiency after withdrawal of treatment and of Cushing's syndrome while on treatment. Adverse effects including striae have been reported with inappropriate use of topical corticosteroids in infants and children.

HPA axis suppression, Cushing's syndrome, linear growth retardation, delayed weight gain, and intracranial hypertension have been reported in pediatric patients receiving topical corticosteroids. Manifestations of adrenal suppression in pediatric patients include low plasma cortisol levels, and absence of response to ACTH stimulation. Manifestations of intracranial hypertension include bulging fontanelles, headaches, and bilateral papilledema.

D

ADVERSE REACTIONS

In controlled clinical trials, the total incidence of adverse reactions associated with the use of desonide was approximately 8%. These were: Stinging and burning approximately 3%, irritation, contact dermatitis, condition worsened, peeling of skin, itching, intense transient erythema, and dryness/scaliness, each less than 2%.

The following additional local adverse reactions have been reported infrequently with other topical corticosteroids, and they may occur more frequently with the use of occlusive dressings, especially with higher potency corticosteroids. These reactions are listed in an approximate decreasing order of occurrence: folliculitis, acneiform eruptions, hypopigmentation, perioral dermatitis, secondary infection, skin atrophy, striae, and miliaria.

DOSAGE AND ADMINISTRATION

Desonide cream, ointment, and lotion should be applied to the affected areas as a thin film 2 or 3 times daily depending on the severity of the condition.

As with other corticosteroids, therapy should be discontinued when control is achieved. If no improvement is seen within 2 weeks, reassessment of diagnosis may be necessary.

Desonide should not be used with occlusive dressings.

SHAKE LOTION WELL BEFORE USING.

PRODUCT LISTING - RATED THERAPEUTICALLY EQUIVALENT

Cream - Topical - 0.05%			
15 gm	$7.96	GENERIC, Copley	38245-0184-70
15 gm	$8.55	GENERIC, Qualitest Products Inc	00603-7731-74
15 gm	$8.69	GENERIC, Taro Pharmaceuticals U.S.A. Inc	51672-9080-01
15 gm	$8.82	GENERIC, Geneva Pharmaceuticals	00781-7230-27
15 gm	$9.05	GENERIC, Watson/Rugby Laboratories Inc	00536-7502-20
15 gm	$9.63	GENERIC, Ivax Corporation	00182-5115-51
15 gm	$9.65	GENERIC, Major Pharmaceuticals Inc	00904-7724-36
15 gm	$12.10	GENERIC, Ivax Corporation	00182-5066-51
15 gm	$12.45	TRIDESILON, Allscripts Pharmaceutical Company	54569-1557-00
15 gm	$12.95	TRIDESILON, Clay-Park Laboratories Inc	45802-0424-35
15 gm	$15.47	GENERIC, Taro Pharmaceuticals U.S.A. Inc	51672-1280-01
15 gm	$21.31	DESOWEN, Galderma Laboratories Inc	00299-5770-15
60 gm	$22.78	GENERIC, Copley	38245-0184-73
60 gm	$25.25	GENERIC, Geneva Pharmaceuticals	00781-7230-35
60 gm	$25.50	GENERIC, Qualitest Products Inc	00603-7731-88
60 gm	$25.50	GENERIC, Major Pharmaceuticals Inc	00904-7724-02
60 gm	$26.10	GENERIC, Ivax Corporation	00182-5115-52
60 gm	$33.45	GENERIC, Ivax Corporation	00182-5066-52
60 gm	$35.90	TRIDESILON, Clay-Park Laboratories Inc	45802-0424-37
60 gm	$39.88	GENERIC, Taro Pharmaceuticals U.S.A. Inc	51672-1280-03
60 gm	$53.81	DESOWEN, Galderma Laboratories Inc	00299-5770-60
90 gm	$37.13	DESOWEN, Galderma Laboratories Inc	00299-5770-90
Lotion - Topical - 0.05%			
60 ml	$32.83	GENERIC, Fougera	00168-0310-02
60 ml	$33.39	GENERIC, Glades Pharmaceuticals	59366-2855-02
120 ml	$50.46	GENERIC, Fougera	00168-0310-04
120 ml	$51.75	GENERIC, Glades Pharmaceuticals	59366-2855-04
Ointment - Topical - 0.05%			
15 gm	$12.95	TRIDESILON, Clay-Park Laboratories Inc	45802-0425-35
15 gm	$14.55	GENERIC, Taro Pharmaceuticals U.S.A. Inc	51672-1281-01
15 gm	$18.17	GENERIC, Fougera	00168-0309-15
15 gm	$21.31	DESOWEN, Galderma Laboratories Inc	00299-5775-15
60 gm	$24.46	FEDERAL UPPER LIMIT, H.C.F.A. F F P	99999-0967-04
60 gm	$35.90	TRIDESILON, Clay-Park Laboratories Inc	45802-0425-37
60 gm	$39.88	GENERIC, Taro Pharmaceuticals U.S.A. Inc	51672-1281-03
60 gm	$45.92	GENERIC, Fougera	00168-0309-60
60 gm	$53.81	DESOWEN, Galderma Laboratories Inc	00299-5775-60

PRODUCT LISTING - EQUIVALENTS NOT AVAILABLE

Cream - Topical - 0.05%			
15 gm	$9.85	GENERIC, Moore, H.L. Drug Exchange Inc	00839-7135-47
15 gm	$9.95	GENERIC, Clay-Park Laboratories Inc	45802-0422-35
15 gm	$15.47	GENERIC, Allscripts Pharmaceutical Company	54569-4884-00
60 gm	$25.50	GENERIC, Clay-Park Laboratories Inc	45802-0422-37
60 gm	$26.31	GENERIC, Moore, H.L. Drug Exchange Inc	00839-7135-50
Lotion - Topical - 0.05%			
59 ml	$36.69	DESOWEN, Galderma Laboratories Inc	00299-5765-02
118 ml	$56.38	DESOWEN, Galderma Laboratories Inc	00299-5765-04
Ointment - Topical - 0.05%			
15 gm	$9.95	GENERIC, Clay-Park Laboratories Inc	45802-0423-35

15 gm	$12.71	GENERIC, Allscripts Pharmaceutical Company	54569-4885-00
60 gm	$25.50	GENERIC, Clay-Park Laboratories Inc	45802-0423-37

Desoximetasone (000968)

For complete prescribing information, refer to the CD-ROM included with the book.

Categories: Dermatosis, corticosteroid-responsive; Pregnancy Category C; FDA Approved 1977 Feb
Drug Classes: Corticosteroids, topical; Dermatologics
Brand Names: Topicort
Foreign Brand Availability: Actiderm (Argentina); Dercason (Indonesia); Desicort (Israel); Dethasone (Korea); Esperson (Bulgaria; Ecuador; Indonesia; Korea; Malaysia; Portugal; Taiwan; Thailand); Flubason (Italy; Spain); Ibaril (Bulgaria; Denmark; Finland; Netherlands; Norway; Sweden); Inerson (Indonesia); Stiedex (England); Topcort (Indonesia); Topicorte (Bahrain; Belgium; Cyprus; Egypt; France; Iran; Iraq; Jordan; Kuwait; Lebanon; Libya; Malaysia; Netherlands; Oman; Portugal; Qatar; Republic-of-Yemen; Saudi-Arabia; Syria; Thailand; United-Arab-Emirates); Topisolon (Austria; Bahamas; Barbados; Belize; Benin; Bermuda; Burkina-Faso; Curacao; Ethiopia; Gambia; Germany; Ghana; Guinea; Guyana; Ireland; Ivory-Coast; Jamaica; Kenya; Liberia; Malawi; Mali; Mauritania; Mauritius; Morocco; Netherland-Antilles; Niger; Nigeria; Senegal; Seychelles; Sierra-Leone; Sudan; Surinam; Sweden; Switzerland; Tanzania; Trinidad; Tunia; Uganda; Zambia; Zimbabwe)

DESCRIPTION

Topicort emollient cream 0.25%, emollient cream 0.05%, gel 0.05%, and ointment 0.25% contain the active synthetic corticosteroid desoximetasone. The topical corticosteroids constitute a class of primarily synthetic steroids used as anti-inflammatory and anti-pruritic agents.

Each gram of Topicort emollient cream 0.25% contains 2.5 mg of desoximetasone in an emollient cream consisting of white petrolatum, purified water, isopropyl myristate, lanolin alcohols, mineral oil, cetostearyl alcohol, aluminum stearate, and magnesium stearate.

Each gram of Topicort emollient cream 0.05% contains 0.5 mg of desoximetasone in an emollient cream consisting of white petrolatum, purified water, isopropyl myristate, lanolin alcohols, mineral oil, cetostearyl alcohol, aluminum stearate, edetate disodium, lactic acid, and magnesium stearate.

Each gram of Topicort gel 0.05% contains 0.5 mg of desoximetasone in a gel consisting of purified water, SD alcohol 40 (20% w/w), isopropyl myristate, carbomer 940, trolamine, edetate disodium, and docusate sodium.

Each gram of Topicort ointment 0.25% contains 2.5 mg of desoximetasone in a base consisting of white petrolatum, propylene glycol, sorbitan sesquioleate, beeswax, fatty alcohol citrate, fatty acid pentaerythritol ester, aluminum stearate, citric acid, and butylated hydroxyanisole.

The chemical name of desoximetasone is pregna-1, 4-diene-3,20-dione, 9-fluoro-11,21-dihydroxy-16-methyl-,(11β,16α)-.

Desoximetasone has the empirical formula $C_{22}H_{29}FO_4$ and a molecular weight of 376.47.
Storage: Store at controlled room temperature (59-86°F).

INDICATIONS AND USAGE

Desoximetasone emollient cream 0.25%, emollient cream 0.05%, gel 0.05%, and ointment 0.25% are indicated for the relief of the inflammatory and pruritic manifestations of corticosteroid-responsive dermatoses.

CONTRAINDICATIONS

Topical corticosteroids are contraindicated in those patients with a history of hypersensitivity to any of the components of the preparation.

DOSAGE AND ADMINISTRATION

Apply a thin film of desoximetasone emollient cream 0.25%, emollient cream 0.05%, gel 0.05% or ointment 0.25% to the affected skin areas twice daily. Rub in gently.

PRODUCT LISTING - RATED THERAPEUTICALLY EQUIVALENT

Cream - Topical - 0.05%

15 gm	$9.90	GENERIC, Major Pharmaceuticals Inc	00904-0765-36
15 gm	$10.00	GENERIC, Geneva Pharmaceuticals	00781-7185-27
15 gm	$18.80	GENERIC, Taro Pharmaceuticals U.S.A. Inc	51672-1271-01
60 gm	$23.55	GENERIC, Major Pharmaceuticals Inc	00904-0765-02
60 gm	$24.00	GENERIC, Geneva Pharmaceuticals	00781-7185-35
60 gm	$50.15	GENERIC, Taro Pharmaceuticals U.S.A. Inc	51672-1271-03

Cream - Topical - 0.25%

15 gm	$12.42	GENERIC, Moore, H.L. Drug Exchange Inc	00839-7665-47
15 gm	$14.75	GENERIC, Major Pharmaceuticals Inc	00904-0764-36
15 gm	$19.49	GENERIC, Qualitest Products Inc	00603-7733-74
15 gm	$23.90	TOPICORT, Southwood Pharmaceuticals Inc	58016-3187-01
15 gm	$24.16	TOPICORT, Physicians Total Care	54868-0976-01
15 gm	$25.56	TOPICORT, Allscripts Pharmaceutical Company	54569-0786-00
15 gm	$25.86	GENERIC, Taro Pharmaceuticals U.S.A. Inc	51672-1270-01
15 gm	$34.26	TOPICORT, Medicis Dermatologics Inc	99207-0011-15
60 gm	$30.24	GENERIC, Moore, H.L. Drug Exchange Inc	00839-7665-50
60 gm	$35.75	GENERIC, Major Pharmaceuticals Inc	00904-0764-02
60 gm	$37.93	FEDERAL UPPER LIMIT, H.C.F.A. F F P	99999-0968-04
60 gm	$47.00	GENERIC, Qualitest Products Inc	00603-7733-88
60 gm	$57.20	TOPICORT, Physicians Total Care	54868-0976-02
60 gm	$62.09	GENERIC, Taro Pharmaceuticals U.S.A. Inc	51672-1270-03
60 gm	$82.28	TOPICORT, Medicis Dermatologics Inc	99207-0011-60

Gel - Topical - 0.05%

15 gm	$25.42	GENERIC, Taro Pharmaceuticals U.S.A. Inc	51672-1261-01
15 gm	$29.75	GENERIC, Taro Pharmaceuticals U.S.A. Inc	99207-0014-15
60 gm	$62.29	GENERIC, Taro Pharmaceuticals U.S.A. Inc	51672-1261-03

Ointment - Topical - 0.25%

15 gm	$15.41	GENERIC, Fougera	00168-0151-15
15 gm	$25.86	GENERIC, Taro Pharmaceuticals U.S.A. Inc	51672-1262-01
15 gm	$49.83	TOPICORT, Physicians Total Care	54868-2662-01
60 gm	$37.09	GENERIC, Fougera	00168-0151-60
60 gm	$56.78	TOPICORT, Physicians Total Care	54868-2662-02
60 gm	$69.77	GENERIC, Taro Pharmaceuticals U.S.A. Inc	51672-1262-03
60 gm	$81.66	TOPICORT, Taro Pharmaceuticals U.S.A. Inc	99207-0025-60

PRODUCT LISTING - EQUIVALENTS NOT AVAILABLE

Cream - Topical - 0.25%

15 gm	$19.31	GENERIC, Southwood Pharmaceuticals Inc	58016-6228-01
15 gm	$19.50	GENERIC, Allscripts Pharmaceutical Company	54569-4486-00
60 gm	$29.75	GENERIC, Aligen Independent Laboratories Inc	00405-0920-56

Gel - Topical - 0.05%

15 gm	$18.44	TOPICORT, Aventis Pharmaceuticals	00039-0014-23
60 gm	$45.22	TOPICORT, Aventis Pharmaceuticals	00039-0014-60
60 gm	$72.91	GENERIC, Taro Pharmaceuticals U.S.A. Inc	99207-0014-60

Dexamethasone (000974)

For related information, see the comparative table section in Appendix A.

Categories: Adrenocortical insufficiency; Anemia, acquired hemolytic; Anemia, congenital hypoplastic; Anemia, erythroblastopenia; Ankylosing spondylitis; Arthritis, gouty; Arthritis, post-traumatic; Arthritis, psoriatic; Arthritis, rheumatoid; Asthma; Berylliosis; Bursitis; Carditis, rheumatic; Chorioretinitis; Choroiditis; Colitis, ulcerative; Conjunctivitis, allergic; Crohn's disease; Dermatitis herpetiformis, bullous; Dermatitis, atopic; Dermatitis, contact; Dermatitis, exfoliative; Dermatitis, seborrheic; Dermatomyositis, systemic; Dermatosis, corticosteroid-responsive; Epicondylitis; Erythema multiforme; Herpes zoster ophthalmicus; Hypercalcemia, secondary to neoplasia; Hypersensitivity reactions; Inflammation, anterior segment, ophthalmic; Inflammation, ophthalmic; Inflammatory bowel disease; Iridocyclitis; Iritis; Keratitis; Leukemia; Loffler's syndrome; Lupus erythematosus, systemic; Lymphoma; Meningitis, tuberculous; Multiple sclerosis; Mycosis fungoides; Nephrotic syndrome; Neuritis, optic; Ophthalmia, sympathetic; Pemphigus; Pneumonitis, aspiration; Polymyositis; Psoriasis; Rhinitis, perennial allergic; Rhinitis, seasonal allergic; Sarcoidosis; Serum sickness; Stevens-Johnson syndrome; Synovitis, secondary to osteoarthritis; Tenosynovitis; Thrombocytopenia, secondary; Thyroiditis, nonsuppurative; Trichinosis; Tuberculosis, disseminated; Tuberculosis, fulminating; Tuberculosis, meningitis; Ulcer, allergic corneal marginal; Uveitis; Pregnancy Category C; FDA Approved 1958 Oct; WHO Formulary
Drug Classes: Corticosteroids; Corticosteroids, ophthalmic; Corticosteroids, topical; Dermatologics; Ophthalmics
Brand Names: Aeroseb-Dex; Decaderm; **Decadron**; Decarex; Decaspray; Dexone; Dms; Hexadrol; Maxidex; Mymethasone
Foreign Brand Availability: Alfalyl (Colombia); Alin (Dominican-Republic; El-Salvador; Mexico; Nicaragua; Panama); Artrosone (Spain); Cetadexon (Indonesia); Corsona (Indonesia); Cortidex (Indonesia); Cortidexason (Germany); Dabu (Japan); Danasone (Indonesia); Decadran (Spain); Decdan (India); Decilone (Philippines); Dectancyl (Bahrain; Cyprus; Egypt; Iran; Iraq; Jordan; Kuwait; Lebanon; Libya; Oman; Qatar; Republic-of-Yemen; Saudi-Arabia; Syria; United-Arab-Emirates); Desalark (Italy); Desigdron (Philippines); Dexacortal (Sweden); Dexalocal (Dominican-Republic; El-Salvador; Guatemala; Honduras; Hong-Kong; Switzerland); Dexame (Japan); Dexamed (Malaysia); Dexametason (Finland); Dexamethason (Hungary); Dexamonozon (Germany); Dexamethasone (Greece; Israel; New-Zealand); Dexano (Thailand); Dexa-P (Thailand); Dexasone (Canada; Hong-Kong; Thailand); Dexasone S (Japan); Dexmethsone (Australia; Hong-Kong); Dexona (Bahrain; Cyprus; Egypt; India; Iran; Iraq; Jordan; Kuwait; Lebanon; Libya; Oman; Qatar; Republic-of-Yemen; Saudi-Arabia; Syria; United-Arab-Emirates); Dextrasone (Malaysia); Dibasona (Mexico); Fortecortin (Austria; Czech-Republic; Germany; Russia; Switzerland); Isopto-Dex (Germany); Isopto-Maxidex (Finland; Norway; Sweden); Loverine (Japan); Mexasone (Singapore); Oftan-Dexa (Finland); Oradexon (Bahrain; Belgium; Benin; Burkina-Faso; Cyprus; Czech-Republic; Egypt; Ethiopia; Finland; Gambia; Ghana; Greece; Guinea; Hungary; Indonesia; Iran; Iraq; Ivory-Coast; Jordan; Kenya; Kuwait; Lebanon; Liberia; Libya; Malawi; Mali; Mauritania; Mauritius; Morocco; Netherlands; Niger; Nigeria; Oman; Peru; Qatar; Republic-of-Yemen; Saudi-Arabia; Senegal; Seychelles; Sierra-Leone; South-Africa; Sudan; Syria; Taiwan; Tanzania; Tunia; Turkey; Uganda; United-Arab-Emirates; Zambia; Zimbabwe); Pidexon (Indonesia); Predni-F (Germany); Santenson (Japan); Santeson (Philippines); Sawasone (Japan); Spersadex (Norway); Thilodexine (Greece); Vexamet (Philippines); Visumetazone (Italy); Wymesone (India)

DESCRIPTION

Glucocorticoids are adrenocortical steroids, both naturally occurring and synthetic, which are readily absorbed from the gastrointestinal tract.

Dexamethasone, a synthetic adrenocortical steroid, is a white to practically white, odorless, crystalline powder. It is stable in air. It is practically insoluble in water. The molecular weight is 392.47. It is designated chemically as 9-fluoro-11β,17,21-trihydroxy-16α-methylpregna-1,4-diene-3,20-dione. The empirical formula is $C_{22}H_{29}FO_5$.

ORAL FORMS

Dexamethasone tablets are supplied in six potencies, 0.25, 0.5, 0.75, 1.5, 4, and 6 mg. Inactive ingredients are calcium phosphate, lactose, magnesium stearate, and starch. Dexamethasone tablets 0.25 mg also contain FD&C yellow 6. Dexamethasone tablets 0.5 mg also contain FD&C yellow 10 and FD&C yellow 6. Dexamethasone tablets 0.75 mg also contain FD&C blue 1. Dexamethasone tablets 1.5 mg also contain FD&C red 40. Dexamethasone tablets 6 mg also contain FD&C blue 1 and iron oxide.

Dexamethasone elixir contains 0.5 mg of dexamethasone in each 5 ml. Benzoic acid, 0.1%, is added as a preservative. It also contains alcohol 5%. Inactive ingredients are FD&C red 40, flavors, glycerin, purified water, and sodium saccharin.

TOPICAL FORMS

The topical corticosteroids constitute a class of primarily synthetic steroids used as anti-inflammatory and anti-pruritic agents.

Topical Aerosol Dexamethasone is a topical steroid preparation, each 25 mg of which contains 10 mg of dexamethasone. The inactive ingredients are isopropyl myristate, and isobutane. Each second of spray dispenses approximately 0.75 mg of dexamethasone.

Dexamethasone cream is a topical steroid preparation containing 0.1% of dexamethasone. Each gram contains 1 mg dexamethasone in Estergel, specially formulated vehicle consisting of gelled isopropyl myristate, wood alcohols, refined lanolin alcohol, microcrystalline wax, anhydrous citric acid, and anhydrous sodium phosphate dibasic.

This emollient gel vehicle is anhydrous, lipophilic, hydrophilic, and moisture retentive. The base largely disappears when rubbed on the skin.

CLINICAL PHARMACOLOGY

ORAL FORMS

Naturally occurring glucocorticoids (hydrocortisone and cortisone), which also have salt-retaining properties, are used as replacement therapy in adrenocortical deficiency states. Their synthetic analogs, including dexamethasone, are primarily used for their potent anti-inflammatory effects in disorders of many organ systems.

Glucocorticoids cause profound and varied metabolic effects. In addition, they modify the body's immune responses to diverse stimuli.

At equipotent anti-inflammatory doses, dexamethasone almost completely lacks the sodium-retaining property of hydrocortisone and closely related derivatives of hydrocortisone.

TOPICAL FORMS

Topical corticosteroids share anti-inflammatory, anti-pruritic, and vasoconstrictive actions.

The mechanism of anti-inflammatory activity of the topical corticosteroids is unclear. Various laboratory methods, including vasoconstrictor assays, are used to compare and predict potencies and/or clinical efficacies of the topical corticosteroids. There is some evidence to suggest that a recognizable correlation exists between vasoconstrictor potency and therapeutic efficacy in man.

Pharmacokinetics

The extent of percutaneous absorption of topical corticosteroids is determined by many factors including the vehicle, the integrity of the epidermal barrier, and the use of occlusive dressings.

Topical corticosteroids can be absorbed from normal intact skin. Inflammation and/or other disease processes in the skin increase percutaneous absorption. Occlusive dressings substantially increase the percutaneous absorption of topical corticosteroids. Thus, occlusive dressings may be a valuable therapeutic adjunct for treatment of resistant dermatoses (see DOSAGE AND ADMINISTRATION).

Once absorbed through the skin, topical corticosteroids are handled through pharmacokinetic pathways similar to systemically administered corticosteroids. Corticosteroids are bound to plasma proteins in varying degrees. Corticosteroids are metabolized primarily in the liver and are then excreted by the kidneys. Some of the topical corticosteroids and their metabolites are also excreted into the bile.

INDICATIONS AND USAGE

ORAL FORMS

Endocrine Disorders: Primary or secondary adrenocortical insufficiency (hydrocortisone or cortisone is the first choice; synthetic analogs may be used in conjunction with mineralocorticoids where applicable; in infancy mineralocorticoid supplementation is of particular importance); congenital adrenal hyperplasia; nonsuppurative thyroiditis; hypercalcemia associated with cancer.

Rheumatic Disorders: As adjunctive therapy for short-term administration (to tide the patient over an acute episode or exacerbation) in:

Psoriatic arthritis; rheumatoid arthritis, including juvenile rheumatoid arthritis (selected cases may require low-dose maintenance therapy); ankylosing spondylitis; acute and subacute bursitis; acute nonspecific tenosynovitis; acute gouty arthritis; post-traumatic osteoarthritis; synovitis of osteoarthritis; epicondylitis.

Collagen Diseases: During an exacerbation or as maintenance therapy in selected cases of—Systemic lupus erythematosus; acute rheumatic carditis.

Dermatologic Diseases: Pemphigus; bullous dermatitis herpetiformis; severe erythema multiforme (stevens-johnson syndrome); exfoliative dermatitis; mycosis fungoides; severe psoriasis; severe seborrheic dermatitis.

Allergic States: Control of severe or incapacitating allergic conditions intractable to adequate trials of conventional treatment: seasonal or perennial allergic rhinitis; bronchial asthma; contact dermatitis; atopic dermatitis; serum sickness; drug hypersensitivity reactions.

Ophthalmic Diseases: Severe acute and chronic allergic and inflammatory processes involving the eye and its adnexa, such as—allergic conjunctivitis; keratitis; allergic corneal marginal ulcers; herpes zoster ophthalmicus; iritis and iridocyclitis; chorioretinitis; anterior segment inflammation; diffuse posterior uveitis and choroiditis; optic neuritis; sympathetic ophthalmia.

Respiratory Diseases: Symptomatic sarcoidosis; loeffler's syndrome not manageable by other means; berylliosis; fulminating or disseminated pulmonary tuberculosis when used concurrently with appropriate antituberculous chemotherapy; aspiration pneumonitis.

Hematologic Disorders: Idiopathic thrombocytopenic purpura in adults; secondary thrombocytopenia in adults; acquired (autoimmune) hemolytic anemia; erythroblastopenic (rbc anemia); congenital (erythroid) hypoplastic anemia.

Neoplastic Disease: For palliative management of: leukemias and lymphomas in adults; acute leukemia of childhood.

Edematous States: To induce a diuresis or remission of proteinuria in the nephrotic syndrome, without uremia, of the idiopathic type or that due to lupus erythematosus.

Gastrointestinal Disease: To tide the patient over a critical period of the disease in: ulcerative colitis; regional enteritis.

Cerebral Edema: Associated with primary or metastatic brain tumor, craniotomy, or head injury. Use in cerebral edema is not a substitute for careful neurosurgical evaluation and definitive management such as neurosurgery or other specific therapy.

Miscellaneous: Tuberculous meningitis with subarachnoid block or impending block when used concurrently with appropriate anti-tuberculous chemotherapy, trichinosis with neurologic or myocardial involvement.

Diagnostic testing of adrenocortical hyperfunction.

TOPICAL FORMS

Topical dexamethasone is indicated for relief of the inflammatory and pruritic manifestations of corticosteroid-responsive dermatoses.

NON-FDA APPROVED INDICATIONS

Although not approved by the FDA, several studies have reported the efficacy of dexamethasone as an antiemetic in cancer chemotherapy.

CONTRAINDICATIONS

ORAL FORMS

Systemic fungal infections.
Hypersensitivity to this drug.

TOPICAL FORMS

Topical corticosteroids are contraindicated in those patients with a history of hypersensitivity to any of the components of the preparation.

WARNINGS

ORAL FORMS

In patients on corticosteroid therapy subjected to unusual stress, increased dosage of rapidly acting corticosteroids before, during, and after the stressful situation is indicated.

Drug-induced secondary adrenocortical insufficiency may result from too rapid withdrawal of corticosteroids and may be minimized by gradual reduction of dosage. This type of relative insufficiency may persist for months after discontinuation of therapy; therefore, in any situation of stress occurring during the period, hormone therapy should be reinstituted. If the patient is receiving steroids already, dosage may have to be increased. Since mineralocorticoid secretion may be impaired, salt and/or a mineralocorticoid should be administered concurrently.

Corticosteroids may mask some signs of infection, and new infections may appear during their use. There may be decreased resistance and inability to localize infection when corticosteroids are used. Moreover, corticosteroids may affect the nitroblue-tetrazolium test for bacterial infection and produce false negative results.

In cerebral malaria, a double-blind trial has shown that the use of corticosteroids is associated with prolongation of come and a higher incidence of pneumonia and gastrointestinal bleeding.

Corticosteroids may activate latent amebiasis. Therefore, it is recommended that latent or active amebiasis be ruled out before initiating corticosteroid therapy in any patient who has spent time in the tropics or any patient with unexplained diarrhea.

Prolonged use of corticosteroids may produce posterior subcapsular cataracts, glaucoma with possible damage to the optic nerves, and may enhance the establishment of secondary ocular infections due to fungi or viruses.

Use in Pregnancy

Since adequate human reproduction studies have not been done with corticosteroids, use of these drugs in pregnancy or in women of childbearing potential requires that the anticipated benefits be weighed against the possible hazards to the mother and embryo or fetus. Infants born of mothers who have received substantial doses of corticosteroids during pregnancy should be carefully observed for signs of hypoadrenalism.

Corticosteroids appear in breast milk and could suppress growth, interfere with endogenous corticosteroid production, or cause other unwanted effects. Mothers taking pharmacologic doses of corticosteroids should be advised not to nurse.

Average and large doses of hydrocortisone or cortisone can cause elevation of blood pressure, salt and water retention, and increased excretion of potassium. These effects are less likely to occur with the synthetic derivatives except when used in large doses. Dietary salt restriction and potassium supplementation may be necessary. All corticosteroids increase calcium excretion.

Administration of live virus vaccines, including smallpox, is contraindicated in individuals receiving immunosuppressive doses of corticosteroids. If inactivated viral or bacterial vaccines are administered to individuals receiving immunosuppressive doses of corticosteroid the expected serum antibody response may not be obtained. However, immunization procedures may be undertaken in patients who are receiving corticosteroids as replacement therapy, e.g., for Addison's disease.

Patients who are on drugs which suppress the immune system are more susceptible to infections than healthy individuals. Chickenpox and measles, for example, can have a more serious or even fatal course in non-immune children or adults on corticosteroids. In such children or adults who have not had these diseases, particular care should be taken to avoid exposure. The risk of developing a disseminated infection varies among individuals and can be related to the dose, route and duration of corticosteroid administration as well as to the underlying disease. If exposed to chickpox, prophylaxis with varicella zoster immune globulin (VZIG) may be indicated. If chickenpox develops, treatment with antiviral agents may be considered. If exposed to measles, prophylaxis with immune globulin (IG) may be indicated (see the respective package inserts for VZIG and IG for complete prescribing information).

The use of dexamethasone tablets or elixir in active tuberculosis should be restricted to those cases of fulminating or disseminated tuberculosis in which the corticosteroid is used for the management of the disease in conjunction with an appropriate antituberculous regimen.

If corticosteroids are indicated in patients with latent tuberculosis or tuberculin reactivity, close observation is necessary as reactivation of the disease may occur. During prolonged corticosteroid therapy, these patients should be receive chemoprophylaxis.

Literature reports suggest an apparent association between corticosteroids' and left ventricular free wall rupture after a recent myocardial infarction; therefore, therapy with corticosteroids should be used with great caution in these patients.

TOPICAL AEROSOL

Avoid spraying in eyes or nose. Contents under pressure. Do not puncture or burn. Keep out of reach of children. Use only as directed. Intentional misuse by deliberately concentrating and inhaling the contents can be harmful or fatal.

Topically applied steroids are absorbed systemically. There may be rare instances in which this absorption results in immunosuppression. Patients who are on drugs which suppress the immune system are more susceptible to infections than healthy individuals.

Chickenpox and measles, for example, can have a more serious or even fatal course in non-immune children (see PRECAUTIONS, Pediatric Use) or adults on corticosteroids. In such children or adults who have not had these diseases, particular care should be taken to avoid exposure. The risk of developing a disseminated infection varies among individuals and can be related to the dose, route, and duration of corticosteroid administration as well as to the underlying disease. If exposed to chickenpox, prophylaxis with varicella zoster immune globulin (VZIG) may be indicated. If chickpox develops, treatment with antiviral agents may be considered. If exposed to measles, prophylaxis with immune globulin (IG) may be indicated (see the respective package inserts for VZIG and IG for complete prescribing information).

PRECAUTIONS

ORAL FORMS

Following prolonged therapy, withdrawal of corticosteroids may result in symptoms of the corticosteroid withdrawal syndrome including fever, myalgia, arthralgia, and malaise. This may occur in patients even without evidence of adrenal insufficiency.

There is an enhanced effect of corticosteroids in patients with hypothyroidism and in those with cirrhosis.

Corticosteroids should be used cautiously in patients with ocular herpes simplex because of possible corneal perforation.

The lowest possible dose of corticosteroids should be used to control the condition under treatment, and when reduction in dosage is possible, the reduction should be gradual.

Psychic derangements may appear when corticosteroids are used, ranging from euphoria, insomnia, mood swings, personality changes, and severe depression instability or psychotic tendencies may be aggravated by corticosteroids.

Aspirin should be used cautiously in conjunction with corticosteroids in hypoprothrombinemia.

Steroids should be used with caution in nonspecific ulcerative colitis, if there is a probability of impending perforation, abscess, or other pyogenic infection, diverticulitis, fresh intestinal anastomoses, active or latent peptic ulcer, renal insufficiency, hypertension, osteoporosis, and myasthenia gravis. Signs of peritoneal irritation following gastrointestinal perforation in patients receiving large doses of corticosteroids may be minimal or absent. Fat embolism has been reported as a possible complication of hypercortisonism.

When large doses are given, some authorities advise that corticosteroids be taken with meals and antacids taken between meals to help to prevent peptic ulcer.

Growth and development of infants and children on prolonged corticosteroid therapy should be carefully observed.

Steroids may increase or decrease motility and number of spermatozoa in some patients.

False-negative results in the dexamethasone suppression test (DST) in patients being treated with indomethacin have been reported. Thus, results of the DST should be interpreted with caution in these patients.

The prothrombin time should be checked frequently in patients who are receiving corticosteroids and cumarin anticoagulants at the same time because of reports that corticosteroids have altered the response to these anticoagulants. Studies have shown that the usual effect produced by adding corticosteroids is inhibition of response to coumarins, although there have been some conflicting reports of potentiation not substantiated by studies.

When corticosteroids are administered concomitantly with potassium-depleting diuretics, patients should be observed closely for development of hypokalemia.

TOPICAL FORMS

General

Systemic absorption of topical corticosteroids has produced reversible hypothalamic-pituitary-adrenal (HPA) axis suppression, manifestations of Cushing's syndrome, hyperglycemia, and glycosuria in some patients.

Conditions which augment systemic absorption include the application of the more potent corticosteroids, use over large surface areas, prolonged use, and the addition of occlusive dressings.

Therefore, patients receiving a large dose of a potent topical corticosteroid applied to a large surface area or under an occlusive dressing should be evaluated periodically for evidence of HPA axis suppression by using urinary free cortisol and ACTH stimulation tests. If HPA axis suppression is noted, an attempt should be made to withdraw the drug, to reduce the frequency of application, or to substitute a less potent corticosteroid.

Recovery of HPA axis function is generally prompt and complete upon discontinuation of the drug. Infrequently, signs and symptoms of corticosteroid withdrawal may occur, requiring supplemental systemic corticosteroids.

Children may absorb proportionally larger amounts of topical corticosteroids and thus be more susceptible to systemic toxicity (see Pediatric Use).

If irritation develops, topical corticosteroids should be discontinued and appropriate therapy instituted.

In the presence of dermatological infections, the use of an appropriate antifungal or antibacterial agent should be instituted. If a favorable response does not occur promptly, the corticosteroid should be discontinued until the infection has been adequately controlled.

The product is not for ophthalmic use. However, if applied to the eyelids or skin near the eyes, the drug may enter the eyes. In patients with a history of herpes simplex keratitis ocular exposure to corticosteroids may lead to a recurrence. Prolonged ocular exposure may cause steroid glaucoma.

A few individuals may be sensitive to one or more of the components of this product. If any reaction indicating sensitivity is observed, discontinue use.

Generally, occlusive dressings should not be used on weeping or exudative lesions.

If occlusive dressing therapy is used, inspect lesions between dressings for development of infection. If infection develops, the technique should be discontinued and appropriate antimicrobial therapy instituted.

When large areas of the body are covered with an occlusive dressing, thermal homeostasis may be impaired. If elevation of body temperature occurs, use of the occlusive dressing should be discontinued.

Information for the Patient

Patients using topical corticosteroids should receive the following information and instructions:

This medication is to be used as directed by the physician. It is for external use only. Avoid contact with the eyes.

Patients should be advised not to use this medication for any disorder other than that for which it was prescribed.

The treated skin area should not be bandaged or otherwise covered or wrapped so as to be occlusive unless directed by the physician.

Patients should report any signs of local adverse reactions, especially under occlusive dressing.

Parents of pediatric patients should be advised not to use tight-fitting diapers or plastic pants on a child being treated in the diaper area, as these garments may constitute occlusive dressings.

Susceptible patients who are on immunosuppressant doses of corticosteroids should be warned to avoid exposure to chickenpox or measles. Patients should also be advised that if they are exposed, medical advice should be sought without delay.

Laboratory Tests

The following tests may be helpful in evaluating the HPA axis suppression:

- Urinary free cortisol test.
- ACTH stimulation test.

Carcinogenesis, Mutagenesis, and Impairment of Fertility

Long-term animal studies have not been performed to evaluate the carcinogenic potential or the effect on fertility of topical corticosteroids.

Studies to determine mutagenicity with prednisolone and hydrocortisone have revealed negative results.

Pregnancy Category C

Corticosteroids are generally teratogenic in laboratory animals when administered systemically at relatively low dosage levels. The more potent corticosteroids have been shown to be teratogenic after dermal application in laboratory animals. There are no adequate and well-controlled studies in pregnant women on teratogenic effects from topically applied corticosteroids. Therefore, topical corticosteroids should be used during pregnancy only if the potential benefit justifies the potential risk to the fetus. Drugs of this class should not be used extensively on pregnant patients, in large amounts, or for prolonged periods of time.

Nursing Mothers

It is not known whether topical administration of corticosteroids could result in sufficient systemic absorption to produce detectable quantities in breast milk. Systemically administered corticosteroids are secreted into breast milk in quantities *not* likely to have a deleterious effect on the infant. Nevertheless, caution should be exercised when topical corticosteroids are administered to a nursing woman.

Pediatric Use

Pediatric patients may demonstrate greater susceptibility to topical corticosteroid-induced HPA axis suppression and Cushing's syndrome than mature patients because of a larger skin surface to body weight ratio.

Hypothalamic-pituitary-adrenal (HPA) axis suppression, Cushing's syndrome, and intracranial hypertension have been reported in children receiving topical corticosteroids. Manifestations of adrenal suppression in children include linear growth retardation, delayed weight gain, low plasma cortisol levels, and absence of response to ACTH stimulation. Manifestations of intracranial hypertension include bulging fontanelles, headaches, and bilateral papilledema.

Administration of topical corticosteroids to children should be limited to the least amount compatible with an effective therapeutic regimen. Chronic corticosteroid therapy may interfere with the growth and development of children.

Topical Aerosol Only

CAUTION: Flammable. Do not use around open flame or while smoking.

DRUG INTERACTIONS

Phenytoin, phenobarbital, ephedrine, and rifampin may enhance the metabolic clearance of corticosteroids, resulting in decreased blood levels and lessened physiologic activity thus requiring adjustment in corticosteroid dosage. These interactions may interfere with dexamethasone suppression tests which should be interpreted with caution during administration of these drugs.

ADVERSE REACTIONS

ORAL FORMS

Fluid and Electrolyte Disturbances: Sodium retention; fluid retention; congestive heart failure in susceptible patients; potassium loss; hypokalemic alkalosis; hypertension.

Musculoskeletal: Muscle weakness; steroid myopathy; loss of muscle mass; osteoporosis; vertebral compression fractures; aseptic necrosis of femoral and humeral heads; pathologic fracture of long bones; tendon rupture.

Gastrointestinal: Peptic ulcer with possible perforation and hemorrhage; perforation of the small and large bowel, particularly in patients with inflammatory bowel disease; pancreatitis; abdominal distention; ulcerative esophagitis.

Dermatologic: Impaired wound healing; thin fragile skin; petechiae and ecchymoses; erythema; increased sweating; may suppress reactions to skin tests; other cutaneous reactions, such as allergic dermatitis, urticaria, angioneurotic edema.

Neurologic: Convulsions; increased intracranial pressure with papilledema (pseudotumor cerebri) usually after treatment; vertigo; headache; psychic disturbances.

Endocrine: Menstrual irregularities; development of cushingoid state; suppression of growth in children; secondary adrenocortical and pituitary unresponsiveness, particularly in times of stress,as in trauma, surgery, or illness; decreased carbohydrate tolerance; manifestations of latent diabetes mellitus; increased requirements for insulin or oral hypoglycemic agents in diabetics; hirsutism.

Ophthalmic: Posterior subcapsular cataracts; increased intraocular pressure; glaucoma; exophthalmos.

Metabolic: Negative nitrogen balance due to protein catabolism.

Cardiovascular: Myocardial rupture following recent myocardial infarction (see WARNINGS).

Other: Hypersensitivity; thromboembolism; weight gain; increased appetite; nausea; malaise.

TOPICAL FORMS

The following adverse reactions are reported infrequently with topical corticosteroids, but may occur more frequently with the use of occlusive dressings. These reactions are listed in an approximate decreasing order of occurrence: Burning; itching; irritation; dryness; folliculitis; hypertrichosis; acneiform eruptions; hypopigmentation; perioral dermatitis; allergic contact dermatitis; maceration of the skin; secondary infection; skin atrophy; striae; miliaria.

DOSAGE AND ADMINISTRATION

ORAL FORMS

FOR ORAL ADMINISTRATION: DOSAGE REQUIREMENTS ARE VARIABLE AND MUST BE INDIVIDUALIZED ON THE BASIS OF THE DISEASE AND THE RESPONSE OF THE PATIENT.

The initial dosage varies from 0.75 to 9 mg a day depending on the disease being treated. In less severe diseases doses lower than 0.75 mg may suffice, while in severe diseases doses higher than 9 mg may be required. The initial dosage should be maintained or adjusted until the patient's response is satisfactory. If satisfactory clinical response does not occur after a reasonable period of time, discontinue dexamethasone tablets or elixir and transfer the patient to other therapy.

After a favorable initial response, the proper maintenance dosage should be determined by decreasing the initial dosage in small amounts to the lowest dosage that maintains an adequate clinical response.

Patients should be observed closely for signs that might require dosage adjustment, including changes in clinical status resulting from remissions or exacerbations of the disease, individual drug responsiveness, and the effect of stress (*e.g.*, surgery, infection, trauma). During stress it may be necessary to increase dosage temporarily.

If the drug is to be stopped after more than a few days of treatment, it usually should be withdrawn gradually.

The following milligram equivalents facilitate changing to dexamethasone from other glucocorticoids (see TABLE 1).

TABLE 1

Dexamethasone	Methylprednisolone and Triamcinolone	Prednisolone and Prednisone	Hydrocortisone	Cortisone
0.75 mg=	4 mg=	5 mg=	20 mg=	25 mg

In acute, self-limited allergic disorders or acute exacerbations of chronic allergic disorders, the following dosage schedule combining parenteral and oral therapy is suggested:

Dexamethasone sodium phosphate injection, 4 mg/ml:

First Day: 1-2 ml, intramuscularly; dexamethasone tablets, 0.75 mg.

Second Day: 4 tablets in 2 divided doses.

Third Day: 4 tablets in 2 divided doses.

Fourth Day: 2 tablets in 2 divided doses.

Fifth Day: 1 tablet.

Sixth Day: 1 tablet.

Seventh Day: No treatment.

Eighth Day: Follow-up visit.

This schedule is designed to ensure adequate therapy during acute episodes, while minimizing the risk of overdosage in chronic cases.

In cerebral edema, dexamethasone sodium phosphate injection is generally administered initially in a dosage of 10 mg intravenously followed by 4 mg every 6 hours intramuscularly until the symptoms of cerebral edema subside. Response is usually noted within 12-24 hours and dosage may be reduced after 2-4 days and gradually discontinued over a period of 5-7 days. For palliative management of patients with recurrent or inoperable brain tumors, maintenance therapy with either dexamethasone sodium phosphate injection or dexamethasone tablets in a dosage of 2 mg two or three times daily may be effective.

Dexamethasone Suppression Tests

Tests for Cushing's syndrome: Give 1.0 mg of dexamethasone orally at 11.00 p.m. Blood is drawn in for plasma cortisol determination at 8.00 a.m. the following morning.

For greater accuracy, give 0.5 mg of dexamethasone orally every 6 hours for 48 hours. Twenty-four hour urine collections are made for determination of 17-hydroxycorticosteroid excretion.

Test to distinguish Cushing's syndrome due to pituitary ACTH excess from Cushing's syndrome due to other causes: Give 2.0 mg of dexamethasone orally 6 hours for 48 hours. Twenty-four hour urine collections are made for determination of 17-hydroxycorticosteroid excretion.

TOPICAL AEROSOL

Patients should be instructed in the correct way to use dexamethasone aerosol spray. The preparation is readily applied, even on hairy areas. It does not have to rubbed into the skin.

Optimal effects will be obtained with dexamethasone aerosol spray when these directions are followed:

Keep the affected area clean to reduce the possibility of infection.

Shake the container *gently* once or twice each time before using. Hold it about 6 inches from the area to be treated. Effective medication may be obtained with the container held either upright or inverted, since it is fitted with a special valve that dispenses approximately the same dosage in either position.

Spray each 4 inch square of affected area for 1 or 2 seconds 3 or 4 times a day, depending on the nature of the condition and the response to therapy.

When a favorable response is obtained, reduce dosage gradually and eventually discontinue.

Occlusive dressings may be used for the management of psoriasis or recalcitrant conditions.

TOPICAL CREAM

Apply to the affected area as a thin film 3 or 4 times daily.

Occlusive dressings may be used for the management of psoriasis or recalcitrant conditions.

Before using this preparation in the ear, clean the aural canal thoroughly and sponge dry. Confirm that the eardrum is intact. With a cotton-tipped applicator, apply a thin coating of the cream to the affected cream to the affected canal area 3 or 4 times a day.

PRODUCT LISTING - RATED THERAPEUTICALLY EQUIVALENT

Elixir - Oral - 0.5 mg/5 ml

100 ml	$7.45	GENERIC, Major Pharmaceuticals Inc	00904-0972-04
100 ml	$7.50	GENERIC, Cmc-Consolidated Midland Corporation	00223-6496-01
100 ml	$9.04	GENERIC, Morton Grove Pharmaceuticals Inc	60432-0466-00
100 ml	$11.08	GENERIC, Alpharma Uspd Makers Of Barre and Nmc	00472-0972-33
100 ml	$17.50	GENERIC, Cmc-Consolidated Midland Corporation	00223-6496-02
240 ml	$9.50	FEDERAL UPPER LIMIT, H.C.F.A. F F P	99999-0974-03
240 ml	$12.74	GENERIC, Geneva Pharmaceuticals	00781-6400-08
240 ml	$15.00	GENERIC, Ivax Corporation	00182-1013-44
240 ml	$15.00	GENERIC, Watson/Schein Pharmaceuticals Inc	00364-7182-76
240 ml	$15.75	GENERIC, Mutual/United Research Laboratories	00677-0601-42
240 ml	$23.29	GENERIC, Major Pharmaceuticals Inc	00904-0972-09
240 ml	$23.50	GENERIC, Alpharma Uspd Makers Of Barre and Nmc	00472-0972-08
240 ml	$23.50	GENERIC, Qualitest Products Inc	00603-1145-56
240 ml	$23.50	GENERIC, Morton Grove Pharmaceuticals Inc	60432-0466-08
240 ml	$27.12	GENERIC, Moore, H.L. Drug Exchange Inc	00839-7997-66

Suspension - Ophthalmic - 0.1%

5 ml	$35.19	MAXIDEX, Alcon Laboratories Inc	00998-0615-05
15 ml	$81.06	MAXIDEX, Alcon Laboratories Inc	00998-0615-15

Tablet - Oral - 0.5 mg

100's	$64.90	DECADRON, Merck & Company Inc	00006-0041-68

Tablet - Oral - 0.75 mg

12's	$10.19	DECADRON 5-12 PAK, Merck & Company Inc	00006-0063-12
100's	$81.14	DECADRON, Merck & Company Inc	00006-0063-68

Tablet - Oral - 1.5 mg

51's	$23.95	GENERIC, Par Pharmaceutical Inc	00095-0086-51
100's	$27.14	GENERIC, Roxane Laboratories Inc	00054-4182-25
100's	$31.99	GENERIC, Roxane Laboratories Inc	00054-8181-25

Tablet - Oral - 4 mg

50's	$117.43	DECADRON, Merck & Company Inc	00006-0097-50

PRODUCT LISTING - RATED NOT THERAPEUTICALLY EQUIVALENT

Tablet - Oral - 0.25 mg

100's	$4.05	GENERIC, Interstate Drug Exchange Inc	00814-2358-14
100's	$4.05	GENERIC, Major Pharmaceuticals Inc	00904-0242-60
100's	$4.25	GENERIC, Moore, H.L. Drug Exchange Inc	00839-6019-06
100's	$4.42	GENERIC, Aligen Independent Laboratories Inc	00405-4313-01
100's	$11.05	GENERIC, Par Pharmaceutical Inc	49884-0083-01

Tablet - Oral - 0.5 mg

50's	$3.45	GENERIC, Circle Pharmaceuticals Inc	00659-2501-05

100's	$6.15	GENERIC, Interstate Drug Exchange Inc	00814-2362-14
100's	$6.72	GENERIC, Aligen Independent Laboratories Inc	00405-4314-01
100's	$6.75	GENERIC, Cmc-Consolidated Midland Corporation	00223-0790-01
100's	$6.82	GENERIC, Moore, H.L. Drug Exchange Inc	00839-6020-06
100's	$8.95	GENERIC, Ivax Corporation	00182-1612-01
100's	$10.99	GENERIC, Major Pharmaceuticals Inc	00904-0243-60
100's	$12.01	GENERIC, Roxane Laboratories Inc	00054-4179-25
100's	$16.49	GENERIC, Roxane Laboratories Inc	00054-8179-25
100's	$21.00	GENERIC, Par Pharmaceutical Inc	49884-0084-01
Tablet - Oral - 0.75 mg			
7's	$1.29	GENERIC, Allscripts Pharmaceutical Company	54569-0322-05
10's	$3.38	GENERIC, Pd-Rx Pharmaceuticals	55289-0903-10
12's	$2.20	GENERIC, Allscripts Pharmaceutical Company	54569-0322-00
12's	$3.50	GENERIC, Vintage Pharmaceuticals Inc	00254-2667-06
12's	$4.50	GENERIC, Major Pharmaceuticals Inc	00904-0244-12
12's	$5.45	GENERIC, First Horizon Pharmaceutical Corporation	60904-0085-27
12's	$7.24	GENERIC, Qualitest Products Inc	00603-3191-11
12's	$7.24	GENERIC, Allscripts Pharmaceutical Company	54569-3110-00
12's	$8.95	GENERIC, Pharma Pac	52959-0392-12
20's	$3.67	GENERIC, Allscripts Pharmaceutical Company	54569-0322-03
20's	$3.71	GENERIC, Pd-Rx Pharmaceuticals	55289-0903-20
21's	$8.01	GENERIC, Pharma Pac	52959-0392-21
28's	$19.54	GENERIC, Pharma Pac	52959-0392-28
100's	$2.05	GENERIC, Global Pharmaceutical Corporation	00115-3100-01
100's	$6.75	GENERIC, Interstate Drug Exchange Inc	00814-2360-14
100's	$7.50	GENERIC, Cmc-Consolidated Midland Corporation	00223-0791-01
100's	$7.64	GENERIC, Aligen Independent Laboratories Inc	00405-4315-01
100's	$7.65	GENERIC, Martec Pharmaceuticals Inc	52555-0064-01
100's	$7.90	GENERIC, Moore, H.L. Drug Exchange Inc	00839-1228-06
100's	$11.95	GENERIC, Major Pharmaceuticals Inc	00904-0244-60
100's	$12.61	GENERIC, Ivax Corporation	00182-0488-01
100's	$14.61	GENERIC, Roxane Laboratories Inc	00054-4180-25
100's	$18.94	GENERIC, Roxane Laboratories Inc	00054-8180-25
100's	$40.00	GENERIC, Par Pharmaceutical Inc	49884-0085-01
Tablet - Oral - 1 mg			
100's	$28.90	GENERIC, Roxane Laboratories Inc	00054-4181-25
100's	$31.21	GENERIC, Roxane Laboratories Inc	00054-8174-25
Tablet - Oral - 1.5 mg			
50's	$10.40	GENERIC, Par Pharmaceutical Inc	49884-0086-03
50's	$12.30	GENERIC, Ivax Corporation	00182-1613-19
100's	$10.50	GENERIC, Interstate Drug Exchange Inc	00814-2364-14
100's	$15.22	GENERIC, Watson/Schein Pharmaceuticals Inc	00364-0399-01
100's	$15.90	GENERIC, Major Pharmaceuticals Inc	00904-0245-60
100's	$76.00	GENERIC, Par Pharmaceutical Inc	49884-0086-01
Tablet - Oral - 2 mg			
6's	$3.00	GENERIC, Allscripts Pharmaceutical Company	54569-0336-01
14's	$6.99	GENERIC, Allscripts Pharmaceutical Company	54569-0336-02
15's	$7.49	GENERIC, Allscripts Pharmaceutical Company	54569-0336-03
100's	$56.60	GENERIC, Roxane Laboratories Inc	00054-4183-25
100's	$59.00	GENERIC, Roxane Laboratories Inc	00054-8176-25
Tablet - Oral - 4 mg			
6's	$4.99	GENERIC, Allscripts Pharmaceutical Company	54569-0324-04
8's	$6.65	GENERIC, Allscripts Pharmaceutical Company	54569-0324-07
12's	$9.98	GENERIC, Allscripts Pharmaceutical Company	54569-0324-06
50's	$8.50	GENERIC, Major Pharmaceuticals Inc	00904-0246-51
50's	$19.00	GENERIC, Ivax Corporation	00182-1614-19
50's	$95.80	GENERIC, Par Pharmaceutical Inc	49884-0087-03
100's	$23.55	GENERIC, Interstate Drug Exchange Inc	00814-2365-14
100's	$24.53	GENERIC, Vangard Labs	00615-1515-01
100's	$28.83	GENERIC, Vangard Labs	00615-1515-13
100's	$32.65	GENERIC, Martec Pharmaceuticals Inc	52555-0066-01
100's	$34.09	GENERIC, Moore, H.L. Drug Exchange Inc	00839-6734-06
100's	$37.17	GENERIC, Ivax Corporation	00182-1614-01
100's	$42.50	GENERIC, Major Pharmaceuticals Inc	00904-0246-60
100's	$47.24	HEXADROL, Organon	00052-0798-91
100's	$50.80	HEXADROL, Organon	00052-0798-90
100's	$58.41	GENERIC, Roxane Laboratories Inc	00054-4184-25
100's	$62.05	GENERIC, Roxane Laboratories Inc	00054-8175-25
100's	$182.00	GENERIC, Par Pharmaceutical Inc	49884-0087-01
100's	$189.90	GENERIC, Mutual/United Research Laboratories	00677-0849-01
Tablet - Oral - 6 mg			
50's	$102.00	GENERIC, Par Pharmaceutical Inc	49884-0129-03
100's	$88.49	GENERIC, Roxane Laboratories Inc	00054-8183-25
100's	$98.88	GENERIC, Roxane Laboratories Inc	00054-4186-25
100's	$193.80	GENERIC, Par Pharmaceutical Inc	49884-0129-01

PRODUCT LISTING - EQUIVALENTS NOT AVAILABLE

Elixir - Oral - 0.5 mg/5 ml			
5 ml x 40	$37.44	GENERIC, Roxane Laboratories Inc	00054-8168-16
20 ml x 40	$34.29	GENERIC, Roxane Laboratories Inc	00054-8177-16
100 ml	$11.08	GENERIC, Allscripts Pharmaceutical Company	54569-1034-00
240 ml	$16.34	GENERIC, Aligen Independent Laboratories Inc	00405-2625-77
500 ml	$17.56	GENERIC, Roxane Laboratories Inc	00054-3177-63
Spray - Topical - 0.01%			
58 gm	$18.61	AEROSEB-DEX, Allergan Inc	00023-0852-90
Tablet - Oral - 0.5 mg			
12's	$6.12	GENERIC, Southwood Pharmaceuticals Inc	58016-0290-12
15's	$7.65	GENERIC, Southwood Pharmaceuticals Inc	58016-0290-15
20's	$10.20	GENERIC, Southwood Pharmaceuticals Inc	58016-0290-20
30's	$15.30	GENERIC, Southwood Pharmaceuticals Inc	58016-0290-30
100's	$51.00	GENERIC, Southwood Pharmaceuticals Inc	58016-0290-00
Tablet - Oral - 0.75 mg			
12's	$2.95	GENERIC, Vangard Labs	00615-0506-52
12's	$9.35	GENERIC, Southwood Pharmaceuticals Inc	58016-0293-12
15's	$11.69	GENERIC, Southwood Pharmaceuticals Inc	58016-0293-15
20's	$15.58	GENERIC, Southwood Pharmaceuticals Inc	58016-0293-20
30's	$23.38	GENERIC, Southwood Pharmaceuticals Inc	58016-0293-30
100's	$77.92	GENERIC, Southwood Pharmaceuticals Inc	58016-0293-00
Tablet - Oral - 1.5 mg			
100's	$15.00	GENERIC, Cmc-Consolidated Midland Corporation	00223-0792-01
Tablet - Oral - 4 mg			
10's	$21.40	GENERIC, Southwood Pharmaceuticals Inc	58016-0781-10
12's	$25.68	GENERIC, Southwood Pharmaceuticals Inc	58016-0781-12
14's	$29.96	GENERIC, Southwood Pharmaceuticals Inc	58016-0781-14
15's	$32.10	GENERIC, Southwood Pharmaceuticals Inc	58016-0781-15
20's	$42.80	GENERIC, Southwood Pharmaceuticals Inc	58016-0781-20
21's	$44.94	GENERIC, Southwood Pharmaceuticals Inc	58016-0781-21
24's	$51.36	GENERIC, Southwood Pharmaceuticals Inc	58016-0781-24
28's	$59.92	GENERIC, Southwood Pharmaceuticals Inc	58016-0781-28
30's	$64.20	GENERIC, Southwood Pharmaceuticals Inc	58016-0781-30
40's	$85.60	GENERIC, Southwood Pharmaceuticals Inc	58016-0781-40
50's	$107.00	GENERIC, Southwood Pharmaceuticals Inc	58016-0781-50
100's	$214.00	GENERIC, Southwood Pharmaceuticals Inc	58016-0781-00

Dexamethasone Acetate *(000975)*

For related information, see the comparative table section in Appendix A.

Categories: Alopecia areata; Anemia, acquired hemolytic; Anemia, congenital hypoplastic; Anemia, erythroblastopenia; Ankylosing spondylitis; Arthritis, gouty; Arthritis, post-traumatic; Arthritis, psoriatic; Arthritis, rheumatoid; Asthma; Berylliosis; Bursitis; Carditis, rheumatic; Chorioretinitis; Choroiditis; Colitis, ulcerative; Conjunctivitis, allergic; Dermatitis herpetiformis, bullous; Dermatitis, atopic; Dermatitis, contact; Dermatitis, exfoliative; Dermatitis, seborrheic; Enteritis, regional; Epicondylitis; Erythema multiforme; Granuloma annulare; Herpes zoster ophthalmicus; Hypercalcemia, secondary to neoplasia; Hyperplasia, congenital adrenal; Hypersensitivity reactions; Inflammation, anterior segment, ophthalmic; Iridocyclitis; Iritis; Keratitis; Leukemia; Lichen planus; Lichen simplex chronicus; Loffler's syndrome; Lupus erythematosus, systemic; Lymphoma; Mycosis fungoides; Necrobiosis lipoidica diabeticorum; Nephrotic syndrome; Neuritis, optic; Ophthalmia, sympathetic; Pemphigus; Pneumonitis, aspiration; Psoriasis; Rhinitis, perennial allergic; Rhinitis, seasonal allergic; Sarcoidosis; Serum sickness; Stevens-Johnson syndrome; Synovitis, secondary to osteoarthritis; Tenosynovitis; Thrombocytopenia, secondary; Thyroiditis, nonsuppurative; Transfusion reaction; Trichinosis; Ulcer, allergic corneal marginal; Uveitis; Pregnancy Category C; FDA Approved 1973 Sep

Drug Classes: Corticosteroids

Brand Names: Adrenocot L.A.; Dalalone; De-Sone La; Deca-Plex La; **Decadron-La**; Decaject-La; Decapan La; Decarex; Decasone R.P.; Dekasol; Dexacen La-8; Dexacorten-La; Dexasone L.A.; Dexim La; Dexone La; Medidex-La; Or-Dex L.A.; Preladron La; Primethasone; Solurex La

Foreign Brand Availability: Decadron Depot (Netherlands); Decadron I.A. (Belgium); Dectancyl (France)

HCFA JCODE(S): J1095 per 8 mg IM

DESCRIPTION

Dexamethasone acetate, a synthetic adrenocortical steroid, is a white to practically white, odorless powder. It is a practically insoluble ester of dexamethasone.

Dexamethasone acetate suspension is present as the monohydrate with the empirical formula: $C_{24}H_{31}FO_6 \cdot H_2O$, and molecular weight, 452.52. Dexamethasone acetate is designated chemically as 21-(acetytaxy)-9-fluoro-11β,17-dihydroxy-16α-methylpregna-1,4-diene-3,20-dione.

Dexamethasone acetate suspension is a sterile white suspension (pH 5.0-7.5) that settles on standing, but is easily resuspended by mild shaking.

Each milliliter contains dexamethasone acetate equivalent to 8 mg dexamethasone. Inactive ingredients per ml: 6.57 mg sodium chloride; 5 mg creatinine; 0.5 mg disodium edetate; 5 mg sodium carboxymethylcellulose: 0.75 mg polysorbate 80; sodium hydroxide to adjust pH; and water for injection, as 1 ml, with 9 mg benzyl alcohol, and 1 mg sodium bisulfite added as preservatives.

CLINICAL PHARMACOLOGY

Dexamethasone acetate suspension is a long-acting, repository adrenocorticosteroid preparation with a prompt onset of action. It is suitable for intramuscular or local injection, but not when an immediate effect of short duration is desired.

Naturally occurring glucocorticoids (hydrocortisone and cortisone), which also have self-retaining properties, are used as replacement therapy in adrenocortical deficiency states. Their synthetic analogs, including dexamethasone, are primarily used for their potent anti-inflammatory effects in disorders of many organ systems.

Glucocorticoids cause profound and varied metabolic effects. In addition, they modify the body's immune responses to diverse stimuli

At equipotent anti-inflammatory doses, dexamethasone almost completely lacks the sodium-retaining property of hydrocortisone.

INDICATIONS AND USAGE

By intramuscular injection when oral therapy is not feasible:

Endocrine Disorders: Congenital adrenal hyperplasia, nonsuppurative thyroiditis, hypercalcemia associated with cancer.

Rheumatic Disorders: *As adjunctive therapy for short-term administration (to tide the patient over an acute episode or exacerbation) in:* Post-traumatic osteoarthritis, synovitis of osteoarthritis, rheumatoid arthritis, including juvenile rheumatoid arthritis (selected cases may require low-dose maintenance therapy), acute and subacute bursitis, epicondylitis, acute nonspecific tenosynovitis, acute gouty arthritis, psoriatic arthritis, ankylosing spondylitis.

Collagen Disease: *During an exacerbation or as maintenance therapy in selected cases of:* Systemic lupus erythematosus, acute rheumatic carditis.

Dermatologic Diseases: Pemphigus, severe erythema multiforme (Stevens-Johnson Syndrome), exfoliative dermatitis, bullous dermatitis herpetiformis, severe seborrheic dermatitis, severe psoriasis, mycosis fungoides.

Allergic States: Control of severe of incapacitating allergic conditions intractable to adequate trails of conventional treatment in bronchial asthma, contact dermatitis, atopic dermatitis, serum sickness, seasonal or perennial allergic rhinitis, drug hypersensitivity reactions, urticarial transfusion reactions.

Ophthalmic Diseases: *Severe acute and chronic allergic and inflammatory processes involving the eye, such as:* Herpes zoster ophthalmicus; iritis, iridocyclitis; chorioretinitis; diffuse posterior uveitis and choroiditis; optic neuritis; sympathetic ophthalmia; anterior segment inflammation; allergic conjunctivitis; keratitis; allergic corneal marginal ulcers.

Gastrointestinal Diseases: *To tide the patient over a critical period of the disease in:* Ulcerative colitis (systemic therapy), regional enteritis (systemic therapy).

Respiratory Diseases: Symptomatic sarcoidosis, berylliosis, loeffler's syndrome not manageable by other means, aspiration pneumonitis.

Hematologic Disorders: Acquired (autoimmune) hemolytic anemia secondary thrombocytopenia in adults, erythroblastopenia (rbc anemia), congenital (erythroid) hypoplastic anemia.

Neoplastic Diseases: *For palliative management of:* Leukemias and lymphomas in adults, acute leukemia of childhood.

Edematous States: To induce diuresis or remission of proteinuria in the nephrotic syndrome, without uremia of the idiopathic type, or that due to lupus erythematosus.

Miscellaneous: Trichinosis with neurologic or myocardial involvement.

By intra-articular or soft tissue injection as adjunctive therapy for short-term administration to tide the patient over an acute episode or exacerbation in:

Synovitis of osteoarthritis
Rheumatoid arthritis
Acute and subacute bursitis
Acute gouty arthritis
Epicondylitis
Acute nonspecific tenosynovitis
Post-traumatic osteoarthritis

By intralesional injection in:

Keroids
Localized hypertrophic, infiltrated, inflammatory lesions of: Lichen planus, psoriatic plaques, granuloma annulare, and lichen simplex chronicus (neurodermatitis)
Discoid lupus erythematosus
Necrobiosis lipoidica diabeticorum
Alopecia aerate
May also be useful in cystic tumors of an aponeurosis of tendon (ganglia)

NON-FDA APPROVED INDICATIONS

Although not approved by the FDA, several studies have reported the efficacy of dexamethasone as an antiemetic in cancer chemotherapy.

CONTRAINDICATIONS

Systemic fungal infections.

Hypersensitivity to any component of this product.

WARNINGS

DO NOT INJECT INTRAVENOUSLY.

In patients on corticosteroid therapy subjected to any unusual stress, increased dosage of rapidly acting corticosteroids before, during, and after the stressful situation is indicated.

Drug-induced secondary adrenocortical insufficiency may result from too rapid withdrawal of corticosteroids and may be minimized by gradual reduction of dosage. This type of relative insufficiency may persist for months after discontinuation of therapy: therefore, in any situation of stress occurring during that period, hormone therapy should be reinstituted. If the patient is receiving steroids already, dosage may have to be increased. since mineralocorticoid secretion may be impaired, salt and/or a mineralocorticoid should be administered concurrently.

Corticosteroids may mask some signs of infection, and new infections may appear during their used. There may be decreased resistance and inability to localize infection when corticosteroids are used. Moreover, corticosteroids may affect the nitroblue-tetrazolium test for bacterial infection and produce false negative results.

Corticosteroids may activate latent amebiasis. Therefore, it is recommended that latent or active amebiasis be ruled out before initiating corticosteroid therapy in any patient who has spent time in the tropics or any patient with unexplained diarrhea.

Prolonged use of corticosteroids may produce posterior subcapsular cataracts, glaucoma with possible damage to the optic nerves, and may enhance the establishment of secondary ocular infections due to fungi or viruses.

Usage In Pregnancy: Since adequate human reproduction studies have not been done with corticosteroids, use of these drugs in pregnancy or in women of childbearing potential requires that the anticipated benefits be weighed against the possible hazards to the mother and embryo or fetus. Infants born of mothers who have received substantial doses of corticosteroids during pregnancy should be carefully observed for signs of hypoadrenalism. Corticosteroids appear in breast milk and could suppress growth, interfere with endogenous corticosteroid production, or cause other unwanted effects. Mothers taking pharmacologic doses of corticosteroids should be advised not to nurse.

Average and large doses of cortisone or hydrocortisone can cause elevation of blood pressure, salt and water retention, and increased excretion of potassium. These effects are less likely to occur with the synthetic derivatives except when used in large doses. Dietary salt restriction and potassium supplementation may be necessary. All corticosteroids increase calcium excretion.

While on corticosteroid therapy patients should not be vaccinated against smallpox. Other immunization procedures should not be undertaken in patients who are on corticosteroids, especially on high doses, because of possible hazards of neurologic complications and lack of antibody response.

If corticosteroids are indicated in patients, with latent tuberculosis or tuberculin reactivity, close observation is necessary as reactivation of the disease may occur. During prolonged corticosteroid therapy, these patients should receive chemoprophylaxis.

Because rare instances of anaphylactoid reactions have occurred in patients receiving parenteral corticosteroid therapy, appropriate precautionary measures should be taken prior to administration, especially when the patient has a history of allergy to any drug.

Repository adrenocorticosteroid preparations may cause atrophy at the site of injection. To minimize the likelihood and/or severity of atrophy, do not inject subcutaneously, avoid injection into the deltoid muscle, and avoid, repeated intramuscular injections into the same site if possible.

Dosage in children under 12 has not been established.

PRECAUTIONS

Dexamethasone acetate suspension is not recommended as initial therapy in acute, life-threatening situations.

This product, like many other steroid formulations, is sensitive to heat. Therefore, if should not be autoclaved when it is desirable to sterilize the exterior of the vial.

Following prolonged therapy, withdrawal of corticosteroids may result in symptoms of the corticosteroid withdrawal syndrome including fever, myalgia, arthralgia, and malaise. This may occur in patients even without evidence of adrenal insufficiency.

There is an enhanced effect of corticosteroids in patients with hypothyroidism and in those with cirrhosis.

Corticosteroids should be used cautiously in patients with ocular herpes simplex for fear of corneal perforation.

Psychic derangements may appear when corticosteroids are used, ranging from euphoria, insomnia, mood swings, personality changes, and severe depression to frank psychotic manifestations. Also, existing emotional instability or psychotic tendencies may be aggravated by corticosteroids.

Aspirin should be used cautiously in conjunction with corticosteroids in hypoprothrombinemia.

Steroids should be used with caution in nonspecific ulcerative colitis, if there is a probability of impending perforation, abscess or other pyogenic infection, also in diverticulitis, fresh intestinal anastomoses, active or latent peptic ulcer, renal insufficiency, hypertension, osteoporosis, and myasthenia gravis. Fat embolism has been reported as a possible complication of hypercortisonism.

When large doses are given, some authorities advise that antacids be administered between meals to help to prevent peptic ulcer.

Growth and development of infants and children on prolonged corticosteroid therapy should be carefully followed.

Steroids may increase or decrease motility and number of spermatozoa in some patients.

Phenytoin, phenobarbital, ephedrine, and rifampin may enhance the metabolic clearance of corticosteroids, resulting in decreased blood levels and lessened physiologic activity, thus requiring adjustment in corticosteroid dosage.

The prothrombin time should be checked frequently in patients who are receiving corticosteroids and coumarin anticoagulants at the same time because of reports that corticosteroids have altered the response to these anticoagulants. Studies have shown that the usual effect produced by adding corticosteroids is inhibition of response to coumarin, although there have been some conflicting reports of potentiation not substantiated by studies.

When corticosteroids are administered concomitantly with potassium-depleting diuretics, patients-should be observed closely for development of hypokalemia.

Intra-articular injection of a corticosteroid may produce systemic as well as local effects.

Appropriate examination of any joint fluid present is necessary to exclude a septic process.

A marked increase in pain accompanied by local swelling, further restriction of joint motion, fever, and malaise is suggestive of septic arthritis. If this complication occurs and the diagnosis of sepsis is confirmed, appropriate antimicrobial therapy should be instituted.

Injection of a steroid into an infected site is to be avoided.

Corticosteroids should not be injected into unstable joints.

Patients should be impressed strongly with the importance of not overusing joints in which symptomatic benefit has been obtained as long as the inflammatory process remains active.

Frequent intra-articular injection may result in damage to joint-tissues.

ADVERSE REACTIONS

Fluid and Electrolyte Disturbances: Sodium retention, fluid retention, congestive heart failure in susceptible patients, potassium loss, hypokalemic alkalosis, hypertension.

Musculoskeletal: Muscle weakness, steroid myopathy, loss of muscle mass, osteoporosis, vertebral compression fractures, aseptic necrosis of femoral and humeral heads, pathologic fracture of long bones, tendon rapture.

Gastrointestinal: Peptic ulcer with possible subsequent perforation and hemorrhage, pancreatitis, abdominal distention, ulcerative esophagitis.

Dermatologic: Impaired wound healing, thin fragile skin, petechiae and ecchymoses, erythema, increased sweating, may suppress reactions to skin tests, other cutaneous reactions, such as allergic dermatitis, urticaria, angioneurotic edema

Neurologic: Convulsions, increased intracranial pressure with papilledema (pseudotumor cerebri) usually after treatment, vertigo, headache.

Endocrine: Menstrual irregularities, development of cushingoid state, suppression of growth in children, secondary adrenocortical and pituitary unresponsiveness, particularly in times of stress, as in trauma, surgery, or illness, decreased carbohydrate tolerance, manifestations of latent diabetes mellitus, increased requirements for insulin or oral hypoglycemic agents in diabetics.

Ophthalmic: Posterior subcapsular cataracts, increased intraocular pressure, glaucoma, exophthalmos.

Metabolic: Negative nitrogen balance due to protein catabolism.

Other: Anaphylactoid or hypersensitivity reactions, thromboembolism, weight gain, increased appetite, nausea, malaise.

D

The Following *Additional* Adverse Reactions are Related to Parenteral Corticosteroid Therapy: Rare instances of blindness associated with intralesional therapy around the face and head;hyperpigmentation or hypopigmentation; subcutaneous and cutaneous atrophy; sterile abscess; postinjection flare (following intra-articular use); charcol-like arthropathy; scarring; induration; inflammation; paresthesia; delayed pain or soreness; muscle twitching, ataxia, hiccups, and nystagmus have been reported in low incidence after injection of dexamethasone acetate suspension.

DOSAGE AND ADMINISTRATION

For intramuscular, intralesional, intra-articular, and soft tissue injection.

Dosage Requirements Are Variable and Must Be Individualized on the Basis of the Disease and the Response of the Patient

Dosages in children under 12 has not been established.

Intramuscular injection: Dosage ranges from 1 to 2 ml, equivalent to 8 to 16 mg of dexamethasone. If further treatment is needed, dosage may be repeated at intervals of 1-3 weeks.

Intralesional injection: The usual dose is 0.1 to 0.2 ml, equivalent to 0.8 to 1.6 mg of dexamethasone, per injection site.

Intra-articular and soft tissue injection: The dose varies, depending on the location and the severity of inflammation. The usual dose is 0.5 to 2 mal, equivalent to 4 to 16 mg of dexamethasone. If further treatment is needed, dosage may be repeated at intervals of 1-3 weeks. Frequent intra-articular injection may result in damage to joint tissues.

PRODUCT LISTING - RATED THERAPEUTICALLY EQUIVALENT

Suspension - Injectable - 8 mg/ml

5 ml	$29.90	GENERIC, Geneva Pharmaceuticals	00781-3008-75

PRODUCT LISTING - RATED NOT THERAPEUTICALLY EQUIVALENT

Suspension - Injectable - 8 mg/ml

5 ml	$3.79	GENERIC, Mcguff Company	49072-0155-10
5 ml	$9.25	GENERIC, Med Tek Pharmaceuticals Inc	52349-0104-05
5 ml	$9.95	GENERIC, C.O. Truxton Inc	00463-1104-05
5 ml	$11.50	GENERIC, Cmc-Consolidated Midland Corporation	00223-7390-05
5 ml	$12.00	GENERIC, Hyrex Pharmaceuticals	00314-0897-75
5 ml	$12.45	GENERIC, Roberts/Hauck Pharmaceutical Corporation	43797-0113-11
5 ml	$12.90	GENERIC, Forest Pharmaceuticals	00785-8045-05
5 ml	$18.20	GENERIC, Pasadena Research Laboratories Inc	00418-4091-31
5 ml	$20.00	GENERIC, Bolan Pharmaceutical Inc	44437-0092-05
5 ml	$21.00	GENERIC, Interstate Drug Exchange Inc	00814-2355-38
5 ml	$29.03	GENERIC, Major Pharmaceuticals Inc	00904-0906-05
5 ml	$29.93	GENERIC, Mutual/United Research Laboratories	00677-0822-20
5 ml	$32.93	GENERIC, General Injectables and Vaccines Inc	52584-0092-05

PRODUCT LISTING - EQUIVALENTS NOT AVAILABLE

Suspension - Injectable - 8 mg/ml

5 ml	$18.62	GENERIC, Moore, H.L. Drug Exchange Inc	00839-6109-25
5 ml	$24.00	GENERIC, Forest Pharmaceuticals	00456-1075-05
5 ml	$27.95	CORTASTAT LA, Clint Pharmaceutical Inc	55553-0092-05
5 ml	$29.95	GENERIC, Legere Pharmaceuticals	25332-0011-05

Suspension - Injectable - 16 mg/ml

1 ml x 10	$66.00	DALALONE D.P., Forest Pharmaceuticals	00456-1097-41
5 ml	$66.00	DALALONE D.P., Forest Pharmaceuticals	00456-1097-05
5 ml	$25.00	DALALONE D.P., Allscripts Pharmaceutical Company	54569-3953-00

Dexamethasone; Tobramycin (000980)

Categories: Burns, ophthalmic; Conjunctivitis, infectious; Dermatosis, corticosteroid-responsive with secondary infection; Foreign body, ophthalmic; Inflammation, cornea; Inflammation, ophthalmic; Trauma, ophthalmic; Uveitis; Pregnancy Category C; FDA Approved 1988 Aug; WHO Formulary

Drug Classes: Anti-infectives, ophthalmic; Corticosteroids, ophthalmic; Ophthalmics

Brand Names: Tobradex

DESCRIPTION

Tobramycin and dexamethasone ophthalmic suspension and ointment are sterile, multiple dose antibiotic and steroid combinations for topical ophthalmic use:.

Tobramycin: *Empirical Formula:* $C_{18}H_{37}N_5O_9$*Chemical Name:* *O*-3-Amino-3-deoxy-α-D-glucopyranosyl-(1→4)-*O*-[2,6-diamino-2,3,6-trideoxy-α-D-*ribo*-hexopyransol-(1→6)]-2-deoxy-L-streptamine.

Dexamethasone: *Empirical Formula:* $C_{22}H_{29}FO_5$*Chemical Name:* 9-Fluoro-11β,17,21-trihydroxy-16α-methylpregna-1,4-dien-3,20-dione.

Each ml of Tobradex Suspension Contains: *Actives:* Tobramycin 0.3% (3 mg) and dexamethasone 0.1% (1 mg). *Preservative:* Benzalkonium chloride 0.01%. *Inactives:* Tyloxapol, edetate disodium, sodium chloride, hydroxyethyl cellulose, sodium sulfate, sulfuric acid and/or sodium hydroxide (to adjust pH) and purified water.

Suspension Storage: Store at 8-27°C (46-80°F). Store suspension upright and shake well before using.

Each Gram of Tobradex Ointment Contains: *Actives:* Tobramycin 0.3% (3 mg) and dexamethasone 0.1% (1 mg). *Preservative:* Chlorobutanol 0.5%. *Inactives:* Mineral Oil and White Petrolatum.

Ointment Storage: Store at 8-27°C (46-80°F).

CLINICAL PHARMACOLOGY

Corticoids suppress the inflammatory response to a variety of agents and they probably delay or slow healing. Since corticoids may inhibit the body's defense mechanism against infection, a concomitant antimicrobial drug may be used when this inhibition is considered to be clinically significant. Dexamethasone is a potent corticoid.

The antibiotic component in the combination (tobramycin) is included to provide action against susceptible organisms. *In vitro* studies have demonstrated that tobramycin is active against susceptible strains of the following microorganisms:

Staphylococci, including *S. aureus* and *S. epidermis* (coagulase-positive and coagulase-negative), including penicillin-resistant strains.

Streptococci, including some of the Group A-beta-hemolytic species, some nonhemolytic species, and some *Streptococcus pneumoniae.*

Pseudomonas aeruginosa, Escherichia Coli, Klebsiella pneumoniae, Enterobacter aerogenes, Proteus mirabilis, Morganella morganii most *Proteus vulgaris* strains, *Haemophilus influenzae* and *H. aegyptius, Moraxella lacunata, Acinetobacter calcoaceticus* and some *Neisseria* species.

Bacterial susceptibility studies demonstrate that in some cases microorganisms resistant to gentamicin remain susceptible to tobramycin.

No data are available on the extent of systemic absorption from dexamethasone and tobramycin ophthalmic suspension or ointment; however, it is known that some systemic absorption can occur with ocularly applied drugs. If the maximum dose of dexamethasone and tobramycin suspension or ointment is given for the first 48 hours (2 drops in each eye every 2 hours) and complete systemic absorption occurs, which is highly unlikely, the daily dose of dexamethasone would be 2.4 mg. The usual physiologic replacement dose id 0.75 mg daily. If dexamethasone and tobramycin ophthalmic suspension is given after the first 48 hours as 2 drops in each eye every 4 hours, the administered dose of dexamethasone would be 1.2 mg daily.

INDICATIONS AND USAGE

Dexamethasone and tobramycin ophthalmic suspension and ointment are indicated for steroid-responsive inflammatory ocular conditions for which a corticosteroid is indicated and where superficial bacterial ocular infection or a risk of bacterial infection exists.

Ocular steroids are indicated in inflammatory conditions of the palpebral and bulbar conjunctiva, cornea and anterior segment of the globe where the inherent risk of steroid use in certain infective conjunctivides is accepted to obtain a diminution in edema and inflammation. They are also indicated in chronic anterior uveitis and corneal injury from chemical, radiation or thermal burns, or penetration of foreign bodies.

The use of a combination drug with an anti-infective component is indicated where the risk of superficial ocular infection is high or where there is an expectation that potentially dangerous numbers of bacteria will be present in the eye.

The particular anti-infective drug in this product is active against the following common bacterial eye pathogens:

Staphylococci, including *S. aureus* and *S. epidermis* (coagulase-positive and coagulase-negative), including penicillin-resistant strains.

Streptococci, including some of the Group A beta-hemolytic species, some nonhemolytic species, and some *Streptococcus pneumoniae.*

Pseudomonas aeruginosa, Escherichia coli, Klebsiella pneumoniae, Enterobacter aerogenes, Proteus mirabilis, Morganella morganii, most *Proteus vulgaris* strains *Haemophilus influenzae* and *H. aegyptius, Moraxella lacunata, Acinetobacter calcoaceticus* and some *Neisseria* species.

CONTRAINDICATIONS

Epithelial herpes simplex keratitis (dendritic keratitis), vaccina, varicella, and many other viral diseases of the cornea and conjunctiva. Mycobacterial infection of the eye. Fungal diseases of ocular structures. Hypersensitivity to a component of the medication.

WARNINGS

NOT FOR INJECTION INTO THE EYE. Sensitivity to topically applied aminoglycosides may occur in some patients. If a sensitivity does occur, discontinue use.

Prolonged use of steroids may result in glaucoma, with damage to the optic nerve, defects in visual acuity and fields of vision, and posterior subcapsular cataract formation. Intraocular pressure should be routinely monitored even though it may be difficult in children and uncooperative patients. Prolonged use may suppress the host response and thus increase the hazard of secondary ocular infections. In those diseases, causing thinning of the cornea or sclera, perforations have been known to occur with the use of topical steroids. In acute purulent conditions of the eye, steroids may mask infection or enhance existing infection.

PRECAUTIONS

GENERAL

The possibility of fungal infections of the cornea should be considered after long-term steroid dosing. As with other antibiotic preparations, prolonged use may result in overgrowth of nonsusceptible organisms, including fungi. If superinfection occurs, appropriate therapy should be initiated. When multiple prescriptions are required, or whenever clinical judgment dictates, the patient should be examined with the aid of magnification, such as slit lamp biomicroscopy and, where, appropriate, fluorescein staining.

Cross-sensitivity to other aminoglycoside antibiotics may occur, if hypersensitivity develops with this product, discontinue use and institute appropriate therapy.

INFORMATION FOR THE PATIENT

Do not touch dropper tip to any surface, as this may contaminate the contents.

CARCINOGENESIS, MUTAGENESIS, AND IMPAIRMENT OF FERTILITY

No studies have been conducted to evaluate the carcinogenic or mutagenic potential. No impairment of fertility was noted in studies of subcutaneous tobramycin in rats at doses of 50 and 100 mg/kg/day.

PREGNANCY CATEGORY C

Corticosteroids have been found to be teratogenic in animal studies. Ocular administration of 0.1% dexamethasone resulted in 15.6% and 32.3% incidence of fetal anomalies in 2 groups of pregnant rabbits. Fetal growth retardation and increased mortality rates have been observed in rats with chronic dexamthasone therapy. Reproduction studies have been performed in rats and rabbits with tobramycin at doses of up to 100 mg/kg/day parenterally and have revealed no evidence of impaired fertility or harm to the fetus. There are no adequate and well controlled studies in pregnant women. Dexamethasone and tobramycin ophthalmic suspension and ointment should be used during pregnancy only if the potential benefit justifies the potential risk to the fetus.

NURSING MOTHERS

Systemically administered corticosteroids appear in human milk and could suppress growth, interfere with endogenous corticosteroid production, or cause other untoward effects. It is not known whether topical administration of corticosteroids could result in sufficient systemic absorption to produce detectable quantities in human milk. Because many drugs are excreted in human milk, caution should be exercised when dexamethasone and tobramycin ophthalmic suspension is administered to a nursing woman.

PEDIATRIC USE

Safety and effectiveness in children have not yet been established.

ADVERSE REACTIONS

Adverse reactions have occurred with steroid/anti-infective combination drugs which can be attributed to the steroid component, the anti-infective component, or the combination. Exact incidence figures are not available. The most frequent adverse reactions to topical ocular tobramycin are hypersensitivity and localized ocular toxicity, including lid itching and swelling, and conjunctival erythema. These reactions occur in less than 4% of patients. Similar reactions may occur with the topical use of other aminoglycoside antibiotics. Other adverse reactions have not been reported; however; if topical ocular tobramycin is administered concomitantly with systemic aminoglycoside antibiotics, care should be taken to monitor the total serum concentration. The reactions due to steroid component are: elevation of intraocular pressure (IOP) with possible development of glaucoma, and infrequent optic nerve damage; posterior subcapsular cataract formation; and delayed wound healing.

SECONDARY INFECTION

The development of secondary infection has occurred after use of combinations containing steroids and antimicrobials. Fungal infections of the cornea are particularly prone to develop coincidentally with long-term applications of steroids. The possibility of fungal invasion must be considered in any persistent corneal ulceration where steroid treatment has been used. Secondary bacterial ocular infection following suppression of host responses also occurs.

DOSAGE AND ADMINISTRATION

SUSPENSION

One (1) or 2 drops instilled into the conjunctival sac(s) every 4-6 hours. During the initial 24-48 hours, the dosage may be increased to 1 or 2 drops every 2 hours. Frequency should be decreased gradually as warranted by improvement in clinical signs. Care should be taken not to discontinue therapy prematurely.

Not more than 20 ml should be prescribed initially and the prescription should not be refilled without further evaluation as outlined in PRECAUTIONS

OINTMENT

Apply a small amount (approximately ½ inch ribbon) into the conjunctival sac(s) up to 3 or 4 times daily.

How to apply dexamethasone and tobramycin opthalmic ointment:

1. Tilt your head back.
2. Place a finger on your cheek just under your eye and gently pull down until a "V" pocket is formed between your eyeball and your lower lid.
3. Place a small amount (about ½ inch) of dexamethasone and tobramycin ophthalmic ointment in the "V" pocket. Do not let the tip of the tube touch your eye.
4. Look downward before closing your eye.

Not more than 8 g should be prescribed initially and the prescription should not be refilled without further evaluation as outlined in PRECAUTIONS.

PRODUCT LISTING - RATED THERAPEUTICALLY EQUIVALENT

Suspension - Ophthalmic - 0.1%;0.3%

Size	Price	Product	NDC
2.50 ml	$18.57	TOBRADEX, Southwood Pharmaceuticals Inc	58016-6527-00
2.50 ml	$19.00	TOBRADEX, Southwood Pharmaceuticals Inc	58016-6527-01
2.50 ml	$19.31	TOBRADEX, Allscripts Pharmaceutical Company	54569-4400-00
2.50 ml	$26.81	TOBRADEX, Alcon Laboratories Inc	00065-0647-25
3 ml	$21.19	TOBRADEX, Physicians Total Care	54868-2789-01
5 ml	$38.25	TOBRADEX, Allscripts Pharmaceutical Company	54569-2285-00
5 ml	$40.19	TOBRADEX, Physicians Total Care	54868-2789-00
5 ml	$49.55	TOBRADEX, Southwood Pharmaceuticals Inc	58016-5014-01
5 ml	$53.56	TOBRADEX, Alcon Laboratories Inc	00065-0647-05
5 ml	$60.53	TOBRADEX, Pharma Pac	52959-0092-01
10 ml	$72.88	TOBRADEX, Allscripts Pharmaceutical Company	54569-4493-00
10 ml	$91.81	TOBRADEX, Pharma Pac	52959-0092-00
10 ml	$102.00	TOBRADEX, Alcon Laboratories Inc	00065-0647-10

PRODUCT LISTING - EQUIVALENTS NOT AVAILABLE

Ointment - Ophthalmic - 0.1%;0.3%

Size	Price	Product	NDC
3.50 gm	$41.50	TOBRADEX, Allscripts Pharmaceutical Company	54569-2590-00
3.50 gm	$44.31	TOBRADEX, Southwood Pharmaceuticals Inc	58016-6073-01
3.50 gm	$58.06	TOBRADEX, Alcon Laboratories Inc	00065-0648-35
3.50 gm	$59.58	TOBRADEX, Pharma Pac	52959-0592-03

Dexmethylphenidate Hydrochloride *(003532)*

Categories: Attention deficit hyperactivity disorder; FDA Approved 2001 Nov; Pregnancy Category C
Drug Classes: Stimulants, central nervous system
Brand Names: Focalin
Cost of Therapy: $28.78 (ADHD; Focalin; 2.5 mg; 2 tablets/day; 30 day supply)

DESCRIPTION

Dexmethylphenidate hydrochloride is the *d-threo*-enantiomer of racemic methylphenidate hydrochloride, which is a 50/50 mixture of the *d-threo-* and *l-threo*-enantiomers. Dexmethylphenidate hydrochloride is a central nervous system (CNS) stimulant, available in three tablet strengths. Each tablet contains dexmethylphenidate hydrochloride 2.5, 5, or 10 mg for oral administration. Dexmethylphenidate hydrochloride is methyl α-phenyl-2-piperidineacetate hydrochloride, (R,R′)-(+)-. Its empirical formula is $C_{14}H_{19}NO_2{\cdot}HCl$. Its molecular weight is 269.77.

Dexmethylphenidate hydrochloride is a white to off white powder. Its solutions are acid to litmus. It is freely soluble in water and in methanol, soluble in alcohol, and slightly soluble in chloroform and in acetone.

Dexmethylphenidate hydrochloride also contains the following inert ingredients: pregelatinized starch, lactose monohydrate, sodium starch glycolate, microcrystalline cellulose, magnesium stearate, and FD&C blue no.1 #5516 aluminum lake (2.5 mg tablets), D&C yellow lake #10 (5 mg tablets); the 10 mg tablet contains no dye.

CLINICAL PHARMACOLOGY

PHARMACODYNAMICS

Dexmethylphenidate HCl is a central nervous system stimulant. Dexmethylphenidate HCl, the more pharmacologically active enantiomer of the *d-* and *l*-enantiomers, is thought to block the reuptake of norepinephrine and dopamine into the presynaptic neuron and increase the release of these monoamines into the extraneuronal space. The mode of therapeutic action in Attention Deficit Hyperactivity Disorder (ADHD) is not known.

PHARMACOKINETICS

Absorption

Dexmethylphenidate HCl is readily absorbed following oral administration of dexmethylphenidate HCl. In patients with ADHD, plasma dexmethylphenidate concentrations increase rapidly, reaching a maximum in the fasted state at about 1 to 1½ hours post-dose. No differences in the pharmacokinetics of dexmethylphenidate HCl were noted following single and repeated twice daily dosing, thus indicating no significant drug accumulation in children with ADHD.

When given to children as capsules in single doses of 2.5, 5, and 10 mg, C_{max} and AUC(0-∞) of dexmethylphenidate were proportional to dose. In the same study, plasma dexmethylphenidate levels were comparable to those achieved following single *dl-threo*-methylphenidate HCl doses given as capsules in twice the total mg amount (equimolar with respect to dexmethylphenidate HCl).

Food Effects

In a single dose study conducted in adults, coadministration of 2 × 10 mg dexmethylphenidate HCl with a high fat breakfast resulted in a dexmethylphenidate T_{max} of 2.9 hours post-dose as compared to 1.5 hours post-dose when given in a fasting state. C_{max} and AUC(0-∞) were comparable in both the fasted and non-fasted states.

Distribution

Plasma dexmethylphenidate concentrations in children decline exponentially following oral administration of dexmethylphenidate HCl.

Metabolism and Excretion

In humans, dexmethylphenidate is metabolized primarily to *d*-α-phenyl-piperidine acetic acid (also known as *d*-ritalinic acid) by de-esterification. This metabolite has little or no pharmacological activity. There is little or no *in vivo* interconversion to the *l-threo-*

enantiomer, based on a finding of minute levels of *l-threo*-methylphenidate being detectable in a few samples in only 2 of 58 children and adults. After oral dosing of radiolabeled racemic methylphenidate in humans, about 90% of the radioactivity was recovered in urine. The main urinary metabolite was ritalinic acid, accountable for approximately 80% of the dose.

In vitro studies showed that dexmethylphenidate did not inhibit cytochrome P450 isoenzymes.

The mean plasma elimination half-life of dexmethylphenidate is approximately 2.2 hours.

SPECIAL POPULATIONS

Gender

Pharmacokinetic parameters were similar for boys and girls (mean age 10 years). In a single dose study conducted in adults, the mean dexmethylphenidate AUC(0-∞) values (adjusted for body weight) following single 2 × 10 mg doses of dexmethylphenidate HCl were 25-35% higher in adult female volunteers (n=6) compared to male volunteers (n=9). Both T_{max} and $T_{1/2}$ were comparable for males and females.

Race

There is insufficient experience with the use of dexmethylphenidate HCl to detect ethnic variations in pharmacokinetics.

Age

The pharmacokinetics of dexmethylphenidate after dexmethylphenidate HCl administration have not been studied in children less than 6 years of age. When single doses of dexmethylphenidate HCl were given to children between the ages of 6-12 years and healthy adult volunteers, C_{max} of dexmethylphenidate was similar, however children showed somewhat lower AUCs compared to the adults.

Renal Insufficiency

There is no experience with the use of dexmethylphenidate HCl in patients with renal insufficiency. After oral administration of radiolabeled racemic methylphenidate in humans, methylphenidate was extensively metabolized and approximately 80% of the radioactivity was excreted in the urine in the form of ritalinic acid. Since very little unchanged drug is excreted in the urine, renal insufficiency is expected to have little effect on the pharmacokinetics of dexmethylphenidate HCl.

Hepatic Insufficiency

There is no experience with the use of dexmethylphenidate HCl in patients with hepatic insufficiency. (See DRUG INTERACTIONS.)

INDICATIONS AND USAGE

Dexmethylphenidate HCl is indicated for the treatment of Attention Deficit Hyperactivity Disorder (ADHD).

The efficacy of dexmethylphenidate HCl in the treatment of ADHD was established in two controlled trials of patients aged 6-17 years of age who met DSM-IV criteria for ADHD.

A diagnosis of ADHD (DSM-IV) implies the presence of hyperactive-impulsive or inattentive symptoms that cause impairment and were present before age 7 years. The symptoms must cause clinically significant impairment, *e.g.,* in social, academic, or occupational functioning, and be present in two or more settings, *e.g.,* school (or work) and at home. The symptoms must not be better accounted for by another mental disorder. For the inattentive type, at least six of the following symptoms must have persisted for at least 6 months: lack of attention to details/careless mistakes; lack of sustained attention; poor listener; failure to follow through on tasks; poor organization; avoids tasks requiring sustained mental effort; loses things; easily distracted; forgetful. For the Hyperactive-Impulsive Type, at least six of the following symptoms must have persisted for at least 6 months: fidgeting/squirming; leaving seat; inappropriate running/climbing; difficulty with quiet activities; "on the go"; excessive talking; blurting answers; can't wait turn; intrusive. The Combined Type requires both inattentive and hyperactive-impulsive criteria to be met.

SPECIAL DIAGNOSTIC CONSIDERATIONS

Specific etiology of this syndrome is unknown, and there is no single diagnostic test. Adequate diagnosis requires the use not only of medical but of special psychological, educational, and social resources. Learning may or may not be impaired. The diagnosis must be based upon a complete history and evaluation of the child and not solely on the presence of the required number of DSM-IV characteristics.

NEED FOR COMPREHENSIVE TREATMENT PROGRAM

Dexmethylphenidate HCl is indicated as an integral part of a total treatment program for ADHD that may include other measures (psychological, educational, social) for patients with this syndrome. Drug treatment may not be indicated for all patients with this syndrome. Stimulants are not intended for use in the patient who exhibits symptoms secondary to environmental factors and/or other primary psychiatric disorders, including psychosis. Appropriate educational placement is essential and psychosocial intervention is often helpful. When remedial measures alone are insufficient, the decision to prescribe stimulant medication will depend upon the physician's assessment of the chronicity and severity of the patient's symptoms.

LONG-TERM USE

The effectiveness of dexmethylphenidate HCl for long-term use, *i.e.,* for more than 6 weeks, has not been systematically evaluated in controlled trials. Therefore, the physician who elects to use dexmethylphenidate HCl for extended periods should periodically re-evaluate the long-term usefulness of the drug for the individual patient (see DOSAGE AND ADMINISTRATION).

CONTRAINDICATIONS

AGITATION

Dexmethylphenidate HCl is contraindicated in patients with marked anxiety, tension, and agitation, since the drug may aggravate these symptoms.

HYPERSENSITIVITY TO METHYLPHENIDATE

Dexmethylphenidate HCl is contraindicated in patients known to be hypersensitive to methylphenidate or other components of the product.

GLAUCOMA

Dexmethylphenidate HCl is contraindicated in patients with glaucoma.

TICS

Dexmethylphenidate HCl is contraindicated in patients with motor tics or with a family history or diagnosis of Tourette's syndrome (see ADVERSE REACTIONS).

MONOAMINE OXIDASE INHIBITORS

Dexmethylphenidate HCl is contraindicated during treatment with monoamine oxidase inhibitors, and also within a minimum of 14 days following discontinuation of a monoamine oxidase inhibitor (hypertensive crises may result).

WARNINGS

DEPRESSION

Dexmethylphenidate HCl should not be used to treat severe depression.

FATIGUE

Dexmethylphenidate HCl should not be used for the prevention or treatment of normal fatigue states.

LONG-TERM SUPPRESSION OF GROWTH

Sufficient data on safety of long-term use of dexmethylphenidate HCl in children are not yet available. Although a causal relationship has not been established, suppression of growth (*i.e.,* weight gain and/or height) has been reported with the long-term use of stimulants in children. Therefore, patients requiring long-term therapy should be carefully monitored. Patients who are not growing or gaining weight as expected should have their treatment interrupted.

PSYCHOSIS

Clinical experience suggests that in psychotic children, administration of methylphenidate may exacerbate symptoms of behavior disturbance and thought disorder.

SEIZURES

There is some clinical evidence that methylphenidate may lower the convulsive threshold in patients with prior history of seizures, in patients with prior EEG abnormalities in the absence of a history of seizures, and, very rarely, in the absence of a history of seizures and no prior EEG evidence of seizures. In the presence of seizures, the drug should be discontinued.

HYPERTENSION AND OTHER CARDIOVASCULAR CONDITIONS

Use cautiously in patients with hypertension. Blood pressure should be monitored at appropriate intervals in all patients taking dexmethylphenidate HCl, especially those with hypertension. In the placebo controlled studies, the mean pulse increase was 2-5 bpm for both dexmethylphenidate HCl and racemic methylphenidate compared to placebo, with mean increases of systolic and diastolic blood pressure of 2-3 mm Hg, compared to placebo. Therefore, caution is indicated in treating patients whose underlying medical conditions might be compromised by increases in blood pressure or heart rate, *e.g.,* those with pre-existing hypertension, heart failure, recent myocardial infarction, or hyperthyroidism.

VISUAL DISTURBANCE

Symptoms of visual disturbances have been encountered in rare cases following use of methylphenidate. Difficulties with accommodation and blurring of vision have been reported.

USE IN CHILDREN UNDER 6 YEARS OF AGE

Dexmethylphenidate HCl should not be used in children under 6 years, since safety and efficacy in this age group have not been established.

DRUG DEPENDENCE

Dexmethylphenidate HCl should be given cautiously to patients with a history of drug dependence or alcoholism. Chronic, abusive use can lead to marked tolerance and psychological dependence with varying degrees of abnormal behavior. Frank psychotic episodes can occur, especially with parenteral abuse. Careful supervision is required during drug withdrawal from abusive use since severe depression may occur. Withdrawal following chronic therapeutic use may unmask symptoms of the underlying disorder that may require follow-up.

PRECAUTIONS

HEMATOLOGIC MONITORING

Periodic CBC, differential, and platelet counts are advised during prolonged therapy.

INFORMATION FOR THE PATIENT

Patient information is printed at the end of this insert. To assure safe and effective use of dexmethylphenidate HCl, the information and instructions provided in the patient information section should be discussed with patients.

CARCINOGENESIS, MUTAGENESIS, AND IMPAIRMENT OF FERTILITY

Lifetime carcinogenicity studies have not been carried out with dexmethylphenidate. In a lifetime carcinogenicity study carried out in B6C3F1 mice, racemic methylphenidate caused an increase in hepatocellular adenomas and, in males only, an increase in hepatoblastomas at a daily dose of approximately 60 mg/kg/day. Hepatoblastoma is a relatively rare rodent malignant tumor type. There was no increase in total malignant hepatic tumors. The mouse strain used is sensitive to the development of hepatic tumors, and the significance of these results to humans is unknown.

Racemic methylphenidate did not cause any increase in tumors in a lifetime carcinogenicity study carried out in F344 rats; the highest dose used was approximately 45 mg/kg/day.

In a 24 week study of racemic methylphenidate in the transgenic mouse strain p53+/-, which is sensitive to genotoxic carcinogens, there was no evidence of carcinogenicity. Mice were fed diets containing the same concentrations as in the lifetime carcinogenicity study; the high-dose group was exposed to 60-74 mg/kg/day of racemic methylphenidate.

Dexmethylphenidate was not mutagenic in the *in vitro* Ames reverse mutation assay, the *in vitro* mouse lymphoma cell forward mutation assay, or the *in vivo* mouse bone marrow micronucleus test.

Racemic methylphenidate was not mutagenic in the *in vitro* Ames reverse mutation assay or in the *in vitro* mouse lymphoma cell forward mutation assay, and was negative *in vivo* in the mouse bone marrow micronucleus assay. However, sister chromatid exchanges and chromosome aberrations were increased, indicative of a weak clastogenic response, in an *in vitro* assay of racemic methylphenidate in cultured Chinese Hamster Ovary (CHO) cells.

Racemic methylphenidate did not impair fertility in male or female mice that were fed diets containing the drug in an 18 week Continuous Breeding study. The study was conducted at doses of up to 160 mg/kg/day.

PREGNANCY CATEGORY C

In studies conducted in rats and rabbits, dexmethylphenidate was administered orally at doses of up to 20 and 100 mg/kg/day, respectively, during the period of organogenesis. No evidence of teratogenic activity was found in either the rat or rabbit study; however, delayed fetal skeletal ossification was observed at the highest dose level in rats. When dexmethylphenidate was administered to rats throughout pregnancy and lactation at doses of up to 20 mg/kg/day, postweaning body weight gain was decreased in male offspring at the highest dose, but no other effects on postnatal development were observed. At the highest doses tested, plasma levels (AUCs) of dexmethylphenidate in pregnant rats and rabbits were approximately 5 and 1 times, respectively, those in adults dosed with the maximum recommended human dose of 20 mg/day.

Racemic methylphenidate has been shown to have teratogenic effects in rabbits when given in doses of 200 mg/kg/day throughout organogenesis.

Adequate and well-controlled studies in pregnant women have not been conducted. Dexmethylphenidate HCl should be used during pregnancy only if the potential benefit justifies the potential risk to the fetus.

NURSING MOTHERS

It is not known whether dexmethylphenidate is excreted in human milk. Because many drugs are excreted in human milk, caution should be exercised if dexmethylphenidate HCl is administered to a nursing woman.

PEDIATRIC USE

The safety and efficacy of dexmethylphenidate HCl in children under 6 years old have not been established. Long-term effects of dexmethylphenidate HCl in children have not been well established (see WARNINGS).

DRUG INTERACTIONS

Methylphenidate may decrease the effectiveness of drugs used to treat hypertension. Because of possible effects on blood pressure, dexmethylphenidate HCl should be used cautiously with pressor agents.

Human pharmacologic studies have shown that racemic methylphenidate may inhibit the metabolism of coumarin anticoagulants, anticonvulsants (*e.g.,* phenobarbital, phenytoin, primidone), and some antidepressants (tricyclics and selective serotonin reuptake inhibitors). Downward dose adjustments of these drugs may be required when given concomitantly with methylphenidate. It may be necessary to adjust the dosage and monitor plasma drug concentration (or, in the case of coumarin, coagulation times), when initiating or discontinuing concomitant methylphenidate.

Serious adverse events have been reported in concomitant use with clonidine, although no causality for the combination has been established. The safety of using methylphenidate in combination with clonidine or other centrally acting alpha-2 agonists has not been systematically evaluated.

ADVERSE REACTIONS

The pre-marketing development program for dexmethylphenidate HCl included exposures in a total of 696 participants in clinical trials (684 patients, 12 healthy adult subjects). These participants received dexmethylphenidate HCl 5, 10, or 20 mg/day. The 684 ADHD patients (ages 6-17 years) were evaluated in two controlled clinical studies, two clinical pharmacology studies, and two uncontrolled long-term safety studies. Safety data on all patients are included in the discussion that follows. Adverse reactions were assessed by collecting adverse events, and results of physical examinations, vital sign and body weight measurements, and laboratory analyses.

Adverse events during exposure were primarily obtained by general inquiry and recorded by clinical investigators using terminology of their own choosing. Consequently, it is not possible to provide a meaningful estimate of the proportion of individuals experiencing adverse events without first grouping similar types of events into a smaller number of standardized event categories. In the tables and tabulations that follow, standard COSTART dictionary terminology has been used to classify reported adverse events.

The stated frequencies of adverse events represent the proportion of individuals who experienced, at least once, a treatment-emergent adverse event of the type listed. An event was considered treatment emergent if it occurred for the first time or worsened while receiving therapy following baseline evaluation.

ADVERSE FINDINGS IN CLINICAL TRIALS WITH DEXMETHYLPHENIDATE HCl

Adverse Events Associated With Discontinuation of Treatment

No dexmethylphenidate HCl-treated patients discontinued due to adverse events in two placebo-controlled trials. Overall, 50 of 684 children treated with dexmethylphenidate HCl (7.3%) experienced an adverse event that resulted in discontinuation. The most common reasons for discontinuation were twitching (described as motor or vocal tics), anorexia, insomnia, and tachycardia (approximately 1% each).

Adverse Events Occurring at an Incidence of 5% or More Among Dexmethylphenidate HCl-Treated Patients

TABLE 1 enumerates treatment-emergent adverse events for two, placebo-controlled, parallel group trials in children with ADHD at dexmethylphenidate HCl doses of 5, 10, and 20 mg/day. The table includes only those events that occurred in 5% or more of patients treated with dexmethylphenidate HCl where the incidence in patients treated with dexmethylphenidate HCl was at least twice the incidence in placebo-treated patients.

The prescriber should be aware that these figures cannot be used to predict the incidence of adverse events in the course of usual medical practice where patient characteristics and other factors differ from those which prevailed in the clinical trials. Similarly, the cited frequencies cannot be compared with figures obtained from other clinical investigations involving different treatments, uses, and investigators. The cited figures, however, do provide the prescribing physician with some basis for estimating the relative contribution of drug and non-drug factors to the adverse event incidence rate in the population studied.

TABLE 1 *Treatment-Emergent Adverse Events* Occurring During Double-Blind Treatment in Clinical Trials of Dexmethylphenidate HCl*

Body System / Preferred Term	Placebo (n=79)	Dexmethylphenidate HCl (n=82)
Body as a Whole		
Abdominal pain	15%	6%
Fever	5%	1%
Digestive System		
Anorexia	6%	1%
Nausea	9%	1%

* Events, regardless of causality, for which the incidence for patients treated with dexmethylphenidate HCl was at least 5% and twice the incidence among placebo-treated patients. Incidence has been rounded to the nearest whole number.

ADVERSE EVENTS WITH OTHER METHYLPHENIDATE HCl PRODUCTS

Nervousness and insomnia are the most common adverse reactions reported with other methylphenidate products. In children, loss of appetite, abdominal pain, weight loss during prolonged therapy, insomnia, and tachycardia may occur more frequently; however, any of the other adverse reactions listed below may also occur.

Other reactions include:

Cardiac: Angina, arrhythmia, palpitations, pulse increased or decreased.

Gastrointestinal: Nausea.

Immune: Hypersensitivity reactions including skin rash, urticaria, fever, arthralgia, exfoliative dermatitis, erythema multiforme with histopathological findings of necrotizing vasculitis, and thrombocytopenic purpura.

Nervous System: Dizziness, drowsiness, dyskinesia, headache, rare reports of Tourette's syndrome, toxic psychosis.

Vascular: Blood pressure increased or decreased, cerebral arteritis and/or occlusion.

Although a definite causal relationship has not been established, the following have been reported in patients taking methylphenidate:

Blood/Lymphatic: Leukopenia and/or anemia.

Hepatobiliary: Abnormal liver function, ranging from transaminase elevation to hepatic coma.

Psychiatric: Transient depressed mood.

Skin/Subcutaneous: Scalp hair loss.

Very rare reports of neuroleptic malignant syndrome (NMS) have been received, and, in most of these, patients were concurrently receiving therapies associated with NMS. In a single report, a 10 year old boy who had been taking methylphenidate for approximately 18 months experienced an NMS-like event within 45 minutes of ingesting his first dose of venlafaxine. It is uncertain whether this case represented a drug-drug interaction, a response to either drug alone, or some other cause.

In children, loss of appetite, abdominal pain, weight loss during prolonged therapy, insomnia, and tachycardia may occur more frequently; however, any of the other adverse reactions listed above may also occur.

DOSAGE AND ADMINISTRATION

Dexmethylphenidate HCl is administered twice daily, at least 4 hours apart. Dexmethylphenidate HCl may be administered with or without food.

Dosage should be individualized according to the needs and responses of the patient.

PATIENTS NEW TO METHYLPHENIDATE

The recommended starting dose of dexmethylphenidate HCl for patients who are not currently taking racemic methylphenidate, or for patients who are on stimulants other than methylphenidate, is 5 mg/day (2.5 mg twice daily).

Dosage may be adjusted in 2.5 to 5 mg increments to a maximum of 20 mg/day (10 mg twice daily). In general, dosage adjustments may proceed at approximately weekly intervals.

PATIENTS CURRENTLY USING METHYLPHENIDATE

For patients currently using methylphenidate, the recommended starting dose of dexmethylphenidate HCl is half the dose of racemic methylphenidate. The maximum recommended dose is 20 mg/day (10 mg twice daily).

MAINTENANCE/EXTENDED TREATMENT

There is no body of evidence available from controlled trials to indicate how long the patient with ADHD should be treated with dexmethylphenidate HCl. It is generally agreed, however, that pharmacological treatment of ADHD may be needed for extended periods. Nevertheless, the physician who elects to use dexmethylphenidate HCl for extended periods in patients with ADHD should periodically re-evaluate the long-term usefulness of the drug for the individual patient with periods off medication to assess the patient's functioning without pharmacotherapy. Improvement may be sustained when the drug is either temporarily or permanently discontinued.

DOSE REDUCTION AND DISCONTINUATION

If paradoxical aggravation of symptoms or other adverse events occur, the dosage should be reduced, or, if necessary, the drug should be discontinued.

If improvement is not observed after appropriate dosage adjustment over a 1 month period, the drug should be discontinued.

D

HOW SUPPLIED

Dexmethylphenidate hydrochloride tablets are available in:

2.5 mg: Blue, D-shaped, embossed "D" on upper convex face and "2.5" on lower convex face.

5 mg: Yellow, D-shaped, embossed "D" on upper convex face and "5" on lower convex face.

10 mg: White, D-shaped, embossed "D" on upper convex face and "10" on lower convex face.

Storage: Store at 25°C (77°F); excursions permitted 15-30°C (59-86°F). Protect from light and moisture.

PRODUCT LISTING - EQUIVALENTS NOT AVAILABLE

Tablet - Oral - 2.5 mg

100's	$47.96	FOCALIN, Mikart Inc	00078-0380-05

Tablet - Oral - 5 mg

100's	$68.38	FOCALIN, Mikart Inc	00078-0381-05

Tablet - Oral - 10 mg

100's	$98.31	FOCALIN, Mikart Inc	00078-0382-05

Diazepam *(001033)*

Categories: Alcohol withdrawal; Anxiety disorder, generalized; Athetosis; Delirium tremens; Muscle spasm; Preanesthesia; Seizures, generalized tonic-clonic; Status epilepticus; Stiff-man syndrome; Tetanus; DEA Class CIV; FDA Approval Pre 1982; Pregnancy Category D; Orphan Drugs; WHO Formulary

Drug Classes: Anxiolytics; Benzodiazepines; Relaxants, skeletal muscle

Brand Names: Dizac; **Valium**; Valrelease

Foreign Brand Availability: Alboral (Mexico); Aliseum (Italy); Amiprol (Argentina); Ansiolin (Italy); Antenex (Australia; New-Zealand); Anxionil (Philippines); Apo-diazepam (Canada); Apozepam (Denmark; Sweden); Armonil (Argentina); Arzepam (Mexico); Assival (Israel); Atensine (Ireland); Azedipamin (Japan); Benzopin (South-Africa); Best (Argentina); Betapam (South-Africa); Calmpose (Benin; Burkina-Faso; Ethiopia; Gambia; Ghana; Guinea; India; Ivory-Coast; Kenya; Liberia; Malawi; Mali; Mauritania; Mauritius; Morocco; Niger; Nigeria; Senegal; Seychelles; Sierra-Leone; South-Africa; Sudan; Tanzania; Tunia; Uganda; Zambia; Zimbabwe); Caudel (Argentina); Desconet (Argentina); Diaceplex (Spain); Dialag (Bahamas; Barbados; Belize; Benin; Bermuda; Burkina-Faso; Curacao; Ethiopia; Gambia; Ghana; Guinea; Guyana; Ivory-Coast; Jamaica; Kenya; Liberia; Malawi; Mali; Mauritania; Mauritius; Morocco; Netherland-Antilles; Niger; Nigeria; Puerto-Rico; Senegal; Seychelles; Sierra-Leone; South-Africa; Sudan; Surinam; Tanzania; Trinidad; Tunia; Uganda; Zambia; Zimbabwe); Dialar (England); Diano (Thailand); Diapam (Finland; Russia; Thailand; Turkey); Diapanil (Mexico); Diapax (Japan); Diapine (Malaysia; Thailand); Diaquel (South-Africa); Diazem (Turkey); Diazemuls (England; Italy; Netherlands); Diazepam (Hong-Kong); Diazepan (Bahrain; Benin; Burkina-Faso; Costa-Rica; Cyprus; Dominican-Republic; Egypt; El-Salvador; Ethiopia; Gambia; Ghana; Guatemala; Guinea; Honduras; Iran; Iraq; Israel; Ivory-Coast; Jordan; Kenya; Kuwait; Lebanon; Liberia; Libya; Malawi; Mali; Mauritania; Mauritius; Morocco; Nicaragua; Niger; Nigeria; Oman; Panama; Qatar; Republic-of-Yemen; Saudi-Arabia; Senegal; Seychelles; Sierra-Leone; South-Africa; Spain; Sudan; Syria; Tanzania; Tunia; Uganda; United-Arab-Emirates; Zambia; Zimbabwe); Diazepin (Indonesia); Dipaz (Ecuador); Dipezona (Argentina); Doval (South-Africa); Drenian (Spain); Ducene (Australia; New-Zealand); Dupin (Taiwan); DZP (Malaysia); Eridan (Italy); Elcion CR (India); Euphorin P (Japan); Gewacalm (Austria); Gradual (Argentina); Gubex (Argentina); Horizon (Japan); Kratium (Bahamas; Barbados; Belize; Benin; Bermuda; Burkina-Faso; Curacao; Ethiopia; Gambia; Ghana; Guinea; Guyana; Ivory-Coast; Jamaica; Kenya; Liberia; Malawi; Mali; Mauritania; Mauritius; Morocco; Netherland-Antilles; Niger; Nigeria; Puerto-Rico; Senegal; Seychelles; Sierra-Leone; South-Africa; Sudan; Surinam; Tanzania; Trinidad; Tunia; Uganda; Zambia; Zimbabwe); Kratium 2 (Hong-Kong); Lembrol (Argentina); Lovium (Indonesia); Mentalium (Indonesia); Nivalen (Bahrain; Benin; Burkina-Faso; Cyprus; Egypt; Ethiopia; Gambia; Ghana; Guinea; Iran; Iraq; Israel; Ivory-Coast; Jordan; Kenya; Kuwait; Lebanon; Liberia; Libya; Malawi; Mali; Mauritania; Mauritius; Morocco; Niger; Nigeria; Oman; Qatar; Republic-of-Yemen; Saudi-Arabia; Senegal; Seychelles; Sierra-Leone; South-Africa; Sudan; Syria; Tanzania; Tunia; Uganda; United-Arab-Emirates; Zambia; Zimbabwe); Noan (Italy); Ortopsique (Mexico); Paceum (Switzerland); Pacitran (Peru); Pax (South-Africa); Paxum (India); Placidox 2 (India); Placidox 5 (India); Placidox 10 (India); Plidan (Argentina); Propam (New-Zealand); Psychopax (Austria; Switzerland); Radizepam (Bahrain; Benin; Burkina-Faso; Cyprus; Egypt; Ethiopia; Gambia; Ghana; Guinea; Iran; Iraq; Israel; Ivory-Coast; Jordan; Kenya; Kuwait; Lebanon; Liberia; Libya; Malawi; Mali; Mauritania; Mauritius; Morocco; Niger; Nigeria; Oman; Qatar; Republic-of-Yemen; Saudi-Arabia; Senegal; Seychelles; Sierra-Leone; South-Africa; Sudan; Syria; Tanzania; Tunia; Uganda; United-Arab-Emirates; Zambia; Zimbabwe); Relanium (Bulgaria; Russia); Reliver (Japan); Reposepan (Peru); Saromet (Argentina); Seduxen (Bahamas; Barbados; Belize; Bermuda; Curacao; Guyana; Jamaica; Netherland-Antilles; Puerto-Rico; Surinam; Trinidad); Simasedan (Argentina); Sipam (Thailand); Sonacon (Japan); Stesolid (Bahrain; Cyprus; Czech-Republic; Denmark; Egypt; England; Finland; Germany; Hungary; Indonesia; Iran; Iraq; Israel; Jordan; Kuwait; Lebanon; Libya; Netherlands; Norway; Oman; Qatar; Republic-of-Yemen; Saudi-Arabia; Sweden; Switzerland; Syria; Taiwan; Thailand; United-Arab-Emirates); Tranquirit (Italy); Trazepam (Philippines); Valaxona (Denmark); Valiquid (Germany); Valpam (Australia); Vatran (Italy); Vazen (Peru); Vivol (Canada)

Cost of Therapy: $24.02 (Anxiety; Valium; 2 mg; 2 tablets/day; 30 day supply)
$1.80 (Anxiety; Generic Tablets; 2 mg; 2 tablets/day; 30 day supply)

HCFA JCODE(S): J3360 up to 5 mg IM, IV

INTRAVENOUS

DESCRIPTION

INJECTABLE SOLUTION

Each ml of Valium contains 5 mg diazepam compounded with 40% propylene glycol, 10% ethyl alcohol, 5% sodium benzoate and benzoic acid as buffers, and 1.5% benzyl alcohol as preservative.

Diazepam is a benzodiazepine derivative. Chemically, diazepam is 7-chloro-1,3-dihydro-1-methyl-5-phenyl-2H-1,4-benzodiazepin-2-one. It is a colorless crystalline compound, insoluble in water and has a molecular weight of 284.74.

INJECTABLE EMULSION

Diazepam is a benzodiazepine derivative identified chemically as 7-chloro-1,3-dihydro-1-methyl-5-phenyl-2H-1,4-benzodiazepin-2-one. It is a colorless crystalline compound, insoluble in water and has a molecular weight of 284.75.

Each ml of Dizac for IV administration only contains 5 mg diazepam, fractionated soybean oil 150 mg, diacetylated monoglycerides 50 mg, fractionated egg yolk phospholipids 12 mg, glycerin 22.0 mg, water for injection, and sodium hydroxide to adjust pH to approximately 8. Dizac is a sterile formulation and contains no preservatives.

STRICT ASEPTIC TECHNIQUE MUST ALWAYS BE MAINTAINED DURING HANDLING. DIZAC INJECTABLE EMULSION IS A SINGLE-USE PARENTERAL PRODUCT, CONTAINS NO ANTIMICROBIAL PRESERVATIVES, AND CAN SUPPORT RAPID GROWTH OF MICROORGANISMS. ALWAYS DISCARD UNUSED PORTION (SEE DOSAGE AND ADMINISTRATION, ASEPTIC GUIDELINES FOR PARENTERAL USE). THERE HAVE BEEN REPORTS IN WHICH FAILURE TO USE ASEPTIC TECHNIQUE WHEN HANDLING OTHER PARENTERAL PRODUCTS (CONTAINING THE SAME VEHICLE) WAS ASSOCIATED WITH MICROBIAL CONTAMINATION OF THE PRODUCT AND WITH FEVER, INFECTION/SEPSIS, OTHER LIFE THREATENING ILLNESSES, AND/OR DEATH. DO NOT USE IF CONTAMINATION IS SUSPECTED.

CLINICAL PHARMACOLOGY

In animals, diazepam appears to act on parts of the limbic system, the thalamus and hypothalamus, and induces calming effects. Diazepam, unlike chlorpromazine and reserpine, has no demonstrable peripheral autonomic blocking action, nor does it produce extrapyramidal side effects; however, animals treated with diazepam do have a transient ataxia at higher doses. Diazepam was found to have transient cardiovascular depressor effects in dogs. Long-term experiments in rats revealed no disturbances of endocrine function. *Injectable Solution Only:* Injections into animals have produced localized irritation of tissue surrounding injection sites and some thickening of veins after intravenous use.

Additional Information for Injectable Emulsion: Injections into animals of diazepam injectable emulsion have produced significantly less localized irritation of tissue surrounding injection sites than has been observed following injection of formulations containing diazepam and propylene glycol.

After a 10 mg intravenous injection of diazepam injectable emulsion, the mean maximum concentration (C_{max}) was 455 ng/ml and was attained at approximately 8 minutes after injection. The mean area under the plasma concentration-time curve (AUC) was 4685 ng/ml/h. The mean absolute bioavailability of diazepam injectable emulsion compared to an intravenous injection of diazepam was 93%. In the same study, the mean maximum concentration of N-desmethyldiazepam, the active metabolite, was 48 ng/ml at approximately 48 hours after the injection. The mean AUC of N-desmethyldiazepam was 5043 ng/ml/h.

In a randomized clinical trial the sedative effect of diazepam injectable emulsion and diazepam injection solution was compared at three different dose levels (0.04, 0.10 and 0.20 mg/kg b.w.). Approximately the same extent of sedation was observed with the 2 formulations indicating that the same dosing recommendations should apply. The data for diazepam injectable emulsion were suggestive of a slightly lower bioavailability for diazepam in females compared to males given this formulation, and in younger patients (age 20-55), a relative potency for females compared to males of roughly 2/3 (see DOSAGE AND ADMINISTRATION). Twenty-three percent (23%) of the patients given diazepam injection solution experienced pain at the site of injection compared to none in the diazepam injectable emulsion group. However, other comparative studies of diazepam injectable emulsion administered intravenously have reported local pain in a range of 0-14% and injection site thrombohlebitis in a range of 0-6%, suggesting that intravenous administration of diazepam injectable emulsion may be associated with some risk of such reactions.

INDICATIONS AND USAGE

Diazepam is indicated for the management of anxiety disorders or for the short-term relief of the symptoms of anxiety. Anxiety or tension associated with the stress of everyday life usually does not require treatment with an anxiolytic.

In acute alcohol withdrawal, diazepam may be useful in the symptomatic relief of acute agitation, tremor, impending or acute delirium tremens and hallucinosis.

As an adjunct prior to endoscopic procedures if apprehension, anxiety or acute stress reactions are present, and to diminish the patient's recall of the procedures (see WARNINGS).

Diazepam is a useful adjunct for the relief of skeletal muscle spasm due to reflex spasm to local pathology (such as inflammation of the muscles or joints, or secondary to trauma); spasticity caused by upper motor neuron disorders (such as cerebral palsy and paraplegia); athetosis; stiff-man syndrome; and tetanus.

Injectable diazepam is a useful adjunct in status epilepticus and severe recurrent convulsive seizures.

Diazepam is a useful premedication (for injectable solution only, the IM route is preferred) for relief of anxiety and tension in patients who are to undergo surgical procedures. Intravenously, prior to cardioversion for the relief of anxiety and tension and to diminish the patient's recall of the procedure.

NON-FDA APPROVED INDICATIONS

Diazepam has been used for the treatment of insomnia and nightmares but these uses are not FDA approved.

CONTRAINDICATIONS

Diazepam is contraindicated in patients with a known hypersensitivity to this drug; acute narrow angle glaucoma; and open angle glaucoma unless patients are receiving appropriate therapy. *Injectable Emulsion Only:* Because the diazepam emulsion vehicle contains soybean oil, diazepam injectable emulsion should not be used in patients with known hypersensitivity to soy protein.

WARNINGS

When used intravenously, the following procedures should be undertaken to reduce the possibility of venous thrombosis, phlebitis, local irritation, swelling, and, rarely, vascular impairment: diazepam should be injected slowly, taking at least 1 minute for each 5 mg (1 ml) given; do not use small veins, such as those on the dorsum of the hand or wrist; extreme care should be taken to avoid intra-arterial administration or extravasation (see CLINICAL PHARMACOLOGY).

Do not mix or dilute diazepam with other solutions or drugs in syringe or infusion container. If it is not feasible to administer diazepam directly IV, it may be injected slowly through the infusion tubing as close as possible to the vein insertion.

Extreme care must be used in administering injectable diazepam by the IV route to the elderly, to very ill patients and to those with limited pulmonary reserve because of the possibility that apnea and/or cardiac arrest may occur. Concomitant use of barbiturates, alcohol or other central nervous system depressants increases depression with increased risk of apnea. Resuscitative equipment including that necessary to support respiration should be readily available.

When diazepam is used with a narcotic analgesic, the dosage of the narcotic should be reduced by at least one-third and administered in small increments. In some cases the use of a narcotic may not be necessary.

Diazepam should not be administered to patients in shock, coma, or in acute alcoholic intoxication with depression of vital sins. As is true of most CNS-acting drugs, patients receiving diazepam should be cautioned against engaging in hazardous occupations requiring complete mental alertness, such as operating machinery or driving a motor vehicle.

Tonic status epilepticus has been precipitated in patients treated with IV diazepam for petit mal status or petit mal variant status.

USE IN PREGNANCY

An increased risk of congenital malformations associated with the use of minor tranquilizers (diazepam, meprobamate and chlordiazepoxide) during the first trimester of pregnancy has been suggested in several studies. Because use of these drugs is rarely a matter of urgency, their use during this period should almost always be avoided. The possibility that a woman of childbearing potential may become pregnant at the time of institution of therapy should be considered. Patients should be advised that if they become pregnant during therapy or intend to become pregnant they should communicate with their physicians about the desirability of discontinuing the drug.

In humans, measurable amounts of diazepam were found in maternal and cord blood, indicating placental transfer of the drug. Until additional information is available, diazepam injectable forms are not recommended for obstetrical use.

PEDIATRIC USE

Efficacy and safety of parenteral diazepam has not been established in the neonate (30 days or less of age).

Prolonged central nervous system depression has been observed in neonates, apparently due to inability to biotransform diazepam into inactive metabolites.

In pediatric use, in order to obtain maximum clinical effect with the minimum amount of drug and thus to reduce the risk of hazardous side effects, such as apnea or prolonged periods of somnolence, it is recommended that the drug be given slowly over a 3 minute period in a dosage not to exceed 0.25 mg/kg. After an interval of 15-30 minutes the initial dosage can be safely repeated. If, however, relief of symptoms is not obtained after a third administration, adjunctive therapy appropriate to the condition being treated is recommended.

Withdrawal symptoms of the barbiturate type have occurred after the discontinuation of benzodiazepines.

ADDITIONAL INFORMATION FOR INJECTABLE EMULSION

STRICT ASEPTIC TECHNIQUE MUST ALWAYS BE MAINTAINED DURING HANDLING. DIAZEPAM INJECTABLE EMULSION IS A SINGLE-USE PARENTERAL PRODUCT, CONTAINS NO ANTIMICROBIAL PRESERVATIVES, AND CAN SUPPORT RAPID GROWTH OF MICROORGANISMS. ALWAYS DISCARD UNUSED PORTION (SEE DOSAGE AND ADMINISTRATION, ASEPTIC GUIDELINES FOR PARENTERAL USE). THERE HAVE BEEN REPORTS IN WHICH FAILURE TO USE ASEPTIC TECHNIQUE WHEN HANDLING OTHER PARENTERAL PRODUCTS (CONTAINING THE SAME VEHICLE) WAS ASSOCIATED WITH MICROBIAL CONTAMINATION OF THE PRODUCT AND WITH FEVER, INFECTION/SEPSIS, OTHER LIFE THREATENING ILLNESSES, AND/OR DEATH. DO NOT USE IF CONTAMINATION IS SUSPECTED.

PRECAUTIONS

Although seizures may be brought under control promptly, a significant proportion of patients experience a return to seizure activity, presumably due to the short-lived effect of diazepam after IV administration. The physician should be prepared to readminister the drug. However, diazepam is not recommended for maintenance, and once seizures are brought under control, consideration should be given to the administration of agents useful in longer term control of seizures.

If diazepam is to be combined with other psychotropic agents or anticonvulsant drugs, careful consideration should be given to the pharmacology of the agents to be employed—particularly with known compounds which may potentiate the action of diazepam, such as phenothiazines, narcotics, barbiturates, MAO inhibitors and other antidepressants. In highly anxious patients with evidence of accompanying depression, particularly those who may have suicidal tendencies, protective measures may be necessary. The usual precautions in treating patients with impaired hepatic function should be observed. Metabolites of diazepam are excreted by the kidney; to avoid their excess accumulation, caution should be exercised in the administration to patients with compromised kidney function.

Since an increase in cough reflex and laryngospasm may occur with peroral endoscopic procedures, the use of a topical anesthetic agent and the availability of necessary countermeasures are recommended. Injectable forms of diazepam have produced hypotension or muscular weakness in some patients, particularly when used with narcotics, barbiturates or alcohol.

FOR INJECTABLE SOLUTION ONLY

Until additional information is available, injectable diazepam in not recommended for obstretical use.

Lower doses (usually 2 -5 mg) should be used for elderly and debilitated patients.

The clearance of diazepam and certain other benzodiazepines can be delayed in association with cimetidine (Tagamet) administration. The clinical significance of this is unclear.

LABOR AND DELIVERY

For Injectable Emulsion Only: In humans, measurable amounts of diazepam were found in maternal and cord blood. indicating placental transfer of the drug. Until additional information is available, injectable diazepam is not recommended for obsterical use.

ADVERSE REACTIONS

Side effects most commonly reported were drowsiness, fatigue and ataxia; venous thrombosis and phlebitis at the site of injection were also reported as common side effects for the injectable solution. Other adverse reactions less frequently reported include:

CNS: Confusion, depression, dysarthria, headache, hypoactivity, slurred speech, syncope, tremor, vertigo.

G.I.: Constipation, nausea.

G.U.: Incontinence, changes in libido, urinary retention.

Cardiovascular: Bradycardia, cardiovascular collapse, hypotension; venous thrombosis and phlebitis at the site of injection are infrequently reported for the injectable emulsion form.

EENT: Blurred vision, diplopia, nystagmus.

Skin: Urticaria, skin rash.

Other: Hiccups, changes in salivation, neutropenia, jaundice. Paradoxical reactions such as acute hyperexcited states, anxiety, hallucinations, increased muscle spasticity, insomnia, rage, sleep disturbances and stimulation have been reported; should these occur, use of the drug should be discontinued. Minor changes in EEG patterns, usually low-voltage fast activity, have been observed in patients during and after diazepam therapy and are of no known significance.

In peroral endoscopic procedures, coughing, depressed respiration, dyspnea, hyperventilation, laryngospasm and pain in throat or chest have been reported.

Because of isolated reports of neutropenia and jaundice, periodic blood counts and liver function tests are advisable during long-term therapy.

DOSAGE AND ADMINISTRATION

INJECTABLE SOLUTION

Dosage should be individualized for maximum beneficial effect. The usual recommended dose in older children and adults ranges from 2 -20 mg IM or IV, depending on the indication and its severity. In some conditions, *e.g.,* tetanus, larger doses may be required (see dosage for specific indications in TABLE 1A). In acute conditions the injection may be repeated within 1 hour although an interval of 3-4 hours is usually satisfactory. Lower doses (usually 2 -5 mg) and slow increase in dosage should be used for elderly or debilitated patients and when other sedative drugs are administered. (See WARNINGS and ADVERSE REACTIONS.)

For dosage in infants above the age of 30 days and children, see the specific indications in TABLE 1B). Facilities for respiratory assistance should be readily available.

Intramuscular

Diazepam injectable solution should be injected deeply into the muscle.

Intravenous Use

(See WARNINGS, particularly for use in children.) The solution or emulsion should be injected slowly, taking at least 1 minute for each 5 mg (1 ml) given. Do not use small veins such as those on the dorsum of the hand or wrist. Extreme care should be taken to avoid intra-arterial administration or extravasation.

Do not mix or dilute diazepam injectable solution with other solutions or drugs in syringe or infusion container. If it is not feasible to administer diazepam directly IV, it may be injected slowly through the infusion tubing as close as possible to vein insertion.

INJECTABLE EMULSION

Diazepam injectable emulsion is intended for intravenous use only and should NOT be administered intramuscularly or subcutaneously. Dosage should be individualized for maximum beneficial effect. The usual recommended dose in older children and adults ranges from 2 -20 mg IV, depending on the indication and its severity.

In some conditions, *e.g.,* tetanus, larger doses may be required (see dosage for specific indications in TABLE 1A). There are data comparing intravenously administered diazepam injectable emulsion in females and males that are suggestive of (1) a slightly lower bioavailability of diazepam for females compared to males, and (2) for younger patients (ages 20-55), a relative potency for females compared to males of roughly ⅔. In acute conditions the injection may be repeated within 1 hour although an interval of 3-4 hours is usually satisfactory. Lower doses (usually 2 -5 mg) and slow increase in dosage should be used for elderly or debilitated patients and when other sedative drugs are administered. (See WARNINGS and ADVERSE REACTIONS.)

For dosage in infants above the age of 30 days and children, see the specific indications in TABLE 1B). Facilities for respiratory assistance should be readily available.

Intravenous Use

(See WARNINGS, particularly for use in children.) The emulsion should be injected slowly, taking at least 1 minute for each each 5 mg (1 ml) given. Do not use small veins, such as those on the dorsum of the hand or wrist. Extreme care should be taken to avoid intra-arterial administration or extravasation.

D

Do not add diazepam injectable emulsion to infusion sets containing polyvinylchloride. Diazepam injectable emulsion is compatible with polyethylene-lined or glass infusion sets and polyethylene/polypropylene plastic syringes. Diazepam injectable emulsion is incompatible with morphine and glycopyrrolate.

Do not mix or dilute diazepam injectable emulsion with other solutions or drugs in syringe or infusion container. If it is not feasible to administer diazepam directly IV, it may be injected slowly through the infusion tubing as close as possible to vein insertion.

Parental drug products should be inspected visually for particulate matter and discoloration prior to administration whenever solution and container permit. Diazepam injectable emulsion must not be administered through filters with a pore size less than 5 microns because this could restrict the flow of diazepam injectable emulsion and/or cause the breakdown of the emulsion. Do not use if there is evidence of separation of the phases of the emulsion.

STRICT ASEPTIC TECHNIQUE MUST ALWAYS BE MAINTAINED DURING HANDLING. DIZAC INJECTABLE EMULSION IS A SINGLE-USE PARENTERAL PRODUCT, CONTAINS NO ANTIMICROBIAL PRESERVATIVES, AND CAN SUPPORT RAPID GROWTH OF MICROORGANISMS. ALWAYS DISCARD UNUSED PORTION (SEE DOSAGE AND ADMINISTRATION, ASEPTIC GUIDELINES FOR PARENTERAL USE). THERE HAVE BEEN REPORTS IN WHICH FAILURE TO USE ASEPTIC TECHNIQUE WHEN HANDLING OTHER PARENTERAL PRODUCTS (CONTAINING THE SAME VEHICLE) WAS ASSOCIATED WITH MICROBIAL CONTAMINATION OF THE PRODUCT AND WITH FEVER, INFECTION/SEPSIS, OTHER LIFE THREATENING ILLNESSES, AND/OR DEATH. DO NOT USE IF CONTAMINATION IS SUSPECTED.

Aseptic Guidelines for Parenteral Use of Diazepam Injectable Emulsion

Diazepam injectable emulsion should be prepared for use just prior to initiation of each individual treatment procedure. Diazepam injectable emulsion should be drawn into sterile syringes immediately after ampules are opened. The syringe(s) should be labeled with appropriate information including the date and time the ampule was opened. Administration should commence promptly and be completed within 6 hours after the ampules have been opened. Diazepam injectable emulsion should be prepared for single patient use only. Any unused portion of diazepam injectable emulsion , reservoirs, dedicated administration tubing and/or solutions containing diazepam injectable emulsion must be discarded after the end of parenteral treatment or at 6 hours, whichever occurs sooner. The IV line should be flushed every 6 hours and at the end of treatment procedure to remove residual diazepam injectable emulsion.

Once the acute symptomatology has been properly controlled with diazepam injectable emulsion, the patient may be placed on therapy with an appropriate oral agent if further treatment is required.

TABLE 1A *Usual Adult Dosage, Diazepam Injectable Solution and Emulsion*

Indication	Usual Adult Dosage
Moderate Anxiety Disorders and Symptoms of Anxiety	2 -5 mg, IV.* Repeat in 3-4 hours, if necessary.
Severe Anxiety Disorders and Symptoms of Anxiety	5 -10 mg, IV.* Repeat in 3-4 hours, if necessary.
Acute Alcohol Withdrawal: As an aid in symptomatic relief of acute agitation tremor, impending or acute delirium tremens and hallucinosis.	10 mg, IV initially,* then 5 -10 mg in 3-4 hours, if necessary.
Endoscopic Procedures: Adjunctively, if apprehension, anxiety or acute stress reactions are present prior to endoscopic procedures. Dosage of narcotics should be reduced by at least a third and in some cases may be omitted. See PRECAUTIONS for peroral procedures.	Titrate IV dosage to desired sedative response, such as slurring of speech, with slow administration immediately prior to the procedure. Generally 10 mg or less is adequate, but up to 20 mg IV may be given, particularly when concomitant narcotics are omitted.†
Muscle Spasm: Associated with local pathology, cerebral palsy, athetosis, stiff-man syndrome or tetanus.	5 -10 mg, IV initially,* then 5 -10 mg in 3-4 hours, if necessary. For tetanus, larger doses may be required.
Status Epilepticus and Severe Recurrent Convulsive Seizures: In the convulsing patient, the IV route is by far preferred. This injection should be administered slowly.‡	5 -10 mg initially IV. This injection may be repeated if necessary at 10-15 minute intervals up to a maximum dose of 30 mg. If necessary, therapy with diazepam may be repeated in 2-4 hours; however, residual active metabolites may persist, and readministration should be made with this consideration. Extreme caution must be exercised with individuals with chronic lung disease or unstable cardiovascular status.
Preoperative Medication: To relieve anxiety and tension. (If atropine, scopolamine or other premedications are desired, they must be administered in separate syringes.)	10 mg, IV before surgery§
Cardioversion: To relieve anxiety and tension and to reduce recall of procedure.	5 -15 mg, IV, within 5-10 minutes prior to the procedure.

* **Injectable Solution Only:** IM route may be used
† **Injectable Solution Only:** If IV cannot be used, 5 -10 mg IM approximately 30 minutes prior to the procedure.
‡ **Injectable Solution Only:** If IV administration is impossible, the IM route may be used.
§ **Injectable Solution Only:** IM is the preferred route

Once the acute symptomology has been properly controlled with injectable diazepam, the patient may be placed on oral therapy with diazepam if further treatment is required.

ANIMAL PHARMACOLOGY

Oral LD_{50} of diazepam is 720 mg/kg in mice and 1240 mg/kg in rats. Intraperitoneal administration of 400 mg/kg to a monkey resulted in death on the sixth day.

TABLE 1B *Dosage Range in Children, Diazepam Injectable Solution and Emulsion*

	IV administration should be made slowly
Muscle Spasm: Associated with local pathology, cerebral palsy, athetosis, stiff-man syndrome or tetanus.	For tetanus in infants over 30 days of age, 1 -2 mg IV* slowly, repeated every 3-4 hours as necessary. In children 5 years or older, 5 -10 mg repeated every 3-4 hours may be required to control tetanus spasms. Respiratory assistance should be available.
Status Epilepticus and Severe Recurrent Convulsive Seizures: In the convulsing patient, the IV route is by far preferred. This injection should be administered slowly. †	Infants over 30 days of age and children under 5 years, 0.2 -0.5 mg slowly every 2-5 minutes up to a maximum of 5 mg IV. Children 5 years or older, 1 mg every 2-5 minutes up to a maximum of 10 mg (slow IV administration). Repeat in 2-4 hours if necessary. EEG monitoring of the seizure may be helpful.

* **Injectable Solution Only:** IM route may be used
† **Injectable Solution Only:** If IV administration is impossible, the IM route may be used.

REPRODUCTION STUDIES

A series of rat reproduction studies was performed with diazepam in oral doses of 1, 10, 80, and 100 mg/kg given for periods ranging from 60-228 days prior to mating. At 100 mg/kg there was a decrease in the number of pregnancies and surviving offspring in these rats. These effects may be attributable to prolonged sedative activity, resulting in lack of interest in mating and lessened maternal nursing and care of the young. Neonatal survival of rats at doses lower than 100 mg/kg was within normal limits. Several neonates, both controls and experimentals, in these rat reproduction studies showed skeletal or other defects. Further studies in rats at doses up to and including 80 mg/kg day did not reveal significant teratological effects on the offspring. Rabbits were maintained on doses of 1, 2, 5 and 8 mg/kg from day 6 through day 18 of gestation. No adverse effects on reproduction and no teratological changes were noted.

HOW SUPPLIED

DIZAC INJECTABLE EMULSION

Contains no preservatives. Discard unused portion.

Storage

Store at or below 25°C (77°F). Do not freeze. It has been demonstrated that Dizac can be exposed to temperature changes between 5–30° C for a period of not more than 4 hours at least 20 times without deterioration of the emulsion quality.

PROTECT FROM LIGHT.

ORAL

DESCRIPTION

Diazepam is a benzodiazepine derivative. Chemically diazepam is 7-chloro-1,3-dihydro-1-methyl-5-phenyl-2H-1,4-benzodiazepin-2-one. It is a colorless crystalline compound, insoluble in water and has a molecular weight of 284.74.

Valium 5-mg tablets contain FD&C yellow no. 6 and D&C yellow no. 10 dyes. Valium 10-mg tablets contain FD&C blue no. 1 dye. Valium 2-mg tablets contain no dye.

CLINICAL PHARMACOLOGY

In animals, diazepam appears to act on parts of the limbic system, the thalamus and hypothalamus, and induces calming effects. Diazepam, unlike chlorpromazine and reserpine, has no demonstrable peripheral autonomic blocking action, nor does it produce extrapyramidal side effects; however, animals treated with diazepam do have a transient ataxia at higher doses. Diazepam was found to have transient cardiovascular depressor effects in dogs. Long-term experiments in rats revealed no disturbances of endocrine function.

Oral LD_{50} of diazepam is 720 mg/kg in mice and 1240 mg/kg in rats. Intraperitoneal administration of 400 mg/kg to a monkey resulted in death on the sixth day.

REPRODUCTION STUDIES

A series of rat reproduction studies was performed with diazepam in oral doses of 1, 10, 80, and 100 mg/kg given for periods ranging from 60-228 days prior to mating. At 100 mg/kg there was a decrease in the number of pregnancies and surviving offspring in these rats. These effects may be attributable to prolonged sedative activity, resulting in lack of interest in mating and lessened maternal nursing and care of the young. Neonatal survival of rats at doses lower than 100 mg/kg was within normal limits. Several neonates, both controls and experimentals, in these rat reproduction studies showed skeletal or other defects. Further studies in rats at doses up to and including 80 mg/kg day did not reveal significant teratological effects on the offspring. Rabbits were maintained on doses of 1, 2, 5 and 8 mg/kg from day 6 through day 18 of gestation. No adverse effects on reproduction and no teratological changes were noted.

In humans, measurable blood levels of diazepam were obtained in maternal and cord blood, indicating placental transfer of the drug.

INDICATIONS AND USAGE

Diazepam is indicated for the management of anxiety disorders or for the short-term relief of the symptoms of anxiety. Anxiety or tension associated with the stress of everyday life usually does not require treatment with an anxiolytic.

In acute alcohol withdrawal, diazepam may be useful in the symptomatic relief of acute agitation, tremor, impending or acute delirium tremens and hallucinosis.

Diazepam is a useful adjunct for the relief of skeletal muscle spasm due to reflex spasm to local pathology (such as inflammation of the muscles or joints, or secondary to trauma); spasticity caused by upper motor neuron disorders (such as cerebral palsy and paraplegia); athetosis; stiff-man syndrome; and tetanus.

Oral diazepam may be used adjunctively in convulsive disorders, although it has not proved useful as the sole therapy.

The effectiveness of diazepam in long-term use, that is, more than 4 months, has not been assessed by systematic clinical studies. The physician should periodically reassess the usefulness of the drug for the individual patient.

NON-FDA APPROVED INDICATIONS

Diazepam has been used for the treatment of insomnia and nightmares but these uses are not FDA approved.

CONTRAINDICATIONS

Diazepam is contraindicated in patients with a known hypersensitivity to this drug and, because of lack of sufficient clinical experience, in children under 6 months of age. It may be used in patients with open angle glaucoma who are receiving appropriate therapy, but is contraindicated in acute narrow angle glaucoma.

WARNINGS

Diazepam is not of value in the treatment of psychotic patients and should not be employed in lieu of appropriate treatment. As is true of most preparations containing CNS-acting drugs, patients receiving diazepam should be cautioned against engaging in hazardous occupations requiring complete mental alertness such as operating machinery or driving a motor vehicle.

As with other agents which have anticonvulsant activity, when diazepam is used as an adjunct in treating convulsive disorders, the possibility of an increase in the frequency and/or severity of grand mal seizures may require an increase in the dosage of standard anticonvulsant medication. Abrupt withdrawal of diazepam in such cases may also be associated with a temporary increase in the frequency and/or severity of seizures.

Since diazepam has a central nervous system depressant effect, patients should be advised against the simultaneous ingestion of alcohol and other CNS-depressant drugs during diazepam therapy.

USE IN PREGNANCY

An increased risk of congenital malformations associated with the use of minor tranquilizers (diazepam, meprobamate and chlordiazepoxide) during the first trimester of pregnancy has been suggested in several studies. Because use of these drugs is rarely a matter of urgency, their use during this period should almost always be avoided. The possibility that a woman of childbearing potential may become pregnant at the time of institution of therapy should be considered. Patients should be advised that if they become pregnant during therapy or intend to become pregnant they should communicate with their physicians about the desirability of discontinuing the drug.

PRECAUTIONS

If diazepam is to be combined with other psychotropic agents or anticonvulsant drugs, careful consideration should be given to the pharmacology of the agents to be employed—particularly with known compounds which may potentiate the action of diazepam, such as phenothiazines, narcotics, barbiturates, MAO inhibitors and other antidepressants. The usual precautions are indicated for severely depressed patients or those in whom there is any evidence of latent depression; particularly the recognition that suicidal tendencies may be present and protective measures may be necessary. The usual precautions in treating patients with impaired renal or hepatic function should be observed.

In elderly and debilitated patients, it is recommended that the dosage be limited to the smallest effective amount to preclude the development of ataxia or oversedation (2 to 2.5 mg once or twice daily, initially, to be increased gradually as needed and tolerated).

The clearance of diazepam and certain other benzodiazepines can be delayed in association with cimetidine (Tagamet) administration. The clinical significance of this is unclear.

INFORMATION FOR THE PATIENT

To assure the safe and effective use of benzodiazepines, patients should be informed that, since benzodiazepines may produce psychological and physical dependence, it is advisable that they consult with their physician before either increasing the dose or abruptly discontinuing this drug.

ADVERSE REACTIONS

Side effects most commonly reported were drowsiness, fatigue and ataxia. Infrequently encountered were confusion, constipation, depression, diplopia, dysarthria, headache, hypotension, incontinence, jaundice, changes in libido, nausea, changes in salivation, skin rash, slurred speech, tremor, urinary retention, vertigo and blurred vision. Paradoxical reactions such as acute hyperexcited states, anxiety, hallucinations, increased muscle spasticity, insomnia, rage, sleep disturbances and stimulation have been reported; should these occur, use of the drug should be discontinued.

Because of isolated reports of neutropenia and jaundice, periodic blood counts and liver function tests are advisable during long-term therapy. Minor changes in EEG patterns, usually low-voltage fast activity, have been observed in patients during and after diazepam therapy and are of no known significance.

DOSAGE AND ADMINISTRATION

Dosage should be individualized for maximum beneficial effect. While the usual daily dosages shown in TABLE 1 will meet the needs of most patients, there will be some who may require higher doses. In such cases dosage should be increased cautiously to avoid adverse effects.

HOW SUPPLIED

VALIUM

For oral administration, round, scored tablets with a cut "V" design—2 mg, white; 5 mg, yellow; 10 mg, blue.

Imprint on Tablets:

2 mg: "2 VALIUM" (front); "ROCHE" (scored side).
5 mg: "5 VALIUM" (front); "ROCHE" (scored side).
10 mg: "10 VALIUM" (front); "ROCHE" (scored side).

TABLE 1 *Usual Daily Dosage, Diazepam Tablets*

	Usual Daily Dose
Adults:	
Management of Anxiety Disorders and Relief of Symptoms of Anxiety.	Depending upon severity of symptoms—2 -10 mg, 2-4 times daily
Symptomatic Relief in Acute Alcohol Withdrawal.	10 mg, 3 or 4 times during the first 24 hours, reducing to 5 mg, 3 or 4 times daily as needed
Adjunctively for Relief of Skeletal Muscle Spasm.	2 -10 mg, 3 or 4 times daily
Adjunctively in Convulsive Disorders.	2 -10 mg, 2-4 times daily
Geriatric Patients, or in the presence of debilitating disease.	2 to 2.5 mg, 1 or 2 times daily initially; increase gradually as needed and tolerated
Children:	
Because of varied responses to CNS-acting drugs, initiate therapy with lowest dose and increase as required. Not for use in children under 6 months.	1 to 2.5 mg, 3 or 4 times daily initially; increase gradually as needed and tolerated

RECTAL

DESCRIPTION

Diastat rectal delivery system is a non-sterile diazepam gel provided in a prefilled, unit-dose, rectal delivery system. Diastat contains 5 mg/ml diazepam, propylene glycol, ethyl alcohol (10%), hydroxypropyl methylcellulose, sodium benzoate, benzyl alcohol (1.5%), benzoic acid and water. Diastat is clear to slightly yellow and has a pH between 6.5-7.2.

Diazepam is a benzodiazepine anticonvulsant with the chemical name 7-chloro-1,3-dihydro-1-methyl-5-phenyl-2H-1,4-benzodiazepin-2-one.

Storage: Store at controlled room temperature 15-30°C (59-86°F).

CLINICAL PHARMACOLOGY

MECHANISM OF ACTION

Although the precise mechanism by which diazepam exerts its antiseizure effects is unknown, animal and *in vitro* studies suggest that diazepam acts to suppress seizures through an interaction with γ-aminobutyric acid (GABA) receptors of the A-type ($GABA_A$). GABA, the major inhibitory neurotransmitter in the central nervous system, acts at this receptor to open the membrane channel allowing chloride ions to flow into neurons. Entry of chloride ions causes an inhibitory potential that reduces the ability of neurons to depolarize to the threshold potential necessary to produce action potentials. Excessive depolarization of neurons is implicated in the generation and spread of seizures. It is believed that diazepam enhances the actions of GABA by causing GABA to bind more tightly to the $GABA_A$ receptor.

PHARMACOKINETICS

Pharmacokinetic information of diazepam following rectal administration was obtained from studies conducted in healthy adult subjects. No pharmacokinetic studies were conducted in pediatric patients. Therefore, information from the literature is used to define pharmacokinetic labeling in the pediatric population.

Diazepam rectal gel is well absorbed following rectal administration, reaching peak plasma concentrations in 1.5 hours. The absolute bioavailability of diazepam rectal gel relative to diazepam injectable solution is 90%. The volume of distribution of diazepam rectal gel is calculated to be approximately 1 L/kg. The mean elimination half-life of diazepam and desmethyldiazepam following administration of a 15 mg dose of diazepam rectal gel was found to be about 46 hours (CV=43%) and 71 hours (CV=37%), respectively. Both diazepam and its major active metabolite desmethyldiazepam bind extensively to plasma proteins (95-98%).

Metabolism and Elimination

It has been reported in the literature that diazepam is extensively metabolized to one major active metabolite (desmethyldiazepam) and two minor active metabolites, 3-hydroxydiazepam (temazepam) and 3-hydroxy-N-diazepam (oxazepam) in plasma. At therapeutic doses, desmethyldiazepam is found in plasma at concentrations equivalent to those of diazepam while oxazepam and temazepam are not usually detectable. The metabolism of diazepam is primarily hepatic and involves demethylation (involving primarily CYP2C19 and CYP3A4) and 3-hydroxylation (involving primarily CYP3A4), followed by glucuronidation. The marked inter-individual variability in the clearance of diazepam reported in the literature is probably attributable to variability of CYP2CI9 (which is known to exhibit genetic polymorphism; about 3-5% of Caucasians have little or no activity and are "poor metabolizers") and CYP3A4. No inhibition was demonstrated in the presence of inhibitors selective for CYP2A6, CYP2C9, CYP2D6, CYP2EI, or CYP1A2, indicating that these enzymes are not significantly involved in metabolism of diazepam.

SPECIAL POPULATIONS

Hepatic Impairment

No pharmacokinetic studies were conducted with diazepam rectal gel in hepatically impaired subjects. Literature review indicates that following administration of 0.1 to 0.15 mg/kg of diazepam intravenously, the half-life of diazepam was prolonged by 2 to 5-fold in subjects with alcoholic cirrhosis (n=24) compared to age-matched control subjects (n=37) with a corresponding decrease in clearance by half; however, the exact degree of hepatic impairment in these subjects was not characterized in this literature (see PRECAUTIONS).

Renal Impairment

The pharmacokinetics of diazepam have not been studied in renally impaired subjects (see PRECAUTIONS).

Pediatrics

No pharmacokinetic studies were conducted with diazepam rectal gel in the pediatric population. However, literature review indicates that following IV administration (0.33 mg/kg), diazepam has a longer half-life in neonates (birth up to 1 month; approximately 50-95 hours) and infants (1 month up to 2 years; about 40-50 hours), whereas it has a shorter half-life in children (2–12 years; approximately 15-21 hours) and adolescents (12-16 years; about 18-20 hours) (see PRECAUTIONS).

Elderly

A study of single dose IV administration of diazepam (0.1 mg/kg) indicates that the elimination half-life of diazepam increases linearly with age, ranging from about 15 hours at 18 years (healthy young adults) to about 100 hours at 95 years (healthy elderly) with a corresponding decrease in clearance of free diazepam (see PRECAUTIONS and DOSAGE AND ADMINISTRATION).

Effect of Gender, Race, and Cigarette Smoking

No targeted pharmacokinetic studies have been conducted to evaluate the effect of gender, race, and cigarette smoking on the pharmacokinetics of diazepam. However, covariate analysis of a population of treated patients following administration of diazepam rectal gel indicated that neither gender nor cigarette smoking had any effect on the pharmacokinetics of diazepam.

INDICATIONS AND USAGE

Diazepam rectal gel is a gel formulation of diazepam intended for rectal administration in the management of selected, refractory, patients with epilepsy, on stable regimens of AEDs, who require intermittent use of diazepam to control bouts of increased seizure activity.

Evidence to support the use of diazepam rectal gel was adduced in two controlled trials (see CLINICAL PHARMACOLOGY) that enrolled patients with partial onset or generalized convulsive seizures who were identified jointly by their caregivers and physicians as suffering intermittent and periodic episodes of markedly increased seizure activity, sometimes heralded by non-convulsive symptoms, that for the individual patient were characteristic and were deemed by the prescriber to be of a kind for which a benzodiazepine would ordinarily be administered acutely. Although these clusters or bouts of seizures differed among patients, for any individual patient the clusters of seizure activity were not only stereotypic but were judged by those conducting and participating in these studies to be distinguishable from other seizures suffered by that patient. The conclusion that a patient experienced such unique episodes of seizure activity was based on historical information.

NON-FDA APPROVED INDICATIONS

Diazepam has been used for the treatment of insomnia and nightmares but these uses are not FDA approved.

CONTRAINDICATIONS

Diazepam rectal gel is contraindicated in patients with a known hypersensitivity to diazepam. Diazepam rectal gel may be used in patients with open angle glaucoma who are receiving appropriate therapy but is contraindicated in acute narrow angle glaucoma.

WARNINGS

GENERAL

Diazepam rectal gel should only be administered by caregivers who in the opinion of the prescribing physician 1) are able to distinguish the distinct cluster of seizures (and/or the events presumed to herald their onset) from the patient's ordinary seizure activity, 2) have been instructed and judged to be competent to administer the treatment rectally, 3) understand explicitly which seizure manifestations may or may not be treated with diazepam rectal gel, and 4) are able to monitor the clinical response and recognize when that response is such that immediate professional medical evaluation is required.

CNS DEPRESSION

Because diazepam rectal gel produces CNS depression, patients receiving this drug who are otherwise capable and qualified to do so should be cautioned against engaging in hazardous occupations requiring mental alertness, such as operating machinery, driving a motor vehicle, or riding a bicycle until they have completely returned to their level of baseline functioning.

Although diazepam rectal gel is indicated for use solely on an intermittent basis, the potential for a synergistic CNS-depressant effect when used simultaneously with alcohol or other CNS depressants must be considered by the prescribing physician, and appropriate recommendations made to the patient and/or caregiver.

Prolonged CNS depression has been observed in neonates treated with diazepam. Therefore, diazepam rectal gel is not recommended for use in children under 6 months of age.

PREGNANCY RISKS

No clinical studies have been conducted with diazepam rectal gel in pregnant women. Data from several sources raise concerns about the use of diazepam during pregnancy.

General Concerns and Considerations About Anticonvulsants

Reports suggest an association between the use of anticonvulsant drugs by women with epilepsy and an elevated incidence of birth defects in children born to these women. Data are more extensive with respect to phenytoin and phenobarbital, but a smaller number of systematic or anecdotal reports suggest a possible similar association with the use of all known anticonvulsant drugs.

The reports suggesting an elevated incidence of birth defects in children of drug-treated epileptic women cannot be regarded as adequate to prove a definite cause and effect relationship. There are intrinsic methodologic problems in obtaining adequate data on drug teratogenicity in humans; the possibility also exists that other factors (*e.g.*, genetic factors or the epileptic condition itself) may be more important than drug therapy in leading to birth defects. The great majority of mothers on anticonvulsant medication deliver normal infants. It is important to note that anticonvulsant drugs should not be discontinued in patients in whom the drug is administered to prevent seizures because of the strong possibility of precipitating *status epilepticus* with attendant hypoxia and threat to life. In individual cases where the severity and frequency of the seizure disorder are such that the removal of medication does not pose a serious threat to the patient, discontinuation of the drug may be considered prior to and during pregnancy, although it cannot be said with any confidence that even mild seizures do not pose some hazards to the developing embryo or fetus.

General Concerns About Benzodiazepines

An increased risk of congenital malformations associated with the use of benzodiazepine drugs has been suggested in several studies.

There may also be non-teratogenic risks associated with the use of benzodiazepines during pregnancy. There have been reports of neonatal flaccidity, respiratory and feeding difficulties, and hypothermia in children born to mothers who have been receiving benzodiazepines late in pregnancy. In addition, children born to mothers receiving benzodiazepines on a regular basis late in pregnancy may be at some risk of experiencing withdrawal symptoms during the postnatal period.

Advice Regarding the Use of Diazepam Rectal Gel in Women of Childbearing Potential

In general, the use of diazepam rectal gel in women of childbearing potential, and more specifically during known pregnancy, should be considered only when the clinical situation warrants the risk to the fetus.

The specific considerations addressed above regarding the use of anticonvulsants in epileptic women of childbearing potential should be weighed in treating or counseling these women.

Because of experience with other members of the benzodiazepine class, diazepam rectal gel is assumed to be capable of causing an increased risk of congenital abnormalities when administered to a pregnant woman during the first trimester. The possibility that a woman of childbearing potential may be pregnant at the time of institution of therapy should be considered. If this drug is used during pregnancy, or if the patient becomes pregnant while taking this drug, the patient should be apprised of the potential hazard to the fetus. Patients should also be advised that if they become pregnant during therapy or intend to become pregnant they should communicate with their physician about the desirability of discontinuing the drug.

WITHDRAWAL SYMPTOMS

Withdrawal symptoms of the barbiturate type have occurred after the discontinuation of regular use of benzodiazepines.

CHRONIC USE

Diazepam rectal gel is not recommended for chronic, daily use as an anticonvulsant because of the potential for development of tolerance to diazepam. Chronic daily use of diazepam may increase the frequency and/or severity of tonic clonic seizures, requiring an increase in the dosage of standard anticonvulsant medication. In such cases, abrupt withdrawal of chronic diazepam may also be associated with a temporary increase in the frequency and/or severity of seizures.

USE IN PATIENTS WITH PETIT MAL STATUS

Tonic *status epilepticus* has been precipitated in patients treated with IV diazepam for petit mal status or petit mal variant status.

PRECAUTIONS

CAUTION IN RENALLY IMPAIRED PATIENTS

Metabolites of diazepam rectal gel are excreted by the kidneys; to avoid their excess accumulation, caution should be exercised in the administration of the drug to patients with impaired renal function.

CAUTION IN HEPATICALLY IMPAIRED PATIENTS

Concomitant liver disease is known to decrease the clearance of diazepam (see CLINICAL PHARMACOLOGY, Special Populations, Hepatic Impairment). Therefore, diazepam rectal gel should be used with caution in patients with liver disease.

PEDIATRIC USE

The controlled trials demonstrating the effectiveness of diazepam rectal gel included children 2 years of age and older. Clinical studies have not been conducted to establish the efficacy and safety of diazepam rectal gel in children under 2 years of age.

USE IN PATIENTS WITH COMPROMISED RESPIRATORY FUNCTION

Diazepam rectal gel should be used with caution in patients with compromised respiratory function related to a concurrent disease process (*e.g.*, asthma, pneumonia) or neurologic damage.

GERIATRIC USE

In elderly patients diazepam rectal gel should be used with caution due to an increase in half-life with a corresponding decrease in the clearance of free diazepam. It is also recommended that the dosage be decreased to reduce the likelihood of ataxia or oversedation.

INFORMATION TO BE COMMUNIATED BY THE PRESCRIBER TO THE CAREGIVER

Prescribers are strongly advised to take all reasonable steps to ensure that caregivers fully understand their role and obligations vis a vis the administration of diazepam rectal gel to individuals in their care. Prescribers should routinely discuss the steps involved. The successful and safe use of diazepam rectal gel depends in large measure on the competence and performance of the caregiver.

Prescribers should advise caregivers that they expect to be informed immediately if a patient develops any new findings which are not typical of the patient's characteristic seizure episode.

INTERFERENCE WITH COGNITIVE AND MOTOR PERFORMANCE

Because benzodiazepines have the potential to impair judgment, thinking, or motor skills, patients should be cautioned about operating hazardous machinery, including automobiles, until they are reasonably certain that diazepam rectal gel therapy does not affect them adversely.

PREGNANCY CATEGORY D

Patients should be advised to notify their physician if they become pregnant or intend to become pregnant during therapy with diazepam rectal gel (see WARNINGS).

LABOR AND DELIVERY

In humans, measurable amounts of diazepam have been found in maternal and cord blood, indicating placental transfer of the drug. Until additional information is available, diazepam rectal gel is not recommended for obstetrical use.

NURSING MOTHERS

Because diazepam and its metabolites may be present in human breast milk for prolonged periods of time after acute use of diazepam rectal gel, patients should be advised not to breast-feed for an appropriate period of time after receiving treatment with diazepam rectal gel.

CONCOMITANT MEDICATION

Although diazepam rectal gel is indicated for use solely on an intermittent basis, the potential for a synergistic CNS-depressant effect when used simultaneously with alcohol or other CNS-depressants must be considered by the prescribing physician, and appropriate recommendations made to the patient and/or caregiver.

CARCINOGENESIS, MUTAGENESIS, AND IMPAIRMENT OF FERTILITY

The carcinogenic potential of rectal diazepam has not been evaluated. In studies in which mice and rats were administered diazepam in the diet at a dose of 75 mg/kg/day (approximately 6 and 12 times, respectively, the maximum recommended human dose [MRHD=1 mg/kg/day] on a mg/m^2 basis) for 80 and 104 weeks, respectively, an increased incidence of liver tumors was observed in males of both species.

The data currently available are inadequate to determine the mutagenic potential of diazepam.

Reproduction studies in rats showed decreases in the number of pregnancies and in the number of surviving offspring following administration of an oral dose of 100 mg/kg/day (approximately 16 times the MRHD on a mg/m^2 basis) prior to and during mating and throughout gestation and lactation. No adverse effects on fertility or offspring viability were noted at a dose of 80 mg/kg/day (approximately 13 times the MRHD on a mg/m^2 basis).

DRUG INTERACTIONS

If diazepam is to be combined with other psychotropic agents or other CNS depressants, careful consideration should be given to the pharmacology of the agents to be employed—particularly with known compounds which may potentiate the action of diazepam, such as phenothiazines, narcotics, barbiturates, MAO inhibitors and other antidepressants.

The clearance of diazepam and certain other benzodiazepines can be delayed in association with cimetidine administration. The clinical significance of this is unclear.

Valproate may potentiate the CNS-depressant effects of diazepam.

There have been no clinical studies or reports in literature to evaluate the interaction of rectally administered diazepam with other drugs. As with all drugs, the potential for interaction by a variety of mechanisms is a possibility.

EFFECT OF OTHER DRUGS ON DIAZEPAM METABOLISM

In vitro studies using human liver preparations suggest that CYP2CI9 and CYP3A4 are the principal isozymes involved in the initial oxidative metabolism of diazepam. Therefore, potential interactions may occur when diazepam is given concurrently with agents that affect CYP2CI9 and CYP3A4 activity. Potential inhibitors of CYP2CI9 (*e.g.*, cimetidine, quinidine, and tranylcypromine) and CYP3A4 (*e.g.*, ketoconazole, troleandomycin, and clotrimazole) could decrease the rate of diazepam elimination, while inducers of CYP2CI9 (*e.g.*, rifampin) and CYP3A4 (*e.g.*, carbamazepine, phenytoin, dexamethasone and phenobarbital) could increase the rate of elimination of diazepam.

EFFECT OF DIAZEPAM ON THE METABOLISM OF OTHER DRUGS

There are no reports as to which isozymes could be inhibited or induced by diazepam. But, based on the fact that diazepam is a substrate for CYP2CI9 and CYP3A4, it is possible that diazepam may interfere with the metabolism of drugs which are substrates for CYP2CI9, (*e.g.*, omeprazole, propranolol, and imipramine) and CYP3A4 (*e.g.*, cyclosporine, paclitaxel, terfenadine, theophylline, and warfarin) leading to a potential drug-drug interaction.

ADVERSE REACTIONS

Diazepam rectal gel adverse event data were collected from double-blind, placebo-controlled studies and open-label studies. The majority of adverse events were mild to moderate in severity and transient in nature.

Two (2) patients who received diazepam rectal gel died 7–15 weeks following treatment; neither of these deaths were deemed related to diazepam rectal gel.

The most frequent adverse event reported to be related to diazepam rectal gel in the two double-blind, placebo-controlled studies was somnolence (23%). Less frequent adverse events were dizziness, headache, pain, abdominal pain, nervousness, vasodilatation, diarrhea, ataxia, euphoria, incoordination, asthma, rhinitis, and rash, which occurred in approximately 2-5% of patients.

Approximately 1.4% of the 573 patients who received diazepam rectal gel in clinical trials of epilepsy discontinued treatment because of an adverse event. The adverse event most frequently associated with discontinuation (occurring in 3 patients) was somnolence. Other adverse events most commonly associated with discontinuation and occurring in 2 patients were hypoventilation and rash. Adverse events occurring in 1 patient were asthenia, hyperkinesia, incoordination, vasodilitation and urticaria. These events were judged to be related to diazepam rectal gel.

In the two domestic double-blind, placebo-controlled, parallel-group studies, the proportion of patients who discontinued treatment because of adverse events was 2% for the group treated with diazepam rectal gel, versus 2% for the placebo group. In the diazepam rectal gel group, the adverse events considered the primary reason for discontinuation were different in the 2 patients who discontinued treatment; 1 discontinued due to rash and 1 discontinued due to lethargy. The primary reason for discontinuation in the patients treated with placebo was lack of effect.

ADVERSE EVENT INCIDENCE IN CONTROLLED CLINICAL TRIALS

TABLE 1 lists treatment-emergent signs and symptoms that occurred in > 1% of patients enrolled in parallel-group, placebo-controlled trials and were numerically more common in the diazepam rectal gel group. Adverse events were usually mild or moderate in intensity.

The prescriber should be aware that these figures, obtained when diazepam rectal gel was added to concurrent antiepileptic drug therapy, cannot be used to predict the frequency of adverse events in the course of usual medical practice when patient characteristics and other factors may differ from those prevailing during clinical studies. Similarly, the cited frequencies cannot be directly compared with figures obtained from other clinical investigations involving different treatments, uses, or investigators. An inspection of these frequencies, however, does provide the prescribing physician with one basis to estimate the relative contribution of drug and non-drug factors to the adverse event incidences in the population studied.

TABLE 1 *Treatment-Emergent Signs and Symptoms That Occurred in >1% of Patients Enrolled in Parallel-Group, Placebo-Controlled Trials and Were Numerically More Common in the Diazepam Rectal Gel Group*

Body System COSTART Term	Diazepam n=101 %	Placebo n=104 %
Body as a Whole		
Headache	5%	4%
Cardiovascular		
Vasodilatation	2%	0%
Digestive		
Diarrhea	4%	<1%
Nervous		
Ataxia	3%	<1%
Dizziness	3%	2%
Euphoria	3%	0%
Incoordination	3%	0%
Somnolence	23%	8%
Respiratory		
Asthma	2%	0%
Skin and Appendages		
Rash	3%	0%

Other events reported by 1% or more of patients treated in controlled trials but equally or more frequent in the placebo group than in the diazepam rectal gel group were abdominal pain, pain, nervousness, and rhinitis. Other events reported by fewer than 1% of patients were infection, anorexia, vomiting, anemia, lymphadenopathy, grand mal convulsion, hyperkinesia, cough increased, pruritus, sweating, mydriasis, and urinary tract infection.

The pattern of adverse events was similar for different age, race and gender groups.

OTHER ADVERSE EVENTS OBSERVED DURING ALL CLINICAL TRIALS

Diazepam rectal gel has been administered to 573 patients with epilepsy during all clinical trials, only some of which were placebo-controlled. During these trials, all adverse events were recorded by the clinical investigators using terminology of their own choosing. To provide a meaningful estimate of the proportion of individuals having adverse events, similar types of events were grouped into a smaller number of standardized categories using modified COSTART dictionary terminology. These categories are used in the listing below. All of the events listed below occurred in at least 1% of the 573 individuals exposed to diazepam rectal gel. All reported events are included except those already listed above, events unlikely to be drug-related, and those too general to be informative. Events are included without regard to determination of a causal relationship to diazepam.

Body as a Whole: Asthenia.

Cardiovascular: Hypotension, vasodilation.

Nervous: Agitation, confusion, convulsion, dysarthria, emotional lability, speech disorder, thinking abnormal, vertigo.

Respiratory: Hiccup.

The following infrequent adverse events were not seen with diazepam rectal gel but have been reported previously with diazepam use: depression, slurred speech, syncope, constipation, changes in libido, urinary retention, bradycardia, cardiovascular collapse, nystagmus, urticaria, neutropenia and jaundice.

Paradoxical reactions such as acute hyperexcited states, anxiety, hallucinations, increased muscle spasticity, insomnia, rage, sleep disturbances and stimulation have been reported with diazepam; should these occur, use of diazepam rectal gel should be discontinued.

DOSAGE AND ADMINISTRATION

This section is intended primarily for the prescriber, however, the prescriber should also be aware of the dosing information and directions for use provided in the patient package insert.

A decision to prescribe diazepam rectal gel involves more than the diagnosis and the selection of the correct dose for the patient.

First, the prescriber must be convinced from historical reports and/or personal observations that the patient exhibits the characteristic identifiable seizure cluster that can be distinguished from the patient's usual seizure activity by the caregiver who will be responsible for administering diazepam rectal gel.

Second, because diazepam rectal gel is only intended for adjunctive use, the prescriber must ensure that the patient is receiving an optimal regimen of standard anti-epileptic drug treatment and is, nevertheless, continuing to experience these characteristic episodes.

Third, because a non-health professional will be obliged to identify episodes suitable for treatment, make the decision to administer treatment upon that identification, administer the drug, monitor the patient, and assess the adequacy of the response to treatment, a major component of the prescribing process involves the necessary instruction of this individual.

Fourth, the prescriber and caregiver must have a common understanding of what is and is not an episode of seizures that is appropriate for treatment, the timing of administration in relation to the onset of the episode, the mechanics of administering the drug, how and what to observe following administration, and what would constitute an outcome requiring immediate and direct medical attention.

D

CALCULATING PRESCRIBED DOSE

The diazepam rectal gel dose should be individualized for maximum beneficial effect. The recommended dose of diazepam rectal gel is 0.2-0.5 mg/kg depending on age. See TABLE 2 for specific recommendations.

TABLE 2 *Recommended Dosage by Age, Rectal Delivery System*

Age (years)	Recommended Dose
2 through 5	0.5 mg/kg
6 through 11	0.3 mg/kg
12 and older	0.2 mg/kg

Because diazepam rectal gel is provided in fixed, unit-doses of 5, 10, 15 and 20 mg, the prescribed dose is obtained by rounding upward to the next available dose. TABLE 3 provides acceptable weight ranges for each dose and age category, such that patients will receive between 90% and 180% of the calculated recommended dose. The safety of this strategy has been established in clinical trials.

TABLE 3 *Weight Ranges for Dosage and Age, Rectal Delivery System*

2 - 5 Years		6 - 11 Years		12+ Years	
0.5 mg/kg		0.3 mg/kg		0.2 mg/kg	
Weight	Dose	Weight	Dose	Weight	Dose
6-11 kg	5 mg	10-18 kg	5 mg	14-27 kg	5 mg
12-22 kg	10 mg	19-37 kg	10 mg	28-50 kg	10 mg
23-33 kg	15 mg	38-55 kg	15 mg	51-75 kg	15 mg
34-44 kg	20 mg	56-74 kg	20 mg	76-111 kg	20 mg

The rectal delivery system includes a plastic applicator with a flexible, molded tip available in two lengths, designated for convenience as Pediatric and Adult. The 2.5, 5.0, and 10.0 mg dosages are available with a 4.4 cm Pediatric tip. The 10.0, 15.0, and 20.0 mg dosages are available with a 6.0 cm Adult tip.

It is important to note that if a 15 mg dose is to be administered to a pediatric patient utilizing the plastic applicator with a pediatric tip, prescriptions must be written for 2 different twin packs, one for the 5 mg dosage and one for the 10 mg dosage.

In elderly and debilitated patients, it is recommended that the dosage be adjusted downward to reduce the likelihood of ataxia or oversedation.

The prescribed dose of diazepam rectal gel should be adjusted by the physician periodically to reflect changes in the patient's age or weight. It is recommended that dosage be reviewed at 6 month intervals.

A 2.5 mg dose is available for use as a supplemental dose. This dose may be prescribed at the discretion of the physician for patients who require more precise dose titration than is achieved using 1 of the 4 standard doses provided. The 2.5 mg dose may also be used as a partial replacement dose for patients who may expel a portion of the first dose.

ADDITIONAL DOSE

The prescriber may wish to prescribe a second dose of diazepam rectal gel. A second dose, when required, may be given 4-12 hours after the first dose.

TREATMENT FREQUENCY

It is recommended that diazepam rectal gel be used to treat no more than five episodes per month and no more than one episode every 5 days.

ANIMAL PHARMACOLOGY

Diazepam has been shown to be teratogenic in mice and hamsters when given orally at single doses of 100 mg/kg or greater (approximately 8 times the maximum recommended human dose [MRHD=1 mg/kg/day] or greater on a mg/m^2 basis). Cleft palate and exencephaly are the most common and consistently reported malformations produced in these species by administration of high, maternally-toxic doses of diazepam during organogenesis. Rodent studies have indicated that prenatal exposure to diazepam doses similar to those used clinically can produce long-term changes in cellular immune responses, brain neurochemistry, and behavior.

PRODUCT LISTING - RATED THERAPEUTICALLY EQUIVALENT

Solution - Injectable - 5 mg/ml

Size	Price	Product	NDC
1 ml x 25	$17.00	GENERIC, Baxter Pharmaceutical Products, Inc	10019-0004-44
2 ml x 10	$6.30	GENERIC, Baxter Pharmaceutical Products, Inc	10019-0005-67
2 ml x 10	$14.37	GENERIC, Abbott Pharmaceutical	00074-1273-12
2 ml x 10	$18.88	GENERIC, Abbott Pharmaceutical	00074-3210-32
2 ml x 10	$19.36	GENERIC, Abbott Pharmaceutical	00074-1273-02
2 ml x 10	$23.34	GENERIC, Sanofi Winthrop Pharmaceuticals	00024-0376-02
2 ml x 10	$25.40	GENERIC, Abbott Pharmaceutical	00074-1273-32
2 ml x 10	$25.90	GENERIC, Esi Lederle Generics	00641-1408-33
2 ml x 10	$26.13	GENERIC, Abbott Pharmaceutical	00074-1273-22
2 ml x 10	$43.50	VALIUM, Roche Laboratories	00140-1931-06
2 ml x 10	$64.03	VALIUM, Roche Laboratories	00140-1933-06
2 ml x 10	$76.30	VALIUM, Roche Laboratories	00004-1933-06
2 ml x 25	$64.00	GENERIC, Esi Lederle Generics	00641-1408-35
2 ml x 25	$70.25	GENERIC, Esi Lederle Generics	00641-0371-25
2 ml x 25	$90.00	GENERIC, Watson/Schein Pharmaceuticals Inc	00364-0825-48
2 ml x 50	$87.60	GENERIC, Abbott Pharmaceutical	00074-3210-01
10 ml	$7.88	GENERIC, Interstate Drug Exchange Inc	00814-2399-40
10 ml	$8.09	GENERIC, Moore, H.L. Drug Exchange Inc	00839-7190-30
10 ml	$9.50	GENERIC, Roberts/Hauck Pharmaceutical Corporation	43797-0014-12
10 ml	$10.00	GENERIC, Dunhall Pharmaceuticals Inc	00217-6805-08
10 ml	$11.88	GENERIC, Esi Lederle Generics	00641-2289-41
10 ml	$18.10	GENERIC, Mutual/United Research Laboratories	00677-1088-21
10 ml	$21.41	VALIUM, Roche Laboratories	00140-1932-06
10 ml	$26.56	VALIUM, Roche Laboratories	00004-1932-09
10 ml x 5	$9.74	GENERIC, Abbott Pharmaceutical	00074-3213-02
10 ml x 25	$175.50	GENERIC, Abbott Pharmaceutical	00074-3213-01

Tablet - Oral - 2 mg

Size	Price	Product	NDC
3's	$3.44	GENERIC, Prescript Pharmaceuticals	00247-0939-03
6's	$3.52	GENERIC, Prescript Pharmaceuticals	00247-0939-06
15's	$3.75	GENERIC, Prescript Pharmaceuticals	00247-0939-15
20's	$14.59	GENERIC, Pd-Rx Pharmaceuticals	55289-0979-20
30's	$4.15	GENERIC, Prescript Pharmaceuticals	00247-0939-30
30's	$16.14	GENERIC, Pd-Rx Pharmaceuticals	55289-0979-30
100's	$3.00	GENERIC, Interstate Drug Exchange Inc	00814-2395-14
100's	$4.23	FEDERAL UPPER LIMIT, H.C.F.A. F F P	99999-1033-02
100's	$4.95	GENERIC, Major Pharmaceuticals Inc	00904-3903-60
100's	$8.51	GENERIC, Moore, H.L. Drug Exchange Inc	00839-7131-06
100's	$8.99	GENERIC, Geneva Pharmaceuticals	00781-1482-01
100's	$10.03	GENERIC, Aligen Independent Laboratories Inc	00405-0068-01
100's	$10.45	GENERIC, Mylan Pharmaceuticals Inc	00378-0271-01
100's	$10.65	GENERIC, Purepac Pharmaceutical Company	00228-2051-10
100's	$12.50	GENERIC, Ivax Corporation	00172-3925-60
100's	$14.04	GENERIC, Watson/Schein Pharmaceuticals Inc	00364-0774-01
100's	$14.04	GENERIC, Watson/Schein Pharmaceuticals Inc	00591-5621-01
100's	$14.70	GENERIC, Auro Pharmaceutical	55829-0831-10
100's	$24.21	GENERIC, Udl Laboratories Inc	51079-0284-20
100's	$24.21	GENERIC, Udl Laboratories Inc	51079-0284-21
100's	$25.25	GENERIC, Geneva Pharmaceuticals	00781-1482-13
100's	$40.04	VALIUM, Roche Laboratories	00140-0004-49
100's	$44.42	VALIUM, Roche Laboratories	00140-0004-50
100's	$70.86	VALIUM, Roche Laboratories	00140-0004-01

Tablet - Oral - 5 mg

Size	Price	Product	NDC
6's	$12.56	GENERIC, Pd-Rx Pharmaceuticals	55289-0091-06
9's	$12.99	GENERIC, Pd-Rx Pharmaceuticals	55289-0091-09
10's	$13.14	GENERIC, Pd-Rx Pharmaceuticals	55289-0091-10
15's	$13.88	GENERIC, Pd-Rx Pharmaceuticals	55289-0091-15
20's	$13.50	VALIUM, Allscripts Pharmaceutical Company	54569-0948-00
21's	$14.74	GENERIC, Pd-Rx Pharmaceuticals	55289-0091-21
25's	$1.93	GENERIC, Circle Pharmaceuticals Inc	00659-3029-25
25's	$14.89	GENERIC, Pd-Rx Pharmaceuticals	55289-0091-97
30's	$10.65	GENERIC, Heartland Healthcare Services	61392-0721-30
30's	$10.65	GENERIC, Heartland Healthcare Services	61392-0721-39
30's	$16.05	GENERIC, Pd-Rx Pharmaceuticals	55289-0091-30
31's	$11.01	GENERIC, Heartland Healthcare Services	61392-0721-31
32's	$11.36	GENERIC, Heartland Healthcare Services	61392-0721-32
45's	$15.98	GENERIC, Heartland Healthcare Services	61392-0721-45
60's	$20.42	GENERIC, Pd-Rx Pharmaceuticals	55289-0091-60
60's	$21.30	GENERIC, Heartland Healthcare Services	61392-0721-60
90's	$24.89	GENERIC, Pd-Rx Pharmaceuticals	55289-0091-90
90's	$31.95	GENERIC, Heartland Healthcare Services	61392-0721-90
100's	$3.38	GENERIC, Interstate Drug Exchange Inc	00814-2396-14
100's	$6.85	GENERIC, Major Pharmaceuticals Inc	00904-3901-60
100's	$7.18	FEDERAL UPPER LIMIT, H.C.F.A. F F P	99999-1033-06
100's	$10.73	GENERIC, Moore, H.L. Drug Exchange Inc	00839-7132-06
100's	$12.95	GENERIC, Geneva Pharmaceuticals	00781-1483-01
100's	$16.35	GENERIC, Mylan Pharmaceuticals Inc	00378-0345-01
100's	$16.65	GENERIC, Purepac Pharmaceutical Company	00228-2052-10
100's	$16.65	GENERIC, Barr Laboratories Inc	00555-0363-02
100's	$16.68	GENERIC, Warner Chilcott Laboratories	00047-0326-24
100's	$16.72	GENERIC, Aligen Independent Laboratories Inc	00405-0069-01
100's	$19.12	GENERIC, Esi Lederle Generics	00005-3129-23
100's	$19.95	GENERIC, Ivax Corporation	00172-3926-60
100's	$21.73	GENERIC, Auro Pharmaceutical	55829-0832-10
100's	$22.01	GENERIC, Watson/Schein Pharmaceuticals Inc	00364-0775-01
100's	$22.01	GENERIC, Watson/Schein Pharmaceuticals Inc	00591-5619-01
100's	$22.87	GENERIC, Major Pharmaceuticals Inc	00904-3901-61

Qty	Price	Product	NDC
100's	$32.14	GENERIC, Udl Laboratories Inc	51079-0285-20
100's	$32.14	GENERIC, Udl Laboratories Inc	51079-0285-21
100's	$33.48	GENERIC, Geneva Pharmaceuticals	00781-1483-13
100's	$61.10	VALIUM, Roche Laboratories	00140-0005-49
100's	$67.48	VALIUM, Roche Laboratories	00140-0005-50
100's	$110.21	VALIUM, Roche Laboratories	00140-0005-01
Tablet - Oral - 10 mg			
2's	$3.41	GENERIC, Prescript Pharmaceuticals	00247-0493-02
3's	$3.44	GENERIC, Prescript Pharmaceuticals	00247-0493-03
6's	$3.52	GENERIC, Prescript Pharmaceuticals	00247-0493-06
6's	$12.68	GENERIC, Pd-Rx Pharmaceuticals	55289-0092-06
7's	$3.54	GENERIC, Prescript Pharmaceuticals	00247-0493-07
10's	$3.62	GENERIC, Prescript Pharmaceuticals	00247-0493-10
12's	$3.67	GENERIC, Prescript Pharmaceuticals	00247-0493-12
14's	$3.73	GENERIC, Prescript Pharmaceuticals	00247-0493-14
20's	$3.88	GENERIC, Prescript Pharmaceuticals	00247-0493-20
20's	$15.01	GENERIC, Pd-Rx Pharmaceuticals	55289-0092-20
25's	$15.83	GENERIC, Pd-Rx Pharmaceuticals	55289-0092-25
30's	$4.15	GENERIC, Prescript Pharmaceuticals	00247-0493-30
30's	$16.68	GENERIC, Pd-Rx Pharmaceuticals	55289-0092-30
30's	$234.00	GENERIC, Medirex Inc	57480-0517-06
60's	$21.74	GENERIC, Pd-Rx Pharmaceuticals	55289-0092-60
90's	$26.64	GENERIC, Pd-Rx Pharmaceuticals	55289-0092-90
100's	$3.75	GENERIC, Interstate Drug Exchange Inc	00814-2397-14
100's	$6.00	GENERIC, Prescript Pharmaceuticals	00247-0493-00
100's	$11.50	GENERIC, Major Pharmaceuticals Inc	00904-3902-60
100's	$14.17	FEDERAL UPPER LIMIT, H.C.F.A. F F P	99999-1033-10
100's	$17.62	GENERIC, Aligen Independent Laboratories Inc	00405-0070-01
100's	$19.71	GENERIC, Moore, H.L. Drug Exchange Inc	00839-7133-06
100's	$19.75	GENERIC, Ivax Corporation	00182-1757-01
100's	$19.99	GENERIC, Geneva Pharmaceuticals	00781-1484-01
100's	$25.25	GENERIC, Esi Lederle Generics	00005-3130-23
100's	$25.41	GENERIC, Major Pharmaceuticals Inc	00904-3902-61
100's	$31.25	GENERIC, Mylan Pharmaceuticals Inc	00378-0477-01
100's	$31.85	GENERIC, Purepac Pharmaceutical Company	00228-2053-10
100's	$31.85	GENERIC, Barr Laboratories Inc	00555-0164-02
100's	$33.00	GENERIC, Ivax Corporation	00172-3927-60
100's	$35.61	GENERIC, Auro Pharmaceutical	55829-0833-10
100's	$38.03	GENERIC, Udl Laboratories Inc	51079-0286-21
100's	$42.19	GENERIC, Watson/Schein Pharmaceuticals Inc	00364-0776-01
100's	$42.19	GENERIC, Watson/Schein Pharmaceuticals Inc	00591-5620-01
100's	$42.50	GENERIC, Udl Laboratories Inc	51079-0286-20
100's	$44.29	GENERIC, Ivax Corporation	00182-1757-89
100's	$44.29	GENERIC, Geneva Pharmaceuticals	00781-1484-13
100's	$101.52	VALIUM, Roche Laboratories	00140-0006-49
100's	$111.77	VALIUM, Roche Laboratories	00140-0006-50
100's	$185.54	VALIUM, Roche Laboratories	00140-0006-01
120's	$11.48	GENERIC, Pd-Rx Pharmaceuticals	55289-0092-98

PRODUCT LISTING - EQUIVALENTS NOT AVAILABLE

Qty	Price	Product	NDC
Concentrate - Oral - 5 mg/ml			
30 ml	$23.52	GENERIC, Roxane Laboratories Inc	00054-3185-44
Gel - Rectal - 5 mg/ml			
0.50 ml x 2	$211.70	DIASTAT PEDIATRIC, Elan Pharmaceuticals	59075-0650-20
0.50 ml x 2	$211.70	DIASTAT PEDIATRIC, Xcel Pharmaceuticals Inc	66490-0650-20
1 ml x 2	$211.70	DIASTAT PEDIATRIC, Elan Pharmaceuticals	59075-0651-20
1 ml x 2	$211.70	DIASTAT PEDIATRIC, Xcel Pharmaceuticals Inc	66490-0651-20
2 ml x 2	$156.00	DIASTAT, Elan Pharmaceuticals	59075-0653-20
2 ml x 2	$211.70	DIASTAT, Xcel Pharmaceuticals Inc	59075-0652-20
2 ml x 2	$211.70	DIASTAT, Xcel Pharmaceuticals Inc	66490-0652-20
3 ml x 2	$211.70	DIASTAT, Elan Pharmaceuticals	59075-0654-20
3 ml x 2	$211.70	DIASTAT, Xcel Pharmaceuticals Inc	66490-0654-20
4 ml x 2	$199.71	DIASTAT, Elan Pharmaceuticals	59075-0655-20
4 ml x 2	$211.70	DIASTAT, Xcel Pharmaceuticals Inc	66490-0655-20
Solution - Injectable - 5 mg/ml			
1 ml x 25	$99.18	GENERIC, Physicians Total Care	54868-4061-00
2 ml	$7.08	GENERIC, Physicians Total Care	54868-2320-02
2 ml	$7.35	GENERIC, Prescript Pharmaceuticals	00247-0294-02
2 ml x 10	$25.88	GENERIC, Allscripts Pharmaceutical Company	54569-2775-00
2 ml x 10	$41.62	GENERIC, Physicians Total Care	54868-4586-00
2 ml x 10	$43.06	GENERIC, Physicians Total Care	54868-2320-01
2 ml x 50	$70.31	GENERIC, Allscripts Pharmaceutical Company	54569-4167-00
10 ml	$11.88	GENERIC, Allscripts Pharmaceutical Company	54569-1413-00
10 ml	$24.26	GENERIC, Physicians Total Care	54868-0617-00
20 ml	$43.39	GENERIC, Prescript Pharmaceuticals	00247-0294-20
Solution - Oral - 5 mg/5 ml			
5 ml x 40	$74.40	GENERIC, Roxane Laboratories Inc	00054-8207-16
10 ml x 40	$104.00	GENERIC, Roxane Laboratories Inc	00054-8208-16
500 ml	$42.67	GENERIC, Roxane Laboratories Inc	00054-3188-63
Tablet - Oral - 2 mg			
12's	$13.66	GENERIC, Southwood Pharmaceuticals Inc	58016-0274-12
20's	$2.06	GENERIC, Allscripts Pharmaceutical Company	54569-0947-03
20's	$6.63	GENERIC, Southwood Pharmaceuticals Inc	58016-0274-20
30's	$3.08	DIAZEPAM, Allscripts Pharmaceutical Company	54569-0947-00
30's	$4.18	GENERIC, Physicians Total Care	54868-2126-04
30's	$9.95	GENERIC, Southwood Pharmaceuticals Inc	58016-0274-30
50's	$6.15	GENERIC, Physicians Total Care	54868-2126-01
50's	$21.00	GENERIC, Pharma Pac	52959-0295-50
100's	$9.81	GENERIC, Physicians Total Care	54868-2126-02
200's	$17.12	GENERIC, Physicians Total Care	54868-2126-03
Tablet - Oral - 5 mg			
2's	$0.33	GENERIC, Allscripts Pharmaceutical Company	54569-4764-00
2's	$3.41	GENERIC, Prescript Pharmaceuticals	00247-0187-02
3's	$3.44	GENERIC, Prescript Pharmaceuticals	00247-0187-03
3's	$4.71	GENERIC, Pharma Pac	52959-0047-03
4's	$2.70	GENERIC, Southwood Pharmaceuticals Inc	58016-0275-04
4's	$3.46	GENERIC, Prescript Pharmaceuticals	00247-0187-04
5's	$7.15	GENERIC, Pharma Pac	52959-0047-05
6's	$1.00	GENERIC, Allscripts Pharmaceutical Company	54569-0949-07
6's	$2.95	GENERIC, Physicians Total Care	54868-0059-08
6's	$3.52	GENERIC, Prescript Pharmaceuticals	00247-0187-06
6's	$4.05	GENERIC, Southwood Pharmaceuticals Inc	58016-0275-06
6's	$7.25	GENERIC, Pharma Pac	52959-0047-06
7's	$3.54	GENERIC, Prescript Pharmaceuticals	00247-0187-07
8's	$5.40	GENERIC, Southwood Pharmaceuticals Inc	58016-0275-08
10's	$1.67	GENERIC, Allscripts Pharmaceutical Company	54569-0949-04
10's	$3.26	GENERIC, Physicians Total Care	54868-0059-06
10's	$3.62	GENERIC, Prescript Pharmaceuticals	00247-0187-10
10's	$6.76	GENERIC, Southwood Pharmaceuticals Inc	58016-0275-10
10's	$7.39	GENERIC, Pharma Pac	52959-0047-10
12's	$3.67	GENERIC, Prescript Pharmaceuticals	00247-0187-12
12's	$8.52	GENERIC, Pharma Pac	52959-0047-12
14's	$3.73	GENERIC, Prescript Pharmaceuticals	00247-0187-14
14's	$9.46	GENERIC, Southwood Pharmaceuticals Inc	58016-0275-14
15's	$2.50	GENERIC, Allscripts Pharmaceutical Company	54569-0949-00
15's	$3.64	GENERIC, Physicians Total Care	54868-0059-09
15's	$3.75	GENERIC, Prescript Pharmaceuticals	00247-0187-15
15's	$10.13	GENERIC, Southwood Pharmaceuticals Inc	58016-0275-15
15's	$10.46	GENERIC, Pharma Pac	52959-0047-15
16's	$10.81	GENERIC, Southwood Pharmaceuticals Inc	58016-0275-16
18's	$12.16	GENERIC, Southwood Pharmaceuticals Inc	58016-0275-18
20's	$3.33	GENERIC, Allscripts Pharmaceutical Company	54569-0949-01
20's	$3.88	GENERIC, Prescript Pharmaceuticals	00247-0187-20
20's	$4.00	GENERIC, Physicians Total Care	54868-0059-01
20's	$13.51	GENERIC, Southwood Pharmaceuticals Inc	58016-0275-20
20's	$13.78	GENERIC, Pharma Pac	52959-0047-20
21's	$3.91	GENERIC, Prescript Pharmaceuticals	00247-0187-21
21's	$14.07	GENERIC, Pharma Pac	52959-0047-21
21's	$14.19	GENERIC, Southwood Pharmaceuticals Inc	58016-0275-21
24's	$16.21	GENERIC, Southwood Pharmaceuticals Inc	58016-0275-24
28's	$4.09	GENERIC, Prescript Pharmaceuticals	00247-0187-28
28's	$18.91	GENERIC, Southwood Pharmaceuticals Inc	58016-0275-28
30's	$4.15	GENERIC, Prescript Pharmaceuticals	00247-0187-30
30's	$4.42	GENERIC, Pharmaceutical Corporation Of America	51655-0801-24
30's	$4.73	GENERIC, Physicians Total Care	54868-0059-02
30's	$5.00	GENERIC, Allscripts Pharmaceutical Company	54569-0949-02
30's	$19.40	GENERIC, Pharma Pac	52959-0047-30
30's	$20.27	GENERIC, Southwood Pharmaceuticals Inc	58016-0275-30
32's	$3.38	GENERIC, Vangard Labs	00615-1533-32
36's	$24.32	GENERIC, Southwood Pharmaceuticals Inc	58016-0275-36
40's	$27.02	GENERIC, Southwood Pharmaceuticals Inc	58016-0275-40
50's	$4.68	GENERIC, Prescript Pharmaceuticals	00247-0187-50
50's	$6.23	GENERIC, Physicians Total Care	54868-0059-05
50's	$8.33	GENERIC, Allscripts Pharmaceutical Company	54569-0949-06
50's	$31.74	GENERIC, Pharma Pac	52959-0047-50
50's	$33.78	GENERIC, Southwood Pharmaceuticals Inc	58016-0275-50
60's	$4.94	GENERIC, Prescript Pharmaceuticals	00247-0187-60
60's	$6.98	GENERIC, Physicians Total Care	54868-0059-00
60's	$9.84	GENERIC, Pharmaceutical Corporation Of America	51655-0801-25
60's	$9.99	GENERIC, Allscripts Pharmaceutical Company	54569-0949-03
60's	$40.53	GENERIC, Southwood Pharmaceuticals Inc	58016-0275-60
90's	$9.22	GENERIC, Physicians Total Care	54868-0059-03
90's	$11.26	GENERIC, Pharmaceutical Corporation Of America	51655-0801-26
90's	$60.80	GENERIC, Southwood Pharmaceuticals Inc	58016-0275-90
100's	$6.00	GENERIC, Prescript Pharmaceuticals	00247-0187-00
100's	$9.97	GENERIC, Physicians Total Care	54868-0059-04
100's	$11.48	GENERIC, Vangard Labs	00615-1533-01
100's	$16.65	GENERIC, Allscripts Pharmaceutical Company	54569-0949-05
100's	$67.55	GENERIC, Southwood Pharmaceuticals Inc	58016-0275-00
120's	$18.68	GENERIC, Pharmaceutical Corporation Of America	51655-0801-82
Tablet - Oral - 10 mg			
1's	$0.32	GENERIC, Allscripts Pharmaceutical Company	54569-0936-06
2's	$0.64	GENERIC, Allscripts Pharmaceutical Company	54569-0936-07

5's	$1.59	GENERIC, Allscripts Pharmaceutical Company	54569-0936-05
6's	$2.71	GENERIC, Physicians Total Care	54868-0988-01
6's	$6.83	GENERIC, Southwood Pharmaceuticals Inc	58016-0273-06
10's	$2.85	GENERIC, Physicians Total Care	54868-0988-02
10's	$11.38	GENERIC, Southwood Pharmaceuticals Inc	58016-0273-10
12's	$13.66	GENERIC, Southwood Pharmaceuticals Inc	58016-0273-12
15's	$4.78	GENERIC, Allscripts Pharmaceutical Company	54569-0936-04
15's	$17.07	GENERIC, Southwood Pharmaceuticals Inc	58016-0273-15
20's	$21.85	GENERIC, Pharma Pac	52959-0306-20
20's	$22.76	GENERIC, Southwood Pharmaceuticals Inc	58016-0273-20
30's	$3.55	GENERIC, Physicians Total Care	54868-0988-00
30's	$6.49	GENERIC, Pharmaceutical Corporation Of America	51655-0833-24
30's	$9.56	GENERIC, Allscripts Pharmaceutical Company	54569-0936-02
30's	$31.60	GENERIC, Pharma Pac	52959-0306-30
30's	$34.14	GENERIC, Southwood Pharmaceuticals Inc	58016-0273-30
40's	$12.74	GENERIC, Allscripts Pharmaceutical Company	54569-0936-09
60's	$11.98	GENERIC, Pharmaceutical Corporation Of America	51655-0833-25
60's	$19.11	GENERIC, Allscripts Pharmaceutical Company	54569-0936-03
60's	$68.28	GENERIC, Southwood Pharmaceuticals Inc	58016-0273-60
90's	$17.47	GENERIC, Pharmaceutical Corporation Of America	51655-0833-26
90's	$28.67	GENERIC, Allscripts Pharmaceutical Company	54569-0936-08
90's	$102.42	GENERIC, Southwood Pharmaceuticals Inc	58016-0273-90
100's	$5.15	GENERIC, Physicians Total Care	54868-0988-05
100's	$31.85	GENERIC, Allscripts Pharmaceutical Company	54569-0936-00
100's	$113.80	GENERIC, Southwood Pharmaceuticals Inc	58016-0273-00
120's	$22.95	GENERIC, Pharmaceutical Corporation Of America	51655-0833-82

Diclofenac (001045)

For related information, see the comparative table section in Appendix A.

Categories: Ankylosing spondylitis; Arthritis, osteoarthritis; Arthritis, rheumatoid; Dysmenorrhea; Inflammation, opthalamic, postoperative; Keratoses, actinic; Pain, mild to moderate; Pain, ophthalmic; Photophobia, postoperative; Pregnancy Category B; FDA Approved 1988 Jul

Drug Classes: Analgesics, non-narcotic; Nonsteroidal anti-inflammatory drugs; Ophthalmics

Brand Names: Cataflam; Diclofenac Sodium; **Voltaren**

Foreign Brand Availability: Abdiflam (Indonesia); Abitren (Israel); Allvoran (Germany); Almiral (Bahamas; Bahrain; Barbados; Belize; Benin; Bermuda; Burkina-Faso; Curacao; Cyprus; Egypt; Ethiopia; Gambia; Ghana; Guinea; Guyana; Hong-Kong; Iran; Iraq; Israel; Ivory-Coast; Jamaica; Jordan; Kenya; Kuwait; Lebanon; Liberia; Libya; Malawi; Malaysia; Mali; Mauritania; Mauritius; Morocco; Netherland-Antilles; Niger; Nigeria; Oman; Puerto-Rico; Qatar; Republic-of-Yemen; Saudi-Arabia; Senegal; Seychelles; Sierra-Leone; Singapore; South-Africa; Sudan; Surinam; Syria; Taiwan; Tanzania; Trinidad; Tunia; Uganda; United-Arab-Emirates; Zambia; Zimbabwe); Almiral SR (Hong-Kong; Malaysia); Alonpin (Japan); Apo-Diclofenac EC (New-Zealand); Arcanafenac (South-Africa); Arthrifen (Philippines); Artren (Colombia; Ecuador); Artrenac (Mexico); Artrites (Colombia); Artrites Retard (Colombia); Berifen (Indonesia); Berifen Gel (Costa-Rica; Dominican-Republic; El-Salvador; Guatemala; Honduras; Nicaragua; Panama); Betaren (Israel); Bolabomin (Japan); Calozan (Costa-Rica; Dominican-Republic; El-Salvador; Guatemala; Honduras; Nicaragua; Panama); Cataflam Drops (Malaysia); Cataflam DD (Ecuador); Catanac (Indonesia); Catas (Korea); Clo-Far (Mexico); Clofec (Thailand); Clonaren (Philippines); Clonodifen (Mexico); Cordralan (Peru); Curinflam (Argentina); DDL plaster (Korea); Declophen (Bahrain; Cyprus; Egypt; Iran; Iraq; Israel; Jordan; Kuwait; Lebanon; Libya; Oman; Qatar; Republic-of-Yemen; Saudi-Arabia; Syria; United-Arab-Emirates); Decrol (Korea); Depain (Korea); Diclax (New-Zealand); Diclax SR (New-Zealand); Diclo-Basan (Switzerland); Diclobene (Austria); Diclofenac (Colombia); Diclofen (Bahrain; Cyprus; Egypt; Iran; Iraq; Israel; Jordan; Kuwait; Lebanon; Libya; Oman; Qatar; Republic-of-Yemen; Saudi-Arabia; Syria; Taiwan; Thailand; United-Arab-Emirates); Diclofen Cremogel (Bahrain; Cyprus; Egypt; Iran; Iraq; Jordan; Kuwait; Lebanon; Libya; Oman; Qatar; Republic-of-Yemen; Saudi-Arabia; Syria; United-Arab-Emirates); Dicloflam (South-Africa); Diclohexal (Australia); Diclomax (India; Republic-Of-Yemen); Diclomol (Thailand); Diclon (Denmark); Dicloran Gel (Benin; Burkina-Faso; Ethiopia; Gambia; Ghana; Guinea; India; Ivory-Coast; Kenya; Liberia; Malawi; Mali; Mauritania; Mauritius; Morocco; Niger; Nigeria; Senegal; Seychelles; Sierra-Leone; Sudan; Tanzania; Tunia; Uganda; Zambia; Zimbabwe); Dicloren (Taiwan); Diclosian (Thailand); Diclotec (Canada); Diclowal (Costa-Rica; Dominican-Republic; El-Salvador; Guatemala; Honduras; Nicaragua; Panama); Dicsnal (Japan); Difen (Thailand); Difena (Taiwan); Difenac (Japan; South-Africa; Thailand); Dioxaflex (Mexico); Doflex (India); Dolaren (Mexico); Dolflam-Retard (Mexico); Doloflam (Philippines); Dolotren (Dominican-Republic; El-Salvador; Guatemala; Honduras; Nicaragua; Panama; Taiwan); Dolotren Gel (Taiwan); Dosanac (Thailand); E (Greece); Ecofenac (Switzerland); Epifenac (Bahrain; Cyprus; Egypt; Iran; Iraq; Jordan; Kuwait; Lebanon; Libya; Oman; Qatar; Republic-of-Yemen; Saudi-Arabia; Syria; United-Arab-Emirates); Fenac (Australia; New-Zealand); Flector (France); Flexagen (South-Africa); Flogofenac (China); Flogozan (Costa-Rica; Dominican-Republic; El-Salvador; Guatemala; Honduras; Nicaragua; Panama); Fortfen SR (South-Africa); Freejex (Korea); Hizemin (Japan); Inac (Singapore); Inac gel (Singapore); Inflamac (Switzerland); Inflanac (Hong-Kong; Malaysia; Thailand); Jonac Gel (India); Klotaren (Indonesia); Lofenac (Thailand); Lotirac (Korea); Magluphen (Austria); Monoflam (Czech-Republic; Germany); Naboal (Japan); Nac Gel (India); Naclof (Ecuador; Hong-Kong; Korea; Philippines; South-Africa; Taiwan; Thailand); Nacoflar (Indonesia); Novo-Difenac (Hong-Kong); Novolten (China); Ofenac (Korea); Olfen (China; Hong-Kong); Olfen Gel (Singapore; Thailand); Olfen Roll-On (Israel); Olfen-75 SR (Hong-Kong); Optanac (Indonesia); Osteoflam (India); Painstop (Taiwan); Panamor (South-Africa); Profenac (Bahrain; Cyprus; Egypt; Iran; Iraq; Jordan; Kuwait; Lebanon; Libya; Oman; Qatar; Republic-of-Yemen; Saudi-Arabia; Syria; United-Arab-Emirates); Relaxyl Gel (India); Remethan (Germany; Singapore); Remethan Gel (Taiwan); Rewodina (Germany; Malaysia; Russia); Rhewlin (Singapore); Rhewlin Forte (Singapore); Rhewlin SR (Singapore); Rolactin (Korea); Savismin (Japan); Staren (Taiwan); Soproxen (Thailand); Sting Gel (Singapore); Taks (Bahrain; Cyprus; Egypt; Iran; Iraq; Israel; Jordan; Kuwait; Lebanon; Libya; Oman; Qatar; Republic-of-Yemen; Saudi-Arabia; Syria; United-Arab-Emirates); Tigen Plaster (Korea); Toraren (Korea); Tsudohmin (Japan); Uniren (Singapore); Valentac (Korea); Voldic (Bahrain; Cyprus; Egypt; Iran; Iraq; Jordan; Kuwait; Lebanon; Libya; Oman; Qatar; Republic-of-Yemen; Saudi-Arabia; Syria; United-Arab-Emirates); Voldic Emulgel (Bahrain; Cyprus; Egypt; Iran; Iraq; Israel; Jordan; Kuwait; Lebanon; Libya; Oman; Qatar; Republic-of-Yemen; Saudi-Arabia; Syria; United-Arab-Emirates); Volero (Korea); Volfenac (Costa-Rica; Dominican-Republic; El-Salvador; Guatemala; Honduras; Nicaragua; Panama); Volta (Thailand); Voltadex Emulgel (Indonesia); Voltalen (New-Zealand); Voltalen Emulgel (New-Zealand); Votalen SR (New-Zealand); Voltaren Emulgel (Australia; Austria; Bahamas; Bahrain; Barbados; Belize; Bermuda; Colombia; Curacao; Cyprus; Czech-Republic; Egypt; Germany; Greece; Guyana; Hong-Kong; Indonesia; Iran; Iraq; Israel; Jamaica; Jordan; Kuwait; Lebanon; Libya; Malaysia; Mexico; Netherland-Antilles; New-Zealand; Oman; Philippines; Puerto-Rico; Qatar; Republic-of-Yemen; Saudi-Arabia; South-Africa; Spain; Surinam; Switzerland; Syria; Taiwan; Trinidad; Turkey; United-Arab-Emirates); Voltaren Forte (Philippines); Voltaren Ofta (Germany; Italy); Voltaren Oftalmico (Colombia); Voltaren Ophta (Canada); Voltaren Ophtha (Australia; Denmark; Israel; New-Zealand; Norway; Switzerland); Voltaren Rapid (Australia; New-Zealand); Voltaren Retard (Colombia; Mexico); Voltaren SR (Hong-Kong; Philippines); Voltarene (France); Voltarene Emulgel (France); Voltarol (England; Ireland); Voltarol Emulgel (England; Ireland); Voren (China; Indonesia; Taiwan); Voren Emulgel (China); Voveran (India); Voveran Emulgel (India); Vurdon (Bahrain; Benin; Burkina-Faso; Cyprus; Egypt; Ethiopia; Gambia; Ghana; Guinea; Iran; Iraq; Israel; Ivory-Coast; Jordan; Kenya; Kuwait; Lebanon; Liberia; Libya; Malawi; Mali; Mauritania; Mauritius; Morocco; Niger; Nigeria; Oman; Qatar; Republic-of-Yemen; Saudi-Arabia; Senegal; Seychelles; Sierra-Leone; South-Africa; Sudan; Syria; Tanzania; Tunia; Uganda; United-Arab-Emirates; Zambia; Zimbabwe); Yuren (Taiwan); Zolterol SR (Singapore)

Cost of Therapy: $168.24 (Primary Dysmenorrhea; Cataflam; 50 mg; 3 tablets/day; 30 day supply)
$76.99 (Osteoarthritis; Voltaren; 50 mg; 2 tablets/day; 30 day supply)
$93.11 (Osteoarthritis; Generic Enteric Coated Tablets; 50 mg; 2 tablets/day; 30 day supply)
$93.75 (Osteoarthritis; Voltaren-XR; 100 mg; 1 tablet/day; 30 day supply)

OPHTHALMIC

DESCRIPTION

Voltaren Ophthalmic (diclofenac sodium ophthalmic solution) 0.1% solution is a sterile, topical, nonsteroidal, anti-inflammatory product for ophthalmic use. Diclofenac sodium is designated chemically as 2-[(2,6-dichlorophenyl)amino] benzeneacetic acid, monosodium salt, with an empirical formula of $C_{14}H_{10}Cl_2NO_2Na$.

Voltaren Ophthalmic is available as a sterile solution which contains diclofenac sodium 0.1% (1 mg/ml). Inactive Ingredients: polyoxyl 35 castor oil, boric acid, tromethamine, sorbic acid (2 mg/ml), edetate disodium (1 mg/ml), and purified water. Diclofenac sodium is a faintly yellow-white to light-beige, slightly hygroscopic crystalline powder. It is freely soluble in methanol, sparingly soluble in water, very slightly soluble in acetonitrile, and insoluble in chloroform and in 0.1 N hydrochloric acid. Its molecular weight is 318.14. Voltaren Ophthalmic 0.1% is an iso-osmotic solution with an osmolality of about 300 mOsmol/1000 g, buffered at approximately pH 7.2. Voltaren Ophthalmic solution has a faint characteristic odor of castor oil.

CLINICAL PHARMACOLOGY

PHARMACODYNAMICS

Diclofenac sodium is one of a series of phenylacetic acids that has demonstrated anti-inflammatory and analgesic properties in pharmacological studies. It is thought to inhibit the enzyme cyclooxygenase, which is essential in the biosynthesis of prostaglandins.

ANIMAL STUDIES

Prostaglandins have been shown in many animal models to be mediators of certain kinds of intraocular inflammation. In studies performed in animal eyes, prostaglandins have been shown to produce disruption of the blood-aqueous humor barrier, vasodilation, increased vascular permeability, leukocytosis, and increased intraocular pressure.

PHARMACOKINETICS

Results from a bioavailability study established that plasma levels of diclofenac following ocular instillation of 2 drops of diclofenac sodium ophthalmic solution to each eye were below the limit of quantification (10 ng/ml) over a 4 hour period. This study suggests that limited, if any, systemic absorption occurs with diclofenac sodium ophthalmic solution.

INDICATIONS AND USAGE

Diclofenac sodium ophthalmic solution is indicated for the treatment of postoperative inflammation in patients who have undergone cataract extraction and for the temporary relief of pain and photophobia in patients undergoing corneal refractive surgery.

NON-FDA APPROVED INDICATIONS

Unlabeled uses of diclofenac ophthalmic solution have included noninfected inflammatory conditions such as chronic conjunctivitis, keratoconjunctivitis, trauma, and to inhibit miosis during cataract surgery.

CONTRAINDICATIONS

Diclofenac sodium ophthalmic solution is contraindicated in patients who are hypersensitive to any component of the medication.

WARNINGS

The refractive stability of patients undergoing corneal refractive procedures and treated with diclofenac has not been established. Patients should be monitored for a year following use in this setting. With some nonsteroidal anti-inflammatory drugs, there exists the potential for increased bleeding time due to interference with thrombocyte aggregation. There have been reports that ocularly applied nonsteroidal anti-inflammatory drugs may cause increased bleeding of ocular tissues (including hyphemas) in conjunction with ocular surgery. There is the potential for cross-sensitivity to acetylsalicylic acid, phenylacetic acid derivatives, and other nonsteroidal anti-inflammatory agents. Therefore, caution should be used when treating individuals who have previously exhibited sensitivities to these drugs.

PRECAUTIONS

GENERAL

It is recommended that diclofenac sodium ophthalmic solution, like other NSAIDs, be used with caution in surgical patients with known bleeding tendencies or who are receiving other medications which may prolong bleeding time. Diclofenac may slow or delay healing. Results from clinical studies indicate that diclofenac sodium ophthalmic solution has no significant effect upon ocular pressure; however, elevations in intraocular pressure may occur following cataract surgery.

INFORMATION FOR THE PATIENT

Except for the use of a bandage hydrogel soft contact lens during the first 3 days following refractive surgery, diclofenac sodium ophthalmic solution should not be used by patients currently wearing soft contact lenses due to adverse events that have occurred in other circumstances.

CARCINOGENESIS, MUTAGENESIS, AND IMPAIRMENT OF FERTILITY

Long-term carcinogenicity studies in rats given diclofenac in oral doses up to 2 mg/kg/day (approximately the human oral dose) revealed no significant increases in tumor incidence. There was a slight increase in benign rat mammary fibroadenomas in mid-dose females (high-dose females had excessive mortality) but the increase was not significant for this common rat tumor. A 2 year carcinogenicity study conducted in mice employing oral diclofenac up to 2 mg/kg/day did not reveal any oncogenic potential. Diclofenac did not show mutagenic potential in various mutagenicity studies including the Ames test. Diclofenac administered to male and female rats at 4 mg/kg/day did not affect fertility.

PREGNANCY

Teratogenic Effects, Pregnancy Category C

Reproduction studies performed in mice at oral doses up to 5000 times (20 mg/kg/day) and in rats and rabbits at oral doses up to 2500 times (10 mg/kg/day) the human topical dose have revealed no evidence of teratogenicity due to diclofenac despite the induction of maternal toxicity and fetal toxicity. In rats, maternally toxic doses were associated with dystocia, prolonged gestation, reduced fetal weights and growth, and reduced fetal survival. Diclofenac has been shown to cross the placental barrier in mice and rats. There are, however, no adequate and well-controlled studies in pregnant women. Because animal reproduction studies are not always predictive of human response, this drug should be used during pregnancy only if clearly needed.

Nonteratogenic Effects

Because of the known effects of prostaglandin biosynthesis-inhibiting drugs on the fetal cardiovascular system (closure of ductus arteriosus), the use of diclofenac sodium ophthalmic solution during late pregnancy should be avoided.

PEDIATRIC USE

Safety and effectiveness in pediatric patients have not been established.

ADVERSE REACTIONS

OCULAR

Transient burning and stinging were reported in approximately 15% of patients across studies with the use of diclofenac sodium ophthalmic solution. In cataract surgery studies, keratitis was reported in up to 28% of patients receiving diclofenac sodium ophthalmic solution, although in many of these cases keratitis was initially noted prior to the initiation of treatment. Elevated intraocular pressure following cataract surgery was reported in approximately 15% of patients undergoing cataract surgery. Lacrimation complaints were reported in approximately 30% of case studies undergoing incisional refractive surgery. The following adverse reactions were reported in approximately 5% or less of the patients: abnormal vision, acute elevated IOP, blurred vision, conjunctivitis, corneal deposits, corneal edema, corneal opacity, corneal lesions, discharge, eyelid swelling, injection, iritis, irritation, itching, lacrimation disorder, and ocular allergy.

SYSTEMIC

The following adverse reactions were reported in 3% or less of the patients: Abdominal pain, asthenia, chills, dizziness, facial edema, fever, headache, insomnia, nausea, pain, rhinitis, viral infection, and vomiting.

D

DOSAGE AND ADMINISTRATION

CATARACT SURGERY

One drop of diclofenac sodium ophthalmic solution should be applied to the affected eye, 4 times daily beginning 24 hours after cataract surgery and continuing throughout the first 2 weeks of the postoperative period.

CORNEAL REFRACTIVE SURGERY

One or two drops of diclofenac sodium ophthalmic solution should be applied to the operative eye within the hour prior to corneal refractive surgery. Within 15 minutes after surgery, 1 or 2 drops should be applied to the operative eye and continued 4 times daily for up to 3 days.

HOW SUPPLIED

Voltaren Ophthalmic 0.1% (1 mg/ml) sterile solution is supplied in dropper-tip, plastic, squeeze bottles containing 2.5 or 5 ml.

STORAGE

Store between 15-30°C (59-86°F). Protect from light.

Dispense in original, unopened container only.

ORAL

DESCRIPTION

Diclofenac, as the sodium or potassium salt, is a benzeneacetic acid derivative, designated chemically as 2-[(2,6-dichlorophenyl)amino] benzeneacetic acid, monosodium or monopotassium salt.

Diclofenac, as the sodium or potassium salt, is a faintly yellowish white to light beige, virtually odorless, slightly hygroscopic crystalline powder. Molecular weights of the sodium and potassium salts are 318.14 and 334.25, respectively. It is freely soluble in methanol, soluble in ethanol, and practically insoluble in chloroform and in dilute acid. Diclofenac sodium is sparingly soluble in water while diclofenac potassium is soluble in water. The n-octanol/water partition coefficient is, for both diclofenac salts, 13.4 at pH 7.4 and 1545 at pH 5.2. Both salts have a single dissociation constant (pKa) of 4.0 ± 0.2 at 25°C in water.

DICLOFENAC POTASSIUM

Diclofenac potassium is available as Cataflam Immediate-Release Tablets of 50 mg for oral administration.

Cataflam Inactive Ingredients: Calcium phosphate, colloidal silicon dioxide, iron oxides, magnesium stearate, microcrystalline cellulose, polyethylene glycol, povidone, sodium starch glycolate, starch, sucrose, talc, titanium dioxide.

DICLOFENAC SODIUM

Diclofenac sodium is available as Voltaren Delayed-Release (enteric-coated) Tablets of 25, 50, and 75 mg for oral administration, and Voltaren-XR Extended-Release Tablets of 100 mg.

Voltaren Inactive Ingredients: Hydroxypropyl methylcellulose, iron oxide, lactose, magnesium stearate, methacrylic acid copolymer, microcrystalline cellulose, polyethylene glycol, povidone, propylene glycol, sodium hydroxide, sodium starch glycolate, talc, titanium dioxide, D&C yellow no. 10 aluminum lake (25 mg tablet only), FD&C blue no. 1 aluminum lake (50 mg tablet only).

Voltaren-XR Inactive Ingredients: Cetyl alcohol, hydroxypropyl methylcellulose, iron oxide, magnesium stearate, polyethylene glycol, polysorbate, povidone, silicon dioxide, sucrose, talc, titanium dioxide.

CLINICAL PHARMACOLOGY

PHARMACODYNAMICS

Diclofenac is a nonsteroidal anti-inflammatory drug (NSAID). In pharmacologic studies, diclofenac has shown anti-inflammatory, analgesic, and antipyretic activity. As with other NSAIDs, its mode of action is not known; its ability to inhibit prostaglandin synthesis, however, may be involved in its anti-inflammatory activity, as well as contribute to its efficacy in relieving pain related to inflammation and primary dysmenorrhea. With regard to its analgesic effect, diclofenac is not a narcotic.

PHARMACOKINETICS

Diclofenac potassium immediate-release tablets, diclofenac sodium delayed-release tablets, and diclofenac sodium extended-release tablets, contain the same therapeutic moiety, diclofenac. They differ in the cationic portion of the salt (see DESCRIPTION), as well as in their release characteristics. Diclofenac potassium immediate-release tablets are formulated to release diclofenac in the stomach. Diclofenac sodium delayed-release (enteric-coated) tablets are in a pharmaceutical formulation that resists dissolution in the low pH of gastric fluid but allows a rapid release of drug in the higher pH-environment of the duodenum. Conversely, diclofenac sodium extended-release tablets are formulated to release drug over a prolonged period. The primary pharmacokinetic difference between the three products is in the pattern of drug release and absorption, as described below and shown in TABLE 1. For this reason, separate sections are provided below to describe the different absorption profiles of diclofenac potassium immediate-release tablets, diclofenac sodium delayed-release tablets, and diclofenac sodium extended-release tablets.

TABLE 1 *Mean (% CV) Pharmacokinetics of Diclofenac Following Single Oral Doses of Diclofenac Potassium Immediate-Release Tablets, Diclofenac Sodium Delayed-Release Tablets, and Diclofenac Sodium Extended-Release Tablets*

	Diclofenac Potassium Immediate-Release Tablets	Diclofenac Sodium Delayed-Release Tablets	Diclofenac Sodium Extended-Release Tablets
Dose (mg)	50	50	100
AUC (ng·h/ml)	1309 (21.7%)	1429 (38.4%)	2079 (33.7%)
C_{max} (ng/ml)	1312 (44.1%)	1417 (22.4%)	417 (40.7%)
T_{max} (h)	1.00 (74.6%)	2.22 (49.8%)	5.25 (28.3%)

ABSORPTION

Under fasting condition, diclofenac is completely absorbed from the gastrointestinal tract. However, due to first-pass metabolism, only about 50% of the absorbed dose is systemically available.

Diclofenac Potassium Immediate-Release Tablets

In some fasting volunteers, measurable plasma levels are observed within 10 minutes of dosing with diclofenac potassium immediate-release tablets. Peak plasma levels are achieved in approximately 1 hour in fasting normal volunteers, with a range from 0.33-2 hours.

The extent of diclofenac absorption is not significantly affected when diclofenac potassium immediate-release tablets is taken with food. However, the rate of absorption is reduced by food, as indicated by a delay in T_{max} and decrease in C_{max} values by approximately 30%. After repeated oral administration of diclofenac potassium immediate-release tablets 50 mg tid no accumulation of diclofenac in plasma occurred.

Diclofenac Sodium Delayed-Release Tablets

Peak plasma levels are achieved in 2 hours in fasting normal volunteers, with a range from 1-4 hours. The area under the plasma concentration curve (AUC) is dose-proportional within the range of 25-150 mg. Peak plasma levels are less than dose-proportional and are approximately 1.0, 1.5, and 2.0 µg/ml for 25, 50, and 75 mg doses, respectively. It should be noted that the administration of several individual diclofenac sodium delayed-release tablets may not yield equivalent results in peak concentration as the administration of one tablet of a higher strength. This is probably due to the staggered gastric emptying of tablets into the duodenum. After repeated oral administration of diclofenac sodium delayed-release 50 mg bid, diclofenac did not accumulate in plasma.

When diclofenac sodium delayed-release is taken with food, there is usually a delay in the onset of absorption of 1-4.5 hours, with delays as long as 10 hours in some patients, and a reduction in peak plasma levels of approximately 40%. The extent of absorption of diclofenac, however, is not significantly affected by food intake.

Diclofenac Sodium Extended-Release Tablets

The extent of diclofenac absorption from the extended-release tablet is not significantly affected when the drug is taken with food, however, food significantly altered the absorption pattern as indicated by a delay of 1-2 hours in T_{max} and a 2-fold increase in C_{max} values. The plasma profile of the extended-release tablet, under fasting conditions, was characterized by multiple peaks and high intersubject variability in blood profiles. In contrast, the plasma profile for the extended-release tablets under fed conditions showed a more consistent absorption pattern with a single peak usually occurring between 5 and 6 hours after the meal.

DISTRIBUTION

Plasma concentrations of diclofenac decline from peak levels in a biexponential fashion, with the terminal phase having a half-life of approximately 2 hours. Clearance and volume of distribution are about 350 ml/min and 550 ml/kg, respectively. More than 99% of diclofenac is reversibly bound to human plasma albumin.

As with other NSAIDs, diclofenac diffuses into and out of the synovial fluid. Diffusion into the joint occurs when plasma levels are higher than those in the synovial fluid, after which the process reverses and synovial fluid levels are higher than plasma levels. It is not known whether diffusion into the joint plays a role in the effectiveness of diclofenac.

METABOLISM AND ELIMINATION

Diclofenac is eliminated through metabolism and subsequent urinary and biliary excretion of the glucuronide and the sulfate conjugates of the metabolites. Approximately 65% of the dose is excreted in the urine, and approximately 35% in the bile.

Conjugates of unchanged diclofenac account for 5-10% of the dose excreted in the urine and for less than 5% excreted in the bile. Little or no unchanged unconjugated drug is excreted. Conjugates of the principal metabolite account for 20-30% of the dose excreted in the urine and for 10-20% of the dose excreted in the bile. Conjugates of three other metabolites together account for 10-20% of the dose excreted in the urine and for small amounts excreted in the bile. The elimination half-life values for these metabolites are shorter than those for the parent drug. Urinary excretion of an additional metabolite (half-life 80 hours) accounts for only 1.4% of the oral dose. The degree of accumulation of diclofenac metabolites is unknown. Some of the metabolites may have activity.

SPECIAL POPULATIONS

A 4 week study, comparing plasma level profiles of diclofenac (diclofenac sodium delayed-release 50 mg bid) in younger (26-46 years) versus older (66-81 years) adults, did not show differences between age groups (10 patients per age group).

Geriatric Population

An 8 day study, comparing the kinetics of diclofenac (100 mg diclofenac sodium extended-release tablets qd) in osteoarthritis patients older than 65 years versus younger than 65 years showed no significant differences between the two groups with respect to peak plasma levels, time to peak levels, or AUC.

Patients With Renal and/or Hepatic Impairment

To date, no differences in the pharmacokinetics of diclofenac have been detected in studies of patients with renal (50 mg intravenously) or hepatic impairment (100 mg oral solution). In patients with renal impairment (n=5, creatinine clearance 3-42 ml/min), AUC values and elimination rates were comparable to those in healthy subjects. In patients with biopsy-confirmed cirrhosis or chronic active hepatitis (variably elevated transaminases and mildly elevated bilirubins, n=10), diclofenac concentrations and urinary elimination values were comparable to those in healthy subjects.

INDIVIDUALIZATION OF DOSAGE

Diclofenac, like other NSAIDs, shows interindividual differences in both pharmacokinetics and clinical response (pharmacodynamics). Consequently, the recommended strategy for initiating therapy is to use a starting dose likely to be effective for the majority of patients and to adjust dosage thereafter based on observation of diclofenac's beneficial and adverse effects.

In patients weighing less than 60 kg (132 lb), or where the severity of the disease, concomitant medication, or other diseases warrant, the maximum recommended total daily dose of diclofenac should be reduced. Experience with other NSAIDs has shown that starting therapy with maximum doses in patients at increased risk due to renal or hepatic disease, low body weight (<60 kg), advanced age, a known ulcer diathesis, or known sensitivity to NSAID effects, is likely to increase frequency of adverse reactions and is not recommended (see PRECAUTIONS).

Osteoarthritis/RheumatoidArthritis/Ankylosing Spondylitis

The usual starting dose of diclofenac potassium immediate-release tablets or diclofenac sodium delayed-release for patients with osteoarthritis, is 100-150 mg/day, using a bid or tid dosing regimen. For patients with osteoarthritis, the usual starting dose of diclofenac sodium extended-release tablets is 100 mg qd. In two variable-dose clinical trials in osteoarthritis using diclofenac sodium delayed-release tablets, of 266 patients started on 100 mg/day, 176 chose to increase the dose to 150 mg/day. Dosages above 200 mg/day have not been studied in patients with osteoarthritis.

For most patients with rheumatoid arthritis, the usual starting dose of diclofenac potassium immediate-release tablets or diclofenac sodium delayed-release tablets is 150 mg/day, using a bid or tid dosing regimen. The usual starting dose of diclofenac sodium extended-release tablets is 100 mg qd. Patients requiring more relief of pain and inflammation may increase the dose to 200 mg/day. In clinical trials, patients receiving 200 mg/day were less likely to drop from the trial due to lack of efficacy than patients receiving 150 mg/day as diclofenac sodium delayed-release tablets or 100 mg/day as diclofenac sodium extended-release tablets. Dosages above 225 mg/day are not recommended in patients with rheumatoid arthritis because of increased risk of adverse events.

The recommended dose of diclofenac sodium delayed-release tablets for patients with ankylosing spondylitis is 100-125 mg/day, using a qid dosing regimen (see DOSAGE AND ADMINISTRATION regarding the 125 mg/day dosing regimen). In a variable-dose clinical trial, of 132 patients started on 75 mg/day, 122 chose to increase the dose to 125 mg/day. Dosages above 125 mg/day have not been studied in patients with ankylosing spondylitis.

Analgesia/Primary Dysmenorrhea

Because of earlier absorption of diclofenac from diclofenac potassium immediate-release tablets, it is the formulation indicated for management of pain and primary dysmenorrhea when prompt onset of pain relief is desired. The results of clinical trials suggest an initial diclofenac potassium immediate-release tablets dose of 50 mg for pain or for primary dysmenorrhea, followed by doses of 50 mg every 8 hours, as needed. With experience, some patients with recurring pain, such as dysmenorrhea, may find that an initial dose of 100 mg of diclofenac potassium immediate-release tablets, followed by 50 mg doses, will provide better relief. After the first day, when the maximum recommended dose may be 200 mg, the total daily dose should generally not exceed 150 mg.

INDICATIONS AND USAGE

Diclofenac potassium immediate-release tablets and diclofenac sodium delayed-release tablets are indicated for the acute and chronic treatment of signs and symptoms of osteoarthritis and rheumatoid arthritis. Diclofenac sodium extended-release tablets are indicated for chronic therapy of osteoarthritis and rheumatoid arthritis. In addition, diclofenac potassium immediate-release tablets and diclofenac sodium delayed-release tablets are indicated for the treatment of ankylosing spondylitis. Only diclofenac potassium immediate-release tablets is indicated for the management of pain and primary dysmenorrhea, when prompt pain relief is desired, because it is formulated to provide earlier plasma concentrations of diclofenac (see CLINICAL PHARMACOLOGY, Pharmacokinetics).

NON-FDA APPROVED INDICATIONS

While not FDA approved indications, diclofenac has also been used in the management of pain and nonrheumatic inflammatory conditions.

CONTRAINDICATIONS

Diclofenac in all oral formulations is contraindicated in patients with known hypersensitivity to diclofenac and diclofenac-containing products. Diclofenac should not be given to patients who have experienced asthma, urticaria, or other allergic-type reactions after taking aspirin or other NSAIDs. Severe, rarely fatal, anaphylactic-like reactions to diclofenac have been reported in such patients (see WARNINGS, Anaphylactoid Reactions, and PRECAUTIONS, General, Pre-Existing Asthma).

WARNINGS

GASTROINTESTINAL EFFECTS

Peptic ulceration and gastrointestinal bleeding have been reported in patients receiving diclofenac. Physicians and patients should therefore remain alert for ulceration and bleeding in patients treated chronically with diclofenac even in the absence of previous GI tract symptoms. It is recommended that patients be maintained on the lowest dose of diclofenac possible, consistent with achieving a satisfactory therapeutic response.

Risk of GI Ulcerations, Bleeding, and Perforation With NSAID Therapy

Serious gastrointestinal toxicity such as bleeding, ulceration, and perforation can occur at any time, with or without warning symptoms, in patients treated chronically with NSAID therapy. Although minor upper gastrointestinal problems, such as dyspepsia, are common, usually developing early in therapy, physicians should remain alert for ulceration and bleeding in patients treated chronically with NSAIDs even in the absence of previous GI tract symptoms. In patients observed in clinical trials of several months to 2 years' duration, symptomatic upper GI ulcers, gross bleeding, or perforation appear to occur in approximately 1% of patients for 3-6 months, and in about 2-4% of patients treated for 1 year. Physicians should inform patients about the signs and/or symptoms of serious GI toxicity and what steps to take if they occur.

Studies to date have not identified any subset of patients not at risk of developing peptic ulceration and bleeding. Except for a prior history of serious GI events and other risk factors known to be associated with peptic ulcer disease, such as alcoholism, smoking, etc., no risk factors (*e.g.*, age, sex) have been associated with increased risk. Elderly or debilitated patients seem to tolerate ulceration or bleeding less well than other individuals, and most spontaneous reports of fatal GI events are in this population. Studies to date are inconclusive concerning the relative risk of various NSAIDs in causing such reactions. High doses of any NSAID probably carry a greater risk of these reactions, although controlled clinical trials showing this do not exist in most cases. In considering the use of relatively large doses (within the recommended dosage range), sufficient benefit should be anticipated to offset the potential increased risk of GI toxicity.

HEPATIC EFFECTS

Elevations of one or more liver tests may occur during diclofenac therapy. These laboratory abnormalities may progress, may remain unchanged, or may be transient with continued therapy. Borderline elevations (*i.e.*, less than 3 times the ULN [=the Upper Limit of the Normal range]), or greater elevations of transaminases occurred in about 15% of diclofenac-treated patients. Of the hepatic enzymes, ALT (SGPT) is the one recommended for the monitoring of liver injury.

In clinical trials, meaningful elevations (*i.e.*, more than 3 times the ULN) of AST (SGOT) (ALT was not measured in all studies) occurred in about 2% of approximately 5700 patients at some time during diclofenac sodium delayed-release tablet treatment. In a large, open, controlled trial, meaningful elevations of ALT and/or AST occurred in about 4% of 3700 patients treated for 2-6 months, including marked elevations (*i.e.*, more than 8 times the ULN) in about 1% of the 3700 patients. In that open-label study, a higher incidence of borderline (less than 3 times the ULN), moderate (3-8 times the ULN), and marked (>8 times the ULN) elevations of ALT or AST was observed in patients receiving diclofenac when compared to other NSAIDs. Transaminase elevations were seen more frequently in patients with osteoarthritis than in those with rheumatoid arthritis (see ADVERSE REACTIONS).

In addition to enzyme elevations seen in clinical trials, postmarketing surveillance has found rare cases of severe hepatic reactions, including liver necrosis, jaundice, and fulminant fatal hepatitis with and without jaundice. Some of these rare reported cases underwent liver transplantation.

Physicians should measure transaminases periodically in patients receiving long-term therapy with diclofenac, because severe hepatotoxicity may develop without a prodrome of distinguishing symptoms. The optimum times for making the first and subsequent transaminase measurements are not known. In the largest US trial (open-label) that involved 3700 patients monitored first at 8 weeks and 1200 patients monitored again at 24 weeks, almost all meaningful elevations in transaminases were detected before patients became symptomatic. In 42 of the 51 patients in all trials who developed marked transaminase elevations, abnormal tests occurred during the first 2 months of therapy with diclofenac. Postmarketing experience has shown severe hepatic reactions can occur at any time during treatment with diclofenac. Cases of drug-induced hepatotoxicity have been reported in the first month, and in some cases, the first 2 months of therapy. Based on these experiences, transaminases should be monitored within 4-8 weeks after initiating treatment with diclofenac (see PRECAUTIONS, Laboratory Tests). As with other NSAIDs, if abnormal liver tests persist or worsen, if clinical signs and/or symptoms consistent with liver disease develop, or if systemic manifestations occur (*e.g.*, eosinophilia, rash, etc.), diclofenac should be discontinued immediately.

To minimize the possibility that hepatic injury will become severe between transaminase measurements, physicians should inform patients of the warning signs and symptoms of hepatotoxicity (*e.g.*, nausea, fatigue, lethargy, pruritus, jaundice, right upper quadrant tenderness, and "flu-like" symptoms), and the appropriate action patients should take if these signs and symptoms appear.

ANAPHYLACTOID REACTIONS

As with other NSAIDs, anaphylactoid reactions may occur in patients without prior exposure to diclofenac. Diclofenac should not be given to patients with the aspirin triad. The triad typically occurs in asthmatic patients who experience rhinitis with or without nasal polyps, or who exhibit severe, potentially fatal bronchospasm after taking aspirin or other nonsteroidal anti-inflammatory drugs. Fatal reactions have been reported in such patients (see CONTRAINDICATIONS, and PRECAUTIONS, General, Pre-Existing Asthma). Emergency help should be sought in cases where an anaphylactoid reaction occurs.

ADVANCED RENAL DISEASE

In cases with advanced kidney disease, treatment with diclofenac, as with other NSAIDs, should only be initiated with close monitoring of the patient's kidney functions (see PRECAUTIONS, General, Renal Effects).

PREGNANCY

In late pregnancy, diclofenac should, as with other NSAIDs, be avoided because it will cause premature closure of the ductus arteriosus (see PRECAUTIONS, Pregnancy, Teratogenic Effects, Pregnancy Category B, and PRECAUTIONS, Labor and Delivery).

PRECAUTIONS

GENERAL

Diclofenac oral formulations should not be used concomitantly with other diclofenac-containing products since they also circulate in plasma as the diclofenac anion.

Fluid Retention and Edema

Fluid retention and edema have been observed in some patients taking diclofenac. Therefore, as with other NSAIDs, diclofenac should be used with caution in patients with a history of cardiac decompensation, hypertension, or other conditions predisposing to fluid retention.

Hematologic Effects

Anemia is sometimes seen in patients receiving diclofenac or other NSAIDs. This may be due to fluid retention, GI blood loss, or an incompletely described effect upon erythropoiesis.

Renal Effects

As a class, NSAIDs have been associated with renal papillary necrosis and other abnormal renal pathology in long-term administration to animals. In oral diclofenac studies in animals, some evidence of renal toxicity was noted. Isolated incidents of papillary necrosis were observed in a few animals at high doses (20-120 mg/kg) in several baboon subacute studies. In patients treated with diclofenac, rare cases of interstitial nephritis and papillary necrosis have been reported (see ADVERSE REACTIONS).

A second form of renal toxicity, generally associated with NSAIDs, is seen in patients with conditions leading to a reduction in renal blood flow or blood volume, where renal prostaglandins have a supportive role in the maintenance of renal perfusion. In these patients, administration of an NSAID results in a dose-dependent decrease in prostaglandin synthesis and, secondarily, in a reduction of renal blood flow, which may precipitate overt renal failure. Patients at greatest risk of this reaction are those with impaired renal function, heart failure, liver dysfunction, those taking diuretics, and the elderly. Discontinuation of NSAID therapy is typically followed by recovery to the pretreatment state.

Cases of significant renal failure in patients receiving diclofenac have been reported from marketing experience, but were not observed in over 4000 patients in clinical trials during which serum creatinine and BUN values were followed serially. There were only 11 patients (0.3%) whose serum creatinine and concurrent serum BUN values were greater than 2.0 mg/dl and 40 mg/dl, respectively, while on diclofenac (mean rise in the 11 patients: creatinine 2.3 mg/dl and BUN 28.4 mg/dl).

Since diclofenac metabolites are eliminated primarily by the kidneys, patients with significantly impaired renal function should be more closely monitored than subjects with normal renal function.

Porphyria

The use of diclofenac in patients with hepatic porphyria should be avoided. To date, 1 patient has been described in whom diclofenac probably triggered a clinical attack of porphyria. The postulated mechanism, demonstrated in rats, for causing such attacks by diclofenac, as well as some other NSAIDs, is through stimulation of the porphyrin precursor delta-aminolevulinic acid (ALA).

Aseptic Meningitis

As with other NSAIDs, aseptic meningitis with fever and coma has been observed on rare occasions in patients on diclofenac therapy. Although it is probably more likely to occur in patients with systemic lupus erythematosus and related connective tissue diseases, it has been reported in patients who do not have an underlying chronic disease. If signs or symptoms of meningitis develop in a patient on diclofenac, the possibility of its being related to diclofenac should be considered.

Pre-Existing Asthma

About 10% of patients with asthma may have aspirin-sensitive asthma. The use of aspirin in patients with aspirin-sensitive asthma has been associated with severe bronchospasm which can be fatal. Since cross-reactivity, including bronchospasm, between aspirin and other nonsteroidal anti-inflammatory drugs has been reported in such aspirin-sensitive patients, diclofenac should not be administered to patients with this form of aspirin sensitivity and should be used with caution in all patients with preexisting asthma.

Other Precautions

The pharmacologic activity of diclofenac may reduce fever and inflammation, thus diminishing their utility as diagnostic signs in detecting underlying conditions.

In order to avoid exacerbation of manifestations of adrenal insufficiency, patients who have been on prolonged corticosteroid treatment should have their therapy tapered slowly rather than discontinued abruptly when diclofenac is added to the treatment program.

Blurred and/or diminished vision, scotomata, and/or changes in color vision have been reported. If a patient develops such complaints while receiving diclofenac, the drug should be discontinued and the patient should have an ophthalmologic examination which includes central visual fields and color vision testing.

INFORMATION FOR THE PATIENT

Diclofenac, like other drugs of its class, is not free of side effects. The side effects of these drugs can cause discomfort and, rarely, more serious side effects, such as gastrointestinal bleeding, and more rarely, liver toxicity (see WARNINGS, Hepatic Effects), which may result in hospitalization and even fatal outcomes.

NSAIDs are often essential agents in the management of arthritis and have a major role in the management of pain, but they also may be commonly employed for conditions that are less serious.

Physicians may wish to discuss with their patients the potential risks (see WARNINGS, PRECAUTIONS, and ADVERSE REACTIONS) and likely benefits of NSAID treatment, particularly when the drugs are used for less serious conditions where treatment without NSAIDs may represent an acceptable alternative to both the patient and physician.

Because serious GI tract ulceration and bleeding can occur without warning symptoms, physicians should follow chronically treated patients for the signs and symptoms of ulceration and bleeding and should inform them of the importance of this follow-up (see WARNINGS, Gastrointestinal Effects, Risk of GI Ulcerations, Bleeding, and Perforation With NSAID Therapy). If diclofenac is used chronically, patients should also be instructed to report any signs and symptoms that might be due to hepatotoxicity of diclofenac; these symptoms may become evident between visits when periodic liver laboratory tests are performed (see WARNINGS, Hepatic Effects, and Laboratory Tests).

D

LABORATORY TESTS

Hepatic Effects

Transaminases and other hepatic enzymes should be monitored in patients treated with NSAIDs. For patients on diclofenac therapy, it is recommended that a determination be made within 4 weeks of initiating therapy and at intervals thereafter. If clinical signs and symptoms consistent with liver disease develop, or if systemic manifestations occur (*e.g.*, eosinophilia, rash, etc.) and abnormal liver tests are detected, persist or worsen, diclofenac should be discontinued immediately.

Hematologic Effects

Patients on long-term treatment with NSAIDs, including diclofenac, should have their hemoglobin or hematocrit checked periodically for signs or symptoms of anemia. Appropriate measures should be taken in case such signs of anemia occur.

PROTEIN BINDING

In vitro, diclofenac interferes minimally or not at all with the protein binding of salicylic acid (20% decrease in binding), tolbutamide, prednisolone (10% decrease in binding), or warfarin. Benzylpenicillin, ampicillin, oxacillin, chlortetracycline, doxycycline, cephalothin, erythromycin, and sulfamethoxazole have no influence *in vitro* on the protein binding of diclofenac in human serum.

DRUG/LABORATORY TEST INTERACTIONS

Effect on Blood Coagulation

Diclofenac increases platelet aggregation time but does not affect bleeding time, plasma thrombin clotting time, plasma fibrinogen, or factors V and VII to XII. Statistically significant changes in prothrombin and partial thromboplastin times have been reported in normal volunteers. The mean changes were observed to be less than 1 second in both instances, however, and are unlikely to be clinically important. Diclofenac is a prostaglandin synthetase inhibitor, however, and all drugs that inhibit prostaglandin synthesis interfere with platelet function to some degree; therefore, patients who may be adversely affected by such an action should be carefully observed.

CARCINOGENESIS, MUTAGENESIS, AND IMPAIRMENT OF FERTILITY

Long-term carcinogenicity studies in rats given diclofenac sodium up to 2 mg/kg/day (or 12 mg/m^2/day, approximately the human dose) have revealed no significant increases in tumor incidence. There was a slight increase in benign mammary fibroadenomas in mid-dose-treated (0.5 mg/kg/day or 3 mg/m^2/day) female rats (high-dose females had excessive mortality), but the increase was not significant for this common rat tumor. A 2 year carcinogenicity study conducted in mice employing diclofenac sodium at doses up to 0.3 mg/kg/day (0.9 mg/m^2/day) in males and 1 mg/kg/day (3 mg/m^2/day) in females did not reveal any oncogenic potential. Diclofenac sodium did not show mutagenic activity in *in vitro* point mutation assays in mammalian (mouse lymphoma) and microbial (yeast, Ames) test systems and was nonmutagenic in several mammalian *in vitro* and *in vivo* tests, including dominant lethal and male germinal epithelial chromosomal studies in mice, and nucleus anomaly and chromosomal aberration studies in Chinese hamsters. Diclofenac sodium administered to male and female rats at 4 mg/kg/day (24 mg/m^2/day) did not affect fertility.

PREGNANCY, TERATOGENIC EFFECTS, PREGNANCY CATEGORY B

Reproduction studies have been performed in mice given diclofenac sodium (up to 20 mg/kg/day or 60 mg/m^2/day) and in rats and rabbits given diclofenac sodium (up to 10 mg/kg/day or 60 mg/m^2/day for rats, and 80 mg/m^2/day for rabbits), and have revealed no evidence of teratogenicity despite the induction of maternal toxicity and fetal toxicity. In rats, maternally toxic doses were associated with dystocia, prolonged gestation, reduced fetal weights and growth, and reduced fetal survival. Diclofenac has been shown to cross the placental barrier in mice and rats. There are, however, no adequate and well-controlled studies in pregnant women. Because animal reproduction studies are not always predictive of human response, this drug should not be used during pregnancy unless the benefits to the mother justify the potential risk to the fetus. Because of the risk to the fetus resulting in premature closure of the ductus arteriosus, diclofenac should be avoided in late pregnancy.

LABOR AND DELIVERY

The effects of diclofenac on labor and delivery in pregnant women are unknown. Because of the known effects of prostaglandin-inhibiting drugs on the fetal cardiovascular system (closure of ductus arteriosus), use of diclofenac during late pregnancy should be avoided and, as with other nonsteroidal anti-inflammatory drugs, it is possible that diclofenac may inhibit uterine contractions and delay parturition.

NURSING MOTHERS

Because of the potential for serious adverse reactions in nursing infants from diclofenac, a decision should be made whether to discontinue nursing or to discontinue the drug, taking into account the importance of the drug to the mother.

PEDIATRIC USE

Safety and effectiveness of diclofenac in pediatric patients have not been established.

GERIATRIC USE

Of the more than 6000 patients treated with diclofenac in US trials, 31% were older than 65 years of age. No overall difference was observed between efficacy, adverse event, or pharmacokinetic profiles of older and younger patients. As with any NSAID, the elderly are likely to tolerate adverse reactions less well than younger patients.

DRUG INTERACTIONS

Aspirin: Concomitant administration of diclofenac and aspirin is not recommended because diclofenac is displaced from its binding sites during the concomitant administration of aspirin, resulting in lower plasma concentrations, peak plasma levels, and AUC values.

Anticoagulants: While studies have not shown diclofenac to interact with anticoagulants of the warfarin type, caution should be exercised, nonetheless, since interactions have been seen with other NSAIDs. Because prostaglandins play an important role in hemostasis, and NSAIDs affect platelet function as well, concurrent therapy with all NSAIDs, including diclofenac, and warfarin requires close monitoring of patients to be certain that no change in their anticoagulant dosage is required.

Digoxin, Methotrexate, Cyclosporine: Diclofenac, like other NSAIDs, may affect renal prostaglandins and increase the toxicity of certain drugs. Ingestion of diclofenac may increase serum concentrations of digoxin and methotrexate and increase cyclosporine's nephrotoxicity. Patients who begin taking diclofenac or who increase their diclofenac dose or any other NSAID while taking digoxin, methotrexate, or cyclosporine may develop toxicity characteristics for these drugs. They should be observed closely, particularly if renal function is impaired. In the case of digoxin, serum levels should be monitored.

Lithium: Diclofenac decreases lithium renal clearance and increases lithium plasma levels. In patients taking diclofenac and lithium concomitantly, lithium toxicity may develop.

Oral Hypoglycemics: Diclofenac does not alter glucose metabolism in normal subjects nor does it alter the effects of oral hypoglycemic agents. There are rare reports, however, from marketing experiences, of changes in effects of insulin or oral hypoglycemic agents in the presence of diclofenac that necessitated changes in the doses of such agents. Both hypo- and hyperglycemic effects have been reported. A direct causal relationship has not been established, but physicians should consider the possibility that diclofenac may alter a diabetic patient's response to insulin or oral hypoglycemic agents.

Diuretics: Diclofenac and other NSAIDs can inhibit the activity of diuretics. Concomitant treatment with potassium-sparing diuretics may be associated with increased serum potassium levels.

Other Drugs: In small groups of patients (7-10/interaction study), the concomitant administration of azathioprine, gold, chloroquine, D-penicillamine, prednisolone, doxycycline, or digitoxin did not significantly affect the peak levels and AUC values of diclofenac. Phenobarbital toxicity has been reported to have occurred in a patient on chronic phenobarbital treatment following the initiation of diclofenac therapy.

ADVERSE REACTIONS

Adverse reaction information is derived from blinded, controlled, and open-label clinical trials, as well as worldwide marketing experience. In the description below, rates of more common events represent clinical study results; rarer events are derived principally from marketing experience and publications, and accurate rate estimates are generally not possible.

In 718 patients treated for shorter periods, *i.e.,* 2 weeks or less, with diclofenac potassium immediate-release tablets, adverse reactions were reported one-half to one-tenth as frequently as by patients treated for longer periods. In a 6-month, double-blind trial comparing diclofenac potassium immediate-release tablets (n=196) versus diclofenac sodium delayed-release tablets (n=197) versus ibuprofen (n=197), adverse reactions were similar in nature and frequency. In controlled clinical trials, the incidence of adverse reactions for diclofenac sodium delayed-release tablets and diclofenac sodium extended-release tablets at comparable doses were similar.

The incidence of common adverse reactions (greater than 1%) is based upon controlled clinical trials in 1543 patients treated up to 13 weeks with diclofenac sodium delayed-release tablets. By far the most common adverse effects were gastrointestinal symptoms, most of them minor, occurring in about 20%, and leading to discontinuation in about 3%, of patients. Peptic ulcer or GI bleeding occurred in clinical trials in 0.6% (95% confidence interval: 0.2-1%) of approximately 1800 patients during their first 3 months of diclofenac treatment and in 1.6% (95% confidence interval: 0.8-2.4%) of approximately 800 patients followed for 1 year.

Gastrointestinal symptoms were followed in frequency by central nervous system side effects such as headache (7%) and dizziness (3%).

Meaningful (exceeding 3 times the Upper Limit of Normal) elevations of ALT (SGPT) or AST (SGOT) occurred at an overall rate of approximately 2% during the first 2 months of diclofenac sodium delayed-release treatment. Unlike aspirin-related elevations, which occur more frequently in patients with rheumatoid arthritis, these elevations were more frequently observed in patients with osteoarthritis (2.6%) than in patients with rheumatoid arthritis (0.7%). Marked elevations (exceeding 8 times the ULN) were seen in 1% of patients treated for 2-6 months (see WARNINGS, Hepatic Effects).

THE FOLLOWING ADVERSE REACTIONS WERE REPORTED IN PATIENTS TREATED WITH DICLOFENAC:

Incidence Greater Than 1% — Causal Relationship Probable:

(All derived from clinical trials.)

*Incidence, 3-9% (incidence of unmarked reactions is 1-3%).

Body as a Whole: Abdominal pain or cramps,* headache,* fluid retention, abdominal distention.

Digestive: Diarrhea,* indigestion,* nausea,* constipation,* flatulence, liver test abnormalities,*PUB, *i.e.*, peptic ulcer, with or without bleeding and/or perforation, or bleeding without ulcer (see above and also WARNINGS).
Nervous System: Dizziness.
Skin and Appendages: Rash, pruritus.
Special Senses: Tinnitus.

Incidence Less Than 1% — Causal Relationship Probable:

(Adverse reactions reported only in worldwide marketing experience or in the literature, not seen in clinical trials, are considered rare and are *italicized.*)

Body as a Whole: Malaise, swelling of lips and tongue, photosensitivity, *anaphylaxis,* anaphylactoid reactions.
Cardiovascular: Hypertension, congestive heart failure.
Digestive: Vomiting, jaundice, melena, *esophageal lesions,* aphthous stomatitis, dry mouth and mucous membranes, bloody diarrhea, hepatitis, *hepatic necrosis, cirrhosis, hepatorenal syndrome,* appetite change, pancreatitis with or without concomitant hepatitis, *colitis.*
Hemic and Lymphatic: Hemoglobin decrease, leukopenia, thrombocytopenia, *eosinophilia, hemolytic anemia, aplastic anemia, agranulocytosis,* purpura, *allergic purpura.*
Metabolic and Nutritional Disorders: Azotemia.
Nervous System: Insomnia, drowsiness, depression, diplopia, anxiety, irritability, *aseptic meningitis, convulsions.*
Respiratory: Epistaxis, asthma, laryngeal edema.
Skin and Appendages: Alopecia, urticaria, eczema, dermatitis, *bullous eruption, erythema multiforme major,* angioedema, *Stevens-Johnson syndrome.*
Special Senses: Blurred vision, taste disorder, reversible and irreversible hearing loss, scotoma.
Urogenital: *Nephrotic syndrome,* proteinuria, *oliguria, interstitial nephritis, papillary necrosis, acute renal failure.*

Incidence Less Than 1% — Causal Relationship Unknown:

(The following reactions have been reported in patients taking diclofenac under circumstances that do not permit a clear attribution of the reaction to diclofenac. These reactions are being included as alerting information to physicians. Adverse reactions reported only in worldwide marketing experience or in the literature, not seen in clinical trials, are considered rare and are italicized.)

Body as a Whole: Chest pain.
Cardiovascular: Palpitations, *flushing,* tachycardia, premature ventricular contractions, myocardial infarction, *hypotension.*
Digestive: *Intestinal perforation.*
Hemic and Lymphatic: *Bruising.*
Metabolic and Nutritional Disorders: Hypoglycemia, *weight loss.*
Nervous System: Paresthesia, memory disturbance, nightmares, tremor, tic, *abnormal coordination, disorientation, psychotic reaction.*
Respiratory: Dyspnea, hyperventilation, edema of pharynx.
Skin and Appendages: Excess perspiration, *exfoliative dermatitis.*
Special Senses: Vitreous floaters, night blindness, amblyopia.
Urogenital: Urinary frequency, nocturia, hematuria, impotence, vaginal bleeding.

DOSAGE AND ADMINISTRATION

Diclofenac may be administered as 50 mg diclofenac potassium immediate-release tablets, as 25, 50, and 75 mg diclofenac sodium delayed-release tablets, or as 100 mg diclofenac sodium extended-release tablets. Diclofenac potassium immediate-release tablets is the formulation indicated for management of acute pain and primary dysmenorrhea when prompt onset of pain relief is desired because of earlier absorption of diclofenac. For the same reason, diclofenac sodium extended-release tablets are not indicated for the management of acute painful conditions and should be used as chronic therapy in patients with osteoarthritis and rheumatoid arthritis.

The dosage of diclofenac should be individualized to the lowest effective dose to minimize adverse effects (see CLINICAL PHARMACOLOGY, Individualization of Dosage).

OSTEOARTHRITIS

The recommended dosage is 100-150 mg/day: Diclofenac potassium immediate-release tablets or diclofenac sodium delayed-release 50 mg bid or tid; or diclofenac sodium delayed-release 75 mg bid. The recommended dosage for chronic therapy with diclofenac sodium extended-release is 100 mg qd. Dosages of diclofenac sodium extended-release tablets of 200 mg daily are not recommended for patients with osteoarthritis. Dosages above 200 mg/day have not been studied in patients with osteoarthritis.

RHEUMATOID ARTHRITIS

The recommended dosage is 100-200 mg/day: Diclofenac potassium immediate-release tablets or diclofenac sodium delayed-release 50 mg tid or qid; or diclofenac sodium delayed-release 75 mg bid. The recommended dosage for chronic therapy with diclofenac sodium extended-release is 100 mg qd. In the rare patient where diclofenac sodium extended-release 100 mg/day is unsatisfactory, the dose may be increased to 100 mg bid if the benefits outweigh the clinical risks. Dosages above 225 mg/day are not recommended in patients with rheumatoid arthritis.

ANKYLOSING SPONDYLITIS

The recommended dosage is 100-125 mg/day: Diclofenac sodium delayed-release 25 mg qid with an extra 25 mg dose at bedtime if necessary. Dosages above 125 mg/day have not been studied in patients with ankylosing spondylitis.

ANALGESIA AND PRIMARY DYSMENORRHEA

The recommended starting dose of diclofenac potassium immediate-release tablets is 50 mg tid. With experience, physicians may find that in some patients an initial dose of 100 mg of diclofenac potassium immediate-release tablets, followed by 50 mg doses, will provide better relief. After the first day, when the maximum recommended dose may be 200 mg, the total daily dose should generally not exceed 150 mg.

HOW SUPPLIED

CATAFLAM TABLETS

50 mg: Light brown, round, biconvex (imprinted "CATAFLAM" on one side and "50" on the other side).

VOLTAREN DELAYED-RELEASE TABLETS

25 mg: Yellow, biconvex, triangular-shaped (imprinted "VOLTAREN 25" on one side).
50 mg: Light brown, biconvex, triangular-shaped (imprinted "VOLTAREN 50" on one side).
75 mg: Light pink, biconvex, triangular-shaped (imprinted "VOLTAREN 75" on one side).

D

VOLTAREN-XR EXTENDED-RELEASE TABLETS

100 mg: Light pink, coated, round, biconvex with beveled edges (imprinted "Voltaren-XR" on one side and "100" on the other side).

STORAGE

Do not store above 30°C (86°F). Protect from moisture. Dispense in *tight* container.

TOPICAL

DESCRIPTION

Solaraze gel, 3%, contains the active ingredient, diclofenac sodium, in a clear, transparent, colorless to slightly yellow gel base. Diclofenac sodium is a white to slightly yellow crystalline powder. It is freely soluble in methanol, soluble in ethanol, sparingly soluble in water, slightly soluble in acetone, and partially insoluble in ether. The chemical name for diclofenac sodium is: Sodium [*o*-(2,6-dichloranilino) phenyl] acetate.

Diclofenac sodium has a molecular weight of 318.13.

Solaraze also contains benzyl alcohol, hyaluronate sodium, polyethylene glycol monomethyl ether, and purified water.

1 g of Solaraze gel contains 30 mg of the active substance, diclofenac sodium.

CLINICAL PHARMACOLOGY

The mechanism of action of diclofenac sodium in the treatment of actinic keratosis (AK) is unknown. The contribution to efficacy of individual components of the vehicle has not been established.

PHARMACOKINETICS

Absorption

When diclofenac sodium gel is applied topically, diclofenac is absorbed into the epidermis. In a study in patients with compromised skin (mainly atopic dermatitis and other dermatitic conditions) of the hands, arms or face, approximately 10% of the applied dose (2 grams of 3% gel over 100 cm^2) of diclofenac was absorbed systemically in both normal and compromised epidermis after 7 days, with 4 times daily applications.

After topical application of 2 g diclofenac sodium gel 3 times daily for 6 days to the calf of the leg in healthy subjects, diclofenac could be detected in plasma. Mean bioavailability parameters were AUC(0-t) 9 ± 19 ng·h/ml (mean ±SD) with a C_{max} of 4 ± 5 ng/ml and a T_{max} of 4.5 ± 8 hours. In comparison, a single oral 75 mg dose of diclofenac sodium delayed-release tablet produced an AUC of 1600 ng·h/ml. Therefore, the systemic bioavailability after topical application of diclofenac sodium gel is lower than after oral dosing.

Blood drawn at the end of treatment from 60 patients with AK lesions treated with diclofenac sodium gel in three adequate and well-controlled clinical trials were assayed for diclofenac levels. Each patient was administered 0.5 g of diclofenac sodium gel twice a day for up to 105 days. There were up to three 5 cm × 5 cm treatment sites per patient on the face, forehead, hands, forearm, and scalp. Serum concentrations of diclofenac were on average at, or below 20 ng/ml. These data indicate that systemic absorption of diclofenac in patients treated topically with diclofenac sodium gel is much lower than that occurring after oral daily dosing of diclofenac sodium.

No information is available on the absorption of diclofenac when diclofenac sodium gel is used under occlusion.

Distribution

Diclofenac binds tightly to serum albumin. The volume of distribution of diclofenac following oral administration is approximately 550 ml/kg.

Metabolism

Biotransformation of diclofenac following oral administration involves conjugation at the carboxyl group of the side chain or single or multiple hydroxylations resulting in several phenolic metabolites, most of which are converted to glucuronide conjugates. Two of these phenolic metabolites are biologically active, however to a much smaller extent than diclofenac. Metabolism of diclofenac following topical administration is thought to be similar to that after oral administration. The small amounts of diclofenac and its metabolites appearing in the plasma following topical administration makes the quantification of specific metabolites imprecise.

Elimination

Diclofenac and its metabolites are excreted mainly in the urine after oral dosing. Systemic clearance of diclofenac from plasma is 263 ± 56 ml/min (mean ±SD). The terminal plasma half-life is 1-2 hours. Four of the metabolites also have short terminal half-lives of 1-3 hours.

INDICATIONS AND USAGE

Diclofenac sodium gel is indicated for the topical treatment of actinic keratoses (AK). Sun avoidance is indicated during therapy.

CONTRAINDICATIONS

Diclofenac sodium gel is contraindicated in patients with a known hypersensitivity to diclofenac, benzyl alcohol, polyethylene glycol monomethyl ether 350 and/or hyaluronate sodium.

WARNINGS

As with other NSAIDs, anaphylactoid reactions may occur in patients without prior exposure to diclofenac. Diclofenac sodium should be given with caution to patients with the aspirin triad. The triad typically occurs in asthmatic patients who experience rhinitis with or without nasal polyps, or who exhibit severe, potentially fatal bronchospasm after taking aspirin or other NSAIDs.

D

PRECAUTIONS

GENERAL

Diclofenac sodium gel should be used with caution in patients with active gastrointestinal ulceration or bleeding and severe renal or hepatic impairments. Diclofenac sodium gel should not be applied to open skin wounds, infections, or exfoliative dermatitis. It should not be allowed to come in contact with the eyes.

The safety of the concomitant use of sunscreens, cosmetics or other topical medications and diclofenac sodium gel is unknown.

INFORMATION FOR THE PATIENT

In clinical studies, localized dermal side effects such as contact dermatitis, exfoliation, dry skin, and rash were found In patients treated with diclofenac sodium gel at a higher incidence than in those with placebo.

Patients should understand the importance of monitoring and follow-up evaluation, the signs and symptoms of dermal adverse reactions, and the possibility of irritant or allergic contact dermatitis. If severe dermal reactions occur, treatment with diclofenac sodium gel may be interrupted until the condition subsides. Exposure to sunlight and the use of sunlamps should be avoided.

Safety and efficacy of the use of diclofenac sodium gel together with other dermal products, including cosmetics, sunscreens, and other topical medications on the area being treated have not been studied.

CARCINOGENESIS, MUTAGENESIS, AND IMPAIRMENT OF FERTILITY

There did not appear to be any increase in drug-related neoplasms following daily topical applications of diclofenac sodium gel for 2 years at concentrations up to 0.035% diclofenac sodium and 2.5% hyaluronate sodium in albino mice. (*Note:* Diclofenac sodium gel contains 3% diclofenac sodium.) When administered orally for 2 years, diclofenac showed no evidence of carcinogenic potential in rats given diclofenac sodium at up to 2 mg/kg/day (3 times the estimated systemic human exposure*), or in mice given diclofenac sodium at up to 0.3 mg/kg/day in males and 1 mg/kg/day in females (25% and 83%, respectively, of the estimated systemic human exposure).

A photococarcinogenicity study with up to 0.035% diclofenac in the diclofenac sodium vehicle gel was conducted in hairless mice at topical doses up to 2.8 mg/kg/day. Median tumor onset was earlier in the 0.035% group (diclofenac sodium gel contains 3% diclofenac sodium).

Diclofenac was not genotoxic in *in vitro* point mutation assays in mammalian mouse lymphoma cells and Ames microbial test systems, or when tested in mammalian *in vivo* assays including dominant lethal and male germinal epithelial chromosomal studies in mice, and nucleus anomaly and chromosomal aberration studies in Chinese hamsters. It was also negative in the transformation assay utilizing BALB/3T3 mouse embryo cells.

Fertility studies have not been conducted with diclofenac sodium gel. Diclofenac sodium showed no evidence of impairment of fertility after oral treatment with 4 mg/kg/day (7 times the estimated systemic human exposure) in male or female rats.

* Based on body surface area and assuming 10% bioavailability following topical application of 2 g diclofenac sodium gel per day (1 mg/kg diclofenac sodium).

PREGNANCY, TERATOGENIC EFFECTS, PREGNANCY CATEGORY B

The safety of diclofenac sodium gel has not been established during pregnancy. However, reproductive studies performed with diclofenac sodium alone at oral doses up to 20 mg/kg/day (15 times the estimated systemic human exposure*) in mice, 10 mg/kg/day (15 times the estimated systemic human exposure) in rats, and 10 mg/kg/day (30 times the estimated systemic human exposure) in rabbits have revealed no evidence of teratogenicity despite the induction of maternal toxicity. In rats, maternally toxic doses were associated with dystocia, prolonged gestation, reduced fetal weights and growth, and reduced fetal survival.

* Based on body surface area and assuming 10% bioavailability following topical application of 2 g diclofenac sodium gel per day (1 mg/kg diclofenac sodium).

Diclofenac has been shown to cross the placental barrier in mice and rats. There are, however, no adequate and well controlled studies in pregnant women. Because animal reproduction studies are not always predictive of human response, this drug should not be used during pregnancy unless the benefits to the mother justify the potential risk to the fetus. Because of the risk to the fetus resulting in premature closure of the ductus arteriosus, diclofenac should be avoided in late pregnancy.

LABOR AND DELIVERY

The effects of diclofenac on labor and delivery in pregnant women are unknown. Because of the known effects of prostaglandin-inhibiting drugs on the fetal cardiovascular system (closure of ductus arteriosus), use of diclofenac during late pregnancy should be avoided and, as with other nonsteroidal anti-inflammatory drugs, it is possible that diclofenac may inhibit uterine contractions and delay parturition.

NURSING MOTHERS

Because of the potential for serious adverse reactions in nursing infants from diclofenac sodium, a decision should be made whether to discontinue nursing or to discontinue the drug, taking into account the importance of the drug to the mother.

PEDIATRIC USE

Actinic keratosis is not a condition seen within the pediatric population. Diclofenac sodium gel should not be used by children.

GERIATRIC USE

Of the 211 subjects treated with diclofenac sodium gel in controlled clinical studies, 143 subjects were 65 and over. Of those 143 subjects, 55 subjects were 75 and over. No overall differences in safety or effectiveness were observed between these subjects and younger subjects, and other reported clinical experience has not identified differences in responses between the elderly and younger patients, but greater sensitivity of some older individuals cannot be ruled out.

DRUG INTERACTIONS

Although the systemic absorption of diclofenac sodium gel is low, concomitant oral administration of other NSAIDs such as aspirin at anti-inflammatory/analgesic doses should be minimized.

ADVERSE REACTIONS

Of the 423 patients evaluable for safety in adequate and well-controlled trials, 211 were treated with diclofenac sodium gel drug product and 212 were treated with vehicle gel. Eighty-seven percent (87%) of the diclofenac sodium gel treated patients (183 patients) and 84% of the vehicle treated patients (178 patients) experienced one or more adverse events (AEs) during the studies. The majority of these reactions were mild to moderate in severity and resolved upon discontinuation of therapy.

Of the 211 patients treated with diclofenac sodium gel, 172 (82%) experienced AEs involving skin and the application site compared to 160 (75%) vehicle treated patients. Application site reactions (ASRs) were the most frequent AEs in both diclofenac sodium gel and vehicle treated groups. Of note, four reactions, *contact dermatitis, rash, dry skin,* and *exfoliation* (scaling) were significantly more prevalent in the diclofenac sodium gel group than in the vehicle treated patients.

Eighteen percent (18%) of diclofenac sodium gel-treated patients and 4% of vehicle-treated patients discontinued from the clinical trials due to adverse events (whether considered related to treatment or not). These discontinuations were mainly due to skin irritation or related cutaneous adverse reactions.

TABLE 4A and TABLE 4B below presents the AEs reported at an incidence of >1% for patients treated with either diclofenac sodium gel or vehicle (60-and 90 day treatment groups) during the Phase 3 studies.

***TABLE 4A** Adverse Events Reported (>1% in any Treatment Group) During Diclofenac Sodium Gel Phase 3 Clinical Trials — Incidences for 60 Day and 90 Day Treatments*

	60 Day Treatment		90 Day Treatment	
	Diclofenac Sodium Gel n=48	Vehicle n=49	Diclofenac Sodium Gel n=114	Vehicle n=114
Body as a Whole	21%	20%	20%	18%
Abdominal pain	2%	0%	1%	0%
Accidental injury	0%	0%	4%	2%
Allergic reaction	0%	0%	1%	3%
Asthenia	0%	0%	2%	0%
Back Pain	4%	0%	2%	2%
Chest Pain	2%	0%	1%	0%
Chills	0%	2%	0%	0%
Flu syndrome	10%	6%	1%	4%
Headache	0%	6%	7%	6%
Infection	4%	6%	4%	5%
Neck pain	0%	0%	2%	0%
Pain	2%	0%	2%	2%
Cardiovascular System	2%	4%	3%	1%
Hypertension	2%	0%	1%	0%
Migraine	0%	2%	1%	0%
Phlebitis	0%	2%	0%	0%
Digestive System	4%	0%	6%	8%
Constipation	0%	0%	0%	2%
Diarrhea	2%	0%	2%	3%
Dyspepsia	2%	0%	3%	4%
Metabolic and Nutritional Disorders	2%	8%	7%	2%
Creatine phosphokinase increased	0%	0%	4%	1%
Creatinine increased	2%	2%	0%	1%
Edema	0%	2%	0%	0%
Hypercholesteremia	0%	2%	1%	0%
Hyperglycemia	0%	2%	1%	0%
SGOT increased	0%	0%	3%	0%
SGPT increased	0%	0%	2%	0%
Musculoskeletal System	4%	0%	3%	4%
Arthralgia	2%	0%	0%	2%
Arthrosis	2%	0%	0%	0%
Myalgia	2%	0%	3%	1%
Nervous System	2%	2%	2%	5%
Anxiety	0%	2%	0%	1%
Dizziness	0%	0%	0%	4%
Hypokinesia	2%	0%	0%	0%

Skin and appendages adverse events reported for diclofenac sodium gel at less than 1% incidence in the Phase 3 studies: Skin hypertrophy, paresthesia, seborrhea, urticaria, application site reactions (skin carcinoma, hypertonia, skin hypertrophy lacrimation disorder, maculopapular rash, purpuric rash, vasodilation).

TABLE 4B *Adverse Events Reported (>1% in any Treatment Group) During Diclofenac Sodium Gel Phase 3 Clinical Trials — Incidences for 60 Day and 90 Day Treatments*

	60 Day Treatment		90 Day Treatment	
	Diclofenac Sodium Gel	Vehicle	Diclofenac Sodium Gel	Vehicle
	n=48	n=49	n=114	n=114
Respiratory System	8%	8%	7%	6%
Asthma	2%	0%	0%	0%
Dyspnea	2%	0%	2%	0%
Pharyngitis	2%	8%	2%	4%
Pneumonia	2%	0%	0%	1%
Rhinitis	2%	2%	2%	2%
Sinusitis	0%	0%	2%	0%
Skin and Appendages	75%	86%	86%	71%
Acne	0%	2%	0%	1%
Application site reaction	75%	71%	84%	70%
Acne	0%	4%	1%	0%
Alopecia	2%	0%	1%	1%
Contact dermatitis	19%	4%	33%	4%
Dry skin	27%	12%	25%	17%
Edema	4%	0%	3%	0%
Exfoliation	6%	4%	24%	13%
Hyperesthesia	0%	0%	3%	1%
Pain	15%	22%	26%	30%
Paresthesia	8%	4%	20%	20%
Photosensitivity reaction	0%	2%	3%	0%
Pruritus	31%	59%	52%	45%
Rash	35%	20%	46%	17%
Vesiculobullous Rash	0%	0%	4%	1%
Contact dematitis	2%	0%	0%	0%
Dry skin	0%	4%	3%	0%
Herpes simplex	0%	2%	0%	0%
Maculopapular rash	0%	2%	0%	0%
Pain	2%	2%	1%	0%
Pruritus	4%	6%	4%	1%
Rash	2%	10%	4%	0%
Skin carcinoma	0%	6%	2%	2%
Skin nodule	0%	2%	0%	0%
Skin ulcer	2%	0%	1%	0%
Special Senses	2%	0%	4%	2%
Conjuctivitis	2%	0%	4%	1%
Eye pain	0%	2%	2%	0%
Urogenital System	0%	0%	4%	5%
Hematuria	0%	0%	2%	1%
Other	0%	0%	0%	3%
Procedure	0%	0%	0%	3%

ADVERSE REACTIONS REPORTED FOR ORAL DICLOFENAC DOSAGE FORM (NOT TOPICAL DICLOFENAC SODIUM GEL)

*Incidence greater than 1% marked with asterisk.

Body as a Whole: Abdominal pain or cramps*, headache*, fluid retention*, abdominal distention*, malaise, swelling of lips and tongue, photosensitivity, anaphylaxis, anaphylactiod reactions, chest pain.

Cardiovascular: Hypertension, congestive heart failure, palpitations, flushing, tachycardia, premature ventricular contractions, myocardial infarction, hypotension.

Digestive: Diarrhea*, indigestion*, nausea*, constipation*, flatulence*, liver test abnormalities*, PUB*, *i.e.,* peptic ulcer, with or without bleeding and/or perforation, or bleeding without ulcer, vomiting, jaundice, melena, esophageal lesions, aphthous stomatitis, dry mouth and mucous membranes, bloody diarrhea, hepatitis, hepatic necrosis, cirrhosis, hepatorenal syndrome, appetite change, pancreatitis with or without concomitant hepatitis, colitis, intestinal perforation.

Hemic and Lymphatic: Hemoglobin decrease, leukopenia, thrombocytopenia, eosinophilia, hemolytic anemia, aplastic anemia, agranulocytosis, purpura, allergic purpura, bruising.

Metabolic and Nutritional Disorders: Azotemia, hypoglycemia, weight loss.

Nervous System: Dizziness*, insomnia, drowsiness, depression, diplopia, anxiety, irritability, aseptic meningitis, convulsions, paresthesia, memory disturbance, nightmares, tremor, tic, abnormal coordination, disorientation, psychotic reaction.

Respiratory: Epistaxis, asthma, laryngeal edema, dyspnea, hyperventilation, edema of pharynx.

Skin and Appendages: Rash*, pruritus*, alopecia, urticaria, eczema, dermatitis, bullous eruption, erythema multiforme major, angioedema, Stevens-Johnson syndrome, excess perspiration, exfoliative dermatitis.

Special Senses: Tinnitus*, blurred vision, taste disorder, reversible and irreversible hearing loss, scotoma, vitreous floaters, night blindness, amblyopia.

Urogenital: Nephrotic syndrome, proteinuria, oliguria, interstitial nephritis, papillary necrosis, acute renal failure, urinary frequency, nocturia, hematuria, impotence, vaginal bleeding.

DOSAGE AND ADMINISTRATION

Diclofenac sodium gel is applied to lesion areas twice daily. It is to be smoothed onto the affected skin gently. The amount needed depends upon the size of the lesion site. Assure that enough diclofenac sodium gel is applied to adequately cover each lesion. Normally 0.5 g of gel is used on each 5 cm × 5 cm lesion site. The recommended duration of therapy is from 60-90 days. Complete healing of the lesion(s) or optimal therapeutic effect may not be evident for up to 30 days following cessation of therapy. Lesions that do not respond to therapy should be carefully re-evaluated and management reconsidered.

HOW SUPPLIED

Solaraze gel is available in tubes of 25 and 50 g. Each gram of gel contains 30 mg of diclofenac sodium.

Storage: Store at controlled room temperatures: 15-30°C (59-86°F) Protect from heat. Avoid freezing.

PRODUCT LISTING - RATED THERAPEUTICALLY EQUIVALENT

Tablet - Oral - Potassium 50 mg

1's	$6.72	CATAFLAM, Pd-Rx Pharmaceuticals	55289-0818-79
15's	$30.49	CATAFLAM, Allscripts Pharmaceutical Company	54569-3823-02
20's	$37.39	CATAFLAM, Southwood Pharmaceuticals Inc	58016-0444-20
20's	$44.38	CATAFLAM, Physicians Total Care	54868-3199-02
20's	$47.43	CATAFLAM, Pharma Pac	52959-0344-20
20's	$80.71	CATAFLAM, Pd-Rx Pharmaceuticals	55289-0818-20
21's	$42.69	CATAFLAM, Allscripts Pharmaceutical Company	54569-3823-01
21's	$49.80	CATAFLAM, Pharma Pac	52959-0344-21
21's	$95.42	CATAFLAM, Pd-Rx Pharmaceuticals	55289-0818-21
25's	$54.44	CATAFLAM, Physicians Total Care	54868-3199-00
25's	$113.62	CATAFLAM, Pd-Rx Pharmaceuticals	55289-0818-25
30's	$56.08	CATAFLAM, Southwood Pharmaceuticals Inc	58016-0444-30
30's	$60.98	CATAFLAM, Allscripts Pharmaceutical Company	54569-3823-00
30's	$63.80	CATAFLAM, Pharma Pac	52959-0344-30
30's	$65.09	CATAFLAM, Physicians Total Care	54868-3199-01
40's	$74.77	CATAFLAM, Southwood Pharmaceuticals Inc	58016-0444-40
60's	$112.16	CATAFLAM, Southwood Pharmaceuticals Inc	58016-0444-60
100's	$155.19	GENERIC, Geneva Pharmaceuticals	00781-1297-01
100's	$155.19	GENERIC, Geneva Pharmaceuticals	00781-5017-01
100's	$156.55	GENERIC, Teva Pharmaceuticals Usa	00093-0948-01
100's	$156.55	GENERIC, Watson Laboratories Inc	52544-0585-01
100's	$156.60	GENERIC, Mylan Pharmaceuticals Inc	00378-2474-01
100's	$186.93	CATAFLAM, Southwood Pharmaceuticals Inc	58016-0444-00
100's	$248.58	CATAFLAM, Novartis Pharmaceuticals	00028-0151-01

Tablet - Oral - 50 mg

100's	$86.25	FEDERAL UPPER LIMIT, H.C.F.A. F F P	99999-1045-02

Tablet, Delayed Release - Oral - 50 mg

100's	$47.48	FEDERAL UPPER LIMIT, H.C.F.A. F F P	99999-1045-03

Tablet, Delayed Release - Oral - 75 mg

100's	$58.50	FEDERAL UPPER LIMIT, H.C.F.A. F F P	99999-1045-06

Tablet, Enteric Coated - Oral - Sodium 25 mg

30's	$24.25	VOLTAREN, Pharma Pac	52959-0416-30
60's	$26.58	GENERIC, Roxane Laboratories Inc	00054-4223-21
60's	$28.00	GENERIC, Geneva Pharmaceuticals	00781-1785-60
100's	$44.30	GENERIC, Roxane Laboratories Inc	00054-4223-25
100's	$46.65	GENERIC, Geneva Pharmaceuticals	00781-1285-01
100's	$46.65	GENERIC, Geneva Pharmaceuticals	00781-1785-01
100's	$47.40	GENERIC, Roxane Laboratories Inc	00054-8223-25
100's	$49.91	GENERIC, Geneva Pharmaceuticals	00781-1285-13
100's	$49.91	GENERIC, Geneva Pharmaceuticals	00781-1785-13
100's	$85.80	VOLTAREN, Novartis Pharmaceuticals	00028-0258-01

Tablet, Enteric Coated - Oral - Sodium 50 mg

10's	$14.48	GENERIC, Pd-Rx Pharmaceuticals	55289-0166-10
14's	$17.10	GENERIC, Pd-Rx Pharmaceuticals	55289-0166-14
14's	$22.73	VOLTAREN, Pd-Rx Pharmaceuticals	55289-0526-14
15's	$19.29	VOLTAREN, Allscripts Pharmaceutical Company	54569-2155-01
15's	$21.42	VOLTAREN, Prescript Pharmaceuticals	00247-0275-15
20's	$27.45	VOLTAREN, Prescript Pharmaceuticals	00247-0275-20
21's	$28.65	VOLTAREN, Prescript Pharmaceuticals	00247-0275-21
25's	$25.59	GENERIC, Pd-Rx Pharmaceuticals	55289-0166-97
28's	$52.92	VOLTAREN, Pd-Rx Pharmaceuticals	55289-0526-28
30's	$33.75	GENERIC, Pd-Rx Pharmaceuticals	55289-0166-30
30's	$38.57	VOLTAREN, Allscripts Pharmaceutical Company	54569-2155-02
30's	$39.48	VOLTAREN, Prescript Pharmaceuticals	00247-0275-30
30's	$44.42	VOLTAREN, Physicians Total Care	54868-0896-02
30's	$44.71	VOLTAREN, Pharma Pac	52959-0161-30
31 x 10	$300.61	GENERIC, Vangard Labs	00615-4506-53
32 x 10	$300.61	GENERIC, Vangard Labs	00615-4506-63
42's	$53.94	VOLTAREN, Prescript Pharmaceuticals	00247-0275-42
42's	$54.00	VOLTAREN, Allscripts Pharmaceutical Company	54569-2155-07
42's	$57.99	VOLTAREN, Pharma Pac	52959-0161-42
42's	$59.96	VOLTAREN, Pd-Rx Pharmaceuticals	55289-0526-42
60's	$51.66	GENERIC, Roxane Laboratories Inc	00054-4221-21
60's	$54.39	GENERIC, Geneva Pharmaceuticals	00781-1787-60
60's	$56.82	GENERIC, Purepac Pharmaceutical Company	00228-2550-06
60's	$56.82	GENERIC, Purepac Pharmaceutical Company	00228-2743-06
60's	$75.62	VOLTAREN, Prescript Pharmaceuticals	00247-0275-60
60's	$87.67	VOLTAREN, Physicians Total Care	54868-0896-03
90's	$111.75	VOLTAREN, Prescript Pharmaceuticals	00247-0275-90
100's	$86.13	GENERIC, Roxane Laboratories Inc	00054-4221-25
100's	$90.68	GENERIC, Geneva Pharmaceuticals	00781-1787-01
100's	$91.60	GENERIC, Teva Pharmaceuticals Usa	00093-8735-01
100's	$91.60	GENERIC, Teva Pharmaceuticals Usa	55953-0735-40
100's	$92.17	GENERIC, Roxane Laboratories Inc	00054-8221-25

Qty	Price	Product	NDC
100's	$94.57	GENERIC, Purepac Pharmaceutical Company	00228-2550-11
100's	$94.57	GENERIC, Purepac Pharmaceutical Company	00228-2743-11
100's	$97.05	GENERIC, Geneva Pharmaceuticals	00781-1287-13
100's	$97.05	GENERIC, Geneva Pharmaceuticals	00781-1787-13
100's	$100.93	GENERIC, Watson Laboratories Inc	52544-0338-01
100's	$139.57	VOLTAREN, Physicians Total Care	54868-0896-01
100's	$179.86	VOLTAREN, Novartis Pharmaceuticals	00028-0262-01
200 x 5	$969.71	GENERIC, Vangard Labs	00615-4506-43

Tablet, Enteric Coated - Oral - Sodium 75 mg

Qty	Price	Product	NDC
10's	$15.45	GENERIC, Pd-Rx Pharmaceuticals	55289-0150-10
10's	$33.42	VOLTAREN, Pd-Rx Pharmaceuticals	55289-0595-10
14's	$22.86	VOLTAREN, Pharma Pac	52959-0318-14
14's	$23.32	VOLTAREN, Allscripts Pharmaceutical Company	54569-2156-07
14's	$25.40	VOLTAREN, Prescript Pharmaceuticals	00247-0065-14
15's	$19.13	GENERIC, Pd-Rx Pharmaceuticals	55289-0150-15
15's	$24.99	VOLTAREN, Allscripts Pharmaceutical Company	54569-2156-02
15's	$26.98	VOLTAREN, Prescript Pharmaceuticals	00247-0065-15
15's	$38.10	VOLTAREN, Pd-Rx Pharmaceuticals	55289-0595-15
20's	$23.78	GENERIC, Pd-Rx Pharmaceuticals	55289-0150-20
20's	$33.32	VOLTAREN, Allscripts Pharmaceutical Company	54569-2156-03
20's	$34.86	VOLTAREN, Prescript Pharmaceuticals	00247-0065-20
20's	$35.15	VOLTAREN, Pharma Pac	52959-0318-20
20's	$49.80	VOLTAREN, Pd-Rx Pharmaceuticals	55289-0595-20
21's	$36.42	VOLTAREN, Prescript Pharmaceuticals	00247-0065-21
28's	$47.46	VOLTAREN, Prescript Pharmaceuticals	00247-0065-28
30's	$33.75	GENERIC, Pd-Rx Pharmaceuticals	55289-0150-30
30's	$49.97	VOLTAREN, Allscripts Pharmaceutical Company	54569-2156-01
30's	$50.60	VOLTAREN, Prescript Pharmaceuticals	00247-0065-30
30's	$51.47	VOLTAREN, Physicians Total Care	54868-0897-04
30's	$51.90	VOLTAREN, Pharma Pac	52959-0318-30
30's	$73.20	VOLTAREN, Pd-Rx Pharmaceuticals	55289-0595-30
31 x 10	$441.66	GENERIC, Vangard Labs	00615-4507-53
32 x 10	$441.66	GENERIC, Vangard Labs	00615-4507-63
40's	$64.52	VOLTAREN, Physicians Total Care	54868-0897-02
42's	$69.51	VOLTAREN, Prescript Pharmaceuticals	00247-0065-42
60's	$62.58	GENERIC, Roxane Laboratories Inc	00054-4222-21
60's	$62.58	GENERIC, Geneva Pharmaceuticals	00781-1789-60
60's	$65.90	GENERIC, Geneva Pharmaceuticals	00781-1289-60
60's	$66.15	GENERIC, Sidmak Laboratories Inc	50111-0547-04
60's	$68.79	GENERIC, Purepac Pharmaceutical Company	00228-2551-06
60's	$68.79	GENERIC, Purepac Pharmaceutical Company	00228-2744-06
60's	$97.85	VOLTAREN, Prescript Pharmaceuticals	00247-0065-60
90's	$145.11	VOLTAREN, Prescript Pharmaceuticals	00247-0065-90
100's	$104.31	GENERIC, Roxane Laboratories Inc	00054-4222-25
100's	$106.46	GENERIC, Geneva Pharmaceuticals	00781-1789-01
100's	$109.82	GENERIC, Ivax Corporation	00182-2619-01
100's	$109.82	GENERIC, Martec Pharmaceuticals Inc	52555-0205-01
100's	$109.85	GENERIC, Teva Pharmaceuticals Usa	00093-8737-01
100's	$111.63	GENERIC, Roxane Laboratories Inc	00054-8222-25
100's	$112.96	GENERIC, Watson/Rugby Laboratories Inc	00536-5738-01
100's	$114.47	GENERIC, Purepac Pharmaceutical Company	00228-2551-11
100's	$114.47	GENERIC, Purepac Pharmaceutical Company	00228-2744-11
100's	$114.47	GENERIC, Watson Laboratories Inc	52544-0339-01
100's	$117.53	GENERIC, Geneva Pharmaceuticals	00781-1289-13
100's	$158.93	VOLTAREN, Physicians Total Care	54868-0897-05
100's	$217.81	VOLTAREN, Novartis Pharmaceuticals	00028-0264-01
180's	$198.68	VOLTAREN, Allscripts Pharmaceutical Company	54569-8538-00
200 x 5	$1424.71	GENERIC, Vangard Labs	00615-4507-43

Tablet, Extended Release - Oral - Sodium 100 mg

Qty	Price	Product	NDC
10's	$33.67	VOLTAREN-XR, Allscripts Pharmaceutical Company	54569-4513-00
20's	$62.89	VOLTAREN-XR, Pharma Pac	52959-0472-20
100's	$281.15	GENERIC, Mylan Pharmaceuticals Inc	00378-0355-01
100's	$281.24	GENERIC, Teva Pharmaceuticals Usa	00093-1041-01
100's	$281.42	GENERIC, Geneva Pharmaceuticals	00781-1381-01
100's	$281.50	GENERIC, Purepac Pharmaceutical Company	00228-2717-11
100's	$437.13	VOLTAREN-XR, Novartis Pharmaceuticals	00028-0205-01

PRODUCT LISTING - EQUIVALENTS NOT AVAILABLE

Solution - Ophthalmic - 0.1%

Qty	Price	Product	NDC
2 ml	$31.74	VOLTAREN OPHTHALMIC, Ciba Vision Ophthalmics	58768-0100-02
2.50 ml	$28.51	VOLTAREN OPHTHALMIC, Pharma Pac	52959-0594-03
2.50 ml	$28.77	VOLTAREN OPHTHALMIC, Allscripts Pharmaceutical Company	54569-4081-00
3 ml	$31.28	VOLTAREN OPHTHALMIC, Physicians Total Care	54868-2584-02
5 ml	$34.38	VOLTAREN OPHTHALMIC, Southwood Pharmaceuticals Inc	58016-6449-01
5 ml	$35.75	GENERIC, Southwood Pharmaceuticals Inc	58016-4046-01
5 ml	$45.14	VOLTAREN OPHTHALMIC, Allscripts Pharmaceutical Company	54569-4082-00
5 ml	$48.73	VOLTAREN OPHTHALMIC, Physicians Total Care	54868-2584-01
5 ml	$51.79	VOLTAREN OPHTHALMIC, Ciba Vision Ophthalmics	58768-0100-05

Tablet - Oral - Potassium 50 mg

Qty	Price	Product	NDC
20's	$31.31	GENERIC, Allscripts Pharmaceutical Company	54569-4770-02
21's	$32.88	GENERIC, Allscripts Pharmaceutical Company	54569-4770-01
28's	$54.60	GENERIC, Pharma Pac	52959-0659-28
30's	$46.97	GENERIC, Allscripts Pharmaceutical Company	54569-4770-00
40's	$75.01	GENERIC, Pharma Pac	52959-0659-40

Tablet, Enteric Coated - Oral - Sodium 25 mg

Qty	Price	Product	NDC
30's	$14.75	GENERIC, Pharma Pac	52959-0377-30
60's	$27.00	GENERIC, Pharma Pac	52959-0377-60

Tablet, Enteric Coated - Oral - Sodium 50 mg

Qty	Price	Product	NDC
10's	$12.10	GENERIC, Southwood Pharmaceuticals Inc	58016-0381-10
14's	$20.75	GENERIC, Pharma Pac	52959-0436-14
15's	$14.19	GENERIC, Allscripts Pharmaceutical Company	54569-4165-01
15's	$18.15	GENERIC, Southwood Pharmaceuticals Inc	58016-0381-15
20's	$24.20	GENERIC, Southwood Pharmaceuticals Inc	58016-0381-20
20's	$29.50	GENERIC, Pharma Pac	52959-0436-20
28's	$41.16	GENERIC, Pharma Pac	52959-0436-28
30's	$28.37	GENERIC, Allscripts Pharmaceutical Company	54569-4165-02
30's	$36.30	GENERIC, Southwood Pharmaceuticals Inc	58016-0381-30
30's	$43.80	GENERIC, Pharma Pac	52959-0436-30
30's	$50.59	GENERIC, Alpharma Uspd Makers Of Barre and Nmc	63874-0334-30
40's	$57.55	GENERIC, Pharma Pac	52959-0436-40
60's	$54.39	GENERIC, Watson Laboratories Inc	00591-0338-60
60's	$54.39	GENERIC, Watson Laboratories Inc	52544-0338-60
60's	$56.74	GENERIC, Allscripts Pharmaceutical Company	54569-4165-03
80's	$96.80	GENERIC, Southwood Pharmaceuticals Inc	58016-0381-80
100's	$105.68	GENERIC, Alpharma Uspd Makers Of Barre and Nmc	63874-0334-01
100's	$121.00	GENERIC, Southwood Pharmaceuticals Inc	58016-0381-00

Tablet, Enteric Coated - Oral - Sodium 75 mg

Qty	Price	Product	NDC
10's	$14.70	GENERIC, Southwood Pharmaceuticals Inc	58016-0382-10
10's	$22.20	GENERIC, Pharma Pac	52959-0423-10
14's	$15.38	GENERIC, Allscripts Pharmaceutical Company	54569-4166-03
14's	$20.58	GENERIC, Southwood Pharmaceuticals Inc	58016-0382-14
14's	$22.47	GENERIC, Pharma Pac	52959-0423-14
15's	$22.05	GENERIC, Southwood Pharmaceuticals Inc	58016-0382-15
20's	$21.97	GENERIC, Allscripts Pharmaceutical Company	54569-4166-01
20's	$25.23	GENERIC, St. Mary'S Mpp	60760-0789-20
20's	$29.40	GENERIC, Southwood Pharmaceuticals Inc	58016-0382-20
20's	$31.52	GENERIC, Pharma Pac	52959-0423-20
21's	$34.15	GENERIC, Pharma Pac	52959-0423-21
28's	$35.28	GENERIC, Southwood Pharmaceuticals Inc	58016-0382-28
28's	$42.66	GENERIC, Pharma Pac	52959-0423-28
30's	$32.96	GENERIC, Allscripts Pharmaceutical Company	54569-4166-02
30's	$44.10	GENERIC, Southwood Pharmaceuticals Inc	58016-0382-30
30's	$45.61	GENERIC, Pharma Pac	52959-0423-30
30's	$60.17	GENERIC, Alpharma Uspd Makers Of Barre and Nmc	63874-0426-30
40's	$50.40	GENERIC, Southwood Pharmaceuticals Inc	58016-0382-40
60's	$58.85	GENERIC, Pharma Pac	52959-0423-60
60's	$68.54	GENERIC, Watson Laboratories Inc	52544-0339-60
60's	$78.07	GENERIC, St. Mary'S Mpp	60760-0789-60
60's	$88.20	GENERIC, Southwood Pharmaceuticals Inc	58016-0382-60
80's	$117.60	GENERIC, Southwood Pharmaceuticals Inc	58016-0382-80
90's	$113.40	GENERIC, Southwood Pharmaceuticals Inc	58016-0382-90
100's	$114.47	GENERIC, Watson Laboratories Inc	00591-0339-01
100's	$136.21	GENERIC, Alpharma Uspd Makers Of Barre and Nmc	63874-0426-01
100's	$147.00	GENERIC, Southwood Pharmaceuticals Inc	58016-0382-00

Tablet, Extended Release - Oral - Sodium 100 mg

Qty	Price	Product	NDC
10's	$31.23	GENERIC, Southwood Pharmaceuticals Inc	58016-0489-10
14's	$43.72	GENERIC, Southwood Pharmaceuticals Inc	58016-0489-14
15's	$46.84	GENERIC, Southwood Pharmaceuticals Inc	58016-0489-15
20's	$62.45	GENERIC, Southwood Pharmaceuticals Inc	58016-0489-20
21's	$65.57	GENERIC, Southwood Pharmaceuticals Inc	58016-0489-21
30's	$93.68	GENERIC, Southwood Pharmaceuticals Inc	58016-0489-30
40's	$124.90	GENERIC, Southwood Pharmaceuticals Inc	58016-0489-40
50's	$156.13	GENERIC, Southwood Pharmaceuticals Inc	58016-0489-50
60's	$187.35	GENERIC, Southwood Pharmaceuticals Inc	58016-0489-60
90's	$281.02	GENERIC, Southwood Pharmaceuticals Inc	58016-0489-90
100's	$312.25	GENERIC, Southwood Pharmaceuticals Inc	58016-0489-00

Diclofenac Sodium; Misoprostol (003382)

For related information, see the comparative table section in Appendix A.

Categories: Arthritis, osteoarthritis; Arthritis, rheumatoid; Pregnancy Category X
Drug Classes: Analgesics, non-narcotic; Gastrointestinals; Nonsteroidal anti-inflammatory drugs; Prostaglandins
Brand Names: Arthrotec
Foreign Brand Availability: Arthrotec 50 (Australia); Artotec (France; Russia); Artrotec (Costa-Rica; Dominican-Republic; El-Salvador; Guatemala; Honduras; Mexico; Nicaragua; Panama; Peru)
Cost of Therapy: $154.26 (Osteoarthritis; Arthotec; 50 mg; 200 µg; 3 tablets/day; 30 day supply)

WARNING

This drug, because of the abortifacient property of the misoprostol component, is contraindicated in women who are pregnant. (See PRECAUTIONS.) Reports, primarily from Brazil, of congenital anomalies and reports of fetal death subsequent to misuse of misoprostol alone, as an abortifacient, have been received. Patients must be advised of the abortifacient property and warned not to give the drug to others. This drug should not be used in women of childbearing potential unless the patient requires nonsteroidal anti-inflammatory drug (NSAID) therapy and is at high risk of developing gastric or duodenal ulceration or for developing complications from gastric or duodenal ulcers associated with the use of the NSAID. (See WARNINGS.) In such patients, diclofenac sodium; misoprostol may be prescribed if the patient:

- **Has had a negative serum pregnancy test within 2 weeks prior to beginning therapy.**
- **Is capable of complying with effective contraceptive measures.**
- **Has received both oral and written warnings of the hazards of misoprostol, the risk of possible contraception failure, and the danger to other women of childbearing potential should the drug be taken by mistake.**
- **Will begin diclofenac sodium; misoprostol only on the second or third day of the next normal menstrual period.**

DESCRIPTION

Arthrotec is a combination product containing diclofenac sodium, a nonsteroidal anti-inflammatory drug (NSAID) with analgesic properties, and misoprostol, a gastrointestinal (GI) mucosal protective prostaglandin E_1 analog. Arthrotec oral tablets are white to off-white, round, biconvex and approximately 11 mm in diameter. Each tablet consists of an enteric-coated core containing 50 mg (Arthrotec 50) or 75 mg (Arthrotec 75) diclofenac sodium surrounded by an outer mantle containing 200 µg misoprostol.

Diclofenac sodium is a phenylacetic acid derivative that is a white to off-white, virtually odorless, crystalline powder. Diclofenac sodium is freely soluble in methanol, soluble in ethanol and practically insoluble in chloroform and in dilute acid. Diclofenac sodium is sparingly soluble in water. Its chemical formula and name are:

$C_{14}H_{10}Cl_2NO_2Na$ [M.W. = 318.14] 2-[(2,6-dichlorophenyl) amino]benzeneacetic acid, monosodium salt.

Misoprostol is a water-soluble, viscous liquid that contains approximately equal amounts of two diastereomers. Its chemical formula and name are: $C_{22}H_{38}O_5$ [M.W. = 382.54] (±)methyl 11α,16-dihydroxy-16-methyl-9-oxoprost-13E-en-1-oate.

Inactive ingredients in Arthrotec include: colloidal silicon dioxide; crospovidone; hydrogenated castor oil; hydroxypropyl methylcellulose; lactose; magnesium stearate; methacrylic acid copolymer; microcrystalline cellulose; povidone (polyvidone) K-30; sodium hydroxide; starch (corn); talc; triethyl citrate.

CLINICAL PHARMACOLOGY

PHARMACODYNAMICS AND PHARMACOKINETICS OF DICLOFENAC SODIUM

Diclofenac sodium is a nonsteroidal anti-inflammatory drug (NSAID). In pharmacologic studies, diclofenac sodium has shown anti-inflammatory, analgesic and antipyretic properties. The mechanism of action of diclofenac sodium, like other NSAIDs, is not completely understood but may be related to prostaglandin synthetase inhibition.

Diclofenac sodium is completely absorbed from the GI tract after fasting, oral administration. The diclofenac sodium in diclofenac sodium; misoprostol is in a pharmaceutical formulation that resists dissolution in the low pH of gastric fluid but allows a rapid release of drug in the higher pH environment of the duodenum. Only 50% of the absorbed dose is systemically available due to first pass metabolism. Peak plasma levels are achieved in 2 hours (range 1-4 hours), and the area under the plasma concentration curve (AUC) is dose proportional within the range of 25 mg to 150 mg. Peak plasma levels are less than dose proportional and are approximately 1.5 and 2.0 µg/ml for 50 mg and 75 mg doses, respectively.

Plasma concentrations of diclofenac sodium decline from peak levels in a biexponential fashion, with the terminal phase having a half-life of approximately 2 hours. Clearance and volume of distribution are about 350 ml/min and 550 ml/kg, respectively. More than 99% of diclofenac sodium is reversibly bound to human plasma albumin.

Diclofenac sodium is eliminated through metabolism and subsequent urinary and biliary excretion of the glucuronide and the sulfate conjugates of the metabolites. Approximately 65% of the dose is excreted in the urine and 35% in the bile.

Conjugates of unchanged diclofenac account for 5-10% of the dose excreted in the urine and for less than 5% excreted in the bile. Little or no unchanged unconjugated drug is excreted. Conjugates of the principal metabolite account for 20-30% of the dose excreted in the urine and for 10-20% of the dose excreted in the bile.

Conjugates of three other metabolites together account for 10-20% of the dose excreted in the urine and for small amounts excreted in the bile. The elimination half-life values for these metabolites are shorter than those for the parent drug. Urinary excretion of an additional metabolite (half-life = 80 hours) accounts for only 1.4% of the oral dose. The degree of accumulation of diclofenac metabolites is unknown. Some of the metabolites may have activity.

PHARMACODYNAMICS AND PHARMACOKINETICS OF MISOPROSTOL

Misoprostol is a synthetic prostaglandin E_1 analog with gastric antisecretory and (in animals) mucosal protective properties. NSAIDs inhibit prostaglandin synthesis. A deficiency of prostaglandins within the gastric and duodenal mucosa may lead to diminishing bicarbonate and mucus secretion and may contribute to the mucosal damage caused by NSAIDs.

Misoprostol can increase bicarbonate and mucus production, but in humans this has been shown at doses 200 µg and above that are also antisecretory. It is therefore not possible to tell whether the ability of misoprostol to prevent gastric and duodenal ulcers is the result of its antisecretory effect, its mucosal protective effect, or both.

In vitro studies on canine parietal cells using tritiated misoprostol acid as the ligand have led to the identification and characterization of specific prostaglandin receptors. Receptor binding is saturable, reversible, and stereospecific. The sites have a high affinity for misoprostol, for its acid metabolite, and for other E type prostaglandins, but not for F or I prostaglandins and other unrelated compounds, such as histamine or cimetidine. Receptor-site affinity for misoprostol correlates well with an indirect index of antisecretory activity. It is likely that these specific receptors allow misoprostol taken with food to be effective topically, despite the lower serum concentrations attained.

Misoprostol produces a moderate decrease in pepsin concentration during basal conditions, but not during histamine stimulation. It has no significant effect on fasting or postprandial gastrin nor intrinsic factor output.

Effects on Gastric Acid Secretion: Misoprostol, over the range of 50-200 µg, inhibits basal and nocturnal gastric acid secretion, and acid secretion in response to a variety of stimuli, including meals, histamine, pentagastrin, and coffee. Activity is apparent 30 minutes after oral administration and persists for at least 3 hours. In general, the effects of 50 µg were modest and shorter lived, and only the 200 µg dose had substantial effects on nocturnal secretion or on histamine- and meal-stimulated secretion.

Orally administered misoprostol is rapidly and extensively absorbed, and it undergoes rapid metabolism to its biologically active metabolite, misoprostol acid. Misoprostol acid in diclofenac sodium; misoprostol reaches a maximum plasma concentration in about 20 minutes and is, thereafter, quickly eliminated with an elimination $T_{1/2}$ of about 30 minutes. There is high variability in plasma levels of misoprostol acid between and within studies, but mean values after single doses show a linear relationship with dose of misoprostol over the range of 200 to 400 µg. No accumulation of misoprostol acid was found in multiple-dose studies, and plasma steady state was achieved within 2 days. The serum protein binding of misoprostol acid is less than 90% and is concentration-independent in the therapeutic range.

After oral administration of radiolabeled misoprostol, about 70% of detected radioactivity appears in the urine. Maximum plasma concentrations of misoprostol acid are diminished when the dose is taken with food, and total availability of misoprostol acid is reduced by use of concomitant antacid. Clinical trials were conducted with concomitant antacid; this effect does not appear to be clinically important.

Pharmacokinetic studies also showed a lack of drug interaction with antipyrine or propranolol given with misoprostol. Misoprostol given for 1 week had no effect on the steady state pharmacokinetics of diazepam when the two drugs were administered 2 hours apart.

PHARMACOKINETICS OF DICLOFENAC SODIUM; MISOPROSTOL

The pharmacokinetics following oral administration of a single dose (see TABLE 1A) or multiple doses of diclofenac sodium; misoprostol to healthy subjects under fasted conditions are similar to the pharmacokinetics of the two individual components.

TABLE 1A *Misoprostol Acid Mean (SD)*

Treatment (n=36)	C_{max} (pg/ml)	T_{max} (h)	AUC(0-4h) (pg·h/ml)
Diclofenac Sodium; Misoprostol 50	441 (137)	0.30 (0.13)	266 (95)
Cytotec	478 (201)	0.30 (0.10)	295 (143)
Diclofenac Sodium; Misoprostol 75	304 (110)	0.26 (0.09)	177 (49)
Cytotec	290 (130)	0.35 (0.12)	176 (58)

SD = Standard deviation of the mean
AUC = Area under the curve
C_{max} = Peak concentration
T_{max} = Time to peak concentration

TABLE 1B *Diclofenac Mean (SD)*

Treatment (n=36)	C_{max} (ng/ml)	T_{max} (h)	AUC(0-4h) (ng·h/ml)
Diclofenac Sodium; Misoprostol 50	1207 (364)	2.4 (1.0)	1380 (272)
Voltaren	1298 (441)	2.4 (1.0)	1357 (290)
Diclofenac Sodium; Misoprostol 75	2025 (2005)	2.0 (1.4)	2773 (1347)
Voltaren	2367 (1318)	1.9 (0.7)	2609 (1185)

SD = Standard deviation of the mean
AUC = Area under the curve
C_{max} = Peak concentration
T_{max} = Time to peak concentration

The rate and extent of absorption of both diclofenac sodium and misoprostol acid from diclofenac sodium; misoprostol 50 and diclofenac sodium; misoprostol 75 are similar to those from diclofenac sodium and misoprostol formulations each administered alone.

Neither diclofenac sodium nor misoprostol acid accumulated in plasma following repeated doses of diclofenac sodium; misoprostol given every 12 hours under fasted conditions. Food decreases the multiple-dose bioavailability profile of diclofenac sodium; misoprostol 50 and diclofenac sodium; misoprostol 75.

D

SPECIAL POPULATIONS

A 4 week study, comparing plasma level profiles of diclofenac (50 mg bid) in younger (26-46 years) versus older (66-81 years) adults, did not show differences between age groups (10 patients per age group). In a multiple-dose (bid) crossover study of 24 people aged 65 years or older, the misoprostol contained in diclofenac sodium; misoprostol did not affect the pharmacokinetics of diclofenac sodium.

Differences in the pharmacokinetics of diclofenac have not been detected in studies of patients with renal (50 mg intravenously) or hepatic impairment (100 mg oral solution). In patients with renal impairment (n=5; creatinine clearance 3-42 ml/min), AUC values and elimination rates were comparable to those in healthy people. In patients with biopsy-confirmed cirrhosis or chronic active hepatitis (variably elevated transaminases and mildly elevated bilirubins, n=10), diclofenac concentrations and urinary elimination values were comparable to those in healthy people.

Pharmacokinetic studies with misoprostol in patients with varying degrees of renal impairment showed an approximate doubling of $T_{½max}$ and AUC compared to healthy people. In people over 64 years of age, the AUC for misoprostol acid is increased.

Misoprostol does not affect the hepatic mixed function oxidase (cytochrome P-450) enzyme system in animals. In a study of people with mild to moderate hepatic impairment, mean misoprostol acid AUC and C_{max} showed approximately double the mean values obtained in healthy people. Three people who had the lowest antipyrine and lowest indocyanine green clearance values had the highest misoprostol acid AUC and C_{max} values.

INDICATIONS AND USAGE

Diclofenac sodium; misoprostol is indicated for treatment of the signs and symptoms of osteoarthritis or rheumatoid arthritis in patients at high risk of developing NSAID-induced gastric and duodenal ulcers and their complications. See WARNINGS, Gastrointestinal (GI) Effects — Risk Of GI Ulceration, Bleeding and Perforation for a list of factors that may increase the risk of NSAID-induced gastric and duodenal ulcers and their complications.

CONTRAINDICATIONS

See BOXED WARNING related to misoprostol.

Diclofenac sodium; misoprostol is contraindicated in patients with hypersensitivity to diclofenac or to misoprostol or other prostaglandins. Diclofenac sodium; misoprostol should not be given to patients who have experienced asthma, urticaria, or other allergic-type reactions after taking aspirin or other NSAIDs. Severe, rarely fatal, anaphylactic-like reactions to diclofenac sodium have been reported.

WARNINGS

MISOPROSTOL

See BOXED WARNING.

DICLOFENAC

Gastrointestinal (GI) Effects — Risk Of GI Ulceration, Bleeding and Perforation

Serious GI toxicity, such as inflammation, bleeding, ulceration and perforation of the stomach, small intestine or large intestine, can occur at any time, with or without warning symptoms, in patients treated with NSAIDs. Minor upper GI problems, such as dyspepsia, are common and may also occur at any time during NSAID therapy. Therefore, physicians and patients should remain alert for ulceration and bleeding, even in the absence of previous GI tract symptoms. Patients should be informed about the signs and/or symptoms and the steps to take if they occur. The utility of periodic laboratory monitoring has not been demonstrated; nor has it been adequately assessed. Only 1 in 5 patients who develop a serious upper GI adverse event on NSAID therapy is symptomatic. It has been demonstrated that upper GI ulcers, gross bleeding, or perforation, caused by NSAIDs, appear to occur in approximately 1% of patients treated for 3-6 months, and in 2-4% of patients treated for 1 year. These trends continue thus, increasing the likelihood of developing a serious GI event at some time during the course of therapy. However, even short-term therapy has risk.

NSAIDs should be prescribed with extreme caution in those with a prior history of ulcer disease or GI bleeding. Most spontaneous reports of fatal GI events are in elderly or debilitated patients and therefore special care should be taken in treating this population. **To minimize the potential risk for an adverse event, the lowest effective dose should be used for the shortest possible duration.** For very highrisk patients, alternate therapies that do not involve NSAIDs should be considered.

Studies have shown that patients with a history of peptic ulcer disease and/or GI bleeding, and who use NSAIDs, have a greater than 10-fold risk for developing a GI bleed than patients with neither of these risk factors. In addition to a past history of ulcer disease, pharmacoepidemiological studies have identified several other conditions or co-therapies that may increase the risk for GI bleeding, such as: treatment with oral corticosteroids, treatment with anticoagulants, longer duration of NSAID therapy, older age, smoking, alcoholism, poor general health and *Helicobacter pylori* positive status.

Hepatic Effects

Elevations of one or more liver tests may occur during diclofenac sodium; misoprostol therapy. These laboratory abnormalities may progress, may remain unchanged, or may be transient with continued therapy. Borderline elevations (*i.e.,* less than 3 times the ULN [ULN=the upper limit of the normal range]), or greater elevations of transaminases occurred in about 15% of diclofenac-treated patients. Of the hepatic enzymes, ALT (SGPT) is the one recommended for the monitoring of liver injury.

In clinical trials, meaningful elevations (ie, more than 3 times the ULN) of AST (SGOT) (ALT was not measured in all studies) occurred in about 2% of approximately 5700 patients at some time during diclofenac treatment. In a large, open, controlled trial, meaningful elevations of ALT and/or AST occurred in about 4% of 3700 patients treated for 2-6 months, including marked elevations (*i.e.,* more than 8 times the ULN) in about 1% of the 3700 patients. In that open-label study, a higher incidence of borderline (less than 3 times the ULN), moderate (3-8 times the ULN), and marked (>8 times the ULN) elevations of ALT or AST was observed in patients receiving diclofenac when compared to other NSAIDs. Transaminase elevations were seen more frequently in patients with osteoarthritis than in those with rheumatoid arthritis.

In addition to enzyme elevations seen in clinical trials, postmarketing surveillance has found rare cases of severe hepatic reactions, including liver necrosis, jaundice, and fulminant fatal hepatitis with and without jaundice. Some of these rare reported cases underwent liver transplantation.

Physicians should measure transaminases periodically in patients receiving long-term therapy with diclofenac, because severe hepatotoxicity may develop without a prodrome of distinguishing symptoms. The optimum times for making the first and subsequent transaminase measurements are not known. In the largest US trial (open-label) that involved 3700 patients monitored first at 8 weeks and 1200 patients monitored again at 24 weeks, almost all meaningful elevations in transaminases were detected before patients became symptomatic. In 42 of the 51 patients in all trials who developed marked transaminase elevations, abnormal tests occurred during the first 2 months of therapy with diclofenac. Postmarketing experience has shown severe hepatic reactions can occur at any time during treatment with diclofenac. Cases of drug-induced hepatotoxicity have been reported in the first month, and in some cases, the first 2 months of therapy. Based on these experiences, transaminases should be monitored within 4 to 8 weeks after initiating treatment with diclofenac (see PRECAUTIONS, Laboratory Tests).

In clinical trials with diclofenac sodium; misoprostol, meaningful elevation of ALT (SGPT, more than 3 times the ULN) occurred in 1.6% of 2184 patients treated with diclofenac sodium; misoprostol and in 1.4% of 1691 patients treated with diclofenac sodium. These increases were generally transient, and enzyme levels returned to within the normal range upon discontinuation of diclofenac sodium; misoprostol therapy. The misoprostol component of diclofenac sodium; misoprostol does not appear to exacerbate the hepatic effects caused by the diclofenac sodium component. As with other NSAID containing products, if abnormal liver tests persist or worsen, if clinical signs and/or symptoms consistent with liver disease develop, or if systemic manifestations occur (*e.g.,* eosinophilia, rash, etc.), diclofenac sodium; misoprostol should be discontinued immediately.

To minimize the possibility that hepatic injury will become severe between transaminase measurements, physicians should inform patients of the warning signs and symptoms of hepatotoxicity (*e.g.,* nausea, fatigue, lethargy, pruritus, jaundice, right upper quadrant tenderness, and "flu-like" symptoms), and the appropriate action patients should take if these signs and symptoms appear.

Anaphylactoid Reactions

As with other NSAID containing products, anaphylactoid reactions may occur in patients without known prior exposure to diclofenac sodium; misoprostol or its components. Diclofenac sodium; misoprostol should not be given to patients with the aspirin triad. The triad typically occurs in asthmatic patients who experience rhinitis with or without nasal polyps, or who exhibit severe, potentially fatal bronchospasm after taking aspirin or other NSAIDs (see CONTRAINDICATIONS and PRECAUTIONS, General, Preexisting Asthma). Emergency help should be sought in cases where an anaphylactoid reaction occurs. Allergic reactions have been reported by less than 0.1% of patients who received diclofenac sodium; misoprostol in clinical trials, and there have been rare reports of anaphylaxis in the marketed use of diclofenac sodium; misoprostol outside of the United States.

Advanced Renal Disease

In patients with advanced kidney disease, treatment with diclofenac sodium; misoprostol is not recommended. If NSAID therapy must be initiated however, close monitoring of the patient's kidney function is advisable (see PRECAUTIONS, General, Renal Effects).

PRECAUTIONS

GENERAL

Diclofenac sodium; misoprostol cannot be used to substitute for corticosteroids or to treat for corticosteroid insufficiency. Abrupt discontinuation of corticosteroids may lead to disease exacerbation. Patients on prolonged corticosteroid therapy should have their therapy tapered slowly if a decision is made to discontinue corticosteroids.

The pharmacological activity of diclofenac sodium; misoprostol in reducing inflammation may diminish the utility of this diagnostic sign in detecting complications of presumed noninfectious, painful conditions.

Renal Effects

Caution should be used when initiating treatment with diclofenac sodium; misoprostol in patients with considerable dehydration. It is advisable to rehydrate patients first and then start therapy with diclofenac sodium; misoprostol. Caution is also recommended in patients with preexisting kidney disease (see WARNINGS, Advanced Renal Disease).

As with other NSAIDs, long-term administration of diclofenac has resulted in renal papillary necrosis and other renal medullary changes. Renal toxicity has also been seen in patients in which renal prostaglandins have a compensatory role in the maintenance of renal perfusion. In these patients, administration of an NSAID may cause a dose-dependent reduction in prostaglandin formation and, secondarily, in renal blood flow, which may precipitate overt renal decompensation. Patients at greatest risk of this reaction are those with impaired renal function, heart failure, or liver dysfunction, those taking diuretics and ACE inhibitors, and the elderly. Discontinuation of NSAID therapy is usually followed by recovery to the pretreatment state.

Diclofenac metabolites are eliminated primarily by the kidneys. The extent to which the metabolites may accumulate in patients with renal failure has not been studied. As with other NSAIDs, metabolites of which are excreted by the kidney, patients with significantly impaired renal function should be more closely monitored.

Hematologic Effects

Anemia is sometimes seen in patients receiving diclofenac or other NSAIDs. This may be due to fluid retention, GI blood loss, or an incompletely described effect upon erythropoiesis. Patients on long-term treatment with NSAIDs, including diclofenac sodium; misoprostol, should have their hemoglobin or hematocrit checked if they exhibit any signs or symptoms of anemia.

All drugs that inhibit the biosynthesis of prostaglandins may interfere to some extent with platelet function and vascular responses to bleeding.

NSAIDs inhibit platelet aggregation and, unlike aspirin, their effect on platelet function is reversible, quantitatively less, and of shorter duration. Diclofenac sodium; misoprostol does not generally affect platelet counts, prothrombin time (PT), or partial thromboplastin time (PTT). Patients receiving diclofenac sodium; misoprostol who may be adversely affected by alterations in platelet function, such as those with coagulation disorders or patients receiving anticoagulants, should be carefully monitored.

Aseptic Meningitis

As with other NSAIDs, aseptic meningitis with fever and coma has been observed on rare occasions in patients on diclofenac therapy. Although it is probably more likely to occur in patients with systemic lupus and related connective tissue diseases, it has been reported in patients who do not have an underlying chronic disease. If signs or symptoms of meningitis develop in a patient on diclofenac, the possibility of its being related to diclofenac should be considered.

Fluid Retention and Edema

Fluid retention and edema have been observed in some patients taking NSAID containing products, including diclofenac sodium; misoprostol. Therefore, as with other NSAID containing products, diclofenac sodium; misoprostol should be used with caution in patients with a history of cardiac decompensation, hypertension, or other conditions predisposing to fluid retention.

Preexisting Asthma

Patients with asthma may have aspirin-sensitive asthma. The use of aspirin in patients with aspirin-sensitive asthma has been associated with severe bronchospasm, which can be fatal. Since cross-reactivity, including bronchospasm, between aspirin and other NSAIDs has been reported in such aspirin-sensitive patients, diclofenac sodium; misoprostol should not be administered to patients with this form of aspirin sensitivity and should be used with caution in patients with preexisting asthma.

Porphyria

The use of diclofenac sodium; misoprostol in patients with hepatic porphyria should be avoided. To date, 1 patient has been described in whom diclofenac sodium probably triggered a clinical attack of porphyria. The postulated mechanism, demonstrated in rats, for causing such attacks by diclofenac sodium, as well as some other NSAIDs, is through stimulation of the porphyrin precursor delta-aminolevulinic acid (ALA).

INFORMATION FOR THE PATIENT

See the Patient Instructions that are distributed with the prescription.

Diclofenac sodium; misoprostol is available only as a unit-of-use package that includes a leaflet containing patient information. The patient should read the leaflet before taking diclofenac sodium; misoprostol and each time the prescription is renewed because the leaflet may have been revised. Keep diclofenac sodium; misoprostol out of the reach of children.

LABORATORY TESTS

Patients on long-term treatment with NSAIDs should have their CBC and a chemistry profile checked periodically. If clinical signs and symptoms consistent with liver or renal disease develop, systemic manifestations occur (*e.g.*, eosinophilia, rash, etc) or if abnormal liver tests persist or worsen, diclofenac sodium; misoprostol should be discontinued.

Effect on Blood Coagulation

Diclofenac sodium impairs platelet aggregation but does not affect bleeding time, plasma thrombin clotting time, plasma fibrinogen, or factors V and VII to XII. Statistically significant changes in prothrombin and partial thromboplastin times have been reported in normal volunteers. The mean changes were observed to be less than 1 second in both instances, however, and are unlikely to be clinically important. Diclofenac sodium is a prostaglandin synthetase inhibitor, however, and all drugs that inhibit prostaglandin synthesis interfere with platelet function to some degree; therefore, patients who may be adversely affected by such an action should be carefully observed. Misoprostol has not been shown to exacerbate the effects of diclofenac on platelet activity.

CARCINOGENESIS, MUTAGENESIS, AND IMPAIRMENT OF FERTILITY

Long-term animal studies to evaluate the potential for carcinogenesis and animal studies to evaluate the effects on fertility have been performed with each component of diclofenac sodium; misoprostol given alone. Diclofenac sodium; misoprostol itself (diclofenac sodium and misoprostol combinations in 250:1 ratio) was not genotoxic in the Ames test, the Chinese hamster ovary cell (CHO/HGPRT) forward mutation test, the rat lymphocyte chromosome aberration test or the mouse micronucleus test.

In a 24 month rat carcinogenicity study, oral misoprostol at doses up to 2.4 mg/kg/day (14.4 mg/m^2/day, 24 times the recommended maximum human dose of 0.6 mg/m^2/day) was not tumorigenic. In a 21 month mouse carcinogenicity study, oral misoprostol at doses up to 16 mg/kg/day (48 mg/m^2/day), 80 times the recommended maximum human dose based on body surface area, was not tumorigenic. Misoprostol, when administered to male and female breeding rats in an oral dose-range of 0.1 to 10 mg/kg/day (0.6 to 60 mg/m^2/day, 1 to 100 times the recommended maximum human dose based on body surface area) produced dose-related pre- and post-implantation losses and a significant decrease in the number of live pups born at the highest dose. These findings suggest the possibility of a general adverse effect on fertility in males and females.

In a 24 month rat carcinogenicity study, oral diclofenac sodium up to 2 mg/kg/day (12 mg/m^2/day) was not tumorigenic. For a 50-kg person of average height (1.46m^2 body surface area), this dose represents 0.08 times the recommended maximum human dose (148 mg/m^2) on a body surface area basis. In a 24 month mouse carcinogenicity study, oral diclofenac sodium at doses up to 0.3 mg/kg/day (0.9 mg/m^2/day, 0.006 times the recommended maximum human dose based on body surface area) in males and 1 mg/kg/day (3 mg/m^2/day, 0.02 times the recommended maximum human dose based on body surface area) in females was not tumorigenic. Diclofenac sodium at oral doses up to 4 mg/kg/day (24 mg/m^2/day, 0.16 times the recommended maximum human dose based on body surface area) was found to have no effect on fertility and reproductive performance of male and female rats.

PREGNANCY CATEGORY X

See BOXED WARNING regarding misoprostol. Diclofenac sodium; misoprostol is contraindicated in pregnancy.

NONTERATOGENIC EFFECTS

Misoprostol may endanger pregnancy (may cause miscarriage) and thereby cause harm to the fetus when administered to a pregnant woman. Misoprostol produces uterine contractions, uterine bleeding, and expulsion of the products of conception. Miscarriages caused by misoprostol may be incomplete. In studies in women undergoing elective termination of pregnancy during the first trimester, misoprostol caused partial or complete expulsion of the products of conception in 11% of the subjects and increased uterine bleeding in 41%.

Reports, primarily from Brazil, of congenital anomalies and reports of fetal death subsequent to misuse of misoprostol alone, as an abortifacient, have been received (see BOXED WARNING). If a woman is or becomes pregnant while taking this drug, the drug should be discontinued and the patient apprised of the potential hazard to the fetus.

The diclofenac sodium component of diclofenac sodium; misoprostol, like other NSAIDs which are prostaglandin-inhibiting drugs, may affect the fetal cardiovascular system causing premature closure of the ductus arteriosus. NSAIDs may also inhibit uterine contractions.

TERATOGENIC EFFECTS

An oral teratology study has been performed in pregnant rabbits at dose combinations (250:1 ratio) up to 10 mg/kg/day diclofenac sodium (120 mg/m^2/day, 0.8 times the recommended maximum human dose based on body surface area) and 0.04 mg/kg/day misoprostol (0.48 mg/m^2/day, 0.8 times the recommended maximum human dose based on body surface area) and has revealed no evidence of teratogenic potential for diclofenac sodium; misoprostol.

Oral teratology studies have been performed in pregnant rats at doses up to 1.6 mg/kg/day (9.6 mg/m^2/day, 16 times the recommended maximum human dose based on body surface area) and pregnant rabbits at doses up to 1.0 mg/kg/day (12 mg/m^2/day, 20 times the recommended maximum human dose based on body surface area) and have revealed no evidence of teratogenic potential for misoprostol.

Oral teratology studies have been performed in pregnant mice at doses up to 20 mg/kg/day (60 mg/m^2/day, 0.4 times the recommended maximum human dose based on body surface area), pregnant rats at doses up to 10 mg/kg/day (60 mg/m^2/day, 0.4 times the recommended maximum human dose based on body surface area) and pregnant rabbits at doses up to 10 mg/kg/day (120 mg/m^2/day, 0.8 times the recommended maximum human dose based on body surface area) and have revealed no evidence of teratogenic potential for diclofenac sodium.

NURSING MOTHERS

Diclofenac sodium has been found in the milk of nursing mothers. It is unlikely that misoprostol is excreted into milk since the drug is rapidly metabolized throughout the body. Excretion of the active metabolite (misoprostol acid) into milk is possible, but has not been studied. Because of the potential for serious adverse reactions in nursing infants, diclofenac sodium; misoprostol is not recommended for use by nursing mothers.

PEDIATRIC USE

Safety and efficacy of diclofenac sodium; misoprostol in patients below the age of 18 years have not been established.

GERIATRIC USE

Approximately 1800 patients treated with diclofenac in US trials and 500 patients treated with diclofenac sodium; misoprostol in multinational trials were older than 65 years of age. No overall differences were observed between efficacy, adverse events or pharmacokinetic profiles of older and younger patients. However, as with any NSAID, the elderly are likely to tolerate adverse events less well than younger patients.

DRUG INTERACTIONS

Aspirin: Concomitant administration of diclofenac sodium; misoprostol and aspirin is not recommended because diclofenac sodium is displaced from its binding sites by aspirin, resulting in lower plasma concentrations, peak plasma levels and AUC values.

Digoxin: Elevated digoxin levels have been reported in patients receiving digoxin and diclofenac sodium. Patients receiving digoxin and diclofenac sodium; misoprostol should be monitored for possible digoxin toxicity.

Antihypertensive Agents: NSAIDs can inhibit the activity of antihypertensives, including ACE inhibitors. Thus, caution should be taken when administering diclofenac sodium; misoprostol with such agents.

Warfarin: The effects of warfarin and NSAIDs on GI bleeding are synergistic, such that users of both drugs together have a risk of serious bleeding greater than users of either drug alone.

Oral Hypoglycemics: Diclofenac sodium does not alter glucose metabolism in healthy people nor does it alter the effects of oral hypoglycemic agents. There are rare reports, however, from marketing experience, of changes in effects of insulin or oral hypoglycemic agents in the presence of diclofenac sodium that necessitated change in the doses of such agents. Both hypo- and hyperglycemic effects have been reported. A direct causal relationship has not been established, but physicians should consider the possibility that diclofenac sodium may alter a diabetic patient's response to insulin or oral hypoglycemic agents.

Methotrexate And Cyclosporine: Diclofenac sodium; misoprostol, like other NSAID containing products, may affect renal prostaglandins and increase the toxicity of certain drugs. Ingestion of diclofenac sodium; misoprostol may increase serum concentrations of methotrexate and increase cyclosporine nephrotoxicity. Patients who begin taking diclofenac sodium; misoprostol or who increase their dose of diclofenac sodium; misoprostol or any other NSAID containing product while taking

D

methotrexate or cyclosporine may develop toxicity characteristic for these drugs. They should be observed closely, particularly if renal function is impaired.

Lithium: NSAIDs have produced an elevation of plasma lithium levels and a reduction in renal lithium clearance. The mean minimum lithium concentration increased 15% and the renal clearance was decreased by approximately 20%. These effects have been attributed to inhibition of renal prostaglandin synthesis by the NSAID. Thus, when NSAIDs and lithium are administered concurrently, subjects should be observed carefully for signs of lithium toxicity.

Antacids: Antacids reduce the bioavailability of misoprostol acid. Antacids may also delay absorption of diclofenac sodium. Magnesium-containing antacids exacerbate misoprostol-associated diarrhea. Thus, it is not recommended that diclofenac sodium; misoprostol be coadministered with magnesium-containing antacids.

Diuretics: The diclofenac sodium component of diclofenac sodium; misoprostol, like other NSAIDs, can inhibit the activity of diuretics. Concomitant therapy with potassium-sparing diuretics may be associated with increased serum potassium levels.

Other Drugs: In small groups of patients (7-10 patients/interaction study), the concomitant administration of azathioprine, gold, chloroquine, D-penicillamine, prednisolone, doxycycline or digitoxin did not significantly affect the peak levels and AUC levels of diclofenac sodium. Phenobarbital toxicity has been reported to have occurred in a patient on chronic phenobarbital treatment following the initiation of diclofenac therapy. *In vitro,* diclofenac interferes minimally with the protein binding of prednisolone (10% decrease in binding). Benzylpenicillin, ampicillin, oxacillin, chlortetracycline, doxycycline, cephalothin, erythromycin, and sulfamethoxazole have no influence, *in vitro,* on the protein binding of diclofenac in human serum.

ADVERSE REACTIONS

ADVERSE REACTIONS ASSOCIATED WITH DICLOFENAC SODIUM; MISOPROSTOL

Adverse reaction information for diclofenac sodium; misoprostol is derived from Phase III multinational controlled clinical trials in over 2000 patients, receiving diclofenac sodium; misoprostol 50 or diclofenac sodium; misoprostol 75, as well as from blinded, controlled trials of diclofenac delayed release tablets and misoprostol tablets.

GASTROINTESTINAL

GI disorders had the highest reported incidence of adverse events for patients receiving diclofenac sodium; misoprostol. These events were generally minor, but led to discontinuation of therapy in 9% of patients on diclofenac sodium; misoprostol and 5% of patients on diclofenac.

TABLE 4

GI Disorder	Diclofenac Sodium; Misoprostol	Diclofenac
Abdominal pain	21%	15%
Diarrhea	19%	11%
Dyspepsia	14%	11%
Nausea	11%	6%
Flatulence	9%	4%

Diclofenac sodium; misoprostol can cause more abdominal pain, diarrhea and other GI symptoms than diclofenac alone.

Diarrhea and abdominal pain developed early in the course of therapy, and were usually self-limited (resolved after 2-7 days). Rare instances of profound diarrhea leading to severe dehydration have been reported in patients receiving misoprostol. Patients with an underlying condition such as inflammatory bowel disease, or those in whom dehydration, were it to occur, would be dangerous, should be monitored carefully if diclofenac sodium; misoprostol is prescribed. The incidence of diarrhea can be minimized by administering diclofenac sodium; misoprostol with food and by avoiding coadministration with magnesium-containing antacids.

GYNECOLOGICAL

Gynecological disorders previously reported with misoprostol use have also been reported for women receiving diclofenac sodium; misoprostol (see below). Postmenopausal vaginal bleeding may be related to diclofenac sodium; misoprostol administration. If it occurs, diagnostic workup should be undertaken to rule out gynecological pathology.

ELDERLY

Overall, there were no significant differences in the safety profile of diclofenac sodium; misoprostol in over 500 patients 65 years of age or older compared with younger patients.

Other adverse experiences reported occasionally or rarely with diclofenac sodium; misoprostol, diclofenac or other NSAIDs, or misoprostol are:

Body as a Whole: Death, fatigue, fever, infection, malaise, sepsis.

Cardiovascular System: Arrhythmia, atrial fibrillation, congestive heart failure, hypertension, hypotension, increased CPK, increased LDH, myocardial infarction, palpitations, phlebitis, premature ventricular contractions, syncope, tachycardia, vasculitis.

Central and Peripheral Nervous System: Coma, convulsions, diplopia, drowsiness, hyperesthesia, hypertonia, hypoesthesia, meningitis, migraine, neuralgia, paresthesia, tremor, vertigo.

Digestive: Anorexia, dry mouth, dysphagia, enteritis, esophageal ulceration, gastroesophageal reflux, GI bleeding, GI neoplasm benign, glossitis, hematemesis, hemorrhoids, intestinal perforation, peptic ulcer, stomatitis and ulcerative stomatitis, tenesmus.

Female Reproductive Disorders: Breast pain, dysmenorrhea, intermenstrual bleeding, leukorrhea, menorrhagia, vaginal hemorrhage.

Hemic and Lymphatic System: Agranulocytosis, aplastic anemia, coagulation time increased, ecchymosis, eosinophilia, epistaxis, hemolytic anemia, leukocytosis, leukopenia, lymphadenopathy, melena, pulmonary embolism, purpura, pancytopenia, rectal bleeding, thrombocythemia, thrombocytopenia.

Hypersensitivity: Angioedema, laryngeal/pharyngeal edema, urticaria.

Liver and Biliary System: Abnormal hepatic function, bilirubinemia, hepatitis, jaundice, liver failure, pancreatitis.

Male Reproductive Disorders: Impotence, perineal pain.

Metabolic and Nutritional: Alkaline phosphatase increased, BUN increased, dehydration, glycosuria, gout, hypercholesterolemia, hyperglycemia, hyperuricemia, hypoglycemia, hyponatremia, periorbital edema, porphyria, weight changes.

Musculoskeletal System: Arthralgia, myalgia.

Psychiatric: Anxiety, asthenia, concentration impaired, confusion, depression, disorientation, dream abnormalities, hallucinations, irritability, malaise, nervousness, paranoia, psychotic reaction, somnolence.

Respiratory System: Asthma, coughing, dyspnea, hyperventilation, pneumonia, respiratory depression.

Skin and Appendages: Acne, alopecia, bruising, erythema multiforme, eczema, exfoliative dermatitis, pemphigoid reaction, photosensitivity, pruritus ani, skin ulceration, Stevens-Johnson syndrome, sweating increased, toxic epidermal necrolysis.

Special Senses: Hearing impairment, taste loss, taste perversion.

Urinary System: Cystitis, dysuria, hematuria, interstitial nephritis, micturition frequency, nocturia, nephrotic syndrome, oliguria/polyuria, papillary necrosis, proteinuria, renal failure, urinary tract infection.

Vision: Amblyopia, blurred vision, conjunctivitis, glaucoma, iritis, lacrimation abnormal, night blindness, vision abnormal.

DOSAGE AND ADMINISTRATION

Diclofenac sodium; misoprostol is administered as diclofenac sodium; misoprostol 50 (50 mg diclofenac sodium/200 μg misoprostol) or as diclofenac sodium; misoprostol 75 (75 mg diclofenac sodium/200 μg misoprostol).

Note: See Special Dosing Considerations.

OSTEOARTHRITIS

The recommended dosage is diclofenac sodium; misoprostol 50 tid. For patients who experience intolerance, diclofenac sodium; misoprostol 75 bid or diclofenac sodium; misoprostol 50 bid can be used, but are less effective in preventing ulcers. This fixed combination product, diclofenac sodium; misoprostol, is not appropriate for patients who would not receive the appropriate does of both ingredients. Doses of the components delivered with these regimens are as follows:

TABLE 5

	Diclofenac Sodium	Misoprostol
Diclofenac Sodium; Misoprostol 50 tid	150 mg/day	600 μg/day
Diclofenac Sodium; Misoprostol 50 bid	100 mg/day	400 μg/day
Diclofenac Sodium; Misoprostol 75 bid	150 mg/day	400 μg/day

RHEUMATOID ARTHRITIS

The recommended dosage is diclofenac sodium; misoprostol 50 tid or qid. For patients who experience intolerance, diclofenac sodium; misoprostol 75 bid or diclofenac sodium; misoprostol 50 bid can be used, but are less effective in preventing ulcers. This fixed combination product, diclofenac sodium; misoprostol, is not appropriate for patients who would not receive the appropriate dose of both ingredients. Doses of the components delivered with these regimens are as follows:

TABLE 6

	Diclofenac Sodium	Misoprostol
Diclofenac Sodium; Misoprostol 50 qid	200 mg/day	800 μg/day
Diclofenac Sodium; Misoprostol 50 tid	150 mg/day	600 μg/day
Diclofenac Sodium; Misoprostol 50 bid	100 mg/day	400 μg/day
Diclofenac Sodium; Misoprostol 75 bid	150 mg/day	400 μg/day

SPECIAL DOSING CONSIDERATIONS

Diclofenac sodium; misoprostol contains misoprostol, which provides protection against gastric and duodenal ulcers. For gastric ulcer prevention, the 200 μg qid and tid regimens are therapeutically equivalent, but more protective than the bid regimen. For duodenal ulcer prevention, the qid regimen is more protective than the tid or bid regimens. However, the qid regimen is less well tolerated than the tid regimen because of usually self-limited diarrhea related to the misoprostol dose (see ADVERSE REACTIONS, Gastrointestinal), and the bid regimen may be better tolerated than tid in some patients.

Dosages may be individualized using the separate products (misoprostol and diclofenac), after which the patient may be changed to the appropriate diclofenac sodium; misoprostol dose. If clinically indicated, misoprostol co-therapy with diclofenac sodium; misoprostol, or use of the individual components to optimize the misoprostol dose and/or frequency of administration, may be appropriate. The total dose of misoprostol should not exceed 800 μg/day, and no more than 200 μg of misoprostol should be administered at any one time. Doses of diclofenac higher than 150 mg/day in osteoarthritis or higher than 225 mg/day in rheumatoid arthritis are not recommended.

For additional information, it may be helpful to refer to the prescribing information for misoprostol tablets and diclofenac tablets.

ANIMAL PHARMACOLOGY

A reversible increase in the number of normal surface gastric epithelial cells occurred in the dog, rat, and mouse during long-term toxicology studies with misoprostol. No such increase has been observed in humans administered misoprostol for up to 1 year. An apparent response of the female mouse to misoprostol in long-term studies at 100-1000 times the human dose was hyperostosis, mainly of the medulla of sternebrae. Hyperostosis did not occur in long-term studies in the dog and rat and has not been seen in humans treated with misoprostol.

HOW SUPPLIED

Arthrotec is supplied as a film-coated tablet in dosage strengths of either 50 mg diclofenac sodium/200 µg misoprostol or 75 mg diclofenac sodium/200 µg misoprostol.

The 50 mg/200 µg dosage strength is a round, biconvex, white to off-white tablet imprinted with four "A's" encircling a "50" in the middle on one side and "SEARLE" and "1411" on the other.

The 75 mg/200 µg dosage strength is a round, biconvex, white to off-white tablet imprinted with four "A's" encircling a "75" in the middle on one side and "SEARLE" and "1421" on the other.

Storage: Store at or below 25°C (77°F), in a dry area.

PRODUCT LISTING - EQUIVALENTS NOT AVAILABLE

Quantity	Price	Product	NDC
Tablet - Oral - 50 mg;200 mcg			
15's	$32.04	ARTHROTEC, Pd-Rx Pharmaceuticals	55289-0406-15
20's	$53.60	ARTHROTEC, Pharma Pac	52959-0531-20
30's	$60.62	ARTHROTEC, Pd-Rx Pharmaceuticals	55289-0406-30
30's	$76.40	ARTHROTEC, Pharma Pac	52959-0531-30
42's	$94.50	ARTHROTEC, Pharma Pac	52959-0531-42
60's	$109.25	ARTHROTEC, Searle	00025-1411-60
60's	$129.10	ARTHROTEC, Pharma Pac	52959-0531-60
90's	$163.88	ARTHROTEC, Searle	00025-1411-90
100's	$171.70	ARTHROTEC, Searle	00025-1411-34
Tablet - Oral - 75 mg;200 mcg			
14's	$40.90	ARTHROTEC, Pharma Pac	52959-0525-14
20's	$58.90	ARTHROTEC, Pharma Pac	52959-0525-20
30's	$54.60	ARTHROTEC, Southwood Pharmaceuticals Inc	58016-0498-30
30's	$87.65	ARTHROTEC, Pharma Pac	52959-0525-30
60's	$109.20	ARTHROTEC, Southwood Pharmaceuticals Inc	58016-0498-60
60's	$109.25	ARTHROTEC, Searle	00025-1421-60
100's	$171.70	ARTHROTEC, Searle	00025-1421-34
100's	$182.00	ARTHROTEC, Southwood Pharmaceuticals Inc	58016-0498-00

Dicloxacillin Sodium *(001046)*

For related information, see the comparative table section in Appendix A.

Categories: Infection, staphylococcal, penicillinase-producing; Pregnancy Category B; FDA Approved 1971 Apr
Drug Classes: Antibiotics, penicillins
Brand Names: Dycill; Dynapen; Maclicine; Orbenin; **Pathocil**; Staphcillin
Foreign Brand Availability: Brispen (Mexico); Cloxydin (Thailand); Dacocilin (Taiwan); Diclex (Thailand); Diclixin (Peru); Diclo (Italy); Diclocil (Australia; Colombia; Costa-Rica; Denmark; Ecuador; El-Salvador; Finland; Greece; Guatemala; Honduras; Hong-Kong; Italy; New-Zealand; Nicaragua; Norway; Panama; Peru; Portugal; Sweden; Thailand); Diclopen-T (Ecuador); Diclox (Thailand); Dicloxin (Thailand); Dicloxman (Thailand); Dicloxno (Thailand); Diloxin (Thailand); Distaph (Australia); H.G. Dicloxacil (Ecuador); Novapen (Italy); Posipen (Costa-Rica; Dominican-Republic; El-Salvador; Guatemala; Honduras; Mexico; Nicaragua; Panama); Staphcillin A (Japan); Ziefmycin (Taiwan)
Cost of Therapy: $14.33 (Infection; Generic Capsule; 250 mg; 4 capsules/day; 10 day supply)

DESCRIPTION

Dicloxacillin sodium is 5-methyl-3-(2,6-dichlorophenyl)-4-isoxazolyl penicillin sodium salt monohydrate, a penicillinase-resistant, acid- resistant, semisynthetic penicillin derived from the penicillin nucleus, 6-aminopenicillanic acid. It is resistant to inactivation by the enzyme penicillinase (beta-lactamase).[1-5]

The structural formula of dicloxacillin sodium is as follows:

$C_{19}H_{16}Cl_2N_3NaO_5 \cdot H_2O$ 510.32 [CAS-13412-64-1] 4-Thia-1-azabicyclo[3.2.0]heptane-2-carboxylic acid,6-[3-(2,6-dichlorophenyl)-5-methyl-4-isoxazolyl[carbonyl]-amino]-3,3-dimethyl-7-oxo-, monosodium salt, monohydrate, [2*S*- (2α,5α,6β)]. *Inactive Ingredients:* 250 mg capsules—FD&C blue no.2, gelatin, lactose, magnesium stearate, red iron oxide, silicon dioxide, sodium lauryl sulfate, titanium dioxide and yellow iron oxide. 500 mg capsules—FD&C blue no. 2, gelatin, magnesium stearate, red iron oxide, silicon dioxide, sodium lauryl sulfate, titanium oxide and yellow iron oxide.

CLINICAL PHARMACOLOGY

MICROBIOLOGY

Penicillinase-resistant penicillins exert a bactericidal action against penicillin-susceptible microorganisms during the state of multiplication.[6] All penicillins inhibit the biosynthesis of the bacterial cell wall.[3,7]

The drugs in this class are highly resistant to inactivation by staphylococcal penicillinase and are active against penicillinase-producing and nonpenicillinase-producing strains of *Staphylococcus aureus.* The penicillinase-resistant penicillins are active *in vitro* against a variety of other bacteria.[3,5,7-17]

SUSCEPTIBILITY TESTING

Quantitative methods of susceptibility testing that require measurements of zone diameters or minimal inhibitory concentrations (MICs) give the most precise estimates of antibiotic susceptibility. One such procedure has been recommended for use with disks to test susceptibility to this class of drugs. Interpretations correlate diameters on the disk test with MIC values.

A penicillinase-resistant class disk may be used to determine microbial susceptibility to cloxacillin, dicloxacillin, methicillin, nafcillin and oxacillin.[18]

Table 1 shows the interpretation of test results for penicillinase-resistant penicillins using the FDA Standard Disk Test Method (formerly Bauer-Kirby-Sherris-Turck method) of disk bacteriological susceptibility testing for staphylococci with a disk containing 5 µg methicillin sodium.

With this procedure, a report from a laboratory of "susceptible" indicates that the infecting organism is likely to respond to therapy. A report of "resistant" indicates that the infecting organism is not likely to respond to therapy. A report of "intermediate" susceptibility suggests that the organism might be susceptible if high doses of the antibiotic are used, or if the infection is confined to tissues and fluids (*e.g.,* urine) in which high antibiotic levels are attained.

In general, all staphylococci should be tested against the penicillin G disk and against the methicillin disk.[18] Routine methods of antibiotic susceptibility testing may fail to detect strains of organisms resistant to the penicillinase-resistant penicillins. For this reason, the use of large inocula and 48 hour incubation periods may be necessary to obtain accurate susceptibility studies with these antibiotics. Bacterial strains which are resistant to one of the penicillinase-resistant penicillins should be considered resistant to all of the drugs in the class.[3,8]

TABLE 1 *Standardized Test Method of Bacteriological Susceptibility Testing Using a Class Disk Containing 5 µg Methicillin Sodium*[18]

Diameter of Zone Indicating "Susceptibility"	Diameter of Zone Indicating "Intermediate"	Diameter of Zone Indicating "Resistant"
At least 14 mm	10-13 mm	Less than 10 mm

PHARMACOKINETICS

Methicillin sodium is readily destroyed by gastric acidity and must be administered by intramuscular or intravenous injections.[8,11,17] The isoxazolyl penicillins (cloxacillin and oxacillin) and nafcillin are more acid resistant and may be administered orally.[3,15,16,19,20] Absorption of the isoxazolyl penicillins after oral administration is rapid but incomplete; peak blood levels are achieved in 1 to 1.5 hours.[3,4,19] In one study, after ingestion of a single 500 mg oral dose, peak serum concentrations range from 5-7 µg/ml for oxacillin, from 7.5-14.4 µg/ml for cloxacillin and from 10-17 µg/ml for dicloxacillin. Oral absorption of nafcillin sodium is irregular and wide individual variations in absorption are observed. One hour after ingestion of a single 1 gram oral dose of nafcillin as the sodium salt, the average serum concentration of 1.19 µg/ml (range 0-3.12 µg/ml) was achieved.[4,20,25]

Oral absorption of cloxacillin, dicloxacillin, oxacillin and nafcillin is delayed when the drugs are administered after meals.[10,14,16,20] Intramuscular injections of nafcillin (1 gram), oxacillin (560 mg) and methicillin sodium (1 gram) produced peak serum levels in 0.5 to 1 hour of 7.61 µg/ml, 15 µg/ml and 17 µg/ml, respectively.[1,8,17,19,25]

Once absorbed, the penicillinase-resistant penicillins bind to serum protein, mainly albumin. The degree of protein binding reported varies with the method of study and the investigator (see TABLE 2).[3,8]

TABLE 2

Penicillin-Resistant Penicillin Percent Protein-Binding ±SD[8]

Drug	%	Drug	%
Methicillin	37.3 ± 7.9	Oxacillin	94.2 ± 2.1
Dicloxacillin	97.9 ± 0.6	Nafcillin	89.9 ± 1.5
Cloxacillin	95.2 ± 0.5		

The penicillinase-resistant penicillins vary in the extent to which they are distributed in the body fluids. With normal doses, insignificant concentrations are found in the cerebrospinal fluid and aqueous humor. Methicillin is found in the pericardial and ascitic fluids. All the drugs in this class are found in therapeutic concentrations in the pleural, bile and amniotic fluids.[3,8,22]

The penicillinase-resistant penicillins are rapidly excreted primarily as unchanged drug in the urine by glomerular filtration and active tubular secretion.[3,26] The elimination half-life for methicillin and oxacillin is about 0.5 hour, for nafcillin less than 1 hour and for dicloxacillin about 0.7 hour.[23,26,27] Nonrenal elimination includes hepatic inactivation and excretion in bile.[3,17,27] Renal clearance of methicillin is delayed in premature infants, neonates and patients with renal insufficiency.[8,28]

INDICATIONS AND USAGE

The penicillinase-resistant penicillins are indicated in the treatment of infections caused by penicillinase-producing staphylococci which have demonstrated susceptibility to the drugs. Cultures and susceptibility tests should be performed initially to determine the causative organisms and their sensitivity to the drug (see CLINICAL PHARMACOLOGY, Susceptibility Testing).[29].

The penicillinase-resistant penicillins may be used to initiate therapy in suspected cases of resistant staphylococcal infections prior to the availability of laboratory test results.[14,29,30] The penicillin-resistant penicillins should not be used in infections caused by organisms susceptible to penicillin G.[16,29,31] If the susceptibility tests indicate that the infection is due to an organism other than a resistant staphylococcus, therapy should not be continued with a penicillinase-resistant penicillin.[30]

CONTRAINDICATIONS

A history of a hypersensitivity (anaphylactic) reaction to any penicillins is a contraindication.

WARNINGS

SERIOUS AND OCCASIONALLY FATAL HYPERSENSITIVITY (ANAPHYLACTIC) REACTIONS HAVE BEEN REPORTED IN PATIENTS ON PENICILLIN THERAPY. THESE REACTIONS ARE MORE LIKELY TO OCCUR IN INDIVIDUALS WITH A HISTORY OF PENICILLIN HYPERSENSITIVITY AND/OR A HISTORY OF SENSITIVITY TO MULTIPLE ALLERGENS. THERE HAVE BEEN REPORTS OF INDIVIDUALS WITH A SENSITIVITY TO MULTIPLE ALLERGENS. THERE HAVE BEEN REPORTS OF INDIVIDUALS WITH A HISTORY OF PENICILLIN HYPERSENSITIVITY WHO HAVE BEEN EXPERIENCED SEVERE REACTIONS WHEN TREATED WITH CEPHALOSPORINS. BEFORE INITIATING THERAPY WITH DYCILL, CAREFUL INQUIRY SHOULD BE MADE CONCERNING PREVIOUS HYPERSENSITIVITY REACTIONS TO PENICILLINS, CEPHALOSPORINS, OR OTHER ALLERGENS. IF AN ALLERGIC REACTION OCCURS, DYCILL SHOULD BE DISCONTINUED AND APPROPRIATE THERAPY INSTITUTED. **SERIOUS ANAPHYLACTIC REACTIONS REQUIRE IMMEDIATE EMERGENCY TREATMENT WITH EPINEPHRINE, OXYGEN, INTRAVENOUS STEROIDS, AND AIRWAY MANAGEMENT, INCLUDING INTUBATION, SHOULD ALSO BE ADMINISTERED AS INDICATED.**

Pseudomembranous colitis has been reported with nearly all antibacterial agents, including Dycill, and may range in severity from mild to life-threatening. Therefore, it is important to consider this diagnosis in patients who present with diarrhea subsequent to the administration of antibacterial agents.

Treatment with antibacterial agents alters the normal flora of the colon and may permit overgrowth of clostridia. Studies indicate that a toxin produced by *Clostridium difficile* is one primary cause of "antibiotic-associated colitis."

After the diagnosis of pseudomembranous colitis usually respond to drug discontinuation alone. In moderate to severe cases, consideration should be given to management with fluids and electrolytes, protein supplementation and treatment with an antibacterial drug clinically effective against *C. difficile* colitis.

PRECAUTIONS

GENERAL

Penicillinase-resistant penicillins should generally not be administered to patients with a history of sensitivity to any penicillin.[30,31,41,42]

Penicillin should be used with caution in individuals with histories of significant allergies and/or asthma.[3] Whenever allergic reactions occur, penicillin should be withdrawn unless, in the opinion of the physician, the condition being treated is life-threatening and amenable only to penicillin therapy. The oral route of administration should not be relied upon in patients with severe illness, or with nausea, vomiting, gastric dilation, cardiospasm or intestinal hypermotility. Occasionally patients will not absorb therapeutic amounts of orally administered penicillin.[25]

The use of antibiotics may results in overgrowth of nonsusceptible organisms.[3,32,43] If new infections due to bacteria or fungi occur, the drug should be discontinued and appropriate measures taken.

INFORMATION FOR THE PATIENT

Patients receiving penicillins should be given the following information and instructions by the physician:

1. Patients should be told that penicillin is an antibacterial agent which will work with the body's natural defenses to control certain types of infections. They should be told that the drug should not be taken if they have had an allergic reaction to any form of penicillin previously, and to inform the physician of any allergies or previous allergic reactions to any drugs they may have had[44] (see WARNINGS).
2. Patients who have previously experienced an anaphylactic reaction to penicillin should be instructed to wear a medical identification tag or bracelet.
3. Because most antibacterial drugs taken by mouth are best absorbed on an empty stomach, patients should be directed, unless circumstances warrant otherwise, to take penicillin 1 hour before meals or 2 hours after eating[36,37] (see CLINICAL PHARMACOLOGY, Pharmacokinetics).
4. Patients should be told to take the entire course of therapy prescribed, even if fever and other symptoms have stopped (see PRECAUTIONS, General).
5. If any of the following reactions occur, stop taking your prescription and notify the physician: shortness of breath, wheezing, skin rash, mouth irritation, black tongue, sore throat, nausea, vomiting, diarrhea, fever, swollen joints, or any unusual bleeding or bruising[36] (see ADVERSE REACTIONS).
6. Do not take any additional medications without physician approval, including nonprescription drugs such as antacids, laxatives or vitamins.[36]
7. Discard and liquid forms of penicillin after 7 days if stored at room temperature or after 14 days if refrigerated.

LABORATORY TESTS

Bacteriologic studies to determine the causative organisms and their susceptibility to the penicillinase-resistant penicillins should be performed (see CLINICAL PHARMACOLOGY, Microbiology). In the treatment of suspected staphylococcal infections, therapy should be changed to another active agent if culture tests fail to demonstrate the presence of staphylococci.[29]

Periodic assessment of organ system function including renal hepatic and hematopoietic should be made during prolonged therapy with the penicillinase-resistant penicillins.[29]

Blood cultures, white blood cell and differential cell counts should be obtained prior to initiation of therapy and at least weekly during therapy with penicillinase-resistant penicillins.[29]

Periodic urinalysis, blood urea nitrogen and creatinine determinations should be performed during therapy with the penicillinase-resistant penicillins and overdosage alterations should be considered if these values become elevated.[29,36] If any impairment of renal function is suspected or known to exist, a reduction in the total dosage should be considered and blood levels monitored to avoid possible neurotoxic reactions[39](see DOSAGE AND ADMINISTRATION).

SGOT and SGPT values should be obtained periodically during therapy to monitor for possible liver function abnormalities.[40,41]

CARCINOGENESIS, MUTAGENESIS, AND IMPAIRMENT OF FERTILITY

No long-term animal studies have been conducted with these drugs.

Studies on reproduction (nafcillin) in rats and rabbits reveal no fetal or maternal abnormalities before conception and continuously through weaning (one generation).

PREGNANCY CATEGORY B

Reproduction studies performed in the mouse, rat and rabbit have revealed no evidence of impaired fertility or harm to the fetus due to the penicillinase-resistant penicillins.[45,46] Human experience with the penicillins during pregnancy has not shown any positive evidence of adverse effects on the fetus. There are, however, no adequate or well-controlled studies in pregnant women showing conclusively that harmful effects of these drugs on the fetus can be excluded.[47,48] Because animal reproduction studies are not always predictive of human response, this drug should be used during pregnancy only if clearly needed.

NURSING MOTHERS

Penicillins are excreted in breast milk.[6,49,50] Caution should be exercised when penicillins are administered to a nursing woman.

PEDIATRIC USE

Because of incompletely developed renal function in newborns penicillinase-resistant penicillins (especially methicillin) may not be completely excreted, with abnormally high blood levels resulting.[28] Frequent blood levels are advisable in this group with dosage adjustments when necessary. All newborns treated with penicillins should be monitored closely for clinical and laboratory evidence of toxic or adverse effects[51] (see DOSAGE AND ADMINISTRATION).

DRUG INTERACTIONS

Tetracycline, a bacteriostatic antibiotic, may antagonize the bactericidal effect of penicillin and concurrent use of these drugs should be avoided.[41,42]

ADVERSE REACTIONS

BODY AS A WHOLE

The reported incidence of allergic reactions to penicillin ranges from 0.7-10%[28,34,52-54] (see WARNINGS). Sensitization is usually the result of treatment but some individuals have had immediate reactions to penicillin when first treated. In such cases, it is thought that the patients may have had prior exposure to the drug via trace amounts present in milk and vaccines.[56]

Two types of allergic reactions to penicillins are noted clinically, immediate and delayed.[52,55,56]

Immediate reactions usually occur within 20 minutes of administration and range in severity from urticaria and pruritus to angioneurotic edema, laryngospasm, bronchospasm, hypotension, vascular collapse and death. Such immediate anaphylactic reactions are very rare (see WARNINGS) and usually occur after parenteral therapy but have occurred in patients receiving oral therapy. Another type of immediate reaction, an accelerated reaction, may occur between 20 minutes and 48 hours after administration and may include urticaria, pruritus and fever. Although laryngeal edema, laryngospasm and hypotension occasionally occur, fatality is uncommon.[34,52,53,55]

Delayed allergic reactions to penicillin therapy usually occur after 48 hours and sometimes as late as 2-4 weeks after initiation of therapy.[56] Manifestations of this type of reaction include serum-sickness-like symptoms (*i.e.*, fever, malaise, urticaria, myalgia, arthralgia, abdominal pain) and various rashes.[20,34,35,53,55] Nausea, vomiting, diarrhea, stomatitis, black or hairy tongue and other symptoms of gastrointestinal irritation may occur, especially during oral penicillin therapy.[3,41]

NERVOUS SYSTEM REACTIONS

Neurotoxic reactions similar to those observed with penicillin G may occur with large intravenous doses of the penicillinase-resistant penicillins, especially with patients with renal insufficiency.[7,39]

UROGENITAL REACTIONS

Renal tubular damage and interstitial nephritis have been associated with the administration of methicillin sodium and infrequently with the administration of nafcillin and oxacillin.[8,38,57-61] Manifestations of this reaction may include rash, fever, eosinophilia, hematuria, proteinuria and renal insufficiency. Methicillin-induced nephropathy does not appear to be dose-related and is generally reversible upon prompt discontinuation of therapy.[7,8,57,59]

METABOLIC REACTIONS

Agranulocytosis, neutropenia and bone marrow depression have been associated with the use of methicillin sodium and nafcillin.[14,62-65]

Hepatotoxicity, characterized by fever, nausea and vomiting associated with abnormal liver function tests, mainly elevated SGOT levels, has been associated with the use of oxacillin.[40,41]

DOSAGE AND ADMINISTRATION

For mild-to-moderate upper-respiratory and localized skin and soft-tissue infections due to sensitive organisms:

Adults and Children Weighing 40 Kg (88 lbs.) or More: 125 mg every 6 hours.

Patients Weighing Less Than 40 Kg (88 lbs.): 12.5 mg/kg/day in equally divided doses every 6 hours.

For more severe infections such as those of the lower respiratory tract or disseminated infections:

Adults and Children Weighing 40 Kg (88 lbs.) or More: 250 mg or higher every 6 hours.

Patients Weighing Less Than 40 Kg (88 lbs.): 25 mg/kg/day or higher in equally divided doses every 6 hours.

Dicloxacillin sodium is best absorbed when taken on an empty stomach, preferably 1-2 hours before meals.

Bacteriologic studies to determine the causative organisms and their sensitivity to the penicillinase-resistant penicillins should always be performed. Duration of therapy varies with the type and severity of infection as well as the overall condition of the patient: therefore, it should be determined by the clinical and bacteriological response of the patient. In severe staphylococcal infections, therapy with penicillinase-resistant penicillins should be continued for at least 14 days.[29] Therapy should be continued for at least 48 hours after the patient has become afebrile, asymptomatic, and cultures are negative. The treatment of endocarditis and osteomyelitis may require a longer term of therapy.

Concurrent administration of the penicillinase-resistant penicillins and probenecid increases and prolongs serum penicillin levels. Probenecid decreases the apparent volume of distribution and slows the rate of excretion by competitively inhibiting renal tubular secretion of penicillin.[6,8,21,25,32,66,67] Penicillin-probenecid therapy is generally limited to those infections where very high serum levels of penicillin are necessary.

Oral preparations of the penicillinase-resistant penicillins should not be used as initial therapy in serious, life-threatening infections[16] see PRECAUTIONS, General. Oral therapy with the penicillinase-resistant penicillins may be used to follow up the previous use of a parenteral agent as soon as the clinical condition warrants.[3]

PRODUCT LISTING - RATED THERAPEUTICALLY EQUIVALENT

Size	Price	Product	NDC
Capsule - Oral - 250 mg			
10's	$5.25	GENERIC, Pd-Rx Pharmaceuticals	55289-0592-10
20's	$10.50	GENERIC, Pd-Rx Pharmaceuticals	55289-0592-20
25's	$9.75	GENERIC, Pd-Rx Pharmaceuticals	55289-0592-97
28's	$12.96	GENERIC, Circle Pharmaceuticals Inc	00659-0113-28
28's	$14.30	GENERIC, Pd-Rx Pharmaceuticals	55289-0592-28
40's	$7.90	GENERIC, Pd-Rx Pharmaceuticals	55289-0149-40
40's	$12.00	GENERIC, Golden State Medical	60429-0059-40
40's	$15.02	GENERIC, Circle Pharmaceuticals Inc	00659-0113-40
40's	$17.19	GENERIC, Pd-Rx Pharmaceuticals	55289-0592-40
100's	$19.00	GENERIC, Raway Pharmacal Inc	00686-0610-20
100's	$35.82	GENERIC, Qualitest Products Inc	00603-3241-21
100's	$38.07	GENERIC, Moore, H.L. Drug Exchange Inc	00839-6178-06
100's	$39.75	GENERIC, Geneva Pharmaceuticals	00781-2220-01
100's	$39.75	GENERIC, Major Pharmaceuticals Inc	00904-2647-60
100's	$41.60	GENERIC, Esi Lederle Generics	00005-3135-23
100's	$42.20	GENERIC, Aligen Independent Laboratories Inc	00405-4322-01
100's	$42.90	GENERIC, Interstate Drug Exchange Inc	00814-2435-14
100's	$66.00	GENERIC, Teva Pharmaceuticals Usa	00093-3123-01
100's	$66.05	GENERIC, Apothecon Inc	59772-6048-01
Capsule - Oral - 500 mg			
20's	$16.50	GENERIC, Pd-Rx Pharmaceuticals	55289-0094-20
30's	$12.97	GENERIC, Pd-Rx Pharmaceuticals	58864-0150-30
30's	$23.18	GENERIC, Pd-Rx Pharmaceuticals	55289-0094-30
30's	$80.13	DYNAPEN, Pd-Rx Pharmaceuticals	55289-0065-30
40's	$31.68	GENERIC, Pd-Rx Pharmaceuticals	55289-0094-40
100's	$36.00	GENERIC, Raway Pharmacal Inc	00686-0611-20
100's	$60.50	GENERIC, Qualitest Products Inc	00603-3242-21
100's	$66.00	GENERIC, Major Pharmaceuticals Inc	00904-2648-60
100's	$66.35	GENERIC, Moore, H.L. Drug Exchange Inc	00839-6614-06
100's	$67.45	GENERIC, Geneva Pharmaceuticals	00781-2225-01
100's	$74.93	GENERIC, Interstate Drug Exchange Inc	00814-2436-14
100's	$75.82	GENERIC, Aligen Independent Laboratories Inc	00405-4323-01
100's	$120.00	GENERIC, Teva Pharmaceuticals Usa	00093-3125-01
100's	$120.11	GENERIC, Apothecon Inc	59772-6058-01
Powder For Reconstitution - Oral - 62.5 mg/5 ml			
100 ml	$10.08	DYNAPEN, Bristol-Myers Squibb	00015-7856-40
200 ml	$16.69	DYNAPEN, Bristol-Myers Squibb	00015-7856-64

PRODUCT LISTING - EQUIVALENTS NOT AVAILABLE

Size	Price	Product	NDC
Capsule - Oral - 250 mg			
4's	$3.78	GENERIC, Prescript Pharmaceuticals	00247-0129-04
6's	$2.52	GENERIC, Allscripts Pharmaceutical Company	54569-0384-05
6's	$3.99	GENERIC, Prescript Pharmaceuticals	00247-0129-06
10's	$9.40	GENERIC, Southwood Pharmaceuticals Inc	58016-0121-10
12's	$4.62	GENERIC, Prescript Pharmaceuticals	00247-0129-12
12's	$11.27	GENERIC, Southwood Pharmaceuticals Inc	58016-0121-12
14's	$13.15	GENERIC, Southwood Pharmaceuticals Inc	58016-0121-14
15's	$14.09	GENERIC, Southwood Pharmaceuticals Inc	58016-0121-15
18's	$16.91	GENERIC, Southwood Pharmaceuticals Inc	58016-0121-18
20's	$5.47	GENERIC, Prescript Pharmaceuticals	00247-0129-20
20's	$8.40	GENERIC, Allscripts Pharmaceutical Company	54569-0384-04
20's	$18.72	GENERIC, Alpharma Uspd Makers Of Barre and Nmc	63874-0108-20
20's	$18.79	GENERIC, Southwood Pharmaceuticals Inc	58016-0121-20
20's	$19.06	GENERIC, Pharma Pac	52959-0048-20
24's	$22.55	GENERIC, Southwood Pharmaceuticals Inc	58016-0121-24
28's	$6.32	GENERIC, Prescript Pharmaceuticals	00247-0129-28
28's	$11.77	GENERIC, Allscripts Pharmaceutical Company	54569-0384-00
28's	$12.77	GENERIC, Pharmaceutical Corporation Of America	51655-0213-29
28's	$26.31	GENERIC, Southwood Pharmaceuticals Inc	58016-0121-28
28's	$27.04	GENERIC, Alpharma Uspd Makers Of Barre and Nmc	63874-0108-28
28's	$27.27	GENERIC, Pharma Pac	52959-0048-28
30's	$6.53	GENERIC, Prescript Pharmaceuticals	00247-0129-30
30's	$28.13	GENERIC, Pharma Pac	52959-0048-30
30's	$28.19	GENERIC, Southwood Pharmaceuticals Inc	58016-0121-30
40's	$7.59	GENERIC, Prescript Pharmaceuticals	00247-0129-40
40's	$16.81	GENERIC, Allscripts Pharmaceutical Company	54569-0384-01
40's	$19.25	GENERIC, Pharmaceutical Corporation Of America	51655-0213-51
40's	$37.58	GENERIC, Southwood Pharmaceuticals Inc	58016-0121-40
40's	$38.25	GENERIC, Pharma Pac	52959-0048-40
41's	$39.08	GENERIC, Pharma Pac	52959-0048-41
100's	$93.95	GENERIC, Southwood Pharmaceuticals Inc	58016-0121-00
Capsule - Oral - 500 mg			
4's	$4.11	GENERIC, Prescript Pharmaceuticals	00247-0104-04
8's	$4.87	GENERIC, Prescript Pharmaceuticals	00247-0104-08
10's	$17.60	GENERIC, Southwood Pharmaceuticals Inc	58016-0122-10
12's	$21.48	GENERIC, Southwood Pharmaceuticals Inc	58016-0122-12
14's	$6.00	GENERIC, Prescript Pharmaceuticals	00247-0104-14
14's	$25.06	GENERIC, Southwood Pharmaceuticals Inc	58016-0122-14
15's	$26.85	GENERIC, Southwood Pharmaceuticals Inc	58016-0122-15
20's	$7.14	GENERIC, Prescript Pharmaceuticals	00247-0104-20
20's	$14.67	GENERIC, Allscripts Pharmaceutical Company	54569-1889-04
20's	$35.80	GENERIC, Southwood Pharmaceuticals Inc	58016-0122-20
20's	$36.40	GENERIC, Alpharma Uspd Makers Of Barre and Nmc	63874-0123-20
20's	$54.57	GENERIC, Pharma Pac	52959-0049-20
21's	$36.96	GENERIC, Southwood Pharmaceuticals Inc	58016-0122-21
24's	$42.24	GENERIC, Southwood Pharmaceuticals Inc	58016-0122-24
28's	$8.65	GENERIC, Prescript Pharmaceuticals	00247-0104-28
28's	$20.54	GENERIC, Allscripts Pharmaceutical Company	54569-1889-00
28's	$50.12	GENERIC, Southwood Pharmaceuticals Inc	58016-0122-28
28's	$74.73	GENERIC, Pharma Pac	52959-0049-28
30's	$9.04	GENERIC, Prescript Pharmaceuticals	00247-0104-30
30's	$53.70	GENERIC, Southwood Pharmaceuticals Inc	58016-0122-30
30's	$79.85	GENERIC, Pharma Pac	52959-0049-30
40's	$10.93	GENERIC, Prescript Pharmaceuticals	00247-0104-40
40's	$29.35	GENERIC, Allscripts Pharmaceutical Company	54569-1889-01
40's	$71.60	GENERIC, Southwood Pharmaceuticals Inc	58016-0122-40
40's	$103.25	GENERIC, Pharma Pac	52959-0049-40
50's	$89.50	GENERIC, Southwood Pharmaceuticals Inc	58016-0122-50
60's	$105.60	GENERIC, Southwood Pharmaceuticals Inc	58016-0122-60
100's	$179.00	GENERIC, Southwood Pharmaceuticals Inc	58016-0122-00

D

Dicyclomine Hydrochloride *(001048)*

Categories: Irritable bowel syndrome; Pregnancy Category B; FDA Approved 1984 Oct
Drug Classes: Anticholinergics; Gastrointestinals
Brand Names: A-Spas; Antispas; **Bentyl**; Bo-Cyclomine; Coochil; Dedoxia; Diciclomina; Dicyclocot; Magesan; Medispaz-Im; Protylol
Foreign Brand Availability: Babyspasmil (Argentina); Balacon (Japan); Bentylol (Canada); Clomin (South-Africa; Thailand); Cyclominol (India); Diclomin (Mexico); Dicomin (Thailand); Dilomin (Philippines); Formulex (Canada); Lomine (Canada); Magesan P (Japan); Medicyclomine (South-Africa); Merbentyl (Australia; England; Ireland; New-Zealand; South-Africa); Nomcramp (South-Africa); Notensyl (Israel); Panakiron (Japan); Respolimin (Japan); Spasmotine (Philippines); Swityl (Taiwan)
Cost of Therapy: $119.88 (Irritable Bowel Syndrome; Bentyl; 20 mg; 8 tablets/day; 30 day supply)
$3.84 (Irritable Bowel Syndrome; Generic tablets; 20 mg; 8 tablets/day; 30 day supply)
HCFA JCODE(S): J0500 up to 20 mg IM

DESCRIPTION

Dicyclomine HCl is an Antispasmodic and Anticholinergic (antimuscarinic) Agent Available in the Following Forms:

1. Bentyl capsules for oral use contain 10 mg dicyclomine HCl. Dicyclomine HCl 10 mg capsules also contain inactive ingredients: calcium sulfate, corn starch, FD&C blue no. 1, FD&C red no. 40, gelatin, lactose, magnesium stearate, pregelatinized corn starch, and titanium dioxide.
2. Bentyl tablets for oral use contain 20 mg dicyclomine HCl. Dicyclomine HCl 20 mg tablets also contain inactive ingredients: acacia, dibasic calcium phosphate, corn starch, FD&C blue no. 1, lactose, magnesium stearate, pregelatinized corn starch, and sucrose.
3. Bentyl syrup for oral use contains 10 mg dicyclomine HCl in each 5 ml (1 teaspoonful). Dicyclomine HCl syrup also contains inactive ingredients: citric acid, D&C red no. 33, FD&C blue no. 1, FD&C red no. 40, FD&C yellow no. 6, flavors, glucose, methylparaben, propylene glycol, propylparaben, saccharin sodium, and water.
4. Dicyclomine HCl injection is a sterile, pyrogen-free, aqueous solution for intramuscular injection (NOT FOR INTRAVENOUS USE).

Bentyl Ampul: *2 ml:* Each ml contains 10 mg dicyclomine HCl in sterile water for injection, made isotonic with sodium chloride.

Bentyl Vial: *10 ml:* Each ml contains 10 mg dicyclomine HCl in sterile water for injection, made isotonic with sodium chloride. A preservative containing 0.5% chlorobutanol hydrous (chloral derivative) has been added.

Chemically, dicyclomine HCl is (bicyclohexyl)-1-carboxylic acid, 2-(diethylamino)ethyl-ester-, HCl. The molecular weight is 345.96 and the molecular formula is $C_{19}H_{35}NO_2 \cdot HCl$.

Dicyclomine HCl occurs as a fine, white, crystalline, practically odorless powder with a bitter taste. It is soluble in water, freely soluble in alcohol and chloroform, and very slightly soluble in ether.

CLINICAL PHARMACOLOGY

Dicyclomine relieves smooth muscle spasm of the gastrointestinal tract. Animal studies indicate that this action is achieved via a dual mechanism: (1) a specific anticholinergic effect (antimuscarinic) at the acetylcholine-receptor sites with approximately 1/8 the milligram potency of atropine (*in vitro*, guinea pig ileum); and (2) a direct effect upon smooth muscle (musculotropic) as evidenced by dicyclomine's antagonism of bradykinin- and histamine-induced spasms of the isolated guinea pig ileum. Atropine did not affect responses to these two agonists. *In vivo* studies in cats and dogs showed dicyclomine to be equally potent against acetylcholine (ACh)- or barium chloride ($BaCl_2$)-induced intestinal spasm while atropine was at least 200 times more potent against effects of ACh than $BaCl_2$. Tests for mydriatic effects in mice showed that dicyclomine was approximately 1/500 as potent as atropine; antisialagogue tests in rabbits showed dicyclomine to be 1/300 as potent as atropine.

D

In humans, dicyclomine is rapidly absorbed after oral administration, reaching peak values within 60-90 minutes. The principal route of elimination is via the urine (79.5% of the dose). Excretion also occurs in the feces, but to a lesser extent (8.4%). Mean half-life of plasma elimination in one study was determined to be approximately 1.8 hours when plasma concentrations were measured for 9 hours after a single dose. In subsequent studies, plasma concentrations were followed for up to 24 hours after a single dose, showing a secondary phase of elimination with a somewhat longer half-life. Mean volume of distribution for a 20 mg oral dose is approximately 3.65 L/kg suggesting extensive distribution in tissues.

In controlled clinical trials involving over 100 patients who received drug, 82% of patients treated for functional bowel/irritable bowel syndrome with dicyclomine HCl at initial doses of 160 mg daily (40 mg qid) demonstrated a favorable clinical response compared with 55% treated with placebo. ($P<0.05$). In these trials, most of the side effects were typically anticholinergic in nature (see TABLE 1) and were reported by 61% of the patients.

TABLE 1

Side Effect	Dicyclomine HCl (40 mg qid)	Placebo
Dry mouth	33%	5%
Dizziness	29%	2%
Blurred vision	27%	2%
Nausea	14%	6%
Light-headedness	11%	3%
Drowsiness	9%	1%
Weakness	7%	1%
Nervousness	6%	2%

Nine percent (9%) of patients were discontinued from the drug because of one or more of these side effects (compared with 2% in the placebo group). In 41% of the patients with side effects, side effects disappeared or were tolerated at the 160 mg daily dose without reduction. A dose reduction from 160 mg daily to an average daily dose of 90 mg was required in 46% of the patients with side effects who then continued to experience a favorable clinical response; their side effects either disappeared or were tolerated. (See ADVERSE REACTIONS.)

INDICATIONS AND USAGE

For the treatment of functional bowel/irritable bowel syndrome.

NON-FDA APPROVED INDICATIONS

Although not approved by the FDA, other uses of dicyclomine include treatment of urinary retention and dyspepsia.

CONTRAINDICATIONS

1. Obstructive uropathy.
2. Obstructive disease of the gastrointestinal tract.
3. Severe ulcerative colitis. (see PRECAUTIONS).
4. Reflux esophagitis.
5. Unstable cardiovascular status in acute hemorrhage.
6. Glaucoma.
7. Myasthenia gravis.
8. Evidence of prior hypersensitivity to dicyclomine HCl or other ingredients of these formulations.
9. Infants less than 6 months of age (see WARNINGS and PRECAUTIONS, Information for the Patient).
10. Nursing Mothers (see WARNINGS and PRECAUTIONS, Information for the Patient).

WARNINGS

In the presence of a high environmental temperature, heat prostration can occur with drug use (fever and heat stroke due to decreased sweating). If symptoms occur, the drug should be discontinued and supportive measures instituted.

Diarrhea may be an early symptom of incomplete intestinal obstruction, especially in patients with ileostomy or colostomy. In this instance, treatment with this drug would be inappropriate and possibly harmful.

Dicyclomine HCl may produce drowsiness or blurred vision. The patient should be warned not to engage in activities requiring mental alertness, such as operating a motor vehicle or other machinery or performing hazardous work while taking this drug.

Psychosis has been reported in sensitive individuals given anticholinergic drugs. CNS signs and symptoms include confusion, disorientation, short-term memory loss, hallucinations, dysarthria, ataxia, coma, euphoria, decreased anxiety, fatigue, insomnia, agitation and mannerisms, and inappropriate affect. These CNS signs and symptoms usually resolve within 12-24 hours after discontinuation of the drug.

There are reports that administration of dicyclomine HCl syrup to infants has been followed by serious respiratory symptoms (dyspnea, shortness of breath, breathlessness, respiratory collapse, apnea, asphyxia), seizures, syncope, pulse rate fluctuations, muscular hypotonia, and coma. Death has been reported. No causal relationship between these effects observed in infants and dicyclomine administration has been established. **Dicyclomine HCl is contraindicated in infants less than 6 months of age and in nursing mothers (see CONTRAINDICATIONS and PRECAUTIONS, Nursing Mothers and Pediatric Use.)**

Safety and efficacy of dicyclomine HCl in pediatric patients have not been established.

PRECAUTIONS

GENERAL

Use With Caution in Patients With:

1. Autonomic neuropathy.
2. Hepatic or renal disease.
3. Ulcerative colitis—large doses may suppress intestinal motility to the point of producing a paralytic ileus and the use of this drug may precipitate or aggravate the serious complication of toxic megacolon (see CONTRAINDICATIONS).
4. Hyperthyroidism.
5. Hypertension.
6. Coronary heart disease.
7. Congestive heart failure.
8. Cardiac tachyarrhythmia.
9. Hiatal hernia (see CONTRAINDICATIONS, Reflux Esophagitis).
10. Known or suspected prostatic hypertrophy.

Investigate any tachycardia before administration of dicyclomine HCl, since it may increase the heart rate.

With overdosage, a curare-like action may occur (*i.e.*, neuromuscular blockade leading to muscular weakness and possible paralysis).

INFORMATION FOR THE PATIENT

Dicyclomine HCl may produce drowsiness or blurred vision. The patient should be warned not to engage in activities requiring mental alertness, such as operating a motor vehicle or other machinery or to perform hazardous work while taking this drug.

Dicyclomine HCl is contraindicated in infants less than 6 months of age and in nursing mothers. (See CONTRAINDICATIONS, WARNINGS, and PRECAUTIONS, Nursing Mothers and Pediatric Use.)

In the presence of a high environmental temperature, heat prostration can occur with drug use (fever and heat stroke due to decreased sweating). If symptoms occur, the drug should be discontinued and a physician contacted.

CARCINOGENESIS, MUTAGENESIS, AND IMPAIRMENT OF FERTILITY

There are no known human data on long-term potential for carcinogenicity or mutagenicity.

Long-term studies in animals to determine carcinogenic potential are not known to have been conducted.

In studies in rats at doses of up to 100 mg/kg/day, dicyclomine HCl produced no deleterious effects on breeding, conception, or parturition.

PREGNANCY, TERATOGENIC EFFECTS, PREGNANCY CATEGORY B

Reproduction studies have been performed in rats and rabbits at doses up to 33 times the maximum recommended human dose based on 160 mg/day (3 mg/kg) and have revealed no evidence of impaired fertility or harm to the fetus due to dicyclomine. Epidemiologic studies in pregnant women with products containing dicyclomine HCl (at doses up to 40 mg/day) have not shown that dicyclomine increases the risk of fetal abnormalities if administered during the first trimester of pregnancy. There are, however, no adequate and well-controlled studies in pregnant women at the recommended doses (80-160 mg day). Because animal reproduction studies are not always predictive of human response, dicyclomine HCl as indicated for functional bowel/irritable bowel syndrome should be used during pregnancy only if clearly needed.

NURSING MOTHERS

Since dicyclomine HCl has been reported to be excreted in human milk, DICYCLOMINE HCL IS CONTRAINDICATED IN NURSING MOTHERS. (See CONTRAINDICATIONS, WARNINGS, Pediatric Use, and ADVERSE REACTIONS.)

PEDIATRIC USE

See CONTRAINDICATIONS, WARNINGS, and PRECAUTIONS, Nursing Mothers. DICYCLOMINE HCL IS CONTRAINDICATED IN INFANTS LESS THAN 6 MONTHS OF AGE.

Safety and effectiveness in pediatric patients have not been established.

DRUG INTERACTIONS

The following agents may increase certain actions or side effects of anticholinergic drugs: Amantadine, antiarrhythmic agents of class I (*e.g.*, quinidine), antihistamines, antipsychotic agents (*e.g.*, phenothiazines), benzodiazepines, MAO inhibitors, narcotic analgesics (*e.g.*, meperidine), nitrates and nitrites, sympathomimetic agents, tricyclic antidepressants, and other drugs having anticholinergic activity.

Anticholinergics antagonize the effects of antiglaucoma agents. Anticholinergic drugs in the presence of increased intraocular pressure may be hazardous when taken concurrently with agents such as corticosteroids. (See also CONTRAINDICATIONS.)

Anticholinergic agents may affect gastrointestinal absorption of various drugs, such as slowly dissolving dosage forms of digoxin; increased serum digoxin concentrations may result. Anticholinergic drugs may antagonize the effects of drugs that alter gastrointestinal motility, such as metoclopramide. Because antacids may interfere with the absorption of anticholinergic agents, simultaneous use of these drugs should be avoided. The inhibiting effects of anticholinergic drugs on gastric hydrochloric acid secretion are antagonized by agents used to treat achlorhydria and those used to test gastric secretion.

ADVERSE REACTIONS

Controlled clinical trials have provided frequency information for reported adverse effects of dicyclomine HCl listed in a decreasing order of frequency. (See CLINICAL PHARMACOLOGY.)

Not all of the following adverse reactions have been reported with dicyclomine HCl. Adverse reactions are included here that have been reported for pharmacologically similar drugs with anticholinergic/antispasmodic action.

Gastrointestinal: Dry mouth, nausea, vomiting, constipation, bloated feeling, abdominal pain, taste loss, anorexia.

Central Nervous System: Dizziness, light-headedness, tingling, headache, drowsiness, weakness, nervousness, numbness, mental confusion and/or excitement (especially in elderly persons), dyskinesia, lethargy, syncope, speech disturbance, insomnia.

Ophthalmologic: Blurred vision, diplopia, mydriasis, cycloplegia, increased ocular tension.

Dermatologic/Allergic: Rash, urticaria, itching, and other dermal manifestations; severe allergic reaction or drug idiosyncrasies including anaphylaxis.

Genitourinary: Urinary hesitancy, urinary retention.

Cardiovascular: Tachycardia, palpitations.

Respiratory: Dyspnea, apnea, asphyxia (see WARNINGS).

Other: Decreased sweating, nasal stuffiness or congestion, sneezing, throat congestion, impotence, suppression of lactation (see PRECAUTIONS, Nursing Mothers).

With the injectable form, there may be a temporary sensation of light-headedness. Some local irritation and focal coagulation necrosis may occur following the IM injection of the drug.

DOSAGE AND ADMINISTRATION

DOSAGE MUST BE ADJUSTED TO INDIVIDUAL PATIENT NEEDS. (See CLINICAL PHARMACOLOGY.)

ADULTS—ORAL

The only oral dose clearly shown to be effective is 160 mg per day (in 4 equally divided doses). Since this dose is associated with a significant incidence of side effects, it is prudent to begin with 80 mg per day (in 4 equally divided doses). Depending upon the patient's response during the first week of therapy, the dose should be increased to 160 mg per day unless side effects limit dosage escalation.

If efficacy is not achieved within 2 weeks or side effects require doses below 80 mg per day, the drug should be discontinued. Documented safety data are not available for doses above 80 mg daily for periods longer than 2 weeks.

ADULTS—INTRAMUSCULAR INJECTION

NOT FOR INTRAVENOUS USE.

The intramuscular dosage form is to be used temporarily when the patient cannot take oral medication. Intramuscular injection is about twice as bioavailable as oral dosage forms; consequently, the recommended intramuscular dose is 80 mg daily (in 4 equally divided doses).

Oral dicyclomine HCl should be started as soon as possible and the intramuscular form should not be used for periods longer than 1 or 2 days.

ASPIRATE THE SYRINGE BEFORE INJECTING TO AVOID INTRAVASCULAR INJECTION. SINCE THROMBOSIS MAY OCCUR IF THE DRUG IS INADVERTENTLY INJECTED INTRAVASCULARLY. Parenteral drug products should be inspected visually for particulate matter and discoloration prior to administration, whenever solution and container permit.

HOW SUPPLIED

STORAGE

Store capsules, tablets, and syrup at controlled room temperature, 15-30°C (59-86°F). Protect syrup from excessive heat. To avoid fading of the tablets, avoid exposure to direct sunlight. Dispense tablets and capsules in a tight, light-resistant container

Store injections at room temperature, preferably below 30°C (86°F).

Protect from freezing.

PRODUCT LISTING - RATED THERAPEUTICALLY EQUIVALENT

Qty	Price	Product	NDC
Capsule - Oral - 10 mg			
20's	$7.28	GENERIC, Pd-Rx Pharmaceuticals	55289-0923-20
30's	$8.78	GENERIC, Pd-Rx Pharmaceuticals	55289-0923-30
100's	$6.40	GENERIC, Major Pharmaceuticals Inc	00904-0193-60
100's	$9.14	GENERIC, Major Pharmaceuticals Inc	00904-0193-61
100's	$12.22	FEDERAL UPPER LIMIT, H.C.F.A. F F P	99999-1048-01
100's	$21.95	GENERIC, Major Pharmaceuticals Inc	00904-7896-60
100's	$22.95	GENERIC, Moore, H.L. Drug Exchange Inc	00839-5100-06
100's	$23.00	GENERIC, Lannett Company Inc	00527-0586-01
100's	$23.10	GENERIC, Aligen Independent Laboratories Inc	00405-4328-01
100's	$23.95	GENERIC, West Ward Pharmaceutical Corporation	00143-3126-01
100's	$24.82	GENERIC, Endo Laboratories Llc	60951-0615-70
100's	$26.37	GENERIC, Mutual/United Research Laboratories	00677-0341-01
100's	$26.38	GENERIC, Mylan Pharmaceuticals Inc	00378-1610-01
100's	$26.38	GENERIC, Watson Laboratories Inc	00591-0794-01
100's	$26.38	GENERIC, Watson Laboratories Inc	52544-0794-01
100's	$26.38	GENERIC, Mova Pharmaceutical Corporation	55370-0854-07
100's	$26.60	GENERIC, Udl Laboratories Inc	51079-0118-20
100's	$35.01	BENTYL, Aventis Pharmaceuticals	00068-0120-61
250's	$10.15	GENERIC, Major Pharmaceuticals Inc	00904-0193-70
Solution - Injectable - 10 mg/ml			
2 ml x 5	$83.70	BENTYL, Allscripts Pharmaceutical Company	54569-2046-00
2 ml x 5	$89.80	BENTYL, Aventis Pharmaceuticals	00068-0809-23
10 ml	$7.50	GENERIC, Keene Pharmaceuticals Inc	00588-5908-70
10 ml	$8.75	GENERIC, Cmc-Consolidated Midland Corporation	00223-7430-10
10 ml	$11.94	GENERIC, Hyrex Pharmaceuticals	00314-0299-70
10 ml	$14.80	GENERIC, Ivax Corporation	00182-0708-63
Syrup - Oral - 10 mg/5 ml			
480 ml	$38.90	BENTYL, Aventis Pharmaceuticals	00068-0125-16
Tablet - Oral - 20 mg			
20's	$9.75	GENERIC, Pd-Rx Pharmaceuticals	55289-0095-20
30's	$1.80	GENERIC, Circle Pharmaceuticals Inc	00659-1612-30
30's	$9.30	GENERIC, Heartland Healthcare Services	61392-0041-30
30's	$9.30	GENERIC, Heartland Healthcare Services	61392-0041-39
30's	$12.30	GENERIC, Pd-Rx Pharmaceuticals	55289-0095-30
30's	$13.18	BENTYL, Allscripts Pharmaceutical Company	54569-0418-00
30's	$15.01	BENTYL, Pharma Pac	52959-0390-30
30's	$16.47	BENTYL, Physicians Total Care	54868-0392-01
31's	$9.61	GENERIC, Heartland Healthcare Services	61392-0041-31
32's	$9.92	GENERIC, Heartland Healthcare Services	61392-0041-32
45's	$13.95	GENERIC, Heartland Healthcare Services	61392-0041-45
60's	$2.38	GENERIC, Circle Pharmaceuticals Inc	00659-1612-60
60's	$18.60	GENERIC, Heartland Healthcare Services	61392-0041-60
60's	$21.75	GENERIC, Pd-Rx Pharmaceuticals	55289-0095-60
90's	$27.90	GENERIC, Heartland Healthcare Services	61392-0041-90
100's	$3.05	GENERIC, Circle Pharmaceuticals Inc	00659-1612-02
100's	$4.50	GENERIC, Interstate Drug Exchange Inc	00814-2447-14
100's	$6.25	GENERIC, Cmc-Consolidated Midland Corporation	00223-0795-01
100's	$7.99	GENERIC, Major Pharmaceuticals Inc	00904-0195-61
100's	$11.85	FEDERAL UPPER LIMIT, H.C.F.A. F F P	99999-1048-02
100's	$29.75	GENERIC, Major Pharmaceuticals Inc	00904-0195-60
100's	$30.50	GENERIC, West Ward Pharmaceutical Corporation	00143-1227-01
100's	$34.84	GENERIC, Udl Laboratories Inc	51079-0119-20
100's	$35.45	GENERIC, Interstate Drug Exchange Inc	55370-0879-07
100's	$35.50	GENERIC, Mylan Pharmaceuticals Inc	00378-1620-01
100's	$35.50	GENERIC, Lannett Company Inc	00527-1282-01
100's	$35.50	GENERIC, Watson Laboratories Inc	00591-0795-01
100's	$35.50	GENERIC, Watson Laboratories Inc	52544-0795-01
100's	$36.50	GENERIC, Endo Laboratories Llc	60951-0616-70
100's	$39.75	GENERIC, Pd-Rx Pharmaceuticals	55289-0395-17
100's	$49.95	BENTYL, Aventis Pharmaceuticals	00068-0123-61
250's	$13.55	GENERIC, Major Pharmaceuticals Inc	00904-0195-70

PRODUCT LISTING - EQUIVALENTS NOT AVAILABLE

Qty	Price	Product	NDC
Capsule - Oral - 10 mg			
2's	$3.56	GENERIC, Prescript Pharmaceuticals	00247-0188-02
3's	$3.67	GENERIC, Prescript Pharmaceuticals	00247-0188-03
4's	$3.78	GENERIC, Prescript Pharmaceuticals	00247-0188-04
6's	$1.58	GENERIC, Allscripts Pharmaceutical Company	54569-0417-07
6's	$3.99	GENERIC, Prescript Pharmaceuticals	00247-0188-06
10's	$2.64	GENERIC, Allscripts Pharmaceutical Company	54569-0417-04
10's	$4.41	GENERIC, Prescript Pharmaceuticals	00247-0188-10
12's	$3.32	GENERIC, Southwood Pharmaceuticals Inc	58016-0702-12
12's	$4.62	GENERIC, Prescript Pharmaceuticals	00247-0188-12
14's	$4.84	GENERIC, Prescript Pharmaceuticals	00247-0188-14
15's	$3.96	GENERIC, Allscripts Pharmaceutical Company	54569-0417-06
15's	$4.94	GENERIC, Prescript Pharmaceuticals	00247-0188-15
20's	$5.47	GENERIC, Prescript Pharmaceuticals	00247-0188-20
24's	$5.89	GENERIC, Prescript Pharmaceuticals	00247-0188-24
30's	$5.36	GENERIC, Southwood Pharmaceuticals Inc	58016-0702-30
30's	$6.53	GENERIC, Prescript Pharmaceuticals	00247-0188-30
30's	$7.91	GENERIC, Allscripts Pharmaceutical Company	54569-0417-00
30's	$19.20	GENERIC, Pharma Pac	52959-0168-30
40's	$7.59	GENERIC, Prescript Pharmaceuticals	00247-0188-40
60's	$15.83	GENERIC, Allscripts Pharmaceutical Company	54569-0417-02
100's	$1.60	GENERIC, Global Pharmaceutical Corporation	00115-3200-01
100's	$2.09	GENERIC, Vangard Labs	00615-0327-01
100's	$13.94	GENERIC, Prescript Pharmaceuticals	00247-0188-00
100's	$21.11	GENERIC, Ivax Corporation	00182-0519-01
100's	$22.05	GENERIC, Huffman Laboratories Division Pharmed Group	54252-0110-01
100's	$26.38	GENERIC, Qualitest Products Inc	00603-3265-21
100's	$26.38	GENERIC, Allscripts Pharmaceutical Company	54569-0417-03
Solution - Injectable - 10 mg/ml			
10 ml	$9.50	DICYCLOCOT, C.O. Truxton Inc	00463-1104-10
10 ml	$9.60	GENERIC, Roberts/Hauck Pharmaceutical Corporation	43797-0008-12
Tablet - Oral - 20 mg			
10's	$3.55	GENERIC, Allscripts Pharmaceutical Company	54569-0419-07
12's	$5.06	GENERIC, Southwood Pharmaceuticals Inc	58016-0703-12
20's	$7.10	GENERIC, Allscripts Pharmaceutical Company	54569-0419-02
20's	$10.63	GENERIC, Pharma Pac	52959-0221-20
30's	$10.65	GENERIC, Allscripts Pharmaceutical Company	54569-0419-00
30's	$12.66	GENERIC, Southwood Pharmaceuticals Inc	58016-0703-30
30's	$13.32	GENERIC, Pharma Pac	52959-0221-30
60's	$21.30	GENERIC, Allscripts Pharmaceutical Company	54569-0419-04

100's	$1.60	GENERIC, Global Pharmaceutical Corporation	00115-3220-01
100's	$30.94	GENERIC, Huffman Laboratories Division Pharmed Group	54252-0111-01
100's	$36.49	GENERIC, Qualitest Products Inc	00603-3266-21
100's	$42.50	GENERIC, Southwood Pharmaceuticals Inc	58016-0703-00

Didanosine *(003060)*

D

For related information, see the comparative table section in Appendix A.

Categories: Infection, human immunodeficiency virus; Pregnancy Category B; FDA Approved 1991 Oct; WHO Formulary
Drug Classes: Antivirals; Nucleoside reverse transcriptase inhibitors
Brand Names: DDI; Dideoxyinosine; **Videx**
Foreign Brand Availability: Bristol-Videx EC (Colombia); Cipladinex 100 (Colombia); Viden DDI (Colombia); Videx EC (Hong-Kong; Israel; Thailand)
Cost of Therapy: $247.69 (HIV; Videx, Chewable; 200 mg; 2 tablets/day; 30 day supply)

WARNING

VIDEX

FATAL AND NONFATAL PANCREATITIS HAVE OCCURRED DURING THERAPY WITH VIDEX USED ALONE OR IN COMBINATION REGIMENS IN BOTH TREATMENT-NAIVE AND TREATMENT-EXPERIENCED PATIENTS, REGARDLESS OF DEGREE OF IMMUNOSUPPRESSION. VIDEX SHOULD BE SUSPENDED IN PATIENTS WITH SUSPECTED PANCREATITIS AND DISCONTINUED IN PATIENTS WITH CONFIRMED PANCREATITIS (SEE WARNINGS, Videx).

LACTIC ACIDOSIS AND SEVERE HEPATOMEGALY WITH STEATOSIS, INCLUDING FATAL CASES, HAVE BEEN REPORTED WITH THE USE OF NUCLEOSIDE ANALOGUES ALONE OR IN COMBINATION, INCLUDING DIDANOSINE AND OTHER ANTIRETROVIRALS. FATAL LACTIC ACIDOSIS HAS BEEN REPORTED IN PREGNANT WOMEN WHO RECEIVED THE COMBINATION OF DIDANOSINE AND STAVUDINE WITH OTHER ANTIRETROVIRAL AGENTS. THE COMBINATION OF DIDANOSINE AND STAVUDINE SHOULD BE USED WITH CAUTION DURING PREGNANCY AND IS RECOMMENDED ONLY IF THE POTENTIAL BENEFIT CLEARLY OUTWEIGHS THE POTENTIAL RISK. (SEE WARNINGS, Videx AND PRECAUTIONS, Videx, Pregnancy, Reproduction, and Fertility — Pregnancy Category B.)

VIDEX EC

FATAL AND NONFATAL PANCREATITIS HAVE OCCURRED DURING THERAPY WITH DIDANOSINE USED ALONE OR IN COMBINATION REGIMENS IN BOTH TREATMENT-NAIVE AND TREATMENT-EXPERIENCED PATIENTS, REGARDLESS OF DEGREE OF IMMUNOSUPPRESSION. VIDEX EC SHOULD BE SUSPENDED IN PATIENTS WITH SUSPECTED PANCREATITIS AND DISCONTINUED IN PATIENTS WITH CONFIRMED PANCREATITIS (SEE WARNINGS, Videx EC).

LACTIC ACIDOSIS AND SEVERE HEPATOMEGALY WITH STEATOSIS, INCLUDING FATAL CASES, HAVE BEEN REPORTED WITH THE USE OF NUCLEOSIDE ANALOGUES ALONE OR IN COMBINATION, INCLUDING DIDANOSINE AND OTHER ANTIRETROVIRALS. FATAL LACTIC ACIDOSIS HAS BEEN REPORTED IN PREGNANT WOMEN WHO RECEIVED THE COMBINATION OF DIDANOSINE AND STAVUDINE WITH OTHER ANTIRETROVIRAL AGENTS. THE COMBINATION OF DIDANOSINE AND STAVUDINE SHOULD BE USED WITH CAUTION DURING PREGNANCY AND IS RECOMMENDED ONLY IF THE POTENTIAL BENEFIT CLEARLY OUTWEIGHS THE POTENTIAL RISK. (SEE WARNINGS, Videx EC AND PRECAUTIONS, Videx EC, Pregnancy, Reproduction, and Fertility — Pregnancy Category B.)

DESCRIPTION

Note: The trade names have been used throughout this monograph for clarity.

VIDEX

Videx is a brand name for didanosine (ddI), a synthetic purine nucleoside analogue active against the Human Immunodeficiency Virus (HIV).

Videx Chewable/Dispersible Buffered Tablets are available for oral administration in strengths of 25, 50, 100, 150, and 200 mg of didanosine. Each tablet is buffered with calcium carbonate and magnesium hydroxide. Videx tablets also contain aspartame, sorbitol, microcrystalline cellulose, polyplasdone, mandarin-orange flavor, and magnesium stearate.

Videx Buffered Powder for Oral Solution is supplied for oral administration in single-dose packets containing 100, 167, or 250 mg of didanosine. Packets of each product strength also contain a citrate-phosphate buffer (composed of dibasic sodium phosphate, sodium citrate, and citric acid) and sucrose.

Videx Pediatric Powder for Oral Solution is supplied for oral administration in 4 or 8 ounce glass bottles containing 2 or 4 g of didanosine, respectively.

Didanosine is also available as an enteric-coated formulation (Videx EC delayed-release capsules). Please consult the prescribing information for Videx EC.

The chemical name for didanosine is 2′,3′-dideoxyinosine.

Didanosine is a white crystalline powder with the molecular formula $C_{10}H_{12}N_4O_3$ and a molecular weight of 236.2. The aqueous solubility of didanosine at 25°C and pH of approximately 6 is 27.3 mg/ml. Didanosine is unstable in acidic solutions. For example, at pH <3 and 37°C, 10% of didanosine decomposes to hypoxanthine in less than 2 minutes.

VIDEX EC

Videx EC is the brand name for an enteric-coated formulation of didanosine (ddI), a synthetic purine nucleoside analogue active against the Human Immunodeficiency Virus (HIV).

Videx EC Delayed-Release Capsules, containing enteric-coated beadlets, are available for oral administration in strengths of 125, 200, 250, and 400 mg of didanosine. The inactive ingredients in the beadlets include carboxymethylcellulose sodium 12, diethyl phthalate, methacrylic acid copolymer, sodium hydroxide, sodium starch glycolate, and talc. The capsule shells contain colloidal silicon dioxide, gelatin, sodium lauryl sulfate, and titanium dioxide. The capsules are imprinted with edible inks.

Didanosine is also available as buffered formulations. Please consult the prescribing information for Videx buffered formulations and Pediatric Powder for Oral Solution for additional information.

The chemical name for didanosine is 2′,3′-dideoxyinosine.

Didanosine is a white crystalline powder with the molecular formula $C_{10}H_{12}N_4O_3$ and a molecular weight of 236.2. The aqueous solubility of didanosine at 25°C and pH of approximately 6 is 27.3 mg/ml. Didanosine is unstable in acidic solutions. For example, at pH <3 and 37°C, 10% of didanosine decomposes to hypoxanthine in less than 2 minutes. In Videx EC, an enteric coating is used to protect didanosine from degradation by stomach acid.

CLINICAL PHARMACOLOGY

VIDEX

Microbiology

Mechanism of Action

Didanosine is a synthetic nucleoside analogue of the naturally occurring nucleoside deoxyadenosine in which the 3′-hydroxyl group is replaced by hydrogen. Intracellularly, didanosine is converted by cellular enzymes to the active metabolite, dideoxyadenosine 5′-triphosphate. Dideoxyadenosine 5′-triphosphate inhibits the activity of HIV-1 reverse transcriptase both by competing with the natural substrate, deoxyadenosine 5′-triphosphate, and by its incorporation into viral DNA causing termination of viral DNA chain elongation.

In Vitro HIV Susceptibility

The *in vitro* anti-HIV-1 activity of didanosine was evaluated in a variety of HIV-1 infected lymphoblastic cell lines and monocyte/macrophage cell cultures. The concentration of drug necessary to inhibit viral replication by 50% (IC_{50}) ranged from 2.5 to 10 μM (1 μM = 0.24 μg/ml) in lymphoblastic cell lines and 0.01 to 0.1 μM in monocyte/macrophage cell cultures. The relationship between *in vitro* susceptibility of HIV to didanosine and the inhibition of HIV replication in humans has not been established.

Drug Resistance

HIV-1 isolates with reduced sensitivity to didanosine have been selected *in vitro* and were also obtained from patients treated with didanosine. Genetic analysis of isolates from didanosine-treated patients showed mutations in the reverse transcriptase gene that resulted in the amino acid substitutions K65R, L74V, and M184V. The L74V mutation was most frequently observed in clinical isolates. Phenotypic analysis of HIV-1 isolates from 60 patients (some with prior zidovudine treatment) receiving 6-24 months of didanosine monotherapy showed that isolates from 10 of 60 patients exhibited an average of a 10-fold decrease in susceptibility to didanosine *in vitro* compared to baseline isolates. Clinical isolates that exhibited a decrease in didanosine susceptibility harbored 1 or more didanosine-associated mutations. The clinical relevance of genotypic and phenotypic changes associated with didanosine therapy has not been established.

Cross-Resistance

HIV-1 isolates from 2 of 39 patients receiving combination therapy for up to 2 years with zidovudine and didanosine exhibited decreased susceptibility to zidovudine, didanosine, zalcitabine, stavudine, and lamivudine *in vitro*. These isolates harbored 5 mutations (A62V, V75I, F77L, F116Y, and Q151M) in the reverse transcriptase gene. The clinical relevance of these observations has not been established.

Pharmacokinetics

The pharmacokinetic parameters of didanosine are summarized in TABLE 1. Didanosine is rapidly absorbed, with peak plasma concentrations generally observed from 0.25-1.50 hours following oral dosing. Increases in plasma didanosine concentrations were dose proportional over the range of 50-400 mg. Steady-state pharmacokinetic parameters did not differ significantly from values obtained after a single dose. Binding of didanosine to plasma proteins *in vitro* was low (<5%). Based on data from *in vitro* and animal studies, it is presumed that the metabolism of didanosine in man occurs by the same pathways responsible for the elimination of endogenous purines.

Effect of Food on Absorption of Didanosine

Didanosine peak plasma concentrations (C_{max}) and area under the plasma concentration time curve (AUC) were decreased by approximately 55% when Videx tablets were administered up to 2 hours after a meal. Administration of Videx tablets up to 30 minutes before a meal did not result in any significant changes in bioavailability. Videx should be taken on an empty stomach, at least 30 minutes before or 2 hours after eating. (See DOSAGE AND ADMINISTRATION, Videx.)

Special Populations

Renal Insufficiency

It is recommended that the Videx dose be modified in patients with reduced creatinine clearance and in patients receiving maintenance hemodialysis (see DOSAGE AND ADMINISTRATION, Videx). Data from two studies indicated that the apparent oral clearance of didanosine decreased and the terminal elimination half-life increased as creatinine clearance decreased (see TABLE 2). Following oral administration, didanosine was not detectable in peritoneal dialysate fluid (n=6); recovery in hemodialysate (n=5) ranged from 0.6-7.4% of the dose over a 3-4 hour dialysis period. The absolute bioavailability of didanosine was not affected in patients requiring dialysis.

TABLE 1 *Mean ±SD Pharmacokinetic Parameters for Didanosine in Adult and Pediatric Patients*

Parameter	Adult Patients*	n	Pediatric Patients† 8 months to 19 years	n	2 weeks to 4 months	n
Oral bioavailability	42 ± 12%	6	25 ± 20%	46	ND	
Apparent volume of distribution‡ (L/m^2)	43.70 ± 8.90	6	28 ± 15	49	ND	
CSF-plasma ratio§	21 ± 0.03%¤	5	46% (range 12-85%)	7	ND	
Systemic clearance‡ (ml/min/m^2)	526 ± 64.7	6	516 ± 184	49	ND	
Renal clearance¶ (ml/min/m^2)	223 ± 85.0	6	240 ± 90	15	ND	
Apparent oral clearance** (ml/min/m^2)	1252 ± 154	6	2064 ± 736	48	1353 ± 759	41
Elimination half-life¶ (h)	1.5 ± 0.4	6	0.8 ± 0.3	60	1.2 ± 0.3	21
Urinary recovery of didanosine¶	18 ± 8%	6	18 ± 10%	15	ND	

CSF = cerebrospinal fluid, ND = not determined.
* Parameter units for adults were converted to the same uints in pediatric patients to facilitate comparisons among populations: mean adult body weight = 70 kg and mean adult body surface area = 1.73 m^2.
† In 1-day-old infants (n=10), the mean ±SD apparent oral clearance was 1523 ± 1176 ml/min/m^2 and half-life was 2.0 ± 0.7 h.
‡ Following IV administration.
§ Following IV administration in adults and IV or oral administration in pediatric patients.
¤ Mean ± SE.
¶ Following oral administration.
** Apparent oral clearance estimate was determined as the ratio of the mean systemic clearance and the mean oral bioavailability estimate.

TABLE 2 *Mean ±SD Pharmacokinetic Parameters for Didanosine Following a Single Oral Dose*

Creatinine Clearance (ml/min)	n	CLCR (ml/min)	CL/F (ml/min)	CLR (ml/min)	T½ (h)
≥90	12	112 ± 22	2164 ± 638	458 ± 164	1.42 ± 0.33
60-90	6	68 ± 8	1566 ± 833	247 ± 153	1.59 ± 0.13
30-59	6	46 ± 8	1023 ± 378	100 ± 44	1.75 ± 0.43
10-29	3	13 ± 5	628 ± 104	20 ± 8	2.0 ± 0.3
Dialysis patients	11	ND	543 ± 174	<10	4.1 ± 1.2

ND = Not determined due to anuria.
CLCR = Creatinine clearance.
CL/F = Apparent oral clearance.
CLR = Renal clearance.

Pediatric Patients

The pharmacokinetics of didanosine have been evaluated in HIV-exposed and infected pediatric patients from birth to 19 years of age (see TABLE 1). Overall, the pharmacokinetics of didanosine in pediatric patients age are similar to those of didanosine in adults. Didanosine plasma concentrations appear to increase in proportion to oral doses ranging from 25-120 mg/m^2 in pediatric patients less than 5 months old and from 80-180 mg/m^2 in children above 8 months old. For information on controlled clinical studies in pediatric patients, see PRECAUTIONS, Videx, Pediatric Use.

Geriatric Patients

Didanosine pharmacokinetics have not been studied in patients over 65 years of age.

Gender

The effects of gender on didanosine pharmacokinetics have not been studied.

Drug Interactions

TABLE 3 and TABLE 4 summarize the effects on AUC and C_{max}, with a 90% or 95% confidence interval (CI) when available, following coadministration of Videx with a variety of drugs. For most of the listed drugs, no clinically significant pharmacokinetic interactions were observed. Clinical recommendations based on drug interaction studies for drugs in bold font are included in DRUG INTERACTIONS, Videx.

VIDEX EC

Microbiology

Mechanism of Action

Didanosine is a synthetic nucleoside analogue of the naturally occurring nucleoside deoxyadenosine in which the 3′-hydroxyl group is replaced by hydrogen. Intracellularly, didanosine is converted by cellular enzymes to the active metabolite, dideoxyadenosine 5′-triphosphate. Dideoxyadenosine 5′-triphosphate inhibits the activity of HIV-1 reverse transcriptase both by competing with the natural substrate, deoxyadenosine 5′-triphosphate, and by its incorporation into viral DNA causing termination of viral DNA chain elongation.

In Vitro HIV Susceptibility

The *in vitro* anti-HIV-1 activity of didanosine was evaluated in a variety of HIV-1 infected lymphoblastic cell lines and monocyte/macrophage cell cultures. The concentration of drug necessary to inhibit viral replication by 50% (IC_{50}) ranged from 2.5 to 10 μM (1 μM = 0.24 μg/ml) in lymphoblastic cell lines and 0.01 to 0.1 μM in monocyte/macrophage cell cultures. The relationship between *in vitro* susceptibility of HIV to didanosine and the inhibition of HIV replication in humans has not been established.

TABLE 3 *Results of Drug Interaction Studies: Effects of Coadministered Drug on Didanosine Plasma AUC and C_{max} Values*

Drug	Didanosine Dosage	n	Didanosine AUC (95% CI)	C_{max} (95% CI)
Drugs with clinical recommendations regarding coadministration (see DRUG INTERACTIONS, Videx)				
Allopurinal				
Renally impaired, 300 mg/day	200 mg single dose	2	inc 312%	inc 232%
Healthy volunteer, 300 mg/day for 7 days	400 mg single dose	14	inc 113%	inc 69%
Ciprofloxacin				
750 mg q12h for 3 days, 2 h before didanosine	200 mg q12h for 3 days	8*	dec 16%	dec 28%
Ganciclovir				
1000 mg q8h, 2 h after didanosine	200 mg q12h	12	inc 111%	NA
Indinavir				
800 mg single dose, simultaneous	200 mg single dose	16	NC	NC
800 mg single dose, 1 h before didanosine	200 mg single dose	16	dec 17% (-27, -7%)†	dec 13% (-28, 5%)†
Ketoconazole				
200 mg/day for 4 days, 2 h before didanosine	375 mg q12h for 4 days	12*	NC	dec 12%
Methadone				
Chronic maintenance dose	200 mg single dose	16, 10‡	dec 57%	dec 66%
Tenofovir§¤				
300 mg once daily 1 h after didanosine	250¶ or 400 mg once daily for 7 days	14	inc 44% (31, 59%)†	inc 28% (11, 48%)†
No clinically significant interaction observed				
Loperamide				
4 mg q6h for 1 day	300 mg single dose	12*	NC	dec 23%
Metoclopramide				
10 mg single dose	300 mg single dose	12*	NC	inc 13%
Ranitidine				
150 mg single dose, 2 h before didanosine	375 mg single dose	12*	inc 14%	inc 13%
Rifabutin				
300 or 600 mg/day for 12 days	167 or 250 mg q12h for 12 days	11	inc 13% (-1, 27%)	inc 17% (-4, 38%)
Ritonavir				
600 mg q12h for 4 days	200 mg q12h for 4 days	12	dec 13% (0, 23%)	dec 16% (5, 26%)
Stavudine				
40 mg q12h for 4 days	100 mg q12h for 4 days	10	NC	NC
Sulfamethoxazole				
1000 mg single dose	200 mg single dose	8*	NC	NC
Trimethoprim				
200 mg single dose	200 mg single dose	8*	NC	inc 17% (-23, 77%)
Zidovudine				
200 mg q8h for 3 days	200 mg q12h for 3days	6*	NC	NC

inc Indicates increase.
dec Indicates decrease.
NC Indicates no change, or mean increase or decrease of <10%.
* HIV-infected patients.
† 90% CI.
‡ Parallel-group design; entries are subjects receiving combination and control regimens, respectively.
§ Tenofovir disoproxil fumarate.
¤ In a drug interaction study with the enteric-coated formulation of didanosine (Videx EC) and tenofovir, the AUC and C_{max} of didanosine each increased 48% when Videx EC was administered in the fasting state 2 hours before tenofovir with a light meal. The AUC and C_{max} of didanosine increased 60% and 64%, respectively, when Videx EC was administered together with tenofovir and a light meal.
¶ Patients less than 60 kg.
NA Not available.

Drug Resistance

HIV-1 isolates with reduced sensitivity to didanosine have been selected *in vitro* and were also obtained from patients treated with didanosine. Genetic analysis of isolates from didanosine-treated patients showed mutations in the reverse transcriptase gene that resulted in the amino acid substitutions K65R, L74V, and M184V. The L74V mutation was most frequently observed in clinical isolates. Phenotypic analysis of HIV-1 isolates from 60 patients (some with prior zidovudine treatment) receiving 6-24 months of didanosine monotherapy showed that isolates from 10 of 60 patients exhibited an average of a 10-fold decrease in susceptibility to didanosine *in vitro* compared to baseline isolates. Clinical isolates that exhibited a decrease in didanosine susceptibility harbored 1 or more didanosine-associated mutations. The clinical relevance of genotypic and phenotypic changes associated with didanosine therapy has not been established.

Cross-Resistance

HIV-1 isolates from 2 of 39 patients receiving combination therapy for up to 2 years with zidovudine and didanosine exhibited decreased susceptibility to zidovudine, didanosine,

D

TABLE 4 *Results of Drug Interaction Studies: Effects of Didanosine on Coadministered Drug Plasma AUC and C_{max} Values*

			Coadministered Drug	
Drug	**Didanosine Dosage**	**n**	**AUC (95% CI)**	**C_{max} (95% CI)**
Drugs with clinical recommendations regarding coadministration (see DRUG INTERACTIONS, Videx)				
Ciprofloxacin				
750 mg q12h for 3 days, 2 h before didanosine	200 mg q12h for 3 days	8*	dec 26%	dec 16%
750 mg single dose	Buffered placebo tablets	12	dec 98%	dec 93%
Delavirdine				
400 mg single dose, simultaneous	125 or 200 mg q12h	12*	dec 32%	dec 53%
400 mg single dose, 1 h before didanosine	125 or 200 mg q12h	12*	inc 20%	inc 18%
Ganciclovir				
1000 mg q8h, 2 h after didanosine	200 mg q12h	12*	dec 21%	NA
Indinavir				
800 mg single dose, simultaneous	200 mg single dose	16	dec 84%	dec 82%
800 mg single dose, 1 h before didanosine	200 mg single dose	16	dec 11%	dec 4%
Ketoconazole				
200 mg/day for 4 days, 2 h before didanosine	375 mg q12h for 4 days	12*	dec 14%	dec 20%
Nelfinavir				
750 mg single dose, 1 h after didanosine	200 mg single dose	10*	inc 12%	NC
No clinically significant interaction observed				
Dapsone				
100 mg single dose	200 mg q12h for 14 days	6*	NC	NC
Ranitidine				
150 mg single dose, 2 h before didanosine	375 mg single dose	12*	dec 16%	NC
Ritonavir				
600 mg q12h for 4 days	200 mg q12h for 4 days	12	NC	NC
Stavudine				
40 mg q12h for 4 days	100 mg q12h for 4 days	10*	NC	inc 17%
Sulfamethoxazole				
1000 mg single dose	200 mg single dose	8*	dec 11% (-17, -4%)	dec 12% (-28, 8%)
Tenofovir†				
300 mg once daily 1 h after didanosine	250‡ or 400 mg once daily for 7 days	14	NC	NC
Trimethoprim				
200 mg single dose	200 mg single dose	8*	inc 10% (-9, 34%)	dec 22% (-59, 49%)
Zidovudine				
200 mg q8h for 3 days	200 mg q12h for 3 days	6*	dec 10% (-27, 11%)	dec 16.5% (-53, 47%)

inc Indicates increase.
dec Indicates decrease.
↔ Indicates no change, or mean increase or decrease of <10%.
* HIV-infected patients.
† Tenofovir disoproxil fumarate.
‡ Patients less than 60 kg.
NA Not available.

zalcitabine, stavudine, and lamivudine *in vitro*. These isolates harbored 5 mutations (A62V, V751, F77L, F116Y, and Q151M) in the reverse transcriptase gene. The clinical relevance of these observations has not been established.

Pharmacokinetics

The pharmacokinetic parameters of didanosine are summarized in TABLE 5. Didanosine is rapidly absorbed, with peak plasma concentrations generally observed from 0.25-1.50 hours following oral dosing with a buffered formulation. Increases in plasma didanosine concentrations were dose proportional over the range of 50-400 mg. Steady-state pharmacokinetic parameters did not differ significantly from values obtained after a single dose. Binding of didanosine to plasma proteins *in vitro* was low (<5%). Based on data from *in vitro* and animal studies, it is presumed that the metabolism of didanosine in man occurs by the same pathways responsible for the elimination of endogenous purines.

Comparison of Didanosine Formulations

In Videx EC, the active ingredient, didanosine, is protected against degradation by stomach acid by the use of an enteric coating on the beadlets in the capsule. The enteric coating dissolves when the beadlets empty into the small intestine, the site of drug absorption. With buffered formulations of didanosine, administration with antacid provides protection from degradation by stomach acid.

In healthy volunteers, as well as subjects infected with HIV, the area under the plasma concentration time curve (AUC) is equivalent for didanosine administered as the Videx EC formulation relative to a buffered tablet formulation. The peak plasma concentration (C_{max}) of didanosine, administered as Videx EC, is reduced approximately 40% relative to

TABLE 5 *Pharmacokinetic Parameters for Didanosine in Adults*

Parameter	Mean ±SD	n
Oral bioavailability*	42 ± 12%	6
Apparent volume of distribution†	1.08 ± 0.22 L/kg	6
CSF-plasma ratio†	21 ± 0.03%‡	5
Systemic clearance†	13.0 ± 1.6 ml/min/kg	6
Renal clearance*	5.5 ± 2.1 ml/min/kg	6
Elimination half-life*	1.5 ± 0.4 h	6
Urinary recovery of didanosine*	18 ± 8%	6

CSF = Cerebrospinal fluid.
* Following oral administration of a buffered formulation.
† Following IV administration.
‡ Mean ±SE.

didanosine buffered tablets. The time to the peak concentration (T_{max}) increases from approximately 0.67 hours for didanosine buffered tablets to 2.0 hours for Videx EC.

Effect of Food on Absorption of Didanosine

In the presence of food, the C_{max} and AUC for Videx EC were reduced by approximately 46% and 19%, respectively, compared to the fasting state. Videx EC should be taken on an empty stomach.

Special Populations

Renal Insufficiency

It is recommended that the Videx EC dose be modified in patients with reduced creatinine clearance and in patients receiving maintenance hemodialysis (see DOSAGE AND ADMINISTRATION, Videx EC). Data from two studies using a buffered formulation of didanosine indicated that the apparent oral clearance of didanosine decreased and the terminal elimination half-life increased as creatinine clearance decreased (see TABLE 6). Following oral administration, didanosine was not detectable in peritoneal dialysate fluid (n=6); recovery in hemodialysate (n=5) ranged from 0.6-7.4% of the dose over a 3-4 hour dialysis period. The absolute bioavailability of didanosine was not affected in patients requiring dialysis.

TABLE 6 *Mean ±SD Pharmacokinetic Parameters for Didanosine Following a Single Oral Dose of a Buffered Formulation*

	Creatinine Clearance (ml/min)				
Parameter	**≥90 (n=12)**	**60-90 (n=6)**	**30-59 (n=6)**	**10-29 (n=3)**	**Dialysis Patients (n=11)**
CLCR (ml/min)	112 ± 22	68 ± 8	46 ± 8	13 ± 5	ND*
CL/F (ml/min)	2164 ± 638	1566 ± 833	1023 ± 378	628 ± 104	543 ± 174
CLR (ml/min)	485 ± 164	247 ± 153	100 ± 44	20 ± 8	<10
T½ (h)	1.42 ± 0.33	1.59 ± 0.13	1.75 ± 0.43	2.0 ± 0.3	4.1 ± 1.2

* ND = Not determined due to anuria.
CLCR = creatinine clearance; CL/F = apparent oral clearance; CLR = renal clearance.

Pediatric Patients

The pharmacokinetics of didanosine administered as Videx EC have not been studied in pediatric patients.

Geriatric Patients

Didanosine pharmacokinetics have not been studied in patients over 65 years of age (see PRECAUTIONS, Videx EC, Geriatric Use).

Gender

The effects of gender on didanosine pharmacokinetics have not been studied.

Drug Interactions

See also DRUG INTERACTIONS, Videx EC.

Videx EC

TABLE 7 and TABLE 8 summarize the effects on AUC and C_{max}, with a 90% confidence interval (CI) when available, following coadministration of Videx EC with a variety of drugs. The only clinically significant pharmacokinetic interaction noted was between Videx EC and tenofovir disoproxil fumarate. Clinical recommendations based on drug interaction studies for drugs in bold font are included in DRUG INTERACTIONS, Videx EC.

Didanosine Buffered Formulations

TABLE 9 and TABLE 10 summarize the effects on AUC and C_{max}, with a 90% or 95% CI when available, following coadministration of buffered formulations of didanosine with a variety of drugs. Except as noted in table footnotes, the results of these studies may be expected to apply to Videx EC. For most of the listed drugs, no clinically significant pharmacokinetic interactions were noted. Clinical recommendations based on drug interaction studies for drugs in bold font are included in DRUG INTERACTIONS, Videx EC.

INDICATIONS AND USAGE

VIDEX

Videx in combination with other antiretroviral agents is indicated for the treatment of HIV-1 infection.

VIDEX EC

Videx EC in combination with other antiretroviral agents is indicated for the treatment of HIV-1 infection in adults.

TABLE 7 *Results of Drug Interaction Studies With Videx EC: Effects of Coadministered Drug on Didanosine Plasma AUC and C_{max} Values**

Drug	Didanosine Dosage	n	AUC of Didanosine (90% CI)	C_{max} of Didansoine (90% CI)
Tenofovir†				
300 mg once daily with a light meal‡	400 mg single dose fasting 2 h before tenofovir	26	inc 48% (31, 67%)	inc 48% (25, 76%)
	400 mg single dose together with tenofovir and a light meal	25	inc 60% (44, 79%)	inc 64% (41, 89%)

inc Indicates increase.
* All studies conducted in healthy volunteers.
† Tenofovir disoproxil fumarate.
‡ 373 kcalories, 8.2 gams fat.

TABLE 8 *Results of Drug Interaction Studies With Videx EC: Effects of Didanosine on Coadministered Drug Plasma AUC and C_{max} Values**

Drug	Didanosine Dosage	n	Coadministered Drug AUC	Coadministered Drug C_{max}
Ciprofloxacin				
750 mg single dose	400 mg single dose	16	NC	NC
Indinavir				
800 mg single dose	400 mg single dose	23	NC	NC
Ketoconazole				
200 mg single dose	400 mg single dose	21	NC	NC
Tenofovir†				
300 mg once daily with a light meal‡	400 mg single dose fasting 2 h before tenofovir	25	NC	NC
300 mg once daily with a light meal‡	400 mg single dose together with tenofovir and a light meal	25	NC	NC

NC Indicates no change, or mean increase or decrease of <10%.
* All studies conducted in healthy volunteers.
† Tenofovir disoproxil fumarate.
‡ 373 kcalories, 8.2 grams fat.

TABLE 9 *Results of Drug Interaction Studies With Buffered Formulations of Didanosine: Effects of Coadministered Drug on Didanosine Plasma AUC and C_{max} Values*

Drug	Didanosine Dosage	n	Didanosine AUC (95% CI)	Didanosine C_{max} (95% CI)
Drugs With Clinical Recommendations Regarding Coadministration*				
Allopurinal				
Renally impaired, 300 mg/day	200 mg single dose	2	inc 312%	inc 232%
Healthy volunteer, 300 mg/day for 7 days	400 mg single dose	14	inc 113%	inc 69%
Ganciclovir				
1000 mg q8h, 2 h after didanosine	200 mg q12h	12	inc 111%	NA
Methadone				
Chronic maintenance dose	200 mg single dose	16, 10†	dec 57%	dec 66%
Tenofovir‡				
300 mg once daily 1 h after didanosine	250§ or 400 mg once daily for 7 days	14	inc 44% (31, 59%)¤	inc 28% (11, 48%)¤
No Clinically Significant Interaction Observed				
Ciprofloxacin				
750 mg q12h for 3 days, 2 h before didanosine	200 mg q12h for 3 days	8¶	dec 16%	dec 28%
Indinavir				
800 mg single dose, simultaneous	200 mg single dose	16	NC	NC
800 mg single dose, 1 h before didanosine	200 mg single dose	16	dec 17% (-27, -7%)¤	dec 13% (-28, 5%)¤
Ketoconazole				
200 mg/day for 4 days, 2 h before didanosine	375 mg q12h for 4 days	12¶	NC	dec 12%
Loperamide				
4 mg q6h for 1 day	300 mg single dose	12¶	NC	dec 23%
Metoclopramide				
10 mg single dose	300 mg single dose	12¶	NC	inc 13%
Ranitidine				
150 mg single dose, 2 h before didanosine	375 mg single dose	12¶	inc 14%	inc 13%
Rifabutin				
300 or 600 mg/day for 12 days	167 or 250 mg q12h for 12 days	11	inc 13% (-1, 27%)	inc 17% (-4, 38%)
Ritonavir				
600 mg q12h for 4 days	200 mg q12h for 4 days	12	dec 13% (0, 23%)	dec 16% (5, 26%)
Stavudine				
40 mg q12h for 4 days	100 mg q12h for 4 days	10	NC	NC
Sulfamethoxazole				
1000 mg single dose	200 mg single dose	8¶	NC	NC
Trimethoprim				
200 mg single dose	200 mg single dose	8¶	NC	inc 17% (-23, 77%)
Zidovudine				
200 mg q8h for 3 days	200 mg q12h for 3days	6¶	NC	NC

inc Indicates increase.
dec Indicates decrease.
NC Indicates no change, or mean increase or decrease of <10%.
* See DRUG INTERACTIONS, Videx EC.
† Parallel-group design; entries are subjects receiving combination and control regimens, respectively.
‡ Tenofovir disoproxil fumarate.
§ Patients less than 60 kg.
¤ 90% CI.
¶ HIV-infected patients.
NA Not available.

CONTRAINDICATIONS

VIDEX

Videx is contraindicated in patients with previously demonstrated clinically significant hypersensitivity to any of the components of the formulations.

VIDEX EC

Videx EC is contraindicated in patients with previously demonstrated clinically significant hypersensitivity to any component of the formulation.

WARNINGS

VIDEX

Pancreatitis

FATAL AND NONFATAL PANCREATITIS HAVE OCCURRED DURING THERAPY WITH VIDEX USED ALONE OR IN COMBINATION REGIMENS IN BOTH TREATMENT-NAIVE AND TREATMENT-EXPERIENCED PATIENTS, REGARDLESS OF DEGREE OF IMMUNOSUPPRESSION. VIDEX SHOULD BE SUSPENDED IN PATIENTS WITH SIGNS OR SYMPTOMS OF PANCREATITIS AND DISCONTINUED IN PATIENTS WITH CONFIRMED PANCREATITIS. PATIENTS TREATED WITH VIDEX IN COMBINATION WITH STAVUDINE, WITH OR WITHOUT HYDROXYUREA, MAY BE AT INCREASED RISK FOR PANCREATITIS.

When treatment with life-sustaining drugs known to cause pancreatic toxicity is required, suspension of Videx therapy is recommended. In patients with risk factors for pancreatitis, Videx should be used with extreme caution and only if clearly indicated. Patients with advanced HIV infection, especially the elderly, are at increased risk of pancreatitis and should be followed closely. Patients with renal impairment may be at greater risk for pancreatitis if treated without dose adjustment.

The frequency of pancreatitis is dose related. In Phase 3 studies, incidence ranged from 1-10% with doses higher than are currently recommended and 1-7% with recommended dose.

In pediatric Phase 1 studies, pancreatitis occurred in 3% (2/60) of patients treated at entry doses below 300 mg/m^2/day and in 13% (5/38) of patients treated at higher doses. In study ACTG 152, pancreatitis occurred in none of the 281 pediatric patients who received didanosine 120 mg/m^2 q12h and in <1% of the 274 pediatric patients who received didanosine 90 mg/m^2 q12h in combination with zidovudine. Videx use should be suspended in pediatric patients with signs or symptoms of pancreatitis and discontinued in pediatric patients with confirmed pancreatitis.

Lactic Acidosis/Severe Hepatomegaly With Steatosis

Lactic acidosis and severe hepatomegaly with steatosis, including fatal cases, have been reported with the use of nucleoside analogues alone or in combination, including didanosine and other antiretrovirals. A majority of these cases have been in women. Obesity and prolonged nucleoside exposure may be risk factors. Fatal lactic acidosis has been reported in pregnant women who received the combination of didanosine and stavudine with other antiretroviral agents. The combination of didanosine and stavudine should be used with caution during pregnancy and is recommended only if the potential benefit clearly outweighs the potential risk (see PRECAUTIONS, Videx, Pregnancy, Reproduction, and Fertility — Pregnancy Category B). Particular caution should be exercised when administering Videx to any patient with known risk factors for liver disease; however, cases have also been reported in patients with no known risk factors. Treatment with Videx should be suspended in any patient who develops clinical or laboratory findings suggestive of symptomatic hyperlactatemia, lactic acidosis, or pronounced hepatotoxicity (which may include hepatomegaly and steatosis even in the absence of marked transaminase elevations).

Retinal Changes and Optic Neuritis

Retinal changes and optic neuritis have been reported in adult and pediatric patients. Periodic retinal examinations should be considered for patients receiving Videx. (See ADVERSE REACTIONS, Videx.)

VIDEX EC

Pancreatitis

FATAL AND NONFATAL PANCREATITIS HAVE OCCURRED DURING THERAPY WITH DIDANOSINE USED ALONE OR IN COMBINATION REGI-

TABLE 10 Results of Drug Interaction Studies With Buffered Formulations of Didanosine: Effects of Didanosine on Coadministered Drug Plasma AUC and C_{max} Values

Drug	Didanosine Dosage	n	Coadministered Drug AUC (95% CI)	Coadministered Drug C_{max} (95% CI)
No Clinically Significant Interaction Observed				
Dapsone				
100 mg single dose	200 mg q12h for 14 days	6*	NC	NC
Delavirdine				
400 mg single dose, simultaneous	125 or 200 mg q12h	12*	dec 32%†	dec 53%†
400 mg single dose, 1 h before didanosine	125 or 200 mg q12h	12*	inc 20%	inc 18%
Ganciclovir				
1000 mg q8h, 2 h after didanosine	200 mg q12h	12*	dec 21%	NA
Nelfinavir				
750 mg single dose, 1 h after didanosine	200 mg single dose	10*	inc 12%	NC
Ranitidine				
150 mg single dose, 2 h before didanosine	375 mg single dose	12*	dec 16%	NC
Ritonavir				
600 mg q12h for 4 days	200 mg q12h for 4 days	12	NC	NC
Stavudine				
40 mg q12h for 4 days	100 mg q12h for 4 days	10*	NC	inc 17%
Sulfamethoxazole				
1000 mg single dose	200 mg single dose	8*	dec 11% (-17, -4%)	dec 12% (-28, 8%)
Tenofovir‡				
300 mg once daily 1 h after didanosine	250§ or 400 mg once daily for 7 days	14	NC	NC
Trimethoprim				
200 mg single dose	200 mg single dose	8*	inc 10% (-9, 34%)	dec 22% (-59, 49%)
Zidovudine				
200 mg q8h for 3 days	200 mg q12h for 3 days	6*	dec 10% (-27, 11%)	dec 16.5% (-53, 47%)

inc Indicates increase.
dec Indicates decrease.
↔ Indicates no change, or mean increase or decrease of <10%.
* HIV-infected patients.
† This result is probably related to the buffer and is not expected to occur with Videx EC.
‡ Tenofovir disoproxil fumarate.
§ Patients less than 60 kg.
NA Not available.

MENS IN BOTH TREATMENT-NAIVE AND TREATMENT-EXPERIENCED PATIENTS, REGARDLESS OF DEGREE OF IMMUNOSUPPRESSION. VIDEX EC SHOULD BE SUSPENDED IN PATIENTS WITH SIGNS OR SYMPTOMS OF PANCREATITIS AND DISCONTINUED IN PATIENTS WITH CONFIRMED PANCREATITIS. PATIENTS TREATED WITH VIDEX EC IN COMBINATION WITH STAVUDINE, WITH OR WITHOUT HYDROXYUREA, MAY BE AT INCREASED RISK FOR PANCREATITIS.

When treatment with life-sustaining drugs known to cause pancreatic toxicity is required, suspension of Videx EC therapy is recommended. In patients with risk factors for pancreatitis, Videx EC should be used with extreme caution and only if clearly indicated. Patients with advanced HIV infection, especially the elderly, are at increased risk of pancreatitis and should be followed closely. Patients with renal impairment may be at greater risk for pancreatitis if treated without dose adjustment.

The frequency of pancreatitis is dose related. In Phase 3 studies with buffered formulations of didanosine, incidence ranged from 1-10% with doses higher than are currently recommended and 1-7% with recommended dose.

Lactic Acidosis/Severe Hepatomegaly With Steatosis

Lactic acidosis and severe hepatomegaly with steatosis, including fatal cases, have been reported with the use of nucleoside analogues alone or in combination, including didanosine and other antiretrovirals. A majority of these cases have been in women. Obesity and prolonged nucleoside exposure may be risk factors. Fatal lactic acidosis has been reported in pregnant women who received the combination of didanosine and stavudine with other antiretroviral agents. The combination of didanosine and stavudine should be used with caution during pregnancy and is recommended only if the potential benefit clearly outweighs the potential risk (see PRECAUTIONS, Videx EC, Pregnancy, Reproduction, and Fertility — Pregnancy Category B). Particular caution should be exercised when administering Videx EC to any patient with known risk factors for liver disease; however, cases have also been reported in patients with no known risk factors. Treatment with Videx EC should be suspended in any patient who develops clinical or laboratory findings suggestive of lactic acidosis or pronounced hepatotoxicity (which may include hepatomegaly and steatosis even in the absence of marked transaminase elevations).

Retinal Changes and Optic Neuritis

Retinal changes and optic neuritis have been reported in patients taking didanosine. Periodic retinal examinations should be considered for patients receiving Videx EC. (See ADVERSE REACTIONS, Videx EC.)

PRECAUTIONS

VIDEX

Frequency of Dosing

The preferred dosing frequency of Videx is twice daily because there is more evidence to support the effectiveness of this dosing frequency. Once-daily dosing should be considered only for adult patients whose management requires once-daily dosing of Videx.

Videx should be taken on an empty stomach, at least 30 minutes before or 2 hours after eating.

Peripheral Neuropathy

Peripheral neuropathy, manifested by numbness, tingling, or pain in the hands or feet, has been reported in patients receiving Videx therapy. Peripheral neuropathy has occurred more frequently in patients with advanced HIV disease, in patients with a history of neuropathy, or in patients being treated with neurotoxic drug therapy, including stavudine (see ADVERSE REACTIONS, Videx).

Fat Redistribution

Redistribution/accumulation of body fat including central obesity, dorsocervical fat enlargement (buffalo hump), peripheral wasting, facial wasting, breast enlargement, and "cushingoid appearance" have been observed in patients receiving antiretroviral therapy. The mechanism and long-term consequences of these events are currently unknown. A causal relationship has not been established.

General

Patients With Phenylketonuria

Videx chewable/dispersible buffered tablets contain the following quantities of phenylalanine:

Phenylalanine per 2 tablet dose: 73 mg
Phenylalanine per tablet: 36.5 mg

Patients on Sodium-Restricted Diets

Videx Buffered Powder for Oral Solution: Each single-dose packet of Videx buffered powder for oral solution contains 1380 mg sodium.

Patients With Renal Impairment

Patients with renal impairment (creatinine clearance <60 ml/min) may be at greater risk of toxicity from Videx due to decreased drug clearance (see CLINICAL PHARMACOLOGY, Videx). A dose reduction is recommended in these patients (see DOSAGE AND ADMINISTRATION, Videx). The magnesium content of each buffered tablet of Videx is 8.6 mEq. This may present an excessive load of magnesium to patients with significant renal impairment, particularly after prolonged dosing.

Patients With Hepatic Impairment

It is unknown if hepatic impairment significantly affects didanosine pharmacokinetics. Therefore, these patients should be monitored closely for evidence of didanosine toxicity.

Hyperuricemia

Videx has been associated with asymptomatic hyperuricemia; treatment suspension may be necessary if clinical measures aimed at reducing uric acid levels fail.

Information for the Patient

See Patient Information Leaflet.

Patients should be informed that a serious toxicity of Videx used alone and in combination regimens, is pancreatitis, which may be fatal.

Patients should be informed that the preferred dosing frequency of Videx is twice daily because there is more evidence to support the effectiveness of this dosing frequency. Once-daily dosing should be considered only for adult patients whose management requires once-daily dosing of Videx.

Patients should also be aware that peripheral neuropathy, manifested by numbness, tingling, or pain in hands or feet, may develop during therapy with Videx. Patients should be counseled that peripheral neuropathy occurs with greatest frequency in patients with advanced HIV disease or a history of peripheral neuropathy, and that dose modification and/or discontinuation of Videx may be required if toxicity develops.

Patients should be informed that when Videx is used in combination with other agents with similar toxicities, the incidence of adverse events may be higher than when Videx is used alone. These patients should be followed closely.

Patients should be cautioned about the use of medications or other substances, including alcohol, that may exacerbate Videx toxicities.

Patients should be advised that to ensure proper acid neutralization in the stomach they must take at least 2 of the appropriate strength Videx tablets at each dose. To reduce the risk of gastrointestinal side effects from excess antacid, patients should take no more than 4 Videx tablets at each dose.

Videx is not a cure for HIV infection, and patients may continue to develop HIV-associated illnesses, including opportunistic infection. Therefore, patients should remain under the care of a physician when using Videx. Patients should be advised that Videx therapy has not been shown to reduce the risk of transmission of HIV to others through sexual contact or blood contamination. Patients should be informed that the long-term effects of Videx are unknown at this time.

Patients should be informed that redistribution or accumulation of body fat may occur in patients receiving antiretroviral therapy and that the cause and long-term health effects of these conditions are not known at this time.

Carcinogenesis and Mutagenesis

Lifetime carcinogenicity studies were conducted in mice and rats for 22 and 24 months, respectively. In the mouse study, initial doses of 120, 800, and 1200 mg/kg/day for each sex were lowered after 8 months to 120, 210, and 210 mg/kg/day for females and 120, 300, and 600 mg/kg/day for males. The two higher doses exceeded the maximally tolerated dose in females and the high dose exceeded the maximally tolerated dose in males. The low dose in females represented 0.68-fold maximum human exposure and the intermediate dose in males represented 1.7-fold maximum human exposure based on relative AUC comparisons. In the rat study, initial doses were 100, 250, and 1000 mg/kg/day, and the high dose was lowered to 500 mg/kg/day after 18 months. The upper dose in male and female rats represented 3-fold maximum human exposure.

Didanosine induced no significant increase in neoplastic lesions in mice or rats at maximally tolerated doses.

Didanosine was positive in the following genetic toxicology assays: (1) the *Escherichia coli* tester strain WP2 uvrA bacterial mutagenicity assay; (2) the L5178Y/TK+/- mouse lymphoma mammalian cell gene mutation assay; (3) the *in vitro* chromosomal aberrations assay in cultured human peripheral lymphocytes; (4) the *in vitro* chromosomal aberrations assay in Chinese Hamster Lung cells; and (5) the BALB/c 3T3 *in vitro* transformation assay. No evidence of mutagenicity was observed in an Ames *Salmonella* bacterial mutagenicity assay or in rat and mouse *in vivo* micronucleus assays.

Pregnancy, Reproduction, and Fertility — Pregnancy Category B

Reproduction studies have been performed in rats and rabbits at doses up to 12 and 14.2 times the estimated human exposure (based upon plasma levels), respectively, and have revealed no evidence of impaired fertility or harm to the fetus due to didanosine. At approximately 12 times the estimated human exposure, didanosine was slightly toxic to female rats and their pups during mid and late lactation. These rats showed reduced food intake and body weight gains but the physical and functional development of the offspring was not impaired and there were no major changes in the F2 generation. A study in rats showed that didanosine and/or its metabolites are transferred to the fetus through the placenta. Animal reproduction studies are not always predictive of human response.

There are no adequate and well-controlled studies of didanosine in pregnant women. Didanosine should be used during pregnancy only if the potential benefit justifies the potential risk.

Fatal lactic acidosis has been reported in pregnant women who received the combination of didanosine and stavudine with other antiretroviral agents. It is unclear if pregnancy augments the risk of lactic acidosis/hepatic steatosis syndrome reported in nonpregnant individuals receiving nucleoside analogues (see WARNINGS, Videx, Lactic Acidosis/Severe Hepatomegaly With Steatosis). **The combination of didanosine and stavudine should be used with caution during pregnancy and is recommended only if the potential benefit clearly outweighs the potential risk.** Health care providers caring for HIV-infected pregnant women receiving didanosine should be alert for early diagnosis of lactic acidosis/hepatic steatosis syndrome.

Antiretroviral Pregnancy Registry: To monitor maternal-fetal outcomes of pregnant women exposed to didanosine and other antiretroviral agents, an Antiretroviral Pregnancy Registry has been established. Physicians are encouraged to register patients by calling 1-800-258-4263.

Nursing Mothers

The Centers for Disease Control and Prevention recommend that HIV-infected mothers not breast-feed their infants to avoid risking postnatal transmission of HIV. A study in rats showed that following oral administration, didanosine and/or its metabolites were excreted into the milk of lactating rats. It is not known if didanosine is excreted in human milk. Because of both the potential for HIV transmission and the potential for serious adverse reactions in nursing infants, **mothers should be instructed not to breast-feed if they are receiving Videx.**

Pediatric Use

Use of Videx in pediatric patients from 2 weeks of age through adolescence is supported by evidence from adequate and well-controlled studies of Videx in adults and pediatric patients (see CLINICAL PHARMACOLOGY, Videx; ADVERSE REACTIONS, Videx; and DOSAGE AND ADMINISTRATION, Videx).

Dosing recommendations for Videx in patients less than 2 weeks of age cannot be made because the pharmacokinetics of didanosine in these children are too variable to determine an appropriate dose.

Geriatric Use

In an Expanded Access Program for patients with advanced HIV infection, patients aged 65 years and older had a higher frequency of pancreatitis (10%) than younger patients (5%) (see WARNINGS, Videx). Clinical studies of didanosine did not include sufficient numbers of subjects aged 65 years and over to determine whether they respond differently than younger subjects. Didanosine is known to be substantially excreted by the kidney, and the risk of toxic reactions to this drug may be greater in patients with impaired renal function. Because elderly patients are more likely to have decreased renal function, care should be taken in dose selection. In addition, renal function should be monitored and dosage adjustments should be made accordingly (see DOSAGE AND ADMINISTRATION, Videx, Dose Adjustment).

VIDEX EC

Dosing

Videx EC should be administered once daily on an empty stomach.

Peripheral Neuropathy

Peripheral neuropathy, manifested by numbness, tingling, or pain in the hands or feet, has been reported in patients receiving didanosine therapy. Peripheral neuropathy has occurred more frequently in patients with advanced HIV disease, in patients with a history of neuropathy, or in patients being treated with neurotoxic drug therapy, including stavudine (see ADVERSE REACTIONS, Videx EC).

Fat Redistribution

Redistribution/accumulation of body fat including central obesity, dorsocervical fat enlargement (buffalo hump), peripheral wasting, facial wasting, breast enlargement, and "cushingoid appearance" have been observed in patients receiving antiretroviral therapy. The mechanism and long-term consequences of these events are currently unknown. A causal relationship has not been established.

General

Patients With Renal Impairment

Patients with renal impairment (creatinine clearance <60 ml/min) may be at greater risk of toxicity from didanosine due to decreased drug clearance (see CLINICAL PHARMACOLOGY, Videx EC). A dose reduction is recommended in these patients (see DOSAGE AND ADMINISTRATION, Videx EC).

Patients With Hepatic Impairment

It is unknown if hepatic impairment significantly affects didanosine pharmacokinetics. Therefore, these patients should be monitored closely for evidence of didanosine toxicity.

Hyperuricemia

Didanosine has been associated with asymptomatic hyperuricemia; treatment suspension may be necessary if clinical measures aimed at reducing uric acid levels fail.

Information for the Patient

See Patient Information Leaflet.

Patients should be informed that a serious toxicity of didanosine, used alone and in combination regimens, is pancreatitis, which may be fatal.

Patients should also be aware that peripheral neuropathy, manifested by numbness, tingling, or pain in hands or feet, may develop during therapy with Videx EC. Patients should be counseled that peripheral neuropathy occurs with greatest frequency in patients with advanced HIV disease or a history of peripheral neuropathy, and that dose modification and/or discontinuation of Videx EC may be required if toxicity develops.

Patients should be informed that when didanosine is used in combination with other agents with similar toxicities, the incidence of adverse events may be higher than when didanosine is used alone. These patients should be followed closely.

Patients should be cautioned about the use of medications or other substances, including alcohol, that may exacerbate Videx EC toxicities.

Videx EC is not a cure for HIV infection, and patients may continue to develop HIV-associated illnesses, including opportunistic infection. Therefore, patients should remain under the care of a physician when using Videx EC. Patients should be advised that Videx EC therapy has not been shown to reduce the risk of transmission of HIV to others through sexual contact or blood contamination. Patients should be informed that the long-term effects of Videx EC are unknown at this time.

Patients should be informed that redistribution or accumulation of body fat may occur in patients receiving antiretroviral therapy and that the cause and long-term health effects of these conditions are not known at this time.

Carcinogenesis and Mutagenesis

Lifetime carcinogenicity studies were conducted in mice and rats for 22 and 24 months, respectively. In the mouse study, initial doses of 120, 800, and 1200 mg/kg/day for each sex were lowered after 8 months to 120, 210, and 210 mg/kg/day for females and 120, 300, and 600 mg/kg/day for males. The two higher doses exceeded the maximally tolerated dose in females and the high dose exceeded the maximally tolerated dose in males. The low dose in females represented 0.68-fold maximum human exposure and the intermediate dose in males represented 1.7-fold maximum human exposure based on relative AUC comparisons. In the rat study, initial doses were 100, 250, and 1000 mg/kg/day, and the high dose was lowered to 500 mg/kg/day after 18 months. The upper dose in male and female rats represented 3-fold maximum human exposure.

Didanosine induced no significant increase in neoplastic lesions in mice or rats at maximally tolerated doses.

Didanosine was positive in the following genetic toxicology assays: (1) the *Escherichia coli* tester strain WP2 uvrA bacterial mutagenicity assay; (2) the L5178Y/TK+/- mouse lymphoma mammalian cell gene mutation assay; (3) the *in vitro* chromosomal aberrations assay in cultured human peripheral lymphocytes; (4) the *in vitro* chromosomal aberrations assay in Chinese Hamster Lung cells; and (5) the BALB/c 3T3 *in vitro* transformation assay. No evidence of mutagenicity was observed in an Ames *Salmonella* bacterial mutagenicity assay or in rat and mouse *in vivo* micronucleus assays.

Pregnancy, Reproduction, and Fertility — Pregnancy Category B

Reproduction studies have been performed in rats and rabbits at doses up to 12 and 14.2 times the estimated human exposure (based upon plasma levels), respectively, and have revealed no evidence of impaired fertility or harm to the fetus due to didanosine. At approximately 12 times the estimated human exposure, didanosine was slightly toxic to female rats and their pups during mid and late lactation. These rats showed reduced food intake and body weight gains but the physical and functional development of the offspring was not impaired, and there were no major changes in the F2 generation. A study in rats showed that didanosine and/or its metabolites are transferred to the fetus through the placenta. Animal reproduction studies are not always predictive of human response.

There are no adequate and well-controlled studies of didanosine in pregnant women. Didanosine should be used during pregnancy only if the potential benefit justifies the potential risk.

Fatal lactic acidosis has been reported in pregnant women who received the combination of didanosine and stavudine with other antiretroviral agents. It is unclear if pregnancy augments the risk of lactic acidosis/hepatic steatosis syndrome reported in nonpregnant individuals receiving nucleoside analogues (see WARNINGS, Videx EC, Lactic Acidosis/Severe Hepatomegaly With Steatosis). **The combination of didanosine and stavudine should be used with caution during pregnancy and is recommended only if the potential benefit clearly outweighs the potential risk.** Healthcare providers caring for HIV-infected pregnant women receiving didanosine should be alert for early diagnosis of lactic acidosis/hepatic steatosis syndrome.

Antiretroviral Pregnancy Registry: To monitor maternal-fetal outcomes of pregnant women exposed to didanosine and other antiretroviral agents, an Antiretroviral Pregnancy Registry has been established. Physicians are encouraged to register patients by calling 1-800-258-4263.

Nursing Mothers

The Centers for Disease Control and Prevention recommend that HIV-infected mothers not breast-feed their infants to avoid risking post-natal transmission of HIV. A study in rats showed that following oral administration, didanosine and/or its metabolites were excreted into the milk of lactating rats. It is not known if didanosine is excreted in human milk. Because of both the potential for HIV transmission and the potential for serious adverse reactions in nursing infants, **mothers should be instructed not to breast-feed if they are receiving Videx EC.**

Pediatric Use

The safety and efficacy of Videx EC in pediatric patients have not been established. Please consult the complete prescribing information for Videx buffered formulations and pediatric powder for oral solution for dosage and administration of didanosine to pediatric patients.

Geriatric Use

In an Expanded Access Program using a buffered formulation of didanosine for the treatment of advanced HIV infection, patients aged 65 years and older had a higher frequency of pancreatitis (10%) than younger patients (5%) (see WARNINGS, Videx EC). Clinical studies of didanosine, including those for Videx EC, did not include sufficient numbers of subjects aged 65 years and over to determine whether they respond differently than younger subjects. Didanosine is known to be substantially excreted by the kidney, and the risk of toxic reactions to this drug may be greater in patients with impaired renal function. Because elderly patients are more likely to have decreased renal function, care should be taken in dose selection. In addition, renal function should be monitored and dosage adjustments should be made accordingly (see DOSAGE AND ADMINISTRATION, Videx EC, Dose Adjustment).

DRUG INTERACTIONS

VIDEX

See also CLINICAL PHARMACOLOGY, Videx, Drug Interactions.

Drug interactions that have been established based on drug interaction studies are listed with the pharmacokinetic results in TABLE 3 and TABLE 4). The clinical recommendations based on the results of these studies are listed in TABLE 13.

TABLE 13 *Established Drug Interactions With Videx*

Drug	Effect	Clinical Comment
Coadministration not recommended based on drug interaction studies (see CLINICAL PHARMACOLOGY, Videx, Drug Interactions for magnitude of interaction)		
Allopurinol	inc didanosine concentration	Coadministration not recommended.
Alteration in dose or regimen recommended based on drug interaction studies (see CLINICAL PHARMACOLOGY, Videx, Drug Interactions for magnitude of interaction)		
Ciprofloxacin	dec ciprofloxacin concentration	Administer Videx at least 2 h after or 6 h before ciprofloxacin.
Delavirdine	dec didanosine concentration	Administer Videx 1 h after delavirdine.
Ganciclovir	inc didanosine concentration	Appropriate doses for this combination, with respect to efficacy and safety, have not been established.
Indinavir	dec indinavir concentration	Administer Videx 1 h after indinavir.
Methadone	dec didanosine concentration	Appropriate doses for this combination, with respect to efficacy and safety, have not been established.
Nelfinavir	No interaction 1 h after didanosine	Administer nelfinavir 1 h after Videx.
Tenofovir disoproxil fumarate	inc didanosine concentration	Appropriate doses for this combination, with respect to efficacy and safety, have not been established. Use with caution and monitor closely for didanosine-associated toxicities (see below).

inc Indicates increase.
dec Indicates decrease.

Coadministration of Videx with drugs that are known to cause pancreatitis may increase the risk of this toxicity (see WARNINGS, Videx, Pancreatitis). Because Videx formulations either contain buffers or are mixed with antacids before administration, interactions may be anticipated with drugs whose absorption can be affected by the level of acidity in the stomach and with drugs that have been demonstrated to interact with antacids containing magnesium, calcium, or aluminum. Predicted drug interactions with Videx are listed in TABLE 14.

Tenofovir Disoproxil Fumarate or Ribavirin

Exposure to didanosine or its active metabolite (dideoxyadenosine 5′-triphosphate) is increased when didanosine is coadministered with either tenofovir (see TABLE 3 and TABLE 13) or ribavirin (see TABLE 14). **Increased exposure may cause or worsen didanosine-related clinical toxicities, including pancreatitis, symptomatic hyperlactatemia/lactic acidosis, and peripheral neuropathy. Coadministration of tenofovir or ribavirin with Videx should be undertaken with caution, and patients should be monitored closely for didanosine-related toxicities. Videx should be suspended if signs or symptoms of pancreatitis, symptomatic hyperlactatemia, or lactic acidosis develop** (see WARNINGS, Videx).

TABLE 14 *Predicted Drug Interactions With Videx*

Drug or Drug Class	Effect	Clinical Comment
Use with caution, risk of adverse reactions may be increased		
Drugs that may cause pancreatic toxicity	inc risk of pancreatitis	Use only with extreme caution.*
Neurotoxic drugs	inc risk of neuropathy	Use with caution.†
Antacids containing magnesium or aluminum	inc side effects associated with antacid components	Use caution with Videx chewable/dispersable buffered tablets and pediatric powder for oral solution.
Ribavirin	inc risk of toxicity	Ribavirin has been shown *in vitro* to increase intracellular triphosphate levels of didanosine. Use with caution and monitor closely for didanosine-associated toxicities (see Tenofovir Disoproxil Fumarate or Ribavirin).
Use with caution, plasma concentrations may be decreased by coadministration with Videx		
Azole antifungals	dec ketoconazole or itraconazole concentration	Administer drugs such as ketoconazole or itraconazole at least 2 h before Videx.
Quinolone antibiotics‡	dec quinolone concentration	Consult package insert of the quinolone.
Tetracycline antibiotics	dec antibiotic concentration	Consult package insert of the tetracycline.

inc Indicates increase.
dec Indicates decrease.
* Only if other drugs are not available and if clearly indicated. If treatment with life-sustaining drugs that cause pancreatic toxicity is required, suspension of Videx is recommended (see WARNINGS, Videx, Pancreatitis).
† See PRECAUTIONS, Videx, Peripheral Neuropathy.
‡ See also ciprofloxacin in TABLE 13.

VIDEX EC

See also CLINICAL PHARMACOLOGY, Videx EC, Drug Interactions.

Drug interactions that have been established based on drug interaction studies are listed with the pharmacokinetic results in TABLE 8, TABLE 9, and TABLE 10). The clinical recommendations based on the results of these studies are listed in TABLE 15.

TABLE 15 *Established Drug Interactions Based on Studies With Videx EC or Studies With Buffered Formulations of Didanosine and Expected to Occur With Videx EC*

Drug	Effect	Clinical Comment
Coadministration not recommended based on drug interaction studies (see CLINICAL PHARMACOLOGY, Videx EC, Drug Interactions for magnitude of interaction)		
Allopurinol	inc didanosine concentration	Coadministration not recommended.
Alteration in dose or regimen recommended based on drug interaction studies (see CLINICAL PHARMACOLOGY, Videx EC, Drug Interactions for magnitude of interaction)		
Ganciclovir	inc didanosine concentration	Appropriate doses for this combination, with respect to efficacy and safety, have not been established.
Methadone	dec didanosine concentration	Appropriate doses for this combination, with respect to efficacy and safety, have not been established.
Tenofovir disoproxil fumarate	inc didanosine concentration	Appropriate doses for this combination, with respect to efficacy and safety, have not been established. Use with caution and monitor closely for didanosine-associated toxicities (see below).

inc Indicates increase.
dec Indicates decrease.

Coadministration of Videx EC with drugs that are known to cause pancreatitis may increase the risk of this toxicity (see WARNINGS, Videx EC, Pancreatitis). Predicted drug interactions with Videx EC are listed in TABLE 16.

Tenofovir Disoproxil Fumarate and Ribavirin

Exposure to didanosine or its active metabolite (dideoxyadenosine 5′-triphosphate) is increased when didanosine is coadministered with either tenofovir (see TABLE 7, TABLE 9, and TABLE 15) or ribavirin (see TABLE 16). Increased exposure may cause or worsen didanosine-related clinical toxicities, including pancreatitis, symptomatic hyperlactatemia/lactic acidosis, and peripheral neuropathy. Coadministration of tenofovir or ribavirin with Videx EC should be undertaken with caution, and patients should be monitored closely for didanosine-related toxicities. Videx EC should be suspended if signs or symptoms of pancreatitis, symptomatic hyperlactatemia, or lactic acidosis develop (see WARNINGS, Videx EC).

ADVERSE REACTIONS

VIDEX

A SERIOUS TOXICITY OF VIDEX IS PANCREATITIS, WHICH MAY BE FATAL (see WARNINGS, Videx). OTHER IMPORTANT TOXICITIES INCLUDE LACTIC ACIDOSIS/SEVERE HEPATOMEGALY WITH STEATOSIS; RETINAL CHANGES

TABLE 16 *Predicted Drug Interactions With Videx EC*

Drug or Drug Class	Effect	Clinical Comment
Use with caution, risk of adverse reactions may be increased		
Drugs that may cause pancreatic toxicity	inc risk of pancreatitis	Use only with extreme caution.*
Neurotoxic drugs	inc risk of neuropathy	Use with caution.†
Ribavirin	inc risk of toxicity	Ribavirin has been shown *in vitro* to increase intracellular triphosphate levels of didanosine and other purine nucleoside analogues. Use with caution and monitor closely for didanosine-associated toxicities (see Tenofovir Disoproxil Fumarate and Ribavirin).

inc Indicates increase.
* Only if other drugs are not available and if clearly indicated. If treatment with life-sustaining drugs that cause pancreatic toxicity is required, suspension of Videx EC is recommended (see WARNINGS, Videx EC, Pancreatitis).
† See PRECAUTIONS, Videx EC, Peripheral Neuropathy.

AND OPTIC NEURITIS; AND PERIPHERAL NEUROPATHY (see WARNINGS, Videx and PRECAUTIONS, Videx).

When Videx is used in combination with other agents with similar toxicities, the incidence of these toxicities may be higher than when Videx is used alone. Thus, patients treated with Videx in combination with stavudine, with or without hydroxyurea, may be at increased risk for pancreatitis, which may be fatal, and hepatotoxicity (see WARNINGS, Videx). Patients treated with Videx in combination with stavudine may also be at increased risk for peripheral neuropathy (see PRECAUTIONS, Videx).

Adults

Selected clinical adverse events that occurred in adult patients in clinical studies with Videx are provided in TABLE 17 and TABLE 18.

TABLE 17 *Selected Clinical Adverse Events From Monotherapy Studies*

	ACTG 116A		ACTG 116B/117	
	Videx	Zidovudine	Videx	Zidovudine
Adverse Events	n=197	n=212	n=298	n=304
Diarrhea	19%	15%	28%	21%
Peripheral neurologic symptoms/ neuropathy	17%	14%	20%	12%
Rash/pruritus	7%	8%	9%	5%
Abdominal pain	13%	8%	7%	8%
Pancreatitis	7%	3%	6%	2%

TABLE 18 *Selected Clinical Adverse Events From Combination Studies*

	AI454-148*		START 2*	
Adverse	Videx + Stavudine + Nelfinavir	Zidovudine + Lamivudine + Nelfinavir	Videx + Stavudine + Indinavir	Zidovudine + Lamivudine + Indinavir
Events	n=482	n=248	n=102	n=103
Diarrhea	70%	60%	45%	39%
Nausea	28%	40%	53%	67%
Headache	21%	30%	46%	37%
Peripheral neurologic symptoms/ neuropathy	26%	6%	21%	10%
Rash	13%	16%	30%	18%
Vomiting	12%	14%	30%	35%
Pancreatitis‡	1%	†	<1%	†

Percentages based on treated subjects.
* Median duration of treatment 48 weeks.
† This event not observed in this study arm.
‡ **Pancreatitis resulting in death was observed in 1 patient who received didanosine plus stavudine plus nelfinavir in Study AI454-148 and in 1 patient who received didanosine plus stavudine plus indinavir in the START 2 study. In addition, pancreatitis resulting in death was observed in 2 of 68 patients who received Videx plus stavudine plus indinavir plus hydroxyurea in an ACTG clinical trial (see WARNINGS, Videx).**

The frequency of pancreatitis is dose related. In Phase 3 studies, incidence ranged from 1-10% with doses higher than are currently recommended and from 1-7% with recommended dose.

Selected laboratory abnormalities in clinical studies with Videx are shown in TABLE 19, TABLE 20, and TABLE 21.

Observed During Clinical Practice

The following events have been identified during postapproval use of Videx. Because they are reported voluntarily from a population of unknown size, estimates of frequency cannot be made. These events have been chosen for inclusion due to their seriousness, frequency of reporting, causal connection to Videx, or a combination of these factors.

Body as a Whole: Alopecia, anaphylactoid reaction, asthenia, chills/fever, pain, and redistribution/accumulation of body fat (see PRECAUTIONS, Videx, Fat Redistribution).

Digestive Disorders: Anorexia, dyspepsia, and flatulence.

TABLE 19 *Selected Laboratory Abnormalities From Monotherapy Studies*

	ACTG 116A		ACTG 116B/117	
	Videx	Zidovudine	Videx	Zidovudine
Parameter	n=197	n=212	n=298	n=304
SGOT (AST) (>5 × ULN)	9%	4%	7%	6%
SGPT (ALT) (>5 × ULN)	9%	6%	6%	6%
Alkaline phosphatase (>5 × ULN)	4%	1%	1%	1%
Amylase (≥1.4 × ULN)	17%	12%	15%	5%
Uric acid (>12 mg/dl)	3%	1%	2%	1%

ULN = Upper limit of normal.

TABLE 20 *Selected Laboratory Abnormalities From Combination Studies (Grades 3-4)*

	AI454-148*		START 2*	
	Videx + Stavudine + Nelfinavir	Zidovudine + Lamivudine + Nelfinavir	Videx + Stavudine + Indinavir	Zidovudine + Lamivudine + Indinavir
Parameter	n=482	n=248	n=102	n=103
Bilirubin (>2.6 × ULN)	<1%	<1%	16%	8%
SGOT (AST) (>5 × ULN)	3%	2%	7%	7%
SGPT (ALT) (>5 × ULN)	3%	3%	8%	5%
GGT (>5 × ULN)	NC	NC	5%	2%
Lipase (>2 × ULN)	7%	2%	5%	5%
Amylase (>2 × ULN)	NC	NC	8%	2%

ULN = Upper limit of normal, NC = Not Collected.
Percentages based on treated subjects.
* Median duration of treatment 48 weeks.

TABLE 21 *Selected Laboratory Abnormalities From Combination Studies (All Grades)*

	AI454-148*		START 2*	
	Videx + Stavudine + Nelfinavir	Zidovudine + Lamivudine + Nelfinavir	Videx + Stavudine + Indinavir	Zidovudine + Lamivudine + Indinavir
Parameter	n=482	n=248	n=102	n=103
Bilirubin	7%	3%	68%	55%
SGOT (AST)	42%	23%	53%	20%
SGPT (ALT)	37%	24%	50%	18%
GGT	NC	NC	28%	12%
Lipase	17%	11%	26%	19%
Amylase	NC	NC	31%	17%

NC = Not Collected.
Percentages based on treated subjects.
* Median duration of treatment 48 weeks.

Exocrine Gland Disorders: Pancreatitis (including fatal cases) (see WARNINGS, Videx), sialoadenitis, parotid gland enlargement, dry mouth, and dry eyes.

Hematologic Disorders: Anemia, leukopenia, and thrombocytopenia.

Liver: Symptomatic hyperlactatemia, lactic acidosis and hepatic steatosis (see WARNINGS, Videx); hepatitis and liver failure.

Metabolic Disorders: Diabetes mellitus, hypoglycemia, and hyperglycemia.

Musculoskeletal Disorders: Myalgia (with or without increases in creatine kinase), rhabdomyolysis including acute renal failure and hemodialysis, arthralgia, and myopathy.

Ophthalmologic Disorders: Retinal depigmentation and optic neuritis (see WARNINGS, Videx).

Pediatric Patients

In clinical trials, 743 pediatric patients between 2 weeks and 18 years of age have been treated with Videx. Adverse events and laboratory abnormalities reported to occur in these patients were generally consistent with the safety profile of didanosine in adults.

In pediatric Phase 1 studies, pancreatitis occurred in 2 of 60 (3%) patients treated at entry doses below 300 mg/m^2/day and in 5 of 38 (13%) patients treated at higher doses. In study ACTG 152, pancreatitis occurred in none of the 281 pediatric patients who received didanosine 120 mg/m^2 q12h and in <1% of the 274 pediatric patients who received didanosine 90 mg/m^2 q12h in combination with zidovudine.

Retinal changes and optic neuritis have been reported in pediatric patients.

VIDEX EC

A SERIOUS TOXICITY OF DIDANOSINE IS PANCREATITIS, WHICH MAY BE FATAL (see WARNINGS, Videx EC). OTHER IMPORTANT TOXICITIES INCLUDE LACTIC ACIDOSIS/SEVERE HEPATOMEGALY WITH STEATOSIS; RETINAL

CHANGES AND OPTIC NEURITIS; AND PERIPHERAL NEUROPATHY (see WARNINGS, Videx EC and PRECAUTIONS, Videx EC).

When didanosine is used in combination with other agents with similar toxicities, the incidence of these toxicities may be higher than when didanosine is used alone. Thus, patients treated with Videx EC in combination with stavudine, with or without hydroxyurea, may be at increased risk for pancreatitis, which may be fatal, and hepatotoxicity (see WARNINGS, Videx EC). Patients treated with Videx EC in combination with stavudine may also be at increased risk for peripheral neuropathy (see PRECAUTIONS, Videx EC).

Selected clinical adverse events that occurred in a study of Videx EC in combination with other antiretroviral agents are provided in TABLE 22.

TABLE 22 *Selected Clinical Adverse Events, Study AI454-152**

Adverse Events	Videx EC + Stavudine + Nelfinavir n=258	Zidovudine/Lamivudine† + Nelfinavir n=253
Diarrhea	57%	58%
Peripheral neurologic symptoms/neuropathy	25%	11%
Nausea	24%	36%
Headache	22%	17%
Rash	14%	12%
Vomiting	14%	19%
Pancreatitis§	<1%	‡

Percentages based on treated patients.
* Median duration of treatment was 62 weeks in the Videx EC + stavudine + nelfinavir group and 61 weeks in the zidovudine/lamivudine + nelfinavir group.
† Zidovudine/lamivudine combination tablet.
‡ This event was not observed in this study arm.
§ **In clinical trials using a buffered formulation of didanosine, pancreatitis resulting in death was observed in 1 patient who received didanosine plus stavudine plus nelfinavir, 1 patient who received didanosine plus stavudine plus indinavir, and 2 of 68 patients who received didanosine plus stavudine plus indinavir plus hydroxyurea. In an early access program, pancreatitis resulting in death was observed in 1 patient who received Videx EC plus stavudine plus hydroxyurea plus ritonavir plus indinavir plus efavirenz** (see WARNINGS, Videx EC).

The frequency of pancreatitis is dose related. In Phase 3 studies with buffered formulations of didanosine, incidence ranged from 1-10% with doses higher than are currently recommended and 1-7% with recommended dose.

Selected laboratory abnormalities that occurred in a study of Videx EC in combination with other antiretroviral agents are shown in TABLE 23.

TABLE 23 *Selected Laboratory Abnormalities, Study AI454-152**

	Videx EC + Stavudine + Nelfinavir n=258		Zidovudine/Lamivudine† + Nelfinavir n=253	
Parameter	Grades 3-4‡	All Grades	Grades 3-4‡	All Grades
SGOT (AST)	5%	46%	5%	19%
SGPT (ALT)	6%	44%	5%	22%
Lipase	5%	23%	2%	13%
Bilirubin	<1%	9%	<1%	3%

Percentages based on treated patients.
* Median duration of treatment was 62 weeks in the Videx EC + stavudine + nelfinavir group and 61 weeks in the zidovudine/lamivudine + nelfinavir group.
† Zidovudine/lamivudine combination tablet.
‡ >5 × ULN for SGOT and SGPT, ≥2.1 × ULN for lipase, and ≥2.6 × ULN for bilirubin (ULN = upper limit of normal).

Observed During Clinical Practice

The following events have been identified during postapproval use of didanosine buffered formulations. Because they are reported voluntarily from a population of unknown size, estimates of frequency cannot be made. These events have been chosen for inclusion due to their seriousness, frequency of reporting, causal connection to didanosine, or a combination of these factors.

Body as a Whole: Abdominal pain, alopecia, anaphylactoid reaction, asthenia, chills/fever, pain, and redistribution/accumulation of body fat (see PRECAUTIONS, Videx EC, Fat Redistribution).

Digestive Disorders: Anorexia, dyspepsia, and flatulence.

Exocrine Gland Disorders: Pancreatitis (including fatal cases) (see WARNINGS, Videx EC), sialoadenitis, parotid gland enlargement, dry mouth, and dry eyes.

Hematologic Disorders: Anemia, leukopenia, and thrombocytopenia.

Liver: Lactic acidosis and hepatic steatosis (see WARNINGS, Videx EC); hepatitis and liver failure.

Metabolic Disorders: Diabetes mellitus, elevated serum alkaline phosphatase level, elevated serum amylase level, elevated serum gamma-glutamyltransferase level, elevated serum uric acid level, hypoglycemia, and hyperglycemia.

Musculoskeletal Disorders: Myalgia (with or without increases in creatine kinase), rhabdomyolysis including acute renal failure and hemodialysis, arthralgia, and myopathy.

Ophthalmologic Disorders: Retinal depigmentation and optic neuritis (see WARNINGS, Videx EC).

DOSAGE AND ADMINISTRATION

VIDEX

Dosage

All Videx formulations should be administered on an empty stomach, at least 30 minutes before or 2 hours after eating. For either a once-daily or twice-daily regimen, patients must take at least 2 of the appropriate strength tablets at each dose to provide adequate buffering and prevent gastric acid degradation of didanosine. Because of the need for adequate buffering, the 200 mg strength tablet should only be used as a component of a once-daily regimen. To reduce the risk of gastrointestinal side effects, patients should take no more than 4 tablets at each dose.

Adults

The preferred dosing frequency of Videx is twice daily because there is more evidence to support the effectiveness of this dosing regimen. Once-daily dosing should be considered only for adult patients whose management requires once-daily dosing of Videx. The daily dose in adult patients is dependent on weight as outlined in TABLE 24.

TABLE 24 *Adult Dosing*

Patient Weight	Videx Tablets*	Videx Buffered Powder†
Preferred dosing		
≥60 kg	200 mg twice daily	250 mg twice daily
<60 kg	125 mg twice daily	167 mg twice daily
Dosing for patients whose management requires once-daily frequency		
≥60 kg	400 mg once daily	†
<60 kg	250 mg once daily	†

* The 200 mg strength tablet should only be used as a component of a once-daily regimen.
† Not suitable for once-daily dosing except for patients with renal impairment. See TABLE 25.

Pediatric Patients

The recommended dose of Videx in pediatric patients between 2 weeks and 8 months of age is 100 mg/m^2 twice daily, and the recommended Videx dose for pediatric patients older than 8 months is 120 mg/m^2 twice daily.

Dosing recommendations for Videx in patients less than 2 weeks of age cannot be made because the pharmacokinetics of didanosine in these children are too variable to determine an appropriate dose. There are no data on once-daily dosing of Videx in pediatric patients.

Dose Adjustment

Clinical and laboratory signs suggestive of pancreatitis should prompt dose suspension and careful evaluation of the possibility of pancreatitis. Videx use should be discontinued in patients with confirmed pancreatitis (see WARNINGS, Videx and Drug Interactions, Videx).

Patients with symptoms of peripheral neuropathy may tolerate a reduced dose of Videx after resolution of the symptoms of peripheral neuropathy upon drug discontinuation. If neuropathy recurs after resumption of Videx, permanent discontinuation of Videx should be considered.

Renal Impairment

In adult patients with impaired renal function, the dose of Videx should be adjusted to compensate for the slower rate of elimination. The recommended doses and dosing intervals of Videx in adult patients with renal insufficiency are presented in TABLE 25.

TABLE 25 *Recommended Dosage of Videx in Renal Impairment*

Creatinine Clearance	≥60 kg Tablet*	≥60 kg Buffered Powder†	<60 kg Tablet*	<60 kg Buffered Powder†
≥60 ml/min	200 mg twice daily‡	250 mg twice daily	125 mg twice daily‡	167 mg twice daily
30-59 ml/min	200 mg once daily or 100 twice daily	100 mg twice daily	150 mg once daily or 75 mg twice daily	100 mg twice daily
10-29 ml/min	150 mg once daily	167 mg once daily	100 mg once daily	100 mg once daily
<10 ml/min	100 mg once daily	100 mg once daily	75 mg once daily	100 mg once daily

* Videx chewable/dispersible buffered tablet. Two Videx tablets must be taken with each dose; different strengths of tablets may be combined to yield the recommended dose.
† Videx buffered powder for oral solution.
‡ 400 mg once daily (≥60 kg) or 250 mg once daily (<60 kg) for patients whose management requires once-daily frequency of administration.

Urinary excretion is also a major route of elimination of didanosine in pediatric patients; therefore, the clearance of didanosine may be altered in children with renal impairment. Although there are insufficient data to recommend a specific dose adjustment of Videx in this patient population, a reduction in the dose and/or an increase in the interval between doses should be considered.

Patients Requiring Continuous Ambulatory Peritoneal Dialysis (CAPD) or Hemodialysis

For patients requiring CAPD or hemodialysis, follow dosing recommendations for patients with creatinine clearance less than 10 ml/min, shown in TABLE 25. It is not necessary to administer a supplemental dose of Videx following hemodialysis.

Hepatic Impairment

See WARNINGS, Videx and PRECAUTIONS, Videx.

Method of Preparation

Videx Chewable/Dispersible Buffered Tablets

Adult Dosing

To provide adequate buffering, at least 2 of the appropriate strength tablets, but no more than 4 tablets, should be thoroughly chewed or dispersed in at least 1 ounce of water prior to consumption (see PRECAUTIONS, Videx, Information for the Patient). To disperse tablets, add 2 tablets to at least 1 ounce of drinking water. Stir until a uniform dispersion forms, and drink the entire dispersion immediately. If additional flavoring is desired, the dispersion may be diluted with 1 ounce of clear apple juice. Stir the further diluted dispersion just prior to consumption. The dispersion with clear apple juice is stable at room temperature, 62-73°F (17-23°C), for up to 1 hour.

Videx Buffered Powder for Oral Solution

1. Open packet carefully and pour contents into a container with approximately 4 ounces of drinking water. Do not mix with fruit juice or other acid-containing liquid.
2. Stir until the powder completely dissolves (approximately 2-3 minutes).
3. Drink the entire solution immediately.

Videx Pediatric Powder for Oral Solution

Prior to dispensing, the pharmacist must constitute dry powder with purified water, to an initial concentration of 20 mg/ml and immediately mix the resulting solution with antacid to a final concentration of 10 mg/ml as follows:

20 mg/ml Initial Solution:

Constitute the product to 20 mg/ml by adding 100 ml or 200 ml of purified water, to the 2 g or 4 g of Videx powder, respectively, in the product bottle.

10 mg/ml Final Admixture:

1. Immediately mix one part of the 20 mg/ml initial solution with one part of either Mylanta Double Strength Liquid, Extra Strength Maalox Plus Suspension, or Maalox TC Suspension for a final dispensing concentration of 10 mg Videx per ml. For patient home use, the admixture should be dispensed in appropriately sized, flint-glass or plastic (HDPE, PET, or PETG) bottles with child-resistant closures. This admixture is stable for 30 days under refrigeration, 36-46°F (2-8°C).
2. Instruct the patient to shake the admixture thoroughly prior to use and to store the tightly closed container in the refrigerator, 36-46°F (2-8°C), up to 30 days.

Handling and Disposal

Spill, Leak, and Disposal Procedure

Avoid generating dust during clean-up of powdered products; use wet mop or damp sponge. Clean surface with soap and water as necessary. Containerize larger spills.

There is no single preferred method of disposal of containerized waste. Disposal options include incineration, landfill, or sewer as dictated by specific circumstances and relevant national, state, and local regulations.

VIDEX EC

Dosage

Adults

Videx EC should be administered on an empty stomach.

Videx EC Delayed-Release Capsules should be swallowed intact.

The recommended daily dose is dependent on body weight and is administered as 1 capsule given on a once-daily schedule as outlined in TABLE 26.

TABLE 26 *Dosing of Videx EC Delayed-Release Capsules*

Patient Weight	Dosage
≥60 kg	400 mg once daily
<60 kg	250 mg once daily

Pediatric Patients

Videx EC has not been studied in pediatric patients. Please consult the complete prescribing information for Videx buffered formulations and Pediatric Powder for Oral Solution for dosage and administration of didanosine to pediatric patients.

Dose Adjustment

Clinical and laboratory signs suggestive of pancreatitis should prompt dose suspension and careful evaluation of the possibility of pancreatitis. Videx EC use should be discontinued in patients with confirmed pancreatitis (see WARNINGS, Videx EC and DRUG INTERACTIONS, Videx EC).

Based on data with buffered didanosine formulations, patients with symptoms of peripheral neuropathy may tolerate a reduced dose of Videx EC after resolution of the symptoms of peripheral neuropathy upon drug interruption. If neuropathy recurs after resumption of Videx EC, permanent discontinuation of Videx EC should be considered.

Renal Impairment

Dosing recommendations for Videx EC and Videx buffered formulations are different for patients with renal impairment. Please consult the complete prescribing information on administration of Videx buffered formulations to patients with renal impairment.

In adult patients with impaired renal function, the dose of Videx EC should be adjusted to compensate for the slower rate of elimination. The recommended doses and dosing intervals of Videx EC in adult patients with renal insufficiency are presented in TABLE 27.

Patients Requiring Continuous Ambulatory Peritoneal Dialysis (CAPD) or Hemodialysis

For patients requiring CAPD or hemodialysis, follow dosing recommendations for patients with creatinine clearance less than 10 ml/min, shown in TABLE 27. It is not necessary to administer a supplemental dose of didanosine following hemodialysis.

Hepatic Impairment

See WARNINGS, Videx EC and PRECAUTIONS, Videx EC.

TABLE 27 *Recommended Dosage of Videx EC in Renal Impairment by Body Weight**

Creatinine Clearance (ml/min)	Dosage ≥60 kg	Dosage <60 kg
≥60	400 mg once daily	250 mg once daily
30-59	200 mg once daily	125 mg once daily
10-29	125 mg once daily	125 mg once daily
<10	125 mg once daily	†

* Based on studies using a buffered formulation of didanosine.
† Not suitable for use in patients <60 kg with CLCR <10 ml/min. An alternate formulation of didanosine should be used.

Handling and Disposal

Disposal options include incineration, landfill, or sewer as dictated by specific circumstances and relevant national, state, and local regulations.

ANIMAL PHARMACOLOGY

VIDEX

Animal Toxicology

Evidence of a dose-limiting skeletal muscle toxicity has been observed in mice and rats (but not in dogs) following long-term (greater than 90 days) dosing with didanosine at doses that were approximately 1.2 to 12 times the estimated human exposure. The relationship of this finding to the potential of Videx to cause myopathy in humans is unclear. However, human myopathy has been associated with administration of Videx and other nucleoside analogues.

VIDEX EC

Animal Toxicology

Evidence of a dose-limiting skeletal muscle toxicity has been observed in mice and rats (but not in dogs) following long-term (greater than 90 days) dosing with didanosine at doses that were approximately 1.2 to 12 times the estimated human exposure. The relationship of this finding to the potential of didanosine to cause myopathy in humans is unclear. However, human myopathy has been associated with administration of didanosine and other nucleoside analogues.

HOW SUPPLIED

VIDEX

Videx Chewable/Dispersible Buffered Tablets

Videx chewable/dispersible buffered tablets are available in:

25 mg: Round, off white to light orange/yellow with a mottled appearance, orange-flavored, tablets embossed with "VIDEX" on one side and "25" on the other.

50 mg: Round, off white to light orange/yellow with a mottled appearance, orange-flavored, tablets embossed with "VIDEX" on one side and "50" on the other.

100 mg: Round, off white to light orange/yellow with a mottled appearance, orange-flavored, tablets embossed with "VIDEX" on one side and "100" on the other.

150 mg: Round, off white to light orange/yellow with a mottled appearance, orange-flavored, tablets embossed with "VIDEX" on one side and "150" on the other.

200 mg: Round, off white to light orange/yellow with a mottled appearance, orange-flavored, tablets embossed with "VIDEX" on one side and "200" on the other.

Storage: The tablets should be stored in tightly closed bottles at 15-30°C (59-86°F). If dispersed in water, the dose may be held for up to 1 hour at ambient temperature.

Videx Buffered Powder for Oral Solution

Videx buffered powder for oral solution is supplied in single-dose, child-resistant foil packets in the following strengths of Videx: 100, 167, or 250 mg. Each product strength provides a sweetened, buffered solution of Videx.

Storage: The packets should be stored at 15-30°C (59-86°F). After dissolving in water, the solution may be stored at ambient room temperature for up to 4 hours.

Videx Pediatric Powder for Oral Solution

Videx pediatric powder for oral solution is supplied in 4 and 8 ounce glass bottles containing 2 or 4 g of Videx, respectively.

Storage: The bottles of powder should be stored at 15-30°C (59-86°F). The Videx admixture may be stored up to 30 days in a refrigerator, 2-8°C (36-46°F). Discard any unused portion after 30 days.

VIDEX EC

Videx EC delayed-release capsules are available in:

125 mg: White, opaque capsule imprinted with "BMS 125 mg" "6671" in tan.

200 mg: White, opaque capsule imprinted with "BMS 200 mg" "6672" in green.

250 mg: White, opaque capsule imprinted with "BMS 250 mg" "6673" in blue.

400 mg: White, opaque capsule imprinted with "BMS 400 mg" "6674" in red.

Storage: The capsules should be stored in tightly closed containers at 25°C (77°F). Excursions between 15 and 30°C (59 and 86°F) are permitted.

PRODUCT LISTING - EQUIVALENTS NOT AVAILABLE

Capsule, Enteric Coated - Oral - 125 mg

30's $97.84 VIDEX, Bristol-Myers Squibb 00087-6671-17

Capsule, Enteric Coated - Oral - 200 mg

30's $156.53 VIDEX EC, Bristol-Myers Squibb 00087-6672-17

Capsule, Enteric Coated - Oral - 250 mg

30's $195.66 VIDEX EC, Bristol-Myers Squibb 00087-6673-17

Capsule, Enteric Coated - Oral - 400 mg

30's $313.06 VIDEX EC, Bristol-Myers Squibb 00087-6674-17

Powder For Reconstitution - Oral - 10 mg/ml

200 ml $40.15 VIDEX, Bristol-Myers Squibb 00087-6632-41

400 ml	$87.66	VIDEX, Bristol-Myers Squibb	00087-6633-41
Powder For Reconstitution - Oral - 100 mg			
30's	$65.57	VIDEX, Bristol-Myers Squibb	00087-6614-43
Powder For Reconstitution - Oral - 167 mg			
30's	$105.58	VIDEX, Bristol-Myers Squibb	00087-6615-43
Powder For Reconstitution - Oral - 250 mg			
30's	$163.95	VIDEX, Bristol-Myers Squibb	00087-6616-43
Tablet, Chewable - Oral - 25 mg			
60's	$31.62	VIDEX, Bristol-Myers Squibb	00087-6650-01
Tablet, Chewable - Oral - 50 mg			
60's	$69.06	VIDEX, Bristol-Myers Squibb	00087-6651-01
Tablet, Chewable - Oral - 100 mg			
12's	$23.78	VIDEX, Allscripts Pharmaceutical Company	54569-4313-01
60's	$118.88	VIDEX, Allscripts Pharmaceutical Company	54569-4313-00
60's	$128.06	VIDEX, Physicians Total Care	54868-2502-00
60's	$138.10	VIDEX, Bristol-Myers Squibb	00087-6652-01
Tablet, Chewable - Oral - 150 mg			
60's	$207.17	VIDEX, Bristol-Myers Squibb	00087-6653-01
Tablet, Chewable - Oral - 200 mg			
60's	$247.69	VIDEX, Allscripts Pharmaceutical Company	54569-4905-00
60's	$276.20	VIDEX, Bristol-Myers Squibb	00087-6665-15

D

Diethylstilbestrol Diphosphate *(001055)*

For complete prescribing information, refer to the CD-ROM included with the book.

Categories: Carcinoma, prostate; Pregnancy Category X; FDA Approved 1955 Sep
Drug Classes: Antineoplastics, hormones/hormone modifiers; Estrogens; Hormones/hormone modifiers
Brand Names: Stilphostrol
Foreign Brand Availability: Honvol (Canada)
HCFA JCODE(S): J9165 250 mg IV

DESCRIPTION

Stilphostrol (diethylstilbestrol diphosphate) is available as tablets containing 50 mg diethylstilbestrol diphosphate, colored white to off-white with grey to tan mottling. Inactive ingredients: corn starch, lactose, magnesium stearate and talc. Stilphostrol is also available for intravenous administration as a sterile solution in 5 ml ampules containing 0.25 gram diethylstilbestrol diphosphate as its sodium salt. The solution is clear, colorless to light straw-colored, with a pH of 9.0-10.5, and may darken with age and exposure to heat and light.

Diethylstilbestrol diphosphate is a phosphoryiated, nonsteroidal estrogen with the chemical name: Diethylstilbestrol 4,4′-Diphosphoric ester, an empirical formula of $C_{18}H_{22}O_8P_2$.

INDICATIONS AND USAGE

Diethylstilbestrol diphosphate is indicated in the treatment of prostatic carcinoma-palliative therapy of advanced disease.

CONTRAINDICATIONS

Estrogens should not be used in men with any of the following conditions:

Known or suspected cancer of the breast except in appropriately selected patients being treated for metastatic disease.

Known or suspected estrogen-dependent neoplasia.

Active thrombophlebitis or thromboembolic disorders.

DIETHYLSTILBESTROL DIPHOSPHATE IS NOT INDICATED IN THE TREATMENT OF ANY DISORDER IN WOMEN.

WARNINGS

Induction of Malignant Neoplasms: Long-term continuous administration of natural and synthetic estrogens in certain animal species increases the frequency of carcinomas of the breast, cervix, vagina, and liver.

Gallbladder Disease: A study has reported a 2- to 3-fold increase in the risk of surgically confirmed gallbladder disease in women receiving postmenopausal estrogens,[2] similar to a 2-fold increase previously noted in users of oral contraceptives.[3,9]

Effects Similar to Those Caused by Estrogen-Progestogen Oral Contraceptives: There are several serious adverse effects of oral contraceptives. It has been shown that there is an increased risk of thrombosis in men receiving estrogens for prostatic cancer and women for postpartum breast engorgement.[4-7]

Thromboembolic Disease: It is now well established that users of oral contraceptives have an increased risk of various thromboembolic and thrombotic vascular diseases, such as thrombophlebitis, pulmonary embolism, stroke, and myocardial infarction.[8-16] Cases of retinal thrombosis, mesenteric thrombosis, and optic neuritis have been reported in oral contraceptive users. There is evidence that the risk of several of these adverse reactions is related to the dose of the drug.[17,18] An increased risk of postsurgery thromboembolic complications has also been reported in users of oral contraceptives [19,20] If feasible, estrogen should be discontinued at least 4 weeks before surgery of the type associated with an increased risk of thromboembolism or during periods of prolonged immobilization. Estrogens should not be used in persons with active thrombophlebitis or thromboembolic disorders. They should be used with caution in patients with cerebral vascular or coronary artery disease and only for those in whom estrogens are clearly indicated. Large doses of estrogen (5 mg conjugated estrogens per day), comparable to those used to treat cancer of the prostrate, have been shown in a large prospective clinical trial in men[21] to increase the risk of nonfatal myocardial infarction, pulmonary embolism and thrombophlebitis. When estrogen doses of this size are used, any of the thromboembolic and thrombotic adverse effects associated with oral contraceptive use should be considered a clear risk.

Hepatic Adenoma: Benign hepatic adenomas appear to be associated with the use of oral contraceptives.[22-24] Although benign, and rare, these may rupture and may cause death through intra-abdominal hemorrhage. Such lesions have not yet been reported in association with other estrogen or progestogen preparations but should be considered in estrogen users having abdominal pain and tenderness, abdominal mass, or hypovolemic shock. Hepatocellular carcinoma has also been reported in women taking estrogen containing oral contraceptives. [23] The relationship of this malignancy to these drugs is not known at this time.

Elevated Blood Pressure: Women using oral contraceptives sometimes experience increased blood pressure which, in most cases, returns to normal on discontinuing the drug. There is now a report that this may occur with use of estrogens in the menopause[25] and blood pressure should be monitored with estrogen use, especially if high doses are used.

Glucose Tolerance: A worsening of gluclose tolerance has been observed in a significant percentage of patients on estrogen-containing oral contraceptives. For this reason, diabetic patients should be carefully observed while receiving estrogen.

Hypercalcemia: Administration of estrogens may lead to severe hypercalcemia in patients with breast cancer and bone metastases. If this occurs, the drug should be stopped and appropriate measures taken to reduce the serum calcium level.

DOSAGE AND ADMINISTRATION

Inoperable, progressing prostatic cancer.

DIETHYLSTILBESTROL DIPHOSPHATE TABLETS 50 MG

Start with 1 tablet three times a day and increase this dose level to 4 or more tablets three times a day, depending on the tolerance of the patient. Maximum daily dose not to exceed one gram.

Alternatively, if relief is not obtained with high oral dosages. Diethylstilbestrol diphosphate may be administered intravenously. Diethylstilbestrol diphosphate solution must be diluted before intravenous infusion.

DIETHYLSTILBESTROL DIPHOSPHATE AMPULES 0.25 GRAM

It is recommended that 0.5 gram (2 ampules) dissolved in approximately 250 ml of normal saline for injection or 5% dextrose for injection be given intravenously the first day, and that each day thereafter one gram (4 ampules) be similarly administered in approximately 250-500 ml of normal saline for injection or 5% dextrose for injection.

The infusion should be administered slowly (20-30 drops per minute) during the first 10-15 minutes and then the rate of flow adjusted so that the entire amount is given in a period of about one hour. This procedure should be followed for 5 days or more depending on the response of the patient. Following the first intensive course of therapy. 0-25-0.5 gram (1 or 2 ampules) may be administered in a similar manner once or twice weekly or maintenance obtained with diethylstilbestrol diphosphate tablets.

STABILITY OF SOLUTION

After reconstitution, if storage is desired, the solution should be kept at room temperature and away from direct light. Under these conditions the solution is stable for about 5 days, so long as cloudiness or evidence of a precipitate has not occurred.

Diflorasone Diacetate *(001057)*

For complete prescribing information, refer to the CD-ROM included with the book.

Categories: Dermatosis, corticosteroid-responsive; Pregnancy Category C; FDA Approved 1977 Sep
Drug Classes: Corticosteroids, topical; Dermatologics
Brand Names: Bexilona; Dermonilo; **Florone**; Florone E; Maxiflor; Psorcon; Sparcort
Foreign Brand Availability: Diacort (Japan); Diflal (Japan); Murode (Spain); Soriflor (Denmark); Sterodelta (Italy)

DESCRIPTION

Not for Ophthalmic Use.

Each gram of florone cream and florone ointment contains 0.5 mg diflorasone diacetate in a cream or ointment base.

Chemically, diflorasone diacetate is 6α,9-difluoro-11β,17,21-trihydroxy-16β-methylpregna-1,4-diene-3,20-dione17,21-diacetate.

Florone cream contains diflorasone diacetate in an emulsified and hydrophilic cream base consisting of propylene glycol, stearic acid, polysorbate 60, sorbitan monostearate and monooleate, sorbic acid, citric acid and water. The corticosteroid is formulated as a solution in the vehicle using 15% propylene glycol to optimize drug delivery.

Florone ointment contains diflorasone diacetate in an emollient, occlusive base consisting of polyoxypropylene 15-stearyl ether, stearic acid, lanolin alcohol and white petrolatum.
Storage: Store at controlled room temperature 15-30°C (59-86°F).

INDICATIONS AND USAGE

Topical corticosteroids are indicated for relief of the inflammatory and pruritic manifestations of corticosteroid responsive dermatoses.

CONTRAINDICATIONS

Topical steroids are contraindicated in those patients with a history of hypersensitivity to any of the components of the preparation.

DOSAGE AND ADMINISTRATION

Topically corticosteroids should be applied to the affected area as a thin film from 1-4 times daily depending on the severity of the condition.

Occlusive dressings may be used for the management of psoriasis or recalcitrant conditions.

If an infection develops, the use of occlusive dressings should be discontinued and appropriate antimicrobial therapy initiated.

PRODUCT LISTING - RATED THERAPEUTICALLY EQUIVALENT

Cream - Topical - 0.05%

Size	Price	Product, Manufacturer	NDC
15 gm	$34.69	GENERIC, Taro Pharmaceuticals U.S.A. Inc	51672-1296-01
15 gm	$35.52	GENERIC, Fougera	00168-0242-15
15 gm	$36.44	PSORCON, Physicians Total Care	54868-2658-00
30 gm	$48.31	GENERIC, Taro Pharmaceuticals U.S.A. Inc	51672-1296-02
30 gm	$48.80	GENERIC, Fougera	00168-0242-30
60 gm	$91.20	GENERIC, Taro Pharmaceuticals U.S.A. Inc	51672-1296-03
60 gm	$92.14	GENERIC, Fougera	00168-0242-60
60 gm	$132.29	PSORCON, Aventis Pharmaceuticals	00066-0069-60

Ointment - Topical - 0.05%

Size	Price	Product, Manufacturer	NDC
15 gm	$37.05	GENERIC, Fougera	00168-0243-15
15 gm	$49.59	GENERIC, Taro Pharmaceuticals U.S.A. Inc	51672-1295-01
30 gm	$40.10	PSORCON, Southwood Pharmaceuticals Inc	58016-3247-01
30 gm	$50.28	GENERIC, Taro Pharmaceuticals U.S.A. Inc	51672-1295-02
30 gm	$50.91	GENERIC, Fougera	00168-0243-30
60 gm	$96.63	GENERIC, Taro Pharmaceuticals U.S.A. Inc	51672-1295-03
60 gm	$97.85	GENERIC, Fougera	00168-0243-60
60 gm	$119.23	PSORCON, Physicians Total Care	54868-2222-01
60 gm	$140.15	PSORCON, Aventis Pharmaceuticals	00066-0071-60

PRODUCT LISTING - EQUIVALENTS NOT AVAILABLE

Cream - Topical - 0.05%

Size	Price	Product, Manufacturer	NDC
15 gm	$40.06	PSORCON E, Aventis Pharmaceuticals	00066-0272-17
30 gm	$43.19	MAXIFLOR, Allergan Inc	00023-0766-30
30 gm	$55.04	PSORCON E, Aventis Pharmaceuticals	00066-0272-31
60 gm	$70.14	MAXIFLOR, Allergan Inc	00023-0766-60
62 gm	$105.75	PSORCON E, Aventis Pharmaceuticals	00066-0272-60

Ointment - Topical - 0.05%

Size	Price	Product, Manufacturer	NDC
15 gm	$40.06	PSORCON E, Aventis Pharmaceuticals	00066-0275-17
30 gm	$43.19	MAXIFLOR, Allergan Inc	00023-0770-30
30 gm	$48.54	FLORONE, Aventis Pharmaceuticals	00066-0075-31
30 gm	$55.04	PSORCON E, Aventis Pharmaceuticals	00066-0275-31
60 gm	$73.65	MAXIFLOR, Allergan Inc	00023-0770-60
60 gm	$105.75	PSORCON E, Aventis Pharmaceuticals	00066-0275-60

Diflunisal *(001058)*

For related information, see the comparative table section in Appendix A.

Categories: Arthritis, osteoarthritis; Arthritis, rheumatoid; Pain, mild to moderate; Pregnancy Category C; FDA Approved 1982 Apr

Drug Classes: Analgesics, non-narcotic; Salicylates

Brand Names: **Dolobid**

Foreign Brand Availability: Adomal (Italy); Analeric (Greece); Ansal (New-Zealand); Biartac (Belgium); Diflonid (Denmark; Norway; Sweden); Diflusal (Belgium); Dolobis (France); Dolocid (Netherlands); Donobid (Denmark; Finland; Norway; Sweden); Dorbid (Brazil); Flovacil (Argentina); Flunidor (Portugal); Fluniget (Austria); Ilacen (Taiwan); Reuflos (Italy); Unisal (Switzerland)

Cost of Therapy: $71.39 (Osteoarthritis; Dolobid; 250 mg; 2 tablets/day; 30 day supply)
$46.66 (Osteoarthritis; Generic Tablets; 250 mg; 2 tablets/day; 30 day supply)

DESCRIPTION

Diflunisal is 2′,4′-difluoro-4-hydroxy-3-biphenylcarboxylic acid. Its empirical formula is $C_{13}H_8F_2O_3$.

Diflunisal has a molecular weight of 250.20. It is a stable, white, crystalline compound with a melting point of 211-213°C. It is practically insoluble in water at neutral or acidic pH. Because it is an organic acid, it dissolves readily in dilute alkali to give a moderately stable solution at room temperature. It is soluble in most organic solvents including ethanol, methanol, and acetone.

Dolobid is available in 250 mg and 500 mg tablets for oral administration. Tablets Dolobid contain the following inactive ingredients: cellulose, FD&C yellow 6, hydroxypropyl cellulose, hydroxypropyl methylcellulose, magnesium stearate, starch, talc, and titanium dioxide.

CLINICAL PHARMACOLOGY

ACTION

Diflunisal is a non-steroidal drug with analgesic, anti-inflammatory, and antipyretic properties. It is a peripherally-acting non-narcotic analgesic drug. Habituation, tolerance, and addiction have not been reported.

Diflunisal is a difluorophenyl derivative of salicylic acid. Chemically, diflunisal differs from aspirin (acetylsalicylic acid) in 2 respects. The first of these 2 is the presence of a difluorophenyl substituent at carbon 1. The second difference is the removal of the 0-acetyl group from the carbon 4 position. Diflunisal is not metabolized to salicylic acid, and the fluorine atoms are not displaced from the difluorophenyl ring structure.

The precise mechanism of the analgesic and anti-inflammatory actions of diflunisal is not known. Diflunisal is a prostaglandin synthetase inhibitor. In animals, prostaglandins sensitize afferent nerves and potentiate the action of bradykinin in inducing pain. Since prostaglandins are known to be among the mediators of pain and inflammation, the mode of action of diflunisal may be due to a decrease of prostaglandins in peripheral tissues.

PHARMACOKINETICS AND METABOLISM

Diflunisal is rapidly and completely absorbed following oral administration with peak plasma concentrations occurring between 2-3 hours. The drug is excreted in the urine as 2 soluble glucuronide conjugates accounting for about 90% of the administered dose. Little or no diflunisal is excreted in the feces. Diflunisal appears in human milk in concentrations of 2-7% of those in plasma. More than 99% of diflunisal in plasma is bound to proteins.

As is the case with salicylic acid, concentration-dependent pharmacokinetics prevail when Diflunisal is administered; a doubling of dosage produces a greater than doubling of drug accumulation. The effect becomes more apparent with repetitive doses. Following single doses, peak plasma concentrations of 41 ± 11 µg/ml (mean ±SD) were observed following 250 mg doses, 87 ± 17 µg/ml were observed following 500 mg and 124 ± 11 µg/ml following single 1000 mg doses. However, following administration of 250 mg bid, a mean peak level of 56 ± 14 µg/ml was observed on day 8, while the mean peak level after 500 mg bid for 11 days was 190 ± 33 µg/ml. In contrast to salicylic acid which has a plasma half-life of 2½ hours, the plasma half-life of diflunisal is 3-4 times longer (8-12 hours), because of a difluorophenyl substituent at carbon 1. Because of its long half-life and nonlinear pharmacokinetics, several days are required for diflunisal plasma levels to reach steady state following multiple doses. For this reason, an initial loading dose is necessary to shorten the time to reach steady state levels, and 2-3 days of observation are necessary for evaluating changes in treatment regimens if a loading dose is not used.

Studies in baboons to determine passage across the blood-brain barrier have shown that only small quantities of diflunisal, under normal or acidotic conditions are transported into the cerebrospinal fluid (CSF). The ratio of blood/CSF concentrations after intravenous doses of 50 mg/kg or oral doses of 100 mg/kg of diflunisal was 100:1. In contrast, oral doses of 500 mg/kg of aspirin resulted in a blood/CSF ratio of 5:1.

MILD TO MODERATE PAIN

Diflunisal is a peripherally-acting analgesic agent with a long duration of action. Diflunisal produces significant analgesia within 1 hour and maximum analgesia within 2-3 hours.

Consistent with its long half-life, clinical effects of diflunisal mirror its pharmacokinetic behavior, which is the basis for recommending a loading dose when instituting therapy. Patients treated with diflunisal, on the first dose, tend to have a slower onset of pain relief when compared with drugs achieving comparable peak effects. However, diflunisal produces longer-lasting responses than the comparative agents.

Comparative single dose clinical studies have established the analgesic efficacy of diflunisal at various dose levels relative to other analgesics. Analgesic effect measurements were derived from hourly evaluations by patients during 8 and 12 hour postdosing observation periods. The following information may serve as a guide for prescribing diflunisal.

Diflunisal 500 mg was comparable in analgesic efficacy to aspirin 650 mg, acetaminophen 600 mg or 650 mg, and acetaminophen 650 mg with propoxyphene napsylate 100 mg. Patients treated with diflunisal had longer lasting responses than the patients treated with the comparative analgesics.

Diflunisal 1000 mg was comparable in analgesic efficacy to acetaminophen 600 mg with codeine 60 mg. Patients treated with diflunisal had longer lasting responses than the patients who received acetaminophen with codeine.

A loading dose of 1000 mg provides faster onset of pain relief, shorter time to peak analgesic effect, and greater peak analgesic effect than an initial 500 mg dose.

In contrast to the comparative analgesics, a significantly greater proportion of patients treated with diflunisal did not remedicate and continued to have a good analgesic effect 8-12 hours after dosing. Seventy-five percent (75%) of patients treated with diflunisal continued to have a good analgesic response at 4 hours. When patients having a good analgesic response at 4 hours were followed, 78% of these patients continued to have a good analgesic response at 8 hours and 64% at 12 hours.

CHRONIC ANTI-INFLAMMATORY THERAPY IN OSTEOARTHRITIS AND RHEUMATOID ARTHRITIS

In the controlled, double-blind clinical trials in which diflunisal (500-1000 mg a day) was compared with anti-inflammatory doses of aspirin (2-4 grams a day), patients treated with diflunisal had a significantly lower incidence of tinnitus and of adverse effects involving the gastrointestinal system than patients treated with aspirin. (See also Effect on Fecal Blood Loss.)

OSTEOARTHRITIS

The effectiveness of diflunisal for the treatment of osteoarthritis was studied in patients with osteoarthritis of the hip and/or knee. The activity of diflunisal was demonstrated by clinical improvement in the signs and symptoms of disease activity.

In a double-blind multicenter study of 12 weeks' duration in which dosages were adjusted according to patient response, diflunisal, 500 or 750 mg daily, was shown to be comparable in effectiveness to aspirin, 2000 or 3000 mg daily. In open-label extensions of this study to 24 or 48 weeks, diflunisal continued to show similar effectiveness and generally was well tolerated.

RHEUMATOID ARTHRITIS

In controlled clinical trials, the effectiveness of diflunisal was established for both acute exacerbations and long-term management of rheumatoid arthritis. The activity of diflunisal was demonstrated by clinical improvement in the signs and symptoms of disease activity.

In a double-blind multicenter study of 12 weeks' duration in which dosages were adjusted according to patient response, diflunisal 500 or 750 mg daily was comparable in effectiveness to aspirin 2600 or 3900 mg daily. In open-label extensions of this study to 52 weeks, diflunisal continued to be effective and was generally well tolerated.

Diflunisal 500, 750, or 1000 mg daily was compared with aspirin 2000, 3000, or 4000 mg daily in a multicenter study of 8 weeks' duration in which dosages were adjusted according to patient response. In this study, diflunisal was comparable in efficacy to aspirin.

In a double-blind multicenter study of 12 weeks' duration in which dosages were adjusted according to patient needs, diflunisal 500 or 750 mg daily and ibuprofen 1600 or 2400 mg daily were comparable in effectiveness and tolerability.

In a double-blind multicenter study of 12 weeks' duration, diflunisal 750 mg daily was comparable in efficacy to naproxen 750 mg daily. The incidence of gastrointestinal adverse effects and tinnitus was comparable for both drugs. This study was extended to 48 weeks on an open-label basis. Diflunisal continued to be effective and generally well tolerated.

In patients with rheumatoid arthritis, diflunisal and gold salts may be used in combination at their usual dosage levels. In clinical studies, diflunisal added to the regimen of gold salts usually resulted in additional symptomatic relief but did not alter the course of the underlying disease.

D

ANTIPYRETIC ACTIVITY

Diflunisal is not recommended for use as an antipyretic agent. In single 250 mg, 500 mg, or 750 mg doses, diflunisal produced measurable but not clinically useful decreases in temperature in patients with fever; however, the possibility that it may mask fever in some patients, particularly with chronic or high doses, should be considered.

URICOSURIC EFFECT

In normal volunteers, an increase in the renal clearance of uric acid and a decrease in serum uric acid was observed when diflunisal was administered at 500 mg or 750 mg daily in divided doses. Patients on long-term therapy taking diflunisal at 500-1000 mg daily in divided doses showed a prompt and consistent reduction across studies in mean serum uric acid levels, which were lowered as much as 1.4 mg%. It is not known whether diflunisal interferes with the activity of other uricosuric agents.

EFFECT ON PLATELET FUNCTION

As an inhibitor of prostaglandin synthetase, diflunisal has a dose-related effect on platelet function and bleeding time. In normal volunteers, 250 mg bid for 8 days had no effect on platelet function, and 500 mg bid, the usual recommended dose, had a slight effect. At 1000 mg bid, which exceeds the maximum recommended dosage, however, diflunisal inhibited platelet function. In contrast to aspirin, these effects of diflunisal were reversible, because of the absence of the chemically labile and biologically reactive 0-acetyl group at the carbon 4 position. Bleeding time was not altered by a dose of 250 mg bid, and was only slightly increased at 500 mg bid. At 1000 mg bid, a greater increase occurred, but was not statistically significantly different from the change in the placebo group.

EFFECT ON FECAL BLOOD LOSS

When diflunisal was given to normal volunteers at the usual recommended dose of 500 mg twice daily, fecal blood loss was not significantly different from placebo. Aspirin at 1000 mg 4 times daily produced the expected increase in fecal blood loss. Diflunisal at 1000 mg twice daily (*NOTE:* Exceeds the recommended dosage) caused a statistically significant increase in fecal blood loss, but this increase was only one-half as large as that associated with aspirin 1300 mg twice daily.

EFFECT ON BLOOD GLUCOSE

Diflunisal did not affect fasting blood sugar in diabetic patients who were receiving tolbutamide or placebo.

INDICATIONS AND USAGE

Diflunisal is indicated for acute or long-term use for symptomatic treatment of the following:

1. Mild to moderate pain.
2. Osteoarthritis.
3. Rheumatoid arthritis.

CONTRAINDICATIONS

Patients who are hypersensitive to this product.

Patients in whom acute asthmatic attacks, urticaria, or rhinitis are precipitated by aspirin or other non-steroidal anti-inflammatory drugs.

WARNINGS

Peptic ulceration and gastrointestinal bleeding have been reported in patients receiving diflunisal. Fatalities have occurred rarely. Gastrointestinal bleeding is associated with higher morbidity and mortality in patients acutely ill with other conditions, the elderly, and patients with hemorrhagic disorders. In patients with active gastrointestinal bleeding or an active peptic ulcer, the physician must weigh the benefits of therapy with diflunisal against possible hazards, institute an appropriate ulcer regimen, and carefully monitor the patient's progress. When diflunisal is given to patients with a history of either upper or lower gastrointestinal tract disease, it should be given only after consulting ADVERSE REACTIONS and under close supervision.

RISK OF GI ULCERATIONS, BLEEDING, AND PERFORATION WITH NSAID THERAPY

Serious gastrointestinal toxicity such as bleeding, ulceration, and perforation, can occur at any time, with or without warning symptoms, in patients treated chronically with NSAID therapy. Although minor upper gastrointestinal problems, such as dyspepsia, are common, usually developing early in therapy, physicians should remain alert for ulceration and bleeding in patients treated chronically with NSAIDs even in the absence of previous GI tract symptoms. In patients observed in clinical trials of several months to 2 years duration, symptomatic upper GI ulcers, gross bleeding or perforation appear to occur in approximately 1% of patients treated for 3-6 months, and in about 2-4% of patients treated for 1 year. Physicians should inform patients about the signs and/or symptoms of serious GI toxicity and what steps to take if they occur.

Studies to date have not identified any subset of patients not at risk of developing peptic ulceration and bleeding. Except for a prior history of serious GI events and other risk factors known to be associated with peptic ulcer disease, such as alcoholism, smoking, etc., no risk factors (*e.g.,* age, sex) have been associated with increased risk. Elderly or debilitated patients seem to tolerate ulceration or bleeding less well than other individuals and most spontaneous reports of fatal GI events are in this population. Studies to date are inconclusive concerning the relative risk of various NSAIDs in causing such reactions. High doses of any NSAID probably carry a greater risk of these reactions, although controlled clinical trials showing this do not exist in most cases. In considering the use of relatively large doses (within the recommended dosage range), sufficient benefit should be anticipated to offset the potential increased risk of GI toxicity.

PRECAUTIONS

GENERAL

Non-steroidal anti-inflammatory drugs, including diflunisal, may mask the usual signs and symptoms of infection. Therefore, the physician must be continually on the alert for this and should use the drug with extra care in the presence of existing infection.

Although diflunisal has less effect on platelet function and bleeding time than aspirin, at higher doses it is an inhibitor of platelet function; therefore, patients who may be adversely affected should be carefully observed when diflunisal is administered. (See CLINICAL PHARMACOLOGY.)

Because of reports of adverse eye findings with agents of this class, it is recommended that patients who develop eye complaints during treatment with diflunisal have ophthalmologic studies.

Peripheral edema has been observed in some patients taking diflunisal. Therefore, as with other drugs in this class, diflunisal should be used with caution in patients with compromised cardiac function, hypertension, or other conditions predisposing to fluid retention.

Acetylsalicylic acid has been associated with Reye syndrome. Because diflunisal is a derivative of salicylic acid, the possibility of its association with Reye syndrome cannot be excluded.

HYPERSENSITIVITY SYNDROME

A potentially life-threatening, apparent hypersensitivity syndrome has been reported. This multisystem syndrome includes constitutional symptoms (fever, chills), and cutaneous findings. (See ADVERSE REACTIONS, Dermatologic.) It may also include involvement of major organs (changes in liver function, jaundice, leukopenia, thrombocytopenia, eosinophilia, disseminated intravascular coagulation, renal impairment, including renal failure), and less specific findings (adenitis, arthralgia, myalgia, arthritis, malaise, anorexia, disorientation). If evidence of hypersensitivity occurs, therapy with diflunisal should be discontinued.

RENAL EFFECTS

As with other non-steroidal anti-inflammatory drugs, long term administration of diflunisal to animals has resulted in renal papillary necrosis and other abnormal renal pathology. In humans, there have been reports of acute interstitial nephritis with hematuria and proteinuria and occasionally nephrotic syndrome.

A second form of renal toxicity has been seen in patients with prerenal and renal conditions leading to a reduction in renal blood flow or blood volume, where the renal prostaglandins have a supportive role in the maintenance of renal perfusion. In these patients administration of an NSAID may cause a dose dependent reduction in prostaglandin formation and may precipitate overt renal decompensation. Patients at greatest risk of this reaction are those with conditions such as renal or hepatic dysfunction, diabetes mellitus, advanced age, extracellular volume depletion from any cause, congestive heart failure, septicemia, pyelonephritis, or concomitant use of any nephrotoxic drug. Diflunisal or other NSAIDs should be given with caution and renal function should be monitored in any patient who may have reduced renal reserve. Discontinuation of NSAID therapy is typically followed by recovery to the pretreatment state.

Since diflunisal is eliminated primarily by the kidneys, patients with significantly impaired renal function should be closely monitored; a lower daily dosage should be anticipated to avoid excessive drug accumulation.

INFORMATION FOR THE PATIENT

Diflunisal, like other drugs of its class, is not free of side effects. The side effects of these drugs can cause discomfort and, rarely, there are more serious side effects such as gastrointestinal bleeding, which may result in hospitalization and even fatal outcomes.

NSAIDs (Non-steroidal Anti-inflammatory Drugs) are often essential agents in the management of arthritis and have a major role in the treatment of pain, but they also may be commonly employed for conditions which are less serious.

Physicians may wish to discuss with their patients the potential risks (see WARNINGS, PRECAUTIONS, and ADVERSE REACTIONS) and likely benefits of NSAID treatment, particularly when the drugs are used for less serious conditions where treatment without NSAIDs may represent an acceptable alternative to both the patient and physician.

LABORATORY TESTS

Liver Function Tests

As with other non-steroidal anti-inflammatory drugs, borderline elevations of one or more liver tests may occur in up to 15% of patients. These abnormalities may progress, may remain essentially unchanged, or may be transient with continued therapy. The SGPT (ALT) test is probably the most sensitive indicator of liver dysfunction. Meaningful (3 times the upper limit of normal) elevations of SGPT or SGOT (AST) occurred in controlled clinical trials in less than 1% of patients. A patient with symptoms and/or signs suggesting liver dysfunction, or in whom an abnormal liver test has occurred, should be evaluated for evidence of the development of more severe hepatic reactions while on therapy with diflunisal. Severe hepatic reactions, including jaundice, have been reported with diflunisal as well as with other non-steroidal anti-inflammatory drugs. Although such reactions are rare, if abnormal liver tests persist or worsen, if clinical signs and symptoms consistent with liver disease develop, or if systemic manifestations occur (*e.g.,* eosinophilia, rash, etc.), diflunisal should be discontinued, since liver reactions can be fatal.

Gastrointestinal

Because serious GI tract ulceration and bleeding can occur without warning symptoms, physicians should follow chronically treated patients for the signs and symptoms of ulceration and bleeding and should inform them of the importance of this follow-up. (See WARNINGS, Risk of GI Ulcerations, Bleeding, and Perforation with NSAID Therapy.)

DRUG/LABORATORY TEST INTERACTIONS

Serum Salicylate Assays: Caution should be used in interpreting the results of serum salicylate assays when diflunisal is present. Salicylate levels have been found to be falsely elevated with some assay methods.

CARCINOGENESIS, MUTAGENESIS, AND IMPAIRMENT OF FERTILITY

Diflunisal did not affect the type or incidence of neoplasia in a 105-week study in the rat given doses up to 40 mg/kg/day (equivalent to approximately 1.3 times the maximum recommended human dose), or in long-term carcinogenic studies in mice given diflunisal at doses up to 80 mg/kg/day (equivalent to approximately 2.7 times the maximum recommended human dose). It was concluded that there was no carcinogenic potential for diflunisal.

Diflunisal passes the placental barrier to a minor degree in the rat. Diflunisal had no mutagenic activity after oral administration in the dominant lethal assay, in the Ames microbial mutagen test or in the V-79 Chinese hamster lung cell assay.

No evidence of impaired fertility was found in reproduction studies in rats at doses up to 50 mg/kg/day.

PREGNANCY CATEGORY C

A dose of 60 mg/kg/day of diflunisal (equivalent to 2 times the maximum human dose) was maternotoxic, embryotoxic, and teratogenic in rabbits. In 3 of 6 studies in rabbits, evidence of teratogenicity was observed at doses ranging from 40-50 mg/kg/day. Teratology studies in mice, at doses up to 45 mg/kg/day, and in rats at doses up to 100 mg/kg/day, revealed no harm to the fetus due to diflunisal. Aspirin and other salicylates have been shown to be teratogenic in a wide variety of species, including the rat and rabbit, at doses ranging from 50-400 mg/kg/day (approximately 1-8 times the human dose). There are no adequate and well controlled studies with diflunisal in pregnant women. Diflunisal should be used during the first two trimesters of pregnancy only if the potential benefit justifies the potential risk to the fetus. The known effect of drugs of this class on the human fetus during the third trimester of pregnancy include: constriction of the ductus arteriosus prenatally, tricuspid incompetence, and pulmonary hypertension; non-closure of the ductus arteriosus postnatally which may be resistant to medical management; myocardial degenerative changes, platelet dysfunction with resultant bleeding, intracranial bleeding, renal dysfunction or failure, renal injury/dysgenesis which may result in prolonged or permanent renal failure, oligohydramnios, gastrointestinal bleeding or perforation, and increased risk of necrotizing enterocolitis. Use during the third trimester of pregnancy is not recommended.

In rats at a dose of 1.5 times the maximum human dose, there was an increase in the average length of gestation. Similar increases in the length of gestation have been observed with aspirin, indomethacin, and phenylbutazone, and may be related to inhibition of prostaglandin synthetase. Drugs of this class may cause dystocia and delayed parturition in pregnant animals.

NURSING MOTHERS

Diflunisal is excreted in human milk in concentrations of 2-7% of those in plasma. Because of the potential for serious adverse reactions in nursing infants from diflunisal, a decision should be made whether to discontinue nursing or to discontinue the drug, taking into account the importance of the drug to the mother.

PEDIATRIC USE

Safety and effectiveness of diflunisal in pediatric patients have not been established. Use of diflunisal in pediatric patients below the age of 12 is not recommended.

The adverse effects observed following diflunisal administration to neonatal animals appear to be species, age, and dose-dependent. At dose levels approximately 3 times the usual human therapeutic dose, both aspirin (200-400 mg/kg/day) and diflunisal (80 mg/kg/day) resulted in death, leukocytosis, weight loss, and bilateral cataracts in neonatal (4- to 5-day-old) beagle puppies after 2-10 doses. Administration of an 80 mg/kg/day dose of diflunisal to 25-day-old puppies resulted in lower mortality, and did not produce cataracts. In newborn rats, a 400 mg/kg/day dose of aspirin resulted in increased mortality and some cataracts, whereas the effects of diflunisal administration at doses up to 140 mg/kg/day were limited to a decrease in average body weight gain.

GERIATRIC USE

As with any NSAID, caution should be exercised in treating the elderly (65 years and older) since advancing age appears to increase the possibility of adverse reactions. Elderly patients seem to tolerate ulceration or bleeding less well than other individuals and many spontaneous reports of fatal GI events are in this population. (See WARNINGS, Risk of GI Ulcerations, Bleeding, and Perforation with NSAID Therapy.)

This drug is known to be substantially excreted by the kidney and the risk of toxic reactions to this drug may be greater in patients with impaired renal function. Because elderly patients are more likely to have decreased renal function, care should be taken in dose selection and it may be useful to monitor renal function. (See Renal Effects.)

DRUG INTERACTIONS

Oral Anticoagulants: In some normal volunteers, the concomitant administration of diflunisal and warfarin, acenocoumarol, or phenprocoumon resulted in prolongation of prothrombin time. This may occur because diflunisal competitively displaces coumarins from protein binding sites. Accordingly, when diflunisal is administered with oral anticoagulants, the prothrombin time should be closely monitored during and for several days after concomitant drug administration. Adjustment of dosage of oral anticoagulants may be required.

Tolbutamide: In diabetic patients receiving diflunisal and tolbutamide, no significant effects were seen on tolbutamide plasma levels or fasting blood glucose.

Hydrochlorothiazide: In normal volunteers, concomitant administration of diflunisal and hydrochlorothiazide resulted in significantly increased plasma levels of hydrochlorothiazide. Diflunisal decreased the hyperuricemic effect of hydrochlorothiazide.

Furosemide: In normal volunteers, the concomitant administration of diflunisal and furosemide had no effect on the diuretic activity of furosemide. Diflunisal decreased the hyperuricemic effect of furosemide.

Antacids: Concomitant administration of antacids may reduce plasma levels of diflunisal. This effect is small with occasional doses of antacids, but may be clinically significant when antacids are used on a continuous schedule.

Acetaminophen: In normal volunteers, concomitant administration of diflunisal and acetaminophen resulted in an approximate 50% increase in plasma levels of acetaminophen. Acetaminophen had no effect on plasma levels of diflunisal. Since acetaminophen in high doses has been associated with hepatotoxicity, concomitant administration of diflunisal and acetaminophen should be used cautiously, with careful monitoring of patients.

Concomitant administration of diflunisal and acetaminophen in dogs, but not in rats, at approximately 2 times the recommended maximum human therapeutic dose of each (40-52 mg/kg/day of diflunisal/acetaminophen), resulted in greater gastrointestinal toxicity than when either drug was administered alone. The clinical significance of these findings has not been established.

Methotrexate: Caution should be used if diflunisal is administered concomitantly with methotrexate. Non-steroidal anti-inflammatory drugs have been reported to decrease the tubular secretion of methotrexate and to potentiate its toxicity.

Cyclosporine: Administration of non-steroidal anti-inflammatory drugs concomitantly with cyclosporine has been associated with an increase in cyclosporine-induced toxicity, possibly due to decreased synthesis of renal prostacyclin. NSAIDs should be used with caution in patients taking cyclosporine, and renal function should be carefully monitored.

NON-STEROIDAL ANTI-INFLAMMATORY DRUGS

The administration of diflunisal to normal volunteers receiving indomethacin decreased the renal clearance and significantly increased the plasma levels of indomethacin. In some patients the combined use of indomethacin and diflunisal has been associated with fatal gastrointestinal hemorrhage. Therefore, indomethacin and diflunisal should not be used concomitantly.

The concomitant use of diflunisal and other NSAIDs is not recommended due to the increased possibility of gastrointestinal toxicity, with little or no increase in efficacy. The following information was obtained from studies in normal volunteers.

Aspirin: In normal volunteers, a small decrease in diflunisal levels was observed when multiple doses of diflunisal and aspirin were administered concomitantly.

Sulindac: The concomitant administration of diflunisal and sulindac in normal volunteers resulted in lowering of the plasma levels of the active sulindac sulfide metabolite by approximately one-third.

Naproxen: The concomitant administration of diflunisal and naproxen in normal volunteers had no effect on the plasma levels of naproxen, but significantly decreased the urinary excretion of naproxen and its glucuronide metabolite. Naproxen had no effect on plasma levels of diflunisal.

ADVERSE REACTIONS

The adverse reactions observed in controlled clinical trials encompass observations in 2427 patients.

Listed below are the adverse reactions reported in the 1314 of these patients who received treatment in studies of 2 weeks or longer. Five hundred thirteen patients were treated for at least 24 weeks, 255 patients were treated for at least 48 weeks, and 46 patients were treated for 96 weeks. In general, the adverse reactions listed below were 2-14 times less frequent in the 1113 patients who received short-term treatment for mild to moderate pain.

Incidence Greater Than 1%:

Gastrointestinal: The most frequent types of adverse reactions occurring with diflunisal are gastrointestinal: these include nausea*, vomiting, dyspepsia*, gastrointestinal pain*, diarrhea*, constipation, and flatulence.

Psychiatric: Somnolence, insomnia.

Central Nervous System: Dizziness.

Special Senses: Tinnitus.

Dermatologic: Rash*.

Miscellaneous: Headache*, fatigue/tiredness.

*Incidence between 3% and 9%. Those reactions occurring in 1-3% are not marked with an asterisk.

Incidence Less Than 1 in 100: The following adverse reactions, occurring less frequently than 1 in 100, were reported in clinical trials or since the drug was marketed. The probability exists of a causal relationship between diflunisal and these adverse reactions.

Dermatologic: Erythema multiforme, exfoliative dermatitis, Stevens-Johnson syndrome, toxic epidermal necrolysis, urticaria, pruritus, sweating, dry mucous membranes, stomatitis, photosensitivity.

Gastrointestinal: Peptic ulcer, gastrointestinal bleeding, anorexia, eructation, gastrointestinal perforation, gastritis. Liver function abnormalities; jaundice, sometimes with fever; cholestasis; hepatitis.

Hematologic: Thrombocytopenia; agranulocytosis; hemolytic anemia.

Genitourinary: Dysuria; renal impairment, including renal failure; interstitial nephritis; hematuria; proteinuria.

Psychiatric: Nervousness, depression, hallucinations, confusion, disorientation.

Central Nervous System: Vertigo; light-headedness; paresthesias.

Special Senses: Transient visual disturbances including blurred vision.

Hypersensitivity Reactions: Acute anaphylactic reaction with bronchospasm; angioedema; flushing. Hypersensitivity vasculitis. Hypersensitivity syndrome. (See PRECAUTIONS.)

Miscellaneous: Asthenia, edema.

D

CAUSAL RELATIONSHIP UNKNOWN

Other reactions have been reported in clinical trials or since the drug was marketed, but occurred under circumstances where a causal relationship could not be established. However, in these rarely reported events, that possibility cannot be excluded. Therefore, these observations are listed to serve as alerting information to physicians.

Respiratory: Dyspnea.
Cardiovascular: Palpitation, syncope.
Musculoskeletal: Muscle cramps.
Genitourinary: Nephrotic syndrome.
Special Senses: Hearing loss.
Miscellaneous: Chest pain.

A rare occurrence of fulminant necrotizing fasciitis, particularly in association with Group A β-hemolytic streptococcus, has been described in persons treated with non-steroidal anti-inflammatory agents, including diflunisal, sometimes with fatal outcome. (See also PRECAUTIONS, General.)

POTENTIAL ADVERSE EFFECTS

In addition, a variety of adverse effects not observed with diflunisal in clinical trials or in marketing experience, but reported with other non-steroidal analgesic/anti-inflammatory agents, should be considered potential adverse effects of diflunisal.

DOSAGE AND ADMINISTRATION

Concentration-dependent pharmacokinetics prevail when diflunisal is administered; a doubling of dosage produces a greater than doubling of drug accumulation. The effect becomes more apparent with repetitive doses.

For mild to moderate pain, an initial dose of 1000 mg followed by 500 mg every 12 hours is recommended for most patients. Following the initial dose, some patients may require 500 mg every 8 hours.

A lower dosage may be appropriate depending on such factors as pain severity, patient response, weight, or advanced age; for example, 500 mg initially, followed by 250 mg every 8-12 hours.

For osteoarthritis and rheumatoid arthritis, the suggested dosage range is 500-1000 mg daily in 2 divided doses. The dosage of diflunisal may be increased or decreased according to patient response.

Maintenance doses higher than 1500 mg a day are not recommended.

Diflunisal may be administered with water, milk or meals. Tablets should be swallowed whole, not crushed or chewed.

HOW SUPPLIED

Dolobid tablets are capsule-shaped, film-coated tablets supplied as follows:

250 mg: Peach colored, coded "DOLOBID" on one side and "MSD 675" on the other.
500 mg: Orange colored, coded "DOLOBID" on one side and "MSD 697" on the other.

PRODUCT LISTING - RATED THERAPEUTICALLY EQUIVALENT

Tablet - Oral - 250 mg			
60's	$47.85	GENERIC, Roxane Laboratories Inc	00054-4210-21
60's	$49.21	GENERIC, Purepac Pharmaceutical Company	00228-2545-06
60's	$49.46	GENERIC, Endo Laboratories Llc	60951-0768-60
60's	$71.39	DOLOBID, Merck & Company Inc	00006-0675-61
100's	$87.25	GENERIC, Roxane Laboratories Inc	00054-8210-25
100's	$98.65	GENERIC, Major Pharmaceuticals Inc	00904-7763-61
Tablet - Oral - 500 mg			
10's	$8.91	GENERIC, Pd-Rx Pharmaceuticals	55289-0460-10
10's	$13.74	DOLOBID, Alpharma Uspd Makers Of Barre and Nmc	63874-0307-10
10's	$14.18	DOLOBID, Allscripts Pharmaceutical Company	54569-0296-06
10's	$19.68	DOLOBID, Pharma Pac	52959-0351-10
15's	$13.37	GENERIC, Pd-Rx Pharmaceuticals	55289-0460-15
15's	$28.65	DOLOBID, Pharma Pac	52959-0351-15
20's	$17.70	GENERIC, Pd-Rx Pharmaceuticals	55289-0460-20
20's	$27.04	DOLOBID, Alpharma Uspd Makers Of Barre and Nmc	63874-0307-20
20's	$37.11	DOLOBID, Pharma Pac	52959-0351-20
24's	$43.04	DOLOBID, Pharma Pac	52959-0351-24
30's	$25.20	GENERIC, Medirex Inc	57480-0479-06
30's	$26.93	GENERIC, Pd-Rx Pharmaceuticals	55289-0460-30
30's	$33.75	GENERIC, Heartland Healthcare Services	61392-0042-30
30's	$42.55	DOLOBID, Allscripts Pharmaceutical Company	54569-0296-07
45's	$50.63	GENERIC, Heartland Healthcare Services	61392-0042-45
60's	$58.25	GENERIC, Aligen Independent Laboratories Inc	00405-4330-31
60's	$58.25	GENERIC, Moore, H.L. Drug Exchange Inc	00839-7764-05
60's	$59.02	GENERIC, Ivax Corporation	00182-1954-26
60's	$60.00	FEDERAL UPPER LIMIT, H.C.F.A. F F P	99999-1058-02
60's	$61.53	GENERIC, Purepac Pharmaceutical Company	00228-2546-06
60's	$65.83	GENERIC, Watson/Rugby Laboratories Inc	00536-5563-08
60's	$67.50	GENERIC, Heartland Healthcare Services	61392-0042-60
60's	$68.89	GENERIC, Roxane Laboratories Inc	00054-4220-21
60's	$73.84	DOLOBID, Alpharma Uspd Makers Of Barre and Nmc	63874-0307-60
60's	$76.59	GENERIC, Endo Laboratories Llc	60951-0769-60
60's	$79.12	GENERIC, Teva Pharmaceuticals Usa	00093-0755-06
60's	$89.26	DOLOBID, Merck & Company Inc	00006-0697-61
90's	$101.25	GENERIC, Heartland Healthcare Services	61392-0042-90
100's	$58.33	GENERIC, Mutual/United Research Laboratories	00677-1460-06
100's	$94.86	GENERIC, Purepac Pharmaceutical Company	00228-2546-10
100's	$104.28	GENERIC, Roxane Laboratories Inc	00054-8220-25
100's	$104.90	GENERIC, Ivax Corporation	00182-1954-89
100's	$122.72	DOLOBID, Alpharma Uspd Makers Of Barre and Nmc	63874-0307-01
100's	$125.00	GENERIC, Medirex Inc	57480-0479-01
100's	$129.23	GENERIC, Teva Pharmaceuticals Usa	00093-0755-01

PRODUCT LISTING - EQUIVALENTS NOT AVAILABLE

Tablet - Oral - 250 mg			
60's	$46.66	GENERIC, West Point Pharma	59591-0195-61
Tablet - Oral - 500 mg			
4's	$4.58	GENERIC, Prescript Pharmaceuticals	00247-0320-04
5's	$4.87	GENERIC, Prescript Pharmaceuticals	00247-0320-05
10's	$6.40	GENERIC, Prescript Pharmaceuticals	00247-0320-10
10's	$11.55	GENERIC, Allscripts Pharmaceutical Company	54569-3658-00
10's	$11.90	GENERIC, Southwood Pharmaceuticals Inc	58016-0194-10
12's	$7.01	GENERIC, Prescript Pharmaceuticals	00247-0320-12
12's	$14.28	GENERIC, Southwood Pharmaceuticals Inc	58016-0194-12
14's	$7.61	GENERIC, Prescript Pharmaceuticals	00247-0320-14
14's	$16.66	GENERIC, Southwood Pharmaceuticals Inc	58016-0194-14
15's	$7.92	GENERIC, Prescript Pharmaceuticals	00247-0320-15
15's	$17.33	GENERIC, Allscripts Pharmaceutical Company	54569-3658-03
15's	$17.85	GENERIC, Southwood Pharmaceuticals Inc	58016-0194-15
15's	$18.75	GENERIC, Pharma Pac	52959-0379-15
16's	$8.22	GENERIC, Prescript Pharmaceuticals	00247-0320-16
20's	$9.45	GENERIC, Prescript Pharmaceuticals	00247-0320-20
20's	$23.10	GENERIC, Allscripts Pharmaceutical Company	54569-3658-01
20's	$23.80	GENERIC, Southwood Pharmaceuticals Inc	58016-0194-20
20's	$24.15	GENERIC, Pharma Pac	52959-0379-20
21's	$24.99	GENERIC, Southwood Pharmaceuticals Inc	58016-0194-21
24's	$28.56	GENERIC, Southwood Pharmaceuticals Inc	58016-0194-24
28's	$33.32	GENERIC, Southwood Pharmaceuticals Inc	58016-0194-28
30's	$12.48	GENERIC, Prescript Pharmaceuticals	00247-0320-30
30's	$34.65	GENERIC, Allscripts Pharmaceutical Company	54569-3658-02
30's	$35.33	GENERIC, Pharma Pac	52959-0379-30
30's	$35.70	GENERIC, Southwood Pharmaceuticals Inc	58016-0194-30
40's	$47.60	GENERIC, Southwood Pharmaceuticals Inc	58016-0194-40
60's	$58.33	GENERIC, West Point Pharma	59591-0196-61
60's	$69.90	GENERIC, St. Mary'S Mpp	60760-0196-60
60's	$71.34	GENERIC, Southwood Pharmaceuticals Inc	58016-0194-60

Digoxin *(001061)*

Categories: Fibrillation, atrial; Heart failure, congestive; Pregnancy Category C; FDA Approved 1954 Nov; WHO Formulary
Drug Classes: Antiarrhythmics; Cardiac glycosides; Inotropes
Brand Names: Cardoxin; Coragoxine; Digon; Lanorale; Lanoxicaps; **Lanoxin**; Lenoxicaps; Natigoxin; Novodigal
Foreign Brand Availability: Cardigox (Belgium); Cardiogoxin (Argentina); Cardioxin (India); Digacin (Germany); Digomal (Italy); Digosin (Japan; Korea); Digoxina (Peru); Digoxine Navtivelle (France); Digoxin-Sandoz (Benin; Burkina-Faso; Ethiopia; Gambia; Ghana; Guinea; Indonesia; Ivory-Coast; Japan; Kenya; Liberia; Malawi; Mali; Mauritania; Mauritius; Morocco; Niger; Nigeria; Senegal; Seychelles; Sierra-Leone; South-Africa; Sudan; Tanzania; Tunia; Uganda; Zambia; Zimbabwe); Digoxin-Zori (Israel); Dilanacin (Cyprus; Egypt; Iraq; Jordan; Sudan); Eudigox (Italy); Fargoxin (Indonesia); Grexin (Thailand); Lanacordin (Spain); Lanacrist (Sweden); Lanicor (Argentina; Austria; Bahamas; Barbados; Belize; Benin; Bermuda; Burkina-Faso; Curacao; Czech-Republic; Ecuador; Ethiopia; Gambia; Germany; Ghana; Greece; Guinea; Guyana; Italy; Ivory-Coast; Jamaica; Kenya; Liberia; Malawi; Mali; Mauritania; Mauritius; Morocco; Netherland-Antilles; Niger; Nigeria; Portugal; Puerto-Rico; Senegal; Seychelles; Sierra-Leone; South-Africa; Sudan; Surinam; Tanzania; Trinidad; Tunia; Uganda; Zambia; Zimbabwe); Lanikor (Russia); Lanitop (Ecuador); Lanoxin PG (New-Zealand); Lenoxin (Germany); Mapluxin (Mexico); Purgoxin (South-Africa); Toloxin (Thailand)
Cost of Therapy: $4.72 (Heart Failure; Lanoxin; 0.25 mg; 1 tablet/day; 30 day supply)
$1.42 (Heart Failure; Generic Tablets; 0.25 mg; 1 tablet/day; 30 day supply)
$9.49 (Heart Failure; Lanoxicaps; 0.2 mg; 1 capsule/day; 30 day supply)
HCFA JCODE(S): J1160 up to 0.5 mg IM, IV

INTRAVENOUS

DESCRIPTION

Note: The trade name has been used throughout this monograph for clarity.

Digoxin is one of the cardiac (or digitalis) glycosides, a closely related group of drugs having in common specific effects on the myocardium. These drugs are found in a number of plants. Digoxin is extracted from the leaves of *Digitalis lanata*. The term "digitalis" is used to designate the whole group of glycosides. The glycosides are composed of two portions: a sugar and a cardenolide (hence "glycosides").

Digoxin is described chemically as (3β,5β,12β)-3-[(*O*-2,6-dideoxy-β-*D*-*ribo*-hexopyranosyl-(1→4)-*O*-2,6-dideoxy-β-*D*-*ribo*-hexopyranosyl-(1→4)-2,6-dideoxy-β-*D*-*ribo*-hexopyranosyl)oxy]-12,14-dihydroxy-card-20(22)-enolide. Its molecular formula is $C_{41}H_{64}O_{14}$ and its molecular weight is 780.95.

Digoxin exists as odorless white crystals that melt with decomposition above 230°C. The drug is practically insoluble in water and in ether; slightly soluble in diluted (50%) alcohol and in chloroform; and freely soluble in pyridine.

Lanoxin injection and Lanoxin injection pediatric are sterile solutions of digoxin for intravenous or intramuscular injection. The vehicle contains 40% propylene glycol and 10% alcohol. The injection is buffered to a pH of 6.8-7.2 with 0.17% sodium phosphate and 0.08% anhydrous citric acid. Each 2 ml ampul of Lanoxin injection contains 500 μg (0.5 mg) digoxin (250 μg [0.25 mg] per ml). Each 1 ml ampul of Lanoxin injection pediatric contains 100 μg (0.1 mg) digoxin. Dilution is not required.

CLINICAL PHARMACOLOGY

MECHANISM OF ACTION

Digoxin inhibits sodium-potassium ATPase, an enzyme that regulates the quantity of sodium and potassium inside cells. Inhibition of the enzyme leads to an increase in the intracellular concentration of sodium and thus (by stimulation of sodium-calcium exchange) an increase in the intracellular concentration of calcium. The beneficial effects of digoxin result from direct actions on cardiac muscle, as well as indirect actions on the cardiovascular system mediated by effects on the autonomic nervous system. The autonomic effects include: (1) a vagomimetic action, which is responsible for the effects of digoxin on the sinoatrial and atrioventricular (AV) nodes; and (2) baroreceptor sensitization, which results in increased afferent inhibitory activity and reduced activity of the sympathetic nervous system and renin-angiotensin system for any given increment in mean arterial pressure. The pharmacologic consequences of these direct and indirect effects are: (1) an increase in the force and velocity of myocardial systolic contraction (positive inotropic action); (2) a decrease in the degree of activation of the sympathetic nervous system and renin-angiotensin system (neurohormonal deactivating effect); and (3) slowing of the heart rate and decreased conduction velocity through the AV node (vagomimetic effect). The effects of digoxin in heart failure are mediated by its positive inotropic and neurohormonal deactivating effects, whereas the effects of the drug in atrial arrhythmias are related to its vagomimetic actions. In high doses, digoxin increases sympathetic outflow from the central nervous system (CNS). This increase in sympathetic activity may be an important factor in digitalis toxicity.

PHARMACOKINETICS

Note: The following data are from studies performed in adults, unless otherwise stated.

Absorption

Comparisons of the systemic availability and equivalent doses for preparations of Lanoxin are shown in TABLE 1.

TABLE 1 *Comparisons of the Systemic Availability and Equivalent Doses for Preparations of Lanoxin*

Product	Absolute Bioavailability	Equivalent Doses (μg)* Among Dosage Forms			
Lanoxin tablets	60-80%	62.5	125	250	500
Lanoxin elixir pediatric	70-85%	62.5	125	250	500
Lanoxicaps	90-100%	50	100	200	400
Lanoxin injection/IV	100%	50	100	200	400

* For example, 125 μg Lanoxin tablets equivalent to 125 μg Lanoxin elixir pediatric equivalent to 100 μg Lanoxicaps equivalent to 100 μg Lanoxin injection/IV.

Distribution

Following drug administration, a 6-8 hour tissue distribution phase is observed. This is followed by a much more gradual decline in the serum concentration of the drug, which is dependent on the elimination of digoxin from the body. The peak height and slope of the early portion (absorption/distribution phases) of the serum concentration-time curve are dependent upon the route of administration and the absorption characteristics of the formulation. Clinical evidence indicates that the early high serum concentrations do not reflect the concentration of digoxin at its site of action, but that with chronic use, the steady-state post-distribution serum concentrations are in equilibrium with tissue concentrations and correlate with pharmacologic effects. In individual patients, these post-distribution serum concentrations may be useful in evaluating therapeutic and toxic effects (see DOSAGE AND ADMINISTRATION, Serum Digoxin Concentrations).

Digoxin is concentrated in tissues and therefore has a large apparent volume of distribution. Digoxin crosses both the blood-brain barrier and the placenta. At delivery, the serum digoxin concentration in the newborn is similar to the serum concentration in the mother. Approximately 25% of digoxin in the plasma is bound to protein. Serum digoxin concentrations are not significantly altered by large changes in fat tissue weight, so that its distribution space correlates best with lean (*i.e.,* ideal) body weight, not total body weight.

Metabolism

Only a small percentage (16%) of a dose of digoxin is metabolized. The end metabolites, which include 3 β-digoxigenin, 3-keto-digoxigenin, and their glucuronide and sulfate conjugates, are polar in nature and are postulated to be formed via hydrolysis, oxidation, and conjugation. The metabolism of digoxin is not dependent upon the cytochrome P-450 system, and digoxin is not known to induce or inhibit the cytochrome P-450 system.

Excretion

Elimination of digoxin follows first-order kinetics (that is, the quantity of digoxin eliminated at any time is proportional to the total body content). Following intravenous administration to healthy volunteers, 50-70% of a digoxin dose is excreted unchanged in the urine. Renal excretion of digoxin is proportional to glomerular filtration rate and is largely independent of urine flow. In healthy volunteers with normal renal function, digoxin has a half-life of 1.5-2.0 days. The half-life in anuric patients is prolonged to 3.5-5 days. Digoxin is not effectively removed from the body by dialysis, exchange transfusion, or during cardiopulmonary bypass because most of the drug is bound to tissue and does not circulate in the blood.

Special Populations

Race differences in digoxin pharmacokinetics have not been formally studied. Because digoxin is primarily eliminated as unchanged drug via the kidney and because there are no important differences in creatinine clearance among races, pharmacokinetic differences due to race are not expected.

The clearance of digoxin can be primarily correlated with renal function as indicated by creatinine clearance. In children with renal disease, digoxin must be carefully titrated based upon clinical response. The Cockcroft and Gault formula for estimation of creatinine clearance includes age, body weight, and gender. TABLE 6 provides the usual daily maintenance dose requirements of Lanoxin injection based on creatinine clearance (per 70 kg).

Plasma digoxin concentration profiles in patients with acute hepatitis generally fell within the range of profiles in a group of healthy subjects.

PHARMACODYNAMICS AND CLINICAL EFFECTS

The times to onset of pharmacologic effect and to peak effect of preparations of Lanoxin are shown in TABLE 2.

TABLE 2 *Times to Onset of Pharmacologic Effect and to Peak Effect of Preparations of Lanoxin*

Product	Time to Onset of Effect*	Time to Peak Effect*
Lanoxin tablets	0.5-2 hours	2-6 hours
Lanoxin elixir pediatric	0.5-2 hours	2-6 hours
Lanoxicaps	0.5-2 hours	2-6 hours
Lanoxin injection/IV	5-30 minutes†	1-4 hours

* Documented for ventricular response rate in atrial fibrillation, inotropic effects and electrocardiographic changes.
† Depending upon rate of infusion.

Hemodynamic Effects

Digoxin produces hemodynamic improvement in patients with heart failure. Short- and long-term therapy with the drug increases cardiac output and lowers pulmonary artery pressure, pulmonary capillary wedge pressure, and systemic vascular resistance. These hemodynamic effects are accompanied by an increase in the left ventricular ejection fraction and a decrease in end-systolic and end-diastolic dimensions.

Chronic Heart Failure

Two 12 week, double-blind, placebo-controlled studies enrolled 178 (RADIANCE trial) and 88 (PROVED trial) adult patients with NYHA class II or III heart failure previously treated with oral digoxin, a diuretic, and an ACE inhibitor (RADIANCE only) and randomized them to placebo or treatment with Lanoxin tablets. Both trials demonstrated better preservation of exercise capacity in patients randomized to Lanoxin. Continued treatment with Lanoxin reduced the risk of developing worsening heart failure, as evidenced by heart failure-related hospitalizations and emergency care and the need for concomitant heart failure therapy. The larger study also showed treatment-related benefits in NYHA class and patients' global assessment. In the smaller trial, these trended in favor of a treatment benefit.

The Digitalis Investigation Group (DIG) main trial was a multicenter, randomized, double-blind, placebo-controlled mortality study of 6801 patients with heart failure and left ventricular ejection fraction ≤0.45. At randomization, 67% were NYHA class I or II, 71% had heart failure of ischemic etiology, 44% had been receiving digoxin, and most were receiving concomitant ACE inhibitor (94%) and diuretic (82%). Patients were randomized to placebo or Lanoxin tablets, the dose of which was adjusted for the patient's age, sex, lean body weight, and serum creatinine (see DOSAGE AND ADMINISTRATION), and followed for up to 58 months (median 37 months). The median daily dose prescribed was 0.25 mg. Overall all-cause mortality was 35% with no difference between groups (95% confidence limits for relative risk of 0.91-1.07). Lanoxin was associated with a 25% reduction in the number of hospitalizations for heart failure, a 28% reduction in the risk of a patient having at least one hospitalization for heart failure, and a 6.5% reduction in total hospitalizations (for any cause).

Use of Lanoxin was associated with a trend to increase time to all-cause death or hospitalization. The trend was evident in subgroups of patients with mild heart failure as well as more severe disease, as shown in TABLE 3A and TABLE 3B. Although the effect on all-cause death or hospitalization was not statistically significant, much of the apparent benefit derived from effects on mortality and hospitalization attributed to heart failure.

TABLE 3A *Subgroup Analyses of Mortality and Hospitalization During the First 2 Years Following Randomization*

		Risk of All-Cause Mortality or All-Cause Hospitalization*		
	n	Placebo	Lanoxin	Relative Risk†
All Patients (EF ≤0.45)	6801	604	593	0.94 (0.88-1.00)
NYHA I/II	4571	549	541	0.96 (0.89-1.04)
EF 0.25-0.45	4543	568	571	0.99 (0.91-1.07)
CTR ≤0.55	4455	561	563	0.98 (0.91-1.06)
NYHA III/IV	2224	719	696	0.88 (0.80-0.97)
EF <0.25	2258	677	637	0.84 (0.76-0.93)
CTR >0.55	2346	687	650	0.85 (0.77-0.94)
EF >0.45‡	987	571	585	1.04 (0.88-1.23)

* Number of patients with an event during the first 2 years per 1000 randomized patients.
† Relative risk (95% confidence interval).
‡ DIG Ancillary Study.

In situations where there is no statistically significant benefit of treatment evident from a trial's primary endpoint, results pertaining to a secondary endpoint should be interpreted cautiously.

Chronic Atrial Fibrillation

In adult patients with chronic atrial fibrillation, digoxin slows rapid ventricular response rate in a linear dose-response fashion from 0.25-0.75 mg/day. Digoxin should not be used for the treatment of multifocal atrial tachycardia.

D

TABLE 3B *Subgroup Analyses of Mortality and Hospitalization During the First 2 Years Following Randomization*

		Risk of HF-Related Mortality or HF-Related Hospitalization*		
	n	Placebo	Lanoxin	Relative Risk†
All Patients (EF ≤0.45)	6801	294	217	0.69 (0.63-0.76)
NYHA I/II	4571	242	178	0.70 (0.62-0.80)
EF 0.25-0.45	4543	244	190	0.74 (0.66-0.84)
CTR ≤0.55	4455	239	180	0.71 (0.63-0.81)
NYHA III/IV	2224	402	295	0.65 (0.57-0.75)
EF <0.25	2258	394	270	0.61 (0.53-0.71)
CTR >0.55	2346	398	287	0.65 (0.57-0.75)
EF >0.45‡	987	179	136	0.72 (0.53-0.99)

* Number of patients with an event during the first 2 years per 1000 randomized patients.
† Relative risk (95% confidence interval).
‡ DIG Ancillary Study.

INDICATIONS AND USAGE

HEART FAILURE

Lanoxin is indicated for the treatment of mild to moderate heart failure. Lanoxin increases left ventricular ejection fraction and improves heart failure symptoms as evidenced by exercise capacity and heart failure-related hospitalizations and emergency care, while having no effect on mortality. Where possible, Lanoxin should be used with a diuretic and an angiotensin-converting enzyme inhibitor, but an optimal order for starting these three drugs cannot be specified.

ATRIAL FIBRILLATION

Lanoxin is indicated for the control of ventricular response rate in patients with chronic atrial fibrillation.

CONTRAINDICATIONS

Digitalis glycosides are contraindicated in patients with ventricular fibrillation or in patients with a known hypersensitivity to digoxin. A hypersensitivity reaction to other digitalis preparations usually constitutes a contraindication to digoxin.

WARNINGS

SINUS NODE DISEASE AND AV BLOCK

Because digoxin slows sinoatrial and AV conduction, the drug commonly prolongs the PR interval. The drug may cause severe sinus bradycardia or sinoatrial block in patients with pre-existing sinus node disease and may cause advanced or complete heart block in patients with pre-existing incomplete AV block. In such patients consideration should be given to the insertion of a pacemaker before treatment with digoxin.

ACCESSORY AV PATHWAY (WOLFF-PARKINSON-WHITE SYNDROME)

After intravenous digoxin therapy, some patients with paroxysmal atrial fibrillation or flutter and a coexisting accessory AV pathway have developed increased antegrade conduction across the accessory pathway bypassing the AV node, leading to a very rapid ventricular response or ventricular fibrillation. Unless conduction down the accessory pathway has been blocked (either pharmacologically or by surgery), digoxin should not be used in such patients. The treatment of paroxysmal supraventricular tachycardia in such patients is usually direct-current cardioversion.

USE IN PATIENTS WITH PRESERVED LEFT VENTRICULAR SYSTOLIC FUNCTION

Patients with certain disorders involving heart failure associated with preserved left ventricular ejection fraction may be particularly susceptible to toxicity of the drug. Such disorders include restrictive cardiomyopathy, constrictive pericarditis, amyloid heart disease, and acute cor pulmonale. Patients with idiopathic hypertrophic subaortic stenosis may have worsening of the outflow obstruction due to the inotropic effects of digoxin.

PRECAUTIONS

USE IN PATIENTS WITH IMPAIRED RENAL FUNCTION

Digoxin is primarily excreted by the kidneys; therefore, patients with impaired renal function require smaller than usual maintenance doses of digoxin (see DOSAGE AND ADMINISTRATION). Because of the prolonged elimination half-life, a longer period of time is required to achieve an initial or new steady-state serum concentration in patients with renal impairment than in patients with normal renal function. If appropriate care is not taken to reduce the dose of digoxin, such patients are at high risk for toxicity, and toxic effects will last longer in such patients than in patients with normal renal function.

USE IN PATIENTS WITH ELECTROLYTE DISORDERS

In patients with hypokalemia or hypomagnesemia, toxicity may occur despite serum digoxin concentrations below 2.0 ng/ml, because potassium or magnesium depletion sensitizes the myocardium to digoxin. Therefore, it is desirable to maintain normal serum potassium and magnesium concentrations in patients being treated with digoxin. Deficiencies of these electrolytes may result from malnutrition, diarrhea, or prolonged vomiting, as well as the use of the following drugs or procedures: diuretics, amphotericin B, corticosteroids, antacids, dialysis, and mechanical suction of gastrointestinal secretions.

Hypercalcemia from any cause predisposes the patient to digitalis toxicity. Calcium, particularly when administered rapidly by the intravenous route, may produce serious arrhythmias in digitalized patients. On the other hand, hypocalcemia can nullify the effects of digoxin in humans; thus, digoxin may be ineffective until serum calcium is restored to normal. These interactions are related to the fact that digoxin affects contractility and excitability of the heart in a manner similar to that of calcium.

USE IN THYROID DISORDERS AND HYPERMETABOLIC STATES

Hypothyroidism may reduce the requirements for digoxin. Heart failure and/or atrial arrhythmias resulting from hypermetabolic or hyperdynamic states (*e.g.*, hyperthyroidism, hypoxia, or arteriovenous shunt) are best treated by addressing the underlying condition. Atrial arrhythmias associated with hypermetabolic states are particularly resistant to digoxin treatment. Care must be taken to avoid toxicity if digoxin is used.

USE IN PATIENTS WITH ACUTE MYOCARDIAL INFARCTION

Digoxin should be used with caution in patients with acute myocardial infarction. The use of inotropic drugs in some patients in this setting may result in undesirable increases in myocardial oxygen demand and ischemia.

USE DURING ELECTRICAL CARDIOVERSION

It may be desirable to reduce the dose of digoxin for 1-2 days prior to electrical cardioversion of atrial fibrillation to avoid the induction of ventricular arrhythmias, but physicians must consider the consequences of increasing the ventricular response if digoxin is withdrawn. If digitalis toxicity is suspected, elective cardioversion should be delayed. If it is not prudent to delay cardioversion, the lowest possible energy level should be selected to avoid provoking ventricular arrhythmias.

LABORATORY TEST MONITORING

Patients receiving digoxin should have their serum electrolytes and renal function (serum creatinine concentrations) assessed periodically; the frequency of assessments will depend on the clinical setting. For discussion of serum digoxin concentrations, see DOSAGE AND ADMINISTRATION.

DRUG/LABORATORY TEST INTERACTIONS

The use of therapeutic doses of digoxin may cause prolongation of the PR interval and depression of the ST segment on the electrocardiogram. Digoxin may produce false positive ST-T changes on the electrocardiogram during exercise testing. These electrophysiologic effects reflect an expected effect of the drug and are not indicative of toxicity.

CARCINOGENESIS, MUTAGENESIS, AND IMPAIRMENT OF FERTILITY

There have been no long-term studies performed in animals to evaluate carcinogenic potential, nor have studies been conducted to assess the mutagenic potential of digoxin or its potential to affect fertility.

PREGNANCY, TERATOGENIC EFFECTS, PREGNANCY CATEGORY C

Animal reproduction studies have not been conducted with digoxin. It is also not known whether digoxin can cause fetal harm when administered to a pregnant woman or can affect reproduction capacity. Digoxin should be given to a pregnant woman only if clearly needed.

NURSING MOTHERS

Studies have shown that digoxin concentrations in the mother's serum and milk are similar. However, the estimated exposure of a nursing infant to digoxin via breast feeding will be far below the usual infant maintenance dose. Therefore, this amount should have no pharmacologic effect upon the infant. Nevertheless, caution should be exercised when digoxin is administered to a nursing woman.

PEDIATRIC USE

Newborn infants display considerable variability in their tolerance to digoxin. Premature and immature infants are particularly sensitive to the effects of digoxin, and the dosage of the drug must not only be reduced but must be individualized according to their degree of maturity. Digitalis glycosides can cause poisoning in children due to accidental ingestion.

GERIATRIC USE

The majority of clinical experience gained with digoxin has been in the elderly population. This experience has not identified differences in response or adverse effects between the elderly and younger patients. However, this drug is known to be substantially excreted by the kidney, and the risk of toxic reactions to this drug may be greater in patients with impaired renal function. Because elderly patients are more likely to have decreased renal function, care should be taken in dose selection, which should be based on renal function, and it may be useful to monitor renal function (see DOSAGE AND ADMINISTRATION).

DRUG INTERACTIONS

Potassium-depleting *diuretics* are a major contributing factor to digitalis toxicity. *Calcium,* particularly if administered rapidly by the intravenous route, may produce serious arrhythmias in digitalized patients. *Quinidine, verapamil, amiodarone, propafenone, indomethacin, itraconazole, alprazolam,* and *spironolactone* raise the serum digoxin concentration due to a reduction in clearance and/or in volume of distribution of the drug, with the implication that digitalis intoxication may result. *Erythromycin* and *clarithromycin* (and possibly other *macrolide antibiotics*) and *tetracycline* may increase digoxin absorption in patients who inactivate digoxin by bacterial metabolism in the lower intestine, so that digitalis intoxication may result. *Propantheline* and *diphenoxylate,* by decreasing gut motility, may increase digoxin absorption. *Antacids, kaolin-pectin, sulfasalazine, neomycin, cholestyramine,* certain *anticancer drugs,* and *metoclopramide* may interfere with intestinal digoxin absorption, resulting in unexpectedly low serum concentrations. *Rifampin* may decrease serum digoxin concentration, especially in patients with renal dysfunction, by increasing the non-renal clearance of digoxin. There have been inconsistent reports regarding the effects of other drugs *(e.g., quinine, penicillamine)* on serum digoxin concentration. *Thyroid* administration to a digitalized, hypothyroid patient may increase the dose requirement of digoxin. Concomitant use of digoxin and *sympathomimetics* increases the risk of cardiac arrhythmias. *Succinylcholine* may cause a sudden extrusion of potassium from muscle cells, and may thereby cause arrhythmias in digitalized patients. Although beta-adrenergic blockers or calcium channel blockers and digoxin may be useful in combination to control atrial fibrillation, their additive effects on AV node conduction can result in advanced or complete heart block.

Due to the considerable variability of these interactions, the dosage of digoxin should be individualized when patients receive these medications concurrently. Furthermore, caution should be exercised when combining digoxin with any drug that may cause a significant deterioration in renal function, since a decline in glomerular filtration or tubular secretion may impair the excretion of digoxin.

ADVERSE REACTIONS

In general, the adverse reactions of digoxin are dose-dependent and occur at doses higher than those needed to achieve a therapeutic effect. Hence, adverse reactions are less common when digoxin is used within the recommended dose range or therapeutic serum concentration range and when there is careful attention to concurrent medications and conditions.

Because some patients may be particularly susceptible to side effects with digoxin, the dosage of the drug should always be selected carefully and adjusted as the clinical condition of the patient warrants. In the past, when high doses of digoxin were used and little attention was paid to clinical status or concurrent medications, adverse reactions to digoxin were more frequent and severe. Cardiac adverse reactions accounted for about one-half, gastrointestinal disturbances for about one-fourth, and CNS and other toxicity for about one-fourth of these adverse reactions. However, available evidence suggests that the incidence and severity of digoxin toxicity has decreased substantially in recent years. In recent controlled clinical trials, in patients with predominantly mild to moderate heart failure, the incidence of adverse experiences was comparable in patients taking digoxin and in those taking placebo. In a large mortality trial, the incidence of hospitalization for suspected digoxin toxicity was 2% in patients taking Lanoxin tablets compared to 0.9% in patients taking placebo. In this trial, the most common manifestations of digoxin toxicity included gastrointestinal and cardiac disturbances; CNS manifestations were less common.

ADULTS

Cardiac: Therapeutic doses of digoxin may cause heart block in patients with pre-existing sinoatrial or AV conduction disorders; heart block can be avoided by adjusting the dose of digoxin. Prophylactic use of a cardiac pacemaker may be considered if the risk of heart block is considered unacceptable. High doses of digoxin may produce a variety of rhythm disturbances, such as first-degree, second-degree (Wenckebach), or third-degree heart block (including asystole); atrial tachycardia with block; AV dissociation; accelerated junctional (nodal) rhythm; unifocal or multiform ventricular premature contractions (especially bigeminy or trigeminy); ventricular tachycardia; and ventricular fibrillation. Digoxin produces PR prolongation and ST segment depression which should not by themselves be considered digoxin toxicity. Cardiac toxicity can also occur at therapeutic doses in patients who have conditions which may alter their sensitivity to digoxin (see WARNINGS and PRECAUTIONS).

Gastrointestinal: Digoxin may cause anorexia, nausea, vomiting, and diarrhea. Rarely, the use of digoxin has been associated with abdominal pain, intestinal ischemia, and hemorrhagic necrosis of the intestines.

CNS: Digoxin can produce visual disturbances (blurred or yellow vision), headache, weakness, dizziness, apathy, confusion, and mental disturbances (such as anxiety, depression, delirium, and hallucination).

Other: Gynecomastia has been occasionally observed following the prolonged use of digoxin. Thrombocytopenia and maculopapular rash and other skin reactions have been rarely observed.

TABLE 4 summarizes the incidence of those adverse experiences listed above for patients treated with Lanoxin tablets or placebo from two randomized, double-blind, placebo-controlled withdrawal trials. Patients in these trials were also receiving diuretics with or without angiotensin-converting enzyme inhibitors. These patients had been stable on digoxin, and were randomized to digoxin or placebo. The results shown in TABLE 4 reflect the experience in patients following dosage titration with the use of serum digoxin concentrations and careful follow-up. These adverse experiences are consistent with results from a large, placebo-controlled mortality trial (DIG trial) wherein over half the patients were not receiving digoxin prior to enrollment.

TABLE 4 *Adverse Experiences In Two Parallel, Double-Blind, Placebo-Controlled Withdrawal Trials (Number of Patients Reporting)*

Adverse Experience	Digoxin Patients (n=123)	Placebo Patients (n=125)
Cardiac		
Palpitation	1	4
Ventricular extrasystole	1	1
Tachycardia	2	1
Heart arrest	1	1
Gastrointestinal		
Anorexia	1	4
Nausea	4	2
Vomiting	2	1
Diarrhea	4	1
Abdominal pain	0	6
CNS		
Headache	4	4
Dizziness	6	5
Mental disturbances	5	1
Other		
Rash	2	1
Death	4	3

INFANTS AND CHILDREN

The side effects of digoxin in infants and children differ from those seen in adults in several respects. Although digoxin may produce anorexia, nausea, vomiting, diarrhea, and CNS disturbances in young patients, these are rarely the initial symptoms of overdosage. Rather, the earliest and most frequent manifestation of excessive dosing with digoxin in infants and children is the appearance of cardiac arrhythmias, including sinus bradycardia. In children, the use of digoxin may produce any arrhythmia. The most common are conduction disturbances or supraventricular tachyarrhythmias, such as atrial tachycardia (with or without block) and junctional (nodal) tachycardia. Ventricular arrhythmias are less common. Sinus bradycardia may be a sign of impending digoxin intoxication, especially in infants, even in the absence of first-degree heart block. Any arrhythmia or alteration in cardiac conduction that develops in a child taking digoxin should be assumed to be caused by digoxin, until further evaluation proves otherwise.

DOSAGE AND ADMINISTRATION

GENERAL

Recommended dosages of digoxin may require considerable modification because of individual sensitivity of the patient to the drug, the presence of associated conditions, or the use of concurrent medications.

Parenteral administration of digoxin should be used only when the need for rapid digitalization is urgent or when the drug cannot be taken orally. Intramuscular injection can lead to severe pain at the injection site, thus intravenous administration is preferred. If the drug must be administered by the intramuscular route, it should be injected deep into the muscle followed by massage. No more than 500 μg (2 ml) should be injected into a single site.

Lanoxin injection and Lanoxin injection pediatric can be administered undiluted or diluted with a 4-fold or greater volume of sterile water for injection, 0.9% sodium chloride injection, or 5% dextrose injection. The use of less than a 4-fold volume of diluent could lead to precipitation of the digoxin. Immediate use of the diluted product is recommended.

If tuberculin syringes are used to measure very small doses, one must be aware of the problem of inadvertent overadministration of digoxin. The syringe should *not* be flushed with the parenteral solution after its contents are expelled into an indwelling vascular catheter.

Slow infusion of Lanoxin injection is preferable to bolus administration. Rapid infusion of digitalis glycosides has been shown to cause systemic and coronary arteriolar constriction, which may be clinically undesirable. Caution is thus advised and Lanoxin injection should probably be administered over a period of 5 minutes or longer. Mixing of Lanoxin injection with other drugs in the same container or simultaneous administration in the same intravenous line is not recommended.

In selecting a dose of digoxin, the following factors must be considered:

The body weight of the patient. Doses should be calculated based upon lean (*i.e.,* ideal) body weight.

The patient's renal function, preferably evaluated on the basis of estimated creatinine clearance.

The patient's age. Infants and children require different doses of digoxin than adults. Also, advanced age may be indicative of diminished renal function even in patients with normal serum creatinine concentration (*i.e.,* below 1.5 mg/dl).

Concomitant disease states, concurrent medications, or other factors likely to alter the pharmacokinetic or pharmacodynamic profile of digoxin (see PRECAUTIONS).

SERUM DIGOXIN CONCENTRATIONS

In general, the dose of digoxin used should be determined on clinical grounds. However, measurement of serum digoxin concentrations can be helpful to the clinician in determining the adequacy of digoxin therapy and in assigning certain probabilities to the likelihood of digoxin intoxication. About two-thirds of adults considered adequately digitalized (without evidence of toxicity) have serum digoxin concentrations ranging from 0.8-2.0 ng/ml. However, digoxin may produce clinical benefits even at serum concentrations below this range. About two-thirds of adult patients with clinical toxicity have serum digoxin concentrations greater than 2.0 ng/ml. However, since one-third of patients with clinical toxicity have concentrations less than 2.0 ng/ml, values below 2.0 ng/ml do not rule out the possibility that a certain sign or symptom is related to digoxin therapy. Rarely, there are patients who are unable to tolerate digoxin at serum concentrations below 0.8 ng/ml. Consequently, the serum concentration of digoxin should always be interpreted in the overall clinical context, and an isolated measurement should not be used alone as the basis for increasing or decreasing the dose of the drug.

To allow adequate time for equilibration of digoxin between serum and tissue, sampling of serum concentrations should be done just before the next scheduled dose of the drug. If this is not possible, sampling should be done at least 6-8 hours after the last dose, regardless of the route of administration or the formulation used. On a once-daily dosing schedule, the concentration of digoxin will be 10-25% lower when sampled at 24 vs 8 hours, depending upon the patient's renal function. On a twice-daily dosing schedule, there will be only minor differences in serum digoxin concentrations whether sampling is done at 8 or 12 hours after a dose.

If a discrepancy exists between the reported serum concentration and the observed clinical response, the clinician should consider the following possibilities:

Analytical problems in the assay procedure.

Inappropriate serum sampling time.

Administration of a digitalis glycoside other than digoxin.

Conditions (described in WARNINGS and PRECAUTIONS) causing an alteration in the sensitivity of the patient to digoxin.

Serum digoxin concentration may decrease acutely during periods of exercise without any associated change in clinical efficacy due to increased binding of digoxin to skeletal muscle.

HEART FAILURE

Adults

Digitalization may be accomplished by either of two general approaches that vary in dosage and frequency of administration, but reach the same endpoint in terms of total amount of digoxin accumulated in the body.

If rapid digitalization is considered medically appropriate, it may be achieved by administering a loading dose based upon projected peak digoxin body stores. Maintenance dose can be calculated as a percentage of the loading dose.

More gradual digitalization may be obtained by beginning an appropriate maintenance dose, thus allowing digoxin body stores to accumulate slowly. Steady-state serum digoxin concentrations will be achieved in approximately 5 half-lives of the drug for the individual patient. Depending upon the patient's renal function, this will take between 1 and 3 weeks.

Infants and Children

In general, divided daily dosing is recommended for infants and young children (under age 10). In the newborn period, renal clearance of digoxin is diminished and suitable dosage adjustments must be observed. This is especially pronounced in the premature infant. Beyond the immediate newborn period, children generally require proportionally larger doses than adults on the basis of body weight or body surface area. Children over 10 years of age require adult dosages in proportion to their body weight. Some researchers have suggested that infants and young children tolerate slightly higher serum concentrations than do adults.

Digitalization may be accomplished by either of two general approaches that vary in dosage and frequency of administration, but reach the same endpoint in terms of total amount of digoxin accumulated in the body.

If rapid digitalization is considered medically appropriate, it may be achieved by administering a loading dose based upon projected peak digoxin body stores. Maintenance dose can be calculated as a percentage of the loading dose.

More gradual digitalization may be obtained by beginning an appropriate maintenance dose, thus allowing digoxin body stores to accumulate slowly. Steady-state serum digoxin concentrations will be achieved in approximately 5 half-lives of the drug for the individual patient. Depending upon the patient's renal function, this will take between 1 and 3 weeks.

Rapid Digitalization With a Loading Dose

Lanoxin injection and Lanoxin injection pediatric are frequently used to achieve rapid digitalization, with conversion to Lanoxin tablets or Lanoxicaps for maintenance therapy. If patients are switched from intravenous to oral digoxin formulations, allowances must be made for differences in bioavailability when calculating maintenance dosages (see TABLE 1 and dosing in TABLE 5 and TABLE 6).

Intramuscular injection of digoxin is extremely painful and offers no advantages unless other routes of administration are contraindicated.

Peak digoxin body stores of 8-12 µg/kg should provide therapeutic effect with minimum risk of toxicity in most patients with heart failure and normal sinus rhythm. Because of altered digoxin distribution and elimination, projected peak body stores for patients with renal insufficiency should be conservative (*i.e.,* 6-10 µg/kg) (see PRECAUTIONS).

The loading dose should be administered in several portions, with roughly half the total given as the first dose. Additional fractions of this planned total dose may be given at 6-8 hour intervals (4-8 hour intervals for infants and children), **with careful assessment of clinical response before each additional dose.** If the patient's clinical response necessitates a change from the calculated loading dose of digoxin, then calculation of the maintenance dose should be based upon the amount actually given.

Additional Information for Lanoxin Injection

A single initial intravenous dose of 400-600 µg (0.4-0.6 mg) of Lanoxin injection usually produces a detectable effect in 5-30 minutes that becomes maximal in 1-4 hours. Additional doses of 100-300 µg (0.1-0.3 mg) may be given cautiously at 6-8 hour intervals until clinical evidence of an adequate effect is noted. The usual amount of Lanoxin injection that a 70 kg patient requires to achieve 8-12 µg/kg peak body stores is 600-1000 µg (0.6-1.0 mg).

Additional Information for Lanoxin Injection Pediatric

Digitalizing and daily maintenance doses for each pediatric age group are given in TABLE 5 and should provide therapeutic effect with minimum risk of toxicity in most patients with heart failure and normal sinus rhythm. These recommendations assume the presence of normal renal function.

TABLE 5 *Usual Digitalizing and Maintenance Dosages for Lanoxin Injection Pediatric in Children With Normal Renal Function Based on Lean Body Weight*

Age	IV Digitalizing* Dose (µg/kg)	Daily IV Maintenance Dose† (µg/kg)
Premature	15-25	20-30% of the IV digitalizing dose‡
Full-term	20-30	
1-24 months	30-50	
2-5 years	25-35	25-35% of the IV digitalizing dose‡
5-10 years	15-30	
Over 10 years	8-12	

* IV digitalizing doses are 80% of oral digitalizing doses.
† Divided daily dosing is recommended for children under 10 years of age.
‡ Projected or actual digitalizing dose providing clinical response.

In children with renal disease, digoxin dosing must be carefully titrated based on clinical response.

Gradual Digitalization With a Maintenance Dose

Lanoxin Injection Pediatric

More gradual digitalization can also be accomplished by beginning an appropriate maintenance dose. The range of percentages provided in TABLE 5 can be used in calculating this dose for patients with normal renal function.

It cannot be overemphasized that these pediatric dosage guidelines are based upon average patient response and substantial individual variation can be expected. Accordingly, ultimate dosage selection must be based upon clinical assessment of the patient.

Maintenance Dosing

Lanoxin Injection

The doses of oral digoxin used in controlled trials in patients with heart failure have ranged from 125-500 µg (0.125-0.5 mg) once daily. In these studies, the digoxin dose has been generally titrated according to the patient's age, lean body weight, and renal function. Therapy is generally initiated at a dose of 250 µg (0.25 mg) once daily in patients under age 70 with good renal function, at a dose of 125 µg (0.125 mg) once daily in patients over age 70 or with impaired renal function, and at a dose of 62.5 µg (0.0625 mg) in patients with marked renal impairment. Doses may be increased every 2 weeks according to clinical response.

In a subset of approximately 1800 patients enrolled in the DIG trial (wherein dosing was based on an algorithm similar to that in TABLE 6) the mean (±SD) serum digoxin concentrations at 1 month and 12 months were 1.01 ± 0.47 ng/ml and 0.97 ± 0.43 ng/ml, respectively.

The maintenance dose should be based upon the percentage of the peak body stores lost each day through elimination.

The following formula has had wide clinical use:

Maintenance Dose = Peak Body Stores (*i.e.,* Loading Dose) × % Daily Loss/100

Where: % Daily Loss = 14 + Ccr/5

(Ccr is creatinine clearance, corrected to 70 kg body weight or 1.73 m^2 body surface area.)

TABLE 6 provides average daily maintenance dose requirements of Lanoxin injection for patients with heart failure based upon lean body weight and renal function.

TABLE 6 *Usual Daily Maintenance Dose Requirements (µg) of Lanoxin Injection for Estimated Peak Body Stores of 10 µg/kg**

Corrected Ccr†	Lean Body Weight 50 kg 110 lb	60 kg 132 lb	70 kg 154 lb	80 kg 176 lb	90 kg 198 lb	100 kg 220 lb	Number of Days Before Steady State Achieved‡
0	75§	75	100	100	125	150	22
10	75	100	100	125	150	150	19
20	100	100	125	150	150	175	16
30	100	125	150	150	175	200	14
40	100	125	150	175	200	225	13
50	125	150	175	200	225	250	12
60	125	150	175	200	225	250	11
70	150	175	200	225	250	275	10
80	150	175	200	250	275	300	9
90	150	200	225	250	300	325	8
100	175	200	250	275	300	350	7

* Daily maintenance doses have been rounded to the nearest 25 µg increment.
† In ml/min per 70 kg. Ccr is creatinine clearance, corrected to 70 kg body weight or 1.73 m^2 body surface area. *For adults,* if only serum creatinine concentrations (Scr) are available, a Ccr (corrected to 70 kg body weight) may be estimated in men as (140 -Age)/Scr. For women, this result should be multiplied by 0.85. *Note: This equation cannot be used for estimating creatinine clearance in infants or children.*
‡ If no loading dose administered.
§ 75 µg = 0.075 mg.

Example: Based on TABLE 6, a patient in heart failure with an estimated lean body weight of 70 kg and a Ccr of 60 ml/min should be given a dose of 175 µg (0.175 mg) daily of Lanoxin injection. If no loading dose is administered, steady-state serum concentrations in this patient should be anticipated at approximately 11 days.

It cannot be overemphasized that dosage guidelines provided are based upon average patient response and substantial individual variation can be expected. Accordingly, ultimate dosage selection must be based upon clinical assessment of the patient.

ATRIAL FIBRILLATION

Peak digoxin body stores larger than the 8-12 µg/kg required for most patients with heart failure and normal sinus rhythm have been used for control of ventricular rate in patients with atrial fibrillation. Doses of digoxin used for the treatment of chronic atrial fibrillation should be titrated to the minimum dose that achieves the desired ventricular rate control without causing undesirable side effects. Data are not available to establish the appropriate resting or exercise target rates that should be achieved.

DOSE ADJUSTMENT WHEN CHANGING PREPARATIONS

The difference in bioavailability between Lanoxin injection or Lanoxicaps and Lanoxin Elixir Pediatric or Lanoxin tablets must be considered when changing patients from one dosage form to another.

Doses of 100 µg (0.1 mg) and 200 µg (0.2 mg) of Lanoxicaps are approximately equivalent to 125 µg (0.125 mg) and 250 µg (0.25 mg) doses of Lanoxin tablets and elixir pediatric, respectively (see TABLE 1).

HOW SUPPLIED

Lanoxin (digoxin) Injection: 500 µg (0.5 mg) in 2 ml (250 µg [0.25 mg] per ml).
Lanoxin (digoxin) Injection Pediatric: 100 µg (0.1 mg) in 1 ml.
Storage: Store at 25°C (77°F); excursions permitted to 15-30°C (59-86°F) and protect from light.

ORAL

DESCRIPTION

Note: The trade name has been used throughout this monograph for clarity.

Lanoxin (digoxin) is one of the cardiac (or digitalis) glycosides, a closely related group of drugs having in common specific effects on the myocardium. These drugs are found in a number of plants. Digoxin is extracted from the leaves of *Digitalis lanata.* The term "digitalis" is used to designate the whole group of glycosides. The glycosides are composed of two portions: a sugar and a cardenolide (hence "glycosides").

Digoxin is described chemically as (3β,5β,12β)-3-[(*O*-2,6-dideoxy-β-*D*-*ribo*-hexopyranosyl-(1→4)-*O*-2,6-dideoxy-β-*D*-*ribo*-hexopyranosyl-(1→4)-2,6-dideoxy-β-*D*-*ribo*-hexopyranosyl)oxy]-12,14-dihydroxy-card-20(22)-enolide. Its molecular formula is $C_{41}H_{64}O_{14}$, and its molecular weight is 780.95.

Digoxin exists as odorless white crystals that melt with decomposition above 230°C. The drug is practically insoluble in water and in ether; slightly soluble in diluted (50%) alcohol and in chloroform; and freely soluble in pyridine.

LANOXICAPS

Lanoxicaps is a stable solution of digoxin enclosed within a soft gelatin capsule for oral use. Each capsule contains the labeled amount of digoxin dissolved in a solvent comprised of polyethylene glycol 400, 8% ethyl alcohol, propylene glycol, and purified water. Inactive ingredients in the capsule shell include FD&C red no. 40 (0.05 mg capsule), D&C yellow no. 10 (0.1 mg and 0.2 mg capsules), FD&C blue no. 1 (0.2 mg capsule), gelatin, glycerin, methylparaben and propylparaben (added as preservatives), purified water, and sorbitol. Capsules are printed with edible ink.

LANOXIN TABLETS

Lanoxin tablets are supplied as 125 µg (0.125 mg) or 250 µg (0.25 mg) tablets for oral administration. Each tablet contains the labeled amount of digoxin and the following inactive ingredients: corn and potato starches, lactose, and magnesium stearate. In addition, the dyes used in the 125 µg (0.125 mg) tablets are D&C yellow no. 10 and FD&C yellow no. 6.

LANOXIN ELIXIR PEDIATRIC

Lanoxin elixir pediatric is a stable solution of digoxin specially formulated for oral use in infants and children. Each ml contains 50 µg (0.05 mg) digoxin. The lime-flavored elixir contains the inactive ingredients alcohol 10%, methylparaben 0.1% (added as a preservative), citric acid, D&C green no. 5 and yellow no. 10, flavor, propylene glycol, sodium phosphate, and sucrose. Each package is supplied with a specially calibrated dropper to facilitate the administration of accurate dosage even in premature infants. Starting at 0.2 ml, this 1 ml dropper is marked in divisions of 0.1 ml, each corresponding to 5 µg (0.005 mg) digoxin.

CLINICAL PHARMACOLOGY

MECHANISM OF ACTION

Digoxin inhibits sodium-potassium ATPase, an enzyme that regulates the quantity of sodium and potassium inside cells. Inhibition of the enzyme leads to an increase in the intracellular concentration of sodium and thus (by stimulation of sodium-calcium exchange) an increase in the intracellular concentration of calcium. The beneficial effects of digoxin result from direct actions on cardiac muscle, as well as indirect actions on the cardiovascular system mediated by effects on the autonomic nervous system. The autonomic effects include: (1) a vagomimetic action, which is responsible for the effects of digoxin on the sinoatrial and atrioventricular (AV) nodes; and (2) baroreceptor sensitization, which results in increased afferent inhibitory activity and reduced activity of the sympathetic nervous system and renin-angiotensin system for any given increment in mean arterial pressure. The pharmacologic consequences of these direct and indirect effects are: (1) an increase in the force and velocity of myocardial systolic contraction (positive inotropic action); (2) a decrease in the degree of activation of the sympathetic nervous system and renin-angiotensin system (neurohormonal deactivating effect); and (3) slowing of the heart rate and decreased conduction velocity through the AV node (vagomimetic effect). The effects of digoxin in heart failure are mediated by its positive inotropic and neurohormonal deactivating effects, whereas the effects of the drug in atrial arrhythmias are related to its vagomimetic actions. In high doses, digoxin increases sympathetic outflow from the central nervous system (CNS). This increase in sympathetic activity may be an important factor in digitalis toxicity.

PHARMACOKINETICS

Absorption

Lanoxicaps

Absorption of digoxin from Lanoxicaps capsules has been demonstrated to be 90-100% complete compared to an identical intravenous dose of digoxin (absolute bioavailability). In comparison, the absolute bioavailability of conventional digoxin tablets has been demonstrated to be 60-80%. The enhanced absorption from Lanoxicaps compared to digoxin tablets and elixir is associated with reduced between-patient and within-patient variability in steady-state serum concentrations. The peak serum concentrations are higher than those observed after tablets. When digoxin tablets or capsules are taken after meals, the rate of absorption is slowed, but the total amount of digoxin absorbed is usually unchanged. When taken with meals high in bran fiber, however, the amount absorbed from an oral dose may be reduced. Comparisons of the systemic availability and equivalent doses for preparations of Lanoxin are shown in TABLE 7.

Lanoxin Tablets

Following oral administration, peak serum concentrations of digoxin occur at 1-3 hours. Absorption of digoxin from Lanoxin tablets has been demonstrated to be 60-80% complete compared to an identical intravenous dose of digoxin (absolute bioavailability) or Lanoxicaps (relative bioavailability). When Lanoxin tablets are taken after meals, the rate of absorption is slowed, but the total amount of digoxin absorbed is usually unchanged. When taken with meals high in bran fiber, however, the amount absorbed from an oral dose may be reduced. Comparisons of the systemic availability and equivalent doses for oral preparations of Lanoxin are shown in TABLE 7.

Lanoxin Elixir Pediatric

Note: The following data are from studies performed in adults, unless otherwise stated. Absorption of digoxin from Lanoxin elixir pediatric formulation has been demonstrated to be 70-85% complete compared to an identical intravenous dose of digoxin (absolute bioavailability). When the elixir is taken after meals, the rate of absorption is slowed, but the total amount of digoxin absorbed is usually unchanged. When taken with meals high in bran fiber, however, the amount absorbed from an oral dose may be reduced. Comparisons of the systemic availability and equivalent doses for preparations of Lanoxin are shown in TABLE 7.

***TABLE 7** Comparisons of the Systemic Availability and Equivalent Doses for Oral Preparations of Lanoxin*

Product	Absolute Bioavailability	Equivalent Doses (µg)* Among Dosage Forms			
Lanoxin tablets	60-80%	62.5	125	250	500
Lanoxin elixir pediatric	70-85%	62.5	125	250	500
Lanoxicaps	90-100%	50	100	200	400
Lanoxin injection/IV	100%	50	100	200	400

* For example, 125 µg Lanoxin tablets equivalent to 125 µg Lanoxin elixir pediatric equivalent to 100 µg Lanoxicaps equivalent to 100 µg Lanoxin injection/IV.

In some patients, orally administered digoxin is converted to inactive reduction products (*e.g.*, dihydrodigoxin) by colonic bacteria in the gut. Data suggest that 1 in 10 patients treated with digoxin tablets will degrade 40% or more of the ingested dose. As a result, certain antibiotics may increase the absorption of digoxin in such patients. Although inactivation of these bacteria by antibiotics is rapid, the serum digoxin concentration will rise at a rate consistent with the elimination half-life of digoxin. The magnitude of rise in serum digoxin concentration relates to the extent of bacterial inactivation, and may be as much as 2-fold in some cases. This phenomenon is minimized with Lanoxicaps because they are rapidly absorbed in the upper gastrointestinal tract.

Distribution

Following drug administration, a 6-8 hour tissue distribution phase is observed. This is followed by a much more gradual decline in the serum concentration of the drug, which is dependent on the elimination of digoxin from the body. The peak height and slope of the early portion (absorption/distribution phases) of the serum concentration-time curve are dependent upon the route of administration and the absorption characteristics of the formulation. Clinical evidence indicates that the early high serum concentrations (particularly high for digoxin capsules) do not reflect the concentration of digoxin at its site of action, but that with chronic use, the steady-state post-distribution serum concentrations are in equilibrium with tissue concentrations and correlate with pharmacologic effects. In individual patients, these post-distribution serum concentrations may be useful in evaluating therapeutic and toxic effects (see DOSAGE AND ADMINISTRATION, Serum Digoxin Concentrations).

Digoxin is concentrated in tissues and therefore has a large apparent volume of distribution. Digoxin crosses both the blood-brain barrier and the placenta. At delivery, the serum digoxin concentration in the newborn is similar to the serum concentration in the mother. Approximately 25% of digoxin in the plasma is bound to protein. Serum digoxin concentrations are not significantly altered by large changes in fat tissue weight, so that its distribution space correlates best with lean (*i.e.*, ideal) body weight, not total body weight.

Metabolism

Only a small percentage (16%) of a dose of digoxin is metabolized. The end metabolites, which include 3 β-digoxigenin, 3-keto-digoxigenin, and their glucuronide and sulfate conjugates, are polar in nature and are postulated to be formed via hydrolysis, oxidation, and conjugation. The metabolism of digoxin is not dependent upon the cytochrome P-450 system, and digoxin is not known to induce or inhibit the cytochrome P-450 system.

Excretion

Elimination of digoxin follows first-order kinetics (that is, the quantity of digoxin eliminated at any time is proportional to the total body content). Following intravenous administration to healthy volunteers, 50-70% of a digoxin dose is excreted unchanged in the urine. Renal excretion of digoxin is proportional to glomerular filtration rate and is largely independent of urine flow. In healthy volunteers with normal renal function, digoxin has a half-life of 1.5-2.0 days. The half-life in anuric patients is prolonged to 3.5 to 5 days. Digoxin is not effectively removed from the body by dialysis, exchange transfusion, or during cardiopulmonary bypass because most of the drug is bound to tissue and does not circulate in the blood.

Special Populations

Race differences in digoxin pharmacokinetics have not been formally studied. Because digoxin is primarily eliminated as unchanged drug via the kidney and because there are no important differences in creatinine clearance among races, pharmacokinetic differences due to race are not expected.

The clearance of digoxin can be primarily correlated with renal function as indicated by creatinine clearance. The Cockcroft and Gault formula for estimation of creatinine clearance includes age, body weight, and gender. TABLE 11 and TABLE 12 provide the usual daily maintenance dose requirements of Lanoxicaps capsules and Lanoxin tablets based on creatinine clearance (per 70 kg).

Plasma digoxin concentration profiles in patients with acute hepatitis generally fell within the range of profiles in a group of healthy subjects.

Lanoxin Elixir Pediatric: In children with renal disease, digoxin must be carefully titrated based on clinical response.

PHARMACODYNAMICS AND CLINICAL EFFECTS

The times to onset of pharmacologic effect and to peak effect of preparations of Lanoxin are shown in TABLE 8.

D

TABLE 8 *Times to Onset of Pharmacologic Effect and to Peak Effect of Preparations of Lanoxin*

Product	Time to Onset of Effect*	Time to Peak Effect*
Lanoxin tablets	0.5-2 hours	2-6 hours
Lanoxin elixir pediatric	0.5-2 hours	2-6 hours
Lanoxicaps	0.5-2 hours	2-6 hours
Lanoxin injection/IV	5-30 minutes†	1-4 hours

* Documented for ventricular response rate in atrial fibrillation, inotropic effects and electrocardiographic changes.
† Depending upon rate of infusion.

Hemodynamic Effects

Digoxin produces hemodynamic improvement in patients with heart failure. Short- and long-term therapy with the drug increases cardiac output and lowers pulmonary artery pressure, pulmonary capillary wedge pressure, and systemic vascular resistance. These hemodynamic effects are accompanied by an increase in the left ventricular ejection fraction and a decrease in end-systolic and end-diastolic dimensions.

Chronic Heart Failure

Two 12 week, double-blind, placebo-controlled studies enrolled 178 (RADIANCE trial) and 88 (PROVED trial) adult patients with NYHA class II or III heart failure previously treated with digoxin, a diuretic, and an ACE inhibitor (RADIANCE only) and randomized them to placebo or treatment with Lanoxin. Both trials demonstrated better preservation of exercise capacity in patients randomized to Lanoxin. Continued treatment with Lanoxin reduced the risk of developing worsening heart failure, as evidenced by heart failure-related hospitalizations and emergency care and the need for concomitant heart failure therapy. The larger study also showed treatment-related benefits in NYHA class and patients' global assessment. In the smaller trial, these trended in favor of a treatment benefit.

The Digitalis Investigation Group (DIG) main trial was a multicenter, randomized, double-blind, placebo-controlled mortality study of 6801 patients with heart failure and left ventricular ejection fraction ≤0.45. At randomization, 67% were NYHA class I or II, 71% had heart failure of ischemic etiology, 44% had been receiving digoxin, and most were receiving concomitant ACE inhibitor (94%) and diuretic (82%). Patients were randomized to placebo or Lanoxin tablets, the dose of which was adjusted for the patient's age, sex, lean body weight, and serum creatinine (see DOSAGE AND ADMINISTRATION), and followed for up to 58 months (median 37 months). The median daily dose prescribed was 0.25 mg. Overall all-cause mortality was 35% with no difference between groups (95% confidence limits for relative risk of 0.91-1.07). Lanoxin was associated with a 25% reduction in the number of hospitalizations for heart failure, a 28% reduction in the risk of a patient having at least one hospitalization for heart failure, and a 6.5% reduction in total hospitalizations (for any cause).

Use of Lanoxin was associated with a trend to increase time to all-cause death or hospitalization. The trend was evident in subgroups of patients with mild heart failure as well as more severe disease, as shown in TABLE 9A and TABLE 9B. Although the effect on all-cause death or hospitalization was not statistically significant, much of the apparent benefit derived from effects on mortality and hospitalization attributed to heart failure.

TABLE 9A *Subgroup Analyses of Mortality and Hospitalization During the First 2 Years Following Randomization*

		Risk of All-Cause Mortality or All-Cause Hospitalization*		
	n	Placebo	Lanoxin	Relative Risk†
All Patients (EF ≤0.45)	6801	604	593	0.94 (0.88-1.00)
NYHA I/II	4571	549	541	0.96 (0.89-1.04)
EF 0.25-0.45	4543	568	571	0.99 (0.91-1.07)
CTR ≤0.55	4455	561	563	0.98 (0.91-1.06)
NYHA III/IV	2224	719	696	0.88 (0.80-0.97)
EF <0.25	2258	677	637	0.84 (0.76-0.93)
CTR >0.55	2346	687	650	0.85 (0.77-0.94)
EF >0.45‡	987	571	585	1.04 (0.88-1.23)

* Number of patients with an event during the first 2 years per 1000 randomized patients.
† Relative risk (95% confidence interval).
‡ DIG Ancillary Study.

In situations where there is no statistically significant benefit of treatment evident from a trial's primary endpoint, results pertaining to a secondary endpoint should be interpreted cautiously.

Chronic Atrial Fibrillation

In adult patients with chronic atrial fibrillation, digoxin slows rapid ventricular response rate in a linear dose-response fashion from 0.25-0.75 mg/day. Digoxin should not be used for the treatment of multifocal atrial tachycardia.

INDICATIONS AND USAGE

HEART FAILURE

Lanoxin is indicated for the treatment of mild to moderate heart failure. Lanoxin increases left ventricular ejection fraction and improves heart failure symptoms as evidenced by exercise capacity and heart failure-related hospitalizations and emergency care, while having no effect on mortality. Where possible, Lanoxin should be used with a diuretic and an angiotensin-converting enzyme inhibitor, but an optimal order for starting these three drugs cannot be specified.

TABLE 9B *Subgroup Analyses of Mortality and Hospitalization During the First 2 Years Following Randomization*

		Risk of HF-Related Mortality or HF-Related Hospitalization*		
	n	Placebo	Lanoxin	Relative Risk†
All Patients (EF ≤0.45)	6801	294	217	0.69 (0.63-0.76)
NYHA I/II	4571	242	178	0.70 (0.62-0.80)
EF 0.25-0.45	4543	244	190	0.74 (0.66-0.84)
CTR ≤0.55	4455	239	180	0.71 (0.63-0.81)
NYHA III/IV	2224	402	295	0.65 (0.57-0.75)
EF <0.25	2258	394	270	0.61 (0.53-0.71)
CTR >0.55	2346	398	287	0.65 (0.57-0.75)
EF >0.45‡	987	179	136	0.72 (0.53-0.99)

* Number of patients with an event during the first 2 years per 1000 randomized patients.
† Relative risk (95% confidence interval).
‡ DIG Ancillary Study.

ATRIAL FIBRILLATION

Lanoxin is indicated for the control of ventricular response rate in patients with chronic atrial fibrillation.

CONTRAINDICATIONS

Digitalis glycosides are contraindicated in patients with ventricular fibrillation or in patients with a known hypersensitivity to digoxin. A hypersensitivity reaction to other digitalis preparations usually constitutes a contraindication to digoxin.

WARNINGS

SINUS NODE DISEASE AND AV BLOCK

Because digoxin slows sinoatrial and AV conduction, the drug commonly prolongs the PR interval. The drug may cause severe sinus bradycardia or sinoatrial block in patients with pre-existing sinus node disease and may cause advanced or complete heart block in patients with pre-existing incomplete AV block. In such patients consideration should be given to the insertion of a pacemaker before treatment with digoxin.

ACCESSORY AV PATHWAY (WOLFF-PARKINSON-WHITE SYNDROME)

After intravenous digoxin therapy, some patients with paroxysmal atrial fibrillation or flutter and a coexisting accessory AV pathway have developed increased antegrade conduction across the accessory pathway bypassing the AV node, leading to a very rapid ventricular response or ventricular fibrillation. Unless conduction down the accessory pathway has been blocked (either pharmacologically or by surgery), digoxin should not be used in such patients. The treatment of paroxysmal supraventricular tachycardia in such patients is usually direct-current cardioversion.

USE IN PATIENTS WITH PRESERVED LEFT VENTRICULAR SYSTOLIC FUNCTION

Patients with certain disorders involving heart failure associated with preserved left ventricular ejection fraction may be particularly susceptible to toxicity of the drug. Such disorders include restrictive cardiomyopathy, constrictive pericarditis, amyloid heart disease, and acute cor pulmonale. Patients with idiopathic hypertrophic subaortic stenosis may have worsening of the outflow obstruction due to the inotropic effects of digoxin.

PRECAUTIONS

USE IN PATIENTS WITH IMPAIRED RENAL FUNCTION

Digoxin is primarily excreted by the kidneys; therefore, patients with impaired renal function require smaller than usual maintenance doses of digoxin (see DOSAGE AND ADMINISTRATION). Because of the prolonged elimination half-life, a longer period of time is required to achieve an initial or new steady-state serum concentration in patients with renal impairment than in patients with normal renal function. If appropriate care is not taken to reduce the dose of digoxin, such patients are at high risk for toxicity, and toxic effects will last longer in such patients than in patients with normal renal function.

USE IN PATIENTS WITH ELECTROLYTE DISORDERS

In patients with hypokalemia or hypomagnesemia, toxicity may occur despite serum digoxin concentrations below 2.0 ng/ml, because potassium or magnesium depletion sensitizes the myocardium to digoxin. Therefore, it is desirable to maintain normal serum potassium and magnesium concentrations in patients being treated with digoxin. Deficiencies of these electrolytes may result from malnutrition, diarrhea, or prolonged vomiting, as well as the use of the following drugs or procedures: diuretics, amphotericin B, corticosteroids, antacids, dialysis, and mechanical suction of gastrointestinal secretions.

Hypercalcemia from any cause predisposes the patient to digitalis toxicity. Calcium, particularly when administered rapidly by the intravenous route, may produce serious arrhythmias in digitalized patients. On the other hand, hypocalcemia can nullify the effects of digoxin in humans; thus, digoxin may be ineffective until serum calcium is restored to normal. These interactions are related to the fact that digoxin affects contractility and excitability of the heart in a manner similar to that of calcium.

USE IN THYROID DISORDERS AND HYPERMETABOLIC STATES

Hypothyroidism may reduce the requirements for digoxin. Heart failure and/or atrial arrhythmias resulting from hypermetabolic or hyperdynamic states (*e.g.,* hyperthyroidism, hypoxia, or arteriovenous shunt) are best treated by addressing the underlying condition. Atrial arrhythmias associated with hypermetabolic states are particularly resistant to digoxin treatment. Care must be taken to avoid toxicity if digoxin is used.

USE IN PATIENTS WITH ACUTE MYOCARDIAL INFARCTION

Digoxin should be used with caution in patients with acute myocardial infarction. The use of inotropic drugs in some patients in this setting may result in undesirable increases in myocardial oxygen demand and ischemia.

USE DURING ELECTRICAL CARDIOVERSION

It may be desirable to reduce the dose of digoxin for 1-2 days prior to electrical cardioversion of atrial fibrillation to avoid the induction of ventricular arrhythmias, but physicians must consider the consequences of increasing the ventricular response if digoxin is withdrawn. If digitalis toxicity is suspected, elective cardioversion should be delayed. If it is not prudent to delay cardioversion, the lowest possible energy level should be selected to avoid provoking ventricular arrhythmias.

LABORATORY TEST MONITORING

Patients receiving digoxin should have their serum electrolytes and renal function (serum creatinine concentrations) assessed periodically; the frequency of assessments will depend on the clinical setting. For discussion of serum digoxin concentrations, see DOSAGE AND ADMINISTRATION.

DRUG/LABORATORY TEST INTERACTIONS

The use of therapeutic doses of digoxin may cause prolongation of the PR interval and depression of the ST segment on the electrocardiogram. Digoxin may produce false positive ST-T changes on the electrocardiogram during exercise testing. These electrophysiologic effects reflect an expected effect of the drug and are not indicative of toxicity.

CARCINOGENESIS, MUTAGENESIS, AND IMPAIRMENT OF FERTILITY

There have been no long-term studies performed in animals to evaluate carcinogenic potential, nor have studies been conducted to assess the mutagenic potential of digoxin or its potential to affect fertility.

PREGNANCY, TERATOGENIC EFFECTS, PREGNANCY CATEGORY C

Animal reproduction studies have not been conducted with digoxin. It is also not known whether digoxin can cause fetal harm when administered to a pregnant woman or can affect reproduction capacity. Digoxin should be given to a pregnant woman only if clearly needed.

NURSING MOTHERS

Studies have shown that digoxin concentrations in the mother's serum and milk are similar. However, the estimated exposure of a nursing infant to digoxin via breast feeding will be far below the usual infant maintenance dose. Therefore, this amount should have no pharmacologic effect upon the infant. Nevertheless, caution should be exercised when digoxin is administered to a nursing woman.

PEDIATRIC USE

Newborn infants display considerable variability in their tolerance to digoxin. Premature and immature infants are particularly sensitive to the effects of digoxin, and the dosage of the drug must not only be reduced but must be individualized according to their degree of maturity. Digitalis glycosides can cause poisoning in children due to accidental ingestion.

GERIATRIC USE

The majority of clinical experience gained with digoxin has been in the elderly population. This experience has not identified differences in response or adverse effects between the elderly and younger patients. However, this drug is known to be substantially excreted by the kidney, and the risk of toxic reactions to this drug may be greater in patients with impaired renal function. Because elderly patients are more likely to have decreased renal function, care should be taken in dose selection, which should be based on renal function, and it may be useful to monitor renal function (see DOSAGE AND ADMINISTRATION).

DRUG INTERACTIONS

Potassium-depleting *diuretics* are a major contributing factor to digitalis toxicity. *Calcium*, particularly if administered rapidly by the intravenous route, may produce serious arrhythmias in digitalized patients. *Quinidine, verapamil, amiodarone, propafenone, indomethacin, itraconazole, alprazolam,* and *spironolactone* raise the serum digoxin concentration due to a reduction in clearance and/or in volume of distribution of the drug, with the implication that digitalis intoxication may result. *Erythromycin* and *clarithromycin* (and possibly other *macrolide antibiotics*) and *tetracycline* may increase digoxin absorption in patients who inactivate digoxin by bacterial metabolism in the lower intestine, so that digitalis intoxication may result. The risk of this interaction may be reduced if digoxin is given as Lanoxicaps (see CLINICAL PHARMACOLOGY, Pharmacokinetics, Absorption). *Propantheline* and *diphenoxylate,* by decreasing gut motility, may increase digoxin absorption. *Antacids, kaolin-pectin, sulfasalazine, neomycin, cholestyramine,* certain *anticancer drugs,* and *metoclopramide* may interfere with intestinal digoxin absorption, resulting in unexpectedly low serum concentrations. *Rifampin* may decrease serum digoxin concentration, especially in patients with renal dysfunction, by increasing the non-renal clearance of digoxin. There have been inconsistent reports regarding the effects of other drugs *[e.g., quinine, penicillamine]* on serum digoxin concentration. *Thyroid* administration to a digitalized, hypothyroid patient may increase the dose requirement of digoxin. Concomitant use of digoxin and *sympathomimetics* increases the risk of cardiac arrhythmias. *Succinylcholine* may cause a sudden extrusion of potassium from muscle cells, and may thereby cause arrhythmias in digitalized patients. Although beta-adrenergic blockers or calcium channel blockers and digoxin may be useful in combination to control atrial fibrillation, their additive effects on AV node conduction can result in advanced or complete heart block.

Due to the considerable variability of these interactions, the dosage of digoxin should be individualized when patients receive these medications concurrently. Furthermore, caution should be exercised when combining digoxin with any drug that may cause a significant deterioration in renal function, since a decline in glomerular filtration or tubular secretion may impair the excretion of digoxin.

ADVERSE REACTIONS

In general, the adverse reactions of digoxin are dose-dependent and occur at doses higher than those needed to achieve a therapeutic effect. Hence, adverse reactions are less common when digoxin is used within the recommended dose range or therapeutic serum concentration range and when there is careful attention to concurrent medications and conditions.

Because some patients may be particularly susceptible to side effects with digoxin, the dosage of the drug should always be selected carefully and adjusted as the clinical condition of the patient warrants. In the past, when high doses of digoxin were used and little attention was paid to clinical status or concurrent medications, adverse reactions to digoxin were more frequent and severe. Cardiac adverse reactions accounted for about one-half, gastrointestinal disturbances for about one-fourth, and CNS and other toxicity for about one-fourth of these adverse reactions. However, available evidence suggests that the incidence and severity of digoxin toxicity has decreased substantially in recent years. In recent controlled clinical trials, in patients with predominantly mild to moderate heart failure, the incidence of adverse experiences was comparable in patients taking digoxin and in those taking placebo. In a large mortality trial, the incidence of hospitalization for suspected digoxin toxicity was 2% in patients taking Lanoxin tablets compared to 0.9% in patients taking placebo. In this trial, the most common manifestations of digoxin toxicity included gastrointestinal and cardiac disturbances; CNS manifestations were less common.

ADULTS

Cardiac: Therapeutic doses of digoxin may cause heart block in patients with pre-existing sinoatrial or AV conduction disorders; heart block can be avoided by adjusting the dose of digoxin. Prophylactic use of a cardiac pacemaker may be considered if the risk of heart block is considered unacceptable. High doses of digoxin may produce a variety of rhythm disturbances, such as first-degree, second-degree (Wenckebach), or third-degree heart block (including asystole); atrial tachycardia with block; AV dissociation; accelerated junctional (nodal) rhythm; unifocal or multiform ventricular premature contractions (especially bigeminy or trigeminy); ventricular tachycardia; and ventricular fibrillation. Digoxin produces PR prolongation and ST segment depression which should not by themselves be considered digoxin toxicity. Cardiac toxicity can also occur at therapeutic doses in patients who have conditions which may alter their sensitivity to digoxin (see WARNINGS and PRECAUTIONS).

Gastrointestinal: Digoxin may cause anorexia, nausea, vomiting, and diarrhea. Rarely, the use of digoxin has been associated with abdominal pain, intestinal ischemia, and hemorrhagic necrosis of the intestines.

CNS: Digoxin can produce visual disturbances (blurred or yellow vision), headache, weakness, dizziness, apathy, confusion, and mental disturbances (such as anxiety, depression, delirium, and hallucination).

Other: Gynecomastia has been occasionally observed following the prolonged use of digoxin. Thrombocytopenia and maculopapular rash and other skin reactions have been rarely observed.

TABLE 10 summarizes the incidence of those adverse experiences listed above for patients treated with Lanoxin tablets or placebo from two randomized, double-blind, placebo-controlled withdrawal trials. Patients in these trials were also receiving diuretics with or without angiotensin-converting enzyme inhibitors. These patients had been stable on digoxin, and were randomized to digoxin or placebo. The results shown in TABLE 10 reflect the experience in patients following dosage titration with the use of serum digoxin concentrations and careful follow-up. These adverse experiences are consistent with results from a large, placebo-controlled mortality trial (DIG trial) wherein over half the patients were not receiving digoxin prior to enrollment.

TABLE 10 *Adverse Experiences In Two Parallel, Double-Blind, Placebo-Controlled Withdrawal Trials (Number of Patients Reporting)*

Adverse Experience	Digoxin Patients (n=123)	Placebo Patients (n=125)
Cardiac		
Palpitation	1	4
Ventricular extrasystole	1	1
Tachycardia	2	1
Heart arrest	1	1
Gastrointestinal		
Anorexia	1	4
Nausea	4	2
Vomiting	2	1
Diarrhea	4	1
Abdominal pain	0	6
CNS		
Headache	4	4
Dizziness	6	5
Mental disturbances	5	1
Other		
Rash	2	1
Death	4	3

INFANTS AND CHILDREN

The side effects of digoxin in infants and children differ from those seen in adults in several respects. Although digoxin may produce anorexia, nausea, vomiting, diarrhea, and CNS disturbances in young patients, these are rarely the initial symptoms of overdosage. Rather, the earliest and most frequent manifestation of excessive dosing with digoxin in infants and children is the appearance of cardiac arrhythmias, including sinus bradycardia. In children, the use of digoxin may produce any arrhythmia. The most common are conduction disturbances or supraventricular tachyarrhythmias, such as atrial tachycardia (with or without block) and junctional (nodal) tachycardia. Ventricular arrhythmias are less common. Sinus bradycardia may be a sign of impending digoxin intoxication, especially in infants, even in the absence of first-degree heart block. Any arrhythmia or alteration in cardiac conduction that develops in a child taking digoxin should be assumed to be caused by digoxin, until further evaluation proves otherwise.

DOSAGE AND ADMINISTRATION

GENERAL

Recommended dosages of digoxin may require considerable modification because of individual sensitivity of the patient to the drug, the presence of associated conditions, or the use of concurrent medications. Due to the more complete absorption of digoxin from soft capsules, recommended oral doses are only 80% of those for tablets and elixir.

Because the significance of the higher peak serum concentrations associated with once daily capsules is not established, divided daily dosing is presently recommended for:

- Infants and children under 10 years of age.
- Patients requiring a daily dose of 300 µg (0.3 mg) or greater.
- Patients with a previous history of digitalis toxicity.
- Patients considered likely to become toxic.
- Patients in whom compliance is not a problem.

Where compliance is considered a problem, single daily dosing may be appropriate.

In selecting a dose of digoxin, the following factors must be considered:

- The body weight of the patient. Doses should be calculated based upon lean (*i.e.,* ideal) body weight.
- The patient's renal function, preferably evaluated on the basis of estimated creatinine clearance.
- The patient's age. Infants and children require different doses of digoxin than adults. Also, advanced age may be indicative of diminished renal function even in patients with normal serum creatinine concentration (*i.e.,* below 1.5 mg/dl).
- Concomitant disease states, concurrent medications, or other factors likely to alter the pharmacokinetic or pharmacodynamic profile of digoxin (see PRECAUTIONS).

SERUM DIGOXIN CONCENTRATIONS

In general, the dose of digoxin used should be determined on clinical grounds. However, measurement of serum digoxin concentrations can be helpful to the clinician in determining the adequacy of digoxin therapy and in assigning certain probabilities to the likelihood of digoxin intoxication. About two-thirds of adults considered adequately digitalized (without evidence of toxicity) have serum digoxin concentrations ranging from 0.8-2.0 ng/ml. However, digoxin may produce clinical benefits even at serum concentrations below this range. About two-thirds of adult patients with clinical toxicity have serum digoxin concentrations greater than 2.0 ng/ml. However, since one-third of patients with clinical toxicity have concentrations less than 2.0 ng/ml, values below 2.0 ng/ml do not rule out the possibility that a certain sign or symptom is related to digoxin therapy. Rarely, there are patients who are unable to tolerate digoxin at serum concentrations below 0.8 ng/ml. Consequently, the serum concentration of digoxin should always be interpreted in the overall clinical context, and an isolated measurement should not be used alone as the basis for increasing or decreasing the dose of the drug.

To allow adequate time for equilibration of digoxin between serum and tissue, sampling of serum concentrations should be done just before the next scheduled dose of the drug. If this is not possible, sampling should be done at least 6-8 hours after the last dose, regardless of the route of administration or the formulation used. On a once-daily dosing schedule, the concentration of digoxin will be 10-25% lower when sampled at 24 vs 8 hours, depending upon the patient's renal function. On a twice-daily dosing schedule, there will be only minor differences in serum digoxin concentrations whether sampling is done at 8 or 12 hours after a dose.

If a discrepancy exists between the reported serum concentration and the observed clinical response, the clinician should consider the following possibilities:

- Analytical problems in the assay procedure.
- Inappropriate serum sampling time.
- Administration of a digitalis glycoside other than digoxin.
- Conditions (described in WARNINGS and PRECAUTIONS) causing an alteration in the sensitivity of the patient to digoxin.
- Serum digoxin concentration may decrease acutely during periods of exercise without any associated change in clinical efficacy due to increased binding of digoxin to skeletal muscle.

HEART FAILURE

Adults

Digitalization may be accomplished by either of two general approaches that vary in dosage and frequency of administration, but reach the same endpoint in terms of total amount of digoxin accumulated in the body.

- If rapid digitalization is considered medically appropriate, it may be achieved by administering a loading dose based upon projected peak digoxin body stores. Maintenance dose can be calculated as a percentage of the loading dose.
- More gradual digitalization may be obtained by beginning an appropriate maintenance dose, thus allowing digoxin body stores to accumulate slowly. Steady-state serum digoxin concentrations will be achieved in approximately 5 half-lives of the drug for the individual patient. Depending upon the patient's renal function, this will take between 1 and 3 weeks.

Rapid Digitalization With a Loading Dose

Peak digoxin body stores of 8-12 µg/kg should provide therapeutic effect with minimum risk of toxicity in most patients with heart failure and normal sinus rhythm. Because of altered digoxin distribution and elimination, projected peak body stores for patients with renal insufficiency should be conservative (*i.e.,* 6-10 µg/kg) (see PRECAUTIONS).

The loading dose should be administered in several portions, with roughly half the total given as the first dose. Additional fractions of this planned total dose may be given at 6-8 hour intervals, **with careful assessment of clinical response before each additional dose.**

If the patient's clinical response necessitates a change from the calculated loading dose of digoxin, then calculation of the maintenance dose should be based upon the amount actually given.

Lanoxicaps and Lanoxin Tablets

A single initial dose of 400-600 µg (0.4-0.6 mg) of Lanoxicaps or 500-750 µg (0.5-0.75 mg) of Lanoxin tablets usually produces a detectable effect in 0.5 to 2 hours that becomes maximal in 2-6 hours. Additional doses of Lanoxicaps of 100-300 µg (0.1-0.3 mg) or Lanoxin tablets of 125-375 µg (0.125-0.375 mg) may be given cautiously at 6-8 hour intervals until clinical evidence of an adequate effect is noted. The usual amount of Lanoxicaps that a 70 kg patient requires to achieve 8-12 µg/kg peak body stores is 600-1000 µg (0.6-1.0 mg). The usual amount of Lanoxin tablets that a 70 kg patient requires to achieve 8-12 µg/kg peak body stores is 750-1250 µg (0.75-1.25 mg).

Lanoxin injection is frequently used to achieve rapid digitalization, with conversion to Lanoxin tablets or Lanoxicaps for maintenance therapy. If patients are switched from intravenous to oral digoxin formulations, allowances must be made for differences in bioavailability when calculating maintenance dosages (see TABLE 7).

Maintenance Dosing

Lanoxicaps and Lanoxin Tablets

The doses of digoxin used in controlled trials in patients with heart failure have ranged from 125-500 µg (0.125-0.5 mg) once daily. In these studies, the digoxin dose has been generally titrated according to the patient's age, lean body weight, and renal function. Therapy is generally initiated at a dose of 250 µg (0.25 mg) once daily in patients under age 70 with good renal function, at a dose of 125 µg (0.125 mg) once daily in patients over age 70 or with impaired renal function, and at a dose of 62.5 µg (0.0625 mg) in patients with marked renal impairment. Doses may be increased every 2 weeks according to clinical response.

In a subset of approximately 1800 patients enrolled in the DIG trial (wherein dosing was based on an algorithm similar to those in TABLE 11 and TABLE 12 the mean (±SD) serum digoxin concentrations at 1 month and 12 months were 1.01 ± 0.47 ng/ml and 0.97 ± 0.43 ng/ml, respectively.

The maintenance dose should be based upon the percentage of the peak body stores lost each day through elimination.

The following formula has had wide clinical use:

Maintenance Dose = Peak Body Stores (*i.e.,* Loading Dose) × % Daily Loss/100

Where: % Daily Loss = 14 + Ccr/5

(Ccr is creatinine clearance, corrected to 70 kg body weight or 1.73 m^2 body surface area)

TABLE 11 and TABLE 12 provide average daily maintenance dose requirements of Lanoxicaps capsules and Lanoxin tablets for patients with heart failure based upon lean body weight and renal function:

TABLE 11 *Usual Daily Maintenance Dose Requirements (µg) of Lanoxicaps Capsules for Estimated Peak Body Stores of 10 µg/kg*

	Lean Body Weight						Number of Days Before Steady State Achieved†
	50 kg	**60 kg**	**70 kg**	**80 kg**	**90 kg**	**100 kg**	
Corrected Ccr*	**110 lb**	**132 lb**	**154 lb**	**176 lb**	**198 lb**	**220 lb**	
0	50‡	100	100	100	150	150	22
10	100	100	100	150	150	150	19
20	100	100	150	150	150	200	16
30	100	150	150	150	200	200	14
40	100	150	150	200	200	250	13
50	150	150	200	200	250	250	12
60	150	150	200	200	250	300	11
70	150	200	200	250	250	300	10
80	150	200	200	250	300	300	9
90	150	200	250	250	300	350	8
100	200	200	250	300	300	350	7

* In ml/min per 70 kg. Ccr is creatinine clearance, corrected to 70 kg body weight or 1.73 m^2 body surface area. *For adults,* if only serum creatinine concentrations (Scr) are available, a Ccr (corrected to 70 kg body weight) may be estimated in men as (140 -Age)/Scr. For women, this result should be multiplied by 0.85. *Note: This equation cannot be used for estimating creatinine clearance in infants or children.*

† If no loading dose administered.

‡ 50 µg = 0.05 mg.

Example: Based on TABLE 11 and TABLE 12, a patient in heart failure with an estimated lean body weight of 70 kg and a Ccr of 60 ml/min, should be given a dose of 200 µg (0.2 mg) daily of Lanoxicaps, usually taken as a divided dose of one 100 µg (0.1 mg) capsule after the morning and evening meals, or a dose of 250 µg (0.25 mg) daily of Lanoxin tablets, usually taken after the morning meal. If no loading dose is administered, steady-state serum concentrations in this patient should be anticipated at approximately 11 days.

INFANTS AND CHILDREN

Lanoxicaps and Lanoxin Tablets

In general, divided daily dosing is recommended for infants and young children (under age 10). (In these patients, where dosage adjustment is frequent and outside the fixed dosages available, Lanoxicaps may not be the formulation of choice.) In the newborn period, renal clearance of digoxin is diminished and suitable dosage adjustments must be observed. This is especially pronounced in the premature infant. Beyond the immediate newborn period, children generally require proportionally larger doses than adults on the basis of body weight or body surface area. Children over 10 years of age require adult dosages in proportion to their body weight. Some researchers have suggested that infants and young children tolerate slightly higher serum concentrations than do adults.

Daily maintenance doses for each age group are given in TABLE 13 and TABLE 14, and should provide therapeutic effects with minimum risk of toxicity in most patients with heart

TABLE 12 *Usual Daily Maintenance Dose Requirements (µg) of Lanoxin Tablets for Estimated Peak Body Stores of 10 µg/kg*

Corrected Ccr*	Lean Body Weight 50 kg 110 lb	60 kg 132 lb	70 kg 154 lb	80 kg 176 lb	90 kg 198 lb	100 kg 220 lb	Number of Days Before Steady State Achieved†
0	62.5‡	125	125	125	187.5	187.5	22
10	125	125	125	187.5	187.5	187.5	19
20	125	125	187.5	187.5	187.5	250	16
30	125	187.5	187.5	187.5	250	250	14
40	125	187.5	187.5	250	250	250	13
50	187.5	187.5	250	250	250	250	12
60	187.5	187.5	250	250	250	375	11
70	187.5	250	250	250	250	375	10
80	187.5	250	250	250	375	375	9
90	187.5	250	250	250	375	500	8
100	250	250	250	375	375	500	7

* In ml/min per 70 kg. Ccr is creatinine clearance, corrected to 70 kg body weight or 1.73 m^2 body surface area. *For adults,* if only serum creatinine concentrations (Scr) are available, a Ccr (corrected to 70 kg body weight) may be estimated in men as (140 − Age)/Scr. For women, this result should be multiplied by 0.85. *Note:* This equation cannot be used for estimating creatinine clearance in infants or children.
† If no loading dose administered.
‡ 62.5 µg = 0.0625 mg.

failure and normal sinus rhythm. These recommendations assume the presence of normal renal function.

TABLE 13 *Usual Digitalizing and Maintenance Dosages for Lanoxicaps in Children With Normal Renal Function Based on Lean Body Weight*

Age	Digitalizing* Dose	Daily Maintenance Dose†
2-5 years	25-35 µg/kg	25-35% of the oral or IV digitalizing dose‡ (µg/kg)
5-10 years	15-30 µg/kg	
Over 10 years	8-12 µg/kg	

* IV digitalizing doses are the same as digitalizing doses of Lanoxicaps.
† Divided daily dosing is recommended for children under 10 years of age.
‡ Projected or actual digitalizing dose providing desired clinical response.

TABLE 14 *Daily Maintenance Doses for Lanoxin Tablets in Children With Normal Renal Function*

Age	Daily Maintenance Dose
2-5 years	10-15 µg/kg
5-10 years	7-10 µg/kg
Over 10 years	3-5 µg/kg

In children with renal disease, digoxin must be carefully titrated based upon clinical response.

It cannot be overemphasized that both the adult and pediatric dosage guidelines provided are based upon average patient response and substantial individual variation can be expected. Accordingly, ultimate dosage selection must be based upon clinical assessment of the patient.

Lanoxin Elixir Pediatric

Lanoxin injection pediatric can be used to achieve rapid digitalization, with conversion to an oral formulation of Lanoxin for maintenance therapy. If patients are switched from intravenous to oral digoxin formulations, allowances must be made for differences in bioavailability when calculating maintenance dosages (see TABLE 7 and TABLE 15).

Digitalizing and daily maintenance doses for each age group are given in TABLE 15, and should provide therapeutic effect with minimum risk of toxicity in most patients with heart failure and normal sinus rhythm. These recommendations assume the presence of normal renal function.

TABLE 15 *Usual Digitalizing and Maintenance Dosages for Lanoxin Elixir Pediatric in Children With Normal Renal Function Based on Lean Body Weight*

Age	Oral Digitalizing* Dose	Daily Maintenance Dose†
Premature	20-30 µg/kg	20-30% of *oral* digitalizing dose‡ (µg/kg)
Full-term	25-35 µg/kg	
1-24 months	35-60 µg/kg	
2-5 years	30-40 µg/kg	25-35% of *oral* digitalizing dose‡ (µg/kg)
5-10 years	20-35 µg/kg	
Over 10 years	10-15 µg/kg	

* IV digitalizing doses are 80% of oral digitalizing doses.
† Divided daily dosing is recommended for children under 10 years of age.
‡ Projected or actual digitalizing dose providing clinical response.

In children with renal disease, digoxin dosing must be carefully titrated based upon desired clinical response.

Gradual Digitalization With a Maintenance Dose

More gradual digitalization can also be accomplished by beginning an appropriate maintenance dose. The range of percentages provided in TABLE 15 can be used in calculating this dose for patients with normal renal function.

It cannot be overemphasized that these pediatric dosage guidelines are based upon average patient response and substantial individual variation can be expected. Accordingly, ultimate dosage selection must be based upon clinical assessment of the patient.

ATRIAL FIBRILLATION

Peak digoxin body stores larger than the 8-12 µg/kg required for most patients with heart failure and normal sinus rhythm have been used for control of ventricular rate in patients with atrial fibrillation. Doses of digoxin used for the treatment of chronic atrial fibrillation should be titrated to the minimum dose that achieves the desired ventricular rate control without causing undesirable side effects. Data are not available to establish the appropriate resting or exercise target rates that should be achieved.

DOSE ADJUSTMENT WHEN CHANGING PREPARATIONS

The absolute bioavailability of the capsule formulation is greater than that of the standard tablets and very near that of the intravenous dosage form. As a result, the doses recommended for Lanoxicaps capsules are the same as those for Lanoxin injection (see TABLE 7). Adjustments in dosage will seldom be necessary when converting a patient from the intravenous formulation to Lanoxicaps. The difference in bioavailability between Lanoxin injection or Lanoxicaps and Lanoxin elixir pediatric or Lanoxin tablets must be considered when changing patients from one dosage form to another.

Doses of 100 µg (0.1 mg) and 200 µg (0.2 mg) of Lanoxicaps are approximately equivalent to 125 µg (0.125 mg) and 250 µg (0.25 mg) doses of Lanoxin tablets and elixir pediatric, respectively (see TABLE 7).

HOW SUPPLIED

LANOXICAPS (DIGOXIN SOLUTION IN CAPSULES)

Lanoxicaps capsules are available as follows:

50 µg (0.05 mg): Imprint "A2C" (red).
100 µg (0.1 mg): Imprint "B2C" (yellow).
200 µg (0.2 mg): Imprint "C2C" (green).

Storage: Store at 25°C (77°F); excursions permitted to 15-30°C (59-86°F) in a dry place and protect from light.

LANOXIN TABLETS

Lanoxin (digoxin) tablets are available as follows:

125 µg (0.125 mg): Scored, imprinted with "LANOXIN" and "Y3B" (yellow).
250 µg (0.25 mg): Scored, imprinted with "LANOXIN"and "X3A" (white).

Storage: Store at 25°C (77°F); excursions permitted to 15-30°C (59-86°F) in a dry place and protect from light.

LANOXIN ELIXIR PEDIATRIC

Lanoxin (digoxin) elixir pediatric is available as 50 µg (0.05 mg) per ml.
Storage: Store at 25°C (77°F); excursions permitted to 15-30°C (59-86°F) and protect from light.

PRODUCT LISTING - RATED THERAPEUTICALLY EQUIVALENT

Elixir - Oral - 0.05 mg/ml

60 ml	$36.44	LANOXIN, Glaxosmithkline	00173-0264-27

Solution - Injectable - 0.1 mg/ml

1 ml x 10	$66.80	LANOXIN, Glaxosmithkline	00173-0262-10

Solution - Injectable - 0.25 mg/ml

1 ml x 10	$23.39	GENERIC, Abbott Pharmaceutical	00074-2169-01
1 ml x 10	$24.34	GENERIC, Abbott Pharmaceutical	00074-2169-31
2 ml	$5.74	LANOXIN, Prescript Pharmaceuticals	00247-0274-02
2 ml x 10	$24.82	GENERIC, Abbott Pharmaceutical	00074-2169-02
2 ml x 10	$25.72	LANOXIN, Allscripts Pharmaceutical Company	54569-1523-00
2 ml x 10	$27.80	LANOXIN, Glaxosmithkline	00173-0260-10
2 ml x 10	$30.88	GENERIC, Abbott Pharmaceutical	00074-2169-32
2 ml x 25	$47.00	GENERIC, Esi Lederle Generics	00641-1410-35
2 ml x 100	$103.96	GENERIC, Esi Lederle Generics	00641-1410-36
2 ml x 100	$113.50	LANOXIN, Glaxosmithkline	00173-0260-35

Tablet - Oral - 0.125 mg

1's	$0.21	LANOXIN, Allscripts Pharmaceutical Company	54569-0483-03
3's	$0.61	LANOXIN, Allscripts Pharmaceutical Company	54569-0483-04
10 x 30	$60.30	GENERIC, Udl Laboratories Inc	51079-0945-24
10's	$2.05	LANOXIN, Allscripts Pharmaceutical Company	54569-0483-05
12's	$1.89	LANOXIN, Southwood Pharmaceuticals Inc	58016-0536-12
15's	$2.36	LANOXIN, Southwood Pharmaceuticals Inc	58016-0536-15
25's	$10.79	LANOXIN, Pd-Rx Pharmaceuticals	55289-0927-97
30's	$4.72	LANOXIN, Southwood Pharmaceuticals Inc	58016-0536-30
30's	$6.15	LANOXIN, Allscripts Pharmaceutical Company	54569-0483-00
30's	$7.19	LANOXIN, Glaxosmithkline	00173-0242-30
30's	$9.00	LANOXIN, Pd-Rx Pharmaceuticals	55289-0927-30
30's	$11.03	LANOXIN, Physicians Total Care	54868-0790-02
31 x 10	$78.53	GENERIC, Vangard Labs	00615-0547-53
60's	$15.51	LANOXIN, Physicians Total Care	54868-0790-05

90's	$10.13	LANOXIN, Allscripts Pharmaceutical Company	54569-8519-00
100's	$15.72	LANOXIN, Southwood Pharmaceuticals Inc	58016-0536-00
100's	$18.94	GENERIC, Bertek Pharmaceuticals Inc	62794-0145-01
100's	$20.51	LANOXIN, Allscripts Pharmaceutical Company	54569-0483-01
100's	$24.03	LANOXIN, Glaxosmithkline	00173-0242-55
100's	$25.07	LANOXIN, Physicians Total Care	54868-0790-03
100's	$27.60	GENERIC, Udl Laboratories Inc	51079-0945-20
100's	$33.55	LANOXIN, Glaxosmithkline	00173-0242-56
100's	$34.19	LANOXIN, Pd-Rx Pharmaceuticals	55289-0927-01
Tablet - Oral - 0.25 mg			
3's	$2.39	LANOXIN, Southwood Pharmaceuticals Inc	58016-0537-03
10 x 30	$60.30	GENERIC, Udl Laboratories Inc	51079-0946-24
10's	$2.05	LANOXIN, Allscripts Pharmaceutical Company	54569-0484-03
10's	$3.10	LANOXIN, Southwood Pharmaceuticals Inc	58016-0537-10
12's	$1.89	LANOXIN, Southwood Pharmaceuticals Inc	58016-0537-12
15's	$2.36	LANOXIN, Southwood Pharmaceuticals Inc	58016-0537-15
25's	$12.17	LANOXIN, Pd-Rx Pharmaceuticals	55289-0098-97
30's	$4.72	LANOXIN, Southwood Pharmaceuticals Inc	58016-0537-30
30's	$6.15	LANOXIN, Allscripts Pharmaceutical Company	54569-0484-00
30's	$7.19	LANOXIN, Glaxosmithkline	00173-0249-30
30's	$8.34	LANOXIN, Physicians Total Care	54868-0683-02
30's	$12.23	LANOXIN, Pd-Rx Pharmaceuticals	55289-0098-30
31 x 10	$78.53	GENERIC, Vangard Labs	00615-0518-53
31 x 10	$78.53	GENERIC, Vangard Labs	00615-0518-63
60's	$15.51	LANOXIN, Physicians Total Care	54868-0683-04
60's	$30.10	LANOXIN, Pd-Rx Pharmaceuticals	55289-0098-60
90's	$10.13	LANOXIN, Allscripts Pharmaceutical Company	54569-8513-00
100's	$15.72	LANOXIN, Southwood Pharmaceuticals Inc	58016-0537-00
100's	$18.94	GENERIC, Bertek Pharmaceuticals Inc	62794-0146-01
100's	$20.51	LANOXIN, Allscripts Pharmaceutical Company	54569-0484-01
100's	$20.97	LANOXIN, Pd-Rx Pharmaceuticals	55289-0098-01
100's	$24.03	LANOXIN, Glaxosmithkline	00173-0249-55
100's	$25.07	LANOXIN, Physicians Total Care	54868-0683-01
100's	$27.60	GENERIC, Udl Laboratories Inc	51079-0946-20
100's	$30.07	LANOXIN, American Health Packaging	62584-0249-01
100's	$33.55	LANOXIN, Glaxosmithkline	00173-0249-56

PRODUCT LISTING - EQUIVALENTS NOT AVAILABLE

Capsule - Oral - 0.05 mg			
100's	$14.70	GENERIC, Alra	51641-0235-01
100's	$17.70	GENERIC, Alra	51641-0235-11
100's	$26.95	LANOXICAPS, Glaxosmithkline	00173-0270-55
Capsule - Oral - 0.1 mg			
30's	$8.11	LANOXICAPS, Glaxosmithkline	00173-0272-30
100's	$29.41	LANOXICAPS, Glaxosmithkline	00173-0272-55
Capsule - Oral - 0.2 mg			
30's	$9.94	LANOXICAPS, Glaxosmithkline	00173-0274-30
100's	$34.21	LANOXICAPS, Glaxosmithkline	00173-0274-55
Elixir - Oral - 0.05 mg/ml			
2 ml x 40	$46.00	GENERIC, Roxane Laboratories Inc	00054-8192-16
5 ml x 40	$68.40	GENERIC, Roxane Laboratories Inc	00054-8193-16
60 ml	$9.63	GENERIC, Bausch and Lomb	24208-0360-67
60 ml	$9.91	GENERIC, Aligen Independent Laboratories Inc	00405-2630-56
60 ml	$10.40	GENERIC, Roxane Laboratories Inc	00054-3192-46
60 ml	$14.00	GENERIC, Liquipharm Inc	54198-0148-02
Tablet - Oral - 0.125 mg			
30's	$5.07	GENERIC, Southwood Pharmaceuticals Inc	58016-0202-30
30's	$5.07	GENERIC, Southwood Pharmaceuticals Inc	58016-0354-30
30's	$6.60	GENERIC, Medirex Inc	57480-0452-06
30's	$6.81	GENERIC, Pd-Rx Pharmaceuticals	55289-0002-30
31 x 10	$78.53	GENERIC, Vangard Labs	00615-0547-63
60's	$6.53	GENERIC, Southwood Pharmaceuticals Inc	58016-0202-60
60's	$6.53	GENERIC, Southwood Pharmaceuticals Inc	58016-0354-60
100's	$4.44	GENERIC, Physicians Total Care	54868-2134-01
100's	$8.65	GENERIC, Alra	51641-0233-01
100's	$9.52	GENERIC, Moore, H.L. Drug Exchange Inc	00839-7641-06
100's	$9.63	GENERIC, Southwood Pharmaceuticals Inc	58016-0202-00
100's	$9.63	GENERIC, Southwood Pharmaceuticals Inc	58016-0354-00
100's	$10.65	GENERIC, Alra	51641-0233-11
100's	$12.50	GENERIC, Amide Pharmaceutical Inc	52152-0145-02
100's	$15.50	GENERIC, Raway Pharmacal Inc	00686-0547-13
100's	$17.25	GENERIC, Amide Pharmaceutical Inc	52152-0145-11
100's	$18.79	GENERIC, Duramed Pharmaceuticals Inc	51285-0916-02
100's	$20.26	GENERIC, Lannett Company Inc	00527-1324-01
Tablet - Oral - 0.25 mg			
3's	$2.40	GENERIC, Pd-Rx Pharmaceuticals	55289-0626-03
25's	$6.60	GENERIC, Pd-Rx Pharmaceuticals	55289-0626-97
30's	$2.25	GENERIC, Circle Pharmaceuticals Inc	00659-1002-30
30's	$2.60	GENERIC, Major Pharmaceuticals Inc	00904-2058-46
30's	$5.07	GENERIC, Southwood Pharmaceuticals Inc	58016-0355-30
30's	$5.07	GENERIC, Southwood Pharmaceuticals Inc	58016-0755-30
30's	$6.60	GENERIC, Medirex Inc	57480-0453-06
30's	$6.81	GENERIC, Pd-Rx Pharmaceuticals	55289-0626-30
30's	$17.22	GENERIC, Pharma Pac	52959-0152-30
32's	$5.88	GENERIC, Vangard Labs	00615-0518-32
60's	$6.53	GENERIC, Southwood Pharmaceuticals Inc	58016-0355-60
60's	$6.53	GENERIC, Southwood Pharmaceuticals Inc	58016-0755-60
60's	$6.98	GENERIC, Pd-Rx Pharmaceuticals	55289-0626-60
100's	$2.00	GENERIC, Vita Elixir Company Inc	00181-0603-00
100's	$4.74	GENERIC, Circle Pharmaceuticals Inc	00659-1002-02
100's	$5.45	GENERIC, Physicians Total Care	54868-0055-02
100's	$9.52	GENERIC, Moore, H.L. Drug Exchange Inc	00839-1247-06
100's	$9.63	GENERIC, Southwood Pharmaceuticals Inc	58016-0355-00
100's	$9.63	GENERIC, Southwood Pharmaceuticals Inc	58016-0755-00
100's	$10.65	GENERIC, Alra	51641-0234-11
100's	$12.50	GENERIC, Amide Pharmaceutical Inc	52152-0146-02
100's	$14.88	GENERIC, Pd-Rx Pharmaceuticals	55289-0626-01
100's	$16.00	GENERIC, Raway Pharmacal Inc	00686-0518-13
100's	$17.25	GENERIC, Amide Pharmaceutical Inc	52152-0146-11
100's	$18.79	GENERIC, Duramed Pharmaceuticals Inc	51285-0915-02
100's	$20.26	GENERIC, Lannett Company Inc	00527-1325-01
Tablet - Oral - 0.5 mg			
100's	$18.50	GENERIC, Amide Pharmaceutical Inc	52152-0147-02
100's	$25.00	LANOXIN, Glaxosmithkline	00173-0253-55

Digoxin Immune Fab (Ovine) *(001062)*

Categories: Toxicity, digoxin; Pregnancy Category C; FDA Pre 1938 Drugs; Orphan Drugs
Drug Classes: Antidotes
Brand Names: **Digibind**; DigiFab
Foreign Brand Availability: Digitalis Antidot (Belgium); Digitalis Antidot BM (Czech-Republic; Germany; Russia; Sweden; Switzerland); Digitalis-Antidot BM (Austria); Digoxin Immune FAB (Ovine) Digibind (Australia)

DESCRIPTION

Digibind, digoxin immune Fab (ovine), is a sterile lyophilized powder of antigen binding fragments (Fab) derived from specific antidigoxin antibodies raised in sheep. Production of antibodies specific for digoxin involves conjugation of digoxin as a hapten to human albumin. Sheep are immunized with this material to produce antibodies specific for the antigenic determinants of the digoxin molecule. The antibody is then papain-digested and digoxin-specific Fab fragments of the antibody are isolated and purified by affinity chromatography. These antibody fragments have a molecular weight of approximately 46,200.

Each vial, which will bind approximately 0.5 mg of digoxin (or digitoxin), contains 38 mg of digoxin-specific Fab fragments derived from sheep plus 75 mg of sorbitol as a stabilizer and 28 mg of sodium chloride. The vial contains no preservatives.

Digibind is administered by intravenous injection after reconstitution with sterile water for injection (4 ml/vial).

CLINICAL PHARMACOLOGY

After intravenous injection of digoxin immune Fab (ovine) in the baboon, digoxin-specific Fab fragments are excreted in the urine with a biological half-life of about 9-13 hours.[1] In humans with normal renal function, the half-life appears to be 15-20 hours.[2] Experimental studies in animals indicate that these antibody fragments have a large volume of distribution in the extracellular space, unlike whole antibody which distributes in a space only about twice the plasma volume.[1] Ordinarily, following administration of digoxin immune Fab (ovine), improvement in signs and symptoms of digitalis intoxication begins within one-half hour or less.[2-5]

The affinity of digoxin immune Fab (ovine) for digoxin is in the range of 10^9 to 10^{11} M^{-1}, which is greater than the affinity of digoxin for (sodium, potassium) ATPase, the presumed receptor for its toxic effects. The affinity of digoxin immune Fab (ovine) for digitoxin is about 10^8 to 10^9 M^{-1}.

Digoxin immune Fab (ovine) binds molecules of digoxin, making them unavailable for binding at their site of action on cells in the body. The Fab fragment-digoxin complex accumulates in the blood, from which it is excreted by the kidney. The net effect is to shift the equilibrium away from binding of digoxin to its receptors in the body, thereby reversing its effects.

INDICATIONS AND USAGE

Digoxin immune Fab (ovine) is indicated for treatment of potentially life-threatening digoxin intoxication.[3] Although designed specifically to treat life-threatening digoxin overdose, it has also been used successfully to treat life-threatening digitoxin overdose.[3] Since human experience is limited and the consequences of repeated exposures are unknown, digoxin immune Fab (ovine) is not indicated for milder cases of digitalis toxicity.

Manifestations of life-threatening toxicity include severe ventricular arrhythmias such as ventricular tachycardia or ventricular fibrillation, or progressive bradyarrhythmias such as severe sinus bradycardia or second or third degree heart block not responsive to atropine.

Ingestion of more than 10 mg of digoxin in previously healthy adults or 4 mg of digoxin in previously healthy children, or ingestion causing steady-state serum concentrations greater than 10 ng/ml, often results in cardiac arrest. Digitalis-induced progressive elevation of the serum potassium concentration also suggests imminent cardiac arrest. If the potassium concentration exceeds 5 mEq/L in the setting of severe digitalis intoxication, therapy with digoxin immune Fab (ovine) is indicated.

NON-FDA APPROVED INDICATIONS

Digoxin immune Fab fragments (divalent) have been used without FDA approval for the treatment of lanatoside C (acute Nerium oleander leaves) intoxication.

CONTRAINDICATIONS

There are no known contraindications to the use of digoxin immune Fab (ovine).

WARNINGS

Suicidal ingestion often involves more than one drug; thus, toxicity from other drugs should not be overlooked.

One should consider the possibility of anaphylactic, hypersensitivity, or febrile reactions. If an anaphylactoid reaction occurs, the drug infusion should be discontinued and appropriate therapy initiated using aminophylline, oxygen, volume expansion, diphenhydramine, corticosteroids, and airway management as indicated. The need for epinephrine should be balanced against its potential risk in the setting of digitalis toxicity.

Since the Fab fragment of the antibody lacks the antigenic determinants of the Fc fragment, it should pose less of an immunogenic threat to patients than does an intact immunoglobulin molecule. Patients with known allergies would be particularly at risk, as would individuals who have previously received antibodies or Fab fragments raised in sheep. Papain is used to cleave the whole antibody into Fab and Fc fragments, and traces of papain or inactivated papain residues may be present in digoxin immune Fab (ovine). Patients with allergies to papain, chymopapain, or other papaya extracts also may be particularly at risk.

Skin testing for allergy was performed during the clinical investigation of digoxin immune Fab (ovine). Only 1 patient developed erythema at the site of skin testing, with no accompanying wheal reaction; this individual had no adverse reaction to systemic treatment with digoxin immune Fab (ovine). Since allergy testing can delay urgently needed therapy, it is not routinely required before treatment of life-threatening digitalis toxicity with digoxin immune Fab (ovine).

Skin testing may be appropriate for high risk individuals, especially patients with known allergies or those previously treated with digoxin immune Fab (ovine).

The intradermal skin test can be performed by:

Diluting 0.1 ml of reconstituted digoxin immune Fab (ovine) (9.5 mg/ml) in 9.9 ml sterile isotonic saline (1:100 dilution, 95 μg/ml).

Injecting 0.1 ml of the 1:100 dilution (9.5 μg) intradermally and observing for an urticarial wheal surrounded by a zone of erythema. The test should be read at 20 minutes.

The scratch test procedure is performed by placing one drop of a 1:100 dilution of digoxin immune Fab (ovine) on the skin and then making a ¼ inch scratch through the drop with a sterile needle. The scratch site is inspected at 20 minutes for an urticarial wheal surrounded by erythema.

If skin testing causes a systemic reaction, a tourniquet should be applied above the site of testing and measures to treat anaphylaxis should be instituted. Further administration of digoxin immune Fab (ovine) should be avoided unless its use is absolutely essential, in which case the patient should be pretreated with corticosteroids and diphenhydramine. The physician should be prepared to treat anaphylaxis.

PRECAUTIONS

GENERAL

Standard therapy for digitalis intoxication includes withdrawal of the drug and correction of factors that may contribute to toxicity, such as electrolyte disturbances, hypoxia, acid-base disturbances, and agents such as catecholamines. Also, treatment of arrhythmias may include judicious potassium supplements, lidocaine, phenytoin, procainamide and/or propranolol; treatment of sinus bradycardia or atrioventricular block may involve atropine or pacemaker insertion. Massive digitalis intoxication can cause hyperkalemia; administration of potassium supplements in the setting of massive intoxication may be hazardous (see Laboratory Tests). After treatment with digoxin immune Fab (ovine), the serum potassium concentration may drop rapidly[2] and must be monitored frequently, especially over the first several hours after digoxin immune Fab (ovine) is given (see Laboratory Tests).

The elimination half-life in the setting of renal failure has not been clearly defined. Patients with renal dysfunction have been successfully treated with digoxin immune Fab (ovine).[4] There is no evidence to suggest the time-course of therapeutic effect is any different in these patients than in patients with normal renal function, but excretion of the Fab fragment-digoxin complex from the body is probably delayed. In patients who are functionally anephric, one would anticipate failure to clear the Fab fragment-digoxin complex from the blood by glomerular filtration and renal excretion. Whether failure to eliminate the Fab fragment-digoxin complex in severe renal failure can lead to reintoxication following release of newly unbound digoxin into the blood is uncertain. Such patients should be monitored for a prolonged period for possible recurrence of digitalis toxicity.

Patients with intrinsically poor cardiac function may deteriorate from withdrawal of the inotropic action of digoxin. Studies in animals have shown that the reversal of inotropic effect is relatively gradual, occurring over hours. When needed, additional support can be provided by use of intravenous inotropes, such as dopamine or dobutamine, or vasodilators. One must be careful in using catecholamines not to aggravate digitalis toxic rhythm disturbances. Clearly, other types of digitalis glycosides should not be used in this setting.

Redigitalization should be postponed, if possible, until the Fab fragments have been eliminated from the body, which may require several days. Patients with impaired renal function may require a week or longer.

LABORATORY TESTS

Digoxin immune Fab (ovine) will interfere with digitalis immunoassay measurements.[6] Thus, the standard serum digoxin concentration measurement can be clinically misleading until the Fab fragment is eliminated from the body.

Serum digoxin or digitoxin concentration should be obtained before administration of digoxin immune Fab (ovine) if at all possible. These measurements may be difficult to interpret if drawn soon after the last digitalis dose, since at least 6-8 hours are required for equilibration of digoxin between serum and tissue. Patients should be closely monitored, including temperature, blood pressure, electrocardiogram, and potassium concentration, during and after administration of digoxin immune Fab (ovine). The total serum digoxin concentration may rise precipitously following administration of digoxin immune Fab (ovine), but this will be almost entirely bound to the Fab fragment and therefore not able to react with receptors in the body.

Potassium concentrations should be followed carefully. Severe digitalis intoxication can cause life-threatening elevation in serum potassium concentration by shifting potassium from inside to outside the cell. The elevation in serum potassium concentration can lead to increased renal excretion of potassium. Thus, these patients may have hyperkalemia with a total body deficit of potassium. When the effect of digitalis is reversed by digoxin immune Fab (ovine), potassium shifts back inside the cell, with a resulting decline in serum potassium concentration.[4] Hypokalemia may thus develop rapidly. For these reasons, serum potassium concentration should be monitored repeatedly, especially over the first several hours after digoxin immune Fab (ovine) is given, and cautiously treated when necessary.

CARCINOGENESIS, MUTAGENESIS, AND IMPAIRMENT OF FERTILITY

There have been no long-term studies performed in animals to evaluate carcinogenic potential.

PREGNANCY CATEGORY C

Animal reproduction studies have not been conducted with digoxin immune Fab (ovine). It is also not known whether digoxin immune Fab (ovine) can cause fetal harm when administered to a pregnant woman or can affect reproduction capacity. Digoxin immune Fab (ovine) should be given to a pregnant woman only if clearly needed.

NURSING MOTHERS

It is not known whether this drug is excreted in human milk. Because many drugs are excreted in human milk, caution should be exercised when digoxin immune Fab (ovine) is administered to a nursing woman.

PEDIATRIC USE

Digoxin immune Fab (ovine) has been successfully used in infants with no apparent adverse sequelae. As in all other circumstances, use of this drug in infants should be based on careful consideration of the benefits of the drug balanced against the potential risk involved.

GERIATRIC USE

Of the 150 subjects in an open-label study of digoxin immune Fab (ovine), 42% were 65 and over, while 21% were 75 and over. In a post-marketing surveillance study that enrolled 717 adults, 84% were 60 and over, and 60% were 70 and over. No overall differences in safety or effectiveness were observed between these subjects and younger subjects, and other reported clinical experience has not identified differences in responses between the elderly and younger patients, but greater sensitivity of some older individuals cannot be ruled out.

The kidney excretes the Fab fragment-digoxin complex, and the risk of digoxin release with recurrence of toxicity is potentially increased when excretion of the complex is slowed by renal failure. However, recurrence of toxicity was reported for only 2.8% of patients in the surveillance study and the only factor associated with recurrence of toxicity was inadequacy of initial dose — not renal function. Calculation of the dose is the same for patients of all ages and for patients with normal and impaired renal function. Because elderly patients are more likely to have decreased renal function, it may be useful to monitor renal function and to observe for possible recurrence of toxicity.

ADVERSE REACTIONS

Allergic reactions to digoxin immune Fab (ovine) have been reported rarely. Patients with a history of allergy, especially to antibiotics, appear to be at particular risk (see WARNINGS). In a few instances, low cardiac output states and congestive heart failure could have been exacerbated by withdrawal of the inotropic effects of digitalis. Hypokalemia may occur from re-activation of (sodium, potassium) ATPase (see Laboratory Tests). Patients with atrial fibrillation may develop a rapid ventricular response from withdrawal of the effects of digitalis on the atrioventricular node.[4]

DOSAGE AND ADMINISTRATION

GENERAL GUIDELINES

The dosage of digoxin immune Fab (ovine) varies according to the amount of digoxin (or digitoxin) to be neutralized. The average dose used during clinical testing was 10 vials.

DOSAGE FOR ACUTE INGESTION OF UNKNOWN AMOUNT

Twenty (20) vials (760 mg) of digoxin immune Fab (ovine) is adequate to treat most life-threatening ingestions in both **adults and children.** However, in children it is important to monitor for volume overload. In general, a large dose of digoxin immune Fab (ovine) has a faster onset of effect but may enhance the possibility of a febrile reaction. The physician may consider administering 10 vials, observing the patient's response, and following with an additional 10 vials if clinically indicated.

DOSAGE FOR TOXICITY DURING CHRONIC THERAPY

For adults, 6 vials (228 mg) usually is adequate to reverse most cases of toxicity. This dose can be used in patients who are in acute distress or for whom a serum digoxin or digitoxin concentration is not available. In infants and small children (≤20 kg) a single vial usually should suffice.

Methods for calculating the dose of digoxin immune Fab (ovine) required to neutralize the known or estimated amount of digoxin or digitoxin in the body are given below (see Dosage Calculation).

When determining the dose for digoxin immune Fab (ovine), the following guidelines should be considered:

Erroneous calculations may result from inaccurate estimates of the amount of digitalis ingested or absorbed or from nonsteady-state serum digitalis concentrations. Inaccurate serum digitalis concentration measurements are a possible source of error. Most serum digoxin assay kits are designed to measure values less than 5 ng/ml. Dilution of samples is required to obtain accurate measures above 5 ng/ml.

Dosage calculations are based on a steady-state volume of distribution of approximately 5 L/kg for digoxin (0.5 L/kg for digitoxin) to convert serum digitalis concentration to the amount of digitalis in the body. The conversion is based on the principle that body load equals drug steady-state serum concentration multiplied by volume of distribution. These volumes are population averages and vary widely among individuals. Many patients may require higher doses for complete neutralization. Doses should ordinarily be rounded up to the next whole vial.

If toxicity has not adequately reversed after several hours or appears to recur, readministration of digoxin immune Fab (ovine) at a dose guided by clinical judgment may be required.

Failure to respond to digoxin immune Fab (ovine) raises the possibility that the clinical problem is not caused by digitalis intoxication. If there is no response to an adequate dose of digoxin immune Fab (ovine), the diagnosis of digitalis toxicity should be questioned.

DOSAGE CALCULATION

Acute Ingestion of Known Amount

Each vial of digoxin immune Fab (ovine) contains 38 mg of purified digoxin-specific Fab fragments which will bind approximately 0.5 mg of digoxin (or digitoxin). Thus one can calculate the total number of vials required by dividing the total digitalis body load in mg by 0.5 mg/vial (see Formula 1).

For toxicity from an acute ingestion, total body load in milligrams will be approximately equal to the amount ingested in milligrams for digoxin capsules and digitoxin, or the amount ingested in milligrams multiplied by 0.80 (to account for incomplete absorption) for digoxin tablets.

TABLE 1 gives dosage estimates in number of vials for **adults and children** who have ingested a single large dose of digoxin and for whom the approximate number of tablets or capsules is known. The dose of digoxin immune Fab (ovine) (in number of vials) represented in TABLE 1 can be approximated using Formula 1.

Formula 1:

Dose (in no. of vials) = (Total digitalis body load in mg) ÷ (0.5 mg of digitalis bound/vial)

TABLE 1 *Approximate Dose of Digoxin Immune Fab (ovine) for Reversal of a Single Large Digoxin Overdose*

Number of Digoxin Tablets or Capsules Ingested*	Dose of Digoxin Immune Fab (ovine) No. of Vials
25	10
50	20
75	30
100	40
150	60
200	80

* 0.25 mg tablets with 80% bioavailability or 0.2 mg digoxin capsules with 100% bioavailability.

Calculations Based on Steady-State Serum Digoxin Concentrations

TABLE 2 gives dosage estimates in number of vials for **adult patients** for whom a steady-state serum digoxin concentration is known. The dose of digoxin immune Fab (ovine) (in number of vials) represented in TABLE 2 can be approximated using Formula 2.

Formula 2:

Dose (in no. of vials) = [(Serum digoxin concentration in ng/ml) (weight in kg)] ÷ 100

TABLE 3 gives dosage estimates in milligrams **for infants and small children** based on the steady-state serum digoxin concentration. The dose of digoxin immune Fab (ovine) represented in TABLE 3 can be estimated by multiplying the dose (in number of vials) calculated from Formula 2 by the amount of digoxin immune Fab (ovine) contained in a vial (38 mg/vial) (see Formula 3). Since infants and small children can have much smaller dosage requirements, it is recommended that the 38 mg vial be reconstituted as directed and administered with a tuberculin syringe. For very small doses, a reconstituted vial can be diluted with 34 ml of sterile isotonic saline to achieve a concentration of 1 mg/ml.

TABLE 2 *Adult Dose Estimate of Digoxin Immune Fab (ovine) (in Number of Vials) From Steady-State Serum Digoxin Concentration*

	Serum Digoxin Concentration (ng/ml)						
Patient Weight	1	2	4	8	12	16	20
40 kg	0.5 V	1 V	2 V	3 V	5 V	7 V	8 V
60 kg	0.5 V	1 V	3 V	5 V	7 V	10 V	12 V
70 kg	1 V	2 V	3 V	6 V	9 V	11 V	14 V
80 kg	1 V	2 V	3 V	7 V	10 V	13 V	16 V
100 kg	1 V	2 V	4 V	8 V	12 V	16 V	20 V

V = vials.

Formula 3:

Dose (in mg) = (Dose [in no. of vials]) (38 mg/vial)

TABLE 3 *Infants and Small Children Dose Estimates of Digoxin Immune Fab (ovine) (in mg) From Steady-State Serum Digoxin Concentration*

	Serum Digoxin Concentration (ng/ml)						
Patient Weight	1	2	4	8	12	16	20
1 kg	0.4* mg	1* mg	1.5* mg	3* mg	5 mg	6 mg	8 mg
3 kg	1* mg	2* mg	5 mg	9 mg	14 mg	18 mg	23 mg
5 kg	2* mg	4 mg	8 mg	15 mg	23 mg	30 mg	38 mg
10 kg	4 mg	8 mg	15 mg	30 mg	46 mg	61 mg	76 mg
20 kg	8 mg	15 mg	30 mg	61 mg	91 mg	122 mg	152 mg

* Dilution of reconstituted vial to 1 mg/ml may be desirable.

Calculation Based on Steady-State Digitoxin Concentration

The dose of digoxin immune Fab (ovine) for digitoxin toxicity can be approximated using Formula 4.

Formula 4:

Dose (in no. of vials) = [(Serum digitoxin concentration in ng/ml) (weight in kg)] ÷ 1000

If the dose based on ingested amount differs substantially from that calculated from the serum digoxin or digitoxin concentration, it may be preferable to use the higher dose.

ADMINISTRATION

The contents in each vial to be used should be dissolved with 4 ml of sterile water for injection, by gentle mixing, to give a clear, colorless, approximately isosmotic solution with a protein concentration of 9.5 mg/ml. Reconstituted product should be used promptly. If it is not used immediately, it may be stored under refrigeration at 2-8°C (36-46°F) for up to 4 hours. The reconstituted product may be diluted with sterile isotonic saline to a convenient volume. Parenteral drug products should be inspected visually for particulate matter and discoloration prior to administration, whenever solution and container permit.

Digoxin immune Fab (ovine), is administered by the intravenous route over 30 minutes. It is recommended that it be infused through a 0.22 micron membrane filter to ensure no undissolved particulate matter is administered. If cardiac arrest is imminent, it can be given as a bolus injection.

HOW SUPPLIED

Digibind is supplied in vials containing 38 mg of purified lyophilized digoxin-specific Fab fragments.

Storage: Refrigerate at 2-8°C (36-46°F). Unreconstituted vials can be stored at up to 30°C (86°F) for a total of 30 days.

PRODUCT LISTING - RATED THERAPEUTICALLY EQUIVALENT

Solution - Injectable - 10 mg/ml

4 ml $758.24 DIGIBIND, Glaxosmithkline 00173-0230-44

PRODUCT LISTING - EQUIVALENTS NOT AVAILABLE

Solution - Injectable - 10 mg/ml

4 ml $400.00 GENERIC, Savage Laboratories 00281-0365-10

Dihydroergotamine Mesylate *(001063)*

Categories: Headache, cluster; Headache, migraine; Pregnancy Category X; FDA Approved 1946 Apr
Drug Classes: Ergot alkaloids and derivatives
Brand Names: D.H.E. 45; Migranal
Foreign Brand Availability: Adhaegon (Austria); Detemes Retard (Austria); Dihydergot (Australia; Belgium; Benin; Burkina-Faso; Czech-Republic; Ethiopia; Gambia; Germany; Ghana; Greece; Guinea; India; Indonesia; Israel; Ivory-Coast; Kenya; Liberia; Malawi; Mali; Mauritania; Mauritius; Morocco; Netherlands; Niger; Nigeria; Norway; Senegal; Seychelles; Sierra-Leone; South-Africa; Spain; Sudan; Switzerland; Tanzania; Tunia; Turkey; Uganda; Zambia; Zimbabwe); Dihydergot Sandoz (Austria); Dihydroergotamine-Sandoz (Canada); Erganton (Germany); Ergont (Germany); Ergovasan (Austria); Ikaran (Belgium; France; Italy; Portugal); Ikaran LP (France); Ikaran Retard (Switzerland); Orstanorm (Finland; Sweden); Poligot (Thailand); Seglor (France; Italy; Taiwan); Seglor Retard (Portugal); Tamik (France; Hong-Kong); Tenuatina (Spain); Verladyn (Germany); Verteblan (Greece)
HCFA JCODE(S): J1110 per 1 mg IM, IV

IM-IV

WARNING

Serious and/or life-threatening peripheral ischemia has been associated with the coadministration of dihydroergotamine with potent CYP 3A4 inhibitors including protease inhibitors and macrolide antibiotics. Because CYP 3A4 inhibition elevates the serum levels of dihydroergotamine, the risk for vasospasm leading to cerebral ischemia and/or ischemia of the extremities is increased. Hence, concomitant use of these medications is contraindicated.

(See also CONTRAINDICATIONS and WARNINGS section.)

DESCRIPTION

Dihydroergotamine mesylate is ergotamine hydrogenated in the 9,10 position as the mesylate salt. Dihydroergotamine mesylate is known chemically as ergotaman-3′,6′,18- trione,9,10 -dihydro -12′-hydroxy-2′-methyl-5′-(phenylmethyl)-, (5′α)-, monomethanesulfonate. Its molecular weight is 679.80 and its empirical formula is $C_{33}H_{37}N_5O_5 \cdot CH_4O_3S$.

D.H.E. 45 (dihydroergotamine mesylate) Injection is a clear, colorless solution supplied in sterile ampuls for IV, IM, or subcutaneous administration containing per ml:

Dihydroergotamine Mesylate: 1 mg
Ethanol, 94% w/w: 6.2% by vol
Glycerin: 15% by wt
Water for Injection, qs to: 1 ml

CLINICAL PHARMACOLOGY

MECHANISM OF ACTION

Dihydroergotamine binds with high affinity to $5\text{-HT}_{1D\alpha}$ and $5\text{-HT}_{1D\beta}$ receptors. It also binds with high affinity to serotonin 5-HT_{1A}, 5-HT_{2A}, and 5-HT_{2C} receptors, noradrenaline α_{2A}, α_{2B} and α, receptors, and dopamine D_{2L} and D_3 receptors.

The therapeutic activity of dihydroergotamine in migraine is generally attributed to the agonist effect at 5-HT_{1D} receptors. Two current theories have been proposed to explain the efficacy of 5-HT_{1D} receptor agonists in migraine. One theory suggests that activation of 5-HT_{1D} receptors located on intracranial blood vessels, including those on arterio-venous anastomoses, leads to vasoconstriction, which correlates with the relief of migraine headache. The alternative hypothesis suggests that activation of 5-HT_{1D} receptors on sensory nerve endings of the trigeminal system results in the inhibition of proinflammatory neuropeptide release.

In addition, dihydroergotamine possesses oxytocic properties. (See CONTRAINDICATIONS.)

PHARMACOKINETICS

Absorption

Absolute bioavailability for the subcutaneous and intramuscular route have not been determined, however, no difference was observed in dihydroergotamine bioavailability from intramuscular and subcutaneous doses. Dihydroergotamine mesylate is poorly bioavailable following oral administration.

Distribution

Dihydroergotamine mesylate is 93% plasma protein bound. The apparent steady-state volume of distribution is approximately 800 liters.

Metabolism

Four dihydroergotamine mesylate metabolites have been identified in human plasma following oral administration. The major metabolite, 8′-β-hydroxydihydroergotamine, exhibits affinity equivalent to its parent for adrenergic and 5-HT receptors and demonstrates equivalent potency in several venoconstrictor activity models, *in vivo* and *in vitro.* The other metabolites, *i.e.*, dihydrolysergic acid, dihydrolysergic amide, and a metabolite formed by oxidative opening of the proline ring are of minor importance. Following nasal administration, total metabolites represent only 20%-30% of plasma AUC. Quantitative pharmacokinetic characterization of the four metabolites has not been performed.

Excretion

The major excretory route of dihydroergotamine is via the bile in the feces. The total body clearance is 1.5 L/min which reflects mainly hepatic clearance. Only 6%-7% of unchanged dihydroergotamine is excreted in the urine after intramuscular injection. The renal clearance (0.1 L/min) is unaffected by the route of dihydroergotamine administration. The decline of plasma dihydroergotamine after intramuscular or intravenous administration is multi-exponential with a terminal half-life of about 9 hours.

Subpopulations

No studies have been conducted on the effect of renal or hepatic impairment, gender, race, or ethnicity on dihydroergotamine pharmacokinetics. Dihydroergotamine mesylate injection is contraindicated in patients with severely impaired hepatic or renal function. (See CONTRAINDICATIONS.)

Interactions

Pharmacokinetic interactions have been reported in patients treated orally with other ergot alkaloids (*e.g.*, increased levels of ergotamine) and macrolide antibiotics, principally troleandomycin, presumably due to inhibition of cytochrome P450 3A metabolism of the alkaloids by troleandomycin. Dihydroergotamine has also been shown to be an inhibitor of cytochrome P450 3A catalyzed reactions and rare reports of ergotism have been obtained from patients treated with dihydroergotamine and macrolide antibiotics (*e.g.*, troleandomycin, clarithromycin, erythromycin), and in patients treated with dihydroergotamine and protease inhibitors (*e.g.*, ritonavir), presumably due to inhibition of cytochrome P450 3A metabolism of ergotamine (see CONTRAINDICATIONS). No pharmacokinetic interactions involving other cytochrome P450 isoenzymes are known.

INDICATIONS AND USAGE

Dihydroergotamine mesylate injection is indicated for the acute treatment of migraine headaches with or without aura and the acute treatment of cluster headache episodes.

NON-FDA APPROVED INDICATIONS

Dihydroergotamine (in conjunction with heparin) has also been used to reduce the risk of post-surgical deep venous thrombosis. This last use, however, is not approved by the FDA.

CONTRAINDICATIONS

There have been a few reports of serious adverse events associated with the coadministration of dihydroergotamine and potent CYP 3A4 inhibitors, such as protease inhibitors and macrolide antibiotics, resulting in vasospasm that led to cerebral ischemia and/or ischemia of the extremities. The use of potent CYP 3A4 inhibitors (ritonavir, nelfinavir, indinavir, erythromycin, clarithromycin, troleandomycin, ketoconazole, itraconazole) with dihydroergotamine is, therefore contraindicated (see WARNINGS, CYP 3A4 Inhibitors).

Dihydroergotamine mesylate injection should not be given to patients with ischemic heart disease (angina pectoris, history of myocardial infarction, or documented silent ischemia) or to patients who have clinical symptoms or findings consistent with coronary artery vasospasm including Prinzmetal's variant angina. (See WARNINGS.)

Because dihydroergotamine mesylate injection may increase blood pressure, it should not be given to patients with uncontrolled hypertension.

Dihydroergotamine mesylate injection, 5-HT_1 agonists (*e.g.*, sumatriptan), ergotamine-containing or ergot-type medications or methysergide should not be used within 24 hours of each other.

Dihydroergotamine mesylate injection should not be administered to patients with hemiplegic or basilar migraine.

In addition to those conditions mentioned above, dihydroergotamine mesylate injection is also contraindicated in patients with known peripheral arterial disease, sepsis, following vascular surgery and severely impaired hepatic or renal function.

Dihydroergotamine mesylate injection may cause fetal harm when administered to a pregnant woman. Dihydroergotamine possesses oxytocic properties and, therefore, should not be administered during pregnancy. If this drug is used during pregnancy, or if the patient becomes pregnant while taking this drug, the patient should be apprised of the potential hazard to the fetus.

There are no adequate studies of dihydroergotamine in human pregnancy, but developmental toxicity has been demonstrated in experimental animals. In embryo-fetal development studies of dihydroergotamine mesylate nasal spray, intranasal administration to pregnant rats throughout the period of organogenesis resulted in decreased fetal body weights and/or skeletal ossification at doses of 0.16 mg/day (associated with maternal plasma dihydroergotamine exposures [AUC] approximately 0.4-1.2 times the exposures in humans receiving the MRDD of 4 mg) or greater. A no effect level for embryo-fetal toxicity was not established in rats. Delayed skeletal ossification was also noted in rabbit fetuses following intranasal administration of 3.6 mg/day (maternal exposures approximately 7 times human exposures at the MRDD) during organogenesis. A no effect level was seen at 1.2 mg/day (maternal exposures approximately 2.5 times human exposures at the MRDD). When dihydroergotamine mesylate nasal spray was administered intranasally to female rats during pregnancy and lactation, decreased body weights and impaired reproductive function (decreased mating indices) were observed in the offspring at doses of 0.16 mg/day or greater. A no effect level was not established. Effects on development occurred at doses below those that produced evidence of significant maternal toxicity in these studies. Dihydroergotamine-induced intrauterine growth retardation has been attributed to reduced uteroplacental blood flow resulting from prolonged vasoconstriction of the uterine vessels and/or increased myometrial tone.

Dihydroergotamine mesylate injection is contraindicated in patients who have previously shown hypersensitivity to ergot alkaloids.

Dihydroergotamine mesylate should not be used by nursing mothers. (See PRECAUTIONS.)

Dihydroergotamine mesylate should not be used with peripheral and central vasoconstrictors because the combination may result in additive or synergistic elevation of blood pressure.

WARNINGS

Dihydroergotamine mesylate injection should only be used where a clear diagnosis of migraine headache has been established.

CYP 3A4 INHIBITORS (E.G., MACROLIDE ANTIBIOTICS AND PROTEASE INHIBITORS)

There have been rare reports of serious adverse events in connection with the coadministration of dihydroergotamine and potent CYP 3A4 inhibitors, such as protease inhibitors and macrolide antibiotics, resulting in vasospasm that led to cerebral ischemia and/or ischemia of the extremities. The use of potent CYP 3A4 inhibitors with dihydroergotamine should therefore be avoided (see CONTRAINDICATIONS). Examples of some of the more potent CYP 3A4 inhibitors include: anti-fungals ketoconazole and itraconazole, the protease inhibitors ritonavir, nelfinavir, and indinavir, and macrolide antibiotics erythromycin, clarithromycin, and troleandomycin. Other less potent CYP 3A4 inhibitors should be administered with caution. Less potent inhibitors include saquinavir, nefazodone, fluconazole, grapefruit juice, fluoxetine, fluvoxamine, zileuton, and clotrimazole. These lists are not exhaustive, and the prescriber should consider the effects on CYP3A4 of other agents being considered for concomitant use with dihydroergotamine.

FIBROTIC COMPLICATIONS

There have been reports of pleural and retroperitoneal fibrosis in patients following prolonged daily use of injectable dihydroergotamine mesylate. Rarely, prolonged daily use of other ergot alkaloid drugs has been associated with cardiac valvular fibrosis. Rare cases have also been reported in association with the use of injectable dihydroergotamine mesylate; however, in those cases, patients also received drugs known to be associated with cardiac valvular fibrosis.

Administration of dihydroergotamine mesylate injection, should not exceed the dosing guidelines and should not be used for chronic daily administration (see DOSAGE AND ADMINISTRATION).

RISK OF MYOCARDIAL ISCHEMIA AND/OR INFARCTION AND OTHER ADVERSE CARDIAC EVENTS

Dihydroergotamine mesylate injection should not be used by patients with documented ischemic or vasospastic coronary artery disease. (See CONTRAINDICATIONS.) It is strongly recommended that dihydroergotamine mesylate injection not be given to patients in whom unrecognized coronary artery disease (CAD) is predicted by the presence of risk factors (*e.g.*, hypertension, hypercholesterolemia, smoker, obesity, diabetes, strong family history of CAD, females who are surgically or physiologically postmenopausal, or males who are over 40 years of age) unless a cardiovascular evaluation provides satisfactory clinical evidence that the patient is reasonably free of coronary artery and ischemic myocardial disease or other significant underlying cardiovascular disease. The sensitivity of cardiac diagnostic procedures to detect cardiovascular disease or predisposition to coronary artery vasospasm is modest, at best. If, during the cardiovascular evaluation, the patient's medical history or electrocardiographic investigations reveal findings indicative of or consistent with coronary artery vasospasm or myocardial ischemia, dihydroergotamine mesylate injection should not be administered. (See CONTRAINDICATIONS.)

For patients with risk factors predictive of CAD who are determined to have a satisfactory cardiovascular evaluation, it is strongly recommended that administration of the first dose of dihydroergotamine mesylate injection take place in the setting of a physician's office or similar medically staffed and equipped facility unless the patient has previously received dihydroergotamine mesylate. Because cardiac ischemia can occur in the absence of clinical symptoms, consideration should be given to obtaining on the first occasion of use an electrocardiogram (ECG) during the interval immediately following dihydroergotamine mesylate injection, in those patients with risk factors.

It is recommended that patients who are intermittent long-term users of dihydroergotamine mesylate injection and who have or acquire risk factors predictive of CAD, as described above, undergo periodic interval cardiovascular evaluation as they continue to use dihydroergotamine mesylate injection.

The systematic approach described above is currently recommended as a method to identify patients in whom dihydroergotamine mesylate injection may be used to treat migraine headaches with an acceptable margin of cardiovascular safety.

CARDIAC EVENTS AND FATALITIES

The potential for adverse cardiac events exists. Serious adverse cardiac events, including acute myocardial infarction, life-threatening disturbances of cardiac rhythm, and death have been reported to have occurred following the administration of dihydroergotamine mesylate injection. Considering the extent of use of dihydroergotamine mesylate in patients with migraine, the incidence of these events is extremely low.

DRUG-ASSOCIATED CEREBROVASCULAR EVENTS AND FATALITIES

Cerebral hemorrhage, subarachnoid hemorrhage, stroke, and other cerebrovascular events have been reported in patients treated with dihydroergotamine mesylate injection; and some have resulted in fatalities. In a number of cases, it appears possible that the cerebrovascular events were primary, the dihydroergotamine mesylate injection having been administered in the incorrect belief that the symptoms experienced were a consequence of migraine, when they were not. It should be noted that patients with migraine may be at increased risk of certain cerebrovascular events (*e.g.*, stroke, hemorrhage, transient ischemic attack).

OTHER VASOSPASM RELATED EVENTS

Dihydroergotamine mesylate injection, like other ergot alkaloids, may cause vasospastic reactions other than coronary artery vasospasm. Myocardial, peripheral vascular, and colonic ischemia have been reported with dihydroergotamine mesylate injection.

Dihydroergotamine mesylate injection associated vasospastic phenomena may also cause muscle pains, numbness, coldness, pallor, and cyanosis of the digits. In patients with compromised circulation, persistent vasospasm may result in gangrene or death. Dihydroergotamine mesylate injection should be discontinued immediately if signs or symptoms of vasoconstriction develop.

INCREASE IN BLOOD PRESSURE

Significant elevation in blood pressure has been reported on rare occasions in patients with and without a history of hypertension treated with dihydroergotamine mesylate injection. Dihydroergotamine mesylate injection is contraindicated in patients with uncontrolled hypertension. (See CONTRAINDICATIONS.)

An 18% increase in mean pulmonary artery pressure was seen following dosing with another 5-HT_1 agonist in a study evaluating subjects undergoing cardiac catheterization.

PRECAUTIONS

GENERAL

Dihydroergotamine mesylate injection may cause coronary artery vasospasm; patients who experience signs or symptoms suggestive of angina following its administration should, therefore, be evaluated for the presence of CAD or a predisposition to variant angina before receiving additional doses. Similarly, patients who experience other symptoms or signs suggestive of decreased arterial flow, such as ischemic bowel syndrome or Raynaud's syndrome following the use of any 5-HT agonist are candidates for further evaluation. (See WARNINGS.)

Fibrotic Complications: See WARNINGS, Fibrotic Complications.

INFORMATION FOR THE PATIENT

To assure safe and effective use of dihydroergotamine mesylate injection, the information and instructions provided in the patient information sheet should be discussed with patients.

Patients should be advised to report to the physician immediately any of the following: numbness or tingling in the fingers and toes, muscle pain in the arms and legs, weakness in the legs, pain in the chest, temporary speeding or slowing of the heart rate, swelling, or itching.

Prior to the initial use of the product by a patient, the prescriber should take steps to ensure that the patient understands how to use the product as provided. See Patient Information Sheet and product packaging.

Administration of dihydroergotamine mesylate injection , should not exceed the dosing guidelines and should not be used for chronic daily administration (see DOSAGE AND ADMINISTRATION).

CARCINOGENESIS, MUTAGENESIS, AND IMPAIRMENT OF FERTILITY

Carcinogenesis

Assessment of the carcinogenic potential of dihydroergotamine mesylate in mice and rats is ongoing.

Mutagenesis

Dihydroergotamine mesylate was clastogenic in two *in vitro* chromosomal aberration assays, the V79 Chinese hamster cell assay with metabolic activation and the cultured human peripheral blood lymphocyte assay. There was no evidence of mutagenic potential when dihydroergotamine mesylate was tested in the presence or absence of metabolic activation in two gene mutation assays (the Ames test and the *in vitro* mammalian Chinese hamster V79/HGPRT assay) and in an assay for DNA damage (the rat hepatocyte unscheduled DNA synthesis test). Dihydroergotamine was not clastogenic in the *in vivo* mouse and hamster micronucleus tests.

Impairment of Fertility

Impairment of fertility was not evaluated for dihydroergotamine mesylate injection. There was no evidence of impairment of fertility in rats given intranasal doses of Dihydroergotamine mesylate nasal spray up to 1.6 mg/day (associated with mean plasma dihydroergotamine mesylate exposures [AUC] approximately 9-11 times those in humans receiving the MRDD of 4 mg).

PREGNANCY CATEGORY X

See CONTRAINDICATIONS.

NURSING MOTHERS

Ergot drugs are known to inhibit prolactin. It is likely that dihydroergotamine mesylate injection is excreted in human milk, but there are no data on the concentration of dihydroergotamine in human milk. It is known that ergotamine is excreted in breast milk and may cause vomiting, diarrhea, weak pulse, and unstable blood pressure in nursing infants. Because of the potential for these serious adverse events in nursing infants exposed to dihydroergotamine mesylate injection, nursing should not be undertaken with the use of dihydroergotamine mesylate injection. (See CONTRAINDICATIONS.)

PEDIATRIC USE

Safety and effectiveness in pediatric patients have not been established.

DRUG INTERACTIONS

Vasoconstrictors: Dihydroergotamine mesylate injection should not be used with peripheral vasoconstrictors because the combination may cause synergistic elevation of blood pressure.

Sumatriptan: Sumatriptan has been reported to cause coronary artery vasospasm, and its effect could be additive with dihydroergotamine mesylate injection. Sumatriptan and dihydroergotamine mesylate injection should not be taken within 24 hours of each other. (See CONTRAINDICATIONS.)

Beta Blockers: Although the results of a clinical study did not indicate a safety problem associated with the administration of dihydroergotamine mesylate injection to subjects already receiving propranolol, there have been reports that propranolol may potentiate the vasoconstrictive action of ergotamine by blocking the vasodilating property of epinephrine.

Nicotine: Nicotine may provoke vasoconstriction in some patients, predisposing to a greater ischemic response to ergot therapy.

CYP 3A4 Inhibitors (e.g., macrolide antibiotics and protease inhibitors): See CONTRAINDICATIONS and WARNINGS.

SSRIs: Weakness, hyperreflexia, and incoordination have been reported rarely when 5-HT_1 agonists have been coadministered with SSRI's (*e.g.*, fluoxetine, fluvoxamine, paroxetine, sertraline). There have been no reported cases from spontaneous reports of drug interaction between SSRI's and dihydroergotamine mesylate injection.

Oral Contraceptives: The effect of oral contraceptives on the pharmacokinetics of dihydroergotamine mesylate injection has not been studied.

ADVERSE REACTIONS

Serious cardiac events, including some that have been fatal, have occurred following use of dihydroergotamine mesylate injection, but are extremely rare. Events reported have included coronary artery vasospasm, transient myocardial ischemia, myocardial infarction, ventricular tachycardia, and ventricular fibrillation. (See CONTRAINDICATIONS, WARNINGS, and PRECAUTIONS.) Fibrotic complications have been reported in association with long term use of injectable dihydroergotamine mesylate (see WARNINGS, Fibrotic Complications).

POST-INTRODUCTION REPORTS

The following events derived from postmarketing experience have been occasionally reported in patients receiving dihydroergotamine mesylate injection: vasospasm, paraesthesia, hypertension, dizziness, anxiety, dyspnea, headache, flushing, diarrhea, rash, increased sweating, and pleural and retroperitoneal fibrosis after long-term use of dihydroergotamine. Extremely rare cases of myocardial infarction and stroke have been reported. A causal relationship has not been established.

Dihydroergotamine mesylate injection is not recommended for prolonged daily use. (See DOSAGE AND ADMINISTRATION.)

DOSAGE AND ADMINISTRATION

Dihydroergotamine mesylate injection should be administered in a dose of 1 ml intravenously, intramuscularly or subcutaneously. The dose can be repeated, as needed, at 1 hour intervals to a total dose of 3 ml for intramuscular or subcutaneous delivery or 2 ml for intravenous delivery in a 24 hour period. The total weekly dosage should not exceed 6 ml. Dihydroergotamine mesylate injection, should not be used for chronic daily administration.

HOW SUPPLIED

D.H.E. 45 Injection is available as a clear, colorless, sterile solution in single 1 ml sterile ampuls containing 1 mg of dihydroergotamine mesylate per ml.

Storage: Store below 25°C (77°F), in light-resistant containers. Do not refrigerate or freeze. To assure constant potency, protect the ampuls from light and heat. Administer only if clear and colorless.

INTRANASAL

WARNING

The solution used in dihydroergotamine mesylate nasal spray (4 mg/ml) is intended for intranasal use and must not be injected.

Serious and/or life-threatening peripheral ischemia has been associated with the coadministration of dihydroergotamine with potent CYP 3A4 inhibitors including protease inhibitors and macrolide antibiotics. Because CYP 3A4 inhibition elevates the serum levels of dihydroergotamine, the risk for vasospasm leading to cerebral ischemia and/or ischemia of the extremities is increased. Hence, concomitant use of these medications is contraindicated.

(See also CONTRAINDICATIONS and WARNINGS.)

DESCRIPTION

Dihydroergotamine mesylate is ergotamine hydrogenated in the 9,10 position as the mesylate salt. Dihydroergotamine mesylate is known chemically as ergotaman-3′,6′,18-trione,9,10-dihydro-12′-hydroxy-2′-methyl-5′-(phenylmethyl)-,(5′α)-, monomethanesulfonate. Its molecular weight is 679.80 and its empirical formula is $C_{33}H_{37}N_5O_5{\cdot}CH_4O_3S$.

Migranal (dihydroergotamine mesylate) Nasal Spray is provided for intranasal administration as a clear, colorless to faintly yellow solution in an amber glass ampul containing:

Dihydroergotamine Mesylate: 4.0 mg
Caffeine, Anhydrous: 10.0 mg
Dextrose, Anhydrous: 50.0 mg
Carbon Dioxide: qs
Water for Injection: 1.0 ml

CLINICAL PHARMACOLOGY

MECHANISM OF ACTION

Dihydroergotamine binds with high affinity to 5-$HT_{1D\alpha}$ and 5-$HT_{1D\beta}$ receptors. It also binds with high affinity to serotonin 5-HT_{1A}, 5-HT_{2A}, and 5-HT_{2C} receptors, noradrenaline α_{2A}, α_{2B} and α_1 receptors, and dopamine D_{2L} and D_3 receptors.

The therapeutic activity of dihydroergotamine in migraine is generally attributed to the agonist effect at 5-HT_{1D} receptors. Two current theories have been proposed to explain the efficacy of 5-HT_{1D} receptor agonists in migraine. One theory suggests that activation of 5-HT_{1D} receptors located on intracranial blood vessels, including those on arterio-venous anastomoses, leads to vasoconstriction, which correlates with the relief of migraine headache. The alternative hypothesis suggests that activation of 5-HT_{1D} receptors on sensory nerve endings of the trigeminal system results in the inhibition of pro-inflammatory neuropeptide release.

In addition, dihydroergotamine possesses oxytocic properties. (See CONTRAINDICATIONS.)

PHARMACOKINETICS

Absorption

Dihydroergotamine mesylate is poorly bioavailable following oral administration. Following intranasal administration, however, the mean bioavailability of dihydroergotamine mesylate is 32% relative to the injectable administration. Absorption is variable, probably reflecting both intersubject differences of absorption and the technique used for self-administration.

Distribution

Dihydroergotamine mesylate is 93% plasma protein bound. The apparent steady-state volume of distribution is approximately 800 liters.

Metabolism

Four dihydroergotamine mesylate metabolites have been identified in human plasma following oral administration. The major metabolite, 8′-β-hydroxydihydroergotamine, exhibits affinity equivalent to its parent for adrenergic and 5-HT receptors and demonstrates equivalent potency in several venoconstrictor activity models, *in vivo* and *in vitro*. The other metabolites, *i.e.*, dihydrolysergic acid, dihydrolysergic amide and a metabolite formed by oxidative opening of the proline ring are of minor importance. Following nasal administration, total metabolites represent only 20-30% of plasma AUC. The systemic clearance of dihydroergotamine mesylate following IV and IM administration is 1.5 L/min. Quantitative pharmacokinetic characterization of the four metabolites has not been performed.

Excretion

The major excretory route of dihydroergotamine is via the bile in the feces. After intranasal administration the urinary recovery of parent drug amounts to about 2% of the administered dose compared to 6% after IM administration. The total body clearance is 1.5 L/min which reflects mainly hepatic clearance. The renal clearance (0.1 L/min) is unaffected by the route of dihydroergotamine administration. The decline of plasma dihydroergotamine is biphasic with a terminal half-life of about 10 hours.

Subpopulations

No studies have been conducted on the effect of renal or hepatic impairment, gender, race, or ethnicity on dihydroergotamine pharmacokinetics. Dihydroergotamine mesylate nasal spray is contraindicated in patients with severely impaired hepatic or renal function. (See CONTRAINDICATIONS.)

Interactions

The pharmacokinetics of dihydroergotamine did not appear to be significantly affected by the concomitant use of a local vasoconstrictor (*e.g.*, fenoxazoline).

Multiple oral doses of the β-adrenoceptor antagonist propranolol, used for migraine prophylaxis, had no significant influence on the C_{max}, T_{max} or AUC of dihydroergotamine doses up to 4 mg.

Pharmacokinetic interactions have been reported in patients treated orally with other ergot alkaloids (*e.g.*, increased levels of ergotamine) and macrolide antibiotics, principally troleandomycin, presumably due to inhibition of cytochrome P450 3A metabolism of the alkaloids by troleandomycin. Dihydroergotamine has also been shown to be an inhibitor of cytochrome P450 3A catalyzed reactions and rare reports of ergotism have been obtained from patients treated with dihydroergotamine and macrolide antibiotics (*e.g.*, troleandomycin, clarithromycin, erythromycin), and in patients treated with dihydroergotamine and protease inhibitors (*e.g.*, ritonavir), presumably due to inhibition of cytochrome P450 3A metabolism of ergotamine (see CONTRAINDICATIONS). No pharmacokinetic interactions involving other cytochrome P450 isoenzymes are known.

INDICATIONS AND USAGE

Dihydroergotamine mesylate nasal spray is indicated for the acute treatment of migraine headaches with or without aura.

Dihydroergotamine mesylate nasal spray is not intended for the prophylactic therapy of migraine or for the management of hemiplegic or basilar migraine.

CONTRAINDICATIONS

There have been a few reports of serious adverse events associated with the coadministration of dihydroergotamine and potent CYP 3A4 inhibitors, such as protease inhibitors and macrolide antibiotics, resulting in vasospasm that led to cerebral ischemia and/or ischemia of the extremities. The use of potent CYP 3A4 inhibitors (ritonavir, nelfinavir, indinavir, erythromycin, clarithromycin, troleandomycin, ketoconazole, itraconazole) with dihydroergotamine is, therefore contraindicated (see WARNINGS, CYP 3A4 Inhibitors).

Dihydroergotamine mesylate nasal spray should not be given to patients with ischemic heart disease (angina pectoris, history of myocardial infarction, or documented silent ischemia) or to patients who have clinical symptoms or findings consistent with coronary artery vasospasm including Prinzmetal's variant angina. (See WARNINGS.)

Because dihydroergotamine mesylate nasal spray may increase blood pressure, it should not be given to patients with uncontrolled hypertension.

Dihydroergotamine mesylate nasal spray, 5-HT_1 agonists (*e.g.*, sumatriptan), ergotamine-containing or ergot-type medications or methysergide should not be used within 24 hours of each other.

Dihydroergotamine mesylate nasal spray should not be administered to patients with hemiplegic or basilar migraine.

In addition to those conditions mentioned above, dihydroergotamine mesylate nasal spray is also contraindicated in patients with known peripheral arterial disease, sepsis, following vascular surgery, and severely impaired hepatic or renal function.

Dihydroergotamine mesylate nasal spray may cause fetal harm when administered to a pregnant woman. Dihydroergotamine possesses oxytocic properties and, therefore, should not be administered during pregnancy. If this drug is used during pregnancy, or if the patient becomes pregnant while taking this drug, the patient should be apprised of the potential hazard to the fetus.

There are no adequate studies of dihydroergotamine in human pregnancy, but developmental toxicity has been demonstrated in experimental animals. In embryofetal development studies of dihydroergotamine mesylate nasal spray, intranasal administration to pregnant rats throughout the period of organogenesis resulted in decreased fetal body weights and/or skeletal ossification at doses of 0.16 mg/day (associated with maternal plasma dihydroergotamine exposures [AUC] approximately 0.4-1.2 times the exposures in humans receiving the MRDD of 4 mg) or greater. A no effect level for embryo-fetal toxicity was not established in rats. Delayed skeletal ossification was also noted in rabbit fetuses following intranasal administration of 3.6 mg/day (maternal exposures approximately 7 times human exposures at the MRDD) during organogenesis. A no effect level was seen at 1.2 mg/day (maternal exposures approximately 2.5 times human exposures at the MRDD). When dihydroergotamine mesylate nasal spray was administered intranasally to female rats during pregnancy and lactation, decreased body weights and impaired reproductive function (decreased mating indices) were observed in the offspring at doses of 0.16 mg/day or greater. A no effect level was not established. Effects on development occurred at doses below those that produced evidence of significant maternal toxicity in these studies. Dihydroergotamine-induced intrauterine growth retardation has been attributed to reduced uteroplacental blood flow resulting from prolonged vasoconstriction of the uterine vessels and/or increased myometrial tone.

Dihydroergotamine mesylate nasal spray is contraindicated in patients who have previously shown hypersensitivity to ergot alkaloids.

Dihydroergotamine mesylate should not be used by nursing mothers. (See PRECAUTIONS.)

Dihydroergotamine mesylate should not be used with peripheral and central vasoconstrictors because the combination may result in additive or synergistic elevation of blood pressure.

WARNINGS

Dihydroergotamine mesylate nasal spray should only be used where a clear diagnosis of migraine headache has been established.

CYP 3A4 INHIBITORS (E.G., MACROLIDE ANTIBIOTICS AND PROTEASE INHIBITORS)

There have been rare reports of serious adverse events in connection with the coadministration of dihydroergotamine and potent CYP 3A4 inhibitors, such as protease inhibitors and macrolide antibiotics, resulting in vasospasm that led to cerebral ischemia and/or and ischemia of the extremities. The use of potent CYP 3A4 inhibitors with dihydroergotamine should therefore be avoided (see CONTRAINDICATIONS). Examples of some of the more potent CYP 3A4 inhibitors include: anti-fungals ketoconazole and itraconazole, the protease inhibitors ritonavir, nelfinavir, and indinavir, and macrolide antibiotics erythromycin, clarithromycin, and troleandomycin. Other less potent CYP 3A4 inhibitors should be administered with caution. Less potent inhibitors include saquinavir, nefazodone, fluconazole, grapefruit juice, fluoxetine, fluvoxamine, zileuton, and clotrimazole. These lists are not exhaustive, and the prescriber should consider the effects on CYP3A4 of other agents being considered for concomitant use with dihydroergotamine.

FIBROTIC COMPLICATIONS

There have been reports of pleural and retroperitoneal fibrosis in patients following prolonged daily use of injectable dihydroergotamine mesylate. Rarely, prolonged daily use of other ergot alkaloid drugs has been associated with cardiac valvular fibrosis. Rare cases have also been reported in association with the use of injectable dihydroergotamine mesylate; however, in those cases, patients also received drugs known to be associated with cardiac valvular fibrosis.

Administration of dihydroergotamine mesylate nasal spray, should not exceed the dosing guidelines and should not be used for chronic daily administration (see DOSAGE AND ADMINISTRATION).

RISK OF MYOCARDIAL ISCHEMIA AND/OR INFARCTION AND OTHER ADVERSE CARDIAC EVENTS

Dihydroergotamine mesylate nasal spray should not be used by patients with documented ischemic or vasospastic coronary artery disease. (See CONTRAINDICATIONS.) It is strongly recommended that dihydroergotamine mesylate nasal spray not be given to patients in whom unrecognized coronary artery disease (CAD) is predicted by the presence of risk factors (*e.g.*, hypertension, hypercholesterolemia, smoker, obesity, diabetes, strong family history of CAD, females who are surgically or physiologically post-menopausal, or males who are over 40 years of age) unless a cardiovascular evaluation provides satisfactory clinical evidence that the patient is reasonably free of coronary artery and ischemic myocardial disease or other significant underlying cardiovascular disease. The sensitivity of cardiac diagnostic procedures to detect cardiovascular disease or predisposition to coronary artery vasospasm is modest, at best. If, during the cardiovascular evaluation, the patient's medical history or electrocardiographic investigations reveal findings indicative of or consistent with coronary artery vasospasm or myocardial ischemia, dihydroergotamine mesylate nasal spray should not be administered. (See CONTRAINDICATIONS.)

For patients with risk factors predictive of CAD who are determined to have a satisfactory cardiovascular evaluation, it is strongly recommended that administration of the first dose of dihydroergotamine mesylate nasal spray take place in the setting of a physician's office or similar medically staffed and equipped facility unless the patient has previously received dihydroergotamine mesylate. Because cardiac ischemia can occur in the absence of clinical symptoms, consideration should be given to obtaining on the first occasion of use an electrocardiogram (ECG) during the interval immediately following dihydroergotamine mesylate nasal spray, in these patients with risk factors.

It is recommended that patients who are intermittent long-term users of dihydroergotamine mesylate nasal spray and who have or acquire risk factors predictive of CAD, as described above, undergo periodic interval cardiovascular evaluation as they continue to use dihydroergotamine mesylate nasal spray.

The systematic approach described above is currently recommended as a method to identify patients in whom dihydroergotamine mesylate nasal spray may be used to treat migraine headaches with an acceptable margin of cardiovascular safety.

CARDIAC EVENTS AND FATALITIES

No deaths have been reported in patients using dihydroergotamine mesylate nasal spray. However, the potential for adverse cardiac events exists. Serious adverse cardiac events, including acute myocardial infarction, life-threatening disturbances of cardiac rhythm, and death have been reported to have occurred following the administration of dihydroergotamine mesylate injection. Considering the extent of use of dihydroergotamine mesylate in patients with migraine, the incidence of these events is extremely low.

DRUG-ASSOCIATED CEREBROVASCULAR EVENTS AND FATALITIES

Cerebral hemorrhage, subarachnoid hemorrhage, stroke, and other cerebrovascular events have been reported in patients treated with dihydroergotamine mesylate injection; and some have resulted in fatalities. In a number of cases, it appears possible that the cerebrovascular events were primary, the dihydroergotamine mesylate injection having been administered in the incorrect belief that the symptoms experienced were a consequence of migraine, when they were not. It should be noted that patients with migraine may be at increased risk of certain cerebrovascular events (*e.g.*, stroke, hemorrhage, transient ischemic attack).

OTHER VASOSPASM RELATED EVENTS

Dihydroergotamine mesylate nasal spray, like other ergot alkaloids, may cause vasospastic reactions other than coronary artery vasospasm. Myocardial and peripheral vascular ischemia have been reported with dihydroergotamine mesylate nasal spray.

Dihydroergotamine mesylate nasal spray associated vasospastic phenomena may also cause muscle pains, numbness, coldness, pallor, and cyanosis of the digits. In patients with compromised circulation, persistent vasospasm may result in gangrene or death, dihydroergotamine mesylate nasal spray should be discontinued immediately if signs or symptoms of vasoconstriction develop.

INCREASE IN BLOOD PRESSURE

Significant elevation in blood pressure has been reported on rare occasions in patients with and without a history of hypertension treated with dihydroergotamine mesylate nasal spray and dihydroergotamine mesylate injection. Dihydroergotamine mesylate nasal spray is contraindicated in patients with uncontrolled hypertension. (See CONTRAINDICATIONS.)

An 18% increase in mean pulmonary artery pressure was seen following dosing with another $5HT_1$ agonist in a study evaluating subjects undergoing cardiac catheterization.

LOCAL IRRITATION

Approximately 30% of patients using dihydroergotamine mesylate nasal spray (compared to 9% of placebo patients) have reported irritation in the nose, throat, and/or disturbances in taste. Irritative symptoms include congestion, burning sensation, dryness, paraesthesia, discharge, epistaxis, pain, or soreness. The symptoms were predominantly mild to moderate in severity and transient. In approximately 70% of the above mentioned cases, the symptoms resolved within 4 hours after dosing with dihydroergotamine mesylate nasal spray. Examinations of the nose and throat in a small subset (n=66) of study participants treated for up to 36 months (range 1-36 months) did not reveal any clinically noticeable injury. Other than this limited number of patients, the consequences of extended and repeated use of dihydroergotamine mesylate nasal spray on the nasal and/or respiratory mucosa have not been systematically evaluated in patients.

Nasal tissue in animals treated with dihydroergotamine mesylate daily at nasal cavity surface area exposures (in mg/mm^2) that were equal to or less than those achieved in humans receiving the maximum recommended daily dose of 0.08 mg/kg/day showed mild mucosal irritation characterized by mucous cell and transitional cell hyperplasia and squamous cell metaplasia. Changes in rat nasal mucosa at 64 weeks were less severe than at 13 weeks. Local effects on respiratory tissue after chronic intranasal dosing in animals have not been evaluated.

PRECAUTIONS

GENERAL

Dihydroergotamine mesylate nasal spray may cause coronary artery vasospasm; patients who experience signs or symptoms suggestive of angina following its administration should, therefore, be evaluated for the presence of CAD or a predisposition to variant angina before receiving additional doses. Similarly, patients who experience other symptoms or signs suggestive of decreased arterial flow, such as ischemic bowel syndrome or Raynaud's syndrome following the use of any 5-HT agonist are candidates for further evaluation. (See WARNINGS.)

Fibrotic Complications: See WARNINGS, Fibrotic Complications.

INFORMATION FOR THE PATIENT

To assure safe and effective use of dihydroergotamine mesylate nasal spray, the information and instructions provided in the patient information sheet should be discussed with patients.

Once the nasal spray applicator has been prepared, it should be discarded (with any remaining drug) after 8 hours.

Patients should be advised to report to the physician immediately any of the following: Numbness or tingling in the fingers and toes, muscle pain in the arms and legs, weakness in the legs, pain in the chest, temporary speeding or slowing of the heart rate, swelling, or itching.

Prior to the initial use of the product by a patient, the prescriber should take steps to ensure that the patient understands how to use the product as provided. See the Patient Instructions that are distributed with the prescription and product packaging.

Administration of dihydroergotamine mesylate nasal spray, should not exceed the dosing guidelines and should not be used for chronic daily administration (see DOSAGE AND ADMINISTRATION).

CARCINOGENESIS, MUTAGENESIS, AND IMPAIRMENT OF FERTILITY

Carcinogenesis

Assessment of the carcinogenic potential of dihydroergotamine mesylate in mice and rats is ongoing.

Mutagenesis

Dihydroergotamine mesylate was clastogenic in two *in vitro* chromosomal aberration assays, the V79 Chinese hamster cell assay with metabolic activation and the cultured human peripheral blood lymphocyte assay. There was no evidence of mutagenic potential when dihydroergotamine mesylate was tested in the presence or absence of metabolic activation in two gene mutation assays (the Ames test and the *in vitro* mammalian Chinese hamster V79/HGPRT assay) and in an assay for DNA damage (the rat hepatocyte unscheduled DNA synthesis test). Dihydroergotamine was not clastogenic in the *in vivo* mouse and hamster micronucleus tests.

Impairment of Fertility

There was no evidence of impairment of fertility in rats given intranasal doses of dihydroergotamine mesylate nasal spray up to 1.6 mg/day (associated with mean plasma dihydroergotamine mesylate exposures [AUC] approximately 9-11 times those in humans receiving the MRDD of 4 mg).

PREGNANCY CATEGORY X

See CONTRAINDICATIONS.

NURSING MOTHERS

Ergot drugs are known to inhibit prolactin. It is likely that dihydroergotamine mesylate nasal spray is excreted in human milk, but there are no data on the concentration of dihydroergotamine in human milk. It is known that ergotamine is excreted in breast milk and may cause vomiting, diarrhea, weak pulse, and unstable blood pressure in nursing infants. Because of the potential for these serious adverse events in nursing infants exposed to dihydroergotamine mesylate nasal spray, nursing should not be undertaken with the use of dihydroergotamine mesylate nasal spray. (See CONTRAINDICATIONS.)

PEDIATRIC USE

Safety and effectiveness in pediatric patients have not been established.

USE IN THE ELDERLY

There is no information about the safety and effectiveness of dihydroergotamine mesylate nasal spray in this population because patients over age 65 were excluded from the controlled clinical trials.

DRUG INTERACTIONS

Vasoconstrictors: Dihydroergotamine mesylate nasal spray should not be used with peripheral vasoconstrictors because the combination may cause synergistic elevation of blood pressure.

Sumatriptan: Sumatriptan has been reported to cause coronary artery vasospasm, and its effect could be additive with dihydroergotamine mesylate nasal spray. Sumatriptan and dihydroergotamine mesylate nasal spray should not be taken within 24 hours of each other. (See CONTRAINDICATIONS.)

Beta Blockers: Although the results of a clinical study did not indicate a safety problem associated with the administration of dihydroergotamine mesylate nasal spray to subjects already receiving propranolol, there have been reports that propranolol may potentiate the vasoconstrictive action of ergotamine by blocking the vasodilating property of epinephrine.

Nicotine: Nicotine may provoke vasoconstriction in some patients, predisposing to a greater ischemic response to ergot therapy.

CYP 3A4 Inhibitors (e.g., macrolide antibiotics and protease inhibitors): See CONTRAINDICATIONS and WARNINGS.

SSRIs: Weakness, hyperreflexia, and incoordination have been reported rarely when $5HT_1$ agonists have been co-administered with SSRI's (*e.g.*, fluoxetine, fluvoxamine, paroxetine, sertraline). There have been no reported cases from spontaneous reports of drug interaction between SSRI's and dihydroergotamine mesylate nasal spray or injection.

Oral Contraceptives: The effect of oral contraceptives on the pharmacokinetics of dihydroergotamine mesylate nasal spray has not been studied.

ADVERSE REACTIONS

During clinical studies and the foreign postmarketing experience with dihydroergotamine mesylate nasal spray there have been no fatalities due to cardiac events.

Serious cardiac events, including some that have been fatal, have occurred following use of the parenteral form of dihydroergotamine mesylate injection, but are extremely rare. Events reported have included coronary artery vasospasm, transient myocardial ischemia, myocardial infarction, ventricular tachycardia, and ventricular fibrillation. (See CONTRAINDICATIONS, WARNINGS, and PRECAUTIONS.)

Fibrotic complications have been reported in association with long term use of injectable dihydroergotamine mesylate (see WARNINGS, Fibrotic Complications).

INCIDENCE IN CONTROLLED CLINICAL TRIALS

Of the 1796 patients and subjects treated with dihydroergotamine mesylate nasal spray doses 2 mg or less in US and foreign clinical studies, 26 (1.4%) discontinued because of adverse events.

The adverse events associated with discontinuation were, in decreasing order of frequency: Rhinitis 13, dizziness 2, facial edema 2, and 1 each due to cold sweats, accidental trauma, depression, elective surgery, somnolence, allergy, vomiting, hypotension, and paraesthesia.

The most commonly reported adverse events associated with the use of dihydroergotamine mesylate nasal spray during placebo-controlled, double-blind studies for the treatment of migraine headache and not reported at an equal incidence by placebo-treated patients were rhinitis, altered sense of taste, application site reactions, dizziness, nausea, and vomiting. The events cited reflect experience gained under closely monitored conditions of clinical trials in a highly selected patient population. In actual clinical practice or in other clinical trials, these frequency estimates may not apply, as the conditions of use, reporting behavior, and the kinds of patients treated may differ.

Dihydroergotamine mesylate nasal spray was generally well tolerated. In most instances these events were transient and self-limited and did not result in patient discontinuation from a study. TABLE 3 summarizes the incidence rates of adverse events reported by at least 1% of patients who received dihydroergotamine mesylate nasal spray for the treatment of migraine headaches during placebo-controlled, double-blind clinical studies and were more frequent than in those patients receiving placebo.

TABLE 3 *Adverse Events Reported by at Least 1% of the Dihydroergotamine Mesylate Nasal Spray Treated Patients and Occurred More Frequently Than in the Placebo-Group in the Migraine Placebo-Controlled Trials*

	Dihydroergotamine Mesylate Nasal Spray n=597	Placebo n=631
Respiratory System		
Rhinitis	26%	7%
Pharyngitis	3%	1%
Sinusitis	1%	1%
Gastrointestinal System		
Nausea	10%	4%
Vomiting	4%	1%
Diarrhea	2%	<1%
Special Senses, Other		
Altered sense of taste	8%	1%
Application Site		
Application site reaction	6%	2%
Central and Peripheral Nervous System		
Dizziness	4%	2%
Somnolence	3%	2%
Paraesthesia	2%	2%
Body as a Whole, General		
Hot flushes	1%	<1%
Fatigue	1%	1%
Asthenia	1%	0%
Autonomic Nervous System		
Mouth dry	1%	1%
Musculoskeletal System		
Stiffness	1%	<1%

OTHER ADVERSE EVENTS DURING CLINICAL TRIALS

In the paragraphs that follow, the frequencies of less commonly reported adverse clinical events are presented. Because the reports include events observed in open and uncontrolled studies, the role of dihydroergotamine mesylate nasal spray in their causation cannot be reliably determined. Furthermore, variability associated with adverse event reporting, the terminology used to describe adverse events, etc., limit the value of the quantitative frequency estimates provided. Event frequencies are calculated as the number of patients who used dihydroergotamine mesylate nasal spray in placebo-controlled trials and reported an event divided by the total number of patients (n=1796) exposed to dihydroergotamine mesylate nasal spray. All reported events are included except those already listed in TABLE 3, those too general to be informative, and those not reasonably associated with the use of the drug. Events are further classified within body system categories and enumerated in order of decreasing frequency using the following definitions: *frequent* adverse events are defined as those occurring in at least 1/100 patients; *infrequent* adverse events are those occurring in 1/100 to 1/1000 patients; and *rare* adverse events are those occurring in fewer than 1/1000 patients.

Skin and Appendages: *Infrequent:* Petechia, pruritus, rash, cold clammy skin; *Rare:* Papular rash, urticaria, herpes simplex.

Musculoskeletal: *Infrequent:* Cramps, myalgia, muscular weakness, dystonia; *Rare:* Arthralgia, involuntary muscle contractions, rigidity.

Central and Peripheral Nervous System: *Infrequent:* Confusion, tremor, hypoesthesia, vertigo; *Rare:* Speech disorder, hyperkinesia, stupor, abnormal gait, aggravated migraine.

Autonomic Nervous System: *Infrequent:* Increased sweating.

Special Senses: *Infrequent:* Sense of smell altered, photophobia, conjunctivitis, abnormal lacrimation, abnormal vision, tinnitus, earache; *Rare:* Eye pain.

Psychiatric: *Infrequent:* Nervousness, euphoria, insomnia, concentration impaired; *Rare:* Anxiety, anorexia, depression.

Gastrointestinal: *Infrequent:* Abdominal pain, dyspepsia, dysphagia, hiccup; *Rare:* Increased salivation, esophagospasm.

Cardiovascular: *Infrequent:* Edema, palpitation, tachycardia; *Rare:* Hypotension, peripheral ischemia, angina.

Respiratory System: *Infrequent:* Dyspnea, upper respiratory tract infections; *Rare:* Bronchospasm, bronchitis, pleural pain, epistaxis.

Urinary System: *Infrequent:* Increased frequency of micturition, cystitis.

Reproductive, Female: *Rare:* Pelvic inflammation, vaginitis.

Body as a Whole — General: *Infrequent:* Feeling cold, malaise, rigors, fever, periorbital edema; *Rare:* Flu-like symptoms, shock, loss of voice, yawning.

Application Site: *Infrequent:* Local anesthesia.

POST-INTRODUCTION REPORTS

Voluntary reports of adverse events temporally associated with dihydroergotamine products used in the management of migraine that have been received since the introduction of the injectable formulation are included in this section save for those already listed above. Because of their source (open and uncontrolled clinical use), whether or not events reported in association with the use of dihydroergotamine are causally related to it cannot be determined.

There have been reports of pleural and retroperitoneal fibrosis in patients following prolonged daily use of injectable dihydroergotamine mesylate. Dihydroergotamine mesylate nasal spray is not recommended for prolonged daily use. (See DOSAGE AND ADMINISTRATION.)

DOSAGE AND ADMINISTRATION

The solution used in dihydroergotamine mesylate nasal spray (4 mg/ml) is intended for intranasal use and must not be injected.

In clinical trials, dihydroergotamine mesylate nasal spray has been effective for the acute treatment of migraine headaches with or without aura. One spray (0.5 mg) of dihydroergotamine mesylate nasal spray should be administered in each nostril. Fifteen (15) minutes later, an additional 1 spray (0.5 mg) of dihydroergotamine mesylate nasal spray should be administered in each nostril, for a total dosage of 4 sprays (2.0 mg) of dihydroergotamine mesylate nasal spray. Studies have shown no additional benefit from acute doses greater than 2.0 mg for a single migraine administration. The safety of doses greater than 3.0 mg in a 24 hour period and 4.0 mg in a 7 day period has not been established.

Dihydroergotamine mesylate nasal spray, should not be used for chronic daily administration.

Prior to administration, the pump must be primed (*i.e.,* squeeze 4 times) before use. (See the Patient Instruction Booklet from manufacturer.)

Once the nasal spray applicator has been prepared, it should be discarded (with any remaining drug in opened ampul) after 8 hours.

HOW SUPPLIED

Migranal Nasal Spray is available (as a clear, colorless to faintly yellow solution) in 1 ml amber glass ampuls containing 4 mg of dihydroergotamine mesylate.

Migranal Nasal Spray is provided in individual kits. The kits consist of 4 unit dose trays, a patient instruction booklet, 1 assembly case, and 1 patient information sheet packed in a carton. Each unit dose tray contains 1 ampul, a nasal spray applicator, and a breaker cap on the ampul.

Storage: Store below 25°C (77°F). Do not refrigerate or freeze.

PRODUCT LISTING - EQUIVALENTS NOT AVAILABLE

Solution - Injectable - 1 mg/ml

1 ml x 10	$441.60	D.H.E. 45, Novartis Pharmaceuticals	00078-0041-01
1 ml x 10	$441.60	D.H.E. 45, Xcel Pharmaceuticals Inc	66490-0041-01

Spray - Nasal - 4 mg/ml

1 ml x 4	$125.78	MIGRANAL, Novartis Pharmaceuticals	00078-0245-98
1 ml x 4	$125.78	MIGRANAL, Xcel Pharmaceuticals Inc	66490-0245-98

Diltiazem Hydrochloride (001069)

For related information, see the comparative table section in Appendix A.

Categories: Angina, chronic stable; Angina, variant; Fibrillation, atrial; Flutter, atrial; Hypertension, essential; Tachycardia, paroxysmal supraventricular; Pregnancy Category C; FDA Approved 1982 Nov

Drug Classes: Antiarrhythmics, class IV; Calcium channel blockers

Brand Names: **Cardizem**; Dilacor XR; Tiazac

Foreign Brand Availability: Adizem-CD (Israel); Altiazem (Bulgaria; Hong-Kong; Italy); Altiazem Retard (Italy); Altiazem RR (Russia); Angiotrofin (Colombia; Mexico); Angiotrofin Retard (Costa-Rica; Dominican-Republic; El-Salvador; Guatemala; Honduras; Mexico; Nicaragua; Panama); Angiozem (Philippines); Angizem (Italy; Thailand); Angoral (Colombia); Anzem (South-Africa); Apo-diltiazem (New-Zealand); Auscard (Australia); Beatizem (Singapore); Bi-Tildiem (France); Calcicard (England); Calnurs (Japan); Cardcal (Australia); Cardiazem (Korea); Cardiben S.R. (Korea); Cardil (Bulgaria; Denmark; Malaysia; Russia; Taiwan); Cardil Retard (Greece); Cardiosta LP (France); Cardium (Hong-Kong; Singapore); Cardizem CD (Australia; Canada; New-Zealand); Cardizem Retard (Denmark; Finland; Sweden); Cardizem SR (Canada); Carex (Argentina); Cartia XT (Taiwan); Cascor XL (Thailand); Cirilen (Ecuador); Cirilen AP (Ecuador); Coras (Australia; New-Zealand); Dazil (Bahrain; Cyprus; Egypt; Iran; Iraq; Israel; Jordan; Kuwait; Lebanon; Libya; Oman; Qatar; Republic-of-Yemen; Saudi-Arabia; Syria; United-Arab-Emirates); Deltazen (France); Diatal (South-Africa); Diladel (Italy); Dilatam (Israel; Philippines; Singapore; South-Africa; Thailand); Dilatam 120 (Israel); Dilatame (Austria); Dilcard (New-Zealand); Dilcardia (Benin; Burkina-Faso; Ethiopia; Gambia; Ghana; Guinea; India; Ivory-Coast; Kenya; Liberia; Malawi; Mali; Mauritania; Mauritius; Morocco; Niger; Nigeria; Senegal; Seychelles; Sierra-Leone; South-Africa; Sudan; Tanzania; Tunia; Uganda; Zambia; Zimbabwe); Dilcor (Denmark); Dilem (Thailand); Dilem SR (Thailand); Dilfar (Portugal); Dilgard (Benin; Burkina-Faso; Ethiopia; Gambia; Ghana; Guinea; Ivory-Coast; Kenya; Liberia; Malawi; Mali; Mauritania; Mauritius; Morocco; Niger; Nigeria; Senegal; Seychelles; Sierra-Leone; Sudan; Tanzania; Tunia; Uganda; Zambia; Zimbabwe); Dilren (Russia); Dilrene (Czech-Republic; France; Hungary); Dilso (Indonesia); Diltahexal (Australia; Germany); Diltam (Ireland); Diltan (Bahamas; Barbados; Belize; Bermuda; Curacao; Guyana; Jamaica; Netherland-Antilles; Puerto-Rico; Surinam; Trinidad); Diltan SR (Bahrain; Cyprus; Egypt; Iran; Iraq; Israel; Jordan; Kuwait; Lebanon; Libya; Oman; Qatar; Republic-of-Yemen; Saudi-Arabia; Syria; United-Arab-Emirates); Diltelan (Korea; Taiwan); Diltiamax (Australia); Diltiasyn (Colombia); Diltime (Benin; Burkina-Faso; Ethiopia; Gambia; Ghana; Guinea; Ivory-Coast; Kenya; Liberia; Malawi; Mali; Mauritania; Mauritius; Morocco; Niger; Nigeria; Senegal; Seychelles; Sierra-Leone; South-Africa; Sudan; Tanzania; Tunia; Uganda; Zambia; Zimbabwe); Dilzem (Australia; Austria; Bahamas; Bahrain; Barbados; Belize; Bermuda; Bulgaria; Curacao; Cyprus; Czech-Republic; Egypt; Finland; Germany; Guyana; Hungary; India; Iran; Iraq; Israel; Jamaica; Jordan; Kuwait; Lebanon; Libya; Netherland-Antilles; New-Zealand; Oman; Philippines; Poland; Puerto-Rico; Qatar; Republic-of-Yemen; Russia; Saudi-Arabia; Surinam; Switzerland; Syria; Thailand; Trinidad; United-Arab-Emirates); Dilzem Retard (Austria; Bahrain; Bulgaria; Cyprus; Czech-Republic; Egypt; Germany; Iran; Iraq; Israel; Jordan; Kuwait; Lebanon; Libya; Oman; Qatar; Republic-of-Yemen; Saudi-Arabia; Syria; United-Arab-Emirates); Dilzem RR (Switzerland); Dilzem SR (China; England; New-Zealand); Dilzene (Italy); Dilzereal 90 Retard (Germany); Dilzicardin (Germany); Dinisor (Spain); Dinisor Retard (Spain); Dodexen (Peru); Dodexen A.P. (Peru); DTM (India); Dyalac (Philippines); Filazem (Philippines); Gadoserin (Japan); Hagen (Taiwan); Helsibon (Japan); Herben (Korea); Herbesser (Indonesia; Japan; Malaysia; Taiwan; Thailand); Herbesser 60 (Malaysia; Thailand); Herbesser R100 (Japan); Herbesser 90 SR (Hong-Kong; Malaysia; Thailand); Herbesser 180 SR (Hong-Kong); Herbesser R200 (Japan); Herbessor (China); Hesor (Taiwan); Iski (India); Iski-90 SR (India); Kaizem CD (India); Lacerol (Dominican-Republic; El-Salvador; Guatemala; Honduras; Nicaragua); Levodex (Israel); Levozem (Israel); Lytelsen (Japan); Masdil (Spain); Miocardie (Taiwan); Mono-Tildiem SR (Singapore); Myonil (Denmark); Myonil Retard (Denmark); Pazeadin (Japan); Presoken (Mexico); Tazem (Taiwan); Tiadil (Portugal); Tilazem (Colombia; Ecuador; Mexico; Peru; South-Africa); Tilazem 90 (South-Africa); Tildiem (Belgium; England; France; Greece; Italy; Malaysia; Netherlands; Switzerland); Tildiem CR (Netherlands); Tildiem LA (England); Tildiem Retard (Greece); Zemtrial (Philippines); Zildem (South-Africa); Ziruvate (Japan)

Cost of Therapy: $81.66 (Angina; Cardizem; 60 mg; 3 tablets/day; 30 day supply)
$97.88 (Hypertension; Cardizem SR; 120 mg; 2 capsules/day; 30 day supply)

INTRAVENOUS

DESCRIPTION

Note: The trade names have been used throughout this monograph for clarity.

Diltiazem hydrochloride is a calcium ion influx inhibitor (slow channel blocker or calcium channel antagonist). Chemically, diltiazem hydrochloride is 1,5-benzothiazepin-4(5H)one,3-(acetyloxy),-5-[2-(dimethylamino)ethyl]-2,3-dihydro-2-(4-methoxyphenyl)-, monohydrochloride,(+)cis-.

Diltiazem hydrochloride is a white to off-white crystalline powder with a bitter taste. It is soluble in water, methanol, and chloroform. It has a molecular weight of 450.98.

CARDIZEM INJECTABLE

Cardizem injectable is a clear, colorless, sterile, nonpyrogenic solution. It has a pH range of 3.7-4.1.

Cardizem injectable is for direct intravenous (IV) bolus injection and continuous IV infusion.

25 mg, 5 ml vial: Each sterile vial contains 25 mg diltiazem hydrochloride, 3.75 mg citric acid, 3.25 mg sodium citrate dihydrate, 357 mg sorbitol solution, and water for injection up to 5 ml. Sodium hydroxide or hydrochloric acid is used for pH adjustment.

50 mg, 10 ml vial: Each sterile vial contains 50 mg diltiazem hydrochloride, 7.5 mg citric acid, 6.5 mg sodium citrate dihydrate, 714 mg sorbitol solution, and water for injection up to 10 ml. Sodium hydroxide or hydrochloric acid is used for pH adjustment.

CARDIZEM LYO-JECT SYRINGE

Cardizem Lyo-Ject syringe, after reconstitution contains a clear, colorless, sterile, nonpyrogenic solution. It has a pH range of 4.0-7.0.

Cardizem Lyo-Ject syringe after reconstitution is for direct IV bolus injection and continuous IV infusion.

Cardizem Lyo-Ject syringe 25 mg syringe is available in a dual chamber, disposable syringe. Chamber 1 contains lyophilized powder comprised of diltiazem HCl 25 mg and mannitol 37.5 mg. Chamber 2 contains sterile diluent composed of 5 ml water for injection with 0.5% benzyl alcohol, and 0.6% sodium chloride.

CARDIZEM MONOVIAL

Cardizem Monovial, after reconstitution in an infusion bag, produces a clear, colorless, sterile, nonpyrogenic solution.

Cardizem Monovial for continuous IV infusion is available in a glass vial with transfer needle set. The vial contains lyophilized powder comprised of diltiazem HCl 100 mg and mannitol 75 mg.

CLINICAL PHARMACOLOGY

MECHANISM OF ACTION

Cardizem inhibits the influx of calcium (Ca^{2+}) ions during membrane depolarization of cardiac and vascular smooth muscle. The therapeutic benefits of Cardizem in supraventricular tachycardias are related to its ability to slow AV nodal conduction time and prolong AV nodal refractoriness. Cardizem exhibits frequency (use) dependent effects on AV nodal conduction such that it may selectively reduce the heart rate during tachycardias involving the AV node with little or no effect on normal AV nodal conduction at normal heart rates.

Cardizem slows the ventricular rate in patients with a rapid ventricular response during atrial fibrillation or atrial flutter. Cardizem converts paroxysmal supraventricular tachycardia (PSVT) to normal sinus rhythm by interrupting the reentry circuit in AV nodal reentrant tachycardias and reciprocating tachycardias, *e.g.*, Wolff-Parkinson-White syndrome (WPW). Cardizem prolongs the sinus cycle length. It has no effect on the sinus node recovery time or on the sinoatrial conduction time in patients without SA nodal dysfunction. Cardizem has no significant electrophysiologic effects on tissues in the heart that are fast sodium channel dependent, *e.g.*, His-Purkinje tissue, atrial and ventricular muscle, and extranodal accessory pathways.

Like other calcium channel antagonists, because of its effect on vascular smooth muscle, Cardizem decreases total peripheral resistance resulting in a decrease in both systolic and diastolic blood pressure.

HEMODYNAMICS

In patients with cardiovascular disease, Cardizem injectable administered intravenously in single bolus doses, followed in some cases by a continuous infusion, reduced blood pressure, systemic vascular resistance, the rate-pressure product, and coronary vascular resistance and increased coronary blood flow. In a limited number of studies of patients with compromised myocardium (severe congestive heart failure, acute myocardial infarction, hypertrophic cardiomyopathy), administration of IV diltiazem produced no significant effect on contractility, left ventricular end diastolic pressure, or pulmonary capillary wedge pressure. The mean ejection fraction and cardiac output/index remained unchanged or increased. Maximal hemodynamic effects usually occurred within 2-5 minutes of an injection. However, in rare instances, worsening of congestive heart failure has been reported in patients with preexisting impaired ventricular function.

PHARMACODYNAMICS

The prolongation of PR interval correlated significantly with plasma diltiazem concentration in normal volunteers using the Sigmoidal E_{max} model. Changes in heart rate, systolic blood pressure, and diastolic blood pressure did not correlate with diltiazem plasma concentration in normal volunteers. Reduction in mean arterial pressure correlated linearly with diltiazem plasma concentration in a group of hypertensive patients.

In patients with atrial fibrillation and atrial flutter, a significant correlation was observed between the percent reduction in HR and plasma diltiazem concentration using the Sigmoidal E_{max} model. Based on this relationship, the mean plasma diltiazem concentration required to produce a 20% decrease in heart rate was determined to be 80 ng/ml. Mean plasma diltiazem concentrations of 130 ng/ml and 300 ng/ml were determined to produce reduction in heart rate of 30% and 40%.

PHARMACOKINETICS AND METABOLISM

Following a single IV injection in healthy male volunteers, Cardizem appears to obey linear pharmacokinetics over a dose range of 10.5-21.0 mg. The plasma elimination half-life is approximately 3.4 hours. The apparent volume of distribution of Cardizem is approximately 305 L. Cardizem is extensively metabolized in the liver with a systemic clearance of approximately 65 L/h.

After constant rate IV infusion to healthy male volunteers, diltiazem exhibits nonlinear pharmacokinetics over an infusion range of 4.8-13.2 mg/h for 24 hours. Over this infusion range, as the dose is increased, systemic clearance decreases from 64-48 L/h while the plasma elimination half-life increases from 4.1-4.9 hours. The apparent volume of distribution remains unchanged (360-391 L). In patients with atrial fibrillation or atrial flutter, diltiazem systemic clearance has been found to be decreased compared to healthy volunteers. In patients administered bolus doses ranges from 2.5-38.5 mg, systemic clearance averaged 36 L/h. In patients administered continuous infusions at 10 mg/h or 15 mg/h for 24 hours, diltiazem systemic clearance averaged 42 L/h and 31 L/h, respectively.

Based on the results of pharmacokinetic studies in healthy volunteers administered different ***oral*** Cardizem formulations, constant rate IV infusions of Cardizem at 3, 5, 7, and 11 mg/h are predicted to produce steady-state plasma diltiazem concentrations equivalent to 120, 180, 240, and 360 mg total daily oral doses of Cardizem tablets or Cardizem SR capsules.

After oral administration, Cardizem undergoes extensive metabolism in man by deacetylation, N-demethylation, and O-demethylation via cytochrome P-450 (oxidative metabolism) in addition to conjugation. Metabolites N-monodesmethyldiltiazem, desacetyldiltiazem, desacetyl-N-monodesmethyldiltiazem, desacetyl-O-desmethyldiltiazem, and desacetyl-N, O-desmethyldiltiazem have been identified in human urine. Following oral administration, 2-4% of the unchanged Cardizem appears in the urine. Drugs which induce or inhibit hepatic microsomal enzymes may alter diltiazem disposition.

Following single IV injection of Cardizem, however, plasma concentration of N-monodesmethyldiltiazem and desacetyldiltiazem, two principal metabolites found in plasma after oral administration, are typically not detected. These metabolites are observed, however, following 24 hour constant rate IV infusion. Total radioactivity measurement following short IV administration in healthy volunteers suggests the presence of other unidentified metabolites which attain higher concentrations than those of diltiazem and are more slowly eliminated; half-life of total radioactivity is about 20 hours compared to 2-5 hours for diltiazem.

Cardizem is 70-80% bound to plasma proteins. *In vitro* studies suggest $alpha_1$-acid glycoprotein binds approximately 40% of the drug at clinically significant concentrations. Albumin appears to bind approximately 30% of the drug, while other constituents bind the remaining bound fraction. Competitive *in vitro* ligand binding studies have shown that ardizem binding is not altered by therapeutic concentration of digoxin, phenytoin, hydrochlorothiazide, indomethacin, phenylbutazone, propranolol, salicylic acid, tolbutamide, or warfarin.

Renal insufficiency, or even end-stage renal disease, does not appear to influence diltiazem disposition following ***oral*** administration. Liver cirrhosis was shown to reduce diltiazem's apparent ***oral*** clearance and prolong its half-life.

INDICATIONS AND USAGE

Cardizem injectable, Cardizem Lyo-Ject syringe, or Cardizem Monovial are indicated for the following:

Atrial Fibrillation or Atrial Flutter: Temporary control of rapid ventricular rate in atrial fibrillation or atrial flutter. It should not be used in patients with atrial fibrillation or atrial flutter associated with an accessory bypass tract such as in Wolff-Parkinson-White (WPW) syndrome or short PR syndrome. In addition, Cardizem injectable or Cardizem Lyo-Ject syringe are indicated for:

Proxysmal Supraventricular Tachycardia: Rapid conversion of paroxysmal supraventricular tachycardias (PSVT) to sinus rhythm. This includes AV nodal reentrant tachycardias and reciprocating tachycardias associated with an extranodal accessory pathyway such as the WPW syndrome or short PR syndrome. Unless otherwise contraindicated, appropriate vagal maneuvers should be attempted prior to administration of Cardizem injectable or Cardizem Lyo-Ject syringe.

The use of Cardizem injectable, Cardizem Lyo-Ject syringe, or Cardizem Monovial should be undertaken with caution when the patient is compromised hemodynamically or is taking other drugs that decrease any or all of the following: peripheral resistance, myocardial filling, myocardial contractility, or electrical impulse propagation in the myocardium.

For either indication and particularly when employing continuous IV infusion, the setting should include continuous monitoring of the ECG and frequent measurement of blood pressure. A defibrillator and emergency equipment should be readily available.

In domestic controlled trials in patients with atrial fibrillation or atrial flutter, bolus administration of Cardizem injectable was effective in reducing heart rate by at least 20% in 95% of patients. Cardizem injectable rarely converts atrial fibrillation or atrial flutter to normal sinus rhythm. Following administration of 1 or 2 IV bolus doses of Cardizem injectable, response usually occurs within 3 minutes and maximal heart rate reduction generally occurs in 2-7 minutes. Heart rate reduction may last from 1-3 hours. If hypotension occurs, it is generally short-lived, but may last from 1-3 hours.

A 24 hour continuous infusion of Cardizem injectable in the treatment of atrial fibrillation or atrial flutter maintained at least a 20% heart rate reduction during the infusion in 83% of patients. Upon discontinuation of infusion, heart rate reduction may last from 0.5 hours to more than 10 hours (median duration 7 hours). Hypotension, if it occurs, may be similarly persistent.

In the controlled clinical trials, 3.2% of patients required some form of intervention (typically, use of IV fluids or the Trendelenburg position) for blood pressure support following Cardizem injectable.

In domestic controlled trials, bolus administration of Cardizem injectable was effective in converting PSVT to normal sinus rhythm in 88% of patients within 3 minutes of the first or second bolus dose.

Symptoms associated with the arrhythmia were improved in conjunction with decreased heart rate or conversion to normal sinus rhythm following administration of Cardizem injectable.

CONTRAINDICATIONS

Injectable forms of diltiazem are contraindicated in:

- Patients with sick sinus syndrome except in the presence of a functioning ventricular pacemaker.
- Patients with second- or third-degree AV block except in the presence of a functioning ventricular pacemaker.
- Patients with severe hypotension or cardiogenic shock.
- Patients who have demonstrated hypersensitivity to the drug.
- IV diltiazem and IV beta-blockers should not be administered together or in close proximity (within a few hours).
- Patients with atrial fibrillation or atrial flutter associated with an accessory bypass tract such as in WPW syndrome or short PR syndrome. As with other agents which slow AV nodal conduction and do not prolong the refractoriness of the accessory pathway (*e.g.,* verapamil, digoxin), in rare instances patients in atrial fibrillation or atrial flutter associated with an accessory bypass tract may experience a potentially life-threatening increase in heart rate accompanied by hypotension when treated with injectable forms of diltiazem. As such, the initial use of injectable forms of diltiazem should be, if possible, in a setting where monitoring and resuscitation capabilities, including DC cardioversion/defibrillation, are present. Once familiarity of the patient's response is established, use in an office setting may be acceptable.
- Patients with ventricular tachycardia. Administration of other calcium channel blockers to patients with wide complex tachycardia (QRS $\geq$0.12 seconds) has resulted in hemodynamic deterioration and ventricular fibrillation. It is important that an accurate pretreatment diagnosis distinguish wide complex QRS tachycardia of supraventricular origin from that of ventricular origin prior to administration of injectable forms of diltiazem.
- In newborns, due to the presence of benzyl alcohol (Cardizem Lyo-Ject syringe only).

WARNINGS

CARDIAC CONDUCTION

Diltiazem prolongs AV nodal conduction and refractoriness that may rarely result in second- or third-degree AV block in sinus rhythm. Concomitant use of diltiazem with agents known to affect cardiac conduction may result in additive effects (see DRUG INTERACTIONS). If high-degree AV block occurs in sinus rhythm, IV diltiazem should be discontinued and appropriate supportive measures instituted.

CONGESTIVE HEART FAILURE

Although diltiazem has a negative inotropic effect in isolated animal tissue preparations, hemodynamic studies in humans with normal ventricular function and in patients with a compromised myocardium, such as severe CHF, acute MI, and hypertrophic cardiomyopathy, have not shown a reduction in cardiac index nor consistent negative effects on contractility (dp/dt). Administration of oral diltiazem in patients with acute myocardial infarction and pulmonary congestion documented by x-ray on admission is contraindicated. Experience with the use of Cardizem injectable in patients with impaired ventricular function is limited. Caution should be exercised when using the drug in such patients.

HYPOTENSION

Decreases in blood pressure associated with Cardizem injectable therapy may occasionally result in symptomatic hypotension (3.2%). The use of IV diltiazem for control of ventricular response in patients with supraventricular arrhythmias should be undertaken with caution when the patient is compromised hemodynamically. In addition, caution should be used in patients taking other drugs that decrease peripheral resistance, intravascular volume, myocardial contractility or conduction.

ACUTE HEPATIC INJURY

In rare instances, significant elevations in enzymes such as alkaline phosphatase, LDH, SGOT, SGPT, and other phenomena consistent with acute hepatic injury have been noted following oral diltiazem. Therefore, the potential for acute hepatic injury exists following administration of IV diltiazem.

VENTRICULAR PREMATURE BEATS (VPBS)

VPBs may be present on conversion of PSVT to sinus rhythm with Cardizem injectable. These VPBs are transient, are typically considered to be benign, and appear to have no clinical significance. Similar ventricular complexes have been noted during cardioversion, other pharmacologic therapy, and during spontaneous conversion of PSVT to sinus rhythm.

PRECAUTIONS

GENERAL

Cardizem is extensively metabolized by the liver and excreted by the kidneys and in bile. The drug should be used with caution in patients with impaired renal or hepatic function (see WARNINGS). High IV dosages (4.5 mg/kg tid) administered to dogs resulted in significant bradycardia and alterations in AV conduction. In subacute and chronic dog and rat studies designed to produce toxicity, high oral doses of diltiazem were associated with hepatic damage. In special subacute hepatic studies, oral doses of 125 mg/kg and higher in rats were associated with histological changes in the liver, which were reversible when the drug was discontinued. In dogs, oral doses of 20 mg/kg were also associated with hepatic changes; however, these changes were reversible with continued dosing.

Dermatologic events progressing to erythema multiforme and/or exfoliative dermatitis have been infrequently reported following oral diltiazem. Therefore, the potential for these dermatologic reactions exists following exposure to IV diltiazem. Should a dermatologic reaction persist, the drug should be discontinued.

CARCINOGENESIS, MUTAGENESIS, AND IMPAIRMENT OF FERTILITY

A 24 month study in rats at oral dosage levels of up to 100 mg/kg/day and a 21 month study in mice at oral dosage levels of up to 30 mg/kg/day showed no evidence of carcinogenicity. There was also no mutagenic response *in vitro* or *in vivo* in mammalian cell assays or *in vitro* in bacteria. No evidence of impaired fertility was observed in a study performed in male and female rats at oral dosages of up to 100 mg/kg/day.

PREGNANCY CATEGORY C

Reproduction studies have been conducted in mice, rats, and rabbits.

Administration of oral doses ranging from 5-10 times greater (on a mg/kg basis) than the daily recommended oral antianginal therapeutic dose has resulted in embryo and fetal lethality. These doses, in some studies, have been reported to cause skeletal abnormalities. In the perinatal/postnatal studies there was some reduction in early individual pup weights and survival rates. There was an increased incidence of stillbirths at doses of 20 times the human oral antianginal dose or greater.

There are no well-controlled studies in pregnant women; therefore, use Cardizem in pregnant women only if the potential benefit justifies the potential risk to the fetus.

NURSING MOTHERS

Diltiazem is excreted in human milk. One report with oral diltiazem suggests that concentrations in breast milk may approximate serum levels. If use of Cardizem is deemed essential, an alternative method of infant feeding should be instituted.

PEDIATRIC USE

Safety and effectiveness in pediatric patients have not been established.

DRUG INTERACTIONS

Due to potential for additive effects, caution is warranted in patients receiving Cardizem injectable, Cardizem Lyo-Ject syringe, or Cardizem Monovial concomitantly with other agent(s) known to affect cardiac contractility and/or SA or AV node conduction (see WARNINGS).

As with all drugs, care should be exercised when treating patients with multiple medications. Cardizem undergoes extensive metabolism by the cytochrome P-450 mixed function oxidase system. Although specific pharmacokinetic drug-drug interaction studies have not been conducted with single IV injection or constant rate IV infusion, coadministration of injectable diltiazem with other agents which primarily undergo the same route of biotransformation may result in competitive inhibition of metabolism.

DIGITALIS

IV diltiazem has been administered to patients receiving either IV or oral digitalis therapy. The combination of the two drugs was well tolerated without serious adverse effects. However, since both drugs affect AV nodal conduction, patients should be monitored for excessive slowing of the heart rate and/or AV block.

BETA-BLOCKERS

IV diltiazem has been administered to patients on chronic oral beta-blocker therapy. The combination of the two drugs was generally well tolerated without serious adverse effects. If IV diltiazem is administered to patients receiving chronic oral beta-blocker therapy, the possibility for bradycardia, AV block, and/or depression of contractility should be considered (see CONTRAINDICATIONS). ***Oral*** administration of diltiazem with propranolol in 5 normal volunteers resulted in increased propranolol levels in all subjects and bioavailability of propranolol was increased approximately 50%. *In vitro*, propranolol appears to be displaced from its binding sites by diltiazem.

ANESTHETICS

The depression of cardiac contractility, conductivity, and automaticity as well as the vascular dilation associated with anesthetics may be potentiated by calcium channel blockers. When used concomitantly, anesthetics and calcium blockers should be titrated carefully.

CYCLOSPORINE

A pharmacokinetic interaction between diltiazem and cyclosporine has been observed during studies involving renal and cardiac transplant patients. In renal and cardiac transplant recipients, a reduction of cyclosporine dose ranging from 15-48% was necessary to maintain cyclosporine trough concentrations similar to those seen prior to the addition of diltiazem. If these agents are to be administered concurrently, cyclosporine concentrations should be monitored, especially when diltiazem therapy is initiated, adjusted or discontinued.

The effect of cyclosporine on diltiazem plasma concentrations has not been evaluated.

CARBAMAZEPINE

Concomitant administration of ***oral*** diltiazem with carbamazepine has been reported to result in elevated plasma levels of carbamazepine (by 40-72%), resulting in toxicity in some cases. Patients receiving these drugs concurrently should be monitored for a potential drug interaction.

ADVERSE REACTIONS

The following adverse reaction rates are based on the use of Cardizem injectable in over 400 domestic clinical trial patients with atrial fibrillation/flutter or PSVT under double-blind or open-label conditions. Worldwide experience in over 1300 patients was similar.

Adverse events reported in controlled and uncontrolled clinical trials were generally mild and transient. Hypotension was the most commonly reported adverse event during clinical trials. Asymptomatic hypotension occurred in 4.3% of patients. Symptomatic hypotension occurred in 3.2% of patients. When treatment for hypotension was required, it generally consisted of administration of saline or placing the patient in the Trendelenburg position. Other events reported in at least 1% of the diltiazem-treated patients were injection site reactions (*e.g.*, itching, burning) 3.9%, vasodilatin (flushing) 1.7%, and arrhythmia (junctional rhythm or isorhythmic dissociation) 1.0%.

In addition, the following events were reported infrequently (less than 1%):

Cardiovascular: Asystole, atrial flutter, AV block first degree, AV block second degree, bradycardia, chest pain, congestive heart failure, sinus pause, sinus node dysfunction, syncope, ventricular arrhythmia, ventricular fibrillation, ventricular tachycardia.

Dermatologic: Pruritus, sweating.

Gastrointestinal: Constipation, elevated SGOT or alkaline phosphatase, nausea, vomiting.

Nervous System: Dizziness, paresthesia.

Other: Amblyopia, asthenia, dry mouth, dyspnea, edema, headache, hyperuricemia.

Although not observed in clinical trials with Cardizem injectable, the following events associated with oral diltiazem may occur:

Cardiovascular: AV block (third degree), bundle branch block, ECG abnormality, palpitations, syncope, tachycardia, ventricular extrasystoles.

Dermatologic: Alopecia, erythema multiforme (including Stevens-Johnson syndrome, toxic epidermal necrolysis), exfoliative dermatitis, leukocytoclastic vasculitis, petechiae, photosensitivity, purpura, rash, urticaria.

Gastrointestinal: Anorexia, diarrhea, dysgeusia, dyspepsia, mild elevations of SGPT and LDH, thirst, weight increase.

Nervous System: Abnormal dreams, amnesia, depression, extrapyramidal symptoms, gait abnormality, hallucinations, insomnia, nervousness, personality change, somnolence, tremor.

Other: Allergic reactions, angioedema (including facial or periorbital edema), CPK elevation, epistaxis, eye irritation, gingival hyperplasia, hemolytic anemia, hyperglycemia, impotence, increased bleeding time, leukopenia, muscle cramps, nasal congestion, nocturia, osteoarticular pain, polyuria, retinopathy, sexual difficulties, thrombocytopenia, tinnitus.

Events such as myocardial infarction have been observed which are not readily distinguishable from the natural history of the disease for the patient.

DOSAGE AND ADMINISTRATION

DIRECT IV SINGLE INJECTIONS (BOLUS)

The initial dose of Cardizem injectable or Cardizem Lyo-Ject syringe (see instructions for reconstitution of Lyo-Ject syringe in blister pack) should be 0.25 mg/kg actual body weight as a bolus administered over 2 minutes (20 mg is a reasonable dose for the average patient). If response is inadequate, a second dose may be administered after 15 minutes. The second bolus dose of Cardizem injectable or Cardizem Lyo-Ject syringe should be 0.35 mg/kg actual body weight administered over 2 minutes (25 mg is a reasonable dose for the average patient). Subsequent IV bolus doses should be individualized for each patient. Patients with low body weights should be dosed on a mg/kg basis. Some patients may response to an initial dose of 0.15 mg/kg, although duration of action may be shorter. Experience with this dose is limited.

CONTINUOUS IV INFUSION

For continued reduction of the heart rate (up to 24 hours) in patients with atrial fibrillation or atrial flutter, an IV infusion of Cardizem injectable, Cardizem Lyo-Ject syringe, or Cardizem Monovial may be administered. (For reconstitution of Cardizem Lyo-Ject syringe or Cardizem Monovial, see instructions contained within packaging.) Immediately following bolus administration of 20 mg (0.25 mg/kg) or 25 mg (0.35 mg/kg) Cardizem injectable or Cardizem Lyo-Ject syringe, and reduction of heart rate, begin an IV infusion of Cardizem injectable, Cardizem Lyo-Ject syringe, or Cardizem Monovial. The recommended initial infusion rate of Cardizem injectable, Cardizem Lyo-Ject syringe, or Cardizem Monovial is 10 mg/h. Some patients may maintain response to an initial rate of 5 mg/h. The infusion rate may be increased in 5 mg/h increments up to 15 mg/h as needed, if further reduction in heart rate is required. The infusion may be maintained for up to 24 hours.

Diltiazem shows dose-dependent, non-linear pharmacokinetics. Duration of infusion longer than 24 hours and infusion rates greater than 15 mg/h have not been studied. Therefore, infusion duration exceeding 24 hours and infusion rates exceeding 15 mg/h are not recommended.

TRANSITION TO FURTHER ANTIARRHYTHMIC THERAPY

Transition to other antiarrhythmic agents following administration of Cardizem injectable is generally safe. However, reference should be made to the respective agent manufacturer's package insert for information relative to dosage and administration.

In controlled clinical trials, therapy with antiarrhythmic agents to maintain reduced heart rate in atrial fibrillation or atrial flutter or for prophylaxis of PSVT was generally started within 3 hours after bolus administration of Cardizem injectable. These antiarrhythmic agents were IV or oral digoxin, Class 1 antiarrhythmics (*e.g.*, quinidine, procainamide), calcium channel blockers, and oral beta-blockers.

Experience in the use of antiarrhythmic agents following maintenance infusion of Cardizem injectable is limited. Patients should be dosed on an individual basis and reference should be made to the respective manufacturer's package insert for information relative to dosage and administration.

HOW SUPPLIED

CARDIZEM INJECTABLE

Cardizem injectable is supplied in 5 ml vials with each vial containing 25 mg of diltiazem HCl (5 mg/ml) and 10 ml vials with each vial containing 50 mg diltiazem HCl (5 mg/ml).
Storage: STORE PRODUCT UNDER REFRIGERATION 2-8°C (36-46°F). DO NOT FREEZE. MAY BE STORED AT ROOM TEMPERATURE FOR UP TO 1 MONTH. DESTROY AFTER 1 MONTH AT ROOM TEMPERATURE. SINGLE-USE CONTAINERS. DISCARD UNUSED PORTION.

CARDIZEM LYO-JECT SYRINGE

Cardizem Lyo-Ject 25 mg syringe is supplied in a single molded nonsterile tray.
Storage: PRODUCT IS TO BE STORED AT ROOM TEMPERATURE 15-30°C (59-86°F). DO NOT FREEZE. RECONSTITUTED MATERIAL IS STABLE FOR 24 HOURS AT CONTROLLED ROOM TEMPERATURE. SINGLE-USE CONTAINERS. DISCARD UNUSED PORTION.

CARDIZEM MONOVIAL

Cardizem Monovial for continuous infusion (100 mg) is supplied in a glass vial with transfer needle set.
Storage: PRODUCT IS TO BE STORED AT ROOM TEMPERATURE 15-30°C (59-86°F). DO NOT FREEZE. RECONSTITUTED MATERIAL IS STABLE FOR 24 HOURS AT CONTROLLED ROOM TEMPERATURE. SINGLE-USE VIAL.

ORAL

DESCRIPTION

Note: The trade names have been used throughout this mongraph for clarity.

CARDIZEM CD CAPSULES

Cardizem is a calcium ion influx inhibitor (slow channel blocker or calcium antagonist). Chemically, diltiazem hydrochloride is 1,5-benzothiazepin-4(5H)one,3-(acetyloxy)-5-[2-(dimethylamino) ethyl]-2,3-dihydro-2-(4-methoxyphenyl)-, monohydrochloride,(+)-cis-.

Diltiazem hydrochloride is a white to off-white crystalline powder with a bitter taste. It is soluble in water, methanol, and chloroform. It has a molecular weight of 450.98. Cardizem CD is formulated as a once-a-day extended release capsule containing either 120, 180, 240, 300, or 360 mg diltiazem hydrochloride. The 120, 180, 240, and 300 mg capsules also contain: black iron oxide, ethylcellulose, FD&C blue no. 1, fumaric acid, gelatin-NF, sucrose, starch, talc, titanium dioxide, white wax, and other ingredients. The 360 mg capsule also contains: black iron oxide, diethyl phthalate, FD&C blue no. 1, gelatin-NF, povidone K17, sodium lauryl sulfate, starch, sucrose, talc, titanium dioxide, and other ingredients.

For oral administration.

CARDIZEM DIRECT COMPRESSION TABLETS

Cardizem is a calcium ion influx inhibitor (slow channel blocker or calcium antagonist). Chemically, diltiazem hydrochloride is 1,5(Benzothiazepin-4(5H)one,3-(acetyloxy)-5-[2-(dimethyl-amino)ethyl]-2,3-dihydro-2-(4-methoxyphenyl)-,monohydrochloride,(+)-cis-.

Diltiazem hydrochloride is a white to off-white crystalline powder with a bitter taste. It is soluble in water, methanol, and chloroform. It has a molecular weight of 450.98. Each tablet of Cardizem contains 30, 60, 90, or 120 mg diltiazem hydrochloride. *Also Contains:* D&C yellow no. 10 aluminum lake, FD&C yellow no. 6 aluminum lake (60 mg and 120 mg), FD&C blue no. 1 aluminum lake (30 mg and 90 mg), hydroxypropyl methylcellulose, lactose, magnesium stearate, methylparaben, microcrystalline cellulose, silicon dioxide and other ingredients.

For oral administration.

CARDIZEM LA EXTENDED RELEASE TABLETS

Once-a-day dosage.

Diltiazem hydrochloride is a calcium ion cellular influx inhibitor (slow channel blocker or calcium antagonist). Chemically, diltiazem hydrochloride is 1,5-benzothiazepin-4(5H)one,3-(acetyloxy)-5-[2-(dimethylamino)ethyl]-2,3-dihydro-2-(4-methoxyphenyl)-, monohydrochloride, (+)-cis-.

Diltiazem hydrochloride is a white to off-white crystalline powder with a bitter taste. It is soluble in water, methanol and chloroform. It has a molecular weight of 450.99. Cardizem LA tablets, for oral administration, are formulated as a once-a-day extended release tablet containing either 120, 180, 240, 300, 360, or 420 mg of diltiazem hydrochloride.

Also contains: Carnauba wax, colloidal silicon dioxide, croscarmellose sodium, hydrogenated vegetable oil, hydroxypropylmethylcellulose, magnesium stearate, microcrystalline cellulose, microcrystalline wax, pregelatinized starch, polyacrylate dispersion 30%, polyethylene glycol, polydextrose, polysorbate, povidone, simethicone, sucrose stearate, talc, titanium dioxide, triacetin.

CARDIZEM SR SUSTAINED RELEASE CAPSULES

Cardizem is a calcium ion influx inhibitor (slow channel blocker or calcium antagonist). Chemically, diltiazem hydrochloride is 1,5(benzothiazepin-4(5H)one,3-(acetyloxy)-5-[2-(dimethylamino)ethyl]-2,3-dihydro-2-(4-methoxyphenyl)-,monohydrochloride,(+)-cis-.

Diltiazem hydrochloride is a white to off-white crystalline powder with a bitter taste. It is soluble in water, methanol, and chloroform. It has a molecular weight of 450.98. Each Cardizem SR sustained release capsule contains either 60, 90, or 120 mg diltiazem hydrochloride.

Also Contains: D&C yellow no. 10, FD&C blue no. 1, FD&C red no. 40, FD&C yellow no. 6, fumaric acid, povidone, starch, sucrose, talc, titanium dioxide, and other ingredients. For oral administration.

CLINICAL PHARMACOLOGY

CARDIZEM CD CAPSULES

The therapeutic effects of Cardizem CD are believed to be related to its ability to inhibit the influx of calcium ions during membrane depolarization of cardiac and vascular smooth muscle.

Mechanism of Action

Hypertension

Cardizem CD produces its antihypertensive effect primarily by relaxation of vascular smooth muscle and the resultant decrease in peripheral vascular resistance. The magnitude of blood pressure reduction is related to the degree of hypertension; thus hypertensive individuals experience an antihypertensive effect, whereas there is only a modest fall in blood pressure in normotensives.

Angina

Cardizem CD has been shown to produce increases in exercise tolerance, probably due to its ability to reduce myocardial oxygen demand. This is accomplished via reductions in heart rate and systemic blood pressure at submaximal and maximal work loads. Diltiazem has been shown to be a potent dilator of coronary arteries, both epicardial and subendocardial. Spontaneous and ergonovine-induced coronary artery spasm are inhibited by diltiazem.

In animal models, diltiazem interferes with the slow inward (depolarizing) current in excitable tissue. It causes excitation-contraction uncoupling in various myocardial tissues without changes in the configuration of the action potential. Diltiazem produces relaxation of coronary vascular smooth muscle and dilation of both large and small coronary arteries at drug levels which cause little or no negative inotropic effect. The resultant increases in coronary blood flow (epicardial and subendocardial) occur in ischemic and nonischemic models and are accompanied by dose-dependent decreases in systemic blood pressure and decreases in peripheral resistance.

Hemodynamic and Electrophysiologic Effects

Like other calcium channel antagonists, diltiazem decreases sinoatrial and atrioventricular conduction in isolated tissues and has a negative inotropic effect in isolated preparations. In the intact animal, prolongation of the AH interval can be seen at higher doses. In man, diltiazem prevents spontaneous and ergonovine-provoked coronary artery spasm. It causes a decrease in peripheral vascular resistance and a modest fall in blood pressure in normotensive individuals and, in exercise tolerance studies in patients with ischemic heart disease, reduces the heart rate-blood pressure product for any given work load. Studies to date, primarily in patients with good ventricular function, have not revealed evidence of a negative inotropic effect; cardiac output, ejection fraction, and left ventricular end diastolic pressure have not been affected. Such data have no predictive value with respect to effects in patients with poor ventricular function, and increased heart failure has been reported in patients with preexisting impairment of ventricular function. There are as yet few data on the interaction of diltiazem and beta-blockers in patients with poor ventricular function. Resting heart rate is usually slightly reduced by diltiazem.

In hypertensive patients, Cardizem CD produces antihypertensive effects both in the supine and standing positions. In a double-blind, parallel, dose-response study utilizing doses ranging from 90 to 540 mg once daily, Cardizem CD lowered supine diastolic blood pressure in an apparent linear manner over the entire dose range studied. The changes in diastolic blood pressure, measured at trough, for placebo, 90 mg, 180 mg, 360 mg, and 540 mg were -2.9, -4.5, -6.1, -95, and -10.5 mm Hg, respectively. Postural hypotension is infrequently noted upon suddenly assuming an upright position. No reflex tachycardia is associated with the chronic antihypertensive effects. Cardizem CD decreases vascular resistance, increases cardiac output (by increasing stroke volume), and produces a slight decrease or no change in heart rate. During dynamic exercise, increases in diastolic pressure are inhibited, while maximum achievable systolic pressure is usually reduced. Chronic therapy with Cardizem CD produces no change or an increase in plasma catecholamines. No increased activity of the rennin-angiotensin-aldosterone axis has been observed. Cardizem CD reduces the renal and peripheral effects of angiotensin II. Hypertensive animal models respond to diltiazem with reductions in blood pressure and increased urinary output and natriuresis without a change in urinary sodium/potassium ratio.

In a double-blind, parallel dose-response study of doses from 60-480 mg once daily, Cardizem CD increased time to termination of exercise in a linear manner over the entire dose range studied. The improvement in time to termination of exercise utilizing a Bruce exercise protocol, measured at trough, for placebo, 60 mg, 120 mg, 240 mg, 360 mg, and 480 mg was 29, 40, 56, 51, 69, and 68 seconds, respectively. As doses of Cardizem CD were increased, overall angina frequency was decreased. Cardizem CD, 180 mg once daily, or placebo was administered in a double-blind study to patients receiving concomitant treatment with long-acting nitrates and/or beta-blockers. A significant increase in time to termination of exercise and a significant decrease in overall angina frequency was observed. In this trial the overall frequency of adverse events in the Cardizem CD treatment group was the same as the placebo group. IV diltiazem in doses of 20 mg prolongs AH conduction time and AV node functional and effective refractory periods by approximately 20%. In a study involving single oral doses of 300 mg of Cardizem in 6 normal volunteers, the average maximum PR prolongation was 14% with no instances of greater than first-degree AV block. Diltiazem-associated prolongation of the AH interval is not more pronounced in patients with first-degree heart block. In patients with sick sinus syndrome, diltiazem significantly prolongs sinus cycle length (up to 50% in some cases).

Chronic oral administration of Cardizem to patients in doses of up to 540 mg/day has resulted in small increases in PR interval, and on occasion produces abnormal prolongation. (See WARNINGS, Cardizem CD Capsules.)

Pharmacokinetics and Metabolism

Diltiazem is well absorbed from the gastrointestinal tract and is subject to an extensive first-pass effect, giving an absolute bioavailability (compared to IV administration) of about 40%. Cardizem undergoes extensive metabolism in which only 2-4% of the unchanged drug appears in the urine. Drugs which induce or inhibit hepatic microsomal enzymes may alter diltiazem disposition.

Total radioactivity measurement following short IV administration in healthy volunteers suggests the presence of other unidentified metabolites, which attain higher concentrations than those of diltiazem and are more slowly eliminated; half-life of total radioactivity is about 20 hours compared to 2-5 hours for diltiazem.

In vitro binding studies show Cardizem is 70-80% bound to plasma proteins. Competitive *in vitro* ligand binding studies have also shown Cardizem binding is not altered by therapeutic concentrations of digoxin, hydrochlorothiazide, phenylbutazone, propranolol, salicylic acid, or warfarin. The plasma elimination half-life following single or multiple drug administration is approximately 3.0-4.5 hours. Desacetyl diltiazem is also present in the plasma at levels of 10-20% of the parent drug and is 25-50% as potent as a coronary vasodilator as diltiazem. Minimum therapeutic plasma diltiazem concentrations appear to be in the range of 50-200 ng/ml. There is a departure from linearity when dose strengths are increased; the half-life is slightly increased with dose. A study that compared patients with normal hepatic function to patients with cirrhosis found an increase in half-life and a 69% increase in bioavailability in the hepatically impaired patients. A single study in 9 patients with severely impaired renal function showed no difference in the pharmacokinetic profile of diltiazem compared to patients with normal renal function.

Cardizem CD Capsules

When compared to a regimen of Cardizem tablets at steady-state, more than 95% of drug is absorbed from the Cardizem CD formulation. A single 360-mg dose of the capsule results in detectable plasma levels within 2 hours and peak plasma levels between 10 and 14 hours; absorption occurs throughout the dosing interval. When Cardizem CD was coadministered with a high fat content breakfast, the extent of diltiazem absorption was not affected. Dose-dumping does not occur. The apparent elimination half-life after single or multiple dosing is 5-8 hours. A departure from linearity similar to that seen with Cardizem tablets and Cardizem SR capsules is observed. As the dose of Cardizem CD capsules is increased from a daily dose of 120-240 mg, there is an increase in the area-under-the-curve of 2.7 times. When the dose is increased from 240-360 mg there is an increase in the area-under-the-curve of 1.6 times.

CARDIZEM DIRECT COMPRESSION TABLETS

The therapeutic effects of Cardizem are believed to be related to its ability to inhibit the influx of calcium ions during membrane depolarization of cardiac and vascular smooth muscle.

Mechanism of Action

Although precise mechanisms of its antianginal actions are still being delineated, Cardizem is believed to act in the following ways:

- ***Angina due to coronary artery spasm:*** Cardizem has been shown to be a potent dilator of coronary arteries both epicardial and subendocardial. Spontaneous and ergonovine-induced coronary artery spasms are inhibited by Cardizem.
- ***Exertional angina:*** Cardizem has been shown to produce increases in exercise tolerance, probably due to its ability to reduce myocardial oxygen demand. This is accomplished via reductions in heart rate and systemic blood pressure at submaximal and maximal exercise workloads.

In animal models, diltiazem interferes with the slow inward (depolarizing) current in excitable tissue. It causes excitation-contraction uncoupling in various myocardial tissues without changes in the configuration of the action potential. Diltiazem produces relaxation of coronary vascular smooth muscle and dilation of both large and small coronary arteries at drug levels which cause little or no negative inotropic effect. The resultant increases in coronary blood flow (epicardial and subendocardial) occur in ischemic and nonischemic models and are accompanied by dose-dependent decreases in systemic blood pressure and decreases in peripheral resistance.

Hemodynamic and Electrophysiologic Effects

Like other calcium antagonists, diltiazem decreases sinoatrial and atrioventricular conduction in isolated tissues and has a negative inotropic effect in isolated preparations. In the intact animal, prolongation of the AH interval can be seen at higher doses.

In man, diltiazem prevents spontaneous and ergonovine-provoked coronary artery spasm. It causes a decrease in peripheral vascular resistance and a modest fall in blood pressure and, in exercise tolerance studies in patients with ischemic heart disease, reduces the heart rate-blood pressure product for any given work load. Studies to date, primarily in patients with good ventricular function, have not revealed evidence of a negative inotropic effect; cardiac output, ejection fraction, and left ventricular end-diastolic pressure have not been affected. There are as yet few data on the interaction of diltiazem and beta-blockers. Resting heart rate is usually unchanged or slightly reduced by diltiazem.

IV diltiazem in doses of 20 mg prolongs AH conduction time and AV node functional and effective refractory periods by approximately 20%. In a study involving single oral doses of 300 mg of Cardizem in 6 normal volunteers, the average maximum PR prolongation was 14% with no instances of greater than first-degree AV block. Diltiazem-associated prolongation of the AH interval is not more pronounced in patients with first-degree heart block. In patients with sick sinus syndrome, diltiazem significantly prolongs sinus cycle length (up to 50% in some cases).

Chronic oral administration of Cardizem in doses of up to 240 mg/day has resulted in small increases in PR interval, but has not usually produced abnormal prolongation.

Pharmacokinetics and Metabolism

Diltiazem is well absorbed from the gastrointestinal tract and is subject to an extensive first-pass effect, giving an absolute bioavailability (compared to IV dosing) of about 40%. Cardizem undergoes extensive metabolism in which 2-4% of the unchanged drug appears in the urine. *In vitro* binding studies show Cardizem is 70-80% bound to plasma proteins. Competitive *in vitro* ligand binding studies have also shown Cardizem binding is not altered by therapeutic concentrations of digoxin, hydrochlorothiazide, phenylbutazone, propranolol, salicylic acid, or warfarin. The plasma elimination half-life following single or multiple drug administration is approximately 3.0-4.5 hours. Desacetyl diltiazem is also present in the plasma at levels of 10-20% of the parent drug and is 25-50% as potent a coronary vasodilator as diltiazem. Minimum therapeutic plasma levels of Cardizem appear to be in the range of 50-200 ng/ml. There is a departure from linearity when dose strengths are increased. A study that compared patients with normal hepatic function to patients with cirrhosis found an increase in half-life and a 69% increase in AUC (area-under-the-plasma concentration versus time curve) in the hepatically impaired patients. A single study in 9 patients with severely impaired renal function showed no difference in the pharmacokinetic profile of diltiazem as compared to patients with normal renal function.

Cardizem Direct Compression Tablets

Diltiazem is absorbed from the tablet formulation to about 98% of a reference solution. Single oral doses of 30-120 mg of Cardizem direct compression tablets result in detectable plasma levels within 30-60 minutes and peak plasma levels 2-4 hours after drug administration. As the dose of Cardizem direct compression tablets is increased from a daily dose of 120 mg (30 mg qid) to 240 mg (60 mg qid) daily, there is an increase in area-under-the curve of 2.3 times. When the dose is increased from 240-360 mg daily, there is an increase in area-under-the-curve of 1.8 times.

CARDIZEM LA EXTENDED RELEASE TABLETS

The therapeutic effects of diltiazem are believed to be related to its ability to inhibit the influx of calcium ions during membrane depolarization of cardiac and vascular smooth muscle.

Mechanism of Action

Diltiazem produces its antihypertensive effect primarily by relaxation of vascular smooth muscle and the resultant decrease in peripheral vascular resistance. The magnitude of blood pressure reduction is related to the degree of hypertension; thus hypertensive individuals experience an antihypertensive effect, whereas there is only a modest fall in blood pressure in normotensives.

Pharmacodynamics and Clinical Studies

In a randomized, double-blind, parallel-group, dose-response study involving 478 patients with essential hypertension, evening doses of Cardizem LA 120, 240, 360, and 540 mg were compared to placebo and to 360 mg administered in the morning. The mean reductions in diastolic blood pressure by ABPM at roughly 24 hours after the morning (4 AM-8AM) or evening (6 PM-10 PM) administration (*i.e.*, the time corresponding to expected trough serum concentrations) are shown in TABLE 1.

TABLE 1 *Mean Change in Trough Diastolic Pressure by ABPM*

Evening Dosing	
120 mg	-2.0
240 mg	-4.4
360 mg	-4.4
540 mg	-8.1
Morning Dosing	
360 mg	-6.4

A second randomized, double-blind, parallel-group, dose-response study (n=258) evaluated Cardizem LA following morning doses of placebo or 120, 180, 300, or 540 mg. Diastolic blood pressure measured by supine office cuff sphygmomanometer at trough (7 AM to 9 AM) decreased in an apparently linear manner over the dosage range studied. Group mean changes for placebo, 120 mg, 180 mg, 300 mg and 540 mg were -2.6, -1.9, -5.4, -6.1 and -8.6 mm Hg respectively.

Whether the time of administration impacts the clinical benefits of antihypertensive treatment is not known.

Postural hypotension is infrequently noted upon suddenly assuming an upright position. No reflex tachycardia is associated with the chronic antihypertensive effects.

Like other calcium channel antagonists, diltiazem decreases sinoatrial and atrioventricular conduction in isolated tissues and has a negative inotropic effect in isolated preparations. In the intact animal, prolongation of the AH interval can be seen at higher doses.

In man, diltiazem prevents spontaneous and ergonovine-provoked coronary artery spasm. It causes a decrease in peripheral vascular resistance and a modest fall in blood pressure in normotensive individuals and, in exercise tolerance studies in patients with ischemic heart disease, reduces the heart rate-blood pressure product for any given work load. Studies to date, primarily in patients with good ventricular function, have not revealed evidence of a negative inotropic effect; cardiac output, ejection fraction, and left ventricular end diastolic pressure have not been affected. Such data has no predictive value with respect to effects in patients with poor ventricular function, and increased heart failure has been reported in patients with preexisting impairment of ventricular function. There are as yet few data on the interaction of diltiazem and beta-blockers in patients with poor ventricular function. Resting heart rate is usually slightly reduced by diltiazem. Diltiazem decreases vascular resistance, increases cardiac output (by increasing stroke volume), and produces a slight decrease or no change in heart rate.

During dynamic exercise, increases in diastolic pressure are inhibited, while maximum achievable systolic pressure is usually reduced. Chronic therapy with diltiazem produces no change or an increase in plasma catecholamines. No increased activity of the renin-angiotensin-aldosterone axis has been observed. Diltiazem reduces the renal and peripheral effects of angiotensin II. Hypertensive animal models respond to diltiazem with reductions in blood pressure and increased urinary output and natriuresis without a change in urinary sodium/potassium ratio.

IV diltiazem HCl in doses of 20 mg prolongs AH conduction time and AV node functional and effective refractory periods by approximately 20%. In a study involving single oral doses of 300 mg of diltiazem HCl in 6 normal volunteers, the average maximum PR prolongation was 14% with no instances of greater than first-degree AV block. Diltiazem associated prolongation of the AH interval is not more pronounced in patients with first-degree heart block. In patients with sick sinus syndrome, diltiazem significantly prolongs sinus cycle length (up to 50% in some cases).

Chronic oral administration of diltiazem HCl to patients in doses of up to 540 mg/day has resulted in small increases in PR interval, and on occasion produces abnormal prolongation. (See WARNINGS, Cardizem LA Extended Release Tablets.)

Pharmacokinetics and Metabolism

Diltiazem is well absorbed from the gastrointestinal tract and is subject to an extensive first-pass effect, giving an absolute bioavailability (compared to IV administration) of about 40%. Diltiazem undergoes extensive metabolism in which only 2-4% of the unchanged drug appears in the urine. Drugs which induce or inhibit hepatic microsomal enzymes may alter diltiazem disposition.

Total radioactivity measurement following short IV administration in healthy volunteers suggests the presence of other unidentified metabolites, which attain higher concentrations than those of diltiazem and are more slowly eliminated; half-life of total radioactivity is about 20 hours compared to 2-5 hours for diltiazem.

In vitro binding studies show diltiazem is 70-80% bound to plasma proteins. Competitive *in vitro* ligand binding studies have also shown diltiazem HCl binding is not altered by therapeutic concentrations of digoxin, hydrochlorothiazide, phenylbutazone, propranolol, salicylic acid, or warfarin. The plasma elimination half-life following single or multiple drug administration is approximately 3.0-4.5 hours. Desacetyl diltiazem is also present in the plasma at levels of 10-20% of the parent drug and is 25-50% as potent as a coronary vasodilator as diltiazem. Minimum therapeutic plasma diltiazem concentrations appear to be in the range of 50-200 ng/ml. There is a departure from linearity when dose strengths are increased; the half-life is slightly increased with dose. A study that compared patients with normal hepatic function to patients with cirrhosis found an increase in half-life and a 69% increase in bioavailability in the hepatically impaired patients. A single study in patients with severely impaired renal function showed no difference in the pharmacokinetic profile of diltiazem compared to patients with normal renal function.

Cardizem LA Tablets

A single 360 mg dose of Cardizem LA results in detectable plasma levels within 3-4 hours and peak plasma levels between 11 and 18 hours; absorption occurs throughout the dosing interval. The apparent elimination half-life for Cardizem LA tablets after single or multiple dosing is 6-9 hours. When Cardizem LA tablets were coadministered with a high fat content breakfast, diltiazem peak and systemic exposures were not affected indicating that the tablet can be administered without regard to food.

As the dose of Cardizem LA tablets is increased from 120-240 mg, area-under-the-curve increases 2.5-fold.

CARDIZEM SR SUSTAINED RELEASE CAPSULES

The therapeutic effects of Cardizem are believed to be related to its ability to inhibit the influx of calcium ions during membrane depolarization of cardiac and vascular smooth muscle.

Mechanism of Action

Cardizem SR produces its antihypertensive effect primarily by relaxation of vascular smooth muscle and the resultant decrease in peripheral vascular resistance. The magnitude of blood pressure reduction is related to the degree of hypertension; thus hypertensive individuals experience an antihypertensive effect, whereas there is only a modest fall in blood pressure in normotensives.

Hemodynamic and Electrophysiologic Effects

Like other calcium antagonists, diltiazem decreases sinoatrial and atrioventricular conduction in isolated tissues and has a negative inotropic effect in isolated preparations. In the intact animal, prolongation of the AH interval can be seen at higher doses.

In man, diltiazem prevents spontaneous and ergonovine-provoked coronary artery spasm. It causes a decrease in peripheral vascular resistance and a modest fall in blood pressure in normotensive individuals and, in exercise tolerance studies in patients with ischemic heart disease, reduces the heart rate-blood pressure product for any given work load. Studies to date, primarily in patients with good ventricular function, have not revealed evidence of a negative inotropic effect; cardiac output, ejection fraction, and left ventricular end diastolic pressure have not been affected. Increased heart failure has, however, been reported in occasional patients with preexisting impairment of ventricular function. There are as yet few data on the interaction of diltiazem and beta-blockers in patients with poor ventricular function. Resting heart rate is usually unchanged or slightly reduced by diltiazem.

Cardizem SR produces antihypertensive effects both in the supine and standing positions. Postural hypotension is infrequently noted upon suddenly assuming an upright position. No reflex tachycardia is associated with the chronic antihypertensive effects. Cardizem SR decreases vascular resistance, increases cardiac output (by increasing stroke volume), and produces a slight decrease or no change in heart rate. During dynamic exercise, increases in diastolic pressure are inhibited while maximum achievable systolic pressure is usually reduced. Heart rate at maximum exercise does not change or is slightly reduced. Chronic therapy with Cardizem produces no change or an increase in plasma catecholamines. No increased activity of the rennin-angiotensin-aldosterone axis has been observed. Cardizem SR antagonizes the renal and peripheral effects of angiotensin II. Hypertensive animal models respond to diltiazem with reductions in blood pressure and increased urinary output and natriuresis without a change in urinary sodium/potassium ratio.

IV diltiazem in doses of 20 mg prolongs AH conduction time and AV node functional and effective refractory periods by approximately 20%. In a study involving single oral doses of 300 mg of Cardizem in 6 normal volunteers, the average maximum PR prolongation was 14% with no instances of greater than first-degree AV block. Diltiazem-associated prolongation of the AH interval is not more pronounced in patients with first-degree heart block. In patients with sick sinus syndrome, diltiazem significantly prolongs sinus cycle length (up to 50% in some cases).

Chronic oral administration of Cardizem in doses of up to 360 mg/day has resulted in small increases in PR interval, and on occasion produces abnormal prolongation. (See WARNINGS, Cardizem SR Sustained Release Capsules.)

Pharmacokinetics and Metabolism

Diltiazem is well absorbed from the gastrointestinal tract and is subject to an extensive first-pass effect, giving an absolute bioavailability (compared to IV administration) of about 40%. Cardizem undergoes extensive metabolism in which 2-4% of the unchanged drug appears in the urine. *In vitro* binding studies show Cardizem is 70-80% bound to plasma proteins. Competitive *in vitro* ligand binding studies have also shown Cardizem binding is not altered by therapeutic concentrations of digoxin, hydrochlorothiazide, phenylbutazone, propranolol, salicylic acid, or warfarin. The plasma elimination half-life following single or multiple drug administration is approximately 3.0-4.5 hours. Desacetyl diltiazem is also present in the plasma at levels of 10-20% of the parent drug and is 25-50% as potent a coronary vasodilator as diltiazem. Minimum therapeutic plasma levels of Cardizem appear to be in the range of 50-200 ng/ml. There is a departure from linearity when dose strengths are increased; the half-life is slightly increased with dose. A study that compared patients with normal hepatic function to patients with cirrhosis found an increase in half-life and a 69% increase in bioavailability in the hepatically impaired patients. A single study in 9 patients with severely impaired renal function showed no difference in the pharmacokinetic profile of diltiazem compared to patients with normal renal function.

Cardizem SR Capsules

Diltiazem is absorbed from the capsule formulation to about 92% of a reference solution at steady-state. A single 120 mg dose of the capsule results in detectable plasma levels within 2-3 hours and peak plasma levels at 6-11 hours. The apparent elimination half-life after single or multiple dosing is 5-7 hours. A departure from linearity similar to that observed with the Cardizem direct compression tablet is observed. As the dose of Cardizem SR is increased from a daily dose of 120 mg (60 mg bid) to 240 mg (120 mg bid) daily, there is an increase in area-under-the curve of 2.6 times. When the dose is increased from 240-360 mg daily, there is an increase in area-under-the-curve of 1.8 times. The average plasma levels of the capsule dose twice daily at steady-state are equivalent to the tablet dosed 4 times daily when the same total daily dose is administered.

INDICATIONS AND USAGE

CARDIZEM CD CAPSULES

Cardizem CD is indicated for the treatment of hypertension. It may be used alone or in combination with other antihypertensive medications.

Cardizem CD is indicated for the management of chronic stable angina and angina due to coronary artery spasm.

CARDIZEM DIRECT COMPRESSION TABLETS

Cardizem is indicated for the management of chronic stable angina and angina due to coronary artery spasm.

CARDIZEM LA EXTENDED RELEASE TABLETS

Cardizem LA is indicated for the treatment of hypertension. It may be used alone or in combination with other antihypertensive medications.

CARDIZEM SR SUSTAINED RELEASE CAPSULES

Cardizem SR is indicated for the treatment of hypertension. It may be used alone or in combination with other antihypertensive medications, such as diuretics.

CONTRAINDICATIONS

CARDIZEM CD CAPSULES

Cardizem is contraindicated in (1) patients with sick sinus syndrome except in the presence of a functioning ventricular pacemaker, (2) patients with second- or third-degree AV block except in the presence of a functioning ventricular pacemaker, (3) patients with hypotension (less than 90 mm Hg systolic), (4) patients who have demonstrated hypersensitivity to the drug, and (5) patients with acute myocardial infarction and pulmonary congestion documented by x-ray on admission.

CARDIZEM DIRECT COMPRESSION TABLETS

Cardizem is contraindicated in (1) patients with sick sinus syndrome except in the presence of a functioning ventricular pacemaker, (2) patients with second- or third-degree AV block except in the presence of a functioning ventricular pacemaker, (3) patients with hypotension (less than 90 mm Hg systolic), (4) patients who have demonstrated hypersensitivity to the drug, and (5) patients with acute myocardial infarction and pulmonary congestion documented by x-ray on admission.

CARDIZEM LA EXTENDED RELEASE TABLETS

Diltiazem is contraindicated in (1) patients with sick sinus syndrome except in the presence of a functioning ventricular pacemaker, (2) patients with second-or third-degree AV block except in the presence of a functioning ventricular pacemaker, (3) patients with hypotension (less than 90 mm Hg systolic), (4) patients who have demonstrated hypersensitivity to the drug, and (5) patients with acute myocardial infarction and pulmonary congestion documented by x-ray on admission.

CARDIZEM SR SUSTAINED RELEASE CAPSULES

Cardizem is contraindicated in (1) patients with sick sinus syndrome except in the presence of a functioning ventricular pacemaker, (2) patients with second- or third-degree AV block except in the presence of a functioning ventricular pacemaker, (3) patients with hypotension (less than 90 mm Hg systolic), (4) patients who have demonstrated hypersensitivity to the drug, and (5) patients with acute myocardial infarction and pulmonary congestion documented by x-ray on admission.

WARNINGS

CARDIZEM CD CAPSULES

Cardiac Conduction

Cardizem prolongs AV node refractory periods without significantly prolonging sinus node recovery time, except in patients with sick sinus syndrome. This effect may rarely result in abnormally slow heart rates (particularly in patients with sick sinus syndrome) or second- or third-degree AV block (13 of 3290 patients or 0.40%). Concomitant use of diltiazem with beta-blockers or digitalis may result in additive effects on cardiac conduction. A patient with Prinzmetal's angina developed periods of asystole (2-5 seconds) after a single dose of 60 mg of diltiazem. (See ADVERSE REACTIONS, Cardizem CD Capsules.)

Congestive Heart Failure

Although diltiazem has a negative inotropic effect in isolated animal tissue preparations, hemodynamic studies in humans with normal ventricular function have not shown a reduction in cardiac index nor consistent negative effects on contractility (dp/dt). An acute study of oral diltiazem in patients with impaired ventricular function (ejection fraction 24% ± 6%) showed improvement in indices of ventricular function without significant decrease in contractile function (dp/dt). Worsening of congestive heart failure has been reported in patients with preexisting impairment of ventricular function. Experience with the use of Cardizem (diltiazem HCl) in combination with beta-blockers in patients with impaired ventricular function is limited. Caution should be exercised when using this combination.

Hypotension

Decreases in blood pressure associated with Cardizem therapy may occasionally result in symptomatic hypotension.

Acute Hepatic Injury

Mild elevations of transaminases with and without concomitant elevation in alkaline phosphatase and bilirubin have been observed in clinical studies. Such elevations were usually transient and frequently resolved even with continued diltiazem treatment. In rare instances, significant elevations in enzymes such as alkaline phosphatase, LDH, SGOT, SGPT, and other phenomena consistent with acute hepatic injury have been noted. These reactions tended to occur early after therapy initiation (1-8 weeks) and have been reversible upon discontinuation of drug therapy. The relationship to Cardizem is uncertain in some cases, but probable in some. (See PRECAUTIONS, Cardizem CD Capsules.)

CARDIZEM DIRECT COMPRESSION TABLETS

Cardiac Conduction

Cardizem prolongs AV node refractory periods without significantly prolonging sinus node recovery time, except in patients with sick sinus syndrome. This effect may rarely result in abnormally slow heart rates (particularly in patients with sick sinus syndrome) or second- or third-degree AV block (6 of 1243 patientsfro 0.48%). Concomitant use of diltiazem with beta-blockers or digitalis may result in additive effects on cardiac conduction. A patient with Prinzmetal's angina developed periods of asystole (2-5 seconds) after a single dose of 60 mg of diltiazem. (See ADVERSE REACTIONS, Cardizem Direct Compression Tablets.)

Congestive Heart Failure

Although diltiazem has a negative inotropic effect in isolated animal tissue preparations, hemodynamic studies in humans with normal ventricular function have not shown a reduction in cardiac index or consistent negative effects on contractility (dp/dt). Experience with the use of Cardizem alone or in combination with beta-blockers in patients with impaired ventricular function is limited. Caution should be exercised when using the drug in such patients.

Hypotension

Decreases in blood pressure associated with Cardizem therapy may occasionally result in symptomatic hypotension.

Acute Hepatic Injury

In rare instances, significant elevations in enzymes such as alkaline phosphatase, LDH, SGOT, SGPT, and other phenomena consistent with acute hepatic injury have been noted. These reactions have been reversible upon discontinuation of drug therapy. The relationship to Cardizem is uncertain in some cases, but probable in some. (See PRECAUTIONS, Cardizem Direct Compression Tablets.)

CARDIZEM LA EXTENDED RELEASE TABLETS

Cardiac Conduction

Diltiazem prolongs AV node refractory periods without significantly prolonging sinus node recovery time, except in patients with sick sinus syndrome. This effect may rarely result in abnormally slow heart rates (particularly in patients with sick sinus syndrome) or second-or third-degree AV block (13 of 3290 patients or 0.40%). Concomitant use of diltiazem with beta-blockers or digitalis may result in additive effects on cardiac conduction. A patient with Prinzmetal's angina developed periods of asystole (2-5 seconds) after a single dose of 60 mg of diltiazem (see ADVERSE REACTIONS, Cardizem LA Extended Release Tablets).

Congestive Heart Failure

Although diltiazem has a negative inotropic effect in isolated animal tissue preparations, hemodynamic studies in humans with normal ventricular function have not shown a reduction in cardiac index nor consistent negative effects on contractility (dp/dt). An acute study of oral diltiazem in patients with impaired ventricular function (ejection fraction 24% ± 6%) showed improvement in indices of ventricular function without significant decrease in contractile function (dp/dt). Worsening of congestive heart failure has been reported in patients with preexisting impairment of ventricular function. Experience with the use of diltiazem in combination with beta-blockers in patients with impaired ventricular function is limited. Caution should be exercised when using this combination.

Hypotension

Decreases in blood pressure associated with diltiazem therapy may occasionally result in symptomatic hypotension.

Acute Hepatic Injury

Mild elevations of transaminases with and without concomitant elevation in alkaline phosphatase and bilirubin have been observed in clinical studies. Such elevations were usually transient and frequently resolved even with continued diltiazem treatment. In rare instances, significant elevations in enzymes such as alkaline phosphatase, LDH, SGOT, SGPT, and other phenomena consistent with acute hepatic injury have been noted. These reactions tended to occur early after therapy initiation (1-8 weeks) and have been reversible upon discontinuation of drug therapy. The relationship to diltiazem is uncertain in some cases, but probable in some. (See PRECAUTIONS, Cardizem LA Extended Release Tablets.)

CARDIZEM SR SUSTAINED RELEASE CAPSULES

Cardiac Conduction

Cardizem prolongs AV node refractory periods without significantly prolonging sinus node recovery time, except in patients with sick sinus syndrome. This effect may rarely result in abnormally slow heart rates (particularly in patients with sick sinus syndrome) or second- or third-degree AV block (9 of 2111 patients for 0.43%). Concomitant use of diltiazem with beta-blockers or digitalis may result in additive effects on cardiac conduction. A patient with Prinzmetal's angina developed periods of asystole (2-5 seconds) after a single dose of 60 mg of diltiazem. (See ADVERSE REACTIONS, Cardizem SR Sustained Release Capsules.)

Congestive Heart Failure

Although diltiazem has a negative inotropic effect in isolated animal tissue preparations, hemodynamic studies in humans with normal ventricular function have not shown a reduction in cardiac index or consistent negative effects on contractility (dp/dt). An acute study of oral diltiazem in patients with impaired ventricular function (ejection fraction 24% ± 6%) showed improvement in indices of ventricular function without significant decrease in contractile function (dp/dt). Experience with the use of Cardizem in combination with beta-blockers in patients with impaired ventricular function is limited. Caution should be exercised when using this combination.

Hypotension

Decreases in blood pressure associated with Cardizem therapy may occasionally result in symptomatic hypotension.

Acute Hepatic Injury

Mild elevations of transaminases with and without concomitant elevation in alkaline phosphatase and bilirubin have been observed in clinical studies. Such elevations were usually transient and frequently resolved even with continued diltiazem treatment. In rare instances, significant elevations in enzymes such as alkaline phosphatase, LDH, SGOT, SGPT, and other phenomena consistent with acute hepatic injury have been noted. These reactions tended to occur early after therapy initiation (1-8 weeks) and have been reversible upon discontinuation of drug therapy. The relationship to Cardizem is uncertain in some cases, but probable in some. (See PRECAUTIONS, Cardizem SR Sustained Release Capsules.)

PRECAUTIONS

CARDIZEM CD CAPSULES

General

Cardizem (diltiazem HCl) is extensively metabolized by the liver and excreted by the kidneys and in bile. As with any drug given over prolonged periods, laboratory parameters of renal and hepatic function should be monitored at regular intervals. The drug should be used with caution in patients with impaired renal or hepatic function. In subacute and chronic dog and rat studies designed to produce toxicity, high doses of diltiazem were associated with hepatic damage. In special subacute hepatic studies, oral doses of 125 mg/kg and higher in rats were associated with histological changes in the liver which were reversible when the drug was discontinued. In dogs, doses of 20 mg/kg were also associated with hepatic changes; however, these changes were reversible with continued dosing.

Dermatological events (see ADVERSE REACTIONS, Cardizem CD Capsules) may be transient and may disappear despite continued use of Cardizem. However, skin eruptions progressing to erythema multiforme and/or exfoliative dermatitis have also been infrequently reported. Should a dermatologic reaction persist, the drug should be discontinued.

Carcinogenesis, Mutagenesis, and Impairment of Fertility

A 24 month study in rats at oral dosage levels of up to 100 mg/kg/day and a 21 month study in mice at oral dosage levels of up to 30 mg/kg/day showed no evidence of carcinogenicity. There was also no mutagenic response *in vitro* or *in vivo* in mammalian cell assays or *in vitro* in bacteria. No evidence of impaired fertility was observed in a study performed in male and female rats at oral dosages of up to 100 mg/kg/day.

Pregnancy Category C

Reproduction studies have been conducted in mice, rats, and rabbits. Administration of doses ranging from 5-10 times greater (on a mg/kg basis) than the daily recommended therapeutic dose has resulted in embryo and fetal lethality. These doses, in some studies, have been reported to cause skeletal abnormalities. In the perinatal/postnatal studies, there was an increased incidence of stillbirths at doses of 20 times the human dose or greater.

There are no well-controlled studies in pregnant women; therefore, use Cardizem in pregnant women only if the potential benefit justifies the potential risk to the fetus.

Nursing Mothers

Diltiazem is excreted in human milk. One report suggests that concentrations in breast milk may approximate serum levels. If use of Cardizem is deemed essential, an alternative method of infant feeding should be instituted.

Pediatric Use

Safety and effectiveness in pediatric patients have not been established.

CARDIZEM DIRECT COMPRESSION TABLETS

General

Cardizem is extensively metabolized by the liver and excreted by the kidneys and in bile. As with any drug given over prolonged periods, laboratory parameters of renal and hepatic function should be monitored at regular intervals. The drug should be used with caution in patients with impaired renal or hepatic function. In subacute and chronic dog and rat studies designed to produce toxicity, high doses of diltiazem were associated with hepatic damage. In special subacute hepatic studies, oral doses of 125 mg/kg and higher in rats were associated with histological changes in the liver, which were reversible when the drug was discontinued. In dogs, doses of 20 mg/kg were also associated with hepatic changes; however, these changes were reversible with continued dosing.

Dermatological events (see ADVERSE REACTIONS, Cardizem Direct Compression Tablets) may be transient and may disappear despite continued use of Cardizem. However, skin eruptions progressing to erythema multiforme and/or exfoliative dermatitis have also been infrequently reported. Should a dermatologic reaction persist, the drug should be discontinued.

Carcinogenesis, Mutagenesis, and Impairment of Fertility

A 24 month study in rats and a 21 month study in mice showed no evidence of carcinogenicity. There was also no mutagenic response in *in vitro* bacterial tests. No intrinsic effect on fertility was observed in rats.

Pregnancy Category C

Reproduction studies have been conducted in mice, rats, and rabbits. Administration of doses ranging from 5-10 times greater (on a mg/kg basis) than the daily recommended therapeutic dose has resulted in embryo and fetal lethality. These doses, in some studies, have been reported to cause skeletal abnormalities. In the perinatal/postnatal studies, there was some reduction in early individual pup weights and survival rates. There was an increased incidence of stillbirths at doses of 20 times the human dose or greater.

There are no well-controlled studies in pregnant women; therefore, use Cardizem in pregnant women only if the potential benefit justifies the potential risk to the fetus.

Nursing Mothers

Diltiazem is excreted in human milk. One report suggests that concentrations in breast milk may approximate serum levels. If use of Cardizem is deemed essential, an alternative method of infant feeding should be instituted.

Pediatric Use

Safety and effectiveness in pediatric patients have not been established.

CARDIZEM LA EXTENDED RELEASE TABLETS

General

Diltiazem HCl is extensively metabolized by the liver and excreted by the kidneys and in bile. As with any drug given over prolonged periods, laboratory parameters of renal and hepatic function should be monitored at regular intervals. The drug should be used with caution in patients with impaired renal or hepatic function.

In subacute and chronic dog and rat studies designed to produce toxicity, high doses of diltiazem were associated with hepatic damage. In special subacute hepatic studies, oral doses of 125 mg/kg and higher in rats were associated with histological changes in the liver, which were reversible when the drug was discontinued. In dogs, doses of 20 mg/kg were also associated with hepatic changes; however, these changes were reversible with continued dosing.

Dermatological events (see ADVERSE REACTIONS, Cardizem LA Extended Release Tablets) may be transient and may disappear despite continued use of diltiazem. However, skin eruptions progressing to erythema multiforme and/or exfoliative dermatitis have also been infrequently reported. Should a dermatologic reaction persist, the drug should be discontinued.

Carcinogenesis, Mutagenesis, and Impairment of Fertility

A 24 month study in rats at oral dosage levels of up to 100 mg/kg/day, and a 21 month study in mice at oral dosage levels of up to 30 mg/kg/day showed no evidence of carcinogenicity. There was also no mutagenic response *in vitro* or *in vivo* in mammalian cell assays or *in vitro* in bacteria. No evidence of impaired fertility was observed in a study performed in male and female rats at oral dosages of up to 100 mg/kg/day.

Pregnancy Category C

Reproduction studies have been conducted in mice, rats, and rabbits. Administration of doses ranging from 4-6 times (depending on species) the upper limit of the optimum dosage range in clinical trials (480 mg qd or 8 mg/kg qd for a 60 kg patient) resulted in embryo and fetal lethality. These studies revealed, in one species or another, a propensity to cause abnormalities of the skeleton, heart, retina, and tongue. Also observed were reductions in early individual pup weights and pup survival, prolonged delivery and increased incident of stillbirths.

There are no well-controlled studies in pregnant women; therefore, use diltiazem in pregnant women only if the potential benefit justifies the potential risk to the fetus.

Nursing Mothers

Diltiazem is excreted in human milk. One report suggests that concentrations in breast milk may approximate serum levels. If use of diltiazem is deemed essential, an alternative method of infant feeding should be instituted.

Pediatric Use

Safety and effectiveness in pediatric patients have not been established.

Geriatric Use

Clinical studies of diltiazem did not include sufficient numbers of subjects aged 65 and over to determine whether they respond differently from younger subjects. Other reported clinical experience has not identified differences in responses between the elderly and younger patients. In general, dose selection for an elderly patient should be cautious, usually starting at the low end of the dosing range, reflecting the greater frequency of decreased hepatic, renal, or cardiac function, and of concomitant disease or other drug therapy.

CARDIZEM SR SUSTAINED RELEASE CAPSULES

General

Cardizem is extensively metabolized by the liver and excreted by the kidneys and in bile. As with any drug given over prolonged periods, laboratory parameters of renal and hepatic function should be monitored at regular intervals. The drug should be used with caution in patients with impaired renal or hepatic function. In subacute and chronic dog and rat studies designed to produce toxicity, high doses of diltiazem were associated with hepatic damage. In special subacute hepatic studies, oral doses of 125 mg/kg and higher in rats were associated with histological changes in the liver which were reversible when the drug was discontinued. In dogs, doses of 20 mg/kg were also associated with hepatic changes; however, these changes were reversible with continued dosing.

Dermatological events (see ADVERSE REACTIONS, Cardizem SR Sustained Release Tablets) may be transient and may disappear despite continued use of Cardizem. However, skin eruptions progressing to erythema multiforme and/or exfoliative dermatitis have also been infrequently reported. Should a dermatologic reaction persist, the drug should be discontinued.

Carcinogenesis, Mutagenesis, and Impairment of Fertility

A 24 month study in rats and a 21 month study in mice showed no evidence of carcinogenicity. There was also no mutagenic response in *in vitro* bacterial tests. No intrinsic effect on fertility was observed in rats.

Pregnancy Category C

Reproduction studies have been conducted in mice, rats, and rabbits. Administration of doses ranging from 5-10 times greater (on a mg/kg basis) than the daily recommended therapeutic dose has resulted in embryo and fetal lethality. These doses, in some studies, have been reported to cause skeletal abnormalities. In the perinatal/postnatal studies, there was some reduction in early individual pup weights and survival rates. There was an increased incidence of stillbirths at doses of 20 times the human dose or greater.

There are no well-controlled studies in pregnant women; therefore, use Cardizem in pregnant women only if the potential benefit justifies the potential risk to the fetus.

Nursing Mothers

Diltiazem is excreted in human milk. One report suggests that concentrations in breast milk may approximate serum levels. If use of Cardizem is deemed essential, an alternative method of infant feeding should be instituted.

Pediatric Use

Safety and effectiveness in pediatric patients have not been established.

DRUG INTERACTIONS

CARDIZEM CD CAPSULES

Due to the potential for additive effects, caution and careful titration are warranted in patients receiving Cardizem concomitantly with other agents known to affect cardiac contractility and/or conduction. (See WARNINGS, Cardizem CD Capsules.) Pharmacologic studies indicate that there may be additive effects in prolonging AV conduction when using beta-blockers or digitalis concomitantly with Cardizem. (See WARNINGS, Cardizem CD Capsules.)

As with all drugs, care should be exercised when treating patients with multiple medications. Cardizem undergoes biotransformation by cytochrome P-450 mixed function oxidase. Coadministration of Cardizem with other agents which follow the same route of biotransformation may result in the competitive inhibition of metabolism. Especially in patients with renal and/or hepatic impairment, dosages of similarly metabolized drugs, particularly those of low therapeutic ratio, may require adjustment when starting or stopping concomitantly administered diltiazem to maintain optimum therapeutic blood levels.

Beta-Blockers

Controlled and uncontrolled domestic studies suggest that concomitant use of Cardizem and beta-blockers is usually well tolerated, but available data are not sufficient to predict the effects of concomitant treatment in patients with left ventricular dysfunction or cardiac conduction abnormalities.

Administration of Cardizem (diltiazem HCl) concomitantly with propranolol in 5 normal volunteers resulted in increased propranolol levels in all subjects and bioavailability of propranolol was increased approximately 50%. *In vitro,* propranolol appears to be displaced from its binding sites by diltiazem. If combination therapy is initiated or withdrawn in conjunction with propranolol, an adjustment in the propranolol dose may be warranted. (See WARNINGS, Cardizem CD Capsules.)

Cimetidine

A study in 6 healthy volunteers has shown a significant increase in peak diltiazem plasma levels (58%) and area-under-the-curve (53%) after a 1 week course of cimetidine at 1200 mg/day and a single dose of diltiazem 60 mg. Ranitidine produced smaller, nonsignificant increases. The effect may be mediated by cimetidine's known inhibition of hepatic cytochrome P-450, the enzyme system responsible for the first-pass metabolism of diltiazem. Patients currently receiving diltiazem therapy should be carefully monitored for a change in pharmacological effect when initiating and discontinuing therapy with cimetidine. An adjustment in the diltiazem dose may be warranted.

Digitalis

Administration of Cardizem with digoxin in 24 healthy male subjects increased plasma digoxin concentrations approximately 20%. Another investigator found no increase in digoxin levels in 12 patients with coronary artery disease. Since there have been conflicting results regarding the effect of digoxin levels, it is recommended that digoxin levels be monitored when initiating, adjusting, and discontinuing Cardizem therapy to avoid possible over- or under-digitalization. (See WARNINGS, Cardizem CD Capsules.)

Anesthetics

The depression of cardiac contractility, conductivity, and automaticity as well as the vascular dilation associated with anesthetics may be potentiated by calcium channel blockers. When used concomitantly, anesthetics and calcium blockers should be titrated carefully.

Cyclosporine

A pharmacokinetic interaction between diltiazem and cyclosporine has been observed during studies involving renal and cardiac transplant patients. In renal and cardiac transplant recipients, a reduction of cyclosporine dose ranging from 15-48% was necessary to maintain cyclosporine trough concentrations similar to those seen prior to the addition of diltiazem. If these agents are to be administered concurrently, cyclosporine concentrations should be monitored, especially when diltiazem therapy is initiated, adjusted, or discontinued.

The effect of cyclosporine on diltiazem plasma concentrations has not been evaluated.

Carbamazepine

Concomitant administration of diltiazem with carbamazepine has been reported to result in elevated serum levels of carbamazepine (40-72% increase), resulting in toxicity in some cases. Patients receiving these drugs concurrently should be monitored for a potential drug interaction.

CARDIZEM DIRECT COMPRESSION TABLETS

Due to the potential for additive effects, caution and careful titration are warranted in patients receiving Cardizem concomitantly with any agents known to affect cardiac contractility and/or conduction. (See WARNINGS, Cardizem Direct Compression Tablets.)

Pharmacologic studies indicate that there may be additive effects in prolonging AV conduction when using beta-blockers or digitalis concomitantly with Cardizem. (See WARNINGS, Cardizem Direct Compression Tablets.)

As with all drugs, care should be exercised when treating patients with multiple medications. Cardizem undergoes biotransformation by cytochrome P-450 mixed function oxidase. Coadministration of Cardizem with other agents which follow the same route of biotransformation may result in the competitive inhibition of metabolism. Especially in patients with renal and/or hepatic impairment, dosages of similarly metabolized drugs, particularly those of low therapeutic ratio, may require adjustment when starting or stopping concomitantly administered diltiazem to maintain optimum therapeutic blood levels.

Beta-Blockers

Controlled and uncontrolled domestic studies suggest that concomitant use of Cardizem and beta-blockers is usually well tolerated. Available data are not sufficient, however, to predict the effects of concomitant treatment, particularly in patients with left ventricular dysfunction or cardiac conduction abnormalities.

Administration of Cardizem concomitantly with propranolol in 5 normal volunteers resulted in increased propranolol levels in all subjects; and bioavailability of propranolol was increased approximately 50%. *In vitro,* propranolol appears to be displaced from its binding sites by diltiazem. If combination therapy is initiated or withdrawn in conjunction with propranolol, an adjustment in the propranolol dose may be warranted. (See WARNINGS, Cardizem Direct Compression Tablets.)

Cimetidine

A study in 6 healthy volunteers has shown a significant increase in peak diltiazem plasma levels (58%) and area-under-the-curve (53%) after a 1 week course of cimetidine at 1200 mg/day and a single dose of diltiazem 60 mg. Ranitidine produced smaller, nonsignificant increases. The effect may be mediated by cimetidine's known inhibition of hepatic cytochrome P-450, the enzyme system responsible for the first-pass metabolism of diltiazem. Patients currently receiving diltiazem therapy should be carefully monitored for a change in pharmacological effect when initiating and discontinuing therapy with cimetidine. An adjustment in the diltiazem dose may be warranted.

Digitalis

Administration of Cardizem with digoxin in 24 healthy male subjects increased plasma digoxin concentrations approximately 20%. Another investigator found no increase in digoxin levels in 12 patients with coronary artery disease. Since there have been conflicting results regarding the effect of digoxin levels, it is recommended that digoxin levels be monitored when initiating, adjusting, and discontinuing Cardizem therapy to avoid possible over- or under-digitalization. (See WARNINGS, Cardizem Direct Compression Tablets.)

Anesthetics

The depression of cardiac contractility, conductivity, and automaticity, as well as the vascular dilation associated with anesthetics may be potentiated by calcium channel blockers. When used concomitantly, anesthetics and calcium blockers should be titrated carefully.

Cyclosporine

A pharmacokinetic interaction between diltiazem and cyclosporine has been observed during studies involving renal and cardiac transplant patients. In renal and cardiac transplant recipients, a reduction of cyclosporine dose ranging from 15-48% was necessary to maintain concentrations similar to those seen prior to the addition of diltiazem. If these agents are to be administered concurrently, cyclosporine concentrations should be monitored, especially when diltiazem therapy is initiated, adjusted or discontinued. The effect of cyclosporine on diltiazem plasma concentrations has not been evaluated.

Carbamazepine

Concomitant administration of diltiazem with carbamazepine has been reported to result in elevated serum levels of carbamazepine (40-72% increase), resulting in toxicity in some cases. Patients receiving these drugs concurrently should be monitored for a potential drug interaction.

CARDIZEM LA EXTENDED RELEASE TABLETS

Due to the potential for additive effects, caution and careful titration are warranted in patients receiving diltiazem concomitantly with other agents known to affect cardiac contractility and/or conduction (See WARNINGS, Cardizem LA Extended Release Tablets). Pharmacologic studies indicate that there may be additive effects in prolonging AV conduction when using beta-blockers or digitalis concomitantly with diltiazem (See WARNINGS, Cardizem LA Extended Release Tablets).

As with all drugs, care should be exercised when treating patients with multiple medications. Diltiazem is both a substrate and an inhibitor of the cytochrome P-450 3A4 enzyme system. Other drugs that are specific substrates, inhibitors, or inducers of this enzyme system may have a significant impact on the efficacy and side effect profile of diltiazem. Patients taking other drugs that are substrates of CYP450, especially patients with renal and/or hepatic impairment, may require dosage adjustment when starting or stopping concomitantly administered diltiazem in order to maintain optimum therapeutic blood levels.

Beta-Blockers

Controlled and uncontrolled domestic studies suggest that concomitant use of diltiazem and beta-blockers is usually well tolerated, but available data are not sufficient to predict the effects of concomitant treatment in patients with left ventricular dysfunction or cardiac conduction abnormalities.

Administration of diltiazem concomitantly with propranolol in 5 normal volunteers resulted in increased propranolol levels in all subjects and bioavailability of propranolol was increased approximately 50%. *In vitro,* propranolol appears to be displaced from its binding sites by diltiazem. If combination therapy is initiated or withdrawn in conjunction with propranolol, an adjustment in the propranolol dose may be warranted (See WARNINGS, Cardizem LA Extended Release Tablets).

Cimetidine

A study in 6 healthy volunteers has shown a significant increase in peak diltiazem plasma levels (58%) and area-under-the-curve (53%) after a 1 week course of cimetidine at 1200 mg/day and a single dose of diltiazem 60 mg. Ranitidine produced smaller, nonsignificant increases. The effect may be mediated by cimetidine's known inhibition of hepatic cytochrome P-450, the enzyme system responsible for the first-pass metabolism of diltiazem. Patients currently receiving diltiazem therapy should be carefully monitored for a change in pharmacological effect when initiating and discontinuing therapy with cimetidine. An adjustment in the diltiazem dose may be warranted.

Digitalis

Administration of diltiazem with digoxin in 24 healthy male subjects increased plasma digoxin concentrations approximately 20%. Another investigator found no increase in digoxin levels in 12 patients with coronary artery disease. Since there have been conflicting results regarding the effect of digoxin levels, it is recommended that digoxin levels be monitored when initiating, adjusting, and discontinuing diltiazem therapy to avoid possible over- or under-digitalization (See WARNINGS, Cardizem LA Extended Release Tablets).

Anesthetics

The depression of cardiac contractility, conductivity, and automaticity, as well as the vascular dilation associated with anesthetics may be potentiated by calcium channel blockers. When used concomitantly, anesthetics and calcium blockers should be titrated carefully.

Benzodiazepines

Studies showed that diltiazem increased the AUC of midazolam and triazolam by 3- to 4-fold and the C_{max} by 2-fold, compared to placebo. The elimination half-life of midazolam and triazolam also increase (1.5- to 2.5-fold) during coadministration with diltiazem. These pharmacokinetic effects seen during diltiazem coadministration can result in increased clinical effects (*e.g.,* prolonged sedation) of both midazolam and triazolam.

Cyclosporine

A pharmacokinetic interaction between diltiazem and cyclosporine has been observed during studies involving renal and cardiac transplant patients. In renal and cardiac transplant recipients, a reduction of cyclosporine dose ranging from 15-48% was necessary to maintain cyclosporine trough concentrations similar to those seen prior to the addition of diltiazem. If these agents are to be administered concurrently, cyclosporine concentrations should be monitored, especially when diltiazem therapy is initiated, adjusted, or discontinued.

The effect of cyclosporine on diltiazem plasma concentrations has not been evaluated.

Carbamazepine

Concomitant administration of diltiazem with carbamazepine has been reported to result in elevated serum levels of carbamazepine (40-72% increase), resulting in toxicity in some cases. Patients receiving these drugs concurrently should be monitored for a potential drug interaction.

Lovastatin

In a 10-subject study, coadministration of diltiazem (120 mg bid diltiazem SR) with lovastatin resulted in a 3-4 times increase in mean lovastatin AUC and C_{max} versus lovastatin alone; no change in pravastatin AUC and C_{max} was observed during diltiazem coadministration. Diltiazem plasma levels were not significantly affected by lovastatin or pravastatin.

Rifampin

Coadministration of rifampin with diltiazem lowered the diltiazem plasma concentrations to undetectable levels. Coadministration of diltiazem with rifampin or any known CYP 3A4 inducer should be avoided when possible, and alternative therapy considered.

CARDIZEM SR SUSTAINED RELEASE CAPSULES

Due to the potential for additive effects, caution and careful titration are warranted in patients receiving Cardizem concomitantly with any agents known to affect cardiac contractility and/or conduction. (See WARNINGS, Cardizem SR Sustained Release Capsules.) Pharmacologic studies indicate that there may be additive effects in prolonging AV conduction when using beta-blockers or digitalis concomitantly with Cardizem. (See WARNINGS, Cardizem SR Sustained Release Capsules.)

As with all drugs, care should be exercised when treating patients with multiple medications. Cardizem undergoes biotransformation by cytochrome P-450 mixed function oxidase. Coadministration of Cardizem with other agents which follow the same route of biotransformation may result in the competitive inhibition of metabolism. Especially in patients with renal and/or hepatic impairment, dosages of similarly metabolized drugs, particularly those of low therapeutic ratio may require adjustment when starting or stopping concomitantly administered diltiazem to maintain optimum therapeutic blood levels.

Beta-Blockers

Controlled and uncontrolled domestic studies suggest that concomitant use of Cardizem and beta-blockers is usually well tolerated, but available data are not sufficient to predict the effects of concomitant treatment in patients with left ventricular dysfunction or cardiac conduction abnormalities.

Administration of Cardizem concomitantly with propranolol in 5 normal volunteers resulted in increased propranolol levels in all subjects and bioavailability of propranolol was increased approximately 50%. *In vitro,* propranolol appears to be displaced from its binding sites by diltiazem. If combination therapy is initiated or withdrawn in conjunction with propranolol, an adjustment in the propranolol dose may be warranted. (See WARNINGS, Cardizem SR Sustained Release Capsules.)

Cimetidine

A study in 6 healthy volunteers has shown a significant increase in peak diltiazem plasma levels (58%) and area-under-the-curve (53%) after a 1 week course of cimetidine at 1200 mg/day and a single dose of diltiazem 60 mg. Ranitidine produced smaller, nonsignificant increases. The effect may be mediated by cimetidine's known inhibition of hepatic cytochrome P-450, the enzyme system responsible for the first-pass metabolism of diltiazem. Patients currently receiving diltiazem therapy should be carefully monitored for a change in pharmacological effect when initiating and discontinuing therapy with cimetidine. An adjustment in the diltiazem dose may be warranted.

Digitalis

Administration of Cardizem with digoxin in 24 healthy male subjects increased plasma digoxin concentrations approximately 20%. Another investigator found no increase in digoxin levels in 12 patients with coronary artery disease. Since there have been conflicting results regarding the effect of digoxin levels, it is recommended that digoxin levels be monitored when initiating, adjusting, and discontinuing Cardizem therapy to avoid possible over- or under-digitalization. (See WARNINGS, Cardizem SR Sustained Release Capsules.)

Anesthetics

The depression of cardiac contractility, conductivity, and automaticity as well as the vascular dilation associated with anesthetics may be potentiated by calcium channel blockers. When used concomitantly, anesthetics and calcium blockers should be titrated carefully.

Cyclosporine

A pharmacokinetic interaction between diltiazem and cyclosporine has been observed during studies involving renal and cardiac transplant patients. In renal and cardiac transplant recipients, a reduction of cyclosporine dose ranging from 15-48% was necessary to maintain cyclosporine trough concentrations similar to those seen prior to the addition of diltiazem. If these agents are to be administered concurrently, cyclosporine concentrations should be monitored, especially when diltiazem therapy is initiated, adjusted or discontinued. The effect of cyclosporine on diltiazem plasma concentrations has not been evaluated.

Carbamazepine

Concomitant administration of diltiazem with carbamazepine has been reported to result in elevated serum levels of carbamazepine (40-72% increase), resulting in toxicity in some cases. Patients receiving these drugs concurrently should be monitored for a potential drug interaction.

ADVERSE REACTIONS

CARDIZEM CD CAPSULES

Serious adverse reactions have been rare in studies carried out to date, but it should be recognized that patients with impaired ventricular function and cardiac conduction abnormalities have usually been excluded from these studies.

The TABLE 2 presents the most common adverse reactions reported in placebo-controlled angina and hypertension trials in patients receiving Cardizem CD up to 360 mg with rates in placebo patients shown for comparison.

TABLE 2 *Cardizem CD Capsule Placebo-Controlled Angina and Hypertension Trials Combined*

Adverse Reactions	Cardizem CD (n=607)	Placebo (n=301)
Headache	5.4%	5.0%
Dizziness	3.0%	3.0%
Bradycardia	3.3%	1.3%
AV block first-degree	3.3%	0.0%
Edema	2.6%	1.3%
ECG abnormality	1.6%	2.3%
Asthenia	1.8%	1.7%

In clinical trials of Cardizem CD capsules, Cardizem tablets, and Cardizem SR capsules involving over 3200 patients, the most common events (*i.e.,* greater than 1%) were edema (4.6%), headache (4.6%), dizziness (3.5%), asthenia (2.6%), first-degree AV block (2.4%), bradycardia (1.7%), flushing (1.4%), nausea (1.4%), and rash (1.2%).

In addition, the following events were reported infrequently (less than 1%) in angina or hypertension trials:

Cardiovascular: Angina, arrhythmia, AV block (second- or third-degree), bundle branch block, congestive heart failure, ECG abnormalities, hypotension, palpitations, syncope, tachycardia, ventricular extrasystoles.

Nervous System: Abnormal dreams, amnesia, depression, gait abnormality, hallucinations, insomnia, nervousness, paresthesia, personality change, somnolence, tinnitus, tremor.

Gastrointestinal: Anorexia, constipation, diarrhea, dry mouth, dysgeusia, dyspepsia, mild elevations of SGOT, SGPT, LDH, and alkaline phosphatase (see WARNINGS, Cardizem CD Capsules, Acute Hepatic Injury), thirst, vomiting, weight increase.

Dermatologic: Petechiae, photosensitivity, pruritus, urticaria.

Other: Amblyopia, CPK increase, dyspnea, epistaxis, eye irritation, hyperglycemia, hyperuricemia, impotence, muscle cramps, nasal congestion, nocturia, osteoarticular pain, polyuria, sexual difficulties.

The following postmarketing events have been reported infrequently in patients receiving Cardizem: allergic reactions, alopecia, angioedema (including facial or periorbital edema), asystole, erythema multiforme (including Stevens-Johnson syndrome, toxic epidermal necrolysis), exfoliative dermatitis, extrapyramidal symptoms, gingival hyperplasia, hemolytic anemia, increased bleeding time, leukopenia, purpura, retinopathy, and thrombocytopenia. In addition, events such as myocardial infarction have been observed which are not readily distinguishable from the natural history of the disease in these patients. A number of well documented cases of generalized rash, some characterized as leukocytoclastic vasculitis, have been reported. However, a definitive cause and effect relationship between these events and Cardizem therapy is yet to be established.

CARDIZEM DIRECT COMPRESSION TABLETS

Serious adverse reactions have been rare in studies carried out to date, but it should be recognized that patients with impaired ventricular function and cardiac conduction abnormalities have usually been excluded.

In domestic placebo-controlled angina trials, the incidence of adverse reactions reported during Cardizem therapy was not greater than that reported during placebo therapy.

The following represent occurrences observed in clinical studies of angina patients. In many cases, the relationship to Cardizem has not been established. The most common occurrences from these studies, as well as their frequency of presentation, are edema (2.4%), headache (2.1%), nausea (1.9%), dizziness (1.5%), rash (1.3%), and asthenia (1.2%).

In addition, the following events were reported infrequently (less than 1%):

Cardiovascular: Angina, arrhythmia, AV block (first-degree), AV block (second- or third-degree — see WARNINGS, Cardizem Direct Compression Tablets, Cardiac Conduction), bradycardia, bundle branch block, congestive heart failure, ECG abnormaility, flushing, hypotension, palpitations, syncope, tachycardia, ventricular extrasystoles.

Nervous System: Abnormal dreams, amnesia, depression, gait abnormality, hallucinations, insomnia, nervousness, paresthesia, personality change, somnolence, tremor.

Gastrointestinal: Anorexia, constipation, diarrhea, dysgeusia, dyspepsia, mild elevations of alkaline phosphatase, SGOT, SGPT, and LDH (see WARNINGS, Cardizem Direct Compression Tablets, Acute Hepatic Injury), thirst, vomiting, weight increase.

Dermatologic: Petechiae, photosensitivity, pruritus, urticaria.

Other: Amblyopia, CPK elevation, dry mouth, dyspnea, epistaxis, eye irritation, hyperglycemia, hyperuricemia, impotence, muscle cramps, nasal congestion, nocturia, osteoarticular pain, polyuria, sexual difficulties, tinnitus.

The following postmarketing events have been reported infrequently in patients receiving Cardizem: allergic reactions, alopecia, angioedema (including facial or periorbital edema), asystole, erythema multiforme (including Stevens-Johnson syndrome, toxic epidermal necrolysis), extrapyramidal symptoms, gingival hyperplasia, hemolytic anemia, increased bleeding time, leukopenia, purpura, retinopathy, and thrombocytopenia. There have been observed cases of a generalized rash, some characterized as leukocytoclastic vasculitis. In addition, events such as myocardial infarction have been observed which are not readily distinguishable from the natural history of the disease in these patients. A definitive cause and effect relationship between these events and Cardizem therapy cannot yet be established. Exfoliative dermatitis (proven by rechallenge) has also been reported.

CARDIZEM LA EXTENDED RELEASE TABLETS

Serious adverse reactions have been rare in studies carried out to date, but it should be recognized that patients with impaired ventricular function and cardiac conduction abnormalities have usually been excluded from these studies.

TABLE 3 presents adverse reactions more common on diltiazem than on placebo (but excluding events with no plausible relationship to treatment), as reported in placebo-controlled hypertension trials in patients receiving a diltiazem HCl extended-release formulation (once-a-day dosing) up to 540 mg.

TABLE 3

Adverse Reactions (MedDRA Term)	Placebo n=120	Diltiazem HCl Extended Release 120-360 mg n=501	Diltiazem HCl Extended Release 540 mg n=123
Oedema lower limb	4 (3%)	24 (5%)	10 (8%)
Sinus congestion	0 (0%)	2 (1%)	2 (2%)
Rash NOS	0 (0%)	3 (1%)	2 (4%)

In clinical trials of other diltiazem formulations involving over 3200 patients, the most common events (*i.e.,* greater than 1%) were edema (4.6%), headache (4.6%), dizziness (3.5%), asthenia (2.6%), first-degree AV block (2.4%), bradycardia (1.7%), flushing (1.4%), nausea (1.4%) and rash (1.2%).

In addition, the following events have been reported infrequently (less than 2%) in hypertension trials with other diltiazem products:

Cardiovascular: Angina, arrhythmia, AV block (second- or third-degree), bundle branch block, congestive heart failure, ECG abnormalities, hypotension, palpitations, syncope, tachycardia, ventricular extrasystoles.

Nervous System: Abnormal dreams, amnesia, depression, gait abnormality, hallucinations, insomnia, nervousness, paresthesia, personality change, somnolence, tinnitus, tremor.

Gastrointestinal: Anorexia, constipation, diarrhea, dry mouth, dysgeusia, mild elevations of SGOT, SGPT, LDH, and alkaline phosphatase (see WARNINGS, Cardizem LA Extended Release Tablets, Acute Hepatic Injury), nausea, thirst, vomiting, weight increase.

Dermatologic: Petechiae, photosensitivity, pruritus.

Other: Albuminuria, allergic reaction, amblyopia, asthenia, CPK increase, crystalluria, dyspnea, ecchymosis, edema, epistaxis, eye irritation, headache, hyperglycemia, hyperuricemia, impotence, muscle cramps, nasal congestion, neck rigidity, nocturia, osteoarticular pain, pain, polyuria, rhinitis, sexual difficulties, gynecomastia.

The following postmarketing events have been reported infrequently in patients receiving diltiazem: allergic reactions, alopecia, angioedema (including facial or periorbital edema), asystole, erythema multiforme (including Stevens-Johnson syndrome, toxic epidermal necrolysis), exfoliative dermatitis, extrapyramidal symptoms, gingival hyperplasia, hemolytic anemia, increased bleeding time, leukopenia, purpura, retinopathy, and thrombocytopenia. In addition, events such as myocardial infarction have been observed which are not readily distinguishable from the natural history of the disease in these patients. A number of well-documented cases of generalized rash, some characterized as leukocytoclastic vasculitis, have been reported. However, a definitive cause and effect relationship between these events and diltiazem therapy is yet to be established.

CARDIZEM SR SUSTAINED RELEASE CAPSULES

Serious adverse reactions have been rare in studies carried out to date, but it should be recognized that patients with impaired ventricular function and cardiac conduction abnormalities have usually been excluded from these studies.

The adverse events described below represent events observed in clinical studies of hypertensive patients receiving either Cardizem direct compression tablets or Cardizem SR sustained release capsules as well as experiences observed in studies of angina and during marketing. The most common events in hypertension studies are shown in TABLE 4 with rates in placebo patients shown for comparison. Less common events are listed by body system; these include any adverse reactions seen in angina studies that were not observed in hypertension studies. In all hypertensive patients studied (over 900), the most common adverse events were edema (9%), headache (8%), dizziness (6%), asthenia (5%), sinus bradycardia (3%), flushing (3%), and first-degree AV block (3%). Only edema and perhaps bradycardia and dizziness were dose related. The most common events observed in clinical studies (over 2100 patients) of angina patients and hypertensive patients receiving Cardizem direct compression tablets or Cardizem SR sustained release capsules were (*i.e.,* greater than 1%) edema (5.4%), headache (4.5%), dizziness (3.4%), asthenia (2.8%), first-degree AV block (1.8%), flushing (1.7%), nausea (1.6%), bradycardia (1.5%), and rash (1.5%).

In addition, the following events were reported infrequently (less tan 1%) with Cardizem SR sustained release capsules or Cardizem direct compression tablets or have been observed in angina or hypertension trials.

Cardiovascular: Angina, arrhythmia, second- or third-degree AV block (see WARNINGS, Cardizem SR Sustained Release Capsules, Cardiac Conduction), bundle branch block, congestive heart failure, syncope, tachycardia, ventricular extrasystoles.

Nervous System: Abnormal dreams, amnesia, depression, gait abnormality, hallucinations, nervousness, paresthesia, personality change, tremor.

Gastrointestinal: Anorexia, diarrhea, dry mouth, dysgeusia, mild elevations of SGOT, SGPT, and LDH (see WARNINGS, Cardizem SR Sustained Release Capsules, Acute Hepatic Injury), thirst, vomiting, weight increase.

Dermatologic: Petechiae, photosensitivity, pruritus, urticaria.

TABLE 4 *Double-Blind Placebo Controlled Hypertension Trials*

Adverse	Diltiazem n=315	Placebo n=211
Headache	38 (12%)	17 (8%)
AV block first-degree	24 (7.6%)	4 (1.9%)
Dizziness	22 (7%)	6 (2.8%)
Edema	19 (6%)	2 (0.9%)
Bradycardia	19 (6%)	3 (1.4%)
ECG abnormality	13 (4.1%)	3 (1.4%)
Asthenia	10 (3.2%)	1 (0.5%)
Constipation	5 (1.6%)	2 (0.9%)
Dyspepsia	4 (1.3%)	1 (0.5%)
Nausea	4 (1.3%)	2 (0.9%)
Palpitations	4 (1.3%)	2 (0.9%)
Polyuria	4 (1.3%)	2 (0.9%)
Somnolence	4 (1.3%)	—
Alk phos increase	3 (1%)	1 (0.5%)
Hypotension	3 (1%)	1 (0.5%)
Insomnia	3 (1%)	1 (0.5%)
Rash	3 (1%)	1 (0.5%)
AV block second-degree	2 (0.6%)	—

Other: Amblyopia, CPK increase, dyspnea, epistaxis, eye irritation, hyperglycemia, hyperuricemia, impotence, muscle cramps, nasal congestion, nocturia, osteoarticular pain, sexual difficulties, tinnitus.

The following postmarketing events have been reported infrequently in patients receiving Cardizem: allergic reactions, alopecia, angioedema (including facial or periorbital edema), asystole, erythema multiforme (including Stevens-Johnson syndrome, toxic epidermal necrolysis), extrapyramidal symptoms, gingival hyperplasia, hemolytic anemia, increased bleeding time, leukopenia, purpura, retinopathy, and thrombocytopenia. There have been observed cases of a generalized rash, some characterized as leukocytoclastic vasculitis. In addition, events such as myocardial infarction have been observed which are not readily distinguishable from the natural history of the disease in these patients. A definitive cause and effect relationship between these events and Cardizem therapy cannot yet be established. Exfoliative dermatitis (proven by rechallenge) has also been reported.

DOSAGE AND ADMINISTRATION

CARDIZEM CD CAPSULES

Patients controlled on diltiazem alone or in combination with other medications may be switched to Cardizem CD capsules at the nearest equivalent total daily dose. Higher doses of Cardizem CD may be needed in some patients. Patients should be closely monitored. Subsequent titration to higher or lower doses may be necessary and should be initiated as clinically warranted. There is limited general clinical experience with doses above 360 mg, but doses to 540 mg have been studied in clinical trials. The incidence of side effects increases as the dose increases with first-degree AV block, dizziness, and sinus bradycardia bearing the strongest relationship to dose.

Hypertension

Dosage needs to be adjusted by titration to individual patient needs. When used as monotherapy, reasonable starting doses are 180-240 mg once daily, although some patients may respond to lower doses. Maximum antihypertensive effect is usually observed by 14 days of chronic therapy; therefore, dosage adjustments should be scheduled accordingly. The usual dosage range studied in clinical trials was 240-360 mg once daily. Individual patients may respond to higher doses of up to 480 mg once daily.

Angina

Dosages for the treatment of angina should be adjusted to each patient's needs, starting with a dose of 120 or 180 mg once daily. Individual patients may respond to higher doses of up to 480 mg once daily. When necessary, titration may be carried out over a 7-14 day period.

Concomitant Use With Other Cardiovascular Agents

Sublingual NTG: May be taken as required to abort acute anginal attacks during Cardizem CD (diltiazem HCl) therapy.

Prophylactic Nitrate Therapy: Cardizem CD may be safely coadministered with short- and long-acting nitrates.

Beta-blockers: See WARNINGS, Cardizem CD Capsules and PRECAUTIONS, Cardizem CD Capsules.

Antihypertensives: Cardizem CD has an additive antihypertensive effect when used with other antihypertensive agents. Therefore, the dosage of Cardizem CD or the concomitant antihypertensives may need to be adjusted when adding one to the other.

CARDIZEM DIRECT COMPRESSION TABLETS

Exertional Angina Pectoris Due to Atherosclerotic Coronary Artery Disease or Angina Pectoris at Rest Due to Coronary Artery Spasm

Dosage must be adjusted to each patient's needs. Starting with 30 mg four times daily, before meals, and at bedtime, dosage should be increased gradually (given in divided doses 3 or 4 times daily) at 1-2 day intervals until optimum response is obtained. Although individual patients may respond to any dosage level, the average optimum dosage range appears to be 180-360 mg/day. There are no available data concerning dosage requirements in patients with impaired renal or hepatic function. If the drug must be used in such patients, titration should be carried out with particular caution.

Concomitant Use With Other Cardiovascular Agents

Sublingual NTG: May be taken as required to abort acute anginal attacks during Cardizem therapy.

Prophylactic Nitrate Therapy: Cardizem may be safely coadministered with short- and long-acting nitrates, but there have been no controlled studies to evaluate the antianginal effectiveness of this combination.

Beta-Blockers: See WARNINGS, Cardizem Direct Compression Tablets and PRECAUTIONS, Cardizem Direct Compression Tablets.

CARDIZEM LA EXTENDED RELEASE TABLETS

Cardizem LA tablets have an extended release formulation intended for once-a-day administration.

Patients controlled on diltiazem alone or in combination with other medications may be switched to Cardizem LA tablets once-a-day at the nearest equivalent total daily dose. Higher doses of Cardizem LA tablets once-a-day dosage may be needed in some patients. Patients should be closely monitored. Subsequent titration to higher or lower doses may be necessary and should be initiated as clinically warranted. There is limited general clinical experience with doses above 360 mg, but the safety and efficacy of doses as high as 540 mg have been studied in clinical trials. The incidence of side effects increases as the dose increases with first-degree AV block, dizziness, and sinus bradycardia bearing the strongest relationship to dose.

The tablet should be swallowed whole and not chewed or crushed.

Hypertension

Dosage needs to be adjusted by titration to individual patient needs. When used as monotherapy, reasonable starting doses are 180-240 mg once daily, although some patients may respond to lower doses. Maximum antihypertensive effect is usually observed by 14 days of chronic therapy; therefore, dosage adjustments should be scheduled accordingly. The dosage range studied in clinical trials was 120-540 mg once daily. The dosage may be titrated to a maximum of 540 mg daily.

Cardizem LA tablets should be taken about the same time once each day either in the morning or at bedtime. The time of dosing should be considered when making dose adjustments based on trough effects.

Concomitant Use With Other Cardiovascular Agents

Sublingual NTG: May be taken as required to abort acute anginal attacks during diltiazem HCl extended-release therapy.

Prophylactic Nitrate Therapy: Diltiazem HCl extended release tablets may be safely coadministered with short-and long-acting nitrates.

Beta-Blockers: See WARNINGS, Cardizem LA Extended Release Tablets and PRECAUTIONS, Cardizem LA Extended Release Tablets.

Antihypertensives: Cardizem LA has an additive antihypertensive effect when used with other antihypertensive agents. Therefore, the dosage of diltiazem HCl extended release tablets or the concomitant antihypertensives may need to be adjusted when adding one to the other.

CARDIZEM SR SUSTAINED RELEASE CAPSULES

Dosages must be adjusted to each patient's needs, starting with 60-120 mg twice daily. Maximum antihypertensive effect is usually observed by 14 days of chronic therapy; therefore, dosage adjustments should be scheduled accordingly. Although individual patients may response to lower doses, the usual optimum dosage range in clinical trials was 240-360 mg/day.

Cardizem SR has an additive antihypertensive effect when used with other antihypertensive agents. Therefore, the dosage of Cardizem SR or the concomitant antihypertensives may need to be adjusted when adding one to the other. See WARNINGS, Cardizem SR Sustained Release Capsules and PRECAUTIONS, Cardizem SR Sustained Release Capsules regarding use with beta-blockers.

HOW SUPPLIED

CARDIZEM CD CAPSULES

120 mg: Light turquoise blue/light turquoise blue capsule imprinted with "cardizem CD" and "120 mg" on one end.

180 mg: Light turquoise blue/blue capsule imprinted with "cardizem CD" and "180 mg" on one end.

240 mg: Blue/blue capsule imprinted with "cardizem CD" and "240 mg" on one end.

300 mg: Light gray/blue capsule imprinted with "cardizem CD" and "300 mg" on one end.

360 mg: Light blue/white capsule imprinted with "cardizem CD" and "360 mg" on one end.

Storage Conditions: Store at 25°C (77°F); excursions permitted to 15-30°C (59-86°F). Avoid excessive humidity.

CARDIZEM DIRECT COMPRESSSION TABLETS

Cardizem direct compression tablets are available as follows:

30 mg: Each green tablet is engraved with "MARION" on one side and "1771" on the other.

60 mg: Each scored, yellow tablet is engraved with "MARION" on one side and "17772" on the other.

90 mg: Each scored, green oblong tablet is engraved with "CARDIZEM" on one side and "90 mg" on the other.

120 mg: Each scored, yellow oblong tablet is engraved with "CARDIZEM" on one side and "120 mg" on the other.

Storage: Store at controlled room temperature 15-30°C (59-86°F).

CARDIZEM LA EXTENDED RELEASE TABLETS

Cardizem LA is supplied as white, capsule-shaped tablets in strengths of 120, 180, 240, 300, 360, and 420 mg debossed with "B" on one side and the diltiazem content (mg) on the other.

Storage Conditions
Store at 25°C (77°F); excursions permitted to 15-30°C (59-86°F).
Avoid excessive humidity and temperatures above 30°C (86°F).
Dispense in tight, light resistant container.

CARDIZEM SR SUSTAINED RELEASE CAPSULES

Cardizem SR sustained release capsules are available as follows:

60 mg: Ivory/brown capsule imprinted with Cardizem logo on one end and "Cardizem SR 60 mg" on the other.

90 mg: Gold/brown capsule imprinted with Cardizem logo on one end and "Cardizem SR 90 mg" on the other.

120 mg: Caramel/brown capsule imprinted with Cardizem logo on one end and "Cardizem SR 120 mg" on the other.

Storage Conditions: Store at controlled room temperature 15-30°C (59-86°F).

PRODUCT LISTING - RATED THERAPEUTICALLY EQUIVALENT

Capsule, Extended Release - Oral - 180 mg/24 Hours

30's	$42.36	GENERIC, Allscripts Pharmaceutical Company	54569-3803-00
30's	$57.04	GENERIC, Physicians Total Care	54868-2148-03
100's	$96.25	GENERIC, Udl Laboratories Inc	51079-0948-08
100's	$106.34	GENERIC, Watson Laboratories Inc	52544-0663-01

Powder For Injection - Intravenous - 25 mg

6's	$166.39	CARDIZEM LYO-JECT, Aventis Pharmaceuticals	00088-1789-17

Powder For Injection - Intravenous - 100 mg

3's	$143.22	CARDIZEM MONOVIAL, Aventis Pharmaceuticals	00088-1788-16

Solution - Intravenous - 5 mg/ml

5 ml	$10.20	GENERIC, Apotex Usa Inc	60505-0704-01
5 ml	$11.00	GENERIC, Bertek Pharmaceuticals Inc	62794-0307-31
5 ml x 6	$60.00	GENERIC, Baxter Pharmaceutical Products, Inc	10019-0510-05
5 ml x 6	$92.79	CARDIZEM, Aventis Pharmaceuticals	00088-1790-32
5 ml x 10	$39.31	GENERIC, Abbott Pharmaceutical	00074-1171-01
5 ml x 10	$43.80	GENERIC, International Medication Systems, Limited	00548-5800-00
5 ml x 10	$47.50	GENERIC, Bedford Laboratories	55390-0565-05
5 ml x 10	$50.00	GENERIC, Baxter Pharmaceutical Products, Inc	10019-0510-01
5 ml x 10	$77.19	GENERIC, Abbott Pharmaceutical	00074-2291-11
5 ml x 10	$87.50	GENERIC, Gensia Sicor Pharmaceuticals Inc	00703-1553-03
5 ml x 10	$100.00	GENERIC, Baxter Pharmaceutical Products, Inc	10019-0510-02
5 ml x 10	$110.00	GENERIC, Bertek Pharmaceuticals Inc	62794-0307-97
5 ml x 10	$120.00	GENERIC, Vha Supply	55390-0566-05
6's	$142.20	CARDIZEM, Aventis Pharmaceuticals	00088-1790-17
10 ml	$20.40	GENERIC, Apotex Usa Inc	60505-0704-02
10 ml	$21.50	GENERIC, Bertek Pharmaceuticals Inc	62794-0309-31
10 ml x 6	$110.28	GENERIC, Baxter Pharmaceutical Products, Inc	10019-0510-10
10 ml x 6	$171.97	CARDIZEM, Aventis Pharmaceuticals	00088-1790-33
10 ml x 10	$78.80	GENERIC, Abbott Pharmaceutical	00074-1171-02
10 ml x 10	$81.30	GENERIC, International Medication Systems, Limited	00548-5802-00
10 ml x 10	$95.00	GENERIC, Bedford Laboratories	55390-0565-10
10 ml x 10	$173.75	GENERIC, Gensia Sicor Pharmaceuticals Inc	00703-1554-03
10 ml x 10	$204.00	GENERIC, Vha Supply	55390-0566-10
10 ml x 10	$215.00	GENERIC, Bertek Pharmaceuticals Inc	62794-0309-97
25 ml x 10	$230.00	GENERIC, Bedford Laboratories	55390-0565-30

Tablet - Oral - 30 mg

10's	$3.23	GENERIC, Pd-Rx Pharmaceuticals	55289-0335-10
25 x 30	$336.60	GENERIC, Sky Pharmaceuticals Packaging, Inc	63739-0079-03
25's	$6.09	GENERIC, Pd-Rx Pharmaceuticals	55289-0335-97
25's	$11.25	GENERIC, Udl Laboratories Inc	51079-0745-19
30 x 20	$271.20	GENERIC, Medirex Inc	57480-0489-06
30's	$13.58	GENERIC, Heartland Healthcare Services	61392-0053-30
30's	$13.58	GENERIC, Heartland Healthcare Services	61392-0053-39
31 x 10	$140.28	GENERIC, Vangard Labs	00615-3548-53
31 x 10	$140.28	GENERIC, Vangard Labs	00615-3548-63
31's	$14.03	GENERIC, Heartland Healthcare Services	61392-0053-31
32's	$14.48	GENERIC, Heartland Healthcare Services	61392-0053-32
45's	$20.36	GENERIC, Heartland Healthcare Services	61392-0053-45
50's	$9.75	GENERIC, Pd-Rx Pharmaceuticals	55289-0335-50
60's	$27.15	GENERIC, Heartland Healthcare Services	61392-0053-60
90's	$32.78	GENERIC, Golden State Medical	60429-0061-90
90's	$40.73	GENERIC, Heartland Healthcare Services	61392-0053-90
100's	$10.19	FEDERAL UPPER LIMIT, H.C.F.A. F F P	99999-1069-04
100's	$13.43	GENERIC, Pd-Rx Pharmaceuticals	55289-0335-01
100's	$34.37	GENERIC, West Point Pharma	59591-0071-68
100's	$34.90	GENERIC, Major Pharmaceuticals Inc	00904-7707-60
100's	$34.90	GENERIC, Major Pharmaceuticals Inc	00904-7714-60
100's	$35.45	GENERIC, Esi Lederle Generics	00005-3333-43
100's	$35.96	GENERIC, Qualitest Products Inc	00603-3319-21
100's	$39.85	GENERIC, Ivax Corporation	00172-4219-60
100's	$39.90	GENERIC, Martec Pharmaceuticals Inc	52555-0465-01
100's	$40.10	GENERIC, Ivax Corporation	00182-1937-01
100's	$41.00	GENERIC, Watson/Rugby Laboratories Inc	00536-3101-21
100's	$42.58	GENERIC, Major Pharmaceuticals Inc	00904-7714-61
100's	$44.94	GENERIC, Udl Laboratories Inc	51079-0745-20
100's	$45.25	GENERIC, Medirex Inc	57480-0489-01
100's	$47.25	GENERIC, Mylan Pharmaceuticals Inc	00378-0023-01
100's	$47.27	GENERIC, Teva Pharmaceuticals Usa	00093-0318-01
100's	$47.27	GENERIC, Watson Laboratories Inc	00591-0775-01
100's	$47.27	GENERIC, Watson Laboratories Inc	52544-0775-01
100's	$55.20	CARDIZEM, Aventis Pharmaceuticals	00088-1771-49
100's	$59.49	CARDIZEM, Aventis Pharmaceuticals	00088-1771-47
270's	$97.31	GENERIC, Golden State Medical	60429-0061-27

Tablet - Oral - 60 mg

25 x 30	$542.70	GENERIC, Sky Pharmaceuticals Packaging, Inc	63739-0080-03
25's	$17.58	GENERIC, Udl Laboratories Inc	51079-0746-19
30's	$21.90	GENERIC, Heartland Healthcare Services	61392-0054-30
30's	$21.90	GENERIC, Heartland Healthcare Services	61392-0054-39
31 x 10	$217.93	GENERIC, Vangard Labs	00615-3549-53
31 x 10	$217.93	GENERIC, Vangard Labs	00615-3549-63
31's	$22.63	GENERIC, Heartland Healthcare Services	61392-0054-31
32's	$23.36	GENERIC, Heartland Healthcare Services	61392-0054-32
45's	$32.85	GENERIC, Heartland Healthcare Services	61392-0054-45
60's	$43.80	GENERIC, Heartland Healthcare Services	61392-0054-60
90's	$51.41	GENERIC, Golden State Medical	60429-0062-90
90's	$65.70	GENERIC, Heartland Healthcare Services	61392-0054-90
100's	$11.14	FEDERAL UPPER LIMIT, H.C.F.A. F F P	99999-1069-09
100's	$26.49	GENERIC, Pd-Rx Pharmaceuticals	55289-0329-01
100's	$53.86	GENERIC, West Point Pharma	59591-0072-68
100's	$54.50	GENERIC, Major Pharmaceuticals Inc	00904-7708-60
100's	$54.50	GENERIC, Major Pharmaceuticals Inc	00904-7715-60
100's	$55.53	GENERIC, Esi Lederle Generics	00005-3334-43
100's	$56.23	GENERIC, Aligen Independent Laboratories Inc	00405-4341-01
100's	$56.23	GENERIC, Qualitest Products Inc	00603-3320-21
100's	$56.77	GENERIC, Geneva Pharmaceuticals	00781-1159-01
100's	$61.47	GENERIC, Major Pharmaceuticals Inc	00904-7715-61
100's	$62.57	GENERIC, Ivax Corporation	00172-4220-60
100's	$62.60	GENERIC, Martec Pharmaceuticals Inc	52555-0466-01
100's	$62.75	GENERIC, Ivax Corporation	00182-1938-01
100's	$69.93	GENERIC, Aligen Independent Laboratories Inc	00405-4347-01
100's	$70.30	GENERIC, Udl Laboratories Inc	51079-0746-20
100's	$74.10	GENERIC, Mylan Pharmaceuticals Inc	00378-0045-01
100's	$74.12	GENERIC, Teva Pharmaceuticals Usa	00093-0319-01
100's	$74.12	GENERIC, Watson Laboratories Inc	52544-0776-01
100's	$89.82	CARDIZEM, Aventis Pharmaceuticals	00088-1772-49
100's	$90.73	CARDIZEM, Physicians Total Care	54868-0671-00
100's	$93.35	CARDIZEM, Aventis Pharmaceuticals	00088-1772-47
120's	$68.42	GENERIC, Golden State Medical	60429-0062-12
270's	$153.20	GENERIC, Golden State Medical	60429-0062-27

Tablet - Oral - 90 mg

25's	$12.90	GENERIC, Pd-Rx Pharmaceuticals	55289-0893-97
30 x 20	$539.80	GENERIC, Medirex Inc	57480-0491-06
30's	$29.82	GENERIC, Heartland Healthcare Services	61392-0055-30
30's	$29.82	GENERIC, Heartland Healthcare Services	61392-0055-39
31's	$30.81	GENERIC, Heartland Healthcare Services	61392-0055-31
32's	$31.81	GENERIC, Heartland Healthcare Services	61392-0055-32
45's	$44.73	GENERIC, Heartland Healthcare Services	61392-0055-45
60's	$59.64	GENERIC, Heartland Healthcare Services	61392-0055-60
90's	$89.46	GENERIC, Heartland Healthcare Services	61392-0055-90
100's	$23.12	FEDERAL UPPER LIMIT, H.C.F.A. F F P	99999-1069-14
100's	$30.92	GENERIC, Vangard Labs	00615-3550-13
100's	$75.65	GENERIC, Aligen Independent Laboratories Inc	00405-4342-01
100's	$75.70	GENERIC, West Point Pharma	59591-0075-68
100's	$76.40	GENERIC, Major Pharmaceuticals Inc	00904-7716-60
100's	$78.04	GENERIC, Esi Lederle Generics	00005-3335-43
100's	$78.66	GENERIC, Qualitest Products Inc	00603-3321-21
100's	$79.74	GENERIC, Geneva Pharmaceuticals	00781-1174-01
100's	$80.01	GENERIC, Aligen Independent Laboratories Inc	00405-4348-01
100's	$85.69	GENERIC, Udl Laboratories Inc	51079-0747-20
100's	$86.29	GENERIC, Major Pharmaceuticals Inc	00904-7716-61
100's	$87.92	GENERIC, Ivax Corporation	00172-4221-60
100's	$87.95	GENERIC, Martec Pharmaceuticals Inc	52555-0467-01
100's	$88.10	GENERIC, Ivax Corporation	00182-1939-01
100's	$89.95	GENERIC, Medirex Inc	57480-0491-01
100's	$90.17	GENERIC, Watson/Rugby Laboratories Inc	00536-3103-21
100's	$101.30	GENERIC, Mylan Pharmaceuticals Inc	00378-0135-01
100's	$101.32	GENERIC, Teva Pharmaceuticals Usa	00093-0320-01
100's	$101.32	GENERIC, Watson Laboratories Inc	52544-0777-01
100's	$118.31	CARDIZEM, Aventis Pharmaceuticals	00088-1791-49
100's	$131.28	CARDIZEM, Aventis Pharmaceuticals	00088-1791-47

Tablet - Oral - 120 mg

30's	$38.78	GENERIC, Heartland Healthcare Services	61392-0056-30
30's	$38.78	GENERIC, Heartland Healthcare Services	61392-0056-39
31's	$40.07	GENERIC, Heartland Healthcare Services	61392-0056-31
32's	$41.37	GENERIC, Heartland Healthcare Services	61392-0056-32
45's	$58.17	GENERIC, Heartland Healthcare Services	61392-0056-45
60's	$77.56	GENERIC, Heartland Healthcare Services	61392-0056-60
90's	$116.34	GENERIC, Heartland Healthcare Services	61392-0056-90
100's	$23.31	FEDERAL UPPER LIMIT, H.C.F.A. F F P	99999-1069-17
100's	$99.00	GENERIC, Aligen Independent Laboratories Inc	00405-4343-01
100's	$99.00	GENERIC, Medirex Inc	57480-0492-01
100's	$99.06	GENERIC, West Point Pharma	59591-0077-68
100's	$99.25	GENERIC, Major Pharmaceuticals Inc	00904-7717-60
100's	$102.13	GENERIC, Esi Lederle Generics	00005-3336-43
100's	$104.40	GENERIC, Geneva Pharmaceuticals	00781-1175-01
100's	$104.60	GENERIC, Major Pharmaceuticals Inc	00904-7717-61
100's	$105.10	GENERIC, Qualitest Products Inc	00603-3322-21
100's	$115.13	GENERIC, Ivax Corporation	00172-4222-60
100's	$115.13	GENERIC, Ivax Corporation	00182-1940-01

Quantity	Price	Product	NDC
100's	$115.25	GENERIC, Watson/Rugby Laboratories Inc	00536-3104-01
100's	$115.25	GENERIC, Martec Pharmaceuticals Inc	52555-0468-01
100's	$136.39	GENERIC, Teva Pharmaceuticals Usa	00093-0321-01
100's	$136.39	GENERIC, Watson/Rugby Laboratories Inc	52544-0778-01
100's	$136.40	GENERIC, Mylan Pharmaceuticals Inc	00378-0525-01
100's	$164.52	CARDIZEM, Aventis Pharmaceuticals	00088-1792-49
100's	$171.84	CARDIZEM, Aventis Pharmaceuticals	00088-1792-47

PRODUCT LISTING - RATED NOT THERAPEUTICALLY EQUIVALENT

Capsule, Extended Release - Oral - 60 mg

Quantity	Price	Product	NDC
30's	$9.71	GENERIC, Physicians Total Care	54868-3214-01
30's	$25.78	GENERIC, Heartland Healthcare Services	61392-0188-30
30's	$25.78	GENERIC, Heartland Healthcare Services	61392-0188-39
31's	$26.64	GENERIC, Heartland Healthcare Services	61392-0188-31
32's	$27.50	GENERIC, Heartland Healthcare Services	61392-0188-32
45's	$38.67	GENERIC, Heartland Healthcare Services	61392-0188-45
60's	$51.56	GENERIC, Heartland Healthcare Services	61392-0188-60
90's	$77.34	GENERIC, Heartland Healthcare Services	61392-0188-90
100's	$29.60	GENERIC, Physicians Total Care	54868-3214-00
100's	$75.48	GENERIC, Mylan Pharmaceuticals Inc	00378-6060-01
100's	$75.60	GENERIC, Udl Laboratories Inc	51079-0924-20
100's	$91.50	CARDIZEM SR, Aventis Pharmaceuticals	00088-1777-49
100's	$109.51	CARDIZEM SR, Aventis Pharmaceuticals	00088-1777-47

Capsule, Extended Release - Oral - 90 mg

Quantity	Price	Product	NDC
30's	$29.08	GENERIC, Heartland Healthcare Services	61392-0189-30
30's	$29.08	GENERIC, Heartland Healthcare Services	61392-0189-39
31's	$30.05	GENERIC, Heartland Healthcare Services	61392-0189-31
32's	$31.02	GENERIC, Heartland Healthcare Services	61392-0189-32
45's	$43.62	GENERIC, Heartland Healthcare Services	61392-0189-45
60's	$58.16	GENERIC, Heartland Healthcare Services	61392-0189-60
60's	$62.89	CARDIZEM SR, Allscripts Pharmaceutical Company	54569-2912-02
90's	$87.24	GENERIC, Heartland Healthcare Services	61392-0189-90
100's	$86.28	GENERIC, Mylan Pharmaceuticals Inc	00378-6090-01
100's	$86.40	GENERIC, Udl Laboratories Inc	51079-0925-20
100's	$104.81	CARDIZEM SR, Aventis Pharmaceuticals	00088-1778-49
100's	$125.13	CARDIZEM SR, Aventis Pharmaceuticals	00088-1778-47

Capsule, Extended Release - Oral - 120 mg

Quantity	Price	Product	NDC
100's	$112.47	GENERIC, Mylan Pharmaceuticals Inc	00378-6120-01
100's	$115.84	GENERIC, Udl Laboratories Inc	51079-0926-20
100's	$136.44	CARDIZEM SR, Aventis Pharmaceuticals	00088-1779-49
100's	$163.13	CARDIZEM SR, Aventis Pharmaceuticals	00088-1779-47

Capsule, Extended Release - Oral - 120 mg/24 Hours

Quantity	Price	Product	NDC
15's	$17.89	TIAZAC, Physicians Total Care	54868-3774-00
30's	$32.67	TIAZAC, Allscripts Pharmaceutical Company	54569-4715-00
30's	$34.65	GENERIC, American Health Packaging	62584-0974-30
30's	$34.90	DILACOR XR, Watson/Rugby Laboratories Inc	52544-0732-30
30's	$36.70	GENERIC, Purepac Pharmaceutical Company	00228-2588-03
30's	$38.15	TIAZAC, Forest Pharmaceuticals	00456-2612-30
30's	$39.86	DILACOR XR, American Health Packaging	62584-0250-30
90's	$97.79	CARTIA XT, Andrx Pharmaceuticals	62037-0597-90
90's	$103.68	TIAZAC, Forest Pharmaceuticals	00456-2612-90
90's	$107.80	GENERIC, Purepac Pharmaceutical Company	00228-2588-09
90's	$107.83	GENERIC, Teva Pharmaceuticals Usa	00093-5112-98
90's	$108.58	DILACOR XR, American Health Packaging	62584-0250-90
90's	$108.81	GENERIC, American Health Packaging	62584-0974-90
100's	$82.00	GENERIC, Udl Laboratories Inc	51079-0947-08
100's	$90.01	GENERIC, Andrx Pharmaceuticals	62037-0548-01
100's	$91.01	GENERIC, Mylan Pharmaceuticals Inc	00378-5220-01
100's	$91.01	GENERIC, Apotex Usa Inc	60505-0014-06
100's	$107.71	DILACOR XR, Watson/Rugby Laboratories Inc	52544-0732-01
100's	$127.19	TIAZAC, Forest Pharmaceuticals	00456-2612-63
100's	$146.11	DILACOR XR, Watson/Rugby Laboratories Inc	52544-0482-01

Capsule, Extended Release - Oral - 180 mg/24 Hours

Quantity	Price	Product	NDC
10 x 10	$135.08	DILACOR XR, Watson Laboratories Inc	52544-0733-44
14's	$18.91	DILACOR XR, Allscripts Pharmaceutical Company	54569-4211-00
15's	$21.34	TIAZAC, Physicians Total Care	54868-3956-02
30's	$39.44	TIAZAC, Allscripts Pharmaceutical Company	54569-4716-00
30's	$41.09	DILACOR XR, Watson/Rugby Laboratories Inc	52544-0733-30
30's	$41.50	TIAZAC, Physicians Total Care	54868-3956-01
30's	$41.79	GENERIC, American Health Packaging	62584-0975-30
30's	$42.61	DILACOR XR, American Health Packaging	62584-0251-30
30's	$45.40	GENERIC, Purepac Pharmaceutical Company	00228-2577-03
30's	$46.08	TIAZAC, Forest Pharmaceuticals	00456-2613-30
60's	$81.82	TIAZAC, Physicians Total Care	54868-3956-00
90's	$118.04	CARTIA XT, Andrx Pharmaceuticals	62037-0598-90
90's	$125.13	TIAZAC, Forest Pharmaceuticals	00456-2613-90
90's	$127.84	DILACOR XR, American Health Packaging	62584-0251-90
90's	$130.10	GENERIC, Purepac Pharmaceutical Company	00228-2577-09
90's	$130.11	GENERIC, American Health Packaging	62584-0975-90
90's	$130.12	GENERIC, Teva Pharmaceuticals Usa	00093-5117-98
100's	$105.98	GENERIC, Andrx Pharmaceuticals	62037-0549-01
100's	$107.15	GENERIC, Mylan Pharmaceuticals Inc	00378-5280-01
100's	$107.15	GENERIC, Apotex Usa Inc	60505-0015-06
100's	$119.08	DILACOR XR, Aventis Pharmaceuticals	00075-0251-00
100's	$126.82	DILACOR XR, Watson/Rugby Laboratories Inc	52544-0733-01
100's	$152.89	TIAZAC, Forest Pharmaceuticals	00456-2613-63
100's	$172.02	DILACOR XR, Watson/Rugby Laboratories Inc	52544-0483-01

Capsule, Extended Release - Oral - 240 mg/24 Hours

Quantity	Price	Product	NDC
30's	$43.95	DILACOR XR, Watson Laboratories Inc	52544-0734-30
30's	$45.58	DILACOR XR, American Health Packaging	62584-0252-30
30's	$55.94	TIAZAC, Allscripts Pharmaceutical Company	54569-4717-00
30's	$58.39	TIAZAC, Physicians Total Care	54868-3958-00
30's	$59.25	GENERIC, American Health Packaging	62584-0976-30
30's	$61.55	GENERIC, Purepac Pharmaceutical Company	00228-2578-03
30's	$65.35	TIAZAC, Forest Pharmaceuticals	00456-2614-30
90's	$136.73	DILACOR XR, American Health Packaging	62584-0252-90
90's	$167.45	CARTIA XT, Andrx Pharmaceuticals	62037-0599-90
90's	$177.55	TIAZAC, Forest Pharmaceuticals	00456-2614-90
90's	$184.55	GENERIC, Purepac Pharmaceutical Company	00228-2578-09
90's	$184.58	GENERIC, American Health Packaging	62584-0976-90
90's	$184.60	GENERIC, Teva Pharmaceuticals Usa	00093-5118-98
100's	$103.70	GENERIC, Udl Laboratories Inc	51079-0949-08
100's	$112.95	GENERIC, Apotex Usa Inc	60505-0016-06
100's	$113.35	GENERIC, Andrx Pharmaceuticals	62037-0550-01
100's	$114.60	GENERIC, Mylan Pharmaceuticals Inc	00378-5340-01
100's	$127.36	DILACOR XR, Aventis Pharmaceuticals	00075-0252-00
100's	$144.46	DILACOR XR, Watson Laboratories Inc	52544-0734-44
100's	$178.98	TIAZAC, Forest Pharmaceuticals	00456-2614-63
100's	$183.99	DILACOR XR, Watson Laboratories Inc	52544-0484-01

Capsule, Extended Release - Oral - 300 mg/24 Hours

Quantity	Price	Product	NDC
30's	$76.76	GENERIC, American Health Packaging	62584-0977-30
30's	$78.24	CARDIZEM CD, Allscripts Pharmaceutical Company	54569-4440-00
30's	$80.65	GENERIC, Purepac Pharmaceutical Company	00228-2579-03
30's	$84.69	TIAZAC, Forest Pharmaceuticals	00456-2615-30
30's	$105.09	CARDIZEM CD, Physicians Total Care	54868-2150-01
90's	$217.03	CARTIA XT, Andrx Pharmaceuticals	62037-0600-90
90's	$230.03	TIAZAC, Forest Pharmaceuticals	00456-2615-90
90's	$230.29	GENERIC, American Health Packaging	62584-0977-90
90's	$239.20	GENERIC, Purepac Pharmaceutical Company	00228-2579-09
90's	$239.24	GENERIC, Teva Pharmaceuticals Usa	00093-5119-98
100's	$258.93	TIAZAC, Forest Pharmaceuticals	00456-2615-63

PRODUCT LISTING - EQUIVALENTS NOT AVAILABLE

Capsule, Extended Release - Oral - 60 mg

Quantity	Price	Product	NDC
30's	$22.01	GENERIC, Allscripts Pharmaceutical Company	54569-3784-00
30's	$25.78	GENERIC, Medirex Inc	57480-0804-06
100's	$69.20	GENERIC, Major Pharmaceuticals Inc	00904-7840-60

Capsule, Extended Release - Oral - 90 mg

Quantity	Price	Product	NDC
30's	$25.17	GENERIC, Allscripts Pharmaceutical Company	54569-3785-00
30's	$29.08	GENERIC, Medirex Inc	57480-0805-06
60's	$50.35	GENERIC, Allscripts Pharmaceutical Company	54569-3785-02
100's	$71.36	GENERIC, Medirex Inc	57480-0805-01
100's	$79.20	GENERIC, Major Pharmaceuticals Inc	00904-7841-60

Capsule, Extended Release - Oral - 120 mg/24 Hours

Quantity	Price	Product	NDC
30's	$33.74	GENERIC, Allscripts Pharmaceutical Company	54569-3786-00
30's	$34.34	DILTIAZEM HYDROCHLORIDE XT, Dixon-Shane Inc	17236-0755-30
30's	$39.00	CARDIZEM LA, Biovail Pharmaceuticals Inc	64455-0100-30
90's	$97.79	DILTIAZEM HYDROCHLORIDE XT, Dixon-Shane Inc	17236-0755-90
100's	$112.46	GENERIC, Allscripts Pharmaceutical Company	54569-3786-01

Capsule, Extended Release - Oral - 180 mg/24 Hours

Quantity	Price	Product	NDC
30's	$25.50	GENERIC, Physicians Total Care	54868-4186-00
30's	$37.95	GENERIC, Compumed Pharmaceuticals	00403-4499-30
30's	$41.27	DILTIAZEM HYDROCHLORIDE XT, Dixon-Shane Inc	17236-0756-30
30's	$41.76	GENERIC, Allscripts Pharmaceutical Company	54569-4913-00
30's	$42.30	CARDIZEM LA, Biovail Pharmaceuticals Inc	64455-0101-30
90's	$118.04	DILTIAZEM HYDROCHLORIDE XT, Dixon-Shane Inc	17236-0756-90
100's	$48.10	GENERIC, Pharma Pac	52959-0072-01

Capsule, Extended Release - Oral - 240 mg/24 Hours

Quantity	Price	Product	NDC
30's	$27.80	GENERIC, Physicians Total Care	54868-4184-00
30's	$45.90	CARDIZEM LA, Biovail Pharmaceuticals Inc	64455-0102-30
30's	$58.59	DILTIAZEM HYDROCHLORIDE XT, Dixon-Shane Inc	17236-0758-30
30's	$59.22	GENERIC, Allscripts Pharmaceutical Company	54569-4914-00
30's	$65.82	GENERIC, Allscripts Pharmaceutical Company	54569-3804-00
30's	$80.51	GENERIC, Physicians Total Care	54868-2149-02
90's	$153.95	GENERIC, Compumed Pharmaceuticals	00403-0021-74

Package	Price	Product	NDC
90's	$167.45	DILTIAZEM HYDROCHLORIDE XT, Dixon-Shane Inc	17236-0758-90
Capsule, Extended Release - Oral - 300 mg/24 Hours			
30's	$75.92	DILTIAZEM HYDROCHLORIDE XT, Dixon-Shane Inc	17236-0759-30
30's	$76.76	GENERIC, Allscripts Pharmaceutical Company	54569-4924-00
90's	$217.03	DILTIAZEM HYDROCHLORIDE XT, Dixon-Shane Inc	17236-0759-90
150's	$498.33	GENERIC, Sky Pharmaceuticals Packaging, Inc	63739-0286-15
Capsule, Extended Release - Oral - 360 mg/24 Hours			
30's	$69.90	CARDIZEM LA, Biovail Pharmaceuticals Inc	64455-0104-30
30's	$86.31	TIAZAC, Forest Pharmaceuticals	00456-2616-30
90's	$234.45	TIAZAC, Forest Pharmaceuticals	00456-2616-90
100's	$274.47	TIAZAC, Forest Pharmaceuticals	00456-2616-63
Capsule, Extended Release - Oral - 420 mg/24 Hours			
30's	$78.90	CARDIZEM LA, Biovail Pharmaceuticals Inc	64455-0105-30
30's	$90.48	TIAZAC, Forest Pharmaceuticals	00456-2617-30
90's	$245.73	TIAZAC, Forest Pharmaceuticals	00456-2617-90
Solution - Intravenous - 5 mg/ml			
25 ml	$23.75	GENERIC, Baxter Pharmaceutical Products, Inc	10019-0510-03
Tablet - Oral - 30 mg			
12's	$5.22	GENERIC, Southwood Pharmaceuticals Inc	58016-0606-12
15's	$6.53	GENERIC, Southwood Pharmaceuticals Inc	58016-0606-15
20's	$8.70	GENERIC, Southwood Pharmaceuticals Inc	58016-0606-20
30's	$4.69	GENERIC, Physicians Total Care	54868-2290-03
30's	$12.33	GENERIC, Allscripts Pharmaceutical Company	54569-3665-01
30's	$13.05	GENERIC, Southwood Pharmaceuticals Inc	58016-0606-30
60's	$8.05	GENERIC, Physicians Total Care	54868-2290-00
90's	$11.41	GENERIC, Physicians Total Care	54868-2290-04
90's	$27.28	GENERIC, Southwood Pharmaceuticals Inc	58016-0606-90
100's	$11.87	GENERIC, Physicians Total Care	54868-2290-02
100's	$39.95	GENERIC, Moore, H.L. Drug Exchange Inc	00839-7748-06
100's	$40.40	GENERIC, Allscripts Pharmaceutical Company	54569-3665-00
100's	$43.50	GENERIC, Southwood Pharmaceuticals Inc	58016-0606-00
Tablet - Oral - 60 mg			
12's	$8.19	GENERIC, Southwood Pharmaceuticals Inc	58016-0607-12
15's	$10.24	GENERIC, Southwood Pharmaceuticals Inc	58016-0607-15
20's	$13.65	GENERIC, Southwood Pharmaceuticals Inc	58016-0607-20
21's	$13.29	GENERIC, Allscripts Pharmaceutical Company	54569-3667-01
30's	$19.39	GENERIC, Allscripts Pharmaceutical Company	54569-3667-02
30's	$20.48	GENERIC, Southwood Pharmaceuticals Inc	58016-0607-30
90's	$61.42	GENERIC, Southwood Pharmaceuticals Inc	58016-0607-90
100's	$12.53	GENERIC, Physicians Total Care	54868-2276-02
100's	$58.98	GENERIC, Moore, H.L. Drug Exchange Inc	00839-7749-06
100's	$64.63	GENERIC, Allscripts Pharmaceutical Company	54569-3667-00
100's	$68.25	GENERIC, Southwood Pharmaceuticals Inc	58016-0607-00
Tablet - Oral - 90 mg			
12's	$11.51	GENERIC, Southwood Pharmaceuticals Inc	58016-0608-12
15's	$14.38	GENERIC, Southwood Pharmaceuticals Inc	58016-0608-15
20's	$19.18	GENERIC, Southwood Pharmaceuticals Inc	58016-0608-20
30's	$28.76	GENERIC, Southwood Pharmaceuticals Inc	58016-0608-30
90's	$86.29	GENERIC, Southwood Pharmaceuticals Inc	58016-0608-90
100's	$20.42	GENERIC, Physicians Total Care	54868-2277-00
100's	$81.93	GENERIC, Moore, H.L. Drug Exchange Inc	00839-7750-06
100's	$95.88	GENERIC, Southwood Pharmaceuticals Inc	58016-0608-00
Tablet - Oral - 120 mg			
100's	$105.64	GENERIC, Moore, H.L. Drug Exchange Inc	00839-7751-06

Dimercaprol *(003517)*

Categories: Toxicity, arsenic; Toxicity, gold; Toxicity, lead; Toxicity, mercury; WHO Formulary
Drug Classes: Antidotes; Chelators
Brand Names: BAL in Oil; BAL; BAL in Oil Ampules

DESCRIPTION

Dimercaprol (2,3-dimercapto-1-propanol) is a colorless or almost colorless liquid, having a disagreeable, mercaptan-like odor. Each 1 ml sterile BAL in Oil contains 100 mg dimercaprol in 200 mg benzyl benzoate and 700 mg peanut oil. The slight sediment which may be noticed in some ampules develops during sterilization. It is not an indication that the solution is deteriorating.

CLINICAL PHARMACOLOGY

Dimercaprol promotes the excretion of arsenic, gold and mercury in cases of poisoning. It is also used in combination with edetate calcium disodium injection to promote the excretion of lead.

INDICATIONS AND USAGE

Dimercaprol is indicated in the treatment of arsenic, gold and mercury poisoning. It is indicated in acute lead poisoning when used concomitantly with edetate calcium disodium injection.

Dimercaprol injection is effective for use in acute poisoning by mercury salts if therapy is begun within 1-2 hours following ingestion. It is not very effective in chronic mercury poisoning.

Dimercaprol injection is of questionable value in poisoning caused by other heavy metals such as antimony and bismuth. It should not be used in iron, cadmium, or selenium poisoning because the resulting dimercaprol-metal complexes are more toxic than the metal alone, especially to the kidneys.

CONTRAINDICATIONS

Dimercaprol is contraindicated in most instances of hepatic insufficiency with the exception of postarsenical jaundice. The drug should be discontinued or used only with extreme caution if acute renal insufficiency develops during therapy.

WARNINGS

There may be local pain at the site of the injection. A reaction apparently peculiar to children is fever which may persist during therapy. It occurs in approximately 30% of children. A transient reduction of the percentage of polymorphonuclear leukocytes may also be observed.

PRECAUTIONS

Because the dimercaprol-metal complex breaks down easily in an acid medium, production of an alkaline urine affords protection to the kidney during therapy. Medicinal iron should not be administered to patients under therapy with dimercaprol.

Data is not available regarding the use of dimercaprol during pregnancy and it should not be used unless judged by the physician to be necessary in the treatment of life threatening acute poisoning.

ADVERSE REACTIONS

One of the most consistent responses to dimercaprol injection is a rise in blood pressure accompanied by tachycardia. This rise is roughly proportional to the dose administered.

Doses larger than those recommended may cause other transitory signs and symptoms in approximate order of frequency as follows:

Nausea, and in some instances, vomiting.
Headache.
A burning sensation in the lips, mouth and throat.
A feeling of constriction, even pain, in the throat, chest, or hands.
Conjuctivitis, lacrimation, blepharal spasm, rhinorrhea, and salivation.
Tingling of the hands.
A burning sensation in the penis.
Sweating of the forehead, hands and other areas.
Abdominal pain.
Occasional appearance of painful sterile abscesses.

Many of the above symptoms are accompanied by a feeling of anxiety, weakness, and unrest and often are relieved by administration of an antihistamine.

DOSAGE AND ADMINISTRATION

By deep intramuscular injection only.

For mild arsenic or gold poisoning, 2.5 mg/kg of body weight 4 times daily for 2 days, two times on the third day, and once daily thereafter for 10 days; for severe arsenic or gold poisoning, 3 mg/kg every 4 hours for 2 days, 4 times on the third day, then twice daily thereafter for 10 days.

For mercury poisoning, 5 mg/kg initially, followed by 2.5 mg/kg one or two times daily for 10 days.

For acute lead encephalopathy 4 mg/kg body weight is given alone in the first dose and thereafter at 4 hour intervals in combination with edetate calcium disodium injection administered at a separate site.

For less severe poisoning the dose can be reduced to 3 mg/kg after the first dose. Treatment is maintained for 2-7 days depending on the clinical response. Successful treatment depends on beginning injections at the earliest possible moment and on the use of adequate amounts at frequent intervals. Other supportive measures should always be used in conjunction with dimercaprol therapy.

PRODUCT LISTING - EQUIVALENTS NOT AVAILABLE

Package	Price	Product	NDC
Solution - Injectable - 10%			
3 ml x 10	$747.60	BAL IN OIL, Taylor Pharmaceuticals	11098-0526-03

Dinoprostone (003051)

For complete prescribing information, refer to the CD-ROM included with the book.

Categories: Abortion; Abortion, spontaneous; Labor, induction; Mole, hydatidiform; Pregnancy Category C; FDA Approved 1977 Aug
Drug Classes: Oxytocics; Prostaglandins; Stimulants, uterine
Brand Names: Cervidil; Prepidil; **Prostin E2**; Prostin E2 Vaginal Suppository; Prostin VR Pediatric
Foreign Brand Availability: Cerviprime (India); Cerviprost (Austria; Czech-Republic; Denmark; Finland; Germany; Italy; Norway; Russia; Switzerland); K-PE (Japan); Minprostin E(2) (Germany); Prandin E2 (South-Africa); Primiprost (India); Propess (France; Hong-Kong; Israel); Prostarmon E (Korea; Taiwan); Prostin E2 Tab (New-Zealand); Prostin E2 Vaginal Cream (Australia); Prostin E2 Vaginal Gel (New-Zealand); Prostin 3 (Singapore); Prostine (France)

D

DESCRIPTION

CERVICAL GEL

Prepidil gel contains dinoprostone as the naturally occurring form of prostaglandin E_2 (PGE_2) and is designated chemically as (5Z,11α,13E,15S)-11,15-Dihydroxy-9-oxo-prosta-5,13-dien-1-oic acid. The molecular formula is $C_{20}H_{32}O_5$ and the molecular weight is 352.5. Dinoprostone occurs as a white to off-white crystalline powder with a melting point within the range of 65-69°C. It is soluble in ethanol, in 25% ethanol in water, and in water to the extent of 130 mg/100 ml. The active constituent of Prepidil gel is dinoprostone 0.5 mg/3 g (2.5 ml gel); other constituents are colloidal silicon dioxide (240 mg/3 g) and triacetin (2760 mg/3 g).

VAGINAL SUPPOSITORY

Prostin E2 vaginal suppository, an oxytocic, contains dinoprostone as the naturally occurring prostaglandin E_2 (PGE_2).

Its chemical name is (5Z,11α,13E,15S)-11,15-Dihydroxy-9-oxo-prosta-5,13-dien-1-oic acid.

The molecular formula is $C_{20}H_{32}O_5$. The molecular weight of dinoprostone is 352.5. Dinoprostone occurs as a white crystalline powder. It has a melting point within the range of 64-71°C. Dinoprostone is soluble in ethanol and in 25% ethanol in water. It is soluble in water to the extent of 130 mg/100 ml.

Each suppository contains 20 mg of dinoprostone in a mixture of glycerides of fatty acids.

INDICATIONS AND USAGE

CERVICAL GEL

Dinoprostone cervical gel is indicated for ripening an unfavorable cervix in pregnant women at or near term with a medical or obstetrical need for labor induction.

VAGINAL SUPPOSITORY

1. Dinoprostone vaginal suppository is indicated for the termination of pregnancy from the 12th through the 20th gestational week as calculated from the first day of the last normal menstrual period.
2. Dinoprostone vaginal suppository is also indicated for evacuation of the uterine contents in the management of missed abortion or intrauterine fetal death up to 28 weeks of gestational age as calculated from the first day of the last normal menstrual period.
3. Dinoprostone vaginal suppository is indicated in the management of nonmetastatic gestational trophoblastic disease (benign hydatidiform mole).

CONTRAINDICATIONS

CERVICAL GEL

Endocervically administered dinoprostone gel is not recommended for the following:

a. Patients in whom oxytocic drugs are generally contraindicated or where prolonged contractions of the uterus are considered inappropriate, such as:
   - Cases with a history of cesarean section or major uterine surgery.
   - Cases in which cephalopelvic disproportion is present.
   - Cases in which there is a history of difficult labor and/or traumatic delivery.
   - Grand multiparae with 6 or more previous term pregnancies cases with non-vertex presentation.
   - Cases with hyperactive or hypertonic uterine patterns.
   - Cases of fetal distress where delivery is not imminent.
   - In obstetric emergencies where the benefit-to-risk ratio for either the fetus or the mother favors surgical intervention.

b. Patients with hypersensitivity to prostaglandins or constituents of the gel.
c. Patients with placenta previa or unexplained vaginal bleeding during this pregnancy.
d. Patients for whom vaginal delivery is not indicated, such as vasa previa or active herpes genitalia.

VAGINAL SUPPOSITORY

1. Hypersensitivity to dinoprostone.
2. Acute pelvic inflammatory disease.
3. Patients with active cardiac, pulmonary, renal, or hepatic disease.

WARNINGS

CERVICAL GEL

FOR HOSPITAL USE ONLY.

Dinoprostone, as with other potent oxytocic agents, should be used only with strict adherence to recommended dosages. Dinoprostone should be administered by physicians in a hospital that can provide immediate intensive care and acute surgical facilities.

VAGINAL SUPPOSITORY

Dinoprostone, as with other potent oxytocic agents, should be used only with strict adherence to recommended dosages. Dinoprostone should be used by medically trained personnel in a hospital which can provide immediate intensive care and acute surgical facilities.

Dinoprostone does not appear to directly affect the fetoplacental unit. Therefore, the possibility does exist that the previable fetus aborted by dinoprostone could exhibit transient life signs. Dinoprostone is not indicated if the fetus *in utero* has reached the stage of viability. Dinoprostone should not be considered a feticidal agent.

Evidence from animal studies has suggested that certain prostaglandins may have some teratogenic potential. Therefore, any failed pregnancy termination with dinoprostone should be completed by some other means.

Dinoprostone vaginal suppository should not be used for extemporaneous preparation of any other dosage form.

Neither the dinoprostone vaginal suppository, as dispensed nor any extemporaneous formulation made from the dinoprostone vaginal suppository should be used for cervical ripening or other indication in the patient with term pregnancy.

DOSAGE AND ADMINISTRATION

CERVICAL GEL

NOTE: USE CAUTION IN HANDLING THIS PRODUCT TO PREVENT CONTACT WITH SKIN. WASH HANDS THOROUGHLY WITH SOAP AND WATER AFTER ADMINISTRATION.

Dinoprostone gel should be brought to room temperature (15-30°C; 59-86°F) just prior to administration. Do not force the warming process by using a water bath or other source of external heat (*e.g.*, microwave oven).

To prepare the product for use, remove the peel-off seal from the end of the syringe. Then remove the protective end cap (to serve as plunger extension) and insert the protective end cap into the plunger stopper assembly in the barrel of syringe. Choose the appropriate length shielded catheter (10 or 20 mm) and aseptically remove the sterile shielded catheter from the package. Careful vaginal examination will reveal the degree of effacement which will regulate the size of the shielded endocervical catheter to be used. That is, the 20 mm endocervical catheter should be used if no effacement is present, and the 10 mm catheter should be used if the cervix is 50% effaced. Firmly attach the catheter hub to the syringe tip as evidenced by a distinct click. Fill the catheter with sterile gel by pushing the plunger assembly to expel air from the catheter prior to administration to the patient.

To properly administer the product, the patient should be in a dorsal position with the cervix visualized using a speculum. Using sterile technique, introduce the gel with the catheter provided into the cervical canal just below the level of the internal os. Administer the contents of the syringe by gentle expulsion and then remove the catheter. The gel is easily extrudable from the syringe. Use the contents of 1 syringe for 1 patient only. No attempt should be made to administer the small amount of gel remaining in the catheter. The syringe, catheter, and any unused package contents should be discarded after use.

Following administration of dinoprostone gel, the patient should remain in the supine position for at least 15-30 minutes to minimize leakage from the cervical canal.

If the desired response is obtained from dinoprostone gel, the recommended interval before giving intravenous oxytocin is 6-12 hours. If there is no cervical/uterine response to the initial dose of dinoprostone gel, repeat dosing may be given. The recommended repeat dose is 0.5 mg dinoprostone with a dosing interval of 6 hours. The need for additional dosing and the interval must be determined by the attending physician based on the course of clinical events. The maximum recommended cumulative dose for a 24 hour period is 1.5 mg of dinoprostone (7.5 ml dinoprostone gel).

VAGINAL SUPPOSITORY

STORE IN A FREEZER NOT ABOVE -20°C (-4°F) BUT BRING TO ROOM TEMPERATURE JUST PRIOR TO USE.

REMOVE FOIL BEFORE USE.

A suppository containing 20 mg of dinoprostone should be inserted high into the vagina. The patient should remain in the supine position for 10 minutes following insertion.

Additional intravaginal administration of each subsequent suppository should be at 3-5 hour intervals until abortion occurs. Within the above recommended intervals administration time should be determined by abortifacient progress, uterine contractility response, and by patient tolerance. Continuous administration of the drug for more than 2 days is not recommended.

PRODUCT LISTING - EQUIVALENTS NOT AVAILABLE

Gel - Vaginal - 0.5 mg/3 Gm

3 gm	$97.96	PREPIDIL, Pharmacia and Upjohn	00009-3359-01
3 gm x 5	$928.70	PREPIDIL, Pharmacia and Upjohn	00009-3359-02

Insert - Vaginal - 0.3 mg/Hr

1's	$210.52	CERVIDIL, Forest Pharmaceuticals	00456-4123-63

Suppository - Vaginal - 20 mg

5's	$614.50	PROSTIN E2, Pharmacia and Upjohn	00009-0827-02
5's	$3163.63	PROSTIN E2, Pharmacia Corporation	00009-0827-03

Diphenhydramine Hydrochloride *(001079)*

Categories: Anaphylaxis, adjunct; Angioedema; Conjunctivitis, allergic; Dermatographism; Motion sickness; Parkinson's disease; Transfusion reaction; Urticaria; Pregnancy Category B; FDA Approved 1946 Mar
Drug Classes: Antihistamines, H1
Brand Names: Allerdryl 50; Allergia-C; Allergina; Amidryl; Banophen; Beldin; Belix; Ben-A-Vance; Ben-Rex; Bena-D-10; **Benadryl**; Benadryl Steri-Dose; Benahist; Benapon; Bendramine; Benoject; Bydramine; Dibenil; Dimidril; Diphen; Diphenacen-50; Diphenhist; Dytuss; Fynex; Genahist; Hydramine; Hydril; Hyrexin; Noradryl; Norafed; Nordryl; Pharm-A-Dry; Restamin; Shodryl; Tega Dryl; Truxadryl; Tusstat; Uad Dryl; Wehdryl
Foreign Brand Availability: Allermin (Japan); Benadryl N (Bulgaria; Czech-Republic); Benocten (Switzerland); Broncho D (Israel); Cathejell (Israel); Dibrondrin (Austria); Difenhydramin (Denmark); Dimiril (India); Dormutil (Germany); Histergan (Bahamas; Bahrain; Barbados; Belize; Benin; Bermuda; Burkina-Faso; Curacao; Cyprus; Egypt; Ethiopia; Gambia; Ghana; Guinea; Guyana; Iran; Iraq; Ivory-Coast; Jamaica; Jordan; Kenya; Kuwait; Lebanon; Liberia; Libya; Malawi; Mali; Mauritania; Mauritius; Morocco; Netherland-Antilles; Niger; Nigeria; Oman; Qatar; Republic-of-Yemen; Saudi-Arabia; Senegal; Seychelles; Sierra-Leone; Sudan; Surinam; Syria; Tanzania; Trinidad; Tunia; Uganda; United-Arab-Emirates; Zambia; Zimbabwe); Nytol (Canada; South-Africa); Nytol Quickgels (Mexico); ratioAllerg (Germany); Resmin (Japan); Tzoali (Mexico); Unisom Sleepgels (Australia; Hong-Kong; New-Zealand); Vena (Japan); Venasmin (Japan)
Cost of Therapy: \$240.90 (Parkinsonism; Benadryl Capsule; 25 mg; 3/day; 365 day supply)
\$0.34 (Nighttime Sleep Aid; Generic Capsules; 50 mg; 1 capsule/day; 30 day supply)
HCFA JCODE(S): J1200 up to 50 mg IV, IM

DESCRIPTION

Diphenhydramine HCl, is an antihistamine drug having the chemical name 2-(Diphenylmethoxy)-N,N-dimethylethylamine hydrochloride and has the empirical formula $C_{17}H_{21}NO \cdot HCl$. It occurs as a white, crystalline powder and is freely soluble in water and alcohol and has a molecular weight of 291.82.

Each diphenhydramine HCl capsule contains 25 mg or 50 mg diphenhydramine HCl for oral administration.

Each Benadryl 25-mg capsule also contains lactose and magnesium stearate. The capsule shell and/or band contains D&C red no. 28; FD&C blue no. 1; FD&C red no. 3; FD&C red no. 40; gelatin; colloidal silicon dioxide; and sodium lauryl sulfate.

Each Benadryl 50-mg capsule also contains confectioner's sugar and talc. The capsule shell and/or band contains FD&C blue no. 1; FD&C red no. 3; gelatin; glyceryl monooleate; colloidal silicon dioxide; sodium lauryl sulfate; and titanium dioxide.

Each 5 ml of diphenhydramine HCl elixir contains 12.5 mg diphenhydramine HCl with 14% alcohol for oral administration.

Diphenhydramine HCl in the parenteral form is a sterile, pyrogen-free solution available in two concentrations: 10 mg and 50 mg of diphenhydramine HCl per ml. The solutions for parenteral use have been adjusted to a pH between 5.0 and 6.0 either with sodium hydroxide or hydrochloric acid. The multidose Steri-Vials contain 0.1 mg/ml benzethonium chloride as a germicidal agent.

Storage: Store capsules and injection at controlled room temperature 15-30°C (59-86°F). Protect from moisture, freezing, and light.

CLINICAL PHARMACOLOGY

Diphenhydramine HCl is an antihistamine with anticholinergic (drying) and sedative effects. Antihistamines appear to compete with histamine for cell receptor sites on effector cells.

Diphenhydramine is widely distributed throughout the body, including the CNS.

CAPSULES AND ELIXER

A single oral dose of diphenhydramine HCl is quickly absorbed with maximum activity occurring in approximately 1 hour. The duration of activity following an average dose of diphenhydramine HCl is from 4-6 hours. Diphenhydramine HCl capsules are widely distributed throughout the body, including the CNS. Little, if any, is excreted unchanged in the urine; most appears as the degradation products of metabolic transformation in the liver, which are almost completely excreted within 24 hours.

INJECTION

Diphenhydramine HCl in the injectable form has a rapid onset of action. Detailed information on the pharmacokinetics of diphenhydramine HCl injection is not available.

INDICATIONS AND USAGE

CAPSULES AND ELIXER

Diphenhydramine HCl in the oral form is effective for the following indications:

Antihistaminic: For allergic conjunctivitis due to foods; mild, uncomplicated allergic skin manifestations of urticaria and angioedema; amelioration of allergic reactions to blood or plasma; dermatographism; as therapy for anaphylactic reactions adjunctive to epinephrine and other standard measures after the acute manifestations have been controlled.

Motion Sickness: For active and prophylactic treatment of motion sickness.

Antiparkinsonism: For parkinsonism (including drug-induced) in the elderly unable to tolerate more potent agents; mild cases of parkinsonism (including drug-induced) in other age groups; in other cases of parkinsonism (including drug-induced) in combination with centrally acting anticholinergic agents.

Nighttime sleep-aid.

INJECTION

Diphenhydramine HCl in the injectable form should only be used when the oral forms are impractical.

CONTRAINDICATIONS

Use in Newborn or Premature Infants: This drug should not be used in newborn or premature infants.

Use in Nursing Mothers: Because of the higher risk of antihistamines for infants generally, and for newborns and prematures in particular, antihistamine therapy is contraindicated in nursing mothers.

Antihistamines are Also Contraindicated in the Following Conditions: Hypersensitivity to diphenhydramine HCl and other antihistamines of similar chemical structure.

INJECTION

Use as a Local Anesthetic: Because of the risk of local necrosis, this drug in the parenteral from should not be used as a local anesthetic.

WARNINGS

Antihistamines should be used with considerable caution in patients with narrow-angle glaucoma, stenosing peptic ulcer, pyloroduodenal obstruction, symptomatic prostatic hypertrophy, or bladder-neck obstruction.

USE IN CHILDREN

In infants and children, especially, antihistamines in overdosage may cause hallucinations, convulsions, or death.

As in adults, antihistamines may diminish mental alertness in children. In the young child, particularly, they may produce excitation.

Use in the Elderly (approximately 60 years or older): Antihistamines are more likely to cause dizziness, sedation, and hypotension in elderly patients.

PRECAUTIONS

GENERAL

Diphenhydramine HCl has an atropine-like action and therefore should be used with caution in patients with a history of lower respiratory disease including asthma, increased intraocular pressure, hyperthyroidism, cardiovascular disease or hypertension.

INFORMATION FOR THE PATIENT

Patients taking diphenhydramine HCl should be advised that this drug may cause drowsiness and has an additive effect with alcohol.

Patients should be warned about engaging in activities requiring mental alertness such as driving a car or operating appliances, machinery, etc.

CARCINOGENESIS, MUTAGENESIS, AND IMPAIRMENT OF FERTILITY

Long-term studies in animals to determine mutagenic and carcinogenic potential have not been performed.

PREGNANCY CATEGORY B

Reproduction studies have been performed in rats and rabbits at doses up to 5 times the human dose and have revealed no evidence of impaired fertility or harm to the fetus due to diphenhydramine HCl. There are, however, no adequate and well-controlled studies in pregnant women. Because animal reproduction studies are not always predictive of human response, this drug should be used during pregnancy only if clearly needed.

INJECTION

Use with caution in patients with lower respiratory disease including asthma.

DRUG INTERACTIONS

Diphenhydramine HCl has additive effects with alcohol and other CNS depressants (hypnotics, sedatives, tranquilizers, etc).

MAO inhibitors prolong and intensify the anticholinergic (drying) effects of antihistamines.

ADVERSE REACTIONS

The Most Frequent Adverse Reactions Are Underscored:

1. ***General:*** Urticaria, drug rash, anaphylactic shock, photosensitivity, excessive perspiration, chills, dryness of mouth, nose, and throat.
2. ***Cardiovascular System:*** Hypotension, headache, palpitations, tachycardia, extrasystoles.
3. ***Hematologic System:*** Hemolytic anemia, thrombocytopenia, agranulocytosis.
4. ***Nervous System:*** Sedation, sleepiness, dizziness, disturbed coordination, fatigue, confusion, restlessness, excitation, nervousness, tremor, irritability, insomnia, euphoria, paresthesia, blurred vision, diplopia, vertigo, tinnitus, acute labyrinthitis, neuritis, convulsions.
5. ***GI System:*** Epigastric distress, anorexia, nausea, vomiting, diarrhea, constipation.
6. ***GU System:*** Urinary frequency, difficult urination, urinary retention, early menses.
7. ***Respiratory System:*** Thickening of bronchial secretions, tightness of chest and wheezing, nasal stuffiness.

DOSAGE AND ADMINISTRATION

DOSAGE SHOULD BE INDIVIDUALIZED ACCORDING TO THE NEEDS AND THE RESPONSE OF THE PATIENT.

CAPSULES

A single oral dose of diphenhydramine HCl is quickly absorbed with maximum activity occurring in approximately 1 hour. The duration of activity following an average dose of diphenhydramine HCl is from 4-6 hours.

Adults: 25-50 mg 3 or 4 times daily. The nighttime sleep-aid dosage is 50 mg at bedtime.

Children (Over 20 lb): 12.5 to 25 mg 3-4 times daily. Maximum daily dosage not to exceed 300 mg. For physicians who wish to calculate the dose on the basis of body weight or surface area, the recommended dosage is 5 mg/kg/24 hours or 150 mg/m^2/24 hours.

Data are not available on the use of diphenhydramine HCl as a nighttime sleep-aid in children under 12 years.

The basis for determining the most effective dosage regimen will be the response of the patient to medication and the condition under treatment.

In motion sickness, full dosage is recommended for prophylactic use, the first dose to be given 30 minutes before exposure to motion and similar doses before meals and upon retiring for the duration of exposure.

ELIXER

A single oral dose of diphenhydramine HCl is quickly absorbed with maximum activity occurring in approximately 1 hour. The duration of activity following an average dose of diphenhydramine HCl is from 4-6 hours.

Children (Over 20 lb): One (1) to 2 teaspoonfuls 3-4 times daily. Maximum daily dosage not to exceed 300 mg.

For physicians who wish to calculate the dose on the basis of body weight or surface area, the recommended dosage is 5 mg/kg/24 hours or 150 mg/m^2/24 hours.

Adults: Two (2) to 4 teaspoonfuls 3-4 times daily. The basis for determining the most effective dosage regimen will be the response of the patient to medication and the condition under treatment.

In motion sickness, full dosage is recommended for prophylactic use, the first dose to be given 30 minutes before exposure to motion and similar doses before meals and upon retiring for the duration of exposure.

INJECTION

Parenteral drug products should be inspected visually for particulate matter and discoloration prior to administration, whenever solution and container permit.

Children: 5 mg/kg/24 h or 150 mg/m^2/24 h. Maximum daily dosage is 300 mg. Divide into 4 doses, administered intravenously or deeply intramuscularly.

Adults: 10-50 mg intravenously or deep intramuscularly, 100 mg if required; maximum daily dosage is 400 mg.

PRODUCT LISTING - RATED THERAPEUTICALLY EQUIVALENT

Capsule - Oral - 25 mg

10's	$4.72	GENERIC, Pd-Rx Pharmaceuticals	55289-0479-10
15's	$5.08	GENERIC, Pd-Rx Pharmaceuticals	55289-0479-15
20's	$5.44	GENERIC, Pd-Rx Pharmaceuticals	55289-0479-20
24's	$5.72	GENERIC, Pd-Rx Pharmaceuticals	55289-0479-24
25's	$6.80	GENERIC, Pd-Rx Pharmaceuticals	55289-0479-97
30's	$1.90	GENERIC, Major Pharmaceuticals Inc	00904-2055-46
30's	$2.54	GENERIC, Pd-Rx Pharmaceuticals	58864-0162-30
30's	$3.11	GENERIC, Heartland Healthcare Services	61392-0220-30
30's	$3.11	GENERIC, Heartland Healthcare Services	61392-0220-39
30's	$6.16	GENERIC, Pd-Rx Pharmaceuticals	55289-0479-30
31's	$3.22	GENERIC, Heartland Healthcare Services	61392-0220-31
32's	$3.32	GENERIC, Heartland Healthcare Services	61392-0220-32
60's	$3.18	GENERIC, Pd-Rx Pharmaceuticals	58864-0162-60
60's	$6.23	GENERIC, Heartland Healthcare Services	61392-0220-60
90's	$9.34	GENERIC, Heartland Healthcare Services	61392-0220-90
100's	$1.04	GENERIC, Global Pharmaceutical Corporation	00115-1110-01
100's	$3.00	GENERIC, Interstate Drug Exchange Inc	00814-2550-14
100's	$6.19	GENERIC, Purepac Pharmaceutical Company	00228-2191-10
100's	$6.32	GENERIC, Aligen Independent Laboratories Inc	00405-4344-01
100's	$6.55	GENERIC, Moore, H.L. Drug Exchange Inc	00839-1278-06
100's	$6.85	GENERIC, Major Pharmaceuticals Inc	00904-2055-61
100's	$11.16	GENERIC, Geneva Pharmaceuticals	00781-2458-13
100's	$11.20	GENERIC, Pd-Rx Pharmaceuticals	55289-0479-01
100's	$13.97	GENERIC, Auro Pharmaceutical	55829-0627-10
250's	$6.75	GENERIC, Interstate Drug Exchange Inc	00814-2550-22

Capsule - Oral - 50 mg

10's	$2.60	GENERIC, Pd-Rx Pharmaceuticals	55289-0100-10
15's	$3.90	GENERIC, Pd-Rx Pharmaceuticals	55289-0100-15
20's	$5.00	GENERIC, Pd-Rx Pharmaceuticals	55289-0100-20
25's	$2.60	GENERIC, Udl Laboratories Inc	51079-0066-19
30's	$1.35	GENERIC, Heartland Healthcare Services	61392-0223-30
30's	$1.35	GENERIC, Heartland Healthcare Services	61392-0223-39
30's	$1.95	GENERIC, Major Pharmaceuticals Inc	00904-2056-46
30's	$2.50	GENERIC, Circle Pharmaceuticals Inc	00659-0703-30
30's	$2.60	GENERIC, Pd-Rx Pharmaceuticals	58864-0163-30
30's	$5.50	GENERIC, Pd-Rx Pharmaceuticals	55289-0100-30
30's	$84.40	GENERIC, Medirex Inc	57480-0322-06
31 x 10	$39.61	GENERIC, Vangard Labs	00615-0369-53
31 x 10	$39.61	GENERIC, Vangard Labs	00615-0369-63
31's	$1.40	GENERIC, Heartland Healthcare Services	61392-0223-31
32's	$1.44	GENERIC, Heartland Healthcare Services	61392-0223-32
40's	$5.46	GENERIC, Pd-Rx Pharmaceuticals	58864-0100-40
60's	$2.70	GENERIC, Heartland Healthcare Services	61392-0223-60
60's	$3.54	GENERIC, Pd-Rx Pharmaceuticals	58864-0163-60
90's	$4.05	GENERIC, Heartland Healthcare Services	61392-0223-90
100's	$1.12	GENERIC, Global Pharmaceutical Corporation	00115-1111-01
100's	$1.75	GENERIC, Raway Pharmacal Inc	00686-0649-01
100's	$3.04	GENERIC, Circle Pharmaceuticals Inc	00659-0703-02
100's	$3.25	GENERIC, Cmc-Consolidated Midland Corporation	00223-0586-01
100's	$3.75	GENERIC, Interstate Drug Exchange Inc	00814-2555-14
100's	$4.56	GENERIC, Richmond Pharmaceuticals	54738-0116-01
100's	$4.56	GENERIC, Richmond Pharmaceuticals	54738-0116-13
100's	$4.83	GENERIC, Watson/Schein Pharmaceuticals Inc	00364-0117-01
100's	$6.14	GENERIC, Moore, H.L. Drug Exchange Inc	00839-1280-06
100's	$6.50	GENERIC, Raway Pharmacal Inc	00686-0369-13
100's	$6.80	GENERIC, Purepac Pharmaceutical Company	00228-2192-10
100's	$6.98	GENERIC, Aligen Independent Laboratories Inc	00405-4345-01
100's	$9.40	GENERIC, Pd-Rx Pharmaceuticals	55289-0100-01
100's	$13.45	GENERIC, Geneva Pharmaceuticals	00781-2498-13
100's	$13.45	GENERIC, Major Pharmaceuticals Inc	00904-2056-61
100's	$13.45	GENERIC, Udl Laboratories Inc	51079-0066-20
100's	$13.62	GENERIC, Barr Laboratories Inc	00555-0059-02
100's	$16.62	GENERIC, Auro Pharmaceutical	55829-0628-10
250's	$8.25	GENERIC, Interstate Drug Exchange Inc	00814-2555-22

Elixir - Oral - 12.5 mg/5 ml

120 ml	$1.64	FEDERAL UPPER LIMIT, H.C.F.A. F F P	99999-1079-12

Solution - Injectable - 10 mg/ml

30 ml	$2.00	GENERIC, C.O. Truxton Inc	00463-1080-30
30 ml	$3.75	GENERIC, Keene Pharmaceuticals Inc	00588-5111-90
30 ml	$4.00	GENERIC, Roberts/Hauck Pharmaceutical Corporation	43797-0121-13
30 ml	$4.75	GENERIC, Major Pharmaceuticals Inc	00904-0013-30
30 ml	$7.35	GENERIC, Interstate Drug Exchange Inc	00814-2570-46
30 ml	$7.87	GENERIC, Moore, H.L. Drug Exchange Inc	00839-5569-36

Solution - Injectable - 50 mg/ml

1 ml x 10	$10.30	GENERIC, Abbott Pharmaceutical	00074-2290-01
1 ml x 10	$12.47	GENERIC, Abbott Pharmaceutical	00074-2290-31
1 ml x 10	$15.24	BENADRYL, Allscripts Pharmaceutical Company	54569-1574-00
1 ml x 10	$16.90	BENADRYL, Parke-Davis	00071-4259-03
1 ml x 10	$18.52	BENADRYL, Physicians Total Care	54868-0554-00
1 ml x 10	$18.60	BENADRYL, Parke-Davis	00071-4259-45
1 ml x 25	$23.50	BENADRYL, Parke-Davis	00071-4259-13
1 ml x 25	$30.00	GENERIC, Esi Lederle Generics	00641-0376-25
1 ml x 25	$86.00	GENERIC, American Pharmaceutical Partners	63323-0664-01
10 ml	$2.50	GENERIC, C.O. Truxton Inc	00463-1089-10
10 ml	$5.75	GENERIC, Roberts/Hauck Pharmaceutical Corporation	43797-0124-12
10 ml	$5.89	GENERIC, General Injectables and Vaccines Inc	52584-0117-10
10 ml	$6.40	GENERIC, Major Pharmaceuticals Inc	00904-0835-10
10 ml	$7.15	GENERIC, Hyrex Pharmaceuticals	00314-0673-70
10 ml	$8.13	GENERIC, Moore, H.L. Drug Exchange Inc	00839-6305-30
10 ml	$8.75	GENERIC, Cmc-Consolidated Midland Corporation	00223-7478-10
10 ml	$9.47	BENADRYL, Allscripts Pharmaceutical Company	54569-3548-00
10 ml	$10.18	BENADRYL, Parke-Davis	00071-4402-10
10 ml	$12.01	BENADRYL, Physicians Total Care	54868-0007-00
30 ml	$4.50	GENERIC, Keene Pharmaceuticals Inc	00588-5112-70

PRODUCT LISTING - EQUIVALENTS NOT AVAILABLE

Capsule - Oral - 25 mg

2's	$3.41	GENERIC, Prescript Pharmaceuticals	00247-0073-02
3's	$3.44	GENERIC, Prescript Pharmaceuticals	00247-0073-03
4's	$3.46	GENERIC, Prescript Pharmaceuticals	00247-0073-04
5's	$3.48	GENERIC, Prescript Pharmaceuticals	00247-0073-05
6's	$3.52	GENERIC, Prescript Pharmaceuticals	00247-0073-06
7's	$3.54	GENERIC, Prescript Pharmaceuticals	00247-0073-07
8's	$3.56	GENERIC, Prescript Pharmaceuticals	00247-0073-08
10's	$3.62	GENERIC, Prescript Pharmaceuticals	00247-0073-10
12's	$3.67	GENERIC, Prescript Pharmaceuticals	00247-0073-12
14's	$3.73	GENERIC, Prescript Pharmaceuticals	00247-0073-14
15's	$1.56	GENERIC, Heartland Healthcare Services	61392-0220-15
15's	$3.75	GENERIC, Prescript Pharmaceuticals	00247-0073-15
16's	$3.78	GENERIC, Prescript Pharmaceuticals	00247-0073-16
20's	$3.88	GENERIC, Prescript Pharmaceuticals	00247-0073-20
20's	$3.96	GENERIC, Dhs Inc	55887-0973-20
21's	$3.91	GENERIC, Prescript Pharmaceuticals	00247-0073-21
24's	$0.85	GENERIC, Perrigo, L. Company	00113-0462-62
24's	$1.50	GENERIC, Logen	00820-0141-24
24's	$2.20	GENERIC, Major Pharmaceuticals Inc	00904-2035-24
24's	$2.35	GENERIC, Qualitest Products Inc	00603-0240-18
24's	$3.09	GENERIC, Mckesson Drug Company	49348-0044-04
24's	$3.99	GENERIC, Prescript Pharmaceuticals	00247-0073-24
25's	$4.01	GENERIC, Prescript Pharmaceuticals	00247-0073-25
30's	$2.69	GENERIC, Perrigo, L. Company	37937-0091-44
30's	$2.69	GENERIC, Mckesson Drug Company	49348-0044-44
30's	$3.40	GENERIC, St. Mary'S Mpp	60760-0330-30
30's	$4.15	GENERIC, Prescript Pharmaceuticals	00247-0073-30
40's	$4.41	GENERIC, Prescript Pharmaceuticals	00247-0073-40
45's	$4.67	GENERIC, Heartland Healthcare Services	61392-0220-45
100's	$2.75	GENERIC, Consolidated Midland Corporation	00223-0585-01
100's	$3.50	GENERIC, Richmond Pharmaceuticals	54738-0115-01
100's	$4.10	GENERIC, Major Pharmaceuticals Inc	00904-5306-60
100's	$4.41	GENERIC, Richmond Pharmaceuticals	54738-0115-13
100's	$4.45	GENERIC, Major Pharmaceuticals Inc	00904-2035-60
100's	$4.50	GENERIC, Dixon-Shane Inc	17236-0516-01
100's	$5.72	GENERIC, Mckesson Drug Company	49348-0044-10
100's	$6.00	GENERIC, Prescript Pharmaceuticals	00247-0073-00

Capsule - Oral - 50 mg

2's	$3.44	GENERIC, Prescript Pharmaceuticals	00247-0120-02
3's	$3.47	GENERIC, Prescript Pharmaceuticals	00247-0120-03
4's	$3.52	GENERIC, Prescript Pharmaceuticals	00247-0120-04
5's	$3.55	GENERIC, Prescript Pharmaceuticals	00247-0120-05
6's	$0.17	GENERIC, Allscripts Pharmaceutical Company	54569-0241-04
6's	$3.60	GENERIC, Prescript Pharmaceuticals	00247-0120-06
6's	$6.75	GENERIC, Pharma Pac	52959-0053-06
7's	$3.64	GENERIC, Prescript Pharmaceuticals	00247-0120-07
8's	$3.68	GENERIC, Prescript Pharmaceuticals	00247-0120-08

10's	$0.29	GENERIC, Allscripts Pharmaceutical Company	54569-0241-05
10's	$3.76	GENERIC, Prescript Pharmaceuticals	00247-0120-10
10's	$8.15	GENERIC, Pharma Pac	52959-0053-10
12's	$3.85	GENERIC, Prescript Pharmaceuticals	00247-0120-12
12's	$8.52	GENERIC, Pharma Pac	52959-0053-12
14's	$3.93	GENERIC, Prescript Pharmaceuticals	00247-0120-14
15's	$0.44	GENERIC, Allscripts Pharmaceutical Company	54569-0241-02
15's	$3.96	GENERIC, Prescript Pharmaceuticals	00247-0120-15
15's	$8.99	GENERIC, Pharma Pac	52959-0053-15
20's	$0.58	GENERIC, Allscripts Pharmaceutical Company	54569-0241-03
20's	$2.52	GENERIC, Pharmaceutical Corporation Of America	51655-0088-52
20's	$4.03	GENERIC, Dhs Inc	55887-0885-20
20's	$4.18	GENERIC, Prescript Pharmaceuticals	00247-0120-20
20's	$9.75	GENERIC, Pharma Pac	52959-0053-20
24's	$4.34	GENERIC, Prescript Pharmaceuticals	00247-0120-24
24's	$4.95	GENERIC, Eon Labs Manufacturing Inc	00185-0649-24
30's	$4.59	GENERIC, Prescript Pharmaceuticals	00247-0120-30
30's	$11.31	GENERIC, Pharma Pac	52959-0053-30
45's	$2.03	GENERIC, Heartland Healthcare Services	61392-0223-45
100's	$4.20	GENERIC, Contract Pharmacal Corporation	10267-0836-01
100's	$4.75	GENERIC, Dixon-Shane Inc	17236-0518-01
100's	$4.85	GENERIC, Moore, H.L. Drug Exchange Inc	00839-7459-06
100's	$7.46	GENERIC, Prescript Pharmaceuticals	00247-0120-00
100's	$9.04	GENERIC, Eon Labs Manufacturing Inc	00185-0649-01
Liquid - Oral - 25 mg/5 ml			
120 ml	$21.99	GENERIC, Cypress Pharmaceutical Inc	63717-0570-04
Solution - Injectable - 10 mg/ml			
30 ml	$8.25	GENERIC, Cmc-Consolidated Midland Corporation	00223-7477-30
Solution - Injectable - 50 mg/ml			
1 ml	$30.00	GENERIC, Cmc-Consolidated Midland Corporation	00223-7478-25
1 ml x 10	$29.35	GENERIC, Allscripts Pharmaceutical Company	54569-2268-00
10 ml	$9.75	BANARIL, Clint Pharmaceutical Inc	55553-0827-10
10 ml	$13.81	GENERIC, Prescript Pharmaceuticals	00247-0289-10
Tablet - Oral - 25 mg			
24's	$2.19	GENERIC, Longs Drug Company	12333-9073-01
30's	$1.75	GENERIC, Pharmaceutical Corporation Of America	51655-0113-24
30's	$1.80	GENERIC, Circle Pharmaceuticals Inc	00659-0729-30
32's	$2.21	GENERIC, Vangard Labs	00615-0368-32
32's	$2.28	GENERIC, Vangard Labs	00615-0369-32
100's	$4.95	GENERIC, Vangard Labs	00615-0368-01
100's	$5.06	GENERIC, Vangard Labs	00615-0369-01
100's	$11.15	GENERIC, Udl Laboratories Inc	51079-0967-20
Tablet - Oral - 50 mg			
30's	$2.90	GENERIC, Pharmaceutical Corporation Of America	51655-0088-24
50's	$4.43	GENERIC, Watson/Rugby Laboratories Inc	00536-3772-06
Tablet, Chewable - Oral - 25 mg			
60's	$55.49	GENERIC, Cypress Pharmaceutical Inc	63717-0571-06

Diphtheria and Tetanus Toxoids and Acellular Pertussis Adsorbed; Hepatitis B (Recombinant) and Inactivated Poliovirus Vaccine Combined *(003581)*

For complete prescribing information, refer to the CD-ROM included with the book.

Categories: Immunization, diptheria; Immunization, hepatitis B; Immunization, pertussis; Immunization, poliomyelitis; Immunization, tetanus; Pregnancy Category C; FDA Approved 2002 Dec
Drug Classes: Vaccines
Brand Names: **Pediarix**

DESCRIPTION

Note: The trade name has been used throughout this monograph for clarity.

Pediarix [diphtheria and tetanus toxoids and acellular pertussis adsorbed, hepatitis B (recombinant) and inactivated poliovirus vaccine combined] is a noninfectious, sterile, multivalent vaccine for intramuscular administration manufactured by SmithKline Beecham Biologicals. It contains diphtheria and tetanus toxoids, 3 pertussis antigens (inactivated pertussis toxin [PT], filamentous hemagglutinin [FHA], and pertactin [69 kiloDalton outer membrane protein]), hepatitis B surface antigen, plus poliovirus Type 1 (Mahoney), Type 2 (MEF-1), and Type 3 (Saukett). The diphtheria toxoid, tetanus toxoid, and pertussis antigens are the same as those in Infanrix (diphtheria and tetanus toxoids and acellular pertussis vaccine adsorbed). The hepatitis B surface antigen is the same as that in Engerix-B [hepatitis B vaccine (recombinant)].

The diphtheria toxin is produced by growing *Corynebacterium diphtheriae* in Fenton medium containing a bovine extract. Tetanus toxin is produced by growing *Clostridium tetani* in a modified Latham medium derived from bovine casein. The bovine materials used in these extracts are sourced from countries which the United States Department of Agriculture (USDA) has determined neither have nor are at risk of bovine spongiform encephalopathy (BSE). Both toxins are detoxified with formaldehyde, concentrated by ultrafiltration, and purified by precipitation, dialysis, and sterile filtration.

The 3 acellular pertussis antigens (PT, FHA, and pertactin) are isolated from *Bordetella pertussis* culture grown in modified Stainer-Scholte liquid medium. PT and FHA are isolated from the fermentation broth; pertactin is extracted from the cells by heat treatment and flocculation. The antigens are purified in successive chromatographic and precipitation steps. PT is detoxified using glutaraldehyde and formaldehyde. FHA and pertactin are treated with formaldehyde.

The hepatitis B surface antigen (HBsAg) is obtained by culturing genetically engineered *Saccharomyces cerevisiae* cells, which carry the surface antigen gene of the hepatitis B virus, in synthetic medium. The surface antigen expressed in the *S. cerevisiae* cells is purified by several physiochemical steps, which include precipitation, ion exchange chromatography, and ultrafiltration. The purified HBsAg undergoes dialysis with cysteine to remove residual thimerosal.

The inactivated poliovirus component of Pediarix is an enhanced potency component. Each of the 3 strains of poliovirus is individually grown in Vero cells, a continuous line of monkey kidney cells, cultivated on microcarriers. Calf serum and lactalbumin hydrolysate are used during Vero cell culture and/or virus culture. Calf serum is sourced from countries the USDA has determined neither have nor are at risk of BSE. After clarification, each viral suspension is purified by ultrafiltration, diafiltration, and successive chromatographic steps, and inactivated with formaldehyde. The 3 purified viral strains are then pooled to form a trivalent concentrate.

The diphtheria, tetanus, and pertussis antigens are individually adsorbed onto aluminum hydroxide; hepatitis B component is adsorbed onto aluminum phosphate. All antigens are then diluted and combined to produce the final formulated vaccine. Each 0.5 ml dose is formulated to contain 25 Lf of diphtheria toxoid, 10 Lf of tetanus toxoid, 25 μg of inactivated PT, 25 μg of FHA, 8 μg of pertactin, 10 μg of HBsAg, 40 D-antigen Units (DU) of Type 1 poliovirus, 8 DU of Type 2 poliovirus, and 32 DU of Type 3 poliovirus.

Diphtheria and tetanus toxoid potency is determined by measuring the amount of neutralizing antitoxin in previously immunized guinea pigs. The potency of the acellular pertussis components (PT, FHA, and pertactin) is determined by enzyme-linked immunosorbent assay (ELISA) on sera from previously immunized mice. Potency of the hepatitis B component is established by HBsAg ELISA. The potency of the inactivated poliovirus component is determined by using the D-antigen ELISA and by a poliovirus neutralizing cell culture assay on sera from previously immunized rats.

Each 0.5 ml dose also contains 2.5 mg of 2-phenoxyethanol as a preservative, 4.5 mg of NaCl, and aluminum adjuvant (not more than 0.85 mg aluminum by assay). Each dose also contains ≤100 μg of residual formaldehyde and ≤100 μg of polysorbate 80 (Tween 80). Thimerosal is used at the early stages of manufacture and is removed by subsequent purification steps to below the analytical limit of detection (<25 ng of mercury/20 μg HBsAg) which upon calculation is <12.5 ng mercury/dose. Neomycin sulfate and polymyxin B are used in the polio vaccine manufacturing process and may be present in the final vaccine at ≤0.05 ng neomycin and ≤0.01 ng polymyxin B/dose. The procedures used to manufacture the HBsAg antigen result in a product that contains ≤5% yeast protein.

The vaccine must be well shaken before administration and is a turbid white suspension after shaking.

INDICATIONS AND USAGE

Pediarix is indicated for active immunization against diphtheria, tetanus, pertussis (whooping cough), all known subtypes of hepatitis B virus, and poliomyelitis caused by poliovirus Types 1, 2, and 3 as a 3 dose primary series in infants born of HBsAg-negative mothers, beginning as early as 6 weeks of age. Pediarix should not be administered to any infant before the age of 6 weeks, or to individuals 7 years of age or older.

Infants born of HBsAg-positive mothers should receive Hepatitis B Immune Globulin (Human) (HBIG) and monovalent hepatitis B vaccine (recombinant) within 12 hours of birth and should complete the hepatitis B vaccination series according to a particular schedule.[36] (See manufacturer's prescribing information for hepatitis B vaccine [recombinant].) (See DOSAGE AND ADMINISTRATION.)

Infants born of mothers of unknown HBsAg status should receive monovalent hepatitis B vaccine (recombinant) within 12 hours of birth and should complete the hepatitis B vaccination series according to a particular schedule.[36] (See manufacturer's prescribing information for hepatitis B vaccine [recombinant].) (See DOSAGE AND ADMINISTRATION.)

Pediarix will not prevent hepatitis caused by other agents, such as hepatitis A, C, and E viruses, or other pathogens known to infect the liver. As hepatitis D (caused by the delta virus) does not occur in the absence of hepatitis B infection, hepatitis D will also be prevented by vaccination with Pediarix.

Hepatitis B has a long incubation period. Vaccination with Pediarix may not prevent hepatitis B infection in individuals who had an unrecognized hepatitis B infection at the time of vaccine administration.

When passive protection against tetanus or diphtheria is required, tetanus immune globulin or diphtheria antitoxin, respectively, should be administered at separate sites.[1]

As with any vaccine, Pediarix may not protect 100% of individuals receiving the vaccine, and is not recommended for treatment of actual infections.

CONTRAINDICATIONS

Hypersensitivity to any component of the vaccine, including yeast, neomycin, and polymyxin B, is a contraindication (see DESCRIPTION).

It is a contraindication to use this vaccine after a serious allergic reaction (*e.g.,* anaphylaxis) temporally associated with a previous dose of this vaccine or with any components of this vaccine. Because of the uncertainty as to which component of the vaccine might be responsible, no further vaccination with any of these components should be given. Alternatively, such individuals may be referred to an allergist for evaluation if further immunizations are to be considered.[1]

In addition, the following events are contraindications to administration of any pertussis-containing vaccine, including Pediarix:[10]

- Encephalopathy (*e.g.,* coma, decreased level of consciousness, prolonged seizures) within 7 days of administration of a previous dose of a pertussis-containing vaccine that is not attributable to another identifiable cause;

- Progressive neurologic disorder, including infantile spasms, uncontrolled epilepsy, or progressive encephalopathy. Pertussis vaccine should not be administered to individuals with such conditions until a treatment regimen has been established and the condition has stabilized.

Pediarix is not contraindicated for use in individuals with HIV infection.[10,37]

WARNINGS

Administration of Pediarix is associated with higher rates of fever relative to separately administered vaccines. In one study that evaluated medically attended fever after the first dose of Pediarix or separately administered vaccines, infants who received Pediarix had a higher rate of medical encounters for fever within the first 4 days following vaccination. In some infants, these encounters included the performance of diagnostic studies to evaluate other causes of fever.

The vial stopper is latex-free. The tip cap and the rubber plunger of the needleless prefilled syringes contain dry natural latex rubber that may cause allergic reactions in latex sensitive individuals.

If any of the following events occur in temporal relation to receipt of whole-cell DTP or a vaccine containing an acellular pertussis component, the decision to give subsequent doses of Pediarix or any vaccine containing a pertussis component should be based on careful consideration of the potential benefits and possible risks:[38,39]

- Temperature of ≥40.5°C (105°F) within 48 hours not due to another identifiable cause;
- Collapse or shock-like state (hypotonic-hyporesponsive episode) within 48 hours;
- Persistent, inconsolable crying lasting ≥3 hours, occurring within 48 hours;
- Seizures with or without fever occurring within 3 days.

When a decision is made to withhold pertussis vaccine, immunization with DT vaccine, hepatitis B vaccine, and IPV should be continued.

If Guillain-Barré syndrome occurs within 6 weeks of receipt of prior vaccine containing tetanus toxoid, the decision to give subsequent doses of Pediarix or any vaccine containing tetanus toxoid should be based on careful consideration of the potential benefits and possible risks.[10]

A committee of the Institute of Medicine (IOM) has concluded that evidence is consistent with a causal relationship between whole-cell DTP vaccine and acute neurologic illness, and under special circumstances, between whole-cell DTP vaccine and chronic neurologic disease in the context of the National Childhood Encephalopathy Study (NCES) report.[40,41] However, the IOM committee concluded that the evidence was insufficient to indicate whether or not whole-cell DTP vaccine increased the overall risk of chronic neurologic disease.[41] Acute encephalopathy and permanent neurologic damage have not been reported causally linked or in temporal association with administration of Pediarix, but the experience with Pediarix is insufficient to rule this out. Encephalopathy has been reported following Infanrix, but data are not sufficient to evaluate a causal relationship.

The decision to administer a pertussis-containing vaccine to children with stable CNS disorders must be made by the physician on an individual basis, with consideration of all relevant factors, and assessment of potential risks and benefits for that individual. The Advisory Committee on Immunization Practices (ACIP) and the Committee on Infectious Diseases of the American Academy of Pediatrics (AAP) have issued guidelines for such children.[38,42] The parent or guardian should be advised of the potential increased risk involved.

A family history of seizures or other CNS disorders is not a contraindication to pertussis vaccine.[38]

For children at higher risk for seizures than the general population, an appropriate antipyretic may be administered at the time of vaccination with a vaccine containing an acellular pertussis component (including Pediarix) and for the ensuing 24 hours according to the respective prescribing information recommended dosage to reduce the possibility of post-vaccination fever.[10,38]

Vaccination should be deferred during the course of a moderate or severe illness with or without fever. Such children should be vaccinated as soon as they have recovered from the acute phase of the illness.[10]

As with other intramuscular injections, Pediarix should not be given to children on anticoagulant therapy unless the potential benefit clearly outweighs the risk of administration.

DOSAGE AND ADMINISTRATION

PREPARATION FOR ADMINISTRATION

Pediarix contains an adjuvant; therefore shake vigorously to obtain a homogeneous, turbid, white suspension. DO NOT USE IF RESUSPENSION DOES NOT OCCUR WITH VIGOROUS SHAKING. Inspect visually for particulate matter or discoloration prior to administration. After removal of the dose, any vaccine remaining in the vial should be discarded.

Pediarix should be administered by intramuscular injection. The preferred sites are the anterolateral aspects of the thigh or the deltoid muscle of the upper arm. The vaccine should not be injected in the gluteal area or areas where there may be a major nerve trunk. Gluteal injections may result in suboptimal hepatitis B immune response. Before injection, the skin at the injection site should be cleaned and prepared with a suitable germicide. After insertion of the needle, aspirate to ensure that the needle has not entered a blood vessel.

Do not administer this product subcutaneously or intravenously.

RECOMMENDED SCHEDULE

The primary immunization series for Pediarix is 3 doses of 0.5 ml, given intramuscularly, at 6-8 week intervals (preferably 8 weeks). The customary age for the first dose is 2 months of age, but it may be given starting at 6 weeks of age.

Pediarix should not be administered to any infant before the age of 6 weeks. Only monovalent hepatitis B vaccine can be used for the birth dose.

Infants born of HBsAg-positive mothers should receive HBIG and hepatitis B vaccine (recombinant) within 12 hours of birth at separate sites and should complete the hepatitis B vaccination series according to a particular schedule.[36] (See manufacturer's prescribing information for hepatitis B vaccine [recombinant].)

Infants born of mothers of unknown HBsAg status should receive hepatitis B vaccine (recombinant) within 12 hours of birth and should complete the hepatitis B vaccination series according to a particular schedule.[36] (See manufacturer's prescribing information for hepatitis B vaccine [recombinant].)

The administration of Pediarix for completion of the hepatitis B vaccination series in infants who were born of HBsAg-positive mothers and who received monovalent hepatitis B vaccine (recombinant) and HBIG has not been studied.

MODIFIED SCHEDULES

Children Previously Vaccinated With 1 or More Doses of Hepatitis B Vaccine

Infants born of HBsAg-negative mothers and who received a dose of hepatitis B vaccine at or shortly after birth may be administered 3 doses of Pediarix according to the recommended schedule. However, data are limited regarding the safety of Pediarix in such infants. There are no data to support the use of a 3 dose series of Pediarix in infants who have previously received more than 1 dose of hepatitis B vaccine. Pediarix may be used to complete a hepatitis B vaccination series in infants who have received 1 or more doses of hepatitis B vaccine (recombinant) and who are also scheduled to receive the other vaccine components of Pediarix. However, the safety and efficacy of Pediarix in such infants have not been studied.

Children Previously Vaccinated With 1 or More Doses of Infanrix

Pediarix may be used to complete the first 3 doses of the DTaP series in infants who have received 1 or 2 doses of Infanrix and are also scheduled to receive the other vaccine components of Pediarix. However, the safety and efficacy of Pediarix in such infants have not been evaluated.

Children Previously Vaccinated With 1 or More Doses of IPV

Pediarix may be used to complete the first 3 doses of the IPV series in infants who have received 1 or 2 doses of IPV and are also scheduled to receive the other vaccine components of Pediarix. However, the safety and efficacy of Pediarix in such infants have not been studied.

INTERCHANGEABILITY OF PEDIARIX AND LICENSED DTAP, IPV, OR RECOMBINANT HEPATITIS B VACCINES

It is recommended that Pediarix be given for all 3 doses because data are limited regarding the safety and efficacy of using acellular pertussis vaccines from different manufacturers for successive doses of the pertussis vaccination series. Pediarix is not recommended for completion of the first 3 doses of the DTaP vaccination series initiated with a DTaP vaccine from a different manufacturer because no data are available regarding the safety or efficacy of using such a regimen.

Pediarix may be used to complete a hepatitis B vaccination series initiated with a licensed hepatitis B vaccine (recombinant) vaccine from a different manufacturer.

Pediarix may be used to complete the first 3 doses of the IPV vaccination series initiated with IPV from a different manufacturer.

ADDITIONAL DOSING INFORMATION

If any recommended dose of pertussis vaccine cannot be given, DT (for pediatric use), hepatitis B (recombinant), and inactivated poliovirus vaccines should be given as needed to complete the series.

Interruption of the recommended schedule with a delay between doses should not interfere with the final immunity achieved with Pediarix. There is no need to start the series over again, regardless of the time elapsed between doses.

The use of reduced volume (fractional doses) is not recommended. The effect of such practices on the frequency of serious adverse events and on protection against disease has not been determined.[10]

Preterm infants should be vaccinated according to their chronological age from birth.[10]

Pediarix is not indicated for use as a booster dose following a 3 dose primary series of Pediarix. Children who have received a 3 dose primary series of Pediarix should receive a fourth dose of IPV at 4-6 years of age and a fourth dose of DTaP vaccine at 15-18 months of age. Because the pertussis antigen components of Infanrix are the same as those components in Pediarix, these children should receive Infanrix as their fourth dose of DTaP. However, data are insufficient to evaluate the safety of Infanrix following 3 doses of Pediarix.

CONCOMITANT VACCINE ADMINISTRATION

In clinical trials, Pediarix was routinely administered, at separate sites, concomitantly with Hib vaccine. Safety data are available following the first dose of Pediarix administered concomitantly, at separate sites, with Hib and pneumococcal conjugate vaccines.

When concomitant administration of other vaccines is required, they should be given with separate syringes and at different injection sites.

PRODUCT LISTING - EQUIVALENTS NOT AVAILABLE

Suspension - Intramuscular - Strength n/a

0.50 ml x 5	$429.15	PEDIARIX, Glaxosmithkline	58160-0841-46
0.50 ml x 10	$858.30	PEDIARIX, Glaxosmithkline	58160-0841-11

Diphtheria Antitoxin *(001086)*

For complete prescribing information, refer to the CD-ROM included with the book.

Categories: Diphtheria; Immunization, diphtheria; FDA Pre 1938 Drugs; WHO Formulary
Drug Classes: Vaccines

DESCRIPTION

Diphtheria antitoxin is a sterile solution of pepsin treated antitoxic substances obtained from the sera of horses immunized against diphtheria toxin with diphtheria toxoid alone or in conjunction with diphtheria toxin. This product is preserved with tricresol 0.4%.

Storage: Store between 2-8°C (35-46°F). Potency not affected by freezing.

INDICATIONS AND USAGE

For prevention or treatment of diphtheria.

Diphtheria antitoxin neutralizes the toxins produced by *Corynebacterium diphtheriae*..

CONTRAINDICATIONS

None known. If diphtheria is present, antitoxin must be given.

DOSAGE AND ADMINISTRATION

CAUTION

A separate, sterile syringe and needle should be used for each individual patient to prevent transmission of hepatitis or other infectious agents from one person to another.

ADMINISTRATION

Intramuscularly or by slow intravenous infusion.

Antitoxin should be warmed to 32-34°C (90-95°F) before injection.

Do not warm above recommended temperature.

DOSAGE[1]

With prophylactic doses the incidence of serum sickness is generally below 10%; with therapeutic dosage a higher incidence should be anticipated, depending upon the amount administered. The incubation period varies from 7-12 days. A short incubation period (accelerated serum sickness) occurs in individuals who have been sensitized by previous serum therapy.

THERAPEUTIC REGIMEN

Perform sensitivity tests.

Give all of the required antitoxin, intramuscularly or intravenously, at once. Each hour's delay increases the dosage requirements and decreases the beneficial effects.

Suggested Ranges Are: Pharyngeal or laryngeal disease of 48 hours' duration, 20,000-40,000 units; nasopharyngeal lesions, 40,000-60,000 units, extensive disease of 3 or more days' duration or any patient with brawny swelling of the neck, 80,000-120,000 units.

Give children the same dose as adults.

In addition, appropriate antimicrobial agents in full therapeutic dosage should be started.

Any person with clinical symptoms of diphtheria should receive diphtheria antitoxin at once without waiting for bacteriologic confirmation of the diagnosis. Observation and supportive treatment should be continued until all local and general symptoms are controlled, or until some other etiologic agent has been identified.

PROPHYLACTIC REGIMEN

All asymptomatic, unimmunized contacts of patients with diphtheria should receive prompt prophylaxis with appropriate antimicrobial therapy with cultures before and after treatment, immunization with diphtheria toxoid, and continued surveillance for seven days.

Close contacts not under surveillance should receive appropriate antimicrobial therapy, immunization with diphtheria toxoid and diphtheria antitoxin.[2] Prior to administering diphtheria antitoxin:

Perform appropriate sensitivity tests.

If sensitivity testing is negative, give 10,000 units intramuscularly.[3] The dose is dependent upon length of time since exposure, the extent of the exposure and the medical condition of the individual.

If sensitivity testing is positive, proceed with desensitization schedule outlined above.

PRODUCT LISTING - EQUIVALENTS NOT AVAILABLE

Powder For Injection - Injectable - 20000 U

1's $331.25 GENERIC, Aventis Pharmaceuticals 49281-0230-89

Diphtheria Tetanus Toxoids (001087)

For complete prescribing information, refer to the CD-ROM included with the book.

Categories: Immunization, diphtheria; Immunization, tetanus; FDA Pre 1938 Drugs; WHO Formulary
Drug Classes: Vaccines

DESCRIPTION

The diphtheria toxoid component is prepared by cultivating a suitable strain of *Corynebacterium diphtheriae* on a modified Mueller's casein hydrolysate medium (J. Immunology 37:103, 1939). The tetanus toxoid component is prepared by cultivating a suitable strain of *Clostridium tetani* on a protein-free semisynthetic medium (Appl. Microbiol. *10:*146, 1962). Formaldehyde is used as the toxoiding (detoxifying) agent for both diphtheria and tetanus toxins. The final product contains no more than 0.02 percent free formaldehyde and contains 0.01 percent thimerosal (mercury derivative) as preservative.

The aluminum content of the final product does not exceed 0.85 mg per 0.5 ml dose.

During processing, hydrochloric acid and sodium hydroxide are used to adjust the pH. Sodium chloride is added to the finished product to control isotonicity.

INDICATIONS AND USAGE

Diphtheria/tetanus is indicated for active immunization against diphtheria and tetanus in infants and children through 6 years of age. Diphtheria and tetanus toxoids and pertussis vaccine are the preferred agents for primary immunization of infants and children through 6 years of age. However, in instances where the pertussis vaccine component of triple antigen is not tolerated, or where the physician prefers to administer pertussis vaccine as a separate course of injections, this pediatric combination of diphtheria and tetanus toxoids may be used.

CONTRAINDICATIONS

An acute respiratory infection or other active infection is reason for deferring administration of routine primary immunizing or recall (booster) doses but *not* emergency recall (booster) doses.

Interruption of the recommended schedule with a delay between doses does not interfere with the final immunity achieved, nor does it necessitate starting the series over again, regardless of the length of time elapsed between doses.[1]

DOSAGE AND ADMINISTRATION

The basic immunizing course consists of 2 (primary) doses of 0.5 ml each, given at an interval of 4-8 weeks, followed by a third (reinforcing) dose of 0.5 ml 6-12 months later. The third (reinforcing) dose is an integral part of the basic immunizing course; basic immunization cannot be considered complete until the third dose has been given. Prolonging the interval between primary immunizing doses, for 6 months or longer, does not interfere with the final immunity. Injections should be given intramuscularly, preferably into the deltoid or midlateral muscles of the thigh. The same muscle site should not be injected more than once during the course of basic immunization.

If active immunization is initiated during the first year of life, a routine recall (booster) dose of 0.5 ml is indicated at 4-6 years of age. Over age 6, the use of Diphtheria/Tetanus (FOR ADULT USE) is recommended for basic immunization and recall (booster) doses.

In event of injury for which tetanus prophylaxis is indicated, an emergency recall (booster) dose of 0.5 ml of the single antigen, tetanus toxoid, should be given:

For clean, minor wounds - if more than TEN (10) years have elapsed since the time of administration of the last recall (booster) dose or the last (reinforcing) dose of the basic immunizing series.

For all other wounds - if more than FIVE (5) years have elapsed since the time of administration of the last recall (booster) dose or the last (reinforcing) dose of the basic immunizing series.

If emergency tetanus prophylaxis is indicated during the period between the second primary dose and the reinforcing dose, a 0.5 ml dose of the single antigen, tetanus toxoid, should be given. If given before 6 months have elapsed, it should be counted as a primary dose; if given after 6 months, it should be regarded as the reinforcing dose.

A 0.5 ml dose of tetanus toxoid *and* an appropriate dose of Tetanus Immune Globulin (Human), given with *separate* syringes and at *different* sites, are indicated at time of injury if:

The past immunization history with tetanus toxoid or the date of the last recall (booster) dose is unknown or of questionable validity.

The interval since the third (reinforcing) dose of the basic immunizing series or the last recall (booster) dose is more than 10 years; AND a delay of more than 24 hours has occurred between the time of injury and initiation of specific tetanus prophylaxis; AND the injury is of the type that could readily lead to fulminating tetanus (for example - compound fracture; extensive burn; crushing, penetrating, or massively contaminated wound; injury causing interruption or impairment of the local blood supply).

Individuals who have received no prior injections, or only 1 prior injection of this product or tetanus toxoid, should be given an adequate dose of Tetanus Immune Globulin (Human) at time of injury.

Upon intimate exposure to diphtheria, an emergency recall (booster) dose of 0.5 ml is indicated.[1]

TECHNIC FOR INJECTION

Before injection, the skin over the site to be injected should be cleansed and prepared with a suitable germicide. After insertion of the needle, aspirate to help avoid inadvertent injection into a blood vessel. Expel the antigen slowly and terminate the dose with a small bubble of air (0.1-0.2 ml). Do not inject intracutaneously or into superficial subcutaneous structures.

PRODUCT LISTING - EQUIVALENTS NOT AVAILABLE

Suspension - Intramuscular - 2 U;5 U/0.5 ml

0.50 ml x 10	$147.60	GENERIC, Aventis Pharmaceuticals	49281-0271-10
5 ml	$37.97	GENERIC, Allscripts Pharmaceutical Company	54569-4927-00
5 ml	$94.25	GENERIC, Allscripts Pharmaceutical Company	54569-1460-00
5 ml	$121.25	GENERIC, Aventis Pharmaceuticals	49281-0271-83
5 ml	$121.25	GENERIC, Aventis Pharmaceuticals	49281-0275-10

Suspension - Intramuscular - 2 U;10 U/0.5 ml

5 ml	$7.50	GENERIC, Sclavo Inc	42021-0211-09

Suspension - Intramuscular - 10 U;5 U/0.5 ml

5 ml	$37.97	GENERIC, Allscripts Pharmaceutical Company	54569-4926-00

Suspension - Intramuscular - 15 U;10 U/0.5 ml

5 ml	$7.50	GENERIC, Sclavo Inc	42021-0210-11

Diphtheria; Pertussis; Tetanus (001089)

For complete prescribing information, refer to the CD-ROM included with the book.

Categories: Immunization, diphtheria; Immunization, pertussis; Immunization, tetanus; Pregnancy Category C; FDA Approved 1991 Jan; WHO Formulary
Drug Classes: Vaccines
Brand Names: Acel-Imune; Daptacel; **DTP Adsorbed**; Infanrix; Tri-Immunol; Tripedia
Foreign Brand Availability: Acelluvax DPT (Israel); Acelluvax DTP (Thailand); Adacel (Canada); Adsorbed DT COQ (Hong-Kong; Taiwan); Anatoxal Di Te Per Berna (Ecuador; Peru); Boostrix (Australia; Israel; New-Zealand); D.T. COQ (Malaysia); Dif per tet all (Italy; Malaysia; Philippines; Thailand); DiTePer Anatoxal Berna Vaccine (Hong-Kong; Malaysia; Philippines); DPT (Taiwan); P.D.T. Vax Purified (Korea); Tripacel (Australia; Hong-Kong; New-Zealand); Tripvac (India)

D

DESCRIPTION

Note: The trade names have been used throughout this monograph for clarity.

TRIPEDIA

Tripedia, Diphtheria and Tetanus Toxoids and Acellular Pertussis Vaccine Adsorbed (DTaP), for intramuscular use, is a sterile preparation of diphtheria and tetanus toxoids adsorbed, with acellular pertussis vaccine in an isotonic sodium chloride solution containing thimerosal as a preservative and sodium phosphate to control pH. After shaking, the vaccine is a homogeneous white suspension. Tripedia vaccine is distributed by Aventis Pasteur Inc. (AvP).

Corynebacterium diphtheriae cultures are grown in a modified Mueller and Miller medium.[2] *Clostridium tetani* cultures are grown in a peptone-based medium containing a bovine extract. The meat used in this medium is US sourced. Both toxins are detoxified with formaldehyde. The detoxified materials are then separately purified by serial ammonium sulfate fractionation and diafiltration.

The acellular pertussis vaccine components are isolated from culture fluids of Phase 1 *Bordetella pertussis* grown in a modified Stainer-Scholte medium.[1] After purification by salt precipitation, ultracentrifugation, and ultrafiltration, preparations containing varying amounts of both pertussis toxin (PT) and filamentous hemagglutinin (FHA) are combined to obtain a 1:1 ratio and treated with formaldehyde to inactivate PT.

The diphtheria and tetanus toxoids are adsorbed using aluminum potassium sulfate (alum). The adsorbed toxoids are combined with acellular pertussis concentrate, and diluted to a final volume using sterile phosphate-buffered physiological saline. The 1 dose vial of vaccine is formulated without preservatives but contains a trace amount of thimerosal [(mercury derivative), (≤0.3 µg mercury/dose)] from the manufacturing process. The multidose (7.5 ml) vial of vaccine contains the preservative thimerosal [(mercury derivative), 25 µg mercury/dose]. Each 0.5 ml dose contains, by assay, not more than 0.170 mg of aluminum and not more than 100 µg (0.02%) of residual formaldehyde. The vaccine contains gelatin and polysorbate 80 (Tween-80), which are used in the production of the pertussis concentrate.

Each 0.5 ml dose is formulated to contain 6.7 Lf of diphtheria toxoid and 5 Lf of tetanus toxoid (both toxoids induce at least 2 units of antitoxin per ml in the guinea pig potency test), and 46.8 µg of pertussis antigens. This is represented in the final vaccine as approximately 23.4 µg of inactivated PT (also referred to as lymphocytosis promoting factor or LPF) and 23.4 µg of FHA. The inactivated acellular pertussis component contributes not more than 50 endotoxin units (EU) to the endotoxin content of 1 ml of DTaP. The potency of the pertussis components is evaluated by measuring the antibody response to PT and FHA in immunized mice using an ELISA system.

Acellular Pertussis Vaccine Concentrates (For Further Manufacturing Use) are produced by The Research Foundation for Microbial Diseases of Osaka University (BIKEN), Osaka, Japan, under US license, and are combined with diphtheria and tetanus toxoids manufactured by AvP. The Tripedia vaccine is filled, labeled, packaged, and released by AvP.

When Tripedia vaccine is used to reconstitute ActHIB the combination vaccine is TriHIBit. Each single 0.5 ml dose of TriHIBit, for the fourth dose only, is formulated to contain 6.7 Lf of diphtheria toxoid, 5 Lf of tetanus toxoid (both toxoids induce at least 2 units of antitoxin per ml in the guinea pig potency test), 46.8 µg of pertussis antigens (approximately 23.4 µg of inactivated PT and 23.4 µg of FHA), 10 µg of purified *Haemophilus influenzae* type b capsular polysaccharide conjugated to 24 µg of inactivated tetanus toxoid, and 8.5% sucrose. (Refer to ActHIB package insert.)

INFANRIX

Infanrix (Diphtheria and Tetanus Toxoids and Acellular Pertussis Vaccine Adsorbed) is a sterile combination of diphtheria and tetanus toxoids and 3 pertussis antigens [inactivated pertussis toxin (PT), filamentous hemagglutinin (FHA), and pertactin (69 kD outer membrane protein)] adsorbed onto aluminum hydroxide. Infanrix is intended for intramuscular injection only. After shaking, the vaccine is a homogeneous white turbid suspension.

Three acellular pertussis antigens (pertussis toxin [PT], filamentous hemagglutinin [FHA], and pertactin) are isolated from Phase 1 *Bordetella pertussis* culture grown in modified Stainer-Scholte liquid medium. PT and FHA are extracted from the fermentation broth by adsorption on hydroxyapatite gel; pertactin is extracted from the cells by heat treatment and flocculation using barium chloride. These antigens are purified in successive chromatographic steps: PT and FHA by hydrophobic, affinity, and size exclusion; pertactin by ion exchange, hydrophobic and size exclusion processes. PT is detoxified using formaldehyde and glutaraldehyde. FHA and pertactin are treated with formaldehyde.

Diphtheria toxin is produced by growing *Corynebacterium diphtheriae* in Linggoud and Fenton medium containing a bovine extract. Tetanus toxin is produced by growing *Clostridium tetani* in a modified Latham medium. Both toxins are detoxified with formaldehyde, concentrated by ultrafiltration, and purified by precipitation, sterile filtration, and dialysis.

Each antigen is individually adsorbed onto aluminum hydroxide. Each 0.5 ml dose contains, by assay, not more than 0.625 mg aluminum. Each 0.5 ml dose is formulated to contain 25 Lf diphtheria toxoid, 10 Lf tetanus toxoid (both toxoids induce at least 2 antitoxin units/ml of serum in the guinea pig potency test), 25 µg PT, 25 µg FHA, and 8 µg pertactin. The potency of the pertussis component is evaluated by measurement of the antibody response to PT, FHA, and pertactin in immunized mice using an ELISA.

Each 0.5 ml dose also contains 2.5 mg 2-phenoxyethanol as a preservative, 4.5 mg sodium chloride, water for injection, and not more than 0.02% (w/v) residual formaldehyde.

The vaccine contains polysorbate 80 (Tween 80) which is used in the production of the pertussis concentrate. The inactivated acellular pertussis components contribute less than 5 endotoxin units (EU) per 0.5 ml dose.

Diphtheria and Tetanus Toxoids adsorbed bulk concentrates for further manufacturing use are produced by Chiron Behring GmbH & Co, Marburg, Germany. The acellular pertussis antigens are manufactured by SmithKline Beecham Biologicals S.A., Rixensart, Belgium. Formulation, filling, testing, packaging, and release of the vaccine are conducted by SmithKline Beecham Biologicals S.A.

DAPTACEL

Daptacel, Diphtheria and Tetanus Toxoids and Acellular Pertussis Vaccine Adsorbed, for intramuscular use, manufactured by Aventis Pasteur Limited, is a sterile suspension of pertussis antigens and diphtheria and tetanus toxoids adsorbed on aluminum phosphate in a sterile isotonic sodium chloride solution. After shaking, the vaccine is a white homogeneous cloudy suspension. Each dose of Daptacel contains the following active ingredients: pertussis toxoid, 10 µg; filamentous hemagglutinin (FHA), 5 µg; pertactin (PRN), 3 µg; fimbriae types 2 and 3, 5 µg; diphtheria toxoid, 15 Lf; tetanus toxoid, 5 Lf.

Other ingredients per dose include 3.3 mg (0.6% v/v) 2-phenoxyethanol as the preservative, 0.33 mg of aluminum as the adjuvant, ≤0.1 mg residual formaldehyde and <50 ng residual glutaraldehyde.

The acellular pertussis vaccine components are produced from *Bordetella pertussis* cultures grown in Stainer-Scholte medium[96] modified by the addition of casamino acids and dimethyl-beta-cyclodextrin. The fimbriae types 2 and 3 are extracted from the bacterial cells and the pertussis toxin, FHA and PRN are prepared from the supernatant. These proteins are purified by sequential filtration, salt-precipitation, ultrafiltration and chromatography. Pertussis toxin is inactivated with glutaraldehyde and FHA is treated with formaldehyde. The individual antigens are adsorbed separately onto aluminum phosphate.

Corynebacterium diphtheriae is grown in modified Mueller's growth medium.[97] After ammonium sulfate fractionation, the diphtheria toxin is detoxified with formalin and diafiltered. *Clostridium tetani* is grown in modified Mueller-Miller casamino acid medium without beef heart infusion.[98] Tetanus toxin is detoxified with formalin and purified by ammonium sulfate fractionation and diafiltration. Diphtheria and tetanus toxoids are individually adsorbed onto aluminum phosphate.

The adsorbed diphtheria, tetanus and acellular pertussis components are combined in a sterile isotonic sodium chloride solution containing 2-phenoxyethanol as preservative.

Both diphtheria and tetanus toxoids induce at least 2 units of antitoxin per ml in the guinea pig potency test. The potency of the acellular pertussis vaccine components is evaluated by the antibody response of immunized mice to pertussis toxin, FHA, PRN and fimbriae types 2 and 3 measured by enzyme-linked immunosorbent assay (ELISA).

INDICATIONS AND USAGE

Diphtheria and Tetanus Toxoids and Acellular Pertussis Vaccine Adsorbed is indicated for active immunization against diphtheria, tetanus, and pertussis (whooping cough) simultaneously in infants and children 6 weeks to 7 years of age (prior to seventh birthday). Because of the substantial risks of complications of the disease, completion of a primary series of pertussis vaccine early in life is strongly recommended.[3] However, in instances where the pertussis vaccine component is contraindicated, Diphtheria and Tetanus Toxoids Adsorbed (For Pediatric Use) (DT) should be used for each of the remaining doses. (See CONTRAINDICATIONS.)

If passive immunization is required, Tetanus Immune Globulin (Human) (TIG) and/or equine Diphtheria Antitoxin should be used.

Children who have had well-documented pertussis (*i.e.,* positive culture for *B. pertussis* or epidemiologic linkage to a culture positive case) should complete the vaccination series with at least DT. Some experts recommend including the pertussis component as well (*i.e.,* administration of DTaP). Although well-documented pertussis disease is likely to confer immunity against pertussis, the duration of such immunity is unknown.[30,31]

Diphtheria and Tetanus Toxoids and Acellular Pertussis Vaccine Adsorbed is not to be used for treatment of *B. pertussis, C. diphtheriae,* or *C. tetani* infections.

As with any vaccine, vaccination with Diphtheria and Tetanus Toxoids and Acellular Pertussis Vaccine Adsorbed may not protect 100% of susceptible individuals.

When Tripedia vaccine is used to reconstitute ActHIB (TriHIBit), the combined vaccines are indicated for the active immunization of children 15-18 months of age who have been immunized previously against diphtheria, tetanus and pertussis with 3 doses consisting of either whole-cell DTP or Tripedia and 3 or fewer doses of ActHIB within the first year of life for the prevention of diphtheria, tetanus, pertussis and invasive diseases caused by *H. influenzae* type b.[1] (Refer to ActHIB package insert.)

CONTRAINDICATIONS

This vaccine is contraindicated in children and adults 7 years of age and older.

Hypersensitivity to any component of the vaccine is a contraindication to further administration (see DESCRIPTION).[99]

The following events after receipt of Diphtheria and Tetanus Toxoids and Acellular Pertussis Vaccine Adsorbed are contraindications to further administration of any pertussis-containing vaccine.[99]

An immediate anaphylactic reaction. Because of uncertainty as to which component of the vaccine may be responsible, no further vaccination with diphtheria, tetanus or pertussis components should be carried out. Alternatively, such individuals may be referred to an allergist for evaluation if further immunizations are to be considered.

Encephalopathy not attributable to another identifiable cause (*e.g.,* an acute, severe central nervous system disorder occurring within 7 days after vaccination and consisting of major alterations in consciousness, unresponsiveness or generalized or focal seizures that persist more than a few hours, without recovery within 24 hours). In such cases, DT vaccine should be administered for the remaining doses in the vaccination schedule.

The decision to administer or delay vaccination because of a current or recent febrile illness depends on the severity of symptoms and on the etiology of the disease. According to the ACIP, all vaccines can be administered to persons with mild illness such as diarrhea, mild upper-respiratory infection with or without low-grade fever, or other low-grade febrile illness.[32,108] However, children with moderate or serious illness should not be immunized until recovered.[3]

Elective immunization procedures should be deferred during an outbreak of poliomyelitis because of the risk of provoking paralysis.[109-111]

WARNINGS

If any of the following events occur in temporal relation to receipt of whole-cell DTP or acellular DTP vaccine, the decision to give subsequent doses of vaccine containing the pertussis component should be carefully considered. There may be circumstances, such as high incidence of pertussis, in which the potential benefits outweigh possible risks, particularly since these events have not been proven to cause permanent sequelae.[3,74] The following events were previously considered contraindications and are now considered precautions by the ACIP:

- **Temperature of ≥40.5°C (105°F) within 48 hours, not due to another identifiable cause.**
- **Collapse or shock-like state (hypotonic-hyporesponsive episode) within 48 hours.**
- **Persistent, inconsolable crying lasting ≥3 hours, occurring within 48 hours.**
- **Convulsions with or without fever, occurring within 3 days.**

Data from approximately 15,000 children participating in German and US studies, suggest that persistent, inconsolable crying lasting at least 3 hours following vaccination with Tripedia vaccine may occur less frequently than has been observed historically for DTP vaccine.[1,35]

In the Italian efficacy trial, the incidence of temperature ≥104°F, crying for 3 hours or more and seizures within 48 hours of vaccination was less than that following administration of whole-cell DTP vaccine manufactured by Connaught Laboratories, Inc. No hypotonic-hyporesponsive episodes were reported after administration of Infanrix in this trial.[70]

When a decision is made to withhold the pertussis component, immunization with DT should be continued.

Diphtheria and Tetanus Toxoids and Acellular Pertussis Vaccine Adsorbed should not be given to children with any coagulation disorder, including thrombocytopenia, that would contraindicate intramuscular injection unless the potential benefit clearly outweighs the risk of administration.

A committee of the Institute of Medicine (IOM) has concluded that evidence is consistent with a causal relationship between DTP and acute neurologic illness, and under special circumstances, between DTP and chronic neurologic disease in the context of the NCES report.[37,38] However, the IOM committee concluded that the evidence was insufficient to indicate whether or not DTP increased the overall risk of chronic neurologic disease.[38] Acute encephalopathy or permanent neurological injury have not been reported in temporal association after administration of Diphtheria and Tetanus Toxoids and Acellular Pertussis Vaccine Adsorbed but the experience with this vaccine is insufficient to rule this out.

Infants and children with recognized possible or potential underlying neurologic conditions seem to be at enhanced risk for the appearance of manifestations of the underlying neurologic disorder within 2 or 3 days following whole-cell pertussis vaccination.[3] Whether to administer Tripedia vaccine to such children must be decided on an individual basis after consideration of the risks and benefits. An important consideration includes the current local incidence of pertussis. The Advisory Committee on Immunization Practices (ACIP) and the American Academy of Pediatrics (AAP) have issued guidelines for such children.[3,30,31]

In the opinion of the manufacturer, seizure disorder in children before or after any immunization with Tripedia is considered a warning against further immunization with this vaccine. The ACIP and AAP recognize certain circumstances in which children with stable central nervous system disorders, including well-controlled seizures or satisfactorily explained single seizures, may receive acellular pertussis vaccine.[30,31]

The decision to administer a pertussis-containing vaccine to such children must be made by the physician on an individual basis, with consideration of all relevant factors, and assessment of potential risks and benefits for that individual. ACIP and AAP have issued guidelines for such children.[3,74,76] The parent or guardian should be advised of the potential increased risk involved.

Some studies suggest that infants and children with a history of convulsions in first-degree family members (*i.e.*, siblings and parents) have a 3.2-fold increased risk for neurologic events compared with those without such histories when given DTP.[27,36] However, a family history of convulsions in parents and siblings is not considered a contraindication to pertussis vaccination by either the AAP or the ACIP. The AAP and ACIP recommend that children with such family histories should receive pertussis vaccine according to the recommended schedule.[3,30,31]

In children with a personal or family history of convulsions, acetaminophen or other appropriate antipyretic should be given at the time of Diphtheria and Tetanus Toxoids and Acellular Pertussis Vaccine Adsorbed vaccination and for the ensuing 24 hours, according to the respective package insert recommended dosage, to reduce the possibility of post-vaccination fever.[3,30,31]

Tripedia vaccine should not be combined through reconstitution with any vaccine for administration to infants younger than 15 months of age. Tripedia vaccine should not be reconstituted with any vaccine other than ActHIB for children 15 months of age or older.

DOSAGE AND ADMINISTRATION

TRIPEDIA

Parenteral drug products should be inspected visually for extraneous particulate matter and/or discoloration prior to administration whenever solution and container permit. If these conditions exist, the vaccine should not be administered.

SHAKE VIAL WELL *before withdrawing each dose.* Inject 0.5 ml of Tripedia vaccine intramuscularly only. The preferred injection sites are the anterolateral aspect of the thigh and the deltoid muscle of the upper arm. The vaccine should not be injected into the gluteal area or areas where there may be a major nerve trunk.

The primary series for children less than 7 years of age is 3 intramuscular doses of 0.5 ml. The customary age for the first dose is 2 months of age but may be given as early as 6 weeks of age and up to the seventh birthday.

Before injection, the skin over the site to be injected should be cleansed with a suitable germicide. After insertion of the needle, aspirate to ensure that the needle has not entered a blood vessel.

Fractional doses (doses <0.5 ml) should not be given. The effect of fractional doses on the frequency of serious adverse events and on efficacy has not been determined.

Do NOT administer this product subcutaneously.

Primary Immunization

The primary series consists of 3 doses administered at intervals of 4-8 weeks. It is recommended that Tripedia vaccine be given for all 3 doses since no interchangeability data on DTaP vaccines exist for the primary series.

Tripedia vaccine may be used to complete the primary series in infants who have received 1 or 2 doses of whole-cell pertussis DTP. However, the safety and efficacy of Tripedia vaccine in such infants has not been evaluated.

Tripedia vaccine should not be combined through reconstitution with any other vaccine for administration to infants younger than 15 months of age. Available serologic data do not support the use of Tripedia vaccine to reconstitute ActHIB (TriHIBit) for primary immunization.

Booster Immunization

When Tripedia vaccine is given for the primary series, a fourth dose is recommended at 15-20 months of age. The interval between the third and fourth dose should be at least 6 months. When Tripedia is given for the first 4 doses, a fifth dose of Tripedia is recommended at 4-6 years of age, preferably prior to school entry.[30,31] If the fourth dose was administered after the fourth birthday, a fifth dose prior to school entry is not necessary.[30,31]

If a child receives whole-cell pertussis DTP for 1 or more doses, Tripedia vaccine may be given to complete the 5-dose series. A fourth dose is recommended at 15-20 months of age. The interval between the third and fourth dose should be at least 6 months. Children 4-6 years of age (up to the seventh birthday) who received all 4 doses by the fourth birthday, including 1 or more doses of whole-cell pertussis DTP, should receive a single dose of Tripedia vaccine before entering kindergarten or elementary school. This dose is not needed if the fourth dose was given on or after the fourth birthday.[30,31]

Tripedia vaccine combined with ActHIB (TriHIBit) by reconstitution may be administered at 15-18 months of age for the fourth dose. (Refer to ActHIB package insert.)

If any recommended dose of pertussis vaccine cannot be given, DT (For Pediatric Use) should be given as needed to complete the series.

PERSONS 7 YEARS OF AGE AND OLDER SHOULD NOT BE IMMUNIZED WITH TRIPEDIA VACCINE.[3,30]

Preterm infants should be vaccinated according to their chronological age from birth.[3,30]

Interruption of the recommended schedule with a delay between doses should not interfere with the final immunity achieved with Tripedia vaccine. There is no need to start the series over again, regardless of the time between doses.

Routine simultaneous administration of DTaP, IPV, Haemophilus b conjugate vaccine, MMR, pneumococcal conjugate vaccine, varicella vaccine, and hepatitis B vaccine is encouraged for children who are the recommended age to receive these vaccines and for whom no specific contraindications exist at the time of the visit, unless, in the judgment of the provider, complete vaccination of the child will not be compromised by administering different vaccines at different visits. Simultaneous administration is particularly important if the child might not return for subsequent vaccinations.[32]

There are no data available on the simultaneous administration of Tripedia, with varicella vaccine, or IPV, or pneumococcal conjugate vaccine.

Data are unavailable to the manufacturer concerning the effects on immune responses to IPV when IPV is given concurrently at separate sites with ActHIB reconstituted with Tripedia (TriHIBit) as a booster.

If passive immunization is needed for tetanus prophylaxis, Tetanus Immune Globulin (Human) (TIG) is the product of choice. It provides longer protection than antitoxin of animal origin and causes few adverse reactions. The currently recommended prophylactic dose of TIG for wounds of average severity is 250 units intramuscularly. When tetanus toxoid and TIG are administered concurrently, separate syringes and separate sites should be used. The ACIP recommends the use of only adsorbed toxoid in this situation.

DAPTACEL

Daptacel is a sterile white homogenous cloudy suspension of acellular pertussis vaccine components and diphtheria and tetanus toxoids adsorbed on aluminum in a sterile isotonic sodium chloride solution and containing 2-phenoxyethanol as preservative. Inspect the vial visually for extraneous particulate matter and/or discoloration before administration. If these conditions exist, the product should not be administered.

JUST BEFORE USE, SHAKE THE VIAL WELL, until a uniform, cloudy suspension results. WITHDRAW AND INJECT A 0.5 ml DOSE. When administering a dose from a rubber-stoppered vial, do not remove either the rubber stopper or the metal seal holding it in place. Aseptic technique must be used for withdrawal of each dose.

Before injection, the skin over the site to be injected should be cleansed with a suitable germicide. After insertion of the needle into the muscle, aspirate to ensure that the needle has not entered a blood vessel.

Administer the vaccine **intramuscularly** (IM). In children younger than 1 year (*i.e.*, infants), the anterolateral aspect of the thigh provides the largest muscle and is the preferred site of injection. In older children, the deltoid muscle is usually large enough for IM injection. The vaccine should not be injected into the gluteal area or areas where there may be a major nerve trunk.[108]

Fractional doses (doses <0.5 ml) should not be given. The effect of fractional doses on the frequency of serious adverse events and on efficacy has not been determined.

Do NOT administer this product intravenously or subcutaneously.

D

Immunization Series
A 0.5 ml dose of Daptacel is approved for administration as a 4 dose series at 2, 4 and 6 months of age, at intervals of 6-8 weeks and at 17-20 months of age. The customary age for the first dose is 2 months of age, but it may be given as early as 6 weeks of age and up to the seventh birthday. The interval between the third and fourth dose should be at least 6 months. It is recommended that Daptacel be given for all doses in the series because no data on the interchangeability of Daptacel with other DTaP vaccines exist. At this time, data are insufficient to establish the frequency of adverse events following a fifth dose of Daptacel in children who have previously received 4 doses of Daptacel.[123]

Daptacel may be used to complete the immunization series in infants who have received 1 or more doses of whole-cell pertussis DTP. However, the safety and efficacy of Daptacel in such infants have not been fully demonstrated.[99]

PERSONS 7 YEARS OF AGE AND OLDER SHOULD NOT BE IMMUNIZED WITH DAPTACEL OR ANY OTHER PERTUSSIS-CONTAINING VACCINES.[32]

Daptacel should not be combined through reconstitution or mixed with any other vaccine.

If any recommended dose of pertussis vaccine cannot be given, DT (For Pediatric Use) should be given as needed to complete the series.

Pre-term infants should be vaccinated according to their chronological age from birth.[108]

Interruption of the recommended schedule with a delay between doses should not interfere with the final immunity achieved with Daptacel. There is no need to start the series over again, regardless of the time between doses.

Simultaneous Vaccine Administration
In clinical trials, Daptacel was routinely administered, at separate sites, concomitantly with 1 or more of the following vaccines: OPV, hepatitis B vaccine and *Haemophilus influenzae* type b vaccine.[107] No safety and immunogenicity data are currently available on the simultaneous administration of pneumococcal conjugate vaccine, MMR vaccine and varicella vaccine and no immunogenicity data are currently available on the simultaneous administration of IPV. Two afebrile seizures, occurring within 24 hours of immunization, have been reported from 2 US trials where Daptacel was given with other concomitant vaccines. When concomitant administration of other vaccines is required, they should be given with different syringes and at different injection sites.

ACIP encourages routine simultaneous administration of DTaP, IPV, *Haemophilus influenzae* type b vaccine, pneumococcal conjugate vaccine, MMR, varicella vaccine and hepatitis B vaccine for children who are the recommended age to receive these vaccines and for whom no specific contraindications exist at the time of the visit, unless, in the judgment of the provider, complete vaccination of the child will not be compromised by administering different vaccines at different visits. Simultaneous administration is particularly important if the child might not return for subsequent vaccinations.[32]

If passive immunization is needed for tetanus prophylaxis, Tetanus Immune Globulin (Human) (TIG) is the product of choice. It provides longer protection than antitoxin of animal origin and is associated with few adverse reactions. The currently recommended prophylactic dose of TIG for wounds of average severity is 250 units intramuscularly. When tetanus toxoid-containing vaccines and TIG and/or Diphtheria Antitoxin are administered concurrently, separate syringes and separate sites should be used.

INFANRIX
Preparation for Administration
Shake the vial or syringe well before use. The vaccine is ready to use without reconstitution. Parenteral drug products should be inspected visually for particulate matter or discoloration prior to administration, whenever solution and container permit. With thorough agitation, Infanrix is a homogeneous white turbid suspension. Discard if it appears otherwise. Since this product is a suspension containing an adjuvant, shake vigorously to obtain a uniform suspension prior to withdrawal from the vial. DO NOT USE IF RESUSPENSION DOES NOT OCCUR WITH VIGOROUS SHAKING. After removal of the 0.5 ml dose, any vaccine remaining in the vial should be discarded.

Infanrix should be administered by intramuscular injection. The preferred sites are the anterolateral aspects of the thigh or the deltoid muscle of the upper arm. The vaccine should not be injected in the gluteal area or areas where there may be a major nerve trunk. Before injection, the skin at the injection site should be cleaned and prepared with a suitable germicide. After insertion of the needle, aspirate to ensure that the needle has not entered a blood vessel.

Do not administer this product subcutaneously.

Primary Immunization
The primary immunization course for children less than 7 years of age is 3 doses of 0.5 ml, given intramuscularly, at 4-8 week intervals (preferably 8 weeks). The customary age for the first dose is 2 months of age, but it may be given starting at 6 weeks of age and up to the seventh birthday. It is recommended that Infanrix be given for all 3 doses since no interchangeability data on acellular DTP vaccines exist for the primary series. Infanrix may be used to complete the primary series in infants who have received 1 or 2 doses of whole-cell DTP vaccine. However, the safety and efficacy of Infanrix in such infants have not been evaluated.

Booster Immunization
When Infanrix is given for the primary series, a fourth dose is recommended at 15-20 months of age. The interval between the third and fourth dose should be at least 6 months. At this time, data are insufficient to establish the frequency of adverse events following a fifth dose of Infanrix in children who have previously received 4 doses of Infanrix.

If a child has received whole-cell DTP vaccine for 1 or more doses, Infanrix may be given to complete the 5-dose series. A fourth dose is recommended at 15-20 months of age. The interval between the third and fourth dose should be at least 6 months. Children 4-6 years of age (up to the seventh birthday) who received all 4 doses by the fourth birthday, including 1 or more doses of whole-cell DTP vaccine, should receive a single dose of Infanrix before entering kindergarten or elementary school. This dose is not needed if the fourth dose was given on or after the fourth birthday.

Additional Dosing Information
If any recommended dose of pertussis vaccine cannot be given, DT (For Pediatric Use) should be given as needed to complete the series.

Interruption of the recommended schedule with a delay between doses should not interfere with the final immunity achieved with Infanrix. There is no need to start the series over again, regardless of the time elapsed between doses.

The use of reduced volume (fractional doses) is not recommended. The effect of such practices on the frequency of serious adverse events and on protection against disease has not been determined.[32]

Preterm infants should be vaccinated according to their chronological age from birth.[32]

For persons 7 years of age or older, Tetanus and Diphtheria Toxoids (Td) For Adult Use should be given for routine booster immunization against tetanus and diphtheria.

Simultaneous Vaccine Administration
In clinical trials, Infanrix was routinely administered, at separate sites, concomitantly with 1 or more of the following vaccines: poliovirus vaccine live oral (OPV), hepatitis B vaccine, and Haemophilus influenzae type b vaccine (Hib).

No data are available on the simultaneous administration of measles, mumps, and rubella vaccine (MMR), varicella vaccine, or inactivated polio virus (IPV) with Infanrix.

When concomitant administration of other vaccines is required, they should be given with different syringes and at different injection sites.

The ACIP encourages routine simultaneous administration of acellular DTP, OPV (or IPV), Hib, MMR, and hepatitis B vaccine for children who are at the recommended age to receive these vaccines and for whom no specific contraindications exist at the time of the visit, unless, in the judgment of the provider, complete vaccination of the child will not be compromised by administering vaccines at different visits. Simultaneous administration is particularly important if the child might not return for subsequent vaccinations.[32]

PRODUCT LISTING - EQUIVALENTS NOT AVAILABLE

Suspension - Intramuscular - Strength n/a

0.50 ml x 10	$220.45	INFANRIX, Allscripts Pharmaceutical Company	54569-4969-00
0.50 ml x 10	$239.74	TRIPEDIA, Aventis Pharmaceuticals	49281-0288-10
0.50 ml x 10	$240.00	INFANRIX, Glaxosmithkline	58160-0840-11
0.50 ml x 25	$614.00	INFANRIX, Glaxosmithkline	58160-0840-50
7.50 ml	$289.69	TRIPEDIA, Allscripts Pharmaceutical Company	54569-4746-00
7.50 ml	$309.63	CERTIVA, Ross Product Division Pharmaceuticals	62448-4012-01
7.50 ml	$317.11	TRIPEDIA, Aventis Pharmaceuticals	49281-0288-15
7.50 ml	$357.06	TRIPEDIA, Aventis Pharmaceuticals	49281-0282-15

Suspension - Intramuscular - 15 U;23 mcg;5 U/0.5 ml

0.50 ml x 5	$123.68	DAPTACEL, Aventis Pharmaceuticals	49281-0286-05

Dipivefrin Hydrochloride *(001088)*

Categories: Glaucoma, open-angle; Pregnancy Category B; FDA Approved 1980 May
Drug Classes: Adrenergic agonists; Ophthalmics
Brand Names: Akpro; **Propine**
Foreign Brand Availability: D Epifrin (Germany); D'Epifrin (Philippines); Difrin (Israel); Diopine (Greece; Mexico; Netherlands; Spain; Switzerland); Diphemin (Switzerland); Dipoquin (Australia); Glaucothil (Austria; Germany); Glaudrops (Spain); Pivalephrine (Japan); Prodren (Israel)
Cost of Therapy: $18.56 (Glaucoma; Propine Ophthalmic Solution; 0.1%; 5 ml; 2 drops/day; variable day supply)
$12.27 (Glaucoma; Generic Ophthalmic Solution; 0.1%; 5 ml; 2 drops/day; variable day supply)

DESCRIPTION

This solution contains dipivefrin hydrochloride in a sterile, isotonic solution. Dipivefrin HCl is a white, crystalline powder, freely soluble in water.
Empirical Formula: $C_{19}H_{29}O_5N \cdot HCl$
Chemical Name: (±)-3.4-Dihydroxy—α—((methylamino) methyl) benzylalcohol 3,4-dipivalate hydrochloride.
Contains: Dipivefrin HCl 0.1% with; benzalkonium chloride 0.005%; edetate disodium; sodium chloride; hydrochloric acid to adjust pH; and purified water.
Storage: Store in tight, light-resistant containers.

CLINICAL PHARMACOLOGY

Dipivefrin HCl is a member of a class of drugs known as prodrugs. Prodrugs are usually not active in themselves and require biotransformation to the parent compound before therapeutic activity is seen. These modifications are undertaken to enhance absorption, decrease side effects and enhance stability and comfort, thus making the parent compound a more useful drug. Enhanced absorption makes the prodrug a more efficient delivery system for the parent drug because less drug will be needed to produce the desired therapeutic response.

Dipivefrin HCl is a prodrug of epinephrine formed by the diesterification of epinephrine and pivalic acid. The addition of pivaloyl groups to the epinephrine molecule enhances its lipophilic character and as a consequence, its penetration into the anterior chamber.

Dipivefrin HCl is converted to epinephrine inside the human eye by enzyme hydrolysis. The liberated epinephrine, an adrenergic agonist, appears to exert its action by decreasing aqueous production and by enhancing outflow facility. The dipivefrin HCl prodrug delivery system is a more efficient way of delivering the therapeutic effects of epinephrine, with fewer side effects than are associated with conventional epinephrine therapy.

The onset of action with 1 drop of dipivefrin HCl occurs about 30 minutes after treatment, with maximum effect seen at about 1 hour.

Using a prodrug means that less drug is needed for therapeutic effect since absorption is enhanced with the prodrug. Dipivefrin HCl at 0.1% dipivefrin was judged less irritating than a 1% solution of epinephrine hydrochloride or bitartrate. In addition, only 8 of 455 patients

(1.8%) treated with dipivefrin HCl reported discomfort due to photophobia, glare or light sensitivity.

INDICATIONS AND USAGE

Dipivefrin HCl is indicated as initial therapy for the control of intraocular pressure in chronic open-angle glaucoma. Patients responding inadequately to other antiglaucoma therapy may respond to addition of dipivefrin HCl.

In controlled and open-label studies of glaucoma, dipivefrin HCl demonstrated a statistically significant intraocular pressure-lowering effect. Patients using dipivefrin HCl twice daily in studies with mean durations of 76-146 days experienced mean pressure reductions ranging from 20-24%.

Therapeutic response to dipivefrin HCl twice daily is somewhat less than 2% epinephrine twice daily. Controlled studies showed statistically significant differences in lowering of intraocular pressure between dipivefrin HCl and 2% epinephrine. In controlled studies in patients with a history of epinephrine intolerance, only 3% of patients treated with dipivefrin HCl exhibited intolerance, while 55% of those treated with epinephrine again developed intolerance.

Therapeutic response to dipivefrin HCl twice daily therapy is comparable to 2% pilocarpine 4 times daily. In controlled clinical studies comparing dipivefrin HCl and 2% pilocarpine, there were no statistically significant differences in the maintenance of IOP levels for the 2 medications. Dipivefrin HCl does not produce miosis or accommodative spasm which cholinergic agents are known to produce. The blurred vision and night blindness often associated with miotic agents are not present with dipivefrin HCl therapy. Patients with cataracts avoid the inability to see around lenticular opacities caused by constricted pupil.

NON-FDA APPROVED INDICATIONS

Dipivefrin has been used without FDA approval to reduce IOP in patients with ocular hypertension and pseudoexfoliative, low-tension, and secondary (*e.g.*, post-angle closure, pigmentary, traumatic, or herpetic) glaucomas.

CONTRAINDICATIONS

Dipivefrin HCl should not be used in patients with narrow angles since any dilation of the pupil may predispose the patient to an attack of angle-closure glaucoma. This product is contraindicated in patients who are hypersensitive to any of its components.

PRECAUTIONS

APHAKIC PATIENTS

Macular edema has been shown to occur in up to 30% of aphakic patients treated with epinephrine. Discontinuation of epinephrine generally results in reversal of the maculopathy.

PREGNANCY CATEGORY B

Reproduction studies have been performed in rats and rabbits at daily oral doses up to 10 mg/kg body weight (5 mg/kg body weight (5 mg/kg in teratogenicity studies), and have revealed no evidence of impaired fertility or harm to the fetus due to dipivefrin HCl. There are, however, no adequate and well-controlled studies in pregnant women. Because animal reproduction studies are not always predictive of human response, this drug should be used during pregnancy only if clearly needed.

NURSING MOTHERS

It is not known whether this drug is excreted in human milk. Because many drugs are excreted in human milk, caution should be exercised when dipivefrin HCl is administered to a nursing woman.

USAGE IN CHILDREN

Clinical studies for safety and efficacy in children have not been done.

ANIMAL STUDIES

Rabbit studies indicated a dose-related incidence of meibomian gland retention cysts following topical administration of both dipivefrin hydrochloride and epinephrine.

ADVERSE REACTIONS

Cardiovascular Effects: Tachycardia, arrhythmias and hypertension have been reported with ocular administration of epinephrine.

Local Effects: The most frequent side effects reported with dipivefrin HCl alone were injection in 6.5% of patients and burning and stinging in 6%. Follicular conjunctivitis, mydriasis and allergic reactions to dipivefrin HCl have been reported infrequently. Epinephrine therapy can lead to adrenochrome deposits in the conjunctiva and cornea.

DOSAGE AND ADMINISTRATION

INITIAL GLAUCOMA THERAPY

The usual dosage of dipivefrin HCl is 1 drop in the eye(s) every 12 hours.

REPLACEMENT WITH DIPIVEFRIN HCl

When patients are being transferred to dipivefrin HCl from antiglaucoma agents other than epinephrine, on the first day continue the previous medication and add 1 drop of dipivefrin HCl in each eye every 12 hours. On the following day, discontinue the previously used antiglaucoma agent and continue with dipivefrin HCl.

In transferring patients from conventional epinephrine therapy to dipivefrin HCl, simply discontinue the epinephrine medication and institute the dipivefrin HCl regimen.

ADDITION OF DIPIVEFRIN HCl

When patients on other antiglaucoma agents require additional therapy, add 1 drop of dipivefrin HCl every 12 hours.

CONCOMITANT THERAPY

For difficult to control patients, the addition of dipivefrin HCl to other agents such as pilocarpine, carbachol, echothiophate iodide or acetazolamide has been shown to be effective.

Note: Not for injection.

PRODUCT LISTING - RATED THERAPEUTICALLY EQUIVALENT

Solution - Ophthalmic - 0.1%

Size	Price	Product	NDC
5 ml	$4.35	FEDERAL UPPER LIMIT, H.C.F.A. F F P	99999-1088-01
5 ml	$14.07	GENERIC, Bausch and Lomb	24208-0540-05
5 ml	$14.10	GENERIC, Pacific Pharma	60758-0087-05
5 ml	$18.56	PROPINE, Southwood Pharmaceuticals Inc	58016-6058-01
5 ml	$25.11	PROPINE, Allergan Inc	00023-9208-05
10 ml	$25.31	GENERIC, Watson/Schein Pharmaceuticals Inc	00364-3040-54
10 ml	$27.18	GENERIC, Bausch and Lomb	24208-0540-10
10 ml	$27.18	GENERIC, Pacific Pharma	60758-0087-10
10 ml	$33.44	PROPINE, Southwood Pharmaceuticals Inc	58016-6438-01
10 ml	$45.60	PROPINE, Allergan Inc	00023-9208-10
15 ml	$41.50	GENERIC, Pacific Pharma	60758-0087-15
15 ml	$41.55	GENERIC, Bausch and Lomb	24208-0540-15
15 ml	$48.63	PROPINE, Southwood Pharmaceuticals Inc	58016-6464-01
15 ml	$71.35	PROPINE, Allergan Inc	00023-9208-15

PRODUCT LISTING - EQUIVALENTS NOT AVAILABLE

Solution - Ophthalmic - 0.1%

Size	Price	Product	NDC
5 ml	$14.10	GENERIC, Falcon Pharmaceuticals, Ltd.	61314-0235-05
10 ml	$26.12	GENERIC, Allscripts Pharmaceutical Company	54569-4307-00
10 ml	$27.20	GENERIC, Falcon Pharmaceuticals, Ltd.	61314-0235-10
15 ml	$41.55	GENERIC, Allscripts Pharmaceutical Company	54569-4376-00
15 ml	$41.60	GENERIC, Falcon Pharmaceuticals, Ltd.	61314-0235-15

Dipyridamole *(001090)*

Categories: Imaging, myocardial, adjunct; Surgery, heart valve, adjunct; Pregnancy Category B; FDA Approved 1986 Dec

Drug Classes: Platelet inhibitors

Brand Names: Dipridacot; Permole; **Persantine**

Foreign Brand Availability: Adezan (Greece); Agilease (Japan); Agremol (Thailand); Anginal (Japan; Taiwan); Anti-Plate 75 (Benin; Burkina-Faso; Ethiopia; Gambia; Ghana; Guinea; Ivory-Coast; Kenya; Liberia; Malawi; Mali; Mauritania; Mauritius; Morocco; Niger; Nigeria; Senegal; Seychelles; Sierra-Leone; Sudan; Tanzania; Tunia; Uganda; Zambia; Zimbabwe); Apo-Dipyridamole FC (Canada); Atlantin (Japan); Atrombin (Finland); Cardoxin (Israel); Cardoxin Forte (Israel); Chilcolan (Japan); Cleridium (France; Philippines); Coronair (Belgium); Coronamole (Japan); Corosan (Italy); Cortab (Indonesia); Dipyridan (Japan); Dipyrol (South-Africa); Dirinol (Mexico); Efosin (Taiwan); Ethrine (Greece); Gulliostin (Japan); Isephanine (Japan); Justpertin (Japan); Lodimol (Mexico); Microbanzol (Japan); Miosen (Spain); Novodil (Italy); Parotin (Taiwan); Permiltin (Japan); Persantin (Argentina; Australia; Austria; Bahamas; Bahrain; Barbados; Belize; Benin; Bermuda; Bulgaria; Burkina-Faso; Curacao; Cyprus; Czech-Republic; Denmark; Egypt; England; Ethiopia; Finland; Gambia; Ghana; Greece; Guinea; Guyana; Hong-Kong; Hungary; India; Indonesia; Iran; Iraq; Ireland; Italy; Ivory-Coast; Jamaica; Jordan; Kenya; Kuwait; Lebanon; Liberia; Libya; Malawi; Malaysia; Mali; Mauritania; Mauritius; Mexico; Morocco; Netherland-Antilles; Netherlands; New-Zealand; Niger; Nigeria; Norway; Oman; Peru; Philippines; Portugal; Qatar; Republic-of-Yemen; Saudi-Arabia; Senegal; Seychelles; Sierra-Leone; South-Africa; Spain; Sudan; Surinam; Sweden; Switzerland; Syria; Taiwan; Tanzania; Thailand; Trinidad; Tunia; Uganda; United-Arab-Emirates; Zambia; Zimbabwe); Persantin 75 (Colombia; Mexico; Peru); Persantin 100 (Australia); Persantin Depot (Austria; Finland); Persantin Forte (Germany); Persantin PL (New-Zealand); Persantin PL Prolonguetas (Mexico); Persantin Prolonguets (Portugal); Persantin Retard (Netherlands); Persantin Retardkapseln (Switzerland); Persantin SR (Australia); Piroan (Japan); Plato (South-Africa); Posanin (Thailand); Prexin (Philippines); Pytazen SR (New-Zealand); Ridamol (Philippines); Rupenol (Taiwan); Sandel (Taiwan); Solantin (Taiwan); Tovincocard (Italy); Trompersantin (Mexico); Vasokor (Indonesia)

Cost of Therapy: $141.25 (Thromboembolism; Persantine; 75 mg; 4 tablets/day; 30 day supply)
$11.70 (Thromboembolism; Generic tablets; 75 mg; 4 tablets/day; 30 day supply)

HCFA JCODE(S): J1245 per 10 mg IV

DESCRIPTION

TABLETS

Dipyridamole tablets is a platelet inhibitor chemically described as 2,6-bis-(diethanolamino)-4,8-dipiperidino-pyrimido-(5,4,-d) pyrimidine.

The molecular formula is $C_{24}H_{40}N_8O_4$.

The molecular weight is 504.62.

Dipyridamole is an odorless yellow crystalline powder, having a bitter taste. It is soluble in dilute acids, methanol and chloroform, and practically insoluble in water.

Dipyridamole tablets for oral administration contain:

Persantine Active Ingredient: Tablets 25, 50, and 75 mg: dipyridamole 25, 50, and 75 mg respectively.

Persantine Inactive Ingredients: Tablets 25, 50, and 75 mg: acacia, carnauba wax, corn starch, FD&C blue no. 1 aluminum lake, D&C yellow no. 10 aluminum lake, D&C red no. 30 aluminum lake, lactose, magnesium stearate, polyethylene glycol, povidone, shellac, sodium benzoate, sucrose, talc, titanium dioxide, white wax.

Storage: Store below 86°F (30°C).

INTRAVENOUS INJECTION

Dipyridamole injection is a coronary vasodilator described as 2,2',2'',2'''-[(4,8-Dipiperidinopyrimido [5,4-*d*]pyrimidine-2,6-diyl)dinitrilo]tetraethanol. The molecular formula is $C_{24}H_{40}N_8O_4$. The molecular weight is 504.64.

Dipyridamole in solution is an odorless, pale yellow liquid which can be diluted in sodium chloride injection or dextrose injection for intravenous administration.

IV dipyridamole as a sterile solution for intravenous administration contains:

Persantine IV Active Ingredient: *Ampules 2 ml:* Dipyridamole 10 mg; *Ampules 10 ml:* Dipyridamole 50 mg; *Vial 10 ml:* Dipyridamole 50 mg.

Persantine IV Inactive Ingredients: *Ampules 2 ml:* Polyethylene glycol 600 100 mg, tartaric acid 4 mg; *Ampules 10 ml:* Polyethylene glycol 600 500 mg, tartaric acid 20 mg; *Vial*

10 ml: Polyethylene glycol 600 500 mg, tartaric acid 20 mg; pH is adjusted to 2.7 ± 0.5 with hydrochloric acid.

Storage: Store between 15-25°C (59-77°F). **Avoid freezing. Protect from light.** Retain in carton until time of use. Discard unused portion.

CLINICAL PHARMACOLOGY

TABLETS

It is believed that platelet reactivity and interaction with prosthetic cardiac valve surfaces, resulting in abnormally shortened platelet survival time, is a significant factor in thromboembolic complications occurring in connection with prosthetic heart valve replacement.

Dipyridamole has been found to lengthen abnormally shortened platelet survival time in a dose-dependent manner.

In three randomized controlled clinical trials involving 854 patients who had undergone surgical placement of a prosthetic heart valve, dipyridamole, in combination with warfarin, decreased the incidence of postoperative thromboembolic events by 62-91% compared to warfarin treatment alone. The incidence of thromboembolic events in patients receiving the combination of dipyridamole and warfarin ranged from 1.2-1.8%. In three additional studies involving 392 patients taking dipyridamole and coumarin-like anticoagulants, the incidence of thromboembolic events ranged from 2.3-6.9%.

In these trials, the coumarin anticoagulant was begun between 24 hours and 4 days postoperatively, and the dipyridamole was begun between 24 hours and 10 days postoperatively. The length of follow-up in these trials varied from 1-2 years.

Dipyridamole does not influence prothrombin time or activity measurements when administered with warfarin.

Mechanism of Action

Dipyridamole is a platelet adhesion inhibitor, although the mechanism of action has not been fully elucidated. The mechanism may relate to inhibition of red blood cell uptake of adenosine, itself an inhibitor of platelet reactivity, phosphodiesterase inhibition leading to increased cyclic-3', 5'-adenosine monophosphate within platelets, and inhibition of thromboxane A_2 formation which is a potent stimulator of platelet activation.

Hemodynamics

In dogs intraduodenal doses of dipyridamole of 0.5-4.0 mg/kg produced dose-related decreases in systemic and coronary vascular resistance leading to decreases in systemic blood pressure and increases in coronary blood flow. Onset of action was in about 24 minutes and effects persisted for about 3 hours.

Similar effects were observed following IV dipyridamole in doses ranging from 0.025-2.0 mg/kg.

In man the same qualitative hemodynamic effects have been observed. However, acute intravenous administration of dipyridamole may worsen regional myocardial perfusion distal to partial occlusion of coronary arteries.

Pharmacokinetics and Metabolism

Following an oral dose of dipyridamole, the average time to peak concentration is about 75 minutes. The decline in plasma concentration following a dose of dipyridamole fits a two-compartment model. The alpha half-life (the initial decline following peak concentration) is approximately 40 minutes. The beta half-life (the terminal decline in plasma concentration) is approximately 10 hours. Dipyridamole is highly bound to plasma proteins. It is metabolized in the liver where it is conjugated as a glucuronide and excreted with the bile.

INTRAVENOUS INJECTION

In a study of 10 patients with angiographically normal or minimally stenosed (less than 25% luminal diameter narrowing) coronary vessels, dipyridamole injection in a dose of 0.56 mg/kg infused over 4 minutes resulted in an average fivefold increase in coronary blood flow velocity compared to resting coronary flow velocity (range 3.8-7 times resting velocity). The mean time to peak flow velocity was 6.5 minutes from the start of the 4 minute infusion (range 2.5-8.7 minutes). Cardiovascular responses to the intravenous administration of dipyridamole when given to patients in the supine position include a mild but significant increase in heart rate of approximately 20% and mild but significant decreases in both systolic and diastolic blood pressure of approximately 2-8%, with vital signs returning to baseline values in approximately 30 minutes.

Mechanism of Action

Dipyridamole is a coronary vasodilator in man. The mechanism of vasodilation has not been fully elucidated, but may result from inhibition of uptake of adenosine, an important mediator of coronary vasodilation. The vasodilatory effects of dipyridamole are abolished by administration of the adenosine receptor antagonist theophylline.

How dipyridamole-induced vasodilation leads to abnormalities in thallium distribution and ventricular function is also uncertain but presumably represents a "steal" phenomenon in which relatively intact vessels dilate, and sustain enhanced flow, leaving reduced pressure and flow across areas of hemodynamically important coronary vascular constriction.

Pharmacokinetics and Metabolism

Plasma dipyridamole concentrations decline in a triexponential fashion following intravenous infusion of dipyridamole, with half-lives averaging 3-12 minutes, 33-62 minutes, and 11.6-15 hours. Two (2) minutes following a 0.568 mg/kg dose of dipyridamole intravenous injection administered as a 4 minute infusion, the mean dipyridamole serum concentration is 4.6±1.3 µg/ml. The average plasma protein binding of dipyridamole is approximately 99%, primarily to a_1-glycoprotein. Dipyridamole is metabolized in the liver to the glucuronic acid conjugate and excreted with the bile. The average total body clearance is 2.3-3.5 ml/min/kg, with an apparent volume of distribution at steady state of 1-2.5 L/kg and a central apparent volume of 3-5 liters.

INDICATIONS AND USAGE

TABLETS

Dipyridamole tablets are indicated as an adjunct to coumarin anticoagulants in the prevention of postoperative thromboembolic complications of cardiac valve replacement.

INTRAVENOUS INJECTION

Dipyridamole injection is indicated as an alternative to exercise in thallium myocardial perfusion imaging for the evaluation of coronary artery disease in patients who cannot exercise adequately.

In a study of about 1100 patients who underwent coronary arteriography and dipyridamole assisted thallium imaging, the results of both tests were interpreted blindly and the sensitivity and specificity of the dipyridamole thallium study in predicting the angiographic outcome were calculated. The sensitivity of the dipyridamole test (true positive dipyridamole divided by the total number of patients with positive angiography) was about 85%. The specificity (true negative divided by the number of patients with negative angiograms) was about 50%.

In a subset of patients who had exercise thallium imaging as well as dipyridamole thallium imaging, sensitivity and specificity of the two tests was almost identical.

CONTRAINDICATIONS

Tablets: None known.

Intravenous Injection: Hypersensitivity to dipyridamole.

WARNINGS

INTRAVENOUS INJECTION

Serious adverse reactions associated with the administration of intravenous dipyridamole have included cardiac death, fatal and non-fatal myocardial infarction, ventricular fibrillation, symptomatic ventricular tachycardia, stroke, transient cerebral ischemia, seizures, anaphylactoid reaction, and bronchospasm. There have been reported cases of asystole, sinus node arrest, sinus node depression, and conduction block. Patients with abnormalities of cardiac impulse formation/conduction or severe coronary artery disease may be at increased risk for these events.

In a study of 3911 patients given intravenous dipyridamole as an adjunct to thallium myocardial perfusion imaging, two types of serious adverse events were reported: 1) four cases of myocardial infarction (0.1%), two fatal (0.05%); and two non-fatal (0.05%); and 2) six cases of severe bronchospasm (0.2%). Although the incidence of these serious adverse events was small (0.3%, 10 of 3911), the potential clinical information to be gained through use of intravenous dipyridamole thallium imaging (see INDICATIONS AND USAGE noting the rate of false positive and false negative results) must be weighed against the risk to the patient. Patients with a history of unstable angina may be at a greater risk for severe myocardial ischemia. Patients with a history of asthma may be at a greater risk for bronchospasm during dipyridamole use.

When thallium myocardial perfusion imaging is performed with intravenous dipyridamole, parenteral aminophylline should be readily available for relieving adverse events such as bronchospasm or chest pain. Vital signs should be monitored during, and for 10-15 minutes following, the intravenous infusion of dipyridamole and an electrocardiographic tracing should be obtained using at least one chest lead. Should severe chest pain or bronchospasm occur, parenteral aminophylline may be administered by slow intravenous injection (50-100 mg over 30-60 seconds) in doses ranging from 50-250 mg. In the case of severe hypotension, the patient should be placed in a supine position with the head tilted down if necessary, before administration of parenteral aminophylline. If 250 mg of aminophylline does not relieve chest pain symptoms within a few minutes, sublingual nitroglycerin may be administered. If chest pain continues despite use of aminophylline and nitroglycerin, the possibility of myocardial infarction should be considered. If the clinical condition of a patient with an adverse event permits a 1 minute delay in the administration of parenteral aminophylline, thallium-201 may be injected and allowed to circulate for one minute before the injection of aminophylline. This will allow initial thallium perfusion imaging to be performed before reversal of the pharmacologic effects of dipyridamole on the coronary circulation.

PRECAUTIONS

GENERAL

Tablets: Dipyridamole should be used with caution in patients with hypotension since it can produce peripheral vasodilation.

Intravenous Injection: See WARNINGS.

CARCINOGENESIS, MUTAGENESIS, AND IMPAIRMENT OF FERTILITY

Tablets

In a 111-week oral study in mice and in a 128-142-week oral study in rats, dipyridamole produced no significant carcinogenic effects at doses of 8, 25 and 75 mg/kg (1, 3.1 and 9.4 times the maximum recommended daily human dose). Mutagenicity testing with dipyridamole was negative. Reproduction studies with dipyridamole revealed no evidence of impaired fertility in rats at dosages up to 60 times the maximum recommended human dose. A significant reduction in number of corpora lutea with consequent reduction in implantations and live fetuses was, however, observed at 155 times the maximum recommended human dose.

Intravenous Injection

In studies in which dipyridamole was administered in the feed at doses of up to 75 mg/kg/day (9.4 times* the maximum recommended daily human oral dose) in mice (up to 128 weeks in males and up to 142 weeks in females) and rats (up to 111 weeks in males and females), there was no evidence of drug-related carcinogenesis. Mutagenicity tests of dipyridamole with bacterial and mammalian cell systems were negative. There was no evidence of impaired fertility when dipyridamole was administered to male and female rats at oral doses up to 500 mg/kg/day (63 times* the maximum recommended daily human oral dose). A significant reduction in number of corpora lutea with consequent reduction in implantations and live fetuses was, however, observed at 1250 mg/kg/day.

PREGNANCY, TERATOGENIC EFFECTS, PREGNANCY CATEGORY B
Tablets

Reproduction studies have been performed in mice at doses up to 125 mg/kg (15.6 times the maximum recommended daily human dose), rats at doses up to 1000 mg/kg (125 times the maximum recommended daily human dose) and rabbits at doses up to 40 mg/kg (5 times the maximum recommended daily human dose) and have revealed no evidence of harm to the fetus due to dipyridamole.

Intravenous Injection

Reproduction studies performed in mice and rats at daily oral doses of up to 125 mg/kg (15.6 times* the maximum recommended daily human oral dose) and in rabbits at daily oral doses of up to 20 mg/kg (2.5 times* the maximum recommended daily human oral dose) have revealed no evidence of impaired embryonic development due to dipyridamole.

Tablets and Intravenous Injection

There are, however, no adequate and well-controlled studies in pregnant women. Because animal reproduction studies are not always predictive of human responses, this drug should be used during pregnancy only if clearly needed.

*Calculation based on assumed body weight of 50 kg.

NURSING MOTHERS

As dipyridamole is excreted in human milk, caution should be exercised when dipyridamole is administered to a nursing woman.

PEDIATRIC USE

Tablets: Safety and effectiveness in children below the age of 12 years has not been established.

Intravenous Injection: Safety and effectiveness in the pediatric population have not been established.

DRUG INTERACTIONS

INTRAVENOUS INJECTION

Oral maintenance theophylline and other xanthine derivatives such as caffeine may abolish the coronary vasodilation induced by intravenous dipyridamole administration. This could lead to a false negative thallium imaging result (see CLINICAL PHARMACOLOGY, Mechanism of Action).

Myasthenia gravis patients receiving therapy with cholinesterase inhibitors may experience worsening of their disease in the presence of dipyridamole.

ADVERSE REACTIONS

TABLETS

Adverse reactions at therapeutic doses are usually minimal and transient. On long-term use of dipyridamole, initial side effects usually disappear. The following reactions were reported in two heart valve replacement trials comparing dipyridamole and warfarin therapy to either warfarin alone or warfarin and placebo (see TABLE 1).

TABLE 1

	Dipyridamole/Warfarin (n=147)	Placebo/Warfarin (n=170)
Dizziness	13.6%	8.2%
Abdominal distress	6.1%	3.5%
Headache	2.3%	0.0
Rash	2.3%	1.1%

Other reactions from uncontrolled studies include diarrhea, vomiting, flushing and pruritus. In addition, angina pectoris has been reported rarely and there have been rare reports of liver dysfunction. On those uncommon occasions when adverse reactions have been persistent or intolerable, they have ceased on withdrawal of the medication.

When dipyridamole was administered concomitantly with warfarin, bleeding was no greater in frequency or severity than that observed when warfarin was administered alone.

INTRAVENOUS INJECTION

Adverse reaction information concerning intravenous dipyridamole is derived from a study of 3911 patients in which intravenous dipyridamole was used as an adjunct to thallium myocardial perfusion imaging and from spontaneous reports of adverse reactions and the published literature.

Serious adverse events (cardiac death, fatal and non-fatal myocardial infarction, ventricular fibrillation, asystole, sinus node arrest, symptomatic ventricular tachycardia, stroke, transient cerebral ischemia, seizures, anaphylactoid reaction, and bronchospasm) are described in WARNINGS.

In the study of 3911 patients, the most frequent adverse reactions were chest pain/angina pectoris (19.7%), electrocardiographic changes (most commonly ST-T changes) (15.9%), headache (12.2%), and dizziness (11.8%).

Adverse reactions occurring in greater than 1% of the patients in the study are shown in TABLE 2.

TABLE 2

	Incidence of Drug-Related Adverse Events
Chest pain/angina pectoris	19.7%
Headache	12.2%
Dizziness	11.8%
Electrocardiographic abnormalities/ST-T changes	7.5%
Electrocardiographic abnormalities/extrasystoles	5.2%
Hypotension	4.6%
Nausea	4.6%
Flushing	3.4%
Electrocardiographic abnormalities/tachycardia	3.2%
Dyspnea	2.6%
Pain unspecified	2.6%
Blood pressure lability	1.6%
Hypertension	1.5%
Paresthesia	1.3%
Fatigue	1.2%

Less common adverse reactions occurring in 1% or less of the patients within the study included:

Cardiovascular System: Electrocardiographic abnormalities unspecified (0.8%), arrhythmia unspecified (0.6%), palpitation (0.3%), ventricular tachycardia (0.2%; see WARNINGS), bradycardia (0.2%), myocardial infarction (0.1%; see WARNINGS), AV block (0.1%), syncope (0.1%), orthostatic hypotension (0.1%), atrial fibrillation (0.1%), supraventricular tachycardia (0.1%), ventricular arrhythmia unspecified (0.03%; see WARNINGS), heart block unspecified (0.03%), cardiomyopathy (0.03%), edema (0.03%).

Central and Peripheral Nervous System: Hypothesia (0.5%), hypertonia (0.3%), nervousness/anxiety (0.2%), tremor (0.1%), abnormal coordination (0.03%), somnolence (0.03%), dysphonia (0.03%), migraine (0.03%), vertigo (0.03%).

Gastrointestinal System: Dyspepsia (1.0%), dry mouth (0.8%), abdominal pain (0.7%), flatulence (0.6%), vomiting (0.4%), eructation (0.1%), dysphagia (0.03%), tenesmus (0.03%), appetite increased (0.03%).

Respiratory System: Pharyngitis (0.3%), bronchospasm (0.2 see WARNINGS), hyperventilation (0.1%), rhinitis (0.1%), coughing (0.03%), pleural pain (0.03%).

Other: Myalgia (0.9%), back pain (0.6%), injection site reaction unspecified (0.4%), diaphoresis (0.4%), asthenia (0.3%), malaise (0.3%), arthralgia (0.3%), injection site pain (0.1%), rigor (0.1%), earache (0.1%), tinnitus (0.1%), vision abnormalities unspecified (0.1%), dysgeusia (0.1%), thirst (0.03%), depersonalization (0.03%), eye pain (0.03%), renal pain (0.03%), perineal pain (0.03%), breast pain (0.03%), intermittent claudication (0.03%), leg cramping (0.03%). In additional postmarketing experience, there have been rare reports of allergic reaction including urticaria, pruritus, dermatitis, and rash.

DOSAGE AND ADMINISTRATION

TABLETS

Adjunctive Use in Prophylaxis of Thromboembolism After Cardiac Valve Replacement

The recommended dose is 75-100 mg four times daily as an adjunct to the usual warfarin therapy. Please note that aspirin is not to be administered concomitantly with coumarin anticoagulants.

INTRAVENOUS INJECTION

The dose of dipyridamole injection as an adjunct to thallium myocardial perfusion imaging should be adjusted according to the weight of the patient. The recommended dose is 0.142 mg/kg/minute (0.57 mg/kg total) infused over 4 minutes. Although the maximum tolerated dose has not been determined, clinical experience suggests that a total dose beyond 60 mg is not needed for any patient.

Prior to intravenous administration, dipyridamole injection should be diluted in at least a 1:2 ratio with 0.45% sodium chloride injection, 0.9% sodium chloride injection, or 5% dextrose injection for a total volume of approximately 20-50 ml. Infusion of undiluted dipyridamole injection may cause local irritation.

Thallium-201 should be injected within 5 minutes following the 4 minute infusion of dipyridamole.

Do not mix dipyridamole injection with other drugs in the same syringe or infusion container.

Parenteral drug products should be inspected visually for particulate matter and discoloration prior to administration, whenever solution and container permit.

PRODUCT LISTING - RATED THERAPEUTICALLY EQUIVALENT

Solution - Intravenous - 5 mg/ml

2 ml x 5	$30.00	GENERIC, Gensia Sicor Pharmaceuticals Inc	00703-1652-02
2 ml x 5	$126.25	PERSANTINE, Dupont Pharmaceuticals	11994-0005-25
2 ml x 5	$148.45	GENERIC, Esi Lederle Generics	00641-1138-34
2 ml x 5	$164.38	PERSANTINE, Dupont Pharmaceuticals	00590-0302-21
2 ml x 5	$164.38	PERSANTINE, Vha Supply	11994-0005-65
2 ml x 10	$29.50	GENERIC, American Pharmaceutical Partners	63323-0613-02
2 ml x 10	$86.30	GENERIC, Abbott Pharmaceutical	00074-2043-02
2 ml x 10	$230.40	GENERIC, Bedford Laboratories	55390-0555-10
10 ml	$115.20	GENERIC, Bedford Laboratories	55390-0555-01
10 ml	$149.90	GENERIC, American Pharmaceutical Partners	63323-0613-10
10 ml x 5	$138.00	GENERIC, Gensia Sicor Pharmaceuticals Inc	00703-1654-02
10 ml x 5	$142.50	GENERIC, Esi Lederle Generics	00641-1139-31
10 ml x 5	$606.00	PERSANTINE, Dupont Pharmaceuticals	11994-0005-05
10 ml x 5	$748.15	GENERIC, Esi Lederle Generics	00641-2569-44
10 ml x 5	$789.00	PERSANTINE, Vha Supply	11994-0005-60
10 ml x 10	$430.23	GENERIC, Abbott Pharmaceutical	00074-2043-10
50 ml	$750.00	PERSANTINE IV, Dupont Pharmaceuticals	00590-0302-54

Tablet - Oral - 25 mg

25's	$4.71	GENERIC, Pd-Rx Pharmaceuticals	55289-0748-97
30's	$4.68	GENERIC, Heartland Healthcare Services	61392-0549-30
30's	$4.69	GENERIC, Heartland Healthcare Services	61392-0549-39
31's	$4.84	GENERIC, Heartland Healthcare Services	61392-0549-31
32's	$5.00	GENERIC, Heartland Healthcare Services	61392-0549-32
45's	$7.03	GENERIC, Heartland Healthcare Services	61392-0549-45

60's	$9.37	GENERIC, Heartland Healthcare Services	61392-0549-60
90's	$14.05	GENERIC, Heartland Healthcare Services	61392-0549-90
100's	$3.75	GENERIC, Interstate Drug Exchange Inc	00814-2605-14
100's	$4.75	GENERIC, Cmc-Consolidated Midland Corporation	00223-0837-01
100's	$4.79	GENERIC, Moore, H.L. Drug Exchange Inc	00839-6327-06
100's	$4.79	GENERIC, Moore, H.L. Drug Exchange Inc	00839-7918-06
100's	$6.27	GENERIC, Purepac Pharmaceutical Company	00228-2193-10
100's	$6.27	GENERIC, Mova Pharmaceutical Corporation	55370-0151-07
100's	$6.28	GENERIC, Aligen Independent Laboratories Inc	00405-5350-01
100's	$6.47	GENERIC, Vangard Labs	00615-1543-01
100's	$6.50	GENERIC, Raway Pharmacal Inc	00686-0068-20
100's	$7.20	GENERIC, Pd-Rx Pharmaceuticals	55289-0748-01
100's	$8.56	GENERIC, Esi Lederle Generics	00005-3743-23
100's	$18.26	GENERIC, Vangard Labs	00615-1543-13
100's	$20.00	GENERIC, Udl Laboratories Inc	51079-0068-20
100's	$22.85	GENERIC, Ivax Corporation	00182-1568-89
100's	$24.22	GENERIC, Auro Pharmaceutical	55829-0235-10
100's	$35.10	GENERIC, Major Pharmaceuticals Inc	00904-1086-60
100's	$39.00	GENERIC, Major Pharmaceuticals Inc	00904-1086-61
100's	$39.26	GENERIC, Barr Laboratories Inc	00555-0252-02
100's	$51.59	PERSANTINE, Physicians Total Care	54868-1288-00
100's	$54.61	PERSANTINE, Boehringer-Ingelheim	00597-0017-01
120's	$18.74	GENERIC, Heartland Healthcare Services	61392-0549-34
Tablet - Oral - 50 mg			
30's	$8.93	GENERIC, Heartland Healthcare Services	61392-0552-30
30's	$8.93	GENERIC, Heartland Healthcare Services	61392-0552-39
31's	$9.22	GENERIC, Heartland Healthcare Services	61392-0552-31
32's	$3.08	GENERIC, Vangard Labs	00615-1573-32
32's	$9.52	GENERIC, Heartland Healthcare Services	61392-0552-32
45's	$13.39	GENERIC, Heartland Healthcare Services	61392-0552-45
60's	$17.85	GENERIC, Heartland Healthcare Services	61392-0552-60
90's	$26.78	GENERIC, Heartland Healthcare Services	61392-0552-90
100's	$7.00	GENERIC, Raway Pharmacal Inc	00686-0069-20
100's	$7.28	GENERIC, Interstate Drug Exchange Inc	00814-2606-14
100's	$7.90	GENERIC, Moore, H.L. Drug Exchange Inc	00839-6494-06
100's	$7.90	GENERIC, Moore, H.L. Drug Exchange Inc	00839-7919-06
100's	$9.68	GENERIC, Pd-Rx Pharmaceuticals	55289-0679-01
100's	$9.92	GENERIC, Vangard Labs	00615-1573-01
100's	$10.34	GENERIC, Purepac Pharmaceutical Company	00228-2183-10
100's	$10.34	GENERIC, Mova Pharmaceutical Corporation	55370-0152-07
100's	$10.38	GENERIC, Aligen Independent Laboratories Inc	00405-5351-01
100's	$11.25	GENERIC, Esi Lederle Generics	00005-3790-23
100's	$16.62	GENERIC, Auro Pharmaceutical	55829-0236-10
100's	$26.00	GENERIC, Geneva Pharmaceuticals	00781-1678-13
100's	$29.75	GENERIC, Udl Laboratories Inc	51079-0069-20
100's	$31.05	GENERIC, Ivax Corporation	00182-1569-89
100's	$56.50	GENERIC, Major Pharmaceuticals Inc	00904-1087-60
100's	$62.95	GENERIC, Barr Laboratories Inc	00555-0285-02
100's	$65.65	GENERIC, Major Pharmaceuticals Inc	00904-1087-61
100's	$87.99	PERSANTINE, Boehringer-Ingelheim	00597-0018-01
200 x 5	$310.23	GENERIC, Vangard Labs	00615-1573-43
Tablet - Oral - 75 mg			
32's	$4.10	GENERIC, Vangard Labs	00615-1574-32
100's	$9.00	GENERIC, Raway Pharmacal Inc	00686-0070-20
100's	$9.75	GENERIC, Interstate Drug Exchange Inc	00814-2607-14
100's	$11.14	GENERIC, Aligen Independent Laboratories Inc	00405-5352-01
100's	$11.19	GENERIC, Moore, H.L. Drug Exchange Inc	00839-6429-06
100's	$11.19	GENERIC, Moore, H.L. Drug Exchange Inc	00839-7920-06
100's	$14.18	GENERIC, Vangard Labs	00615-1574-01
100's	$15.02	GENERIC, Purepac Pharmaceutical Company	00228-2185-10
100's	$15.02	GENERIC, Mova Pharmaceutical Corporation	55370-0154-07
100's	$19.88	GENERIC, Esi Lederle Generics	00005-3791-23
100's	$24.22	GENERIC, Auro Pharmaceutical	55829-0237-10
100's	$63.10	GENERIC, Udl Laboratories Inc	51079-0070-20
100's	$67.18	GENERIC, Ivax Corporation	00182-1570-89
100's	$73.20	GENERIC, Major Pharmaceuticals Inc	00904-1088-60
100's	$83.00	GENERIC, Barr Laboratories Inc	00555-0286-02
100's	$86.33	GENERIC, Major Pharmaceuticals Inc	00904-1088-61
100's	$117.71	PERSANTINE, Boehringer-Ingelheim	00597-0019-01

PRODUCT LISTING - EQUIVALENTS NOT AVAILABLE

Tablet - Oral - 25 mg			
100's	$5.20	GENERIC, Major Pharmaceuticals Inc	00904-1083-60
100's	$8.15	GENERIC, Aligen Independent Laboratories Inc	00405-4350-01
100's	$17.95	GENERIC, Allscripts Pharmaceutical Company	54569-0466-00
Tablet - Oral - 50 mg			
100's	$8.50	GENERIC, Major Pharmaceuticals Inc	00904-1085-60
100's	$10.82	GENERIC, Aligen Independent Laboratories Inc	00405-4351-01
100's	$28.95	GENERIC, Allscripts Pharmaceutical Company	54569-0468-01
Tablet - Oral - 75 mg			
100's	$11.25	GENERIC, Major Pharmaceuticals Inc	00904-1084-60
100's	$18.82	GENERIC, Aligen Independent Laboratories Inc	00405-4352-01
100's	$41.75	GENERIC, Allscripts Pharmaceutical Company	54569-0470-00

Dirithromycin *(003229)*

For complete prescribing information, refer to the CD-ROM included with the book.

For related information, see the comparative table section in Appendix A.

Categories: Bronchitis, chronic, acute exacerbation; Infection, lower respiratory tract; Infection, skin and skin structures; Infection, upper respiratory tract; Pharyngitis; Tonsillitis; FDA Approved 1995 Jun; Pregnancy Category C
Drug Classes: Antibiotics, macrolides
Brand Names: **Dynabac**; Nortron
Foreign Brand Availability: Onzayt (Philippines)
Cost of Therapy: $61.05 (Infection; Dynabac; 250 mg; 2 tablets/day; 7 day supply)

DESCRIPTION

Dynabac contain the semi-synthetic macrolide antibiotic dirithromycin for oral administration. It is a pro-drug which is converted non-enzymatically during intestinal absorption into the microbiologically active moiety erythromycylamine.

Chemically, dirithromycin is designated (9*S*)-9-deoxo-11-deoxy-9,11-[imino[(1R)-2-(2-methoxyethoxy)-ethylidene]oxy] erythromycin and has the molecular formula $C_{42}H_{78}N_2O_{14}$. Its molecular weight is 835.09.

Chemically, erythromycylamine is designated 9-(*S*)-9-amino-9-deoxoerythromycin and has a molecular formula of $C_{37}H_{70}N_2O_{12}$. Its molecular weight is 743.97.

Dirithromycin is a basic compound. The free base is poorly soluble in water and readily soluble in polar organic solvents. Dirithromycin is hydrolyzed to erythromycylamine in acidic aqueous solutions; hydrolysis is virtually complete within 2 hours.

Dynabac tablets are enteric coated to protect the contents from gastric acid and to permit absorption of the antibiotic in the small intestine. Each enteric-coated tablet contains dirithromycin equivalent to 250 mg and the following inactive ingredients: microcrystalline cellulose, croscarmellose sodium, magnesium carbonate, magnesium stearate, sodium starch glycolate, hydroxypropyl cellulose, hydroxypropyl methylcellulose, polyethylene glycol, propylene glycol, benzyl alcohol, methacrylic acid copolymer, titanium dioxide, triethyl citrate, and talc.

INDICATIONS AND USAGE

Dirithromycin is indicated for the treatment of individuals age 12 years and older with mild-to-moderate infections caused by susceptible strains of the designated microorganisms in the specific conditions listed below. **Dirithromycin should not be used in patients with known, suspected, or potential bacteremias as serum levels are inadequate to provide antibacterial coverage of the blood stream.**

ACUTE BACTERIAL EXACERBATIONS OF CHRONIC BRONCHITIS

Due to *Moraxella catarrhalis* or *Streptococcus pneumoniae.*

Note

Because the safety and efficacy of dirithromycin in the treatment of respiratory disease secondary to *H. influenzae* have not been demonstrated, dirithromycin is NOT indicated for the empiric treatment of acute bacterial exacerbations of chronic or secondary bacterial infection of acute bronchitis. Infections known, suspected, or considered potentially to be caused by *Haemophilus* species should be treated by an antibacterial agent indicated for such treatment.

SECONDARY BACTERIAL INFECTION OF ACUTE BRONCHITIS

Due to *Moraxella catarrhalis* or *Streptococcus pneumoniae.* (See Note above.)

COMMUNITY-ACQUIRED PNEUMONIA

Due to *Legionella pneumophila, Mycoplasma pneumoniae* or *Streptococcus pneumoniae.*

PHARYNGITIS/TONSILLITIS

Due to *Streptococcus pyogenes.*

Note

The usual drug of choice in the treatment and prevention of streptococcal infections and the prophylaxis of rheumatic fever is penicillin. Dirithromycin generally is effective in the eradication of *S. pyogenes* from the nasopharynx; however, data establishing the efficacy of dirithromycin in the subsequent prevention of rheumatic fever are not available at present.

UNCOMPLICATED SKIN AND SKIN STRUCTURE INFECTIONS

Due to *Staphylococcus aureus* (methicillin-susceptible strains). (Abscesses usually require surgical drainage.)

Note

Because the safety and efficacy of dirithromycin in the treatment of uncomplicated skin and skin structure infections due to *S. pyogenes* have not been demonstrated, dirithromycin is NOT indicated for the empiric treatment of uncomplicated skin and skin structure infections. Infections known, suspected, or potentially caused by *S. pyogenes* should be treated with an antibacterial agent indicated for such treatment.

CONTRAINDICATIONS

Dirithromycin is contraindicated in patients with known hypersensitivity to dirithromycin, erythromycin, or any other macrolide antibiotic.

WARNINGS

In a prospective study involving 6 healthy male volunteers, dirithromycin did not affect the metabolism of terfenadine. These 6 volunteers received terfenadine alone (60 mg twice daily) for 8 days, followed by terfenadine in combination with dirithromycin (500 mg once daily) for 10 days. (Both drugs were thus dosed to steady state.) The pharmacokinetics of terfenadine and its acid metabolite and the electrocardiographic QTc interval were measured during both periods: with terfenadine alone, and with terfenadine plus dirithromycin. In 5 men, terfenadine levels were undetectable (<5 ng/ml) throughout the study; in 1 man, the C_{max} of terfenadine was 8.1 ng/ml with terfenadine alone and 7.2 ng/ml with terfenadine plus dirithromycin. The mean C_{max}, T_{max} and AUC of the acid metabolite of terfenadine were not significantly changed. The mean QTc interval (milliseconds) was 369 with terfenadine alone and 367 with terfenadine plus dirithromycin.

Serious cardiac dysrhythmias, some resulting in death, have occurred in patients receiving terfenadine concomitantly with other macrolide antibiotics. In addition, most macrolides are contraindicated in patients receiving terfenadine therapy who have pre-existing cardiac abnormalities (arrhythmia, bradycardia, QTc interval prolongation, ischemic heart disease, congestive heart failure, etc.) or electrolyte disturbances. Until further use data are available, it is prudent to monitor the terfenadine levels when dirithromycin and terfenadine are coadministered. (See terfenadine monograph.)

Dirithromycin should not be used in patients with known, suspected, or potential bacteremias as serum levels are inadequate to provide antibacterial coverage of the blood stream.

Pseudomembranous colitis has been reported with nearly all antibacterial agents, including dirithromycin, and may range in severity from mild to life-threatening. Therefore, it is important to consider this diagnosis in patients who present with diarrhea subsequent to the administration of antibacterial agents.

Treatment with antibacterial agents alters the normal flora of the colon and may permit overgrowth of clostridia. Studies indicate that a toxin produced by *Clostridium difficile* is a primary cause of "antibiotic-associated colitis".

After the diagnosis of pseudomembranous colitis has been established, therapeutic measures should be initiated. Mild cases of pseudomembranous colitis usually respond to discontinuation of the drug alone. In moderate-to-severe cases, consideration should be given to management with fluids and electrolytes, protein supplementation, and treatment with an antibacterial drug clinically effective against *C. difficile* colitis.

DOSAGE AND ADMINISTRATION

Dirithromycin should be administered with food or within 1 hour of having eaten. Dirithromycin tablets should not be cut, crushed, or chewed.

TABLE 9 *Recommended Dosage Schedule for Dirithromycin (12 years of age and older)*

Infection (mild to moderate severity)	Dose	Frequency	Duration (days)
Acute bacterial exacerbations of chronic bronchitis due to *Moraxella catarrhalis* or *Streptococcus pneumoniae*	500 mg	q day	7
NOT FOR EMPIRIC THERAPY (See INDICATIONS AND USAGE.)			
Secondary bacterial infection of acute bronchitis due to *M. catarrhalis* or *S. pneumoniae*	500 mg	q day	7
NOT FOR EMPIRIC THERAPY (See INDICATIONS AND USAGE.)			
Community-acquired pneumonia due to *Legionella pneumophila, Mycoplasma pneumoniae* or *S. pneumoniae*	500 mg	q day	14
Pharyngitis/tonsillitis due to *Streptococcus pyogenes*	500 mg	q day	10
Uncomplicated skin and skin structure infections due to *Staphylococcus aureus* (methicillin susceptible)	500 mg	q day	7
NOT FOR EMPIRIC THERAPY (See INDICATIONS AND USAGE.)			

PRODUCT LISTING - EQUIVALENTS NOT AVAILABLE

Tablet, Enteric Coated - Oral - 250 mg

10 x 3	$94.40	DYNABAC, Sanofi Winthrop Pharmaceuticals	00024-0490-10
10 x 3	$130.83	DYNABAC, Muro Pharmaceuticals Inc	00451-0490-10
60's	$261.66	DYNABAC, Muro Pharmaceuticals Inc	00451-0490-60

Disopyramide Phosphate *(001093)*

Categories: Arrhythmia, ventricular; Tachycardia, ventricular; Pregnancy Category C; FDA Approved 1977 Aug
Drug Classes: Antiarrhythmics, class IA
Brand Names: **Norpace**; Norpace CR
Foreign Brand Availability: Dimodan (Mexico); Dirytmin (Belgium; Netherlands; Sweden); Disofarin (Mexico); Durbis (Denmark; Finland; Norway; Sweden; Switzerland); Durbis Retard (Finland; Norway; Sweden); Isorythm (France); Lispine (Japan); Norpace Retard (Czech-Republic; Finland; Hong-Kong; Indonesia; New-Zealand; Philippines; South-Africa); Norpaso (Argentina); Pyramide (New-Zealand); Ritmodan (Italy; Portugal); Ritmoforine (Netherlands); Rythmical (Israel); Rythmodan (Australia; Austria; Bahrain; Belgium; Canada; China; Cyprus; Czech-Republic; Ecuador; Egypt; England; France; Greece; Indonesia; Iran; Iraq; Ireland; Japan; Jordan; Kuwait; Lebanon; Libya; Netherlands; New-Zealand; Oman; Qatar; Republic-of-Yemen; Russia; Saudi-Arabia; South-Africa; Syria; United-Arab-Emirates); Rythmodan Retard (New-Zealand; South-Africa); Rythmodan LA (Canada); Rythmodul (Germany); Rytmilen (Bulgaria; Russia)
Cost of Therapy: $137.77 (Arrhythmia; Norpace; 150 mg; 4 capsules/day; 30 day supply)
$34.54 (Arrhythmia; Generic Capsules; 150 mg; 4 capsules/day; 30 day supply)
$137.70 (Arrhythmia; Norpace CR; 150 mg; 4 capsules/day; 30 day supply)
$135.60 (Arrhythmia; Generic Extended-Release Capsules; 150 mg; 4 capsules/day; 30 day supply)

D

DESCRIPTION

Norpace (disopyramide phosphate) is an antiarrhythmic drug available for oral administration in immediate-release and controlled-release capsules containing 100 or 150 mg of disopyramide base, present as the phosphate. The base content of the phosphate salt is 77.6%.

Disopyramide phosphate is freely soluble in water, and the free base (pKa 10.4) has an aqueous solubility of 1 mg/ml. The chloroform: water partition coefficient of the base is 3.1 at pH 7.2.

Disopyramide phosphate is a racemic mixture of *d*- and *l*-isomers. This drug is not chemically related to other antiarrhythmic drugs.

Norpace CR (controlled-release) capsules are designed to afford a gradual and consistent release of disopyramide. Thus, for maintenance therapy, disopyramide phosphate controlled-release provides the benefit of less-frequent dosing (every 12 hours) as compared with the every 6 hour dosage schedule of immediate-release disopyramide phosphate capsules.

Inactive ingredients of Norpace include corn starch, edible ink, FD&C red no. 3, FD&C yellow no. 6, gelatin, lactose, talc, and titanium dioxide; the 150 mg capsule also contains FD&C blue no. 1.

Inactive ingredients of Norpace CR include corn starch, D&C yellow no. 10, edible ink, ethylcellulose, FD&C blue no. 1, gelatin, shellac, sucrose, talc, and titanium dioxide, the 150 mg capsule also contains FD&C red no. 3 and FD&C yellow no. 6.

CLINICAL PHARMACOLOGY

MECHANISM OF ACTION

Disopyramide phosphate is a Type 1 antiarrhythmic drug (*i.e.*, similar to procainamide and quinidine). *In animal studies* disopyramide phosphate decreases the rate of diastolic depolarization (phase 4) in cells with augmented automaticity, decreases the upstroke velocity (phase 0) and increases the action potential duration of normal cardiac cells, decreases the disparity in refractoriness between infarcted and adjacent normally perfused myocardium, and has no effect on alpha- or beta-adrenergic receptors.

ELECTROPHYSIOLOGY

In man, disopyramide phosphate at therapeutic plasma levels shortens the sinus node recovery time, lengthens the effective refractory period of the atrium, and has a minimal effect on the effective refractory period of the AV node. Little effect has been shown on AV-nodal and His-Purkinje conduction times or QRS duration. However, prolongation of conduction in accessory pathways occurs.

HEMODYNAMICS

At recommended oral doses, disopyramide phosphate rarely produces significant alterations of blood pressure in patients without congestive heart failure (see WARNINGS). With intravenous disopyramide phosphate, either increases in systolic/diastolic or decreases in systolic blood pressure have been reported, depending on the infusion rate and the patient population. Intravenous disopyramide phosphate may cause cardiac depression with an approximate mean 10% reduction of cardiac output, which is more pronounced in patients with cardiac dysfunction.

ANTICHOLINERGIC ACTIVITY

The *in vitro* anticholinergic activity of disopyramide phosphate is approximately 0.06% that of atropine; however, the usual dose for disopyramide phosphate is 150 mg every 6 hours and for disopyramide phosphate controlled-release 300 mg every 12 hours, compared to 0.4-0.6 mg for atropine (see WARNINGS, Anticholinergic Activity and ADVERSE REACTIONS, Anticholinergic for anticholinergic side effects).

PHARMACOKINETICS

Following oral administration of immediate-release disopyramide phosphate, it is rapidly and almost completely absorbed, and peak plasma levels are usually attained within 2 hours. The usual therapeutic plasma levels of disopyramide base are 2-4 μg/ml, and at these concentrations protein binding varies from 50-65%. Because of concentration-dependent protein binding, it is difficult to predict the concentration of the free drug when total drug is measured.

The mean plasma half-life of disopyramide in healthy humans is 6.7 hours (range of 4-10 hours). In 6 patients with impaired renal function (creatinine clearance less than 40 ml/min), disopyramide half-life values were 8-18 hours.

After the oral administration of 200 mg of disopyramide to 10 cardiac patients with borderline to moderate heart failure, the time to peak serum concentration of 2.3 ± 1.5 hours (mean ±SD) was increased, and the mean peak serum concentration of 4.8 ± 1.6 μg/ml was higher than in healthy volunteers. After intravenous administration in these same patients, the mean elimination half-life was 9.7 ± 4.2 hours (range in healthy volunteers of 4.4-7.8 hours). In a second study of the oral administration of disopyramide to 7 patients with heart disease, including left ventricular dysfunction, the mean plasma half-life was slightly prolonged to 7.8 ± 1.9 hours (range of 5 to 9.5 hours).

In healthy men, about 50% of a given dose of disopyramide is excreted in the urine as the unchanged drug, about 20% as the mono-N-dealkylated metabolite, and 10% as the other metabolites. The plasma concentration of the major metabolite is approximately one-tenth that of disopyramide. Altering the urinary pH in man does not affect the plasma half-life of disopyramide.

In a crossover study in healthy subjects, the bioavailability of disopyramide from disopyramide phosphate controlled-release capsules was similar to that from the immediate-release capsules. With a single 300 mg oral dose, peak disopyramide plasma concentrations of 3.23 ± 0.75 μg/ml (mean ±SD) at 2.5 ± 2.3 hours were obtained with two 150 mg immediate-release capsules and 2.22 ± 0.47 μg/ml at 4.9 ± 1.4 hours with two 150 mg disopyramide phosphate controlled-release capsules. The elimination half-life of disopyramide was 8.31 ± 1.83 hours with the immediate-release capsules and 11.65 ± 4.72 hours with disopyramide phosphate controlled-release capsules. The amount of disopyramide and mono-N-dealkylated metabolite excreted in the urine in 48 hours was 128 and 48 mg, respectively, with the immediate-release capsules, and 112 and 33 mg, respectively, with disopyramide phosphate controlled-release capsules. The differences in the urinary excretion of either constituent were not statistically significant.

Following multiple doses, steady-state plasma levels of between 2 and 4 μg/ml were attained following either 150 mg every 6 hour dosing with immediate-release capsules or 300 mg every 12 hour dosing with disopyramide phosphate controlled-release capsules.

DRUG INTERACTIONS

Effects of Other Drugs On Disopyramide Pharmacokinetics

In vitro metabolic studies indicated that disopyramide is metabolized by cytochrome P450 3A4 and that inhibitors of this enzyme may result in elevation of plasma levels of disopyramide. Although specific drug interaction studies have not been done, cases of life-threatening interactions have been reported for disopyramide when given with clarithromycin and erythromycin.

INDICATIONS AND USAGE

Disopyramide phosphate and disopyramide phosphate controlled-release are indicated for the treatment of documented ventricular arrhythmias, such as sustained ventricular tachycardia, that, in the judgment of the physician, are life-threatening. Because of the proarrhythmic effects of disopyramide phosphate and disopyramide phosphate controlled-release, their use with lesser arrhythmias is generally not recommended. Treatment of patients with asymptomatic ventricular premature contractions should be avoided.

Initiation of disopyramide phosphate or disopyramide phosphate controlled-release treatment, as with other antiarrhythmic agents used to treat life-threatening arrhythmias, should be carried out in the hospital. Disopyramide phosphate controlled-release should not be used initially if rapid establishment of disopyramide plasma levels is desired.

Antiarrhythmic drugs have not been shown to enhance survival in patients with ventricular arrhythmias.

NON-FDA APPROVED INDICATIONS

Although not FDA approved, disopyramide is used for the treatment of paroxysmal supraventricular tachycardia, or SVT (including paroxysmal SVT associated with the Wolff-Parkinson-White syndrome), hypertrophic obstructive cardiomyopathy (reducing subaortic pressure gradient and improving clinical symptoms), and neuromediated (vasodepressor) syncope.

CONTRAINDICATIONS

Disopyramide phosphate and disopyramide phosphate controlled-release are contraindicated in the presence of cardiogenic shock, preexisting second- or third-degree AV block (if no pacemaker is present), congenital Q-T prolongation, or known hypersensitivity to the drug.

WARNINGS

Mortality

In the National Heart, Lung and Blood Institute's Cardiac Arrhythmia Suppression Trial (CAST), a long-term, multi-center, randomized, double-blind study in patients with asymptomatic non-life-threatening ventricular arrhythmias who had had a myocardial infarction more than 6 days but less than 2 years previously, an excessive mortality or non-fatal cardiac arrest rate (7.7%) was seen in patients treated with encainide or flecainide compared with that seen in patients assigned to carefully matched placebo-treated groups (3.0%). The average duration of treatment with encainide or flecainide in this study was 10 months.

The applicability of the CAST results to other populations (*e.g.,* those without recent myocardial infarctions) is uncertain. Considering the known proarrhythmic properties of disopyramide phosphate or disopyramide phosphate controlled-release and the lack of evidence of improved survival for any antiarrhythmic drug in patients without life-threatening arrhythmias, the use of disopyramide phosphate or disopyramide phosphate controlled-release as well as other antiarrhythmic agents should be reserved for patients with life-threatening ventricular arrhythmias.

NEGATIVE INOTROPIC PROPERTIES

Heart Failure/Hypotension

Disopyramide phosphate or disopyramide phosphate controlled-release may cause or worsen congestive heart failure or produce severe hypotension as a consequence of its negative inotropic properties. Hypotension has been observed primarily in patients with primary cardiomyopathy or inadequately compensated congestive heart failure. Disopyramide phosphate or disopyramide phosphate controlled-release should not be used in patients with uncompensated or marginally compensated congestive heart failure or hypotension unless the congestive heart failure or hypotension is secondary to cardiac arrhythmia. Patients with a history of heart failure may be treated with disopyramide phosphate or disopyramide phosphate controlled-release, but careful attention must be given to the maintenance of cardiac function, including optimal digitalization. If hypotension occurs or congestive heart failure worsens, disopyramide phosphate or disopyramide phosphate controlled-release should be discontinued and, if necessary, restarted at a lower dosage only after adequate cardiac compensation has been established.

QRS Widening

Although it is unusual, significant widening (greater than 25%) of the QRS complex may occur during disopyramide phosphate or disopyramide phosphate controlled-release administration; in such cases disopyramide phosphate or disopyramide phosphate controlled-release should be discontinued.

Q-T Prolongation

As with other Type 1 antiarrhythmic drugs, prolongation of the Q-T interval (corrected) and worsening of the arrhythmia, including ventricular tachycardia and ventricular fibrillation, may occur. Patients who have evidenced prolongation of the Q-T interval in response to quinidine may be at particular risk. As with other Type 1A antiarrhythmics, disopyramide phosphate has been associated with torsade de pointes.

If a Q-T prolongation of greater than 25% is observed and if ectopy continues, the patient should be monitored closely, and consideration be given to discontinuing disopyramide phosphate or disopyramide phosphate controlled-release.

Hypoglycemia

In rare instances significant lowering of blood glucose values has been reported during disopyramide phosphate administration. The physician should be alert to this possibility, especially in patients with congestive heart failure, chronic malnutrition, hepatic, renal or other diseases, or drugs (*e.g.,* beta adrenoceptor blockers, alcohol) which could compromise preservation of the normal glucoregulatory mechanisms in the absence of food. In these patients the blood glucose levels should be carefully followed.

CONCOMITANT ANTIARRHYTHMIC THERAPY

The concomitant use of disopyramide phosphate or disopyramide phosphate controlled-release with other Type 1A antiarrhythmic agents (such as quinidine or procainamide), Type 1C antiarrhythmics (such as encainide, flecainide or propafenone), and/or propranolol should be reserved for patients with life-threatening arrhythmias who are demonstratably unresponsive to single-agent antiarrhythmic therapy. Such use may produce serious negative inotropic effects, or may excessively prolong conduction. This should be considered particularly in patients with any degree of cardiac decompensation or those with a prior history thereof. Patients receiving more than one antiarrhythmic drug must be carefully monitored.

HEART BLOCK

If first-degree heart block develops in a patient receiving disopyramide phosphate or disopyramide phosphate controlled-release, the dosage should be reduced. If the block persists despite reduction of dosage, continuation of the drug must depend upon weighing the benefit being obtained against the risk of higher degrees of heart block. Development of second- or third-degree AV block or unifascicular, bifascicular, or trifascicular block requires discontinuation of disopyramide phosphate or disopyramide phosphate controlled-release therapy, unless the ventricular rate is adequately controlled by a temporary or implanted ventricular pacemaker.

ANTICHOLINERGIC ACTIVITY

Because of its anticholinergic activity, disopyramide phosphate should not be used in patients with glaucoma, myasthenia gravis, or urinary retention unless adequate overriding measures are taken; these consist of the topical application of potent miotics (*e.g.,* pilocarpine) for patients with glaucoma, and catheter drainage or operative relief for patients with urinary retention. Urinary retention may occur in patients of either sex as a consequence of disopyramide phosphate or disopyramide phosphate controlled-release administration, but males with benign prostatic hypertrophy are at particular risk. In patients with a family history of glaucoma, intraocular pressure should be measured before initiating disopyramide phosphate or disopyramide phosphate controlled-release therapy. Disopyramide phosphate should be used with special care in patients with myasthenia gravis since its anticholinergic properties could precipitate a myasthenic crisis in such patients.

PRECAUTIONS

GENERAL

Atrial Tachyarrhythmias

Patients with atrial flutter or fibrillation should be digitalized prior to disopyramide phosphate or disopyramide phosphate controlled-release administration to ensure that drug-induced enhancement of AV conduction does not result in an increase of ventricular rate beyond physiologically acceptable limits.

Conduction Abnormalities

Care should be taken when prescribing disopyramide phosphate or disopyramide phosphate controlled-release for patients with sick sinus syndrome (bradycardia-tachycardia syndrome), Wolff-Parkinson-White syndrome (WPW), or bundle branch block. The effect of disopyramide phosphate in these conditions is uncertain at present.

Cardiomyopathy

Patients with myocarditis or other cardiomyopathy may develop significant hypotension in response to the usual dosage of disopyramide phosphate, probably due to cardiodepressant mechanisms. Therefore, a loading dose of disopyramide phosphate should not be given to such patients, and initial dosage and subsequent dosage adjustments should be made under close supervision (see DOSAGE AND ADMINISTRATION).

Renal Impairment

More than 50% of disopyramide is excreted in the urine unchanged. Therefore disopyramide phosphate dosage should be reduced in patients with impaired renal function (see DOSAGE AND ADMINISTRATION). The electrocardiogram should be carefully monitored for prolongation of PR interval, evidence of QRS widening, or other signs of overdosage.

Disopyramide phosphate controlled-release is not recommended for patients with severe renal insufficiency (creatinine clearance 40 ml/min or less).

Hepatic Impairment

Hepatic impairment also causes an increase in the plasma half-life of disopyramide. Dosage should be reduced for patients with such impairment. The electrocardiogram should be carefully monitored for signs of overdosage.

Patients with cardiac dysfunction have a higher potential for hepatic impairment; this should be considered when administering disopyramide phosphate or disopyramide phosphate controlled-release.

Potassium Imbalance

Antiarrhythmic drugs may be ineffective in patients with hypokalemia, and their toxic effects may be enhanced in patients with hyperkalemia. Therefore, potassium abnormalities should be corrected before starting disopyramide phosphate or disopyramide phosphate controlled-release therapy.

CARCINOGENESIS, MUTAGENESIS, AND IMPAIRMENT OF FERTILITY

Eighteen (18) months of disopyramide phosphate administration to rats, at oral doses up to 400 mg/kg/day (about 30 times the usual daily human dose of 600 mg/day, assuming a patient weight of at least 50 kg), revealed no evidence of carcinogenic potential. An evaluation of mutagenic potential by Ames test was negative. Disopyramide phosphate, at doses up to 250 mg/kg/day, did not adversely affect fertility of rats.

PREGNANCY, TERATOGENIC EFFECTS, PREGNANCY CATEGORY C

Disopyramide phosphate was associated with decreased numbers of implantation sites and decreased growth and survival of pups when administered to pregnant rats at 250 mg/kg/day (20 or more times the usual daily human dose of 12 mg/kg, assuming a patient weight of at least 50 kg), a level at which weight gain and food consumption of dams were also reduced. Increased resorption rates were reported in rabbits at 60 mg/kg/day (5 or more times the usual daily human dose). Effects on implantation, pup growth, and survival were not evaluated in rabbits. There are no adequate and well-controlled studies in pregnant women. Disopyramide phosphate or disopyramide phosphate controlled-release should be used during pregnancy only if the potential benefit justifies the potential risk to the fetus.

Nonteratogenic Effects: Disopyramide phosphate has been reported to stimulate contractions of the pregnant uterus. Disopyramide has been found in human fetal blood.

LABOR AND DELIVERY

It is not known whether the use of disopyramide phosphate or disopyramide phosphate controlled-release during labor or delivery has immediate or delayed adverse effects on the fetus, or whether it prolongs the duration of labor or increases the need for forceps delivery or other obstetric intervention.

NURSING MOTHERS

Studies in rats have shown that the concentration of disopyramide and its metabolites is between 1 and 3 times greater in milk than it is in plasma. Following oral administration, disopyramide has been detected in human milk at a concentration not exceeding that in plasma. Because of the potential for serious adverse reactions in nursing infants from disopyramide phosphate or disopyramide phosphate controlled-release, a decision should be made whether to discontinue nursing or to discontinue the drug, taking into account the importance of the drug to the mother.

PEDIATRIC USE

Safety and effectiveness in pediatric patients have not been established (see DOSAGE AND ADMINISTRATION).

GERIATRIC USE

Clinical studies of disopyramide phosphate/disopyramide phosphate controlled-release did not include sufficient numbers of subjects aged 65 and over to determine whether they respond differently from younger subjects. Other reported clinical experience has not identified differences in responses between the elderly and younger patients. In general, dose selection for an elderly patient should be cautious, usually starting at the low end of the dosing range, reflecting the greater frequency of decreased hepatic, renal, or cardiac function, and of concomitant disease or other drug therapy. Because of its anticholinergic activity, disopyramide phosphate should not be used in patients with glaucoma, urinary retention, or benign prostatic hypertrophy (medical conditions commonly associated with the elderly) unless adequate overriding measures are taken (see WARNINGS, Anticholinergic Activity). In the event of increased anticholinergic side effects, plasma levels of disopyramide should be monitored and the dose of the drug adjusted accordingly. A reduction of the dose by one-third, from the recommended 600-400 mg/day, would be reasonable, without changing the dosing interval. This drug is known to be substantially excreted by the kidney, and the risk of toxic reactions to this drug may be greater in patients with impaired renal function. Because elderly patients are more likely to have decreased renal function, care should be taken in dose selection, and it may be useful to monitor renal function (see Renal Impairment and DOSAGE AND ADMINISTRATION).

DRUG INTERACTIONS

If phenytoin or other hepatic enzyme inducers are taken concurrently with disopyramide phosphate or disopyramide phosphate controlled-release, lower plasma levels of disopyramide may occur. Monitoring of disopyramide plasma levels is recommended in such concurrent use to avoid ineffective therapy. Other antiarrhythmic drugs (*e.g.,* quinidine, procainamide, lidocaine, propranolol) have occasionally been used concurrently with disopyramide phosphate. Excessive widening of the QRS complex and/or prolongation of the Q-T interval may occur in these situations (see WARNINGS). In healthy subjects, no significant drug-drug interaction was observed when disopyramide phosphate was coadministered with either propranolol or diazepam. Concomitant administration of disopyramide phosphate and quinidine resulted in slight increases in plasma disopyramide levels and slight decreases in plasma quinidine levels. Disopyramide phosphate does not increase serum digoxin levels.

Until data on possible interactions between verapamil and disopyramide phosphate are obtained, disopyramide should not be administered within 48 hours before or 24 hours after verapamil administration.

Although potent inhibitors of cytochrome P450 3A4 (*e.g.,* ketoconazole) have not been studied clinically, *in vitro* studies have shown that erythromycin and oleandomycin inhibit the metabolism of disopyramide. Cases of life-threatening interactions have been reported for disopyramide when given with clarithromycin and erythromycin indicating that coadministration of disopyramide with inhibitors of cytochrome P450 3A4 could result in potentially fatal interaction.

ADVERSE REACTIONS

The adverse reactions which were reported in disopyramide phosphate clinical trials encompass observations in 1500 patients, including 90 patients studied for at least 4 years. The most serious adverse reactions are hypotension and congestive heart failure. The most common adverse reactions, which are dose dependent, are associated with the anticholinergic properties of the drug. These may be transitory, but may be persistent or can be severe. Urinary retention is the most serious anticholinergic effect.

The following reactions were reported in 10-40% of patients:

Anticholinergic: Dry mouth (32%), urinary hesitancy (14%), constipation (11%).

The following reactions were reported in 3-9% of patients:

Anticholinergic: Blurred vision, dry nose/eyes/throat.

Genitourinary: Urinary retention, urinary frequency and urgency.

Gastrointestinal: Nausea, pain/bloating/gas.

General: Dizziness, general fatigue/muscle weakness, headache, malaise, aches/pains.

The following reactions were reported in 1-3% of patients:

Genitourinary: Impotence.

Cardiovascular: Hypotension with or without congestive heart failure, increased congestive heart failure (see WARNINGS), cardiac conduction disturbances (see WARNINGS), edema/weight gain, shortness of breath, syncope, chest pain.

Gastrointestinal: Anorexia, diarrhea, vomiting.

Dermatologic: Generalized rash/dermatoses, itching.

Central Nervous System: Nervousness.

Other: Hypokalemia, elevated cholesterol/triglycerides.

The following reactions were reported in less than 1%: Depression, insomnia, dysuria, numbness/tingling, elevated liver enzymes, AV block, elevated BUN, elevated creatinine, decreased hemoglobin/hematocrit.

Hypoglycemia has been reported in association with disopyramide phosphate administration (see WARNINGS).

Infrequent occurrences of reversible cholestatic jaundice, fever, and respiratory difficulty have been reported in association with disopyramide therapy, as have rare instances of thrombocytopenia, reversible agranulocytosis, and gynecomastia. Some cases of LE (lupus erythematosus) symptoms have been reported; most cases occurred in patients who had been switched to disopyramide from procainamide following the development of LE symptoms. Rarely, acute psychosis has been reported following disopyramide phosphate therapy, with prompt return to normal mental status when therapy was stopped. The physician should be aware of these possible reactions and should discontinue disopyramide phosphate or disopyramide phosphate controlled-release therapy promptly if they occur.

DOSAGE AND ADMINISTRATION

The dosage of disopyramide phosphate or disopyramide phosphate controlled-release must be individualized for each patient on the basis of response and tolerance. The usual adult dosage of disopyramide phosphate or disopyramide phosphate controlled-release is 400-800 mg/day given in divided doses. The recommended dosage for most adults is 600 mg/day given in divided doses (either 150 mg every 6 hours for immediate-release disopyramide phosphate or 300 mg every 12 hours for disopyramide phosphate controlled-release). For patients whose body weight is less than 110 pounds (50 kg), the recommended dosage is 400 mg/day given in divided doses (either 100 mg every 6 hours for immediate-release disopyramide phosphate or 200 mg every 12 hours for disopyramide phosphate controlled-release). In the event of increased anticholinergic side effects, plasma levels of disopyramide should be monitored and the dose of the drug adjusted accordingly. A reduction of the dose by one-third, from the recommended 600-400 mg/day, would be reasonable, without changing the dosing interval.

For patients with cardiomyopathy or possible cardiac decompensation, a loading dose, as discussed below, should not be given, and initial dosage should be limited to 100 mg of immediate-release disopyramide phosphate every 6-8 hours. Subsequent dosage adjustments should be made gradually, with close monitoring for the possible development of hypotension and/or congestive heart failure (see WARNINGS).

For patients with moderate renal insufficiency (creatinine clearance greater than 40 ml/min) or hepatic insufficiency, the recommended dosage is 400 mg/day given in divided doses (either 100 mg every 6 hours for immediate-release disopyramide phosphate or 200 mg every 12 hours for disopyramide phosphate controlled-release).

For patients with severe renal insufficiency (C_{cr} 40 ml/min or less), the recommended dosage regimen of immediate-release disopyramide phosphate is 100 mg at intervals shown in TABLE 1, with or without an initial loading dose of 150 mg.

For patients in whom rapid control of ventricular arrhythmia is essential, an initial loading dose of 300 mg of immediate-release disopyramide phosphate (200 mg for patients whose body weight is less than 110 pounds) is recommended, followed by the appropriate maintenance dosage. Therapeutic effects are usually attained 30 minutes to 3 hours after administration of a 300 mg loading dose. If there is no response or evidence of toxicity within 6 hours of the loading dose, 200 mg of immediate-release disopyramide phosphate every 6 hours may be prescribed instead of the usual 150 mg. If there is no response to this dosage within 48 hours, either disopyramide phosphate should then be discontinued or the physician should consider hospitalizing the patient for careful monitoring while subsequent

TABLE 1 *Immediate-Release Disopyramide Phosphate Dosage Interval for Patients with Renal Insufficiency**

Creatinine Clearance (ml/min)	40-30	30-15	<15
Approximate maintenance-dosing interval	q8h	q12h	q24h

* Dosing schedules are for disopyramide phosphate immediate-release capsules; disopyramide phosphate controlled-release is not recommended for patients with severe renal insufficiency.

immediate-release disopyramide phosphate doses of 250 or 300 mg every 6 hours are given. A limited number of patients with severe refractory ventricular tachycardia have tolerated daily doses of disopyramide phosphate up to 1600 mg/day (400 mg every 6 hours), resulting in disopyramide plasma levels up to 9 µg/ml. If such treatment is warranted, it is essential that patients be hospitalized for close evaluation and continuous monitoring.

Disopyramide phosphate should not be used initially if rapid establishment of disopyramide plasma levels is desired.

TRANSFERRING TO DISOPYRAMIDE PHOSPHATE OR DISOPYRAMIDE PHOSPHATE CONTROLLED-RELEASE

The following dosage schedule based on theoretical considerations rather than experimental data is suggested for transferring patients with normal renal function from either quinidine sulfate or procainamide therapy (Type 1 antiarrhythmic agents) to disopyramide phosphate or disopyramide phosphate controlled-release therapy:

Disopyramide phosphate or disopyramide phosphate controlled-release should be started using the regular maintenance schedule **without a loading dose** 6-12 hours after the last dose of quinidine sulfate or 3-6 hours after the last dose of procainamide.

In patients in whom withdrawal of quinidine sulfate or procainamide is likely to produce life-threatening arrhythmias, the physician should consider hospitalization of the patient. When transferring a patient from immediate-release disopyramide phosphate to disopyramide phosphate controlled-release, the maintenance schedule of disopyramide phosphate controlled-release may be started 6 hours after the last dose of immediate-release disopyramide phosphate.

PEDIATRIC DOSAGE

Controlled clinical studies have not been conducted in pediatric patients; however, the suggested dosage table (TABLE 2) is based on published clinical experience.

Total daily dosage should be divided and equal doses administered orally every 6 hours or at intervals according to individual patient needs. Disopyramide plasma levels and therapeutic response must be monitored closely. Patients should be hospitalized during the initial treatment period, and dose titration should start at the lower end of the ranges provided in TABLE 2.

TABLE 2 *Suggested Total Daily Dosage**

Age (years)	Disopyramide (mg/kg body weight/day)
Under 1	10-30
1-4	10-20
4-12	10-15
12-18	6-15

* Dosage is expressed in milligrams (mg) of disopyramide base. Since disopyramide phosphate 100 mg capsules contain 100 mg of disopyramide base, the pharmacist can readily prepare a 1-10 mg/ml liquid suspension by adding the entire contents of disopyramide phosphate capsules to cherry syrup. (Prepare cherry syrup as follows: cherry juice, 475 ml; sucrose 800 g; alcohol 20 ml; purified water, sufficient quantity to make 1000 ml). The resulting suspension, when refrigerated, is stable for 1 month and should be thoroughly shaken before the measurement of each dose. The suspension should be dispensed in an amber glass bottle with a child-resistant closure.

Disopyramide phosphate controlled-release capsules should not be used to prepare the above suspension.

HOW SUPPLIED

NORPACE

Norpace is supplied in hard gelatin capsules containing either 100 o 150 mg of disopyramide base, present as the phosphate.

100 mg Capsules: White and orange, with markings "SEARLE", "2752", "NORPACE", and "100 MG".

150 mg Capsules: Brown and orange, with markings "SEARLE", "2762", "NORPACE", and "150 MG".

Storage: Store at 25°C (77°F); excursions permitted to 15-30°C (59-86°F).

NORPACE CR

Norpace CR Controlled-Release is supplied as specially prepared controlled-release beads in hard gelatin capsules containing either 100 o 150 mg of disopyramide base, present as the phosphate.

100 mg Capsules: White and light green, with markings "SEARLE", "2732", "NORPACE CR", and "100 mg".

150 mg Capsules: Brown and light green, with markings "SEARLE", "2742", "NORPACE CR", and "150 mg".

Storage: Store at 25°C (77°F); excursions permitted to 15-30°C (59-86°F).

PRODUCT LISTING - RATED THERAPEUTICALLY EQUIVALENT

Capsule - Oral - 100 mg

100's	$12.38	GENERIC, Us Trading Corporation	56126-0330-11
100's	$17.40	GENERIC, Interstate Drug Exchange Inc	00814-2614-14
100's	$17.81	GENERIC, Vangard Labs	00615-0392-13
100's	$19.00	GENERIC, Raway Pharmacal Inc	00686-0296-20
100's	$22.30	GENERIC, Aligen Independent Laboratories Inc	00405-4357-01
100's	$22.88	GENERIC, Moore, H.L. Drug Exchange Inc	00839-7091-06
100's	$22.89	GENERIC, Caremark Inc	00339-5681-12
100's	$23.95	GENERIC, Major Pharmaceuticals Inc	00904-2482-60
100's	$24.09	GENERIC, Qualitest Products Inc	00603-3408-21
100's	$28.05	GENERIC, Major Pharmaceuticals Inc	00904-2482-61
100's	$34.60	GENERIC, Auro Pharmaceutical	55829-0631-10
100's	$36.20	GENERIC, Geneva Pharmaceuticals	00781-2110-13
100's	$57.84	GENERIC, Watson/Schein Pharmaceuticals Inc	00364-0739-01
100's	$64.27	GENERIC, Watson/Schein Pharmaceuticals Inc	00364-0739-90
100's	$69.41	GENERIC, Teva Pharmaceuticals Usa	00093-3127-01
100's	$69.41	GENERIC, Watson/Schein Pharmaceuticals Inc	00591-5560-01
100's	$97.23	NORPACE, Searle	00025-2752-31

Capsule - Oral - 150 mg

100's	$19.43	GENERIC, Interstate Drug Exchange Inc	00814-2615-14
100's	$21.00	GENERIC, Raway Pharmacal Inc	00686-0297-20
100's	$23.90	GENERIC, Vangard Labs	00615-0393-13
100's	$26.35	GENERIC, Aligen Independent Laboratories Inc	00405-4358-01
100's	$27.48	GENERIC, Caremark Inc	00339-5683-12
100's	$27.66	GENERIC, Moore, H.L. Drug Exchange Inc	00839-7092-06
100's	$28.00	GENERIC, Major Pharmaceuticals Inc	00904-2483-60
100's	$28.50	GENERIC, Ivax Corporation	00182-1744-01
100's	$28.78	GENERIC, Qualitest Products Inc	00603-3409-21
100's	$32.93	GENERIC, Major Pharmaceuticals Inc	00904-2483-61
100's	$40.44	GENERIC, Auro Pharmaceutical	55829-0632-10
100's	$42.45	GENERIC, Geneva Pharmaceuticals	00781-2115-13
100's	$66.30	GENERIC, Major Pharmaceuticals Inc	00904-2489-60
100's	$68.32	GENERIC, Watson/Schein Pharmaceuticals Inc	00364-0740-01
100's	$75.91	GENERIC, Watson/Schein Pharmaceuticals Inc	00364-0740-90
100's	$81.98	GENERIC, Teva Pharmaceuticals Usa	00093-3129-01
100's	$81.98	GENERIC, Watson/Schein Pharmaceuticals Inc	00591-5561-01
100's	$114.81	NORPACE, Searle	00025-2762-31

Capsule, Extended Release - Oral - 100 mg

100's	$57.56	GENERIC, Caremark Inc	00339-5845-12
100's	$57.56	GENERIC, Ethex Corporation	58177-0003-04
100's	$85.93	NORPACE CR, Searle	00025-2732-34
100's	$117.08	NORPACE CR, Searle	00025-2732-31

Capsule, Extended Release - Oral - 150 mg

100's	$113.00	GENERIC, Ethex Corporation	58177-0002-04
100's	$114.75	NORPACE CR, Physicians Total Care	54868-0692-00
100's	$116.47	NORPACE CR, Searle	00025-2742-34
100's	$138.39	NORPACE CR, Searle	00025-2742-31

PRODUCT LISTING - EQUIVALENTS NOT AVAILABLE

Capsule - Oral - 100 mg

100's	$13.50	GENERIC, Cmc-Consolidated Midland Corporation	00223-0842-01

Divalproex Sodium *(001096)*

Categories: Bipolar affective disorder; Headache, migraine, prophylaxis; Mania; Seizures, absence; Seizures, complex partial; Pregnancy Category D; FDA Approved 1983 Mar

Drug Classes: Anticonvulsants

Brand Names: **Depakote**; Depakote Sprinkle

Foreign Brand Availability: Epival (Canada); Valcote (Colombia; Peru)

Cost of Therapy: $62.55 (Migraine; Depakote Delayed-Release; 250 mg; 2 tablets/day; 30 day supply)
$93.83 (Mania; Depakote Delayed-Release; 250 mg; 3 tablets/day; 30 day supply)
$116.96 (Epilepsy; Depakote ER; 500 mg; 2 tablets/day; 30 day supply)

WARNING

HEPATIC FAILURE RESULTING IN FATALITIES HAS OCCURRED IN PATIENTS RECEIVING VALPROIC ACID AND ITS DERIVATIVES. EXPERIENCE HAS INDICATED THAT CHILDREN UNDER THE AGE OF TWO YEARS ARE AT A CONSIDERABLY INCREASED RISK OF DEVELOPING FATAL HEPATOTOXICITY, ESPECIALLY THOSE ON MULTIPLE ANTICONVULSANTS, THOSE WITH CONGENITAL METABOLIC DISORDERS, THOSE WITH SEVERE SEIZURE DISORDERS ACCOMPANIED BY MENTAL RETARDATION, AND THOSE WITH ORGANIC BRAIN DISEASE. WHEN DIVALPROEX SODIUM IS USED IN THIS PATIENT GROUP, IT SHOULD BE USED WITH EXTREME CAUTION AND AS A SOLE AGENT. THE BENEFITS OF THERAPY SHOULD BE WEIGHED AGAINST THE RISKS. ABOVE THIS AGE GROUP, EXPERIENCE IN EPILEPSY HAS INDICATED THAT THE INCIDENCE OF FATAL HEPATOTOXICITY DECREASES CONSIDERABLY IN PROGRESSIVELY OLDER PATIENT GROUPS.

THESE INCIDENTS USUALLY HAVE OCCURRED DURING THE FIRST SIX MONTHS OF TREATMENT. SERIOUS OR FATAL HEPATOTOXICITY MAY BE PRECEDED BY NON-SPECIFIC SYMPTOMS SUCH AS MALAISE, WEAKNESS, LETHARGY, FACIAL EDEMA, ANOREXIA, AND VOMITING. IN PATIENTS WITH EPILEPSY, A LOSS OF SEIZURE CONTROL MAY ALSO OCCUR. PATIENTS SHOULD BE MONITORED CLOSELY FOR APPEARANCE OF THESE SYMPTOMS. LIVER FUNCTION TESTS SHOULD BE PERFORMED

WARNING — Cont'd

PRIOR TO THERAPY AND AT FREQUENT INTERVALS THEREAFTER, ESPECIALLY DURING THE FIRST SIX MONTHS.

TERATOGENICITY: VALPROATE CAN PRODUCE TERATOGENIC EFFECTS SUCH AS NEURAL TUBE DEFECTS (*e.g.*, SPINA BIFIDA), ACCORDINGLY, THE USE OF DIVALPROEX SODIUM IN WOMEN OF CHILDBEARING POTENTIAL REQUIRES THAT THE BENEFITS OF ITS USE BE WEIGHED AGAINST THE RISK OF INJURY TO THE FETUS. THIS IS ESPECIALLY IMPORTANT WHEN THE TREATMENT OF A SPONTANEOUSLY REVERSIBLE CONDITION NOT ORDINARILY ASSOCIATED WITH PERMANENT INJURY OR RISK OF DEATH (*e.g.*, MIGRAINE) IS CONTEMPLATED. (SEE WARNINGS and PRECAUTIONS, Information for the Patient.)

DESCRIPTION

Divalproex sodium is a stable co-ordination compound comprised of sodium valproate and valproic acid in a 1:1 molar relationship and formed during the partial neutralization of valproic acid with 0.5 equivalent of sodium hydroxide. Chemically it is designated as sodium hydrogen bis (2-propylpentanoate).

Divalproex sodium occurs as a white powder with a characteristic odor.

Depakote tablets and Sprinkle capsules are antiepileptics for oral administration.

Depakote Sprinkle Capsules: Depakote sprinkle capsules contain specially coated particles of divalproex sodium equivalent to 125 mg of valproic acid in a hard gelatin capsule. *Inactive Ingredients:* Cellulosic polymers, D&C red no. 28, FD&C blue no. 1, gelatin, iron oxide, magnesium stearate, silica gel, titanium dioxide and triethyl citrate.

Depakote Tablets: Depakote tablets are supplied in three dosage strengths containing divalproex sodium equivalent to 125 mg, 250 mg, or 500 mg of valproic acid. *Inactive Ingredients:* Cellulosic polymers, diacetylated monoglycerides, povidone, pregelatinized starch (contains corn starch), silica gel, talc, titanium dioxide and vanillin.

In Addition, Individual Tablets Contain: *125 mg Tablets:* FD&C blue no. 1 and FD&C red no. 40. *250 mg Tablets:* FD&C yellow no. 6 and iron oxide. *500 mg Tablets:* D&C red no. 30, FD&C blue no. 2, and iron oxide.

CLINICAL PHARMACOLOGY

PHARMACODYNAMICS

Divalproex sodium dissociates to the valproate ion in the gastrointestinal tract. The mechanisms by which valproate exerts its therapeutic effects have not been established. It has been suggested that its activity in epilepsy is related to increased brain concentrations of gamma-aminobutyric acid (GABA).

PHARMACOKINETICS

Absorption/Bioavailability

Equivalent oral doses of divalproex sodium products and valproic acid capsules deliver equivalent quantities of valproate ion systemically. Although the rate of valproate ion absorption may vary with the formulation administered (liquid, solid, or sprinkle), the conditions of use (*e.g.*, fasting or postprandial) and the method of administration (*e.g.*, whether the contents of the capsule are sprinkled on food or the capsule is taken intact), these differences should be of minor clinical importance under the steady state conditions achieved in chronic use in the treatment of epilepsy.

However, it is possible that differences among the various valproate products in T_{max} and C_{max} could be important upon initiation of treatment. For example, in single dose studies, the effect of feeding had a greater influence on the rate of absorption of the tablet (increase in T_{max} from 4-8 hours) than on the absorption of the sprinkle capsules (increase in T_{max} from 3.3-4.8 hours).

While the absorption rate from the GI tract and fluctuation in valproate plasma concentrations vary with dosing regimen and formulation, the efficacy of valproate as an anticonvulsant in chronic use is unlikely to be affected. Experience employing dosing regimens from once-a-day to four-times-a-day, as well as studies in primate epilepsy models involving constant rate infusion, indicate that total daily systemic bioavailability (extent of absorption) is the primary determinant of seizure control and that differences in the ratios of plasma peak to trough concentrations between valproate formulations are inconsequential from a practical clinical standpoint. Whether or not rate of absorption influences the efficacy of valproate as an antimanic or antimigraine agent is unknown.

Co-administration of oral valproate products with food and substitution among the various divalproex sodium and valproic acid formulations should cause no clinical problems in the management of patients with epilepsy. (See DOSAGE AND ADMINISTRATION.) Nonetheless, any changes in dosage administration, or the addition or discontinuance of concomitant drugs should ordinarily be accompanied by close monitoring of clinical status and valproate plasma concentrations.

Distribution

Protein Binding

The plasma protein binding of valproate is concentration dependent and the free fraction increases from approximately 10% at 40 μg/ml to 18.5% at 130 μg/ml. Protein binding of valproate is reduced in the elderly, in patients with chronic hepatic diseases, in patients with renal impairment, and in the presence of other drugs (*e.g.*, aspirin). Conversely, valproate may displace certain protein-bound drugs (*e.g.*, phenytoin, carbamazepine, warfarin, and tolbutamide). (See DRUG INTERACTIONS for more detailed information on the pharmacokinetic interactions of valproate with other drugs.)

CNS Distribution

Valproate concentrations in cerebrospinal fluid (CSF) approximate unbound concentrations in plasma (about 10% of total concentration).

Metabolism

Valproate is metabolized almost entirely by the liver. In adult patients on monotherapy, 30-50% of an administered dose appears in urine as a glucuronide conjugate. Mitochondrial β-oxidation is the other major metabolic pathway, typically accounting for over 40% of the dose. Usually, less than 15-20% of the dose is eliminated by other oxidative mechanisms. Less than 3% of an administered dose is excreted unchanged in urine.

The relationship between dose and total valproate concentration is nonlinear; concentration does not increase proportionally with the dose, but rather, increases to a lesser extent due to saturable plasma protein binding. The kinetics of unbound drug are linear.

Elimination

Mean plasma clearance and volume of distribution for total valproate are 0.56 L/h/1.73 m^2 and 11 L/1.73 m^2, respectively. Mean plasma clearance and volume of distribution for free valproate are 4.6 L/h/1.73 m^2 and 92 L/h/1.73 m^2. Mean terminal half-life for valproate monotherapy ranged from 9-16 hours following oral dosing regimens of 250-1000 mg.

The estimates cited apply primarily to patients who are not taking drugs that affect hepatic metabolizing enzyme systems. For example, patients taking enzyme-inducing antiepileptic drugs (carbamazepine, phenytoin, and phenobarbital) will clear valproate more rapidly. Because of these changes in valproate clearance, monitoring of antiepileptic concentrations should be intensified whenever concomitant antiepileptics are introduced or withdrawn.

D

Special Populations

Effect of Age

Neonates: Children within the first 2 months of life have a markedly decreased ability to eliminate valproate compared to older children and adults. This is a result of reduced clearance (perhaps due to delay in development of glucuronosyltransferase and other enzyme systems involved in valproate elimination) as well as increased volume of distribution (in part due to decreased plasma protein binding). For example, in one study, the half-life in children under 10 days ranged from 10-67 hours compared to a range of 7-13 hours in children greater than 2 months.

Children: Pediatric patients (*i.e.*, between 3 months and 10 years) have 50% higher clearances expressed on weight (*i.e.*, ml/min/kg) than do adults. Over the age of 10 years, children have pharmacokinetic parameters that approximate those of adults.

Elderly: The capacity of elderly patients (age range: 69-89 years) to eliminate valproate has been shown to be reduced compared to younger adults (age range: 22-26 years). Intrinsic clearance is reduced by 39%; the free fraction is increased by 44%. Accordingly, the initial dosage should be reduced in the elderly. (See DOSAGE AND ADMINISTRATION.)

Effect of Gender

There are no differences in the body surface area adjusted unbound clearance between males and females (4.8 ± 0.17 and 4.7 ± 0.07 L/h per 1.73m^2, respectively).

Effect of Race

The effects of race on the kinetics of valproate have not been studied.

Effect of Disease

Liver Disease: (See BOXED WARNING, CONTRAINDICATIONS, and WARNINGS.) Liver disease impairs the capacity to eliminate valproate. In one study, the clearance of free valproate was decreased by 50% in 7 patients with cirrhosis and by 16% in 4 patients with acute hepatitis, compared with 6 healthy subjects. In that study, the half-life of valproate was increased from 12-18 hours. Liver disease is also associated with decreased albumin concentrations and larger unbound fractions (2-2.6 fold increases) of valproate. Accordingly, monitoring of total concentrations may be misleading since free concentrations may be substantially elevated in patients with hepatic disease whereas total concentrations may appear to be normal.

Renal Disease: A slight reduction (27%) in the unbound clearance of valproate has been reported in patients with renal failure (creatinine clearance $<$10 ml/minute); however, hemodialysis typically reduces valproate concentrations by about 20%. Therefore, no dosage adjustment appears to be necessary in patients with renal failure. Protein binding in these patients is substantially reduced; thus, monitoring total concentrations may be misleading.

PLASMA LEVELS AND CLINICAL EFFECT

The relationship between plasma concentration and clinical response is not well documented. One contributing factor is the nonlinear, concentration dependent protein binding of valproate which affects the clearance of the drug. Thus, monitoring of total serum valproate cannot provide a reliable index of the bioactive valproate species.

For example, because the plasma protein binding of valproate is concentration dependent, the free fraction increases from approximately 10% at 40 μg/ml to 18.5% at 130 μg/ml. Higher than expected free fractions occur in the elderly, in hyperlipidemic patients, and in patients with hepatic and renal diseases.

Epilepsy: The therapeutic range in epilepsy is commonly considered to be 50-100 μg/ml of total valproate, although some patients may be controlled with lower or higher plasma concentrations.

Mania: In placebo-controlled trials of acute mania, patients were dosed to clinical response with trough plasma concentrations between 50 and 125 μg/ml (see DOSAGE AND ADMINISTRATION).

INDICATIONS AND USAGE

MANIA

Divalproex sodium is indicated for the treatment of the manic episodes associated with bipolar disorder. A manic episode is a distinct period of abnormally and persistently elevated, expansive, or irritable mood. Typical symptoms of mania include pressure of speech, motor hyperactivity, reduced need for sleep, flight of ideas, grandiosity, poor judgement, aggressiveness, and possible hostility.

The efficacy of divalproex sodium was established in 3 week trials with patients meeting DSM-III-R criteria for bipolar disorder who were hospitalized for acute mania.

The safety and effectiveness of divalproex sodium for long-term use in mania (*i.e.*, more than 3 weeks) has not been systematically evaluated in controlled clinical trials. Therefore, physicians who elect to use divalproex sodium for extended periods of time should continually re-evaluate the long term usefulness of the drug for the individual patient.

EPILEPSY

Divalproex sodium is indicated as monotherapy and adjunctive therapy in the treatment of patients with complex partial seizures that occur either in isolation or in association with other types of seizures. Divalproex sodium is also indicated for use as sole and adjunctive therapy in the treatment of simple and complex absence seizures, and adjunctively in patients with multiple seizure types that include absence seizures.

Simple absence is defined as very brief clouding of the sensorium or loss of consciousness, accompanied by certain generalized epileptic discharges without other detectable clinical signs. Complex absence is the term used when other signs are also present.

MIGRAINE

Divalproex sodium is indicated for the prophylaxis of migraine headaches. There is no evidence that divalproex sodium is useful in the acute treatment of migraine headaches. Because valproic acid may be a hazard to the fetus, divalproex sodium should be considered for women of childbearing potential only after this risk has been thoroughly discussed with the patient and weighed against the potential benefits of treatment (see WARNINGS, Use in Pregnancy and PRECAUTIONS, Information for the Patient).

See WARNINGS FOR STATEMENT REGARDING FATAL HEPATIC DYSFUNCTION.

NON-FDA APPROVED INDICATIONS

Divalproex sodium has also shown efficacy in the treatment of borderline personality disorder. One small study (n=14) has reported that divalproex sodium may be beneficial to patients with autism spectrum disorders. However, these uses have not been approved by the FDA and further clinical trials are needed.

CONTRAINDICATIONS

DIVALPROEX SODIUM SHOULD NOT BE ADMINISTERED TO PATIENTS WITH HEPATIC DISEASE OR SIGNIFICANT HEPATIC DYSFUNCTION.

Divalproex sodium is contraindicated in patients with known hypersensitivity to the drug.

WARNINGS

Hepatic failure resulting in fatalities has occurred in patients receiving valproic acid. These incidents usually have occurred during the first 6 months of treatment. Serious or fatal hepatotoxicity may be preceded by non-specific symptoms such as malaise, weakness, lethargy, facial edema, anorexia, and vomiting. In patients with epilepsy, a loss of seizure control may also occur. Patients should be monitored closely for appearance of these symptoms. Liver function tests should be performed prior to therapy and at frequent intervals thereafter, especially during the first 6 months. However, physicians should not rely totally on serum biochemistry since these tests may not be abnormal in all instances, but should also consider the results of careful interim medical history and physical examination.

Caution should be observed when administering divalproex sodium products to patients with a prior history of hepatic disease. Patients on multiple anticonvulsants, children, those with congenital metabolic disorders, those with severe seizure disorders accompanied by mental retardation, and those with organic brain disease may be at particular risk. Experience has indicated that children under the age of 2 years are at a considerably increased risk of developing fatal hepatotoxicity, especially those with the aforementioned conditions. When divalproex sodium is used in this patient group, it should be used with extreme caution and as a sole agent. The benefits of therapy should be weighed against the risks. Above this age group, experience in epilepsy has indicated that the incidence of fatal hepatotoxicity decreases considerably in progressively older patient groups.

The drug should be discontinued immediately in the presence of significant hepatic dysfunction, suspected or apparent. In some cases, hepatic dysfunction has progressed in spite of discontinuation of drug.

The frequency of adverse effects (particularly elevated liver enzymes and thrombocytopenia (see PRECAUTIONS) may be dose-related. In a clinical trial of divalproex sodium as monotherapy in patients with epilepsy, 34/126 patients (27%) receiving approximately 50 mg/kg/day on average, had at least one value of platelets $\leq 75 \times 10^9$/L. Approximately half of these patients had treatment discontinued, with return of platelet counts to normal. In the remaining patients, platelet counts normalized with continued treatment. In this study, the probability of thrombocytopenia appeared to increase significantly at total valproate concentrations of $\geq$110 μg/ml (females) or $\geq$135 μg/ml (males). The therapeutic benefit which may accompany the higher doses should therefore be weighed against the possibility of a greater incidence of adverse effects.

USE IN PREGNANCY

ACCORDING TO PUBLISHED AND UNPUBLISHED REPORTS, VALPROIC ACID MAY PRODUCE TERATOGENIC EFFECTS IN THE OFFSPRING OF HUMAN FEMALES RECEIVING THE DRUG DURING PREGNANCY.

THERE ARE MULTIPLE REPORTS IN THE CLINICAL LITERATURE WHICH INDICATE THAT THE USE OF ANTIEPILEPTIC DRUGS DURING PREGNANCY RESULTS IN AN INCREASED INCIDENCE OF BIRTH DEFECTS IN THE OFFSPRING. ALTHOUGH DATA ARE MORE EXTENSIVE WITH RESPECT TO TRIMETHADIONE, PARAMETHADIONE, PHENYTOIN, AND PHENOBARBITAL, REPORTS INDICATE A POSSIBLE SIMILAR ASSOCIATION WITH THE USE OF OTHER ANTIEPILEPTIC DRUGS.

THE INCIDENCE OF NEURAL TUBE DEFECTS IN THE FETUS MAY BE INCREASED IN MOTHERS RECEIVING VALPROATE DURING THE FIRST TRIMESTER OF PREGNANCY. THE CENTERS FOR DISEASE CONTROL (CDC) HAS ESTIMATED THE RISK OF VALPROIC ACID EXPOSED WOMEN HAVING CHILDREN WITH SPINA BIFIDA TO BE APPROXIMATELY 1-2%.

OTHER CONGENITAL ANOMALIES (*e.g.,* CRANIOFACIAL DEFECTS, CARDIOVASCULAR MALFORMATIONS, AND ANOMALIES INVOLVING VARIOUS BODY SYSTEMS), COMPATIBLE AND INCOMPATIBLE WITH LIFE, HAVE BEEN REPORTED. SUFFICIENT DATA TO DETERMINE THE INCIDENCE OF THESE CONGENITAL ANOMALIES IS NOT AVAILABLE.

THE HIGHER INCIDENCE OF CONGENITAL ANOMALIES IN ANTIEPILEPTIC DRUG-TREATED WOMEN WITH SEIZURE DISORDERS CANNOT BE REGARDED AS A CAUSE AND EFFECT RELATIONSHIP. THERE ARE INTRINSIC METHODOLOGIC PROBLEMS IN OBTAINING ADEQUATE DATA ON DRUG TERATOGENICITY IN HUMANS; GENETIC FACTORS OR THE EPILEPTIC CONDITION ITSELF, MAY BE MORE IMPORTANT THAN DRUG THERAPY IN CONTRIBUTING TO CONGENITAL ANOMALIES.

PATIENTS TAKING VALPROATE MAY DEVELOP CLOTTING ABNORMALITIES. A PATIENT WHO HAD LOW FIBRINOGEN WHEN TAKING MULTIPLE ANTICONVULSANTS INCLUDING VALPROATE GAVE BIRTH TO AN INFANT WITH AFIBRINOGENEMIA WHO SUBSEQUENTLY DIED OF HEMORRHAGE. IF VALPROATE IS USED IN PREGNANCY, THE CLOTTING PARAMETERS SHOULD BE MONITORED CAREFULLY.

HEPATIC FAILURE, RESULTING IN THE DEATH OF A NEWBORN AND OF AN INFANT, HAVE BEEN REPORTED FOLLOWING THE USE OF VALPROATE DURING PREGNANCY.

Animal studies have demonstrated valproate-induced teratogenicity. Increased frequencies of malformations, as well as intrauterine growth retardation and death, have been observed in mice, rats, rabbits, and monkeys following prenatal exposure to valproate. Malformations of the skeletal system are the most common structural abnormalities produced in experimental animals, but neural tube closure defects have been seen in mice exposed to maternal plasma valproate concentrations exceeding 230 μg/ml (2.3 times the upper limit of the human therapeutic range) during susceptible periods of embryonic development. Administration of an oral dose of 200 mg/kg/day or greater (50% of the maximum human daily dose or greater on an mg/m^2 basis) to pregnant rats during organogenesis produced malformations (skeletal, cardiac, and urogenital) and growth retardation in the offspring. These doses resulted in peak maternal plasma valproate levels of approximately 340 μg/ml or greater (3.4 times the upper limit of the human therapeutic range or greater). Behavioral deficits have been reported in the offspring of rats given a dose of 200 mg/kg/day throughout most of the pregnancy. An oral dose of 350 mg/kg/day (approximately 2 times the maximum human daily dose on a mg/m^2 basis) produced skeletal and visceral malformations in rabbits exposed during organogenesis. Skeletal malformations, growth retardation, and death were observed in rhesus monkeys following administration of an oral dose of 200 mg/kg/day (equal to the maximum human daily dose on a mg/m^2 basis) during organogenesis. This dose resulted in peak maternal plasma valproate levels of approximately 280 μg/ml (2.8 times the upper limit of the human therapeutic range).

The prescribing physician will wish to weigh the benefits of therapy against the risks in treating or counseling women of childbearing potential. If this drug is used during pregnancy, or if the patient becomes pregnant while taking this drug, the patient should be apprised of the potential hazard to the fetus.

Antiepileptic drugs should not be discontinued abruptly in patients in whom the drug is administered to prevent major seizures because of the strong possibility of precipitating status epilepticus with attendant hypoxia and threat to life. In individual cases where the severity and frequency of the seizure disorder are such that the removal of medication does not pose a serious threat to the patient, discontinuation of the drug may be considered prior to and during pregnancy, although it cannot be said with any confidence that even minor seizures do not pose some hazard to the developing embryo or fetus.

Tests to detect neural tube and other defects using current accepted procedures should be considered a part of routine prenatal care in childbearing women receiving valproate.

PRECAUTIONS

HEPATIC DYSFUNCTION

See BOXED WARNING, CONTRAINDICATIONS, and WARNINGS.

GENERAL

Because of reports of thrombocytopenia (see WARNINGS), inhibition of the secondary phase of platelet aggregation, and abnormal coagulation parameters (*e.g.,* low fibrinogen), platelet counts and coagulation tests are recommended before initiating therapy and at periodic intervals. It is recommended that patients receiving divalproex sodium be monitored for platelet count, and coagulation parameters prior to planned surgery. In a clinical trial of divalproex sodium as monotherapy in patients with epilepsy, 34/126 patients (27%) receiving approximately 50 mg/kg/day on average, had at least one value of platelets $\leq 75 \times 10^9$/L. Approximately half of these patients had treatment discontinued, with return of platelet counts to normal. In the remaining patients, platelet counts normalized with continued treatment. In this study, the probability of thrombocytopenia appeared to increase significantly at total valproate concentrations of $\geq$110 μg/ml (females) or $\geq$135 μg/ml (males). Evidence of hemorrhage, bruising or a disorder of hemostasis/coagulation is an indication for reduction of the dosage or withdrawal of therapy.

Hyperammonemia with or without lethargy or coma has been reported and may be present in the absence of abnormal liver function tests. Asymptomatic elevations of ammonia are more common and when present require more frequent monitoring. If clinically significant symptoms occur, divalproex sodium therapy should be modified or discontinued.

Since divalproex sodium may interact with concurrently administered drugs which are capable of enzyme induction, periodic plasma concentration determinations of valproate and concomitant drugs are recommended during the early course of therapy. (See DRUG INTERACTIONS.)

Valproate is partially eliminated in the urine as a keto-metabolite which may lead to a false interpretation of the urine ketone test.

There have been reports of altered thyroid function tests associated with valproate. The clinical significance of these is unknown.

Suicidal ideation may be a manifestation of certain psychiatric disorders, and may persist until significant remission of symptoms occurs. Close supervision of high risk patients should accompany initial drug therapy.

INFORMATION FOR THE PATIENT

Since divalproex sodium products may produce CNS depression, especially when combined with another CNS depressant (*e.g.,* alcohol), patients should be advised not to engage in hazardous activities, such as driving an automobile or operating dangerous machinery, until it is known that they do not become drowsy from the drug.

MIGRAINE PATIENTS

Since divalproex sodium has been associated with certain types of birth defects, female patients of child-bearing age considering the use of divalproex sodium for the prevention of migraine should be advised to read the Patient Instructions that are distributed with the prescription.

CARCINOGENESIS, MUTAGENESIS, AND IMPAIRMENT OF FERTILITY

Carcinogenesis

Valproic acid was administered to Sprague Dawley rats and ICR (HA/ICR) mice at doses of 0, 80, and 170 mg/kg/day (approximately 10-50% of the maximum human daily dose on a mg/m^2 basis) for two years. A variety of neoplasms were observed in both species. The chief findings were a statistically significant increase in the incidence of subcutaneous fibrosarcomas in high dose male rats receiving valproic acid and a statistically significant dose-related trend for benign pulmonary adenomas in male mice receiving valproic acid. The significance of these findings for humans is unknown.

Mutagenesis

Valproate was not mutagenic in an *in vitro* bacterial assay (Ames test), did not produce dominant lethal effects in mice, and did not increase chromosome aberration frequency in an *in vivo* cytogenic study in rats. Increased frequencies of sister chromatid exchange (SCE) have been reported in a study of epileptic children taking valproate, but this association was not observed in another study conducted in adults. There is some evidence that increased SCE frequencies may be associated with epilepsy. The biological significance of increase in SCE frequency is not known.

Impairment of Fertility

Chronic toxicity studies in juvenile and adult rats and dogs demonstrated reduced spermatogenesis and testicular atrophy at oral doses of 400 mg/kg/day or greater in rats (approximately equivalent to or greater than the maximum human daily dose on a mg/m^2 basis) and 150 mg/kg/day or greater in dogs (approximately 1.4 times the maximum human daily dose or greater on a mg/m^2 basis). Segment I fertility studies in rats have shown doses up to 350 mg/kg/day (approximately equal to the maximum human daily dose on a mg/m^2 dose) for 60 days to have no effect on fertility. THE EFFECT OF VALPROATE ON TESTICULAR DEVELOPMENT AND ON SPERM PRODUCTION AND FERTILITY IN HUMANS IS UNKNOWN.

PREGNANCY CATEGORY D

See WARNINGS.

NURSING MOTHERS

Valproate is excreted in breast milk. Concentrations in breast milk have been reported to be 1-10% of serum concentrations. It is not known what effect this would have on a nursing infant. Consideration should be given to discontinuing nursing when divalproex sodium is administered to a nursing woman.

PEDIATRIC USE

Experience has indicated that pediatric patients under the age of 2 years are at a considerably increased risk of developing fatal hepatotoxicity, especially those with the aforementioned conditions (see BOXED WARNING). When divalproex sodium is used in this patient group, it should be used with extreme caution and as a sole agent. The benefits of therapy should be weighed against the risks. Above the age of 2 years, experience in epilepsy has indicated that the incidence of fatal hepatotoxicity decreases considerably in progressively older patient groups.

Younger children, especially those receiving enzyme-inducing drugs, will require larger maintenance doses to attain targeted total and unbound valproic acid concentrations.

The variability in free fraction limits the clinical usefulness of monitoring total serum valproic acid concentrations. Interpretation of valproic acid concentrations in children should include consideration of factors that affect hepatic metabolism and protein binding.

The safety and effectiveness of divalproex sodium for the treatment of acute mania has not been studied in individuals below the age of 18 years.

The safety and effectiveness of divalproex sodium for the prophylaxis of migraines has not been studied in individuals below the age of 16 years.

The basic toxicology and pathologic manifestations of valproate sodium in neonatal (4-day old) and juvenile (14-day old) rats are similar to those seen in young adult rats. However, additional findings, including renal alterations in juvenile rats and renal alterations and retinal dysplasia in neonatal rats, have been reported. These findings occurred at 240 mg/kg/day, a dosage approximately equivalent to the human maximum recommended daily dose on a mg/m^2 basis. They were not seen at 90 mg/kg, or 40% of the maximum human daily dose on a mg/m^2 basis.

GERIATRIC USE

No patients above the age of 65 years were enrolled in double-blind prospective clinical trials of mania associated with bipolar illness. In a case review study of 583 patients, 72 patients (12%) were greater than 65 years of age. A higher percentage of patients above 65 years of age reported accidental injury, infection, pain, somnolence, and tremor. Discontinuation of valproate was occasionally associated with the latter two events. It is not clear whether these events indicate additional risk or whether they result from preexisting medical illness and concomitant medication use among these patients.

In a double-blind, multicenter trial of valproate, in elderly patients with dementia, doses were increased by 125 mg/day to a target dose of 20 mg/kg/day. Patients experienced a significant increase in somnolence and discontinuations for somnolence compared to placebo. In some patients these events were also associated with reduced nutritional intake and weight loss. There was a trend for the patients who experienced these events to have lower albumin concentrations, valproate clearance, and to be older than patients who better tolerated a given dose. In elderly patients, dosage should be increased more slowly and with monitoring for possible adverse events. (See DOSAGE AND ADMINISTRATION.)

There is insufficient information available to discern the safety and effectiveness of divalproex sodium for the prophylaxis of migraines in patients over 65.

DRUG INTERACTIONS

EFFECTS OF CO-ADMINISTERED DRUGS ON VALPROATE CLEARANCE

Drugs that affect the level of expression of hepatic enzymes, particularly those that elevate levels of glucuronosyltransferases, may increase the clearance of valproate. For example, phenytoin, carbamazepine, and phenobarbital (or primidone) can double the clearance of valproate. Thus, patients on monotherapy will generally have longer half-lives and higher concentrations than patients receiving polytherapy with antiepilepsy drugs.

In contrast, drugs that are inhibitors of cytochrome P450 isozymes (*e.g.,* antidepressants) may be expected to have little effect on valproate clearance because cytochrome P450 microsomal medicated oxidation is a relatively minor secondary metabolic pathway compared to glucuronidation and beta-oxidation.

Because of these changes in valproate clearance, monitoring of valproate and concomitant drug concentrations should be increased whenever enzyme inducing drugs are introduced or withdrawn.

The following list provides information about the potential for an influence of several commonly prescribed medications on valproate pharmacokinetics. The list is not exhaustive, nor could it be, since new interactions are continuously being reported.

Drugs for Which a Potentially Important Interaction Has Been Observed

Aspirin: A study involving the co-administration of aspirin at antipyretic doses (11-16 mg/kg) with valproate to pediatric patients (n=6) revealed a decrease in protein binding and an inhibition of metabolism of valproate. Valproate free fraction was increased 4-fold in the presence of aspirin compared to valproate alone. The β-oxidation pathway consisting of 2-E-valproic acid, 3-OH-valproic acid, and 3-keto valproic acid was decreased from 25% of total metabolites excreted on valproate alone to 8.3% in the presence of aspirin. Caution should be observed if valproate and aspirin are to be co-administered.

Felbamate: A study involving the co-administration of 1200 mg/day of felbamate with valproate to patients with epilepsy (n=10) revealed an increase in mean valproate peak concentration by 35% (from 86-115 μg/ml) compared to valproate alone. Increasing the felbamate dose to 2400 mg/day increased the mean valproate peak concentration to 133 μg/ml (another 16% increase). A decrease in valproate dosage may be necessary when felbamate therapy is initiated.

Rifampin: A study involving the administration of a single dose of valproate (7 mg/kg) 36 hours after 5 nights of daily dosing with rifampin (600 mg) revealed a 40% increase in the oral clearance of valproate. Valproate dosage adjustment may be necessary when it is co-administered with rifampin.

Drugs for Which Either No Interaction or a Likely Clinically Unimportant Interaction Has Been Observed

Antacids: A study involving the co-administration of valproate 500 mg with commonly administered antacids (Maalox, Trisogel, and Titralac—160 mEq doses) did not reveal any effect on the extent of absorption of valproate.

Chlorpromazine: A study involving the administration of 100-300 mg/day of chlorpromazine to schizophrenic patients already receiving valproate (200 mg bid) revealed a 15% increase in trough plasma levels of valproate.

Haloperidol: A study involving the administration of 6-10 mg/day of haloperidol to schizophrenic patients already receiving valproate (200 mg bid) revealed no significant changes in valproate trough plasma levels.

Cimetidine and Ranitidine: Cimetidine and ranitidine do not affect the clearance of valproate.

EFFECTS OF VALPROATE ON OTHER DRUGS

Valproate has been found to be a weak inhibitor of some P450 isozymes, epoxide hydrase, and glucuronyl tranferases.

The following list provides information about the potential for an influence of valproate co-administration on the pharmacokinetics or pharmacodynamics of several commonly prescribed medications. The list is not exhaustive, since new interactions are continuously being reported.

Drugs for Which a Potentially Important Valproate Interaction Has Been Observed

Carbamazepine/Carbamazepine-10,11-Epoxide: Serum levels of carbamazepine (CBZ) decreased 17% while that of carbamazepine-10,11-epoxide (CBZ-E) increased by 45% upon co-administration of valproate and CBZ to epileptic patients.

Clonazepam: The concomitant use of valproic acid and clonazepam may induce absence status in patients with a history of absence type seizures.

Diazepam: Valproate displaces diazepam from its plasma albumin binding sites and inhibits its metabolism. Co-administration of valproate (1500 mg daily) increased the free fraction of diazepam (10 mg) by 90% in healthy volunteers (n=6). Plasma clearance and volume of distribution for free diazepam were reduced by 25% and 20%, respectively, in the presence of valproate. The elimination half-life of diazepam remained unchanged upon addition of valproate.

Ethosuximide: Valproate inhibits the metabolism of ethosuximide. Administration of a single ethosuximide dose of 500 mg with valproate (800-1600 mg/day) to healthy volunteers (n=6) was accompanied by a 25% increase in elimination half-life of ethosuximide and a 15% decrease in its total clearance as compared to ethosuximide alone. Patients receiving valproate and ethosuximide, especially along with other anticonvulsants, should be monitored for alterations in serum concentrations of both drugs.

Lamotrigine: In a steady-state study involving 10 healthy volunteers, the elimination half-life of lamotrigine increased from 26-70 hours with valproate co-administration

D

(a 165% increase). The dose of lamotrigine should be reduced when co-administered with valproate.

Phenobarbital: Valproate was found to inhibit the metabolism of phenobarbital. Co-administration of valproate (250 mg bid for 14 days) with phenobarbital to normal subjects (n=6) resulted in a 50% increase in half-life and a 30% decrease in plasma clearance of phenobarbital (60 mg single-dose). The fraction of phenobarbital dose excreted unchanged increased by 50% in presence of valproate. There is evidence for severe CNS depression, with or without significant elevations of barbiturate or valproate serum concentrations. All patients receiving concomitant barbiturate therapy should be closely monitored for neurologic toxicity. Serum barbiturate concentrations should be obtained, if possible, and the barbiturate dosage decreased, if appropriate.

Primidone: Primidone is metabolized to a barbiturate, may be involved in a similar interaction with valproate.

Phenytoin: Valproate displaces phenytoin from its plasma albumin binding sites and inhibits its hepatic metabolism. Co-administration of valproate (400 mg tid) with phenytoin (250 mg) in normal volunteers (n=7) was associated with a 60% increase in the free fraction of phenytoin. Total plasma clearance and apparent volume of distribution of phenytoin increased 30% in the presence of valproate. Both the clearance and apparent volume of distribution of free phenytoin were reduced by 25%.

In patients with epilepsy, there have been reports of breakthrough seizures occurring with the combination of valproate and phenytoin. The dosage of phenytoin should be adjusted as required by the clinical situation.

Tolbutamide: From *in vitro* experiments, the unbound fraction of tolbutamide was increased from 20-50% when added to plasma samples taken from patients treated with valproate. The clinical relevance of this displacement is unknown.

Warfarin: In an *in vitro* study, valproate increased the unbound fraction of warfarin by up to 32.6%. The therapeutic relevance of this is unknown; however, coagulation tests should be monitored if divalproex sodium therapy is instituted in patients taking anticoagulants.

Zidovudine: In 6 patients who were seropositive for HIV, the clearance of zidovudine (100 mg q8h) was decreased by 38% after administration of valproate (250 or 500 mg q8h); the half-life of zidovudine was unaffected.

Drugs for Which Either No Interaction or a Likely Clinically Unimportant Interaction Has Been Observed

Acetaminophen: Valproate had no effect on any of the pharmacokinetic parameters of acetaminophen when it was concurrently administered to three epileptic patients.

Amitriptyline/Nortriptyline: Administration of a single oral 50 mg dose of amitriptyline to 15 normal volunteers (10 males and 5 females) who received valproate (500 mg bid) resulted in a 21% decrease in plasma clearance of amitriptyline and a 34% decrease in the net clearance of nortriptyline. Rare postmarketing reports of concurrent use of valproate and amitriptyline resulting in an increased amitriptyline level have been received. Concurrent use of valproate and amitriptyline has rarely been associated with toxicity. Monitoring of amitrytyline levels should be considered for patients taking valproate concomitantly with amitriptyline.

Clozapine: In psychotic patients (n=11), no interaction was observed when valproate was co-administered with clozapine.

Lithium: Co-administration of valproate (500 mg bid) and lithium carbonate (300 mg tid) to normal male volunteers (n=16) had no effect on the steady-state kinetics of lithium.

Lorazepam: Concomitant administration of valproate (500 mg bid) and lorazepam (1 mg bid) in normal male volunteers (n=9) was accompanied by a 17% decrease in the plasma clearance of lorazepam.

Oral Contraceptive Steroids: Administration of a single dose of ethinyloestradiol (50 µg)/levonorgestrel (250 µg) to 6 women on valproate (200 mg bid) therapy for 2 months did not reveal any pharmacokinetic interaction.

ADVERSE REACTIONS

MANIA

The incidence of treatment-emergent events has been ascertained based on combined data from two placebo-controlled clinical trials of divalproex sodium in the treatment of manic episodes associated with bipolar disorder. The adverse events were usually mild or moderate in intensity, but sometimes were serious enough to interrupt treatment. In clinical trials, the rates of premature termination due to intolerance were not statistically different between placebo, divalproex sodium, and lithium carbonate. A total of 4%, 8%, and 11% of patients discontinued therapy due to intolerance in the placebo, divalproex sodium, and lithium carbonate groups, respectively.

TABLE 5 summarizes those adverse events reported for patients in these trials where the incidence rate in divalproex sodium-treated group was greater than 5% and greater than the placebo incidence, or where the incidence in the divalproex sodium-treated group was statistically greater than the placebo group. Vomiting was the only event that was reported by significantly ($p \leq 0.05$) more patients receiving divalproex sodium compared to placebo.

The following additional adverse events were reported by greater than 1% but not more than 5% of the 89 divalproex sodium-treated patients in controlled clinical trials.

Body as a Whole: Chest pain, chills, chills and fever, fever, neck pain, and neck rigidity.

Cardiovascular System: Hypertension, hypotension, palpitations, postural hypotension, tachycardia, and vasodialation.

Digestive System: Anorexia, fecal incontinence, flatulence, gastroenteritis, glossitis, and periodontal abscess.

Hemic and Lymphatic System: Ecchymosis.

Metabolic and Nutritional Disorders: Edema, and peripheral edema.

Musculoskeletal System: Arthralgia, arthrosis, leg cramps, and twitching.

Nervous System: Abnormal dreams, abnormal gait, agitation, ataxia, catatonic reaction, confusion, depression, diplopia, dysarthria, hallucinations, hypertonia, hypokinesia, insomnia, paresthesia, reflexes increased, tardive dyskinesia, thinking abnormalities, and vertigo.

TABLE 5 *Adverse Events Reported by >5% of Divalproex Sodium-Treated Patients During Placebo-Controlled Trials of Acute Mania**

Adverse Event	Divalproex Sodium (n=89)	Placebo (n=97)
Nausea	22%	15%
Somnolence	19%	12%
Dizziness	12%	4%
Vomiting	12%	3%
Asthenia	10%	7%
Abdominal Pain	9%	8%
Dyspepsia	9%	8%
Rash	6%	3%

* The following adverse events occured at an equal or greater incidence for placebo than for divalproex sodium: back pain, headache, constipation, diarrhea, tremor, and pharyngitis.

Respiratory System: Dyspnea, and rhinitis.

Skin and Appendages: Alopecia, discoid lupus erythematosis, dry skin, furunculosis, masculopapular rash, and seborrhea.

Special Senses: Amblyopia, conjunctivitis, deafness, dry eyes, ear pain, and tinnitus.

Urogenital System: Dysmenorrhea, dysuria, and urinary incontinence.

MIGRAINE

Based on two placebo-controlled clinical trials and their long term extension, divalproex sodium was generally well tolerated with most adverse events rated as mild to moderate in severity. Of the 202 patients exposed to divalproex sodium in the placebo-controlled trials, 17% discontinued for intolerance. This is compared to a rate of 5% for the 81 placebo patients. Including the long term extension study, the adverse events reported as the primary reason for discontinuation by ≥1% of 248 divalproex sodium-treated patients were alopecia (6%), nausea and/or vomiting (5%), weight gain (2%), tremor (2%), somnolence (1%), elevated SGOT and/or SGPT (1%), and depression (1%).

TABLE 6 includes those adverse events reported for patients in the placebo-controlled trials where the incidence rate in the divalproex sodium-treated group was greater than 5% and was greater than that for placebo patients.

TABLE 6 *Adverse Events Reported by >5% of Divalproex Sodium-Treated Patients During Migraine Placebo-Controlled Trials with a Greater Incidence Than Patients Taking Placebo**

Body System/Event	Divalproex Sodium (n=202)	Placebo (n=81)
Gastrointestinal System		
Nausea	31%	10%
Dyspepsia	13%	9%
Diarrhea	12%	7%
Vomiting	11%	1%
Abdominal pain	9%	4%
Increased appetite	6%	4%
Nervous System		
Asthenia	20%	9%
Somnolence	17%	5%
Dizziness	12%	6%
Tremor	9%	0%
Other		
Weight gain	8%	2%
Back pain	8%	6%
Alopecia	7%	1%

* The following adverse events occurred in at least 5% of divalproex sodium-treated patients and at an equal or greater incidence for placebo than for divalproex sodium: flu syndrome and pharyngitis.

The following additional adverse events were reported by greater than 1% but not more than 5% of the 202 divalproex sodium-treated patients in the controlled clinical trials.

Body as a Whole: Chest pain, chills, face edema, fever, and malaise.

Cardiovascular System: Vasodilation.

Digestive System: Anorexia, constipation, dry mouth, flatulence, gastrointestinal disorder (unspecified), and stomatitis.

Hemic and Lymphatic System: Ecchymosis.

Metabolic and Nutritional Disorders: Peripheral edema, SGOT increase, and SGPT increase.

Musculoskeletal System: Leg cramps and myalgia.

Nervous System: Abnormal dreams, amnesia, confusion, depression, emotional lability, insomnia, nervousness, paresthesia, speech disorder, thinking abnormalities, and vertigo.

Respiratory System: Cough increased, dyspnea, rhinitis, and sinusitis.

Skin and Appendages: Pruritus and rash.

Special Senses: Conjunctivitis, ear disorder, taste perversion, and tinnitus.

Urogenital System: Cystitis, metrorrhagia, and vaginal hemorrhage.

EPILEPSY

Based on a placebo-controlled trial of adjunctive therapy for treatment of complex partial seizures, divalproex sodium was generally well tolerated with most adverse events rated as mild to moderate in severity. Intolerance was the primary reason for discontinuation in the divalproex sodium-treated patients (6%), compared to 1% of the placebo-treated patients.

TABLE 7 lists treatment-emergent adverse events which were reported by ≥5% of divalproex sodium-treated patients and for which the incidence was greater than in the placebo group, in the placebo-controlled trial of adjunctive therapy for treatment of complex partial seizures. Since patients were also treated with other antiepilepsy drugs, it is not possible, in most cases, to determine whether the following adverse events can be ascribed to divalproex sodium alone, or the combination of divalproex sodium and other antiepilepsy drugs.

***TABLE 7** Adverse Events Reported by ≥5% of Patients Treated with Divalproex Sodium During Placebo-Controlled Trial of Adjunctive Therapy for Complex Partial Seizures*

Body System/Event	Divalproex Sodium (n=77)	Placebo (n=70)
Body as a Whole		
Headache	31%	21%
Asthenia	27%	7%
Fever	6%	4%
Gastrointestinal System		
Nausea	48%	14%
Vomiting	27%	7%
Abdominal pain	23%	6%
Diarrhea	13%	6%
Anorexia	12%	0%
Dyspepsia	8%	4%
Constipation	5%	1%
Nervous System		
Somnolence	27%	11%
Tremor	25%	6%
Dizziness	25%	13%
Diplopia	16%	9%
Amblyopia/blurred vision	12%	9%
Ataxia	8%	1%
Nystagmus	8%	1%
Emotional lability	6%	4%
Thinking abnormal	6%	0%
Amnesia	5%	1%
Respiratory System		
Flu syndrome	12%	9%
Infection	12%	6%
Bronchitis	5%	1%
Rhinitis	5%	4%
Other		
Alopecia	6%	1%
Weight loss	6%	0%

TABLE 8 lists treatment-emergent adverse events which were reported by ≥5% of patients in the high dose divalproex sodium group, and for which the incidence was greater than in the low dose group, in a controlled trial of divalproex sodium monotherapy treatment of complex partial seizures. Since patients were being titrated off another antiepilepsy drug during the first portion of the trial, it is not possible, in many cases, to determine whether the following adverse events can be ascribed to divalproex sodium alone, or the combination of divalproex sodium and other antiepilepsy drugs.

***TABLE 8** Adverse Events Reported by ≥5% of Patients in the High Dose Group in the Controlled Trial of Divalproex Sodium Monotherapy for Complex Partial Seizures**

Body System/Event	High Dose (n=131)	Low Dose (n=134)
Body as a Whole		
Asthenia	21%	10%
Digestive System		
Nausea	34%	26%
Diarrhea	23%	19%
Vomiting	23%	15%
Abdominal pain	12%	9%
Anorexia	11%	4%
Dyspepsia	11%	10%
Hemic/Lymphatic System		
Thrombocytopenia	24%	1%
Ecchymosis	5%	4%
Metabolic/Nutritional		
Weight gain	9%	4%
Peripheral edema	8%	3%
Nervous System		
Tremor	57%	19%
Somnolence	30%	18%
Dizziness	18%	13%
Insomnia	15%	9%
Nervousness	11%	7%
Amnesia	7%	4%
Nystagmus	7%	1%
Depression	5%	4%
Respiratory System		
Infection	20%	13%
Pharyngitis	8%	2%
Dyspnea	5%	1%
Skin and Appendages		
Alopecia	24%	13%
Special Senses		
Amblyopia/blurred vision	8%	4%
Tinnitus	7%	1%

* Headache was the only adverse that occurred in ≥5% of patients in the high dose group and at equal or greater incidence in the low dose group.

The following additional adverse events were reported by greater than 1% but less than 5% of the 358 patients treated with divalproex sodium in the controlled trials of complex partial seizures.

Body as a Whole: Back pain, chest pain, and malaise.

Cardiovascular System: Tachycardia, hypertension, and palpitation.

Digestive System: Increased appetite, flatulence, hematemesis, eructation, pancreatitis, and periodontal abscess.

Hemic and Lymphatic System: Petechia.

Metabolic and Nutritional Disorders: SGOT increased, and SGPT increased.

Musculoskeletal System: Myalgia, twitching, arthralgia, leg cramps, and myasthenia.

Nervous System: Anxiety, confusion, abnormal gait, paresthesia, hypertonia, incoordination, abnormal dreams, and personality disorder.

Respiratory System: Sinusitis, cough increased, pneumonia, and epistaxis.

Skin and Appendages: Rash, pruritus, and dry skin.

Special Senses: Taste perversion, abnormal vision, deafness, and otitis media.

Urogenital System: Urinary incontinence, vaginitis, dysmenorrhea, amenorrhea, and urinary frequency.

D

OTHER PATIENT POPULATIONS

Adverse events that have been reported with all dosage forms of valproate from epilepsy trials, spontaneous reports, and other sources are listed below by body system.

Gastrointestinal: The most commonly reported side effects at the initiation of therapy are nausea, vomiting, and indigestion. These effects are usually transient and rarely require discontinuation of therapy. Diarrhea, abdominal cramps, and constipation have been reported. Both anorexia with some weight loss and increased appetite with weight gain have also been reported. The administration of delayed-release divalproex sodium may result in reduction of gastrointestinal side effects in some patients.

CNS Effects: Sedative effects have occurred in patients receiving valproate alone but occur most often in patients receiving combination therapy. Sedation usually abates upon reduction of other antiepileptic medication. Tremor (may be dose-related), hallucinations, ataxia, headache, nystagmus, diplopia, asterixis, "spots before eyes", dysarthria, dizziness, confusion, hypesthesia, vertigo, incoordination, and parkinsonism. Rare cases of coma have occurred in patients receiving valproate alone or in conjunction with phenobarbital. In rare instances encephalopathy with fever has developed shortly after the introduction of valproate monotherapy without evidence of hepatic dysfunction or inappropriate plasma levels; all patients recovered after the drug was withdrawn.

Several reports have noted reversible cerebral atrophy and dementia in association with valproate therapy.

Dermatologic: Transient hair loss, skin rash, photosensitivity, generalized pruritus, erythema multiforme, and Stevens-Johnson syndrome. Rare cases of toxic epidermal necrolysis have been reported including a fatal case in a 6 month old infant taking valproate and several other concomitant medications. An additional case of toxic epidermal necrosis resulting in death was reported in a 35 year old patient with AIDS taking several concomitant medications and had with a history of multiple cutaneous drug reactions.

Psychiatric: Emotional upset, depression, psychosis, aggression, hyperactivity, hostility, and behavioral deterioration.

Musculoskeletal: Weakness.

Hematologic: Thrombocytopenia and inhibition of the secondary phase of platelet aggregation may be reflected in altered bleeding time, petechiae, bruising, hematoma formation, epistaxis, and frank hemorrhage (see PRECAUTIONS, General and DRUG INTERACTIONS). Relative lymphocytosis, macrocytosis, hypofibrinogenemia, leukopenia, eosinophilia, anemia including macrocytic with or without folate deficiency, bone marrow suppression, pancytopenia, aplastic anemia, and acute intermittent porphyria.

Hepatic: Minor elevations of transaminases (*e.g.*, SGOT and SGPT) and LDH are frequent and appear to be dose-related. Occasionally, laboratory test results include increases in serum bilirubin and abnormal changes in other liver function tests. These results may reflect potentially serious hepatotoxicity (see WARNINGS).

Endocrine: Irregular menses, secondary amenorrhea, breast enlargement, galactorrhea, and parotid gland swelling. Abnormal thyroid function tests (see PRECAUTIONS).

There have been rare spontaneous reports of polycystic ovary disease. A cause and effect relationship has not been established.

Pancreatic: Acute pancreatitis including fatalities.

Metabolic: Hyperammonemia (see PRECAUTIONS), hyponatremia, and inappropriate ADH secretion. There have been rare reports on Fanconi's syndrome occurring chiefly in children. Decreased carnitine concentrations have been reported although the clinical relevance is undetermined. Hyperglycemia has occurred and was associated with a fatal outcome in a patient with preexistent nonketotic hyperglycinemia.

Genitourinary: Enuresis and urinary tract infection.

Special Senses: Hearing loss, either reversible or irreversible, has been reported; however, a cause and effect relationship has not been established. Ear pain has also been reported.

Other: Anaphylaxis, edema of the extremities, lupus erythematosus, bone pain, cough increased, pneumonia, otitis media, bradycardia, cutaneous vasculitis, and fever.

DOSAGE AND ADMINISTRATION

MANIA

Divalproex sodium tablets are administered orally. The recommended initial dose is 750 mg daily in divided doses. The dose should be increased as rapidly as possible to achieve the lowest therapeutic dose which produces the desired clinical effect or the desired range of plasma concentrations. In placebo-controlled clinical trials of acute mania, patients were dosed to a clinical response with a trough plasma concentration between 50 and 125 μg/ml. Maximum concentrations were generally achieved within 14 days. The maximum recommended dose is 60 mg/kg/day.

There is no body of evidence available from controlled trials to guide a clinician in the longer term management of a patient who improves during divalproex sodium treatment of an acute manic episode. While it is generally agreed that pharmacological treatment beyond an acute response in mania is desirable, both for maintenance of the initial response and for prevention of new manic episodes, there are no systematically obtained data to support the benefits of divalproex sodium in such longer-term treatment. Although there are no efficacy data that specifically address longer-term antimanic treatment with divalproex sodium, the safety of divalproex sodium in long-term use is supported by data from record reviews involving approximately 360 patients treated with divalproex sodium for greater than 3 months.

EPILEPSY

Divalproex sodium tablets are administered orally. Divalproex sodium has been studied as monotherapy and adjunctive therapy in complex partial seizures, and in simple and complex absence seizures in adults and adolescents. As the divalproex sodium dosage is titrated upward, concentrations of phenobarbital, carbamazepine, and/or phenytoin may be affected (see DRUG INTERACTIONS).

Complex Partial Seizures

For adults and children 10 years of age and older.

Monotherapy (initial therapy)

Divalproex sodium has not been systematically studied as initial therapy. Patients should initiate therapy at 10-15 mg/kg/day. The dosage should be increased by 5-10 mg/kg/week to achieve optimal clinical response. Ordinarily, optimal clinical response is achieved at daily doses below 60 mg/kg/day. If satisfactory clinical response has not been achieved, plasma levels should be measured to determine whether or not they are in the usually accepted therapeutic range (50-100 μg/ml). No recommendation regarding the safety of valproate for use at doses above 60 mg/kg/day can be made.

The probability of thromocytopenia increases significantly at total trough valproate plasma concentrations above 100 μg/ml in females and 135 μg/ml in males. The benefit of improved seizure control with higher doses should be weighed against the possibility of a greater incidence of adverse reactions.

Conversion to Monotherapy

Patients should initiate therapy at 10-15 mg/kg/day. The dosage should be increased by 5-10 mg/kg/week to achieve optimal clinical response. Ordinarily, optimal clinical response is achieved at daily doses below 60 mg/kg/day. If satisfactory clinical response has not been achieved, plasma levels should be measured to determine whether or not they are in the usually accepted therapeutic range (50-100 μg/ml). No recommendation regarding the safety of valproate for use at doses above 60 mg/kg/day can be made. Concomitant antiepilepsy drug (AED) dosage can ordinarily be reduced by approximately 25% every 2 weeks. This reduction may be started at initiation of divalproex sodium therapy, or delayed by 1-2 weeks if there is a concern that seizures are likely to occur with a reduction. The speed and duration of withdrawal of the concomitant AED can be highly variable, and patients should be monitored closely during this period for increased seizure frequency.

Adjunctive Therapy

Divalproex sodium may be added to the patient's regimen at a dosage of 10-15 mg/kg/day. The dosage may be increased by 5-10 mg/kg/week to achieve optimal clinical response. Ordinarily, optimal clinical response is achieved at daily doses below 60 mg/kg/day. If satisfactory clinical response has not been achieved, plasma levels should be measured to determine whether or not they are in the usually accepted therapeutic range (50-100 μg/ml). No recommendation regarding the safety of valproate for use at doses above 60 mg/kg/day can be made. If the total daily dose exceeds 250 mg, it should be given in divided doses.

In a study of adjunctive therapy for complex partial seizures in which patients were receiving either carbamazepine or phenytoin in addition to divalproex sodium, no adjustment of carbamazepine or phenytoin dosage was needed. However, since valproate may interact with these or other concurrently administered AEDs as well as other drugs. (See DRUG INTERACTIONS), periodic plasma concentration determinations of concomitant AEDs are recommended during the early course of therapy (see DRUG INTERACTIONS.)

Simple and Complex Absence Seizures

The recommended initial dose is 15 mg/kg/day, increasing at one week intervals by 5-10 mg/kg/day until seizures are controlled or side effects preclude further increases. The maximum recommended dosage is 60 mg/kg/day. If the total daily dose exceeds 250 mg, it should be given in divided doses.

A good correlation has not been established between daily dose, serum concentrations, and therapeutic effect. However, therapeutic valproate serum concentrations for most patients with absence seizures is considered to range from 50-100 μg/ml. Some patients may be controlled with lower or higher serum concentrations (see CLINICAL PHARMACOLOGY).

As the divalproex sodium dosage is titrated upward, blood concentrations of phenobarbital and/or phenytoin may be affected (see PRECAUTIONS).

Antiepilepsy drugs should not be abruptly discontinued in patients in whom the drug is administered to prevent major seizures because of the strong possibility of precipitating status elipticus with attendant hypoxia and threat to life.

In epileptic patients previously receiving divalproex sodium (valproic acid) therapy, divalproex sodium tablets should be initiated at the same daily dose and dosing schedule. After the patient is stabilized on divalproex sodium tablets, a dosing schedule of 2 or 3 times a day may be elected in selected patients.

MIGRAINE

Divalproex sodium tablets are administered orally. The recommended starting dose is 250 mg twice daily. Some patients may benefit from doses up to 1000 mg/day. In the clinical trials, there was no evidence that higher doses led to greater efficacy.

GENERAL DOSING ADVICE

Dosing in Elderly Patients

Due to a decrease in unbound clearance of valproate, the starting dose should be reduced; the ultimate therapeutic dose should be achieved on the basis of clinical response.

Dose-Related Adverse Events

The frequency of adverse effects (particularly elevated liver enzymes and thrombocytopenia) may be dose-related. The probability of thrombocytopenia appears to increase significantly at total valproate concentrations of ≥110 μg/ml (females) or ≥135 μg/ml (males) (see PRECAUTIONS). The benefit of improved therapeutic effect with higher doses should be weighed against the possibility of a greater incidence of adverse reactions.

GI Irritation

Patients who experience GI irritation may benefit from administration of the drug with food or by slowly building up the dose from an initial low level.

HOW SUPPLIED

Depakote tablets are available as 125 mg tablets (salmon pink-colored), 250 mg tablets (peach-colored), and 500 mg tablets (lavender-colored).

Storage: Store tablets and capsules below 30°C (86°F).

PRODUCT LISTING - EQUIVALENTS NOT AVAILABLE

Capsule, Enteric Coated - Oral - 125 mg

100's	$53.38	DEPAKOTE SPRINKLES, Abbott Pharmaceutical	00074-6114-13
100's	$58.06	DEPAKOTE SPRINKLES, Abbott Pharmaceutical	00074-6114-11

Tablet, Enteric Coated - Oral - 125 mg

100's	$53.09	DEPAKOTE, Abbott Pharmaceutical	00074-6212-13
100's	$57.76	DEPAKOTE, Abbott Pharmaceutical	00074-6212-11

Tablet, Enteric Coated - Oral - 250 mg

30's	$26.60	DEPAKOTE, Allscripts Pharmaceutical Company	54569-0261-00
100's	$104.26	DEPAKOTE, Abbott Pharmaceutical	00074-6214-13
100's	$111.63	DEPAKOTE, Abbott Pharmaceutical	00074-6214-11

Tablet, Enteric Coated - Oral - 500 mg

100's	$192.29	DEPAKOTE, Abbott Pharmaceutical	00074-6215-13
100's	$204.29	DEPAKOTE, Abbott Pharmaceutical	00074-6215-11

Tablet, Extended Release - Oral - 250 mg

100's	$104.25	DEPAKOTE ER, Abbott Pharmaceutical	00074-3826-13

Tablet, Extended Release - Oral - 500 mg

100's	$183.40	DEPAKOTE ER, Abbott Pharmaceutical	00074-7126-13
100's	$194.93	DEPAKOTE ER, Abbott Pharmaceutical	00074-7126-11

Dobutamine Hydrochloride *(001099)*

Categories: Decompensation, cardiac; Pregnancy Category B; FDA Approved 1978 Jul
Drug Classes: Adrenergic agonists; Inotropes
Brand Names: Dobutamine Hcl In Dextrose; Dobutamine Hcl W/Dextrose; **Dobutrex**
Foreign Brand Availability: Butamine (Israel); Cardiject (India); Cardiomin (Philippines); Dobuject (China; Czech-Republic; Denmark; Finland; Indonesia; Israel; Korea; Mexico; Russia; Singapore; Sweden; Thailand); Dobumine (Korea); Dobutamin Giulini (Germany); Dobutamin Hexal (Germany); Dobutamina (Ecuador); Dobutamin-Ratiopharm (Germany); Inotrex (Greece; Portugal); Inotrop (Indonesia); Oxiken (Mexico)
HCFA JCODE(S): J1250 per 250 mg IV

DESCRIPTION

Dobutamine in 5% dextrose injection is a sterile, nonpyrogenic, prediluted solution of dobutamine hydrochloride and dextrose in water for injection. It is administered by intravenous infusion.

Each 100 ml contains dobutamine HCl equivalent to 50, 100, 200, or 400 mg of dobutamine; dextrose, hydrous 5 g in water for injection, with sodium metabisulfite 25 mg and edetate disodium, dihydrate 10 mg added as stabilizers; osmolar concentration, respectively, 260, 263, 270, or 284 mOsmol/L (calc.). The pH is 3.0 (2.5-5.5). May contain hydrochloric acid and/or sodium hydroxide for pH adjustment. Dobutamine in 5% dextrose injection is oxygen sensitive.

Dobutamine HCl is chemically designated (±)-4-[2-[[3-(p-hydroxyphenyl)-1-methylpropyl]amino]ethyl]-pyrocatechol HCl. It is a synthetic catecholamine.

Dextrose, USP is chemically designated D-glucose monohydrate ($C_{16}H_{12}O_6 \cdot H_2O$), a hexose sugar freely soluble in water.

Water for injection is chemically designated H_2O.

The flexible plastic container is fabricated from a specially formulated nonplasticized, thermoplastic co-polyester (CR3). Water can permeate from inside the container into the overwrap but not in amounts sufficient to affect the solution significantly. Solutions inside the plastic container also can leach out certain of its chemical components in very small amounts before the expiration period has attained. However, the safety of the plastic has been confirmed by tests in animals according to USP biological standards for plastic containers.

CLINICAL PHARMACOLOGY

Dobutamine is a direct-acting inotropic agent whose primary activity results from stimulation of the β-receptors of the heart while producing comparatively mild chronotropic, hypertensive, arrhythmogenic, and vasodilative effects. It does not cause the release of endogenous norepinephrine, as does dopamine. In animal studies, dobutamine produces less increase in heart rate and less decrease in peripheral vascular resistance for a given inotropic effect than does isoproterenol.

In patients with depressed cardiac function, both dobutamine and isoproterenol increase the cardiac output to a similar degree. In the case of dobutamine, this increase is usually not accompanied by marked increases in heart rate (although tachycardia is occasionally observed), and the cardiac stroke volume is usually increased. In contrast, isoproterenol increases the cardiac index primarily by increasing the heart rate while stroke volume changes little or declines.

Facilitation of atrioventricular conduction has been observed in human electrophysiologic studies and in patients with atrial fibrillation.

Systemic vascular resistance is usually decreased with administration of dobutamine. Occasionally, minimum vasoconstriction has been observed.

Most clinical experience with dobutamine is short-term-not more than several hours in duration. In the limited number of patients who were studied for 24, 48, and 72 hours, a persistent increase in cardiac output occurred in some, whereas output returned toward baseline values in others.

The onset of action of dobutamine in 5% dextrose injection is within 1 or 2 minutes; however, as much as 10 minutes may be required to obtain the peak effect of a particular infusion rate.

The plasma half-life of dobutamine in humans is 2 minutes. The principal routes of metabolism are methylation of the catechol and conjugation. In human urine, the major excretion products are the conjugates of dobutamine and 3-O-methyl dobutamine. The 3-O-methyl derivative of dobutamine is inactive.

Alteration of synaptic concentrations of catecholamines with either reserpine or tricyclic antidepressants does not alter the actions of dobutamine in animals, which indicates that the actions of dobutamine are not dependent on presynaptic mechanisms.

INDICATIONS AND USAGE

Dobutamine in 5% dextrose injection is indicated when parenteral therapy is necessary for inotropic support in the short-term treatment of adults with cardiac decompensation due to depressed contractility resulting either from organic heart disease or from cardiac surgical procedures.

In patients who have atrial fibrillation with rapid ventricular response, a digitalis preparation should be used prior to institution of therapy with dobutamine.

NON-FDA APPROVED INDICATIONS

Although not approved by the FDA to treat congestive heart failure (CHF), there are data to show sustained improvement of cardiac function in patients with CHF after short-term (72 hour) dobutamine infusion. Dobutamine is also used without FDA approval when combined with magnetic resonance imaging or echocardiography ("stress echocardiography") for the diagnosis of coronary artery disease.

CONTRAINDICATIONS

Dobutamine in 5% dextrose injection is contraindicated in patients with idiopathic hypertrophic subaortic stenosis and in patients who have shown previous manifestations of hypersensitivity to dobutamine.

Dextrose solutions without electrolytes should not be administered simultaneously blood through the same infusion set because of the possibility that pseudoagglutination of red cells may occur.

WARNINGS

1. ***Increase in Heart Rate or Blood Pressure:*** Dobutamine HCl may cause a marked increase in heart rate or blood pressure, especially systolic pressure. Approximately 10% of patients in clinical studies have had rate increases of 30 beats/minute or more, and about 7.5% have had a 50 mm Hg or greater increase in systolic pressure. Usually, reduction of dosage promptly reverses these effects. Because dobutamine facilitates atrioventricular conduction, patients with a trial fibrillation are at risk of developing rapid ventricular response. Patients with preexisting hypertension appear to face an increased risk of developing an exaggerated pressor response.
2. ***Ectopic Activity:*** Dobutamine may precipitate or exacerbate ventricular ectopic activity, but it rarely has caused ventricular tachycardia.
3. ***Hypersensitivity:*** Reactions suggestive of hypersensitivity associated with administration of dobutamine in 5% dextrose injection, including skin rash, fever, eosinophilia, and bronchospasm, have been reported occasionally. Addictive medications should not be delivered via this solution.
4. Dobutamine in 5% dextrose injection contains sodium bisulfite, a sulfite that may cause allergic-type reactions, including anaphylactic symptoms and life-threatening or less severe asthmatic episodes in certain susceptible people. The overall prevalence of sulfite sensitivity in the general population is unknown and probably low. Sulfite sensitivity is seen more frequently in asthmatic than in nonasthmatic people.

PRECAUTIONS

1. During the administration of dobutamine in 5% dextrose injection solution, as with any adrenergic agent, ECG and blood pressure should be continuously monitored. In addition, pulmonary wedge pressure and cardiac output should be monitored whenever possible to aid in the safe and effective infusion of dobutamine in 5% dextrose injection.
2. Hypovolemia should be corrected with suitable volume expanders before treatment with dobutamine in 5% dextrose injection is instituted.
3. Animal studies indicated that dobutamine may be ineffective if the patient has recently received a β-blocking drug. In such a case, peripheral vascular resistance may increase.
4. No improvement may be observed in the presence of marked mechanical obstruction, such as severe valvular aortic stenosis.
5. Dobutamine, like other β-agonists, can produced a mild reduction in serum potassium concentration, rarely to hypokalemic levels. Accordingly, consideration should be given to monitoring serum potassium.
6. Excess administration of potassium-free solutions may result in significant hypokalemia. The intravenous administration of these solutions can cause fluid and/or solute overloading resulting in dilution of serum electrolyte concentrations, overhydration, congested states or pulmonary edema.
7. Avoid bolus administration of the drug. (See DOSAGE AND ADMINISTRATION.) Clinical evaluation and periodic laboratory determinations are necessary to monitor changes in fluid balance, electrolyte concentrations and acid-base balance during prolonged parenteral therapy or whenever the condition of the patient warrants such elevation. Solutions containing dextrose should be used with caution in patients with known subclinical or overt diabetes mellitus.
8. Dobutamine in 5% dextrose injection may exhibit a pink color that, if present, will increase with time. This color change is due to slight oxidation of the drug, but there is no significant loss of potency during the time of administration. Do not administer unless solution is clear and container is undamaged. Discard unused portion.

USAGE FOLLOWING ACUTE MYOCARDIAL INFARCTION

Clinical experience with dobutamine following myocardial infarction has been insufficient to establish the safety of drug for this use. There is concern that any agent that increases contractile force and heart rate may increase the size of an infarction by intensifying ischemia, but it is not known whether dobutamine does so.

CARCINOGENESIS, MUTAGENESIS, AND IMPAIRMENT OF FERTILITY

Studies to evaluate the carcinogenic or mutagenic potential of dobutamine or the potential of the drug to affect fertility adversely have not been performed.

PREGNANCY CATEGORY B

Reproduction studies performed in rats and rabbits have revealed no evidence of harm to the fetus due to dobutamine. The drug, however, has not been administered to pregnant women and should be used only when the expected benefits clearly outweigh the potential risks to the fetus.

PEDIATRIC USE

The safety and effectiveness of dobutamine in 5% dextrose injection for use in children have not been studied.

DRUG INTERACTIONS

There was no evidence of drug interactions in clinical studies in which dobutamine HCl was administered concurrently with other drugs, including digitalis preparations, furosemide, spironolactone, lidocaine, glyceryl trinitrate, isosorbide dinitrate, morphine, atropine, heparin, protamine, potassium chloride, folic acid, and acetaminophen. Preliminary studies indicate that the concomitant use of dobutamine and nitroprusside results in a higher cardiac output and, usually, a lower pulmonary wedge pressure than when either drug is used alone.

ADVERSE REACTIONS

INCREASED HEART RATE, BLOOD PRESSURE, AND VENTRICULAR ECTOPIC ACTIVITY

A 10-20 mm increase in systolic blood pressure and an increase in heart rate of 5-15 beats/minute have been noted in most patients (see WARNINGS regarding exaggerated chronotropic and pressor effects). Approximately 5% of patients have had increased premature ventricular beats during infusions. These effects are dose related.

HYPOTENSION

Precipitous decreases in blood pressure have occasionally been described in association with dobutamine therapy. Decreasing the dose or discontinuing the infusion typically results in rapid return of blood pressure to baseline values. In rare cases, however, intervention may be required and reversibility may not be immediate.

REACTIONS AT SITES OF INTRAVENOUS INFUSION

Phlebitis has occasionally been reported. Local inflammatory changes have been described following inadvertent infiltration.

MISCELLANEOUS UNCOMMON EFFECTS

The following adverse effects have been reported in 1-3% of patients: nausea, headache, anginal pain, nonspecific chest pain, palpitations, and shortness of breath.

Administration of dobutamine, like other catecholamines, can produce a mild reduction in serum potassium concentrations, rarely to hypokalemic levels (see PRECAUTIONS.)

LONGER-TERM SAFETY

Infusions of up to 72 hours have revealed no adverse effects other than those seen with shorter infusions.

DOSAGE AND ADMINISTRATION

Do NOT add sodium bicarbonate or other alkalinizing substance, since dobutamine is inactivated in alkaline solution. Dobutamine in 5% dextrose injection is administered only intravenously via a suitable catheter or needle infusion. The less concentrated 0.5 mg/ml solution may be preferred when fluid expansion is not a problem. The more concentrated 1 mg/ml, 2 mg/ml, or 4 mg/ml solutions may be preferred in patients with fluid retention or when a slower rate of infusion is desired.

RECOMMENDED DOSAGE

The rate of infusion needed to increase cardiac output usually ranged from 2.5-15 μg/kg/min. On rare occasions, infusion rates up to 40 μg/kg/min have been required to obtain the desired effect.

RATE OF ADMINISTRATION

When administering dobutamine (or any potent medication) by continuous intravenous infusion, it is advisable to use a precision volume control IV set.

Each patient must be individually titrated to the desired hemodynamic response to dobutamine. The rate of administration and the duration of therapy should be adjusted according to the patient's response as determined by heart rate, presence of ectopic activity, blood pressure, urine flow, and, whenever possible, measurement of central venous or pulmonary wedge pressure and cardiac output.

As with all potent intravenously administered drugs, care should be taken to control the rate of infusion so as to avoid inadvertent administration of a bolus of the drug.

Parenteral drug products should be visually inspected for particulate matter and discoloration prior to administration, whenever solution and container permit (see PRECAUTIONS and TABLE 1 through TABLE 4B.

TABLE 1 *Dobutamine Infusion Rate (ml/h) Chart Using 500 µg/ml Concentration*

	Patient Body Weight (kg)									
*	30	40	50	60	70	80	90	100	110	120
2.5	9	12	15	18	21	24	27	30	33	36
5	18	24	30	36	42	48	54	60	66	72
7.5	27	36	45	54	63	72	81	90	99	108
10	36	48	60	72	84	96	108	120	132	144
12.5	45	60	75	90	105	120	135	150	165	180
15	54	72	90	108	126	144	162	180	198	216
17.5	63	84	105	126	147	168	189	210	231	252

* Infusion rate (µg/kg/min).

TABLE 2 *Dobutamine Infusion Rate (ml/h) Chart Using 1000 µg/ml Concentration*

	Patient Body Weight (kg)									
*	30	40	50	60	70	80	90	100	110	120
2.5	4.5	6	7.5	9	10.5	12	13.5	15	16.5	18
5	9	12	15	18	21	24	27	30	33	36
7.5	13.5	18	22.5	27	31.5	36	40.5	45	49.5	54
10	18	24	30	36	42	48	54	60	66	72
12.5	22.5	30	37.5	45	52.5	60	67.5	75	82.5	90
15	27	36	45	54	63	72	81	90	99	108
17.5	31.5	42	52.5	63	73.5	84	94.5	105	115.5	126

* Infusion rate (µg/kg/min).

TABLE 3A *Dobutamine Infusion Rate (ml/h) Chart Using 2000 µg/ml Concentration*

	Patient Body Weight (kg)				
Infusion rate (µg/kg/min)	30	40	50	60	70
2.5	2.25	3	3.75	4.5	5.25
5	4.5	6	7.5	9	10.5
7.5	6.75	9	11.25	13.5	15.75
10	9	12	15	18	21
12.5	11.25	15	18.75	22.5	26.25
15	13.5	18	22.5	27	31.5
17.5	15.75	21	26.25	31.5	36.75

TABLE 3B *Dobutamine Infusion Rate (ml/h) Chart Using 2000 µg/ml Concentration*

	Patient Body Weight (kg)				
Infusion rate (µg/kg/min)	80	90	100	110	120
2.5	6	6.75	7.5	8.25	9
5	12	13.5	15	16.5	18
7.5	18	20.25	22.5	24.75	27
10	24	27	30	33	36
12.5	30	33.75	37.5	41.25	45
15	36	40.5	45	49.5	54
17.5	42	47.25	52.5	57.75	63

TABLE 4A *Dobutamine Infusion Rate (ml/h) Chart Using 4000 µg/ml Concentration*

	Patient Body Weight (kg)				
Infusion rate (µg/kg/min)	30	40	50	60	70
2.5	1.125	1.5	1.875	2.25	2.625
5	2.25	3	3.75	4.5	5.25
7.5	3.375	4.5	5.625	6.75	7.875
10	4.5	6	7.5	9	10.5
12.5	5.625	7.5	9.375	11.25	13.125
15	6.75	9	11.25	13.5	15.75
17.5	7.875	10.5	13.125	15.75	18.375

INSTRUCTIONS FOR USE

To Open: Tear outer wrap at notch and remove solution container. Some opacity of the plastic due to moisture absorption during the sterilization process may be observed. This is normal and does not affect the solution quality or safety. The opacity will diminish gradually.

PREPARATION FOR ADMINISTRATION (USE ASEPTIC TECHNIQUE)

1. Close flow control clamp of administration set.
2. Remove cover from outlet port at bottom of container.
3. Insert piercing pin of administration set into port with a twisting motion until the set is firmly seated. *Note:* See full directions on administration set carton.

TABLE 4B *Dobutamine Infusion Rate (ml/h) Chart Using 4000 µg/ml Concentration*

	Patient Body Weight (kg)				
Infusion rate (µg/kg/min)	80	90	100	110	120
2.5	3	3.375	3.75	4.125	4.5
5	6	6.75	7.5	8.25	9
7.5	9	10.125	11.25	12.375	13.5
10	12	13.5	15	16.5	18
12.5	15	16.875	18.75	20.625	22.5
15	18	20.25	22.5	24.75	27
17.5	21	23.625	26.25	28.875	31.5

4. Suspend container from hanger.
5. Squeeze and release drip chamber to establish proper fluid level in chamber.
6. Open flow control clamp and clear air from set. Close clamp.
7. Attach set to venipuncture device. If device is not indwelling, prime and make venipuncture.
8. Regulate rate of administration with flow control clamp.

WARNING: Do not use flexible container in series connections.

HOW SUPPLIED

Dobutamine in 5% Dextrose Injection is supplied in 250 and 500 ml LifeCare flexible containers.

Exposure of pharmaceutical products to heat should be minimized.

Avoid excessive heat. Protect from freezing. It is recommended that the product be stored at room temperature (25°C); however, brief exposure up to 40°C does not adversely affect the product.

PRODUCT LISTING - RATED THERAPEUTICALLY EQUIVALENT

Solution - Intravenous - 5%;50 mg/100 ml

250 ml x 12	$731.70	GENERIC, Abbott Pharmaceutical	00074-2345-32
500 ml x 12	$535.50	GENERIC, Abbott Pharmaceutical	00074-2345-34

Solution - Intravenous - 5%;100 mg/100 ml

250 ml x 12	$244.39	GENERIC, Abbott Pharmaceutical	00074-2346-32
250 ml x 18	$894.96	GENERIC, Baxter I.V. Systems Division	00338-1073-02
500 ml x 12	$710.52	GENERIC, Baxter I.V. Systems Division	00338-1073-03
500 ml x 12	$732.74	GENERIC, Abbott Pharmaceutical	00074-2346-34

Solution - Intravenous - 5%;200 mg/100 ml

250 ml x 12	$366.37	GENERIC, Abbott Pharmaceutical	00074-2347-32
250 ml x 18	$1549.26	GENERIC, Baxter I.V. Systems Division	00338-1075-02

Solution - Intravenous - 5%;400 mg/100 ml

250 ml x 12	$488.49	GENERIC, Abbott Pharmaceutical	00074-3724-32
250 ml x 18	$2617.65	GENERIC, Baxter I.V. Systems Division	00338-1077-02

Solution - Intravenous - 12.5 mg/ml

20 ml	$9.87	GENERIC, Abbott Pharmaceutical	00074-2344-01
20 ml	$9.89	GENERIC, Abbott Pharmaceutical	00074-3440-10
20 ml	$21.00	GENERIC, Bedford Laboratories	55390-0560-20
20 ml	$51.88	GENERIC, Lilly, Eli and Company	00702-7375-01
20 ml x 10	$49.88	GENERIC, Abbott Pharmaceutical	00074-2025-20
20 ml x 10	$59.38	GENERIC, Lilly, Eli and Company	00702-7375-10
20 ml x 10	$92.39	GENERIC, Abbott Pharmaceutical	00074-2344-02
20 ml x 10	$120.00	DOBUTREX, Lilly, Eli and Company	00002-7175-10
20 ml x 10	$120.00	DOBUTREX, Lilly, Eli and Company	00002-7375-10
20 ml x 10	$122.13	GENERIC, Abbott Pharmaceutical	00074-3440-20
20 ml x 10	$169.20	GENERIC, Gensia Sicor Pharmaceuticals Inc	00703-1815-03
20 ml x 10	$210.00	GENERIC, Bedford Laboratories	55390-0560-90
20 ml x 25	$68.75	GENERIC, Baxter Pharmaceutical Products, Inc	10019-0184-20
40 ml x 10	$79.80	GENERIC, Abbott Pharmaceutical	00074-2025-54
40 ml x 10	$234.00	GENERIC, Sanofi Winthrop Pharmaceuticals	00024-0594-01
100 ml	$14.35	GENERIC, Abbott Pharmaceutical	00074-4729-01

PRODUCT LISTING - EQUIVALENTS NOT AVAILABLE

Solution - Intravenous - 5%;100 mg/100 ml

250 ml x 18	$601.88	GENERIC, Lilly, Eli and Company	00002-7496-01
500 ml x 12	$596.64	GENERIC, Baxter I.V. Systems Division	00338-1071-03

Solution - Intravenous - 5%;200 mg/100 ml

250 ml x 18	$216.00	GENERIC, Lilly, Eli and Company	00002-7498-01

Solution - Intravenous - 5%;400 mg/100 ml

250 ml	$126.88	GENERIC, B. Braun/Mcgaw Inc	00264-9823-59
250 ml x 18	$337.50	GENERIC, Lilly, Eli and Company	00002-7500-01

Solution - Intravenous - 12.5 mg/ml

20 ml x 10	$31.30	GENERIC, American Regent Laboratories Inc	00517-2075-10

Docetaxel (003205)

Categories: Carcinoma, breast; Carcinoma, lung; FDA Approved 1996 May; Pregnancy Category D
Drug Classes: Antineoplastics, antimitotics
Brand Names: Taxotere
Foreign Brand Availability: Doxotel (Thailand); Dexotel (India); Oncodocel (Colombia); Taxoter (Russia)
HCFA JCODE(S): J9170 20 mg IV

WARNING

Docetaxel for injection concentrate should be administered under the supervision of a qualified physician experienced in the use of antineoplastic agents. Appropriate management of complications is possible only when adequate diagnostic and treatment facilities are readily available.

The incidence of treatment-related mortality associated with docetaxel therapy is increased in patients with abnormal liver function, in patients receiving higher doses, and in patients with non-small cell lung carcinoma and a history of prior treatment with platinum-based chemotherapy who receive docetaxel as a single agent at a dose of 100 mg/m^2 (see WARNINGS).

Docetaxel should generally not be given to patients with bilirubin >upper limit of normal (ULN), or to patients with SGOT and/or SGPT >1.5 × ULN concomitant with alkaline phosphatase >2.5 × ULN. Patients with elevations of bilirubin or abnormalities of transaminase concurrent with alkaline phosphatase are at increased risk for the development of Grade 4 neutropenia, febrile neutropenia, infections, severe thrombocytopenia, severe stomatitis, severe skin toxicity, and toxic death. Patients with isolated elevations of transaminase >1.5 × ULN also had a higher rate of febrile neutropenia Grade 4 but did not have an increased incidence of toxic death. Bilirubin, SGOT or SGPT, and alkaline phosphatase values should be obtained prior to each cycle of docetaxel therapy and reviewed by the treating physician.

Docetaxel therapy should not be given to patients with neutrophil counts of <1500 cells/mm^3. In order to monitor the occurrence of neutropenia, which may be severe and result in infection, frequent blood cell counts should be performed on all patients receiving docetaxel.

Severe hypersensitivity reactions characterized by hypotension and/or bronchospasm, or generalized rash/erythema occurred in 2.2% (2/92) of patients who received the recommended 3 day dexamethasone premedication. Hypersensitivity reactions requiring discontinuation of the docetaxel infusion were reported in 5 patients who did not receive premedication. These reactions resolved after discontinuation of the infusion and the administration of appropriate therapy. Docetaxel must not be given to patients who have a history of severe hypersensitivity reactions to docetaxel or to other drugs formulated with polysorbate 80 (see WARNINGS).

Severe fluid retention occurred in 6.5% (6/92) of patients despite use of a 3 day dexamethasone premedication regimen. It was characterized by 1 or more of the following events: poorly tolerated peripheral edema, generalized edema, pleural effusion requiring urgent drainage, dyspnea at rest, cardiac tamponade, or pronounced abdominal distention (due to ascites) (see PRECAUTIONS).

DESCRIPTION

Docetaxel is an antineoplastic agent belonging to the taxoid family. It is prepared by semisynthesis beginning with a precursor extracted from the renewable needle biomass of yew plants. The chemical name for docetaxel is (2R,3S)-N-carboxy-3-phenylisoserine,N-*tert*-butyl ester,13-ester with 5β-20-epoxy-1,2α,4,7β,10β,13α-hexahydroxytax-11-en-9-one 4-acetate 2-benzoate, trihydrate.

Docetaxel is a white to almost-white powder with an empirical formula of $C_{43}H_{53}NO_{14}\cdot 3H_2O$, and a molecular weight of 861.9. It is highly lipophilic and practically insoluble in water. Taxotere (docetaxel) for injection concentrate is a clear yellow to brownish-yellow viscous solution. Taxotere is sterile, non-pyrogenic, and is available in single-dose vials containing 20 mg (0.5 ml) or 80 mg (2.0 ml) docetaxel (anhydrous). Each ml contains 40 mg docetaxel (anhydrous) and 1040 mg polysorbate 80.

Taxotere for injection concentrate requires dilution prior to use. A sterile, non-pyrogenic, single-dose diluent is supplied for that purpose. The diluent for Taxotere contains 13% ethanol in water for injection, and is supplied in 1.5 ml (to be used with 20 mg Taxotere for injection concentrate) and 6.0 ml (to be used with 80 mg Taxotere for injection concentrate) vials.

CLINICAL PHARMACOLOGY

Docetaxel is an antineoplastic agent that acts by disrupting the microtubular network in cells that is essential for mitotic and interphase cellular functions. Docetaxel binds to free tubulin and promotes the assembly of tubulin into stable microtubules while simultaneously inhibiting their disassembly. This leads to the production of microtubule bundles without normal function and to the stabilization of microtubules, which results in the inhibition of mitosis in cells. Docetaxel's binding to microtubules does not alter the number of protofilaments in the bound microtubules, a feature which differs from most spindle poisons currently in clinical use.

HUMAN PHARMACOKINETICS

The pharmacokinetics of docetaxel have been evaluated in cancer patients after administration of 20-115 mg/m^2 in Phase 1 studies. The area under the curve (AUC) was dose proportional following doses of 70-115 mg/m^2 with infusion times of 1-2 hours. Docetaxel's pharmacokinetic profile is consistent with a three-compartment pharmacokinetic model, with half-lives for the α, β, and γ phases of 4 minutes, 36 minutes, and 11.1 hours, respectively. The initial rapid decline represents distribution to the peripheral compartments and the late (terminal) phase is due, in part, to a relatively slow efflux of docetaxel from the peripheral compartment. Mean values for total body clearance and steady state volume of distribution were 21 L/h/m^2 and 113 L, respectively. Mean total body clearance for Japanese patients dosed at the range of 10-90 mg/m^2 was similar to that of European/American populations dosed at 100 mg/m^2, suggesting no significant difference in the elimination of docetaxel in the 2 populations.

A study of ^{14}C-docetaxel was conducted in 3 cancer patients. Docetaxel was eliminated in both the urine and feces following oxidative metabolism of the *tert*-butyl ester group, but fecal excretion was the main elimination route. Within 7 days, urinary and fecal excretion accounted for approximately 6% and 75% of the administered radioactivity, respectively. About 80% of the radioactivity recovered in feces is excreted during the first 48 hours as 1 major and 3 minor metabolites with very small amounts (less than 8%) of unchanged drug.

A population pharmacokinetic analysis was carried out after docetaxel treatment of 535 patients dosed at 100 mg/m^2. Pharmacokinetic parameters estimated by this analysis were very close to those estimated from Phase 1 studies. The pharmacokinetics of docetaxel were not influenced by age or gender and docetaxel total body clearance was not modified by pretreatment with dexamethasone. In patients with clinical chemistry data suggestive of mild to moderate liver function impairment (SGOT and/or SGPT >1.5 times the upper limit of normal [ULN] concomitant with alkaline phosphatase >2.5 times ULN), total body clearance was lowered by an average of 27%, resulting in a 38% increase in systemic exposure (AUC). This average, however, includes a substantial range and there is, at present, no measurement that would allow recommendation for dose adjustment in such patients. Patients with combined abnormalities of transaminase and alkaline phosphatase should, in general, not be treated with docetaxel.

Clearance of docetaxel in combination therapy with cisplatin was similar to that previously observed following monotherapy with docetaxel. The pharmacokinetic profile of cisplatin in combination therapy with docetaxel was similar to that observed with cisplatin alone.

In vitro studies showed that docetaxel is about 94% protein bound, mainly to α_1-acid glycoprotein, albumin, and lipoproteins. In 3 cancer patients, the *in vitro* binding to plasma proteins was found to be approximately 97%. Dexamethasone does not affect the protein binding of docetaxel.

In vitro drug interaction studies revealed that docetaxel is metabolized by the CYP3A4 isoenzyme, and its metabolism can be inhibited by CYP3A4 inhibitors, such as ketoconazole, erythromycin, troleandomycin, and nifedipine. Based on *in vitro* findings, it is likely that CYP3A4 inhibitors and/or substrates may lead to substantial increases in docetaxel blood concentrations. No clinical studies have been performed to evaluate this finding (see PRECAUTIONS).

INDICATIONS AND USAGE

BREAST CANCER

Docetaxel is indicated for the treatment of patients with locally advanced or metastatic breast cancer after failure of prior chemotherapy.

NON-SMALL CELL LUNG CANCER

Docetaxel, as a single agent, is indicated for the treatment of patients with locally advanced or metastatic non-small cell lung cancer after failure of prior platinum-based chemotherapy.

Docetaxel in combination with cisplatin is indicated for the treatment of patients with unresectable, locally advanced or metastatic non-small cell lung cancer who have not previously received chemotherapy for this condition.

CONTRAINDICATIONS

Docetaxel is contraindicated in patients who have a history of severe hypersensitivity reactions to docetaxel or to other drugs formulated with polysorbate 80.

Docetaxel should not be used in patients with neutrophil counts of <1500 cells/mm^3.

WARNINGS

Docetaxel should be administered under the supervision of a qualified physician experienced in the use of antineoplastic agents. Appropriate management of complications is possible only when adequate diagnostic and treatment facilities are readily available.

TOXIC DEATHS

Breast Cancer

Docetaxel administered at 100 mg/m^2 was associated with deaths considered possibly or probably related to treatment in 2.0% (19/965) of metastatic breast cancer patients, both previously treated and untreated, with normal baseline liver function and in 11.5% (7/61) of patients with various tumor types who had abnormal baseline liver function (SGOT and/or SGPT >1.5 times ULN together with AP >2.5 times ULN). Among patients dosed at 60 mg/m^2, mortality related to treatment occurred in 0.6% (3/481) of patients with normal liver function, and in 3 of 7 patients with abnormal liver function. Approximately half of these deaths occurred during the first cycle. Sepsis accounted for the majority of the deaths.

Non-Small Cell Lung Cancer

Docetaxel administered at a dose of 100 mg/m^2 in patients with locally advanced or metastatic non-small cell lung cancer who had a history of prior platinum-based chemotherapy was associated with increased treatment-related mortality (14% and 5% in 2 randomized, controlled studies). There were 2.8% treatment-related deaths among the 176 patients treated at the 75 mg/m^2 dose in the randomized trials. Among patients who experienced treatment-related mortality at the 75 mg/m^2 dose level, 3 of 5 patients had a PS of 2 at study entry (see BOXED WARNING and DOSAGE AND ADMINISTRATION).

Premedication Regimen

All patients should be premedicated with oral corticosteroids such as dexamethasone 16 mg/day (*e.g.*, 8 mg bid) for 3 days starting 1 day prior to docetaxel to reduce the severity of fluid retention and hypersensitivity reactions (see DOSAGE AND ADMINISTRATION). This regimen was evaluated in 92 patients with metastatic breast cancer previously treated with chemotherapy given docetaxel at a dose of 100 mg/m^2 every 3 weeks.

Hypersensitivity Reactions

Patients should be observed closely for hypersensitivity reactions, especially during the first and second infusions. Severe hypersensitivity reactions characterized by hypotension and/or bronchospasm, or generalized rash/erythema occurred in 2.2% of the 92 patients premedicated with 3 day corticosteroids. Hypersensitivity reactions requiring discontinuation of the docetaxel infusion were reported in 5 out of 1260 patients with various tumor types who did not receive premedication, but in 0/92 patients premedicated with 3 day corticosteroids. Patients with a history of severe hypersensitivity reactions should not be rechallenged with docetaxel.

Hematologic Effects

Neutropenia (<2000 neutrophils/mm^3) occurs in virtually all patients given 60-100 mg/m^2 of docetaxel and Grade 4 neutropenia (<500 cells/mm^3) occurs in 85% of patients given 100 mg/m^2 and 75% of patients given 60 mg/m^2. Frequent monitoring of blood counts is, therefore, essential so that dose can be adjusted. Docetaxel should not be administered to patients with neutrophils <1500 cells/mm^3.

Febrile neutropenia occurred in about 12% of patients given 100 mg/m^2 but was very uncommon in patients given 60 mg/m^2. Hematologic responses, febrile reactions and infections, and rates of septic death for different regimens are dose related.

Three breast cancer patients with severe liver impairment (bilirubin >1.7 times ULN) developed fatal gastrointestinal bleeding associated with severe drug-induced thrombocytopenia.

Hepatic Impairment

See BOXED WARNING.

Fluid Retention

See BOXED WARNING.

Pregnancy

Docetaxel can cause fetal harm when administered to pregnant women. Studies in both rats and rabbits at doses ≥0.3 and 0.03 mg/kg/day, respectively (about 1/50 and 1/300 the daily maximum recommended human dose on a mg/m^2 basis), administered during the period of organogenesis, have shown that docetaxel is embryotoxic and fetotoxic (characterized by intrauterine mortality, increased resorption, reduced fetal weight, and fetal ossification delay).

The doses indicated above also caused maternal toxicity.

There are no adequate and well-controlled studies in pregnant women using docetaxel. If docetaxel is used during pregnancy, or if the patient becomes pregnant while receiving this drug, the patient should be apprised of the potential hazard to the fetus or potential risk for loss of the pregnancy. Women of childbearing potential should be advised to avoid becoming pregnant during therapy with docetaxel.

PRECAUTIONS

GENERAL

Responding patients may not experience an improvement in performance status on therapy and may experience worsening. The relationship between changes in performance status, response to therapy, and treatment-related side effects has not been established.

HEMATOLOGIC EFFECTS

In order to monitor the occurrence of myelotoxicity, it is recommended that frequent peripheral blood cell counts be performed on all patients receiving docetaxel. Patients should not be retreated with subsequent cycles of docetaxel until neutrophils recover to a level >1500 cells/mm^3 and platelets recover to a level >100,000 cells/mm^3.

A 25% reduction in the dose of docetaxel for injection concentrate is recommended during subsequent cycles following severe neutropenia (<500 cells/mm^3) lasting 7 days or more, febrile neutropenia, or a Grade 4 infection in a docetaxel cycle (see DOSAGE AND ADMINISTRATION).

HYPERSENSITIVITY REACTIONS

Hypersensitivity reactions may occur within a few minutes following initiation of a docetaxel infusion. If minor reactions such as flushing or localized skin reactions occur, interruption of therapy is not required. More severe reactions, however, require the immediate discontinuation of docetaxel and aggressive therapy. All patients should be premedicated with an oral corticosteroid prior to the initiation of the infusion of docetaxel (see BOXED WARNING and WARNINGS, Premedication Regimen).

CUTANEOUS

Localized erythema of the extremities with edema followed by desquamation has been observed. In case of severe skin toxicity, an adjustment in dosage is recommended (see DOSAGE AND ADMINISTRATION). The discontinuation rate due to skin toxicity was 1.6% (15/965) for metastatic breast cancer patients. Among 92 breast cancer patients premedicated with 3 day corticosteroids, there were no cases of severe skin toxicity reported and no patient discontinued docetaxel due to skin toxicity.

FLUID RETENTION

Severe fluid retention has been reported following docetaxel therapy (see BOXED WARNING and WARNINGS, Premedication Regimen). Patients should be premedicated with oral corticosteroids prior to each docetaxel administration to reduce the incidence and severity of fluid retention (see DOSAGE AND ADMINISTRATION). Patients with pre-existing effusions should be closely monitored from the first dose for the possible exacerbation of the effusions.

When fluid retention occurs, peripheral edema usually starts in the lower extremities and may become generalized with a median weight gain of 2 kg.

Among 92 breast cancer patients premedicated with 3 day corticosteroids, moderate fluid retention occurred in 27.2% and severe fluid retention in 6.5%. The median cumulative dose to onset of moderate or severe fluid retention was 819 mg/m^2. Nine (9) of 92 (9.8%) of patients discontinued treatment due to fluid retention: 4 patients discontinued with severe fluid retention; the remaining 5 had mild or moderate fluid retention. The median cumulative dose to treatment discontinuation due to fluid retention was 1021 mg/m^2. Fluid retention was completely, but sometimes slowly, reversible with a median of 16 weeks from the last infusion of docetaxel to resolution (range: 0-42+ weeks). Patients developing peripheral edema may be treated with standard measures, *e.g.*, salt restriction, oral diuretic(s).

NEUROLOGIC

Severe neurosensory symptoms (paresthesia, dysesthesia, pain) were observed in 5.5% (53/965) of metastatic breast cancer patients, and resulted in treatment discontinuation in 6.1%. When these symptoms occur, dosage must be adjusted. If symptoms persist, treatment should be discontinued (see DOSAGE AND ADMINISTRATION). Patients who experienced neurotoxicity in clinical trials and for whom follow-up information on the complete resolution of the event was available had spontaneous reversal of symptoms with a median of 9 weeks from onset (range: 0-106 weeks). Severe peripheral motor neuropathy mainly manifested as distal extremity weakness occurred in 4.4% (42/965).

ASTHENIA

Severe asthenia has been reported in 14.9% (144/965) of metastatic breast cancer patients but has led to treatment discontinuation in only 1.8%. Symptoms of fatigue and weakness may last a few days up to several weeks and may be associated with deterioration of performance status in patients with progressive disease.

INFORMATION FOR THE PATIENT

For additional information, see the Patient Information leaflet accompanying your prescription.

CARCINOGENESIS, MUTAGENESIS, AND IMPAIRMENT OF FERTILITY

No studies have been conducted to assess the carcinogenic potential of docetaxel. Docetaxel has been shown to be clastogenic in the *in vitro* chromosome aberration test in CHO-K_1 cells and in the *in vivo* micronucleus test in the mouse, but it did not induce mutagenicity in the Ames test or the CHO/HGPRT gene mutation assays. Docetaxel produced no impairment of fertility in rats when administered in multiple IV doses of up to 0.3 mg/kg (about 1/50 the recommended human dose on a mg/m^2 basis), but decreased testicular weights were reported. This correlates with findings of a 10 cycle toxicity study (dosing once every 21 days for 6 months) in rats and dogs in which testicular atrophy or degeneration was observed at IV doses of 5 mg/kg in rats and 0.375 mg/kg in dogs (about 1/3 and 1/15 the recommended human dose on a mg/m^2 basis, respectively). An increased frequency of dosing in rats produced similar effects at lower dose levels.

PREGNANCY CATEGORY D

See WARNINGS.

NURSING MOTHERS

It is not known whether docetaxel is excreted in human milk. Because many drugs are excreted in human milk, and because of the potential for serious adverse reactions in nursing infants from docetaxel, mothers should discontinue nursing prior to taking the drug.

PEDIATRIC USE

The safety and effectiveness of docetaxel in pediatric patients have not been established.

DRUG INTERACTIONS

There have been no formal clinical studies to evaluate the drug interactions of docetaxel with other medications. *In vitro* studies have shown that the metabolism of docetaxel may be modified by the concomitant administration of compounds that induce, inhibit, or are metabolized by cytochrome P450 3A4, such as cyclosporine, terfenadine, ketoconazole, erythromycin, and troleandomycin. Caution should be exercised with these drugs when treating patients receiving docetaxel as there is a potential for a significant interaction.

ADVERSE REACTIONS

The adverse reactions are described separately for docetaxel 100 mg/m^2, the maximum dose approved for breast cancer, and 75 mg/m^2, the dose approved for advanced non-small cell lung carcinoma after prior platinum-based chemotherapy and in combination with cisplatin for treatment of patients with non-small cell lung carcinoma who have not previously received chemotherapy for this condition.

DOCETAXEL 100 MG/M^2

Adverse drug reactions occurring in at least 5% of patients are compared for 3 populations who received docetaxel administered at 100 mg/m^2 as a 1 hour infusion every 3 weeks: 2045 patients with various tumor types and normal baseline liver function tests; the subset of 965 patients with locally advanced or metastatic breast cancer, both previously treated and untreated with chemotherapy, who had normal baseline liver function tests; and an additional 61 patients with various tumor types who had abnormal liver function tests at baseline. These reactions were described using COSTART terms and were considered possibly or probably related to docetaxel. At least 95% of these patients did not receive hematopoietic support. The safety profile is generally similar in patients receiving docetaxel for the treatment of breast cancer and in patients with other tumor types.

HEMATOLOGIC

See WARNINGS.

Reversible marrow suppression was the major dose-limiting toxicity of docetaxel. The median time to nadir was 7 days, while the median duration of severe neutropenia (<500 cells/mm^3) was 7 days. Among 2045 patients with solid tumors and normal baseline LFTs, severe neutropenia occurred in 75.4% and lasted for more than 7 days in 2.9% of cycles.

Febrile neutropenia (<500 cells/mm^3 with fever >38°C with IV antibiotics and/or hospitalization) occurred in 11% of patients with solid tumors, in 12.3% of patients with metastatic breast cancer, and in 9.8% of 92 breast cancer patients premedicated with 3 day corticosteroids.

Severe infectious episodes occurred in 6.1% of patients with solid tumors, in 6.4% of patients with metastatic breast cancer, and in 5.4% of 92 breast cancer patients premedicated with 3 day corticosteroids.

TABLE 8 *Summary of Adverse Events in Patients Receiving Docetaxel at 100 mg/m²*

Adverse Event	All Tumor Types Normal LFTs* n=2045	All Tumor Types Elevated LFTs† n=61	Breast Cancer Normal LFTs* n=965
Hematologic			
Neutropenia			
<2000 cells/mm³	95.5%	96.4%	98.5%
<500 cells/mm³	75.4%	87.5%	85.9%
Leukopenia			
<4000 cells/mm³	95.6%	98.3%	98.6%
<1000 cells/mm³	31.6%	46.6%	43.7%
Thrombocytopenia			
<100,000 cells/mm³	8.0%	24.6%	9.2%
Anemia			
<11 g/dl	90.4%	91.8%	93.6%
<8 g/dl	8.8%	31.1%	7.7%
Febrile neutropenia‡	11.0%	26.2%	12.3%
Septic Death	1.6%	4.9%	1.4%
Non-Septic Death	0.6%	6.6%	0.6%
Infections			
Any	21.6%	32.8%	22.2%
Severe	6.1%	16.4%	6.4%
Fever in Absence of Infection			
Any	31.2%	41.0%	35.1%
Severe	2.1%	8.2%	2.2%
Hypersensitivity Reactions			
Regardless of premedication			
Any	21.0%	19.7%	17.6%
Severe	4.2%	9.8%	2.6%
With 3 day premedication	n=92	n=3	n=92
Any	15.2%	33.3%	15.2%
Severe	2.2%	0%	2.2%
Fluid Retention			
Regardless of premedication			
Any	47.0%	39.3%	59.7%
Severe	6.9%	8.2%	8.9%
With 3 day premedication	n=92	n=3	n=92
Any	64.1%	66.7%	64.1%
Severe	6.5%	33.3%	6.5%
Neurosensory			
Any	49.3%	34.4%	58.3%
Severe	4.3%	0%	5.5%
Cutaneous			
Any	47.6%	54.1%	47.0%
Severe	4.8%	9.8%	5.2%
Nail Changes			
Any	30.6%	23.0%	40.5%
Severe	2.5%	4.9%	3.7%
Gastrointestinal			
Nausea	38.8%	37.7%	42.1%
Vomiting	22.3%	23.0%	23.4%
Diarrhea	38.7%	32.8%	42.6%
Severe	4.7%	4.9%	5.5%
Stomatitis			
Any	41.7%	49.2%	51.7%
Severe	5.5%	13.0%	7.4%
Alopecia	75.8%	62.3%	74.2%
Asthenia			
Any	61.8%	52.5%	66.3%
Severe	12.8%	24.6%	14.9%
Myalgia			
Any	18.9%	16.4%	21.1%
Severe	1.5%	1.6%	1.8%
Arthralgia	9.2%	6.6%	8.2%
Infusion Site Reactions	4.4%	3.3%	4.0%

*** Normal Baseline LFTs: Transaminases ≤1.5 times ULN or alkaline phosphatase ≤2.5 times ULN or isolated elevations of transaminases or alkaline phosphatase up to 5 times ULN.**
† Elevated Baseline LFTs: SGOT and/or SGPT >1.5 times ULN concurrent with alkaline phosphatase >2.5 times ULN.
‡ Febrile Neutropenia: ANC Grade 4 with fever >38°C with IV antibiotics and/or hospitalization.

Thrombocytopenia (<100,000 cells/mm³) associated with fatal gastrointestinal hemorrhage has been reported.

HYPERSENSITIVITY REACTIONS

Severe hypersensitivity reactions are discussed in BOXED WARNING, WARNINGS, and PRECAUTIONS. Minor events, including flushing, rash with or without pruritus, chest tightness, back pain, dyspnea, drug fever, or chills, have been reported and resolved after discontinuing the infusion and appropriate therapy.

FLUID RETENTION

See BOXED WARNING, WARNINGS, Premedication Regimen, and PRECAUTIONS.

CUTANEOUS

Severe skin toxicity is discussed in PRECAUTIONS. Reversible cutaneous reactions characterized by a rash including localized eruptions, mainly on the feet and/or hands, but also on the arms, face, or thorax, usually associated with pruritus, have been observed. Eruptions generally occurred within 1 week after docetaxel infusion, recovered before the next infusion, and were not disabling.

Severe nail disorders were characterized by hypo- or hyperpigmentation, and occasionally by onycholysis (in 0.8% of patients with solid tumors) and pain.

NEUROLOGIC

See PRECAUTIONS.

GASTROINTESTINAL

Gastrointestinal reactions (nausea and/or vomiting and/or diarrhea) were generally mild to moderate. Severe reactions occurred in 3-5% of patients with solid tumors and to a similar extent among metastatic breast cancer patients. The incidence of severe reactions was 1% or less for the 92 breast cancer patients premedicated with 3 day corticosteroids.

Severe stomatitis occurred in 5.5% of patients with solid tumors, in 7.4% of patients with metastatic breast cancer, and in 1.1% of the 92 breast cancer patients premedicated with 3 day corticosteroids.

CARDIOVASCULAR

Hypotension occurred in 2.8% of patients with solid tumors; 1.2% required treatment. Clinically meaningful events such as heart failure, sinus tachycardia, atrial flutter, dysrhythmia, unstable angina, pulmonary edema, and hypertension occurred rarely. 8.1% (7/86) of metastatic breast cancer patients receiving docetaxel 100 mg/m² in a randomized trial and who had serial left ventricular ejection fractions assessed developed deterioration of LVEF by ≥10% associated with a drop below the institutional lower limit of normal.

INFUSION SITE REACTIONS

Infusion site reactions were generally mild and consisted of hyperpigmentation, inflammation, redness or dryness of the skin, phlebitis, extravasation, or swelling of the vein.

HEPATIC

In patients with normal LFTs at baseline, bilirubin values greater than the ULN occurred in 8.9% of patients. Increases in SGOT or SGPT >1.5 times the ULN, or alkaline phosphatase >2.5 times ULN, were observed in 18.9% and 7.3% of patients, respectively. While on docetaxel, increases in SGOT and/or SGPT >1.5 times ULN concomitant with alkaline phosphatase >2.5 times ULN occurred in 4.3% of patients with normal LFTs at baseline. (Whether these changes were related to the drug or underlying disease has not been established.)

MONOTHERAPY WITH DOCETAXEL FOR UNRESECTABLE, LOCALLY ADVANCED OR METASTATIC NSCLC PREVIOUSLY TREATED WITH PLATINUM-BASED CHEMOTHERAPY

Docetaxel 75 mg/m²

Treatment emergent adverse drug reactions are shown in TABLE 9. Included in TABLE 9 are safety data for a total of 176 patients with non-small cell lung carcinoma and a history of prior treatment with platinum-based chemotherapy who were treated in 2 randomized, controlled trials. These reactions were described using NCI Common Toxicity Criteria regardless of relationship to study treatment, except for the hematologic toxicities or otherwise noted.

COMBINATION THERAPY WITH DOCETAXEL IN CHEMOTHERAPY NAÏVE ADVANCED UNRESECTABLE OR METASTATIC NSCLC

TABLE 10 presents safety data from 2 arms of an open label, randomized controlled trial (TAX326) that enrolled patients with unresectable stage IIIB or IV non-small cell lung cancer and no history of prior chemotherapy. Adverse reactions were described using the NCI Common Toxicity Criteria except where otherwise noted.

Deaths within 30 days of last study treatment occurred in 31 patients (7.6%) in the docetaxel + cisplatin arm and 37 patients (9.3%) in the vinorelbine + cisplatin arm. Deaths within 30 days of last study treatment attributed to study drug occurred in 9 patients (2.2%) in the docetaxel + cisplatin arm and 8 patients (2.0%) in the vinorelbine + cisplatin arm.

The second comparison in the study, vinorelbine + cisplatin versus docetaxel + carboplatin (which did not demonstrate a superior survival associated with docetaxel) demonstrated a higher incidence of thrombocytopenia, diarrhea, fluid retention, hypersensitivity reactions, skin toxicity, alopecia and nail changes on the docetaxel + carboplatin arm, while a higher incidence of anemia, neurosensory toxicity, nausea, vomiting, anorexia and asthenia was observed on the vinorelbine + cisplatin arm.

POST-MARKETING EXPERIENCES

The following adverse events have been identified from clinical trials and/or post-marketing surveillance. Because they are reported from a population of unknown size, precise estimates of frequency cannot be made.

Body as a whole: Diffuse pain, chest pain, radiation recall phenomenon.
Cardiovascular: Atrial fibrillation, deep vein thrombosis, ECG abnormalities, thrombophlebitis, pulmonary embolism, syncope, tachycardia, myocardial infarction.
Cutaneous: Rare cases of bullous eruption such as erythema multiforme or Stevens-Johnson syndrome. Multiple factors may have contributed to the development of these effects.
Gastrointestinal: Abdominal pain, anorexia, constipation, duodenal ulcer, esophagitis, gastrointestinal hemorrhage. Rare occurrences of dehydration as a consequence to gastrointestinal events, gastrointestinal perforation, ischemic colitis, colitis, intestinal obstruction, ileus, and neutropenic enterocolitis have been reported.
Hematologic: Bleeding episodes.
Hepatic: Rare cases of hepatitis have been reported.
Neurologic: Confusion, rare cases of seizures or transient loss of consciousness have been observed, sometimes appearing during the infusion of the drug.
Ophthalmologic: Conjunctivitis, lacrimation or lacrimation with or without conjunctivitis. Rare cases of lacrimal duct obstruction resulting in excessive tearing have been reported primarily in patients receiving other anti-tumor agents concomitantly.
Respiratory: Dyspnea, acute pulmonary edema, acute respiratory distress syndrome, interstitial pneumonia.
Urogenital: Renal insufficiency.

DOSAGE AND ADMINISTRATION

BREAST CANCER

The recommended dose of docetaxel is 60-100 mg/m² administered intravenously over 1 hour every 3 weeks.

TABLE 9 *Treatment Emergent Adverse Events Regardless of Relationship to Treatment in Patients Receiving Docetaxel as Monotherapy for Non-Small Cell Lung Cancer Previously Treated With Platinum-Based Chemotherapy**

Adverse Event	Docetaxel 75 mg/m² n=176	Best Supportive Care n=49	Vinorelbine/ Ifosfamide n=119
Neutropenia			
Any	84.1%	14.3%	83.2%
Grade 3/4	65.3%	12.2%	57.1%
Leukopenia			
Any	83.5%	6.1%	89.1%
Grade 3/4	49.4%	0%	42.9%
Thrombocytopenia			
Any	8.0%	0%	7.6%
Grade 3/4	2.8%	0%	1.7%
Anemia			
Any	91.0%	55.1%	90.8%
Grade 3/4	9.1%	12.2%	14.3%
Febrile Neutropenia†	6.3%	NA†	0.8%
Infection			
Any	33.5%	28.6%	30.3%
Grade 3/4	10.2%	6.1%	9.2%
Treatment Related Mortality	2.8%	NA†	3.4%
Hypersensitivity Reactions			
Any	5.7%	0%	0.8%
Grade 3/4	2.8%	0%	0%
Fluid Retention			
Any	33.5%	ND‡	22.7%
Severe	2.8%	-	3.4%
Neurosensory			
Any	23.3%	14.3%	28.6%
Grade 3/4	1.7%	6.1%	5.0%
Neuromotor			
Any	15.9%	8.2%	10.1%
Grade 3/4	4.5%	6.1%	3.4%
Skin			
Any	19.9%	6.1%	16.8%
Grade 3/4	0.6%	2.0%	0.8%
Gastrointestinal			
Nausea			
Any	33.5%	30.6%	31.1%
Grade 3/4	5.1%	4.1%	7.6%
Vomiting			
Any	21.6%	26.5%	21.8%
Grade 3/4	2.8%	2.0%	5.9%
Diarrhea			
Any	22.7%	6.1%	11.8%
Grade 3/4	2.8%	0%	4.2%
Alopecia	56.3%	34.7%	49.6%
Asthenia			
Any	52.8%	57.1%	53.8%
Severe‡	18.2%	38.8%	22.7%
Stomatitis			
Any	26.1%	6.1%	7.6%
Grade 3/4	1.7%	0%	0.8%
Pulmonary			
Any	40.9%	49.0%	45.4%
Grade 3/4	21.0%	28.6%	18.5%
Nail Disorder			
Any	11.4%	0%	1.7%
Severe‡	1.1%	0%	0%
Myalgia			
Any	6.3%	0%	2.5%
Severe‡	0%	0%	0%
Arthralgia			
Any	3.4%	2.0%	1.7%
Severe‡	0%	0%	0.8%
Taste Perversion			
Any	5.7%	0%	0%
Severe‡	0.6%	0%	0%

*** Normal Baseline LFTs: Transaminases ≤1.5 times ULN or alkaline phosphatase ≤2.5 times ULN or isolated elevations of transaminases or alkaline phosphatase up to 5 times ULN.**
† Febrile Neutropenia: ANC Grade 4 with fever >38°C with IV antibiotics and/or hospitalization.
‡ COSTART term and grading system.
NA = Not Applicable.
ND = Not Done.

NON-SMALL CELL LUNG CANCER

For treatment after failure of prior platinum-based chemotherapy, docetaxel was evaluated as monotherapy, and the recommended dose is 75 mg/m² administered intravenously over 1 hour every 3 weeks. A dose of 100 mg/m² in patients previously treated with chemotherapy was associated with increased hematologic toxicity, infection, and treatment-related mortality in randomized, controlled trials (see BOXED WARNING and WARNINGS).

For chemotherapy-naïve patients, docetaxel was evaluated in combination with cisplatin. The recommended dose of docetaxel is 75 mg/m² administered intravenously over 1 hour immediately followed by cisplatin 75 mg/m² over 30-60 minutes every 3 weeks.

PREMEDICATION REGIMEN

All patients should be premedicated with oral corticosteroids such as dexamethasone 16 mg/day (*e.g.*, 8 mg bid) for 3 days starting 1 day prior to docetaxel administration in order to reduce the incidence and severity of fluid retention as well as the severity of hypersensitivity reactions (see BOXED WARNING, WARNINGS, and PRECAUTIONS).

TABLE 10 *Adverse Events Regardless of Relationship to Treatment in Chemotherapy Naïve Advanced Non-Small Cell Lung Cancer Patients Receiving Docetaxel in Combination With Cisplatin*

Adverse Event	Docetaxel 75 mg/m² + Cisplatin 75 mg/m² n=406	Vinorelbine 25 mg/m² + Cisplatin 100 mg/m² n=396
Neutropenia		
Any	91%	90%
Grade 3/4	74%	78%
Febrile Neutropenia	5%	5%
Thrombocytopenia		
Any	15%	15%
Grade 3/4	3%	4%
Anemia		
Any	89%	94%
Grade 3/4	7%	25%
Infection		
Any	35%	37%
Grade 3/4	8%	8%
Fever in Absence of Infection		
Any	33%	29%
Grade 3/4	<1%	1%
Hypersensitivity Reaction*		
Any	12%	4%
Grade 3/4	3%	<1%
Fluid Retention†		
Any	54%	42%
All severe or life-threatening events	2%	2%
Pleural effusion		
Any	23%	22%
All severe or life-threatening events	2%	2%
Peripheral edema		
Any	34%	18%
All severe or life-threatening events	<1%	<1%
Weight gain		
Any	15%	9%
All severe or life-threatening events	<1%	<1%
Neurosensory		
Any	47%	42%
Grade 3/4	4%	4%
Neuro-motor		
Any	19%	17%
Grade 3/4	3%	6%
Skin		
Any	16%	14%
Grade 3/4	<1%	1%
Nausea		
Any	72%	76%
Grade 3/4	10%	17%
Vomiting		
Any	55%	61%
Grade 3/4	8%	16%
Diarrhea		
Any	47%	25%
Grade 3/4	7%	3%
Anorexia†		
Any	42%	40%
All severe or life-threatening events	5%	5%
Stomatitis		
Any	24%	21%
Grade 3/4	2%	1%
Alopecia		
Any	75%	42%
Grade 3	<1%	0%
Asthenia†		
Any	74%	75%
All severe or life-threatening events	12%	14%
Nail Disorder†		
Any	14%	<1%
All severe events	<1%	0%
Myalgia†		
Any	18%	12%
All severe events	<1%	<1%

* Replaces NCI term "Allergy".
† COSTART term and grading system.

DOSAGE ADJUSTMENTS DURING TREATMENT

Breast Cancer

Patients who are dosed initially at 100 mg/m² and who experience either febrile neutropenia, neutrophils <500 cells/mm³ for more than 1 week, or severe or cumulative cutaneous reactions during docetaxel therapy should have the dosage adjusted from 100 mg/m² to 75 mg/m². If the patient continues to experience these reactions, the dosage should either be decreased from 75 mg/m² to 55 mg/m² or the treatment should be discontinued. Conversely, patients who are dosed initially at 60 mg/m² and who do not experience febrile neutropenia, neutrophils <500 cells/mm³ for more than 1 week, severe or cumulative cutaneous reactions, or severe peripheral neuropathy during docetaxel therapy may tolerate higher doses. Patients who develop ≥Grade 3 peripheral neuropathy should have docetaxel treatment discontinued entirely.

Non-Small Cell Lung Cancer

Monotherapy With Docetaxel for NSCLC Treatment After Failure of Prior Platinum Based Chemotherapy

Patients who are dosed initially at 75 mg/m^2 and who experience either febrile neutropenia, neutrophils <500 cells/mm^3 for more than 1 week, severe or cumulative cutaneous reactions, or other Grade 3/4 non-hematological toxicities during docetaxel treatment should have treatment withheld until resolution of the toxicity and then resumed at 55 mg/m^2. Patients who develop ≥Grade 3 peripheral neuropathy should have docetaxel treatment discontinued entirely.

Combination Therapy With Docetaxel for Chemotherapy Naive NSCLC

For patients who are dosed initially at docetaxel 75 mg/m^2 in combination with cisplatin, and whose nadir of platelet count during the previous course of therapy is <25,000 cells/mm^3, in patients who experience febrile neutropenia, and in patients with serious non-hematologic toxicities, the docetaxel dosage in subsequent cycles should be reduced to 65 mg/m^2. In patients who require a further dose reduction, a dose of 50 mg/m^2 is recommended. For cisplatin dosage adjustments, see manufacturers' prescribing information.

Special Populations

Hepatic Impairment

Patients with bilirubin >ULN should generally not receive docetaxel. Also, patients with SGOT and/or SGPT >1.5 × ULN concomitant with alkaline phosphatase >2.5 × ULN should generally not receive docetaxel.

Children

The safety and effectiveness of docetaxel in pediatric patients below the age of 16 years have not been established.

Elderly

See PRECAUTIONS, Geriatric Use.

In general, dose selection for an elderly patient should be cautious, reflecting the greater frequency of decreased hepatic, renal, or cardiac function and of concomitant disease or other drug therapy in elderly patients.

PREPARATION AND ADMINISTRATION PRECAUTIONS

Docetaxel is a cytotoxic anticancer drug and, as with other potentially toxic compounds, caution should be exercised when handling and preparing docetaxel solutions. The use of gloves is recommended. Please refer to HOW SUPPLIED, Handling and Disposal.

If docetaxel concentrate, initial diluted solution, or final dilution for infusion should come into contact with the skin, immediately and thoroughly wash with soap and water. If docetaxel concentrate, initial diluted solution, or final dilution for infusion should come into contact with mucosa, immediately and thoroughly wash with water.

Docetaxel for injection concentrate requires two dilutions prior to administration.

The initial diluted solution may be used immediately or stored either in the refrigerator or at room temperature for a maximum of 8 hours.

The final docetaxel dilution for infusion should be administered intravenously as a 1 hour infusion under ambient room temperature and lighting conditions.

Contact of the docetaxel concentrate with plasticized PVC equipment or devices used to prepare solutions for infusion is not recommended. In order to minimize patient exposure to the plasticizer DEHP (di-2-ethylhexyl phthalate), which may be leached from PVC infusion bags or sets, the final docetaxel dilution for infusion should be stored in bottles (glass, polypropylene) or plastic bags (polypropylene, polyolefin) and administered through polyethylene-lined administration sets.

STABILITY

Docetaxel infusion solution, if stored between 2 and 25°C (36 and 77°F) is stable for 4 hours. Fully prepared docetaxel infusion solution (in either 0.9% sodium chloride solution or 5% dextrose solution) should be used within 4 hours (including the 1 hour IV administration).

HOW SUPPLIED

Taxotere for injection concentrate is supplied in a single-dose vial as a sterile, pyrogen-free, non-aqueous, viscous solution with an accompanying sterile, non-pyrogenic, diluent (13% ethanol in water for injection) vial. The following strengths are available:

Taxotere (docetaxel) 80 mg concentrate for infusion: 80 mg docetaxel in 2 ml polysorbate 80 and diluent for docetaxel 80 mg. Thirteen percent (13%) (w/w) ethanol in water for injection.

Taxotere (docetaxel) 20 mg concentrate for infusion: 20 mg docetaxel in 0.5 ml polysorbate 80 and diluent for docetaxel 20 mg. Thirteen percent 13% (w/w) ethanol in water for injection.

Storage: Store between 2 and 25°C (36 and 77°F). Retain in the original package to protect from bright light. Freezing does not adversely affect the product.

HANDLING AND DISPOSAL

Procedures for proper handling and disposal of anticancer drugs should be considered. Several guidelines on this subject have been published[1-7]. There is no general agreement that all of the procedures recommended in the guidelines are necessary or appropriate.

PRODUCT LISTING - EQUIVALENTS NOT AVAILABLE

Solution - Intravenous - 40 mg/ml

0.50 ml	$376.75	TAXOTERE, Aventis Pharmaceuticals	00075-8001-20
2 ml	$1506.96	TAXOTERE, Aventis Pharmaceuticals	00075-8001-80

Docusate Sodium (001104)

Categories: Constipation; FDA Pre 1938 Drugs
Drug Classes: Laxatives
Brand Names: Prenate-90
Foreign Brand Availability: Colace (Canada; Ireland); Coloxyl (Australia; New-Zealand); Cusate (Thailand); Jamylene (France); Lambanol (Italy); Laxadine (Indonesia); Norgalax (Bahrain; Belgium; Cyprus; Egypt; Iran; Iraq; Jordan; Kuwait; Lebanon; Libya; Oman; Qatar; Republic-of-Yemen; Russia; Saudi-Arabia; Syria; United-Arab-Emirates); Regutol (Bahrain; Cyprus; Egypt; Iran; Iraq; Jordan; Kuwait; Lebanon; Libya; Oman; Qatar; Republic-of-Yemen; Saudi-Arabia; Syria; United-Arab-Emirates); Selax (Canada); Soflax (Canada); Softon (Hong-Kong); Tirolaxo (Spain)

D

DESCRIPTION

Colace (docusate sodium) is a stool softner.

Colace capsules, 50 mg, contain the following:

Active ingredient: Contains 50 mg of docusate sodium.

Inactive ingredients: Polyethylene glycol 400, gelatin, glycerin, sorbitol, propylene glycol, FD&C red no. 40, D&C red no. 33.

Colace capsules, 100 mg, contain the following:

Active ingredient: Contains 100 mg of docusate sodium.

Inactive ingredients: Polyethylene glycol 400, gelatin, glycerin, sorbitol, propylene glycol, methylparaben, titanium dioxide, FD&C red no. 40, D&C red no. 33, propylparaben, FD&C yellow no. 6.

Colace liquid, 1%, contains the following:

Active ingredient: Each ml contains 10 mg of docusate sodium.

Inactive ingredients: Citric acid, D&C red no. 33, methylparaben, poloxamer, polyethylene glycol, propylene glycol, propylparaben, sodium citrate, vanillin, and purified water.

Colace syrup, 20 mg/5 ml, contains the following:

Active ingredient: Each 5 ml contains 20 mg of docusate sodium.

Inactive ingredients: Alcohol (not more than 1%), citric acid, D&C red no. 33, FD&C red no. 40, flavor (natural), menthol, methylparaben, peppermint oil, poloxamer, polyethylene glycol, propylparaben, sodium citrate, sucrose, and purified water.

CLINICAL PHARMACOLOGY

Docusate sodium, a surface-active agent, helps to keep stools soft for easy, natural passage and is not a stimulant laxative, thus, not habit forming. Useful in constipation due to hard stools, in painful anorectal conditions, in cardiac and other conditions in which maximum ease of passage is desirable to avoid difficult or painful defecation, and when peristaltic stimulants are contraindicated.

INDICATIONS AND USAGE

NON-FDA APPROVED INDICATIONS

Although not an FDA approved use, docusate liquid has been used in emergency departments for the removal of cerumen when visualization of the tympanic membrane is necessary.

CONTRAINDICATIONS

There are no known contraindications to docusate sodium.

WARNINGS

Do not use when abdominal pain, nausea, or vomiting are present, unless directed by a doctor.

As with any drug, pregnant or nursing women should seek the advice of a health professional before using this product.

ADVERSE REACTIONS

The incidence of side effects — none of a serious nature — is exceedingly small. Bitter taste, throat irritation, and nausea (primarily associated with the use of the syrup and liquid) are the main side effects reported. Rash has occurred.

DOSAGE AND ADMINISTRATION

ORALLY

Suggested Daily Dosage:

Adults and older children: 50-200 mg.

Children 6-12: 40-120 mg liquid.

Children 3-6 years of age: 2 ml one to three times daily.

Infants and children under 3 years of age: As prescribed by physician.

The higher doses are recommended for initial therapy. Dosage should be adjusted to individual response. The effect on stools is usually apparent 1-3 days after the first dose. Docusate sodium liquid or syrup may be given in a 6-8 oz glass of milk or fruit juice or in infant's formula to prevent throat irritation.

FOR RETENTION OR FLUSHING ENEMAS

Add 5-10 ml (1-2 teaspoons) of docusate sodium liquid to enema fluid.

HOW SUPPLIED

COLACE CAPSULES

Colace capsules are supplied in 50 and 100 mg strengths.

Storage: Store at controlled room temperature 15-30°C (59-86°F).

COLACE LIQUID

Colace liquid, 1% solution; 10 mg/ml is supplied in16 fl oz and 30 ml bottles with a calibrated dropper.

COLACE SYRUP
Colace syrup, 20 mg/5 ml teaspoon; contains not more than 1% alcohol, is supplied in 8 and 16 fl oz bottles.

Dofetilide *(003482)*

Categories: Fibrillation, atrial; Flutter, atrial; FDA Approved 1999 Oct; Pregnancy Category C
Drug Classes: Antiarrhythmics, class III
Foreign Brand Availability: Tikosyn (Austria; Belgium; Bulgaria; Czech-Republic; Denmark; England; Finland; France; Germany; Greece; Hungary; Ireland; Italy; Netherlands; Norway; Poland; Portugal; Slovenia; Spain; Sweden; Switzerland; Turkey)
Cost of Therapy: $118.01 (Atrial Fibrillation/Atrial Flutter; Tikosyn; 500 µg; 2 capsules/day; 30 day supply)

D

WARNING

To minimize the risk of induced arrhythmia, patients initiated or re-initiated on dofetilide should be placed for a minimum of 3 days in a facility that can provide calculations of creatinine clearance, continuous electrocardiographic monitoring, and cardiac resuscitation. For detailed instructions regarding dose selection, see DOSAGE AND ADMINISTRATION. Dofetilide is available only to hospitals and prescribers who have received appropriate dofetilide dosing and treatment initiation education, see DOSAGE AND ADMINISTRATION.

DESCRIPTION

Dofetilide is an antiarrhythmic drug with Class III (cardiac action potential duration prolonging) properties. Its empirical formula is $C_{19}H_{27}N_3O_5S_2$ and it has a molecular weight of 441.6.

The chemical name for dofetilide is N-[4-[2-[methyl[2-[4-[(methylsulfonyl)amino]phenoxy]ethyl]amino]ethyl]phenyl]- methanesulfonamide.

Dofetilide is a white to off-white powder. It is very slightly soluble in water and propan-2-ol and is soluble in 0.1 M aqueous sodium hydroxide, acetone and aqueous 0.1 M hydrochloric acid.

Tikosyn capsules contain the following inactive ingredients: Microcrystalline cellulose, corn starch, colloidal silicon dioxide and magnesium stearate. Tikosyn is supplied for oral administration in 3 dosage strengths: 125 µg (0.125 mg) orange and white capsules, 250 µg (0.25 mg) peach capsules, and 500 µg (0.5 mg) peach and white capsules.

CLINICAL PHARMACOLOGY

MECHANISM OF ACTION

Dofetilide shows Vaughan Williams Class III antiarrhythmic activity. The mechanism of action is blockade of the cardiac ion channel carrying the rapid component of the delayed rectifier potassium current, I_{Kr}. At concentrations covering several orders of magnitude, dofetilide blocks only I_{Kr} with no relevant block of the other repolarizing potassium currents (*e.g.*, I_{Ks}, I_{K1}). At clinically relevant concentrations dofetilide has no effect on sodium channels (associated with Class I effect), adrenergic alpha receptors, or adrenergic beta receptors.

ELECTROPHYSIOLOGY

Dofetilide increases the monophasic action potential duration in a predictable, concentration-dependent manner, primarily due to delayed repolarization. This effect, and the related increase in effective refractory period, is observed in the atria and ventricles in both resting and paced electrophysiology studies. The increase in QT interval observed on the surface ECG is a result of prolongation of both effective and functional refractory periods in the His-Purkinje system and the ventricles.

Dofetilide did not influence cardiac conduction velocity and sinus node function in a variety of studies in patients with or without structural heart disease. This is consistent with a lack of effect of dofetilide on the PR interval and QRS width in patients with pre-existing heart block and/or sick sinus syndrome.

In patients, dofetilide terminates induced re-entrant tachyarrhythmias (*e.g.*, atrial fibrillation/flutter and ventricular tachycardia) and prevents their re-induction. Dofetilide does not increase the electrical energy required to convert electrically-induced ventricular fibrillation, and it significantly reduces the defibrillation threshold in patients with ventricular tachycardia and ventricular fibrillation undergoing implantation of a cardioverter-defibrillator device.

HEMODYNAMICS

In hemodynamic studies, dofetilide had no effect on cardiac output, cardiac index, stroke volume index, or systemic vascular resistance in patients with ventricular tachycardia, mild to moderate congestive heart failure or angina and either normal or low left ventricular ejection fraction. There was no evidence of a negative inotropic effect related to dofetilide therapy in patients with atrial fibrillation. There was no increase in heart failure in patients with significant left ventricular dysfunction. In the overall clinical program, dofetilide did not affect blood pressure. Heart rate was decreased by 4-6 bpm in studies in patients.

PHARMACOKINETICS

Absorption and Distribution

The oral bioavailability of dofetilide is >90%, with maximal plasma concentrations occurring at about 2-3 hours in the fasted state. Oral bioavailability is unaffected by food or antacid. The terminal half life of dofetilide is approximately 10 hours; steady state plasma concentrations are attained within 2-3 days, with an accumulation index of 1.5-2.0. Plasma concentrations are dose proportional. Plasma protein binding of dofetilide is 60-70%, is independent of plasma concentration, and is unaffected by renal impairment. Volume of distribution is 3 L/kg.

Metabolism and Excretion

Approximately 80% of a single dose of dofetilide is excreted in urine, of which approximately 80% is excreted as unchanged dofetilide with the remaining 20% consisting of inactive or minimally active metabolites. Renal elimination involves both glomerular filtration and active tubular secretion (via the cation transport system, a process that can be inhibited by cimetidine, trimethoprim, prochlorperazine, megestrol and ketoconazole). *In vitro* studies with human liver microsomes show that dofetilide can be metabolized by CYP3A4, but it has a low affinity for this isoenzyme. Metabolites are formed by N-dealkylation and N-oxidation. There are no quantifiable metabolites circulating in plasma, but 5 metabolites have been identified in urine.

PHARMACOKINETICS IN SPECIAL POPULATIONS

Renal Impairment

In volunteers with varying degrees of renal impairment and patients with arrhythmias, the clearance of dofetilide decreases with decreasing creatinine clearance. As a result, and as seen in clinical studies, the half-life of dofetilide is longer in patients with lower creatinine clearances. **Because increase in QT interval and the risk of ventricular arrhythmias are directly related to plasma concentrations of dofetilide, dosage adjustment based on calculated creatinine clearance is critically important** (see DOSAGE AND ADMINISTRATION). Patients with severe renal impairment (creatinine clearance <20 ml/min) were not included in clinical or pharmacokinetic studies (see CONTRAINDICATIONS).

Hepatic Impairment

There was no clinically significant alteration in the pharmacokinetics of dofetilide in volunteers with mild to moderate hepatic impairment (Child-Pugh class A and B) compared to age- and weight-matched healthy volunteers. Patients with severe hepatic impairment were not studied.

Patients With Heart Disease

Population pharmacokinetic analyses indicate that the plasma concentration of dofetilide in patients with supraventricular and ventricular arrhythmias, ischemic heart disease, or congestive heart failure are similar to those of healthy volunteers, after adjusting for renal function.

Elderly

After correction for renal function, clearance of dofetilide is not related to age.

Women

A population pharmacokinetic analysis showed that women have approximately 12-18% lower dofetilide oral clearances than men (14-22% greater plasma dofetilide levels), after correction for weight and creatinine clearance. In females, as in males, renal function was the single most important factor influencing dofetilide clearance. In normal female volunteers, hormone replacement therapy (a combination of conjugated estrogens and medroxyprogesterone) did not increase dofetilide exposure.

DRUG-DRUG INTERACTIONS

See DRUG INTERACTIONS.

Dose-Response and Concentration Response for Increase in QT Interval

Increase in QT interval is directly related to dofetilide dose and plasma concentration. The relationship in normal volunteers between dofetilide plasma concentrations and change in QTc is linear, with a positive slope of approximately 15-25 milliseconds/(ng/ml) after the first dose and approximately 10-15 milliseconds/(ng/ml) at Day 23 (reflecting a steady state of dosing). A linear relationship between mean QTc increase and dofetilide dose was also seen in patients with renal impairment, in patients with ischemic heart disease, and in patients with supraventricular and ventricular arrhythmias.

INDICATIONS AND USAGE

MAINTENANCE OF NORMAL SINUS RHYTHM (DELAY IN AF/AFL RECURRENCE)

Dofetilide is indicated for the maintenance of normal sinus rhythm (delay in time to recurrence of atrial fibrillation/atrial flutter [AF/AFl]) in patients with atrial fibrillation/atrial flutter of greater than 1 week duration who have been converted to normal sinus rhythm. Because dofetilide can cause life threatening ventricular arrhythmias, it should be reserved for patients in whom atrial fibrillation/atrial flutter is highly symptomatic.

In general, antiarrhythmic therapy for atrial fibrillation/atrial flutter aims to prolong the time in normal sinus rhythm. Recurrence is expected in some patients.

CONVERSION OF ATRIAL FIBRILLATION/FLUTTER

Dofetilide is indicated for the conversion of atrial fibrillation and atrial flutter to normal sinus rhythm.

Dofetilide has not been shown to be effective in patients with paroxysmal atrial fibrillation.

CONTRAINDICATIONS

Dofetilide is contraindicated in patients with congenital or acquired long QT syndromes. Dofetilide should not be used in patients with a baseline QT interval or QTc >440 milliseconds (500 milliseconds in patients with ventricular conduction abnormalities). Dofetilide is also contraindicated in patients with severe renal impairment (calculated creatinine clearance <20 ml/min).

The concomitant use of verapamil or the cation transport system inhibitors cimetidine, trimethoprim (alone or in combination with sulfamethoxazole) or ketoconazole with dofetilide is contraindicated (see DRUG INTERACTIONS), as each of these drugs cause a substantial increase in dofetilide plasma concentrations. In addition, other known inhibitors of the renal cation transport system such as prochlorperazine and megestrol should not be used in patients on dofetilide.

Dofetilide is also contraindicated in patients with a known hypersensitivity to the drug.

WARNINGS

VENTRICULAR ARRHYTHMIA

Dofetilide can cause serious ventricular arrhythmias, primarily torsade de pointes (TdP) type ventricular tachycardia, a polymorphic ventricular tachycardia associated with QT interval prolongation. QT interval prolongation is directly related to dofetilide plasma concentration. Factors such as reduced creatinine clearance or certain dofetilide drug interactions will increase dofetilide plasma concentration. The risk of TdP can be reduced by controlling the plasma concentration through adjustment of the initial dofetilide dose according to creatinine clearance and by monitoring the ECG for excessive increases in the QT interval.

Treatment with dofetilide must therefore be started only in patients placed for a minimum of 3 days in a facility that can provide electrocardiographic monitoring and in the presence of personnel trained in the management of serious ventricular arrhythmias. Calculation of the creatinine clearance for all patients must precede administration of the first dose of dofetilide. For detailed instructions regarding dose selection, see DOSAGE AND ADMINISTRATION.

The risk of dofetilide induced ventricular arrhythmia was assessed in 3 ways in clinical studies: (1) by description of the QT interval and its relation to the dose and plasma concentration of dofetilide; (2) by observing the frequency of TdP in dofetilide treated patients according to dose; (3) by observing the overall mortality rate in patients with atrial fibrillation and in patients with structural heart disease.

Relation of QT Interval to Dose

The QT interval increases linearly with increasing dofetilide dose.

Frequency of Torsade de Pointes

In the supraventricular arrhythmia population (patients with AF and other supraventricular arrhythmias) the overall incidence of torsade de pointes was 0.8%. The frequency of TdP by dose is shown in TABLE 4. There were no cases of TdP on placebo.

TABLE 4 *Summary of Torsade de Pointes in Patients Randomized to Dofetilide by Dose; Patients With Supraventricular Arrhythmias*

Dofetilide Dose	Number of Patients	Torsade de Pointes
<250 μg bid	217	0
250 μg bid	388	1 (0.3%)
>250-500 μg bid	703	6 (0.9%)
>500 μg bid	38	4 (10.5%)
All doses	1346	11 (0.8%)

As shown in TABLE 5, the rate of TdP was reduced when patients were dosed according to their renal function (see CLINICAL PHARMACOLOGY, Pharmacokinetics in Special Populations, Renal Impairment, and DOSAGE AND ADMINISTRATION).

TABLE 5 *Incidence of Torsade de Pointes Before and After Introduction of Dosing According to Renal Function*

Population	Total n/N %	Before n/N %	After n/N %
Supreventricular arrhythmias	11/1346 (0.8%)	6/193 (3.1%)	5/1153 (0.4%)
DIAMOND CHF	25/762 (3.3%)	7/148 (4.7%)	18/614 (2.9%)
DIAMOND MI	7/749 (0.9%)	3/101 (3.0%)	4/648 (0.6%)
DIAMOND AF	4/249 (1.6%)	0/43 (0%)	4/206 (1.9%)

The majority of the episodes of TdP occurred within the first 3 days of dofetilide therapy (10/11 events in the studies of patients with supraventricular arrhythmias; 19/25 and 4/7 events in DIAMOND CHF and DIAMOND MI, respectively; 2/4 events in the DIAMOND AF subpopulation).

Mortality

In a pooled survival analysis of patients in the supraventricular arrhythmia population (low prevalence of structural heart disease), deaths occurred in 0.9% (12/1346) of patients receiving dofetilide and 0.4% (3/677) in the placebo group. Adjusted for duration of therapy, primary diagnosis, age, gender, and prevalence of structural heart disease, the point estimate of the hazard ratio for the pooled studies (dofetilide/placebo) was 1.1 (95% CI: 0.3, 4.3). The DIAMOND CHF and MI trials examined mortality in patients with structural heart disease (ejection fraction ≤35%). In these large, double-blind studies, deaths occurred in 36% (541/1511) of dofetilide patients and 37% (560/1517) of placebo patients. In an analysis of 506 DIAMOND patients with atrial fibrillation/flutter at baseline, 1 year mortality on dofetilide was 31% vs 32% on placebo.

Because of the small number of events, an excess mortality due to dofetilide cannot be ruled out with confidence in the pooled survival analysis of placebo-controlled trials in patients with supraventricular arrhythmias. However, it is reassuring that in 2 large placebo-controlled mortality studies in patients with significant heart disease (DIAMOND CHF/MI), there were no more deaths in dofetilide-treated patients than in patients given placebo.

DRUG-DRUG INTERACTIONS

See CONTRAINDICATIONS.

Because there is a linear relationship between dofetilide plasma concentration and QTc, concomitant drugs that interfere with the metabolism or renal elimination of dofetilide may increase the risk of arrhythmia (torsade de pointes). Dofetilide is metabolized to a small degree by the CYP3A4 isoenzyme of the cytochrome P450 system and an inhibitor of this system could increase systemic dofetilide exposure. More important, dofetilide is eliminated by cationic renal secretion, and 3 inhibitors of this process have been shown to increase systemic dofetilide exposure. The magnitude of the effect on renal elimination by cimetidine, trimethoprim and ketoconazole (all contraindicated concomitant uses with dofetilide) suggests that all renal cation transport inhibitors should be contraindicated.

USE WITH DRUGS THAT PROLONG QT INTERVAL AND ANTIARRHYTHMIC AGENTS

The use of dofetilide in conjunction with other drugs that prolong the QT interval has not been studied and is not recommended. Such drugs include phenothiazines, cisapride, bepridil, tricyclic antidepressants, and certain oral macrolides. Class I or Class III antiarrhythmic agents should be withheld for at least 3 half-lives prior to dosing with dofetilide. In clinical trials, dofetilide was administered to patients previously treated with oral amiodarone only if serum amiodarone levels were below 0.3 mg/L or amiodarone had been withdrawn for at least 3 months.

PRECAUTIONS

RENAL IMPAIRMENT

The overall systemic clearance of dofetilide is decreased and plasma concentration increased with decreasing creatinine clearance. The dose of dofetilide must be adjusted based on creatinine clearance (see DOSAGE AND ADMINISTRATION). Patients undergoing dialysis were not included in clinical studies, and appropriate dosing recommendations for these patients are unknown. There is no information about the effectiveness of hemodialysis in removing dofetilide from plasma.

HEPATIC IMPAIRMENT

After adjustment for creatinine clearance, no additional dose adjustment is required for patients with mild or moderate hepatic impairment. Patients with severe hepatic impairment have not been studied. Dofetilide should be used with particular caution in these patients.

CARDIAC CONDUCTION DISTURBANCES

Animal and human studies have not shown any adverse effects of dofetilide on conduction velocity. No effect on AV nodal conduction following dofetilide treatment was noted in normal volunteers and in patients with first-degree heart block. Patients with sick sinus syndrome or with second- or third-degree heart block were not included in the Phase 3 clinical trials unless a functioning pacemaker was present. Dofetilide has been used safely in conjunction with pacemakers (53 patients in DIAMOND studies, 136 in trials in patients with ventricular and supraventricular arrhythmias).

POTASSIUM-DEPLETING DIURETICS

Hypokalemia or hypomagnesemia may occur with administration of potassium-depleting diuretics, increasing the potential for torsade de pointes. Potassium levels should be within the normal range prior to administration of dofetilide and maintained in the normal range during administration of dofetilide.

INFORMATION FOR THE PATIENT

Please refer patient to the patient package insert.

Prior to initiation of dofetilide therapy, the patient should be advised to read the patient package insert and reread it each time therapy is renewed in case the patient's status has changed. The patient should be fully instructed on the need for compliance with the recommended dosing of dofetilide and the potential for drug interactions, and the need for periodic monitoring of QTc and renal function to minimize the risk of serious abnormal rhythms.

Medications and Supplements

Assessment of patients' medication history should include all over-the-counter, prescription and herbal/natural preparations with emphasis on preparations that may affect the pharmacokinetics of dofetilide such as cimetidine, trimethoprim alone or in combination with sulfamethoxazole, prochlorperazine, megestrol, ketoconazole, other cardiovascular drugs (especially verapamil), phenothiazines, and tricyclic antidepressants (see WARNINGS). See also CONTRAINDICATIONS. If a patient is taking dofetilide and requires anti-ulcer therapy, omeprazole, ranitidine or antacids (aluminum and magnesium hydroxides) should be used as alternatives to cimetidine, as these agents have no effect on the pharmacokinetics of dofetilide. Patients should be instructed to notify their health care providers of any change in over-the-counter, prescription or supplement use. If a patient is hospitalized or is prescribed a new medication for any condition, the patient must inform the health care provider of ongoing dofetilide therapy. Patients should also check with their health care provider and/or pharmacist prior to taking a new over-the-counter preparation.

Electrolyte Imbalance

If patients experience symptoms that may be associated with altered electrolyte balance, such as excessive or prolonged diarrhea, sweating, or vomiting or loss of appetite or thirst, these conditions should immediately be reported to their health care provider.

Dosing Schedule

Patients should be instructed NOT to double the next dose if a dose is missed. The next dose should be taken at the usual time.

DRUG/LABORATORY TEST INTERACTIONS

None known.

CARCINOGENESIS, MUTAGENESIS, AND IMPAIRMENT OF FERTILITY

Dofetilide had no genotoxic effects, with or without metabolic activation, based on the bacterial mutation assay and tests of cytogenetic aberrations *in vivo* in mouse bone marrow and *in vitro* in human lymphocytes. Rats and mice treated with dofetilide in the diet for 2 years showed no evidence of an increased incidence of tumors compared to controls. The highest dofetilide dose administered for 24 months was 10 mg/kg/day to rats and 20 mg/kg/day to mice. Mean dofetilide AUCs(0-24h) at these doses were about 26 and 10 times, respectively, the maximum likely human AUC.

There was no effect on mating or fertility when dofetilide was administered to male and female rats at doses as high as 1.0 mg/kg/day, a dose that would be expected to provide a mean dofetilide AUC(0-24h) about 3 times the maximum likely human AUC. Increased incidences of testicular atrophy and epididymal oligospermia and a reduction in testicular weight were, however, observed in other studies in rats. Reduced testicular weight and increased incidence of testicular atrophy were also consistent findings in dogs and mice. The no effect doses for these findings in chronic administration studies in these 3 species (3, 0.1 and 6 mg/kg/day) were associated with mean dofetilide AUCs that were about 4, 1.3 and 3 times the maximum likely human AUC, respectively.

PREGNANCY CATEGORY C

Dofetilide has been shown to adversely affect *in utero* growth and survival of rats and mice when orally administered during organogenesis at doses of ≥2 or more mg/kg/day. Other than an increased incidence of non-ossified 5th metacarpal, and the occurrence of hydroureter and hydronephroses at doses as low as 1 mg/kg/day in the rat, structural anomalies associated with drug treatment were not observed in either species at doses below 2 mg/kg/day. The clearest drug-effect associations were for sternebral and vertebral anomalies in both species; cleft palate, adactyly, levocardia, dilation of cerebral ventricles, hydroureter, hydronephroses, and unossified metacarpal in the rat; and increased incidence of unossified calcaneum in the mouse. The "no observed adverse effect dose" in both species was 0.5 mg/kg/day. The mean dofetilide AUCs(0-24h) at this dose in the rat and mouse are estimated to be about equal to the maximum likely human AUC and about half the likely human AUC, respectively. There are no adequate and well controlled studies in pregnant women. Therefore, dofetilide should only be administered to pregnant women where the benefit to the patient justifies the potential risk to the fetus.

D

NURSING MOTHERS

There is no information on the presence of dofetilide in breast milk. Patients should be advised not to breast feed an infant if they are taking dofetilide.

GERIATRIC USE

Of the total number of patients in clinical studies of dofetilide, 46% were 65-89 years old. No overall differences in safety, effect on QTc, or effectiveness were observed between elderly and younger patients. Because elderly patients are more likely to have decreased renal function with a reduced creatinine clearance, care must be taken in dose selection. (See DOSAGE AND ADMINISTRATION.)

USE IN WOMEN

Female patients constituted 32% of the patients in the placebo-controlled trials of dofetilide. As with other drugs that cause torsade de pointes, dofetilide was associated with a greater risk of torsade de pointes in female patients than in male patients. During the dofetilide clinical development program the risk of torsade de pointes in females was approximately 3 times the risk in males. Unlike torsade de pointes, the incidence of other ventricular arrhythmias was similar in female patients receiving dofetilide and patients receiving placebo. Although no study specifically investigated this risk, in post-hoc analyses, no increased mortality was observed in females on dofetilide compared to females on placebo.

PEDIATRIC USE

The safety and effectiveness of dofetilide in children (<18 years old) has not been established.

DRUG INTERACTIONS

DRUG-DRUG INTERACTIONS

Cimetidine: See CONTRAINDICATIONS. Concomitant use of cimetidine is contraindicated. Cimetidine at 400 mg bid (the usual prescription dose) co-administered with dofetilide (500 µg bid) for 7 days has been shown to increase dofetilide plasma levels by 58%. Cimetidine at doses of 100 mg bid (OTC dose) resulted in a 13% increase in dofetilide plasma levels (500 µg single dose). No studies have been conducted at intermediate doses of cimetidine. If a patient requires dofetilide and anti-ulcer therapy, it is suggested that omeprazole, ranitidine, or antacids (aluminum and magnesium hydroxides) be used as alternatives to cimetidine, as these agents have no effect on the pharmacokinetic profile of dofetilide.

Verapamil: See CONTRAINDICATIONS.) Concomitant use of verapamil is contraindicated. Co-administration of dofetilide with verapamil resulted in increases in dofetilide peak plasma levels of 42%, although overall exposure to dofetilide was not significantly increased. In an analysis of the supraventricular arrhythmia and DIAMOND patient populations, the concomitant administration of verapamil with dofetilide was associated with a higher occurrence of torsade de pointes.

Ketoconazole: See CONTRAINDICATIONS. Concomitant use of ketoconazole is contraindicated. Ketoconazole at 400 mg daily (the maximum approved prescription dose) co-administered with dofetilide (500 µg bid) for 7 days has been shown to increase dofetilide C_{max} by 53% in males and 97% in females, and AUC by 41% in males and 69% in females.

Trimethoprim Alone or in Combination With Sulfamethoxazole: (see CONTRAINDICATIONS) Concomitant use of trimethoprim alone or in combination with sulfamethoxazole is contraindicated. Trimethoprim 160 mg in combination with 800 mg sulfamethoxazole co-administered bid with dofetilide (500 µg bid) for 4 days has been shown to increase dofetilide AUC by 103% and C_{max} by 93%.

POTENTIAL DRUG INTERACTIONS

Dofetilide is eliminated in the kidney by cationic secretion. Inhibitors of renal cationic secretion are contraindicated with dofetilide. In addition, drugs that are actively secreted via this route (*e.g.*, triamterene, metformin and amiloride) should be co-administered with care as they might increase dofetilide levels.

Dofetilide is metabolized to a small extent by the CYP3A4 isoenzyme of the cytochrome P450 system. Inhibitors of the CYP3A4 isoenzyme could increase systemic dofetilide exposure. Inhibitors of this isoenzyme (*e.g.*, macrolide antibiotics, azole antifungal agents, protease inhibitors, serotonin reuptake inhibitors, amiodarone, cannabinoids, diltiazem, grapefruit juice, nefazadone, norfloxacin, quinine, zafirlukast) should be cautiously coadministered with dofetilide as they can potentially increase dofetilide levels. Dofetilide is not an inhibitor of CYP3A4 nor of other cytochrome P450 isoenzymes (*e.g.*, CYP2C9, CYP2D6) and is not expected to increase levels of drugs metabolized by CYP3A4.

OTHER DRUG INTERACTION INFORMATION

Digoxin: Studies in healthy volunteers have shown that dofetilide does not affect the pharmacokinetics of digoxin. In patients, the concomitant administration of digoxin with dofetilide was associated with a higher occurrence of torsade de pointes. It is not clear whether this represents an interaction with dofetilide or the presence of more severe structural heart disease in patients on digoxin; structural heart disease is a known risk factor for arrhythmia. No increase in mortality was observed in patients taking digoxin as concomitant medication.

Other Drugs: In healthy volunteers, amlodipine, phenytoin, glyburide, ranitidine, omeprazole, hormone replacement therapy (a combination of conjugated estrogens and medroxyprogesterone), antacid (aluminum and magnesium hydroxides) and theophylline did not affect the pharmacokinetics of dofetilide. In addition, studies in healthy volunteers have shown that dofetilide does not affect the pharmacokinetics or pharmacodynamics of warfarin, or the pharmacokinetics of propranolol (40 mg twice daily), phenytoin, theophylline, or oral contraceptives.

Population pharmacokinetic analyses were conducted on plasma concentration data from 1445 patients in clinical trials to examine the effects of concomitant medications on clearance or volume of distribution of dofetilide. Concomitant medications were grouped as ACE inhibitors, oral anticoagulants, calcium channel blockers, beta blockers, cardiac glycosides, inducers of CYP3A4, substrates and inhibitors of CYP3A4, substrates and inhibitors of P-glycoprotein, nitrates, sulphonylureas, loop diuretics, potassium sparing diuretics, thiazide diuretics, substrates and inhibitors of tubular organic cation transport, and QTc-prolonging drugs. Differences in clearance between patients on these medications (at any occasion in the study) and those off medications varied between -16% and +3%. The mean clearances of dofetilide were 16 and 15% lower in patients on thiazide diuretics and inhibitors of tubular organic cation transport, respectively.

ADVERSE REACTIONS

The dofetilide clinical program involved approximately 8600 patients in 130 clinical studies of normal volunteers and patients with supraventricular and ventricular arrhythmias. Dofetilide was administered to 5194 patients, including 2 large, placebo-controlled mortality trials (DIAMOND CHF and DIAMOND MI) in which 1511 patients received dofetilide for up to 3 years.

In the following section, adverse reaction data for cardiac arrhythmias and non-cardiac adverse reactions are presented separately for patients included in the supraventricular arrhythmia development program and for patients included in the DIAMOND CHF and MI mortality trials.

In studies of patients with supraventricular arrhythmias a total of 1346 and 677 patients were exposed to dofetilide and placebo for 551 and 207 patient years, respectively. A total of 8.7% of patients in the dofetilide groups were discontinued from clinical trials due to adverse events compared to 8.0% in the placebo groups. The most frequent reason for discontinuation (>1%) was ventricular tachycardia (2.0% on dofetilide vs 1.3% on placebo). The most frequent adverse events were headache, chest pain, and dizziness.

SERIOUS ARRHYTHMIAS AND CONDUCTION DISTURBANCES

Torsade de pointes is the only arrhythmia that showed a dose-response relationship to dofetilide treatment. It did not occur in placebo treated patients. The incidence of torsade de pointes in patients with supraventricular arrhythmias was 0.8% (11/1346) (see WARNINGS). The incidence of torsade de pointes in patients who were dosed according to the recommended dosing regimen (see DOSAGE AND ADMINISTRATION) was 0.8% (4/525). TABLE 6 shows the frequency by randomized dose of serious arrhythmias and conduction disturbances reported as adverse events in patients with supraventricular arrhythmias.

TABLE 6 *Incidence of Serious Arrhythmias and Conduction Disturbances in Patients With Supraventricular Arrhythmias*

	Dofetilide Dose (bid)				
	<250 µg	250 µg	>250-500 µg	>500 µg	Placebo
Arrhythmia Event:	n=217	n=388	n=703	n=38	n=677
Ventricular arrhythmias*†	3.7%	2.6%	3.4%	15.8%	2.7%
Ventricular fibrillation	0	0.3%	0.4%	2.6%	0.1%
Ventricular tachycardia†	3.7%	2.6%	3.3%	13.2%	2.5%
Torsade de pointes	0	0.3%	0.9%	10.5%	0
Various forms of block					
AV block	0.9%	1.5%	0.4%	0	0.3%
Bundle branch block	0	0.5%	0.1%	0	0.1%
Heart block	0	0.5%	0.1%	0	0.1%

* Patients with more than one arrhythmia are counted only once in this category.
† Ventricular arrhythmias and ventricular tachycardia include all cases of torsade de pointes.

In the DIAMOND trials a total of 1511 patients were exposed to dofetilide for 1757 patient years. The incidence of torsade de pointes was 3.3% in CHF patients and 0.9% in patients with a recent MI.

TABLE 7 shows the incidence of serious arrhythmias and conduction disturbances reported as adverse events in the DIAMOND subpopulation that had AF at entry to these trials.

OTHER ADVERSE REACTIONS

TABLE 8 presents other adverse events reported with a frequency of >2% on dofetilide and reported numerically more frequently on dofetilide than on placebo in the studies of patients with supraventricular arrhythmias.

TABLE 7 *Incidence of Serious Arrhythmias and Conduction Disturbances in Patients with AF at Entry to the DIAMOND Studies*

	Dofetilide n=249	Placebo n=257
Ventricular arrhythmias*†	14.5%	13.6%
Ventricular fibrilation	4.8%	3.1%
Ventricular tachycardia†	12.4%	11.3%
Torsade de pointes	1.6%	0
Various forms of block		
AV block	0.8%	2.7%
(Left) bundle branch block	0	0.4%
Heart block	1.2%	0.8%

* Patients with more than one arrhythmia are counted only once in this category.
† Ventricular arrhythmias and ventricular tachycardia include all cases of torsade de pointes.

TABLE 8 *Frequency of Adverse Events Occurring at >2% on Dofetilide, and Numerically More Frequently on Dofetilide than Placebo in Patients With Supraventricular Arrhythmias*

Adverse Event	Dofetilide	Placebo
Headache	11%	9%
Chest pain	10%	7%
Dizziness	8%	6%
Respiratory tract infection	7%	5%
Dyspnea	6%	5%
Nausea	5%	4%
Insomnia	4%	2%
Flu syndrome	4%	3%
Accidental injury	3%	1%
Back pain	3%	2%
Procedure (medical/surgical/health service)	3%	2%
Diarrhea	3%	2%
Rash	3%	2%
Abdominal pain	3%	2%

Adverse events reported at a rate >2% but no more frequently on dofetilide than on placebo were: Angina pectoris, anxiety, arthralgia, asthenia, atrial fibrillation, complications (application, injection, incision, insertion, or device), hypertension, pain, palpitation, peripheral edema, supraventricular tachycardia, sweating, urinary tract infection, ventricular tachycardia.

The following adverse events have been reported with a frequency of ≤2% and numerically more frequently with dofetilide than placebo in patients with supraventricular arrhythmias: Angioedema, bradycardia, cerebral ischemia, cerebrovascular accident, edema, facial paralysis, flaccid paralysis, heart arrest, increased cough, liver damage, migraine, myocardial infarct, paralysis, paresthesia, sudden death, and syncope.

The incidences of clinically significant laboratory test abnormalities in patients with supraventricular arrhythmias were similar for patients on dofetilide and those on placebo. No clinically relevant effects were noted in serum alkaline phosphatase, serum GGT, LDH, AST, ALT, total bilirubin, total protein, blood urea nitrogen, creatinine, serum electrolytes (calcium, chloride, glucose, magnesium, potassium, sodium) or creatine kinase. Similarly, no clinically relevant effects were observed in hematologic parameters.

In the DIAMOND population, adverse events other than those related to the post-infarction and heart failure patient population were generally similar to those seen in the supraventricular arrhythmia groups.

DOSAGE AND ADMINISTRATION

- Therapy with dofetilide must be initiated (and, if necessary, re-initiated) in a setting that provides continuous electrocardiographic (ECG) monitoring and in the presence of personnel trained in the management of serious ventricular arrhythmias. Patients should continue to be monitored in this way for a minimum of 3 days. Additionally, patients should not be discharged within 12 hours of electrical or pharmacological conversion to normal sinus rhythm.
- **The dose of dofetilide must be individualized according to calculated creatinine clearance and QTc. (QT interval should be used if the heart rate is <60 beats per minute. There are no data on use of dofetilide when the heart rate is <50 beats per minute.)** The usual recommended dose of dofetilide is 500 μg bid, as modified by the dosing algorithm described below. For consideration of a lower dose, see Special Considerations below.
- Patients with atrial fibrillation should be anticoagulated according to usual medical practice prior to electrical or pharmacological cardioversion. Anticoagulant therapy may be continued after cardioversion according to usual medical practice for the treatment of people with AF. Hypokalemia should be corrected before initiation of dofetilide therapy (see WARNINGS, Ventricular Arrhythmia).
- Patients to be discharged on dofetilide therapy from an in-patient setting as described above must have an adequate supply of dofetilide, at the patient's individualized dose, to allow uninterrupted dosing until the patient receives the first outpatient supply.
- Dofetilide is distributed only to those hospitals and other appropriate institutions confirmed to have received applicable dosing and treatment initiation education programs. Inpatient and subsequent outpatient discharge and refill prescriptions are filled only upon confirmation that the prescribing physician has received applicable dosing and treatment initiation education programs. For this purpose, a list for use by pharmacists is maintained containing hospitals and physicians who have received one of the education programs.

INSTRUCTIONS FOR INDIVIDUALIZED DOSE INITIATION

Initiation of Dofetilide Therapy

Step 1.*Electrocardiographic Assessment:* Prior to administration of the first dose, the QTc must be determined using an average of 5-10 beats. If the QTc is >440 milliseconds (500 milliseconds in patients with ventricular conduction abnormalities), dofetilide is contraindicated. If heart rate is less than 60 beats per minute, QT interval should be used. Patients with heart rates <50 beats per minute have not been studied.

Step 2. *Calculation of Creatinine Clearance:* Prior to the administration of the first dose, the patient's creatinine clearance must be calculated using the following formula:

Creatinine clearance (male) = [(140-age) × body weight in kg]/[72 × serum creatinine (mg/dl)]

Creatinine clearance (female) = [(140-age) × body weight in kg × 0.85]/[72 × serum creatinine (mg/dl)]

When serum creatinine is given in mmol/L, divide the value by 88.4 (1 mg/dl = 88.4 mmol/L).

Step 3. *Starting Dose:* The starting dose of dofetilide is determined as indicated in TABLE 9.

TABLE 9

Calculated Creatinine Clearance	Dofetilide Dose
>60 ml/min	500 μg twice daily
40-60 ml/min	250 μg twice daily
20-<40 ml/min	125 μg twice daily
<20 ml/min	Dofetilide is contraindicated in these patients

Step 4. Administer the adjusted dofetilide dose and begin continuous ECG monitoring.

Step 5. At 2-3 hours after administering the first dose of dofetilide, determine the QTc. If the QTc has increased by greater than 15% compared to the baseline established in **Step 1** OR if the QTc is >500 milliseconds (550 milliseconds in patients with ventricular conduction abnormalities), subsequent dosing should be adjusted as indicated in TABLE 10.

TABLE 10

If the Starting Dose Based on Creatinine Clearance is:	Then the Adjusted Dose (for QTc Prolongation) is:
500 μg twice daily	250 μg twice daily
250 μg twice daily	125 μg twice daily
125 μg twice daily	125 μg once a day

Step 6. At 2-3 hours after each subsequent dose of dofetilide, determine the QTc (for in-hospital doses 2-5). No further down titration of dofetilide based on QTc is recommended.

Note: If at any time after the second dose of dofetilide is given, the QTc is >500 milliseconds (550 milliseconds in patients with ventricular conduction abnormalities) dofetilide should be discontinued.

Step 7. Patients are to be continuously monitored by ECG for a minimum of 3 days, or for a minimum of 12 hours after electrical or pharmacological conversion to normal sinus rhythm, whichever is greater.

MAINTENANCE OF DOFETILIDE THERAPY

Renal function and QTc should be re-evaluated every 3 months or as medically warranted. If QTc exceeds 500 milliseconds (550 milliseconds in patients with ventricular conduction abnormalities), dofetilide therapy should be discontinued and patients should be carefully monitored until QTc returns to baseline levels. If renal function deteriorates, adjust dose as described in Initiation of Dofetilide Therapy, Step 3.

SPECIAL CONSIDERATIONS

Consideration of a Dose Lower Than That Determined by the Algorithm

The dosing algorithm shown above should be used to determine the individualized dose of dofetilide. In clinical trials, the highest dose of 500 μg bid of dofetilide as modified by the dosing algorithm led to greater effectiveness than lower doses of 125 or 250 μg bid as modified by the dosing algorithm. The risk of torsade de pointes, however, is related to dose as well as to patient characteristics (see WARNINGS). Physicians, in consultation with their patients, may therefore in some cases choose doses lower than determined by the algorithm. It is critically important that if at any time this lower dose is increased, the patient needs to be rehospitalized for 3 days. Previous toleration of higher doses does not eliminate the need for rehospitalization.

The maximum recommended dose in patients with a calculated creatinine clearance greater than 60 ml/min is 500 μg bid; doses greater than 500 μg bid have been associated with an increased incidence of torsade de pointes.

A patient who misses a dose should NOT double the next dose. The next dose should be taken at the usual time.

Cardioversion

If patients do not convert to normal sinus rhythm within 24 hours of initiation of dofetilide therapy, electrical conversion should be considered. Patients continuing on dofetilide after successful electrical cardioversion should continue to be monitored by electrocardiography for 12 hours post cardioversion, or a minimum of 3 days after initiation of dofetilide therapy, whichever is greater.

SWITCH TO DOFETILIDE FROM CLASS I OR OTHER CLASS III ANTIARRHYTHMIC THERAPY

Before initiating dofetilide therapy, previous antiarrhythmic therapy should be withdrawn under careful monitoring for a minimum of 3 plasma half-lives. Because of the unpredictable pharmacokinetics of amiodarone, dofetilide should not be initiated following amiodarone therapy until amiodarone plasma levels are below 0.3 μg/ml or until amiodarone has been withdrawn for at least 3 months.

STOPPING DOFETILIDE PRIOR TO ADMINISTRATION OF POTENTIALLY INTERACTING DRUGS

If dofetilide needs to be discontinued to allow dosing of other potentially interacting drug(s), a washout period of at least 2 days should be followed before starting the other drug(s).

HOW SUPPLIED

Tikosyn 125 μg (0.125 mg) capsules are supplied as No. 4 capsules with a light orange cap and white body, printed with "TKN 125 PFIZER".

Tikosyn 250 μg (0.25 mg) capsules are supplied as No. 4 capsules, peach cap and body, printed with "TKN 250 PFIZER".

Tikosyn 500 μg (0.5 mg) capsules are supplied as No. 2 capsules, peach cap and white body, printed with "TKN 500 PFIZER".

STORAGE

Store at controlled room temperature, 15-30°C (59-86°F).

PROTECT FROM MOISTURE AND HUMIDITY.

Dispense in tight containers.

PRODUCT LISTING - EQUIVALENTS NOT AVAILABLE

Capsule - Oral - 125 mcg			
14's	$0.01	TIKOSYN, Pfizer U.S. Pharmaceuticals	00069-5800-61
40's	$78.68	TIKOSYN, Pfizer U.S. Pharmaceuticals	00069-5800-43
60's	$114.58	TIKOSYN, Pfizer U.S. Pharmaceuticals	00069-5800-60
Capsule - Oral - 250 mcg			
14's	$0.01	TIKOSYN, Pfizer U.S. Pharmaceuticals	00069-5810-61
40's	$78.68	TIKOSYN, Pfizer U.S. Pharmaceuticals	00069-5810-43
60's	$118.01	TIKOSYN, Pfizer U.S. Pharmaceuticals	00069-5810-60
Capsule - Oral - 500 mcg			
14's	$0.01	TIKOSYN, Pfizer U.S. Pharmaceuticals	00069-5820-61
40's	$78.68	TIKOSYN, Pfizer U.S. Pharmaceuticals	00069-5820-43
60's	$118.01	TIKOSYN, Pfizer U.S. Pharmaceuticals	00069-5820-60

Dolasetron Mesylate *(003362)*

Categories: Nausea, postoperative; Nausea, secondary to cancer chemotherapy; Vomiting, postoperative; Vomiting, secondary to cancer chemotherapy; Pregnancy Category B; FDA Approved 1997 Oct
Drug Classes: Antiemetics/antivertigo; Serotonin receptor antagonists
Brand Names: Anzemet
Foreign Brand Availability: Anemet (Germany); Zamanon (South-Africa)
Cost of Therapy: $73.31 (Nausea and Vomiting; Anzemet; 100 mg; 1 tablet; 1 day supply)
$173.16 (Nausea and Vomiting; Anzemet Injection; 20 mg/ml; 100 mg; 1 day supply)
HCFA JCODE(S): J1260 1 mg IV

INTRAVENOUS

DESCRIPTION

Dolasetron mesylate is an antinauseant and antiemetic agent. Chemically, dolasetron mesylate is (2α,6α,8α,9aβ)-octahydro-3-oxo-2,6-methano-2*H*-quinolizin-8-yl-1*H*-indole-3-carboxylate monomethanesulfonate, monohydrate. It is a highly specific and selective serotonin subtype 3 ($5\text{-}HT_3$) receptor antagonist both *in vitro* and *in vivo*.

The empirical formula is $C_{19}H_{20}N_2O_3{\cdot}CH_3SO_3H{\cdot}H_2O$, with a molecular weight of 438.50. Approximately 74% of dolasetron mesylate monohydrate is dolasetron base.

Dolasetron mesylate monohydrate is a white to off-white powder that is freely soluble in water and propylene glycol, slightly soluble in ethanol, and slightly soluble in normal saline.

Anzemet injection is a clear, colorless, nonpyrogenic, sterile solution for intravenous administration. Each milliliter of Anzemet injection contains 20 mg of dolasetron mesylate and 38.2 mg mannitol with an acetate buffer in water for injection. The pH of the resulting solution is 3.2–3.8.

CLINICAL PHARMACOLOGY

Dolasetron mesylate and its active metabolite, hydrodolasetron (MDL 74,156), are selective serotonin $5\text{-}HT_3$ receptor antagonists not shown to have activity at other known serotonin receptors and with low affinity for dopamine receptors. The serotonin $5\text{-}HT_3$ receptors are located on the nerve terminals of the vagus in the periphery and centrally in the chemoreceptor trigger zone of the area postrema. It is thought that chemotherapeutic agents produce nausea and vomiting by releasing serotonin from the enterochromaffin cells of the small intestine, and that the released serotonin then activates $5\text{-}HT_3$ receptors located on vagal efferents to initiate the vomiting reflex.

Acute, usually reversible, ECG changes (PR and QTc prolongation; QRS widening), caused by dolasetron mesylate, have been observed in healthy volunteers and in controlled clinical trials. The active metabolites of dolasetron may block sodium channels, a property unrelated to its ability to block $5\text{-}HT_3$ receptors. QTc prolongation is primarily due to QRS widening. Dolasetron appears to prolong both depolarization and, to a lesser extent, repolarization time. The magnitude and frequency of the ECG changes increased with dose (related to peak plasma concentrations of hydrodolasetron but not the parent compound). These ECG interval prolongations usually returned to baseline within 6–8 hours, but in some patients were present at 24 hour follow up. Dolasetron mesylate administration has little or no effect on blood pressure.

In healthy volunteers (n=64), dolasetron mesylate in single intravenous doses up to 5 mg/kg produced no effect on pupil size or meaningful changes in EEG tracings. Results from neuropsychiatric tests revealed that dolasetron mesylate did not alter mood or concentration. Multiple daily doses of dolasetron have had no effect on colonic transit in humans. Dolasetron mesylate has no effect on plasma prolactin concentrations.

PHARMACOKINETICS IN HUMANS

Intravenous dolasetron mesylate is rapidly eliminated ($T_{1/2}$ <10 min) and completely metabolized to the most clinically relevant species, hydrodolasetron.

The reduction of dolasetron to hydrodolasetron is mediated by a ubiquitous enzyme, carbonyl reductase. Cytochrome P-450 (CYP)IID6 is primarily responsible for the subsequent hydroxylation of hydrodolasetron and both CYPIIIA and flavin monooxygenase are responsible for the N-oxidation of hydrodolasetron.

Hydrodolasetron is excreted in the urine unchanged (53.0% of administered intravenous dose). Other urinary metabolites include hydroxylated glucuronides and N-oxide.

Hydrodolasetron appeared rapidly in plasma, with a maximum concentration occurring approximately 0.6 hours after the end of intravenous treatment, and was eliminated with a mean half-life of 7.3 hours (%CV=24) and an apparent clearance of 9.4 ml/min/kg (%CV=28) in 24 adults. Hydrodolasetron is eliminated by multiple routes, including renal excretion and, after metabolism, mainly glucuronidation, and hydroxylation. Hydrodolasetron exhibits linear pharmacokinetics over the intravenous dose range of 50–200 mg and they are independent of infusion rate. Doses lower than 50 mg have not been studied. Two-thirds (2/3) of the administered dose is recovered in the urine and 1/3 in the feces. Hydrodolasetron is widely distributed in the body with a mean apparent volume of distribution of 5.8 L/kg (%CV=25, n=24) in adults.

Sixty-nine (69) to 77% of hydrodolasetron is bound to plasma protein. In a study with ^{14}C labeled dolasetron, the distribution of radioactivity to blood cells was not extensive. The binding of hydrodolasetron to α_1-acid glycoprotein is approximately 50%. The pharmacokinetics of hydrodolasetron are linear and similar in men and women.

The pharmacokinetics of hydrodolasetron, in special and targeted patient populations following intravenous administration of dolasetron mesylate injection, are summarized in TABLE 1. The pharmacokinetics of hydrodolasetron are similar in adult healthy volunteers and in adult cancer patients receiving chemotherapeutic agents. The apparent clearance of hydrodolasetron in pediatric and adolescent patients is 1.4 times to 2–fold higher than in adults. The apparent clearance of hydrodolasetron is not affected by age in adult cancer patients. Following intravenous administration, the apparent clearance of hydrodolasetron remains unchanged with severe hepatic impairment and decreases 47% with severe renal impairment. No dose adjustment is necessary for elderly patients or for patients with hepatic or renal impairment.

In a pharmacokinetic study in pediatric cancer patients (ages 3–11, n=25; ages 12–17, n=21) given a single 0.6, 1.2, 1.8, or 2.4 mg/kg dose of dolasetron mesylate injection intravenously, apparent clearance values were highest and half-lives were lowest in the youngest age group. For the 3–11 and the 12–17 year age groups, all receiving doses between 0.6–2.4 mg/kg, mean apparent clearances are 2 and 1.3 times greater, respectively, than for healthy adults receiving the same range of doses.

Thirty-two (32) pediatric cancer patients ages 3–11 years (n=19) and 12–17 years (n=13), received 0.6, 1.2, or 1.8 mg dolasetron mesylate injection diluted with either apple or apple-grape juice and administered orally. In this study, the mean apparent clearances were 3 times greater in the younger pediatric group and 1.8 times greater in the older pediatric group than those observed in healthy adult volunteers. Across this spectrum of pediatric patients, maximum plasma concentrations were 0.6–0.7 times those observed in healthy adults receiving similar doses.

In a pharmacokinetic study in 18 pediatric patients (2–11 years of age) undergoing surgery with general anesthesia and administered a single 1.2 mg/kg intravenous dose of dolasetron mesylate injection, mean apparent clearance was greater (40%) and terminal half-life shorter (36%) for hydrodolasetron than in healthy adults receiving the same dose.

For 12 pediatric patients, ages 2–12 years receiving 1.2 mg/kg dolasetron mesylate injection diluted in apple or apple-grape juice and administered orally, the mean apparent clearance was 34% greater and half-life was 21% shorter than in healthy adults receiving the same dose.

INDICATIONS AND USAGE

Dolasetron mesylate injection is indicated for the following:

1. **The prevention of nausea and vomiting associated with initial and repeat courses of emetogenic cancer chemotherapy, including high dose cisplatin.**
2. **The prevention of postoperative nausea and vomiting.** As with other antiemetics, routine prophylaxis is not recommended for patients in whom there is little expectation that nausea and/or vomiting will occur postoperatively. In patients where nausea and/or vomiting must be avoided postoperatively, dolasetron mesylate injection is recommended even where the incidence of postoperative nausea and/or vomiting is low.
3. **The treatment of postoperative nausea and/or vomiting.**

CONTRAINDICATIONS

Dolasetron mesylate injection is contraindicated in patients known to have hypersensitivity to the drug.

WARNINGS

Dolasetron mesylate can cause ECG interval changes (PR, QTc, JT prolongation and QRS widening). These changes are related in magnitude and frequency to blood levels of the active metabolite. These changes are self-limiting with declining blood levels. Some patients have interval prolongations for 24 hours or longer. Interval prolongation could lead to cardiovascular consequences, including heart block or cardiac arrhythmias. These have rarely been reported.

A cardiac conduction abnormality observed on an intra-operative cardiac rhythm monitor (interpreted as complete heart block) was reported in a 61-year-old woman who received 200 mg dolasetron mesylate for the prevention of postoperative nausea and vomiting. This patient was also taking verapamil. A similar event also interpreted as complete heart block was reported in one patient receiving placebo.

A 66-year-old man with Stage IV non-Hodgkins lymphoma died suddenly 6 hours after receiving 1.8 mg/kg (119 mg) intravenous dolasetron mesylate injection. This patient had

TABLE 1 *Pharmacokinetic Values for Plasma Hydrodolasetron Following Intravenous Administration of Dolasetron Mesylate Injection**

Age	Age (years)	Dose	CL_{app} (ml/min/kg)	T½ (h)	C_{max} (ng/ml)
Young healthy volunteers (n=24)	19-40	100 mg	9.4 (28%)	7.3 (24%)	320 (25%)
Elderly healthy volunteers (n=15)	65-75	2.4 mg/kg	8.3 (30%)	6.9 (22%)	620 (31%)
Cancer patients					
Adults (n=273)	19-87	0.6-3.0 mg/kg	10.2 (34%)†	7.5 (43%)†	505 (26%)‡
Adolescents (n=21)	12-17	0.6-3.0 mg/kg	12.5 (37%)	5.5 (31%)	562 (45%)§
Children (n=25)	3-11	0.6-2.4 mg/kg	19.2 (30%)	4.4 (24%)	505 (100%)¤
Pediatric surgery patients (n=18)	2-11	1.2 mg/kg	13.1 (47%)	4.8 (23%)	255 (22%)
Patients with sever renal impairment (n=12) (creatinine clearance ≤10 ml/min)	28-74	200 mg	5.0 (33%)	10.9 (30%)	867 (31%)
Patients with Severe Hepatic Impairment (n=3)	42-52	150 mg	9.6 (19%)	11.7 (22%)	396 (45%)

CL_{app} = apparent clearance; T½ = terminal elimination half-life; () = Coefficient of variation in %.
* Mean values.
† Results from population kinetic study.
‡ Results from adult cancer study (dose=1.8 mg/kg, n=8).
§ Results from adolescents (dose=1.8 mg/kg, n=7).
¤ Results from children (dose=1.8 mg/kg, n=5).

other potential risk factors including substantial exposure to doxorubicin and concomitant cyclophosphamide.

PRECAUTIONS

GENERAL

Dolasetron should be administered with caution in patients who have or may develop prolongation of cardiac conduction intervals, particularly QTc. These include patients with hypokalemia or hypomagnesemia, patients taking diuretics with potential for inducing electrolyte abnormalities, patients with congenital QT syndrome, patients taking anti-arrhythmic drugs or other drugs which lead to QT prolongation, and cumulative high dose anthracycline therapy.

Cross hypersensitivity reactions have been reported in patients who received other selective 5-HT_3 receptor antagonists. These reactions have not been seen with dolasetron mesylate.

CARCINOGENESIS, MUTAGENESIS, AND IMPAIRMENT OF FERTILITY

In a 24 month carcinogenicity study, there was a statistically significant ($P<0.001$) increase in the incidence of combined hepatocellular adenomas and carcinomas in male mice treated with 150 mg/kg/day and above. In this study, mice (CD-1) were treated orally with dolasetron mesylate 75, 150 or 300 mg/kg/day (225, 450 or 900 mg/m^2/day). For a 50 kg person of average height (1.46 m^2 body surface area), these doses represent 3.4, 6.8 and 13.5 times the recommended clinical dose (66.6 mg/m^2, intravenous) on a body surface area basis. No increase in liver tumors was observed at a dose of 75 mg/kg/day in male mice and at doses up to 300 mg/kg/day in female mice.

In a 24 month rat (Sprague-Dawley) carcinogenicity study, oral dolasetron mesylate was not tumorigenic at doses up to 150 mg/kg/day (900 mg/m^2/day, 13.5 times the recommended human dose based on body surface area) in male rats and 300 mg/kg/day (1800 mg/m^2/day, 27 times the recommended human dose based on body surface area) in female rats.

Dolasetron mesylate was not genotoxic in the Ames test, the rat lymphocyte chromosomal aberration test, the Chinese hamster ovary (CHO) cell (HGPRT) forward mutation test, the rat hepatocyte unscheduled DNA synthesis (UDS) test or the mouse micronucleus test.

Dolasetron mesylate was found to have no effect on fertility and reproductive performance at oral doses up to 100 mg/kg/day (600 mg/m^2/day, 9 times the recommended human dose based on body surface area) in female rats and up to 400 mg/kg/day (2400 mg/m^2/day, 36 times the recommended human dose based on body surface area) in male rats.

PREGNANCY, TERATOGENIC EFFECTS, PREGNANCY CATEGORY B

Teratology studies have not revealed evidence of impaired fertility or harm to the fetus due to dolasetron mesylate. These studies have been performed in pregnant rats at intravenous doses up to 60 mg/kg/day (5.4 times the recommended human dose based on body surface area) and pregnant rabbits at intravenous doses up to 20 mg/kg/day (3.2 times the recommended human dose based on body surface area). There are, however, no adequate and well-controlled studies in pregnant women. Because animal reproduction studies are not always predictive of human response, this drug should be used during pregnancy only if clearly needed.

NURSING MOTHERS

It is not known whether dolasetron mesylate is excreted in human milk. Because many drugs are excreted in human milk, caution should be exercised when dolasetron mesylate injection is administered to a nursing woman.

PEDIATRIC USE

Four open-label, noncomparative pharmacokinetic studies have been performed in a total of 108 pediatric patients receiving emetogenic chemotherapy or undergoing surgery with general anesthesia. These patients received dolasetron mesylate injection either intravenously or orally in juice. Pediatric patients from 2–17 years of age participated in these trials, which included intravenous dolasetron mesylate injection doses of 0.6, 1.2, 1.8, or 2.4 mg/kg, and oral doses of 0.6, 1.2, or 1.8 mg/kg. There is no experience in pediatric patients under 2 years of age. Overall, dolasetron mesylate injection was well tolerated in these pediatric patients. Efficacy information collected in pediatric patients receiving cancer chemotherapy are consistent with those obtained in adults. No efficacy information was collected in the pediatric postoperative nausea and vomiting studies.

USE IN ELDERLY PATIENTS

Dosage adjustment is not needed in patients over 65. Effectiveness in prevention of nausea and vomiting in elderly patients was no different than in younger age groups.

D

DRUG INTERACTIONS

The potential for clinically significant drug-drug interactions posed by dolasetron and hydrodolasetron appears to be low for drugs commonly used in chemotherapy or surgery, because hydrodolasetron is eliminated by multiple routes. See PRECAUTIONS, General for information about potential interaction with other drugs that prolong the QTc interval. Blood levels of hydrodolasetron increased 24% when dolasetron was coadministered with cimetidine (nonselective inhibitor of cytochrome P-450) for 7 days, and decreased 28% with coadministration of rifampin (potent inducer of cytochrome P-450) for 7 days.

Dolasetron mesylate injection has been safely coadministered with drugs used in chemotherapy and surgery. As with other agents which prolong ECG intervals, caution should be exercised in patients taking drugs which prolong ECG intervals, particularly QTc.

In patients taking furosemide, nifedipine, diltiazem, ACE inhibitors, verapamil, glyburide, propranolol, and various chemotherapy agents, no effect was shown on the clearance of hydrodolasetron. Clearance of hydrodolasetron decreased by about 27% when dolasetron mesylate was administered intravenously concomitantly with atenolol. Dolasetron mesylate did not influence anesthesia recovery time in patients. Dolasetron mesylate did not inhibit the antitumor activity of four chemotherapeutic agents (cisplatin, 5-fluorouracil, doxorubicin, cyclophosphamide) in four murine models.

ADVERSE REACTIONS

CHEMOTHERAPY PATIENTS

In controlled clinical trials, 2265 adult patients received dolasetron mesylate injection. The overall adverse event rates were similar with 1.8 mg/kg dolasetron mesylate injection and ondansetron or granisetron. Patients were receiving concurrent chemotherapy, predominantly high-dose (≥50 mg/m^2) cisplatin. Following is a combined listing of all adverse events reported in ≥2% of patients in these controlled trials (TABLE 4).

TABLE 4 *Adverse Events ≥2% From Chemotherapy-Induced Nausea and Vomiting Studies*

Event	Dolasetron Mesylate Injection 1.8 mg/kg (n=695)	Ondansetron/Granisetron* (n=356)
Headache	169 (24.3%)	73 (20.5%)
Diarrhea	86 (12.4%)	25 (7.0%)
Fever	30 (4.3%)	18 (5.1%)
Fatigue	25 (3.6%)	12 (3.4%)
Hepatic function abnormal†	25 (3.6%)	12 (3.4%)
Abdominal pain	22 (3.2%)	7 (2.0%)
Hypertension	20 (2.9%)	9 (2.5%)
Pain	17 (2.4%)	7 (2.0%)
Dizziness	15 (2.2%)	7 (2.0%)
Chills/shivering	14 (2.0%)	6 (1.7%)

* Ondansetron 32 mg intravenous, granisetron 3 mg intravenous.
† Includes events coded as SGOT-and/or SGPT-increased (see also Liver and Biliary System.

POSTOPERATIVE PATIENTS

In controlled clinical trials with 2550 adult patients, headache and dizziness were reported more frequently with 12.5 mg dolasetron mesylate injection than with placebo. Rates of other adverse events were similar. Following is a listing of all adverse events reported in ≥2% of patients receiving either placebo or 12.5 mg dolasetron mesylate injection for the prevention or treatment of postoperative nausea and vomiting in controlled clinical trials (TABLE 5).

TABLE 5 *Adverse Events ≥2% From Placebo-Controlled Postoperative Nausea and Vomiting Studies*

Event	Dolasetron Mesylate Injection 12.5 mg (n=615)	Placebo (n=739)
Headache	58 (9.4%)	51 (6.9%)
Dizziness	34 (5.5%)	23 (3.1%)
Drowsiness	15 (2.4%)	18 (2.4%)
Pain	15 (2.4%)	21 (2.8%)
Urinary retention	12 (2.0%)	16 (2.2%)

In clinical trials, the following infrequently reported adverse events, assessed by investigators as treatment-related or causality unknown, occurred following oral or intravenous administration of dolasetron mesylate to adult patients receiving concomitant cancer chemotherapy or surgery:

Cardiovascular: Hypotension; *Rarely:* Edema, peripheral edema. *The following events also occurred rarely and with a similar frequency as placebo and/or active comparator:* Mobitz I AV block, chest pain, orthostatic hypotension, myocardial ischemia, syncope, severe bradycardia, and palpitations. See PRECAUTIONS for information on potential effects on ECG.

In addition, the following asymptomatic treatment-emergent ECG changes were seen at rates less than or equal to those for active or placebo controls: Bradycardia, tachycardia, T wave change, ST-T wave change, sinus arrhythmia, extrasystole (APCs or VPCs), poor R-wave progression, bundle branch block (left and right), nodal arrhythmia, U wave change, atrial flutter/fibrillation.

Furthermore, severe hypotension, bradycardia and syncope have been reported immediately or closely following IV administration.

Dermatologic: Rash, increased sweating.

Gastrointestinal System: Constipation, dyspepsia, abdominal pain, anorexia; *Rarely:* Pancreatitis.

Hearing, Taste and Vision: Taste perversion, abnormal vision; *Rarely:* Tinnitus, photophobia.

Hematologic: *Rarely:* Hematuria, epistaxis, prothrombin time prolonged, PTT increased, anemia, purpura/hematoma, thrombocytopenia.

Hypersensitivity: *Rarely:* Anaphylactic reaction, facial edema, urticaria.

Liver and Biliary System: Transient increases in AST (SGOT) and/or ALT (SGPT) values have been reported as adverse events in less than 1% of adult patients receiving dolasetron mesylate in clinical trials. The increases did not appear to be related to dose or duration of therapy and were not associated with symptomatic hepatic disease. Similar increases were seen with patients receiving active comparator. *Rarely:* Hyperbilirubinemia, increased GGT.

Metabolic and Nutritional: *Rarely:* Alkaline phosphatase increased.

Musculoskeletal: *Rarely:* Myalgia, arthralgia.

Nervous System: Flushing, vertigo, paraesthesia, tremor; *Rarely:* Ataxia, twitching.

Psychiatric: Agitation, sleep disorder, depersonalization; *Rarely:* Confusion, anxiety, abnormal dreaming.

Respiratory System: *Rarely:* Dyspnea, bronchospasm.

Urinary System: *Rarely:* Dysuria, polyuria, acute renal failure.

Vascular (extracardiac): Local pain or burning on IV administration; *Rarely:* Peripheral ischemia, thrombophlebitis/phlebitis.

DOSAGE AND ADMINISTRATION

The recommended dose of dolasetron mesylate injection should not be exceeded.

PREVENTION OF CANCER CHEMOTHERAPY-INDUCED NAUSEA AND VOMITING

Adults

The recommended intravenous dosage of dolasetron mesylate injection from clinical trial results is 1.8 mg/kg given as a single dose approximately 30 minutes before chemotherapy (see Administration). Alternatively, for most patients, a fixed dose of 100 mg can be administered over 30 seconds.

Pediatric Patients

The recommended intravenous dosage in pediatric patients 2–16 years of age is 1.8 mg/kg given as a single dose approximately 30 minutes before chemotherapy, up to a maximum of 100 mg (see Administration). Safety and effectiveness in pediatric patients under 2 years of age have not been established.

Dolasetron mesylate injection mixed in apple or apple-grape juice may be used for oral dosing of pediatric patients. When dolasetron mesylate injection is administered orally, the recommended dosage in pediatric patients 2–16 years of age is 1.8 mg/kg up to a maximum 100 mg dose given within 1 hour before chemotherapy.

The diluted product may be kept up to 2 hours at room temperature before use.

Use in the Elderly, in Renal Failure Patients, or in Hepatically Impaired Patients

No dosage adjustment is recommended.

PREVENTION OR TREATMENT OF POSTOPERATIVE NAUSEA AND/OR VOMITING

Adults

The recommended intravenous dosage of dolasetron mesylate injection is 12.5 mg given as a single dose approximately 15 minutes before the cessation of anesthesia (prevention) or as soon as nausea or vomiting presents (treatment).

Pediatric Patients

The recommended intravenous dosage in pediatric patients 2–16 years of age is 0.35 mg/kg, with a maximum dose of 12.5 mg, given as a single dose approximately 15 minutes before the cessation of anesthesia or as soon as nausea or vomiting presents.

Safety and effectiveness in pediatric patients under 2 years of age have not been established.

Dolasetron mesylate injection mixed in apple or apple-grape juice may be used for oral dosing of pediatric patients. When dolasetron mesylate injection is administered orally, the recommended oral dosage in pediatric patients 2–16 years of age is 1.2 mg/kg up to a maximum 100 mg dose given within 2 hours before surgery. The diluted product may be kept up to 2 hours at room temperature before use.

Use in the Elderly, in Renal Failure Patients, or in Hepatically Impaired Patients

No dosage adjustment is recommended.

ADMINISTRATION

Dolasetron mesylate injection can be safely infused intravenously as rapidly as 100 mg/30 seconds or diluted in a compatible intravenous solution (see Stability) to 50 ml and infused over a period of up to 15 minutes. Dolasetron mesylate injection should not be mixed with other drugs. Flush the infusion line before and after administration of dolasetron mesylate injection.

STABILITY

After dilution, dolasetron mesylate injection is stable under normal lighting conditions at room temperature for 24 hours or under refrigeration for 48 hours with the following compatible intravenous fluids: 0.9% sodium chloride injection, 5% dextrose injection, 5% dextrose and 0.45% sodium chloride injection, 5% dextrose and lactated Ringer's injection, lactated Ringer's injection, and 10% mannitol injection. Although dolasetron mesylate injection is chemically and physically stable when diluted as recommended, sterile precautions should be observed because diluents generally do not contain preservative. After dilution, do not use beyond 24 hours, or 48 hours if refrigerated.

Parenteral drug products should be inspected visually for particulate matter and discoloration before administration whenever solution and container permit.

HOW SUPPLIED

Anzemet injection (dolasetron mesylate injection) is supplied in single-use ampuls and vials as a clear, colorless solution.

Storage: Store at controlled room temperature 20-25°C (68-77°F). Protect from light.

ORAL

DESCRIPTION

Dolasetron mesylate is an antinauseant and antiemetic agent. Chemically, dolasetron mesylate is (2α,6α,8α,9aβ)-octahydro-3-oxo-2,6-methano-2*H*-quinolizin-8-yl-l*H*-indole-3-carboxylate monomethanesulfonate, monohydrate. It is a highly specific and selective serotonin subtype 3 (5-HT_3) receptor antagonist both *in vitro* and *in vivo*.

The empirical formula is $C_{19}H_{20}N_2O_3 \cdot CH_3SO_3H \cdot H_2O$, with a molecular weight of 438.50. Approximately 74% of dolasetron mesylate monohydrate is dolasetron base.

Dolasetron mesylate monohydrate is a white to off-white powder that is freely soluble in water and propylene glycol, slightly soluble in ethanol, and slightly soluble in normal saline.

Each Anzemet tablet for oral administration contains dolasetron mesylate (as the monohydrate) and also contains the inactive ingredients: carnauba wax, croscarmellose sodium, hydroxypropyl methylcellulose, lactose, magnesium stearate, polyethylene glycol, polysorbate 80, pregelatinized starch, synthetic red iron oxide, titanium dioxide, and white wax. The tablets are printed with black ink, which contains lecithin, pharmaceutical glaze, propylene glycol, and synthetic black iron oxide.

CLINICAL PHARMACOLOGY

Dolasetron mesylate and its active metabolite, hydrodolasetron (MDL 74,156), are selective serotonin 5-HT_3 receptor antagonists not shown to have activity at other known serotonin receptors and with low affinity for dopamine receptors. The serotonin 5-HT_3 receptors are located on the nerve terminals of the vagus in the periphery and centrally in the chemoreceptor trigger zone of the area postrema. It is thought that chemotherapeutic agents produce nausea and vomiting by releasing serotonin from the enterochromaffin cells of the small intestine, and that the released serotonin then activates 5-HT_3 receptors located on vagal efferents to initiate the vomiting reflex.

Acute, usually reversible, ECG changes (PR and QTc prolongation; QRS widening), caused by dolasetron mesylate, have been observed in healthy volunteers and in controlled clinical trials. The active metabolites of dolasetron may block sodium channels, a property unrelated to its ability to block 5-HT_3 receptors. QTc prolongation is primarily due to QRS widening. Dolasetron appears to prolong both depolarization and, to a lesser extent, repolarization time. The magnitude and frequency of the ECG changes increased with dose (related to peak plasma concentrations of hydrodolasetron but not the parent compound). These ECG interval prolongations usually returned to baseline within 6–8 hours, but in some patients were present at 24 hour follow up. Dolasetron mesylate administration has little or no effect on blood pressure.

In healthy volunteers (n=64), dolasetron mesylate in single intravenous doses up to 5 mg/kg produced no effect on pupil size or meaningful changes in EEG tracings. Results from neuropsychiatric tests revealed that dolasetron mesylate did not alter mood or concentration. Multiple daily doses of dolasetron have had no effect on colonic transit in humans. Dolasetron has no effect on plasma prolactin concentrations.

PHARMACOKINETICS IN HUMANS

Oral dolasetron is well absorbed, although parent drug is rarely detected in plasma due to rapid and complete metabolism to the most clinically relevant species, hydrodolasetron.

The reduction of dolasetron to hydrodolasetron is mediated by a ubiquitous enzyme, carbonyl reductase. Cytochrome P-450 (CYP)IID6 is primarily responsible for the subsequent hydroxylation of hydrodolasetron and both CYPIIIA and flavin monooxygenase are responsible for the N-oxidation of hydrodolasetron.

Hydrodolasetron is excreted in the urine unchanged (61.0% of administered oral dose). Other urinary metabolites include hydroxylated glucuronides and N-oxide.

Hydrodolasetron appears rapidly in plasma, with a maximum concentration occurring approximately 1 hour after dosing, and is eliminated with a mean half-life of 8.1 hours (%CV=18%) and an apparent clearance of 13.4 ml/min/kg (%CV=29%) in 30 adults. The apparent absolute bioavailability of oral dolasetron, determined by the major active metabolite hydrodolasetron, is approximately 75%. Orally administered dolasetron intravenous solution and tablets are bioequivalent. Food does not affect the bioavailability of dolasetron taken by mouth.

Hydrodolasetron is eliminated by multiple routes, including renal excretion and, after metabolism, mainly, glucuronidation and hydroxylation. Two-thirds (2/3) of the administered dose is recovered in the urine and 1/3 in the feces. Hydrodolasetron is widely distributed in the body with a mean apparent volume of distribution of 5.8 L/kg (%CV=25%, n=24) in adults.

Sixty-nine (69) to 77% of hydrodolasetron is bound to plasma protein. In a study with ^{14}C labeled dolasetron, the distribution of radioactivity to blood cells was not extensive. Approximately 50% of hydrodolasetron is bound to α_1-acid glycoprotein. The pharmacokinetics of hydrodolasetron are linear and similar in men and women.

The pharmacokinetics of hydrodolasetron, in special and targeted patient populations following oral administration of dolasetron, are summarized in TABLE 6. The pharmacokinetics of hydrodolasetron are similar in adult healthy volunteers and in adult cancer patients receiving chemotherapeutic agents. The apparent clearance following oral administration of hydrodolasetron is approximately 1.6- to 3.4-fold higher in children and adolescents than in adults. The clearance following oral administration of hydrodolasetron is not affected by age in adult cancer patients. The apparent oral clearance of hydrodolasetron decreases 42% with severe hepatic impairment and 44% with severe renal impairment. No dose adjustment is necessary for elderly patients or for patients with hepatic or renal impairment.

The pharmacokinetics of dolasetron mesylate tablets have not been studied in the pediatric population. However, the following pharmacokinetic data are available on intravenous dolasetron mesylate injection administered orally to children.

Thirty-two (32) pediatric cancer patients ages 3–11 years (n=19) and 12–17 years (n=13), received 0.6, 1.2, or 1.8 mg dolasetron mesylate injection diluted with either apple or apple-grape juice and administered orally. In this study, the mean apparent clearances of hydrodolasetron were 3 times greater in the younger pediatric group and 1.8 times greater in the older pediatric group than those observed in healthy adult volunteers. Across this spectrum of pediatric patients, maximum plasma concentrations were 0.6–0.7 times those observed in healthy adults receiving similar doses.

For 12 pediatric patients, ages 2–12 years receiving 1.2 mg/kg dolasetron mesylate injection diluted in apple or apple-grape juice and administered orally, the mean apparent clearance was 34% greater and half-life was 21% shorter than in healthy adults receiving the same dose.

***TABLE 6** Pharmacokinetic Values for Plasma Hydrodolasetron Following Oral Administration of Dolasetron Mesylate**

	Age (years)	Dose	CL_{app} (ml/min/kg)	T½ (h)	C_{max} (ng/ml)
Young healthy volunteers (n=30)	19-45	200 mg	13.4 (29%)	8.1 (18%)	556 (28%)
Elderly healthy volunteers (n=15)	65-75	2.4 mg/kg	9.5 (36%)	7.2 (32%)	662 (28%)
Cancer patients					
Adults (n=61)†	24-84	25-200 mg/kg	12.9 (49%)	7.9 (43%)	—‡
Adolescents (n=13)	12-17	0.6-1.8 mg/kg	26.5 (67%)	6.4 (30%)	374§ (32%)
Children (n=19)	3-11	0.6-1.8 mg/kg	44.2 (49%)	5.5 (39%)	217¤ (67%)
Pediatric surgery patients (n=11)	2-12	1.2 mg/kg	20.8 (49%)	5.9 (24%)	159 (32%)
Patients with severe renal impairment (n=12) (creatinine clearance ≤10 ml/min)	28-74	200 mg	7.2 (48%)	10.7 (29%)	701 (21%)
Patients with severe hepatic impairment (n=3)	42-52	150 mg	8.8 (57%)	11.0 (36%)	410 (12%)

CL_{app} = apparent clearance; T½ = terminal elimination half-life; () = Coefficient of variation in %.
* Mean values.
† Analyzed by nonlinear mixed effect modeling with data pooled across dose strengths.
‡ Sampling times did not allow calculation.
§ Results from adolescents (dose=1.8 mg/kg, n=3).
¤ Results from children (dose=1.8 mg/kg, n=7).

INDICATIONS AND USAGE

Dolasetron mesylate tablets are indicated for:

The prevention of nausea and vomiting associated with moderately emetogenic cancer chemotherapy, including initial and repeat courses.

The prevention of postoperative nausea and vomiting.

CONTRAINDICATIONS

Dolasetron mesylate tablets are contraindicated in patients known to have hypersensitivity to the drug.

WARNINGS

Dolasetron mesylate can cause ECG interval changes (PR, QTc, JT prolongation and QRS widening). These changes are related in magnitude and frequency to blood levels of the active metabolite. These changes are self-limiting with declining blood levels. Some patients have interval prolongations for 24 hours or longer. Interval prolongation could lead to cardiovascular consequences, including heart block or cardiac arrhythmias. These have rarely been reported.

A cardiac conduction abnormality observed on an intra-operative cardiac rhythm monitor (interpreted as complete heart block) was reported in a 61-year-old woman who received 200 mg dolasetron mesylate for the prevention of postoperative nausea and vomiting. This patient was also taking verapamil. A similar event also interpreted as complete heart block was reported in one patient receiving placebo.

A 66-year-old man with Stage IV non-Hodgkins lymphoma died suddenly 6 hours after receiving 1.8 mg/kg (119 mg) intravenous dolasetron mesylate injection. This patient had other potential risk factors including substantial exposure to doxorubicin and concomitant cyclophosphamide.

PRECAUTIONS

GENERAL

Dolasetron should be administered with caution in patients who have or may develop prolongation of cardiac conduction intervals, particularly QTc. These include patients with hypokalemia or hypomagnesemia, patients taking diuretics with potential for inducing electrolyte abnormalities, patients with congenital QT syndrome, patients taking anti-arrhythmic drugs or other drugs which lead to QT prolongation, and cumulative high dose anthracycline therapy.

Cross hypersensitivity reactions have been reported in patients who received other selective 5-HT_3 receptor antagonists. These reactions have not been seen with dolasetron mesylate.

CARCINOGENESIS, MUTAGENESIS, AND IMPAIRMENT OF FERTILITY

In a 24 month carcinogenicity study, there was a statistically significant ($P<0.001$) increase in the incidence of combined hepatocellular adenomas and carcinomas in male mice treated with 150 mg/kg/day and above. In this study, mice (CD-1) were treated orally with dolasetron mesylate 75, 150 or 300 mg/kg/day (225, 450 or 900 mg/m²/day). For a 50 kg person of average height (1.46 m² body surface area), these doses represent 3, 6, and 12 times the recommended clinical dose (74 mg/m²) on a body surface area basis. No increase in liver tumors was observed at a dose of 75 mg/kg/day in male mice and at doses up to 300 mg/kg/day in female mice.

In a 24 month rat (Sprague-Dawley) carcinogenicity study, oral dolasetron mesylate was not tumorigenic at doses up to 150 mg/kg/day (900 mg/m²/day, 12 times the recommended human dose based on body surface area) in male rats and 300 mg/kg/day (1800 mg/m²/day, 24 times the recommended human dose based on body surface area) in female rats.

Dolasetron mesylate was not genotoxic in the Ames test, the rat lymphocyte chromosomal aberration test, the Chinese hamster ovary (CHO) cell (HGPRT) forward mutation test, the rat hepatocyte unscheduled DNA synthesis (UDS) test or the mouse micronucleus test.

Dolasetron mesylate was found to have no effect on fertility and reproductive performance at oral doses up to 100 mg/kg/day (600 mg/m²/day, 8 times the recommended human dose based on body surface area) in female rats and up to 400 mg/kg/day (2400 mg/m²/day, 32 times the recommended human dose based on body surface area) in male rats.

PREGNANCY, TERATOGENIC EFFECTS, PREGNANCY CATEGORY B

Teratology studies have not revealed evidence of impaired fertility or harm to the fetus due to dolasetron mesylate. These studies have been performed in pregnant rats at oral doses up to 100 mg/kg/day (8 times the recommended human dose based on body surface area) and pregnant rabbits at oral doses up to 100 mg/kg/day (16 times the recommended human dose based on body surface area). There are, however, no adequate and well-controlled studies in pregnant women. Because animal reproduction studies are not always predictive of human response, this drug should be used during pregnancy only if clearly needed.

NURSING MOTHERS

It is not known whether dolasetron mesylate is excreted in human milk. Because many drugs are excreted in human milk, caution should be exercised when dolasetron mesylate tablets are administered to a nursing woman.

PEDIATRIC USE

Dolasetron mesylate tablets are expected to be as safe and effective as when dolasetron mesylate injection is given orally to pediatric patients. Dolasetron mesylate tablets are recommended for children old enough to swallow tablets (see CLINICAL PHARMACOLOGY, Pharmacokinetics in Humans).

ELDERLY

Dosage adjustment is not needed in patients over 65. Effectiveness in prevention of nausea and vomiting in elderly patients was no different than in younger age groups.

DRUG INTERACTIONS

The potential for clinically significant drug-drug interactions posed by dolasetron and hydrodolasetron appears to be low for drugs commonly used in chemotherapy or surgery, because hydrodolasetron is eliminated by multiple routes. See PRECAUTIONS, General for information about potential interaction with other drugs that prolong the QTc interval. Blood levels of hydrodolasetron increased 24% when dolasetron was coadministered with cimetidine (nonselective inhibitor of cytochrome P-450) for 7 days, and decreased 28% with coadministration of rifampin (potent inducer of cytochrome P-450) for 7 days.

Dolasetron mesylate has been safely coadministered with drugs used in chemotherapy and surgery. As with other agents which prolong ECG intervals, caution should be exercised in patients taking drugs which prolong ECG intervals, particularly QTc.

In patients taking furosemide, nifedipine, diltiazem, ACE inhibitors, verapamil, glyburide, propranolol, and various chemotherapy agents, no effect was shown on the clearance of hydrodolasetron Clearance of hydrodolasetron decreased by about 27% when dolasetron mesylate was administered intravenously concomitantly with atenolol. Dolasetron mesylate did not influence anesthesia recovery time in patients. Dolasetron mesylate did not inhibit the antitumor activity of four chemotherapeutic agents (cisplatin, 5-fluorouracil, doxorubicin, cyclophosphamide) in four murine models.

ADVERSE REACTIONS

CHEMOTHERAPY PATIENTS

In controlled clinical trials, 943 adult cancer patients received dolasetron mesylate tablets. These patients were receiving concurrent chemotherapy, predominantly cyclophosphamide and doxorubicin regimens. The following adverse events were reported in ≥2% of patients receiving either dolasetron mesylate 25 or 100 mg tablets for prevention of cancer chemotherapy induced nausea and vomiting in controlled clinical trials (TABLE 9).

***TABLE 9** Adverse Events ≥2% From Chemotherapy-Induced Nausea and Vomiting Studies*

	Dolasetron Mesylate	
	25 mg	100 mg
Event	(n=235)	(n=227)
Headache	42 (17.9%)	52 (22.9%)
Fatigue	6 (2.6%)	13 (5.7%)
Diarrhea	5 (2.1%)	12 (5.3%)
Bradycardia	12 (5.1%)	9 (4.0%)
Dizziness	3 (1.3%)	7 (3.1%)
Pain	0	7 (3.1%)
Tachycardia	7 (3.0%)	6 (2.6%)
Dyspepsia	7 (3.0%)	5 (2.2%)
Chills/shivering	3 (1.3%)	5 (2.2%)

D

POSTOPERATIVE PATIENTS

In controlled clinical trials, 936 adult female patients have received oral dolasetron mesylate for the prevention of postoperative nausea and vomiting. Following is a listing of all adverse events reported in ≥2% of patients receiving either placebo or dolasetron mesylate for prevention of postoperative nausea and vomiting in controlled clinical trials (TABLE 10).

TABLE 10 *Adverse Events ≥2% from Placebo-Controlled Postoperative Nausea and Vomiting Studies*

Event	Dolasetron Mesylate 100 mg (n=228)	Placebo (n=231)
Headache	16 (7.0%)	11 (4.8%)
Hypotension	12 (5.3%)	15 (6.5%)
Dizziness	10 (4.4%)	0 (0.0%)
Fever	8 (3.5%)	7 (3.0%)
Pruritus	7 (3.1%)	8 (3.5%)
Oliguria	6 (2.6%)	3 (1.3%)
Hypertension	5 (2.2%)	7 (3.0%)
Tachycardia	5 (2.2%)	2 (0.9%)

In clinical trials, the following infrequently reported adverse events, assessed by investigators as treatment-related or causality unknown, occurred following oral or intravenous administration of dolasetron mesylate to adult patients receiving concomitant cancer chemotherapy or surgery:

Cardiovascular: Hypotension; *Rarely:* Edema, peripheral edema. *The following events also occurred rarely and with a similar frequency as placebo and/or active comparator:* Mobitz I AV block, chest pain, orthostatic hypotension, myocardial ischemia, syncope, severe bradycardia, and palpitations. See PRECAUTIONS for information on potential effects on ECG.

In addition, the following asymptomatic treatment-emergent ECG changes were seen at rates less than or equal to those for active or placebo controls: Bradycardia, T wave change, ST-T wave change, sinus arrhythmia, extrasystole (APCs or VPCs), poor R-wave progression, bundle branch block (left and right), nodal arrhythmia, U wave change, atrial flutter/fibrillation.

Furthermore, severe hypotension, bradycardia and syncope have been reported immediately or closely following IV administration.

Dermatologic: Rash, increased sweating.

Gastrointestinal System: Constipation, dyspepsia, abdominal pain, anorexia; *Rarely:* Pancreatitis.

Hearing, Taste and Vision: Taste perversion, abnormal vision; *Rarely:* Tinnitus, photophobia.

Hematologic: Rarely: Hematuria, epistaxis, prothrombin time prolonged, PTT increased, anemia, purpura/hematoma, thrombocytopenia.

Hypersensitivity: Rarely: Anaphylactic reaction, facial edema, urticaria.

Liver and Biliary System: Transient increases in AST (SGOT) and/or ALT (SGPT) values have been reported as adverse events in less than 1% of adult patients receiving dolasetron mesylate in clinical trials. The increases did not appear to be related to dose or duration of therapy and were not associated with symptomatic hepatic disease. Similar increases were seen with patients receiving active comparator. *Rarely:* Hyperbilirubinemia, increased GGT.

Metabolic and Nutritional: Rarely: Alkaline phosphatase increased.

Musculoskeletal: Rarely: Myalgia, arthralgia.

Nervous System: Flushing, vertigo, paraesthesia, tremor; *Rarely:* Ataxia, twitching.

Psychiatric: Agitation, sleep disorder, depersonalization; *Rarely:* Confusion, anxiety, abnormal dreaming.

Respiratory System: Rarely: Dyspnea, bronchospasm.

Urinary System: Rarely: Dysuria, polyuria, acute renal failure.

Vascular (extracardiac): Local pain or burning on IV administration; *Rarely:* Peripheral ischemia, thrombophlebitis/phlebitis.

DOSAGE AND ADMINISTRATION

The recommended doses of dolasetron mesylate tablets should not be exceeded.

PREVENTION OF CANCER CHEMOTHERAPY-INDUCED NAUSEA AND VOMITING

Adults: The recommended oral dosage of dolasetron mesylate (dolasetron mesylate) is 100 mg given within 1 hour before chemotherapy.

Pediatric patients: The recommended oral dosage in pediatric patients 2–16 years of age is 1.8 mg/kg given within 1 hour before chemotherapy, up to a maximum of 100 mg. Safety and effectiveness in pediatric patients under 2 years of age have not been established.

Use in the elderly, renal failure patients, or hepatically impaired patients: No dosage adjustment is recommended. (See CLINICAL PHARMACOLOGY, Pharmacokinetics in Humans.)

PREVENTION OF POSTOPERATIVE NAUSEA AND VOMITING

Adults: The recommended oral dosage of dolasetron mesylate is 100 mg within 2 hours before surgery.

Pediatric patients: The recommended oral dosage in pediatric patients 2–16 years of age is 1.2 mg/kg given within 2 hours before surgery, up to a maximum of 100 mg. Safety and effectiveness in pediatric patients under 2 years of age have not been established.

Use in the elderly, renal failure patients, or hepatically impaired patients: No dosage adjustment is recommended. (See CLINICAL PHARMACOLOGY, Pharmacokinetics in Humans.)

HOW SUPPLIED

50 mg: Light pink, film coated, round tablet imprinted with "ANZEMET 50" on one side.
100 mg: Pink, film coated, elongated oval tablet imprinted with "100" on one side and "ANZEMET" on the other.

Storage: Store at controlled room temperature 20-25°C (68-77°F). Protect from light.

PRODUCT LISTING - EQUIVALENTS NOT AVAILABLE

Solution - Intravenous - 20 mg/ml

0.62 ml x 6	$117.15	ANZEMET, Abbott Pharmaceutical	00074-1208-65
0.62 ml x 6	$140.22	ANZEMET, Aventis Pharmaceuticals	00088-1208-65
0.62 ml x 10	$233.70	ANZEMET, Aventis Pharmaceuticals	00088-1208-69
2 ml x 10	$195.30	ANZEMET, Aventis Pharmaceuticals	00088-1208-76
5 ml	$173.16	ANZEMET, Aventis Pharmaceuticals	00088-1206-32

Tablet - Oral - 50 mg

5's	$249.00	ANZEMET, Aventis Pharmaceuticals	00088-1202-29
5's	$287.60	ANZEMET, Aventis Pharmaceuticals	00088-1202-05
10's	$575.27	ANZEMET, Aventis Pharmaceuticals	00088-1202-43

Tablet - Oral - 100 mg

5's	$366.54	ANZEMET, Allscripts Pharmaceutical Company	54569-4870-00
5's	$381.20	ANZEMET, Aventis Pharmaceuticals	00088-1203-05
5's	$381.20	ANZEMET, Aventis Pharmaceuticals	00088-1203-29
10's	$762.41	ANZEMET, Aventis Pharmaceuticals	00088-1203-43

Donepezil Hydrochloride *(003311)*

Categories: Alzheimer's disease; Pregnancy Category C; FDA Approved 1996 Nov
Drug Classes: Cholinesterase inhibitors
Brand Names: Aricept
Foreign Brand Availability: Asenta (Israel); Eranz (Colombia; Mexico); Memorit (Israel)
Cost of Therapy: $148.88 (Dementia, Alzheimer's; Aricept; 5 mg; 1 tablet/day; 30 day supply)

DESCRIPTION

Donepezil hydrochloride is a reversible inhibitor of the enzyme acetylcholinesterase, known chemically as (±)-2,3-dihydro-5,6-dimethoxy-2-[[1-(phenylmethyl)-4-piperidinyl] methyl]-1*H*-inden-1-one hydrochloride. Donepezil hydrochloride is commonly referred to in the pharmacological literature as E2020. It has an empirical formula of $C_{24}H_{29}NO_3HCl$ and a molecular weight of 415.96. Donepezil hydrochloride is a white crystalline powder and is freely soluble in chloroform, soluble in water and in glacial acetic acid, slightly soluble in ethanol and in acetonitrile, and practically insoluble in ethyl acetate and in n-hexane.

Aricept is available for oral administration in film-coated tablets containing 5 or 10 mg of donepezil hydrochloride. Inactive ingredients are lactose monohydrate, corn starch, microcrystalline cellulose, hydroxypropyl cellulose, and magnesium stearate. The film coating contains talc, polyethylene glycol, hydroxypropyl methylcellulose, and titanium dioxide. Additionally, the 10 mg tablet contains yellow iron oxide (synthetic) as a coloring agent.

CLINICAL PHARMACOLOGY

Current theories on the pathogenesis of the cognitive signs and symptoms of Alzheimer's disease attribute some of them to a deficiency of cholinergic neurotransmission.

Donepezil HCl is postulated to exert its therapeutic effect by enhancing cholinergic function. This is accomplished by increasing the concentration of acetylcholine through reversible inhibition of its hydrolysis by acetylcholinesterase. If this proposed mechanism of action is correct, donepezil's effect may lessen as the disease process advances and fewer cholinergic neurons remain functionally intact. There is no evidence that donepezil alters the course of the underlying dementing process.

PHARMACOKINETICS

Donepezil is well absorbed with a relative oral bioavailability of 100%. It reaches peak plasma concentrations in 3-4 hours. Pharmacokinetics are linear over a dose range of 1-10 mg given once daily. Neither food nor time of administration (morning vs evening dose) influences the rate or extent of absorption. The elimination half-life of donepezil is about 70 hours, and the mean apparent plasma clearance (Cl/F) is 0.13 L/h/kg. Following multiple-dose administration, donepezil accumulates in plasma by 4- to 7-fold, and steady state is reached within 15 days. The steady state volume of distribution is 12 L/kg. Donepezil is approximately 96% bound to human plasma proteins, mainly to albumins (about 75%) and $alpha_1$-acid glycoprotein (about 21%) over the concentration range of 2-1000 ng/ml.

Donepezil is both excreted in the urine intact and extensively metabolized to 4 major metabolites, 2 of which are known to be active, and a number of minor metabolites, not all of which have been identified. Donepezil is metabolized by CYP 450 isoenzymes 2D6 and 3A4 and undergoes glucuronidation. Following administration of ^{14}C-labeled donepezil, plasma radioactivity, expressed as a percent of the administered dose, was present primarily as intact donepezil (53%) and as 6-O-desmethyl donepezil (11%), which has been reported to inhibit AChE to the same extent as donepezil *in vitro* and was found in plasma at concentrations equal to about 20% of donepezil. Approximately 57% and 15% of the total radioactivity was recovered in urine and feces, respectively, over a period of 10 days, while 28% remained unrecovered, with about 17% of the donepezil dose recovered in the urine as unchanged drug.

SPECIAL POPULATIONS

Hepatic Disease

In a study of 10 patients with stable alcoholic cirrhosis, the clearance of donepezil HCl was decreased by 20% relative to 10 healthy age- and sex-matched subjects.

Renal Disease

In a study of 4 patients with moderate to severe renal impairment (CLCR <22 ml/min/1.73 m^2) the clearance of donepezil HCl did not differ from 4 age- and sex-matched healthy subjects.

Age

No formal pharmacokinetic study was conducted to examine age-related differences in the pharmacokinetics of donepezil HCl. However, mean plasma donepezil HCl concentrations measured during therapeutic drug monitoring of elderly patients with Alzheimer's disease are comparable to those observed in young healthy volunteers.

Gender and Race

No specific pharmacokinetic study was conducted to investigate the effects of gender and race on the disposition of donepezil HCl. However, retrospective pharmacokinetic analysis indicates that gender and race (Japanese and Caucasians) did not affect the clearance of donepezil HCl.

DRUG-DRUG INTERACTIONS

Drugs Highly Bound to Plasma Proteins

Drug displacement studies have been performed *in vitro* between this highly-bound drug (96%) and other drugs such as furosemide, digoxin, and warfarin. Donepezil HCl at concentrations of 0.3-10 μg/ml did not affect the binding of furosemide (5 μg/ml), digoxin (2 ng/ml), and warfarin (3 μg/ml) to human albumin. Similarly, the binding of donepezil HCl to human albumin was not affected by furosemide, digoxin, and warfarin.

Effect of Donepezil HCl on the Metabolism of Other Drugs

No *in vivo* clinical trials have investigated the effect of donepezil HCl on the clearance of drugs metabolized by CYP 3A4 (*e.g.*, cisapride, terfenadine) or by CYP 2D6 (*e.g.*, imipramine). However, *in vitro* studies show a low rate of binding to these enzymes (mean Ki about 50-130 μM), that, given the therapeutic plasma concentrations of donepezil (164 nM), indicates little likelihood of interference.

Whether donepezil HCl has any potential for enzyme induction is not known.

Formal pharmacokinetic studies evaluated the potential of donepezil HCl for interaction with theophylline, cimetidine, warfarin, and digoxin. No significant effects on the pharmacokinetics of these drugs were observed.

Effect of Other Drugs on the Metabolism of Donepezil HCl

Ketoconazole and quinidine, inhibitors of CYP 450, 3A4 and 2D6, respectively, inhibit donepezil metabolism *in vitro*. Whether there is a clinical effect of these inhibitors is not known. Inducers of CYP 2D6 and CYP 3A4 (*e.g.*, phenytoin, carbamazepine, dexamethasone, rifampin, and phenobarbital) could increase the rate of elimination of donepezil HCl.

Formal pharmacokinetic studies demonstrated that the metabolism of donepezil HCl is not significantly affected by concurrent administration of digoxin or cimetidine.

INDICATIONS AND USAGE

Donepezil HCl is indicated for the treatment of mild to moderate dementia of the Alzheimer's type.

CONTRAINDICATIONS

Donepezil HCl is contraindicated in patients with known hypersensitivity to donepezil HCl or to piperidine derivatives.

WARNINGS

ANESTHESIA

Donepezil HCl, as a cholinesterase inhibitor, is likely to exaggerate succinylcholine-type muscle relaxation during anesthesia.

CARDIOVASCULAR CONDITIONS

Because of their pharmacological action, cholinesterase inhibitors may have vagotonic effects on the sinoatrial and atrioventricular nodes. This effect may manifest as bradycardia or heart block in patients both with and without known underlying cardiac conduction abnormalities. Syncopal episodes have been reported in association with the use of donepezil HCl.

GASTROINTESTINAL CONDITIONS

Through their primary action, cholinesterase inhibitors may be expected to increase gastric acid secretion due to increased cholinergic activity. Therefore, patients should be monitored closely for symptoms of active or occult gastrointestinal bleeding, especially those at increased risk for developing ulcers (*e.g.*, those with a history of ulcer disease or those receiving concurrent nonsteroidal antiinflammatory drugs [NSAIDS]). Clinical studies of donepezil HCl have shown no increase, relative to placebo, in the incidence of either peptic ulcer disease or gastrointestinal bleeding.

Donepezil HCl, as a predictable consequence of its pharmacological properties, has been shown to produce diarrhea, nausea, and vomiting. These effects, when they occur, appear more frequently with the 10 mg/day dose than with the 5 mg/day dose. In most cases, these effects have been mild and transient, sometimes lasting 1-3 weeks, and have resolved during continued use of donepezil HCl.

GENITOURINARY

Although not observed in clinical trials of donepezil HCl, cholinomimetics may cause bladder outflow obstruction.

NEUROLOGICAL CONDITIONS

Seizures: Cholinomimetics are believed to have some potential to cause generalized convulsions. However, seizure activity also may be a manifestation of Alzheimer's disease.

PULMONARY CONDITIONS

Because of their cholinomimetic actions, cholinesterase inhibitors should be prescribed with care to patients with a history of asthma or obstructive pulmonary disease.

PRECAUTIONS

CARCINOGENESIS, MUTAGENESIS, AND IMPAIRMENT OF FERTILITY

Carcinogenicity studies of donepezil have not been completed.

Donepezil was not mutagenic in the Ames reverse mutation assay in bacteria. In the chromosome aberration test in cultures of Chinese hamster lung (CHL) cells, some clastogenic effects were observed. Donepezil was not clastogenic in the *in vivo* mouse micronucleus test.

Donepezil had no effect on fertility in rats at doses of up to 10 mg/kg/day [approximately 8 times the maximum recommended human dose (MRHD) on a mg/m^2 basis].

PREGNANCY CATEGORY C

Teratology studies conducted in pregnant rats at doses of up to 16 mg/kg/day (approximately 13 times the MRHD on a mg/m^2 basis) and in pregnant rabbits at doses of up to 10 mg/kg/day (approximately 16 times the MRHD on a mg/m^2 basis) did not disclose any evidence for a teratogenic potential of donepezil. However, in a study in which pregnant rats were given up to 10 mg/kg/day (approximately 8 times the MRHD on a mg/m^2 basis) from day 17 of gestation through day 20 postpartum, there was a slight increase in stillbirths and a slight decrease in pup survival through day 4 postpartum at this dose; the next lower dose tested was 3 mg/kg/day. There are no adequate or well-controlled studies in pregnant women. Donepezil HCl should be used during pregnancy only if the potential benefit justifies the potential risk to the fetus.

NURSING MOTHERS

It is not known whether donepezil is excreted in human breast milk. Donepezil HCl has no indication for use in nursing mothers.

PEDIATRIC USE

There are no adequate and well-controlled trials to document the safety and efficacy of donepezil HCl in any illness occurring in children.

DRUG INTERACTIONS

DRUG-DRUG INTERACTIONS

See CLINICAL PHARMACOLOGY, Pharmacokinetics, Drug-Drug Interactions.

EFFECT OF DONEPEZIL HCl ON THE METABOLISM OF OTHER DRUGS

No *in vivo* clinical trials have investigated the effect of donepezil HCl on the clearance of drugs metabolized by CYP 3A4 (*e.g.*, cisapride, terfenadine) or by CYP 2D6 (*e.g.*, imipramine). However, *in vitro* studies show a low rate of binding to these enzymes (mean Ki about 50-130 μM), that, given the therapeutic plasma concentrations of donepezil (164 nM), indicates little likelihood of interference.

Whether donepezil HCl has any potential for enzyme induction is not known.

EFFECT OF OTHER DRUGS ON THE METABOLISM OF DONEPEZIL HCl

Ketoconazole and quinidine, inhibitors of CYP 450, 3A4 and 2D6, respectively, inhibit donepezil metabolism *in vitro*. Whether there is a clinical effect of these inhibitors is not known. Inducers of CYP 2D6 and CYP 3A4 (*e.g.*, phenytoin, carbamazepine, dexamethasone, rifampin, and phenobarbital) could increase the rate of elimination of donepezil HCl.

USE WITH ANTICHOLINERGICS

Because of their mechanism of action, cholinesterase inhibitors have the potential to interfere with the activity of anticholinergic medications.

USE WITH CHOLINOMIMETICS AND OTHER CHOLINESTERASE INHIBITORS

A synergistic effect may be expected when cholinesterase inhibitors are given concurrently with succinylcholine, similar neuromuscular blocking agents or cholinergic agonists such as bethanechol.

ADVERSE REACTIONS

ADVERSE EVENTS LEADING TO DISCONTINUATION

The rates of discontinuation from controlled clinical trials of donepezil HCl due to adverse events for the donepezil HCl 5 mg/day treatment groups were comparable to those of placebo-treatment groups at approximately 5%. The rate of discontinuation of patients who received 7 day escalations from 5-10 mg/day was higher at 13%.

The most common adverse events leading to discontinuation, defined as those occurring in at least 2% of patients and at twice the incidence seen in placebo patients, are shown in TABLE 1.

TABLE 1 *Most Frequent Adverse Events Leading to Withdrawal From Controlled Clinical Trials by Dose Group*

Dose Group	Placebo	Donepezil HCl 5 mg/day	Donepezil HCl 10 mg/day
Patients Randomized	355	350	315
Event/% Discontinuing			
Nausea	1%	1%	3%
Diarrhea	0%	<1%	3%
Vomiting	<1%	<1%	2%

MOST FREQUENT ADVERSE CLINICAL EVENTS SEEN IN ASSOCIATION WITH THE USE OF DONEPEZIL HCl

The most common adverse events, defined as those occurring at a frequency of at least 5% in patients receiving 10 mg/day and twice the placebo rate, are largely predicted by donepezil HCl's cholinomimetic effects. These include nausea, diarrhea, insomnia, vomiting, muscle cramp, fatigue, and anorexia. These adverse events were often of mild intensity and transient, resolving during continued donepezil HCl treatment without the need for dose modification.

There is evidence to suggest that the frequency of these common adverse events may be affected by the rate of titration. An open-label study was conducted with 269 patients who received placebo in the 15 and 30 week studies. These patients were titrated to a dose of 10 mg/day over a 6 week period. The rates of common adverse events were lower than those seen in patients titrated to 10 mg/day over 1 week in the controlled clinical trials and were comparable to those seen in patients on 5 mg/day.

See TABLE 2 for a comparison of the most common adverse events following 1 and 6 week titration regimens.

TABLE 2 *Comparison of Rates of Adverse Events in Patients Titrated to 10 mg/day Over 1 and 6 Weeks*

	No Titration		1 Week Titration	6 Week Titration
	Placebo	5 mg/day	10 mg/day	10 mg/day
Adverse Event	(n=315)	(n=311)	(n=315)	(n=269)
Nausea	6%	5%	19%	6%
Diarrhea	5%	8%	15%	9%
Insomnia	6%	6%	14%	6%
Fatigue	3%	4%	8%	3%
Vomiting	3%	3%	8%	5%
Muscle cramps	2%	6%	8%	3%
Anorexia	2%	3%	7%	3%

ADVERSE EVENTS REPORTED IN CONTROLLED TRIALS

The events cited reflect experience gained under closely monitored conditions of clinical trials in a highly selected patient population. In actual clinical practice, or in other clinical trials, these frequency estimates may not apply, as the conditions of use, reporting behavior, and the kinds of patients treated may differ. TABLE 3 lists treatment emergent signs and symptoms that were reported in at least 2% of patients in placebo-controlled trials who received donepezil HCl, and for which the rate of occurrence was greater for donepezil HCl assigned patients than placebo assigned patients. In general, adverse events occurred more frequently in female patients and with advancing age.

TABLE 3 *Adverse Events Reported in Controlled Clinical Trials in at Least 2% of Patients Receiving Donepezil HCl and at Higher Frequency Than Placebo-Treated Patients*

Body System / Adverse Event	Placebo (n=355)	Donepezil HCl (n=747)
Patients With Any Adverse Event	72%	74%
Body as a Whole		
Headache	9%	10%
Pain, various locations	8%	9%
Accident	6%	7%
Fatigue	3%	5%
Cardiovascular System		
Syncope	1%	2%
Digestive System		
Nausea	6%	11%
Diarrhea	5%	10%
Vomiting	3%	5%
Anorexia	2%	4%
Hemic and Lymphatic System		
Ecchymosis	3%	4%
Metabolic and Nutritional Systems		
Weight decrease	1%	3%
Musculoskeletal System		
Muscle cramps	2%	6%
Arthritis	1%	2%
Nervous System		
Insomnia	6%	9%
Dizziness	6%	8%
Depression	<1%	3%
Abnormal dreams	0%	3%
Somnolence	<1%	2%
Urogenital System		
Frequent urination	1%	2%

OTHER ADVERSE EVENTS OBSERVED DURING CLINICAL TRIALS

Donepezil HCl has been administered to over 1700 individuals during clinical trials worldwide. Approximately 1200 of these patients have been treated for at least 3 months, and more than 1000 patients have been treated for at least 6 months. Controlled and uncontrolled trials in the US included approximately 900 patients. In regards to the highest dose of 10 mg/day, this population includes 650 patients treated for 3 months, 475 patients treated for 6 months, and 116 patients treated for over 1 year. The range of patient exposure is from 1 to 1214 days.

Treatment emergent signs and symptoms that occurred during 3 controlled clinical trials and 2 open-label trials in the United States were recorded as adverse events by the clinical investigators using terminology of their own choosing. To provide an overall estimate of the proportion of individuals having similar types of events, the events were grouped into a smaller number of standardized categories using a modified COSTART dictionary, and event frequencies were calculated across all studies. These categories are used in the listing below. The frequencies represent the proportion of 900 patients from these trials who experienced that event while receiving donepezil HCl. All adverse events occurring at least twice are included, except for those already listed in TABLE 2, TABLE 3, COSTART terms too general to be informative, or events less likely to be drug caused. Events are classified by body system and listed using the following definitions: *Frequent Adverse Events:* Those occurring in at least 1/100 patients; *Infrequent Adverse Events:* Those occurring in 1/100 to 1/1000 patients. These adverse events are not necessarily related to donepezil HCl treatment and, in most cases, were observed at a similar frequency in placebo-treated patients in the controlled studies. No important additional adverse events were seen in studies conducted outside the US.

Body as a Whole: *Frequent:* Influenza, chest pain, toothache; *Infrequent:* Fever, edema face, periorbital edema, hernia hiatal, abscess, cellulitis, chills, generalized coldness, head fullness, listlessness.

Cardiovascular System: *Frequent:* Hypertension, vasodilation, atrial fibrillation, hot flashes, hypotension; *Infrequent:* Angina pectoris, postural hypotension, myocardial infarction, AV block (first degree), congestive heart failure, arteritis, bradycardia, peripheral vascular disease, supraventricular tachycardia, deep vein thrombosis.

Digestive System: *Frequent:* Fecal incontinence, gastrointestinal bleeding, bloating, epigastric pain; *Infrequent:* Eructation, gingivitis, increased appetite, flatulence, periodontal abscess, cholelithiasis, diverticulitis, drooling, dry mouth, fever sore, gastritis, irritable colon, tongue edema, epigastric distress, gastroenteritis, increased transaminases, hemorrhoids, ileus, increased thirst, jaundice, melena, polydypsia, duodenal ulcer, stomach ulcer.

Endocrine System: *Infrequent:* Diabetes mellitus, goiter.

Hemic and Lymphatic System: *Infrequent:* Anemia, thrombocythemia, thrombocytopenia, eosinophilia, erythrocytopenia.

Metabolic and Nutritional Disorders: *Frequent:* Dehydration; *Infrequent:* Gout, hypokalemia, increased creatine kinase, hyperglycemia, weight increase, increased lactate dehydrogenase.

Musculoskeletal System: *Frequent:* Bone fracture; *Infrequent:* Muscle weakness, muscle fasciculation.

Nervous System: *Frequent:* Delusions, tremor, irritability, paresthesia, aggression, vertigo, ataxia, increased libido, restlessness, abnormal crying, nervousness, aphasia; *Infrequent:* Cerebrovascular accident, intracranial hemorrhage, transient ischemic attack, emotional lability, neuralgia, coldness (localized), muscle spasm, dysphoria, gait abnormality, hypertonia, hypokinesia, neurodermatitis, numbness (localized), paranoia, dysarthria, dysphasia, hostility, decreased libido, melancholia, emotional withdrawal, nystagmus, pacing.

Respiratory System: *Frequent:* Dyspnea, sore throat, bronchitis; *Infrequent:* Epistaxis, post nasal drip, pneumonia, hyperventilation, pulmonary congestion, wheezing, hypoxia, pharyngitis, pleurisy, pulmonary collapse, sleep apnea, snoring.

Skin and Appendages: *Frequent:* Pruritus, diaphoresis, urticaria; *Infrequent:* Dermatitis, erythema, skin discoloration, hyperkeratosis, alopecia, fungal dermatitis, herpes zoster, hirsutism, skin striae, night sweats, skin ulcers.

Special Senses: *Frequent:* Cataract, eye irritation, vision blurred; *Infrequent:* Dry eyes, glaucoma, earache, tinnitus, blepharitis, decreased hearing, retinal hemorrhage, otitis externa, otitis media, bad taste, conjunctival hemorrhage, ear buzzing, motion sickness, spots before eyes.

Urogenital System: *Frequent:* Urinary incontinence, nocturia; *Infrequent:* Dysuria, hematuria, urinary urgency, metrorrhagia, cystitis, enuresis, prostate hypertrophy, pyelonephritis, inability to empty bladder, breast fibroadenosis, fibrocystic breast, mastitis, pyuria, renal failure, vaginitis.

POSTINTRODUCTION REPORTS

Voluntary reports of adverse events temporally associated with donepezil HCl that have been received since market introduction and are not listed above, and where there is inadequate data to determine the causal relationship with the drug include: abdominal pain, agitation, cholecystitis, confusion, convulsions, hallucinations, heart block (all types), hemolytic anemia, hepatitis, hyponatremia, neuroleptic malignant syndrome, pancreatitis, and rash.

DOSAGE AND ADMINISTRATION

The dosages of donepezil HCl shown to be effective in controlled clinical trials are 5 and 10 mg administered once per day.

The higher dose of 10 mg did not provide a statistically significantly greater clinical benefit than 5 mg. There is a suggestion, however, based upon order of group mean scores and dose trend analyses of data from these clinical trials, that a daily dose of 10 mg of donepezil HCl might provide additional benefit for some patients. Accordingly, whether or not to employ a dose of 10 mg is a matter of prescriber and patient preference.

Evidence from the controlled trials indicates that the 10 mg dose, with a 1 week titration, is likely to be associated with a higher incidence of cholinergic adverse events than the 5 mg dose. In open-label trials using a 6 week titration, the frequency of these same adverse events was similar between the 5 and 10 mg dose groups. Therefore, because steady state is not achieved for 15 days and because the incidence of untoward effects may be influenced by the rate of dose escalation, treatment with a dose of 10 mg should not be contemplated until patients have been on a daily dose of 5 mg for 4-6 weeks.

Donepezil HCl should be taken in the evening, just prior to retiring. Donepezil HCl can be taken with or without food.

HOW SUPPLIED

Aricept is supplied as film-coated, round tablets containing either 5 or 10 mg of donepezil HCl.

5 mg: The 5 mg tablets are white. The strength in mg ("5") is debossed on one side and "ARICEPT" is debossed on the other side.

10 mg: The 10 mg tablets are yellow. The strength in mg ("10") is debossed on one side and "ARICEPT" is debossed on the other side.

Storage: Store at controlled room temperature, 15-30°C (59-86°F).

PRODUCT LISTING - EQUIVALENTS NOT AVAILABLE

Tablet - Oral - 5 mg

30's	$148.89	ARICEPT, Pfizer U.S. Pharmaceuticals	62856-0245-30
90's	$446.68	ARICEPT, Pfizer U.S. Pharmaceuticals	62856-0245-90
100's	$496.28	ARICEPT, Pfizer U.S. Pharmaceuticals	62856-0245-41

Tablet - Oral - 10 mg

30's	$148.89	ARICEPT, Pfizer U.S. Pharmaceuticals	62856-0246-30
90's	$446.68	ARICEPT, Pfizer U.S. Pharmaceuticals	62856-0246-90
100's	$496.28	ARICEPT, Pfizer U.S. Pharmaceuticals	62856-0246-41

Dopamine Hydrochloride *(001108)*

Categories: Heart failure, congestive; Hypotension, secondary to low cardiac output; Perfusion, organ; Shock; Pregnancy Category C; FDA Approved 1974 Feb; WHO Formulary
Drug Classes: Adrenergic agonists; Inotropes
Brand Names: Dopamine HCl; **Intropin**
Foreign Brand Availability: Cardiopal (Colombia); Cardiosteril (Germany); Catabon (Japan); Docard (Israel; Philippines); Dopamex (Thailand); Dopamin (Bulgaria; Norway); Dopamin AWD (Germany; Hungary); Dopamin Braun (Switzerland); Dopamin Guilini (Austria; Germany; Indonesia); Dopamin Leopold (Austria); Dopamin Natterman (Austria; Bulgaria; Germany); Dopamina (Spain); Dopamine (France; Netherlands); Dopamine Injection (Australia); Dopaminex (Thailand); Dopaminum (Poland); Dopinga (India); Dopmin (Bulgaria; Czech-Republic; Denmark; Finland; Malaysia; Taiwan; Turkey); Dopmin E (Russia); Drynalken (Mexico); Dynatra (Belgium); Dynos (South-Africa); Giludop (Denmark; Sweden; Turkey); Inopan (Korea); Inopin (Thailand); Inotropin (Mexico); Intropin IV (Hong-Kong; Malaysia); Uramin (Taiwan)

WARNING

Full-strength dopamine HCl injection must be diluted prior to adminstration.

DESCRIPTION

Dopamine HCl is available in both full-strength and diluted forms. For the sake of clarity in this monograph, the information for these different forms will be presented as "Full-Strength" and "Prediluted" when differentiation between forms is necessary.

FULL-STRENGTH FORMS

Dopamine, a sympathomimetic amine vasopressor, is the naturally occurring immediate precursor of norepinephrine. Dopamine HCl is a white to off-white crystalline powder, which may have a slight odor of hydrochloric acid. It is freely soluble in water and soluble in alcohol. Dopamine HCl is sensitive to alkalies, iron salts, and oxidizing agents. Chemically it is designated as 4-(2-aminoethyl) pyrocatechol hydrochloride, its molecular formula is $C_8H_{11}NO_2 \cdot HCl$, and the molecular weight is 189.64.

Dopamine HCl injection is a clear, practically colorless, sterile, pyrogen-free, aqueous solution of dopamine HCl for intravenous infusion after dilution. Each milliliter of the 40 mg/ml preparation contains 40 mg of dopamine HCl (equivalent to 32.31 mg of dopamine base). Each milliliter of the 80 mg/ml preparation contains 80 mg of dopamine HCl (equivalent to 64.62 mg of dopamine base). *Each Milliliter of Both Preparations Contains the Following:* Sodium metabisulfite 9 mg added as an antioxidant; citric acid, anhydrous 10 mg; and sodium citrate, dihydrate 5 mg added as a buffer. May contain additional citric acid and/or sodium citrate for pH adjustment. pH is 3.3 (2.5-5.0).

Dopamine HCl must be diluted in an appropriate, sterile parenteral solution before intravenous administration (see DOSAGE AND ADMINISTRATION).

PREDILUTED FORMS

Dopamine HCl in 5% dextrose injection is a sterile, nonpyrogenic, prediluted solution of dopamine HCl in 5% dextrose injection. It is administered by intravenous infusion.

Each 100 milliliters contains dopamine HCl 80 mg (0.8 mg/ml), 160 mg (1.6 mg/ml) or 320 mg (3.2 mg/ml) and dextrose, hydrous 5 g in water for injection, with sodium metabisulfite added 50 mg as a stabilizer; osmolar concentration, respectively 261, 269, or 286 mOsmol/L (calc.), pH 3.8 (2.5-4.5). May contain hydrochloric acid and/or sodium hydroxide for pH adjustment.

Dopamine administered intravenously is a myocardial inotropic agent, which also may increase mesenteric and renal blood flow plus urinary output.

Dopamine HCl is chemically designated 3, 4-dihydroxyphenethylamine HCl ($C_8H_{11}NO_2 \cdot HCl$), a white crystalline powder freely soluble in water. Dopamine (also referred to as 3-hydroxytramine) is a naturally occurring endogenous catecholamine precursor of norepinephrine.

Dextrose is chemically designated D-glucose monohydrate ($C_6H_{12}O_6 \cdot H_2O$), a hexose sugar freely soluble in water. Water for injection is chemically designated H_2O.

The flexible plastic container is fabricated from a specially formulated nonplasticized, thermoplastic co-polyester (CR3). Water can permeate from inside the container into the overwrap but not in amounts sufficient to affect the solution significantly. Solutions inside the plastic container also can leach out certain of its chemical components in very small amounts before the expiration period is attained. However, the safety of the plastic has been confirmed by tests in animals according to USP biological standards for plastic containers.

CLINICAL PHARMACOLOGY

FULL STRENGTH FORMS

Dopamine is a natural catecholamine formed by the decarboxylation of 3,4-dihydroxyphenylalanine (DOPA). It is a precursor to norepinephrine in noradrenergic nerves and is also a neurotransmitter in certain areas of the central nervous system, especially in the nigrostriatal tract, and in a few peripheral sympathetic nerves.

Dopamine produces positive chronotropic and inotropic effects on the myocardium, resulting in increased heart rate and cardiac contractility. This is accomplished directly by exerting an agonist action on beta-adrenoceptors and indirectly by causing release of norepinephrine from storage sites in sympathetic nerve endings.

Dopamine's onset of action occurs within 5 minutes of intravenous administration, and with dopamine's plasma half-life of about 2 minutes, the duration of action is less than 10 minutes. However, if monoamine oxidase (MAO) inhibitors are present, the duration may increase to 1 hour. The drug is widely distributed in the body but does not cross the blood-brain barrier to a significant extent. Dopamine is metabolized in the liver, kidney and plasma by MAO and catechol-O-methyltransferase to the inactive compounds homovanillic acid (HVA) and 3,4-dihydroxyphenylacetic acid. About 25% of the dose is taken up into specialized neurosecretory vesicles (the adrenergic nerve terminals), where it is hydroxylated to form norepinephrine. It has been reported that about 80% of the drug is excreted in the urine within 24 hours, primarily as HVA and its sulfate and glucuronide conjugates and as 3,4-dihydroxyphenylacetic acid. A very small portion is excreted unchanged.

The predominant effects of dopamine are dose-related, although it should be noted that actual response of an individual patient will largely depend on the clinical status of the patient at the time the drug is administered. At low rates of infusion (0.5 to 2 μg/kg/min) dopamine causes vasodilation that is presumed to be due to a specific agonist action on dopamine receptors (distinct from alpha- and beta-adrenoceptors) in the renal, mesenteric, coronary and intracerebral vascular beds. At these dopamine receptors, haloperidol is an antagonist. The vasodilation in these vascular beds is accompanied by increased glomerular filtration rate, renal blood flow, sodium excretion and urine flow. Hypotension sometimes occurs. An increase in urinary output produced by dopamine is usually not associated with a decrease in osmolality of the urine.

At intermediate rates of infusion (2-10 μg/kg/min), dopamine acts to stimulate the $beta_1$-adrenoceptors, resulting in improved myocardial contractility, increased SA rate and enhanced impulse conduction in the heart. There is little, if any, stimulation of the $beta_2$-adrenoceptors (peripheral vasodilation). Dopamine causes less increase in myocardial oxygen consumption than isoproterenol, and its use is not usually associated with a tachyarrhythmia. Clinical studies indicate that it usually increases systolic and pulse pressure with either no effect or a slight increase in diastolic pressure. Blood flow to the peripheral vascular beds may decrease while mesenteric flow increases due to increased cardiac output. Total peripheral resistance (alpha effects) at low and intermediate doses is usually unchanged.

At higher rates of infusion (10-20 μg/kg/min), there is some effect on alpha-adrenoceptors, with consequent vasoconstrictor effects and a rise in blood pressure. The vasoconstrictor effects are first seen in the skeletal muscle vascular beds, but with increasing doses, they are also evident in the renal and mesenteric vessels. At very high rates of infusion (above 20 μg/kg/min), stimulation of alpha-adrenoceptors predominates and vasoconstriction may compromise the circulation of the limbs and override the dopaminergic effects of dopamine, reversing renal dilation and natruresis.

PREDILUTED FORMS

Dopamine exhibits an inotropic action on the myocardium, resulting in increased cardiac output. It causes less increase in myocardial oxygen consumption than isoproterenol and the effect of dopamine usually is not associated with tachyarrhythmia. Reported clinical studies have revealed that the drug usually increases systolic and pulse pressure without any or only a minor elevating effect on diastolic pressure. Total peripheral resistance at low and intermediate doses is usually unchanged. Blood flow to peripheral vascular beds may decrease while mesenteric blood flow is increased. The drug also has been reported to produce dilation of the renal vasculature which is accompanied by increases in glomerular filtration rate, renal blood flow and sodium excretion. Increased urinary output produced by dopamine is usually not associated with decreased urine osmolality.

Solutions containing carbohydrate in the form of dextrose restore blood glucose levels and provide calories. Carbohydrate in the form of dextrose may aid in minimizing liver glycogen depletion and exerts a protein-sparing action. Dextrose injected parenterally undergoes oxidation to carbon dioxide and water.

Water is an essential constituent of all body tissues and accounts for approximately 70% of total body weight. Average normal adult daily requirement ranges from 2-3 L (1.0-1.5 L each for insensible water loss due to perspiration and urine production.)

Water balance is maintained by various regulatory mechanisms. Water distribution depends primarily on the concentration of electrolytes and sodium (Na^+) plays a major role in maintaining physiologic equilibrium.

The reported clearance rate of dopamine in critically ill infants and children has ranged from 46-168 ml/kg/min, with the higher values seen in the younger patients. The apparent volume of distribution in neonates is reported as 0.6 to 4 L/kg, leading to an elimination half-life of 5-11 minutes.

INDICATIONS AND USAGE

Dopamine HCl injection is indicated for the correction of hemodynamic imbalances present in shock due to myocardial infarction, trauma, endotoxic septicemia, open heart surgery, renal failure and chronic cardiac decompensation as in refractory congestive failure.

When indicated, restoration of circulatory volume should be instituted or completed with a suitable plasma expander or whole blood, prior to administration of prediluted dopamine HCl.

Patients most likely to respond to dopamine are those whose physiological parameters (such as urine flow, myocardial function and blood pressure) have not undergone extreme deterioration. Reports indicate that the shorter the time between onset of signs and symptoms and initiation of therapy with volume restoration and dopamine, the better the prognosis.

POOR PERFUSION OF VITAL ORGANS

Although urine flow is apparently one of the better diagnostic signs for monitoring vital organ perfusion, the physician also should observe the patient for signs of reversal of mental confusion or coma. Loss of pallor, increase in toe temperature or adequacy of nail bed capillary filling also may be observed as indices of adequate dosage. Reported studies indicate that when dopamine is administered before urine flow has decreased to approximately 0.3 ml/minute, prognosis is more favorable.

However, it has been observed that in some oliguric or anuric patients, administration of the drug has produced an increase in urine flow which may reach normal levels. The drug may also increase urine flow in patients whose output is within normal limits and thus may help in reducing the degree of pre-existing fluid accumulation. Conversely, at higher than optimal doses for a given patient, urinary flow may decrease, requiring a reduction of dosage. Concurrent administration of dopamine and diuretic agents may produce an additive or potentiating effect.

LOW CARDIAC OUTPUT

Dopamine's direct inotropic effect on the myocardium which increases cardiac output at low or moderate doses is related to a favorable prognosis. Increased output has been associated with unchanged or decreased systemic vascular resistance (SVR). The association of static or decreased SVR with low or moderate increases in cardiac output is regarded as a reflection of differential effects on specific vascular beds, with increased resistance in peripheral beds (*e.g.,* femoral), and concurrent decreases in mesenteric and renal vascular beds. Redistribution of blood flow parallels these changes so that an increase in cardiac output is accompanied by an increase in mesenteric and renal blood flow. In many instances the renal fraction of the total cardiac output has been found to increase. Increase in cardiac output produced by dopamine is not associated with substantial decreases in systemic vascular resistance as may occur with isoproterenol.

HYPOTENSION

Low to moderate doses of dopamine, which have little effect on SVR can be used to manage hypotension due to inadequate cardiac output. At high therapeutic doses, dopamine's alpha-adrenergic action becomes more prominent and thus may correct hypotension due to diminished SVR. As in other circulatory decompensation states, prognosis is better in patients whose blood pressure and urine flow have not undergone extreme deterioration. Therefore, it is suggested the physician administer dopamine as soon as a definite trend toward decreased systolic and diastolic pressure becomes apparent.

NON-FDA APPROVED INDICATIONS

Non-approved uses of dopamine include the treatment of congestive heart failure and improving renal blood flow and kidney function in patients with acute renal failure and hepatorenal syndrome.

CONTRAINDICATIONS

Dopamine HCl should not be used in patients with pheochromocytoma.

Dopamine HCl should not be administered in the presence of uncorrected tachyarrhythmias or ventricular fibrillation.

WARNINGS

Dopamine HCl and dopamine HCl in 5% dextrose contain sodium metabisulfite, a sulfite that may cause allergic-type reactions including anaphylactic symptoms and life-threatening or less severe asthmatic episodes in certain susceptible people. The overall prevalence of sulfite sensitivity in the general population is unknown and probably low. Sulfite sensitivity is seen more frequently in asthmatic than in nonasthmatic people.

Do NOT add any alkalinizing substance, since dopamine is inactivated in alkaline solution.

Patients who have been receiving monoamine oxidase (MAO) inhibitors prior to the administration of dopamine should receive substantially reduced dosage of the latter. (See DRUG INTERACTIONS.)

Additional Information for Prediluted Form: Additive medications should not be delivered via this solution.

PRECAUTIONS

GENERAL

Solutions containing dextrose should be used with caution in patients with known subclinical or overt diabetes mellitus.

Fluid and Electrolyte Balance

Prediluted Only: Excess administration of potassium-free solutions may result in significant hypokalemia.

The intravenous administration of these solutions can cause fluid and/or solute overloading resulting in dilution of serum electrolyte concentrations, overhydration, congested states or pulmonary edema.

Careful Monitoring Required

Close monitoring of the following indices—urine flow, cardiac output, and blood pressure (and, for full-strength forms, pulmonary wedge pressure)— during dopamine infusion is necessary as in the case of any adrenergic agent.

Hypoxia, Hypercapnia, Acidosis

These conditions, which may also reduce the effectiveness and/or increase the incidence of adverse effects of dopamine, must be identified and corrected prior to, or concurrently with, administration of dopamine HCl.

Ventricular Arrhythmias

If an increased number of ectopic beats are observed the dose should be reduced if possible.

Hypotension

At lower infusion rates, if hypotension occurs, the infusion rate should be rapidly increased until adequate blood pressure is obtained. If hypotension persists, dopamine HCl should be discontinued and a more potent vasoconstrictor agent such as norepinephrine should be administered.

Occlusive Vascular Disease

Patients with a history of occlusive vascular disease (*e.g.,* arteriosclerosis, arterial embolism, Raynaud's disease, cold injury such as frostbite, diabetic endarteritis and Buerger's disease) should be closely monitored for any changes in color or temperature of the skin of the extremities. If a change in skin color or temperature occurs and is thought to be the result of compromised circulation to the extremities, the benefits of continued dopamine infusion should be weighed against the risk of possible necrosis. These changes may be reversed by either decreasing the rate or discontinuing the infusion entirely.

Extravasation

Dopamine HCl should be infused into a large vein whenever possible to prevent the possibility of infiltration of perivascular tissue adjacent to the infusion site. Extravasation may cause necrosis and sloughing of surrounding tissue. Large veins of the antecubital fossa are preferred to veins in the dorsum of the hand or ankle. Less suitable infusion sites should be used only when larger veins are unavailable and the patient's condition requires immediate attention. The physician should switch to a more suitable site as soon as possible and the infusion site in use should be continuously monitored for free flow. *Additional Information for Prediluted Forms:* Administration into an umbilical arterial catheter is not recommended.

IMPORTANT—Antidote for Peripheral Ischemia: To prevent sloughing and necrosis in ischemic areas, the area should be infiltrated as soon as possible with 10-15 ml of 0.9% sodium chloride injection containing from 5-10 mg of phentolamine mesylate, an adrenergic blocking agent. A syringe with a fine hypodermic needle should be used, and the solution liberally infiltrated throughout the ischemic area. Sympathetic blockade with phentolamine causes immediate and conspicuous local hyperemic changes if the area is infiltrated within 12 hours. Therefore, phentolamine mesylate should be given as soon as possible after the extravasation is noted. *Additional Information for Prediluted Forms:* Pediatric dosage of phentolamine mesylate should be 0.1-0.2 mg/kg up to a maximum of 10 mg per dose.

Laboratory Tests

Infusion of dopamine suppresses pituitary secretion of thyroid-stimulating hormone, growth hormone, and prolactin.

Weaning

When discontinuing the infusion, it may be necessary to gradually decrease the dose of dopamine HCl while expanding blood volume with IV fluids, since sudden cessation may result in marked hypotension.

Additional Information for Full-Strength Forms

Hypovolemia

Prior to treatment with dopamine HCl, hypovolemia should be fully corrected, if possible, with either whole blood or plasma as indicated. Monitoring of central venous pressure or left ventricular filling pressure may be helpful in detecting and treating hypovolemia.

Decreased Pulse Pressure

If a disproportionate increase in diastolic blood pressure and a marked decrease in pulse pressure are observed in patients receiving dopamine HCl, the rate of infusion should be decreased and the patient observed carefully for further evidence of predominant vasoconstrictor activity, unless such an effect is desired.

CARCINOGENESIS, MUTAGENESIS, AND IMPAIRMENT OF FERTILITY

Prediluted Forms Only

Long-term animal studies have not been performed to evaluate the carcinogenic potential of dopamine HCl.

Dopamine HCl at doses approaching maximal solubility showed no clear genotoxic potential in the Ames test. Although there was a reproducible dose-dependent increase in the number of revertant colonies with strains TA100 and TA98, both with and without metabolic activation, the small increase was considered inconclusive evidence of mutagenicity. In the L5178Y TK$^{+/-}$ mouse lymphoma assay, dopamine HCl at the highest concentrations used of 750 μg/ml without metabolic activation, and 3000 μg/ml with activation, was toxic and associated with increases in mutant frequencies when compared to untreated and solvent controls; at the lower concentrations no increases over controls were noted.

No clear evidence of clastogenic potential was reported in the *in vivo* mouse or male rat bone marrow micronucleus test when the animals were treated intravenously with up to 224 mg/kg and 30 mg/kg of dopamine HCl, respectively.

PREGNANCY, TERATOGENIC EFFECTS, PREGNANCY CATEGORY C

Full-Strength Forms

Animal studies have revealed no evidence of teratogenic effects due to dopamine. However, in one study, administration of dopamine HCl to pregnant rats resulted in a decreased survival rate of the newborn and a potential for cataract formation in the survivors. There are no adequate and well-controlled studies in pregnant women and it is not known if dopamine crosses the placental barrier. Because animal reproduction studies are not always predictive of human response, this drug should be used during pregnancy only if, in the judgement of the physician, the potential benefit justifies the potential risk to the fetus.

Prediluted Forms

Teratogenicity studies in rats and rabbits at dopamine HCl dosages up to 6 mg/kg/day intravenously during organogenesis produced no detectable teratogenic or embryotoxic effects, although maternal toxicity consisting of mortalities, decreased body weight gain, and pharmacotoxic signs were observed in rats. In a published study, dopamine HCl administered at 10 mg/kg subcutaneously for 30 days, markedly prolonged metestrus and increased mean pituitary and ovary weights in female rats. Similar administration to pregnant rats throughout gestation or for 5 days starting on gestation day 10 or 15 resulted in decreased body weight gains, increased mortalities and slight increases in cataract formation among the offspring. There are no adequate and well-controlled studies in pregnant women, and it is not known if dopamine HCl crosses the placental barrier. Dopamine HCl should be used during pregancy only if the potential benefit justifies the potential risk to the fetus.

LABOR AND DELIVERY

In obstetrics, if vasopressor drugs are used to correct hypotension or are added to a local anesthetic solution the interaction with some oxytocic drugs may cause severe hypertension, and for the full-strength forms, may even cause rupture of a cerebral blood vessel to occur during the postpartum period.

NURSING MOTHERS

It is not known whether this drug is excreted in human milk. Because many drugs are excreted in human milk, caution should be exercised when dopamine HCl is administered to a nursing mother.

PEDIATRIC USE

Full-Strength Forms

Safety and effectiveness in pediatric patients have not been established. Dopamine HCl has been used in a limited number of pediatric patients, but such use has been inadequate to fully define proper dosage and limitations for use.

Prediluted Forms

Dopamine infusions have been used in patients for every age from birth onwards. There are scattered reports of infusion rates in neonates up to 125 μg/kg/min, but most reports in pediatric patients describe dosing that is similar (on a μg/kg/min basis) to that used in adults. Except for vasoconstrictive effects caused by inadvertant infusion of dopamine into the umbilical artery, adverse effects unique to the pediatric populations have not been identified, nor have adverse effects identified in adults been found to be more common in pediatric patients.

GERIATRIC USE

Prediluted Forms

Clinical studies of dopamine injection did not include sufficient numbers of subjects aged 65 and over to determine whether they respond differently from younger subjects. Other reported clinical experience has not identified differences in responses between the elderly and younger patients. In general, dose selection for an elderly patient should be cautious, usually starting at the low end of the dosing range, reflecting the frequency of decreased hepatic, renal or cardiac function, and of concomitant disease or other drug therapy.

DRUG INTERACTIONS

Cyclopropane or halogenated hydrocarbon anesthetics increase cardiac autonomic irritability and may sensitize the myocardium to the action of certain intravenously administered catecholamines, such as dopamine. This interaction appears to be related both to pressor activity and to the beta-adrenergic stimulating properties of these catecholamines, and may produce ventricular arrhythmias and hypertension. Therefore, EXTREME CAUTION should be exercised when administering dopamine HCl to patients receiving cycloproprane or halogenated hydrocarbon anesthetics. Results of studies in animals indicate that dopamine-induced ventricular arrythmias during anesthesia can be reversed by propranolol.

Because dopamine is metabolized by monoamine oxidase (MAO), inhibition of this enzyme prolongs and potentiates the effect of dopamine. Patients who have been treated with MAO inhibitors within 2-3 weeks prior to the administration of dopamine should receive initial doses of dopamine HCl no greater than one-tenth (1/10) the usual dose.

Concurrent administration of low-dose dopamine HCl and diuretic agents may produce an additive or potentiating effect on urine flow.

Tricyclic antidepressants may potentiate the cardiovascular effects of adrenergic agents.

Cardiac effects of dopamine are antagonized by beta-adrenergic blocking agents, such as propranolol and metoprolol. The peripheral vasoconstriction caused by high doses of dopamine HCl is antagonized by alpha-adrenergic blocking agents. Dopamine-induced renal and mesenteric vasodilation is not antagonized by either alpha- or beta-adrenergic blocking agents.

Butyrophenones (such as haloperidol) and phenothiazines can suppress the dopaminergic renal and mesenteric vasodilation induced with low-dose dopamine infusion.

The concomitant use of vasopressors, vasoconstricting agents (such as ergonovine) and some oxytocic drugs may result in severe hypertension (see PRECAUTIONS, Labor and Delivery).

Administration of phenytoin to patients receiving dopamine HCl has been reported to lead to hypotension and bradycardia. It is suggested that in patients receiving dopamine HCl, alternatives to phenytoin should be considered if anticonvulsant therapy is needed.

ADVERSE REACTIONS

The following adverse reactions have been observed, but there are not enough data to support an estimate of their frequency.

Cardiovascular System: Ventricular arrhythmia (at very high doses), ectopic beats, tachycardia, anginal pain, palpitation, cardiac conduction abnormalities, widened QRS complex, bradycardia, hypotension, hypertension, vasoconstriction.

Respiratory System: Dyspnea.

Gastrointestinal System: Nausea, vomiting.

Metabolic/Nutritional System: Azotemia.

Central Nervous System: Headache, anxiety.

Dermatologic System: Piloerection.

Other: Gangrene of the extremities has occurred when high doses were administered for prolonged periods or in patients with occlusive vascular disease receiving low doses of dopamine HCl.

DOSAGE AND ADMINISTRATION

FULL STRENGTH FORMS

WARNING: This is a potent drug. It must be diluted before administration to patient. Dopamine HCl injection is administered (only after dilution) by intravenous infusion.

Suggested Dilution

For the 40 mg/ml preparation, transfer by aseptic technique the contents containing either 5 ml, 200 mg, or 10 ml, 400 mg of dopamine HCl to either a 250 ml or 500 ml bottle of one of the sterile IV solutions listed below. For the 80 mg/ml preparation, transfer by aseptic technique the contents containing 10 ml, 800 mg of dopamine HCl to a 250 ml, 500 ml, or 1000 ml bottle of one of the following sterile IV solutions:

0.9% sodium chloride injection.
5% dextrose injection.
5% dextrose and 0.9% sodium chloride injection.
5% dextrose and 0.45% sodium chloride injection.
5% dextrose and lactated ringer's injection.
Sodium lactate injection 1/6 Molar.
Lactated ringer's injection.

The resultant dilutions are summarized in TABLE 1.

TABLE 1

Concentration of Dopamine HCl	40 mg/ml		80 mg/ml
Volume of Dopamine HCl Injection	5 ml	10 ml	10 ml
250 ml bottle of IV solution	800 μg/ml	1600 μg/ml	3200 μg/ml
500 ml bottle of IV solution	400 μg/ml	800 μg/ml	1600 μg/ml
1000 ml bottle of IV solution	200 μg/ml	400 μg/ml	800 μg/ml

Dopamine HCl injection has been found to be stable for a minimum of 24 hours after dilution in the foregoing IV solutions. However, as with all IV admixtures, dilution should be made just prior to administration.

Do NOT add dopamine HCl to sodium bicarbonate injection or other alkaline IV solutions, since the drug is inactivated in alkaline solution.

Rate of Administration

Dopamine HCl injection, after dilution, is administered intravenously by infusion via a suitable IV catheter or needle. When administering dopamine HCl (or any potent medication) by continuous intravenous infusion, it is advisable to use a precision volume control IV set. Each patient must be individually titrated to the desired hemodynamic or renal response to dopamine.

In titrating to the desired increase in systolic blood pressure, the optimum dosage rate for renal response may be exceeded, thus necessitating a reduction in rate after the hemodynamic condition is stabilized.

Administration at rates greater than 50 μg/kg/min have safely been used in advanced circulatory decompensation states. If unnecessary fluid expansion is of concern, adjustment of drug concentration may be preferred over increasing the flow rate of a less concentrated dilution.

Suggested Regimen

1. When appropriate, increase blood volume with whole blood or plasma until central venous pressure is 10-15 cm H_2O or pulmonary wedge pressure is 14-18 mm Hg.
2. Begin infusion of diluted solution at doses of 2-5 μg/kg/min of dopamine HCl in patients who are likely to respond to modest increments of heart force and renal perfusion.

In more seriously ill patients, begin infusion of diluted solution at doses of 5 μg/kg/min of dopamine HCl and increase gradually using 5-10 μg/kg/min increments up to 20-50 μg/kg/min as needed. If doses in excess of 50 μg/kg/min are required, it is advisable to check urine output frequently. Should urinary flow begin to decrease in the absence of hypotension, reduction of dopamine dosage should be considered. Multiclinic trials have shown that more than 50 percent of patients have been satisfactorily maintained on doses less than 20 μg/kg/min.

In patients who do not respond to these doses with adequate arterial pressures or urine flow, additional increments of dopamine may be given in an effort to produce an appropriate arterial pressure and central perfusion.

3. Treatment of all patients requires constant evaluation of therapy in terms of blood volume, augmentation of cardiac contractility, and distribution of peripheral perfusion. Dosage of dopamine should be adjusted according to the patient's response, with particular attention to diminution of established urine flow rate, increasing tachycardia or development of new dysrhythmias as indices for decreasing or temporarily suspending the dosage.
4. As with all potent intravenously administered drugs, care should be taken to control the rate of administration to avoid inadvertent administration of a bolus of drug.

Parenteral drug products should be inspected visually for particulate matter and discoloration prior to administration, whenever solution and container permit.

PREDILUTED FORMS

Do NOT administer if solution is darker than slightly yellow or discolored in any other way. Do NOT administer unless solution is clear and container is undamaged. Discard unused portion.

Dextrose solutions without electrolytes should not be administered simultaneously with blood through the same infusion set because of the possibility that pseudoagglutination of red cells may occur.

Do NOT add sodium bicarbonate or other alkalinizing substance, since dopamine is inactivated in alkaline solution.

Dopamine HCl in 5% dextrose injection should be infused into a large vein whenever possible to prevent the infiltration of perivascular tisse adjacent to the infusion site. Extravasation may cause necrosis and sloughing of the surrounding tissue. Large veins of the antecubital fossa are preferred to veins of the dorsum of the hand or ankle. Less suitable infusion sites should be used only when larger veins are unavailable and the patient's condition requires immediate attention. The physician should switch to a more suitable site as soon as possible and the infusion site in use should be continuously monitored for free flow.

The less concentrated 800 μg/ml solution may be preferred when fluid expansion is not a problem. The more concentrated 1600 μg/ml or 3200 μg/ml solutions, may be preferred in patients with fluid retension or when a slower rate of infusion is desired.

Rate of Administration

Administration into an umbilical artery catheter is not recommended.

Dopamine in 5% dextrose injection should not be infused through ordinary IV apparatus, regulated only by gravity and mechanical clamps. Only an infusion pump, preferably a volumetric pump, should be used.

Each patient must be individually titrated to the desired hemodynamic or renal response to dopamine.

In titrating to the desired increase in systolic blood pressure, the optimum dosage rate for renal response may be exceeded, thus necessitating a reduction in rate after the hemodynamic condition is stabilized.

If a disproportionate rise in diastolic pressure (*i.e.*, a marked decrease in pulse pressure) is observed in patients receiving dopamine, the infusion rate should be decreased and the patient observed carefully for further evidence of predominant vasoconstrictor activity, unless such an effect is desired.

Administration rates greater than 50 μg/kg/min have safely been used in adults in advanced circulatory decompensation states. If unnecessary fluid expansion is of concern, adjustment of drug concentration may be preferred over increasing the flow rate of a less concentrated dilution.

Suggested Regimen

1. When appropriate, increase blood volume with whole blood or plasma until central venous pressure is 10-15 cm H_2O or pulmonary wedge pressure is 14-18 mm Hg.
2. Begin infusion of dopamine HCl solution at doses of 2-5 μg/kg/min in adult or pediatric patients who are likely to respond to modest increments of heart force and renal perfusion.

In more seriously ill patients, begin infusion of dopamine HCl at doses of 5 μg/kg/min and increase gradually, using 5-10 μg/kg/min increments, up to a rate of 20-50 μg/kg/min as needed. If doses in excess of 50 μg/kg/min are required, check urine output frequently. Should urinary flow begin to decrease in the absence of hypotention, reduction of dopamine dosage should be considered. More than 50% of adult patients have been satisfactorily maintained on doses less than 20 μg/kg/min.

In patients who do not respond to these doses with adequate arterial pressures or urine flow, additional increments of dopamine may be given in an effort to produce an appropriate arterial pressure and central perfusion.

3. Treatment of all patients requires constant evaluation of therapy in terms of blood volume, augmentation of cardiac contractility, urine flow, cardiac output, blood pressure, and distribution of peripheral perfusion.

Dosage of dopamine should be adjusted according to the patient's response. Diminution of establishing urine flow rate, increasing tachycardia or development of new dysrhythmias are reasons to consider decreasing or temporarily suspending the dosage.

4. As with all potent intravenously administered drugs, care should be taken to control the rate of infusion so as to avoid inadvertant administration of a bolus of the drug.

TABLE 2 *800 μg/ml Dosing Chart for Dopamine (ml/h) Infusion Rate*

Infusion Rate (μg/kg/min)	Patient Body Weight (kg) 10	20	30	40	50	60	70	80	90	100
2.5	1.9	3.8	5.6	7.5	9.4	11.3	13.1	15	16.9	18.8
5	3.8	7.5	11.3	15	18.8	22.5	26.3	30	33.8	37.5
10	7.5	15	22.5	30	37.5	45	52.5	60	67.5	75
15	11.3	22.5	33.8	45	56.3	67.5	78.8	90	101.3	112.5
20	15	30	45	60	75	90	105	120	135	150
25	18.8	37.5	56.3	75	93.8	112.5	131.3	150	168.8	187.5
30	22.5	45	67.5	90	112.5	135	157.5	180	202.5	225
35	26.3	52.5	78.8	105	131.3	157.5	183.8	210	236.3	262.5
40	30	60	90	120	150	180	210	240	270	300
45	33.8	67.5	101.3	135	168.8	202.5	236.3	270	303.8	337.5
50	37.5	75	112.5	150	187.5	225	262.5	300	337.5	375

TABLE 3 *1600 μg/ml Dosing Chart for Dopamine (ml/h) Infusion Rate*

Infusion Rate (μg/kg/min)	Patient Body Weight (kg) 10	20	30	40	50	60	70	80	90	100
2.5	0.9	1.9	2.8	3.8	4.7	5.6	6.6	7.5	8.4	9.4
5	1.9	3.8	5.6	7.5	9.4	11.3	13.1	15	16.9	18.8
10	3.8	7.5	11.3	15	18.8	22.5	26.3	30	33.8	37.5
15	5.6	11.3	16.9	22.5	28.1	33.8	39.4	45	50.6	56.3
20	7.5	15	22.5	30	37.5	45	52.5	60	67.5	75
25	9.4	18.8	28.1	37.5	46.9	56.3	65.6	75	84.4	93.8
30	11.3	22.5	33.8	45	56.3	67.5	78.8	90	101.3	112.5
35	13.1	26.3	39.4	52.5	65.6	78.8	91.9	105	118.1	131.3
40	15	30	45	60	75	90	105	120	135	150
45	16.9	33.8	50.6	67.5	84.4	101.3	118.1	135	151.9	168.8
50	18.8	37.5	56.3	75	93.8	112.5	131.3	150	168.8	187.5

TABLE 4 *3200 μg/ml Dosing Chart for Dopamine (ml/h) Infusion Rate*

Infusion Rate (μg/kg/min)	Patient Body Weight (kg) 10	20	30	40	50	60	70	80	90	100
2.5	0.5	0.9	1.4	1.9	2.3	2.8	3.3	3.8	4.2	4.7
5	0.9	1.9	2.8	3.8	4.7	5.6	6.6	7.5	8.4	9.4
10	1.9	3.8	5.6	7.5	9.4	11.3	13.1	15	16.9	18.8
15	2.8	5.6	8.4	11.3	14.1	16.9	19.7	22.5	25.3	28.1
20	3.8	7.5	11.3	15	18.8	22.5	26.3	30	33.8	37.5
25	4.7	9.4	14.1	18.8	23.4	28.1	32.8	37.5	42.2	46.9
30	5.6	11.3	16.9	22.5	28.1	33.8	39.4	45	50.6	56.3
35	6.6	13.1	19.7	26.3	32.8	39.4	45.9	52.5	59.1	65.6
40	7.5	15	22.5	30	37.5	45	52.5	60	67.5	75
45	8.4	16.9	25.3	33.8	42.2	50.6	59.1	67.5	75.9	84.4
50	9.4	18.8	28.1	37.5	46.9	56.3	65.6	75	84.4	93.8

Parenteral drug products should be visually inspected for particulate matter and discoloration prior to administration, whenever solution and container permit.

Instructions for Use

To Open: Tear outer wrap at notch and remove solution container. Some opacity of the plastic due to moisture absorption during the sterilzation process may be observed. This is normal and does not affect the solution quality or safety. The opacity will diminish gradually.

Preparation for Administration (use aseptic technique)

1. Close flow control clamp of administration set.
2. Remove cover from outlet port at bottom of container.
3. Insert piercing pin of administration set into port with a twisting motion until the set is firmly seated. *NOTE:* See full directions on administration set carton.
4. Suspend container from hanger.
5. Squeeze and release drip chamber to establish proper fluid level in chamber.
6. Open flow control clamp and clear air from set. Close clamp.
7. Attach set to venipuncture device. If device is not indwelling, prime and make venipuncture.
8. Regulate rate of administration with an infusion pump, preferably a volumetric pump.

HOW SUPPLIED

Avoid contact with alkalies (including sodium bicarbonate), oxidizing agents or iron salts.
NOTE: Do not use the injection if it is darker than slightly yellow or discolored in any other way.

FULL-STRENGTH FORMS

Storage: Store at controlled room temperature, 15-30°C (59-86°F).

PREDILUTED FORMS

Dopamine HCl in 5% dextrose injection is supplied as 200, 400, or 800 mg dopamine HCl in either 250 and 500 ml LifeCare flexible containers.

Storage: Exposure of pharmaceutical products to heat should be minimized. Avoid excessive heat. Protect from freezing. It is recommended that the product be stored at room temperature (25°C); however, brief exposure up to 40°C does not adversely affect the product.

PRODUCT LISTING - RATED THERAPEUTICALLY EQUIVALENT

Solution - Intravenous - 5%;80 mg/100 ml

250 ml	$21.11	GENERIC, B. Braun/Mcgaw Inc	00264-1442-55
250 ml x 12	$105.00	GENERIC, B. Braun/Mcgaw Inc	00264-5144-20
250 ml x 12	$173.88	GENERIC, Abbott Pharmaceutical	00074-7808-22
250 ml x 18	$347.33	GENERIC, Baxter I.V. Systems Division	00338-1005-02
500 ml	$30.64	GENERIC, B. Braun/Mcgaw Inc	00264-1441-55
500 ml x 12	$212.18	GENERIC, Abbott Pharmaceutical	00074-7808-24
500 ml x 12	$213.04	GENERIC, Abbott Pharmaceutical	00074-4141-03
500 ml x 12	$340.56	GENERIC, Baxter I.V. Systems Division	00338-1005-03
500 ml x 12	$357.00	GENERIC, B. Braun/Mcgaw Inc	00264-5144-10

Solution - Intravenous - 5%;160 mg/100 ml

250 ml	$31.56	GENERIC, B. Braun/Mcgaw Inc	00264-1482-55
250 ml x 12	$194.51	GENERIC, Abbott Pharmaceutical	00074-4142-02
250 ml x 12	$225.58	GENERIC, Abbott Pharmaceutical	00074-7809-22
250 ml x 12	$367.80	GENERIC, B. Braun/Mcgaw Inc	00264-5148-20
250 ml x 18	$510.84	GENERIC, Baxter I.V. Systems Division	00338-1007-02
500 ml	$48.44	GENERIC, B. Braun/Mcgaw Inc	00264-1481-55
500 ml x 12	$262.20	GENERIC, Abbott Pharmaceutical	00074-7809-24
500 ml x 12	$313.93	GENERIC, Abbott Pharmaceutical	00074-4142-03
500 ml x 12	$517.68	GENERIC, Baxter I.V. Systems Division	00338-1007-03
500 ml x 12	$564.60	GENERIC, B. Braun/Mcgaw Inc	00264-5148-10

Solution - Intravenous - 5%;320 mg/100 ml

250 ml	$48.44	GENERIC, B. Braun/Mcgaw Inc	00264-1492-55
250 ml x 12	$247.81	GENERIC, Abbott Pharmaceutical	00074-7810-22
250 ml x 12	$255.00	GENERIC, B. Braun/Mcgaw Inc	00264-5149-20
250 ml x 12	$295.40	GENERIC, Abbott Pharmaceutical	00074-4155-02
250 ml x 18	$776.70	GENERIC, Baxter I.V. Systems Division	00338-1009-02

Solution - Intravenous - 40 mg/ml

5 ml x 10	$34.90	GENERIC, Abbott Pharmaceutical	00074-5819-16
5 ml x 10	$49.90	GENERIC, Astra-Zeneca Pharmaceuticals	00186-0638-01
5 ml x 10	$64.80	GENERIC, Abbott Pharmaceutical	00074-5819-01
5 ml x 25	$22.86	GENERIC, Abbott Pharmaceutical	00074-5820-10
5 ml x 25	$54.75	GENERIC, American Regent Laboratories Inc	00517-1805-25
10 ml x 10	$102.40	GENERIC, Astra-Zeneca Pharmaceuticals	00186-0639-01
10 ml x 10	$300.10	GENERIC, Abbott Pharmaceutical	00074-9105-18
10 ml x 25	$39.19	GENERIC, Abbott Pharmaceutical	00074-9104-20
10 ml x 25	$81.25	GENERIC, Cmc-Consolidated Midland Corporation	00223-7484-05
10 ml x 25	$142.00	GENERIC, Cmc-Consolidated Midland Corporation	00223-7485-05
10 ml x 25	$623.70	GENERIC, Abbott Pharmaceutical	00074-9105-01
100 ml	$61.25	INTROPIN, Dupont Pharmaceuticals	00590-0040-06

Solution - Intravenous - 80 mg/ml

5 ml x 10	$83.10	GENERIC, Astra-Zeneca Pharmaceuticals	00186-0641-01
5 ml x 25	$102.25	GENERIC, American Regent Laboratories Inc	00517-1905-25
10 ml x 10	$61.26	GENERIC, Abbott Pharmaceutical	00074-4266-18
10 ml x 25	$80.45	GENERIC, Abbott Pharmaceutical	00074-4265-01
10 ml x 25	$172.00	GENERIC, Cmc-Consolidated Midland Corporation	00223-7486-05
10 ml x 25	$181.25	GENERIC, Cmc-Consolidated Midland Corporation	00223-7487-05
10 ml x 25	$998.70	GENERIC, Abbott Pharmaceutical	00074-4266-01

Solution - Intravenous - 160 mg/ml

5 ml x 10	$110.00	GENERIC, Astra-Zeneca Pharmaceuticals	00186-0642-01
5 ml x 25	$203.50	GENERIC, American Regent Laboratories Inc	00517-1305-25

PRODUCT LISTING - EQUIVALENTS NOT AVAILABLE

Solution - Intravenous - 40 mg/ml

5 ml	$9.70	GENERIC, Allscripts Pharmaceutical Company	54569-4223-00
5 ml x 25	$26.00	GENERIC, Raway Pharmacal Inc	00686-1805-25

Solution - Intravenous - 80 mg/ml

5 ml x 25	$31.00	GENERIC, Raway Pharmacal Inc	00686-1405-25

Solution - Intravenous - 160 mg/ml

5 ml x 25	$49.00	GENERIC, Raway Pharmacal Inc	00686-1305-25

Dornase Alfa *(003180)*

Categories: Cystic fibrosis; Recombinant DNA Origin; FDA Approved 1993 Dec; Pregnancy Category B; Orphan Drugs
Drug Classes: Enzymes, respiratory; Mucolytics
Brand Names: Deoxyribonuclease; DNase; **Pulmozyme**

DESCRIPTION

Dornase alfa inhalation solution is a sterile, clear, colorless, highly purified solution of recombinant human deoxyribonuclease I (rhDNase), an enzyme which selectively cleaves DNA. The protein is produced by genetically engineered Chinese Hamster Ovary (CHO) cells containing DNA encoding for the native human protein, deoxyribonuclease I (DNase). Fermentation is carried out in a nutrient medium containing the antibiotic gentamicin, 100-200 mg/L. However, the presence of the antibiotic is not detectable in the final product. The product is purified by tangential flow filtration and column chromatography. The purified glycoprotein contains 260 amino acids with an approximate molecular weight of 37,000 daltons.[1] The primary amino acid sequence is identical to that of the native human enzyme.

Dornase alfa inhalation solution is administered by inhalation of an aerosol mist produced by a compressed air driven nebulizer system. Each dornase alfa single-use ampule will deliver 2.5 ml of the solution to the nebulizer bowl. The aqueous solution contains 1.0 mg/ml dornase alfa, 0.15 mg/ml calcium chloride dihydrate and 8.77 mg/ml sodium chloride. The solution contains no preservative. The nominal pH of the solution is 6.3.

CLINICAL PHARMACOLOGY

GENERAL

In cystic fibrosis (CF) patients, retention of viscous purulent secretions in the airways contributes both to reduced pulmonary function and to exacerbations of infection.[2,3]

Purulent pulmonary secretions contain very high concentrations of extracellular DNA released by degenerating leukocytes that accumulate in response to infection.[4] *In vitro*, dornase alfa hydrolyzes the DNA in sputum of CF patients and reduces sputum viscoelasticity.[1]

PHARMACOKINETICS

When 2.5 mg dornase alfa was administered by inhalation to 18 CF patients, mean sputum concentrations of 3 μg/ml DNase were measurable within 15 minutes. Mean sputum concentrations declined to an average of 0.6 μg/ml 2 hours following inhalation. Inhalation of up to 10 mg TID of dornase alfa by 4 CF patients for 6 consecutive days, did not result in a significant elevation of serum concentrations of DNase above normal endogenous levels.[5,6] After administration of up to 2.5 mg of dornase alfa twice daily for 6 months to 321 CF patients, no accumulation of serum DNase was noted.

Dornase alfa, 2.5 mg by inhalation, was administered daily to 98 patients aged 3 months to ≤10 years, and bronchoalveolar lavage (BAL) fluid was obtained within 90 minutes of the first dose. BAL DNase concentrations were detectable in all patients but showed a broad range, from 0.007-1.8 μg/ml. Over an average of 14 days of exposure, serum DNase concentrations (mean ±SD) increased by 1.3 ± 1.3 ng/ml for the 3 months to <5 year age group and by 0.8 ± 1.2 ng/ml for the 5 to ≤10 year age group. The relationship between BAL or serum DNase concentration and adverse experiences and clinical outcomes is unknown.

INDICATIONS AND USAGE

Daily administration of dornase alfa in conjunction with standard therapies is indicated in the management of cystic fibrosis patients to improve pulmonary function.

Safety and efficacy of daily administration have not been demonstrated in patients for longer than 12 months.

NON-FDA APPROVED INDICATIONS

Dornase alfa has been studied in the treatment of acute chronic bronchitis, although this use is not approved by the FDA. Dornase alfa has also been used to effectively treat atelectasis in asthma and CF. In the treatment of patients with chronic obstructive pulmonary disease, a phase III trial was halted after an interim analysis revealed a higher mortality rate in the active over the placebo group (10.3% vs 9.5%, respectively, n=3700).

CONTRAINDICATIONS

Dornase alfa is contraindicated in patients with known hypersensitivity to dornase alfa, Chinese hamster ovary cell products, or any component of the product.

WARNINGS

None.

PRECAUTIONS

GENERAL

Dornase alfa should be used in conjunction with standard therapies for CF.

INFORMATION FOR THE PATIENT

Dornase alfa must be stored in the refrigerator at 2-8°C (36-46°F) and protected from strong light. It should be kept refrigerated during transport and should not be exposed to room temperatures for a total time of 24 hours. The solution should be discarded if it is cloudy or discolored. Dornase alfa contains no preservative and, once opened, the entire contents of the ampule must be used or discarded. Patients should be instructed in the proper use and maintenance of the nebulizer and compressor system used in its delivery.

Dornase alfa should not be diluted or mixed with other drugs in the nebulizer. Mixing of dornase alfa with other drugs could lead to adverse physicochemical and/or functional changes in dornase alfa or the admixed compound.

CARCINOGENESIS, MUTAGENESIS, AND IMPAIRMENT OF FERTILITY

Carcinogenesis

Lifetime studies in Sprague Dawley rats showed no carcinogenic effect when dornase alfa was administered at doses up to 246 μg/kg body weight per day.

Dornase alfa was administered to rats as an aerosol for up to 30 min/day, daily for 2 years, with resulting lower respiratory tract doses of up to 246 μg/kg/day, which represents up to a 28.8-fold multiple of the clinical dose. There was no increase in the development of benign or malignant neoplasms and no occurrence of unusual tumor types in rats after lifetime exposure.

Mutagenesis

Ames tests using 6 different tester strains of bacteria (four of *S. typhimurium* and two of *E. coli*) at concentrations up to 5000 μg/plate, a cytogenic assay using human peripheral blood lymphocytes at concentrations up to 2000 μg/plate, and a mouse lymphoma assay at concentrations up to 1000 mg/plate, with and without metabolic activation, revealed no evidence of mutagenesis potential. Dornase alfa was tested in a micronucleus (*in vivo*) assay for its potential to produce chromosome damage in bone marrow cells of mice following a bolus intravenous dose of 10 mg/kg on 2 consecutive days. No evidence of chromosomal damage was noted.

Impairment of Fertility

In studies with rats receiving up to 10 mg/kg/day, a dose representing systemic exposures greater than 600 times that expected following the recommended human dose, fertility and reproductive performance of both males and females was not affected.

PREGNANCY CATEGORY B

Reproduction studies have been performed in rats and rabbits with intravenous doses up to 10 mg/kg/day, representing systemic exposures greater than 600 times that expected following the recommended human dose. These studies have revealed no evidence of impaired fertility, harm to the fetus, or effects on development due to dornase alfa. There are, however, no adequate and well-controlled studies in pregnant women. Because animal reproductive studies are not always predictive of the human response, this drug should be used during pregnancy only if clearly needed.

NURSING MOTHERS

It is not known whether dornase alfa is excreted in human milk. Small amounts of dornase alfa were detected in maternal milk of cynomolgus monkeys when administered a bolus dose (100 μg/kg) of dornase alfa followed by a 6 hour intravenous infusion (80 μg/kg/h). Little or no measurable dornase alfa would be expected in human milk after chronic aerosol administration of recommended doses. Because many drugs are excreted in human milk, caution should still be exercised when dornase alfa is administered to a nursing woman.

PEDIATRIC USE

Because of the limited experience with the administration of Pulmozyme to patients younger than 5 years of age, its use should be considered only for those patients in whom there is a potential for benefit in pulmonary function or in risk of respiratory tract infection.

DRUG INTERACTIONS

Clinical trials have indicated that dornase alfa can be effectively and safely used in conjunction with standard cystic fibrosis therapies including oral, inhaled and/or parenteral antibiotics, bronchodilators, enzyme supplements, vitamins, oral and inhaled corticosteroids, and analgesics. No formal drug interaction studies have been performed.

ADVERSE REACTIONS

Patients have been exposed to dornase alfa for up to 12 months in clinical trials.

In a randomized, placebo-controlled clinical trial in patients with FVC ≥40% of predicted, over 600 patients received dornase alfa once or twice daily for 6 months; most adverse events were not more common on dornase alfa than on placebo and probably reflected the sequelae of the underlying lung disease. In most cases events that were increased were mild, transient in nature, and did not require alterations in dosing. Few patients experienced adverse events resulting in permanent discontinuation from dornase alfa, and the discontinuation rate was similar for placebo (2%) and dornase alfa (3%). Events that were more frequent (greater than 3%) in dornase alfa treated patients than in placebo-treated patients are listed in TABLE 2A and TABLE 2B.

In a randomized, placebo-controlled trial of patients with advanced disease (FVC <40% of predicted) the safety profile for most adverse events was similar to that reported for the trial in patients with mild to moderate disease. For this study, adverse events that were reported with a higher frequency (greater than 3%) in the dornase alfa treated patients, are also listed in TABLE 2A and TABLE 2B.

Events observed at similar rates in dornase alfa inhalation solution and placebo treated patients with FVC ≥40% predicted:

Body as a Whole: Abdominal pain, asthenia, fever, flu syndrome, malaise, sepsis.

Digestive System: Intestinal obstruction, gall bladder disease, liver disease, pancreatic disease.

Metabolic Nutritional System: Diabetes mellitus, hypoxia, weight loss.

Respiratory System: Apnea, bronchiectasis, bronchitis, change in sputum, cough increase, dyspnea, hemoptysis, lung function decrease, nasal polyps, pneumonia, pneumothorax, rhinitis, sinusitis, sputum increase, wheeze.

Mortality rates observed in controlled trials were similar for the placebo and dornase alfa. Causes of death were consistent with progression of cystic fibrosis and included apnea,

TABLE 2A *Adverse Events Increased 3% or More in Dornase Alfa Treated Patients Over Placebo in CF Clinical Trials*

Mild to Moderate CF Patients (FVC ≥40% of predicted) — Treated for 24 Weeks

		Dornase Alfa	
	Placebo	qd	bid
Adverse Event*	n=325	n=322	n=321
Voice alteration	7%	12%	16%
Pharyngitis	33%	36%	40%
Rash	7%	10%	12%
Laryngitis	1%	3%	4%
Chest pain	16%	18%	21%
Conjunctivitis	2%	4%	5%
Fever	Difference was less than 3% for this adverse event in the Trial in mild to moderate CF patients.		
Dyspnea (when reported as serious)	Difference was less than 3% for this adverse event in the Trial in mild to moderate CF patients.		

* Of any severity or seriousness.
Difference was less than 3% for this adverse event in the Trial in mild to moderate CF patients.

TABLE 2B *Adverse Events Increased 3% or More in Dornase Alfa Treated Patients Over Placebo in CF Clinical Trials*

Advanced CF Patients (FVC <40% of predicted) — Treated for 12 Weeks

	Placebo	Dornase Alfa qd
Adverse Event*	n=159	n=161
Voice alteration	6%	18%
Pharyngitis	28%	32%
Rash	1%	3%
Laryngitis	1%	3%
Chest pain	23%	25%
Conjunctivitis	0%	1%
Rhinitis	24%	30%
FVC decrease of ≥10% of predicted†	17%	22%
Fever	28%	32%
Dyspepsia	0%	3%
Dyspnea (when reported as serious)	12%‡	17%‡

* Of any severity or seriousness.
† Total reports of dyspnea (regardless of severity or seriousness) had a difference of less than 3% for the Trial in advanced CF patients.
‡ Total reports of dyspnea (regardless of severity or seriousness) had a difference of less than 3% for the Trial in advanced CF patients.

cardiac arrest, cardiopulmonary arrest, cor pulmonale, heart failure, massive hemoptysis, pneumonia, pneumothorax, and respiratory failure.

The safety of dornase alfa, 2.5 mg by inhalation, was studied with 2 weeks of daily administration in 98 patients with cystic fibrosis (65 aged 3 months to <5 years, 33 aged 5 to ≤10 years). The Pari Baby reusable nebulizer (which uses a facemask instead of a mouthpiece) was utilized in patients unable to demonstrate the ability to inhale or exhale orally throughout the entire treatment period (54/65, 83% of the younger and 2/33, 6% of the older patients). The number of patients reporting cough was higher in the younger age group as compared to the older age group (29/65, 45% compared to 10/33, 30%) as was the number reporting moderate to severe cough (24/65, 37% as compared to 6/33, 18%). Other events tended to be of mild to moderate severity. The number of patients reporting rhinitis was higher in the younger age group as compared to the older age group (23/65, 35% compared to 9/33, 27%) as was the number reporting rash (4/65, 6% as compared to 0/33). The nature of adverse events was similar to that seen in the larger trials of dornase alfa.

ALLERGIC REACTIONS

There have been no reports of anaphylaxis attributed to the administration of dornase alfa to date. Skin rash and urticaria have been observed, and were mild and transient in nature. Within all of the studies, a small percentage (average of 2-4%) of patients treated with dornase alfa developed serum antibodies to dornase alfa. None of these patients developed anaphylaxis, and the clinical significance of serum antibodies to dornase alfa is unknown.

DOSAGE AND ADMINISTRATION

The recommended dose for use in most cystic fibrosis patients is one 2.5 mg single-use ampule inhaled once daily using a recommended nebulizer. Some patients may benefit from twice daily administration. Clinical trials have been performed with the following nebulizers and compressors: the disposable jet nebulizer Hudson T Up-draft II and disposable jet nebulizer Marquest Acorn II in conjunction with a Pulmo-Aide compressor, and the reusable Pari LC Jet+ nebulizer, in conjunction with the Pari Proneb compressor. Safety and efficacy have been demonstrated only with these recommended nebulizer systems.

No clinical data are currently available that support the safety and efficacy of administration of dornase alfa with other nebulizer systems. That patient should follow the manufacturer's instructions on the use and maintenance of the equipment.

Dornase alfa should not be diluted or mixed with other drugs in the nebulizer. Mixing of dornase alfa with other drugs could lead to adverse physiochemical and/or functional changes in dornase alfa or the admixed compound.

HOW SUPPLIED

Pulmozyne inhalation solution is supplied in single-use ampules. Each ampule delivers 2.5 ml of a sterile, clear, colorless, aqueous solution containing 1.0 mg/ml dornase alfa, 0.15 mg/ml calcium chloride dihydrate and 8.77 mg/ml sodium chloride with no preservative. The nominal pH of the solution is 6.3.

Storage: Dornase alfa inhalation solution should be stored under refrigeration 2-8°C (36-46°F). Ampules should be protected from strong light. Do not use beyond the expiration date stamped on the ampule. Unused ampules should be stored in their protective foil pouch under refrigeration.

PRODUCT LISTING - EQUIVALENTS NOT AVAILABLE

Solution - Inhalation - 2.5 mg/2.5 ml

2 ml x 30	$1439.70	PULMOZYME, Genentech	50242-0100-40
3 ml	$34.37	PULMOZYME, Genentech	50242-0100-39

Dorzolamide Hydrochloride *(003235)*

Categories: Glaucoma, open-angle; Hypertension, ocular; FDA Approved 1994 Dec; Pregnancy Category C
Drug Classes: Carbonic anhydrase inhibitors; Ophthalmics
Brand Names: Trusopt
Cost of Therapy: $23.85 (Glaucoma; Trusopt Ophthalmic Solution; 2%; 5 ml; 3 drops/day; variable day supply)

DESCRIPTION

Trusopt (dorzolamide HCl ophthalmic solution) is a carbonic anhydrase inhibitor formulated for topical ophthalmic use.

Dorzolamide HCl is described chemically as: (4*S*-*trans*)-4-(ethylamino)-5,6-dihydro-6-methyl-4*H*-thieno[2,3-*b*]thiopyran-2-sulfonamide 7,7-dioxide monohydrochloride. Dorzolamide HCl is optically active.

Its empirical formula is $C_{10}H_{16}N_2O_4S_3 \cdot HCl$.

Dorzolamide HCl has a molecular weight of 360.9 and a melting point of about 264°C. It is a white to off-white, crystalline powder, which is soluble in water and slightly soluble in methanol and ethanol.

Trusopt sterile ophthalmic solution is supplied as a sterile, isotonic, buffered, slightly viscous, aqueous solution of Trusopt. The pH of the solution is approximately 5.6, and the osmolarity is 260-330 mOsM. Each ml of Trusopt 2% contains 20 mg dorzolamide (22.3 mg of dorzolamide HCl). Inactive ingredients are hydroxyethyl cellulose, mannitol, sodium citrate dihydrate, sodium hydroxide (to adjust pH) and water for injection. Benzalkonium chloride 0.0075% is added as a preservative.

CLINICAL PHARMACOLOGY

MECHANISM OF ACTION

Carbonic anhydrase (CA) is an enzyme found in many tissues of the body including the eye. It catalyzes the reversible reaction involving the hydration of carbon dioxide and the dehydration of carbonic acid. In humans, carbonic anhydrase exists as a number of isoenzymes, the most active being carbonic anhydrase II (CA-II), found primarily in red blood cells (RBCs), but also in other tissues. Inhibition of carbonic anhydrase in the ciliary processes of the eye decreases aqueous humor secretion, presumably by slowing the formation of bicarbonate ions with subsequent reduction in sodium and fluid transport. The result is a reduction in intraocular pressure (IOP).

Dorzolamide HCl ophthalmic solution contains dorzolamide HCl, an inhibitor of human carbonic anhydrase II. Following topical ocular administration, dorzolamide HCl reduces elevated intraocular pressure. Elevated intraocular pressure is a major risk factor in the pathogenesis of optic nerve damage and glaucomatous visual field loss.

PHARMACOKINETICS AND PHARMACODYNAMICS

When topically applied, dorzolamide reaches the systemic circulation. To assess the potential for systemic carbonic anhydrase inhibition following topical administration, drug and metabolite concentrations in RBCs and plasma and carbonic anhydrase inhibition in RBCs were measured. Dorzolamide accumulates in RBCs during chronic dosing as a result of binding to CA-II. The parent drug forms a single N-desethyl metabolite, which inhibits CA-II less potently than the parent drug but also inhibits CA-I. The metabolite also accumulates in RBCs where it binds primarily to CA-I. Plasma concentrations of dorzolamide and metabolite are generally below the assay limit of quantitation (15nM). Dorzolamide binds moderately to plasma proteins (approximately 33%). Dorzolamide is primarily excreted unchanged in the urine; the metabolite also is excreted in urine. After dosing is stopped, dorzolamide washes out of RBCs nonlinearly, resulting in a rapid decline of drug concentration initially, followed by a slower elimination phase with a half-life of about 4 months.

To simulate the systemic exposure after long-term topical ocular administration, dorzolamide was given orally to 8 healthy subjects for up to 20 weeks. The oral dose of 2 mg bid closely approximates the amount of drug delivered by topical ocular administration of dorzolamide HCl 2% tid. Steady state was reached within 8 weeks. The inhibition of CA-II and total carbonic anhydrase activities was below the degree of inhibition anticipated to be necessary for a pharmacological effect on renal function and respiration in healthy individuals.

INDICATIONS AND USAGE

Dorzolamide HCl ophthalmic solution is indicated in the treatment of elevated intraocular pressure in patients with ocular hypertension or open-angle glaucoma.

NON-FDA APPROVED INDICATIONS

Dorzolamide has also been used to prevent postsurgical elevations in IOP after cataract extraction; however, it is not approved by the FDA for this purpose.

CONTRAINDICATIONS

Dorzolamide HCl is contraindicated in patients who are hypersensitive to any component of this product.

WARNINGS

Dorzolamide HCl is a sulfonamide and although administered topically is absorbed systemically. Therefore, the same types of adverse reactions that are attributable to sulfonamides may occur with topical administration with dorzolamide HCl. Fatalities have occurred, although rarely, due to severe reactions to sulfonamides including Stevens-Johnson syndrome, toxic epidermal necrolysis, fulminant hepatic necrosis, agranulocytosis, aplastic anemia, and other blood dyscrasias. Sensitization may recur when a sulfonamide is readministered irrespective of the route of administration. If signs of serious reactions or hypersensitivity occur, discontinue the use of this preparation.

PRECAUTIONS

GENERAL

The management of patients with acute angle-closure glaucoma requires therapeutic interventions in addition to ocular hypotensive agents. Dorzolamide HCl has not been studied in patients with acute angle-closure glaucoma.

Dorzolamide HCl has not been studied in patients with severe renal impairment (CRCL <30 ml/min). Because dorzolamide HCl and its metabolite are excreted predominantly by the kidney, dorzolamide HCl is not recommended in such patients.

Dorzolamide HCl has not been studied in patients with hepatic impairment and should therefore be used with caution in such patients.

In clinical studies, local ocular adverse effects, primarily conjunctivitis and lid reactions, were reported with chronic administration of dorzolamide HCl. Many of these reactions had the clinical appearance and course of an allergic-type reaction that resolved upon discontinuation of drug therapy. If such reactions are observed, dorzolamide HCl should be discontinued and the patient evaluated before considering restarting the drug. (See ADVERSE REACTIONS.)

There is a potential for an additive effect on the known systemic effects of carbonic anhydrase inhibition in patients receiving an oral carbonic anhydrase inhibitor and dorzolamide HCl. The concomitant administration of dorzolamide HCl and oral carbonic anhydrase inhibitors is not recommended.

There have been reports of bacterial keratitis associated with the use of multiple dose containers of topical ophthalmic products. These containers had been inadvertently contaminated by patients who, in most cases, had a concurrent corneal disease or a disruption of the ocular epithelial surface.

Choroidal detachment has been reported with administration of aqueous suppressant therapy (*e.g.,* dorzolamide) after filtration procedures.

INFORMATION FOR THE PATIENT

Dorzolamide HCl is a sulfonamide and although administered topically is absorbed systemically. Therefore the same types of adverse reactions that are attributable to sulfonamides may occur with topical administration. Patients should be advised that if serious or unusual reactions or signs of hypersensitivity occur, they should discontinue the use of the product (see WARNINGS).

Patients should be advised that if they develop any ocular reactions, particularly conjunctivitis and lid reactions, they should discontinue use and seek their physician's advice.

Patients should be instructed to avoid allowing the tip of the dispensing container to contact the eye or surrounding structures.

Patients should also be instructed that ocular solutions, if handled improperly or if the tip of the dispensing container contacts the eye or surrounding structures, can become contaminated by common bacteria known to cause ocular infections. Serious damage to the eye and subsequent loss of vision may result from using contaminated solutions.

Patients also should be advised that if they have ocular surgery or develop an intercurrent ocular condition (*e.g.,* trauma or infection), they should immediately seek their physician's advice concerning the continued use of the present multidose container.

If more than one topical ophthalmic drug is being used, the drugs should be administered at least 10 minutes apart.

Patients should be advised that dorzolamide HCl contains benzalkonium chloride which may be absorbed by soft contact lenses. Contact lenses should be removed prior to administration of the solution. Lenses may be reinserted 15 minutes following dorzolamide HCl administration.

CARCINOGENESIS, MUTAGENESIS, AND IMPAIRMENT OF FERTILITY

In a 2 year study of dorzolamide HCl administered orally to male and female Sprague-Dawley rats, urinary bladder papillomas were seen in male rats in the highest dosage group of 20 mg/kg/day (250 times the recommended human ophthalmic dose). Papillomas were not seen in rats given oral doses equivalent to approximately 12 times the recommended human ophthalmic dose. No treatment-related tumors were seen in a 21 month study in female and male mice given oral doses up to 75 mg/kg/day (~900 times the recommended human ophthalmic dose).

The increased incidence of urinary bladder papillomas seen in the high-dose male rats is a class-effect of carbonic anhydrase inhibitors in rats. Rats are particularly prone to developing papillomas in response to foreign bodies, compounds causing crystalluria, and diverse sodium salts.

No changes in bladder urothelium were seen in dogs given oral dorzolamide HCl for 1 year at 2 mg/kg/day (25 times the recommended human ophthalmic dose) or monkeys dosed topically to the eye at 0.4 mg/kg/day (~5 times the recommended human ophthalmic dose) for 1 year.

The following tests for mutagenic potential were negative: (1) *in vivo* (mouse) cytogenetic assay; (2) *in vitro* chromosomal aberration assay; (3) alkaline elution assay; (4) V-79 assay; and (5) Ames test.

In reproduction studies of dorzolamide HCl in rats, there were no adverse effects on the reproductive capacity of males or females at doses up to 188 or 94 times, respectively, the recommended human ophthalmic dose.

PREGNANCY, TERATOGENIC EFFECTS, PREGNANCY CATEGORY C

Developmental toxicity studies with dorzolamide HCl in rabbits at oral doses of ≥2.5 mg/kg/day (31 times the recommended human ophthalmic dose) revealed malformations of the vertebral bodies. These malformations occurred at doses that caused metabolic acidosis with decreased body weight gain in dams and decreased fetal weights. No treatment-related malformations were seen at 1.0 mg/kg/day (13 times the recommended human ophthalmic dose). There are no adequate and well-controlled studies in pregnant women. Dorzolamide HCl should be used during pregnancy only if the potential benefit justifies the potential risk to the fetus.

NURSING MOTHERS

In a study of dorzolamide HCl in lactating rats, decreases in body weight gain of 5-7% in offspring at an oral dose of 7.5 mg/kg/day (94 times the recommended human ophthalmic dose) were seen during lactation. A slight delay in postnatal development (incisor eruption, vaginal canalization and eye openings), secondary to lower fetal body weight, was noted.

It is not known whether this drug is excreted in human milk. Because many drugs are excreted in human milk and because of the potential for serious adverse reactions in nursing infants from dorzolamide HCl, a decision should be made whether to discontinue nursing or to discontinue the drug, taking into account the importance of the drug to the mother.

PEDIATRIC USE

Safety and effectiveness in pediatric patients have not been established.

GERIATRIC USE

No overall differences in safety or effectiveness have been observed between elderly and younger patients.

DRUG INTERACTIONS

Although acid-base and electrolyte disturbances were not reported in the clinical trials with dorzolamide HCl, these disturbances have been reported with oral carbonic anhydrase inhibitors and have, in some instances, resulted in drug interactions (*e.g.,* toxicity associated with high-dose salicylate therapy). Therefore, the potential for such drug interactions should be considered in patients receiving dorzolamide HCl.

ADVERSE REACTIONS

CONTROLLED CLINICAL TRIALS

The most frequent adverse events associated with dorzolamide HCl were ocular burning, stinging, or discomfort immediately following ocular administration (approximately one-third of patients). Approximately one-quarter of patients noted a bitter taste following administration. Superficial punctate keratitis occurred in 10-15% of patients and signs and symptoms of ocular allergic reaction in approximately 10%. Events occurring in approximately 1-5% of patients were conjunctivitis and lid reactions (see PRECAUTIONS, General), blurred vision, eye redness, tearing, dryness, and photophobia. Other ocular events and systemic events were reported infrequently, including headache, nausea, asthenia/fatigue; and, rarely, skin rashes, urolithiasis, and iridocyclitis.

CLINICAL PRACTICE

The following adverse events have occurred either at low incidence (<1%) during clinical trials or have been reported during the use of dorzolamide HCl in clinical practice where these events were reported voluntarily from a population of unknown size and frequency of occurrence cannot be determined precisely. They have been chosen for inclusion based on factors such as seriousness, frequency of reporting, possible causal connection to dorzolamide HCl, or a combination of these factors: signs and symptoms of systemic allergic reactions including angioedema, bronchospasm, pruritus, and urticaria; dizziness, paresthesia; ocular pain, transient myopia, choroidal detachment following filtration surgery, eyelid crusting; dyspnea; contact dermatitis, epistaxis, dry mouth and throat irritation.

DOSAGE AND ADMINISTRATION

The dose is 1 drop of dorzolamide HCl ophthalmic solution in the affected eye(s) 3 times daily.

Dorzolamide HCl may be used concomitantly with other topical ophthalmic drug products to lower intraocular pressure. If more than 1 topical ophthalmic drug is being used, the drugs should be administered at least 10 minutes apart.

HOW SUPPLIED

Trusopt ophthalmic solution is a slightly opalescent, nearly colorless, slightly viscous solution.

Storage: Store Trusopt ophthalmic solution at 15-30°C (59-86°F). Protect from light.

PRODUCT LISTING - EQUIVALENTS NOT AVAILABLE

Solution - Ophthalmic - 2%

5 ml	$23.85	TRUSOPT, Southwood Pharmaceuticals Inc	58016-6565-05
5 ml	$25.04	TRUSOPT, Allscripts Pharmaceutical Company	54569-4193-00
5 ml	$25.69	TRUSOPT, Merck & Company Inc	00006-3519-03
5 ml	$27.48	TRUSOPT, Merck & Company Inc	00006-3519-35
5 ml	$28.87	TRUSOPT, Physicians Total Care	54868-3593-01
10 ml	$50.10	TRUSOPT, Allscripts Pharmaceutical Company	54569-4159-00
10 ml	$51.40	TRUSOPT, Merck & Company Inc	00006-3519-10
10 ml	$54.99	TRUSOPT, Merck & Company Inc	00006-3519-36
10 ml	$57.17	TRUSOPT, Physicians Total Care	54868-3593-00

Dorzolamide Hydrochloride; Timolol Maleate (003417)

For complete prescribing information, refer to the CD-ROM included with the book.

Categories: Glaucoma, open-angle; Hypertension, ocular; FDA Approved 1998 Apr; Pregnancy Category C
Drug Classes: Antiadrenergics, beta blocking; Carbonic anhydrase inhibitors; Ophthalmics
Foreign Brand Availability: Cosopt (Canada; Hong-Kong; Israel; Korea; Mexico; New-Zealand; Philippines; Singapore; South-Africa; Taiwan; Thailand); Timpilo (Australia; Austria; Belgium; Czech-Republic; Denmark; France; Germany; Greece; Hungary; Netherlands; New-Zealand; Russia; Sweden; Switzerland)
Cost of Therapy: $46.90 (Glaucoma; Cosopt Ophthalmic Solution; 2%; 0.5%; 5 ml; 2 drops/day; variable day supply)

D

DESCRIPTION

Note: The trade name has been used throughout this monograph for clarity.
Cosopt (dorzolamide hydrochloride-timolol maleate ophthalmic solution) is the combination of a topical carbonic anhydrase inhibitor and a topical beta-adrenergic receptor blocking agent.

Dorzolamide hydrochloride is described chemically as: (4*S-trans*)-4-(ethylamino)-5,6-dihydro-6-methyl-4*H*-thieno[2,3-*b*]thiopyran-2-sulfonamide 7,7-dioxide monohydrochloride. Dorzolamide hydrochloride is optically active.

Its empirical formula is $C_{10}H_{16}N_2O_4S_3 \cdot HCl$.

Dorzolamide hydrochloride has a molecular weight of 360.91. It is a white to off-white, crystalline powder, which is soluble in water and slightly soluble in methanol and ethanol.

Timolol maleate is described chemically as: (-)-1-(*tert*-butylamino)-3-[(4-morpholino-1,2,5-thiadiazol-3-yl)oxy]-2-propanol maleate (1:1) (salt). Timolol maleate possesses an asymmetric carbon atom in its structure and is provided as the levo-isomer.

Its molecular formula is $C_{13}H_{24}N_4O_3S \cdot C_4H_4O_4$.

Timolol maleate has a molecular weight of 432.50. It is a white, odorless, crystalline powder which is soluble in water, methanol, and alcohol. Timolol maleate is stable at room temperature.

Cosopt is supplied as a sterile, isotonic, buffered, slightly viscous, aqueous solution. The pH of the solution is approximately 5.65, and the osmolarity is 242-323 mOsM. Each ml of Cosopt contains 20 mg dorzolamide (22.26 mg of dorzolamide hydrochloride) and 5 mg timolol (6.83 mg timolol maleate). Inactive ingredients are sodium citrate, hydroxyethyl cellulose, sodium hydroxide, mannitol, and water for injection. Benzalkonium chloride 0.0075% is added as a preservative.

INDICATIONS AND USAGE

Cosopt is indicated for the reduction of elevated intraocular pressure in patients with open-angle glaucoma or ocular hypertension who are insufficiently responsive to beta-blockers (failed to achieve target IOP determined after multiple measurements over time). The IOP-lowering of Cosopt bid was slightly less than that seen with the concomitant administration of 0.5% timolol bid and 2.0% dorzolamide tid.

CONTRAINDICATIONS

Cosopt is contraindicated in patients with (1) bronchial asthma; (2) a history of bronchial asthma; (3) severe chronic obstructive pulmonary disease (see WARNINGS); (4) sinus bradycardia; (5) second or third degree atrioventricular block; (6) overt cardiac failure (see WARNINGS); (7) cardiogenic shock; or (8) hypersensitivity to any component of this product.

WARNINGS

SYSTEMIC EXPOSURE

Cosopt contains dorzolamide, a sulfonamide, and timolol maleate, a beta-adrenergic blocking agent; and although administered topically, is absorbed systemically. Therefore, the same types of adverse reactions that are attributable to sulfonamides and/or systemic administration of beta-adrenergic blocking agents may occur with topical administration. For example, severe respiratory reactions and cardiac reactions, including death due to bronchospasm in patients with asthma, and rarely death in association with cardiac failure, have been reported following systemic or ophthalmic administration of timolol maleate (see CONTRAINDICATIONS). Fatalities have occurred, although rarely, due to severe reactions to sulfonamides including Stevens-Johnson syndrome, toxic epidermal necrolysis, fulminant hepatic necrosis, agranulocytosis, aplastic anemia, and other blood dyscrasias. Sensitization may recur when a sulfonamide is readministered irrespective of the route of administration. If signs of serious reactions or hypersensitivity occur, discontinue the use of this preparation.

CARDIAC FAILURE

Sympathetic stimulation may be essential for support of the circulation in individuals with diminished myocardial contractility, and its inhibition by beta-adrenergic receptor blockade may precipitate more severe failure.

In patients without a history of cardiac failure continued depression of the myocardium with beta-blocking agents over a period of time can, in some cases, lead to cardiac failure. At the first sign or symptom of cardiac failure, Cosopt should be discontinued.

OBSTRUCTIVE PULMONARY DISEASE

Patients with chronic obstructive pulmonary disease (*e.g.*, chronic bronchitis, emphysema) of mild or moderate severity, bronchospastic disease, or a history of bronchospastic disease (other than bronchial asthma or a history of bronchial asthma, in which Cosopt is contraindicated [see CONTRAINDICATIONS]) should, in general, not receive beta-blocking agents, including Cosopt.

MAJOR SURGERY

The necessity or desirability of withdrawal of beta-adrenergic blocking agents prior to major surgery is controversial. Beta-adrenergic receptor blockade impairs the ability of the heart to respond to beta-adrenergically mediated reflex stimuli. This may augment the risk of general anesthesia in surgical procedures. Some patients receiving beta-adrenergic receptor blocking agents have experienced protracted severe hypotension during anesthesia. Difficulty in restarting and maintaining the heartbeat has also been reported. For these reasons, in patients undergoing elective surgery, some authorities recommend gradual withdrawal of beta-adrenergic receptor blocking agents.

If necessary during surgery, the effects of beta-adrenergic blocking agents may be reversed by sufficient doses of adrenergic agonists.

DIABETES MELLITUS

Beta-adrenergic blocking agents should be administered with caution in patients subject to spontaneous hypoglycemia or to diabetic patients (especially those with labile diabetes) who are receiving insulin or oral hypoglycemic agents. Beta-adrenergic receptor blocking agents may mask the signs and symptoms of acute hypoglycemia.

THYROTOXICOSIS

Beta-adrenergic blocking agents may mask certain clinical signs (*e.g.*, tachycardia) of hyperthyroidism. Patients suspected of developing thyrotoxicosis should be managed carefully to avoid abrupt withdrawal of beta-adrenergic blocking agents that might precipitate a thyroid storm.

DOSAGE AND ADMINISTRATION

The dose is 1 drop of Cosopt in the affected eye(s) 2 times daily.

If more than 1 topical ophthalmic drug is being used, the drugs should be administered at least 10 minutes apart.

PRODUCT LISTING - EQUIVALENTS NOT AVAILABLE

Solution - Ophthalmic - 2%;0.5%

5 ml	$42.75	COSOPT, Allscripts Pharmaceutical Company	54569-4744-00
5 ml	$46.90	COSOPT, Merck & Company Inc	00006-3628-35
10 ml	$85.50	COSOPT, Allscripts Pharmaceutical Company	54569-4745-00
10 ml	$93.84	COSOPT, Merck & Company Inc	00006-3628-36

Doxazosin Mesylate (003007)

Categories: Hyperplasia, benign prostatic; Hypertension, essential; Pregnancy Category B; FDA Approved 1990 Nov; WHO Formulary
Drug Classes: Antiadrenergics, alpha blocking; Antiadrenergics, peripheral
Brand Names: Cardura
Foreign Brand Availability: Alfadil (Sweden); Cadex (Israel); Cadil (Korea); Cardenalin (Japan); Cardil (Korea); Cardoral (Israel); Cardoxan (New-Zealand); Cardular (Germany); Cardular PP (Germany); Cardular Uro (Germany); Cardura XL (Hong-Kong); Cardura-XL S.R. (Korea); Carduran (Colombia; Denmark; Norway; Philippines; Spain); Dedralen (Italy); Diblocin (Germany); Diblocin PP (Germany); Diblocin Uro (Germany); Dophilin (Taiwan); Dosan (New-Zealand); Doxaben (Taiwan); Doxacard (India); Doxagamma (Germany); Doxaloc (Israel); Doxasyn (Hong-Kong); Jutalar (Germany); Kaltensif (Indonesia); Kinxasen (Taiwan); Pencor (Thailand); Supressin (Austria); Uriduct (Germany); Zoxan LP (France)
Cost of Therapy: $34.65 (Hypertension; Cardura; 1 mg; 1 tablet/day; 30 day supply)

DESCRIPTION

Doxazosin mesylate is a quinazoline compound that is a selective inhibitor of the $alpha_1$ subtype of alpha adrenergic receptors. The chemical name of doxazosin mesylate is 1-(4-amino-6,7-dimethoxy-2-quinazolinyl)-4-(1,4-benzodioxan-2-ylcarbonyl) piperazine methanesulfonate. The empirical formula for doxazosin mesylate is $C_{23}H_{25}N_5O_5 \cdot CH_4O_3S$ and the molecular weight is 547.6.

Cardura is freely soluble in dimethylsulfoxide, soluble in dimethylformamide, slightly soluble in methanol, ethanol, and water (0.8% at 25°C), and very slightly soluble in acetone and methylene chloride. Doxazosin mesylate is available as colored tablets for oral use and contains 1 mg (white), 2 mg (yellow), 4 mg (orange) and 8 mg (green) of doxazosin as the free base.

The inactive ingredients for all tablets are: Microcrystalline cellulose, lactose, sodium starch glycolate, magnesium stearate and sodium lauryl sulfate. The 2 mg tablet contains D&C yellow 10 and FD&C yellow 6; the 4 mg tablet contains FD&C yellow 6; the 8 mg tablet contains FD&C blue 10 and D&C yellow 10.

CLINICAL PHARMACOLOGY

PHARMACODYNAMICS

Benign Prostatic Hyperplasia (BPH)

Benign prostatic hyperplasia (BPH) is a common cause of urinary outflow obstruction in aging males. Severe BPH may lead to urinary retention and renal damage. A static and a dynamic component contribute to the symptoms and reduced urinary flow rate associated with BPH. The static component is related to an increase in prostate size caused, in part, by a proliferation of smooth muscle cells in the prostatic stroma. However, the severity of BPH symptoms and the degree of urethral obstruction do not correlate well with the size of the prostate. The dynamic component of BPH is associated with an increase in smooth muscle tone in the prostate and bladder neck. The degree of tone in this area is mediated by the $alpha_1$ adrenoceptor, which is present in high density in the prostatic stroma, prostatic capsule and bladder neck. Blockade of the $alpha_1$ receptor decreases urethral resistance and may relieve the obstruction and BPH symptoms. In the human prostate, doxazosin mesylate antagonizes phenylephrine ($alpha_1$ agonist)-induced contractions, *in vitro*, and binds with high affinity to the $alpha_{1c}$ adrenoceptor. The receptor subtype is thought to be the predominant functional type in the prostate. Doxazosin mesylate acts within 1-2 weeks to decrease the severity of BPH symptoms and improve urinary flow rate. Since $alpha_1$ adrenoceptors are of low density in the urinary bladder (apart from the bladder neck), doxazosin mesylate should maintain bladder contractility.

The efficacy of doxazosin mesylate was evaluated extensively in over 900 patients with BPH in double-blind, placebo-controlled trials. Doxazosin mesylate treatment was superior to placebo in improving patient symptoms and urinary flow rate. Significant relief with doxazosin mesylate was seen as early as 1 week into the treatment regimen, with doxazosin mesylate treated patients (n=173) showing a significant ($p < 0.01$) increase in maximum flow rate of 0.8 ml/sec compared to a decrease of 0.5 ml/sec in the placebo group (n=41). In long-term studies improvement was maintained for up to 2 years of treatment. In 66-71% of patients, improvements above baseline were seen in both symptoms and maximum urinary flow rate.

In three placebo-controlled studies of 14-16 weeks duration obstructive symptoms (hesitation, intermittency, dribbling, weak urinary stream, incomplete emptying of the bladder) and irritative symptoms (nocturia, daytime frequency, urgency, burning) of BPH were evaluated at each visit by patient-assessed symptom questionnaires. The bothersomeness of symptoms was measured with a modified Boyarsky questionnaire. Symptom severity/frequency was assessed using a modified Boyarsky questionnaire or an AUA-based questionnaire. Uroflowmetric evaluations were performed at times of peak (2-6 hours post-dose) and/or trough (24 hours post-dose) plasma concentrations of doxazosin mesylate.

The results from the three placebo-controlled studies (n=609) showing significant efficacy with 4 and 8 mg doxazosin are summarized in TABLE 1A and TABLE 1B. In all three studies, doxazosin mesylate resulted in statistically significant relief of obstructive and irritative symptoms compared to placebo. Statistically significant improvements of 2.3-3.3 ml/sec in maximum flow rate were seen with doxazosin mesylate in Studies 1 and 2, compared to 0.1-0.7 ml/sec with placebo.

TABLE 1A *Summary of Effectiveness Data in Placebo-Controlled Trials*

		Symptom Score*	
	n	Mean Baseline	Mean† Change
Study 1 (titration to maximum dose of 8 mg)‡			
Placebo	47	15.6	-2.3
Doxazosin mesylate	49	14.5	-4.9¤
Study 2 (titration to fixed dose — 14 weeks)§			
Placebo	37	20.7	-2.5
Doxazosin mesylate 4 mg	38	21.2	-5.0¤
Doxazosin mesylate 8 mg	42	19.9	-4.2¶
Study 3 (titration to fixed dose — 12 weeks)			
Placebo	47	14.9	-4.7
Doxazosin mesylate 4 mg	46	16.6	-6.1¶

* AUA questionnaire (range 0-30) in Studies 1 and 3. Modified Boyarsky Questionnaire (range 7-39) in Study 2.
† Change is to endpoint.
‡ 36 patients received a dose of 8 mg doxazosin mesylate.
§ Study in hypertensives with BPH.
¤ $p < 0.01$ compared to placebo mean change.
¶ $p < 0.05$ compared to placebo mean change.

TABLE 1B *Summary of Effectiveness Data in Placebo-Controlled Trials*

		Maximum Flow Rate (ml/sec)	
	n	Mean Baseline	Mean* Change
Study 1 (titration to maximum dose of 8 mg)†			
Placebo	41	9.7	+0.7
Doxazosin mesylate	41	9.8	+2.9§
Study 2 (titration to fixed dose — 14 weeks)‡			
Placebo	30	10.6	+0.1
Doxyzosin mesylate 4 mg	32	9.8	+2.3¤
Doxyzosin mesylate 8 mg	36	10.5	+3.3§
Study 3 (titration to fixed dose — 12 weeks)			
Placebo	44	9.9	+2.1
Doxyzosin mesylate 4 mg	46	9.6	+2.6

* Change is to fixed-dose efficacy phase. 22-26 hours post-dose for Studies 1 and 3 and 2-6 hours post-dose for Study 2.
† 36 patients received a dose of 8 mg doxazosin mesylate.
‡ Study in hypertensives with BPH.
§ $p < 0.01$ compared to placebo mean change.
¤ $p < 0.05$ compared to placebo mean change.

In one fixed dose study (study 2) doxazosin mesylate therapy (4-8 mg, once daily) resulted in a significant and sustained improvement in maximum urinary flow rate of 2.3-3.3 ml/sec (see TABLE 1A and TABLE 1B) compared to placebo (0.1 ml/sec). In this study, the only study in which weekly evaluations were made, significant improvement with doxazosin mesylate versus placebo was seen after 1 week. The proportion of patients who responded with a maximum flow rate improvement of ≥3 ml/sec was significantly larger with doxazosin mesylate (34-42%) than placebo (13-17%). A significantly greater improvement was also seen in average flow rate with doxazosin mesylate (1.6 ml/sec) than with placebo (0.2 ml/sec).

In BPH patients (n=450) treated for up to 2 years in open-label studies, doxazosin mesylate therapy resulted in significant improvement above baseline in urinary flow rates and BPH symptoms. The significant effects of doxazosin mesylate were maintained over the entire treatment period.

Although blockade of $alpha_1$ adrenoceptors also lowers blood pressure in hypertensive patients with increased peripheral vascular resistance, doxazosin mesylate treatment of normotensive men with BPH did not result in a clinically significant blood pressure lowering effect (TABLE 2). The proportion of normotensive patients with a sitting systolic blood pressure less than 90 mm Hg and/or diastolic blood pressure less than 60 mm Hg at any time during treatment with doxazosin mesylate 1-8 mg once daily was 6.7% with doxazosin and not significantly different (statistically) from that with placebo (5%).

TABLE 2 *Mean Changes in Blood Pressure From Baseline to the Mean of the Final Efficacy Phase in Normotensives (diastolic BP <90 mm Hg) in Two Double-Blind, Placebo-Controlled US Studies With Doxazosin Mesylate 1-8 mg Once Daily*

	Placebo (n=85)		Doxazosin Mesylate (n=183)	
	Baseline	Change	Baseline	Change
Sitting BP (mm Hg)				
Systolic	128.4	-1.4	128.8	-4.9*
Diastolic	79.2	-1.2	79.6	-2.4*
Standing BP (mm Hg)				
Systolic	128.5	-0.6	128.5	-5.3*
Diastolic	80.5	-0.7	80.4	-2.6*

* $p \leq 0.05$ compared to placebo.

Hypertension

The mechanism of action of doxazosin mesylate is selective blockade of the $alpha_1$ (postjunctional) subtype of adrenergic receptors. Studies in normal human subjects have shown that doxazosin competitively antagonized the pressor effects of phenylephrine (an $alpha_1$ agonist) and the systolic pressor effect of norepinephrine. Doxazosin and prazosin have similar abilities to antagonize phenylephrine. The antihypertensive effect of doxazosin mesylate results from a decrease in systemic vascular resistance. The parent compound doxazosin is primarily responsible for the antihypertensive activity. The low plasma concentrations of known active and inactive metabolites of doxazosin (2-piperazinyl, 6′- and 7′-hydroxy and 6- and 7-O-desmethyl compounds) compared to parent drug indicate that the contribution of even the most potent compound (6′-hydroxy) to the antihypertensive effect of doxazosin in man is probably small. The 6′- and 7′-hydroxy metabolites have demonstrated antioxidant properties at concentrations of 5 μM, *in vitro*.

Administration of doxazosin mesylate results in a reduction in systemic vascular resistance. In patients with hypertension there is little change in cardiac output. Maximum reductions in blood pressure usually occur 2-6 hours after dosing and are associated with a small increase in standing heart rate. Like other $alpha_1$-adrenergic blocking agents, doxazosin has a greater effect on blood pressure and heart rate in the standing position.

In a pooled analysis of placebo-controlled hypertension studies with about 300 hypertensive patients per treatment group, doxazosin, at doses of 1-16 mg given once daily, lowered blood pressure at 24 hours by about 10/8 mm Hg compared to placebo in the standing position and about 9/5 mm Hg in the supine position. Peak blood pressure effects (1-6 hours) were larger by about 50-75% (*i.e.*, trough values were about 55-70% of peak effect), with the larger peak-trough differences seen in systolic pressures. There was no apparent difference in the blood pressure response of Caucasians and blacks or of patients above and below age 65. In these predominantly normocholesterolemic patients doxazosin produced small reductions in total serum cholesterol (2-3%), LDL cholesterol (4%), and a similarly small increase in HDL/total cholesterol ratio (4%). The clinical significance of these findings is uncertain. In the same patient population, patients receiving doxazosin mesylate gained a mean of 0.6 kg compared to a mean loss of 0.1 kg for placebo patients.

PHARMACOKINETICS

After oral administration of therapeutic doses, peak plasma levels of doxazosin mesylate occur at about 2-3 hours. Bioavailability is approximately 65%, reflecting first pass metabolism of doxazosin by the liver. The effect of food on the pharmacokinetics of doxazosin mesylate was examined in a crossover study with 12 hypertensive subjects. Reductions of 18% in mean maximum plasma concentration and 12% in the area under the concentration-time curve occurred when doxazosin mesylate was administered with food. Neither of these differences was statistically or clinically significant.

Doxazosin mesylate is extensively metabolized in the liver, mainly by O-demethylation of the quinazoline nucleus or hydroxylation of the benzodioxan moiety. Although several active metabolites of doxazosin have been identified, the pharmacokinetics of these metabolites have not been characterized. In a study of 2 subjects administered radiolabelled doxazosin 2 mg orally and 1 mg intravenously on 2 separate occasions, approximately 63% of the dose was eliminated in the feces and 9% of the dose was found in the urine. On average only 4.8% of the dose was excreted as unchanged drug in the feces and only a trace of the total radioactivity in the urine was attributed to unchanged drug. At the plasma concentrations achieved by therapeutic doses approximately 98% of the circulating drug is bound to plasma proteins.

Plasma elimination of doxazosin is biphasic, with a terminal elimination half-life of about 22 hours. Steady-state studies in hypertensive patients given doxazosin doses of 2-16 mg once daily showed linear kinetics and dose proportionality. In two studies, following the administration of 2 mg orally once daily, the mean accumulation ratios (steady-state AUC versus first dose AUC) were 1.2 and 1.7. Enterohepatic recycling is suggested by secondary peaking of plasma doxazosin concentrations.

In a crossover study in 24 normotensive subjects, the pharmacokinetics and safety of doxazosin were shown to be similar with morning and evening dosing regimens. The area under the curve after morning dosing was, however, 11% less than that after evening dosing and the time to peak concentration after evening dosing occurred significantly later than that after morning dosing (5.6 hours vs 3.5 hours).

The pharmacokinetics of doxazosin mesylate in young (<65 years) and elderly (≥65 years) subjects were similar for plasma half-life values and oral clearance. Pharmacokinetic studies in elderly patients and patients with renal impairment have shown no significant alterations compared to younger patients with normal renal function. Administration of a single 2 mg dose to patients with cirrhosis (Child-Pugh Class A) showed a 40% increase in exposure to doxazosin. There are only limited data on the effects of drugs known to influence the hepatic metabolism of doxazosin [*e.g.*, cimetidine (see DRUG INTERACTIONS)]. As with any drug wholly metabolized by the liver, use of doxazosin mesylate in patients with altered liver function should be undertaken with caution.

In two placebo-controlled studies, of normotensive and hypertensive BPH patients, in which doxazosin was administered in the morning and the titration interval was 2 weeks and 1 week, respectively, trough plasma concentrations of doxazosin mesylate were similar in the 2 populations. Linear kinetics and dose proportionality were observed.

INDICATIONS AND USAGE

BENIGN PROSTATIC HYPERPLASIA (BPH)

Doxazosin mesylate is indicated for the treatment of both the urinary outflow obstruction and obstructive and irritative symptoms associated with BPH: obstructive symptoms (hesitation, intermittency, dribbling, weak urinary stream, incomplete emptying of the bladder) and irritative symptoms (nocturia, daytime frequency, urgency, burning). Doxazosin mesylate may be used in all BPH patients whether hypertensive or normotensive. In patients with hypertension and BPH, both conditions were effectively treated with doxazosin mesylate monotherapy. Doxazosin mesylate provides rapid improvement in symptoms and urinary flow rate in 66-71% of patients. Sustained improvements with doxazosin mesylate were seen in patients treated for up to 14 weeks in double-blind studies and up to 2 years in open-label studies.

HYPERTENSION

Doxazosin mesylate is also indicated for the treatment of hypertension. Doxazosin mesylate may be used alone or in combination with diuretics, beta-adrenergic blocking agents, calcium channel blockers or angiotensin-converting enzyme inhibitors.

CONTRAINDICATIONS

Doxazosin mesylate is contraindicated in patients with a known sensitivity to quinazolines (*e.g.*, prazosin, terazosin), doxaosin, or any of the inert ingredients.

WARNINGS

SYNCOPE AND "FIRST-DOSE" EFFECT

Doxazosin, like other alpha-adrenergic blocking agents, can cause marked hypotension, especially in the upright position, with syncope and other postural symptoms such as dizziness. Marked orthostatic effects are most common with the first dose but can also occur when there is a dosage increase, or if therapy is interrupted for more than a few days. To decrease the likelihood of excessive hypotension and syncope, it is essential that treatment be initiated with the 1 mg dose. The 2, 4, and 8 mg tablets are not for initial therapy. Dosage should then be adjusted slowly (see DOSAGE AND ADMINISTRATION) with evaluations and increases in dose every 2 weeks to the recommended dose. Additional antihypertensive agents should be added with caution.

Patients being titrated with doxazosin should be cautioned to avoid situations where injury could result should syncope occur, during both the day and night.

In an early investigational study of the safety and tolerance of increasing daily doses of doxazosin in normotensives beginning at 1 mg/day, only 2 of 6 subjects could tolerate more than 2 mg/day without experiencing symptomatic postural hypotension. In another study of 24 healthy normotensive male subjects receiving initial doses of 2 mg/day of doxazosin, 7 (29%) of the subjects experienced symptomatic postural hypotension between 0.5 and 6 hours after the first dose necessitating termination of the study. In this study, 2 of the normotensive subjects experienced syncope. Subsequent trials in hypertensive patients always began doxazosin dosing at 1 mg/day resulting in a 4% incidence of postural side effects at 1 mg/day with no cases of syncope.

In multiple dose clinical trials in hypertension involving over 1500 hypertensive patients with dose titration every 1-2 weeks, syncope was reported in 0.7% of patients. None of these events occurred at the starting dose of 1 mg and 1.2% (8/664) occurred at 16 mg/day.

In placebo-controlled, clinical trials in BPH, 3 out of 665 patients (0.5%) taking doxazosin reported syncope. Two (2) of the patients were taking 1 mg doxazosin, while 1 patient was taking 2 mg doxazosin when syncope occurred. In the open-label, long-term extension follow-up of approximately 450 BPH patients, there were 3 reports of syncope (0.7%). One (1) patient was taking 2 mg, 1 patient was taking 8 mg and 1 patient was taking 12 mg when syncope occurred. In a clinical pharmacology study, 1 subject receiving 2 mg experienced syncope.

If syncope occurs, the patient should be placed in a recumbent position and treated supportively as necessary.

PRIAPISM

Rarely (probably less frequently than once in every several thousand patients), $alpha_1$ antagonists, including doxazosin, have been associated with priapism (painful penile erection, sustained for hours and unrelieved by sexual intercourse or masturbation). Because this condition can lead to permanent impotence if not promptly treated, patients must be advised about the seriousness of the condition (see PRECAUTIONS, Information for the Patient).

PRECAUTIONS

GENERAL

Prostate Cancer

Carcinoma of the prostate causes many of the symptoms associated with BPH and the two disorders frequently co-exist. Carcinoma of the prostate should therefore be ruled out prior to commencing therapy with doxazosin mesylate.

Orthostatic Hypotension

While syncope is the most severe orthostatic effect of doxazosin mesylate, other symptoms of lowered blood pressure, such as dizziness, lightheadedness, or vertigo can occur, especially at initiation of therapy or at the time of dose increases.

Hypertension

These symptoms were common in clinical trials in hypertension, occurring in up to 23% of all patients treated and causing discontinuation of therapy in about 2%.

In placebo-controlled titration trials in hypertension, orthostatic effects were minimized by beginning therapy at 1 mg/day and titrating every 2 weeks to 2, 4, or 8 mg/day. There was an increased frequency of orthostatic effects in patients given 8 mg or more, 10%, compared to 5% at 1-4 mg and 3% in the placebo group.

Benign Prostatic Hyperplasia

In placebo-controlled trials in BPH, the incidence of orthostatic hypotension with doxazosin was 0.3% and did not increase with increasing dosage (to 8 mg/day). The incidence of discontinuations due to hypotensive or orthostatic symptoms was 3.3% with doxazosin and 1% with placebo. The titration interval in these studies was 1-2 weeks.

Patients in occupations in which orthostatic hypotension could be dangerous should be treated with particular caution. As $alpha_1$ antagonists can cause orthostatic effects, it is important to evaluate standing blood pressure 2 minutes after standing and patients should be advised to exercise care when arising from a supine or sitting position.

If hypotension occurs, the patient should be placed in the supine position and, if this measure is inadequate, volume expansion with intravenous fluids or vasopressor therapy may be used. A transient hypotensive response is not a contraindication to further doses of doxazosin mesylate.

INFORMATION FOR THE PATIENT

Refer to the Patient Instructions that are distributed with the prescription for complete instructions.

Patients should be made aware of the possibility of syncopal and orthostatic symptoms, especially at the initiation of therapy, and urged to avoid driving or hazardous tasks for 24 hours after the first dose, after a dosage increase, and after interruption of therapy when treatment is resumed. They should be cautioned to avoid situations where injury could result should syncope occur during initiation of doxazosin therapy. They should also be advised of the need to sit or lie down when symptoms of lowered blood pressure occur, although these symptoms are not always orthostatic, and to be careful when rising from a sitting or lying position. If dizziness, lightheadedness, or palpitations are bothersome they should be reported to the physician, so that dose adjustment can be considered. Patients should also be told that drowsiness or somnolence can occur with doxazosin mesylate or any selective $alpha_1$ adrenoceptor antagonist, requiring caution in people who must drive or operate heavy machinery.

Patients should be advised about the possibility of priapism as a result of treatment with $alpha_1$ antagonists. Patients should know that this adverse event is very rare. If they experience priapism, it should be brought to immediate medical attention for if not treated promptly it can lead to permanent erectile dysfunction (impotence).

DRUG/LABORATORY TEST INTERACTIONS

Doxazosin mesylate does not affect the plasma concentration of prostate specific antigen in patients treated for up to 3 years. Both doxazosin, an $alpha_1$ inhibitor, and finasteride, a 5-alpha reductase inhibitor, are highly protein bound and hepatically metabolized. There is no definitive controlled clinical experience on the concomitant use of $alpha_1$ inhibitors and 5-alpha reductase inhibitors at this time.

IMPAIRED LIVER FUNCTION

Doxazosin mesylate should be administered with caution to patients with evidence of impaired hepatic function or to patients receiving drugs known to influence hepatic metabolism (see CLINICAL PHARMACOLOGY).

LEUKOPENIA/NEUTROPENIA

Analysis of hematologic data from hypertensive patients receiving doxazosin mesylate in controlled hypertension clinical trials showed that the mean WBC (n=474) and mean neutrophil counts (n=419) were decreased by 2.4% and 1.0%, respectively, compared to placebo, a phenomenon seen with other alpha blocking drugs. In BPH patients the incidence of clinically significant WBC abnormalities was 0.4% (2/459) with doxazosin mesylate and 0% (0/147) with placebo, with no statistically significant difference between the 2 treatment groups. A search through a data base of 2400 hypertensive patients and 665 BPH patients revealed 4 hypertensives in which drug-related neutropenia could not be ruled out and 1 BPH patient in which drug related leukopenia could not be ruled out. Two hypertensives had a single low value on the last day of treatment. Two hypertensives had stable, non-progressive neutrophil counts in the $1000/mm^3$ range over periods of 20 and 40 weeks. One BPH patient had a decrease from a WBC count of $4800/mm^3$ to $2700/mm^3$ at the end of the study; there was no evidence of clinical impairment. In cases where follow-up was available the WBCs and neutrophil counts returned to normal after discontinuation of doxazosin mesylate. No patients became symptomatic as a result of the low WBC or neutrophil counts.

CARDIAC TOXICITY IN ANIMALS

An increased incidence of myocardial necrosis or fibrosis was displayed by Sprague-Dawley rats after 6 months of dietary administration at concentrations calculated to provide 80 mg doxazosin/kg/day and after 12 months of dietary administration at concentrations calculated to provide 40 mg doxazosin/kg/day (AUC exposure in rats 8 times the human AUC exposure with a 12 mg/day therapeutic dose). Myocardial fibrosis was observed in both rats and mice treated in the same manner with 40 mg doxazosin/kg/day for 18 months (exposure 8 times human AUC exposure in rats and somewhat equivalent to human C_{max} exposure in mice). No cardiotoxicity was observed at lower doses (up to 10 or 20 mg/kg/day, depending on the study) in either species. These lesions were not observed after 12 months of oral dosing in dogs at maximum doses of 20 mg/kg/day [maximum plasma concentrations (C_{max}) in dogs 14 times the C_{max} exposure in humans receiving a 12 mg/day therapeutic dose] and in Wistar rats at doses of 100 mg/kg/day (C_{max} exposures 15 times human C_{max} exposure with a 12 mg/day therapeutic dose). There is no evidence that similar lesions occur in humans.

CARCINOGENESIS, MUTAGENESIS, AND IMPAIRMENT OF FERTILITY

Chronic dietary administration (up to 24 months) of doxazosin mesylate at maximally tolerated doses of 40 mg/kg/day in rats and 120 mg/kg/day in mice revealed no evidence of carcinogenic potential. The highest doses evaluated in the rat and mouse studies are associated with AUCs (a measure of systemic exposure) that are 8 times and 4 times, respectively, the human AUC at a dose of 16 mg/day.

Mutagenicity studies revealed no drug- or metabolite-related effects at either chromosomal or subchromosomal levels.

Studies in rats showed reduced fertility in males treated with doxazosin at oral doses of 20 (but not 5 or 10) mg/kg/day, about 4 times the AUC exposures obtained with a 12 mg/day human dose. This effect was reversible within 2 weeks of drug withdrawal. There have been no reports of any effects of doxazosin on male fertility in humans.

PREGNANCY, TERATOGENIC EFFECTS, PREGNANCY CATEGORY C

Studies in pregnant rabbits and rats at daily oral doses of up to 41 and 20 mg/kg, respectively (plasma drug concentrations 10 and 4 times human C_{max} and AUC exposures with a 12 mg/day therapeutic dose), have revealed no evidence of harm to the fetus. A dosage regimen of 82 mg/kg/day in the rabbit was associated with reduced fetal survival. There are no adequate and well-controlled studies in pregnant women. Because animal reproduction studies are not always predictive of human response, doxazosin mesylate should be used during pregnancy only if clearly needed.

Radioactivity was found to cross the placenta following oral administration of labelled doxazosin to pregnant rats.

NONTERATOGENIC EFFECTS

In peri-postnatal studies in rats, postnatal development at maternal doses of 40 or 50 mg/kg/day of doxazosin (8 times human AUC exposure with a 12 mg/day therapeutic dose) was delayed as evidenced by slower body weight gain and slightly later appearance of anatomical features and reflexes.

NURSING MOTHERS

Studies in lactating rats given a single oral dose of 1 mg/kg of [2-^{14}C]-doxazosin mesylate indicate that doxazosin accumulates in rat breast milk with a maximum concentration about 20 times greater than the maternal plasma concentration. It is not known whether this drug is excreted in human milk. Because many drugs are excreted in human milk, caution should be exercised when doxazosin mesylate is administered to a nursing mother.

PEDIATRIC USE

The safety and effectiveness of doxazosin mesylate as an antihypertensive agent have not been established in children.

USE IN ELDERLY

The safety and effectiveness profile of doxazosin mesylate in BPH was similar in the elderly (age ≥65 years) and younger (age <65 years) patients.

DRUG INTERACTIONS

Most (98%) of plasma doxazosin is protein bound. *In vitro* data in human plasma indicate that doxazosin mesylate has no effect on protein binding of digoxin, warfarin, phenytoin or indomethacin. There is no information on the effect of other highly plasma protein bound drugs on doxazosin binding. Doxazosin mesylate has been administered without any evidence of an adverse drug interaction to patients receiving thiazide diuretics, beta-blocking agents, and nonsteroidal anti-inflammatory drugs. In a placebo-controlled trial in normal volunteers, the administration of a single 1 mg dose of doxazosin on day 1 of a 4 day regimen of oral cimetidine (400 mg twice daily) resulted in a 10% increase in mean AUC of doxazosin (p=0.006), and a slight but not statistically significant increase in mean C_{max} and mean half-life of doxazosin. The clinical significance of this increase in doxazosin AUC is unknown.

In clinical trials, doxazosin mesylate tablets have been administered to patients on a variety of concomitant medications; while no formal interaction studies have been conducted, no interactions were observed. Doxazosin mesylate tablets have been used with the following drugs or drug classes:

- Analgesic/anti-inflammatory (*e.g.*, acetaminophen, aspirin, codeine and codeine combinations, ibuprofen, indomethacin).
- Antibiotics (*e.g.*, erythromycin, trimethoprim and sulfamethoxazole, amoxicillin).
- Antihistamines (*e.g.*, chlorpheniramine).
- Cardiovascular agents (*e.g.*, atenolol, hydrochlorothiazide, propranolol).
- Corticosteroids.
- Gastrointestinal agents (*e.g.*, antacids).
- Hypoglycemics and endocrine drugs.
- Sedatives and tranquilizers (*e.g.*, diazepam).
- Cold and flu remedies.

ADVERSE REACTIONS

BENIGN PROSTATIC HYPERPLASIA

The incidence of adverse events has been ascertained from worldwide clinical trials in 965 BPH patients. The incidence rates presented in TABLE 3 are based on combined data from seven placebo-controlled trials involving once daily administration of doxazosin mesylate in doses of 1-16 mg in hypertensives and 0.5-8 mg in normotensives. The adverse events when the incidence in the doxazosin mesylate group was at least 1% are summarized in TABLE 3. No significant difference in the incidence of adverse events compared to placebo was seen except for dizziness, fatigue, hypotension, edema and dyspnea. Dizziness and dyspnea appeared to be dose-related.

In these placebo-controlled studies of 665 doxazosin mesylate patients, treated for a mean of 85 days, additional adverse reactions have been reported. These are less than 1% and not distinguishable from those that occurred in the placebo group.

Adverse reactions with an incidence of less than 1% but of clinical interest are (doxazosin mesylate versus placebo):

Cardiovascular System: Angina pectoris (0.6% vs 0.7%), postural hypotension (0.3% vs 0.3%), syncope (0.5% vs 0.0%), tachycardia (0.9% vs 0.0%).

Urogenital System: Dysuria (0.5% vs 1.3%).

Psychiatric Disorders: Libido decreased (0.8% vs 0.3%).

***TABLE 3** Adverse Reactions During Placebo-Controlled Studies — Benign Prostatic Hyperplasia*

Body System	Doxazosin Mesylate (n=665)	Placebo (n=300)
Body as a Whole		
Back pain	1.8%	2.0%
Chest pain	1.2%	0.7%
Fatigue	8.0%*	1.7%
Headache	9.9%	9.0%
Influenza-like symptoms	1.1%	1.0%
Pain	2.0%	1.0%
Cardiovascular System		
Hypotension	1.7%*	0.0%
Palpitation	1.2%	0.3%
Digestive System		
Abdominal pain	2.4%	2.0%
Diarrhea	2.3%	2.0%
Dyspepsia	1.7%	1.7%
Nausea	1.5%	0.7%
Metabolic and Nutritional Disorders		
Edema	2.7%*	0.7%
Nervous System		
Dizziness†	15.6%*	9.0%
Mouth dry	1.4%	0.3%
Somnolence	3.0%	1.0%
Respiratory System		
Dyspnea	2.6%*	0.3%
Respiratory disorder	1.1%	0.7%
Special Senses		
Vision abnormal	1.4%	0.7%
Urogenital System		
Impotence	1.1%	1.0%
Urinary tract infection	1.4%	2.3%
Skin & Appendages		
Sweating increased	1.1%	1.0%
Psychiatric Disorders		
Anxiety	1.1%	0.3%
Insomnia	1.2%	0.3%

* p ≤0.05 for treatment differences.
† Includes vertigo.

The safety profile in patients treated for up to 3 years was similar to that in the placebo-controlled studies.

The majority of adverse experiences with doxazosin mesylate were mild.

HYPERTENSION

Doxazosin mesylate has been administered to approximately 4000 hypertensive patients, of whom 1679 were included in the hypertension clinical development program. In that program, minor adverse effects were frequent, but led to discontinuation of treatment in only 7% of patients. In placebo-controlled studies adverse effects occurred in 49% and 40% of patients in the doxazosin and placebo groups, respectively, and led to discontinuation in 2% of patients in each group. The major reasons for discontinuation were postural effects (2%), edema, malaise/fatigue, and some heart rate disturbance, each about 0.7%.

In controlled hypertension clinical trials directly comparing doxazosin mesylate to placebo there was no significant difference in the incidence of side effects, except for dizziness (including postural), weight gain, somnolence and fatigue/malaise. Postural effects and edema appeared to be dose related. The prevalence rates presented below are based on combined data from placebo-controlled studies involving once daily administration of doxazosin at doses ranging from 1-16 mg. TABLE 4 summarizes those adverse experiences (possibly/probably related) reported for patients in these hypertension studies where the prevalence rate in the doxazosin group was at least 0.5% or where the reaction is of particular interest.

Additional adverse reactions have been reported, but these are, in general, not distinguishable from symptoms that might have occurred in the absence of exposure to doxazosin. The following adverse reactions occurred with a frequency of between 0.5% and 1%: syncope, hypoesthesia, increased sweating, agitation, increased weight. The following additional adverse reactions were reported by <0.5% of 3960 patients who received doxazosin in controlled or open, short- or long-term clinical studies; including international studies.

Cardiovascular System: Angina pectoris, myocardial infarction, cerebrovascular accident.

Autonomic Nervous System: Pallor.

Metabolic: Thirst, gout, hypokalemia.

Hematopoietic: Lymphadenopathy, purpura.

Reproductive System: Breast pain.

Skin Disorders: Alopecia, dry skin, eczema.

Central Nervous System: Paresis, tremor, twitching, confusion, migraine, impaired concentration.

Psychiatric: Paroniria, amnesia, emotional lability, abnormal thinking, depersonalization.

Special Senses: Parosmia, earache, taste perversion, photophobia, abnormal lacrimation.

Gastrointestinal System: Increased appetite, anorexia, fecal incontinence, gastroenteritis.

Respiratory System: Bronchospasm, sinusitis, coughing, pharyngitis.

Urinary System: Renal calculus.

General Body System: Hot flushes, back pain, infection, fever/rigors, decreased weight, influenza-like symptoms.

Doxazosin mesylate has not been associated with any clinically significant changes in routine biochemical tests. No clinically relevant adverse effects were noted on serum potassium, serum glucose, uric acid, blood urea nitrogen, creatinine or liver function tests.

TABLE 4 *Adverse Reactions During Placebo-Controlled Studies — Hypertension*

	Doxazosin (n=339)	Placebo (n=336)
Cardiovascular System		
Dizziness	19%	9%
Vertigo	2%	1%
Postural hypotension	0.3%	0%
Edema	4%	3%
Palpitation	2%	3%
Arrhythmia	1%	0%
Hypotension	1%	0%
Tachycardia	0.3%	1%
Peripheral ischemia	0.3%	0%
Skin & Appendages		
Rash	1%	1%
Pruritus	1%	1%
Musculoskeletal System		
Arthralgia/arthritis	1%	0%
Muscle weakness	1%	0%
Myalgia	1%	0%
Central & Peripheral Nervous System		
Headache	14%	16%
Paresthesia	1%	1%
Kinetic disorders	1%	0%
Ataxia	1%	0%
Hypertonia	1%	0%
Muscle cramps	1%	0%
Autonomic		
Mouth dry	2%	2%
Flushing	1%	0%
Special Senses		
Vision abnormal	2%	1%
Conjunctivitis/eye pain	1%	1%
Tinnitus	1%	0.3%
Psychiatric		
Somnolence	5%	1%
Nervousness	2%	2%
Depression	1%	1%
Insomnia	1%	1%
Sexual dysfunction	2%	1%
Gastrointestinal		
Nausea	3%	4%
Diarrhea	2%	3%
Constipation	1%	1%
Dyspepsia	1%	1%
Flatulence	1%	1%
Abdominal pain	0%	2%
Vomiting	0%	1%
Respiratory		
Rhinitis	3%	1%
Dyspnea	1%	1%
Epistaxis	1%	0%
Urinary		
Polyuria	2%	0%
Urinary incontinence	1%	0%
Micturition frequency	0%	2%
General		
Fatigue/malaise	12%	6%
Chest pain	2%	2%
Asthenia	1%	1%
Face edema	1%	0%
Pain	2%	2%

Doxazosin mesylate has been associated with decreases in white blood cell counts (see PRECAUTIONS).

In post-marketing experience the following additional adverse reactions have been reported:

Autonomic Nervous System: Priapism.
Central Nervous System: Hypoesthesia.
Endocrine System: Gynecomastia.
Gastrointestinal System: Vomiting.
General Body System: Allergic reaction.
Heart Rate/Rhythm: Bradycardia.
Hematopoietic: Leukopenia, thrombocytopenia.
Liver/Biliary System: Hepatitis, hepatitis cholestatic.
Respiratory System: Bronchospasm aggravated.
Skin Disorders: Urticaria.
Urinary System: Hematuria, micturition disorder, micturition frequency, nocturia.

DOSAGE AND ADMINISTRATION

DOSAGE MUST BE INDIVIDUALIZED. The initial dosage of doxazosin mesylate in patients with hypertension and/or BPH is 1 mg given once daily in the AM or PM. This starting dose is intended to minimize the frequency of postural hypotension and first dose syncope associated with doxazosin mesylate. Postural effects are most likely to occur between 2 and 6 hours after a dose. Therefore blood pressure measurements should be taken during this time period after the first dose and with each increase in dose. If doxazosin mesylate administration is discontinued for several days, therapy should be restarted using the initial dosing regimen.

BENIGN PROSTATIC HYPERPLASIA (1-8 MG ONCE DAILY)

The initial dosage of doxazosin mesylate is 1 mg, given once daily in the AM or PM. Depending on the individual patient's urodynamics and BPH symptomatology, dosage may then be increased to 2 mg and thereafter to 4 mg and 8 mg once daily, the maximum recommended dose for BPH. The recommended titration interval is 1-2 weeks. Blood pressure should be evaluated routinely in these patients.

HYPERTENSION (1-16 MG ONCE DAILY)

The initial dosage of doxazosin mesylate is 1 mg given once daily. Depending on the individual patient's standing blood pressure response (based on measurements taken at 2-6 hours post-dose and 24 hours post-dose), dosage may then be increased to 2 mg and thereafter if necessary to 4, 8 and 16 mg to achieve the desired reduction in blood pressure. **Increases in dose beyond 4 mg increase the likelihood of excessive postural effects including syncope, postural dizziness/vertigo and postural hypotension. At a titrated dose of 16 mg once daily the frequency of postural effects is about 12% compared to 3% for placebo.**

HOW SUPPLIED

Cardura is available as colored tablets for oral administration. Each tablet contains doxazosin mesylate equivalent to 1 mg (white), 2 mg (yellow), 4 mg (orange) or 8 mg (green) of the active constituent, doxazosin.

Cardura Tablets are available as 1 mg (white), 2 mg (yellow), 4 mg (orange) and 8 mg (green) scored tablets.

Recommended Storage: Store below 30°C (86°F).

PRODUCT LISTING - RATED THERAPEUTICALLY EQUIVALENT

Tablet - Oral - 1 mg

30's	$29.16	GENERIC, Ethex Corporation	58177-0266-22
30's	$30.81	CARDURA, Allscripts Pharmaceutical Company	54569-4864-00
30's	$35.98	CARDURA, Physicians Total Care	54868-1768-01
100's	$59.18	FEDERAL UPPER LIMIT, H.C.F.A. F F P	99999-3007-01
100's	$87.72	GENERIC, Geneva Pharmaceuticals	00781-5001-01
100's	$91.92	GENERIC, Ivax Corporation	00172-3685-60
100's	$92.33	GENERIC, Ethex Corporation	58177-0266-04
100's	$92.35	GENERIC, Mylan Pharmaceuticals Inc	00378-4021-01
100's	$92.35	GENERIC, Udl Laboratories Inc	51079-0957-20
100's	$92.44	GENERIC, Teva Pharmaceuticals Usa	00093-8120-01
100's	$92.44	GENERIC, Watson/Schein Pharmaceuticals Inc	00591-0639-01
100's	$92.44	GENERIC, Par Pharmaceutical Inc	49884-0552-01
100's	$94.90	GENERIC, Apotex Usa Inc	60505-0093-00
100's	$95.27	GENERIC, Purepac Pharmaceutical Company	00228-2642-11
100's	$115.49	CARDURA, Pfizer U.S. Pharmaceuticals	00049-2750-66
100's	$118.93	CARDURA, Pfizer U.S. Pharmaceuticals	00049-2750-41

Tablet - Oral - 2 mg

30's	$29.45	GENERIC, Ethex Corporation	58177-0267-22
30's	$30.81	CARDURA, Allscripts Pharmaceutical Company	54569-4865-00
30's	$35.98	CARDURA, Physicians Total Care	54868-2151-01
30's	$41.63	CARDURA, Pd-Rx Pharmaceuticals	55289-0277-30
60's	$70.78	CARDURA, Physicians Total Care	54868-2151-00
100's	$59.18	FEDERAL UPPER LIMIT, H.C.F.A. F F P	99999-3007-02
100's	$91.92	GENERIC, Ivax Corporation	00172-3686-60
100's	$92.33	GENERIC, Major Pharmaceuticals Inc	00904-5523-60
100's	$92.33	GENERIC, Ethex Corporation	58177-0267-04
100's	$92.34	GENERIC, Geneva Pharmaceuticals	00781-5002-01
100's	$92.35	GENERIC, Mylan Pharmaceuticals Inc	00378-4022-01
100's	$92.35	GENERIC, Udl Laboratories Inc	51079-0958-20
100's	$92.44	GENERIC, Teva Pharmaceuticals Usa	00093-8121-01
100's	$92.44	GENERIC, Watson Laboratories Inc	00591-0640-01
100's	$92.44	GENERIC, Par Pharmaceutical Inc	49884-0553-01
100's	$92.44	GENERIC, Watson Laboratories Inc	52544-0640-01
100's	$94.90	GENERIC, Apotex Usa Inc	60505-0094-00
100's	$95.27	GENERIC, Purepac Pharmaceutical Company	00228-2643-11
100's	$98.17	GENERIC, Major Pharmaceuticals Inc	00904-5523-61
100's	$115.49	CARDURA, Pfizer U.S. Pharmaceuticals	00049-2760-66
100's	$116.59	CARDURA, Physicians Total Care	54868-2151-02
100's	$118.93	CARDURA, Pfizer U.S. Pharmaceuticals	00049-2760-41

Tablet - Oral - 4 mg

30's	$30.51	GENERIC, Ethex Corporation	58177-0268-22
30's	$33.31	CARDURA, Allscripts Pharmaceutical Company	54569-3250-00
30's	$37.71	CARDURA, Physicians Total Care	54868-2640-01
100's	$62.10	FEDERAL UPPER LIMIT, H.C.F.A. F F P	99999-3007-03
100's	$96.49	GENERIC, Ivax Corporation	00172-3687-60
100's	$96.92	GENERIC, Geneva Pharmaceuticals	00781-5003-01
100's	$96.92	GENERIC, Major Pharmaceuticals Inc	00904-5524-60
100's	$96.92	GENERIC, Ethex Corporation	58177-0268-04
100's	$96.95	DOXAZOSIN MESYLATE, Mylan Pharmaceuticals Inc	00378-4024-01
100's	$96.95	GENERIC, Udl Laboratories Inc	51079-0959-20
100's	$97.00	GENERIC, Par Pharmaceutical Inc	49884-0554-01
100's	$97.03	DOXAZOSIN MESYLATE, Teva Pharmaceuticals Usa	00093-8122-01
100's	$97.03	GENERIC, Watson Laboratories Inc	00591-0641-01
100's	$97.03	GENERIC, Watson Laboratories Inc	52544-0641-01
100's	$99.89	GENERIC, Apotex Usa Inc	60505-0095-00
100's	$100.10	GENERIC, Purepac Pharmaceutical Company	00228-2644-11
100's	$101.70	GENERIC, Major Pharmaceuticals Inc	00904-5524-61
100's	$118.03	CARDURA, Pfizer U.S. Pharmaceuticals	00049-2770-41
100's	$121.21	CARDURA, Pfizer U.S. Pharmaceuticals	00049-2770-66

Tablet - Oral - 8 mg

30's	$33.96	CARDURA, Allscripts Pharmaceutical Company	54569-3297-01
30's	$39.53	CARDURA, Physicians Total Care	54868-3419-00
100's	$65.18	FEDERAL UPPER LIMIT, H.C.F.A. F F P	99999-3007-04
100's	$101.32	GENERIC, Ivax Corporation	00172-3688-60
100's	$101.78	GENERIC, Geneva Pharmaceuticals	00781-5004-01

100's	$101.80	GENERIC, Mylan Pharmaceuticals Inc	00378-4028-01
100's	$101.90	GENERIC, Teva Pharmaceuticals Usa	00093-8123-01
100's	$101.90	GENERIC, Watson/Schein Pharmaceuticals Inc	00591-0642-01
100's	$101.90	GENERIC, Par Pharmaceutical Inc	49884-0555-01
100's	$101.90	GENERIC, Watson Laboratories Inc	52544-0642-01
100's	$104.70	GENERIC, Apotex Usa Inc	60505-0096-00
100's	$105.13	GENERIC, Purepac Pharmaceutical Company	00228-2645-11
100's	$123.93	CARDURA, Pfizer U.S. Pharmaceuticals	00049-2780-41
100's	$127.29	CARDURA, Pfizer U.S. Pharmaceuticals	00049-2780-66

PRODUCT LISTING - EQUIVALENTS NOT AVAILABLE

Tablet - Oral - 1 mg

100's	$92.33	GENERIC, Major Pharmaceuticals Inc	00904-5522-60
100's	$92.44	GENERIC, Watson Laboratories Inc	52544-0639-01
100's	$97.19	GENERIC, Major Pharmaceuticals Inc	00904-5522-61

Tablet - Oral - 8 mg

100's	$101.77	GENERIC, Ethex Corporation	58177-0269-04
100's	$101.78	GENERIC, Major Pharmaceuticals Inc	00904-5525-60

Doxepin Hydrochloride *(001111)*

For related information, see the comparative table section in Appendix A.

Categories: Anxiety; Depression; Dermatitis, atopic; Lichen simplex chronicus; Pregnancy Category B, Topical; Pregnancy Category C, Oral; FDA Approved 1969 Sep
Drug Classes: Antidepressants, tricyclic; Dermatologics
Brand Names: Adapin; Alopam; **Sinequan**; Sinquane; Xepin; Zonalon
Foreign Brand Availability: Anten (New-Zealand); Aponal (Germany); Deptran (Australia); Doneurin (Germany); Doxal (Finland); Expan (Colombia); Gilex (Israel); Mareen (Germany); Quitaxon (Belgium; Benin; Burkina-Faso; Denmark; Ethiopia; France; Gambia; Ghana; Guinea; Ivory-Coast; Kenya; Liberia; Malawi; Mali; Mauritania; Mauritius; Morocco; Niger; Nigeria; Portugal; Senegal; Seychelles; Sierra-Leone; Sudan; Tanzania; Tunia; Uganda; Zambia; Zimbabwe); Sinquan (Denmark; Germany; Switzerland); Zonalon Cream (Israel)
Cost of Therapy: $39.02 (Depression; Sinequan; 75 mg; 1 capsule/day; 30 day supply)
$10.73 (Depression; Generic Capsules; 75 mg; 1 capsule/day; 30 day supply)

ORAL

DESCRIPTION

Sinequan is one of a class of psychotherapeutic agents known as dibenzoxepin tricyclic compounds. The molecular formula of the compound is $C_{19}H_{21}NO{\cdot}HCl$ having a molecular weight of 316. It is a white crystalline solid readily soluble in water, lower alcohols and chloroform.

Inert ingredients for the capsule formulations are: hard gelatin capsules (which may contain blue 1, red 3, red 40, yellow 10, and other inert ingredients); magnesium stearate; sodium lauryl sulfate; starch.

Inert ingredients for the oral concentrate formulation are: glycerin; methylparaben; peppermint oil; propylparaben; water.

Chemically, doxepin hydrochloride is a dibenzoxepin derivative and is the first of a family of tricyclic psychotherapeutic agents. Specifically, it is an isomeric mixture of 1-Propanamine, 3-dibenz[b,e]oxepin-11(6H)ylidene-N,N-dimethyl-,hydrochloride.

CLINICAL PHARMACOLOGY

MECHANISM OF ACTION

The mechanism of action of doxepin HCl is not definitely known. It is not a central nervous system stimulant nor a monoamine oxidase inhibitor. The current hypothesis is that the clinical effects are due, at least in part, to influences on the adrenergic activity at the synapses so that deactivation of norepinephrine by reuptake into the nerve terminals is prevented. Animal studies suggest that doxepin HCl does not appreciably antagonize the antihypertensive action of guanethidine. In animal studies anticholinergic, antiserotonin and antihistamine effects on smooth muscle have been demonstrated. At higher than usual clinical doses, norepinephrine response was potentiated in animals. This effect was not demonstrated in humans.

At clinical dosages up to 150 mg/day, doxepin HCl can be given to man concomitantly with guanethidine and related compounds without blocking the antihypertensive effect. At dosages above 150 mg/day blocking of the antihypertensive effect of these compounds has been reported.

Doxepin HCl is virtually devoid of euphoria as a side effect. Characteristic of this type of compound, doxepin HCl has not been demonstrated to produce the physical tolerance or psychological dependence associated with addictive compounds.

INDICATIONS AND USAGE

Doxepin HCl is Recommended for the Treatment of:

- Psychoneurotic patients with depression and/or anxiety.
- Depression and/or anxiety associated with alcoholism (not to be taken concomitantly with alcohol).
- Depression and/or anxiety associated with organic disease (the possibility of drug interaction should be considered if the patient is receiving other drugs concomitantly).
- Psychotic depressive disorders with associated anxiety including involutional depression and manic-depressive disorders.

The target symptoms of psychoneurosis that respond particularly well to doxepin HCl include anxiety, tension, depression, somatic symptoms and concerns, sleep disturbances, guilt, lack of energy, fear, apprehension and worry.

Clinical experience has shown that doxepin HCl is safe and well tolerated even in the elderly patient. Owing to lack of clinical experience in the pediatric population, doxepin HCl is not recommended for use in children under 12 years of age.

NON-FDA APPROVED INDICATIONS

Doxepin has also been used in the treatment of urinary incontinence, neuropathic pain, primary insomnia, and chronic pain although these uses are not explicitly approved by the FDA.

CONTRAINDICATIONS

Doxepin HCl is contraindicated in individuals who have shown hypersensitivity to the drug. Possibility of cross sensitivity with other dibenzoxepines should be kept in mind.

Doxepin HCl is contraindicated in patients with glaucoma or a tendency to urinary retention. These disorders should be ruled out, particularly in older patients.

WARNINGS

The once-a-day dosage regimen of doxepin HCl in patients with intercurrent illness or patients taking other medications should be carefully adjusted. This is especially important in patients receiving other medications with anticholinergic effects.

USAGE IN GERIATRICS

The use of doxepin HCl on a once-a-day dosage regimen in geriatric patients should be adjusted carefully based on the patient's condition (see PRECAUTIONS, Geriatric Use).

USE IN PREGNANCY

Reproduction studies have been performed in rats, rabbits, monkeys and dogs and there was no evidence of harm to the animal fetus. The relevance to humans is not known. Since there is no experience in pregnant women who have received this drug, safety in pregnancy has not been established. There has been a report of apnea and drowsiness occurring in a nursing infant whose mother was taking doxepin HCl.

USE IN CHILDREN

The use of doxepin HCl in children under 12 years of age is not recommended because safe conditions for its use have not been established.

PRECAUTIONS

DROWSINESS

Since drowsiness may occur with the use of this drug, patients should be warned of the possibility and cautioned against driving a car or operating dangerous machinery while taking the drug. Patients should also be cautioned that their response to alcohol may be potentiated.

Sedating drugs may cause confusion and oversedation in the elderly; elderly patients generally should be started on low doses of doxepin HCl and observed closely. (See Geriatric Use.)

SUICIDE

Since suicide is an inherent risk in any depressed patient and may remain so until significant improvement has occurred, patients should be closely supervised during the early course of therapy. Prescriptions should be written for the smallest feasible amount.

PSYCHOSIS

Should increased symptoms of psychosis or shift to manic symptomatology occur, it may be necessary to reduce dosage or add a major tranquilizer to the dosage regimen.

GERIATRIC USE

A determination has not been made whether controlled clinical studies of doxepin HCl included sufficient numbers of subjects aged 65 and over to define a difference in response from younger subjects. Other reported clinical experience has not identified differences in responses between the elderly and younger patients. In general, dose selection for an elderly patient should be cautious, usually starting at the low end of the dosing range, reflecting the greater frequency of decreased hepatic, renal or cardiac function, and of concomitant disease or other drug therapy.

The extent of renal excretion of doxepin HCl has not been determined. Because elderly patients are more likely to have decreased renal function, care should be taken in dose selections.

Sedating drugs may cause confusion and oversedation in the elderly; elderly patients generally should be started on low doses of doxepin HCl and observed closely. (See WARNINGS.)

DRUG INTERACTIONS

DRUGS METABOLIZED BY P450 2D6

The biochemical activity of the drug metabolizing isozyme cytochrome P450 2D6 (debrisoquin hydroxylase) is reduced in a subset of the Caucasian population (about 7-10% of Caucasians are so-called "poor metabolizers"); reliable estimates of the prevalence of reduced P450 2D6 isozyme activity among Asian, African and other populations are not yet available. Poor metabolizers have higher than expected plasma concentrations of tricyclic antidepressants (TCAs) when given usual doses. Depending on the fraction of drug metabolized by P450 2D6, the increase in plasma concentration may be small, or quite large (8-fold increase in plasma AUC of the TCA).

In addition, certain drugs inhibit the activity of this isozyme and make normal metabolizers resemble poor metabolizers. An individual who is stable on a given dose of TCA may become abruptly toxic when given one of these inhibiting drugs as concomitant therapy. The drugs that inhibit cytochrome P450 2D6 include some that are not metabolized by the enzyme (quinidine; cimetidine) and many that are substrates for P450 2D6 (many other antidepressants, phenothiazines, and the Type 1C antiarrhythmics propafenone and flecainide). While all the selective serotonin reuptake inhibitors (SSRIs), *e.g.*, fluoxetine, sertraline, and paroxetine, inhibit P450 2D6, they may vary in the extent of inhibition. The extent to which SSRI-TCA interactions may pose clinical problems will depend on the degree of inhibition and the pharmacokinetics of the SSRI involved. Nevertheless, caution is indicated in the coadministration of TCAs with any of the SSRIs and also in switching from one class to the other. Of particular importance, sufficient time must elapse before initiating TCA treatment in a patient being withdrawn from fluoxetine, given the long half-life of the parent and active metabolite (at least 5 weeks may be necessary).

Concomitant use of tricyclic antidepressants with drugs that can inhibit cytochrome P450 2D6 may require lower doses than usually prescribed for either the tricyclic antidepressant or the other drug. Furthermore, whenever one of these other drugs is withdrawn from co-therapy, an increased dose of tricyclic antidepressant may be required. It is desirable to monitor TCA plasma levels whenever a TCA is going to be co-administered with another drug known to be an inhibitor of P450 2D6.

D

MAO INHIBITORS

Serious side effects and even death have been reported following the concomitant use of certain drugs with MAO inhibitors. Therefore, MAO inhibitors should be discontinued at least 2 weeks prior to the cautious initiation of therapy with doxepin HCl. The exact length of time may vary and is dependent upon the particular MAO inhibitor being used, the length of time it has been administered, and the dosage involved.

CIMETIDINE

Cimetidine has been reported to produce clinically significant fluctuations in steady-state serum concentrations of various tricyclic antidepressants. Serious anticholinergic symptoms (*i.e.,* severe dry mouth, urinary retention and blurred vision) have been associated with elevations in the serum levels of tricyclic antidepressant when cimetidine therapy is initiated. Additionally, higher than expected tricyclic antidepressant levels have been observed when they are begun in patients already taking cimetidine. In patients who have been reported to be well controlled on tricyclic antidepressants receiving concurrent cimetidine therapy, discontinuation of cimetidine has been reported to decrease established steady-state serum tricyclic antidepressant levels and compromise their therapeutic effects.

ALCOHOL

It should be borne in mind that alcohol ingestion may increase the danger inherent in any intentional or unintentional doxepin HCl overdosage. This is especially important in patients who may use alcohol excessively.

TOLAZAMIDE

A case of severe hypoglycemia has been reported in a Type II diabetic patient maintained on tolazamide (1 gm/day) 11 days after the addition of doxepin (75 mg/day).

ADVERSE REACTIONS

NOTE: Some of the adverse reactions noted below have not been specifically reported with doxepin HCl use. However, due to the close pharmacological similarities among the tricyclics, the reactions should be considered when prescribing doxepin HCl.

Anticholinergic Effects: Dry mouth, blurred vision, constipation, and urinary retention have been reported. If they do not subside with continued therapy, or become severe, it may be necessary to reduce the dosage.

Central Nervous System Effects: Drowsiness is the most commonly noticed side effect. This tends to disappear as therapy is continued. Other infrequently reported CNS side effects are confusion, disorientation, hallucinations, numbness, paresthesias, ataxia, extrapyramidal symptoms, seizures, tardive dyskinesia, and tremor.

Cardiovascular: Cardiovascular effects including hypotension, hypertension, and tachycardia have been reported occasionally.

Allergic: Skin rash, edema, photosensitization, and pruritis have occasionally occurred.

Hematologic: Eosinophilia has been reported in a few patients. There have been occasional reports of bone marrow depression manifesting as agranulocytosis, leukopenia, thrombocytopenia, and purpura.

Gastrointestinal: Nausea, vomiting, indigestion, taste disturbances, diarrhea, anorexia, and aphthous stomatitis have been reported. (See Anticholinergic Effects.)

Endocrine: Raised or lowered libido, testicular swelling, gynecomastia in males, enlargement of breasts and galactorrhea in the female, raising or lowering of blood sugar levels and syndrome of inappropriate antidiuretic hormone secretion have been reported with tricyclic administration.

Other: Dizziness, tinnitus, weight gain, sweating, chills, fatigue, weakness, flushing, jaundice, alopecia, headache, exacerbation of asthma, and hyperpyrexia (in association with chlorpromazine) have been occasionally observed as adverse effects.

WITHDRAWAL SYMPTOMS

The possibility of development of withdrawal symptoms upon abrupt cessation of treatment after prolonged doxepin HCl administration should be borne in mind. These are not indicative of addiction and gradual withdrawal of medication should not cause these symptoms.

DOSAGE AND ADMINISTRATION

For most patients with illness of mild to moderate severity, a starting daily dose of 75 mg is recommended. Dosage may subsequently be increased or decreased at appropriate intervals and according to individual response. The usual optimum dose range is 75-150 mg/day.

In more severely ill patients higher doses may be required with subsequent gradual increase to 300 mg/day if necessary. Additional therapeutic effect is rarely to be obtained by exceeding a dose of 300 mg/day.

In patients with very mild symptomatology or emotional symptoms accompanying organic disease, lower doses may suffice. Some of these patients have been controlled on doses as low as 25-50 mg/day.

The total daily dosage of doxepin HCl may be given on a divided or once-a-day dosage schedule. If the once-a-day schedule is employed, the maximum recommended dose is 150 mg/day. This dose may be given at bedtime. **The 150 mg capsule strength is intended for maintenance therapy only and is not recommended for initiation of treatment.**

Anti-anxiety effect is apparent before the antidepressant effect. Optimal antidepressant effect may not be evident for 2-3 weeks.

HOW SUPPLIED

SINEQUAN CAPSULES

Sinequan is available as capsules containing doxepin HCl equivalent to: 10, 25, 50, 75, 100, and 150 mg.

SINEQUAN ORAL CONCENTRATE

Sinequan oral concentrate is available in 120 ml bottles with an accompanying dropper calibrated at 5, 10, 15, 20, and 25 mg. Each ml contains doxepin HCl equivalent to 10 mg doxepin. Just prior to administration, Sinequan oral concentrate should be diluted with approximately 120 ml of water, whole or skimmed milk, or orange, grapefruit, tomato, prune or pineapple juice. Sinequan oral concentrate is not physically compatible with a number of carbonated beverages. For those patients requiring antidepressant therapy who are on methadone maintenance, Sinequan oral concentrate and methadone syrup can be mixed together with Gatorade, lemonade, orange juice, sugar water, Tang, or water; but not with grape juice. Preparation and storage of bulk dilutions is not recommended.

TOPICAL

DESCRIPTION

FOR TOPICAL DERMATOLOGIC USE ONLY — NOT FOR OPHTHALMIC, ORAL, OR INTRAVAGINAL USE.

Zonalon cream, 5% is a topical cream. Each gram contains: 50 mg of doxepin hydrochloride (equivalent to 44.3 mg of doxepin).

Doxepin hydrochloride is one of a class of agents known as dibenzoxepin tricyclic antidepressant compounds. It is an isomeric mixture of N,N-dimethyldibenz(*b,e*)oxepin-$\Delta^{11(6H),\gamma}$-propylamine hydrochloride.

Doxepin hydrochloride has an empirical formula of $C_{19}H_{21}NO{\cdot}HCl$ and a molecular weight of 316.

Zonalon cream also contains sorbitol, cetyl alcohol, isopropyl myristate, glyceryl stearate, PEG-100 stearate, petrolatum, benzyl alcohol, titanium dioxide and purified water.

CLINICAL PHARMACOLOGY

Although doxepin HCl does have H1 and H2 histamine receptor blocking actions, the exact mechanism by which doxepin exerts its antipruritic effect is unknown. Doxepin HCl cream can produce drowsiness which may reduce awareness, including awareness of pruritic symptoms. In 19 pruritic eczema patients treated with doxepin HCl cream, plasma doxepin concentrations ranged from nondetectable to 47 ng/ml from percutaneous absorption. Plasma levels from topical application of doxepin HCl cream can result in CNS and other systemic side effects.

Once absorbed into the systemic circulation, doxepin undergoes hepatic metabolism that results in conversion to pharmacologically-active desmethyldoxepin. Further glucuronidation results in urinary excretion of the parent drug and its metabolites. Desmethyldoxepin has a half-life that ranges from 28-52 hours and is not affected by multiple dosing. Plasma levels of both doxepin and desmethyldoxepin are highly variable and are poorly correlated with dosage. Wide distribution occurs in body tissues including lungs, heart, brain, and liver. Renal disease, genetic factors, age, and other medications affect the metabolism and subsequent elimination of doxepin. (See DRUG INTERACTIONS.)

INDICATIONS AND USAGE

Doxepin HCl cream is indicated for the short-term (up to 8 days) management of moderate pruritis in adult patients with atopic dermatitis or lichen simplex chronicus. (See DOSAGE AND ADMINISTRATION.)

CONTRAINDICATIONS

Because doxepin HCl has an anticholinergic effect and because significant plasma levels of doxepin are detectable after topical doxepin HCl cream application, the use of doxepin HCl cream is contraindicated in patients with untreated narrow angle glaucoma or a tendency to urinary retention.

Doxepin HCl cream is contraindicated in individuals who have shown previous sensitivity to any of its components.

WARNINGS

Drowsiness occurs in over 20% of patients treated with doxepin HCl cream, especially in patients receiving treatment to greater than 10% of their body surface area. **Patients should be warned about the possibility of sedation and cautioned against driving a motor vehicle or operating hazardous machinery while being treated with doxepin HCl cream.**

The sedating effects of alcoholic beverages, antihistamines, and other CNS depressants may be potentiated when doxepin HCl cream is used.

If excessive drowsiness occurs it may be necessary to reduce the frequency of applications, the amount of cream applied, and/or the percentage of body surface area treated, or discontinue the drug. However, the efficacy with reduced frequency of applications has not been established.

Keep this product away from the eyes.

PRECAUTIONS

GENERAL

Drowsiness

Since drowsiness may occur with the use of doxepin HCl cream, patients should be warned of the possibility and cautioned against driving a car or operating dangerous machinery while using this drug. Patients should also be cautioned that their response to alcohol may be potentiated.

Sedating drugs may cause confusion and oversedation in the elderly; elderly patients generally should be observed closely for confusion and oversedation when started on doxepin HCl cream. (See Geriatric Use.)

Use Under Occlusion

Occlusive dressings may increase the absorption of most topical drugs; therefore, occlusive dressings should not be utilized with doxepin HCl cream.

Contact Sensitization

Use of doxepin HCl cream can cause Type IV hypersensitivity reactions (contact sensitization) to doxepin.

CARCINOGENESIS, MUTAGENESIS, AND IMPAIRMENT OF FERTILITY

Carcinogenesis, mutagenesis, and impairment of fertility studies have not been conducted with doxepin HCl.

PREGNANCY CATEGORY B

Reproduction studies have been performed in which doxepin was orally administered to rats and rabbits at doses up to 0.6 and 1.2 times, respectively, the estimated exposure to doxepin that results from use of 16 g of doxepin HCl cream per day (four applications of 4 g of cream per day; dose multiples reflect comparisons made following normalization of the data on the basis of body surface area estimates) and have revealed no evidence of harm to rat or rabbit fetuses due to doxepin. There are, however, no adequate and well-controlled studies in pregnant women. Because animal reproduction studies are not always predictive of human response, this drug should be used during pregnancy only if clearly needed.

NURSING MOTHERS

Doxepin is excreted in human milk after oral administration. It is possible that doxepin may also be excreted in human milk following topical application of doxepin HCl cream.

One case has been reported of apnea and drowsiness in a nursing infant whose mother was taking an oral dosage form of doxepin HCl.

Because of the potential for serious adverse reactions in nursing infants from doxepin, a decision should be made whether to discontinue nursing or to discontinue taking the drug, taking into account the importance of the drug to the mother.

PEDIATRIC USE

The use of doxepin HCl cream in pediatric patients is not recommended. Safe conditions for use of doxepin HCl cream in children have not been established. One case has been reported of a 2.5 year old child who developed somnolence, grand mal seizure, respiratory depression, ECG abnormalities, and coma after treatment with doxepin HCl cream. A total of 27 g had been applied over 3 days for eczema. He was treated with supportive care, activated charcoal, and systemic alkalization and recovered.

GERIATRIC USE

Clinical studies of doxepin HCl cream did not include sufficient numbers of subjects aged 65 and over to determine whether they respond differently from younger subjects. Other reported clinical experience has not identified differences in responses between the elderly and younger patients. In general, dose selection for an elderly patient should be cautious, usually starting at the low end of the dosing range, reflecting the greater frequency of decreased hepatic, renal or cardiac function, and of concomitant disease or other drug therapy.

The extent of renal excretion of doxepin has not been determined. Because elderly patients are more likely to have decreased renal function, care should be taken in dose selections.

Sedating drugs may cause confusion and oversedation in the elderly; elderly patients generally should be observed closely for confusion and oversedation when started on doxepin HCl cream. (See WARNINGS.) An 80-year old male nursing home patient developed probable systemic anticholinergic toxicity which included urinary retention and delirium after doxepin HCl cream had been applied to his arms, legs and back 3 times daily for 2 days.

DRUG INTERACTIONS

Studies have not been performed examining drug interactions with doxepin HCl cream. However, since plasma levels of doxepin following topical application of doxepin HCl cream can reach levels obtained with oral doxepin HCl therapy, the following drug interactions are possible following topical doxepin HCl cream application.

DRUGS METABOLIZED BY P450 2D6

The biochemical activity of the drug metabolizing isozyme cytochrome P450 2D6 (debrisoquin hydroxylase) is reduced in a subset of the Caucasian population (about 7-10% of Caucasians are socalled "poor metabolizers"); reliable estimates of the prevalence of reduced P450 2D6 isozyme activity among Asian, African and other populations are not yet available. Poor metabolizers have higher than expected plasma concentrations of tricyclic antidepressants (TCAs) when given usual doses. Depending on the fraction of drug metabolized by P450 2D6, the increase in plasma concentration may be small, or quite large (8-fold increase in plasma AUC of the TCA).

In addition, certain drugs inhibit the activity of this isozyme and make normal metabolizers resemble poor metabolizers. An individual who is stable on a given dosage regimen of a TCA may become abruptly toxic when given one of these inhibiting drugs as concomitant therapy. The drugs that inhibit cytochrome P450 2D6 include some that are not metabolized by the enzyme (quinidine; cimetidine) and many that are substrates for P450 2D6 (many other antidepressants, phenothiazines, and the Type 1C antiarrhythmics propafenone and flecainide). While all the selective serotonin reuptake inhibitors (SSRIs), *e.g.*, fluoxetine, sertraline, and paroxetine, inhibit P450 2D6, they may vary in the extent of inhibition. The extent to which SSRI-TCA interactions may pose clinical problems will depend on the degree of inhibition and the pharmacokinetics of the SSRI involved. Nevertheless, caution is indicated in the coadministration of TCAs with any of the SSRIs. Of particular importance, sufficient time must elapse before initiating TCA treatment in a patient being withdrawn from fluoxetine, given the long half-life of the parent and active metabolite (at least 5 weeks may be necessary).

Concomitant use of tricyclic antidepressants with drugs that can inhibit cytochrome P450 2D6 may require lower doses than usually prescribed for either the tricyclic antidepressant or the other drug. It is desirable to monitor TCA plasma levels whenever a TCA is going to be coadministered with another drug known to be an inhibitor of P450 2D6.

MAO INHIBITORS

Serious side effects and even death have been reported following the concomitant use of certain drugs with MAO inhibitors. Therefore, MAO inhibitors should be discontinued at least 2 weeks prior to the cautious initiation of therapy with doxepin HCl cream. The exact length of time may vary and is dependent upon the particular MAO inhibitor being used, the length of time it has been administered, and the dosage involved.

CIMETIDINE

Serious anticholinergic symptomes (*i.e.*, severe dry mouth, urinary retention and blurred vision) have been associated with elevations in the serum levels of tricyclic antidepressant when cimetidine therapy is initiated. Additionally, higher than expected tricyclic antidepressant levels have been observed when they are begun in patients already taking cimetidine.

ALCOHOL

Alcohol ingestion may exacerbate the potential sedative effects of doxepin HCl cream. This is especially important in patients who may use alcohol excessively.

TOLAZAMIDE

A case of severe hypoglycemia has been reported in a Type II diabetic patient maintained on tolazamide (1 gm/day) 11 days after the addition of oral doxepin (75 mg/day).

ADVERSE REACTIONS

CONTROLLED CLINICAL TRIALS

Systemic Adverse Effects

In controlled clinical trials of patients treated with doxepin HCl cream, the most common systemic adverse effect reported was drowsiness. Drowsiness occurred in 71 of 330 (22%) of patients treated with doxepin HCl cream compared to 7 of 334 (2%) of patients treated with vehicle cream. Drowsiness resulted in the premature discontinuation of the drug in approximately 5% of patients treated with doxepin HCl cream in controlled clinical trials.

Local Site Adverse Effects

In controlled clinical trials of patients treated with doxepin HCl cream, the most common local site adverse effect reported was burning and/or stinging at the site of application. These occurred in 76 of 330 (23%) of patients treated with doxepin HCl cream compared to 54 of 334 (16%) of patients treated with vehicle cream. Most of these reactions were categorized as "mild"; however, approximately 25% of patients who reported burning and/or stinging reported the reaction as "severe." Four patients treated with doxepin HCl cream withdrew from the study because of the burning and/or stinging.

TABLE 1 presents the adverse events reported at an incidence of ≥1% in either doxepin HCl or vehicle cream treatment groups during the trials.

TABLE 1

Adverse Event	Doxepin HCl n=330	Vehicle n=334
Burning/stinging	76 (23.0%)	54 (16.2%)
Drowsiness	71 (21.5%)	7 (2.1%)
Dry mouth*	32 (9.7%)	4 (1.2%)
Pruritis†	13 (3.9%)	20 (6.0%)
Fatigue/tiredness	10 (3.0%)	5 (1.5%)
Exacerbated exzema	10 (3.0%)	8 (2.4%)
Other application site reaction‡	10 (3.0%)	16 (4.8%)
Dizziness§	7 (2.1%)	3 (0.9%)
Mental/emotional changes	6 (1.8%)	1 (0.3%)
Taste perversion¤	5 (1.5%)	1 (0.3%)
Edema	4 (1.2%)	1 (0.3%)
Headache	3 (0.9%)	14 (4.2%)

* Includes reports of "dry lips", "dry throat", and "thirst".
† Includes reports of "pruritis exacerbated".
‡ Includes report of "increased irritation at application site".
§ Includes reports of "lightheadedness" and "dizziness/vertigo".
¤ Includes reports of "bitter taste" and "metallic taste in mouth".

Adverse events occurring in 0.5 to $<1.0\%$ of doxepin HCl cream treated patients in the controlled clinical trials included: nervousness/anxiety, tongue numbness, fever, and nausea.

POST-MARKETING EXPERIENCE

Twenty-six (26) cases of allergic contact dermatitis have been reported in patients using doxepin HCl cream, 20 of which were documented by positive patch test to doxepin 5% cream.

DOSAGE AND ADMINISTRATION

A thin film of doxepin HCl cream should be applied 4 times each day with at least a 3-4 hour interval between applications. There are no data to establish the safety and effectiveness of doxepin HCl cream when used for greater than 8 days. Chronic use beyond 8 days may result in higher systemic levels and should be avoided. Use of doxepin HCl cream for longer than 8 days may result in an increased likelihood of contact sensitization.

The risk for sedation may increase with greater body surface area application of doxepin HCl cream (see WARNINGS). Clinical experience has shown that drowsiness is significantly more common in patients applying doxepin HCl cream to over 10% of body surface area; therefore, patients with greater than 10% of body surface area (see WARNINGS) affected should be particularly cautioned concerning possible drowsiness and other systemic adverse effects of doxepin. If excessive drowsiness occurs, it may be necessary to do one or more of the following: reduce the body surface area treated, reduce the number of applications per day, reduce the amount of cream applied, or discontinue the drug.

Occlusive dressings may increase the absorption of most topical drugs; therefore, occlusive dressings should not be utilized with doxepin cream.

HOW SUPPLIED

Zonalon cream is available in 30 and 45 g tubes.

Storage: Store at or below 27°C (80°F).

PRODUCT LISTING - RATED THERAPEUTICALLY EQUIVALENT

Capsule - Oral - 10 mg

Package	Price	Product	NDC
100's	$6.41	GENERIC, Us Trading Corporation	56126-0345-11
100's	$8.91	FEDERAL UPPER LIMIT, H.C.F.A. F F P	99999-1111-23
100's	$12.95	GENERIC, Dixon-Shane Inc	17236-0375-01
100's	$13.00	GENERIC, Martec Pharmaceuticals Inc	52555-0294-01
100's	$13.56	GENERIC, Moore, H.L. Drug Exchange Inc	00839-7892-06
100's	$13.95	GENERIC, Ivax Corporation	00182-1325-01
100's	$15.00	GENERIC, Raway Pharmacal Inc	00686-0436-20
100's	$19.57	GENERIC, Vangard Labs	00615-0395-13
100's	$24.40	GENERIC, Dixon-Shane Inc	17236-0375-11
100's	$24.81	GENERIC, American Health Packaging	62584-0686-01
100's	$25.35	GENERIC, Major Pharmaceuticals Inc	00904-1260-60
100's	$25.75	GENERIC, Geneva Pharmaceuticals	00781-2800-13
100's	$25.86	GENERIC, Major Pharmaceuticals Inc	00904-1260-61
100's	$31.52	GENERIC, Watson/Schein Pharmaceuticals Inc	00364-2113-01
100's	$31.52	GENERIC, Watson/Schein Pharmaceuticals Inc	00591-5629-01
100's	$31.52	GENERIC, Watson Laboratories Inc	52544-0695-01
100's	$31.58	GENERIC, Martec Pharmaceuticals Inc	52555-0447-01
100's	$31.60	GENERIC, Mylan Pharmaceuticals Inc	00378-1049-01
100's	$32.45	GENERIC, Udl Laboratories Inc	51079-0436-20
100's	$36.40	GENERIC, Par Pharmaceutical Inc	49884-0217-01
100's	$43.18	SINEQUAN, Pfizer U.S. Pharmaceuticals	00049-5340-66
100's	$125.62	GENERIC, Dixon-Shane Inc	17236-0375-10

Capsule - Oral - 25 mg

Package	Price	Product	NDC
30's	$4.94	GENERIC, Prescript Pharmaceuticals	00247-1232-30
30's	$11.67	GENERIC, Heartland Healthcare Services	61392-0727-30
30's	$11.67	GENERIC, Heartland Healthcare Services	61392-0727-39
31's	$12.06	GENERIC, Heartland Healthcare Services	61392-0727-31
32's	$12.45	GENERIC, Heartland Healthcare Services	61392-0727-32
45's	$17.51	GENERIC, Heartland Healthcare Services	61392-0727-45
60's	$23.34	GENERIC, Heartland Healthcare Services	61392-0727-60
90's	$35.02	GENERIC, Heartland Healthcare Services	61392-0727-90
100's	$7.77	GENERIC, Us Trading Corporation	56126-0346-11
100's	$10.50	GENERIC, Mova Pharmaceutical Corporation	55370-0530-07
100's	$13.25	GENERIC, Dixon-Shane Inc	17236-0356-01
100's	$13.30	GENERIC, Martec Pharmaceuticals Inc	52555-0295-01
100's	$13.49	GENERIC, Moore, H.L. Drug Exchange Inc	00839-7221-06
100's	$14.25	GENERIC, Ivax Corporation	00182-1326-01
100's	$15.50	GENERIC, Raway Pharmacal Inc	00686-0437-20
100's	$18.22	FEDERAL UPPER LIMIT, H.C.F.A. F F P	99999-1111-27
100's	$30.66	GENERIC, Dixon-Shane Inc	17236-0356-11
100's	$30.77	GENERIC, American Health Packaging	62584-0687-01
100's	$31.71	GENERIC, Geneva Pharmaceuticals	00781-2801-13
100's	$32.85	GENERIC, Major Pharmaceuticals Inc	00904-1261-60
100's	$36.50	GENERIC, Major Pharmaceuticals Inc	00904-1261-61
100's	$41.60	GENERIC, Mylan Pharmaceuticals Inc	00378-3125-01
100's	$41.60	GENERIC, Martec Pharmaceuticals Inc	52555-0448-01
100's	$41.61	GENERIC, Watson/Schein Pharmaceuticals Inc	00364-2114-01
100's	$41.61	GENERIC, Watson Laboratories Inc	00591-2114-01
100's	$41.61	GENERIC, Watson/Schein Pharmaceuticals Inc	00591-5630-01
100's	$41.61	GENERIC, Watson Laboratories Inc	52544-0696-01
100's	$42.85	GENERIC, Udl Laboratories Inc	51079-0437-20
100's	$46.95	GENERIC, Par Pharmaceutical Inc	49884-0218-01
100's	$55.71	SINEQUAN, Pfizer U.S. Pharmaceuticals	00049-5350-66

Capsule - Oral - 50 mg

Package	Price	Product	NDC
7's	$3.81	GENERIC, Prescript Pharmaceuticals	00247-1177-07
30's	$5.34	GENERIC, Prescript Pharmaceuticals	00247-1177-30
30's	$8.64	GENERIC, Pd-Rx Pharmaceuticals	55289-0018-30
30's	$13.02	GENERIC, Heartland Healthcare Services	61392-0728-30
30's	$13.02	GENERIC, Heartland Healthcare Services	61392-0728-39
31's	$13.45	GENERIC, Heartland Healthcare Services	61392-0728-31
32's	$13.89	GENERIC, Heartland Healthcare Services	61392-0728-32
45's	$19.53	GENERIC, Heartland Healthcare Services	61392-0728-45
60's	$26.04	GENERIC, Heartland Healthcare Services	61392-0728-60
90's	$39.06	GENERIC, Heartland Healthcare Services	61392-0728-90
100's	$9.23	GENERIC, Us Trading Corporation	56126-0347-11
100's	$14.47	FEDERAL UPPER LIMIT, H.C.F.A. F F P	99999-1111-29
100's	$14.75	GENERIC, Mova Pharmaceutical Corporation	55370-0531-07
100's	$18.90	GENERIC, Dixon-Shane Inc	17236-0357-01
100's	$19.24	GENERIC, Moore, H.L. Drug Exchange Inc	00839-7894-06
100's	$19.50	GENERIC, Raway Pharmacal Inc	00686-0438-20
100's	$19.95	GENERIC, Ivax Corporation	00182-1327-01
100's	$42.74	GENERIC, Dixon-Shane Inc	17236-0357-11
100's	$43.26	GENERIC, American Health Packaging	62584-0688-01
100's	$46.29	GENERIC, Major Pharmaceuticals Inc	00904-1262-60
100's	$46.76	GENERIC, Major Pharmaceuticals Inc	00904-1262-61
100's	$55.20	GENERIC, Mylan Pharmaceuticals Inc	00378-4250-01
100's	$55.20	GENERIC, Martec Pharmaceuticals Inc	52555-0296-01
100's	$55.20	GENERIC, Martec Pharmaceuticals Inc	52555-0449-04
100's	$55.21	GENERIC, Watson Laboratories Inc	00591-5631-01
100's	$55.21	GENERIC, Watson Laboratories Inc	52544-0697-01
100's	$56.86	GENERIC, Udl Laboratories Inc	51079-0438-20
100's	$66.10	GENERIC, Par Pharmaceutical Inc	49884-0219-01
100's	$78.40	SINEQUAN, Pfizer U.S. Pharmaceuticals	00049-5360-66

Capsule - Oral - 75 mg

Package	Price	Product	NDC
30's	$5.63	GENERIC, Pd-Rx Pharmaceuticals	55289-0258-30
30's	$6.13	GENERIC, Prescript Pharmaceuticals	00247-1233-30
30's	$20.88	GENERIC, Heartland Healthcare Services	61392-0729-30
30's	$20.88	GENERIC, Heartland Healthcare Services	61392-0729-39
31's	$21.58	GENERIC, Heartland Healthcare Services	61392-0729-31
32's	$22.27	GENERIC, Heartland Healthcare Services	61392-0729-32
45's	$31.32	GENERIC, Heartland Healthcare Services	61392-0729-45
60's	$41.76	GENERIC, Heartland Healthcare Services	61392-0729-60
90's	$62.64	GENERIC, Heartland Healthcare Services	61392-0729-90
100's	$11.85	GENERIC, Us Trading Corporation	56126-0348-11
100's	$20.52	FEDERAL UPPER LIMIT, H.C.F.A. F F P	99999-1111-31
100's	$35.75	GENERIC, Dixon-Shane Inc	17236-0358-01
100's	$36.95	GENERIC, Ivax Corporation	00182-1328-01
100's	$43.27	GENERIC, Moore, H.L. Drug Exchange Inc	00839-7895-06
100's	$68.43	GENERIC, Dixon-Shane Inc	17236-0358-11
100's	$73.31	GENERIC, Major Pharmaceuticals Inc	00904-1263-61
100's	$76.75	GENERIC, Major Pharmaceuticals Inc	00904-1263-60
100's	$88.83	ADAPIN, Lotus Biochemical Corporation	59417-0361-71
100's	$91.55	GENERIC, Watson/Schein Pharmaceuticals Inc	00364-2116-01
100's	$91.55	GENERIC, Watson/Schein Pharmaceuticals Inc	00591-5632-01
100's	$91.60	GENERIC, Mylan Pharmaceuticals Inc	00378-5375-01
100's	$94.25	GENERIC, Udl Laboratories Inc	51079-0645-20
100's	$109.65	GENERIC, Par Pharmaceutical Inc	49884-0220-01
100's	$130.06	SINEQUAN, Pfizer U.S. Pharmaceuticals	00049-5390-66

Capsule - Oral - 100 mg

Package	Price	Product	NDC
30's	$6.53	GENERIC, Prescript Pharmaceuticals	00247-0773-30
30's	$23.31	GENERIC, Heartland Healthcare Services	61392-0730-30
30's	$23.31	GENERIC, Heartland Healthcare Services	61392-0730-39
31's	$24.09	GENERIC, Heartland Healthcare Services	61392-0730-31
32's	$24.86	GENERIC, Heartland Healthcare Services	61392-0730-32
45's	$34.97	GENERIC, Heartland Healthcare Services	61392-0730-45
60's	$46.62	GENERIC, Heartland Healthcare Services	61392-0730-60
90's	$12.88	GENERIC, Prescript Pharmaceuticals	00247-0773-90
90's	$69.93	GENERIC, Heartland Healthcare Services	61392-0730-90
100's	$13.94	GENERIC, Prescript Pharmaceuticals	00247-0773-00
100's	$14.42	GENERIC, Us Trading Corporation	56126-0349-11
100's	$21.00	GENERIC, Raway Pharmacal Inc	00686-0651-20
100's	$27.50	GENERIC, Raway Pharmacal Inc	00686-0465-20
100's	$28.85	GENERIC, Mova Pharmaceutical Corporation	55370-0532-07
100's	$41.74	FEDERAL UPPER LIMIT, H.C.F.A. F F P	99999-1111-24
100's	$42.05	GENERIC, Dixon-Shane Inc	17236-0359-01
100's	$42.30	GENERIC, Martec Pharmaceuticals Inc	52555-0332-01
100's	$42.65	GENERIC, Moore, H.L. Drug Exchange Inc	00839-7224-06
100's	$42.65	GENERIC, Moore, H.L. Drug Exchange Inc	00839-7896-06
100's	$42.95	GENERIC, Ivax Corporation	00182-1329-01
100's	$76.64	GENERIC, Dixon-Shane Inc	17236-0359-11
100's	$77.83	GENERIC, Ivax Corporation	00182-1329-89
100's	$83.69	GENERIC, Major Pharmaceuticals Inc	00904-1264-60
100's	$92.99	GENERIC, Major Pharmaceuticals Inc	00904-1264-61
100's	$96.84	ADAPIN, Lotus Biochemical Corporation	59417-0359-71
100's	$99.80	GENERIC, Mylan Pharmaceuticals Inc	00378-6410-01
100's	$99.82	GENERIC, Watson/Schein Pharmaceuticals Inc	00364-2117-01
100's	$99.82	GENERIC, Watson/Schein Pharmaceuticals Inc	00591-5633-01
100's	$102.79	GENERIC, Udl Laboratories Inc	51079-0651-20
100's	$119.50	GENERIC, Par Pharmaceutical Inc	49884-0221-01
100's	$141.80	SINEQUAN, Pfizer U.S. Pharmaceuticals	00049-5380-66

Capsule - Oral - 150 mg

Package	Price	Product	NDC
50's	$80.40	ADAPIN, Lotus Biochemical Corporation	59417-0370-65
50's	$106.11	GENERIC, Par Pharmaceutical Inc	49884-0222-03
50's	$117.73	SINEQUAN, Pfizer U.S. Pharmaceuticals	00049-5370-50
100's	$36.47	GENERIC, Us Trading Corporation	56126-0401-11
100's	$52.45	GENERIC, Major Pharmaceuticals Inc	00904-1265-60
100's	$55.50	GENERIC, Dixon-Shane Inc	17236-0655-01
100's	$58.25	GENERIC, Moore, H.L. Drug Exchange Inc	00839-7509-06
100's	$59.85	GENERIC, Ivax Corporation	00182-1878-01
100's	$207.98	GENERIC, Par Pharmaceutical Inc	49884-0222-01

Concentrate - Oral - 10 mg/ml

Package	Price	Product	NDC
120 ml	$13.74	FEDERAL UPPER LIMIT, H.C.F.A. F F P	99999-1111-32
120 ml	$14.90	GENERIC, Moore, H.L. Drug Exchange Inc	00839-7470-65
120 ml	$16.81	GENERIC, Ivax Corporation	00182-6043-71
120 ml	$18.25	GENERIC, Morton Grove Pharmaceuticals Inc	60432-0651-04
120 ml	$18.75	GENERIC, Silarx Pharmaceuticals Inc	54838-0512-40
120 ml	$23.70	GENERIC, Teva Pharmaceuticals Usa	00093-9612-12
120 ml	$23.70	GENERIC, Copley	38245-0612-14
120 ml	$32.45	SINEQUAN, Pfizer U.S. Pharmaceuticals	00049-5100-47

PRODUCT LISTING - EQUIVALENTS NOT AVAILABLE

Capsule - Oral - 10 mg

10's	$5.26	GENERIC, Pharma Pac	52959-0541-10
20's	$9.99	GENERIC, Pharma Pac	52959-0541-20
30's	$7.41	GENERIC, Heartland Healthcare Services	61392-0726-30
30's	$7.41	GENERIC, Heartland Healthcare Services	61392-0726-39
30's	$9.45	GENERIC, Southwood Pharmaceuticals Inc	58016-0663-30
30's	$9.48	GENERIC, Allscripts Pharmaceutical Company	54569-2462-00
30's	$10.90	GENERIC, Pharma Pac	52959-0537-30
30's	$13.81	GENERIC, Pharma Pac	52959-0541-30
31's	$7.66	GENERIC, Heartland Healthcare Services	61392-0726-31
32's	$7.90	GENERIC, Heartland Healthcare Services	61392-0726-32
45's	$11.12	GENERIC, Heartland Healthcare Services	61392-0726-45
60's	$14.82	GENERIC, Heartland Healthcare Services	61392-0726-60
60's	$18.90	GENERIC, Southwood Pharmaceuticals Inc	58016-0663-60
90's	$22.23	GENERIC, Heartland Healthcare Services	61392-0726-90
90's	$28.35	GENERIC, Southwood Pharmaceuticals Inc	58016-0663-90

Capsule - Oral - 25 mg

10's	$5.05	GENERIC, Southwood Pharmaceuticals Inc	58016-0833-10
14's	$7.07	GENERIC, Southwood Pharmaceuticals Inc	58016-0833-14
15's	$7.58	GENERIC, Southwood Pharmaceuticals Inc	58016-0833-15
20's	$10.10	GENERIC, Southwood Pharmaceuticals Inc	58016-0833-20
21's	$10.61	GENERIC, Southwood Pharmaceuticals Inc	58016-0833-21
30's	$11.15	GENERIC, Allscripts Pharmaceutical Company	54569-2179-00
30's	$15.15	GENERIC, Southwood Pharmaceuticals Inc	58016-0833-30
40's	$20.20	GENERIC, Southwood Pharmaceuticals Inc	58016-0833-40
50's	$18.84	GENERIC, Allscripts Pharmaceutical Company	54569-2179-01
50's	$25.25	GENERIC, Southwood Pharmaceuticals Inc	58016-0833-50
60's	$30.30	GENERIC, Southwood Pharmaceuticals Inc	58016-0833-60
90's	$45.45	GENERIC, Southwood Pharmaceuticals Inc	58016-0833-90
100's	$50.50	GENERIC, Southwood Pharmaceuticals Inc	58016-0388-00

Capsule - Oral - 50 mg

10's	$7.10	GENERIC, Southwood Pharmaceuticals Inc	58016-0834-10
14's	$9.94	GENERIC, Southwood Pharmaceuticals Inc	58016-0834-14
15's	$10.65	GENERIC, Southwood Pharmaceuticals Inc	58016-0834-15
20's	$14.20	GENERIC, Southwood Pharmaceuticals Inc	58016-0834-20
21's	$14.91	GENERIC, Southwood Pharmaceuticals Inc	58016-0834-21
30's	$16.56	GENERIC, Allscripts Pharmaceutical Company	54569-1696-01
30's	$21.30	GENERIC, Southwood Pharmaceuticals Inc	58016-0834-30
30's	$21.75	GENERIC, Pharma Pac	52959-0662-30
40's	$28.40	GENERIC, Southwood Pharmaceuticals Inc	58016-0834-40
50's	$35.50	GENERIC, Southwood Pharmaceuticals Inc	58016-0834-50
60's	$42.60	GENERIC, Southwood Pharmaceuticals Inc	58016-0834-60
90's	$63.90	GENERIC, Southwood Pharmaceuticals Inc	58016-0834-90
100's	$55.20	GENERIC, Allscripts Pharmaceutical Company	54569-1696-00
100's	$71.00	GENERIC, Southwood Pharmaceuticals Inc	58016-0834-00

Concentrate - Oral - 10 mg/ml

120 ml	$13.00	GENERIC, Raway Pharmacal Inc	00686-0612-14

Cream - Topical - 5%

30 gm	$28.33	ZONALON, Physicians Total Care	54868-3494-00
30 gm	$42.55	ZONALON, Bioglan Pharmaceutical Inc	62436-0523-30
45 gm	$49.96	PRUDOXIN, Healthpoint	00064-3600-45
45 gm	$57.37	ZONALON, Bioglan Pharmaceutical Inc	62436-0523-45

Doxercalciferol *(003471)*

For complete prescribing information, refer to the CD-ROM included with the book.

Categories: Hypoparathyroidism, secondary; Dialysis, adjunct; FDA Approved 1999 Jun; Pregnancy Category B
Drug Classes: Vitamins/minerals
Brand Names: Hectorol
Cost of Therapy: $107.38 (Secondary Hyperparathyroidis; Hectorol; 2.5 μg; 12 capsules/week; 30 day supply)

DESCRIPTION

Doxercalciferol is a synthetic vitamin D analog that undergoes metabolic activation *in vivo* to form 1α,25-dihydroxyvitamin D_2 (1α,25-$(OH)_2D_2$), a naturally occurring, biologically active form of vitamin D_2.

Hectorol soft gelatin capsules contain 2.5 μg doxercalciferol. Each capsule also contains butylated hydroxyanisole (BHA), ethanol, and fractionated triglyceride of coconut oil. Gelatin capsule shells contain glycerin, D&C yellow no. 10, and titanium dioxide.

Hectorol injection is available as a sterile, clear, colorless, aqueous solution for intravenous injection. Each ml of solution contains doxercalciferol, 2 μg; Tween Polysorbate 20, 4 mg; sodium chloride, 1.5 mg; sodium ascorbate, 10 mg, sodium phosphate, dibasic 7.6 mg; sodium phosphate, monobasic 1.8 mg; and disodium edetate, 1.1 mg.

Doxercalciferol is a colorless crystalline compound with a calculated molecular weight of 412.66 and a molecular formula of $C_{28}H_{44}O_2$. It is soluble in oils and organic solvents, but is relatively insoluble in water. Chemically, doxercalciferol is (1α,3β,5Z,7E,22E)-9,10-secoergosta-5,7,10(19)22-tetraene-1,3-diol.

Other names frequently used for doxercalciferol are 1α-OH-D_2, 1α-hydroxyvitamin D_2, and 1α-hydroxyergocalciferol.

INDICATIONS AND USAGE

Doxercalciferol is indicated for the reduction of elevated iPTH levels in the management of secondary hyperparathyroidism in patients undergoing chronic renal dialysis.

CONTRAINDICATIONS

Doxercalciferol should not be given to patients with a tendency towards hypercalcemia or evidence of vitamin D toxicity.

WARNINGS

Overdosage of any form of vitamin D, including doxercalciferol, is dangerous. Progressive hypercalcemia due to overdosage of vitamin D and its metabolites may be so severe as to require emergency attention. Acute hypercalcemia may exacerbate tendencies for cardiac arrhythmias and seizures and will affect the action of digitalis drugs. Chronic hypercalcemia can lead to generalized vascular calcification and other soft-tissue calcification. The serum calcium times serum phosphorus (Ca × P) product should not be allowed to exceed 70. Radiographic evaluation of suspect anatomical regions may be useful in the early detection of this condition.

Since doxercalciferol is a precursor for 1α,25-$(OH)_2D_2$, a potent metabolite of vitamin D, pharmacologic doses of vitamin D and its derivatives should be withheld during doxercalciferol treatment to avoid possible additive effects and hypercalcemia.

Oral calcium-based or other non-aluminum containing phosphate binders and a low phosphate diet should be used to control serum phosphorus levels in patients undergoing dialysis. Uncontrolled serum phosphorus exacerbates secondary hyperparathyroidism and can lessen the effectiveness of doxercalciferol in reducing blood PTH levels. After initiating doxercalciferol therapy, the dose of phosphate binders should be decreased to correct persistent mild hypercalcemia (10.6-11.2 mg/dl for 3 consecutive determinations) or increased to correct persistent mild hyperphosphatemia (7.0-8.0 mg/dl for 3 consecutive determinations).

Magnesium containing antacids and doxercalciferol should not be used concomitantly in patients on chronic renal dialysis because such use may lead to the development of hypermagnesemia.

DOSAGE AND ADMINISTRATION

The optimal dose of doxercalciferol must be carefully determined for each patient.

CAPSULES

The recommended initial dose of doxercalciferol is 10.0 μg administered 3 times weekly at dialysis (approximately every other day). The initial dose should be adjusted, as needed, in order to lower blood iPTH into the range of 150-300 pg/ml. The dose may be increased at 8 week intervals by 2.5 μg if iPTH is not lowered by 50% and fails to reach the target range. The maximum recommended dose of doxercalciferol is 20 μg administered 3 times a week at dialysis for a total of 60 μg/week. Drug administration should be suspended if iPTH falls below 100 pg/ml and restarted 1 week later at a dose that is at least 2.5 μg lower than the last administered dose. During titration, iPTH, serum calcium, and serum phosphorus levels should be obtained weekly. If hypercalcemia, hyperphosphatemia, or a serum calcium times serum phosphorus product greater than 70 is noted, the drug should be immediately suspended until these parameters are appropriately lowered. Then, the drug should be restarted at a dose that is at least 2.5 μg lower.

Dosing must be individualized and based on iPTH levels with monitoring of serum calcium and serum phosphorus levels. The following is a suggested approach in dose titration (see TABLE 7 and TABLE 8).

TABLE 7 *Initial Dosing*

iPTH Level	Doxercalciferol Dose
>400 pg/ml	10.0 μg 3 times per week at dialysis.

TABLE 8 *Dose Titration*

iPTH Level	Doxercalciferol Dose
Decreased by <50% and above 300 pg/ml	Increase by 2.5 μg at 8 week intervals as necessary
150-300 pg/ml	Maintain
<100 pg/ml	Suspend for 1 week, then resume at a dose that is at least 2.5 μg lower

INJECTION

The recommended initial dose of doxercalciferol is 4.0 μg administered as a bolus dose 3 times weekly at the end of dialysis (approximately every other day). The initial dose should be adjusted, as needed, in order to lower blood iPTH into the range of 150-300 pg/ml. The dose may be increased at 8 week intervals by 1.0-2.0 μg if iPTH is not lowered by 50% and fails to reach the target range. Dosages higher than 18 μg weekly have not been studied. Drug administration should be suspended if iPTH falls below 100 pg/ml and restarted 1 week later at a dose which is at least 1.0 μg lower than the last administered dose. During titration, iPTH, serum calcium, and serum phosphorus levels should be obtained weekly. If hypercalcemia, hyperphosphatemia, or a serum calcium times phosphorus product greater than 70 is noted, the drug should be immediately suspended until these parameters are appropriately lowered. Then, the drug should be restarted at a dose which is 1.0 μg lower.

Dosing must be individualized and based on iPTH levels with monitoring of serum calcium and serum phosphorus levels. The following is a suggested approach in dose titration (see TABLE 9 and TABLE 10).

TABLE 9 *Initial Dosing*

PTH Level	Doxercalciferol Dose
>400 pg/ml	4.0 μg 3 times per week at the end of dialysis, or approximately every other day.

TABLE 10 *Dose Titration*

PTH Level	Doxercalciferol Dose
Decreased by <50% and above 300 pg/ml	Increase by 1.0-2.0 μg at 8 week intervals as necessary
150-300 pg/ml	Maintain
<100 pg/ml	Suspend for 1 week, then resume at a dose that is at least 1.0 μg lower

Discard unused portion.

PRODUCT LISTING - EQUIVALENTS NOT AVAILABLE

D

Capsule - Oral - 2.5 mcg

50's $111.85 HECTOROL, Bone Care International 64894-0825-50

Solution - Injectable - 2 mcg/ml

1 ml x 50 $578.79 HECTOROL, Berlex Laboratories 64894-0820-50

2 ml x 50 $964.65 HECTOROL, Berlex Laboratories 64894-0840-50

Doxorubicin Hydrochloride *(001112)*

Categories: Carcinoma, bladder; Carcinoma, breast; Carcinoma, lung; Carcinoma, gastric; Carcinoma, ovarian; Carcinoma, thyroid; Leukemia, acute lymphoblastic; Leukemia, acute myeloblastic; Lymphoma; Lymphoma, Hodgkin's; Neuroblastoma; Osteosarcoma; Sarcoma, soft tissue; Wilms' tumor; FDA Approved 1974 Aug; Pregnancy Category D; WHO Formulary
Drug Classes: Antineoplastics, antibiotics
Brand Names: Adiblastine; Adriablastine; Adriablatina; Adriacin; **Adriamycin**; Adriamycin Rdf; Adriblastina; Adriblatina; Doxil; Doxorubicin Hcl; Farmablastina; Rubex
Foreign Brand Availability: Adriablastina (Colombia)
HCFA JCODE(S): J9000 10 mg IV

WARNING

FOR INTRAVENOUS USE ONLY

Severe local tissue necrosis will occur if there is extravasation during administration (see DOSAGE AND ADMINISTRATION). Doxorubicin must not be given by the intramuscular or subcutaneous route.

Myocardial toxicity manifested in its most severe form by potentially fatal congestive heart failure may occur either during therapy or months to years after termination of therapy. The probability of developing impaired myocardial function based on a combined index of signs, symptoms and decline in left ventricular ejection fraction (LVEF) is estimated to be 1-2% at a total cumulative dose of 300 mg/m^2 of doxorubicin, 3-5% at a dose of 400 mg/m^2, 5-8% at 450 mg/m^2 and 6-20% at 500 mg/m^2*. The risk of developing CHF increases rapidly with increasing total cumulative doses of doxorubicin in excess of 450 mg/m^2. This toxicity may occur at lower cumulative doses in patients with prior mediastinal irradiation or on concurrent cyclophosphamide therapy or with pre-existing heart disease. Pediatric patients are at increased risk for developing delayed cardiotoxicity.

Secondary acute myelogenous leukemia (AML) has been reported in patients treated with anthracyclines, including doxorubicin (see ADVERSE REACTIONS). The occurrence of refractory secondary leukemia is more common when such drugs are given in combination with DNA-damaging antineoplastic agents, when patients have been heavily pretreated with cytotoxic drugs, or when doses of anthracyclines have been escalated. The rate of developing treatment-related leukemia was estimated in an analysis of 1474 breast cancer patients who received adjuvant treatment with doxorubicin-containing regimens (*i.e.,* FAC) in clinical trials. The estimated risk of developing treatment-related leukemia at 10 years was 2.5% for the 810 patients receiving radiotherapy plus chemotherapy and 0.5% for the 664 patients receiving chemotherapy alone. The overall risk was estimated at 1.5% at 10 years for the entire patient population. Pediatric patients are also at risk of developing secondary AML.

Dosage should be reduced in patients with impaired hepatic function.

Severe myelosuppression may occur.

Doxorubicin should be administered only under the supervision of a physician who is experienced in the use of cancer chemotherapeutic agents.

***Data on file at Pharmacia & Upjohn.**

DESCRIPTION

Doxorubicin is a cytotoxic anthracycline antibiotic isolated from cultures of *Streptomyces peucetius* var. *caesius*.

Doxorubicin consists of a naphthacenequinone nucleus linked through a glycosidic bond at ring atom 7 to an amino sugar, daunosamine.

Chemically, doxorubicin HCl is: 5,12-Naphthacenedione, 10-[(3-amino-2,3,6-trideoxy-α-L-*lyxo*-hexopyranosyl)oxy]-7,8,9,10-tetrahydro-6,8,11-trihydroxy-8-(hydroxylacetyl)-1-methoxy-, hydrochloride (8S-*cis*)-.

The molecular formula is $C_{27}H_{29}NO_{11}$·HCl. The molecular weight is 579.99.

Doxorubicin binds to nucleic acids, presumably by specific intercalation of the planar anthracycline nucleus with the DNA double helix. The anthracycline ring is lipophilic, but the saturated end of the ring system contains abundant hydroxyl groups adjacent to the amino sugar, producing a hydrophilic center. The molecule is amphoteric, containing acidic functions in the ring phenolic groups and a basic function in the sugar amino group. It binds to cell membranes as well as plasma proteins.

ADRIAMYCIN RDF

Adriamycin RDF for injection is a sterile red-orange lyophilized powder for intravenous use only, is available in 10, 20, and 50 mg single dose vials and a 150 mg multidose vial.

Each **10 mg single dose vial** contains 10 mg of doxorubicin HCl, 50 mg of lactose, (hydrous) and 1 mg of methylparaben (added to enhance dissolution) as a sterile red-orange lyophilized powder.

Each **20 mg single dose vial** contains 20 mg of doxorubicin HCl, 100 mg of lactose (hydrous) and 2 mg of methylparaben (added to enhance dissolution) as a sterile red-orange lyophilized powder.

Each **50 mg single dose vial** contains 50 mg of doxorubicin HCl, 250 mg of lactose (hydrous) and 5 mg of methylparaben (added to enhance dissolution) as a sterile red-orange lyophilized powder.

Each **150 mg multidose vial** contains 150 mg of doxorubicin HCl, 750 mg of lactose (hydrous) and 15 mg of methylparaben (added to enhance dissolution) as a sterile red-orange lyophilized powder.

ADRIAMYCIN PFS

Adriamycin PFS injection is a sterile parenteral, isotonic solution for intravenous use only, containing no preservative, available in 5 ml (10 mg), 10 ml (20 mg), 25 ml (50 mg), and 37.5 ml (75 mg) single dose glass vials and a 100 ml (200 mg) multidose glass vial. Adriamycin PFS is also available in 5 ml (10 mg), 10 ml (20 mg), and 25 ml (50 mg) single dose Cytosafe vials and 75 ml (150 mg) and 100 ml (200 mg) multidose Cytosafe vials.

Each ml contains doxorubicin HCl 2 mg, and the following inactive ingredients: sodium chloride 0.9% and water for injection qs. Hydrochloric acid is used to adjust the pH to a target pH of 3.0.

CLINICAL PHARMACOLOGY

The cytotoxic effect of doxorubicin on malignant cells and its toxic effects on various organs are thought to be related to nucleotide base intercalation and cell membrane lipid binding activities of doxorubicin. Intercalation inhibits nucleotide replication and action of DNA and RNA polymerases. The interaction of doxorubicin with topoisomerase II to form DNA-cleavable complexes appears to be an important mechanism of doxorubicin cytocidal activity. Doxorubicin cellular membrane binding may effect a variety of cellular functions. Enzymatic electron reduction of doxorubicin by a variety of oxidases, reductases and dehydrogenases generate highly reactive species including the hydroxyl free radical OH·. Free radical formation has been implicated in doxorubicin cardiotoxicity by means of Cu (II) and Fe (III) reduction at the cellular level. Cells treated with doxorubicin have been shown to manifest the characteristic morphologic changes associated with apoptosis or programmed cell death. Doxorubicin-induced apoptosis may be an integral component of the cellular mechanism of action relating to therapeutic effects, toxicities, or both.

Animal studies have shown activity in a spectrum of experimental tumors, immunosuppression, carcinogenic properties in rodents, induction of a variety of toxic effects, including delayed and progressive cardiac toxicity, myelosuppression in all species and atrophy to testes in rats and dogs.

Pharmacokinetic studies, determined in patients with various types of tumors undergoing either single or multi-agent therapy have shown that doxorubicin follows a multiphasic disposition after IV injection. The initial distributive half-life of approximately 5.0 minutes suggests rapid tissue uptake of doxorubicin, while its slow elimination from tissues is reflected by a terminal half-life of 20-48 hours. Steady-state distribution volumes exceed 20-30 L/kg and are indicative of extensive drug uptake into tissues. Plasma clearance is in the range of 8-20 ml/min/kg and is predominately by metabolism and biliary excretion. Approximately 40% of the dose appears in the bile in 5 days, while only 5-12% of the drug and its metabolites appear in the urine during the same time period. Binding of doxorubicin and its major metabolite, doxorubicinol to plasma proteins is about 74-76% and is independent of plasma concentration of doxorubicin up to 2 μM. Enzymatic reduction at the 7 position and cleavage of the daunosamine sugar yields aglycones which are accompanied by free radical formation, the local production of which may contribute to the cardiotoxic activity of doxorubicin. Disposition of doxorubicinol (DOX-OL) in patients is formation rate limited. The terminal half-life of DOX-OL is similar to doxorubicin. The relative exposure of DOX-OL, compared to doxorubicin ranges between 0.4-0.6. In urine, <3% of the dose was recovered as DOX-OL over 7 days.

A published clinical study involving 6 men and 21 women with no prior anthracycline therapy reported a significantly higher median doxorubicin clearance in the men compared to the women (113 vs 45 L/h). However, the terminal half-life of doxorubicin was longer in men compared to the women (54 vs 35 hours).

In 4 patients, dose-dependent pharmacokinetics have been shown for doxorubicin in the dose range of 30-70 mg/m^2. Systemic clearance of doxorubicin is significantly reduced in obese women with ideal body weight greater than 130%. There was a significant reduction in clearance without any change in volume of distribution in obese patients when compared with normal patients with less than 115% ideal body weight. The clearance of doxorubicin and doxorubicinol was also reduced in patients with impaired hepatic function. Doxorubicin was excreted in the milk of 1 lactating patient, with peak milk concentration at 24 hours after treatment being approximately 4.4-fold greater than the corresponding plasma concentration. Doxorubicin was detectable in the milk up to 72 hours after therapy with 70 mg/m^2 of doxorubicin given as a 15 minute intravenous infusion and 100 mg/m^2 of cisplatin as a 26 hour intravenous infusion. The peak concentration of doxorubicinol in milk at 24 hours was 0.2 μM and AUC up to 24 hours was 16.5 μM·h, while the AUC for doxorubicin was 9.9 μM·h.

Following administration of 10-75 mg/m^2 doses of doxorubicin to 60 children and adolescents ranging from 2 months to 20 years of age, doxorubicin clearance averaged 1443 ± 114 ml/min/m^2. Further analysis demonstrated that clearance in 52 children greater than 2 years of age (1540 ml/min/m^2) was increased compared with adults. However, clearance in infants younger than 2 years of age (813 ml/min/m^2) was decreased compared with older children and approached the range of clearance values determined in adults.

Doxorubicin does not cross the blood brain barrier.

INDICATIONS AND USAGE

Doxorubicin HCl has been used successfully to produce regression in disseminated neoplastic conditions such as acute lymphoblastic leukemia, acute myeloblastic leukemia, Wilms' tumor, neuroblastoma, soft tissue and bone sarcomas, breast carcinoma, ovarian carcinoma, transitional cell bladder carcinoma, thyroid carcinoma, gastric carcinoma,

Hodgkin's disease, malignant lymphoma and bronchogenic carcinoma in which the small cell histologic type is the most responsive compared to other cell types.

CONTRAINDICATIONS

Doxorubicin therapy should not be started in patients who have marked myelosuppression induced by previous treatment with other antitumor agents or by radiotherapy. Doxorubicin treatment is contraindicated in patients who received previous treatment with complete cumulative doses of doxorubicin, daunorubicin, idarubicin, and/or other anthracyclines and anthracenes.

WARNINGS

Special attention must be given to the cardiotoxicity induced by doxorubicin. Irreversible myocardial toxicity, manifested in its most severe form by life-threatening or fatal congestive heart failure, may occur either during therapy or months to years after termination of therapy. The probability of developing impaired myocardial function, based on a combined index of signs, symptoms and decline in left ventricular ejection fraction (LVEF) is estimated to be 1-2% at a total cumulative dose of 300 mg/m^2 of doxorubicin, 3-5% at a dose of 400 mg/m^2, 5-8% at a dose of 450 mg/m^2 and 6-20% at a dose of 500 mg/m^2 given in a schedule of a bolus injection once every 3 weeks (data on file at Pharmacia & Upjohn). In a retrospective review by Von Hoff *et al.,* the probability of developing congestive heart failure was reported to be 5/168 (3%) at a cumulative dose of 430 mg/m^2 of doxorubicin, 8/110 (7%) at 575 mg/m^2 and 3/14 (21%) at 728 mg/m^2. The cumulative incidence of CHF was 2.2%. In a prospective study of doxorubicin in combination with cyclophosphamide, fluorouracil and/or vincristine in patients with breast cancer or small cell lung cancer, the cumulative incidence of congestive heart failure was 5-6%. The probability of CHF at various cumulative doses of doxorubicin was 1.5% at 300 mg/m^2, 4.9% at 400 mg/m^2, 7.7% at 450 mg/m^2 and 20.5% at 500 mg/m^2.

Cardiotoxicity may occur at lower doses in patients with prior mediastinal irradiation, concurrent cyclophosphamide therapy exposure at an early age and advanced age. Data also suggest that pre-existing heart disease is a co-factor for increased risk of doxorubicin cardiotoxicity. In such cases, cardiac toxicity may occur at doses lower than the respective recommended cumulative dose of doxorubicin. Studies have suggested that concomitant administration of doxorubicin and calcium channel entry blockers may increase the risk of doxorubicin cardiotoxicity. The total dose of doxorubicin administered to the individual patient should also take into account previous or concomitant therapy with related compounds such as daunorubicin, idarubicin and mitoxantrone. Cardiomyopathy and/or congestive heart failure may be encountered several months or years after discontinuation of doxorubicin therapy.

The risk of congestive heart failure and other acute manifestations of doxorubicin cardiotoxicity in pediatric patients may be as much or lower than in adults. Pediatric patients appear to be at particular risk for developing delayed cardiac toxicity in that doxorubicin induced cardiomyopathy impairs myocardial growth as pediatric patients mature, subsequently leading to possible development of congestive heart failure during early adulthood. As many as 40% of pediatric patients may have subclinical cardiac dysfunction and 5-10% of pediatric patients may develop congestive heart failure on long-term follow-up. This late cardiac toxicity may be related to the dose of doxorubicin. The longer the length of follow-up the greater the increase in the detection rate.

Treatment of doxorubicin induced congestive heart failure includes the use of digitalis, diuretics, after load reducers such as angiotensin I converting enzyme (ACE) inhibitors, low salt diet, and bed rest. Such intervention may relieve symptoms and improve the functional status of the patient.

MONITORING CARDIAC FUNCTION

In adult patients severe cardiac toxicity may occur precipitously without antecedent ECG changes. Cardiomyopathy induced by anthracyclines is usually associated with very characteristic histopathologic changes on an endomyocardial biopsy (EM biopsy), and a decrease of left ventricular ejection fraction (LVEF), as measured by multi-gated radionuclide angiography (MUGA scans) and/or echocardiogram (ECHO), from pretreatment baseline values. However, it has not been demonstrated that monitoring of the ejection fraction will predict when individual patients are approaching their maximally tolerated cumulative dose of doxorubicin. Cardiac function should be carefully monitored during treatment to minimize the risk of cardiac toxicity. A baseline cardiac evaluation with an ECG, LVEF, and/or an echocardiogram (ECHO) is recommended especially in patients with risk factors for increased cardiac toxicity (pre-existing heart disease, mediastinal irradiation, or concurrent cyclophosphamide therapy). Subsequent evaluations should be obtained at a cumulative dose of doxorubicin of at least 400 mg/m^2 and periodically thereafter during the course of therapy. Pediatric patients are at increased risk for developing delayed cardiotoxicity following doxorubicin administration and therefore a follow-up cardiac evaluation is recommended periodically to monitor for this delayed cardiotoxicity.

In adults, a 10% decline in LVEF to below the lower limit of normal or an absolute LVEF of 45%, or a 20% decline in LVEF at any level is indicative of deterioration in cardiac function. In pediatric patients, deterioration in cardiac function during or after the completion of therapy with doxorubicin is indicated by a drop in fractional shortening (FS) by an absolute value of $\geq$10 percentile units or below 29%, and a decline in LVEF of 10 percentile units or an LVEF below 55%. In general, if test results indicate deterioration in cardiac function associated with doxorubicin, the benefit of continued therapy should be carefully evaluated against the risk of producing irreversible cardiac damage.

Acute life-threatening arrhythmias have been reported to occur during or within a few hours after doxorubicin administration.

There is a high incidence of bone marrow depression, primarily of leukocytes, requiring careful hematologic monitoring. With the recommended dose schedule, leukopenia is usually transient, reaching its nadir 10-14 days after treatment with recovery usually occurring by the 21st day. White blood counts as low as 1000/mm^3 are to be expected during treatment with appropriate doses of doxorubicin. Red blood cell and platelet levels should also be monitored since they may be depressed. Hematologic toxicity may require dose reduction or suspension or delay of doxorubicin therapy. Persistent severe myelosuppression may result in superinfection or hemorrhage.

Doxorubicin may potentiate the toxicity of other anticancer therapies. Exacerbation of cyclophosphamide induced hemorrhagic cystitis and enhancement of the hepatotoxicity of 6-mercaptopurine have been reported. Radiation induced toxicity to the myocardium, mucosae, skin and liver have been reported to be increased by the administration of doxorubicin. Pediatric patients receiving concomitant doxorubicin and actinomycin-D have manifested acute "recall" pneumonitis at variable times after local radiation therapy.

Since metabolism and excretion of doxorubicin occurs predominantly by the hepatobiliary route, toxicity to recommended doses of doxorubicin can be enhanced by hepatic impairment; therefore, prior to the individual dosing, evaluation of hepatic function is recommended using conventional laboratory tests such as SGOT, SGPT, alkaline phosphatase and bilirubin. (See DOSAGE AND ADMINISTRATION.)

Necrotizing colitis manifested by typhlitis (cecal inflammation), bloody stools and severe and sometimes fatal infections have been associated with a combination of doxorubicin given by IV push daily for 3 days and cytarabine given by continuous infusion daily for 7 or more days.

On IV administration of doxorubicin, extravasation may occur with or without an accompanying stinging or burning sensation, even if blood returns well on aspiration of the infusion needle (see DOSAGE AND ADMINISTRATION). If any signs or symptoms of extravasation have occurred, the injection or infusion should be immediately terminated and restarted in another vein.

PREGNANCY CATEGORY D

Safe use of doxorubicin in pregnancy has not been established. Doxorubicin is embryotoxic and teratogenic in rats and embryotoxic and abortifacient in rabbits. There are no adequate and well-controlled studies in pregnant women. If doxorubicin is to be used during pregnancy, or if the patient becomes pregnant during therapy, the patient should be apprised of the potential hazard to the fetus. Women of childbearing age should be advised to avoid becoming pregnant.

PRECAUTIONS

GENERAL

Doxorubicin is not an anti-microbial agent.

INFORMATION FOR THE PATIENT

Doxorubicin HCl imparts a red coloration to the urine for 1-2 days after administration, and patients should be advised to expect this during active therapy.

LABORATORY TESTS

Initial treatment with doxorubicin requires observation of the patient and periodic monitoring of complete blood counts, hepatic function tests, and radionuclide left ventricular ejection fraction (see WARNINGS).

Like other cytotoxic drugs, doxorubicin may induce "tumor lysis syndrome" and hyperuricemia in patients with rapidly growing tumors. Appropriate supportive and pharmacologic measures may prevent or alleviate this complication.

CARCINOGENESIS, MUTAGENESIS, AND IMPAIRMENT OF FERTILITY

Formal long-term carcinogenicity studies have not been conducted with doxorubicin. Doxorubicin and related compounds have been shown to have mutagenic and carcinogenic properties when tested in experimental models (including bacterial systems, mammalian cells in culture, and female Sprague-Dawley rats).

The possible adverse effect on fertility in males and females in humans or experimental animals have not been adequately evaluated. Testicular atrophy was observed in rats and dogs.

Treatment-related acute myelogenous leukemia has been reported in patients treated with doxorubicin-containing adjuvant chemotherapy regimens (see ADVERSE REACTIONS, Hematologic). The exact role of doxorubicin has not been elucidated. Pediatric patients treated with doxorubicin or other topoisomerase II inhibitors are at a risk for developing acute myelogenous leukemia and other neoplasms. The extent of increased risk associated with doxorubicin has not been precisely quantified.

PREGNANCY CATEGORY D

See WARNINGS.

NURSING MOTHERS

Because of the potential for serious adverse reactions in nursing infants from doxorubicin, mothers should be advised to discontinue nursing during doxorubicin therapy.

PEDIATRIC USE

Pediatric patients are at increased risk for developing delayed cardiotoxicity. Follow-up cardiac evaluations are recommended periodically to monitor for this delayed cardiotoxicity (see WARNINGS).

Doxorubicin, as a component of intensive chemotherapy regimens administered to pediatric patients, may contribute to prepubertal growth failure. It may also contribute to gonadal impairment, which is usually temporary.

DRUG INTERACTIONS

Paclitaxel: Two published studies report that initial administration of paclitaxel infused over 24 hours followed by doxorubicin administered over 48 hours resulted in a significant decrease in doxorubicin clearance with more profound neutropenic and stomatitis episodes than the reverse sequence of administration.

Progesterone: In a published study, progesterone was given intravenously to patients with advanced malignancies (ECOG PS <2) at high doses (up to 10 g over 24 hours) concomitantly with a fixed doxorubicin dose (60 mg/m^2) via bolus. Enhanced doxorubicin-induced neutropenia and thrombocytopenia were observed.

Verapamil: A study of the effects of verapamil on the acute toxicity of doxorubicin in mice revealed higher initial peak concentrations of doxorubicin in the heart with a higher incidence and severity of degenerative changes in cardiac tissue resulting in a shorter survival.

Cyclosporine: The addition of cyclosporine to doxorubicin may result in increases in AUC for both doxorubicin and doxorubicinol possibly due to a decrease in clearance of parent drug and a decrease in metabolism of doxorubicinol. Literature reports suggest that adding cyclosporine to doxorubicin results in more profound and prolonged hematologic toxicity than doxorubicin alone. Coma and/or seizures have also been described.

Literature reports have also described the following drug interactions: Phenobarbital increases the elimination of doxorubicin, phenytoin levels may be decreased by doxorubicin, streptozocin may inhibit hepatic metabolism of doxorubicin, and administration of live vaccines to immunosuppressed patients including those undergoing cytotoxic chemotherapy may be hazardous.

ADVERSE REACTIONS

Dose limiting toxicities of therapy are myelosuppression and cardiotoxicity.

Other Reactions Reported Are:

Cardiotoxicity: (See WARNINGS.)

Cutaneous: Reversible complete alopecia occurs in most cases. Hyperpigmentation of nailbeds and dermal crease, primarily in pediatric patients, and onycholysis have been reported in a few cases. Recall of skin reaction due to prior radiotherapy has occurred with doxorubicin administration.

Gastrointestinal: Acute nausea and vomiting occurs frequently and may be severe. This may be alleviated by antiemetic therapy. Mucositis (stomatitis and esophagitis) may occur 5-10 days after administration. The effect may be severe leading to ulceration and represents a site of origin for severe infections. The dosage regimen consisting of administration of doxorubicin on 3 successive days results in greater incidence and severity of mucositis. Ulceration and necrosis of the colon, especially the cecum, may occur leading to bleeding or severe infections which can be fatal. This reaction has been reported in patients with acute non-lymphocytic leukemia treated with a 3 day course of doxorubicin combined with cytarabine. Anorexia and diarrhea have been occasionally reported.

Vascular: Phlebosclerosis has been reported especially when small veins are used or a single vein is used for repeated administration. Facial flushing may occur if the injection is given too rapidly.

Local: Severe cellulitis, vesication and tissue necrosis will occur if extravasation of doxorubicin occurs during administration. Erythematous streaking along the vein proximal to the site of injection had been reported (see DOSAGE AND ADMINISTRATION).

Hematologic: The occurrence of secondary acute myeloid leukemia with or without a preleukemic phase has been reported in patients concurrently treated with doxorubicin in association with DNA-damaging antineoplastic agents. Such cases could have a short (1-3 years) latency period. An analysis of 1474 breast cancer patients who received adjuvant doxorubicin treatment in clinical trials, showed a 10 year estimated risk of developing treatment-related leukemia at 2.5% (95% confidence interval [CI], 1.0-5.1%) for the 810 patients receiving radiotherapy plus chemotherapy and 0.5% (95% CI, 0.1-2.4%) for the 664 patients receiving chemotherapy alone. The overall risk was 1.5% (95% CI, 0.7-2.9%) at 10 years for the entire patient population. Pediatric patients are also at risk of developing secondary acute myeloid leukemia.

Hypersensitivity: Fever, chills and urticaria have been reported occasionally. Anaphylaxis may occur. A case of apparent cross sensitivity to lincomycin has been reported.

Neurological: Peripheral neurotoxicity in the form of local-regional sensory and/or motor disturbances have been reported in patients treated intra-arterially with doxorubicin, mostly in combination with cisplatin. Animal studies have demonstrated seizures and coma in rodents and dogs treated with intra-carotid doxorubicin. Seizures and coma have been reported in patients treated with doxorubicin in combination with cisplatin or vincristine.

Other: Conjunctivitis and lacrimation occur rarely.

DOSAGE AND ADMINISTRATION

Care in the administration of doxorubicin HCl will reduce the chance of perivenous infiltration (see WARNINGS). It may also decrease the chance of local reactions such as urticaria and erythematous streaking. On IV administration of doxorubicin, extravasation may occur with or without an accompanying burning or stinging sensation, even if blood returns well on aspiration of the infusion needle. If any signs or symptoms of extravasation have occurred, the injection or infusion should be immediately terminated and restarted in another vein. If extravasation is suspected, intermittent application of ice to the site for 15 minutes qid × 3 days may be useful. The benefit of local administration of drugs has not been clearly established. Because of the progressive nature of extravasation reactions, close observation and plastic surgery consultation is recommended. Blistering, ulceration and/or persistent pain are indications for wide excision surgery, followed by split-thickness skin grafting.

The most commonly used dose schedule when used as a single agent is 60-75 mg/m^2 as a single IV injection administered at 21 day intervals. The lower dosage should be given to patients with inadequate marrow reserves due to old age, or prior therapy, or neoplastic marrow infiltration. Doxorubicin HCl has been used concurrently with other approved chemotherapeutic agents. Evidence is available that in some types of neoplastic disease combination chemotherapy is superior to single agents. The benefits and risks of such therapy continue to be elucidated. When used in combination with other chemotherapy drugs, the most commonly used dosage of doxorubicin is 40-60 mg/m^2 given as a single intravenous injection every 21-28 days. Doxorubicin dosage must be reduced in case of hyperbilirubinemia as found in TABLE 1.

TABLE 1

Plasma Bilirubin Concentration	Dosage Reduction
1.2-3.0 mg/dl	50%
3.1-5.0 mg/dl	75%

RECONSTITUTION DIRECTIONS

Doxorubicin HCl 10, 20, 50, and 150 mg vials should be reconstituted with 5, 10, 25, and 75 ml, respectively, of sodium chloride injection, (0.9%), to give a final concentration of 2 mg/ml of doxorubicin HCl. An appropriate volume of air should be withdrawn from the vial during reconstitution to avoid excessive pressure buildup. Bacteriostatic diluents are not recommended.

After adding the diluent, the vial should be shaken and the contents allowed to dissolve. The reconstituted solution is stable for 7 days at room temperature and under normal room light (100 foot-candles) and 15 days under refrigeration (2-8°C). It should be protected from exposure to sunlight. Discard any of the unused solution from the 10, 20, and 50 mg single dose vials. Unused solutions of the multiple dose vial remaining beyond the recommended storage times should be discarded.

It is recommended that doxorubicin HCl be slowly administered into the tubing of a freely running IV infusion of sodium chloride injection or 5% dextrose injection. The tubing should be attached to a Butterfly needle inserted preferably into a large vein. If possible, avoid veins over joints or in extremities with compromised venous or lymphatic drainage. The rate of administration is dependent on the size of the vein, and the dosage. However, the dose should be administered in not less than 3-5 minutes. Local erythematous streaking along the vein as well as facial flushing may be indicative of too rapid an administration. A burning or stinging sensation may be indicative of perivenous infiltration and the infusion should be immediately terminated and restarted in another vein. Perivenous infiltration may occur painlessly.

Doxorubicin should not be mixed with heparin or fluorouracil since it has been reported that these drugs are incompatible to the extent that a precipitate may form. Until specific compatibility data are available, it is not recommended that doxorubicin be mixed with other drugs.

Parenteral drug products should be inspected visually for particulate matter and discoloration prior to administration, whenever solution and container permit.

HANDLING AND DISPOSAL

Skin reactions associated with doxorubicin have been reported. Skin accidentally exposed to doxorubicin should be rinsed copiously with soap and warm water, and if the eyes are involved, standard irrigation techniques should be used immediately. The use of goggles, gloves, and protective gowns is recommended during preparation and administration of the drug.

Procedures for proper handling and disposal of anti-cancer drugs should be considered. Several guidelines on this subject have been published.[1-7] There is no general agreement that all the procedures recommended in the guidelines are necessary or appropriate.

Caregivers of pediatric patients receiving doxorubicin should be counseled to take precautions (such as wearing latex gloves) to prevent contact with the patient's urine and other body fluids for at least 5 days after each treatment.

HOW SUPPLIED

ADRIAMYCIN RDF POWDER FOR INJECTION

Single and Multidose Vials

Adriamycin RDF Powder for Injection is available in 10, 20, and 50 mg single dose vials. It is also available in a 150 mg multidose vial.

Storage: Store at controlled room temperature, 15-30°C (59-86°F). Protect from light. Retain in carton until time of use. The single dose vials contain no preservative. Discard unused portion of single dose vials.

Reconstituted Solution Stability

After adding the diluent, the vial should be shaken and the contents allowed to dissolve. The reconstituted solution is stable for 7 days at room temperature and under normal room light (100 foot-candles) and 15 days under refrigeration (2-8°C). It should be protected from exposure to sunlight. Discard any unused solution from the 10, 20, and 50 mg single dose vials. Unused solutions of the multiple dose vial remaining beyond the recommended storage times should be discarded.

ADRIAMYCIN PFS INJECTION

Single Dose Glass Vials

Sterile single use only, contains no preservative.

Adriamycin PFS Injection in single dose glass vials is available as follows:

10 mg vial, 2 mg/ml, 5 ml.
20 mg vial, 2 mg/ml, 10 ml.
50 mg vial, 2 mg/ml, 25 ml.
75 mg vial, 2 mg/ml, 37.5 ml.

Storage: Store refrigerated, 2-8°C (36-46°F). Protect from light. Retain in carton until time of use. Discard unused portion.

Multidose Glass Vials

Adriamycin PFS Injection is also available in a 200 mg, 2 mg/ml, 100 ml sterile multidose vial which contains no preservative.

Storage: Store refrigerated, 2-8°C (36-46°F). Protect from light. Retain in carton until contents are used.

Single Dose Cytosafe Vials

Sterile single use only polypropylene vials, contains no preservative.

Adriamycin PFS Injection in single dose Cytosafe vials is available as follows:

10 mg vial, 2 mg/ml, 5 ml.
20 mg vial, 2 mg/ml, 10 ml.
50 mg vial, 2 mg/ml, 25 ml.

Storage: Store refrigerated, 2-8°C (36-46°F). Protect from light. Retain in carton until time of use. Discard unused portion.

Multidose Cytosafe Vials
Sterile multidose polypropylene vials, contains no preservative.

Adriamycin PFS Injection is also available in multidose Cytosafe vials as follows:
150 mg, 2 mg/ml, 75 ml.
200 mg, 2 mg/ml, 100 ml.

Storage: Store refrigerated, 2-8°C (36-46°F). Protect from light. Retain in carton until contents are used.

PRODUCT LISTING - RATED THERAPEUTICALLY EQUIVALENT

Powder For Injection - Injectable - 10 mg

1's	$44.40	GENERIC, Baxter Pharmaceutical Products, Inc	10019-0920-01
1's	$53.64	ADRIAMYCIN RDF, Pharmacia and Upjohn	00013-1086-91
10's	$137.50	GENERIC, Bedford Laboratories	55390-0231-10
10's	$151.30	GENERIC, Gensia Sicor Pharmaceuticals Inc	00703-5043-03
10's	$450.70	GENERIC, Vha Supply	55390-0241-10
10's	$450.75	GENERIC, Chiron Therapeutics	00702-0231-10
10's	$473.50	GENERIC, Chiron Therapeutics	00702-0235-10

Powder For Injection - Injectable - 20 mg

1's	$92.00	ADRIAMYCIN RDF, Pharmacia and Upjohn	00013-1096-94
1's	$107.28	ADRIAMYCIN RDF, Pharmacia and Upjohn	00013-1096-91
6's	$568.20	GENERIC, Chiron Therapeutics	00702-0236-06
10's	$540.98	GENERIC, Chiron Therapeutics	00702-0232-06
10's	$901.60	GENERIC, Bedford Laboratories	55390-0232-10
10's	$901.60	GENERIC, Bedford Laboratories	55390-0242-10

Powder For Injection - Injectable - 50 mg

1's	$67.50	GENERIC, Bedford Laboratories	55390-0233-01
1's	$125.18	ADRIAMYCIN RDF, Physicians Total Care	54868-3131-00
1's	$190.00	GENERIC, Vha Supply	55390-0243-01
1's	$197.15	RUBEX, Bristol-Myers Squibb	00015-3352-22
1's	$222.00	GENERIC, Baxter Pharmaceutical Products, Inc	10019-0921-02
1's	$225.40	GENERIC, Chiron Therapeutics	00702-0233-01
1's	$236.74	GENERIC, Chiron Therapeutics	00702-0237-01
1's	$268.18	ADRIAMYCIN RDF, Pharmacia Corporation	00013-1106-79

Solution - Injectable - 2 mg/ml

5 ml	$56.34	ADRIAMYCIN PFS, Pharmacia Corporation	00013-1236-91
5 ml x 10	$137.50	GENERIC, Bedford Laboratories	55390-0235-10
5 ml x 10	$168.00	GENERIC, Abbott Pharmaceutical	00074-5043-03
5 ml x 10	$473.50	GENERIC, Vha Supply	55390-0245-10
10 ml	$112.66	ADRIAMYCIN PFS, Pharmacia and Upjohn	00013-1146-91
10 ml	$112.66	ADRIAMYCIN PFS, Pharmacia Corporation	00013-1246-91
10 ml x 10	$275.00	GENERIC, Bedford Laboratories	55390-0236-10
10 ml x 10	$947.00	GENERIC, Vha Supply	00702-0236-10
10 ml x 10	$947.00	GENERIC, Bedford Laboratories	55390-0246-10
25 ml	$67.50	GENERIC, Bedford Laboratories	55390-0237-01
25 ml	$83.13	GENERIC, Gensia Sicor Pharmaceuticals Inc	00703-5046-01
25 ml	$236.74	GENERIC, Vha Supply	55390-0247-01
25 ml	$281.68	ADRIAMYCIN PFS, Pharmacia and Upjohn	00013-1156-79
25 ml	$281.68	ADRIAMYCIN PFS, Pharmacia Corporation	00013-1256-79
37.50 ml	$422.51	ADRIAMYCIN PFS, Pharmacia and Upjohn	00013-1176-87
50 ml	$84.00	GENERIC, Abbott Pharmaceutical	00074-5046-01
100 ml	$275.00	GENERIC, Bedford Laboratories	55390-0238-01
100 ml	$332.50	GENERIC, Gensia Sicor Pharmaceuticals Inc	00703-5040-01
100 ml	$336.00	GENERIC, Abbott Pharmaceutical	00074-5040-01
100 ml	$945.98	GENERIC, Vha Supply	55390-0248-01
100 ml	$1017.96	GENERIC, Astra-Zeneca Pharmaceuticals	00186-1532-81
100 ml	$1104.13	ADRIAMYCIN PFS, Pharmacia and Upjohn	00013-1166-83
100 ml	$1104.13	ADRIAMYCIN PFS, Pharmacia Corporation	00013-1266-83

PRODUCT LISTING - EQUIVALENTS NOT AVAILABLE

Powder For Injection - Injectable - 75 mg

1's	$184.01	ADRIAMYCIN PFS, Pharmacia and Upjohn	00013-1176-01

Powder For Injection - Injectable - 100 mg

1's	$394.29	RUBEX, Bristol-Myers Squibb	00015-3353-22

Powder For Injection - Injectable - 150 mg

1's	$788.04	ADRIAMYCIN RDF, Pharmacia Corporation	00013-1116-83

Solution - Injectable - 2 mg/ml

75 ml	$845.03	ADRIAMYCIN PFS, Pharmacia Corporation	00013-1286-83

Doxorubicin, Liposomal *(003276)*

Categories: Carcinoma, ovarian; Sarcoma, Kaposi's; Recombinant DNA Origin; FDA Approved 1995 Nov; Pregnancy Category D; Orphan Drugs

Drug Classes: Antineoplastics, antibiotics

Brand Names: **Doxil**

Foreign Brand Availability: A.D.Mycin (Korea); Adriablastin (Austria; Hungary; Switzerland); Adriablastina (Czech-Republic; Greece; Portugal); Adriablastina R.D. (Thailand); Adriacin (Japan); Adriamicine (Russia); Adriamycin (Australia; China; Czech-Republic; Denmark; England; Finland; Hong-Kong; Ireland; Malaysia; New-Zealand; Norway; Sweden; Thailand); Adriamycin P.F.S. (Korea); Adriamycin PFS (Canada); Adriamycin RD (Indonesia); Adriamycin R.D.F. (Korea); Adriamycin RDF (Canada); Adriblastin (Russia); Adriblastine (France); Adriblastina (Bahrain; Belgium; Benin; Bulgaria; Burkina-Faso; Costa-Rica; Cyprus; Dominican-Republic; Egypt; El-Salvador; Ethiopia; Gambia; Ghana; Guatemala; Guinea; Honduras; Iran; Iraq; Italy; Ivory-Coast; Jordan; Kenya; Kuwait; Lebanon; Liberia; Libya; Malawi; Mali; Mauritania; Mauritius; Morocco; Netherlands; Nicaragua; Niger; Nigeria; Oman; Panama; Peru; Philippines; Qatar; Republic-of-Yemen; Saudi-Arabia; Senegal; Seychelles; Sierra-Leone; South-Africa; Sudan; Syria; Taiwan; Tanzania; Tunia; Turkey; Uganda; United-Arab-Emirates; Zambia; Zimbabwe); Adriblastina CS (Colombia); Adriblastina PFS (Israel); Adrim (India; Philippines); Adrimedac (Germany); Adrubicin (Korea); Amminac (Thailand); Caelyx (Australia; Austria; Belgium; Bulgaria; Canada; Czech-Republic; Denmark; England; Finland; France; Germany; Greece; Hong-Kong; Hungary; Ireland; Israel; Italy; Mexico; Netherlands; Norway; Peru; Philippines; Poland; Portugal; Singapore; Slovenia; South-Africa; Spain; Sweden; Switzerland; Taiwan; Thailand; Turkey); Carcinocin (Indonesia); Doxolem (Costa-Rica; Dominican-Republic; El-Salvador; Guatemala; Honduras; Mexico; Nicaragua; Panama; Thailand); Doxor Lyo (Taiwan); Doxorubin (New-Zealand; Thailand); Doxorubicin (India); Doxorubicin Meiji (India); Ifadox (Mexico); Farmiblastina (Spain); Myocet (Austria; Belgium; Bulgaria; Czech-Republic; Denmark; England; Finland; France; Germany; Greece; Hungary; Ireland; Italy; Netherlands; Norway; Poland; Portugal; Slovenia; Spain; Sweden; Switzerland; Turkey); Rubidox (Philippines)

D

WARNING

Note: The trade name was used throughout this monograph for clarity.

Experience with Doxil (doxorubicin HCl liposome injection) at high cumulative doses is too limited to have established its effects on the myocardium. It should therefore be assumed that Doxil will have myocardial toxicity similar to conventional formulations of doxorubicin HCl. Irreversible myocardial toxicity leading to congestive heart failure often unresponsive to cardiac supportive therapy may be encountered as the total dosage of doxorubicin HCl approaches 550 mg/m². Prior use of other anthracyclines or anthracenediones will reduce the total dose of doxorubicin HCl that can be given without cardiac toxicity. Cardiac toxicity also may occur at lower cumulative doses in patients with prior mediastinal irradiation or who are receiving concurrent cyclophosphamide therapy.

Doxil should be administered to patients with a history of cardiovascular disease only when the benefit outweighs the risk to the patient.

Acute infusion-related reactions including, but not limited to, flushing, shortness of breath, facial swelling, headache, chills, back pain, tightness in the chest or throat, and/or hypotension have occurred in up to 10% of patients treated with Doxil. In most patients, these reactions resolve over the course of several hours to a day once the infusion is terminated. In some patients, the reaction has resolved with slowing of the infusion rate. Serious and sometimes life-threatening or fatal allergic/anaphylactoid-like infusion reactions have been reported. Medications to treat such reactions, as well as emergency equipment, should be available for immediate use. Doxil should be administered at an initial rate of 1 mg/min to minimize the risk of infusion reactions. (See WARNINGS, Infusion Reactions.)

Severe myelosuppression may occur. (See WARNINGS, Myelosuppression.)

Dosage should be reduced in patients with impaired hepatic function. (See DOSAGE AND ADMINISTRATION.)

Accidental substitution of Doxil for doxorubicin HCl has resulted in severe side effects. Doxil should not be substituted for doxorubicin HCl on a mg per mg basis. (See DESCRIPTION and DOSAGE AND ADMINISTRATION.)

Doxil should be administered only under the supervision of a physician who is experienced in the use of cancer chemotherapeutic agents.

DESCRIPTION

FOR INTRAVENOUS INFUSION ONLY.

Doxil (doxorubicin hydrochloride liposome injection) is doxorubicin hydrochloride encapsulated in Stealth liposomes for intravenous (IV) administration.

Note: Liposomal encapsulation can substantially affect a drug's functional properties relative to those of the unencapsulated drug. In addition, different liposomal drug products may vary from one another in the chemical composition and physical form of the liposomes. Such differences can substantially affect the functional properties of liposomal drug products. DO NOT SUBSTITUTE.

Doxorubicin is a cytotoxic anthracycline antibiotic isolated from *Streptomyces peucetius* var. *caesius*.

Doxorubicin hydrochloride, which is the established name for (8*S*,10*S*)-10-[(3-amino-2,3,6-trideoxy-α-L-*lyxo*-hexopyranosyl)oxy]-8-glycolyl-7,8,9,10-tetrahydro-6,8,11-trihydroxy-1-methoxy-5,12-naphthacenedione hydrochloride.

The molecular formula of the drug is $C_{27}H_{29}NO_{11}$·HCl; its molecular weight is 579.99.

Doxil is provided as a sterile, translucent, red liposomal dispersion in 10 or 30 ml glass, single use vials. Each vial contains 20 or 50 mg doxorubicin hydrochloride at a concentration of 2 mg/ml and a pH of 6.5. The Stealth liposome carriers are composed of N-(carbonyl-methoxypolyethylene glycol 2000)-1,2-distearoyl-*sn*-glycero-3-phosphoethanolamine sodium salt (MPEG-DSPE), 3.19 mg/ml; fully hydrogenated soy phosphatidylcholine (HSPC), 9.58 mg/ml; and cholesterol, 3.19 mg/ml. Each ml also contains ammonium sulfate, approximately 2 mg; histidine as a buffer; hydrochloric acid and/or sodium hydroxide for pH control; and sucrose to maintain isotonicity. Greater than 90% of the drug is encapsulated in the Stealth liposomes.

CLINICAL PHARMACOLOGY

MECHANISM OF ACTION

The active ingredient of Doxil is doxorubicin HCl. The mechanism of action of doxorubicin HCl is thought to be related to its ability to bind DNA and inhibit nucleic acid synthesis. Cell structure studies have demonstrated rapid cell penetration and perinuclear chromatin binding, rapid inhibition of mitotic activity and nucleic acid synthesis, and induction of mutagenesis and chromosomal aberrations.

Doxil is doxorubicin HCl encapsulated in long-circulating Stealth liposomes. Liposomes are microscopic vesicles composed of a phospholipid bilayer that are capable of encapsulating active drugs. The Stealth liposomes of Doxil liposome are formulated with surface-bound methoxypolyethylene glycol (MPEG), a process often referred to as pegylation, to protect liposomes from detection by the mononuclear phagocyte system (MPS) and to increase blood circulation time.

Stealth liposomes have a half-life of approximately 55 hours in humans. They are stable in blood, and direct measurement of liposomal doxorubicin shows that at least 90% of the drug (the assay used cannot quantify less than 5-10% free doxorubicin) remains liposome-encapsulated during circulation.

It is hypothesized that because of their small size (ca. 100 nm) and persistence in the circulation, the pegylated Doxil liposomes are able to penetrate the altered and often compromised vasculature of tumors. This hypothesis is supported by studies using colloidal gold-containing Stealth liposomes, which can be visualized microscopically. Evidence of penetration of Stealth liposomes from blood vessels and their entry and accumulation in tumors has been seen in mice with C-26 colon carcinoma tumors and in transgenic mice with Kaposi's sarcoma-like lesions. Once the Stealth liposomes distribute to the tissue compartment, the encapsulated doxorubicin HCl becomes available. The exact mechanism of release is not understood.

PHARMACOKINETICS

The plasma pharmacokinetics of Doxil were evaluated in 42 patients with AIDS-related Kaposi's sarcoma (KS) who received single doses of 10 or 20 mg/m^2 administered by a 30 minute infusion. Twenty-three (23) of these patients received single doses of both 10 and 20 mg/m^2 with a 3 week wash-out period between doses. The pharmacokinetic parameter values of Doxil, given for total doxorubicin (mostly liposomally bound), are presented in TABLE 1.

TABLE 1 *Pharmacokinetic Parameters of Doxil in AIDS Patients With Kaposi's Sarcoma (n=23)*

Parameter	Dose 10 mg/m^2	20 mg/m^2
Peak plasma concentration (μg/ml)	4.12 ± 0.215	8.34 ± 0.49
Plasma clearance (L/h/m^2)	0.056 ± 0.01	0.041 ± 0.004
Steady-state volume of distribution (L/m^2)	2.83 ± 0.145	2.72 ± 0.120
AUC (μg/ml·h)	277 ± 32.9	590 ± 58.7
First phase (λ_1) half-life (h)	4.7 ± 1.1	5.2 ±1.4
Second phase (λ_2) half-life (h)	52.3 ± 5.6	55.0 ± 4.8

Mean ± Standard Error.

Doxil displayed linear pharmacokinetics over the range of 10-20 mg/m^2. Disposition occurred in 2 phases after Doxil administration, with a relatively short first phase (~5 hours) and a prolonged second phase (~55 hours) that accounted for the majority of the area under the curve (AUC).

The pharmacokinetics of Doxil at a 50 mg/m^2 dose is reported to be nonlinear. At this dose, the elimination half-life of Doxil is expected to be longer and the clearance lower compared to a 20 mg/m^2 dose. The exposure (AUC) is thus expected to be more than proportional at a 50 mg/m^2 dose when compared with the lower doses.

Distribution

In contrast to the pharmacokinetics of doxorubicin, which displays a large volume of distribution, ranging from 700-1100 L/m^2, the small steady state volume of distribution of Doxil shows that Doxil is confined mostly to the vascular fluid volume. Plasma protein binding of Doxil has not been determined; the plasma protein binding of doxorubicin is approximately 70%.

Metabolism

Doxorubicinol, the major metabolite of doxorubicin, was detected at very low levels (range: of 0.8-26.2 ng/ml) in the plasma of patients who received 10 or 20 mg/m^2 Doxil.

Excretion

The plasma clearance of Doxil was slow, with a mean clearance value of 0.041 L/h/m^2 at a dose of 20 mg/m^2. This is in contrast to doxorubicin, which displays a plasma clearance value ranging from 24-35 L/h/m^2.

Because of its slower clearance, the AUC of Doxil, primarily representing the circulation of liposome-encapsulated doxorubicin, is approximately 2-3 orders of magnitude larger than the AUC for a similar dose of conventional doxorubicin HCl as reported in the literature.

Special Populations

The pharmacokinetics of Doxil have not been separately evaluated in women, in members of different ethnic groups, or in individuals with renal or hepatic insufficiency.

Drug-Drug Interactions

Although the patient populations for the current indications are on various medications, drug-drug interactions between Doxil and other drugs, including antiviral agents, have not been evaluated.

TISSUE DISTRIBUTION

Kaposi's sarcoma lesions and normal skin biopsies were obtained at 48 and 96 hours postinfusion of 20 mg/m^2 Doxil in 11 patients. The concentration of Doxil in KS lesions was a median of 19 (range, 3-53) times higher than in normal skin at 48 hours posttreatment; however, this was not corrected for likely differences in blood content between KS lesions and normal skin. The corrected ratio may lie between 1 and 22 times. Thus, higher concentrations of Doxil are delivered to KS lesions than to normal skin.

INDICATIONS AND USAGE

Doxil (doxorubicin HCl liposome injection) is indicated for:

The treatment of metastatic carcinoma of the ovary in patients with disease that is refractory to both paclitaxel- and platinum-based chemotherapy regimens. Refractory disease is defined as disease that has progressed while on treatment, or within 6 months of completing treatment.

The treatment of AIDS-related Kaposi's sarcoma in patients with disease that has progressed on prior combination chemotherapy or in patients who are intolerant to such therapy.

These indications are based on objective tumor response rates. No results are available from controlled trials that demonstrate a clinical benefit resulting from this treatment, such as improvement in disease-related symptoms or increased survival.

NON-FDA APPROVED INDICATIONS

Doxorubicin liposomal has been investigated alone or as an adjunct for its activity against advanced nonovarian gynecologic cancer, solid tumors, metastatic head and neck cancer, hormone-refractory prostate cancer, glioblastomas, metastatic brain tumors, and metastatic breast cancer; however, none of these uses is approved by the FDA.

CONTRAINDICATIONS

Doxil is contraindicated in patients who have a history of hypersensitivity reactions to a conventional formulation of doxorubicin HCl or the components of Doxil.

Doxil is contraindicated in nursing mothers.

WARNINGS

CARDIAC TOXICITY

Experience with large cumulative doses of Doxil is limited. Doxil's cardiac risk and its risk compared to conventional doxorubicin formulations have not been adequately evaluated. At present, therefore, warnings related to the use of conventional formulation doxorubicin HCl should be observed.

Special attention must be given to the cardiac toxicity exhibited by doxorubicin HCl. Acute left ventricular failure can occur with doxorubicin, particularly in patients who have received total doxorubicin dosage exceeding the currently recommended limit of 550 mg/m^2. Lower (400 mg/m^2) doses appear to cause heart failure in patients who have received radiotherapy to the mediastinal area or concomitant therapy with other potentially cardiotoxic agents such as cyclophosphamide.

Caution should be observed in patients who have received other anthracyclines, and the total dose of doxorubicin HCl given should take into account any previous or concomitant therapy with other anthracyclines or related compounds. Congestive heart failure and/or cardiomyopathy may be encountered after discontinuation of therapy. Patients with a history of cardiovascular disease should be administered Doxil only when the potential benefit of treatment outweighs the risk.

Cardiac function should be carefully monitored in patients treated with Doxil. The most definitive test for anthracycline myocardial injury is endomyocardial biopsy. Other methods, such as echocardiography or gated radionuclide scans, have been used to monitor cardiac function during anthracycline therapy. Any of these methods should be employed to monitor potential cardiac toxicity during Doxil therapy. If these test results indicate possible cardiac injury associated with Doxil therapy, the benefit of continued therapy must be carefully weighed against the risk of myocardial injury. (See ADVERSE REACTIONS.)

In the AIDS-KS studies, 68 (9.6%) patients experienced cardiac-related adverse events. In 30 patients (4.3%), the event was thought to be possibly or probably related to Doxil. Nine cases of possibly or probably related cardiomyopathy and/or congestive heart failure were reported. Seven (1.0%) of the possibly or probably related cardiac events were severe. These severe events included arrhythmia (nonspecific), cardiomyopathy, heart failure, pericardial effusion, and tachycardia. Three patients discontinued study due to cardiac events.

MYELOSUPPRESSION

In ovarian cancer patients, myelosuppression was generally moderate and reversible. Anemia was the most common hematologic adverse event (52.6%), followed by leukopenia (WBC <4000 mm^3; 42.2%), thrombocytopenia (24.2%), and neutropenia (19.0%) (see TABLE 5).

In ovarian cancer patients, 3.3% received G-CSF (or GM-CSF) to support their blood counts. (See DOSAGE AND ADMINISTRATION, Dose Modification Guidelines.)

In AIDS-KS patients, who often present with baseline myelosuppression due to such factors as their HIV disease or concomitant medications, myelosuppression appears to be the dose-limiting adverse event, at the recommended dose of 20 mg/m^2 (see TABLE 7). Leukopenia is the most common adverse event experienced in this population; anemia and thrombocytopenia can also be expected. Sepsis occurred in 5% of patients; for 0.7% of patients the event was considered possibly or probably related to Doxil. Eleven patients (1.6%) discontinued study because of bone marrow suppression or neutropenia.

In all patients, because of the potential for bone marrow suppression, careful hematologic monitoring is required during use of Doxil, including white blood cell, neutrophil, platelet counts, and Hgb/Hct. With the recommended dosage schedule, leukopenia is usually transient. Hematologic toxicity may require dose reduction or delay or suspension of Doxil therapy. Persistent severe myelosuppression may result in superinfection, neutropenic fever, or hemorrhage. Development of sepsis in the setting of neutropenia has resulted in discontinuation of treatment and in rare cases, death.

Doxil may potentiate the toxicity of other anticancer therapies. In particular, hematologic toxicity may be more severe when Doxil is administered in combination with other agents that cause bone marrow suppression.

INFUSION REACTIONS

Acute infusion-related reactions characterized by flushing, shortness of breath, facial swelling, headache, chills, chest pain, back pain, tightness in the chest and throat, fever, tachycardia, pruritus, rash, cyanosis, syncope, bronchospasm, asthma, apnea, and/or hypotension have occurred in up to 10% of patients treated with Doxil. In most patients, these reactions resolve over the course of several hours to a day once the infusion is terminated. In some patients, the reaction resolves when the rate of infusion is slowed.

Serious and sometimes life-threatening or fatal allergic/anaphylactoid-like infusion reactions have been reported. Medications to treat such reactions, as well as emergency equipment, should be available for immediate use.

The majority of infusion-related events occurred during the first infusion. Similar reactions have not been reported with conventional doxorubicin and they presumably represent a reaction to the Doxil liposomes or one of its surface components.

The initial rate of infusion should be 1 mg/min to help minimize the risk of infusion reactions. (See DOSAGE AND ADMINISTRATION.)

PALMAR-PLANTAR ERYTHRODYSESTHESIA

In ovarian cancer patients, 37.4% of patients experienced PPE (developed palmar-plantar skin eruptions characterized by swelling, pain, erythema and, for some patients, desquamation of the skin on the hands and the feet), with 16.4% of the patients reporting Grade 3 or 4 events. Thirteen (3.5%) of the ovarian cancer patients discontinued treatment due to PPE or other skin toxicity. (See definitions of PPE grades in DOSAGE AND ADMINISTRATION, Dose Modification Guidelines.)

Among 705 patients with AIDS-related Kaposi's sarcoma treated with Doxil at 20 mg/m^2, 24 (3.4%) developed PPE, with 3 (0.9%) discontinuing.

PPE was generally seen after 2 or 3 cycles of treatment but may occur earlier. In most patients the reaction is mild and resolves in 1-2 weeks so that prolonged delay of therapy need not occur. However, dose modification may be required to manage PPE. (See DOSAGE AND ADMINISTRATION, Dose Modification Guidelines.) The reaction can be severe and debilitating in some patients and may require discontinuation of treatment.

PREGNANCY CATEGORY D

Doxil can cause fetal harm when administered to a pregnant woman. Doxil is embryotoxic at doses of 1 mg/kg/day in rats and is embryotoxic and abortifacient at 0.5 mg/kg/day in rabbits (both doses are about one-eighth the 50 mg/m^2 human dose on a mg/m^2 basis). Embryotoxicity was characterized by increased embryo-fetal deaths and reduced live litter sizes.

There are no adequate and well-controlled studies in pregnant women. If Doxil is to be used during pregnancy, or if the patient becomes pregnant during therapy, the patient should be apprised of the potential hazard to the fetus. If pregnancy occurs in the first few months following treatment with Doxil, the prolonged half-life of the drug must be considered. Women of childbearing potential should be advised to avoid pregnancy.

TOXICITY POTENTIATION

The doxorubicin in Doxil may potentiate the toxicity of other anticancer therapies. Exacerbation of cyclophosphamide-induced hemorrhagic cystitis and enhancement of the hepatotoxicity of 6-mercaptopurine have been reported with the conventional formulation of doxorubicin HCl. Radiation-induced toxicity to the myocardium, mucosae, skin, and liver have been reported to be increased by the administration of doxorubicin HCl.

INJECTION SITE EFFECTS

Doxil is not a vesicant, but should be considered an irritant and precautions should be taken to avoid extravasation. With intravenous administration of Doxil, extravasation may occur with or without an accompanying stinging or burning sensation, even if blood returns well on aspiration of the infusion needle. (See DOSAGE AND ADMINISTRATION.) If any signs or symptoms of extravasation have occurred, the infusion should be immediately terminated and restarted in another vein. The application of ice over the site of extravasation for approximately 30 minutes may be helpful in alleviating the local reaction. **Doxil must not be given by the intramuscular or subcutaneous route.**

In studies with rabbits, lesions that were induced by subcutaneous injection of Doxil were minor and reversible compared to more severe and irreversible lesions and tissue necrosis that were induced after subcutaneous injection of conventional doxorubicin HCl.

HEPATIC IMPAIRMENT

The pharmacokinetics of Doxil has not been adequately evaluated in patients with hepatic impairment. Doxorubicin is eliminated in large part by the liver. Thus, Doxil dosage should be reduced in patients with impaired hepatic function. (See DOSAGE AND ADMINISTRATION.)

Prior to Doxil administration, evaluation of hepatic function is recommended using conventional clinical laboratory tests such as SGOT, SGPT, alkaline phosphatase and bilirubin. (See DOSAGE AND ADMINISTRATION.)

CARCINOGENESIS, MUTAGENESIS, IMPAIRMENT OF FERTILITY

Secondary acute myelogenous leukemia has been reported in patients treated with topoisomerase II inhibitors, including anthracyclines.

Although no studies have been conducted with Doxil, doxorubicin HCl and related compounds have been shown to have mutagenic and carcinogenic properties when tested in experimental models.

Stealth liposomes without drug were negative when tested in Ames, mouse lymphoma and chromosomal aberration assays *in vitro,* and mammalian micronucleus assay *in vivo.*

The possible adverse effects on fertility in males and females in humans or experimental animals have not been adequately evaluated. However, Doxil resulted in mild to moderate ovarian and testicular atrophy in mice after a single dose of 36 mg/kg (about twice the 50 mg/m^2 human dose on a mg/m^2 basis). Decreased testicular weights and hypospermia were present in rats after repeat doses ≥0.25 mg/kg/day (about one-thirtieth the 50 mg/m^2 human dose on a mg/m^2 basis), and diffuse degeneration of the seminiferous tubules and a marked decrease in spermatogenesis were observed in dogs after repeat doses of 1 mg/kg/day (about one-half the 50 mg/m^2 human dose on a mg/m^2 basis).

PRECAUTIONS

GENERAL

Patients receiving therapy with Doxil should be monitored by a physician experienced in the use of cancer chemotherapeutic agents. Most adverse events are manageable with dose reductions or delays. (See DOSAGE AND ADMINISTRATION, Dose Modification Guidelines.)

LABORATORY TESTS

Complete blood counts, including platelet counts, should be obtained frequently and at a minimum prior to each dose of Doxil.

PREGNANCY CATEGORY D

See WARNINGS.

NURSING MOTHERS

It is not known whether this drug is excreted in human milk. Because many drugs, including anthracyclines, are excreted in human milk and because of the potential for serious adverse reactions in nursing infants from Doxil, mothers should discontinue nursing prior to taking this drug.

PEDIATRIC USE

The safety and effectiveness of Doxil in pediatric patients have not been established.

GERIATRIC USE

Of the 373 ovarian cancer patients, 29% were 60-69 years old, while 22.8% were 70 years and over. No overall differences were observed between these subjects and younger subjects, but greater sensitivity of some older individuals cannot be ruled out. There are insufficient data for a comparative evaluation of efficacy according to age.

RADIATION THERAPY

Recall of skin reaction due to prior radiotherapy has occurred with Doxil administration.

INFORMATION FOR THE PATIENT

Patients and patients' caregivers should be informed of the expected adverse effects of Doxil, particularly hand-foot syndrome, stomatitis, and neutropenia and its complications of neutropenic fever, infection, and sepsis.

Hand-foot syndrome (palmar-plantar erythrodysesthesia): Patients who experience tingling or burning, redness, flaking, bothersome swelling, small blisters, or small sores on the palms of their hands or soles of their feet (symptoms of hand-foot syndrome) should notify their physician.

Stomatitis: Patients who experience painful redness, swelling, or sores in the mouth (symptoms of stomatitis) should notify their physician.

Fever and neutropenia: Patients who develop a fever of 100.5°F or higher should notify their physician.

Nausea, vomiting, tiredness, weakness, rash, or mild hair loss: Patients who develop any of these symptoms should notify their physician.

DRUG INTERACTIONS

No formal drug interaction studies have been conducted with Doxil. Until specific compatibility data are available, it is not recommended that Doxil be mixed with other drugs. Doxil may interact with drugs known to interact with the conventional formulation of doxorubicin HCl.

ADVERSE REACTIONS

OVARIAN CANCER PATIENTS

Safety data are available from 373 ovarian cancer patients treated with Doxil in 4 clinical studies. The patient population was predominantly white (93.6%) with a median age of 60 years. Patients received a median cycle dose of 50 mg/m^2 administered with a median cycle length of 29.5 days. They remained on study drug for a median of 56 days and received a median cumulative dose of 137.5 mg/m^2. Patients received a median of 3 cycles of Doxil, although some patients remained on study drug for a prolonged period, with 46 patients (12.3%) receiving more than 10 cycles of treatment.

Adverse events (AEs) were reported in all but 2 of the 361 patients who had at least 1 AE form collected. A total of 3124 AEs were reported, an average of 8.6 AEs per patient. Most (91.7%) patients had AEs that were considered related to study drug.

TABLE 5 *Hematology Data Reported in Ovarian Cancer Patients*

	% Ovarian Patients (n=373)
Neutropenia	
<1000/mm^3	19.0%
<500/mm^3	8.3%
Febrile neutropenia	0.3%
Anemia	
<10 g/dl	52.6%
<8 g/dl	25.0%
RBC trasfusions	12.9%
Epoetin alpha support*	2.1%
Thrombocytopenia	
<150,000/mm^3	24.2%
<25,000/mm^3	1.1%
Platelet transfusions*	1.4%

* From concomitant medication or transfusion logs, not reported as AEs.

The following additional (not in TABLE 6) adverse events were observed in ovarian cancer patients with doses administered every 4 weeks; only events considered at least possibly drug-related by investigators are included.

TABLE 6 *Drug Related Non-Hematologic Adverse Events Reported in ≥5% of Ovarian Cancer Patients*

Non-Hematologic Adverse Event	% Ovarian Patients (n=361)
Palmar-Plantar Erythrodysesthesia	
All grades	37.4%
Grade 3 & 4	16.4%
Stomatitis	
All grades	37.4%
Grade 3 & 4	7.7%
Nausea	
All grades	37.7%
Grade 3 & 4	4.2%
Asthenia	33.0%
Vomiting	22.4%
Rash	21.6%
Alopecia	15.2%
Constipation	12.7%
Anorexia	11.9%
Mucous membrane disorder	11.6%
Diarrhea	10.0%
Abdominal pain	8.0%
Paresthesia	7.8%
Pain	7.2%
Fever	6.9%
Pharyngitis	5.5%
Dry skin	5.5%
Headache	5.3%

Incidence 1-5%:

Body as a Whole: Allergic reaction, chills, infection, chest pain, back pain, abdomen enlarged, malaise.

Digestive System: Dyspepsia, oral moniliasis, mouth ulceration, esophagitis, dysphagia.

Metabolic and Nutritional System: Peripheral edema, dehydration.

Musculoskeletal System: Myalgia.

Nervous System: Somnolence, dizziness, depression, insomnia, anxiety.

Respiratory System: Dyspnea, cough increased, rhinitis.

Cutaneous: Pruritus, skin discoloration, skin disorder, vesiculobullous rash, maculopapular rash, exfoliative dermatitis, herpes zoster, sweating.

Special Senses: Conjunctivitis, taste perversion.

Incidence Less Than 1%:

Body as a Whole: Cellulitis, anaphylactoid reaction, ascites, flu syndrome, neck pain, moniliasis, injection site pain, face edema, chills and fever, pelvic pain, chest pain substernal, injection site inflammation.

Cardiovascular System: Hypertension, angina pectoris, pericardial effusion, postural hypotension, hypotension, palpitation, syncope, shock, bradycardia, arrhythmia, phlebitis, tachycardia, cardiomegaly, heart failure, hemorrhage.

Digestive System: Gingivitis, eructation, increased salivation, melena, gastrointestinal hemorrhage, proctitis, jaundice, ileus, periodontal abscess, flatulence, aphthous stomatitis, gastritis, glossitis, gum hemorrhage.

Hemic and Lymphatic System: Hypochromic anemia, lymphadenopathy, ecchymosis, petechia.

Metabolic/Nutritional Disorders: SGOT increase, creatinine increase, hypocalcemia, hyperglycemia, hypokalemia, hypermagnesemia, hyponatremia, weight gain, bilirubinemia, generalized edema, cachexia, hypochloremia.

Musculoskeletal System: Arthralgia, bone pain, myasthenia.

Nervous System: Peripheral neuritis, incoordination, thinking abnormal, confusion, hypertonia, nervousness, hyperesthesia, hypesthesia, neuropathy, ataxia.

Respiratory System: Pleural effusion, asthma, hiccup, pneumothorax, laryngitis, sinusitis, voice alteration, epistaxis, pneumonia.

Skin and Appendages: Skin ulcer, herpes simplex, contact dermatitis, fungal dermatitis, furunculosis, skin nodule, urticaria, acne.

Special Senses: Amblyopia, blepharitis, parosmia, taste loss.

Urogenital System: Urinary tract infection, leukorrhea, cystitis, nocturia, dysuria, breast pain, mastitis, oliguria, vaginitis, kidney function abnormal, vaginal hemorrhage, hydronephrosis, vaginal moniliasis.

AIDS-KS PATIENTS

Information on adverse events is based on the experience reported in 753 patients with AIDS-related KS enrolled in four studies. The majority of patients were treated with 20 mg/m^2 of Doxil every 2-3 weeks. The median time on study was 127 days and ranged from 1-811 days. The median cumulative dose was 120 mg/m^2 and ranged from 3.3-798.6 mg/m^2. Twenty-six patients (3.0%) received cumulative doses of greater than 450 mg/m^2.

Of these 753 patients, 61.2% were considered poor risk for KS tumor burden, 91.5% poor for immune system, and 46.9% for systemic illness; 36.2% were poor risk for all 3 categories. Patients' median CD4 count was 21.0 cells/mm^3, with 50.8% of patients having less than 50 cells/mm^3. The mean absolute neutrophil count at study entry was approximately 3000 cells/mm^3.

Patients received a variety of potentially myelotoxic drugs in combination with Doxil. Of the 693 patients with concomitant medication information, 58.7% were on 1 or more antiretroviral medications; 34.9% patients were on zidovudine (AZT), 20.8% on didanosine (ddI), 16.5% on zalcitabine (ddC), and 9.5% on stavudine (D4T). A total of 85.1% patients were on PCP prophylaxis, most (54.4%) on sulfamethoxazole/trimethoprim. Eighty-five percent (85%) of patients were receiving antifungal medications, primarily fluconazole (75.8%). Seventy-two percent (72%) of patients were receiving antivirals, 56.3% acyclovir, 29% ganciclovir, and 16% foscarnet. In addition, 47.8% patients received colony stimulating factors (sargramostim/filgrastim) sometime during their course of treatment.

Of the 753 patients enrolled in the Doxil clinical trials, adverse event information was available for 705 patients. In many instances it was difficult to determine whether adverse events resulted from Doxil, from concomitant therapy, or from the patients' underlying disease(s).

Eighty-three percent (83%) of the patients reported adverse events that were considered to be possibly or probably related to the treatment with Doxil.

Adverse reactions only infrequently (5%) led to discontinuation of treatment. Those that did so included bone marrow suppression, cardiac adverse events, infusion-related reactions, toxoplasmosis, palmar-plantar erythrodysesthesia, pneumonia, cough/dyspnea, fatigue, optic neuritis, progression of a non-KS tumor, allergy to penicillin, and unspecified reasons.

TABLE 7 *Hematology Data Reported in AIDS-KS Patients*

	Refractory or Intolerant AIDS-KS Patients (n=74)	Total AIDS-KS Patients (n=720)
Neutropenia		
<1000/mm^3	34 (45.9%)	352 (48.9%)
<500/mm^3	8 (10.8%)	96 (13.3%)
Anemia		
<10 g/dl	43 (58.1%)	399 (55.4%)
<8 g/dl	12 (16.2%)	131 (18.2%)
Thrombocytopenia		
<150,000/mm^3	45 (60.8%)	439 (60.9%)
<25,000/mm^3	1 (1.4%)	30 (4.2%)

TABLE 8 *Probably and Possibly Drug-Related Non-Hematologic Adverse Events Reported in ≥5% of AIDS-KS Patients*

Adverse Event	Refractory or Intolerant AIDS-KS Patients (n=77)	Total AIDS-KS Patients (n=705)
Nausea	14 (18.2%)	119 (16.9%)
Asthenia	5 (6.5%)	70 (9.9%)
Fever	6 (7.8%)	64 (9.1%)
Alopecia	7 (9.1%)	63 (8.9%)
Alkaline phosphatase increase	1 (1.3%)	55 (7.8%)
Vomiting	6 (7.8%)	55 (7.8%)
Hypochromic anemia	4 (5.2%)	69 (9.8%)
Diarrhea	4 (5.2%)	55 (7.8%)
Stomatitis	4 (5.2%)	48 (6.8%)
Oral moniliasis	1 (1.3%)	39 (5.5%)

The following additional (not in TABLE 8) adverse events were observed in AIDS-KS patients; only events considered at least possibly drug-related by investigators are included.

Incidence 1-5%:

Body as a Whole: Headache, back pain, infection, allergic reaction, chills.

Cardiovascular: Chest pain, hypotension, tachycardia.

Cutaneous: Herpes simplex, rash, itching.

Digestive System: Mouth ulceration, glossitis, constipation, aphthous stomatitis, anorexia, dysphagia, abdominal pain.

Hematologic: Hemolysis, increased prothrombin time.

Metabolic/Nutritional: SGPT increase, weight loss, hypocalcemia, hyperbilirubinemia, hyperglycemia.

Other: Dyspnea, albuminuria, pneumonia, retinitis, emotional lability, dizziness, somnolence.

Incidence Less Than 1%:

Body as a Whole: Face edema, cellulitis, sepsis, abscess, radiation injury, flu syndrome, moniliasis, hypothermia, injection site hemorrhage, injection site pain, cryptococcosis, ascites.

Cardiovascular System: Thrombophlebitis, cardiomyopathy, pericardial effusion, hemorrhage, palpitation, syncope, bundle branch block, congestive heart failure, cardiomegaly, heart arrest, migraine, thrombosis, ventricular arrhythmia.

Digestive System: Dyspepsia, cholestatic jaundice, gastritis, gingivitis, ulcerative proctitis, colitis, esophageal ulcer, esophagitis, gastrointestinal hemorrhage, hepatic failure, leukoplakia of mouth, pancreatitis, ulcerative stomatitis, hepatitis, hepatosplenomegaly, increased appetite, jaundice, sclerosing cholangitis, tenesmus, fecal impaction.

Endocrine System: Diabetes mellitus.

Hemic and Lymphatic System: Eosinophilia, lymphadenopathy, lymphangitis, lymphedema, petechia, thromboplastin decrease.

Metabolic/Nutritional Disorders: Lactic dehydrogenase increase, hypernatremia, creatinine increase, BUN increase, dehydration, edema, hypercalcemia, hyperkalemia, hyperlipemia, hyperuricemia, hypoglycemia, hypokalemia, hypolipemia, hypomagnesemia, hyponatremia, hypophosphatemia, hypoproteinemia, ketosis, weight gain.

Musculoskeletal System: Myalgia, arthralgia, bone pain, myositis.

Nervous System: Paresthesia, insomnia, peripheral neuritis, depression, neuropathy, anxiety, convulsion, hypotonia, acute brain syndrome, confusion, hemiplegia, hypertonia, hypokinesia, vertigo.

Respiratory System: Pleural effusion, asthma, bronchitis, cough increase, hyperventilation, pharyngitis, pneumothorax, rhinitis, sinusitis.

Skin and Appendages: Maculopapular rash, skin ulcer, skin discoloration, herpes zoster, exfoliative dermatitis, cutaneous moniliasis, erythema multiforme, erythema nodosum, furunculosis, psoriasis, pustular rash, skin necrosis, urticaria, vesiculobullous rash.

Special Senses: Otitis media, taste perversion, abnormal vision, blindness, conjunctivitis, eye pain, optic neuritis, tinnitus, visual field defect.
Urogenital System: Hematuria, balanitis, cystitis, dysuria, genital edema, glycosuria, kidney failure.

DOSAGE AND ADMINISTRATION

OVARIAN CANCER PATIENTS

Doxil should be administered intravenously at a dose of 50 mg/m^2 (doxorubicin HCl equivalent) at an initial rate of 1 mg/min to minimize the risk of infusion reactions. If no infusion-related AEs are observed, the rate of infusion can be increased to complete administration of the drug over 1 hour. The patient should be dosed once every 4 weeks, for as long as the patient does not progress, shows no evidence of cardiotoxicity (see WARNINGS), and continues to tolerate treatment. A minimum of 4 courses is recommended because median time to response in clinical trials was 4 months. To manage adverse events such as PPE, stomatitis, or hematologic toxicity the doses may be delayed or reduced (see Dose Modification Guidelines). Pretreatment with or concomitant use of antiemetics should be considered.

AIDS-KS PATIENTS

Doxil should be administered intravenously at a dose of 20 mg/m^2 (doxorubicin HCl equivalent) over 30 minutes, once every 3 weeks, for as long as patients respond satisfactorily and tolerate treatment.

GENERAL

Do not administer as a bolus injection or an undiluted solution. Rapid infusion may increase the risk of infusion-related reactions. (See WARNINGS, Infusion Reactions.)

Each 10 ml vial contains 20 mg doxorubicin HCl at a concentration of 2 mg/ml.

Each 30 ml vial contains 50 mg doxorubicin HCl at a concentration of 2 mg/ml.

Until specific compatibility data are available, it is not recommended that Doxil be mixed with other drugs.

Doxil should be considered an irritant and precautions should be taken to avoid extravasation. With intravenous administration of Doxil, extravasation may occur with or without an accompanying stinging or burning sensation, even if blood returns well on aspiration of the infusion needle. If any signs or symptoms of extravasation have occurred the infusion should be immediately terminated and restarted in another vein. The application of ice over the site of extravasation for approximately 30 minutes may be helpful in alleviating the local reaction. **Doxil must not be given by the intramuscular or subcutaneous route.**

DOSE MODIFICATION GUIDELINES

Doxil exhibits nonlinear pharmacokinetics at 50 mg/m^2; therefore, dose adjustments may result in a non-proportional greater change in plasma concentration and exposure to the drug. (See CLINICAL PHARMACOLOGY, Pharmacokinetics.)

Patients should be carefully monitored for toxicity. Adverse events, such as PPE, hematologic toxicities, and stomatitis may be managed by dose delays and adjustments. Following the first appearance of a Grade 2 or higher adverse event, the dosing should be adjusted or delayed as described in the Recommended Dose Modification Guidelines. Once the dose has been reduced, it should not be increased at a later time.

Recommended Dose Modification Guidelines

Palmar-Plantar Erythrodysesthesia

Toxicity Grade 1:
Mild erythema, swelling, or desquamation not interfering with daily activities.
Dose Adjustment: **Redose unless patient has experienced previous Grade 3 or 4 toxicity.** If so, delay up to 2 weeks and decrease dose by 25%. Return to original dose interval.

Toxicity Grade 2:
Erythema, desquamation, or swelling interfering with, but not precluding normal physical activities; small blisters or ulcerations less than 2 cm in diameter.
Dose Adjustment: **Delay dosing up to 2 weeks or until resolved to Grade 0-1.** If after 2 weeks there is no resolution, Doxil should be discontinued.

Toxicity Grade 3:
Blistering, ulceration, or swelling interfering with walking or normal daily activities; cannot wear regular clothing.
Dose Adjustment: **Delay dosing up to 2 weeks or until resolved to Grade 0-1.** Decrease dose by 25% and return to original dose interval. If after 2 weeks there is no resolution, Doxil should be discontinued.

Toxicity Grade 4:
Diffuse or local process causing infectious complications, or a bed ridden state or hospitalization.
Dose Adjustment: **Delay dosing up to 2 weeks or until resolved to Grade 0-1.** Decrease dose by 25% and return to original dose interval. If after 2 weeks there is no resolution, Doxil should be discontinued.

Hematological Toxicity

Grade 1:
ANC: 1,500-1,900
Platelets: 75,000-150,000
Modification: Resume treatment with no dose reduction.

Grade 2:
ANC: 1,000 to <1,500
Platelets: 50,000 to <75,000
Modification: Wait until ANC ≥1,500 and platelets ≥75,000; redose with no dose reduction.

Grade 3:
ANC: 500-999
Platelets: 25,000 to <50,000
Modification: Wait until ANC ≥1,500 and platelets ≥75,000; redose with no dose reduction.

Grade 4:
ANC: <500
Platelets: <25,000
Modification: Wait until ANC ≥1,500 and platelets ≥75,000; redose at 25% dose reduction or continue full dose with cytokine support.

Stomatitis

Toxicity Grade 1:
Painless ulcers, erythema, or mild soreness.
Dose Adjustment: **Redose unless patient has experienced previous Grade 3 or 4 toxicity.** If so, delay up to 2 weeks and decrease dose by 25%. Return to original dose interval.

Toxicity Grade 2:
Painful erythema, edema, or ulcers, but can eat.
Dose Adjustment: **Delay dosing up to 2 weeks or until resolved to Grade 0-1.** If after 2 weeks there is no resolution, Doxil should be discontinued.

Toxicity Grade 3:
Painful erythema, edema, or ulcers, and cannot eat.
Dose Adjustment: **Delay dosing up to 2 weeks or until resolved to Grade 0-1.** Decrease dose by 25% and return to original dose interval. If after 2 weeks there is no resolution, Doxil should be discontinued.

Toxicity Grade 4:
Requires parenteral or enteral support.
Dose Adjustment: **Delay dosing up to 2 weeks or until resolved to Grade 0-1.** Decrease dose by 25% and return to original dose interval. If after 2 weeks there is no resolution, Doxil should be discontinued.

PATIENTS WITH IMPAIRED HEPATIC FUNCTION

Limited clinical experience exists in treating hepatically impaired patients with Doxil. Based on experience with doxorubicin HCl, it is recommended that Doxil dosage be reduced if the bilirubin is elevated as follows: serum bilirubin 1.2-3.0 mg/dl give ½ normal dose, >3 mg/dl give ¼ normal dose.

PREPARATION FOR IV ADMINISTRATION

The appropriate dose of Doxil, up to a maximum of 90 mg, must be diluted in 250 ml of 5% dextrose injection prior to administration. Aseptic technique must be strictly observed since no preservative or bacteriostatic agent is present in Doxil. Diluted Doxil should be refrigerated at 2-8°C (36-46°F) and administered within 24 hours.

Do not use with in-line filters.

Do not mix with other drugs.

Do not use with any diluent other than 5% dextrose injection.

Do not use any bacteriostatic agent, such as benzyl alcohol.

Doxil is not a clear solution but a translucent, red liposomal dispersion.

Parenteral drug products should be inspected visually for particulate matter and discoloration prior to administration, whenever solution and container permit. Do not use if a precipitate or foreign matter is present.

STORAGE AND STABILITY

Refrigerate unopened vials of Doxil at 2-8°C (36-46°F). Avoid freezing. Prolonged freezing may adversely affect liposomal drug products; however, short-term freezing (less than 1 month) does not appear to have a deleterious effect on Doxil.

PROCEDURE FOR PROPER HANDLING AND DISPOSAL

Caution should be exercised in the handling and preparation of Doxil.

The use of gloves is required.

If Doxil comes into contact with skin or mucosa, immediately wash thoroughly with soap and water.

Doxil should be considered an irritant and precautions should be taken to avoid extravasation. With intravenous administration of Doxil, extravasation may occur with or without an accompanying stinging or burning sensation, even if blood returns well on aspiration of the infusion needle. If any signs or symptoms of extravasation have occurred, the infusion should be immediately terminated and restarted in another vein. Doxil must not be given by the intramuscular or subcutaneous route.

Doxil should be handled and disposed of in a manner consistent with other anticancer drugs. Several guidelines on this subject exist.[2-8]

HOW SUPPLIED

Doxil injection is supplied as a sterile, translucent, red liposomal dispersion in 10 or 30 ml glass, single use vials.

Each vial contains 20 or 50 mg doxorubicin HCl at a concentration of 2 mg/ml.

Storage: Refrigerate at 2-8°C. Avoid freezing. Prolonged freezing may adversely affect liposomal drug products; however, short-term freezing (less than 1 month) does not appear to have a deleterious effect on Doxil.

PRODUCT LISTING - EQUIVALENTS NOT AVAILABLE

Dispersion - Intravenous - 2 mg/ml

10 ml	$828.38	DOXIL, Alza	17314-9600-01
25 ml	$2070.94	DOXIL, Alza	17314-9600-02

Doxycycline (001113)

Categories: Acne vulgaris; Actinomycosis; Amebiasis, adjunct; Anthrax; Bartonellosis; Brucellosis; Chancroid; Cholera; Conjunctivitis, inclusion; Gonorrhea; Granuloma inguinale; Infection, endocervical; Infection, genital tract; Infection, lower respiratory tract; Infection, rectal; Infection, sexually transmitted; Infection, upper respiratory tract; Infection, urinary tract; Listeriosis; Lymphogranuloma venereum; Malaria, prophylaxis; Periodontitis; Plague; Psittacosis; Q fever; Relapsing fever; Rickettsialpox; Rocky mountain spotted fever; Shigellosis; Syphilis; Tick fever; Trachoma; Tularemia; Typhus fever; Urethritis; Vincent's infection; Yaws; Pregnancy Category D; FDA Approved 1967 Dec; WHO Formulary

Drug Classes: Antibiotics, tetracyclines

Brand Names: Doxy; Doxy-100; Doxychel; Doxycycline Hyclate; Doxycycline Monohydrate; Monodox; **Vibramycin**; Vibramycin Calcium; Vibramycin Hyclate; Vibramycin Monohydrate

D

Foreign Brand Availability: Amermycin (Thailand); Atrax (Philippines); Azudoxat (Germany); Bactidox (Germany); Banndoclin (Indonesia); Basedillin (Japan); Bassado (Italy); Biocolyn (Philippines); Biodoxi (India); Bronmycin (Malaysia); Cloran (Korea); Cyclidox (South-Africa); Dagracycline (Netherlands); Dentistar (Korea); Deoxymykoin (Czech-Republic); Doinmycin (Taiwan); Doryx (Australia; China; New-Zealand; Singapore); Dosil (Spain); Dotur (Costa-Rica; Dominican-Republic; El-Salvador; Guatemala; Honduras; Nicaragua; Panama); Doxaciclin (Japan); Doxat (Bahrain; Cyprus; Egypt; Iran; Iraq; Israel; Jordan; Kuwait; Lebanon; Libya; Oman; Qatar; Republic-of-Yemen; Saudi-Arabia; Syria; United-Arab-Emirates); Doxibiotic (Israel); Doxilin (Singapore); Doximed (Finland); Doximycin (Czech-Republic; Finland); Doxin (Indonesia; Philippines; Thailand); Doxine (New-Zealand; Singapore); Doxi-Sergo (Spain); Doxsig (Australia); Doxy-1 (India); Doxycin (Canada); Doxycline (Thailand); Doxycycline (Belgium); Doxylag (Bahamas; Bahrain; Barbados; Belize; Benin; Bermuda; Burkina-Faso; Curacao; Cyprus; Egypt; Ethiopia; Gambia; Ghana; Guinea; Guyana; Iran; Iraq; Israel; Ivory-Coast; Jamaica; Jordan; Kenya; Kuwait; Lebanon; Liberia; Libya; Malawi; Mali; Mauritania; Mauritius; Morocco; Netherland-Antilles; Niger; Nigeria; Oman; Puerto-Rico; Qatar; Republic-of-Yemen; Saudi-Arabia; Senegal; Seychelles; Sierra-Leone; South-Africa; Sudan; Surinam; Syria; Tanzania; Trinidad; Tunia; Uganda; United-Arab-Emirates; Zambia; Zimbabwe); Doxylin (Australia; Israel; New-Zealand; Norway; Thailand); Doxymycin (Netherlands; South-Africa; Taiwan); Doxytec (Canada); Doxytrim (Israel); Dumoxin (Bahrain; Cyprus; Denmark; Egypt; Finland; Indonesia; Iran; Iraq; Israel; Jordan; Kuwait; Lebanon; Libya; Netherlands; Norway; Oman; Qatar; Republic-of-Yemen; Saudi-Arabia; Syria; Thailand; United-Arab-Emirates); Esdoxin (Japan); Etidoxina (Colombia); Gewacyclin (Austria); Granudoxy (France); Ibralene (Philippines); Idocyklin (Sweden); Interdoxin (Indonesia); Lydox (India); Magdrin (Japan); Medomycin (Bahamas; Barbados; Belize; Benin; Bermuda; Burkina-Faso; Curacao; Ethiopia; Gambia; Ghana; Guinea; Guyana; Hong-Kong; Ivory-Coast; Jamaica; Kenya; Liberia; Malawi; Malaysia; Mali; Mauritania; Mauritius; Morocco; Netherland-Antilles; Niger; Nigeria; Puerto-Rico; Senegal; Seychelles; Sierra-Leone; South-Africa; Sudan; Surinam; Taiwan; Tanzania; Thailand; Trinidad; Tunia; Uganda; Zambia; Zimbabwe); Miradin (Italy); Monocin (Korea); Paldomycin (Japan); Periostat (England; Ireland; Israel); Radox (Bahrain; Benin; Burkina-Faso; Cyprus; Egypt; Ethiopia; Gambia; Ghana; Guinea; Iran; Iraq; Israel; Ivory-Coast; Jordan; Kenya; Kuwait; Lebanon; Liberia; Libya; Malawi; Mali; Mauritania; Mauritius; Morocco; Niger; Nigeria; Oman; Qatar; Republic-of-Yemen; Saudi-Arabia; Senegal; Seychelles; Sierra-Leone; South-Africa; Sudan; Syria; Tanzania; Tunia; Uganda; United-Arab-Emirates; Zambia; Zimbabwe); Remycin (Taiwan); Roximycin (Japan); Serodoxy (Korea); Servidoxine (Ecuador); Servidoxyne (Malaysia; Philippines; Thailand); Siadocin (Thailand); Siclidon (Indonesia); Sigadoxin (Austria; Portugal; Switzerland); Supracyclin (Austria; Switzerland); Supramycina (Ecuador); Tenutan (Bahamas; Barbados; Belize; Bermuda; Curacao; Guyana; Jamaica; Netherland-Antilles; Puerto-Rico; Surinam; Trinidad); Tolexine (France); Tolexine Ge (France); Torymycin (Thailand); Tsurupioxin (Japan); Unidox (Bahrain; Cyprus; Egypt; Iran; Iraq; Israel; Jordan; Kuwait; Lebanon; Libya; Oman; Qatar; Republic-of-Yemen; Saudi-Arabia; Syria; United-Arab-Emirates); Veemycin (Thailand); Viadoxin (Indonesia); Vibrabiotic (Greece); Vibradox (Denmark; Portugal); Vibracina (Spain); Vibramicina (Argentina; Colombia; Costa-Rica; Dominican-Republic; Ecuador; El-Salvador; Guatemala; Honduras; Mexico; Nicaragua; Panama; Peru; Portugal); Vibramycin-N (Korea); Vibramycine (Belgium; France); Vibra-S (Netherlands); Vibra-Tabs (Australia; Canada; Finland); Vibratab (Hungary); Vibraveineuse (France); Vibravenos (Germany); Vibravenos SF (Israel); Viradoxyl-N (Korea); Wanmycin (Hong-Kong; Malaysia); Zadorin (Bahamas; Bahrain; Barbados; Belize; Benin; Bermuda; Burkina-Faso; Costa-Rica; Curacao; Cyprus; Dominican-Republic; Ecuador; Egypt; El-Salvador; Ethiopia; Gambia; Ghana; Guatemala; Guinea; Guyana; Honduras; Hong-Kong; Iran; Iraq; Israel; Ivory-Coast; Jamaica; Jordan; Kenya; Kuwait; Lebanon; Liberia; Libya; Malawi; Mali; Mauritania; Mauritius; Morocco; Netherland-Antilles; Nicaragua; Niger; Nigeria; Oman; Panama; Puerto-Rico; Qatar; Republic-of-Yemen; Saudi-Arabia; Senegal; Seychelles; Sierra-Leone; South-Africa; Sudan; Surinam; Syria; Tanzania; Trinidad; Tunia; Uganda; United-Arab-Emirates; Zambia; Zimbabwe)

Cost of Therapy: $51.39 (Gonorrhea; Vibramycin; 100 mg; 2 capsules/day; 7 day supply)
$1.78 (Gonorrhea; Generic capsules; 100 mg; 2 capsules/day; 7 day supply)
$110.12 (Malaria Prophylaxis; Vibramycin; 100 mg; 1 capsule/day; 30 day supply)
$59.81 (Periodontitis; Periostat; 20 mg; 2 capsules/day; 30 day supply)

DENTAL

DESCRIPTION

SUBGINGIVAL APPLICATION

The Atridox product is a subgingival controlled-release product composed of a 2 syringe mixing system. Syringe A contains 450 mg of the Atrigel Delivery System, which is a bioabsorbable, flowable polymeric formulation composed of 36.7% poly(DL-lactide) (PLA) dissolved in 63.3% *N*-methyl-2-pyrrolidone (NMP). Syringe B contains doxycycline hyclate which is equivalent to 42.5 mg doxycycline. The constituted product is a pale yellow to yellow viscous liquid with a concentration of 10.0% of doxycycline hyclate. Upon contact with the crevicular fluid, the liquid product solidifies and then allows for controlled release of drug for a period of 7 days.

Doxycycline is a broad-spectrum antibiotic synthetically derived from oxytetracycline. The empirical formula is: $(C_{22}H_{24}N_2O_8 \cdot HCl)_2 \cdot C_2H_6O \cdot H_2O$.

CAPSULES

Periostat is available as a 20 mg capsule formulation of doxycycline hyclate for oral administration.

Doxycycline is synthetically derived from oxytetracycline.

Doxyclycline hyclate capsules have a molecular weight of 1025.89. The chemical designation for doxycycline is 4-(dimethylamino)-1,4,4a,5,5a,6,11,12a-octahydro-3,5,10,12,12a-pentahydroxy-6-methyl-1,11-dioxo-2-naphthacenecarboxamide monohydrochloride, compound with ethyl alcohol (2:1), monohydrate.

Doxycycline hyclate is a light-yellow crystalline powder which is soluble in water.

Inert ingredients in the formulation are: Hard gelatin capsules; magnesium stearate; and microcrystalline cellulose. Each capsule contains doxycycline hyclate equivalent to 20 mg of doxycycline.

The empirical formula is: $(C_{22}H_{24}N_2O_8 \cdot HCl)_2 \cdot C_2H_6O \cdot H_2O$.

CLINICAL PHARMACOLOGY

SUBGINGIVAL APPLICATION

Microbiology

Doxycycline is a broad-spectrum semisynthetic tetracycline.[1]

Doxycycline is bacteriostatic, inhibiting bacterial protein synthesis due to disruption of transfer RNA and messenger RNA at ribosomal sites.[1] *In vitro* testing has shown that *Porphyromonas gingivalis, Prevotella intermedia, Campylobacter rectus,* and *Fusobacterium nucleatum,* which are associated with periodontal disease, are susceptible to doxycycline at concentrations ≤6.0 μg/ml.[2] A single-center, single-blind, randomized, clinical study in 45 subjects with periodontal disease demonstrated that a single treatment with doxycycline hyclate resulted in the reduction in the numbers of *P. gingivalis, P. intermedia, C. rectus, F. nucleatum, Bacteroides forsythus,* and *E. corrodens* in subgingival plaque samples. Levels of aerobic and anaerobic bacteria were also reduced after treatment with doxycycline hyclate. The clinical significance of these findings, however, is not known. During these studies, no overgrowth of opportunistic organisms such as gram-negative bacilli and yeast were observed. However, as with other antibiotic preparations, doxycycline hyclate therapy may result in the overgrowth of nonsusceptible organisms including fungi. (See PRECAUTIONS.)

Pharmacokinetics

In a clinical pharmacokinetic study, subjects were randomized to receive either doxycycline hyclate covered with Coe-Pak periodontal dressing (n=13), doxycycline hyclate covered with Octyldent periodontal adhesive (n=13), or oral doxycycline (n=5) (according to package dosing instructions). The doxycycline release characteristics in gingival crevicular fluid (GCF), saliva, and serum were evaluated.

Doxycycline levels in GCF peaked (~1500 μg/ml and ~2000 μg/ml for Coe-Pak and Octyldent groups, respectively) 2 hours following treatment with doxycycline hyclate. These levels remained above 1000 μg/ml through 18 hours, at which time the levels began to decline gradually. However, local levels of doxycycline remained well above the minimum inhibitory concentration (MIC_{90}) for periodontal pathogens (≤6.0 μg/ml)[2] through Day 7. In contrast, subjects receiving oral doxycycline had peak GCF levels of ~2.5 μg/ml at 12 hours following the initial oral dosing with levels declining at ~0.2 μg/ml by Day 7. High variability was observed for doxycycline levels in GCF for both oral and doxycycline hyclate subgingival application treatment groups.

The maximum concentration of doxycycline in saliva was achieved at 2 hours after both treatments with doxycycline hyclate, with means of 4.05 μg/ml and 8.78 μg/ml and decreased to 0.36 μg/ml and 0.23 μg/ml at Day 7 for the Coe-Pak group and the Octyldent group, respectively.

CAPSULES

After oral administration, doxycycline hyclate is rapidly and nearly completely absorbed from the gastrointestinal tract. Doxycycline is eliminated with a half-life of approximately 18 hours by renal and fecal excretion of unchanged drug.

Mechanism of Action

Doxycycline has been shown to inhibit collagenase activity *in vitro*.[1] Additional studies have shown that doxycycline reduces the elevated collagenase activity in the gingival crevicular fluid of patients with adult periodontitis.[2,3] The clinical significance of these findings is not known.

Microbiology

Doxycycline is a member of the tetracycline class of antibiotics. The dosage of doxycycline achieved with this product during administration is well below the concentration required to inhibit microorganisms commonly associated with adult periodontitis. Clinical studies with this product demonstrated no effect on total anaerobic and facultative bacteria in plaque samples from patients administered this dose regimen for 9-18 months. This product **should not** be used for reducing the numbers of or eliminating those microorganisms associated with periodontitis.

Pharmacokinetics

The pharmacokinetics of doxycycline following oral administration of doxycycline hyclate were investigated in 3 volunteer studies involving 87 adults. Additionally, doxycycline pharmacokinetics have been characterized in numerous scientific publications.[4] Pharmacokinetic parameters for doxycycline hyclate following single oral doses and at steady-state in healthy subjects are presented in TABLE 1.

TABLE 1 *Pharmacokinetic Parameters for Doxycycline Hyclate Capsules*

	n	C_{max} (ng/ml)	T_{max} (h)	Cl/F (L/h)	T½ (h)
Single dose 20 mg	42	400 ± 142	1.5 (0.5–4.0)	3.80 ± 0.85	18.4 ± 5.38
Steady-state 20 mg bid	30	790 ± 285	2 (0.98–12.0)	3.76 ± 1.06	Not determined

Absorption

Doxycycline is virtually completely absorbed after oral administration. Following 20 mg doxycycline, twice a day, in healthy volunteers, the mean peak concentration in plasma was 790 ng/ml and the average steady-state concentration was 482 ng/ml. The effect of food on the absorption of doxycycline from doxycycline hyclate has not been studied.

Distribution

Doxycycline is greater than 90% bound to plasma proteins. Its apparent volume of distribution is variously reported as between 52.6 and 134 L.[4,6]

Metabolism

Major metabolites of doxycycline have not been identified. However, enzyme inducers such as barbiturates, carbamazepine, and phenytoin decrease the half-life of doxycycline.

Excretion

Doxycycline is excreted in the urine and feces as unchanged drug. It is variously reported that between 29% and 55.4% of an administered dose can be accounted for in the urine by 72 hours.[5,6] Half-life averaged 18 hours in subjects receiving a single 20 mg doxycycline dose.

Special Populations

Geriatric

Doxycycline pharmacokinetics have not been evaluated in geriatric patients.

Pediatric

Doxycycline pharmacokinetics have not been evaluated in pediatric patients (see WARNINGS).

Gender

A study was conducted in 42 subjects where doxycycline pharmacokinetics were compared in men and women. It was observed that C_{max} was approximately 1.7-fold higher in women than in men. There were no apparent differences in other pharmacokinetic parameters.

Race

Differences in doxycycline pharmacokinetics among racial groups have not been evaluated.

Renal Insufficiency

Studies have shown no significant difference in serum half-life of doxycycline in patients with normal and severely impaired renal function. Hemodialysis does not alter the half-life of doxycycline.

Hepatic Insufficiency

Doxycycline pharmacokinetics have not been evaluated in patients with hepatic insufficiency.

Drug Interactions

See DRUG INTERACTIONS.

INDICATIONS AND USAGE

SUBGINGIVAL APPLICATION

Doxycycline hyclate is indicated for use in the treatment of chronic adult periodontitis for a gain in clinical attachment, reduction in probing depth, and reduction in bleeding on probing.

CAPSULES

Doxycycline hyclate is indicated for use as an adjunct to scaling and root planing to promote attachment level gain and to reduce pocket depth in patients with adult periodontitis.

CONTRAINDICATIONS

Doxycycline hyclate should not be used in patients who are hypersensitive to doxycycline or any other drug in the tetracycline class.

WARNINGS

THE USE OF DRUGS OF THE TETRACYCLINE CLASS DURING TOOTH DEVELOPMENT (LAST HALF OF PREGNANCY, INFANCY, AND CHILDHOOD TO THE AGE OF 8 YEARS) MAY CAUSE PERMANENT DISCOLORATION OF THE TEETH. This adverse reaction is more common during long-term use of the drugs, but has been observed following repeated short-term courses. Enamel hypoplasia has also been reported. TETRACYCLINE DRUGS, THEREFORE, SHOULD NOT BE USED IN THIS AGE GROUP, OR IN PREGNANT WOMEN, UNLESS OTHER DRUGS ARE NOT LIKELY TO BE EFFECTIVE OR ARE CONTRAINDICATED.

All tetracyclines form a stable calcium complex in any bone forming tissue. A decrease in fibula growth rate has been observed in premature infants given oral tetracyclines in doses of 25 mg/kg every 6 hours. This reaction was shown to be reversible when the drug was discontinued.

Doxycycline can cause fetal harm when administered to a pregnant woman. Results of animal studies indicate that tetracyclines cross the placenta, are found in fetal tissues, and can have toxic effects on the developing fetus (often related to retardation of skeletal development). Evidence of embryotoxicity has also been noted in animals treated early in pregnancy. If any tetracyclines are used during pregnancy, or if the patient becomes pregnant while taking this drug, the patient should be apprised of the potential hazard to the fetus.

The catabolic action of the tetracyclines may cause an increase in BUN. Studies to date indicate that this does not occur with the use of doxycycline in patients with impaired renal function.

Photosensitivity manifested by an exaggerated sunburn reaction has been observed in some individuals taking tetracyclines. Patients apt to be exposed to direct sunlight or ultraviolet light should be advised that this reaction can occur with tetracycline drugs, and treatment of the capsules should be discontinued at the first evidence of skin erythema.

PRECAUTIONS

SUBGINGIVAL APPLICATION

General

Doxycycline hyclate has not been clinically tested in pregnant women.

Doxycycline hyclate has not been clinically evaluated in patients with conditions involving extremely severe periodontal defects with very little remaining periodontium.

Doxycycline hyclate has not been clinically tested for use in the regeneration of alveolar bone, either in preparation for or in conjunction with the placement of endosseous (dental) implants or in the treatment of failing implants.

Doxycycline hyclate has not been clinically tested in immunocompromised patients (such as patients immunocompromised by diabetes, chemotherapy, radiation therapy, or infection with HIV).

As with other antibiotic preparations, doxycycline hyclate therapy may result in overgrowth of nonsusceptible organisms, including fungi.[1] The effects of prolonged treatment, greater than 6 months, have not been studied.

Doxycycline hyclate should be used with caution in patients with a history of or predisposition to oral candidiasis. The safety and effectiveness of doxycycline hyclate have not been established for the treatment of periodontitis in patients with coexistent oral candidiasis.

Information for the Patient

Mechanical oral hygiene procedures (*i.e.,* tooth brushing, flossing) should be avoided on any treated areas for 7 days.

Avoid excessive sunlight or artificial ultraviolet light while receiving doxycycline.

Doxycycline may decrease the effectiveness of birth control pills.

Carcinogenesis, Mutagenesis, and Impairment of Fertility

Long-term studies in animals to evaluate carcinogenic potential of doxycycline have not been conducted. However, there has been evidence of oncogenic activity in rats in studies with the related antibiotics, oxytetracycline (adrenal and pituitary tumors), and minocycline (thyroid tumors). Likewise, although mutagenicity studies of doxycycline have not been conducted, positive results in *in vitro* mammalian cell assays have been reported for related antibiotics (tetracycline, oxytetracycline). Doxycycline administered orally at dosage levels as high as 250 mg/kg/day had no apparent effect on the fertility of female rats. Effect on male fertility has not been studied.

Pregnancy Category D

See WARNINGS.

Nursing Mothers

Tetracyclines appear in breast milk following oral administration. It is not known whether doxycycline is excreted in human milk following use of doxycycline hyclate. Because of the potential for serious adverse reactions in nursing infants from doxycycline, a decision should be made whether to discontinue nursing or to discontinue the drug, taking into account the importance of the drug to the mother. (See WARNINGS.)

Pediatric Use

The safety and effectiveness of doxycycline hyclate in pediatric patients have not been established. Oral doses of doxycycline in children up to 8 years of age have caused permanent discoloration of teeth.

CAPSULES

While no overgrowth by opportunistic microorganisms such as yeast were noted during clinical studies, as with other antimicrobials, doxycycline hyclate therapy may result in overgrowth of nonsusceptible microorganisms including fungi.

The use of tetracyclines may increase the incidence of vaginal candidiasis.

Doxycycline hyclate should be used with caution in patients with a history or predisposition to oral candidiasis. The safety and effectiveness of doxycycline hyclate has not been established for the treatment of periodontitis in patients with coexistent oral candidiasis.

If superinfection is suspected, appropriate measures should be taken.

Laboratory Tests

In long term therapy, periodic laboratory evaluations of organ systems, including hematopoietic, renal, and hepatic studies should be performed.

Drug/Laboratory Test Interactions

False elevations of urinary catecholamine levels may occur due to interference with the fluorescence test.

Carcinogenesis, Mutagenesis, and Impairment of Fertility

Doxycycline hyclate has not been evaluated for carcinogenic potential in long-term animal studies. Evidence of oncogenic activity was obtained in studies with related compounds (*i.e.,* oxytetracycline [adrenal and pituitary tumors] and minocycline [thyroid tumors]).

Doxycycline hyclate demonstrated no potential to cause genetic toxicity in an *in vitro* point mutation study with mammalian cells (CHO/HGPRT forward mutation assay) or in an *in vivo* micronucleus assay conducted in CD-1 mice. However, data from an *in vitro* assay with CHO cells for potential to cause chromosomal aberrations suggest that doxycycline hyclate is a weak clastogen.

Oral administration of doxycycline hyclate to male and female Sprague-Dawley rats adversely affected fertility and reproductive performance, as evidenced by increased time for mating to occur, reduced sperm motility, velocity, and concentration, abnormal sperm morphology, and increased pre- and post-implantation losses. Doxycycline hyclate induced reproductive toxicity at all dosages that were examined in this study, as even the lowest dosage tested (50 mg/kg/day) induced a statistically significant reduction in sperm velocity. Note that 50 mg/kg/day is approximately 10 times the amount of doxycycline hyclate contained in the recommended daily dose of doxycycline hyclate for a 60 kg human when compared on the basis of body surface area estimates (mg/m^2). Although doxycycline impairs the fertility of rats when administered at sufficient dosage, the effect of doxycycline hyclate on human fertility is unknown.

Pregnancy, Teratogenic Effects, Pregnancy Category D

(See WARNINGS.) Results from animal studies indicate that doxycycline crosses the placenta and is found in fetal tissues.

Nonteratogenic Effects: (See WARNINGS.)

Labor and Delivery

The effect of tetracyclines on labor and delivery is unknown.

Nursing Mothers

Tetracyclines are excreted in human milk. Because of the potential for serious adverse reactions in nursing infants from doxycycline, the use of doxycycline hyclate in nursing mothers is contraindicated. (See WARNINGS.)

Pediatric Use

The use of doxycycline hyclate in infancy and childhood is contraindicated. (See WARNINGS.)

DRUG INTERACTIONS

CAPSULES

Because tetracyclines have been shown to depress plasma prothrombin activity, patients who are on anticoagulant therapy may require downward adjustment of their anticoagulant dosage.

Since bacteriostatic antibiotics, such as the tetracycline class of antibiotics, may interfere with the bactericidal action of members of the β-lactam (*e.g.*, penicillin) class of antibiotics, it is not advisable to administer these antibiotics concomitantly.

Absorption of tetracyclines is impaired by antacids containing aluminum, calcium, or magnesium and by iron-containing preparations. Absorption is also impaired by bismuth subsalicylate.

Barbiturates, carbamazepine, and phenytoin decrease the half-life of doxycycline.

The concurrent use of tetracycline and Penthrane (methoxy-fluorane) has been reported to result in fatal renal toxicity.

Concurrent use of tetracycline may render oral contraceptives less effective.

ADVERSE REACTIONS

SUBGINGIVAL APPLICATION

In clinical trials involving a total of 1436 patients, adverse experiences from all causalities were monitored across treatment groups.

In the Circulatory System category, 10 subjects (1.6%) in the doxycycline hyclate group were reported as having "unspecified essential hypertension". Only 1 subject (0.2%) in the Vehicle group, and none in the Scaling and Root Planing or Oral Hygiene groups were reported to have "unspecified essential hypertension". In all cases, the event occurred anywhere from 13-134 days post treatment. There is no known association of oral administration of doxycycline with essential hypertension.

Two patients in the polymer vehicle group and none in the doxycycline hyclate group (0.2% for both groups combined) reported adverse events consistent with a localized allergic response.

Sex, age, race and smoking status did not appear to be correlated with adverse events.

TABLE 3 lists the incidence of treatment-emergent adverse events from all-causalities, across all treatment groups, occurring in ≥1% of the entire study population.

TABLE 3

Body System Verbatim Terms	Doxycycline n=609	Vehicle n=413	OH n=204	SRP n=210
Circulatory				
High blood pressure	1.6%	0.2%	0.0%	0.0%
Digestive				
Gum discomfort, pain or soreness; loss of attachment; increased pocket depth	18.1%	23.0%	20.1%	21.0%
Toothache, pressure sensitivity	14.3%	14.3%	10.3%	18.1%
Periodontal abscess, exudate, infection, drainage, extreme mobility, suppuration	9.9%	10.9%	10.3%	8.6%
Thermal tooth sensitivity	7.7%	8.5%	4.4%	6.7%
Gum inflammation, swelling, sensitivity	4.1%	5.8%	5.4%	5.7%
Soft tissue erythema, sore mouth, unspecified pain	4.3%	5.3%	2.7%	6.2%
Indigestion, upset stomach, stomach ache	3.6%	4.1%	2.9%	3.8%
Diarrhea	3.3%	2.4%	1.0%	1.0%
Tooth mobility, bone loss	2.0%	0.7%	0.5%	2.4%
Periapical abscess, lesion	1.5%	1.9%	1.0%	0.5%
Aphthous ulcer, canker sores	0.7%	1.7%	1.0%	1.4%
Fistula	0.8%	1.5%	1.5%	1.0%
Endodontic abscess, pulpitis	1.5%	1.5%	0.0%	0.5%
Jaw pain	1.1%	0.5%	1.0%	1.9%
Tooth loss	0.8%	1.5%	1.5%	0.0%
Bleeding gums	1.0%	0.7%	0.0%	2.4%
Genitourinary				
Premenstrual tension syndrome	4.4%	3.1%	2.5%	3.3%
Ill-Defined Conditions				
Headache	27.3%	28.1%	23.5%	23.8%
Cough	3.6%	6.1%	2.9%	2.4%
Sleeplessness	3.4%	1.5%	2.0%	2.9%
Body aches, soreness	1.6%	1.2%	1.5%	1.4%
Nausea and vomiting	1.8%	0.7%	2.5%	0.5%
Fever	1.0%	1.9%	1.0%	1.9%
Injury & Poisoning				
Broken tooth	5.1%	4.1%	4.9%	5.7%
Mental				
Tension headache	1.8%	0.7%	0.0%	1.0%
Musculoskeletal				
Muscle aches	6.4%	4.6%	4.9%	3.3%
Backaches	3.6%	5.3%	2.5%	6.2%
Pain in arms or legs	1.5%	2.2%	2.0%	2.4%
Lower back pain	1.6%	1.7%	0.5%	2.9%
Neck pain	1.3%	1.7%	1.0%	1.9%
Shoulder pain	1.0%	1.0%	1.5%	1.0%
Nervous System				
Ear infection	1.6%	1.9%	2.0%	0.0%
Respiratory				
Common cold	25.5%	25.2%	18.1%	16.7%
Flu, respiratory	6.1%	9.0%	3.9%	6.7%
Stuffy head, post nasal drip, congestion	5.6%	7.7%	2.9%	4.8%
Sore throat	5.7%	6.5%	2.0%	3.3%
Sinus infection	5.3%	2.7%	1.0%	1.9%
Flu	2.8%	2.9%	2.9%	3.3%
Bronchitis	2.3%	1.9%	1.5%	1.0%
Allergies	1.0%	1.0%	1.0%	1.9%
Skin & Subcutaneous Tissue				
Skin infection or inflammation	1.3%	1.0%	1.0%	1.0%

CAPSULES

Adverse Reactions in Clinical Trials of Doxycycline Hyclate

In clinical trials of adult patients with periodontal disease 213 patients received doxycycline hyclate 20 mg bid over a 9-12 month period. The most frequent adverse reactions occurring in studies involving treatment with doxycycline hyclate or placebo are listed in TABLE 4.

TABLE 4 *Incidence (%) of Adverse Reactions in Doxycycline Hyclate Capsules Clinical Trials*

Adverse Reaction	Doxycycline Hyclate 20 mg bid (n=213)	Placebo (n=215)
Headache	55 (26%)	56 (26%)
Common cold	47 (22%)	46 (21%)
Flu symptoms	24 (11%)	40 (19%)
Tooth ache	14 (7%)	28 (13%)
Periodontal abscess	8 (4%)	21 (10%)
Tooth disorder	13 (6%)	19 (9%)
Nausea	17 (8%)	12 (6%)
Sinusitis	7 (3%)	18 (8%)
Injury	11 (5%)	18 (8%)
Dyspepsia	13 (6%)	5 (2%)
Sore throat	11 (5%)	13 (6%)
Joint pain	12 (6%)	8 (4%)
Diarrhea	12 (6%)	8 (4%)
Sinus congestion	11 (5%)	11 (5%)
Coughing	9 (4%)	11 (5%)
Sinus headache	8 (4%)	8 (4%)
Rash	8 (4%)	6 (3%)
Back pain	7 (3%)	8 (4%)
Back ache	4 (2%)	9 (4%)
Menstrual cramp	9 (4%)	5 (2%)
Acid indigestion	8 (4%)	7 (3%)
Pain	8 (4%)	5 (2%)
Infection	4 (2%)	6 (3%)
Gum pain	1 (1%)	6 (3%)
Bronchitis	7 (3%)	5 (2%)
Muscle pain	2 (1%)	6 (3%)

Note: Percentages are based on total number of study participants in each treatment group.

Adverse Reactions for Tetracyclines

The following adverse reactions have been observed in patients receiving tetracyclines:

Gastrointestinal: Anorexia, nausea, vomiting, diarrhea, glossitis, dysphagia, enterocolitis, and inflammatory lesions (with vaginal candidiasis) in the anogenital region. Hepatoxicity has been reported rarely. Rare instances of esophagitis and esophageal ulcerations have been reported in patients receiving the capsule forms of the drugs in the tetracycline class. Most of these patients took medications immediately before going to bed. (See DOSAGE AND ADMINISTRATION.)

Skin: Maculopapular and erythematous rashes. Exfoliative dermatitis has been reported but is uncommon. (For information concerning photosensitivity, see WARNINGS.)

Renal Toxicity: Rise in BUN has been reported and is apparently dose related. (See WARNINGS.)

Hypersensitivity Reactions: Urticaria, angioneurotic edema, anaphylaxis, anaphylactoid purpura, serum sickness, pericarditis, and exacerbation of systemic lupus erythematosus.

Blood: Hemolytic anemia, thrombocytopenia, neutropenia, and eosinophilia have been reported.

DOSAGE AND ADMINISTRATION

SUBGINGIVAL APPLICATION

Preparation for Use

1. Remove the pouched product from refrigeration at least 15 minutes prior to mixing.
2. Couple Syringe A (liquid delivery system) and Syringe B (drug powder).
3. Inject the liquid contents of Syringe A (indicated by purple stripe) into Syringe B (doxycycline powder) and then push the contents back into Syringe A. This entire operation is 1 mixing cycle.
4. Complete 100 mixing cycles at a pace of 1 cycle/second using brisk strokes. **If immediate use is desired, skip to step 7.**
5. If necessary, the coupled syringes can be stored in the resealable pouch at room temperature for a maximum of 3 days.
6. After storage, perform an additional 10 mixing cycles just prior to use. **Continue with immediate use instructions.**
7. The contents will be in **Syringe A** (indicated by purple stripe). Hold the coupled syringes vertically with **Syringe A** at the bottom. Pull back on the **Syringe A** plunger and allow the contents to flow down the barrel for several seconds.
8. Uncouple the 2 syringes and attach the blunt cannula to **Syringe A. Product is now ready for application.**

Product Administration

Doxycycline hyclate does not require local anesthesia for placement. Bend the cannula to resemble a periodontal probe and explore the periodontal pocket in a manner similar to periodontal probing. Keeping the cannula tip near the base of the pocket, express the product into the pocket until the formulation reaches the top of the gingival margin. Withdraw the cannula tip from the pocket. In order to separate the tip from the formulation, turn the tip of the cannula towards the tooth, press the tip against the tooth surface, and pinch the string of formulation from the tip of the cannula. Variations on this technique may be needed to achieve separation between doxycycline hyclate and cannula.

If desired, using an appropriate dental instrument, doxycycline hyclate may be packed into the pocket. Dipping the edge of the instrument in water before packing will help keep doxycycline hyclate from sticking to the instrument, and will help speed coagulation of doxycycline hyclate. A few drops of water dripped onto the surface of doxycycline hyclate once in the pocket will also aid in coagulation. If necessary, add more doxycycline hyclate as described above and pack it into the pocket until the pocket is full.

Cover the pockets containing doxycycline hyclate with either Coe-Pak periodontal dressing or Octyldent dental adhesive.

Application of doxycycline hyclate may be repeated 4 months after initial treatment.

CAPSULES

THE DOSAGE OF DOXYCYCLINE HYCLATE CAPSULES DIFFERS FROM THAT OF DOXYCYCLINE USED TO TREAT INFECTIONS. EXCEEDING THE RECOMMENDED DOSAGE MAY RESULT IN AN INCREASED INCIDENCE OF SIDE EFFECTS INCLUDING THE DEVELOPMENT OF RESISTANT MICROORGANISMS.

Doxycycline hyclate 20 mg twice daily as an adjunct following scaling and root planing may be administered for up to 9 months. Safety beyond 12 months and efficacy beyond 9 months have not been established.

Doxycycline hyclate should be administered at least 1 hour prior to morning and evening meals.

Administration of adequate amounts of fluid along with the capsules is recommended to wash down the drug and reduce the risk of esophageal irritation and ulceration. (See ADVERSE REACTIONS.)

HOW SUPPLIED

SUBGINGIVAL APPLICATION

Atridox is available in a pouch containing a doxycycline hyclate syringe (50 mg), an ATRIGEL Delivery System syringe (450 mg), and a blunt cannula.

Each Atridox syringe system is intended for use in only 1 patient. Do not use if pouch has been previously opened or damaged.

Atridox is a variable dose product dependent on the size, shape, and number of pockets being treated.

Dosage Information

The final blended product is 500 mg of formulation containing 50.0 mg of doxycycline hyclate (10.0% doxycycline hyclate).
Storage: Store at 2-8°C (36-46°F).

CAPSULES

Periostat (white capsule imprinted with "Periostat") containing doxycycline hyclate equivalent to 20 mg doxycycline.
Storage: All products are to be stored at controlled room temperatures of 15-30°C (59-86°F) and dispensed in tight, light-resistant containers.

INTRAVENOUS

DESCRIPTION

FOR INTRAVENOUS USE ONLY

Vibramycin (doxycycline hyclate for injection) Intravenous is a broad-spectrum antibiotic synthetically derived from oxytetracycline, and is available as Vibramycin Hyclate (doxycycline hydrochloride hemiethanolate hemihydrate). The chemical designation of this light-yellow crystalline powder is alpha-6-deoxy-5-oxytetracycline. Doxycycline has a high degree of lipoid solubility and a low affinity for calcium binding. It is highly stable in normal human serum.

CLINICAL PHARMACOLOGY

ACTIONS

Doxycycline is primarily bacteriostatic and thought to exert its antimicrobial effect by the inhibition of protein synthesis. Doxycycline is active against a wide range of gram-positive and gram-negative organisms.

The drugs in the tetracycline class have closely similar antimicrobial spectra and cross resistance among them is common. Microorganisms may be considered susceptible to doxycycline (likely to respond to doxycycline therapy) if the minimum inhibitory concentration (MIC) is not more than 4.0 μg/ml. Microorganisms may be considered intermediate (harboring partial resistance) if the MIC is 4.0-12.5 μg/ml and resistant (not likely to respond to therapy) if the MIC is greater than 12.5 μg/ml.

Susceptibility plate testing: If the Kirby-Bauer method of disc susceptibility testing is used, a 30 μg doxycycline disc should give a zone of at least 16 mm when tested against a doxycycline-susceptible bacterial strain. A tetracycline disc may be used to determine microbial susceptibility. If the Kirby-Bauer method of disc susceptibility testing is used, a 30 μg tetracycline disc should give a zone of at least 19 mm when tested against a tetracycline-susceptible bacterial strain.

Tetracyclines are readily absorbed and are bound to plasma proteins in varying degree. They are concentrated by the liver in the bile, and excreted in the urine and feces at high concentrations and in a biologically active form.

Following a single 100 mg dose administered in a concentration of 0.4 mg/ml in a 1 hour infusion, normal adult volunteers average a peak of 2.5 μg/ml, while 200 mg of a concentration of 0.4 mg/ml administered over 2 hours averaged a peak of 3.6 μg/ml.

Excretion of doxycycline by the kidney is about 40%/72 hours in individuals with normal function (creatinine clearance about 75 ml/min.). This percentage excretion may fall as low as 1-5%/72 hours in individuals with severe renal insufficiency (creatinine clearance below 10 ml/min.). Studies have shown no significant difference in serum half-life of doxycycline (range 18-22 hours) in individuals with normal and severely impaired renal function.

Hemodialysis does not alter this serum half-life of doxycycline.

INDICATIONS AND USAGE

Doxycycline is indicated in infections caused by the following microorganisms:

Rickettsiae (Rocky Mountain spotted fever, typhus fever, and the typhus group, Q fever, rickettsialpox and tick fevers).

Mycoplasma pneumoniae (PPLO, Eaton Agent).

Agents of psittacosis and ornithosis.

Agents of lymphogranuloma venereum and granuloma inguinale.

The spirochetal agent of relapsing fever *(Borrelia recurrentis).*

The following gram-negative microorganisms:

Haemophilus ducreyi (chancroid), *Pasteurella pestis* and *Pasteurella tularensis, Bartonella bacilliformis, Bacteroides* species, *Vibrio comma* and *Vibrio fetus, Brucella* species (in conjunction with streptomycin).

Because many strains of the following groups of microorganisms have been shown to be resistant to tetracyclines, culture and susceptibility testing are recommended.

Doxycycline is indicated for treatment of infections caused by the following gram-negative microorganisms when bacteriologic testing indicates appropriate susceptibility to the drug:

Escherichia coli, Enterobacter aerogenes (formerly *Aerobacter aerogenes*), *Shigella* species, *Mima* species and *Herellea* species, *Haemophilus influenzae* (respiratory infections), *Klebsiella* species (respiratory and urinary infections).

Doxycycline is indicated for treatment of infections caused by the following gram-positive microorganisms when bacteriologic testing indicates appropriate susceptibility to the drug:

Streptococcus species: Up to 44% of strains of *Streptococcus pyogenes* and 74% of *Streptococcus faecalis* have been found to be resistant to tetracycline drugs. Therefore, tetracyclines should not be used for streptococcal disease unless the organism has been demonstrated to be sensitive.

For upper respiratory infections due to group A beta-hemolytic streptococci, penicillin is the usual drug of choice, including prophylaxis of rheumatic fever.

***Diplococcus pneumoniae, Staphylococcus aureus,* respiratory skin and soft tissue infections.** Tetracyclines are not the drugs of choice in the treatment of any type of staphylococcal infections.

Anthrax due to Bacillus anthracis, including inhalational anthrax (post-exposure): To reduce the incidence or progression of disease following exposure to aerosolized Bacillus anthracis.

When penicillin is contraindicated, doxycycline is an alternative drug in the treatment of infections due to:

Neisseria gonorrhoeae and N. meningitidis, Treponema pallidum and Treponema pertenue (syphilis and yaws), Listeria monocytogenes, Clostridium species, Fusobacterium fusiforme (Vincent's infection), Actinomyces species.

In acute intestinal amebiasis, doxycycline may be a useful adjunct to amebicides.

Doxycycline is indicated in the treatment of trachoma, although the infectious agent is not always eliminated, as judged by immunofluorescence.

CONTRAINDICATIONS

This drug is contraindicated in persons who have shown hypersensitivity to any of the tetracyclines.

WARNINGS

THE USE OF DRUGS OF THE TETRACYCLINE CLASS DURING TOOTH DEVELOPMENT (LAST HALF OF PREGNANCY, INFANCY AND CHILDHOOD TO THE AGE OF 8 YEARS) MAY CAUSE PERMANENT DISCOLORATION OF THE TEETH (YELLOW-GRAY-BROWN). This adverse reaction is more common during long-term use of the drugs but has been observed following repeated short-term courses. Enamel hypoplasia has also been reported. TETRACYCLINE DRUGS, THEREFORE, SHOULD NOT BE USED IN THIS AGE GROUP, EXCEPT FOR ANTHRAX, INCLUDING INHALATIONAL ANTHRAX (POST-EXPOSURE), UNLESS OTHER DRUGS ARE NOT LIKELY TO BE EFFECTIVE OR ARE CONTRAINDICATED.

Photosensitivity manifested by an exaggerated sunburn reaction has been observed in some individuals taking tetracyclines. Patients apt to be exposed to direct sunlight or ultraviolet light, should be advised that this reaction can occur with tetracycline drugs, and treatment should be discontinued at the first evidence of skin erythema.

The antianabolic action of the tetracyclines may cause an increase in BUN. Studies to date indicate that this does not occur with the use of doxycycline in patients with impaired renal function.

USE IN PREGNANCY

(See above WARNINGS about use during tooth development.)

Doxycycline hyclate for injection has not been studied in pregnant patients. It should not be used in pregnant women unless, in the judgment of the physician, it is essential for the welfare of the patient.

Results of animal studies indicate that tetracyclines cross the placenta, are found in fetal tissues and can have toxic effects on the developing fetus (often related to retardation of skeletal development). Evidence of embryotoxicity has also been noted in animals treated early in pregnancy.

USE IN CHILDREN

The use of doxycycline hyclate for injection in children under 8 years is not recommended because safe conditions for its use have not been established.

(See above WARNINGS about use during tooth development.)

As with other tetracyclines, doxycycline forms a stable calcium complex in any bone-forming tissue. A decrease in the fibula growth rate has been observed in prematures given oral tetracycline in doses of 25 mg/kg every 6 hours. This reaction was shown to be reversible when the drug was discontinued.

Tetracyclines are present in the milk of lactating women who are taking a drug in this class.

PRECAUTIONS

As with other antibiotic preparations, use of this drug may result in overgrowth of nonsusceptible organisms, including fungi. If superinfection occurs, the antibiotic should be discontinued and appropriate therapy instituted.

In venereal diseases when coexistent syphilis is suspected, a dark field examination should be done before treatment is started and the blood serology repeated monthly for at least 4 months.

Because tetracyclines have been shown to depress plasma prothrombin activity, patients who are on anticoagulant therapy may require downward adjustment of their anticoagulant dosage.

In long-term therapy, periodic laboratory evaluation of organ systems, including hematopoietic, renal, and hepatic studies should be performed.

All infections due to group A beta-hemolytic streptococci should be treated for at least 10 days.

Since bacteriostatic drugs may interfere with the bactericidal action of penicillin, it is advisable to avoid giving tetracycline in conjunction with penicillin.

ADVERSE REACTIONS

Gastrointestinal: Anorexia, nausea, vomiting, diarrhea, glossitis, dysphagia, enterocolitis, and inflammatory lesions (with monilial overgrowth) in the anogenital region. Hepatotoxicity has been reported rarely. These reactions have been caused by both the oral and parenteral administration of tetracyclines.

Skin: Maculopapular and erythematous rashes. Exfoliative dermatitis has been reported but is uncommon. Photosensitivity is discussed above. (See WARNINGS.)

Renal Toxicity: Rise in BUN has been reported and is apparently dose related. (See WARNINGS.)

Hypersensitivity Reactions: Urticaria, angioneurotic edema, anaphylaxis, anaphylactoid purpura, pericarditis and exacerbation of systemic lupus erythematosus.

Bulging fontanels in infants and benign intracranial hypertension in adults have been reported in individuals receiving full therapeutic dosages. These conditions disappeared rapidly when the drug was discontinued.

Blood: Hemolytic anemia, thrombocytopenia, neutropenia and eosinophilia have been reported.

When given over prolonged periods, tetracyclines have been reported to produce brown-black microscopic discoloration of thyroid glands. No abnormalities of thyroid function studies are known to occur.

DOSAGE AND ADMINISTRATION

Note: Rapid administration is to be avoided. Parenteral therapy is indicated only when oral therapy is not indicated. Oral therapy should be instituted as soon as possible. If intravenous therapy is given over prolonged periods of time, thrombophlebitis may result.

THE USUAL DOSAGE AND FREQUENCY OF ADMINISTRATION OF VIBRAMYCIN IV (100-200 mg/day) DIFFERS FROM THAT OF THE OTHER TETRACYCLINES (1-2 g/day). EXCEEDING THE RECOMMENDED DOSAGE MAY RESULT IN AN INCREASED INCIDENCE OF SIDE EFFECTS.

Studies to date have indicated that doxycycline at the usual recommended doses does not lead to excessive accumulation of the antibiotic in patients with renal impairment.

ADULTS

The usual dosage of doxycycline hyclate for injection is 200 mg on the first day of treatment administered in 1 or 2 infusions. Subsequent daily dosage is 100-200 mg depending upon the severity of infection, with 200 mg administered in 1 or 2 infusions.

In the treatment of primary and secondary syphilis, the recommended dosage is 300 mg daily for at least 10 days.

In the treatment of inhalational anthrax (post-exposure) the recommended dose is 100 mg of doxycycline, twice a day. Parenteral therapy is only indicated when oral therapy is not indicated and should not be continued over a prolonged period of time. Oral therapy should be instituted as soon as possible. Therapy must continue for a total of 60 days.

FOR CHILDREN ABOVE 8 YEARS OF AGE

The recommended dosage schedule for children weighing 100 lb or less is 2 mg/lb of body weight on the first day of treatment, administered in 1 or 2 infusions. Subsequent daily dosage is 1-2 mg/lb of body weight given as 1 or 2 infusions, depending on the severity of the infection. For children over 100 lb the usual adult dose should be used (see WARNINGS, Use in Children).

In the treatment of inhalational anthrax (post-exposure) the recommended dose is 1 mg/lb (2.2 mg/kg) of body weight, twice a day in children weighing less than 100 lb (45 kg). Parenteral therapy is only indicated when oral therapy is not indicated and should not be continued over a prolonged period of time. Oral therapy should be instituted as soon as possible. Therapy must continue for a total of 60 days.

GENERAL

The duration of infusion may vary with the dose (100-200 mg/day), but is usually 1-4 hours. A recommended minimum infusion time for 100 mg of a 0.5 mg/ml solution is 1 hour. Therapy should be continued for at least 24-48 hours after symptoms and fever have subsided. The therapeutic antibacterial serum activity will usually persist for 24 hours following recommended dosage.

Intravenous solutions should not be injected intramuscularly or subcutaneously. Caution should be taken to avoid the inadvertent introduction of the intravenous solution into the adjacent soft tissue.

PREPARATION OF SOLUTION

To prepare a solution containing 10 mg/ml, the contents of the vial should be reconstituted with 10 ml (for the 100 mg/vial container) or 20 ml (for the 200 mg/vial container) of sterile water for injection or any of the 10 intravenous infusion solutions listed below. Each 100 mg of doxycycline hyclate for injection (*i.e.,* withdraw entire solution from the 100 mg vial) is further diluted with 100-1000 ml of the intravenous solutions listed below. Each 200 mg of doxycycline hyclate for injection (*i.e.,* withdraw entire solution from the 200 mg vial) is further diluted with 200-2000 ml of the following intravenous solutions:

- Sodium chloride injection
- 5% Dextrose injection
- Ringer's injection
- Invert sugar, 10% in water
- Lactated Ringer's injection
- Dextrose 5% in lactated Ringer's
- Normosol-M in D5-W (Abbott)
- Normosol-R in D5-W (Abbott)
- Plasma-Lyte 56 in 5% dextrose (Travenol)
- Plasma-Lyte 148 in 5% dextrose (Travenol)

This will result in desired concentrations of 0.1-1.0 mg/ml. Concentrations lower than 0.1 mg/ml or higher than 1.0 mg/ml are not recommended.

STABILITY

Doxycycline hyclate for injection is stable for 48 hours in solution when diluted with sodium chloride injection, or 5% dextrose injection, to concentrations between 1.0 mg/ml and 0.1 mg/ml and stored at 25°C. Doxycycline hyclate for injection in these solutions is stable under fluorescent light for 48 hours, but must be protected from direct sunlight during storage and infusion. Reconstituted solutions (1.0 to 0.1 mg/ml) may be stored up to 72 hours prior to start of infusion if refrigerated and protected from sunlight and artificial light. Infusion must then be completed within 12 hours. Solutions must be used within these time periods or discarded.

Doxycycline hyclate for injection, when diluted with Ringer's injection, or invert sugar, 10% in water, or Normosol-M in D5-W (Abbott), or Normosol-R in D5-W (Abbott), or Plasma-Lyte 56 in 5% dextrose (Travenol), or Plasma-Lyte 148 in 5% dextrose (Travenol) to a concentration between 1.0 mg/ml and 0.1 mg/ml, must be completely infused within 12 hours after reconstitution to ensure adequate stability. During infusion, the solution must be protected from direct sunlight. Reconstituted solutions (1.0 to 0.1 mg/ml) may be stored up to 72 hours prior to start of infusion if refrigerated and protected from sunlight and artificial light. Infusion must then be completed within 12 hours. Solutions must be used within these time periods or discarded.

When diluted with lactated Ringer's injection, or dextrose 5% in lactated Ringer's, infusion of the solution (ca. 1.0 mg/ml) or lower concentrations (not less than 0.1 mg/ml) must be completed within 6 hours after reconstitution to ensure adequate stability. During infusion, the solution must be protected from direct sunlight. Solutions must be used within this time period or discarded.

Solutions of doxycycline hyclate for injection at a concentration of 10 mg/ml in sterile water for injection, when frozen immediately after reconstitution are stable for 8 weeks when stored at -20°C. If the product is warmed, care should be taken to avoid heating it after the thawing is complete. Once thawed the solution should not be refrozen.

HOW SUPPLIED

Vibramycin (doxycycline hyclate for injection) Intravenous is available as a sterile powder in a vial containing doxycycline hyclate equivalent to 100 mg of doxycycline with 480 mg of ascorbic acid; and in individually packaged vials containing doxycycline hyclate equivalent to 200 mg of doxycycline with 960 mg of ascorbic acid.

ORAL

DESCRIPTION

Vibramycin is a broad-spectrum antibiotic synthetically derived from oxytetracycline, and is available as Vibramycin Monohydrate (doxycycline monohydrate); Vibramycin Hyclate and Vibra-Tabs (doxycycline hydrochloride hemiethanolate hemihydrate); and Vibramycin Calcium (doxycycline calcium) for oral administration.

The molecular formula of doxycycline monohydrate is $C_{22}H_{24}N_2O_8 \cdot H_2O$ and a molecular weight of 462.46. The chemical designation for doxycycline is 4-(Dimethylamino)-1,4,4a,5,5a,6,11,12a-octahydro-3,5,10,12,12a-pentahydroxy-6-methyl-1,11-dioxo-2-naphthacenecarboxamide monohydrate. The molecular formula for doxycycline hydrochloride hemiethanolate hemihydrate is $(C_{22}H_{24}N_2O_8 \cdot HCl)_2 \cdot C_2H_6O \cdot H_2O$ and the molecular weight is 1025.89. Doxycycline is a light-yellow crystalline powder. Doxycycline hyclate is soluble in water, while doxycycline monohydrate is very slightly soluble in water.

Doxycycline has a high degree of lipoid solubility and a low affinity for calcium binding. It is highly stable in normal human serum. Doxycycline will not degrade into an epianhydro form.

Inert ingredients in the syrup formulation are: Apple flavor; butylparaben; calcium chloride; carmine; glycerin; hydrochloric acid; magnesium aluminum silicate; povidone; propylene glycol; propylparaben; raspberry flavor; simethicone emulsion; sodium hydroxide; sodium metabisulfite; sorbitol solution; water.

Inert ingredients in the capsule formulations are: Hard gelatin capsules (which may contain blue 1 and other inert ingredients); magnesium stearate; microcrystalline cellulose; sodium lauryl sulfate.

Inert ingredients for the oral suspension formulation are: Carboxymethylcellulose sodium; blue 1; methylparaben; microcrystalline cellulose; propylparaben; raspberry flavor; red 28; simethicone emulsion; sucrose.

Inert ingredients for the tablet formulation are: Ethylcellulose; hydroxypropyl methylcellulose; magnesium stearate; microcrystalline cellulose; propylene glycol; sodium lauryl sulfate; talc; titanium dioxide; yellow 6 lake.

CLINICAL PHARMACOLOGY

Tetracyclines are readily absorbed and are bound to plasma proteins in varying degree. They are concentrated by the liver in the bile, and excreted in the urine and feces at high concentrations and in a biologically active form. Doxycycline is virtually completely absorbed after oral administration.

Following a 200 mg dose, normal adult volunteers averaged peak serum levels of 2.6 μg/ml of doxycycline at 2 hours decreasing to 1.45 μg/ml at 24 hours. Excretion of doxycycline by the kidney is about 40%/72 hours in individuals with normal function (creatinine clearance about 75 ml/min). This percentage excretion may fall as low as 1-5%/72 hours in individuals with severe renal insufficiency (creatinine clearance below 10 ml/min). Studies have shown no significant difference in serum half-life of doxycycline (range 18-22 hours) in individuals with normal and severely impaired renal function.

Hemodialysis does not alter serum half-life.

Results of animal studies indicate that tetracyclines cross the placenta and are found in fetal tissues.

MICROBIOLOGY

The tetracyclines are primarily bacteriostatic and are thought to exert their antimicrobial effect by the inhibition of protein synthesis. The tetracyclines, including doxycycline, have a similar antimicrobial spectrum of activity against a wide range of gram-positive and gram-negative organisms. Cross-resistance of these organisms to tetracyclines is common.

GRAM-NEGATIVE BACTERIA

Neisseria gonorrhoeae
Calymmatobacterium granulomatis
Haemophilus ducreyi
Haemophilus influenzae
Yersinia pestis (formerly *Pasteurella pestis*)
Francisella tularensis (formerly *Pasteurella tularensis*)
Vibrio cholerae (formerly *Vibrio comma*)
Bartonella bacilliformis
Brucella species

Because many strains of the following groups of gram-negative microorganisms have been shown to be resistant to tetracyclines, culture and susceptibility testing are recommended:

Escherichia coli
Klebsiella species
Enterobacter aerogenes
Shigella species
Acinetobacter species (formerly *Mima* species and *Herellea* species)
Bacteroides species

GRAM-POSITIVE BACTERIA

Because many strains of the following groups of gram-positive microorganisms have been shown to be resistant to tetracycline, culture and susceptibility testing are recommended. Up to 44% of strains of *Streptococcus pyogenes* and 74% of *Streptococcus faecalis* have been found to be resistant to tetracycline drugs. Therefore, tetracycline should not be used for streptococcal disease unless the organism has been demonstrated to be susceptible.

Streptococcus pyogenes
Streptococcus pneumoniae
Enterococcus group (*Streptococcus faecalis* and *Streptococcus faecium*)
Alpha-hemolytic streptococci (viridans group)

OTHER MICROORGANISMS

Rickettsiae
Clostridium species
Chlamydia psittaci
Fusobacterium fusiforme
Chlamydia trachomatis
Actinomyces species
Mycoplasma pneumoniae
Bacillus anthracis
Ureaplasma urealyticum
Propionbacterium acnes
Borrelia recurrentis
Entamoeba species
Treponema pallidum
Balantidium coli
Treponema pertenue
Plasmodium falciparum

Doxycycline has been found to be active against the asexual erythrocytic forms of *Plasmodium falciparum* but not against the gametocytes of *P. falciparum*. The precise mechanism of action of the drug is not known.

SUSCEPTIBILITY TESTING

Diffusion Techniques

Quantitative methods that require measurement of zone diameters give the most precise estimate of the susceptibility of bacteria to antimicrobial agents. One such standard procedure[1] which has been recommended for use with disks to test susceptibility of organisms to doxycycline uses the 30 μg tetracycline-class disk or the 30 μg doxycycline disk. Interpretation involves the correlation of the diameter obtained in the disk test with the minimum inhibitory concentration (MIC) for tetracycline or doxycycline, respectively.

Reports from the laboratory giving results of the standard single-disk susceptibility test with a 30 μg tetracycline-class disk or the 30 μg doxycycline disk should be interpreted according to the criteria in TABLE 9.

A report of "Susceptible" indicates that the pathogen is likely to be inhibited by generally achievable blood levels. A report of "Intermediate" suggests that the organism would be susceptible if a high dosage is used or if the infection is confined to tissues and fluids in which high antimicrobial levels are attained. A report of "Resistant" indicates that achievable concentrations are unlikely to be inhibitory, and other therapy should be selected.

Standardized procedures require the use of laboratory control organisms. The 30 μg tetracycline-class disk or the 30 μg doxycycline disk should give the zone diameters in TABLE 10.

TABLE 9

Zone Diameter		
Tetracycline	Doxycycline	Interpretation
≥19 mm	≥16 mm	Susceptible
15-18 mm	13-15 mm	Intermediate
≤14 mm	≤12 mm	Resistant

TABLE 10

	Zone Diameter	
Organism	Tetracycline	Doxycycline
E. coli ATCC 25922	18-25 mm	18-24 mm
S. aureus ATCC 25923	19-28 mm	23-29 mm

Dilution Techniques

Use a standardized dilution method[2] (broth, agar, microdilution) or equivalent with tetracycline powder. The MIC values obtained should be interpreted according to the criteria found in TABLE 11.

TABLE 11

MIC	Interpretation
≤4 μg/ml	Susceptible
8 μg/ml	Intermediate
≥16 μg/ml	Resistant

As with standard diffusion techniques, dilution methods require the use of laboratory control organisms. Standard tetracycline powder should provide the MIC values found in TABLE 12.

TABLE 12

Organism	MIC
E. coli ATCC 25922	1.0-4.0 μg/ml
S. aureus ATCC 29213	0.25-1.0 μg/ml
E. faecalis ATCC 29212	8-32 μg/ml
P. aeruginosa ATCC 27853	8-32 μg/ml

INDICATIONS AND USAGE

TREATMENT

Doxycycline is indicated for the treatment of the following infections:

Rocky mountain spotted fever, typhus fever and the typhus group, Q fever, rickettsialpox, and tick fevers caused by Rickettsiae.
Respiratory tract infections caused by *Mycoplasma pneumoniae.*
Lymphogranuloma venereum caused by *Chlamydia trachomatis.*
Psittacosis (ornithosis) caused by *Chlamydia psittaci.*
Trachoma caused by *Chlamydia trachomatis,* although the infectious agent is not always eliminated as judged by immunofluorescence.
Inclusion conjunctivitis caused by *Chlamydia trachomatis.*
Uncomplicated urethral, endocervical or rectal infections in adults caused by *Chlamydia trachomatis.*
Nongonococcal urethritis caused by *Ureaplasma urealyticum.*
Relapsing fever due to *Borrelia recurrentis.*

Doxycycline is also indicated for the treatment of infections caused by the following gram-negative microorganisms:

Chancroid caused by *Haemophilus ducreyi.*
Plague due to *Yersinia pestis* (formerly *Pasteurella pestis*).
Tularemia due to *Francisella tularensis* (formerly *Pasteurella tularensis*).
Cholera caused by *Vibrio cholerae* (formerly *Vibrio comma*).
Campylobacter fetus infections caused by *Campylobacter fetus* (formerly *Vibrio fetus*).
Brucellosis due to *Brucella* species (in conjunction with streptomycin).
Bartonellosis due to *Bartonella bacilliformis.*
Granuloma inguinale caused by *Calymmatobacterium granulomatis.*

Because many strains of the following groups of microorganisms have been shown to be resistant to doxycycline, culture and susceptibility testing are recommended.

Doxycycline is indicated for treatment of infections caused by the following gram-negative microorganisms, when bacteriologic testing indicates appropriate susceptibility to the drug:

Escherichia coli.
Enterobacter aerogenes (formerly *Aerobacter aerogenes*).
Shigella species.
Acinetobacter species (formerly *Mima* species and *Herellea* species).
Respiratory tract infections caused by *Haemophilus influenzae.*
Respiratory tract and urinary tract infections caused by *Klebsiella* species.

Doxycycline is indicated for treatment of infections caused by the following gram-positive microorganisms when bacteriologic testing indicates appropriate susceptibility to the drug:

Upper respiratory tract infections caused by *Streptococcus pneumoniae* (formerly *Diplococcus pneumoniae*).

Anthrax due to *Bacillus anthracis,* including inhalational anthrax (post-exposure):

To reduce the incidence or progression of disease following exposure to aerosolized *Bacillus anthracis.*

When penicillin is contraindicated, doxycycline is an alternative drug in the treatment of the following infections:

- Uncomplicated gonorrhea caused by *Neisseria gonorrhoeae.*
- Syphilis caused by *Treponema pallidum.*
- Yaws caused by *Treponema pertenue.*
- Listeriosis due to *Listeria monocytogenes.*
- Vincent's infection caused by *Fusobacterium fusiforme.*
- Actinomycosis caused by *Actinomyces israelii.*
- Infections caused by *Clostridium* species.
- In acute intestinal amebiasis, doxycycline may be a useful adjunct to amebicides.
- In severe acne, doxycycline may be useful adjunctive therapy.

PROPHYLAXIS

Doxycycline is indicated for the prophylaxis of malaria due to *Plasmodium falciparum* in short-term travelers (<4 months) to areas with chloroquine and/or pyrimethamine-sulfadoxine resistant strains. See DOSAGE AND ADMINISTRATION and PRECAUTIONS, Information for the Patient.

CONTRAINDICATIONS

This drug is contraindicated in persons who have shown hypersensitivity to any of the tetracyclines.

WARNINGS

THE USE OF DRUGS OF THE TETRACYCLINE CLASS DURING TOOTH DEVELOPMENT (LAST HALF OF PREGNANCY, INFANCY AND CHILDHOOD TO THE AGE OF 8 YEARS) MAY CAUSE PERMANENT DISCOLORATION OF THE TEETH (YELLOW-GRAY-BROWN). This adverse reaction is more common during long-term use of the drugs, but it has been observed following repeated short-term courses. Enamel hypoplasia has also been reported. TETRACYCLINE DRUGS, THEREFORE, SHOULD NOT BE USED IN THIS AGE GROUP, EXCEPT FOR ANTHRAX, INCLUDING INHALATIONAL ANTHRAX (POST-EXPOSURE), UNLESS OTHER DRUGS ARE NOT LIKELY TO BE EFFECTIVE OR ARE CONTRAINDICATED.

Pseudomembranous colitis has been reported with nearly all antibacterial agents, including doxycycline, and may range in severity from mild to life-threatening. Therefore, it is important to consider this diagnosis in patients who present with diarrhea subsequent to the administration of antibacterial agents.

Treatment with antibacterial agents alters the normal flora of the colon and may permit overgrowth of clostridia. Studies indicate that a toxin produced by *Clostridium difficile* is a primary cause of "antibiotic-associated colitis".

After the diagnosis of pseudomembranous colitis has been established, therapeutic measures should be initiated. Mild cases of pseudomembranous colitis usually respond to discontinuation of the drug alone. In moderate to severe cases, consideration should be given to management with fluids and electrolytes, protein supplementation and treatment with an antibacterial drug clinically effective against *Clostridium difficile* colitis.

All tetracyclines form a stable calcium complex in any bone-forming tissue. A decrease in fibula growth rate has been observed in prematures given oral tetracycline in doses of 25 mg/kg every 6 hours. This reaction was shown to be reversible when the drug was discontinued.

Results of animal studies indicate that tetracyclines cross the placenta, are found in fetal tissues, and can have toxic effects on the developing fetus (often related to retardation of skeletal development). Evidence of embryotoxicity has also been noted in animals treated early in pregnancy. If any tetracycline is used during pregnancy or if the patient becomes pregnant while taking this drug, the patient should be apprised of the potential hazard to the fetus.

The antianabolic action of the tetracyclines may cause an increase in BUN. Studies to date indicate that this does not occur with the use of doxycycline in patients with impaired renal function.

Photosensitivity manifested by an exaggerated sunburn reaction has been observed in some individuals taking tetracyclines. Patients apt to be exposed to direct sunlight or ultraviolet light should be advised that this reaction can occur with tetracycline drugs, and treatment should be discontinued at the first evidence of skin erythema.

Doxycycline syrup contains sodium metabisulfite, a sulfite that may cause allergic-type reactions including anaphylactic symptoms and life-threatening or less severe asthmatic episodes in certain susceptible people. The overall prevalence of sulfite sensitivity in the general population is unknown and probably low. Sulfite sensitivity is seen more frequently in asthmatic than in non-asthmatic people.

PRECAUTIONS

GENERAL

As with other antibiotic preparations, use of this drug may result in overgrowth of nonsusceptible organisms, including fungi. If superinfection occurs, the antibiotic should be discontinued and appropriate therapy instituted.

Bulging fontanels in infants and benign intracranial hypertension in adults have been reported in individuals receiving tetracyclines. These conditions disappeared when the drug was discontinued.

Incision and drainage or other surgical procedures should be performed in conjunction with antibiotic therapy, when indicated.

Doxycycline offers substantial but not complete suppression of the asexual blood stages of *Plasmodium* strains.

Doxycycline does not suppress *P. falciparum's* sexual blood stage gametocytes. Subjects completing this prophylactic regimen may still transmit the infection to mosquitoes outside endemic areas.

INFORMATION FOR THE PATIENT

Patients taking doxycycline for malaria prophylaxis should be advised:

- That no present-day antimalarial agent, including doxycycline, guarantees protection against malaria.
- To avoid being bitten by mosquitoes by using personal protective measures that help avoid contact with mosquitoes, especially from dusk to dawn (*e.g.,* staying in well-screened areas, using mosquito nets, covering the body with clothing, and using an effective insect repellent.
- ***That Doxycycline Prophylaxis:***
  - Should begin 1-2 days before travel to the malarious area.
  - Should be continued daily while in the malarious area and after leaving the malarious area.
  - Should be continued for 4 further weeks to avoid development of malaria after returning from an endemic area.
  - Should not exceed 4 months.

All patients taking doxycycline should be advised:

- To avoid excessive sunlight or artificial ultraviolet light while receiving doxycycline and to discontinue therapy if phototoxicity (*e.g.,* skin eruption, etc.) occurs. Sunscreen or sunblock should be considered. (See WARNINGS.)
- To drink fluids liberally along with doxycycline to reduce the risk of esophageal irritation and ulceration. (See ADVERSE REACTIONS.)
- That the absorption of tetracyclines is reduced when taken with foods, especially those which contain calcium. However, the absorption of doxycycline is not markedly influenced by simultaneous ingestion of food or milk. (See DRUG INTERACTIONS.)
- That the absorption of tetracyclines is reduced when taking bismuth subsalicylate (see DRUG INTERACTIONS).
- That the use of doxycycline might increase the incidence of vaginal candidiasis.

LABORATORY TESTS

In venereal disease, when co-existent syphilis is suspected, dark field examinations should be done before treatment is started and the blood serology repeated monthly for at least 4 months.

In long-term therapy, periodic laboratory evaluation of organ systems, including hematopoietic, renal, and hepatic studies, should be performed.

DRUG/LABORATORY TEST INTERACTIONS

False elevations of urinary catecholamine levels may occur due to interference with the fluorescence test.

CARCINOGENESIS, MUTAGENESIS, AND IMPAIRMENT OF FERTILITY

Long-term studies in animals to evaluate carcinogenic potential of doxycycline have not been conducted. However, there has been evidence of oncogenic activity in rats in studies with the related antibiotics, oxytetracycline (adrenal and pituitary tumors), and minocycline (thyroid tumors).

Likewise, although mutagenicity studies of doxycycline have not been conducted, positive results in *in vitro* mammalian cell assays have been reported for related antibiotics (tetracycline, oxytetracycline).

Doxycycline administered orally at dosage levels as high as 250 mg/kg/day had no apparent effect on the fertility of female rats. Effect on male fertility has not been studied.

PREGNANCY, TERATOGENIC EFFECTS, PREGNANCY CATEGORY D

There are no adequate and well-controlled studies on the use of doxycycline in pregnant women. The vast majority of reported experience with doxycycline during human pregnancy is short-term, first trimester exposure. There are no human data available to assess the effects of long-term therapy of doxycycline in pregnant women such as that proposed for treatment of anthrax exposure. An expert review of published data on experiences with doxycycline use during pregnancy by TERIS — the Teratogen Information System — concluded that therapeutic doses during pregnancy are unlikely to pose a substantial teratogenic risk (the quantity and quality of data were assessed as limited to fair), but the data are insufficient to state that there is no risk[3]. A case-control study (18,515 mothers of infants with congenital anomalies and 32,804 mothers of infants with no congenital anomalies) shows a weak but marginally statistically significant association with total malformations and use of doxycycline anytime during pregnancy. Sixty-three (0.19%) of the controls and 56 (0.30%) of the cases were treated with doxycycline. This association was not seen when the analysis was confined to maternal treatment during the period of organogenesis (*i.e.,* in the second and third months of gestation) with the exception of a marginal relationship with neural tube defect based on only 2 exposed cases[4].

A small prospective study of 81 pregnancies describes 43 pregnant women treated for 10 days with doxycycline during early first trimester. All mothers reported their exposed infants were normal at 1 year of age[5].

Nonteratogenic Effects: (See WARNINGS.)

LABOR AND DELIVERY

The effect of tetracyclines on labor and delivery is unknown.

NURSING MOTHERS

Tetracyclines are excreted in human milk; however, the extent of absorption of tetracyclines, including doxycycline, by the breastfed infant is not known. Short-term use by lactating women is not necessarily contraindicated; however, the effects of prolonged exposure to doxycycline in breast milk are unknown[6]. Because of the potential for serious adverse reactions in nursing infants from doxycycline, a decision should be made whether to discontinue nursing or to discontinue the drug, taking into account the importance of the drug to the mother. (See WARNINGS.)

PEDIATRIC USE

See WARNINGS and DOSAGE AND ADMINISTRATION.

DRUG INTERACTIONS

Because tetracyclines have been shown to depress plasma prothrombin activity, patients who are on anticoagulant therapy may require downward adjustment of their anticoagulant dosage.

Since bacteriostatic drugs may interfere with the bactericidal action of penicillin, it is advisable to avoid giving tetracyclines in conjunction with penicillin.

Absorption of tetracyclines is impaired by antacids containing aluminum, calcium, or magnesium, and iron-containing preparations.

Absorption of tetracycline is impaired by bismuth subsalicylate.

Barbiturates, carbamazepine, and phenytoin decrease the half-life of doxycycline.

The concurrent use of tetracycline and methoxyflurane has been reported to result in fatal renal toxicity.

Concurrent use of tetracycline may render oral contraceptives less effective.

ADVERSE REACTIONS

Due to oral doxycycline's virtually complete absorption, side effects of the lower bowel, particularly diarrhea, have been infrequent.

The following adverse reactions have been observed in patients receiving tetracyclines:

Gastrointestinal: Anorexia, nausea, vomiting, diarrhea, glossitis, dysphagia, enterocolitis, and inflammatory lesions (with monilial overgrowth) in the anogenital region. Hepatotoxicity has been reported rarely. These reactions have been caused by both the oral and parenteral administration of tetracyclines. Rare instances of esophagitis and esophageal ulcerations have been reported in patients receiving capsule and tablet forms of the drugs in the tetracycline class. Most of these patients took medications immediately before going to bed. (See DOSAGE AND ADMINISTRATION.)

Skin: Maculopapular and erythematous rashes. Exfoliative dermatitis has been reported but is uncommon. Photosensitivity is discussed above. (See WARNINGS.)

Renal Toxicity: Rise in BUN has been reported and is apparently dose related. (See WARNINGS.)

Hypersensitivity Reactions: Urticaria, angioneurotic edema, anaphylaxis, anaphylactoid purpura, serum sickness, pericarditis, and exacerbation of systemic lupus erythematosus.

Blood: Hemolytic anemia, thrombocytopenia, neutropenia, and eosinophilia have been reported.

Other: Bulging fontanels in infants and intracranial hypertension in adults. See PRECAUTIONS, General.

When given over prolonged periods, tetracyclines have been reported to produce brown-black microscopic discoloration of the thyroid gland. No abnormalities of thyroid function studies are known to occur.

DOSAGE AND ADMINISTRATION

THE USUAL DOSAGE AND FREQUENCY OF ADMINISTRATION OF DOXYCYCLINE DIFFERS FROM THAT OF THE OTHER TETRACYCLINES. EXCEEDING THE RECOMMENDED DOSAGE MAY RESULT IN AN INCREASED INCIDENCE OF SIDE EFFECTS.

Adults: The usual dose of oral doxycycline is 200 mg on the first day of treatment (administered 100 mg every 12 hours) followed by a maintenance dose of 100 mg/day. The maintenance dose may be administered as a single dose or as 50 mg every 12 hours.

In the management of more severe infections (particularly chronic infections of the urinary tract), 100 mg every 12 hours is recommended.

For Children Above 8 Years of Age: The recommended dosage schedule for children weighing 100 lb or less is 2 mg/lb of body weight divided into 2 doses on the first day of treatment, followed by 1 mg/lb of body weight given as a single daily dose or divided into 2 doses, on subsequent days. For more severe infections up to 2 mg/lb of body weight may be used. For children over 100 lb the usual adult dose should be used.

The therapeutic antibacterial serum activity will usually persist for 24 hours following recommended dosage.

When used in streptococcal infections, therapy should be continued for 10 days.

Administration of adequate amounts of fluid along with capsule and tablet forms of drugs in the tetracycline class is recommended to wash down the drugs and reduce the risk of esophageal irritation and ulceration. (See ADVERSE REACTIONS.)

If gastric irritation occurs, it is recommended that doxycycline be given with food or milk. The absorption of doxycycline is not markedly influenced by simultaneous ingestion of food or milk.

Studies to date have indicated that administration of doxycycline at the usual recommended doses does not lead to excessive accumulation of the antibiotic in patients with renal impairment.

Uncomplicated gonococcal infections in adults (except anorectal infections in men): 100 mg, by mouth, twice a day for 7 days. As an alternate single visit dose, administer 300 mg stat followed in 1 hour by a second 300 mg dose. The dose may be administered with food, including milk or carbonated beverage, as required.

Uncomplicated urethral, endocervical, or rectal infection in adults caused by Chlamydia trachomatis: 100 mg by mouth twice a day for 7 days.

Nongonococcal urethritis (NGU) caused by C. trachomatis or U. urealyticum: *100 mg by mouth twice a day for 7 days.*

Syphilis — Early: *Patients who are allergic to penicillin should be treated with doxycycline 100 mg by mouth twice a day for 2 weeks.*

Syphilis of More Than 1 Year's Duration: *Patients who are allergic to penicillin should be treated with doxycycline 100 mg by mouth twice a day for 4 weeks.*

Acute Epididymo-Orchitis Caused by N. gonorrhoeae: *100 mg, by mouth, twice a day for at least 10 days.*

Acute Epididymo-Orchitis Caused by C. trachomatis: *100 mg, by mouth, twice a day for at least 10 days.*

For Prophylaxis of Malaria: *For adults, the recommended dose is 100 mg daily. For children over 8 years of age, the recommended dose is 2 mg/kg given once daily up to the adult dose. Prophylaxis should begin 1-2 days before travel to the malarious area. Prophylaxis should be continued daily during travel in the malarious area and for 4 weeks after the traveler leaves the malarious area.*

Inhalational Anthrax (post-exposure):

Adults: *100 mg of doxycycline, by mouth, twice a day for 60 days.*

Children: *Weighing less than 100 lb (45 kg); 1 mg/lb (2.2 mg/kg) of body weight, by mouth, twice a day for 60 days. Children weighing 100 lb or more should receive the adult dose.*

ANIMAL PHARMACOLOGY

Hyperpigmentation of the thyroid has been produced by members of the tetracycline class in the following species: in rats by oxytetracycline, doxycycline, tetracycline PO_4, and methacycline; in minipigs by doxycycline, minocycline, tetracycline PO_4, and methacycline; in dogs by doxycycline and minocycline; in monkeys by minocycline.

Minocycline, tetracycline PO_4, methacycline, doxycycline, tetracycline base, oxytetracycline HCl, and tetracycline HCl were goitrogenic in rats fed a low iodine diet. This goitrogenic effect was accompanied by high radioactive iodine uptake. Administration of minocycline also produced a large goiter with high radioiodine uptake in rats fed a relatively high iodine diet.

Treatment of various animal species with this class of drugs has also resulted in the induction of thyroid hyperplasia in the following: in rats and dogs (minocycline); in chickens (chlortetracycline); and in rats and mice (oxytetracycline). Adrenal gland hyperplasia has been observed in goats and rats treated with oxytetracycline.

HOW SUPPLIED

CAPSULES

Vibramycin Hyclate (doxycycline hyclate) is available in:

50 mg: White and light blue and are imprinted with "VIBRA" on one half and "PFIZER 094" on the other half.

100 mg: Light blue and are imprinted with "VIBRA" on one half and "PFIZER 095" on the other half.

Storage: Store below 30°C (86°F) and dispense in tight, light-resistant containers.

TABLETS

Vibra-Tabs (doxycycline hyclate) is available in:

100 mg: Salmon colored film-coated tablets imprinted on one side with "VIBRA-TABS" and "PFIZER 099" on the other side.

Storage: Store below 30°C (86°F) and dispense in tight, light-resistant containers.

ORAL SUSPENSION

Vibramycin Calcium Syrup (doxycycline calcium) is available as a raspberry-apple flavored oral suspension. Each teaspoonful (5 ml) contains doxycycline calcium equivalent to 50 mg of doxycycline: 1 pint (473 ml) bottles.

Vibramycin Monohydrate (doxycycline monohydrate) is available as a raspberry-flavored, dry powder for oral suspension. When reconstituted, each teaspoonful (5 ml) contains doxycycline monohydrate equivalent to 25 mg of doxycycline: 2 oz (60 ml) bottles.

Storage: Store below 30°C (86°F) and dispense in tight, light-resistant containers.

PRODUCT LISTING - RATED THERAPEUTICALLY EQUIVALENT

Package	Price	Product, Manufacturer	NDC
Capsule - Oral - Hyclate 50 mg			
16's	$4.14	GENERIC, Pd-Rx Pharmaceuticals	55289-0502-16
30's	$23.78	GENERIC, Heartland Healthcare Services	61392-0731-30
30's	$23.78	GENERIC, Heartland Healthcare Services	61392-0731-39
31's	$24.57	GENERIC, Heartland Healthcare Services	61392-0731-31
32's	$25.37	GENERIC, Heartland Healthcare Services	61392-0731-32
45's	$35.67	GENERIC, Heartland Healthcare Services	61392-0731-45
50's	$9.00	GENERIC, West Ward Pharmaceutical Corporation	00143-3141-50
50's	$9.50	GENERIC, Dunhall Pharmaceuticals Inc	00217-0804-50
50's	$12.60	GENERIC, Watson/Schein Pharmaceuticals Inc	00364-2032-50
50's	$13.23	GENERIC, Moore, H.L. Drug Exchange Inc	00839-1288-04
50's	$14.65	GENERIC, Martec Pharmaceuticals Inc	52555-0433-00
50's	$15.86	GENERIC, Purepac Pharmaceutical Company	00228-2194-05
50's	$15.93	GENERIC, Aligen Independent Laboratories Inc	00405-4378-50
50's	$19.95	GENERIC, Major Pharmaceuticals Inc	00904-0427-51
50's	$37.35	GENERIC, Watson/Schein Pharmaceuticals Inc	00591-5535-50
50's	$37.35	GENERIC, Watson/Rugby Laboratories Inc	52544-0500-50
50's	$37.75	GENERIC, Mylan Pharmaceuticals Inc	00378-0145-89
50's	$37.80	GENERIC, Mutual/United Research Laboratories	00677-0598-02
50's	$37.80	GENERIC, Mutual Pharmaceutical Co Inc	53489-0118-02
50's	$41.01	GENERIC, Ivax Corporation	00172-2984-48
50's	$41.01	GENERIC, Qualitest Products Inc	00603-3480-19
50's	$110.39	VIBRAMYCIN HYCLATE, Pfizer U.S. Pharmaceuticals	00069-0940-50
60's	$9.54	GENERIC, Pd-Rx Pharmaceuticals	55289-0235-60
60's	$47.56	GENERIC, Heartland Healthcare Services	61392-0731-60
90's	$71.34	GENERIC, Heartland Healthcare Services	61392-0731-90
100's	$15.25	GENERIC, Raway Pharmacal Inc	00686-0148-20
100's	$32.20	GENERIC, Major Pharmaceuticals Inc	00904-0427-61
100's	$51.53	GENERIC, Watson/Schein Pharmaceuticals Inc	00364-2032-90
100's	$145.10	GENERIC, Par Pharmaceutical Inc	49884-0726-01
Capsule - Oral - Hyclate 100 mg			
2's	$5.25	GENERIC, Pd-Rx Pharmaceuticals	55289-0107-02
2's	$5.25	GENERIC, Pd-Rx Pharmaceuticals	55289-0866-02
6's	$8.82	GENERIC, Pd-Rx Pharmaceuticals	55289-0107-06
10's	$10.35	GENERIC, Pd-Rx Pharmaceuticals	55289-0107-10
12's	$10.41	GENERIC, Pd-Rx Pharmaceuticals	55289-0107-12

14's	$3.14	GENERIC, Pd-Rx Pharmaceuticals	58864-0190-14
14's	$6.60	GENERIC, West Ward Pharmaceutical Corporation	00143-3142-14
14's	$10.50	GENERIC, Pd-Rx Pharmaceuticals	55289-0107-14
14's	$11.58	GENERIC, Pd-Rx Pharmaceuticals	55289-0866-14
14's	$17.00	GENERIC, Dixon-Shane Inc	17236-0527-14
14's	$73.94	VIBRAMYCIN, Pd-Rx Pharmaceuticals	55289-0043-14
20's	$3.68	GENERIC, Pd-Rx Pharmaceuticals	58864-0190-20
20's	$13.29	GENERIC, Pd-Rx Pharmaceuticals	55289-0107-20
20's	$14.34	GENERIC, Pd-Rx Pharmaceuticals	55289-0866-20
20's	$18.26	GENERIC, Dhs Inc	55887-0979-20
20's	$27.20	GENERIC, St. Mary'S Mpp	60760-0562-20
21's	$19.07	GENERIC, Dhs Inc	55887-0979-21
28's	$14.22	GENERIC, Pd-Rx Pharmaceuticals	55289-0107-28
28's	$25.43	GENERIC, Dhs Inc	55887-0979-28
28's	$34.00	GENERIC, Dixon-Shane Inc	17236-0527-28
30's	$4.58	GENERIC, Pd-Rx Pharmaceuticals	58864-0190-30
30's	$18.00	GENERIC, Pd-Rx Pharmaceuticals	55289-0107-30
30's	$27.24	GENERIC, Dhs Inc	55887-0979-30
30's	$57.69	GENERIC, Heartland Healthcare Services	61392-0732-30
30's	$57.69	GENERIC, Heartland Healthcare Services	61392-0732-39
31's	$59.62	GENERIC, Heartland Healthcare Services	61392-0732-31
32's	$61.54	GENERIC, Heartland Healthcare Services	61392-0732-32
40's	$17.01	GENERIC, Pd-Rx Pharmaceuticals	55289-0107-40
45's	$86.54	GENERIC, Heartland Healthcare Services	61392-0732-45
50's	$18.70	GENERIC, Mova Pharmaceutical Corporation	55370-0813-05
50's	$21.65	GENERIC, Martec Pharmaceuticals Inc	52555-0434-00
50's	$23.50	GENERIC, Watson/Schein Pharmaceuticals Inc	00364-2033-50
50's	$24.82	GENERIC, Aligen Independent Laboratories Inc	00405-4377-50
50's	$25.25	GENERIC, Moore, H.L. Drug Exchange Inc	00839-1289-04
50's	$25.35	GENERIC, West Ward Pharmaceutical Corporation	00143-3142-50
50's	$29.65	GENERIC, Parmed Pharmaceuticals Inc	00349-1008-50
50's	$65.75	GENERIC, Major Pharmaceuticals Inc	00904-0428-51
50's	$66.43	GENERIC, Dixon-Shane Inc	17236-0527-55
50's	$67.10	GENERIC, Mylan Pharmaceuticals Inc	00378-0148-89
50's	$67.10	GENERIC, Mutual/United Research Laboratories	00677-0562-02
50's	$67.10	GENERIC, Mutual Pharmaceutical Co Inc	53489-0119-02
50's	$68.47	GENERIC, Watson Laboratories Inc	00591-0498-50
50's	$68.47	GENERIC, Watson Laboratories Inc	00591-5440-50
50's	$68.47	GENERIC, Watson Laboratories Inc	52544-0498-50
50's	$70.21	GENERIC, Ivax Corporation	00172-2985-48
50's	$70.21	GENERIC, Qualitest Products Inc	00603-3481-19
50's	$118.45	GENERIC, Par Pharmaceutical Inc	49884-0727-03
50's	$225.30	VIBRAMYCIN, Pfizer U.S. Pharmaceuticals	00069-0950-50
56's	$20.40	GENERIC, Pd-Rx Pharmaceuticals	55289-0107-56
60's	$21.48	GENERIC, Pd-Rx Pharmaceuticals	55289-0107-60
60's	$115.39	GENERIC, Heartland Healthcare Services	61392-0732-60
90's	$173.08	GENERIC, Heartland Healthcare Services	61392-0732-90
100's	$12.02	GENERIC, Us Trading Corporation	56126-0019-11
100's	$12.71	GENERIC, Pd-Rx Pharmaceuticals	55289-0107-01
100's	$21.00	GENERIC, Raway Pharmacal Inc	00686-0522-20
100's	$39.93	GENERIC, Pd-Rx Pharmaceuticals	55289-0107-17
100's	$55.50	GENERIC, West Ward Pharmaceutical Corporation	00143-3142-25
100's	$60.15	GENERIC, Ivax Corporation	00182-1035-89
100's	$123.13	GENERIC, Vangard Labs	00615-0385-13
100's	$134.20	GENERIC, Udl Laboratories Inc	51079-0522-20
100's	$580.00	GENERIC, Watson Laboratories Inc	00591-5440-05

Capsule - Oral - Monohydrate 50 mg

100's	$118.74	GENERIC, Watson Laboratories Inc	52544-0309-01
100's	$130.61	GENERIC, Eon Labs Manufacturing Inc	00185-0805-01

Capsule - Oral - Monohydrate 100 mg

50's	$96.92	GENERIC, Watson Laboratories Inc	52544-0310-50
50's	$106.61	GENERIC, Eon Labs Manufacturing Inc	00185-0810-53
100's	$213.23	GENERIC, Eon Labs Manufacturing Inc	00185-0810-01
250's	$465.80	GENERIC, Watson Laboratories Inc	52544-0310-25
250's	$512.39	GENERIC, Eon Labs Manufacturing Inc	00185-0810-52
250's	$512.39	GENERIC, Par Pharmaceutical Inc	49884-0727-04

Capsule - Oral - 50 mg

50's	$4.20	FEDERAL UPPER LIMIT, H.C.F.A. F F P	99999-1113-11

Capsule - Oral - 100 mg

50's	$5.25	FEDERAL UPPER LIMIT, H.C.F.A. F F P	99999-1113-09

Capsule, Enteric Coated - Oral - Hyclate 100 mg

50's	$102.50	GENERIC, Major Pharmaceuticals Inc	00904-0429-51
50's	$124.45	GENERIC, Purepac Pharmaceutical Company	00228-2598-07
50's	$152.94	DORYX, Warner Chilcott Laboratories	00430-0838-19

Powder For Injection - Injectable - 100 mg

5's	$73.75	GENERIC, American Pharmaceutical Partners	63323-0130-10
10's	$147.50	GENERIC, Bedford Laboratories	55390-0100-10

Tablet - Oral - Hyclate 100 mg

2's	$0.92	GENERIC, Allscripts Pharmaceutical Company	54569-3074-06
14's	$3.24	GENERIC, Pd-Rx Pharmaceuticals	58864-0189-14
14's	$4.55	GENERIC, Versapharm Inc	61748-0111-14
20's	$3.80	GENERIC, Pd-Rx Pharmaceuticals	58864-0189-20
20's	$4.40	GENERIC, Major Pharmaceuticals Inc	00904-0428-95
20's	$10.07	GENERIC, Golden State Medical	60429-0069-20
30's	$4.76	GENERIC, Pd-Rx Pharmaceuticals	58864-0189-30
50's	$9.75	GENERIC, Interstate Drug Exchange Inc	00814-2660-08
50's	$12.83	GENERIC, Moore, H.L. Drug Exchange Inc	00839-6641-04
50's	$15.00	GENERIC, Dunhall Pharmaceuticals Inc	00217-0805-50
50's	$17.70	GENERIC, Mova Pharmaceutical Corporation	55370-0814-05
50's	$19.39	GENERIC, Watson/Schein Pharmaceuticals Inc	00364-2063-50
50's	$21.65	GENERIC, Martec Pharmaceuticals Inc	52555-0229-00
50's	$25.00	GENERIC, Marin Pharmaceutical	12539-0484-53
50's	$25.01	GENERIC, Aligen Independent Laboratories Inc	00405-4379-50
50's	$27.00	GENERIC, Bristol-Myers Squibb	00003-0812-40
50's	$29.85	GENERIC, Esi Lederle Generics	00005-3116-18
50's	$31.21	GENERIC, Ivax Corporation	00172-3626-48
50's	$65.75	GENERIC, Major Pharmaceuticals Inc	00904-0430-51
50's	$67.10	GENERIC, Mylan Pharmaceuticals Inc	00378-0167-89
50's	$67.10	GENERIC, Mutual/United Research Laboratories	00677-0799-02
50's	$67.10	GENERIC, Mutual Pharmaceutical Co Inc	53489-0120-02
50's	$68.47	GENERIC, Watson/Schein Pharmaceuticals Inc	00591-5553-50
50's	$68.47	GENERIC, Qualitest Products Inc	00603-3482-19
50's	$68.47	GENERIC, Watson/Rugby Laboratories Inc	52544-0499-50
50's	$225.30	VIBRA-TABS, Pfizer U.S. Pharmaceuticals	00069-0990-50
100's	$15.55	GENERIC, Raway Pharmacal Inc	00686-0554-20
100's	$32.82	GENERIC, Major Pharmaceuticals Inc	00904-0428-61
100's	$52.15	GENERIC, Ivax Corporation	00182-1535-89
100's	$55.40	GENERIC, Udl Laboratories Inc	51079-0554-20
100's	$119.86	GENERIC, Auro Pharmaceutical	55829-0662-10
100's	$138.40	GENERIC, Major Pharmaceuticals Inc	00904-0430-61

Tablet - Oral - 100 mg

50's	$5.85	FEDERAL UPPER LIMIT, H.C.F.A. F F P	99999-1113-13

PRODUCT LISTING - EQUIVALENTS NOT AVAILABLE

Capsule - Oral - Hyclate 50 mg

20's	$15.10	GENERIC, Allscripts Pharmaceutical Company	54569-0147-02
50's	$6.30	GENERIC, Interstate Drug Exchange Inc	00814-2663-08
50's	$10.00	GENERIC, Cmc-Consolidated Midland Corporation	00223-0871-00
50's	$37.74	GENERIC, Allscripts Pharmaceutical Company	54569-0147-01
100's	$19.50	GENERIC, Cmc-Consolidated Midland Corporation	00223-0871-01

Capsule - Oral - Hyclate 100 mg

1's	$3.41	GENERIC, Prescript Pharmaceuticals	00247-0006-01
2's	$3.46	GENERIC, Prescript Pharmaceuticals	00247-0006-02
3's	$3.52	GENERIC, Prescript Pharmaceuticals	00247-0006-03
4's	$2.10	GENERIC, Allscripts Pharmaceutical Company	54569-1840-04
4's	$3.56	GENERIC, Prescript Pharmaceuticals	00247-0006-04
5's	$3.62	GENERIC, Prescript Pharmaceuticals	00247-0006-05
6's	$2.91	GENERIC, Southwood Pharmaceuticals Inc	58016-0156-06
6's	$3.67	GENERIC, Prescript Pharmaceuticals	00247-0006-06
6's	$8.34	GENERIC, Pharma Pac	52959-0055-06
7's	$3.39	GENERIC, Southwood Pharmaceuticals Inc	58016-0156-07
7's	$3.73	GENERIC, Prescript Pharmaceuticals	00247-0006-07
8's	$3.78	GENERIC, Prescript Pharmaceuticals	00247-0006-08
10's	$3.88	GENERIC, Prescript Pharmaceuticals	00247-0006-10
10's	$8.87	GENERIC, Southwood Pharmaceuticals Inc	58016-0156-10
10's	$8.87	GENERIC, Southwood Pharmaceuticals Inc	58016-0161-10
10's	$12.06	GENERIC, Pharma Pac	52959-0055-10
11's	$3.94	GENERIC, Prescript Pharmaceuticals	00247-0006-11
11's	$14.74	GENERIC, Allscripts Pharmaceutical Company	54569-1840-07
12's	$3.99	GENERIC, Prescript Pharmaceuticals	00247-0006-12
12's	$10.64	GENERIC, Southwood Pharmaceuticals Inc	58016-0156-12
12's	$10.64	GENERIC, Southwood Pharmaceuticals Inc	58016-0161-12
12's	$16.08	GENERIC, Allscripts Pharmaceutical Company	54569-1840-03
14's	$4.09	GENERIC, Prescript Pharmaceuticals	00247-0006-14
14's	$12.40	GENERIC, Southwood Pharmaceuticals Inc	58016-0161-14
14's	$12.41	GENERIC, Southwood Pharmaceuticals Inc	58016-0156-14
14's	$16.34	GENERIC, Pharma Pac	52959-0055-14
14's	$17.23	GENERIC, Pharmaceutical Corporation Of America	51655-0186-84
15's	$4.15	GENERIC, Prescript Pharmaceuticals	00247-0006-15
15's	$13.29	GENERIC, Southwood Pharmaceuticals Inc	58016-0161-15
15's	$13.30	GENERIC, Southwood Pharmaceuticals Inc	58016-0156-15
15's	$17.48	GENERIC, Pharma Pac	52959-0055-15
16's	$14.19	GENERIC, Southwood Pharmaceuticals Inc	58016-0156-16
16's	$14.19	GENERIC, Southwood Pharmaceuticals Inc	58016-0161-16
17's	$4.26	GENERIC, Prescript Pharmaceuticals	00247-0006-17
18's	$15.96	GENERIC, Southwood Pharmaceuticals Inc	58016-0161-18
20's	$4.41	GENERIC, Prescript Pharmaceuticals	00247-0006-20
20's	$10.50	GENERIC, Allscripts Pharmaceutical Company	54569-1840-01
20's	$17.73	GENERIC, Southwood Pharmaceuticals Inc	58016-0156-20
20's	$17.73	GENERIC, Southwood Pharmaceuticals Inc	58016-0161-20
20's	$20.37	GENERIC, Pharma Pac	52959-0055-20
20's	$23.40	GENERIC, Pharmaceutical Corporation Of America	51655-0186-52
21's	$4.47	GENERIC, Prescript Pharmaceuticals	00247-0006-21
21's	$18.61	GENERIC, Southwood Pharmaceuticals Inc	58016-0161-21
21's	$18.62	GENERIC, Southwood Pharmaceuticals Inc	58016-0156-21

Qty	Price	Manufacturer	NDC
24's	$21.28	GENERIC, Southwood Pharmaceuticals Inc	58016-0156-24
24's	$21.28	GENERIC, Southwood Pharmaceuticals Inc	58016-0161-24
28's	$4.84	GENERIC, Prescript Pharmaceuticals	00247-0006-28
28's	$24.82	GENERIC, Southwood Pharmaceuticals Inc	58016-0156-28
28's	$24.82	GENERIC, Southwood Pharmaceuticals Inc	58016-0161-28
28's	$28.34	GENERIC, Pharma Pac	52959-0055-28
30's	$4.94	GENERIC, Prescript Pharmaceuticals	00247-0006-30
30's	$26.60	GENERIC, Southwood Pharmaceuticals Inc	58016-0156-30
30's	$30.24	GENERIC, Pharma Pac	52959-0055-30
40's	$20.99	GENERIC, Allscripts Pharmaceutical Company	54569-1840-00
40's	$35.46	GENERIC, Southwood Pharmaceuticals Inc	58016-0156-40
40's	$35.46	GENERIC, Southwood Pharmaceuticals Inc	58016-0161-40
42's	$5.58	GENERIC, Prescript Pharmaceuticals	00247-0006-42
50's	$6.00	GENERIC, Prescript Pharmaceuticals	00247-0006-50
50's	$44.33	GENERIC, Southwood Pharmaceuticals Inc	58016-0161-50
56's	$6.32	GENERIC, Prescript Pharmaceuticals	00247-0006-56
60's	$53.20	GENERIC, Southwood Pharmaceuticals Inc	58016-0156-60
60's	$53.20	GENERIC, Southwood Pharmaceuticals Inc	58016-0161-60
100's	$88.60	GENERIC, Southwood Pharmaceuticals Inc	58016-0156-00
100's	$91.11	GENERIC, Pharma Pac	52959-0055-00
Capsule - Oral - Monohydrate 50 mg			
100's	$118.74	GENERIC, Watson Laboratories Inc	52544-0410-01
100's	$161.24	MONODOX, Oclassen Pharmaceuticals Inc	55515-0260-06
Capsule - Oral - Monohydrate 100 mg			
50's	$96.92	GENERIC, Watson Laboratories Inc	52544-0411-50
50's	$131.62	MONODOX, Oclassen Pharmaceuticals Inc	55515-0259-04
250's	$465.80	GENERIC, Watson Laboratories Inc	52544-0411-25
250's	$632.58	MONODOX, Oclassen Pharmaceuticals Inc	55515-0259-07
Capsule - Oral - 20 mg			
100's	$80.94	PERIOSTAT, Collagenex Pharmaceuticals	27280-0007-01
Capsule, Enteric Coated - Oral - Hyclate 75 mg			
60's	$155.99	DORYX, Warner Chilcott Laboratories	00430-0836-20
Powder For Reconstitution - Oral - 25 mg/5 ml			
60 ml	$13.74	VIBRAMYCIN MONOHYDRATE, Pfizer U.S. Pharmaceuticals	00069-0970-65
Syrup - Oral - 50 mg/5 ml			
480 ml	$208.49	VIBRAMYCIN CALCIUM, Pfizer U.S. Pharmaceuticals	00069-0971-93
Tablet - Oral - Hyclate 100 mg			
6's	$3.33	GENERIC, Allscripts Pharmaceutical Company	54569-3074-00
7's	$3.88	GENERIC, Allscripts Pharmaceutical Company	54569-0118-02
8's	$4.44	GENERIC, Allscripts Pharmaceutical Company	54569-3074-01
10's	$1.68	GENERIC, Circle Pharmaceuticals Inc	00659-0132-10
10's	$5.54	GENERIC, Allscripts Pharmaceutical Company	54569-0118-00
14's	$7.76	GENERIC, Allscripts Pharmaceutical Company	54569-0118-01
15's	$8.32	GENERIC, Allscripts Pharmaceutical Company	54569-3074-02
20's	$3.26	GENERIC, Circle Pharmaceuticals Inc	00659-0132-20
20's	$11.09	GENERIC, Allscripts Pharmaceutical Company	54569-0118-03
20's	$18.65	GENERIC, Pharma Pac	52959-0474-20
28's	$15.52	GENERIC, Allscripts Pharmaceutical Company	54569-0118-05
30's	$16.63	GENERIC, Allscripts Pharmaceutical Company	54569-0118-06
50's	$9.45	GENERIC, Interstate Drug Exchange Inc	00814-2665-08
50's	$12.50	GENERIC, Cmc-Consolidated Midland Corporation	00223-0872-05
50's	$19.95	GENERIC, Edwards Pharmaceuticals Inc	00485-0041-50
50's	$25.00	GENERIC, Marin Pharmaceutical	12539-0743-53
50's	$68.47	GENERIC, Watson Laboratories Inc	00591-0499-50
60's	$33.26	GENERIC, Allscripts Pharmaceutical Company	54569-0118-08
100's	$55.44	GENERIC, Allscripts Pharmaceutical Company	54569-0118-09
Tablet - Oral - Monohydrate 50 mg			
100's	$186.91	GENERIC, Bioglan Pharmaceutical Inc	62436-0728-01
Tablet - Oral - Monohydrate 100 mg			
50's	$152.59	GENERIC, Bioglan Pharmaceutical Inc	62436-0729-03
250's	$733.27	GENERIC, Bioglan Pharmaceutical Inc	62436-0729-04
Tablet - Oral - 20 mg			
100's	$99.69	PERIOSTAT, Collagenex Pharmaceuticals	64682-0008-02

Dronabinol *(001116)*

Categories: Anorexia, secondary to HIV; Nausea, secondary to cancer chemotherapy; Vomiting, secondary to cancer chemotherapy; Pregnancy Category B; DEA Class CII; FDA Approved 1985 May; Orphan Drugs
Drug Classes: Antiemetics/antivertigo
Brand Names: Marezine; **Marinol**
Cost of Therapy: \$2065.48 (Nausea and Vomiting; Marinol; 10 mg; 4 capsules/day; 30 day supply)
\$216.25 (Apetite Stimulation; Marinol; 2.5 mg; 2 capsules/day; 30 day supply)

DESCRIPTION

Dronabinol is a cannabinoid designated chemically as (6aR-trans)-6a,7,8,10a-tetrahydro-6,6,9-trimethyl-3-pentyl-6H-dibenzo[b,d]pyran-1-ol.

The empirical formula is $C_{21}H_{30}O_2$. The molecular weight is 314.47.

Dronabinol, delta-9-tetrahydrocannabinol (delta-9-THC), is naturally occurring and has been extracted from *Cannabis sativa L.* (marijuana).

Dronabinol is also chemically synthesized and is a light-yellow resinous oil that is sticky at room temperature and hardens upon refrigeration. Dronabinol is insoluble in water and is formulated in sesame oil. It has a pKa of 10.6 and an octanol-water partition coefficient: 6000:1 at pH 7.

CAPSULES FOR ORAL ADMINISTRATION

Marinol is supplied as round, soft gelatin capsules containing either 2.5, 5, or 10 mg dronabinol. Each Marinol capsule is formulated with the following inactive ingredients: sesame oil, gelatin, glycerin, methylparaben, propylparaben, FD&C yellow no. 6 (5 mg and 10 mg), and titanium dioxide.

D

CLINICAL PHARMACOLOGY

Dronabinol is an orally active cannabinoid which, like other cannabinoids, has complex effects on the central nervous system (CNS), including central sympathomimetic activity. Cannabinoid receptors have been discovered in neural tissues. These receptors may play a role in mediating the effects of dronabinol and other cannabinoids.

PHARMACODYNAMICS

Dronabinol-induced sympathomimetic activity may result in tachycardia and/or conjunctival injection. Its effects on blood pressure are inconsistent, but occasional subjects have experienced orthostatic hypotension and/or syncope upon abrupt standing.

Dronabinol also demonstrates reversible effects on appetite, mood, cognition, memory, and perception. These phenomena appear to be dose-related, increasing in frequency with higher dosages, and subject to great interpatient variability.

After oral administration, dronabinol has an onset of action of approximately 0.5 to 1 hours and peak effect at 2-4 hours. Duration of action for psychoactive effects is 4-6 hours, but the appetite stimulant effect of dronabinol may continue for 24 hours or longer after administration.

Tachyphylaxis and tolerance develop to some of the pharmacologic effects of dronabinol and other cannabinoids with chronic use, suggesting an indirect effect on sympathetic neurons. In a study of the pharmacodynamics of chronic dronabinol exposure, healthy male volunteers (n=12) received 210 mg/day dronabinol, administered orally in divided doses, for 16 days. An initial tachycardia induced by dronabinol was replaced successively by normal sinus rhythm and then bradycardia. A decrease in supine blood pressure, made worse by standing, was also observed initially. These volunteers developed tolerance to the cardiovascular and subjective adverse CNS effects of dronabinol within 12 days of treatment initiation.

Tachyphylaxis and tolerance do not, however, appear to develop to the appetite stimulant effect of dronabinol. In studies involving patients with Acquired Immune Deficiency Syndrome (AIDS), the appetite stimulant effect of dronabinol has been sustained for up to five months in clinical trials, at dosages ranging from 2.5 to 20 mg/day.

PHARMACOKINETICS

Absorption and Distribution

Dronabinol is almost completely absorbed (90-95%) after single oral doses. Due to the combined effects of first pass hepatic metabolism and high lipid solubility, only 10-20% of the administered dose reaches the systemic circulation. Dronabinol has a large apparent volume of distribution, approximately 10 L/kg, because of its lipid solubility. The plasma protein binding of dronabinol and its metabolites is approximately 97%.

The elimination phase of dronabinol can be described using a two compartment model with an initial (alpha) half-life of about 4 hours and a terminal (beta) half-life of 25-36 hours. Because of its large volume of distribution, dronabinol and its metabolites may be excreted at low levels for prolonged periods of time.

Metabolism

Dronabinol undergoes extensive first-pass hepatic metabolism, primarily by microsomal hydroxylation, yielding both active and inactive metabolites. Dronabinol and its principal active metabolite, 11-OH-delta-9-THC, are present in approximately equal concentrations in plasma. Concentrations of both parent drug and metabolite peak at approximately 2-4 hours after oral dosing and decline over several days. Values for clearance average about 0.2 L/kg-h, but are highly variable due to the complexity of cannabinoid distribution.

Elimination

Dronabinol and its biotransformation products are excreted in both feces and urine. Biliary excretion is the major route of elimination with about half of a radiolabeled oral dose being recovered from the feces within 72 hours as contrasted with 10-15% recovered from urine. Less than 5% of an oral dose is recovered unchanged in the feces.

Following single dose administration, low levels of dronabinol metabolites have been detected for more than 5 weeks in the urine and feces.

In a study of dronabinol involving AIDS patients, urinary cannabinoid/creatinine concentration ratios were studied biweekly over a six week period. The urinary cannabinoid/creatinine ratio was closely correlated with dose. No increase in the cannabinoid/creatinine ratio was observed after the first two weeks of treatment, indicating that steady-state cannabinoid levels had been reached. This conclusion is consistent with prediction based on the observed terminal half-life of dronabinol.

Special Populations

The pharmacokinetic profile of dronabinol has not been investigated in either pediatric or geriatric patients.

INDICATIONS AND USAGE

Dronabinol is Indicated for the Treatment of:

1. Anorexia associated with weight loss in patients with AIDS.
2. Nausea and vomiting associated with cancer chemotherapy in patients who have failed to respond adequately to conventional antiemetic treatments.

CONTRAINDICATIONS

Dronabinol is contraindicated in any patient who has a history of hypersensitivity to any cannabinoid or sesame oil.

WARNINGS

Dronabinol is a medication with a potential for abuse. Physicians and pharmacists should use the same care in prescribing and accounting for dronabinol as they would with morphine or other drugs controlled under Schedule II (CII) of the Controlled Substances Act. Because of the risk of diversion, it is recommended that prescriptions be limited to the amount necessary for the period between clinic visits.

Patients receiving treatment with dronabinol should be specifically warned not to drive, operate machinery, or engage in any hazardous activity until it is established that they are able to tolerate the drug and to perform such tasks safely.

PRECAUTIONS

GENERAL

The risk/benefit ratio of dronabinol use should be carefully evaluated in patients with the following medical conditions because of individual variation in response and tolerance to the effects of dronabinol.

Dronabinol should be used with caution in patients with cardiac disorders because of occasional hypotension, possible hypertension, syncope, or tachycardia (see CLINICAL PHARMACOLOGY).

Dronabinol should be used with caution in patients with a history of substance abuse, including alcohol abuse or dependence, because they may be more prone to abuse dronabinol as well. Multiple substance abuse is common and marijuana, which contains the same active compound, is a frequently abused substance.

Dronabinol should be used with caution and careful psychiatric monitoring in patients with mania, depression, or schizophrenia because dronabinol may exacerbate these illnesses.

Dronabinol should be used with caution in patients receiving concomitant therapy with sedatives, hypnotics, or other psychoactive drugs because of the potential for additive or synergistic CNS effects.

Dronabinol should be used with caution in pregnant patients, nursing mothers, or pediatric patients because it has not been studied in these patient populations.

Dronabinol should be used with caution for treatment of anorexia and weight loss in elderly patients with AIDS because they may be more sensitive to the psychoactive effects and because its use in these patients has not been studied.

INFORMATION FOR THE PATIENT

Patients receiving treatment with dronabinol should be alerted to the potential for additive central nervous system depression if dronabinol is used concomitantly with alcohol or other CNS depressants such as benzodiazepines and barbiturates.

Patients receiving treatment with dronabinol should be specifically warned not to drive, operate machinery, or engage in any hazardous activity until it is established that they are able to tolerate the drug and to perform such tasks safely.

Patients using dronabinol should be advised of possible changes in mood and other adverse behavioral effects of the drug so as to avoid panic in the event of such manifestations. Patients should remain under the supervision of a responsible adult during initial use of dronabinol and following dosage adjustments.

CARCINOGENESIS, MUTAGENESIS, AND IMPAIRMENT OF FERTILITY

Carcinogenicity studies have not been performed with dronabinol. Mutagenicity testing of dronabinol was negative in an Ames test. In a long-term study (77 days) in rats, oral administration of dronabinol at doses of 30-150 mg/m^2, equivalent to 0.3-1.5 times maximum recommended human dose (MRHD) of 90 mg/m^2/day in cancer patients or 2-10 times MRHD of 15 mg/m^2/day in AIDS patients, reduced ventral prostate, seminal vesicle and epididymal weights and caused a decrease in seminal fluid volume. Decreases in spermatogenesis, number of developing germ cells, and number of Leydig cells in the testis were also observed. However, sperm count, mating success, and testosterone levels were not affected. The significance of these animal findings in humans is not known.

PREGNANCY CATEGORY C

Reproduction studies with dronabinol have been performed in mice at 15-450 mg/m^2, equivalent to 0.2 to 5 times maximum recommended human dose (MRHD) of 90 mg/m^2/day in cancer patients or 1-30 times MRHD of 15 mg/m^2/day in AIDS patients, and in rats at 74-295 mg/m^2 (equivalent to 0.8 to 3 times MRHD of 90 mg/m^2 in cancer patients or 5-20 times MRHD of 15 mg/m^2/day in AIDS patients). These studies have revealed no evidence of teratogenicity due to dronabinol. At these dosages in mice and rats, dronabinol decreased maternal weight gain and number of viable pups and increased fetal mortality and early resorptions. Such effects were dose dependent and less apparent at lower doses which produced less maternal toxicity. There are no adequate and well-controlled studies in pregnant women. Dronabinol should be used only if the potential benefit justifies the potential risk to the fetus.

NURSING MOTHERS

Use of dronabinol is not recommended in nursing mothers since, in addition to the secretion of HIV virus in breast milk, dronabinol is concentrated in and secreted in human breast milk and is absorbed by the nursing baby.

DRUG INTERACTIONS

In studies involving patients with AIDS and/or cancer, dronabinol has been co-administered with a variety of medications (*e.g.,* cytotoxic agents, anti-infective agents, sedatives, or opioid analgesics) without resulting in any clinically significant drug/drug interactions. Although no drug/drug interactions were discovered during the clinical trials of dronabinol, cannabinoids may interact with other medication through both metabolic and pharmacodynamic mechanisms. Dronabinol is highly protein bound to plasma proteins, and therefore, might displace other protein-bound drugs. Although this displacement has not been confirmed *in vivo,* practitioners should monitor patients for a change in dosage requirements when administering dronabinol to patients receiving other highly protein-bound drugs. Published reports of drug/drug interactions involving cannabinoids are summarized in TABLE 2.

TABLE 2

Concomitant Drug	Clinical Effect(s)
Amphetamines, cocaine, other sympathomimetic agents	Additive hypertension, tachycardia, possibly cardiotoxicity
Atropine, scopolamine, antihistamines, other anticholinergic agents	Additive or super-additive tachycardia, drowsiness
Amitriptyline, amoxapine, desipramine, other tricyclic antidepressants	Additive tachycardia, hypertension, drowsiness
Barbiturates, benzodiazepines, ethanol, lithium, opioids, buspirone, antihistamines, muscle relaxants, other CNS depressants	Additive drowsiness and CNS depression
Disulfiram	A reversible hypomanic reaction was reported in a 28 y/o man who smoked marijuana; confirmed by dechallenge and rechallenge.
Fluoxetine	A 21 y/o female with depression and bulimia receiving 20 mg/day fluoxetine × 4 weeks became hypomanic after smoking marijuana; symptoms resolved after 4 days.
Antipyrine, barbiturates	Decreased clearance of these agents, presumably via competitive inhibition of metabolism
Theophylline	Increased theophylline metabolism reported with smoking of marijuana; effect similar to that following smoking tobacco

ADVERSE REACTIONS

Adverse experiences information summarized below was derived from well-controlled clinical trials conducted in the US and US territories involving 474 patients exposed to dronabinol. Studies of AIDS-related weight loss included 157 patients receiving dronabinol at a dose of 2.5 mg twice daily and 67 receiving placebo. Studies of different durations were combined by considering the first occurrence of events during the first 28 days. Studies of nausea and vomiting related to cancer chemotherapy included 317 patients receiving dronabinol and 68 receiving placebo.

A cannabinoid dose-related "high" (easy laughing, elation and heightened awareness) has been reported by patients receiving dronabinol in both the antiemetic (24%) and the lower dose appetite stimulant clinical trials (8%).

The most frequently reported adverse experiences in patients with AIDS during placebo-controlled clinical trials involved the CNS and were reported by 33% of patients receiving dronabinol. About 25% of patients reported a minor CNS adverse event during the first 2 weeks and about 4% reported such an event each week for the next 6 weeks thereafter.

PROBABLY CAUSALLY RELATED: INCIDENCE GREATER THAN 1%

Rates derived from clinical trials in AIDS-related anorexia (n=157) and chemotherapy-related nausea (n=317). Rates were generally higher in the anti-emetic use (given in parentheses).

Body as a Whole: Asthenia.
Cardiovascular: Palpitations, tachycardia, vasodilation/facial flush.
Digestive: Abdominal pain*, nausea*, vomiting*.
Nervous System: (Amnesia), anxiety/nervousness, (ataxia), confusion, depersonalization, dizziness*, euphoria*, (hallucination), paranoid reaction*, somnolence*, thinking abnormal.

* Incidence of events 3-10%.

PROBABLY CAUSALLY RELATED: INCIDENCE LESS THAN 1%

Event rates derived from clinical trials in AIDS-related anorexia (n=157) and chemotherapy-related nausea (n=317).

Cardiovascular: Conjunctivitis*, hypotension*.
Digestive: Diarrhea*, fecal incontinence.
Musculoskeletal: Myalgias.
Nervous System: Depression, nightmares, speech difficulties, tinnitus.
Skin and Appendages: Flushing*.
Special Senses: Vision difficulties.

* Incidence of events 0.3-1%.

CAUSAL RELATIONSHIP UNKNOWN: INCIDENCE LESS THAN 1%

The clinical significance of the association of these events with dronabinol treatment is unknown, but they are reported as alerting information for the clinician.

Body as a Whole: Chills, headache, malaise.
Digestive: Anorexia, hepatic enzyme elevation.
Respiratory: Cough, rhinitis, sinusitis.
Skin and Appendages: Sweating.

DOSAGE AND ADMINISTRATION

APPETITE STIMULATION

Initially, 2.5 mg dronabinol should be administered orally twice daily (b.i.d.), before lunch and supper. For patients unable to tolerate this 5 mg/day dosage of dronabinol, the dosage can be reduced to 2.5 mg/day administered as a single dose in the evening or at bedtime. If clinically indicated and in the absence of significant adverse effects, the dosage may be gradually increased to a maximum of 20 mg/day dronabinol, administered in divided oral doses. Caution should be exercised in escalating the dosage of dronabinol because of the increased frequency of dose-related adverse experiences at higher dosages (see PRECAUTIONS).

ANTIEMETIC

Dronabinol is best administered at an initial dose of 5 mg/m^2, given 1-3 hours prior to the administration of chemotherapy, then every 2-4 hours after chemotherapy is given, for a total of 4-6 doses/day. Should the 5 mg/m^2 dose prove to be ineffective, and in the absence of significant side effects, the dose may be escalated by 2.5 mg/m^2 increments to a maximum of 15 mg/m^2 per dose. Caution should be exercised in dose escalation, however, as the incidence of disturbing psychiatric symptoms increases significantly at maximum dose (see PRECAUTIONS).

SAFETY AND HANDLING

Dronabinol should be packaged in a well-closed container and stored in a cool environment between 8-15°C (46-59°F). Protect from freezing. No particular hazard to health care workers handling the capsules has been identified.

Access to abusable drugs such as dronabinol presents an occupational hazard for addiction in the health care industry. Routine procedures for handling controlled substances developed to protect the public may not be adequate to protect health-care workers. Implementation of more effective accounting procedures and measures to appropriately restrict access to drugs of this class may minimize the risk of self-administration by health-care providers.

HOW SUPPLIED

Marinol Capsules (dronabinol solution in sesame oil in soft gelatin capsules): *2.5 mg:* White. *5 mg:* Dark brown. *10 mg:* Orange.

PRODUCT LISTING - EQUIVALENTS NOT AVAILABLE

Capsule - Oral - 2.5 mg			
60's	$216.25	MARINOL, Roxane Laboratories Inc	00054-2601-21
60's	$270.20	MARINOL, Roxane Laboratories Inc	00051-0021-21
Capsule - Oral - 5 mg			
25's	$187.54	MARINOL, Roxane Laboratories Inc	00054-2602-11
25's	$234.31	MARINOL, Roxane Laboratories Inc	00051-0022-11
Capsule - Oral - 10 mg			
60's	$1032.74	MARINOL, Unimed Pharmaceuticals	00051-0023-21

Droperidol *(001117)*

Categories: Nausea; Vomiting; Pregnancy Category C; FDA Approved 1970 Jun
Drug Classes: Anesthetics, general; Antiemetics/antivertigo; Anxiolytics; Sedatives/hypnotics
Brand Names: **Inapsine**
Foreign Brand Availability: Dehidrobenzoperidol (Portugal; Spain); Dehydrobenzperidol (Austria; Bahrain; Belgium; Cyprus; Czech-Republic; Denmark; Egypt; Finland; Germany; Iran; Iraq; Jordan; Kuwait; Lebanon; Libya; Mexico; Netherlands; Oman; Qatar; Republic-of-Yemen; Saudi-Arabia; Switzerland; Syria; Taiwan; Thailand; Turkey; United-Arab-Emirates); Droleptan (Australia; Bahrain; Cyprus; Egypt; England; France; Iran; Iraq; Jordan; Kuwait; Lebanon; Libya; New-Zealand; Oman; Qatar; Republic-of-Yemen; Saudi-Arabia; Syria; United-Arab-Emirates); Droperol (India); Inapsin (South-Africa); Sintodian (Italy)
HCFA JCODE(S): J1790 up to 5 mg IM, IV

WARNING

FOR INTRAVENOUS OR INTRAMUSCULAR USE ONLY

Cases of QT prolongation and/or torsades de pointes have been reported in patients receiving droperidol at doses at or below recommended doses. Some cases have occurred in patients with no known risk factors for QT prolongation and some cases have been fatal.

Due to its potential for serious proarrhythmic effects and death, droperidol should be reserved for use in the treatment of patients who fail to show an acceptable response to other adequate treatments, either because of insufficient effectiveness or the inability to achieve an effective dose due to intolerable adverse effects from those drugs (see WARNINGS, ADVERSE REACTIONS, CONTRAINDICATIONS, and PRECAUTIONS).

Cases of QT prolongation and serious arrhythmias (*e.g.,* torsades de pointes) have been reported in patients treated with droperidol. Based on these reports, all patients should undergo a 12-lead ECG prior to administration of droperidol to determine if a prolonged QT interval (*i.e.,* QTc greater than 440 milliseconds for males or 450 milliseconds for females) is present. If there is a prolonged QT interval, droperidol should NOT be administered. For patients in whom the potential benefit of droperidol treatment is felt to outweigh the risks of potentially serious arrhythmias, ECG monitoring should be performed prior to treatment and continued for 2-3 hours after completing treatment to monitor for arrhythmias.

Droperidol is contraindicated in patients with known or suspected QT prolongation, including patients with congenital long QT syndrome.

Droperidol should be administered with extreme caution to patients who may be at risk for development of prolonged QT syndrome (*e.g.,* congestive heart failure, bradycardia, use of a diuretic, cardiac hypertrophy, hypokalemia, hypomagnesemia, or administration of other drugs known to increase the QT interval). Other risk factors may include age over 65 years, alcohol abuse, and use of agents such as benzodiazepines, volatile anesthetics, and IV opiates. Droperidol should be initiated at a low dose and adjusted upward, with caution, as needed to achieve the desired effect.

DESCRIPTION

Inapsine contains droperidol, a neuroleptic (tranquilizer) agent. Inapsine injection is available in ampoules and vials. Each milliliter contains 2.5 mg of droperidol in an aqueous solution adjusted to pH 3.4 ± 0.4 with lactic acid. Droperidol is chemically identified as 1-(1-[3-(p-fluorobenzoyl)propyl]-1,2,3,6-tetrahydro-4-pyridyl)-2-benzimidazolinone with a molecular weight of 379.43.

The molecular formula of droperidol is $C_{22}H_{22}FN_3O_2$, the partition coefficient in n-octanol:water is 3.46, and the pKa is 7.46.

Droperidol injection is a sterile, non-pyrogenic aqueous solution for intravenous or intramuscular injection.

CLINICAL PHARMACOLOGY

Droperidol produces marked tranquilization and sedation. It allays apprehension and provides a state or mental detachment and indifference while maintaining a state of reflex alertness.

Droperidol produces an antiemetic effect as evidenced by the antagonism of apomorphine in dogs. It lowers the incidence of nausea and vomiting during surgical procedures and provides antiemetic protection in the postoperative period.

Droperidol potentiates other CNS depressants. It produces mild alpha-adrenergic blockade, peripheral vascular dilatation and reduction of the pressor effect of epinephrine. It can produce hypotension and decreased peripheral vascular resistance and may decrease pulmonary arterial pressure (particularly if it is abnormally high). It may reduce the incidence of epinephrine-induced arrhythmias, but it does not prevent other cardiac arrhythmias.

The onset of action of single intramuscular and intravenous doses is from 3-10 minutes following administration, although the peak effect may not be apparent for up to 30 minutes. The duration of the tranquilizing and sedative effects generally is 2-4 hours, although alteration of alertness may persist for as long as 12 hours.

INDICATIONS AND USAGE

Droperidol is indicated to reduce the incidence of nausea and vomiting associated with surgical and diagnostic procedures.

NON-FDA APPROVED INDICATIONS

Unlabeled indications of droperidol include treatment of hiccups, chemotherapy-induced nausea and vomiting, use during endotracheal intubation, and to control agitation in psychotic patients and patients with Meniere's disease.

CONTRAINDICATIONS

Droperidol is contraindicated in patients with known or suspected QT prolongation (*i.e.,* QTc interval greater than 440 milliseconds for males or 450 milliseconds for females). This would include patients with congenital long QT syndrome.

Droperidol is contraindicated in patients with known hypersensitivity to the drug.

Droperidol is not recommended for any use other than the treatment of perioperative nausea and vomiting in patients for whom other treatments are ineffective or inappropriate (see WARNINGS).

WARNINGS

Droperidol should be administered with extreme caution in the presence of risk factors for development of prolonged QT syndrome, such as: (1) clinically significant bradycardia (less than 50 bpm), (2) any clinically significant cardiac disease, (3) treatment with Class I and Class III antiarrhythmics, (4) treatment with monoamine oxidase inhibitors (MAOIs), (5) concomitant treatment with other drug products known to prolong the QT interval (see DRUG INTERACTIONS), and (6) electrolytes imbalance, in particular hypokalemia and hypomagnesemia, or concomitant treatment with drugs (*e.g.,* diuretics) that may cause electrolyte imbalance.

EFFECTS ON CARDIAC CONDUCTION

A dose-dependent prolongation of the QT interval was observed within 10 minutes of droperidol administration in a study of 40 patients without known cardiac disease who underwent extracranial head and neck surgery. Significant QT prolongation was observed at all three dose levels evaluated, with 0.1, 0.175, and 0.25 mg/kg associated with prolongation of median QTc by 37, 44, and 59 milliseconds, respectively.

Case of QT prolongation and serious arrhythmias (*e.g.,* torsade de pointes, ventricular arrhythmias, cardiac arrest, and death) have been observed during post-marketing treatment with droperidol. Some cases have occurred in patients with no known risk factors and at doses at or below recommended doses. There has been at least one case of nonfatal torsade de pointes confirmed by rechallenge.

Based on these reports, all patients should undergo a 12-lead ECG prior to administration of droperidol to determine if a prolonged QT interval (*i.e.,* QTc interval greater than 440 milliseconds for males or 450 milliseconds for females) is present. If there is a prolonged QT interval, droperidol should NOT be administered. For patients in whom the potential benefit of droperidol treatment is felt to outweigh the risks of potentially serious arrhythmias, ECG monitoring should be performed prior to treatment and continued for 2-3 hours after completing treatment to monitor for arrhythmias.

FLUIDS AND OTHER COUNTERMEASURES TO MANAGE HYPOTENSION SHOULD BE READILY AVAILABLE.

As with other CNS depressant drugs, patients who receive droperidol should have appropriate surveillance.

It is recommended that opioids, when required, initially be used in reduced doses.

As with other neuroleptic agents, very rare reports of neuroleptic malignant syndrome (altered consciousness, muscle rigidity and autonomic instability) have occurred in patients who have received droperidol.

Since it may be difficult to distinguish neuroleptic malignant syndrome from malignant hyperpyrexia in the perioperative period, prompt treatment with dantrolene should be considered if increases in temperature, heart rate or carbon dioxide production occur.

PRECAUTIONS

GENERAL

The initial dose of droperidol should be appropriately reduced in elderly, debilitated and other poor-risk patients. The effect of the initial dose should be considered in determining incremental doses.

Certain forms of conduction anesthesia, such as spinal anesthesia and some peridural anesthetics, can alter respiration by blocking intercostal nerves and can cause peripheral vasodilatation and hypotension because of sympathetic blockade. Through other mechanisms (see CLINICAL PHARMACOLOGY), droperidol can also alter circulation. Therefore, when droperidol is used to supplement these forms of anesthesia, the anesthetist should be familiar with the physiological alterations involved, and be prepared to manage them in the patients elected for these forms of anesthesia.

If hypotension occurs, the possibility of hypovolemia should be considered and managed with appropriate parenteral fluid therapy. Repositioning the patient to improve venous return to the heart should be considered when operative conditions permit. It should be noted that in spinal and peridural anesthesia, tilting the patient into a head-down position may result in a higher level of anesthesia than is desirable, as well as impair venous return to the heart. Care should be exercised in moving and positioning of patients because of a possibility of orthostatic hypotension. If volume expansion with fluids plus these other countermeasures do not correct the hypotension, then the administration of pressor agents other than epinephrine should be considered. Epinephrine may paradoxically decrease the blood pressure in patients treated with droperidol due to the alpha-adrenergic blocking action of droperidol.

Since droperidol may decrease pulmonary arterial pressure, this fact should be considered by those who conduct diagnostic or surgical procedures where interpretation of pulmonary arterial pressure measurements might determine final management of the patient.

Vital signs and ECG should be monitored routinely.

When the EEG is used for postoperative monitoring, it may be found that the EEG pattern returns to normal slowly.

IMPAIRED HEPATIC OR RENAL FUNCTION

Droperidol should be administered with caution to patients with liver and kidney dysfunction because of the importance of these organs in the metabolism and excretion of drugs.

PHEOCHROMOCYTOMA

In patients with diagnosed/suspected pheochromocytoma, severe hypotension and tachycardia have been observed after the administration of droperidol.

CARCINOGENESIS, MUTAGENESIS, AND IMPAIRMENT OF FERTILITY

No carcinogenicity studies have been carried out with droperidol. The micronucleus test in female rats revealed no mutagenic effects in single oral doses as high as 160 mg/kg. An oral study in rats (Segment I) revealed no impairment of fertility in either males or females at 0.63, 2.5 and 10 mg/kg doses (approximately 2, 9 and 36 times maximum recommended human IV/IM dosage).

PREGNANCY CATEGORY C

Droperidol administered intravenously has been shown to cause a slight increase in mortality of the newborn rat at 4.4 times the upper human dose. At 44 times the upper human dose, mortality rate was comparable to that for control animals. Following intramuscular administration, increased mortality of the offspring at 1.8 times the upper human dose is attributed to CNS depression in the dams who neglected to remove placentae from their offspring. Droperidol has not been shown to be teratogenic in animals. There are no adequate and well-controlled studies in pregnant women. Droperidol should be used during pregnancy only if the potential benefit justifies the potential risk to the fetus.

LABOR AND DELIVERY

There are insufficient data to support the use of droperidol in labor and delivery. Therefore, such use is not recommended.

NURSING MOTHERS

It is not known whether droperidol is excreted in human milk. Because many drugs are excreted in human milk, caution should be exercised when droperidol is administered to a nursing mother.

PEDIATRIC USE

The safety of droperidol in children younger than 2 years of age has not been established.

DRUG INTERACTIONS

POTENTIALLY ARRHYTHMOGENIC AGENTS

Any drug known to have the potential to prolong the QT interval should not be used together with droperidol. Possible pharmacodynamic interactions can occur between droperidol and potentially arrhythmogenic agents such as Class I or Class III antiarrhythmics, antihistamines that prolong the QT interval, antimalarials, calcium channel blockers, neuroleptics that prolong the QT interval, and antidepressants.

Caution should be used when patients are taking concomitant drugs known to induce hypokalemia or hypomagnesemia as they may precipitate QT prolongation and interact with droperidol. These would include diuretics, laxatives, supraphysiological use of steroid hormones with mineralocorticoid potential.

CNS DEPRESSANT DRUGS

Other CNS depressant drugs (*e.g.*, barbiturates, tranquilizers, opioids and general anesthetics) have additive or potentiating effects with droperidol. When patients have received such drugs, the dose of droperidol required will be less than usual. Following the administration of droperidol, the dose of other CNS depressant drugs should be reduced.

ADVERSE REACTIONS

QT interval prolongation, torsade de pointes, cardiac arrest and ventricular tachycardia have been reported in patients treated with droperidol. Some of these cases were associated with death. Some cases occurred in patients with no known risk factors, and some were associated with droperidol doses at or below recommended doses.

Physicians should be alert to palpitations, syncope, or other symptoms suggestive of episodes of irregular cardiac rhythm in patients taking droperidol and promptly evaluate such cases (see WARNINGS, Effects on Cardiac Conduction).

The most common somatic adverse reactions reported to occur with droperidol are mild to moderate hypotension and tachycardia, but these effects usually subside without treatment. If hypotension occurs and is severe or persists, the possibility of hypovolemia should be considered and managed with appropriate parenteral fluid therapy.

The most common behavioral adverse effects of droperidol include dysphoria, postoperative drowsiness, restlessness, hyperactivity and anxiety, which can either be the result of an inadequate dosage (lack of adequate treatment effect) or of an adverse drug reaction (part of the symptom complex of akathisia).

Care should be taken to search for extrapyramidal signs and symptoms (dystonia, akathisia, oculogyric crisis) to differentiate these different clinical conditions. When extrapyramidal symptoms are the cause, they can usually be controlled with anticholinergic agents.

Postoperative hallucinatory episodes (sometimes associated with transient periods of mental depression) have also been reported.

Other less common adverse reactions include anaphylaxis, dizziness, chills and/or shivering, laryngospasm, and bronchospasm.

Elevated blood pressure, with or without pre-existing hypertension, has been reported following administration of droperidol combined with fentanyl citrate or other parenteral analgesics. This might be due to unexplained alterations in sympathetic activity following large doses; however, it is also frequently attributed to anesthetic or surgical stimulation during light anesthesia.

DOSAGE AND ADMINISTRATION

Dosage should be individualized. Some of the factors to be considered in determining the dose are age, body weight, physical status, underlying pathological condition, use of other drugs, type of anesthesia to be used and the surgical procedure involved.

Vital signs and ECG should be monitored routinely.

Adult Dosage: The maximum recommended initial dose of droperidol is 2.5 mg IM or slow IV. Additional 1.25 mg doses of droperidol may be administered to achieve the desired effect. However, additional doses should be administered with caution, and only if the potential benefit outweighs the potential risk.

Children's Dosage: For children 2-12 years of age, the maximum recommended initial dose is 0.1 mg/kg, taking into account the patient's age and other clinical factors. However, additional doses should be administered with caution and only if the potential benefit outweighs the potential risk.

See WARNINGS and PRECAUTIONS for use of droperidol with other CNS depressants and in patients with altered response.

Parenteral drug products should be inspected visually for particulate matter and discoloration prior to administration, whenever solution and container permit. If such abnormalities are observed, the drug should not be administered.

HOW SUPPLIED

Inapsine is available in 1 and 2 ml ampoules and vials.

Storage: PROTECT FROM LIGHT. STORE AT ROOM TEMPERATURE 15-25°C (59-77°F).

PRODUCT LISTING - RATED THERAPEUTICALLY EQUIVALENT

Solution - Injectable - 2.5 mg/ml

1 ml x 10	$45.90	INAPSINE, Akorn Inc	11098-0010-01
2 ml x 10	$12.59	GENERIC, Abbott Pharmaceutical	00074-2269-02
2 ml x 10	$15.32	GENERIC, Abbott Pharmaceutical	00074-2269-32
2 ml x 10	$16.25	GENERIC, Faulding Pharmaceutical Company	61703-0206-07
2 ml x 10	$16.63	GENERIC, Abbott Pharmaceutical	00074-1187-01
2 ml x 10	$18.76	GENERIC, Abbott Pharmaceutical	00074-2269-11
2 ml x 10	$34.38	GENERIC, Solo Pak Medical Products Inc	39769-0123-03
2 ml x 10	$42.50	GENERIC, American Regent Laboratories Inc	00517-9702-10
2 ml x 10	$57.30	INAPSINE, Akorn Inc	11098-0010-02
2 ml x 25	$106.25	GENERIC, American Regent Laboratories Inc	00517-9702-25
5 ml	$35.00	GENERIC, Dupont Pharmaceuticals	00590-5981-61
5 ml x 10	$54.00	GENERIC, Astra-Zeneca Pharmaceuticals	00186-1221-03
20 ml	$44.86	GENERIC, Dupont Pharmaceuticals	00590-5981-53

Drospirenone; Ethinyl Estradiol *(003523)*

Categories: Contraception; FDA Approved 2001 May; Pregnancy Category X
Drug Classes: Contraceptives; Estrogens; Progestins
Brand Names: Yasmin
Cost of Therapy: $33.00 (Contraception; Yasmin; 3 mg; 0.03 mg; 1 tablet/day; 28 day supply)

DESCRIPTION

Note: The trade name has been used throughout this monograph for clarity.

PATIENTS SHOULD BE COUNSELED THAT THIS PRODUCT DOES NOT PROTECT AGAINST HIV INFECTION (AIDS) AND OTHER SEXUALLY TRANSMITTED DISEASES.

Yasmin provides an oral contraceptive regimen consisting of 21 active film coated tablets each containing 3.0 mg of drospirenone and 0.030 mg of ethinyl estradiol and 7 inert film coated tablets. The inactive ingredients are lactose monohydrate, corn starch, modified starch, povidone 25000, magnesium stearate, hydroxylpropylmethyl cellulose, macrogol 6000, talc, titanium dioxide, ferric oxide pigment, yellow. The inert film coated tablets contain lactose monohydrate, corn starch, povidone 25000, magnesium stearate, hydroxylpropylmethyl cellulose, talc, titanium dioxide.

Drospirenone (6R,7R,8R,9S,10R,13S,14S,15S,16S,17S)-1,3′,4′,6,6a,7,8,9,10,11,12,13,14,15,15a,16-hexadecahydro-10,13-dimethylspiro-[17H-dicyclopropa-6,7:15,16]cyclopenta[a]phenanthrene-17,2′(5H)-furan]-3,5′(2H)-dione) is a synthetic progestational compound and has a molecular weight of 366.5 and a molecular formula of $C_{24}H_{30}O_3$. Ethinyl estradiol (19-nor-17alpha-pregna 1,3,5(10)-triene-20-yne-3,17-diol) is a synthetic estrogenic compound and has a molecular weight of 296.4 and a molecular formula of $C_{20}H_{24}O_2$.

CLINICAL PHARMACOLOGY

PHARMACODYNAMICS

Combination oral contraceptives (COCs) act by suppression of gonadotropins. Although the primary mechanism of this action is inhibition of ovulation, other alterations include changes in the cervical mucus (which increases the difficulty of sperm entry into the uterus) and the endometrium (which reduces the likelihood of implantation).

Drospirenone is a spironolactone analogue with antimineralocorticoid activity. Preclinical studies in animals and *in vitro* have shown that drospirenone has no androgenic, estrogenic, glucocorticoid, and antiglucocorticoid activity. Preclinical studies in animals have also shown that drospirenone has antiandrogenic activity.

PHARMACOKINETICS

Absorption

The absolute bioavailability of drospirenone (DRSP) from a single entity tablet is about 76%. The absolute bioavailability of ethinyl estradiol (EE) is approximately 40% as a result of presystemic conjugation and first-pass metabolism. The absolute bioavailabilty of Yasmin which is a combination tablet of drospirenone and ethinyl estradiol has not been evaluated. Serum concentrations of DRSP and EE reached peak levels within 1-3 hours after administration of Yasmin. After single dose administration of Yasmin, the relative bioavailability, compared to a suspension, was 107% and 117% for DRSP and EE, respectively.

The pharmacokinetics of DRSP are dose proportional following single doses ranging from 1-10 mg. Following daily dosing of Yasmin, steady state DRSP concentrations were observed after 10 days. There was about 2- to 3-fold accumulation in serum C_{max} and AUC(0-24h) values of DRSP following multiple dose administration of Yasmin (see TABLE 1).

For EE, steady-state conditions are reported during the second half of a treatment cycle. Following daily administration of Yasmin serum C_{max} and AUC(0-24h) values of EE accumulate by a factor of about 1.5-2.0.

TABLE 1 *Table of Mean Pharmacokinetic Parameters of Yasmin*

(Drospirenone 3 mg and Ethinyl Estradiol 0.030 mg)

Cycle/Day	No. of Subjects	C_{max} (ng/ml)	T_{max} (hours)	AUC(0-24h) (ng·h/ml)	T½ (hours)
		Drospirenone Mean (% CV) Values			
1/1	12	36.9 (13)	1.7 (47)	288 (25)	NA
1/21	12	87.5 (59)	1.7 (20)	827 (23)	30.9 (44)
6/21	12	84.2 (19)	1.8 (19)	930 (19)	32.5 (38)
9/21	12	81.3 (19)	1.6 (38)	957 (23)	31.4 (39)
13/21	12	78.7 (18)	1.6 (26)	968 (24)	31.1 (36)
		Ethinyl Estradiol Mean (% CV) Values			
		(pg/ml)	**(hours)**	**(pg·h/ml)**	**(hours)**
1/1	11	53.5 (43)	1.9 (45)	280.3 (87)	NA
1/21	11	92.1 (35)	1.5 (40)	461.3 (94)	NA
6/21	11	99.1 (45)	1.5 (47)	346.4 (74)	NA
9/21	11	87.0 (43)	1.5 (42)	485.3 (92)	NA
13/21	10	90.5 (45)	1.6 (38)	469.5 (83)	NA

NA = Not available.

Effect of Food

The rate of absorption of DRSP and EE following single administration of 2 Yasmin tablets was slower under fed conditions with the serum C_{max} being reduced about 40% for both components. The extent of absorption of DRSP, however, remained unchanged. In contrast the extent of absorption of EE was reduced by about 20% under fed conditions.

Distribution

DRSP and EE serum levels decline in two phases. The apparent volume of distribution of DRSP is approximately 4 L/kg and that of EE is reported to be approximately 4-5 L/kg.

DRSP does not bind to sex hormone binding globulin (SHBG) or corticosteroid binding globulin (CBG) but binds about 97% to other serum proteins. Multiple dosing over 3 cycles resulted in no change in the free fraction (as measured at trough levels). EE is reported to be highly but non-specifically bound to serum albumin (approximately 98.5%) and induces an increase in the serum concentrations of both SHBG and CBG. EE induced effects on SHBG and CBG were not affected by variation of the DRSP dosage in the range of 2-3 mg.

Metabolism

The two main metabolites of DRSP found in human plasma were identified to be the acid form of DRSP generated by opening of the lactone ring and the 4,5-dihydrodrospirenone-3-sulfate. These metabolites were shown not to be pharmacologically active. In *in vitro* studies with human liver microsomes, DRSP was metabolized only to a minor extent mainly by cytochrome P450 3A4 (CYP3A4).

EE has been reported to be subject to presystemic conjugation in both small bowel mucosa and the liver. Metabolism occurs primarily by aromatic hydroxylation but a wide variety of hydroxylated and methylated metabolites are formed. These are present as free metabolites and as conjugates with glucuronide and sulfate. CYP3A4 in the liver are responsible for the 2-hydroxylation which is the major oxidative reaction. The 2-hydroxy metabolite is further transformed by methylation and glucuronidation prior to urinary and fecal excretion.

Excretion

DRSP serum levels are characterized by a terminal disposition phase half-life of approximately 30 hours after both single and multiple dose regimens. Excretion of DRSP was nearly complete after 10 days and amounts excreted were slightly higher in feces compared to urine. DRSP was extensively metabolized and only trace amounts of unchanged DRSP were excreted in urine and feces. At least 20 different metabolites were observed in urine and feces. About 38-47% of the metabolites in urine were glucuronide and sulfate conjugates. In feces, about 17-20% of the metabolites were excreted as glucuronides and sulfates.

For EE the terminal disposition phase half-life has been reported to be approximately 24 hours. EE is not excreted unchanged. EE is excreted in the urine and feces as glucuronide and sulfate conjugates and undergoes enterohepatic circulation.

Special Populations

Race

The effect of race on the disposition of Yasmin has not been evaluated.

Hepatic Dysfunction

Yasmin is contraindicated in patients with hepatic dysfunction **(also see BOLDED WARNING).**

Renal Insufficiency

Yasmin is contraindicated in patients with renal insufficiency **(also see BOLDED WARNING).**

The effect of renal insufficiency on the pharmacokinetics of DRSP (3 mg daily for 14 days) and the effect of DRSP on serum potassium levels were investigated in female subjects (n=28, age 30-65) with normal renal function and mild and moderate renal impairment. All subjects were on a low potassium diet. During the study 7 subjects continued the use of potassium sparing drugs for the treatment of the underlying illness. On the 14th day (steady-state) of DRSP treatment, the serum DRSP levels in the group with mild renal impairment (creatinine clearance CLCR, 50-80 ml/min) were comparable to those in the group with normal renal function (CLCR, >80 ml/min). The serum DRSP levels were on average 37% higher in the group with moderate renal impairment (CLCR, 30-50 ml/min) compared to those in the group with normal renal function. DRSP treatment was well tolerated by all groups. DRSP treatment did not show any clinically significant effect on serum potassium concentration. Although hyperkalemia was not observed in the study, in 5 of the 7 subjects who continued use of potassium sparing drugs during the study, mean serum potassium levels increased by up to 0.33 mEq/L. Therefore, potential exists for hyperkalemia to occur in subjects with renal impairment whose serum potassium is in the upper reference range, and who are concomitantly using potassium sparing drugs.

NON-CONTRACEPTIVE HEALTH BENEFITS

The following non-contraceptive health benefits related to the use of oral contraceptives are supported by epidemiological studies which largely utilized oral contraceptive formulations containing doses exceeding 0.035 mg of ethinyl estradiol or 0.05 mg mestranol.

Effects on menses:

Increased menstrual cycle regularity.
Decreased blood loss and decreased incidence of iron-deficiency anemia.
Decreased incidence of dysmenorrhea.

Effects related to inhibition of ovulation:

Decreased incidence of functional ovarian cysts.
Decreased incidence of ectopic pregnancies.

Effects from long-term use:

Decreased incidence of fibroadenomas and fibrocystic disease of the breast.
Decreased incidence of acute pelvic inflammatory disease.
Decreased incidence of endometrial cancer.
Decreased incidence of ovarian cancer.

INDICATIONS AND USAGE

Yasmin is indicated for the prevention of pregnancy in women who elect to use an oral contraceptive.

Oral contraceptives are highly effective. TABLE 2 lists the typical accidental pregnancy rates for users of combination oral contraceptives and other methods of contraception. The efficacy of these contraceptive methods, except sterilization, depends upon the reliability with which they are used. Correct and consistent use of methods can result in lower failure rates.

In clinical efficacy studies of Yasmin of up to 2 years duration, 2629 subjects completed 33,160 cycles of use without any other contraception. The mean age of the subjects was 25.5 ± 4.7 years. The age range was 16-37 years. The racial demographic was: 83% Caucasians, 1% Hispanic, 1% Black, <1% Asian, <1% other, <1% missing data, 14% not inquired and <1% unspecified. Pregnancy rates in the clinical trials were less than 1 per 100 woman-years of use.

CONTRAINDICATIONS

Yasmin should not be used in women who have the following:

- Renal insufficiency.
- Hepatic dysfunction.
- Adrenal insufficiency.
- Thrombophlebitis or thromboembolic disorders.
- A past history of deep-vein thrombophlebitis or thromboembolic disorders.
- Cerebral-vascular or coronary-artery disease.
- Known or suspected carcinoma of the breast.
- Carcinoma of the endometrium or other known or suspected estrogen-dependent neoplasia.
- Undiagnosed abnormal genital bleeding.
- Cholestatic jaundice of pregnancy or jaundice with prior pill use.
- Liver tumor (benign or malignant) or active liver disease.
- Known or suspected pregnancy.
- Heavy smoking (>15 cigarettes per day) and over age 35.

D

TABLE 2 *Percentage of Women Experiencing an Unintended Pregnancy During the First Year of Typical Use and First Year of Perfect Use of Contraception and the Percentage Continuing Use at the End of the First Year*

United States

Method	% of Women Experiencing an Accidnetal Pregnancy within the First Year of Use		% of Women Continuing
	Typical Use*	Perfect Use†	Use at 1 Year‡
(1)	(2)	(3)	(4)
Chance§	85%	85%	
Spermicides¤	26%	6%	40%
Periodic abstinence	25%		63%
Calendar		9%	
Ovulation method		3%	
Sympto-thermal¶		2%	
Post-ovulation		1%	
Withdrawal	19%	4%	
Cap**			
Parous women	40%	26%	42%
Nulliparous women	20%	9%	56%
Sponge			
Parous women	40%	20%	42%
Nulliparous women	20%	9%	56%
Diaphragm**	20%	6%	56%
Condom††			
Female (Reality)	21%	5%	56%
Male	14%	3%	61%
Pill	5%		71%
Progesterin only		0.5%	
Comibined		0.1%	
IUD			
Progesterone T	2.0%	1.5%	81%
Copper T 380A	0.8%	0.6%	78%
Lng 20	0.1%	0.1%	81%
Depo Provera	0.3%	0.3%	70%
Norplant and Norplant-2	0.05%	0.05%	88%
Female sterilization	0.5%	0.5%	100%
Male sterilization	0.15%	0.10%	100%

Emergency Contraceptive Pills: Treatment initiated within 72 hours after unprotected intercourse reduces the risk of pregnancy by at least 75%.‡‡

Lactational Amenorrhea Method: LAM is highly effective, *temporary* method of contraception.§§

* Among *typical* couples who initiate use of a method (not necessarily for the first time), the percentage who experience an accidental pregnancy during the first year if they do not stop use for any other reason.

† Among couples who initiate use of a method (not necessarily for the first time) and who use it *perfectly* (both consistently and correctly), the percentage who experience an accidental pregnancy during the first year if they do not stop use for any reason.

‡ Among couples attempting to avoid pregnancy, the percentage who continue to use a method for 1 year.

§ The percents becoming pregnant in columns (2) and (3) are based on data from populations where contraception is not used and from women who cease using contraception in order to become pregnant. Among such populations, about 89% become pregnant within 1 year. This estimate was lowered slightly (to 85%) to represent the percentage who would become pregnant within 1 year among women now relying on reversible methods of contraception if they abandoned contraception altogether.

¤ Foams, creams, gels, vaginal suppositories, and vaginal film.

¶ Cervical mucus (ovulation) method supplemented by calendar in the pre-ovulatory and basal body temperature in the post-ovulatory phases.

** With spermicidal cream or jelly.

†† Without spermicides.

‡‡ The treatment schedule is one dose within 72 hours after unprotected intercourse, and a second dose 12 hours after the first dose. The Food and Drug Administration has declared the following brands of oral contraceptives to be safe and effective for emergency contraception: Ovral (1 dose is 2 white pills), Alesse (1 dose is 5 pink pills), Nordette or Levlen (1 dose is 2 light-orange pills), Lo/Ovral (1 dose is 4 white pills), Triphasil or Tri-Levlen (1 dose is 4 yellow pills).

§§ However, to maintain effective protection against pregnancy, another method of contraception must be used as soon as menstruation resumes, the frequency or duration of breastfeeds is reduced, bottle feeds are introduced, or the baby reaches 6 months of age.

Source: Trussell J, Contraceptive efficacy. In Hatcher RA, Trussell J, Stewart F, Cates W, Stewart GK, Kowal D, Guest F, Contraceptive Technology: Seventeenth Revised Edition. New York NY: Irvington Publishers, 1998.

WARNINGS

Cigarette smoking increases the risk of serious cardiovascular side effects from oral contraceptive use. This risk increases with age and with heavy smoking (15 or more cigarettes per day) and is quite marked in women over 35 years of age. Women who use oral contraceptives should be strongly advised not to smoke.

Yasmin contains 3 mg of the progestin drospirenone that has antimineralocorticoid activity, including the potential for hyperkalemia in high-risk patients, comparable to a 25 mg dose of spironolactone. Yasmin should not be used in patients with conditions that predispose to hyperkalemia (*i.e.,* renal insufficiency, hepatic dysfunction and adrenal insufficiency). Women receiving daily, long-term treatment for chronic conditions or diseases with medications that may increase serum potassium, should have their serum potassium level checked during the first treatment cycle. Drugs that may increase serum potassium include ACE inhibitors, angiotensin-II receptor antagonists, potassium-sparing diuretics, heparin, aldosterone antagonists, and NSAIDs.

The use of oral contraceptives is associated with increased risks of several serious conditions including myocardial infarction, thromboembolism, stroke, hepatic neoplasia, gallbladder disease, and hypertension, although the risk of serious morbidity or mortality is very small in healthy women without underlying risk factors. The risk of morbidity and mortality increases significantly in the presence of other underlying risk factors such as hypertension, hyperlipidemias, obesity and diabetes.

Practitioners prescribing oral contraceptives should be familiar with the following information relating to these risks.

The information contained in this package insert is based principally on studies carried out in patients who used oral contraceptives with higher formulations of estrogens and progestogens than those in common use today. The effect of long-term use of the oral contraceptives with lower formulations of both estrogens and progestogens remains to be determined.

Throughout this labeling, epidemiologic studies reported are of two types: retrospective or case control studies and prospective or cohort studies. Case control studies provide a measure of the relative risk of a disease, namely, a ratio of the incidence of a disease among oral contraceptive users to that among nonusers. The relative risk does not provide information on the actual clinical occurrence of a disease. Cohort studies provide a measure of attributable risk, which is the difference in the incidence of disease between oral contraceptive users and nonusers. The attributable risk does provide information about the actual occurrence of a disease in the population. For further information, the reader is referred to a text on epidemiologic methods.

THROMBOEMBOLIC DISORDERS AND OTHER VASCULAR PROBLEMS

Myocardial Infarction

An increased risk of myocardial infarction has been attributed to oral contraceptive use. This risk is primarily in smokers or women with other underlying risk factors for coronary-artery disease such as hypertension, hypercholesterolemia, morbid obesity, and diabetes. The relative risk of heart attack for current oral contraceptive users has been estimated to be 2-6. The risk is very low under the age of 30.

Smoking in combination with oral contraceptive use has been shown to contribute substantially to the incidence of myocardial infarctions in women in their mid-thirties or older with smoking accounting for the majority of excess cases. Mortality rates associated with circulatory disease have been shown to increase substantially in smokers over the age of 35 and nonsmokers over the age of 40 (TABLE 3) among women who use oral contraceptives.

Oral contraceptives may compound the effects of well-known risk factors, such as hypertension, diabetes, hyperlipidemias, age and obesity. In particular, some progestogens are known to decrease HDL cholesterol and cause glucose intolerance, while estrogens may create a state of hyperinsulinism. Oral contraceptives have been shown to increase blood pressure among users (see Elevated Blood Pressure). Similar effects on risk factors have been associated with an increased risk of heart disease. Oral contraceptives must be used with caution in women with cardiovascular disease risk factors.

TABLE 3* *Circulatory Disease Mortality Rates Per 100,000 Woman-Years By Age Smoking Status and Oral Contraceptive Use*

Age	Ever-Users		Control	
	Non-Smokers	Smokers	Non-Smokers	Smokers
15-24	0.0	10.5	0.0	0.0
25-34	4.4	14.2	2.7	4.2
35-44	21.5	63.4	6.4	15.2
45+	52.4	206.7	11.4	27.9

* Adapted from P.M. Layde and V. Beral.

Thromboembolism

An increased risk of thromboembolic and thrombotic disease associated with the use of oral contraceptives is well established. Case control studies have found the relative risk of users compared to nonusers to be 3 for the first episode of superficial venous thrombosis, 4-11 for deep vein thrombosis or pulmonary embolism, and 1.5 to 6 for women with predisposing conditions for venous thromboembolic disease. Cohort studies have shown the relative risk to be somewhat lower, about 3 for new cases and about 4.5 for new cases requiring hospitalization. The risk of thromboembolic disease due to oral contraceptives is not related to length of use and disappears after pill use is stopped.

A 2- to 4-fold increase in the relative risk of post-operative thromboembolic complications has been reported with the use of oral contraceptives. The relative risk of venous thrombosis in women who have predisposing conditions is twice that of women without such medical conditions. If feasible, oral contraceptives should be discontinued from at least 4 weeks prior to and for 2 weeks after elective surgery of a type associated with an increase in risk of thromboembolism and during and following prolonged immobilization. Since the immediate postpartum period is also associated with an increased risk of thromboembolism, oral contraceptives should be started no earlier than 4-6 weeks after delivery.

Cerebrovascular Diseases

Oral contraceptives have been shown to increase both the relative and attributable risks of cerebrovascular events (thrombotic and hemorrhagic strokes), although, in general, the risk is greatest among older (>35 years), hypertensive women who also smoke. Hypertension was found to be a risk factor, for both users and nonusers, for both types of strokes, while smoking interacted to increase the risk for hemorrhagic strokes.

In a large study, the relative risk of thrombotic strokes has been shown to range from 3 for normotensive users to 14 for users with severe hypertension. The relative risk of hemorrhagic stroke is reported to be 1.2 for nonsmokers who used oral contraceptives, 2.6 for smokers who did not use oral contraceptives, 7.6 for smokers who used oral contraceptives, 1.8 for normotensive users and 25.7 for users with severe hypertension. The attributable risk is also greater in older women.

Dose-Related Risk of Vascular Disease From Oral Contraceptives

A positive association has been observed between the amount of estrogen and progestogen in oral contraceptives and the risk of vascular disease. A decline in serum high-density lipoproteins (HDL) has been reported with many progestational agents. A decline in serum high-density lipoproteins has been associated with an increased incidence of ischemic heart disease. Because estrogens increase HDL cholesterol, the net effect of an oral contraceptive depends on a balance achieved between doses of estrogen and progestogen and the nature and absolute amount of progestogen used in the contraceptive. The amount of both hormones should be considered in the choice of an oral contraceptive.

Minimizing exposure to estrogen and progestogen is in keeping with good principles of therapeutics. For any particular estrogen/progestogen combination, the dosage regimen prescribed should be one which contains the least amount of estrogen and progestogen that is compatible with a low failure rate and the needs of the individual patient. New acceptors of oral contraceptive agents should be started on preparations containing the lowest estrogen content which provides satisfactory results in the individual.

Persistence of Risk of Vascular Disease

There are two studies which have shown persistence of risk of vascular disease for ever-users of oral contraceptives. In a study in the US, the risk of developing myocardial infarction after discontinuing oral contraceptives persists for at least 9 years for women aged 40-49 years who had used oral contraceptives for 5 or more years, but this increased risk was not demonstrated in other age groups. In another study in Great Britain, the risk of developing cerebrovascular disease persisted for at least 6 years after discontinuation of oral contraceptives, although excess risk was very small. However, both studies were performed with oral contraceptive formulations containing 50 μg or higher of estrogens.

ESTIMATES OF MORTALITY FROM CONTRACEPTIVE USE

One study gathered data from a variety of sources which have estimated the mortality rate associated with different methods of contraception at different ages (TABLE 4). These estimates include the combined risk of death associated with contraceptive methods plus the risk attributable to pregnancy in the event of method failure. Each method of contraception has its specific benefits and risks. The study concluded that with the exception of oral contraceptive users 35 and older who smoke and 40 and older who do not smoke, mortality associated with all methods of birth control is below that associated with childbirth.

The observation of a possible increase in risk of mortality with age for oral contraceptive users is based on data gathered in the 1970's — but not reported until 1983. However, current clinical practice involves the use of lower estrogen dose formulations combined with careful restriction of oral contraceptive use to women who do not have the various risk factors listed in this labeling.

Because of these changes in practice and, also, because of some limited new data which suggest that the risk of cardiovascular disease with the use of oral contraceptives may now be less than previously observed, the Fertility and Maternal Health Drugs Advisory Committee was asked to review the topic in 1989. The Committee concluded that although cardiovascular disease risks may be increased with oral contraceptive use after age 40 in healthy nonsmoking women (even with the newer low-dose formulations), there are greater potential health risks associated with pregnancy in older women and with the alternative surgical and medical procedures which may be necessary if such women do not have access to effective and acceptable means of contraception.

Therefore, the Committee recommended that the benefits of oral contraceptive use by healthy nonsmoking women over 40 may outweigh the possible risks. Of course, women of all ages who take oral contraceptives, should take the lowest possible dose formulation that is effective.

***TABLE 4** Annual Number of Birth-Related or Method-Related Deaths Associated With Control of Fertility Per 100,000 Nonsterile Women, By Fertility-Control Method According To Age*

Method of Control and Outcome	15-19	20-24	25-29	30-34	35-39	40-44
No fertility control methods*	7.0	7.4	9.1	14.8	25.7	28.2
Oral contraceptives non-smoker†	0.3	0.5	0.9	1.9	13.8	31.6
Oral contraceptives smoker†	2.2	3.4	6.6	13.5	51.1	117.2
IUD†	0.8	0.8	1.0	1.0	1.4	1.4
Condom*	1.1	1.6	0.7	0.2	0.3	0.4
Diaphragm/spermicide*	1.9	1.2	1.2	1.3	2.2	2.8
Periodic abstinence*	2.5	1.6	1.6	1.7	2.9	3.6

* Deaths are birth related.
† Deaths are method related.
Adapted from H.W. Ory, *Family Planning Perspectives,* 15:57-63, 1983.

CARCINOMA OF THE REPRODUCTIVE ORGANS AND BREASTS

Numerous epidemiological studies have been performed on the incidence of breast, endometrial, ovarian and cervical cancer in women using oral contraceptives.

The risk of having breast cancer diagnosed may be slightly increased among current and recent users of COCs. However this excess risk appears to decrease over time after COC discontinuation and by 10 years after cessation the increased risk disappears. The risk does not appear to increase with duration of use and no consistent relationships have been found with dose or type of steroid. Most studies show a similar pattern of risk with COC use regardless of a woman's reproductive history or her family breast cancer history. Some studies have found a small increase in risk for women who first use COCs before age 20.

Breast cancers diagnosed in current or previous OC users tend to be less clinically advanced than in nonusers.

Women who currently have or have had breast cancer should not use oral contraceptives because breast cancer is a hormonally-sensitive tumor.

Some studies suggest that oral contraceptive use has been associated with an increase in the risk of cervical intraepithelial neoplasia in some populations of women. However, there continues to be controversy about the extent to which such findings may be due to differences in sexual behavior and other factors.

In spite of many studies of the relationship between oral contraceptive use and breast and cervical cancers, a cause-and-effect relationship has not been established.

HEPATIC NEOPLASIA

Benign hepatic adenomas are associated with oral contraceptive use, although the incidence of benign tumors is rare in the US. Indirect calculations have estimated the attributable risk to be in the range of 3.3 cases/100,000 for users, a risk that increases after 4 or more years of use. Rupture of rare, benign, hepatic adenomas may cause death through intra-abdominal hemorrhage.

Studies from Britain have shown an increased risk of developing hepatocellular carcinoma in long-term (>8 years) oral contraceptive users. However, these cancers are extremely rare in the US and the attributable risk (the excess incidence) of liver cancers in oral contraceptive users approaches less than one per million users.

OCULAR LESIONS

There have been clinical case reports of retinal thrombosis associated with the use of oral contraceptives. Oral contraceptives should be discontinued if there is unexplained partial or complete loss of vision; onset of proptosis or diplopia; papilledema; or retinal vascular lesions. Appropriate diagnostic and therapeutic measures should be undertaken immediately.

ORAL CONTRACEPTIVE USE BEFORE OR DURING EARLY PREGNANCY

Extensive epidemiological studies have revealed no increased risk of birth defects in women who have used oral contraceptives prior to pregnancy. Studies also do not suggest a teratogenic effect, particularly in so far as cardiac anomalies and limb-reduction defects are concerned, when taken inadvertently during early pregnancy.

The administration of oral contraceptives to induce withdrawal bleeding should not be used as a test for pregnancy. Oral contraceptives should not be used during pregnancy to treat threatened or habitual abortion.

It is recommended that for any patient who has missed two consecutive periods, pregnancy should be ruled out before continuing oral contraceptive use. If the patient has not adhered to the prescribed dosing schedule, the possibility of pregnancy should be considered at the time of the first missed period. Oral contraceptive use should be discontinued if pregnancy is confirmed.

GALLBLADDER DISEASE

Earlier studies have reported an increased lifetime relative risk of gallbladder surgery in users of oral contraceptives and estrogens. More recent studies, however, have shown that the relative risk of developing gallbladder disease among oral contraceptive users may be minimal. The recent findings of minimal risk may be related to the use of oral contraceptive formulations containing lower hormonal doses of estrogens and progestogens.

CARBOHYDRATE AND LIPID METABOLIC EFFECTS

Oral contraceptives have been shown to cause glucose intolerance in a significant percentage of users. Oral contraceptives containing greater than 75 μg of estrogens cause hyperinsulinism, while lower doses of estrogen cause less glucose intolerance. Progestogens increase insulin secretion and create insulin resistance, this effect varying with different progestational agents. However, in the nondiabetic woman, oral contraceptives appear to have no effect on fasting blood glucose. Because of these demonstrated effects, prediabetic and diabetic women should be carefully observed while taking oral contraceptives.

A small proportion of women will have persistent hypertriglyceridemia while on the pill. As discussed earlier (see Thromboembolic Disorders and Other Vascular Problems: Myocardial Infarction and Dose-Related Risk of Vascular Disease From Oral Contraceptives), changes in serum triglycerides and lipoprotein levels have been reported in oral contraceptive users.

ELEVATED BLOOD PRESSURE

An increase in blood pressure has been reported in women taking oral contraceptives and this increase is more likely in older oral contraceptive users and with continued use. Data from the Royal College of General Practitioners and subsequent randomized trials have shown that the incidence of hypertension increases with increasing concentrations of progestogens.

Women with a history of hypertension or hypertension-related diseases, or renal disease should be encouraged to use another method of contraception. If women with hypertension elect to use oral contraceptives, they should be monitored closely, and if significant elevation of blood pressure occurs, oral contraceptives should be discontinued. For most women, elevated blood pressure will return to normal after stopping oral contraceptives and there is no difference in the occurrence of hypertension among ever- and never-users.

HEADACHE

The onset or exacerbation of migraine or development of headache with a new pattern which is recurrent, persistent or severe requires discontinuation of oral contraceptives and evaluation of the cause.

BLEEDING IRREGULARITIES

Breakthrough bleeding and spotting are sometimes encountered in patients on oral contraceptives, especially during the first 3 months of use. Nonhormonal causes should be considered and adequate diagnostic measures taken to rule out malignancy or pregnancy in the event of breakthrough bleeding, as in the case of any abnormal vaginal bleeding. If pathology has been excluded, time or a change to another formulation may solve the problem. In the event of amenorrhea, pregnancy should be ruled out.

Some women may encounter post-pill amenorrhea or oligomenorrhea, especially when such a condition was pre-existent.

PRECAUTIONS

GENERAL

Patients should be counseled that this product does not protect against HIV infection (AIDS) and other sexually transmitted diseases.

PHYSICAL EXAMINATION AND FOLLOW-UP

It is good medical practice for all women to have annual history and physical examinations, including women using oral contraceptives. The physical examination, however, may be deferred until after initiation of oral contraceptives if requested by the woman and judged appropriate by the clinician. The physical examination should include special reference to blood pressure, breasts, abdomen and pelvic organs, including cervical cytology and relevant laboratory tests. In case of undiagnosed, persistent or recurrent abnormal vaginal bleeding, appropriate measures should be conducted to rule out malignancy. Women with a strong family history of breast cancer or who have breast nodules should be monitored with particular care.

LIPID DISORDERS

Women who are being treated for hyperlipidemias should be followed closely if they elect to use oral contraceptives. Some progestogens may elevate LDL levels and may render the control of hyperlipidemias more difficult.

LIVER FUNCTION

If jaundice develops in any woman receiving oral contraceptives, the medication should be discontinued. Steroid hormones may be poorly metabolized in patients with impaired liver function.

FLUID RETENTION

Oral contraceptives may cause some degree of fluid retention. They should be prescribed with caution, and only with careful monitoring, in patients with conditions which might be aggravated by fluid retention.

EMOTIONAL DISORDERS

Women with a history of depression should be carefully observed and the drug discontinued if depression recurs to a serious degree.

CONTACT LENSES

Contact-lens wearers who develop visual changes or changes in lens tolerance should be assessed by an ophthalmologist.

INTERACTIONS WITH LABORATORY TESTS

Certain endocrine- and liver-function tests and blood components may be affected by oral contraceptives:

- Increased prothrombin and factors VII, VIII, IX and X; decreased antithrombin 3; increased norepinephrine-induced platelet aggregability.
- Increased thyroid-binding globulin (TBG) leading to increased circulating total thyroid hormone, as measured by protein-bound iodine (PBI), T4 by column or by radioimmunoassay. Free T3 resin uptake is decreased, reflecting the elevated TBG, free T4 concentration is unaltered.
- Other binding proteins may be elevated in serum.
- Sex-hormone-binding globulins are increased and result in elevated levels of total circulating sex steroids and corticoids; however, free or biologically active levels remain unchanged.
- Triglycerides may be increased.
- Glucose tolerance may be decreased.
- Serum folate levels may be depressed by oral contraceptive therapy. This may be of clinical significance if a woman becomes pregnant shortly after discontinuing oral contraceptives.

CARCINOGENESIS, MUTAGENESIS, AND IMPAIRMENT OF FERTILITY

In a 24 month oral carcinogenicity study in mice dosed with 10 mg/kg/day drospirenone alone or 1 + 0.01, 3 + 0.03 and 10 + 0.1 mg/kg/day of drospirenone and ethinyl estradiol, 0.1 to 2 times the exposure (AUC of drospirenone) of women taking a contraceptive dose, there was an increase in carcinomas of the harderian gland in the group that received the high dose of drospirenone alone. In a similar study in rats given 10 mg/kg/day drospirenone alone or 0.3 + 0.003, 3 + 0.03 and 10 + 0.1 mg/kg/day drospirenone and ethinyl estradiol, 0.8 to 10 times the exposure of women taking a contraceptive dose, there was an increased incidence of benign and total (benign and malignant) adrenal gland pheochromocytomas in the group receiving the high dose of drospirenone. Drospirenone was not mutagenic in a number of *in vitro* (Ames, Chinese Hamster Lung gene mutation and chromosomal damage in human lymphocytes) and *in vivo* (mouse micronucleus) genotoxicity tests. Drospirenone increased unscheduled DNA synthesis in rat hepatocytes and formed adducts with rodent liver DNA but not with human liver DNA. See WARNINGS.

PREGNANCY CATEGORY X

See CONTRAINDICATIONS and WARNINGS.

Estrogens and progestins should not be used during pregnancy. Fourteen (14) pregnancies that occurred with Yasmin exposure *in utero* (none with more than a single cycle of exposure) have been identified. One (1) infant was born with esophageal atresia. A causal association with Yasmin is unknown.

A teratology study in pregnant rats given drospirenone orally at doses of 5, 15 and 45 mg/kg/day, 6-50 times the human exposure based on AUC of drospirenone, resulted in an increased number of fetuses with delayed ossification of bones of the feet in the two higher doses. A similar study in rabbits dosed orally with 1, 30 and 100 mg/kg/day drospirenone, 2-27 times the human exposure, resulted in an increase in fetal loss and retardation of fetal development (delayed ossification of small bones, multiple fusions of ribs) at the high dose only. When drospirenone was administered with ethinyl estradiol (100:1) during late pregnancy (the period of genital development) at doses of 5, 15 and 45 mg/kg, there was a dose dependent increase in feminization of male rat fetuses. In a study in 36 cynomolgous monkeys, no teratogenic or feminization effects were observed with orally administered drospirenone and ethinyl estradiol (100:1) at doses up to 10 mg/kg/day drospirenone, 30 times the human exposure.

NURSING MOTHERS

Small amounts of oral contraceptive steroids have been identified in the milk of nursing mothers, and a few adverse effects on the child have been reported, including jaundice and breast enlargement. In addition, oral contraceptives given in the postpartum period may interfere with lactation by decreasing the quantity and quality of breast milk. If possible, the nursing mother should be advised not to use oral contraceptives but to use other forms of contraception until she has completely weaned her child.

After oral administration of Yasmin about 0.02% of the drospirenone dose was excreted into the breast milk of postpartum women within 24 hours. This results in a maximal daily dose of about 3 μg drospirenone in an infant.

PEDIATRIC USAGE

Safety and efficacy of Yasmin have been established in women of reproductive age. Safety and efficacy are expected to be the same for postpubertal adolescents under the age of 16 and for users 16 years and older. Use of this product before menarche is not indicated.

INFORMATION FOR THE PATIENT

See the Patient Labeling that is distributed with the prescription.

DRUG INTERACTIONS

EFFECTS OF OTHER DRUGS ON COMBINED HORMONAL CONTRACEPTIVES

Rifampin. Metabolism of ethinyl estradiol and some progestins (*e.g.*, norethindrone) is increased by rifampin. A reduction in contraceptive effectiveness and an increase in menstrual irregularities have been associated with concomitant use of rifampin.

Anticonvulsants. Anticonvulsants such as phenobarbital, phenytoin, and carbamazepine have been shown to increase the metabolism of ethinyl estradiol and/or some progestins, which could result in a reduction of contraceptive effectiveness.

Antibiotics. Pregnancy while taking combined hormonal contraceptives has been reported when the combined hormonal contraceptives were administered with antimicrobials such as ampicillin, tetracycline, and griseofulvin. However, clinical pharmacokinetic studies have not demonstrated any consistent effects of antibiotics (other than rifampin) on plasma concentrations of synthetic steroids.

Atorvastatin. Coadministration of atorvastatin and an oral contraceptive increased AUC values for norethindrone and ethinyl estradiol by approximately 30% and 20%, respectively.

St. John's Wort. Herbal products containing St. John's Wort (hypericum perforatum) may induce hepatic enzymes (cytochrome P450) and p-glycoprotein transporter and may reduce the effectiveness of oral contraceptives and emergency contraceptive pills. This may also result in breakthrough bleeding.

Other. Ascorbic acid and acetominophen may increase plasma concentrations of some synthetic estrogens, possibly by inhibition of conjugation. A reduction in contraceptive effectiveness and an increased incidence of menstrual irregularities has been suggested with phenylbutazone.

EFFECTS OF DROSPIRENONE ON OTHER DRUGS

Metabolic Interactions

Metabolism of DRSP and potential effects of DRSP on hepatic cytochrome P450 (CYP) enzymes have been investigated in *in vitro* and *in vivo* studies (see CLINICAL PHARMACOLOGY, Pharmacokinetics, Metabolism). In *in vitro* studies DRSP did not affect turnover of model substrates of CYP1A2 and CYP2D6, but had an inhibitory influence on the turnover of model substrates of CYP1A1, CYP2C9, CYP2C19 and CYP3A4 with CYP2C19 being the most sensitive enzyme. The potential effect of DRSP on CYP2C19 activity was investigated in a clinical pharmacokinetic study using omeprazole as a marker substrate. In the study with 24 postmenopausal women [including 12 women with homozygous (wild type) CYP2C19 genotype and 12 women with heterozygous CYP2C19 genotype] the daily oral administration of 3 mg DRSP for 14 days did not affect the oral clearance of omeprazole (40 mg, single oral dose). Based on the available results of *in vivo* and *in vitro* studies it can be concluded that, at clinical dose level, DRSP shows little propensity to interact to a significant extent with cytochrome P450 enzymes.

Interactions With Drugs That Have the Potential to Increase Serum Potassium

There is a potential for an increase in serum potassium in women taking Yasmin with other drugs **(see BOLDED WARNING).** Of note, occasional or chronic use of NSAID medication was not restricted in any of the Yasmin clinical trials.

A drug-drug interaction study of DRSP 3 mg/estradiol (E2) 1 mg versus placebo was performed in 24 mildly hypertensive postmenopausal women taking enalapril meleate 10 mg twice daily. Potassium levels were obtained every other day for a total of 2 weeks in all subjects. Mean serum potassium levels in the DRSP/E2 treatment group relative to baseline were 0.22 mEq/L higher than those in the placebo group. Serum potassium concentrations also were measured at multiple timepoints over 24 hours at baseline and on Day 14. On Day 14, the ratios for serum potassium C_{max} and AUC in the DRSP/E2 group to those in the placebo group were 0.955 (90% CI: 0.914, 0.999) and 1.010 (90% CI: 0.944, 1.080), respectively. No patient in either treatment group developed hyperkalemia (serum potassium concentrations >5.5 mEq/L).

EFFECTS OF COMBINED HORMONAL CONTRACEPTIVES ON OTHER DRUGS

Combined oral contraceptives containing ethinyl estradiol may inhibit the metabolism of other compounds. Increased plasma concentrations of cyclosporine, prednisolone, and theophylline have been reported with concomitant administration of oral contraceptives. In addition, oral contraceptives may induce the conjugation of other compounds. Decreased plasma concentrations of acetaminophen and increased clearance on temazepam, salicylic acid, morphine, and clofibric acid have been noted when these drugs were administered with oral contraceptives.

ADVERSE REACTIONS

An increased risk of the following serious adverse reactions has been associated with the use of oral contraceptives (see WARNINGS): Thrombophlebitis, arterial thromboembolism, pulmonary embolism, myocardial infarction, cerebral hemorrhage, cerebral thrombosis, hypertension, gallbladder disease, hepatic adenomas or benign liver tumors.

There is evidence of an association between the following conditions and the use of oral contraceptives, although additional confirmatory studies are needed: Mesenteric thrombosis, retinal thrombosis.

The following adverse reactions have been reported in patients receiving oral contraceptives and are believed to be drug-related: Nausea; vomiting; gastrointestinal symptoms (such as abdominal cramps and bloating); breakthrough bleeding; spotting; change in menstrual flow; amenorrhea; temporary infertility after discontinuation of treatment; edema; melasma which may persist; breast changes: tenderness, enlargement, secretion; change in weight (increase or decrease); change in cervical erosion and secretion; diminution in lactation when given immediately postpartum; cholestatic jaundice; migraine; rash (allergic); mental depression; reduced tolerance to carbohydrates; vaginal candidiasis; change in corneal curvature (steepening); Intolerance to contact lenses.

The following adverse reactions have been reported in users of oral contraceptives and a causal association has been neither confirmed nor refuted: Acne, Budd-Chiari syndrome, cataracts, changes in appetite, changes in libido, colitis, cystitis-like syndrome, dizziness, erythema multiforme, erythema nodosum, headache, hemolytic uremic syndrome, hemorrhagic eruption, hirsutism, impaired renal function, loss of scalp hair, nervousness, porphyria, pre-menstrual syndrome, vaginitis.

The following are the most common adverse events reported with use of Yasmin during the clinical trials, occurring in >1% of subjects and which may or may not be drug related: Headache, menstrual disorder, breast pain, abdominal pain, nausea, leukorrhea, flu syndrome, acne, vaginal moniliasis, depression, diarrhea, asthenia, dysmenorrhea, back pain, infection, pharyngitis, intermenstrual bleeding, migraine, vomiting, dizziness, nervousness, vaginitis, sinusitis, cystitis, bronchitis, gastroenteritis, allergic reaction, urinary tract infection, pruritus, emotional lability, surgery, rash, upper respiratory infection.

DOSAGE AND ADMINISTRATION

To achieve maximum contraceptive effectiveness, Yasmin (drospirenone and ethinyl estradiol) must be taken exactly as directed at intervals not exceeding 24 hours.

Yasmin consists of 21 tablets of a monophasic combined hormonal preparation plus 7 inert tablets. The dosage of Yasmin is one yellow tablet daily for 21 consecutive days followed by 7 white inert tablets per menstrual cycle. A patient should begin to take Yasmin either on the first day of her menstrual period (Day 1 Start) or on the first Sunday after the onset of her menstrual period (Sunday Start).

DAY 1 START

During the first cycle of Yasmin use, the patient should be instructed to take one yellow Yasmin daily, beginning on day one (1) of her menstrual cycle. (The first day of menstruation is day one.) She should take one yellow Yasmin daily for 21 consecutive days, followed by one white inert tablet daily on menstrual cycle days 22-28. It is recommended that Yasmin be taken at the same time each day, preferably after the evening meal or at bedtime. If Yasmin is first taken later than the first day of the menstrual cycle, Yasmin should not be considered effective as a contraceptive until after the first 7 consecutive days of product administration. The possibility of ovulation and conception prior to initiation of medication should be considered.

SUNDAY START

During the first cycle of Yasmin use, the patient should be instructed to take one yellow Yasmin daily, beginning on the first Sunday after the onset of her menstrual period. She should take one yellow Yasmin daily for 21 consecutive days, followed by one white inert tablet daily on menstrual cycle days 22-28. It is recommended that Yasmin be taken at the same time each day, preferably after the evening meal or at bedtime. Yasmin should not be considered effective as a contraceptive until after the first 7 consecutive days of product administration. The possibility of ovulation and conception prior to initiation of medication should be considered.

The patient should begin her next and all subsequent 28 day regimens of Yasmin on the same day of the week that she began her first regimen, following the same schedule. She should begin taking her yellow tablets on the next day after ingestion of the last white tablet, regardless of whether or not a menstrual period has occurred or is still in progress. Anytime a subsequent cycle of Yasmin is started later than the day following administration of the last white tablet, the patient should use another method of contraception until she has taken a yellow Yasmin daily for 7 consecutive days.

When switching from another oral contraceptive, Yasmin should be started on the same day that a new pack of the previous oral contraceptive would have been started.

Withdrawal bleeding usually occurs within 3 days following the last white tablet. If spotting or breakthrough bleeding occurs while taking Yasmin, the patient should be instructed to continue taking her Yasmin as instructed and by the regimen described above. She should be instructed that this type of bleeding is usually transient and without significance; however, if the bleeding is persistent or prolonged, the patient should be advised to consult her physician.

Although the occurrence of pregnancy is unlikely if Yasmin is taken according to directions, if withdrawal bleeding does not occur, the possibility of pregnancy must be considered. If the patient has not adhered to the prescribed dosing schedule (missed one or more active tablets or started taking them on a day later than she should have), the probability of pregnancy should be considered at the time of the first missed period and appropriate diagnostic measures taken before the medication is resumed. If the patient has adhered to the prescribed regimen and misses two consecutive periods, pregnancy should be ruled out before continuing the contraceptive regimen.

The risk of pregnancy increases with each active yellow tablet missed. For additional patient instructions regarding missed pills, see the "WHAT TO DO IF YOU MISS PILLS" section in the DETAILED PATIENT LABELING which is distributed with the prescription. If breakthrough bleeding occurs following missed tablets, it will usually be transient and of no consequence. If the patient misses one or more white tablets, she should still be protected against pregnancy provided she begins taking yellow tablets again on the proper day.

In the nonlactating mother, Yasmin may be initiated 4 weeks postpartum, for contraception. When the tablets are administered in the postpartum period, the increased risk of thromboembolic disease associated with the postpartum period must be considered. (See CONTRAINDICATIONS, WARNINGS, and PRECAUTIONS concerning thromboembolic disease.)

HOW SUPPLIED

Yasmin 28 tablets (drospirenone and ethinyl estradiol) are available in packages of 3 blister packs. Each pack contains 21 active yellow round, unscored, film coated tablets each containing 3 mg drospirenone and 0.03 mg ethinyl estradiol, and 7 inert white round, unscored, film coated tablets.

Storage: Store at 25°C (77°F); excursions permitted to 15-30°C (59-86°F).

PRODUCT LISTING - EQUIVALENTS NOT AVAILABLE

Tablet - Oral - 3 mg;0.03 mg

28 x 3 $99.00 YASMIN, Berlex Laboratories 50419-0402-03

Drotrecogin alfa (003536)

Categories: Septicemia; FDA Approved 2001 Nov; Pregnancy Category C
Drug Classes: Thrombolytics
Brand Names: Xigris

DESCRIPTION

Xigris [drotrecogin alfa (activated)] is a recombinant form of human Activated Protein C. An established human cell line possessing the complementary DNA for the inactive human Protein C zymogen secretes the protein into the fermentation medium. Fermentation is carried out in a nutrient medium containing the antibiotic geneticin sulfate. Geneticin sulfate is not detectable in the final product. Human Protein C is enzymatically activated by cleavage with thrombin and subsequently purified.

Drotrecogin alfa (activated) is a serine protease with the same amino acid sequence as human plasma-derived Activated Protein C. Drotrecogin alfa (activated) is a glycoprotein of approximately 55 kilodalton molecular weight, consisting of a heavy chain and a light chain linked by a disulfide bond. Drotrecogin alfa (activated) and human plasma-derived Activated Protein C have the same sites of glycosylation, although some differences in the glycosylation structures exist.

Xigris is supplied as a sterile, lyophilized, white to off-white powder for intravenous infusion. The 5 and 20 mg vials of Xigris contain 5.3 mg and 20.8 mg of drotrecogin alfa (activated), respectively. The 5 and 20 mg vials of Xigris also contain 40.3 and 158.1 mg of sodium chloride, 10.9 and 42.9 mg of sodium citrate, and 31.8 and 124.9 mg of sucrose, respectively.

CLINICAL PHARMACOLOGY

GENERAL PHARMACOLOGY

Activated Protein C exerts an antithrombotic effect by inhibiting Factors Va and VIIIa. *In vitro* data indicate that Activated Protein C has indirect profibrinolytic activity through its ability to inhibit plasminogen activator inhibitor-1 (PAI-1) and limiting generation of activated thrombin-activatable-fibrinolysis-inhibitor. Additionally, *in vitro* data indicate that Activated Protein C may exert an anti-inflammatory effect by inhibiting human tumor necrosis factor production by monocytes, by blocking leukocyte adhesion to selectins, and by limiting the thrombin-induced inflammatory responses within the microvascular endothelium.

PHARMACODYNAMICS

The specific mechanisms by which drotrecogin alfa exerts its effect on survival in patients with severe sepsis are not completely understood. In patients with severe sepsis, drotrecogin alfa infusions of 48 or 96 hours produced dose-dependent declines in D-dimer and IL-6. Compared to placebo, drotrecogin alfa-treated patients experienced more rapid declines in D-dimer, PAI-1 levels, thrombin-antithrombin levels, prothrombin F1.2, IL-6, more rapid increases in protein C and antithrombin levels, and normalization of plasminogen. As assessed by infusion duration, the maximum observed pharmacodynamic effect of drotrecogin alfa (activated) on D-dimer levels occurred at the end of 96 hours of infusion for the 24 μg/kg/h treatment group.

HUMAN PHARMACOKINETICS

Drotrecogin alfa and endogenous Activated Protein C are inactivated by endogenous plasma protease inhibitors. Plasma concentrations of endogenous Activated Protein C in healthy subjects and patients with severe sepsis are usually below detection limits.

In patients with severe sepsis, drotrecogin alfa infusions of 12-30 μg/kg/h rapidly produce steady state concentrations (C^{ss}) that are proportional to infusion rates. In the Phase 3 trial, the median clearance of drotrecogin alfa was 40 L/h (interquartile range of 27-52 L/h). The median C^{ss} of 45 ng/ml (interquartile range of 35-62 ng/ml) was attained within 2 hours after starting infusion. In the majority of patients, plasma concentrations of drotrecogin alfa fell below the assay's quantitation limit of 10 ng/ml within 2 hours after stopping infusion. Plasma clearance of drotrecogin alfa in patients with severe sepsis is approximately 50% higher than that in healthy subjects.

SPECIAL POPULATIONS

In adult patients with severe sepsis, small differences were detected in the plasma clearance of drotrecogin alfa with regard to age, gender, hepatic dysfunction or renal dysfunction. Dose adjustment is not required based on these factors alone or in combination (see PRECAUTIONS).

End Stage Renal Disease

Patients with end stage renal disease requiring chronic renal replacement therapy were excluded from the Phase 3 study. In patients without sepsis undergoing hemodialysis (n=6), plasma clearance (mean ±SD) of drotrecogin alfa administered on non-dialysis days was 30 ± 8 L/h. Plasma clearance of drotrecogin alfa was 23 ± 4 L/h in patients without sepsis undergoing peritoneal dialysis (n=5). These clearance rates did not meaningfully differ from those in normal healthy subjects (28 ± 9 L/h) (n=190).

Pediatrics

Safety and efficacy have not been established in pediatric patients with severe sepsis (see INDICATIONS AND USAGE), therefore no dosage recommendation can be made. The pharmacokinetics of a dose of 24 μg/kg/h of drotrecogin alfa appear to be similar in pediatric and adult patients with severe sepsis.

D

Drug-Drug Interactions

Formal drug interactions studies have not been conducted.

INDICATIONS AND USAGE

Drotrecogin alfa is indicated for the reduction of mortality in adult patients with severe sepsis (sepsis associated with acute organ dysfunction) who have a high risk of death (*e.g.*, as determined by APACHE II.

Efficacy has not been established in adult patients with severe sepsis and lower risk of death. Safety and efficacy have not been established in pediatric patients with severe sepsis.

CONTRAINDICATIONS

Drotrecogin alfa increases the risk of bleeding. Drotrecogin alfa is contraindicated in patients with the following clinical situations in which bleeding could be associated with a high risk of death or significant morbidity:

- Active internal bleeding.
- Recent (within 3 months) hemorrhagic stroke.
- Recent (within 2 months) intracranial or intraspinal surgery, or severe head trauma.
- Trauma with an increased risk of life-threatening bleeding.
- Presence of an epidural catheter.
- Intracranial neoplasm or mass lesion or evidence of cerebral herniation.

Drotrecogin alfa is contraindicated in patients with known hypersensitivity to drotrecogin alfa (activated) or any component of this product.

WARNINGS

Bleeding is the most common serious adverse effect associated with drotrecogin alfa therapy. Each patient being considered for therapy with drotrecogin alfa should be carefully evaluated and anticipated benefits weighed against potential risks associated with therapy.

Certain conditions, many of which led to exclusion from the Phase 3 trial, are likely to increase the risk of bleeding with drotrecogin alfa therapy. Therefore, for patients with severe sepsis who have one or more of the following conditions, the increased risk of bleeding should be carefully considered when deciding whether to use drotrecogin alfa therapy:

- Concurrent therapeutic heparin (≥15 units/kg/h).
- Platelet count <30,000 × 10^6/L, even if the platelet count is increased after transfusions.
- Prothrombin time-INR >3.0.
- Recent (within 6 weeks) gastrointestinal bleeding.
- Recent administration (within 3 days) of thrombolytic therapy.
- Recent administration (within 7 days) of oral anticoagulants or glycoprotein IIb/IIIa inhibitors.
- Recent administration (within 7 days) of aspirin >650 mg per day or other platelet inhibitors.
- Recent (within 3 months) ischemic stroke (see CONTRAINDICATIONS).
- Intracranial arteriovenous malformation or aneurysm.
- Known bleeding diathesis.
- Chronic severe hepatic disease.
- Any other condition in which bleeding constitutes a significant hazard or would be particularly difficult to manage because of its location.

Should clinically important bleeding occur, immediately stop the infusion of drotrecogin alfa. Continued use of other agents affecting the coagulation system should be carefully assessed. Once adequate hemostasis has been achieved, continued use of drotrecogin alfa may be reconsidered.

Drotrecogin alfa should be discontinued 2 hours prior to undergoing an invasive surgical procedure or procedures with an inherent risk of bleeding. Once adequate hemostasis has been achieved, initiation of drotrecogin alfa may be reconsidered 12 hours after major invasive procedures or surgery or restarted immediately after uncomplicated less invasive procedures.

PRECAUTIONS

LABORATORY TESTS

Most patients with severe sepsis have a coagulopathy that is commonly associated with prolongation of the activated partial thromboplastin time (APTT) and the prothrombin time (PT). Drotrecogin alfa may variably prolong the APTT. Therefore, the APTT cannot be reliably used to assess the status of the coagulopathy during drotrecogin alfa infusion. Drotrecogin alfa has minimal effect on the PT and the PT can be used to monitor the status of the coagulopathy in these patients.

IMMUNOGENICITY

As with all therapeutic proteins, there is a potential for immunogenicity. The incidence of antibody development in patients receiving drotrecogin alfa has not been adequately determined, as the assay sensitivity is inadequate to reliably detect all potential antibody responses. One patient in the Phase 2 trial developed antibodies to drotrecogin alfa without clinical sequelae. One patient in the Phase 3 trial who developed antibodies to drotrecogin alfa developed superficial and deep vein thrombi during the study, and died of multi-organ failure on day 36 post-treatment but the relationship of this event to antibody is not clear.

Drotrecogin alfa has not been readministered to patients with severe sepsis.

DRUG/LABORATORY TEST INTERACTION

Because drotrecogin alfa may affect the APTT assay, drotrecogin alfa present in plasma samples may interfere with one-stage coagulation assays based on the APTT (such as factor VIII, IX, and XI assays). This interference may result in an apparent factor concentration that is lower than the true concentration. Drotrecogin alfa present in plasma samples does not interfere with one-stage factor assays based on the PT (such as factor II, V, VII, and X assays).

CARCINOGENESIS, MUTAGENESIS, AND IMPAIRMENT OF FERTILITY

Long-term studies in animals to evaluate potential carcinogenicity of drotrecogin alfa have not been performed.

Drotrecogin alfa was not mutagenic in an *in vivo* micronucleus study in mice or in an *in vitro* chromosomal aberration study in human peripheral blood lymphocytes with or without rat liver metabolic activation.

The potential of drotrecogin alfa to impair fertility has not been evaluated in male or female animals.

PREGNANCY CATEGORY C

Animal reproductive studies have not been conducted with drotrecogin alfa. It is not known whether drotrecogin alfa can cause fetal harm when administered to a pregnant woman or can affect reproduction capacity. Drotrecogin alfa should be given to pregnant women only if clearly needed.

NURSING MOTHERS

It is not known whether drotrecogin alfa is excreted in human milk or absorbed systemically after ingestion. Because many drugs are excreted in human milk, and because of the potential for adverse effects on the nursing infant, a decision should be made whether to discontinue nursing or discontinue the drug, taking into account the importance of the drug to the mother.

PEDIATRIC USE

The safety and effectiveness of drotrecogin alfa have not been established in the age group newborn (38 weeks gestational age) to 18 years. The efficacy of drotrecogin alfa in adult patients with severe sepsis and high risk of death cannot be extrapolated to pediatric patients with severe sepsis.

GERIATRIC USE

In clinical studies evaluating 1821 patients with severe sepsis, approximately 50% of the patients were 65 years or older. No overall differences in safety or effectiveness were observed between these patients and younger patients.

DRUG INTERACTIONS

Drug interactions with drotrecogin alfa have not been studied in patients with severe sepsis. Caution should be employed when drotrecogin alfa is used with other drugs that affect hemostasis (see CLINICAL PHARMACOLOGY, WARNINGS). Approximately 2/3 of the patients in the Phase 3 study received prophylactic low dose heparin. Concomitant use of prophylactic low dose heparin did not appear to affect safety. Its effect on the efficacy of drotrecogin alfa has not been evaluated in a randomized controlled clinical trial.

ADVERSE REACTIONS

BLEEDING

Bleeding is the most common adverse reaction associated with drotrecogin alfa.

In the Phase 3 study, serious bleeding events were observed during the 28 day study period in 3.5% of drotrecogin alfa-treated and 2.0% of placebo-treated patients, respectively. The difference in serious bleeding between drotrecogin alfa and placebo occurred primarily during the infusion period and is shown in TABLE 2.[1] Serious bleeding events were defined as any intracranial hemorrhage, any life-threatening bleed, any bleeding event requiring the administration of ≥3 units of packed red blood cells per day for 2 consecutive days, or any bleeding event assessed as a serious adverse event.

***TABLE 2** Number of Patients Experiencing a Serious Bleeding Event by Site of Hemorrhage During the Study Drug Infusion Period* in PROWESS[1]*

	Drotrecogin alfa n=850	Placebo n=840
Total	20 (2.4%)	8 (1.0%)
Site of Hemorrhage		
Gastrointestinal	5	4
Intra-abdominal	2	3
Intra-thoracic	4	0
Retroperitoneal	3	0
Intracranial	2	0
Genitourinary	2	0
Skin/soft tissue	1	0
Other	1	1

* Study drug infusion period is defined as the date of initiation of study drug to the date of study drug discontinuation plus the next calendar day.

† Patients requiring the administration of ≥3 units of packed red blood cells per day for 2 consecutive days without an identified site of bleeding.

In PROWESS, 2 cases of intracranial hemorrhage (ICH) occurred during the infusion period for drotrecogin alfa-treated patients and no cases were reported in the placebo patients. The incidence of ICH during the 28 day study period was 0.2% for drotrecogin alfa-treated patients and 0.1% for placebo-treated patients. ICH has been reported in patients receiving drotrecogin alfa in non-placebo controlled trials with an incidence of approximately 1% during the infusion period. The risk of ICH may be increased in patients with risk factors for bleeding such as severe coagulopathy and severe thrombocytopenia (see WARNINGS).

In PROWESS, 25% of the drotrecogin alfa-treated patients and 18% of the placebo-treated patients experienced at least one bleeding event during the 28 day study period. In both treatment groups, the majority of bleeding events were ecchymoses or gastrointestinal tract bleeding.

OTHER ADVERSE REACTIONS

Patients administered drotrecogin alfa as treatment for severe sepsis experience many events which are potential sequelae of severe sepsis and may or may not be attributable to drotrecogin alfa therapy. In clinical trials, there were no types of non-bleeding adverse events suggesting a causal association with drotrecogin alfa.

DOSAGE AND ADMINISTRATION

Drotrecogin alfa should be administered intravenously at an infusion rate of 24 μg/kg/h for a total duration of infusion of 96 hours. Dose adjustment based on clinical or laboratory parameters is not recommended (see PRECAUTIONS).

If the infusion is interrupted, drotrecogin alfa should be restarted at the 24 μg/kg/h infusion rate. Dose escalation or bolus doses of drotrecogin alfa are not recommended.

In the event of clinically important bleeding, immediately stop the infusion (see WARNINGS).

Preparation and administration instructions: Use aseptic technique.

Use appropriate aseptic technique during the preparation of drotrecogin alfa for intravenous administration.

Calculate the dose and the number of drotrecogin alfa vials needed. Each drotrecogin alfa vial contains 5 or 20 mg of drotrecogin alfa. The vial contains an excess of drotrecogin alfa to facilitate delivery of the label amount.

Prior to administration, 5 mg vials must be reconstituted with 2.5 ml sterile water for injection, and 20 mg vials of drotrecogin alfa must be reconstituted with 10 ml of sterile water for injection. The resulting concentration of the solution is approximately 2 mg/ml of drotrecogin alfa. Slowly add the sterile water for injection to the vial and avoid inverting or shaking the vial. Gently swirl each vial until the powder is completely dissolved.

The solution of reconstituted drotrecogin alfa must be further diluted with sterile 0.9% sodium chloride injection. Slowly withdraw the appropriate amount of reconstituted drotrecogin alfa solution from the vial. Add the reconstituted drotrecogin alfa into a prepared infusion bag of sterile 0.9% sodium chloride injection. When adding the drotrecogin alfa into the infusion bag, direct the stream to the side of the bag to minimize the agitation of the solution. Gently invert the infusion bag to obtain a homogeneous solution. Do not transport the infusion bag between locations using mechanical delivery systems.

Because drotrecogin alfa contains no antibacterial preservatives, the intravenous solution should be prepared immediately upon reconstitution of the drotrecogin alfa in the vial(s). If the vial of reconstituted drotrecogin alfa is not used immediately, it may be held at controlled room temperature 15-30°C (59-86°F), but must be used within 3 hours. Intravenous administration must be completed within 12 hours after the intravenous solution is prepared.

Parenteral drug products should be inspected visually for particulate matter and discoloration prior to administration.

When using an intravenous infusion pump to administer the drug, the solution of reconstituted drotrecogin alfa is typically diluted into an infusion bag containing sterile 0.9% sodium chloride injection to a final concentration of between 100 and 200 μg/ml.

When using a syringe pump to administer the drug, the solution of reconstituted drotrecogin alfa is typically diluted with sterile 0.9% sodium chloride injection to a final concentration of between 100 and 1000 μg/ml. When administering drotrecogin alfa at low concentrations (less than approximately 200 μg/ml) at low flow rates (less than approximately 5 ml/h), the infusion set must be primed for approximately 15 minutes at a flow rate of approximately 5 ml/h.

Drotrecogin alfa should be administered via a dedicated intravenous line or a dedicated lumen of a multilumen central venous catheter. The ONLY other solutions that can be administered through the same line are 0.9% sodium chloride injection, lactated Ringer's injection, dextrose, or dextrose and saline mixtures.

Avoid exposing drotrecogin alfa solutions to heat and/or direct sunlight. No incompatibilities have been observed between drotrecogin alfa and glass infusion bottles or infusion bags and syringes made of polyvinylchloride, polyethylene, polypropylene, or polyolefin.

HOW SUPPLIED

Xigris is available in 5 mg and 20 mg single-use vials containing sterile, preservative-free, lyophilized drotrecogin alfa (activated).

Storage: Xigris should be stored in a refrigerator 2-8°C (36-46°F). Do not freeze. Protect unreconstituted vials of Xigris from light. Retain in carton until time of use. Do not use beyond the expiration date stamped on the vial.

PRODUCT LISTING - EQUIVALENTS NOT AVAILABLE

Powder For Injection - Intravenous - 5 mg

1's $262.50 XIGRIS, Lilly, Eli and Company 00002-7559-01

Powder For Injection - Intravenous - 20 mg

1's $1050.00 XIGRIS, Lilly, Eli and Company 00002-7561-01

Dutasteride (003562)

Categories: Hyperplasia, benign prostatic; Pregnancy Category X; FDA Approved 2001 Nov
Drug Classes: 5-alpha-reductase inhibitors; Antiandrogens; Hormones/hormone modifiers
Brand Names: **Avodart**
Cost of Therapy: $78.00 (BPH; Avodart; 0.5 mg; 1 capsule/day; 30 day supply)

D

DESCRIPTION

Dutasteride is a synthetic 4-azasteroid compound that is a selective inhibitor of both the type 1 and type 2 isoforms of steroid 5α-reductase (5AR), an intracellular enzyme that converts testosterone to 5α-dihydrotestosterone (DHT).

Dutasteride is chemically designated as (5α,17β)-N-{2,5 bis(trifluoromethyl)phenyl}-3-oxo-4-azaandrost-1-ene-17-carboxamide. The empirical formula of dutasteride is $C_{27}H_{30}F_6N_2O_2$, representing a molecular weight of 528.5.

Dutasteride is a white to pale yellow powder with a melting point of 242-250°C. It is soluble in ethanol (44 mg/ml), methanol (64 mg/ml) and polyethylene glycol 400 (3 mg/ml), but it is insoluble in water.

Avodart soft gelatin capsules for oral administration contain 0.5 mg of the active ingredient dutasteride in yellow capsules with red print. Each capsule contains 0.5 mg dutasteride dissolved in a mixture of mono-di-glycerides of caprylic/capric acid and butylated hydroxytoluene. The inactive excipients in the capsule shell are gelatin (from certified BSE-free bovine sources), glycerin, and ferric oxide (yellow). The soft gelatin capsules are printed with edible red ink.

CLINICAL PHARMACOLOGY

PHARMACODYNAMICS

Mechanism of Action

Dutasteride inhibits the conversion of testosterone to 5α-dihydrotestosterone (DHT). DHT is the androgen primarily responsible for the initial development and subsequent enlargement of the prostate gland. Testosterone is converted to DHT by the enzyme 5α-reductase, which exists as 2 isoforms, type 1 and type 2. The type 2 isoenzyme is primarily active in the reproductive tissues while the type 1 isoenzyme is also responsible for testosterone conversion in the skin and liver.

Dutasteride is a competitive and specific inhibitor of both type 1 and type 2 5α-reductase isoenzymes, with which it forms a stable enzyme complex. Dissociation from this complex has been evaluated under *in vitro* and *in vivo* conditions and is extremely slow. Dutasteride does not bind to the human androgen receptor.

Effect on DHT and Testosterone

The maximum effect of daily doses of dutasteride on the reduction of DHT is dose dependent and is observed within 1-2 weeks. After 1 and 2 weeks of daily dosing with dutasteride 0.5 mg, median serum DHT concentrations were reduced by 85% and 90%, respectively. In patients with BPH treated with dutasteride 0.5 mg/day for 2 years, the median decrease in serum DHT was 94% at 1 year and 93% at 2 years. The median increase in serum testosterone was 19% at both 1 and 2 years but remained within the physiologic range.

In BPH patients treated with 5 mg/day of dutasteride or placebo for up to 12 weeks prior to transurethral resection of the prostate, mean DHT concentrations in prostatic tissue were significantly lower in the dutasteride group compared with placebo (784 and 5793 pg/g, respectively, $p < 0.001$). Mean prostatic tissue concentrations of testosterone were significantly higher in the dutasteride group compared with placebo (2073 and 93 pg/g, respectively, $p < 0.001$).

Adult males with genetically inherited type 2 5α-reductase deficiency also have decreased DHT levels. These 5α-reductase deficient males have a small prostate gland throughout life and do not develop BPH. Except for the associated urogenital defects present at birth, no other clinical abnormalities related to 5α-reductase deficiency have been observed in these individuals.

Other Effects

Plasma lipid panel and bone mineral density were evaluated following 52 weeks of dutasteride 0.5 mg once daily in healthy volunteers. There was no change in bone mineral density as measured by dual energy x-ray absorptiometry (DEXA) compared with either placebo or baseline. In addition, the plasma lipid profile (*i.e.*, total cholesterol, low density lipoproteins, high density lipoproteins, and triglycerides) was unaffected by dutasteride. No clinically significant changes in adrenal hormone responses to ACTH stimulation were observed in a subset population (n=13) of the 1 year healthy volunteer study.

PHARMACOKINETICS

Absorption

Following administration of a single 0.5 mg dose of a soft gelatin capsule, time to peak serum concentrations (T_{max}) of dutasteride occurs within 2-3 hours. Absolute bioavailability in 5 healthy subjects is approximately 60% (range 40-94%). When the drug is administered with food, the maximum serum concentrations were reduced by 10-15%. This reduction is of no clinical significance.

Distribution

Pharmacokinetic data following single and repeat oral doses show that dutasteride has a large volume of distribution (300-500 L). Dutasteride is highly bound to plasma albumin (99.0%) and alpha-1 acid glycoprotein (96.6%).

In a study of healthy subjects (n=26) receiving dutasteride 0.5 mg/day for 12 months, semen dutasteride concentrations averaged 3.4 ng/ml (range 0.4 to 14 ng/ml) at 12 months and, similar to serum, achieved steady-state concentrations at 6 months. On average, at 12 months, 11.5% of serum dutasteride concentrations partitioned into semen.

Metabolism and Elimination

Dutasteride is extensively metabolized in humans. While not all metabolic pathways have been identified, *in vitro* studies showed that dutasteride is metabolized by the CYP3A4 isoenzyme to 2 minor mono-hydroxylated metabolites. Dutasteride is not metabolized *in vitro* by human cytochrome P450 isoenzymes CYP1A2, CYP2C9, CYP2C19, and CYP2D6 at 2000 ng/ml (50-fold greater than steady-state serum concentrations). In human serum, following dosing to steady state, unchanged dutasteride, 3 major metabolites (4′-hydroxydutasteride, 1,2-dihydrodutasteride, and 6-hydroxydutasteride) and 2 minor metabolites (6,4′-dihydroxydutasteride and 15-hydroxydutasteride), as assessed by mass spectrometric response, have been detected. The absolute stereochemistry of the hydroxyl additions in the 6 and 15 positions is not known. *In vitro,* 4′-hydroxydutasteride and 1,2-dihydrodutasteride metabolites are much less potent than dutasteride against both isoforms of human 5AR. The activity of 6β-hydroxydutasteride is comparable to that of dutasteride.

D

Dutasteride and its metabolites were excreted mainly in feces. As a percent of dose, there was approximately 5% unchanged dutasteride (~1% to ~15%) and 40% as dutasteride-related metabolites (~2% to ~90%). Only trace amounts of unchanged dutasteride were found in urine (<1%). Therefore, on average, the dose unaccounted for approximated 55% (range 5-97%).

The terminal elimination half-life of dutasteride is approximately 5 weeks at steady state. The average steady-state serum dutasteride concentration was 40 ng/ml following 0.5 mg/day for 1 year. Following daily dosing, dutasteride serum concentrations achieve 65% of steady-state concentration after 1 month and approximately 90% after 3 months. Due to the long half-life of dutasteride, serum concentrations remain detectable (greater than 0.1 ng/ml) for up to 4-6 months after discontinuation of treatment.

SPECIAL POPULATIONS

Pediatric

Dutasteride pharmacokinetics have not been investigated in subjects less than 18 years of age.

Geriatric

No dose adjustment is necessary in the elderly. The pharmacokinetics and pharmacodynamics of dutasteride were evaluated in 36 healthy male subjects between the ages of 24 and 87 years following administration of a single 5 mg dose of dutasteride. In this single-dose study, dutasteride half-life increased with age (approximately 170 hours in men 20-49 years of age, approximately 260 hours in men 50-69 years of age, and approximately 300 hours in men over 70 years of age). Of 2167 men treated with dutasteride in the 3 pivotal studies, 60% were age 65 and over and 15% were age 75 and over. No overall differences in safety or efficacy were observed between these patients and younger patients.

Gender

Dutasteride is not indicated for use in women (see WARNINGS and PRECAUTIONS). The pharmacokinetics of dutasteride in women have not been studied.

Race

The effect of race on dutasteride pharmacokinetics has not been studied.

Renal Impairment

The effect of renal impairment on dutasteride pharmacokinetics has not been studied. However, less than 0.1% of a steady-state 0.5 mg dose of dutasteride is recovered in human urine, so no adjustment in dosage is anticipated for patients with renal impairment.

Hepatic Impairment

The effect of hepatic impairment on dutasteride pharmacokinetics has not been studied. Because dutasteride is extensively metabolized, exposure could be higher in hepatically impaired patients (see PRECAUTIONS, Use in Hepatic Impairment).

DRUG INTERACTIONS

In vitro drug metabolism studies reveal that dutasteride is metabolized by human cytochrome P450 isoenzyme CYP3A4. In a human mass balance analysis (n=8), dutasteride was extensively metabolized. Less than 20% of the dose was excreted unchanged in the feces. No clinical drug interaction studies have been performed to evaluate the impact of CYP3A4 enzyme inhibitors on dutasteride pharmacokinetics. However, based on the *in vitro* data, blood concentrations of dutasteride may increase in the presence of inhibitors of CYP3A4 such as ritonavir, ketoconazole, verapamil, diltiazem, cimetidine, and ciprofloxacin. Dutasteride is not metabolized *in vitro* by human cytochrome P450 isoenzymes CYP1A2, CYP2C9, CYP2C19, and CYP2D6 at 2000 ng/ml (50-fold greater than steady-state serum concentrations).

Clinical drug interaction studies have shown no pharmacokinetic or pharmacodynamic interactions between dutasteride and tamsulosin, terazosin, warfarin, digoxin, and cholestyramine (see DRUG INTERACTIONS).

Dutasteride does not inhibit the *in vitro* metabolism of model substrates for the major human cytochrome P450 isoenzymes (CYP1A2, CYP2C9, CYP2C19, CYP2D6, and CYP3A4) at a concentration of 1000 ng/ml, 25 times greater than steady-state serum concentrations in humans.

INDICATIONS AND USAGE

Dutasteride is indicated for the treatment of symptomatic benign prostatic hyperplasia (BPH) in men with an enlarged prostate to:

- Improve symptoms.
- Reduce the risk of acute urinary retention.
- Reduce the risk of the need for BPH-related surgery.

CONTRAINDICATIONS

Dutasteride is contraindicated for use in women and children.

Dutasteride is contraindicated for patients with known hypersensitivity to dutasteride, other 5α-reductase inhibitors, or any component of the preparation.

WARNINGS

EXPOSURE OF WOMEN — RISK TO MALE FETUS

Dutasteride is absorbed through the skin. Therefore, women who are pregnant or may be pregnant should not handle dutasteride soft gelatin capsules because of the possibility of absorption of dutasteride and the potential risk of a fetal anomaly to a male fetus (see CONTRAINDICATIONS). In addition, women should use caution whenever handling dutasteride soft gelatin capsules. If contact is made with leaking capsules, the contact area should be washed immediately with soap and water.

PRECAUTIONS

GENERAL

Lower urinary tract symptoms of BPH can be indicative of other urological diseases, including prostate cancer. Patients should be assessed to rule out other urological diseases prior to treatment with dutasteride. Patients with a large residual urinary volume and/or severely diminished urinary flow may not be good candidates for 5α-reductase inhibitor therapy and should be carefully monitored for obstructive uropathy.

BLOOD DONATION

Men being treated with dutasteride should not donate blood until at least 6 months have passed following their last dose. The purpose of this deferred period is to prevent administration of dutasteride to a pregnant female transfusion recipient.

USE IN HEPATIC IMPAIRMENT

The effect of hepatic impairment on dutasteride pharmacokinetics has not been studied. Because dutasteride is extensively metabolized and has a half-life of approximately 5 weeks at steady state, caution should be used in the administration of dutasteride to patients with liver disease.

USE WITH POTENT CYP3A4 INHIBITORS

Although dutasteride is extensively metabolized, no metabolically-based drug interaction studies have been conducted. The effect of potent CYP3A4 inhibitors has not been studied. Because of the potential for drug-drug interactions, care should be taken when administering dutasteride to patients taking potent, chronic CYP3A4 enzyme inhibitors (*e.g.*, ritonavir).

EFFECTS ON PSA AND PROSTATE CANCER DETECTION

Digital rectal examinations, as well as other evaluations for prostate cancer, should be performed on patients with BPH prior to initiating therapy with dutasteride and periodically thereafter.

Dutasteride reduces total serum PSA concentration by approximately 40% following 3 months of treatment and approximately 50% following 6, 12, and 24 months of treatment. This decrease is predictable over the entire range of PSA values, although it may vary in individual patients. Therefore, for interpretation of serial PSAs in a man taking dutasteride, a new baseline PSA concentration should be established after 3-6 months of treatment, and this new value should be used to assess potentially cancer-related changes in PSA. To interpret an isolated PSA value in a man treated with dutasteride for 6 months or more, the PSA value should be doubled for comparison with normal values in untreated men.

INFORMATION FOR THE PATIENT

Physicians should instruct their patients to read the Information for Patient leaflet that accompanies the prescription before starting therapy with dutasteride and to reread it upon prescription renewal for new information regarding the use of dutasteride.

Dutasteride soft gelatin capsules should not be handled by a woman who is pregnant or who may become pregnant because of the potential for absorption of dutasteride and the subsequent potential risk to a developing male fetus (see CONTRAINDICATIONS and WARNINGS, Exposure of Women — Risk to Male Fetus).

Physicians should inform patients that ejaculate volume might be decreased in some patients during treatment with dutasteride. This decrease does not appear to interfere with normal sexual function. In clinical trials, impotence and decreased libido, considered by the investigator to be drug-related, occurred in a small number of patients treated with dutasteride or placebo (see TABLE 1).

Men treated with dutasteride should not donate blood until at least 6 months have passed following their last dose to prevent pregnant women from receiving dutasteride through blood transfusion (see PRECAUTIONS, Blood Donation).

DRUG/LABORATORY TEST INTERACTIONS

Effects on PSA

PSA levels generally decrease in patients treated with dutasteride as the prostate volume decreases. In approximately one-half of the subjects, a 20% decrease in PSA is seen within the first month of therapy. After 6 months of therapy, PSA levels stabilize to a new baseline that is approximately 50% of the pre-treatment value. Results of subjects treated with dutasteride for up to 2 years indicate this 50% reduction in PSA is maintained. Therefore, a new baseline PSA concentration should be established after 3-6 months of treatment with dutasteride (see Effects on PSA and Prostate Cancer Detection).

Hormone Levels

In healthy volunteers, 52 weeks of treatment with dutasteride 0.5 mg/day (n=26) resulted in no clinically significant change compared with placebo (n=23) in sex hormone binding globulin, estradiol, luteinizing hormone, follicle-stimulating hormone, thyroxine (free T4), and dehydroepiandrosterone. Statistically significant, baseline-adjusted mean increases compared with placebo were observed for total testosterone at 8 weeks (97.1 ng/dl, $p < 0.003$) and thyroid-stimulating hormone (TSH) at 52 weeks (0.4 μIU/ml, $p < 0.05$). The median percentage changes from baseline within the dutasteride group were 17.9% for testosterone at 8 weeks and 12.4% for TSH at 52 weeks. The mean levels of testosterone and TSH had returned to baseline at the 24 week post-treatment follow-up period in the group of subjects with available data at the visit. In BPH patients treated with dutasteride in a large

Phase 3 trial, there was a median percent increase in luteinizing hormone of 12% at 6 months and 19% at both 12 and 24 months.

Reproductive Function

The effects of dutasteride 0.5 mg/day on reproductive function were evaluated in normal volunteers aged 18-52 (n=26) throughout 52 weeks of treatment. Semen characteristics were evaluated at 3 timepoints and indicated no clinically meaningful changes in sperm concentration, sperm motility, or sperm morphology. A 0.8 ml (25%) mean decrease in ejaculate volume with a concomitant reduction in total sperm per ejaculate was observed at 52 weeks, but remained within the normal range. At the 24 week post-treatment follow-up visit, mean values for both parameters had returned to baseline in the group of subjects with available data at that visit.

CNS TOXICITY

In rats and dogs, repeated oral administration of dutasteride resulted in some animals showing signs of non-specific, reversible, centrally-mediated toxicity, without associated histopathological changes at exposure 425- and 315-fold the expected clinical exposure (of parent drug), respectively.

CARCINOGENESIS, MUTAGENESIS, AND IMPAIRMENT OF FERTILITY

Carcinogenesis

In a 2 year carcinogenicity study in B6C3F1 mice, at doses of 3, 35, 250, and 500 mg/kg/day for males and 3, 35, and 250 mg/kg/day for females. An increased incidence of benign hepatocellular adenomas was noted at 250 mg/kg/day (290-fold the expected clinical exposure to a 0.5 mg daily dose) in females only. Two of the 3 major metabolites have been detected in mice. The exposure to these metabolites in mice is either lower than in humans or is not known.

In a 2 year carcinogenicity study in Han Wistar rats, at doses of 1.5, 7.5, and 53 mg/kg/day for males and 0.8, 6.3, and 15 mg/kg/day for females there was an increase in Leydig cell adenomas in the testes at 53 mg/kg/day (135-fold the expected clinical exposure). An increased incidence of Leydig cell hyperplasia was present at 7.5 mg/kg/day (52-fold the expected clinical exposure) and 53 mg/kg/day in male rats. A positive correlation between proliferative changes in the Leydig cells and an increase in circulating luteinizing hormone levels has been demonstrated with 5α-reductase inhibitors and is consistent with an effect on the hypothalamic-pituitary-testicular axis following 5α-reductase inhibition. At tumorigenic doses in rats, luteinizing hormone levels in rats were increased by 167%. In this study, the major human metabolites were tested for carcinogenicity at approximately 1-3 times the expected clinical exposure.

Mutagenesis

Dutasteride was tested for genotoxicity in a bacterial mutagenesis assay (Ames test), a chromosomal aberration assay in CHO cells, and a micronucleus assay in rats. The results did not indicate any genotoxic potential of the parent drug. Two major human metabolites were also negative in either the Ames test or an abbreviated Ames test.

Impairment of Fertility

Treatment of sexually mature male rats with dutasteride at doses of 0.05, 10, 50, and 500 mg/kg/day (0.1- to 110-fold the expected clinical exposure of parent drug) for up to 31 weeks resulted in dose- and time-dependent decreases in fertility, reduced cauda epididymal (absolute) sperm counts but not sperm concentration (at 50 and 500 mg/kg/day), reduced weights of the epididymis, prostate and seminal vesicles, and microscopic changes in the male reproductive organs. The fertility effects were reversed by recovery week 6 at all doses, and sperm counts were normal at the end of a 14 week recovery period. The 5α-reductase-related changes consisted of cytoplasmic vacuolation of tubular epithelium in the epididymides and decreased cytoplasmic content of epithelium, consistent with decreased secretory activity in the prostate and seminal vesicles. The microscopic changes were no longer present at recovery week 14 in the low-dose group and were partly recovered in the remaining treatment groups. Low levels of dutasteride (0.6 to 17 ng/ml) were detected in the serum of untreated female rats mated to males dosed at 10, 50, or 500 mg/kg/day for 29-30 weeks.

In a fertility study in female rats, oral administration of dutasteride at doses of 0.05, 2.5, 12.5, and 30 mg/kg/day resulted in reduced litter size, increased embryo resorption and feminization of male fetuses (decreased anogenital distance) at doses of ≥2.5 mg/kg/day (2- to 10-fold the clinical exposure of parent drug in men). Fetal body weights were also reduced at ≥0.05 mg/kg/day in rats (<0.02-fold the human exposure).

PREGNANCY CATEGORY X

See CONTRAINDICATIONS.

Dutasteride is contraindicated for use in women. Dutasteride has not been studied in women because preclinical data suggest that the suppression of circulating levels of dihydrotestosterone may inhibit the development of the external genital organs in a male fetus carried by a woman exposed to dutasteride.

In an intravenous embryo-fetal development study in the rhesus monkey (12/group), administration of dutasteride at 400, 780, 1325, or 2010 ng/day on gestation days 20-100 did not adversely affect development of male external genitalia. Reduction of fetal adrenal weights, reduction in fetal prostate weights, and increases in fetal ovarian and testis weights were observed in monkeys treated with the highest dose. Based on the highest measured semen concentration of dutasteride in treated men (14 ng/ml) these doses represent 0.8 to 16 times based on blood levels of parent drug (32 to 186 times based on a ng/kg daily dose) the potential maximum exposure of a 50 kg human female to 5 ml semen daily from a dutasteride-treated man, assuming 100% absorption. Dutasteride is highly bound to proteins in human semen (>96%), potentially reducing the amount of dutasteride available for vaginal absorption.

In an embryo-fetal development study in female rats, oral administration of dutasteride at doses of 0.05, 2.5, 12.5, and 30 mg/kg/day resulted in feminization of male fetuses (decreased anogenital distance) and male offspring (nipple development, hypospadias, and distended preputial glands) at all doses (0.07- to 111-fold the expected male clinical exposure). An increase in stillborn pups was observed at 30 mg/kg/day, and reduced fetal body weight was observed at doses ≥2.5 mg/kg/day (15- to 111-fold the expected clinical exposure). Increased incidences of skeletal variations considered to be delays in ossification associated with reduced body weight were observed at doses of 12.5 and 30 mg/kg/day (56- to 111-fold the expected clinical exposure).

In an oral pre- and post-natal development study in rats, dutasteride doses of 0.05, 2.5, 12.5, or 30 mg/kg/day were administered. Unequivocal evidence of feminization of the genitalia (*i.e.,* decreased anogenital distance, increased incidence of hypospadias, nipple development) of F1 generation male offspring occurred at doses ≥2.5 mg/kg/day (14- to 90-fold the expected clinical exposure in men). At a daily dose of 0.05 mg/kg/day (0.05-fold the expected clinical exposure), evidence of feminization was limited to a small, but statistically significant, decrease in anogenital distance. Doses of 2.5 to 30 mg/kg/day resulted in prolonged gestation in the parental females and a decrease in time to vaginal patency for female offspring and decrease prostate and seminal vesicle weights in male offspring. Effects on newborn startle response were noted at doses greater than or equal to 12.5 mg/kg/day. Increased stillbirths were noted at 30 mg/kg/day.

D

Feminization of male fetuses is an expected physiological consequence of inhibition of the conversion of testosterone to DHT by a 5α-reductase inhibitors. These results are similar to observations in male infants with genetic 5α-reductase deficiency.

In the rabbit, embryo-fetal study doses of 30, 100, and 200 mg/kg (28- to 93-fold the expected clinical exposure in men) were administered orally on days 7-29 of pregnancy to encompass the late period of external genitalia development. Histological evaluation of the genital papilla of fetuses revealed evidence of feminization of the male fetus at all doses. A second embryo-fetal study in rabbits at doses of 0.05, 0.4, 3.0, and 30 mg/kg/day (0.3- to 53-fold the expected clinical exposure) also produced evidence of feminization of the genitalia in male fetuses at all doses. It is not known whether rabbits or rhesus monkeys produce any of the major human metabolites.

NURSING MOTHERS

Dutasteride is not indicated for use in women. It is not known whether dutasteride is excreted in human breast milk.

PEDIATRIC USE

Dutasteride is not indicated for use in the pediatric population. Safety and effectiveness in the pediatric population have not been established.

GERIATRIC USE

Of 2167 male subjects treated with dutasteride in 3 clinical studies, 60% were 65 and over and 15% were 75 and over. No overall differences in safety or efficacy were observed between these subjects and younger subjects. Other reported clinical experience has not identified differences in responses between the elderly and younger patients.

DRUG INTERACTIONS

Care should be taken when administering dutasteride to patients taking potent, chronic CYP3A4 inhibitors (see PRECAUTIONS, Use With Potent CYP3A4 Inhibitors).

Dutasteride does not inhibit the *in vitro* metabolism of model substrates for the major human cytochrome P450 isoenzymes (CYP1A2, CYP2C9, CYP2C19, CYP2D6, and CYP3A4) at a concentration of 1000 ng/ml, 25 times greater than steady-state serum concentrations in humans. *In vitro* studies demonstrate that dutasteride does not displace warfarin, diazepam, or phenytoin from plasma protein binding sites, nor do these model compounds displace dutasteride.

Digoxin: In a study of 20 healthy volunteers, dutasteride did not alter the steady-state pharmacokinetics of digoxin when administered concomitantly at a dose of 0.5 mg/day for 3 weeks.

Warfarin: In a study of 23 healthy volunteers, 3 weeks of treatment with dutasteride 0.5 mg/day did not alter the steady-state pharmacokinetics of the S- or R-warfarin isomers or alter the effect of warfarin on prothrombin time when administered with warfarin.

Alpha Adrenergic Blocking Agents: In a single sequence, cross-over study in healthy volunteers, the administration of tamsulosin or terazosin in combination with dutasteride had no effect on the steady-state pharmacokinetics of either alpha adrenergic blocker. The percent change in DHT concentrations was similar for dutasteride alone compared with the combination treatment.

A clinical trial was conducted in which dutasteride and tamsulosin were administered concomitantly for 24 weeks followed by 12 weeks of treatment with either the dutasteride and tamsulosin combination or dutasteride monotherapy. Results from the second phase of the trial revealed no excess of serious adverse events or discontinuations due to adverse events in the combination group compared to the dutasteride monotherapy group.

Calcium Channel Antagonists: In a population PK analysis, a decrease in clearance of dutasteride was noted when coadministered with the CYP3A4 inhibitors verapamil (-37%, n=6) and diltiazem (-44%, n=5). In contrast, no decrease in clearance was seen when amlodipine, another calcium channel antagonist that is not a CYP3A4 inhibitor, was coadministered with dutasteride (+7%, n=4).

The decrease in clearance and subsequent increase in exposure to dutasteride in the presence of verapamil and diltiazem is not considered to be clinically significant. No dose adjustment is recommended.

Cholestyramine: Administration of a single 5 mg dose of dutasteride followed 1 hour later by 12 g cholestyramine did not affect the relative bioavailability of dutasteride in 12 normal volunteers.

Other Concomitant Therapy: Although specific interaction studies were not performed with other compounds, approximately 90% of the subjects in the 3 Phase 3 pivotal efficacy studies receiving dutasteride were taking other medications concomitantly. No clinically significant adverse interactions could be attributed to the combination of dutasteride and concurrent therapy when dutasteride was coadministered with anti-hyperlipidemics, angiotensin-converting enzyme (ACE) inhibitors, beta-adrenergic blocking agents, calcium channel blockers, corticosteroids, diuretics, nonsteroidal anti-inflammatory drugs (NSAIDs), phosphodiesterase Type V inhibitors, and quinolone antibiotics.

ADVERSE REACTIONS

Most adverse reactions were mild or moderate and generally resolved while on treatment in both the dutasteride and placebo groups. The most common adverse events leading to withdrawal in both treatment groups were associated with the reproductive system.

Over 4300 male subjects with BPH were randomly assigned to receive placebo or 0.5 mg daily doses of dutasteride in 3 identical, placebo-controlled Phase 3 treatment studies. Of this group, 2167 male subjects were exposed to dutasteride, including 1772 exposed for 1 year and 1510 exposed for 2 years. The population was aged 47-94 years (mean age 66 years) and greater than 90% Caucasian. Over the 2 year treatment period, 376 subjects (9% of each treatment group) were withdrawn from the studies due to adverse experiences, most commonly associated with the reproductive system. Withdrawals due to adverse events considered by the investigator to have a reasonable possibility of being caused by the study medication occurred in 4% of the subjects receiving dutasteride and in 3% of the subjects receiving placebo. TABLE 1 summarizes clinical adverse reactions that were reported by the investigator as drug-related in at least 1% of subjects receiving dutasteride and at a higher incidence than subjects receiving placebo.

TABLE 1 *Drug-Related Adverse Events* Reported in ≥1% Subjects Over a 24 Month Period and More Frequently in the Dutasteride Group Than the Placebo Group (Pivotal Studies Pooled)*

	Adverse Event Onset			
Adverse Event	**Month 0-6**	**Month 7-12**	**Month 13-18**	**Month 19-34**
Dutasteride	**(n=2167)**	**(n=1901)**	**(n=1725)**	**(n=1605)**
Placebo	**(n=2158)**	**(n=1922)**	**(n=1714)**	**(n=1555)**
Impotence				
Dutasteride	4.7%	1.4%	1.0%	0.8%
Placebo	1.7%	1.5%	0.5%	0.9%
Decreased Libido				
Dutasteride	3.0%	0.7%	0.3%	0.3%
Placebo	1.4%	0.6%	0.2%	0.1%
Ejaculation Disorder				
Dutasteride	1.4%	0.5%	0.5%	0.1%
Placebo	0.5%	0.3%	0.1%	0.0%
Gynecomastia†				
Dutasteride	0.5%	0.8%	1.1%	0.6%
Placebo	0.2%	0.3%	0.3%	0.1%

*** A drug-related adverse event is one considered by the investigator to have a reasonable possibility of being caused by the study medication. In assessing causality, investigators were asked to select from 1 of 2 options: reasonably related to study medication or unrelated to study medication.**

† Includes breast tenderness and breast enlargement.

LONG-TERM TREATMENT

The incidence of most drug-related sexual adverse events (impotence, decreased libido, and ejaculation disorder) decreased with duration of treatment. The incidence of drug-related gynecomastia remained constant over the treatment period (see TABLE 1). The relationship between long-term use of dutasteride and male breast neoplasia is currently unknown.

DOSAGE AND ADMINISTRATION

The recommended dose of dutasteride is 1 capsule (0.5 mg) taken orally once a day. The capsules should be swallowed whole. Dutasteride may be administered with or without food.

No dosage adjustment is necessary for subjects with renal impairment or for the elderly (see CLINICAL PHARMACOLOGY, Special Populations: Geriatric and Renal Impairment). Due to the absence of data in patients with hepatic impairment, no dosage recommendation can be made (see PRECAUTIONS, General).

HOW SUPPLIED

Avodart soft gelatin capsules 0.5 mg are oblong, opaque, dull yellow, gelatin capsules imprinted with "GX CE2" in red ink on one side.

STORAGE AND HANDLING

Store at 25°C (77°F); excursions permitted to 15-30°C (59-86°F).

Dutasteride is absorbed through the skin. Dutasteride soft gelatin capsules should not be handled by women who are pregnant or who may become pregnant because of the potential for absorption of dutasteride and the subsequent potential risk to a developing male fetus (see CLINICAL PHARMACOLOGY, Pharmacokinetics; WARNINGS, Exposure of Women — Risk to Male Fetus; and PRECAUTIONS: Information for the Patient, and Pregnancy Category X).

Econazole Nitrate *(001127)*

Categories: Candidiasis; Tinea corporis; Tinea cruris; Tinea pedis; Tinea versicolor; Pregnancy Category C; FDA Approved 1982 Dec

Drug Classes: Antifungals, topical; Dermatologics

Brand Names: Spectazole

Foreign Brand Availability: Amicel (Italy); Bismultin (Greece); Derma-Coryl (Bahrain; Cyprus; Egypt; Iran; Iraq; Jordan; Kuwait; Lebanon; Libya; Oman; Qatar; Republic-of-Yemen; Saudi-Arabia; Syria; United-Arab-Emirates); Dermazole (Hong-Kong; Singapore); Econol (India); Econ (Thailand); Ecostatin (Canada; England; Ireland; New-Zealand); Ecotam (Spain); Ecreme (New-Zealand); Epi-Pevaryl (Germany); Fungazol (Korea); Gyno-Coryl (Bahrain; Cyprus; Egypt; Iran; Iraq; Jordan; Kuwait; Lebanon; Libya; Oman; Qatar; Republic-of-Yemen; Saudi-Arabia; Syria; United-Arab-Emirates); Micolak (Mexico); Micolis (Ecuador; Peru); Micos (Italy); Micostyl (Mexico); Palavale (Japan); Penicomb (Greece); Pevaryl (Austria; Bahrain; Belgium; Benin; Bulgaria; Burkina-Faso; Cyprus; Czech-Republic; Denmark; England; Ethiopia; Finland; France; Gambia; Ghana; Guinea; Hong-Kong; Hungary; Italy; Ivory-Coast; Jordan; Kenya; Liberia; Malawi; Malaysia; Mali; Mauritania; Mauritius; Morocco; Netherlands; New-Zealand; Niger; Nigeria; Norway; Philippines; Portugal; Senegal; Seychelles; Sierra-Leone; South-Africa; Spain; Sudan; Sweden; Switzerland; Tanzania; Tunia; Uganda; Zambia; Zimbabwe)

Cost of Therapy: $14.64 (Tinea Pedis; Spectazole Cream; 1%; 1/day; 28 day supply)
$15.49 (Tinea Pedis; Spectazole Cream; 1%; 15 g; 1 application/day; variable day supply)

DESCRIPTION

Spectazole cream contains the antifungal agent, econazole nitrate 1%, in a water-miscible base consisting of pegoxol 7 stearate, peglicol 5 oleate, mineral oil, benzoic acid, butylated hydroxyanisole, and purified water. The white to off-white soft cream is for topical use only.

Chemically, econazole nitrate is 1-[2-{(4-chloro-phenyl)methoxy}-2-(2,4-dichlorophenyl)ethyl]-1H-imidazole mononitrate.

CLINICAL PHARMACOLOGY

After topical application to the skin of normal subjects, systemic absorption of econazole nitrate is extremely low. Although most of the applied drug remains on the skin surface, drug concentrations were found in the stratum corneum which, by far, exceeded the minimum inhibitory concentration for dermatophytes. Inhibitory concentrations were achieved in the epidermis and as deep as the middle region of the dermis. Less that 1% of the applied dose was recovered in the urine and feces.

MICROBIOLOGY

Econazole nitrate has been shown to be active against most strains of the following microorganisms, both *in vitro* and in clinical infections as described in INDICATIONS AND USAGE.

Dermatophytes:

- *Epidermophyton floccosum.*
- *Microsporum audouini.*
- *Microsporum canis.*
- *Microsporum gypseum.*
- *Trichophyton mentagrophytes.*
- *Trichophyton rubrum.*
- *Trichophyton tonsurans.*

Yeasts:

- *Candida albicans.*
- *Malassezia furfur.*

Econazole nitrate exhibits broad-spectrum antifungal activity against the following organisms *in vitro*, **but the clinical significance of these data is unknown.**

Dermatophytes:

- *Trichophyton verrucosum.*

Yeasts:

- *Candida guillermondii.*
- *Candida parapsilosis.*
- *Candida tropicalis.*

INDICATIONS AND USAGE

Econazole nitrate cream is indicated for topical application in the treatment of tinea pedis, tinea cruris, and tinea corporis caused by *Trichophyton rubrum, Trichophyton mentagrophytes, Trichophyton tonsurans, Microsporum canis, Microsporum audouini, Microsporum gypseum* and *Epidermophyton floccosum,* in the treatment of cutaneous candidiasis, and in the treatment of tinea versicolor.

CONTRAINDICATIONS

Econazole nitrate cream is contraindicated in individuals who have shown hypersensitivity to any of its ingredients.

WARNINGS

Econazole nitrate is not for ophthalmic use.

PRECAUTIONS

General: If a reaction suggesting sensitivity or chemical irritation should occur, use of the medication should be discontinued.

For external use only. Avoid introduction of econazole nitrate cream into the eyes.

Carcinogenicity Studies: Long-term animal studies to determine carcinogenic potential have not been performed.

Fertility (reproduction): Oral administration of econazole nitrate in rats has been reported to produce prolonged gestation. Intravaginal administration in humans has not shown prolonged gestation or other adverse reproductive effects attributable to econazole nitrate therapy.

Pregnancy Category C: Econazole nitrate has not been shown to be teratogenic when administered orally to mice, rabbits or rats. Fetotoxic or embryotoxic effects were observed in Segment I oral studies with rats receiving 10-40 times the human dermal dose. Similar effects were observed in Segment II of Segment III studies with mice, rabbits and/or rats receiving oral doses 80 or 40 times the human dermal dose.

Econazole should be used in the first trimester of pregnancy only when the physician considers it essential to the welfare of the patient. The drug should be used during the second and third trimesters of pregnancy only if clearly needed.

Nursing Mothers: It is not known whether econazole nitrate is excreted in human milk. Following oral administration of econazole nitrate to lactating rats, econazole and/or metabolites were excreted in milk and were found in nursing pups. Also, in lactating rats receiving large oral doses (40-80 times the human dermal dose), there was a reduction in post partum viability of pups and survival to weaning; however, at these high doses, maternal toxicity was present and may have been a contributing factor. Caution should be exercised when econazole nitrate is administered to a nursing woman.

ADVERSE REACTIONS

During clinical trials, approximately 3% of patients treated with econazole nitrate 1% cream reported side effects thought possibly to be due to the drug, consisting mainly of burning, itching, stinging and erythema. One case of pruritic rash has also been reported.

DOSAGE AND ADMINISTRATION

Sufficient econazole nitrate cream should be applied to cover affected areas once daily in patients with tinea pedis, tinea cruris, tinea corporis, and tinea versicolor, and twice daily (morning and evening) in patients with cutaneous candidiasis.

Early relief of symptoms is experienced by the majority of patients and clinical improvement may be seen fairly soon after treatment is begun; however, candidal infections and tinea cruris and corporis should be treated for 2 weeks and tinea pedis for one month in order to reduce the possibility of recurrence. If a patient shows no clinical improvement after the treatment period, the diagnosis should be redetermined. Patients with tinea versicolor usually exhibit clinical and mycological clearing after two weeks of treatment.

HOW SUPPLIED

Storage: Store Spectazole cream below 86°F.

PRODUCT LISTING - EQUIVALENTS NOT AVAILABLE

Cream - Topical - 1%

Size	Price	Product	NDC
15 gm	$15.49	SPECTAZOLE, Allscripts Pharmaceutical Company	54569-2639-00
15 gm	$17.50	GENERIC, Fougera	00168-0312-15
15 gm	$17.60	GENERIC, Taro Pharmaceuticals U.S.A. Inc	51672-1303-01
15 gm	$17.81	SPECTAZOLE, Physicians Total Care	54868-2241-01
15 gm	$19.56	SPECTAZOLE, Janssen Pharmaceuticals	00062-5460-02
30 gm	$27.36	SPECTAZOLE, Allscripts Pharmaceutical Company	54569-1628-01
30 gm	$30.92	GENERIC, Fougera	00168-0312-30
30 gm	$30.93	GENERIC, Taro Pharmaceuticals U.S.A. Inc	51672-1303-02
30 gm	$34.55	SPECTAZOLE, Janssen Pharmaceuticals	00062-5460-01
85 gm	$62.64	SPECTAZOLE, Physicians Total Care	54868-2241-03
85 gm	$63.06	GENERIC, Fougera	00168-0312-85
85 gm	$63.06	GENERIC, Taro Pharmaceuticals U.S.A. Inc	51672-1303-08
85 gm	$70.46	SPECTAZOLE, Janssen Pharmaceuticals	00062-5460-03

Efavirenz *(003418)*

For related information, see the comparative table section in Appendix A.

Categories: Infection, human immunodeficiency virus; FDA Approved 1998 Sep; Pregnancy Category C; WHO Formulary
Drug Classes: Antivirals; Non-nucleoside reverse transcriptase inhibitors
Foreign Brand Availability: Efavir (India); Stocrin (Australia; Austria; Belgium; Bulgaria; Colombia; Czech-Republic; Denmark; England; Finland; France; Germany; Greece; Hong-Kong; Hungary; Ireland; Israel; Italy; Mexico; Netherlands; New-Zealand; Norway; Peru; Poland; Portugal; Singapore; Slovenia; South-Africa; Spain; Sweden; Switzerland; Taiwan; Thailand; Turkey); Sustiva (Austria; Belgium; Bulgaria; Canada; Czech-Republic; Denmark; England; Finland; France; Germany; Greece; Hungary; Ireland; Italy; Netherlands; Norway; Poland; Portugal; Slovenia; Spain; Sweden; Switzerland; Turkey)
Cost of Therapy: $431.65 (HIV; Sustiva; 200 mg; 3 capsules/day; 30 day supply)

DESCRIPTION

Efavirenz is an HIV-1 specific, non-nucleoside, reverse transcriptase inhibitor (NNRTI).

Efavirenz is chemically described as (S)-6-chloro-4-(cyclopropylethynyl)-1,4-dihydro-4-(trifluoromethyl)-2H-3,1-benzoxazin-2-one.

Its empirical formula is $C_{14}H_9ClF_3NO_2$.

Efavirenz is a white to slightly pink crystalline powder with a molecular mass of 315.68. It is practically insoluble in water (<10 µg/ml).

CAPSULES

Sustiva is available as capsules for oral administration containing either 50, 100, or 200 mg of efavirenz and the following inactive ingredients: lactose monohydrate, magnesium stearate, sodium lauryl sulfate, and sodium starch glycolate. The capsule shell contains the following inactive ingredients and dyes: gelatin, sodium lauryl sulfate, titanium dioxide and/or yellow iron oxide. The capsule shells may also contain silicon dioxide. The capsules are printed with ink containing carmine 40 blue, FD&C blue no. 2 and titanium dioxide.

TABLETS

Sustiva is available as film-coated tablets for oral administration containing 600 mg of efavirenz and the following inactive ingredients: croscarmellose sodium, hydroxypropyl cellulose, lactose monohydrate, magnesium stearate, microcrystalline cellulose, and sodium lauryl sulfate. The film coating contains Opadry Yellow and Opadry Clear. The tablets are polished with carnauba wax and printed with purple ink, Opacode WB.

CLINICAL PHARMACOLOGY

MICROBIOLOGY

Mechanism of Action

Efavirenz is a non-nucleoside reverse transcriptase (RT) inhibitor of human immunodeficiency virus type 1 (HIV-1). Efavirenz activity is mediated predominantly by noncompetitive inhibition of HIV-1 RT. HIV-2 RT and human cellular DNA polymerases alpha, beta, gamma, and delta are not inhibited by efavirenz.

In Vitro HIV Susceptibility

The clinical significance of *in vitro* susceptibility of HIV-1 to efavirenz has not been established. The *in vitro* antiviral activity of efavirenz was assessed in lymphoblastoid cell lines, peripheral blood mononuclear cells (PBMCs) and macrophage/monocyte cultures. The 90-95% inhibitory concentration (IC_{90-95}) of efavirenz for wild type laboratory adapted strains and clinical isolates ranged from 1.7 to 25 nM. Efavirenz demonstrated synergistic activity against HIV-1 in cell culture when combined with zidovudine (ZDV), didanosine, or indinavir (IDV).

E

Resistance

HIV-1 isolates with reduced susceptibility to efavirenz (>380-fold increase in IC_{90}) compared to baseline can emerge *in vitro*. Phenotypic (n=26) changes in evaluable HIV-1 isolates and genotypic (n=104) changes in plasma virus from selected patients treated with efavirenz in combination with IDV, or with ZDV plus lamivudine were monitored. One or more RT mutations at amino acid positions 98, 100, 101, 103, 106, 108, 188, 190 and 225, were observed in 102 of 104 patients with a frequency of at least 9% compared to baseline. The mutation at RT amino acid position 103 (lysine to asparagine) was the most frequently observed (≥90%). A mean loss in susceptibility (IC_{90}) to efavirenz of 47-fold was observed in 26 clinical isolates. Five clinical isolates were evaluated for both genotypic and phenotypic changes from baseline. Decreases in efavirenz susceptibility (range from 9 to >312-fold increase in IC_{90}) were observed for these isolates *in vitro* compared to baseline. All 5 isolates possessed at least one of the efavirenz-associated RT mutations. The clinical relevance of phenotypic and genotypic changes associated with efarivenz therapy is under evaluation.

Cross-Resistance

Rapid emergence of HIV-1 strains that are cross-resistant to non-nucleoside RT inhibitors has been observed *in vitro*. Thirteen clinical isolates previously characterized as efavirenz-resistant were also phenotypically resistant to nevirapine and delavirdine *in vitro* compared to baseline. Clinically derived ZDV-resistant HIV-1 isolates tested *in vitro* retained susceptibility to efavirenz. Cross-resistance between efavirenz and HIV protease inhibitors is unlikely because of the different enzyme targets involved.

PHARMACOKINETICS

Absorption

Peak efavirenz plasma concentrations of 1.6-9.1 µM were attained by 5 hours following single oral doses of 100-1600 mg administered to uninfected volunteers. Dose-related increases in C_{max} and AUC were seen for doses up to 1600 mg; the increases were less than proportional suggesting diminished absorption at higher doses.

In HIV-infected patients at steady-state, mean C_{max}, mean C_{min}, and mean AUC were dose proportional following 200, 400, and 600 mg daily doses. Time-to-peak plasma concentrations were approximately 3-5 hours and steady-state plasma concentrations were reached in 6-10 days. In 35 patients receiving efavirenz 600 mg once daily, steady-state C_{max} was 12.9 ± 3.7 µM (mean ± SD), steady-state C_{min} was 5.6 ± 3.2 µM, and AUC was 184 ± 73 µM·h.

Effect of Food on Oral Absorption

Capsules

Administration of a single 600 mg dose of efavirenz capsules with a high fat/high caloric meal (894 kcal, 54 g fat, 54% calories from fat) or a reduced fat/normal caloric meal (440 kcal, 2 g fat, 4% calories from fat) was associated with a mean increase of 22% and 17% in efavirenz AUC(∞) and a mean increase of 39% and 51% in efavirenz C_{max}, respectively, relative to the exposures achieved when given under fasted conditions. (See DOSAGE AND ADMINISTRATION and PRECAUTIONS, Information for the Patient.)

Tablets

Administration of a single 600 mg efavirenz tablet with a high fat/high caloric meal (approximately 1000 kcal, 500-600 kcal from fat) was associated with a 28% increase in mean AUC(∞) of efavirenz and a 79% increase in mean C_{max} of efavirenz relative to the exposures achieved under fasted conditions. (See DOSAGE AND ADMINISTRATION and PRECAUTIONS, Information for the Patient.)

Distribution

Efavirenz is highly bound (approximately 99.5-99.75%) to human plasma proteins, predominantly albumin. In HIV-1 infected patients (n=9) who received efavirenz 200-600 mg once daily for at least 1 month, cerebrospinal fluid concentrations ranged from 0.26-1.19% (mean 0.69%) of the corresponding plasma concentration. This proportion is approximately 3-fold higher than the non-protein-bound (free) fraction of efavirenz in plasma.

Metabolism

Studies in humans and *in vitro* studies using human liver microsomes have demonstrated that efavirenz is principally metabolized by the cytochrome P450 system to hydroxylated metabolites with subsequent glucuronidation of these hydroxylated metabolites. These metabolites are essentially inactive against HIV-1. The *in vitro* studies suggest that CYP3A4 and CYP2B6 are the major isozymes responsible for efavirenz metabolism.

Efavirenz has been shown to induce P450 enzymes, resulting in the induction of its own metabolism. Multiple doses of 200-400 mg/day for 10 days resulted in a lower than predicted extent of accumulation (22-42% lower) and a shorter terminal half-life of 40-55 hours (single dose half-life 52-76 hours).

Elimination

Efavirenz has a terminal half-life of 52-76 hours after single doses and 40-55 hours after multiple doses. A 1 month mass balance/excretion study was conducted using 400 mg/day with a ^{14}C-labeled dose administered on Day 8. Approximately 14-34% of the radiolabel was recovered in the urine and 16-61% was recovered in the feces. Nearly all of the urinary excretion of the radiolabeled drug was in the form of metabolites. Efavirenz accounted for the majority of the total radioactivity measured in feces.

SPECIAL POPULATIONS

Hepatic Impairment

The pharmacokinetics of efavirenz have not been adequately studied in patients with hepatic impairment (see PRECAUTIONS, General).

Renal Impairment

The pharmacokinetics of efavirenz have not been studied in patients with renal insufficiency; however, less than 1% of efavirenz is excreted unchanged in the urine, so the impact of renal impairment on efavirenz elimination should be minimal.

Gender and Race

The pharmacokinetics of efavirenz in patients appear to be similar between men and women and among the racial groups studied.

Geriatric

See PRECAUTIONS, Geriatric Use.

Pediatrics

See PRECAUTIONS, Pediatric Use.

DRUG INTERACTIONS

See also CONTRAINDICATIONS and DRUG INTERACTIONS.

Efavirenz has been shown *in vivo* to cause hepatic enzyme induction, thus increasing the biotransformation of some drugs metabolized by CYP3A4. *In vitro* studies have shown that efavirenz inhibited P450 isozymes 2C9, 2C19, and 3A4 with Ki values (8.5-17 μM) in the range of observed efavirenz plasma concentrations. In *in vitro* studies, efavirenz did not inhibit CYP2E1 and inhibited CYP2D6 and CYP1A2 (Ki values 82-160 μM) only at concentrations well above those achieved clinically. The effects on CYP3A4 activity are expected to be similar between 200, 400, and 600 mg doses of efavirenz. Coadministration of efavirenz with drugs primarily metabolized by 2C9, 2C19 and 3A4 isozymes may result in altered plasma concentrations of the coadministered drug. Drugs which induce CYP3A4 activity would be expected to increase the clearance of efavirenz resulting in lowered plasma concentrations.

Drug interaction studies were performed with efavirenz and other drugs likely to be coadministered or drugs commonly used as probes for pharmacokinetic interaction. The effects of coadministration of efavirenz on the AUC and C_{max} are summarized in TABLE 1 and TABLE 2. For information regarding clinical recommendations see DRUG INTERACTIONS.

TABLE 1 *Effect of Efavirenz on Coadministered Drug Plasma C_{max} and AUC*

				Coadministered Drug (% change)	
Coadministered Drug	**Dose**	**Efavirenz Dose**		**C_{max} (mean [90% CI])**	**AUC (mean [90% CI])**
Indinavir	800 mg q8h × 14 days	200 mg × 14 days	n=17	dec (16%) [-10-35%]	dec (31%) [13-45%]
Nelfinavir	750 mg q8h × 7 days	600 mg × 7 days	n=10	inc (21%) [10-33%]	inc (20%) [8-34%]
Metabolite AG-1402				dec (40%) [30-48%]	dec (37%) [25-48%]
Ritonavir	500 mg q12h × 8 days After AM dose	600 mg × 10 days	n=11	inc (24%) [12-38%]	inc (18%) [6-33%]
	After PM dose			NC	NC
Saquinavir SGC*	1200 mg q8h × 10 days	600 mg × 10 days	n=12	dec (50%) [28-66%]	dec (62%) [45-74%]
Lamivudine	150 mg q12h × 14 days	600 mg × 14 days	n=9	NC	NC
Zidovudine	300 mg q12h × 14 days	600 mg × 14 days	n=9	NC	NC
Azithromycin	600 mg single dose	400 mg × 7 days	n=14	inc (22%) [4-42%]	NC
Clarithromycin	500 mg q12h × 7 days	400 mg × 7 days	n=11	dec (26%) [15-35%]	dec (39%) [30-46%]
14-OH metabolite				inc (49%) [32-69%]	inc (34%) [18-53%]
Fluconazole	200 mg × 7 days	400 mg × 7 days	n=10	NC	NC
Ritabutin	300 mg qd × 14 days	600 mg × 14 days	n=9	dec (32%) [15-46%]	dec (38%) [28-47%]
Cetirizine	10 mg single dose	600 mg × 10 days	n=11	dec (24%) [18-30%]	NC
Ethinyl estradiol	50 μg single dose	400 mg × 10 days	n=13	NC	inc (37%) [25-51%]
Lorazepam	2 mg single dose	600 mg × 10 days	n=12	inc (16%) [2-32%]	inc (7%) [1-14%]
Methadone	Stable maintenance 35-100 mg daily	600 mg × 14-21 days	n=11	dec (45%) [25-59%]	dec (52%) [33-66%]

inc = Indicates increase; dec = Indicates decrease; NC = Indicates no change.
* Soft gelatin capsule.

TABLE 2 *Effect of Coadministered Drug on Efavirenz Plasma C_{max} and AUC*

				Efavirenz (% change)	
Coadministered Drug	**Dose**	**Efavirenz Dose**		**C_{max} (mean [90% CI])**	**AUC (mean [90% CI])**
Indinavir	800 mg q8h × 14 days	200 mg × 14 days	n=11	NC	NC
Nelfinavir	750 mg q8h × 7 days	600 mg × 7 days	n=10	NC	NC
Ritonavir	500 mg q12h × 8 days	600 mg × 10 days	n=9	inc (14%) [4-26%]	inc (21%) [10-34%]
Saquinavir SGC*	1200 mg q8h × 10 days	600 mg × 10 days	n=13	dec (13%) [5-20%]	dec (12%) [4-19%]
Azithromycin	600 mg single dose	400 mg × 7 days	n=14	NC	NC
Clarithromycin	500 mg q12h × 7 days	400 mg × 7 days	n=12	inc (11%) [3-19%]	NC
Fluconazole	200 mg × 7 days	400 mg × 7 days	n=10	NC	inc (16%) [6-26%]
Rifabutin	300 mg qd × 14 days	600 mg × 14 days	n=11	NC	NC
Rifampin	600 mg × 7 days	600 mg × 7 days	n=12	dec (20%) [11-28%]	dec (26%) [15-36%]
Aluminum hydroxide 400 mg, magnesium hydroxide 400 mg, plus simethicone 40 mg	30 ml single dose	400 mg single dose	n=17	NC	NC
Cetirizine	10 mg single dose	600 mg × 10 days	n=11	NC	dec (8%) [4-11%]
Ethinyl estradiol	50 μg single dose	400 mg × 10 days	n=13	NC	NC
Famotidine	40 mg single dose	400 mg single dose	n=17	NC	NC

inc = Indicates increase; dec = Indicates decrease; NC = Indicates no change.
* Soft gelatin capsule.

INDICATIONS AND USAGE

Efavirenz in combination with other antiretroviral agents is indicated for the treatment of HIV-1 infection. This indication is based on two clinical trials of at least 1 year duration that demonstrated prolonged suppression of HIV-RNA.

CONTRAINDICATIONS

Efavirenz is contraindicated in patients with clinically significant hypersensitivity to any of its components.

Efavirenz should not be administered concurrently with astemizole, cisapride, midazolam, triazolam, or ergot derivatives because competition for CYP3A4 by efavirenz could result in inhibition of metabolism of these drugs and create the potential for serious and/or life-threatening adverse events (*e.g.*, cardiac arrhythmias, prolonged sedation or respiratory depression).

WARNINGS

ALERT: Find out about medicines that should NOT be taken with efavirenz. This statement is also included on the product's bottle labels. (See CONTRAINDICATIONS and DRUG INTERACTIONS

Efavirenz must not be used as a single agent to treat HIV or added on as a sole agent to a failing regimen. As with all other non-nucleoside reverse transcriptase inhibitors, resistant virus emerges rapidly when efavirenz is administered as monotherapy. The choice of new antiretroviral agents to be used in combination with efavirenz should take into consideration the potential for viral cross-resistance.

PSYCHIATRIC SYMPTOMS

Serious psychiatric adverse experiences have been reported in patients treated with efavirenz. In controlled trials of 1008 patients treated with regimens containing efavirenz for an average of 1.6 years and 635 patients treated with control regimens for an average of 1.3 years, the frequency of specific serious psychiatric events among patients who received efavirenz or control regimens, respectively, were: severe depression (1.6%, 0.6%), suicidal ideation (0.6%, 0.3%), non-fatal suicide attempts (0.4%, 0%), aggressive behavior (0.4%, 0.3%), paranoid reactions (0.4%, 0.3%) and manic reactions (0.1%, 0%). Patients with a history of psychiatric disorders appear to be at greater risk of these serious psychiatric adverse experiences, with the frequency of each of the above events ranging from 0.3% for manic reactions to 2.0% for both severe depression and suicidal ideation. There have also been occasional post-marketing reports of death by suicide, delusions and psychosis-like behavior, although a causal relationship to the use of efavirenz cannot be determined from these reports. Patients with serious psychiatric adverse experiences should seek immediate medical evaluation to assess the possibility that the symptoms may be related to the use of efavirenz, and if so, to determine whether the risks of continued therapy outweigh the benefits (see ADVERSE REACTIONS).

NERVOUS SYSTEM SYMPTOMS

Fifty-three percent (53%) of patients receiving efavirenz in controlled trials reported central nervous system symptoms compared to 25% of patients receiving control regimens. These symptoms included, but were not limited to, dizziness (28.1%), insomnia (16.3%), impaired concentration (8.3%), somnolence (7.0%), abnormal dreams (6.2%) and hallucinations (1.2%). These symptoms were severe in 2.0% of patients and 2.1% of patients discontinued therapy as a result. These symptoms usually begin during the first or second day of therapy and generally resolve after the first 2-4 weeks of therapy. After 4 weeks of therapy, the prevalence of nervous system symptoms of at least moderate severity ranged from 5-9% in patients treated with regimens containing efavirenz and from 3-5% in patients treated with a control regimen. Patients should be informed that these common symptoms were likely to improve with continued therapy and were not predictive of subsequent onset of the less frequent psychiatric symptoms (see Psychiatric Symptoms). Dosing at bedtime may improve the tolerability of these nervous system symptoms (see ADVERSE REACTIONS and DOSAGE AND ADMINISTRATION).

Patients receiving efavirenz should be alerted to the potential for additive central nervous system effects when efavirenz is used concomitantly with alcohol or psychoactive drugs.

Patients who experience central nervous system symptoms such as dizziness, impaired concentration and/or drowsiness should avoid potentially hazardous tasks such as driving or operating machinery.

DRUG INTERACTIONS

Concomitant use of efavirenz and St. John's wort (*hypericum perforatum*) or St. John's wort-containing products is not recommended. Coadministration of non-nucleoside reverse transcriptase inhibitors (NNRTIs), including efavirenz, with St. John's wort is expected to substantially decrease NNRTI concentrations and may result in suboptimal levels of efavirenz and lead to loss of virologic response and possible resistance to efavirenz or to the class of NNRTIs.

REPRODUCTIVE RISK POTENTIAL

Malformations have been observed in fetuses from efavirenz-treated monkeys that received doses which resulted in plasma drug concentrations similar to those in humans given 600 mg/day (see PRECAUTIONS, Pregnancy Category C); therefore, pregnancy should be avoided in women receiving efavirenz. Barrier contraception should always be used in combination with other methods of contraception (*e.g.,* oral or other hormonal contraceptives). Women of childbearing potential should undergo pregnancy testing prior to initiation of efavirenz.

PRECAUTIONS

GENERAL

Skin Rash

In controlled clinical trials, 26% (266/1008) of patients treated with 600 mg efavirenz experienced new onset skin rash compared with 17% (111/635) of patients treated in control groups. Rash associated with blistering, moist desquamation, or ulceration occurred in 0.9% (9/1008) of patients treated with efavirenz. The incidence of Grade 4 rash (*e.g.,* erythema multiforme, Stevens-Johnson Syndrome) in patients treated with efavirenz in all studies and expanded access was 0.1%. The median time to onset of rash in adults was 11 days and the median duration, 16 days. The discontinuation rate for rash in clinical trials was 1.7% (17/1008). Efavirenz should be discontinued in patients developing severe rash associated with blistering, desquamation, mucosal involvement or fever. Appropriate antihistamines and/or corticosteroids may improve the tolerability and hasten the resolution of rash.

Rash was reported in 26 of 57 pediatric patients (46%) treated with efavirenz capsules. One pediatric patient experienced Grade 3 rash (confluent rash with fever), and 2 patients had Grade 4 rash (erythema multiforme). The median time to onset of rash in pediatric patients was 8 days. Prophylaxis with appropriate antihistamines prior to initiating therapy with efavirenz in pediatric patients should be considered (see ADVERSE REACTIONS).

Liver Enzymes

In patients with known or suspected history of Hepatitis B or C infection and in patients treated with other medications associated with liver toxicity, monitoring of liver enzymes is recommended. In patients with persistent elevations of serum transaminases to greater than 5 times the upper limit of the normal range, the benefit of continued therapy with efavirenz needs to be weighed against the unknown risks of significant liver toxicity (see ADVERSE REACTIONS, Laboratory Abnormalities).

Because of the extensive cytochrome P450-mediated metabolism of efavirenz and limited clinical experience in patients with hepatic impairment, caution should be exercised in administering efavirenz to these patients.

Cholesterol

Monitoring of cholesterol and triglycerides should be considered in patients treated with efavirenz (see ADVERSE REACTIONS).

Fat Redistribution

Redistribution/accumulation of body fat including central obesity, dorsocervical fat enlargement (buffalo hump), peripheral wasting, facial wasting, breast enlargement, and "cushingoid appearance" have been observed in patients receiving antiretrovial therapy. The mechanism and long-term consequences of these events are currently unknown. A casual relationship has not been established.

INFORMATION FOR THE PATIENT

A statement to patients and healthcare providers is included on the product's bottle labels: **ALERT: Find out about medicines that should NOT be taken with efavirenz.** A Patient Package Insert (PPI) for efavirenz is available for patient information.

Patients should be informed that efavirenz is not a cure for HIV infection and that they may continue to develop opportunistic infections and other complications associated with HIV disease. Patients should be told that there are currently no data demonstrating that efavirenz therapy can reduce the risk of transmitting HIV to others through sexual contact or blood contamination.

Patients should be advised to take efavirenz every day as prescribed. Efavirenz must always be used in combination with other antiretroviral drugs. Patients should should be advised to take efavirenz on an empty stomach, preferably at bedtime. Taking efavirenz with food increases efavirenz concentrations and may increase the frequency of adverse events. Dosing at bedtime may improve the tolerability of nervous system symptoms (see ADVERSE REACTIONS and DOSAGE AND ADMINISTRATION). Patients should remain under the care of a physician while taking efavirenz.

Patients should be informed that central nervous system symptoms including dizziness, insomnia, impaired concentration, drowsiness and abnormal dreams are commonly reported during the first weeks of therapy with efavirenz. Dosing at bedtime may improve the tolerability of these symptoms, and these symptoms are likely to improve with continued therapy. Patients should be alerted to the potential for additive central nervous system effects when efavirenz is used concomitantly with alcohol or psychoactive drugs. Patients should be instructed that if they experience these symptoms they should avoid potentially hazardous tasks such as driving or operating machinery (see WARNINGS, Nervous System Symptoms). In clinical trials, patients who develop central nervous system symptoms were not more likely to subsequently develop psychiatric symptoms (see WARNINGS, Psychiatric Symptoms).

Patients should also be informed that serious psychiatric symptoms including severe depression, suicide attempts, aggressive behavior, delusions, paranoia and psychosis-like symptoms have also been infrequently reported in patients receiving efavirenz. Patients should be informed that if they experience severe psychiatric adverse experiences they should seek immediate medical evaluation to assess the possibility that the symptoms may be related to the use of efavirenz, and if so, to determine whether discontinuation of efavirenz may be required. Patients should also inform their physician of any history of mental illness or substance abuse (see WARNINGS, Psychiatric Symptoms).

Patients should be informed that another common side effect is rash. These rashes usually go away without any change in treatment. In a small number of patients, rash may be serious. Patients should be advised that they should contact their physician promptly if they develop a rash.

Because malformations have been observed in fetuses from efavirenz-treated animals, instructions should be given to avoid pregnancy in women receiving efavirenz. Women should be advised to notify their physician if they become pregnant while taking efavirenz. A reliable form of barrier contraception should always be used in combination with other methods of contraception, including oral or other hormonal contraception because the effects of efavirenz on hormonal contraceptives are not fully characterized.

Efavirenz may interact with some drugs; therefore, patients should be advised to report to their doctor the use of any prescription, non-prescription medication or herbal products, particularly St. John's wort.

Patients should be informed that redistribution or accumulation of body fat may occur in patients receiving antiretrovial therapy and that the cause and long-term health effects of these conditions are not known at this time.

CARCINOGENESIS, MUTAGENESIS, AND IMPAIRMENT OF FERTILITY

Long-term carcinogenicity studies of efavirenz in rats and mice are in progress.

Efavirenz was not mutagenic or genotoxic in *in vitro* and *in vivo* genotoxicity assays which included bacterial mutation assays in *S. typhimurium* and *E. coli,* mammalian mutation assays in Chinese Hamster Ovary cells, chromosomal aberration assays in human peripheral blood lymphocytes or Chinese Hamster Ovary cells, and an *in vivo* mouse bone marrow micronucleus assay.

Efavirenz did not impair mating or fertility of male or female rats, and did not affect sperm of treated male rats. The reproductive performance of offspring born to female rats given efavirenz was not affected. As a result of the rapid clearance of efavirenz in rats, systemic drug exposures achieved in these studies were equivalent to or below those achieved in humans given therapeutic doses of efavirenz.

PREGNANCY CATEGORY C

Malformations have been observed in 3 of 20 fetuses/infants from efavirenz-treated cynomolgus monkeys (versus 0 of 20 concomitant controls) in a developmental toxicity study. The pregnant monkeys were dosed throughout pregnancy (post coital days 20-150) with efavirenz 60 mg/kg daily, a dose which resulted in plasma drug concentrations similar to those in humans given 600 mg/day of efavirenz. Anencephaly and unilateral anophthalmia were observed in 1 fetus, microophthalmia was observed in another fetus, and cleft palate was observed in a third fetus. Efavirenz crosses the placenta in cynomolgus monkeys and produces fetal blood concentrations similar to maternal blood concentrations. Because teratogenic effects have been seen in primates at efavirenz exposures similar to those seen in the clinic at the recommended dose, pregnancy should be avoided in women receiving efavirenz. Barrier contraception should always be used in combination with other methods of contraception (*e.g.,* oral or other hormonal contraceptives). Women of childbearing potential should undergo pregnancy testing prior to initiation of efavirenz (see WARNINGS, Reproductive Risk Potential).

Efavirenz has been shown to cross the placenta in rats and rabbits and produces fetal blood concentrations of efavirenz similar to maternal concentrations. An increase in fetal resorptions was observed in rats at efavirenz doses that produced peak plasma concentrations and AUC values in female rats equivalent to, or lower than those achieved in humans given 600 mg once daily of efavirenz. Efavirenz produced no reproductive toxicities when given to pregnant rabbits at doses that produced peak plasma concentrations similar to, and AUC values approximately half of those achieved in humans given 600 mg once daily of efavirenz.

There are no adequate and well-controlled studies in pregnant women. Efavirenz should be used during pregnancy only if the potential benefit justifies the potential risk to the fetus, such as in pregnant women without other therapeutic options.

Antiretroviral Pregnancy Registry: To monitor fetal outcomes of pregnant women exposed to efavirenz, an Antiretroviral Pregnancy Registry has been established. Physicians are encouraged to register patients by calling 800-258-4263.

NURSING MOTHERS

The Centers for Disease Control and Prevention recommend that HIV-infected mothers not breast-feed their infants to avoid risking postnatal transmission of HIV. Although it is not known if efavirenz is secreted in human milk, efavirenz is secreted into the milk of lactating rats. Because of the potential for HIV transmission and the potential for serious adverse effects in nursing infants, **mothers should be instructed not to breast-feed if they are receiving efavirenz.**

E

PEDIATRIC USE

ACTG 382 is an ongoing open-label study in 57 NRTI-experienced pediatric patients to characterize the safety, pharmacokinetics, and antiviral activity of efavirenz in combination with nelfinavir (20-30 mg/kg tid) and NRTIs. Mean age was 8 years (range 3-16). Efavirenz has not been studied in pediatric patients below 3 years of age or who weigh less than 13 kg. At 48 weeks, the type and frequency of adverse experiences was generally similar to that of adult patients with the exception of a higher incidence of rash which was reported in 46% (26/57) of pediatric patients compared to 26% of adults, and a higher frequency of Grade 3 or 4 rash reported in 5% (3/57) of pediatric patients compared to 0.9% of adults (see TABLE 7).

The starting dose of efavirenz was 600 mg once daily adjusted to body size, based on weight, targeting AUC levels in the range of 190-380 μM·h. The pharmacokinetics of efavirenz in pediatric patients were similar to the pharmacokinetics in adults who received 600 mg daily doses of efavirenz. In 48 pediatric patients receiving the equivalent of a 600 mg dose of efavirenz, steady-state C_{max} was 14.2 ± 5.8 μM (mean ± SD), steady-state C_{min} was 5.6 ± 4.1 μM, and AUC was 218 ± 104 μM·h.

GERIATRIC USE

Clinical studies of efavirenz did not include sufficient numbers of subjects aged 65 and over to determine whether they respond differently from younger subjects. In general, dose selection for an elderly patient should be cautious, reflecting the greater frequency of decreased hepatic, renal, or cardiac function and of concomitant disease or other therapy.

DRUG INTERACTIONS

See also CONTRAINDICATIONS and CLINICAL PHARMACOLOGY, Drug Interactions.

Efavirenz has been shown *in vivo* to induce CYP3A4. Other compounds that are substrates of CYP3A4 may have decreased plasma concentrations when coadministered with efavirenz. *In vitro* studies have demonstrated that efavirenz inhibits 2C9, 2C19 and 3A4 isozymes in the range of observed efavirenz plasma concentrations. Coadministration of efavirenz with drugs primarily metabolized by these isozymes may result in altered plasma concentrations of the coadministered drug. Therefore, appropriate dose adjustments may be necessary for these drugs.

Drugs which induce CYP3A4 activity (*e.g.,* phenobarbital, rifampin, rifabutin) would be expected to increase the clearance of efavirenz resulting in lowered plasma concentrations. Drug interactions with efavirenz are summarized in TABLE 5A, TABLE 5B, and TABLE 5C.

TABLE 5A *Drugs That Should Not Be Coadministered With Efavirenz**

Drug Class	Drugs Within Class Not To Be Coadministered With Efavirenz
Antihistamines	Astemizole
Benzodiazepines	Midazolam, triazolam
GI motility agents	Cisapride
Anti-migraine	Ergot derivatives

* See TABLE 1 and TABLE 2.

OTHER DRUGS

Based on the results of drug interaction studies (see TABLE 1 and TABLE 2), no dosage adjustment is recommended when efavirenz is given with the following: aluminum/magnesium hydroxide antacids, azithromycin, cetirizine, famotidine, fluconazole, lamivudine, lorazepam, nelfinavir, and zidovudine.

Specific drug interaction studies have not been performed with efavirenz and NRTIs other than lamivudine and zidovudine. Clinically significant interactions would not be expected since the NRTIs are metabolized via a different route than efavirenz and would be unlikely to compete for the same metabolic enzymes and elimation pathways.

ADVERSE REACTIONS

The most significant adverse events observed in patients treated with efavirenz are nervous system symptoms, psychiatric symptoms, and rash.

NERVOUS SYSTEM SYMPTOMS

Fifty-three percent (53%) of patients receiving efavirenz reported central nervous system symptoms (see WARNINGS, Nervous System Symptoms). TABLE 6 lists the frequency of the symptoms of different degrees of severity, and gives the discontinuation rates, in clinical trials for 1 or more of the following nervous system symptoms: dizziness, insomnia, impaired concentration, somnolence, abnormal dreaming, euphoria, confusion, agitation, amnesia, hallucinations, stupor, abnormal thinking, and depersonalization. The frequencies of specific central and peripheral nervous system symptoms are provided in TABLE 8A and TABLE 8B.

PSYCHIATRIC SYMPTOMS

Serious psychiatric adverse experiences have been reported in patients treated with efavirenz. In controlled trials the frequency of specific serious psychiatric symptoms among patients who received efavirenz or control regimens, respectively, were: severe depression (1.6%, 0.6%), suicidal ideation (0.6%, 0.3%), non-fatal suicide attempts (0.4%, 0%), aggressive behavior (0.4%, 0.3%), paranoid reactions (0.4%, 0.3%) and manic reactions (0.1%, 0%) (see WARNINGS, Psychiatric Symptoms). Additional psychiatric symptoms observed at a frequency of >2% among patients treated with efavirenz or control regimens, respectively, in controlled clinical trials were depression (15.8%, 13.1%), anxiety (11.1%, 7.6%), and nervousness (6.3%, 2.0%).

SKIN RASH

Rashes are usually mild-to-moderate maculopapular skin eruptions that occur within the first 2 weeks of initiating therapy with efavirenz. In most patients, rash resolves with continuing efavirenz therapy within 1 month. Efavirenz can be reinitiated in patients interrupting therapy because of rash. Use of appropriate antihistamines and/or corticosteroids may be considered when efavirenz is restarted. Efavirenz should be discontinued in patients developing severe rash associated with blistering, desquamation, mucosal involvement or fever. The frequency of rash by NCI grade and the discontinuation rates as a result of rash are provided in TABLE 7.

TABLE 5B *Drugs That Should not be Coadministered With Efavirenz: Established Drug Interactions**

Drug Name	Effect	Clinical Comment
Clarithromycin	Decrease (dec) clarithromycin concentration. Increase (inc) 14-OH metabolite concentration.	Plasma concentrations decreased by efavirenz; clinical significance unknown. In uninfected volunteers, 46% developed rash while receiving efavirenz and clairthromycin. No dose adjustment of efavirenz is recommended when given with clarithromycin. Alternatives to clarithromycin, such as azithromycin, should be considered (see Other Drugs). Other macrolide antibiotics, such as erythromycin, have not been studied in combination with efavirenz.
Indinavir	dec indinavir concentration	Increase indinavir dose from 800 mg to 1000 mg every 8 hours.
Methadone	dec methadone concentration	Coadministration in HIV-infected individuals with a history of injection drug use resulted in decreased plasma levels of methadone and signs of opiate withdrawal. Methadone dose was increased by a mean of 22% to alleviate withdrawal symptoms. Patients should be monitored for signs of withdrawal and their methadone dose increased as required to alleviate withdrawal symptoms.
Ethinyl estradiol	inc ethinyl estradiol concentration	Plasma concentrations increased by efavirenz; clinical significance unknown. Because the potential interaction of efavirenz with oral contraceptives has not been fully characterized, a reliable method of barrier contraception should be used in addition to oral contraceptives.
Rifabutin	dec rifabutin concentration	Increase daily dose of rifabutin by 50%. Consider doubling the rifabutin dose in regimens where rifabutin is given 2 or 3 times a week.
Rifampin	dec efavirenz concentration	Clinical significance of reduced efavirenz concentrations unknown.
Ritonavir	inc ritonavir concentration. inc efavirenz concentration.	Combination was associated with a higher frequency of adverse clinical experiences (*e.g.,* dizziness, nausea, paresthesia) and laboratory abnormalities (elevated liver ensymes). Monitoring of liver enzymes is recommended when efavirenz is used in combination with ritonavir.
Saquinavir	dec saquinavir concentration	Should not be used as sole protease inhibitor in combination with efavirenz.

* See TABLE 1 and TABLE 2.

TABLE 5C *Other Potentially Clinically Significant Drug or Herbal Product Interactions With Efavirenz*†*

Anticoagulants: Warfarin	Plasma concentrations and effects potentially increased or decreased by efavirenz.
Anticonvulsants: Phenytoin, Phenobarbital, Carbamazepine	Potential for reduction in anticonvulsant and/or efavirenz plasma levels; periodic monitoring of anticonvulsant plasma levels should be conducted.
Antifungals: Itraconazole, Ketaconazole	Drug interaction studies with efavirenz and these imidazole and triazole antifungals have not been conducted. Efavirenz has the potential to decrease plasma concentrations of itraconazole and ketoconazole.
Anti-HIV Protease Inhibitors:	No pharmacokinetic data are available.
Saquinavir/ritonavir combination Amprenavir	Efavirenz has the potential to decrease serum concentrations of amprenavir.
Non-nucleoside reverse transcriptase inhibitors	No studies have been performed with other NNRTIs.
St. John's Wort *(hypericum perforatum)*	Expected to substantially decrease plasma levels of efavirenz; has not been studied in combination with efavirenz.

* See TABLE 1 and TABLE 2.
† This table is not all-inclusive.

As seen in TABLE 7, rash is more common in pediatric patients and more often of higher grade (*i.e.,* more severe) (see PRECAUTIONS, General).

Experience with efavirenz in patients who discontinued other antiretroviral agents of the NNRTI class is limited. Nineteen (19) patients who discontinued nevirapine because of rash have been treated with efavirenz. Nine (9) of these patients developed mild-to-moderate rash while receiving therapy with efavirenz, and 2 of these patients discontinued because of rash.

A few cases of pancreatitis have been described, although a causal relationship with efavirenz has not been established. Asymptomatic increases in serum amylase levels were observed in a significantly higher number of patients treated with efavirenz 600 mg than in control patients (see Laboratory Abnormalities).

TABLE 6 *Percent of Patients With 1 or More Selected Nervous System Symptoms*†*

Percent of Patients With:	Efavirenz 600 mg Once Daily (n=1008)	Control Groups (n=635)
Symptoms of any severity	52.7%	24.6%
Mild symptoms‡	33.3%	15.6%
Moderate symptoms§	17.4%	7.7%
Severe symptoms¤	2.0%	1.3%
Treatment discontinuation as a result of symptoms	2.1%	1.1%

* Includes events reported regardless of causality.
† Data from Study 006 and three Phase 2/3 studies.
‡ "Mild" = Symptoms which do not interfere with patient's daily activities.
§ "Moderate" = Symptoms which may interfere with daily activities.
¤ "Severe" = Events which interrupt patient's usual daily activities.

TABLE 7 *Percent of Patients With Treatment-Emergent Rash*†*

	Description of Rash Grade‡	Efavirenz 600 mg Once Daily Adults (n=1008)	Efavirenz Pediatric Patients (n=57)	Control Groups Adults (n=635)
Rash of any grade	—	26.3%	45.6%	17.5%
Grade 1 rash	Erythema, pruritus	10.7%	8.8%	9.8%
Grade 2 rash	Diffuse maculopapular rash, dry desquamation	14.7%	31.6%	7.4%
Grade 3 rash	Vesiculation, moist desquamation, ulceration	0.8%	1.8%	0.3%
Grade 4 rash	Erythema multiforme, Stevens-Johnson Syndrome, toxic epidermal necrolysis, necrosis requiring surgery, exfoliative dermatitis	0.1%	3.5%	0.0%
Treatment discontinuation as a result of rash	—	1.7%	8.8%	0.3%

* Includes events reported regardless of causality.
† Data from Study 006 and three Phase 2/3 studies.
‡ NCI grading system.

Drug-related clinical adverse experiences of moderate or severe intensity observed in ≥2% of patients in two controlled clinical trials are presented in TABLE 8A and TABLE 8B.

TABLE 8A *Percent of Patients With Treatment-Emergent* Adverse Events of Moderate or Severe Intensity Reported in ≥2% of Patients in Study 006*

	Study 006 LAM, NNRTI and Protease Inhibitor Naive Patients		
Adverse Event	**Efavirenz†+ ZDV/ LAM (n=412)**	**Efavirenz†+ Indinavir (n=415)**	**Indinavir + ZDV/ LAM (n=401)**
Body as a Whole			
Fatigue	7%	5%	8%
Pain	1%	1%	5%
Central and Peripheral Nervous System			
Dizziness	8%	8%	3%
Headache	7%	4%	4%
Concentration impaired	5%	2%	0%
Insomnia	6%	7%	3%
Abnormal dreams	3%	1%	0%
Somnolence	3%	2%	2%
Anorexia	1%	0%	1%
Gastrointestinal			
Nausea	12%	7%	25%
Vomiting	7%	6%	14%
Diarrhea	6%	8%	6%
Dyspepsia	3%	3%	5%
Abdominal pain	1%	2%	4%
Psychiatric			
Anxiety	1%	3%	0%
Depression	2%	1%	0%
Nervousness	2%	2%	0%
Skin and Appendages			
Rash	13%	20%	7%
Pruritus	0%	1%	1%
Increased sweating	2%	1%	0%

* Includes adverse events at least possibly related to study drug or of unknown relationship for Study 006.
† Efavirenz provided as 600 mg once daily.

TABLE 8B *Percent of Patients With Treatment-Emergent* Adverse Events of Moderate or Severe Intensity Reported in ≥2% of Patients in Study ACTG 364*

	Study ACTG 364 NRTI-Experienced, NNRTI and Protease Inhibitor Naive Patients		
Adverse Event	**Efavirenz†+ Nelfinavir + NRTIs (n=64)**	**Efavirenz†+ NRTIs (n=65)**	**Nelfinavir + NRTIs (n=66)**
Body as a Whole			
Fatigue	0%	2%	3%
Pain	13%	6%	17%
Central and Peripheral Nervous System			
Dizziness	2%	6%	6%
Headache	5%	2%	3%
Concentration impaired	0%	0%	0%
Insomnia	0%	0%	2%
Abnormal dreams	—	—	—
Somnolence	0%	0%	0%
Anorexia	0%	2%	2%
Gastrointestinal			
Nausea	3%	2%	2%
Vomiting	—	—	—
Diarrhea	14%	3%	9%
Dyspepsia	0%	0%	2%
Abdominal pain	3%	3%	3%
Psychiatric			
Anxiety	—	—	—
Depression	3%	0%	5%
Nervousness	2%	0%	2%
Skin and Appendages			
Rash	9%	5%	9%
Pruritus	9%	5%	9%
Increased sweating	0%	0%	0%

* Includes all adverse events regardless of relationship to study drug for Study ACTG 364.
† Efavirenz provided as 600 mg once daily.
— Not specified.

In Study 006, lipodystrophy was reported in 2.3% of patients treated with efavirenz + IDV, 0.7% of patients treated with efavirenz + ZDV + LAM and 1.0% of patients treated with IDV + ZDV + LAM.

Clinical adverse experience observed in ≥10% of 57 pediatric patients aged 3-16 years who received efavirenz capsules, nelfinavir, and 1 or more NRTIs were: rash (46%), diarrhea/loose stools (39%), fever (21%), cough (16%), dizziness/lightheaded/fainting (16%), ache/pain/discomfort (14%), nausea/vomiting (12%), and headache (11%). The incidence of nervous system symptoms was 18% (10/57). One patient experienced Grade 3 rash, 2 patients had Grade 4 rash, and 5 patients (9%) discontinued because of rash (see also PRECAUTIONS: Skin Rash and Pediatric Use).

POST-MARKETING EXPERIENCE

Body as a Whole: Allergic reactions, asthenia, redistribution/accumulation of body fat (see PRECAUTIONS, Fat Redistribution).

Central and Peripheral Nervous System: Abnormal coordination, ataxia, convulsions, hypoesthesia, paresthesia, neuropathy, tremor.

Endocrine: Gynecomastia.

Gastrointestinal: Constipation, malabsorption.

Cardiovascular: Flushing, palpitations.

Liver and Biliary System: Hepatic enzyme increase, hepatic failure, hepatitis.

Metabolic and Nutritional: Hypercholesterolemia, hypertriglyceridemia.

Musculoskeletal: Arthralgia, myalgia, myopathy.

Psychiatric: Aggressive reactions, agitation, delusions, emotional lability, mania, neurosis, paranoia, psychosis, suicide.

Respiratory: Dyspnea.

Skin and Appendages: Erythema multiforme, nail disorders, skin discoloration, Stevens-Johnson Syndrome.

Special Senses: Abnormal vision, tinnitus.

LABORATORY ABNORMALITIES

Liver Enzymes

Among 1008 patients treated with 600 mg efavirenz in controlled clinical trials, 3% developed AST levels and 3% developed ALT levels greater than 5 times the upper limit of normal. Similar elevations of AST and ALT were seen in patients treated with control regimens.

Liver function tests should be monitored in patients with a prior history of Hepatitis B and/or C. In 156 patients treated with 600 mg of efavirenz who were seropositive for Hepatitis B and/or C, 7% developed AST levels and 8% developed ALT levels greater than 5 times the upper limit of normal. In 91 patients seropositive for Hepatitis B and/or C treated with control regimens, 5% developed AST elevations and 4% developed ALT elevations to these levels. Elevations of GGT to greater than 5 times the upper limit of the normal range were observed in 4% of all patients treated with 600 mg of efavirenz and in 10% of patients seropositive for Hepatitis B or C. In patients treated with control regimens, the incidence of GGT elevations to this level was 1.5-2%, irrespective of Hepatitis B or C serology. Isolated elevations of GGT in patients receiving efavirenz may reflect enzyme induction not associated with liver toxicity (see PRECAUTIONS, General).

Lipids

Increases in total cholesterol of 10-20% have been observed in some uninfected volunteers receiving efavirenz. In patients treated with efavirenz + ZDV + LAM, increases in non-fasting total cholesterol and HDL of approximately 20% and 25%, respectively, were observed. In patients treated with efavirenz + IDV, increases in non-fasting cholesterol and

HDL of approximately 40% and 35%, respectively, were observed. The effects of efavirenz on triglycerides and LDL were not well-characterized since samples were taken from non-fasting patients. The clinical significance of these findings is unknown (see PRECAUTIONS, General).

Serum Amylase

Asymptomatic elevations in serum amylase greater than 1.5 times the upper limit of normal were seen in 10% of patients treated with efavirenz and in 6% of patients treated with control regimens. The clinical significance of asymptomatic increases in serum amylase is unknown (see ADVERSE REACTIONS).

Cannabinoid Test Interaction

Efavirenz does not bind to cannabinoid receptors. False-positive urine cannabinoid test results have been observed in non-HIV-infected volunteers receiving efavirenz when the Microgenics CEDIA DAU Multi-Level THC assay was used for screening. Negative results were obtained when more specific confirmatory testing was performed with gas chromatography/mass spectrometry.

Of the three assays analyzed (Microgenics CEDIA DAU Multi-Level THC assay, Cannabinoid Enzyme Immunoassay [Diagnostic Reagents, Inc.], and AxSYM Cannabinoid Assay [Abbott Laboratories]), only the Microgenics CEDIA DAU Multi-Level THC assay showed false-positive results. The other two assays provided true-negative results. The effects of efavirenz on cannabinoid screening tests other than these three are unknown. The manufacturers of cannabinoid assays should be contacted for additional information regarding the use of their assays with patients receiving efavirenz.

DOSAGE AND ADMINISTRATION

ADULTS

The recommended dosage of efavirenz is 600 mg orally, once daily, in combination with a protease inhibitor and/or nucleoside analogue reverse transcriptase inhibitors (NRTIs). It is recommended that efavirenz be taken on an empty stomach preferably at bedtime. The increased efavirenz concentrations observed following administration of efavirenz with food may lead to an increase in frequency of adverse events (see CLINICAL PHARMACOLOGY, Effect of Food on Oral Absorption). Dosing at bedtime may improve the tolerability of nervous system symptoms (see WARNINGS, Nervous System Symptoms; PRECAUTIONS, Information for the Patient; and ADVERSE REACTIONS).

CONCOMITANT ANTIRETROVIRAL THERAPY

Efavirenz must be given in combination with other antiretroviral medications (see CLINICAL PHARMACOLOGY, Drug Interactions; DRUG INTERACTIONS; and INDICATIONS AND USAGE).

PEDIATRIC PATIENTS

It is recommended that efavirenz be taken on an empty stomach, preferably at bedtime. TABLE 9 describes the recommended dose of efavirenz for pediatric patients 3 years of age or older and weighing between 10 and 40 kg. The recommended dosage of efavirenz for pediatric patients weighing greater than 40 kg is 600 mg, once daily.

TABLE 9 *Pediatric Dose to be Administered Once Daily*

Body Weight		Efavirenz Dose
10 to <15 kg	22 to <33 lb	200 mg
15 to <20 kg	33 to <44 lb	250 mg
20 to <25 kg	44 to <55 lb	300 mg
25 to <32.5 kg	55 to <71.5 lb	350 mg
32.5 to <40 kg	71.5 to <88 lb	400 mg
≥40 kg	≥88 lb	600 mg

HOW SUPPLIED

Capsules

Sustiva capsules are available as follows:

200 mg: Gold color, reverse printed with "SUSTIVA" on the body and imprinted "200 mg" on the cap.

100 mg: White, reverse printed with "SUSTIVA" on the body and imprinted "100 mg" on the cap.

50 mg: Gold color and white, printed with "SUSTIVA" on the gold color cap and reverse printed "50 mg" on the white body.

Tablets

Sustiva tablets are available as follows:

600 mg: Yellow, capsular-shaped, film-coated tablets, with "SUSTIVA" printed on both sides.

Storage: Sustiva capsules and tablets should be stored at 25°C (77°F); excursions permitted to 15-30°C (59-86°F).

PRODUCT LISTING - RATED THERAPEUTICALLY EQUIVALENT

Capsule - Oral - 50 mg
30's $36.02 SUSTIVA, Dupont Pharmaceuticals 00056-0470-30

Capsule - Oral - 100 mg
30's $71.94 SUSTIVA, Dupont Pharmaceuticals 00056-0473-30

Capsule - Oral - 200 mg
90's $431.65 SUSTIVA, Dupont Pharmaceuticals 00056-0474-92

PRODUCT LISTING - EQUIVALENTS NOT AVAILABLE

Tablet - Oral - 600 mg
30's $449.64 SUSTIVA, Bristol-Myers Squibb 00056-0510-30

Eletriptan (003584)

For related information, see the comparative table section in Appendix A.

Categories: Headache, migraine; Pregnancy Category C; FDA Approved 2002 Dec
Drug Classes: Serotonin receptor agonists
Brand Names: **Relpax**
Foreign Brand Availability: Relert (Israel)
Cost of Therapy: $15.80 (Migraine Headache; Relpax; 40 mg; 1 tablet/day; 1 day supply)

DESCRIPTION

Relpax tablets contain eletriptan hydrobromide, which is a selective 5-hydroxytryptamine 1B/1D (5-HT1B/1D) receptor agonist. Eletriptan is chemically designated as 3-[[(R)-1-Methyl-2-pyrrolidinyl]methyl]-5-[2-(phenylsulfonyl)ethyl]indole, monohydrobromide.

The empirical formula is $C_{22}H_{26}N_2O_2S \cdot HBr$, representing a molecular weight of 463.40. Eletriptan hydrobromide is a white to light pale colored powder that is readily soluble in water.

Each Relpax tablet for oral administration contains 24.2 or 48.5 mg of eletriptan hydrobromide equivalent to 20 mg or 40 mg of eletriptan, respectively. Each tablet also contains the inactive ingredients microcrystalline cellulose, lactose, croscarmellose sodium, magnesium stearate, titanium dioxide, hydroxypropyl methylcellulose, triacetin and FD&C yellow no. 6 aluminum lake.

CLINICAL PHARMACOLOGY

MECHANISM OF ACTION

Eletriptan binds with high affinity to 5-HT_{1B}, 5-HT_{1D} and 5-HT_{1F} receptors, has modest affinity for 5-HT_{1A}, 5-HT_{1E}, 5-HT_{2B} and 5-HT_7 receptors, and little or no affinity for 5-HT_{2A}, 5-HT_{2C}, 5-HT_3, 5-HT_4, 5-HT_{5A} and 5-HT_6 receptors. Eletriptan has no significant affinity or pharmacological activity at adrenergic alpha_1, alpha_2, or beta; dopaminergic D_1 or D_2; muscarinic; or opioid receptors.

Two theories have been proposed to explain the efficacy of 5-HT receptor agonists in migraine. One theory suggests that activation of 5-HT_1 receptors located on intracranial blood vessels, including those on the arteriovenous anastomoses, leads to vasoconstriction, which is correlated with the relief of migraine headache. The other hypothesis suggests that activation of 5-HT_1 receptors on sensory nerve endings in the trigeminal system results in the inhibition of pro-inflammatory neuropeptide release.

In the anesthetized dog, eletriptan has been shown to reduce carotid arterial blood flow, with only a small increase in arterial blood pressure at high doses. While the effect on blood flow was selective for the carotid arterial bed, decreases in coronary artery diameter were observed. Eletriptan has also been shown to inhibit trigeminal nerve activity in the rat.

PHARMACOKINETICS

Absorption

Eletriptan is well absorbed after oral administration with peak plasma levels occurring approximately 1.5 hours after dosing to healthy subjects. In patients with moderate to severe migraine the median T_{max} is 2.0 hours. The mean absolute bioavailability of eletriptan is approximately 50%. The oral pharmacokinetics are slightly more than dose proportional over the clinical dose range. The AUC and C_{max} of eletriptan are increased by approximately 20-30% following oral administration with a high fat meal.

Distribution

The volume of distribution of eletriptan following IV administration is 138 L. Plasma protein binding is moderate and approximately 85%.

Metabolism

The N-demethylated metabolite of eletriptan is the only known active metabolite. This metabolite causes vasoconstriction similar to eletriptan in animal models. Though the half-life of the metabolite is estimated to be about 13 hours, the plasma concentration of the N-demethylated metabolite is 10-20% of parent drug and is unlikely to contribute significantly to the overall effect of the parent compound.

In vitro studies indicate that eletriptan is primarily metabolized by cytochrome P-450 enzyme CYP3A4 (see WARNINGS, DOSAGE AND ADMINISTRATION; and CLINICAL PHARMACOLOGY, Drug Interactions).

Elimination

The terminal elimination half-life of eletriptan is approximately 4 hours. Mean renal clearance (CLR) following oral administration is approximately 3.9 L/h. Non-renal clearance accounts for about 90% of the total clearance.

SPECIAL POPULATIONS

Age

The pharmacokinetics of eletriptan are generally unaffected by age.

Eletriptan has been given to only 50 patients over the age of 65. Blood pressure was increased to a greater extent in elderly subjects than in young subjects. The pharmacokinetic disposition of eletriptan in the elderly is similar to that seen in younger adults (see PRECAUTIONS).

There is a statistically significant increased half-life (from about 4.4-5.7 hours) between elderly (65-93 years of age) and younger adult subjects (18-45 years of age) (see PRECAUTIONS).

Gender

The pharmacokinetics of eletriptan are unaffected by gender.

Race

A comparison of pharmacokinetic studies run in western countries with those run in Japan have indicated an approximate 35% reduction in the exposure of eletriptan in Japanese male volunteers compared to western males. Population pharmacokinetic analysis of two clinical studies indicates no evidence of pharmacokinetic differences between Caucasians and non Caucasian patients.

Menstrual Cycle

In a study of 16 healthy females, the pharmacokinetics of eletriptan remained consistent throughout the phases of the menstrual cycle.

Renal Impairment

There was no significant change in clearance observed in subjects with mild, moderate or severe renal impairment, though blood pressure elevations were observed in this population (see WARNINGS).

Hepatic Impairment

The effects of severe hepatic impairment on eletriptan metabolism have not been evaluated. Subjects with mild or moderate hepatic impairment demonstrated an increase in both AUC (34%) and half-life. The C_{max} was increased by 18% (see PRECAUTIONS and DOSAGE AND ADMINISTRATION).

DRUGINTERACTIONS

CYP3A4 Inhibitors

In vitro studies have shown that eletriptan is metabolized by the CYP3A4 enzyme. A clinical study demonstrated about a 3-fold increase in C_{max} and about a 6-fold increase in the AUC of eletriptan when combined with ketoconazole. The half-life increased from 5-8 hours and the T_{max} increased from 2.8-5.4 hours. Another clinical study demonstrated about a 2-fold increase in C_{max} and about a 4-fold increase in AUC when erythromycin was coadministered with eletriptan. It has also been shown that coadministration of verapamil and eletriptan yields about a 2-fold increase in C_{max} and about a 3-fold increase in AUC of eletriptan, and that coadministration of fluconazole and eletriptan yields about a 1.4-fold increase in C_{max} and about a 2-fold increase in AUC of eletriptan.

Eletriptan should not be used within at least 72 hours of treatment with the following potent CYP3A4 inhibitors: ketoconazole, itraconazole, nefazodone, troleandomycin, clarithromycin, ritonavir and nelfinavir. Eletriptan should not be used within 72 hours with drugs that have demonstrated potent CYP3A4 inhibition and have this potent effect described in the CONTRAINDICATIONS, WARNINGS or PRECAUTIONS sections of their labeling (see WARNINGS and DOSAGE AND ADMINISTRATION).

Propranolol

The C_{max} and AUC of eletriptan were increased by 10 and 33% respectively in the presence of propranolol. No interactive increases in blood pressure were observed. No dosage adjustment appears to be needed for patients taking propranolol (see PRECAUTIONS).

The Effect of Eletriptan on Other Drugs

The effect of eletriptan on enzymes other than cytochrome P-450 has not been investigated. *In vitro* human liver microsome studies suggest that eletriptan has little potential to inhibit CYP1A2, 2C9, 2E1 and 3A4 at concentrations up to 100 μM. While eletriptan has an effect on CYP2D6 at high concentration, this effect should not interfere with metabolism of other drugs when eletriptan is used at recommended doses. There is no *in vitro* or *in vivo* evidence that clinical doses of eletriptan will induce drug metabolizing enzymes. Therefore, eletriptan is unlikely to cause clinically important drug interactions mediated by these enzymes.

INDICATIONS AND USAGE

Eletriptan hydrobromide is indicated for the acute treatment of migraine with or without aura in adults.

Eletriptan hydrobromide is not intended for the prophylactic therapy of migraine or for use in the management of hemiplegic or basilar migraine (see CONTRAINDICATIONS). Safety and effectiveness of eletriptan hydrobromide tablets have not been established for cluster headache, which is present in an older, predominantly male population.

CONTRAINDICATIONS

Eletriptan hydrobromide tablets should not be given to patients with ischemic heart disease (*e.g.*, angina pectoris, history of myocardial infarction, or documented silent ischemia) or to patients who have symptoms, or findings consistent with ischemic heart disease, coronary artery vasospasm, including Prinzmetal's variant angina, or other significant underlying cardiovascular disease (see WARNINGS).

Eletriptan hydrobromide tablets should not be given to patients with cerebrovascular syndromes including (but not limited to) strokes of any type as well as transient ischemic attacks (see WARNINGS).

Eletriptan hydrobromide tablets should not be given to patients with peripheral vascular disease including (but not limited to) ischemic bowel disease (see WARNINGS).

Because eletriptan hydrobromide tablets may increase blood pressure, it should not be given to patients with uncontrolled hypertension (see WARNINGS).

Eletriptan hydrobromide tablets should not be administered to patients with hemiplegic or basilar migraine.

Eletriptan hydrobromide tablets should not be used within 24 hours of treatment with another 5-HT_1 agonist, an ergotamine-containing or ergot-type medication such as dihydroergotamine (DHE) or methysergide.

Eletriptan hydrobromide tablets should not be used in patients with known hypersensitivity to eletriptan or any of its inactive ingredients.

Eletriptan hydrobromide tablets should not be given to patients with severe hepatic impairment.

WARNINGS

Eletriptan hydrobromide tablets should only be used where a clear diagnosis of migraine has been established.

CYP3A4 INHIBITORS

Eletriptan should not be used within at least 72 hours of treatment with the following potent CYP3A4 inhibitors: ketoconazole, itraconazole, nefazodone, troleandomycin, clarithromycin, ritonavir, and nelfinavir. Eletriptan should not be used within 72 hours with drugs that have demonstrated potent CYP3A4 inhibition and have this potent effect described in the CONTRAINDICATIONS, WARNINGS or PRECAUTIONS sections of their labeling (see CLINICAL PHARMACOLOGY, Drug Interactions; and DOSAGE AND ADMINISTRATION).

In a coronary angiographic study of rapidly infused intravenous eletriptan to concentrations exceeding those achieved with 80 mg oral eletriptan in the presence of potent CYP3A4 inhibitors, a small dose-related decrease in coronary artery diameter similar to that seen with a 6 mg subcutaneous dose of sumatriptan was observed.

RISK OF MYOCARDIAL ISCHEMIA AND/OR INFARCTION AND OTHER CARDIAC EVENTS

Because of the potential of 5-HT_1 agonists to cause coronary vasospasm, eletriptan should not be given to patients with documented ischemic or vasospastic coronary artery disease (CAD) (see CONTRAINDICATIONS). It is strongly recommended that eletriptan not be given to patients in whom unrecognized CAD is predicted by the presence of risk factors (*e.g.*, hypertension, hypercholesterolemia, smoker, obesity, diabetes, strong family history of CAD, female with surgical or physiological menopause, or male over 40 years of age) unless a cardiovascular evaluation provides satisfactory clinical evidence that the patient is reasonably free of coronary artery and ischemic myocardial disease or other significant underlying cardiovascular disease. The sensitivity of cardiac diagnostic procedures to detect cardiovascular disease or predisposition to coronary artery vasospasm is modest, at best. If, during the cardiovascular evaluation, the patient's medical history, electrocardiographic, or other investigations reveal findings indicative of, or consistent with coronary artery vasospasm or myocardial ischemia, eletriptan should not be administered (see CONTRAINDICATIONS).

For patients with risk factors predictive of CAD, who are determined to have a satisfactory cardiovascular evaluation, it is strongly recommended that administration of the first dose of eletriptan take place in the setting of a physician's office or similar medically staffed and equipped facility unless the patient has previously received eletriptan. Because cardiac ischemia can occur in the absence of clinical symptoms, consideration should be given to obtaining on the first occasion of use an electrocardiogram (ECG) during the interval immediately following administration of eletriptan hydrobromide tablets, in these patients with risk factors.

It is recommended that patients who are intermittent long-term users of 5-HT_1 agonists including eletriptan hydrobromide tablets, and who have or acquire risk factors predictive of CAD, as described above, undergo periodic cardiovascular evaluation as they continue to use eletriptan hydrobromide tablets.

The systematic approach described above is intended to reduce the likelihood that patients with unrecognized cardiovascular disease will be inadvertently exposed to eletriptan.

CARDIAC EVENTS AND FATALITIES ASSOCIATED WITH 5-HT_1 AGONISTS

Serious adverse cardiac events, including acute myocardial infarction, life-threatening disturbances of cardiac rhythm, and death have been reported within a few hours following the administration of other 5-HT_1 agonists. Considering the extent of use of 5-HT_1 agonists in patients with migraine, the incidence of these events is extremely low.

Premarketing Experience With Eletriptan Among the 7143 Unique Individuals Who Received Eletriptan During Pre-Marketing Clinical Trials

In a clinical pharmacology study, in subjects undergoing diagnostic coronary angiography, a subject with a history of angina, hypertension and hypercholesterolemia, receiving IV eletriptan (C_{max} of 127 ng/ml equivalent to 60 mg oral eletriptan), reported chest tightness and experienced angiographically documented coronary vasospasm with no ECG changes of ischemia. There was also one report of atrial fibrillation in a patient with a past history of atrial fibrillation.

Postmarketing Experience With Eletriptan

There was one report of myocardial infarction and death in a patient with cardiovascular risk factors (hypertension, hyperlipidemia, strong family history of CAD) in association with inappropriate concomitant use of eletriptan and sumatriptan. The uncontrolled nature of postmarketing surveillance, however, makes it impossible to determine definitively if the case was actually caused by eletriptan or to reliably assess causation in individual cases.

CEREBROVASCULAR EVENTS AND FATALITIES ASSOCIATED WITH 5-HT_1 AGONISTS

Cerebral hemorrhage, subarachnoid hemorrhage, stroke, and other cerebrovascular events have been reported in patients treated with 5-HT_1 agonists, and some have resulted in fatalities. In a number of cases, it appears possible that the cerebrovascular events were primary, the agonist having been administered in the incorrect belief that the symptoms experienced were a consequence of migraine, when they were not. It should be noted that patients with migraine may be at increased risk of certain cerebrovascular events (*e.g.*, stroke, hemorrhage, and transient ischemic attack).

OTHER VASOSPASM-RELATED EVENTS

5-HT_1 agonists may cause vasospastic reactions other than coronary artery vasospasm. Both peripheral vascular ischemia and colonic ischemia with abdominal pain and bloody diarrhea have been reported with 5-HT_1 agonists.

INCREASE IN BLOOD PRESSURE

Significant elevation in blood pressure, including hypertensive crisis, has been reported on rare occasion in patients receiving 5-HT_1 agonists with and without a history of hypertension. In clinical pharmacology studies, oral eletriptan (at doses of 60 mg or more) was shown to cause small, transient dose-related increases in blood pressure, predominantly diastolic, consistent with its mechanism of action and with other 5-$HT_{1B/1D}$ agonists. The effect was more pronounced in renally impaired and elderly subjects. A single patient with hepatic cirrhosis received eletriptan 80 mg and experienced a blood pressure of 220/96 mm Hg 5 hours after dosing. The treatment related event persisted for 7 hours.

Eletriptan is contraindicated in patients with uncontrolled hypertension (see CONTRAINDICATIONS).

An 18% increase in mean pulmonary artery pressure was seen following dosing with another 5-HT_1 agonist in a study evaluating subjects undergoing cardiac catheterization.

PRECAUTIONS

GENERAL

As with other 5-HT_1 agonists, sensations of tightness, pain, pressure and heaviness have been reported after treatment with eletriptan in the precordium, throat, and jaw. Events that are localized to the chest, throat, neck and jaw have not been associated with arrhythmias or ischemic ECG changes in clinical trials; in a clinical pharmacology study of subjects undergoing diagnostic coronary angiography, 1 subject with a history of angina, hypertension and hypercholesterolemia, receiving IV eletriptan, reported chest tightness and experienced angiographically documented coronary vasospasm with no ECG changes of ischemia. Because 5-HT_1 agonists may cause coronary artery vasospasm, patients who experience signs or symptoms suggestive of angina following dosing should be evaluated for the presence of CAD or a predisposition to Prinzmetal's variant angina before receiving additional doses of medication, and should be monitored electrocardiographically if dosing is resumed and similar symptoms recur. Similarly, patients who experience other symptoms or signs suggestive of decreased arterial flow, such as ischemic bowel syndrome or Raynaud's syndrome following the use of any 5-HT_1 agonist are candidates for further evaluation (see CONTRAINDICATIONS and WARNINGS).

HEPATICALLY IMPAIRED PATIENTS

The effects of severe hepatic impairment on eletriptan metabolism was not evaluated. Subjects with mild or moderate hepatic impairment demonstrated an increase in both AUC (34%) and half-life. The C_{max} was increased by 18%. Eletriptan should not be used in patients with severe hepatic impairment. No dose adjustment is necessary in mild to moderate impairment (see DOSAGE AND ADMINISTRATION).

BINDING TO MELANIN-CONTAINING TISSUES

In rats treated with a single IV (3 mg/kg) dose of radiolabeled eletriptan, elimination of radioactivity from the retina was prolonged, suggesting that eletriptan and/or its metabolites may bind to the melanin of the eye. Because there could be accumulation in melanin-rich tissues over time, this raises the possibility that eletriptan could cause toxicity in these tissues after extended use. Although no systematic monitoring of ophthalmologic function was undertaken in clinical trials, and no specific recommendations for ophthalmologic monitoring are offered, prescribers should be aware of the possibility of long-term ophthalmologic effects.

CORNEAL OPACITIES

Transient corneal opacities were seen in dogs receiving oral eletriptan at 5 mg/kg and above. They were observed during the first week of treatment, but were not present thereafter despite continued treatment. Exposure at the no-effect dose level of 2.5 mg/kg was approximately equal to that achieved in humans at the maximum recommended daily dose.

INFORMATION FOR THE PATIENT

Additional information for patients is provided in the Patient's Instructions that are distributed with the prescription.

LABORATORY TESTS

No specific laboratory tests are recommended.

DRUG/LABORATORY TEST INTERACTIONS

Eletriptan hydrobromide tablets are not known to interfere with commonly employed clinical laboratory tests.

CARCINOGENESIS

Lifetime carcinogenicity studies, 104 weeks in duration, were carried out in mice and rats by administering eletriptan in the diet. In rats, the incidence of testicular interstitial cell adenomas was increased at the high dose of 75 mg/kg/day. The estimated exposure (AUC) to parent drug at that dose was approximately 6 times that achieved in humans receiving the maximum recommended daily dose (MRDD) of 80 mg, and at the no-effect dose of 15 mg/kg/day it was approximately 2 times the human exposure at the MRDD. In mice, the incidence of hepatocellular adenomas was increased at the high dose of 400 mg/kg/day. The exposure to parent drug (AUC) at that dose was approximately 18 times that achieved in humans receiving the MRDD, and the AUC at the no-effect dose of 90 mg/kg/day was approximately 7 times the human exposure at the MRDD.

MUTAGENESIS

Eletriptan was not mutagenic in bacterial or mammalian cell assays *in vitro*, testing negative in the Ames reverse mutation test and the hypoxanthine-guanine phosphoribosyl transferase (HGPRT) mutation test in Chinese hamster ovary cells. It was not clastogenic in two *in vivo* mouse micronucleus assays. Results were equivocal in *in vitro* human lymphocyte clastogenicity tests, in which the incidence of polyploidy was increased in the absence of metabolic activation (-S9 conditions), but not in the presence of metabolic activation.

IMPAIRMENT OF FERTILITY

In a rat fertility and early embryonic development study, doses tested were 50, 100 and 200 mg/kg/day, resulting in systemic exposures to parent drug in rats, based on AUC, that were 4, 8 and 16 times MRDD, respectively, in males and 7, 14 and 28 times MRDD, respectively, in females. There was a prolongation of the estrous cycle at the 200 mg/kg/day dose due to an increase in duration of estrus, based on vaginal smears. There were also dose-related, statistically significant decreases in mean numbers of corpora lutea per dam at all 3 doses, resulting in decreases in mean numbers of implants and viable fetuses per dam. This suggests a partial inhibition of ovulation by eletriptan. There was no effect on fertility of males and no other effect on fertility of females.

PREGNANCY CATEGORY C

In reproductive toxicity studies in rats and rabbits, oral administration of eletriptan was associated with developmental toxicity (decreased fetal and pup weights and an increased incidence of fetal structural abnormalities). Effects on fetal and pup weights were observed at doses that were, on a mg/m^2 basis, 6-12 times greater than the clinical maximum recommended daily dose (MRDD) of 80 mg. The increase in structural alterations occurred in the rat and rabbit at doses that, on a mg/m^2 basis, were 12 times greater than (rat) and approximately equal to (rabbit) the MRDD.

When pregnant rats were administered eletriptan during the period of organogenesis at doses of 10, 30 or 100 mg/kg/day, fetal weights were decreased and the incidences of vertebral and sternebral variations were increased at 100 mg/kg/day (approximately 12 times the MRDD on a mg/m^2 basis). The 100 mg/kg dose was also maternally toxic, as evidenced by decreased maternal body weight gain during gestation. The no-effect dose for developmental toxicity in rats exposed during organogenesis was 30 mg/kg, which is approximately 4 times the MRDD on a mg/m^2 basis.

When doses of 5, 10 or 50 mg/kg/day were given to New Zealand White rabbits throughout organogenesis, fetal weights were decreased at 50 mg/kg, which is approximately 12 times the MRDD on a mg/m^2 basis. The incidences of fused sternebrae and vena cava deviations were increased in all treated groups. Maternal toxicity was not produced at any dose. A no-effect dose for developmental toxicity in rabbits exposed during organogenesis was not established, and the 5 mg/kg dose is approximately equal to the MRDD on a mg/m^2 basis.

There are no adequate and well-controlled studies in pregnant women; therefore, eletriptan should be used during pregnancy only if the potential benefit justifies the potential risk to the fetus.

NURSING MOTHERS

Eletriptan is excreted in human breast milk. In one study of 8 women given a single dose of 80 mg, the mean total amount of eletriptan in breast milk over 24 hours in this group was approximately 0.02% of the administered dose. The ratio of eletriptan mean concentration in breast milk to plasma was 1:4, but there was great variability. The resulting eletriptan concentration-time profile was similar to that seen in the plasma over 24 hours, with very low concentrations of drug (mean 1.7 ng/ml) still present in the milk 18-24 hours post dose. The N-desmethyl active metabolite was not measured in the breast milk. Caution should be exercised when eletriptan hydrobromide is administered to nursing women.

PEDIATRIC USE

Safety and effectiveness of eletriptan hydrobromide tablets in pediatric patients have not been established; therefore, eletriptan hydrobromide is not recommended for use in patients under 18 years of age.

The efficacy of eletriptan hydrobromide tablets (40 mg) in patients 11-17 was not established in a randomized, placebo-controlled trial of 274 adolescent migraineurs. Adverse events observed were similar in nature to those reported in clinical trials in adults. Postmarketing experience with other triptans includes a limited number of reports that describe pediatric patients who have experienced clinically serious adverse events that are similar in nature to those reported rarely in adults. Long-term safety of eletriptan was studied in 76 adolescent patients who received treatment for up to 1 year. A similar profile of adverse events to that of adults was observed. The long-term safety of eletriptan in pediatric patients has not been established.

GERIATRIC USE

Eletriptan has been given to only 50 patients over the age of 65. Blood pressure was increased to a greater extent in elderly subjects than in young subjects. The pharmacokinetic disposition of eletriptan in the elderly is similar to that seen in younger adults (see CLINICAL PHARMACOLOGY). In clinical trials, there were no apparent differences in efficacy or the incidence of adverse events between patients under 65 years of age and those 65 and above (n=50).

There is a statistically significantly increased half-life (from about 4.4-5.7 hours) between elderly (65-93 years of age) and younger adult subjects (18-45 years of age) (see CLINICAL PHARMACOLOGY).

DRUG INTERACTIONS

ERGOT-CONTAINING DRUGS

Ergot-containing drugs have been reported to cause prolonged vasospastic reactions. Because these effects may be additive, use of ergotamine-containing or ergot-type medications (like dihydroergotamine [DHE] or methysergide) and eletriptan within 24 hours of each other is not recommended (see CONTRAINDICATIONS).

CYP3A4 INHIBITORS

Eletriptan is metabolized primarily by CYP3A4 (see WARNINGS regarding use with potent CYP3A4 inhibitors).

MONOAMINE OXIDASE INHIBITORS

Eletriptan is not a substrate for monoamine oxidase (MAO) enzymes, therefore there is no expectation of an interaction between eletriptan and MAO inhibitors.

PROPRANOLOL

The C_{max} and AUC of eletriptan were increased by 10 and 33% respectively in the presence of propranolol. No interactive increases in blood pressure were observed. No dosage adjustment appears to be needed for patients taking propranolol (see CLINICAL PHARMACOLOGY).

OTHER 5-HT$_1$ AGONISTS

Concomitant use of other 5-HT$_1$ agonists within 24 hours of eletriptan hydrobromide treatment is not recommended (see CONTRAINDICATIONS).

ADVERSE REACTIONS

Serious cardiac events, including some that have been fatal, have occurred following the use of 5-HT$_1$ agonists. These events are extremely rare and most have been reported in patients with risk factors predictive of CAD. Events reported have included coronary artery vasospasm, transient myocardial ischemia, myocardial infarction, ventricular tachycardia, and ventricular fibrillation (see CONTRAINDICATIONS, WARNINGS and PRECAUTIONS).

INCIDENCE IN CONTROLLED CLINICAL TRIALS

Among 4597 patients who treated the first migraine headache with eletriptan hydrobromide in short-term placebo-controlled trials, the most common adverse events reported with treatment with eletriptan hydrobromide were asthenia, nausea, dizziness, and somnolence. These events appear to be dose related.

In long-term open-label studies where patients were allowed to treat multiple migraine attacks for up to 1 year, 128 (8.3%) out of 1544 patients discontinued treatment due to adverse events.

TABLE 2 lists adverse events that occurred in the subset of 5125 migraineurs who received eletriptan doses of 20, 40 and 80 mg or placebo in worldwide placebo-controlled clinical trials. The events cited reflect experience gained under closely monitored conditions of clinical trials in a highly selected patient population. In actual clinical practice or in other clinical trials, those frequency estimates may not apply, as the conditions of use, reporting behavior, and the kinds of patients treated may differ.

Only adverse events that were more frequent in an eletriptan hydrobromide treatment group compared to the placebo group with an incidence greater than or equal to 2% are included in TABLE 2.

TABLE 2 *Adverse Experience Incidence in Placebo-Controlled Migraine Clinical Trials: Events Reported by ≥2% Patients Treated With Eletriptan Hydrobromide and More Than Placebo*

		Eletriptan Hydrobromide		
	Placebo	20 mg	40 mg	80 mg
Adverse Event Type	(n=988)	(n=431)	(n=1774)	(n=1932)
Atypical Sensations				
Paresthesia	2%	3%	3%	4%
Flushing/feeling of warmth	2%	2%	2%	2%
Pain and Pressure Sensations				
Chest — tightness/pain/pressure	1%	1%	2%	4%
Abdominal — pain/discomfort/ stomach pain/ cramps/pressure	1%	1%	2%	2%
Digestive				
Dry mouth	2%	2%	3%	4%
Dyspepsia	1%	1%	2%	2%
Dysphagia — throat tightness/ difficulty swallowing	0.2%	1%	2%	2%
Nausea	5%	4%	5%	8%
Neurological				
Dizziness	3%	3%	6%	7%
Somnolence	4%	3%	6%	7%
Headache	3%	4%	3%	4%
Other				
Asthenia	3%	4%	5%	10%

Eletriptan hydrobromide is generally well-tolerated. Across all doses, most adverse reactions were mild and transient. The frequency of adverse events in clinical trials did not increase when up to 2 doses of eletriptan hydrobromide were taken within 24 hours. The incidence of adverse events in controlled clinical trials was not affected by gender, age, or race of the patients. Adverse event frequencies were also unchanged by concomitant use of drugs commonly taken for migraine prophylaxis (*e.g.,* SSRIs, beta blockers, calcium channel blockers, tricyclic antidepressants), estrogen replacement therapy and oral contraceptives.

OTHER EVENTS OBSERVED IN ASSOCIATION WITH THE ADMINISTRATION OF ELETRIPTAN HYDROBROMIDE TABLETS

In the paragraphs that follow, the frequencies of less commonly reported adverse clinical events are presented. Because the reports include events observed in open studies, the role of eletriptan hydrobromide tablets in their causation cannot be reliably determined. Furthermore, variability associated with adverse event reporting, the terminology used to describe adverse events, etc., limit the value of the quantitative frequency estimates provided. Event frequencies are calculated as the number of patients reporting an event divided by the total number of patients (n=4719) exposed to eletriptan hydrobromide. All reported events are included except those already listed in TABLE 2, those too general to be informative, and those not reasonably associated with the use of the drug. Events are further classified within body system categories and enumerated in order of decreasing frequency using the following definitions: *Frequent:* Those occurring in at least 1/100 patients; *Infrequent:* Those occurring in 1/100 to 1/1000 patients; and *Rare:* Those occurring in fewer than 1/1000 patients.

General: *Frequent:* Back pain, chills and pain. *Infrequent:* Face edema and malaise. *Rare:* Abdomen enlarged, abscess, accidental injury, allergic reaction, fever, flu syndrome, halitosis, hernia, hypothermia, lab test abnormal, moniliasis, rheumatoid arthritis and shock.

Cardiovascular: *Frequent:* Palpitation. *Infrequent:* Hypertension, migraine, peripheral vascular disorder and tachycardia. *Rare:* Angina pectoris, arrhythmia, atrial fibrillation, AV block, bradycardia, hypotension, syncope, thrombophlebitis, cerebrovascular disorder, vasospasm and ventricular arrhythmia.

Digestive: *Infrequent:* Anorexia, constipation, diarrhea, eructation, esophagitis, flatulence, gastritis, gastrointestinal disorder, glossitis, increased salivation and liver function tests abnormal. *Rare:* Gingivitis, hematemesis, increased appetite, rectal disorder, stomatitis, tongue disorder, tongue edema and tooth disorder.

Endocrine: *Rare:* Goiter, thyroid adenoma and thyroiditis.

Hemic and Lymphatic: *Rare:* Anemia, cyanosis, leukopenia, lymphadenopathy, monocytosis and purpura.

Metabolic: *Infrequent:* Creatine phosphokinase increased, edema, peripheral edema and thirst. *Rare:* Alkaline phosphatase increased, bilirubinemia, hyperglycemia, weight gain and weight loss.

Musculoskeletal: *Infrequent:* Arthralgia, arthritis, arthrosis, bone pain, myalgia and myasthenia. *Rare:* Bone neoplasm, joint disorder, myopathy and tenosynovitis.

Neurological: *Frequent:* Hypertonia, hypesthesia and vertigo. *Infrequent:* Abnormal dreams, agitation, anxiety, apathy, ataxia, confusion, depersonalization, depression, emotional lability, euphoria, hyperesthesia, hyperkinesia, incoordination, insomnia, nervousness, speech disorder, stupor, thinking abnormal and tremor. *Rare:* Abnormal gait, amnesia, aphasia, catatonic reaction, dementia, diplopia, dystonia, hallucinations, hemiplegia, hyperalgesia, hypokinesia, hysteria, manic reaction, neuropathy, neurosis, oculogyric crisis, paralysis, psychotic depression, sleep disorder and twitching.

Respiratory: *Frequent:* Pharyngitis. *Infrequent:* Asthma, dyspnea, respiratory disorder, respiratory tract infection, rhinitis, voice alteration and yawn. *Rare:* Bronchitis, choking sensation, cough increased, epistaxis, hiccup, hyperventilation, laryngitis, sinusitis and sputum increased.

Skin and Appendages: *Frequent:* Sweating. *Infrequent:* Pruritus, rash and skin disorder. *Rare:* Alopecia, dry skin, eczema, exfoliative dermatitis, maculopapular rash, psoriasis, skin discoloration, skin hypertrophy and urticaria.

Special Senses: *Infrequent:* Abnormal vision, conjunctivitis, ear pain, eye pain, lacrimation disorder, photophobia, taste perversion and tinnitus. *Rare:* Abnormality of accommodation, dry eyes, ear disorder, eye hemorrhage, otitis media, parosmia and ptosis.

Urogenital: *Infrequent:* Impotence, polyuria, urinary frequency and urinary tract disorder. *Rare:* Breast pain, kidney pain, leukorrhea, menorrhagia, menstrual disorder and vaginitis.

DOSAGE AND ADMINISTRATION

In controlled clinical trials, single doses of 20 and 40 mg were effective for the acute treatment of migraine in adults. A greater proportion of patients had a response following a 40 mg dose than following a 20 mg dose. Individuals may vary in response to doses of eletriptan hydrobromide tablets. The choice of dose should therefore be made on an individual basis. An 80 mg dose, although also effective, was associated with an increased incidence of adverse events. Therefore, the maximum recommended single dose is 40 mg.

If after the initial dose, headache improves but then returns, a repeat dose may be beneficial. If a second dose is required, it should be taken at least 2 hours after the initial dose. If the initial dose is ineffective, controlled clinical trials have not shown a benefit of a second dose to treat the same attack. The maximum daily dose should not exceed 80 mg.

The safety of treating an average of more than 3 headaches in a 30 day period has not been established.

CYP3A4 INHIBITORS

Eletriptan is metabolized by the CYP3A4 enzyme. Eletriptan should not be used within at least 72 hours of treatment with the following potent CYP3A4 inhibitors: ketoconazole, itraconazole, nefazodone, troleandomycin, clarithromycin, ritonavir and nelfinavir. Eletriptan should not be used within 72 hours with drugs that have demonstrated potent CYP3A4 inhibition and have this potent effect described in the CONTRAINDICATIONS, WARNINGS, or PRECAUTIONS sections of their labeling (see WARNINGS and CLINICAL PHARMACOLOGY, Drug Interactions).

HEPATIC IMPAIRMENT

The drug should not be given to patients with severe hepatic impairment since the effect of severe hepatic impairment on eletriptan metabolism was not evaluated. No dose adjustment is necessary in mild to moderate impairment (see CLINICAL PHARMACOLOGY, CONTRAINDICATIONS and PRECAUTIONS).

HOW SUPPLIED

Relpax tablets of 20 and 40 mg eletriptan (base) as the hydrobromide are available as follows:

20 mg: Orange, round, convex shaped, film-coated tablets identified with "REP20" on one side and "Pfizer" on the reverse.

40 mg: Orange, round, convex shaped, film-coated tablets identified with "REP40" on one side and "Pfizer" on the reverse.

Storage: Store at 25°C (77°F); excursions permitted to 15-30°C (59-86°F).

PRODUCT LISTING - EQUIVALENTS NOT AVAILABLE

Tablet - Oral - 20 mg

6 x 2 $189.60 RELPAX, Pfizer U.S. Pharmaceuticals 00049-2330-34

Tablet - Oral - 40 mg

6 x 2 $189.60 RELPAX, Pfizer U.S. Pharmaceuticals 00049-2340-34

Emedastine Difumarate (003394)

Categories: Conjunctivitis, allergic; Pregnancy Category B; FDA Approved 1997 Dec
Drug Classes: Antihistamines, H1; Antihistamines, ophthalmic; Ophthalmics
Brand Names: Emadine
Foreign Brand Availability: Daren (Japan); Remicut (Japan)
Cost of Therapy: $53.13 (Allergic Conjunctivitis; Emadine Ophthalmic Solution; 0.05%; 5 ml; 4 drops/day; variable day supply)

DESCRIPTION

Emedastine difumarate ophthalmic solution 0.05% is a sterile ophthalmic solution containing emedastine, a relatively selective, H_1-receptor antagonist for topical administration to the eyes. Emedastine difumarate is a white, crystalline, water-soluble fine powder with a molecular weight of 534.57.

The chemical name for emedastine difumarate is 1H-Benzlmidazole, 1-(2-ethoxyethyl)-2-(hexahydro-4-methyl-1H-1,4-diazepin-1-yl), (E)-2-butenadioate (1:2).

Each ml of emadine contains: *Active:* 0.884 mg emedastine difumarate equivalent to 0.5 mg emedastine. *Preservative:* Benzalkonium chloride 0.01%. *Inactives:* Tromethamine; sodium chloride; hydroxypropyl methylcellulose; hydrochloric acid/sodium hydroxide (adjust pH); and purified water. It has a pH of approximately 7.4 and an osmolality of approximately 300 mOam/kg.

Storage: Store at 4-30°C (39-86°F)

CLINICAL PHARMACOLOGY

Emedastine is a relatively selective, histamine H_1 antagonist. *In vitro* examinations of emedastine's affinity for histamine receptors (H_1:Kl=1.3 nM, H_2: Kl=49,067 nM, and H_3: Kl=12,430 nM) demonstrate relative selectivity for the H_1 histamine receptor. *In vivo* studies have shown concentration-dependent inhibition of histamine-stimulated vascular permeability in the conjunctiva following topical ocular administration. Emedastine appears to be devoid of affects on adrenergic, dopaminergic and serotonin receptors.

Following topical administration in man, emedastine was shown to have low systemic exposure. In a study involving 10 normal volunteers dosed bilaterally twice daily for 16 days with emedastine ophthalmic solution 0.05%, plasma concentrations of the parent compound were generally below the quantitation limit of the assay (<0.3 ng/ml). Samples in which emedastine was quantifiable ranged from 0.30-0.49 ng/ml. The elimination half-life of oral emedastine in plasma is 3-4 hours. Approximately 44% of the oral dose is recovered in the urine over 24 hours with only 3.6% of the dose excreted as parent drug. Two primary metabolites, 5- and 6-hydroxyemedastine, are excreted in the urine as both free and conjugated forms. The 5'-oxoanaloges of 5- and 6-hydroxyemedastine and the N-oxide are also formed as minor metabolites.

In an environmental study, patients with allergic conjunctivitis were treated with emedastine difumarate for six weeks. The results demonstrated that emedastine difumarate provides relief of the signs and symptoms of allergic conjunctivitis.

In conjunctival antigen challenge studies, in which subjects were challenged with antigen both initially and up to four hours after dosing, emedastine difumarate was demonstrated to be significantly more effective than placebo in preventing ocular itching associated with allergic conjunctivitis.

INDICATIONS AND USAGE

Emedastine difumarate ophthalmic solution 0.05% is indicated for the temporary relief of the signs and symptoms of allergic conjunctivitis.

CONTRAINDICATIONS

Emedastine difumarate ophthalmic solution is contraindicated in persons with a known hypersensitivity to emedastine difumarate or any of the solution's components.

WARNINGS

Emedastine difumarate ophthalmic solution is for topical use only and not for injection or oral use.

PRECAUTIONS

INFORMATION FOR THE PATIENT

To prevent contaminating the dropper tip and solution, care should be taken not to touch the eyelids or surrounding areas with the dropper tip of the bottle. Keep the bottle tightly closed when not in use. Do not use if the solution has become discolored.

Patients should be advised not to wear a contact lens if their eye is red. Emedastine difumarate ophthalmic solution should not be used to treat contact lens related irritation. The preservative in emedastine difumarate ophthalmic solution, benzalkonium chloride, may be absorbed by soft contact lenses. Patients who wear soft contact lenses and whose eyes are not red, should be instructed to wait at least ten minutes after instilling emedastine difumarate ophthalmic solution before they insert their contact lenses.

CARCINOGENESIS, MUTAGENESIS, AND IMPAIRMENT OF FERTILITY

Emedastine difumarate demonstrated no carcinogenicity effects in lifetime studies in mice and rats at dietary doses more than 80,000 times and more than 26,000 times the maximum recommended ocular human use level of 0.002 mg/kg/day for a 50 kg adult, respectively. Higher dose levels were not tested. Emedastine difumarate was determined to be nonmutagenic in an *in vitro* bacterial reverse mutation (Ames) test, an *in vitro* modification of the Ames test, an *in vitro* mammalian chromosome aberration test, an *in vitro* mammalian forward mutation test, an *in vitro* mammalian DNA repair synthesis test, an *in vivo* mammalian sister chromatid exchange test and an *in vivo* mouse micronucleus test. There was no evidence of impaired fertility or reproductive capacity in rats at 15,000 times the maximum recommended ocular human use level.

PREGNANCY CATEGORY B

Teratology and peri- and post-natal studies have been conducted with emedastine difumarate in rats and rabbits. At 15,000 times the maximum recommended ocular human use level, emedastine difumarate was shown not to be teratogenic in rats and rabbits and no effects on peri/post-natal development were observed in rats. However, at 70,000 times the maximum recommended ocular human use level, emedastine difumarate was shown to increase the incidence of external, visceral and skeletal anomalies in rats. There are, however, no adequate and well controlled studies in pregnant women. Because animal studies are not always predictive of human response, this drug should be used during pregnancy only if clearly needed.

NURSING MOTHERS

Emedastine has been identified in breast milk in rats following oral administration. It is not known whether topical ocular administration could result in sufficient systemic absorption to produce detectable quantities in breast milk. Nevertheless, caution should be exercised when emedastine difumarate ophthalmic solution is administered to a nursing mother.

PEDIATRIC USE

Safety and effectiveness in pediatric patients below the age of 3 years have not been established.

ADVERSE REACTIONS

In controlled clinical studies of emedastine difumarate ophthalmic solution lasting for 42 days, the most frequent adverse reaction was headache 11%. The following adverse experiences were reported in less than 5% of patients: Abnormal dreams, asthenia, bad taste, blurred vision, burning or stinging, corneal infiltrates, corneal staining, dermatitis, discomfort, dry eye, foreign body sensation, hyperemia, keratitis, pruritus, rhinitis, sinusitis and tearing. Some of these events were similar to the underlying disease being studied.

DOSAGE AND ADMINISTRATION

The recommended dose is one drop in the affected eye up to four times daily.

PRODUCT LISTING - EQUIVALENTS NOT AVAILABLE

Solution - Ophthalmic - 0.05%
5 ml $53.13 EMADINE, Alcon Laboratories Inc 00065-0325-05

Emtricitabine (003604)

Categories: Infection, human immunodeficiency virus; Pregnancy Category B; FDA Approved 2003 Jul
Drug Classes: Antivirals; Nucleoside reverse transcriptase inhibitors
Brand Names: Emtriva

WARNING

LACTIC ACIDOSIS AND SEVERE HEPATOMEGALY WITH STEATOSIS, INCLUDING FATAL CASES, HAVE BEEN REPORTED WITH THE USE OF NUCLEOSIDE ANALOGUES ALONE OR IN COMBINATION WITH OTHER ANTIRETROVIRALS (SEE WARNINGS).

DESCRIPTION

Emtriva is the brand name of emtricitabine, a synthetic nucleoside analogue with activity against human immunodeficiency virus type 1 (HIV-1) reverse transcriptase.

The chemical name of emtricitabine is 5-fluoro-1-(2*R*,5*S*)-[2-(hydroxymethyl)-1,3-oxathiolan-5-yl]cytosine. Emtricitabine is the (-) nantiomer of a thio analogue of cytidine, which differs from other cytidine analogues in that it has a fluorine in the 5-position.

It has a molecular formula of $C_8H_{10}FN_3O_3S$ and a molecular weight of 247.24.

Emtricitabine is a white to off-white powder with a solubility of approximately 112 mg/ml in water at 25°C. The log P for emtricitabine is -0.43 and the pKa is 2.65.

Emtriva capsules are for oral administration. Each capsule contains 200 mg of emtricitabine and the inactive ingredients, crospovidone, magnesium stearate, microcrystalline cellulose and povidone.

CLINICAL PHARMACOLOGY

MICROBIOLOGY

Mechanism of Action

Emtricitabine, a synthetic nucleoside analog of cytosine. is phosphorylated by cellular enzymes to form emtricitabine 5'-triphosphate. Emtricitabine 5'-triphosphate inhibits the activity of the HIV-1 reverse transcriptase by competing with the natural substrate deoxycytidine 5'-triphosphate and by being incorporated into nascent viral DNA which results in chain termination. Emtricitabine 5'-triphosphate is a weak inhibitor of mammalian DNA polymerase α, β, ϵ and mitochondrial DNA polymerase γ.

Antiviral Activity In Vitro

The *in vitro* antiviral activity of emtricitabine against laboratory and clinical isolates of HIV was assessed in lymphoblastoid cell lines, the MAGI-CCR5 cell line, and peripheral blood mononuclear cells. The 50% inhibitory concentration (IC_{50}) value for emtricitabine was in the range of 0.0013-0.64 μM (0.0003-0.158 μg/ml). In drug combination studies of emtricitabine with nucleoside reverse transcriptase inhibitors (abacavir, lamivudine, stavudine, tenofovir, zalcitabine, zidovudine), non-nucleoside reverse transcriptase inhibitors (delavirdine, efavirenz, nevirapine), and protease inhibitors (amprenavir, nelfinavir, ritonavir, saquinavir), additive to synergistic effects were observed. Most of the drug combinations have not been studied in humans. Emtricitabine displayed antiviral activity *in vitro* against HIV-1 clades A, C, D, E, F, and G (IC_{50} values ranged from 0.007-0.075 μM) and showed strain specific activity against HIV-2 (IC_{50} values ranged from 0.007-1.5 μM).

Drug Resistance
Emtricitabine-resistant isolates of HIV have been selected *in vitro.* Genotypic analysis of these isolates showed that the reduced susceptibility to emtricitabine was associated with a mutation in the HIV reverse transcriptase gene at codon 184 which resulted in an amino acid substitution of methionine by valine or isoleucine (M184V/I).

Emtricitabine-resistant isolates of HIV have been recovered from some patients treated with emtricitabine alone or in combination with other antiretroviral agents. In a clinical study, viral isolates from 37.5% of treatment-naive patients with virologic failure showed reduced susceptibility to emtricitabine. Genotypic analysis of these isolates showed that the resistance was due to M184V/I mutations in the HIV reverse transcriptase gene.

Cross Resistance
Cross-resistance among certain nucleoside analogue reverse transcriptase inhibitors has been recognized. Emtricitabine-resistant isolates (M184V/I) were cross-resistant to lamivudine and zalcitabine but retained sensitivity to abacavir, didanosine, stavudine, tenofovir, zidovudine, and NNRTIs (delavirdine, efavirenz, and nevirapine). HIV-1 isolates containing the K65R mutation, selected *in vivo* by abacavir, didanosine, tenofovir, and zalcitabine, demonstrated reduced susceptibility to inhibition by emtricitabine. Viruses harboring mutations conferring reduced susceptibility to stavudine and zidovudine (M41 L, D67N, K70R, L210W, T215Y/F, K219Q/E) or didanosine (L74V) remained sensitive to emtricitabine. HIV-1 containing the K103N mutation associated with resistance to NNRTIs was susceptible to emtricitabine.

PHARMACODYNAMICS
The *in vivo* activity of emtricitabine was evaluated in two clinical trials in which 101 patients were administered 25-400 mg/day of emtricitabine as monotherapy for 10-14 days. A dose-related antiviral effect was observed, with a median decrease from baseline in plasma HIV-1 RNA of 1.3 $\log_{10}$ at a dose of 25 mg qd and 1.7 $\log_{10}$ to 1.9 $\log_{10}$ at a dose of 200 mg qd or bid.

PHARMACOKINETICS
The pharmacokinetics of emtricitabine were evaluated in healthy volunteers and HIV-infected individuals. Emtricitabine pharmacokinetics are similar between these populations.

Absorption
Emtricitabine is rapidly and extensively absorbed following oral administration with peak plasma concentrations occurring at 1-2 hours post-dose. Following multiple dose oral administration of emtricitabine to 20 HIV-infected subjects, the (mean ± SD) steady-state plasma emtricitabine peak concentration (C_{max}) was 1.8 ± 0.7 μg/ml and the area under the plasma concentration-time curve over a 24 hour dosing interval (AUC) was 10.0 ± 3.1 h·μg/ml. The mean steady state plasma trough concentration at 24 hours post-dose was 0.09 μg/ml. The mean absolute bioavailability of emtricitabine was 93%.

The multiple dose pharmacokinetics of emtricitabine are dose proportional over a dose range of 25-200 mg.

Effects of Food on Oral Absorption
Emtricitabine may be taken with or without food. Emtricitabine systemic exposure (AUC) was unaffected while C_{max} decreased by 29% when emtricitabine was administered with food (an approximately 1000 kcal high-fat meal).

Distribution
In vitro binding of emtricitabine to human plasma proteins was <4% and independent of concentration over the range of 0.02-200 μg/ml. At peak plasma concentration, the mean plasma to blood drug concentration ratio was ~1.0 and the mean semen to plasma drug concentration ratio was ~4.0.

Metabolism
In vitro studies indicate that emtricitabine is not an inhibitor of human CYP450 enzymes. Following administration of ^{14}C-emtricitabine, complete recovery of the dose was achieved in urine (~86%) and feces (~14%). Thirteen percent (13%) of the dose was recovered in urine as three putative metabolites. The biotransformation of emtricitabine includes oxidation of the thiol moiety to form the 3′-sulfoxide diastereomers (~9% of dose) and conjugation with glucuronic acid to form 2′-O-glucuronide (~4% of dose). No other metabolites were identifiable.

Elimination
The plasma emtricitabine half-life is approximately 10 hours. The renal clearance of emtricitabine is greater than the estimated creatinine clearance, suggesting elimination by both glomerular filtration and active tubular secretion. There may be competition for elimination with other compounds that are also renally eliminated.

Special Populations
The pharmacokinetics of emtricitabine were similar in male and female patients and no pharmacokinetic differences due to race have been identified.

The pharmacokinetics of emtricitabine have not been fully evaluated in children or in the elderly.

The pharmacokinetics of emtricitabine have not been studied in patients with hepatic impairment, however, emtricitabine is not metabolized by liver enzymes, so the impact of liver impairment should be limited.

The pharmacokinetics of emtricitabine are altered in patients with renal impairment (see PRECAUTIONS). In patients with creatinine clearance <50 ml/min or with end-stage renal disease (ESRD) requiring dialysis, C_{max} and AUC of emtricitabine were increased due to a reduction in renal clearance (TABLE 1). It is recommended that the dosing interval for emtricitabine be modified in patients with creatinine clearance <50 ml/min or in patients with ESRD who require dialysis (see DOSAGE AND ADMINISTRATION).

TABLE 1 *Mean ± SD Pharmacokinetic Parameters in Patients With Varying Degrees of Renal Function*

	Creatine Clearance (ml/min)				
	>80 (n=6)	50-80 (n=6)	30-49 (n=6)	<30 (n=5)	ESRD*<30 (n=5)
Baseline creatine clearance (ml/min)	107 ± 21	59.8 ± 6.5	40.9 ± 5.1	22.9 ± 5.3	8.8 ± 1.4
C_{max} (μg/ml)	2.2 ± 0.6	3.8 ± 0.9	3.2 ± 0.6	2.8 ± 0.7	2.8 ± 0.5
AUC (h·μg/ml)	11.8 ± 2.9	19.9 ± 1.1	25.0 ± 5.7	34.0 ± 2.1	53.2 ± 9.9
CL/F (ml/min)	302 ± 94	168 ± 10	138 ± 28	99 ± 6	64 ± 12
CLR (ml/min)	213.3 ± 89.0	121.4 ± 39.0	68.6 ± 32.1	29.5 ± 11.4	—

* ESRD patients requiring dialysis.
— = Not applicable.

Hemodialysis
Hemodialysis treatment removes approximately 30% of the emtricitabine dose over a 3 hour dialysis period starting within 1.5 hours of emtricitabine dosing (blood flow rate of 400 ml/min and a dialysate flow rate of 600 ml/min). It is not known whether emtricitabine can be removed by peritoneal dialysis.

Drug Interactions
At concentrations up to 14-fold higher than those observed *in vivo,* emtricitabine did not inhibit *in vitro* drug metabolism mediated by any of the following human CYP450 isoforms: CYP1A2, CYP2A6, CYP2B6, CYP2C9, CYP2C19, CYP2D6 and CYP3A4. Emtricitabine did not inhibit the enzyme responsible for glucuronidation (uridine-5′-disphosphoglucuronyl transferase). Based on the results of these *in vitro* experiments and the known elimination pathways of emtricitabine, the potential for CYP450 mediated interactions involving emtricitabine with other medicinal products is low.

Emtricitabine has been evaluated in healthy volunteers in combination with tenofovir disoproxil fumarate (DF), indinavir, famciclovir, and stavudine. TABLE 2 and TABLE 3 summarize the pharmacokinetic effects of coadministered drug on emtricitabine pharmacokinetics and effects of emtricitabine on the pharmacokinetics of coadministered drug.

TABLE 2 *Drug Interactions: Change in Pharmacokinetic Parameters for Emtricitabine in the Presence of the Coadministered Drug**

Coadministered Drug			% Change of Emtricitabine Pharmacokinetic Parameters† (90% CI)		
Dose of Coadministed Drug	Emtricitabine Dose	n	C_{max}	AUC	C_{min}
Tenofovir DF					
300 mg once daily × 7 days	200 mg once daily × 7 days	17	NE	NE	inc 20 (inc 12 to inc 29)
Indinavir					
800 mg × 1	200 mg × 1	12	NE	NE	NA
Famciclovir					
500 mg × 1	200 mg × 1	12	NE	NE	NA
Stavudine					
40 mg × 1	200 × 1	6	NE	NE	NA

* All interaction studies conducted in healthy volunteers.
† inc = increase; dec = decrease; NE = no effect; NA = not applicable.

TABLE 3 *Drug Interactions: Change in Pharmacokinetic Parameters for Coadministered Drug in the Presence of Emtricitabine**

Coadministered Drug			% Change of Coadministered Drug Pharmacokinetic Parameters† (90% CI)		
Dose of Coadministed Drug	Emtricitabine Dose	n	C_{max}	AUC	C_{min}
Tenofovir					
300 mg once daily × 7 days	200 mg once daily × 7 days	17	NE	NE	NE
Indinavir					
800 mg × 1	200 mg × 1	12	NE	NE	NA
Famciclovir					
500 mg × 1	200 mg × 1	12	NE	NE	NA
Stavudine					
40 mg × 1	200 × 1	6	NE	NE	NA

* All interaction studies conducted in healthy volunteers.
† inc = increase; dec = decrease; NE = no effect; NA = not applicable.

INDICATIONS AND USAGE

Emtricitabine is indicated, in combination with other antiretroviral agents, for the treatment of HIV-1 infection in adults.

This indication is based on analyses of plasma HIV-1 RNA levels and CD4 cell counts from controlled studies of 48 weeks duration in antiretroviral-naive patients and antiretroviral-treatment-experienced patients who were virologically suppressed on an HIV treatment regimen.

In antiretroviral-treatment-experienced patients, the use of emtricitabine may be considered for adults with HIV strains that are expected to be susceptible to emtricitabine as assessed by genotypic or phenotypic testing. (See CLINICAL PHARMACOLOGY, Microbiology: Drug Resistance and Cross Resistance.)

CONTRAINDICATIONS

Emtricitabine is contraindicated in patients with previously demonstrated hypersensitivity to any of the components of the products.

WARNINGS

LACTIC ACIDOSIS/SEVERE HEPATOMEGALY WITH STEATOSIS

Lactic acidosis and severe hepatomegaly with steatosis, including fatal cases, have been reported with the use of nucleoside, analogues alone or in combination, including emtricitabine and other antiretrovirals. A majority of these cases have been in women. Obesity and prolonged nucleoside exposure may be risk factors. However, cases have also been reported in patients with no known risk factors. Treatment with emtricitabine should be suspended in any patient who develops clinical or laboratory findings suggestive of lactic acidosis or pronounced hepatotoxicity (which may include hepatomegaly and steatosis even in the absence of marked transaminase elevations).

POST TREATMENT EXACERBATION OF HEPATITIS

It is recommended that all patients with HIV be tested for the presence of chronic hepatitis B virus (HBV) before initiating antiretroviral therapy. Emtricitabine is not indicated for the treatment of chronic HBV infection and the safety and efficacy of emtricitabine have not been established in patients co-infected with HBV and HIV. Exacerbations of hepatitis B have been reported in patients after the discontinuation of emtricitabine. Patients co-infected with HIV and HBV should be closely monitored with both clinical and laboratory follow-up for at least several months after stopping treatment.

PRECAUTIONS

PATIENTS WITH IMPAIRED RENAL FUNCTION

Emtricitabine is principally eliminated by the kidney. Reduction of the dosage of emtricitabine is recommended for patients with impaired renal function (see CLINICAL PHARMACOLOGY and DOSAGE AND ADMINISTRATION).

FAT REDISTRIBUTION

Redistribution/accumulation of body fat including central obesity, dorsocervical fat enlargement (buffalo hump), peripheral wasting, facial wasting, breast enlargement, and "cushingoid appearance" have been observed in patients receiving antiretroviral therapy. The mechanism and long-term consequences of these events are unknown. A causal relationship has not been established.

INFORMATION FOR THE PATIENT

Emtricitabine is not a cure for HIV infection and patients may continue to experience illnesses associated with HIV infection, including opportunistic infections. Patients should remain under the care of a physician when using emtricitabine.

Patients should be advised that:

- The use of emtricitabine has not been shown to reduce the risk of transmission of HIV to others through sexual contact or blood contamination.
- The long-term effects of emtricitabine are unknown.
- Emtricitabine capsules are for oral ingestion only.
- It is important to take emtricitabine with combination therapy on a regular dosing schedule to avoid missing doses.
- Redistribution or accumulation of body fat may occur in patients receiving antiretroviral therapy and that the cause and long-term health effects of these conditions are not known.

CARCINOGENESIS, MUTAGENESIS, AND IMPAIRMENT OF FERTILITY

Carcinogenesis

Long-term carcinogenicity studies of emtricitabine in rats and mice are in progress.

Mutagenesis

Emtricitabine was not genotoxic in the reverse mutation bacterial test (Ames test), mouse lymphoma or mouse micronucleus assays.

Impairment of Fertility

Emtricitabine did not affect fertility in male rats at approximately 140-fold or in male and female mice at approximately 60-fold higher exposures (AUC) than in humans given the recommended 200 mg daily dose. Fertility was normal in the offspring of mice exposed daily from before birth *(in utero)* through sexual maturity at daily exposures (AUC) of approximately 60-fold higher than human exposures at the recommended 200 mg daily dose.

PREGNANCY CATEGORY B

The incidence of fetal variations and malformations was not increased in embryofetal toxicity studies performed with emtricitabine in mice at exposures (AUC) approximately 60-fold higher and in rabbits at approximately 120-fold higher than human exposures at the recommended daily dose. There are, however, no adequate and well-controlled studies in pregnant women. Because animal reproduction studies are not always predictive of human response, emtricitabine should be used during pregnancy only if clearly needed.

Antiretroviral Pregnancy Registry: To monitor fetal outcomes of pregnant women exposed to emtricitabine, an antiretroviral Pregnancy Registry has been established. Healthcare providers are encouraged to register patients by calling 1-800-258-4263.

NURSING MOTHERS

The Centers for Disease Control and Prevention recommend that HIV-infected mothers not breast-feed their infants to avoid risking postnatal transmission of HIV. It is not known whether emtricitabine is secreted into human milk. Because of both the potential for HIV transmission and the potential for serious adverse reactions in nursing infants, **mothers should be instructed not to breast-feed if they are receiving emtricitabine.**

PEDIATRIC USE

Safety and effectiveness in pediatric patients have not been established.

GERIATRIC USE

Clinical studies of emtricitabine did not contain sufficient numbers of subjects aged 65 years and over to determine whether they respond differently from younger subjects. In general, dose selection for the elderly patient should be cautious, keeping in mind the greater frequency of decreased hepatic, renal, or cardiac function, and of concomitant disease or other drug therapy (see PRECAUTIONS, Patients With Impaired Renal Function and DOSAGE AND ADMINISTRATION).

DRUG INTERACTIONS

The potential for drug interactions with emtricitabine has been studied in combination with indinavir, stavudine, famciclovir, and tenofovir disoproxil fumarate. There were no clinically significant drug interactions for any of these drugs (see CLINICAL PHARMACOLOGY, Pharmacokinetics, Drug Interactions).

ADVERSE REACTIONS

More than 2000 adult patients with HIV infection have been treated with emtricitabine alone or in combination with other antiretroviral agents for periods of 10 days to 200 weeks in Phase 1-111 clinical trials.

Assessment of adverse reactions is based on data from studies 301A and 303 in which 571 treatment naive (301A) and 440 treatment experienced (303) patients received emtricitabine 200 mg (n=580) or comparator drug (n=431) for 48 weeks.

The most common adverse events that occurred in patients receiving emtricitabine with other antiretroviral agents in clinical trials were headache, diarrhea, nausea, and rash, which were generally of mild to moderate severity. Approximately 1% of patients discontinued participation in the clinical studies due to these events. All adverse events were reported with similar frequency in emtricitabine and control treatment groups with the exception of skin discoloration which was reported with higher frequency in the emtricitabine treated group.

Skin discoloration, manifested by hyperpigmentation on the palms and/or soles was generally mild and asymptomatic. The mechanism and clinical significance are unknown.

A summary of emtricitabine treatment emergent clinical adverse events in studies 301A and 303 is provided in TABLE 6A and TABLE 6B.

TABLE 6A *Selected Treatment-Emergent Adverse Events (All Grades, Regardless of Causality) Reported in ≥3% of Emtricitabine-Treated Patients in Study 303 (0-48 Weeks)*

Adverse Event	Emtricitabine + ZDV/d4T + NNRTI/PI (n=294)	Lamivudine + ZDV/d4T + NNRTI/PI (n=146)
Body as a Whole		
Abdominal pain	8%	11%
Asthenia	16%	10%
Headache	13%	6%
Digestive System		
Diarrhea	23%	18%
Dyspepsia	4%	5%
Nausea	18%	12%
Vomiting	9%	7%
Musculoskeletal		
Arthralgia	3%	4%
Myalgia	4%	4%
Nervous System		
Abnormal dreams	2%	<1%
Depressive disorders	6%	10%
Dizziness	4%	5%
Insomnia	7%	3%
Neuropathy/peripheral neuritis	4%	3%
Paresthesia	5%	7%
Respiratory		
Increased cough	14%	11%
Rhinitis	18%	12%
Skin		
Rash event*	17%	14%

* Rash event includes rash, pruritus, maculopapular rash, urticaria, vesiculobullous rash, pustular rash, and allergic reaction.

LABORATORY ABNORMALITIES

Laboratory abnormalities in these studies occurred with similar frequency in the emtricitabine and comparator groups. A summary of Grade 3 and 4 laboratory abnormalities is provided in TABLE 7A and TABLE 7B.

DOSAGE AND ADMINISTRATION

For adults 18 years of age and older. the dose of emtricitabine is 200 mg once daily taken orally with or without food.

DOSE ADJUSTMENT IN PATIENTS WITH RENAL IMPAIRMENT

Significantly increased drug exposures were seen when emtricitabine was administered to patients with renal impairment, (see CLINICAL PHARMACOLOGY, Pharmacokinetics, Special Populations). Therefore, the dosing interval of emtricitabine should be adjusted in patients with baseline creatinine clearance <50 ml/min using the guidelines in TABLE 8. The safety and effectiveness of these dosing interval adjustment guidelines have not been clinically evaluated. Therefore, clinical response to treatment and renal function should be closely monitored in these patients.

TABLE 6B *Selected Treatment-Emergent Adverse Events (All Grades, Regardless of Causality) Reported in ≥3% of Emtricitabine-Treated Patients in Study 301A (0-48 Weeks)*

Adverse Event	Emtricitabine + Didanosine + Efavirenz (n=286)	Stavudine + Didanosine + Efavirenz (n=285)
Body as a Whole		
Abdominal pain	14%	17%
Asthenia	12%	17%
Headache	22%	25%
Digestive System		
Diarrhea	23%	32%
Dyspepsia	8%	12%
Nausea	13%	23%
Vomiting	9%	12%
Musculoskeletal		
Arthralgia	5%	6%
Myalgia	6%	3%
Nervous System		
Abnormal dreams	11%	19%
Depressive disorders	9%	13%
Dizziness	25%	26%
Insomnia	16%	21%
Neuropathy/peripheral neuritis	4%	13%
Paresthesia	6%	12%
Respiratory		
Increased cough	14%	8%
Rhinitis	12%	10%
Skin		
Rash event*	30%	33%

* Rash event includes rash, pruritus, maculopapular rash, urticaria, vesiculobullous rash, pustular rash, and allergic reaction.

TABLE 7A *Treatment-Emergent Grade 3/4 Laboratory Abnormalities Reported in ≥1% of Emtricitabine-Treated Patients in Study 303*

	Emtricitabine + ZDV/d4T + NNRTI/PI (n=294)	Lamivudine + ZDV/d4T + NNRTI/PI (n=146)
Percentage with Grade 3 or Grade 4 laboratory abnormality	31%	28%
ALT (>5.0 × ULN*)	2%	1%
AST (>5.0 × ULN)	3%	<1%
Bilirubin (>2.5 × ULN)	1%	2%
Creatine kinase (>4.0 × ULN)	11%	14%
Neutrophils (<750 mm^3)	5%	3%
Pancreatic amylase (>2.0 × ULN)	2%	2%
Serum amylase (>2.0 × ULN)	2%	2%
Serum glucose (<40 or >250 mg/dl)	3%	3%
Serum lipase (>2.0 × ULN)	<1%	<1%
Triglycerides (>750 mg/dl)	10%	8%

* ULN = upper limit of normal.

TABLE 7B *Treatment-Emergent Grade 3/4 Laboratory Abnormalities Reported in ≥1% of Emtricitabine-Treated Patients in Study 301A*

	Emtricitabine + Didanosine + Efavirenz (n=286)	Stavudine + Didanosine + Efavirenz (n=285)
Percentage with Grade 3 or Grade 4 laboratory abnormality	34%	38%
ALT (>5.0 × ULN*)	5%	6%
AST (>5.0 × ULN)	6%	9%
Bilirubin (>2.5 × ULN)	<1%	<1%
Creatine kinase (>4.0 × ULN)	12%	11%
Neutrophils (<750 mm^3)	5%	7%
Pancreatic amylase (>2.0 × ULN)	<1%	1%
Serum amylase (>2.0 × ULN)	5%	10%
Serum glucose (<40 or >250 mg/dl)	2%	3%
Serum lipase (>2.0 × ULN)	1%	2%
Triglycerides (>750 mg/dl)	9%	6%

* ULN = upper limit of normal.

TABLE 8 *Dosing Interval Adjustment in Patients With Renal Impairment*

	Creatine Clearance (ml/min)			
	≥50	30-49	15-29	<15*†
Recommended dose and dosing interval	200 mg every 24 hours	200 mg every 48 hours	200 mg every 72 hours	200 mg every 96 hours

* Including patients requiring hemodialysis.
† Hemodialysis Patients: If dosing on day of dialysis, give dose after dialysis.

HOW SUPPLIED

Emtriva is available as capsules. Emtriva capsules, 200 mg, are size 1 hard gelatin capsules with a blue cap and white body, printed with "200 mg" in black on the cap and "GILEAD" and the corporate logo in black on the body.

Storage: Store at 25°C (77°F); excursions permitted to 15-30°C (59-86°F).

Enalapril Maleate *(001138)*

For related information, see the comparative table section in Appendix A.

Categories: Heart failure, congestive; Hypertension, essential; Left ventricular dysfunction, asymptomatic; Pregnancy Category C; FDA Approved 1985 Dec

Drug Classes: Angiotensin converting enzyme inhibitors

Brand Names: **Vasotec**

Foreign Brand Availability: Acetensil (Spain); Alapren (South-Africa); Alphapril (Australia); Alphrin (Korea); Amprace (Australia; New-Zealand); Analept (Bulgaria; Greece); Anapril (Hong-Kong; Singapore); Auspril (Australia); Beartec (Korea); Benalipril (Germany); Biocronil (Colombia); BQL (Benin; Burkina-Faso; Ethiopia; Gambia; Ghana; Guinea; India; Ivory-Coast; Kenya; Liberia; Malawi; Mali; Mauritania; Mauritius; Morocco; Niger; Nigeria; Senegal; Seychelles; Sierra-Leone; Sudan; Tanzania; Tunia; Uganda; Zambia; Zimbabwe); Controlvas (Spain); Converten (India); Convertin (Israel); Corprilor (Singapore); Ednyt (Bahamas; Barbados; Belize; Bermuda; Curacao; Guyana; Jamaica; Netherland-Antilles; Puerto-Rico; Surinam; Trinidad); Elfonal (Korea); EnaABZ (Germany); Enahexal (New-Zealand); Enaladil (Mexico); Enalapril (Germany; Spain); Enaloc (Finland); Enalpapril (Israel); Enam (China); Enap (Singapore); Enapren (Italy); Enapril (Thailand); Enaprin (Korea); Enaril (Korea; Thailand); Enatec (Bahamas; Barbados; Belize; Bermuda; Curacao; Guyana; Jamaica; Netherland-Antilles; Puerto-Rico; Surinam; Trinidad); Envas (India); Glioten (Colombia; Ecuador; Mexico; Peru); Hytrol (India); Innovace (England; Ireland); Inoprilat (Indonesia); Invoril (Benin; Burkina-Faso; China; Ethiopia; Gambia; Ghana; Guinea; India; Ivory-Coast; Kenya; Liberia; Malawi; Mali; Mauritania; Mauritius; Morocco; Niger; Nigeria; Senegal; Seychelles; Sierra-Leone; Singapore; Sudan; Tanzania; Thailand; Tunia; Uganda; Zambia; Zimbabwe); Kenopril (Mexico); Lapril (Thailand); Lenipril (Korea); Lepril (Korea); Lotrial (Costa-Rica; Dominican-Republic; Ecuador; El-Salvador; Guatemala; Honduras; Nicaragua; Panama; Peru); Lowtril (Korea); Meipril (Indonesia); Naprilene (Italy); Naritec (Korea; Thailand); Nuril (India); Pres (Germany); Presil (Colombia); Renaton (Korea); Renavace (Japan); Renitec (Australia; Austria; Belgium; Benin; Bulgaria; Burkina-Faso; China; Colombia; Czech-Republic; Denmark; Ecuador; Ethiopia; Finland; France; Gambia; Ghana; Greece; Guinea; Hong-Kong; Hungary; Ivory-Coast; Kenya; Liberia; Malawi; Malaysia; Mali; Mauritania; Mauritius; Mexico; Morocco; Netherlands; New-Zealand; Niger; Nigeria; Norway; Peru; Philippines; Portugal; Senegal; Seychelles; Sierra-Leone; South-Africa; Spain; Sudan; Sweden; Taiwan; Tanzania; Thailand; Tunia; Turkey; Uganda; Zambia; Zimbabwe); Renitek (Russia); Reniten (Switzerland); Renivace (Indonesia); Repantril (Indonesia); Sintec (Taiwan); Tenace (Indonesia); Unaril (Taiwan); Unipril (Colombia); Vasopress (Philippines); Xanef (Germany)

Cost of Therapy: $26.40 (Hypertension; Vasotec; 5 mg; 1 tablet/day; 30 day supply)

INTRAVENOUS

WARNING

USE IN PREGNANCY.

When used in pregnancy during the second and third trimesters, ACE inhibitors can cause injury and even death to the developing fetus. When pregnancy is detected, enalaprilat IV should be discontinued as soon as possible. See WARNINGS, Fetal/Neonatal Morbidity and Mortality.

DESCRIPTION

Vasotec IV (enalaprilat) is a sterile aqueous solution for intravenous administration. Enalaprilat is an angiotensin converting enzyme inhibitor. It is chemically described as (*S*)-1-[*N*-(1-carboxy-3-phenylpropyl)-L-alanyl]-L-proline dihydrate. Its empirical formula is $C_{18}H_{24}N_2O_5 \cdot 2H_2O$.

Enalaprilat is a white to off-white, crystalline powder with a molecular weight of 384.43. It is sparingly soluble in methanol and slightly soluble in water.

Each milliliter of Vasotec IV contains 1.25 mg enalaprilat (anhydrous equivalent); sodium chloride to adjust tonicity; sodium hydroxide to adjust pH; water for injection, qs; with benzyl alcohol, 9 mg, added as a preservative.

CLINICAL PHARMACOLOGY

Enalaprilat, an angiotensin-converting enzyme (ACE) inhibitor when administered intravenously, is the active metabolite of the orally administered pro-drug, enalapril maleate. Enalaprilat is poorly absorbed orally.

MECHANISM OF ACTION

Intravenous enalaprilat, or oral enalapril, after hydrolysis to enalaprilat, inhibits ACE in human subjects and animals. ACE is a peptidyl dipeptidase that catalyzes the conversion of angiotensin 1 to the vasoconstrictor substance, angiotensin 2. Angiotensin 2 also stimulates aldosterone secretion by the adrenal cortex. Inhibition of ACE results in decreased plasma angiotensin 2, which leads to decreased vasopressor activity and to decreased aldosterone secretion. Although the latter decrease is small, it results in small increases of serum potassium. In hypertensive patients treated with enalapril alone for up to 48 weeks, mean increases in serum potassium of approximately 0.2 mEq/L were observed. In patients treated with enalapril plus a thiazide diuretic, there was essentially no change in serum potassium. (See PRECAUTIONS.) Removal of angiotensin 2 negative feedback on renin secretion leads to increased plasma renin activity.

ACE is identical to kininase, an enzyme that degrades bradykinin. Whether increased levels of bradykinin, a potent vasodepressor peptide, play a role in the therapeutic effects of enalaprilat remains to be elucidated.

While the mechanism through which enalaprilat lowers blood pressure is believed to be primarily suppression of the renin-angiotensin-aldosterone system, enalaprilat has antihypertensive activity even in patients with low-renin hypertension. In clinical studies, black hypertensive patients (usually a low-renin hypertensive population) had a smaller average response to enalaprilat monotherapy than non-black patients.

PHARMACOKINETICS AND METABOLISM

Following intravenous administration of a single dose, the serum concentration profile of enalaprilat is polyexponential with a prolonged terminal phase, apparently representing a small fraction of the administered dose that has been bound to ACE. The amount bound does not increase with dose, indicating a saturable site of binding. The effective half-life for accumulation of enalaprilat, as determined from oral administration of multiple doses of enalapril maleate, is approximately 11 hours. Excretion of enalaprilat is primarily renal with more than 90% of an administered dose recovered in the urine as unchanged drug within 24 hours. Enalaprilat is poorly absorbed following oral administration.

The disposition of enalaprilat in patients with renal insufficiency is similar to that in patients with normal renal function until the glomerular filtration rate is 30 ml/min or less. With glomerular filtration rate ≤30 ml/min, peak and trough enalaprilat levels increase, time to peak concentration increases and time to steady state may be delayed. The effective half-life of enalaprilat is prolonged at this level of renal insufficiency. (See DOSAGE AND ADMINISTRATION.) Enalaprilat is dialyzable at the rate of 62 ml/min.

E

Studies in dogs indicate that enalaprilat does not enter the brain, and that enalapril crosses the blood-brain barrier poorly, if at all. Multiple doses of enalapril maleate in rats do not result in accumulation in any tissues. Milk in lactating rats contains radioactivity following administration of ^{14}C enalapril maleate. Radioactivity was found to cross the placenta following administration of labeled drug to pregnant hamsters.

PHARMACODYNAMICS

Enalaprilat IV results in the reduction of both supine and standing systolic and diastolic blood pressure, usually with no orthostatic component. Symptomatic postural hypotension is therefore infrequent, although it might be anticipated in volume-depleted patients (see WARNINGS). The onset of action usually occurs within 15 minutes of administration with the maximum effect occurring within 1-4 hours. The abrupt withdrawal of enalaprilat has not been associated with a rapid increase in blood pressure.

The duration of hemodynamic effects appears to be dose-related. However, for the recommended dose, the duration of action in most patients is approximately 6 hours.

Following administration of enalapril, there is an increase in renal blood flow; glomerular filtration rate is usually unchanged. The effects appear to be similar in patients with renovascular hypertension.

INDICATIONS AND USAGE

Enalaprilat IV is indicated for the treatment of hypertension when oral therapy is not practical.

Enalaprilat IV has been studied with only one other antihypertensive agent, furosemide, which showed approximately additive effects on blood pressure. Enalapril, the pro-drug of enalaprilat, has been used extensively with a variety of other antihypertensive agents, without apparent difficulty except for occasional hypotension.

In using enalaprilat IV, consideration should be given to the fact that another angiotensin converting enzyme inhibitor, captopril, has caused agranulocytosis, particularly in patients with renal impairment or collagen vascular disease, and that available data are insufficient to show that enalaprilat IV does not have a similar risk. (See WARNINGS.)

In considering use of enalaprilat IV, it should be noted that in controlled clinical trials ACE inhibitors have an effect on blood pressure that is less in black patients than in non-blacks. In addition, it should be noted that black patients receiving ACE inhibitors have been reported to have a higher incidence of angioedema compared to non-blacks. (See WARNINGS, Anaphylactoid and Possibly Related Reactions, Angioedema.)

NON-FDA APPROVED INDICATIONS

Although enalapril is not approved by the FDA for the treatment or prevention of diabetic nephropathy, it and some other ACE inhibitors have been shown to decrease proteinuria and preserve renal function in patients with hypertension and diabetes mellitus better than other antihypertensive agents. More recently, enalapril has been shown to decrease the progression of nephropathy in normotensive patients with Type 2 diabetes mellitus.

CONTRAINDICATIONS

Enalaprilat IV is contraindicated in patients who are hypersensitive to any component of this product and in patients with a history of angioedema related to previous treatment with an angiotensin converting enzyme inhibitor and in patients with hereditary or idiopathic angioedema.

WARNINGS

HYPOTENSION

Excessive hypotension is rare in uncomplicated hypertensive patients but is a possible consequence of the use of enalaprilat especially in severely salt/volume depleted persons such as those treated vigorously with diuretics or patients on dialysis. Patients at risk for excessive hypotension, sometimes associated with oliguria and/or progressive azotemia, and rarely with acute renal failure and/or death, include those with the following conditions or characteristics: heart failure, hyponatremia, high dose diuretic therapy, recent intensive diuresis or increase in diuretic dose, renal dialysis, or severe volume and/or salt depletion of any etiology. It may be advisable to eliminate the diuretic, reduce the diuretic dose or increase salt intake cautiously before initiating therapy with enalaprilat IV in patients at risk for excessive hypotension who are able to tolerate such adjustments. (See DRUG INTERACTIONS, ADVERSE REACTIONS, and DOSAGE AND ADMINISTRATION.) In patients with heart failure, with or without associated renal insufficiency, excessive hypotension has been observed and may be associated with oliguria and/or progressive azotemia, and rarely with acute renal failure and/or death. Because of the potential for an excessive fall in blood pressure especially in these patients, therapy should be followed closely whenever the dose of enalaprilat is adjusted and/or diuretic is increased. Similar considerations may apply to patients with ischemic heart or cerebrovascular disease, in whom an excessive fall in blood pressure could result in a myocardial infarction or cerebrovascular accident.

If hypotension occurs, the patient should be placed in the supine position and, if necessary, receive an intravenous infusion of normal saline. A transient hypotensive response is not a contraindication to further doses, which usually can be given without difficulty once the blood pressure has increased after volume expansion.

ANAPHYLACTOID AND POSSIBLY RELATED REACTIONS

Presumably because angiotensin-converting enzyme inhibitors affect the metabolism of eicosanoids and polypeptides, including endogenous bradykinin, patients receiving ACE inhibitors (including enalaprilat IV) may be subject to a variety of adverse reactions, some of them serious.

Angioedema

Angioedema of the face, extremities, lips, tongue, glottis and/or larynx has been reported in patients treated with angiotensin converting enzyme inhibitors, including enalaprilat. This may occur at any time during treatment. In such cases enalaprilat IV should be promptly discontinued and appropriate therapy and monitoring should be provided until complete and sustained resolution of signs and symptoms has occurred. In instances where swelling has been confined to the face and lips the condition has generally resolved without treatment, although antihistamines have been useful in relieving symptoms. Angioedema associated with laryngeal edema may be fatal. **Where there is involvement of the tongue, glottis or larynx, likely to cause airway obstruction, appropriate therapy, *e.g.,* subcutaneous epinephrine solution 1:1000 (0.3-0.5 ml) and/or measures necessary to ensure a patent airway, should be promptly provided.** (See ADVERSE REACTIONS.)

Patients with a history of angioedema unrelated to ACE inhibitor therapy may be at increased risk of angioedema while receiving an ACE inhibitor (see also INDICATIONS AND USAGE and CONTRAINDICATIONS).

Anaphylactoid Reactions During Desensitization

Two (2) patients undergoing desensitizing treatment with hymenoptera venom while receiving ACE inhibitors sustained life-threatening anaphylactoid reactions. In the same patients, these reactions were avoided when ACE inhibitors were temporarily withheld, but they reappeared upon inadvertent rechallenge.

Anaphylactoid Reactions During Membrane Exposure

Anaphylactoid reactions have been reported in patients dialyzed with high-flux membranes and treated concomitantly with an ACE inhibitor. Anaphylactoid reactions have also been reported in patients undergoing low-density lipoprotein apheresis with dextran sulfate absorption.

NEUTROPENIA/AGRANULOCYTOSIS

Another angiotensin converting enzyme inhibitor, captopril, has been shown to cause agranulocytosis and bone marrow depression, rarely in uncomplicated patients but more frequently in patients with renal impairment especially if they also have a collagen vascular disease. Available data from clinical trials of enalapril are insufficient to show that enalapril does not cause agranulocytosis in similar rates. Marketing experience has revealed cases of neutropenia, or agranulocytosis in which a causal relationship to enalapril cannot be excluded. Periodic monitoring of white blood cell counts in patients with collagen vascular disease and renal disease should be considered.

HEPATIC FAILURE

Rarely, ACE inhibitors have been associated with a syndrome that starts with cholestatic jaundice and progresses to fulminant hepatic necrosis, and (sometimes) death. The mechanism of this syndrome is not understood. Patients receiving ACE inhibitors who develop jaundice or marked elevations of hepatic enzymes should discontinue the ACE inhibitor and receive appropriate medical follow-up.

FETAL/NEONATAL MORBIDITY AND MORTALITY

ACE inhibitors can cause fetal and neonatal morbidity and death when administered to pregnant women. Several dozen cases have been reported in the world literature. When pregnancy is detected, ACE inhibitors should be discontinued as soon as possible.

The use of ACE inhibitors during the second and third trimesters of pregnancy has been associated with fetal and neonatal injury, including hypotension, neonatal skull hypoplasia, anuria, reversible or irreversible renal failure, and death. Oligohydramnios has also been reported, presumably resulting from decreased fetal renal function; oligohydramnios in this setting has been associated with fetal limb contractures, craniofacial deformation, and hypoplastic lung development. Prematurity, intrauterine growth retardation, and patent ductus arteriosus have also been reported, although it is not clear whether these occurrences were due to the ACE-inhibitor exposure.

These adverse effects do not appear to have resulted from intrauterine ACE-inhibitor exposure that has been limited to the first trimester. Mothers whose embryos and fetuses are exposed to ACE inhibitors only during the first trimester should be so informed. Nonetheless, when patients become pregnant, physicians should make every effort to discontinue the use of enalaprilat IV as soon as possible.

Rarely (probably less often than once in every thousand pregnancies), no alternative to ACE inhibitors will be found. In these rare cases, the mothers should be apprised of the potential hazards to their fetuses, and serial ultrasound examinations should be performed to assess the intraamniotic environment.

If oligohydramnios is observed, enalaprilat IV should be discontinued unless it is considered lifesaving for the mother. Contraction stress testing (CST), a non-stress test (NST), or biophysical profiling (BPP) may be appropriate, depending upon the week of pregnancy. Patients and physicians should be aware, however, that oligohydramnios may not appear until after the fetus has sustained irreversible injury.

Infants with histories of *in utero* exposure to ACE inhibitors should be closely observed for hypotension, oliguria, and hyperkalemia. If oliguria occurs, attention should be directed toward support of blood pressure and renal perfusion. Exchange transfusion or dialysis may be required as means of reversing hypotension and/or substituting for disordered renal function. Enalapril, which crosses the placenta, has been removed from neonatal circulation by peritoneal dialysis with some clinical benefit, and theoretically may be removed by exchange transfusion, although there is no experience with the latter procedure.

No teratogenic effects of oral enalapril were seen in studies of pregnant rats and rabbits. On a body surface area basis, the doses used were 57 and 12 times, respectively, the maximum recommended human daily dose (MRHDD).

PRECAUTIONS

GENERAL

Aortic Stenosis/Hypertrophic Cardiomyopathy

As with all vasodilators, enalapril should be given with caution to patients with obstruction in the outflow tract of the left ventricle.

Impaired Renal Function

As a consequence of inhibiting the renin-angiotensin-aldosterone system, changes in renal function may be anticipated in susceptible individuals. In patients with severe heart failure whose renal function may depend on the activity of the renin-angiotensin-aldosterone system, treatment with angiotensin converting enzyme inhibitors, including enalapril or enalaprilat, may be associated with oliguria and/or progressive azotemia and rarely with acute renal failure and/or death.

In clinical studies in hypertensive patients with unilateral or bilateral renal artery stenosis, increases in blood urea nitrogen and serum creatinine were observed in 20% of patients receiving enalapril. These increases were almost always reversible upon discontinuation of enalapril or enalaprilat and/or diuretic therapy. In such patients renal function should be monitored during the first few weeks of therapy.

Some hypertensive patients with no apparent pre-existing renal vascular disease have developed increases in blood urea and serum creatinine, usually minor and transient, especially when enalaprilat has been given concomitantly with a diuretic. This is more likely to occur in patients with pre-existing renal impairment. Dosage reduction of enalaprilat and/or discontinuation of the diuretic may be required.

Evaluation of the hypertensive patient should always include assessment of renal function. (See DOSAGE AND ADMINISTRATION.)

Hyperkalemia

Elevated serum potassium (greater than 5.7 mEq/L) was observed in approximately 1% of hypertensive patients in clinical trials receiving enalapril. In most cases these were isolated values which resolved despite continued therapy. Hyperkalemia was a cause of discontinuation of therapy in 0.28% of hypertensive patients. Risk factors for the development of hyperkalemia include renal insufficiency, diabetes mellitus, and the concomitant use of potassium-sparing agents or potassium supplements, which should be used cautiously, if at all, with enalaprilat IV. (See DRUG INTERACTIONS.)

Cough

Presumably due to the inhibition of the degradation of endogenous bradykinin, persistent nonproductive cough has been reported with all ACE inhibitors, always resolving after discontinuation of therapy. ACE inhibitor-induced cough should be considered in the differential diagnosis of cough.

Surgery/Anesthesia

In patients undergoing major surgery or during anesthesia with agents that produce hypotension, enalapril may block angiotensin 2 formation secondary to compensatory renin release. If hypotension occurs and is considered to be due to this mechanism, it can be corrected by volume expansion.

CARCINOGENESIS, MUTAGENESIS, AND IMPAIRMENT OF FERTILITY

Carcinogenicity studies have not been done with enalaprilat IV.

Enalaprilat IV is the bioactive form of its ethyl ester, enalapril maleate. There was no evidence of a tumorigenic effect when enalapril was administered for 106 weeks to male and female rats at doses up to 90 mg/kg/day or for 94 weeks to male and female mice at doses up to 90 and 180 mg/kg/day, respectively. These doses are 26 times (in rats and female mice) and 13 times (in male mice) the maximum recommended human daily dose (MRHDD) when compared on a body surface area basis.

Enalaprilat IV was not mutagenic in the Ames microbial mutagen test with or without metabolic activation. Enalapril showed no drug-related changes in the following genotoxicity studies: rec-assay, reverse mutation assay with *E. coli,* sister chromatid exchange with cultured mammalian cells, the micronucleus test with mice, and in an *in vivo* cytogenic study using mouse bone marrow. There were no adverse effects on reproductive performance of male and female rats treated with up to 90 mg/kg/day of enalapril (26 times the MRHDD when compared on a body surface area basis).

PREGNANCY CATEGORIES C (FIRST TRIMESTER) AND D (SECOND AND THIRD TRIMESTERS)

See WARNINGS, Fetal/Neonatal Morbidity and Mortality.

NURSING MOTHERS

Enalapril and enalaprilat have been detected in human breast milk. Because of the potential for serious adverse reactions in nursing infants from enalapril, a decision should be made whether to discontinue nursing or to discontinue enalaprilat IV, taking into account the importance of the drug to the mother.

PEDIATRIC USE

Safety and effectiveness in pediatric patients have not been established.

DRUG INTERACTIONS

HYPOTENSION — PATIENTS ON DIURETIC THERAPY

Patients on diuretics and especially those in whom diuretic therapy was recently instituted, may occasionally experience an excessive reduction of blood pressure after initiation of therapy with enalaprilat. The possibility of hypotensive effects with enalaprilat can be minimized by administration of an intravenous infusion of normal saline, discontinuing the diuretic or increasing the salt intake prior to initiation of treatment with enalaprilat. If it is necessary to continue the diuretic, provide close medical supervision for at least 1 hour after the initial dose of enalaprilat. (See WARNINGS.)

AGENTS CAUSING RENIN RELEASE

The antihypertensive effect of enalaprilat IV appears to be augmented by antihypertensive agents that cause renin release (*e.g.,* diuretics).

NON-STEROIDAL ANTI-INFLAMMATORY AGENTS

In some patients with compromised renal function who are being treated with non-steroidal anti-inflammatory drugs, the coadministration of enalapril may result in a further deterioration of renal function. These effects are usually reversible.

OTHER CARDIOVASCULAR AGENTS

Enalaprilat IV has been used concomitantly with digitalis, beta adrenergic-blocking agents, methyldopa, nitrates, calcium-blocking agents, hydralazine, and prazosin without evidence of clinically significant adverse interactions.

AGENTS INCREASING SERUM POTASSIUM

Enalaprilat IV attenuates potassium loss caused by thiazide-type diuretics. Potassium-sparing diuretics (*e.g.,* spironolactone, triamterene, or amiloride), potassium supplements, or potassium-containing salt substitutes may lead to significant increases in serum potassium. Therefore, if concomitant use of these agents is indicated because of demonstrated hypokalemia, they should be used with caution and with frequent monitoring of serum potassium.

LITHIUM

Lithium toxicity has been reported in patients receiving lithium concomitantly with drugs which cause elimination of sodium, including ACE inhibitors. A few cases of lithium toxicity have been reported in patients receiving concomitant enalapril and lithium and were reversible upon discontinuation of both drugs. It is recommended that serum lithium levels be monitored frequently if enalapril is administered concomitantly with lithium.

ADVERSE REACTIONS

Enalaprilat IV has been found to be generally well tolerated in controlled clinical trials involving 349 patients (168 with hypertension, 153 with congestive heart failure and 28 with coronary artery disease). The most frequent clinically significant adverse experience was hypotension (3.4%), occurring in 8 patients (5.2%) with congestive heart failure, 3 (1.8%) with hypertension and 1 with coronary artery disease. Other adverse experiences occurring in greater than 1% of patients were: headache (2.9%) and nausea (1.1%).

Adverse experiences occurring in 0.5-1.0% of patients in controlled clinical trials included: myocardial infarction, fatigue, dizziness, fever, rash and constipation.

Angioedema: Angioedema has been reported in patients receiving enalaprilat, with an incidence higher in black than in non-black patients. Angioedema associated with laryngeal edema may be fatal. If angioedema of the face, extremities, lips, tongue, glottis and/or larynx occurs, treatment with enalaprilat should be discontinued and appropriate therapy instituted immediately. (See WARNINGS.)

Cough: See PRECAUTIONS, General, Cough.

ENALAPRIL MALEATE

Since enalapril is converted to enalaprilat, those adverse experiences associated with enalapril might also be expected to occur with enalaprilat IV.

The following adverse experiences have been reported with enalapril and, within each category, are listed in order of decreasing severity:

Body as a Whole: Syncope, orthostatic effects, anaphylactoid reactions (see WARNINGS, Anaphylactoid and Possibly Related Reactions, Anaphylactoid Reactions During Membrane Exposure), chest pain, abdominal pain, asthenia.

Cardiovascular: Cardiac arrest; myocardial infarction or cerebrovascular accident, possibly secondary to excessive hypotension in high risk patients (see WARNINGS, Hypotension); pulmonary embolism and infarction; pulmonary edema; rhythm disturbances including atrial tachycardia and bradycardia; atrial fibrillation; orthostatic hypotension; angina pectoris; palpitation, Raynaud's phenomenon.

Digestive: Ileus, pancreatitis, hepatic failure, hepatitis (hepatocellular [proven on rechallenge] or cholestatic jaundice) (see WARNINGS, Hepatic Failure), melena, diarrhea, vomiting, dyspepsia, anorexia, glossitis, stomatitis, dry mouth.

Hematologic: Rare cases of neutropenia, thrombocytopenia, and bone marrow depression.

Musculoskeletal: Muscle cramps.

Nervous/Psychiatric: Depression, vertigo, confusion, ataxia, somnolence, insomnia, nervousness, peripheral neuropathy (*e.g.,* paresthesia, dysesthesia), dream abnormality.

Respiratory: Bronchospasm, dyspnea, pneumonia, bronchitis, cough, rhinorrhea, sore throat and hoarseness, asthma, upper respiratory infection, pulmonary infiltrates, eosinophilic pneumonitis.

Skin: Exfoliative dermatitis, toxic epidermal necrolysis, Stevens-Johnson syndrome, pemphigus, herpes zoster, erythema multiforme, urticaria, pruritus, alopecia, flushing, diaphoresis, photosensitivity.

Special Senses: Blurred vision, taste alteration, anosmia, tinnitus, conjunctivitis, dry eyes, tearing.

Urogenital: Renal failure, oliguria, renal dysfunction (see PRECAUTIONS and DOSAGE AND ADMINISTRATION), urinary tract infection, flank pain, gynecomastia, impotence.

Miscellaneous: *A symptom complex has been reported which may include some or all of the following:* A positive ANA, an elevated erythrocyte sedimentation rate, arthralgia/arthritis, myalgia/myositis, fever, serositis, vasculitis, leukocytosis, eosinophilia, photosensitivity, rash and other dermatologic manifestations.

Hypotension
Combining the results of clinical trials in patients with hypertension or congestive heart failure, hypotension (including postural hypotension, and other orthostatic effects) was reported in 2.3% of patients following the initial dose of enalapril or during extended therapy. In the hypertensive patients, hypotension occurred in 0.9% and syncope occurred in 0.5% of patients. Hypotension or syncope was a cause for discontinuation of therapy in 0.1% of hypertensive patients. (See WARNINGS.)

Fetal/Neonatal Morbidity and Mortality
See WARNINGS, Fetal/Neonatal Morbidity and Mortality.

CLINICAL LABORATORY TEST FINDINGS

Serum Electrolytes
Hyperkalemia (see PRECAUTIONS), hyponatremia.

Creatinine, Blood Urea Nitrogen
In controlled clinical trials minor increases in blood urea nitrogen and serum creatinine, reversible upon discontinuation of therapy, were observed in about 0.2% of patients with essential hypertension treated with enalapril alone. Increases are more likely to occur in patients receiving concomitant diuretics or in patients with renal artery stenosis. (See PRECAUTIONS.)

Hematology
Small decreases in hemoglobin and hematocrit (mean decreases of approximately 0.3 g percent and 1.0 vol percent, respectively) occur frequently in hypertensive patients treated with enalapril but are rarely of clinical importance unless another cause of anemia coexists. In clinical trials, less than 0.1% of patients discontinued therapy due to anemia. Hemolytic anemia, including cases of hemolysis in patients with G-6-PD deficiency, has been reported; a causal relationship to enalapril cannot be excluded.

Liver Function Tests
Elevations of liver enzymes and/or serum bilirubin have occurred (see WARNINGS, Hepatic Failure).

DOSAGE AND ADMINISTRATION

FOR INTRAVENOUS ADMINISTRATION ONLY.

The dose in hypertension is 1.25 mg every 6 hours administered intravenously over a 5 minute period. A clinical response is usually seen within 15 minutes. Peak effects after the first dose may not occur for up to 4 hours after dosing. The peak effects of the second and subsequent doses may exceed those of the first.

No dosage regimen for enalaprilat IV has been clearly demonstrated to be more effective in treating hypertension than 1.25 mg every 6 hours. However, in controlled clinical studies in hypertension, doses as high as 5 mg every 6 hours were well tolerated for up to 36 hours. There has been inadequate experience with doses greater than 20 mg/day.

In studies of patients with hypertension, enalaprilat IV has not been administered for periods longer than 48 hours. In other studies, patients have received enalaprilat IV for as long as 7 days.

The dose for patients being converted to enalaprilat IV from oral therapy for hypertension with enalapril maleate is 1.25 mg every 6 hours. For conversion from intravenous to oral therapy, the recommended initial dose of tablets enalapril (enalapril maleate) is 5 mg once a day with subsequent dosage adjustments as necessary.

PATIENTS ON DIURETIC THERAPY
For patients on diuretic therapy the recommended starting dose for hypertension is 0.625 mg administered intravenously over a 5 minute period; also see Patients at Risk of Excessive Hypotension. A clinical response is usually seen within 15 minutes. Peak effects after the first dose may not occur for up to 4 hours after dosing, although most of the effect is usually apparent within the first hour. If after 1 hour there is an inadequate clinical response, the 0.625 mg dose may be repeated. Additional doses of 1.25 mg may be administered at 6 hour intervals.

For conversion from intravenous to oral therapy, the recommended initial dose of tablets enalaprilat for patients who have responded to 0.625 mg of enalaprilat every 6 hours is 2.5 mg once a day with subsequent dosage adjustment as necessary.

DOSAGE ADJUSTMENT IN RENAL IMPAIRMENT
The usual dose of 1.25 mg of enalaprilat every 6 hours is recommended for patients with a creatinine clearance >30 ml/min (serum creatinine of up to approximately 3 mg/dl). For patients with creatinine clearance ≤30 ml/min (serum creatinine ≥3 mg/dl), the initial dose is 0.625 mg. (See WARNINGS.)

If after 1 hour there is an inadequate clinical response, the 0.625 mg dose may be repeated. Additional doses of 1.25 mg may be administered at 6 hour intervals.

For dialysis patients, see Patients at Risk of Excessive Hypotension.

For conversion from intravenous to oral therapy, the recommended initial dose of tablets enalaprilat is 5 mg once a day for patients with creatinine clearance >30 ml/min and 2.5 mg once daily for patients with creatinine clearance ≤30 ml/min. Dosage should then be adjusted according to blood pressure response.

PATIENTS AT RISK OF EXCESSIVE HYPOTENSION
Hypertensive patients at risk of excessive hypotension include those with the following concurrent conditions or characteristics: heart failure, hyponatremia, high dose diuretic therapy, recent intensive diuresis or increase in diuretic dose, renal dialysis, or severe volume and/or salt depletion of any etiology (see WARNINGS). Single doses of enalaprilat as low as 0.2 mg have produced excessive hypotension in normotensive patients with these diagnoses. Because of the potential for an extreme hypotensive response in these patients, therapy should be started under very close medical supervision. The starting dose should be no greater than 0.625 mg administered intravenously over a period of no less than 5 minutes and preferably longer (up to 1 hour).

Patients should be followed closely whenever the dose of enalaprilat is adjusted and/or diuretic is increased.

ADMINISTRATION
Enalaprilat IV should be administered as a slow intravenous infusion, as indicated above. It may be administered as provided or diluted with up to 50 ml of a compatible diluent.

Parenteral drug products should be inspected visually for particulate matter and discoloration prior to use whenever solution and container permit.

COMPATIBILITY AND STABILITY
Enalaprilat IV as supplied and mixed with the following intravenous diluents has been found to maintain full activity for 24 hours at room temperature:

5% dextrose injection
0.9% sodium chloride injection
0.9% sodium chloride injection in 5% dextrose
5% dextrose in lactated Ringer's injection
McGaw Isolyte E

HOW SUPPLIED

Vasotec IV, 1.25 mg/ml, is a clear, colorless solution and is supplied in vials containing 1 and 2 ml.
Storage: Store below 30°C (86°F).

ORAL

WARNING
USE IN PREGNANCY.
When used in pregnancy during the second and third trimesters, ACE inhibitors can cause injury and even death to the developing fetus. When pregnancy is detected, enalapril maleate should be discontinued as soon as possible. See WARNINGS, Fetal/Neonatal Morbidity and Mortality.

DESCRIPTION

Vasotec (enalapril maleate) is the maleate salt of enalapril, the ethyl ester of a long-acting angiotensin converting enzyme inhibitor, enalaprilat. Enalapril maleate is chemically described as (*S*)-1-[*N*-[1-(ethoxycarbonyl)-3-phenylpropyl]-L-alanyl]-L-proline,(*Z*)-2-butenedioate salt (1:1). Its empirical formula is $C_{20}H_{28}N_2O_5{\cdot}C_4H_4O_4$.

Enalapril maleate is a white to off-white, crystalline powder with a molecular weight of 492.53. It is sparingly soluble in water, soluble in ethanol, and freely soluble in methanol.

Enalapril is a pro-drug; following oral administration, it is bioactivated by hydrolysis of the ethyl ester to enalaprilat, which is the active angiotensin converting enzyme inhibitor.

Enalapril maleate is supplied as 2.5, 5, 10, and 20 mg tablets for oral administration. In addition to the active ingredient enalapril maleate, each tablet contains the following inactive ingredients: lactose, magnesium stearate, starch, and other ingredients. The 2.5, 10, and 20 mg tablets also contain iron oxides.

CLINICAL PHARMACOLOGY

MECHANISM OF ACTION
Enalapril, after hydrolysis to enalaprilat, inhibits angiotensin-converting enzyme (ACE) in human subjects and animals. ACE is a peptidyl dipeptidase that catalyzes the conversion of angiotensin 1 to the vasoconstrictor substance, angiotensin 2. Angiotensin 2 also stimulates aldosterone secretion by the adrenal cortex. The beneficial effects of enalapril in hypertension and heart failure appear to result primarily from suppression of the renin-angiotensin-aldosterone system. Inhibition of ACE results in decreased plasma angiotensin 2, which leads to decreased vasopressor activity and to decreased aldosterone secretion. Although the latter decrease is small, it results in small increases of serum potassium. In hypertensive patients treated with enalapril maleate alone for up to 48 weeks, mean increases in serum potassium of approximately 0.2 mEq/L were observed. In patients treated with enalapril maleate plus a thiazide diuretic, there was essentially no change in serum potassium. (See PRECAUTIONS.) Removal of angiotensin 2 negative feedback on renin secretion leads to increased plasma renin activity.

ACE is identical to kininase, an enzyme that degrades bradykinin. Whether increased levels of bradykinin, a potent vasodepressor peptide, play a role in the therapeutic effects of enalapril maleate remains to be elucidated.

While the mechanism through which enalapril maleate lowers blood pressure is believed to be primarily suppression of the renin-angiotensin-aldosterone system, enalapril maleate is antihypertensive even in patients with low-renin hypertension. Although enalapril maleate was antihypertensive in all races studied, black hypertensive patients (usually a low-renin hypertensive population) had a smaller average response to enalapril monotherapy than non-black patients.

PHARMACOKINETICS AND METABOLISM
Following oral administration of enalapril maleate, peak serum concentrations of enalapril occur within about 1 hour. Based on urinary recovery, the extent of absorption of enalapril is approximately 60%. Enalapril absorption is not influenced by the presence of food in the gastrointestinal tract. Following absorption, enalapril is hydrolyzed to enalaprilat, which is a more potent angiotensin converting enzyme inhibitor than enalapril; enalaprilat is poorly absorbed when administered orally. Peak serum concentrations of enalaprilat occur 3-4 hours after an oral dose of enalapril maleate. Excretion of enalapril maleate is primarily renal. Approximately 94% of the dose is recovered in the urine and feces as enalaprilat or enalapril. The principal components in urine are enalaprilat, accounting for about 40% of the dose, and intact enalapril. There is no evidence of metabolites of enalapril, other than enalaprilat.

The serum concentration profile of enalaprilat exhibits a prolonged terminal phase, apparently representing a small fraction of the administered dose that has been bound to ACE.

The amount bound does not increase with dose, indicating a saturable site of binding. The effective half-life for accumulation of enalaprilat following multiple doses of enalapril maleate is 11 hours.

The disposition of enalapril and enalaprilat in patients with renal insufficiency is similar to that in patients with normal renal function until the glomerular filtration rate is 30 ml/min or less. With glomerular filtration rate ≤30 ml/min, peak and trough enalaprilat levels increase, time to peak concentration increases and time to steady state may be delayed. The effective half-life of enalaprilat following multiple doses of enalapril maleate is prolonged at this level of renal insufficiency. (See DOSAGE AND ADMINISTRATION.) Enalaprilat is dialyzable at the rate of 62 ml/min.

Studies in dogs indicate that enalapril crosses the blood-brain barrier poorly, if at all; enalaprilat does not enter the brain. Multiple doses of enalapril maleate in rats do not result in accumulation in any tissues. Milk of lactating rats contains radioactivity following administration of ^{14}C-enalapril maleate. Radioactivity was found to cross the placenta following administration of labeled drug to pregnant hamsters.

PHARMACODYNAMICS AND CLINICAL EFFECTS

Hypertension

Administration of enalapril maleate to patients with hypertension of severity ranging from mild to severe results in a reduction of both supine and standing blood pressure usually with no orthostatic component. Symptomatic postural hypotension is therefore infrequent, although it might be anticipated in volume-depleted patients. (See WARNINGS.)

In most patients studied, after oral administration of a single dose of enalapril, onset of antihypertensive activity was seen at 1 hour with peak reduction of blood pressure achieved by 4-6 hours.

At recommended doses, antihypertensive effects have been maintained for at least 24 hours. In some patients the effects may diminish toward the end of the dosing interval (see DOSAGE AND ADMINISTRATION).

In some patients achievement of optimal blood pressure reduction may require several weeks of therapy.

The antihypertensive effects of enalapril maleate have continued during long-term therapy. Abrupt withdrawal of enalapril maleate has not been associated with a rapid increase in blood pressure.

In hemodynamic studies in patients with essential hypertension, blood pressure reduction was accompanied by a reduction in peripheral arterial resistance with an increase in cardiac output and little or no change in heart rate. Following administration of enalapril maleate, there is an increase in renal blood flow; glomerular filtration rate is usually unchanged. The effects appear to be similar in patients with renovascular hypertension.

When given together with thiazide-type diuretics, the blood pressure lowering effects of enalapril maleate are approximately additive.

In a clinical pharmacology study, indomethacin or sulindac was administered to hypertensive patients receiving enalapril maleate. In this study there was no evidence of a blunting of the antihypertensive action of enalapril maleate.

Heart Failure

In trials in patients treated with digitalis and diuretics, treatment with enalapril resulted in decreased systemic vascular resistance, blood pressure, pulmonary capillary wedge pressure and heart size, and increased cardiac output and exercise tolerance. Heart rate was unchanged or slightly reduced, and mean ejection fraction was unchanged or increased. There was a beneficial effect on severity of heart failure as measured by the New York Heart Association (NYHA) classification and on symptoms of dyspnea and fatigue. Hemodynamic effects were observed after the first dose, and appeared to be maintained in uncontrolled studies lasting as long as 4 months. Effects on exercise tolerance, heart size, and severity and symptoms of heart failure were observed in placebo-controlled studies lasting from 8 weeks to over 1 year.

Heart Failure, Mortality Trials

In a multicenter, placebo-controlled clinical trial, 2569 patients with all degrees of symptomatic heart failure and ejection fraction ≤35% were randomized to placebo or enalapril and followed for up to 55 months (SOLVD-Treatment). Use of enalapril was associated with an 11% reduction in all-cause mortality and a 30% reduction in hospitalization for heart failure. Diseases that excluded patients from enrollment in the study included severe stable angina (>2 attacks/day), hemodynamically significant valvular or outflow tract obstruction, renal failure (creatinine >2.5 mg/dl), cerebral vascular disease (*e.g.*, significant carotid artery disease), advanced pulmonary disease, malignancies, active myocarditis and constrictive pericarditis. The mortality benefit associated with enalapril does not appear to depend upon digitalis being present.

A second multicenter trial used the SOLVD protocol for study of asymptomatic or minimally symptomatic patients. SOLVD-Prevention patients, who had left ventricular ejection fraction ≤35% and no history of symptomatic heart failure, were randomized to placebo (n=2117) or enalapril (n=2111) and followed for up to 5 years. The majority of patients in the SOLVD-Prevention trial had a history of ischemic heart disease. A history of myocardial infarction was present in 80% of patients, current angina pectoris in 34%, and a history of hypertension in 37%. No statistically significant mortality effect was demonstrated in this population. Enalapril-treated subjects had 32% fewer first hospitalizations for heart failure, and 32% fewer total heart failure hospitalizations. Compared to placebo, 32% fewer patients receiving enalapril developed symptoms of overt heart failure. Hospitalizations for cardiovascular reasons were also reduced. There was an insignificant reduction in hospitalizations for any cause in the enalapril treatment group (for enalapril versus placebo, respectively, 1166 vs 1201 first hospitalizations, 2649 vs 2840 total hospitalizations), although the study was not powered to look for such an effect.

The SOLVD-Prevention trial was not designed to determine whether treatment of asymptomatic patients with low ejection fraction would be superior, with respect to preventing hospitalization, to closer follow-up and use of enalapril at the earliest sign of heart failure. However, under the conditions of follow-up in the SOLVD-Prevention trial (every 4 months at the study clinic; personal physician as needed), 68% of patients on placebo who were hospitalized for heart failure had no prior symptoms recorded which would have signaled initiation of treatment.

The SOLVD-Prevention trial was also not designed to show whether enalapril modified the progression of underlying heart disease.

In another multicenter, placebo-controlled trial (CONSENSUS) limited to patients with NYHA Class IV congestive heart failure and radiographic evidence of cardiomegaly, use of enalapril was associated with improved survival. The results are shown in TABLE 1.

TABLE 1

Survival (%)	Enalapril Maleate (n=127)	Placebo (n=126)
6 months	74%	56%
1 year	64%	48%

In both CONSENSUS and SOLVD-Treatment trials, patients were also usually receiving digitalis, diuretics, or both.

CLINICAL PHARMACOLOGY IN PEDIATRIC PATIENTS

A multiple dose pharmacokinetic study was conducted in 40 hypertensive male and female pediatric patients aged 2 months to ≤16 years following daily oral administration of 0.07-0.14 mg/kg enalapril maleate. At steady state, the mean effective half-life for accumulation of enalaprilat was 14 hours and the mean urinary recovery of total enalapril and enalaprilat in 24 hours was 68% of the administered dose. Conversion of enalapril to enalaprilat was in the range of 63-76%. The overall results of this study indicate that the pharmacokinetics of enalapril in hypertensive children aged 2 months to ≤16 years are consistent across the studied age groups and consistent with pharmacokinetic historic data in healthy adults.

In a clinical study involving 110 hypertensive pediatric patients 6-16 years of age, patients who weighed <50 kg received either 0.625, 2.5, or 20 mg of enalapril daily and patients who weighed ≥50 kg received either 1.25, 5, or 40 mg of enalapril daily. Enalapril administration once daily lowered trough blood pressure in a dose-dependent manner. The dose-dependent antihypertensive efficacy of enalapril was consistent across all subgroups (age, Tanner stage, gender, race). However, the lowest doses studied, 0.625 and 1.25 mg, corresponding to an average of 0.02 mg/kg once daily, did not appear to offer consistent antihypertensive efficacy. In this study, enalapril maleate was generally well tolerated.

In the above pediatric studies, enalapril maleate was given as tablets of enalapril maleate and for those children and infants who were unable to swallow tablets or who required a lower dose than is available in tablet form, enalapril was administered in a suspension formulation (see DOSAGE AND ADMINISTRATION, Preparation of Suspension).

INDICATIONS AND USAGE

HYPERTENSION

Enalapril maleate is indicated for the treatment of hypertension.

Enalapril maleate is effective alone or in combination with other antihypertensive agents, especially thiazide-type diuretics. The blood pressure lowering effects of enalapril maleate and thiazides are approximately additive.

HEART FAILURE

Enalapril maleate is indicated for the treatment of symptomatic congestive heart failure, usually in combination with diuretics and digitalis. In these patients enalapril maleate improves symptoms, increases survival, and decreases the frequency of hospitalization (see CLINICAL PHARMACOLOGY, Pharmacodynamics and Clinical Effects, Heart Failure, Mortality Trials for details and limitations of survival trials).

ASYMPTOMATIC LEFT VENTRICULAR DYSFUNCTION

In clinically stable asymptomatic patients with left ventricular dysfunction (ejection fraction (≤35%), enalapril maleate decreases the rate of development of overt heart failure and decreases the incidence of hospitalization for heart failure. (See CLINICAL PHARMACOLOGY, Pharmacodynamics and Clinical Effects, Heart Failure, Mortality Trials for details and limitations of survival trials.)

In using enalapril maleate consideration should be given to the fact that another angiotensin converting enzyme inhibitor, captopril, has caused agranulocytosis, particularly in patients with renal impairment or collagen vascular disease, and that available data are insufficient to show that enalapril maleate does not have a similar risk. (See WARNINGS.)

In considering use of enalapril maleate, it should be noted that in controlled clinical trials ACE inhibitors have an effect on blood pressure that is less in black patients than in non-blacks. In addition, it should be noted that black patients receiving ACE inhibitors have been reported to have a higher incidence of angioedema compared to non-blacks. (See WARNINGS, Anaphylactoid and Possibly Related Reactions, Angioedema.)

NON-FDA APPROVED INDICATIONS

Although enalapril is not approved by the FDA for the treatment or prevention of diabetic nephropathy, it and some other ACE inhibitors have been shown to decrease proteinuria and preserve renal function in patients with hypertension and diabetes mellitus better than other antihypertensive agents. More recently, enalapril has been shown to decrease the progression of nephropathy in normotensive patients with Type 2 diabetes mellitus.

CONTRAINDICATIONS

Enalapril maleate is contraindicated in patients who are hypersensitive to this product and in patients with a history of angioedema related to previous treatment with an angiotensin converting enzyme inhibitor and in patients with hereditary or idiopathic angioedema.

WARNINGS

ANAPHYLACTOID AND POSSIBLY RELATED REACTIONS

Presumably because angiotensin-converting enzyme inhibitors affect the metabolism of eicosanoids and polypeptides, including endogenous bradykinin, patients receiving ACE inhibitors (including enalapril maleate) may be subject to a variety of adverse reactions, some of them serious.

Angioedema
Angioedema of the face, extremities, lips, tongue, glottis and/or larynx has been reported in patients treated with angiotensin converting enzyme inhibitors, including enalapril maleate. This may occur at any time during treatment. In such cases enalapril maleate should be promptly discontinued and appropriate therapy and monitoring should be provided until complete and sustained resolution of signs and symptoms has occurred. In instances where swelling has been confined to the face and lips the condition has generally resolved without treatment, although antihistamines have been useful in relieving symptoms. Angioedema associated with laryngeal edema may be fatal. **Where there is involvement of the tongue, glottis or larynx, likely to cause airway obstruction, appropriate therapy, *e.g.*, subcutaneous epinephrine solution 1:1000 (0.3-0.5 ml) and/or measures necessary to ensure a patent airway, should be promptly provided.** (See ADVERSE REACTIONS.)

Patients with a history of angioedema unrelated to ACE inhibitor therapy may be at increased risk of angioedema while receiving an ACE inhibitor (see also INDICATIONS AND USAGE and CONTRAINDICATIONS).

E

Anaphylactoid Reactions During Desensitization
Two (2) patients undergoing desensitizing treatment with hymenoptera venom while receiving ACE inhibitors sustained life-threatening anaphylactoid reactions. In the same patients, these reactions were avoided when ACE inhibitors were temporarily withheld, but they reappeared upon inadvertent rechallenge.

Anaphylactoid Reactions During Membrane Exposure
Anaphylactoid reactions have been reported in patients dialyzed with high-flux membranes and treated concomitantly with an ACE inhibitor. Anaphylactoid reactions have also been reported in patients undergoing low-density lipoprotein apheresis with dextran sulfate absorption.

HYPOTENSION
Excessive hypotension is rare in uncomplicated hypertensive patients treated with enalapril maleate alone. Patients with heart failure given enalapril maleate commonly have some reduction in blood pressure, especially with the first dose, but discontinuation of therapy for continuing symptomatic hypotension usually is not necessary when dosing instructions are followed; caution should be observed when initiating therapy. (See DOSAGE AND ADMINISTRATION.) Patients at risk for excessive hypotension, sometimes associated with oliguria and/or progressive azotemia, and rarely with acute renal failure and/or death, include those with the following conditions or characteristics: heart failure, hyponatremia, high dose diuretic therapy, recent intensive diuresis or increase in diuretic dose, renal dialysis, or severe volume and/or salt depletion of any etiology. It may be advisable to eliminate the diuretic (except in patients with heart failure), reduce the diuretic dose or increase salt intake cautiously before initiating therapy with enalapril maleate in patients at risk for excessive hypotension who are able to tolerate such adjustments. (See DRUG INTERACTIONS and ADVERSE REACTIONS.) In patients at risk for excessive hypotension, therapy should be started under very close medical supervision and such patients should be followed closely for the first 2 weeks of treatment and whenever the dose of enalapril and/or diuretic is increased. Similar considerations may apply to patients with ischemic heart or cerebrovascular disease, in whom an excessive fall in blood pressure could result in a myocardial infarction or cerebrovascular accident.

If excessive hypotension occurs, the patient should be placed in the supine position and, if necessary, receive an intravenous infusion of normal saline. A transient hypotensive response is not a contraindication to further doses of enalapril maleate, which usually can be given without difficulty once the blood pressure has stabilized. If symptomatic hypotension develops, a dose reduction or discontinuation of enalapril maleate or concomitant diuretic may be necessary.

NEUTROPENIA/AGRANULOCYTOSIS
Another angiotensin converting enzyme inhibitor, captopril, has been shown to cause agranulocytosis and bone marrow depression, rarely in uncomplicated patients but more frequently in patients with renal impairment especially if they also have a collagen vascular disease. Available data from clinical trials of enalapril are insufficient to show that enalapril does not cause agranulocytosis at similar rates. Marketing experience has revealed cases of neutropenia or agranulocytosis in which a causal relationship to enalapril cannot be excluded. Periodic monitoring of white blood cell counts in patients with collagen vascular disease and renal disease should be considered.

HEPATIC FAILURE
Rarely, ACE inhibitors have been associated with a syndrome that starts with cholestatic jaundice and progresses to fulminant hepatic necrosis, and (sometimes) death. The mechanism of this syndrome is not understood. Patients receiving ACE inhibitors who develop jaundice or marked elevations of hepatic enzymes should discontinue the ACE inhibitor and receive appropriate medical follow-up.

FETAL/NEONATAL MORBIDITY AND MORTALITY
ACE inhibitors can cause fetal and neonatal morbidity and death when administered to pregnant women. Several dozen cases have been reported in the world literature. When pregnancy is detected, ACE inhibitors should be discontinued as soon as possible.

The use of ACE inhibitors during the second and third trimesters of pregnancy has been associated with fetal and neonatal injury, including hypotension, neonatal skull hypoplasia, anuria, reversible or irreversible renal failure, and death. Oligohydramnios has also been reported, presumably resulting from decreased fetal renal function; oligohydramnios in this setting has been associated with fetal limb contractures, craniofacial deformation, and hypoplastic lung development. Prematurity, intrauterine growth retardation, and patent ductus arteriosus have also been reported, although it is not clear whether these occurrences were due to the ACE-inhibitor exposure.

These adverse effects do not appear to have resulted from intrauterine ACE-inhibitor exposure that has been limited to the first trimester. Mothers whose embryos and fetuses are exposed to ACE inhibitors only during the first trimester should be so informed. Nonetheless, when patients become pregnant, physicians should make every effort to discontinue the use of enalapril maleate as soon as possible.

Rarely (probably less often than once in every thousand pregnancies), no alternative to ACE inhibitors will be found. In these rare cases, the mothers should be apprised of the potential hazards to their fetuses, and serial ultrasound examinations should be performed to assess the intraamniotic environment.

If oligohydramnios is observed, enalapril maleate should be discontinued unless it is considered lifesaving for the mother. Contraction stress testing (CST), a non-stress test (NST), or biophysical profiling (BPP) may be appropriate, depending upon the week of pregnancy. Patients and physicians should be aware, however, that oligohydramnios may not appear until after the fetus has sustained irreversible injury.

Infants with histories of *in utero* exposure to ACE inhibitors should be closely observed for hypotension, oliguria, and hyperkalemia. If oliguria occurs, attention should be directed toward support of blood pressure and renal perfusion. Exchange transfusion or dialysis may be required as means of reversing hypotension and/or substituting for disordered renal function. Enalapril, which crosses the placenta, has been removed from neonatal circulation by peritoneal dialysis with some clinical benefit, and theoretically may be removed by exchange transfusion, although there is no experience with the latter procedure.

No teratogenic effects of enalapril were seen in studies of pregnant rats and rabbits. On a body surface area basis, the doses used were 57 and 12 times, respectively, the maximum recommended human daily dose (MRHDD).

PRECAUTIONS

GENERAL

Aortic Stenosis/Hypertrophic Cardiomyopathy
As with all vasodilators, enalapril should be given with caution to patients with obstruction in the outflow tract of the left ventricle.

Impaired Renal Function
As a consequence of inhibiting the renin-angiotensin-aldosterone system, changes in renal function may be anticipated in susceptible individuals. In patients with severe heart failure whose renal function may depend on the activity of the renin-angiotensin-aldosterone system, treatment with angiotensin converting enzyme inhibitors, including enalapril maleate, may be associated with oliguria and/or progressive azotemia and rarely with acute renal failure and/or death.

In clinical studies in hypertensive patients with unilateral or bilateral renal artery stenosis, increases in blood urea nitrogen and serum creatinine were observed in 20% of patients. These increases were almost always reversible upon discontinuation of enalapril and/or diuretic therapy. In such patients renal function should be monitored during the first few weeks of therapy.

Some patients with hypertension or heart failure with no apparent pre-existing renal vascular disease have developed increases in blood urea and serum creatinine, usually minor and transient, especially when enalapril maleate has been given concomitantly with a diuretic. This is more likely to occur in patients with pre-existing renal impairment. Dosage reduction and/or discontinuation of the diuretic and/or enalapril maleate may be required.

Evaluation of patients with hypertension or heart failure should always include assessment of renal function. (See DOSAGE AND ADMINISTRATION.)

Hyperkalemia
Elevated serum potassium (greater than 5.7 mEq/L) was observed in approximately 1% of hypertensive patients in clinical trials. In most cases these were isolated values which resolved despite continued therapy. Hyperkalemia was a cause of discontinuation of therapy in 0.28% of hypertensive patients. In clinical trials in heart failure, hyperkalemia was observed in 3.8% of patients but was not a cause for discontinuation.

Risk factors for the development of hyperkalemia include renal insufficiency, diabetes mellitus, and the concomitant use of potassium-sparing diuretics, potassium supplements and/or potassium-containing salt substitutes, which should be used cautiously, if at all, with enalapril maleate. (See DRUG INTERACTIONS.)

Cough
Presumably due to the inhibition of the degradation of endogenous bradykinin, persistent nonproductive cough has been reported with all ACE inhibitors, always resolving after discontinuation of therapy. ACE inhibitor-induced cough should be considered in the differential diagnosis of cough.

Surgery/Anesthesia
In patients undergoing major surgery or during anesthesia with agents that produce hypotension, enalapril may block angiotensin 2 formation secondary to compensatory renin release. If hypotension occurs and is considered to be due to this mechanism, it can be corrected by volume expansion.

INFORMATION FOR THE PATIENT

Angioedema
Angioedema, including laryngeal edema, may occur at any time during treatment with angiotensin converting enzyme inhibitors, including enalapril. Patients should be so advised and told to report immediately any signs or symptoms suggesting angioedema (swelling of face, extremities, eyes, lips, tongue, difficulty in swallowing or breathing) and to take no more drug until they have consulted with the prescribing physician.

Hypotension
Patients should be cautioned to report lightheadedness, especially during the first few days of therapy. If actual syncope occurs, the patients should be told to discontinue the drug until they have consulted with the prescribing physician.

All patients should be cautioned that excessive perspiration and dehydration may lead to an excessive fall in blood pressure because of reduction in fluid volume. Other causes of volume depletion such as vomiting or diarrhea may also lead to a fall in blood pressure; patients should be advised to consult with the physician.

Hyperkalemia

Patients should be told not to use salt substitutes containing potassium without consulting their physician.

Neutropenia

Patients should be told to report promptly any indication of infection (*e.g.*, sore throat, fever) which may be a sign of neutropenia.

Pregnancy

Female patients of childbearing age should be told about the consequences of second- and third-trimester exposure to ACE inhibitors, and they should also be told that these consequences do not appear to have resulted from intrauterine ACE-inhibitor exposure that has been limited to the first trimester. These patients should be asked to report pregnancies to their physicians as soon as possible.

Note: As with many other drugs, certain advice to patients being treated with enalapril is warranted. This information is intended to aid in the safe and effective use of this medication. It is not a disclosure of all possible adverse or intended effects.

CARCINOGENESIS, MUTAGENESIS, AND IMPAIRMENT OF FERTILITY

There was no evidence of a tumorigenic effect when enalapril was administered for 106 weeks to male and female rats at doses up to 90 mg/kg/day or for 94 weeks to male and female mice at doses up to 90 and 180 mg/kg/day, respectively. These doses are 26 times (in rats and female mice) and 13 times (in male mice) the maximum recommended human daily dose (MRHDD) when compared on a body surface area basis.

Neither enalapril maleate nor the active diacid was mutagenic in the Ames microbial mutagen test with or without metabolic activation. Enalapril was also negative in the following genotoxicity studies: rec-assay, reverse mutation assay with *E. coli*, sister chromatid exchange with cultured mammalian cells, and the micronucleus test with mice, as well as in an *in vivo* cytogenic study using mouse bone marrow.

There were no adverse effects on reproductive performance of male and female rats treated with up to 90 mg/kg/day of enalapril (26 times the MRHDD when compared on a body surface area basis).

PREGNANCY CATEGORIES C (FIRST TRIMESTER) AND D (SECOND AND THIRD TRIMESTERS)

See WARNINGS, Fetal/Neonatal Morbidity and Mortality.

NURSING MOTHERS

Enalapril and enalaprilat have been detected in human breast milk. Because of the potential for serious adverse reactions in nursing infants from enalapril, a decision should be made whether to discontinue nursing or to discontinue enalapril maleate, taking into account the importance of the drug to the mother.

PEDIATRIC USE

Antihypertensive effects of enalapril maleate have been established in hypertensive pediatric patients age 1 month to 16 years. Use of enalapril maleate in these age groups is supported by evidence from adequate and well-controlled studies of enalapril maleate in pediatric and adult patients as well as by published literature in pediatric patients. (See CLINICAL PHARMACOLOGY, Clinical Pharmacology in Pediatric Patients; and DOSAGE AND ADMINISTRATION.)

Enalapril maleate is not recommended in neonates and in pediatric patients with glomerular filtration rate <30 ml/min/1.73 m^2, as no data are available.

DRUG INTERACTIONS

HYPOTENSION — PATIENTS ON DIURETIC THERAPY

Patients on diuretics and especially those in whom diuretic therapy was recently instituted, may occasionally experience an excessive reduction of blood pressure after initiation of therapy with enalapril. The possibility of hypotensive effects with enalapril can be minimized by either discontinuing the diuretic or increasing the salt intake prior to initiation of treatment with enalapril. If it is necessary to continue the diuretic, provide close medical supervision after the initial dose for at least 2 hours and until blood pressure has stabilized for at least an additional hour. (See WARNINGS and DOSAGE AND ADMINISTRATION.)

AGENTS CAUSING RENIN RELEASE

The antihypertensive effect of enalapril maleate is augmented by antihypertensive agents that cause renin release (*e.g.*, diuretics).

NON-STEROIDAL ANTI-INFLAMMATORY AGENTS

In some patients with compromised renal function who are being treated with non-steroidal anti-inflammatory drugs, the coadministration of enalapril may result in a further deterioration of renal function. These effects are usually reversible.

OTHER CARDIOVASCULAR AGENTS

Enalapril maleate has been used concomitantly with beta adrenergic-blocking agents, methyldopa, nitrates, calcium-blocking agents, hydralazine, prazosin, and digoxin without evidence of clinically significant adverse interactions.

AGENTS INCREASING SERUM POTASSIUM

Enalapril maleate attenuates potassium loss caused by thiazide-type diuretics. Potassium-sparing diuretics (*e.g.*, spironolactone, triamterene, or amiloride), potassium supplements, or potassium-containing salt substitutes may lead to significant increases in serum potassium. Therefore, if concomitant use of these agents is indicated because of demonstrated hypokalemia, they should be used with caution and with frequent monitoring of serum potassium. Potassium sparing agents should generally not be used in patients with heart failure receiving enalapril maleate.

LITHIUM

Lithium toxicity has been reported in patients receiving lithium concomitantly with drugs which cause elimination of sodium, including ACE inhibitors. A few cases of lithium toxicity have been reported in patients receiving concomitant enalapril maleate and lithium and were reversible upon discontinuation of both drugs. It is recommended that serum lithium levels be monitored frequently if enalapril is administered concomitantly with lithium.

ADVERSE REACTIONS

Enalapril maleate has been evaluated for safety in more than 10,000 patients, including over 1000 patients treated for 1 year or more. Enalapril maleate has been found to be generally well tolerated in controlled clinical trials involving 2987 patients.

For the most part, adverse experiences were mild and transient in nature. In clinical trials, discontinuation of therapy due to clinical adverse experiences was required in 3.3% of patients with hypertension and in 5.7% of patients with heart failure. The frequency of adverse experiences was not related to total daily dosage within the usual dosage ranges. In patients with hypertension the overall percentage of patients treated with enalapril maleate reporting adverse experiences was comparable to placebo.

HYPERTENSION

Adverse experiences occurring in greater than 1% of patients with hypertension treated with enalapril maleate in controlled clinical trials are shown in TABLE 2. In patients treated with enalapril maleate, the maximum duration of therapy was 3 years; in placebo treated patients the maximum duration of therapy was 12 weeks.

TABLE 2

	Enalapril Maleate Incidence (discontinuation) (n=2314)	Placebo Incidence (n=230)
Body as a Whole		
Fatigue	3.0% (<0.1%)	2.6%
Orthostatic effects	1.2% (<0.1%)	0.0%
Asthenia	1.1% (0.1%)	0.9%
Digestive		
Diarrhea	1.4% (<0.1%)	1.7%
Nausea	1.4% (0.2%)	1.7%
Nervous/Psychiatric		
Headache	5.2% (0.3%)	9.1%
Dizziness	4.3% (0.4%)	4.3%
Respiratory		
Cough	1.3% (0.1%)	0.9%
Skin		
Rash	1.4% (0.4%)	0.4%

HEART FAILURE

Adverse experiences occurring in greater than 1% of patients with heart failure treated with enalapril maleate are shown in TABLE 3. The incidences represent the experiences from both controlled and uncontrolled clinical trials (maximum duration of therapy was approximately 1 year). In the placebo treated patients, the incidences reported are from the controlled trials (maximum duration of therapy is 12 weeks). The percentage of patients with severe heart failure (NYHA Class IV) was 29% and 43% for patients treated with enalapril maleate and placebo, respectively.

TABLE 3

	Enalapril Maleate Incidence (discontinuation) (n=673)	Placebo Incidence (n=339)
Body as a Whole		
Orthostatic effects	2.2% (0.1%)	0.3%
Syncope	2.2% (0.1%)	0.9%
Chest pain	2.1% (0.0%)	2.1%
Fatigue	1.8% (0.0%)	1.8%
Abdominal pain	1.6% (0.4%)	2.1%
Asthenia	1.6% (0.1%)	0.3%
Cardiovascular		
Hypotension	6.7% (1.9%)	0.6%
Orthostatic hypotension	1.6% (0.1%)	0.3%
Angina pectoris	1.5% (0.1%)	1.8%
Myocardial infarction	1.2% (0.3%)	1.8%
Digestive		
Diarrhea	2.1% (0.1%)	1.2%
Nausea	1.3% (0.1%)	0.6%
Vomiting	1.3% (0.0%)	0.9%
Nervous/Psychiatric		
Dizziness	7.9% (0.6%)	0.6%
Headache	1.8% (0.1%)	0.9%
Vertigo	1.6% (0.1%)	1.2%
Respiratory		
Cough	2.2% (0.0%)	0.6%
Bronchitis	1.3% (0.0%)	0.9%
Dyspnea	1.3% (0.1%)	0.4%
Pneumonia	1.0% (0.0%)	2.4%
Skin		
Rash	1.3% (0.0%)	2.4%
Urogenital		
Urinary tract infection	1.3% (0.0%)	2.4%

Other serious clinical adverse experiences occurring since the drug was marketed or adverse experiences occurring in 0.5-1.0% of patients with hypertension or heart failure in clinical trials are listed below and, within each category, are in order of decreasing severity.

Body as a Whole: Anaphylactoid reactions (see WARNINGS, Anaphylactoid and Possibly Related Reactions).

Cardiovascular: Cardiac arrest; myocardial infarction or cerebrovascular accident, possibly secondary to excessive hypotension in high risk patients (see WARNINGS, Hypotension); pulmonary embolism and infarction; pulmonary edema; rhythm disturbances including atrial tachycardia and bradycardia; atrial fibrillation; palpitation, Raynaud's phenomenon.

Digestive: Ileus, pancreatitis, hepatic failure, hepatitis (hepatocellular [proven on rechallenge] or cholestatic jaundice) (see WARNINGS, Hepatic Failure), melena, anorexia, dyspepsia, constipation, glossitis, stomatitis, dry mouth.

Hematologic: Rare cases of neutropenia, thrombocytopenia and bone marrow depression.

Musculoskeletal: Muscle cramps.

Nervous/Psychiatric: Depression, confusion, ataxia, somnolence, insomnia, nervousness, peripheral neuropathy (*e.g.*, paresthesia, dysesthesia), dream abnormality.

Respiratory: Bronchospasm, rhinorrhea, sore throat and hoarseness, asthma, upper respiratory infection, pulmonary infiltrates, eosinophilic pneumonitis.

Skin: Exfoliative dermatitis, toxic epidermal necrolysis, Stevens-Johnson syndrome, pemphigus, herpes zoster, erythema multiforme, urticaria, pruritus, alopecia, flushing, diaphoresis, photosensitivity.

Special Senses: Blurred vision, taste alteration, anosmia, tinnitus, conjunctivitis, dry eyes, tearing.

Urogenital: Renal failure, oliguria, renal dysfunction (see PRECAUTIONS and DOSAGE AND ADMINISTRATION), flank pain, gynecomastia, impotence.

Miscellaneous: *A symptom complex has been reported which may include some or all of the following:* A positive ANA, an elevated erythrocyte sedimentation rate, arthralgia/arthritis, myalgia/myositis, fever, serositis, vasculitis, leukocytosis, eosinophilia, photosensitivity, rash and other dermatologic manifestations.

ANGIOEDEMA

Angioedema has been reported in patients receiving enalapril maleate, with an incidence higher in black than in non-black patients. Angioedema associated with laryngeal edema may be fatal. If angioedema of the face, extremities, lips, tongue, glottis and/or larynx occurs, treatment with enalapril maleate should be discontinued and appropriate therapy instituted immediately. (See WARNINGS.)

HYPOTENSION

In the hypertensive patients, hypotension occurred in 0.9% and syncope occurred in 0.5% of patients following the initial dose or during extended therapy. Hypotension or syncope was a cause for discontinuation of therapy in 0.1% of hypertensive patients. In heart failure patients, hypotension occurred in 6.7% and syncope occurred in 2.2% of patients. Hypotension or syncope was a cause for discontinuation of therapy in 1.9% of patients with heart failure. (See WARNINGS.)

FETAL/NEONATAL MORBIDITY AND MORTALITY

See WARNINGS, Fetal/Neonatal Morbidity and Mortality.

COUGH

See PRECAUTIONS, General, Cough.

PEDIATRIC PATIENTS

The adverse experience profile for pediatric patients appear to be similar to that seen in adult patients.

CLINICAL LABORATORY TEST FINDINGS

Serum Electrolytes

Hyperkalemia (see PRECAUTIONS), hyponatremia.

Creatinine, Blood Urea Nitrogen

In controlled clinical trials minor increases in blood urea nitrogen and serum creatinine, reversible upon discontinuation of therapy, were observed in about 0.2% of patients with essential hypertension treated with enalapril maleate alone. Increases are more likely to occur in patients receiving concomitant diuretics or in patients with renal artery stenosis. (See PRECAUTIONS.) In patients with heart failure who were also receiving diuretics with or without digitalis, increases in blood urea nitrogen or serum creatinine, usually reversible upon discontinuation of enalapril maleate and/or other concomitant diuretic therapy, were observed in about 11% of patients. Increases in blood urea nitrogen or creatinine were a cause for discontinuation in 1.2% of patients.

Hematology

Small decreases in hemoglobin and hematocrit (mean decreases of approximately 0.3 g percent and 1.0 vol percent, respectively) occur frequently in either hypertension or congestive heart failure patients treated with enalapril maleate but are rarely of clinical importance unless another cause of anemia coexists. In clinical trials, less than 0.1% of patients discontinued therapy due to anemia. Hemolytic anemia, including cases of hemolysis in patients with G-6-PD deficiency, has been reported; a causal relationship to enalapril cannot be excluded.

Liver Function Tests

Elevations of liver enzymes and/or serum bilirubin have occurred (see WARNINGS, Hepatic Failure).

DOSAGE AND ADMINISTRATION

HYPERTENSION

In patients who are currently being treated with a diuretic, symptomatic hypotension occasionally may occur following the initial dose of enalapril maleate. The diuretic should, if possible, be discontinued for 2-3 days before beginning therapy with enalapril maleate to reduce the likelihood of hypotension. (See WARNINGS.) If the patient's blood pressure is not controlled with enalapril maleate alone, diuretic therapy may be resumed.

If the diuretic cannot be discontinued an initial dose of 2.5 mg should be used under medical supervision for at least 2 hours and until blood pressure has stabilized for at least an additional hour. (See WARNINGS and DRUG INTERACTIONS.)

The recommended initial dose in patients not on diuretics is 5 mg once a day. Dosage should be adjusted according to blood pressure response. The usual dosage range is 10-40 mg/day administered in a single dose or 2 divided doses. In some patients treated once daily, the antihypertensive effect may diminish toward the end of the dosing interval. In such patients, an increase in dosage or twice daily administration should be considered. If blood pressure is not controlled with enalapril maleate alone, a diuretic may be added.

Concomitant administration of enalapril maleate with potassium supplements, potassium salt substitutes, or potassium-sparing diuretics may lead to increases of serum potassium (see PRECAUTIONS).

DOSAGE ADJUSTMENT IN HYPERTENSIVE PATIENTS WITH RENAL IMPAIRMENT

The usual dose of enalapril is recommended for patients with a creatinine clearance >30 ml/min (serum creatinine of up to approximately 3 mg/dl). For patients with creatinine clearance ≤30 ml/min (serum creatinine ≥3 mg/dl), the first dose is 2.5 mg once daily. The dosage may be titrated upward until blood pressure is controlled or to a maximum of 40 mg daily (see TABLE 4).

TABLE 4

Renal Status	Creatinine-Clearance	Initial Dose (mg/day)
Normal renal function	>80 ml/min	5 mg
Mild impairment	≤80 >30 ml/min	5 mg
Moderate to severe impairment	≤30 ml/min	2.5 mg
Dialysis patients*	—	2.5 mg on dialysis days†

* See WARNINGS, Anaphylactoid and Possibly Related Reactions, Anaphylactoid Reactions During Membrane Exposure.
† Dosage on nondialysis days should be adjusted depending on the blood pressure response.

HEART FAILURE

Enalapril maleate is indicated for the treatment of symptomatic heart failure, usually in combination with diuretics and digitalis. In the placebo-controlled studies that demonstrated improved survival, patients were titrated as tolerated up to 40 mg, administered in 2 divided doses.

The recommended initial dose is 2.5 mg. The recommended dosing range is 2.5-20 mg given twice a day. Doses should be titrated upward, as tolerated, over a period of a few days or weeks. The maximum daily dose administered in clinical trials was 40 mg in divided doses.

After the initial dose of enalapril maleate, the patient should be observed under medical supervision for at least 2 hours and until blood pressure has stabilized for at least an additional hour. (See WARNINGS and DRUG INTERACTIONS.) If possible, the dose of any concomitant diuretic should be reduced which may diminish the likelihood of hypotension. The appearance of hypotension after the initial dose of enalapril maleate does not preclude subsequent careful dose titration with the drug, following effective management of the hypotension.

ASYMPTOMATIC LEFT VENTRICULAR DYSFUNCTION

In the trial that demonstrated efficacy, patients were started on 2.5 mg twice daily and were titrated as tolerated to the targeted daily dose of 20 mg (in divided doses).

After the initial dose of enalapril maleate, the patient should be observed under medical supervision for at least 2 hours and until blood pressure has stabilized for at least an additional hour. (See WARNINGS and DRUG INTERACTIONS.) If possible, the dose of any concomitant diuretic should be reduced which may diminish the likelihood of hypotension. The appearance of hypotension after the initial dose of enalapril maleate does not preclude subsequent careful dose titration with the drug, following effective management of the hypotension.

DOSAGE ADJUSTMENT IN PATIENTS WITH HEART FAILURE AND RENAL IMPAIRMENT OR HYPONATREMIA

In patients with heart failure who have hyponatremia (serum sodium less than 130 mEq/L) or with serum creatinine greater than 1.6 mg/dl, therapy should be initiated at 2.5 mg daily under close medical supervision. (See Heart Failure; WARNINGS; and DRUG INTERACTIONS.) The dose may be increased to 2.5 mg bid, then 5 mg bid and higher as needed, usually at intervals of 4 days or more if at the time of dosage adjustment there is not excessive hypotension or significant deterioration of renal function. The maximum daily dose is 40 mg.

PEDIATRIC HYPERTENSIVE PATIENTS

The usual recommended starting dose is 0.08 mg/kg (up to 5 mg) once daily. Dosage should be adjusted according to blood pressure response. Doses above 0.58 mg/kg (or in excess of 40 mg) have not been studied in pediatric patients.

See CLINICAL PHARMACOLOGY, Clinical Pharmacology in Pediatric Patients.

Enalapril maleate is not recommended in neonates and in pediatric patients with glomerular filtration rate <30 ml/min/1.73 m^2, as no data are available.

PREPARATION OF SUSPENSION (FOR 200 ML OF A 1.0 MG/ML SUSPENSION)

Add 50 ml of Bicitra to a polyethylene terephthalate (PET) bottle containing ten 20 mg tablets of enalapril maleate and shake for at least 2 minutes. Let concentrate stand for 60 minutes. Following the 60 minute hold time, shake the concentrate for an additional minute. Add 150 ml of Ora-Sweet SF to the concentrate in the PET bottle and shake the suspension to disperse the ingredients. The suspension should be refrigerated at 2-8°C (36-46°F) and can be stored for up to 30 days. Shake the suspension before each use.

HOW SUPPLIED

Vasotec tablets are available as follows:

2.5 mg: Yellow, biconvex barrel shaped, scored, compressed tablets with code "MSD 14" on one side and "VASOTEC" on the other.

5 mg: White, barrel shaped, scored, compressed tablets, with code "MSD 712" on one side and "VASOTEC" on the other.

10 mg: Salmon, barrel shaped, compressed tablets, with code "MSD 713" on one side and "VASOTEC" on the other.

20 mg: Peach, barrel shaped, compressed tablets, with code "MSD 714" on one side and "VASOTEC" on the other.

STORAGE

Store below 30°C (86°F) and avoid transient temperatures above 50°C (122°F). Keep container tightly closed. Protect from moisture.

Dispense in a tight container, if product package is subdivided.

PRODUCT LISTING - RATED THERAPEUTICALLY EQUIVALENT

Solution - Intravenous - 1.25 mg/ml

1 ml	$3.84	GENERIC, Abbott Pharmaceutical	00074-2122-01
1 ml	$5.64	GENERIC, Baxter Pharmaceutical Products, Inc	10019-0095-03
1 ml	$5.88	GENERIC, Baxter Pharmaceutical Products, Inc	10019-0092-03
1 ml	$15.30	GENERIC, Faulding Pharmaceutical Company	61703-0237-44
1 ml	$16.68	VASOTEC, Merck & Company Inc	00006-3824-01
1 ml x 10	$37.50	GENERIC, Bedford Laboratories	55390-0010-10
1 ml x 10	$47.38	GENERIC, Abbott Pharmaceutical	00074-2109-31
2 ml	$7.68	GENERIC, Abbott Pharmaceutical	00074-2122-02
2 ml	$11.28	GENERIC, Baxter Pharmaceutical Products, Inc	10019-0095-04
2 ml	$11.75	GENERIC, Baxter Pharmaceutical Products, Inc	10019-0092-04
2 ml	$30.65	GENERIC, Faulding Pharmaceutical Company	61703-0237-16
2 ml	$33.43	VASOTEC, Merck & Company Inc	00006-3508-04
2 ml	$33.43	VASOTEC, Merck & Company Inc	00006-3824-04
2 ml x 10	$75.00	GENERIC, Bedford Laboratories	55390-0011-10

Tablet - Oral - 2.5 mg

12 x 90	$1011.69	VASOTEC, Merck & Company Inc	00006-0014-94
30's	$28.20	VASOTEC, Allscripts Pharmaceutical Company	54569-3258-01
30's	$30.47	VASOTEC, Physicians Total Care	54868-2280-00
60's	$59.73	VASOTEC, Physicians Total Care	54868-2280-02
90's	$84.31	VASOTEC, Biovail Pharmaceuticals Inc	64455-0140-90
100's	$76.86	GENERIC, Ivax Corporation	00172-4195-60
100's	$78.86	GENERIC, Ivax Corporation	00172-4195-10
100's	$79.04	GENERIC, Ranbaxy Laboratories	63304-0522-01
100's	$80.28	GENERIC, Geneva Pharmaceuticals	00781-1229-01
100's	$80.30	GENERIC, Mylan Pharmaceuticals Inc	00378-1051-01
100's	$80.30	GENERIC, Udl Laboratories Inc	51079-0950-20
100's	$80.35	GENERIC, Watson/Rugby Laboratories Inc	00364-2698-01
100's	$80.35	GENERIC, Watson/Schein Pharmaceuticals Inc	00591-0668-01
100's	$80.35	GENERIC, Par Pharmaceutical Inc	49884-0591-01
100's	$80.35	GENERIC, Watson Laboratories Inc	52544-0668-01
100's	$80.36	GENERIC, Purepac Pharmaceutical Company	00228-2658-11
100's	$80.37	GENERIC, Teva Pharmaceuticals Usa	00093-0026-01
100's	$80.37	GENERIC, Eon Labs Manufacturing Inc	00185-0114-01
100's	$80.90	GENERIC, Taro Pharmaceuticals U.S.A. Inc	51672-4037-01
100's	$84.51	GENERIC, Geneva Pharmaceuticals	00781-1229-13
100's	$93.68	VASOTEC, Merck & Company Inc	00006-0014-68

Tablet - Oral - 5 mg

3's	$7.84	VASOTEC, Pd-Rx Pharmaceuticals	55289-0622-03
10's	$11.82	VASOTEC, Allscripts Pharmaceutical Company	54569-0606-03
12 x 90	$1285.33	VASOTEC, Merck & Company Inc	00006-0712-94
30's	$30.10	VASOTEC, Compumed Pharmaceuticals	00403-2241-30
30's	$33.00	VASOTEC, Southwood Pharmaceuticals Inc	58016-0572-30
30's	$33.78	VASOTEC, Physicians Total Care	54868-1090-05
30's	$35.46	VASOTEC, Allscripts Pharmaceutical Company	54569-0606-00
30's	$42.15	VASOTEC, Pd-Rx Pharmaceuticals	55289-0622-30
60's	$61.12	VASOTEC, Allscripts Pharmaceutical Company	54569-0606-02
60's	$66.00	VASOTEC, Southwood Pharmaceuticals Inc	58016-0572-60
60's	$66.36	VASOTEC, Physicians Total Care	54868-1090-06
90's	$99.00	VASOTEC, Southwood Pharmaceuticals Inc	58016-0572-90
90's	$107.11	VASOTEC, Biovail Pharmaceuticals Inc	64455-0141-90
100's	$88.00	VASOTEC, Compumed Pharmaceuticals	00403-2241-01
100's	$97.64	GENERIC, Ivax Corporation	00172-4196-60
100's	$99.40	GENERIC, Major Pharmaceuticals Inc	00904-5502-60
100's	$99.64	GENERIC, Ivax Corporation	00172-4196-10
100's	$100.41	GENERIC, Ranbaxy Laboratories	63304-0523-01
100's	$102.00	GENERIC, Mylan Pharmaceuticals Inc	00378-1052-01
100's	$102.00	GENERIC, Geneva Pharmaceuticals	00781-1231-01
100's	$102.00	GENERIC, Udl Laboratories Inc	51079-0951-20
100's	$102.10	GENERIC, Purepac Pharmaceutical Company	00228-2659-11
100's	$102.10	GENERIC, Par Pharmaceutical Inc	49884-0592-01
100's	$102.10	GENERIC, Watson Laboratories Inc	52544-0669-01
100's	$102.11	GENERIC, Teva Pharmaceuticals Usa	00093-0027-01
100's	$102.11	GENERIC, Eon Labs Manufacturing Inc	00185-0127-01
100's	$102.72	GENERIC, Taro Pharmaceuticals U.S.A. Inc	51672-4038-01
100's	$106.25	GENERIC, Geneva Pharmaceuticals	00781-1231-13
100's	$109.25	VASOTEC, Physicians Total Care	54868-1090-01
100's	$110.00	VASOTEC, Southwood Pharmaceuticals Inc	58016-0572-00
100's	$118.19	VASOTEC, Allscripts Pharmaceutical Company	54569-0606-01
100's	$119.01	VASOTEC, Merck & Company Inc	00006-0712-68

Tablet - Oral - 10 mg

12 x 90	$1349.45	VASOTEC, Merck & Company Inc	00006-0713-94
30's	$34.80	VASOTEC, Southwood Pharmaceuticals Inc	58016-0569-30
30's	$37.16	VASOTEC, Allscripts Pharmaceutical Company	54569-0607-00
30's	$40.95	VASOTEC, Physicians Total Care	54868-0620-01
30's	$42.15	VASOTEC, Pd-Rx Pharmaceuticals	55289-0483-30
60's	$64.17	VASOTEC, Allscripts Pharmaceutical Company	54569-0607-03
60's	$69.60	VASOTEC, Southwood Pharmaceuticals Inc	58016-0569-60
60's	$80.70	VASOTEC, Physicians Total Care	54868-0620-05
90's	$104.40	VASOTEC, Southwood Pharmaceuticals Inc	58016-0569-90
90's	$112.45	VASOTEC, Biovail Pharmaceuticals Inc	64455-0142-90
100's	$102.52	GENERIC, Ivax Corporation	00172-4197-60
100's	$104.37	GENERIC, Major Pharmaceuticals Inc	00904-5503-60
100's	$104.52	GENERIC, Ivax Corporation	00172-4197-10
100's	$105.42	GENERIC, Ranbaxy Laboratories	63304-0524-01
100's	$107.10	GENERIC, Mylan Pharmaceuticals Inc	00378-1053-01
100's	$107.10	GENERIC, Geneva Pharmaceuticals	00781-1232-01
100's	$107.10	GENERIC, Udl Laboratories Inc	51079-0952-20
100's	$107.20	GENERIC, Watson/Schein Pharmaceuticals Inc	00591-0670-01
100's	$107.20	GENERIC, Par Pharmaceutical Inc	49884-0593-01
100's	$107.20	GENERIC, Watson Laboratories Inc	52544-0670-01
100's	$107.21	GENERIC, Teva Pharmaceuticals Usa	00093-0028-01
100's	$107.21	GENERIC, Purepac Pharmaceutical Company	00228-2660-11
100's	$107.22	GENERIC, Eon Labs Manufacturing Inc	00185-0147-01
100's	$107.85	GENERIC, Taro Pharmaceuticals U.S.A. Inc	51672-4039-01
100's	$111.34	GENERIC, Geneva Pharmaceuticals	00781-1232-13
100's	$114.67	VASOTEC, Physicians Total Care	54868-0620-03
100's	$116.00	VASOTEC, Southwood Pharmaceuticals Inc	58016-0569-00
100's	$123.85	VASOTEC, Allscripts Pharmaceutical Company	54569-0607-01
100's	$124.95	VASOTEC, Merck & Company Inc	00006-0713-68

Tablet - Oral - 20 mg

12 x 90	$1920.10	VASOTEC, Merck & Company Inc	00006-0714-94
30's	$49.50	VASOTEC, Southwood Pharmaceuticals Inc	58016-0571-30
30's	$49.86	VASOTEC, Physicians Total Care	54868-0541-01
30's	$52.27	VASOTEC, Allscripts Pharmaceutical Company	54569-0612-00
60's	$98.55	VASOTEC, Physicians Total Care	54868-0541-03
60's	$99.00	VASOTEC, Southwood Pharmaceuticals Inc	58016-0571-60
90's	$148.50	VASOTEC, Southwood Pharmaceuticals Inc	58016-0571-90
100's	$145.87	GENERIC, Ivax Corporation	00172-4198-60
100's	$147.87	GENERIC, Ivax Corporation	00172-4198-10
100's	$149.99	GENERIC, Ranbaxy Laboratories	63304-0525-01
100's	$152.37	GENERIC, Geneva Pharmaceuticals	00781-1233-01
100's	$152.40	GENERIC, Mylan Pharmaceuticals Inc	00378-1054-01
100's	$152.40	GENERIC, Udl Laboratories Inc	51079-0953-20
100's	$152.50	GENERIC, Par Pharmaceutical Inc	49884-0594-01
100's	$152.50	GENERIC, Watson Laboratories Inc	52544-0671-01
100's	$152.53	GENERIC, Purepac Pharmaceutical Company	00228-2661-11
100's	$152.54	GENERIC, Teva Pharmaceuticals Usa	00093-0029-01
100's	$152.54	GENERIC, Eon Labs Manufacturing Inc	00185-0214-01
100's	$153.37	GENERIC, Taro Pharmaceuticals U.S.A. Inc	51672-4040-01
100's	$165.00	VASOTEC, Southwood Pharmaceuticals Inc	58016-0571-00
100's	$177.79	VASOTEC, Merck & Company Inc	00006-0714-68
100's	$178.49	GENERIC, Major Pharmaceuticals Inc	00904-5504-60

PRODUCT LISTING - EQUIVALENTS NOT AVAILABLE

Tablet - Oral - 5 mg

100's	$102.10	GENERIC, Watson/Rugby Laboratories Inc	00364-2701-01
100's	$102.10	GENERIC, Watson/Schein Pharmaceuticals Inc	00591-0669-01

Tablet - Oral - 10 mg

100's	$107.20	GENERIC, Watson/Rugby Laboratories Inc	00364-2727-01

Tablet - Oral - 20 mg

90's	$160.01	VASOTEC, Biovail Pharmaceuticals Inc	64455-0143-90
100's	$152.50	GENERIC, Watson/Rugby Laboratories Inc	00364-2734-01
100's	$152.50	GENERIC, Watson/Schein Pharmaceuticals Inc	00591-0671-01

Enalapril Maleate; Felodipine *(003325)*

For complete prescribing information, refer to the CD-ROM included with the book.

Categories: Hypertension, essential; Pregnancy Category C, 1st Trimester; Pregnancy Category D, 2nd & 3rd Trimesters; FDA Approved 1996 Dec
Drug Classes: Angiotensin converting enzyme inhibitors; Calcium channel blockers
Brand Names: Lexxel
Cost of Therapy: $46.69 (Hypertension; Lexxel; 5 mg; 2.5 mg; 1 tablet/day; 30 day supply)

E

WARNING

Note: The trade name has been used throughout this monograph for clarity.

USE IN PREGNANCY

When used in pregnancy during the second and third trimesters, ACE inhibitors can cause injury and even death to the developing fetus. When pregnancy is detected, Lexxel should be discontinued as soon as possible. See WARNINGS, Fetal/Neonatal Morbidity and Mortality.

DESCRIPTION

Lexxel (enalapril maleate-felodipine ER) is a combination product, consisting of an outer layer of enalapril maleate surrounding a core tablet of an extended-release felodipine formulation.

Enalapril maleate is the maleate salt of enalapril, the ethyl ester of a long-acting angiotensin converting enzyme inhibitor, enalaprilat. Enalapril maleate is chemically described as (S)-1-[N-[1-(ethoxycarbonyl)-3-phenylpropyl]-L-alanyl]-L-proline, (Z)-2-butenedioate salt (1:1). Its empirical formula is $C_{20}H_{28}N_2O_5 \cdot C_4H_4O_4$.

Enalapril maleate is a white to off-white, crystalline powder with a molecular weight of 492.53. It is sparingly soluble in water, soluble in ethanol, and freely soluble in methanol.

Felodipine, a calcium channel blocker, is a dihydropyridine derivative that is chemically described as ± ethyl methyl 4-(2,3-dichlorophenyl)-1,4-dihydro-2,6-dimethyl-3,5-pyridinedicarboxylate. Its empirical formula is $C_{18}H_{19}Cl_2NO_4$.

Felodipine is a slightly yellowish, crystalline powder with a molecular weight of 384.26. It is insoluble in water and is freely soluble in dichloromethane and ethanol. Felodipine is a racemic mixture; however, S-felodipine is the more biologically active enantiomer.

Lexxel is available for oral use in two tablet combinations of enalapril maleate with felodipine as an extended-release formulation: Lexxel 5-2.5, containing 5 mg of enalapril maleate and 2.5 mg of felodipine ER and Lexxel 5-5, containing 5 mg of enalapril maleate and 5 mg of felodipine ER.

Inactive ingredients include: Propyl gallate, polyoxyl 40 hydrogenated castor oil, cellulose compounds, lactose, aluminum silicate, sodium stearyl fumarate, carnauba wax, and iron oxides.

The tablets are imprinted with an ink of synthetic red iron oxide (Lexxel 5-2.5) or synthetic black iron oxide (Lexxel 5-5) which contains pharmaceutical glaze in SD-45, n-butyl alcohol, propylene glycol, isopropyl alcohol, ammonium hydroxide, and simethicone (Lexxel 5-2.5) and methyl alcohol (Lexxel 5-5).

INDICATIONS AND USAGE

Lexxel is indicated for the treatment of hypertension.

This fixed combination drug is not indicated for the initial therapy of hypertension. (See DOSAGE AND ADMINISTRATION.)

In using Lexxel, consideration should be given to the fact that another angiotensin converting enzyme inhibitor, captopril, has caused agranulocytosis, particularly in patients with renal impairment or collagen vascular disease, and that available data are insufficient to show that enalapril (a component of Lexxel) does not have a similar risk. (See WARNINGS, Neutropenia/Agranulocytosis.)

In considering use of Lexxel, it should be noted that black patients receiving ACE inhibitors have been reported to have a higher incidence of angioedema compared to nonblacks. (See WARNINGS, Anaphylactoid and Possibly Related Reactions, Angioedema.)

CONTRAINDICATIONS

Lexxel is contraindicated in patients who are hypersensitive to any component of this product. Because of the enalapril component, Lexxel is contraindicated in patients with a history of angioedema related to previous treatment with an angiotensin converting enzyme inhibitor and in patients with hereditary or idiopathic angioedema.

WARNINGS

ANAPHYLACTOID AND POSSIBLY RELATED REACTIONS

Presumably because angiotensin-converting enzyme inhibitors affect the metabolism of eicosanoids and polypeptides, including endogenous bradykinin, patients receiving ACE inhibitors (including Lexxel) may be subject to a variety of adverse reactions, some of them serious.

Angioedema

Angioedema of the face, extremities, lips, tongue, glottis, and/or larynx has been reported in patients treated with angiotensin converting enzyme inhibitors, including enalapril. This may occur at any time during treatment. In such cases Lexxel should be promptly discontinued, and appropriate therapy and monitoring should be provided until complete and sustained resolution of signs and symptoms has occurred. In instances where swelling has been confined to the face and lips the condition has generally resolved without treatment, although antihistamines have been useful in relieving symptoms. Angioedema associated with laryngeal edema may be fatal. **Where there is involvement of the tongue, glottis or larynx, likely to cause airway obstruction, appropriate therapy, *e.g.*, subcutaneous epinephrine solution 1:1000 (0.3-0.5 ml) and/or measures necessary to ensure a patent airway, should be promptly provided.**

Patients with a history of angioedema unrelated to ACE inhibitor therapy may be at increased risk of angioedema while receiving an ACE inhibitor (see also INDICATIONS AND USAGE and CONTRAINDICATIONS).

Anaphylactoid Reactions During Desensitization

Two patients undergoing desensitizing treatment with hymenoptera venom while receiving ACE inhibitors sustained life-threatening anaphylactoid reactions. In the same patients, these reactions were avoided when ACE inhibitors were temporarily withheld, but they reappeared upon inadvertent rechallenge.

Anaphylactoid Reactions During Membrane Exposure

Anaphylactoid reactions have been reported in patients dialyzed with high-flux membranes and treated concomitantly with an ACE inhibitor. Anaphylactoid reactions have also been reported in patients undergoing low-density lipoprotein apheresis with dextran sulfate absorption.

HYPOTENSION

Lexxel can occasionally cause symptomatic hypotension.

Excessive hypotension is rare in uncomplicated hypertensive patients treated with enalapril alone. Patients at risk for excessive hypotension, sometimes associated with oliguria and/or progressive azotemia, and rarely with acute renal failure and/or death, include those with the following conditions or characteristics: heart failure, hyponatremia, high dose diuretic therapy, recent intensive diuresis or increase in diuretic dose, renal dialysis, or severe volume and/or salt depletion of any etiology. It may be advisable to eliminate the diuretic (except in patients with heart failure), reduce the diuretic dose or increase salt intake cautiously before initiating therapy with enalapril maleate in patients at risk for excessive hypotension who are able to tolerate such adjustments. In patients at risk for excessive hypotension, therapy should be started under very close medical supervision and such patients should be followed closely for the first 2 weeks of treatment and whenever the dose of enalapril and/or diuretic is increased. Similar considerations may apply to patients with ischemic heart or cerebrovascular disease, in whom an excessive fall in blood pressure could result in a myocardial infarction or cerebrovascular accident.

If excessive hypotension occurs, the patient should be placed in the supine position and, if necessary, receive an intravenous infusion of normal saline. A transient hypotensive response is not a contraindication to further doses of enalapril maleate, which usually can be given without difficulty once the blood pressure has stabilized. If symptomatic hypotension develops, a dose reduction or discontinuation of enalapril or diuretic may be necessary.

Felodipine, like other calcium channel blockers, may occasionally precipitate significant hypotension and rarely syncope. It may lead to reflex tachycardia which in susceptible individuals may precipitate angina pectoris.

NEUTROPENIA/AGRANULOCYTOSIS

Another angiotensin converting enzyme inhibitor, captopril, has been shown to cause agranulocytosis and bone marrow depression, rarely in uncomplicated patients but more frequently in patients with renal impairment, especially if they also have a collagen vascular disease. Available data from clinical trials of enalapril are insufficient to show that enalapril does not cause agranulocytosis at similar rates. Marketing experience has revealed cases of neutropenia or agranulocytosis in which a causal relationship to enalapril cannot be excluded. Periodic monitoring of white blood cell counts in patients with collagen vascular disease and renal disease should be considered.

HEPATIC FAILURE

Rarely, ACE inhibitors have been associated with a syndrome that starts with cholestatic jaundice and progresses to fulminant hepatic necrosis and (sometimes) death.

The mechanism of this syndrome is not understood. Patients receiving ACE inhibitors who develop jaundice or marked elevations of hepatic enzymes should discontinue the ACE inhibitor and receive appropriate medical follow-up.

FETAL/NEONATAL MORBIDITY AND MORTALITY

ACE inhibitors can cause fetal and neonatal morbidity and death when administered to pregnant women. Several dozen cases have been reported in the world literature. When pregnancy is detected, Lexxel should be discontinued as soon as possible.

The use of ACE inhibitors during the second and third trimesters of pregnancy has been associated with fetal and neonatal injury, including hypotension, neonatal skull hypoplasia, anuria, reversible or irreversible renal failure, and death. Oligohydramnios has also been reported, presumably resulting from decreased fetal renal function; oligohydramnios in this setting has been associated with fetal limb contractures, craniofacial deformation, and hypoplastic lung development. Prematurity, intrauterine growth retardation, and patent ductus arteriosus have also been reported, although it is not clear whether these occurrences were due to the ACE-inhibitor exposure.

These adverse effects do not appear to have resulted from intrauterine ACE-inhibitor exposure that has been limited to the first trimester. Mothers whose embryos and fetuses are exposed to ACE inhibitors only during the first trimester should be so informed. Nonetheless, when patients become pregnant, physicians should make every effort to discontinue the use of Lexxel as soon as possible.

Rarely (probably less often than once in every thousand pregnancies), no alternative to ACE inhibitors will be found. In these rare cases, the mothers should be apprised of the potential hazards to their fetuses, and serial ultrasound examinations should be performed to assess the intra-amniotic environment.

If oligohydramnios is observed, Lexxel should be discontinued unless it is considered lifesaving for the mother. Contraction stress testing (CST), a non-stress test (NST), or biophysical profiling (BPP) may be appropriate, depending upon the week of pregnancy. Patients and physicians should be aware, however, that oligohydramnios may not appear until after the fetus has sustained irreversible injury.

Infants with histories of *in utero* exposure to ACE inhibitors should be closely observed for hypotension, oliguria, and hyperkalemia. If oliguria occurs, attention should be directed toward support of blood pressure and renal perfusion. Exchange transfusion or dialysis may be required as means of reversing hypotension and/or substituting for disordered renal function. Enalapril, which crosses the placenta, has been removed from neonatal circulation by peritoneal dialysis with some clinical benefit, and theoretically may be removed by exchange transfusion, although there is no experience with the latter procedure.

No teratogenic effects of enalapril were seen in studies of pregnant rats and rabbits. On a body surface area basis, the doses used were 57 times and 12 times, respectively, the maximum recommended human daily dose (MRHDD).

In rats administered the combination of enalapril and felodipine (enalapril [E]=1.9; felodipine [F]=2.5 mg/kg/day), an increased incidence of fetuses with dilated renal pelvis/ureter was observed.

However, there was no evidence of this effect in the offspring postweaning. In mice, with doses of E=23, F=30 mg/kg/day or greater, there was an increased incidence of both early and late *in utero* deaths. Other than a transient and slight decrease in body weight gain in the first generation offspring, there were no adverse effects in offspring with regard to sexual maturation, behavioral development, fertility or fecundity.

Enalapril-felodipine given to pregnant mice (enalapril 20.8, felodipine 27 mg/kg/day) and rats (enalapril = 17.3, felodipine = 22.5 mg/kg/day) produced plasma levels (C_{max} and AUC values) of enalapril/enalaprilat that were 76- to 418-fold greater and plasma levels of felodipine that were 151- to 433-fold greater than those expected in humans (non-pregnant) at the dose to be used in humans.

DOSAGE AND ADMINISTRATION

Lexxel is an effective treatment for hypertension. This fixed combination drug is not indicated for initial therapy of hypertension.

The recommended initial dose of enalapril maleate for hypertension in patients not receiving diuretics is 5 mg once a day. The usual dosage range of enalapril maleate for hypertension is 10-40 mg/day administered in a single dose or two divided doses. In some patients treated once daily with enalapril, the antihypertensive effect may diminish toward the end of the dosing interval. In such patients, an increase in dosage or twice daily administration should be considered. The recommended initial dose of felodipine ER is 5 mg once a day with a usual dosage range of 2.5-10 mg once a day. In elderly or hepatically impaired patients, the recommended initial dose of felodipine is 2.5 mg. When Lexxel is taken with food, the peak concentration of felodipine is almost doubled, and the trough (24 hour) concentration is approximately halved.

In clinical trials of enalapril-felodipine ER combination therapy using enalapril doses of 5-20 mg and felodipine ER doses of 2.5-10 mg once daily, the antihypertensive effects increased with increasing doses of each component in all patient groups.

The hazards (see WARNINGS) of enalapril are generally independent of dose; those of felodipine are a mixture of dose-dependent phenomena (primarily peripheral edema) and dose-independent phenomena, the former much more common than the latter. Therapy with any combination of enalapril and felodipine will thus be associated with both sets of dose-independent hazards.

Rarely, the dose-independent hazards associated with enalapril or felodipine are serious. To minimize dose-independent hazards, it is usually appropriate to begin therapy with Lexxel only after a patient has failed to achieve the desired antihypertensive effect with one or the other monotherapy.

Replacement therapy: Although the felodipine component of Lexxel has not been shown to be bioequivalent to the available extended-release felodipine (Plendil), patients receiving enalapril and felodipine from separate tablets once a day may instead wish to receive the tablets of Lexxel containing the same component doses.

Therapy guided by clinical effect: A patient whose blood pressure is not adequately controlled with felodipine (or another dihydropyridine) or enalapril (or another ACE inhibitor) alone may be switched to combination therapy with Lexxel, initially 1 tablet daily, usually Lexxel 5-5. If blood pressure control is inadequate after a week or two, the dose may be increased to 2 tablets Lexxel 5-5 administered once daily. The next incremental effect can be achieved with 4 tablets Lexxel administered once daily. If control remains unsatisfactory, consider addition of a thiazide diuretic.

Use in patients with metabolic impairments: Regimens of therapy with Lexxel need not be adjusted for renal function as long as the patient's creatinine clearance is >30 ml/min/1.73 m^2 (serum creatinine roughly ≤3 mg/dl or 265 μmol/L). In patients with more severe renal impairment, the recommended initial dose of enalapril is 2.5 mg.

Lexxel should regularly be taken either without food or with a light meal. Lexxel should be swallowed whole and not divided, crushed or chewed.

PRODUCT LISTING - EQUIVALENTS NOT AVAILABLE

Tablet, Extended Release - Oral - 5 mg;2.5 mg

30's	$43.14	LEXXEL, Astra-Zeneca Pharmaceuticals	00186-0002-31
100's	$129.41	LEXXEL, Astra-Zeneca Pharmaceuticals	00186-0002-28

Tablet, Extended Release - Oral - 5 mg;5 mg

30's	$46.69	LEXXEL, Astra-Zeneca Pharmaceuticals	00186-0001-31
100's	$126.00	LEXXEL, Astra-Zeneca Pharmaceuticals	61113-0001-28
100's	$155.64	LEXXEL, Astra-Zeneca Pharmaceuticals	00186-0001-68

Enalapril Maleate; Hydrochlorothiazide *(001139)*

Categories: Hypertension, essential; Pregnancy Category C; FDA Approved 1986 Oct
Drug Classes: Angiotensin converting enzyme inhibitors; Diuretics, thiazide and derivatives
Brand Names: **Vaseretic**
Foreign Brand Availability: Acesistem (Italy); Angiozide (Bahrain; Cyprus; Egypt; Iran; Iraq; Jordan; Kuwait; Lebanon; Libya; Oman; Qatar; Republic-of-Yemen; Saudi-Arabia; Syria; United-Arab-Emirates); Co-Renitec (Austria; Bahrain; Belgium; Benin; Burkina-Faso; Cyprus; Czech-Republic; Egypt; Ethiopia; France; Gambia; Ghana; Greece; Guinea; Hong-Kong; Iran; Iraq; Ivory-Coast; Jordan; Kenya; Kuwait; Lebanon; Liberia; Libya; Malawi; Mali; Mauritania; Mauritius; Mexico; Morocco; New-Zealand; Niger; Nigeria; Oman; Qatar; Republic-of-Yemen; Saudi-Arabia; Senegal; Seychelles; Sierra-Leone; South-Africa; Sudan; Syria; Tanzania; Tunia; Uganda; United-Arab-Emirates; Zambia; Zimbabwe); Co-Reniten (Switzerland); Corenitec (Denmark; Netherlands); Ecaprinil-D (Costa-Rica; Dominican-Republic; El-Salvador; Guatemala; Honduras; Nicaragua; Panama); Enace-D (India); Enap HL (Singapore); Innozide (England; Ireland); Invozide (India); Lotrial D (Ecuador; Peru); Naprizide (Israel); Pres Plus (Germany); Renacor (Germany); Renidur (Portugal); Renitec Comp (Norway); Tenazide (Indonesia); Uniretic (Colombia); Vasoretic (Italy)
Cost of Therapy: $37.49 (Hypertension; Vaseretic; 5 mg; 12.5 mg; 1 tablet/day; 30 day supply)

E

DESCRIPTION

Vaseretic combines an angiotensin converting enzyme inhibitor, enalapril maleate, and a diuretic, hydrochlorothiazide.

FOR COMPLETE PRESCRIBING INFORMATION, REFER TO ENALAPRIL MALEATE AND HYCROCHLOROTHIAZIDE .

INDICATIONS AND USAGE

Vaseretic is indicated for the treatment of hypertension in patients for whom combination therapy is appropriate.

This fixed dose combination is not indicated for initial therapy. Patients already receiving a diuretic when enalapril is initiated, or given a diuretic and enalapril simultaneously, can develop symptomatic hypotension. In the initial titration of the individual entities, it is important, if possible, to stop the diuretic for several days before starting enalapril or, if this is not possible, begin enalapril at a low initial dose (see DOSAGE AND ADMINISTRATION**). This fixed dose combination is not suitable for titration but may be substituted for the individual components if the titrated doses are the same as those in the combination.**

In using Vaseretic, consideration should be given to the fact that another angiotensin converting enzyme inhibitor, captopril, has caused agranulocytosis, particularly in patients with renal impairment or collagen vascular disease, and that available data are insufficient to show that enalapril does not have a similar risk.

NON-FDA APPROVED INDICATIONS

Enalapril hydrochlorothiazide is also used without FDA approval for the treatment of congestive heart failure.

DOSAGE AND ADMINISTRATION

DOSAGE MUST BE INDIVIDUALIZED. THE FIXED COMBINATION IS NOT FOR INITIAL THERAPY. THE DOSE OF 'VASERETIC' SHOULD BE DETERMINED BY THE TITRATION OF THE INDIVIDUAL COMPONENTS.

Once the patient has been successfully titrated with the individual components as described below, Vaseretic (one or two 10-25 tablets once daily) may be substituted if the titrated doses are the same as those in the fixed combination. (See INDICATIONS AND USAGE.)

Patients usually do not require doses in excess of 50 mg of hydrochlorothiazide daily; when combined with other antihypertensive agents. Therefore, since each tablet of Vaseretic includes 25 mg of hydrochlorothiazide, the daily dosage of Vaseretic should not exceed two tablets. If further blood pressure control is indicated, additional doses of enalapril or other non-diuretic antihypertensive agents should be considered.

For enalapril monotherapy the recommended initial dose in patients not on diuretics is 5 mg of enalapril once a day. Dosage should be adjusted according to blood pressure response. The usual dosage range of enalapril is 10-40 mg/day administered in a single dose or 2 divided doses. In some patients treated once daily, the antihypertensive effects may diminish toward the end of the dosing interval. In such patients, an increase in dosage or twice daily administration should be considered. If blood pressure is not controlled with enalapril alone, a diuretic may be added.

In patients who are currently being treated with a diuretic, symptomatic hypotension occasionally may occur following the initial dose of enalapril. The diuretic should, if possible, be discontinued for 2-3 days before beginning therapy with enalapril to reduce the likelihood of hypotension. If the patient's blood pressure is not controlled with enalapril alone, diuretic therapy may be resumed.

If the diuretic cannot be discontinued an initial dose of 2.5 mg of enalapril should be used under medical supervision for at least 2 hours and until blood pressure has stabilized for at least an additional hour.

Concomitant administration of Vaseretic with potassium supplements, potassium salt substitutes, or potassium sparing agents may lead to increases of serum potassium.

Dosage Adjustment in Renal Impairment: The usual dose of Vaseretic is recommended for patients with a creatinine clearance >30 ml/min (serum creatinine of up to approximately 3 mg/dl).

When concomitant diuretic therapy is required in patients with severe renal impairment, a loop diuretic, rather than a thiazide diuretic is preferred for use with enalapril; therefore, for patients with severe renal dysfunction the enalapril maleate-hydrochlorothiazide combination tablet is not recommended.

HOW SUPPLIED

Tablets Vaseretic 10-25, are rust, squared capsule-shaped, compressed tablets, coded "MSD 720" on one side and "Vaseretic" on the other. Each tablet contains 10 mg of enalapril maleate and 25 mg of hydrochlorothiazide.

Storage: Store below 30°C (86°F) and avoid transient temperatures above 50°C (122°F). Keep container tightly closed. Protect from moisture. Dispense in a tight container, if product package is subdivided.

PRODUCT LISTING - RATED THERAPEUTICALLY EQUIVALENT

Tablet - Oral - 5 mg;12.5 mg

100's	$107.10	GENERIC, Mylan Pharmaceuticals Inc	00378-0712-01
100's	$107.20	GENERIC, Par Pharmaceutical Inc	49884-0686-01
100's	$107.21	GENERIC, Teva Pharmaceuticals Usa	00093-1044-01
100's	$107.22	GENERIC, Eon Labs Manufacturing Inc	00185-0151-01
100's	$109.60	GENERIC, Taro Pharmaceuticals U.S.A. Inc	51672-4045-01
100's	$124.95	VASERETIC 5-12.5, Biovail Pharmaceuticals Inc	64455-0145-01

Tablet - Oral - 10 mg;25 mg

90's	$99.97	VASERETIC 10-25, Allscripts Pharmaceutical Company	54569-8595-00
100's	$119.30	GENERIC, Mylan Pharmaceuticals Inc	00378-0723-01
100's	$119.39	GENERIC, Eon Labs Manufacturing Inc	00185-0172-01
100's	$119.40	GENERIC, Teva Pharmaceuticals Usa	00093-1052-01
100's	$119.40	GENERIC, Par Pharmaceutical Inc	49884-0687-01
100's	$122.05	GENERIC, Taro Pharmaceuticals U.S.A. Inc	51672-4046-01
100's	$139.16	VASERETIC 10-25, Biovail Pharmaceuticals Inc	64455-0146-01

PRODUCT LISTING - EQUIVALENTS NOT AVAILABLE

Tablet - Oral - 5 mg;12.5 mg

100's	$124.95	VASERETIC 5-12.5, Merck & Company Inc	00006-0173-68

Tablet - Oral - 10 mg;25 mg

100's	$139.16	VASERETIC 10-25, Merck & Company Inc	00006-0720-68

Enalaprilat *(001140)*

For related information, see the comparative table section in Appendix A.

Categories: Heart failure, congestive; Hypertension, essential; Pregnancy Category C; FDA Approved 1988 Feb
Drug Classes: Angiotensin converting enzyme inhibitors
Brand Names: Vasotec-IV

DESCRIPTION

For Full Prescribing Information, Please Refer to Enalapril Maleate.

Enfuvirtide *(003587)*

For related information, see the comparative table section in Appendix A.

Categories: Infection, human immunodeficiency virus; Pregnancy Category B; FDA Approved 2003 Mar
Drug Classes: Antivirals; Fusion inhibitors
Brand Names: Fuzeon

DESCRIPTION

Enfuvirtide is an inhibitor of the fusion of HIV-1 with CD4+ cells. Enfuvirtide is a linear 36-amino acid synthetic peptide with the N-terminus acetylated and the C-terminus is a carboxamide. It is composed of naturally occurring L-amino acid residues.

Enfuvirtide is a white to off-white amorphous solid. It has negligible solubility in pure water and the solubility increases in aqueous buffers (pH 7.5) to 85-142 g/100 ml. The empirical formula of enfuvirtide is $C_{204}H_{301}N_{51}O_{64}$, and the molecular weight is 4492. It has the following primary amino acid sequence:

CH_3CO-Tyr-Thr-Ser-Leu-Ile-His-Ser-Leu-Ile-Glu-Glu-Ser-Gln-Asn-Gln-Gln-Glu-Lys-Asn-Glu-Gln-Glu-Leu-Leu-Glu-Leu-Asp-Lys-Trp-Ala-Ser-Leu-Trp-Asn-Trp-Phe-NH_2.

The drug product, Fuzeon for injection, is a white to off-white, sterile, lyophilized powder. Each single-use vial contains 108 mg of enfuvirtide for the delivery of 90 mg. Prior to subcutaneous (SC) administration, the contents of the vial are reconstituted with 1.1 ml of sterile water for injection giving a volume of approximately 1.2 ml to provide the delivery of 1 ml of the solution. Each 1 ml of the reconstituted solution contains approximately 90 mg of enfuvirtide with approximate amounts of the following excipients: 22.55 mg of mannitol, 2.39 mg of sodium carbonate (anhydrous), and sodium hydroxide and hydrochloric acid for pH adjustment as needed. The reconstituted solution has an approximate pH of 9.0.

CLINICAL PHARMACOLOGY

MICROBIOLOGY

Mechanism of Action

Enfuvirtide interferes with the entry of HIV-1 into cells by inhibiting fusion of viral and cellular membranes. Enfuvirtide binds to the first heptad-repeat (HR1) in the gp41 subunit of the viral envelope glycoprotein and prevents the conformational changes required for the fusion of viral and cellular membranes.

Antiviral Activity In Vitro

The *in vitro* antiviral activity of enfuvirtide was assessed by infecting different CD4+ cell types with laboratory and clinical isolates of HIV-1. The IC_{50} (50% inhibitory concentration) for enfuvirtide in laboratory and primary isolates representing HIV-1 clades A to G ranged from 4-280 nM (18-1260 ng/ml). The IC_{50} for baseline clinical isolates ranged from 0.089 to 107 nM (0.4 to 480 ng/ml) by the cMAGI assay (n=130) and from 1.56 to 1680 nM (7-7530 ng/ml) by a recombinant phenotypic entry assay (n=612). Enfuvirtide was similarly active *in vitro* against R5, X4, and dual tropic viruses. Enfuvirtide has no activity against HIV-2.

Enfuvirtide exhibited additive to synergistic effects in cell culture assays when combined with individual members of various antiretroviral classes, including zidovudine, lamivudine, nelfinavir, indinavir, and efavirenz.

Drug Resistance

HIV-1 isolates with reduced susceptibility to enfuvirtide have been selected *in vitro*. Genotypic analysis of the *in vitro*-selected resistant isolates showed mutations that resulted in amino acid substitutions at the enfuvirtide binding HR1 domain positions 36-38 of the HIV-1 envelope glycoprotein gp41. Phenotypic analysis of site-directed mutants in positions 36-38 in an HIV-1 molecular clone showed a 5- to 684-fold decrease in susceptibility to enfuvirtide.

In clinical trials, HIV-1 isolates with reduced susceptibility to enfuvirtide have been recovered from subjects treated with enfuvirtide in combination with other antiretroviral agents. Posttreatment HIV-1 virus from 185 subjects exhibited decreases in susceptibility to enfuvirtide ranging from 4- to 422-fold relative to their respective baseline virus and exhibited genotypic changes in gp41 amino acids 36-45. Substitutions in this region were observed with decreasing frequency at amino acid positions 38, 43, 36, 40, 42, and 45.

Cross-Resistance

HIV-1 clinical isolates resistant to nucleoside analogue reverse transcriptase inhibitors (NRTI), non-nucleoside analogue reverse transcriptase inhibitors (NNRTI), and protease inhibitors (PI) were susceptible to enfuvirtide in cell culture.

PHARMACOKINETICS

The pharmacokinetic properties of enfuvirtide were evaluated in HIV-1 infected adult and pediatric patients.

Absorption

Following a 90 mg single SC injection of enfuvirtide into the abdomen in 12 HIV-1 infected subjects, the mean (±SD) C_{max} was 4.59 ± 1.5 μg/ml, AUC was 55.8 ± 12.1 μg·h/ml and the median T_{max} was 8 hours (ranged from 3-12 h). The absolute bioavailability [using a 90 mg intravenous (IV) dose as a reference] was 84.3% ± 15.5%. Following 90 mg bid dosing of enfuvirtide subcutaneously in combination with other antiretroviral agents in 11 HIV-1 infected subjects, the mean (±SD) steady-state C_{max} was 5.0 ± 1.7 μg/ml, C_{trough} was 3.3 ± 1.6 μg/ml, AUC(0-12h) was 48.7 ± 19.1 μg·h/ml, and the median T_{max} was 4 hours (ranged from 4-8 h).

Absorption of the 90 mg dose was comparable when injected into the subcutaneous tissue of the abdomen, thigh or arm.

Distribution

The mean (±SD) steady-state volume of distribution after IV administration of a 90 mg dose of enfuvirtide (n=12) was 5.5 ± 1.1 L.

Enfuvirtide is approximately 92% bound to plasma proteins in HIV-infected plasma over a concentration range of 2-10 μg/ml. It is bound predominantly to albumin and to a lower extent to α-1 acid glycoprotein.

Metabolism/Elimination

As a peptide, enfuvirtide is expected to undergo catabolism to its constituent amino acids, with subsequent recycling of the amino acids in the body pool.

Mass balance studies to determine elimination pathway(s) of enfuvirtide have not been performed in humans.

In vitro studies with human microsomes and hepatocytes indicate that enfuvirtide undergoes hydrolysis to form a deamidated metabolite at the C-terminal phenylalanine residue, M3. The hydrolysis reaction is not NADPH dependent. The M3 metabolite is detected in human plasma following administration of enfuvirtide, with an AUC ranging from 2.4 to 15% of the enfuvirtide AUC.

Following a 90 mg single SC dose of enfuvirtide (n=12) the mean ±SD elimination half-life of enfuvirtide is 3.8 ± 0.6 h and the mean ±SD apparent clearance was 24.8 ± 4.1 ml/h/kg. Following 90 mg bid dosing of enfuvirtide subcutaneously in combination with other antiretroviral agents in 11 HIV-1 infected subjects, the mean ±SD apparent clearance was 30.6 ± 10.6 ml/h/kg.

SPECIAL POPULATIONS

Hepatic Insufficiency

Formal pharmacokinetic studies of enfuvirtide have not been conducted in patients with hepatic impairment.

Renal Insufficiency

Formal pharmacokinetic studies of enfuvirtide have not been conducted in patients with renal insufficiency. However, analysis of plasma concentration data from subjects in clinical trials indicated that the clearance of enfuvirtide is not affected in patients with creatinine clearance greater than 35 ml/min. The effect of creatinine clearance less than 35 ml/min on enfuvirtide clearance is unknown.

Gender and Weight

Gender

Analysis of plasma concentration data from subjects in clinical trials indicated that the clearance of enfuvirtide is 20% lower in females than males after adjusting for body weight.

Weight

Enfuvirtide clearance decreases with decreased body weight irrespective of gender. Relative to the clearance of a 70 kg male, a 40 kg male will have 20% lower clearance and a 110 kg male will have a 26% higher clearance. Relative to a 70 kg male, a 40 kg female will have a 36% lower clearance and a 110 kg female will have the same clearance.

No dose adjustment is recommended for weight or gender.

Race

Analysis of plasma concentration data from subjects in clinical trials indicated that the clearance of enfuvirtide was not different in Blacks compared to Caucasians. Other pharmacokinetic studies suggest no difference between Asians and Caucasians after adjusting for body weight.

Pediatric Patients

The pharmacokinetics of enfuvirtide have been studied in 18 pediatric subjects aged 6-16 years at a dose of 2 mg/kg. Enfuvirtide pharmacokinetics were determined in the presence of concomitant medications including antiretroviral agents. A dose of 2 mg/kg bid (maximum 90 mg bid) provided enfuvirtide plasma concentrations similar to those obtained in adult patients receiving 90 mg bid.

In the 18 pediatric subjects receiving the 2 mg/kg bid dose, the mean ±SD steady-state AUC was 53.6 ± 21.4 µg·h/ml, C_{max} was 5.9 ± 2.2 µg/ml, C_{trough} was 3.0 ± 1.5 µg/ml, and apparent clearance was 40 ± 14 ml/h/kg.

Geriatric Patients

The pharmacokinetics of enfuvirtide have not been studied in patients over 65 years of age.

DRUG INTERACTIONS

Influence of Enfuvirtide on the Metabolism of Concomitant Drugs

Based on the results from an *in vitro* human microsomal study, enfuvirtide is not an inhibitor of CYP450 enzymes. In an *in vivo* human metabolism study (n=12), enfuvirtide at the recommended dose of 90 mg bid did not alter the metabolism of CYP3A4, CYP2D6, CYP1A2, CYP2C19 or CYP2E1 substrates.

Influence of Concomitant Drugs on the Metabolism of Enfuvirtide

In separate pharmacokinetic interaction studies, coadministration of ritonavir (n=12), saquinavir/ritonavir (n=12), and rifampin (n=12) did not result in clinically significant pharmacokinetic interactions with enfuvirtide (see TABLE 1).

***TABLE 1** Effect of Ritonavir, Saquinavir/Ritonavir, and Rifampin on the Steady-State Pharmacokinetics of Enfuvirtide (90 mg bid)**

Coadministered Drug	Dose of Coadministered Drug	n	% Change of Enfuvirtide Pharmacokinetic Parameters† (90% CI) C_{max}	AUC	C_{trough}
Ritonavir	200 mg, q12h, 4 days	12	inc 24 (inc 9 to inc 41)	inc 22 (inc 8 to inc 37)	inc 14 (inc 2 to inc 28)
Saquinavir/ Ritonavir	1000/100 mg, q12h, 4 days	12	NE	inc 14 (inc 5 to inc 24)	inc 26 (inc 17 to inc 35)
Rifampin	600 mg, qd, 10 days	12	NE	NE	dec 15 (dec 22 to dec 7)

* All studies were performed in HIV-1+ subjects using a sequential crossover design.
† inc = Increase; dec = Decrease; NE = No effect (inc or dec <10%).

INDICATIONS AND USAGE

Enfuvirtide in combination with other antiretroviral agents is indicated for the treatment of HIV-1 infection in treatment-experienced patients with evidence of HIV-1 replication despite ongoing antiretroviral therapy.

This indication is based on analyses of plasma HIV-1 RNA levels and CD4 cell counts in controlled studies of enfuvirtide of 24 weeks duration. Subjects enrolled were treatment-experienced adults; many had advanced disease. There are no studies of enfuvirtide in antiretroviral naive patients. There are no results from controlled trials evaluating the effect of enfuvirtide on clinical progression of HIV-1.

CONTRAINDICATIONS

Enfuvirtide is contraindicated in patients with known hypersensitivity to enfuvirtide or any of its components (see WARNINGS).

WARNINGS

LOCAL INJECTION SITE REACTIONS

The most common adverse events associated with enfuvirtide use are local injection site reactions. Manifestations may include pain and discomfort, induration, erythema, nodules and cysts, pruritus, and ecchymosis. Nine percent (9%) of patients had local reactions that required analgesics or limited usual activities (see ADVERSE REACTIONS). Reactions are often present at more than 1 injection site. Patients must be familiar with the enfuvirtide injection instructions in order to know how to inject enfuvirtide appropriately and how to monitor carefully for signs or symptoms of cellulitis or local infection.

PNEUMONIA

An increased rate of bacterial pneumonia was observed in subjects treated with enfuvirtide in the Phase 3 clinical trials compared to the control arm (see ADVERSE REACTIONS). It is unclear if the increased incidence of pneumonia is related to enfuvirtide use. However, because of this finding, patients with HIV infection should be carefully monitored for signs and symptoms of pneumonia, especially if they have underlying conditions which may predispose them to pneumonia. Risk factors for pneumonia included low initial CD4 cell count, high initial viral load, IV drug use, smoking, and a prior history of lung disease (see ADVERSE REACTIONS).

HYPERSENSITIVITY REACTIONS

Hypersensitivity reactions have been associated with enfuvirtide therapy and may recur on re-challenge. Hypersensitivity reactions have included individually and in combination: rash, fever, nausea and vomiting, chills, rigors, hypotension, and elevated serum liver transaminases. Other adverse events that may be immune mediated and have been reported in subjects receiving enfuvirtide include primary immune complex reaction, respiratory distress glomerulonephritis, and Guillain-Barre syndrome. Patients developing signs and symptoms suggestive of a systemic hypersensitivity reaction should discontinue enfuvirtide and should seek medical evaluation immediately. Therapy with enfuvirtide should not be restarted following systemic signs and symptoms consistent with a hypersensitivity reaction. Risk factors that may predict the occurrence or severity of hypersensitivity to enfuvirtide have not been identified (see ADVERSE REACTIONS).

PRECAUTIONS

NON-HIV INFECTED INDIVIDUALS

There is a theoretical risk that enfuvirtide use may lead to the production of anti-enfuvirtide antibodies which cross react with HIV gp41. This could result in a false positive HIV test with an ELISA assay; a confirmatory western blot test would be expected to be negative. Enfuvirtide has not been studied in non-HIV infected individuals.

INFORMATION FOR THE PATIENT

To assure safe and effective use of enfuvirtide, the following information and instructions should be given to patients:

- Patients should be informed that injection site reactions occur commonly. Patients must be familiar with the enfuvirtide Injection Instructions for instructions on how to appropriately inject enfuvirtide and how to carefully monitor for signs or symptoms of cellulitis or local infection. Patients should be instructed when to contact their healthcare provider about these reactions.
- Patients should be made aware that an increased rate of bacterial pneumonia was observed in subjects treated with enfuvirtide in Phase 3 clinical trials compared to the control arm. Patients should be advised to seek medical evaluation immediately if they develop signs or symptoms suggestive of pneumonia (cough with fever, rapid breathing, shortness of breath) (see WARNINGS).
- Patients should be advised of the possibility of a hypersensitivity reaction to enfuvirtide. Patients should be advised to discontinue therapy and immediately seek medical evaluation if they develop signs/symptoms of hypersensitivity (see WARNINGS).
- Enfuvirtide is not a cure for HIV-1 infection and patients may continue to contract illnesses associated with HIV-1 infection. The long-term effects of enfuvirtide are unknown at this time. Enfuvirtide therapy has not been shown to reduce the risk of transmitting HIV-1 to others through sexual contact or blood contamination.
- Enfuvirtide must be taken as part of a combination antiretroviral regimen. Use of enfuvirtide alone may lead to rapid development of virus resistant to enfuvirtide and possibly other agents of the same class.
- Patients and caregivers must be instructed in the use of aseptic technique when administering enfuvirtide in order to avoid injection site infections. Appropriate training for enfuvirtide reconstitution and self-injection must be given by a healthcare provider, including a careful review of the enfuvirtide Patient Package Insert and enfuvirtide Injection Instructions. The first injection should be performed under the supervision of an appropriately qualified healthcare provider. It is recommended that the patient and/or caregiver's understanding and use of aseptic self-injection techniques and procedures be periodically re-evaluated.
- Patients should contact their healthcare provider for any questions regarding the administration of enfuvirtide. Patients should be told not to reuse needles or syringes, and be instructed in safe disposal procedures including the use of a puncture-resistant container for disposal of used needles and syringes. Patients must be instructed on the safe disposal of full containers as per local requirements. Caregivers who experience an accidental needlestick after patient injection should contact a healthcare provider immediately.
- Patients should inform their healthcare provider if they are pregnant, plan to become pregnant or become pregnant while taking this medication.
- Patients should inform their healthcare provider if they are breast-feeding.
- Patients should not change the dose or dosing schedule of enfuvirtide or any antiretroviral medication without consulting their healthcare provider.
- Patients should contact their healthcare provider immediately if they stop taking enfuvirtide or any other drug in their antiretroviral regimen.
- Patients should be told that they can obtain more information on the self-administration of Fuzeon at www.FUZEON.com or by calling 1-877-4-FUZEON (1-877-438-9366).

Patients should be advised that no studies have been conducted on the ability to drive or operate machinery while taking enfuvirtide. If patients experience dizziness while taking enfuvirtide, they should be advised to talk to their healthcare provider before driving or operating machinery.

CARCINOGENESIS, MUTAGENESIS, AND IMPAIRMENT OF FERTILITY

Carcinogenesis

Long-term animal carcinogenicity studies of enfuvirtide have not been conducted.

Mutagenesis

Enfuvirtide was neither mutagenic nor clastogenic in a series of *in vivo* and *in vitro* assays including the Ames bacterial reverse mutation assay, a mammalian cell forward gene mutation assay in AS52 Chinese Hamster ovary cells or an *in vivo* mouse micronucleus assay.

Impairment of Fertility

Enfuvirtide produced no adverse effects on fertility in male or female rats at doses of up to 30 mg/kg/day administered by SC injection (1.6 times the maximum recommended adult human daily dose on a m^2 basis).

PREGNANCY CATEGORY B

Reproduction studies have been performed in rats and rabbits at doses up to 27 times and 3.2 times the adult human dose on a m^2 basis. The animal studies revealed no evidence of harm

E

to the fetus from enfuvirtide. There are no adequate and well-controlled studies in pregnant women. Because animal reproduction studies are not always predictive of human response, this drug should be used during pregnancy only if clearly needed.

ANTIRETROVIRAL PREGNANCY REGISTRY

To monitor maternal-fetal outcomes of pregnant women exposed to enfuvirtide and other antiretroviral drugs, an Antiretroviral Pregnancy Registry has been established. Physicians are encouraged to register patients by calling 1-800-258-4263.

NURSING MOTHERS

The Centers for Disease Control and Prevention recommends that HIV-infected mothers not breast-feed their infants to avoid the risk of postnatal transmission of HIV. It is not known whether enfuvirtide is excreted in human milk. Because of both the potential for HIV transmission and the potential for serious adverse reactions in nursing infants, **mothers should be instructed not to breast-feed if they are receiving enfuvirtide.**

Studies where radio-labeled ^{3}H-enfuvirtide was administered to lactating rats indicated that radioactivity was present in the milk. It is not known whether the radioactivity in the milk was from radio-labeled enfuvirtide or from radiolabeled metabolites of enfuvirtide (*i.e.*, amino acids and peptide fragments).

PEDIATRIC USE

The safety and pharmacokinetics of enfuvirtide have not been established in pediatric subjects below 6 years of age. Limited efficacy data is available in pediatric subjects 6 years of age and older.

Thirty-five (35) HIV-1 infected pediatric subjects ages 6-16 years have received enfuvirtide in two open-label, single-arm clinical trials. Adverse experiences were similar to those observed in adult patients.

Study T20-204 was an open-label, multicenter trial that evaluated the safety, and antiviral activity of enfuvirtide in treatment-experienced pediatric subjects. Eleven (11) subjects from 6-12 years were enrolled (median age of 9 years). Median baseline CD4 cell count was 509 cells/μL and the median baseline HIV-1 RNA was 4.5 $\log_{10}$ copies/ml.

Ten (10) of the 11 study subjects completed 48 weeks of chronic therapy. By Week 48, 6/11 (55%) subjects had ≥1 $\log_{10}$ decline in HIV-1 RNA and 4/11 (36%) subjects were below 400 copies/ml of HIV-1 RNA. The median changes from baseline in HIV-1 RNA and CD4 cell count were -1.48 $\log_{10}$ copies/ml and 122 cells/μL, respectively.

Study T20-310 is an ongoing, open-label, multicenter trial evaluating the pharmacokinetics, safety, and antiviral activity of enfuvirtide in treatment-experienced pediatric subjects and adolescents. Twenty-four (24) subjects from 6-16 years were enrolled (median age of 13 years). Median baseline CD4 cell count was 143 cells/μL and the median baseline HIV-1 RNA was 5.0 $\log_{10}$ copies/ml. The evaluation of the antiviral activity is ongoing.

GERIATRIC USE

Clinical studies of enfuvirtide did not include sufficient numbers of subjects aged 65 and over to determine whether they respond differently from younger subjects.

DRUG INTERACTIONS

CYP450 METABOLIZED DRUGS

Results from *in vitro* and *in vivo* studies suggest that enfuvirtide is unlikely to have significant drug interactions with concomitantly administered drugs metabolized by CYP450 enzymes (see CLINICAL PHARMACOLOGY).

ANTIRETROVIRAL AGENTS

No drug interactions with other antiretroviral medications have been identified that would warrant alteration of either the enfuvirtide dose or the dose of the other antiretroviral medication.

ADVERSE REACTIONS

The overall safety profile of enfuvirtide is based on 1188 subjects who received at least 1 dose of enfuvirtide during various clinical trials. This includes 1153 adults, 608 of whom received the recommended dose for greater than 24 weeks, and 35 pediatric subjects.

Assessment of treatment-emergent adverse events is based on the pooled data from the two Phase 3 studies T20-301 and T20-302.

LOCAL INJECTION SITE REACTIONS

Local injection site reactions were the most frequent adverse events associated with the use of enfuvirtide. In Phase 3 clinical studies (T20-301 and T20-302), 98% of subjects had at least 1 local injection site reaction (ISR). Three percent (3%) of subjects discontinued treatment with enfuvirtide because of ISRs. Eighty-six percent (86%) of subjects experienced their first ISR during the initial week of treatment. The majority of ISRs were associated with mild to moderate pain at the injection site, erythema, induration, and the presence of nodules or cysts. For most subjects the severity of signs and symptoms associated with ISRs did not change during the 24 weeks of treatment. In 17% of subjects an individual ISR lasted for longer than 7 days. Because of the frequency and duration of individual ISRs, 23% of subjects had 6 or more ongoing ISRs at any given time. Individual signs and symptoms characterizing local ISRs are summarized in TABLE 4. Infection at the injection site (including abscess and cellulitis) was reported in 1% of subjects.

OTHER ADVERSE EVENTS

Hypersensitivity reactions have been attributed to enfuvirtide (≤1%) and in some cases have recurred upon re-challenge (see WARNINGS).

The events most frequently reported in subjects receiving enfuvirtide + background regimen, excluding injection site reactions, were diarrhea (26.8%), nausea (20.1%), and fatigue (16.1%). These events were also commonly observed in subjects that received background regimen alone: diarrhea (33.5%), nausea (23.7%), and fatigue (17.4%).

Treatment-emergent adverse events (% of subjects), excluding ISRs, from Phase 3 studies are summarized for adult subjects, regardless of severity and causality, in TABLE 5. Only events occurring in ≥2% of subjects and at a higher rate in subjects treated with enfuvirtide are summarized in TABLE 5; events that occurred at a higher rate in the control arms are not displayed.

***TABLE 4** Summary of Individual Signs/Symptoms Characterizing Local Injection Site Reactions to Enfuvirtide in Studies T20-301 and T20-302 Combined n=663 (% of Subjects)*

Event Category	Any Severity Grade	% of Events Comprising Grade 3 Reactions	% of Events Comprising Grade 4 Reactions
Pain/discomfort*	95%	9%	0%
Induration†	89%	41%	16%
Erythema‡	89%	22%	10%
Nodules and cysts§	76%	26%	0%
Pruritus¤	62%	4%	NA
Ecchymosis¶	48%	8%	5%

* Grade 3 = severe pain requiring analgesics (or narcotic analgesics for ≤72 hours) and/or limiting usual activities; Grade 4 = severe pain requiring hospitalization or prolongation of hospitalization, resulting in death, or persistent or significant disability/incapacity, or life-threatening, or medically significant.
† Grade 3 = ≥25 mm but <50 mm; Grade 4 = ≥50 mm average diameter.
‡ Grade 3 = ≥50 mm but <85 mm average diameter; Grade 4 = ≥85 mm average diameter.
§ Grade 3 = ≥3 cm; Grade 4 = if draining.
¤ Grade 3 = refractory to topical treatment or requiring oral or parenteral treatment; Grade 4 = not applicable.
¶ Grade 3 = >3 cm but ≤5 cm; Grade 4 = >5 cm.

***TABLE 5** Percentage of Patients With Selected Treatment-Emergent Adverse Events* Reported in ≥2% of Adult Patients and Occurring More Frequently in Patients Treated With Enfuvirtide (Pooled Studies T20-301/T20-302 at 24 Weeks)*

Adverse Event (by System Organ Class)	Enfuvirtide + Background Regimen n=663	Background Regimen n=334
Nervous System Disorders		
Peripheral neuropathy	8.9%	6.3%
Taste disturbance	2.4%	1.5%
Psychiatric Disorders		
Insomnia	11.3%	8.7%
Depression	8.6%	7.2%
Anxiety	5.7%	3.0%
Respiratory, Thoracic, and Mediastinal Disorders		
Cough	7.4%	5.4%
Infections		
Sinusitis	6.2%	2.1%
Herpes simplex	5.0%	3.9%
Skin papilloma	4.2%	1.5%
Influenza	3.9%	1.8%
General		
Weight decreased	6.5%	5.1%
Appetite decreased	6.3%	2.4%
Asthenia	5.7%	4.2%
Anorexia	2.6%	1.8%
Influenza-like illness	2.3%	0.9%
Skin and Subcutaneous Tissue Disorders		
Pruritus nos	5.1%	4.2%
Musculoskeletal, Connective Tissue, and Bone Disorders		
Myalgia	5.0%	2.4%
Gastrointestinal Disorders		
Constipation	3.9%	2.7%
Abdominal pain upper	3.0%	2.7%
Pancreatitis	2.4%	0.9%
Eye Disorders		
Conjunctivitis	2.4%	0.9%
Blood and Lymphatic System Disorders		
Lymphadenopathy	2.3%	0.3%

* Excludes injection site reactions.

An increased rate of bacterial pneumonia was observed in subjects treated with enfuvirtide in the Phase 3 clinical trials compared to the control arm (4.68 pneumonia events per 100 patient-years versus 0.61 events per 100 patient-years, respectively). Approximately half of the study subjects with pneumonia required hospitalization. One subject death in the enfuvirtide arm was attributed to pneumonia. Risk factors for pneumonia included low initial CD4 lymphocyte count, high initial viral load, IV drug use, smoking, and a prior history of lung disease. It is unclear if the increased incidence of pneumonia was related to enfuvirtide use. However, because of this finding patients with HIV infection should be carefully monitored for signs and symptoms of pneumonia, especially if they have underlying conditions which may predispose them to pneumonia (see WARNINGS).

LESS COMMON EVENTS

The following adverse events have been reported in 1 or more subjects; however, a causal relationship to enfuvirtide has not been established.

Immune System Disorders: Worsening abacavir hypersensitivity reaction.
Renal and Urinary Disorders: Renal insufficiency (glomerulonephritis); renal failure.
Blood and Lymphatic Disorders: Thrombocytopenia; neutropenia, and fever.
Endocrine and Metabolic: Hyperglycemia.
Infections and Infestations: Pneumonia.
Nervous System Disorders: Guillain-Barre syndrome (fatal); sixth nerve palsy.

LABORATORY ABNORMALITIES

TABLE 6 shows the treatment-emergent laboratory abnormalities that occurred in at least 2% of subjects and more frequently in those receiving enfuvirtide + background regimen than background regimen alone from studies T20-301 and T20-302.

TABLE 6 *Percentage of Treatment-Emergent Laboratory Abnormalities That Occurred in ≥2% of Adult Patients and More Frequently in Patients Receiving Enfuvirtide (Pooled Studies T20-301 and T20-302 at 24 Weeks)*

Laboratory Parameters	Grading	Enfuvirtide + Background Regimen n=663	Background Regimen n=334
Eosinophilia			
1-2 × ULN (0.7 × 10^9/L)	0.7-1.4 × 10^9/L	8.3%	1.5%
>2 × ULN (0.7 × 10^9/L)	>1.4 × 10^9/L	1.8%	0.9%
Amylase (U/L)			
Grade 3	>2-5 × ULN	6.2%	3.6%
Grade 4	>5 × ULN or clinical pancreatitis	0.9%	0.6%
Lipase (U/L)			
Grade 3	>2-5 × ULN	5.9%	3.6%
Grade 4	>5 × ULN	2.3%	1.8%
Triglycerides (mmol/L)			
Grade 3	>1000 mg/dl	8.9%	7.2%
ALT			
Grade 3	>5-10 × ULN	3.5%	2.1%
Grade 4	>10 × ULN	0.9%	0.6%
AST			
Grade 3	>5-10 × ULN	3.6%	3.0%
Grade 4	>10 × ULN	1.2%	0.6%
Creatine Phosphokinase (U/L)			
Grade 3	>5-10 × ULN	5.9%	3.6%
Grade 4	>10 × ULN	2.3%	3.6%
GGT (U/L)			
Grade 3	>5-10 × ULN	3.5%	3.3%
Grade 4	>10 × ULN	2.4%	1.8%
Hemoglobin (g/dl)			
Grade 3	6.5-7.9 g/dl	1.5%	0.9%
Grade 4	<6.5 g/dl	0.6%	0.6%

ADVERSE EVENTS IN PEDIATRIC PATIENTS

Enfuvirtide has been studied in 35 pediatric subjects 6-16 years of age with duration of enfuvirtide exposure ranging from 1 dose to 48 weeks. Adverse experiences seen during clinical trials were similar to those observed in adult subjects.

DOSAGE AND ADMINISTRATION

ADULTS

The recommended dose of enfuvirtide is 90 mg (1 ml) twice daily injected subcutaneously into the upper arm, anterior thigh or abdomen. Each injection should be given at a site different from the preceding injection site, and only where there is no current injection site reaction from an earlier dose. Enfuvirtide should not be injected into moles, scar tissue, bruises or the navel. Additional detailed information regarding the administration of enfuvirtide is described in the enfuvirtide Injection Instructions that are distributed with the prescription.

PEDIATRIC PATIENTS

No data are available to establish a dose recommendation of enfuvirtide in pediatric patients below the age of 6 years. In pediatric patients 6-16 years of age, the recommended dosage of enfuvirtide is 2 mg/kg twice daily up to a maximum dose of 90 mg twice daily injected subcutaneously into the upper arm, anterior thigh or abdomen. Each injection should be given at a site different from the preceding injection site and only where there is no current injection site reaction from an earlier dose. Enfuvirtide should not be injected into moles, scar tissue, bruises or the navel. TABLE 7 contains dosing guidelines for enfuvirtide based on body weight. Weight should be monitored periodically and the enfuvirtide dose adjusted accordingly.

TABLE 7 *Pediatric Dosing Guidelines*

Weight		Dose per bid Injection	Injection Volume (90 mg Enfuvirtide per ml)
11.0-15.5 kg	24-34 lbs	27 mg/dose	0.3 ml
15.6-20.0 kg	>34 to 44 lbs	36 mg/dose	0.4 ml
20.1-24.5 kg	>44 to 54 lbs	45 mg/dose	0.5 ml
24.6-29.0 kg	>54 to 64 lbs	54 mg/dose	0.6 ml
29.1-33.5 kg	>64 to 74 lbs	63 mg/dose	0.7 ml
33.6-38.0 kg	>74 to 84 lbs	72 mg/dose	0.8 ml
38.1-42.5 kg	>84 to 94 lbs	81 mg/dose	0.9 ml
≥42.6 kg	>94 lbs	90 mg/dose	1.0 ml

DIRECTIONS FOR USE

For more detailed instructions, see enfuvirtide Injection Instructions that are distributed with the prescription.

Subcutaneous Administration

Enfuvirtide must only be reconstituted with 1.1 ml of sterile water for injection. After adding sterile water, the vial should be gently tapped for 10 seconds and then gently rolled between the hands to avoid foaming and to ensure all particles of drug are in contact with the liquid and no drug remains on the vial wall. The vial should then be allowed to stand until the powder goes completely into solution, which could take up to 45 minutes. Reconstitution time can be reduced by gently rolling the vial between the hands until the product is completely dissolved. Before the solution is withdrawn for administration, the vial should be inspected visually to ensure that the contents are fully dissolved in solution, and that the solution is clear, colorless and without bubbles or particulate matter. If there is evidence of particulate matter, the vial must not be used and should be returned to the pharmacy.

Enfuvirtide contains no preservatives. Once reconstituted, enfuvirtide should be injected immediately or kept refrigerated in the original vial until use. Reconstituted enfuvirtide must be used within 24 hours. The subsequent dose of enfuvirtide can be reconstituted in advance and must be stored in the refrigerator in the original vial and used within 24 hours. Refrigerated reconstituted solution should be brought to room temperature before injection and the vial should be inspected visually again to ensure that the contents are fully dissolved in solution and that the solution is clear, colorless, and without bubbles or particulate matter.

The reconstituted solution should be injected subcutaneously in the upper arm, abdomen or anterior thigh. The injection should be given at a site different from the preceding injection site and only where there is no current injection site reaction. Also, do not inject into moles, scar tissue, bruises or the navel. A vial is suitable for single use only; unused portions must be discarded (see enfuvirtide Injection Instructions that are distributed with the prescription).

Patients should contact their healthcare provider for any questions regarding the administration of enfuvirtide. Information about the self-administration of Fuzeon may also be obtained by calling the toll-free number 1-877-4-FUZEON (1-877-438-9366) or at the Fuzeon website, www.FUZEON.com. Patients should be taught to recognize the signs and symptoms of injection site reactions and instructed when to contact their healthcare provider about these reactions.

HOW SUPPLIED

Fuzeon (enfuvirtide) for injection is a white to off-white, sterile, lyophilized powder and it is packaged in a single-use clear glass vial containing 108 mg of enfuvirtide for the delivery of approximately 90 mg/1 ml when reconstituted with 1.1 ml of sterile water for injection.

Storage: Store at 25°C (77°F); excursions permitted to 15-30°C (59-86°F).

Reconstituted solution should be stored under refrigeration at 2-8°C (36-46°F) and used within 24 hours.

Enoxaparin Sodium *(003160)*

For related information, see the comparative table section in Appendix A.

Categories: Ischemia, myocardial; Thrombosis, deep vein; Thrombosis, deep vein, prophylaxis; Embolism, pulmonary, prophylaxis; Pregnancy Category B; FDA Approved 1993 Mar
Drug Classes: Anticoagulants
Brand Names: Clexane; Heparin, Low Weight; **Lovenox**
Foreign Brand Availability: Clexane Forte (Israel); Clexane 40 (South-Africa); Klexane (Canada; Denmark; Finland; Norway; Sweden)
Cost of Therapy: $256.90 (Deep Vein Thrombosis; Lovenox Injection; 30 mg/syringe; 2 syringes/day; 7 day supply)
HCFA JCODE(S): J1650 30 mg SC

WARNING

SPINAL/EPIDURAL HEMATOMAS

When neuraxial anesthesia (epidural/spinal anesthesia) or spinal puncture is employed, patients anticoagulated or scheduled to be anticoagulated with low molecular weight heparins or heparinoids for prevention of thromboembolic complications are at risk of developing an epidural or spinal hematoma which can result in long-term or permanent paralysis.

The risk of these events is increased by the use of indwelling epidural catheters for administration of analgesia or by the concomitant use of drugs affecting hemostasis such as non-steroidal anti-inflammatory drugs (NSAIDs), platelet inhibitors, or other anticoagulants. The risk also appears to be increased by traumatic or repeated epidural or spinal puncture.

Patients should be frequently monitored for signs and symptoms of neurological impairment. If neurologic compromise is noted, urgent treatment is necessary.

The physician should consider the potential benefit versus risk before neuraxial intervention in patients anticoagulated or to be anticoagulated for thromboprophylaxis (see also WARNINGS, Hemorrhage and DRUG INTERACTIONS).

DESCRIPTION

Lovenox injection is a sterile solution containing enoxaparin sodium, a low molecular weight heparin.

Lovenox injection is available in two concentrations: 100 and 150 mg/ml of enoxaparin sodium in water for injection.

Lovenox injection 100 mg/ml concentration: Contains 10 mg enoxaparin sodium (or approximate anti-Factor Xa activity of 1000 IU [with reference to the WHO First International Low Molecular Weight Heparin Reference Standard]) per 0.1 ml water for injection.

Lovenox injection 150 mg/ml concentration: Contains 15 mg enoxaparin sodium (or appropriate anti-Factor Xa activity of 1500 IU [with reference to the WHO First International Low Molecular Weight Heparin Reference Standard]) per 0.1 ml water for injection.

The solutions are preservative-free and intended for use only as a single-dose injection. (See DOSAGE AND ADMINISTRATION and HOW SUPPLIED for dosage unit descriptions.) The pH of the injection is 5.5-7.5. Nitrogen is used in the headspace to inhibit oxidation.

Enoxaparin is obtained by alkaline degradation of heparin benzyl ester derived from porcine intestinal mucosa. Its structure is characterized by a 2-O-sulfo-4-enepyranosuronic acid group at the non-reducing end and a 2-N,6-O-disulfo-D-glucosamine at the reducing end of the chain. The substance is the sodium salt. The average molecular weight is about 4500 daltons.

The molecular weight distribution is:

***<2000 daltons:** ≤20%*
***2000-8000 daltons:** ≥68%*
***>8000 daltons:** ≤18%*

CLINICAL PHARMACOLOGY

Enoxaparin is a low molecular weight heparin which has antithrombotic properties. In humans, enoxaparin given at a dose of 1.5 mg/kg subcutaneously (SC) is characterized by a higher ratio of anti-Factor Xa to anti-Factor IIa activity (mean ±SD, 14.0 ± 3.1) (based on areas under anti-Factor activity versus time curves) compared to the ratios observed for heparin (mean ±SD, 1.22 ± 0.13). Increases of up to 1.8 times the control values were seen in the thrombin time (TT) and the activated partial thromboplastin time (aPTT). Enoxaparin at a 1 mg/kg dose (100 mg/ml concentration), administered SC every 12 hours to patients in a large clinical trial resulted in aPTT values of 45 seconds or less in the majority of patients (n=1607).

PHARMACODYNAMICS

Conducted using 100 mg/ml concentration.

Maximum anti-Factor Xa and anti-thrombin (anti-Factor IIa) activities occur 3-5 hours after SC injection of enoxaparin. Mean peak anti-Factor Xa activity was 0.16 IU/ml (1.58 µg/ml) and 0.38 IU/ml (3.83 µg/ml) after the 20 mg and the 40 mg clinically tested SC doses, respectively. Mean (n=46) peak anti-Factor Xa activity was 1.1 IU/ml at steady state in patients with unstable angina receiving 1 mg/kg SC every 12 hours for 14 days. Mean absolute bioavailability of enoxaparin, given SC, based on anti-Factor Xa activity is 92% in healthy volunteers. The volume of distribution of anti-Factor Xa activity is about 6 L. Following intravenous (IV) dosing, the total body clearance of enoxaparin is 26 ml/min. After IV dosing of enoxaparin labeled with the gamma-emitter, ^{99m}Tc, 40% of radioactivity and 8-20% of anti-Factor Xa activity were recovered in urine in 24 hours. Elimination half-life based on anti-Factor Xa activity was 4.5 hours after SC administration. Following a 40 mg SC once a day dose, significant anti-Factor Xa activity persists in plasma for about 12 hours.

Following SC dosing, the apparent clearance (CL/F) of enoxaparin is approximately 15 ml/min. Apparent clearance and A_{max} derived from anti-Factor Xa values following single SC dosing (40 and 60 mg) were slightly higher in males than in females. The source of the gender difference in these parameters has not been conclusively identified, however, body weight may be a contributing factor.

Apparent clearance and A_{max} derived from anti-Factor Xa values following single and multiple SC dosing in elderly subjects were close to those observed in young subjects. Following once a day SC dosing of 40 mg enoxaparin, the Day 10 mean area under anti-Factor Xa activity versus time curve (AUC) was approximately 15% greater than the mean Day 1 AUC value. In subjects with moderate renal impairment (creatinine clearance 30-80 ml/min), anti-Factor Xa CL/F values were similar to those in healthy subjects. However, mean CL/F values of subjects with severe renal impairment (creatinine clearance <30 ml/min), were approximately 30% lower than the mean CL/F value of control group subjects. (See PRECAUTIONS.)

Although not studied clinically, the 150 mg/ml concentration of enoxaparin sodium is projected to result in anticoagulant activities similar to those of 100 and 200 mg/ml concentrations at the same enoxaparin dose. When a daily 1.5 mg/kg SC injection of enoxaparin sodium was given to 25 healthy male and female subjects using a 100 or 200 mg/ml concentration the following pharmacokinetic profiles were obtained (see TABLE 1).

TABLE 1 *Pharmacokinetic Parameters* After 5 Days of 1.5 mg/kg SC Once Daily Doses of Enoxaparin Sodium Using 100 or 200 mg/ml Concentrations*

	Anti-Xa	Anti-IIa	Heptest	aPTT
A_{max} (IU/ml or Δ sec)				
100 mg/ml	1.37 (±0.23)	0.23 (±0.05)	104.5 (±16.6)	19.3 (±4.7)
200 mg/ml	1.45 (±0.22)	0.26 (±0.05)	110.9 (±17.1)	22 (±6.7)
90% CI	102-110%		102-111%	
T_{max}†(h)				
100 mg/ml	3 (2-6)	4 (2-5)	2.5 (2-4.5)	3 (2-4.5)
200 mg/ml	3.5 (2-6)	4.5 (2.5-6)	3.3 (2-5)	3 (2-5)
AUC(ss) (h·IU/ml or h·Δ sec)				
100 mg/ml	14.26 (±2.93)	1.54 (±0.61)	1321 (±219)	
200 mg/ml	15.43 (±2.96)	1.77 (±0.67)	1401 (±227)	
90% CI	105-112%		103-109%	

* Means ±SD at Day 5 and 90% Confidence Interval (CI) of the ratio.
† Median (range).

INDICATIONS AND USAGE

Enoxaparin sodium injection is indicated for the prevention of DVT, which may lead to pulmonary embolism:

In patients undergoing abdominal surgery who are at risk for thromboembolic complications.

In patients undergoing hip replacement surgery, during and following hospitalization.

In patients undergoing knee replacement surgery.

In medical patients who are at risk for thromboembolic complications due to severely restricted mobility during acute illness.

Enoxaparin sodium injection is indicated for the prophylaxis of ischemic complications of unstable angina and non-Q-wave myocardial infarction, when concurrently administered with aspirin.

Enoxaparin sodium injection is indicated for:

The **inpatient treatment** of acute DVT **with or without pulmonary embolism,** when administered in conjunction with warfarin sodium.

The **outpatient treatment** of acute DVT **without pulmonary embolism** when administered in conjunction with warfarin sodium.

See DOSAGE AND ADMINISTRATION, Adult Dosage for appropriate dosage regimens.

CONTRAINDICATIONS

Enoxaparin sodium injection is contraindicated in patients with active major bleeding, in patients with thrombocytopenia associated with a positive *in vitro* test for anti-platelet antibody in the presence of enoxaparin sodium, or in patients with hypersensitivity to enoxaparin sodium.

Patients with known hypersensitivity to heparin or pork products should not be treated with enoxaparin sodium injection.

WARNINGS

Enoxaparin sodium injection is not intended for intramuscular administration.

Enoxaparin sodium injection cannot be used interchangeably (unit for unit) with heparin or other low molecular weight heparins as they differ in their manufacturing process, molecular weight distribution, anti-Xa and anti-IIa activities, units, and dosage. Each of these medicines has its own instructions for use.

Enoxaparin sodium injection should be used with extreme caution in patients with history of heparin-induced thrombocytopenia.

HEMORRHAGE

Enoxaparin sodium injection, like other anticoagulants, should be used with extreme caution in conditions with increased risk of hemorrhage, such as bacterial endocarditis, congenital or acquired bleeding disorders, active ulcerative and angiodysplastic gastrointestinal disease, hemorrhagic stroke, or shortly after brain, spinal, or ophthalmological surgery, or in patients treated concomitantly with platelet inhibitors.

Cases of epidural or spinal hematomas have been reported with the associated use of enoxaparin sodium injection and spinal/epidural anesthesia or spinal puncture resulting in long-term or permanent paralysis. The risk of these events is higher with the use of post-operative indwelling epidural catheters or by the concomitant use of additional drugs affecting hemostasis such as NSAIDs (see BOXED WARNING, ADVERSE REACTIONS, Ongoing Safety Surveillance and DRUG INTERACTIONS).

Major hemorrhages, including retroperitoneal and intracranial bleeding have been reported. Some of these cases have been fatal.

Bleeding can occur at any site during therapy with enoxaparin sodium injection. An unexplained fall in hematocrit or blood pressure should lead to a search for a bleeding site.

THROMBOCYTOPENIA

Thrombocytopenia can occur with the administration of enoxaparin sodium injection.

Moderate thrombocytopenia (platelet counts between 100,000/mm^3 and 50,000/mm^3) occurred at a rate of 1.3% in patients given enoxaparin sodium injection, 1.2% in patients given heparin, and 0.7% in patients given placebo in clinical trials.

Platelet counts less than 50,000/mm^3 occurred at a rate of 0.1% in patients given enoxaparin sodium injection, in 0.2% in patients given heparin, and 0.4% of patients given placebo in the same trials.

Thrombocytopenia of any degree should be monitored closely. If the platelet count falls below 100,000/mm^3, enoxaparin sodium injection should be discontinued. Cases of heparin-induced thrombocytopenia with thrombosis have also been observed in clinical practice. Some of these cases were complicated by organ infarction, limb ischemia, or death.

PROSTHETIC HEART VALVES

The use of enoxaparin sodium injection is not recommended for thromboprophylaxis in patients with prosthetic heart valves. Cases of prosthetic heart valve thrombosis have been reported in patients with prosthetic valves who have received enoxaparin for thromboprophylaxis. Some of these cases were pregnant women in whom thrombosis led to maternal deaths and fetal deaths. Pregnant women with prosthetic heart valves may be at higher risk for thromboembolism (see PRECAUTIONS, Pregnancy Category B).

PRECAUTIONS

GENERAL

Enoxaparin sodium injection should not be mixed with other injections or infusions.

Enoxaparin sodium injection should be used with care in patients with a bleeding diathesis, uncontrolled arterial hypertension or a history of recent gastrointestinal ulceration, diabetic retinopathy, and hemorrhage. Elderly patients and patients with renal insufficiency may show delayed elimination of enoxaparin. Enoxaparin sodium injection should be used with care in these patients. Adjustment of enoxaparin sodium dose may be considered for low weight (<45 kg) patients and/or for patients with severe renal impairment (creatinine clearance <30 ml/min).

If thromboembolic events occur despite enoxaparin sodium injection prophylaxis, appropriate therapy should be initiated.

LABORATORY TESTS

Periodic complete blood counts, including platelet count, and stool occult blood tests are recommended during the course of treatment with enoxaparin sodium injection. When administered at recommended prophylaxis doses, routine coagulation tests such as Prothrombin Time (PT) and Activated Partial Thromboplastin Time (aPTT) are relatively insensitive measures of enoxaparin sodium injection activity and, therefore, unsuitable for monitoring. Anti-Factor Xa may be used to monitor the anticoagulant effect of enoxaparin sodium injection in patients with significant renal impairment. If during enoxaparin sodium injection therapy abnormal coagulation parameters or bleeding should occur, anti-Factor Xa levels may be used to monitor the anticoagulant effects of enoxaparin sodium injection (see CLINICAL PHARMACOLOGY, Pharmacodynamics).

CARCINOGENESIS, MUTAGENESIS, AND IMPAIRMENT OF FERTILITY

No long-term studies in animals have been performed to evaluate the carcinogenic potential of enoxaparin. Enoxaparin was not mutagenic in *in vitro* tests, including the Ames test, mouse lymphoma cell forward mutation test, and human lymphocyte chromosomal aberration test and the *in vivo* rat bone marrow chromosomal aberration test. Enoxaparin was found to have no effect on fertility or reproductive performance of male and female rats at SC doses up to 20 mg/kg/day or 141 mg/m^2/day. The maximum human dose in clinical trials was 2.0 mg/kg/day or 78 mg/m^2/day (for an average body weight of 70 kg, height of 170 cm, and body surface area of 1.8 m^2).

PREGNANCY CATEGORY B

Teratogenic Effects

Teratology studies have been conducted in pregnant rats and rabbits at SC doses of enoxaparin up to 30 mg/kg/day or 211 mg/m^2/day and 410 mg/m^2/day, respectively. There was no evidence of teratogenic effects or fetotoxicity due to enoxaparin. There are, however, no adequate and well-controlled studies in pregnant women. Because animal reproduction studies are not always predictive of human response, this drug should be used during pregnancy only if clearly needed.

There have been reports of congenital anomalies in infants born to women who received enoxaparin during pregnancy including cerebral anomalies, limb anomalies, hypospadias, peripheral vascular malformation, fibrotic dysplasia, and cardiac defect. A cause and effect relationship has not been established nor has the incidence been shown to be higher than in the general population.

Nonteratogenic Effects

There have been post-marketing reports of fetal death when pregnant women received enoxaparin sodium injection. Causality for these cases has not been determined. Pregnant women receiving anticoagulants, including enoxaparin, are at increased risk for bleeding. Hemorrhage can occur at any site and may lead to death of mother and/or fetus. Pregnant women receiving enoxaparin should be carefully monitored. Pregnant women and women of child-bearing potential should be apprised of the potential hazard to the fetus and the mother if enoxaparin is administered during pregnancy.

In a clinical study of pregnant women with prosthetic heart valves given enoxaparin (1 mg/kg bid) to reduce the risk of thromboembolism, 2 of 7 women developed clots resulting in blockage of the valve and leading to maternal and fetal death. There are postmarketing reports of prosthetic valve thrombosis in pregnant women with prosthetic heart valves while receiving enoxaparin for thromboprophylaxis. These events resulted in maternal death or surgical interventions. The use of enoxaparin sodium injection is not recommended for thromboprophylaxis in pregnant women with prosthetic heart valves (see WARNINGS, Prosthetic Heart Valves).

NURSING MOTHERS

It is not known whether this drug is excreted in human milk. Because many drugs are excreted in human milk, caution should be exercised when enoxaparin sodium injection is administered to nursing women.

PEDIATRIC USE

Safety and effectiveness of enoxaparin sodium injection in pediatric patients has not been established.

GERIATRIC USE

Over 2800 patients, 65 years and older, have received enoxaparin sodium injection in pivotal clinical trials. The efficacy of enoxaparin sodium injection in the elderly (≥65 years) was similar to that seen in younger patients (<65 years). The incidence of bleeding complications was similar between elderly and younger patients when 30 mg every 12 hours or 40 mg once a day doses of enoxaparin sodium injection were employed. The incidence of bleeding complications was higher in elderly patients as compared to younger patients when enoxaparin sodium injection was administered at doses of 1.5 mg/kg once a day or 1 mg/kg every 12 hours. The risk of enoxaparin sodium injection-associated bleeding increased with age. Serious adverse events increased with age for patients receiving enoxaparin sodium injection. Other clinical experience (including postmarketing surveillance and literature reports) has not revealed additional differences in the safety of enoxaparin sodium injection between elderly and younger patients. Careful attention to dosing intervals and concomitant medications (especially antiplatelet medications) is advised. Monitoring of geriatric patients with low body weight (<45 kg) and those predisposed to decreased renal function should be considered. (See CLINICAL PHARMACOLOGY and PRECAUTIONS: General and Laboratory Tests.)

DRUG INTERACTIONS

Unless really needed, agents which may enhance the risk of hemorrhage should be discontinued prior to initiation of enoxaparin sodium injection therapy. These agents include medications such as: anticoagulants, platelet inhibitors including acetylsalicylic acid, salicylates, NSAIDs (including ketorolac tromethamine), dipyridamole, or sulfinpyrazone. If co-administration is essential, conduct close clinical and laboratory monitoring (see PRECAUTIONS, Laboratory Tests).

ADVERSE REACTIONS

HEMORRHAGE

The incidence of major hemorrhagic complications during enoxaparin sodium injection treatment has been low.

The rates of major bleeding events that have been reported during clinical trials with enoxaparin sodium injection are listed in TABLES 13-17.

Injection site hematomas during the extended prophylaxis period after hip replacement surgery occurred in 9% of the enoxaparin sodium injection patients versus 1.8% of the placebo patients.

***TABLE 13** Major Bleeding Episodes Following Abdominal and Colorectal Surgery**

	Dosing Regimen	
	Enoxaparin	**Heparin**
Indications	**40 mg qd SC**	**5000 U q8h SC**
Abdominal surgery	n=555 23 (4%)	n=560 16 (3%)
Colorectal surgery	n=673 28 (4%)	n=674 21 (3%)

* Bleeding complications were considered major: (1) if the hemorrhage caused a significant clinical event, or (2) if accompanied by a hemoglobin decreased ≥2 g/dl or transfusion of 2 or more units of blood products. Retroperitoneal, intraocular, and intracranial hemorrhages were always considered major.

***TABLE 14** Major Bleeding Episodes Following Hip or Knee Replacement Surgery**

	Dosing Regimen		
	Enoxaparin		**Heparin**
Indications	**40 mg qd SC**	**30 mg q12h SC**	**15,000 U/24h SC**
Hip Replacement Surgery Without Extended Prophylaxis†		n=786 31 (4%)	n=541 32 (6%)
Hip Replacement Surgery With Extended Prophylaxis			
Perioperative Period‡	n=288 4 (2%)		
Extended Prophylaxis Period§	n=221 0 (0%)		
Knee Replacement Surgery Without Extended Prophylaxis†		n=294 3 (1%)	n=225 3 (1%)

* Bleeding complications were considered major: (1) if the hemorrhage caused a significant clinical event, or (2) if accompanied by a hemoglobin decreased ≥2 g/dl or transfusion of 2 or more units of blood products. Retroperitoneal and intracranial hemorrhages were always considered major. In the knee replacement surgery trials, intraocular hemorrhages were also considered major hemorrhages.

† Enoxaparin sodium injection 30 mg every 12 hours SC initiated 12-24 hours after surgery and continued for up to 14 days after surgery.

‡ Enoxaparin sodium injection 40 mg SC once a day initiated up to 12 hours prior to surgery and continued for up to 7 days after surgery.

§ Enoxaparin sodium injection 40 mg SC once a day for up to 21 days after discharge.

Note: At no time point were the 40 mg once a day preoperative and the 30 mg every 12 hours postoperative hip replacement surgery prophylactic regimens compared in clinical trials.

***TABLE 15** Major Bleeding Episodes in Medical Patients With Severely Restricted Mobility During Acute Illness**

	Dosing Regimen		
	Enoxaparin†		**Placebo†**
Indications	**20 mg qd SC**	**40 mg qd SC**	
Medical patients during acute illness	n=351 1 (<1%)	n=360 3 (<1%)	n=362 2 (<1%)

* Bleeding complications were considered major: (1) if the hemorrhage caused a significant clinical event, (2) if the hemorrhage caused a decrease in hemoglobin of ≥2 g/dl or transfusion of 2 or more units of blood products. Retroperitoneal and intracranial hemorrhages were always considered major although none were reported during the trial.

† The rates represent major bleeding on study medication up to 24 hours after last dose.

***TABLE 16** Major Bleeding Episodes in Unstable Angina and Non-Q-Wave Myocardial Infarction*

	Dosing Regimen	
	Enoxaparin*	**Heparin***
Indication	**1 mg/kg q12h SC**	**aPTT Adjusted IV Therapy**
Unstable angina and non-Q-wave MI†‡	n=1578 17 (1%)	n=1529 18 (1%)

* The rates represent major bleeding on study medication up to 12 hours after dose.

† Aspirin therapy was administered concurrently (100-325 mg/day).

‡ Bleeding complications were considered major: (1) if the hemorrhage caused a significant clinical event, or (2) if accompanied by a hemoglobin decrease by ≥3 g/dl or transfusion of 2 or more units of blood products. Intraocular, retroperitoneal, and intracranial hemorrhages were always considered major.

THROMBOCYTOPENIA

See WARNINGS, Thrombocytopenia.

ELEVATIONS OF SERUM AMINOTRANSFERASES

Asymptomatic increases in aspartate (AST [SGOT]) and alanine (ALT [SGPT]) aminotransferase levels greater than 3 times the upper limit of normal of the laboratory reference range have been reported in up to 6.1% and 5.9% of patients, respectively, during treatment with enoxaparin sodium injection. Similar significant increases in aminotransferase levels have also been observed in patients and healthy volunteers treated with heparin and other low

TABLE 17 *Major Bleeding Episodes in DVT With or Without Pulmonary Embolism Treatment**

	Dosing Regimen†		
	Enoxaparin		Heparin
Indications	1.5 mg/kg qd SC	1 mg/kg q12h SC	aPTT Adjusted IV Therapy
Treatment of DVT and PE	n=298	n=559	n=554
	5 (2%)	9 (2%)	9 (2%)

* Bleeding complications were considered major: (1) if the hemorrhage caused a significant clinical event, or (2) if accompanied by a hemoglobin decrease ≥2 g/dl or transfusion of 2 or more units of blood products. Retroperitoneal, intraocular, and intracranial hemorrhages were always considered major.
† All patients also received warfarin sodium (dose-adjusted according to PT to achieve an INR of 2.0-3.0) commencing within 72 hours of enoxaparin sodium injection or standard heparin therapy and continuing for up to 90 days.

molecular weight heparins. Such elevations are fully reversible and are rarely associated with increases in bilirubin.

Since aminotransferase determinations are important in the differential diagnosis of myocardial infarction, liver disease, and pulmonary emboli, elevations that might be caused by drugs like enoxaparin sodium injection should be interpreted with caution.

LOCAL REACTIONS

Mild local irritation, pain, hematoma, ecchymosis, and erythema may follow SC injection of enoxaparin sodium injection.

OTHER

Other adverse effects that were thought to be possibly or probably related to treatment with enoxaparin sodium injection, heparin, or placebo in clinical trials with patients undergoing hip or knee replacement surgery, abdominal or colorectal surgery, or treatment for DVT and that occurred at a rate of at least 2% in the enoxaparin sodium injection group, are provided in TABLE 18, TABLE 19A, TABLE 19B, and TABLE 20.

TABLE 18 *Adverse Events Occurring at ≥2% Incidence in Enoxaparin Sodium Injection Treated Patients* Undergoing Abdominal or Colorectal Surgery*

	Enoxaparin		Heparin	
	40 mg qd SC		5000 U q8h SC	
	n=1228		n=1234	
Adverse Event	Severe	Total	Severe	Total
Hemorrhage	<1%	7%	<1%	6%
Anemia	<1%	3%	<1%	3%
Ecchymosis	0%	3%	0%	3%

* Excluding unrelated adverse events.

TABLE 19A *Adverse Events Occurring at ≥2% Incidence in Enoxaparin Sodium Injection Treated Patients* Undergoing Hip or Knee Replacement Surgery*

	Enoxaparin		Enoxaparin		Enoxaparin	
	40 mg qd SC		40 mg qd SC		30 mg q12h SC	
	Perioperative Period		Extended Prophylaxis Period			
	n=288†		n=131‡		n=1080	
Adverse Event	Severe	Total	Severe	Total	Severe	Total
Fever	0%	8%	0%	0%	<1%	5%
Hemorrhage	<1%	13%	0%	5%	<1%	4%
Nausea					<1%	3%
Anemia	0%	16%	0%	<2%	<1%	2%
Edema					<1%	2%
Peripheral edema	0%	6%	0%	0%	<1%	3%

* Excluding unrelated adverse events.
† Data represents enoxaparin sodium injection 40 mg SC once a day initiated up to 12 hours prior to surgery in 288 hip replacement surgery patients who received enoxaparin sodium injection peri-operatively in an unblinded fashion in one clinical trial.
‡ Data represents enoxaparin sodium injection 40 mg SC once a day given in a blinded fashion as extended prophylaxis at the end of the peri-operative period in 131 of the original 288 hip replacement surgery patients for up to 21 days in one clinical trial.

ADVERSE EVENTS IN ENOXAPARIN SODIUM INJECTION TREATED PATIENTS WITH UNSTABLE ANGINA OR NON-Q-WAVE MYOCARDIAL INFARCTION

Non-hemorrhagic clinical events reported to be related to enoxaparin sodium injection therapy occurred at an incidence of ≤1%.

Non-major hemorrhagic episodes, primarily injection site ecchymoses and hematomas, were more frequently reported in patients treated with SC enoxaparin sodium injection than in patients treated with IV heparin.

Serious adverse events with enoxaparin sodium injection or heparin in a clinical trial in patients with unstable angina or non-Q-wave myocardial infarction that occurred at a rate of at least 0.5% in the enoxaparin sodium injection group, are provided in TABLE 21 (irrespective of relationship to drug therapy).

TABLE 19B *Adverse Events Occurring at ≥2% Incidence in Enoxaparin Sodium Injection Treated Patients* Undergoing Hip or Knee Replacement Surgery*

	Heparin		Placebo	
	15,000 U/24h SC		q12h SC	
	n=766		n=115	
Adverse Event	Severe	Total	Severe	Total
Fever	<1%	4%	0%	3%
Hemorrhage	1%	4%	0%	3%
Nausea	<1%	2%	0%	2%
Anemia	2%	5%	<1%	7%
Edema	<1%	2%	0%	2%
Peripheral edema	<1%	4%	0%	3%

* Excluding unrelated adverse events.

TABLE 20 *Adverse Events Occurring at ≥2% Incidence in Enoxaparin Sodium Injection Treated Medical Patients* With Severely Restricted Mobility During Acute Illness*

	Enoxaparin	Placebo
	40 mg qd SC	qd SC
Adverse Event	n=360	n=362
Dyspnea	3.3%	5.2%
Thrombocytopenia	2.8%	2.8%
Confusion	2.2%	1.1%
Diarrhea	2.2%	1.7%
Nausea	2.5%	1.7%

* Excluding unrelated and unlikely adverse events.

TABLE 21 *Serious Adverse Events Occurring at ≥0.5% Incidence in Enoxaparin Sodium Injection Treated Patients With Unstable Angina or Non-Q-Wave Myocardial Infarction*

	Enoxaparin	Heparin
	1 mg/kg q12h SC	aPTT Adjusted IV Therapy
Adverse Event	n=1578	n=1529
Atrial fibrillation	11 (0.70%)	3 (0.20%)
Heart failure	15 (0.95%)	11 (0.72%)
Lung edema	11 (0.70%)	11 (0.72%)
Pneumonia	13 (0.82%)	9 (0.59%)

TABLE 22 *Adverse Events Occurring at ≥2% Incidence in Enoxaparin Sodium Injection Treated Patients* Undergoing Treatment of DVT With or Without Pulmonary Embolism*

	Enoxaparin				Heparin	
	1.5 mg/kg qd SC		1 mg/kg q12h SC		aPTT Adjusted IV Therapy	
	n=298		n=559		n=544	
Adverse Event	Severe	Total	Severe	Total	Severe	Total
Injection site hemorrhage	0%	5%	0%	3%	<1%	<1%
Injection site pain	0%	2%	0%	2%	0%	0%
Hematuria	0%	2%	0%	<1%	<1%	2%

* Excluding unrelated adverse events.

ONGOING SAFETY SURVEILLANCE

Since 1993, there have been more than 80 reports of epidural or spinal hematoma formation with concurrent use of enoxaparin sodium injection and spinal/epidural anesthesia or spinal puncture. The majority of patients had a post-operative indwelling epidural catheter placed for analgesia or received additional drugs affecting hemostasis such as NSAIDs. Many of the epidural or spinal hematomas caused neurologic injury, including long-term or permanent paralysis. Because these events were reported voluntarily from a population of unknown size, estimates of frequency cannot be made.

Other Ongoing Safety Surveillance Reports

Local reactions at the injection site (*i.e.*, skin necrosis, nodules, inflammation, oozing), systemic allergic reactions (*i.e.*, pruritus, urticaria, anaphylactoid reactions), vesiculobullous rash, purpura, thrombocytosis, and thrombocytopenia with thrombosis (see WARNINGS, Thrombocytopenia). Very rare cases of hyperlipidemia have been reported, with one case of hyperlipidemia, with marked hypertriglyceridemia, reported in a diabetic pregnant woman; causality has not been determined.

DOSAGE AND ADMINISTRATION

All patients should be evaluated for a bleeding disorder before administration of enoxaparin sodium injection, unless the medication is needed urgently. Since coagulation parameters

are unsuitable for monitoring enoxaparin sodium injection activity, routine monitoring of coagulation parameters is not required (see PRECAUTIONS, Laboratory Tests).
Note: Lovenox injection is available in two concentrations: 100 and 150 mg/ml of enoxaparin sodium in water for injection.

ADULT DOSAGE

Abdominal Surgery

In patients undergoing abdominal surgery who are at risk for thromboembolic complications, the recommended dose of enoxaparin sodium injection is **40 mg once a day** administered by SC injection with the initial dose given 2 hours prior to surgery. The usual duration of administration is 7-10 days; up to 12 days administration has been well tolerated in clinical trials.

Hip or Knee Replacement Surgery

In patients undergoing hip or knee replacement surgery, the recommended dose of enoxaparin sodium injection is **30 mg every 12 hours** administered by SC injection. Provided that hemostasis has been established, the initial dose should be given 12-24 hours after surgery. For hip replacement surgery, a dose of **40 mg once a day** SC, given initially 12 (±3) hours prior to surgery, may be considered. Following the initial phase of thromboprophylaxis in hip replacement surgery patients, continued prophylaxis with enoxaparin sodium injection 40 mg once a day administered by SC injection for 3 weeks is recommended. The usual duration of administration is 7-10 days; up to 14 days administration has been well tolerated in clinical trials.

Medical Patients During Acute Illness

In medical patients at risk for thromboembolic complications due to severely restricted mobility during acute illness, the recommended dose of enoxaparin sodium injection is **40 mg once a day** administered by SC injection. The usual duration of administration is 6-11 days; up to 14 days of enoxaparin sodium injection has been well tolerated in the controlled clinical trial.

Unstable Angina and Non-Q-Wave Myocardial Infarction

In patients with unstable angina or non-Q-wave myocardial infarction, the recommended dose of enoxaparin sodium injection is **1 mg/kg** administered SC **every 12 hours** in conjunction with oral aspirin therapy (100-325 mg once daily). Treatment with enoxaparin sodium injection should be prescribed for a minimum of 2 days and continued until clinical stabilization. To minimize the risk of bleeding following vascular instrumentation during the treatment of unstable angina, adhere precisely to the intervals recommended between enoxaparin sodium injection doses. The vascular access sheath for instrumentation should remain in place for 6-8 hours following a dose of enoxaparin sodium injection. The next scheduled dose should be given no sooner than 6-8 hours after sheath removal. The site of the procedure should be observed for signs of bleeding or hematoma formation. The usual duration of treatment is 2-8 days; up to 12.5 days of enoxaparin sodium injection has been well tolerated in clinical trials.

Treatment of DVT With or Without Pulmonary Embolism

In **outpatient treatment,** patients with acute DVT without pulmonary embolism who can be treated at home, the recommended dose of enoxaparin sodium injection is **1 mg/kg every 12 hours** administered SC. In **inpatient (hospital) treatment,** patients with acute DVT with pulmonary embolism or patients with acute DVT without pulmonary embolism (who are not candidates for outpatient treatment), the recommended dose of enoxaparin sodium injection is **1 mg/kg every 12 hours** administered SC **or 1.5 mg/kg once a day** administered SC at the same time every day. In both outpatient and inpatient (hospital) treatments, warfarin sodium therapy should be initiated when appropriate (usually within 72 hours of enoxaparin sodium injection). Enoxaparin sodium injection should be continued for a minimum of 5 days and until a therapeutic oral anticoagulant effect has been achieved (International Normalization Ratio 2.0-3.0). The average duration of administration is 7 days; up to 17 days enoxaparin sodium injection administration has been well tolerated in controlled clinical trials.

ADMINISTRATION

Enoxaparin injection is a clear, colorless to pale yellow sterile solution, and as with other parenteral drug products, should be inspected visually for particulate matter and discoloration prior to administration.

When using enoxaparin sodium injection ampules, to assure withdrawal of the appropriate volume of drug, the use of a tuberculin syringe or equivalent is recommended.

Enoxaparin sodium injection is administered by SC injection. It must not be administered by intramuscular injection. Enoxaparin sodium injection is intended for use under the guidance of a physician. Patients may self-inject only if their physician determines that it is appropriate and with medical follow-up, as necessary. Proper training in subcutaneous injection technique (with or without the assistance of an injection device) should be provided.

Subcutaneous Injection Technique

Patients should be lying down and enoxaparin sodium injection administered by deep SC injection. To avoid the loss of drug when using the 30 and 40 mg prefilled syringes, do not expel the air bubble from the syringe before the injection. Administration should be alternated between the left and right anterolateral and left and right posterolateral abdominal wall. The whole length of the needle should be introduced into a skin fold held between the thumb and forefinger; the skin fold should be held throughout the injection. To minimize bruising, do not rub the injection site after completion of the injection. An automatic injector, Lovenox EasyInjector, is available for patients to administer enoxaparin sodium injection packaged in 30 and 40 mg prefilled syringes. Please see directions accompanying the Lovenox EasyInjector automatic injection device.

HOW SUPPLIED

Lovenox Injection is available in two concentrations (see TABLE 23).
Storage: Store at controlled room temperature: 15-25°C (59-77°F).

TABLE 23

Dosage Unit	Strength*	Anti-Xa Activity†	Syringe Label Color
100 mg/ml Concentration			
Ampules	30 mg/0.3 ml	3000 IU	Medium Blue
Prefilled syringes‡	30 mg/0.3 ml	3000 IU	Medium Blue
Prefilled syringes‡	40 mg/0.4 ml	4000 IU	Yellow
Graduated prefilled syringes‡	60 mg/0.6 ml	6000 IU	Orange
Graduated prefilled syringes‡	80 mg/0.8 ml	8000 IU	Brown
Graduated prefilled syringes‡	100 mg/1 ml	10,000 IU	Black
150 mg/ml Concentration			
Graduated prefilled syringes‡	120 mg/0.8 ml	12,000 IU	Purple
Graduated prefilled syringes‡	150 mg/1 ml	15,000 IU	Navy Blue

* Strength represents the number of mg of enoxaparin sodium in water for injection. Lovenox Injection ampules, 30 and 40 mg prefilled syringes, and 60, 80, and 100 mg graduated prefilled syringes each contain **10 mg enoxaparin sodium per 0.1 ml water for injection.** The 120 and 150 mg graduated prefilled syringes each contain **15 mg enoxaparin sodium per 0.1 ml water for injection.**

† Approximate anti-Factor Xa activity based on reference to the WHO First International Low Molecular Weight Heparin Reference Standard

‡ Each Lovenox Injection syringe and graduated prefilled syringe is affixed with a 27 gauge × ½ inch needle.

PRODUCT LISTING - EQUIVALENTS NOT AVAILABLE

Solution - Subcutaneous - 100 mg/ml

0.30 ml x 10	$183.50	LOVENOX, Aventis Pharmaceuticals	00075-0624-03
0.30 ml x 10	$192.60	LOVENOX, Aventis Pharmaceuticals	00075-0624-30
0.40 ml x 10	$256.90	LOVENOX, Aventis Pharmaceuticals	00075-0620-40
0.60 ml x 10	$385.80	LOVENOX, Aventis Pharmaceuticals	00075-0621-60
0.80 ml x 10	$514.40	LOVENOX, Aventis Pharmaceuticals	00075-0622-80
1 ml x 10	$642.90	LOVENOX, Aventis Pharmaceuticals	00075-0623-00
3 ml	$192.65	LOVENOX, Aventis Pharmaceuticals	00075-0626-03

Solution - Subcutaneous - 150 mg/ml

0.80 ml x 10	$771.80	LOVENOX, Aventis Pharmaceuticals	00075-2912-01
1 ml x 10	$964.80	LOVENOX, Aventis Pharmaceuticals	00075-2915-01

Entacapone *(003454)*

Categories: Parkinson's disease; Pregnancy Category C; FDA Approved 1999 Oct
Drug Classes: Antiparkinson agents; Dopaminergics
Foreign Brand Availability: Comtade (Colombia); Comtan (Australia; Austria; Belgium; Bulgaria; Czech-Republic; Denmark; England; Finland; France; Germany; Greece; Hong-Kong; Hungary; Indonesia; Ireland; Israel; Italy; Mexico; Netherlands; New-Zealand; Norway; Philippines; Poland; Portugal; Slovenia; South-Africa; Spain; Sweden; Switzerland; Thailand; Turkey); Comtess (Austria; Belgium; Bulgaria; Czech-Republic; Denmark; England; Finland; France; Germany; Greece; Hungary; Ireland; Italy; Netherlands; Norway; Poland; Portugal; Slovenia; Spain; Sweden; Switzerland; Turkey)
Cost of Therapy: $171.82 (Parkinsonism; Comtan; 200 mg; 3 tablets/day; 30 day supply)

DESCRIPTION

Comtan is available as tablets containing 200 mg entacapone.

Entacapone is an inhibitor of catechol-*O*-methyltransferase (COMT), used in the treatment of Parkinson's disease as an adjunct to carbidopa; levodopa therapy. It is a nitrocatechol-structured compound with a relative molecular mass of 305.29. The chemical name of entacapone is (E)-2-cyano-3-(3,4-dihydroxy-5-nitrophenyl)-N,N-diethyl-2-propenamide. Its empirical formula is $C_{14}H_{15}N_3O_5$.
Inactive Ingredients: Microcrystalline cellulose, mannitol, croscarmellose sodium, hydrogenated vegetable oil, hydroxypropyl methylcellulose, polysorbate 80, glycerol 85%, sucrose, magnesium stearate, yellow iron oxide, red oxide, and titanium dioxide.

CLINICAL PHARMACOLOGY

MECHANISM OF ACTION

Entacapone is a selective and reversible inhibitor of catechol-*O*-methyltransferase (COMT).

In mammals, COMT is distributed throughout various organs with the highest activities in the liver and kidney. COMT also occurs in the heart, lung, smooth and skeletal muscles, intestinal tract, reproductive organs, various glands, adipose tissue, skin, blood cells, and neuronal tissues, especially in glial cells. COMT catalyzes the transfer of the methyl group of S-adenosyl-L-methionine to the phenolic group of substrates that contain a catechol structure. Physiological substrates of COMT include dopa, catecholamines (dopamine, norepinephrine, and epinephrine) and their hydroxylated metabolites. The function of COMT is the elimination of biologically active catechols and some other hydroxylated metabolites. In the presence of a decarboxylase inhibitor, COMT becomes the major metabolizing enzyme for levodopa, catalyzing the metabolism to 3-methoxy-4-hydroxy-L-phenylalanine (3-OMD) in the brain and periphery.

The mechanism of action of entacapone is believed to be through its ability to inhibit COMT and alter the plasma pharmacokinetics of levodopa. When entacapone is given in conjunction with levodopa and an aromatic amino acid decarboxylase inhibitor, such as carbidopa, plasma levels of levodopa are greater and more sustained than after administration of levodopa and an aromatic amino acid decarboxylase inhibitor alone. It is believed that at a given frequency of levodopa administration, these more sustained plasma levels of levodopa result in more constant dopaminergic stimulation in the brain, leading to greater effects on the signs and symptoms of Parkinson's disease. The higher levodopa levels also lead to increased levodopa adverse effects, sometimes requiring a decrease in the dose of levodopa.

In animals, while entacapone enters the CNS to a minimal extent, it has been shown to inhibit central COMT activity. In humans, entacapone inhibits the COMT enzyme in peripheral tissues. The effects of entacapone on central COMT activity in humans have not been studied.

PHARMACODYNAMICS

COMT Activity in Erythrocytes

Studies in healthy volunteers have shown that entacapone reversibly inhibits human erythrocyte catechol-*O*-methyltransferase (COMT) activity after oral administration. There was a linear correlation between entacapone dose and erythrocyte COMT inhibition, the maximum inhibition being 82% following an 800 mg single dose. With a 200 mg single dose of entacapone, maximum inhibition of erythrocyte COMT activity is on average 65% with a return to baseline level within 8 hours.

EFFECT ON THE PHARMACOKINETICS OF LEVODOPA AND ITS METABOLITES

When 200 mg entacapone is administered together with carbidopa; levodopa, it increases the area under the curve (AUC) of levodopa by approximately 35% and the elimination half life of levodopa is prolonged from 1.3 hours to 2.4 hours. In general, the average peak levodopa plasma concentration and the time of its occurrence (T_{max} of 1 hour) are unaffected. The onset of effect occurs after the first administration and is maintained during long-term treatment. Studies in Parkinson's disease patients suggest that the maximal effect occurs with 200 mg entacapone. Plasma levels of 3-OMD are markedly and dose-dependently decreased by entacapone when given with carbidopa; levodopa.

PHARMACOKINETICS OF ENTACAPONE

Entacapone pharmacokinetics are linear over the dose range of 5-800 mg, and are independent of carbidopa; levodopa coadministration. The elimination of entacapone is biphasic, with an elimination half-life of 0.4-0.7 hours based on the β-phase and 2.4 hours based on the γ-phase. The γ-phase accounts for approximately 10% of the total AUC. The total body clearance after iv administration is 850 ml/min. After a single 200 mg dose of entacapone, the C_{max} is approximately 1.2 μg/ml.

Absorption

Entacapone is rapidly absorbed, with a T_{max} of approximately 1 hour. The absolute bioavailability following oral administration is 35%. Food does not affect the pharmacokinetics of entacapone.

Distribution

The volume of distribution of entacapone at steady state after IV injection is small (20 L). Entacapone does not distribute widely into tissues due to its high plasma protein binding. Based on *in vitro* studies, the plasma protein binding of entacapone is 98% over the concentration range of 0.4-50 μg/ml. Entacapone binds mainly to serum albumin.

Metabolism and Elimination

Entacapone is almost completely metabolized prior to excretion, with only a very small amount (0.2% of dose) found unchanged in urine. The main metabolic pathway is isomerization to the *cis*-isomer, followed by direct glucuronidation of the parent and *cis*-isomer; the glucuronide conjugate is inactive. After oral administration of a ^{14}C-labeled dose of entacapone, 10% of labeled parent and metabolite is excreted in urine and 90% in feces.

Special Populations

Entacapone pharmacokinetics are independent of age. No formal gender studies have been conducted. Racial representation in clinical trials was largely limited to Caucasians (there were only 4 blacks in one US trial and no Asians in any of the clinical trials); no conclusions can therefore be reached about the effect of entacapone on groups other than Caucasian.

Hepatic Impairment

A single 200 mg dose of entacapone, without levodopa/dopa decarboxylase inhibitor coadministration, showed approximately 2-fold higher AUC and C_{max} values in patients with a history of alcoholism and hepatic impairment (n=10) compared to normal subjects (n=10). All patients had biopsy-proven liver cirrhosis caused by alcohol. According to Child-Pugh grading 7 patients with liver disease had mild hepatic impairment and 3 patients had moderate hepatic impairment. As only about 10% of the entacapone dose is excreted in urine as parent compound and conjugated glucuronide, biliary excretion appears to be the major route of excretion of this drug. Consequently, entacapone should be administered with care to patients with biliary obstruction.

Renal Impairment

The pharmacokinetics of entacapone have been investigated after a single 200 mg entacapone dose, without levodopa/dopa decarboxylase inhibitor coadministration, in a specific renal impairment study. There were three groups: normal subjects (n=7; creatinine clearance >1.12 ml/sec/1.73 m^2) moderate impairment (n=10; creatinine clearance ranging from 0.60-0.89 ml/sec/1.73 m^2), and severe impairment (n=7; creatinine clearance ranging from 0.20-0.44 ml/sec/1.73 m^2). No important effects of renal function on the pharmacokinetics of entacapone were found.

INDICATIONS AND USAGE

Entacapone is indicated as an adjunct to carbidopa; levodopa to treat patients with idiopathic Parkinson's Disease who experience the signs and symptoms of end-of-dose "wearing-off".

Entacapone's effectiveness has not been systematically evaluated in patients with idiopathic Parkinson's Disease who do not experience end-of-dose "wearing-off".

CONTRAINDICATIONS

Entacapone tablets are contraindicated in patients who have demonstrated hypersensitivity to the drug or its ingredients.

WARNINGS

Monoamine oxidase (MAO) and COMT are the two major enzyme systems involved in the metabolism of catecholamines. It is theoretically possible, therefore, that the combination of entacapone and a non-selective MAO inhibitor (*e.g.*, phenelzine and tranylcypromine) would result in inhibition of the majority of the pathways responsible for normal catecholamine metabolism. For this reason, patients should ordinarily not be treated concomitantly with entacapone and a non-selective MAO inhibitor.

Entacapone can be taken concomitantly with a selective MAO-B inhibitor (*e.g.*, selegiline).

DRUGS METABOLIZED BY CATECHOL-O-METHYLTRANSFERASE (COMT)

When a single 400 mg dose of entacapone was given together with intravenous isoprenaline (isoproterenol) and epinephrine without coadministered levodopa/dopa decarboxylase inhibitor, the overall mean maximal changes in heart rate during infusion were about 50% and 80% higher than with placebo, for isoprenaline and epinephrine, respectively.

Therefore, drugs known to be metabolized by COMT, such as isoproterenol, epinephrine, norepinephrine, dopamine, dobutamine, alpha-methyldopa, apomorphine, isoetherine, and bitolterol should be administered with caution in patients receiving entacapone regardless of the route of administration (including inhalation), as their interaction may result in increased heart rates, possibly arrhythmias, and excessive changes in blood pressure.

Ventricular tachycardia was noted in one 32-year-old healthy male volunteer in an interaction study after epinephrine infusion and oral entacapone administration. Treatment with propranolol was required. A causal relationship to entacapone administration appears probable but cannot be attributed with certainty.

PRECAUTIONS

HYPOTENSION/SYNCOPE

Dopaminergic therapy in Parkinson's disease patients has been associated with orthostatic hypotension. Entacapone enhances levodopa bioavailability and, therefore, might be expected to increase the occurrence of orthostatic hypotension. In entacapone clinical trials, however, no differences from placebo were seen for measured orthostasis or symptoms of orthostasis. Orthostatic hypotension was documented at least once in 2.7% and 3.0% of the patients treated 200 mg entacapone and placebo respectively. A total of 4.3% and 4.0% of the patients treated with 200 mg entacapone and placebo, respectively, reported orthostatic symptoms at some time during their treatment and also had at least one episode of orthostatic hypotension documented (however, the episode of orthostatic symptoms itself was not accompanied by vital sign measurements). Neither baseline treatment with dopamine agonists or selegiline, nor the presence of orthostasis at baseline, increased the risk of orthostatic hypotension in patients treated with entacapone compared to patients on placebo.

In the large controlled trials, approximately 1.2% and 0.8% of 200 mg entacapone and placebo patients, respectively, reported at least one episode of syncope. Reports of syncope were generally more frequent in patients in both treatment groups who had an episode of documented hypotension (although the episodes of syncope, obtained by history, were themselves not documented with vital sign measurement).

DIARRHEA

In clinical trials, diarrhea developed in 60 of 603 (10.0%) and 16 of 400 (4.0%) of patients treated with 200 mg entacapone and placebo, respectively. In patients treated with entacapone, diarrhea was generally mild to moderate in severity (8.6%) but was regarded as severe in 1.3%. Diarrhea resulted in withdrawal in 10 of 603 (1.7%) patients, (1.2%) with mild and moderate diarrhea, and 3 (0.5%) with severe diarrhea. Diarrhea generally resolved after discontinuation of entacapone. Two patients with diarrhea were hospitalized. Typically, diarrhea presents within 4-12 weeks after entacapone is started, but it may appear as early as the first week and as late as many months after the initiation of treatment.

HALLUCINATIONS

Dopaminergic therapy in Parkinson's disease patients has been associated with hallucinations. In clinical trials, hallucinations developed in approximately 4% of patients treated with 200 mg entacapone or placebo. Hallucinations led to drug discontinuation and premature withdrawal from clinical trials in 0.8% and 0% of patients treated with 200 mg entacapone and placebo, respectively. Hallucinations led to hospitalization in 1.0% and 0.3% of patients in the 200 mg entacapone and placebo groups, respectively.

DYSKINESIA

Entacapone may potentiate the dopaminergic side effects of levodopa and may cause and/or exacerbate preexisting dyskinesia. Although decreasing the dose of levodopa may ameliorate this side effect, many patients in controlled trials continued to experience frequent dyskinesias despite a reduction in their dose of levodopa. The rates of withdrawal for dyskinesia were 1.5% and 0.8% for 200 mg entacapone and placebo, respectively.

EVENTS REPORTED WITH DOPAMINERGIC THERAPY

The events listed below are rare events known to be associated with the use of drugs that increase dopaminergic activity, although they are most often associated with the use of direct dopamine agonists.

Rhabdomyolysis

Cases of severe rhabdomyolysis have been reported with entacapone use. The complicated nature of these cases makes it impossible to determine what role, if any, entacapone played in their pathogenesis. Severe prolonged motor activity including dyskinesia may account for rhabdomyolysis. One case, however, included fever and alteration of consciousness. It is therefore possible that the rhabdomyolysis may be a result of the syndrome described in Hyperpyrexia and Confusion.

Hyperpyrexia and Confusion

Cases of a symptom complex resembling the neuroleptic malignant syndrome characterized by elevated temperature, muscular rigidity, altered consciousness, and elevated CPK have been reported in association with the rapid dose reduction or withdrawal of other dopaminergic drugs. Several cases with similar signs and symptoms have been reported in association with entacapone therapy, although no information about dose manipulation is available. The complicated nature of these cases makes it difficult to determine what role, if any, entacapone may have played in their pathogenesis. No cases have been reported following the abrupt withdrawal or dose reduction of entacapone treatment during clinical studies.

Prescribers should exercise caution when discontinuing entacapone treatment. When considered necessary, withdrawal should proceed slowly. If a decision is made to discontinue treatment with entacapone, recommendations include monitoring the patient closely and adjusting other dopaminergic treatments as needed. This syndrome should be considered in the differential diagnosis for any patient who develops a high fever or severe rigidity. Tapering entacapone has not been systematically evaluated.

Fibrotic Complications

Cases of retroperitoneal fibrosis, pulmonary infiltrates, pleural effusion, and pleural thickening have been reported in some patients treated with ergot derived dopaminergic agents. These complications may resolve when the drug is discontinued, but complete resolution does not always occur. Although these adverse events are believed to be related to the ergoline structure of these compounds, whether other, nonergot derived drugs (*e.g.,* entacapone) that increase dopaminergic activity can cause them is unknown. It should be noted that the expected incidence of fibrotic complications is so low that even if entacapone caused these complications at rates similar to those attributable to other dopaminergic therapies, it is unlikely that it would have been detected in a cohort of the size exposed to entacapone. Four cases of pulmonary fibrosis were reported during clinical development of entacapone; 3 of these patients were also treated with pergolide and one with bromocriptine. The duration of treatment with entacapone ranged from 7-17 months.

RENAL TOXICITY

In a 1 year toxicity study, entacapone (plasma exposure 20 times that in humans receiving the maximum recommended daily dose of 1600 mg) caused an increased incidence in male rats of nephrotoxicity that was characterized by regenerative tubules, thickening of basement membranes, infiltration of mononuclear cells and tubular protein casts. These effects were not associated with changes in clinical chemistry parameters, and there is no established method for monitoring for the possible occurrence of these lesions in humans. Although this toxicity could represent a species-specific effect, there is not yet evidence that this is so.

HEPATIC IMPAIRMENT

Patients with hepatic impairment should be treated with caution. The AUC and C_{max} of entacapone approximately doubled in patients with documented liver disease compared to controls. (See CLINICAL PHARMACOLOGY, Pharmacokinetics of Entacapone and DOSAGE AND ADMINISTRATION.)

INFORMATION FOR THE PATIENT

Patients should be instructed to take entacapone only as prescribed.

Patients should be informed that hallucinations can occur.

Patients should be advised that they may develop postural (orthostatic) hypotension with or without symptoms such as dizziness, nausea, syncope, and sweating. Hypotension may occur more frequently during initial therapy. Accordingly, patients should be cautioned against rising rapidly after sitting or lying down, especially if they have been doing so for prolonged periods, and especially at the initiation of treatment with entacapone.

Patients should be advised that they should neither drive a car nor operate other complex machinery until they have gained sufficient experience on entacapone to gauge whether or not it affects their mental and/or motor performance adversely. Because of the possible additive sedative effects, caution should be used when patients are taking other CNS depressants in combination with entacapone.

Patients should be informed that nausea may occur, especially at the initiation of treatment with entacapone.

Patients should be advised of the possibility of an increase in dyskinesia.

Patients should be advised that treatment with entacapone may cause a change in the color of their urine (a brownish orange discoloration) that is not clinically relevant. In controlled trials, 10% of patients treated with entacapone reported urine discoloration compared to 0% of placebo patients.

Although entacapone has not been shown to be teratogenic in animals, it is always given in conjunction with carbidopa; levodopa, which is known to cause visceral and skeletal malformations in the rabbit. Accordingly, patients should be advised to notify their physicians if they become pregnant or intend to become pregnant during therapy (see Pregnancy Category C).

Entacapone is excreted into maternal milk in rats. Because of the possibility that entacapone may be excreted into human maternal milk, patients should be advised to notify their physicians if they intend to breastfeed or are breastfeeding an infant.

LABORATORY TESTS

Entacapone is a chelator of iron. The impact of entacapone on the body's iron stores is unknown; however, a tendency towards decreasing serum iron concentrations was noted in clinical trials. In a controlled clinical study serum ferritin levels (as marker of iron deficiency and subclinical anemia) were not changed with entacapone compared to placebo after 1 year of treatment and there was no difference in rates of anemia or decreased hemoglobin levels.

SPECIAL POPULATIONS

Patients with hepatic impairment should be treated with caution (see INDICATIONS AND USAGE and DOSAGE AND ADMINISTRATION).

CARCINOGENESIS

Two year carcinogenicity studies of entacapone were conducted in mice and rats. Rats were treated once daily by oral gavage with entacapone doses of 20, 90, or 400 mg/kg. An increased incidence of renal tubular adenomas and carcinomas was found in male rats treated with the highest dose of entacapone. Plasma exposures (AUC) associated with this dose were approximately 20 times higher than estimated plasma exposures of humans receiving the maximum recommended daily dose of entacapone (MRDD = 1600 mg). Mice were treated once daily by oral gavage with doses of 20, 100, or 600 mg/kg of entacapone (0.05, 0.3, and 2 times the MRDD for humans on a mg/m^2 basis). Because of a high incidence of premature mortality in mice receiving the highest dose of entacapone, the mouse study is not an adequate assessment of carcinogenicity. Although no treatment related tumors were observed in animals receiving the lower doses, the carcinogenic potential of entacapone has not been fully evaluated. The carcinogenic potential of entacapone administered in combination with carbidopa; levodopa has not been evaluated.

MUTAGENESIS

Entacapone was mutagenic and clastogenic in the *in vitro* mouse lymphoma/thymidine kinase assay in the presence and absence of metabolic activation, and was clastogenic in cultured human lymphocytes in the presence of metabolic activation. Entacapone, either alone or in combination with carbidopa; levodopa, was not clastogenic in the *in vivo* mouse micronucleus test or mutagenic in the bacterial reverse mutation assay (Ames test).

IMPAIRMENT OF FERTILITY

Entacapone did not impair fertility or general reproductive performance in rats treated with up to 700 mg/kg/day (plasma AUCs 28 times those in humans receiving the MRDD). Delayed mating, but no fertility impairment, was evident in female rats treated with 700 mg/kg/day of entacapone.

PREGNANCY CATEGORY C

In embryofetal development studies, entacapone was administered to pregnant animals throughout organogenesis at doses of up to 1000 mg/kg/day in rats and 300 mg/kg/day in rabbits. Increased incidences of fetal variations were evident in litters from rats treated with the highest dose, in the absence of overt signs of maternal toxicity. The maternal plasma drug exposure (AUC) associated with this dose was approximately 34 times the estimated plasma exposure in humans receiving the maximum recommended daily dose (MRDD) of 1600 mg. Increased frequencies of abortions and late/total resorptions and decreased fetal weights were observed in the litters of rabbits treated with maternotoxic doses of 100 mg/kg/day (plasma AUCs 0.4 times those in humans receiving the MRDD) or greater. There was no evidence of teratogenicity in these studies.

However, when entacapone was administered to female rats prior to mating and during early gestation, an increased incidence of fetal eye anomalies (macrophthalmia, microphthalmia, anophthalmia) was observed in the litters of dams treated with doses of 160 mg/kg/day (plasma AUCs 7 times those in humans receiving the MRDD) or greater, in the absence of maternotoxicity. Administration of up to 700 mg/kg/day (plasma AUCs 28 times those in humans receiving the MRDD) to female rats during the latter part of gestation and throughout lactation, produced no evidence of developmental impairment in the offspring.

Entacapone is always given concomitantly with carbidopa; levodopa, which is known to cause visceral and skeletal malformations in rabbits. The teratogenic potential of entacapone in combination with carbidopa; levodopa was not assessed in animals.

There is no experience from clinical studies regarding the use of entacapone in pregnant women. Therefore, entacapone should be used during pregnancy only if the potential benefit justifies the potential risk to the fetus.

NURSING MOTHERS

In animal studies, entacapone was excreted into maternal rat milk.

It is not known whether entacapone is excreted in human milk. Because many drugs are excreted in human milk, caution should be exercised when entacapone is administered to a nursing woman.

PEDIATRIC USE

There is no identified potential use of entacapone in pediatric patients.

DRUG INTERACTIONS

In vitro studies of human CYP enzymes showed that entacapone inhibited the CYP enzymes 1A2, 2A6, 2C9, 2C19, 2D6, 2E1, and 3A only at very high concentrations (IC50 from 200 to over 1000 μM; an oral 200 mg dose achieves a highest level of approximately 5 μM in people); these enzymes would therefore not be expected to be inhibited in clinical use.

PROTEIN BINDING

Entacapone is highly protein bound (98%). *In vitro* studies have shown no binding displacement between entacapone and other highly bound drugs, such as warfarin, salicylic acid, phenylbutazone, and diazepam.

DRUGS METABOLIZED BY CATECHOL-O-METHYLTRANSFERASE (COMT)

See WARNINGS.

HORMONE LEVELS

Levodopa is known to depress prolactin secretion and increase growth hormone levels. Treatment with entacapone coadministered with levodopa/dopa decarboxylase inhibitor does not change these effects.

EFFECT OF ENTACAPONE ON THE METABOLISM OF OTHER DRUGS

See WARNINGS regarding concomitant use of entacapone and non-selective MAO inhibitors.

No interaction was noted with the MAO-B inhibitor selegiline in two multiple-dose interaction studies when entacapone was coadministered with a levodopa/dopa decarboxylase inhibitor (n=29). More than 600 Parkinson's disease patients in clinical trials have used selegiline in combination with entacapone and levodopa/dopa decarboxylase inhibitor.

As most entacapone excretion is via the bile, caution should be exercised when drugs known to interfere with biliary excretion, glucuronidation, and intestinal beta-glucuronidase are given concurrently with entacapone. These include probenecid, cholestyramine, and some antibiotics (*e.g.*, erythromycin, rifampicin, ampicillin, and chloramphenicol).

No interaction with the tricyclic antidepressant imipramine was shown in a single-dose study with entacapone without coadministered levodopa/dopa-decarboxylase inhibitor.

ADVERSE REACTIONS

During the pre-marketing development of entacapone, 1450 patients with Parkinson's Disease were treated with entacapone. Included were patients with fluctuating symptoms, as well as those with stable responses to levodopa therapy. All patients received concomitant treatment with levodopa preparations, however, and were similar in other clinical aspects.

The most commonly observed adverse events (>5%) in the double-blind, placebo-controlled trials (n=1003) associated with the use of entacapone and not seen at an equivalent frequency among the placebo-treated patients were: dyskinesia/hyperkinesia, nausea, urine discoloration, diarrhea, and abdominal pain.

Approximately 14% of the 603 patients given entacapone in the double-blind, placebo-controlled trials discontinued treatment due to adverse events compared to 9% of the 400 patients who received placebo. The most frequent causes of discontinuation in decreasing order are: psychiatric reasons (2% vs 1%), diarrhea (2% vs 0%), dyskinesia/hyperkinesia (2% vs 1%), nausea (2% vs 1%), abdominal pain (1% vs 0%), and aggravation of Parkinson's Disease symptoms (1% vs 1%).

ADVERSE EVENT INCIDENCE IN CONTROLLED CLINICAL STUDIES

TABLE 4 lists treatment emergent adverse events that occurred in at least 1% of patients treated with entacapone participating in the double-blind, placebo-controlled studies and that were numerically more common in the entacapone group, compared to placebo. In these studies, either entacapone or placebo was added to carbidopa; levodopa (or benserazide; levodopa).

***TABLE 4** Summary of Patients with Adverse Events after Start of Trial Drug Administration at Least 1% in Entacapone Group and Greater Than Placebo*

System Organ Class / Preferred Term	Entacapone (n=603)	Placebo (n=400)
Skin and Appendages Disorders		
Sweating increased	2%	1%
Musculo-Skeletal System Disorders		
Back pain	2%	1%
Central and Peripheral Nervous System Disorders		
Dyskinesia	25%	15%
Hyperkinesia	10%	5%
Hypokinesia	9%	8%
Dizziness	8%	6%
Special Senses — Other Disorders		
Taste perversion	1%	0%
Psychiatric Disorders		
Anxiety	2%	1%
Somnolence	2%	0%
Agitation	1%	0%
Gastrointestinal System Disorders		
Nausea	14%	8%
Diarrhea	10%	4%
Abdominal pain	8%	4%
Constipation	6%	4%
Vomiting	4%	1%
Mouth dry	3%	0%
Dyspepsia	2%	1%
Flatulence	2%	0%
Gastritis	1%	0%
Gastro-intestinal disorders nos	1%	0%
Respiratory System Disorders		
Dyspnea	3%	1%
Platelet, Bleeding, and Clotting Disorders		
Purpura	2%	1%
Urinary System Disorders		
Urine discoloration	10%	0%
Body as a Whole — General Disorders		
Back pain	4%	2%
Fatigue	6%	4%
Asthenia	2%	1%
Resistance Mechanism Disorders		
Infection bacterial	1%	0%

The prescriber should be aware that these figures cannot be used to predict the incidence of adverse events in the course of usual medical practice where patient characteristics and other factors differ from those that prevailed in the clinical studies. Similarly, the cited frequencies cannot be compared with figures obtained from other clinical investigations involving different treatments, uses, and investigators. The cited figures do, however, provide the prescriber with some basis for estimating the relative contribution of drug and nondrug factors to the adverse events observed in the population studied.

EFFECTS OF GENDER AND AGE ON ADVERSE REACTIONS

No differences were noted in the rate of adverse events attributable to entacapone by age or gender.

DOSAGE AND ADMINISTRATION

The recommended dose of entacapone is one 200 mg tablet administered concomitantly with each carbidopa; levodopa dose to a maximum of 8 times daily. Clinical experience with daily doses above 1600 mg is limited.

Entacapone should always be administered in association with carbidopa; levodopa. Entacapone has no antiparkinsonian effect of its own.

In clinical trials, the majority of patients required a decrease in daily levodopa dose if their daily dose of levodopa had been ≥800 mg, or if patients had moderate or severe dyskinesias before beginning treatment.

To optimize an individual patient's response, reductions in daily levodopa dose or extending the interval between doses may be necessary. In clinical trials, the average reduction in daily levodopa dose was about 25% in those patients requiring a levodopa dose reduction. (More than 58% of patients with levodopa doses above 800 mg daily required such a reduction.)

Entacapone can be combined with both the immediate and sustained release formulations of carbidopa; levodopa.

Entacapone may be taken with or without food (see CLINICAL PHARMACOLOGY).

PATIENTS WITH IMPAIRED HEPATIC FUNCTION

Patients with hepatic impairment should be treated with caution. The AUC and C_{max} of entacapone approximately doubled in patients with documented liver disease compared to controls. However, these studies were conducted with single-dose entacapone without levodopa/dopa decarboxylase inhibitor coadministration, and therefore the effects of liver disease on the kinetics of chronically administered entacapone have not been evaluated (see CLINICAL PHARMACOLOGY, Pharmacokinetics of Entacapone).

WITHDRAWING PATIENTS FROM ENTACAPONE

Rapid withdrawal or abrupt reduction in the entacapone dose could lead to emergence of signs and symptoms of Parkinson's disease, and may lead to hyperpyrexia and confusion, a symptom complex resembling the neuroleptic malignant syndrome (see PRECAUTIONS, Events Reported With Dopaminergic Therapy). This syndrome should be considered in the differential diagnosis for any patient who develops a high fever or severe rigidity. If a decision is made to discontinue treatment with entacapone, patients should be monitored closely and other dopaminergic treatments should be adjusted as needed. Although tapering entacapone has not been systematically evaluated, it seems prudent to withdraw patients slowly if the decision to discontinue treatment is made.

HOW SUPPLIED

Comtan is supplied as 200 mg film-coated tablets for oral administration. The oval-shaped tablets are brownish-orange, unscored, and embossed "COMTAN" on one side.

Storage: Store at 25°C (77°F) excursions permitted to 15-30°C (59-86°F).

PRODUCT LISTING - EQUIVALENTS NOT AVAILABLE

Tablet - Oral - 200 mg

100's $190.91 COMTAN, Novartis Pharmaceuticals 00078-0327-05

Epinephrine *(001166)*

For related information, see the comparative table section in Appendix A.

Categories: Anaphylaxis; Anesthesia, local, adjunct; Anesthesia, spinal, adjunct; Angioedema; Asthma; Cardiac arrest; Glaucoma, open-angle; Rhinitis, allergic; Serum sickness; Urticaria; Uterine contraction, inhibition; Pregnancy Category C; FDA Approved 1951 Jun; WHO Formulary

Drug Classes: Adrenergic agonists; Bronchodilators; Inotropes; Ophthalmics

Brand Names: Adrenalin Chloride; Ana-Guard; Epifrin; **Epipen**; Glaucon; Philip; Racepinephrine; Sus-Phrine

Foreign Brand Availability: Adrenalin (Bulgaria; Canada; Finland; Norway; Sweden; Turkey); Adrenalin Medihaler (Denmark; Finland); Adrenalina (Italy); Adrenalina Sintetica (Switzerland); Adrenaline (Greece; Russia); Adrenaline Injection (Australia; New-Zealand); Adrenaline Aguettant (France); Adrenalini Bitarticas (Indonesia); Bosmin (Taiwan); Epipen Junior (Israel); Epipen Jr. 0.15mg Adrenaline Auto-Injector (Australia); Eppy (Bulgaria; Italy; South-Africa; Sweden); Eppy "N" (Israel); Eppystabil (Austria); Isopto Epinal (Spain); L-Adrenalin (Austria); Medihaler-Iso (Benin; Burkina-Faso; Ethiopia; Gambia; Ghana; Guinea; Ivory-Coast; Kenya; Liberia; Malawi; Mali; Mauritania; Mauritius; Morocco; Niger; Nigeria; Senegal; Seychelles; Sierra-Leone; Sudan; Tanzania; Tunia; Uganda; Zambia; Zimbabwe); Simplene (England; Ireland; South-Africa); Suprarenin (Austria); Weimer Adrenaline (Hong-Kong; Philippines); Weradren (Philippines)

HCFA JCODE(S): J0170 up to 1 ml ampule SC, IM; J7640 2.25%, per ml INH

IM-SC

DESCRIPTION

Note: The trade names have been used throughout this monograph for clarity.

ADRENALIN INJECTION

A sterile solution intended for subcutaneous or intramuscular injection. When diluted, it may also be administered intracardially or intravenously. Each milliliter contains 1 mg Adrenalin (epinephrine) as the hydrochloride dissolved in water for injection, with sodium chloride added for isotonicity. The ampoules contain not more than 0.1% sodium bisulfite as an antioxidant, and the air in the ampoule has been displaced by nitrogen. The Steri-Vials contain 0.5% Chlorobutanol (chloroform derivative) as a preservative and not more than 0.15% sodium bisulfite as an antioxidant. Epinephrine is the active principle of the adrenal medulla, chemically described as (--)-3,4-dihydroxy-alpha-[(methylamino)methyl] benzyl alcohol.

EPIPEN AND EPIPEN JR

The EpiPen and Epipen Jr auto-injectors contain 2 ml epinephrine injection for emergency intramuscular use. Each EpiPen auto-injector delivers **a single dose** of 0.3 mg epinephrine from epinephrine injection, 1:1000 (0.3 ml) in a sterile solution.

Each EpiPen Jr auto-injector delivers **a single dose** of 0.15 mg epinephrine from epinephrine injection, 1:2000 (0.3 ml) in a sterile solution.

For stability purposes, approximately 1.7 ml remains in the auto-injector after activation and cannot be used.

Each 0.3 ml in EpiPen contains 0.3 mg epinephrine, 1.8 mg sodium chloride, 0.5 mg sodium metabisulfite, hydrochloric acid to adjust pH, and water for injection. The pH range is 2.2-5.0. Each 0.3 ml in EpiPen Jr contains 0.15 mg epinephrine, 1.8 mg sodium chloride, 0.5 mg sodium metabisulfite, hydrochloric acid to adjust pH, and water for injection. The pH range is 2.2-5.0.

Epinephrine is a sympathomimetic catecholamine. Chemically, epinephrine is B-(3,4-dihydroxyphenyl)-a-methylaminoethanol.

It deteriorates rapidly on exposure to air or light, turning pink from oxidation to adrenochrome and brown from the formation of melanin. Epinephrine solutions which show evidence of discoloration should be replaced.

CLINICAL PHARMACOLOGY

ADRENALIN INJECTION

Adrenalin is a sympathomimetic drug. It activates an adrenergic receptive mechanism on effector cells and imitates all actions of the sympathetic nervous system except those on the arteries of the face and sweat glands. Epinephrine acts on both alpha and beta receptors and is the most potent alpha receptor activator.

EPIPEN AND EPIPEN JR

Epinephrine is a sympathomimetic drug, acting on both alpha and beta receptors. It is the drug of choice for the emergency treatment of severe allergic reactions (Type I) to insect stings or bites, foods, drugs, and other allergens. It can also be used in the treatment of idiopathic or exercise-induced anaphylaxis. Epinephrine when given subcutaneously or intramuscularly has a rapid onset and short duration of action. The strong vasoconstrictor action of epinephrine through its effect on alpha adrenergic receptors acts quickly to counter vasodilation and increased vascular permeability which can lead to loss of intravascular fluid volume and hypotension during anaphylactic reactions. Epinephrine through its action on beta receptors on bronchial smooth muscle causes bronchial smooth muscle relaxation which alleviates wheezing and dyspnea. Epinephrine also alleviates pruritis, urticaria, and angioedema and may be effective in relieving gastrointestinal and genitourinary symptoms associated with anaphylaxis.

INDICATIONS AND USAGE

ADRENALIN INJECTION

In general, the most common uses of epinephrine are to relieve respiratory distress due to bronchospasm, to provide rapid relief of hypersensitivity reactions to drugs and other allergens, and to prolong the action of infiltration anesthetics. Its cardiac effects may be of use in restoring cardiac rhythm in cardiac arrest due to various causes, but it is not used in cardiac failure or in hemorrhagic, traumatic, or cardiogenic shock.

Epinephrine is used as a hemostatic agent. It is also used in treating mucosal congestion of hay fever, rhinitis, and acute sinusitis; to relieve bronchial asthmatic paroxysms; in syncope due to complete heart block or carotid sinus hypersensitivity; for symptomatic relief of serum sickness, urticaria, angioneurotic edema; for resuscitation in cardiac arrest following anesthetic accidents; in simple (open angle) glaucoma; for relaxation of uterine musculature and to inhibit uterine contractions. Epinephrine injection can be utilized to prolong the action of intraspinal and local anesthetics (see CONTRAINDICATIONS, Adrenalin Injection).

EPIPEN AND EPIPEN JR

Epinephrine is indicated in the emergency treatment of allergic reactions (anaphylaxis) to insect stings or bites, foods, drugs and other allergens as well as idiopathic or exercise-induced anaphylaxis. The EpiPen and EpiPen Jr auto-injectors are intended for immediate self-administration by a person with a history of an anaphylactic reaction. Such reactions may occur within minutes after exposure and consist of flushing, apprehension, syncope, tachycardia, thready or unobtainable pulse associated with a fall in blood pressure, convulsions, vomiting, diarrhea and abdominal cramps, involuntary voiding, wheezing, dyspnea due to laryngeal spasm, pruritis, rashes, uticaria or angioedema. The EpiPen and EpiPen Jr are designed as emergency supportive therapy only and are not a replacement or substitute for immediate medical or hospital care.

CONTRAINDICATIONS

ADRENALIN INJECTION

Epinephrine is contraindicated in narrow angle (congestive) glaucoma, shock, during general anesthesia with halogenated hydrocarbons or cyclopropane and in individuals with organic brain damage. Epinephrine is also contraindicated with local anesthesia of certain areas, *e.g.*, fingers, toes, because of the danger of vasoconstriction producing sloughing of tissue; in labor because it may delay the second stage; in cardiac dilatation and coronary insufficiency.

EPIPEN AND EPIPEN JR

There are no absolute contraindications to the use of epinephrine in a life-threatening situation.

WARNINGS

ADRENALIN INJECTION

Administer with caution to elderly people; to those with cardiovascular disease, hypertension, diabetes, or hyperthyroidism; in psychoneurotic individuals; and in pregnancy.

Patients with long-standing bronchial asthma and emphysema who have developed degenerative heart disease should be administered the drug with extreme caution.

Overdosage or inadvertent intravenous injection of epinephrine may cause cerebrovascular hemorrhage resulting from the sharp rise in blood pressure.

Fatalities may also result from pulmonary edema because of the peripheral constriction and cardiac stimulation produced. Rapidly acting vasodilators, such as nitrites, or alpha blocking agents may counteract the marked pressor effects of epinephrine.

Epinephrine is the preferred treatment for serious allergic or other emergency situations even though this product contains sodium bisulfite, a sulfite that may in other products cause allergic-type reactions including anaphylactic symptoms or life-threatening or less severe asthmatic episodes in certain susceptible persons. The alternatives to using epinephrine in a life-threatening situation may not be satisfactory. The presence of a sulfite in this product should not deter administration of the drug for treatment of serious allergic or other emergency situations.

EPIPEN AND EPIPEN JR

Epinephrine is light sensitive and should be stored in the tube provided. Store at room temperature (15-30°C/59-86°F). Do not refrigerate. Before using, check to make sure the solution in the auto-injector is not discolored. Replace the auto-injector if the solution is discolored or contains a precipitate. Avoid possible inadvertent intravascular administration. EpiPen and EpiPen Jr should **only** be injected into the anterolateral aspect of the thigh. DO NOT INJECT INTO BUTTOCK.

Large doses or accidental intravenous injection of epinephrine may result in cerebral hemorrhage due to sharp rise in blood pressure. DO NOT INJECT INTRAVENOUSLY. Rapidly acting vasodilators can counteract the marked pressor effects of epinephrine.

Epinephrine is the preferred treatment for serious allergic or other emergency situations even though this product contains sodium metabisulfite, a sulfite that may in other products cause allergic-type reactions including anaphylactic symptoms or life-threatening or less severe asthmatic episodes in certain susceptible persons. The alternatives to using epinephrine in a life-threatening situation may not be satisfactory. The presence of a sulfite in this product should not deter administration of the drug for treatment of serious allergic or other emergency situations.

Accidental injection into the hands or feet may result in loss of blood flow to the affected area and should be avoided. If there is an accidental injection into these areas, advise the patient to go immediately to the nearest emergency room for treatment. EpiPen and EpiPen Jr should **only** be injected into the anterolateral aspect of the thigh.

E

PRECAUTIONS

ADRENALIN INJECTION

General

Adrenalin should be protected from exposure to light. Do not remove ampoules or syringes from carton until ready to use. The solution should not be used if it is pinkish or darker than slightly yellow or if it contains a precipitate.

Epinephrine is readily destroyed by alkalies and oxidizing agents. In the latter category are oxygen, chlorine, bromine, iodine, permanganates, chromates, nitrites, and salts of easily reducible metals, especially iron.

Usage in Pregnancy, Pregnancy Category C

Adrenalin has been shown to be teratogenic in rats when given in doses about 25 times the human dose. There are no adequate and well-controlled studies in pregnant women. Adrenalin should be used during pregnancy only if the potential benefit justifies the potential risk to the fetus.

EPIPEN AND EPIPEN JR

Epinephrine is essential for the treatment of anaphylaxis. Patients with a history of severe allergic reactions (anaphylaxis) to insect stings or bites, foods, drugs, and other allergens as well as idiopathic and exercise-induced anaphylaxis should be carefully instructed about the circumstances under which this life-saving medication should be used. It must be clearly determined that the patient is at risk of future anaphylaxis, since the following risks may be associated with epinephrine administration (see DOSAGE AND ADMINISTRATION, EpiPen and Epipen Jr).

Epinephrine is ordinarily administered with extreme caution to patients who have heart disease. Use of epinephrine with drugs that may sensitize the heart to arrhythmias, *e.g.*, digitalis, mercurial diuretics, or quinidine, ordinarily is not recommended. Anginal pain may be induced by epinephrine in patients with coronary insufficiency.

The effects of epinephrine may be potentiated by tricyclic antidepressants and monoamine oxidase inhibitors.

Some patients may be at greater risk of developing adverse reactions after epinephrine administration. These include: hyperthyroid individuals, individuals with cardiovascular disease, hypertension, or diabetes, elderly individuals, pregnant women, pediatric patients under 30 kg (66 lb) body weight using EpiPen, and pediatric patients under 15 kg (33 lb) body weight using EpiPen Jr.

Despite these concerns, epinephrine is essential for the treatment of anaphylaxis. Therefore, patients with these conditions, and/or any other person who might be in a position to administer EpiPen or EpiPen Jr to a patient experiencing anaphylaxis should be carefully instructed in regard to the circumstances under which this life-saving medication should be used.

Carcinogenesis, Mutagenesis, and Impairment of Fertility

Studies of epinephrine in animals to evaluate the carcinogenic and mutagenic potential or the effect on fertility have not been conducted. This should not prevent the use of this life-saving medication under the conditions noted under INDICATIONS AND USAGE, EpiPen and Epipen Jr and as indicated under PRECAUTIONS , EpiPen and Epipen Jr.

Usage in Pregnancy, Pregnancy Category C

Epinephrine has been shown to be teratogenic in rats when given in doses about 25 times the human dose. There are no adequate and well-controlled studies in pregnant women. Epinephrine should be used during pregnancy only if the potential benefit justifies the potential risk to the fetus.

Pediatric Use

Epinephrine may be given safely to pediatric patients at a dosage appropriate to body weight (see DOSAGE AND ADMINISTRATION, EpiPen and Epipen Jr).

DRUG INTERACTIONS

ADRENALIN INJECTION

Use of epinephrine with excessive doses of digitalis, mercurial diuretics, or other drugs that sensitize the heart to arrhythmias is not recommended. Anginal pain may be induced when coronary insufficiency is present.

The effects of epinephrine may be potentiated by tricyclic antidepressants; certain antihistamines, *e.g.*, diphenhydramine, tripelennamine, d-chlorpheniramine; and sodium l-thyroxine.

ADVERSE REACTIONS

ADRENALIN INJECTION

Transient and minor side effects of anxiety, headache, fear, and palpitations often occur with therapeutic doses, especially in hyperthyroid individuals. Repeated local injections can result in necrosis at sites of injection from vascular constriction. "Epinephrine-fastness" can occur with prolonged use.

EPIPEN AND EPIPEN JR

Side effects of epinephrine may include palpitations, tachycardia, sweating, nausea and vomiting, respiratory difficulty, pallor, dizziness, weakness, tremor, headache, apprehension, nervousness and anxiety.

Cardiac arrhythmias may follow administration of epinephrine.

DOSAGE AND ADMINISTRATION

ADRENALIN INJECTION

Parenteral drug products should be inspected visually for particulate matter and discoloration whenever solution and container permit.

Vial and contents must be discarded 30 days after initial use.

Subcutaneously or intramuscularly: 0.2 to 1 ml (mg). Start with a small dose and increase if required.

Note: The subcutaneous is the preferred route of administration. If given intramuscularly, injection into the buttocks should be avoided.

For bronchial asthma and certain allergic manifestations, *e.g.,* angioedema, urticaria, serum sickness, anaphylactic shock, use epinephrine subcutaneously. For bronchial asthma in pediatric patients, administer 0.01 mg/kg or 0.3 mg/m^2 to a maximum of 0.5 mg subcutaneously, repeated every 4 hours if required.

For cardiac resuscitation: A dose of 0.5 ml (0.5 mg) diluted to 10 ml with sodium chloride injection can be administered intravenously or intracardially to restore myocardial contractility. External cardiac massage should follow intracardial administration to permit the drug to enter coronary circulation. The drug should be used secondarily to unsuccessful attempts with physical or electromechanical methods.

Ophthalmologic use (for producing conjunctival decongestion, to control hemorrhage, produce mydriasis and reduce intraocular pressure): Use a concentration of 1:10,000 (0.1 mg/ml) to 1:1,000 (1 mg/ml).

Intraspinal use (Amp 88): Usual dose is 0.2-0.4 ml (0.2-0.4 mg) added to anesthetic spinal fluid mixture (may prolong anesthetic action by limiting absorption).

For use with local anesthetic: Epinephrine 1:100,000 (0.01 mg/ml) to 1:20,000 (0.05 mg/ml) is the usual concentration employed with local anesthetics.

EPIPEN AND EPIPEN JR

A physician who prescribes EpiPen or EpiPen Jr should take appropriate steps to insure that the patient (or parent) understands the indications and use of this device thoroughly. The physician should review with the patient or any other person who might be in a position to administer EpiPen or EpiPen Jr to a patient experiencing anaphylaxis, in detail, the patient instructions and operation of the EpiPen or EpiPen Jr auto-injector. Inject the delivered dose of the EpiPen auto-injector (0.3 ml epinephrine injection, 1:1000) or the EpiPen Jr auto injector (0.3ml epinephrine injection, 1:2000) intramuscularly into the anterolateral aspect of the thigh, through clothing if necessary. See detailed Directions for Use on the Patient Instructions which are distributed with the prescription.

Usual epinephrine adult dose for allergic emergencies is 0.3 mg. For pediatric use, the appropriate dosage may be 0.15 or 0.30 mg depending upon the body weight of the patient. A dosage of 0.01 mg/kg body weight is recommended. EpiPen Jr, which provides a dosage of 0.15 mg, may be more appropriate for patients weighing less than 30 kg. However, the prescribing physician has the option of prescribing more or less than these amounts, based on careful assessment of each individual patient and recognizing the life-threatening nature of the reactions for which this drug is being prescribed. The physician should consider using other forms of injectable epinephrine if doses lower than 0.15 mg are felt to be necessary.

Each EpiPen or EpiPen Jr contains a single dose of epinephrine. With severe persistent anaphylaxis, repeat injections with an additional EpiPen may be necessary.

Parenteral drug products should be periodically inspected visually by the patient for particulate matter or discoloration and should be replaced if these are present.

HOW SUPPLIED

ADRENALIN INJECTION

Amp 88: Sterile solution containing 1 mg Adrenalin (epinephrine) as the hydrochloride in each 1 ml ampoule (1:1000). For intramuscular or subcutaneous use. When diluted, it may also be administered intracardially, intravenously, or intraspinally.

S.V. 11: Sterile solution containing 1 mg Adrenalin (epinephrine) as the hydrochloride (1:1000). For intramuscular or subcutaneous use. When diluted, it may also be administered intracardially or intravenously. Supplied in a 30 ml Steri-Vial (rubber-diaphragm-capped vial).

Storage

Store between 15 and 25°C (59 and 77°F).
Protect from light and freezing.

EPIPEN AND EPIPEN JR

EpiPen auto-injectors (epinephrine injections, 1:1000, 0.3 ml) are available in individual cartons, and as EpiPen 2-Pak, a pack that contains two EpiPen auto-injectors (epinephrine injections, 1:1000, 0.3 ml) and one EpiPen trainer device.

EpiPen Jr auto-injectors (epinephrine injection, 1:2000, 0.3 ml) are available in individual cartons, and as EpiPen Jr 2-Pak, a pack that contains two EpiPen Jr auto-injectors (epinephrine injections, 1:2000, 0.3 ml) and one EpiPen trainer device.

Storage:

Store in a dark place at room temperature (15-30°C/59-86°F). Do not refrigerate. Contains no latex.

INHALATION

DESCRIPTION

Note: The trade names have been used throughout this monograph for clarity.

Each ml contains 10 mg Adrenalin (epinephrine) as the hydrochloride, dissolved in sodium chloride-citrate buffer solution with 0.2 mg Phemerol (benzethonium chloride) as a preservative and not more than 0.2% sodium bisulfite as an antioxidant.

INDICATIONS AND USAGE

For temporary relief of shortness of breath, tightness of chest, and wheezing due to bronchial asthma. The inhalation of Adrenalin Chloride solution 1:100 eases breathing for asthma patients by reducing spasms of bronchial muscles.

WARNINGS

Adrenalin Chloride solution 1:100 is supplied for use by oral (not nasal) inhalation only. Because of the relatively high concentration, Adrenalin Chloride solution 1:100 is not suitable for hypodermic injection.

Do not use this product unless a diagnosis of asthma has been made by a physician.

Do not use this product if you have heart disease, high blood pressure, thyroid disease, or difficulty in urination due to enlargement of the prostate gland unless directed by a physician.

Do not use this product if you have ever been hospitalized for asthma or if you are taking any prescription drug for asthma unless directed by a physician.

Drug interaction precaution: Do not use this product if you are presently taking a prescription drug for high blood pressure or depression without first consulting your physician. **Do not use this product more frequently or at higher doses than recommended unless directed by a physician.** Excessive use may cause nervousness and rapid heart beat and, possibly, adverse effects on the heart.

Do not continue to use this product but seek medical assistance immediately if symptoms are not relieved within 20 minutes or become worse.

Do not use the inhalation solution if it is pinkish or darker than slightly yellow or if it contains a precipitate.

As with any drug, if you are pregnant or nursing a baby, seek the advice of a health professional before using this product.

DOSAGE AND ADMINISTRATION

For relief of bronchial congestion in asthma, Adrenalin Chloride solution 1:100 should be applied with a glass or plastic nebulizer capable of delivering a very fine spray, and which will work with a very small amount of solution.

Approximately 10 drops (not more) of Adrenalin Chloride solution 1:100 are placed in the reservoir of the nebulizer, the nozzle of which is placed just inside the partially opened mouth. As the bulb is squeezed once or twice the patient inhales deeply, drawing the vaporized solution into the lungs. Treatment should be started at the first symptoms. Rinsing the mouth with water immediately after using Adrenalin Chloride solution 1:100 will help prevent the sensation of dryness of mouth and throat which may otherwise follow.

Inhalation dosage for adults, children, and adolescents 4 years of age and older: 1-3 inhalations not more often than every 3 hours. The use of this product by children and adolescents should be supervised by an adult.

Pediatric patients under 4 years of age: Consult a physician.

When the nebulizer contains any liquid and is not in use, it should be stoppered and kept in an upright position. Because of oxidation, Adrenalin Chloride solution 1:100 will turn pink to brown when exposed to air. Light, heat, alkalies, and certain metals (*e.g.,* copper, iron, zinc) will also promote deterioration. A discolored inhalation solution or one containing a precipitate should not be used.

HOW SUPPLIED

Adrenalin Chloride solution 1:100 (epinephrine inhalation solution), for oral inhalation use. Supplied in bottles containing ¼ fluid ounce (7.5 ml) each.

Storage: Store between 15 and 25°C (59 and 77°F). Protect from light and freezing.

OPHTHALMIC

DESCRIPTION

Note: The trade names have been used throughout this monograph for clarity.

Epifrin (epinephrine) sterile ophthalmic solution is a topical sympathomimetic agent for ophthalmic use.

Chemical Name: 1,2-benzenediol,4-[1-hydroxy-2-(methylamino)ethyl]-, (R)-.

Contains:

Active: Epinephrine, 0.5%, 1%, 2%

Preservative: Benzalkonium chloride

Inactives: Sodium metabisulfite; edetate disodium; hydrochloric acid; and purified water.

CLINICAL PHARMACOLOGY

Epinephrine is an adrenergic agonist that stimulates α- and β-adrenergic receptors. The capacity of Epifrin to decrease the aqueous inflow in open-angle glaucoma has been well documented. Studies have also shown that prolonged topical epinephrine therapy offers significant improvement in the coefficient of aqueous outflow.

Epifrin is effective alone in reducing intraocular pressure and is particularly useful in combination with miotics or beta-adrenergic blocking agents for the difficult-to-control patients. The addition of Epifrin to the patient's regimen often provides better control of intraocular pressure than the original agent alone.

INDICATIONS AND USAGE

Epifrin is indicated for the treatment of chronic simple glaucoma.

CONTRAINDICATIONS

Epifrin should not be used in patients who have had an attack of narrow-angle glaucoma, since dilation of the pupil may trigger an acute attack. Do not use if hypersensitive to any ingredient.

WARNINGS

Epifrin should be used with caution in patients with a narrow angle, since dilation of the pupil may trigger an acute attack of narrow-angle glaucoma.

Use with caution in patients with hypertensive cardiovascular disease or coronary artery disease.

Epinephrine has been reported to produce reversible macular edema in some aphakic patients and should be used with caution in these patients.

Contains sodium metabisulfite, a sulfite that may cause allergic-type reactions, including anaphylactic symptoms and life-threatening or less severe asthmatic episodes in certain susceptible people. The overall prevalence of sulfite sensitivity in the general population is unknown and probably low. Sulfite sensitivity is seen more frequently in asthmatic than in nonasthmatic people.

PRECAUTIONS

GENERAL

Epinephrine in any form is relatively uncomfortable upon instillation. However, discomfort lessens as the concentration of epinephrine decreases. Epifrin is not for injection.

CARCINOGENESIS, MUTAGENESIS, AND IMPAIRMENT OF FERTILITY

No studies have been conducted in animals or in humans to evaluate the potential of these effects.

PREGNANCY CATEGORY C

Animal reproduction studies have not been conducted with epinephrine. It is also not known whether epinephrine can cause fetal harm when administered to a pregnant woman or if it can affect reproduction capacity. Epinephrine should be given to a pregnant woman only if clearly needed.

PEDIATRIC USE

Safety and effectiveness in pediatric patients have not been established.

ADVERSE REACTIONS

Undesirable reactions to topical epinephrine include eye pain or ache, browache, headache, conjunctival hyperemia and allergic lid reactions.

Adrenochrome deposits in the conjunctiva and cornea after prolonged epinephrine therapy have been reported. Topical epinephrine has been reported to produce reversible macular edema in some aphakic patients.

DOSAGE AND ADMINISTRATION

The usual dosage is 1 drop in the affected eye(s) once or twice daily. However, the dosage should be adjusted to meet the needs of the individual patients. This is made easier with Epifrin sterile ophthalmic solution available in three strengths.

HOW SUPPLIED

Epifrin is available on prescription only in plastic dropper bottles containing 15 ml of a 0.5%, 1% or 2% solution.

Note: Protect from light and excessive heat. If the solution discolors or a precipitate forms, it should be discarded.

PRODUCT LISTING - RATED THERAPEUTICALLY EQUIVALENT

Solution - Injectable - 0.1 mg/ml

Size	Price	Product	NDC
10 ml x 10	$25.89	GENERIC, Abbott Pharmaceutical	00074-4921-18
10 ml x 10	$26.40	GENERIC, Abbott Pharmaceutical	00074-4921-34
10 ml x 10	$34.32	GENERIC, Abbott Pharmaceutical	00074-4901-18
10 ml x 10	$124.08	GENERIC, Abbott Pharmaceutical	00074-4921-01
10 ml x 10	$130.86	GENERIC, Abbott Pharmaceutical	00074-4921-23
10 ml x 10	$139.20	GENERIC, Abbott Pharmaceutical	00074-4901-01
10 ml x 25	$343.80	GENERIC, Abbott Pharmaceutical	00074-4921-33

Solution - Injectable - 1 mg/ml

Size	Price	Product	NDC
1 ml x 25	$16.03	GENERIC, Abbott Pharmaceutical	00074-7241-01

PRODUCT LISTING - EQUIVALENTS NOT AVAILABLE

Solution - Injectable - 0.1 mg/ml

Size	Price	Product	NDC
1 ml x 100	$119.44	GENERIC, Allscripts Pharmaceutical Company	54569-1673-01
10 ml	$13.75	GENERIC, Allscripts Pharmaceutical Company	54569-1673-00
10 ml x 10	$29.64	GENERIC, Abbott Pharmaceutical	00074-4320-01
10 ml x 10	$53.20	GENERIC, International Medication Systems, Limited	00548-3316-00
10 ml x 25	$122.00	GENERIC, International Medication Systems, Limited	00548-1016-00
10 ml x 25	$131.25	GENERIC, International Medication Systems, Limited	00548-2016-00
10 ml x 25	$170.00	GENERIC, International Medication Systems, Limited	00548-1014-00

Solution - Injectable - 0.15 mg

Size	Price	Product	NDC
1's	$42.48	EPIPEN JR AUTO-INJECTOR, Allscripts Pharmaceutical Company	54569-1391-00
1's	$52.38	EPIPEN JR AUTO-INJECTOR, Dey Laboratories	49502-0501-01
2's	$100.31	EPIPEN JR AUTO-INJECTOR, Dey Laboratories	49502-0501-02

Solution - Injectable - 0.3 mg

Size	Price	Product	NDC
1's	$32.34	EPIPEN AUTO INJECTOR, Allscripts Pharmaceutical Company	54569-1392-00
1's	$52.38	EPIPEN AUTO INJECTOR, Dey Laboratories	49502-0500-01
2's	$100.31	EPIPEN AUTO INJECTOR, Dey Laboratories	49502-0500-02

Solution - Injectable - 1 mg/ml

Size	Price	Product	NDC
1 ml	$3.74	GENERIC, Prescript Pharmaceuticals	00247-0259-01
1 ml x 6	$132.90	ANA-GUARD, Hollister Incorporated	65044-9984-06
1 ml x 10	$9.60	GENERIC, Pro Metic Pharma	62174-0537-07
1 ml x 10	$16.88	ADRENALIN, Allscripts Pharmaceutical Company	54569-1578-00
1 ml x 10	$23.40	GENERIC, Allscripts Pharmaceutical Company	54569-1422-00
1 ml x 10	$24.15	ADRENALIN, Physicians Total Care	54868-1363-00
1 ml x 10	$25.10	ADRENALIN, Monarch Pharmaceuticals Inc	61570-0418-81
1 ml x 25	$12.25	GENERIC, American Regent Laboratories Inc	00517-1061-25
1 ml x 25	$14.50	GENERIC, Esi Lederle Generics	00641-1420-35
1 ml x 25	$22.50	GENERIC, Cmc-Consolidated Midland Corporation	00223-7520-05
1 ml x 25	$38.98	GENERIC, Allscripts Pharmaceutical Company	54569-3075-00
1 ml x 25	$109.50	GENERIC, American Regent Laboratories Inc	00517-1071-25
1 ml x 25	$110.00	GENERIC, Raway Pharmacal Inc	00686-1071-25
1 ml x 50	$39.00	GENERIC, Raway Pharmacal Inc	00686-1061-25
1 ml x 100	$60.00	GENERIC, Cmc-Consolidated Midland Corporation	00223-7520-01
1's	$19.87	ANA-GUARD, Bayer	00026-9984-01
1's	$124.25	ANA-GUARD, Bayer	00026-9984-06
5 ml	$5.27	GENERIC, Prescript Pharmaceuticals	00247-0259-05
10 ml	$7.19	GENERIC, Prescript Pharmaceuticals	00247-0259-10
10's	$534.48	GENERIC, Abbott Pharmaceutical	00074-3096-05
30 ml	$1.20	GENERIC, Veratex Corporation	17022-1442-07
30 ml	$5.98	GENERIC, International Medication Systems, Limited	00548-9061-00
30 ml	$9.25	GENERIC, American Regent Laboratories Inc	00517-1130-01
30 ml	$12.56	ADRENALIN, Southwood Pharmaceuticals Inc	58016-3177-01
30 ml	$17.60	GENERIC, King Pharmaceuticals Inc	60793-0401-11
30 ml	$18.57	ADRENALIN, Allscripts Pharmaceutical Company	54569-1547-00

Solution - Ophthalmic - 0.5%

Size	Price	Product	NDC
15 ml	$46.36	EPIFRIN, Allergan Inc	11980-0119-15

Solution - Ophthalmic - 1%

Size	Price	Product	NDC
15 ml	$49.69	EPIFRIN, Allergan Inc	11980-0122-15

Solution - Ophthalmic - 2%

Size	Price	Product	NDC
15 ml	$54.36	EPIFRIN, Allergan Inc	11980-0058-15

Solution - Topical - 1:100

Size	Price	Product	NDC
7.50 ml	$29.06	ADRENALIN, TOPICAL, Monarch Pharmaceuticals Inc	61570-0301-41

Suspension - Subcutaneous - 5 mg/ml

Size	Price	Product	NDC
0.30 ml x 10	$55.50	GENERIC, Forest Pharmaceuticals	00456-0664-39
5 ml	$38.50	GENERIC, Forest Pharmaceuticals	00456-0664-05
5 ml	$44.34	GENERIC, Prescript Pharmaceuticals	00247-0316-05
25's	$124.00	GENERIC, Forest Pharmaceuticals	00456-0664-34

Epinephrine Bitartrate; Prilocaine Hydrochloride *(003121)*

Categories: Anesthesia, local; FDA Approval Pre 1982
Drug Classes: Anesthetics, local
Brand Names: Citanest Forte
Foreign Brand Availability: Citanest Adrenalin (Finland; Sweden)

DESCRIPTION

For Complete Prescribing Information See: PRILOCAINE HYDROCHLORIDE

Epinephrine; Lidocaine Hydrochloride (001171)

Categories: Anesthesia, local; Pregnancy Category B; FDA Approved 1985 Jan; WHO Formulary
Drug Classes: Anesthetics, local
Brand Names: Alphacaine HCl w Epinephrine; Iontocaine; Lidocaton; Lignospan; Norocaine; Octocaine; **Xylocaine w Epinephrine**
Foreign Brand Availability: Pisacaina 2% con epifrina (Mexico); Roxicaina (Colombia); Xilonest al 1% con epinefrina (Peru); Xilonest al 2% con epinefrina (Peru); Xylanaest Mit Epinephrin (Austria); Xylocain Adrenalin (Finland; Sweden; Switzerland); Xylocain-Adrenalin (Norway); Xylocain-Epinephrin (Austria); Xylocaine with Adrenaline (Australia; Benin; Burkina-Faso; Ethiopia; Gambia; Ghana; Guinea; India; Ivory-Coast; Kenya; Liberia; Malawi; Mali; Mauritania; Mauritius; Morocco; New-Zealand; Niger; Nigeria; Philippines; Senegal; Seychelles; Sierra-Leone; Sudan; Taiwan; Tanzania; Tunia; Uganda; Zambia; Zimbabwe); Xylocaine w Adrenaline (Hong-Kong)

E

DESCRIPTION

For Full Prescribing Information, See Lidocaine Hydrochloride.

PRODUCT LISTING - RATED THERAPEUTICALLY EQUIVALENT

Solution - Injectable - 1:100000;1%

10 ml x 5	$13.50	XYLOCAINE HCL WITH EPINEPHRINE, Astra-Zeneca Pharmaceuticals	00186-0115-12
20 ml	$16.95	XYLOCAINE HCL WITH EPINEPHRINE, Astra-Zeneca Pharmaceuticals	00186-0115-01
20 ml x 25	$38.59	GENERIC, Abbott Pharmaceutical	00074-3178-01
30 ml x 25	$45.42	GENERIC, Abbott Pharmaceutical	00074-3178-02
50 ml	$5.44	XYLOCAINE HCL WITH EPINEPHRINE, Allscripts Pharmaceutical Company	54569-1507-01
50 ml	$6.73	XYLOCAINE HCL WITH EPINEPHRINE, Physicians Total Care	54868-1796-00
50 ml x 5	$30.75	XYLOCAINE HCL WITH EPINEPHRINE, Astra-Zeneca Pharmaceuticals	00186-0150-01
50 ml x 25	$81.64	GENERIC, Abbott Pharmaceutical	00074-3178-03

Solution - Injectable - 1:100000;2%

2 ml x 100	$42.00	XYLOCAINE WITH EPINEPHRINE DENTAL CARTRIDGES, Astra-Zeneca Pharmaceuticals	00186-0175-14
20 ml	$3.05	XYLOCAINE HCL WITH EPINEPHRINE, Allscripts Pharmaceutical Company	54569-3597-00
20 ml	$3.94	XYLOCAINE HCL WITH EPINEPHRINE, Physicians Total Care	54868-1797-00
20 ml x 5	$17.25	XYLOCAINE HCL WITH EPINEPHRINE, Astra-Zeneca Pharmaceuticals	00186-0125-01
20 ml x 25	$44.23	GENERIC, Abbott Pharmaceutical	00074-3182-01
30 ml x 25	$98.27	GENERIC, Abbott Pharmaceutical	00074-3182-02
50 ml	$6.18	XYLOCAINE HCL WITH EPINEPHRINE, Allscripts Pharmaceutical Company	54569-2625-00
50 ml x 5	$35.00	XYLOCAINE HCL WITH EPINEPHRINE, Astra-Zeneca Pharmaceuticals	00186-0160-01
50 ml x 25	$114.30	GENERIC, Abbott Pharmaceutical	00074-3182-03

Solution - Injectable - 1:200000;0.5%

50 ml	$30.15	XYLOCAINE HCL WITH EPINEPHRINE, Astra-Zeneca Pharmaceuticals	00186-0140-01
50 ml x 25	$76.30	GENERIC, Abbott Pharmaceutical	00074-3177-01

Solution - Injectable - 1:200000;1%

10 ml x 5	$33.45	XYLOCAINE-MPF-EPINEPHRINE, Astra-Zeneca Pharmaceuticals	00186-0114-12
30 ml	$11.80	XYLOCAINE-MPF-EPINEPHRINE, Physicians Total Care	54868-4043-00
30 ml	$58.00	XYLOCAINE-MPF-EPINEPHRINE, Astra-Zeneca Pharmaceuticals	00186-0114-01
30 ml x 5	$29.75	GENERIC, Abbott Pharmaceutical	00074-3179-01
30 ml x 5	$60.30	XYLOCAINE-MPF-EPINEPHRINE, Astra-Zeneca Pharmaceuticals	00186-0114-91
30 ml x 5	$62.30	XYLOCAINE-MPF-EPINEPHRINE, Astra-Zeneca Pharmaceuticals	00186-0260-02
30 ml x 5	$66.30	XYLOCAINE-MPF-EPINEPHRINE, Astra-Zeneca Pharmaceuticals	00186-0260-92

Solution - Injectable - 1:200000;1.5%

5 ml x 10	$32.89	GENERIC, Abbott Pharmaceutical	00074-1209-01
30 ml x 5	$39.48	GENERIC, Abbott Pharmaceutical	00074-3181-01
30 ml x 5	$40.00	GENERIC, Abbott Pharmaceutical	00074-3180-02

Solution - Injectable - 1:200000;2%

20 ml x 5	$41.50	GENERIC, Abbott Pharmaceutical	00074-3183-01
20 ml x 5	$72.70	XYLOCAINE-MPF-EPINEPHRINE, Astra-Zeneca Pharmaceuticals	00186-0250-02
20 ml x 5	$75.90	XYLOCAINE-MPF-EPINEPHRINE, Astra-Zeneca Pharmaceuticals	00186-0122-91
20 ml x 5	$77.55	XYLOCAINE-MPF-EPINEPHRINE, Astra-Zeneca Pharmaceuticals	00186-0122-01

PRODUCT LISTING - EQUIVALENTS NOT AVAILABLE

Kit - Injectable - 1:50000;2%

10's	$372.60	SADDLE BLOCK-22, Abbott Pharmaceutical	00074-4792-01
10's	$383.04	SADDLE BLOCK-25, Abbott Pharmaceutical	00074-4795-01
10's	$385.80	SADDLE BLOCK-26, Abbott Pharmaceutical	00074-4745-01

Kit - Injectable - 1:200000;1.5%

10's	$457.78	GENERIC, Abbott Pharmaceutical	00074-4808-20
10's	$533.00	GENERIC, Abbott Pharmaceutical	00074-8284-20
10's	$539.36	GENERIC, Abbott Pharmaceutical	00074-4769-20
10's	$548.63	GENERIC, Abbott Pharmaceutical	00074-4810-20
10's	$584.20	GENERIC, Abbott Pharmaceutical	00074-4775-20

Solution - Injectable - 1:100000;1%

30 ml	$5.26	GENERIC, Allscripts Pharmaceutical Company	54569-2215-01
30 ml	$5.98	GENERIC, Prescript Pharmaceuticals	00247-0051-30
50 ml	$7.73	GENERIC, Prescript Pharmaceuticals	00247-0051-50

Solution - Injectable - 1:200000;1.5%

5 ml x 10	$25.30	XYLOCAINE-MPF-EPINEPHRINE, Astra-Zeneca Pharmaceuticals	00186-0265-03
10 ml x 5	$37.75	XYLOCAINE-MPF-EPINEPHRINE, Astra-Zeneca Pharmaceuticals	00186-0117-12
30 ml	$67.05	XYLOCAINE-MPF-EPINEPHRINE, Astra-Zeneca Pharmaceuticals	00186-0117-01
30 ml x 5	$67.90	XYLOCAINE-MPF-EPINEPHRINE, Astra-Zeneca Pharmaceuticals	00186-0117-91
30 ml x 5	$71.50	XYLOCAINE-MPF-EPINEPHRINE, Astra-Zeneca Pharmaceuticals	00186-0265-02

Solution - Injectable - 1:200000;2%

10 ml x 5	$44.05	XYLOCAINE-MPF-EPINEPHRINE, Astra-Zeneca Pharmaceuticals	00186-0122-12

Epirubicin Hydrochloride (003443)

For complete prescribing information, refer to the CD-ROM included with the book.

Categories: Carcinoma, breast; Pregnancy Category D; FDA Approved 1999 Sep; Orphan Drugs
Drug Classes: Antineoplastics, antibiotics
Brand Names: **Ellence**; Farmorubicin RD
Foreign Brand Availability: Binarin (Mexico); EPI-cell (Germany); Epilem (Mexico; Thailand); Farmorubicin (Austria; Bahrain; Bulgaria; Cyprus; Czech-Republic; Denmark; Egypt; Finland; Germany; Greece; Hungary; Iran; Iraq; Israel; Japan; Jordan; Kuwait; Lebanon; Libya; Mexico; Norway; Oman; Qatar; Republic-of-Yemen; Russia; Saudi-Arabia; South-Africa; Sweden; Switzerland; Syria; Turkey; United-Arab-Emirates); Farmorubicin PFS (Bulgaria); Farmorubicina (Italy; Peru; Portugal; Spain); Farmorubicina CS (Colombia); Farmorubicina R.D. (Costa-Rica; Dominican-Republic; El-Salvador; Guatemala; Honduras; Nicaragua; Panama); Farmorubicine (Belgium; France; Netherlands); Pharmorubicin (Australia; Canada; England; Hong-Kong; Ireland; Malaysia; New-Zealand; Philippines); Pharmorubicin PDF (Korea); Pharmorubicin PFS (Canada; Taiwan); Pharmorubucin RD (China); Pharmorubicin R.D.F. (Korea); Pharmorubicin RDS (Canada)

WARNING

SEVERE LOCAL TISSUE NECROSIS WILL OCCUR IF THERE IS EXTRAVASATION DURING ADMINISTRATION. EPIRUBICIN MUST NOT BE GIVEN BY THE INTRAMUSCULAR OR SUBCUTANEOUS ROUTE.

MYOCARDIAL TOXICITY, MANIFESTED IN ITS MOST SEVERE FORM BY POTENTIALLY FATAL CONGESTIVE HEART FAILURE (CHF), MAY OCCUR EITHER DURING THERAPY WITH EPIRUBICIN OR MONTHS TO YEARS AFTER TERMINATION OF THERAPY. THE PROBABILITY OF DEVELOPING CLINICALLY EVIDENT CHF IS ESTIMATED AS APPROXIMATELY 0.9% AT A CUMULATIVE DOSE OF 550 MG/M^2, 1.6% AT 700 MG/M^2, AND 3.3% AT 900 MG/M^2. IN THE ADJUVANT TREATMENT OF BREAST CANCER, THE MAXIMUM CUMULATIVE DOSE USED IN CLINICAL TRIALS WAS 720 MG/M^2. THE RISK OF DEVELOPING CHF INCREASES RAPIDLY WITH INCREASING TOTAL CUMULATIVE DOSES OF EPIRUBICIN IN EXCESS OF 900 MG/M^2; THIS CUMULATIVE DOSE SHOULD ONLY BE EXCEEDED WITH EXTREME CAUTION. ACTIVE OR DORMANT CARDIOVASCULAR DISEASE, PRIOR OR CONCOMITANT RADIOTHERAPY TO THE MEDIASTINAL/PERICARDIAL AREA, PREVIOUS THERAPY WITH OTHER ANTHRACYCLINES OR ANTHRACENEDIONES, OR CONCOMITANT USE OF OTHER CARDIOTOXIC DRUGS MAY INCREASE THE RISK OF CARDIAC TOXICITY. CARDIAC TOXICITY WITH EPIRUBICIN HCL MAY OCCUR AT LOWER CUMULATIVE DOSES WHETHER OR NOT CARDIAC RISK FACTORS ARE PRESENT.

SECONDARY ACUTE MYELOGENOUS LEUKEMIA (AML) HAS BEEN REPORTED IN PATIENTS WITH BREAST CANCER TREATED WITH ANTHRACYCLINES, INCLUDING EPIRUBICIN. THE OCCURRENCE OF REFRACTORY SECONDARY LEUKEMIA IS MORE COMMON WHEN SUCH DRUGS ARE GIVEN IN COMBINATION WITH DNA-DAMAGING ANTINEOPLASTIC AGENTS, WHEN PATIENTS HAVE BEEN HEAVILY PRETREATED WITH CYTOTOXIC DRUGS, OR WHEN DOSES OF ANTHRACYCLINES HAVE BEEN ESCALATED. THE CUMULATIVE RISK OF DEVELOPING TREATMENT-RELATED AML, IN 3846 PATIENTS WITH BREAST CANCER WHO RECEIVED ADJUVANT TREATMENT WITH EPIRUBICIN-CONTAINING REGIMENS, WAS ESTIMATED AS 0.2% AT 3 YEARS AND 0.8% AT 5 YEARS.

DOSAGE SHOULD BE REDUCED IN PATIENTS WITH IMPAIRED HEPATIC FUNCTION (SEE DOSAGE AND ADMINISTRATION).

SEVERE MYELOSUPPRESSION MAY OCCUR.

EPIRUBICIN SHOULD BE ADMINISTERED ONLY UNDER THE SUPERVISION OF A PHYSICIAN WHO IS EXPERIENCED IN THE USE OF CANCER CHEMOTHERAPEUTIC AGENTS.

DESCRIPTION

Epirubicin HCl injection is an anthracycline cytotoxic agent intended for intravenous administration. Ellence is supplied as a sterile, clear, red solution and is available in polypropylene vials containing 50 and 200 mg of epirubicin HCl as a preservative-free, ready-to-use solution. Each milliliter of solution contains 2 mg of epirubicin HCl. *Inactive*

Ingredients: Sodium chloride and water for injection. The pH of the solution has been adjusted to 3.0 with hydrochloric acid.

Epirubicin HCl is the 4′-epimer of doxorubicin and is a semi-synthetic derivative of daunorubicin. The chemical name is (8S-*cis*)-10-[(3-amino-2,3,6-trideoxy-α-L-*arabino*-hexopyranosyl)oxy]-7,8,9,10-tetrahydro-6,8,11-trihydroxy-8-(hydroxyacetyl)-1-methoxy-5,12-naphthacenedione hydrochloride. The active ingredient is a red-orange hygroscopic powder, with the empirical formula $C_{27}H_{29}NO_{11}HCl$ and a molecular weight of 579.95.

INDICATIONS AND USAGE

Epirubicin HCl injection is indicated as a component of adjuvant therapy in patients with evidence of axillary node tumor involvement following resection of primary breast cancer.

NON-FDA APPROVED INDICATIONS

The drug has been reported to have efficacy in the treatment of small cell lung cancer, non-small cell lung cancer, non-Hodgkin's lymphoma, Hodgkin's disease, gastric cancer, bladder cancer, ovarian cancer, prostatic cancer, and primary hepatocelluar carcinoma. However, these uses have not been approved by the FDA and further clinical trials for these indications are needed.

CONTRAINDICATIONS

Patients should not be treated with epirubicin HCl injection if they have any of the following conditions: baseline neutrophil count <1500 cells/mm^3; severe myocardial insufficiency or recent myocardial infarction; previous treatment with anthracyclines up to the maximum cumulative dose; hypersensitivity to epirubicin, other anthracyclines, or anthracenediones; or severe hepatic dysfunction (see WARNINGS and DOSAGE AND ADMINISTRATION).

WARNINGS

Epirubicin HCl injection should be administered only under the supervision of qualified physicians experienced in the use of cytotoxic therapy. Initial treatment with epirubicin HCl should be preceded by a careful baseline assessment of blood counts; serum levels of total bilirubin, AST, and creatinine; and cardiac function as measured by left ventricular ejection function (LVEF). Patients should be carefully monitored during treatment for possible clinical complications due to myelosuppression. Supportive care may be necessary for the treatment of severe neutropenia and severe infectious complications. Monitoring for potential cardiotoxicity is also important, especially with greater cumulative exposure to epirubicin.

HEMATOLOGIC TOXICITY

A dose-dependent, reversible leukopenia and/or neutropenia is the predominant manifestation of hematologic toxicity associated with epirubicin and represents the most common acute dose-limiting toxicity of this drug. In most cases, the WBC nadir is reached 10-14 days from drug administration. Leukopenia/neutropenia is usually transient, with WBC and neutrophil counts generally returning to normal values by Day 21 after drug administration. As with other cytotoxic agents, epirubicin HCl at the recommended dose in combination with cyclophosphamide and fluorouracil can produce severe leukopenia and neutropenia. Severe thrombocytopenia and anemia may also occur. Clinical consequences of severe myelosuppression include fever, infection, septicemia, septic shock, hemorrhage, tissue hypoxia, symptomatic anemia, or death. If myelosuppressive complications occur, appropriate supportive measures (*e.g.,* intravenous antibiotics, colony-stimulating factors, transfusions) may be required. Myelosuppression requires careful monitoring. Total and differential white blood cell (WBC), red blood cell (RBC), and platelet counts should be assessed before and during each cycle of therapy with epirubicin HCl.

CARDIAC FUNCTION

Cardiotoxicity is a known risk of anthracycline treatment. Anthracycline-induced cardiac toxicity may be manifested by early (or acute) or late (delayed) events. Early cardiac toxicity of epirubicin consists mainly of sinus tachycardia and/or ECG abnormalities such as non-specific ST-T wave changes, but tachyarrhythmias, including premature ventricular contractions and ventricular tachycardia, bradycardia, as well as atrioventricular and bundle-branch block have also been reported. These effects do not usually predict subsequent development of delayed cardiotoxicity, are rarely of clinical importance, and are generally not considered an indication for the suspension of epirubicin treatment. Delayed cardiac toxicity results from a characteristic cardiomyopathy that is manifested by reduced LVEF and/or signs and symptoms of congestive heart failure (CHF) such as tachycardia, dyspnea, pulmonary edema, dependent edema, hepatomegaly, ascites, pleural effusion, gallop rhythm. Life-threatening CHF is the most severe form of anthracycline-induced cardiomyopathy. This toxicity appears to be dependent on the cumulative dose of epirubicin HCl and represents the cumulative dose-limiting toxicity of the drug. If it occurs, delayed cardiotoxicity usually develops late in the course of therapy with epirubicin HCl or within 2-3 months after completion of treatment, but later events (several months to years after treatment termination) have been reported.

In a retrospective survey, including 9144 patients, mostly with solid tumors in advanced stages, the probability of developing CHF increased with increasing cumulative doses of epirubicin HCl. The estimated risk of epirubicin-treated patients developing clinically evident CHF was 0.9% at a cumulative dose of 550 mg/m^2, 1.6% at 700 mg/m^2, and 3.3% at 900 mg/m^2. The risk of developing CHF in the absence of other cardiac risk factors increased steeply after an epirubicin cumulative dose of 900 mg/m^2.

In another retrospective survey of 469 epirubicin-treated patients with metastatic or early breast cancer, the reported risk of CHF was comparable to that observed in the larger study of over 9000 patients.

Given the risk of cardiomyopathy, a cumulative dose of 900 mg/m^2 epirubicin HCl should be exceeded only with extreme caution. Risk factors (active or dormant cardiovascular disease, prior or concomitant radiotherapy to the mediastinal/pericardial area, previous therapy with other anthracyclines or anthracenediones, concomitant use of other drugs with the ability to suppress cardiac contractility) may increase the risk of cardiac toxicity. Although not formally tested, it is probable that the toxicity of epirubicin and other anthracyclines or anthracenediones is additive. Cardiac toxicity with epirubicin HCl may occur at lower cumulative doses whether or not cardiac risk factors are present.

Although endomyocardial biopsy is recognized as the most sensitive diagnostic tool to detect anthracycline-induced cardiomyopathy, this invasive examination is not practically performed on a routine basis. Electrocardiogram (ECG) changes such as dysrhythmias, a reduction of the QRS voltage, or a prolongation beyond normal limits of the systolic time interval may be indicative of anthracycline-induced cardiomyopathy, but ECG is not a sensitive or specific method for following anthracycline-related cardiotoxicity. The risk of serious cardiac impairment may be decreased through regular monitoring of LVEF during the course of treatment with prompt discontinuation of epirubicin HCl at the first sign of impaired function. The preferred method for repeated assessment of cardiac function is evaluation of LVEF measured by multi-gated radionuclide angiography (MUGA) or echocardiography (ECHO). A baseline cardiac evaluation with an ECG and a MUGA scan or an ECHO is recommended, especially in patients with risk factors for increased cardiac toxicity. Repeated MUGA or ECHO determinations of LVEF should be performed, particularly with higher, cumulative anthracycline doses. The technique used for assessment should be consistent through follow-up. In patients with risk factors, particularly prior anthracycline or anthracenedione use, the monitoring of cardiac function must be particularly strict and the risk-benefit of continuing treatment with epirubicin HCl in patients with impaired cardiac function must be carefully evaluated.

E

SECONDARY LEUKEMIA

The occurrence of secondary acute myelogenous leukemia, with or without a preleukemic phase, has been reported in patients treated with anthracyclines. Secondary leukemia is more common when such drugs are given in combination with DNA-damaging antineoplastic agents, when patients have been heavily pretreated with cytotoxic drugs, or when doses of the anthracyclines have been escalated. These leukemias can have a short 1-3 year latency period. An analysis of 3844 patients who received adjuvant treatment with epirubicin in controlled clinical trials showed a cumulative risk of secondary acute myelogenous leukemia of about 0.2% (approximate 95% CI, 0.05 to 0.4) at 3 years and approximately 0.8% (approximate 95% CI, 0.3-1.2) at 5 years. Epirubicin HCl is mutagenic, clastogenic, and carcinogenic in animals.

LIVER FUNCTION

The major route of elimination of epirubicin is the hepatobiliary system. Serum total bilirubin and AST levels should be evaluated before and during treatment with epirubicin HCl. Patients with elevated bilirubin or AST may experience slower clearance of drug with an increase in overall toxicity. Lower doses are recommended in these patients (see DOSAGE AND ADMINISTRATION). Patients with severe hepatic impairment have not been evaluated; therefore, epirubicin should not be used in this patient population.

RENAL FUNCTION

Serum creatinine should be assessed before and during therapy. Dosage adjustment is necessary in patients with serum creatinine >5 mg/dl (see DOSAGE AND ADMINISTRATION). Patients undergoing dialysis have not been studied.

TUMOR-LYSIS SYNDROME

As with other cytotoxic agents, epirubicin HCl may induce hyperuricemia as a consequence of the extensive purine catabolism that accompanies drug-induced rapid lysis of highly chemosensitive neoplastic cells (tumor lysis syndrome). Other metabolic abnormalities may also occur. While not generally a problem in patients with breast cancer, physicians should consider the potential for tumor-lysis syndrome in potentially susceptible patients and should consider monitoring serum uric acid, potassium, calcium phosphate, and creatinine immediately after initial chemotherapy administration. Hydration, urine alkalinization, and prophylaxis with allopurinol to prevent hyperuricemia may minimize potential complications of tumor-lysis syndrome.

DOSAGE AND ADMINISTRATION

Epirubicin HCl injection is administered to patients by intravenous infusion. Epirubicin HCl is given in repeated 3-4 week cycles. The total dose of epirubicin HCl may be given on Day 1 of each cycle or divided equally and given on Days 1 and 8 of each cycle. The recommended dosages of epirubicin HCl are as follows.

STARTING DOSES

The recommended starting dose of epirubicin HCl is 100-120 mg/m^2. The following regimens shown in TABLE 6 were used in the trials supporting use of epirubicin HCl as a component of adjuvant therapy in patients with axillary-node positive breast cancer.

TABLE 6

Regimen	Drug	Dose
CEF-120:	Cyclophosphamide	75 mg/m^2 PO D 1-14
	Epirubicin HCl	60 mg/m^2 IV D 1, 8
	5-Fluorouracil	500 mg/m^2 IV D 1, 8
	Repeated every 28 days for 6 cycles	
FEC-100:	5-Fluorouracil	500 mg/m^2
	Epirubicin HCl	100 mg/m^2
	Cyclophosphamide	500 mg/m^2
	All drugs administered intravenously on day 1 and repeated every 21 days for 6 cycles	

Patients administered the 120 mg/m^2 regimen of epirubicin HCl also received prophylactic antibiotic therapy with trimethoprim-sulfamethoxazole (*e.g.,* Septra, Bactrim) or a fluoroquinolone.

Bone Marrow Dysfunction

Consideration should be given to administration of lower starting doses (75-90 mg/m^2) for heavily pretreated patients, patients with pre-existing bone marrow depression, or in the presence of neoplastic bone marrow infiltration (see WARNINGS).

Hepatic Dysfunction

Definitive recommendation regarding use of epirubicin HCl in patients with hepatic dysfunction are not available because patients with hepatic abnormalities were excluded from participation in adjuvant trials of FEC-100/CEF-120 therapy. In patients with elevated serum AST or serum total bilirubin concentrations, the following dose reductions were recommended in the clinical trials, although few patients experienced hepatic impairment.

Bilirubin 1.2-3 mg/dl or AST 2-4 times upper limit of normal ½ of recommended starting dose.

Bilirubin >3 mg/dl or AST >4 times upper limit of normal ¼ of recommended starting dose.

Renal Dysfunction

While no specific dose recommendation can be made based on the limited available data in patients with renal impairment, lower doses should be considered in patients with severe renal impairment (serum creatinine >5 mg/dl).

E

DOSE MODIFICATION

Dosage adjustments after the first treatment cycle should be made based on hematologic and nonhematologic toxicities. Patients experiencing during treatment cycle nadir platelet counts <50,000/mm^3, absolute neutrophil counts (ANC) <250/mm^3, neutropenic fever, or Grades 3/4 nonhematologic toxicity should have the Day 1 dose in subsequent cycles reduced to 75% of the Day 1 dose given in the current cycle. Day 1 chemotherapy in subsequent courses of treatment should be delayed until platelet counts are ≥100,000/mm^3, ANC ≥1500/mm^3, and nonhematologic toxicities have recovered to ≤Grade 1.

For patients receiving a divided dose of epirubicin HCl (Day 1 and Day 8), the Day 8 dose should be 75% of Day 1 if platelet counts are 75,000-100,000/mm^3 and ANC is 1000-1499/mm^3. If Day 8 platelet counts are <75,000/mm^3, ANC <1000/mm^3, or Grade 3/4 nonhematologic toxicity has occurred, the Day 8 dose should be omitted.

PREPARATION FOR ADMINISTRATION PRECAUTIONS

Parenteral drug products should be inspected visually for particulate matter and discoloration prior to administration, whenever solution and container permit.

Protective Measures

The following protective measures should be taken when handling epirubicin HCl.

Personnel should be trained in appropriate techniques for reconstitution and handling.

Pregnant staff should be excluded from working with this drug.

Personnel handling epirubicin HCl should wear protective clothing: goggles, gowns, and disposable gloves and masks.

A designated area should be defined for syringe preparation (preferably under a laminar flow system), with the work surface protected by disposable, plastic-backed, absorbent paper.

All items used for reconstitution, administration or cleaning (including gloves) should be placed in high-risk, waste-disposal bags for high temperature incineration.

Spillage or leakage should be treated with dilute sodium hypochlorite (1% available chlorine) solution, preferably by soaking, and then water. All contaminated and cleaning materials should be placed in high-risk, waste-disposal bags for incineration. Accidental contact with the skin or eyes should be treated immediately by copious lavage with water, or soap and water, or sodium bicarbonate solution; medical attention should be sought.

Incompatibilities

Prolonged contact with any solution of an alkaline pH should be avoided as it will result in hydrolysis of the drug. Epirubicin HCl should not be mixed with heparin or fluorouracil due to chemical incompatibility that may lead to precipitation.

Epirubicin HCl can be used in combination with other antitumor agents, but it is not recommended that it be mixed with other drugs in the same syringe.

PREPARATION OF INFUSION SOLUTION

Epirubicin HCl is provided as a preservative-free, ready-to-use solution.

Intravenous administration of epirubicin HCl should be performed with caution. It is recommended that epirubicin HCl be administered into the tubing of a freely flowing intravenous infusion (0.9% sodium chloride or 5% glucose solution) over a period of 3-5 minutes. This technique is intended to minimize the risk of thrombosis or perivenous extravasation, which could lead to severe cellulitis, vescication, or tissue necrosis. A direct push injection is not recommended due to the risk of extravasation, which may occur even in the presence of adequate blood return upon needle aspiration. Venous sclerosis may result from injection into small vessels or repeated injections into the same vein. Epirubicin HCl should be used within 24 hours of first penetration of the rubber stopper. Discard any unused solution.

PRODUCT LISTING - EQUIVALENTS NOT AVAILABLE

Injection - Intravenous - 2 mg/ml

25 ml	$757.66	ELLENCE, Pharmacia and Upjohn	00009-5091-01
100 ml	$3030.64	ELLENCE, Pharmacia and Upjohn	00009-5093-01

Eplerenone (003570)

Categories: Hypertension, essential; Pregnancy Category B; FDA Approved 2002 Sep
Drug Classes: Selective aldosterone receptor antagonist
Brand Names: Inspra

DESCRIPTION

Inspra contains eplerenone, a blocker of aldosterone binding at the mineralocorticoid receptor.

Eplerenone is chemically described as Pregn-4-ene-7,21-dicarboxylic acid,9,11-epoxy-17-hydroxy-3-oxo-,γ-lactone, methyl ester, (7α,11α,17α)-. Its empirical formula is $C_{24}H_{30}O_6$ and it has a molecular weight of 414.50.

Eplerenone is an odorless, white to off-white crystalline powder. It is very slightly soluble in water, with its solubility essentially pH independent. The octanol/water partition coefficient of eplerenone is approximately 7.1 at pH 7.0.

Inspra for oral administration contains 25, 50, or 100 mg of eplerenone and the following inactive ingredients: lactose, microcrystalline cellulose, croscarmellose sodium, hydroxypropyl methylcellulose, sodium lauryl sulfate, talc, magnesium stearate, titanium dioxide, polyethylene glycol, polysorbate 80, and iron oxide yellow and iron oxide red (25 mg tablet) and iron oxide red (50 and 100 mg tablets).

CLINICAL PHARMACOLOGY

MECHANISM OF ACTION

Eplerenone binds to the mineralocorticoid receptor and blocks the binding of aldosterone, a component of the renin-angiotensin-aldosterone-system (RAAS). Aldosterone synthesis, which occurs primarily in the adrenal gland, is modulated by multiple factors, including angiotensin II and non-RAAS mediators such as adrenocorticotropic hormone (ACTH) and potassium. Aldosterone binds to mineralocorticoid receptors in both epithelial (*e.g.*, kidney) and nonepithelial (*e.g.*, heart, blood vessels, and brain) tissues and increases blood pressure through induction of sodium reabsorption and possibly other mechanisms.

Eplerenone has been shown to produce sustained increases in plasma renin and serum aldosterone, consistent with inhibition of the negative regulatory feedback of aldosterone on renin secretion. The resulting increased plasma renin activity and aldosterone circulating levels do not overcome the effect of eplerenone on blood pressure.

Eplerenone has relative selectivity in binding to recombinant human mineralocorticoid receptors compared to its binding to recombinant human glucocorticoid, progesterone and androgen receptors.

PHARMACOKINETICS

General

Eplerenone is cleared predominantly by cytochrome P450 3A4 (CYP3A4) metabolism, with an elimination half-life of 4-6 hours. Steady state is reached within 2 days.

Absorption is not affected by food. Inhibitors of CYP3A4 (*e.g.*, ketoconazole, saquinavir) increase blood levels of eplerenone.

Absorption and Distribution

Mean peak plasma concentrations of eplerenone are reached approximately 1.5 hours following oral administration. The absolute bioavailability of eplerenone is unknown. Both peak plasma levels (C_{max}) and area under the curve (AUC) are dose proportional over doses of 25-100 mg and less than proportional at doses above 100 mg.

The plasma protein binding of eplerenone is about 50% and is primarily bound to alpha 1-acid glycoproteins. In healthy subjects and patients with hypertension, the apparent volume of distribution at steady state ranged from 43-90 L. Eplerenone does not preferentially bind to red blood cells.

Metabolism and Excretion

Eplerenone metabolism is primarily mediated via CYP3A4. No active metabolites of eplerenone have been identified in human plasma.

Less than 5% of an eplerenone dose is recovered as unchanged drug in the urine and feces. Following a single oral dose of radiolabeled drug, approximately 32% of the dose was excreted in the feces and approximately 67% was excreted in the urine. The elimination half-life of eplerenone is approximately 4-6 hours. The apparent plasma clearance is approximately 10 L/h.

Special Populations

Age, Gender, and Race

The pharmacokinetics of eplerenone at a dose of 100 mg once daily have been investigated in the elderly (≥65 years), in males and females, and in blacks. The pharmacokinetics of eplerenone did not differ significantly between males and females. At steady state, elderly subjects had increases in C_{max} (22%) and AUC (45%) compared with younger subjects (18-45 years). At steady state, C_{max} was 19% lower and AUC was 26% lower in blacks. (See DOSAGE AND ADMINISTRATION.)

Renal Insufficiency

The pharmacokinetics of eplerenone were evaluated in patients with varying degrees of renal insufficiency and in patients undergoing hemodialysis. Compared with control subjects, steady-state AUC and C_{max} were increased by 38% and 24%, respectively, in patients with severe renal impairment and were decreased by 26% and 3%, respectively, in patients undergoing hemodialysis. No correlation was observed between plasma clearance of eplerenone and creatinine clearance. Eplerenone is not removed by hemodialysis. (See WARNINGS, Hyperkalemia.)

Hepatic Insufficiency

The pharmacokinetics of eplerenone 400 mg have been investigated in patients with moderate (Child-Pugh Class B) hepatic impairment and compared with normal subjects. Steady-state C_{max} and AUC of eplerenone were increased by 3.6% and 42%, respectively. (See DOSAGE AND ADMINISTRATION.)

Drug-Drug Interactions

Also see DRUG INTERACTIONS.

Drug-drug interactions studies were conducted with a 100 mg dose of eplerenone.

Eplerenone is metabolized primarily by CYP3A4. A potent inhibitor of CYP3A4 (ketoconazole) caused increased exposure of about 5-fold while less potent CYP3A4 inhibitors (erythromycin, saquinavir, verapamil, and fluconazole) gave approximately 2-fold increases. Grapefruit juice caused only a small increase (about 25%) in exposure. (See PRECAUTIONS and DOSAGE AND ADMINISTRATION.)

Eplerenone is not an inhibitor of CYP1A2, CYP3A4, CYP2C19, CYP2C9, or CYP2D6. Eplerenone did not inhibit the metabolism of chloroxazone, diclofenac, methylphenidate, losartan, amiodarone, dexamethasone, mephobarbital, phenytoin, phenacetin, dextromethorphan, metoprolol, tolbutaminde, amlodipine, astemizole, cisapride, diazepam, 17α-ethinylestradiol, fluoxetine, lovastatin, methylprednisolone, midazolam, nifedipine, simvastatin, triazolam, verapamil, glyburide, and warfarin *in vitro*. Eplerenone is not a substrate or an inhibitor of P-Glycoprotein at clinically relevant doses.

No clinically significant drug-drug pharmacokinetic interactions were observed when eplerenone was administered with digoxin, warfarin, midazolam, cisapride, cyclosporine, simvastatin, or oral contraceptives (norethindrone/ethinyl estradiol). St. Johns Wort (a CYP3A4 inducer) caused a small (about 30%) decrease in eplerenone AUC.

No significant changes in eplerenone pharmacokinetics were observed when eplerenone was administered with aluminum and magnesium-containing antacids.

INDICATIONS AND USAGE

Eplerenone is indicated for the treatment of hypertension. Eplerenone may be used alone or in combination with other antihypertensive agents.

CONTRAINDICATIONS

Eplerenone is contraindicated in patients with the following conditions:

- Serum potassium >5.5 meq/L.
- Type 2 diabetes with microalbuminuria.
- Serum creatinine >2.0 mg/dl in males or >1.8 mg/dl in females.
- Creatinine clearance <50 ml/min.

Eplerenone is also contraindicated in patients treated concomitantly with the following medications:

- Potassium supplements or potassium-sparing diuretics (amiloride, spironolactone, or triamterene).
- Strong inhibitors of CYP450 3A4 (*e.g.*, ketoconazole, itraconazole).

(See also CLINICAL PHARMACOLOGY, Drug-Drug Interaction; WARNINGS, Hyperkalemia; DRUG INTERACTIONS; and ADVERSE REACTIONS, Clinical Laboratory Test Findings, Potassium.)

WARNINGS

HYPERKALEMIA

The principal risk of eplerenone is hyperkalemia. Hyperkalemia can cause serious, sometimes fatal arrhythmias. This risk can be minimized by patient selection, avoidance of certain concomitant treatments, and monitoring. For patient selection and avoidance of certain concomitant medications, see CONTRAINDICATIONS; DRUG INTERACTIONS; and ADVERSE REACTIONS, Clinical Laboratory Test Findings. Periodic monitoring is recommended in patients at risk for the development of hyperkalemia (including patients receiving concomitant ACE inhibitors or angiotensin II receptor antagonists) until the effect of eplerenone is established. During the clinical trials serum potassium levels were monitored every 2 weeks for the first 1-2 months and then monthly thereafter.

PRECAUTIONS

IMPAIRED HEPATIC FUNCTION

In 16 subjects with mild-to-moderate hepatic impairment who received 400 mg of eplerenone no elevations of serum potassium above 5.5 mmol/L were observed. The mean increase in serum potassium was 0.12 meq/L in patients with hepatic impairment and 0.13 meq/L in normal controls. The use of eplerenone in patients with severe hepatic impairment has not been evaluated. (See DOSAGE AND ADMINISTRATION and CLINICAL PHARMACOLOGY, Pharmacokinetics, Special Populations.)

IMPAIRED RENAL FUNCTION

See CONTRAINDICATIONS.

INFORMATION FOR THE PATIENT

Patients receiving eplerenone should be informed not to use potassium supplements, salt substitutes containing potassium, or contraindicated drugs without consulting the prescribing physician (see CONTRAINDICATIONS).

PREGNANCY CATEGORY B

There are no adequate and well-controlled studies in pregnant women. Eplerenone should be used during pregnancy only if the potential benefit justifies the potential risk to the fetus.

Teratogenic Effects

Embryo-fetal development studies were conducted with doses up to 1000 mg/kg/day in rats and 300 mg/kg/day in rabbits (exposures up to 32 and 31 times the human AUC for the 100 mg/day therapeutic dose, respectively). No teratogenic effects were seen in rats or rabbits, although decreased body weight in maternal rabbits and increased rabbit fetal resorptions and post-implantation loss were observed at the highest administered dosage. Because animal reproduction studies are not always predictive of human response, eplerenone should be used during pregnancy only if clearly needed.

NURSING MOTHERS

The concentration of eplerenone in human breast milk after oral administration is unknown. However preclinical data show that eplerenone and/or metabolites are present in rat breast milk (0.85:1 [milk:plasma] AUC ratio) obtained after a single oral dose. Peak concentrations in plasma and milk were obtained from 0.5 to 1 hour after dosing. Rat pups exposed by this route developed normally. Because many drugs are excreted in human milk and because of the unknown potential for adverse effects on the nursing infant, a decision should be made whether to discontinue nursing or discontinue the drug, taking into account the importance of the drug to the mother.

PEDIATRIC USE

The safety and effectiveness of eplerenone has not been established in pediatric patients.

GERIATRIC USE

Of the total number of subjects in clinical studies of eplerenone, 1123 (23%) were 65 and over, while 212 (4%) were 75 and over. No overall differences in safety or effectiveness were observed between elderly subjects and younger subjects. Other reported clinical experience has not identified differences in responses between the elderly and younger patients, but greater sensitivity of some older individuals cannot be ruled out.

CARCINOGENESIS, MUTAGENESIS, AND IMPAIRMENT OF FERTILITY

Eplerenone was non-genotoxic in a battery of assays including *in vitro* bacterial mutagenesis (Ames test in *Salmonella* spp. and *E. coli*), *in vitro* mammalian cell mutagenesis (mouse lymphoma cells), *in vitro* chromosomal aberration (Chinese hamster ovary cells), *in vivo* rat bone marrow micronucleus formation, and *in vivo/ex vivo* unscheduled DNA synthesis in rat liver.

There was no drug-related tumor response in heterozygous P53 deficient mice when tested for 6 months at dosages up to 1000 mg/kg/day (systemic AUC exposures up to 9 times the exposure in humans receiving the 100 mg/day therapeutic dose). Statistically significant increases in benign thyroid tumors were observed after 2 years in both male and female rats when administered eplerenone 250 mg/kg/day (highest dose tested) and in male rats only at 75 mg/kg/day. These dosages provided systemic AUC exposures approximately 2-12 times higher than the average human therapeutic exposure at 100 mg/day. Repeat dose administration of eplerenone to rats increases the hepatic conjugation and clearance of thyroxin, which results in increased levels of TSH by a compensatory mechanism. Drugs that have produced thyroid tumors by this rodentspecific mechanism have not shown a similar effect in humans.

Male rats treated with eplerenone at 1000 mg/kg/day for 10 weeks (AUC 17 times that at the 100 mg/day human therapeutic dose) had decreased weights of seminal vesicles and epididymides and slightly decreased fertility. Dogs administered eplerenone at dosages of 15 mg/kg/day and higher (AUC 5 times that at the 100 mg/day human therapeutic dose) had dose-related prostate atrophy. The prostate atrophy was reversible after daily treatment for 1 year at 100 mg/kg/day. Dogs with prostate atrophy showed no decline in libido, sexual performance, or semen quality. Testicular weight and histology were not affected by eplerenone in any test animal species at any dosage.

DRUG INTERACTIONS

INHIBITORS OF CYP450 3A4

Eplerenone metabolism is predominantly mediated via CYP3A4. A pharmacokinetic study evaluating the administration of a single dose of eplerenone 100 mg with ketoconazole 200 mg bid, a potent inhibitor of the CYP3A4 pathway, showed a 1.7-fold increase in C_{max} of eplerenone and a 5.4-fold increase in AUC of eplerenone. Eplerenone should not be used with strong inhibitors of CYP450 3A4 (*e.g.*, ketoconazole, itraconazole). (See CONTRAINDICATIONS.)

Administration of eplerenone with other CYP3A4 inhibitors (*e.g.*, erythromycin 500 mg bid, verapamil 240 mg qd, saquinavir 1200 mg tid, fluconazole 200 mg qd) resulted in increases in C_{max} of eplerenone ranging from 1.4- to 1.6-fold and AUC from 2.0- to 2.9-fold. (See CLINICAL PHARMACOLOGY, Drug-Drug Interactions and DOSAGE AND ADMINISTRATION.)

ACE INHIBITORS AND ANGIOTENSIN II RECEPTOR ANTAGONISTS

The addition of eplerenone 50-100 mg to ACE inhibitors and angiontensin II receptor antagonists increased mean serum potassium slightly (about 0.09-0.13 meq/L). In a study in diabetics with microalbuminuria eplerenone 200 mg combined with the ACE inhibitor enalapril 10 mg increased the frequency of hyperkalemia (serum potassium >5.5 meq/L) from 17% on enalapril alone to 38% (see CONTRAINDICATIONS). Because the concomitant use of another mineralocorticoid receptor blocker and ACE inhibitors or angiotensin II antagonists has led to clinically relevant hyperkalemia, caution should be used in administering eplerenone with these drugs.

LITHIUM

A drug interaction study of eplerenone with lithium has not been conducted. Lithium toxicity has been reported in patients receiving lithium concomitantly with diuretics and ACE inhibitors. Serum lithium levels should be monitored frequently if eplerenone is administered concomitantly with lithium.

NONSTEROIDAL ANTI-INFLAMMATORY DRUGS (NSAIDS)

A drug interaction study of eplerenone with an NSAID has not been conducted. The administration of other potassium-sparing antihypertensives with NSAIDs has been shown to reduce the antihypertensive effect in some patients and result in severe hyperkalemia in patients with impaired renal function. Therefore, when eplerenone and NSAIDs are used concomitantly, patients should be observed to determine whether the desired effect on blood pressure is obtained.

ADVERSE REACTIONS

Eplerenone has been evaluated for safety in 3091 patients treated for hypertension. A total of 690 patients were treated for over 6 months and 106 patients were treated for over 1 year.

In placebo-controlled studies, the overall rates of adverse events were 47% with eplerenone and 45% with placebo. Adverse events occurred at a similar rate regardless of age, gender, or race. Therapy was discontinued due to an adverse event in 3% of patients treated with eplerenone and 3% of patients given placebo. The most common reasons for discontinuation of eplerenone were headache, dizziness, angina pectoris/myocardial infarction, and increased GGT. The adverse events that were reported at a rate of at least 1% of patients and at a higher rate in patients treated with eplerenone in daily doses of 25-400 mg versus placebo are shown in TABLE 1.

Gynecomastia and abnormal vaginal bleeding were reported with eplerenone but not with placebo. The rates of these sex hormone related adverse events are shown in TABLE 2. The rates increased slightly with increasing duration of therapy. In females, abnormal vaginal bleeding was also reported in 0.8% of patients on antihypertensive medications (other than spironolactone) in active control arms of the studies with eplerenone.

TABLE 1 *Rates (%) of Adverse Events Occurring in Placebo-Controlled Studies in ≥1% of Patients Treated With Eplerenone (25-400 mg) and at a More Frequent Rate Than in Placebo-Treated Patients*

	Eplerenone (n=945)	Placebo (n=372)
Metabolic		
Hypercholesterolemia	1%	0%
Hypertriglyceridemia	1%	0%
Digestive		
Diarrhea	2%	1%
Abdominal pain	1%	0%
Urinary		
Albuminuria	1%	0%
Respiratory		
Coughing	2%	1%
Central/Peripheral Nervous System		
Dizziness	3%	2%
Body as a Whole		
Fatigue	2%	1%
Influenza-like symptoms	2%	1%

Note: Adverse events that are too general to be informative or are very common in the treated population are excluded.

TABLE 2 *Rates of Sex Hormone Related Adverse Events With Eplerenone in Clinical Studies*

	Rates in Males		Rates in Females	
	Gynecomastia	Mastodynia	Either	Abnormal Vaginal Bleeding
All controlled studies	0.5%	0.8%	1.0%	0.6%
Controlled studies lasting ≥6 months	0.7%	1.3%	1.6%	0.8%
Open label, long term study	1.0%	0.3%	1.0%	2.1%

CLINICAL LABORATORY TEST FINDINGS

Serum Electrolytes

Potassium

In placebo-controlled fixed-dose studies, the mean increases in serum potassium were dose related and are shown in TABLE 3 along with the frequencies of values >5.5 meq/L.

TABLE 3 *Changes in Serum Potassium in the Placebo-Controlled, Fixed-Dose Studies of Eplerenone*

Daily Dosage	n	Mean Change meq/L	>5.5 meq/L
Placebo	194	0	1%
25	97	0.08	0%
50	245	0.14	0%
100	193	0.09	1%
200	139	0.19	1%
400	104	104	8.7%

Patients with both Type 2 diabetes and microalbuminuria are at increased risk of developing persistent hyperkalemia. In a study in such patients taking eplerenone 200 mg, the frequencies of maximum serum potassium levels >5.5 meq/L were 33% with eplerenone given alone and 38% when eplerenone was given with enalapril.

Rates of hyperkalemia increased with decreasing renal function. In all studies serum potassium elevations >5.5 meq/L were observed in 10.4% of patients treated with eplerenone with baseline calculated creatinine clearance <70 ml/min, 5.6% of patients with baseline creatinine clearance of 70-100 ml/min, and 2.6% of patients with baseline creatinine clearance of >100 ml/min.

Sodium

Serum sodium decreased in a dose-related manner. Mean decreases ranged from 0.7 meq/L at 50 mg daily to 1.7 meq/L at 400 mg daily. Decreases in sodium (<135 meq/L) were reported for 2.3% of patients administered eplerenone and 0.6% of placebo-treated patients.

Triglycerides

Serum triglycerides increased in a dose-related manner. Mean increases ranged from 7.1 mg/dl at 50 mg daily to 26.6 mg/dl at 400 mg daily. Increases in triglycerides (above 252 mg/dl) were reported for 15% of patients administered eplerenone and 12% of placebo-treated patients.

Cholesterol

Serum cholesterol increased in a dose-related manner. Mean changes ranged from a decrease of 0.4 mg/dl at 50 mg daily to an increase of 11.6 mg/dl at 400 mg daily. Increases in serum cholesterol values greater than 200 mg/dl were reported for 0.3% of patients administered eplerenone and 0% of placebo-treated patients.

Liver Function Tests

Serum alanine aminotransferase (ALT) and gamma glutamyl transpeptidase (GGT) increased in a dose-related manner. Mean increases ranged from 0.8 U/L at 50 mg daily to 4.8 U/L at 400 mg daily for ALT and 3.1 U/L at 50 mg daily to 11.3 U/L at 400 mg daily for GGT. Increases in ALT levels greater than 120 U/L (3 times upper limit of normal) were reported for 15/2259 patients administered eplerenone and 1/351 placebo-treated patients. Increases in ALT levels greater than 200 U/L (5 times upper limit of normal) were reported for 5/2259 of patients administered eplerenone and 1/351 placebo-treated patients. Increases of ALT greater than 120 U/L and bilirubin greater than 1.2 mg/dl were reported 1/2259 patients administered eplerenone and 0/351 placebo-treated patients. Hepatic failure was not reported in patients receiving eplerenone.

BUN/Creatinine

Serum creatinine increased in a dose-related manner. Mean increases ranged from 0.01 mg/dl at 50 mg daily to 0.03 mg/dl at 400 mg daily. Increases in blood urea nitrogen to greater than 30 mg/dl and serum creatinine to greater than 2 mg/dl were reported for 0.5% and 0.2%, respectively, of patients administered eplerenone and 0% of placebo-treated patients.

Uric Acid

Increases in uric acid to greater than 9 mg/dl were reported in 0.3% of patients administered eplerenone and 0% of placebo-treated patients.

DOSAGE AND ADMINISTRATION

Eplerenone may be used alone or in combination with other antihypertensive agents. The recommended starting dose of eplerenone is 50 mg administered once daily. The full therapeutic effect of eplerenone is apparent within 4 weeks. For patients with an inadequate blood pressure response to 50 mg once daily the dosage of eplerenone should be increased to 50 mg twice daily. Higher dosages of eplerenone are not recommended either because they have no greater effect on blood pressure than 100 mg or because they are associated with an increased risk of hyperkalemia.

No adjustment of the starting dose is recommended for the elderly or for patients with mild-to-moderate hepatic impairment. For patients receiving weak CYP3A4 inhibitors, such as erythromycin, saquinavir, verapamil, and fluconazole the starting dose should be reduced to 25 mg once daily (see CONTRAINDICATIONS).

HOW SUPPLIED

Inspra tablets are supplied as follows:

25 mg: Yellow diamond biconvex film-coated tablets. They are debossed with "PHA" on one side and "1710" on the other.

50 mg: Pink diamond biconvex film-coated tablets. They are debossed with "PHA" on one side and "1720" on the other.

100 mg: Red diamond biconvex film-coated tablets. They are debossed with "PHA" on one side and "1730" on the other.

Storage: Store at 25°C (77°F); excursions permitted to 15-30°C (59-86°F).

Epoetin Alfa *(001173)*

Categories: Anemia, secondary to cancer chemotherapy; Anemia, secondary to renal failure; Surgery, prevention of blood transfusions; Anemia, secondary to zidovudine therapy; Pregnancy Category C; Recombinant DNA Origin; FDA Approved 1989 Jun; Orphan Drugs

Drug Classes: Hematopoietic agents; Hormones/hormone modifiers

Brand Names: E.P.O.; **Epogen**; Eprex; Erythropoietin; Procrit

Foreign Brand Availability: Epoade (Japan); Epokine (Philippines); Epoxitin (Italy); Erypo (Austria; Germany; Switzerland); Espo (Japan); Neorecormon (Austria; Belgium; Bulgaria; Czech-Republic; Denmark; England; Finland; France; Germany; Greece; Hungary; Ireland; Italy; Netherlands; Norway; Poland; Portugal; Slovenia; Spain; Sweden; Switzerland; Turkey)

Cost of Therapy: $504.72 (Anemia; Epogen Injection; 3000 u/ml; 1 ml; 3 injections/week; 28 day supply)
$274.28 (Anemia; Procrit Injection; 3000 u/ml; 1 ml; 3 injections/week; 28 day supply)

DESCRIPTION

Erythropoietin is a glycoprotein which stimulates red blood cell production. It is produced in the kidney and stimulates the division and differentiation of committed erythroid progenitors in the bone marrow. Epogen, a 165 amino acid glycoprotein manufactured by recombinant DNA technology, has the same biological effects as endogenous erythropoietin.[1] It has a molecular weight of 30,400 daltons and is produced by mammalian cells into which the human erythropoietin gene has been introduced. The product contains the identical amino acid sequence of isolated natural erythropoietin.

Epogen is formulated as a sterile, colorless liquid in an isotonic sodium chloride/sodium citrate buffered solution for intravenous (IV) or subcutaneous (SC) administration.

Epogen Single-Dose, Preservative-Free Vial: Each 1 ml of solution contains 2000, 3000, 4000 or 10,000 Units of epoetin alfa, 2.5 mg albumin (human), 5.8 mg sodium citrate, 5.8 mg sodium chloride, and 0.06 mg citric acid in water for injection (pH 6.9 ± 0.3). This formulation contains no preservative.

Epogen Multidose, Preserved Vial: 2 ml (20,000 Units, 10,000 Units/ml). Each 1 ml of solution contains 10,000 Units of epoetin alfa, 2.5 mg albumin (human), 1.3 mg sodium citrate, 8.2 mg sodium chloride, 0.11 mg citric acid, and 1% benzyl alcohol as preservative in water for injection (pH 6.1 ± 0.3).

Epogen Multidose, Preserved Vial: 1 ml (20,000 Units/ml). Each 1 ml of solution contains 20,000 Units of epoetin alfa, 2.5 mg albumin (human), 1.3 mg sodium citrate, 8.2 mg chloride, 0.11 mg citric acid, and 1% benzyl alcohol as preservative in water for injection (pH 6.1 ± 0.3).

Storage: Store at 2-8°C (36-46°F). Do not freeze or shake.

CLINICAL PHARMACOLOGY

CHRONIC RENAL FAILURE PATIENTS

Endogenous production of erythropoietin is normally regulated by the level of tissue oxygenation. Hypoxia and anemia generally increase the production of erythropoietin, which in turn stimulates erythropoiesis.[2] In normal subjects, plasma erythropoietin levels range from 0.01 to 0.03 Units/ml,[2,3] and increase up to 100- to 1000-fold during hypoxia or anemia.[2,3] In contrast, in patients with chronic renal failure (CRF), production of erythropoietin is impaired, and this erythropoietin deficiency is the primary cause of their anemia.[3,4]

Chronic renal failure is the clinical situation in which there is a progressive and usually irreversible decline in kidney function. Such patients may manifest the sequelae of renal dysfunction, including anemia, but do not necessarily require regular dialysis. Patients with end-stage renal disease (ESRD) are those patients with CRF who require regular dialysis or kidney transplantation for survival.

Epoetin alfa has been shown to stimulate erythropoiesis in anemic patients with CRF, including both patients on dialysis and those who do not require regular dialysis.[4-13] The first evidence of a response to the 3 times weekly administration of epoetin alfa is an increase in the reticulocyte count within 10 days, followed by increases in the red cell count, hemoglobin, and hematocrit, usually within 2-6 weeks.[4,5] *Because of the length of time required for erythropoiesis — several days for erythroid progenitors to mature and be released into the circulation — a clinically significant increase in hematocrit is usually not observed in less than 2 weeks and may require up to 6 weeks in some patients.* Once the hematocrit reaches the target range (30-36%), that level can be sustained by epoetin alfa therapy in the absence of iron deficiency and concurrent illnesses.

The rate of hematocrit increase varies between patients and is dependent upon the dose of epoetin alfa, within a therapeutic range of approximately 50-300 Units/kg three times weekly.[4] A greater biologic response is not observed at doses exceeding 300 Units/kg three times weekly.[6] Other factors affecting the rate and extent of response include availability of iron stores, the baseline hematocrit, and the presence of concurrent medical problems.

ZIDOVUDINE-TREATED HIV-INFECTED PATIENTS

Responsiveness to epoetin alfa in HIV-infected patients is dependent upon the endogenous serum erythropoietin level prior to treatment. Patients with endogenous serum erythropoietin levels ≤500 mUnits/ml, and who are receiving a dose of zidovudine ≤4200 mg/week, may respond to epoetin alfa therapy. Patients with endogenous serum erythropoietin levels >500 mUnits/ml do not appear to respond to epoetin alfa therapy. In a series of four clinical trials involving 255 patients, 60-80% of HIV-infected patients treated with zidovudine had endogenous serum erythropoietin levels ≤500 mUnits/ml.

Response to epoetin alfa in zidovudine-treated HIV-infected patients is manifested by reduced transfusion requirements and increased hematocrit.

CANCER PATIENTS ON CHEMOTHERAPY

Anemia in cancer patients may be related to the disease itself or the effect of concomitantly administered chemotherapeutic agents. Epoetin alfa has been shown to increase hematocrit and decrease transfusion requirements after the first month of therapy (months 2 and 3), in anemic cancer patients undergoing chemotherapy.

A series of clinical trials enrolled 131 anemic cancer patients who were receiving cyclic cisplatin- or non cisplatin-containing chemotherapy. Endogenous baseline serum erythropoietin levels varied among patients in these trials with approximately 75% (n=83/110) having endogenous serum erythropoietin levels ≤132 mUnits/ml, and approximately 4% (n=4/110) of patients having endogenous serum erythropoietin levels >500 mUnits/ml. In general, patients with lower baseline serum erythropoietin levels responded more vigorously to epoetin alfa than patients with higher baseline erythropoietin levels. Although no specific serum erythropoietin level can be stipulated above which patients would be unlikely to respond to epoetin alfa therapy, treatment of patients with grossly elevated serum erythropoietin levels (*e.g.*,>200 mUnits/ml) is not recommended.

PHARMACOKINETICS

Intravenously administered Epoetin alfa is eliminated at a rate consistent with first order kinetics with a circulating half-life ranging from approximately 4-13 hours in patients with CRF. Within the therapeutic dose range, detectable levels of plasma erythropoietin are maintained for at least 24 hours.[7] After subcutaneous administration of epoetin alfa to patients with CRF, peak serum levels are achieved within 5-24 hours after administration and decline slowly thereafter. There is no apparent difference in half-life between patients not on dialysis whose serum creatinine levels were greater than 3, and patients maintained on dialysis.

In normal volunteers, the half-life of intravenously administered epoetin alfa is approximately 20% shorter than the half-life in CRF patients. The pharmacokinetics of epoetin alfa have not been studied in HIV-infected patients.

INDICATIONS AND USAGE

TREATMENT OF ANEMIA OF CHRONIC RENAL FAILURE PATIENTS

Epoetin alfa is indicated in the treatment of anemia associated with chronic renal failure, including patients on dialysis (end-stage renal disease) and patients not on dialysis. Epoetin alfa is indicated to elevate or maintain the red blood cell level (as manifested by the hematocrit or hemoglobin determinations) and to decrease the need for transfusions in these patients.

Non-dialysis patients with symptomatic anemia considered for therapy should have a hematocrit less than 30%.

Epoetin alfa is not intended for patients who require immediate correction of severe anemia. Epoetin alfa may obviate the need for maintenance transfusions but is not a substitute for emergency transfusion.

Prior to initiation of therapy, the patient's iron stores should be evaluated. Transferrin saturation should be at least 20% and ferritin at least 100 ng/ml. Blood pressure should be adequately controlled prior to initiation of epoetin alfa therapy, and must be closely monitored and controlled during therapy.

Epoetin alfa should be administered under the guidance of a qualified physician (see DOSAGE AND ADMINISTRATION).

TREATMENT OF ANEMIA IN ZIDOVUDINE-TREATED HIV-INFECTED PATIENTS

Epoetin alfa is indicated for the treatment of anemia related to therapy with zidovudine in HIV-infected patients. Epoetin alfa is indicated to elevate or maintain the red blood cell level (as manifested by the hematocrit or hemoglobin determinations) and to decrease the need for transfusions in these patients. Epoetin alfa is not indicated for the treatment of anemia in HIV-infected patients due to other factors such as iron or folate deficiencies, hemolysis or gastrointestinal bleeding, which should be managed appropriately.

Epoetin alfa, at a dose of 100 Units/kg three times per week, is effective in decreasing the transfusion requirement and increasing the red blood cell level of anemic, HIV-infected patients treated with zidovudine, when the endogenous serum erythropoietin level is ≤500 mUnits/ml and when patients are receiving a dose of zidovudine ≤4200 mg/week.

TREATMENT OF ANEMIA IN CANCER PATIENTS ON CHEMOTHERAPY

Epoetin alfa is indicated for the treatment of anemia in patients with non-myeloid malignancies where anemia is due to the effect of concomitantly administered chemotherapy. Epoetin alfa is indicated to decrease the need for transfusions in patients who will be receiving concomitant chemotherapy for a minimum of 2 months. Epoetin alfa is not indicated for the treatment of anemia in cancer patients due to other factors such as iron or folate deficiencies, hemolysis or gastrointestinal bleeding which should be managed appropriately.

REDUCTION OF ALLOGENEIC BLOOD TRANSFUSION IN SURGERY PATIENTS

Epoetin alfa is indicated for the treatment of anemic patients (hemoglobin >10 to ≤13 g/dl) scheduled to undergo elective, noncardiac, nonvascular surgery to reduce the need for allogeneic blood transfusions.[14-16] Epoetin alfa is indicated for patients at high risk for perioperative transfusions with significant, anticipated blood loss. Epoetin alfa is not indicated for anemic patients who are willing to donate autologous blood. The safety of the perioperative use of epoetin alfa has been studied only in patients who are receiving anticoagulant prophylaxis.

E

NON-FDA APPROVED INDICATIONS

Although not FDA approved, epoetin alfa has been used to treat anemia associated with chronic disease.

CONTRAINDICATIONS

Epoetin alfa is contraindicated in patients with:

Uncontrolled hypertension.

Known hypersensitivity to mammalian cell-derived products.

Known hypersensitivity to albumin (human).

WARNINGS

PEDIATRIC USE

The multidose preserved formulation contains benzyl alcohol. Benzyl alcohol has been reported to be associated with and increased incidence of neurological and other complications in premature infants which are sometimes fatal. The safety and effectiveness of epoetin alfa in pediatric patients have not been established.

THROMBOTIC EVENTS AND INCREASED MORTALITY

A randomized, prospective trial of 1265 hemodialysis patients with clinically evident cardiac disease (ischemic heart disease or congestive heart failure) was conducted in which patients were assigned to epoetin alfa treatment targeted to a maintenance hematocrit of either 42 ± 3% or 30 ± 3%. Increased mortality was observed in 634 patients randomized to a target hematocrit of 42% [221 deaths (35% mortality)] compared to 631 patients targeted to remain at a hematocrit of 30% [185 deaths (29%mortality)]. The reason for increased mortality observed in these studies is unknown, however the incidence of non-fatal myocardial infarctions (3.1% vs 2.3%), vascular access thromboses (39% vs 29%), and all other thrombotic events (22% vs 18%) were also higher in the group randomized to achieve a hematocrit of 42%.

Increased mortality was also observed in a randomized placebo-controlled study of epoetin alfa in patients who did not have CRF who were undergoing coronary artery bypass surgery (7 deaths in 126 patients randomized to epoetin alfa versus no deaths among 56 patients receiving placebo). Four (4) of these deaths occurred during the period of study drug administration and all 4 deaths were associated with thrombotic events. While the extent of the population affected in unknown, in patients at risk of thrombosis, the anticipated benefits of epoetin alfa treatment should be weighed against the potential for increased risks associated with therapy.

CHRONIC RENAL FAILURE PATIENTS

Hypertension

Patients with uncontrolled hypertension should not be treated with epoetin alfa; blood pressure should be controlled adequately before initiation of therapy. Up to 80% of patients with CRF have a history of hypertension.[25] Although there does not appear to be any direct pressor effects of epoetin alfa, blood pressure may rise during epoetin alfa therapy. During the early phase of treatment when the hematocrit is increasing, approximately 25% of patients on dialysis may require initiation of, or increases in, antihypertensive therapy. Hypertensive encephalopathy and seizures have been observed in patients with CRF treated with epoetin alfa.

Special care should be taken to closely monitor and aggressively control blood pressure in epoetin alfa-treated patients. Patients should be advised as to the importance of compliance with antihypertensive therapy and dietary restrictions. If blood pressure is difficult to control by initiation of appropriate measures, the hematocrit may be reduced by decreasing or withholding the dose of epoetin alfa. A clinically significant decrease in hematocrit may not be observed for several weeks.

It is recommended that the dose of epoetin alfa be decreased if the hematocrit increase exceeds 4 points in any 2 week period, because of the possible association of excessive rate of rise of hematocrit with an exacerbation of hypertension.

In CRF patients on hemodialysis with clinically evident ischemic heart disease or congestive heart failure, the hematocrit should be managed carefully, not to exceed 36% (see Thrombotic Events).

Seizures

Seizures have occurred in patients with CRF participating in epoetin alfa clinical trials.

In patients on dialysis, there was a higher incidence of seizures during the first 90 days of therapy (occurring in approximately 2.5% of patients) as compared with later time points.

Given the potential for an increased risk of seizures during the first 90 days of therapy, blood pressure and the presence of premonitory neurologic symptoms should be monitored closely. Patients should be cautioned to avoid potentially hazardous activities such as driving or operating heavy machinery during this period.

While the relationship between seizures and the rate of rise of hematocrit is uncertain, *it is recommended that the dose of epoetin alfa be decreased if the hematocrit increase exceeds 4 points in any 2 week period.*

Thrombotic Events

During hemodialysis, patients treated with epoetin alfa may require increased anticoagulation with heparin to prevent clotting of the artificial kidney (see ADVERSE REACTIONS for more information about thrombotic events).

Other thrombotic events (*e.g.*, myocardial infarction, cerebrovascular accident, transient ischemic attack) have occurred in clinical trials at an annualized rate of less than 0.04 events per patient year of epoetin alfa therapy. These trials were conducted in patients with CRF (whether on dialysis or not) in whom the target hematocrit was 32-40%. However, the risk of thrombotic events, including vascular access thrombosis, was significantly increased in patients with ischemic heart disease or congestive heart failure receiving epoetin alfa therapy with the goal of reaching a normal hematocrit (42%) as compared to a target hematocrit of 30%. Patients with pre-existing cardiovascular disease should be monitored closely.

E

Zidovudine-Treated HIV-Infected Patients

In contrast to CRF patients, epoetin alfa therapy has not been linked to exacerbation of hypertension, seizures, and thrombotic events in HIV-infected patients.

PRECAUTIONS

GENERAL

The parenteral administration of any biologic product should be attended by appropriate precautions in case allergic or other untoward reactions occur (see CONTRAINDICATIONS). In clinical trials, while transient rashes were occasionally observed concurrently with epoetin alfa therapy, no serious allergic or anaphylactic reactions were reported. See ADVERSE REACTIONS for more information regarding allergic reactions.

The safety and efficacy of epoetin alfa therapy have not been established in patients with a known history of a seizure disorder or underlying hematologic disease (*e.g.*, sickle cell anemia, myelodysplastic syndromes, or hypercoagulable disorders).

In some female patients, menses have resumed following epoetin alfa therapy; the possibility of pregnancy should be discussed and the need for contraception evaluated.

Hematology

Exacerbation of porphyria has been observed rarely in epoetin alfa-treated patients with CRF. However, epoetin alfa has not caused increased urinary excretion of porphyrin metabolites in normal volunteers, even in the presence of a rapid erythropoietic response. Nevertheless, epoetin alfa should be used with caution in patients with known porphyria.

In preclinical studies in dogs and rats, but not in monkeys, epoetin alfa therapy was associated with subclinical bone marrow fibrosis. Bone marrow fibrosis is a known complication of CRF in humans and may be related to secondary hyperparathyroidism or unknown factors. The incidence of bone marrow fibrosis was not increased in a study of patients on dialysis who were treated with epoetin alfa for 12-19 months, compared to the incidence of bone marrow fibrosis in a matched group of patients who had not been treated with epoetin alfa.

Hematocrit in CRF patients should be measured twice a week; zidovudine-treated HIV-infected and cancer patients should have hematocrit measured once a week until hematocrit has been stabilized, and measured periodically thereafter.

Delayed or Diminished Response

If the patient fails to respond or to maintain a response to doses within the recommended dosing range, the following etiologies should be considered and evaluated:

Iron Deficiency: Virtually all patients will eventually require supplemental iron therapy (see Iron Evaluation).
Underlying infectious, inflammatory, or malignant processes.
Occult blood loss.
Underlying hematologic disease (*i.e.*, thalassemia, refractory anemia, or other myelodysplastic disorders).
Vitamin Deficiencies: Folic acid or vitamin B12.
Hemolysis.
Aluminum intoxication.
Osteitis fibrosa cystica.

Iron Evaluation

During epoetin alfa therapy, absolute or functional iron deficiency may develop. Functional iron deficiency, with normal ferritin levels but low transferrin saturation, is presumably due to the inability to mobilize iron stores rapidly enough to support increased erythropoiesis. Transferrin saturation should be at least 20% and ferritin should be at least 100 ng/ml.

Prior to and during epoetin alfa therapy, the patient's iron status, including transferrin saturation (serum iron divided by iron binding capacity) and serum ferritin, should be evaluated. Virtually all patients will eventually require supplemental iron to increase or maintain transferrin saturation to levels which will adequately support epoetin alfa-stimulated erythropoiesis. All surgery patients being treated with epoetin alfa should receive adeqate iron supplementation throughout the course of therapy in oder to support erythropoesis and avoid depletion of iron stores.

CARCINOGENESIS, MUTAGENESIS, AND IMPAIRMENT OF FERTILITY

Carcinogenic potential of epoetin alfa has not been evaluated. Epoetin alfa does not induce bacterial gene mutation (Ames Test), chromosomal aberrations in mammalian cells, micronuclei in mice, or gene mutation at the HGPRT locus. In female rats treated intravenously with epoetin alfa, there was a trend for slightly increased fetal wastage at doses of 100 and 500 Units/kg.

PREGNANCY CATEGORY C

Epoetin alfa has been shown to have adverse effects in rats when given in doses 5 times the human dose. There are no adequate and well-controlled studies in pregnant women. Epoetin alfa should be used during pregnancy only if potential benefit justifies the potential risk to the fetus.

In studies in female rats, there were decreases in body weight gain, delays in appearance of abdominal hair, delayed eyelid opening, delayed ossification, and decreases in the number of caudal vertebrae in the F1 fetuses of the 500 Units/kg group. In female rats treated intravenously, there was a trend for slightly increased fetal wastage at doses of 100 and 500 Units/kg. Epoetin alfa has not shown any adverse effect at doses as high as 500 Units/kg in pregnant rabbits (from day 6 to 18 of gestation).

NURSING MOTHERS

Postnatal observations of the live offspring (F1 generation) of female rats treated with epoetin alfa during gestation and lactation revealed no effect of epoetin alfa at doses of up to 500 Units/kg. There were, however, decreases in body weight gain, delays in appearance of abdominal hair, eyelid opening, and decreases in the number of caudal vertebrae in the F1 fetuses of the 500 Units/kg group. There were no epoetin alfa-related effects on the F2 generation fetuses.

It in not known whether epoetin alfa is excreted in human milk. Because many drugs are excreted in human milk, caution should be exercised when epoetin alfa is administered to a nursing woman.

PEDIATRIC USE

The safety and effectiveness of epoetin alfa in children have not been established (see WARNINGS).

CHRONIC RENAL FAILURE PATIENTS

Patients With CRF Not Requiring Dialysis

Blood pressure and hematocrit should be monitored no less frequently than for patients maintained on dialysis. Renal function and fluid and electrolyte balance should be closely monitored, as an improved sense of well-being may obscure the need to initiate dialysis in some patients.

Hematology

Sufficient time should be allowed to determine a patient's responsiveness to a dosage of epoetin alfa before adjusting the dose. Because of the time required for erythropoiesis and the red cell half-life, an interval of 2-6 weeks may occur between the time of a dose adjustment (initiation, increase, decrease, or discontinuation) and a significant change in hematocrit.

In order to avoid reaching the suggested target hematocrit too rapidly, or exceeding the suggested target range (hematocrit of 30-36%), the guidelines for dose and frequency of dose adjustments (see DOSAGE AND ADMINISTRATION) should be followed.

For patients who respond to epoetin alfa with a rapid increase in hematocrit (*e.g.*, more than 4 points in any 2 week period), the dose of epoetin alfa should be reduced because of the possible association of excessive rate of rise of hematocrit with an exacerbation of hypertension.

The elevated bleeding time characteristic of CRF decreases toward normal after correction of anemia in epoetin alfa-treated patients. Reduction of bleeding time also occurs after correction of anemia by transfusion.

Laboratory Monitoring

The hematocrit should be determined twice a week until it has stabilized in the suggested target range and the maintenance dose has been established. After any dose adjustment, the hematocrit should also be determined twice weekly for at least 2-6 weeks until it has been determined that the hematocrit has stabilized in response to the dose change. The hematocrit should then be monitored at regular intervals.

A complete blood count with differential and platelet count should be performed regularly. During clinical trials, modest increases were seen in platelets and while blood cell counts. While these changes were statistically significant, they were not clinically significant and the values remained within normal ranges.

In patients with CRF, serum chemistry values [including blood urea nitrogen (BUN), uric acid, creatinine, phosphorus, and potassium] should be monitored regularly. During clinical trials in patients on dialysis, modest increases were seen in BUN, creatinine, phosphorus, and potassium. In some patients with CRF not on dialysis, treated with epoetin alfa, modest increases in serum uric acid and phosphorus were observed. While changes were statistically significant, the values remained within the ranges normally seen in patients with CRF.

Diet

As the hematocrit increases and patients experience an improved sense of well-being and quality of life, the importance of compliance with dietary and dialysis prescriptions should be reinforced. In particular, hyperkalemia is not uncommon in patients with CRF. In US studies in patients on dialysis, hyperkalemia has occurred at an annualized rate of approximately 0.11 episodes per patient-year of epoetin alfa therapy, often in association with poor compliance to medication, dietary, and/or dialysis prescriptions.

Dialysis Management

Therapy with epoetin alfa results in an increase in hematocrit and a decrease in plasma volume which could affect dialysis efficiency. In studies to date, the resulting increase in hematocrit did not appear to adversely affect dialyzer function[9,10] or the efficiency of high flux hemodialysis.[11] During hemodialysis, patients treated with epoetin alfa may require increased anticoagulation with heparin to prevent clotting of the artificial kidney.

Patients who are marginally dialyzed may require adjustments in their dialysis prescription. As with all patients on dialysis, the serum chemistry values [including blood urea nitrogen (BUN), creatinine, phosphorus, and potassium] in epoetin alfa-treated patients should be monitored regularly to assure the adequacy of the dialysis prescription.

Information for the Patient

In those situations in which the physician determines that a home dialysis patient can safely and effectively self-administer epoetin alfa, the patient should be instructed as to the proper dosage and administration. Home dialysis patients should be referred to the full "Information for Home Dialysis Patients" section; it is not a disclosure of all possible effects. Patients should be informed of the signs and symptoms of allergic drug reaction and advised of appropriate actions. If home use is prescribed for a home dialysis patient, the patient should be thoroughly instructed in the importance of proper disposal and cautioned against the reuse of needles, syringes, or drug product. A puncture-resistant container for the disposal of used syringes and needles should be available to the patient. The full container should be disposed of according to the directions provided by the physician.

Renal Function

In patients with CRF not on dialysis, renal function and fluid and electrolyte balance should be closely monitored, as an improved sense of well-being may obscure the need to initiate dialysis in some patients. In patients with CRF not on dialysis, placebo-controlled studies of progression of renal dysfunction over periods of greater than 1 year have not been completed. In shorter term trials in patients with CRF not on dialysis, changes in creatinine and creatinine clearance were not significantly different in epoetin alfa-treated patients, compared with placebo-treated patients. Analysis of the slope of 1/serum creatinine versus time plots in these patients indicates no significant change in the slope after the initiation of epoetin alfa therapy.

ZIDOVUDINE-TREATED HIV-INFECTED PATIENTS

Hypertension

Exacerbation of hypertension has not been observed in zidovudine-treated HIV-infected patients treated with epoetin alfa. However, epoetin alfa should be withheld in these patients if pre-existing hypertension is uncontrolled, and should not be started until blood pressure is controlled. In double-blind studies, a single seizure has been experienced by an epoetin alfa-treated patient.[19]

CANCER PATIENTS ON CHEMOTHERAPY

Hypertension

Hypertension, associated with a significant increase in hematocrit, has been noted rarely in epoetin alfa-treated cancer patients. Nevertheless, blood pressure in epoetin alfa-treated patients should be monitored carefully, particularly in patients with an underlying history of hypertension or cardiovascular disease.

Seizures

In double-blind, placebo-controlled trials, 3.2% (n=2/63) of epoetin alfa-treated patients and 2.9% (n=2/68) of placebo-treated patients had seizures. Seizures in 1.6% (n=1/63) of epoetin alfa-treated patients occurred in the context of a significant increase in blood pressure and hematocrit from baseline values. However, both epoetin alfa- treated patients also had underlying CNS pathology which may have been related to seizure activity.

Thrombotic Events

In double-blind, placebo-controlled trials, 3.2% (n=2/63) of epoetin alfa-treated patients and 11.8% (n=8/68) of placebo-treated patients had thrombotic events (*e.g.*, pulmonary embolism, cerebrovascular accident).

Growth Factor Potential

Epoetin alfa is a growth factor that primarily stimulates red cell production. However, the possibility that epoetin alfa can act as a growth factor for any tumor type, particularly myeloid malignancies, cannot be excluded.

SURGERY PATIENTS

Thrombotic/Vascular Events

In perioperative clinical trials with orthopedic patients, the overall incidence of thrombotic/vascular events was similar in epoetin alfa and placebo-treated patients who had a pretreatment hemoglobin of >10 to ≤13 g/dl. In patients with a hemoglobin of >13 g/dl treated with 300 Units/kg of epoetin alfa, and he possibility that epoetin alfa treatment may be associated with an increased risk of postoperative thrombotic/vascular events cannot be excluded.[14-16]

In one study in which epoetin alfa was administered in the perioperative period to patients undergoing coronary artery bypass graft surgery, there were 7 deaths in the group treated with epoetin alfa (n=126) and no deaths in the placebo-treated group. Among the 7 deaths in the patients treated with epoetin alfa, 4 were at the time of therapy (between study day 2 and 8). The 4 deaths at the time of therapy (3%) were associated with thrombotic/vascular events. A causative role in epoetin alfa cannot be excluded (see WARNINGS).

Hypertension

Blood pressure may rise in the perioperative period in patients being treated with epoetin alfa. Therefore, blood pressure should be monitored carefully.

DRUG INTERACTIONS

No evidence of interaction of epoetin alfa with other drugs was observed in the course of clinical trials.

ADVERSE REACTIONS

CHRONIC RENAL FAILURE PATIENTS

Epoetin alfa is generally well-tolerated. The adverse events reported are frequent sequelae of CRF and are not necessarily attributable to epoetin alfa therapy. In double-blind, placebo-controlled studies involving over 300 patients with CRF, the events reported in greater than 5% of epoetin alfa-treated patients during the blinded phase can be seen in TABLE 3.

Significant adverse events of concern in patients with CRF treated in double-blind, placebo-controlled trials occurred in patients during the blinded phase of the studies as seen in TABLE 4.

TABLE 3

Event	Epoetin alfa-Treated Patients (n=200)	Placebo-Treated Patients (n=135)
Hypertension	24%	19%
Headache	16%	12%
Arthralgias	11%	6%
Nausea	11%	9%
Edema	9%	10%
Fatigue	9%	14%
Diarrhea	9%	6%
Vomiting	8%	5%
Chest pain	7%	9%
Skin reaction (administration site)	7%	12%
Asthenia	7%	12%
Dizziness	7%	13%
Clotted access	7%	2%

TABLE 4

Seizure	1.1%	1.1%
CVA/TIA	0.4%	0.6%
MI	0.4%	1.1%
Death	0	1.7%

In the US epoetin alfa studies in patients on dialysis (over 567 patients), the incidence (number of events per patient-year) of the most frequently reported adverse events were: hypertension (0.75), headache (0.40), tachycardia (0.31), nausea/vomiting (0.26), clotted vascular access (0.25), shortness of breath (0.14), hyperkalemia (0.11), and diarrhea (0.11). Other reported events occurred at a rate of less than 0.10 events per patient per year.

Events reported to have occurred within several hours of administration of epoetin alfa were rare, mild, and transient, and included injection site stinging in dialysis patients and flu-like symptoms such as arthralgias and myalgias.

In all studies analyzed to date, epoetin alfa administration was generally well-tolerated, irrespective of the route of administration.

Hypertension

Increases in blood pressure have been reported in clinical trials, often during the first 90 days of therapy. On occasion, hypertensive encephalopathy and seizures have been observed in patients with CRF treated with epoetin alfa. When data from all patients in the US Phase 3 multicenter trial were analyzed, there was an apparent trend of more reports of hypertensive adverse events in patients on dialysis with a faster rate of rise of hematocrit (greater than 4 hematocrit points in any 2 week period). However, in a double-blind, placebo-controlled trial, hypertensive adverse events were not reported at an increased rate in the epoetin alfa-treated group (150 units/kg three times weekly) relative to the placebo group.

Seizures

There have been 47 seizures in 1010 patients on dialysis treated with epoetin alfa in clinical trials, with an exposure of 986 patient-years for a rate of approximately 0.048 events per patient-year. However, there appeared to be a higher rate of seizures during the first 90 days of therapy (occurring in approximately 2.5% of patients) when compared to subsequent 90-day periods. The baseline incidence of seizures in the untreated dialysis population is difficult to determine; it appears to be in the range of 5-10% per patient-year.[26-28]

Thrombotic Events

In clinical trials where the maintenance hematocrit was 35 ± 3% on epoetin alfa, clotting of the vascular access (A-V- shunt) has occurred at an annualized rate of about 0.25 events per patient-year, and other thrombotic events (*e.g.*, myocardial infarction, cerebrovascular accident, transient ischemic attack, and pulmonary embolism) occurred at a rate of less than 0.04 events per patient-year. In a separate study of 1111 untreated dialysis patients, clotting of the vascular access occurred at a rate of 0.50 events per-patient-year. However, in CRF patients on hemodialysis who also had clinically evident ischemic heart disease or congestive heart failure, the risk of A-V shunt thrombosis was higher (39% vs 29%), p <0.001), and myocardial infarctions, vascular ischemic events, and venous thrombosis were increased, in patients targeted to a hematocrit of 42 ± 3% compared to those maintained at 30 ± 3% (see WARNINGS).

In patients treated with commercial epoetin alfa, there have been rare reports of serious or unusual thrombo-embolic events including migratory thrombophlebitis, microvascular thrombosis, pulmonary embolus, and thrombosis of the retinal artery, and temporal and renal veins. A causal relationship has not been established.

Allergic Reactions

There have been no reports of serious allergic reactions or anaphylaxis associated with epoetin alfa administration during clinical trials. Skin rashes and urticaria have been observed rarely and when reported have generally been mild and transient in nature.

There have been rare reports of potentially serious allergic reactions including urticaria with associated respiratory symptoms or circumoral edema or urticaria alone. Most reactions occurred in situations where a causal relationship could not be established. Symptoms recurred with rechallenge in a few instances, suggesting that allergic reactivity may occasionally be associated with epoetin alfa therapy.

There has been no evidence for development of antibodies to erythropoietin in patients tested to date, including those receiving epoetin alfa for over 4 years. Nevertheless, if an anaphylactoid reaction occurs, epoetin alfa should be immediately discontinued and appropriate therapy initiated.

ZIDOVUDINE-TREATED HIV-INFECTED PATIENTS

Adverse events reported in clinical trials with epoetin alfa in zidovudine-treated HIV-infected patients were consistent with the progression of HIV infection. In double-blind, placebo-controlled studies of 3 months duration involving approximately 300 zidovudine-treated HIV-infected patients, adverse events with an incidence of ≥10% in either epoetin alfa-treated patients or placebo-treated patients as seen in TABLE 5.

TABLE 5 *Epoetin alfa, Adverse Reactions*

Event	Epoetin alfa-Treated Patients (n=144)	Placebo-Treated Patients (n=153)
Pyrexia	38%	29%
Fatigue	25%	31%
Headache	19%	14%
Cough	18%	14%
Diarrhea	16%	18%
Rash	16%	8%
Congestion, respiratory	15%	10%
Nausea	15%	12%
Shortness of breath	14%	13%
Asthenia	11%	14%
Skin reaction, medication site	10%	7%
Dizziness	9%	10%

There were no statistically significant differences between treatment groups in the incidence of the above events.

In the 297 patients studied, epoetin alfa was not associated with significant increases in opportunistic infections or mortality.[22] In 71 patients from this group treated with epoetin alfa at 150 Units/kg three times weekly, serum p24 antigen levels did not appear to increase.[25] Preliminary data showed no enhancement of HIV replication in infected cell lines *in vitro*.[19]

Peripheral white blood cell and platelet counts are unchanged following epoetin alfa therapy.

Allergic Reactions

Two zidovudine-treated HIV-infected patients had urticarial reactions within 48 hours of their first exposure to study medication. One (1) patient was treated with epoetin alfa and 1 was treated with placebo (epoetin alfa vehicle alone). Both patients had positive immediate skin tests against their study medication with a negative saline control. The basis for this apparent pre-existing hypersensitivity to components of the epoetin alfa formulation is unknown, but may be related to HIV-induced immunosuppression or prior exposure to blood products.

Seizures

In double-blind and open label trials of epoetin alfa in zidovudine-treated HIV-infected patients, 10 patients have experienced seizures.[22] In general, these seizures appear to be related to underlying pathology such as meningitis or cerebral neoplasms, not epoetin alfa therapy.

CANCER PATIENTS ON CHEMOTHERAPY

Adverse experiences reported in clinical trials with epoetin alfa in cancer patients were consistent with the underlying disease state. In double-blind, placebo-controlled studies of up to 3 months duration involving 131 cancer patients, adverse events with an incidence >10% in either epoetin alfa-treated or placebo-treated patients can be seen in TABLE 6.

TABLE 6 *Percent of Patients Reporting Event*

Event	Epoetin alfa-Treated Patients (n=63)	Placebo-Treated Patients (n=68)
Pyrexia	29%	19%
Diarrhea	21%*	7%
Nausea	17%†	32%
Vomiting	17%	15%
Edema	17%‡	1%
Asthenia	13%	16%
Fatigue	13%	15%
Shortness of breath	13%	9%
Paresthesia	11%	6%
Upper respiratory infection	11%	4%
Dizziness	5%	12%
Trunk pain	3%§	16%

* p=0.041
† p=0.069
‡ p=0.0016
§ p=0.017

Although some statistically significant differences between epoetin alfa- and placebo-treated patients were noted, the overall safety profile of epoetin alfa appeared to be consistent with the disease process of advanced cancer. During double-blind and subsequent open-label therapy in which patients (n=72 for total epoetin alfa exposure) were treated for up to 32 weeks with doses as high as 927 Units/kg, the adverse experience profile of epoetin alfa was consistent with the progression of advanced cancer.

Based on comparable survival data and on the percentage of epoetin alfa- and placebo-treated patients who discontinued therapy due to death, disease progression, or adverse experiences (22% and 13%, respectively; p=0.25), the clinical outcome in the epoetin alfa- and placebo-treated patients appeared to be similar. Available data from animal tumor models and measurement of proliferation of solid tumor cells from clinical biopsy specimens in response to epoetin alfa suggest that epoetin alfa does not potentiate tumor growth. Nevertheless, as a growth factor, the possibility that epoetin alfa may potentiate growth of some tumors, particularly myeloid tumors, cannot be excluded. A randomized controlled Phase 4 study is currently ongoing to further evaluate this issue.

The mean peripheral white blood cell count was unchanged following epoetin alfa therapy compared to the corresponding value in the placebo-treated group.

SURGERY PATIENTS

Adverse events with an incidence of ≥10% are shown in TABLE 7.

TABLE 7 *Percent of Patients Reporting Event*

	Epoetin alfa			Epoetin alfa	
	300 U/kg	100 U/kg	Placebo	600 U/kg	300 U/kg
Event	(n=112)*	(n=101)*	(n=103)*	(n=73)†	(n=72) †
Pyrexia	51%	50%	60%	47%	42%
Nausea	48%	43%	45%	45%	58%
Constipation	43%	42%	43%	51%	53%
Skin reaction, medication site	25%	19%	22%	26%	29%
Vomiting	22%	12%	14%	21%	29%
Skin pain	18%	18%	17%	5%	4%
Pruritus	16%	16%	14%	14%	22%
Insomnia	13%	16%	13%	21%	18%
Headache	13%	11%	9%	10%	19%
Dizziness	12%	9%	12%	11%	21%
Urinary tract infection	12%	3%	11%	11%	8%
Hypertension	10%	11%	10%	5%	10%
Diarrhea	10%	7%	12%	10%	6%
Deep venous thrombosis	10%	3%	5%	0%‡	0%‡
Dyspepsia	9%	11%	6%	7%	8%
Anxiety	7%	2%	11%	11%	4%
Edema	6%	11%	8%	11%	7%

* Study including patients undergoing orthopedic surgery treated with epoetin alfa or placebo for 15 days
† Study including patients undergoing orthopedic surgery treated with epoetin alfa 600 Units/kg weekly × 4 or 300 Units/kg daily × 15
‡ Determined by clinical symptoms

Thrombotic/Vascular Events

In three double-blind, placebo-controlled orthopedic surgery studies, the rate of deep venous thrombosis (DVT) was similar among epoetin alfa and placebo-treated patients in the recommended population of patients with a pretreatment hemoglobin of >10 to ≤13 g/dl.[14,16,24]

However, in 2 of 3 orthopedic surgery studies the overall rate (all pretreatment hemoglobin groups combined) of DVTs detected by postoperative ultrasonography and /or surveillance venography was higher in the group treated with epoetin alfa than in the placebo-treated group (11% vs 6%). This finding was attributable to the difference in DVT rates observed in the subgroup of patients with pretreatment hemoglobin >13 g/dl. However, the incidence of DVTs was within the range of that reported in the literature for orthopedic surgery patients.

In the orthopedic surgery study of patients with pretreatment hemoglobin of >10 to ≤13 g/dl which compared two dosing regimens (600 Units/kg weekly × 4 and 300 Units/kg daily × 15), 4 subjects in the 600 Units/kg weekly epoetin alfa group (5%) and no subjects in the 300 Units/kg daily group had a thrombotic vascular event during the study period.[15]

In a study examining the use of epoetin alfa in 182 patients scheduled for coronary artery bypass graft surgery 23% of patients treated with epoetin alfa and 29% treated with placebo experienced thrombotic/vascular events. There were 4 deaths among the epoetin alfa-treated patients that were associated with a thrombotic/vascular event. A causative role of epoetin alfa cannot be excluded (see WARNINGS).

DOSAGE AND ADMINISTRATION

CHRONIC RENAL FAILURE PATIENTS

Starting doses of epoetin alfa over the range of 50-100 Units/kg three times weekly have been shown to be safe and effective in increasing hematocrit and eliminating transfusion dependency in patients with CRF. The dose of epoetin alfa should be reduced as the hematocrit approaches 36% or increases by more than 4 points in any 2 week period. The dosage of epoetin alfa must be individualized to maintain the hematocrit within the suggested target range. At the physician's discretion, the suggested target hematocrit range may be expanded to achieve maximal patient benefit.

Epoetin alfa may be given either as an intravenous or subcutaneous injection. In patients on hemodialysis, epoetin alfa usually has been administered as an IV bolus 3 times weekly While the administration of epoetin alfa is independent of the dialysis procedure, epoetin alfa may be administered into the venous line at the end of the dialysis procedure to obviate the need for additional venous access. In patients with CRF not on dialysis, epoetin alfa may be given either as an IV or subcutaneous injection.

Patients who have been judged competent by their physicians to self-administer epoetin alfa without medical or other supervision may give themselves either an IV or SC injection. TABLE 8 provides general therapeutic guidelines for patients with CRF.

TABLE 8

Starting dose:	50-100 Units/kg T.I.W.; IV or subcutaneous
Reduce dose when:	1. Hct. approaches 36% or, 2. Hct. increases >4 points in any 2 week period
Increase dose if:	Hct. does not increase by 5-6 points after 8 weeks of therapy, and hct. is below suggested target range.
Maintenance dose:	Individually titrate
Suggested target Hct. range:	30-36%

During therapy, hematological parameters should be monitored regularly (see PRECAUTIONS, Laboratory Monitoring).

Pre-Therapy Iron Evaluation

Prior to and during epoetin alfa therapy, the patient's iron stores, including transferrin saturation (serum iron divided by iron binding capacity) and serum ferritin, should be evaluated. Transferrin saturation should be at least 20%, and ferritin should be at least 100 ng/ml. Virtually all patients will eventually require supplemental iron to increase or maintain transferrin saturation to levels that will adequately support epoetin alfa-stimulated erythropoiesis.

Dose Adjustment

Following epoetin alfa therapy, a period of time is required for erythroid progenitors to mature and be released into circulation resulting in an eventual increase in hematocrit. Additionally, red blood cell survival time affects hematocrit and may vary due to uremia. As a result, the time required to elicit a clinically significant change in hematocrit (increase or decrease) following any dose adjustment may be at 2-6 weeks.

Dose adjustment should not be made more frequently than once a month, unless clinically indicated. After any dose adjustment, the hematocrit should be determined twice weekly for at least 2-6 weeks (see PRECAUTIONS, Laboratory Monitoring).

- If the hematocrit is increasing and approaching 36%, the dose should be reduced to maintain the suggested target hematocrit range. If the reduced dose does not stop the rise in hematocrit, and it exceeds 36%, doses should be temporarily withheld until the hematocrit begins to decrease, at which point therapy should be reinitiated at a lower dose.
- At any time, if the hematocrit increases by more than 4 points in a 2 week period, the dose should be immediately decreased. After the dose reduction, the hematocrit should be monitored twice weekly for 2-6 weeks, and further dose adjustments should be made as outlined in Maintenance Dose.
- If a hematocrit increase of 5-6 points is not achieved after an 8 week period and iron stores are adequate (see Delayed or Diminished Response), the dose of epoetin alfa may be incrementally increased. Further increases may be made at 4-6 week intervals until the desired response is attained.

Maintenance Dose

The maintenance dose must be individualized for each patient on dialysis. In the US Phase 3 multicenter trial in patients on hemodialysis, the median maintenance dose was 75 Units/kg three times weekly, with a range from 12.5 to 525 Units/kg three times weekly Almost 10% of the patients required a dose of 25 Units/kg, or less, and approximately 10% of the patients required more than 200 Units/kg three times weekly to maintain their hematocrit in the suggested target range.

If the hematocrit remains below, or falls below, the suggested target range, iron stores should be re-evaluated. If the transferrin saturation is less than 20%, supplemental iron should be administered. If the transferrin saturation is greater than 20%, the dose of epoetin alfa may be increased. Such dose increases should not be made more frequently than once a month, unless clinically indicated, as the response time of the hematocrit to a dose increase can be 2-6 weeks. Hematocrit should be measured twice weekly for 2-6 weeks following dose increases. In patients with CRF not on dialysis, the maintenance dose must also be individualized. Epoetin alfa doses of 75-150 Units/kg per week have been shown to maintain hematocrits of 36-38% for up to 6 months.

Delayed or Diminished Response

Over 95% of patients with CRF responded with clinically significant increases in hematocrit, and virtually all patients were transfusion-independent within approximately 2 months of initiation of epoetin alfa therapy.

If a patient fails to respond or maintain a response, other etiologies should be considered and evaluated as clinically indicated. See PRECAUTIONS for discussion of delayed or diminished response.

ZIDOVUDINE-TREATED HIV-INFECTED PATIENTS

Prior to beginning epoetin alfa, it is recommended that the endogenous serum erythropoietin level be determined (prior to transfusion). Available evidence suggests that patients receiving zidovudine with endogenous serum erythropoietin levels >500 mUnits/ml are unlikely to respond to therapy with epoetin alfa.

Starting Dose

For patients with serum erythropoietin levels ≤500 mUnits/ml who are receiving a dose of zidovudine ≤4200 mg/week, the recommended starting dose of epoetin alfa is 100 Units/kg as an intravenous or subcutaneous injection 3 times weekly for 8 weeks.

Increase Dose

During the dose adjustment phase of therapy, the hematocrit should be monitored weekly. If the response is not satisfactory in terms of reducing transfusion requirements or increasing hematocrit after 8 weeks of therapy, the dose of epoetin alfa can be increased by 50-100 Units/kg three times weekly Response should be evaluated every 4-8 weeks thereafter and the dose adjusted accordingly by 50-100 Units/kg increments three times weekly If patients have not responded satisfactorily to an epoetin alfa dose of 300 Units/kg three times weekly, it is unlikely that they will respond to higher doses of epoetin alfa.

Maintenance Dose

After attainment of the desired response (*i.e.*, reduced transfusion requirements or increased hematocrit), the dose of epoetin alfa should be titrated to maintain the response based on factors such as variations in zidovudine dose and the presence of intercurrent infectious or inflammatory episodes. If the hematocrit exceeds 40%, the dose should be discontinued until the hematocrit drops to 36%. The dose should be reduced by 25% when treatment is resumed and then titrated to maintain the desired hematocrit.

CANCER PATIENTS ON CHEMOTHERAPY

Baseline endogenous serum erythropoietin levels varied among patients in these trials with approximately 75% (n=83/110) having endogenous serum erythropoietin levels <132 mUnits/ml, and approximately 4% (n=4/110) of patients having endogenous serum erythropoietin levels >500 mUnits/ml. In general, patients with lower baseline serum erythropoietin levels responded more vigorously to epoetin alfa than patients with higher erythropoietin levels. Although no specific serum erythropoietin level can be stipulated above which patients would be unlikely to respond to epoetin alfa therapy, treatment of patients with grossly elevated serum erythropoietin levels (*e.g.*, >200 mUnits/ml) is not recommended. The hematocrit should be monitored on a weekly basis in patients receiving epoetin alfa therapy until hematocrit becomes stable.

Starting Dose

The recommended starting dose of epoetin alfa is 150 Units/kg subcutaneously 3 times weekly

Dose Adjustment

If the response is not satisfactory in terms of reducing transfusion requirements or increasing hematocrit after 8 weeks of therapy, the dose of epoetin alfa can be increased up to 300 Units/kg three times weekly If patients have not responded satisfactorily to an epoetin alfa dose of 300 Units/kg three times weekly, it is unlikely that they will respond to higher doses of epoetin alfa. If the hematocrit exceeds 40%, the dose of epoetin alfa should be withheld until the hematocrit falls to 36%. The dose of epoetin alfa should be reduced by 25% when treatment is resumed and titrated to maintain the desired hematocrit. If the initial dose of epoetin alfa includes a very rapid hematocrit response (*e.g.*, an increase of more than 4 percentage points in any 2 week period), the dose of epoetin alfa should be reduced.

SURGERY PATIENTS

Prior to initializing treatment with epoetin alfa, a hemoglobin should be obtained to establish that it is >10 to ≤13 g/dl.[14] The recommended dose of epoetin alfa is 300 Units/kg/day subcutaneously for 10 days before surgery, on the day of surgery, and for 4 days after surgery.

An alternate dose schedule is 600 Units/kg epoetin alfa subcutaneously in once weekly doses (21, 14, and 7 days before surgery) plus a fourth dose on the day of surgery.[15]

All patients should receive adequate iron supplementation. Iron supplementation should be initiated no later than the beginning of treatment with epoetin alfa and should continue throughout the course of therapy.

PRODUCT LISTING - EQUIVALENTS NOT AVAILABLE

Solution - Injectable - 2000 U/ml			
1 ml	$26.92	EPOGEN, Amgen	55513-0126-01
1 ml x 6	$160.26	PROCRIT, Ortho Biotech Inc	59676-0302-01
1 ml x 10	$280.40	EPOGEN, Amgen	55513-0126-10
1 ml x 25	$667.75	PROCRIT, Ortho Biotech Inc	59676-0302-02
Solution - Injectable - 3000 U/ml			
1 ml	$40.38	EPOGEN, Amgen	55513-0267-01
1 ml x 6	$240.42	PROCRIT, Ortho Biotech Inc	59676-0303-01
1 ml x 10	$420.60	EPOGEN, Amgen	55513-0267-10
1 ml x 25	$1001.75	PROCRIT, Ortho Biotech Inc	59676-0303-02
Solution - Injectable - 4000 U/ml			
1 ml	$53.83	EPOGEN, Amgen	55513-0148-01
1 ml x 6	$320.52	PROCRIT, Ortho Biotech Inc	59676-0304-01
1 ml x 10	$560.80	EPOGEN, Amgen	55513-0148-10
1 ml x 25	$1335.50	PROCRIT, Ortho Biotech Inc	59676-0304-02
Solution - Injectable - 10000 U/ml			
1 ml	$134.59	EPOGEN, Amgen	55513-0144-01
1 ml	$139.12	PROCRIT, Physicians Total Care	54868-2523-00
1 ml x 6	$801.36	PROCRIT, Ortho Biotech Inc	59676-0310-01
1 ml x 6	$831.79	PROCRIT, Physicians Total Care	54868-2523-01
1 ml x 10	$1402.00	EPOGEN, Amgen	55513-0144-10
1 ml x 25	$3339.00	PROCRIT, Ortho Biotech Inc	59676-0310-02
2 ml	$228.00	PROCRIT, Ortho Biotech Inc	59676-0312-00
2 ml	$269.18	EPOGEN, Amgen	55513-0283-01
2 ml x 6	$1602.72	PROCRIT, Ortho Biotech Inc	59676-0312-01
2 ml x 10	$2804.00	EPOGEN, Amgen	55513-0283-10
Solution - Injectable - 20000 U/ml			
1 ml	$289.46	EPOGEN, Amgen	55513-0478-01
1 ml x 6	$1602.72	PROCRIT, Janssen Pharmaceuticals	59676-0320-01
1 ml x 10	$3015.30	EPOGEN, Amgen	55513-0478-10
Solution - Injectable - 40000 U/ml			
1 ml	$568.00	EPOGEN, Amgen	55513-0823-01
1 ml x 4	$2136.96	PROCRIT, Janssen Pharmaceuticals	59676-0340-01
1 ml x 10	$5916.60	EPOGEN, Amgen	55513-0823-10

Eprosartan Mesylate (003496)

For related information, see the comparative table section in Appendix A.

Categories: Hypertension, essential; FDA Approved 1999 Nov; Pregnancy Category C, 1st Trimester; Pregnancy Category D, 2nd & 3rd Trimesters
Drug Classes: Angiotensin II receptor antagonists
Brand Names: Teveten
Cost of Therapy: $37.50 (Hypertension; Teveten; 600 mg; 1 tablet/day; 30 day supply)

WARNING

USE IN PREGNANCY

When used in pregnancy during the second and third trimesters, drugs that act directly on the renin-angiotensin system can cause injury and even death to the developing fetus. When pregnancy is

E

> **WARNING — Cont'd**
> **detected, eprosartan mesylate should be discontinued as soon as possible (see WARNINGS, Fetal/Neonatal Morbidity and Mortality).**

E

DESCRIPTION

Teveten tablet is a non-biphenyl non-tetrazole angiotensin II receptor (AT_1) antagonist. A selective non-peptide molecule, eprosartan mesylate is chemically described as the monomethanesulfonate of (*E*)-2-butyl-1-(*p*-carboxybenzyl)-α-2-thienylmethylimidazole-5-acrylic acid.

Its empirical formula is $C_{23}H_{24}N_2O_4S{\cdot}CH_4O_3S$ and molecular weight is 520.625.

Eprosartan mesylate is a white to off-white free-flowing crystalline powder that is insoluble in water, freely soluble in ethanol, and melts between 248 and 250°C.

Teveten tablets are available as aqueous film-coated tablets containing eprosartan mesylate equivalent to 400 mg or 600 mg eprosartan zwitterion (pink, oval, non-scored tablets or white, non-scored, capsule-shaped tablets, respectively).

INACTIVE INGREDIENTS

The 400 mg tablet contains the following: croscarmellose sodium, hydroxypropyl methylcellulose, iron oxide red, iron oxide yellow, lactose monohydrate, magnesium stearate, microcrystalline cellulose, polyethylene glycol, polysorbate 80, pregelatinized starch, titanium dioxide. The 600 mg tablet contains crospovidone, hydroxypropyl methylcellulose, lactose monohydrate, magnesium stearate, microcrystalline cellulose, polyethylene glycol, polysorbate 80, pregelatinized starch, titanium dioxide.

CLINICAL PHARMACOLOGY

MECHANISM OF ACTION

Angiotensin II (formed from angiotensin I in a reaction catalyzed by angiotensin-converting enzyme [kininase II]), a potent vasoconstrictor, is the principal pressor agent of the renin-angiotensin system. Angiotensin II also stimulates aldosterone synthesis and secretion by the adrenal cortex, cardiac contraction, renal resorption of sodium, activity of the sympathetic nervous system, and smooth muscle cell growth. Eprosartan blocks the vasoconstrictor and aldosterone-secreting effects of angiotensin II by selectively blocking the binding of angiotensin II to the AT_1 receptor found in many tissues (*e.g.*, vascular smooth muscle, adrenal gland). There is also an AT_2 receptor found in many tissues but it is not known to be associated with cardiovascular homeostasis. Eprosartan does not exhibit any partial agonist activity at the AT_1 receptor. Its affinity for the AT_1 receptor is 1000 times greater than for the AT_2 receptor. *In vitro* binding studies indicate that eprosartan is a reversible, competitive inhibitor of the AT_1 receptor.

Blockade of the AT_1 receptor removes the negative feedback of angiotensin II on renin secretion, but the resulting increased plasma renin activity and circulating angiotensin II do not overcome the effect of eprosartan on blood pressure.

Eprosartan mesylate tablets do not inhibit kininase II, the enzyme that converts angiotensin I to angiotensin II and degrades bradykinin; whether this has clinical relevance is not known. It does not bind to or block other hormone receptors or ion channels known to be important in cardiovascular regulation.

PHARMACOKINETICS

General

Absolute bioavailability following a single 300 mg oral dose of eprosartan is approximately 13%. Eprosartan plasma concentrations peak at 1-2 hours after an oral dose in the fasted state. Administering eprosartan with food delays absorption, and causes variable changes (<25%) in C_{max} and AUC values which do not appear clinically important. Plasma concentrations of eprosartan increase in a slightly less than dose-proportional manner over the 100-800 mg dose range. The terminal elimination half-life of eprosartan following oral administration is typically 5-9 hours. Eprosartan does not significantly accumulate with chronic use.

Metabolism and Excretion

Eprosartan is eliminated by biliary and renal excretion, primarily as unchanged compound. Less than 2% of an oral dose is excreted in the urine as a glucuronide. There are no active metabolites following oral and intravenous dosing with [^{14}C] eprosartan in human subjects. Eprosartan was the only drug-related compound found in the plasma and feces. Following intravenous [^{14}C] eprosartan, about 61% of the material is recovered in the feces and about 37% in the urine. Following an oral dose of [^{14}C] eprosartan, about 90% is recovered in the feces and about 7% in the urine. Approximately 20% of the radioactivity excreted in the urine was an acyl glucuronide of eprosartan with the remaining 80% being unchanged eprosartan.

Distribution

Plasma protein binding of eprosartan is high (approximately 98%) and constant over the concentration range achieved with therapeutic doses.

The pooled population pharmacokinetic analysis from two Phase 3 trials of 299 men and 172 women with mild to moderate hypertension (aged 20-93 years) showed that eprosartan exhibited a population mean oral clearance (CL/F) for an average 60-year-old patient of 48.5 L/h. The population mean steady-state volume of distribution (Vss/F) was 308 liters. Eprosartan pharmacokinetics were not influenced by weight, race, gender or severity of hypertension at baseline. Oral clearance was shown to be a linear function of age with CL/F decreasing 0.62 L/h for every year increase.

SPECIAL POPULATIONS

Pediatric

Eprosartan pharmacokinetics have not been investigated in patients younger than 18 years of age.

Geriatric

Following single oral dose administration of eprosartan to healthy elderly men (aged 68-78 years), AUC, C_{max}, and T_{max} eprosartan values increased, on average by approximately 2-fold, compared to healthy young men (aged 20-39 years) who received the same dose. The extent of plasma protein binding was not influenced by age.

Gender

There was no difference in the pharmacokinetics and plasma protein binding between men and women following single oral dose administration of eprosartan.

Race

A pooled population pharmacokinetic analysis of 442 Caucasian and 29 non-Caucasian hypertensive patients showed that oral clearance and steady-state volume of distribution were not influenced by race.

Renal Insufficiency

Following administration of 600 mg once daily, there was an almost 2-fold increase in AUC and a 50 and 30% increase in C_{max} in moderate and severe renal impairment. The unbound eprosartan fractions increased by 35 and 59% in patients with moderate and severe renal impairment. No initial dosing adjustment is generally necessary in patients with moderate and severe renal impairment, with maximum dose not exceeding 600 mg daily. Eprosartan was poorly removed by hemodialysis (CL_{HD} <1 L/h). (See DOSAGE AND ADMINISTRATION.)

Hepatic Insufficiency

Eprosartan AUC (but not C_{max}) values increased, on average, by approximately 40% in men with decreased hepatic function compared to healthy men after a single 100 mg oral dose of eprosartan. Hepatic disease was defined as a documented clinical history of chronic hepatic abnormality diagnosed by liver biopsy, liver/spleen scan or clinical laboratory tests. The extent of eprosartan plasma protein binding was not influenced by hepatic dysfunction. No dosage adjustment is necessary for patients with hepatic impairment (see DOSAGE AND ADMINISTRATION).

DRUG INTERACTIONS

Concomitant administration of eprosartan and digoxin had no effect on single oral-dose digoxin pharmacokinetics. Concomitant administration of eprosartan and warfarin had no effect on steady-state prothrombin time ratios (INR) in healthy volunteers. Concomitant administration of eprosartan and glyburide in diabetic patients did not affect 24 hour plasma glucose profiles. Eprosartan pharmacokinetics were not affected by concomitant administration of ranitidine. Eprosartan did not inhibit human cytochrome P450 enzymes CYP1A, 2A6, 2C9/8, 2C19, 2D6, 2E and 3A *in vitro*. Eprosartan is not metabolized by the cytochrome P450 system; eprosartan steady-state concentrations were not affected by concomitant administration of ketoconazole or fluconazole, potent inhibitors of CYP3A and 2C9, respectively.

PHARMACODYNAMICS AND CLINICAL EFFECTS

Eprosartan inhibits the pharmacologic effects of angiotensin II infusions in healthy adult men. Single oral doses of eprosartan from 10-400 mg have been shown to inhibit the vasopressor, renal vasoconstrictive and aldosterone secretory effects of infused angiotensin II with complete inhibition evident at doses of 350 mg and above. Eprosartan inhibits the pressor effects of angiotensin II infusions. A single oral dose of 350 mg of eprosartan inhibits pressor effects by approximately 100% at peak, with approximately 30% inhibition persisting for 24 hours. The absence of angiotensin II AT_1 agonist activity has been demonstrated in healthy adult men. In hypertensive patients treated chronically with eprosartan, there was a 2-fold rise in angiotensin II plasma concentration and a 2-fold rise in plasma renin activity, while plasma aldosterone levels remained unchanged. Serum potassium levels also remained unchanged in these patients.

Achievement of maximal blood pressure response to a given dose in most patients may take 2-3 weeks of treatment. Onset of blood pressure reduction is seen within 1-2 hours of dosing with few instances of orthostatic hypotension. Blood pressure control is maintained with once or twice daily dosing over a 24 hour period. Discontinuing treatment with eprosartan does not lead to a rapid rebound increase in blood pressure.

There was no change in mean heart rate in patients treated with eprosartan in controlled clinical trials.

Eprosartan increases mean effective renal plasma flow (ERPF) in salt-replete and salt-restricted normal subjects. A dose-related increase in ERPF of 25-30% occurred in salt-restricted normal subjects, with the effect plateauing between 200 and 400 mg doses. There was no change in ERPF in hypertensive patients and patients with renal insufficiency on normal salt diets. Eprosartan did not reduce glomerular filtration rate in patients with renal insufficiency or in patients with hypertension, after 7 days and 28 days of dosing, respectively. In hypertensive patients and patients with chronic renal insufficiency, eprosartan did not change fractional excretion of sodium and potassium.

Eprosartan (1200 mg once daily for 7 days or 300 mg twice daily for 28 days) had no effect on the excretion of uric acid in healthy men, patients with essential hypertension or those with varying degrees of renal insufficiency.

There were no effects on mean levels of fasting triglycerides, total cholesterol, HDL cholesterol, LDL cholesterol or fasting glucose.

INDICATIONS AND USAGE

Eprosartan mesylate tablets are indicated for the treatment of hypertension. It may be used alone or in combination with other antihypertensives such as diuretics and calcium channel blockers.

CONTRAINDICATIONS

Eprosartan mesylate tablets are contraindicated in patients who are hypersensitive to this product or any of its components.

WARNINGS

FETAL/NEONATAL MORBIDITY AND MORTALITY

Drugs that act directly on the renin-angiotensin system can cause fetal and neonatal morbidity and death when administered to pregnant women. Several dozen cases have been reported in the world literature in patients who were taking angiotensin-converting enzyme inhibitors. When pregnancy is detected, eprosartan mesylate tablets should be discontinued as soon as possible.

The use of drugs that act directly on the renin-angiotensin system during the second and third trimesters of pregnancy has been associated with fetal and neonatal injury, including hypotension, neonatal skull hypoplasia, anuria, reversible or irreversible renal failure, and death. Oligohydramnios has also been reported, presumably resulting from decreased fetal renal function; oligohydramnios in this setting has been associated with fetal limb contractures, craniofacial deformation, and hypoplastic lung development. Prematurity, intrauterine growth retardation, and patent ductus arteriosus have also been reported, although it is not clear whether these occurrences were due to exposure to the drug.

These adverse effects do not appear to have resulted from intrauterine drug exposure that has been limited to the first trimester. Mothers whose embryos and fetuses are exposed to an angiotensin II receptor antagonist only during the first trimester should be so informed. Nonetheless, when patients become pregnant, physicians should advise the patient to discontinue the use of eprosartan as soon as possible.

Rarely (probably less often than once in every thousand pregnancies), no alternative to a drug acting on the renin-angiotensin system will be found. In these rare cases, the mothers should be apprised of the potential hazards to their fetuses, and serial ultrasound examinations should be performed to assess the intra-amniotic environment.

If oligohydramnios is observed, eprosartan mesylate tablets should be discontinued unless it is considered life-saving for the mother. Contraction stress testing (CST), a nonstress test (NST) or biophysical profiling (BPP) may be appropriate, depending upon the week of pregnancy. Patients and physicians should be aware, however, that oligohydramnios may not appear until after the fetus has sustained irreversible injury.

Infants with histories of *in utero* exposure to an angiotensin II receptor antagonist should be closely observed for hypotension, oliguria, and hyperkalemia. If oliguria occurs, attention should be directed toward support of blood pressure and renal perfusion. Exchange transfusion or dialysis may be required as means of reversing hypotension and/or substituting for disordered renal function.

Eprosartan mesylate has been shown to produce maternal and fetal toxicities (maternal and fetal mortality, low maternal body weight and food consumption, resorptions, abortions and litter loss) in pregnant rabbits given oral doses as low as 10 mg eprosartan/kg/day. No maternal or fetal adverse effects were observed at 3 mg/kg/day; this oral dose yielded a systemic exposure (AUC) to unbound eprosartan 0.8 times that achieved in humans given 400 mg bid. No adverse effects on *in utero* or postnatal development and maturation of offspring were observed when eprosartan mesylate was administered to pregnant rats at oral doses up to 1000 mg eprosartan/kg/day (the 1000 mg eprosartan/kg/day dose in non-pregnant rats yielded systemic exposure to unbound eprosartan approximately 0.6 times the exposure achieved in humans given 400 mg bid).

HYPOTENSION IN VOLUME- AND/OR SALT-DEPLETED PATIENTS

In patients with an activated renin-angiotensin system, such as volume- and/or salt-depleted patients (*e.g.*, those being treated with diuretics), symptomatic hypotension may occur. These conditions should be corrected prior to administration of eprosartan mesylate tablets, or the treatment should start under close medical supervision. If hypotension occurs, the patient should be placed in the supine position and, if necessary, given an intravenous infusion of normal saline. A transient hypotensive response is not a contraindication to further treatment, which usually can be continued without difficulty once the blood pressure has stabilized.

PRECAUTIONS

RISK OF RENAL IMPAIRMENT

As a consequence of inhibiting the renin-angiotensin-aldosterone system, changes in renal function have been reported in susceptible individuals treated with angiotensin II antagonists; in some patients, these changes in renal function were reversible upon discontinuation of therapy. In patients whose renal function may depend on the activity of the renin-angiotensin-aldosterone system (*e.g.*, patients with severe congestive heart failure), treatment with angiotensin-converting enzyme inhibitors and angiotensin II receptor antagonists has been associated with oliguria and/or progressive azotemia and (rarely) with acute renal failure and/or death. Eprosartan mesylate tablets would be expected to behave similarly.

In studies of ACE inhibitors in patients with unilateral or bilateral renal artery stenosis, increases in serum creatinine or BUN have been reported. Similar effects have been reported with angiotensin II antagonists; in some patients, these effects were reversible upon discontinuation of therapy.

INFORMATION FOR THE PATIENT

Pregnancy

Female patients of childbearing age should be told about the consequences of second- and third-trimester exposure to drugs that act on the renin-angiotensin system, and they should also be told that these consequences do not appear to have resulted from intrauterine drug exposure that has been limited to the first trimester. These patients should be asked to report pregnancies to their physicians as soon as possible so that treatment may be discontinued under medical supervision.

CARCINOGENESIS, MUTAGENESIS, AND IMPAIRMENT OF FERTILITY

Eprosartan mesylate was not carcinogenic in dietary restricted rats or *ad libitum* fed mice dosed at 600 mg and 2000 mg eprosartan/kg/day, respectively, for up to 2 years. In male and female rats, the systemic exposure (AUC) to unbound eprosartan at the dose evaluated was only approximately 20% of the exposure achieved in humans given 400 mg bid. In mice, the systemic exposure (AUC) to unbound eprosartan was approximately 25 times the exposure achieved in humans given 400 mg bid.

Eprosartan mesylate was not mutagenic *in vitro* in bacteria or mammalian cells (mouse lymphoma assay). Eprosartan mesylate also did not cause structural chromosomal damage *in vivo* (mouse micronucleus assay). In human peripheral lymphocytes *in vitro*, eprosartan mesylate was equivocal for clastogenicity with metabolic activation, and was negative without metabolic activation. In the same assay, eprosartan mesylate was positive for polyploidy with metabolic activation and equivocal for polyploidy without metabolic activation.

Eprosartan mesylate had no adverse effects on the reproductive performance of male or female rats at oral doses up to 1000 mg eprosartan/kg/day. This dose provided systemic exposure (AUC) to unbound eprosartan approximately 0.6 times the exposure achieved in humans given 400 mg bid.

PREGNANCY CATEGORY C (FIRST TRIMESTER) AND D (SECOND AND THIRD TRIMESTERS)

See WARNINGS, Fetal/Neonatal Morbidity and Mortality.

NURSING MOTHERS

Eprosartan is excreted in animal milk; it is not known whether eprosartan is excreted in human milk. Because many drugs are excreted in human milk and because of the potential for serious adverse reactions in nursing infants from eprosartan, a decision should be made whether to discontinue nursing or to discontinue the drug, taking into account the importance of the drug to the mother.

PEDIATRIC USE

Safety and effectiveness in pediatric patients have not been established.

GERIATRIC USE

Of the total number of patients receiving eprosartan mesylate tablets in clinical studies, 29% (681 of 2334) were 65 years and over, while 5% (124 of 2334) were 75 years and over. Based on the pooled data from randomized trials, the decrease in diastolic blood pressure and systolic blood pressure with eprosartan mesylate tablets was slightly less in patients ≥65 years of age compared to younger patients. In a study of only patients over the age of 65, eprosartan mesylate tablets at 200 mg twice daily (and increased optionally up to 300 mg twice daily) decreased diastolic blood pressure on average by 3 mm Hg (placebo corrected). Adverse experiences were similar in younger and older patients.

DRUG INTERACTIONS

Eprosartan has been shown to have no effect on the pharmacokinetics of digoxin and the pharmacodynamics of warfarin and glyburide. Thus, no dosing adjustments are necessary during concomitant use with these agents. Because eprosartan is not metabolized by the cytochrome P450 system, inhibitors of CYP450 enzyme would not be expected to affect its metabolism, and ketoconazole and fluconazole, potent inhibitors of CYP3A and 2C9, respectively, have been shown to have no effect on eprosartan pharmacokinetics. Ranitidine also has no effect on eprosartan pharmacokinetics.

Eprosartan (up to 400 mg bid or 800 mg qd) doses have been safely used concomitantly with a thiazide diuretic (hydrochlorothiazide). Eprosartan doses of up to 300 mg bid have been safely used concomitantly with sustained-release calcium channel blockers (sustained-release nifedipine) with no clinically significant adverse interactions.

ADVERSE REACTIONS

Eprosartan mesylate tablets have been evaluated for safety in more than 3300 healthy volunteers and patients worldwide, including more than 1460 patients treated for more than 6 months, and more than 980 patients treated for 1 year or longer. Eprosartan mesylate tablets were well tolerated at doses up to 1200 mg daily. Most adverse events were of mild or moderate severity and did not require discontinuation of therapy. The overall incidence of adverse experiences and the incidences of specific adverse events reported with eprosartan were similar to placebo.

Adverse experiences were similar in patients regardless of age, gender, or race. Adverse experiences were not dose-related.

In placebo-controlled clinical trials, about 4% of 1202 of patients treated with eprosartan mesylate tablets discontinued therapy due to clinical adverse experiences, compared to 6.5% of 352 patients given placebo.

ADVERSE EVENTS OCCURRING AT AN INCIDENCE OF 1% OR MORE AMONG EPROSARTAN-TREATED PATIENTS

TABLE 1 list adverse events that occurred at an incidence of 1% or more among eprosartan-treated patients who participated in placebo-controlled trials of 8-13 weeks' duration, using doses of 25-400 mg twice daily, and 400-1200 mg once daily. The overall incidence of adverse events reported with eprosartan mesylate tablets (54.4%) was similar to placebo (52.8%).

The following adverse events were also reported at a rate of 1% or greater in patients treated with eprosartan, but were as, or more, frequent in the placebo group: headache, myalgia, dizziness, sinusitis, diarrhea, bronchitis, dependent edema, dyspepsia, chest pain.

Facial edema was reported in 5 patients receiving eprosartan. Angioedema has been reported with other angiotensin II antagonists.

In addition to the adverse events above, potentially important events that occurred in at least 2 patients/subjects exposed to eprosartan or other adverse events that occurred in <1% of patients in clinical studies are listed below. It cannot be determined whether events were causally related to eprosartan:

Body as a Whole: Alcohol intolerance, asthenia, substernal chest pain, peripheral edema, fatigue, fever, hot flushes, influenza-like symptoms, malaise, rigors, pain.

Cardiovascular: Angina pectoris, bradycardia, abnormal ECG, specific abnormal ECG, extrasystoles, atrial fibrillation, hypotension (including orthostatic hypotension), tachycardia, palpitations.

Gastrointestinal: Anorexia, constipation, dry mouth, esophagitis, flatulence, gastritis, gastroenteritis, gingivitis, nausea, periodontitis, toothache, vomiting.

Hematologic: Anemia, purpura.

Liver and Biliary: Increased SGOT, increased SGPT.

TABLE 1 *Adverse Events Reported by ≥1% of Patients Receiving Eprosartan Mesylate Tablets and Were More Frequent on Eprosartan Than Placebo*

Event	Eprosartan (n=1202)	Placebo (n=352)
Body as a Whole		
Infection viral	2%	1%
Injury	2%	1%
Fatigue	2%	1%
Gastrointestinal		
Abdominal pain	2%	1%
Metabolic and Nutritional		
Hypertriglyceridemia	1%	0%
Musculoskeletal		
Arthralgia	2%	1%
Nervous System		
Depression	1%	0%
Respiratory		
Upper respiratory tract infection	8%	5%
Rhinitis	4%	3%
Pharyngitis	4%	3%
Coughing	4%	3%
Urogenital		
Urinary tract infection	1%	0%

E

Metabolic and Nutritional: Increased creatine phosphokinase, diabetes mellitus, glycosuria, gout, hypercholesterolemia, hyperglycemia, hyperkalemia, hypokalemia, hyponatremia.
Musculoskeletal: Arthritis, aggravated arthritis, arthrosis, skeletal pain, tendinitis, back pain.
Nervous System/Psychiatric: Anxiety, ataxia, insomnia, migraine, neuritis, nervousness, paresthesia, somnolence, tremor, vertigo.
Resistance Mechanism: Herpes simplex, otitis externa, otitis media, upper respiratory tract infection.
Respiratory: Asthma, epistaxis.
Skin and Appendages: Eczema, furunculosis, pruritus, rash, maculopapular rash, increased sweating.
Special Senses: Conjunctivitis, abnormal vision, xerophthalmia, tinnitus.
Urinary: Albuminuria, cystitis, hematuria, micturition frequency, polyuria, renal calculus, urinary incontinence.
Vascular: Leg cramps, peripheral ischemia.

LABORATORY TEST FINDINGS

In placebo-controlled studies, clinically important changes in standard laboratory parameters were rarely associated with administration of eprosartan mesylate tablets. Patients were rarely withdrawn from eprosartan mesylate tablets because of laboratory test results.

CREATININE, BLOOD UREA NITROGEN

Minor elevations in creatinine and in BUN occurred in 0.6% and 1.3%, respectively, of patients taking eprosartan mesylate tablets and 0.9% and 0.3%, respectively, of patients given placebo in controlled clinical trials. Two (2) patients were withdrawn from clinical trials for elevations in serum creatinine and BUN, and 3 additional patients were withdrawn for increases in serum creatinine.

LIVER FUNCTION TESTS

Minor elevations of ALAT, ASAT, and alkaline phosphatase occurred for comparable percentages of patients taking eprosartan mesylate tablets or placebo in controlled clinical trials. An elevated ALAT of >3.5 × ULN occurred in 0.1% of patients taking eprosartan mesylate tablets (1 patient) and in no patient given placebo in controlled clinical trials. Four patients were withdrawn from clinical trials for an elevation in liver function tests.

HEMOGLOBIN

A greater than 20% decrease in hemoglobin was observed in 0.1% of patients taking eprosartan mesylate tablets (1 patient) and in no patient given placebo in controlled clinical trials. Two patients were withdrawn from clinical trials for anemia.

LEUKOPENIA

A WBC count of $\leq 3.0 \times 10^3/mm^3$ occurred in 0.3% of patients taking eprosartan mesylate tablets and in 0.3% of patients given placebo in controlled clinical trials. One patient was withdrawn from clinical trials for leukopenia.

NEUTROPENIA

A neutrophil count of $\leq 1.5 \times 10^3/mm^3$ occurred in 1.3% of patients taking eprosartan mesylate tablets and in 1.4% of patients given placebo in controlled clinical trials. No patient was withdrawn from any clinical trials for neutropenia.

THROMBOCYTOPENIA

A platelet count of $\leq 100 \times 10^9/L$ occurred in 0.3% of patients taking eprosartan mesylate tablets (1 patient) and in no patient given placebo in controlled clinical trials. Four patients receiving eprosartan mesylate tablets in clinical trials were withdrawn for thrombocytopenia. In one case, thrombocytopenia was present prior to dosing with eprosartan mesylate tablets.

SERUM POTASSIUM

A potassium value of ≥5.6 mmol/L occurred in 0.9% of patients taking eprosartan mesylate tablets and 0.3% of patients given placebo in controlled clinical trials. One (1) patient was withdrawn from clinical trials for hyperkalemia and 3 for hypokalemia.

DOSAGE AND ADMINISTRATION

The usual recommended starting dose of eprosartan mesylate tablets is 600 mg once daily when used as monotherapy in patients who are not volume-depleted (see WARNINGS, Hypotension in Volume- and/or Salt-Depleted Patients). Eprosartan mesylate tablets can be administered once or twice daily with total daily doses ranging from 400-800 mg. There is limited experience with doses beyond 800 mg/day.

If the antihypertensive effect measured at trough using once daily dosing is inadequate, a twice-a-day regimen at the same total daily dose or an increase in dose may give a more satisfactory response. Achievement of maximum blood pressure reduction in most patients may take 2-3 weeks.

Eprosartan mesylate tablets may be used in combination with other antihypertensive agents such as thiazide diuretics or calcium channel blockers if additional blood-pressure-lowering effect is required. Discontinuation of treatment with eprosartan does not lead to a rapid rebound increase in blood pressure.

ELDERLY, HEPATICALLY IMPAIRED OR RENALLY IMPAIRED PATIENTS

No initial dosing adjustment is generally necessary for elderly or hepatically impaired patients or those with renal impairment. No initial dosing adjustment is generally necessary in patients with moderate and severe renal impairment, with maximum dose not exceeding 600 mg daily.

Eprosartan mesylate tablets may be taken with or without food.

HOW SUPPLIED

Teveten tablets are available as aqueous film-coated tablets as follows:

400 mg: Pink, non-scored, oval tablets, debossed with "SOLVAY" on one side and "5044" on the other.

600 mg: White, non-scored, capsule-shaped tablets, debossed with "SOLVAY" on one side and "5046" on the other.

Storage: Store at controlled room temperature 20-25°C (68-77°F).

PRODUCT LISTING - EQUIVALENTS NOT AVAILABLE

Tablet - Oral - 400 mg

50's	$51.08	TEVETEN, Unimed Pharmaceuticals	00051-5044-42
100's	$103.13	TEVETEN, Biovail Pharmaceuticals Inc	00051-5044-01
100's	$103.13	TEVETEN, Biovail Pharmaceuticals Inc	64455-0130-01

Tablet - Oral - 600 mg

50's	$67.93	TEVETEN, Unimed Pharmaceuticals	00051-5046-42
100's	$137.14	TEVETEN, Biovail Pharmaceuticals Inc	00051-5046-01
100's	$137.14	TEVETEN, Biovail Pharmaceuticals Inc	64455-0131-01

Eprosartan Mesylate; Hydrochlorothiazide *(003589)*

For complete prescribing information, refer to the CD-ROM included with the book.

Categories: Hypertension, essential; Pregnancy Category C, 1st Trimester; Pregnancy Category D, 2nd & 3rd Trimesters; FDA Approved 2001 Nov
Drug Classes: Angiotensin II receptor antagonists; Diuretics, thiazide and derivatives
Brand Names: **Teveten HCT**
Cost of Therapy: $43.20 (Hypertension; Teveten HCT; 600 mg/12.5 mg; 1 tablet/day; 30 day supply)

WARNING

USE IN PREGNANCY

When used in pregnancy during the second and third trimesters, drugs that act directly on the renin-angiotensin system can cause injury and even death to the developing fetus. When pregnancy is detected, eprosartan mesylate; hydrochlorothiazide tablets should be discontinued as soon as possible. See WARNINGS, Fetal/Neonatal Morbidity and Mortality.

DESCRIPTION

Eprosartan mesylate; hydrochlorothiazide 600/12.5 and 600/25 combines an angiotensin II receptor (AT_1 subtype) antagonist and a diuretic, hydrochlorothiazide. Eprosartan mesylate is a non-biphenyl non-tetrazole angiotensin II receptor (AT_1) antagonist. A selective non-peptide molecule, eprosartan mesylate is chemically described as the monomethanesulfonate of *(E)*-2-butyl-1-(*p*-carboxybenzyl)-α-2-thienylmethylimidazole-5-acrylic acid. Its empirical formula is $C_{23}H_{24}N_2O_4S{\cdot}CH_4O_3S$ and molecular weight is 520.625.

Eprosartan mesylate is a white to off-white free-flowing crystalline powder that is insoluble in water, freely soluble in ethanol, and melts between 248 and 250°C. Hydrochlorothiazide is 6-chloro-3,4-dihydro-2 *H* 1,2,4-benzothiadiazine-7-sulfonamide 1,1-dioxide. Its empirical formula is $C_7H_8ClN_3O_4S_2$.

Hydrochlorothiazide is a white, or practically white, crystalline powder with a molecular weight of 297.74, which is slightly soluble in water, but freely soluble in sodium hydroxide solution. Eprosartan mesylate; hydrochlorothiazide is available for oral administration in film-coated, non-scored, capsule-shaped tablet combinations of eprosartan mesylate and hydrochlorothiazide. Eprosartan mesylate; hydrochlorothiazide 600/12.5 contains 735.8 mg of eprosartan mesylate (equivalent to 600 mg eprosartan) and 12.5 mg hydrochlorothiazide in a butterscotch-colored tablet. Eprosartan mesylate; hydrochlorothiazide 600/25 contains 735.8 mg of eprosartan mesylate (equivalent to 600 mg eprosartan) and 25 mg hydrochlorothiazide in a brick-red tablet. *Inactive ingredients of both tablets:* Microcrystalline cellulose, lactose monohydrate, pregelatinized starch, crospovidone, magnesium stearate, and purified water. *Ingredients of the OPADRY OY-R-3736 butterscotch film coating:* Hypromellose, polyethylene glycol 400, titanium dioxide, iron oxide black, and iron oxide yellow. *Ingredients of the OPADRY II 33G24616 pink film coating:* Hypromellose, lactose monohydrate, macrogol/PEG 3000, triacetin, titanium dioxide, iron oxide red, and iron oxide yellow.

INDICATIONS AND USAGE

Eprosartan mesylate; hydrochlorothiazide is indicated for the treatment of hypertension. It may be used alone or in combination with other antihypertensives such as calcium channel blockers. This fixed dose combination is not indicated for initial therapy (see DOSAGE AND ADMINISTRATION).

CONTRAINDICATIONS

Eprosartan mesylate; hydrochlorothiazide is contraindicated in patients who are hypersensitive to this product or any of its components. Because of the hydrochlorothiazide component, this product is contraindicated in patients with anuria or hypersensitivity to other sulfonamide-derived drugs.

WARNINGS

FETAL/NEONATAL MORBIDITY AND MORTALITY

Drugs that act directly on the renin-angiotensin system can cause fetal and neonatal morbidity and death when administered to pregnant women. Several dozen cases have been reported in the world literature in patients who were taking angiotensin-converting enzyme inhibitors. When pregnancy is detected, eprosartan mesylate; hydrochlorothiazide should be discontinued as soon as possible. The use of drugs that act directly on the renin-angiotensin system during the second and third trimesters of pregnancy has been associated with fetal and neonatal injury, including hypotension, neonatal skull hypoplasia, anuria, reversible or irreversible renal failure, and death. Oligohydramnios has also been reported, presumably resulting from decreased fetal renal function; oligohydramnios in this setting has been associated with fetal limb contractures, craniofacial deformation, and hypoplastic lung development. Prematurity, intrauterine growth retardation, and patent ductus arteriosus have also been reported, although it is not clear whether these occurrences were due to exposure to the drug. These adverse effects do not appear to have resulted from intrauterine drug exposure that has been limited to the first trimester. Mothers whose embryos and fetuses are exposed to an angiotensin II receptor antagonist only during the first trimester should be so informed. Nonetheless, when patients become pregnant, physicians should advise the patient to discontinue the use of eprosartan as soon as possible. Rarely (probably less often than once in every thousand pregnancies), no alternative to a drug acting on the renin-angiotensin system will be found. In these rare cases, the mothers should be apprised of the potential hazards to their fetuses, and serial ultrasound examinations should be performed to assess the intra-amniotic environment. If oligohydramnios is observed, eprosartan mesylate; hydrochlorothiazide should be discontinued unless it is considered life-saving for the mother. Contraction stress testing (CST), a non-stress test (NST) or biophysical profiling (BPP) may be appropriate, depending upon the week of pregnancy. Patients and physicians should be aware, however, that oligohydramnios may not appear until after the fetus has sustained irreversible injury. Infants with histories of *in utero* exposure to an angiotensin II receptor antagonist should be closely observed for hypotension, oliguria, and hyperkalemia. If oliguria occurs, attention should be directed toward support of blood pressure and renal perfusion. Exchange transfusion or dialysis may be required as means of reversing hypotension and/or substituting for disordered renal function. Eprosartan mesylate, alone or in combination with hydrochlorothiazide, has been shown to produce maternal and fetal toxicities (maternal and fetal mortality, low maternal body weight and food consumption, resorptions, abortions and litter loss) in pregnant rabbits given oral doses as low as 10 mg eprosartan and 3 mg hydrochlorothiazide/kg/day. No maternal or fetal adverse effects were observed in rabbits at 3 mg eprosartan/kg/day alone or in combination with 1 mg/kg/day of hydrochlorothiazide; this oral dose yielded a systemic exposure (AUC) to unbound eprosartan approximately equal to the human systemic exposure achieved with the dose of eprosartan mesylate contained in the maximum recommended human dose of eprosartan mesylate; hydrochlorothiazide (600 mg eprosartan/day). No adverse effects on *in utero* or postnatal development and maturation of offspring were observed when eprosartan mesylate was administered to pregnant rats at oral doses up to 1000 mg eprosartan/kg/day (the 1000 mg eprosartan/kg/day dose in non-pregnant rats yielded systemic exposure to unbound eprosartan approximately 0.8 times the exposure achieved in humans given 600 mg/day). Thiazides cross the placental barrier and appear in cord blood. There is a risk of fetal or neonatal juandice, thrombocytopenia, and possibly other adverse reactions that have occurred in adults.

HYPOTENSION IN VOLUME- AND/OR SALT-DEPLETED PATIENTS

In patients with an activated renin-angiotensin system, such as volume- and/or salt-depleted patients (*e.g.,* those being treated with diuretics), symptomatic hypotension may occur. These conditions should be corrected prior to administration of eprosartan mesylate; hydrochlorothiazide, or the treatment should start under close medical supervision. If hypotension occurs, the patient should be placed in the supine position and, if necessary, given an IV infusion of normal saline. A transient hypotensive response is not a contraindication to further treatment, which usually can be continued without difficulty once the blood pressure has stabilized.

HYDROCHLOROTHIAZIDE

Impaired Hepatic Function

Thiazides should be used with caution in patients with impaired hepatic function or progressive liver disease, since minor alterations of fluid and electrolyte balance may precipitate hepatic coma.

Hypersensitivity Reactions

Hypersensitivity reactions to hydrochlorothiazide may occur in patients with or without a history of allergy or bronchial asthma, but are more likely in patients with such a history.

Systemic Lupus Erythematosus

Thiazide diuretics have been reported to cause exacerbation or activation of systemic lupus erythematosus. *Lithium Interaction:* Lithium generally should not be given with thiazides.

DOSAGE AND ADMINISTRATION

The usual recommended starting dose of eprosartan is 600 mg once daily when used as monotherapy in patients who are not volume-depleted (see WARNINGS, Hypotension in Volume- and/or Salt-Depleted Patients). Eprosartan can be administered once or twice daily and total daily doses ranging from 400-800 mg. There is limited experience with doses beyond 800 mg/day. If the antihypertensive effect measured at trough using once daily monotherapy dosing is inadequate, a twice-a-day regimen at the same total daily dose or an increase in dose may give a more satisfactory response. Achievement of maximum blood pressure reduction in most patients may take 2-3 weeks. HCTZ is effective in doses of 12.5-50 mg once daily. To minimize dose-independent side effects, it is usually appropriate to begin combination therapy only after a patient has failed to achieve the desired effect with monotherapy. The side effects (see WARNINGS) of eprosartan are generally rare and apparently independent of dose; those of hydrochlorothiazide are a mixture of dose-dependent (primarily hypokalemia) and dose-independent (*e.g.,* pancreatitis) phenomena, the former much more common than the latter. Therapy with any combination of eprosartan and hydrochlorothiazide will be associated with both sets of dose-independent side effects.

REPLACEMENT THERAPY

Eprosartan mesylate; hydrochlorothiazide may be substituted for the individual components. The usual recommended dose of eprosartan mesylate; hydrochlorothiazide is 600 mg/12.5 mg once daily when used as combination therapy in patients who are not volume-depleted (see WARNINGS, Hypotension in Volume-and/or Salt-Depleted Patients). If the antihypertensive effect measured at trough using eprosartan mesylate; hydrochlorothiazide 600/12.5 is inadequate, patients may be titrated to eprosartan mesylate; hydrochlorothiazide 600/25 once daily. Higher doses have not been studied in combination. Achievement of maximum blood pressure reduction in most patients may take 2-3 weeks. If the patient under treatment with eprosartan mesylate; hydrochlorothiazide requires additional blood pressure control at trough, or to maintain a twice a day dosing schedule of monotherapy, 300 mg eprosartan mesylate may be added as evening dose. Eprosartan mesylate; hydrochlorothiazide may be used in combination with other antihypertensive agents such as calcium channel blockers if additional blood-pressure-lowering effect is required. Discontinuation of treatment with eprosartan does not lead to a rapid rebound increase in blood pressure.

Elderly, Hepatically Impaired or Renally Impaired Patients

No initial dosing adjustment is generally necessary for elderly or hepatically impaired patients or those with renal impairment. No initial dosing adjustment is generally necessary in patients with moderate and severe renal impairment with maximum dose not exceeding 600 mg daily. Eprosartan mesylate; hydrochlorothiazide may be taken with or without food.

PRODUCT LISTING - EQUIVALENTS NOT AVAILABLE

Tablet - Oral - 600 mg;12.5 mg

100's	$144.00	TEVETEN HCT, Biovail Pharmaceuticals Inc	64455-0132-01

Tablet - Oral - 600 mg;25 mg

100's	$144.00	TEVETEN HCT, Biovail Pharmaceuticals Inc	64455-0133-01

Eptifibatide (003405)

Categories: Coronary syndrome, acute; FDA Approved 1998 May; Pregnancy Category B
Drug Classes: Platelet inhibitors
Foreign Brand Availability: Integrilin (Austria; Belgium; Bulgaria; Canada; Colombia; Czech-Republic; Denmark; England; Finland; France; Germany; Greece; Hong-Kong; Hungary; Ireland; Israel; Italy; Netherlands; Norway; Poland; Portugal; Singapore; Slovenia; South-Africa; Spain; Sweden; Switzerland; Turkey)

DESCRIPTION

For Intravenous Administration.

Eptifibatide is a cyclic heptapeptide containing six amino acids and one mercaptopropionyl (des-amino cysteinyl) residue. An interchain disulfide bridge is formed between the cysteine amide and the mercaptopropionyl moieties. Chemically it is N^6-(aminoiminomethyl)-N^2-(3-mercapto-1-oxopropyl-L-lysylglycyl-L-α-aspartyl-L-tryptophyl-L-prolyl-L-cysteinamide, cyclic (1$\rightarrow$6)-disulfide. Eptifibatide binds to the platelet receptor glycoprotein (GP) IIb/IIIa of human platelets and inhibits platelet aggregation.

The eptifibatide peptide is produced by solution-phase peptide synthesis, and is purified by preparative reverse-phase liquid chromatography and lyophilized. The molecular formula is $C_{35}H_{49}N_{11}O_9S_2$. The molecular weight is 831.96.

Integrilin (eptifibatide) injection is a clear, colorless, sterile, non-pyrogenic solution for intravenous (IV) use. Each 10 ml vial contains 2 mg/ml of eptifibatide and each 100 ml vial contains either 0.75 mg/ml or 2 mg/ml of eptifibatide. Each vial of either size also contains 5.25 mg/ml citric acid and sodium hydroxide to adjust the pH to 5.25.

CLINICAL PHARMACOLOGY

MECHANISM OF ACTION

Eptifibatide reversibly inhibits platelet aggregation by preventing the binding of fibrinogen, von Willebrand factor, and other adhesive ligands to GP IIb/IIIa. When administered intravenously, eptifibatide inhibits *ex vivo* platelet aggregation in a dose- and concentration-dependent manner. Platelet aggregation inhibition is reversible following cessation of the eptifibatide infusion; this is thought to result from dissociation of eptifibatide from the platelet.

PHARMACODYNAMICS

Infusion of eptifibatide into baboons caused a dose-dependent inhibition of *ex vivo* platelet aggregation, with complete inhibition of aggregation achieved at infusion rates greater than 5.0 μg/kg/min. In a baboon model that is refractory to aspirin and heparin, doses of eptifibatide that inhibit aggregation prevented acute thrombosis with only a modest prolongation (2- to 3-fold) of the bleeding time. Platelet aggregation in dogs was also inhibited by infusions of eptifibatide, with complete inhibition at 2.0 μg/kg/min. This infusion dose completely inhibited canine coronary thrombosis induced by coronary artery injury (Folts model).

Human pharmacodynamic data were obtained in healthy subjects and in patients presenting with unstable angina (UA) or non-Q-wave myocardial infarction (NQMI) and/or undergoing percutaneous coronary interventions. Studies in healthy subjects enrolled only males; patient studies enrolled approximately one-third women. In these studies, eptifibatide inhibited *ex vivo* platelet aggregation induced by adenosine diphosphate (ADP) and other agonists in a dose- and concentration-dependent manner. The effect of eptifibatide was observed immediately after administration of a 180 μg/kg intravenous bolus. TABLE 1 shows the effects of dosing regimens of eptifibatide used in the IMPACT II and PURSUIT studies on *ex vivo* platelet aggregation induced by 20 μM ADP in PPACK-anticoagulated platelet-rich plasma and on bleeding time. The effects of the dosing regimen used in ESPRIT on platelet aggregation have not been studied.

E

TABLE 1 *Platelet Inhibition and Bleeding Time*

	IMPACT II 135/0.5*	PURSUIT 180/2.0†
Inhibition of platelet aggregation 15 minutes after bolus	69%	84%
Inhibition of platelet aggregation at steady state	40-50%	>90%
Bleeding-time prolongation at steady state	<5×	<5×
Inhibition of platelet aggregation 4 hours after infusion discontinuation	<30%	<50%
Bleeding-time prolongation 6 hours after infusion discontinuation	1×	1.4×

* 135 μg/kg bolus followed by a continuous infusion of 0.5 μg/kg/min.
† 180 μg/kg bolus followed by a continuous infusion of 2.0 μg/kg/min.

The eptifibatide dosing regimen used in the ESPRIT study included two 180 μg/kg bolus doses given 10 minutes apart combined with a continuous 2.0 μg/kg/min infusion.

When administered alone, eptifibatide has no measurable effect on prothrombin time (PT) or activated partial thromboplastin time (aPTT).

There were no important differences between men and women or between age groups in the pharmacodynamic properties of eptifibatide. Differences among ethnic groups have not been assessed.

PHARMACOKINETICS

The pharmacokinetics of eptifibatide are linear and dose-proportional for bolus doses ranging from 90 to 250 μg/kg and infusion rates from 0.5 to 3.0 μg/kg/min. Plasma elimination half-life is approximately 2.5 hours. Administration of a single bolus combined with an infusion produces an early peak level, followed by a small decline prior to attaining steady state (within 4-6 hours). When PCI is performed, this decline can be prevented by administering a second 180 μg/kg bolus 10 minutes after the first. The extent of eptifibatide binding to human plasma protein is about 25%.

EXCRETION AND METABOLISM

Clearance in patients with coronary artery disease is 55-58 ml/kg/h. In healthy subjects, renal clearance accounts for approximately 50% of total body clearance, with the majority of the drug excreted in the urine as eptifibatide, deamidated eptifibatide, and other, more polar metabolites. No major metabolites have been detected in human plasma. Clinical studies have included 2418 patients with serum creatinine between 1.0 and 2.0 mg/dl (for the 180 μg/kg bolus and the 2.0 μg/kg/min infusion) and 7 patients with serum creatinine between 2.0 and 4.0 mg/dl (for the 135 μg/kg bolus and the 0.5 μg/kg/min infusion), without dose adjustment; another 8 patients with serum creatinine between 2.0 and 4.0 mg/dl were enrolled in the ESPRIT study and received the full 180/180 μg/kg double bolus regimen with an infusion adjusted down from 2.0 to 1.0 μg/kg/min. No data are available in patients with more severe degrees of renal impairment, but plasma eptifibatide levels are expected to be higher in such patients (see WARNINGS).

SPECIAL POPULATIONS

Patients in clinical studies were older than the subjects in clinical pharmacology studies, and they had lower total body eptifibatide clearance and higher eptifibatide plasma levels.

Clinical studies were conducted in patients aged 20-94 years with coronary artery disease without dose adjustment for age. Limited data are available on lighter weight (<50 kg) patients over 75 years of age. Men and women showed no important differences in the pharmacokinetics of eptifibatide.

INDICATIONS AND USAGE

Eptifibatide is indicated:

- For the treatment of patients with acute coronary syndrome (UA/NQMI), including patients who are to be managed medically and those undergoing percutaneous coronary intervention (PCI). In this setting, eptifibatide has been shown to decrease the rate of a combined endpoint of death or new myocardial infarction.
- For the treatment of patients undergoing PCI, including those undergoing intracoronary stenting. In this setting, eptifibatide has been shown to decrease the rate of a combined endpoint of death, new myocardial infarction, or need for urgent intervention.

In the IMPACT II, PURSUIT and ESPRIT studies of eptifibatide, most patients received heparin and aspirin.

NON-FDA APPROVED INDICATIONS

Although not FDA approved, the use of eptifibatide prior to coronary artery bypass grafting (CABG) has been investigated during the PURSUIT trial. Another non-FDA approved use of the drug has been as a pre-treatment for patients undergoing coronary stent placement, such as the patients enrolled in the ESPRIT trial. Of note from the ESPRIT trial was the novel dosing of eptifibatide given as a 180 mcg/kg double bolus 10 minutes apart, followed by a 2 mcg/kg continuous infusion for 18 to 24 hours. Both trials produced positive results, which were maintained over a 6 month period.

CONTRAINDICATIONS

Treatment with eptifibatide is contraindicated in patients with:

- A history of bleeding diathesis, or evidence of active abnormal bleeding within the previous 30 days.
- Severe hypertension (systolic blood pressure >200 mm Hg or diastolic blood pressure >110 mm Hg) not adequately controlled on antihypertensive therapy.
- Major surgery within the preceding 6 weeks.
- History of stroke within 30 days or any history of hemorrhagic stroke.
- Current or planned administration of another parenteral GP IIb/IIIa inhibitor.
- Dependency on renal dialysis.
- Known hypersensitivity to any component of the product.

WARNINGS

BLEEDING

Bleeding is the most common complication encountered during eptifibatide therapy. Administration of eptifibatide is associated with an increase in major and minor bleeding, as classified by the criteria of the Thrombolysis in Myocardial Infarction Study group (TIMI), (see ADVERSE REACTIONS). Most major bleeding associated with eptifibatide has been at the arterial access site for cardiac catheterization or from the gastrointestinal or genitourinary tract.

In patients undergoing percutaneous coronary interventions, patients receiving eptifibatide experience an increased incidence of major bleeding compared to those receiving placebo without a significant increase in transfusion requirement. Special care should be employed to minimize the risk of bleeding among these patients (see PRECAUTIONS). If bleeding cannot be controlled with pressure, infusion of eptifibatide and concomitant heparin should be stopped immediately.

RENAL INSUFFICIENCY

Eptifibatide is cleared in part by the kidney and its plasma concentration is expected to increase with decreasing renal function (DOSAGE AND ADMINISTRATION). There has been no clinical experience in patients with a serum creatinine >4.0 mg/dl.

PLATELET COUNT <100,000/MM³

Because it is an inhibitor of platelet aggregation, caution should be exercised when administering eptifibatide to patients with a platelet count <100,000/mm³; there has been no clinical experience with eptifibatide initiated in patients with a platelet count <100,000/mm³.

PRECAUTIONS

BLEEDING PRECAUTIONS

Care of the Femoral Artery Access Site in Patients Undergoing Percutaneous Coronary Intervention (PCI)

In patients undergoing PCI, treatment with eptifibatide is associated with an increase in major and minor bleeding at the site of arterial sheath placement. After PCI, eptifibatide infusion should be continued until hospital discharge or up to 18-24 hours, whichever comes first. Heparin use is discouraged after the PCI procedure. Early sheath removal is encouraged while eptifibatide is being infused. Prior to removing the sheath, it is recommended that heparin be discontinued for 3-4 hours and an aPTT of <45 seconds or ACT <150 seconds be achieved. In any case, both heparin and eptifibatide should be discontinued and sheath hemostasis should be achieved at least 2-4 hours before hospital discharge.

Use of Thrombolytics, Anticoagulants, and Other Antiplatelet Agents

In the IMPACT II, PURSUIT and ESPRIT studies, eptifibatide was used concomitantly with heparin and aspirin. In the ESPRIT study, clopidogrel or ticlopidine were used routinely starting the day of PCI. Because eptifibatide inhibits platelet aggregation, caution should be employed when it is used with other drugs that affect hemostasis, including thrombolytics, oral anticoagulants, non-steroidal anti-inflammatory drugs, and dipyridamole. To avoid potentially additive pharmacologic effects, concomitant treatment with other inhibitors of platelet receptor GP IIb/IIIa should be avoided.

There is only a small experience with concomitant use of eptifibatide and thrombolytics. In a study of 180 patients with acute myocardial infarction (AMI), eptifibatide (in regimens up to a bolus of 180 μg/kg followed by a continuous infusion of 0.75 μg/kg/min for 24 hours) was administered concomitantly with the approved "accelerated" regimen of alteplase, a thrombolytic agent. The studied regimens of eptifibatide did not increase the incidence of major bleeding or transfusion compared to the incidence seen when alteplase was given alone.

In the IMPACT II study, 15 patients received a thrombolytic agent in conjunction with the 135/0.5 dosing regimen, 2 of whom experienced a major bleed. In the PURSUIT study, 40 patients who received eptifibatide at the 180/2.0 dosing regimen received a thrombolytic agent, 10 of whom experienced a major bleed.

In another AMI study involving 181 patients, eptifibatide (in regimens up to a bolus of 180 μg/kg followed by a continuous infusion of up to 2.0 μg/kg/min for up to 72 hours) was administered concomitantly with streptokinase (1.5 million units over 60 minutes), another thrombolytic agent. At the highest studied infusion rates (1.3 μg/kg/min and 2.0 μg/kg/min), eptifibatide was associated with an increase in the incidence of bleeding and transfusions compared to the incidence seen when streptokinase was given alone.

These limited data on the use of eptifibatide in patients receiving thrombolytic agents do not allow an estimate of the bleeding risk associated with concomitant use of thrombolytics. Systemic thrombolytic therapy should be used with caution in patients who have received eptifibatide.

Minimization of Vascular and Other Trauma

Arterial and venous punctures, intramuscular injections, and the use of urinary catheters, nasotracheal intubation, and nasogastric tubes should be minimized. When obtaining intravenous access, non-compressible sites (*e.g.*, subclavian or jugular veins) should be avoided.

LABORATORY TESTS

Before infusion of eptifibatide, the following laboratory tests should be performed to identify pre-existing hemostatic abnormalities: hematocrit or hemoglobin, platelet count, serum creatinine, and PT/aPTT. In patients undergoing PCI, the activated clotting time (ACT) should also be measured.

Maintaining Target aPTT and ACT

The aPTT should be maintained between 50 and 70 seconds unless PCI is to be performed. In patients treated with heparin, bleeding can be minimized by close monitoring of the aPTT. TABLE 6 displays the risk of major bleeding according to the maximum aPTT attained within 72 hours in the PURSUIT study.

TABLE 6 *Major Bleeding by Maximal aPTT Within 72 Hours in the PURSUIT Study*

Maximum aPTT (seconds)	Placebo	Eptifibatide 180/1.3*	Eptifibatide 180/2.0
<50	44/721 (6.1%)	21/244 (8.6%)	44/743 (5.9%)
50-70†	92/908 (10.1%)	28/259 (10.8%)	99/883 (11.2%)
>70	281/2786 (10.0%)	99/891 (11.1%)	345/2811 (12.3%)

* Administered only until the first interim analysis.
† (Recommended.)

The ESPRIT study stipulated a target ACT of 200-300 seconds during PCI. Patients receiving eptifibatide 180/2.0/180 (mean ACT 284 seconds) experienced an increased incidence of bleeding relative to placebo (mean ACT 276 seconds), primarily at the femoral artery access site. At these lower ACTs, bleeding was less than previously reported with eptifibatide in the PURSUIT and IMPACT II studies.

The aPTT or ACT should be checked prior to arterial sheath removal. The sheath should not be removed unless the aPTT is <45 seconds or the ACT is <150 seconds.

Thrombocytopenia

If the patient experiences a confirmed platelet decrease to <100,000/mm^3, eptifibatide and heparin should be discontinued and the condition appropriately monitored and treated.

RENAL INSUFFICIENCY

Based on results of the PURSUIT and ESPRIT studies and the fact that the drug is cleared equally by renal and nonrenal mechanisms, dose adjustment is unnecessary for patients with mild to moderate renal impairment (serum creatinine <2.0 mg/dl). For patients with serum creatinine between 2.0 mg/dl and 4.0 mg/dl, the infusion dose should be reduced to 1.0 µg/kg/min while the bolus dose(s) should remain unchanged. Plasma eptifibatide levels are expected to be higher in patients with more severe renal impairment, but no data are available for such patients or for patients on renal dialysis. *In vitro* studies have indicated that eptifibatide may be cleared from plasma by dialysis.

GERIATRIC USE

The PURSUIT and IMPACT II clinical studies enrolled patients up to the age of 94 years (45% were age 65 and over; 12% were age 75 and older). There was no apparent difference in efficacy between older and younger patients treated with eptifibatide. The incidence of bleeding complications was higher in the elderly in both placebo and eptifibatide groups, and the incremental risk of eptifibatide-associated bleeding was greater in the older patients. No dose adjustment was made for elderly patients, but patients over 75 years of age had to weigh at least 50 kg to be enrolled in the PURSUIT study; no such limitation was stipulated in the ESPRIT study (see also ADVERSE REACTIONS).

CARCINOGENESIS, MUTAGENESIS, AND IMPAIRMENT OF FERTILITY

No long-term studies in animals have been performed to evaluate the carcinogenic potential of eptifibatide. Eptifibatide was not genotoxic in the Ames test, the mouse lymphoma cell (L 5178Y, TK$^{+/-}$) forward mutation test, the human lymphocyte chromosome aberration test, or the mouse micronucleus test. Administered by continuous intravenous infusion at total daily doses up to 72 mg/kg/day (about 4 times the recommended maximum daily human dose on a body surface area basis), eptifibatide had no effect on fertility and reproductive performance of male and female rats.

PREGNANCY CATEGORY B

Teratology studies have been performed by continuous intravenous infusion of eptifibatide in pregnant rats at total daily doses of up to 72 mg/kg/day (about 4 times the recommended maximum daily human dose on a body surface area basis) and in pregnant rabbits at total daily doses of up to 36 mg/kg/day (also about 4 times the recommended maximum daily human dose on a body surface area basis). These studies revealed no evidence of harm to the fetus due to eptifibatide. There are, however, no adequate and well-controlled studies in pregnant women with eptifibatide. Because animal reproduction studies are not always predictive of human response, eptifibatide should be used during pregnancy only if clearly needed.

PEDIATRIC USE

Safety and effectiveness of eptifibatide in pediatric patients have not been studied.

NURSING MOTHERS

It is not known whether eptifibatide is excreted in human milk. Because many drugs are excreted in human milk, caution should be exercised when eptifibatide is administered to a nursing mother.

ADVERSE REACTIONS

A total of 16,782 patients were treated in the Phase 3 clinical trials (PURSUIT, ESPRIT and IMPACT II). These 16,782 patients had a mean age of 62 years (range 20-94 years). Eighty-nine percent (89%) of the patients were Caucasian, with the remainder being predominantly Black (5%) and Hispanic (5%). Sixty-eight percent (68%) were men. Because of the different regimens used in PURSUIT, IMPACT II and ESPRIT, data from the three studies were not pooled.

BLEEDING

The incidences of bleeding events and transfusions in the PURSUIT, IMPACT II and ESPRIT studies are shown in TABLE 7A, TABLE 7B, and TABLE 7C. Bleeding was classified as major or minor by the criteria of the TIMI study group. Major bleeding events consisted of intracranial hemorrhage and other bleeding that led to decreases in hemoglobin greater than 5 g/dl. Minor bleeding events included spontaneous gross hematuria, spontaneous hematemesis, other observed blood loss with a hemoglobin decrease of more than 3 g/dl, and other hemoglobin decreases that were greater than 4 g/dl but less than 5 g/dl. In patients who received transfusions, the corresponding loss in hemoglobin was estimated through an adaptation of the method of Landefeld *et al.*

TABLE 7A *Bleeding Events and Transfusions in the PURSUIT Study*

	Placebo	Eptifibatide 180/1.3*	Eptifibatide 180/2.0
Patients	4696	1472	4679
Major bleeding†	425 (9.3%)	152 (10.5%)	498 (10.8%)
Minor bleeding†	347 (7.6%)	152 (10.5%)	604 (13.1%)
Requiring transfusions‡	490 (10.4%)	188 (12.8%)	601 (12.8%)

Note: Denominator is based on patients for whom data are available.
* Administered only until the first interim analysis.
† For major and minor bleeding, patients are counted only once according to the most severe classification.
‡ Includes transfusions of whole blood, packed red blood cells, fresh frozen plasma, cryoprecipitate, platelets, and autotransfusion during the initial hospitalization.

TABLE 7B *Bleeding Events and Transfusions in the ESPRIT Study*

	Placebo	Eptifibatide 180/2.0/180
Patients	1024	1040
Major bleeding*	4 (0.4%)	13 (1.3%)
Minor bleeding*	18 (2.0%)	29 (3.0%)
Requiring transfusions†	11 (1.1%)	16 (1.5%)

Note: Denominator is based on patients for whom data are available.
* For major and minor bleeding, patients are counted only once according to the most severe classification.
† Includes transfusions of whole blood, packed red blood cells, fresh frozen plasma, cryoprecipitate, platelets, and autotransfusion during the initial hospitalization.

TABLE 7C *Bleeding Events and Transfusions in the IMPACT II Study*

	Placebo	Eptifibatide 135/0.5	Eptifibatide 135/0.75
Patients	1285	1300	1286
Major bleeding†	55 (4.5%)	55 (4.4%)	58 (4.7%)
Minor bleeding†	115 (9.3%)	146 (11.7%)	177 (14.2%)
Requiring transfusions‡	66 (5.1%)	71 (5.5%)	74 (5.8%)

Note: denominator is based on patients for whom data are available.
* Administered only until the first interim analysis.
† For major and minor bleeding, patients are counted only once according to the most severe classification.
‡ Includes transfusions of whole blood, packed red blood cells, fresh frozen plasma, cryoprecipitate, platelets, and autotransfusion during the initial hospitalization.

The majority of major bleeding events in the ESPRIT study occurred at the vascular access site (1 and 8 patients, or 0.1% and 0.8% in the placebo and eptifibatide groups, respectively). Bleeding at "other" locations occurred in 0.2% and 0.4% of patients, respectively.

In the PURSUIT study, the greatest increase in major bleeding in eptifibatide-treated patients compared to placebo-treated patients was also associated with bleeding at the femoral artery access site (2.8% vs 1.3%). Oropharyngeal (primarily gingival), genito-urinary, gastrointestinal, and retroperitoneal bleeding were also seen more commonly in eptifibatide-treated patients compared to placebo-treated patients.

Among patients experiencing a major bleed in the IMPACT II study, an increase in bleeding on eptifibatide versus placebo was observed only for the femoral artery access site (3.2% vs 2.8%).

TABLE 8 displays the incidence of TIMI major bleeding according to the cardiac procedures carried out in the PURSUIT study. The most common bleeding complications were related to cardiac revascularization (CABG-related or femoral artery access site bleeding). A corresponding table for ESPRIT is not presented as every patient underwent PCI in the ESPRIT study and only 11 patients underwent CABG.

TABLE 8 *Major Bleeding by Procedures in the PURSUIT Study*

	Placebo	Eptifibatide 180/1.3*	Eptifibatide 180/2.0
Patients	4577	1451	4604
Overall incidence of major bleeding	425 (9.3%)	152 (10.5%)	498 (10.8%)
Breakdown by procedure:			
CABG	375 (8.2%)	123 (8.5%)	377 (8.2%)
Angioplasty without CABG	27 (0.6%)	16 (1.1%)	64 (1.4%)
Angiography without angioplasty or CABG	11 (0.2%)	7 (0.5%)	29 (0.6%)
Medical therapy only	12 (0.3%)	6 (0.4%)	28 (0.6%)

Denominators are based on the total number of patients whose TIMI classification was resolved.
* Administered only until the first interim analysis.

E

In the PURSUIT and ESPRIT studies, the risk of major bleeding with eptifibatide increased as patient weight decreased. This relationship was most apparent for patients weighing less than 70 kg.

Bleeding adverse events resulting in discontinuation of study drug were more frequent among patients receiving eptifibatide than placebo (4.6% vs 0.9% in ESPRIT, 8% vs 1% in PURSUIT, 3.5% vs 1.9% in IMPACT II).

INTRACRANIAL HEMORRHAGE AND STROKE

Intracranial hemorrhage was rare in the PURSUIT, IMPACT II and ESPRIT clinical studies. In the PURSUIT study, 3 patients in the placebo group, 1 patient in the group treated with eptifibatide 180/1.3 and 5 patients in the group treated with eptifibatide 180/2.0 experienced a hemorrhagic stroke. The overall incidence of stroke was 0.5% in patients receiving eptifibatide 180/1.3, 0.7% in patients receiving eptifibatide 180/2.0, and 0.8% in placebo patients.

In the IMPACT II study, intracranial hemorrhage was experienced by 1 patient treated with eptifibatide 135/0.5, 2 patients treated with eptifibatide 135/0.75 and 2 patients in the placebo group. The overall incidence of stroke was 0.5% in patients receiving 135/0.5 eptifibatide, 0.7% in patients receiving eptifibatide 135/0.75 and 0.7% in the placebo group.

In the ESPRIT study, there were 3 hemorrhagic strokes, 1 in the placebo group and 2 in the eptifibatide group. In addition there was 1 case of cerebral infarction in the eptifibatide group.

THROMBOCYTOPENIA

In the PURSUIT and IMPACT II studies, the incidence of thrombocytopenia ($<$100,000/mm^3 or $\geq$50% reduction from baseline) and the incidence of platelet transfusions were similar between patients treated with eptifibatide and placebo. In the ESPRIT study, the incidence was 0.6% in the placebo group and 1.2% in the eptifibatide group.

ALLERGIC REACTIONS

In the PURSUIT study, anaphylaxis was reported in 7 patients receiving placebo (0.15%) and 7 patients receiving eptifibatide 180/2.0 (0.16%). In the IMPACT II study, anaphylaxis was reported in 1 patient (0.08%) on placebo and in no patients on eptifibatide. In the IMPACT II study, 2 patients (1 patient [0.04%] receiving eptifibatide and 1 patient [0.08%] receiving placebo) discontinued study drug because of allergic reactions. In the ESPRIT study, there were no cases of anaphylaxis reported. There were 3 patients who suffered an allergic reaction, 1 on placebo and 2 on eptifibatide. In addition, 1 patient in the placebo group was diagnosed with urticaria.

The potential for development of antibodies to eptifibatide has been studied in 433 subjects. Eptifibatide was non-antigenic in 412 patients receiving a single administration of eptifibatide (135 μg/kg bolus followed by a continuous infusion of either 0.5 μg/kg/min or 0.75 μg/kg/min), and in 21 subjects to whom eptifibatide (135 μg/kg bolus followed by a continuous infusion of 0.75 μg/kg/min) was administered twice, 28 days apart. In both cases, plasma for antibody detection was collected approximately 30 days after each dose. The development of antibodies to eptifibatide at higher doses has not been evaluated.

OTHER ADVERSE REACTIONS

In the PURSUIT and ESPRIT studies, the incidence of serious non-bleeding adverse events was similar in patients receiving placebo or eptifibatide (19% and 19%, respectively in PURSUIT; 6% and 7%, respectively in ESPRIT). In PURSUIT, the only serious non-bleeding adverse event that occurred at a rate of at least 1% and was more common with eptifibatide than placebo (7% vs 6%) was hypotension. Most of the serious non-bleeding events consisted of cardiovascular events typical of an unstable angina population. In the IMPACT II study, serious non-bleeding events that occurred in greater than 1% of patients were uncommon and similar in incidence between placebo- and eptifibatide-treated patients.

Discontinuation of study drug due to adverse events other than bleeding was uncommon in the PURSUIT, IMPACT II and ESPRIT studies, with no single event occurring in >0.5% of the study population (except for "other" in the ESPRIT study). In the PURSUIT study, non-bleeding adverse events leading to discontinuation occurred in the eptifibatide and placebo groups in the following body systems with an incidence of $\geq$0.1%: cardiovascular system (0.3% and 0.3%), digestive system (0.1% and 0.1%), hemic/lymphatic system (0.1% and 0.1%), nervous system (0.3% and 0.4%), urogenital system (0.1% and 0.1%), and whole body system (0.2% and 0.2%). In the ESPRIT study, the following non-bleeding adverse events leading to discontinuation occurred in the eptifibatide and placebo groups with an incidence of $\geq$0.1%: "other" (1.2% and 1.1%). In the IMPACT II study, non-bleeding adverse events leading to discontinuation occurred in the 135/0.5 eptifibatide and placebo groups in the following body systems with an incidence of $\geq$0.1%: whole body (0.3% and 0.1%), cardiovascular system (1.4% and 1.4%), digestive system (0.2% and 0%), hemic/lymphatic system (0.2% and 0%), nervous system (0.3% and 0.2%), and respiratory system (0.1% and 0.1%).

POST-MARKETING EXPERIENCE

The following adverse events have been reported in post-marketing experience, primarily with eptifibatide in combination with heparin and aspirin: cerebral, GI and pulmonary hemorrhage. Fatal bleeding events have been reported.

DOSAGE AND ADMINISTRATION

The safety and efficacy of eptifibatide has been established in clinical studies that employed concomitant use of heparin and aspirin. Different dose regimens of eptifibatide were used in the major clinical studies.

ACUTE CORONARY SYNDROME

The recommended adult dosage of eptifibatide in patients with acute coronary syndrome with a serum creatinine <2.0 mg/dl is an intravenous bolus of 180 μg/kg as soon as possible following diagnosis, followed by a continuous infusion of 2.0 μg/kg/min until hospital discharge or initiation of CABG surgery, up to 72 hours. If a patient is to undergo a percutaneous coronary intervention (PCI) while receiving eptifibatide, the infusion should be continued up to hospital discharge, or for up to 18-24 hours after the procedure, whichever comes first, allowing for up to 96 hours of therapy. Patients weighing more than 121 kg should receive a maximum bolus of 22.6 mg followed by a maximum infusion rate of 15 mg/hour.

The recommended adult dosage of eptifibatide in patients with acute coronary syndrome with serum creatinine between 2.0 and 4.0 mg/dl is an intravenous bolus of 180 μg/kg as soon as possible following diagnosis, immediately followed by a continuous infusion of 1.0 μg/kg/min. Patients with serum creatinine between 2.0 and 4.0 mg/dl and weighing more than 121 kg should receive a maximum bolus of 22.6 mg followed by a maximum infusion rate of 7.5 mg/hour.

PERCUTANEOUS CORONARY INTERVENTION (PCI)

The recommended adult dosage of eptifibatide in patients with a serum creatinine <2.0 mg/dl initiated at the time of PCI is an intravenous bolus of 180 μg/kg administered immediately before the initiation of PCI followed by a continuous infusion of 2.0 μg/kg/min and a second 180 μg/kg bolus 10 minutes after the first bolus. Infusion should be continued until hospital discharge, or for up to 18-24 hours, whichever comes first. A minimum of 12 hours of infusion is recommended. Patients weighing more than 121 kg should receive a maximum of 22.6 mg per bolus followed by a maximum infusion rate of 15 mg/hour.

The recommended adult dose of eptifibatide in patients with a serum creatinine between 2.0 and 4.0 mg/dl initiated at the time of PCI is an intravenous bolus of 180 μg/kg administered immediately before the initiation of the procedure, immediately followed by a continuous infusion of 1.0 μg/kg/min and a second 180 μg/kg bolus administered 10 minutes after the first. Patients with a serum creatinine between 2.0 and 4.0 mg/dl and weighing more than 121 kg should receive a maximum of 22.6 mg per bolus followed by a maximum infusion rate of 7.5 mg/hour.

In patients who undergo coronary artery bypass graft surgery, eptifibatide infusion should be discontinued prior to surgery.

ASPIRIN AND HEPARIN DOSING RECOMMENDATIONS

In the clinical trials that showed eptifibatide to be effective, most patients received concomitant aspirin and heparin. The recommended aspirin and heparin doses to be used are as follows:

Acute Coronary Syndrome

Aspirin

160-325 mg po initially and daily thereafter.

Heparin

Target aPTT 50-70 seconds during medical management.

- If weight $\geq$70 kg, 5000 U bolus followed by infusion of 1000 U/h.
- If weight <70 kg, 60 U/kg bolus followed by infusion of 12 U/kg/h. Target ACT 200-300 seconds during PCI.
- If heparin is initiated prior to PCI, additional boluses during PCI to maintain an ACT target of 200-300 seconds.
- Heparin infusion after the PCI is discouraged.

PCI

Aspirin

160-325 mg po 1-24 hours prior to PCI and daily thereafter.

Heparin

Target ACT 200-300 seconds.

- 60 U/kg bolus initially in patients not treated with heparin within 6 hours prior to PCI.
- Additional boluses during PCI to maintain ACT within target.
- Heparin infusion after the PCI is strongly discouraged. Patients requiring thrombolytic therapy should have eptifibatide infusions stopped.

Instructions for Administration:

1. Like other parenteral drug products, eptifibatide solutions should be inspected visually for particulate matter and discoloration prior to administration, whenever solution and container permit.
2. Eptifibatide may be administered in the same intravenous line as alteplase, atropine, dobutamine, heparin, lidocaine, meperidine, metoprolol, midazolam, morphine, nitroglycerin, or verapamil. Eptifibatide should not be administered through the same intravenous line as furosemide.
3. Eptifibatide may be administered in the same IV line with 0.9% NaCl or 0.9% NaCl/5% dextrose. With either vehicle, the infusion may also contain up to 60 mEq/L of potassium chloride. No incompatibilities have been observed with intravenous administration sets. No compatibility studies have been performed with PVC bags.
4. The bolus dose(s) of eptifibatide should be withdrawn from the 10 ml vial into a syringe. The bolus dose(s) should be administered by IV push.

5. Immediately following the bolus dose administration, a continuous infusion of eptifibatide should be initiated. When using an intravenous infusion pump, eptifibatide should be administered undiluted directly from the 100 ml vial. The 100 ml vial should be spiked with a vented infusion set. Care should be taken to center the spike within the circle on the stopper top.

Eptifibatide is to be administered by volume according to patient weight. Patients should receive eptifibatide according to TABLE 9.

TABLE 9 *Eptifibatide Dosing Charts by Weight*

Patient Weight		180 µg/kg Bolus Vol. (2 mg/ml vial)	2.0 µg/kg/min Infusion Volume (2 mg/ml vial)	2.0 µg/kg/min Infusion Volume (0.75 mg/ml vial)	1.0 µg/kg/min Infusion Volume (2 mg/ml vial)	1.0 µg/kg/min Infusion Volume (0.75 mg/ml vial)
(kg)	(lb)	(ml)	(ml/h)	(ml/h)	(ml/h)	(ml/h)
37-41	81-91	3.4	2.0	6.0	1.0	3.0
42-46	92-102	4.0	2.5	7.0	1.3	3.5
47-53	103-117	4.5	3.0	8.0	1.5	4.0
54-59	118-130	5.0	3.5	9.0	1.8	4.5
60-65	131-143	5.6	3.8	10.0	1.9	5.0
66-71	144-157	6.2	4.0	11.0	2.0	5.5
72-78	158-172	6.8	4.5	12.0	2.3	6.0
79-84	173-185	7.3	5.0	13.0	2.5	6.5
85-90	186-198	7.9	5.3	14.0	2.7	7.0
91-96	199-212	8.5	5.6	15.0	2.8	7.5
97-103	213-227	9.0	6.0	16.0	3.0	8.0
104-109	228-240	9.5	6.4	17.0	3.2	8.5
110-115	241-253	10.2	6.8	18.0	3.4	9.0
116-121	254-267	10.7	7.0	19.0	3.5	9.5
>121	>267	11.3	7.5	20.0	3.7	10.0

HOW SUPPLIED

Integrilin (eptifibatide) injection is supplied as a sterile solution in 10 ml vials containing 20 mg of eptifibatide and 100 ml vials containing either 75 mg of eptifibatide or 200 mg of eptifibatide.

STORAGE

Vials should be stored refrigerated at 2-8°C (36-46°F). Vials may be transferred to room temperature storage [25°C (77°F) with excursions permitted between 15-30°C (59-86°F)] for a period not to exceed 2 months.

Do not use beyond the labeled expiration date. Protect from light until administration. Discard any unused portion left in the vial.

PRODUCT LISTING - EQUIVALENTS NOT AVAILABLE

Solution - Intravenous - 0.75 mg/ml
100 ml $211.25 INTEGRELIN, Schering Corporation 00085-1136-01
Solution - Intravenous - 2 mg/ml
10 ml $67.50 INTEGRELIN, Schering Corporation 00085-1177-01
100 ml $562.50 INTEGRELIN, Schering Corporation 00085-1177-02

Ertapenem *(003544)*

Categories: Abortion, septic; Endomyometritis; Infection, gynecologic; Infection, intra-abdominal; Infection, lower respiratory tract; Infection, skin and skin structures; Infection, urinary tract; Pneumonia; Pyelonephritis; FDA Approved 2001 Nov; Pregnancy Category B
Drug Classes: Antibiotics, carbapenems
Brand Names: Invanz
Cost of Therapy: $499.80 (Infections; Invanz Injection; 1 g; 1 g/day; 10 day supply)

DESCRIPTION

For Intravenous or Intramuscular Use.

Invanz (ertapenem for injection) is a sterile, synthetic, parenteral, 1-β methyl-carbapenem that is structurally related to beta-lactam antibiotics.

Chemically, ertapenem is described as [4*R*-[3(3*S**,5*S**),4α,5β,6β(*R**)]]-3-[[5-[[(3-carboxyphenyl)amino]carbonyl]-3-pyrrolidinyl]thio]-6-(1-hydroxyethyl)-4-methyl-7-oxo-1-azabicyclo[3.2.0]hept-2-ene-2-carboxylic acid monosodium salt. Its molecular weight is 497.50. The empirical formula is $C_{22}H_{24}N_3O_7SNa$.

Ertapenem sodium is a white to off-white hygroscopic, weakly crystalline powder. It is soluble in water and 0.9% sodium chloride solution, practically insoluble in ethanol, and insoluble in isopropyl acetate and tetrahydrofuran.

Invanz is supplied as sterile lyophilized powder for intravenous infusion after reconstitution with appropriate diluent (see DOSAGE AND ADMINISTRATION, Preparation of Solution) and transfer to 50 ml 0.9% sodium chloride injection or for intramuscular injection following reconstitution with 1% lidocaine hydrochloride. Each vial contains 1.046 g ertapenem sodium, equivalent to 1 g ertapenem. The sodium content is approximately 137 mg (approximately 6.0 mEq).

Each vial of Invanz contains the following inactive ingredients: 175 mg sodium bicarbonate and sodium hydroxide to adjust pH to 7.5.

CLINICAL PHARMACOLOGY

PHARMACOKINETICS

Average plasma concentration (µg/ml) of ertapenem following a single 30 minute infusion of a 1 g intravenous (IV) dose and administration of a single 1 g intramuscular (IM) dose in healthy young adults are presented in TABLE 1.

The area under the plasma concentration-time curve (AUC) of ertapenem increased less-than dose-proportional based on total ertapenem concentrations over the 0.5 to 2 g dose,

TABLE 1 *Plasma Concentrations of Ertapenem After Single Dose Administration*

	Average Plasma Concentrations 1 g IV*	Average Plasma Concentrations 1 g IM
0.5 hours	155 µg/ml	33 µg/ml
1 hour	115 µg/ml	53 µg/ml
2 hours	83 µg/ml	67 µg/ml
4 hours	48 µg/ml	57 µg/ml
6 hours	31 µg/ml	40 µg/ml
8 hours	20 µg/ml	27 µg/ml
12 hours	9 µg/ml	13 µg/ml
18 hours	3 µg/ml	4 µg/ml
24 hours	1 µg/ml	2 µg/ml

* Infused at a constant rate over 30 minutes.

whereas the AUC increased greater-than dose proportional based on unbound ertapenem concentrations. Ertapenem exhibits non-linear pharmacokinetics due to concentration-dependent plasma protein binding at the proposed therapeutic dose. (See Distribution.)

There is no accumulation of ertapenem following multiple IV or IM 1 g daily doses in healthy adults.

Absorption

Ertapenem, reconstituted with 1% lidocaine HCl injection (in saline without epinephrine), is almost completely absorbed following IM administration at the recommended dose of 1 g. The mean bioavailability is approximately 90%. Following 1 g daily IM administration, mean peak plasma concentrations (C_{max}) are achieved in approximately 2.3 hours (T_{max}).

Distribution

Ertapenem is highly bound to human plasma proteins, primarily albumin. In healthy young adults, the protein binding of ertapenem decreases as plasma concentrations increase, from approximately 95% bound at an approximate plasma concentration of <100 µg/ml to approximately 85% bound at an approximate plasma concentration of 300 µg/ml.

The apparent volume of distribution at steady state (Vss) of ertapenem is approximately 8.2 liters.

The concentrations of ertapenem achieved in suction-induced skin blister fluid at each sampling point on the third day of 1 g once daily IV doses are presented in TABLE 2. The ratio of AUC(0-24) in skin blister fluid/AUC(0-24) in plasma is 0.61.

TABLE 2 *Concentrations (µg/ml) of Ertapenem in Skin Blister Fluid at Each Sampling Point on the Third Day of 1 g Once Daily IV Doses*

0.5 h	1 h	2 h	4 h	8 h	12 h	24 h
7	12	17	24	24	21	8

The concentration of ertapenem in breast milk from 5 lactating women with pelvic infections (5-14 days postpartum) was measured at random time points daily for 5 consecutive days following the last 1 g dose of IV therapy (3-10 days of therapy). The concentration of ertapenem in breast milk within 24 hours of the last dose of therapy in all 5 women ranged from <0.13 (lower limit of quantitation) to 0.38 µg/ml; peak concentrations were not assessed. By day 5 after discontinuation of therapy, the level of ertapenem was undetectable in the breast milk of 4 women and below the lower limit of quantitation (<0.13 µg/ml) in 1 woman.

Metabolism

In healthy young adults, after infusion of 1 g IV radiolabeled ertapenem, the plasma radioactivity consists predominantly (94%) of ertapenem. The major metabolite of ertapenem is the inactive ring-opened derivative formed by hydrolysis of the beta-lactam ring.

In vitro studies in human liver microsomes indicate that ertapenem does not inhibit metabolism mediated by any of the following cytochrome P450 (CYP) isoforms: 1A2, 2C9, 2C19, 2D6, 2E1 and 3A4. (See DRUG INTERACTIONS.)

In vitro studies indicate that ertapenem does not inhibit P-glycoprotein-mediated transport of digoxin or vinblastine and that ertapenem is not a substrate for P-glycoprotein-mediated transport. (See DRUG INTERACTIONS.)

Elimination

Ertapenem is eliminated primarily by the kidneys. The mean plasma half-life in healthy young adults is approximately 4 hours and the plasma clearance is approximately 1.8 L/hour.

Following the administration of 1 g IV radiolabeled ertapenem to healthy young adults, approximately 80% is recovered in urine and 10% in feces. Of the 80% recovered in urine, approximately 38% is excreted as unchanged drug and approximately 37% as the ring-opened metabolite.

In healthy young adults given a 1 g IV dose, the mean percentage of the administered dose excreted in urine was 17.4% during 0-2 hours postdose, 5.4% during 4-6 hours postdose, and 2.4% during 12-24 hours postdose.

SPECIAL POPULATIONS

Renal Insufficiency

Total and unbound fractions of ertapenem pharmacokinetics were investigated in 26 adult subjects (31-80 years of age) with varying degrees of renal impairment. Following a single 1 g IV dose of ertapenem, the unbound AUC increased 1.5-fold and 2.3-fold in subjects with mild renal insufficiency (CLCR 60-90 ml/min/1.73 m^2) and moderate renal insufficiency (CLCR 31-59 ml/min/1.73 m^2), respectively, compared with healthy young subjects (25-45 years of age). No dosage adjustment is necessary in patients with CLCR ≥31 ml/min/1.73 m^2. The unbound AUC increased 4.4-fold and 7.6-fold in subjects with advanced renal insufficiency (CLCR 5-30 ml/min/1.73 m^2) and end-stage renal insufficiency (CLCR <10 ml/min/1.73 m²), respectively, compared with healthy young subjects. The effects of renal insufficiency on AUC of total drug were of smaller magnitude. The recommended dose of ertapenem in patients with CLCR ≤30 ml/min/1.73 m² is 0.5 g every 24 hours. Following a single 1 g IV dose given immediately prior to a 4 hour hemodialysis session in 5 patients with end-stage renal insufficiency, approximately 30% of the dose was recovered in the dialysate. A supplementary dose of 150 mg is recommended if ertapenem is administered within 6 hours prior to hemodialysis. (See DOSAGE AND ADMINISTRATION.)

Hepatic Insufficiency

The pharmacokinetics of ertapenem in patients with hepatic insufficiency have not been established. However, ertapenem does not appear to undergo hepatic metabolism based on *in vitro* studies and approximately 10% of an administered dose is recovered in the feces. (See PRECAUTIONS and DOSAGE AND ADMINISTRATION.)

E

Gender

The effect of gender on the pharmacokinetics of ertapenem was evaluated in healthy male (n=8) and healthy female (n=8) subjects. The differences observed could be attributed to body size when body weight was taken into consideration. No dose adjustment is recommended based on gender.

Geriatric Patients

The impact of age on the pharmacokinetics of ertapenem was evaluated in healthy male (n=7) and healthy female (n=7) subjects ≥65 years of age. The total and unbound AUC increased 37% and 67%, respectively, in elderly adults relative to young adults. These changes were attributed to age-related changes in creatinine clearance. No dosage adjustment is necessary for elderly patients with normal (for their age) renal function.

Pediatric Patients

The pharmacokinetics of ertapenem in pediatric patients have not been established.

MICROBIOLOGY

Ertapenem has *in vitro* activity against gram-positive and gram-negative aerobic and anaerobic bacteria. The bactericidal activity of ertapenem results from the inhibition of cell wall synthesis and is mediated through ertapenem binding to penicillin binding proteins (PBPs). In *Escherichia coli,* it has strong affinity toward PBPs 1a, 1b, 2, 3, 4 and 5 with preference for PBPs 2 and 3. Ertapenem is stable against hydrolysis by a variety of beta-lactamases, including penicillinases, and cephalosporinases and extended spectrum beta-lactamases. Ertapenem is hydrolyzed by metallo-beta-lactamases.

Ertapenem has been shown to be active against most strains of the following microorganisms *in vitro* and in clinical infections (see INDICATIONS AND USAGE):

Aerobic Gram-Positive Microorganisms:

Staphylococcus aureus (methicillin susceptible strains only), *Streptococcus agalactiae, Streptococcus pneumoniae* (penicillin susceptible strains only), *Streptococcus pyogenes.*

Note: Methicillin-resistant staphylococci and *Enterococcus* spp. are resistant to ertapenem.

Aerobic Gram-Negative Microorganisms:

Escherichia coli, Haemophilus influenzae (Beta-lactamase negative strains only), *Klebsiella pneumoniae, Moraxella catarrhalis.*

Anaerobic Microorganisms:

Bacteroides fragilis, Bacteroides distasonis, Bacteroides ovatus, Bacteroides thetaiotaomicron, Bacteroides uniformis, Clostridium clostridioforme, Eubacterium lentum, Peptostreptococcus species, *Porphyromonas asaccharolytica, Prevotella bivia.*

The following *in vitro* data are available, **but their clinical significance is unknown.**

At least 90% of the following microorganisms exhibit an *in vitro* minimum inhibitory concentration (MIC) less than or equal to the susceptible breakpoint for ertapenem; however, the safety and effectiveness of ertapenem in treating clinical infections due to these microorganisms have not been established in adequate and well-controlled clinical studies:

Aerobic Gram-Positive Microorganisms:

Streptococcus pneumoniae (penicillin-intermediate strains only).

Aerobic Gram-Negative Microorganisms:

Citrobacter freundiiCitrobacter koseri, Enterobacter aerogenes, Enterobacter cloacae, Haemophilus influenzae (Beta-lactamase positive strains), *Haemophilus parainfluenzae, Klebsiella oxytoca* (excluding ESBL producing strains), *Morganella morganii, Proteus mirabilis, Proteus vulgaris, Serratia marcescens.*

Anaerobic microorganisms:

Clostridium perfringens, Fusobacterium spp.

Susceptibility Testing

When available, the results of *in vitro* susceptibility tests should be provided to the physician as periodic reports which describe the susceptibility profile of nosocomial and community-acquired pathogens. These reports should aid the physician in selecting the most effective antimicrobial.

Dilution Techniques

Quantitative methods are used to determine antimicrobial minimum inhibitory concentrations (MICs). These MICs provide estimates of the susceptibility of bacteria to antimicrobial compounds. The MICs should be determined using a standardized procedure. Standardized procedures are based on a broth dilution method[1,4] or equivalent with standardized inoculum concentrations and standardized concentrations of ertapenem powder. The MIC values should be interpreted according to the criteria in TABLE 3.

Note: *Staphylococcus* spp. can be considered susceptible to ertapenem if the penicillin MIC is ≤0.12 μg/ml. If the penicillin MIC is >0.12 μg/ml, then test oxacillin. *Staphylococcus aureus* can be considered susceptible to ertapenem if the oxacillin MIC is ≤2.0 μg/ml and resistant to ertapenem if the oxacillin MIC is ≥4.0 μg/ml. Coagulase negative staphylococci can be considered susceptible to ertapenem if the oxacillin MIC is ≤0.25 μg/ml and resistant to ertapenem if the oxacillin MIC ≥0.5 μg/ml.

TABLE 3 *For Testing Enterobacteriaceae and Staphylococcus spp.:*

MIC (μg/ml)	Interpretation
≤2.0	Susceptible (S)
4.0	Intermediate (I)
≥8.0	Resistant (R)

TABLE 4 *For Testing Haemophilus spp.*:*

MIC (μg/ml)	Interpretation†
≤0.5	Susceptible (S)

* This interpretive standard is applicable only to broth microdilution susceptibility tests with *Haemophilus* spp. using *Haemophilus* Test Medium (HTM)[1] inoculated with a direct colony suspension and incubated in ambient air at 35°C for 20-24 hours.

† The current absence of data in resistant strains precludes defining any results other than "Susceptible". Strains yielding MIC results suggestive of a "nonsusceptible" category should be submitted to a reference laboratory for further testing.

TABLE 5 *For Testing Streptococcus pneumoniae*†:*

MIC (μg/ml)	Interpretation‡
≤1.0	Susceptible (S)

* This interpretive standard is applicable only to broth microdilution susceptibility tests using cation-adjusted Mueller-Hinton broth with 2-5% lysed horse blood inoculated with direct colony suspension and incubated in ambient air at 35°C for 20-24 hours.

† *Streptococcus pneumoniae* that are susceptible to penicillin (penicillin MIC ≤0.06 μg/ml) can be considered susceptible to ertapenem. Testing of ertapenem against penicillin-intermediate or penicillin-resistant isolates is not recommended since reliable interpretive criteria for ertapenem are not available.

‡ The current absence of data in resistant strains precludes defining any results other than "Susceptible". Strains yielding MIC results suggestive of a "nonsusceptible" category should be submitted to a reference laboratory for further testing.

TABLE 6 *For Testing Streptococcus spp. Other Than Streptococcus pneumoniae*†:*

MIC (μg/ml)	Interpretation‡
≤1.0	Susceptible (S)

* This interpretive standard is applicable only to broth microdilution susceptibility tests using cation-adjusted Mueller-Hinton broth with 2-5% lysed horse blood inoculated with direct colony suspension and incubated in ambient air at 35°C for 20-24 hours.

† *Streptococcus* spp. that are susceptible to penicillin (MIC ≤0.12 μg/ml) can be considered susceptible to ertapenem. Testing of ertapenem against penicillin-intermediate or penicillin-resistant isolates is not recommended since reliable interpretive criteria for ertapenem are not available.

‡ The current absence of data in resistant strains precludes defining any results other than "Susceptible". Strains yielding MIC results suggestive of a "nonsusceptible" category should be submitted to a reference laboratory for further testing.

A report of "Susceptible" indicates that the pathogen is likely to be inhibited if the antimicrobial compound in blood reaches the concentrations usually achievable. A report of "Intermediate" indicates that the result should be considered equivocal, and, if the microorganism is not fully susceptible to alternative, clinically feasible drugs, the test should be repeated. This category implies possible clinical applicability in body sites where the drug is physiologically concentrated or in situations where high dosage of drug can be used. This category also provides a buffer zone which prevents small uncontrolled technical factors from causing major discrepancies in interpretation. A report of "Resistant" indicates that the pathogen is not likely to be inhibited if the antimicrobial compound in the blood reaches the concentrations usually achievable; other therapy should be selected.

Standardized susceptibility test procedures require the use of laboratory control microorganisms to control the technical aspects of the laboratory procedures. Quality control microorganisms are specific strains of organisms with intrinsic biological properties. QC strains are very stable strains which will give a standard and repeatable susceptibility pattern. The specific strains used for microbiological quality control are not clinically significant. Standard ertapenem powder should provide the following MIC values.

TABLE 7

Microorgansim	ATCC	MIC Range (μg/ml)
Enterococcus faecalis	29212	4.0-16.0
Escherichia coli	25922	0.004-0.016
*Haemophilus influenzae**	49766	0.016-0.06
Pseudomonas aeruginosa	27853	2.0-8.0
Staphylococcus aureus	29213	0.06-0.25
Streptococcus pneumoniae†	49619	0.03-0.25

* This quality control range is applicable to only *H. influenzae* ATCC 49766 tested by the broth microdilution procedure using HTM[1] inoculated with a direct colony suspension and incubated in ambient air at 35°C for 20-24 hours.

† This quality control range is applicable to only *S. pneumoniae* ATCC 49619 tested by a broth microdilution procedure using cation-adjusted Mueller-Hinton broth with 2-5% lysed horse blood inoculated with a direct colony suspension and incubated in ambient air at 35°C for 20-24 hours.

Diffusion Techniques

Quantitative methods that require measurement of zone diameters also provide reproducible estimates of the susceptibility of bacteria to antimicrobial compounds. One such standardized procedure[2,4] requires the use of standardized inoculum concentrations. This procedure uses paper disks impregnated with 10 μg ertapenem to test the susceptibility of microorganisms to ertapenem.

Reports from the laboratory providing results of the standard single-disk susceptibility test with a 10 μg ertapenem disk should be interpreted according to the criteria in TABLE 8.

TABLE 8 For Testing Enterobacteriaceae or Staphylococcus spp.:

Zone Diameter (mm)	Interpretation
≥19	Susceptible (S)
16-18	Intermediate (I)
≤15	Resistant (R)

Note: *Staphylococcus* spp. can be considered susceptible to ertapenem if the penicillin (10 U disk) zone is ≥29 mm. If the penicillin zone is ≤28 mm, then test oxacillin by disk diffusion (1 μg disk). *Staphylococcus aureus* can be considered susceptible to ertapenem if the oxacillin (1 μg disk) zone is ≥13 mm and resistant to ertapenem if the oxacillin zone is ≤10 mm. Coagulase negative staphylococci can be considered susceptible to ertapenem if the oxacillin zone is ≥18 mm and resistant to ertapenem if the oxacillin (1 μg disk) zone is ≤17 mm.

TABLE 9 For Testing Haemophilus spp.*:

Zone Diameter (mm)	Interpretation†
≥19	Susceptible (S)

* This zone diameter standard is applicable only to tests performed by disk diffusion with *Haemophilus* spp. using HTM[2] inoculated with a direct colony suspension and incubated in 5% CO_2 at 35°C for 16-18 hours.

† The current absence of data in resistant strains precludes defining any results other than "Susceptible". Strains yielding MIC results suggestive of a "nonsusceptible" category should be submitted to a reference laboratory for further testing.

TABLE 10 For Testing Streptococcus pneumoniae*†:

Zone Diameter (mm)	Interpretation‡
≥19	Susceptible (S)

* These zone diameter standards apply only to tests performed using Mueller-Hinton agar supplemented with 5% sheep blood inoculated with a direct colony suspension and incubated in 5% CO_2 at 35°C for 20-24 hours.

† *Streptococcus pneumoniae* that is susceptible to penicillin (1 μg oxacillin disk zone diameter ≥20 mm), can be considered susceptible to ertapenem. Isolates with 1 μg oxacillin zone diameter ≤19 mm should be tested against ertapenem using an MIC method.

‡ The current absence of data in resistant strains precludes defining any results other than "Susceptible". Strains yielding MIC results suggestive of a "nonsusceptible" category should be submitted to a reference laboratory for further testing.

TABLE 11 For Testing Streptococcus spp. other than Streptococcus pneumoniae*†:

Zone Diameter (mm)	Interpretation‡
≥19	Susceptible (S)

* These zone diameter standards apply only to tests performed using Mueller-Hinton agar supplemented with 5% sheep blood inoculated with a direct colony suspension and in ambient air at 35°C for 20-24 hours.

† Beta-hemolytic *Streptococcus* spp. that are susceptible to penicillin (10 units penicillin disk zone diameter ≥24 mm), can be considered susceptible to ertapenem. Isolates with 10 units penicillin disk zone diameter <24 mm should be tested against ertapenem using an MIC method. Penicillin disk diffusion interpretive criteria are not available for viridans group streptococci and they should not be tested against ertapenem.

‡ The current absence of data in resistant strains precludes defining any results other than "Susceptible". Strains yielding MIC results suggestive of a "nonsusceptible" category should be submitted to a reference laboratory for further testing.

Interpretation should be as stated above for results using dilution techniques. Interpretation involves correlation of the diameter obtained in the disk test with the MIC for ertapenem.

As with standardized dilution techniques, diffusion methods require the use of laboratory control microorganisms that are used to control the technical aspects of the laboratory procedures. Quality control microorganisms are specific strains of organisms with intrinsic biological properties. QC strains are very stable strains that will give a standard and repeatable susceptibility pattern. The specific strains used for microbiological quality control are not clinically significant. For the diffusion technique, the 10 μg ertapenem disk should provide the following zone diameters in these laboratory quality control strains:

Anaerobic Techniques

For anaerobic bacteria, the susceptibility to ertapenem as MICs can be determined by standardized test methods.[3] The MIC values obtained should be interpreted according to the criteria in TABLE 13.

Interpretation is identical to that stated above for results using dilution techniques.

As with other susceptibility techniques, the use of laboratory control microorganisms is required to control the technical aspects of the laboratory standardized procedures. Standardized ertapenem powder should provide the MIC values shown in TABLE 14.

TABLE 12

Microorgansim	ATCC	Zone Diameter Range (mm)
Escherichia coli	25922	29-36
*Haemophilus influenzae**	49766	27-33
Pseudomonas aeruginosa	27853	13-21
Staphylococcus aureus	25923	24-31
Streptococcus pneumoniae†	49619	28-35

* This quality control range is applicable to *Haemophilus influenzae* ATCC 49766 tested by disk diffusion using HTM[2] agar inoculated with a direct colony suspension and incubated in 5% CO_2 at 35°C for 16-18 hours.

† This quality control range is applicable to *Streptococcus pneumoniae* ATCC 49619 tested by diffusion using Mueller-Hinton agar supplemented with 5% sheep blood inoculated with a direct colony suspension and incubated in 5% CO_2 at 35°C for 20-24 hours.

TABLE 13

MIC (μg/ml)	Interpretation
≤4.0	Susceptible (S)
8.0	Intermediate (I)
≥16.0	Resistant (R)

TABLE 14

Microorgansim	ATCC	MIC* (μg/ml)
Bacteroides fragilis	25285	0.06-0.25
Bacteroides thetaiotaomicron	29741	0.25-1.0
Eubacterium lentum	43055	05-2.0

* These quality control ranges are applicable only to agar dilution using *Brucella* agar supplemented with hemin, vitamin K1 and 5% defibrinated or laked sheep blood inoculated with a direct colony suspension or a 6-24 hour fresh culture in enriched thioglycollate medium and incubated in an anaerobic jar or chamber at 35-37°C for 42-48 hours.

INDICATIONS AND USAGE

Ertapenem for injection is indicated for the treatment of adult patients with the following moderate to severe infections caused by susceptible strains of the designated microorganisms. (See DOSAGE AND ADMINISTRATION.)

Complicated intra-abdominal infections due to *Escherichia coli, Clostridium clostridioforme, Eubacterium lentum, Peptostreptococcus* species, *Bacteroides fragilis, Bacteroides distasonis, Bacteroides ovatus, Bacteroides thetaiotaomicron,* or *Bacteroides uniformis.*

Complicated skin and skin structure infections due to *Staphylococcus aureus* (methicillin susceptible strains only), *Streptococcus pyogenes, Escherichia coli,* or *Peptostreptococcus* species.

Community acquired pneumonia due to *Streptococcus pneumoniae* (penicillin susceptible strains only) including cases with concurrent bacteremia, *Haemophilus influenzae* (beta-lactamase negative strains only), or *Moraxella catarrhalis.*

Complicated urinary tract infections including pyelonephritis due to *Escherichia coli,* including cases with concurrent bacteremia, or *Klebsiella pneumoniae.*

Acute pelvic infections including postpartum endomyometritis, septic abortion and post surgical gynecologic infections due to *Streptococcus agalactiae, Escherichia coli, Bacteroides fragilis, Porphyromonas asaccharolytica, Peptostreptococcus species,* or *Prevotella bivia.*

Appropriate specimens for bacteriological examination should be obtained in order to isolate and identify the causative organisms and to determine their susceptibility to ertapenem. Therapy with ertapenem for injection may be initiated empirically before results of these tests are known; once results become available, antimicrobial therapy should be adjusted accordingly.

CONTRAINDICATIONS

Ertapenem for injection is contraindicated in patients with known hypersensitivity to any component of this product or to other drugs in the same class or in patients who have demonstrated anaphylactic reactions to beta-lactams.

Due to the use of lidocaine HCl as a diluent, ertapenem for injection administered intramuscularly is contraindicated in patients with a known hypersensitivity to local anesthetics of the amide type. (Refer to the prescribing information for lidocaine HCl.)

WARNINGS

SERIOUS AND OCCASIONALLY FATAL HYPERSENSITIVITY (ANAPHYLACTIC) REACTIONS HAVE BEEN REPORTED IN PATIENTS RECEIVING THERAPY WITH BETA-LACTAMS. THESE REACTIONS ARE MORE LIKELY TO OCCUR IN INDIVIDUALS WITH A HISTORY OF SENSITIVITY TO MULTIPLE ALLERGENS. THERE HAVE BEEN REPORTS OF INDIVIDUALS WITH A HISTORY OF PENICILLIN HYPERSENSITIVITY WHO HAVE EXPERIENCED SEVERE HYPERSENSITIVITY REACTIONS WHEN TREATED WITH ANOTHER BETA-LACTAM. BEFORE INITIATING THERAPY WITH ERTAPENEM FOR INJECTION, CAREFUL INQUIRY SHOULD BE MADE CONCERNING PREVIOUS HYPERSENSITIVITY REACTIONS TO PENICILLINS, CEPHALOSPORINS, OTHER BETA-LACTAMS AND OTHER ALLERGENS. IF AN ALLERGIC REACTION TO ERTAPENEM FOR INJECTION OCCURS, DISCONTINUE THE DRUG IMMEDIATELY. **SERIOUS ANAPHYLACTIC REACTIONS REQUIRE IMMEDIATE EMERGENCY TREATMENT WITH EPINEPHRINE, OXYGEN, IV STEROIDS, AND AIRWAY MANAGEMENT, INCLUDING INTUBATION. OTHER THERAPY MAY ALSO BE ADMINISTERED AS INDICATED.**

Seizures and other CNS adverse experiences have been reported during treatment with ertapenem for injection. (See PRECAUTIONS and ADVERSE REACTIONS.)

Pseudomembranous colitis has been reported with nearly all antibacterial agents, including ertapenem, and may range in severity from mild to life-threatening. Therefore, it is important to consider this diagnosis in patients who present with diarrhea subsequent to the administration of antibacterial agents.

Treatment with antibacterial agents alters the normal flora of the colon and may permit overgrowth of clostridia. Studies indicate that a toxin produced by *Clostridium difficile* is a primary cause of "antibiotic-associated colitis".

After the diagnosis of pseudomembranous colitis has been established, therapeutic measures should be initiated. Mild cases of pseudomembranous colitis usually respond to drug discontinuation alone. In moderate to severe cases, consideration should be given to management with fluids and electrolytes, protein supplementation and treatment with an antibacterial drug clinically effective against *Clostridium difficile* colitis.

Lidocaine HCl is the diluent for IM administration of ertapenem for injection. Refer to the prescribing information for lidocaine HCl.

E

PRECAUTIONS

GENERAL

During clinical investigations in adult patients treated with ertapenem for injection (1 g once a day), seizures, irrespective of drug relationship, occurred in 0.5% of patients during study therapy plus 14 day follow-up period. (See ADVERSE REACTIONS.) These experiences have occurred most commonly in patients with CNS disorders (*e.g.*, brain lesions or history of seizures) and/or compromised renal function. Close adherence to the recommended dosage regimen is urged, especially in patients with known factors that predispose to convulsive activity. Anticonvulsant therapy should be continued in patients with known seizure disorders. If focal tremors, myoclonus, or seizures occur, patients should be evaluated neurologically, placed on anticonvulsant therapy if not already instituted, and the dosage of ertapenem for injection re-examined to determine whether it should be decreased or the antibiotic discontinued. Dosage adjustment of ertapenem for injection is recommended in patients with reduced renal function. (See DOSAGE AND ADMINISTRATION.)

As with other antibiotics, prolonged use of ertapenem for injection may result in overgrowth of non-susceptible organisms. Repeated evaluation of the patient's condition is essential. If superinfection occurs during therapy, appropriate measures should be taken.

Caution should be taken when administering ertapenem for injection intramuscularly to avoid inadvertent injection into a blood vessel. (See DOSAGE AND ADMINISTRATION.)

Lidocaine HCl is the diluent for IM administration of ertapenem for injection. Refer to the prescribing information for lidocaine HCl for additional precautions.

LABORATORY TESTS

While ertapenem for injection possesses toxicity similar to the beta-lactam group of antibiotics, periodic assessment of organ system function, including renal, hepatic, and hematopoietic, is advisable during prolonged therapy.

CARCINOGENESIS, MUTAGENESIS, AND IMPAIRMENT OF FERTILITY

No long-term studies in animals have been performed to evaluate the carcinogenic potential of ertapenem.

Ertapenem was neither mutagenic nor genotoxic in the following *in vitro* assays: alkaline elution/rat hepatocyte assay, chromosomal aberration assay in Chinese hamster ovary cells, and TK6 human lymphoblastoid cell mutagenesis assay; and in the *in vivo* mouse micronucleus assay.

In mice and rats, IV doses of up to 700 mg/kg/day (for mice, approximately 3 times the recommended human dose of 1 g based on body surface area and for rats, approximately 1.2 times the human exposure at the recommended dose of 1 g based on plasma AUCs) resulted in no effects on mating performance, fecundity, fertility, or embryonic survival.

PREGNANCY, TERATOGENIC EFFECTS, PREGNANCY CATEGORY B

In mice and rats given IV doses of up to 700 mg/kg/day (for mice, approximately 3 times the recommended human dose of 1 g based on body surface area and for rats, approximately 1.2 times the human exposure at the recommended dose of 1 g based on plasma AUCs), there was no evidence of developmental toxicity as assessed by external, visceral, and skeletal examination of the fetuses. However, in mice given 700 mg/kg/day, slight decreases in average fetal weights and an associated decrease in the average number of ossified sacrocaudal vertebrae were observed. Ertapenem crosses the placental barrier in rats.

There are, however, no adequate and well-controlled studies in pregnant women. Because animal reproduction studies are not always predictive of human response, this drug should be used during pregnancy only if clearly needed.

NURSING MOTHERS

Ertapenem is excreted in human breast milk. (See CLINICAL PHARMACOLOGY, Pharmacokinetics, Distribution.) Caution should be exercised when ertapenem for injection is administered to a nursing woman. Ertapenem for injection should be administered to nursing mothers only when the expected benefit outweighs the risk.

LABOR AND DELIVERY

Ertapenem for injection has not been studied for use during labor and delivery.

PEDIATRIC USE

Safety and effectiveness in pediatric patients have not been established. Therefore, use in patients under 18 years of age is not recommended.

GERIATRIC USE

Of the 1835 patients in Phase 2b/3 studies treated with ertapenem for injection, approximately 26% were 65 and over, while approximately 12% were 75 and over. No overall differences in safety or effectiveness were observed between these patients and younger patients. Other reported clinical experience has not identified differences in responses between the elderly and younger patients, but greater sensitivity of some older individuals cannot be ruled out.

This drug is known to be substantially excreted by the kidney, and the risk of toxic reactions to this drug may be greater in patients with impaired renal function. Because elderly patients are more likely to have decreased renal function, care should be taken in dose selection, and it may be useful to monitor renal function. (See DOSAGE AND ADMINISTRATION.)

HEPATIC INSUFFICIENCY

The pharmacokinetics of ertapenem in patients with hepatic insufficiency have not been established. Of the total number of patients in clinical studies, 37 patients receiving ertapenem 1 g daily and 36 patients receiving comparator drugs were considered to have Child-Pugh Class A, B, or C liver impairment. The incidence of adverse experiences in patients with hepatic impairment was similar between the ertapenem group and the comparator groups.

DRUG INTERACTIONS

When ertapenem is coadministered with probenecid (500 mg po every 6 hours), probenecid competes for active tubular secretion and reduces the renal clearance of ertapenem. Based on total ertapenem concentrations, probenecid increased the AUC by 25% and reduced the plasma and renal clearances by 20% and 35%, respectively. The half-life increased from 4.0 to 4.8 hours. Because of the small effect on half-life, the coadministration with probenecid to extend the half-life of ertapenem is not recommended.

In vitro studies indicate that ertapenem does not inhibit P-glycoprotein-mediated transport of digoxin or vinblastine and that ertapenem is not a substrate for P-glycoprotein-mediated transport. *In vitro* studies in human liver microsomes indicate that ertapenem does not inhibit metabolism mediated by any of the following 6 cytochrome P450 (CYP) isoforms: 1A2, 2C9, 2C19, 2D6, 2E1 and 3A4. Drug interactions caused by inhibition of P-glycoprotein-mediated drug clearance or CYP-mediated drug clearance with the listed isoforms are unlikely. (See CLINICAL PHARMACOLOGY, Pharmacokinetics: Distribution and Metabolism.)

Other than with probenecid, no specific clinical drug interaction studies have been conducted.

ADVERSE REACTIONS

Clinical studies enrolled 1954 patients treated with ertapenem; in some of the clinical studies, parenteral therapy was followed by a switch to an appropriate oral antimicrobial. Most adverse experiences reported in these clinical studies were described as mild to moderate in severity. Ertapenem was discontinued due to adverse experiences in 4.7% of patients. TABLE 15 shows the incidence of adverse experiences reported in ≥1.0% of patients in these studies. The most common drug-related adverse experiences in patients treated with ertapenem for injection, including those who were switched to therapy with an oral antimicrobial, were diarrhea (5.5%), infused vein complication (3.7%), nausea (3.1%), headache (2.2%), vaginitis in females (2.1%), phlebitis/thrombophlebitis (1.3%), and vomiting (1.1%).

In patients treated for complicated intra-abdominal infections, death occurred in 4.7% (15/316) of patients receiving ertapenem and 2.6% (8/307) of patients receiving comparator drug. These deaths occurred in patients with significant co-morbidity and/or severe baseline infections. Deaths were considered unrelated to study drugs by investigators.

In clinical studies, seizure was reported during study therapy plus 14 day follow-up period in 0.5% of patients treated with ertapenem, 0.3% of patients treated with piperacillin/tazobactam and 0% of patients treated with ceftriaxone. (See PRECAUTIONS.)

Additional adverse experiences that were reported with ertapenem for injection with an incidence >1% within each body system are listed below:

Body as a Whole: Abdominal distention, pain, chills, septicemia, septic shock, dehydration, gout, malaise, necrosis, candidiasis, weight loss, facial edema, injection site induration, injection site pain, flank pain, and syncope.

Cardiovascular System: Heart failure, hematoma, cardiac arrest, bradycardia, arrhythmia, atrial fibrillation, heart murmur, ventricular tachycardia, asystole, and subdural hemorrhage.

Digestive System: Gastrointestinal hemorrhage, anorexia, flatulence, *C. difficile* associated diarrhea, stomatitis, dysphagia, hemorrhoids, ileus, cholelithiasis, duodenitis, esophagitis, gastritis, jaundice, mouth ulcer, pancreatitis, and pyloric stenosis.

Nervous System & Psychiatric: Nervousness, seizure (see WARNINGS and PRECAUTIONS), tremor, depression, hypesthesia, spasm, paresthesia, aggressive behavior, and vertigo.

Respiratory System: Pleural effusion, hypoxemia, bronchoconstriction, pharyngeal discomfort, epistaxis, pleuritic pain, asthma, hemoptysis, hiccups, and voice disturbance.

Skin & Skin Appendage: Sweating, dermatitis, desquamation, flushing, and urticaria.

Special Senses: Taste perversion.

Urogenital System: Renal insufficiency, oliguria/anuria, vaginal pruritus, hematuria, urinary retention, bladder dysfunction, vaginal candidiasis, and vulvovaginitis.

ADVERSE LABORATORY CHANGES

Laboratory adverse experiences that were reported during therapy in ≥1.0% of patients treated with ertapenem for injection in clinical studies are presented in TABLE 16. Drug-related laboratory adverse experiences that were reported during therapy in ≥1.0% of patients treated with ertapenem for injection, including those who were switched to therapy with an oral antimicrobial, in clinical studies were ALT increased (6.0%), AST increased (5.2%), serum alkaline phosphatase increased (3.4%), platelet count increased (2.8%), and eosinophils increased (1.1%). Ertapenem was discontinued due to laboratory adverse experiences in 0.3% of patients.

Additional laboratory adverse experiences that were reported during therapy in >0.1% but <1.0% of patients treated with ertapenem for injection in clinical studies

TABLE 15 *Incidence (%) of Adverse Experiences Reported During Study Therapy Plus 14 Day Follow-Up in ≥1.0% of Patients Treated With Ertapenem in Clinical Studies*

Adverse Events	Ertapenem* 1 g daily (n=802)	PIP/TAZ* 3.375 g q6h (n=774)	Ertapenem† 1 g daily (n=1162)	Ceftriaxone† 1 or 2 g daily (n=942)
Local:				
Extravasation	1.9%	1.7%	0.7%	1.1%
Infused vein complication	7.1%	7.9%	5.4%	6.7%
Phlebitis/ thrombophlebitis	1.9%	2.7%	1.6%	2.0%
Systemic:				
Asthenia/fatigue	1.2%	0.9%	1.2%	1.1%
Death	2.5%	1.6%	1.3%	1.6%
Edema/swelling	3.4%	2.5%	2.9%	3.3%
Fever	5.0%	6.6%	2.3%	3.4%
Abdominal pain	3.6%	4.8%	4.3%	3.9%
Chest pain	1.5%	1.4%	1.0%	2.5%
Hypertension	1.6%	1.4%	0.7%	1.0%
Hypotension	2.0%	1.4%	1.0%	1.2%
Tachycardia	1.6%	1.3%	1.3%	0.7%
Acid regurgitation	1.6%	0.9%	1.1%	0.6%
Oral candidiasis	0.1%	1.3%	1.4%	1.9%
Constipation	4.0%	5.4%	3.3%	3.1%
Diarrhea	10.3%	12.1%	9.2%	9.8%
Dyspepsia	1.1%	0.6%	1.0%	1.6%
Nausea	8.5%	8.7%	6.4%	7.4%
Vomiting	3.7%	5.3%	4.0%	4.0%
Leg pain	1.1%	0.5%	0.4%	0.3%
Anxiety	1.4%	1.3%	0.8%	1.2%
Altered mental status‡	5.1%	3.4%	3.3%	2.5%
Dizziness	2.1%	3.0%	1.5%	2.1%
Headache	5.6%	5.4%	6.8%	6.9%
Insomnia	3.2%	5.2%	3.0%	4.1%
Cough	1.6%	1.7%	1.3%	0.5%
Dyspnea	2.6%	1.8%	1.0%	2.4%
Pharyngitis	0.7%	1.4%	1.1%	0.6%
Rales/rhonchi	1.1%	1.0%	0.5%	1.0%
Respiratory distress	1.0%	0.4%	0.2%	0.2%
Erythema	1.6%	1.7%	1.2%	1.2%
Pruritus	2.0%	2.6%	1.0%	1.9%
Rash	2.5%	3.1%	2.3%	1.5%
Vaginitis	1.4%	1.0%	3.3%	3.7%

* Includes Phase 2b/3 Complicated intra-abdominal infections, Complicated skin and skin structure infections, and Acute pelvic infections studies.
† Includes Phase 2b/3 Community acquired pneumonia and Complicated urinary tract infections, and Phase 2a studies.
‡ Includes agitation, confusion, disorientation, decreased mental acuity, changed mental status, somnolence, stupor.
PIP/TAZ Piperacillin/tazobactam.

TABLE 16 *Incidence* (%) of Specific Laboratory Adverse Experiences Reported During Study Therapy Plus 14 Day Follow-Up in ≥1.0% of Patients Treated With Ertapenem in Clinical Studies*

Adverse Laboratory Experiences	Ertapenem‡ 1 g daily (n=766)†	PIP/TAZ‡ 3.375 g q6h (n=755)†	Ertapenem§ 1 g daily (n=1122)†	Ceftriaxone§ 1 or 2 g daily (n=920)†
ALT increased	8.8%	7.3%	8.3%	6.9%
AST increased	8.4%	8.3%	7.1%	6.5%
Serum albumin decreased	1.7%	1.5%	0.9%	1.6%
Serum alkaline phosphatase increased	6.6%	7.2%	4.3%	2.8%
Serum creatinine increased	1.1%	2.7%	0.9%	1.2%
Serum glucose increased	1.2%	2.3%	1.7%	2.0%
Serum potassium decreased	1.7%	2.8%	1.8%	2.4%
Serum potassium increased	1.3%	0.5%	0.5%	0.7%
Total serum bilirubin increased	1.7%	1.4%	0.6%	1.1%
Eosinophils increased	1.1%	1.1%	2.1%	1.8%
Hematocrit decreased	3.0%	2.9%	3.4%	2.4%
Hemoglobin decreased	4.9%	4.7%	4.5%	3.5%
Platelet count decreased	1.1%	1.2%	1.1%	1.0%
Platelet count increased	6.5%	6.3%	4.3%	3.5%
Segmented neutrophils decreased	1.0%	0.3%	1.5%	0.8%
Prothrombin time increased	1.2%	2.0%	0.3%	0.9%
WBC decreased	0.8%	0.7%	1.5%	1.4%
Urine RBCs increased	2.5%	2.9%	1.1%	1.0%
Urine WBCs increased	2.5%	3.2%	1.6%	1.1%

* Number of patients with laboratory adverse experiences/Number of patients with the laboratory test.
† Number of patients with one or more laboratory tests.
‡ Includes Phase 2b/3 Complicated intra-abdominal infections, Complicated skin and skin structure infections and Acute pelvic infections studies.
§ Includes Phase 2b/3 Community acquired pneumonia and Complicated urinary tract infections, and Phase 2a studies.
PIP/TAZ Piperacillin/tazobactam.

include: Increases in BUN, direct and indirect serum bilirubin, serum sodium, monocytes, PTT, urine epithelial cells; decreases in serum bicarbonate.

DOSAGE AND ADMINISTRATION

The dose of ertapenem for injection in adults is 1 g given once a day.

Ertapenem for injection may be administered by IV infusion for up to 14 days or IM injection for up to 7 days. When administered intravenously, ertapenem for injection should be infused over a period of 30 minutes.

Intramuscular administration of ertapenem for injection may be used as an alternative to IV administration in the treatment of those infections for which IM therapy is appropriate.

DO NOT MIX OR CO-INFUSE ERTAPENEM FOR INJECTION WITH OTHER MEDICATIONS. DO NOT USE DILUENTS CONTAINING DEXTROSE (α-D-GLUCOSE).

TABLE 17 presents dosage guidelines for ertapenem for injection.

TABLE 17 *Dosage Guidelines for Adults With Normal Renal Function* and Body Weight*

Infection†	Daily Dose (IV or IM)	Recommended Duration of Total Antimicrobial Treatment
Complicated intra-abdominal infections	1 g	5-14 days
Complicated skin and skin structure infections	1 g	7-14 days
Community acquired pneumonia	1 g	10-14 days‡
Complicated urinary tract infections, including pyleonephritis	1 g	10-14 days‡
Acute pelvic infections including postpartum endomyometritis, septic abortion and post surgical gynecologic infections	1 g	3-10 days

* Defined as creatinine clearance >90 ml/min/1.73 m^2.
† Due to the designated pathogens (see INDICATIONS AND USAGE).
‡ Duration includes a possible switch to an appropriate oral therapy, after at least 3 days of parenteral therapy, once clinical improvement has been demonstrated.

PATIENTS WITH RENAL INSUFFICIENCY

Ertapenem for injection may be used for the treatment of infections in patients with renal insufficiency. In patients whose creatinine clearance is >30 ml/min/1.73 m^2, no dosage adjustment is necessary. Patients with advanced renal insufficiency (creatinine clearance ≤30 ml/min/1.73 m^2) and end-stage renal insufficiency (creatinine clearance ≤10 ml/min/1.73 m^2) should receive 500 mg daily.

PATIENTS ON HEMODIALYSIS

When patients on hemodialysis are given the recommended daily dose of 500 mg of ertapenem for injection within 6 hours prior to hemodialysis, a supplementary dose of 150 mg is recommended following the hemodialysis session. If ertapenem for injection is given at least 6 hours prior to hemodialysis, no supplementary dose is needed. There are no data in patients undergoing peritoneal dialysis or hemofiltration.

When only the serum creatinine is available, the following formula (Cockcroft and Gault equation: Cockcroft DW, Gault MH. Prediction of creatinine clearance from serum creatinine. Nephron 1976) may be used to estimate creatinine clearance. The serum creatinine should represent a steady state of renal function.

Males: [(weight in kg) × (140 - age in years)] ÷ [(72) × serum creatinine (mg/100 ml)]

Females: (0.85) × (value calculated for males)

PATIENTS WITH HEPATIC INSUFFICIENCY

No dose adjustment recommendations can be made in patients with impaired hepatic function. (See CLINICAL PHARMACOLOGY, Special Populations, Hepatic Insufficiency and PRECAUTIONS.)

No dosage adjustment is recommended based on age or gender. (See CLINICAL PHARMACOLOGY, Special Populations.)

PREPARATION OF SOLUTION

Preparation for Intravenous Administration

DO NOT MIX OR CO-INFUSE ERTAPENEM FOR INJECTION WITH OTHER MEDICATIONS. DO NOT USE DILUENTS CONTAINING DEXTROSE (α-D-GLUCOSE).

ERTAPENEM FOR INJECTION MUST BE RECONSTITUTED AND THEN DILUTED PRIOR TO ADMINISTRATION.

1. Reconstitute the contents of a 1 g vial of ertapenem for injection with 10 ml of one of the following: water for injection, 0.9% sodium chloride injection or bacteriostatic water for injection.
2. Shake well to dissolve and immediately transfer contents of the reconstituted vial to 50 ml of 0.9% sodium chloride injection.
3. Complete the infusion within 6 hours of reconstitution.

Preparation for Intramuscular Administration

ERTAPENEM FOR INJECTION MUST BE RECONSTITUTED PRIOR TO ADMINSTRATION.

1. Reconstitute the contents of a 1 g vial of ertapenem for injection with 3.2 ml of 1.0% lidocaine HCl injection (refer to the prescribing information for lidocaine HCl) (**without epinephrine**). Shake vial thoroughly to form solution.
2. Immediately withdraw the contents of the vial and administer by deep IM injection into a large muscle mass (such as the gluteal muscles or lateral part of the thigh).
3. The reconstituted IM solution should be used within 1 hour after preparation. **NOTE: THE RECONSTITUTED SOLUTION SHOULD NOT BE ADMINISTERED INTRAVENOUSLY.**

Parenteral drug products should be inspected visually for particulate matter and discoloration prior to use, whenever solution and container permit. Solutions of ertapenem for injection range from colorless to pale yellow. Variations of color within this range do not affect the potency of the product.

ANIMAL PHARMACOLOGY

In repeat-dose studies in rats, treatment-related neutropenia occurred at every dose-level tested, including the lowest dose (2 mg/kg, 12 mg/m^2).

Studies in rabbits and Rhesus monkeys were inconclusive with regard to the effect on neutrophil counts.

HOW SUPPLIED

Invanz is supplied as a sterile lyophilized powder in single dose vials containing ertapenem for IV infusion or for IM injection in vials as 1 g ertapenem equivalent.

STORAGE AND STABILITY

Before reconstitution: Do not store lyophilized powder above 25°C (77°F).

Reconstituted and infusion solutions: The reconstituted solution, immediately diluted in 0.9% sodium chloride injection (see DOSAGE AND ADMINISTRATION, Preparation of Solution), **may be stored at room temperature (25°C) and used within 6 hours or stored for 24 hours under refrigeration (5°C) and used within 4 hours after removal from refrigeration. Solutions of ertapenem for injection should not be frozen.**

PRODUCT LISTING - EQUIVALENTS NOT AVAILABLE

Powder For Injection - Injectable - 1 Gm

10's $499.80 INVANZ, Merck & Company Inc 00006-3843-71

Erythromycin *(001179)*

For related information, see the comparative table section in Appendix A.

Categories: Acne vulgaris; Amebiasis, intestinal; Conjunctivitis, infectious; Diphtheria; Endocarditis, prevention; Erythrasma; Infection, endocervical; Infection, gynecologic; Infection, lower respiratory tract; Infection, ophthalmic; Infection, rectal; Infection, skin and skin structures; Infection, upper respiratory tract; Infection, urethra; Legionnaires' disease; Pelvic inflammatory disease; Pertussis; Pneumonia; Rheumatic fever, prophylaxis; Syphilis; Pregnancy Category B; FDA Approved 1964 Jun; WHO Formulary

Drug Classes: Antibiotics, macrolides; Anti-infectives, ophthalmic; Anti-infectives, topical; Ophthalmics

Brand Names: A T S; Akne-Mycin; C-Solve-2; Del-Mycin; E-Base; ETS; Emgel; Erycette; Erygel; Erythra-Derm; **Ilotycin**; PCE; Romycin; Sansac; Staticin; T-Stat

Foreign Brand Availability: Abboticin (Denmark; Finland; Norway; Sweden); Abboticine (Denmark; Finland; Norway; Sweden); Abomacetin (Japan); Acneryne (Belgium); Acnesol (India); Aknederm Ery Gel (Germany); Aknemycin (Austria; Belgium; Germany); Deripil (Spain); E-Mycin (Bahrain; Cyprus; Egypt; Hong-Kong; India; Iran; Iraq; Israel; Jordan; Kuwait; Lebanon; Libya; Malaysia; Oman; Qatar; Republic-of-Yemen; Saudi-Arabia; Syria; United-Arab-Emirates); Emu-V (New-Zealand; South-Africa); Emu-Ve (Argentina); Emuvin (Austria); Emycin (Korea); Erimycin-T (Thailand); Eritrocina (Italy); Eritromicina (Colombia); Ermycin (Bahamas; Bahrain; Barbados; Belize; Bermuda; Curacao; Cyprus; Egypt; Guyana; Iran; Iraq; Israel; Jamaica; Jordan; Kuwait; Lebanon; Libya; Netherland-Antilles; Oman; Puerto-Rico; Qatar; Republic-of-Yemen; Saudi-Arabia; Surinam; Syria; Trinidad; United-Arab-Emirates); Eros (Indonesia); Eryacne (Australia; France; Hong-Kong; New-Zealand; Singapore; Thailand); Eryacnen (Ecuador); Ery-B (Taiwan); Eryc (Australia; Bahamas; Barbados; Belize; Bermuda; Bulgaria; China; Curacao; Czech-Republic; Guyana; Hungary; Israel; Jamaica; Korea; Netherland-Antilles; Netherlands; New-Zealand; Puerto-Rico; Russia; Surinam; Trinidad); Eryc-125 (Canada); Eryc-250 (Canada); Eryc LD (Australia); Erycen (England; Ireland); Erycin (Denmark; Philippines); Erycinum (Austria); Eryderm (Bahrain; Belgium; Cyprus; Egypt; Iran; Iraq; Israel; Jordan; Kuwait; Lebanon; Libya; Malaysia; Mexico; Netherlands; Oman; Qatar; Republic-of-Yemen; Russia; Saudi-Arabia; South-Africa; Switzerland; Syria; United-Arab-Emirates); Erydermer (Germany); Ery-Diolan (Bahrain; Cyprus; Egypt; Iran; Iraq; Israel; Jordan; Kuwait; Lebanon; Libya; Oman; Qatar; Republic-of-Yemen; Saudi-Arabia; Syria; United-Arab-Emirates); Eryhexal (Germany; Russia); Erymax (Belgium; Benin; Burkina-Faso; Ethiopia; Finland; Gambia; Ghana; Guinea; Ivory-Coast; Kenya; Liberia; Malawi; Mali; Mauritania; Mauritius; Morocco; Niger; Nigeria; Norway; Philippines; Senegal; Seychelles; Sierra-Leone; South-Africa; Sudan; Sweden; Tanzania; Tunia; Uganda; Zambia; Zimbabwe); Ery-maxin (Austria); Erymed (Indonesia); Erysafe (India); Ery-Tab (Bahamas; Barbados; Belize; Bermuda; Curacao; Guyana; Jamaica; Netherland-Antilles; Puerto-Rico; Surinam; Thailand; Trinidad); Erytab (Israel); Erythrocin (Hong-Kong; India; Turkey); Erythromid (Canada; Ireland; South-Africa); Erythromycin (Denmark; Hungary; India); Erythro-Teva (Israel); Erytop (Germany); Erytrarco (Switzerland); Erytrociclin (Italy); Etinycine (China); Etrolate (Thailand); Ilotycin T.S. (South-Africa); Inderm Gel (Germany); Latotryd (Mexico); Lederpax (Mexico); Mephamycin (Bahrain; Cyprus; Egypt; Iran; Iraq; Israel; Jordan; Kuwait; Lebanon; Libya; Oman; Qatar; Republic-of-Yemen; Saudi-Arabia; Syria; United-Arab-Emirates); Monomycin (Germany); Oftamolets (Argentina); Oftalmolosa Cusi Eritromicina (Spain); Paediathrocin (Germany); Pantodrin (Spain); Pantomicina (Argentina; Ecuador); Primacine (Indonesia); Robimycin (Benin; Burkina-Faso; Ethiopia; Gambia; Ghana; Guinea; Ivory-Coast; Kenya; Liberia; Malawi; Mali; Mauritania; Mauritius; Morocco; Niger; Nigeria; Senegal; Seychelles; Sierra-Leone; South-Africa; Sudan; Tanzania; Tunia; Uganda; Zambia; Zimbabwe); Sans-acne (Canada; Mexico); Skid Gel E (Germany); Stiemycin (Benin; Burkina-Faso; Costa-Rica; Dominican-Republic; England; Ethiopia; Gambia; Ghana; Guatemala; Guinea; Hong-Kong; Ireland; Ivory-Coast; Kenya; Korea; Liberia; Malawi; Malaysia; Mali; Mauritania; Mauritius; Morocco; New-Zealand; Nicaragua; Niger; Nigeria; Panama; Philippines; Senegal; Seychelles; Sierra-Leone; South-Africa; Sudan; Tanzania; Thailand; Tunia; Uganda; Zambia; Zimbabwe); Stimycine (France)

Cost of Therapy: $5.98 (Infection; E-Mycin; 250 mg; 4 tablets/day; 10 day supply)
$12.63 (Infection; E-Mycin; 333 mg; 3 tablets/day; 10 day supply)
$7.47 (Infection; Generic Tablets; 333 mg; 3 tablets/day; 10 day supply)

DESCRIPTION

Erythromycin is produced from a strain of *Saccaropolyspora erythraea* (formerly *Streptomyces erythraeus*) and belongs to the macrolide group of antibiotics. It is basic and readily forms salts with acids but it is the base which is microbiologically active. Chemically, erythromicin is $C_{37}H_{67}NO_{13}$.

The chemical name for Erythromycin is (3*R**, 4*S**, 5*S**, 6*R**, 7*R**, 9*R**, 11*R**, 12*R**, 13*S**, 14*R**)-4-[(2, 6-Dideoxy-3-C-methyl-3-*O*-methyl-α-L-*ribo*-hexopyranosyl)oxy]-14-ethyl-7, 12, 13-trihydroxy-3, 5, 7, 9, 11, 13-hexamethyl-6- [[3, 4, 6-trideoxy-3-(dimethylamino)-β-D-*xylo*-hexopyranosyl]oxy]oxacyclotetradecane-2, 10-dione.

Erythromycin Delayed-Release Capsules: Erythromycin has the molecular weight of 733.94. The base is white to off-white crystals or powder slightly soluble in water, soluble in alcohol, in chloroform, and in ether. It is odorless or practically odorless. Erythromycin delayed-release tablets are specially enteric-coated to protect the contents from the inactivating effects of gastric acidity and to permit efficient absorption of the antibiotic in the small intestine.

Erythromycin delayed-release capsules contain enteric-coated pellets of erythromycin base for oral administration. Each Erythromycin delayed-release capsule contains 250 mg of erythromycin base. *Also Contains:* Croscarmellose sodium, nonpareil seeds; povidone: FD&C yellow no. 6 aluminum lake and other ingredients. The capsule shell contains gelatin, titanium dioxide; FD&C yellow no. 6.

Topical: Erythromycin topical solution contains 20 mg of erythromycin base in a vehicle consisting of alcohol (66%), propylene glycol, and citric acid to adjust pH.

Pledgets: Each ml of expressible liquid contains 20 mg erythromycin in a base of alcohol (68.5%) (denatured with *tert*-butyl alcohol and denatonium benzoate), propylene glycol and citric acid to adjust pH. Each pledget is filled to contain 0.8 ml of erythromycin topical sollution.

CLINICAL PHARMACOLOGY

Orally administered erythromycin base and its salts are readily absorbed in the microbiologically active form. Interindividual variations in the absorption of erythromycin are, however, observed, and some patients do not achieve acceptable serum levels. Erythromycin is largely bound to plasma proteins, and the freely dissociating bound fraction after administration of erythromycin base represents 90% of the total erythromycin absorbed. After absorption, erythromycin diffuses readily into most body fluids. In the absence of meningeal inflammation, low concentrations are normally achieved in the spinal fluid, but the passage of the drug across the blood-brain barrier increases in meningitis. Erythromycin is excreted in breast milk. The drug crosses the placental barrier, but fetal plasma levels are low. Erythromycin is not removed by peritoneal dialysis or hemodialysis.

In the presence of normal hepatic function erythromycin is concentrated in the liver and is excreted in the bile; the effect of hepatic dysfunction on biliary excretion of erythromycin is not known. After oral administration, less than 5% of the administered dose can be recovered in the active form in the urine.

The enteric coating of pellets in erythromycin delayed-release capsules protects the erythromycin base from inactivation by gastric acidity. Because of their small size and enteric coating, the pellets readily pass intact from the stomach to the small intestine and dissolve efficiently to allow absorption of erythromycin in a uniform manner. After administration of a single dose of a 250 mg erythromycin delayed-release capsules, peak serum levels in the range of 1.13-1.68 μg/ml are attained in approximately 3 hours and decline to 0.30-0.42 μg/ml in 6 hours. Optimal conditions for stability in the presence of gastric secretion and for complete absorption are attained when erythromycin delayed-release capsules is taken on an empty stomach.

Pledgets: The exact mechanism by which erythmromycin reduces lesions of acne vulgaris is not fully known: however, the effect appears to be due in part to the antibacterial activity of the drug.

MICROBIOLOGY

Erythromycin acts by inhibition of protein synthesis in susceptible organisms by reversibly binding to 50 S ribosomal subunits, thereby inhibiting translocation of aminoacyl transfer-RNA and inhibiting polypeptide synthesis. It does not affect nucleic acid synthesis. Antagonism has been demonstrated *in vitro* between erythromycin, clindamycin, lincomycin, and chloramphenicol. Many strains of *Haemophilus influenzae* are resistant to erythromycin alone, but are susceptible to erythromycin and sulfonamides together. Staphylococci resistant to erythromycin may emerge during a course of erythromycin therapy. Specimens should be obtained for culture and susceptibility testing.

Erythromycin is usually active against the following organisms *in vitro* and in clinical infections:

Streptococcus pyogenes (group A Beta-hemolytic streptococci), Alpha-hemolytic streptococci (viridans group), *Staphylococcus aureus* (resistant organisms may emerge during treatment), *Streptococcus pneumoniae, Mycoplasma pneumoniae, Treponema pallidum, Corynebacterium diphtheriae, Corynebacterium minutissimum, Entamoeba histolytica, Listeria monocytogenes, Neisseria gonorrhoeae, Bordetella pertussis, Legionella pneumophila* (agent of Legionnaires' disease), *Ureaplasma urealyticum, Chlamydia trachomatis.*

SUSCEPTIBILITY TESTING

Quantitative methods that require measurement of zone diameters give the most precise estimates of antibiotic susceptibility. One such standardized single disc procedure has been recommended for use with discs to test susceptibility to erythromycin.[1]

Interpretation involves correlation of the zone diameters obtained in the disc test with minimal inhibitory concentration (MIC) values for erythromycin.

Reports from the laboratory giving results of the standardized single-disc susceptibility test using a 15 μg erythromycin disc should be interpreted according to the following criteria:

Susceptible organisms produce zones of 18 mm or greater indicating that the tested organism is likely to respond to therapy.

Resistant organisms produce zones of 13 mm or less, indicating that other therapy should be selected.

Organisms of intermediate susceptibility produce zones of 14-17 mm. The "intermediate" category provides a "buffer zone" which should prevent small, uncontrolled technical factors from causing major discrepancies in interpretations; thus when a zone diameter falls within the "intermediate" range, the results may be considered equivocal. If alternate drugs are not available, confirmation by dilution tests may be indicated.

Standardized procedures require the use of control organisms. The 15 μg erythromycin disc should give some diameter between 22 and 30 mm for *S. aureus* ATCC 25923 control strain.

A bacterial isolate may be considered susceptible if the MIC value[2] for erythromycin is not more than 2 μg/ml. Organisms are considered resistant if the MIC is 8 μg/ml or higher.

The MIC of erythromycin for *S. aureus* ATCC 29213 control strain should be between 0.12 and 0.5 μg/ml.

INDICATIONS AND USAGE

ERYTHROMYCIN DELAYED-RELEASE CAPSULES

Erythromycin delayed-release capsules are indicated in the treatment of infections caused by susceptible strains of the designated microorganisms in the diseases listed below:

Upper Respiratory Tract Infection: Upper respiratory tract infections of mild to moderate degree caused by *Streptococcus pyogenes* (group A beta-hemolytic streptococci); *Strepto-*

coccus pneumoniae (Diplococcus pneumoniae); Haemophilus influenzae (when used concomitantly with adequate doses of sulfonamides, since many strains of *H. influenzae* are not susceptible at the erythromycin concentrations ordinarily achieved). See appropriate sulfonamide labeling for prescribing information.
Lower Respiratory Tract Infection: Lower respiratory tract infections of mild to moderate severity caused by *Streptococcus pyogenes* (group A beta-hemolytic streptococci); *Streptococcus pneumoniae (Diplococcus pneumoniae).*
Respiratory Tract Infection: Respiratory tract infections due to *Mycoplasma pneumoniae.*
Pertussis: Pertussis (whooping cough) caused by *Bordetella pertussis.* Erythromycin is effective in eliminating the organism from the nasopharynx of infected individuals, rendering them noninfectious. Some clinical studies suggest that erythromycin may be helpful in the prophylaxis of pertussis in exposed susceptible individuals.
Diphtheria: As an adjunct to antitoxin in infections due to *Corynebacterium diphtheriae,* to prevent establishment of carriers and to eradicate the organism in carriers.
Erythrasma: In the treatment of infections due to *Corynebacterium minutissimum.*
Intestinal Amebiasis: Intestinal amebiasis caused by *Entamoeba histolytica* (oral erythromycins only). Extraenteric amebiasis requires treatment with other agents.
Acute Pelvic Inflammatory Disease: Acute pelvic inflammatory disease caused by *Neisseria gonorrhoeae.* Erythromycin lactobionate for injection, USP followed by erythromycin base orally, as an alternative drug in treatment of acute inflammatory disease caused by *N. gonorrhoeae* in female patients with a history of sensitivity to penicillin. Before treatment of gonorrhoeae, patients who are suspected of also having syphilis should have a microscopic examination for *Treponema pallidum* (by immunofluorescence or dark field) before receiving erythromycin and monthly serologic tests for a minimum of 4 months thereafter.
Infection: Infections due to *Listeria monocytogenes, Moraxella (Branhamella) catahalis.*
Skin and Soft Tissue Infection: Skin and soft tissue infections of mild to moderate severity caused by *Streptococcus pyogenes* and *Staphylococcus aureus* (resistant staphylococci may emerge during treatment).
Primary Syphilis: Primary syphilis caused by *Treponema pallidum.* Erythromycin (oral forms only) is an alternate choice of treatment for primary syphilis in patients allergic to the penicillins. In treatment of primary syphilis, spinal fluid should be examined before treatment and as part of the follow-up after therapy.
Erythromycins are indicated for treatment of the following infections caused by *Chlamydia trachomatis:* Conjunctivitis of the newborn, pneumonia of infancy, urogenital infections during pregnancy. When tetracyclines are contraindicated or not tolerated, erythromycin is indicated for the treatment of uncomplicated urethral, endocervical, or rectal infections in adults due to *Chlamydia trachomatis.*[4]
Nongonococcal Urethritis: Erythromycin is indicated for the treatment of nongonococcal urethritis caused by *Ureaplasma urealyticum* when tetracyclines are contraindicated or not tolerated.[4]
Legionnaires' Disease: Legionnaires' disease caused by *Legionella pneumophila.* Although no controlled clinical efficacy studies have been conducted, *in vitro* and limited preliminary clinical data suggest that erythromycin may be effective in treating Legionnaires' disease.
Therapy with erythromycin should be monitored by bacteriological studies and by clinical response (see CLINICAL PHARMACOLOGY, Microbiology).
Prevention of Initial Attacks of Rheumatic Fever: Penicillin is considered by the American Heart Association to be the drug of choice in the prevention of initial attacks of rheumatic fever (treatment of group A beta-hemolytic streptococcal infections of the upper respiratory tract).[5] Erythromycin is indicated for the treatment of penicillin-allergic patients. The therapeutic dose should be administered for 10 days.
Prevention of Recurrent Attacks of Rheumatic Fever: Penicillin or sulfonamides are considered by the American Heart Association to be the drug of choice in the prevention of recurrent attacks of rheumatic fever. In patients allergic to penicillin and sulfonamides, oral erythromycin is recommended by the American Heart Association in the long-term prophylaxis of streptoccal pharyngitis (for the prevention of recurrent attacks of rheumatic fever).[5]
Prevention of Bacterial Endocarditis: Although no controlled clinical efficacy trials have been conducted, oral erythromycin has been recommended by the American Heart Association for the prevention of bacterial endocarditis in penicillin-allergic patients with most congenital cardiac malformations, rheumatic or other acquired valvular dysfunction, idiopathic hypertrophic, subaortic stenosis (HSS), previous history of bacterial endocarditis and mitral valve prolapse with insufficiency when they undergo dental procedures and surgical procedures of the upper respiratory tract. [5]

TOPICAL

Pledgets are indicated for the topical control of acne vulgaris.

CONTRAINDICATIONS

Erythromycin is contraindicated in patients with known hypersensitivity to this antibiotic.
Erythromycin is contraindicated in patients taking terfenadine, astemizole, or cisapride. (See DRUG INTERACTIONS.)

TOPICAL

Ery 2% Pads are contraindicated in those individuals who have shown hypersensitivity to any of its components.

WARNINGS

There have been reports of hepatic dysfunction, including increased liver enzymes, and hepatocellular and/or cholestatic hepatitis, with or without jaundice, occurring in patients receiving oral erythromycin products.
There have been reports suggesting that erythromycin does not reach the fetus in adequate concentration to prevent congenital syphilis. Infants born to women treated during pregnancy with oral erythromycin for early syphilis should be treated with an appropriate penicillin regimen.
Pseudomembranous colitis has been reported with nearly all antibacterial agents, including erythromycin, and may range in severity from mild to life threatening. Therefore, it is important to consider this diagnosis in patients who present with diarrhea subsequent to the administration of antibacterial agents.
Treatment with antibacterial agents alters the normal flora of the colon and may permit overgrowth of clostridia. Studies indicate that a toxin produced by *Clostridium difficile* is one primary cause of "antibiotic-associated colitis".
After the diagnosis of pseudomembranous colitis has been established, therapeutic measures should be initiated. Mild cases of pseudomembranous colitis usually respond to discontinuation of the drug alone. In moderate to severe cases, consideration should be given to management with fluids and electrolytes, protein supplementation, and treatment with an antibacterial clinically effective against *Clostridium difficile* colitis.
Rhabdomyolysis with or without renal impairment has been reported in seriously ill patients receiving erythromycin concomitantly with lovastatin. Therefore, patients receiving concomitant lovastatin and erythromycin should be carefully monitored for creatine kinase (CK) and serum transaminase levels. (See package insert for lovastatin.)

PRECAUTIONS

GENERAL

Delayed Release Capsules: Erythromycin is principally excreted by the liver. Caution should be exercised when erythromycin is administered to patients with impaired hepatic function (see CLINICAL PHARMACOLOGY and WARNINGS).
There have been reports that erythromycin may aggravate the weakness of patients with myasthenia gravis.
Prolonged or repeated use of erythromycin may result in an overgrowth of nonsusceptible bacteria or fungi. If superinfection occurs, erythromycin should be discontinued and appropriate therapy instituted.
When indicated, incision and drainage or other surgical procedures should be performed in conjunction with antibiotic therapy.
Topical: The use of antibiotic agents may be associated with the overgrowth of antibiotic-resistant organisms. If this occurs, administration of the drug should be discontinued and appropriate measures taken.
Pledgets: For topical use only; not for opthalmic use. Concommitant topical acne therapy should be used with caution because a possible cumulative irritancy effect may occur, especially with the use of peeling, desquamating, or abrasive agents. Avoid contact with eyes and all mucous membranes.

INFORMATION FOR THE PATIENT

Topical: This form of Erythromycin is for external use only and should be kept away from the eyes, nose, mouth, and other mucous membranes. Concomitant topical acne therapy should be used with caution because a cumulative irritant effect may occur, especially with the use of peeling, desquamating, or abrasive agents.
Pledgets: Patients using Ery 2% pads should receive the following information and instructions:

1. This medication is to be used as directed by the physician. It is for external use only. Avoid contact with eyes, nose, mouth, and all mucous membranes.
2. This medication should not be used for any disorder other than that for which it was prescribed.
3. Patients should not use any other topical acne medication unless otherwise directed by their physician.
4. Patients should report to their physician any signs of local adverse reactions.

LABORATORY TESTS

Delayed Release Capsules: Erythromycin may interfere with AGT (SGOT) determinations if azonefast violet B or diphenylhydrazine colormetric determinations are used. Erythromycin interferes with the fluorometric determination of urinary catecholamines.

CARCINOGENESIS, MUTAGENESIS, AND IMPAIRMENT OF FERTILITY

Long-term (2 year) oral studies conducted in rats with erythromycin ethyl succinate and erythromycin base did not provide evidence of tumorigenicity. There was no apparent effect on male or female fertility in rats fed erythromycin (base) at levels up to 0.25 %of diet.
Pledgets: No animal studies have been performed to evaluate the carcinogenic and mutagenic potential or effects on fertility of topical erythromycin.

PREGNANCY CATEGORY B

Delayed Release Capsules: There is no evidence of teratogenicity or any other adverse effect on reproduction in female rats fed erythromycin base (up to 0.25 percent of diet) prior to and during mating, during gestation, and through weaning of two successive litters. There are, however, no adequate and well-controlled studies in pregnant women. Because animal reproduction studies are not always predictive of human response, this drug should be used during pregnancy only if clearly needed. Erythromycin has been reported to cross the placental barrier in humans, but fetal plasma levels are generally low.
Topical: Animal reproduction studies have not been conducted with this drug. It is also not known whether erythromycin can cause fetal harm when administered to a pregnant woman or can affect reproduction capacity. Erythromycin should be given to a pregnant women only when clearly needed.

LABOR AND DELIVERY

The effect of erythromycin on labor and delivery is unknown.

NURSING MOTHERS

Delayed Release Capsules: Erythromycin is excreted in breast milk; therefore, caution should be exercised when erythromycin is administered to a nursing woman.
Topical: It is not known whether erythromycin is excreted in human milk after topical application. However, erythromycin is excreted in human milk following oral and parenteral erythromycin administration. Caution should be exercised when erythromycin is administered to a nursing woman.

PEDIATRIC USE

Delayed Release Capsules: See INDICATIONS AND USAGE and DOSAGE AND ADMINISTRATION.

Pledgets: Safety and effectiveness of this product in pediatric patients have not been established.

DRUG INTERACTIONS

Erythromycin use in patients who are receiving high doses of theophylline may be associated with an increase in serum theophylline levels and potential theophylline toxicity. In case of theophylline toxicity and/or elevated serum theophylline levels, the dose of theophylline should be reduced while the patient is receiving concomitant erythromycin therapy.

Concomitant administration of erythromycin and digoxin has been reported to result in elevated digoxin serum levels.

There have been reports of increased anticoagulant effects when erythromycin and oral anticoagulants were used concomitantly. Increased anticoagulation effects due to interactions of erythromycin with various oral anticoagulents may be more pronounced in the elderly.

Concurrent use of erythromycin and ergotamine or dihydroergotamine has been associated in some patients with acute ergot toxicity characterized by severe peripheral vasospasm and dysesthesia.

Erythromycin has been reported to decrease the clearance of triazolam and midazolam and thus may increase the pharmacologic effect of these benzodiazepines.

The use of erythromycin in patients concurrently taking drugs metabolized by the cytochrome P450 system may be associated with elevations in serum levels of these other drugs. There have been reports of interactions of erythromycin with carbamazepine, cyclosporine, tacrolimus, hexobarbital, phenytoin, alfentanil, cisapride, disopyramide, lovastatin, bromocriptine, valproate, terfenadine, and astemizole. Serum concentrations of drugs metabolized by the cytochrome P450 system should be monitored closely in patients concurrently receiving erythromycin.

Erythromycin has been reported to significantly alter the metabolism of nonsedating antihistamines terfenadine and astemizole when taken concomitantly. Rare cases of serious cardiovascular adverse events, including electrocardiographic QT/QT$_c$ interval prolongation, cardiac arrest, torsades de pointes, and other ventricular arrhythmias have been observed (see CONTRAINDICATIONS). In addition, deaths have been reported rarely with concomitant administration of terfenadine and erythromycin.

There have been postmarketing reports of drug interactions when erythromycin is coadministered with cisapride, resulting in QT prolongation, cardiac arrythmias, ventricular tachycardia, ventricular fibrulation, and torsades de pointes, most likely due to inhibition of hepatic metabolism of cisapride by erythromycin. Fatalities have been reported. (See CONTRAINDICATIONS.)

Patients receiving concomitant lovastatin and erythromycin should be carefully monitored; cases of rhabdomyolysis have been reported in seriously ill patients.

ADVERSE REACTIONS

DELAYED-RELEASE CAPSULES

The most frequent side effects of oral erythromycin preparations are gastrointestinal and are dose-related. They include nausea, vomiting, abdominal pain, diarrhea and anorexia. Symptoms of hepatitis, hepatic dysfunction and/or abnormal liver function test results may occur (see WARNINGS).

Onset of pseudomembranous colitis symptoms may occur during or after antibiotic treatment (see WARNINGS).

Rarely, erythromycin has been associated with the production of ventricular arrhythmias, including ventricular tachycardia and torsades de pointes, in individuals with prolonged QT intervals. There have been isolated reports of other cardiovascular symptoms such as chest pain, dizziness, and palpitations; however, a cause and effect relationship has not been established.

Allergic reactions ranging from urticaria to anaphylaxis have occurred. Skin reactions ranging from mile eruptions to erythema multiforme, Stevens-Johnson syndrome, and toxic epidermal necrolysis have been reported rarely.

There have been isolated reports of reversible hearing loss occurring chiefly in patients with renal insufficiency and in patients receiving high doses of erythromycin.

TOPICAL

The following local adverse reactions have been reported occasionally: peeling, dryness, itching, erythema, and oiliness. Irritation of the eyes and tenderness of the skin have also been reported with topical use of erythromycin. Generalized urticarial reactions, possibly related to the use of erythromycin, which required systemic steroid therapy have been reported.

Of a total of 90 patients exposed to this form during clinical effectiveness studied, 17 experienced some type of adverse effect. These included dry skin, scaly skin, pruritus, irritation of the eye, and burning sensation.

DOSAGE AND ADMINISTRATION

DELAYED-RELEASE CAPSULES

Erythromycin delayed-release capsules, are well absorbed and may be given without regard to meals. Optimum blood levels are obtained in a fasting state (administration at least one half hour and preferably two hours before or after a meal); however, blood levels obtained upon administration of enteric-coated erythromycin products in the presence of food are still above minimal inhibitory concentrations (MICs) of most organisms for which erythromycin is indicated.

Adults: The usual dose is 250 mg every 6 hours taken 1 hour before meals. If twice a day dosage is desired, the recommended dose is 500 mg every 12 hours. The 333 mg tablet is recommended if dosage is desired every 8 hours. Dosage may be increased up to 4 g/day, according to the severity of the infection. Twice a day dosing is not recommended when doses larger than 1 g daily are administered.

Children: Age, weight, and severity of the infection are important factors in determining the proper dosage. The usual dosage is 30-50 mg/kg/day in divided doses. For the treatment of more severe infections, this dose may be doubled but should not exceed 4 mg/day.

Streptococcal Infections: A therapeutic dosage of oral erythromycin should be administered for at least 10 days. For continuous prophylaxis against recurrences of streptococcal infections in persons with a history of rheumatic heart disease, the dose is 250 mg twice a day. The American Heart Assocation suggests a dosage of 250 mg of erythromycin orally, twice a day in long-term prophylaxis of streptococcal upper respiratory tract infections for the prevention of recurring attacks of rheumatic fever in patients allergic to penicillin and sulfonamides.[4]

For the prevention of bacterial endocarditis in penicillin-allergic patients with valvular heart disease who are to undergo dental procedures or surgical procedures of the upper respiratory tract, the adult dose is 1 g orally (20 mg/kg for children) 1 hour prior to the procedure and then 500 mg (10 mg/kg for children) orally 6 hours later [3] (see INDICATIONS AND USAGE).

Primary Syphilis: 30-40 g given in divided doses over a period of 10-15 days.

Intestinal Amebiasis: 250 mg 4 times daily for 10-14 days for adults; 30-50 mg/kg/day in divided doses for 10-14 days for children.

Legionnaires' Disease: Although optimal doses have not been established, doses utilized in reported clinical data were those recommended above (1-4 g daily in divided doses).

For Conjunctivitis of the Newborn Caused by *Chlamydia trachomatis:* Oral erytromycin suspension 50 mg/kg/day in 4 divided doses for at least 2 weeks. [2]

For Pneumonia of Infancy Caused by *Chlamydia trachomatis:* Although the optimal duration of therapy has not been established, the recommended therapy is oral erythromycin suspension 50 mg/kg/day in 4 divided doses for at least 3 weeks. [2]

Urogenital Infections During Pregnancy Due to *Chlamydia trachomatis:* Although the optimal dose and duration of therapy have not been established, the suggested treatment is erythromycin 500 mg, by mouth, 4 times a day on an empty stomach for at least 7 days. For women who cannot tolerate this regimen, a decreased dose of 250 mg, by mouth, 4 times a day should be used for at least 14 days. [4]

For Adults With Uncomplicated Urethral, Endocervical, or Rectal Infections Caused by *Chlamydia trachomatis* in whom Tetracyclines are Contraindicated or not Tolerated: 500 mg, by mouth, 4 times a day for at least 7 days. [4]

Pertussis: Although optimum dosage and duration of therapy have not been established, doses of erythromycin utilized in reported clinical studies were 40-50 mg/kg/day, given in divided doses for 5-14 days.

Nongonococcal Urethritis Due to *Ureaplasma urealyticum,* When Tetracycline is Contraindicated or not Tolerated: 500 mg of erythromycin, orally, four times daily for at least 7 days[4].

Acute Pelvic Inflammatory Disease Due to *N gonorrhoeae:* 500 mg IV of erythromycin lactobionate for injection every 6 hours for 3 days followed by 250 mg of erythromycin, orally every 6 hours for 7 days.

TOPICAL

Pledgets: The Ery 2% pad should be rubbed over the affected area twice a day after skin is thoroughly washed with warm water and soap and patted dry. Acne lesions on the face neck, shoulder, chest and back may be treated in this manner. Additional pledgets may be used, if needed. Each pledget should be used once and discarded. Close jar tightly after each use.

Topical Liquid: Erythromycin topical solution should be applied to the affected area twice a day after the skin is thoroughly washed with warm water and soap and patted dry. Moisten the applicator or a pad with the solution, then rub over the affected area. Acne lesions of the face, neck, shoulder, chest, and back may be treated in this manner.

HOW SUPPLIED

Pledgets: Ery 2% Pads are available in a plastic jar containing 60 pledgets. Each pledget is filled to contain 0.8 ml of erythromycin topical sollution. Keep jar tightly closed. Store at controlled room temperature between 15° and 30°C (59° and 86°F).

Storage: Store at a room temperature between 15° and 30°C (59° and 86°F).

PRODUCT LISTING - RATED THERAPEUTICALLY EQUIVALENT

Capsule, Delayed Rel Pellets - Oral - 250 mg			
100's	$18.89	FEDERAL UPPER LIMIT, H.C.F.A. F F P	99999-1179-16
Capsule, Enteric Coated - Oral - 250 mg			
20's	$8.68	GENERIC, Dhs Inc	55887-0855-20
20's	$19.82	GENERIC, Dhs Inc	55887-0746-20
20's	$20.66	ERYC, Pd-Rx Pharmaceuticals	55289-0111-20
28's	$7.51	GENERIC, Dhs Inc	55887-0855-28
28's	$21.38	ERYC, Pd-Rx Pharmaceuticals	55289-0111-28
30's	$13.02	GENERIC, Dhs Inc	55887-0855-30
40's	$21.88	ERYC, Prescript Pharmaceuticals	00247-0390-40
40's	$31.68	ERYC, Pd-Rx Pharmaceuticals	55289-0111-40
40's	$33.10	ERYC, Pharma Pac	52959-0341-40
56's	$38.07	GENERIC, Dhs Inc	55887-0746-56
56's	$39.86	ERYC, Pd-Rx Pharmaceuticals	55289-0111-56
60's	$41.84	ERYC, Pharma Pac	52959-0341-60
80's	$56.24	ERYC, Pd-Rx Pharmaceuticals	55289-0111-80
100's	$24.23	GENERIC, Moore, H.L. Drug Exchange Inc	00839-7602-06
100's	$25.25	GENERIC, Major Pharmaceuticals Inc	00904-2465-60
100's	$25.25	GENERIC, Major Pharmaceuticals Inc	00904-7743-60
100's	$25.77	GENERIC, Abbott Pharmaceutical	00074-6301-13
100's	$26.65	GENERIC, Barr Laboratories Inc	00555-0584-02
100's	$28.05	GENERIC, Aligen Independent Laboratories Inc	00405-4399-01
100's	$28.80	GENERIC, Qualitest Products Inc	00603-3548-21
100's	$30.65	GENERIC, Parmed Pharmaceuticals Inc	00349-8974-01
100's	$56.45	ERYC, Warner Chilcott Laboratories	00430-0696-24
Gel - Topical - 2%			
27 gm	$30.07	GENERIC, Elan Pharmaceuticals	51479-0440-01

30 gm	$24.73	GENERIC, Qualitest Products Inc	00603-7735-78
30 gm	$24.73	GENERIC, Glades Pharmaceuticals	59366-2462-03
30 gm	$25.19	GENERIC, Fougera	00168-0216-30
30 gm	$29.94	ERYGEL, Merz Pharmaceuticals	00259-4312-30
30 gm	$32.02	A/T/S, Medicis Dermatologics Inc	99207-0018-30
30 gm	$32.63	ERYGEL, Allscripts Pharmaceutical Company	54569-1767-01
50 gm	$45.85	GENERIC, Elan Pharmaceuticals	51479-0440-02
60 gm	$40.74	GENERIC, Qualitest Products Inc	00603-7735-88
60 gm	$40.74	GENERIC, Glades Pharmaceuticals	59366-2462-05
60 gm	$44.34	GENERIC, Fougera	00168-0216-60
60 gm	$56.30	ERYGEL, Merz Pharmaceuticals	00259-4312-60

Ointment - Ophthalmic - 0.5%

1 gm x 50	$97.00	GENERIC, Bausch and Lomb	24208-0910-19
1 gm x 50	$208.50	GENERIC, Fougera	00168-0070-11
3.50 gm	$3.06	GENERIC, Major Pharmaceuticals Inc	00904-2990-38
3.50 gm	$4.15	GENERIC, Aligen Independent Laboratories Inc	00405-0945-08
3.50 gm	$4.35	GENERIC, Ivax Corporation	00182-5116-31
3.50 gm	$4.39	GENERIC, Moore, H.L. Drug Exchange Inc	00839-6767-43
3.50 gm	$4.40	GENERIC, Qualitest Products Inc	00603-7137-70
3.50 gm	$4.90	GENERIC, Akorn Inc	17478-0070-35
3.50 gm	$4.95	GENERIC, Major Pharmaceuticals Inc	00904-7926-38
3.50 gm	$5.21	GENERIC, Fougera	00168-0070-38
3.50 gm	$5.62	GENERIC, Bausch and Lomb	24208-0910-55
3.50 gm	$5.63	GENERIC, Ocusoft	54799-0540-35
3.50 gm x 24	$125.04	GENERIC, Fougera	00168-0070-39

Solution - Topical - 1.5%

60 ml	$5.25	GENERIC, Major Pharmaceuticals Inc	00904-2844-03
60 ml	$28.36	STATICIN, Bristol-Myers Squibb	00072-8000-60
100 ml	$6.25	GENERIC, Cmc-Consolidated Midland Corporation	00223-6145-01

Solution - Topical - 2%

59 ml	$30.34	ERYMAX, Merz Pharmaceuticals	00023-0540-02
60 ml	$3.95	GENERIC, Syosset Laboratories Company	47854-0669-20
60 ml	$4.12	FEDERAL UPPER LIMIT, H.C.F.A. F F P	99999-1179-10
60 ml	$5.25	GENERIC, Paddock Laboratories Inc	00574-0014-02
60 ml	$5.30	GENERIC, Qualitest Products Inc	00603-7737-52
60 ml	$6.00	GENERIC, Raway Pharmacal Inc	00686-1244-02
60 ml	$6.88	GENERIC, Bausch and Lomb	24208-0421-60
60 ml	$6.88	GENERIC, Bausch and Lomb	24208-0551-67
60 ml	$6.90	GENERIC, Clay-Park Laboratories Inc	45802-0038-46
60 ml	$6.95	GENERIC, Moore, H.L. Drug Exchange Inc	00839-7023-64
60 ml	$6.95	GENERIC, Morton Grove Pharmaceuticals Inc	60432-0671-60
60 ml	$6.97	GENERIC, Major Pharmaceuticals Inc	00904-2845-03
60 ml	$7.00	GENERIC, Alpharma Uspd Makers Of Barre and Nmc	00472-1244-92
60 ml	$7.49	GENERIC, Geneva Pharmaceuticals	00781-7013-61
60 ml	$7.50	GENERIC, Ivax Corporation	00182-1561-43
60 ml	$7.53	GENERIC, Fougera	00168-0215-60
60 ml	$17.47	GENERIC, Abbott Pharmaceutical	00074-2698-02
60 ml	$19.88	GENERIC, Bioglan Pharmaceutical Inc	62436-0701-01
60 ml	$22.52	GENERIC, Bristol-Myers Squibb	00072-8300-60
60 ml	$27.93	A/T/S, Aventis Pharmaceuticals	00039-0016-60
60 ml	$31.42	A/T/S, Medicis Dermatologics Inc	99207-0019-60
100 ml	$4.80	GENERIC, Cmc-Consolidated Midland Corporation	00223-6146-01

Swab - Topical - 2%

60's	$18.05	GENERIC, Glades Pharmaceuticals	59366-2828-06
60's	$21.31	GENERIC, Ivax Corporation	00172-3621-49
60's	$25.34	GENERIC, Bristol-Myers Squibb	00072-8303-60
60's	$26.04	ERYCETTE, Southwood Pharmaceuticals Inc	58016-3205-01
60's	$26.07	GENERIC, Glades Pharmaceuticals	59366-2878-06
60's	$30.70	ERYCETTE, Janssen Pharmaceuticals	00062-1185-01

Tablet, Coated Particles - Oral - 333 mg

100's	$24.90	GENERIC, Major Pharmaceuticals Inc	00904-2474-60
100's	$31.10	GENERIC, Major Pharmaceuticals Inc	00904-2472-60

Tablet, Enteric Coated - Oral - 250 mg

4's	$1.16	ERY-TAB, Allscripts Pharmaceutical Company	54569-3563-03
6's	$2.85	E-MYCIN, Pd-Rx Pharmaceuticals	55289-0120-06
20's	$5.80	ERY-TAB, Allscripts Pharmaceutical Company	54569-3563-01
20's	$5.89	E-MYCIN, Allscripts Pharmaceutical Company	54569-0123-00
20's	$6.96	GENERIC, Pd-Rx Pharmaceuticals	55289-0645-20
20's	$8.99	ERY-TAB, Pharma Pac	52959-0060-20
28's	$5.06	ERY-TAB, Southwood Pharmaceuticals Inc	58016-0162-28
28's	$8.12	ERY-TAB, Allscripts Pharmaceutical Company	54569-3563-05
28's	$8.24	E-MYCIN, Allscripts Pharmaceutical Company	54569-0123-02
28's	$11.16	GENERIC, Pd-Rx Pharmaceuticals	55289-0645-28
28's	$11.21	E-MYCIN, Pharma Pac	52959-0057-28
28's	$11.59	ERY-TAB, Pharma Pac	52959-0060-28
30's	$5.48	ERY-TAB, Southwood Pharmaceuticals Inc	58016-0162-30
30's	$7.55	ERY-TAB, Abbott Pharmaceutical	00074-6304-30
30's	$8.70	ERY-TAB, Allscripts Pharmaceutical Company	54569-3563-02
30's	$8.83	E-MYCIN, Allscripts Pharmaceutical Company	54569-0123-03
30's	$11.88	ERY-TAB, Pharma Pac	52959-0060-30
30's	$11.97	GENERIC, Pd-Rx Pharmaceuticals	55289-0645-30
40's	$6.30	ERY-TAB, Southwood Pharmaceuticals Inc	58016-0162-40
40's	$11.60	ERY-TAB, Allscripts Pharmaceutical Company	54569-3563-04
40's	$11.78	E-MYCIN, Allscripts Pharmaceutical Company	54569-0123-05
40's	$12.01	E-MYCIN, Pharma Pac	52959-0057-40
40's	$14.04	ERY-TAB, Pharma Pac	52959-0060-40
40's	$17.38	GENERIC, Pd-Rx Pharmaceuticals	55289-0645-40
56's	$16.24	ERY-TAB, Allscripts Pharmaceutical Company	54569-3563-00
56's	$16.80	ERY-TAB, Pharma Pac	52959-0060-56
56's	$18.75	GENERIC, Pd-Rx Pharmaceuticals	55289-0645-56
80's	$23.31	GENERIC, Pd-Rx Pharmaceuticals	55289-0645-80
100's	$14.94	E-MYCIN, Southwood Pharmaceuticals Inc	58016-0140-00
100's	$25.18	ERY-TAB, Abbott Pharmaceutical	00074-6304-13
100's	$30.65	GENERIC, Ivax Corporation	00182-1398-01
100's	$39.90	GENERIC, Pd-Rx Pharmaceuticals	55289-0645-01

E

Tablet, Enteric Coated - Oral - 333 mg

6's	$3.15	GENERIC, Pd-Rx Pharmaceuticals	55289-0915-06
9's	$3.89	E-MYCIN, Allscripts Pharmaceutical Company	54569-0129-09
15's	$7.43	GENERIC, Pd-Rx Pharmaceuticals	55289-0915-15
15's	$7.50	E-MYCIN, Pharma Pac	52959-0058-15
15's	$8.75	ERY-TAB, Pharma Pac	52959-0061-15
18's	$10.16	ERY-TAB, Pharma Pac	52959-0061-18
20's	$13.40	E-MYCIN, Pharma Pac	52959-0058-20
21's	$9.08	E-MYCIN, Allscripts Pharmaceutical Company	54569-0129-03
21's	$10.08	ERY-TAB, Pd-Rx Pharmaceuticals	55289-0525-21
21's	$11.21	ERY-TAB, Dhs Inc	55887-0955-21
21's	$11.48	ERY-TAB, Pharma Pac	52959-0061-21
21's	$12.74	E-MYCIN, Pd-Rx Pharmaceuticals	54569-0813-21
21's	$14.02	E-MYCIN, Pharma Pac	52959-0058-21
24's	$8.25	GENERIC, Pd-Rx Pharmaceuticals	55289-0915-24
24's	$14.48	ERY-TAB, Pharma Pac	52959-0061-24
28's	$14.21	ERY-TAB, Pharma Pac	52959-0061-28
30's	$10.13	GENERIC, Pd-Rx Pharmaceuticals	55289-0915-30
30's	$12.86	ERY-TAB, Dhs Inc	55887-0955-30
30's	$12.98	E-MYCIN, Allscripts Pharmaceutical Company	54569-0129-02
30's	$14.36	ERY-TAB, Pd-Rx Pharmaceuticals	55289-0525-30
30's	$15.17	ERY-TAB, Pharma Pac	52959-0061-30
30's	$18.11	E-MYCIN, Pd-Rx Pharmaceuticals	54569-0813-30
30's	$18.95	E-MYCIN, Pharma Pac	52959-0058-30
40's	$13.88	ERY-TAB, Pd-Rx Pharmaceuticals	55289-0525-40
40's	$18.28	ERY-TAB, Pharma Pac	52959-0061-40
40's	$23.60	E-MYCIN, Pharma Pac	52959-0058-40
42's	$19.00	ERY-TAB, Pd-Rx Pharmaceuticals	55289-0525-42
42's	$22.98	ERY-TAB, Pharma Pac	52959-0061-42
63's	$23.00	ERY-TAB, Pd-Rx Pharmaceuticals	55289-0525-63
100's	$31.04	GENERIC, Moore, H.L. Drug Exchange Inc	00839-7656-06
100's	$33.74	GENERIC, Moore, H.L. Drug Exchange Inc	00839-7660-06
100's	$35.22	GENERIC, Aligen Independent Laboratories Inc	00405-4398-01
100's	$37.06	ERY-TAB, Abbott Pharmaceutical	00074-6320-13

Tablet, Enteric Coated - Oral - 500 mg

20's	$9.45	ERY-TAB, Allscripts Pharmaceutical Company	54569-2508-01
20's	$15.54	ERY-TAB, Pharma Pac	52959-0062-20
28's	$12.53	ERY-TAB, Pd-Rx Pharmaceuticals	55289-0217-28
28's	$13.23	ERY-TAB, Allscripts Pharmaceutical Company	54569-2508-00
28's	$17.63	ERY-TAB, Pharma Pac	52959-0062-28
30's	$14.17	ERY-TAB, Allscripts Pharmaceutical Company	54569-2508-04
30's	$19.22	ERY-TAB, Pharma Pac	52959-0062-30
40's	$14.78	ERY-TAB, Pd-Rx Pharmaceuticals	55289-0217-40
40's	$18.90	ERY-TAB, Allscripts Pharmaceutical Company	54569-2508-03
40's	$24.01	ERY-TAB, Pharma Pac	52959-0062-40
56's	$32.33	ERY-TAB, Pharma Pac	52959-0062-56
100's	$42.50	ERY-TAB, Abbott Pharmaceutical	00074-6321-13

PRODUCT LISTING - EQUIVALENTS NOT AVAILABLE

Capsule, Enteric Coated - Oral - 250 mg

1's	$3.48	GENERIC, Prescript Pharmaceuticals	00247-0110-01
4's	$3.88	GENERIC, Prescript Pharmaceuticals	00247-0110-04
8's	$4.41	GENERIC, Prescript Pharmaceuticals	00247-0110-08
10's	$4.68	GENERIC, Prescript Pharmaceuticals	00247-0110-10
12's	$3.23	GENERIC, Allscripts Pharmaceutical Company	54569-2281-04
12's	$4.94	GENERIC, Prescript Pharmaceuticals	00247-0110-12
12's	$6.27	GENERIC, Southwood Pharmaceuticals Inc	58016-0123-12
15's	$7.83	GENERIC, Southwood Pharmaceuticals Inc	58016-0123-15
20's	$5.40	GENERIC, Allscripts Pharmaceutical Company	54569-2281-02
20's	$6.00	GENERIC, Prescript Pharmaceuticals	00247-0110-20
20's	$10.45	GENERIC, Southwood Pharmaceuticals Inc	58016-0123-20
20's	$11.00	GENERIC, Pharma Pac	52959-0064-20
21's	$6.13	GENERIC, Prescript Pharmaceuticals	00247-0110-21
24's	$6.53	GENERIC, Prescript Pharmaceuticals	00247-0110-24
24's	$12.54	GENERIC, Southwood Pharmaceuticals Inc	58016-0123-24
28's	$5.10	GENERIC, Pharmaceutical Corporation Of America	51655-0674-29

Size	Price	Product, Manufacturer	NDC
28's	$7.06	GENERIC, Prescript Pharmaceuticals	00247-0110-28
28's	$7.51	GENERIC, Allscripts Pharmaceutical Company	54569-2281-00
28's	$14.63	GENERIC, Southwood Pharmaceuticals Inc	58016-0123-28
28's	$14.95	GENERIC, Pharma Pac	52959-0064-28
30's	$7.33	GENERIC, Prescript Pharmaceuticals	00247-0110-30
30's	$8.10	GENERIC, Allscripts Pharmaceutical Company	54569-2281-03
30's	$15.68	GENERIC, Southwood Pharmaceuticals Inc	58016-0123-30
40's	$8.65	GENERIC, Prescript Pharmaceuticals	00247-0110-40
40's	$10.80	GENERIC, Allscripts Pharmaceutical Company	54569-2281-01
40's	$11.49	GENERIC, Pharmaceutical Corporation Of America	51655-0674-51
40's	$16.95	GENERIC, Pharma Pac	52959-0064-40
40's	$20.90	GENERIC, Southwood Pharmaceuticals Inc	58016-0123-40
56's	$10.76	GENERIC, Prescript Pharmaceuticals	00247-0110-56
100's	$52.25	GENERIC, Southwood Pharmaceuticals Inc	58016-0123-00
Gel - Topical - 2%			
30 gm	$21.26	GENERIC, Allscripts Pharmaceutical Company	54569-4810-00
Ointment - Ophthalmic - 0.5%			
1 gm x 50	$92.00	GENERIC, Raway Pharmacal Inc	00686-0070-11
3.50 gm	$2.75	GENERIC, Cmc-Consolidated Midland Corporation	00223-4288-03
3.50 gm	$3.50	GENERIC, Raway Pharmacal Inc	00686-0070-38
3.50 gm	$4.50	GENERIC, Sidmak Laboratories Inc	50111-0820-21
3.50 gm	$4.90	GENERIC, Allscripts Pharmaceutical Company	54569-1193-00
3.50 gm	$5.52	GENERIC, Miza Pharmaceutcials Dba Optopics Laboratories Corporation	51394-0479-35
3.50 gm	$6.08	GENERIC, Prescript Pharmaceuticals	00247-0276-81
3.50 gm	$6.81	GENERIC, Southwood Pharmaceuticals Inc	58016-6086-01
3.50 gm	$8.49	GENERIC, Pharma Pac	52959-0301-00
Solution - Topical - 2%			
60 ml	$5.25	GENERIC, Aligen Independent Laboratories Inc	00405-2825-56
60 ml	$9.46	GENERIC, Allscripts Pharmaceutical Company	54569-1883-02
60 ml	$9.65	GENERIC, Southwood Pharmaceuticals Inc	58016-3129-01
60 ml	$10.36	GENERIC, Dermol Pharmaceuticals Inc	50744-0100-20
60 ml	$14.11	GENERIC, Roberts Pharmaceutical Corporation	54092-0316-60
60 ml	$19.08	GENERIC, Medicis Dermatologics Inc	99207-0550-02
60 ml	$20.99	GENERIC, Bioglan Pharmaceutical Inc	62436-0701-02
60 ml	$24.74	ERYMAX, Merz Pharmaceuticals	00259-0540-02
118 ml	$43.74	ERYMAX, Merz Pharmaceuticals	00259-0540-04
Swab - Topical - 2%			
60's	$18.05	GENERIC, Glades Pharmaceuticals	59366-2838-60
Tablet - Oral - 250 mg			
40's	$6.60	GENERIC, Pharmaceutical Corporation Of America	51655-0519-51
40's	$8.22	GENERIC, Allscripts Pharmaceutical Company	54569-2433-00
40's	$13.26	GENERIC, Pd-Rx Pharmaceuticals	55289-0075-40
56's	$11.51	GENERIC, Allscripts Pharmaceutical Company	54569-2433-02
56's	$16.02	GENERIC, Pd-Rx Pharmaceuticals	55289-0075-56
100's	$14.78	GENERIC, Abbott Pharmaceutical	00074-6326-13
100's	$20.56	GENERIC, Abbott Pharmaceutical	00074-6326-11
Tablet - Oral - 500 mg			
6's	$1.63	GENERIC, Allscripts Pharmaceutical Company	54569-2502-01
12's	$3.26	GENERIC, Allscripts Pharmaceutical Company	54569-2502-03
14's	$3.80	GENERIC, Allscripts Pharmaceutical Company	54569-2502-05
20's	$11.25	GENERIC, Pd-Rx Pharmaceuticals	55289-0025-20
28's	$7.60	GENERIC, Allscripts Pharmaceutical Company	54569-2502-00
28's	$14.64	GENERIC, Pd-Rx Pharmaceuticals	55289-0025-28
30's	$8.15	GENERIC, Allscripts Pharmaceutical Company	54569-2502-06
30's	$16.88	GENERIC, Pd-Rx Pharmaceuticals	55289-0025-30
100's	$27.15	GENERIC, Abbott Pharmaceutical	00074-6227-13
Tablet, Coated Particles - Oral - 333 mg			
18's	$18.64	PCE DISPERTAB, Southwood Pharmaceuticals Inc	58016-0145-18
21's	$47.48	PCE DISPERTAB, Pd-Rx Pharmaceuticals	55289-0426-21
30's	$49.25	PCE DISPERTAB, Allscripts Pharmaceutical Company	54569-0157-02
30's	$53.16	PCE DISPERTAB, Pd-Rx Pharmaceuticals	55289-0426-30
60's	$108.63	PCE DISPERTAB, Abbott Pharmaceutical	00074-6290-60
100 ml	$42.50	GENERIC, Cmc-Consolidated Midland Corporation	00223-6141-01
Tablet, Coated Particles - Oral - 500 mg			
10's	$27.45	PCE DISPERTAB, Pharma Pac	52959-0240-10
15's	$32.22	PCE DISPERTAB, Physicians Total Care	54868-1774-00
20's	$36.88	PCE DISPERTAB, Southwood Pharmaceuticals Inc	58016-0663-20
20's	$42.57	PCE DISPERTAB, Physicians Total Care	54868-1774-02
20's	$43.31	PCE DISPERTAB, Allscripts Pharmaceutical Company	54569-2952-01
20's	$55.26	PCE DISPERTAB, Pd-Rx Pharmaceuticals	55289-0027-20
100's	$238.79	PCE DISPERTAB, Abbott Pharmaceutical	00074-3389-13
Tablet, Enteric Coated - Oral - 250 mg			
1's	$3.46	GENERIC, Prescript Pharmaceuticals	00247-0007-01
2's	$3.56	GENERIC, Prescript Pharmaceuticals	00247-0007-02
3's	$3.68	GENERIC, Prescript Pharmaceuticals	00247-0007-03
4's	$3.79	GENERIC, Prescript Pharmaceuticals	00247-0007-04
5's	$3.89	GENERIC, Prescript Pharmaceuticals	00247-0007-05
6's	$4.00	GENERIC, Prescript Pharmaceuticals	00247-0007-06
8's	$4.22	GENERIC, Prescript Pharmaceuticals	00247-0007-08
10's	$4.44	GENERIC, Prescript Pharmaceuticals	00247-0007-10
12's	$4.66	GENERIC, Prescript Pharmaceuticals	00247-0007-12
15's	$4.98	GENERIC, Prescript Pharmaceuticals	00247-0007-15
16's	$5.09	GENERIC, Prescript Pharmaceuticals	00247-0007-16
20's	$5.53	GENERIC, Prescript Pharmaceuticals	00247-0007-20
21's	$5.64	GENERIC, Prescript Pharmaceuticals	00247-0007-21
28's	$6.39	GENERIC, Prescript Pharmaceuticals	00247-0007-28
30's	$6.61	GENERIC, Prescript Pharmaceuticals	00247-0007-30
32's	$6.82	GENERIC, Prescript Pharmaceuticals	00247-0007-32
40's	$7.69	GENERIC, Prescript Pharmaceuticals	00247-0007-40
56's	$9.44	GENERIC, Prescript Pharmaceuticals	00247-0007-56
60's	$9.87	GENERIC, Prescript Pharmaceuticals	00247-0007-60
100's	$14.21	GENERIC, Prescript Pharmaceuticals	00247-0007-00
Tablet, Enteric Coated - Oral - 333 mg			
2's	$3.69	GENERIC, Prescript Pharmaceuticals	00247-0008-02
3's	$3.87	GENERIC, Prescript Pharmaceuticals	00247-0008-03
4's	$4.05	GENERIC, Prescript Pharmaceuticals	00247-0008-04
5's	$4.21	GENERIC, Prescript Pharmaceuticals	00247-0008-05
6's	$4.39	GENERIC, Prescript Pharmaceuticals	00247-0008-06
9's	$4.91	GENERIC, Prescript Pharmaceuticals	00247-0008-09
10's	$5.07	GENERIC, Prescript Pharmaceuticals	00247-0008-10
12's	$5.19	E-MYCIN, Southwood Pharmaceuticals Inc	58016-0184-12
15's	$5.93	GENERIC, Prescript Pharmaceuticals	00247-0008-15
15's	$6.49	E-MYCIN, Southwood Pharmaceuticals Inc	58016-0184-15
15's	$7.62	ERY-TAB, Southwood Pharmaceuticals Inc	58016-0126-15
15's	$7.79	E-MYCIN, Southwood Pharmaceuticals Inc	58016-0184-18
18's	$6.45	GENERIC, Prescript Pharmaceuticals	00247-0008-18
18's	$9.15	ERY-TAB, Southwood Pharmaceuticals Inc	58016-0126-18
20's	$6.80	GENERIC, Prescript Pharmaceuticals	00247-0008-20
20's	$10.13	ERY-TAB, Southwood Pharmaceuticals Inc	58016-0126-20
21's	$6.96	GENERIC, Prescript Pharmaceuticals	00247-0008-21
21's	$10.68	ERY-TAB, Southwood Pharmaceuticals Inc	58016-0126-21
24's	$7.48	GENERIC, Prescript Pharmaceuticals	00247-0008-24
24's	$10.38	E-MYCIN, Southwood Pharmaceuticals Inc	58016-0184-24
28's	$14.24	ERY-TAB, Southwood Pharmaceuticals Inc	58016-0126-28
30's	$8.52	GENERIC, Prescript Pharmaceuticals	00247-0008-30
30's	$12.98	E-MYCIN, Southwood Pharmaceuticals Inc	58016-0184-30
30's	$15.26	ERY-TAB, Southwood Pharmaceuticals Inc	58016-0126-30
40's	$17.30	E-MYCIN, Southwood Pharmaceuticals Inc	58016-0184-40
42's	$10.58	GENERIC, Prescript Pharmaceuticals	00247-0008-42
42's	$21.35	ERY-TAB, Southwood Pharmaceuticals Inc	58016-0126-42
60's	$30.51	ERY-TAB, Southwood Pharmaceuticals Inc	58016-0126-60
100's	$20.56	GENERIC, Prescript Pharmaceuticals	00247-0008-00
100's	$43.25	E-MYCIN, Southwood Pharmaceuticals Inc	58016-0184-00
100's	$50.85	ERY-TAB, Southwood Pharmaceuticals Inc	58016-0126-00
Tablet, Enteric Coated - Oral - 500 mg			
2's	$3.86	GENERIC, Prescript Pharmaceuticals	00247-0175-02
3's	$4.11	GENERIC, Prescript Pharmaceuticals	00247-0175-03
4's	$4.36	GENERIC, Prescript Pharmaceuticals	00247-0175-04
7's	$5.12	GENERIC, Prescript Pharmaceuticals	00247-0175-07
9's	$5.62	GENERIC, Prescript Pharmaceuticals	00247-0175-09
10's	$5.87	GENERIC, Prescript Pharmaceuticals	00247-0175-10
12's	$6.38	GENERIC, Prescript Pharmaceuticals	00247-0175-12
14's	$6.88	GENERIC, Prescript Pharmaceuticals	00247-0175-14
20's	$8.39	GENERIC, Prescript Pharmaceuticals	00247-0175-20
21's	$8.65	GENERIC, Prescript Pharmaceuticals	00247-0175-21
28's	$10.40	GENERIC, Prescript Pharmaceuticals	00247-0175-28
30's	$10.91	GENERIC, Prescript Pharmaceuticals	00247-0175-30
40's	$13.42	GENERIC, Prescript Pharmaceuticals	00247-0175-40
56's	$17.46	GENERIC, Prescript Pharmaceuticals	00247-0175-56

Erythromycin Ethylsuccinate *(001182)*

Categories: Amebiasis, intestinal; Conjunctivitis, infectious; Diphtheria; Endocarditis, prevention; Erythrasma; Infection, endocervical; Infection, gynecologic; Infection, lower respiratory tract; Infection, ophthalmic; Infection, rectal; Infection, skin and skin structures; Infection, upper respiratory tract; Infection, urethra; Legionnaires' disease; Pelvic inflammatory disease; Pertussis; Pneumonia; Rheumatic fever, prophylaxis; Syphilis; Pregnancy Category B; FDA Approved 1964 Sep; WHO Formulary

Drug Classes: Antibiotics, macrolides

Brand Names: **EES**; Eryped; Erythro; Pediamycin; Ro-Mycin

Foreign Brand Availability: Abboticin Novum (Denmark; Finland); Abboticine (France); Ambamida (Argentina); Apo-Erythro-ES (Canada); Baknyl (Ecuador); Bannthrocin (Indonesia); E-Mycin (Australia; New-Zealand); E.E.S. (Malaysia; Taiwan); EES-200 (Canada); EES-400 (Canada); EES 400 (Bahamas; Barbados; Belize; Bermuda; Curacao; Guyana; Hong-Kong; Jamaica; Netherland-Antilles; Surinam; Trinidad); EES Granules (Bahamas; Barbados; Belize; Bermuda; Curacao; Guyana; Jamaica; Netherland-Antilles; Surinam; Trinidad); ERA (New-Zealand); ERA I.M. (New-Zealand); ESE (Portugal); Eriecu (Ecuador); Eritrazon (Portugal); Eritrocina (Portugal); Eritrolag (Benin; Burkina-Faso; Ethiopia; Gambia; Ghana; Guinea; Ivory-Coast; Kenya; Liberia; Malawi; Mali; Mauritania; Mauritius; Morocco; Niger; Nigeria; Senegal; Seychelles; Sierra-Leone; Sudan; Tanzania; Tunia; Uganda; Zambia; Zimbabwe); Eritrowel (Mexico); Ermysin (Finland); Ery (France); Ery-Maxin (Austria); Eryromycen (Japan); Eryson (Malaysia); Erythro-DS (Japan); Erythrocin (Austria; Bahamas; Barbados; Belize; Bermuda; Curacao; Germany; Guyana; Hong-Kong; India; Jamaica; Netherland-Antilles; Surinam; Switzerland; Thailand; Trinidad); Erythrocin ES 500 (Switzerland); Erythrocin I.M. (Australia; Bulgaria); Erythrocine (Belgium; France; Netherlands); Erythrodar (Bahrain; Cyprus; Egypt; Iran; Iraq; Jordan; Kuwait; Lebanon; Libya; Oman; Qatar; Republic-of-Yemen; Saudi-Arabia; Syria; United-Arab-Emirates); Erythrogenat TS (Germany); Erythrogram (France); Erythrol (Israel); Erythromycin-Ratiopharm TS (Czech-Republic); Erythroped (England; Ireland; Israel; South-Africa); Erytran (Switzerland); Esinol (Japan); Esmycin (Japan); Etromycin (Czech-Republic); Kemothrocin (Indonesia); Malocin (Thailand); Minotin (Japan); Monomycin (Austria; Switzerland); Paediathrocin (Germany); Pantomicina (Argentina; Costa-Rica; Dominican-Republic; Ecuador; El-Salvador; Guatemala; Honduras; Mexico; Nicaragua; Panama; Peru; Spain); Pentate (Japan); Servitrocin (Hong-Kong); Succin (South-Africa)

Cost of Therapy: $7.46 (Infection; E.E.S.-400 Filmtab; 400 mg; 4 tablets/day; 10 day supply)

DESCRIPTION

Erythromycin is produced by a strain of *Streptomyces erythraeus* and belongs to the macrolide group of antibiotics. It is basic and readily forms salts with acids. The base, the stearate salt, and the esters are poorly soluble in water. Erythromycin ethylsuccinate is an ester of erythromycin suitable for oral administration.

The granules are intended for reconstitution with water. When reconstituted, they are palatable cherry-flavored suspensions.

The pleasant tasting, fruit-flavored liquids are supplied ready for administration.

Granules and ready-made suspensions are intended primarily for pediatric use but can also be used in adults.

The Filmtab tablets are intended primarily for adults or older children.

Inactive Ingredients *E.E.S. 200 Liquid:* FD&C red no. 40, methylparaben, polysorbate 60, propylparaben, sodium citrate, sucrose, water, xanthan gum and natural and artificial flavors. *E.E.S 400 Liquid:* D&C yellow no. 10, FD&C yellow no. 6, methylparaben, polysorbate 60, propylparaben, sodium citrate, sucrose, water, xanthan gum and natural and artificial flavors. *E.E.S. Granules:* Citric acid, FD&C red no. 3, magnesium aluminum silicate, sodium carboxymethylcellulose, sodium citrate, sucrose and artificial flavor. *E.E.S. 400 Filmtab Tablets:* Cellulosic polymers, confectioner's sugar (contains corn starch), corn starch, D&C red no. 30, D&C yellow no. 10, FD&C red no. 40, magnesium stearate, polacrilin potassium, polyethylene glycol, propylene glycol, sodium citrate, sorbic acid, sorbitan monooleate, titanium dioxide and vitamin E.

Storage: Store tablets and granules (prior to mixing) below 30°C (86°F).

CLINICAL PHARMACOLOGY

MICROBIOLOGY

Biochemical tests demonstrate that erythromycin inhibits protein synthesis of the pathogen without directly affecting nucleic acid synthesis. Antagonism has been demonstrated between clindamycin and erythromycin.

Note: Many strains of *Hemophilus influenzae* are resistant to erythromycin alone, but are susceptible to erythromycin and sulfonamides together. Staphylococci resistant to erythromycin may emerge during a course of erythromycin therapy. Culture and susceptibility testing should be performed.

Disc Susceptibility Tests: Quantitative methods that require measurement of zone diameters give the most precise estimates of antibiotic susceptibility. One recommended procedure (21 CFR section 460.1) uses erythromycin class discs for testing susceptibility; interpretations correlate zone diameters of this disc test with MIC values for erythromycin. With this procedure, a report from the laboratory of "susceptible" indicates that the infecting organism is likely to respond to therapy. A report of "resistant" indicates, that the infective organism is not likely to respond to therapy. A report of "intermediate susceptibility" suggests that the organism would be susceptible if higher doses were used.

Erythromycin binds to the 50 S ribosomal subunits of susceptible bacteria and suppresses protein synthesis.

Orally administered erythromycin ethylsuccinate suspensions and Filmtab tablets are readily and reliably absorbed. Comparable serum levels of erythromycin are achieved in the fasting and nonfasting states.

Erythromycin diffuses readily into most body fluids. Only low concentrations are normally achieved in the spinal fluid, but passage of the drug across the blood-brain barrier increases in meningitis. In the presence of normal hepatic function, erythromycin is concentrated in the liver and excreted in the bile; the effect of hepatic dysfunction on excretion of erythromycin by the liver into the bile is not known. Less than 5% of the orally administered dose of erythromycin is excreted in active form in the urine.

Erythromycin crosses the placental barrier and is excreted in breast milk.

INDICATIONS AND USAGE

Streptococcus pyogenes: *(Group A beta hemolytic streptococcus):* Upper and lower respiratory tract, skin, and soft tissue infections of mild to moderate severity.

Injectable benzathine penicillin G is considered by the American Heart Association to be the drug of choice in the treatment and prevention of streptococcal pharyngitis and in long-term prophylaxis of rheumatic fever.

When oral medication is preferred for treatment of the above conditions, penicillin G, V, or erythromycin are alternate drugs of choice.

When oral medication is given, the importance of strict adherence by the patient to the prescribed dosage regimen must be stressed. A therapeutic dose should be administered for at least 10 days.

Alpha-hemolytic streptococci **(viridans group):** Although no controlled clinical efficacy trials have been conducted, oral erythromycin has been suggested by the American Heart Association and American Dental Association for use in a regimen for prophylaxis against bacterial endocarditis in patients hypersensitive to penicillin who have congenital heart disease, or rheumatic or other acquired valvular heart disease when they undergo dental procedures and surgical procedures of the upper respiratory tract.[1] Erythromycin is not suitable prior to genitourinary or gastrointestinal tract surgery. *Note:* When selecting antibiotics for the prevention of bacterial endocarditis the physician or dentist should read the full joint statement of the American Heart Association and the American Dental Association.[1]

Staphylococcus aureus: Acute infections of skin and soft tissue of mild to moderate severity. Resistant organisms may emerge during treatment.

Streptococcus pneumoniae (Diplococcus pneumoniae): Upper respiratory tract infections (*e.g.*, otitis media, pharyngitis) and lower respiratory tract infections (*e.g.*, pneumonia) of mild to moderate degree.

Mycoplasma pneumoniae: (Eaton agent, PPLO): For respiratory infections due to this organism.

Hemophilus influenzae: For upper respiratory tract infections of mild to moderate severity when used concomitantly with adequate doses of sulfonamides. (See sulfonamide labeling for appropriate prescribing information.)The concomitant use of the sulfonamides is necessary since not all strains of *Hemophilus influenzae* are susceptible to erythromycin at the concentrations of the antibiotic achieved with usual therapeutic doses.

Chlamydia trachomatis: For the treatment of urethritis in adult males due to *Chlamydia trachomatis.*

Ureaplasma urealyticum: For the treatment of urethritis in adult males due to *Ureaplasma urealyticum.*

Treponema pallidum: Erythromycin is an alternate choice of treatment for primary syphilis in patients allergic to the penicillins. In treatment of primary syphilis, spinal fluid examinations should be done before treatment and as part of follow-up after therapy.

Corynebacterium diphtheriae: As an adjunct to antitoxin, to prevent establishment of carriers, and to eradicate the organism in carriers.

Corynebacterium minutissimum: For the treatment of erythrasma.

Entamoeba histolytica: In the treatment of intestinal amebiasis only. Extraenteric amebiasis requires treatment with other agents.

Listeria monocytogenes: Infections due to this organism.

Bordetella pertussis: Erythromycin is effective in eliminating the organism from the nasopharynx of infected individuals, rendering them non-infectious. Some clinical studies suggests that erythromycin may be helpful in the prophylaxis of pertussis in exposed susceptible individuals.

Legionnaires' Disease: Although no controlled clinical efficacy studies have been conducted, *in vitro* and limited preliminary clinical data suggest that erythromycin may be effective in treating Legionnaires' Disease.

CONTRAINDICATIONS

Erythromycin is contraindicated in patients with known hypersensitivity to this antibiotic.

Erythromycin is contraindicated in patients taking terfenadine, astemizole, or cisapride. (See DRUG INTERACTIONS.)

WARNINGS

There have been reports of hepatic dysfunction, including increased liver enzymes, and hepatocellular and/or cholestatic hepatitis, with or without jaundice, occurring in patients receiving oral erythromycin products.

There have been reports suggesting that erythromycin does not reach the fetus in adequate concentration to prevent congenital syphilis. Infants born to women treated during pregnancy with oral erythromycin for early syphilis should be treated with an appropriate penicillin regimen.

Pseudomembranous colitis has been reported with nearly all antibacterial agents, including erythromycin, and may range in severity from mild to life threatening. Therefore, it is important to consider this diagnosis in patients who present with diarrhea subsequent to the administration of antibacterial agents.

Treatment with antibacterial agents alters the normal flora of the colon and may permit overgrowth of clostridia. Studies indicate that a toxin produced by *Clostridium difficile* is a primary cause of "antibiotic-associated colitis".

After the diagnosis of pseudomembranous colitis has been established, therapeutic measures should be initiated. Mild cases of pseudomembranous colitis usually respond to discontinuation of the drug alone. In moderate to severe cases, consideration should be given to management with fluids and electrolytes, protein supplementation, and treatment with an antibacterial clinically effective against *Clostridium difficile* colitis.

Rhabdomyolysis with or without renal impairment has been reported in seriously ill patients receiving erythromycin concomitantly with lovastatin. Therefore, patients receiving concomitant lovastatin and erythromycin should be carefully monitored for creatine kinase (CK) and serum transaminase levels. (See package insert for lovastatin.)

PRECAUTIONS

GENERAL

Erythromycin is principally excreted by the liver. Caution should be exercised when erythromycin is administered to patients with impaired hepatic function. (See CLINICAL PHARMACOLOGY and WARNINGS.)

There have been reports that erythromycin may aggravate the weakness of patients with myasthenia gravis.

Prolonged or repeated use of erythromycin may result in an overgrowth of nonsusceptible bacteria or fungi. If superinfection occurs, erythromycin should be discontinued and appropriate therapy instituted.

When indicated, incision and drainage or other surgical procedures should be performed in conjunction with antibiotic therapy.

LABORATORY TESTS

Erythromycin interferes with the fluorometric determination of urinary catecholamines.

CARCINOGENESIS, MUTAGENESIS, AND IMPAIRMENT OF FERTILITY

Long-term (2-year) oral studies conducted in rats with erythromycin base did not provide evidence of tumorigenicity. Mutagenicity studies have not been conducted. There was no apparent effect on male or female fertility in rats fed erythromycin (base) at levels up to 0.25% of diet.

PREGNANCY CATEGORY B

There is no evidence of teratogenicity or any other adverse effect on reproduction in female rats fed erythromycin base (up to 0.25% of diet) prior to and during mating, during gestation, and through weaning of two successive litters. There are, however, no adequate and well-controlled studies in pregnant women. Because animal reproduction studies are not always predictive of human response, this drug should be used during pregnancy only if clearly needed. Erythromycin has been reported to cross the placental barrier in humans, but fetal plasma levels are generally low.

LABOR AND DELIVERY

The effect of erythromycin on labor and delivery is unknown.

NURSING MOTHERS

Erythromycin is excreted in breast milk, therefore, caution should be exercised when erythromycin is administered to a nursing woman.

PEDIATRIC USE

See INDICATIONS AND USAGE and DOSAGE AND ADMINISTRATION.

DRUG INTERACTIONS

Erythromycin use in patients who are receiving high doses of theophylline may be associated with an increase in serum theophylline levels and potential theophylline toxicity. In case of theophylline toxicity and/or elevated serum theophylline levels, the dose of theophylline should be reduced while the patient is receiving concomitant erythromycin therapy.

Concomitant administration of erythromycin and digoxin has been reported to result in elevated digoxin serum levels.

There have been reports of increased anticoagulant effects when erythromycin and oral anticoagulants were used concomitantly. Increased anticoagulation effects due to interactions of erythromycin with various oral anticoagulants may be more pronounced in the elderly.

Concurrent use of erythromycin and ergotamine or dihydroergotamine has been associated in some patients with acute ergot toxicity characterized by severe peripheral vasospasm and dysesthesia.

Erythromycin has been reported to decrease the clearance of triazolam and midazolam and thus may increase the pharmacologic effect of these benzodiazepines.

The use of erythromycin in patients concurrently taking drugs metabolized by the cytochrome P450 system may be associated with elevations in serum levels of these other drugs. There have been reports of interactions of erythromycin with carbamazepine, cyclosporine, tacrolimus, hexobarbital, phenytoin, alfentanil, cisapride, disopyramide, lovastatin, bromocriptine, valproate, terfenadine, and astemizole. Serum concentrations of drugs metabolized by the cytochrome P450 system should be monitored closely in patients concurrently receiving erythromycin.

Erythromycin has been reported to significantly alter the metabolism of nonsedating antihistamines terfenadine and astemizole when taken concomitantly. Rare cases of serious cardiovascular adverse events, including electrocardiographic QT/QTc interval prolongation, cardiac arrest, torsades de pointes, and other ventricular arrhythmias have been observed. (See CONTRAINDICATIONS.) In addition, deaths have been reported rarely with concomitant administration of terfenadine and erythromycin.

There have been postmarketing reports of drug interactions when erythromycin is coadministered with cisapride, resulting in QT prolongation, cardiac arrythmias, ventricular tachycardia, ventricular fibrulation, and torsades de pointes, most like due to inhibition of hepatic metabolism of cisapride by erythromycin. Fatalities have been reported. (See CONTRAINDICATIONS.)

Patients receiving concomitant lovastatin and erythromycin should be carefully monitored; cases of rhabdomyolysis have been reported in seriously ill patients.

ADVERSE REACTIONS

The most frequent side effects of oral erythromycin preparations are gastrointestinal and are dose-related. They include nausea, vomiting, abdominal pain, diarrhea and anorexia. Symptoms of hepatitis, hepatic dysfunction and/or abnormal liver function test results may occur (See WARNINGS.)

Onset of pseudomembranous colitis symptoms may occur during or after antibiotic treatment. (See WARNINGS.)

Rarely, erythromycin has been associated with the production of ventricular arrhythmias, including ventricular tachycardia and torsades de pointes, in individuals with prolonged QT intervals. There have been isolated reports of other cardiovascular symptoms such as chest pain, dizziness, and palpitations; however, a cause and effect relationship has not been established.

Allergic reactions ranging from urticaria to anaphylaxis have occurred. Skin reactions ranging from mile eruptions to erythema multiforme, Stevens-Johnson syndrome, and toxic epidermal necrolysis have been reported rarely.

There have been isolated reports of reversible hearing loss occurring chiefly in patients with renal insufficiency and in patients receiving high doses of erythromycin.

DOSAGE AND ADMINISTRATION

Erythromycin ethylsuccinate suspensions and Filmtab tablets may be administered without regard to meals.

Children: Age, weight, and severity of the infection are important factors in determining the proper dosage. In mild to moderate infections the usual dosage of erythromycin ethylsuccinate for children is 30-50 mg/kg/day in equally divided doses every 6 hours. For more severe infections this dosage may be doubled. If twice-a-day dosage is desired, one-half of the total daily dose may be given every 12 hours. Doses may also be given three times daily by administering one-third of the total daily dose every 8 hours.

The dosage schedule found in TABLE 1 is suggested for mild to moderate infections:

TABLE 1

Body Weight	Total Daily Dose
Under 10 lb	30-50 mg/kg/day 15-25 mg/lb/day
10-15 lb	200 mg
16-25 lb	400 mg
26-50 lb	800 mg
51-100 lb	1200 mg
Over 100 lb	1600 mg

ADULTS

400 mg erythromycin ethylsuccinate every 6 hours is the usual dose. Dosage may be increased up to 4 g per day according to the severity of the infection. If twice-a-day dosage is desired, one-half of the total daily dose may be given every 12 hours. Doses may also be given three times daily by administering one-third of the total daily dose every 8 hours.

For adult dosage calculation, use a ratio of 400 mg of erythromycin activity as the ethylsuccinate to 250 mg of erythromycin activity as the stearate, base or estolate.

In the treatment of streptococcal infections, a therapeutic dosage of erythromycin ethylsuccinate should be administered for at least 10 days. In continuous prophylaxis against recurrences of streptococcal infections in persons with a history of rheumatic heart disease, the usual dosage is 400 mg twice a day.

For prophylaxis against bacterial endocarditis[1] in patients with congenital heart disease, or rheumatic or other acquired valvular heart disease when undergoing dental procedures or surgical procedures of the upper respiratory tract, give 1.6 g (20 mg/kg for children) orally 1½ to 2 hours before the procedure, and then, 800 mg (10 mg/kg for children) orally every 6 hours for 8 doses.

For Treatment of Urethritis due to *C. trachomatis* or *U. urealyticum*: 800 mg three times a day for 7 days.

For Treatment of Primary Syphilis: *Adults:* 48-64 g given in divided doses over a period of 10-15 days.

For Intestinal Amebiasis: *Adults:* 400 mg four times daily for 10-14 days. *Children:* 30-50 mg/kg/day in divided doses for 10-14 days.

For Use in Pertussis: Although optimal dosage and duration have not been established, doses of erythromycin utilized in reported clinical studies were 40-50 mg/kg/day, given in divided doses for 5-14 days.

For Treatment of Legionnaires' Disease: Although optimal doses have not been established, doses utilized in reported clinical data were those recommended above (1.6-4 g daily in divided doses).

PRODUCT LISTING - RATED THERAPEUTICALLY EQUIVALENT

Granule For Reconstitution - Oral - Ethylsuccinate 200 mg/5 ml

100 ml	$6.95	GENERIC, Cmc-Consolidated Midland Corporation	00223-6142-10
100 ml	$7.41	GENERIC, Moore, H.L. Drug Exchange Inc	00839-6362-73
100 ml	$8.65	GENERIC, Major Pharmaceuticals Inc	00904-2653-04
100 ml	$8.74	ERYPED, Abbott Pharmaceutical	00074-6302-13
100 ml	$8.83	E.E.S. GRANULES, Abbott Pharmaceutical	00074-6369-02
100 ml	$23.50	GENERIC, Cmc-Consolidated Midland Corporation	00223-6142-01
200 ml	$14.08	GENERIC, Moore, H.L. Drug Exchange Inc	00839-6362-78
200 ml	$15.61	E.E.S. GRANULES, Abbott Pharmaceutical	00074-6369-10
200 ml	$15.61	E.E.S. GRANULES, Allscripts Pharmaceutical Company	54569-0128-00
200 ml	$16.27	ERYPED, Abbott Pharmaceutical	00074-6302-53
200 ml	$16.30	GENERIC, Major Pharmaceuticals Inc	00904-2653-08
480 ml	$13.01	GENERIC, Logen	00820-0117-38

Suspension - Oral - Ethylsuccinate 200 mg/5 ml

100 ml	$4.77	E.E.S.-200, Abbott Pharmaceutical	00074-6306-13
100 ml	$4.78	E.E.S.-200, Allscripts Pharmaceutical Company	54569-3057-00
100 ml	$7.00	GENERIC, Ivax Corporation	00182-1530-70
100 ml	$7.01	GENERIC, Barr Laboratories Inc	00555-0215-22
200 ml	$12.95	GENERIC, Ivax Corporation	00182-1530-73
200 ml	$12.95	GENERIC, Barr Laboratories Inc	00555-0215-23
480 ml	$19.04	GENERIC, Alpharma Uspd Makers Of Barre and Nmc	00472-0971-16
480 ml	$20.76	GENERIC, Abbott Pharmaceutical	00074-3747-16
480 ml	$20.76	E.E.S.-200, Abbott Pharmaceutical	00074-6306-16
480 ml	$20.93	GENERIC, Major Pharmaceuticals Inc	00904-2462-16
480 ml	$21.46	GENERIC, Moore, H.L. Drug Exchange Inc	00839-6482-69
480 ml	$22.84	GENERIC, Qualitest Products Inc	00603-1206-58
480 ml	$23.50	GENERIC, Ivax Corporation	00182-1371-40

Suspension - Oral - Ethylsuccinate 400 mg/5 ml

100 ml	$8.57	E.E.S.-400, Abbott Pharmaceutical	00074-6373-13

100 ml	$8.58	E.E.S.-400, Allscripts Pharmaceutical Company	54569-0132-00
480 ml	$33.39	GENERIC, Alpharma Uspd Makers Of Barre and Nmc	00472-0974-16
480 ml	$37.25	GENERIC, Moore, H.L. Drug Exchange Inc	00839-6568-69
480 ml	$38.67	GENERIC, Abbott Pharmaceutical	00074-3748-16
480 ml	$38.67	E.E.S.-400, Abbott Pharmaceutical	00074-6373-16
480 ml	$39.74	GENERIC, Major Pharmaceuticals Inc	00904-2463-16
480 ml	$41.00	GENERIC, Qualitest Products Inc	00603-1207-58
480 ml	$42.48	GENERIC, Ivax Corporation	00182-1773-40

Tablet - Oral - Ethylsuccinate 400 mg

3's	$2.48	GENERIC, Pd-Rx Pharmaceuticals	55289-0110-03
9's	$7.58	GENERIC, Pd-Rx Pharmaceuticals	55289-0110-09
12's	$2.59	E.E.S.-400 FILMTAB, Southwood Pharmaceuticals Inc	58016-0167-12
15's	$3.24	E.E.S.-400 FILMTAB, Southwood Pharmaceuticals Inc	58016-0167-15
20's	$4.32	E.E.S.-400 FILMTAB, Southwood Pharmaceuticals Inc	58016-0167-20
20's	$5.39	E.E.S.-400 FILMTAB, Allscripts Pharmaceutical Company	54569-0127-05
20's	$7.20	GENERIC, Pd-Rx Pharmaceuticals	55289-0110-20
21's	$5.66	E.E.S.-400 FILMTAB, Allscripts Pharmaceutical Company	54569-0127-00
28's	$12.66	GENERIC, Dhs Inc	55887-0849-28
28's	$13.90	GENERIC, Pd-Rx Pharmaceuticals	55289-0110-28
30's	$5.19	GENERIC, Circle Pharmaceuticals Inc	00659-0114-30
30's	$6.48	E.E.S.-400 FILMTAB, Southwood Pharmaceuticals Inc	58016-0167-30
30's	$8.09	E.E.S.-400 FILMTAB, Allscripts Pharmaceutical Company	54569-0127-02
30's	$8.42	GENERIC, Pd-Rx Pharmaceuticals	55289-0110-30
30's	$13.59	GENERIC, Dhs Inc	55887-0849-30
40's	$6.95	GENERIC, Circle Pharmaceuticals Inc	00659-0114-40
40's	$10.78	E.E.S.-400 FILMTAB, Allscripts Pharmaceutical Company	54569-0127-03
40's	$12.44	E.E.S.-400 FILMTAB, Southwood Pharmaceuticals Inc	58016-0167-40
40's	$13.28	GENERIC, Pd-Rx Pharmaceuticals	55289-0110-40
40's	$15.02	GENERIC, Dhs Inc	55887-0849-40
40's	$82.44	GENERIC, Major Pharmaceuticals Inc	00904-2464-39
56's	$13.08	GENERIC, Pd-Rx Pharmaceuticals	55289-0110-56
100's	$18.66	GENERIC, Us Trading Corporation	56126-0387-11
100's	$20.75	GENERIC, Geneva Pharmaceuticals	00781-1873-01
100's	$21.60	E.E.S.-400 FILMTAB, Southwood Pharmaceuticals Inc	58016-0167-00
100's	$22.36	GENERIC, Barr Laboratories Inc	00555-0259-02
100's	$22.45	GENERIC, Major Pharmaceuticals Inc	00904-2464-60
100's	$23.24	GENERIC, Abbott Pharmaceutical	00074-2589-13
100's	$23.24	E.E.S.-400 FILMTAB, Abbott Pharmaceutical	00074-5729-13
100's	$25.77	GENERIC, Moore, H.L. Drug Exchange Inc	00839-6588-06
100's	$26.75	GENERIC, Qualitest Products Inc	00603-3552-21
100's	$26.95	GENERIC, Ivax Corporation	00182-1489-01
100's	$26.95	GENERIC, Mylan Pharmaceuticals Inc	00378-6400-01
100's	$26.96	E.E.S.-400 FILMTAB, Abbott Pharmaceutical	00074-5729-11
100's	$27.75	GENERIC, Interstate Drug Exchange Inc	00814-2995-14

Tablet, Chewable - Oral - Ethylsuccinate 200 mg

40's	$21.65	ERYPED, Abbott Pharmaceutical	00074-6314-40
40's	$25.46	ERYPED, Southwood Pharmaceuticals Inc	58016-0362-40

PRODUCT LISTING - EQUIVALENTS NOT AVAILABLE

Granule For Reconstitution - Oral - Ethylsuccinate 100 mg/2.5 ml

50 ml	$6.85	ERYPED, Abbott Pharmaceutical	00074-6303-50

Granule For Reconstitution - Oral - Ethylsuccinate 200 mg/5 ml

100 ml	$7.70	GENERIC, Southwood Pharmaceuticals Inc	58016-1017-03
100 ml	$7.70	ERYPED 200, Southwood Pharmaceuticals Inc	58016-1036-01
100 ml	$15.50	GENERIC, Pharma Pac	52959-0310-01
200 ml	$14.02	GENERIC, Southwood Pharmaceuticals Inc	58016-1018-06
200 ml	$14.02	ERYPED 200, Southwood Pharmaceuticals Inc	58016-1037-06
200 ml	$19.25	GENERIC, Pharma Pac	52959-0310-02

Granule For Reconstitution - Oral - Ethylsuccinate 400 mg/5 ml

60 ml	$8.00	ERYPED, Abbott Pharmaceutical	00074-6305-60
100 ml	$10.95	GENERIC, Cmc-Consolidated Midland Corporation	00223-6143-10
100 ml	$11.85	ERYPED 400, Southwood Pharmaceuticals Inc	58016-1038-01
100 ml	$13.44	ERYPED, Abbott Pharmaceutical	00074-6305-13
100 ml	$13.44	ERYPED 400, Allscripts Pharmaceutical Company	54569-0134-00
100 ml	$16.94	GENERIC, Prescript Pharmaceuticals	00247-0056-00
100 ml	$42.50	GENERIC, Cmc-Consolidated Midland Corporation	00223-6143-01
200 ml	$21.62	ERYPED 400, Southwood Pharmaceuticals Inc	58016-1039-06
200 ml	$25.02	ERYPED, Abbott Pharmaceutical	00074-6305-53
200 ml	$25.03	ERYPED 400, Allscripts Pharmaceutical Company	54569-0135-00
200 ml	$30.54	GENERIC, Prescript Pharmaceuticals	00247-0056-79
480 ml	$22.46	GENERIC, Logen	00820-0118-38

Suspension - Oral - Ethylsuccinate 200 mg/5 ml

5 ml	$3.48	GENERIC, Prescript Pharmaceuticals	00247-0396-05
10 ml	$3.62	GENERIC, Prescript Pharmaceuticals	00247-0396-10
25 ml	$4.02	GENERIC, Prescript Pharmaceuticals	00247-0396-25
60 ml	$4.98	GENERIC, Prescript Pharmaceuticals	00247-0396-60
90 ml	$5.79	GENERIC, Prescript Pharmaceuticals	00247-0396-90
100 ml	$6.05	GENERIC, Prescript Pharmaceuticals	00247-0396-00
100 ml	$6.95	GENERIC, Raway Pharmacal Inc	00686-0965-39
100 ml	$7.83	GENERIC, Allscripts Pharmaceutical Company	54569-2821-00
100 ml	$15.39	GENERIC, Alpharma Uspd Makers Of Barre and Nmc	63874-0159-10
120 ml	$6.59	GENERIC, Prescript Pharmaceuticals	00247-0396-77
200 ml	$8.75	GENERIC, Prescript Pharmaceuticals	00247-0396-79
200 ml	$14.07	GENERIC, Allscripts Pharmaceutical Company	54569-2187-00
200 ml	$17.54	GENERIC, Alpharma Uspd Makers Of Barre and Nmc	63874-0159-20
240 ml	$9.84	GENERIC, Prescript Pharmaceuticals	00247-0396-95

Suspension - Oral - Ethylsuccinate 400 mg/5 ml

60 ml	$6.00	GENERIC, Prescript Pharmaceuticals	00247-0395-60
90 ml	$7.33	GENERIC, Prescript Pharmaceuticals	00247-0395-90
100 ml	$5.95	GENERIC, Raway Pharmacal Inc	00686-0970-39
100 ml	$7.76	GENERIC, Prescript Pharmaceuticals	00247-0395-00
100 ml	$12.30	GENERIC, Pharma Pac	52959-0305-00
100 ml	$18.52	GENERIC, Alpharma Uspd Makers Of Barre and Nmc	63874-0160-10
120 ml	$8.65	GENERIC, Prescript Pharmaceuticals	00247-0395-77
200 ml	$12.18	GENERIC, Prescript Pharmaceuticals	00247-0395-79
200 ml	$21.00	GENERIC, Pharma Pac	52959-0305-01
200 ml	$28.33	GENERIC, Alpharma Uspd Makers Of Barre and Nmc	63874-0160-20
480 ml	$39.05	GENERIC, Alpharma Uspd Makers Of Barre and Nmc	63874-0160-48

Tablet - Oral - Ethylsuccinate 400 mg

2's	$3.78	GENERIC, Prescript Pharmaceuticals	00247-0116-02
3's	$0.86	GENERIC, Allscripts Pharmaceutical Company	54569-2507-09
3's	$3.99	GENERIC, Prescript Pharmaceuticals	00247-0116-03
4's	$4.20	GENERIC, Prescript Pharmaceuticals	00247-0116-04
5's	$1.43	GENERIC, Allscripts Pharmaceutical Company	54569-3531-02
5's	$4.41	GENERIC, Prescript Pharmaceuticals	00247-0116-05
6's	$3.47	GENERIC, Southwood Pharmaceuticals Inc	58016-0127-06
6's	$4.62	GENERIC, Prescript Pharmaceuticals	00247-0116-06
8's	$4.62	GENERIC, Southwood Pharmaceuticals Inc	58016-0127-08
9's	$5.26	GENERIC, Prescript Pharmaceuticals	00247-0116-09
10's	$5.78	GENERIC, Southwood Pharmaceuticals Inc	58016-0127-10
14's	$8.09	GENERIC, Southwood Pharmaceuticals Inc	58016-0127-14
15's	$6.53	GENERIC, Prescript Pharmaceuticals	00247-0116-15
20's	$5.72	GENERIC, Allscripts Pharmaceutical Company	54569-2507-07
20's	$7.59	GENERIC, Prescript Pharmaceuticals	00247-0116-20
20's	$11.55	GENERIC, Southwood Pharmaceuticals Inc	58016-0127-20
21's	$6.01	GENERIC, Allscripts Pharmaceutical Company	54569-2507-05
21's	$7.80	GENERIC, Prescript Pharmaceuticals	00247-0116-21
21's	$11.72	GENERIC, Pharma Pac	52959-0063-21
21's	$12.13	GENERIC, Southwood Pharmaceuticals Inc	58016-0127-21
24's	$13.86	GENERIC, Southwood Pharmaceuticals Inc	58016-0127-24
28's	$8.01	GENERIC, Allscripts Pharmaceutical Company	54569-2507-03
28's	$9.28	GENERIC, Prescript Pharmaceuticals	00247-0116-28
28's	$12.35	GENERIC, Alpharma Uspd Makers Of Barre and Nmc	63874-0110-28
28's	$14.43	GENERIC, Pharma Pac	52959-0063-28
28's	$16.17	GENERIC, Southwood Pharmaceuticals Inc	58016-0127-28
30's	$8.59	GENERIC, Allscripts Pharmaceutical Company	54569-2507-04
30's	$9.71	GENERIC, Prescript Pharmaceuticals	00247-0116-30
30's	$15.12	GENERIC, Pharma Pac	52959-0063-30
30's	$17.32	GENERIC, Southwood Pharmaceuticals Inc	58016-0127-30
40's	$11.45	GENERIC, Allscripts Pharmaceutical Company	54569-2507-02
40's	$11.82	GENERIC, Prescript Pharmaceuticals	00247-0116-40
40's	$16.32	GENERIC, Alpharma Uspd Makers Of Barre and Nmc	63874-0110-40
40's	$17.49	GENERIC, Pharma Pac	52959-0063-40
40's	$23.10	GENERIC, Southwood Pharmaceuticals Inc	58016-0127-40
42's	$24.26	GENERIC, Southwood Pharmaceuticals Inc	58016-0127-42
50's	$28.88	GENERIC, Southwood Pharmaceuticals Inc	58016-0127-50
60's	$34.65	GENERIC, Southwood Pharmaceuticals Inc	58016-0127-60
100's	$27.50	GENERIC, Cmc-Consolidated Midland Corporation	00223-0912-01
100's	$31.20	GENERIC, Alpharma Uspd Makers Of Barre and Nmc	63874-0110-01

Erythromycin Ethylsuccinate; Sulfisoxazole Acetyl (001181)

Categories: Infection, ear, middle; Pregnancy Category C; FDA Approved 1989 Sep
Drug Classes: Antibiotics, macrolides; Antibiotics, sulfonamides
Brand Names: Erythromycin W/Sulfisoxazole; Eryzole; **Pediazole**; Sulfimycin
Foreign Brand Availability: Erisul (Colombia)
Cost of Therapy: $27.46 (Otitis Media; Pediazole Suspension; 200 mg; 600 mg/5 ml; 20 ml/day; 10 day supply)
$23.15 (Otitis Media; Generic Suspension; 200 mg; 600 mg/5 ml; 20 ml/day; 10 day supply)

DESCRIPTION

This product is a combination of erythromycin ethylsuccinate and sulfisoxazole acetyl. When reconstituted with water as directed on the label, the granules form a white, strawberry-banana flavor suspension that provides the equivalent of 200 mg of erythromycin activity and the equivalent of 600 mg of sulfisoxazole per teaspoonful (5 ml).

Erythromycin is produced by a strain of *S. erythraea* and belongs to the macrolide group of antibiotics. It is basic and readily forms salts and esters. Erythromycin ethylsuccinate is the 2′-ethylsuccinyl ester of erythromycin. It is essentially a tasteless form of the antibiotic suitable for oral administration, particularly in suspension dosage forms. The chemical name is erythromycin 2′-(ethylsuccinate).

Sulfisoxazole acetyl or N^1-acetyl sulfisoxazole is an ester of sulfisoxazole. Chemically, sulfisoxazole is N-(3,4-Dimethyl-5-isoxazolyl)-N-sulfanilylacetamide.

Inactive Ingredients: Citric acid, magnesium aluminum silicate, poloxamer, sodium carboxymethylcellulose, sodium citrate, sucrose, and artificial flavoring.

CLINICAL PHARMACOLOGY

Orally administered erythromycin ethylsuccinate suspensions are readily and reliably absorbed. Erythromycin ethylsuccinate products have demonstrated rapid and consistent absorption in both fasting and nonfasting conditions. Higher serum concentrations are obtained when these products are given with food. Bioavailability data are available from Ross Products Division. Erythromycin is largely bound to plasma proteins. After absorption, erythromycin diffuses readily into most body fluids. In the absence of meningeal inflammation, low concentrations are normally achieved in the spinal fluid, but the passage of the drug across the blood-brain barrier increases in meningitis. Erythromycin crosses the placental barrier and is excreted in human milk. Erythromycin is not removed by peritoneal dialysis or hemodialysis.

In the presence of normal hepatic function, erythromycin is concentrated in the liver and is excreted in the bile; the effect of hepatic dysfunction on biliary excretion of erythromycin is not known. After oral administration, less than 5% of the administered dose can be recovered in the active form in the urine.

Wide variation in blood levels may result following identical doses of sulfonamide. Blood levels should be measured in patients receiving these drugs for serious infections. Free sulfonamide blood levels of 50-150 μg/ml may be considered therapeutically effective for most infections, with blood levels of 120-150 μg/ml being optimal for serious infections. The maximum sulfonamide level should be 200 μg/ml, because adverse reactions occur more frequently above this concentration.

Following oral administration, sulfisoxazole is rapidly and completely absorbed; the small intestine is the major site of absorption, but some of the drug is absorbed from the stomach. Sulfonamides are present in the blood as free, conjugated (acetylated and possibly other forms), and protein-bound forms. The amount present as "free" drug is considered to be the therapeutically active form. Approximately 85% of a dose of sulfisoxazole is bound to plasma proteins, primarily to albumin; 65-72% of the unbound portion is in the non-acetylated form.

Maximum plasma concentrations of intact sulfisoxazole following a single 2 g oral dose of sulfisoxazole to healthy adult volunteers ranged from 127-211 μg/ml (mean, 169 μg/ml), and the time of peak plasma concentration ranged from 1-4 hours (mean, 2.5 hours). The elimination half-life of sulfisoxazole ranged from 4.6-7.8 hours after oral administration. The elimination of sulfisoxazole has been shown to be slower in elderly subjects (63-75 years) with diminished renal function (creatine clearance 37-68 ml/min).[1] After multiple-dose oral administration of 500 mg qid to healthy volunteers, the average steady-state plasma concentrations of intact sulfisoxazole ranged from 49.9-88.8 μg/ml (mean, 63.4 μg/ml).[2]

Sulfisoxazole and its acetylated metabolites are excreted primarily by the kidneys through glomerular filtration. Concentrations of sulfisoxazole are considerably higher in the urine than in the blood. The mean urinary recovery following oral administration of sulfisoxazole is 97% within 48 hours; 52% of this is intact drug, and the remainder is the N^4-acetylated metabolite.

Sulfisoxazole is distributed only in extracellular body fluids. it is excreted in human milk. It readily crosses the placental barrier. In healthy subjects, cerebrospinal fluid concentrations of sulfisoxazole vary; in patients with meningitis, however, concentrations of free drug in cerebrospinal fluid as high as 94 μg/ml have been reported.

MICROBIOLOGY

The drug has been formulated to contain sulfisoxazole for concomitant use with erythromycin.

Erythromycin acts by inhibition of protein synthesis by binding 50 S ribosomal subunits of susceptible organisms. It does not affect nucleic acid synthesis. Antagonism has been demonstrated *in vitro* between erythromycin and clindamycin, lincomycin, and chloramphenicol.

The sulfonamides are bacteriostatic agents, and the spectrum of activity is similar for all. Sulfonamides inhibit bacterial synthesis of dihydrofolic acid by preventing the condensation of the pteridine with*para*-aminobenzoic acid through competitive inhibition of the enzyme dihydropteroate synthetase. Resistant strains have altered dihydropterase synthetase with reduced affinity for sulfonamides or produce increased quantities of *para*-aminobenzoic acid.

SUSCEPTIBILITY TESTING

Quantitative methods that require measurement of zone diameter give the most precise estimates of the susceptibility of bacteria to antimicrobial agents. One such standardized single-disc procedure[3] has been recommended for use with discs to test susceptibility to erythromycin and sulfisoxazole. Interpretation involves correlation of the zone diameters obtained in the disc test with minimal inhibitory concentration (MIC) values for erythromycin.

If the standardized procedure of disc susceptibility is used, a 15 μg erythromycin disc should give a zone diameter of at least 18 mm when tested against an erythromycin-susceptible bacterial strain and a 250-300 μg sulfisoxazole disc should give a zone diameter of at least 17 mm when tested against a sulfisoxazole-susceptible bacterial strain.

In vitro sulfonamide susceptibility tests are not always reliable because media containing excessive amounts of thymidine are capable of reversing the inhibitory effect of sulfonamides, which may result in false resistant reports. The tests must be carefully coordinated with bacteriological and clinical responses. When the patient is already taking sulfonamides, follow-up cultures should have aminobenzoic acid added to the isolation media but not to subsequent susceptibility test media.

INDICATIONS AND USAGE

For treatment of ACUTE OTITIS MEDIA in children that is caused by susceptible strains of *Hemophilus influenzae.*

CONTRAINDICATIONS

Patients with a known hypersensitivity to either of its components, children younger than 2 months of age, pregnant women *at term,* and mothers nursing infants less than 2 months of age.

Use in pregnant women at term, in children less than 2 months of age, and in mothers nursing infants less than 2 months of age is contraindicated because sulfonamides may promote kernicterus in the newborn by displacing bilirubin from plasma proteins.

Erythromycin is contraindicated in patients taking terfenadine. (See DRUG INTERACTIONS.)

WARNINGS

FATALITIES ASSOCIATED WITH THE ADMINISTRATION OF SULFONAMIDES, ALTHOUGH RARE, HAVE OCCURRED DUE TO SEVERE REACTIONS INCLUDING STEVENS-JOHNSON SYNDROME, TOXIC EPIDERMAL NECROLYSIS, FULMINANT HEPATIC NECROSIS, AGRANULOCYTOSIS, APLASTIC ANEMIA, AND OTHER BLOOD DYSCRASIAS.

SULFONAMIDES, INCLUDING SULFONAMIDE-CONTAINING PRODUCTS SUCH AS PEDIAZOLE, SHOULD BE DISCONTINUED AT THE FIRST APPEARANCE OF SKIN RASH OR ANY SIGN OF ADVERSE REACTION. In rare instances, a skin rash may be followed by a more severe reaction, such as Stevens-Johnson syndrome, toxic epidermal necrolysis, hepatic necrosis, and serious blood disorders. (See PRECAUTIONS.)

Clinical signs such as sore throat, fever, pallor, rash, purpura, or jaundice may be early indications of serious reactions.

There have been reports of hepatic dysfunction, with or without jaundice, occurring in patients receiving oral erythromycin products.

Cough, shortness of breath, and pulmonary infiltrates are hypersensitivity reactions of the respiratory tract that have been reported in association with sulfonamide treatment.

The sulfonamides should not be used for the treatment of group A beta-hemolytic streptococcal infections. In an established infection, they will not eradicate the streptococcus, and, therefore, will not prevent sequelae such as rheumatic fever.

Pseudomembranous colitis has been reported with nearly all antibacterial agents, including this drug, and may range in severity from mild to life-threatening. Therefore, it is important to consider this diagnosis in patients who present with diarrhea subsequent to the administration of antibacterial agents.

Treatment with antibacterial agents alters the normal flora of the colon and may permit overgrowth of clostridia. Studies indicate that a toxin produced by *Clostridium difficile* is one primary cause of "antibiotic-associated colitis."

After diagnosis of pseudomembranous colitis has been established, therapeutic measures should be initiated. Mild cases of pseudomembranous colitis usually respond to drug discontinuation alone. In moderate to severe cases, consideration should be given to management with fluids and electrolytes, protein supplementation, and treatment with an antibacterial drug clinically effective against *Clostridium difficile* colitis.

There have been reports suggesting that erythromycin does not reach the fetus in adequate concentration to prevent congenital syphilis. Infants born to women treated during pregnancy with erythromycin for early syphilis should be treated with an appropriate penicillin regimen.

Rhabdomyolysis with or without renal impairment has been reported in seriously ill patients receiving erythromycin concomitantly with lovastatin. Therefore, patients receiving concomitant lovastatin and erythromycin should be carefully monitored for creatine kinase (CK) and serum transaminase levels. (See prescribing information for lovastatin.)

PRECAUTIONS

GENERAL

Erythromycin is principally excreted by the liver. Caution should be exercised in administering the antibiotic to patients with impaired hepatic function. (See CLINICAL PHARMACOLOGY and WARNINGS.)

Prolonged or repeated use of erythromycin may result in an overgrowth of nonsusceptible bacteria or fungi. If superinfection occurs, erythromycin should be discontinued and appropriate therapy instituted.

There have been reports that erythromycin may aggravate the weakness of patients with myasthenia gravis.

When indicated, incision and drainage or other surgical procedures should be performed in conjunction with antibiotic therapy.

Sulfonamides should be given with caution to patients with impaired renal or hepatic function and to those with severe allergy or bronchial asthma. In glucose-6-phosphate dehydrogenase-deficient individuals, hemolysis may occur; this reaction is frequently dose-related.

INFORMATION FOR THE PATIENT

Patients should maintain an adequate fluid intake to prevent crystalluria and stone formation.

LABORATORY TESTS

Complete blood counts should be done frequently in patients receiving sulfonamides. If a significant reduction in the count of any formed blood element is noted, the drug should be discontinued. Urinalysis with careful microscopic examination and renal function tests should be performed during therapy, particularly for those patients with impaired renal function. Blood levels should be measured in patients receiving a sulfonamide for serious infections. (See INDICATIONS AND USAGE.)

DRUG/LABORATORY TEST INTERACTIONS

Erythromycin interferes with the fluorometric determination of urinary catecholamines.

CARCINOGENESIS, MUTAGENESIS, AND IMPAIRMENT OF FERTILITY

Carcinogenesis

The drug has not undergone adequate trials relating to carcinogenicity; each component, however, has been evaluated separately. Long-term (21 month) oral studies conducted in rats with erythromycin ethylsuccinate did not provide evidence of tumorigenicity. Sulfisoxazole was not carcinogenic in either sex when administered to mice by gavage for 103 weeks at dosages up to approximately 18 times the recommended human dose or to rats at 4 times the human dose. Rats appear to be especially susceptible to the goitrogenic effects of sulfonamides, and long-term administration of sulfonamides has resulted in thyroid malignancies in this species.

Mutagenesis

There are no studies available that adequately evaluate the mutagenic potential of the drug or either of its components. However, sulfisoxazole was not observed to be mutagenic in *E. coli* Sd-4-73 when tested in the absence of a metabolic activating system. There was no apparent effect on male or female fertility in rats fed erythromycin (base) at levels up to 0.25% of diet.

Impairment of Fertility

The drug has not undergone adequate trials relating to impairment of fertility. In a reproduction study in rats given 7 times the human dose per day of sulfisoxazole, no effects were observed regarding mating behavior, conception rate or fertility index (percent pregnant).

PREGNANCY, TERATOGENIC EFFECTS, PREGNANCY CATEGORY C

At dosages 7 times the human daily dose, sulfisoxazole was not teratogenic in either rats or rabbits. However, in two other teratogenicity studies, cleft palates developed in both rats and mice after administration of 5-9 times the human therapeutic dose of sulfisoxazole.

There is no evidence of teratogenicity or any other adverse effect on reproduction in female rats fed erythromycin base (up to 0.25% of diet) prior to and during mating, during gestation, and through weaning of two successive litters. There are, however, no adequate and well-controlled studies in pregnant women. Because animal reproduction studies are not always predictive of human response, this drug should be used during pregnancy only if clearly needed. Erythromycin has been reported to cross the placental barrier in humans, but fetal plasma levels are generally low.

There are no adequate or well-controlled studies of the drug in either laboratory animals or in pregnant women. It is not known whether the drug can cause fetal harm when administered to a pregnant woman prior to term or can affect reproduction capacity. The drug should be used during pregnancy only if potential benefit justifies potential risk to the fetus. **Nonteratogenic Effects:** Kernicterus may occur in the newborn as a result of treatment of a pregnant woman *at term* with sulfonamides. (See CONTRAINDICATIONS.)

LABOR AND DELIVERY

The effects of erythromycin and sulfisoxazole on labor and delivery are unknown.

NURSING MOTHERS

Both erythromycin and sulfisoxazole are excreted in human milk. **Because of the potential for the development of kernicterus in neonates due to the displacement of bilirubin from plasma proteins by sulfisoxazole, a decision should be made whether to discontinue nursing or discontinue the drug, taking into account the importance of the drug to the mother.** (See CONTRAINDICATIONS.)

PEDIATRIC USE

See INDICATIONS AND USAGE and DOSAGE AND ADMINISTRATION. Not for use in children under 2 months of age. (See CONTRAINDICATIONS.)

DRUG INTERACTIONS

Erythromycin use in patients who are receiving high doses of theophylline may be associated with an increase of serum theophylline levels and potential theophylline toxicity. In case of theophylline toxicity and/or elevated serum theophylline levels, the dose of theophylline should be reduced while the patient is receiving concomitant erythromycin therapy.

Concomitant administration of erythromycin and digoxin has been reported to result in elevated digoxin serum levels.

There have been reports of increased anticoagulant effects when erythromycin and oral anticoagulants were used concomitantly. Increased anticoagulation effects due to this drug may be more pronounced in the elderly.

Concurrent use of erythromycin and ergotamine or dihydroergotamine has been associated in some patients with acute ergot toxicity characterized by severe peripheral vasospasm and dysesthesia.

Erythromycin has been reported to decrease the clearance of triazolam and midazolam and thus may increase the pharmacologic effect of these benzodiazepines.

The use of erythromycin in patients concurrently taking drugs metabolized by the cytochrome P450 system may be associated with elevations of serum levels of these other drugs. There have been reports of interactions of erythromycin with carbamazepine, cyclosporine, hexobarbital, phenytoin, alfentanil, disopyramide, lovastatin, and bromocriptine. Serum concentrations of drugs metabolized by the cytochrome P450 system should be monitored closely in patients concurrently receiving erythromycin.

Erythromycin significantly alters the metabolism of terfenadine when taken concomitantly. Rare cases of serious cardiovascular adverse events, including death, cardiac arrest, torsades de pointes, and other ventricular arrhythmias, have been observed. (See CONTRAINDICATIONS.)

It has been reported that sulfisoxazole may prolong the prothrombin time in patients who are receiving the anticoagulant warfarin. This interaction should be kept in mind when the drug is given to patients already on the anticoagulant therapy, and the coagulation time should be reassessed.

It has been proposed that sulfisoxazole competes with thiopental for plasma protein binding. In one study involving 48 patients, intravenous sulfisoxazole resulted in a decrease in the amount of thiopental required for anesthesia and in a shortening of the awakening time. It is not known whether chronic oral doses of sulfisoxazole have a similar effect. Until more is known about this interaction, physicians should be aware that patients receiving sulfisoxazole might require less thiopental for anesthesia.

Sulfonamides can displace methotrexate from plasma protein binding sites, thus increasing free methotrexate concentrations. Studies in man have shown sulfisoxazole infusions to decrease plasma protein-bound methotrexate by one fourth.

Sulfisoxazole can also potentiate the blood-sugar-lowering activity of sulfonylureas.

ADVERSE REACTIONS

ERYTHROMYCIN ETHYLSUCCINATE

The most frequent side effects of oral erythromycin preparations are gastrointestinal and are dose-related. They include nausea, vomiting, abdominal pain, diarrhea and anorexia. Symptoms of hepatic dysfunction and/or abnormal liver-function test results may occur. (See WARNINGS.) Pseudomembranous colitis has been rarely reported in association with erythromycin therapy.

Allergic reactions ranging from urticaria and mild skin eruptions to anaphylaxis have occurred.

There have been isolated reports of reversible hearing loss occurring chiefly in patients with renal insufficiency and in patients receiving high doses of erythromycin.

Onset of pseudomembranous colitis symptoms may occur during or after antibiotic treatment. (See WARNINGS.)

SULFISOXAZOLE ACETYL

Included in this listing that follows are adverse reactions that have been reported with other sulfonamide products; pharmacologic similarities require that each of the reactions be considered with the drug's administration.

Allergic/Dermatologic: Anaphylaxis, erythema multiforme (Stevens-Johnson syndrome), toxic epidermal necrolysis (Lyell's syndrome), exfoliative dermatitis, angioedema, arteritis, vasculitis, allergic myocarditis, serum sickness, rash, urticaria, pruritus, photosensitivity, and conjunctival and scleral injection. In addition, periarteritis nodosa and systemic lupus erythematosus has been reported. (See WARNINGS.)

Cardiovascular: Tachycardia, palpitations, syncope, and cyanosis. Rarely, erythromycin has been associated with the production of ventricular arrhythmias, including ventricular tachycardia and torsade de pointes, in individuals with prolonged QT intervals.

Endocrine: The sulfonamides bear certain chemical similarities to some goitrogens, diuretics (acetazolamide and the thiazides) and oral hypoglycemic agents. Cross-sensitivity may exist with these agents. Developments of goiter, diuresis, and hypoglycemia have occurred rarely in patients receiving sulfonamides.

Gastrointestinal: Hepatitis, hepatocellular necrosis, jaundice, pseudomembranous colitis, nausea, emesis, anorexia, abdominal pain, diarrhea, gastrointestinal hemorrhage, melena, flatulence, glossitis, stomatitis, salivary gland enlargement, and pancreatitis. Onset of pseudomembranous colitis symptoms may occur during or after treatment with sulfisoxazole, a component of this drug. (See WARNINGS.) The sulfisoxazole acetyl component of this drug has been reported to cause increased elevation of liver-associated enzymes in patients with hepatitis.

Genitourinary: Crystalluria, hematuria, BUN and creatinine elevations, nephritis, and toxic nephrosis with oliguria and anuria. Acute renal failure and urinary retention have also been reported. The frequency of renal complications, commonly associated with some sulfonamides, is lower in patients receiving the more soluble sulfonamides such as sulfisoxazole.

Hematologic: Leukopenia, agranulocytosis, aplastic anemia, thrombocytopenia, purpura, hemolytic anemia, eosinophilia, clotting disorders including hypoprothrombinemia and hypofibrinogenemia, sulfhemoglobinemia, and methemoglobinemia.

Neurologic: Headache, dizziness, peripheral neuritis, paresthesia, convulsions, tinnitus, vertigo, ataxia, and intracranial hypertension.

Psychiatric: Psychosis, hallucinations, disorientation, depression, and anxiety.

Respiratory: Cough, shortness of breath, and pulmonary infiltrates. (See WARNINGS.)

Vascular: Angioedema, arteritis, and vasculitis.

Miscellaneous: Edema (including periorbital), pyrexia, drowsiness, weakness, fatigue, lassitude, rigors, flushing, hearing loss, insomnia, and pneumonitis.

DOSAGE AND ADMINISTRATION

THIS DRUG SHOULD NOT BE ADMINISTERED TO INFANTS UNDER 2 MONTHS OF AGE BECAUSE OF CONTRAINDICATIONS OF SYSTEMIC SULFONAMIDES IN THIS AGE GROUP.

For Acute Otitis Media in Children: The dose of erythromycin ethylsuccinate w/ sulfisoxazole acetyl can be calculated based on the erythromycin component (50 mg/kg/day) or the sulfisoxazole component (150 mg/kg/day to a maximum of 6 g/day). The total daily dose of erythromycin ethylsuccinate w/ sulfisoxazole acetyl should be administered in equally divided doses 3 or 4 times a day for 10 days. Erythromycin ethylsuccinate w/ sulfisoxazole acetyl may be administered without regard to meals.

The following approximate dosage schedules are recommended for using erythromycin ethylsuccinate w/ sulfisoxazole acetyl:

Children: Two months of age or older. (See TABLE 2A and TABLE 2B.)

TABLE 2A

Four-Times-a-Day Schedule

Weight	Dose — every 6 hours
Less than 8 kg (<18 lb)	Adjust dosage by body weight
8 kg (18 lb)	½ teaspoonful (2.5 ml)
16 kg (35 lb)	1 teaspoonful (5 ml)
24 kg (53 lb)	1 ½ teaspoonfuls (7.5 ml)
Over 32 kg (over 70 lb)	2 teaspoonfuls (10 ml)

TABLE 2B

Three-Times-a-Day Schedule

Weight	Dose - every 8 hours
Less than 6 kg (<13 lb)	Adjust dosage by body weight
6 kg (13 lb)	½ teaspoonful (2.5 ml)
12 kg (26 lb)	1 teaspoonful (5 ml)
18 kg (40 lb)	1½ teaspoonfuls (7.5 ml)
24 kg (53 lb)	2 teaspoonfuls (10 ml)
Over 30 kg (over 65 lb)	2½ teaspoonfuls (12.5 ml)

Recommended storage: Before mixing, store below 86°F (30°C).

PRODUCT LISTING - RATED THERAPEUTICALLY EQUIVALENT

Granule For Reconstitution - Oral - 200 mg;600 mg/5 ml

Size	Price	Product	NDC
100 ml	$11.00	GENERIC, Moore, H.L. Drug Exchange Inc	00839-7514-73
100 ml	$11.90	GENERIC, Mutual/United Research Laboratories	00677-1303-27
100 ml	$11.95	GENERIC, Major Pharmaceuticals Inc	00904-2475-04
100 ml	$12.50	GENERIC, Geneva Pharmaceuticals	00781-7043-46
100 ml	$12.70	GENERIC, Barr Laboratories Inc	00555-0445-22
100 ml	$12.75	GENERIC, Alra	51641-0111-64
100 ml	$12.77	GENERIC, Abbott Pharmaceutical	00074-7156-13
100 ml	$14.96	PEDIAZOLE, Physicians Total Care	54868-0302-01
100 ml	$16.06	PEDIAZOLE, Southwood Pharmaceuticals Inc	58016-4114-01
100 ml	$17.75	PEDIAZOLE, Abbott Pharmaceutical	00074-8030-13
150 ml	$17.30	GENERIC, Major Pharmaceuticals Inc	00904-2475-07
150 ml	$17.40	GENERIC, Qualitest Products Inc	00603-6563-66
150 ml	$17.81	GENERIC, Moore, H.L. Drug Exchange Inc	00839-7514-75
150 ml	$18.50	GENERIC, Geneva Pharmaceuticals	00781-7043-55
150 ml	$18.80	GENERIC, Barr Laboratories Inc	00555-0445-21
150 ml	$18.85	GENERIC, Alra	51641-0111-66
150 ml	$18.88	GENERIC, Abbott Pharmaceutical	00074-7156-43
150 ml	$26.37	PEDIAZOLE, Abbott Pharmaceutical	00074-8030-43
150 ml	$26.38	PEDIAZOLE, Allscripts Pharmaceutical Company	54569-1026-00
200 ml	$23.25	GENERIC, Major Pharmaceuticals Inc	00904-2475-08
200 ml	$24.50	GENERIC, Geneva Pharmaceuticals	00781-7043-48
200 ml	$24.78	GENERIC, Barr Laboratories Inc	00555-0445-23
200 ml	$24.80	GENERIC, Alra	51641-0111-68
200 ml	$24.82	GENERIC, Abbott Pharmaceutical	00074-7156-53
200 ml	$25.30	GENERIC, Mutual/United Research Laboratories	00677-1303-29
200 ml	$25.38	GENERIC, Moore, H.L. Drug Exchange Inc	00839-7514-78
200 ml	$27.46	PEDIAZOLE, Southwood Pharmaceuticals Inc	58016-4113-01
200 ml	$28.48	PEDIAZOLE, Physicians Total Care	54868-0302-02
200 ml	$33.62	PEDIAZOLE, Abbott Pharmaceutical	00074-8030-55
200 ml	$33.62	PEDIAZOLE, Allscripts Pharmaceutical Company	54569-8021-00
200 ml	$34.63	PEDIAZOLE, Abbott Pharmaceutical	00074-8030-53
250 ml	$41.38	PEDIAZOLE, Abbott Pharmaceutical	00074-8030-73

PRODUCT LISTING - EQUIVALENTS NOT AVAILABLE

Granule For Reconstitution - Oral - 200 mg;600 mg/5 ml

Size	Price	Product	NDC
100 ml	$8.65	GENERIC, Prescript Pharmaceuticals	00247-0009-00
100 ml	$12.70	GENERIC, Allscripts Pharmaceutical Company	54569-2000-00
100 ml	$15.95	GENERIC, Southwood Pharmaceuticals Inc	58016-1023-03
100 ml	$17.45	GENERIC, Southwood Pharmaceuticals Inc	58016-1023-01
150 ml	$11.29	GENERIC, Prescript Pharmaceuticals	00247-0009-78
150 ml	$18.80	GENERIC, Allscripts Pharmaceutical Company	54569-2001-00
150 ml	$20.95	GENERIC, Pharma Pac	52959-0164-06
150 ml	$23.30	GENERIC, Southwood Pharmaceuticals Inc	58016-1024-01
200 ml	$13.94	GENERIC, Prescript Pharmaceuticals	00247-0009-79
200 ml	$24.78	GENERIC, Allscripts Pharmaceutical Company	54569-2002-00
200 ml	$25.50	GENERIC, Pharma Pac	52959-0164-03
200 ml	$30.50	GENERIC, Southwood Pharmaceuticals Inc	58016-1025-01

Erythromycin Stearate *(001185)*

Categories: Amebiasis, intestinal; Conjunctivitis, infectious; Diphtheria; Endocarditis, prevention; Erythrasma; Infection, endocervical; Infection, gynecologic; Infection, lower respiratory tract; Infection, ophthalmic; Infection, rectal; Infection, skin and skin structures; Infection, upper respiratory tract; Infection, urethra; Legionnaires' disease; Pelvic inflammatory disease; Pertussis; Pneumonia; Rheumatic fever, prophylaxis; Syphilis; Pregnancy Category B; FDA Approved 1964 Jun; WHO Formulary

Drug Classes: Antibiotics, macrolides

Brand Names: Emestid; Erimit; Erimycin; Erymid; **Erythrocin Stearate**; My-E; Pocin; Tomcin; Wyamycin S

Foreign Brand Availability: Abboticin (Finland); Apo-Erythro-S (Canada); Arcanamycin (South-Africa); Baknyl (Ecuador); Bannthrocin (Indonesia); Cetathrocin (Indonesia); Duramycin (Indonesia); Elocin (Thailand); Emu-V E (Benin; Burkina-Faso; Ethiopia; Gambia; Ghana; Guinea; Ivory-Coast; Kenya; Liberia; Malawi; Mali; Mauritania; Mauritius; Morocco; Niger; Nigeria; Senegal; Seychelles; Sierra-Leone; South-Africa; Sudan; Tanzania; Tunia; Uganda; Zambia; Zimbabwe); ERA (New-Zealand); Eribus (Mexico); Eriecu (Ecuador); Eritrocina (Portugal); Eritrolag (Bahamas; Bahrain; Barbados; Belize; Benin; Bermuda; Burkina-Faso; Curacao; Cyprus; Egypt; Ethiopia; Gambia; Ghana; Guinea; Guyana; Iran; Iraq; Israel; Ivory-Coast; Jamaica; Jordan; Kenya; Kuwait; Lebanon; Liberia; Libya; Malawi; Mali; Mauritania; Mauritius; Morocco; Netherland-Antilles; Niger; Nigeria; Oman; Puerto-Rico; Qatar; Republic-of-Yemen; Saudi-Arabia; Senegal; Seychelles; Sierra-Leone; South-Africa; Sudan; Surinam; Syria; Tanzania; Trinidad; Tunia; Uganda; United-Arab-Emirates; Zambia; Zimbabwe); Eritromicina (Colombia); Eromel (South-Africa); Erotab (Malaysia); Erycin (Taiwan; Thailand); Erymycin AF (South-Africa); Erytab-S (Malaysia); Eryth-Mycin (Thailand); Erythrocin (Australia; Austria; Bahamas; Bahrain; Barbados; Belize; Bermuda; Canada; Curacao; Cyprus; Egypt; England; Germany; Greece; Guyana; Hong-Kong; Iran; Iraq; Israel; Jamaica; Jordan; Kuwait; Lebanon; Libya; Netherland-Antilles; New-Zealand; Oman; Philippines; Puerto-Rico; Qatar; Republic-of-Yemen; Saudi-Arabia; South-Africa; Surinam; Syria; Taiwan; Trinidad; United-Arab-Emirates); Erythrocine (Netherlands); Erythrogenat (Germany); Erythromil (Austria; Belgium; Bulgaria; Czech-Republic; Denmark; England; Finland; France; Germany; Greece; Hungary; Ireland; Italy; Netherlands; Norway; Poland; Portugal; Slovenia; Spain; Sweden; Switzerland; Turkey); Erythromycin (Germany); Erythromycine (Bulgaria); Erythromycinum (Netherlands); Erythropen (Greece); Erythro-Teva (Israel); Etrotab (Malaysia); Galentromicina (Mexico); Kemothrocin (Indonesia); Pantomicina (Costa-Rica; Dominican-Republic; Ecuador; El-Salvador; Guatemala; Honduras; Mexico; Nicaragua; Panama; Peru; Spain); Roug-mycin (Greece); Rythocin (Thailand); Servitrocin (Hong-Kong; Philippines); Urycin (Taiwan)

Cost of Therapy: $4.39 (Infection; Generic Tablets; 500 mg; 2 tablets/day; 10 day supply)

DESCRIPTION

Erythromycin is produced by a strain of *Streptomyces erythraeus* and belongs to the macrolide group of antibiotics. It is basic and readily forms salts with acids. The base, the stearate salt, and the esters are poorly soluble in water, and are suitable for oral administration.

Erythrocin Stearate Filmtab tablets contain the stearate salt of the antibiotic in a unique film coating. *Inactive ingredients for the 250 mg tablet:* Cellulosic polymers, corn starch, D&C red no. 7, polacrilin potassium, polyethylene glycol, povidone, propylene glycol, sodium carboxymethylcellulose, sodium citrate, sorbic acid, sorbitan monooleate and titanium dioxide. *Inactive ingredients for the 500 mg tablet:* Cellulosic polymers, corn starch, FD&C red no. 3, magnesium hydroxide, polacrilin potassium, povidone, propylene glycol, sorbitan monooleate, titanium dioxide and vanillin.

Storage: Store below 30°C (86°F).

CLINICAL PHARMACOLOGY

MICROBIOLOGY

Biochemical tests demonstrate that erythromycin inhibits protein synthesis of the pathogen without directly affecting nucleic acid synthesis. Antagonism has been demonstrated between clindamycin and erythromycin.

Note: Many strains of *Hemophilus influenzae* are resistant to erythromycin alone, but are susceptible to erythromycin and sulfonamides together. Staphylococci resistant to erythromycin may emerge during a course of erythromycin therapy. Culture and susceptibility testing should be performed.

Disc Susceptibility Tests: Quantitative methods that require measurement of zone diameters give the most precise estimates of antibiotic susceptibility. One recommended procedure (21 CFR section 460.1) uses erythromycin class discs for testing susceptibility; interpretations correlate zone diameters of this disc test with MIC values for erythromycin. With this procedure, a report from the laboratory of "susceptible" indicates that the infecting organism is likely to respond to therapy. A report of "resistant" indicates that the infective organism is not likely to respond to therapy. A report of "intermediate susceptibility" suggests that the organism would be susceptible if higher doses were used.

Erythromycin binds to the 50 S ribosomal subunits of susceptible bacteria and suppresses protein synthesis.

Orally administered erythrocin stearate tablets are readily and reliably absorbed. Optimal serum levels of erythromycin are reached when the drug is taken in the fasting state or immediately before meals.

Erythromycin diffuses readily into most body fluids. Only low concentrations are normally achieved in the spinal fluid, but passage of the drug across the blood-brain barrier increases in meningitis. In the presence of normal hepatic function, erythromycin is concentrated in the liver and excreted in the bile; the effect of hepatic dysfunction on excretion of erythromycin by the liver into the bile is not known. Less than 5 percent of the orally administered dose of erythromycin is excreted in active form in the urine.

Erythromycin crosses the placental barrier and is excreted in breast milk.

INDICATIONS AND USAGE

Streptococcus pyogenes **(Group A beta Hemolytic** ***Streptococcus*****):** Upper and lower respiratory tract, skin, and soft tissue infections of mild to moderate severity.

Injectable benzathine penicillin G is considered by the American Heart Association to be the drug of choice in the treatment and prevention of streptococcal pharyngitis and in long-term prophylaxis of rheumatic fever.

When oral medication is preferred for treatment of the above conditions, penicillin G, V, or erythromycin are alternate drugs of choice.

When oral medication is given, the importance of strict adherence by the patient to the prescribed dosage regimen must be stressed. A therapeutic dose should be administered for at least 10 days.

Alpha-hemolytic Streptococci (Viridans Group): Although no controlled clinical efficacy trials have been conducted, oral erythromycin has been suggested by the American Heart Association and American Dental Association for use in a regimen for prophylaxis against bacterial endocarditis in patients hypersensitive to penicillin who have congenital heart disease, or rheumatic or other acquired valvular heart disease when they undergo dental procedures and surgical procedures of the upper respiratory tract.[1] Erythromycin is not suitable prior to genitourinary or gastrointestinal tract surgery. *Note:* When selecting antibiotics for the prevention of bacterial endocarditis the physician or dentist should read the full joint statement of the American Heart Association and the American Dental Association.[1]

Staphylococcus aureus: Acute infections of skin and soft tissue of mild to moderate severity. Resistant organisms may emerge during treatment.

Streptococcus pneumoniae (Diplococcus pneumoniae): Upper respiratory tract infections (*e.g.,* otitis media, pharyngitis) and lower respiratory tract infections (*e.g.,* pneumonia) of mild to moderate degree.

***Mycoplasma pneumoniae* (Eaton agent, PPLO):** For respiratory infections due to this organism.

Hemophilus influenzae: For upper respiratory tract infections of mild to moderate severity when used concomitantly with adequate doses of sulfonamides. (See sulfonamide prescribing information.) The concomitant use of the sulfonamides is necessary since not all strains of *Hemophilus influenzae* are susceptible to erythromycin at the concentrations of the antibiotic achieved with usual therapeutic doses.

Chlamydia trachomatis: Erythromycin is indicated for treatment of the following infections caused by *Chlamydia trachomatis* conjunctivitis of the newborn, pneumonia of infancy and urogenital infections during pregnancy. When tetracyclines are contraindicated or not tolerated, erythromycin is indicated for the treatment of uncomplicated urethral, endocervical, or rectal infections in adults due to *Chlamydia trachomatis.*[2]

Treponema pallidum: Erythromycin is an alternate choice of treatment for primary syphilis in patients allergic to the penicillins. In treatment of primary syphilis, spinal fluid examinations should be done before treatment and as part of follow-up after therapy.

Corynebacterium diphtheriae: As an adjunct to antitoxin, to prevent establishment of carriers, and to eradicate the organism in carriers.

Corynebacterium minutissimum: For the treatment of erythrasma.

Entamoeba histolytica: In the treatment of intestinal amebiasis only. Extra-enteric amebiasis requires treatment with other agents.

Listeria monocytogenes: Infections due to this organism.

Neisseria gonorrhoeae: Erythromycin lactobionate for injection in conjunction with erythromycin stearate orally, as an alternative drug in treatment of acute pelvic inflammatory disease caused by *N. gonorrhoeae* in female patients with a history of sensitivity to penicillin. Before treatment of gonorrhea, patients who are suspected of also having syphilis should have a microscopic examination for *T. pallidum* (by immunofluorescence or darkfield) before receiving erythromycin, and monthly serologic tests for a minimum of 4 months.

Bordetella pertussis: Erythromycin is effective in eliminating the organism from the nasopharynx of infected individuals, rendering them non-infectious. Some clinical studies suggests that erythromycin may be helpful in the prophylaxis of pertussis in exposed susceptible individuals.

Legionnaires' Disease: Although no controlled clinical efficacy studies have been conducted, *in vitro* and limited preliminary clinical data suggest that erythromycin may be effective in treating Legionnaires' Disease.

CONTRAINDICATIONS

Erythromycin is contraindicated in patients with known hypersensitivity to this antibiotic.

WARNINGS

There have been reports of hepatic dysfunction with or without jaundice, occurring in patients receiving oral erythromycin products.

PRECAUTIONS

GENERAL

Erythromycin is principally excreted by the liver. Caution should be exercised when erythromycin is administered to patients with impaired hepatic function. (See CLINICAL PHARMACOLOGY and WARNINGS.)

Prolonged or repeated use of erythromycin may result in an overgrowth of nonsusceptible bacteria or fungi. If superinfection occurs, erythromycin should be discontinued and appropriate therapy instituted.

When indicated, incision and drainage or other surgical procedures should be performed in conjunction with antibiotic therapy.

LABORATORY TESTS

Erythromycin interferes with the fluorometric determination of urinary catecholamines.

CARCINOGENESIS, MUTAGENESIS, AND IMPAIRMENT OF FERTILITY

Long-term (2 year) oral studies conducted in rats with erythromycin base did not provide evidence of tumorigenicity. Mutagenicity studies have not been conducted. There was no apparent effect on male or female fertility in rats fed erythromycin (base) at levels up to 0.25% of diet.

PREGNANCY CATEGORY B

There is no evidence of teratogenicity or any other adverse effect on reproduction in female rats fed erythromycin base (up to 0.25% of diet) prior to and during mating, during gestation, and through weaning of two successive litters. There are, however, no adequate and well-controlled studies in pregnant women. Because animal reproduction studies are not always predictive of human response, this drug should be used during pregnancy only if clearly needed. Erythromycin has been reported to cross the placental barrier in humans, but fetal plasma levels are generally low.

LABOR AND DELIVERY

The effect of erythromycin on labor and delivery is unknown.

NURSING MOTHERS

Erythromycin is excreted in breast milk, therefore, caution should be exercised when erythromycin is administered to a nursing woman.

PEDIATRIC USE

See INDICATIONS AND USAGE and DOSAGE AND ADMINISTRATION.

DRUG INTERACTIONS

Erythromycin use in patients who are receiving high doses of theophylline may be associated with an increase in serum theophylline levels and potential theophylline toxicity. In case of theophylline toxicity and/or elevated serum theophylline levels, the dose of theophylline should be reduced while the patient is receiving concomitant erythromycin therapy.

Concomitant administration of erythromycin and digoxin has been reported to result in elevated digoxin serum levels.

There have been reports of increased anticoagulant effects when erythromycin and oral anticoagulants were used concomitantly.

Concurrent use of erythromycin and ergotamine or dihydroergotamine has been associated in some patients with acute ergot toxicity characterized by severe peripheral vasospasm and dysesthesia.

Erythromycin has been reported to decrease the clearance of triazolam and thus may increase the pharmacologic effect of triazolam.

The use of erythromycin in patients concurrently taking drugs metabolized by the cytochrome P450 system may be associated with elevations in serum erythromycin with carbamazepine, cyclosporine, hexobarbital and phenytoin. Serum concentrations of drugs metabolized by the cytochrome P450 system should be monitored closely in patients concurrently receiving erythromycin.

Troleandomycin significantly alters the metabolism of terfenadine when taken concomitantly; therefore, observe caution when erythromycin and terfenadine are used concurrently.

Patients receiving concomitant lovastatin and erythromycin should be carefully monitored; cases of rhabdomyolysis have been reported in seriously ill patients.

ADVERSE REACTIONS

The most frequent side effects of oral erythromycin preparations are gastrointestinal and are dose-related. They include nausea, vomiting, abdominal pain, diarrhea and anorexia. Symptoms of hepatic dysfunction and/or abnormal liver function test results may occur (see WARNINGS.) Pseudomembranous colitis has been rarely reported in association with erythromycin therapy.

There have been isolated reports of transient central nervous system side effects including confusion, hallucinations, seizures, and vertigo; however, a cause and effect relationship has not been established.

Occasional case reports of cardiac arrhythmias such as ventricular tachycardia have been documented in patients receiving erythromycin therapy. There have been isolated reports of other cardiovascular symptoms such as chest pain, dizziness, and palpitations; however, a cause and effect relationship has not been established.

Allergic reactions ranging from urticaria and mild skin eruptions to anaphylaxis have occurred.

There have been isolated reports of reversible hearing loss occurring chiefly in patients with renal insufficiency and in patients receiving high doses of erythromycin.

DOSAGE AND ADMINISTRATION

Optimal serum levels of erythromycin are reached when erythrocin stearate (erythromycin stearate) is taken in the fasting state or immediately before meals.

Adults: The usual adult dosage is 250 mg every 6 hours; or 500 mg every 12 hours, taken in the fasting state or immediately before meals. Up to 4 g/day may be administered, depending upon the severity of the infection.

Children: Age, weight, and severity of the infection are important factors in determining the proper dosage. For the treatment of mild to moderate infections, the usual dosage is 30-50 mg/kg/day in 3 or 4 divided doses. When dosage is desired on a twice-a-day schedule, one-half of the total daily dose may be taken every 12 hours in the fasting state or immediately before meals. For the treatment of more severe infections the total daily dose may be doubled.

In the treatment of streptococcal infections, a therapeutic dosage of erythromycin should be administered for at least 10 days. In continuous prophylaxis of streptococcal infections in persons with a history of rheumatic heart disease, the dose is 250 mg twice a day.

For prophylaxis against bacterial endocarditis[1] in patients with congenital heart disease, or rheumatic or other acquired valvular heart disease when undergoing dental procedures or surgical procedures of the upper respiratory tract, give 1 g (20 mg/kg for children) orally 1½ to 2 hours before the procedure, and then, 500 mg (10 mg/kg for children) orally every 6 hours for 8 doses.

For conjunctivitis of the newborn caused by *Chlamydia trachomatis:* Oral erythromycin suspension 50 mg/kg/day in 4 divided doses for at least 2 weeks.[2]

For pneumonia of infancy caused by *Chlamydia Trachomatis:* Although the optimal duration of therapy has not been established, the recommended therapy is oral erythromycin suspension 50 mg/kg/day in 4 divided doses for at least 3 weeks.[2]

E

For urogenital infections during pregnancy due to *Chlamydia Trachomatis:* Although the optimal dose and duration of therapy have not been established, the suggested treatment is erythromycin 500 mg, by mouth, 4 times a day on an empty stomach for at least 7 days. For women who cannot tolerate this regimen, a decreased dose of 250 mg, by mouth, 4 times a day should be used for at least 14 days.[2]

For Adults with uncomplicated urethral, endocervical, or rectal infections caused by *Chlamydia Trachomatis* in whom tetracyclines are contraindicated or not tolerated: 500 mg, by mouth, 4 times a day for at least 7 days.[2]

For treatment of primary syphilis: 30 to 40 g given in divided doses over a period of 10-15 days.

For treatment of acute pelvic inflammatory disease caused by *N. Gonorrhoeae:* 500 mg Erythrocin Lactobionate-IV (erythromycin lactobionate for injection) every 6 hours for 3 days, followed by 250 mg erythromycin stearate every 6 hours for 7 days.

For intestinal amebiasis: *Adults:* 250 mg four times daily for 10-14 days. *Children:* 30-50 mg/kg/day in divided doses for 10-14 days.

For use in pertussis: Although optimal dosage and duration have not been established, doses of erythromycin utilized in reported clinical studies were 40-50 mg/kg/day, given in divided doses for 5-14 days.

For treatment of Legionnaires' disease: Although optimal doses have not been established, doses utilized in reported clinical data were 1-4 g daily in divided doses.

PRODUCT LISTING - RATED THERAPEUTICALLY EQUIVALENT

Tablet - Oral - Stearate 250 mg

Qty	Price	Product	NDC
4's	$0.70	ERYTHROCIN STEARATE FILMTAB, Allscripts Pharmaceutical Company	54569-0124-09
4's	$2.63	GENERIC, Pd-Rx Pharmaceuticals	55289-0112-04
6's	$1.07	ERYTHROCIN STEARATE FILMTAB, Allscripts Pharmaceutical Company	54569-0124-07
10's	$4.12	GENERIC, Pd-Rx Pharmaceuticals	55289-0112-10
12's	$2.14	ERYTHROCIN STEARATE FILMTAB, Allscripts Pharmaceutical Company	54569-0124-00
15's	$5.40	GENERIC, Pd-Rx Pharmaceuticals	55289-0112-15
20's	$3.57	ERYTHROCIN STEARATE FILMTAB, Allscripts Pharmaceutical Company	54569-0124-01
20's	$6.57	GENERIC, Pd-Rx Pharmaceuticals	55289-0112-20
25's	$9.78	GENERIC, Pd-Rx Pharmaceuticals	55289-0112-97
28's	$3.35	GENERIC, Circle Pharmaceuticals Inc	00659-0129-28
28's	$4.40	GENERIC, Pharmaceutical Corporation Of America	51655-0098-29
28's	$5.00	ERYTHROCIN STEARATE FILMTAB, Allscripts Pharmaceutical Company	54569-0124-02
28's	$5.94	GENERIC, Pd-Rx Pharmaceuticals	58864-0199-28
28's	$8.55	GENERIC, Pd-Rx Pharmaceuticals	55289-0112-28
28's	$11.86	ERYTHROCIN STEARATE FILMTAB, Pharma Pac	52959-0427-28
30's	$4.90	GENERIC, Heartland Healthcare Services	61392-0113-30
30's	$4.90	GENERIC, Heartland Healthcare Services	61392-0113-39
30's	$5.36	ERYTHROCIN STEARATE FILMTAB, Allscripts Pharmaceutical Company	54569-0124-05
30's	$5.91	GENERIC, Physicians Total Care	54868-0413-04
31's	$5.06	GENERIC, Heartland Healthcare Services	61392-0113-31
32's	$5.52	GENERIC, Heartland Healthcare Services	61392-0113-32
40's	$4.35	GENERIC, Circle Pharmaceuticals Inc	00659-0129-40
40's	$5.25	GENERIC, Pd-Rx Pharmaceuticals	58864-0199-40
40's	$5.60	GENERIC, Pharmaceutical Corporation Of America	51655-0098-51
40's	$7.13	GENERIC, Physicians Total Care	54868-0413-02
40's	$7.14	ERYTHROCIN STEARATE FILMTAB, Allscripts Pharmaceutical Company	54569-0124-03
40's	$10.67	GENERIC, Pd-Rx Pharmaceuticals	55289-0112-40
40's	$15.15	ERYTHROCIN STEARATE FILMTAB, Pharma Pac	52959-0427-40
40's	$32.20	GENERIC, Med-Pro Inc	53978-5029-06
45's	$7.34	GENERIC, Heartland Healthcare Services	61392-0113-45
56's	$9.50	GENERIC, Pd-Rx Pharmaceuticals	58864-0199-56
56's	$11.60	GENERIC, Pd-Rx Pharmaceuticals	55289-0112-56
60's	$9.79	GENERIC, Heartland Healthcare Services	61392-0113-60
60's	$10.71	ERYTHROCIN STEARATE FILMTAB, Allscripts Pharmaceutical Company	54569-0124-06
90's	$14.69	GENERIC, Heartland Healthcare Services	61392-0113-90
100's	$9.00	GENERIC, C.O. Truxton Inc	00463-5012-01
100's	$12.44	GENERIC, Us Trading Corporation	56126-0397-11
100's	$14.18	GENERIC, Pd-Rx Pharmaceuticals	55289-0112-01
100's	$14.58	ERYTHROCIN STEARATE FILMTAB, Abbott Pharmaceutical	00074-6346-20
100's	$14.92	GENERIC, Aligen Independent Laboratories Inc	00405-4411-01
100's	$15.50	GENERIC, Major Pharmaceuticals Inc	00904-2458-60
100's	$15.75	GENERIC, Interstate Drug Exchange Inc	00814-2970-14
100's	$15.85	GENERIC, Ivax Corporation	00182-0538-01
100's	$16.86	GENERIC, Seneca Pharmaceuticals	47028-0013-01
100's	$17.85	ERYTHROCIN STEARATE FILMTAB, Allscripts Pharmaceutical Company	54569-0124-08
100's	$18.16	GENERIC, Mylan Pharmaceuticals Inc	00378-0106-01
100's	$18.16	GENERIC, Moore, H.L. Drug Exchange Inc	00839-5079-06
120's	$16.44	GENERIC, Pd-Rx Pharmaceuticals	55289-0112-98
120's	$19.16	GENERIC, Physicians Total Care	54868-0413-08

Tablet - Oral - Stearate 500 mg

Qty	Price	Product	NDC
2's	$2.63	GENERIC, Pd-Rx Pharmaceuticals	55289-0705-02
6's	$1.66	ERYTHROCIN STEARATE FILMTAB, Allscripts Pharmaceutical Company	54569-3347-00
6's	$3.00	GENERIC, Pd-Rx Pharmaceuticals	55289-0705-06
9's	$2.48	ERYTHROCIN STEARATE FILMTAB, Allscripts Pharmaceutical Company	54569-3347-02
15's	$4.14	ERYTHROCIN STEARATE FILMTAB, Allscripts Pharmaceutical Company	54569-0125-04
15's	$5.64	GENERIC, Pd-Rx Pharmaceuticals	55289-0705-15
16's	$5.33	GENERIC, Pd-Rx Pharmaceuticals	55289-0705-16
20's	$5.52	ERYTHROCIN STEARATE FILMTAB, Allscripts Pharmaceutical Company	54569-3347-01
20's	$8.70	GENERIC, Pd-Rx Pharmaceuticals	55289-0705-20
20's	$9.03	GENERIC, Dhs Inc	55887-0747-20
21's	$5.80	ERYTHROCIN STEARATE FILMTAB, Allscripts Pharmaceutical Company	54569-0125-00
28's	$7.73	ERYTHROCIN STEARATE FILMTAB, Allscripts Pharmaceutical Company	54569-0125-05
28's	$15.96	GENERIC, Pd-Rx Pharmaceuticals	55289-0705-28
30's	$8.28	ERYTHROCIN STEARATE FILMTAB, Allscripts Pharmaceutical Company	54569-0125-01
30's	$12.83	GENERIC, Pd-Rx Pharmaceuticals	55289-0705-30
40's	$8.99	GENERIC, Circle Pharmaceuticals Inc	00659-0116-40
40's	$11.04	ERYTHROCIN STEARATE FILMTAB, Allscripts Pharmaceutical Company	54569-0125-02
40's	$19.44	GENERIC, Pd-Rx Pharmaceuticals	55289-0705-40
56's	$19.32	GENERIC, Pd-Rx Pharmaceuticals	55289-0705-56
60's	$16.56	ERYTHROCIN STEARATE FILMTAB, Allscripts Pharmaceutical Company	54569-0125-03
100's	$21.96	GENERIC, Us Trading Corporation	56126-0391-11
100's	$24.39	GENERIC, Warner Chilcott Laboratories	00047-0919-24
100's	$24.67	GENERIC, Geneva Pharmaceuticals	00781-1850-01
100's	$25.60	GENERIC, Major Pharmaceuticals Inc	00904-2459-60
100's	$26.00	GENERIC, Ivax Corporation	00182-0539-01
100's	$26.35	ERYTHROCIN STEARATE FILMTAB, Abbott Pharmaceutical	00074-6316-13
100's	$27.60	ERYTHROCIN STEARATE FILMTAB, Allscripts Pharmaceutical Company	54569-0125-06
100's	$28.80	GENERIC, Qualitest Products Inc	00603-3554-21
100's	$28.85	GENERIC, Mylan Pharmaceuticals Inc	00378-0107-01
100's	$40.84	GENERIC, Moore, H.L. Drug Exchange Inc	00839-5185-06

PRODUCT LISTING - EQUIVALENTS NOT AVAILABLE

Tablet - Oral - Stearate 250 mg

Qty	Price	Product	NDC
8's	$1.23	GENERIC, Southwood Pharmaceuticals Inc	58016-0124-08
10's	$1.54	GENERIC, Southwood Pharmaceuticals Inc	58016-0124-10
12's	$1.85	GENERIC, Southwood Pharmaceuticals Inc	58016-0124-12
14's	$2.16	GENERIC, Southwood Pharmaceuticals Inc	58016-0124-14
15's	$2.31	GENERIC, Southwood Pharmaceuticals Inc	58016-0124-15
16's	$2.47	GENERIC, Southwood Pharmaceuticals Inc	58016-0124-16
20's	$3.08	GENERIC, Southwood Pharmaceuticals Inc	58016-0124-20
21's	$3.24	GENERIC, Southwood Pharmaceuticals Inc	58016-0124-21
24's	$3.70	GENERIC, Southwood Pharmaceuticals Inc	58016-0124-24
28's	$4.31	GENERIC, Southwood Pharmaceuticals Inc	58016-0124-28
30's	$4.62	GENERIC, Southwood Pharmaceuticals Inc	58016-0124-30
40's	$6.16	GENERIC, Southwood Pharmaceuticals Inc	58016-0124-40
50's	$7.71	GENERIC, Southwood Pharmaceuticals Inc	58016-0124-50
56's	$8.63	GENERIC, Southwood Pharmaceuticals Inc	58016-0124-56
56's	$13.00	GENERIC, Pharmaceutical Corporation Of America	51655-0098-95
60's	$9.25	GENERIC, Southwood Pharmaceuticals Inc	58016-0124-60
100's	$13.25	GENERIC, Cmc-Consolidated Midland Corporation	00223-0914-01
100's	$14.94	GENERIC, Vangard Labs	00615-0124-01
100's	$15.41	GENERIC, Southwood Pharmaceuticals Inc	58016-0124-00
100's	$21.28	GENERIC, Vangard Labs	00615-0124-13
120's	$18.49	GENERIC, Southwood Pharmaceuticals Inc	58016-0124-02

Tablet - Oral - Stearate 500 mg

Qty	Price	Product	NDC
3's	$2.93	GENERIC, Southwood Pharmaceuticals Inc	58016-0125-03
6's	$3.36	GENERIC, Southwood Pharmaceuticals Inc	58016-0125-06
9's	$5.04	GENERIC, Southwood Pharmaceuticals Inc	58016-0125-09
10's	$5.60	GENERIC, Southwood Pharmaceuticals Inc	58016-0125-10
12's	$6.72	GENERIC, Southwood Pharmaceuticals Inc	58016-0125-12
14's	$7.84	GENERIC, Southwood Pharmaceuticals Inc	58016-0125-14
15's	$8.40	GENERIC, Southwood Pharmaceuticals Inc	58016-0125-15
20's	$11.20	GENERIC, Southwood Pharmaceuticals Inc	58016-0125-20
21's	$8.94	GENERIC, Circle Pharmaceuticals Inc	00659-0116-21
21's	$11.76	GENERIC, Southwood Pharmaceuticals Inc	58016-0125-21
24's	$13.44	GENERIC, Southwood Pharmaceuticals Inc	58016-0125-24
28's	$12.32	GENERIC, Pharmaceutical Corporation Of America	51655-0152-29
28's	$16.80	GENERIC, Southwood Pharmaceuticals Inc	58016-0125-28
30's	$7.79	GENERIC, Circle Pharmaceuticals Inc	00659-0116-30
30's	$17.95	GENERIC, Southwood Pharmaceuticals Inc	58016-0125-30
40's	$15.99	GENERIC, Pharma Pac	52959-0504-40
40's	$22.40	GENERIC, Southwood Pharmaceuticals Inc	58016-0125-40
60's	$33.60	GENERIC, Southwood Pharmaceuticals Inc	58016-0125-60
100's	$27.75	GENERIC, Interstate Drug Exchange Inc	00814-2975-14
100's	$27.93	GENERIC, Vangard Labs	00615-0180-01
100's	$56.00	GENERIC, Southwood Pharmaceuticals Inc	58016-0125-00

Escitalopram Oxalate (003568)

For related information, see the comparative table section in Appendix A.

Categories: Depression; Pregnancy Category C; FDA Approved 2002 Aug
Drug Classes: Antidepressants, serotonin specific reuptake inhibitors
Brand Names: Lexapro
Foreign Brand Availability: Cipralex (England; Ireland)

DESCRIPTION

Lexapro (escitalopram oxalate) is an orally administered selective serotonin reuptake inhibitor (SSRI). Escitalopram is the pure S-enantiomer (single isomer) of the racemic bicyclic phthalane derivative citalopram. Escitalopram oxalate is designated S-(+)-1-[3-(dimethylamino)propyl]-1-(*p*-fluorophenyl)-5-phthalancarbonitrile oxalate.

The molecular formula is $C_{20}H_{21}FN_2O{\cdot}C_2H_2O_4$ and the molecular weight is 414.40.

Escitalopram oxalate occurs as a fine white to slightly yellow powder and is freely soluble in methanol and dimethyl sulfoxide (DMSO), soluble in isotonic saline solution, sparingly soluble in water and ethanol, slightly soluble in ethyl acetate, and insoluble in heptane.

Lexapro (escitalopram oxalate) is available as tablets or as an oral solution.

TABLETS

Lexapro tablets are film coated, round tablets containing escitalopram oxalate in strengths equivalent to 5, 10, or 20 mg escitalopram base. The 10 and 20 mg tablets are scored. The tablets also contain the following inactive ingredients: talc, croscarmellose sodium, microcrystalline cellulose/colloidal silicon dioxide, and magnesium stearate. The film coating contains hydroxypropyl methyl cellulose, titanium dioxide, and polyethylene glycol.

ORAL SOLUTION

Lexapro oral solution contains escitalopram oxalate equivalent to 1 mg/ml escitalopram base. It also contains the following inactive ingredients: sorbitol, purified water, citric acid, sodium citrate, malic acid, glycerin, propylene glycol, methylparaben, propylparaben, and natural peppermint flavor.

CLINICAL PHARMACOLOGY

PHARMACODYNAMICS

The mechanism of antidepressant action of escitalopram, the S-enantiomer of racemic citalopram, is presumed to be linked to potentiation of serotonergic activity in the central nervous system resulting from its inhibition of CNS neuronal reuptake of serotonin (5-HT). *In vitro* and *in vivo* studies in animals suggest that escitalopram is a highly selective serotonin reuptake inhibitor (SSRI) with minimal effects on norepinephrine and dopamine neuronal reuptake. Escitalopram is at least 100-fold more potent than the R-enantiomer with respect to inhibition of 5-HT reuptake and inhibition of 5-HT neuronal firing rate. Tolerance to a model of antidepressant effect in rats was not induced by long-term (up to 5 weeks) treatment with escitalopram. Escitalopram has no or very low affinity for serotonergic ($5\text{-}HT_{1\text{-}7}$) or other receptors including alpha- and beta-adrenergic, dopamine ($D_{1\text{-}5}$), histamine ($H_{1\text{-}3}$), muscarinic ($M_{1\text{-}5}$), and benzodiazepine receptors. Escitalopram also does not bind to or has low affinity for various ion channels including Na^+, K^+, Cl^- and Ca^{++} channels. Antagonism of muscarinic, histaminergic and adrenergic receptors has been hypothesized to be associated with various anticholinergic, sedative and cardiovascular side effects of other psychotropic drugs.

PHARMACOKINETICS

The single- and multiple-dose pharmacokinetics of escitalopram are linear and dose-proportional in a dose range of 10-30 mg/day. Biotransformation of escitalopram is mainly hepatic, with a mean terminal half-life of about 27-32 hours. With once daily dosing, steady state plasma concentrations are achieved within approximately 1 week. At steady state, the extent of accumulation of escitalopram in plasma in young healthy subjects was 2.2-2.5 times the plasma concentrations observed after a single dose. The tablet and the oral solution dosage forms of escitalopram oxalate are bioequivalent.

Absorption and Distribution

Following a single oral dose (20 mg tablet or solution) of escitalopram, peak blood levels occur at about 5 hours. Absorption of escitalopram is not affected by food.

The absolute bioavailability of citalopram is about 80% relative to an intravenous dose, and the volume of distribution of citalopram is about 12 L/kg. Data specific on escitalopram are unavailable.

The binding of escitalopram to human plasma proteins is approximately 56%.

Metabolism and Elimination

Following oral administrations of escitalopram, the fraction of drug recovered in the urine as escitalopram and S-demethylcitalopram (S-DCT) is about 8% and 10%, respectively. The oral clearance of escitalopram is 600 ml/min, with approximately 7% of that due to renal clearance.

Escitalopram is metabolized to S-DCT and S-didemethylcitalopram (S-DDCT). In humans, unchanged escitalopram is the predominant compound in plasma. At steady state, the concentration of the escitalopram metabolite S-DCT in plasma is approximately one-third that of escitalopram. The level of S-DDCT was not detectable in most subjects. *In vitro* studies show that escitalopram is at least 7 and 27 times more potent than S-DCT and S-DDCT, respectively, in the inhibition of serotonin reuptake, suggesting that the metabolites of escitalopram do not contribute significantly to the antidepressant actions of escitalopram. S-DCT and S-DDCT also have no or very low affinity for serotonergic ($5\text{-}HT_{1\text{-}7}$) or other receptors including alpha- and beta-adrenergic, dopamine ($D_{1\text{-}5}$), histamine ($H_{1\text{-}3}$), muscarinic ($M_{1\text{-}5}$), and benzodiazepine receptors. S-DCT and S-DDCT also do not bind to various ion channels including Na^+, K^+, Cl^- and Ca^{++} channels.

In vitro studies using human liver microsomes indicated that CYP3A4 and CYP2C19 are the primary isozymes involved in the N-demethylation of escitalopram.

Population Subgroups

Age

Escitalopram pharmacokinetics in subjects ≥65 years of age were compared to younger subjects in a single-dose and a multiple-dose study. Escitalopram AUC and half-life were increased by approximately 50% in elderly subjects, and C_{max} was unchanged. 10 mg is the recommended dose for elderly patients (see DOSAGE AND ADMINISTRATION).

Gender

In a multiple-dose study of escitalopram (10 mg/day for 3 weeks) in 18 male (9 elderly and 9 young) and 18 female (9 elderly and 9 young) subjects, there were no differences in AUC, C_{max} and half-life between the male and female subjects. No adjustment of dosage on the basis of gender is needed.

E

Reduced Hepatic Function

Citalopram oral clearance was reduced by 37% and half-life was doubled in patients with reduced hepatic function compared to normal subjects. 10 mg is the recommended dose of escitalopram for most hepatically impaired patients (see DOSAGE AND ADMINISTRATION).

Reduced Renal Function

In patients with mild to moderate renal function impairment, oral clearance of citalopram was reduced by 17% compared to normal subjects. No adjustment of dosage for such patients is recommended. No information is available about the pharmacokinetics of escitalopram in patients with severely reduced renal function (creatinine clearance <20 ml/min).

Drug-Drug Interactions

In vitro enzyme inhibition data did not reveal an inhibitory effect of escitalopram on CYP3A4, -1A2, -2C9, -2C19, and -2E1. Based on *in vitro* data, escitalopram would be expected to have little inhibitory effect on *in vivo* metabolism mediated by these cytochromes. While *in vivo* data to address this question are limited, results from drug interaction studies suggest that escitalopram, at a dose of 20 mg, has no 3A4 inhibitory effect and a modest 2D6 inhibitory effect. See DRUG INTERACTIONS for more detailed information on available drug interaction data.

INDICATIONS AND USAGE

Escitalopram oxalate is indicated for the treatment of major depressive disorder.

The efficacy of escitalopram oxalate in the treatment of major depressive disorder was established, in part, on the basis of extrapolation from the established effectiveness of racemic citalopram, of which escitalopram is the active isomer. In addition, the efficacy of escitalopram was shown in an 8 week controlled trial of outpatients whose diagnoses corresponded most closely to the DSM-IV category of major depressive disorder (see CLINICAL PHARMACOLOGY).

A major depressive episode (DSM-IV) implies a prominent and relatively persistent (nearly every day for at least 2 weeks) depressed or dysphoric mood that usually interferes with daily functioning, and includes at least 5 of the following 9 symptoms: depressed mood, loss of interest in usual activities, significant change in weight and/or appetite, insomnia or hypersomnia, psychomotor agitation or retardation, increased fatigue, feelings of guilt or worthlessness, slowed thinking or impaired concentration, a suicide attempt or suicidal ideation.

The efficacy of escitalopram oxalate in hospitalized patients with major depressive disorders has not been adequately studied.

The efficacy of escitalopram oxalate in maintaining a response, in patients with major depressive disorder who responded during an 8 week acute treatment phase while taking escitalopram oxalate and were then observed for relapse during a period of up to 36 weeks, was demonstrated in a placebo-controlled trial. Nevertheless, the physician who elects to use escitalopram oxalate for extended periods should periodically re-evaluate the long-term usefulness of the drug for the individual patient (see DOSAGE AND ADMINISTRATION).

CONTRAINDICATIONS

Concomitant use in patients taking monoamine oxidase inhibitors (MAOIs) is contraindicated (see WARNINGS).

Escitalopram oxalate is contraindicated in patients with a hypersensitivity to escitalopram or citalopram or any of the inactive ingredients in escitalopram oxalate.

WARNINGS

POTENTIAL FOR INTERACTION WITH MONOAMINE OXIDASE INHIBITORS

In patients receiving serotonin reuptake inhibitor drugs in combination with a monoamine oxidase inhibitor (MAOI), there have been reports of serious, sometimes fatal, reactions including hyperthermia, rigidity, myoclonus, autonomic instability with possible rapid fluctuations of vital signs, and mental status changes that include extreme agitation progressing to delirium and coma. These reactions have also been reported in patients who have recently discontinued SSRI treatment and have been started on a MAOI. Some cases presented with features resembling neuroleptic malignant syndrome. Furthermore, limited animal data on the effects of combined use of SSRIs and MAOIs suggest that these drugs may act synergistically to elevate blood pressure and evoke behavioral excitation. Therefore, it is recommended that escitalopram oxalate should not be used in combination with a MAOI, or within 14 days of discontinuing treatment with a MAOI. Similarly, at least 14 days should be allowed after stopping escitalopram oxalate before starting a MAOI.

PRECAUTIONS

GENERAL

Hyponatremia

One case of hyponatremia has been reported in association with escitalopram oxalate treatment. Several cases of hyponatremia or SIADH (syndrome of inappropriate antidiuretic hormone secretion) have been reported in association with racemic citalopram. All patients with these events have recovered with discontinuation of escitalopram or citalopram and/or medical intervention. Hyponatremia and SIADH have also been reported in association with other marketed drugs effective in the treatment of major depressive disorder.

Activation of Mania/Hypomania

In placebo-controlled trials of escitalopram oxalate, activation of mania/hypomania was reported in 1 (0.1%) of 715 patients treated with escitalopram oxalate and in none of the 592 patients treated with placebo. Activation of mania/hypomania has also been reported in a small proportion of patients with major affective disorders treated with racemic citalopram and other marketed drugs effective in the treatment of major depressive disorder. As with all drugs effective in the treatment of major depressive disorder, escitalopram oxalate should be used cautiously in patients with a history of mania.

E

Seizures

Although anticonvulsant effects of racemic citalopram have been observed in animal studies, escitalopram oxalate has not been systematically evaluated in patients with a seizure disorder. These patients were excluded from clinical studies during the product's premarketing testing. In clinical trials of escitalopram oxalate, no seizures occurred in subjects exposed to escitalopram oxalate. Like other drugs effective in the treatment of major depressive disorder, escitalopram oxalate should be introduced with care in patients with a history of seizure disorder.

Suicide

The possibility of a suicide attempt is inherent in major depressive disorder and may persist until significant remission occurs. Close supervision of high risk patients should accompany initial drug therapy. As with all drugs effective in the treatment of major depressive disorder, prescriptions for escitalopram oxalate should be written for the smallest quantity of tablets consistent with good patient management, in order to reduce the risk of overdose.

Interference With Cognitive and Motor Performance

In studies in normal volunteers, racemic citalopram in doses of 40 mg/day did not produce impairment of intellectual function or psychomotor performance. Because any psychoactive drug may impair judgement, thinking, or motor skills, however, patients should be cautioned about operating hazardous machinery, including automobiles, until they are reasonably certain that escitalopram oxalate therapy does not affect their ability to engage in such activities.

Use in Patients With Concomitant Illness

Clinical experience with escitalopram oxalate in patients with certain concomitant systemic illnesses is limited. Caution is advisable in using escitalopram oxalate in patients with diseases or conditions that produce altered metabolism or hemodynamic responses.

Escitalopram oxalate has not been systematically evaluated in patients with a recent history of myocardial infarction or unstable heart disease. Patients with these diagnoses were generally excluded from clinical studies during the product's premarketing testing.

In subjects with hepatic impairment, clearance of racemic citalopram was decreased and plasma concentrations were increased. The recommended dose of escitalopram oxalate in hepatically impaired patients is 10 mg/day (see DOSAGE AND ADMINISTRATION).

Because escitalopram is extensively metabolized, excretion of unchanged drug in urine is a minor route of elimination. Until adequate numbers of patients with severe renal impairment have been evaluated during chronic treatment with escitalopram oxalate, however, it should be used with caution in such patients (see DOSAGE AND ADMINISTRATION).

INFORMATION FOR THE PATIENT

Physicians are advised to discuss the following issues with patients for whom they prescribe escitalopram oxalate.

In studies in normal volunteers, racemic citalopram in doses of 40 mg/day did not impair psychomotor performance. The effect of escitalopram oxalate on psychomotor coordination, judgment, or thinking has not been systematically examined in controlled studies.

Because psychoactive drugs may impair judgment, thinking or motor skills, patients should be cautioned about operating hazardous machinery, including automobiles, until they are reasonably certain that escitalopram oxalate therapy does not affect their ability to engage in such activities.

Patients should be told that, although citalopram has not been shown in experiments with normal subjects to increase the mental and motor skill impairments caused by alcohol, the concomitant use of escitalopram oxalate and alcohol in depressed patients is not advised.

Patients should be made aware that escitalopram is the active isomer of citalopram hydrobromide and that the 2 medications should not be taken concomitantly.

Patients should be advised to inform their physician if they are taking, or plan to take, any prescription or over-the-counter drugs, as there is a potential for interactions.

Patients should be advised to notify their physician if they become pregnant or intend to become pregnant during therapy.

Patients should be advised to notify their physician if they are breast feeding an infant.

While patients may notice improvement with escitalopram oxalate therapy in 1-4 weeks, they should be advised to continue therapy as directed.

LABORATORY TESTS

There are no specific laboratory tests recommended.

CONCOMITANT ADMINISTRATION WITH RACEMIC CITALOPRAM

Citalopram: Since escitalopram is the active isomer of racemic citalopram, the 2 agents should not be coadministered.

CARCINOGENESIS, MUTAGENESIS, AND IMPAIRMENT OF FERTILITY

Carcinogenesis

Racemic citalopram was administered in the diet to NMRI/BOM strain mice and COBS WI strain rats for 18 and 24 months, respectively. There was no evidence for carcinogenicity of racemic citalopram in mice receiving up to 240 mg/kg/day. There was an increased incidence of small intestine carcinoma in rats receiving 8 or 24 mg/kg/day racemic citalopram. A no-effect dose for this finding was not established. The relevance of these findings to humans is unknown.

Mutagenesis

Racemic citalopram was mutagenic in the *in vitro* bacterial reverse mutation assay (Ames test) in 2 of 5 bacterial strains (Salmonella TA98 and TA1537) in the absence of metabolic activation. It was clastogenic in the *in vitro* Chinese hamster lung cell assay for chromosomal aberrations in the presence and absence of metabolic activation. Racemic citalopram was not mutagenic in the *in vitro* mammalian forward gene mutation assay (HPRT) in mouse lymphoma cells or in a coupled *in vitro/in vivo* unscheduled DNA synthesis (UDS) assay in rat liver. It was not clastogenic in the *in vitro* chromosomal aberration assay in human lymphocytes or in 2 *in vivo* mouse micronucleus assays.

Impairment of Fertility

When racemic citalopram was administered orally to male and female rats prior to and throughout mating and gestation at doses of 16/24 (males/females), 32, 48, and 72 mg/kg/day, mating was decreased at all doses, and fertility was decreased at doses ≥32 mg/kg/day. Gestation duration was increased at 48 mg/kg/day.

PREGNANCY CATEGORY C

In a rat embyro/fetal development study, oral administration of escitalopram (56, 112 or 150 mg/kg/day) to pregnant animals during the period of organogenesis resulted in decreased fetal body weight and associated delays in ossification at the 2 higher doses (approximately ≥56 times the maximum recommended human dose [MRHD] of 20 mg/day on a body surface area [mg/m^2] basis. Maternal toxicity (clinical signs and decreased body weight gain and food consumption), mild at 56 mg/kg/day, was present at all dose levels. The developmental no effect dose of 56 mg/kg/day is approximately 28 times the MRHD on a mg/m^2 basis. No teratogenicity was observed at any of the doses tested (as high as 75 times the MRHD on a mg/m^2 basis).

When female rats were treated with escitalopram (6, 12, 24, or 48 mg/kg/day) during pregnancy and through weaning, slightly increased offspring mortality and growth retardation were noted at 48 mg/kg/day which is approximately 24 times the MRHD on a mg/m^2 basis. Slight maternal toxicity (clinical signs and decreased body weight gain and food consumption) was seen at this dose. Slightly increased offspring mortality was seen at 24 mg/kg/day. The no effect dose was 12 mg/kg/day which is approximately 6 times the MRHD on a mg/m^2 basis.

In animal reproduction studies, racemic citalopram has been shown to have adverse effects on embryo/fetal and postnatal development, including teratogenic effects, when administered at doses greater than human therapeutic doses.

In two rat embryo/fetal development studies, oral administration of racemic citalopram (32, 56, or 112 mg/kg/day) to pregnant animals during the period of organogenesis resulted in decreased embryo/fetal growth and survival and an increased incidence of fetal abnormalities (including cardiovascular and skeletal defects) at the high dose. This dose was also associated with maternal toxicity (clinical signs, decreased BW gain). The developmental no effect dose was 56 mg/kg/day. In a rabbit study, no adverse effects on embryo/fetal development were observed at doses of racemic citalopram of up to 16 mg/kg/day. Thus, teratogenic effects of racemic citalopram were observed at a maternally toxic dose in the rat and were not observed in the rabbit.

When female rats were treated with racemic citalopram (4.8, 12.8, or 32 mg/kg/day) from late gestation through weaning, increased offspring mortality during the first 4 days after birth and persistent offspring growth retardation were observed at the highest dose. The no effect dose was 12.8 mg/kg/day. Similar effects on offspring mortality and growth were seen when dams were treated throughout gestation and early lactation at doses ≥24 mg/kg/day. A no effect dose was not determined in that study.

There are no adequate and well-controlled studies in pregnant women; therefore, escitalopram should be used during pregnancy only if the potential benefit justifies the potential risk to the fetus.

LABOR AND DELIVERY

The effect of escitalopram oxalate on labor and delivery in humans is unknown.

NURSING MOTHERS

Racemic citalopram, like many other drugs, is excreted in human breast milk. There have been two reports of infants experiencing excessive somnolence, decreased feeding, and weight loss in association with breast feeding from a citalopram-treated mother; in one case, the infant was reported to recover completely upon discontinuation of citalopram by its mother and, in the second case, no follow up information was available. The decision whether to continue or discontinue either nursing or escitalopram oxalate therapy should take into account the risks of citalopram exposure for the infant and the benefits of escitalopram oxalate treatment for the mother.

PEDIATRIC USE

Safety and effectiveness in pediatric patients have not been established.

GERIATRIC USE

Approximately 6% of the 715 patients receiving escitalopram in controlled trials of escitalopram oxalate in major depressive disorder were 60 years of age or older; elderly patients in these trials received daily doses of escitalopram oxalate between 10 and 20 mg. The number of elderly patients in these trials was insufficient to adequately assess for possible differential efficacy and safety measures on the basis of age. Nevertheless, greater sensitivity of some elderly individuals to effects of escitalopram oxalate cannot be ruled out.

In two pharmacokinetic studies, escitalopram half-life was increased by approximately 50% in elderly subjects as compared to young subjects and C_{max} was unchanged (see CLINICAL PHARMACOLOGY). 10 mg/day is the recommended dose for elderly patients (see DOSAGE AND ADMINISTRATION).

Of 4422 patients in clinical studies of racemic citalopram, 1357 were 60 and over, 1034 were 65 and over, and 457 were 75 and over. No overall differences in safety or effectiveness were observed between these subjects and younger subjects, and other reported clinical experience has not identified differences in responses between the elderly and younger patients, but again, greater sensitivity of some elderly individuals cannot be ruled out.

DRUG INTERACTIONS

CNS Drugs: Given the primary CNS effects of escitalopram, caution should be used when it is taken in combination with other centrally acting drugs.

Alcohol: Although racemic citalopram did not potentiate the cognitive and motor effects of alcohol in a clinical trial, as with other psychotropic medications, the use of alcohol by patients taking escitalopram oxalate is not recommended.

Monoamine Oxidase Inhibitors (MAOIs): See CONTRAINDICATIONS and WARNINGS.

Cimetidine: In subjects who had received 21 days of 40 mg/day racemic citalopram, combined administration of 400 mg/day cimetidine for 8 days resulted in an increase in citalopram AUC and C_{max} of 43% and 39%, respectively. The clinical significance of these findings is unknown.

Digoxin: In subjects who had received 21 days of 40 mg/day racemic citalopram, combined administration of citalopram and digoxin (single dose of 1 mg) did not significantly affect the pharmacokinetics of either citalopram or digoxin.

Lithium: Coadministration of racemic citalopram (40 mg/day for 10 days) and lithium (30 mmol/day for 5 days) had no significant effect on the pharmacokinetics of citalopram or lithium. Nevertheless, plasma lithium levels should be monitored with appropriate adjustment to the lithium dose in accordance with standard clinical practice. Because lithium may enhance the serotonergic effects of escitalopram, caution should be exercised when escitalopram oxalate and lithium are coadministered.

Sumatriptan: There have been rare postmarketing reports describing patients with weakness, hyperreflexia, and incoordination following the use of a selective serotonin reuptake inhibitor (SSRI) and sumatriptan. If concomitant treatment with sumatriptan and an SSRI (*e.g.*, fluoxetine, fluvoxamine, paroxetine, sertraline, citalopram, escitalopram) is clinically warranted, appropriate observation of the patient is advised.

Theophylline: Combined administration of racemic citalopram (40 mg/day for 21 days) and the CYP1A2 substrate theophylline (single dose of 300 mg) did not affect the pharmacokinetics of theophylline. The effect of theophylline on the pharmacokinetics of citalopram was not evaluated.

Warfarin: Administration of 40 mg/day racemic citalopram for 21 days did not affect the pharmacokinetics of warfarin, a CYP3A4 substrate. Prothrombin time was increased by 5%, the clinical significance of which is unknown.

Carbamazepine: Combined administration of racemic citalopram (40 mg/day for 14 days) and carbamazepine (titrated to 400 mg/day for 35 days) did not significantly affect the pharmacokinetics of carbamazepine, a CYP3A4 substrate. Although trough citalopram plasma levels were unaffected, given the enzyme inducing properties of carbamazepine, the possibility that carbamazepine might increase the clearance of escitalopram should be considered if the 2 drugs are coadministered.

Triazolam: Combined administration of racemic citalopram (titrated to 40 mg/day for 28 days) and the CYP3A4 substrate triazolam (single dose of 0.25 mg) did not significantly affect the pharmacokinetics of either citalopram or triazolam.

Ketoconazole: Combined administration of racemic citalopram (40 mg) and ketoconazole (200 mg) decreased the C_{max} and AUC of ketoconazole by 21% and 10%, respectively, and did not significantly affect the pharmacokinetics of citalopram.

Ritonavir: Combined administration of a single dose of ritonavir (600 mg), both a CYP3A4 substrate and a potent inhibitor of CYP3A4, and escitalopram (20 mg) did not affect the pharmacokinetics of either ritonavir or escitalopram.

CYP3A4 and -2C19 Inhibitors: *In vitro* studies indicated that CYP3A4 and -2C19 are the primary enzymes involved in the metabolism of escitalopram. However, coadministration of escitalopram (20 mg) and ritonavir (600 mg), a potent inhibitor of CYP3A4, did not significantly affect the pharmacokinetics of escitalopram. Because escitalopram is metabolized by multiple enzyme systems, inhibition of a single enzyme may not appreciably decrease escitalopram clearance.

Drugs Metabolized by Cytochrome P4502D6: *In vitro* studies did not reveal an inhibitory effect of escitalopram on CYP2D6. In addition, steady state levels of racemic citalopram were not significantly different in poor metabolizers and extensive CYP2D6 metabolizers after multiple-dose administration of citalopram, suggesting that coadministration, with escitalopram, of a drug that inhibits CYP2D6, is unlikely to have clinically significant effects on escitalopram metabolism. However, there are limited *in vivo* data suggesting a modest CYP2D6 inhibitory effect for escitalopram, *i.e.*, coadministration of escitalopram (20 mg/day for 21 days) with the tricyclic antidepressant desipramine (single dose of 50 mg), a substrate for CYP2D6, resulted in a 40% increase in C_{max} and a 100% increase in AUC of desipramine. The clinical significance of this finding is unknown. Nevertheless, caution is indicated in the coadministration of escitalopram and drugs metabolized by CYP2D6.

Metoprolol: Administration of 20 mg/day escitalopram oxalate for 21 days resulted in a 50% increase in C_{max} and 82% increase in AUC of the beta-adrenergic blocker metoprolol (given in a single dose of 100 mg). Increased metoprolol plasma levels have been associated with decreased cardioselectivity. Coadministration of escitalopram oxalate and metoprolol had no clinically significant effects on blood pressure or heart rate.

Electroconvulsive Therapy (ECT): There are no clinical studies of the combined use of ECT and escitalopram.

ADVERSE REACTIONS

Adverse event information for escitalopram oxalate was collected from 715 patients with major depressive disorder who were exposed to escitalopram and from 592 patients who were exposed to placebo in double-blind, placebo-controlled trials. An additional 284 patients were newly exposed to escitalopram in open-label trials.

Adverse events during exposure were obtained primarily by general inquiry and recorded by clinical investigators using terminology of their own choosing. Consequently, it is not possible to provide a meaningful estimate of the proportion of individuals experiencing adverse events without first grouping similar types of events into a smaller number of standardized event categories. In the tables and tabulations that follow, standard World Health Organization (WHO) terminology has been used to classify reported adverse events.

The stated frequencies of adverse events represent the proportion of individuals who experienced, at least once, a treatment-emergent adverse event of the type listed. An event was considered treatment-emergent if it occurred for the first time or worsened while receiving therapy following baseline evaluation.

ADVERSE EVENTS ASSOCIATED WITH DISCONTINUATION OF TREATMENT

Among the 715 depressed patients who received escitalopram oxalate in placebo-controlled trials, 6% discontinued treatment due to an adverse event, as compared to 2% of 592 patients receiving placebo. In two fixed dose studies, the rate of discontinuation for adverse events in patients receiving 10 mg/day escitalopram oxalate was not significantly different from the rate of discontinuation for adverse events in patients receiving placebo. The rate of discontinuation for adverse events in patients assigned to a fixed dose of 20 mg/day escitalopram oxalate was 10% which was significantly different from the rate of discontinuation for adverse events in patients receiving 10 mg/day escitalopram oxalate (4%) and placebo (3%). Adverse events that were associated with the discontinuation of at least 1% of patients treated with escitalopram oxalate, and for which the rate was at least twice the placebo rate, were nausea (2%) and ejaculation disorder (2% of male patients).

INCIDENCE OF ADVERSE EVENTS IN PLACEBO-CONTROLLED CLINICAL TRIALS

TABLE 1 enumerates the incidence, rounded to the nearest percent, of treatment emergent adverse events that occurred among 715 depressed patients who received escitalopram oxalate at doses ranging from 10-20 mg/day in placebo-controlled trials. Events included are those occurring in 2% or more of patients treated with escitalopram oxalate and for which the incidence in patients treated with escitalopram oxalate was greater than the incidence in placebo-treated patients.

The prescriber should be aware that these figures cannot be used to predict the incidence of adverse events in the course of usual medical practice where patient characteristics and other factors differ from those which prevailed in the clinical trials. Similarly, the cited frequencies cannot be compared with figures obtained from other clinical investigations involving different treatments, uses, and investigators. The cited figures, however, do provide the prescribing physician with some basis for estimating the relative contribution of drug and non-drug factors to the adverse event incidence rate in the population studied.

The most commonly observed adverse events in escitalopram oxalate patients (incidence of approximately 5% or greater and approximately twice the incidence in placebo patients) were insomnia, ejaculation disorder (primarily ejaculatory delay), nausea, sweating increased, fatigue, and somnolence (see TABLE 1).

TABLE 1 *Treatment-Emergent Adverse Events: Incidence in Placebo-Controlled Clinical Trials**

Body System/ Adverse Event	Escitalopram Oxalate (n=715)	Placebo (n=592)
Autonomic Nervous System Disorders		
Dry mouth	6%	5%
Sweating increased	5%	2%
Central & Peripheral Nervous System Disorders		
Dizziness	5%	3%
Gastrointestinal Disorders		
Nausea	15%	7%
Diarrhea	8%	5%
Constipation	3%	1%
Indigestion	3%	1%
Abdominal pain	2%	1%
General		
Influenza-like symptoms	5%	4%
Fatigue	5%	2%
Psychiatric Disorders		
Insomnia	9%	4%
Somnolence	6%	2%
Appetite decreased	3%	1%
Libido decreased	3%	1%
Respiratory System Disorders		
Rhinitis	5%	4%
Sinusitis	3%	2%
Urogenital		
Ejaculation disorder†‡	9%	<1%
Impotence‡	3%	<1%
Anorgasmia§	2%	<1%

* Events reported by at least 2% of patients treated with escitalopram oxalate are reported, except for the following events which had an incidence on placebo ≥escitalopram oxalate: headache, upper respiratory tract infection, back pain, pharyngitis, inflicted injury, anxiety.
† Primarily ejaculatory delay.
‡ Denominator used was for males only (n=225 escitalopram oxalate; n=188 placebo).
§ Denominator used was for females only (n=490 escitalopram oxalate; n=404 placebo).

DOSE DEPENDENCY OF ADVERSE EVENTS

The potential dose dependency of common adverse events (defined as an incidence rate of ≥5% in either the 10 or 20 mg escitalopram oxalate groups) was examined on the basis of the combined incidence of adverse events in two fixed dose trials. The overall incidence rates of adverse events in 10 mg escitalopram oxalate treated patients (66%) was similar to that of the placebo treated patients (61%), while the incidence rate in 20 mg/day escitalopram oxalate treated patients was greater (86%). TABLE 2 shows common adverse events that occurred in the 20 mg/day escitalopram oxalate group with an incidence that was approximately twice that of the 10 mg/day escitalopram oxalate group and approximately twice that of the placebo group.

TABLE 2 *Incidence of Common Adverse Events* in Patients Receiving Placebo, 10 mg/day Escitalopram Oxalate, or 20 mg/day Escitalopram Oxalate*

Adverse Event	Placebo (n=311)	Escitalopram Oxalate 10 mg/day (n=310)	20 mg/day (n=125)
Insomnia	4%	7%	14%
Diarrhea	5%	6%	14%
Dry mouth	3%	4%	9%
Somnolence	1%	4%	9%
Dizziness	2%	4%	7%
Sweating increased	<1%	3%	8%
Constipation	1%	3%	6%
Fatigue	2%	2%	6%
Indigestion	1%	2%	6%

* Adverse events with an incidence rate of at least 5% in either of the escitalopram oxalate groups and with an incidence rate in the 20 mg/day escitalopram oxalate group that was approximately twice that of the 10 mg/day escitalopram oxalate group and the placebo group.

MALE AND FEMALE SEXUAL DYSFUNCTION WITH SSRIS

Although changes in sexual desire, sexual performance and sexual satisfaction often occur as manifestations of a psychiatric disorder, they may also be a consequence of pharmacologic treatment. In particular, some evidence suggests that selective serotonin reuptake inhibitors (SSRIs) can cause such untoward sexual experiences.

Reliable estimates of the incidence and severity of untoward experiences involving sexual desire, performance and satisfaction are difficult to obtain, however, in part because patients and physicians may be reluctant to discuss them. Accordingly, estimates of the incidence of untoward sexual experience and performance cited in product labeling are likely to underestimate their actual incidence.

TABLE 3 shows the incidence rates of sexual side effects in patients with major depressive disorder in placebo controlled trials.

TABLE 3 *Incidence of Sexual Side Effects in Placebo-Controlled Clinical Trials*

Adverse Event	Escitalopram Oxalate	Placebo
	In Males Only	
	(n=225)	(n=188)
Ejaculation disorder (primarily ejaculatory delay)	9%	<1%
Decreased libido	4%	2%
Impotence	3%	<1%
	In Females Only	
	(n=490)	(n=404)
Decreased libido	2%	<1%
Anorgasmia	2%	<1%

There are no adequately designed studies examining sexual dysfunction with escitalopram treatment.

Priapism has been reported with all SSRIs.

While it is difficult to know the precise risk of sexual dysfunction associated with the use of SSRIs, physicians should routinely inquire about such possible side effects.

VITAL SIGN CHANGES

Escitalopram oxalate and placebo groups were compared with respect to (1) mean change from baseline in vital signs (pulse, systolic blood pressure, and diastolic blood pressure) and (2) the incidence of patients meeting criteria for potentially clinically significant changes from baseline in these variables. These analyses did not reveal any clinically important changes in vital signs associated with escitalopram oxalate treatment. In addition, a comparison of supine and standing vital sign measures in subjects receiving escitalopram oxalate indicated that escitalopram oxalate treatment is not associated with orthostatic changes.

WEIGHT CHANGES

Patients treated with escitalopram oxalate in controlled trials did not differ from placebo-treated patients with regard to clinically important change in body weight.

LABORATORY CHANGES

Escitalopram oxalate and placebo groups were compared with respect to (1) mean change from baseline in various serum chemistry, hematology, and urinalysis variables and (2) the incidence of patients meeting criteria for potentially clinically significant changes from baseline in these variables. These analyses revealed no clinically important changes in laboratory test parameters associated with escitalopram oxalate treatment.

ECG CHANGES

Electrocardiograms from escitalopram oxalate (n=625), racemic citalopram (n=351), and placebo (n=527) groups were compared with respect to (1) mean change from baseline in various ECG parameters and (2) the incidence of patients meeting criteria for potentially clinically significant changes from baseline in these variables. These analyses revealed (1) a decrease in heart rate of 2.2 bpm for escitalopram oxalate and 2.7 bpm for racemic citalopram, compared to an increase of 0.3 bpm for placebo and (2) an increase in QTc interval of 3.9 millisecond for escitalopram oxalate and 3.7 millisecond for racemic citalopram, compared to 0.5 millisecond for placebo. Neither escitalopram oxalate nor racemic citalopram were associated with the development of clinically significant ECG abnormalities.

OTHER EVENTS OBSERVED DURING THE PREMARKETING EVALUATION OF ESCITALOPRAM OXALATE

Following is a list of WHO terms that reflect treatment-emergent adverse events, as defined in the introduction to ADVERSE REACTIONS, reported by the 999 patients treated with escitalopram oxalate for periods of up to 1 year in double-blind or open-label clinical trials during its premarketing evaluation. All reported events are included except those already listed in TABLE 1, those occurring in only 1 patient, event terms that are so general as to be uninformative, and those that are unlikely to be drug related. It is important to emphasize that, although the events reported occurred during treatment with escitalopram oxalate, they were not necessarily caused by it.

Events are further categorized by body system and listed in order of decreasing frequency according to the following definitions: *Frequent* adverse events are those occurring on 1 or more occasions in at least 1/100 patients; *infrequent* adverse events are those occurring in less than 1/100 patients but at least 1/1000 patients.

Cardiovascular: *Frequent:* Palpitation, hypertension. *Infrequent:* Bradycardia, tachycardia, ECG abnormal, flushing, varicose vein.

Central and Peripheral Nervous System Disorders: *Frequent:* Paresthesia, light-headed feeling, migraine, tremor, vertigo. *Infrequent:* Shaking, dysequilibrium, tics, restless legs, carpal tunnel syndrome, twitching, faintness, hyperreflexia, muscle contractions involuntary, muscular tone increased.

Gastrointestinal Disorders: *Frequent:* Vomiting, flatulence, heartburn, tooth ache, gastroenteritis, abdominal cramp, gastroesophageal reflux. *Infrequent:* Bloating, increased stool frequency, abdominal discomfort, dyspepsia, belching, gagging, gastritis, hemorrhoids.

General: *Frequent:* Allergy, pain in limb, hot flushes, fever, chest pain. *Infrequent:* Edema of extremities, chills, malaise, syncope, tightness of chest, leg pain, edema, asthenia, anaphylaxis.

Hemic and Lymphatic Disorders: *Infrequent:* Bruise, anemia, nosebleed, hematoma.

Metabolic and Nutritional Disorders: *Frequent:* Increased weight, decreased weight. *Infrequent:* Bilirubin increased, gout, hypercholesterolemia, hyperglycemia.

Musculoskeletal System Disorders: *Frequent:* Arthralgia, neck/shoulder pain, muscle cramp, myalgia. *Infrequent:* Jaw stiffness, muscle stiffness, arthritis, muscle weakness, arthropathy, back discomfort, joint stiffness, jaw pain.

Psychiatric Disorders: *Frequent:* Dreaming abnormal, yawning, appetite increased, lethargy, irritability, concentration impaired. *Infrequent:* Agitation, jitteriness, apathy, panic reaction, restlessness aggravated, nervousness, forgetfulness, suicide attempt, depression aggravated, feeling unreal, excitability, emotional lability, crying abnormal, depression, anxiety attack, depersonalization, suicidal tendency, bruxism, confusion, carbohydrate craving, amnesia, tremulousness nervous, auditory hallucination.

Reproductive Disorders/Female (% based on female subjects only: n=658): *Frequent:* Menstrual cramps. *Infrequent:* Menstrual disorder, menorrhagia, spotting between menses, pelvic inflammation.

Respiratory System Disorders: *Frequent:* Bronchitis, sinus congestion, coughing, sinus headache, nasal congestion. *Infrequent:* Asthma, breath shortness, laryngitis, pneumonia, tracheitis.

Skin and Appendages Disorders: *Frequent:* Rash. *Infrequent:* Acne, pruritus, eczema, alopecia, dry skin, folliculitis, lipoma, furunculosis, dermatitis.

Special Senses: *Frequent:* Vision blurred, ear ache, tinnitus. *Infrequent:* Taste alteration, eye irritation, conjunctivitis, vision abnormal, visual disturbance, dry eyes, eye infection, pupils dilated.

Urinary System Disorders: *Frequent:* Urinary tract infection, urinary frequency. *Infrequent:* Kidney stone, dysuria, urinary urgency.

EVENTS REPORTED SUBSEQUENT TO THE MARKETING OF RACEMIC CITALOPRAM

Although no causal relationship to racemic citalopram treatment has been found, the following adverse events have been reported to be temporally associated with racemic citalopram treatment and were not observed during the premarketing evaluation of escitalopram or citalopram: acute renal failure, akathisia, allergic reaction, anaphylaxis, angioedema, choreoathetosis, delirium, dyskinesia, ecchymosis, epidermal necrolysis, erythema multiforme, gastrointestinal hemorrhage, grand mal convulsions, hemolytic anemia, hepatic necrosis, myoclonus, neuroleptic malignant syndrome, nystagmus, pancreatitis, priapism, prolactinemia, prothrombin decreased, QT prolonged, rhabdomyolysis, serotonin syndrome, spontaneous abortion, thrombocytopenia, thrombosis, Torsades de pointes, ventricular arrhythmia, and withdrawal syndrome.

DOSAGE AND ADMINISTRATION

INITIAL TREATMENT

The recommended dose of escitalopram oxalate is 10 mg once daily. A fixed dose trial of escitalopram oxalate demonstrated the effectiveness of both 10 mg and 20 mg of escitalopram oxalate, but failed to demonstrate a greater benefit of 20 mg over 10 mg. If the dose is increased to 20 mg, this should occur after a minimum of 1 week.

Escitalopram oxalate should be administered once daily, in the morning or evening, with or without food.

SPECIAL POPULATIONS

10 mg/day is the recommended dose for most elderly patients and patients with hepatic impairment.

No dosage adjustment is necessary for patients with mild or moderate renal impairment. Escitalopram oxalate should be used with caution in patients with severe renal impairment.

MAINTENANCE TREATMENT

It is generally agreed that acute episodes of major depressive disorder require several months or longer of sustained pharmacological therapy beyond response to the acute episode. Systematic evaluation of continuing escitalopram oxalate 10 or 20 mg/day for periods of up to 36 weeks in patients with major depressive disorder who responded while taking escitalopram oxalate during an 8 week acute treatment phase demonstrated a benefit of such maintenance treatment. Nevertheless, patients should be periodically reassessed to determine the need for maintenance treatment.

SWITCHING PATIENTS TO OR FROM A MONOAMINE OXIDASE INHIBITOR

At least 14 days should elapse between discontinuation of an MAOI and initiation of escitalopram oxalate therapy. Similarly, at least 14 days should be allowed after stopping escitalopram oxalate before starting a MAOI (see CONTRAINDICATIONS and WARNINGS).

ANIMAL PHARMACOLOGY

RETINAL CHANGES IN RATS

Pathologic changes (degeneration/atrophy) were observed in the retinas of albino rats in the 2 year carcinogenicity study with racemic citalopram. There was an increase in both incidence and severity of retinal pathology in both male and female rats receiving 80 mg/kg/day. Similar findings were not present in rats receiving 24 mg/kg/day of racemic citalopram for 2 years, in mice receiving up to 240 mg/kg/day of racemic citalopram for 18 months, or in dogs receiving up to 20 mg/kg/day of racemic citalopram for 1 year.

Additional studies to investigate the mechanism for this pathology have not been performed, and the potential significance of this effect in humans has not been established.

CARDIOVASCULAR CHANGES IN DOGS

In a 1 year toxicology study, 5 of 10 beagle dogs receiving oral racemic citalopram doses of 8 mg/kg/day died suddenly between weeks 17 and 31 following initiation of treatment. Sudden deaths were not observed in rats at doses of racemic citalopram up to 120 mg/kg/day, which produced plasma levels of citalopram and its metabolites demethylcitalopram and didemethylcitalopram (DDCT) similar to those observed in dogs at 8 mg/kg/day. A subsequent intravenous dosing study demonstrated that in beagle dogs, racemic DDCT caused QT prolongation, a known risk factor for the observed outcome in dogs.

HOW SUPPLIED

Lexapro tablets are supplied as:

5 mg: White to off-white, round, non-scored film coated. Imprint "FL" on one side of the tablet and "5" on the other side.

10 mg: White to off-white, round, scored film coated. Imprint on scored side with "F" on the left side and "L" on the right side. Imprint on the non-scored side with "10".

20 mg: White to off-white, round, scored film coated. Imprint on scored side with "F" on the left side and "L" on the right side. Imprint on the non-scored side with "20".

Lexapro oral solution is supplied as:

5 mg/5 ml: Peppermint flavor - (240 ml).

Storage: Store at 25°C (77°F); excursions permitted to 15-30°C (59-86°F).

PRODUCT LISTING - EQUIVALENTS NOT AVAILABLE

Solution - Oral - 5 mg/5 ml

240 ml	$106.09	LEXAPRO, Forest Pharmaceuticals	00456-2101-08

Tablet - Oral - 10 mg

10 x 10	$226.83	LEXAPRO, Forest Pharmaceuticals	00456-2010-63
100's	$222.35	LEXAPRO, Forest Pharmaceuticals	00456-2010-01

Tablet - Oral - 20 mg

10 x 10	$236.68	LEXAPRO, Forest Pharmaceuticals	00456-2020-63
100's	$232.04	LEXAPRO, Forest Pharmaceuticals	00456-2020-01

Esmolol Hydrochloride *(001186)*

For related information, see the comparative table section in Appendix A.

Categories: Hypertension, intraoperative; Hypertension, postoperative; Tachycardia, intraoperative; Tachycardia, postoperative; Tachycardia, supraventricular; Pregnancy Category C; FDA Approved 1986 Dec
Drug Classes: Antiadrenergics, beta blocking; Antiarrhythmics, class II
Brand Names: Brevibloc
Foreign Brand Availability: Miniblock (India)

DESCRIPTION

NOT FOR DIRECT INTRAVENOUS INJECTION. AMPUL MUST BE DILUTED PRIOR TO ITS INFUSION. (SEE DOSAGE AND ADMINISTRATION.)

Esmolol hydrochloride is a beta$_1$-selective (cardioselective) adrenergic receptor blocking agent with a very short duration of action (elimination half-life is approximately 9 minutes).

The chemical name for esmolol hydrochloride is (±)-methyl p-[2-hydroxy-3-(isopropylamino)propoxy]hydrocinnamate hydrochloride.

Esmolol hydrochloride has the empirical formula $C_{16}H_{26}NO_4Cl$ and a molecular weight of 331.8. It has one asymmetric center and exists as an enantiomeric pair.

Esmolol hydrochloride is a white to off-white crystalline powder. It is a relatively hydrophilic compound which is very soluble in water and freely soluble in alcohol. Its partition coefficient (octanol/water) at pH 7.0 is 0.42 compared to 17.0 for propranolol.

Brevibloc injection is a clear, colorless to light yellow, sterile, nonpyrogenic solution.

2.5 g, 10 ml ampul: Each ml contains 250 mg esmolol hydrochloride in 25% propylene glycol, 25% alcohol and water for injection; buffered with 17.0 mg sodium acetate, and 0.00715 ml glacial acetic acid. Sodium hydroxide and/or hydrochloric acid added, as necessary, to adjust pH to 3.5-5.5.

100 mg, 10 ml single dose vial: Each ml contains 10 mg esmolol hydrochloride and water for injection, buffered with 2.8 mg Sodium Acetate, and 0.546 mg glacial acetic acid. Sodium hydroxide and/or hydrochloric acid added, as necessary, to adjust pH to 4.5-5.5.

Storage: Store at controlled room temperature 15-30°C (59-86°F). Freezing does not adversely affect the product, but exposure to elevated temperatures should be avoided.

CLINICAL PHARMACOLOGY

Esmolol HCl is a beta$_1$-selective (cardioselective) adrenergic receptor blocking agent with rapid onset, a very short duration of action, and no significant intrinsic sympathomimetic or membrane stabilizing activity at therapeutic dosages. Its elimination half-life after intravenous infusion is approximately 9 minutes. Esmolol HCl inhibits the beta$_1$ receptors located chiefly in cardiac muscle, but this preferential effect is not absolute and at higher doses it begins to inhibit beta$_2$ receptors located chiefly in the bronchial and vascular musculature.

PHARMACOKINETICS AND METABOLISM

Esmolol HCl is rapidly metabolized by hydrolysis of the ester linkage, chiefly by the esterases in the cytosol of red blood cells and not by plasma cholinesterases or red cell membrane acetylcholinesterase. Total body clearance in man was found to be about 20 L/kg/h, which is greater than cardiac output; thus the metabolism of esmolol HCl is not limited by the rate of blood flow to metabolizing tissues such as the liver or affected by hepatic or renal blood flow. Esmolol HCl has a rapid distribution half-life of about 2 minutes and an elimination half-life of about 9 minutes.

Using an appropriate loading dose, steady-state blood levels of esmolol HCl for dosages from 50-300 μg/kg/min (0.05-0.3 mg/kg/min) are obtained within 5 minutes. (Steady-state is reached in about 30 minutes without the loading dose.) Steady-state blood levels of esmolol HCl increase linearly over this dosage range and elimination kinetics are dose-independent over this range. Steady-state blood levels are maintained during infusion but decrease rapidly after termination of the infusion. Because of its short half-life, blood levels of esmolol HCl can be rapidly altered by increasing or decreasing the infusion rate and rapidly eliminated by discontinuing the infusion.

Consistent with the high rate of blood-based metabolism of esmolol HCl, less than 2% of the drug is excreted unchanged in the urine. Within 24 hours of the end of infusion, approximately 73-88% of the dosage has been accounted for in the urine as the acid metabolite of esmolol HCl.

Metabolism of esmolol HCl results in the formation of the corresponding free acid and methanol. The acid metabolite has been shown in animals to have about 1/1500th the activity of esmolol and in normal volunteers its blood levels do not correspond to the level of beta-blockade. The acid metabolite has an elimination half-life of about 3.7 hours and is excreted in the urine with a clearance approximately equivalent to the glomerular filtration rate. Excretion of the acid metabolite is significantly decreased in patients with renal disease, with the elimination half-life increased to about 10-fold that of normals, and plasma levels considerably elevated.

Methanol blood levels, monitored in subjects receiving esmolol HCl for up to 6 hours at 300 μg/kg/min (0.3 mg/kg/min) and 24 hours at 150 μg/kg/min (0.15 mg/kg/min), approximated endogenous levels and were less than 2% of levels usually associated with methanol toxicity.

Esmolol HCl has been shown to be 55% bound to human plasma protein, while the acid metabolite is only 10% bound.

PHARMACODYNAMICS

Clinical pharmacology studies in normal volunteers have confirmed the beta blocking activity of esmolol HCl , showing reduction in heart rate at rest and during exercise, and attenuation of isoproterenol-induced increases in heart rate. Blood levels of esmolol HCl have been shown to correlate with extent of beta blockade. After termination of infusion, substantial recovery from beta blockade is observed in 10-20 minutes.

In human electrophysiology studies, esmolol HCl produced effects typical of a beta blocker: a decrease in the heart rate, increase in sinus cycle length, prolongation of the sinus node recovery time, prolongation of the AH interval during normal sinus rhythm and during atrial pacing, and an increase in antegrade Wenckebach cycle length.

In patients undergoing radionuclide angiography, esmolol HCl, at dosages of 200 μg/kg/min (0.2 mg/kg/min), produced reductions in heart rate, systolic blood pressure, rate pressure product, left and right ventricular ejection fraction and cardiac index at rest, which were similar in magnitude to those produced by intravenous propranolol (4 mg). During exercise, esmolol HCl produced reductions in heart rate, rate pressure product and cardiac index which were also similar to those produced by propranolol, but produced a significantly larger fall in systolic blood pressure. In patients undergoing cardiac catheterization, the maximum therapeutic dose of 300 μg/kg/min (0.3 mg/kg/min) of esmolol HCl produced similar effects, and, in addition, there were small, clinically insignificant, increases in the left ventricular end diastolic pressure and pulmonary capillary wedge pressure. At 30 minutes after the discontinuation of esmolol HCl infusion, all of the hemodynamic parameters had returned to pretreatment levels.

The relative cardioselectivity of esmolol HCl was demonstrated in 10 mildly asthmatic patients. Infusions of esmolol HCl [100, 200 and 300 μg/kg/min (0.1, 0.2 and 0.3 mg/kg/min)] produced no significant increases in specific airway resistance compared to placebo. At 300 μg/kg/min (0.3 mg/kg/min), esmolol HCl produced slightly enhanced bronchomotor sensitivity to dry air stimulus. These effects were not clinically significant, and esmolol HCl was well tolerated by all patients. Six (6) of the patients also received intravenous propranolol, and at a dosage of 1 mg, two experienced significant, symptomatic bronchospasm requiring bronchodilator treatment. One other propranolol-treated patient also experienced dry air-induced bronchospasm. No adverse pulmonary effects were observed in patients with COPD who received therapeutic dosages of esmolol HCl for treatment of supraventricular tachycardia (51 patients) or in perioperative settings (32 patients).

SUPRAVENTRICULAR TACHYCARDIA

In two multicenter, randomized, double-blind, controlled comparisons of esmolol HCl with placebo and propranolol, maintenance doses of 50 to 300 μg/kg/min (0.05 to 0.3 mg/kg/min) of esmolol HCl were found to be more effective than placebo and about as effective as propranolol, 3-6 mg given by bolus injections, in the treatment of supraventricular tachycardia, principally atrial fibrillation and atrial flutter. The majority of these patients developed their arrhythmias postoperatively. About 60-70% of the patients treated with esmolol HCl had a desired therapeutic effect (either a 20% reduction in heart rate, a decrease in heart rate to less than 100 bpm, or, rarely, conversion to NSR) and about 95% of those who responded did so at a dosage of 200 µg/kg/min (0.2 mg/kg/min) or less. The average effective dosage of esmolol HCl was approximately 100-115 µg/kg/min (0.1-0.115 mg/kg/min) in the two studies. Other multicenter baseline-controlled studies gave essentially similar results. In the comparison with propranolol, about 50% of patients in both the esmolol HCl and propranolol groups were on concomitant digoxin. Response rates were slightly higher with both beta-blockers in the digoxin-treated patients.

In all studies significant decreases of blood pressure occurred in 20-50% of patients, identified either as adverse reaction reports by investigators, or by observation of systolic pressure less than 90 mmHg or diastolic pressure less than 50 mmHg. The hypotension was symptomatic (mainly diaphoresis or dizziness) in about 12% of patients, and therapy was discontinued in about 11% of patients, about half of whom were symptomatic. In comparison to propranolol, hypotension was about three times as frequent with esmolol HCl, 53% vs. 17%. The hypotension was rapidly reversible with decreased infusion rate or after discontinuation of therapy with esmolol HCl. For both esmolol HCl and propranolol, hypotension was reported less frequently in patients receiving concomitant digoxin.

E

INDICATIONS AND USAGE

SUPRAVENTRICULAR TACHYCARDIA

Esmolol HCl is indicated for the rapid control of ventricular rate in patients with atrial fibrillation or atrial flutter in perioperative, postoperative, or other emergent circumstances where short term control of ventricular rate with a short-acting agent is desirable. Esmolol HCl is also indicated in noncompensatory sinus tachycardia where, in the physician's judgement, the rapid heart rate requires specific intervention. Esmolol HCl is not intended for use in chronic settings where transfer to another agent is anticipated.

INTRAOPERATIVE AND POSTOPERATIVE TACHYCARDIA AND/OR HYPERTENSION

Esmolol HCl is indicated for the treatment of tachycardia and hypertension that occur during induction and tracheal intubation, during surgery, on emergence from anesthesia, and in the postoperative period, when in the physician's judgment such specific intervention is considered indicated.

Use of esmolol HCl to prevent such events is not recommended.

CONTRAINDICATIONS

Esmolol HCl is contraindicated in patients with sinus bradycardia, heart block greater than first degree, cardiogenic shock or overt heart failure (see WARNINGS).

WARNINGS

HYPOTENSION

In clinical trials 20-50% of patients treated with esmolol HCl have experienced hypotension, generally defined as systolic pressure less than 90 mmHg and/or diastolic pressure less than 50 mmHg. About 12% of the patients have been symptomatic (mainly diaphoresis or dizziness). Hypotension can occur at any dose but is dose-related so that doses beyond 200 µg/kg/min (0.2 mg/kg/min) are not recommended. Patients should be closely monitored, especially if pretreatment blood pressure is low. Decrease of dose or termination of infusion reverses hypotension, usually within 30 minutes.

CARDIAC FAILURE

Sympathetic stimulation is necessary in supporting circulatory function in congestive heart failure, and beta blockade carries the potential hazard of further depressing myocardial contractility and precipitating more severe failure. Continued depression of the myocardium with beta blocking agents over a period of time can, in some cases, lead to cardiac failure. At the first sign or symptom of impending cardiac failure, esmolol HCl should be withdrawn. Although withdrawal may be sufficient because of the short elimination half-life of esmolol HCl, specific treatment may also be considered. The use of esmolol HCl for control of ventricular response in patients with supraventricular arrhythmias should be undertaken with caution when the patient is compromised hemodynamically or is taking other drugs that decrease any or all of the following: peripheral resistance, myocardial filling, myocardial contractility, or electrical impulse propagation in the myocardium. Despite the rapid onset and offset of esmolol HCl's effects, several cases of death have been reported in complex clinical states where esmolol HCl was presumably being used to control ventricular rate.

INTRAOPERATIVE AND POSTOPERATIVE TACHYCARDIA AND/OR HYPERTENSION

Esmolol HCl should not be used as the treatment for hypertension in patients in whom the increased blood pressure is primarily due to the vasoconstriction associated with hypothermia.

BRONCHOSPASTIC DISEASES

PATIENTS WITH BRONCHOSPASTIC DISEASES SHOULD, IN GENERAL, NOT RECEIVE BETA BLOCKERS. Because of its relative $beta_1$ selectivity and titratability, esmolol HCl may be used with caution in patients with bronchospastic diseases. However, since $beta_1$ selectivity is not absolute, esmolol HCl should be carefully titrated to obtain the lowest possible effective dose. In the event of bronchospasm, the infusion should be terminated immediately; a $beta_2$ stimulating agent may be administered if conditions warrant but should be used with particular caution as patients already have rapid ventricular rates.

DIABETES MELLITUS AND HYPOGLYCEMIA

Esmolol HCl should be used with caution in diabetic patients requiring a beta blocking agent. Beta blockers may mask tachycardia occurring with hypoglycemia, but other manifestations such as dizziness and sweating may not be significantly affected.

PRECAUTIONS

GENERAL

Infusion concentrations of 20 mg/ml were associated with more serious venous irritation, including thrombophlebitis, than concentrations of 10 mg/ml. Extravasation of 20 mg/ml may lead to a serious local reaction and possible skin necrosis. Concentrations greater than 10 mg/ml or infusion into small veins or through a butterfly catheter should be avoided.

Because the acid metabolite of esmolol HCl is primarily excreted unchanged by the kidney, esmolol HCl should be administered with caution to patients with impaired renal function. The elimination half-life of the acid metabolite was prolonged ten-fold and the plasma level was considerably elevated in patients with end-stage renal disease.

Care should be taken in the intravenous administration of esmolol HCl as sloughing of the skin and necrosis have been reported in association with infiltration and extravasation of intravenous infusions.

CARCINOGENESIS, MUTAGENESIS, AND IMPAIRMENT OF FERTILITY

Because of its short term usage no carcinogenicity, mutagenicity or reproductive performance studies have been conducted with esmolol HCl.

PREGNANCY CATEGORY C

Teratogenicity studies in rats at intravenous dosages of esmolol HCl up to 3000 µg/kg/min (3 mg/kg/min) (10 times the maximum human maintenance dosage) for 30 minutes daily produced no evidence of maternal toxicity, embryotoxicity or teratogenicity, while a dosage of 10,000 µg/kg/min (10 mg/kg/min) produced maternal toxicity and lethality. In rabbits, intravenous dosages up to 1000 µg/kg/min (1 mg/kg/min) for 30 minutes daily produced no evidence of maternal toxicity, embryotoxicity or teratogenicity, while 2500 µg/kg/min (2.5 mg/kg/min) produced minimal maternal toxicity and increased fetal resorptions.

Although there are no adequate and well-controlled studies in pregnant women. Esmolol HCl should be used during pregnancy only if the potential benefit justifies the potential risk to the fetus.

NURSING MOTHERS

It is not known whether esmolol HCl is excreted in human milk, however, caution should be exercised when esmolol HCl is administered to a nursing woman.

PEDIATRIC USE

The safety and effectiveness of esmolol HCl in children have not been established.

DRUG INTERACTIONS

Catecholamine-depleting drugs, (*e.g.*, reserpine), may have an additive effect when given with beta blocking agents. Patients treated concurrently with esmolol HCl and a catecholamine depletor should therefore be closely observed for evidence of hypotension or marked bradycardia, which may result in vertigo, syncope, or postural hypotension.

A study of interaction between esmolol HCl and warfarin showed that concomitant administration of esmolol HCl and warfarin does not alter warfarin plasma levels. Esmolol HCl concentrations were equivocally higher when given with warfarin, but this is not likely to be clinically important.

When digoxin and esmolol HCl were concomitantly administered intravenously to normal volunteers, there was a 10-20% increase in digoxin blood levels at some time points. Digoxin did not affect esmolol HCl pharmacokinetics. When intravenous morphine and esmolol HCl were concomitantly administered in normal subjects, no effect on morphine blood levels was seen, but esmolol HCl steady-state blood levels were increased by 46% in the presence of morphine. No other pharmacokinetic parameters were changed.

The effect of esmolol HCl on the duration of succinylcholine-induced neuromuscular blockade was studied in patients undergoing surgery. The onset of neuromuscular blockade by succinylcholine was unaffected by esmolol HCl, but the duration of neuromuscular blockade was prolonged from 5 minutes to 8 minutes.

Although the interactions observed in these studies do not appear to be of major clinical importance, esmolol HCl should be titrated with caution in patients being treated concurrently with digoxin, morphine, succinylcholine or warfarin.

While taking beta-blockers, patients with a history of severe anaphylactic reaction to a variety of allergens may be more reactive to repeated challenge, either accidental, diagnostic, or therapeutic. Such patients may be unresponsive to the usual doses of epinephrine used to treat allergic reaction.

Caution should be exercised when considering the use of esmolol HCl and Verapamil in patients with depressed myocardial function. Fatal cardiac arrests have occurred in patients receiving both drugs. Additionally, esmolol HCl should not be used to control supraventricular tachycardia in the presence of agents which are vasoconstrictive and inotropic such as dopamine, epinephrine, and norepinephrine because of the danger of blocking cardiac contractility when systemic vascular resistance is high.

ADVERSE REACTIONS

The following adverse reaction rates are based on use of esmolol HCl in clinical trials involving 369 patients with supraventricular tachycardia and over 600 intraoperative and postoperative patients enrolled in clinical trials. Most adverse effects observed in controlled clinical trial settings have been mild and transient. The most important adverse effect has been hypotension (see WARNINGS). Deaths have been reported in post-marketing experience occurring during complex clinical states where esmolol HCl was presumably being used simply to control ventricular rate (see WARNINGS, Cardiac Failure).

Cardiovascular: Symptomatic hypotension (diaphoresis, dizziness) occurred in 12% of patients, and therapy was discontinued in about 11%, about half of whom were symptomatic. Asymptomatic hypotension occurred in about 25% of patients. Hypotension resolved during esmolol HCl infusion in 63% of these patients and within 30 minutes after discontinuation of infusion in 80% of the remaining patients. Diaphoresis accompanied hypotension in 10% of patients. Peripheral ischemia occurred in approximately 1% of patients. Pallor, flushing, bradycardia (heart rate less than 50 beats per minute), chest pain, syncope, pulmonary edema and heart block have each been reported in less than 1% of patients. In two patients without supraventricular tachycardia but with serious coronary artery disease (post inferior myocardial infarction or unstable angina), severe bradycardia/sinus pause/asystole has developed, reversible in both cases with discontinuation of treatment.

Central Nervous System: Dizziness has occurred in 3% of patients; somnolence in 3%, confusion, headache, and agitation in about 2%, and fatigue in about 1% of patients. Paresthesia, asthenia, depression, abnormal thinking, anxiety, anorexia, and lightheadedness were reported in less than 1% of patients. Seizures were also reported in less than 1% of patients, with one death.

Respiratory: Bronchospasm, wheezing, dyspnea, nasal congestion, rhonchi, and rales have each been reported in less than 1% of patients.

Gastrointestinal: Nausea was reported in 7% of patients. Vomiting has occurred in about 1% of patients. Dyspepsia, constipation, dry mouth, and abdominal discomfort have each occurred in less than 1% of patients. Taste perversion has also been reported.

Skin (infusion site): Infusion site reactions including inflammation and induration were reported in about 8% of patients. Edema, erythema, skin discoloration, burning at the infusion site, thrombophlebitis, and local skin necrosis from extravasation have each occurred in less than 1% of patients.

Miscellaneous: *Each of the following has been reported in less than 1% of patients:* Urinary retention, speech disorder, abnormal vision, midscapular pain, rigors, and fever.

DOSAGE AND ADMINISTRATION

2.5 G AMPUL

THE 2.5 g AMPUL IS NOT FOR DIRECT INTRAVENOUS INJECTION. THIS DOSAGE FORM IS A CONCENTRATED, POTENT DRUG WHICH MUST BE DILUTED PRIOR TO ITS INFUSION. ESMOLOL HCl SHOULD NOT BE ADMIXED WITH SODIUM BICARBONATE. ESMOLOL HCl SHOULD NOT BE MIXED WITH OTHER DRUGS PRIOR TO DILUTION IN A SUITABLE INTRAVENOUS FLUID. (See Compatibility With Commonly Used Intravenous Fluids.)

Dilution: Aseptically prepare a 10 mg/ml infusion, by adding two 2.5 g ampuls to a 500 ml container, or one 2.5 g ampul to a 250 ml container, of a compatible intravenous solution listed below. (Remove overage prior to dilution as appropriate.) This yields a final concentration of 10 mg/ml. The diluted solution is stable for at least 24 hours at room temperature. *Note:* Concentrations of esmolol HCl greater than 10 mg/ml are likely to produce irritation on continued infusion (see PRECAUTIONS). Esmolol HCl has, however, been well tolerated when administered via a central vein.

100 MG VIAL

This dosage form is prediluted to provide a ready-to-use 10 mg/ml concentration recommended for esmolol HCl intravenous administration. It may be used to administer the appropriate esmolol HCl loading dosage infusions by hand-held syringe while the maintenance infusion is being prepared.

When using the 100 mg vial, a loading dose of 0.5 mg/kg/min for a 70 kg patient would be 3.5 ml.

SUPRAVENTRICULAR TACHYCARDIA

In the treatment of supraventricular tachycardia, responses to esmolol HCl usually (over 95%) occur within the range of 50 to 200 μg/kg/min (0.05 to 0.2 mg/kg/min). The average effective dosage is approximately 100 μg/kg/min (0.1 mg/kg/min) although dosages as low as 25 μg/kg/min (0.025 mg/kg/min) have been adequate in some patients. Dosages as high as 300 μg/kg/min (0.3 mg/kg/min) have been used, but these provide little added effect and an increased rate of adverse effects, and are not recommended. Dosage of esmolol HCl in supraventricular tachycardia must be individualized by titration in which each step consists of a loading dosage followed by a maintenance dosage.

To initiate treatment of a patient with supraventricular tachycardia, administer a loading infusion of 500 μg/kg/min (0.5 mg/kg/min) over 1 minute followed by a 4 minute maintenance infusion of 50 μg/kg/min (0.05 mg/kg/min). If an adequate therapeutic effect is observed over the 5 minutes of drug administration, maintain the maintenance infusion dosage with periodic adjustments up or down as needed. If an adequate therapeutic effect is not observed, the same loading dosage is repeated over 1 minute followed by an increased maintenance rate infusion of 100 μg/kg/min (0.1 mg/kg/min).

Continue titration procedure as above, repeating the original loading infusion of 500 μg/kg/min (0.5 mg/kg/min) over 1 minute, but increasing the maintenance infusion rate over the subsequent 4 minutes by 50 μg/kg/min (0.05 mg/kg/min) increments. As the desired heart rate or blood pressure is approached, omit subsequent loading doses and titrate the maintenance dosage up or down to endpoint. Also, if desired, increase the interval between steps from 5-10 minutes (see TABLE 1).

This specific dosage regimen has not been studied intraoperatively and, because of the time required for titration, may not be optimal for intraoperative use.

The safety of dosages above 300 μg/kg/min (0.3 mg/kg/min) has not been studied.

In the event of an adverse reaction, the dosage of esmolol HCl may be reduced or discontinued. If a local infusion site reaction develops, an alternate infusion site should be used and caution should be taken to prevent extravasation. The use of butterfly needles should be avoided.

Abrupt cessation of esmolol HCl in patients has not been reported to produce the withdrawal effects which may occur with abrupt withdrawal of beta blockers following chronic use in coronary artery disease (CAD) patients. However, caution should still be used in abruptly discontinuing infusions of esmolol HCl in CAD patients.

After achieving an adequate control of the heart rate and a stable clinical status in patients with supraventricular tachycardia, transition to alternative antiarrhythmic agents such as propranolol, digoxin, or verapamil, may be accomplished. A recommended guideline for such a transition is given below but the physician should carefully consider the labeling instructions for the alternative agent selected (see TABLE 2).

The dosage of esmolol HCl should be reduced as follows:

1. Thirty minutes following the first dose of the alternative agent, reduce the infusion rate of esmolol HCl by one-half (50%).

TABLE 1

Time	Loading Dose (over 1 minute)		Maintenance Dosage (over 4 minutes)	
(minutes)	μg/kg/min	mg/kg/min	μg/kg/min	mg/kg/min
0-1	500	0.5		
1-5			50	0.05
5-6	500	0.5		
6-10			100	0.1
10-11	500	0.5		
11-15			150	0.15
15-16	—	—		
16-20			200*	0.2*
20-(24 hr)			Maintenance dose titrated to heart rate or other clinical endpoint.	

* As the desired heart rate or endpoint is approached, the loading infusion may be omitted and the maintenance infusion titrated to 300 μg/kg/min (0.3 mg/kg/min) or downward as appropriate. Maintenance dosages above 200 μg/kg/min (0.2 mg/kg/min) have not been shown to have significantly increased benefits. The interval between titration steps may be increased.

TABLE 2

Alternative Agent	Dosage
Propranolol HCl	10-20 mg q 4-6 h
Digoxin	0.125-0.5 mg q 6 h (po or IV)
Verapamil	80 mg q 6 h

2. Following the second dose of the alternative agent, monitor the patient's response and if satisfactory control is maintained for the first hour, discontinue esmolol HCl.

The use of infusions of esmolol HCl up to 24 hours has been well documented; in addition, limited data from 24-48 hours (n=48) indicate that esmolol HCl is well tolerated up to 48 hours.

INTRAOPERATIVE AND POSTOPERATIVE TACHYCARDIA AND/OR HYPERTENSION

In the intraoperative and postoperative settings it is not always advisable to slowly titrate the dose of esmolol HCl to a therapeutic effect. Therefore, two dosing options are presented: immediate control dosing and a gradual control when the physician has time to titrate.

1. ***Immediate Control:*** For intraoperative treatment of tachycardia and/or hypertension give an 80 mg approximately 1 mg/kg) bolus dose over 30 seconds followed by a 150 μg/kg/min infusion, if necessary. Adjust the infusion rate as required up to 300 μg/kg/min to maintain desired heart rate and/or blood pressure.
2. ***Gradual Control:*** For postoperative tachycardia and hypertension, the dosing schedule is the same as that used in supraventricular tachycardia. To initiate treatment, administer a loading dosage infusion of 500 μg/kg/min of esmolol HCl for 1 minute followed by a 4 minute maintenance infusion of 50 μg/kg/min. If an adequate therapeutic effect is not observed within 5 minutes, repeat the same loading dosage and follow with a maintenance infusion increased to 100 μg/kg/min (see CLINICAL PHARMACOLOGY, Supraventricular Tachycardia).

Note: Higher doses (250-300 μg/kg/min) may be required for adequate control of blood pressure than those required for the treatment of atrial fibrillation, flutter and sinus tachycardia. One third of the postoperative hypertensive patients required these higher doses.

COMPATIBILITY WITH COMMONLY USED INTRAVENOUS FLUIDS

Esmolol HCl injection was tested for compatibility with 10 commonly used intravenous fluids at a final concentration of 10 mg esmolol HCl per ml.

Esmolol HCl injection was found to be compatible with the following solutions and was stable for at least 24 hours at controlled room temperature or under refrigeration:

- Dextrose (5%) injection.
- Dextrose (5%) in lactated Ringer's injection.
- Dextrose (5%) in Ringer's injection.
- Dextrose (5%) and sodium chloride (0.45%) injection.
- Dextrose (5%) and sodium chloride (0.9%) injection.
- Lactated Ringer's injection.
- Potassium chloride (40 mEq/L) in dextrose (5%) injection.
- Sodium chloride (0.45%) injection.
- Sodium chloride (0.9%) injection.

Esmolol HCl injection was NOT compatible with sodium bicarbonate (5%) injection.

Note: Parenteral drug products should be inspected visually for particulate matter and discoloration prior to administration, whenever solution and container permit.

PRODUCT LISTING - EQUIVALENTS NOT AVAILABLE

Solution - Intravenous - 10 mg/ml

10 ml x 25	$574.75	BREVIBLOC, Baxter Pharmaceutical Products, Inc	10019-0015-01
250 ml	$1021.90	BREVIBLOC, Baxter Pharmaceutical Products, Inc	10019-0055-61

Solution - Intravenous - 250 mg/ml

10 ml x 10	$1007.40	BREVIBLOC, Baxter Pharmaceutical Products, Inc	10019-0025-18

Esomeprazole Magnesium (000692)

Categories: Ulcer, duodenal; Gastroesophageal Reflux Disease; Esophagitis, erosive; FDA Approved 2001 Feb; Pregnancy Category B
Drug Classes: Gastrointestinals; Proton pump inhibitors
Brand Names: Nexium
Foreign Brand Availability: Esoprax (Colombia); Inexium (France); Sompraz (India)
Cost of Therapy: $284.54 (Infection; Fortaz Injection; 1 g; 2 g/day; 10 day supply)

DESCRIPTION

The active ingredient in Nexium delayed-release capsules is bis(5-methoxy-2-[(S)-[(4-methoxy-3,5-dimethyl-2-pyridinyl)methyl]sulfinyl]-1*H*-benzimidazole-1-yl) magnesium trihydrate, a compound that inhibits gastric acid secretion. Esomeprazole is the S-isomer of omeprazole, which is a mixture of the S- and R-isomers. Its empirical formula is $(C_{17}H_{18}N_3O_3S)_2Mg \cdot 3H_2O$ with molecular weight of 767.2 as a trihydrate and 713.1 on an anhydrous basis.

The magnesium salt is a white to slightly colored crystalline powder. It contains 3 moles of water of solvation and is slightly soluble in water.

The stability of esomeprazole magnesium is a function of pH; it rapidly degrades in acidic media, but it has acceptable stability under alkaline conditions. At pH 6.8 (buffer), the half-life of the magnesium salt is about 19 hours at 25°C and about 8 hours at 37°C.

Nexium is supplied as delayed-release capsules for oral administration. Each delayed-release capsule contains 20 or 40 mg of esomeprazole (present as 22.3 or 44.5 mg esomeprazole magnesium trihydrate) in the form of enteric-coated pellets with the following inactive ingredients: glyceryl monostearate 40-50, hydroxypropyl cellulose, hypromellose, magnesium stearate, methacrylic acid copolymer type C, polysorbate 80, sugar spheres, talc, and triethyl citrate. The capsule shells have the following inactive ingredients: gelatin, FD&C blue no. 1, FD&C red no. 40, D&C red no. 28, titanium dioxide, shellac, ethyl alcohol, isopropyl alcohol, n-butyl alcohol, propylene glycol, sodium hydroxide, polyvinyl pyrrolidone, and D&C yellow no. 10.

CLINICAL PHARMACOLOGY

PHARMACOKINETICS

Absorption

Esomeprazole magnesium delayed-release capsules contain an enteric-coated pellet formulation of esomeprazole magnesium. After oral administration peak plasma levels (C_{max}) occur at approximately 1.5 hours (T_{max}). The C_{max} increases proportionally when the dose is increased, and there is a 3-fold increase in the area under the plasma concentration-time curve (AUC) from 20-40 mg. At repeated once-daily dosing with 40 mg, the systemic bioavailability is approximately 90% compared to 64% after a single dose of 40 mg. The mean exposure (AUC) to esomeprazole increases from 4.32 μmol·h/L on Day 1 to 11.2 μmol·h/L on Day 5 after 40 mg once daily dosing.

The AUC after administration of a single 40 mg dose of esomeprazole is decreased by 43-53% after food intake compared to fasting conditions. Esomeprazole should be taken at least 1 hour before meals.

The pharmacokinetic profile of esomeprazole was determined in 36 patients with symptomatic gastroesophageal reflux disease following repeated once daily administration of 20 and 40 mg capsules of esomeprazole magnesium over a period of 5 days. The results are shown in TABLE 1.

TABLE 1 *Pharmacokinetic Parameters of Esomeprazole Magnesium Following Oral Dosing for 5 Days*

Parameter	Esomeprazole Magnesium 40 mg	Esomeprazole Magnesium 20 mg
AUC	12.6 μmol·h/L	4.2 μmol·h/L
Coefficient of variation	42%	59%
C_{max}	4.7 μmol/L	2.1 μmol/L
T_{max}	1.6 h	1.6 h
T½	1.5 h	1.2 h

Values represent the geometric mean, except the T_{max}, which is the arithmetic mean.

Distribution

Esomeprazole is 97% bound to plasma proteins. Plasma protein binding is constant over the concentration range of 2-20 μmol/L. The apparent volume of distribution at steady state in healthy volunteers is approximately 16 L.

Metabolism

Esomeprazole is extensively metabolized in the liver by the cytochrome P450 (CYP) enzyme system. The metabolites of esomeprazole lack antisecretory activity. The major part of esomeprazole's metabolism is dependent upon the CYP2C19 isoenzyme, which forms the hydroxy and desmethyl metabolites. The remaining amount is dependent on CYP3A4 which forms the sulphone metabolite. CYP2C19 isoenzyme exhibits polymorphism in the metabolism of esomeprazole, since some 3% of Caucasians and 15-20% of Asians lack CYP2C19 and are termed Poor metabolizers. At steady state, the ratio of AUC in Poor metabolizers to AUC in the rest of the population (Extensive metabolizers) is approximately 2.

Following administration of equimolar doses, the S- and R-isomers are metabolized differently by the liver, resulting in higher plasma levels of the S- than of the R-isomer.

Excretion

The plasma elimination half-life of esomeprazole is approximately 1-1.5 hours. Less than 1% of parent drug is excreted in the urine. Approximately 80% of an oral dose of esomeprazole is excreted as inactive metabolites in the urine, and the remainder is found as inactive metabolites in the feces.

SPECIAL POPULATIONS

Geriatric

The AUC and C_{max} values were slightly higher (25% and 18%, respectively) in the elderly as compared to younger subjects at steady state. Dosage adjustment based on age is not necessary.

Pediatric

The pharmacokinetics of esomeprazole have not been studied in patients <18 years of age.

Gender

The AUC and C_{max} values were slightly higher (13%) in females than in males at steady state. Dosage adjustment based on gender is not necessary.

Hepatic Insufficiency

The steady state pharmacokinetics of esomeprazole obtained after administration of 40 mg once daily to 4 patients each with mild (Child Pugh A), moderate (Child Pugh Class B), and severe (Child Pugh Class C) liver insufficiency were compared to those obtained in 36 male and female GERD patients with normal liver function. In patients with mild and moderate hepatic insufficiency, the AUCs were within the range that could be expected in patients with normal liver function. In patients with severe hepatic insufficiency the AUCs were 2-3 times higher than in the patients with normal liver function. No dosage adjustment is recommended for patients with mild to moderate hepatic insufficiency (Child Pugh Classes A and B). However, in patients with severe hepatic insufficiency (Child Pugh Class C) a dose of 20 mg once daily should not be exceeded (see DOSAGE AND ADMINISTRATION).

Renal Insufficiency

The pharmacokinetics of esomeprazole in patients with renal impairment are not expected to be altered relative to healthy volunteers as less than 1% of esomeprazole is excreted unchanged in urine.

COMBINATION THERAPY WITH ANTIMICROBIALS

Esomeprazole magnesium 40 mg once daily was given in combination with clarithromycin 500 mg twice daily and amoxicillin 1000 mg twice daily for 7 days to 17 healthy male and female subjects. The mean steady state AUC and C_{max} of esomeprazole increased by 70% and 18%, respectively during triple combination therapy compared to treatment with esomeprazole alone. The observed increase in esomeprazole exposure during co-administration with clarithromycin and amoxicillin is not expected to produce significant safety concerns.

The pharmacokinetic parameters for clarithromycin and amoxicillin were similar during triple combination therapy and administration of each drug alone. However, the mean AUC and C_{max} for 14-hydroxyclarithromycin increased by 19% and 22%, respectively, during triple combination therapy compared to treatment with clarithromycin alone. This increase in exposure to 14-hydroxyclarithromycin is not considered to be clinically significant.

PHARMACODYNAMICS

Mechanism of Action

Esomeprazole is a proton pump inhibitor that suppresses gastric acid secretion by specific inhibition of the H^+/K^+-ATPase in the gastric parietal cell. The S- and R-isomers of omeprazole are protonated and converted in the acidic compartment of the parietal cell forming the active inhibitor, the achiral sulphenamide. By acting specifically on the proton pump, esomeprazole blocks the final step in acid production, thus reducing gastric acidity. This effect is dose-related up to a daily dose of 20-40 mg and leads to inhibition of gastric acid secretion.

Antisecretory Activity

The effect of esomeprazole on intragastric pH was determined in patients with symptomatic gastroesophageal reflux disease in two separate studies. In the first study of 36 patients, esomeprazole magnesium 40 and 20 mg capsules were administered over 5 days. The results are shown in TABLE 2.

TABLE 2 *Effect on Intragastric pH on Day 5 (n=36)*

Parameter	Esomeprazole Magnesium 40 mg	Esomeprazole Magnesium 20 mg
% Time Gastric pH >4†	70%* (16.8 h)	53% (12.7 h)
Coefficient of variation	26%	37%
Median 24 Hour pH	4.9*	4.1
Coefficient of variation	16%	27%

* p <0.01 esomeprazole magnesium 40 mg versus esomeprazole magnesium 20 mg.
† Gastric pH was measured over a 24 hour period.

In a second study, the effect on intragastric pH of esomeprazole magnesium 40 mg administered once daily over a 5 day period was similar to the first study, (% time with pH >4 was 68% or 16.3 hours).

Serum Gastrin Effects

The effect of esomeprazole magnesium on serum gastrin concentrations was evaluated in approximately 2700 patients in clinical trials up to 8 weeks and in over 1300 patients for up to 6-12 months. The mean fasting gastrin level increased in a dose-related manner. This increase reached a plateau within 2-3 months of therapy and returned to baseline levels within 4 weeks after discontinuation of therapy.

Enterochromaffin-Like (ECL) Cell Effects

In 24 month carcinogenicity studies of omeprazole in rats, a dose-related significant occurrence of gastric ECL cell carcinoid tumors and ECL cell hyperplasia was observed in both male and female animals (see PRECAUTIONS, Carcinogenesis, Mutagenesis, and Impairment of Fertility). Carcinoid tumors have also been observed in rats subjected to fundectomy or long-term treatment with other proton pump inhibitors or high doses of H_2-receptor antagonists.

Human gastric biopsy specimens have been obtained from more than 3000 patients treated with omeprazole in long-term clinical trials. The incidence of ECL cell hyperplasia in these studies increased with time; however, no case of ECL cell carcinoids, dysplasia, or neoplasia has been found in these patients.

In over 1000 patients treated with esomeprazole magnesium (10, 20 or 40 mg/day) up to 6-12 months, the prevalence of ECL cell hyperplasia increased with time and dose. No patient developed ECL cell carcinoids, dysplasia, or neoplasia in the gastric mucosa.

Endocrine Effects

Esomeprazole magnesium had no effect on thyroid function when given in oral doses of 20 or 40 mg for 4 weeks. Other effects of esomeprazole magnesium on the endocrine system were assessed using omeprazole studies. Omeprazole given in oral doses of 30 or 40 mg for 2-4 weeks had no effect on carbohydrate metabolism, circulating levels of parathyroid hormone, cortisol, estradiol, testosterone, prolactin, cholecystokinin or secretin.

MICROBIOLOGY

Esomeprazole magnesium, amoxicillin and clarithromycin triple therapy has been shown to be active against most strains of *Helicobacter pylori (H. pylori) in vitro* and in clinical infections as described in INDICATIONS AND USAGE.

Helicobacter

Helicobacter pylori

Susceptibility testing of *H. pylori* isolates was performed for amoxicillin and clarithromycin using agar dilution methodology, and minimum inhibitory concentrations (MICs) were determined.

Pretreatment Resistance

Clarithromycin pretreatment resistance rate (MIC ≥1 μg/ml) to *H. pylori* was 15% (66/445) at baseline in all treatment groups combined. A total of >99% (394/395) of patients had *H. pylori* isolates which were considered to be susceptible (MIC ≤0.25 μg/ml) to amoxicillin at baseline. One patient had a baseline *H. pylori* isolate with an amoxicillin MIC = 0.5 μg/ml.

Clarithromycin Susceptibility Test Results and Clinical/Bacteriologic Outcomes

The baseline *H. pylori* clarithromycin susceptibility results and the *H. pylori* eradication results at the Day 38 visit are shown in TABLE 3.

TABLE 3 Clarithromycin Susceptibility Test Results and Clinical/Bacteriological Outcomes* for Triple Therapy†

Clarithromycin Pretreatment Results		*H. pylori* Negative (Eradicated)	*H. pylori* Positive (Not Eradicated) Post-Treatment Susceptibility Results S‡	I‡	R‡	No MIC
Susceptible‡	182	162	4	0	2	14
Intermediate‡	1	1	0	0	0	0
Resistant‡	29	13	1	0	13	2

* Includes only patients with pretreatment and post-treatment clarithromycin susceptibility test results.
† Esomeprazole magnesium 40 mg once daily/amoxicillin 1000 mg twice daily/clarithromycin 500 mg twice daily for 10 days.
‡ Susceptible (S) MIC ≤0.25 μg/ml, Intermediate (I) MIC = 0.5 μg/ml, Resistant (R) MIC ≥1.0 μg/ml.

Patients not eradicated of *H. pylori* following esomeprazole magnesium/amoxicillin/clarithromycin triple therapy will likely have clarithromycin resistant *H. pylori* isolates. Therefore, clarithromycin susceptibility testing should be done, when possible. Patients with clarithromycin resistant *H. pylori* should not be re-treated with a clarithromycin-containing regimen.

Amoxicillin Susceptibility Test Results and Clinical/Bacteriological Outcomes

In the esomeprazole magnesium/amoxicillin/clarithromycin clinical trials, 83% (176/212) of the patients in the esomeprazole magnesium/amoxicillin/clarithromycin treatment group who had pretreatment amoxicillin susceptible MICs (≤0.25 μg/ml) were eradicated of *H. pylori*, and 17% (36/212) were not eradicated of *H. pylori*. Of the 36 patients who were not eradicated of *H. pylori* on triple therapy, 16 had no post-treatment susceptibility test results and 20 had post-treatment *H. pylori* isolates with amoxicillin susceptible MICs. Fifteen (15) of the patients who were not eradicated of *H. pylori* on triple therapy also had post-treatment *H. pylori* isolates with clarithromycin resistant MICs. There were no patients with *H. pylori* isolates who developed treatment emergent resistance to amoxicillin.

Susceptibility Test for Helicobacter pylori

The reference methodology for susceptibility testing of *H. pylori* is agar dilution MICs. One to three microliters (1-3 μl) of an inoculum equivalent to a No. 2 McFarland standard (1×10^7 to 1×10^8 CFU/ml for *H. pylori*) are inoculated directly onto freshly prepared antimicrobial containing Mueller-Hinton agar plates with 5% aged defibrinated sheep blood (≥2 weeks old). The agar dilution plates are incubated at 35°C in a microaerobic environment produced by a gas generating system suitable for *Campylobacter*. After 3 days of incubation, the MICs are recorded as the lowest concentration of antimicrobial agent required to inhibit growth of the organism. The clarithromycin and amoxicillin MIC values should be interpreted according to the criteria in TABLE 4.

Standardized susceptibility test procedures require the use of laboratory control microorganisms to control the technical aspects of the laboratory procedures. Standard clarithromycin and amoxicillin powders should provide the MIC values in TABLE 5.

TABLE 4

MIC	Interpretation
Clarithromycin*	
≤0.25 μg/ml	Susceptible (S)
0.5 μg/ml	Intermediate (I)
≥1.0 μg/ml	Resistant (R)
Amoxicillin*†	
≤0.25 μg/ml	Susceptible (S)

* These are breakpoints for the agar dilution methodology and they should not be used to interpret results obtained using alternative methods.
† There were not enough organisms with MICs >0.25 μg/ml to determine a resistance breakpoint.

TABLE 5

Microorganisms	Antimicrobial Agent	MIC*
H. pylori ATCC 43504	Clarithromycin	0.016-0.12 μg/ml
H. pylori ATCC 43504	Amoxicillin	0.016-0.12 μg/ml

* These are quality control ranges for the agar dilution methodology and they should not be used to control test results obtained using alternative methods.

INDICATIONS AND USAGE

TREATMENT OF GASTROESOPHAGEAL REFLUX DISEASE (GERD)

Healing of Erosive Esophagitis

Esomeprazole magnesium is indicated for the short-term treatment (4-8 weeks) in the healing and symptomatic resolution of diagnostically confirmed erosive esophagitis. For those patients who have not healed after 4-8 weeks of treatment, an additional 4-8 week course of esomeprazole magnesium may be considered.

Maintenance of Healing of Erosive Esophagitis

Esomeprazole magnesium is indicated to maintain symptom resolution and healing of erosive esophagitis. Controlled studies do not extend beyond 6 months.

Symptomatic Gastroesophageal Reflux Disease

Esomeprazole magnesium is indicated for treatment of heartburn and other symptoms associated with GERD.

H. PYLORI ERADICATION TO REDUCE THE RISK OF DUODENAL ULCER RECURRENCE

Triple Therapy (esomeprazole magnesium plus amoxicillin and clarithromycin)

Esomeprazole magnesium, in combination with amoxicillin and clarithromycin, is indicated for the treatment of patients with *H. pylori* infection and duodenal ulcer disease (active or history of within the past 5 years) to eradicate *H. pylori*. Eradication of *H. pylori* has been shown to reduce the risk of duodenal ulcer recurrence. (See DOSAGE AND ADMINISTRATION.)

In patients who fail therapy, susceptibility testing should be done. If resistance to clarithromycin is demonstrated or susceptibility testing is not possible, alternative antimicrobial therapy should be instituted. (See CLINICAL PHARMACOLOGY, Microbiology and the clarithromycin prescribing information, CLINICAL PHARMACOLOGY, Microbiology.)

CONTRAINDICATIONS

Esomeprazole magnesium is contraindicated in patients with known hypersensitivity to any component of the formulation or to substituted benzimidazoles.

Clarithromycin is contraindicated in patients with a known hypersensitivity to any macrolide antibiotic.

Concomitant administration of clarithromycin with pimozide is contraindicated. There have been post-marketing reports of drug interactions when clarithromycin and/or erythromycin are co-administered with pimozide resulting in cardiac arrhythmias (QT prolongation, ventricular tachycardia, ventricular fibrillation, and torsade de pointes) most likely due to inhibition of hepatic metabolism of pimozide by erythromycin and clarithromycin. Fatalities have been reported. (Please refer to full prescribing information for clarithromycin.)

Amoxicillin is contraindicated in patients with a known hypersensitivity to any penicillin. (Please refer to full prescribing information for amoxicillin.)

WARNINGS

CLARITHROMYCIN SHOULD NOT BE USED IN PREGNANT WOMEN EXCEPT IN CLINICAL CIRCUMSTANCES WHERE NO ALTERNATIVE THERAPY IS APPROPRIATE. IF PREGNANCY OCCURS WHILE TAKING CLARITHROMYCIN, THE PATIENT SHOULD BE APPRISED OF THE POTENTIAL HAZARD TO THE FETUS. (See WARNINGS in prescribing information for clarithromycin.)

AMOXICILLIN

Serious and occasionally fatal hypersensitivity (anaphylactic) reactions have been reported in patients on penicillin therapy. These reactions are more apt to occur in individuals with a history of penicillin hypersensitivity and/or a history of sensitivity to multiple allergens.

There have been well documented reports of individuals with a history of penicillin hypersensitivity reactions who have experienced severe hypersensitivity reactions when treated with a cephalosporin. Before initiating therapy with any penicillin, careful inquiry should be made concerning previous hypersensitivity reactions to penicillins, cephalosporins, and other allergens. If an allergic reaction occurs, amoxicillin should be discontinued and the appropriate therapy instituted.

SERIOUS ANAPHYLACTIC REACTIONS REQUIRE IMMEDIATE EMERGENCY TREATMENT WITH EPINEPHRINE. OXYGEN, INTRAVENOUS STEROIDS, AND AIRWAY MANAGEMENT, INCLUDING INTUBATION, SHOULD ALSO BE ADMINISTERED AS INDICATED.

Pseudomembranous colitis has been reported with nearly all antibacterial agents, including clarithromycin and amoxicillin, and may range in severity from mild to life threatening. Therefore, it is important to consider this diagnosis in patients who present with diarrhea subsequent to the administration of antibacterial agents.

Treatment with antibacterial agents alters the normal flora of the colon and may permit overgrowth of clostridia. Studies indicate that a toxin produced by *Clostridium difficile* is a primary cause of "antibiotic-associated colitis".

After the diagnosis of pseudomembranous colitis has been established, therapeutic measures should be initiated. Mild cases of pseudomembranous colitis usually respond to discontinuation of the drug alone. In moderate to severe cases, consideration should be given to management with fluids and electrolytes, protein supplementation, and treatment with an antibacterial drug clinically effective against *Clostridium difficile* colitis.

PRECAUTIONS

GENERAL

Symptomatic response to therapy with esomeprazole magnesium does not preclude the presence of gastric malignancy.

Atrophic gastritis has been noted occasionally in gastric corpus biopsies from patients treated long-term with omeprazole, of which esomeprazole magnesium is an enantiomer.

INFORMATION FOR THE PATIENT

Patients should be informed of the following: Esomeprazole magnesium delayed-release capsules should be taken at least 1 hour before meals.

For patients who have difficulty swallowing capsules, 1 tablespoon of applesauce can be added to an empty bowl and the esomeprazole magnesium delayed-release capsule can be opened, and the pellets inside the capsule carefully emptied onto the applesauce. The pellets should be mixed with the applesauce and then swallowed immediately. The applesauce used should not be hot and should be soft enough to be swallowed without chewing. The pellets should not be chewed or crushed. The pellet/applesauce mixture should not be stored for future use.

Antacids may be used while taking esomeprazole magnesium.

CARCINOGENESIS, MUTAGENESIS, AND IMPAIRMENT OF FERTILITY

The carcinogenic potential of esomeprazole was assessed using omeprazole studies. In two 24 month oral carcinogenicity studies in rats, omeprazole at daily doses of 1.7, 3.4, 13.8, 44.0 and 140.8 mg/kg/day (about 0.7-57 times the human dose of 20 mg/day expressed on a body surface area basis) produced gastric ECL cell carcinoids in a dose-related manner in both male and female rats; the incidence of this effect was markedly higher in female rats, which had higher blood levels of omeprazole. Gastric carcinoids seldom occur in the untreated rat. In addition, ECL cell hyperplasia was present in all treated groups of both sexes. In one of these studies, female rats were treated with 13.8 mg omeprazole/kg/day (about 5.6 times the human dose on a body surface area basis) for 1 year, then followed for an additional year without the drug. No carcinoids were seen in these rats. An increased incidence of treatment-related ECL cell hyperplasia was observed at the end of 1 year (94% treated vs 10% controls). By the second year the difference between treated and control rats was much smaller (46% vs 26%) but still showed more hyperplasia in the treated group. Gastric adenocarcinoma was seen in one rat (2%). No similar tumor was seen in male or female rats treated for 2 years. For this strain of rat no similar tumor has been noted historically, but a finding involving only one tumor is difficult to interpret. A 78 week mouse carcinogenicity study of omeprazole did not show increased tumor occurrence, but the study was not conclusive.

Esomeprazole was negative in the Ames mutation test, in the *in vivo* rat bone marrow cell chromosome aberration test, and the *in vivo* mouse micronucleus test. Esomeprazole, however, was positive in the *in vitro* human lymphocyte chromosome aberration test. Omeprazole was positive in the *in vitro* human lymphocyte chromosome aberration test, the *in vivo* mouse bone marrow cell chromosome aberration test, and the *in vivo* mouse micronucleus test.

The potential effects of esomeprazole on fertility and reproductive performance were assessed using omeprazole studies. Omeprazole at oral doses up to 138 mg/kg/day in rats (about 56 times the human dose on a body surface area basis) was found to have no effect on reproductive performance of parental animals.

PREGNANCY, TERATOGENIC EFFECTS, PREGNANCY CATEGORY B

Teratology studies have been performed in rats at oral doses up to 280 mg/kg/day (about 57 times the human dose on a body surface area basis) and in rabbits at oral doses up to 86 mg/kg/day (about 35 times the human dose on a body surface area basis) and have revealed no evidence of impaired fertility or harm to the fetus due to esomeprazole. There are, however, no adequate and well-controlled studies in pregnant women. Because animal reproduction studies are not always predictive of human response, this drug should be used during pregnancy only if clearly needed.

Teratology studies conducted with omeprazole in rats at oral doses up to 138 mg/kg/day (about 56 times the human dose on a body surface area basis) and in rabbits at doses up to 69 mg/kg/day (about 56 times the human dose on a body surface area basis) did not disclose any evidence for a teratogenic potential of omeprazole. In rabbits, omeprazole in a dose range of 6.9-69.1 mg/kg/day (about 5.5-56 times the human dose on a body surface area basis) produced dose-related increases in embryo-lethality, fetal resorptions, and pregnancy disruptions. In rats, dose-related embryo/fetal toxicity and postnatal developmental toxicity were observed in offspring resulting from parents treated with omeprazole at 13.8-138.0 mg/kg/day (about 5.6-56 times the human doses on a body surface area basis). There are no adequate and well-controlled studies in pregnant women. Sporadic reports have been received of congenital abnormalities occurring in infants born to women who have received omeprazole during pregnancy.

Amoxicillin

Pregnancy Category B. See full prescribing information for amoxicillin before using in pregnant women.

Clarithromycin

Pregnancy Category C. See WARNINGS and full prescribing information for clarithromycin before using in pregnant women.

NURSING MOTHERS

The excretion of esomeprazole in milk has not been studied. However, omeprazole concentrations have been measured in breast milk of a woman following oral administration of 20 mg. Because esomeprazole is likely to be excreted in human milk, because of the potential for serious adverse reactions in nursing infants from esomeprazole, and because of the potential for tumorigenicity shown for omeprazole in rat carcinogenicity studies, a decision should be made whether to discontinue nursing or to discontinue the drug, taking into account the importance of the drug to the mother.

PEDIATRIC USE

Safety and effectiveness in pediatric patients have not been established.

GERIATRIC USE

Of the total number of patients who received esomeprazole magnesium in clinical trials, 778 were 65-74 years of age and 124 patients were ≥75 years of age.

No overall differences in safety and efficacy were observed between the elderly and younger individuals, and other reported clinical experience has not identified differences in responses between the elderly and younger patients, but greater sensitivity of some older individuals cannot be ruled out.

DRUG INTERACTIONS

Esomeprazole is extensively metabolized in the liver by CYP2C19 and CYP3A4.

In vitro and *in vivo* studies have shown that esomeprazole is not likely to inhibit CYPs 1A2, 2A6, 2C9, 2D6, 2E1 and 3A4. No clinically relevant interactions with drugs metabolized by these CYP enzymes would be expected. Drug interaction studies have shown that esomeprazole does not have any clinically significant interactions with phenytoin, warfarin, quinidine, clarithromycin or amoxicillin. Post-marketing reports of changes in prothrombin measures have been received among patients on concomitant warfarin and esomeprazole therapy. Increases in INR and prothrombin time may lead to abnormal bleeding and even death. Patients treated with proton pump inhibitors and warfarin concomitantly may need to be monitored for increases in INR and prothrombin time.

Esomeprazole may potentially interfere with CYP2C19, the major esomeprazole metabolizing enzyme. Coadministration of esomeprazole 30 mg and diazepam, a CYP2C19 substrate, resulted in a 45% decrease in clearance of diazepam. Increased plasma levels of diazepam were observed 12 hours after dosing and onwards. However, at that time, the plasma levels of diazepam were below the therapeutic interval, and thus this interaction is unlikely to be of clinical relevance.

Esomeprazole inhibits gastric acid secretion. Therefore, esomeprazole may interfere with the absorption of drugs where gastric pH is an important determinant of bioavailability (*e.g.*, ketoconazole, iron salts and digoxin).

Coadministration of oral contraceptives, diazepam, phenytoin, or quinidine did not seem to change the pharmacokinetic profile of esomeprazole.

COMBINATION THERAPY WITH CLARITHROMYCIN

Co-administration of esomeprazole, clarithromycin, and amoxicillin has resulted in increases in the plasma levels of esomeprazole and 14-hydroxyclarithromycin. (See CLINICAL PHARMACOLOGY, Combination Therapy With Antimicrobials.)

Concomitant administration of clarithromycin with pimozide is contraindicated. (See clarithromycin prescribing information.)

ADVERSE REACTIONS

The safety of esomeprazole magnesium was evaluated in over 10,000 patients (aged 18-84 years) in clinical trials worldwide including over 7400 patients in the US and over 2600 patients in Europe and Canada. Over 2900 patients were treated in long-term studies for up to 6-12 months. In general, esomeprazole magnesium was well tolerated in both short and long-term clinical trials.

The safety in the treatment of healing of erosive esophagitis was assessed in four randomized comparative clinical trials, which included 1240 patients on esomeprazole magnesium 20 mg, 2434 patients on esomeprazole magnesium 40 mg, and 3008 patients on omeprazole 20 mg daily. The most frequently occurring adverse events (≥1%) in all three groups was headache (5.5, 5.0, and 3.8, respectively) and diarrhea (no difference among the three groups). Nausea, flatulence, abdominal pain, constipation, and dry mouth occurred at similar rates among patients taking esomeprazole magnesium or omeprazole.

Additional adverse events that were reported as possibly or probably related to esomeprazole magnesium with an incidence <1% are listed below by body system:

Body as a Whole: Abdomen enlarged, allergic reaction, asthenia, back pain, chest pain, chest pain substernal, facial edema, peripheral edema, hot flushes, fatigue, fever, flu-like disorder, generalized edema, leg edema, malaise, pain, rigors.

Cardiovascular: Flushing, hypertension, tachycardia.

Endocrine: Goiter.

Gastrointestinal: Bowel irregularity, constipation aggravated, dyspepsia, dysphagia, dysplasia GI, epigastric pain, eructation, esophageal disorder, frequent stools, gastroenteritis, GI hemorrhage, GI symptoms not otherwise specified, hiccup, melena, mouth disorder, pharynx disorder, rectal disorder, serum gastrin increased, tongue disorder, tongue edema, ulcerative stomatitis, vomiting.

Hearing: Earache, tinnitus.

Hematologic: Anemia, anemia hypochromic, cervical lymphoadenopathy, epistaxis, leukocytosis, leukopenia, thrombocytopenia.

Hepatic: Bilirubinemia, hepatic function abnormal, SGOT increased, SGPT increased.

Metabolic/Nutritional: Glycosuria, hyperuricemia, hyponatremia, increased alkaline phosphatase, thirst, vitamin B12 deficiency, weight increase, weight decrease.

Musculoskeletal: Arthralgia, arthritis aggravated, arthropathy, cramps, fibromyalgia syndrome, hernia, polymyalgia rheumatica.

Nervous System/Psychiatric: Anorexia, apathy, appetite increased, confusion, depression aggravated, dizziness, hypertonia, nervousness, hypoesthesia, impotence, insomnia, migraine, migraine aggravated, paresthesia, sleep disorder, somnolence, tremor, vertigo, visual field defect.

Reproductive: Dysmenorrhea, menstrual disorder, vaginitis.

Respiratory: Asthma aggravated, coughing, dyspnea, larynx edema, pharyngitis, rhinitis, sinusitis.

Skin and Appendages: Acne, angioedema, dermatitis, pruritus, pruritus ani, rash, rash erythematous, rash maculo-papular, skin inflammation, sweating increased, urticaria.

Special Senses: Otitis media, parosmia, taste loss, taste perversion.

Urogenital: Abnormal urine, albuminuria, cystitis, dysuria, fungal infection, hematuria, micturition frequency, moniliasis, genital moniliasis, polyuria.

Visual: Conjunctivitis, vision abnormal.

Endoscopic findings that were reported as adverse events include: Duodenitis, esophagitis, esophageal stricture, esophageal ulceration, esophageal varices, gastric ulcer, gastritis, hernia, benign polyps or nodules, Barrett's esophagus, and mucosal discoloration.

The incidence of treatment-related adverse events during 6 month maintenance treatment was similar to placebo. There were no differences in types of related adverse events seen during maintenance treatment up to 12 months compared to short-term treatment.

Two placebo-controlled studies were conducted in 710 patients for the treatment of symptomatic gastroesophageal reflux disease. The most common adverse events that were reported as possibly or probably related to esomeprazole magnesium were diarrhea (4.3%), headache (3.8%), and abdominal pain (3.8%).

POST-MARKETING REPORTS

There have been spontaneous reports of adverse events with post-marketing use of esomeprazole. These reports have included rare cases of anaphylactic reaction.

Other adverse events not observed with esomeprazole magnesium, but occurring with omeprazole can be found in the omeprazole prescribing information, ADVERSE REACTIONS section.

COMBINATION TREATMENT WITH AMOXICILLIN AND CLARITHROMYCIN

In clinical trials using combination therapy with esomeprazole magnesium plus amoxicillin and clarithromycin, no adverse events peculiar to these drug combinations were observed. Adverse events that occurred have been limited to those that had been observed with either esomeprazole magnesium, amoxicillin, or clarithromycin alone.

The most frequently reported drug-related adverse events for patients who received triple therapy for 10 days were diarrhea (9.2%), taste perversion (6.6%), and abdominal pain (3.7%). No treatment-emergent adverse events were observed at higher rates with triple therapy than were observed with esomeprazole magnesium alone.

For more information on adverse events with amoxicillin or clarithromycin, refer to their prescribing information, ADVERSE REACTIONS sections.

LABORATORY EVENTS

The following potentially clinically significant laboratory changes in clinical trials, irrespective of relationship to esomeprazole magnesium, were reported in ≤1% of patients: Increased creatinine, uric acid, total bilirubin, alkaline phosphatase, ALT, AST, hemoglobin, white blood cell count, platelets, serum gastrin, potassium, sodium, thyroxine and thyroid stimulating hormone (see CLINICAL PHARMACOLOGY, Pharmacodynamics, Endocrine Effects for further information on thyroid effects). Decreases were seen in hemoglobin, white blood cell count, platelets, potassium, sodium, and thyroxine.

In clinical trials using combination therapy with esomeprazole magnesium plus amoxicillin and clarithromycin, no additional increased laboratory abnormalities particular to these drug combinations were observed.

For more information on laboratory changes with amoxicillin or clarithromycin, refer to their prescribing information, ADVERSE REACTIONS sections.

DOSAGE AND ADMINISTRATION

The recommended adult dosages are outlined in TABLE 9. Esomeprazole magnesium delayed-release capsules should be swallowed whole and taken at least 1 hour before eating.

For patients who have difficulty swallowing capsules, 1 tablespoon of applesauce can be added to an empty bowl and the esomeprazole magnesium delayed-release capsule can be opened, and the pellets inside the capsule carefully emptied onto the applesauce. The pellets should be mixed with the applesauce and then swallowed immediately. The applesauce used should not be hot and should be soft enough to be swallowed without chewing. The pellets should not be chewed or crushed. The pellet/applesauce mixture should not be stored for future use.

The pellets have also been shown *in vitro* to remain intact when exposed to tap water, orange juice, apple juice and yogurt.

Please refer to amoxicillin and clarithromycin full prescribing information for CONTRAINDICATIONS, WARNINGS and dosing in elderly and renally-impaired patients.

SPECIAL POPULATIONS

Geriatric

No dosage adjustment is necessary. (See CLINICAL PHARMACOLOGY, Pharmacokinetics.)

Renal Insufficiency

No dosage adjustment is necessary. (See CLINICAL PHARMACOLOGY, Pharmacokinetics.)

Hepatic Insufficiency

No dosage adjustment is necessary in patients with mild to moderate liver impairment (Child Pugh Classes A and B). For patients with severe liver impairment (Child Pugh Class C), a dose of 20 mg of esomeprazole magnesium should not be exceeded (See CLINICAL PHARMACOLOGY, Pharmacokinetics.)

TABLE 9 *Recommended Adult Dosage Schedule of Esomeprazole Magnesium*

Indication	Dose	Frequency
Gastroesophageal Reflux Disease (GERD)		
Healing of erosive esophagitis	20 or 40 mg	Once daily for 4-8 weeks*
Maintenance of healing of erosive esophagitis	20 mg	Once daily†
Sympotmatic gastroesophageal reflux disease	20 mg	Once daily for 4 weeks‡
H. pylori **Eradication to Reduce the Risk of Duodenal Ulcer Recurrence**		
Triple Therapy:		
Esomeprazole	40 mg	Once daily for 10 days
Amoxicillin	1000 mg	Twice daily for 10 days
Clarithromycin	500 mg	Twice daily for 10 days

* The majority of patients are healed within 4-8 weeks. For patients who do not heal after 4-8 weeks, an additional 4-8 weeks of treatment may be considered.
† Controlled studies did not extend beyond 6 months.
‡ If symptoms do not resolve completely after 4 weeks, an additional 4 weeks of treatment may be considered.

Gender

No dosage adjustment is necessary. (See CLINICAL PHARMACOLOGY, Pharmacokinetics.)

HOW SUPPLIED

Nexium delayed-release capsules are available in:

20 mg: Opaque, hard gelatin, amethyst colored capsules with two radial bars in yellow on the cap and "20 mg" in yellow on the body.

40 mg: Opaque, hard gelatin, amethyst colored capsules with three radial bars in yellow on the cap and "40 mg" in yellow on the body.

Storage: Store at 25°C (77°F); excursions permitted to 15-30°C (59-86°F). Keep container tightly closed. Dispense in a tight container if the product package is subdivided.

PRODUCT LISTING - EQUIVALENTS NOT AVAILABLE

Capsule, Enteric Coated - Oral - 20 mg

30's	$132.63	NEXIUM, Astra-Zeneca Pharmaceuticals	00186-5020-31
90's	$397.88	NEXIUM, Astra-Zeneca Pharmaceuticals	00186-5020-54
100's	$399.66	NEXIUM, Astra-Zeneca Pharmaceuticals	00186-5020-68
100's	$399.66	NEXIUM, Astra-Zeneca Pharmaceuticals	00186-5022-28

Capsule, Enteric Coated - Oral - 40 mg

30's	$132.63	NEXIUM, Astra-Zeneca Pharmaceuticals	00186-5040-31
90's	$397.88	NEXIUM, Astra-Zeneca Pharmaceuticals	00186-5040-54
100's	$399.66	NEXIUM, Astra-Zeneca Pharmaceuticals	00186-5040-68
100's	$442.08	NEXIUM, Astra-Zeneca Pharmaceuticals	00186-5042-28

Estazolam (003009)

Categories: Insomnia; Pregnancy Category X; DEA Class CIV; FDA Approved 1990 Dec
Drug Classes: Benzodiazepines; Sedatives/hypnotics
Brand Names: Evrodin; Nuctulon; **Prosom**; Sedarest
Foreign Brand Availability: Domnamid (Denmark); Esilgan (Indonesia; Italy; Philippines); Eszo 2 (Taiwan); Eurodin (Japan; Taiwan); Kainever (Portugal); Nuctalon (France); Tasedan (Mexico)
Cost of Therapy: $13.49 (Insomnia; Prosom; 1 mg; 1 tablet/day; 10 day supply)
$8.88 (Insomnia; Generic Tablets; 1 mg; 1 tablet/day; 10 day supply)

DESCRIPTION

Estazolam, a triazolobenzodiazepine derivative, is an oral hypnotic agent. Estazolam occurs as a fine, white, odorless powder that is soluble in alcohol and practically insoluble in water. The chemical name for estazolam is 8-chloro-6-phenyl-4H-s-triazolo(4,3-a) (1,4)benzodiazepine. The empirical formula is $C_{16}H_{11}ClN_4$.

Estazolam tablets are scored and contain either 1 or 2 mg of estazolam.

Inactive Ingredients: *1 mg Tablets:* Corn starch, lactose and stearic acid. *2 mg Tablets:* Corn starch, iron oxide, lactose and stearic acid.

Storage: Store below 30°C (86°F).

CLINICAL PHARMACOLOGY

PHARMACOKINETICS

Estazolam tablets have been found to be equivalent in absorption to an orally administered solution of estazolam. Independent of concentration, estazolam in plasma is 93% protein bound.

In healthy subjects who received up to 3 times the recommended dose of estazolam, peak estazolam plasma concentrations occurred within 2 hours after dosing (range 0.5-6.0 hours) and were proportional to the administered dose, suggesting linear pharmacokinetics over the dosage range tested.

The range of estimates for the elimination half-life of estazolam varied from 10-24 hours. The clearance of benzodiazepines is accelerated in smokers compared to nonsmokers and there is evidence that this occurs with estazolam. This decrease in half-life, presumably due to enzyme induction by smoking, is consistent with other drugs with similar hepatic clearance characteristics. In all subjects, and at all doses, the mean elimination half-life appeared to be independent of the dose.

In a small study (n=8), using various doses in older subjects (59-68 years), peak estazolam concentrations were found to be similar to those observed in younger subjects with a mean elimination half-life of 18.4 hours (range 13.5-34.6 hours).

Estazolam is extensively metabolized and the metabolites are excreted primarily in the urine. Less than 5% of a 2 mg dose of estazolam is excreted unchanged in the urine with only 4% of the dose appearing in the feces. 4'-hydroxy estazolam is the major metabolite in plasma with concentrations approaching 12% of those of the parent 8 hours after administration. While it and the lesser metabolite, 1-oxo-estazolam have some pharmacologic activity, their low potencies and low concentrations preclude any significant contribution to the hypnotic effect of estazolam.

POSTULATED RELATIONSHIP BETWEEN ELIMINATION RATE OF BENZODIAZEPINE HYPNOTICS AND THEIR PROFILE OF COMMON UNTOWARD EFFECTS

The type and duration of hypnotic effects and the profile of unwanted effects during administration of benzodiazepine drugs may be influenced by the biologic half-life of administered drug and any active metabolites formed. When half-lives are long, drug or metabolites may accumulate during periods of nightly administration and be associated with impairments of cognitive and/or motor performance during waking hours; the possibility of interaction with other psychoactive drugs or alcohol will be enhanced. In contrast, if half-lives are short, drug and metabolites will be cleared before the next dose is ingested, and carry-over effects related to excessive sedation or CNS depression should be minimal or absent. However, during nightly use for an extended period, pharmacodynamic tolerance or adaptation to some effects of benzodiazepine hypnotics may develop. If the drug has a short elimination half-life, it is possible that a relative deficiency of the drug or its active metabolites (*i.e.*, in relationship to the receptor site) may occur at some point in the interval between each night's use. This sequence of events may account for two clinical findings reported to occur after several weeks of nightly use of rapidly eliminated benzodiazepine hypnotics, namely, increased wakefulness during the last third of the night, and the appearance of increased signs of daytime anxiety in selected patients.

CONTROLLED TRIALS SUPPORTING EFFICACY

In three 7 night, double- blind, parallel-group trials comparing estazolam 1 and/or 2 mg with placebo in adult outpatients with chronic insomnia, estazolam 2 mg was consistently superior to placebo on subjective measures of sleep induction (latency) and sleep maintenance (duration, number of awakenings, depth and quality of sleep) in all three studies; estazolam 1 mg was similarly superior to placebo on all measures of sleep maintenance, however, it significantly improved sleep induction in only one of two studies utilizing the 1 mg dose. In a similarly designed trial comparing estazolam 0.5 mg and 1 mg with placebo in geriatric outpatients with chronic insomnia, only the 1 mg estazolam dose was consistently superior to placebo on sleep induction (latency) and on only one measure of sleep maintenance (*i.e.*, duration of sleep).

In a single night, double-blind, parallel-group trial comparing estazolam 2 mg and placebo in patients admitted for elective surgery and requiring sleep medications, estazolam was superior to placebo on subjective measures of sleep induction and maintenance.

In a 12-week, double-blind, parallel-group trial including a comparison of estazolam 2 mg and placebo in adult outpatients with chronic insomnia, estazolam was superior to placebo on subjective measures of sleep induction (latency) and maintenance (duration, number of awakenings, total wake time during sleep) at week 2, but resulted in persistent improvement over 12 weeks only for sleep duration and total wake time during sleep. Following withdrawal at week 12, rebound insomnia was seen at the first withdrawal week, but there was no difference between drug and placebo by the second withdrawal week in all parameters except for latency, for which normalization did not occur until the fourth withdrawal week.

Adult outpatients with chronic insomnia were evaluated in a sleep laboratory trial comparing 4 doses of estazolam (0.25, 0.50, 1.0 and 2.0 mg) and placebo, each administered for 2 nights in a crossover design. The higher estazolam doses were superior to placebo on most EEG measures of sleep induction and maintenance, especially at the 2 mg dose, but only for sleep duration on subjective measures of sleep.

INDICATIONS AND USAGE

Estazolam is indicated for the short-term management of insomnia characterized by difficulty in falling asleep, frequent nocturnal awakenings, and/or early morning awakenings. Both outpatient studies and a sleep laboratory study have shown that estazolam administered at bedtime improved sleep induction and sleep maintenance. (See CLINICAL PHARMACOLOGY.)

Because insomnia is often transient and intermittent, the prolonged administration of estazolam is generally not necessary nor recommended. Since insomnia may be a symptom of several other disorders, the possibility that the complaint may be related to a condition for which there is a more specific treatment should be considered.

There is evidence to support the ability of estazolam to enhance the duration and quality of sleep for intervals up to 12 weeks. (See CLINICAL PHARMACOLOGY.)

CONTRAINDICATIONS

Benzodiazepines may cause fetal damage when administered during pregnancy. An increased risk of congenital malformations associated with the use of diazepam and chlordiazepoxide during the first trimester of pregnancy has been suggested in several studies.

Transplacental distribution has resulted in neonatal CNS depression and also withdrawal phenomena following the ingestion of therapeutic doses of a benzodiazepine hypnotic during the last weeks of pregnancy.

Estazolam is contraindicated in pregnant women. If there is a likelihood of the patient becoming pregnant while receiving estazolam she should be warned of the potential risk to the fetus. Patients should be instructed to discontinue the drug prior to becoming pregnant. The possibility that a woman of childbearing potential may be pregnant at the time of institution of therapy should be considered.

WARNINGS

Estazolam, like other benzodiazepines, has CNS-depressant effects. For this reason, patients should be cautioned against engaging in hazardous occupations requiring complete mental alertness such as operating machinery or driving a motor vehicle after ingesting the drug, including potential impairment of the performance of such activities that may occur the day following ingestion of estazolam. Patients should also be cautioned about possible combined effects with alcohol and other CNS-depressant drugs.

As with all benzodiazepines, amnesia, paradoxical reactions (*e.g.*, excitement, agitation, etc.), and other adverse behavioral effects may occur unpredictably.

There have been reports of withdrawal signs and symptoms of the type associated with withdrawal from CNS depressant drugs following the rapid decrease or the abrupt discontinuation of benzodiazepines.

PRECAUTIONS

GENERAL

Impaired motor and/or cognitive performance attributable to the accumulation of benzodiazepines and their active metabolites following several days of repeated use at their recommended doses is a concern in certain vulnerable patients (*e.g.*, those especially sensitive to the effects of benzodiazepines or those with a reduced capacity to metabolize and eliminate them). (See DOSAGE AND ADMINISTRATION.)

Elderly or debilitated patients and those with impaired renal or hepatic function should be cautioned about these risks and advised to monitor themselves for signs of excessive sedation or impaired conditions.

Estazolam appears to cause dose-related respiratory depression that is ordinarily not clinically relevant at recommended doses in patients with normal respiratory function. However, patients with compromised respiratory function may be at risk and should be monitored appropriately. As a class, benzodiazepines have the capacity to depress respiratory drive; there are insufficient data available, however, to characterize their relative potency in depressing respiratory drive at clinically recommended doses.

As with other benzodiazepines, estazolam should be administered with caution to patients exhibiting signs or symptoms of depression. Suicidal tendencies may be present in such patients and protective measures may be required. Intentional overdosage is more common in this group of patients; therefore, the least amount of drug that is feasible should be prescribed for the patient at any one time.

INFORMATION FOR THE PATIENT

To assure the safe and effective use of estazolam, the following information and instructions should be given to patients:

1. Inform your physician about any alcohol consumption and medicine you are taking now, including drugs you may buy without a prescription. Alcohol should not be used during treatment with hypnotics.
2. Inform your physician if you are planning to become pregnant, if you are pregnant, or if you become pregnant while you are taking this medicine.
3. You should not take this medicine if you are nursing as the drug may be excreted in breast milk.
4. Until you experience how this medicine affects you, do not drive a car, operate potentially dangerous machinery, or engage in hazardous occupations requiring complete mental alertness after taking this medicine.
5. Since benzodiazepines may produce psychological and physical dependence, you should not increase the dose before consulting with your physician. In addition, since the abrupt discontinuation of estazolam may be associated with a temporary worsening of sleep, you should consult your physician before abruptly discontinuing doses of 2 mg per night or more.

LABORATORY TESTS

Laboratory tests are not ordinarily required otherwise healthy patients. When treatment with estazolam tablets is protracted, periodic blood counts, urinalysis, and blood chemistry analyses are advisable.

CARCINOGENESIS, MUTAGENESIS, AND IMPAIRMENT OF FERTILITY

Two (2) year carcinogenicity studies were conducted in mice and rats at dietary doses of 0.8, 3, 10 mg/kg/day and 0.5, 2, and 10 mg/kg/day, respectively. Evidence of tumorigenicity was not observed in either study. Hyperplastic liver nodules were increased in female mice given the mid and high dose levels. The significance of such nodules in mice is not known at this time.

In vitro and *in vivo* mutagenicity tests including the Ames test, DNA repair in B. subtilis, *in vivo* cytogenetics in mice and rats, and the dominant lethal test in mice did not show a mutagenic potential for estazolam.

Fertility in male and female rats was not affected by doses up to 30 times the usual recommended human dose.

PREGNANCY CATEGORY X

Teratogenic Effects: (See CONTRAINDICATIONS.)

Non-Teratogenic Effects: The child born of a mother who is taking benzodiazepines may be at some risk for withdrawal symptoms from the drug during the postnatal period. Neonatal flaccidity has been reported in an infant born of a mother who received benzodiazepines during pregnancy.

LABOR AND DELIVERY

Estazolam has no established use in labor or delivery.

NURSING MOTHERS

Human studies have not been conducted; however, studies in lactating rats indicate that estazolam and/or its metabolites are secreted in the milk. The use of estazolam in nursing mothers is not recommended.

PEDIATRIC USE

Safety and effectiveness in children below the age of 18 have not been established.

GERIATRIC USE

Approximately 18% of individuals participating in the premarketing clinical trials of estazolam were 60 years of age or older. Overall, the adverse event profile did not differ substantively from that observed in younger individuals. Care should be exercised when prescribing benzodiazepines to small or debilitated elderly patients (See DOSAGE AND ADMINISTRATION.)

DRUG INTERACTIONS

If estazolam is given concomitantly with other drugs acting on the central nervous system, careful consideration should be given to the pharmacology of the agents to be employed. The action of the benzodiazepines may be potentiated by anticonvulsants, antihistamines, alcohol, barbiturates, monoamine oxidase inhibitors, narcotics, phenothiazines, psychotropic medications, or other drugs that produce CNS depression. Smokers have an increased clearance of benzodiazepines as compared to nonsmokers; this was seen in studies with estazolam (See CLINICAL PHARMACOLOGY.)

ADVERSE REACTIONS

COMMONLY OBSERVED

The most commonly observed adverse events associated with the use of estazolam and not seen at an equivalent incidence among placebo treated patients were somnolence, hypokinesia, dizziness and abnormal coordination.

ASSOCIATED WITH DISCONTINUATION OF TREATMENT

Approximately 3% of 1277 patients who received estazolam in US premarketing clinical trials discontinued treatment because of an adverse clinical event.

The only event commonly associated with discontinuation, accounting for 1.3% of the total, was somnolence.

INCIDENCE IN CONTROLLED CLINICAL TRIALS

The table enumerates adverse events that occurred at an incidence of 1% or greater among patients with insomnia who received estazolam in 7 night, placebo-controlled trials. Events reported by investigators were classified into standard dictionary (COSTART) terms for the purpose of establishing event frequencies. Event frequencies reported were not corrected for the occurrence of these events at baseline. The frequencies were obtained from data pooled across 6 studies: estazolam, n=685; placebo, n=433. The prescriber should be aware that these figures cannot be used to predict the incidence of side effects in the course of usual medical practice, in which patient characteristics and other factors differ from those that prevailed in these 6 clinical trials. Similarly, the cited frequencies cannot be compared with figures obtained from other clinical investigators involving related drug products and uses, since each group of drug trials is conducted under a different set of conditions. However, the cited figures provide the physician with a basis of estimating the relative contribution of drug and nondrug factors to the incidence of side effects in the population studied.

TABLE 1 *Incidence of Adverse Experiences in Placebo-Controlled Clinical Studies*

Body System/Adverse Event*	Percentage of Patients Reporting: Estazolam (n=685)	Placebo (n=433)
Body as a Whole		
Headache	16%	27%
Asthenia	11%	8%
Malaise	5%	5%
Lower extremity pain	3%	2%
Back pain	2%	2%
Body Pain	2%	2%
Abdominal pain	1%	2%
Chest pain	1%	1%
Digestive System		
Nausea	4%	5%
Dyspepsia	2%	2%
Musculoskeletal System		
Stiffness	1%	—
Nervous System		
Somnolence	42%	27%
Hypokinesia	8%	4%
Nervousness	8%	11%
Dizziness	7%	3%
Coordination abnormal	4%	1%
Hangover	3%	2%
Confusion	2%	—
Depression	2%	3%
Dream abnormal	2%	2%
Thinking abnormal	2%	1%
Respiratory System		
Cold Symptoms	3%	5%
Pharyngitis	1%	2%
Skin and Appendages		
Pruritus	1%	—

* Events reported by at least 1% of estazolam patients are included

OTHER ADVERSE EVENTS

During clinical trials conducted by Abbott, some of which were not placebo-controlled, estazolam was administered to approximately 1300 patients. Untoward events associated with this exposure were recorded by clinical investigators using terminology of their own choosing. To provide a meaningful estimate of the proportion of individuals experiencing adverse events, similar types of untoward events must be grouped into a smaller number of standardized event categories. In the tabulations that follow, a standard COSTART dictionary terminology has been used to classify reported adverse events. The frequencies presented, therefore, represent the proportion of the 1277 individuals exposed to estazolam who experienced an event of the type cited on at least one occasion while receiving estazolam. All reported events are included except those already listed in the previous table, those COSTART terms so general as to be uninformative, and those events where a drug cause was remote. Events are further classified within body system categories and enumerated in order of decreasing frequency using the following definitions: frequent adverse events are defined as those occurring on one or more occasions in at least 1/100 patients; infrequent adverse events are those occurring in 1/100 to 1/1000 patients; rare events are those occurring in less than 1/1000 patients. It is important to emphasize that, although the events reported did occur during treatment with estazolam, they were not necessarily caused by it.

Body as a Whole: *Infrequent:* Allergic reaction, chills, fever, neck pain, upper extremity pain. *Rare:* Edema, jaw pain, swollen breast.

Cardiovascular System: *Infrequent:* Flushing, palpitation. *Rare:* Arrhythmia, syncope.

Digestive System: *Frequent:* Constipation, dry mouth. *Infrequent:* Decreased appetite, flatulence, gastritis, increased appetite, vomiting. *Rare:* Enterocolitis, melena, ulceration of the mouth.

Endocrine System: *Rare:* Thyroid nodule.

Hematologic and Lymphatic System: *Rare:* Leukopenia, purpura, swollen lymph nodes.

Metabolic/Nutritional Disorders: *Infrequent:* Thirst. *Rare:* Increased SGOT, weight gain, weight loss.

Musculoskeletal System: *Infrequent:* Arthritis, muscle spasm, myalgia. *Rare:* Arthralgia.

Nervous System: *Frequent:* Anxiety. *Infrequent:* Agitation, amnesia, apathy, emotional lability, euphoria, hostility, paresthesia, seizure, sleep disorder, stupor, twitch. *Rare:* Ataxia, circumoral paresthesia, decreased libido, decreased reflexes, hallucinations, neuritis, nystagmus, tremor.

Minor changes in EEG patterns, usually low-voltage fast activity, have been observed in patients during estazolam therapy or withdrawal and are of no known clinical significance.

Respiratory System: *Infrequent:* Asthma, cough, dyspnea, rhinitis, sinusitis. *Rare:* Epistaxis, hyperventilation, laryngitis.

Skin and Appendages: *Infrequent:* Rash, sweating, urticaria. *Rare:* Acne, dry skin.

Special Senses: *Infrequent:* Abnormal vision, ear pain, eye irritation, eye pain, eye swelling, perverse taste, photophobia, tinnitus. *Rare:* Decreased hearing, diplopia, scotomata.

Urogenital System: *Infrequent:* Frequent urination, menstrual cramps, urinary hesitancy, urinary urgency, vaginal discharge/itching. *Rare:* Hematuria, nocturia, oliguria, penile discharge, urinary incontinence.

POSTINTRODUCTION REPORTS

Voluntary reports from non-US postmarketing experience of estazolam have included rare occurrences of the following events: photosensitivity; agranulocytosis. Because of the uncontrolled nature of these spontaneous reports, a casual relationship to estazolam treatment has not been determined.

DOSAGE AND ADMINISTRATION

The recommended initial dose for adults is 1 mg at bedtime; however, some patients may need a 2 mg dose. In healthy elderly patients 1 mg is also the appropriate starting dose, but increases should be initiated with particular care. In small or debilitated older patients, a starting dose of 0.5 mg, while only marginally effective in the overall elderly population, should be considered.

PRODUCT LISTING - RATED THERAPEUTICALLY EQUIVALENT

Tablet - Oral - 1 mg

100's	$59.25	FEDERAL UPPER LIMIT, H.C.F.A. F F P	99999-3009-01
100's	$88.78	GENERIC, Watson Laboratories Inc	00591-0744-01
100's	$88.78	GENERIC, Watson Laboratories Inc	52544-0744-01
100's	$89.00	GENERIC, Teva Pharmaceuticals Usa	00093-0129-01
100's	$89.00	GENERIC, Ivax Corporation	00172-4036-60

Tablet - Oral - 2 mg

100's	$64.49	FEDERAL UPPER LIMIT, H.C.F.A. F F P	99999-3009-02
100's	$98.92	GENERIC, Watson Laboratories Inc	00591-0745-01
100's	$98.92	GENERIC, Watson Laboratories Inc	52544-0745-01
100's	$99.00	GENERIC, Teva Pharmaceuticals Usa	00093-0130-01
100's	$99.00	GENERIC, Ivax Corporation	00172-4037-60

PRODUCT LISTING - EQUIVALENTS NOT AVAILABLE

Tablet - Oral - 1 mg

100's	$101.71	PROSOM, Abbott Pharmaceutical	00074-3735-11
100's	$134.90	PROSOM, Abbott Pharmaceutical	00074-3735-13

Tablet - Oral - 2 mg

100's	$113.10	PROSOM, Abbott Pharmaceutical	00074-3736-11
100's	$150.29	PROSOM, Abbott Pharmaceutical	00074-3736-13

Estradiol (001188)

Categories: Atrophy, vaginal; Atrophy, vulvar; Carcinoma, breast; Carcinoma, prostate; Castration, female; Hypoestrogenism; Hypogonadism, female; Kraurosis vulvae; Menopause; Osteoporosis, prevention; Ovarian failure, primary; Urethritis, atrophic; Vaginitis, atrophic; Pregnancy Category X; FDA Approval Pre 1982; FDA Approved 1975 Jul

Drug Classes: Estrogens; Hormones/hormone modifiers

Brand Names: Alora; Climara; Estrace; **Estraderm**; Estring; Fempatch; Vivelle

Foreign Brand Availability: Aerodiol (France; Hong-Kong; Sweden); Climara Forte (New-Zealand); Climaderm (Colombia; Mexico); Dermestril (China; Germany; Israel; Italy); Dermestril Septem (France); Divigel (Singapore; Thailand); Estracomb TTS (Hong-Kong); Estraderm MX (Australia); Estraderm TTS (Austria; Bahamas; Bahrain; Barbados; Belgium; Belize; Benin; Bermuda; Bulgaria; Burkina-Faso; Colombia; Curacao; Cyprus; Czech-Republic; Egypt; England; Ethiopia; France; Gambia; Germany; Ghana; Greece; Guinea; Guyana; Hungary; Indonesia; Iran; Iraq; Israel; Italy; Ivory-Coast; Jamaica; Japan; Jordan; Kenya; Korea; Kuwait; Lebanon; Liberia; Libya; Malawi; Malaysia; Mali; Mauritania; Mauritius; Morocco; Netherland-Antilles; Netherlands; New-Zealand; Niger; Nigeria; Oman; Philippines; Portugal; Puerto-Rico; Qatar; Republic-of-Yemen; Russia; Saudi-Arabia; Senegal; Seychelles; Sierra-Leone; South-Africa; Spain; Sudan; Surinam; Switzerland; Syria; Taiwan; Tanzania; Trinidad; Tunia; Turkey; Uganda; United-Arab-Emirates; Zambia; Zimbabwe); Estran (Korea); Estrapak 50 (Ecuador); Estreva (Germany; Italy); Estrifam (Germany); Estrofem (Austria; Belgium; Benin; Bulgaria; Burkina-Faso; China; Czech-Republic; Denmark; Ethiopia; Finland; France; Gambia; Ghana; Guinea; Hong-Kong; Israel; Ivory-Coast; Kenya; Korea; Liberia; Malawi; Mali; Mauritania; Mauritius; Morocco; Netherlands; New-Zealand; Niger; Nigeria; Philippines; Senegal; Seychelles; Sierra-Leone; Singapore; South-Africa; Sudan; Switzerland; Taiwan; Tanzania; Thailand; Tunia; Uganda; Zambia; Zimbabwe); Estrofem 2 (Thailand); Estrofem Forte (Benin; Burkina-Faso; Ethiopia; Gambia; Ghana; Guinea; Ivory-Coast; Kenya; Liberia; Malawi; Mali; Mauritania; Mauritius; Morocco; Niger; Nigeria; Senegal; Seychelles; Sierra-Leone; South-Africa; Sudan; Tanzania; Tunia; Uganda; Zambia; Zimbabwe); Evafilm (France); Evorel (Israel; Mexico); Fem 7 (Hong-Kong; Singapore); Fematrix (China; England; Ireland); Femtran (New-Zealand); Femsept (France); Femseven (England; Indonesia; Ireland); Ginedisc (Colombia; Mexico; Peru); GynPolar (Germany); Lindisc (Colombia); Meno-MPA (Israel); Menorest (Colombia; Germany; Italy; South-Africa); Menoring (England; Ireland); Oesclim (China; France); Oestring (Sweden); Oestrodose (Israel); Oestrogel (China); Progynon (Sweden); Progynova (Norway); Sandrena Gel (Australia; Germany); Sisare Gel (Germany); Systen (Mexico); Thais (France); Tradelia (Germany); Vagifem (Austria; Belgium; Bulgaria; Denmark; England; Ireland; Italy; Singapore; Sweden; Switzerland; Thailand); Zumenon (Australia; Austria; Belgium; England; Ireland; Netherlands)

Cost of Therapy: $6.36 (Menopause; Generic Tablets; 1 mg; 1 tablet/day; 21 day supply)

ORAL

WARNING

ESTROGENS HAVE BEEN REPORTED TO INCREASE THE RISK OF ENDOMETRIAL CARCINOMA IN POSTMENOPAUSAL WOMEN: **CLOSE CLINICAL SURVEILLANCE OF ALL WOMEN TAKING ESTROGENS IS IMPORTANT. ADEQUATE DIAGNOSTIC MEASURES, INCLUDING ENDOMETRIAL SAMPLING WHEN INDICATED, SHOULD BE UNDERTAKEN TO RULE OUT MALIGNANCY IN ALL CASES OF UNDIAGNOSED PERSISTENT OR RECURRING ABNORMAL VAGINAL BLEEDING. THERE IS NO EVIDENCE THAT "NATURAL" ESTROGENS ARE MORE OR LESS HAZARDOUS THAN "SYNTHETIC" ESTROGENS AT EQUIESTROGENIC DOSES.**

ESTROGENS SHOULD NOT BE USED DURING PREGNANCY: **THERE IS NO INDICATION FOR ESTROGEN THERAPY DURING PREGNANCY OR DURING THE IMMEDIATE POSTPARTUM PERIOD. ESTROGENS ARE INEFFECTIVE FOR THE PREVENTION OR TREATMENT OF THREATENED OR HABITUAL ABORTION. ESTROGENS ARE NOT INDICATED FOR THE PREVENTION OF POSTPARTUM BREAST ENGORGEMENT. ESTROGEN THERAPY DURING PREGNANCY IS ASSOCIATED WITH AN INCREASED RISK OF CONGENITAL DEFECTS IN THE REPRODUCTIVE ORGANS OF THE FETUS, AND POSSIBLY OTHER BIRTH DEFECTS. STUDIES OF WOMEN WHO RECEIVED DIETHYLSTILBESTROL (DES) DURING PREGNANCY HAVE SHOWN THAT FEMALE OFFSPRING HAVE AN INCREASED RISK OF VAGINAL ADENOSIS, SQUAMOUS CELL DYSPLASIA OF THE UTERINE CERVIX, AND CLEAR CELL VAGINAL CANCER LATER IN LIFE; MALE OFFSPRING HAVE AN INCREASED RISK OF UROGENITAL ABNORMALITIES AND POSSIBLY TESTICULAR CANCER LATER IN LIFE. THE 1985 DES TASK FORCE CONCLUDED THAT THE USE OF DES DURING PREGNANCY IS ASSOCIATED WITH A SUBSEQUENT INCREASED RISK OF BREAST CANCER IN THE MOTHERS, ALTHOUGH A CAUSAL RELATIONSHIP REMAINS UNPROVEN AND THE OBSERVED LEVEL OF EXCESS RISK IS SIMILAR TO THAT FOR A NUMBER OF OTHER BREAST CANCER RISK FACTORS.**

DESCRIPTION

Note: The trade name has been used throughout this monograph for clarity.

Estrace tablets for oral administration contain 0.5, 1 or 2 mg of micronized estradiol per tablet. Estradiol (17β-estradiol) is a white, crystalline, solid, chemically described as estra-1,3,5(10)-triene-3,17β-diol. Its molecular formula is $C_{18}H_{24}O_2$ and its molecular weight is 272.39.

Estrace tablets contain the following inactive ingredients:

0.5 mg: Acacia, dibasic calcium phosphate, lactose, magnesium stearate, colloidal silicon dioxide, starch (corn), and talc.

1 mg: Acacia, D&C red no. 27 (aluminum lake), dibasic calcium phosphate, FD&C blue no. 1 (aluminum lake), lactose, magnesium stearate, colloidal silicon dioxide, starch (corn), and talc.

2 mg: Acacia, dibasic calcium phosphate, FD&C blue no. 1 (aluminum lake), FD&C yellow no. 5 (tartrazine) (aluminum lake), lactose, magnesium stearate, colloidal silicon dioxide, starch (corn), and talc.

CLINICAL PHARMACOLOGY

Estrogen drug products act by regulating the transcription of a limited number of genes. Estrogens diffuse through cell membranes, distribute themselves throughout the cell, and bind to and activate the nuclear estrogen receptor, a DNA-binding protein which is found in estrogen-responsive tissues. The activated estrogen receptor binds to specific DNA sequences, or hormone-response elements, which enhance the transcription of adjacent genes and in turn lead to the observed effects. Estrogen receptors have been identified in tissues of the reproductive tract, breast, pituitary, hypothalamus, liver, and bone of women.

Estrogens are important in the development and maintenance of the female reproductive system and secondary sex characteristics. By a direct action, they cause growth and development of the uterus, fallopian tubes, and vagina. With other hormones, such as pituitary hormones and progesterone, they cause enlargement of the breasts through promotion of ductal growth, stromal development, and the accretion of fat. Estrogens are intricately involved with other hormones, especially progesterone, in the processes of the ovulatory menstrual cycle and pregnancy, and affect the release of pituitary gonadotropins. They also contribute to the shaping of the skeleton, maintenance of tone and elasticity of urogenital structures, changes in the epiphyses of the long bones that allow for the pubertal growth spurt and its termination, and pigmentation of the nipples and genitals.

Estrogens occur naturally in several forms. The primary source of estrogen in normally cycling adult women is the ovarian follicle, which secretes 70-500 µg of estradiol daily, depending on the phase of the menstrual cycle. This is converted primarily to estrone, which circulates in roughly equal proportion to estradiol, and to small amounts of estriol. After menopause, most endogenous estrogen is produced by conversion of androstenedione, secreted by the adrenal cortex, to estrone by peripheral tissues. Thus, estrone — especially in its sulfate ester form — is the most abundant circulating estrogen in postmenopausal women. Although circulating estrogens exist in a dynamic equilibrium of metabolic interconversions, estradiol is the principal intracellular human estrogen and is substantially more potent than estrone or estriol at the receptor.

Estrogens used in therapy are well absorbed through the skin, mucous membranes, and gastrointestinal tract. When applied for a local action, absorption is usually sufficient to cause systemic effects. When conjugated with aryl and alkyl groups for parenteral administration, the rate of absorption of oily preparations is slowed with a prolonged duration of action, such that a single intramuscular injection of estradiol valerate or estradiol cypionate is absorbed over several weeks.

Administered estrogens and their esters are handled within the body essentially the same as endogenous hormones. Metabolic conversion of estrogens occurs primarily in the liver (first pass effect), but also at local target tissue sites. Complex metabolic processes result in a dynamic equilibrium of circulating conjugated and unconjugated estrogenic forms which are continually interconverted, especially between estrone and estradiol and between esterified and unesterified forms. Although naturally-occurring estrogens circulate in the blood largely bound to sex hormone-binding globulin and albumin, only unbound estrogens enter target tissue cells. A significant proportion of the circulating estrogen exists as sulfate conjugates, especially estrone sulfate, which serves as a circulating reservoir for the formation of more active estrogenic species. A certain proportion of the estrogen is excreted into the bile and then reabsorbed from the intestine. During this enterohepatic recirculation, estrogens are desulfated and resulfated and undergo degradation through conversion to less active estrogens (estriol and other estrogens), oxidation to nonestrogenic substances (catecholestrogens, which interact with catecholamine metabolism, especially in the central nervous system), and conjugation with glucuronic acids (which are then rapidly excreted in the urine).

When given orally, naturally-occurring estrogens and their esters are extensively metabolized (first pass effect) and circulate primarily as estrone sulfate, with smaller amounts of other conjugated and unconjugated estrogenic species. This results in limited oral potency. By contrast, synthetic estrogens, such as ethinyl estradiol and the nonsteroidal estrogens, are degraded very slowly in the liver and other tissues, which results in their high intrinsic potency. Estrogen drug products administered by non-oral routes are not subject to first-pass metabolism, but also undergo significant hepatic uptake, metabolism, and enterohepatic recycling.

INDICATIONS AND USAGE

Estradiol tablets are indicated in the:

Treatment of moderate to severe vasomotor symptoms associated with the menopause. There is no adequate evidence that estrogens are effective for nervous symptoms or depression which might occur during menopause and they should not be used to treat these conditions.

Treatment of vulval and vaginal atrophy.

Treatment of hypoestrogenism due to hypogonadism, castration or primary ovarian failure.

Treatment of breast cancer (for palliation only) in appropriately selected women and men with metastatic disease.

Treatment of advanced androgen-dependent carcinoma of the prostate (for palliation only).

Prevention of osteoporosis.

Since estrogen administration is associated with risk, selection of patients should ideally be based on prospective identification of risk factors for developing osteoporosis. Unfortunately, there is no certain way to identify those women who will develop osteoporotic fractures. Most prospective studies of efficacy for this indication have been carried out in white menopausal women, without stratification by other risk factors, and tend to show a universally salutary effect on bone. Thus, patient selection must be individualized based on the balance of risks and benefits. A more favorable risk/benefit ratio exists in a hysterectomized woman because she has no risk of endometrial cancer (see BOXED WARNING).

Estrogen replacement therapy reduces bone resorption and retards or halts postmenopausal bone loss. Case-control studies have shown an approximately 60% reduction in hip and wrist fractures in women whose estrogen replacement was begun within a few years of menopause. Studies also suggest that estrogen reduces the rate of vertebral fractures. Even when started as late as 6 years after menopause, estrogen prevents further loss of bone mass for as long as the treatment is continued. The results of a 2 year, randomized, placebo-controlled, double-blind, dose-ranging study have shown that treatment with 0.5 mg estradiol daily for 23 days (of a 28 day cycle) prevents vertebral bone mass loss in postmenopausal women. When estrogen therapy is discontinued, bone mass declines at a rate comparable to the immediate postmenopausal period. There is no evidence that estrogen replacement therapy restores bone mass to premenopausal levels.

At skeletal maturity there are sex and race differences in both the total amount of bone present and its density, in favor of men and blacks. Thus, women are at higher risk than men because they start with less bone mass and, for several years following natural or induced menopause, the rate of bone mass decline is accelerated. White and Asian women are at higher risk than black women.

Early menopause is one of the strongest predictors for the development of osteoporosis. In addition, other factors affecting the skeleton which are associated with osteoporosis include genetic factors (small build, family history), and endocrine factors (nulliparity, thyrotoxicosis, hyperparathyroidism, Cushing's syndrome, hyperprolactinemia, Type 1 diabetes), lifestyle (cigarette smoking, alcohol abuse, sedentary exercise habits) and nutrition (below average body weight, dietary calcium intake).

The mainstays of prevention and management of osteoporosis are estrogen, an adequate lifetime calcium intake, and exercise. Postmenopausal women absorb dietary calcium less efficiently than premenopausal women and require an average of 1500 mg/day of elemental calcium to remain in neutral calcium balance. By comparison, premenopausal women require about 1000 mg/day and the average calcium intake in the USA is 400-600 mg/day. Therefore, when not contraindicated, calcium supplementation may be helpful.

Weight-bearing exercise and nutrition may be important adjuncts to the prevention and management of osteoporosis. Immobilization and prolonged bed rest produce rapid bone loss, while weight-bearing exercise has been shown both to reduce bone loss and to increase bone mass. The optimal type and amount of physical activity that would prevent osteoporosis have not been established, however in two studies, an hour of walking and running exercise twice or 3 times weekly significantly increased lumbar spine bone mass.

NON-FDA APPROVED INDICATIONS

Other estrogens have been used for treatment of gastrointestinal bleeding in patients with renal failure and gastrointestinal bleeding related to arteriovenous malformations.

CONTRAINDICATIONS

Estrogens should not be used in individuals with any of the following conditions:

Known or suspected pregnancy (see BOXED WARNING). Estrogens may cause fetal harm when administered to a pregnant woman.

Undiagnosed abnormal genital bleeding.

Known or suspected cancer of the breast except in appropriately selected patients being treated for metastatic disease.

Known or suspected estrogen-dependent neoplasia.

Active thrombophlebitis or thromboembolic disorders.

WARNINGS

INDUCTION OF MALIGNANT NEOPLASMS

Endometrial Cancer

The reported endometrial cancer risk among unopposed estrogen users is about 2- to 12-fold greater than in non-users, and appears dependent on duration of treatment and on estrogen dose. Most studies show no significant increased risk associated with use of estrogens for less than 1 year. The greatest risk appears associated with prolonged use — with increased risks of 15- to 24-fold for 5-10 years or more. In three studies, persistence of risk was demonstrated for 8 to over 15 years after cessation of estrogen treatment. In one study a significant decrease in the incidence of endometrial cancer occurred 6 months after estrogen withdrawal. Concurrent progestin therapy may offset this risk but the overall health impact in postmenopausal women is not known (see PRECAUTIONS).

Breast Cancer

While the majority of studies have not shown an increased risk of breast cancer in women who have ever used estrogen replacement therapy, some have reported a moderately increased risk (relative risks of 1.3 to 2) in those taking higher doses or those taking lower doses for prolonged periods of time, especially in excess of 10 years. Other studies have not shown this relationship.

Congenital Lesions With Malignant Potential

Estrogen therapy during pregnancy is associated with an increased risk of fetal congenital reproductive tract disorders, and possibly other birth defects. Studies of women who received DES during pregnancy have shown that female offspring have an increased risk of vaginal adenosis, squamous cell dysplasia of the uterine cervix, and clear cell vaginal cancer later in life; male offspring have an increased risk of urogenital abnormalities and possibly testicular cancer later in life. Although some of these changes are benign, others are precursors of malignancy.

GALLBLADDER DISEASE

Two studies have reported a 2- to 4-fold increase in the risk of gallbladder disease requiring surgery in women receiving postmenopausal estrogens.

CARDIOVASCULAR DISEASE

Large doses of estrogen (5 mg conjugated estrogens per day), comparable to those used to treat cancer of the prostate and breast, have been shown in a large prospective clinical trial in men to increase the risks of nonfatal myocardial infarction, pulmonary embolism, and thrombophlebitis. These risks cannot necessarily be extrapolated from men to women. However, to avoid the theoretical cardiovascular risk to women caused by high estrogen doses, the dose for estrogen replacement therapy should not exceed the lowest effective dose.

ELEVATED BLOOD PRESSURE

Occasional blood pressure increases during estrogen replacement therapy have been attributed to idiosyncratic reactions to estrogens. More often, blood pressure has remained the same or has dropped. One study showed that postmenopausal estrogen users have higher blood pressure than nonusers. Two other studies showed slightly lower blood pressure among estrogen users compared to nonusers. Postmenopausal estrogen use does not increase the risk of stroke. Nonetheless, blood pressure should be monitored at regular intervals with estrogen use.

HYPERCALCEMIA

Administration of estrogens may lead to severe hypercalcemia in patients with breast cancer and bone metastases. If this occurs, the drug should be stopped and appropriate measures taken to reduce the serum calcium level.

PRECAUTIONS

GENERAL

Addition of a Progestin

Studies of the addition of a progestin for 7 or more days of a cycle of estrogen administration have reported a lowered incidence of endometrial hyperplasia which would otherwise be induced by estrogen treatment. Morphological and biochemical studies of endometrium suggest that 10-14 days of progestin are needed to provide maximal maturation of the endometrium and to eliminate any hyperplastic changes. There are possible additional risks which may be associated with the inclusion of progestins in estrogen replacement regimens. These include: (1) adverse effects on lipoprotein metabolism (lowering HDL and raising LDL) which may diminish the possible cardioprotective effect of estrogen therapy (see Drug/Laboratory Test Interactions); (2) impairment of glucose tolerance; and (3) possible enhancement of mitotic activity in breast epithelial tissue (although few epidemiological data are available to address this point). The choice of progestin, its dose, and its regimen may be important in minimizing these adverse effects, but these issues will remain to be clarified.

E

Physical Examination

A complete medical and family history should be taken prior to the initiation of any estrogen therapy. The pretreatment and periodic physical examinations should include special reference to blood pressure, breasts, abdomen, and pelvic organs, and should include a Papanicolaou smear. As a general rule, estrogen should not be prescribed for longer than 1 year without reexamining the patient.

Hypercoagulability

Some studies have shown that women taking estrogen replacement therapy have hypercoagulability, primarily related to decreased antithrombin activity. This effect appears dose- and duration-dependent and is less pronounced than that associated with oral contraceptive use. Also, postmenopausal women tend to have increased coagulation parameters at baseline compared to premenopausal women. There is some suggestion that low dose postmenopausal mestranol may increase the risk of thromboembolism, although the majority of studies (of primarily conjugated estrogens users) report no such increase. There is insufficient information on hypercoagulability in women who have had previous thromboembolic disease.

Familial Hyperlipoproteinemia

Estrogen therapy may be associated with massive elevations of plasma triglycerides leading to pancreatitis and other complications in patients with familial defects of lipoprotein metabolism.

Fluid Retention

Because estrogens may cause some degree of fluid retention, conditions which might be exacerbated by this factor, such as asthma, epilepsy, migraine, and cardiac or renal dysfunction, require careful observation.

Uterine Bleeding and Mastodynia

Certain patients may develop undesirable manifestations of estrogenic stimulation, such as abnormal uterine bleeding and mastodynia.

Impaired Liver Function

Estrogens may be poorly metabolized in patients with impaired liver function and should be administered with caution.

Estrace 2 mg tablets contain FD&C yellow no. 5 (tartrazine) which may cause allergic-type reactions (including bronchial asthma) in certain susceptible individuals. Although the overall incidence of FD&C yellow no. 5 (tartrazine) sensitivity in the general population is low, it is frequently seen in patients who also have aspirin hypersensitivity.

INFORMATION FOR THE PATIENT

See the Patient Instructions that are distributed with the prescription for the vaginal cream, oral tablets, and transdermal system.

LABORATORY TESTS

Estrogen administration should generally be guided by clinical response at the smallest dose, rather than laboratory monitoring, for relief of symptoms for those indications in which symptoms are observable. For prevention of osteoporosis, however, see DOSAGE AND ADMINISTRATION.

DRUG/LABORATORY TEST INTERACTIONS

Accelerated prothrombin time, partial thromboplastin time, and platelet aggregation time; increased platelet count; increased factors II, VII antigen, VIII antigen, VIII coagulant activity, IX, X, XII, VII-X complex, II-VII-X complex, and beta-thromboglobulin; decreased levels of anti-factor Xa and antithrombin III, decreased antithrombin III activity; increased levels of fibrinogen and fibrinogen activity; increased plasminogen antigen and activity.

Increased thyroid-binding globulin (TBG) leading to increased circulating total thyroid hormone, as measured by protein-bound iodine (PBI), T_4 levels (by column or by radioimmunoassay) or T_3 levels by radioimmunoassay. T_3 resin uptake is decreased, reflecting the elevated TBG. Free T_4 and free T_3 concentrations are unaltered.

Other binding proteins may be elevated in serum, *i.e.,* corticosteroid binding globulin (CBG), sex hormone-binding globulin (SHBG), leading to increased circulating corticosteroids and sex steroids, respectively. Free or biologically active hormone concentrations are unchanged. Other plasma proteins may be increased (angiotensinogen/renin substrate, alpha-1-antitrypsin, ceruloplasmin).

Increased plasma HDL and HDL-2 subfraction concentrations, reduced LDL cholesterol concentration, increased triglycerides levels.

Impaired glucose tolerance.

Reduced response to metyrapone test.

Reduced serum folate concentration.

CARCINOGENESIS, MUTAGENESIS, AND IMPAIRMENT OF FERTILITY
Long-term continuous administration of natural and synthetic estrogens in certain animal species increases the frequency of carcinomas of the breast, uterus, cervix, vagina, testis, and liver (see CONTRAINDICATIONS and WARNINGS).

PREGNANCY, TERATOGENIC EFFECTS, PREGNANCY CATEGORY X
Estrogens should not be used during pregnancy (see CONTRAINDICATIONS and BOXED WARNING).

NURSING MOTHERS
As a general principle, the administration of any drug to nursing mothers should be done only when clearly necessary since many drugs are excreted in human milk. In addition, estrogen administration to nursing mothers has been shown to decrease the quantity and quality of the milk.

E

PEDIATRIC USE
Safety and effectiveness in pediatric patients have not been established. Large and repeated doses of estrogen over an extended period of time have been shown to accelerate epiphyseal closure, resulting in short adult stature if treatment is initiated before the completion of physiologic puberty in normally developing children. In patients in whom bone growth is not complete, periodic monitoring of bone maturation and effects on epiphyseal centers is recommended.

Estrogen treatment of prepubertal children also induces premature breast development and vaginal cornification, and may potentially induce vaginal bleeding in girls. In boys, estrogen treatment may modify the normal pubertal process. All other physiological and adverse reactions shown to be associated with estrogen treatment of adults could potentially occur in the pediatric population, including thromboembolic disorders and growth stimulation of certain tumors. Therefore, estrogens should only be administered to pediatric patients when clearly indicated and the lowest effective dose should always be utilized.

ADVERSE REACTIONS

The following additional adverse reactions have been reported with estrogen therapy (see WARNINGS regarding induction of neoplasia, adverse effects on the fetus, increased incidence of gallbladder disease, cardiovascular disease, elevated blood pressure, and hypercalcemia).

Genitourinary System: Changes in vaginal bleeding pattern and abnormal withdrawal bleeding or flow; breakthrough bleeding, spotting; increase in size of uterine leiomyomata; vaginal candidiasis; change in amount of cervical secretion.
Breasts: Tenderness, enlargement.
Gastrointestinal: Nausea; vomiting; abdominal cramps; bloating; cholestatic jaundice; increased incidence of gallbladder disease.
Skin: Chloasma or melasma which may persist when drug is discontinued; erythema multiforme; erythema nodosum; hemorrhagic eruption; loss of scalp hair; hirsutism.
Eyes: Steepening of corneal curvature; intolerance to contact lenses.
Central Nervous System: Headache; migraine; dizziness; mental depression; chorea.
Miscellaneous: Increase or decrease in weight; reduced carbohydrate tolerance; aggravation of porphyria; edema; changes in libido.

DOSAGE AND ADMINISTRATION

For treatment of moderate to severe vasomotor symptoms, vulval and vaginal atrophy associated with the menopause, the lowest dose and regimen that will control symptoms should be chosen and medication should be discontinued as promptly as possible: attempts to discontinue or taper medication should be made at 3-6 month intervals.

The usual initial dosage range is 1-2 mg daily of estradiol adjusted as necessary to control presenting symptoms. The minimal effective dose for maintenance therapy should be determined by titration. Administration should be cyclic (*e.g.,* 3 weeks on and 1 week off).

For treatment of female hypoestrogenism due to hypogonadism, castration, or primary ovarian failure: Treatment is usually initiated with a dose of 1-2 mg daily of estradiol, adjusted as necessary to control presenting symptoms; the minimal effective dose for maintenance therapy should be determined by titration.

For treatment of breast cancer, for palliation only, in appropriately selected women and men with metastatic disease: Suggested dosage is 10 mg three times daily for a period of at least 3 months.

For treatment of advanced androgen-dependent carcinoma of the prostate, for palliation only: Suggested dosage is 1-2 mg three times daily. The effectiveness of therapy can be judged by phosphatase determinations as well as by symptomatic improvement of the patient.

For the prevention of osteoporosis: Therapy with estradiol tablets to prevent postmenopausal bone loss should be initiated as soon as possible after menopause. A daily dosage of 0.5 mg should be administered cyclically (*i.e.,* 23 days on and 5 days off). The dosage may be adjusted if necessary to control concurrent menopausal symptoms. Discontinuation of estrogen replacement therapy may re-establish the natural rate of bone loss.

HOW SUPPLIED

Estrace tablets are available as follows:

0.5 mg: Round, white scored tablets imprinted with "021" and "MJ" on one side.
1 mg: Round, lavender scored tablets imprinted with "755" and "MJ" on one side.
2 mg: Round, turquoise scored tablets imprinted with "756" and "MJ" on one side.

Storage: Store at controlled room temperature 15-30°C (59-86°F). Dispense in a tight, light-resistant container using a child-resistant closure.

TRANSDERMAL

WARNING

Climara:

ESTROGENS INCREASE THE RISK OF ENDOMETRIAL CANCER. Close clinical surveillance of all women taking estrogens is important. Adequate diagnostic measures, including endometrial sampling when indicated, should be undertaken to rule out malignancy in all cases of undiagnosed persistent or recurring abnormal vaginal bleeding. There is currently no evidence that the use of natural estrogens results in a different endometrial risk profile than synthetic estrogens of equivalent estrogen doses.

There is no indication for estrogen therapy during pregnancy or during the immediate postpartum period. Estrogens are ineffective for the prevention or treatment of threatened or habitual abortion. Estrogens are not indicated for the prevention of postpartum breast engorgement.

Estraderm:

ESTROGENS HAVE BEEN REPORTED TO INCREASE THE RISK OF ENDOMETRIAL CARCINOMA IN POSTMENOPAUSAL WOMEN.

Close clinical surveillance of all women taking estrogens is important. Adequate diagnostic measures, including endometrial sampling when indicated, should be undertaken to rule out malignancy in all cases of undiagnosed persistent or recurring abnormal vaginal bleeding. There is no evidence that "natural" estrogens are more or less hazardous than "synthetic" estrogens at equiestrogenic doses.

ESTROGENS SHOULD NOT BE USED DURING PREGNANCY.

Estrogen therapy during pregnancy is associated with an increased risk of congenital defects in the reproductive organs of the fetus, and possibly other birth defects. Studies of women who received diethylstilbestrol (DES) during pregnancy have shown that female offspring have an increased risk of vaginal adenosis, squamous cell dysplasia of the uterine cervix, and clear cell vaginal cancer later in life; male offspring have an increased risk of urogenital abnormalities and possible testicular cancer later in life. The 1985 DES Task Force concluded that use of DES during pregnancy is associated with a subsequent increased risk of breast cancer in the mothers, although a causal relationship remains unproven and the observed level of excess risk is similar to that for a number of other breast cancer risk factors.

There is no indication for estrogen therapy during pregnancy. Estrogens are ineffective for the prevention or treatment of threatened or habitual abortion. Estrogens are not indicated for the prevention of postpartum breast engorgement.

DESCRIPTION

Note: The trade name has been used throughout this monograph for clarity.

CLIMARA
Climara , estradiol transdermal system, is designed to release 1β-estradiol continuously upon application to intact skin. Four (6.5, 12.5, 18.75 and 25.0 cm^2) systems are available to provide nominal *in vivo* delivery of 0.025, 0.05, 0.075 or 0.1 mg respectively of estradiol per day. The period of use is 7 days. Each system has a contact surface area of either 6.5, 12.5, 18.75 or 25.0 cm^2, and contains 2.0, 3.8, 5.7 or 7.6 mg of estradiol respectively. The composition of the systems per unit area is identical.

Estradiol (17β-estradiol) is a white, crystalline powder, chemically described as estra-1,3,5(10)-triene-3,17β-diol. It has an empirical formula of $C_{18}H_{24}O_2$ and molecular weight of 272.37.

The Climara system comprises two layers. Proceeding from the visible surface toward the surface attached to the skin, these layers are (1) a translucent polyethylene film, and (2) an acrylate adhesive matrix containing estradiol. A protective liner (3) of siliconized or fluoropolymer-coated polyester film is attached to the adhesive surface and must be removed before the system can be used.

The active component of the system is 17β-estradiol. The remaining components of the system (acrylate copolymer adhesive, fatty acid esters, and polyethylene backing) are pharmacologically inactive.

ESTRADERM
Estraderm (estradiol transdermal system) is designed to release estradiol through a rate-limiting membrane continuously upon application to intact skin.

Two systems are available to provide nominal *in vivo* delivery of 0.05 or 0.1 mg of estradiol per day via skin of average permeability (interindividual variation in skin permeability is approximately 20%). Each corresponding system having an active surface area of 10 or 20 cm^2 contains 4 or 8 mg of estradiol and 0.3 or 0.6 ml of alcohol, respectively. The composition of the systems per unit area is identical.

Estradiol is a white, crystalline powder, chemically described as estra-1,3,5(10)-triene3,17β-diol.

The Estraderm system comprises four layers. Proceeding from the visible surface toward the surface attached to the skin, these layers are (1) a transparent polyester film, (2) a drug reservoir of estradiol and alcohol gelled with hydroxypropyl cellulose, (3) an ethylene-vinyl acetate copolymer membrane, and (4) an adhesive formulation of light mineral oil and polyisobutylene. A protective liner (5) of siliconized polyethylene terephthalate film is attached to the adhesive surface and must be removed before the system can be used.

The active component of the system is estradiol. The remaining components of the system are pharmacologically inactive. Alcohol is also released from the system during use.

CLINICAL PHARMACOLOGY

CLIMARA
The Climara system provides systemic estrogen replacement therapy by releasing 17β-estradiol, the major estrogenic hormone secreted by the human ovary.

Estrogens are largely responsible for the development and maintenance of the female reproductive system and secondary sexual characteristics. Although circulating estrogens exist in a dynamic equilibrium of metabolic interconversions, estradiol is the principal intracellular human estrogen and is substantially more potent than its metabolites, estrone and estriol at the receptor level. The primary source of estrogen in normally cycling adult women is the ovarian follicle, which secretes 70-500 μg of estradiol daily, depending on the phase of the menstrual cycle. After menopause, most endogenous estrogen is produced by conversion of androstenedione, secreted by the adrenal cortex, to estrone by peripheral tissues. Thus, estrone and the sulfate conjugated form, estrone sulfate, are the most abundant circulating estrogens in postmenopausal women.

Estrogens act through binding to nuclear receptors in estrogen-responsive tissues. To date, two estrogen receptors have been identified. These vary in proportion from tissue to tissue.

Circulating estrogens modulate the pituitary secretion of the gonadotropins luteininizing hormone (LH) and follicle stimulating hormone (FSH) through a negative feedback mechanism and estrogen replacement therapy acts to reduce the elevated levels of these hormones seen in postmenopausal women.

A 2 year clinical trial enrolled a total of 175 healthy, hysterectomized, postmenopausal, nonosteoporotic (*i.e.*, lumbar spine bone mineral density >0.9 g/cm^2) women at 10 study centers in the US. 129 subjects were allocated to receive active treatment with 4 different doses of 17 β-estradiol patches (6.5, 12.5, 15, 25 cm^2) and 46 subjects were allocated to receive placebo patches. 77% of the randomized subjects (100 on active drug and 34 on placebo) contributed data to the analysis of percent change of A-P spine bone mineral density (BMD), the primary efficacy variable. A statistically significant overall treatment effect at each timepoint was noted, implying bone preservation for all active treatment groups at all timepoints, as opposed to bone loss for placebo at all timepoints.

Percent change in BMD of the total hip was also statistically significantly different from placebo for all active treatment groups. The results of the measurements of biochemical markers supported the finding of efficacy for all doses of transdermal estradiol. Serum osteocalcin levels decreased, indicative of a decrease in bone formation, at all timepoints for all active treatment doses, statistically significantly different from placebo (which generally rose). Urinary deoxypyridinoline and pyridinoline changes also suggested a decrease in bone turnover for all active treatment groups.

Pharmacokinetics

Transdermal administration of Climara produces mean serum concentrations of estradiol comparable to those produced by premenopausal women in the early follicular phase of the ovulatory cycle. The pharmacokinetics of estradiol following application of the Climara system were investigated in 197 healthy postmenopausal women in 6 studies. In 5 of the studies Climara system was applied to the abdomen and in a sixth study application to the buttocks and abdomen were compared.

Absorption

The Climara transdermal delivery system continuously releases estradiol which is transported across intact skin leading to sustained circulating levels of estradiol during a 7 day treatment period. The systemic availability of estradiol after transdermal administration is about 20 times higher than that after oral administration. This difference is due to the absence of first pass metabolism when estradiol is given by the transdermal route.

In a bioavailability study, the Climara 6.5 cm^2 was studied with the Climara 12.5 cm^2 as reference.

Dose proportionality was demonstrated for the Climara 6.5 cm^2 transdermal system as compared to the Climara 2.5 cm^2 transdermal system in a 2 week crossover study with a 1 week washout period between the two transdermal systems in 24 postmenopausal women.

Dose proportionality was also demonstrated for the Climara system (12.5 cm^2 and 25 cm^2) in a 1 week study conducted in 54 postmenopausal women. The mean steady state levels (C_{avg}) of the estradiol during the application of Climara 25 cm^2 and 12.5 cm^2 on the abdomen were about 80 and 40 pg/ml, respectively.

In a 3 week multiple application study in 24 postmenopausal women, the 25.0 cm^2 Climara system produced average peak estradiol concentrations (C_{max}) of approximately 100 pg/ml. Trough values at the end of each wear interval (C_{min}) were approximately 35 pg/ml. Nearly identical serum curves were seen each week, indicating little or no accumulation of estradiol in the body. Serum estrone peak and trough levels were 60 and 40 pg/ml, respectively.

In a single-dose, randomized, crossover study conducted to compare the effect of site of application, 38 postmenopausal women wore a single Climara 25 cm^2 system for 1 week on the abdomen and buttocks. C_{max} and C_{avg} values were, respectively, 25% and 17% higher with the buttock application than with the abdomen application.

TABLE 1 provides a summary of estradiol pharmacokinetic parameters determined during evaluation of Climara.

TABLE 1 *Pharmacokinetic Summary — Mean Estradiol Values*

	Climara Delivery Rate			
	0.025	0.05	0.1	0.1
Surface area (cm^2)	6.5	12.5	25	25
Application site	Abdomen	Abdomen	Abdomen	Buttock
No. of subjects	24	102	139	38
Dosing	Single	Single	Single	Single
C_{max} (pg/ml)	32	71	147	174
C_{min} (pg/ml)	17	29	60	71
C_{avg} (pg/ml)	22	41	87	106

The relative standard deviation of each pharmacokinetic parameter after application to the abdomen averaged 50%, which is indicative of the considerable intersubject variability associated with transdermal drug delivery. The relative standard deviation of each pharmacokinetic parameter after application to the buttock was lower than that after application to the abdomen (*e.g.*, for C_{max} 39% vs 62%, and for C_{avg} 35% vs 48%).

Distribution

The distribution of exogenous estrogens is similar to that of endogenous estrogens. Estrogens are widely distributed in the body and are generally found in higher concentrations in the sex hormone target organs. Estradiol and other naturally occurring estrogens are bound mainly to sex hormone binding globulin (SHBG), and to lesser degree to albumin.

Metabolism

Exogenous estrogens are metabolized in the same manner as endogenous estrogens. Circulating estrogens exist in a dynamic equilibrium of metabolic interconversions. These transformations take place mainly in the liver. Estradiol is converted reversibly to estrone, and both can be converted to estriol, which is the major urinary metabolite. Estrogens also undergo enterohepatic recirculation via sulfate and glucuronide conjugation in the liver, biliary secretion of conjugates into the intestine, and hydrolysis in the gut followed by reabsorption. In postmenopausal women a significant portion of the circulating estrogens exist as sulfate conjugates, especially estrone sulfate, which serves as a circulating reservoir for the formation of more active estrogens.

Excretion

Estradiol, estrone and estriol are excreted in the urine along with glucuronide and sulfate conjugates. After removal of the Climara system, serum estradiol levels decline in about 12 hours to preapplication levels with an apparent half-life of approximately 4 hours.

Special Populations

Geriatric: There have not been sufficient numbers of geriatric patients involved in clinical studies utilizing Climara to determine whether those over 65 years of age differ from younger subjects in their response to Climara.

Pediatric: No pharmacokinetic study for Climara has been conducted in a pediatric population.

Gender: Climara is indicated for use in women only.

Race: No studies were done to determine the effect of race on the pharmacokinetics of Climara.

Patients With Renal Impairment: Total estradiol serum levels are higher in postmenopausal women with end stage renal disease (ESRD) receiving maintenance hemodialysis than in normal subjects at baseline and following oral doses of estradiol. Therefore, conventional transdermal estradiol doses used in individuals with normal renal function may be excessive for postmenopausal women with ESRD receiving maintenance hemodialysis.

Patients With Hepatic Impairment: Estrogens may be poorly metabolized in patients with impaired liver function and should be administered with caution.

Drug Interactions: No drug interaction studies have been conducted.

Adhesion

An open-label study of adhesion potentials of placebo transdermal systems that correspond to the 6.5 cm^2 and 12.5 cm^2 sizes of Climara was conducted in 112 healthy women of 45-75 years of age. Each woman applied both transdermal systems weekly, on the upper outer abdomen, for 3 consecutive weeks. It should be noted that lower abdomen and upper quadrant of the buttock are the approved sites of application for Climara.

The adhesion assessment was done visually on days 2, 4, 5, 6, 7 of each week of transdermal system wear. A total of 1654 adhesion observations were conducted for 333 transdermal systems of each size.

Of these observations, approximately 90% showed essentially no lift for both the 6.5 cm^2 and 12.5 cm^2 transdermal systems. Of the total number of transdermal systems applied, approximately 5% showed complete detachment for each size.

Adhesion potentials of the 18.75 cm^2 and 25.0 cm^2 sizes of transdermal systems (0.075 mg/day and 0.1 mg/day) have not been studied.

ESTRADERM

The Estraderm system releases estradiol, the major estrogenic hormone secreted by the human ovary. Although circulating estrogens exist in a dynamic equilibrium of metabolic interconversions, estradiol is the principal intracellular human estrogen and is substantially more potent than estrone or estriol at the receptor level.

Estraderm provides systemic estrogen replacement therapy. Estrogen receptors have been identified in tissues of the reproductive tract, breast, pituitary, hypothalamus, liver, and in the bone of women. Among numerous effects, estradiol is largely responsible for the development and maintenance of the female reproductive system and of secondary sexual characteristics. By a direct action, it causes growth and development of the vagina, uterus, and fallopian tubes. With other hormones, such as pituitary hormones and progesterone, they cause enlargement of the breasts through promotion of ductal growth, stromal development, and the accretion of fat. Estrogens contribute to the shaping of the skeleton, to the maintenance of tone and elasticity of urogenital structures, to changes in the epiphyses of the long bones that allow for the pubertal growth spurt and its termination, to the growth of axillary and pubic hair, and to the pigmentation of the nipples and genitals.

Estrogens are intricately involved with other hormones, especially progesterone, in the processes of the ovulatory menstrual cycle and pregnancy and affect the release of pituitary gonadotropins.

Loss of ovarian estradiol secretion after menopause can result in instability of thermoregulation, causing hot flushes associated with sleep disturbance and excessive sweating, and urogenital atrophy, causing dyspareunia and urinary incontinence. Estradiol replacement therapy alleviates many of these symptoms of estradiol deficiency in the menopausal woman.

Transdermal administration produces therapeutic serum levels of estradiol with lower circulating levels of estrone and estrone conjugates and requires smaller total doses than does oral therapy. Because estradiol has a short half-life (~1 hour), transdermal administration of estradiol allows a rapid decline in blood levels after an Estraderm system is removed, *e.g.*, in a cycling regimen.

In a study using transdermally administered estradiol, 0.1 mg daily, plasma levels increased by 66 pg/ml, resulting in an average plasma level of 73 pg/ml. There were no significant increases in the concentration of renin substrate or other hepatic proteins (sex hormone-binding globulin, thyroxine-binding globulin, and corticosteroid-binding globulin).

Pharmacokinetics

Administration of Estraderm produces mean serum concentrations of estradiol comparable to those produced by daily oral administration of estradiol at about 20 times the daily transdermal dose. In single-application studies in 14 postmenopausal women using Estraderm systems that provided 0.05 and 0.1 mg of exogenous estradiol per day, these systems produced increased blood levels within 4 hours and maintained respective mean serum estradiol concentrations of 32 and 67 pg/ml above baseline over the application period. At the same time, increases in estrone serum concentration averaged only 9 and 27 pg/ml above baseline, respectively. Serum concentrations of estradiol and estrone returned to preapplication levels within 24 hours after removal of the system. The estimated daily urinary output of estradiol conjugates increased 5-10 times the baseline values and returned to near baseline within 2 days after removal of the system.

By comparison, estradiol (2 mg/day) administered orally to postmenopausal women resulted in increases in mean serum concentration of 59 pg/ml of estradiol and 302 pg/ml of estrone above baseline on the third consecutive day of dosing. Urinary output of estradiol conjugates after oral administration increased to about 100 times the baseline values and did not approach baseline until 7-8 days after the last dose.

In a 3 week multiple-application study of 14 postmenopausal women in which Estraderm 0.05 was applied twice weekly, the mean increments in steady-state serum concentration were 30 pg/ml for estradiol and 12 pg/ml for estrone. Urinary output of estradiol conjugates returned to baseline within 3 days after removal of the last (6th) system, indicating little or no estrogen accumulation in the body.

INDICATIONS AND USAGE

CLIMARA

Climara is indicated in the:

Treatment of moderate to severe vasomotor symptoms associated with the menopause.

Treatment of vulvar and vaginal atrophy.

Treatment of hypoestrogenism due to hypogonadism, castration or primary ovarian failure.

Prevention of postmenopausal osteoporosis (loss of bone mass). The mainstays of prevention of postmenopausal osteoporosis are weight bearing exercise, an adequate calcium and vitamin D intake, and when indicated, estrogen. Postmenopausal women absorb dietary calcium less efficiently than premenopausal women and require an average of 1500 mg/day of elemental calcium to remain in neutral calcium balance. The average calcium intake in the US is 400-600 mg/day. Therefore, when not contraindicated, calcium supplementation may be helpful for women with suboptimal dietary intake.

Estrogen replacement therapy reduces bone resorption and retards or halts postmenopausal bone loss. Studies have shown an approximately 60% reduction in hip and wrist fractures in women whose estrogen replacement was begun within a few years of menopause. Studies also suggest that estrogen reduces the rate of vertebral fractures. Even when started as late as 6 years after menopause, estrogen prevents further loss of bone mass for as long as treatment is continued. When estrogen therapy is discontinued, bone mass declines at a rate comparable to the immediate postmenopausal period.

Early menopause is one of the strongest predictors for the development of osteoporosis in all women. Other factors associated with osteoporosis include genetic factors, lifestyle and nutrition.

ESTRADERM

Estraderm (estradiol transdermal system) is indicated in the following:

Treatment of moderate-to-severe vasomotor symptoms associated with menopause. There is no adequate evidence that estrogens are effective for nervous symptoms or depression that might occur during menopause, and they should not be used to treat these conditions.

Treatment of atrophic vaginitis and kraurosis vulvae.

Treatment of atrophic urethritis.

Treatment of hypoestrogenism due to hypogonadism, castration, or primary ovarian failure.

Prevention of osteoporosis (loss of bone mass). The mainstays of prevention and management of osteoporosis are estrogen, an adequate lifetime calcium intake, and exercise. Estrogen replacement therapy is the most effective single modality for the prevention of postmenopausal osteoporosis in women. Estrogen replacement therapy reduces bone resorption and retards or halts postmenopausal bone loss. Case-controlled studies have shown an approximately 60% reduction in hip and wrist fractures in women whose estrogen replacement was begun within a few years of menopause. Studies also suggest that estrogen reduces the rate of vertebral fractures. Even when started as late as 6 years after menopause, estrogen prevents further loss of bone mass for as long as treatment is continued. When estrogen therapy is discontinued, bone mass declines at a rate comparable to the immediate postmenopausal period. A well-controlled, double-blind, prospective trial conducted at the Mayo Clinic has demonstrated that treatment with Estraderm prevents bone loss in postmenopausal women at a dosage of 0.05 mg/day.

Treatment with Estraderm 0.05 mg showed full maintenance of bone density with a slight (0.8%), but not significant, increase. Placebo treatment resulted in a significant loss of more than 6% below baseline vertebral bone mass. Patients using either Estraderm 0.1 or 0.05 mg had significantly greater bone densities than those using placebo.

Women are at higher risk than men because they have less bone mass, and for several years following natural or induced menopause, the rate of bone mass decline is accelerated. Early menopause is one of the strongest predictors for the development of osteoporosis. In addition, other factors affecting the skeleton that are associated with osteoporosis include race (white and Asian women are at higher risk than black women); genetic factors (small build, family history); endocrine factors (nulliparity, thyrotoxicosis, hyperparathyroidism, Cushing's syndrome, hyperprolactinemia, Type 1 diabetes); life-style (cigarette smoking, alcohol abuse, sedentary habits); and nutrition (below-average body weight, dietary calcium intake). Calcium deficiency has been implicated in the pathogenesis of the disease. Therefore, when not contraindicated, it is recommended that postmenopausal women receive calcium supplementation.

Immobilization and prolonged bed rest produce rapid bone loss, while weight-bearing exercise has been shown both to reduce bone loss and to increase bone mass. The optimal type and amount of physical activity that would prevent osteoporosis have not been established.

NON-FDA APPROVED INDICATIONS

Other estrogens have been used for treatment of gastrointestinal bleeding in patients with renal failure and gastrointestinal bleeding related to arteriovenous malformations.

CONTRAINDICATIONS

CLIMARA

Estrogens should not be used in individuals with any of the following conditions:

Known or suspected pregnancy (PRECAUTIONS, Climara). Estrogens may cause fetal harm when administered to a pregnant woman.

Undiagnosed abnormal genital bleeding.

Known or suspected cancer of the breast except in appropriately selected patients being treated for metastatic disease.

Known or suspected estrogen-dependent neoplasia.

Active thrombophlebitis or thromboembolic disorders.

Climara should not be used in patients hypersensitive to its ingredients.

ESTRADERM

Patients with known hypersensitivity to any of the components of the therapeutic system should not use Estraderm.

Estrogens should not be used in women with any of the following conditions:

Known or suspected pregnancy (see BOXED WARNING, Estraderm). Estrogen may cause fetal harm when administered to a pregnant woman.

Known or suspected cancer of the breast.

Known or suspected estrogen-dependent neoplasia.

Undiagnosed abnormal genital bleeding.

Active thrombophlebitis or thromboembolic disorders, or a documented history of these conditions.

WARNINGS

CLIMARA

Induction of Neoplasms

Endometrial Cancer

The reported endometrial cancer risk among unopposed estrogen users is about 2- to 12-fold greater than in non-users, and appears dependent on duration of treatment and on estrogen dose. Most studies show no significant increased risk associated with use of estrogens for less than 1 year. The greatest risk appears associated with prolonged use, with increased risks of 15- to 24-fold for 5-10 years or more, and this risk has been shown to persist for at least 8-15 years after estrogen therapy is discontinued.

Breast Cancer

While some epidemiologic studies suggest a very modest increase in breast cancer risk for estrogen alone versus non-users, other studies have not shown any increased risk. The addition of progestin to estrogen may increase the risk for breast cancer over that noted in non-hormone users more significantly (by about 24-40%), although this is based solely on epidemiologic studies, and definitive conclusions await prospective, controlled clinical trials.

Women without a uterus who require hormone replacement should receive estrogen-alone therapy, and should not be exposed unnecessarily to progestins. Women with a uterus who are candidates for short-term combination estrogen/progestin therapy (for relief of vasomotor symptoms) are not felt to be at a substantially increased risk for breast cancer. Women with a uterus who are candidates for long-term use of estrogen/progestin therapy should be advised of potential benefits and risks (including the potential for an increased risk of breast cancer). All women should receive yearly breast exams by a health-care provider and perform monthly self-breast examinations. In addition, mammography examinations should be scheduled as suggested by providers based on patient age and risk factors.

Thromboembolic Disorders

The physician should be aware of the possibility of thrombotic disorders (thrombophlebitis, retinal thrombosis, cerebral embolism, and pulmonary embolism) during estrogen replacement therapy and be alert to their earliest manifestations. Should any of these occur or be suspected, estrogen replacement therapy should be discontinued immediately. Patients who have risk factors for thrombotic disorders should be kept under careful observation.

Venous Thromboembolism

Several epidemiologic studies have found an increased risk of venous thromboembolism (VTE) in users of estrogen replacement therapy (ERT) who did not have predisposing conditions for VTE, such as past history of cardiovascular disease or a recent history of pregnancy, surgery, trauma, or serious illness. The increased risk was found only in current ERT users; it did not persist in former users. The risk appeared to be higher in the first year of use and decreased thereafter. The findings were similar for ERT alone or with added progestin and pertain to commonly used oral and transdermal doses, with a possible dose-dependent effect on risk. The studies found the VTE risk to be about 1 case per 10,000 women per year among women not using ERT and without predisposing conditions. The risk in current ERT users was increased to 2-3 cases per 10,000 women per year.

Cerebrovascular Disease

Embolic cerebrovascular events have been reported in women receiving postmenopausal estrogens.

Cardiovascular Disease

Large doses of estrogen (5 mg conjugated estrogens per day), comparable to those used to treat cancer of the prostate and breast, have been shown in a large prospective clinical trial in men to increase the risks of nonfatal myocardial infarction, pulmonary embolism, and thrombophlebitis.

Gallbladder Disease

A 2- to 4-fold increase in the risk of gallbladder disease requiring surgery in women receiving postmenopausal estrogens has been reported.

Hypercalcemia

Administration of estrogens may lead to severe hypercalcemia in patients with breast cancer and bone metastases. If this occurs, the drug should be stopped and appropriate measures taken to reduce the serum calcium level.

ESTRADERM

Induction of Malignant Neoplasms

Breast Cancer

While some epidemiologic studies suggest a very modest increase in breast cancer risk for estrogen alone users versus non-users, other studies have not shown any increased risk. The addition of progestin to estrogen may increase the risk for breast cancer over that noted in non-hormone users more significantly (by about 24-40%), although this is based solely on epidemiologic studies, and definitive conclusions await prospective, controlled clinical trials.

Women without a uterus who require hormone replacement should receive estrogen-alone therapy, and should not be exposed unnecessarily to progestins. Women with a uterus who are candidates for short-term combination estrogen/progestin therapy (for relief of vasomotor symptoms) are not felt to be at a substantially increased risk for breast cancer. Women with a uterus who are candidates for long-term use of estrogen/progestin therapy should be advised of potential benefits and risks (including the potential for an increased risk of breast cancer). All women should receive yearly breast exams by a healthcare provider and perform monthly breast self-examinations. In addition, mammography examinations should be scheduled as suggested by providers based on patient age and risk factors.

The reported endometrial cancer risk among unopposed estrogen users is about 2- to 12-fold greater than in non-users and appears dependent on duration of treatment and on estrogen dose. Most studies show no significant increased risk associated with use of estrogens for less than 1 year. The greatest risk appears associated with prolonged use with increased risks of 15- to 24-fold for 5-10 years or more. In three studies, persistence of risk was demonstrated for 8 to over 15 years after cessation of estrogen treatment. In one study, a significant decrease in the incidence of endometrial cancer occurred 6 months after estrogen withdrawal. Concurrent progestin therapy may offset this risk, but the overall health impact in postmenopausal women is not known (see PRECAUTIONS, Estraderm).

Estrogen therapy during pregnancy is associated with an increased risk of fetal congenital reproductive tract disorders. In female offspring, there is an increased risk of vaginal adenosis, squamous cell dysplasia of the cervix, and clear cell vaginal cancer later in life; in males, urogenital and possibly testicular abnormalities. Although some of these changes are benign, it is not known whether they are precursors of malignancy.

Gallbladder Disease

Two studies have reported a 2- to 4-fold increase in the risk of surgically confirmed gallbladder disease in postmenopausal women receiving oral estrogen replacement therapy, similar to the 2-fold increase previously noted in users of oral contraceptives.

Cardiovascular Disease

Large doses of oral estrogen (5 mg conjugated estrogens per day), comparable to those used to treat cancer of the prostate and breast, have been shown in a large prospective clinical trial in men to increase the risk of nonfatal myocardial infarction, pulmonary embolism, and thrombophlebitis. It cannot necessarily be extrapolated from men to women. However, to avoid the theoretical cardiovascular risk to women caused by high estrogen doses, the dose for estrogen replacement therapy should not exceed the lowest effective dose.

Elevated Blood Pressure

Occasional blood pressure increases during postmenopausal estrogen replacement therapy have been attributed to idiosyncratic reactions to estrogens. More often, blood pressure has remained the same or has dropped. Postmenopausal estrogen use does not increase the risk of stroke; nonetheless, blood pressure should be monitored at regular intervals with estrogen use, especially if high doses are used. Ethinyl estradiol and conjugated estrogens have been shown to increase renin substrate. In contrast to these oral estrogens, transdermally administered estradiol does not affect renin substrate.

Hypercalcemia

Administration of estrogen may lead to severe hypercalcemia in patients with breast cancer and bone metastases. If this occurs, the drug should be stopped and appropriate measures taken to reduce the serum calcium level.

PRECAUTIONS

CLIMARA

General

Addition of a Progestin When a Woman Has Not Had a Hysterectomy

Studies of the addition of a progestin for 10 or more days of a cycle of estrogen administration or daily with estrogen in a continuous regimen, have reported a lowered incidence of endometrial hyperplasia than would be induced by estrogen treatment alone. Endometrial hyperplasia may be a precursor to endometrial cancer.

There are, however, possible risks that may be associated with the use of progestins in estrogen replacement regimens. These include: (a) adverse effects on lipoprotein metabolism (*e.g.,* lowering HDL and raising LDL) and (b) impairment of glucose tolerance. The choice of progestin, its dose, and its regimen may be important in minimizing these adverse effects.

Cardiovascular Risk

The effects of estrogen replacement on the risk of cardiovascular disease have not been adequately studied. However, data from the Heart and Estrogen/Progestin Replacement Study (HERS), a controlled clinical trial of secondary prevention of 2763 postmenopausal women with documented heart disease, demonstrated no benefit. During an average follow-up of 4.1 years, treatment with oral conjugated estrogen plus medroxyprogesterone acetate did not reduce the overall rate of coronary heart disease (CHD) events in postmenopausal women with established coronary disease. There were more CHD events in the hormone treated group than in the placebo group in year 1, but fewer events in years 3-5.

Elevated Blood Pressure

In a small number of case reports, substantial increases in blood pressure during estrogen replacement therapy have been attributed to idiosyncratic reactions to estrogens. In a large, randomized, placebo-controlled clinical trial, a generalized effect of estrogen therapy on blood pressure was not seen.

Familial Hyperlipoproteinemia

In patients with familial defects of lipoprotein metabolism, estrogen therapy may be associated with elevations of plasma triglycerides leading to pancreatitis and other complications.

Impaired Liver Function

Estrogens may be poorly metabolized in patients with impaired liver function.

Hypothyroidism

Estrogen administration leads to increased thyroid-binding globulin (TBG) levels. Patients with normal thyroid function can compensate for the increased TBG by making more thyroid hormone, thus maintaining free T_4 and T_3 serum concentrations in the normal range. Patients dependent on thyroid hormone replacement therapy, however, may require increased doses in order to maintain their free thyroid hormone levels in an acceptable range.

Fluid Retention

Because estrogens may cause some degree of fluid retention, conditions which might be influenced by this factor, such as asthma, epilepsy, migraine and cardiac or renal dysfunction, warrant careful observation when estrogens are prescribed.

Exacerbation of Endometriosis

Endometriosis may be exacerbated with administration of estrogen therapy.

Hypocalcemia

Estrogens should be used with caution in individuals with severe hypocalcemia.

Information for the Patient

See text of Patient Information which accompanies prescription.

Laboratory Tests

Estrogen administration should generally be guided by clinical response at the smallest dose, rather than laboratory monitoring, for relief of symptoms for those indications in which symptoms are observable.

Drug/Laboratory Test Interactions

Accelerated prothrombin time, partial thromboplastin time, and platelet aggregation time; increased platelet count; increased factors II, VII antigen, VIII antigen, VIII coagulant activity, IX, X, XII, VII-X complex, II-VII-X complex, and betathromboglobulin; decreased levels of anti-factor Xa and antithrombin III, decreased antithrombin III activity; increased levels of fibrinogen and fibrinogen activity; increased plasminogen antigen and activity.

Increased thyroid-binding globulin (TBG) leading to increased circulating total thyroid hormone, as measured by protein-bound iodine (PBI), T_4 levels (by column or by radioimmunoassay) or T_3 levels by radioimmunoassay. T_3 resin uptake is decreased, reflecting the elevated TBG. Free T_4 and free T_3 concentrations are unaltered.

Other binding proteins may be elevated in serum, *i.e.,* corticosteroid binding globulin (CBG), sex hormone-binding globulin (SHBG), leading to increased circulating corticosteroids and sex steroids respectively. Free or biologically active hormone concentrations are unchanged. Other plasma proteins may be increased (angiotensinogen/renin substrate, alpha-1-antitrypsin, ceruloplasmin).

Increased plasma HDL and HDL-2 subfraction concentrations, reduced LDL cholesterol concentration, increased triglycerides levels.

Impaired glucose tolerance.

Reduced response to metyrapone test.

Reduced serum folate concentration.

Carcinogenesis, Mutagenesis, and Impairment of Fertility

See CONTRAINDICATIONS, Climara.

Long-term continuous administration of natural and synthetic estrogens in certain animal species increases the frequency of carcinomas of the breast, uterus, cervix, vagina, testis, and liver.

Pregnancy Category X

Climara should not be used during pregnancy. See CONTRAINDICATIONS, Climara.

Nursing Mothers

The administration of any drug to nursing mothers should be done only when clearly necessary since many drugs are excreted in human milk. In addition, estrogen administration to nursing mothers has been shown to decrease the quantity and quality of the milk. Estrogens are not indicated for the prevention of postpartum breast engorgement.

Pediatric Use
Estrogen replacement therapy has been used for the induction of puberty in adolescents with some forms of pubertal delay. Safety and effectiveness in pediatric patients have not otherwise been established.

Large and repeated doses of estrogen over an extended time period have been shown to accelerate epiphyseal closure, which could result in short adult stature if treatment is initiated before the completion of physiologic puberty in normally developing children. If estrogen is administered to patients whose bone growth is not complete, periodic monitoring of bone maturation and effects on epiphyseal centers is recommended during estrogen administration.

Estrogen treatment of prepubertal girls also induces premature breast development and vaginal cornification, and may induce vaginal bleeding. In boys, estrogen treatment may modify the normal pubertal process and induce gynecomastia. (See INDICATIONS AND USAGE, Climara and DOSAGE AND ADMINISTRATION, Climara.)

E

Geriatric Use
There have not been sufficient numbers of geriatric patients involved in clinical studies utilizing Climara to determine whether those over 65 years of age differ from younger subjects in their response to Climara.

ESTRADERM
General
Addition of a Progestin
Studies of the addition of a progestin for 10 or more days of a cycle of estrogen administration have reported a lowered incidence of endometrial hyperplasia than would be induced by estrogen treatment alone. Morphologic and biochemical studies of endometria suggest that 10-14 days of progestin are needed to provide maximal maturation of the endometrium and to reduce the likelihood of hyperplastic changes. There are possible additional risks that may be associated with the use of progestins in estrogen replacement regimens. These include (1) adverse effects on lipoprotein metabolism (lowering HDL and raising LDL), which could diminish the purported cardioprotective effect of estrogen therapy (see PRECAUTIONS, Estraderm); (2) impairment of glucose tolerance; and (3) possible enhancement of mitotic activity in breast epithelial tissue, although few epidemiologic data are available to address this point (see PRECAUTIONS, Estraderm). The choice of progestin, its dose, and its regimen may be important in minimizing these adverse effects, but these issues will require further study before they are clarified.

Cardiovascular Risk
The effects of estrogen replacement on the risk of cardiovascular disease have not been adequately studied. However, data from the Heart and Estrogen/Progestin Replacement Study (HERS), a controlled clinical trial of secondary prevention of 2763 postmenopausal women with documented heart disease, demonstrated no benefit. During an average follow-up of 4.1 years, treatment with oral conjugated estrogen plus medroxyprogesterone acetate did not reduce the overall rate of coronary heart disease (CHD) events in postmenopausal women with established coronary disease. There were more CHD events in the hormone treated group than in the placebo group in year 1, but fewer events in years 3-5.

Physical Examination
A complete medical and family history should be taken prior to the initiation of any estrogen therapy. The pretreatment and periodic physical examinations should include special reference to blood pressure, breasts, abdomen, and pelvic organs and should include a Papanicolaou smear. As a general rule, estrogen should not be prescribed for longer than 1 year without another physical examination being performed.

Hypercoagulability
Some studies have shown that women taking estrogen replacement therapy have hypercoagulability, primarily related to decreased antithrombin activity. This effect appears dose- and duration-dependent and is less pronounced than that associated with oral contraceptive use. Also, postmenopausal women tend to have increased coagulation parameters at baseline compared to premenopausal women. Epidemiological studies, which employed primarily orally administered estrogen products, have suggested that hormone replacement therapy (HRT) may be associated with an increased relative risk of developing venous thromboembolism (VTE), *i.e.,* deep venous thrombosis or pulmonary embolism. Risk/benefit should therefore be carefully weighed in consultation with the patient when prescribing either oral or transdermal HRT to women with a risk factor for VTE.

Familial Hyperlipoproteinemia
Estrogen therapy may be associated with massive elevations of plasma triglycerides, leading to pancreatitis and other complications in patients with familial defects of lipoprotein metabolism.

Fluid Retention
Because estrogens may cause some degree of fluid retention, conditions that might be influenced by this factor, such as asthma, epilepsy, migraine, and cardiac or renal dysfunction, require careful observation.

Uterine Bleeding and Mastodynia
Certain patients may develop undesirable manifestations of estrogenic stimulation, such as abnormal uterine bleeding and mastodynia.

Impaired Liver Function
Estrogens may be poorly metabolized in patients with impaired liver function and should be administered with caution.

Information for the Patient
See text of the Patient Package Insert, which accompanies the prescription.

Laboratory Tests
Estrogen administration should generally be guided by clinical response at the smallest dose, rather than laboratory monitoring, for relief of symptoms for those indications in which symptoms are observable. For prevention and treatment of osteoporosis, however, see DOSAGE AND ADMINISTRATION, Estraderm. Tests used to measure adequacy of estrogen replacement therapy include serum estrone and estradiol levels and suppression of serum gonadotropin levels.

Drug/Laboratory Test Interactions
Some of these drug/laboratory test interactions have been observed only with estrogen-progestin combinations (oral contraceptives):

- Accelerated prothrombin time, partial thromboplastin time, and platelet aggregation time; increased platelet count; increased factors II, VII antigen, VIII antigen, VIII coagulant activity, IX, X, XII, VII-X complex, II-VII-X complex, and beta-thromboglobulin; decreased levels of antifactor Xa and antithrombin III; decreased antithrombin III activity; increased levels of fibrinogen and fibrinogen activity; increased plasminogen antigen and activity.
- Increased thyroid-binding globulin (TBG) leading to increased circulating total thyroid hormone, as measured by T_4 levels determined either by column or by radioimmunoassay. Free T_3 resin uptake is decreased, reflecting the elevated TBG; free T_4 and free T_3 concentrations are unaltered.
- Other binding proteins may be elevated in serum, *i.e.,* corticosteroid-binding globulin (CBG), sex hormone-binding globulin (SHBG), leading to increased circulating corticosteroids and sex steroids respectively. Free or biologically active hormone concentrations are unchanged. Other plasma proteins may be increased (angiotensinogen/renin substrate, alpha-1-antitrypsin, ceruloplasmin).
- Increased plasma HDL and HDL-2 subfraction concentrations, reduced LDL cholesterol concentration, increased triglyceride levels.
- Impaired glucose tolerance.
- Reduced response to metyrapone test.
- Reduced serum folate concentration.

Carcinogenesis, Mutagenesis, and Impairment of Fertility
Long-term, continuous administration of natural and synthetic estrogens in certain animal species increases the frequency of carcinomas of the breast, cervix, vagina, testis, and liver (see CONTRAINDICATIONS, Estraderm and BOXED WARNING, Estraderm).

Pregnancy Category X
Estrogens should not be used during pregnancy (see CONTRAINDICATIONS, Estraderm and BOXED WARNING, Estraderm).

Nursing Mothers
As a general principle, the administration of any drug to nursing mothers should be done only when clearly necessary since many drugs are excreted in human milk.

Pediatric Use
The safety and effectiveness in pediatric patients have not been established.

ADVERSE REACTIONS

CLIMARA
Because clinical trials are conducted under widely varying conditions, adverse reaction rates observed in the clinical trials of a drug cannot be directly compared to rates in the clinical trials of another drug and may not reflect the rates observed in practice. The adverse reaction information from clinical trials does, however, provide a basis for identifying the adverse events that appear to be related to drug use and for approximating rates.

See WARNINGS, Climara regarding induction of neoplasia, increased incidence of gallbladder disease, cardiovascular disease, and hypercalcemia; see PRECAUTIONS, Climara regarding cardiovascular risk and elevated blood pressure.

The most commonly reported adverse reaction to the Climara system in clinical trials was skin irritation at the application site. In two well-controlled clinical studies, the overall rate of discontinuation due to skin irritation at the application site was 6.8%: 7.9% for the 12.5 cm^2 system and 5.3% for the 25.0 cm^2 system compared with 11.5% for the placebo system. Patients with known skin irritation to the patch were excluded from participation in the studies. Additional adverse reactions have been reported with estrogen therapy (see TABLE 3).

ESTRADERM
See BOXED WARNING, Estraderm regarding induction of neoplasia, adverse effects on the fetus, gallbladder disease, cardiovascular disease, elevated blood pressure, and hypercalcemia.

The most commonly reported adverse reaction to Estraderm in clinical trials was redness and irritation at the application site. This occurred in about 17% of the women treated and caused approximately 2% to discontinue therapy. Reports of rash have been rare. There have also been rare reports of severe systemic allergic reactions.

The following additional adverse reactions have been reported with estrogen therapy:

- ***Genitourinary System:*** Changes in vaginal bleeding pattern and abnormal withdrawal bleeding or flow; breakthrough bleeding; spotting; increase in size of uterine leiomyomata; vaginal candidiasis; change in amount of cervical secretion.
- ***Breasts:*** Tenderness, enlargement.
- ***Gastrointestinal:*** Nausea, vomiting; abdominal cramps, bloating; cholestatic jaundice; gallbladder disease.
- ***Skin:*** Chloasma or melasma that may persist when drug is discontinued; erythema multiforme; erythema nodosum; hemorrhagic eruption; loss of scalp hair; hirsutism.
- ***Eyes:*** Steepening of corneal curvature; intolerance to contact lenses.
- ***CNS:*** Headache, migraine, dizziness; mental depression; chorea.
- ***Miscellaneous:*** Increase or decrease in weight; reduced carbohydrate tolerance; aggravation of porphyria; edema; changes in libido.

TABLE 3 *Summary of Most Frequently Reported Adverse Experiences/Medical Events (≥5%) by Treatment Groups*

Adverse Event	Climara (mg/day)			
	0.025	0.05	0.1	Placebo
Body System	(n=219)	(n=201)	(n=194)	(n=72)
Body as a Whole	21%	39%	37%	29%
Headache	5%	18%	13%	10%
Pain	1%	8%	11%	7%
Back pain	4%	8%	9%	6%
Edema	0.5%	13%	10%	6%
Gastrointestinal	9%	21%	29%	18%
Abdominal pain	0.0%	11%	16%	8%
Nausea	1%	5%	6%	3%
Flatulence	1%	3%	7%	1%
Musculoskeletal	7%	9%	11%	4%
Arthralgia	1%	5%	5%	3%
Psychiatric	13%	10%	11%	1%
Depression	1%	5%	8%	0%
Reproductive	12%	18%	41%	11%
Breast pain	5%	8%	29%	4%
Leukorrhea	1%	6%	7%	1%
Respiratory	15%	26%	29%	14%
URTI	6%	17%	17%	8%
Pharyngitis	0.5%	3%	7%	3%
Sinusitis	4%	4%	5%	3%
Rhinitis	2%	4%	6%	1%
Skin & Appendages	19%	12%	12%	15%
Pruritus	0.5%	6%	3%	6%

DOSAGE AND ADMINISTRATION

CLIMARA

The adhesive side of the Climara system should be placed on a clean, dry area of the lower abdomen or the upper quadrant of the buttock. *The Climara system should not be applied to the breasts.* The sites of application must be rotated, with an interval of at least 1 week allowed between applications to a particular site. The area selected should not be oily, damaged, or irritated. The waistline should be avoided, since tight clothing may rub and remove the system. Application to areas where sitting would dislodge the system should also be avoided. The system should be applied immediately after opening the pouch and removing the protective liner. The system should be pressed firmly in place with the fingers for about 10 seconds, making sure there is good contact, especially around the edges. If the system lifts, apply pressure to maintain adhesion. In the event that a system should fall off, a new system should be applied for the remainder of the 7 day dosing interval. Only one system should be worn at any one time during the 7 day dosing interval. Swimming, bathing, or using a sauna while using the Climara system has not been studied, and these activities may decrease the adhesion of the system and the delivery of estradiol.

Initiation of Therapy

Four (6.5, 12.5, 18.75 and 25.0 cm^2) Climara systems are available.

For the treatment of vasomotor symptoms, treatment should be initiated with the 6.5 cm^2 (0.025 mg/day) Climara system applied to the skin once weekly. The dose should be adjusted as necessary to control symptoms. Clinical responses (relief of symptoms) at the lowest effective dose should be the guide for establishing administration of the Climara system, especially in women with an intact uterus. Attempts to taper or discontinue the medication should be made at 3-6 month intervals. In women who are not currently taking oral estrogens, treatment with the Climara system can be initiated at once.

In women who are currently taking oral estrogen, treatment with the Climara system can be initiated 1 week after withdrawal of oral therapy or sooner if symptoms reappear in less than 1 week.

For the prevention of postmenopausal osteoporosis, the minimum dose that has been shown to be effective is the 6.5 cm^2 (0.025 mg/day) Climara system. Response to therapy can be assessed by biochemical markers and measurement of bone mineral density.

ESTRADERM

The adhesive side of the Estraderm system should be placed on a clean, dry area of the skin on the trunk of the body (including the buttocks and abdomen). The site selected should be one that is not exposed to sunlight. *Estraderm should not be applied to the breasts.* The Estraderm system should be replaced twice weekly. The sites of application must be rotated, with an interval of at least 1 week allowed between applications to a particular site. The area selected should not be oily, damaged, or irritated. The waistline should be avoided, since tight clothing may rub the system off. The system should be applied immediately after opening the pouch and removing the protective liner. The system should be pressed firmly in place with the palm of the hand for about 10 seconds, making sure there is good contact, especially around the edges. In the unlikely event that a system should fall off, the same system may be reapplied. If necessary, a new system may be applied. In either case, the original treatment schedule should be continued.

Initiation of Therapy

Estraderm is currently available in two dosage forms — 0.05 mg and 0.1 mg. For treatment of moderate-to-severe vasomotor symptoms, atrophic vaginitis, and atrophic urethritis associated with menopause, initiate therapy with Estraderm 0.05 applied to the skin twice weekly. The lowest dose that will control symptoms should be chosen, and medication should be discontinued as promptly as possible. Attempts to discontinue or taper medication given only for these menopausal symptoms should be made at 3-6 month intervals.

Prophylactic therapy with Estraderm to prevent postmenopausal bone loss should be initiated with the 0.05 mg/day dosage as soon as possible after menopause. The dosage may be adjusted if necessary. Discontinuation of estrogen replacement therapy may reestablish bone loss at a rate comparable to the immediate postmenopausal period.

In women not currently taking oral estrogens, treatment with Estraderm may be initiated at once. In women who are currently taking oral estrogen, treatment with Estraderm should be initiated 1 week after withdrawal of oral hormone replacement therapy, or sooner if menopausal symptoms reappear in less than 1 week.

Therapeutic Regimen

Estraderm therapy may be given continuously in patients who do not have an intact uterus. In those patients with an intact uterus, Estraderm may be given on a cyclic schedule (*e.g.*, 3 weeks on drug followed by 1 week off drug).

HOW SUPPLIED

CLIMARA

Climara (estradiol transdermal system) is available as follows:

0.025 mg/day: Each 6.5 cm^2 system contains 2.0 mg of estradiol.
0.05 mg/day: Each 12.5 cm^2 system contains 3.8 mg of estradiol.
0.075 mg/day: Each 18.75 cm^2 system contains 5.7 mg of estradiol.
0.1 mg/day: Each 25.0 cm^2 system contains 7.6 mg of estradiol.

Storage: Do not store above 3°C (86°F). Do not store unpouched. Apply immediately upon removal from the protective pouch.

ESTRADERM

Estraderm estradiol transdermal system is available in the following dosage strengths:

0.05 mg/day: Each 10 cm^2 system contains 4 mg of estradiol for nominal (see DESCRIPTION, Estraderm) delivery of 0.05 mg of estradiol per day.

0.1 mg/day: Each 20 cm^2 system contains 8 mg of estradiol for nominal (see DESCRIPTION, Estraderm) delivery of 0.1 mg of estradiol per day.

Storage

Do not store above 30°C (86°F).

Do not store unpouched. Apply immediately upon removal from the protective pouch.

VAGINAL

WARNING

Vaginal Cream and Ring

ESTROGENS HAVE BEEN REPORTED TO INCREASE THE RISK OF ENDOMETRIAL CARCINOMA IN POSTMENOPAUSAL WOMEN: **Close clinical surveillance of all women taking estrogens is important. Adequate diagnostic measures, including endometrial sampling when indicated, should be undertaken to rule out malignancy in all cases of undiagnosed persistent or recurring abnormal vaginal bleeding. There is no evidence that "natural" estrogens are more or less hazardous than "synthetic" estrogens at equiestrogenic doses.**

ESTROGENS SHOULD NOT BE USED DURING PREGNANCY: **There is no indication for estrogen therapy during pregnancy or during the immediate postpartum period. Estrogens are ineffective for the prevention or treatment of threatened or habitual abortion. Estrogens are not indicated for the prevention of postpartum breast engorgement. Estrogen therapy during pregnancy is associated with an increased risk of congenital defects in the reproductive organs of the fetus, and possibly other birth defects. Studies of women who received diethylstilbestrol (DES) during pregnancy have shown that female offspring have an increased risk of vaginal adenosis, squamous cell dysplasia of the uterine cervix, and clear cell vaginal cancer later in life; male offspring have an increased risk of urogenital abnormalities and possibly testicular cancer later in life. The 1985 DES Task Force concluded that the use of DES during pregnancy is associated with a subsequent increased risk of breast cancer in the mothers, although a causal relationship remains unproven and the observed level of excess risk is similar to that for a number of other breast cancer risk factors.**

Vaginal Tablets

ESTROGENS HAVE BEEN REPORTED TO INCREASE THE RISK OF ENDOMETRIAL CARCINOMA.

Three independent, case controlled studies have reported an increased risk of endometrial cancer in postmenopausal women exposed to exogenous estrogens for more than 1 year. This risk was independent of the other known risk factors for endometrial cancer. These studies are further supported by the finding that incident rates of endometrial cancer have increased sharply since 1969 in eight different areas of the US with population-based cancer-reporting systems, an increase which may be related to the rapidly expanding use of estrogens during the last decade. The three case-controlled studies reported that the risk of endometrial cancer in estrogen users was about 4.5-13.9 times greater in nonusers. The risk appears to depend on both duration of treatment and on estrogen dose. In view of these findings, when estrogens are used for the treatment of menopausal symptoms, the lowest dose that will control symptoms should be utilized and medication should be discontinued as soon as possible. When prolonged treatment is medically indicated, the patient should be reassessed, on at least a semi-annual basis, to determine the need for continued therapy.

Close clinical surveillance of all women taking estrogens is important. In all cases of undiagnosed persistent or reoccurring abnormal vaginal bleeding, adequate diagnostic measures should be undertaken to rule out malignancy.

There is no evidence at present that "natural" estrogens are more or less hazardous than "synthetic" estrogens at equi-estrogenic doses.

DESCRIPTION

Note: The trade name has been used throughout this monograph for clarity.

VAGINAL CREAM

Estradiol (17β-estradiol) is a white, crystalline solid, chemically described as estra-1,3,5(10)-triene-3,17β diol.

It has an empirical formula of $C_{18}H_{24}O_2$ and molecular weight of 272.37.

Estrace vaginal cream contains 0.1 mg estradiol per gram in a nonliquefying base containing purified water, propylene glycol, stearyl alcohol, white ceresin wax, glyceryl monostearate, hydroxypropyl methylcellulose, 2208-4000 cps, sodium lauryl sulfate, methylparaben, edetate disodium and *tertiary*-butylhydroquinone.

VAGINAL RING

Estring is a slightly opaque ring with a whitish core containing a drug reservoir of 2 mg estradiol. Estradiol, silicone polymers and barium sulfate are combined to form the ring. When placed in the vagina, Estring releases estradiol, approximately 7.5 µg/24 hours, in a consistent stable manner over 90 days. *Estring has the following dimensions:* Outer diameter 55 mm; cross-sectional diameter 9 mm; core diameter 2 mm. One (1) Estring should be inserted into the upper third of the vaginal vault, to be worn continuously for 3 months.

Estradiol is chemically described as estra-1,3,5(10)-triene-3,17β-diol. The molecular formula of estradiol is $C_{18}H_{24}O_2$.

The molecular weight of estradiol is 272.39.

E

VAGINAL TABLETS

Vagifem is a small, white, film-coated tablet containing 25.8 µg of estradiol hemihydrate equivalent to 25 µg of estradiol.

Each tablet contains the following inactive ingredients: Hydroxypropyl methylcellulose, lactose monohydrate, maize starch, and magnesium stearate. The film coating contains hydroxypropyl methylcellulose and polyethylene glycol. Each white tablet is 6 mm in diameter and is placed in a disposable applicator. Each tablet-filled applicator is packaged separately in a blister pack.

17β-estradiol hemihydrate is a white, almost white or colorless crystalline solid, chemically described as estra-1,3,5 (10)-triene-3,17 diol.

The chemical formula is $C_{18}H_{24}O_2 \cdot \frac{1}{2}H_2O$ with a molecular weight of 281.4.

CLINICAL PHARMACOLOGY

VAGINAL CREAM

Estrogen drug products act by regulating the transcription of a limited number of genes. Estrogens diffuse through cell membranes, distribute themselves throughout the cell, and bind to and activate the nuclear estrogen receptor, a DNA-binding protein which is found in estrogen-responsive tissues. The activated estrogen receptor binds to specific DNA sequences, or hormone-response elements, which enhance the transcription of adjacent genes and in turn lead to the observed effects. Estrogen receptors have been identified in tissues of the reproductive tract, breast, pituitary, hypothalamus, liver, and bone of women.

Estrogens are important in the development and maintenance of the female reproductive system and secondary sex characteristics. By a direct action, they cause growth and development of the uterus, fallopian tubes, and vagina. With other hormones, such as pituitary hormones and progesterone, they cause enlargement of the breasts through promotion of ductal growth, stromal development, and the accretion of fat. Estrogens are intricately involved with other hormones, especially progesterone, in the processes of the ovulatory menstrual cycle and pregnancy, and affect the release of pituitary gonadotropins. They also contribute to the shaping of the skeleton, maintenance of tone and elasticity of urogenital structures, changes in the epiphyses of the long bones that allow for the pubertal growth spurt and its termination, and pigmentation of the nipples and genitals.

Estrogens occur naturally in several forms. The primary source of estrogen in normally cycling adult women is the ovarian follicle, which secretes 70-500 µg of estradiol daily, depending on the phase of the menstrual cycle. This is converted primarily to estrone, which circulates in roughly equal proportion to estradiol, and to small amounts of estriol. After menopause, most endogenous estrogen is produced by conversion of androstenedione, secreted by the adrenal cortex, to estrone by peripheral tissues. Thus, estrone — especially in its sulfate ester form — is the most abundant circulating estrogen in postmenopausal women. Although circulating estrogens exist in a dynamic equilibrium of metabolic interconversions, estradiol is the principal intracellular human estrogen and is substantially more potent than estrone or estriol at the receptor.

Estrogens used in therapy are well absorbed through the skin, mucous membranes, and gastrointestinal tract. When applied for a local action, absorption is usually sufficient to cause systemic effects. When conjugated with aryl and alkyl groups for parenteral administration, the rate of absorption of oily preparations is slowed with a prolonged duration of action, such that a single intramuscular injection of estradiol valerate or estradiol cypionate is absorbed over several weeks.

Administered estrogens and their esters are handled within the body essentially the same as endogenous hormones. Metabolic conversion of estrogens occurs primarily in the liver (first pass effect), but also at local target tissue sites. Complex metabolic processes result in a dynamic equilibrium of circulating conjugated and unconjugated estrogenic forms which are continually interconverted, especially between estrone and estradiol and between esterified and non-esterified forms. Although naturally-occurring estrogens circulate in the blood largely bound to sex hormone-binding globulin and albumin, only unbound estrogens enter target tissue cells. A significant proportion of the circulating estrogen exists as sulfate conjugates, especially estrone sulfate, which serves as a circulating reservoir for the formation of more active estrogenic species. A certain proportion of the estrogen is excreted into the bile and then reabsorbed from the intestine. During this enterohepatic recirculation, estrogens are desulfated and resulfated and undergo degradation through conversion to less active estrogens (estriol and other estrogens), oxidation to nonestrogenic substances (catecholestrogens, which interact with catecholamine metabolism, especially in the central nervous system), and conjugation with glucuronic acids (which are then rapidly excreted in the urine).

When given orally, naturally-occurring estrogens and their esters are extensively metabolized (first pass effect) and circulate primarily as estrone sulfate, with smaller amounts of other conjugated and unconjugated estrogenic species. This results in limited oral potency. By contrast, synthetic estrogens, such as ethinyl estradiol and the nonsteroidal estrogens, are degraded very slowly in the liver and other tissues, which results in their high intrinsic potency. Estrogen drug products administered by non-oral routes are not subject to first-pass metabolism, but also undergo significant hepatic uptake, metabolism, and enterohepatic recycling.

VAGINAL RING

Pharmacokinetics

Absorption

Estrogens used in therapeutics are well absorbed through the skin, mucous membranes, and the gastrointestinal (GI) tract. The vaginal delivery of estrogens circumvents first-pass metabolism possibly reducing the induction of several other hepatic proteins.

In a Phase 1 study of 14 postmenopausal women, the insertion of estradiol vaginal ring rapidly increased serum estradiol (E_2) levels attesting to the rapid absorption of estradiol via the vaginal mucosa. The time to attain peak serum estradiol levels (T_{max}) was 0.5 to 1 hour. Peak serum estradiol concentrations post-initial burst declined rapidly over the next 24 hours and were virtually indistinguishable from the baseline mean (range: 5-22 pg/ml). Serum levels of estradiol and estrone (E_1) over the following 12 weeks during which the ring was maintained in the vaginal vault remained relatively unchanged (see TABLE 4).

The initial estradiol peak post-application of the second ring in the same women resulted in ~38% lower C_{max}, apparently due to reduced systemic absorption via the revitalized vaginal epithelium. The relative systemic exposure from the initial peak of estradiol accounted for approximately 4% of the total estradiol exposure over the 12 week period.

The constant and stable release of estradiol from the estradiol vaginal ring was demonstrated in a Phase 2 study of 166-222 postmenopausal women who inserted up to 4 rings consecutively at 3 month intervals. Low dose systemic delivery of estradiol from the estradiol vaginal ring resulted in mean steady state serum estradiol estimates of 7.8, 7.0, 7.0, 8.1 pg/ml at weeks 12, 24, 36, and 48, respectively. Similar reproducibility is also seen in levels of estrone. Lower systemic exposure to estradiol and estrone is further supported by serum levels measured during a pivotal Phase 3 study.

In postmenopausal women, mean dose of estradiol systemically absorbed unchanged from the estradiol vaginal ring is ~8% [95% CI: 2.8-12.8%] of the daily amount released locally. Low systemic exposure to estradiol and estrone resulting from the estradiol vaginal ring should elicit lower estrogen-dependent effects.

Distribution

Circulating, unbound estrogens are known to modulate pharmacological response. Estrogens circulate in blood bound to sex-hormone binding globulin (SHBG) and albumin. A dynamic equilibrium exists between the conjugated and the unconjugated forms of estradiol and estrone, which undergo rapid interconversion.

Metabolism

Exogenously delivered or endogenously derived estrogens are primarily metabolized in the liver to estrone and estriol, which are also found in the systemic circulation. Estrogen metabolites are primarily excreted in the urine as glucuronides and sulphates. Of the several estrogen metabolites, urinary estrone and estrone sulphate (E_1S), post-estradiol vaginal ring use, are in the normal postmenopausal range.

Excretion

Mean percent dose excreted in the 24 hour urine as estradiol, 4 and 12 weeks post-application of the estradiol vaginal ring in a Phase 1 study was 5% and 8%, respectively, of the daily released amount.

Drug-Drug Interactions

No formal *drug-drug* interactions studies have been done with the estradiol vaginal ring. It is anticipated that lower exposure to systemic estrogens may reduce the potential for drug interactions thus maintaining the benefit to risk ratio of concomitant drugs.

TABLE 4 *Pharmacokinetic Mean Estimates Following Estradiol Vaginal Ring Application*

Estrogen	C_{max}	$C_{ss\text{-}48\,h}$	$C_{ss\text{-}4w}$	$C_{ss\text{-}12w}$
Estradiol (E_2)	63.2* pg/ml	11.2 pg/ml	9.5 pg/ml	8.0 pg/ml
Baseline-adjusted E_2†	55.6 pg/ml	3.6 pg/ml	2.0 pg/ml	0.4 pg/ml
Estrone (E_1)	66.3 pg/ml	52.5 pg/ml	43.8 pg/ml	47.0 pg/ml
Baseline-adjusted E_1	20.0 pg/ml	6.2 pg/ml	-2.4 pg/ml	0.8 pg/ml

* n=14.
† Based on means.

Pharmacodynamics

In vivo, estrogens diffuse through cell membranes, distribute throughout the cell, bind to and activate the estrogen receptors, thereby eliciting their biological effects. Estrogen receptors have been identified in tissues of the reproductive tract, breast, pituitary, hypothalamus, liver, and bone of women. The estradiol vaginal ring delivers estradiol constantly at a mean rate of ~7.5 µg/24 hours for a period of up to 90 days. Its use in postmenopausal patients in Phase 1 and 2 studies showed no apparent effects on systemic levels of hepatic protein SHBG, or FSH. Lowering of the pretreatment vaginal pH from a mean of 6.0 to a mean of 4.6 (as found in fertile women) over the 12-48 week treatment period, and improvements evident in the vaginal mucosal epithelium seen in all studies attest to the local dynamic effects of estrogens.

VAGINAL TABLETS

In vivo estrogens diffuse through cell membranes, distribute throughout the cell, bind to and activate the estrogen receptors, thereby eliciting their biological effects. Estrogen receptors have been identified in tissue of the reproductive tract, breast, pituitary, hypothalamus, liver, and bone of women. The estrogen contained in estradiol vaginal tablets, 17 β-estradiol is chemically and biologically identical to the endogenous human 17 β-estradiol and is, therefore, classified as a human estrogen. Estrogens regulate growth, differentiation and functioning of many different tissues within and outside of the reproductive system. Estrogens are intricately involved with other hormones, especially progesterone, and during the ovulatory phase of the menstrual cycle cause proliferation of the endometrium. Most of the activity of estrogens appear to be exerted via estrogen receptors in target cells of tissues of the woman's reproductive tract: breast, pituitary, hypothalamus, brain, liver, and bone. The steroid-receptor complex is bound to the cell's DNA and induces synthesis of specific proteins. Maturation of the vaginal epithelium is dependent on estrogen as it increases the number of superficial and intermediate cells as compared with basal cells. Estrogen keeps the pH of the vagina at approximately 4.5 which enhances normal bacterial flora, predominately, *Lactobacillus döderlein*.

Pharmacokinetics

Absorption

Estrogen drug products are well absorbed through the skin, mucous membranes, and the gastrointestinal (GI) tract. The vaginal delivery of estrogens circumvents first-pass metabolism.

A single-center, randomized, double-blind comparison study conducted in the US showed that vaginal application of estradiol vaginal tablets over a 12 week course demonstrated a mean C_{max} of estradiol of 50 pg/ml and that there was no significant accumulation of estradiol as measured by the AUC(0-24) (see TABLE 5).

TABLE 5 *Mean (±SD) Pharmacokinetic Parameters for Estradiol (uncorrected for base line)*

PK Parameter	Timepoint Day 1	Day 14	Day 84
AUC (pg·h/ml)	538 (±265)	567 (±246)	563 (±341)
C_{max} (pg/ml)	51 (±34)	47 (±21)	49 (±27)

Distribution

Circulating, unbound estrogens are known to modulate pharmacological response. Estrogens circulate in the blood bound to sex-hormone binding globulin (SHBG) and albumin. A dynamic equilibrium exists between the conjugated and the unconjugated forms of estradiol and estrone, which undergo rapid interconversion.

Metabolism

Exogenously-delivered or endogenously-derived estrogens are primarily metabolized in the liver to estrone and estriol, which are also found in the systemic circulation. Estradiol vaginal tablet intravaginal administration avoids first-pass metabolism that occurs with oral estrogens.

The levels of E_1 seen during 12 weeks of estradiol vaginal tablet administration do not show any accumulation of E_1, and the observed values are within the postmenopausal range (see TABLE 6).

TABLE 6 *Mean (±SD) Pharmacokinetic Parameters For Estrone (uncorrected for base line)*

E1:	Timepoint Day 1	Day 14	Day 84
AUC (pg·h/ml)	649 (±230)	744 (±267)	681 (±271)
C_{max} (pg/ml)	35 (±12)	39 (±13)	35 (±12)

Excretion

Estrogen metabolites are primarily excreted in the urine as glucuronides and sulfates.

Drug-Drug Interactions

No formal *drug-drug* interaction studies have been done with estradiol vaginal tablets.

INDICATIONS AND USAGE

VAGINAL CREAM

Estradiol vaginal cream is indicated in the treatment of vulval and vaginal atrophy.

VAGINAL RING

Estradiol vaginal ring is indicated for the treatment of urogenital symptoms associated with postmenopausal atrophy of the vagina (such as dryness, burning, pruritus and dyspareunia) and/or the lower urinary tract (urinary urgency and dysuria).

VAGINAL TABLETS

Estradiol vaginal tablets are indicated for the treatment of atrophic vaginitis.

CONTRAINDICATIONS

VAGINAL CREAM

Estrogens should not be used in individuals with any of the following conditions:

Known or suspected pregnancy (see BOXED WARNING and PRECAUTIONS). Estrogens may cause fetal harm when administered to a pregnant woman.

Undiagnosed abnormal genital bleeding.

Known or suspected cancer of the breast.

Known or suspected estrogen-dependent neoplasia, *e.g.*, endometrial carcinoma for the vaginal tablets.

Active thrombophlebitis or thromboembolic disorders.

VAGINAL RING

Estrogens should not be used in individuals with any of the following conditions:

Known or suspected pregnancy (see BOXED WARNING and PRECAUTIONS). Estrogens may cause fetal harm when administered to a pregnant woman.

Undiagnosed abnormal genital bleeding.

Known or suspected cancer of the breast.

Known or suspected estrogen-dependent neoplasia, *e.g.*, endometrial carcinoma for the vaginal tablets.

The estradiol vaginal ring should not be used in patients hypersensitive to any of its ingredients.

VAGINAL TABLETS

Estrogens should not be used in individuals with any of the following conditions:

Known or suspected pregnancy (see BOXED WARNING and PRECAUTIONS). Estrogens may cause fetal harm when administered to a pregnant woman.

Undiagnosed abnormal genital bleeding.

Known or suspected cancer of the breast.

Known or suspected estrogen-dependent neoplasia, *e.g.*, endometrial carcinoma for the vaginal tablets.

Active thrombophlebitis or thromboembolic disorders.

Porphyria.

Hypersensitivity to any estradiol vaginal tablet constituents.

A past history of thrombophlebitis, thrombosis, or thromboembolic disorders associated with previous estrogen use (except when used in treatment of breast malignancy).

WARNINGS

VAGINAL CREAM

Induction of Malignant Neoplasms

Endometrial Cancer

The reported endometrial cancer risk among unopposed estrogen users is about 2- to 12-fold greater than in non-users, and appears dependent on duration of treatment and on estrogen dose. Most studies show no significant increased risk associated with use of estrogens for less than 1 year. The greatest risk appears associated with prolonged use — with increased risks of 15- to 24-fold for 5-10 years or more. In three studies, persistence of risk was demonstrated for 8 to over 15 years after cessation of estrogen treatment. In one study a significant decrease in the incidence of endometrial cancer occurred 6 months after estrogen withdrawal. Concurrent progestin therapy may offset this risk but the overall health impact in postmenopausal women is not known (see PRECAUTIONS).

Breast Cancer

While the majority of studies have not shown an increased risk of breast cancer in women who have ever used estrogen replacement therapy, some have reported a moderately increased risk (relative risks of 1.3-2.0) in those taking higher doses or those taking lower doses for prolonged periods of time, especially in excess of 10 years. Other studies have not shown this relationship.

Congenital Lesions With Malignant Potential

Estrogen therapy during pregnancy is associated with an increased risk of fetal congenital reproductive tract disorders, and possibly other birth defects. Studies of women who have received DES during pregnancy have shown that female offspring have an increased risk of vaginal adenosis, squamous cell dysplasia of the uterine cervix, and clear cell vaginal cancer later in life; male offspring have an increased risk of urogenital abnormalities and possibly testicular cancer later in life. Although some of these changes are benign, others are precursors of malignancy.

Gallbladder Disease

Two studies have reported a 2- to 4-fold increase in the risk of gallbladder disease requiring surgery in women receiving postmenopausal estrogens.

Cardiovascular Disease

Large doses of estrogen (5 mg conjugated estrogens per day), comparable to those used to treat cancer of the prostate and breast, have been shown in a large prospective clinical trial in men to increase the risks of nonfatal myocardial infarction, pulmonary embolism, and thrombophlebitis. These risks cannot necessarily be extrapolated from men to women. However, to avoid the theoretical cardiovascular risk to women caused by high estrogen doses, the dose for estrogen replacement therapy should not exceed the lowest effective dose.

Elevated Blood Pressure

Occasional blood pressure increases during estrogen replacement therapy have been attributed to idiosyncratic reactions to estrogens. More often, blood pressure has remained the same or has dropped. One study showed that postmenopausal estrogen users have higher blood pressure than nonusers. Two other studies showed slightly lower blood pressure among estrogen users compared to nonusers. Postmenopausal estrogen use does not increase the risk of stroke. Nonetheless, blood pressure should be monitored at regular intervals with estrogen use.

Hypercalcemia

Administration of estrogens may lead to severe hypercalcemia in patients with breast cancer and bone metastases. If this occurs, the drug should be stopped and appropriate measures taken to reduce the serum calcium level.

VAGINAL RING

Breast Cancer

While the majority of studies have not shown an increased risk of breast cancer in women who have ever used estrogen replacement therapy, some have reported a moderately increased risk (relative risks of 1.3-2.0) in those taking higher doses or those taking lower doses for prolonged periods of time, especially in excess of 10 years. Other studies have not shown this relationship.

Other

Congenital lesions with malignant potential, gallbladder disease, cardiovascular disease, elevated blood pressure, and hypercalcemia have been associated with systemic estrogen treatment.

VAGINAL TABLETS

Induction of Malignant Neoplasm

Long-term, continuous administration of natural and synthetic estrogens in certain animal species increases the frequency of carcinomas of the breast, cervix, vagina, and liver. There are now reports that estrogens increase risk of carcinoma of the endometrium in humans (see BOXED WARNING).

At the present time there is no satisfactory evidence that estrogens given to postmenopausal women increase the risk of cancer of the breast, although a recent long-term follow-up of a single physician's practice has raised this possibility. Because of the animal data, there is a need for caution in prescribing estrogens for women with a strong family history of breast cancer or who have breast nodules, fibrocystic disease, or abnormal mammograms.

Gallbladder Disease

A recent study has reported a 2- to 3-fold increase in the risk of surgically confirmed gallbladder disease in women receiving postmenopausal estrogens, similar to the 2-fold increase previously noted in users of oral contraceptives.

Effects Similar to Those Caused by Estrogen-Progestogen Oral Contraceptives

There are several serious adverse effects of oral contraceptives, most of which have not, up to now, been documented as consequences of postmenopausal estrogen therapy. This may reflect the comparatively low doses of estrogens used in postmenopausal women. It would be expected that the larger doses of estrogen used to treat prostatic or breast cancer are more likely to result in these adverse effects, and, in fact, it has been shown that there is an increased risk of thrombosis in men receiving estrogens for prostatic cancer.

Thromboembolic Disease

It is now well established that users of oral contraceptives have an increased risk of various thromboembolic and thrombotic vascular diseases, such as thrombophlebitis, pulmonary embolism, stroke, and myocardial infarction. Cases of retinal thrombosis, mesenteric thrombosis, and optic neuritis have been reported in oral-contraceptive users. There is evidence that the risk of several of these adverse reactions is related to the dose of the drug. An increased risk of post-surgery thromboembolic complications has also been reported in users of oral contraceptives. If feasible, estrogen should be discontinued at least 4 weeks before surgery of the type associated with an increased risk of thromboembolism, or during periods of prolonged immobilization.

While an increased rate of thromboembolism and thrombotic disease in postmenopausal users of estrogens has not been found, this does not rule out the possibility that such an increase may be present, or that subgroups of women who have underlying risk factors, or who are receiving large doses of estrogens, may have increased risk. Therefore, estrogens should not be used (except in treatment of malignancy) in a person with a history of such disorders in association with estrogen use. They should be used with caution in patients with cerebral vascular or coronary artery disease and only for those in whom estrogens are clearly needed.

Large doses of estrogens (5 mg conjugated estrogens per day), comparable to those used to treat cancer of the prostate and breast, have been shown in a large prospective clinical trial in men, to increase the risk of nonfatal myocardial infraction, pulmonary embolism, and thrombophlebitis. When estrogen doses of this size are used, any of the thromboembolic and thrombotic adverse effects associated with oral contraceptive use should be considered a clear risk.

Hepatic Adenoma

Benign hepatic adenomas appear to be associated with the oral contraceptives. Although benign, and rare, these may rupture and may cause death through intra-abdominal hemorrhage. Such lesions have not yet been reported in association with other estrogen or progestogen preparations but should be considered in estrogen users having abdominal pain and tenderness, abdominal mass, or hypovolemic shock. Hepatocellular carcinoma has also been reported in women taking estrogen-containing oral contraceptives. The relationship of this malignancy to these drugs is not known at this time.

Elevated Blood Pressure

Women using oral contraceptives sometimes experience increased blood pressure which, in most cases, returns to normal on discontinuing the drug. There is now a report that this may occur with the use of estrogens in the menopause and blood pressure should be monitored with estrogen use, especially if high doses are used.

Glucose Tolerance

A worsening of glucose tolerance has been observed in a significant percentage of patients on estrogen-containing oral contraceptives. For this reason, diabetic patients should be carefully observed while using estrogens.

Hypercalcemia

Administration of estrogens may lead to severe hypercalcemia in patients with breast cancer and bone metastases. If this occurs, the drug should be stopped and appropriate measures taken to reduce the serum calcium level.

Rare Event

Trauma induced by the estradiol vaginal tablet applicator may occur, especially in patients with severely atrophic vaginal mucosa.

PRECAUTIONS

VAGINAL CREAM

General

Addition of a Progestin

Studies of the addition of a progestin for 7 or more days of a cycle of estrogen administration have reported a lowered incidence of endometrial hyperplasia which would otherwise be induced by estrogen treatment. Morphological and biochemical studies of endometrium suggest that 10-14 days of progestin are needed to provide maximal maturation of the endometrium and to eliminate any hyperplastic changes. There are possible additional risks which may be associated with the inclusion of progestins in estrogen replacement regimens. *These Include:* (1) adverse effects on lipoprotein metabolism (lowering HDL and raising LDL) which may diminish the possible cardioprotective effect of estrogen therapy (see Drug-Drug and Drug-Laboratory Interactions); (2) impairment of glucose tolerance; and (3) possible enhancement of mitotic activity in breast epithelial tissue (although few epidemiological data are available to address this point). The choice of progestin, its dose, and its regimen may be important in minimizing these adverse effects, but these issues remain to be clarified.

Physical Examination

A complete medical and family history should be taken prior to the initiation of any estrogen therapy. The pretreatment and periodic physical examinations should include special reference to blood pressure, breasts, abdomen, and pelvic organs, and should include a Papanicolaou smear. As a general rule, estrogen should not be prescribed for longer than 1 year without reexamining the patient.

Hypercoagulability

Some studies have shown that women taking estrogen replacement therapy have hypercoagulability, primarily related to decreased antithrombin activity. This effect appears dose- and duration-dependent and is less pronounced than that associated with oral contraceptive use. Also, postmenopausal women tend to have increased coagulation parameters at baseline compared to premenopausal women. There is some suggestion that low dose postmenopausal mestranol may increase the risk of thromboembolism, although the majority of studies (of primarily conjugated estrogens users) report no such increase. There is insufficient information on hypercoagulability in women who have had previous thromboembolic disease.

Familial Hyperlipoproteinemia

Estrogen therapy may be associated with massive elevations of plasma triglycerides leading to pancreatitis and other complications in patients with familial defects of lipoprotein metabolism.

Fluid Retention

Because estrogens may cause some degree of fluid retention, conditions which might be exacerbated by this factor, such as asthma, epilepsy, migraine, and cardiac or renal dysfunction, require careful observation.

Uterine Bleeding and Mastodynia

Certain patients may develop undesirable manifestations of estrogenic stimulation, such as abnormal uterine bleeding and mastodynia.

Impaired Liver Function

Estrogens may be poorly metabolized in patients with impaired liver function and should be administered with caution.

Information for the Patient

See the Patient Instructions that are distributed with the prescription for complete instructions.

Advise patients that the number of doses per tube of estradiol vaginal cream will vary with dosage requirements and patient handling.

Laboratory Tests

Estrogen administration should generally be guided by clinical response at the smallest dose, rather than laboratory monitoring, for relief of symptoms for those indications in which symptoms are observable. For prevention of osteoporosis, however, see DOSAGE AND ADMINISTRATION for oral estradiol tablets.

Drug-Drug and Drug-Laboratory Interactions

Accelerated prothrombin time, partial thromboplastin time, and platelet aggregation time; increased platelet count; increased factors II, VII antigen, VIII antigen, VIII coagulant activity, IX, X, XII, VII-X complex, II-VII-X complex, and beta-thromboglobulin; decreased levels of anti-factor Xa and antithrombin III, decreased antithrombin III activity; increased levels of fibrinogen and fibrinogen activity; increased plasminogen antigen and activity.

Increased thyroid-binding globulin (TBG) leading to increased circulating total thyroid hormone, as measured by protein-bound iodine (PBI), T_4 levels (by column or by radioimmunoassay) or T_3 levels by radioimmunoassay. T_3 resin uptake is decreased, reflecting the elevated TBG. Free T_4 and free T_3 concentrations are unaltered.

Other binding proteins may be elevated in serum, *i.e.,* corticosteroid binding globulin (CBG), sex hormone-binding globulin (SHBG), leading to increased circulating corticosteroids and sex steroids, respectively. Free or biologically active hormone concentrations are unchanged. Other plasma proteins may be increased (angiotensinogen/renin substrate, alpha-1-antitrypsin, ceruloplasmin).

Increased plasma HDL and HDL-2 subfraction concentrations, reduced LDL cholesterol concentration, increased triglycerides levels.

Impaired glucose tolerance.

Reduced response to metyrapone test.

Reduced serum folate concentration.

Carcinogenesis, Mutagenesis, and Impairment of Fertility

Long-term continuous administration of natural and synthetic estrogens in certain animal species increases the frequency of carcinomas of the breast, uterus, (cervix: for the estradiol vaginal ring and cream only), vagina, and liver (see CONTRAINDICATIONS and WARNINGS).

Pregnancy Category X
Estrogens should not be used during pregnancy (see CONTRAINDICATIONS and BOXED WARNING).

Nursing Mothers
As a general principle, administration of any drug to nursing mothers should be done only when clearly necessary since many drugs are excreted in human milk. In addition, estrogen administration to nursing mothers has been shown to decrease the quantity and quality of the milk.

Pediatric Use
Safety and effectiveness in pediatric patients have not been established. Large and repeated doses of estrogen over an extended period of time have been shown to accelerate epiphyseal closure, resulting in short adult stature if treatment is initiated before the completion of physiologic puberty in normally developing children. In patients in whom bone growth is not complete, periodic monitoring of bone maturation and effects on epiphyseal centers is recommended.

Estrogen treatment of prepubertal children also induces premature breast development and vaginal cornification, and may potentially induce vaginal bleeding in girls. In boys, estrogen treatment may modify the normal pubertal process. All other physiological and adverse reactions shown to be associated with estrogen treatment of adults could potentially occur in the pediatric population, including thromboembolic disorders and growth stimulation of certain tumors. Therefore, estrogens should only be administered to pediatric patients when clearly indicated and the lowest effective dose should always be utilized.

VAGINAL RING
General
Use of Progestins
It is common practice with systemic administration of estrogen to add progestin for 10 or more days during a cycle to lower the incidence of endometrial proliferation or hyperplasia. From the available clinical data, it seems unlikely that the estradiol vaginal ring would have adverse effects on the endometrium. Furthermore, addition of progestins to a patient being treated with the estradiol vaginal ring is not expected to result in vaginal bleeding.

Physical Examination
A complete medical and family history should be taken prior to the initiation of any estrogen therapy. The pretreatment and periodic physical examinations should include special reference to blood pressure, breasts, abdomen, and pelvic organs and should include a Papanicolaou smear. As a general rule, estrogen should not be prescribed for longer than 1 year without reexamining the patient.

Uterine Bleeding and Mastodynia
Although uncommon with the estradiol vaginal ring, certain patients may develop undesirable manifestations of estrogenic stimulation, such as abnormal uterine bleeding and mastodynia.

Liver Disease
Estradiol should be used with caution in patients with impaired liver function.

Location of the Estradiol Vaginal Ring
Some women have experienced moving or gliding of the estradiol vaginal ring within the vagina. Instances of the estradiol vaginal ring being expelled from the vagina in connection with moving the bowels, strain, or constipation have been reported. If this occurs, the estradiol vaginal ring can be rinsed in lukewarm water and reinserted into the vagina by the patient.

Vaginal Irritation
The estradiol vaginal ring may not be suitable for women with narrow, short, or stenosed vaginas. Narrow vagina, vaginal stenosis, prolapse, and vaginal infections are conditions that make the vagina more susceptible to estradiol vaginal ring-caused irritation or ulceration. Women with signs or symptoms of vaginal irritation should alert their physician.

Vaginal Infection
Vaginal infection is generally more common in postmenopausal women due to the lack of the normal flora of fertile women, especially lactobacillus, and the subsequent higher pH. Vaginal infections should be treated with appropriate antimicrobial therapy before initiation of the estradiol vaginal ring. If a vaginal infection develops during use of the estradiol vaginal ring, then the estradiol vaginal ring should be removed and reinserted only after the infection has been appropriately treated.

Other
Hypercoagulability and hyperlipidemia have been reported in women on other types of estrogen replacement therapy but, these have not been seen with estradiol vaginal ring patients.

Fluid retention is another known risk factor with estrogen therapy and may be harmful to patients with asthma, epilepsy, migraine, and cardiac or renal dysfunction.

Estradiol vaginal ring treatment has not been associated with any indication of increase in body weight up to 48 weeks of treatment.

Information for the Patient
See the Patient Instructions that are distributed with the prescription for complete instructions.

Advise patients that the number of doses per tube of estradiol vaginal cream will vary with dosage requirements and patient handling.

Drug-Drug and Drug-Laboratory Interactions
It is recommended that the estradiol vaginal ring be removed during treatment with other vaginally administered preparations.

Drug-drug and drug-laboratory interactions have been reported with estrogen administration overall, but were not observed in clinical trials with the estradiol vaginal ring. However, the possibility of the following interactions should be considered when treating patients with the estradiol vaginal ring.

Accelerated prothrombin time, partial thromboplastin time, and platelet aggregation time; increased platelet count; increased factors II, VII antigen, VIII antigen, VIII coagulant activity, IX, X, XII, VII-X complex, II-VII-X complex, and beta-thromboglobulin; decreased levels of anti-factor Xa and antithrombin III, decreased antithrombin III activity; increased levels of fibrinogen and fibrinogen activity; increased plasminogen antigen and activity.

Increased plasma HDL and HDL-2 subfraction concentrations, reduced LDL cholesterol concentration, increased triglycerides levels.

Carcinogenesis, Mutagenesis, and Impairment of Fertility
Long-term continuous administration of natural and synthetic estrogens in certain animal species increases the frequency of carcinomas of the breast, uterus, (cervix: for the estradiol vaginal ring and cream only), vagina, and liver (see CONTRAINDICATIONS and WARNINGS).

Pregnancy Category X
Estrogens should not be used during pregnancy (see CONTRAINDICATIONS and BOXED WARNING).

Nursing Mothers
This product is not intended for nursing mothers. As a general principle, the administration of any drug to nursing mothers should be done only when clearly necessary since many drugs are excreted in human milk. In addition, estrogen administration to nursing mothers has been shown to decrease the quantity and quality of the milk.

VAGINAL TABLETS
General
A complete medical and family history should be taken prior to the initiation of any estrogen therapy. The pretreatment and periodic physical examinations should include special references to blood pressure, breast, abdomen, and pelvic organs, and should include a Papanicolaou smear. As a general rule, estrogens should not be prescribed for longer than 1 year without another physical exam being performed.

Fluid Retention
Because estrogens may cause some degree of fluid retention, conditions which might be influenced by this factor, such as asthma, epilepsy, migraine, and cardiac and renal dysfunction, require careful observation.

Familial Hyperlipoproteinemia
Estrogen therapy may be associated with massive elevations of plasma triglycerides leading to pancreatitis and other complications in patients with familial defects of lipoprotein metabolism.

Certain patients may develop undesirable manifestations of excessive estrogenic stimulation, such as abnormal or excessive uterine bleeding, mastodynia, etc.

Prolonged administration of unopposed estrogen therapy has been reported to increase the risk of endometrial hyperplasia in some patients.

Preexisting uterine leiomyomata may increase in size during estrogen use.

The pathologist should be advised of estrogen therapy when relevant specimens are submitted.

Patients with a history of jaundice during pregnancy have an increased risk of recurrence of jaundice while receiving estrogen-containing oral-contraceptive therapy. If jaundice develops in any patient receiving estrogen, the medication should be discontinued while the cause is investigated.

Estrogens may be poorly metabolized in patients with impaired liver function and should be administered with caution in such patients.

Because estrogens influence the metabolism of calcium and phosphorus, they should be used with caution in patients with metabolic bone diseases that are associated with hypercalcemia or in patients with renal insufficiency.

Because of the effects of estrogens on epiphyseal closure, they should be used judiciously in young patients in whom bone growth is not yet complete.

Insertion of the Estradiol Vaginal Tablet Applicator
Patients with severely atrophic vaginal mucosa should be instructed to exercise care during insertion of the applicator. After gynecological surgery, any vaginal applicator should be used with caution and only if clearly indicated.

Vaginal Infection
Vaginal infection is generally more common in postmenopausal women due to the lack of normal flora seen in fertile women, especially lactobacilla; hence the subsequent higher pH. Vaginal infections should be treated with appropriate antimicrobial therapy before initiation of estradiol vaginal tablet therapy.

Information for the Patient
See the Patient Instructions that are distributed with the prescription for complete instructions.

Advise patients that the number of doses per tube of estradiol vaginal cream will vary with dosage requirements and patient handling.

Drug-Drug and Drug-Laboratory Interactions
Certain endocrine and liver function tests may be affected by estrogen-containing oral contraceptives.

The following similar changes may be expected with larger doses of estrogens:

Increased prothrombin and factors VII, VIII, IX, and X, decreased antithrombin III; increased norepinephrine induced platelet aggregability.

Increased thyroid binding globulin (TBG) leading to increased circulating total thyroid hormone, as measured by PBI, T_4 by column, or T_4 by radioimmunoassay. Free T_4 resin uptake is decreased, reflecting the elevated TBG, free T_4 concentration is unaltered.

Impaired glucose tolerance.

Reduced response to metyrapone test.

Reduced serum folate concentration.

Increased serum triglyceride and phospholipid concentration.

Carcinogenesis, Mutagenesis, and Impairment of Fertility

Long-term continuous administration of natural and synthetic estrogens in certain animal species increases the frequency of carcinomas of the breast, uterus, (cervix: for the estradiol vaginal ring and cream only), vagina, and liver (see CONTRAINDICATIONS and WARNINGS).

E

Pregnancy Category X

Estrogens are not indicated for use during pregnancy or the immediate postpartum period. Estrogens are ineffective for the prevention or treatment of threatened or habitual abortion. Treatment with diethylstilbesterol (DES) during pregnancy has been associated with an increased risk of congenital defects and cancer in the reproductive organs of the fetus, and possibly other birth defects. The use of DES during pregnancy has also been associated with a subsequent increased risk of breast cancer in the mothers.

Nursing Mothers

As a general principle, administration of any drug to nursing mothers should be done only when clearly necessary since many drugs are excreted in human milk. In addition, estrogen administration to nursing mothers has been shown to decrease the quantity and quality of the milk. Estrogens are not indicated for the prevention of postpartum breast engorgement.

Pediatric Use

Safety and effectiveness in pediatric patients have not been established.

Geriatric Use

Clinical studies of estradiol vaginal tablets did not include sufficient numbers of subjects aged 65 and over to determine whether they respond differently from younger subjects. Other reported clinical experience has not identified differences in responses between the elderly and younger patients. In general, dose selection for an elderly patient should be cautious, usually starting at the low end of the dosing range, reflecting the greater frequency of decreased hepatic renal, or cardiac function, and of concomitant disease or other drug therapy.

ADVERSE REACTIONS

VAGINAL CREAM

The following additional adverse reactions have been reported with estrogen therapy (see WARNINGS regarding induction of neoplasia, adverse effects on the fetus, increased incidence of gallbladder disease, cardiovascular disease, elevated blood pressure, and hypercalcemia):

Genitourinary System: Changes in vaginal bleeding pattern and abnormal withdrawal bleeding or flow; breakthrough bleeding, spotting; increase in size of uterine leiomyomata; vaginal candidiasis; change in amount of cervical secretion.

Breasts: Tenderness, enlargement.

Gastrointestinal: Nausea, vomiting; abdominal cramps, bloating; cholestatic jaundice; increased incidence of gallbladder disease.

Skin: Chloasma or melasma which may persist when drug is discontinued; erythema multiforme; erythema nodosum; hemorrhagic eruption; loss of scalp hair; hirsutism.

Eyes: Steepening of corneal curvature; intolerance to contact lenses.

Central Nervous System: Headache, migraine, dizziness; mental depression; chorea.

Miscellaneous: Increase or decrease in weight; reduced carbohydrate tolerance; aggravation of porphyria; edema; changes in libido.

VAGINAL RING

The biological safety of the silicone elastomer has been studied in various *in vitro* and *in vivo* test models. The results show that the silicone elastomer is non-toxic, non-pyrogenic, non-irritating, and non-sensitizing. Long-term implantation induced encapsulation equal to or less than the negative control (polyethylene) used in the USP test. No toxic reaction or tumor formation was observed with the silicone elastomer.

In general, estradiol vaginal ring was well tolerated. In the two pivotal controlled studies, discontinuation of treatment due to an adverse event was required by 5.4% of patients receiving the estradiol vaginal ring and 3.9% of patients receiving conjugated estrogens vaginal cream. The most common reasons for withdrawal from estradiol vaginal ring treatment due to an adverse event were vaginal discomfort and gastrointestinal symptoms.

The adverse events reported with a frequency of 3% or greater in the two pivotal controlled studies by patients receiving the estradiol vaginal ring or conjugated estrogens vaginal cream are listed in TABLE 9.

Other adverse events (listed alphabetically) occurring at a frequency of 1-3% in the two pivotal controlled studies by patients receiving the estradiol vaginal ring include: Anxiety, bronchitis, chest pain, cystitis, dermatitis, diarrhea, dyspepsia, dysuria, flatulence, gastritis, genital eruption, genital pruritus, hemorrhoids, leg edema, migraine, otitis media, skin hypertrophy, syncope, toothache, tooth disorder, urinary incontinence.

The following additional adverse events were reported at least once by patients receiving the estradiol vaginal ring in the worldwide clinical program, which includes controlled and uncontrolled studies. A causal relationship with the estradiol vaginal ring has not been established:

Body as a Whole: Allergic reaction.

TABLE 9 *Adverse Events Reported by 3% or More of Patients Receiving Either the Estradiol Vaginal Ring or Conjugated Estrogens Vaginal Cream in Two Pivotal Controlled Studies*

Adverse Event	Estradiol Vaginal Ring (n=257)	Conjugated Estrogens Vaginal Cream (n=129)
Musculoskeletal		
Back pain	6%	8%
Arthritis	4%	2%
Arthralgia	3%	5%
Skeletal pain	2%	4%
CNS/Peripheral Nervous System		
Headache	13%	16%
Psychiatric		
Insomnia	4%	0%
Gastrointestinal		
Abdominal pain	4%	2%
Nausea	3%	2%
Respiratory		
Upper respiratory tract infection	5%	6%
Sinusitis	4%	3%
Pharyngitis	1%	3%
Urinary		
Urinary tract infection	2%	7%
Female Reproductive		
Leukorrhea	7%	3%
Vaginitis	5%	2%
Vaginal discomfort/pain	5%	5%
Vaginal hemorrhage	4%	5%
Asymptomatic genital bacterial growth	4%	6%
Breast pain	1%	7%
Resistance Mechanisms		
Genital moniliasis	6%	7%
Body as a Whole		
Flu-like symptoms	3%	2%
Hot flushes	2%	3%
Allergy	1%	4%
Miscellaneous		
Family stress	2%	3%

CNS/Peripheral Nervous System: Dizziness.

Gastrointestinal: Enlarged abdomen, vomiting.

Metabolic/Nutritional Disorders: Weight decrease or increase.

Psychiatric: Depression, decreased libido, nervousness.

Reproductive: Breast engorgement, breast enlargement, intermenstrual bleeding, genital edema, vulval disorder.

Skin/Appendages: Pruritus, pruritus ani.

Urinary: Micturition frequency, urethral disorder.

Vascular: Thrombophlebitis.

Vision: Abnormal vision.

VAGINAL TABLETS

Adverse events that generally have been mild: Vaginal spotting, vaginal discharge, allergic reaction, and skin rash. Adverse events with an incidence of 5% or greater are reported for two comparative trials. Data for patients receiving either estradiol vaginal tablets or placebo in the double blind study are listed in TABLE 10, and data for patients receiving estradiol vaginal tablets in the open label comparator study are listed in TABLE 11.

TABLE 10 *Adverse Events Reported in 5% or Greater Number of Patients Receiving Estradiol Vaginal Tablets in the Placebo Controlled Trial*

Adverse Event	Estradiol Vaginal Tablets (n=91)	Placebo (n=47)
Headache	9%	6%
Abdominal pain	7%	4%
Upper respiratory tract infection	5%	4%
Moniliasis genital	5%	2%
Back pain	7%	6%

TABLE 11 *Adverse Events Reported in 5% or Greater Number of Patients Receiving Estradiol Vaginal Tablets in the Open Label Study*

Adverse Event	Estradiol (n=80)
Pruritus genital	6%
Headache	10%
Upper respiratory tract infection	11%

Other adverse events that occurred in 3-5% of estradiol vaginal tablet subjects included: Allergy, bronchitis, dyspepsia, haematuria, hot flashes, insomnia, pain, sinusitis, vaginal discomfort, vaginitis. A causal relationship to estradiol vaginal tablets has not been established.

DOSAGE AND ADMINISTRATION

VAGINAL CREAM

For treatment of vulval and vaginal atrophy associated with the menopause, the lowest dose and regimen that will control symptoms should be chosen and medication should be discontinued as promptly as possible.

Attempts to discontinue or taper medication should be made at 3-6 month intervals.

Usual Dosage

The usual dosage range is 2-4 g (marked on the applicator) daily for 1 or 2 weeks, then gradually reduced to ½ initial dosage for a similar period. A maintenance dosage of 1 g, 1-3 times a week, may be used after restoration of the vaginal mucosa has been achieved.

Note: The number of doses per tube will vary with dosage requirements and patient handling.

Patients with intact uteri should be monitored closely for signs of endometrial cancer and appropriate diagnostic measures should be taken to rule out malignancy in the event of persistent or recurring abnormal vaginal bleeding.

VAGINAL RING

One (1) estradiol vaginal ring is to be inserted as deeply as possible into the upper one-third of the vaginal vault. The ring is to remain in place continuously for 3 months, after which it is to be removed and, if appropriate, replaced by a new ring. The need to continue treatment should be assessed at 3 or 6 month intervals.

Should the ring be removed or fall out at any time during the 90 day treatment period, the ring should be rinsed in lukewarm water and re-inserted by the patient, or, if necessary, by a physician or nurse.

Retention of the ring for greater than 90 days does not represent overdosage but will result in progressively greater underdosage with the attendant risk of loss of efficacy and increasing risk of vaginal infections and/or erosions.

VAGINAL TABLETS

The estradiol vaginal tablet is gently inserted into the vagina as far as it can comfortably go without force, using the supplied applicator.

Initial Dose: One (1) estradiol vaginal tablet, inserted vaginally, once daily for 2 weeks. It is advisable to have the patient administer treatment at the same time each day.

Maintenance Dose: One (1) estradiol vaginal tablet, inserted vaginally, twice weekly.

The need to continue therapy should be assessed by the physician with the patient. Attempts to discontinue or taper medication should be made at 3-6 month intervals.

HOW SUPPLIED

ESTRACE VAGINAL CREAM

Storage: Store at room temperature. Protect from temperatures in excess of 40°C (104°F).

ESTRING VAGINAL RING

Each Estring is individually packaged in a heat-sealed rectangular pouch consisting of three layers, from outside to inside: polyester, aluminum foil, and low density polyethylene, respectively. The pouch is provided with a tear-off notch on one side.

Storage: Store at controlled room temperature 15-30°C (59-86°F).

VAGIFEM VAGINAL TABLETS

Storage: Store at 25°C (77°F); excursions permitted to 15-30°C (59-86°F).

PRODUCT LISTING - RATED THERAPEUTICALLY EQUIVALENT

Size	Price	Product	NDC
Film, Extended Release - Transdermal - 0.05 mg/24 Hours Weekly			
4's	$26.25	GENERIC, Mylan Pharmaceuticals Inc	00378-3350-99
4's	$27.25	CLIMARA, Allscripts Pharmaceutical Company	54569-4711-00
4's	$33.63	CLIMARA, Berlex Laboratories	50419-0451-04
Film, Extended Release - Transdermal - 0.1 mg/24 Hours Weekly			
4's	$26.25	GENERIC, Mylan Pharmaceuticals Inc	00378-3352-99
4's	$28.69	CLIMARA, Allscripts Pharmaceutical Company	54569-4367-01
4's	$33.63	CLIMARA, Berlex Laboratories	50419-0452-04
24's	$153.00	CLIMARA, Allscripts Pharmaceutical Company	54569-4367-00
Solution - Intramuscular - Cypionate 5 mg/ml			
5 ml	$20.30	DEPO-ESTRADIOL, Allscripts Pharmaceutical Company	54569-2580-00
5 ml	$27.90	DEPO-ESTRADIOL, Pharmacia and Upjohn	00009-0271-01
10 ml	$5.50	GENERIC, Keene Pharmaceuticals Inc	00588-5017-70
10 ml	$6.50	GENERIC, Roberts/Hauck Pharmaceutical Corporation	43797-0110-12
10 ml	$7.44	GENERIC, Pasadena Research Laboratories Inc	00418-6541-41
10 ml	$7.59	GENERIC, Moore, H.L. Drug Exchange Inc	00839-5575-30
10 ml	$8.00	GENERIC, Bolan Pharmaceutical Inc	44437-0254-10
10 ml	$8.25	GENERIC, Interstate Drug Exchange Inc	00814-3020-40
10 ml	$8.50	GENERIC, Cmc-Consolidated Midland Corporation	00223-7602-10
10 ml	$9.40	GENERIC, Hyrex Pharmaceuticals	00314-0855-70
10 ml	$10.00	GENERIC, Ivax Corporation	00182-0662-63
10 ml	$10.00	GENERIC, Forest Pharmaceuticals	00456-1021-10
10 ml	$14.00	GENERIC, Clint Pharmaceutical Inc	55553-0254-10
10 ml	$15.52	GENERIC, Compumed Pharmaceuticals	00403-2862-18
10 ml	$15.52	GENERIC, Allscripts Pharmaceutical Company	54569-3009-00
Solution - Intramuscular - Valerate 10 mg/ml			
5 ml	$34.70	DELESTROGEN, Bristol-Myers Squibb	00003-0330-52
5 ml	$60.43	DELESTROGEN, Bristol-Myers Squibb	00003-0330-50
10 ml	$6.25	GENERIC, Med Tek Pharmaceuticals Inc	52349-0105-10
10 ml	$6.50	GENERIC, Roberts/Hauck Pharmaceutical Corporation	43797-0011-12
10 ml	$6.95	GENERIC, Cmc-Consolidated Midland Corporation	00223-7605-10
10 ml	$7.45	GENERIC, Major Pharmaceuticals Inc	00904-2909-10
Solution - Intramuscular - Valerate 20 mg/ml			
5 ml	$80.31	DELESTROGEN, Bristol-Myers Squibb	00003-0343-50
10 ml	$7.50	GENERIC, Keene Pharmaceuticals Inc	00588-5012-70
10 ml	$8.95	GENERIC, Major Pharmaceuticals Inc	00904-2910-10
10 ml	$9.95	GENERIC, Roberts/Hauck Pharmaceutical Corporation	43797-0012-12
10 ml	$10.75	GENERIC, Compumed Pharmaceuticals	00403-0651-18
10 ml	$13.95	GENERIC, Cmc-Consolidated Midland Corporation	00223-7606-10
10 ml	$14.25	GENERIC, Pasadena Research Laboratories Inc	00418-0451-41
10 ml	$14.25	GENERIC, Forest Pharmaceuticals	00456-0784-10
10 ml	$15.66	GENERIC, Hyrex Pharmaceuticals	00314-0782-70
10 ml	$19.40	GENERIC, Ivax Corporation	00182-1805-63
10 ml	$45.68	GENERIC, Allscripts Pharmaceutical Company	54569-1852-01
Solution - Intramuscular - Valerate 40 mg/ml			
5 ml	$114.40	DELESTROGEN, Allscripts Pharmaceutical Company	54569-1394-00
5 ml	$141.25	DELESTROGEN, Bristol-Myers Squibb	00003-0251-50
5 ml x 10	$797.75	DELESTROGEN, Bristol-Myers Squibb	00003-0251-51
10 ml	$10.50	GENERIC, Keene Pharmaceuticals Inc	00588-5014-70
10 ml	$12.60	GENERIC, Major Pharmaceuticals Inc	00904-2911-10
10 ml	$12.95	GENERIC, Roberts/Hauck Pharmaceutical Corporation	43797-0013-12
10 ml	$14.25	GENERIC, Pasadena Research Laboratories Inc	00418-0461-41
10 ml	$14.93	GENERIC, Interstate Drug Exchange Inc	00814-3035-40
10 ml	$16.95	GENERIC, Cmc-Consolidated Midland Corporation	00223-7607-10
10 ml	$18.00	GENERIC, Bolan Pharmaceutical Inc	44437-0444-70
10 ml	$23.94	GENERIC, Primedics Laboratories	00684-0132-10
10 ml	$26.14	GENERIC, Hyrex Pharmaceuticals	00314-0784-70
10 ml	$75.79	GENERIC, Allscripts Pharmaceutical Company	54569-3007-00
Tablet - Oral - 0.5 mg			
100's	$17.91	FEDERAL UPPER LIMIT, H.C.F.A. F F P	99999-1188-01
100's	$22.81	GENERIC, Moore, H.L. Drug Exchange Inc	00839-8076-06
100's	$22.81	GENERIC, Major Pharmaceuticals Inc	00904-5177-60
100's	$23.05	GENERIC, Caremark Inc	00339-6073-12
100's	$23.27	GENERIC, Martec Pharmaceuticals Inc	52555-0649-01
100's	$23.96	GENERIC, Geneva Pharmaceuticals	00781-1897-01
100's	$23.98	GENERIC, Ivax Corporation	00182-2648-01
100's	$24.35	GENERIC, Barr Laboratories Inc	00555-0899-02
100's	$24.38	GENERIC, Watson Laboratories Inc	52544-0528-01
100's	$24.60	GENERIC, Martec Pharmaceuticals Inc	52555-0716-01
100's	$24.75	GENERIC, Duramed Pharmaceuticals Inc	51285-0501-02
100's	$25.50	GENERIC, Mylan Pharmaceuticals Inc	00378-1452-01
100's	$25.50	GENERIC, Watson Laboratories Inc	00591-0528-01
100's	$25.50	GENERIC, Esi Lederle Generics	59911-5879-02
100's	$27.34	GENERIC, Fielding Company	00421-0768-01
Tablet - Oral - 1 mg			
30's	$13.23	ESTRACE, Allscripts Pharmaceutical Company	54569-0802-01
30's	$26.16	ESTRACE, Pd-Rx Pharmaceuticals	55289-0101-30
50's	$46.61	ESTRACE, Pd-Rx Pharmaceuticals	55289-0101-50
90's	$30.74	ESTRACE, Allscripts Pharmaceutical Company	54569-8528-00
100's	$19.32	FEDERAL UPPER LIMIT, H.C.F.A. F F P	99999-1188-02
100's	$30.27	GENERIC, Qualitest Products Inc	00603-3557-21
100's	$30.39	GENERIC, Moore, H.L. Drug Exchange Inc	00839-8077-06
100's	$30.39	GENERIC, Major Pharmaceuticals Inc	00904-5178-60
100's	$31.00	GENERIC, Martec Pharmaceuticals Inc	52555-0650-01
100's	$31.92	GENERIC, Geneva Pharmaceuticals	00781-1898-01
100's	$31.95	GENERIC, Ivax Corporation	00182-2649-01
100's	$32.47	GENERIC, Barr Laboratories Inc	00555-0886-02
100's	$32.88	GENERIC, Caremark Inc	00339-6074-12
100's	$33.00	GENERIC, Martec Pharmaceuticals Inc	52555-0717-01
100's	$33.60	GENERIC, Duramed Pharmaceuticals Inc	51285-0502-02
100's	$34.50	GENERIC, Mylan Pharmaceuticals Inc	00378-1454-01
100's	$34.50	GENERIC, Watson Laboratories Inc	00591-0487-01
100's	$34.50	GENERIC, Watson Laboratories Inc	52544-0487-01
100's	$34.50	GENERIC, Esi Lederle Generics	59911-5880-02
100's	$36.69	GENERIC, Fielding Company	00421-1259-01
100's	$36.69	GENERIC, Fielding Company	66500-0259-01
100's	$64.01	ESTRACE, Bristol-Myers Squibb	00087-0755-01
Tablet - Oral - 1.5 mg			
100's	$50.83	GENERIC, Fielding Company	00421-0158-01
Tablet - Oral - 2 mg			
30's	$32.10	ESTRACE, Pd-Rx Pharmaceuticals	55289-0396-30
90's	$44.87	ESTRACE, Allscripts Pharmaceutical Company	54569-8577-00
100's	$30.60	FEDERAL UPPER LIMIT, H.C.F.A. F F P	99999-1188-03
100's	$44.38	GENERIC, Moore, H.L. Drug Exchange Inc	00839-8078-06
100's	$44.38	GENERIC, Major Pharmaceuticals Inc	00904-5179-60
100's	$45.27	GENERIC, Martec Pharmaceuticals Inc	52555-0651-01
100's	$46.62	GENERIC, Geneva Pharmaceuticals	00781-1899-01
100's	$46.65	GENERIC, Ivax Corporation	00182-2650-01
100's	$47.45	GENERIC, Barr Laboratories Inc	00555-0887-02
100's	$47.66	GENERIC, Caremark Inc	00339-6075-12
100's	$48.25	GENERIC, Duramed Pharmaceuticals Inc	51285-0504-02
100's	$48.27	GENERIC, Martec Pharmaceuticals Inc	52555-0718-01
100's	$49.50	GENERIC, Mylan Pharmaceuticals Inc	00378-1458-01
100's	$49.50	GENERIC, Watson Laboratories Inc	00591-0488-01
100's	$49.50	GENERIC, Watson Laboratories Inc	52544-0488-01
100's	$49.50	GENERIC, Esi Lederle Generics	59911-5882-02

100's	$53.25	GENERIC, Fielding Company	00421-0748-01
100's	$93.48	ESTRACE, Bristol-Myers Squibb	00087-0756-01

PRODUCT LISTING - RATED NOT THERAPEUTICALLY EQUIVALENT

Film, Extended Release - Transdermal - 0.025 mg/24 Hours Twice Weekly

8's	$30.83	ESCLIM, Women First Healthcare	64248-0310-01

Film, Extended Release - Transdermal - 0.025 mg/24 Hours Weekly

4's	$33.63	CLIMARA, Berlex Laboratories	50419-0454-04

Film, Extended Release - Transdermal - 0.0375 mg/24 Hours Twice Weekly

8 x 3	$96.03	VIVELLE-DOT, Novartis Pharmaceuticals	00078-0343-45
8 x 6	$192.06	VIVELLE, Novartis Pharmaceuticals	00083-2325-62
8's	$25.68	VIVELLE-DOT, Novartis Pharmaceuticals	00078-0343-42
8's	$31.13	ESCLIM, Women First Healthcare	64248-0320-01
8's	$32.01	VIVELLE, Novartis Pharmaceuticals	00083-2325-08

Film, Extended Release - Transdermal - 0.05 mg/24 Hours Twice Weekly

8 x 3	$94.90	ALORA, Watson/Rugby Laboratories Inc	52544-0471-23
8 x 3	$97.83	VIVELLE-DOT, Novartis Pharmaceuticals	00078-0344-45
8 x 6	$204.90	ESTRADERM, Novartis Pharmaceuticals	00083-2310-62
8's	$18.38	ESTRADERM, Novartis Pharmaceuticals	00083-2310-08
8's	$20.64	ESTRADERM, Southwood Pharmaceuticals Inc	58016-3182-01
8's	$20.66	ALORA, Procter and Gamble Pharmaceuticals	00149-0491-04
8's	$24.60	VIVELLE, Physicians Total Care	54868-3795-00
8's	$25.58	ESTRADERM, Allscripts Pharmaceutical Company	54569-0804-00
8's	$26.16	VIVELLE-DOT, Novartis Pharmaceuticals	00078-0344-42
8's	$31.73	ESCLIM, Women First Healthcare	64248-0330-01
8's	$32.61	VIVELLE, Novartis Pharmaceuticals	00083-2326-08
8's	$32.61	ALORA, Watson Laboratories Inc	52544-0471-08
8's	$195.66	VIVELLE, Novartis Pharmaceuticals	00083-2326-62

Film, Extended Release - Transdermal - 0.075 mg/24 Hours Twice Weekly

8 x 3	$99.90	VIVELLE-DOT, Novartis Pharmaceuticals	00078-0345-45
8 x 6	$199.80	VIVELLE, Novartis Pharmaceuticals	00083-2327-62
8's	$25.08	VIVELLE, Physicians Total Care	54868-3797-00
8's	$26.72	VIVELLE-DOT, Novartis Pharmaceuticals	00078-0345-42
8's	$32.31	GENERIC, Women First Healthcare	64248-0340-01
8's	$33.30	VIVELLE, Novartis Pharmaceuticals	00083-2327-08
8's	$33.30	ALORA, Watson Laboratories Inc	52544-0472-08

Film, Extended Release - Transdermal - 0.075 mg/24 Hours Weekly

4's	$33.63	CLIMARA, Berlex Laboratories	50419-0453-04

Film, Extended Release - Transdermal - 0.1 mg/24 Hours Twice Weekly

8 x 3	$102.00	VIVELLE-DOT, Novartis Pharmaceuticals	00078-0346-45
8 x 6	$204.00	VIVELLE, Novartis Pharmaceuticals	00083-2328-62
8 x 6	$219.60	ESTRADERM, Novartis Pharmaceuticals	00083-2320-62
8's	$20.04	ESTRADERM, Novartis Pharmaceuticals	00083-2320-08
8's	$25.56	VIVELLE, Physicians Total Care	54868-3796-00
8's	$27.28	VIVELLE-DOT, Novartis Pharmaceuticals	00078-0346-42
8's	$32.31	ESCLIM, Women First Healthcare	64248-0350-01
8's	$34.00	VIVELLE, Novartis Pharmaceuticals	00083-2328-08
8's	$34.00	ALORA, Watson Laboratories Inc	52544-0473-08

PRODUCT LISTING - EQUIVALENTS NOT AVAILABLE

Cream - Vaginal - 0.1 mg/Gm

12 gm x 4	$87.32	ESTRACE VAGINAL CREAM, Bristol-Myers Squibb	00087-0754-15
12 gm x 4	$87.36	ESTRACE VAGINAL CREAM, Warner Chilcott Laboratories	00430-3754-11
42.50 gm	$39.49	ESTRACE VAGINAL CREAM, Prescript Pharmaceuticals	00247-0244-85
42.50 gm	$44.19	ESTRACE VAGINAL CREAM, Bristol-Myers Squibb	00087-0754-03
42.50 gm	$44.19	ESTRACE VAGINAL CREAM, Bristol-Myers Squibb	00087-0754-42
42.50 gm	$57.34	ESTRACE VAGINAL CREAM, Warner Chilcott Laboratories	00430-3754-14

Film, Extended Release - Transdermal - 0.025 mg/24 Hours Twice Weekly

1's	$3.35	VIVELLE, Novartis Pharmaceuticals	00078-0348-62
8 x 3	$95.25	VIVELLE-DOT, Novartis Pharmaceuticals	00078-0365-45
8 x 6	$190.56	VIVELLE, Novartis Pharmaceuticals	00078-0348-44
8's	$30.49	VIVELLE-DOT, Novartis Pharmaceuticals	00078-0365-42
8's	$31.76	VIVELLE, Novartis Pharmaceuticals	00078-0348-42

Ring - Vaginal - 2 mg

1's	$108.60	ESTRING, Pharmacia and Upjohn	00013-2150-36

Solution - Intramuscular - Cypionate 5 mg/ml

10 ml	$8.98	GENERIC, Hauser, A.F. Inc	52637-0332-10

Solution - Intramuscular - Valerate 10 mg/ml

5 ml	$60.43	DELESTROGEN, Monarch Pharmaceuticals Inc	61570-0180-01

Solution - Intramuscular - Valerate 20 mg/ml

5 ml	$85.14	DELESTROGEN, Monarch Pharmaceuticals Inc	61570-0181-01
5 ml x 10	$480.70	DELESTROGEN, Bristol-Myers Squibb	00003-0343-51
10 ml	$29.95	MENAVAL-20, Legere Pharmaceuticals	25332-0117-10

Solution - Intramuscular - Valerate 40 mg/ml

10 ml	$29.75	CLINAGEN LA 40, Clint Pharmaceutical Inc	55553-0244-10

Tablet - Oral - 0.5 mg

100's	$25.40	GENERIC, Apothecon Inc	59772-0025-03
100's	$48.04	ESTRACE, Bristol-Myers Squibb	00087-0021-41

Tablet - Oral - 1 mg

30's	$8.12	GENERIC, Prescript Pharmaceuticals	00247-0242-30
30's	$10.35	GENERIC, Allscripts Pharmaceutical Company	54569-4907-00
100's	$34.25	GENERIC, Apothecon Inc	59772-0026-03

Tablet - Oral - 1.5 mg

100's	$50.83	GENERIC, Fielding Company	66500-0158-01

Tablet - Oral - 2 mg

21's	$8.64	GENERIC, Prescript Pharmaceuticals	00247-0243-21
30's	$10.89	GENERIC, Prescript Pharmaceuticals	00247-0243-30
30's	$14.85	GENERIC, Allscripts Pharmaceutical Company	54569-4908-00
100's	$49.10	GENERIC, Apothecon Inc	59772-0027-03
100's	$49.95	GENERIC, Pharma Pac	52959-0323-00

Tablet - Vaginal - 25 mcg

8's	$22.90	VAGIFEM, Pharmacia and Upjohn	00009-5173-03
15's	$39.11	VAGIFEM, Pharmacia and Upjohn	00009-5173-02
18's	$51.55	VAGIFEM, Pharmacia and Upjohn	00009-5173-04

Estradiol Acetate *(003593)*

Categories: Atrophy, vaginal; Atrophy, vulvar; Menopause; Pregnancy Category X; FDA Approved 2003 Mar
Drug Classes: Estrogens; Hormones/hormone modifiers
Brand Names: Femring
Cost of Therapy: $95.63 (Menopause; Femring; 0.05 mg/24 hr; 1 ring; 90 day supply)

WARNING

ESTROGENS INCREASE THE RISK OF ENDOMETRIAL CANCER

Close clinical surveillance of all women taking estrogens is important. Adequate diagnostic measures, including endometrial sampling when indicated, should be undertaken to rule out malignancy in all cases of undiagnosed persistent or recurring abnormal vaginal bleeding. There is no evidence that the use of "natural" estrogens results in a different endometrial risk profile than synthetic estrogens at equivalent estrogen doses.

CARDIOVASCULAR AND OTHER RISKS

Estrogens with and without progestins should not be used for the prevention of cardiovascular disease.

The Women's Health Initiative (WHI) study reported increased risks of myocardial infarction, stroke, invasive breast cancer, pulmonary emboli, and deep vein thrombosis in postmenopausal women during 5 years of treatment with conjugated equine estrogens (0.625 mg) combined with medroxyprogesterone acetate (2.5 mg) relative to placebo. Other doses of conjugated estrogens with medroxyprogesterone acetate, and other combinations of estrogens and progestins were not studied in the WHI and, in the absence of comparable data, these risks should be assumed to be similar. Because of these risks, estrogens with or without progestins should be prescribed at the lowest effective doses and for the shortest duration consistent with treatment goals and risks for the individual woman.

DESCRIPTION

Femring (estradiol acetate vaginal ring) is an off-white, soft, flexible ring with a central core containing estradiol acetate.

Femring is made of cured silicone elastomer composed of dimethyl polysiloxane silanol, silica (diatomaceous earth), normal propyl orthosilicate, stannous octoate; barium sulfate and estradiol acetate. The rings have the following dimensions: outer diameter 56 mm, cross-sectional diameter 7.6 mm, core diameter 2 mm.

Femring is available in 2 strengths: Femring 0.05 mg/day has a central core that contains 12.4 mg of estradiol acetate, which releases at a rate equivalent to 0.05 mg of estradiol per day for 3 months. Femring 0.10 mg/day has a central core that contains 24.8 mg of estradiol acetate, which releases at a rate equivalent to 0.10 mg of estradiol per day for 3 months.

Estradiol acetate is chemically described as estra-1,3,5(10)-triene-3,17β-diol-3-acetate. The molecular formula of estradiol acetate is $C_{20}H_{26}O_3$.

The molecular weight of estradiol acetate is 314.41.

CLINICAL PHARMACOLOGY

Endogenous estrogens are largely responsible for the development and maintenance of the female reproductive systems and secondary sexual characteristics. Although circulating estrogens exist in a dynamic equilibrium of metabolic interconversions, estradiol is the principal intracellular human estrogen and is substantially more potent than its metabolites, estrone and estriol, at the receptor level. The primary source of estrogen in normally cycling adult women is the ovarian follicle, which secretes 70-500 µg of estradiol daily, depending on the phase of the menstrual cycle. After menopause, most endogenous estrogen is produced by conversions of androstendione, secreted by the adrenal cortex, to estrone by peripheral tissues. Thus, estrone and the sulfate conjugated form, estrone sulfate, are the most abundant circulating estrogens in postmenopausal women.

Estrogens act through binding to nuclear receptors in estrogen-responsive tissues. To date, two estrogen receptors have been identified. These vary in proportion from tissue to tissue.

Circulating estrogens modulate the pituitary secretion of the gonadotropins, luteinizing hormone (LH) and follicle stimulating hormone (FSH) through a negative feedback mechanism. Estrogens act to reduce the elevated levels of these gonadotropins seen in postmenopausal women.

PHARMACOKINETICS

Estradiol acetate is rapidly hydrolyzed to estradiol.

Absorption

Drug delivery from estradiol acetate vaginal ring is rapid for the first hour and then declines to a relatively constant rate for the remainder of the 3 month dosing interval. *In vitro* studies have shown that this initial release is higher as the rings age upon storage. Estradiol acetate and estradiol are rapidly absorbed through the vaginal mucosa as evidenced by T_{max} values for estradiol of less than 1 hour. Following C_{max}, serum estradiol concentrations decrease rapidly such that by 24-48 hours postdose, serum estradiol concentrations are relatively constant through the end of the 3 month dosing interval.

Following administration of estradiol acetate vaginal ring (0.05 mg/day estradiol), average serum estradiol concentration was 40.6 pg/ml; the corresponding apparent *in vivo* estradiol delivery rate was 0.052 mg/day. Following administration of estradiol acetate vaginal ring (0.10 mg/day estradiol), average serum estradiol concentration was 76 pg/ml; apparent *in vivo* delivery rate was 0.097 mg/day. Results are summarized in TABLE 1 below.

***TABLE 1** Summary of Mean (% RSD)* Pharmacokinetic Parameters for Estradiol Acetate*

Dose (as Estradiol)	n	C_{max} (pg/ml)	T_{max} (h)	C_{avg} (pg/ml)
		0.05 mg/day		
Estradiol†	25	1129 (25)	0.9 (41)	40.6 (26)
Estrone†	25	141 (25)	6.2 (84)	35.9 (21)
Estrone sulfate†	25	2365 (44)	9.3 (39)	494.6 (48)
		0.10 mg/day		
Estradiol‡	12	1665 (23)	0.7 (90)	—
Estradiol§	11	—	—	76.0 (24)
Estrone§	11	—	—	45.7 (25)

* Relative Standard Deviation
† Study 1
‡ Study 2
§ Study 3
— Not determined

Consistent with the avoidance of first pass metabolism achieved by vaginal estradiol administration, serum estradiol concentrations were slightly higher than estrone concentrations.

Distribution

The distribution of exogenous estrogens is similar to that of endogenous estrogens. Estrogens are widely distributed in the body and are generally found in higher concentrations in the sex hormone target organs. Estrogens circulate in blood largely bound to sex hormone binding globulin (SHBG) and albumin.

Metabolism

Exogenous estrogens are metabolized in the same manner as endogenous estrogens. Circulating estrogens exist in a dynamic equilibrium of metabolic interconversions. These transformations take place mainly in the liver. Estradiol is converted reversibly to estrone, and both can be converted to estriol, which is the major urinary metabolite. Estrogens also undergo enterohepatic recirculation via sulfate and glucuronide conjugation in the liver, biliary secretion of conjugates into the intestine, and hydrolysis in the gut followed by reabsorption. In postmenopausal women, a significant portion of the circulating estrogens exist as sulfate conjugates, especially estrone sulfate, which serves as a circulating reservoir for the formation of more active estrogens.

Excretion

Estradiol, estrone, and estriol are excreted in the urine along with glucuronide and sulfate conjugates.

SPECIAL POPULATIONS

No pharmacokinetic studies were conducted in special populations, including patients with renal or hepatic impairment.

DRUG INTERACTIONS

In vitro and *in vivo* studies have shown that estrogens are metabolized partially by cytochrome P450 3A4 (CYP3A4). Therefore, inducers or inhibitors of CYP3A4 may affect estrogen drug metabolism. Inducers of CYP3A4 such as St. John's Wort preparations (Hypericum perforatum), phenobarbital, carbamazepine and rifampin may reduce plasma concentrations of estrogens, possibly resulting in a decrease in therapeutic effects and/or changes in the uterine bleeding profile. Inhibitors of CYP3A4 such as erythromycin, clarithromycin, ketoconazole, itraconazole, ritonavir and grapefruit juice may increase plasma concentrations of estrogens and may result in side effects.

INDICATIONS AND USAGE

Estradiol acetate vaginal ring therapy is indicated in the:

- Treatment of moderate to severe vasomotor symptoms associated with the menopause.
- Treatment of moderate to severe symptoms of vulvar and vaginal atrophy associated with the menopause. When prescribing solely for the treatment of symptoms of vulvar and vaginal atrophy, other vaginal products should be considered.

CONTRAINDICATIONS

Estrogens should not be used in individuals with any of the following conditions:

- Undiagnosed abnormal genital bleeding.
- Known, suspected, or history of cancer of the breast except in appropriately selected patients being treated for metastatic disease.
- Known or suspected estrogen-dependent neoplasia.
- Active deep vein thrombosis, pulmonary embolism or a history of these conditions.
- Active or recent (*e.g.*, within the past year) arterial thromboembolic disease (*e.g.*, stroke, myocardial infarction).
- Estradiol acetate vaginal ring should not be used in patients with known hypersensitivity to any of its components.
- Known or suspected pregnancy. There is no indication for estradiol acetate vaginal ring in pregnancy. There appears to be little or no increased risk of birth defects in women who have used estrogens and progestins from oral contraceptives inadvertently during early pregnancy. (See PRECAUTIONS.)

WARNINGS

See BOXED WARNING.

The use of unopposed estrogens in women who have a uterus is associated with an increased risk of endometrial cancer.

CARDIOVASCULAR DISORDERS

Estrogen and estrogen/progestin therapy have been associated with an increased risk of cardiovascular events such as myocardial infarction and stroke, as well as venous thrombosis and pulmonary embolism (venous thromboembolism or VTE). Should any of these occur or be suspected, estrogens should be discontinued immediately.

Risk factors for cardiovascular disease (*e.g.*, hypertension, diabetes mellitus, tobacco use, hypercholesterolemia and obesity) should be managed appropriately.

Coronary Heart Disease and Stroke

In the Women's Health Initiative study (WHI), an increase in the number of myocardial infarctions and stroke has been observed in women receiving CE compared to placebo. These observations are preliminary and the study is continuing.

In the CE/MPA substudy of WHI, an increased risk of coronary heart disease (CHD) events (defined as nonfatal myocardial infarction and CHD death) was observed in women receiving CE/MPA compared to women receiving placebo (37 vs 30 per 10,000 person-years). The increase in risk was observed in Year 1 and persisted.

In the same substudy of WHI, an increased risk of stroke was observed in women receiving CE/MPA compared to women receiving placebo (29 vs 21 per 10,000 person-years). The increase in risk was observed after the first year and persisted.

In postmenopausal women with documented heart disease (n=2763, average age 66.7 years) a controlled, clinical trial of secondary prevention of cardiovascular disease (Heart and Estrogen/progestin Replacement Study; HERS), treatment with CE/MPA (0.625 mg/2.5 mg per day) demonstrated no benefit. During an average follow-up of 4.1 years, treatment with CE/MPA did not reduce the overall rate of CHD events in postmenopausal women with established coronary heart disease. There were more CHD events in the CE/MPAtreated group than in the placebo group in Year 1 but not during the subsequent years. Two thousand three hundred and twenty one (2321) women from the original HERS trial agreed to participate in an open label extension of HERS, HERS II. Average follow-up in HERS II was an additional 2.7 years, for a total of 6.8 years overall. Rates of CHD events were comparable among women in the CE/MPA group and the placebo group in HERS, HERS II and overall.

Large doses of estrogen (5 mg conjugated estrogens per day), comparable to those used to treat cancer of the prostate and breast, have been shown in a large prospective clinical trial in men to increase the risks of nonfatal myocardial infarction, pulmonary embolism and thrombophlebitis.

Venous Thromboembolism (VTE)

In the Women's Health Initiative study (WHI), an increase in VTE has been observed in women receiving CE compared to placebo. These observations are preliminary and the study is continuing.

In the CE/MPA substudy of WHI, a 2-fold greater rate of VTE, including deep venous thrombosis and pulmonary embolism, was observed in women receiving CE/MPA compared to women receiving placebo. The rate of VTE was 34 per 10,000 woman-years in the CE/MPA group compared to 16 per 10,000 woman-years in the placebo group. The increase in VTE risk was observed during the first year and persisted.

If feasible, estrogens should be discontinued at least 4-6 weeks before surgery of the type associated with an increased risk of thromboembolism or during periods of prolonged immobilization.

MALIGNANT NEOPLASMS

Endometrial Cancer

The use of unopposed estrogens in women with intact uteri has been associated with an increased risk of endometrial cancer. The reported endometrial cancer risk among unopposed estrogen users is about 2- to 12- fold greater than in nonusers, and appears dependent on duration of treatment and on estrogen dose. Most studies show no significant increased risk associated with use of estrogens for less than 1 year. The greatest risk appears associated with prolonged use, with increased risks of 15- to 24-fold for 5-10 years or more, and this risk has been shown to persist for at least 8-15 years after estrogen therapy is discontinued.

Clinical surveillance of all women taking estrogen/progestin combinations is important. Adequate diagnostic measures, including endometrial sampling when indicated, should be undertaken to rule out malignancy in all cases of undiagnosed persistent or recurring abnormal vaginal bleeding. There is no evidence that the use of natural estrogens results in a different endometrial risk profile than synthetic estrogens of equivalent estrogen dose. Adding a progestin to estrogen therapy has been shown to reduce the risk of endometrial hyperplasia which may be a precursor to endometrial cancer.

Breast Cancer

Estrogen and estrogen/progestin therapy in postmenopausal women has been associated with an increased risk of breast cancer. In the CE/MPA substudy of the Women's Health Initiative study (WHI), a 26% increase of invasive breast cancer (38 vs 30 per 10,000 woman-years) after an average of 5.2 years of treatment was observed in women receiving CE/MPA compared to women receiving placebo. The increased risk of breast cancer became apparent after 4 years on CE/MPA. The women reporting prior postmenopausal use of estrogen and/or estrogen with progestin had a higher relative risk for breast cancer associated with CE/MPA than those who had never used these hormones.

In the WHI, no increased risk of breast cancer in CE-treated women compared to placebo was reported after an average of 5.2 years of therapy. These data are preliminary and that substudy of WHI is continuing.

Epidemiologic studies have reported an increased risk of breast cancer in association with increasing duration of postmenopausal treatment with estrogens with or without a progestin. This association was reanalyzed in original data from 51 studies that involved treatment with various doses and types of estrogens, with and without progestins. In the reanalysis, an increased risk of having breast cancer diagnosed became apparent after about 5 years of continued therapy and subsided after treatment had been discontinued for 5 years or longer. Some later studies have suggested that postmenopausal treatment with estrogens and progestin increase the risk of breast cancer more than treatment with estrogen alone.

A postmenopausal woman without a uterus who requires estrogen should receive estrogen-alone therapy and should not be exposed unnecessarily to progestins. All postmenopausal women should receive yearly breast exams by a healthcare provider and perform monthly breast self-examinations. In addition, mammography examinations should be scheduled based on patient age and risk factors.

GALLBLADDER DISEASE

E

A 2- to 4-fold increase in the risk of gallbladder disease requiring surgery in postmenopausal women receiving estrogens has been reported.

HYPERCALCEMIA

Estrogen administration may lead to severe hypercalcemia in patients with breast cancer and bone metastases. If hypercalcemia occurs, use of the drug should be stopped and appropriate measures taken to reduce the serum calcium level.

VISUAL ABNORMALITIES

Retinal vascular thrombosis has been reported in patients receiving estrogens. Discontinue medication pending examination if there is sudden partial or complete loss of vision, or a sudden onset of proptosis, diplopia or migraine. If examination reveals papilledema or retinal vascular lesions, estrogens should be discontinued.

PRECAUTIONS

GENERAL

Addition of a Progestin When a Woman Has Not Had a Hysterectomy

Studies of the addition of a progestin for 10 or more days of a cycle of estrogen administration, or daily with estrogen in a continuous regimen, have reported a lowered incidence of endometrial hyperplasia than would be induced by estrogen treatment alone. Endometrial hyperplasia may be a precursor to endometrial cancer.

There are, however, possible risks that may be associated with the use of progestins with estrogens compared to estrogen-alone regimens. These include: (a) A possible increased risk of breast cancer; (b) Adverse effects on lipoprotein metabolism (*e.g.*, lowering HDL, raising LDL); (c) Impairment of glucose tolerance.

Elevated Blood Pressure

In a small number of case reports, substantial increases in blood pressure have been attributed to idiosyncratic reactions to estrogens. In a large, randomized, placebo-controlled clinical trial, a generalized effect of estrogen therapy on blood pressure was not seen. Blood pressure should be monitored at regular intervals with estrogen use.

Familial Hyperlipoproteinemia

In patients with familial defects of lipoprotein metabolism, estrogen therapy may be associated with elevations of plasma triglycerides leading to pancreatitis and other complications.

Impaired Liver Function and a Past History of Cholestatic Jaundice

Estrogens may be poorly metabolized in patients with impaired liver function. For patients with a history of cholestatic jaundice associated with past estrogen use or with pregnancy, caution should be exercised and in the case of recurrence, medication should be discontinued.

Hypothyroidism

Estrogen administration leads to increased thyroid-binding globulin (TBG) levels. Patients with normal thyroid function can compensate for the increased TBG by making more thyroid hormone, thus maintaining free T^4 and T^3 serum concentrations in the normal range. Patients dependent on thyroid hormone replacement therapy who are also receiving estrogens may require increased doses of their thyroid replacement therapy. These patients should have thyroid function monitored in order to maintain their free thyroid hormone levels in an acceptable range.

Fluid Retention

Because estrogens may cause some degree of fluid retention, patients with conditions that might be influenced by this factor, such as cardiac or renal dysfunction, warrant careful observation when estrogens are prescribed.

Hypocalcemia

Estrogens should be used with caution in individuals with severe hypocalcemia.

Ovarian Cancer

Use of estrogen-only products, in particular for 10 or more years, has been associated with an increased risk of ovarian cancer in some epidemiological studies. Other studies did not show a significant association. Data are insufficient to determine whether there is an increased risk with estrogen/progestin combination therapy in postmenopausal women.

Exacerbation of Endometriosis

Endometriosis may be exacerbated with administration of estrogen therapy.

Exacerbation of Other Conditions

Estrogens may cause an exacerbation of asthma, diabetes mellitus, epilepsy, migraine or porphyria and should be used with caution in women with these conditions.

Vaginal Use and Expulsion

Estradiol acetate vaginal ring may not be suitable for women with conditions that make the vagina more susceptible to vaginal irritation or ulceration, or make expulsions more likely, such as narrow vagina, vaginal stenosis, vaginal infection, cervical prolapse, rectoceles and cystoceles. If local treatment of a vaginal infection is required, estradiol acetate vaginal ring can remain in place during treatment.

INFORMATION FOR THE PATIENT

Physicians are advised to discuss the Patient Information leaflet with patients for whom they prescribe estradiol acetate vaginal ring.

LABORATORY TESTS

Estrogen administration should be initiated at the lowest dose for the approved indication and then guided by clinical response, rather than by serum hormone levels (*e.g.*, estradiol, FSH).

DRUG/LABORATORY TEST INTERACTIONS

Accelerated prothrombin time, partial thromboplastin time, and platelet aggregation time; increased platelet count; increased factors II, VII antigen, VIII antigen, VIII coagulant activity, IX, X, XII, VII-X complex, II-VIIX complex, and beta-thromboglobulin; decreased levels of anti-factor Xa and antithrombin III, decreased antithrombin III activity; increased levels of fibrinogen and fibrinogen activity; increased plasminogen antigen and activity.

Increased thyroid-binding globulin (TBG) levels leading to increased circulating total thyroid hormone levels as measured by protein-bound iodine (PBI), T^4 levels (by column or by radioimmunoassay) or T^3 levels by radioimmunoassay. T^3 resin uptake is decreased, reflecting the elevated TBG. Free T^4 and free T^3 concentrations are unaltered. Patients with normal thyroid function will be able to compensate for the increased TBG levels, but patients on thyroid replacement therapy may require higher doses of thyroid hormone.

Other binding proteins may be elevated in serum (*i.e.*, corticosteroid binding globulin (CBG), sex hormonebinding globulin (SHBG)) leading to increased circulating corticosteroids and sex steroids, respectively. Free or biologically active hormone concentrations are unchanged. Other plasma proteins may be increased (angiotensinogen/renin substrate, alpha-1-antitrypsin, ceruloplasmin).

Increased plasma HDL and HDL_2 cholesterol subfraction concentrations, reduced LDL cholesterol concentration, increased triglyceride levels.

Impaired glucose tolerance.

Reduced response to metyrapone test.

CARCINOGENESIS, MUTAGENESIS, AND IMPAIRMENT OF FERTILITY

Long-term continuous administration of natural and synthetic estrogens in certain animal species increases the frequency of carcinomas of the breast, uterus, cervix, vagina, testis, and liver. (See BOXED WARNING, CONTRAINDICATIONS, and WARNINGS.)

Estradiol acetate was assayed for mutation in four histidine-requiring strains of *Salmonella typhimurium* and in two tryptophan-requiring strains of *Escherichia coli.* Estradiol acetate did not induce mutation in any of the bacterial strains tested under the conditions employed.

PREGNANCY

Estrogens should not be used in pregnancy. (See CONTRAINDICATIONS.)

NURSING MOTHERS

Estrogen administration to nursing mothers has been shown to decrease the quantity and quality of the breast milk. Detectable amounts of estrogens have been identified in the milk of mothers receiving this drug. Caution should be exercised when estradiol acetate vaginal ring is prescribed for a nursing mother.

PEDIATRIC USE

Estradiol acetate vaginal ring is not indicated for use in children.

GERIATRIC USE

There have not been sufficient numbers of geriatric patients involved in studies utilizing estradiol acetate vaginal ring to determine whether those over 65 years of age differ from younger subjects in their response to estradiol acetate vaginal ring.

ADVERSE REACTIONS

See BOXED WARNING, WARNINGS, and PRECAUTIONS.

Because clinical trials are conducted under widely varying conditions, adverse reaction rates observed in the clinical trial of a drug cannot be directly compared to rates in the clinical trials of another drug and may not reflect the rates observed in practice. The adverse reaction information from clinical trials does, however, provide a basis for identifying the adverse events that may be related to drug use and for approximate rates.

In a 13 week clinical trial that included 225 postmenopausal women treated with estradiol acetate vaginal ring and 108 women treated with placebo vaginal rings, adverse events that occurred at a rate of ≥2% are summarized in TABLE 5.

The following additional adverse reactions have been reported with estrogens:

Genitourinary System: Changes in vaginal bleeding pattern and abnormal withdrawal bleeding or flow; spotting; increase in size of uterine leiomyomata; change in amount of cervical secretion; changes in cervical ectropion; ovarian cancer; endometrial hyperplasia; endometrial cancer.

Breasts: Enlargement, pain, nipple discharge, galactorrhea; fibrocystic breast changes; breast cancer.

Cardiovascular: Deep and superficial venous thrombosis; pulmonary embolism; thrombophlebitis; myocardial infarction; stroke; increase in blood pressure.

Gastrointestinal: Vomiting, abdominal cramps; cholestatic jaundice; increased incidence of gallbladder disease; pancreatitis.

Skin: Chloasma or melasma which may persist when drug is discontinued; erythema multiforme; erythema nodosum; hemorrhagic eruption; loss of scalp hair; hirsutism; pruritis, rash.

TABLE 5 *Incidence of AEs Occurring in ≥2% of Subjects Presented in Descending Frequency of Preferred Term*

Adverse Event	Placebo n=108	Estradiol 0.05 mg/day n=113	Estradiol 0.10 mg/day n=112
Headache (NOS)	10 (9.3%)	8 (7.1%)	11 (9.8%)
Intermenstrual bleeding	2 (1.9%)	9 (8.0%)	11 (9.8%)
Vaginal candidiasis	3 (2.8%)	7 (6.2%)	12 (10.7%)
Breast tenderness	2 (1.9%)	7 (6.2%)	12 (10.7%)
Back pain	4 (3.7%)	7 (6.2%)	4 (3.6%)
Genital disorder female (NOS)	9 (8.3%)	3 (2.7%)	3 (2.7%)
Upper respiratory tract infection (NOS)	6 (5.6%)	5 (4.4%)	4 (3.6%)
Abdominal distension	3 (2.8%)	8 (7.1%)	3 (2.7%)
Vaginal discharge	9 (8.3%)	2 (1.8%)	3 (2.7%)
Vulvovaginitis (NOS)	7 (6.5%)	6 (5.3%)	1 (0.9%)
Nausea	5 (4.6%)	3 (2.7%)	2 (1.8%)
Arthralgia	4 (3.7%)	2 (1.8%)	2 (1.8%)
Sinusitis (NOS)	2 (1.9%)	2 (1.8%)	4 (3.6%)
Uterine pain	1 (0.9%)	2 (1.8%)	5 (4.5%)
Nasopharyngitis	3 (2.8%)	2 (1.8%)	2 (1.8%)
Pain in limb	3 (2.8%)	1 (0.9%)	3 (2.7%)
Urinary tract infection (NOS)	2 (1.9%)	1 (0.9%)	4 (3.6%)
Vaginal irritation	4 (3.7%)	1 (0.9%)	2 (1.8%)

AE = Adverse event.
NOS = Not otherwise specified.

Eyes: Retinal vascular thrombosis; steepening of corneal curvature; intolerance to contact lenses.

Central Nervous System: Migraine; dizziness; mental depression; chorea; nervousness; mood disturbances; irritability; exacerbation of epilepsy.

Miscellaneous: Increase or decrease in weight; reduced carbohydrate tolerance; aggravation of porphyria; edema; leg cramps; changes in libido; anaphylactoid/anaphylactic reactions including urticaria and angioedema; hypocalcemia; exacerbation of asthma; increased triglycerides.

DOSAGE AND ADMINISTRATION

When estrogen is prescribed for a postmenopausal woman with a uterus, progestin should also be initiated to reduce the risk of endometrial cancer. A woman without a uterus does not need progestin. Use of estrogen, alone or in combination with a progestin, should be limited to the shortest duration consistent with treatment goals and risks for the individual woman. Patients should be reevaluated periodically as clinically appropriate (*e.g.*, 3-6 month intervals) to determine if treatment is still necessary (see BOXED WARNING and WARNINGS). For women who have a uterus, adequate diagnostic measures, such as endometrial sampling, when indicated, should be undertaken to rule out malignancy in cases of undiagnosed persistent or recurring abnormal vaginal bleeding.

Two doses of estradiol acetate vaginal ring are available, 0.05 and 0.10 mg/day, for the treatment of moderate to severe vasomotor symptoms and/or moderate to severe symptoms of vulvar and vaginal atrophy associated with the menopause.

Patients should be started at the lowest dose.

Femring should remain in place for 3 months and then be replaced by a new Femring.

HOW SUPPLIED

Each Femring (estradiol acetate vaginal ring) is individually packaged.

Femring 0.05 and 0.10 mg/day (estradiol acetate vaginal ring) are available in single units.

Storage: Store at 25°C (77°F); excursions permitted to 15-30°C (59-86°F).

Estradiol Cypionate; Medroxyprogesterone Acetate *(003510)*

Categories: Contraception; FDA Approved 2000 Oct; Pregnancy Category X
Drug Classes: Contraceptives; Estrogens; Hormones/hormone modifiers; Progestins
Brand Names: **Lunelle**
Cost of Therapy: $26.99 (Contraception; Lunelle Injection; 5 mg; 25 mg/0.5 ml; 1 injection; 28 day supply)

DESCRIPTION

Lunelle monthly contraceptive injection contains medroxyprogesterone acetate and estradiol cypionate as its active ingredients. The chemical name for medroxyprogesterone acetate is pregn-4-ene-3,20-dione,17-(acetyloxy)-6-methyl-,(6α)-. The empirical formula is $C_{24}H_{34}O_4$ and its molecular weight is 386.53. Medroxyprogesterone acetate is a white to off-white, odorless crystalline powder that is stable in air and melts between 200 and 210°C. It is freely soluble in chloroform, soluble in acetone and dioxane, sparingly soluble in alcohol and methanol, slightly soluble in ether, and practically insoluble in water. The chemical name for estradiol cypionate is estra-1,3,5,(10)-triene-3,17-diol,(17β)-,17-cyclopentanepropanoate. Estradiol cypionate is a white to off-white crystalline powder that melts between 149 and 153°C. It is soluble in alcohol, acetone, chloroform, and dioxane; sparingly soluble in vegetable oils; and practically insoluble in water. The empirical formula is $C_{26}H_{36}O_3$ and its molecular weight is 396.57.

Lunelle monthly contraceptive injection is available as a 0.5 ml aqueous suspension and contains 25 mg medroxyprogesterone acetate and 5 mg estradiol cypionate. Inactive ingredients are 0.9 mg methylparaben, 14.28 mg polyethylene glycol, 0.95 mg polysorbate 80, 0.1 mg propylparaben, 4.28 mg sodium chloride, and sterile water for injection.

CLINICAL PHARMACOLOGY

Estradiol cypionate; medroxyprogesterone acetate monthly contraceptive injection when administered at the recommended dose to women every month inhibits the secretion of gonadotropins, which, in turn, prevents follicular maturation and ovulation. Although the primary mechanism of this action is inhibition of ovulation, other possible mechanisms of action include thickening and a reduction in volume of cervical mucus (which decrease sperm penetration) and thinning of the endometrium (which may reduce the likelihood of implantation).

PHARMACOKINETICS

Steady-state pharmacokinetic parameters of medroxyprogesterone acetate (MPA) and 17β-estradiol (E_2), the parent active moiety of estradiol cypionate (E_2C), following the third monthly injection of estradiol cypionate; medroxyprogesterone acetate monthly contraceptive injection are shown in TABLE 1.

TABLE 1 *Pharmacokinetic Parameters of Medroxyprogesterone Acetate (MPA) and Estradiol (17β-E_2) after the 3rd Monthly Injection of Estradiol Cypionate; Medroxyprogesterone Acetate Monthly Contraceptive Injection in 14 Surgically Sterile Women*

	MPA Mean	MPA Min	MPA Max
C_{max} (ng/ml)	1.25	0.94	2.17
T_{max} (day)	3.5	1.0	10.0
AUC(0-28) (ng·day/ml)	21.51	14.44	27.00
AUC(0-∞) (ng·day/ml)	33.65	22.02	49.09
T½ (day)	14.7	6.2	36.0
	17β-E_2 Mean	**17β-E_2 Min**	**17β-E_2 Max**
C_{max} (ng/ml)	0.25	0.14	0.48
T_{max} (day)	2.1	1.0	7.0
AUC(0-28) (ng·day/ml)	2.74	1.65	3.56
AUC(0-∞) (ng·day/ml)	2.99	1.65	3.89
T½ (day)	8.4	2.6	20.4

C_{max} = peak serum concentration; T_{max} = time when C_{max} is observed; AUC(0-28) = area under the concentration-time curve over 28 days; T½ = terminal half-life; 1 nanogram = 10^3 picogram.

Absorption

Absorption of MPA and E_2 from the injection site is prolonged after an intramuscular injection of estradiol cypionate; medroxyprogesterone acetate monthly contraceptive injection. The time to maximum plasma concentration (T_{max}) typically occurs within 1-10 days postinjection for MPA and 1-7 days postinjection for E_2. The peak concentrations (C_{max}) generally range from 0.94-2.17 ng/ml for MPA and from 140-480 pg/ml for E_2.

Effect of Injection Site

AUC(0-28) for MPA values were statistically significantly higher following injection of estradiol cypionate; medroxyprogesterone acetate monthly contraceptive injection into the arm as compared to the anterior thigh (average increase was approximately 25%). The mean MPA C_{max} was higher but not statistically significant (average increase 6-12%) when estradiol cypionate; medroxyprogesterone acetate monthly contraceptive injection was injected into the arm compared with the C_{max} observed after injection into the hip or the anterior thigh. However, the average MPA trough (C_{min}) concentrations and the half-lives were comparable for the three injection sites. E_2 concentrations were not measured.

Distribution

Plasma protein binding of MPA averages 86%. MPA binding occurs primarily to serum albumin; no binding of MPA occurs with sex-hormone-binding globulin (SHBG). Estrogens circulate in blood bound to albumin, SHBG, α1-glycoproteins, and transcortin. Estradiol is primarily bound to SHBG and albumin and approximately 3% remains unbound. Unbound estrogens are known to modulate pharmacologic response.

Metabolism

MPA is extensively metabolized. Its metabolism primarily involves ring A and/or side-chain reduction, loss of the acetyl group, hydroxylation in the 2-, 6-, and 21-positions or a combination of these positions, resulting in numerous derivatives. E_2C undergoes ester hydrolysis after intramuscular injection of estradiol cypionate; medroxyprogesterone acetate monthly contraceptive injection, releasing the parent, active compound E_2. Exogenously delivered or endogenously derived E_2 is primarily metabolized to estrone and estriol, both of which are metabolized to their sulfate and glucuronide forms.

Elimination

Residual MPA concentrations at the end of a monthly injection of estradiol cypionate; medroxyprogesterone acetate monthly contraceptive injection are generally below 0.5 ng/ml, consistent with its apparent elimination half-life of 15 days. Most MPA metabolites are excreted in the urine as glucuronide conjugates with only small amounts excreted as sulfates. Following the peak concentration, serum E_2 levels typically decline to 100 pg/ml by day 14 and are consistent with the apparent elimination half-life of 7-8 days. Estrogen metabolites are primarily excreted in the urine as glucuronides and sulfates.

Return of Ovulation

Return of ovulation correlated to some extent with MPA AUC(0-84 days). Additionally, body weight and site of injection affected the AUC of MPA. AUC(0-28) values are significantly higher when estradiol cypionate; medroxyprogesterone acetate monthly contraceptive injection is injected into the arm compared to the anterior thigh muscle and into women with BMI ≤28 kg/m^2 compared to those with BMI >28 kg/m^2. Consequently, return of ovulation may be delayed in women with BMI ≤28 kg/m^2 who receive an injection in the arm.

PHARMACOKINETICS IN SUBPOPULATIONS

Race

The pharmacokinetics of MPA and E_2 has been evaluated in different populations in separate studies. With the exception of one study in Thai women that demonstrated relatively higher C_{max} and shorter T_{max} values indicating more rapid absorption of both MPA and E_2, the pharmacokinetics of MPA and E_2 after the administration of estradiol cypionate; medroxyprogesterone acetate monthly contraceptive injection were similar in women from various ethnic backgrounds. Although pharmacokinetic differences were observed, the contraceptive efficacy was similar among all women of all ethnic backgrounds studied. Following discontinuation, ovulation returned earlier in Thai women.

E

Pediatric

Safety and efficacy of estradiol cypionate; medroxyprogesterone acetate monthly contraceptive injection have been established in women of reproductive age. Safety and efficacy are expected to be the same for postpubertal adolescents under 16 years of age and users 16 years of age and older. Use of this product before menarche is not indicated.

Geriatric

Estradiol cypionate; medroxyprogesterone acetate monthly contraceptive injection is intended for use in healthy women desiring contraception; studies in geriatric women have not been conducted.

Effect of Body Weight

No dosage adjustment is necessary based on body weight. The effect of body weight on the pharmacokinetics of MPA was assessed in a subset of women (n=77, body mass index ranged from 18-45.5 kg/m^2) enrolled in a Phase 3 trial. AUC(0-28) values for MPA were significantly higher in thinner women with body mass index ≤28 kg/m^2 (average increase was approximately 20%) when compared to that in heavier women with body mass index >28 kg/m^2. The mean MPA C_{max} was higher (average increase 42%) in thin/normal women with body mass index ≤28 kg/m^2 compared with heavier women with body mass index >28 kg/m^2. The range of MPA trough (C_{min}) concentrations and the half-lives were comparable for both groups.

Hepatic Insufficiency

No formal studies have evaluated the effect of hepatic disease on the disposition of estradiol cypionate; medroxyprogesterone acetate monthly contraceptive injection. However, steroid hormones may be poorly metabolized in patients with impaired liver function. (See CONTRAINDICATIONS.)

Renal Insufficiency

No formal studies have evaluated the effect of renal disease on the pharmacokinetics of estradiol cypionate; medroxyprogesterone acetate monthly contraceptive injection. However, since both steroidal components of estradiol cypionate; medroxyprogesterone acetate monthly contraceptive injection are almost exclusively eliminated by hepatic metabolism, no dosage adjustment is necessary in women with renal dysfunction.

DRUG-DRUG INTERACTIONS

No formal drug-drug interaction studies were conducted with estradiol cypionate; medroxyprogesterone acetate monthly contraceptive injection. Aminoglutethimide administered concomitantly with estradiol cypionate; medroxyprogesterone acetate monthly contraceptive injection may significantly depress the serum concentrations of MPA. Users of estradiol cypionate; medroxyprogesterone acetate monthly contraceptive injection should be warned of the possibility of decreased efficacy with the use of this or any related drugs. (See DRUG INTERACTIONS.)

INDICATIONS AND USAGE

Estradiol cypionate; medroxyprogesterone acetate monthly contraceptive injection is indicated for the prevention of pregnancy.

The efficacy of estradiol cypionate; medroxyprogesterone acetate monthly contraceptive injection is dependent on adherence to the recommended dosage schedule (*e.g.*, intramuscular injections every 28-30 days, not to exceed 33 days). To ensure that estradiol cypionate; medroxyprogesterone acetate monthly contraceptive injection is not administered inadvertently to a pregnant woman, the first injection should be given during the first 5 days of a normal menstrual period. Estradiol cypionate; medroxyprogesterone acetate monthly contraceptive injection should be administered no earlier than 4 weeks after delivery if not breastfeeding or 6 weeks after delivery if breastfeeding (see PRECAUTIONS, Nursing Mothers).

Several clinical trials of estradiol cypionate; medroxyprogesterone acetate monthly contraceptive injection have reported 12 month failure rates of <1% by Life Table analysis. Pregnancy rates for various contraceptive methods are typically reported for the first year of use and are shown in TABLE 2.

TABLE 2 *Percentage of Women Experiencing an Unintended Pregnancy During the First Year of Typical Use and the First Year of Perfect Use of Contraception and the Percentage Continuing Use at the End of the First Year: US**

Method	% of Women Experiencing an Unintended Pregnancy Within the First Year of Use		% of Women Continuing
	Typical Use‡	Perfect Use§	Use at 1 Year†
(1)	(2)	(3)	(4)
Chance¤	85	85	
Spermicides¶	26	6	40
Periodic abstinence	25		63
Calendar		9	
Ovulation method		3	
Symptothermal**		2	
Postovulation		1	
Cap‡‡			
Parous women	40	26	42
Nulliparous women	20	9	56
Sponge			
Parous women	40	20	42
Nulliparous women	20	9	56
Diaphragm††	20	6	56
Withdrawl	19	4	
Condom‡‡			
Female (Reality)	21	5	56
Male	14	3	61
Pill	5		71
Progestin only		0.5	
Combined		0.1	
IUD			
Progesterone T	2.0	1.5	81
Copper T380A	0.8	0.6	78
LNg 20	0.1	0.1	81
Depo-Provera	0.3	0.3	70
Norplant & Norplant-2	0.05	0.05	88
Female sterilization	0.5	0.5	100
Male sterilization	0.15	0.10	100
Emergency contraceptive pills	Treatment initiated within 72 hours after unprotected intercourse reduces the risk of pregnancy by at least 75%.§§		
Lactational amenorrhea method	LAM is a highly effective, temporary method of contraception.¤¤		

* Adapted from Hatcher *et al.*, 1998.
† Among couples attempting to avoid pregnancy, the percentage who continue to use a method for 1 year.
‡ Among *typical* couples who initiate use of a method (not necessarily for the first time), the percentage who experience an accidental pregnancy during the first year if they do not stop use for any other reason.
§ Among couples who initiate use of a method (not necessarily for the first time) and who use it *perfectly* (both consistently and correctly), the percentage who experience an accidental pregnancy during the first year if they do not stop use for any other reason.
¤ The percentages becoming pregnant in columns (2) and (3) are based on data from populations where contraception is not used and from women who cease using contraception in order to become pregnant. Among such populations, about 89% become pregnant within 1 year. This estimate was lowered slightly (to 85%) to represent the percentages who would become pregnant within 1 year among women now relying on reversible methods of contraception if they abandoned contraception altogether.
¶ Foams, creams, gels, vaginal suppositories, and vaginal film.
** Cervical mucus (ovulation) method supplemented by calendar in the pre-ovulatory and basal body temperature in the post-ovulatory phases.
†† With spermicidal cream or jelly.
‡‡ Without spermicides.
§§ The treatment schedule is one dose within 72 hours after unprotected intercourse, and a second dose 12 hours after the first dose. The Food and Drug Administration has declared the following brands of oral contraceptives to be safe and effective for emergency contraception: Ovral (1 dose is 2 white pills), Alesse (1 dose is 5 pink pills), Nordette or Levlen (1 dose 4 light-orange pills), Lo/Ovral (1 dose is 4 white pills), Triphasil or Tri-Levlen (1 dose is 4 yellow pills).
¤¤ However, to maintain effective protection against pregnancy, another method of contraception must be used as soon as menstruation resumes, the frequency or duration of breastfeeds is reduced, bottle feeds are introduced, or the baby reaches 6 months of age.

CONTRAINDICATIONS

The information contained in this package insert is based not only on information specific to estradiol cypionate; medroxyprogesterone acetate monthly contraceptive injection, but also on studies carried out in women who used injectable progestin-only contraceptives (medroxyprogesterone acetate) or oral contraceptives with higher doses of both estrogens and progestogens than those in common use today. The effect of long-term use of hormonal contraceptives with formulations having lower doses of both estrogens and progestogens remains to be determined.

Estradiol cypionate; medroxyprogesterone acetate monthly contraceptive injection should not be used in women with any of the following conditions or circumstances:

- Known or suspected pregnancy.
- Thrombophlebitis or thromboembolic disorders.
- A past history of deep-vein thrombophlebitis or thromboembolic disorders.
- Cerebral vascular or coronary artery disease.
- Undiagnosed abnormal genital bleeding.
- Liver dysfunction or disease, such as history of hepatic adenoma or carcinoma; history of cholestatic jaundice of pregnancy or jaundice with prior hormonal contraceptive use including severe pruritus of pregnancy.
- Carcinoma of the endometrium, breast, or other known or suspected estrogen-dependent neoplasia.
- Known hypersensitivity to any of the ingredients contained in estradiol cypionate; medroxyprogesterone acetate monthly contraceptive injection.
- Heavy smoking (≥15 cigarettes per day) and over age 35.
- Severe hypertension.
- Diabetes with vascular involvement.
- Headaches with focal neurological symptoms.
- Valvular heart disease with complications.

WARNINGS

Cigarette smoking increases the risk of serious cardiovascular side effects from contraceptives containing estrogen. This risk increases with age and with heavy smoking (15 or more cigarettes per day) and is quite marked in women over 35 years of age. Women who use estradiol cypionate; medroxyprogesterone acetate monthly contraceptive injection should be strongly advised not to smoke.

The use of oral contraceptives is associated with increased risks of several serious conditions including myocardial infarction, thromboembolism, stroke, hepatic neoplasia, and gallbladder disease, although the risk of serious morbidity or mortality is very small in healthy women without underlying risk factors. The risk of morbidity and mortality increases significantly in the presence of other underlying risk factors such as hypertension, hyperlipidemias, obesity, and diabetes.

Practitioners prescribing estradiol cypionate; medroxyprogesterone acetate monthly contraceptive injection should be familiar with the following information relating to these risks.

Throughout this labeling, epidemiological studies reported are of two types: retrospective or case control studies and prospective or cohort studies. Case control studies provide a measure of the relative risk of a disease, namely, a ratio of the incidence of a disease among oral contraceptive users to that among nonusers. The relative risk does not provide information on the actual clinical occurrence of a disease. Cohort studies provide a measure of attributable risk, which is the difference in the incidence of disease between oral contraceptive users and nonusers. The attributable risk does provide information about the actual occurrence of a disease in the population. For further information, the reader is referred to a text on epidemiological methods.

THROMBOEMBOLIC DISORDERS AND OTHER VASCULAR PROBLEMS

Myocardial Infarction

An increased risk of myocardial infarction has been attributed to oral contraceptive use. This risk is primarily in smokers or women with other underlying risk factors for coronary artery disease such as hypertension, hypercholesterolemia, morbid obesity, and diabetes. The relative risk of heart attack for current oral contraceptive users has been estimated to be two to six. The risk is very low in women under the age of 30.

Smoking in combination with oral contraceptive use has been shown to contribute substantially to the incidence of myocardial infarctions in women in their mid-thirties or older with smoking accounting for the majority of excess cases. Mortality rates associated with circulatory disease have been shown to increase substantially in smokers over 35 years of age and older and non-smokers over 40 years of age who use oral contraceptives (see TABLE 3).

TABLE 3 *Circulatory Disease Mortality Rates per 100,000 Women Years by Age Smoking Status and Oral Contraceptive Use**

Age	Ever-Users		Controls	
(years)	Non-Smokers	Smokers	Non-Smokers	Smokers
15-24	0.0	10.5	0.0	0.0
25-34	4.4	14.2	2.7	4.2
35-44	21.5	63.4	6.4	15.2
45+	52.4	206.7	11.4	27.9

* Adapted from Layde PM, Beral V., 1981.

Oral contraceptives may compound the effects of well-known risk factors, such as hypertension, diabetes, hyperlipidemias, age, and obesity. In particular, some progestogens are known to decrease high density lipoproteins (HDL) cholesterol and cause glucose intolerance, while estrogens may create a state of hyperinsulinism. Oral contraceptives have been shown to increase blood pressure among users (see Elevated Blood Pressure). Similar effects on risk factors have been associated with an increased risk of heart disease. Estradiol cypionate; medroxyprogesterone acetate monthly contraceptive injection must be used with caution in women with cardiovascular disease risk factors.

Thromboembolism

An increased risk of thromboembolic and thrombotic diseases associated with the use of oral contraceptives is well established. Case control studies have found the relative risk of users compared with non-users to be 3 for the first episode of superficial venous thrombosis, 4 to 11 for deep vein thrombosis or pulmonary embolism, and 1.5 to 6 for women with predisposing conditions for venous thromboembolic disease. Cohort studies have shown the relative risk to be somewhat lower, about 3 for new cases and about 4.5 for new cases requiring hospitalization. The risk of thromboembolic disease due to oral contraceptives is not related to length of use and disappears after pill use is stopped.

A 2- to 4-fold increase in relative risk of post-operative thromboembolic complications has been reported with the use of oral contraceptives. The relative risk of venous thrombosis in women who have predisposing conditions is twice that of women without such medical conditions. If feasible, oral contraceptives should be discontinued at least 4 weeks prior to and for 2 weeks after elective surgery of a type associated with an increase in risk of thromboembolism and during and following prolonged immobilization. Since the immediate postpartum period is also associated with an increased risk of thromboembolism, oral contraceptives and other combined hormonal contraceptives such as estradiol cypionate; medroxyprogesterone acetate monthly contraceptive injection, should be started no earlier than 4 weeks after delivery.

The clinician should be alert to the earliest manifestations of thrombotic disorders (thrombophlebitis, pulmonary embolism, cerebrovascular disorders, and retinal thrombosis). Should any of these occur or be suspected, estradiol cypionate; medroxyprogesterone acetate monthly contraceptive injection should not be readministered.

Cerebrovascular Disease

Oral contraceptives have been shown to increase both the relative and attributable risks of cerebrovascular events (thrombotic and hemorrhagic strokes), although, in general, the risk is greatest among older (>35 years), hypertensive women who also smoke. Hypertension was found to be a risk factor for both users and nonusers, for both types of strokes, while smoking interacted to increase the risk for hemorrhagic stroke.

The relative risk of thrombotic strokes has been shown to range from 3 for normotensive users to 14 for users with severe hypertension. The relative risk of hemorrhagic stroke is reported to be 1.2 for non-smokers who used oral contraceptives, 2.6 for smokers who did not use oral contraceptives, 7.6 for smokers who used oral contraceptives, 1.8 for normotensive users, and 25.7 for users with severe hypertension. The attributable risk is also greater in older women.

Dose-Related Risk of Vascular Disease

A positive association has been observed between the amount of estrogen and progestogen in oral contraceptives and the risk of vascular disease. A decline in serum HDL has been reported with many progestational agents. A decline in serum HDL has been associated with an increased incidence of ischemic heart disease. Because estrogens increase HDL cholesterol, the net effect of an oral contraceptive depends on a balance achieved between doses of estrogen and progestogen and the type of progestogens used in the contraceptives. The activity and amount of both hormones should be considered in the choice of a hormonal contraceptive.

Persistence of Risk of Vascular Disease

There are two studies which have shown persistence of risk of vascular disease for ever-users of oral contraceptives. In a study in the US, the risk of developing myocardial infarction after discontinuing oral contraceptives persists for at least 9 years for women 40-49 years who had used oral contraceptives for 5 or more years, but this increased risk was not demonstrated in other age groups. In another study in Great Britain, the risk of developing cerebrovascular disease persisted for at least 6 years after discontinuation of oral contraceptives, although excess risk was very small. However, both studies were performed with oral contraceptive formulations containing 50 µg or more of estrogen.

ESTIMATES OF MORTALITY FROM CONTRACEPTIVE USE

One study gathered data from a variety of sources that have estimated the mortality rate associated with different methods of contraception at different ages (see TABLE 4). These estimates include the combined risk of death associated with contraceptive methods plus the risk attributable to pregnancy in the event of method failure. Each method of contraception has its specific benefits and risks. The study concluded that with the exception of oral contraceptive users 35 years and older who smoke and oral contraceptive users 40 years and older who do not smoke, mortality associated with all methods of birth control is low and below that associated with childbirth.

The observation of a possible increase in risk of mortality with age for oral contraceptive users is based on data gathered in the 1970s, but not reported until 1983. However, current clinical practice involves the use of lower estrogen-dose formulations combined with careful restriction of oral contraceptive use to women who do not have the various risk factors listed in this labeling.

Because of these changes in practice and because of some limited new data that suggest the risk of cardiovascular disease with the use of oral contraceptives may now be less than previously observed, the Fertility and Maternal Health Drugs Advisory Committee was asked to review the topic in 1989. The Committee concluded that although cardiovascular disease risk may be increased with oral contraceptive use after age 40 in healthy non-smoking women (even with the newer low-dose formulations), there are also greater potential health risks associated with pregnancy in older women and with the alternative surgical and medical procedures that may be necessary if such women do not have access to effective and acceptable means of contraception. Therefore, the Committee recommended that the benefits of oral contraceptive use by healthy non-smoking women over age 40 may outweigh the possible risks. Women of all ages who take oral contraceptives should take a product which contains the lowest amount of estrogen and progestogen that is effective.

TABLE 4 *Annual Number of Birth-Related or Method-Related Deaths Associated With Control of Fertility per 100,000 Nonsterile Women, by Fertility Control Method According to Age**

Method of Control & Outcome	Range of Ages (years)					
	15-19	20-24	25-29	30-34	35-39	40-44
No fertility control†	7.0	7.4	9.1	14.8	25.7	28.2
Oral contraceptives (non-smoker)‡	0.3	0.5	0.9	1.9	13.8	31.6
Oral contraceptives (smoker)‡	2.2	3.4	6.6	13.5	51.1	117.2
IUD‡	0.8	0.8	1.0	1.0	1.4	1.4
Condom†	1.1	1.6	0.7	0.2	0.3	0.4
Diaphragm/spermicide†	1.9	1.2	1.2	1.3	2.2	2.8
Periodic abstinence	2.5	1.6	1.6	1.7	2.9	3.6

* Adapted from Ory HW. 1983.
† Deaths are birth-related.
‡ Deaths are method-related.

CARCINOMA OF THE REPRODUCTIVE ORGANS AND BREASTS

Numerous epidemiological studies have been performed on the incidence of breast, endometrial, ovarian, and cervical cancer in women using oral contraceptives. Although the risk of breast cancer may be slightly increased among current and recent users of combined oral contraceptives, this excess risk decreases over time after product discontinuation, and by 10 years after cessation the increased risk disappears. In addition, breast cancers diagnosed in current or ever oral contraceptive users tend to be less invasive than in non-users.

The risk of breast cancer does not increase with duration of use, and no relationships have been found with dose or type of steroid. The patterns of risk are also similar regardless of a woman's reproductive history or her family breast cancer history. The sub-group for whom risk has been found to be significantly elevated is women who first used combined oral contraceptives before age 20, but because breast cancer is so rare at these young ages, the number of cases attributable to this early combined oral contraceptive use is extremely small.

Women who currently have or have had breast cancer should not use combined hormonal contraceptives because breast cancer is a hormonally sensitive tumor.

Long-term case-controlled surveillance of users of depot medroxyprogesterone acetate (DMPA) found slight or no increased overall risk of breast cancer. A pooled analysis from two case-control studies, the World Health Organization (WHO) Study and the New Zealand Study, reported the relative risk of breast cancer for women who had ever used DMPA as 1.1. Overall, there was no increase in risk with increasing duration of use of DMPA. The relative risk of breast cancer for women of all ages who had initiated use of DMPA within the previous 5 years was estimated to be 2.0.

E

The WHO Study, a component of the pooled analysis described above, showed an increased relative risk of 2.19 of breast cancer associated with use of DMPA in women whose first exposure to drug was within the previous 4 years and who were under 35 years of age. However, the overall relative risk for ever-users of DMPA was only 1.2.

Some studies suggest that oral contraceptive use has been associated with an increase in the risk of cervical intraepithelial neoplasia in some populations of women. However, there continues to be controversy about the extent to which such findings may be due to differences in sexual behavior and other factors.

A statistically insignificant increase in relative risk estimates of invasive squamous-cell cervical cancer has been associated with the use of DMPA in women who were first exposed before the age of 35 years. The overall, nonsignificant relative rate of invasive squamous-cell cervical cancer in women who ever used DMPA was estimated to be 1.11. No trends in risk with duration of use or times since initial or most recent exposure were observed.

In spite of many studies of the relationship between oral contraceptive use and breast and cervical cancers, a cause and effect relationship has not been established. No long-term studies have been conducted with estradiol cypionate; medroxyprogesterone acetate monthly contraceptive injection to evaluate risk for carcinoma of the reproductive organs.

HEPATIC NEOPLASIA

Benign hepatic adenomas are associated with oral contraceptive use, although the incidence of benign tumors is rare in the US. Indirect calculations have estimated the attributable risk to be in the range of 3.3 cases per 100,000 cases for users, a risk that increases after 4 or more years of use. Rupture of benign, hepatic adenomas may cause death through intra-abdominal hemorrhage.

Studies from Britain have shown an increased risk of developing hepatocellular carcinoma in long-term (>8 years) oral contraceptive users. However, these cancers are extremely rare in the US and the attributable risk (the excess incidence) of liver cancers in oral contraceptive users approaches less than one per million users.

OCULAR LESIONS

There have been clinical case reports of retinal thrombosis associated with the use of oral contraceptives. Estradiol cypionate; medroxyprogesterone acetate monthly contraceptive injection should be discontinued if there is unexplained partial or complete loss of vision, onset of proptosis or diplopia, papilledema, or retinal vascular lesions. Appropriate diagnostic and therapeutic measures should be undertaken immediately.

HORMONAL CONTRACEPTIVE USE BEFORE OR DURING PREGNANCY

The use of hormonal contraceptives during pregnancy is not indicated.

Extensive epidemiological studies have revealed no increased risk of birth defects in women who have used oral contraceptives prior to pregnancy. Studies also do not suggest a teratogenic effect, particularly in so far as cardiac anomalies and limb reduction defects are concerned, when oral contraceptives are taken inadvertently during early pregnancy.

Pregnancies occurring in women receiving injectable progestin-only contraceptives are uncommon. Neonates from unexpected pregnancies that occurred 1-2 months after injection of DMPA may be at an increased risk of low birth weight, which, in turn, is associated with an increased risk of neonatal death. A significant increase in incidence of polysyndactyly and chromosomal anomalies was observed among infants of users of DMPA, the former being most pronounced in women under 30 years of age. The unrelated nature of these defects, the lack of confirmation from other studies, the distant preconceptual exposure to DMPA, and the chance effects due to multiple statistical comparisons, make a causal association unlikely.

Neonates exposed to MPA in utero and followed to adolescence, showed no evidence of any adverse effects on their health including their physical, intellectual, sexual or social development.

Several reports suggest an association between intrauterine exposure to progestational drugs in the first trimester of pregnancy and genital abnormalities in male and female fetuses. The risk of hypospadias (5-8 per 1000 male births in the general population) may be approximately doubled with exposure to these drugs. There are insufficient data to quantify the risk to exposed female fetuses, but because some of these drugs induce mild virilization of the external genitalia of the female fetus and because of the increased association of hypospadias in the male fetus, these drugs should be avoided during pregnancy.

Unexpected pregnancies occurring in women receiving estradiol cypionate; medroxyprogesterone acetate monthly contraceptive injection are uncommon and have not shown congenital malformations or other adverse events.

The administration of combined hormonal contraceptives, such as estradiol cypionate; medroxyprogesterone acetate monthly contraceptive injection, to induce withdrawal bleeding should not be used as a test for pregnancy. Estradiol cypionate; medroxyprogesterone acetate monthly contraceptive injection should not be used during pregnancy to treat threatened or habitual abortion. It is recommended that for any patient who has missed 2 consecutive periods, pregnancy should be considered before initiating or continuing estradiol cypionate; medroxyprogesterone acetate monthly contraceptive injection. If the patient has exceeded the prescribed injection interval (>33 days) for estradiol cypionate; medroxyprogesterone acetate monthly contraceptive injection, the possibility of pregnancy should be ruled out before another injection is administered.

GALLBLADDER DISEASE

Combined hormonal contraceptives may worsen existing gallbladder disease and may accelerate the development of this disease in previously asymptomatic women. Women with a history of combined hormonal contraceptive-related cholestasis are more likely to have the condition recur with subsequent combined hormonal contraceptive use.

In a study of 782 women taking estradiol cypionate; medroxyprogesterone acetate monthly contraceptive injection for up to 15 cycles, cholecystitis and cholelithiasis were the only serious adverse events judged to be possibly related to the study drug. They were reported as an adverse event in 5 subjects, and 3 subjects required cholecystectomy.

CARBOHYDRATE AND LIPID METABOLIC EFFECTS

Combined hormonal or progestin-only contraceptives have been shown to cause glucose intolerance in some users. However, in the nondiabetic woman, combined hormonal contraceptives appear to have no effect on fasting blood glucose. Pre-diabetic and diabetic patients should be carefully observed while receiving therapy with estradiol cypionate; medroxyprogesterone acetate monthly contraceptive injection.

A small proportion of women may have persistent hypertriglyceridemia while using oral contraceptives. Changes in serum triglycerides and lipoprotein levels have been reported in oral contraceptive users.

ELEVATED BLOOD PRESSURE

An increase in blood pressure has been reported in women taking oral contraceptives and this increase is more likely in older oral contraceptive users and with continued use. Data from the Royal College of General Practitioners and subsequent randomized trials have shown that the incidence of hypertension increases with increasing concentrations of progestogens. In a US clinical study, no increase in mean blood pressure was observed over 15 months use of estradiol cypionate; medroxyprogesterone acetate monthly contraceptive injection.

Women with a history of hypertension or hypertension-related diseases, or renal disease should be encouraged to use another method of contraception. If women elect to use combined hormonal contraceptives such as estradiol cypionate; medroxyprogesterone acetate monthly contraceptive injection, they should be monitored closely and if significant elevation of blood pressure occurs, estradiol cypionate; medroxyprogesterone acetate monthly contraceptive injection should be discontinued. For most women, elevated blood pressure will return to normal after stopping oral contraceptives, and there is no difference in the occurrence of hypertension among former and never users.

HEADACHE

The onset or exacerbation of migraine or development of headache with a new pattern which is recurrent, persistent, or severe requires evaluation of the cause before further injections of estradiol cypionate; medroxyprogesterone acetate monthly contraceptive injection are given.

BLEEDING IRREGULARITIES

Most women using estradiol cypionate; medroxyprogesterone acetate monthly contraceptive injection (58.6%) experienced alteration of menstrual bleeding patterns, including 4.1% amenorrhea, after 1 year of use. Altered bleeding patterns include frequent bleeding, irregular bleeding, prolonged bleeding, infrequent bleeding, and amenorrhea. As women continued using estradiol cypionate; medroxyprogesterone acetate monthly contraceptive injection, the percent experiencing frequent or prolonged bleeding decreased, while the percent experiencing amenorrhea increased. The percent of women experiencing irregular bleeding remained fairly constant at approximately 30% throughout the first year of use.

Regardless of the bleeding pattern, subsequent injections should be given 1 month (28-30 days, not to exceed 33 days) after the previous injection, unless discontinuation is medically indicated.

If abnormal bleeding associated with estradiol cypionate; medroxyprogesterone acetate monthly contraceptive injection persists or is severe, appropriate investigation should be instituted to rule out the possibility of organic pathology, and appropriate treatment should be instituted when necessary. In the event of amenorrhea, pregnancy should be ruled out.

BONE MINERAL DENSITY CHANGES

Use of injectable progestogen-only methods may be considered among the risk factors for development of osteoporosis. The rate of bone loss is greatest in the early years of use and then subsequently approaches the normal rate of age related fall. Formal studies on the effect of bone mineral density changes in women receiving estradiol cypionate; medroxyprogesterone acetate monthly contraceptive injection have not been conducted.

ANAPHYLAXIS AND ANAPHYLACTOID REACTION

Anaphylaxis and anaphylactoid reactions have been reported with the components of estradiol cypionate; medroxyprogesterone acetate monthly contraceptive injection. Allergic reactions occurring in women using estradiol cypionate; medroxyprogesterone acetate monthly contraceptive injection have been mainly dermatologic, not respiratory, in nature. If an anaphylactic reaction occurs appropriate therapy should be instituted. Serious anaphylactic reactions require emergency medical treatment.

PRECAUTIONS

GENERAL

Patients should be counseled that this product does not protect against HIV infection (AIDS) and other sexually transmitted diseases.

Physical Examination

It is good medical practice for all women to have an annual history and physical examination, including women using combined hormonal contraceptives. The physical examination should include special reference to blood pressure, breasts, abdomen and pelvic organs, including cervical cytology, and relevant laboratory tests. In case of undiagnosed, persistent, or recurrent abnormal vaginal bleeding, appropriate measures should be conducted to rule out malignancy. Women with a strong family history of breast cancer or who have breast nodules should be monitored with particular care.

Weight Change

In a study of 782 women using estradiol cypionate; medroxyprogesterone acetate monthly contraceptive injection for up to 15 cycles, 5.7% of participants discontinued due to weight gain. Weight gain was the most common adverse event leading to discontinuation of the drug. Women gained an average of 4 pounds during the first year and an additional 2 pounds during the second year of estradiol cypionate; medroxyprogesterone acetate monthly contraceptive injection use. The range of weight change during the first year of estradiol cypionate; medroxyprogesterone acetate monthly contraceptive injection use was 48 pounds lost to 49 pounds gained. TABLE 5 shows the range of weight changes seen for women continuing use up to 24 cycles.

TABLE 5

Weight Change	12 Cycles (n=469)	15 Cycles (n=433)	24 Cycles (n=111)
Lost >20 pounds	1%	2%	5%
Lost >10 to 20 pounds	6%	6%	7%
Gained >10 to 20 pounds	19%	24%	14%
Gained >20 pounds	5%	7%	23%

Lipid Disorders

Women who are being treated for hyperlipidemias should be followed closely if they use combined hormonal contraceptives. Some progestogens may elevate LDL levels and may render the control of hyperlipidemias more difficult.

Liver Function

If jaundice develops in any woman receiving combined hormonal contraceptives, the medication should be discontinued. Steroid hormones may be poorly metabolized in patients with impaired liver function.

Fluid Retention

Progestogens and/or estrogens may cause some degree of fluid retention; therefore, caution should be used in treating any patient with a pre-existing medical condition that might be adversely affected by fluid retention.

Contact Lenses

Contact lens wearers who develop visual changes or changes in lens tolerance should be assessed by an ophthalmologist.

Emotional Disorders

Patients becoming significantly depressed while taking combined hormonal contraceptives should stop the medication and use an alternative method of contraception in an attempt to determine whether the symptom is drug related. Women with a history of depression should be carefully observed and consideration should be given to the discontinuation of estradiol cypionate; medroxyprogesterone acetate monthly contraceptive injection if depression recurs to a serious degree.

CARCINOGENESIS, MUTAGENESIS, AND IMPAIRMENT OF FERTILITY

See WARNINGS.

PREGNANCY CATEGORY X

See CONTRAINDICATIONS and WARNINGS.

RETURN OF OVULATION AND FERTILITY

Ovulation (signaled by a rise in serum progesterone concentrations ≥4.7 ng/ml) was observed 63-112 days after the third monthly injection of estradiol cypionate; medroxyprogesterone acetate monthly contraceptive injection in 11 of 14 women participating in a pharmacodynamic study. The remaining 3 women had not ovulated by day 85 and were lost to follow-up.

In a study of 21 women who received estradiol cypionate; medroxyprogesterone acetate monthly contraceptive injection for 3 months, 52% ovulated during the first post-treatment month, and 71% during the second post-treatment month. In another study of 10 women receiving long-term administration (2 years of treatment) of estradiol cypionate; medroxyprogesterone acetate monthly contraceptive injection, 60% ovulated by the third post-treatment month.

A study of 70 women who discontinued estradiol cypionate; medroxyprogesterone acetate monthly contraceptive injection to become pregnant demonstrated that more than 50% achieved fertility within 6 months after discontinuation, and 83% did so by 1 year.

NURSING MOTHERS

The effects of estradiol cypionate; medroxyprogesterone acetate monthly contraceptive injection in nursing mothers have not been evaluated and are unknown. However, estrogen administration to nursing mothers has been shown to decrease the quantity and quality of breast milk. Small amounts of combined hormonal contraceptive steroids have been identified in the milk of nursing mothers and a few adverse effects on the child have been reported, including jaundice and breast enlargement. Long-term follow-up of children whose mothers used combined hormonal contraceptives while breastfeeding has shown no deleterious effects. However, women who are breastfeeding should not start taking combined hormonal contraceptives until 6 weeks postpartum.

PEDIATRIC USE

Safety and efficacy of estradiol cypionate; medroxyprogesterone acetate monthly contraceptive injection have been established in women of reproductive age. Safety and efficacy are expected to be the same for postpubertal adolescents under 16 years of age and users 16 years of age and older. Use of this product before menarche is not indicated.

INFORMATION FOR THE PATIENT

Patients should be given a copy of the patient labeling prior to administration of estradiol cypionate; medroxyprogesterone acetate monthly contraceptive injection.

Patients should be advised that the contraceptive efficacy of estradiol cypionate; medroxyprogesterone acetate monthly contraceptive injection depends on receiving injections monthly (28-30 days, not to exceed 33 days). The injection schedule must be measured by the number of days, not by bleeding episodes. It is recommended that for any patient who has missed 2 consecutive menstrual periods, pregnancy should be considered before initiating or continuing estradiol cypionate; medroxyprogesterone acetate monthly contraceptive injection. Thereafter, a woman who has continued amenorrhea while using estradiol cypionate; medroxyprogesterone acetate monthly contraceptive injection and who has received her injections according to the recommended dosing schedule may continue to receive subsequent injections each month after the previous injection (not to exceed 33 days), unless discontinuation is medically indicated. All patients presenting for a follow-up injection of estradiol cypionate; medroxyprogesterone acetate monthly contraceptive injection after day 33 should use a barrier method of contraception and should not receive another injection of estradiol cypionate; medroxyprogesterone acetate monthly contraceptive injection until pregnancy has been ruled out.

Patients should be advised that menstrual bleeding patterns are likely be disrupted with use of estradiol cypionate; medroxyprogesterone acetate monthly contraceptive injection. A few patients may experience amenorrhea. Irregular bleeding that occurs after a regular bleeding pattern has emerged should be investigated. In the presence of excessive or prolonged bleeding, other causes should be investigated and consideration should be given to alternative methods of contraception.

Patients should be counseled that this product does not protect against HIV infection (AIDS) and other sexually transmitted diseases.

DRUG INTERACTIONS

EFFECTS OF OTHER DRUGS ON MPA

Aminoglutethamide may decrease the serum concentration of MPA. Users of estradiol cypionate; medroxyprogesterone acetate monthly contraceptive injection should be informed of the possibility of decreased effectiveness with the use of this or any related drug. (See CLINICAL PHARMACOLOGY, Drug-Drug Interactions.)

EFFECTS OF OTHER DRUGS ON COMBINED HORMONAL CONTRACEPTIVES

Rifampin: Metabolism of some synthetic estrogens (*e.g.,* ethinyl estradiol) and progestins (*e.g.,* norethindrone) is increased by rifampin. A reduction in contraceptive effectiveness and an increase in menstrual irregularities have been associated with concomitant use of rifampin.

Anticonvulsants: Anticonvulsants such as phenobarbital, phenytoin, and carbamazepine have been shown to increase the metabolism of some synthetic estrogens and progestins, which could result in a reduction of contraceptive effectiveness.

Antibiotics: Pregnancy while taking oral contraceptives has been reported when the oral contraceptives were administered with antimicrobials such as ampicillin, tetracycline, and griseofulvin. However, clinical pharmacokinetic studies have not demonstrated any consistent effects of antibiotics (other than rifampin) on plasma concentrations of synthetic steroids.

Herbal Products Herbal products containing St. John's Wort (hypericum perforatum) may induce hepatic enzymes (cytochrome P450) and p-glycoprotein transporter and may reduce the effectiveness of contraceptive steroids. This may also result in breakthrough bleeding.

Other: Ascorbic acid and acetominophen may increase plasma concentrations of some synthetic estrogens, possibly by inhibition of conjugation. A reduction in contraceptive effectiveness and an increased incidence of menstrual irregularities has been suggested with phenylbutazone.

EFFECTS OF COMBINED HORMONAL CONTRACEPTIVES ON OTHER DRUGS

Combined hormonal contraceptives containing some synthetic estrogens (*e.g.,* ethinyl estradiol) may inhibit the metabolism of other compounds. Increased plasma concentrations of cyclosporine, prednisolone and theophylline have been reported with concomitant administration of oral contraceptives. In addition, oral contraceptives may induce the conjugation of other compounds. Decreased plasma concentrations of acetominophen and increased clearance of temazepam, salicylic acid, morphine and clofibric acid have been noted when these drugs were administered with oral contraceptives.

DRUG INTERACTIONS WITH LABORATORY TESTS

Certain endocrine and liver function tests and blood components may be affected by combined hormonal contraceptives:

Increased prothrombin and factors VII, VIII, IX, and X; decreased antithrombin 3; increased norepinephrine-induced platelet aggregability.

Increased thyroid binding globulin (TBG) leading to increased circulating total thyroid hormone, as measured by protein-bound iodine (PBI). T4 by column or by radioimmunoassay. Free T3 resin uptake is decreased, reflecting the elevated TBG, free T4 concentration is unaltered.

Other binding proteins may be elevated in serum.

Sex-hormone-binding globulins are increased and result in elevated levels of total circulating sex steroids and corticoids: however, free or biologically active levels remain unchanged.

Triglycerides may be increased.

Glucose tolerance may be decreased.

Serum folate levels may be depressed by combined hormonal contraceptive therapy. This may be of clinical significance if a woman becomes pregnant shortly after discontinuing combined hormonal contraceptives.

The pathologist should be advised of progestogen and estrogen therapy when relevant tissue specimens are submitted.

The following laboratory tests may be affected by progestins including estradiol cypionate; medroxyprogesterone acetate monthly contraceptive injection:

Plasma and urinary steroid levels are decreased (*e.g.,* progesterone, estradiol, pregnanediol, testosterone, cortisol).

Gonadotropin levels are decreased.

Sex-hormone-binding-globulin concentrations are decreased.

Sulfobromophthalein and other liver function test values may be increased.

ADVERSE REACTIONS

An increased risk of the following serious adverse reactions has been associated with the use of combined hormonal contraceptives: (See CONTRAINDICATIONS and WARNINGS.) Arterial thromboembolism, cerebral hemorrhage, cerebral thrombosis, gallbladder disease, hepatic adenomas or benign liver tumors, hypertension, myocardial infarction, pulmonary embolism, and thrombophlebitis.

The following adverse reactions have been reported in patients receiving estradiol cypionate; medroxyprogesterone acetate monthly contraceptive injection and are believed to be drug-related: Abdominal pain, acne, alopecia, amenorrhea, asthenia, breast tenderness/pain, decreased libido, depression, dizziness, dysmenorrhea, emotional lability, enlarged abdomen, headache, menorrhagia, metrorrhagia, nausea, nervousness, vaginal moniliasis, vulvovaginal disorder, and weight gain.

There is evidence of an association between the following conditions and the use of combined hormonal contraceptives, although additional confirmatory studies are needed: Mesenteric thrombosis, and retinal thrombosis.

The following additional adverse reactions have been reported in users of combined hormonal contraceptives, and are believed to be drug-related: Anaphylactic reactions, breast changes: enlargement and secretion, cervical changes, cholestatic jaundice, corneal curvature changes (*i.e.,* steepening), diminution in lactation when given immediately postpartum, edema, intolerance to contact lenses, melasma that may persist, migraine, rash (allergic), reduced carbohydrate tolerance, temporary infertility after treatment discontinuation, and weight decrease.

The following additional adverse reactions have been reported in users of combined hormonal contraceptives, and the association has been neither confirmed nor refuted: Budd-Chiari syndrome, cataracts, changes in appetite, changes in libido, colitis, cystitis-like syndrome, erythema multiforme, erythema nodosum, hemolytic uremic syndrome, hemorrhagic eruption, hirsutism, impaired renal function, premenstrual syndrome, porphyria, and vaginitis.

The most frequent adverse events (reported by 1% or more patients) leading to discontinuation in various trials of women using estradiol cypionate; medroxyprogesterone acetate monthly contraceptive injection were: Weight gain, menorrhagia, amenorrhea, metrorrhagia, vaginal spotting, emotional lability, acne, breast tenderness/pain, headache, dysmenorrhea, nausea, and depression.

DOSAGE AND ADMINISTRATION

Estradiol cypionate; medroxyprogesterone acetate monthly contraceptive injection is effective for contraception during the first cycle of use when administered as recommended.

The recommended dose of estradiol cypionate; medroxyprogesterone acetate monthly contraceptive injection is 0.5 ml administered by intramuscular injection, into the deltoid, gluteus maximus, or anterior thigh. The aqueous suspension must be vigorously shaken just before use to ensure a uniform suspension of 25 mg medroxyprogesterone acetate and 5 mg estradiol cypionate.

First Injection:

- Within first 5 days of the onset of a normal menstrual period, **or**
- Within 5 days of a complete first trimester abortion, **or**
- No earlier than 4 weeks postpartum if not breastfeeding
- No earlier than 6 weeks postpartum if breastfeeding.

Second and Subsequent Injections:

Monthly (28-30 days) after previous injection, not to exceed 33 days.

If the patient has not adhered to the prescribed schedule (greater than 33 days since last injection), pregnancy should be considered and she should not receive another injection until pregnancy is ruled out.

Shortening the injection interval could lead to a change in menstrual pattern.

Do not use bleeding episodes to guide the injection schedule.

SWITCHING FROM OTHER METHODS OF CONTRACEPTION

When switching from other contraceptive methods, estradiol cypionate; medroxyprogesterone acetate monthly contraceptive injection should be given in a manner that ensures continuous contraceptive coverage based upon the mechanism of action of both methods, *e.g.,* patients switching from oral contraceptives should have their first injection of estradiol cypionate; medroxyprogesterone acetate monthly contraceptive injection within 7 days after taking their last active pill.

HOW SUPPLIED

Lunelle monthly contraceptive injection (25 mg medroxyprogesterone acetate and 5 mg estradiol cypionate per 0.5 ml sterile aqueous injectable suspension) is available in a vial containing enough product to deliver 0.5 ml for single-dose administration.

Storage: Store at 25°C (77°F); excursions permitted to 15-30°C (59-86°F).

PRODUCT LISTING - EQUIVALENTS NOT AVAILABLE

Suspension - Intramuscular - 5 mg;25 mg/0.5 ml

0.50 ml	$26.99	LUNELLE, Pharmacia Corporation	00009-3484-04
0.50 ml	$26.99	LUNELLE, Pharmacia Corporation	00009-3484-06
0.50 ml x 25	$674.75	LUNELLE, Pharmacia Corporation	00009-3484-05

Estradiol-17β; Norgestimate *(003459)*

Categories: Atrophy, vaginal; Atrophy, vulvar; Menopause; Osteoporosis, prevention; Vaginitis, atrophic; FDA Approved 1999 Oct; Pregnancy Category X

Drug Classes: Estrogens; Hormones/hormone modifiers; Progestins

Brand Names: **Ortho-Prefest**

Cost of Therapy: $152.57 (Menopause; Ortho-Prefest; biphasic; 1 tablet/day; 30 day supply)

DESCRIPTION

The Ortho-Prefest regimen provides for a single oral tablet to be taken once daily. The pink tablet containing 1.0 mg estradiol is taken on days 1-3 of therapy; the white tablet containing 1.0 mg estradiol and 0.09 mg norgestimate is taken on days 4-6 of therapy. This pattern is then repeated continuously to produce the constant estrogen/intermittent progestogen regimen of Ortho-Prefest.

The estrogenic component of Ortho-Prefest is 17β-estradiol. It is a white, crystalline solid, chemically described as estra-1,3,5(10)-triene-3,17β-diol. It has an empirical formula of $C_{18}H_{24}O_2$ and molecular weight of 272.39.

The progestational component of Ortho-Prefest is micronized norgestimate, a white powder which is chemically described as (17α)-17-(Acetyloxyl)-13-ethyl-18,19-dinorpregn-4-en-20-yn-3-one3-oxime. It has an empirical formula of $C_{23}H_{31}NO_3$ and a molecular weight of 369.50.

Each tablet for oral administration contains 1.0 mg estradiol alone or 1.0 mg estradiol and 0.09 mg of norgestimate, and the following inactive ingredients: croscarmellose sodium, microcrystalline cellulose, magnesium stearate, ferric oxide red, and lactose monohydrate.

CLINICAL PHARMACOLOGY

Estrogens are important in the development and maintenance of the female reproductive system and secondary sex characteristics. By a direct action, they cause growth and development of the uterus, fallopian tubes, and vagina. With other hormones, such as pituitary hormones and progesterone, they cause enlargement of the breasts through promotion of ductal growth, stromal development, and the accretion of fat. Estrogens are intricately involved with other hormones, especially progesterone, in the processes of the ovulatory menstrual cycle and pregnancy and affect the release of pituitary gonadotropins. They also contribute to the shaping of the skeleton, maintenance of tone and elasticity of urogenital structures, changes in the epiphyses of the long bones that allow for the pubertal growth spurt and its termination, and pigmentation of the nipples and genitals.

Although circulating estrogens exist in a dynamic equilibrium of metabolic interconversions, estradiol is the principal intracellular human estrogen and is substantially more potent than its metabolites, estrone, and estriol at the receptor level. The primary source of estrogen in adult women with normal menstrual cycles is the ovarian follicle, which secretes 70-500 μg of estradiol daily, depending on the phase of the menstrual cycle. After menopause, most endogenous estrogens are produced by conversion of androstenedione, secreted by the adrenal cortex, to estrone by the peripheral tissues. Thus, estrone and the sulfate conjugated form, estrone sulfate, are the most abundant circulating estrogens in postmenopausal women.

Circulating estrogens modulate the pituitary secretion of the gonadotropins, luteinizing hormone (LH) and follicle stimulating hormone (FSH) through a negative feedback mechanism and estrogen replacement therapy acts to reduce the elevated levels of these hormones seen in postmenopausal women.

Norgestimate is a derivative of 19-nortestosterone and binds to androgen and progestogen receptors, similar to that of the natural hormone progesterone; it does not bind to estrogen receptors. Progestins counter the estrogenic effects by decreasing the number of nuclear estradiol receptors and suppressing epithelial DNA synthesis in endometrial tissue.

PHARMACOKINETICS

Absorption

Estradiol reaches its peak serum concentration (C_{max}) at approximately 7 hours in postmenopausal women receiving estradiol-17β; norgestimate (see TABLE 1). Norgestimate is completely metabolized; it's primary active metabolite, 17-deacetylnorgestimate, reaches C_{max} at approximately 2 hours after dose (see TABLE 1). Upon coadministration of estradiol-17β; norgestimate with a high fat meal, the C_{max} values for estrone and estrone sulfate were increased by 14% and 24% respectively, and the C_{max} for 17-deacetylnorgestimate was decreased by 16%. The AUC values for these analytes were not significantly affected by food.

Distribution

The distribution of exogenous estrogens is similar to that of endogenous estrogens. Estrogens are widely distributed in the body and are generally found in higher concentrations in the sex hormone target organs. Estradiol is bound mainly to sex hormone binding globulin (SHBG), and to albumin. 17-deacetylnorgestimate, the primary active metabolite of norgestimate, does not bind to SHBG but to other serum proteins. The percent protein binding of 17-deacetylnorgestimate is approximately 99%.

Metabolism

Exogenous estrogens are metabolized in the same manner as endogenous estrogens. Circulating estrogens exist in a dynamic equilibrium of metabolic interconversions. These transformations take place mainly in the liver. Estradiol is converted reversibly to estrone, and both can be converted to estriol, which is the major urinary metabolite. Estrogens also undergo enterohepatic recirculation via sulfate and glucuronide conjugation in the liver, biliary secretion of conjugates into the intestine, and hydrolysis in the gut followed by reabsorption. In postmenopausal women a significant portion of the circulating estrogens exist as sulfate conjugates, especially estrone sulfate, which serves as a circulating reservoir for the formation of more active estrogens. Norgestimate is extensively metabolized by first-pass mechanisms in gastrointestinal tract and/or liver. Norgestimate's primary active metabolite is 17-deacetylnorgestimate.

TABLE 1 *Mean Pharmacokinetic Parameters of E_2, E_1, E_1S, and 17d-NGM* Following Single and Multiple Dosing of Estradiol-17β; Norgestimate*

			First Dose		Multiple Dose	
Analyte	**Parameter†**	**Units**	**E_2**	**E_2/NGM**	**E_2**	**E_2/NGM**
E_2	C_{max}	pg/ml	27.4	39.3	49.7	46.2
	T_{max}	h	7	7	7	7
	AUC(0-24 h)	pg·h/ml	424	681	864	779
E_1	C_{max}	pg/ml	210	285	341	325
	T_{max}	h	6	6	7	6
	AUC(0-24 h)	pg·h/ml	2774	4153	5429	4957
E_1S	C_{max}	ng/ml	11.1	13.9	14.9	14.5
	T_{max}	h	5	4	6	5
	AUC(0-24 h)	ng·h/ml	135	180	198	198
17d-NGM	C_{max}	pg/ml	NA	515	NA	643
	T_{max}	h	NA	2	NA	2
	AUC(0-24 h)	pg·h/ml	NA	2146	NA	5322
	T½	h	NA	37	NA	NA

* E_2 = 17β-Estradiol, E_1 = Estrone, E_1S = Estrone Sulfate, 17d-NGM = 17-deacetylnorgestimate. Baseline uncorrected data are reported for E_2, E_1, and E_1S.
† C_{max} = peak serum concentration, T_{max} = time to reach peak serum concentration, AUC(0-24 h) = area under serum concentration vs. time curve from 0 to 24 hours after dose, T½ = half-life.
NA = Not available or not applicable.

Excretion

Estradiol, estrone, and estriol are excreted in the urine along with glucuronide and sulfate conjugates. Norgestimate metabolites are eliminated in the urine and feces. The half-life (T½) of estradiol and 17-deacetylnorgestimate in postmenopausal women receiving estradiol-17β; norgestimate is approximately 16 and 37 hours, respectively.

SPECIAL POPULATIONS

Pediatric

Estradiol-17β; norgestimate is not indicated in children.

Geriatric

Estradiol-17β; norgestimate has not been studied in geriatric patients

Gender

Estradiol-17β; norgestimate is indicated in women only.

Effects of Race, Age, and Body Weight

The effects of race, age, and body weight on the pharmacokinetics of 17β-estradiol, norgestimate, and their metabolites were evaluated in 164 healthy postmenopausal women (100 Caucasians, 61 Hispanics, 2 Blacks, and 1 Asian). No significant pharmacokinetic difference was observed between the Caucasian and the Hispanic postmenopausal women. No significant difference due to age (40-66 years) was observed. No significant difference due to body weight was observed in women in the 60-80 kg weight range. Women with body weight higher than 80 kg, however, had approximately 40% lower peak serum levels of 17-deacetylnorgestimate, 30% lower AUC values for 17-deacetylnorgestimate and 30% lower C_{max} values for norgestrel. The clinical relevance of these observations is unknown.

Renal Insufficiency

It has been reported in the literature that at both baseline and after estradiol ingestion, postmenopausal women with end stage renal disease (ESRD) had higher free serum estradiol levels than the control subjects. No pharmacokinetic study with norgestimate or a hormone combination with norgestimate has been conducted in postmenopausal women with ESRD.

Hepatic Insufficiency

No pharmacokinetic study for estradiol-17β; norgestimate has been conducted in postmenopausal women with hepatic impairment.

DRUG-DRUG INTERACTIONS

Estradiol, norgestimate, and their metabolites inhibit a variety of P450 enzymes in human liver microsomes. However, the clinical and toxicological consequences of such interaction are likely to be insignificant because, under the recommended dosing regimen, the *in vivo* concentrations of these steroids, even at the peak serum levels, are relatively low compared to the inhibitory constant (Ki). Results of a subset population (n=24) from a clinical study conducted in 36 healthy postmenopausal women indicated that the steady state serum estradiol levels during the estradiol plus norgestimate phase of the regimen may be lower by 12-18% as compared with estradiol administered alone. The serum estrone levels may decrease by 4% and the serum estrone sulfate levels may increase by 17% during the estradiol plus norgestimate phase as compared with estradiol administered alone. The clinical relevance of these observations is unknown.

INDICATIONS AND USAGE

Estradiol-17β; norgestimate therapy is indicated in women with an intact uterus for the:

Treatment of moderate to severe vasomotor symptoms associated with menopause.
Treatment of vulvar and vaginal atrophy.
Prevention of osteoporosis.

Most prospective studies of efficacy for this indication have been carried out in white post-menopausal women, without stratification by other risk factors, and tend to show a universally beneficial effect on bone. Since estrogen administration is associated with risk, patient selection must be individualized based on the balance of risks and benefits.

Case-control studies have shown an approximately 60% reduction in hip and wrist fractures in women whose estrogen replacement was begun within a few years after menopause. Studies also suggest that estrogen reduces the rate of vertebral fractures. When estrogen therapy is discontinued, bone mass declines at a rate comparable to the immediate postmenopausal period.

White and Asian women are at higher risk for osteoporosis than Black women, and thin women are at higher risk than heavier women, who generally have higher endogenous estrogen levels. Early menopause is one of the strongest predictors for the development of osteoporosis. Other factors associated with osteoporosis include genetic factors (small build, family history), lifestyle (cigarette smoking, alcohol abuse, sedentary exercise habits), and nutrition (below average body weight and dietary calcium intake).

The mainstays of prevention and management of osteoporosis are weight-bearing exercise, adequate lifetime calcium intake, and, when indicated, estrogen. Postmenopausal women absorb dietary calcium less efficiently than premenopausal women and require an average of 1500 mg/day of elemental calcium to remain in neutral calcium balance. The average calcium intake in the USA is 400-600 mg/day. Therefore, when not contraindicated, calcium supplementation may be helpful for women with suboptimal dietary intake.

NON-FDA APPROVED INDICATIONS

Although not FDA approved, estradiol-norgestimate may be appropriate therapy for treatment of atrophic urethritis in postmenopausal women with an intact uterus.

CONTRAINDICATIONS

Estrogens/progestins should not be used in individuals with any of the following conditions:

- Known or suspected pregnancy.
- Undiagnosed abnormal genital bleeding.
- Known or suspected cancer of the breast.
- Known or suspected estrogen-dependent neoplasia.
- Active or past history of thrombophlebitis or thromboembolic disorders.
- Hypersensitivity to any components of this product.

WARNINGS

BASED ON EXPERIENCE WITH ESTROGENS AND/OR PROGESTINS

Induction of Malignant Neoplasms

Endometrial Cancer

The reported endometrial cancer risk among unopposed estrogen users is about 2- to 12-fold greater than in non-users, and appears dependent on duration of treatment and on estrogen dose. Most studies show no significant increased risk associated with the use of estrogens for less than 1 year. The greatest risk appears associated with prolonged use, with increased risks of 15- to 24-fold for 5-10 years or more, and this risk has been shown to persist for at least 8-15 years after estrogen therapy is discontinued. Using progestin therapy together with estrogen therapy significantly reduces but does not eliminate this risk.

Appropriate diagnostic measures should be undertaken to rule out malignancy in all cases of undiagnosed, persistent, or recurring abnormal vaginal bleeding.

Breast Cancer

Some studies have reported an increase in the risk of breast cancer in postmenopausal women receiving hormone replacement therapy. A meta-analysis of 51 clinical studies suggests that this increased risk is comparable to that observed in women with every year of delay of natural menopause. This increased risk decreases after cessation of use of hormone replacement therapy and is not apparent 5 years following cessation of treatment. Breast cancers found in current or recent users of hormone replacement therapy are more likely to be localized to the breast than those in non-users. Concurrent progestin use does not appear to protect against this risk. Therefore, a careful appraisal of the risk/benefit ratio should be undertaken before the initiation of long-term treatment.

Women on hormone replacement therapy should have regular examinations and should be instructed in breast self-examination, and women over the age of 50 should have regular mammograms.

Venous Thromboembolism

Epidemiologic studies have reported an increased risk of venous thromboembolism (VTE) in users of estrogen replacement therapy (ERT) who did not have predisposing conditions for VTE, such as past history of cardiovascular disease or a recent history of pregnancy, surgery, trauma, or serious illness. The increased risk was found only in current ERT users; it did not persist in former users. The findings were similar for ERT alone or with added progestin and pertain to commonly used ERT types and doses, including 0.625 mg or more per day orally of conjugated estrogens, 1 mg or more per day orally of estradiol, and 50 μg or more per day or transdermal estradiol. The studies found the VTE risk to be about 1 case per 10,000 women per year among women not using ERT and without predisposing conditions. The risk in current ERT users was increased to 2-3 cases per 10,000 women per year.

Cardiovascular Disease

Large doses of estrogens (5 mg conjugated estrogens per day), comparable to those used to treat cancer of the prostate and breast, have been shown to increase the risks of nonfatal myocardial infarction, pulmonary embolism, and thrombophlebitis in a large prospective clinical trial in men.

Hypercalcemia

Administration of estrogens may lead to severe hypercalcemia in patients with breast cancer and bone metastases. If this occurs, the drugs should be stopped and appropriate measures taken to reduce the serum calcium level.

Gallbladder Disease

A 2- to 4-fold increase in the risk of gallbladder disease requiring surgery in women receiving postmenopausal estrogens has been reported.

PRECAUTIONS

GENERAL

Based on Experience with Estrogens and/or Progestins

Addition of a Progestin When a Women Has Not Had a Hysterectomy

Studies of the addition of a progestin for 10 or more days of a cycle of estrogen administration, or daily with estrogen in a continuous regimen, have reported a lowered incidence of endometrial hyperplasia than would be induced by estrogen treatment alone.

There are, however, possible risks that may be associated with the use of progestins in estrogen replacement regimens. These include:

- Adverse effects on lipoprotein metabolism (lowering HDL and raising LDL).
- Impairment of glucose tolerance.
- Possible enhancement of mitotic activity in breast epithelial tissue. There is minimal epidemiological data available to address this point.

The choice of progestin, its dose, and its regimen may be important in minimizing these adverse effects.

E

Elevated Blood Pressure

Occasional increases in blood pressure during estrogen replacement therapy have been attributed to idiosyncratic reactions to estrogens in a small number of case reports. A generalized effect of estrogen therapy on blood pressure was not found in the one randomized, placebo-controlled study that has been reported. This effect was also not observed in clinical studies with estradiol-17β; norgestimate.

Familial Hyperlipoproteinemia

Estrogen therapy may be associated with elevations of plasma triglycerides leading to pancreatitis and other complications in patients with familial defects of lipoprotein metabolism.

Impaired Liver Function

Estrogens may be poorly metabolized in patients with impaired liver function.

DRUG/LABORATORY TEST INTERACTIONS

Accelerated prothrombin time, partial thromboplastin time, and platelet aggregation time; increased platelet count; increased factors II, VII antigen, VIII antigen, VIII coagulant activity, IX, X, XII, VII-X complex, II-VII-X complex, and beta-thromboglobulin; decreased levels of anti-factor Xa and antithrombin III, decreased antithrombin III activity; increased levels of fibrinogen and fibrinogen activity; increased plasminogen antigen and activity.

Increased thyroid-binding globulin (TBG) leading to increased circulating total thyroid hormone, as measured by protein-bound iodine (PBI), T4 levels (by column or by radioimmunoassay) or T3 levels by radioimmunoassay. T3 resin uptake is decreased, reflecting the elevated TBG. Free T4 and free T3 concentrations are unaltered.

Other binding proteins may be elevated in serum, *i.e.*, corticosteroid binding globulin (CBG), sex hormone-binding globulin (SHBG), leading to increased circulating corticosteroids and sex steroids respectively. Free or biologically active hormone concentrations are unchanged. Other plasma proteins may be increased (angiotensinogen/renin substrate, alpha-1-antitrypsin, ceruloplasmin).

Increased plasma HDL and HDL-2 subfraction concentrations, reduced LDL cholesterol concentration, increased triglycerides levels.

Impaired glucose tolerance. For this reason, diabetic patients should be carefully observed while receiving estrogen/progestin therapy.

Reduced response to metyrapone test.

Reduced serum folate concentration.

CARCINOGENESIS, MUTAGENESIS, AND IMPAIRMENT OF FERTILITY

Long-term continuous administration of natural and synthetic estrogens in certain animal species increases the frequency of carcinomas of the breasts, uterus, cervix, vagina, testis, and liver. (See CONTRAINDICATIONS and WARNINGS.)

PREGNANCY CATEGORY X

Estradiol-17β; norgestimate should not be used during pregnancy. (See CONTRAINDICATIONS.)

NURSING MOTHERS

As a general principle, the administration of any drug to nursing mothers should be done only when clearly necessary since many drugs are excreted in human milk. Estrogen administration to nursing mothers has been shown to decrease the quantity and quality of the milk. Estrogens are not indicated for the prevention of postpartum breast engorgement.

ADVERSE REACTIONS

In four 12 month trials that included 579 healthy postmenopausal women treated with estradiol-17β; norgestimate the following treatment-emergent adverse events occurred at a rate ≥5% (see TABLE 6).

The following additional adverse reactions have been reported with estrogen therapy (see WARNINGS and PRECAUTIONS regarding induction of neoplasia, increased incidence of gallbladder disease, cardiovascular disease, elevated blood pressure, and hypercalcemia).

Genitourinary System: Changes in vaginal bleeding pattern and abnormal withdrawal bleeding or flow; breakthrough bleeding, spotting; increase in size of uterine leiomyomata; vaginal candidiasis; change in amount of cervical secretion.

Breasts: Tenderness, enlargement, galactorrhea.

Gastrointestinal: Cholestatic jaundice, nausea, vomiting; abdominal cramps, bloating, increased incidence of gall bladder disease.

Skin: Chloasma or melasma; which may persist when drug is discontinued; erythema multiforme; erythema nodosum; hemorrhagic eruption; loss of scalp hair; hirsutism.

Central Nervous System: Headache, migraine, dizziness; mental depression; chorea.

Eyes: Steepening of corneal curvature; intolerance to contact lenses.

Miscellaneous: Increase or decrease in weight; reduced carbohydrate tolerance; aggravation of porphyria; edema; changes in libido.

TABLE 6 *All Treatment-Emergent Adverse Events Regardless of Drug Relationship Reported at a Frequency of ≥5% With Estradiol-17β; Norgestimate*

Four 12 month clinical trials

	Estradiol-17β; Norgestimate (n=579)	
Body as a Whole		
Back pain	69	(12%)
Fatigue	32	(6%)
Influenza-like symptoms	64	(11%)
Pain	37	(6%)
Digestive System		
Abdominal pain	70	(12%)
Flatulence	29	(5%)
Nausea	34	(6%)
Tooth disorder	27	(5%)
Musculoskeletal System		
Arthralgia	51	(9%)
Myalgia	30	(5%)
Nervous System		
Dizziness	27	(5%)
Headache	132	(23%)
Psychiatric Disorders		
Depression	27	(5%)
Reproductive System		
Breast pain	92	(16%)
Dysmenorrhea	48	(8%)
Vaginal bleeding (all)	52	(9%)
Vaginitis	42	(7%)
Resistance Mechanism Disorders		
Viral infection	35	(6%)
Respiratory System		
Coughing	28	(5%)
Pharyngitis	38	(7%)
Sinusitis	44	(8%)
Upper respiratory-tract infection	121	(21%)

DOSAGE AND ADMINISTRATION

Estradiol-17β; norgestimate regimen consists of the daily administration of a single tablet containing 1 mg estradiol (pink color) for 3 days followed by a single tablet of 1 mg estradiol combined with 0.09 mg norgestimate (white color) for 3 days. This regimen is repeated continuously without interruption.

For treatment of moderate to severe vasomotor symptoms and vulvar and vaginal atrophy associated with menopause, the patient should start with the first tablet in the first row, and place the weekday schedule sticker which starts with the weekday of first tablet intake in the appropriate space. After all tablets from the blister card have been used, the first tablet from a new blister card should be taken on the following day. This dose may not be the lowest effective dose for treatment of vulvar and vaginal atrophy. Patients should be re-evaluated at 3 month to 6 month intervals to determine if treatment for symptoms is still necessary.

For prevention of osteoporosis, the patient should start with the first tablet in the first row, and place the weekday schedule sticker which starts with the weekday of first tablet intake in the appropriate space. After all tablets from the blister card have been used, the first tablet from a new blister card should be taken on the following day. This dose may not be the lowest effective dose for the prevention of osteoporosis.

MISSED TABLETS

If a tablet is missed for 1 or more days, therapy should be resumed with the next available tablet. The patient should continue to take only 1 tablet each day in sequence.

HOW SUPPLIED

Ortho-Prefest is available as two separate, round-shaped tablets for oral administration supplied in a blister card with the following configuration: 3 pink tablets, followed by 3 white tablets for a total of 30 tablets per blister card.

Each blister card contains 15 tablets of each of the following components:

1 mg Estradiol: Pink tablets embossed with "1" and "J-C" on one side and "E2" and "O-M" on the other side.

1 mg Estradiol/0.09 mg Norgestimate: White tablets embossed with "1/90" and "J-C" on one side and "E2/N" and "O-M" on the other side.

Storage: This product is stable for 18 months. Store at 25°C (77°F); excursions permitted to 15-30°C (59-86°F).

PRODUCT LISTING - EQUIVALENTS NOT AVAILABLE

Tablet - Oral - Biphasic

30 x 6	$188.88	ORTHO-PREFEST, Ortho Mcneil Pharmaceutical	00062-1840-15
30's	$31.48	ORTHO-PREFEST, Ortho Mcneil Pharmaceutical	00062-1840-01

Estradiol; Norethindrone Acetate (003416)

Categories: Atrophy, vaginal; Atrophy, vulvar; Castration, female; Hypoestrogenism; Menopause; Osteoporosis, prevention; Ovarian failure, primary; Vaginitis, atrophic; FDA Approved 1998 Aug; Pregnancy Category X
Drug Classes: Estrogens; Hormones/hormone modifiers; Progestins
Brand Names: CombiPatch
Foreign Brand Availability: Activelle (France; Hong-Kong; Israel; Korea; Singapore; South-Africa; Taiwan; Thailand); Cliane (Indonesia; Korea; New-Zealand); Covina (Taiwan); Estalis continuous (Australia); Estalis Sequi (Australia); Estracomb (Bahrain; Colombia; Cyprus; Egypt; Iran; Iraq; Jordan; Kuwait; Lebanon; Libya; Oman; Qatar; Republic-of-Yemen; Saudi-Arabia; Syria; United-Arab-Emirates); Estragest TTS (Bahrain; Cyprus; Egypt; Germany; Iran; Iraq; Jordan; Kuwait; Lebanon; Libya; Oman; Qatar; Republic-of-Yemen; Saudi-Arabia; Syria; United-Arab-Emirates); Eveprem (Korea); Eviclin (Korea); Evorel Cont (Israel); Evorelconti (Mexico); Evorel Sequi (Israel); Kliogest (China; Korea; Singapore); Kliovance (Australia); Meno-Net (Israel); Novofem (England; Ireland); Tri-Sequens (Colombia; Korea; Singapore); Trisequens (France)
Cost of Therapy: $26.09 (Menopause; Activella; 1 mg; 0.5 mg; 1 tablet/day; day supply)
$31.19 (Menopause; CombiPatch Transdermal; 0.05 mg; 0.14 mg/24 h; 2 patches/week; 28 day supply)

ORAL

DESCRIPTION

Activella is a single tablet containing an estrogen, estradiol (E_2), and a progestin, norethindrone acetate (NETA), for oral administration. Each tablet contains 1 mg estradiol and 0.5 mg norethindrone acetate and the following excipients: lactose monohydrate, starch (corn), copovidone, talc, magnesium stearate, hydroxypropyl methylcellulose and triacetin.

Estradiol (E_2) is a white or almost white crystalline powder. Its chemical name is estra-1,3,5(10)-triene-3,17β-diol hemihydrate with the empirical formula of $C_{18}H_{24}O_2 \cdot ½H_2O$ and a molecular weight of 281.4.

Norethindrone acetate (NETA) is a white or yellowish-white crystalline powder. Its chemical name is 17β-acetoxy-19-nor-17α-pregn-4-en-20-yn-3-one with the empirical formula of $C_{22}H_{28}O_3$ and molecular weight of 340.5.

CLINICAL PHARMACOLOGY

Estrogen drug products act by regulating the transcription of a limited number of genes. Estrogens diffuse through cell membranes and bind to and activate the nuclear estrogen receptor, a DNA-binding protein that is found in estrogen-responsive tissues. The activated estrogen receptor binds to specific DNA sequences, or hormone-response elements, that enhance the transcription of adjacent genes and in turn lead to the observed effects. Estrogen receptors have been identified in tissues of the reproductive tract, breast, pituitary, hypothalamus, liver, and bone in women.

Estrogens are largely responsible for the development and maintenance of the female reproductive system and secondary sexual characteristics. Although circulating estrogens exist in a dynamic equilibrium of metabolic interconversions, estradiol is the principal intracellular human estrogen and is substantially more potent than its metabolites, estrone and estriol, at the receptor level. The primary source of estrogen in normally cycling adult women is the ovarian follicle, which secretes 70,500 μg of estradiol daily, depending on the phase of the menstrual cycle. After menopause, most endogenous estrogen is produced by conversion in peripheral tissues of androstenedione which is secreted by the adrenal cortex, to estrone. Thus, estrone and the sulfate conjugated form, estrone sulfate, are the most abundant circulating estrogens in postmenopausal women.

Circulating estrogens modulate the pituitary secretion of the gonadotropins, luteinizing hormone (LH), and follicle-stimulating hormone (FSH) through a negative feedback mechanism, and estrogen replacement therapy acts to reduce the elevated levels of these hormones seen in postmenopausal women.

Progestin compounds enhance cellular differentiation and generally oppose the actions of estrogens by decreasing estrogen receptor levels, increasing local metabolism of estrogens to less active metabolites, or inducing gene products that blunt cellular responses to estrogen. Progestins exert their effects in target cells by binding to specific progesterone receptors that interact with progesterone response elements in target genes. Progesterone receptors have been identified in the female reproductive tract, breast, pituitary, hypothalamus, and central nervous system. Progestins produce similar endometrial changes to those of the naturally occurring hormone progesterone.

The use of unopposed estrogen therapy has been associated with an increased risk of endometrial hyperplasia, a possible precursor of endometrial adenocarcinoma. The addition of a progestin, in adequate doses and appropriate duration, to an estrogen replacement regimen reduces the incidence of endometrial hyperplasia, and the attendant risk of carcinoma in women with intact uterus.

PHARMACOKINETICS

Absorption

Estradiol is well absorbed through the gastrointestinal tract. Following oral administration of estradiol; norethindrone acetate tablets, peak plasma estradiol concentrations are reached slowly within 5-8 hours. When given orally, estradiol is extensively metabolized (first-pass effect) to estrone sulfate, with smaller amounts of other conjugated and unconjugated estrogens. After oral administration, norethindrone acetate is rapidly absorbed and transformed to norethindrone. It undergoes first-pass metabolism in the liver and other enteric organs, and reaches a peak plasma concentration within 0.5-1.5 hours. The oral bioavailability of estradiol and norethindrone following administration of estradiol; norethindrone acetate tablets when compared to a combination oral solution is 53% and 100%, respectively. The pharmacokinetic parameters of estradiol (E_2), estrone (E_1), and norethindrone (NET) following single oral administration of estradiol; norethindrone acetate tablets in 25 volunteers are summarized in TABLE 1.

Following continuous dosing with once-daily administration of estradiol; norethindrone acetate tablets, serum levels of estradiol, estrone, and norethindrone reached steady-state within 2 weeks with an accumulation of 33-47% above levels following single dose administration.

TABLE 1 *Pharmacokinetic Parameters After a Single Dose of Estradiol; Norethindrone Acetate Tablets in Healthy Postmenopausal Women (n=25)*

	Mean‡ ±SD
Estradiol* (E_2)	
AUC(0-72h) (pg/ml·h)	1053 ± 310
C_{max} (pg/ml)	34.6 ± 10.8
T_{max} (h)	6.8 ± 2.9
T½ (h)§	13.2 ± 4.7
Estrone* (E_1)	
AUC(0-72h) (pg/ml·h)	5223 ± 1618
C_{max} (pg/ml)	251.1 ± 91.0
T_{max} (h)	5.7 ± 1.4
T½ (h)§	12.2 ± 4.6
Norethindrone (NET)	
AUC(0-72h) (pg/ml·h)	23681 ± 9023†
C_{max} (pg/ml)	5308 ± 1510
T_{max} (h)	1.0 ± 0.0
T½ (h)	11.4 ± 2.7

AUC = Area under the curve.
C_{max} = Maximum plasma concentration.
T_{max} = Time at maximum plasma concentration.
T½ = Half-life.
SD = Standard deviation.
* Baseline unadjusted data.
† (n=23).
‡ Arithmetic mean.
§ Baseline adjusted data.

Distribution

The distribution of exogenous estrogens is similar to that of endogenous estrogens. Estrogens are widely distributed in the body and are generally found in higher concentrations in the sex hormone target organs. Estradiol circulates in the blood bound to sex-hormone-binding globulin (SHBG) (37%) and to albumin (61%), while only approximately 1-2% is unbound. Norethindrone also binds to a similar extent to SHBG (36%) and to albumin (61%).

Metabolism and Excretion

Estradiol

Exogenous estrogens are metabolized in the same manner as endogenous estrogens. Circulating estrogens exist in a dynamic equilibrium of metabolic interconversions. These transformations take place mainly in the liver. Estradiol is converted reversibly to estrone, and both can be converted to estriol, which is the major urinary metabolite. Estrogens also undergo enterohepatic recirculation via sulfate and glucuronide conjugation in the liver, biliary secretion of conjugates into the intestine, and hydrolysis in the gut followed by reabsorption. In postmenopausal women, a significant portion of the circulating estrogens exist as sulfate conjugates, especially estrone sulfate, which serves as a circulating reservoir for the formation of more active estrogens. The half-life of estradiol following single dose administration of estradiol; norethindrone acetate tablets is 12-14 hours.

Norethindrone Acetate

The most important metabolites of norethindrone are isomers of 5α-dihydro-norethindrone and tetrahydro-norethindrone, which are excreted mainly in the urine as sulfate or glucuronide conjugates. The terminal half-life of norethindrone is about 8-11 hours.

Drug-Drug Interactions

Coadministration of estradiol with norethindrone acetate did not elicit any apparent influence on the pharmacokinetics of norethindrone. Similarly, no relevant interaction of norethindrone on the pharmacokinetics of estradiol was found within the NETA dose range investigated in a single dose study.

Drug-Food Interactions

A single-dose study in 24 healthy postmenopausal women was conducted to investigate any potential impact of administration of estradiol; norethindrone acetate tablets with and without food. Administration of estradiol; norethindrone acetate tablets with food did not modify the bioavailability of estradiol, although increases in AUC(0-72) of 19% and decreases in C_{max} of 36% for norethindrone were seen.

INDICATIONS AND USAGE

Estradiol; norethindrone acetate tablets therapy is indicated in women with an intact uterus for the:

Treatment of moderate to severe vasomotor symptoms associated with the menopause. There is no adequate evidence that estrogens are effective for nervous symptoms or depression that might occur during menopause and they should not be used to treat these conditions.

Treatment of vulvar and vaginal atrophy.

Prevention of postmenopausal osteoporosis.

Most prospective studies of efficacy for the osteoporosis prevention indication have been carried out in white post-menopausal women, without stratification by other risk factors, and tend to show a universally beneficial effect on bone. Since estrogen administration is associated with risk, patient selection must be individualized based on the balance of risks and benefits.

Case-control studies have shown an approximately 60% reduction in hip and wrist fractures in women whose estrogen replacement was begun within a few years after menopause. Studies also suggest that estrogen reduces the rate of vertebral fractures. When estrogen therapy is discontinued, bone mass declines at a rate comparable to the immediate post-menopausal period.

White and Asian women are at higher risk for osteoporosis than black women, and thin women are at a higher risk than heavier women, who generally have higher endogenous estrogen levels. Early menopause is one of the strongest predictors for the development of osteoporosis. Other factors associated with osteoporosis include genetic factors (small build, family history), lifestyle (cigarette smoking, alcohol abuse, sedentary exercise habits) and nutrition (below average body weight and dietary calcium intake). The mainstays of prevention and management of osteoporosis are weight-bearing exercise, adequate calcium intake, and, when indicated, estrogen. Postmenopausal women absorb dietary calcium less efficiently than premenopausal women and require an average of 1500 mg/day of elemental calcium to remain in neutral calcium balance. The average calcium intake in the US is 400-600 mg/day. Therefore, when not contraindicated, calcium supplementation may be helpful for women with suboptimal dietary intake.

CONTRAINDICATIONS

Estrogens/progestins combined should not be used in women under any of the following conditions or circumstances:

- Known or suspected pregnancy, including use for missed abortions or as a diagnostic test for pregnancy. Estrogen or progestin may cause fetal harm when administered to a pregnant woman.
- Known or suspected breast cancer, or past history of breast cancer associated with the use of estrogens.
- Known or suspected estrogen-dependent neoplasia, *e.g.*, endometrial cancer.
- Abnormal genital bleeding of unknown etiology.
- Known or suspected active deep venous thrombosis, thromboembolic disorders or stroke or past history of these conditions associated with estrogen use.
- Liver dysfunction or disease.
- Hypersensitivity to any of the components of estradiol; norethindrone acetate tablets.

WARNINGS

ALL WARNINGS BELOW PERTAIN TO THE USE OF THIS COMBINATION PRODUCT.

BASED ON EXPERIENCE WITH ESTROGENS AND/OR PROGESTINS

Induction of Malignant Neoplasms

Endometrial Cancer

The reported endometrial cancer risk among unopposed estrogen users is about 2- to 12-fold greater than in non-users, and appears dependent on duration of treatment and on estrogen dose. There is no significant increased risk associated with the use of estrogens for less than 1 year. The greatest risk appears to be associated with prolonged use with increased risks of 15- to 24-fold with 5 or more years of use. In 3 studies, persistence of risk was demonstrated for 8 to over 15 years after cessation of estrogen treatment. In one study, a significant decrease in the incidence of endometrial cancer occurred 6 months after withdrawal. Progestins taken with estrogens have been shown to significantly reduce, but not eliminate, the risk of endometrial cancer associated with estrogen use. In a large clinical trial, the incidence of endometrial hyperplasia with estradiol; norethindrone acetate tablets was 0.4% (one simple hyperplasia without atypia) compared to 14.6% with 1 mg estradiol unopposed.

Clinical surveillance of all women taking estrogen/progestin combinations is important. Adequate diagnostic measures, including endometrial sampling when indicated, should be undertaken to rule out malignancy in all cases of undiagnosed persistent or recurring abnormal vaginal bleeding. There is no evidence that "natural" estrogens are more or less hazardous than "synthetic" estrogens at equivalent estrogen doses.

Breast Cancer

While the majority of studies have not shown an increased risk of breast cancer in women who have ever used estrogen replacement therapy, some have reported a moderately increased risk (relative risks of 1.3-2.0) in those taking higher doses, or in those taking lower doses for prolonged periods of time, especially in excess of 10 years.

While the effects of added progestins on the risk of breast cancer are also unknown, available epidemiological evidence suggest that progestins do not reduce, and may enhance, the moderately increased breast cancer risk that has been reported with prolonged estrogen replacement therapy.

In a 1-year trial among 1176 women who received either unopposed 1 mg estradiol or a combination of 1 mg estradiol plus 1 of 3 different doses of NETA, (0.1, 0.25 and 0.5 mg), 7 new cases of breast cancer were diagnosed, 2 of which occurred among the group of 295 estradiol; norethindrone acetate tablets-treated women.

Women on hormone replacement therapy should have regular breast examinations and should be instructed in breast self-examination, and women over the age of 40 should have regular mammograms.

Congenital Lesions With Malignant Potential

Estrogen therapy during pregnancy is associated with an increased risk of fetal congenital reproductive tract disorders, and possible other birth defects. Studies of women who received diethylstilbestrol (DES) during pregnancy have shown that female offspring have an increased risk of vaginal adenosis, squamous cell dysplasia of the uterine cervix, and clear cell vaginal cancer later in life; male offspring have an increased risk of urogenital abnormalities and possibly testicular cancer later in life. Although some of these changes are benign, others are precursors of malignancy.

Cardiovascular Disease

Large doses of estrogens (5 mg conjugated estrogen per day), comparable to those used to treat cancer of the prostate and breast, have been shown in a large prospective clinical trial in men to increase the risk of nonfatal myocardial infarction, pulmonary embolism, and thrombophlebitis. These risks cannot necessarily be extrapolated from men to women or from unopposed estrogen to combination estrogen/progestin therapy. However, to avoid the theoretical cardiovascular risk to women caused by high estrogen doses, the dose for estrogen replacement therapy should not exceed the lowest effective dose.

Hypercalcemia

Administration of estrogens may lead to severe hypercalcemia in patients with breast cancer and bone metastases. If this occurs, the drugs should be stopped and appropriate measures taken to reduce the serum calcium level.

Effects During Pregnancy

Use in pregnancy is not recommended.

Gallbladder Disease

Two studies have reported a 2- to 4-fold increase in the risk of surgically confirmed gallbladder disease in women receiving postmenopausal estrogens. Among the 1516 women treated in clinical trials with 1 mg estradiol alone or in combination with several doses of NETA, 3 women had surgically confirmed cholelithiasis, none of them on estradiol; norethindrone acetate tablets treatment.

Elevated Blood Pressure

Occasional blood pressure increases during estrogen replacement therapy have been attributed to idiosyncratic reactions to estrogens. More often, blood pressure has remained the same or has dropped. One study showed that postmenopausal estrogen users have higher blood pressure than non-users. Two other studies showed slightly lower blood pressure among estrogen users compared to non-users. Postmenopausal estrogen use does not increase the risk of stroke. Nonetheless, blood pressure should be monitored at regular intervals with estrogen use.

Thromboembolic Disorders

The physician should be alert to the earliest manifestations of thrombotic disorders (thrombophlebitis, cerebrovascular disorders, pulmonary embolism, and retinal thrombosis). Should any of these occur or be suspected, the drugs should be discontinued immediately. In a 1 year study where 295 women were exposed to estradiol; norethindrone acetate tablets, there were 2 cases of deep vein thromboses reported.

Visual Abnormalities

Discontinue medication pending examination if there is a sudden partial or complete loss of vision, or a sudden onset of proptosis, diplopia, or migraine. If examinations reveal papilledema or retinal vascular lesions, medication should be withdrawn.

PRECAUTIONS

GENERAL

Based on Experience With Estrogens and/or Progestins

Cardiovascular Risk

A causal relationship between estrogen replacement therapy and reduction of cardiovascular disease in postmenopausal women has not been proven. Furthermore, the effect of added progestins on this putative benefit is not yet known.

In recent years, many published studies have suggested that there may be a cause-effect relationship between postmenopausal oral estrogen replacement therapy without added progestins and a decrease in cardiovascular disease in women. Although most of the observational studies that assessed this statistical association have reported a 20-50% reduction in coronary heart disease risk and associated mortality in estrogen takers, the following should be considered when interpreting these reports. Because only one of these studies was randomized and it was too small to yield statistically significant results, all relevant studies were subject to selection bias. Thus, the apparently reduced risk of coronary artery disease cannot be attributed with certainty to estrogen replacement therapy. It may instead have been caused by life-style and medical characteristics of the women studied with the result that healthier women were selected for estrogen therapy. In general, treated women were of higher socioeconomic and educational status, more slender, more physically active, more likely to have undergone surgical menopause, and less likely to have diabetes than the untreated women. Although some studies attempted to control for these selection factors, it is common for properly designed randomized trials to fail to confirm benefits suggested by less rigorous study designs. Thus, ongoing and future large-scale randomized trials may fail to confirm this apparent benefit.

Current medical practice often includes the use of concomitant progestin therapy in women with intact uterus. While the effects of added progestins on the risk of ischemic heart disease are not known, all available progestins attenuate at least some of the favorable effects of estrogens on HDL levels, although they maintain the favorable effect of estrogens on LDL levels.

The safety data regarding estradiol; norethindrone acetate tablets were obtained primarily from clinical trials and epidemiologic studies of postmenopausal Caucasian women, who were at generally low risk of cardiovascular disease and higher than average risk for osteoporosis. The safety profile of estradiol; norethindrone acetate tablets derived from these study populations cannot necessarily be extrapolated to other populations of diverse racial and/or demographic composition. When considering prescribing estradiol; norethindrone acetate tablets, physicians are advised to weigh the potential benefits and risks of therapy as applicable to each individual patient.

Use in Hysterectomized Women

Existing data do not support the use of the combination of estrogen and progestin in postmenopausal women without a uterus. Risks that may be associated with the inclusion of progestin in estrogen replacement regimens include deterioration in glucose tolerance, and less favorable effects on lipid metabolism compared to the effects of estrogen alone. The effects of estradiol; norethindrone acetate tablets on glucose tolerance and lipid metabolism have been studied (see Drug/Laboratory Test Interactions).

Physical Examination

A complete medical and family history should be taken prior to the initiation of any estrogen/progestin therapy. The pretreatment and periodic physical examinations should include special reference to blood pressure, breasts, abdomen, and pelvic organs, and should include a Papanicolaou smear. As a general rule, estrogen should not be prescribed for longer than 1 year without another physical examination being performed.

Fluid Retention

Because estrogens/progestins may cause some degree of fluid retention, conditions that might be influenced by this factor, such as asthma, epilepsy, migraine, and cardiac or renal dysfunction, require careful observation.

Uterine Bleeding

Certain patients may develop abnormal uterine bleeding. In cases of undiagnosed abnormal uterine bleeding, adequate diagnostic measures are indicated (see WARNINGS).

Pathology

The pathologist should be advised of estrogen/progestin therapy when relevant specimens are submitted.

Based on Experience With Estrogens

Familial Hyperlipoproteinemia

Estrogen therapy may be associated with massive elevations of plasma triglycerides leading to pancreatitis and other complications in patients with familial defects in lipoprotein metabolism.

Hypercoagulability

Some studies have shown that women taking estrogen replacement therapy have hypercoagulability primarily related to decreased antithrombin activity. This effect appears dose- and duration-dependent and is less pronounced than that associated with oral contraceptive use. Also, postmenopausal women tend to have changes in levels of coagulation parameters at baseline compared to premenopausal women. Epidemiological studies have suggested that estrogen use is associated with a higher relative risk of developing venous thromboembolism, *i.e.,* deep vein thrombosis or pulmonary embolism. The studies found a 2- to 3-fold higher risk for estrogen users compared to non-users. There is insufficient information on hypercoagulability in women who have had previous thromboembolic disease. The effects of estradiol; norethindrone acetate tablets (n=40) compared to placebo (n=40) on selected clotting factors were evaluated in a 12 month study with postmenopausal women. Estradiol; norethindrone acetate tablets decreased factor VII, plasminogen activator inhibitor-1, and, to a lesser extent, antithrombin III activity, compared to placebo. Fibrinogen remained unchanged during estradiol; norethindrone acetate tablets treatment in comparison with an increase over time in the placebo group.

Mastodynia

Certain patients may develop undesirable manifestations of estrogenic stimulation such as mastodynia. In clinical trials, less than one-fifth of the women treated with estradiol; norethindrone acetate tablets reported breast tenderness or breast pain. The majority of the cases were reported as breast tenderness, primarily during the initial months of the treatment.

Based on Experience With Progestins

Impaired Glucose Tolerance

Diabetic patients should be carefully observed while receiving estrogen/progestin therapy. The effects of estradiol; norethindrone acetate tablets on glucose tolerance have been studied (see Drug/Laboratory Test Interactions).

Depression

Patients who have a history of depression should be observed and the drugs discontinued if the depression recurs to a serious degree.

INFORMATION FOR THE PATIENT

See text of Patient Package Insert which accompanies the prescribing information.

DRUG/LABORATORY TEST INTERACTIONS

The following interactions have been observed with estrogen therapy, and/or estradiol; norethindrone acetate tablets:

Estradiol; norethindrone acetate tablets decreases factor VII, plasminogen activator inhibitor-1, and, to a lesser extent, antithrombin III activity.

Estrogen therapy increases thyroid-binding globulin (TBG) leading to increased circulating total thyroid hormone, as measured by protein-bound iodine (PBI), T_4 levels (by column or by radioimmunoassay) or T_3 levels by radioimmunoassay. T_3 resin uptake is decreased, reflecting the elevated TBG. Free T_4 and free T_3 concentrations are unaltered.

Estrogen therapy may elevate other binding proteins in serum *i.e.,* corticosteroid-binding globulin (CBG), sex-hormone-binding globulin (SHBG), leading to increased circulating corticosteroids and sex steroids respectively. Free or biologically active hormone concentrations are unchanged. Other plasma proteins may be increased (angiotensinogen/renin substrate, alpha-1-antitrypsin, ceruloplasmin). In a 12 month clinical trial, SHBG (sex-hormone-binding globulin) was found to increase with estradiol; norethindrone acetate tablets.

Estrogen therapy increases plasma HDL and HDL-2 subfraction concentrations, reduces LDL cholesterol concentration, and increases triglyceride levels.

Estradiol; norethindrone acetate tablets treatment of healthy postmenopausal women does not decrease glucose tolerance when assessed by an oral glucose tolerance test; the insulin response decreases without any increase in the glucose serum levels. Estradiol; norethindrone acetate tablets treatment does not deteriorate insulin sensitivity in healthy postmenopausal women when assessed by an hyperinsulinemic euglycemic clamp.

Estrogen therapy reduces response to metyrapone test.

Estrogen therapy reduces serum folate concentration.

CARCINOGENESIS, MUTAGENESIS, AND IMPAIRMENT OF FERTILITY

Long-term continuous administration of natural and synthetic estrogens in certain animal species increases the frequency of carcinomas of the breast, uterus, cervix, vagina, testis, and liver. (See CONTRAINDICATIONS and WARNINGS.)

PREGNANCY CATEGORY X

Estrogens/progestins should not be used during pregnancy. (See CONTRAINDICATIONS and WARNINGS.)

NURSING MOTHERS

Detectable amounts of estradiol and norethindrone acetate have been identified in the milk of mothers receiving these products and has been reported to decrease the quantity and the quality of the milk. As a general principle, the administration of any drug to nursing mothers should be done only when clearly necessary since many drugs are excreted in human milk.

E

PEDIATRIC USE

Safety and effectiveness in pediatric patients have not been established.

GERIATRIC USE

Clinical studies of estradiol; norethindrone acetate tablets did not include sufficient number of subjects aged 65 and over to determine if they responded differently from younger subjects. Other reported clinical experience has not identified differences in responses between elderly and younger subjects. In general, dose selection for an elderly patient should be cautious, usually starting at the low end of the dosing range, reflecting the greater frequency of decreased hepatic, renal, or cardiac function, and of concomitant disease or other drug therapy.

ADVERSE REACTIONS

(See WARNINGS regarding induction of neoplasia, adverse effects on the fetus, increased incidence of gallbladder disease, elevated blood pressure, thromboembolic disorders, cardiovascular disease, visual abnormalities, and hypercalcemia and PRECAUTIONS regarding cardiovascular disease.)

Adverse events reported by investigators in the Phase 3 studies regardless of causality assessment are shown in TABLE 5A, TABLE 5B, and TABLE 5C.

TABLE 5A *All Treatment-Emergent Adverse Events Regardless of Relationship Reported at a Frequency of ≥5% With Estradiol; Norethindrone Acetate Tablets*

Endometrial Hyperplasia Study (12 Months)

	E_2; NETA Tablets (n=295)	1 mg E_2 (n=296)
Body as a Whole		
Back pain	6%	5%
Headache	16%	16%
Digestive System		
Nausea	3%	5%
Gastroenteritis	2%	2%
Nervous System		
Insomnia	6%	4%
Emotional lability	1%	1%
Respiratory System		
Upper respiratory tract infection	18%	15%
Sinusitis	7%	11%
Metabolic and Nutritional		
Weight increase	0%	0%
Urogenital System		
Breast pain	24%	10%
Post-menopausal bleeding	5%	15%
Uterine fibroid	5%	4%
Ovarian cyst	3%	2%
Resistance Mechanism		
Infection viral	4%	6%
Moniliasis Genital	4%	7%
Secondary Terms		
Injury accidental	4%	3%
Other events	2%	3%

The following adverse reactions have been reported with estrogen and/or progestin therapy:

Genitourinary System: Changes in vaginal bleeding pattern and abnormal withdrawal bleeding or flow, breakthrough bleeding, spotting, increase in size of uterine leiomyomata, vaginal candidiasis, changes in amount of cervical secretion, premenstrual-like syndrome, cystitis-like syndrome.

Breasts: Tenderness, enlargement.

Gastrointestinal: Nausea, vomiting, changes in appetite, cholestatic jaundice, abdominal pain, flatulence, bloating, increased incidence of gallbladder disease.

Skin: Chloasma or melasma that may persist when drug is discontinued, erythema multiforme, erythema nodosum, hemorrhagic eruption, loss of scalp hair, hirsutism, itching, skin rash and pruritus.

Cardiovascular: Changes in blood pressure, cerebrovascular accidents, deep venous thrombosis and pulmonary embolism.

CNS: Headache, migraine, dizziness, depression, chorea, insomnia, nervousness.

Eyes: Steepening of corneal curvature, intolerance to contact lenses.

Miscellaneous: Increase or decrease in weight, aggravation of porphyria, edema, changes in libido, fatigue, allergic reactions, back pain, arthralgia, myalgia.

DOSAGE AND ADMINISTRATION

Estradiol; norethindrone acetate tablets therapy consists of a single tablet to be taken once daily.

TABLE 5B *All Treatment-Emergent Adverse Events Regardless of Relationship Reported at a Frequency of ≥5% with Estradiol; Norethindrone Acetate Tablets*

Vasomotor Symptoms Study (3 Months)

	E_2; NETA Tablets (n=29)	Placebo (n=34)
Body as a Whole		
Back pain	3%	3%
Headache	17%	18%
Digestive System		
Nausea	10%	0%
Gastroenteritis	0%	0%
Nervous System		
Insomnia	3%	3%
Emotional lability	0%	0%
Respiratory System		
Upper respiratory tract infection	10%	6%
Sinusitis	7%	0%
Metabolic and Nutritional		
Weight increase	0%	0%
Urogenital System		
Breast pain	21%	0%
Post-menopausal bleeding	10%	3%
Uterine fibroid	0%	0%
Ovarian cyst	7%	0%
Resistance Mechanism		
Infection viral	0%	3%
Moniliasis genital	0%	0%
Secondary Terms		
Injury accidental	3%	0%
Other events	3%	0%

TABLE 5C *All Treatment-Emergent Adverse Events Regardless of Relationship Reported at a Frequency of ≥5% with Estradiol; Norethindrone Acetate Tablets*

Osteoporosis Study (2 Years)

	E_2; NETA Tablets (n=47)	Placebo (n=48)
Body as a Whole		
Back pain	6%	4%
Headache	11%	6%
Digestive System		
Nausea	11%	0%
Gastroenteritis	6%	4%
Nervous System		
Insomnia	0%	8%
Emotional lability	6%	0%
Respiratory System		
Upper respiratory tract infection	15%	19%
Sinusitis	15%	10%
Metabolic and Nutritional		
Weight increase	9%	6%
Urogenital System		
Breast pain	17%	8%
Post-menopausal bleeding	11%	0%
Uterine fibroid	4%	8%
Ovarian cyst	0%	8%
Resistance Mechanism		
Infection viral	6%	6%
Moniliasis genital	6%	0%
Secondary Terms		
Injury accidental	17%*	4%*
Other events	6%	4%

* Including one upper extremity fracture in each group.

For the treatment of moderate to severe vasomotor symptoms associated with the menopause, treatment of vulvar and vaginal atrophy, and the prevention of postmenopausal osteoporosis - Estradiol; norethindrone acetate tablets 1 mg E_2/0.5 mg NETA daily. The doses of 17β-estradiol and norethindrone acetate in estradiol; norethindrone acetate tablets may not be the lowest effective dose-combination for the prevention of osteoporosis.

Treated patients with an intact uterus should be monitored closely for signs of endometrial cancer, and appropriate diagnostic measures should be taken to rule out malignancy in the event of persistent or recurring abnormal vaginal bleeding.

HOW SUPPLIED

Activella, 1 mg estradiol and 0.5 mg norethindrone acetate, is a white, film-coated tablet, engraved with "NOVO 288" on one side and the APIS bull on the other. It is round, 6 mm in diameter and bi-convex.

Storage: Store in a dry place protected from light. Store at 25°C (77°F), excursions permitted to 15-30°C (59-86°F).

TRANSDERMAL

DESCRIPTION

CombiPatch estradiol; norethindrone acetate transdermal system, is an adhesive-based matrix transdermal patch designed to release both 17β-estradiol (E_2) and norethindrone acetate (NETA), a progestational agent, continuously upon application to intact skin.

Two systems are available, providing the following delivery rates of estradiol and norethindrone acetate (see TABLE 6).

TABLE 6

System Size	E_2	NETA	Nominal Delivery Rate* E_2/NETA
9 cm^2 round	0.62 mg	2.7 mg	0.05/0.14 mg/day
16 cm^2 round	0.51 mg	4.8 mg	0.05/0.25 mg/day

* Based on *in vivo/in vitro* flux data, delivery of both components per day via skin of average permeability (interindividual variation in skin permeability is approximately 20%).

Estradiol (17 β-estradiol) is a white to creamy white, odorless, crystalline powder, chemically described as estra-1,3,5(10)-triene-3,17β-diol. The molecular weight of estradiol is 272.39 and the molecular formula is $C_{18}H_{24}O_2$.

Norethindrone acetate is a white to creamy white, odorless, crystalline powder, chemically described as 17-hydroxy-19-nor-17α-pregn-4-en-20-yn-3-one acetate. The molecular weight of norethindrone acetate is 340.47 and the molecular formula is $C_{22}H_{28}O_3$.

CombiPatch is an alcohol-free, adhesive-based matrix transdermal drug delivery system comprised of three layers. Proceeding from the visible surface toward the surface attached to the skin, these layers are a backing, an adhesive layer, and a protective liner. The adhesive matrix containing estradiol and norethindrone acetate is applied to a backing of polyester/ethylene vinyl acetate laminate film on one side and is protected on the other side by a transparent fluoropolymer-coated release liner. The transparent release liner must be removed before the system can be used. Each system is enclosed in a heat-sealed pouch.

STORAGE

Prior to dispensing to the patient store refrigerated 2-8°C (36-46°F). After dispensing to the patient, CombiPatch can be stored at room temperature below 25°C (77°F) for up to 3 months.

CLINICAL PHARMACOLOGY

The active components of the system are estradiol and norethindrone acetate. The remaining components of the system are pharmacologically inactive: a silicone and acrylic-based multipolymeric adhesive, povidone, oleic acid, and dipropylene glycol.

Estrogens are largely responsible for the development and maintenance of the female reproductive system and secondary sexual characteristics. Although circulating estrogens exist in a dynamic equilibrium of metabolic interconversions, estradiol is the principal intracellular human estrogen and is substantially more potent than its metabolites, estrone and estriol at the receptor level. The primary source of estrogen in normally cycling adult women is the ovarian follicle, which secretes 70-500 µg of estradiol daily, depending on the phase of the menstrual cycle. After menopause, most endogenous estrogen is produced by conversion of androstenedione, secreted by the adrenal cortex to estrone by peripheral tissues. Thus, estrone and the sulfate conjugated form, estrone sulfate, are the most abundant circulating estrogens in postmenopausal women.

Circulating estrogens modulate the pituitary secretion of the gonadotropins, luteinizing hormone (LH), and follicle stimulating hormone (FSH) through a negative feedback mechanism and estrogen replacement therapy acts to reduce the elevated levels of these hormones seen in postmenopausal women.

ABSORPTION

Estradiol

Estrogens used in hormone replacement therapy are well absorbed through the skin, mucous membranes, and gastrointestinal tract. Administration of the estradiol; norethindrone acetate transdermal system every 3-4 days in postmenopausal women produces average steady-state estradiol serum concentrations of 45-50 pg/ml, which are equivalent to the normal ranges observed at the early follicular phase in premenopausal women. These concentrations are achieved within 12-24 hours following the estradiol; norethindrone acetate transdermal system application. Minimal fluctuations in serum estradiol concentrations are observed following the estradiol; norethindrone acetate transdermal system application, indicating consistent hormone delivery over the application interval.

In one study, serum concentrations of estradiol were measured in 40 healthy, postmenopausal women throughout 3 consecutive estradiol; norethindrone acetate transdermal system applications to the abdomen (each dose was applied for three 3.5 day periods). The corresponding pharmacokinetic parameters are summarized in TABLE 7.

TABLE 7 *Mean (SD) Serum Estradiol and Estrone Concentrations (pg/ml) at Steady-State [Uncorrected for Baseline Levels]*

System Size	Dose E_2/NETA	C_{max}	C_{min}	C_{avg}
Estradiol				
9 cm^2	0.05/0.14 mg/day	71 (32)	27 (17)	45 (21)
16 cm^2	0.05/0.25 mg/day	71 (30)	37 (17)	50 (21)
Estrone				
9 cm^2	0.05/0.14 mg/day	72 (23)	49 (19)	54 (19)
16 cm^2	0.05/0.25 mg/day	78 (22)	58 (22)	60 (18)

NORETHINDRONE

Progestins used in hormone replacement therapy are well absorbed through the skin, mucous membranes, and gastrointestinal tract. Norethindrone steady state concentrations are attained within 24 hours of application of the the estradiol; norethindrone acetate transdermal system. Minimal fluctuations in serum norethindrone concentrations are observed following the estradiol; norethindrone acetate transdermal system treatment, indicating consistent hormone delivery over the application interval. Serum concentrations of norethindrone increase linearly with increasing doses of norethindrone acetate.

In one study, serum concentrations of norethindrone were measured in 40 healthy, postmenopausal women throughout three consecutive estradiol; norethindrone acetate transdermal system applications to the abdomen (each dose was applied for three 3.5 day periods). The corresponding pharmacokinetic parameters are summarized in TABLE 8.

TABLE 8 *Mean (SD) Serum Norethindrone Concentrations (pg/ml) at Steady-State*

System Size	Dose E_2/NETA	C_{max}	C_{min}	C_{avg}
9 cm^2	0.05/0.14 mg/day	617 (341)	386 (137)	489 (244)
16 cm^2	0.05/0.25 mg/day	1060 (543)	686 (306)	840 (414)

DISTRIBUTION

Estradiol

Estradiol circulates in the blood bound to sex hormone binding globulin (SHBG) and, to a lesser extent, albumin.

Norethindrone

In plasma, norethindrone is bound approximately 90% to SHBG and albumin.

METABOLISM AND EXCRETION

Estradiol

Transdermally delivered estradiol is metabolized only to a small extent by the skin and bypasses the first-pass effect seen with orally administered estrogen products. Therapeutic estradiol serum levels with lower circulating levels of estrone and estrone conjugates are achieved with smaller transdermal doses (daily and total) as compared to oral therapy, and more closely approximate premenopausal concentrations.

Estradiol has a short elimination half-life of approximately 2-3 hours; therefore, a rapid decline in serum levels is observed after the estradiol; norethindrone acetate transdermal system is removed. Within 4-8 hours serum estradiol concentrations return to untreated, postmenopausal levels (<20 pg/ml)

Concentration data from Phase 2 and 3 studies indicate that the pharmacokinetics of estradiol did not change over time, suggesting no evidence of the accumulation of estradiol following extended patch wear periods (up to 1 year).

Norethindrone

Norethindrone acetate is hydrolyzed to the active moiety, norethindrone, in most tissues including skin and blood. Norethindrone is primarily metabolized in the liver; however, transdermal administration significantly decreases metabolism because hepatic first-pass effect is avoided.

The elimination half-life of norethindrone is reported to be 6-8 hours. Norethindrone serum concentrations diminish rapidly and are less than 50 pg/ml within 48 hours after removal of the estradiol; norethindrone acetate transdermal system.

Concentration data from Phase 2 and 3 studies indicate that the pharmacokinetics of norethindrone did not change over time, suggesting no evidence of the accumulation of norethindrone following extended patch wear periods (up to 1 year).

ADHESION

Averaging across six clinical trials lasting 3 months to 1 year, of 1287 patients treated the estradiol; norethindrone acetate transdermal system completely adhered to the skin nearly 90% of the time over the 3-4 day wear period. Less than 2% of the patients required reapplication or replacement of systems due to lifting or detachment. Only 2 patients (0.2%) discontinued therapy during clinical trials due to adhesion failure.

SPECIAL POPULATIONS

The estradiol; norethindrone acetate transdermal system has been studied only in postmenopausal women.

INDICATIONS AND USAGE

In women with an intact uterus, estradiol; norethindrone acetate transdermal system is indicated for the following:

- Treatment of moderate-to-severe vasomotor symptoms associated with menopause.
- Treatment of vulvar and vaginal atrophy.
- Treatment of hypoestrogenism due to hypogonadism, castration, or primary ovarian failure.

CONTRAINDICATIONS

Estrogens/progestins combined should not be used in women under any of the following conditions or circumstances:

- Known or suspected pregnancy, including use for or as a diagnostic test for pregnancy. Estrogen or progestin may cause fetal harm when administered to a pregnant woman.
- Known or suspected cancer of the breast.
- Known or suspected estrogen-dependent neoplasia.
- Undiagnosed abnormal genital bleeding.
- Active thrombophlebitis, thromboembolic disorders, or stroke.
- Known hypersensitivity to estrogen, progestin, or to any estradiol; norethindrone acetate transdermal system components.

WARNINGS

ALL WARNINGS BELOW PERTAIN TO THE USE OF THIS COMBINATION PRODUCT.

INDUCTION OF MALIGNANT NEOPLASMS

Endometrial Cancer

The reported endometrial cancer risk among users of unopposed estrogen is about 2- to 12-fold or greater than in nonusers, and appears dependent on duration of treatment and on estrogen dose. Most studies show no significant increased risk associated with the use of estrogens for less than 1 year. The greatest risk appears to be associated with prolonged use—with increased risks of 15- to 24-fold for 5 years or more. In 3 studies, persistence of risk was demonstrated for 8 to over 15 years after cessation of estrogen treatment. In one study a significant decrease in the incidence of endometrial cancer occurred 6 months after estrogen withdrawal. Other studies demonstrated a reduced risk of endometrial cancer or the risk returning to pre-estrogen treatment levels when a progestin was administered in combination with estrogen replacement therapy.

Clinical trials demonstrated that when progestin was administered with estrogen, as in the estradiol; norethindrone acetate transdermal system system, versus estrogen therapy alone, there is a markedly reduced incidence of endometrial hyperplasia (≤1% vs. ≥20% respectively), a possible precursor of endometrial cancer.

Breast Cancer

Some studies have reported a moderately increased risk of breast cancer (relative risk 1.3-2.0) in women on estrogen replacement therapy taking high doses, or in those taking low doses for prolonged periods of time, especially in excess of 10 years. The majority of studies, however, have not shown an association between breast cancer and women who have ever used estrogen replacement therapy. There is no conclusive evidence that concurrent progestin use alters the risk of breast cancer in long-term users of estrogen. (See PRECAUTIONS.)

Congenital Lesions With Malignant Potential

Estrogen therapy during pregnancy is associated with an increased risk of fetal congenital reproductive tract disorders, and possibly other birth defects. Studies of women who received DES during pregnancy have shown that female offspring have an increased risk of vaginal adenosis, squamous cell dysplasia of the uterine cervix, and clear cell vaginal cancer later in life, male offspring have an increased risk of urogenital abnormalities and possibly testicular cancer later in life. Although some of these changes are benign, others are precursors of malignancy.

Cardiovascular Disease

Large doses of estrogen (5 mg conjugated estrogens per day), comparable to those used to treat cancer of the prostate and breast, have been shown in a large prospective clinical trial in men to increase the risk of nonfatal myocardial infarction, pulmonary embolism, and thrombophlebitis. These risks cannot necessarily be extrapolated from men to women or from unopposed estrogen to combination estrogen/progestin therapy. However, to avoid the theoretical cardiovascular risk associated with high estrogen doses, the dose for estrogen replacement therapy should not exceed the lowest effective dose.

Hypercalcemia

Administration of estrogens may lead to severe hypercalcemia in patients with breast cancer and bone metastases. If this occurs, the estradiol; norethindrone acetate transdermal system should be discontinued and appropriate measures should be taken to reduce the serum calcium level.

Thromboembolic Disorders

The physician should be alerted to the earliest manifestations of thrombotic disorders (thrombophlebitis, cerebrovascular disorders, pulmonary embolism, and retinal thrombosis). Should any of these occur or be suspected, the estradiol; norethindrone acetate transdermal system should be discontinued immediately.

Visual Abnormalities

If there is sudden partial or complete loss of vision, or a sudden onset of proptosis, diplopia, or migraine, the estradiol; norethindrone acetate transdermal system should be discontinued. If examination reveals papilledema or retinal vascular lesions, the estradiol; norethindrone acetate transdermal system should be discontinued.

PRECAUTIONS

GENERAL

Based on experience with estrogens and/or progestins:

Endometrial cancer: Progestins taken with estrogen drugs significantly reduce, but do not eliminate the risk of endometrial cancer that is associated with the use of estrogen. Close clinical surveillance of all women taking estrogens is important. Adequate diagnostic measures, including endometrial sampling when appropriate, should be undertaken to rule out malignancy in all cases of undiagnosed, persistent, or recurring abnormal vaginal bleeding. There is no evidence at present that "natural" estrogens are more or less hazardous than "synthetic" estrogens at equi-estrogenic doses.

Use in women who have undergone hysterectomy: Existing data do not support the use of the combination of estrogen and progestin in postmenopausal women without a uterus. (See Addition of a progestin.)

Addition of a progestin: There are possible risks that may be associated with the co-administration of a progestin in estrogen-based hormone replacement therapy. These risks, which include adverse effects on carbohydrate metabolism and impairment of glucose tolerance, have not been observed in the estradiol; norethindrone acetate transdermal system clinical trials.

The possible enhancement of mitotic activity in breast epithelial tissue has also been reported with oral progestin therapy. While the effects of added progestins on the risk of breast cancer are unknown, available epidemiological evidence suggests that progestins do not reduce, and may enhance, the moderately increased breast cancer incidence that has been reported with prolonged estrogen replacement therapy. (See WARNINGS.)

Physical examination: A complete medical and family history should be taken before initiation of any estrogen therapy and periodically thereafter. The physical examinations should include special reference to blood pressure, breasts, abdomen, and pelvic organs, as well as a cervical Papanicolaou test. Generally, estrogen should not be prescribed for longer than 1 year without another physical examination being performed.

CARDIOVASCULAR EFFECTS

A causal relationship between estrogen replacement therapy and the reduction of cardiovascular disease in postmenopausal women has not been proven. Furthermore, the effect of added progestins on this putative benefit is not yet known.

In recent years, many published studies have suggested that there may be a cause-effect relationship between postmenopausal oral estrogen replacement therapy without added progestins and a decrease in cardiovascular disease in women. Although many of the observational studies which assessed this statistical association have reported a 20-50% reduction in coronary heart disease risk and associated mortality in estrogen users, the following should be considered when interpreting these reports:

- Because only one of these studies was randomized and it was too small to yield statistically significant results, all relevant studies were subject to selection bias. Thus, the apparently reduced risk of coronary artery disease cannot be attributed with certainty to estrogen replacement therapy. It instead may have been caused by life-style and medical characteristics of the women studied with the result that healthier women were selected for estrogen therapy. In general, treated women were of higher socioeconomic and educational status, more slender, more physically active, more likely to have undergone surgical menopause, and less likely to have diabetes than the untreated women. Although some studies attempted to control for these selection factors, it is common for properly designed randomized trials to fail to confirm benefits suggested by less rigorous study designs. Thus, ongoing and future large scale randomized trials may fail to confirm this apparent benefit.
- Current medical practice often includes the use of concomitant progestin therapy in women with intact uteri. (See PRECAUTIONS and WARNINGS.) While the effects of added progestins on the risk of ischemic heart disease are not known, all available progestins, reverse the favorable effects of estrogens on HDL levels as observed with the estradiol; norethindrone acetate transdermal system, although the norethindrone acetate in the estradiol; norethindrone acetate transdermal system maintained the favorable effects of estrogens on LDL levels.

E

GALLBLADDER DISEASE

There is a reported 2- to 4-fold increase in the risk of surgically confirmed gallbladder disease in postmenopausal women receiving oral estrogens. Similar increases in gallbladder disease have not been reported with transdermal estradiol. Transdermal estrogen therapy does not increase biliary cholesterol saturation index, therefore, the risk may be diminished.

ELEVATED BLOOD PRESSURE

Occasional, reversible blood pressure increases during oral estrogen replacement therapy have been attributed to idiosyncratic reactions to estrogens. More often, however, blood pressure has remained the same or has decreased.

Theoretically, in estrogen and progestin therapy, blood pressure elevations could be the result of increased renin substrate or angiotensin II levels, although these increases have not been reported in transdermal therapy.

Studies with the estradiol; norethindrone acetate transdermal system showed no clinically significant changes in blood pressure among patients taking the estradiol; norethindrone acetate transdermal system. Nonetheless, blood pressure should be monitored at regular intervals with estrogen use.

FLUID RETENTION

Because estrogens and/or progestins may cause some degree of fluid retention, careful observation is required when conditions that might be influenced by this factor are present (*e.g.*, asthma, epilepsy, migraine, and cardiac or renal dysfunction).

UTERINE BLEEDING AND MASTODYNIA

Certain patients may develop undesirable manifestations of estrogenic stimulation, such as abnormal uterine bleeding or mastodynia. In cases of undiagnosed abnormal bleeding, transvaginal ultrasonography or endometrial tissue sampling is generally appropriate, but evaluation should be based on the individual patient. (See WARNINGS.)

COLLECTION OF PATHOLOGICAL SPECIMENS

The pathologist should be advised of estrogen/progestin therapy when relevant specimens are submitted.

BASED ON EXPERIENCE WITH ESTROGENS OR PROGESTINS

Hypercoagulability

Recent retrospective case-controlled studies have reported an increased risk of venous thromboembolism (VTE) among current users of estrogen replacement therapy versus non-users. This risk appears dose-duration dependent and is less pronounced than that associated with oral contraceptives. Although these studies found that estrogen use was associated with an increase in the relative risk of VTE, the absolute risk was low because of the infrequency of this event.

Because of the occasional occurrence of thrombotic disorders (thrombophlebitis, pulmonary embolism, retinal thrombosis, cerebrovascular disorders) and because there is insufficient information on hypercoagulability in women who have had previous thromboembolic disease, the benefit-risk of prescribing hormone replacement therapy should be reviewed individually for women with a past history of deep vein thrombosis or a family history of idiopathic thrombosis. The physician should be alert to the earliest manifestations of these disorders.

Familial Hyperlipoproteinemia

Oral estrogen therapy may be associated with elevations of plasma triglycerides leading to pancreatitis and other complications in patients with familial defects of lipoprotein metabolism. Data from experience with the estradiol; norethindrone acetate transdermal system and other transdermal estradiols regarding lipoproteins consistently show a reduction in triglycerides in postmenopausal women. Nonetheless, patients with familial hyperlipoproteinemia should be monitored closely when on estrogen therapy.

INFORMATION FOR THE PATIENT

See the Patient Package Insert which accompanies the prescribing information.

IMPAIRED LIVER FUNCTION

Estrogens may be poorly metabolized in patients with impaired liver function. Although transdermally administered estrogen therapy avoids first-pass hepatic metabolism, estrogens should still be administered with caution in such patients.

LABORATORY TESTS

Estrogen administration should generally be guided by clinical response at the smallest dose, rather than laboratory monitoring, for relief of symptoms for those indications in which symptoms are observable.

CARCINOGENESIS, MUTAGENESIS, AND IMPAIRMENT OF FERTILITY

Long-term continuous administration of natural and synthetic estrogens in certain animal species increases the frequency of carcinomas of the breast, cervix, vagina, and liver. Long-term continuous administration of natural and synthetic progestins increases the frequency of benign liver tumors in male mice, but not in male or female rats. (See CONTRAINDICATIONS and WARNINGS.)

Norethindrone acetate was not mutagenic in a battery of *in vitro* or *in vivo* genetic toxicity assays.

PREGNANCY CATEGORY X

Estrogens should not be used during pregnancy. Estrogen therapy during pregnancy is associated with an increased risk of congenital defects in the reproductive organs of the fetus, and possibly other birth defects. Studies of women who received diethylstilbestrol (DES) during pregnancy have shown that the female offspring have an increased risk of vaginal adenosis, squamous cell dysplasia of the uterine cervix, and clear cell vaginal cancer later in life; male offspring have an increased risk of urogenital abnormalities and possibly testicular cancer later in life. Although some of these changes are benign, others are precursors of malignancy. The 1985 DES Task Force concluded that use of DES during pregnancy is associated with subsequent increased risk of breast cancer in the mother, although a causal relationship remains unproven and the observed level of excess risk is similar to that for a number of other breast cancer risk factors.

Several reports also suggest an association between intrauterine exposure to progestational drugs in the first trimester of pregnancy and genital abnormalities in male and female fetuses. The risk of hypospadias, 5 to 8 per 1000 male births in the general population, may be approximately doubled with exposure to these drugs. There are insufficient data to quantify the risk to exposed female fetuses; some of these drugs induce mild virilization of the external genitalia of the female fetus.

NURSING MOTHERS

Detectable amounts of estradiol and norethindrone have been identified in the milk of mothers receiving these products and has been reported to decrease the quantity and quality of the milk. As a general principle the administration of any drug to nursing mothers should be done only when clearly necessary since many drugs are excreted in human milk.

DRUG INTERACTIONS

The following laboratory tests may be altered by the use of estrogens or estrogen-progestin combination drugs (such as the estradiol; norethindrone acetate transdermal system):

- Prothrombin time, activated partial thromboplastin time and platelet aggregation time, increased platelet count; increased factors II, VII antigen, VIII antigen, VIII coagulation activity, IX, X, XII, VII-X complex, II-VII-X complex, and beta-thromboglobulin; decreased levels of anti-Factor Xa and antithrombin III, decreased antithrombin III activity increased levels of fibrinogen activity; increased plasminogen antigen and activity.
- Increased thyroid-binding globulin (TBG) leading to increased circulating total thyroid hormone, as measured by protein-bound iodine (PBI), T4 levels (by column or by radioimmunoassay) or T3 levels (by radioimmunoassay). T3 resin uptake is decreased, reflecting elevated TBG. Free T4 and free T3 concentrations are unaltered.
- Other binding proteins may be altered in serum, *i.e.*, increased corticosteroid binding globulin (CBG), leading to increased circulating corticosteroids, decreased SHBG. Free or biologically active hormone concentrations are unchanged. Other plasma proteins may be increased (angiotensinogen/renin substrate, alpha-1-antitrypsin, ceruloplasmin).
- Decreased serum total cholesterol, HDL-C and HDL_2-C subfraction, LDL-C, and triglycerides concentrations.
- Reduced response to metyrapone test.
- Reduced serum folate concentration.
- Increased sulfobromophthalein retention.

ADVERSE REACTIONS

See WARNINGS, and PRECAUTIONS regarding potential adverse effects on the fetus, induction of malignant neoplasms, cardiovascular disease, hypercalcemia, visual abnormalities, and adverse effects similar to those of oral contraceptives, including thromboembolism (see TABLE 15 and TABLE 16).

DOSAGE AND ADMINISTRATION

INITIATION OF THERAPY

Treatment of postmenopausal symptoms is usually initiated during the menopausal stage when vasomotor symptoms occur.

Women not currently using continuous estrogen or combination estrogen/progestin therapy may start therapy with the estradiol; norethindrone acetate transdermal system at any time. However, women currently using continuous estrogen or combination estrogen/progestin therapy should compare the current cycle of therapy, before initiating the estradiol; norethindrone acetate transdermal system therapy. Women often experience withdrawal bleeding at the completion of the cycle. The first day of this bleeding would be an appropriate time to begin the estradiol; norethindrone acetate transdermal system therapy.

TABLE 15 *All Treatment Emergent Study Events Regardless of Relationship Reported at a Frequency of ≥5% with the Estradiol; Norethindrone Acetate Transdermal System Vasomotor Symptom Studies*

	E_2; NETA Transdermal System		
	0.05/0.14 mg/day*	0.05/0.25 mg/day*	Placebo
	n=113	n=112	n=107
Body as a Whole	46%	48%	41%
Abdominal pain	7%	6%	4%
Accidental injury	4%	5%	8%
Asthenia	8%	12%	4%
Back pain	11%	9%	5%
Flu syndrome	9%	5%	7%
Headache	18%	20%	20%
Pain	6%	4%	9%
Digestive	19%	23%	24%
Diarrhea	4%	5%	7%
Dyspepsia	1%	5%	5%
Flatulence	4%	5%	4%
Nausea	11%	8%	7%
Nervous	16%	28%	28%
Depression	3%	5%	9%
Insomnia	3%	6%	7%
Nervousness	3%	5%	1%
Respiratory	24%	38%	26%
Pharyngitis	4%	10%	2%
Respiratory disorder	7%	12%	7%
Rhinitis	7%	13%	9%
Sinusitis	4%	9%	9%
Skin and Appendages	8%	17%	16%
Application site reaction	2%	6%	4%
Urogenital	54%	63%	28%
Breast pain	25%	31%	7%
Dysmenorrhea	20%	21%	5%
Leukorrhea	5%	5%	3%
Menstrual disorder	6%	12%	2%
Papanicolaou smear suspicious	8%	4%	5%
Vaginitis	6%	13%	5%

* Represents mg of estradiol NETA delivered daily by each system.

THERAPEUTIC REGIMENS

Combination estrogen/progestin regimens are indicated for women with an intact uterus. Two estradiol; norethindrone acetate (17 β-estradiol/NETA) transdermal delivery systems are available: 0.05 mg estradiol with 0.14 mg NETA per day (9 cm^2) and 0.05 mg estradiol with 0.25 mg NETA per day (16 cm^2). For all regimens, women should be reevaluated at 3-6 month intervals to determine if changes in hormone replacement therapy or if continued hormone replacement therapy is appropriate.

Continuous Combined Regimen

An estradiol; norethindrone acetate transdermal system 0.05 mg estradiol/0.14 mg NETA per day (9 cm^2) matrix transdermal system is worn continuously on the lower abdomen. Additionally, a dose of 0.05 mg estradiol/0.25 mg NETA (16 cm^2 system) is available if a greater progestin dose is desired. A new system should be applied twice weekly during a 28 day cycle. Irregular bleeding may occur particularly in the first 6 months, but generally decreases with time and often to an amennorheic state.

Continuous Sequential Regimen

The estradiol; norethindrone acetate transdermal system can be applied as a sequential regimen in combination with an estradiol-only transdermal delivery system.

In this treatment regimen an 0.05 mg/day (nominal delivery rate) estradiol-only transdermal system is worn for the first 14 days of a 28 day cycle, replacing the system twice weekly according to product directions. For the remaining 14 days of the 28 day cycle, the estradiol; norethindrone acetate transdermal system 0.05 mg estradiol/0.14 mg NETA per day (9 cm^2) transdermal system should be applied to the lower abdomen. Additionally, a dose of 0.05 mg estradiol/0.25 mg NETA (16 cm^2 system) is available if a greater progestin dose is desired. The estradiol; norethindrone acetate system should be replaced twice weekly during this period in the cycle. Women should be advised that monthly withdrawal bleeding often occurs.

APPLICATION OF THE SYSTEM

Site Selection

Estradiol; norethindrone acetate transdermal system should be placed on a smooth (fold free), clean, dry area of the skin on the lower abdomen. The estradiol; norethindrone acetate transdermal system **should not be applied to or near the breasts.** The area selected should not be oily (which can impair adherence of the system), damaged, or irritated. The waistline should be avoided, since tight clothing may rub the system off or modify drug delivery. The sites of application must be rotated, with an interval of at least 1 week allowed between applications to the same site.

Application

After opening the pouch, remove one side of the protective liner, taking care not to touch the adhesive part of the transdermal delivery system with the fingers. Immediately apply the transdermal delivery system to a smooth (fold free) area of skin on the lower abdomen. Remove the second side of the protective liner and press the system firmly in place with the hand for at least 10 seconds, making sure there is good contact, especially around the edges.

Care should be taken that the system does not become dislodged during bathing and other activities. If a system should fall off, the same system may be reapplied to another area of the lower abdomen. If necessary a new transdermal system may be applied, in which case the original treatment schedule should be continued. **Only one system should be worn at any one time during the 3-4 day dosing interval.**

TABLE 16 *All Treatment Emergent Study Events Regardless of Relationship Reported at a Frequency of ≥5% With the Estradiol; Norethindrone Acetate Transdermal System*

Endometrial Hyperplasia Studies

	E_2; NETA Transdermal System		E_2-only Transdermal System
	0.05/0.14 mg/day	0.05/0.25 mg/day*	0.05 mg/day
	n=325	n=312	n=318
Body as a Whole	61%	60%	59%
Abdominal pain	12%	14%	16%
Accidental injury	10%	11%	8%
Asthenia	10%	13%	11%
Back pain	15%	14%	13%
Flu syndrome	14%	10%	7%
Headache	25%	17%	21%
Infection	5%	3%	3%
Pain	19%	15%	13%
Digestive	42%	32%	31%
Constipation	2%	5%	3%
Diarrhea	14%	9%	7%
Dyspepsia	8%	6%	5%
Flatulence	7%	5%	6%
Nausea	8%	12%	11%
Tooth disorder	6%	4%	1%
Metabolic and Nutritional Disorders	12%	13%	11%
Peripheral edema	6%	6%	5%
Musculoskeletal	17%	17%	15%
Arthralgia	6%	6%	5%
Nervous	33%	30%	28%
Depression	8%	9%	8%
Dizziness	6%	7%	5%
Insomnia	8%	6%	4%
Nervousness	5%	6%	3%
Respiratory	45%	43%	40%
Bronchitis	5%	3%	4%
Pharyngitis	9%	9%	8%
Respiratory disorder	13%	9%	13%
Rhinitis	19%	22%	17%
Sinusitis	10%	12%	12%
Skin and Appendages	38%	37%	31%
Acne	4%	5%	4%
Application site reaction	20%	23%	17%
Rash	6%	5%	3%
Urogenital	71%	79%	74%
Breast enlargement	2%	7%	2%
Breast pain	34%	48%	40%
Dysmenorrhea	30%	31%	19%
Leukorrhea	10%	8%	9%
Menorrhagia	2%	5%	9%
Menstrual disorder	17%	19%	14%
Vaginal hemorrhage	3%	6%	12%
Vaginitis	9%	13%	13%

* Represents mg of estradiol/NETA delivered daily by each system.

Once in place, the transdermal system should not be exposed to the sun for prolonged periods of time.

REMOVAL OF THE SYSTEM

Removal of the system should be done carefully and slowly to avoid irritation of the skin. Should any adhesive remain on the skin after removal of the system, allow the area to dry for 15 minutes. Then gently rubbing the area with an oil-based cream or lotion should remove the adhesive residue.

PRODUCT LISTING - EQUIVALENTS NOT AVAILABLE

Film, Extended Release - Transdermal - 0.05 mg;0.14 mg/24 Hours

8 x 3	$116.28	COMBIPATCH, Novartis Pharmaceuticals	00078-0377-45
8's	$33.60	COMBIPATCH, Novartis Pharmaceuticals	00078-0377-42

Film, Extended Release - Transdermal - 0.05 mg;0.25 mg/24 Hours

8 x 3	$119.07	COMBIPATCH, Novartis Pharmaceuticals	00078-0378-45
8's	$34.44	COMBIPATCH, Novartis Pharmaceuticals	00078-0378-42

Tablet - Oral - 1 mg;0.5 mg

28 x 5	$149.21	ACTIVELLA, Pharmacia and Upjohn	00009-5174-01
28's	$26.09	ACTIVELLA, Pharmacia and Upjohn	00009-5174-02

Estramustine Phosphate Sodium *(001195)*

Categories: Carcinoma, prostate; FDA Approved 1981 Dec
Drug Classes: Antineoplastics, alkylating agents; Hormones/hormone modifiers
Brand Names: Emcyt
Foreign Brand Availability: Cellmustin (Germany); Estracyt (Austria; Bahrain; Belgium; Bulgaria; Cyprus; Czech-Republic; Denmark; Egypt; England; France; Greece; Hong-Kong; Hungary; Iran; Iraq; Italy; Japan; Jordan; Kuwait; Lebanon; Libya; Malaysia; Netherlands; Norway; Oman; Portugal; Qatar; Republic-of-Yemen; Saudi-Arabia; South-Africa; Spain; Sweden; Switzerland; Syria; United-Arab-Emirates); Multosin (Germany); Prostamustin (Germany)
Cost of Therapy: $912.16 (Prostate Cancer; Emcyt; 140 mg; 7 capsules/day; 30 day supply)

DESCRIPTION

Estramustine phosphate sodium, an antineoplastic agent, is an off-white powder readily soluble in water. Emcyt capsules are white and opaque, each containing estramustine phosphate sodium as the disodium salt monohydrate equivalent to 140 mg estramustine phosphate, for oral administration. Each capsule also contains magnesium stearate, silicon dioxide, sodium lauryl sulfate and talc. Gelatin capsule shells contain the following pigment: titanium dioxide.

Chemically, estramustine phosphate sodium is estra-1,3,5(10)-triene-3, 17-diol(17β)-, 3-[bis(2-chloroethyl)carbamate] 17-(dihydrogen phosphate), disodium salt, monohydrate. It is also referred to as estradiol 3-[bis(2-chloroethyl)carbamate)] 17-(dihydrogen phosphate), disodium salt, monohydrate.

Estramustine phosphate sodium has an empiric formula of $C_{23}H_{30}Cl_2NNa_2O_6P{\cdot}H_2O$, a calculated molecular weight of 582.4.

CLINICAL PHARMACOLOGY

Estramustine phosphate is a molecule combining estradiol and nornitrogen mustard by a carbamate link. The molecule is phosphorylated to make it water soluble.

Estramustine phosphate taken orally is readily dephosphorylated during absorption, and the major metabolites in plasma are estramustine, the estrone analog, estradiol and estrone.

Prolonged treatment with estramustine phosphate produces elevated total plasma concentrations of estradiol that fall within ranges similar to the elevated estradiol levels found in prostatic cancer patients given conventional estradiol therapy. Estrogenic effects, as demonstrated by changes in circulating levels of steroids and pituitary hormones, are similar in patients treated with either estramustine phosphate or conventional estradiol.

The metabolic urinary patterns of the estradiol moiety of estramustine phosphate and estradiol itself are very similar, although the metabolites derived from estramustine phosphate are excreted at a slower rate.

E

INDICATIONS AND USAGE

Estramustine phosphate sodium is indicated in the palliative treatment of patients with metastatic and/or progressive carcinoma of the prostate.

NON-FDA APPROVED INDICATIONS

Estramustine in combination with either vinblastine or docetaxel have shown efficacy in the treatment of hormone refractory prostate cancer. Preliminary data also suggest that the combination of estramustine with paclitaxel may be useful in the treatment of advanced breast cancer. However, use in the treatment of hormone refractory prostate cancer and advanced breast cancer have not been approved by the FDA and further clinical trials are needed.

CONTRAINDICATIONS

Estramustine phosphate sodium should not be used in patients with any of the following conditions:

1. Known hypersensitivity to either estradiol or to nitrogen mustard.
2. Active thrombophlebitis or thromboembolic disorders, except in those cases where the actual tumor mass is the cause of the thromboembolic phenomenon and the physician feels the benefits of therapy may outweigh the risks.

WARNINGS

It has been shown that there is an increased risk of thrombosis, including fatal and nonfatal myocardial infarction, in men receiving estrogens for prostatic cancer. Estramustine phosphate sodium should be used with caution in patients with a history of thrombophlebitis, thrombosis or thromboembolic disorders, especially if they were associated with estrogen therapy. Caution should also be used in patients with cerebral vascular or coronary artery disease.

Glucose Tolerance: Because glucose tolerance may be decreased, diabetic patients should be carefully observed while receiving estramustine phosphate sodium.

Elevated Blood Pressure: Because hypertension may occur, blood pressure should be monitored periodically.

PRECAUTIONS

GENERAL

Fluid Retention: Exacerbation of preexisting or incipient peripheral edema or congestive heart disease has been seen in some patients receiving therapy with estramustine phosphate sodium. Other conditions which might be influenced by fluid retention, such as epilepsy, migraine or renal dysfunction, require careful observation.

Estramustine phosphate sodium may be poorly metabolized in patients with impaired liver function and should be administered with caution in such patients.

Because estramustine phosphate sodium may influence the metabolism of calcium and phosphorus, it should be used with caution in patients with metabolic bone diseases that are associated with hypercalcemia or in patients with renal insufficiency.

Gynecomastia and impotence are known estrogenic effects.

Allergic reactions and angioedema at times involving the airway have been reported.

INFORMATION FOR THE PATIENT

Because of the possibility of mutagenic effects, patients should be advised to use contraceptive measures.

LABORATORY TESTS

Certain endocrine and liver function tests may be affected by estrogen-containing drugs. Estramustine phosphate sodium may depress testosterone levels. Abnormalities of hepatic enzymes and of bilirubin have occurred in patients receiving estramustine phosphate sodium. Such tests should be done at appropriate intervals during therapy and repeated after the drug has been withdrawn for two months.

FOOD/DRUG INTERACTION

Milk, milk products and calcium-rich foods or drugs may impair the absorption of estramustine phosphate sodium.

CARCINOGENESIS, MUTAGENESIS, AND IMPAIRMENT OF FERTILITY

Long-term continuous administration of estrogens in certain animal species increases the frequency of carcinomas of the breast and liver. Compounds structurally similar to estramustine phosphate sodium are carcinogenic in mice. Carcinogenic studies of estramustine phosphate sodium have not been conducted in man. Although testing by the Ames method failed to demonstrate mutagenicity for estramustine phosphate sodium, it is known that both estradiol and nitrogen mustard are mutagenic. For this reason and because some patients who had been impotent while on estrogen therapy have regained potency while taking estramustine phosphate sodium, the patient should be advised to use contraceptive measures.

ADVERSE REACTIONS

In a randomized, double-blind trial comparing therapy with estramustine phosphate sodium in 93 patients (11.5-15.9 mg/kg/day) or diethylstilbestrol (DES) in 93 patients (3.0 mg/day), the following adverse effects were reported (see TABLE 1).

TABLE 1 *Estramustine Phosphate Sodium, Adverse Reactions*

	Estramustine phosphate sodium n=93	DES n=93
Cardiovascular-Respiratory		
Cardiac arrest	0	2
Cerebrovascular accident	2	0
Myocardial infarction	3	1
Thrombophlebitis	3	7
Pulmonary emboli	2	5
Congestive heart failure	3	2
Edema	19	17
Dyspnea	11	3
Leg cramps	8	11
Upper respiratory discharge	1	1
Hoarseness	1	0
Gastrointestinal		
Nausea	15	8
Diarrhea	12	11
Minor gastrointestinal upset	11	6
Anorexia	4	3
Flatulence	2	0
Vomiting	1	1
Gastrointestinal bleeding	1	0
Burning throat	1	0
Thirst	1	0
Integumentary		
Rash	1	4
Pruritus	2	2
Dry skin	2	0
Pigment changes	0	3
Easy bruising	3	0
Flushing	1	0
Night sweats	0	1
Fingertip — Peeling skin	1	0
Thinning hair	1	1
Breast Changes		
Tenderness	66	64
Enlargement		
Mild	60	54
Moderate	10	16
Marked	0	5
Miscellaneous		
Lethargy alone	4	3
Depression	0	2
Emotional lability	2	0
Insomnia	3	0
Headache	1	1
Anxiety	1	0
Chest pain	1	1
Hot flashes	0	1
Pain in eyes	0	1
Tearing of eyes	1	1
Tinnitus	0	1
Laboratory Abnormalities		
Hematologic		
Leukopenia	4	2
Thrombopenia	1	2
Hepatic		
Bilirubin alone	1	5
Bilirubin and LDH	0	1
Bilirubin and SGOT	2	1
Bilirubin, LDH and SGOT	2	0
LDH and/or SGOT	31	28
Miscellaneous		
Hypercalcemia - Transient	0	1

DOSAGE AND ADMINISTRATION

The recommended daily dose is 14 mg/kg of body weight (*i.e.,* one 140 mg capsule for each 10 kg or 22 lb of body weight), given in 3 or 4 divided doses. Most patients in studies in the US have been treated at a dosage range of 10 to 16 mg/kg/day.

Patients should be instructed to take estramustine phosphate sodium at least 1 hour before or 2 hours after meals. Estramustine phosphate sodium should be swallowed with water. Milk, milk products and calcium-rich foods or drugs (such as calcium-containing antacids) must not be taken simultaneously with estramustine phosphate sodium.

Patients should be treated for 30-90 days before the physician determines the possible benefits of continued therapy. Therapy should be continued as long as the favorable response lasts. Some patients have been maintained on therapy for more than 3 years at doses ranging from 10-16 mg/kg of body weight per day.

Procedures for proper handling and disposal of anticancer drugs should be considered. Several guidelines on this subject have been published.[1-7] There is no general agreement that all of the procedures recommended in the guidelines are necessary or appropriate.

HOW SUPPLIED

Emcyt capsules are white and opaque, each containing estramustine phosphate sodium as the disodium salt monohydrate equivalent to 140 mg estramustine phosphate.
Note: Emcyt should be stored in the refrigerator at 2-8°C (36-46°F).

PRODUCT LISTING - EQUIVALENTS NOT AVAILABLE

Capsule - Oral - 140 mg
100's $509.91 EMCYT, Pharmacia and Upjohn 00013-0132-02

Estrogens, Conjugated *(001197)*

Categories: Atrophy, vaginal; Atrophy, vulvar; Carcinoma, breast, adjunct; Carcinoma, prostate; Hypoestrogenism; Hypogonadism, female; Kraurosis vulvae; Menopause; Osteoporosis, prevention; Ovarian failure, primary; Vaginitis, atrophic; Pregnancy Category X; FDA Approved 1942 May
Drug Classes: Estrogens; Hormones/hormone modifiers
Brand Names: Azumon; Conjugated Estrogens; Conjugen; Emopremarin; Mannest; Menopak-E; Ovest; **Premarin**
Foreign Brand Availability: Ayerogen (Venezuela); Ayerogen Crema Vaginal (Ecuador); C.E.S. (Canada); Climarest (Germany); Dagynil (Netherlands; Taiwan); Equin (Hong-Kong; Spain); Estranova (Peru); Eyzu (Taiwan); Femavit (Germany); Hyphorin (Japan); Menpoz (Philippines); Neo-Menovar (Argentina); Oestro-Feminal (Czech-Republic; Ecuador; Germany); Premarin Crema V (Mexico); Premarin Crema Vaginal (Colombia); Premarin Creme (Australia; New-Zealand; South-Africa); Premarin Vaginal Creme (Bahamas; Bahrain; Barbados; Belize; Bermuda; Curacao; Cyprus; Egypt; Guyana; Hong-Kong; Iran; Iraq; Israel; Jamaica; Jordan; Kuwait; Lebanon; Libya; Malaysia; Netherland-Antilles; Oman; Philippines; Puerto-Rico; Qatar; Republic-of-Yemen; Saudi-Arabia; Surinam; Syria; Taiwan; Thailand; Trinidad; United-Arab-Emirates); Premarina (Sweden); Presomen (Czech-Republic; Germany); Prevagin-Premaril (Israel); Romeda (Japan); Sefac (Japan); Srogen (Korea); Sukingpo (Taiwan); Sultrona (Mexico); Transannon (Switzerland); Trepova (Mexico)
Cost of Therapy: $22.05 (Menopause; Premarin; 1.25 mg; 1 tablet/day; 30 day supply)
HCFA JCODE(S): J1410 per 25 mg IV, IM

INTRAVENOUS

WARNING

ESTROGENS HAVE BEEN REPORTED TO INCREASE THE RISK OF ENDOMETRIAL CARCINOMA: Three independent, case-controlled studies have reported an increased risk of endometrial cancer in postmenopausal women exposed to exogenous estrogens for more than 1 year.[1-3] This risk was independent of the other known risk factors for endometrial cancer. These studies are further supported by the finding that incidence rates of endometrial cancer have increased sharply since 1969 in 8 different areas of the US with population-based cancer-reporting systems, an increase which may be related to the rapidly expanding use of estrogens during the last decade.[4] The 3 case-controlled studies reported that the risk of endometrial cancer in estrogen users was about 4.5-13.9 times greater than in non-users. The risk appears to depend on both duration of treatment[1] and on estrogen dose.[3] In view of these findings, when estrogens are used for the treatment of menopausal symptoms, the lowest dose that will control symptoms should be utilized and medication should be discontinued as soon as possible. When prolonged treatment is medically indicated, the patient should be reassessed, on at least a semiannual basis, to determine the need for continued therapy. Although the evidence must be considered preliminary, one study suggests that cyclic administration of low doses of estrogen may carry less risk than continuous administration.[3] It therefore appears prudent to utilize such a regimen. Close clinical surveillance of all women taking estrogens is important. In all cases of undiagnosed persistent or recurring abnormal vaginal bleeding, adequate diagnostic measures should be undertaken to rule out malignancy. There is no evidence at present that "natural" estrogens are more or less hazardous than "synthetic" estrogens at equiestrogenic doses.

ESTROGENS SHOULD NOT BE USED DURING PREGNANCY. The use of female sex hormones, both estrogens and progestogens, during early pregnancy may seriously damage the offspring. It has been shown that females exposed *in utero* to diethylstilbestrol, a nonsteroidal estrogen, have an increased risk of developing, in later life, a form of vaginal or cervical cancer that is ordinarily extremely rare.[5,6] This risk has been estimated as not greater than 4/1000 exposures.[7] Furthermore, a high percentage of such exposed women (from 30-90%) have been found to have vaginal adenosis,[8-12] epithelial changes of the vagina and cervix. Although these changes are histologically benign, it is not known whether they are precursors of malignancy. Although similar data are not available with the use of other estrogens, it cannot be presumed they would not induce similar changes. Several reports suggest an association between intrauterine exposure to female sex hormones and congenital anomalies, including congenital heart defects and limb-reduction defects.[13-16] One case-controlled study[16] estimated a 4.7-fold increased risk of limb-reduction defects in infants exposed *in utero* to sex hormones (oral contraceptives, hormone withdrawal tests for pregnancy, or attempted treatment for threatened abortion). Some of these exposures were very short and involved only a few days of treatment. The data suggest that the risk of limb-reduction defects in exposed fetuses is somewhat less than 1/1000. In the past, female sex hormones have been used during pregnancy in an attempt to treat threatened or habitual abortion. There is considerable evidence that estrogens are ineffective for these indications, and there is no evidence from well-controlled studies that progestogens are effective for these uses. If conjugated estrogens is used during pregnancy, or if the patient becomes pregnant while taking this drug, she should be apprised of the potential risks to the fetus, and the advisability of pregnancy continuation.

DESCRIPTION

Conjugated estrogens is a mixture of estrogens, obtained exclusively from natural sources, occurring as the sodium salts of water-soluble estrogen sulfates blended to represent the average composition of material derived from pregnant mares' urine. It is a mixture of sodium estrone sulfate and sodium equilin sulfate. It contains as concomitant components, as sodium sulfate conjugates, 17 α-dihydroequilin, 17 α-estradiol, and 17 β-dihydroequilenin.

Each Secule vial contains 25 mg of conjugated estrogens, in a sterile lyophilized cake which also contains lactose 200 mg, sodium citrate 12.2 mg, and simethicone 0.2 mg. The pH is adjusted with sodium hydroxide or hydrochloric acid. A sterile diluent (5 ml) containing 2% benzyl alcohol in sterile water is provided for reconstitution. The reconstituted solution is suitable for intravenous or intramuscular injection.

CLINICAL PHARMACOLOGY

Estrogen drug products act by regulating the transcription of a limited number of genes. Estrogens diffuse through cell membranes, distribute themselves throughout the cell, and bind to and activate the nuclear estrogen receptor, a DNA-binding protein which is found in estrogen-responsive tissues. The activated estrogen receptor binds to specific DNA sequences, or hormone-response elements, which enhance the transcription of adjacent genes and in turn lead to the observed effects. Estrogen receptors have been identified in tissues of the reproductive tract, breast, pituitary, hypothalamus, liver, and bone of women.

Estrogens are important in the development and maintenance of the female reproductive system and secondary sex characteristics. By a direct action, they cause growth and development of the uterus, fallopian tubes, and vagina. With other hormones, such as pituitary hormones and progesterone, they cause enlargement of the breasts through promotion of ductal growth, stromal development, and the accretion of fat. Estrogens are intricately involved with other hormones, especially progesterone, in the processes of the ovulatory menstrual cycle and pregnancy, and affect the release of pituitary gonadotropins. They also contribute to the shaping of the skeleton, maintenance of tone and elasticity of urogenital structures, changes in the epiphyses of the long bones that allow for the pubertal growth spurt and its termination, and pigmentation of the nipples and genitals.

Estrogens occur naturally in several forms. The primary source of estrogen in normally cycling adult women is the ovarian follicle, which secretes 70-500 μg of estradiol daily, depending on the phase of the menstrual cycle. This is converted primarily to estrone, which circulates in roughly equal proportion to estradiol, and to small amounts of estriol. After menopause, most endogenous estrogen is produced by conversion of androstenedione, secreted by the adrenal cortex, to estrone by peripheral tissues. Thus, estrone, especially in its sulfate ester form, is the most abundant circulating estrogen in postmenopausal women. Although circulating estrogens exist in a dynamic equilibrium of metabolic interconversions, estradiol is the principal intracellular human estrogen and is substantially more potent than estrone or estriol at the receptor.

INFORMATION REGARDING LIPID EFFECTS

The results of a clinical trial conducted in a 97% Caucasian population at low risk for cardiovascular disease show that conjugated estrogens significantly increases HDL-C and the HDL_2-C subfraction and significantly decreases LDL-C.

TABLE 1 summarizes mean percent changes from baseline lipid parameter values after 1 year of treatment with conjugated estrogens.

TABLE 1 *Mean Percent Change From Baseline Lipid Profile Values After 1 Year of Treatment*

Lipid Parameter	Conjugated Estrogens 0.625 mg Dose
Total Cholesterol	0.2
HDL-C	14.1*
HDL_2-C	70.8*
LDL-C	-7.7*
Triglycerides	39.4*

* Significantly ($p \leq 0.05$) different from baseline value.

PHARMACOKINETICS

Absorption

Conjugated estrogens used in therapy are soluble in water and are well absorbed from the gastrointestinal tract after release from the drug formulation. Maximum plasma concentrations of the various conjugated and unconjugated estrogens are attained within 4-10 hours after oral administration.

Estrogens used in therapy are also well absorbed through the skin and mucous membranes. When applied for a local action, absorption is usually sufficient to cause systemic effects. When conjugated with aryl and alkyl groups for parenteral administration, the rate of absorption of oily preparations is slowed with a prolonged duration of action, such that a single intramuscular injection of estradiol valerate or estradiol cypionate is absorbed over several weeks.

Distribution

Although naturally-occurring estrogens circulate in the blood largely bound to sex hormone-binding globulin (SHBG) and albumin, only unbound estrogens enter target tissue cells. (Conjugated estrogens bind mainly to albumin; unconjugated estrogens bind to both albumin and SHBG.) The apparent terminal-phase disposition half-life ($T_{1/2}$) of the various estrogens is prolonged by the slow absorption from conjugated estrogens and ranges from 10-24 hours.

Metabolism

Administered estrogens and their esters are handled within the body essentially the same as the endogenous hormones. Metabolic conversion of estrogens occurs primarily in the liver (first-pass effect), but also at local target tissue sites. Complex metabolic processes result in a dynamic equilibrium of circulating conjugated and unconjugated estrogenic forms which are continually interconverted, especially between estrone and estradiol and between esterified and nonesterified forms. A significant proportion of the circulating estrogen exists as sulfate conjugates, especially estrone sulfate, which serves as a circulating reservoir for the formation of more active estrogenic species. A certain proportion of the estrogen is excreted into the bile, then reabsorbed from the intestine and returned to the liver through the portal venous system. During this enterohepatic recirculation, estrogens are desulfated and resulfated and undergo degradation through conversion to less active estrogens (estriol and other estrogens), oxidation to nonestrogenic substances (catecholestrogens, which interact with catecholamine metabolism, especially in the central nervous system), and conjugation with glucuronic acids (which are then rapidly excreted in the urine).

When given orally, naturally-occurring estrogens and their esters are extensively metabolized (first-pass effect) and circulate primarily as estrone sulfate, with smaller amounts of other conjugated and unconjugated estrogenic species. This results in limited oral potency. By contrast, synthetic estrogens, such as ethinyl estradiol and the nonsteroidal estrogens, are degraded very slowly in the liver and other tissues, which results in their high intrinsic potency. Estrogen drug products administered by non-oral routes are not subject to first-pass metabolism, but also undergo significant hepatic uptake, metabolism, and enterohepatic recycling.

Excretion

Water-soluble estrogen conjugates are strongly acidic and are ionized in body fluids, which favor excretion through the kidneys since tubular reabsorption is minimal.

E

TABLE 2A *Pharmacokinetic Parameters for Conjugated Estrogens*

Pharmakokinetic Profile of Unconjugated Estrogens Following a Dose of 2 × 0.625 mg

Drug	C_{max} (pg/ml)	T_{max} (h)	T½ (h)	AUC (pg·h/ml)
Estrone	139	8.8	28.0	5016
Baseline-adjusted estrone	120	8.8	17.4	2956
Equilin	66	7.9	13.6	1210

TABLE 2B *Pharmacokinetic Parameters for Conjugated Estrogens*

Pharmakokinetic Profile of Conjugated Estrogens Following a Dose of 2 × 0.625 mg

Drug	C_{max} (ng/ml)	T_{max} (h)	T½ (h)	AUC (ng·h/ml)
Total estrone	7.3	7.3	15.0	134
Baseline-adjusted total estrone	7.1	7.3	13.6	122
Total equilin	5.0	6.2	10.1	65

INDICATIONS AND USAGE

Estrogen drug products are indicated in the:

1. Treatment of moderate to severe vasomotor symptoms associated with the menopause. There is no adequate evidence that estrogens are effective for nervous symptoms or depression which might occur during menopause and they should not be used to treat these conditions.
2. Treatment of vulvar and vaginal atrophy.
3. Treatment of hypoestrogenism due to hypogonadism, castration, or primary ovarian failure.
4. Treatment of breast cancer (for palliation only) in appropriately selected women and men with metastatic disease.
5. Treatment of advanced androgen-dependent carcinoma of the prostate (for palliation only).
6. Prevention of osteoporosis. Since estrogen administration is associated with risk, selection of patients ideally should be based on prospective identification of risk factors for developing osteoporosis. Unfortunately, there is no certain way to identify those women who will develop osteoporotic fractures. Most prospective studies of efficacy for this indication have been carried out in white menopausal women, without stratification by other risk factors, and tend to show a universally salutary effect on bone. Thus, patient selection must be individualized based on the balance of risks and benefits. A more favorable risk/benefit ratio exists in a hysterectomized woman because she has no risk of endometrial cancer (see BOXED WARNING).

Estrogen replacement therapy reduces bone resorption and retards or halts postmenopausal bone loss. Case-control studies have shown an approximately 60% reduction in hip and wrist fractures in women whose estrogen replacement was begun within a few years of menopause. Studies also suggest that estrogen reduces the rate of vertebral fractures. Even when started as late as 6 years after menopause, estrogen prevents further loss of bone mass for as long as the treatment is continued. When estrogen therapy is discontinued, bone mass declines at a rate comparable to the immediate postmenopausal period. There is no evidence that estrogen replacement therapy restores bone mass to premenopausal levels.

At skeletal maturity there are sex and race differences in both the total amount of bone present and its density, in favor of men and Blacks. Thus, women are at higher risk than men because they start with less bone mass and, for several years following natural or induced menopause, the rate of bone mass decline is accelerated. White and Asian women are at higher risk than Black women.

Early menopause is one of the strongest predictors for the development of osteoporosis. In addition, other factors affecting the skeleton which are associated with osteoporosis include genetic factors (small build, family history), endocrine factors (nulliparity, thyrotoxicosis, hyperparathyroidism, Cushing's syndrome, hyperprolactinemia, Type 1 diabetes), lifestyle (cigarette smoking, alcohol abuse, sedentary exercise habits), and nutrition (below average body weight, dietary calcium intake).

The mainstays of prevention and management of osteoporosis are estrogen, an adequate lifetime calcium intake, and exercise. Postmenopausal women absorb dietary calcium less efficiently than premenopausal women and require an average of 1500 mg/day of elemental calcium to remain in neutral calcium balance. By comparison, premenopausal women require about 1000 mg/day and the average calcium intake in the US is 400-600 mg/day. Therefore, when not contraindicated, calcium supplementation may be helpful.

Weight-bearing exercise and nutrition may be important adjuncts to the prevention and management of osteoporosis. Immobilization and prolonged bed rest produce rapid bone loss, while weight-bearing exercise has been shown both to reduce bone loss and to increase bone mass. The optimal type and amount of physical activity that would prevent osteoporosis have not been established, however in 2 studies an hour of walking and running exercises 2 or 3 times weekly significantly increased lumbar spine bone mass.

Intravenous conjugated estrogens are indicated in the treatment of abnormal uterine bleeding due to hormonal imbalance in the absence of organic pathology.

NON-FDA APPROVED INDICATIONS

Although not FDA approved, conjugated estrogens have been used for the treatment of atrophic urethritis, gastrointestinal bleeding in patients with renal failure and gastrointestinal bleeding related to arteriovenous malformations.

CONTRAINDICATIONS

Estrogens should not be used in individuals with any of the following conditions:

1. Known or suspected pregnancy (see BOXED WARNING). Estrogens may cause fetal harm when administered to a pregnant woman.
2. Undiagnosed abnormal genital bleeding.
3. Known or suspected cancer of the breast except in appropriately selected patients being treated for metastatic disease.
4. Known or suspected estrogen-dependent neoplasia.
5. Active thrombophlebitis or thromboembolic disorders. There is insufficient information regarding women who have had previous thromboembolic disease.
6. Conjugated estrogens should not be used in patients hypersensitive to their ingredients.

WARNINGS

INDUCTION OF MALIGNANT NEOPLASMS

Long-term, continuous administration of natural and synthetic estrogens in certain animal species increases the frequency of carcinomas of the breast, cervix, vagina, and liver. There are now reports that estrogens increase the risk of carcinoma of the endometrium in humans (see BOXED WARNING). At the present time there is no satisfactory evidence that estrogens given to postmenopausal women increase the risk of cancer of the breast,[17] although a recent long-term follow-up of a single physician's practice has raised this possibility.[18] Because of the animal data, there is a need for caution in prescribing estrogens for women with a strong family history of breast cancer, or who have breast nodules, fibrocystic disease, or abnormal mammograms.

GALLBLADDER DISEASE

A recent study has reported a 2- to 3-fold increase in the risk of surgically confirmed gallbladder disease in women receiving postmenopausal estrogens,[17] similar to the 2-fold increase previously noted in users of oral contraceptives.[19,24a]

EFFECTS SIMILAR TO THOSE CAUSED BY ESTROGEN-PROGESTOGEN ORAL CONTRACEPTIVES

There are several serious adverse effects of oral contraceptives, most of which have not, up to now, been documented as consequences of postmenopausal estrogen therapy. This may reflect the comparatively low doses of estrogen used in postmenopausal women. It would be expected that the larger doses of estrogen used to treat prostatic or breast cancer are more likely to result in these adverse effects, and, in fact, it has been shown that there is an increased risk of thrombosis in men receiving estrogens for prostatic cancer.[20-23]

Thromboembolic Disease: It is now well established that users of oral contraceptives have an increased risk of various thromboembolic and thrombotic vascular diseases, such as thrombophlebitis, pulmonary embolism, stroke, and myocardial infarction.[24-31] Cases of retinal thrombosis, mesenteric thrombosis, and optic neuritis have been reported in oral-contraceptive users. There is evidence that the risk of several of these adverse reactions is related to the dose of the drug.[32,33] An increased risk of postsurgery thromboembolic complications has also been reported in users of oral contraceptives.[34,35] If feasible, estrogen should be discontinued at least 4 weeks before surgery of the type associated with an increased risk of thromboembolism, or during periods of prolonged immobilization. While an increased rate of thromboembolic and thrombotic disease in postmenopausal users of estrogens has not been found,[17-36] this does not rule out the possibility that such an increase may be present, or that subgroups of women who have underlying risk factors, or who are receiving relatively large doses of estrogens, may have increased risk. Therefore, estrogens should not be used in persons with active thrombophlebitis or thromboembolic disorders, and they should not be used (except in treatment of malignancy) in persons with a history of such disorders in association with estrogen use. They should be used with caution in patients with cerebral vascular or coronary artery disease and only for those in whom estrogens are clearly needed. Large doses of estrogen (5 mg conjugated estrogens/day), comparable to those used to treat cancer of the prostate and breast, have been shown in a large prospective clinical trial in men[37] to increase the risk of nonfatal myocardial infarction, pulmonary embolism, and thrombophlebitis. When estrogen doses of this size are used, any of the thromboembolic and thrombotic adverse effects associated with oral-contraceptive use should be considered a clear risk.

Hepatic Adenoma: Benign hepatic adenomas appear to be associated with the use of oral contraceptives.[38-40] Although benign and rare, these may rupture and may cause death through intra-abdominal hemorrhage. Such lesions have not yet been reported in association with other estrogen or progestogen preparations but should be considered in estrogen users having abdominal pain and tenderness, abdominal mass, or hypovolemic shock. Hepatocellular carcinoma has also been reported in women taking estrogen-containing oral contraceptives.[39] The relationship of this malignancy to these drugs is not known at this time.

Glucose Tolerance: A worsening of glucose tolerance has been observed in a significant percentage of patients on estrogen-containing oral contraceptives. For this reason, diabetic patients should be carefully observed while receiving estrogen.

HYPERCALCEMIA

Administration of estrogens may lead to severe hypercalcemia in patients with breast cancer and bone metastases. If this occurs, the drug should be stopped and appropriate measures taken to reduce the serum calcium level.

PRECAUTIONS

GENERAL

A complete medical and family history should be taken prior to the initiation of any estrogen therapy. The pretreatment and periodic physical examinations should include special reference to blood pressure, breasts, abdomen, and pelvic organs, and should include a Pap smear. As a general rule, estrogens should not be prescribed for longer than 1 year without another physical examination being performed.

Fluid Retention

Because estrogens may cause some degree of fluid retention, conditions which might be influenced by this factor, such as asthma, epilepsy, migraine, and cardiac or renal dysfunction require careful observation.

Familial Hyperlipoproteinemia

Estrogen therapy may be associated with massive elevations of plasma triglycerides leading to pancreatitis and other complications in patients with familial defects of lipoprotein metabolism.

Certain patients may develop undesirable manifestations of excessive estrogenic stimulation, such as abnormal or excessive uterine bleeding, mastodynia, etc.

DRUG/LABORATORY TEST INTERACTIONS

Certain endocrine and liver function tests may be affected by estrogen-containing oral contraceptives.

The following similar changes may be expected with larger doses of estrogen:

1. Increased sulfobromophthalein retention.
2. Increased prothrombin and factors VII, VIII, IX, and X; decreased antithrombin;[3] increased norepinephrine-induced platelet aggregability.
3. Increased thyroid-binding globulin (TBG) leading to increased circulating total thyroid hormone, as measured by PBI, T4 by column, or T4 by radioimmunoassay. Free T3 resin uptake is decreased, reflecting the elevated TBG; free T4 concentration is unaltered.
4. Impaired glucose tolerance.
5. Decreased pregnanediol excretion.
6. Reduced response to metyrapone test.
7. Reduced serum folate concentration.
8. Increased serum triglyceride and phospholipid concentration.

CARCINOGENESIS, MUTAGENESIS, AND IMPAIRMENT OF FERTILITY

See WARNINGS.

PREGNANCY CATEGORY X

See CONTRAINDICATIONS and BOXED WARNING.

NURSING MOTHERS

It is not known whether this drug is excreted in human milk. Because many drugs are excreted in human milk and because of the potential for serious adverse reactions in nursing infants from estrogens, a decision should be made whether to discontinue nursing or to discontinue the drug, taking into account the importance of the drug to the mother.

PEDIATRIC USE

Safety and effectiveness in children have not been established.

ADVERSE REACTIONS

The following additional adverse reactions have been reported with estrogen therapy (see WARNINGS regarding induction of neoplasia, adverse effects on the fetus, increased incidence of gallbladder disease, cardiovascular disease, elevated blood pressure, and hypercalcemia; see PRECAUTIONS regarding cardiovascular risk):

Genitourinary System: Changes in vaginal bleeding pattern and abnormal withdrawal bleeding or flow; breakthrough bleeding, spotting; increase in size of uterine leiomyomata; vaginal candidiasis, change in amount of cervical secretion.

Breasts: Tenderness, enlargement.

Gastrointestinal: Nausea, vomiting, abdominal cramps, bloating, cholestatic jaundice, increased incidence of gallbladder disease, pancreatitis.

Skin: Chloasma or melasma that may persist when drug is discontinued, erythema multiforme, erythema nodosum, hemorrhagic eruption, loss of scalp hair, hirsutism.

Cardiovascular: Venous thromboembolism, pulmonary embolism.

Eyes: Steepening of corneal curvature, intolerance to contact lenses.

Central Nervous System: Headache, migraine, dizziness, mental depression, chorea.

Miscellaneous: Increase or decrease in weight, reduced carbohydrate tolerance, aggravation of porphyria, edema, changes in libido.

DOSAGE AND ADMINISTRATION

ABNORMAL UTERINE BLEEDING DUE TO HORMONAL IMBALANCE

One 25 mg injection, intravenously or intramuscularly. Intravenous use is preferred since more rapid response can be expected from this mode of administration.

Repeat in 6-12 hours if necessary. The use of conjugated estrogens intravenous for injection does not preclude the advisability of other appropriate measures.

The usual precautionary measures governing intravenous administration should be adhered to. Injection should be made SLOWLY to obviate the occurrence of flushes.

Infusion of conjugated estrogens intravenous for injection with other agents is not generally recommended. In emergencies, however, when an infusion has already been started it may be expedient to make the injection into the tubing just distal to the infusion needle. If so used, compatibility of solutions must be considered.

COMPATIBILITY OF SOLUTIONS

Conjugated estrogens intravenous is compatible with normal saline, dextrose, and invert sugar solutions. IT IS NOT COMPATIBLE WITH PROTEIN HYDROLYSATE, ASCORBIC ACID, OR ANY SOLUTION WITH AN ACID pH.

Treated patients with an intact uterus should be monitored closely for signs of endometrial cancer, and appropriate diagnostic measures should be taken to rule out malignancy in the event of persistent or recurring abnormal vaginal bleeding.

HOW SUPPLIED

PREMARIN INJECTION

Each Package Provides:

One Secule vial containing 25 mg of conjugated estrogens for injection (also lactose 200 mg, sodium citrate 12.2 mg, and simethicone 0.2 mg). The pH is adjusted with sodium hydroxide or hydrochloric acid.

One 5 ml ampul sterile diluent with 2% benzyl alcohol in sterile water.

Premarin intravenous for injection is prepared by cryodesication.

Storage Before Reconstitution: Store package in refrigerator, 2-8°C (36-46°F).

E

ORAL

WARNING

ESTROGENS INCREASE THE RISK OF ENDOMETRIAL CANCER: Close clinical surveillance of all women taking estrogens is important. Adequate diagnostic measures, including endometrial sampling when indicated, should be undertaken to rule out malignancy in all cases of undiagnosed persistent or recurring abnormal vaginal bleeding. There is no evidence that the use of "natural" estrogens results in a different endometrial risk profile than synthetic estrogens of equivalent estrogen dose.

CARDIOVASCULAR AND OTHER RISKS: Estrogens with or without progestins should not be used for the prevention of cardiovascular disease.

The Women's Health Initiative (WHI) reported increased risks of myocardial infarction, stroke, invasive breast cancer, pulmonary emboli, and deep vein thrombosis in postmenopausal women during 5 years of treatment with conjugated equine estrogens (0.625 mg) combined with medroxyprogesterone acetate (2.5 mg) relative to placebo. Other doses of conjugated estrogens and medroxyprogesterone acetate, and other combinations of estrogens and progestins were not studied in the WHI and, in the absence of comparable data, these risks should be assumed to be similar. Because of these risks, estrogens with or without progestins should be prescribed at the lowest effective doses and for the shortest duration consistent with treatment goals and risks for the individual woman.

DESCRIPTION

Premarin for oral administration contains a mixture of conjugated equine estrogens obtained exclusively from natural sources, occurring as the sodium salts of water-soluble estrogen sulfates blended to represent the average composition of material derived from pregnant mares' urine. It is a mixture of sodium estrone sulfate and sodium equilin sulfate. It contains as concomitant components, as sodium sulfate conjugates, 17 α-dihydroequilin, 17 α-estradiol, and 17 β-dihydroequilin. Tablets for oral administration are available in 0.3, 0.625, 0.9, 1.25, and 2.5 mg strengths of conjugated estrogens.

Premarin tablets contain the following inactive ingredients: Calcium phosphate tribasic, calcium sulfate, carnauba wax, cellulose, glyceryl monooleate, lactose, magnesium stearate, methylcellulose, pharmaceutical glaze, polyethylene glycol, stearic acid, sucrose, titanium dioxide. *0.3 mg tablets also contain:* D&C yellow no. 10, FD&C blue no. 1, FD&C blue no. 2, FD&C yellow no. 6; *0.625 mg tablets also contain:* FD&C blue no. 2, D&C red no. 27, FD&C red no. 40; *0.9 mg tablets also contain:* D&C red no. 6, D&C red no. 7; *1.25 mg tablets also contain:* Black iron oxide, D&C yellow no. 10, FD&C yellow no. 6; *2.5 mg tablets also contain:* FD&C blue no. 2, D&C red no. 7.

CLINICAL PHARMACOLOGY

Endogenous estrogens are largely responsible for the development and maintenance of the female reproductive system and secondary sexual characteristics. Although circulating estrogens exist in a dynamic equilibrium of metabolic interconversions, estradiol is the principal intracellular human estrogen and is substantially more potent than its metabolites, estrone and estriol, at the receptor level.

The primary source of estrogen in normally cycling adult women is the ovarian follicle, which secretes 70-500 micrograms of estradiol daily, depending on the phase of the menstrual cycle. After menopause, most endogenous estrogen is produced by conversion of androstenedione, secreted by the adrenal cortex, to estrone by peripheral tissues. Thus, estrone and the sulfate-conjugated form, estrone sulfate, are the most abundant circulating estrogen in postmenopausal women.

Estrogens act through binding to nuclear receptors in estrogen-responsive tissues. To date, two estrogen receptors have been identified. These vary in proportion from tissue to tissue.

Circulating estrogens modulate the pituitary secretion of the gonadotropins, luteinizing hormone (LH) and follicle stimulating hormone (FSH) through a negative feedback mechanism. Estrogens act to reduce the elevated levels of these gonadotropins seen in postmenopausal women.

PHARMACOKINETICS

Absorption

Conjugated estrogens are soluble in water and are well absorbed from the gastrointestinal tract after release from the drug formulation. The Premarin tablet releases conjugated estrogens slowly over several hours. The pharmacokinetic profile of unconjugated and conjugated estrogens following a dose of 2 × 0.625 mg is provided in TABLE 3A and TABLE 3B.

Distribution

The distribution of exogenous estrogens is similar to that of endogenous estrogens. Estrogens are widely distributed in the body and are generally found in higher concentration in the sex hormone target organs. Estrogens circulate in the blood largely bound to sex hormone-binding globulin (SHBG) and albumin.

Metabolism

Exogenous estrogens are metabolized in the same manner as endogenous estrogens. Circulating estrogens exist in a dynamic equilibrium of metabolic interconversions. These transformations take place mainly in the liver. Estradiol is converted reversibly to estrone, and both can be converted to estriol, which is the major urinary metabolite. Estrogens also undergo enterohepatic recirculation via sulfate and glucuronide conjugation in the liver, biliary secretion of conjugates into the intestine, and hydrolysis in the gut followed by reabsorption. In postmenopausal women a significant portion of the circulating estrogens exists as sulfate conjugates, especially estrone sulfate, which serves as a circulating reservoir for the formation of more active estrogens.

E

Excretion

Estradiol, estrone, and estriol are excreted in the urine along with glucuronide and sulfate conjugates.

TABLE 3A *Pharmacokinetic Parameters for Conjugated Estrogens — Pharmacokinetic Profile of Unconjugated Estrogens Following a Dose of 2 × 0.625 mg**

Drug	C_{max} (pg/ml)	T_{max} (h)	T½† (h)	AUC (pg·h/ml)
Estrone	139 (37)	8.8 (20)	28.0 (13)	5016 (34)
Baseline-adjusted estrone	120 (42)	8.8 (20)	17.4 (37)	2956 (39)
Equilin	66 (42)	7.9 (19)	13.6 (52)	1210 (37)

* Mean (Coefficient of Variation, %)
† T½ = terminal-phase disposition half-life (0.693/γ_2)

TABLE 3B *Pharmacokinetic Parameters for Conjugated Estrogens — Pharmacokinetic Profile of Conjugated Estrogens Following a Dose of 2 × 0.625 mg**

Drug	C_{max} (ng/ml)	T_{max} (h)	T½† (h)	AUC (ng·h/ml)
Total estrone	7.3 (41)	7.3 (51)	15.0 (25)	134 (42)
Baseline-adjusted total estrone	7.1 (41)	7.3 (25)	13.6 (27)	122 (39)
Total equilin	5.0 (42)	6.2 (26)	10.1 (27)	65 (45)

* Mean (Coefficient of Variation, %)
† T½ = terminal-phase disposition half-life (0.693/γ_2)

SPECIAL POPULATIONS

No pharmacokinetic studies were conducted in special populations, including patients with renal or hepatic impairment.

DRUG INTERACTIONS

Data from a single-dose drug-drug interaction study involving conjugated estrogens and medroxyprogesterone acetate indicate that the pharmacokinetic dispositions of both drugs are not significantly altered. No other clinical drug-drug interaction studies have been conducted with conjugated estrogens.

In vitro and *in vivo* studies have shown that estrogens are metabolized partially by cytochrome P450 3A4 (CYP3A4). Therefore, inducers or inhibitors of CYP3A4 may affect estrogen drug metabolism. Inducers of CYP3A4 such as St. John's Wort preparations (Hypericum perforatum), phenobarbital, carbamazepine, and rifampin may reduce plasma concentrations of estrogens, possibly resulting in a decrease in therapeutic effects and/or changes in the uterine bleeding profile. Inhibitors of CYP3A4 such as erythromycin, clarithromycin, ketoconazole, itraconazole, ritonavir and grapefruit juice may increase plasma concentrations of estrogens and may result in side effects.

INDICATIONS AND USAGE

Conjugated estrogens therapy is indicated in the:

- Treatment of moderate to severe vasomotor symptoms associated with the menopause.
- Treatment of moderate to severe symptoms of vulvar and vaginal atrophy associated with the menopause. When prescribing solely for the treatment of symptoms of vulvar and vaginal atrophy, topical vaginal products should be considered.
- Treatment of hypoestrogenism due to hypogonadism, castration or primary ovarian failure.
- Treatment of breast cancer (for palliation only) in appropriately selected women and men with metastatic disease.
- Treatment of advanced androgen-dependent carcinoma of the prostate (for palliation only).
- Prevention of postmenopausal osteoporosis. When prescribing solely for the prevention of postmenopausal osteoporosis, therapy should only be considered for women at significant risk of osteoporosis and non-estrogen medications should be carefully considered.

The mainstays for decreasing the risk of postmenopausal osteoporosis are weight bearing exercise, adequate calcium and vitamin D intake, and when indicated, pharmacologic therapy. Postmenopausal women require an average of 1500 mg/day of elemental calcium. Therefore, when not contraindicated, calcium supplementation may be helpful for women with suboptimal dietary intake. Vitamin D supplementation of 400-800 IU/day may also be required to ensure adequate daily intake in postmenopausal women.

NON-FDA APPROVED INDICATIONS

Although not FDA approved, conjugated estrogens have been used for the treatment of atrophic urethritis, gastrointestinal bleeding in patients with renal failure and gastrointestinal bleeding related to arteriovenous malformations.

CONTRAINDICATIONS

Estrogens should not be used in individuals with any of the following conditions:

- Undiagnosed abnormal genital bleeding.
- Known, suspected, or history of cancer of the breast except in appropriately selected patients being treated for metastatic disease.
- Known or suspected estrogen-dependent neoplasia.
- Active deep vein thrombosis, pulmonary embolism or a history of these conditions.
- Active or recent (*e.g.*, within past year) arterial thromboembolic disease (*e.g.*, stroke, myocardial infarction).
- Conjugated estrogens tablets should not be used in patients with known hypersensitivity to their ingredients.
- Known or suspected pregnancy. There is no indication for conjugated estrogens in pregnancy. There appears to be little or no increased risk of birth defects in women who have used estrogen and progestins from oral contraceptives inadvertently during pregnancy. (See PRECAUTIONS.)

WARNINGS

See BOXED WARNING.

The use of unopposed estrogens in women who have a uterus is associated with an increased risk of endometrial cancer.

CARDIOVASCULAR DISORDERS

Estrogen and estrogen/progestin therapy have been associated with an increased risk of cardiovascular events such as myocardial infarction and stroke, as well as venous thrombosis and pulmonary embolism (venous thromboembolism or VTE). Should any of these occur or be suspected, estrogens should be discontinued immediately.

Risk factors for cardiovascular disease (*e.g.*, hypertension, diabetes mellitus, tobacco use, hypercholesterolemia, and obesity) should be managed appropriately.

Coronary Heart Disease and Stroke

In the conjugated estrogens substudy of the Women's Health Initiative (WHI), an increase in the number of myocardial infarctions and strokes has been observed in women receiving conjugated estrogens compared to placebo. These observations are preliminary, and the study is continuing.

In the Prempro substudy of WHI, an increased risk of coronary heart disease (CHD) events (defined as non-fatal myocardial infarction and CHD death) was observed in women receiving Prempro compared to women receiving placebo (37 vs 30/10,000 person-years). The increase in risk was observed in Year 1 and persisted.

In the same substudy of the WHI, an increased risk of stroke was observed in women receiving Prempro compared to women receiving placebo (29 vs 21/10,000 person-years). The increase in risk was observed after the first year and persisted.

In postmenopausal women with documented heart disease (n=2763, average age 66.7 years) a controlled clinical trial of secondary prevention of cardiovascular disease (Heart and Estrogen/progestin Replacement Study; HERS) treatment with Prempro (0.625 mg conjugated equine estrogen plus 2.5 mg medroxyprogesterone acetate per day) demonstrated no cardiovascular benefit. During an average follow-up of 4.1 years, treatment with Prempro did not reduce the overall rate of CHD events in postmenopausal women with established coronary heart disease. There were more CHD events in the Prempro-treated group than in the placebo group in Year 1, but not during the subsequent years. Two thousand three hundred and twenty one (2321) women from the original HERS trial agreed to participate in an open label extension of HERS, HERS II. Average follow-up in HERS II was an additional 2.7 years, for a total of 6.8 years overall. Rates of CHD events were comparable among women in the Prempro group and the placebo group in HERS, HERS II, and overall.

Large doses of estrogen (5 mg conjugated estrogens per day), comparable to those used to treat cancer of the prostate and breast, have been shown in a large prospective clinical trial in men to increase the risks of nonfatal myocardial infarction, pulmonary embolism, and thrombophlebitis.

Venous Thromboembolism (VTE)

In the conjugated estrogens substudy of the Women's Health Initiative (WHI), an increase in VTE has been observed in women receiving conjugated estrogens compared to placebo. These observations are preliminary, and the study is continuing.

In the Prempro substudy of WHI, a 2-fold greater rate of VTE, including deep venous thrombosis and pulmonary embolism, was observed in women receiving Prempro compared to women receiving placebo. The rate of VTE was 34/10,000 woman-years in the Prempro group compared to 16/10,000 woman-years in the placebo group. The increase in VTE risk was observed during the first year and persisted.

If feasible, estrogens should be discontinued at least 4-6 weeks before surgery of the type associated with an increased risk of thromboembolism, or during periods of prolonged immobilization.

MALIGNANT NEOPLASMS

Endometrial Cancer

The use of unopposed estrogens in women with intact uteri has been associated with an increased risk of endometrial cancer. The reported endometrial cancer risk among unopposed estrogen users is about 2- to 12-fold greater than in non-users, and appears dependent on duration of treatment and on estrogen dose. Most studies show no significant increased risk associated with use of estrogens for less than 1 year. The greatest risk appears associated with prolonged use, with increased risks of 15- to 24-fold for 5-10 years or more and this risk has been shown to persist for at least 8-15 years after estrogen therapy is discontinued.

Clinical surveillance of all women taking estrogen/progestin combinations is important. Adequate diagnostic measures, including endometrial sampling when indicated, should be undertaken to rule out malignancy in all cases of undiagnosed persistent or recurring abnormal vaginal bleeding. There is no evidence that the use of natural estrogens results in a different endometrial risk profile than synthetic estrogens of equivalent estrogen dose. Adding a progestin to postmenopausal estrogen therapy has been shown to reduce the risk of endometrial hyperplasia, which may be a precursor to endometrial cancer.

Breast Cancer

Estrogen and estrogen/progestin therapy in postmenopausal women have been associated with an increased risk of breast cancer. In the Prempro substudy of the Women's Health Initiative study (WHI), a 26% increase of invasive breast cancer (38 vs 30/10,000 woman-years) after an average of 5.2 years of treatment was observed in women receiving Prempro compared to women receiving placebo. The increased risk of breast cancer became apparent after 4 years on Prempro. The women reporting prior postmenopausal use of estrogen and/or estrogen with progestin had a higher relative risk for breast cancer associated with Prempro than those who had never used these hormones.

In the conjugated estrogens substudy of WHI, no increased risk of breast cancer in estrogen-treated women compared to placebo was reported after an average of 5.2 years of therapy. These data are preliminary and that substudy of WHI is continuing.

Epidemiologic studies have reported an increased risk of breast cancer in association with increasing duration of postmenopausal treatment with estrogens, with or without progestin. This association was reanalyzed in original data from 51 studies that involved treatment with various doses and types of estrogens, with and without progestin. In the reanalysis, an increased risk of having breast cancer diagnosed became apparent after about 5 years of continued treatment, and subsided after treatment had been discontinued for about 5 years. Some later studies have suggested that treatment with estrogen and progestin increases the risk of breast cancer more than treatment with estrogen alone.

A postmenopausal woman without a uterus who requires estrogen should receive estrogen-alone therapy, and should not be exposed unnecessarily to progestins. All postmenopausal women should receive yearly breast exams by a healthcare provider and perform monthly breast self-examinations. In addition, mammography examinations should be scheduled based on patient age and risk factors.

GALLBLADDER DISEASE

A 2- to 4-fold increase in the risk of gallbladder disease requiring surgery in postmenopausal women receiving postmenopausal estrogens has been reported.

HYPERCALCEMIA

Estrogen administration may lead to severe hypercalcemia in patients with breast cancer and bone metastases. If hypercalcemia occurs, use of the drug should be stopped and appropriate measures taken to reduce the serum calcium level.

VISUAL ABNORMALITIES

Retinal vascular thrombosis has been reported in patients receiving estrogens. Discontinue medication pending examination if there is sudden partial or complete loss of vision, or a sudden onset of proptosis, diplopia, or migraine. If examination reveals papilledema or retinal vascular lesions, estrogens should be discontinued.

PRECAUTIONS

GENERAL

Addition of a Progestin When a Woman Has Not Had a Hysterectomy

Studies of the addition of a progestin for 10 or more days of a cycle of estrogen administration or daily with estrogen in a continuous regimen have reported a lowered incidence of endometrial hyperplasia than would be induced by estrogen treatment alone. Endometrial hyperplasia may be a precursor to endometrial cancer.

There are, however, possible risks that may be associated with the use of progestins with estrogens compared to estrogen-alone regimens. These include a possible increased risk of breast cancer, adverse effects on lipoprotein metabolism (*e.g.,* lowering HDL, raising LDL) and impairment of glucose tolerance.

Elevated Blood Pressure

In a small number of case reports, substantial increases in blood pressure have been attributed to idiosyncratic reactions to estrogens. In a large, randomized, placebo-controlled clinical trial, a generalized effect of estrogen therapy on blood pressure was not seen. Blood pressure should be monitored at regular intervals with estrogen use.

Familial Hyperlipoproteinemia

In patients with familial defects of lipoprotein metabolism, estrogen therapy may be associated with elevations of plasma triglycerides leading to pancreatitis and other complications.

Impaired Liver Function and Past History of Cholestatic Jaundice

Estrogens may be poorly metabolized in patients with impaired liver function. For patients with a history of cholestatic jaundice associated with past estrogen use or with pregnancy, caution should be exercised and in the case of recurrence, medication should be discontinued.

Hypothyroidism

Estrogen administration leads to increased thyroid-binding globulin (TBG) levels. Patients with normal thyroid function can compensate for the increased TBG by making more thyroid hormone, thus maintaining free T4 and T3 serum concentrations in the normal range. Patients dependent on thyroid hormone replacement therapy who are also receiving estrogens may require increased doses of their thyroid replacement therapy. These patients should have their thyroid function monitored in order to maintain their free thyroid hormone levels in an acceptable range.

Fluid Retention

Because estrogens may cause some degree of fluid retention, patients with conditions that might be influenced by this factor, such as a cardiac or renal dysfunction, warrant careful observation when estrogens are prescribed.

Hypocalcemia

Estrogens should be used with caution in individuals with severe hypocalcemia.

Ovarian Cancer

Use of estrogen-only products, in particular for 10 or more years, has been associated with an increased risk of ovarian cancer in some epidemiological studies. Other studies did not show a significant association. Data are insufficient to determine whether there is an increased risk with combined estrogen/progestin therapy in postmenopausal women.

Exacerbation of Endometriosis

Endometriosis may be exacerbated with administration of estrogen therapy.

Exacerbation of Other Conditions

Estrogen therapy may cause an exacerbation of asthma, diabetes mellitus, epilepsy, migraine or porphyria and should be used with caution in patients with these conditions.

INFORMATION FOR THE PATIENT

Physicians are advised to discuss the contents of the Patient Information leaflet that is included with the prescription with patients for whom they prescribe conjugated estrogens.

LABORATORY TESTS

Estrogen administration should be guided by clinical response at the lowest dose for the treatment of postmenopausal moderate to severe vasomotor symptoms and moderate to severe symptoms of postmenopausal vulvar and vaginal atrophy. Laboratory parameters may be useful in guiding dosage for the treatment of hypoestrogenism due to hypogonadism, castration and primary ovarian failure.

DRUG/LABORATORY TEST INTERACTIONS

- Accelerated prothrombin time, partial thromboplastin time, and platelet aggregation time; increased platelet count; increased factors II, VII antigen, VIII antigen, VIII coagulant activity, IX, X, XII, VII-X complex, II-VII-X complex, and β-thromboglobulin; decreased levels of anti-factor Xa and antithrombin III, decreased antithrombin III activity; increased levels of fibrinogen and fibrinogen activity; increased plasminogen antigen and activity.
- Increased thyroid binding globulin (TBG) leading to increased circulating total thyroid hormone levels, as measured by protein-bound iodine (PBI), T4 levels (by column or by radioimmunoassay) or T3 levels by radioimmunoassay. T3 resin uptake is decreased, reflecting the elevated TBG. Free T4 and free T3 concentrations are unaltered. Patients on thyroid replacement therapy may require higher doses of thyroid hormone.
- Other binding proteins may be elevated in serum, *i.e.,* corticosteroid binding globulin (CBG), sex hormone-binding globulin (SHBG), leading to increased circulating corticosteroids and sex steroids, respectively. Free or biologically active hormone concentrations are unchanged. Other plasma proteins may be increased (angiotensinogen/renin substrate, alpha-1-antitrypsin, ceruloplasmin).
- Increased plasma HDL and HDL_2 subfraction concentrations, reduced LDL cholesterol concentration, increased triglyceride levels.
- Impaired glucose tolerance.
- Reduced response to metyrapone test.

CARCINOGENESIS, MUTAGENESIS, AND IMPAIRMENT OF FERTILITY

Long-term continuous administration of natural and synthetic estrogens in certain animal species increases the frequency of carcinomas of the breast, uterus, cervix, vagina, testis, and liver. (See BOXED WARNING, CONTRAINDICATIONS, and WARNINGS.)

PREGNANCY

Conjugated estrogens should not be used during pregnancy. (See CONTRAINDICATIONS and BOXED WARNING.)

NURSING MOTHERS

Estrogen administration to nursing mothers has been shown to decrease the quantity and quality of breast milk. Detectable amounts of estrogens have been identified in the milk of mothers receiving the drug. Caution should be exercised when conjugated estrogens is administered to a nursing woman.

PEDIATRIC USE

Estrogen therapy has been used for the induction of puberty in adolescents with some forms of pubertal delay. Safety and effectiveness in pediatric patients have not otherwise been established.

Large and repeated doses of estrogen over an extended time period have been shown to accelerate epiphyseal closure, which could result in short adult stature if treatment is initiated before the completion of physiologic puberty in normally developing children. If estrogen is administered to patients whose bone growth is not complete, periodic monitoring of bone maturation and effects on epiphyseal centers is recommended during estrogen administration.

Estrogen treatment of prepubertal girls also induces premature breast development and vaginal cornification, and may induce vaginal bleeding. In boys, estrogen treatment may modify the normal pubertal process and induce gynecomastia. See INDICATIONS AND USAGE and DOSAGE AND ADMINISTRATION.

GERIATRIC USE

Of the total number of subjects in the Prempro substudy of the Women's Health Initiative study, 44% (n=7320) were 65 years and over, while 6.6% (n=1095) were 75 and over. No significant differences in safety were observed between subjects 65 years and over compared to younger subjects. There was a higher incidence of stroke and invasive breast cancer in women 75 and over compared to younger subjects.

With respect to efficacy in the approved indications, there have not been sufficient numbers of geriatric patients involved in studies utilizing conjugated estrogens to determine whether those over 65 years of age differ from younger subjects in their response to conjugated estrogens.

ADVERSE REACTIONS

See BOXED WARNING, WARNINGS, and PRECAUTIONS.

The following additional adverse reactions have been reported with estrogen therapy and/or progestin therapy:

Genitourinary System: Changes in vaginal bleeding pattern and abnormal withdrawal bleeding or flow; breakthrough bleeding, spotting; increase in size of uterine leiomyomata; vaginitis, including vaginal candidiasis; change in amount of cervical secretion; change in cervical ectropion; ovarian cancer; endometrial hyperplasia; endometrial cancer.

Breasts: Tenderness, enlargement, pain, discharge, galactorrhea; fibrocystic breast changes; breast cancer.

Cardiovascular: Deep and superficial venous thrombosis; pulmonary embolism; thrombophlebitis; myocardial infarction; stroke; increase in blood pressure.

Gastrointestinal: Nausea, vomiting; abdominal cramps, bloating; cholestatic jaundice; increased incidence of gallbladder disease; pancreatitis.

Skin: Chloasma or melasma that may persist when drug is discontinued; erythema multiforme; erythema nodosum; hemorrhagic eruption; loss of scalp hair; hirsutism; pruritus, rash.

Eyes: Retinal vascular thrombosis; steepening of corneal curvature; intolerance to contact lenses.

Central Nervous System: Headache; migraine; dizziness; mental depression; chorea; nervousness; mood disturbances; irritability; exacerbation of epilepsy.

Miscellaneous: Increase or decrease in weight; reduced carbohydrate tolerance; aggravation of porphyria; edema; arthralgias; leg cramps; changes in libido; anaphylactoid/anaphylactic reactions including urticaria and angioedema; hypocalcemia; exacerbation of asthma; increased triglycerides.

DOSAGE AND ADMINISTRATION

When estrogen is prescribed for a postmenopausal woman with a uterus, progestin should also be initiated to reduce the risk of endometrial cancer. A woman without a uterus does not need progestin. Use of estrogen, alone or in combination with a progestin, should be limited to the shortest duration consistent with treatment goals and risks for the individual woman. Patients should be re-evaluated periodically as clinically appropriate (*e.g.,* at 3-6 month intervals) to determine if treatment is still necessary (see BOXED WARNING and WARNINGS). For women who have a uterus, adequate diagnostic measures, such as endometrial sampling, when indicated, should be undertaken to rule out malignancy in cases of undiagnosed persistent or recurring abnormal vaginal bleeding.

For treatment of moderate to severe vasomotor symptoms and/or moderate to severe symptoms of vulvar and vaginal atrophy associated with the menopause:

Patients should be started at the lowest dose.

Conjugated estrogens therapy may be given continuously with no interruption in therapy, or in cyclical regimens (regimens such as 25 days on drug followed by 5 days off drug) as is medically appropriate on an individualized basis.

For prevention of postmenopausal osteoporosis.

0.625 mg daily.

Conjugated estrogens therapy may be given continuously with no interruption in therapy, or in cyclical regimens (regimens such as 25 days on drug followed by 5 days off drug) as is medically appropriate on an individualized basis. When using conjugated estrogens solely for the prevention of postmenopausal osteoporosis, alternative non-estrogen treatments should be carefully considered.

For treatment of female hypoestrogenism due to hypogonadism, castration, or primary ovarian failure:

Female hypogonadism — 0.3-0.625 mg daily, administered cyclically (*e.g.,* 3 weeks on and 1 week off). Doses are adjusted depending on the severity of symptoms and responsiveness of the endometrium.

In clinical studies of delayed puberty due to female hypogonadism, breast development was induced by doses as low as 0.15 mg. The dosage may be gradually titrated upward at 6-12 month intervals as needed to achieve appropriate bone age advancement and eventual epiphyseal closure. Clinical studies suggest that doses of 0.15 mg, 0.3 mg, and 0.6 mg are associated with mean ratios of bone age advancement to chronological age progression ($\Delta BA/\Delta CA$) of 1.1, 1.5, and 2.1, respectively. (Conjugated estrogens in the dose strength of 0.15 mg is not available commercially). Available data suggest that chronic dosing with 0.625 mg is sufficient to induce artificial cyclic menses with sequential progestin treatment and to maintain bone mineral density after skeletal maturity is achieved.

Female castration or primary ovarian failure — 1.25 mg daily, cyclically. Adjust dosage, upward or downward, according to severity of symptoms and response of the patient. For maintenance, adjust dosage to lowest level that will provide effective control.

For treatment of breast cancer, for palliation only, in appropriately selected women and men with metastatic disease:

Suggested dosage is 10 mg three times daily for a period of at least 3 months.

For treatment of advanced androgen-dependent carcinoma of the prostate, for palliation only:

1.25-2.5 mg three times daily. The effectiveness of therapy can be judged by phosphatase determinations as well as by symptomatic improvement of the patient.

HOW SUPPLIED

PREMARIN:

2.5 mg: Each oval purple tablet contains 2.5 mg of conjugated estrogens.

1.25 mg: Each oval yellow tablet contains 1.25 mg of conjugated estrogens.

0.9 mg: Each oval white tablet contains 0.9 mg of conjugated estrogens.

0.625 mg: Each oval maroon tablet contains 0.625 mg of conjugated estrogens.

0.3 mg: Each oval green tablet contains 0.3 mg of conjugated estrogens.

Storage: Store at room temperature (approximately 25°C). Dispense in a well-closed container.

VAGINAL

WARNING

ESTROGENS HAVE BEEN REPORTED TO INCREASE THE RISK OF ENDOMETRIAL CARCINOMA. Three independent, case-controlled studies have reported an increased risk of endometrial cancer in postmenopausal women exposed to exogenous estrogens for more than 1 year.[1-3] This risk was independent of the other known risk factors for endometrial cancer. These studies are further supported by the finding that incidence rates of endometrial cancer have increased sharply since 1969 in 8 different areas of the US with population-based cancer-reporting systems, an increase which may be related to the rapidly expanding use of estrogens during the last decade.[4] The 3 case-controlled studies reported that the risk of endometrial cancer in estrogen users was about 4.5-13.9 times greater than in non-users. The risk appears to depend on both duration of treatment[1] and on estrogen dose.[3] In view of these findings, when estrogens are used for the treatment of menopausal symptoms, the lowest dose that will control symptoms should be utilized and medication should be discontinued as soon as possible. When prolonged treatment is medically indicated, the patient should be reassessed, on at least a semiannual basis, to determine the need for continued therapy. Although the evidence must be considered preliminary, one study suggests that cyclic administration of low doses of estrogen may carry less risk than continuous administration.[3] It therefore appears prudent to utilize such a regimen. Close clinical surveillance of all women taking estrogens is important. In all cases of undiagnosed persistent or recurring abnormal vaginal bleeding, adequate diagnostic measures should be undertaken to rule out malignancy.

There is no evidence at present that "natural" estrogens are more or less hazardous than "synthetic" estrogens at equiestrogenic doses.

ESTROGENS SHOULD NOT BE USED DURING PREGNANCY. The use of female sex hormones, both estrogens and progestogens, during early pregnancy may seriously damage the offspring. It has been shown that females exposed *in utero* to diethylstilbestrol, a nonsteroidal estrogen, have an increased risk of developing, in later life, a form of vaginal or cervical cancer that is ordinarily extremely rare.[5,6] This risk has been estimated as not greater than 4/1000 exposures.[7] Furthermore, a high percentage of such exposed women (from 30-90%) have been found to have vaginal adenosis,[8-12] epithelial changes of the vagina and cervix. Although these changes are histologically benign, it is not known whether they are precursors of malignancy. Although similar data are not available with the use of other estrogens, it cannot be presumed they would not induce similar changes. Several reports suggest an association between intrauterine exposure to female sex hormones and congenital anomalies, including congenital heart defects and limb-reduction defects.[13-16] One case-controlled study[16] estimated a 4.7-fold increased risk of limb-reduction defects in infants exposed *in utero* to sex hormones (oral contraceptives, hormone withdrawal tests for pregnancy, or attempted treatment for threatened abortion). Some of these exposures were very short and involved only a few days of treatment. The data suggest that the risk of limb-reduction defects in exposed fetuses is somewhat less than 1/1000. In the past, female sex hormones have been used during pregnancy in an attempt to treat threatened or habitual abortion. There is considerable evidence that estrogens are ineffective for these indications, and there is no evidence from well-controlled studies that progestogens are effective for these uses.

If conjugated estrogens is used during pregnancy, or if the patient becomes pregnant while taking this drug, she should be apprised of the potential risks to the fetus, and the advisability of pregnancy continuation.

DESCRIPTION

Each gram of Premarin (conjugated estrogens) vaginal cream contains 0.625 mg conjugated estrogens in a nonliquifying base containing cetyl esters wax, cetyl alcohol, white wax, glyceryl monostearate, propylene glycol monostearate, methyl stearate, benzyl alcohol, sodium lauryl sulfate, glycerin, and mineral oil. Conjugated estrogens vaginal cream is applied intravaginally. Premarin is a mixture of estrogens obtained exclusively from natural sources, occurring as the sodium salts of water-soluble estrogen sulfates blended to represent the average composition of material derived from pregnant mares' urine. It contains estrone, equilin, and 17 α-dihydroequilin, together with smaller amounts of 17 α-estradiol, equilenin, and 17 α-dihydroequilenin as salts of their sulfate esters.

CLINICAL PHARMACOLOGY

Estrogens are important in the development and maintenance of the female reproductive system and secondary sex characteristics. They promote growth and development of the vagina, uterus, and fallopian tubes, and enlargement of the breasts. Indirectly, they contribute to the shaping of the skeleton, maintenance of tone and elasticity of urogenital structures, changes in the epiphyses of the long bones that allow for the pubertal growth spurt and its termination, growth of axillary and pubic hair, and pigmentation of the nipples and genitals. Decline of estrogenic activity at the end of the menstrual cycle can bring on menstruation, although the cessation of progesterone secretion is the most important factor in the mature ovulatory cycle. However, in the preovulatory or nonovulatory cycle, estrogen is the primary determinant in the onset of menstruation. Estrogens also affect the release of pituitary gonadotropins.

The pharmacologic effects of conjugated estrogens are similar to those of endogenous estrogens. They are soluble in water and may be absorbed from mucosal surfaces after local administration.

In responsive tissues (female genital organs, breasts, hypothalamus, pituitary) estrogens enter the cell and are transported into the nucleus. As a result of estrogen action, specific RNA and protein synthesis occurs.

Metabolism and inactivation occur primarily in the liver. Some estrogens are excreted into the bile; however, they are reabsorbed from the intestine and returned to the liver through the portal venous system. Water-soluble estrogen conjugates are strongly acidic and, therefore, ionized in body fluids, which favor excretion through the kidneys since tubular reabsorption is minimal.

INDICATIONS AND USAGE

Conjugated estrogens vaginal cream is indicated in the treatment of atrophic vaginitis and kraurosis vulvae.

Conjugated estrogens vaginal cream HAS NOT BEEN SHOWN TO BE EFFECTIVE FOR ANY PURPOSE DURING PREGNANCY AND ITS USE MAY CAUSE SEVERE HARM TO THE FETUS (SEE BOXED WARNING).

NON-FDA APPROVED INDICATIONS

Although not FDA approved, conjugated estrogens vaginal cream has been used for the treatment of atrophic urethritis.

CONTRAINDICATIONS

Estrogens should not be used in women with any of the following conditions:

1. Known or suspected cancer of the breast except in appropriately selected patients being treated for metastatic disease.
2. Known or suspected estrogen-dependent neoplasia.
3. Known or suspected pregnancy (see BOXED WARNING).
4. Undiagnosed abnormal genital bleeding.
5. Active thrombophlebitis or thromboembolic disorders.
6. A past history of thrombophlebitis, thrombosis, or thromboembolic disorders associated with previous estrogen use (except when used in treatment of breast malignancy).

Conjugated estrogens vaginal cream should not be used in patients hypersensitive to its ingredients.

WARNINGS

INDUCTION OF MALIGNANT NEOPLASMS

Long-term, continuous administration of natural and synthetic estrogens in certain animal species increases the frequency of carcinomas of the breast, cervix, vagina, and liver. There are now reports that estrogens increase the risk of carcinoma of the endometrium in humans (see BOXED WARNING).

At the present time there is no satisfactory evidence that estrogens given to postmenopausal women increase the risk of cancer of the breast,[17] although a recent long-term follow-up of a single physician's practice has raised this possibility.[18] Because of the animal data, there is a need for caution in prescribing estrogens for women with a strong family history of breast cancer or who have breast nodules, fibrocystic disease, or abnormal mammograms.

GALLBLADDER DISEASE

A study has reported a 2- to 3-fold increase in the risk of surgically confirmed gallbladder disease in women receiving postmenopausal estrogens,[17] similar to the 2-fold increase previously noted in users of oral contraceptives.[19,24a]

EFFECTS SIMILAR TO THOSE CAUSED BY ESTROGEN-PROGESTOGEN ORAL CONTRACEPTIVES

There are several serious adverse effects of oral contraceptives, some of which have not, up to now, been documented as consequences of postmenopausal estrogen therapy. This may reflect the comparatively low doses of estrogen used in postmenopausal women. It would be expected that the larger doses of estrogen used to treat prostatic or breast cancer are more likely to result in these adverse effects, and, in fact, it has been shown that there is an increased risk of thrombosis in men receiving estrogens for prostatic cancer.[20-23]

Thromboembolic Disease

It is now well established that users of oral contraceptives have an increased risk of various thromboembolic and thrombotic vascular diseases, such as thrombophlebitis, pulmonary embolism, stroke, and myocardial infarction.[24-31] Cases of retinal thrombosis, mesenteric thrombosis, and optic neuritis have been reported in oral contraceptive users. There is evidence that the risk of several of these adverse reactions is related to the dose of the drug.[32,33] An increased risk of postsurgery thromboembolic complications has also been reported in users of oral contraceptives.[34,35] If feasible, estrogen should be discontinued at least 4 weeks before surgery of the type associated with an increased risk of thromboembolism, or during periods of prolonged immobilization.

In some studies, women on estrogen replacement therapy, given alone or in combination with a progestin, have been reported to have an increased risk of thrombophlebitis, and/or thromboembolic disease. The physician should be aware of the possibility of thrombotic disorders (thrombophlebitis, retinal thrombosis, cerebral embolism, and pulmonary embolism) during estrogen replacement therapy and be alert to their earliest manifestations. Should any of these occur or be suspected, estrogen replacement therapy should be discontinued immediately. Patients who have risk factors for thrombotic disorders should be kept under careful observation. Subgroups of women who have underlying risk factors, or who are receiving relatively large doses of estrogens, may have increased risk. Therefore, estrogens should not be used in persons with active thrombophlebitis or thromboembolic disorders, and they should not be used (except in treatment of malignancy) in persons with a history of such disorders in association with estrogen use. They should be used with caution in patients with cerebral vascular or coronary artery disease and only for those in whom estrogens are clearly needed.

Large doses of estrogen (5 mg conjugated estrogens/day), comparable to those used to treat cancer of the prostate and breast, have been shown in a large prospective clinical trial in men[36] to increase the risk of nonfatal myocardial infarction, pulmonary embolism, and thrombophlebitis. When estrogen doses of this size are used, any of the thromboembolic and thrombotic adverse effects associated with oral contraceptives or estrogen replacement therapy should be considered a clear risk.

Hepatic Adenoma

Benign hepatic adenomas appear to be associated with the use of oral contraceptives.[37-39] Although benign, and rare, these may rupture and may cause death through intra-abdominal hemorrhage. Such lesions have not yet been reported in association with other estrogen or progestogen preparations but should be considered in estrogen users having abdominal pain and tenderness, abdominal mass, or hypovolemic shock. Hepatocellular carcinoma has also been reported in women taking estrogen-containing oral contraceptives.[38] The relationship of this malignancy to these drugs is not known at this time.

Elevated Blood Pressure

Women using oral contraceptives sometimes experience increased blood pressure which, in most cases, returns to normal on discontinuing the drug. There is now a report that this may occur with use of estrogens in the menopause[40] and blood pressure should be monitored with estrogen use, especially if high doses are used.

Glucose Tolerance

A worsening of glucose tolerance has been observed in a significant percentage of patients on estrogen-containing oral contraceptives. For this reason, diabetic patients should be carefully observed while receiving estrogen.

HYPERCALCEMIA

Administration of estrogens may lead to severe hypercalcemia in patients with breast cancer and bone metastases. If this occurs, the drug should be stopped and appropriate measures taken to reduce the serum calcium level.

PRECAUTIONS

GENERAL

A complete medical and family history should be taken prior to the initiation of any estrogen therapy. The pretreatment and periodic physical examinations should include special reference to blood pressure, breasts, abdomen, and pelvic organs, and should include a Pap smear. As a general rule, estrogens should not be prescribed for longer than 1 year without another physical examination being performed.

Fluid Retention: Because estrogens may cause some degree of fluid retention, conditions which might be influenced by this factor, such as asthma, epilepsy, migraine, and cardiac or renal dysfunction, require careful observation.

Familial Hyperlipoproteinemia: Estrogen therapy may be associated with massive elevations of plasma triglycerides leading to pancreatitis and other complications in patients with familial defects of lipoprotein metabolism.

Certain patients may develop undesirable manifestations of excessive estrogenic stimulation, such as abnormal or excessive uterine bleeding, mastodynia, etc.

Prolonged administration of unopposed estrogen therapy has been reported to increase the risk of endometrial hyperplasia in some patients.

Oral contraceptives appear to be associated with an increased incidence of mental depression.[24a] Although it is not clear whether this is due to the estrogenic or progestogenic component of the contraceptive, patients with a history of depression should be carefully observed.

Pre-existing uterine leiomyomata may increase in size during estrogen use.

The pathologist should be advised of estrogen therapy when relevant specimens are submitted.

Patients with a past history of jaundice during pregnancy have an increased risk of recurrence of jaundice while receiving estrogen-containing oral-contraceptive therapy. If jaundice develops in any patient receiving estrogen, the medication should be discontinued while the cause is investigated.

Estrogens may be poorly metabolized in patients with impaired liver function and should be administered with caution in such patients.

Because estrogens influence the metabolism of calcium and phosphorus, they should be used with caution in patients with metabolic bone diseases that are associated with hypercalcemia or in patients with renal insufficiency.

Because of the effects of estrogens on epiphyseal closure, they should be used judiciously in young patients in whom bone growth is not yet complete.

Barrier Contraceptives: Conjugated estrogens vaginal cream exposure has been reported to weaken latex condoms. The potential for conjugated estrogens vaginal cream to weaken and contribute to the failure of condoms, diaphragms, or cervical caps made of latex or rubber should be considered.

Concomitant Progestin Use: The lowest effective dose appropriate for the specific indication should be utilized. Studies of the addition of a progestin for 7 or more days of a cycle of estrogen administration have reported a lowered incidence of endometrial hyperplasia. Morphological and biochemical studies of the endometrium suggest that 10-13 days of progestin are needed to provide maximal maturation of the endometrium and to eliminate any hyperplastic changes. Whether this will provide protection from endometrial carcinoma has not been clearly established. There are possible additional risks which may be associated with the inclusion of progestin in estrogen replacement regimens. If concomitant progestin therapy is used, potential risks may include adverse effects on carbohydrate and lipid metabolism. The choice of progestin and dosage may be important in minimizing these adverse effects.

DRUG/LABORATORY TEST INTERACTIONS

Certain endocrine and liver function tests may be affected by estrogen-containing oral contraceptives.

The following similar changes may be expected with larger doses of estrogen:

a. Increased sulfobromophthalein retention.
b. Increased prothrombin and factors VII, VIII, IX, and X; decreased antithrombin III; increased norepinephrine-induced platelet aggregability.

c. Increased thyroid-binding globulin (TBG) leading to increased circulating total thyroid hormone, as measured by PBI, T4 by column, or T4 by radioimmunoassay. Free T3 resin uptake is decreased, reflecting the elevated TBG; free T4 concentration is unaltered.
d. Impaired glucose tolerance.
e. Decreased pregnanediol excretion.
f. Reduced response to metyrapone test.
g. Reduced serum folate concentration.
h. Increased serum triglyceride and phospholipid concentration.

CARCINOGENESIS, MUTAGENESIS, AND IMPAIRMENT OF FERTILITY

See WARNINGS for information on carcinogenesis.

PREGNANCY CATEGORY X

See CONTRAINDICATIONS and BOXED WARNING.

E

NURSING MOTHERS

It is not known whether this drug is excreted in human milk. Because many drugs are excreted in human milk and because of the potential for serious adverse reactions in nursing infants from estrogens, a decision should be made whether to discontinue nursing or to discontinue the drug, taking into account the importance of the drug to the mother.

PEDIATRIC USE

Safety and effectiveness in pediatric patients have not been established.

ADVERSE REACTIONS

See WARNINGS regarding induction of neoplasia, adverse effects on the fetus, increased incidence of gallbladder disease, and adverse effects similar to those of oral contraceptives, including thromboembolism.

The following additional adverse reactions have been reported with estrogenic therapy, including oral contraceptives:

Genitourinary System: Breakthrough bleeding, spotting, change in menstrual flow; dysmenorrhea; premenstrual-like syndrome; amenorrhea during and after treatment; increase in size of uterine fibromyomata; vaginal candidiasis; change in cervical erosion and in degree of cervical secretion; cystitis-like syndrome.

Breasts: Tenderness, enlargement, secretion.

Gastrointestinal: Nausea, vomiting, abdominal cramps, bloating; cholestatic jaundice, pancreatitis.

Skin: Chloasma or melasma which may persist when drug is discontinued; erythema multiforme; erythema nodosum; hemorrhagic eruption; loss of scalp hair; hirsutism.

Cardiovascular: Venous thromboembolism, pulmonary embolism.

Eyes: Steepening of corneal curvature; intolerance to contact lenses.

CNS: Headache, migraine, dizziness; mental depression; chorea.

Miscellaneous: Increase or decrease in weight; reduced carbohydrate tolerance; aggravation of porphyria; edema; changes in libido.

DOSAGE AND ADMINISTRATION

Given cyclically for short-term use only:

- For treatment of atrophic vaginitis, or kraurosis vulvae.
- The lowest dose that will control symptoms should be chosen and medication should be discontinued as promptly as possible.
- Administration should be cyclic (*e.g.,* 3 weeks on and 1 week off).
- Attempts to discontinue or taper medication should be made at 3-6 month intervals.

Usual Dosage Range: ½-2 g daily, intravaginally, depending on the severity of the condition. Treated patients with an intact uterus should be monitored closely for signs of endometrial cancer, and appropriate diagnostic measures should be taken to rule out malignancy in the event of persistent or recurring abnormal vaginal bleeding.

HOW SUPPLIED

Premarin Vaginal Cream: Each gram contains 0.625 mg conjugated estrogens.
Storage: Store at room temperature (approximately 25°C).

PRODUCT LISTING - EQUIVALENTS NOT AVAILABLE

Cream with Applicator - Vaginal - 0.625 mg/Gm

Size	Price	Product	NDC
42 gm	$39.92	PREMARIN VAGINAL, Prescript Pharmaceuticals	00247-0252-85
42 gm	$61.73	PREMARIN VAGINAL, Wyeth-Ayerst Laboratories	00046-0872-01
42 gm	$68.69	PREMARIN VAGINAL, Wyeth-Ayerst Laboratories	00046-0872-93
42.50 gm	$52.89	PREMARIN VAGINAL, Allscripts Pharmaceutical Company	54569-0981-00
43 gm	$51.08	PREMARIN VAGINAL, Physicians Total Care	54868-3391-01
45 gm	$56.84	PREMARIN VAGINAL, Physicians Total Care	54868-0454-00

Powder For Injection - Intravenous - 25 mg

Size	Price	Product	NDC
1's	$58.00	PREMARIN INTRAVENOUS, Wyeth-Ayerst Laboratories	00046-0749-05

Tablet - Oral - Synthetic 0.3 mg

Size	Price	Product	NDC
100's	$68.29	CENESTIN, Duramed Pharmaceuticals Inc	51285-0441-02

Tablet - Oral - Synthetic 0.625 mg

Size	Price	Product	NDC
100's	$86.58	CENESTIN, Duramed Pharmaceuticals Inc	51285-0442-02

Tablet - Oral - Synthetic 0.9 mg

Size	Price	Product	NDC
100's	$104.06	CENESTIN, Duramed Pharmaceuticals Inc	51285-0443-02

Tablet - Oral - Synthetic 1.25 mg

Size	Price	Product	NDC
100's	$120.15	CENESTIN, Duramed Pharmaceuticals Inc	51285-0444-02

Tablet - Oral - 0.3 mg

Size	Price	Product	NDC
10's	$6.13	PREMARIN, Southwood Pharmaceuticals Inc	58016-0744-10
12's	$7.35	PREMARIN, Southwood Pharmaceuticals Inc	58016-0744-12
14's	$8.58	PREMARIN, Southwood Pharmaceuticals Inc	58016-0744-14
15's	$9.19	PREMARIN, Southwood Pharmaceuticals Inc	58016-0744-15
20's	$12.25	PREMARIN, Southwood Pharmaceuticals Inc	58016-0744-20
30's	$16.32	PREMARIN, Physicians Total Care	54868-2702-00
30's	$18.38	PREMARIN, Southwood Pharmaceuticals Inc	58016-0744-30
30's	$18.90	PREMARIN, Pd-Rx Pharmaceuticals	55289-0123-30
75's	$21.23	PREMARIN, Allscripts Pharmaceutical Company	54569-8517-01
90's	$25.48	PREMARIN, Allscripts Pharmaceutical Company	54569-8517-00
100's	$47.48	PREMARIN, Allscripts Pharmaceutical Company	54569-0811-01
100's	$61.25	PREMARIN, Southwood Pharmaceuticals Inc	58016-0744-00
100's	$75.88	PREMARIN, Wyeth-Ayerst Laboratories	00046-0868-81

Tablet - Oral - 0.625 mg

Size	Price	Product	NDC
7's	$8.25	PREMARIN, Pd-Rx Pharmaceuticals	55289-0943-07
10's	$8.19	PREMARIN, Southwood Pharmaceuticals Inc	58016-0948-10
12's	$9.83	PREMARIN, Southwood Pharmaceuticals Inc	58016-0948-12
14's	$11.46	PREMARIN, Southwood Pharmaceuticals Inc	58016-0948-14
15's	$12.28	PREMARIN, Southwood Pharmaceuticals Inc	58016-0948-15
20's	$16.38	PREMARIN, Southwood Pharmaceuticals Inc	58016-0948-20
25's	$19.79	PREMARIN, Physicians Total Care	54868-0451-00
25's	$21.75	PREMARIN, Pd-Rx Pharmaceuticals	55289-0943-25
30's	$19.29	PREMARIN, Allscripts Pharmaceutical Company	54569-0812-05
30's	$23.51	PREMARIN, Physicians Total Care	54868-0451-02
30's	$24.56	PREMARIN, Southwood Pharmaceuticals Inc	58016-0948-30
30's	$25.49	PREMARIN, Prescript Pharmaceuticals	00247-0251-30
30's	$25.50	PREMARIN, Pd-Rx Pharmaceuticals	55289-0943-30
30's	$29.88	PREMARIN, Pharma Pac	52959-0223-30
50's	$32.15	PREMARIN, Allscripts Pharmaceutical Company	54569-0812-02
50's	$38.38	PREMARIN, Physicians Total Care	54868-0451-01
50's	$40.94	PREMARIN, Southwood Pharmaceuticals Inc	58016-0948-50
60's	$23.67	PREMARIN, Allscripts Pharmaceutical Company	54569-8500-02
60's	$31.68	PREMARIN, Pharmaceutical Corporation Of America	51655-0452-25
60's	$47.62	PREMARIN, Prescript Pharmaceuticals	00247-0251-60
75's	$29.59	PREMARIN, Allscripts Pharmaceutical Company	54569-8006-00
75's	$29.59	PREMARIN, Allscripts Pharmaceutical Company	54569-8500-01
75's	$48.22	PREMARIN, Allscripts Pharmaceutical Company	54569-0812-01
90's	$35.51	PREMARIN, Allscripts Pharmaceutical Company	54569-8006-02
90's	$35.51	PREMARIN, Allscripts Pharmaceutical Company	54569-8500-00
90's	$69.76	PREMARIN, Prescript Pharmaceuticals	00247-0251-90
100's	$39.45	PREMARIN, Allscripts Pharmaceutical Company	54569-8006-01
100's	$55.76	PREMARIN, Pharma Pac	52959-0223-00
100's	$64.29	PREMARIN, Allscripts Pharmaceutical Company	54569-0812-00
100's	$70.83	PREMARIN, Physicians Total Care	54868-0451-03
100's	$77.14	PREMARIN, Prescript Pharmaceuticals	00247-0251-00
100's	$81.88	PREMARIN, Southwood Pharmaceuticals Inc	58016-0948-00
100's	$96.19	PREMARIN, Wyeth-Ayerst Laboratories	00046-0867-81
100's	$96.19	PREMARIN, Wyeth-Ayerst Laboratories	00046-0867-99
100's	$96.19	PREMARIN, Wyeth-Ayerst Laboratories	00046-3867-81

Tablet - Oral - 0.9 mg

Size	Price	Product	NDC
30's	$23.21	PREMARIN, Prescript Pharmaceuticals	00247-0249-30
30's	$23.27	PREMARIN, Allscripts Pharmaceutical Company	54569-0849-01
75's	$35.05	PREMARIN, Allscripts Pharmaceutical Company	54569-8518-01
90's	$42.06	PREMARIN, Allscripts Pharmaceutical Company	54569-8518-00
100's	$69.53	PREMARIN, Prescript Pharmaceuticals	00247-0249-00
100's	$77.58	PREMARIN, Allscripts Pharmaceutical Company	54569-0849-00
100's	$90.93	PREMARIN, Physicians Total Care	54868-0365-00
100's	$115.63	PREMARIN, Wyeth-Ayerst Laboratories	00046-0864-81

Tablet - Oral - 1.25 mg

Size	Price	Product	NDC
10's	$11.36	PREMARIN, Southwood Pharmaceuticals Inc	58016-0983-10
12's	$13.64	PREMARIN, Southwood Pharmaceuticals Inc	58016-0983-12

14's	$15.91	PREMARIN, Southwood Pharmaceuticals Inc	58016-0983-14
15's	$17.04	PREMARIN, Southwood Pharmaceuticals Inc	58016-0983-15
20's	$22.73	PREMARIN, Southwood Pharmaceuticals Inc	58016-0983-20
25's	$25.00	PREMARIN, Physicians Total Care	54868-0453-00
25's	$26.25	PREMARIN, Pd-Rx Pharmaceuticals	55289-0047-25
28's	$32.15	PREMARIN, Prescript Pharmaceuticals	00247-0250-28
30's	$26.89	PREMARIN, Allscripts Pharmaceutical Company	54569-0813-01
30's	$29.77	PREMARIN, Physicians Total Care	54868-0453-02
30's	$32.42	PREMARIN, Pd-Rx Pharmaceuticals	55289-0047-30
30's	$34.09	PREMARIN, Southwood Pharmaceuticals Inc	58016-0983-30
30's	$34.21	PREMARIN, Prescript Pharmaceuticals	00247-0250-30
42's	$45.38	PREMARIN, Pd-Rx Pharmaceuticals	55289-0047-42
60's	$32.39	PREMARIN, Allscripts Pharmaceutical Company	54569-8505-02
75's	$40.49	PREMARIN, Allscripts Pharmaceutical Company	54569-8505-01
90's	$48.59	PREMARIN, Allscripts Pharmaceutical Company	54569-8014-00
90's	$48.59	PREMARIN, Allscripts Pharmaceutical Company	54569-8505-00
90's	$73.21	PREMARIN, Physicians Total Care	54868-0453-01
90's	$83.37	PREMARIN, Pd-Rx Pharmaceuticals	55289-0047-90
90's	$86.95	PREMARIN, Physicians Total Care	54868-0453-05
100's	$88.90	PREMARIN, Pharma Pac	52959-0222-00
100's	$89.63	PREMARIN, Allscripts Pharmaceutical Company	54569-0813-00
100's	$96.48	PREMARIN, Physicians Total Care	54868-0453-04
100's	$106.22	PREMARIN, Prescript Pharmaceuticals	00247-0250-00
100's	$113.63	PREMARIN, Southwood Pharmaceuticals Inc	58016-0983-00
100's	$133.50	PREMARIN, Wyeth-Ayerst Laboratories	00046-0866-81
100's	$133.50	PREMARIN, Wyeth-Ayerst Laboratories	00046-0866-99
Tablet - Oral - 2.5 mg			
100's	$158.76	PREMARIN, Physicians Total Care	54868-0452-03
100's	$179.83	PREMARIN, Wyeth-Ayerst Laboratories	00046-0865-81

Estrogens, Conjugated; Medroxyprogesterone Acetate *(003239)*

Categories: Atrophy, vaginal; Atrophy, vulvar; Menopause; Osteoporosis, prevention; Pregnancy Category X; FDA Approved 1994 Dec

Drug Classes: Estrogens; Hormones/hormone modifiers; Progestins

Brand Names: Premarin MPA; Premphase; **Prempro**

Foreign Brand Availability: Climarest plus (Germany); Climatrol (Peru); Climatrol HT (Colombia); Climatrol HT Continuo (Colombia); Climatrol HT Continuo Plus (Colombia); Climatrol HT Plus (Colombia); Climopax (Germany); Menoprem Continuous (Australia); Plentiva (Korea; Taiwan); Plentiva Cycle (Korea; Taiwan); Premaril Plus (Israel); Premarin Pak (Mexico); Premelle (Colombia; Hong-Kong; Korea; Peru; Philippines; Singapore; South-Africa; Taiwan; Thailand); Premelle Cycle 5 (Singapore; Thailand); Prempak (Argentina; Bolivia; Brazil; Canada; Chile; CIS; Colombia; Costa-Rica; Dominican-Republic; Ecuador; El-Salvador; Guatemala; Honduras; Hong-Kong; Mexico; Nicaragua; Panama; Paraguay; Peru; Philippines; Thailand; Uruguay; Venezuela)

Cost of Therapy: $20.93 (Menopause; Prempro; 0.625 mg; 2.5 mg; 1 tablet/day; 28 day supply)

DESCRIPTION

Note: The trade names have been used throughout this monograph for clarity.

Prempro therapy consists of a single tablet containing 0.625 mg of the conjugated estrogens found in Premarin tablets and 2.5 or 5 mg of medroxyprogesterone acetate (MPA) for oral administration.

Premphase therapy consists of 2 separate tablets, a maroon Premarin tablet containing 0.625 mg of conjugated estrogens that is taken orally on days 1-14 and a light-blue tablet containing 0.625 mg of the conjugated estrogens found in Premarin tablets and 5 mg of medroxyprogesterone acetate (MPA) that is taken orally on days 15-28.

The conjugated equine estrogens found in Premarin tablets are a mixture of sodium estrone sulfate and sodium equilin sulfate. They contain as concomitant components, as sodium sulfate conjugates, 17α-dihydroequilin, 17α-estradiol and 17β-dihydroequilin.

Medroxyprogesterone acetate (MPA) is a derivative of progesterone. It is a white to off-white, odorless, crystalline powder, stable in air, melting between 200 and 210°C. It is freely soluble in chloroform, soluble in acetone and in dioxane, sparingly soluble in alcohol and in methanol, slightly soluble in ether, and insoluble in water. The chemical name for MPA is pregn-4-ene-3,20-dione, 17-(acetyloxy)-6-methyl-,(6α)-. Its molecular formula is $C_{24}H_{34}O_4$, with a molecular weight of 386.53.

PREMPRO

2.5 mg

Each peach tablet for oral administration contains 0.625 mg conjugated estrogens, 2.5 mg of medroxyprogesterone acetate and the following inactive ingredients: calcium phosphate tribasic, calcium sulfate, carnauba wax, cellulose, glyceryl monooleate, lactose, magnesium stearate, methylcellulose, pharmaceutical glaze, polyethylene glycol, sucrose, povidone, titanium dioxide, red ferric oxide.

5 mg

Each light-blue tablet for oral administration contains 0.625 mg conjugated estrogens, 5 mg of medroxyprogesterone acetate and the following inactive ingredients: calcium phosphate tribasic, calcium sulfate, carnauba wax, cellulose, glyceryl monooleate, lactose, magnesium stearate, methylcellulose, pharmaceutical glaze, polyethylene glycol, sucrose, povidone, titanium dioxide, FD&C blue no. 2.

PREMPHASE

Each maroon Premarin tablet for oral administration contains 0.625 mg of conjugated estrogens and the following inactive ingredients: calcium phosphate tribasic, calcium sulfate, carnauba wax, cellulose, glyceryl monooleate, lactose, magnesium stearate, methylcellulose, pharmaceutical glaze, polyethylene glycol, stearic acid, sucrose, titanium dioxide, FD&C blue no. 2, D&C red no. 27, FD&C red no. 40. These tablets comply with USP Drug Release Test 1.

Each light-blue tablet for oral administration contains 0.625 mg of conjugated estrogens and 5 mg of medroxyprogesterone acetate and the following inactive ingredients: calcium phosphate tribasic, calcium sulfate, carnauba wax, cellulose, glyceryl monooleate, lactose, magnesium stearate, methylcellulose, pharmaceutical glaze, polyethylene glycol, sucrose, povidone, titanium dioxide, FD&C blue no. 2.

E

CLINICAL PHARMACOLOGY

Endogenous estrogens are largely responsible for the development and maintenance of the female reproductive system and secondary sexual characteristics.

Although circulating estrogens exist in a dynamic equilibrium of metabolic interconversions, estradiol is the principal intracellular human estrogen and is substantially more potent than its metabolites, estrone and estriol at the receptor level. The primary source of estrogen in normally cycling adult women is the ovarian follicle, which secretes 70-500 μg of estradiol daily, depending on the phase of the menstrual cycle. After menopause, most endogenous estrogen is produced by conversion of androstenedione, secreted by the adrenal cortex, to estrone by peripheral tissues. Thus, estrone and the sulfate-conjugated form, estrone sulfate, are the most abundant circulating estrogens in postmenopausal women.

Estrogens act through binding to nuclear receptors in estrogen-responsive tissues. To date, two estrogen receptors have been identified. These vary in proportion from tissue to tissue.

Circulating estrogens modulate the pituitary secretion of gonadotropins, luteinizing hormone (LH) and follicle stimulating hormone (FSH) through a negative feedback mechanism. Postmenopausal estrogen therapy acts to reduce the elevated levels of these gonadotropins seen in postmenopausal women.

Parenterally administered medroxyprogesterone acetate (MPA) inhibits gonadotropin production, which in turn prevents follicular maturation and ovulation, although available data indicate that this does not occur when the usually recommended oral dosage is given as single daily doses. MPA may achieve its beneficial effect on the endometrium in part by decreasing nuclear estrogen receptors and suppression of epithelial DNA synthesis in endometrial tissue. Androgenic and anabolic effects of MPA have been noted, but the drug is apparently devoid of significant estrogenic activity.

PHARMACOKINETICS

Absorption

Conjugated estrogens are soluble in water and are well absorbed from the gastrointestinal tract after release from the drug formulation. However, Prempro and Premphase contain a formulation of medroxyprogesterone acetate (MPA) that is immediately released and conjugated estrogens that are slowly released over several hours. MPA is well absorbed from the gastrointestinal tract. TABLE 1A and TABLE 1B summarize the mean pharmacokinetic parameters for unconjugated and conjugated estrogens, and medroxyprogesterone acetate following administration of 0.625 mg/2.5 mg and 0.625 mg/5 mg tablets to healthy postmenopausal women.

Food-Effect

Single dose studies in healthy, postmenopausal women were conducted to investigate any potential drug interaction when Prempro or Premphase is administered with a high fat breakfast. Administration with food decreased the C_{max} of total estrone by 18-34% and increased total equilin C_{max} by 38% compared to the fasting state, with no other effect on the rate or extent of absorption of other conjugated or unconjugated estrogens. Administration with food approximately doubles MPA C_{max} and increases MPA AUC by approximately 20-30%.

Dose Proportionality

The C_{max} and AUC values for MPA observed in two separate pharmacokinetic studies conducted with Prempro or Premphase 2 × 0.625 mg/2.5 mg and 2 × 0.625 mg/5 mg tablets exhibited nonlinear dose proportionality; doubling the MPA dose from 2 × 2.5 to 2 × 5.0 mg increased the mean C_{max} and AUC by 3.2 and 2.8 folds, respectively. The apparent clearance (Cl/F) of MPA obtained with 2 × 0.625 mg/5 mg tablets was lower than that observed with 2 × 0.625 mg/2.5 mg tablets.

Distribution

The distribution of exogenous estrogens is similar to that of endogenous estrogens. Estrogens are widely distributed in the body and are generally found in higher concentrations in the sex hormone target organs. Estrogens circulate in the blood largely bound to sex hormone binding globulin (SHBG) and albumin. MPA is approximately 90% bound to plasma proteins but does not bind to SHBG.

Metabolism

Exogenous estrogens are metabolized in the same manner as endogenous estrogens. Circulating estrogens exist in a dynamic equilibrium of metabolic interconversions. These transformations take place mainly in the liver. Estradiol is converted reversibly to estrone, and both can be converted to estriol, which is the major urinary metabolite. Estrogens also undergo enterohepatic recirculation via sulfate and glucuronide conjugation in the liver, biliary secretion of conjugates into the intestine, and hydrolysis in the gut followed by resorption. In postmenopausal women a significant proportion of the circulating estrogens exists as sulfate conjugates, especially estrone sulfate, which serves as a circulating reservoir for the formation of more active estrogens. Metabolism and elimination of MPA occurs primarily in the liver via hydroxylation, with subsequent conjugation and elimination in the urine.

TABLE 1A *Pharmacokinetic Parameters For Unconjugated and Conjugated Estrogen (CE)*

PK Parameter/Geometric Mean (SD)	C_{max}	T_{max}	T½	AUC
2 × 0.625 mg CE/2.5 mg MPA Combination Tablets (n=54)				
Unconjugated Estrogens				
Estrone	175 (41)*	7.6 h (1.8)	31.6 h (7.4)	5358 (1840)†
BA—Estrone	159 (41)*	7.6 h (1.8)	16.9 h (5.8)	3313 (1310)†
Equilin	71 (22)*	5.8 h (2.0)	9.9 h (3.5)	951 (413)†
Conjugated Estrogens				
Total estrone	6.6 (2.5)‡	6.1 h (1.7)	20.7 h (7.0)	116 (68)§
BA—Total estrone	6.4 (2.5)‡	6.1 h (1.7)	15.4 h (5.2)	100 (57)§
Total equilin	5.1 (2.3)‡	4.6 h (1.6)	11.4 h (2.9)	50 (35)§
2 × 0.625 mg CE/5 mg MPA Combination Tablets (n=51)				
Unconjugated Estrogens				
Estrone	124 (53)*	10 h (3.5)	62.2 h (85.2)	6303 (2542)†
BA—Estrone	104 (51)*	10 h (3.5)	26.0 h (25.9)	3136 (1598)†
Equilin	54 (23)*	8.9 h (3.0)	15.5 h (8.2)	1179 (540)†
Conjugated Estrogens				
Total estrone	6.3 (3.0)‡	9.1 h (2.6)	23.6 h (8.4)	151 (63)§
BA—Total estrone	6.2 (3.0)‡	9.1 h (2.6)	20.6 h (7.3)	139 (56)§
Total equilin	4.2 (2.2)‡	7.0 h (2.5)	17.2 h (22.6)	72 (36)§

* C_{max} measured in pg/ml.
† AUC measured in pg·h/ml.
‡ C_{max} measured in ng/ml.
§ AUC measured in ng·h/ml.
BA = baseline adjusted, C_{max} = peak plasma concentration, T_{max} = time peak concentration occurs, T½ = terminal-phase disposition half-life (0.693/λz), AUC = total area under the curve.

TABLE 1B *Pharmacokinetic Parameters For Medroxyprogesterone Acetate (MPA)*

PK Parameter Geometric Mean (SD)	C_{max} (ng/ml)	T_{max} (h)	T½ (h)	CL/F (L/h/kg)
2 × 0.625 mg CE/2.5 mg MPA Combination Tablets (n=54)				
MPA	1.5 (0.6)	2.8 (1.5)	37.6 (11.2)	2.3 (0.7)
2 × 0.625 mg CE/5 mg MPA Combination Tablets (n=51)				
MPA	4.8 (1.5)	2.4 (1.2)	46.3 (18.0)	1.6 (0.5)

CL/F = apparent oral clearance.

Excretion

Estradiol, estrone, and estriol are excreted in the urine along with glucuronide and sulfate conjugates. Most metabolites of MPA are excreted as glucuronide conjugates with only minor amounts excreted as sulfates.

Special Populations

No pharmacokinetic studies were conducted in special populations, including patients with renal or hepatic impairment.

Drug Interactions

Data from a single-dose drug-drug interaction study involving conjugated estrogens and medroxyprogesterone acetate indicate that the pharmacokinetic disposition of both drugs is not altered when the drugs are coadministered. No other clinical drug-drug interaction studies have been conducted with conjugated estrogens.

In vitro and *in vivo* studies have shown that estrogens are metabolized partially by cytochrome P450 3A4 (CYP3A4). Therefore, inducers or inhibitors of CYP3A4 may affect estrogen drug metabolism. Inducers of CYP3A4 such as St. John's Wort preparations (Hypericum perforatum), phenobarbital, carbamazepine, and rifampicin may reduce plasma concentrations of estrogens, possibly resulting in a decrease in therapeutic effects and/or changes in the uterine bleeding profile. Inhibitors of CYP3A4 such as erythromycin, clarithromycin, ketoconazole, itraconazole, ritonavir and grapefruit juice may increase plasma concentrations of estrogens and may result in side effects.

INDICATIONS AND USAGE

Prempro or Premphase therapy is indicated in women with an intact uterus for the:

Treatment of moderate to severe vasomotor symptoms associated with the menopause.
Treatment of vulvar and vaginal atrophy.
Prevention of postmenopausal osteoporosis.

Prempro and Premphase are not indicated and should not be used to prevent coronary heart disease (see WARNINGS).

Because of the potential increased risks of cardiovascular events, breast cancer and venous thromboembolic events, use of Prempro or Premphase should be limited to the shortest duration consistent with treatment goals and risks for the individual woman, and should be periodically reevaluated. When used solely for the prevention of postmenopausal osteoporosis, alternative treatments should be carefully considered. (See WARNINGS.)

Postmenopausal estrogen therapy reduces bone resorption and retards postmenopausal bone loss. Case-control studies have shown an approximately 60% reduction in hip and wrist fractures in women whose estrogen therapy was begun within a few years of menopause. Studies also suggest that estrogen reduces the rate of vertebral fractures. Even when started as late as 6 years after menopause, estrogen may prevent further loss of bone mass for as long as the treatment is continued. When estrogen therapy is discontinued, bone mass declines at a rate comparable to that of the immediate postmenopausal period.

The mainstays of prevention of postmenopausal osteoporosis are weight-bearing exercise, adequate calcium and vitamin D intake, and when indicated, pharmacologic therapy. Postmenopausal women absorb dietary calcium less efficiently than premenopausal women and require an average of 1500 mg/day of elemental calcium to remain in neutral calcium balance. The average calcium intake in the USA is 400-600 mg/day. Therefore, when not contraindicated, calcium supplementation may be helpful for women with suboptimal dietary intake. Vitamin D supplementation of 400-800 IU/day may also be required to ensure adequate daily intake in postmenopausal women.

Early menopause is one of the strongest predictors for the development of osteoporosis. In addition, other factors affecting the skeleton that are associated with osteoporosis include genetic factors (small build, family history), endocrine factors (nulliparity, thyrotoxicosis, hyperparathyroidism, Cushing's syndrome, hyperprolactinemia, type I diabetes), lifestyle (cigarette smoking, alcohol abuse, sedentary exercise habits) and nutrition (below average body weight, dietary calcium intake).

CONTRAINDICATIONS

Estrogens/progestins combined should not be used in women under any of the following conditions or circumstances:

Known or suspected pregnancy. Estrogen or progestin may cause fetal harm when administered to a pregnant woman. (See PRECAUTIONS.)
Undiagnosed abnormal genital bleeding.
Known or suspected cancer of the breast.
Known or suspected estrogen-dependent neoplasia.
Active deep vein thrombosis/pulmonary embolism or a history of these conditions.
Active or recent arterial thromboembolic disease (*e.g.*, stroke, myocardial infarction).
Liver dysfunction or disease.
Prempro or Premphase therapy should not be used in patients hypersensitive to the ingredients contained in the tablets.

WARNINGS

In a subset of the Women's Health Initiative study, Prempro was reported to increase the risks of cardiovascular events, breast cancer and venous thromboembolic events. Therefore, the use of postmenopausal estrogen/progestin therapy, including Prempro and Premphase, should be limited to the shortest duration consistent with treatment goals and risks for the individual woman, and should be periodically reevaluated. When used solely for the prevention of postmenopausal osteoporosis, alternative treatments should be carefully considered.

CARDIOVASCULAR DISORDERS

Postmenopausal estrogen/progestin therapy has been associated with an increased risk of cardiovascular events such as myocardial infarction and stroke, as well as venous thrombosis and pulmonary embolism (venous thromboembolism or VTE).

Should any of these occur or be suspected, estrogen/progestin therapy should be discontinued immediately. Patients who have risk factors for thrombotic disorders should be kept under careful observation.

Coronary Heart Disease and Stroke

In the Prempro subset of the Women's Health Initiative study (WHI), an increased risk of coronary heart disease (CHD) events (defined as non-fatal myocardial infarction and CHD death) was observed in women receiving Prempro compared to women receiving placebo (37 vs 30 per 10,000 person-years). The increase in risk was observed in Year 1 and persisted.

In the same subset of WHI, an increased risk of stroke was observed in women receiving Prempro compared to women receiving placebo (29 vs 21 per 10,000 person-years). The increase in risk was observed after the first year and persisted.

In postmenopausal women with documented heart disease (n=2763, average age 66.7 years) a controlled clinical trial of secondary prevention of cardiovascular disease (Heart and Estrogen/Progestin Replacement Study; HERS) treatment with Prempro (0.625 mg conjugated equine estrogens plus 2.5 mg medroxyprogesterone acetate per day) demonstrated no cardiovascular benefit. During an average follow-up of 4.1 years, treatment with Prempro did not reduce the overall rate of CHD events in postmenopausal women with established coronary heart disease. There were more CHD events in the Prempro-treated group than in the placebo group in Year 1, but not during the subsequent years. Two thousand three hundred and twenty one (2321) women from the original HERS trial agreed to participate in an open label extension of HERS, HERS II. Average follow-up in HERS II was an additional 2.7 years, for a total of 6.8 years overall. Rates of CHD events were comparable among women in the Prempro group and the placebo group in HERS, HERS II, and overall.

Large doses of estrogen (5 mg conjugated estrogens per day), comparable to those used to treat cancer of the prostate and breast, have been shown in a large prospective clinical trial in men to increase the risk of nonfatal myocardial infarction, pulmonary embolism, and thrombophlebitis.

Venous Thromboembolism (VTE)

In the Prempro subset of WHI a 2-fold greater rate of VTE, including deep venous thrombosis and pulmonary embolism, was observed in women receiving Prempro compared to women receiving placebo. The rate of VTE was 34/10,000 woman-years in the Prempro group compared to 16/10,000 woman-years in the placebo group. The increase in VTE risk was observed during the first year and persisted.

If feasible, estrogens should be discontinued at least 4-6 weeks before surgery of the type associated with an increased risk of thromboembolism, or during periods of prolonged immobilization.

MALIGNANT NEOPLASMS

Breast Cancer

Long-term postmenopausal estrogen/progestin therapy has been associated with an increased risk of breast cancer.

In the Prempro subset of the Women's Health Initiative study, a 26% increase of invasive breast cancer (38 vs 30 per 10,000 woman-years) after an average of 5.2 years of treatment was observed in women receiving Prempro compared to women receiving placebo. The increased risk of breast cancer became apparent after 4 years on Prempro. The women reporting prior postmenopausal hormone use had a higher relative risk for breast cancer associated with Prempro than those who had never used postmenopausal hormones.

A reanalysis of original data from 51 epidemiological studies (not necessarily including Prempro or Premphase) reported an increase in the probability of having breast cancer diagnosed in women currently or recently using postmenopausal hormone (estrogen and/or estrogen/progestin) therapy. The authors estimate that among 1000 women who begin hormone therapy at age 50 and continue for 5, 10, or 15 years, the additional number of cases of breast cancer that would occur by age 70 would be 2 cases, 6 cases and 12 cases, respectively. The probability of a diagnosis of breast cancer approached normal by 5 years after stopping postmenopausal hormone therapy. Additional epidemiological studies suggest that the addition of progestins increases the risk of breast cancer compared to the use of estrogens alone.

Women without a uterus who require postmenopausal hormone therapy should receive estrogen-alone therapy and should not be exposed unnecessarily to progestins. Women with a uterus who are candidates for use of postmenopausal estrogen/progestin therapy should be advised of potential benefits and risks (including the potential for an increased risk of breast cancer). All women should receive yearly breast exams by a healthcare provider and perform monthly breast self-examinations. In addition, mammography examinations should be scheduled as suggested by providers based on patient age and risk factors.

Endometrial Cancer

The reported endometrial cancer risk among users of unopposed estrogen was about 2- to 12-fold greater than in nonusers and appears dependent on duration of treatment and on estrogen dose. Most studies show no significant increased risk associated with the use of estrogens for less than 1 year. The greatest risk appears associated with prolonged use, with increased risks of 15- to 24-fold for 5 years or more, and this risk has been shown to persist for at least 8-15 years after estrogen therapy is discontinued.

Clinical surveillance of all women taking estrogen/progestin combinations is important. Adequate diagnostic measures, including endometrial sampling when indicated, should be undertaken to rule out malignancy in all cases of undiagnosed persistent or recurring abnormal vaginal bleeding. There is no evidence that the use of natural estrogens results in a different endometrial risk profile than synthetic estrogens of equivalent estrogen dose.

Endometrial hyperplasia (a possible precursor of endometrial cancer) has been reported in a large clinical trial to occur at a rate of approximately 1% or less with Prempro or Premphase. In this large clinical trial, only a single case of endometrial cancer was reported to occur among women taking combination Premarin/medroxyprogesterone acetate therapy.

Ovarian Cancer

The association between postmenopausal estrogen therapy and ovarian cancer was evaluated in several case-control and cohort studies. Two large cohort studies suggested an increased risk of ovarian cancer associated with long-term postmenopausal estrogen-only therapy, particularly for 10 or more years of use. In one of these studies, the baseline incidence among untreated postmenopausal women was reported to be 4.4 cases per 10,000 woman-years, compared to 6.5 cases per 10,000 woman-years among women using postmenopausal estrogen therapy. Other epidemiologic studies of postmenopausal estrogen therapy and ovarian cancer did not show a significant association. Data are insufficient to determine whether there is an increased risk with postmenopausal estrogen/progestin therapy.

GALLBLADDER DISEASE

A 2- to 4-fold increase in the risk of gallbladder disease requiring surgery in postmenopausal women receiving estrogens has been reported.

HYPERCALCEMIA

Estrogen administration may lead to severe hypercalcemia in patients with breast cancer and bone metastases. If hypercalcemia occurs, use of the drug should be stopped and appropriate measures taken to reduce the serum calcium level.

VISUAL ABNORMALITIES

Retinal vascular thrombosis has been reported in patients receiving estrogens. Discontinue medication pending examination if there is sudden partial or complete loss of vision, or a sudden onset of proptosis, diplopia, or migraine. If examination reveals papilledema or retinal vascular lesions, Prempro or Premphase should be discontinued.

PRECAUTIONS

GENERAL

Addition of a Progestin When a Woman Has Not Had a Hysterectomy

Studies of the addition of a progestin for 10 or more days of a cycle of estrogen administration, or daily with estrogen in a continuous regimen, have reported a lowered incidence of endometrial hyperplasia than would be induced by estrogen treatment alone. Endometrial hyperplasia may be a precursor to endometrial cancer.

There are, however, possible risks that may be associated with the use of progestins in postmenopausal hormone therapy regimens compared to estrogen-alone regimens. These include an increased risk of breast cancer (see WARNINGS, Malignant Neoplasms), adverse effects on lipoprotein metabolism (*e.g.*, lowering HDL, raising LDL) and impairment of glucose tolerance.

Elevated Blood Pressure

In a small number of case reports, substantial increases in blood pressure during postmenopausal estrogen therapy have been attributed to idiosyncratic reactions to estrogens. In a large, randomized, placebo-controlled clinical trial, a generalized effect of estrogen therapy on blood pressure was not seen. Blood pressure should be monitored at regular intervals with estrogen use.

Familial Hyperlipoproteinemia

In patients with familial defects of lipoprotein metabolism, estrogen therapy may be associated with elevations of plasma triglycerides leading to pancreatitis and other complications.

Impaired Liver Function and Past History of Cholestatic Jaundice

Estrogens may be poorly metabolized in patients with impaired liver function. For patients with a history of cholestatic jaundice associated with past estrogen use or with pregnancy, caution should be exercised and in the case of recurrence, medication should be discontinued.

Hypothyroidism

Estrogen administration leads to increased thyroid-binding globulin (TBG) levels. Patients with normal thyroid function can compensate for the increased TBG by making more thyroid hormone, thus maintaining free T_4 and T_3 serum concentrations in the normal range. Patients dependent on thyroid hormone replacement therapy who are also receiving estrogens may require increased doses of their thyroid replacement therapy. These patients should have their thyroid function monitored in order to maintain their free thyroid hormone levels in an acceptable range.

E

Fluid Retention

Because estrogens/progestins may cause some degree of fluid retention, patients with conditions that might be influenced by this factor, such as cardiac or renal dysfunction, warrant careful observation when estrogens are prescribed.

Hypocalcemia

Estrogens should be used with caution in individuals with severe hypocalcemia.

Exacerbation of Endometriosis

Endometriosis may be exacerbated with administration of estrogen therapy.

Exacerbation of Other Conditions

Postmenopausal estrogen therapy may cause an exacerbation of asthma, diabetes mellitus, epilepsy, migraine or porphyria and should be used with caution in women with these conditions.

INFORMATION FOR THE PATIENT

See text of Patient Information distributed with the prescription.

LABORATORY TESTS

Estrogen administration should generally be guided by clinical response at the lowest dose for the treatment of vasomotor symptoms and vulvar and vaginal atrophy.

DRUG/LABORATORY TEST INTERACTIONS

Accelerated prothrombin time, partial thromboplastin time, and platelet aggregation time; increased platelet count; increased factors II, VII antigen, VIII coagulant activity, IX, X, XII, VII-X complex, II-VII-X complex, and beta-thromboglobulin; decreased levels of anti-factor Xa and antithrombin III, decreased antithrombin III activity; increased levels of fibrinogen and fibrinogen activity; increased plasminogen antigen and activity.

Increased thyroid-binding globulin (TBG) leading to increased circulating total thyroid hormone, as measured by protein-bound iodine (PBI), T_4 levels (by column or by radioimmunoassay) or T_3 levels by radioimmunoassay. T_3 resin uptake is decreased, reflecting the elevated TBG. Free T_4 and T_3 concentrations are unaltered.

Other binding proteins may be elevated in serum, *i.e.*, corticosteroid binding globulin (CBG), sex hormone-binding globulin (SHBG), leading to increased circulating corticosteroids and sex steroids, respectively. Free or biologically active hormone concentrations are unchanged. Other plasma proteins may be increased (angiotensinogen/renin substrate, alpha-1-antitrypsin, ceruloplasmin).

Increased plasma HDL and HDL-2 cholesterol subfraction concentrations, reduced LDL cholesterol concentration, increased triglyceride levels.

Impaired glucose tolerance.

Reduced response to metyrapone test.

Reduced serum folate concentration.

Aminoglutethimide administered concomitantly with medroxyprogesterone acetate (MPA) may significantly depress the bioavailability of MPA.

CARCINOGENESIS, MUTAGENESIS, AND IMPAIRMENT OF FERTILITY

Long-term continuous administration of natural and synthetic estrogens in certain animal species increases the frequency of carcinomas of the breasts, uterus, cervix, vagina, testis, and liver. (See CONTRAINDICATIONS and WARNINGS.)

In a 2 year oral study of medroxyprogesterone acetate (MPA) in which female rats were exposed to dosages of up to 5000 µg/kg/day in their diets (50 times higher — based on AUC values — than the level observed experimentally in women taking 10 mg of MPA), a dose-related increase in pancreatic islet cell tumors (adenomas and carcinomas) occurred. Pancreatic tumor incidence was increased at 1000 and 5000 µg/kg/day, but not at 200 µg/kg/day.

A decreased incidence of spontaneous mammary gland tumors was observed in all 3 MPA-treated groups, compared to controls, in the 2 year rat study. The mechanism for the decreased incidence of mammary gland tumors observed in the MPA-treated rats may be linked to the significant decrease in serum prolactin concentration observed in rats.

Beagle dogs treated with MPA developed mammary nodules, some of which were malignant. Although nodules occasionally appeared in control animals, they were intermittent in nature, whereas the nodules in the drug-treated animals were larger, more numerous, persistent, and there were some breast malignancies with metastases. It is known that progestogens stimulate synthesis and release of growth hormone in dogs. The growth hormone, along with the progestogen, stimulates mammary growth and tumors. In contrast, growth hormone in humans is not increased, nor does growth hormone have any significant mammotrophic role. No pancreatic tumors occurred in dogs.

PREGNANCY CATEGORY X

Prempro and Premphase should not be used during pregnancy. (See CONTRAINDICATIONS.)

NURSING MOTHERS

The administration of any drug to nursing mothers should be done only when clearly necessary since many drugs are excreted in human milk. In addition, estrogen administration to nursing mothers has been shown to decrease the quantity and quality of the milk. Detectable amounts of progestin have been identified in the milk of mothers receiving the drug. The effect of this on the nursing infant has not been determined. Prempro and Premphase are not indicated for the prevention of postpartum breast engorgement.

PEDIATRIC USE

Prempro and Premphase are not indicated in children.

E

GERIATRIC USE

There have not been sufficient numbers of geriatric patients involved in studies utilizing Premarin and medroxyprogesterone acetate to determine whether those over 65 years of age differ from younger subjects in their response to Prempro or Premphase.

ADVERSE REACTIONS

Because clinical trials are conducted under widely varying conditions, adverse reaction rates observed in the clinical trials of a drug cannot be directly compared to rates in the clinical trials of another drug and may not reflect the rates observed in practice. The adverse reaction information from clinical trials does, however, provide a basis for identifying the adverse events that appear to be related to drug use and for approximating rates.

See WARNINGS regarding cardiovascular disorders (including myocardial infarction, stroke and venous thromboembolism), malignant neoplasms (including breast cancer, endometrial cancer and ovarian cancer), gallbladder disease, hypercalcemia and visual abnormalities. See PRECAUTIONS regarding elevated blood pressure, familial hyperlipoproteinemia, impaired liver function and past history of cholestatic jaundice, hypothyroidism, fluid retention, hypocalcemia, exacerbation of endometriosis and other conditions.

In a 1 year clinical trial that included 678 women treated with Prempro, 351 women treated with Premphase, and 347 women treated with Premarin, the following adverse events occurred at a rate ≥5% (see TABLE 8).

TABLE 8 *All Treatment Emergent Study Events Regardless of Drug Relationship Reported at a Frequency ≥5%*

	Prempro (continuous)		Premphase (sequential)	Premarin
	0.625 mg/2.5 mg (n=340)	0.625 mg/5.0 mg (n=338)	0.625 mg/5.0 mg (n=351)	0.625 mg daily (n=347)
Body as a Whole				
Abdominal pain	16%	21%	23%	17%
Accidental injury	5%	4%	5%	5%
Asthenia	6%	8%	10%	8%
Back pain	14%	13%	16%	14%
Flu syndrome	10%	13%	12%	14%
Headache	36%	28%	37%	38%
Infection	16%	16%	18%	14%
Pain	11%	13%	12%	13%
Pelvic pain	4%	5%	5%	5%
Digestive System				
Diarrhea	6%	6%	5%	10%
Dyspepsia	6%	6%	5%	5%
Flatulence	8%	9%	8%	5%
Nausea	11%	9%	11%	11%
Metabolic and Nutritional				
Peripheral edema	4%	4%	3%	5%
Musculoskeletal System				
Arthralgia	9%	7%	9%	7%
Leg cramps	3%	4%	5%	4%
Nervous System				
Depression	6%	11%	11%	10%
Dizziness	5%	3%	4%	6%
Hypertonia	4%	3%	3%	7%
Respiratory System				
Pharyngitis	11%	11%	13%	12%
Rhinitis	8%	6%	8%	7%
Sinusitis	8%	7%	7%	5%
Skin and Appendages				
Pruritus	10%	8%	5%	4%
Rash	4%	6%	4%	3%
Urogenital System				
Breast pain	33%	38%	32%	12%
Cervix disorder	4%	4%	5%	5%
Dysmenorrhea	8%	5%	13%	5%
Leukorrhea	6%	5%	9%	8%
Vaginal hemorrhage	2%	1%	3%	6%
Vaginitis	7%	7%	5%	3%

The following adverse reactions also have been reported with estrogen and/or progestin therapy:

Genitourinary System: Changes in vaginal bleeding pattern and abnormal withdrawal bleeding or flow, breakthrough bleeding, spotting, change in amount of cervical secretion, premenstrual-like syndrome, cystitis-like syndrome, increase in size of uterine leiomyomata, vaginal candidiasis, amenorrhea, changes in cervical erosion, ovarian cancer.

Breasts: Tenderness, enlargement, galactorrhea, discharge, fibrocystic breast changes.

Gastrointestinal: Nausea, cholestatic jaundice, changes in appetite, vomiting, abdominal cramps, bloating, increased incidence of gallbladder disease, pancreatitis.

Skin: Chloasma or melasma that may persist when drug is discontinued, erythema multiforme, erythema nodosum, hemorrhagic eruption, loss of scalp hair, hirsutism, itching, urticaria, pruritus, generalized rash, rash (allergic) with and without pruritus, acne.

Cardiovascular: Change in blood pressure, deep and superficial venous thrombosis/thrombophlebitis, pulmonary embolism, myocardial infarction, cerebral thrombosis and embolism.

CNS: Headache, dizziness, mental depression, mood disturbances, anxiety, irritability, nervousness, migraine, chorea, insomnia, somnolence.

Eyes: Neuro-ocular lesions, *e.g.*, retinal thrombosis and optic neuritis, steepening of corneal curvature, intolerance of contact lenses.

Miscellaneous: Increase or decrease in weight, edema, changes in libido, fatigue, backache, reduced carbohydrate tolerance, aggravation of porphyria, pyrexia, anaphylactoid/anaphylactic reactions including urticaria and angioedema.

DOSAGE AND ADMINISTRATION

Use of postmenopausal estrogen/progestin therapy should be limited to the shortest duration consistent with treatment goals and risks for the individual woman, and should be periodically reevaluated. (See WARNINGS.)

PREMPRO

Prempro therapy consists of a single tablet to be taken once daily.

For treatment of moderate-to-severe vasomotor symptoms and/or vulvar and vaginal atrophy associated with the menopause, patients should be started at the lowest effective dose: Prempro 0.625 mg/2.5 mg daily. Patients should be reevaluated at 3-6 month intervals to determine if treatment for symptoms is still necessary.

Adequate diagnostic measures, including endometrial sampling when indicated, should be undertaken to rule out malignancy in cases of undiagnosed persistent or recurring abnormal vaginal bleeding. In patients where bleeding or spotting remains a problem, after appropriate evaluation, consideration should be given to increasing the medroxyprogesterone acetate (MPA) dose to Prempro 0.625 mg/5 mg daily. This dose should be periodically reassessed by the healthcare provider.

For prevention of postmenopausal osteoporosis: Prempro 0.625 mg/2.5 mg daily. When used solely for the prevention of postmenopausal osteoporosis, alternative treatments should be carefully considered. In patients where bleeding or spotting remains a problem, after appropriate evaluation, consideration should be given to increasing the MPA dose to Prempro 0.625 mg/5 mg daily. This dose should be periodically reassessed by the healthcare provider.

Patients should be monitored closely for signs of endometrial cancer, and appropriate diagnostic measures should be taken to rule out malignancy in the event of persistent or recurring abnormal vaginal bleeding.

PREMPHASE

Premphase therapy consists of 2 separate tablets; one maroon 0.625 mg Premarin tablet taken daily on Days 1-14 and one light-blue tablet, containing 0.625 mg conjugated estrogens and 5 mg of medroxyprogesterone acetate, taken on days 15-28.

For treatment of moderate to severe vasomotor symptoms and/or vulvar and vaginal atrophy associated with the menopause: Patients should be reevaluated at 3-6 month intervals to determine if treatment for symptoms is still necessary. Adequate diagnostic measures, including endometrial sampling when indicated, should be undertaken to rule out malignancy in cases of undiagnosed persistent or recurring abnormal vaginal bleeding.

For prevention of postmenopausal osteoporosis: When Premphase is used solely for the prevention of postmenopausal osteoporosis, alternative treatments should be carefully considered.

Patients should be monitored closely for signs of endometrial cancer, and appropriate diagnostic measures should be taken to rule out malignancy in the event of persistent or recurring abnormal vaginal bleeding.

HOW SUPPLIED

PREMPRO

Prempro therapy consists of a single tablet to be taken once daily.

0.625 mg/2.5 mg: One EZ DIAL dispenser contains 28 oval, peach tablets containing 0.625 mg of the conjugated estrogens found in Premarin tablets and 2.5 mg of medroxyprogesterone acetate for oral administration.

0.625 mg/5 mg: One EZ DIAL dispenser contains 28 oval, light-blue tablets containing 0.625 mg of the conjugated estrogens found in Premarin tablets and 5 mg of medroxyprogesterone acetate for oral administration.

Storage: Store at controlled room temperature 20-25°C (68-77°F).

PREMPHASE

Premphase therapy consists of 2 separate tablets; 1 maroon Premarin tablet taken daily on days 1-14 and 1 light-blue tablet taken on days 15-28.

0.625 mg; 0.625 mg/5 mg: One EZ DIAL dispenser contains 14 oval, maroon Premarin tablets containing 0.625 mg of conjugated estrogens and 14 oval, light-blue tablets that contain 0.625 mg of the conjugated estrogens found in Premarin tablets and 5 mg of medroxyprogesterone acetate (MPA) for oral administration.

Storage: Store at controlled room temperature 20-25°C (68-77°F).

PRODUCT LISTING - EQUIVALENTS NOT AVAILABLE

Tablet - Oral - Biphasic

28 x 3 $109.56 PREMPHASE, Wyeth-Ayerst Laboratories 00046-2573-06

28's	$18.38	PREMPHASE, Wyeth-Ayerst Laboratories	00046-2573-01
28's	$24.00	PREMPHASE, Allscripts Pharmaceutical Company	54569-4673-00
28's	$26.29	PREMPHASE, Wyeth-Ayerst Laboratories	00046-2573-05
28's	$27.78	PREMPHASE, Physicians Total Care	54868-3800-00
Tablet - Oral - 0.625 mg;2.5 mg			
28 x 3	$118.38	PREMPRO, Wyeth-Ayerst Laboratories	00046-0875-06
28's	$17.88	PREMPRO, Wyeth-Ayerst Laboratories	00046-2572-01
28's	$19.20	PREMPRO, Wyeth-Ayerst Laboratories	00046-0875-01
28's	$26.26	PREMPRO, Allscripts Pharmaceutical Company	54569-4618-00
28's	$33.08	PREMPRO, Wyeth-Ayerst Laboratories	00046-0875-05
Tablet - Oral - 0.625 mg;5 mg			
28 x 3	$118.38	PREMPRO, Wyeth-Ayerst Laboratories	00046-0975-06
28's	$21.60	PREMPRO, Wyeth-Ayerst Laboratories	00046-0975-05
28's	$26.26	PREMPRO, Allscripts Pharmaceutical Company	54569-4925-00
28's	$31.18	PREMPRO, Physicians Total Care	54868-3799-00

Estrogens, Esterified; Methyltestosterone *(001201)*

Categories: Menopause; Pregnancy Category X; DEA Class CIII; FDA Approved 1965 Sept
Drug Classes: Estrogens; Hormones/hormone modifiers
Brand Names: **Estratest**
Brand Names: Estratest H.S.
Cost of Therapy: $33.99 (Menopause; Estratest; 1.25 mg; 2.5 mg; 1 tablet/day; 28 day supply)

WARNING

ESTROGENS HAVE BEEN REPORTED TO INCREASE THE RISK OF ENDOMETRIAL CARCINOMA: Three independent case control studies have reported an increased risk of endometrial cancer in postmenopausal women exposed to exogenous estrogens for prolonged periods.[1-3] This risk was independent of the other known risk factors for endometrial cancer. These studies are further supported by the finding that incidence rates of endometrial cancer have increased sharply since 1969 in eight different areas of the United States with population-based cancer reporting systems, an increase which may be related to the rapidly expanding use of estrogens during the last decade.[4]

The three case control studies reported that the risk of endometrial cancer in estrogen users was about 4.5-13.9 times greater than in nonusers. The risk appears to depend on both duration of treatment, and on estrogen dose.[3] In view of these findings, when estrogens are used for the treatment of menopausal symptoms, the lowest dose that will control symptoms should be utilized and medication should be discontinued as soon as possible. When prolonged treatment is medically indicated, the patient should be reassessed on at least a semiannual basis to determine the need for continued therapy. Although the evidence must be considered preliminary, one study suggests that cyclic administration of low doses of estrogen may carry less risk than continuous administration,[3] it therefore appears prudent to utilize such a regimen.

Close clinical surveillance of all women taking estrogens is important. In all cases of undiagnosed persistent or recurring abnormal vaginal bleeding, adequate diagnostic measures should be undertaken to rule out malignancy.

There is no evidence at present that "natural" estrogens are more or less hazardous than "synthetic" estrogens at equiestrogenic doses.

ESTROGENS SHOULD NOT BE USED DURING PREGNANCY: The use of female sex hormones, both estrogens and progestogens, during early pregnancy may seriously damage the offspring. It has been shown that females exposed *in utero* to diethylstilbestrol, a non-steroidal estrogen, have an increased risk of developing in later life a form of vaginal or cervical cancer that is ordinarily extremely rare.[5,6] This risk has been estimated as not greater than 4 per 1000 exposures.[7] Furthermore, a high percentage of such exposed women (from 30-90%) have been found to have vaginal adenosis,[8-12] epithelial changes of the vagina and cervix. Although these changes are histologically benign, it is not known whether they are precursors of malignancy. Although similar data are not available with the use of other estrogens, it cannot be presumed they would not induce similar changes.

Several reports suggest an association between intrauterine exposure to female sex hormones and congenital anomalies, including congenital heart defects and limb reduction defects.[13-16] One case control study[16] estimated a 4.7-fold increased risk of limb reduction defects in infants exposed *in utero* to sex hormones (oral contraceptives, hormone withdrawal tests for pregnancy, or attempted treatment for threatened abortion). Some of these exposures were very short and involved only a few days of treatment. The data suggest that the risk of limb reduction defects in exposed fetuses is somewhat less than 1 per 1000.

In the past, female sex hormones have been used during pregnancy in an attempt to treat threatened or habitual abortion. There is considerable evidence that estrogens are ineffective for these indications, and there is no evidence from well controlled studies that progestogens are effective for these uses.

If estrogens, esterified; methyltestosterone or estrogens, esterified; methyltestosterone half strength is used during pregnancy, or if the patient becomes pregnant while taking this drug, she should be apprised of the potential risks to the fetus, and the advisability of pregnancy continuation.

DESCRIPTION

ESTERIFIED ESTROGENS

Esterified estrogens is a mixture of the sodium salts of the sulfate esters of the estrogenic substances, principally estrone, that are of the type excreted by pregnant mares. Esterified estrogens contain not less than 75.0% and not more than 85.0% of sodium estrone sulfate, and not less than 6.0% and not more than 15.0% of sodium equilin sulfate, in such proportion that the total of these two components is not less than 90.0%. *Category:* Estrogens.

METHYLTESTOSTERONE

Methyltestosterone is an androgen. Androgens are derivatives of cyclopentanoperhydrophenanthrene. Endogenous androgens are C-19 steroids with a side chain at C-17, and with two angular methyl groups. Testosterone is the primary endogenous androgen. Fluoxymesterone and methyltestosterone are synthetic derivatives of testosterone.

Methyltestosterone is a white to light yellow crystalline substance that is virtually insoluble in water but soluble in organic solvents. It is stable in air but decomposes in light.

The empirical formula for methyltestosterone is $C_{20}H_{30}O_2$. The molecular weight is 302.46. The chemical name is Androst-e-en-3-one, 17-hydroxy-17-methyl-,(17b)-

ESTRATEST

Each dark green, capsule shaped, sugar-coated oral tablet contains 1.25 mg of esterified estrogens and 2.5 mg of methyltestosterone.

Estratest H.S. (Half-Strength)

Each light green, capsule shaped, sugar-coated oral tablet contains: 0.625 mg of esterified estrogens and 1.25 mg of methyltestosterone.

Estratest and Estratest H.S. tablets contain the following inactive ingredients: Acacia, calcium carbonate, citric acid, gelatin, lactose (anhydrous), magnesium stearate, methylparaben, microcrystalline cellulose, pharmaceutical glaze, povidone, propylparaben, sodium benzoate, sodium bicarbonate, sodium carboxymethylcellulose, sorbic acid, sucrose, starch (corn), talc, titanium dioxide, tribasic calcium phosphate, and other minor ingredients. *Estratest tablets also contain:* FD&C blue no. 1 lake, FD&C yellow no. 6 lake, and FD&C yellow no. 10 lake. *Estratest H.S. tablets also contain:* FD&C yellow no. 10 lake FD&C blue no. 1 lake, and FD&C blue no. 2 lake.

CLINICAL PHARMACOLOGY

ESTROGENS

Estrogens are important in the development and maintenance of the female reproductive system and secondary sex characteristics. They promote growth and development of the vagina, uterus, and fallopian tubes, and enlargement of the breasts. Indirectly, they contribute to the shaping of the skeleton, maintenance of tone and elasticity of urogenital structures, changes in the epiphyses of the long bones that allow for the pubertal growth spurt and its termination, growth of axillary and pubic hair, and pigmentation of the nipples and genitals. Decline of estrogenic activity at the end of the menstrual cycle can bring on menstruation, although the cessation of progesterone secretion is the most important factor in the mature ovulatory cycle. However, in the preovulatory or nonovulatory cycle, estrogen is the primary determinant in the onset of menstruation. Estrogens also affect the release of pituitary gonadotropins.

The pharmacologic effects of esterified estrogens are similar to those of endogeneous estrogens. They are soluble in water and are well absorbed from the gastrointestinal tract.

In responsive tissues (female genital organs, breasts, hypothalamus, pituitary) estrogens enter the cell and are transported into the nucleus. As a result of estrogen action, specific RNA and protein synthesis occurs.

Pharmacokinetics

Metabolism and inactivation occur primarily in the liver. Some estrogens are excreted into the bile; however they are reabsorbed from the intestine and returned to the liver through the portal venous system. Water soluble esterified estrogens are strongly acidic and are ionized in body fluids, which favor excretion through the kidneys since tubular reabsorption is minimal.

ANDROGENS

Endogenous androgens are responsible for the normal growth and development of the male sex organs and for maintenance of secondary sex characteristics. These effects include the growth and maturation of prostate, seminal vesicles, penis, and scrotum; the development of male hair distribution, such as beard, pubic, chest, and axillary hair, laryngeal enlargement, vocal cord thickening, alterations in body musculature, and fat distribution. Drugs in this class also cause retention of nitrogen, sodium, potassium, phosphorus, and decreased urinary excretion of calcium. Androgens have been reported to increase protein anabolism and decrease protein catabolism. Nitrogen balance is improved only when there is sufficient intake of calories and protein. Androgens are responsible for the growth spurt of adolescence and for the eventual termination of linear growth which is brought about by fusion of the epiphyseal growth centers. In children, exogenous androgens accelerate linear growth rates, but may cause a disproportionate advancement in bone maturation. Use over long periods may result in fusion of the epiphyseal growth centers and termination of growth process. Androgens have been reported to stimulate the production of red blood cells by enhancing the production of erythropoietic stimulating factor.

Pharmacokinetics

Testosterone given orally is metabolized by the gut and 44% is cleared by the liver in the first pass. Oral doses as high as 400 mg per day are needed to achieve clinically effective blood levels for full replacement therapy. The synthetic androgens (methyltestosterone and fluoxymesterone) are less extensively metabolized by the liver and have longer half-lives. They are more suitable than testosterone for oral administration.

Testosterone in plasma is 98% bound to a specific testosterone estradiol binding globulin, and about 2% is free. Generally, the amount of this sex-hormone binding globulin in the plasma will determine the distribution of testosterone between free and bound forms, and the free testosterone concentration will determine its half-life.

About 90% of a dose of testosterone is excreted in the urine as glucuronic and sulfuric acid conjugates of testosterone and its metabolites; about 6% of a dose is excreted in the feces, mostly in the unconjugated form. Inactivation of testosterone occurs primarily in the liver. Testosterone is metabolized to various 17-keto steroids through two different pathways. There are considerable variations of the half-life of testosterone as reported in the literature, ranging from 10 to 100 minutes.

In many tissues the activity of testosterone appears to depend on reduction to dihydrotestosterone, which binds to cytosol receptor proteins. The steroid-receptor complex is transported to the nucleus where it initiates transcription events and cellular changes related to androgen action.

INDICATIONS AND USAGE

Estrogens, esterified; methyltestosterone and estrogens, esterified; methyltestosterone H.S. are indicated in the treatment of moderate to severe vasomotor symptoms associated with the menopause in those patients not improved by estrogens alone.

There is no evidence that estrogens are effective for nervous symptoms or depression without associated vasomotor symptoms, and they should not be used to treat such conditions.

E

ESTROGENS, ESTERIFIED; METHYLTESTOSTERONE AND ESTROGENS, ESTERIFIED; METHYLTESTOSTERONE H.S. HAVE NOT BEEN SHOWN TO BE EFFECTIVE FOR ANY PURPOSE DURING PREGNANCY AND ITS USE MAY CAUSE SEVERE HARM TO THE FETUS (SEE BOXED WARNING).

NON-FDA APPROVED INDICATIONS

Although not FDA approved, methyltestosterone has been used in combination with estrogen to enhance libido in female patients.

CONTRAINDICATIONS

Estrogens should not be used in women with any of the following conditions:

1. Known or suspected cancer of the breast except in appropriately selected patients being treated for metastatic disease.
2. Known or suspected estrogen-dependent neoplasia.
3. Known or suspected pregnancy (see BOXED WARNING).
4. Undiagnosed abnormal genital bleeding.
5. Active thrombophlebitis or thromboembolic disorders.
6. A past history of thrombophlebitis, thrombosis, or thromboembolic disorders associated with previous estrogen use (except when in treatment of breast malignancy).

Methyltestosterone should not be used in:

1. The presence of severe liver damage.
2. Pregnancy and in breast-feeding mothers because of the possibility of masculinization of the female fetus or breast-fed infant.

WARNINGS

ASSOCIATED WITH ESTROGENS

Induction of Malignant Neoplasms

Long term continuous administration of natural and synthetic estrogens in certain animal species increases the frequency of carcinomas of the breast, cervix, vagina, and liver. There is now evidence that estrogens increase the risk of carcinoma of the endometrium in humans (see BOXED WARNING).

At the present time there is no satisfactory evidence that estrogens given to postmenopausal women increase the risk of cancer of the breast,[18] although a recent long-term follow-up of a single physician's practice has raised this possibility.[18a] Because of the animal data, there is a need for caution in prescribing estrogens for women with a strong family history of breast cancer or who have breast nodules, fibrocystic disease, or abnormal mammograms.

Gallbladder Disease

A recent study has reported a 2- to 3-fold increase in the risk of surgically confirmed gallbladder disease in women receiving postmenopausal estrogens,[18] similar to the 2-fold increase previously noted in users of oral contraceptives.[19-24] In the case of oral contraceptives the increased risk appeared after 2 years of use.[24]

Effects Similar to Those Caused by Estrogen-Progestogen Oral Contraceptives

There are several serious adverse effects of oral contraceptives, most of which have not, up to now, been documented as consequences of postmenopausal estrogen therapy. This may reflect the comparatively low doses of estrogen used in postmenopausal women. It would be expected that the larger doses of estrogen used to treat prostatic or breast cancer or postpartum breast engorgement are more likely to result in these adverse effects, and, in fact, it has been shown that there is an increased risk of thrombosis in men receiving estrogens for prostatic cancer and women for postpartum breast engorgement.[20-23]

Thromboembolic Disease

It is now well established that users of oral contraceptives have an increased risk of various thromboembolic and thrombotic vascular diseases, such as thrombophlebitis, pulmonary embolism, stroke, and myocardial infarction.[24-31] Cases of retinal thrombosis, mesenteric thrombosis, and optic neuritis have been reported in oral contraceptive users. There is evidence that the risk of several of these adverse reactions is related to the dose of the drug.[32,33] An increased risk of postsurgery thromboembolic complications has also been reported in users of oral contraceptives.[34,35] If feasible, estrogen should be discontinued at least 4 weeks before surgery of the type associated with an increased risk of thromboembolism, or during periods of prolonged immobilization.

While an increased rate of thromboembolic and thrombotic disease in postmenopausal users of estrogens has not been found,[18-36] this does not rule out the possibility that such an increase may be present or that subgroups of women who have underlying risk factors or who are receiving relatively large doses of estrogens may have increased risk. Therefore estrogens should not be used in persons with active thrombophlebitis or thromboembolic disorders, and they should not be used (except in treatment of malignancy) in persons with a history of such disorders in association with estrogen use. They should be used with caution in patients with cerebral vascular or coronary artery disease and only for those in whom estrogens are clearly needed.

Large doses of estrogen (5 mg esterified estrogens per day), comparable to those used to treat cancer of the prostate and breast, have been shown in a large prospective clinical trial in men[37] to increase the risk of nonfatal myocardial infarction, pulmonary embolism and thrombophlebitis. When estrogen doses of this size are used, any of the thromboembolic and thrombotic adverse effects associated with oral contraceptive use should be considered a clear risk.

Hepatic Adenoma

Benign hepatic adenomas appear to be associated with the use of oral contraceptives.[38-40] Although benign and rare, these may rupture and may cause death through intra-abdominal hemorrhage. Such lesions have not yet been reported in association with other estrogen or progestogen preparations but should be considered in estrogen users having abdominal pain and tenderness, abdominal mass, or hypovolemic shock. Hepatocellular carcinoma has also been reported in women taking estrogen-containing oral contraceptives.[39] The relationship of this malignancy to these drugs is not known at this time.

Elevated Blood Pressure

Increased blood pressure is not uncommon in women using oral contraceptives. There is now a report that this may occur with use of estrogens in the menopause[41] and blood pressure should be monitored with estrogen use, especially if high doses are used.

Glucose Tolerance

A worsening of glucose tolerance has been observed in a significant percentage of patients of estrogen-containing oral contraceptives. For this reason, diabetic patients should be carefully observed while receiving estrogens.

Hypercalcemia

Administration of estrogens may lead to severe hypercalcemia in patients with breast cancer and bone metastases. If this occurs, the drug should be stopped and appropriate measures taken to reduce the serum calcium level.

ASSOCIATED WITH METHYLTESTOSTERONE

In patients with breast cancer, androgen therapy may cause hypercalcemia by stimulating osteolysis. In this case the drug should be discontinued.

Prolonged use of high doses of androgens has been associated with the development of peliosis hepatis and hepatic neoplasms including hepatocellular carcinoma. (See PRECAUTIONS, Carcinogenesis). Peliosis hepatis can be a life-threatening or fatal complication.

Cholestatic hepatitis and jaundice occur with 17-alpha-alkylandrogen sat a relatively low dose. If cholestatic hepatitis with jaundice appears or if liver function tests become abnormal, the androgen should be discontinued and the etiology should be determined. Drug-induced jaundice is reversible when the medication is discontinued.

Edema with or without heart failure may be a serious complication in patients with preexisting cardiac, renal, or hepatic disease. In addition to discontinuation of the drug, diuretic therapy may be required.

PRECAUTIONS

GENERAL

Associated With Estrogens

1. A complete medical and family history should be taken prior to the initiation of any estrogen therapy. The pretreatment and periodic physical examinations should include special reference to blood pressure, breasts, abdomen, and pelvic organs, and should include a Papanicolaou smear. As a general rule, estrogens should not be prescribed for longer than 1 year without another physical examination being performed.
2. ***Fluid Retention:*** Because estrogens may cause some degree of fluid retention, conditions which might be influenced by this factor such as asthma, epilepsy, migraine, and cardiac or renal dysfunction, require careful observation.
3. Certain patients may develop undesirable manifestations of excessive estrogenic stimulation, such as abnormal or excessive uterine bleeding, mastodynia, etc.
4. Oral contraceptives appear to be associated with an increased incidence of mental depression.[24] Although it is not clear whether this is due to the estrogenic or progestogenic component of the contraceptive, patients with a history of depression should be carefully observed.
5. Preexisting uterine leiomyomata may increase in size during estrogen use.
6. The pathologist should be advised of estrogen therapy when relevant specimens are submitted.
7. Patients with a past history of jaundice during pregnancy have an increased risk of recurrence of jaundice while receiving estrogen-containing oral contraceptive therapy. If jaundice develops in any patient receiving estrogen, the medication should be discontinued while the cause is investigated.
8. Estrogens may be poorly metabolized in patients with impaired liver function and they should be administered with caution in such patients.
9. Because estrogens influence the metabolism of calcium and phosphorus, they should be used with caution in patients with metabolic bone diseases that are associated with hypercalcemia or in patients with renal insufficiency.
10. Because of the effects of estrogens on epiphyseal closure, they should be used judiciously in young patients in whom bone growth is not complete.
11. Certain endocrine and liver function tests may be affected by estrogen-containing oral contraceptives. The following similar changes may be expected with larger doses of estrogen:
    a. Increased sulfobromophthalein retention.
    b. Increased prothrombin and factors VII, VIII, IX and X; decreased antithrombin 3: increased norepinephrine-induced platelet aggregability.
    c. Increased thyroid binding (TBG) leading to increased circulating total thyroid hormone, as measured by PBI, T_4 by column, or T_4 by radioimmunoassay. Free T_3 resin uptake is decreased, reflecting the elevated TBG; free T_4 concentration is unaltered.
    d. Impaired glucose tolerance.
    e. Decreased pregnanediol excretion.
    f. Reduced response to metyrapone test.
    g. Reduced serum folate concentration.
    h. Increased serum triglyceride and phospholipid concentration.

Associated With Methyltestosterone

1. Women should be observed for signs of virilization (deepening of the voice, hirsutism, acne, clitoromegaly, and menstrual irregularities). Discontinuation of drug therapy at the time of evidence of mild virilism is necessary to prevent irreversible virilization. Such virilization is usual following androgen use at high doses.
2. Prolonged dosage of androgen may result in sodium and fluid retention. This may present a problem, especially in patients with compromised cardiac reserve or renal disease.
3. Hypersensitivity may occur rarely.
4. PBI may be decreased in patients taking androgens.
5. Hypercalcemia may occur. If this does occur, the drug should be discontinued.

INFORMATION FOR THE PATIENT

Associated With Methyltestosterone

The physician should instruct patients to report any of the following side effects of androgens:

Women: Hoarseness, acne, changes in menstrual periods, or more hair on the face.
All Patients: Any nausea, vomiting, changes in skin color or ankle swelling.

LABORATORY TESTS

Associated With Methyltestosterone

1. Women with disseminated breast carcinoma should have frequent determination of urine and serum calcium levels during the course of androgen therapy (see WARNINGS).
2. Because of the hepatotoxicity associated with the use of 17-alphaalkylated androgens, liver function tests should be obtained periodically.
3. Hemoglobin and hematocrit should be checked periodically for polycythemia in patients who are receiving high doses of androgens.

DRUG/LABORATORY TEST INTERACTIONS

Associated With Methyltestosterone

Androgens may decrease levels of thyroxine-binding globulin, resulting in decreased T_4 serum levels and increased resin uptake of T_3 and T_4. Free thyroid hormone levels remain unchanged, however, and there is no clinical evidence of thyroid dysfunction.

CARCINOGENESIS

Associated With Methyltestosterone

Animal Data

Testosterone has been tested by subcutaneous injection and implantation in mice and rats. The implant induced cervical-uterine tumors in mice, which metastasized in some cases. There is suggestive evidence that injection of testosterone into some strains of female mice increases their susceptibility to hepatoma. Testosterone is also known to increase the number of tumors and decrease the degree of differentiation of chemically induced carcinomas of the liver in rats.

Human Data

There are rare reports of hepatocellular carcinoma in patients receiving long-term therapy with androgens in high doses. Withdrawal of the drugs did not lead to regression of the tumors in all cases.

Geriatric patients treated with androgens may be at increased risk for the development of prostatic hypertrophy and prostatic carcinoma.

PREGNANCY, TERATOGENIC EFFECTS, PREGNANCY CATEGORY X

See CONTRAINDICATIONS.

NURSING MOTHERS

Associated With Esterified Estrogens

As a general principle, the administration of any drug to nursing mothers should be done only when clearly necessary since many drugs are excreted in human milk.

Associated With Methyltestosterone

It is not known whether androgens are excreted in human milk. Because many drugs are excreted in human milk and because of the potential for serious adverse reactions in nursing infants from androgens, a decision should be made whether to discontinue nursing or to discontinue the drug, taking into account the importance of the drug to the mother.

DRUG INTERACTIONS

ASSOCIATED WITH METHYLTESTOSTERONE

Anticoagulants: C-17 substituted derivatives of testosterone, such as methandrostenolone, have been reported to decrease the anticoagulant requirements of patients receiving oral anticoagulants. Patients receiving oral anticoagulant therapy require close monitoring, especially when androgens are started or stopped.

Oxyphenbutazone: Concurrent administration of oxyphenbutazone and androgens may result in elevated serum levels of oxyphenbutazone.

Insulin: In diabetic patients the metabolic effects of androgens may decrease blood glucose and insulin requirements.

ADVERSE REACTIONS

ASSOCIATED WITH ESTROGENS

(See WARNINGS regarding induction of neoplasia, adverse effects on the fetus, increased incidence of gallbladder disease, and adverse effects similar to those of oral contraceptives, including thromboembolism.)

The following additional adverse reactions have been reported with estrogenic therapy, including oral contraceptives:

Genitourinary System: Breakthrough bleeding, spotting, change in menstrual flow, dysmenorrhea, premenstrual-like syndrome, amenorrhea during and after treatment, increase in size of uterine fibromyomata, vaginal candidiasis, change in cervical erosion and in degree of cervical secretion, cystitis-like syndrome.

Breasts: Tenderness, enlargement, secretion.

Gastrointestinal: Nausea, vomiting, abdominal cramps, bloating, cholestatic jaundice.

Skin: Chloasma or melasma which may persist when drug is discontinued, erythema multiforme, erythema nodosum, hemorrhagic eruption, loss of scalp hair, hirsutism.

Eyes: Steepening of corneal curvature, intolerance to contact lenses.

CNS: Headache, migraine, dizziness, mental depression, chorea.

Miscellaneous: Increase or decrease in weight, reduced carbohydrate tolerance, aggravation of porphyria, edema, changes in libido.

ASSOCIATED WITH METHYLTESTOSTERONE

Endocrine and urogenital:

1. ***Female:*** The most common side effects of androgen therapy are amenorrhea and other menstrual irregularities, inhibition of gonadotropin secretion, and virilization, including deepening of the voice and clitoral enlargement. The latter usually is not reversible after androgens are discontinued. When administered to a pregnant woman androgens cause virilization of external genitalia of the female fetus.
2. ***Skin and Appendages:*** Hirsutism, male pattern of baldness, and acne.
3. ***Fluid and Electrolyte Disturbances:*** Retention of sodium, chloride, water, potassium, calcium, and inorganic phosphates.
4. ***Gastrointestinal:*** Nausea, cholestatic jaundice, alterations in liver function test, rarely hepatocellular neoplasms, and peliosis hepatis (see WARNINGS).
5. ***Hematologic:*** Suppression of clotting factors II, V, VII, and X, bleeding in patients on concomitant anticoagulant therapy, and polycythemia.
6. ***Nervous System:*** Increased or decreased libido, headache, anxiety, depression, and generalized paresthesia.
7. ***Metabolic:*** Increased serum cholesterol.
8. ***Miscellaneous:*** Inflammation and pain at the site of intramuscular injection or subcutaneous implantation of testosterone containing pellets, stomatitis with buccal preparations, and rarely anaphylactoid reactions.

DOSAGE AND ADMINISTRATION

GIVEN CYCLICALLY FOR SHORT-TERM USE ONLY

For treatment of moderate to severe vasomotor symptoms associated with the menopause in patients not improved by estrogen alone.

The lowest dose that will control symptoms should be chosen and medication should be discontinued as promptly as possible.

Administration should be cyclic (*e.g.*, 3 weeks on and 1 week off). Attempts to discontinue or taper medication should be made at 3-6 month intervals.

Usual Dosage Range: 1 tablet of esterified estrogens; methyltestosterone or 1-2 tablets of esterified estrogens; methyltestosterone half-strength daily as recommended by the physician.

Treated patients with an intact uterus should be monitored closely for signs of endometrial cancer and appropriate diagnostic measures should be taken to rule out malignancy in the event of persistent or recurring abnormal vaginal bleeding.

HOW SUPPLIED

Estratest: Imprinted "SOLVAY 1026". Dark green, capsule shaped, sugar-coated oral tablets containing 1.25 mg of esterified estrogens and 2.5 mg of methyltestosterone.

Estratest H.S. "Half-Strength": Imprinted "SOLVAY 1023". Light green, capsule shaped, sugar-coated oral tablets containing 0.625 mg of esterified estrogens and 1.25 mg of methyltestosterone.

Storage: Store at controlled room temperature, 15-30°C (59-86°F).

PRODUCT LISTING - EQUIVALENTS NOT AVAILABLE

Tablet - Oral - 0.625 mg;1.25 mg

30's	$27.87	ESTRATEST H.S., Allscripts Pharmaceutical Company	54569-4354-01
100's	$63.25	GENERIC, Sage Pharmaceuticals	59243-0560-01
100's	$131.80	GENERIC, Medi-Hut Inc	66576-0230-01
100's	$148.09	ESTRATEST H.S., Solvay Pharmaceuticals Inc	00032-1023-01

Tablet - Oral - 1.25 mg;2.5 mg

100's	$79.00	GENERIC, Sage Pharmaceuticals	59243-0570-01
100's	$161.35	GENERIC, Medi-Hut Inc	66576-0231-01
100's	$181.31	ESTRATEST, Solvay Pharmaceuticals Inc	00032-1026-01

Estropipate *(001204)*

Categories: Atrophy, vaginal; Atrophy, vulvar; Hypogonadism, female; Menopause; Osteoporosis, prevention; Ovarian failure, primary; Vaginitis, atrophic; Castration, female; Pregnancy Category X; FDA Approved 1977 Jun
Drug Classes: Estrogens; Hormones/hormone modifiers
Brand Names: Harmonet; **Ogen**; Ortho-Est
Foreign Brand Availability: Esgen (Korea); Genoral (Australia); Harmogen (England; Ireland); Sultrex (Argentina)
Cost of Therapy: $17.36 (Menopause; Generic tablets; 1.25 mg; 1 tablet/day; 28 day supply)

WARNING

ESTROGENS HAVE BEEN REPORTED TO INCREASE THE RISK OF ENDOMETRIAL CARCINOMA IN POST-MENOPAUSAL WOMEN.

Close clinical surveillance of all women taking estrogens is important. Adequate diagnostic measures, including endometrial sampling when indicated, should be undertaken to rule out malignancy in all cases of undiagnosed persistent or recurring abnormal vaginal bleeding. There is no evidence that "natural" estrogens are more or less hazardous than "synthetic" estrogens at equi-estrogenic doses.

> **WARNING — Cont'd**
>
> **ESTROGENS SHOULD NOT BE USED DURING PREGNANCY.**
>
> **There is no indication for estrogen therapy during pregnancy or during the immediate postpartum period. Estrogens are ineffective for the prevention or treatment of threatened, or habitual abortion. Estrogens are not indicated for the prevention of postpartum breast engorgement.**
>
> **Estrogen therapy during pregnancy is associated with an increased risk of congenital defects in the reproductive organs of the fetus, and possibly other birth defects. Studies of women who received diethylstilbestrol (DES) during pregnancy have shown that female offspring have an increased risk of vaginal adenosis, squamous cell dysplasia of the uterine cervix, and clear cell vaginal cancer later in life; male offspring have an increased risk of urogenital abnormalities and possibly testicular cancer later in life. The 1985 DES Task Force concluded that use of DES during pregnancy is associated with a subsequent increased risk of breast cancer in the mothers, although a causal relationship remains unproven and the observed level of excess risk is similar to that for a number of other breast cancer risk factors.**

DESCRIPTION

TABLETS AND VAGINAL CREAM

Estropipate (formerly piperazine estrone sulfate), is a natural estrogenic substance prepared from purified crystalline estrone, solubilized as the sulfate and stabilized with piperazine. It is appreciably soluble in water and has almost no odor or taste — properties which are ideally suited for oral administration. The amount of piperazine in estropipate is not sufficient to exert a pharmacological action. Its addition ensures solubility, stability, and uniform potency of the estrone sulfate. Chemically estropipate is represented by estra-1,3,5(10)-trien-17-one,3-(sulfooxy)-, compound with piperazine (1:1). The molecular weight is 436.56.

TABLETS

Estropipate is available as tablets for oral administration containing either 0.75 mg (Ogen 0.625), 1.5 mg (Ogen 1.25) or 3 mg (Ogen 2.5) estropipate. (Calculated as sodium estrone sulfate 0.625 mg, 1.25 mg, and 2.5 mg, respectively).

Inactive Ingredients: *Each Tablet Contains:* Colloidal silicon dioxide, dibasic potassium phosphate, hydrogenated vegetable oil wax, hydroxypropyl cellulose, lactose, magnesium stearate, microcrystalline cellulose, sodium starch glycolate and tromethamine. *Ogen 0.625 Tablet Also Contains:* D&C yellow no. 10 and FD&C yellow no 6. *Ogen 1.25 Tablet Also Contains:* FD&C yellow no. 6. *Ogen 2.5 Tablet Also Contains:* FD&C blue no 2.

VAGINAL CREAM

Each gram of ogen vaginal cream contains 1.5 mg estropipate in a base composed of the following ingredients: Glycerin, mineral oil, glyceryl monostearate, polyethylene glycol ether complex of higher fatty alcohols, cetyl alcohol, anhydrous lanolin, sodium biphosphate, cis-N-(3-chloroallyl) hexaminium chloride, propylparaben, methylparaben, piperazine hexahydrate, citric acid and water.

CLINICAL PHARMACOLOGY

Estrogen drug products act by regulating the transcription of a limited number of genes. Estrogens diffuse through cell membranes, distribute themselves throughout the cell, and bind to and activate the nuclear estrogen receptor, a DNA-binding protein which is found in estrogen responsive tissues. The activated estrogen receptor binds to specific DNA sequences, or hormone-response elements, which enhance the transcription of adjacent genes and in turn lead to the observed effects. Estrogen receptors have been identified in tissues of the reproductive tract, breast, pituitary, hypothalamus, liver, and bone of women.

Estrogens are important in the development and maintenance of the female reproductive system and secondary sex characteristics. By a direct action, they cause growth and development of the uterus, fallopian tubes, and vagina. With other hormones, such as pituitary hormones and progesterone, they cause enlargement of the breasts through promotion of ductal growth, stromal development, and the accretion of fat. Estrogens are intricately involved with other hormones, especially progesterone, in the processes of the ovulatory menstrual cycle and pregnancy, and affect the release of pituitary gonadotropins. They also contribute to the shaping of the skeleton, maintenance of tone and elasticity of urogenital structures, changes in the epiphyses of the long bones that allow for the pubertal growth spurt and its termination, and pigmentation of the nipples and genitals.

Estrogens occur naturally in several forms. The primary source of estrogen in normally cycling adult women is the ovarian follicle, which secretes 70-500 μg of estradiol daily, depending on the phase of the menstrual cycle. This is converted primarily to estrone, which circulates in roughly equal proportion to estradiol, and to small amounts of estriol. After menopause, most endogenous estrogen is produced by conversion of androstenedione, secreted by the adrenal cortex, to estrone by peripheral tissues. Thus, estrone — especially in its sulfate ester form — is the most abundant circulating estrogen in postmenopausal women. Although circulating estrogens exist in a dynamic equilibrium of metabolic interconversions, estradiol is the principal intracellular human estrogen and is substantially more potent than estrone or estriol at the receptor.

Estrogens used in therapy are well absorbed through the skin, mucous membranes, and gastrointestinal tract. When applied for a local action, absorption is usually sufficient to cause systemic effects. When conjugated with aryl and alkyl groups for parenteral administration, the rate of absorption of oily preparations is slowed with a prolonged duration of action, such that a single intramuscular injection of estradiol valerate or estradiol cypionate is absorbed over several weeks.

Administered estrogens and their esters are handled within the body essentially the same as the endogenous hormones. Metabolic conversion of estrogens occurs primarily in the liver (first pass effect), but also at local target tissue sites. Complex metabolic processes result in a dynamic equilibrium of circulating conjugated and unconjugated estrogenic forms which are continually interconverted, especially between estrone and estradiol and between esterified and unesterified forms. Although naturally-occurring estrogens circulate in the blood largely bound to sex hormone-binding globulin and albumin, only unbound estrogens enter target tissue cells. A significant proportion of the circulating estrogen exists as sulfate conjugates, especially estrone sulfate, which serves as a circulating reservoir for the formation of more active estrogenic species. A certain proportion of the estrogen is excreted into the bile and then reabsorbed from the intestine. During this enterohepatic recirculation, estrogens are desulfated and resulfated and undergo degradation through conversion to less active estrogens (estriol and other estrogens), oxidation to nonestrogenic substances (catecholestrogens, which interact with catecholamine metabolism, especially in the central nervous system), and conjugation with glucuronic acids (which are then rapidly excreted in the urine).

When given orally, naturally-occurring estrogens and their esters are extensively metabolized (first pass effect) and circulate primarily as estrone sulfate, with smaller amounts of other conjugated and unconjugated estrogenic species. This results in limited oral potency. By contrast, synthetic estrogens, such as ethinyl estradiol and the nonsteroidal estrogens, are degraded very slowly in the liver and other tissues, which results in their high intrinsic potency. Estrogen drug products administered by non-oral routes are not subject to first-pass metabolism, but also undergo significant hepatic uptake, metabolism, and enterohepatic recycling.

INDICATIONS AND USAGE

TABLETS

Estrogen drug products are indicated in the:

1. Treatment of moderate to severe vasomotor symptoms associated with the menopause. There is no adequate evidence that estrogens are effective for nervous symptoms or depression which might occur during menopause and they should not be used to treat these conditions.
2. Treatment of vulval and vaginal atrophy.
3. Treatment of hypoestrogenism due to hypogonadism, castration or primary ovarian failure.
4. Prevention of osteoporosis.

Since estrogen administration is associated with risk, selection of patients should ideally be based on prospective identification of risk factors for developing osteoporosis. Unfortunately, there is no certain way to identify those women who will develop osteoporotic fractures. Most prospective studies of efficacy for this indication have been carried out in white menopausal women, without stratification by other risk factors, and tend to show a universally salutary effect on bone. Thus, patient selection must be individualized based on the balance of risks and benefits. A more favorable risk/benefit ratio exists in a hysterectomized woman because she has no risk of endometrial cancer (see BOXED WARNING).

Estrogen replacement therapy reduces bone resorption and retards or halts postmenopausal bone loss. Case-control studies have shown an approximately 60% reduction in hip and wrist fractures in women whose estrogen replacement has begun within a few years of menopause. Studies also suggest that estrogen reduces the rate of vertebral fractures. Even when started as late as 6 years after menopause, estrogen prevents further loss of bone mass for as long as the treatment is continued. The results of a double-blind, placebo-controlled 2 year study have shown that treatment with 1 tablet of estropipate 0.625 daily for 25 days (of a 31 day cycle per month) prevents vertebral bone mass loss in postmenopausal women. When estrogen therapy is discontinued, bone mass declines at a rate comparable to the immediate postmenopausal period. There is no evidence that estrogen replacement therapy restores bone mass to premenopausal levels.

At skeletal maturity there are sex and race differences in both the total amount of bone present and its density, in favor of men and blacks. Thus, women are at higher risk than men because they start with less bone mass and, for several years following natural or induced menopause, the rate of bone mass decline is accelerated. White and Asian women are at higher risk than black women.

Early menopause is one of the strongest predictors for the development of osteoporosis. In addition, other factors affecting the skeleton which are associated with osteoporosis include genetic factors (small build, family history), endocrine factors (nulliparity, thyrotoxicosis, hyperparathyroidism, Cushing's syndrome, hyperprolactinemia, Type I diabetes), lifestyle (cigarette smoking, alcohol abuse, sedentary exercise habits) and nutrition (below average body weight, dietary calcium intake).

The mainstays of prevention and management of osteoporosis are estrogen, an adequate lifetime calcium intake, and exercise. Postmenopausal women absorb dietary calcium less efficiently than premenopausal women and require an average of 1500 mg/day of elemental calcium to remain in neutral calcium balance. By comparison, premenopausal women require about 1000 mg/day and the average calcium intake in the USA is 400-600 mg/day. Therefore, when not contraindicated, calcium supplementation may be helpful.

Weight-bearing exercise and nutrition may be important adjuncts to the prevention and management of osteoporosis. Immobilization and prolonged bed rest produce rapid bone loss, while weight-bearing exercise has been shown both to reduce bone loss and increase bone mass. The optimal type and amount of physical activity that would prevent osteoporosis have not been established, however in two studies an hour of walking and running exercises 2 or 3 times weekly significantly increased lumbar spine bone mass.

VAGINAL CREAM

Estropipate vaginal cream is indicated for the treatment of vulval and vaginal atrophy.

NON-FDA APPROVED INDICATIONS

Although not FDA approved, estropipate has been used for the treatment of atrophic urethritis. Other estrogens have been used for treatment of abnormal uterine bleeding, gastrointestinal bleeding in patients with renal failure, gastrointestinal bleeding related to arteriovenous malformations, and for the palliative treatment of metastatic breast cancer and androgen-dependent prostate cancer.

CONTRAINDICATIONS

Estrogens should not be used in individuals with any of the following conditions:

1. Known or suspected pregnancy (see BOXED WARNING). Estrogens may cause fetal harm when administered to a pregnant woman.
2. Undiagnosed abnormal genital bleeding.
3. Known or suspected cancer of the breast except in appropriately selected patients being treated for metastatic disease.

4. Known or suspected estrogen-dependent neoplasia.
5. Active thrombophlebitis or thromboembolic disorders.

Vaginal Cream: Estropipate vaginal cream is contraindicated in patients hypersensitive to its ingredients.

WARNINGS

INDUCTION OF MALIGNANT NEOPLASMS

Endometrial Cancer

The reported endometrial cancer risk among unopposed estrogen users is about 2- to 12-fold greater than in nonusers, and appears dependent on duration of treatment and on estrogen dose. Most studies show no significant increased risk associated with the use of estrogens for less than 1 year. The greatest risk appears associated with prolonged use — with increased risks of 15- to 24-fold for 5-10 years or more. In 3 studies, persistence of risk was demonstrated for 8 to over 15 years after cessation of estrogen treatment. In one study a significant decrease in the incidence of endometrial cancer occurred 6 months after estrogen withdrawal. Concurrent progestin therapy may offset this risk but the overall health impact in postmenopausal women is not known (see PRECAUTIONS).

Breast Cancer

While the majority of studies have not shown an increased risk of breast cancer in women who have ever used estrogen replacement therapy, some have reported a moderately increased risk (relative risks of 1.3-2.0) in those taking higher doses or those taking lower doses for prolonged periods of time, especially in excess of 10 years. Other studies have not shown this relationship.

Congenital Lesions with Malignant Potential

Estrogen therapy during pregnancy is associated with an increased risk of fetal congenital reproductive tract disorders, and possibly other birth defects. Studies of women who received DES during pregnancy have shown that female offspring have an increased risk of vaginal adenosis, squamous cell dysplasia of the uterine cervix, and clear cell vaginal cancer later in life; male offspring have an increased risk of urogenital abnormalities and possibly testicular cancer later in life. Although some of these changes are benign, others are precursors of malignancy.

GALLBLADDER DISEASE

Two studies have reported a 2- to 4-fold increase in the risk of gallbladder disease requiring surgery in women receiving postmenopausal estrogens.

CARDIOVASCULAR DISEASE

Large doses of estrogen (5 mg conjugated estrogens per day), comparable to those used to treat cancer of the prostate and breast, have been shown in a large prospective clinical trial in men to increase the risks of nonfatal myocardial infarction, pulmonary embolism, and thrombophlebitis. These risks cannot necessarily be extrapolated from men to women. However, to avoid the theoretical cardiovascular risk to women caused by high estrogen doses, the dose for estrogen replacement therapy should not exceed the lowest effective dose.

ELEVATED BLOOD PRESSURE

Occasional blood pressure increases during estrogen replacement therapy have been attributed to idiosyncratic reactions to estrogens. More often, blood pressure has remained the same or has dropped. One study showed that postmenopausal estrogen users have higher blood pressure than nonusers. Two other studies showed slightly lower blood pressure among estrogen users compared to nonusers. Postmenopausal estrogen use does not increase the risk of stroke. Nonetheless, blood pressure should be monitored at regular intervals with estrogen use.

HYPERCALCEMIA

Administration of estrogens may lead to severe hypercalcemia in patients with breast cancer and bone metastases. If this occurs, the drug should be stopped and appropriate measures taken to reduce the serum calcium level.

PRECAUTIONS

GENERAL

Addition of a Progestin

Studies of the addition of a progestin for 7 or more days of a cycle of estrogen administration have reported a lowered incidence of endometrial hyperplasia which would otherwise be induced by estrogen treatment. Morphological and biochemical studies of endometrium suggest that 10-14 days of progestin are needed to provide maximal maturation of the endometrium and to eliminate any hyperplastic changes. There are possible additional risks which may be associated with the inclusion of progestins in estrogen replacement regimens. These include: (1) adverse effects on lipoprotein metabolism (lowering HDL and raising LDL) which may diminish the possible cardioprotective effect of estrogen therapy (see PRECAUTIONS, Drug/Laboratory Test Interactions), (2) impairment of glucose tolerance; and (3) possible enhancement of miotic activity in breast epithelial tissue (although few epidemiological data are available to address this point). The choice of progestin, its dose, and its regimen may be important in minimizing these adverse effects, but these issues remain to be clarified.

Physical Examination

A complete medical and family history should be taken prior to the initiation of any estrogen therapy. The pretreatment and periodic physical examinations should include special reference to blood pressure, breasts, abdomen, and pelvic organs, and should include a Papanicolaou smear. As a general rule, estrogen should not be prescribed for longer than 1 year without reexamining the patient.

Hypercoagulability

Some studies have shown that women taking estrogen replacement therapy have hypercoagulability, primarily related to decreased antithrombin activity. This effect appears dose- and duration-dependent and is less pronounced than that associated with oral contraceptive use. Also, postmenopausal women tend to have increased coagulation parameters at baseline compared to premenopausal women. There is some suggestion that low dose postmenopausal mestranol may increase the risk of thromboembolism, although the majority of studies (of primarily conjugated estrogens users) report no such increase. There is insufficient information on hypercoagulability in women who have had previous thromboembolic disease.

Familial Hyperlipoproteinemia

Estrogen therapy may be associated with massive elevations of plasma triglycerides leading to pancreatitis and other complications in patients with familial defects of lipoprotein metabolism.

Fluid Retention

Because estrogens may cause some degree of fluid retention, conditions which might be exacerbated by this factor, such as asthma, epilepsy, migraine, and cardiac or renal dysfunction, require careful observation.

Uterine Bleeding and Mastodynia

Certain patients may develop undesirable manifestations of estrogenic stimulation, such as abnormal uterine bleeding and mastodynia.

Impaired Liver Function

Estrogen may be poorly metabolized in patients with impaired liver function and should be administered with caution.

INFORMATION FOR THE PATIENT

See the Patient Instructions that are distributed with the prescription for complete instructions.

LABORATORY TESTS

Estrogen administration should generally be guided by clinical response at the smallest dose, rather than laboratory monitoring, for relief of symptoms for those indications in which symptoms are observable. For prevention and treatment of osteoporosis, however, see DOSAGE AND ADMINISTRATION.

DRUG/LABORATORY TEST INTERACTIONS

Accelerated prothrombin time, partial thromboplastin time, and platelet aggregation time; increased platelet count; increased factors II, VII antigen, VIII antigen, VIII coagulant activity, IX, X, XII, VII-X complex, II-VII-X complex, and beta-thromboglobulin; decreased levels of anti-factor Xa and antithrombin III, decreased antithrombin III activity; increased levels of fibrinogen and fibrinogen activity; increased plasminogen antigen and activity.

Increased thyroid-binding globulin (TBG) leading to increased circulating total thyroid hormone, as measured by protein-bound iodine (PBI), T4 levels (by column or by radioimmunoassay) or T3 levels by radioimmunoassay. T3 resin uptake is decreased, reflecting the elevated TBG. Free T4 and free T3 concentrations are unaltered.

Other binding proteins may be elevated in serum, *i.e.,* corticosteroid binding globulin (CBG), sex hormone-binding globulin (SHBG), leading to increased circulating corticosteroids and sex steroids respectively. Free or biologically active hormone concentrations are unchanged. Other plasma proteins may be increased (angiotensinogen/renin substrate, alpha-1-antitrypsin, ceruloplasmin).

Increased plasma HDL and HDL-2 subfraction concentrations, reduced LDL cholesterol concentration, increased triglycerides levels.

Impaired glucose intolerance.

Reduced response to metyrapone test.

Reduced serum folate concentration.

CARCINOGENESIS, MUTAGENESIS, AND IMPAIRMENT OF FERTILITY

Long-term continuous administration of natural and synthetic estrogens in certain animal species increases the frequency of carcinomas of the breast, uterus, cervix, vagina, testis, and liver. See CONTRAINDICATIONS and WARNINGS.

PREGNANCY CATEGORY X

Estrogens should not be used during pregnancy. See CONTRAINDICATIONS and BOXED WARNING.

NURSING MOTHERS

As a general principle, the administration of any drug to nursing mothers should be done only when clearly necessary since many drugs are excreted in human milk. In addition, estrogen administration to nursing mothers has been shown to decrease the quantity and quality of the milk.

ADVERSE REACTIONS

VAGINAL CREAM

Hypersensitivity reactions, systemic effects such as breast tenderness, and rarely, withdrawal bleeding, have occurred with the use of topical estrogens. Local irritation (especially when prior inflammation is present) has occurred at inititation of therapy.

TABLETS AND VAGINAL CREAM

The following additional adverse reactions have been reported with estrogen therapy (see WARNINGS regarding induction of neoplasia, adverse effects on the fetus, increased incidence of gallbladder disease, cardiovascular disease, elevated blood pressure, and hypercalcemia).

Genitourinary System: Changes in vaginal bleeding pattern and abnormal withdrawal bleeding or flow, breakthrough bleeding, spotting; increase in size of uterine leiomyomata; vaginal candidiasis; change in amount of cervical secretion.

Breast: Tenderness, enlargement.

Gastrointestinal: Nausea, vomiting; abdominal cramps, bloating; cholestatic jaundice; increased incidence of gallbladder disease.

Skin: Chloasma or melasma that may persist when drug is discontinued; erythema multiforme; erythema nodosum; hemorrhagic eruption; loss of scalp hair; hirsutism.

Eyes: Steepening of corneal curvature; intolerance to contact lenses.

Central Nervous System: Headache, migraine, dizziness; mental depression; chorea.

Miscellaneous: Increase or decrease in weight; reduced carbohydrate tolerance; aggravation of porphyria; edema; changes in libido.

DOSAGE AND ADMINISTRATION

TABLETS

1. For treatment of moderate to severe vasomotor symptoms, vulval and vaginal atrophy associated with the menopause, the lowest dose and regimen that will control symptoms should be chosen and medication should be discontinued as promptly as possible.

Attempts to discontinue or taper medication should be made at 3-6 month intervals.

Usual Dosage Ranges:

Vasomotor Symptoms: One (1) estropipate 0.75 mg tablet to 2 estropipate 3.0 mg tablet per day. The lowest dose that will control symptoms should be chosen. If the patient has not menstruated within the last 2 months or more, cyclic administration is started arbitrarily. If the patient is menstruating, cyclic administration is started on day 5 of bleeding.

Vulval and Vaginal Atrophy: One (1) estropipate 0.75 mg tablet to 2 estropipate 3.0 tablet daily, depending upon the tissue response of the individual patient. The lowest dose that will control symptoms should be chosen. Administer cyclically.

2. For treatment of female hypoestrogenism due to hypogonadism, castration, or primary ovarian failure.

Usual Dosage Ranges:

Female Hypogonadism: a daily dose of 1 estropipate 1.5 mg tablet to 3 estropipate 3.0 mg tablets may be given for the first 3 weeks of a theoretical cycle, followed by a rest period of 8-10 days. The lowest dose that will control symptoms should be chosen. If bleeding does not occur by the end of this period, the same dosage schedule is repeated. The number of courses of estrogen therapy necessary to produce bleeding may vary depending on the responsiveness of the endometrium. If satisfactory withdrawal bleeding does not occur, an oral progestogen may be given in addition to estrogen during the third week of the cycle.

Female Castration or Primary Ovarian Failure: a daily dose of 1 estropipate 1.5 mg tablet to 3 estropipate 3.0 mg tablets may be given for the first 3 weeks of a theoretical cycle, followed by a rest period of 8-10 days. Adjust dosage upward or downward according to severity of symptoms and response of the patient. For maintenance, adjust dosage to lowest level that will provide effective control.

Treated patients with an intact uterus should be monitored closely for signs of endometrial cancer and appropriate diagnostic measures should be taken to rule out malignancy in the event of persistent or recurring abnormal vaginal bleeding.

3. For prevention of osteoporosis, A daily dose of 1 estropipate 0.75 mg tablet for 25 days of a 31 day cycle per month.

VAGINAL CREAM

For treatment of vulval and vaginal atrophy associated with the menopause, the lowest dose and regimen that will control symptoms should be chosen and medication should be discontinued as promptly as possible.

Attempts to discontinue or taper medication should be made at 3-6 month intervals.

Usual Dosage Range: Intravaginally, 2-4 g of estropipate vaginal cream daily, depending upon the severity of the condition.

HOW SUPPLIED

TABLETS

Ogen tablets are available in the following strengths:

0.625: 0.75 mg estropipate, yellow tablets.

1.25: 1.5 mg estropipate, peach-colored tablets.

2.5: 3 mg estropipate, blue tablets.

Storage: Store below 25°C (77°F).

VAGINAL CREAM

Ogen vaginal cream contains 1.5 mg estropipate per gram and is available in packages containing a 1½ oz (42.5 g) tube with one plastic applicator calibrated at 1, 2, 3, and 4 g levels.

Storage: Store below 30°C (86°F).

PRODUCT LISTING - RATED THERAPEUTICALLY EQUIVALENT

Tablet - Oral - 0.625 mg

Package	Price	Product	NDC
90's	$43.72	OGEN, Allscripts Pharmaceutical Company	54569-8525-00
100's	$29.73	GENERIC, Duramed Pharmaceuticals Inc	51285-0875-02
100's	$41.28	GENERIC, Barr Laboratories Inc	00555-0727-02
100's	$42.74	GENERIC, Ivax Corporation	00182-1976-01
100's	$42.80	GENERIC, Caremark Inc	00339-5981-12
100's	$43.05	GENERIC, Aligen Independent Laboratories Inc	00405-4413-01
100's	$43.12	GENERIC, Qualitest Products Inc	00603-3559-21
100's	$43.15	GENERIC, Watson Laboratories Inc	00591-0414-01
100's	$43.15	GENERIC, Watson Laboratories Inc	52544-0414-01
100's	$45.93	GENERIC, Mutual/United Research Laboratories	00677-1508-01
100's	$45.97	GENERIC, Geneva Pharmaceuticals	00781-1543-01
100's	$46.90	GENERIC, Duramed Pharmaceuticals Inc	51285-0010-02
100's	$47.00	GENERIC, Mylan Pharmaceuticals Inc	00378-4551-01
100's	$54.75	ORTHO-EST, Physicians Total Care	54868-3672-00
100's	$79.65	OGEN, Physicians Total Care	54868-1262-00
100's	$80.34	ORTHO-EST, Women First Healthcare	64248-0101-01
100's	$87.20	OGEN, Pharmacia Corporation	00009-3772-01

Tablet - Oral - 0.75 mg

Package	Price	Product	NDC
100's	$27.54	FEDERAL UPPER LIMIT, H.C.F.A. F F P	99999-1204-02

Tablet - Oral - 1.25 mg

Package	Price	Product	NDC
30's	$25.34	ORTHO-EST, Physicians Total Care	54868-3673-01
90's	$61.07	OGEN, Allscripts Pharmaceutical Company	54569-8551-00
100's	$54.90	ORTHO-EST, Janssen Pharmaceuticals	00062-1800-01
100's	$57.14	GENERIC, Duramed Pharmaceuticals Inc	51285-0011-02
100's	$57.14	GENERIC, Duramed Pharmaceuticals Inc	51285-0876-02
100's	$57.67	GENERIC, Barr Laboratories Inc	00555-0728-02
100's	$60.14	GENERIC, Aligen Independent Laboratories Inc	00405-4414-01
100's	$61.19	GENERIC, Caremark Inc	00339-5983-12
100's	$61.36	GENERIC, Ivax Corporation	00182-1977-01
100's	$62.00	GENERIC, Watson/Schein Pharmaceuticals Inc	00364-2601-01
100's	$62.00	GENERIC, Watson Laboratories Inc	52544-0415-01
100's	$64.22	GENERIC, Geneva Pharmaceuticals	00781-1553-01
100's	$65.00	GENERIC, Mylan Pharmaceuticals Inc	00378-4553-01
100's	$74.54	ORTHO-EST, Physicians Total Care	54868-3673-00
100's	$100.12	ORTHO-EST, Women First Healthcare	64248-0102-01
100's	$111.60	OGEN, Physicians Total Care	54868-1261-00
100's	$121.80	OGEN, Pharmacia Corporation	00009-3773-01

Tablet - Oral - 1.5 mg

Package	Price	Product	NDC
100's	$34.50	FEDERAL UPPER LIMIT, H.C.F.A. F F P	99999-1204-03
100's	$62.00	GENERIC, Watson Laboratories Inc	00591-0415-01

Tablet - Oral - 2.5 mg

Package	Price	Product	NDC
100's	$100.35	GENERIC, Qualitest Products Inc	00603-3561-21
100's	$100.39	GENERIC, Barr Laboratories Inc	00555-0729-02
100's	$100.39	GENERIC, Watson Laboratories Inc	52544-0416-01
100's	$105.06	GENERIC, Caremark Inc	00339-5985-12
100's	$106.30	GENERIC, Ivax Corporation	00182-1978-01
100's	$108.00	GENERIC, Mylan Pharmaceuticals Inc	00378-4555-01
100's	$111.77	GENERIC, Geneva Pharmaceuticals	00781-1563-01
100's	$212.01	OGEN, Pharmacia Corporation	00009-3774-01

Tablet - Oral - 3 mg

Package	Price	Product	NDC
100's	$86.22	FEDERAL UPPER LIMIT, H.C.F.A. F F P	99999-1204-01
100's	$100.39	GENERIC, Watson Laboratories Inc	00591-0416-01

PRODUCT LISTING - EQUIVALENTS NOT AVAILABLE

Tablet - Oral - 0.625 mg

Package	Price	Product	NDC
100's	$70.15	GENERIC, Pharma Pac	52959-0326-10

Etanercept (003424)

Categories: Arthritis, rheumatoid; Arthritis, psoriatic; FDA Approved 1998 Nov; Pregnancy Category B; Orphan Drugs

Drug Classes: Disease modifying antirheumatic drugs; Immunomodulators; Tumor necrosis factor modulators

Foreign Brand Availability: Enbrel (Austria; Belgium; Bulgaria; Colombia; Czech-Republic; Denmark; England; Finland; France; Germany; Greece; Hungary; Ireland; Italy; Mexico; Netherlands; New-Zealand; Norway; Philippines; Poland; Portugal; Slovenia; Spain; Sweden; Switzerland; Turkey)

Cost of Therapy: $275.00 (Rheumatoid Arthritis; Enbrel; ; 2 injections/week; variable day supply)

DESCRIPTION

Note: The trade name has been used throughout this monograph for clarity.

Enbrel (etanercept) is a dimeric fusion protein consisting of the extracellular ligand-binding portion of the human 75 kilodalton (p75) tumor necrosis factor receptor (TNFR) linked to the Fc portion of human IgG1. The Fc component of etanercept contains the C_H2 domain, the C_H3 domain and hinge region, but not the C_H1 domain of IgG1. Etanercept is produced by recombinant DNA technology in a Chinese hamster ovary (CHO) mammalian cell expression system. It consists of 934 amino acids and has an apparent molecular weight of approximately 150 kilodaltons.

Enbrel is supplied as a sterile, white, preservative-free, lyophilized powder for parenteral administration after reconstitution with 1 ml of the supplied sterile bacteriostatic water for injection (BWFI) (containing 0.9% benzyl alcohol). Reconstitution with the supplied BWFI yields a multiple-use, clear, and colorless solution of Enbrel with a pH of 7.4 ± 0.3. Each vial of Enbrel contains 25 mg etanercept, 40 mg mannitol, 10 mg sucrose, and 1.2 mg tromethamine.

CLINICAL PHARMACOLOGY

GENERAL

Etanercept binds specifically to tumor necrosis factor (TNF) and blocks its interaction with cell surface TNF receptors. TNF is a naturally occurring cytokine that is involved in normal inflammatory and immune responses. It plays an important role in the inflammatory processes of rheumatoid arthritis (RA), polyarticular-course juvenile rheumatoid arthritis (JRA), and the resulting joint pathology.[1,2] Elevated levels of TNF are found in the synovial fluid of RA patients and in both the synovium and psoriatic plaques of patients with psoriatic arthritis.[3,4]

Two distinct receptors for TNF (TNFRs), a 55 kilodalton protein (p55) and a 75 kilodalton protein (p75), exist naturally as monomeric molecules on cell surfaces and in soluble forms.[5] Biological activity of TNF is dependent upon binding to either cell surface TNFR.

Etanercept is a dimeric soluble form of the p75 TNF receptor that can bind to two TNF molecules. It inhibits the activity of TNF *in vitro* and has been shown to affect several animal models of inflammation, including murine collagen-induced arthritis.[6,7] Etanercept inhibits binding of both TNFα and TNFβ (lymphotoxin alpha [LTα]) to cell surface TNFRs, rendering TNF biologically inactive.[7] Cells expressing transmembrane TNF that bind Enbrel are not lysed *in vitro* in the presence or absence of complement.[7]

Etanercept can also modulate biological responses that are induced or regulated by TNF, including expression of adhesion molecules responsible for leukocyte migration (*i.e.*, E-selectin and to a lesser extent intercellular adhesion molecule-1 [ICAM-1]), serum levels of cytokines (*e.g.*, IL-6), and serum levels of matrix metalloproteinase-3 (MMP-3 or stromelysin).[7]

PHARMACOKINETICS

After administration of 25 mg of Enbrel by a single subcutaneous (SC) injection to 25 patients with RA, a mean ± standard deviation half-life of 102 ± 30 hours was observed with a clearance of 160 ± 80 ml/h. A maximum serum concentration (C_{max}) of 1.1 ± 0.6 μg/ml and time to C_{max} of 69 ± 34 hours was observed in these patients following a single 25 mg dose. After 6 months of twice weekly 25 mg doses in these same RA patients, the mean C_{max} was 2.4 ± 1.0 μg/ml (n=23). Patients exhibited a 2- to 7-fold increase in peak serum concentrations and approximately 4-fold increase in AUC(0-72 h) (range 1- to 17-fold) with repeated dosing. Serum concentrations in patients with RA have not been measured for periods of dosing that exceed 6 months.

Pharmacokinetic parameters were not different between men and women and did not vary with age in adult patients. No formal pharmacokinetic studies have been conducted to examine the effects of renal or hepatic impairment on Enbrel disposition or potential interactions with methotrexate.

Patients with JRA (ages 4-17 years) were administered 0.4 mg/kg of Enbrel twice weekly for up to 18 weeks. The mean serum concentration after repeated SC dosing was 2.1 μg/ml, with a range of 0.7-4.3 μg/ml. Limited data suggests that the clearance of Enbrel is reduced slightly in children ages 4-8 years. The pharmacokinetics of Enbrel in children <4 years of age have not been studied.

INDICATIONS AND USAGE

Enbrel is indicated for reducing signs and symptoms and inhibiting the progression of structural damage in patients with moderately to severely active rheumatoid arthritis. Enbrel can be used in combination with methotrexate in patients who do not respond adequately to methotrexate alone.

Enbrel is indicated for reducing signs and symptoms of moderately to severely active polyarticular-course juvenile rheumatoid arthritis in patients who have had an inadequate response to one or more DMARDs.

Enbrel is indicated for reducing signs and symptoms of active arthritis in patients with psoriatic arthritis. Enbrel can be used in combination with methotrexate in patients who do not respond adequately to methotrexate alone.

NON-FDA APPROVED INDICATIONS

While not FDA approved indications, etanercept is being evaluated in clinical trials in Wegener's granulomatosis, ankylosing spondylitis, psoriasis, and juvenile spondyloarthropathies.

CONTRAINDICATIONS

Enbrel should not be administered to patients with sepsis or with known hypersensitivity to Enbrel or any of its components.

WARNINGS

INFECTIONS

IN POST-MARKETING REPORTS, SERIOUS INFECTIONS AND SEPSIS, INCLUDING FATALITIES, HAVE BEEN REPORTED WITH THE USE OF ENBREL. MANY OF THE SERIOUS INFECTIONS HAVE OCCURRED IN PATIENTS ON CONCOMITANT IMMUNOSUPPRESSIVE THERAPY THAT, IN ADDITION TO THEIR UNDERLYING DISEASE, COULD PREDISPOSE THEM TO INFECTIONS. RARE CASES OF TUBERCULOSIS (TB) HAVE BEEN OBSERVED IN PATIENTS TREATED WITH TNF ANTAGONISTS, INCLUDING ENBREL. PATIENTS WHO DEVELOP A NEW INFECTION WHILE UNDERGOING TREATMENT WITH ENBREL SHOULD BE MONITORED CLOSELY. ADMINISTRATION OF ENBREL SHOULD BE DISCONTINUED IF A PATIENT DEVELOPS A SERIOUS INFECTION OR SEPSIS. TREATMENT WITH ENBREL SHOULD NOT BE INITIATED IN PATIENTS WITH ACTIVE INFECTIONS INCLUDING CHRONIC OR LOCALIZED INFECTIONS. PHYSICIANS SHOULD EXERCISE CAUTION WHEN CONSIDERING THE USE OF ENBREL IN PATIENTS WITH A HISTORY OF RECURRING INFECTIONS OR WITH UNDERLYING CONDITIONS WHICH MAY PREDISPOSE PATIENTS TO INFECTIONS, SUCH AS ADVANCED OR POORLY CONTROLLED DIABETES (see PRECAUTIONS and ADVERSE REACTIONS, Infections).

NEUROLOGIC EVENTS

Treatment with Enbrel and other agents that inhibit TNF have been associated with rare cases of new onset or exacerbation of central nervous system demyelinating disorders, some presenting with mental status changes and some associated with permanent disability. Cases of transverse myelitis, optic neuritis, multiple sclerosis and new onset or exacerbation of seizure disorders have been observed in association with Enbrel therapy. The causal relationship to Enbrel therapy remains unclear. While no clinical trials have been performed evaluating Enbrel therapy in patients with multiple sclerosis, other TNF antagonists administered to patients with multiple sclerosis have been associated with increases in disease activity.[15,16] Prescribers should exercise caution in considering the use of Enbrel in patients with preexisting or recent-onset central nervous system demyelinating disorders (see ADVERSE REACTIONS).

HEMATOLOGIC EVENTS

Rare reports of pancytopenia including aplastic anemia, some with a fatal outcome, have been reported in patients treated with Enbrel . The causal relationship to Enbrel therapy remains unclear. Although no high risk group has been identified, caution should be exercised in patients being treated with Enbrel who have a previous history of significant hematologic abnormalities. All patients should be advised to seek immediate medical attention if they develop signs and symptoms suggestive of blood dyscrasias or infection (*e.g.*, persistent fever, bruising, bleeding, pallor) while on Enbrel. Discontinuation of Enbrel therapy should be considered in patients with confirmed significant hematologic abnormalities.

PRECAUTIONS

GENERAL

Allergic reactions associated with administration of Enbrel during clinical trials have been reported in <2% of patients. If an anaphylactic reaction or other serious allergic reaction occurs, administration of Enbrel should be discontinued immediately and appropriate therapy initiated.

INFORMATION FOR THE PATIENT

If a patient or caregiver is to self-administer Enbrel, he/she should be instructed in injection techniques and how to measure the correct dose to help ensure the proper administration of Enbrel (see the instruction sheet that is distributed with the prescription for more information). The first injection should be performed under the supervision of a qualified health care professional. The patient's or caregiver's ability to self-inject subcutaneously should be assessed. A puncture-resistant container for disposal of needles and syringes should be used. Patients and caregivers should be instructed in the technique as well as proper syringe and needle disposal, and be cautioned against reuse of these items. If the product is intended for multiple-use, additional syringes, needles, and alcohol swabs will be required.

IMMUNOSUPPRESSION

Anti-TNF therapies, including Enbrel, affect host defenses against infections and malignancies since TNF mediates inflammation and modulates cellular immune responses. In a study of 49 patients with RA treated with Enbrel, there was no evidence of depression of delayed-type hypersensitivity, depression of immunoglobulin levels, or change in enumeration of effector cell populations. The impact of treatment with Enbrel on the development and course of malignancies, as well as active and/or chronic infections is not fully understood (see WARNINGS, ADVERSE REACTIONS, Infections and ADVERSE REACTIONS, Malignancies). The safety and efficacy of Enbrel in patients with immunosuppression or chronic infections have not been evaluated.

IMMUNIZATIONS

Most psoriatic arthritis patients receiving Enbrel were able to mount effective B-cell immune responses to pneumococcal polysaccharide vaccine, but titers in aggregate were moderately lower and fewer patients had 2-fold rises in titres compared to patients not receiving Enbrel. The clinical significance of this is unknown. Patients receiving Enbrel may receive concurrent vaccinations, except for live vaccines. No data are available on the secondary transmission of infection by live vaccines in patients receiving Enbrel (see Immunosuppression).

It is recommended that JRA patients, if possible, be brought up to date with all immunizations in agreement with current immunization guidelines prior to initiating Enbrel therapy. Patients with a significant exposure to varicella virus should temporarily discontinue Enbrel therapy and be considered for prophylactic treatment with Varicella Zoster Immune Globulin.

AUTOANTIBODY FORMATION

Treatment with Enbrel may result in the formation of autoimmune antibodies (see ADVERSE REACTIONS, Autoantibodies). In post-marketing experience, rare spontaneous adverse event reports have described patients with rheumatoid factor positive RA who have developed additional autoantibodies in conjunction with rashes compatible with subacute cutaneous lupus or discoid lupus by clinical presentation and biopsy.

CARCINOGENESIS, MUTAGENESIS, AND IMPAIRMENT OF FERTILITY

Long-term animal studies have not been conducted to evaluate the carcinogenic potential of Enbrel or its effect on fertility. Mutagenesis studies were conducted *in vitro* and *in vivo*, and no evidence of mutagenic activity was observed.

PREGNANCY CATEGORY B

Developmental toxicity studies have been performed in rats and rabbits at doses ranging from 60- to 100-fold higher than the human dose and have revealed no evidence of harm to the fetus due to Enbrel. There are, however, no studies in pregnant women. Because animal reproduction studies are not always predictive of human response, this drug should be used during pregnancy only if clearly needed.

NURSING MOTHERS

It is not known whether Enbrel is excreted in human milk or absorbed systemically after ingestion. Because many drugs and immunoglobulins are excreted in human milk, and because of the potential for serious adverse reactions in nursing infants from Enbrel, a decision should be made whether to discontinue nursing or to discontinue the drug.

GERIATRIC USE

A total of 197 RA patients ages 65 years or older have been studied in clinical trials. No overall differences in safety or effectiveness were observed between these patients and younger patients. Because there is a higher incidence of infections in the elderly population in general, caution should be used in treating the elderly.

PEDIATRIC USE

Enbrel is indicated for treatment of polyarticular-course juvenile rheumatoid arthritis in patients who have had an inadequate response to one or more DMARDs. For issues relevant to pediatric patients, in addition to other sections of the label, see also WARNINGS; PRECAUTIONS, Immunizations; and ADVERSE REACTIONS. Enbrel has not been studied in children <4 years of age.

DRUG INTERACTIONS

Specific drug interaction studies have not been conducted with Enbrel.

ADVERSE REACTIONS

ADVERSE REACTIONS IN ADULT PATIENTS WITH RA OR PSORIATIC ARTHRITIS

Enbrel has been studied in approximately 1200 patients with RA, followed for up to 36 months and in 157 patients with psoriatic arthritis for 6 months. The proportion of patients who discontinued treatment due to adverse events was approximately 4% in both Enbrel and placebo-treated patients. The vast majority of these patients were treated with the recommended dose of 25 mg SC twice weekly.

INJECTION SITE REACTIONS

In controlled trials, approximately 37% of patients treated with Enbrel developed injection site reactions. All injection site reactions were described as mild to moderate (erythema and/or itching, pain, or swelling) and generally did not necessitate drug discontinuation. Injection site reactions generally occurred in the first month and subsequently decreased in frequency. The mean duration of injection site reactions was 3-5 days. Seven percent (7%) of patients experienced redness at a previous injection site when subsequent injections were given. In post-marketing experience, injection site bleeding and bruising have also been observed in conjunction with Enbrel therapy.

E

INFECTIONS

In controlled trials, there were no differences in rates of infection among RA and psoriatic arthritis patients treated with Enbrel and those treated with placebo or MTX. The most common type of infection was upper respiratory infection, which occurred at a rate of approximately 20% among both Enbrel- and placebo-treated patients.

In placebo-controlled trials in RA and psoriatic arthritis, no increase in the incidence of serious infections was observed (approximately 1% in both placebo and Enbrel-treated groups). In all clinical trials in RA, 50 of 1197 subjects exposed to Enbrel for up to 36 months experienced serious infections, including pyelonephritis, bronchitis, septic arthritis, abdominal abscess, cellulitis, osteomyelitis, wound infection, pneumonia, foot abscess, leg ulcer, diarrhea, sinusitis, and sepsis. Serious infections, including sepsis and death, have also been reported during post-marketing use of Enbrel. Some have occurred within a few weeks after initiating treatment with Enbrel. Many of the patients had underlying conditions (*e.g.*, diabetes, congestive heart failure, history of active or chronic infections) in addition to their rheumatoid arthritis. (See WARNINGS.) Data from a sepsis clinical trial not specifically in patients with RA suggest that Enbrel treatment may increase mortality in patients with established sepsis.[17]

In post-marketing experience, infections have been observed with various pathogens including viral, bacterial, fungal, and protozoal organisms. Infections have been noted in all organ systems and have been reported in patients receiving Enbrel alone or in combination with immunosuppressive agents.

MALIGNANCIES

Seventeen malignancies of various types were observed in 1197 RA patients treated in clinical trials with Enbrel for up to 36 months. The observed rates and incidences were similar to those expected for the population studied.

IMMUNOGENICITY

Patients with RA or psoriatic arthritis were tested at multiple timepoints for antibodies to Enbrel. Antibodies to the TNF receptor portion or other protein components of the Enbrel drug product, all non-neutralizing, were detected at least once in sera of <5% of adult patients with rheumatoid arthritis or psoriatic arthritis. No apparent correlation of antibody development to clinical response or adverse events was observed. Results from JRA patients were similar to those seen in adult RA patients treated with Enbrel. The long-term immunogenicity of Enbrel is unknown.

The data reflect the percentage of patients whose test results were considered positive for antibodies to Enbrel in an ELISA assay, and are highly dependent on the sensitivity and specificity of the assay. Additionally, the observed incidence of antibody positivity in an assay may be influenced by several factors including sample handling, concomitant medications, and underlying disease. For these reasons, comparison of the incidence of antibodies to Enbrel with the incidence of antibodies to other products may be misleading.

AUTOANTIBODIES

Patients had serum samples tested for autoantibodies at multiple timepoints. In Studies I and II, the percentage of patients evaluated for antinuclear antibodies (ANA) who developed new positive ANA (titer =1:40) was higher in patients treated with Enbrel (11%) than in placebo-treated patients (5%). The percentage of patients who developed new positive anti-double-stranded DNA antibodies was also higher by radioimmunoassay (15% of patients treated with Enbrel compared to 4% of placebo-treated patients) and by crithidia lucilae assay (3% of patients treated with Enbrel compared to none of placebo-treated patients). The proportion of patients treated with Enbrel who developed anticardiolipin antibodies was similarly increased compared to placebo-treated patients. In Study III, no pattern of increased autoantibody development was seen in Enbrel patients compared to MTX patients.

No patients in placebo- and active-controlled trials developed clinical signs suggestive of a lupus-like syndrome. The impact of long-term treatment with Enbrel on the development of autoimmune diseases is unknown. In post-marketing experience, very rare spontaneous adverse event reports have described patients with rheumatoid factor positive and/or erosive RA who have developed additional autoantibodies in conjunction with rash after Enbrel therapy.

OTHER ADVERSE REACTIONS

TABLE 5 summarizes events reported in at least 3% of all patients with higher incidence in patients treated with Enbrel compared to controls in placebo-controlled RA trials (including the combination methotrexate trial) and relevant events from Study III. Adverse events in the psoriatic arthritis trial were similar to those reported in RA clinical trials.

In controlled trials of RA and psoriatic arthritis, rates of serious adverse events were seen at a frequency of approximately 5% among Enbrel- and control-treated patients. Among patients with RA in placebo-controlled, active-controlled, and open-label trials of Enbrel, malignancies (see Malignancies) and infections (see Infections) were the most common serious adverse events observed. Other infrequent serious adverse events observed in RA and psoriatic arthritis clinical trials are listed by body system below:

Cardiovascular: Heart failure, myocardial infarction, myocardial ischemia, hypertension, hypotension, deep vein thrombosis, thrombophlebitis.
Digestive: Cholecystitis, pancreatitis, gastrointestinal hemorrhage.
Musculoskeletal: Bursitis, polymyositis.
Nervous: Cerebral ischemia, depression, multiple sclerosis (see WARNINGS).
Respiratory: Dyspnea, pulmonary embolism.
Urogenital: Membranous glomerulonephropathy.

In a randomized controlled trial in which 51 patients with RA received Enbrel 50 mg twice weekly and 25 patients received Enbrel 25 mg twice weekly, the following serious adverse events were observed in the 50 mg twice weekly arm: gastrointestinal bleeding, normal pressure hydrocephalous, seizure, and stroke. No serious adverse events were observed in the 25 mg arm.

TABLE 5 *Percent of RA Patients Reporting Adverse Events in Controlled Clinical Trials**

	Placebo Controlled		Active Controlled (Study III)	
Event	Placebo† (n=152)	Enbrel (n=349)	MTX (n=217)	Enbrel (n=415)
Injection site reaction	10%	37%	7%	34%
Infection (total)‡	32%	35%	72%	64%
Non-upper respiratory infection (non-URI)‡	32%	38%	60%	51%
Upper respiratory infection (URI)‡	16%	29%	39%	31%
Headache	13%	17%	27%	24%
Nausea	10%	9%	29%	15%
Rhinitis	8%	12%	14%	16%
Dizziness	5%	7%	11%	8%
Pharyngitis	5%	7%	9%	6%
Cough	3%	6%	6%	5%
Asthenia	3%	5%	12%	11%
Abdominal pain	3%	5%	10%	10%
Rash	3%	5%	23%	14%
Peripheral edema	3%	2%	4%	8%
Respiratory disorder	1%	5%	NA	NA
Dyspepsia	1%	4%	10%	11%
Sinusitis	2%	3%	3%	5%
Vomiting	—	3%	8%	5%
Mouth ulcer	1%	2%	14%	6%
Alopecia	1%	1%	12%	6%
Pneumonitis ("MTX lung")	—	—	2%	0%

* Includes data from the 6 month study in which patients received concurrent MTX therapy.
† The duration of exposure for patients receiving placebo was less than the Enbrel-treated patients.
‡ Infection (total) includes data from all three placebo-controlled trials. Non-URI and URI include data only from the two placebo-controlled trials where infections were collected separately from adverse evnets (placebo n=110, Enbrel n=213).

ADVERSE REACTIONS IN PATIENTS WITH JRA

In general, the adverse events in pediatric patients were similar in frequency and type as those seen in adult patients (see WARNINGS and other sections under ADVERSE REACTIONS). Differences from adults and other special considerations are discussed in the following paragraphs.

Severe adverse reactions reported in 69 JRA patients ages 4-17 years included varicella (see also PRECAUTIONS, Immunizations), gastroenteritis, depression/personality disorder, cutaneous ulcer, esophagitis/gastritis, group A streptococcal septic shock, Type I diabetes mellitus, and soft tissue and post-operative wound infection.

Forty-three of 69 (62%) children with JRA experienced an infection while receiving Enbrel during 3 months of study (part 1 open-label), and the frequency and severity of infections was similar in 58 patients completing 12 months of open-label extension therapy. The types of infections reported in JRA patients were generally mild and consistent with those commonly seen in outpatient pediatric populations. Two JRA patients developed varicella infection and signs and symptoms of aseptic meningitis which resolved without sequelae.

The following adverse events were reported more commonly in 69 JRA patients receiving 3 months of Enbrel compared to the 349 adult RA patients in placebo-controlled trials. These included headache (19% of patients, 1.7 events per patient year), nausea (9%, 1.0 events per patient year), abdominal pain (19%, 0.74 events per patient year), and vomiting (13%, 0.74 events per patient year).

In post-marketing experience, the following additional serious adverse events have been reported in pediatric patients: abscess with bacteremia, optic neuritis, pancytopenia, seizures, tuberculous arthritis, urinary tract infection (see WARNINGS), coagulopathy, cutaneous vasculitis, and transaminase elevations. The frequency of these events and their causal relationship to Enbrel therapy are unknown.

ADVERSE REACTION INFORMATION FROM SPONTANEOUS REPORTS

Adverse events have been reported during post-approval use of Enbrel. Because these events are reported voluntarily from a population of uncertain size, it is not always possible to reliably estimate their frequency or establish a causal relationship to Enbrel exposure.

Additional adverse events are listed by body system below:

Body as a Whole: Angioedema, fatigue, fever, flu syndrome, generalized pain, weight gain.
Cardiovascular: Chest pain, vasodilation (flushing).
Digestive: Altered sense of taste, anorexia, diarrhea, dry mouth, intestinal perforation.
Hematologic/Lymphatic: Adenopathy, anemia, aplastic anemia, leukopenia, pancytopenia, thrombocytopenia, (see WARNINGS).
Musculoskeletal: Joint pain.

Nervous: Paresthesias, stroke, seizures and central nervous system events suggestive of multiple sclerosis or isolated demyelinating conditions such as transverse myelitis or optic neuritis (see WARNINGS).
Ocular: Dry eyes, ocular inflammation.
Respiratory: Dyspnea, interstitial lung disease, pulmonary disease, worsening of prior lung disorder.
Skin: Cutaneous vasculitis, pruritis, subcutaneous nodules, urticaria.

DOSAGE AND ADMINISTRATION

ADULT RA AND PSORIATIC ARTHRITIS PATIENTS

The recommended dose of Enbrel for adult patients with rheumatoid arthritis or psoriatic arthritis is 25 mg given twice weekly as a subcutaneous injection 72-96 hours apart. Methotrexate, glucocorticoids, salicylates, nonsteroidal anti-inflammatory drugs (NSAIDs), or analgesics may be continued during treatment with Enbrel. Based on a study of 50 mg Enbrel twice weekly in patients with RA that suggested higher incidence of adverse reactions but similar ACR response rates, doses higher than 25 mg twice weekly are not recommended (see ADVERSE REACTIONS).

JRA PATIENTS

The recommended dose of Enbrel for pediatric patients ages 4-17 years with active polyarticular-course JRA is 0.4 mg/kg (up to a maximum of 25 mg per dose) given twice weekly as a subcutaneous injection 72-96 hours apart. Glucocorticoids, nonsteroidal anti-inflammatory drugs (NSAIDs), or analgesics may be continued during treatment with Enbrel.

Concurrent use with methotrexate and higher doses of Enbrel have not been studied in pediatric patients.

PREPARATION OF ENBREL

Enbrel is intended for use under the guidance and supervision of a physician. Patients may self-inject only if their physician determines that it is appropriate and with medical follow-up, as necessary, after proper training in how to measure the correct dose and in injection technique.

Note: The needle cover of the diluent syringe contains dry natural rubber (latex), which should not be handled by persons sensitive to this substance.

Enbrel should be reconstituted aseptically with 1 ml of the supplied sterile bacteriostatic water for injection (0.9% benzyl alcohol) giving a solution of 1.0 ml containing 25 mg of Enbrel. During reconstitution of Enbrel, the diluent should be injected very slowly into the vial. Some foaming will occur. This is normal. To avoid excessive foaming, do not shake or vigorously agitate. The contents should be swirled gently during dissolution. Generally, dissolution of Enbrel takes less than 10 minutes. Reconstitution with the supplied BWFI yields a multiple-use, preservative solution that expires 14 days after reconstitution. For pediatric patients to be treated with less than a 25 mg dose, write the date in the area marked "Mixing Date:" on the supplied sticker and attach the sticker to the vial immediately after reconstitution. Contents of one vial of Enbrel solution should not be mixed with, or transferred into the contents of another vial of Enbrel. No other medications should be added to solutions containing Enbrel, and do not reconstitute Enbrel with other diluents.

Do not filter reconstituted solution during preparation or administration.

Visually inspect the solution for particulate matter and discoloration prior to administration. The solution should not be used if discolored or cloudy, or if particulate matter remains.

ADMINISTRATION OF ENBREL

Withdraw the solution into a syringe, removing only the dose to be given from the vial. Some foam or bubbles may remain in the vial.

Rotate sites for injection (thigh, abdomen, or upper arm). New injections should be given at least 1 inch from an old site and never into areas where the skin is tender, bruised, red, or hard. See the instruction sheet that is distributed with the prescription for detailed information on injection site selection and dose administration.

STORAGE AND STABILITY

Do not use a dose tray beyond the expiration date stamped on the carton, dose tray label, vial label, or diluent syringe label. The dose tray containing Enbrel (sterile powder) must be refrigerated at 2-8°C (36-46°F). DO NOT FREEZE.

Reconstituted solutions of Enbrel prepared with the supplied bacteriostatic water for injection (0.9% benzyl alcohol) may be stored for up to 14 days if refrigerated at 2-8°C (36-46°F). Discard reconstituted solution after 14 days. **PRODUCT STABILITY AND STERILITY CANNOT BE ASSURED AFTER 14 DAYS.**

HOW SUPPLIED

Enbrel is supplied in a carton containing four dose trays. Each dose tray contains one 25 mg vial of etanercept, one syringe containing 1 ml sterile bacteriostatic water for injection (0.9% benzyl alcohol), one plunger, two alcohol swabs, and a dating sticker for the vial of Enbrel.

PRODUCT LISTING - EQUIVALENTS NOT AVAILABLE

Powder For Injection - Subcutaneous - 25 mg

1's	$155.70	ENBREL, Immunex Corporation	58406-0425-41
4's	$653.30	ENBREL, Immunex Corporation	58406-0425-34

Ethambutol Hydrochloride *(001206)*

For complete prescribing information, refer to the CD-ROM included with the book.

Categories: Tuberculosis; FDA Approved 1967 Nov; Pregnancy Category B; WHO Formulary
Drug Classes: Antimycobacterials
Brand Names: **Myambutol**
Foreign Brand Availability: Althocin (Greece); Ambutol (Malaysia); Apo-Ethambutol (New-Zealand); Arbutol (Indonesia); Blomison (Greece); Clobutol (Portugal); Combutol (India); Conbutol (Thailand); Corsabutol (Indonesia); EMB (Germany); Ebutol (Japan); Esanbutol (Japan); Etapiam (Italy); Ethambin-PIN (Philippines); Ethbutol (Thailand); Etibi (Austria; Canada; Indonesia; Italy); Interbutol (Philippines); Lambutol (Thailand); Mycobutol (Benin; Burkina-Faso; Ethiopia; Gambia; Ghana; Guinea; Ivory-Coast; Kenya; Liberia; Malawi; Mali; Mauritania; Mauritius; Morocco; Niger; Nigeria; Senegal; Seychelles; Sierra-Leone; Sudan; Tanzania; Tunia; Uganda; Zambia; Zimbabwe); Mycrol (South-Africa); Odetol (Philippines); Servambutol (Peru); Stambutol (Finland); Tambutol (Korea); Tibigon (Indonesia); Tibitol (India); Tibutol (Peru); Tobutol (Thailand)
Cost of Therapy: $119.10 (Tuberculosis; Myambutol; 400 mg; 2 tablets/day; 30 day supply)

E

DESCRIPTION

Myambutol (ethambutol hydrochloride) is an oral chemotherapeutic agent which is specifically effective against actively growing microorganisms of the genus *Mycobacterium*, including *M. tuberculosis.*

Myambutol 100 and 400 mg tablets contain the following inactive ingredients: gelatin, hydroxypropyl methylcellulose, magnesium stearate, sodium lauryl sulfate, sorbitol, stearic acid, sucrose, titanium dioxide and other ingredients.

INDICATIONS AND USAGE

Ethambutol HCl is indicated for the treatment of pulmonary tuberculosis. It should not be used as the sole antituberculous drug, but should be used in conjunction with at least one other antituberculous drug. Selection of the companion drug should be based on clinical experience, considerations of comparative safety and appropriate *in vitro* susceptibility studies. In patients who have not received previous antituberculous therapy, *i.e.*, initial treatment, the most frequently used regimens have been the following:

Ethambutol HCl plus isoniazid.
Ethambutol HCl plus isoniazid plus streptomycin.

In patients who have received previous antituberculous therapy, mycobacterial resistance to other drugs used in initial therapy is frequent. Consequently, in such retreatment patients, ethambutol should be combined with at least one of the second line drugs not previously administered to the patient and to which bacterial susceptibility has been indicated by appropriate *in vitro* studies.

Antituberculous drugs used with ethambutol have included cycloserine, ethionamide, pyrazinamide, viomycin and other drugs. Isoniazid, aminosalicylic acid, and streptomycin have also been used in multiple drug regimens.

Alternating drug regimens have also been utilized.

NON-FDA APPROVED INDICATIONS

Ethambutol is also used, although not FDA approved, in the treatment of nontuberculous mycobacterial infections (M. kansasii and M. avium-intracellulare complex). It has been recommended by the U.S. Public Health Service and Infectious Diseases Society of America (USPHS/IDSA) task force on prevention of opportunistic infections for use in HIV-infected patients for the prophylaxis of recurrent mycobacterium avium-intracellulare complex.

CONTRAINDICATIONS

Ethambutol HCl is contraindicated in patients who are known to be hypersensitive to this drug. It is also contraindicated in patients with known optic neuritis unless clinical judgement determines that it may be used.

DOSAGE AND ADMINISTRATION

Ethambutol HCl should not be used alone, in initial treatment or in retreatment.

Ethambutol HCl should be administered on a once every 24 hour basis only.

Absorption is not significantly altered by administration with food. Therapy, in general, should be continued until bacteriological conversion has become permanent and maximal clinical improvement has occurred.

Ethambutol HCl is not recommended for use in pediatric patients under 13 years of age since safe conditions for use have not been established.

INITIAL TREATMENT

In patients who have not received previous antituberculous therapy, administer ethambutol 15 mg/kg (7 mg/lb) of body weight, as a single oral dose once every 24 hours. In the more recent studies, isoniazid has been administered concurrently in a single, daily, oral dose.

RETREATMENT

In patients who have received previous antituberculous therapy, administer ethambutol 25 mg/kg (11 mg/lb) of body weight, as a single oral dose once every 24 hours. Concurrently administer at least one other antituberculous drug to which the organisms have been demonstrated to be susceptible by appropriate *in vitro* tests. Suitable drugs usually consist of those not previously used in the treatment of the patient. After 60 days of ethambutol administration, decrease the dose to 15 mg/kg (7 mg/lb) of body weight, and administer as a single oral dose once every 24 hours.

During the period when a patient is on a daily dose of 25 mg/kg, monthly eye examinations are advised.

See TABLE 2 and TABLE 3 for easy selection of proper weight-dose tablet(s).

TABLE 2 *Weight-Dose Table — 15 mg/kg (7 mg/lb) Schedule*

Weight Range		Daily Dose
Under 85 lb	Under 37 kg	500 mg
85-94.5 lb	37-43 kg	600 mg
95-109.5 lb	43-50 kg	700 mg
110-124.5 lb	50-57 kg	800 mg
125-139.5 lb	57-64 kg	900 mg
140-154.5 lb	64-71 kg	1000 mg
155-169.5 lb	71-79 kg	1100 mg
170-184.5 lb	79-84 kg	1200 mg
185-199.5 lb	84-90 kg	1300 mg
200-214.5 lb	90-97 kg	1400 mg
215 lb and over	Over 97 kg	1500 mg

TABLE 3 *Weight-Dose Table — 25 mg/kg (11 mg/lb) Schedule*

Weight Range		Daily Dose
Under 85 lb	Under 38 kg	900 mg
85-92.5 lb	38-42 kg	1000 mg
93-101.5 lb	42-45.5 kg	1100 mg
102-109.5 lb	45.5-50 kg	1200 mg
110-118.5 lb	50-54 kg	1300 mg
119-128.5 lb	54-58 kg	1400 mg
129-136.5 lb	58-62 kg	1500 mg
137-146.5 lb	62-67 kg	1600 mg
147-155.5 lb	67-71 kg	1700 mg
156-164.5 lb	71-75 kg	1800 mg
165-173.5 lb	75-79 kg	1900 mg
174-182.5 lb	79-83 kg	2000 mg
183-191.5 lb	83-87 kg	2100 mg
192-199.5 lb	87-91 kg	2200 mg
200-209.5 lb	91-95 kg	2300 mg
210-218.5 lb	95-99 kg	2400 mg
219 lb and over	Over 99 kg	2500 mg

PRODUCT LISTING - RATED THERAPEUTICALLY EQUIVALENT

Tablet - Oral - 100 mg

100's	$59.33	MYAMBUTOL, Dura Pharmaceuticals	51479-0046-01
100's	$59.33	MYAMBUTOL, Allscripts Pharmaceutical Company	54569-4084-00

Tablet - Oral - 400 mg

30's	$67.24	MYAMBUTOL, Physicians Total Care	54868-2876-02
40's	$71.42	MYAMBUTOL, Allscripts Pharmaceutical Company	54569-3070-01
60's	$106.68	GENERIC, Versapharm Inc	61748-0014-06
60's	$110.78	MYAMBUTOL, Allscripts Pharmaceutical Company	54569-3070-00
90's	$160.02	GENERIC, Versapharm Inc	61748-0014-09
100's	$177.92	GENERIC, Versapharm Inc	61748-0014-01
100's	$178.63	GENERIC, Barr Laboratories Inc	00555-0923-02
100's	$198.50	MYAMBUTOL, Dura Pharmaceuticals	51479-0047-01
100's	$198.50	MYAMBUTOL, Dura Pharmaceuticals	51479-0047-04
100's	$208.56	MYAMBUTOL, Physicians Total Care	54868-2876-00

PRODUCT LISTING - EQUIVALENTS NOT AVAILABLE

Tablet - Oral - 100 mg

100's	$59.21	GENERIC, Versapharm Inc	61748-0011-01

Tablet - Oral - 400 mg

100's	$177.92	GENERIC, Versapharm Inc	61748-0014-11

Ethinyl Estradiol *(001216)*

Categories: Carcinoma, breast; Carcinoma, prostate; Hypogonadism, female; Menopause; Pregnancy Category X; FDA Approved 1943 Jun; WHO Formulary
Drug Classes: Estrogens; Hormones/hormone modifiers
Brand Names: Estinyl; Feminone; Mikrofollin
Foreign Brand Availability: Estinyl Oestradiol (France); Esto (Korea); Ethinylestradiolum (Netherlands); Etinilestradiolo (Italy); Ginormon (Portugal); Lynoral (India; Indonesia; Netherlands); Progynon C (Austria; Germany)
Cost of Therapy: $10.44 (Menopause; Estinyl; 0.02 mg; 1 tablet/day; 28 day supply)

WARNING

1. ESTROGENS HAVE BEEN REPORTED TO INCREASE THE RISK RATIO OF ENDOMETRIAL CARCINOMA.

Three independent case control studies have reported an increased risk ratio of endometrial cancer in postmenopausal women exposed to exogenous estrogens for prolonged periods. This risk ratio was independent of the other risk factors for endometrial cancer. These studies are further supported by the report that incidence rates of endometrial cancer have increased sharply since 1969 in eight different areas of the US with population-based cancer reporting systems, an increase which may be related to the rapidly expanding use of estrogens during the last decade.

The three case control studies reported that the risk ratio of endometrial cancer in estrogen users was about 4.5 to 13.9 times greater than in nonusers. The risk ratio appears to depend on both duration of treatment and on estrogen dose. In view of these reports, when estrogens are used for the treatment of menopausal symptoms, the lowest dose that will control symptoms should be utilized and medication should be discontinued as soon as possible. When prolonged treatment is medically indicated, the patient should be reassessed on at least a semi-annual basis to determine the need for continued therapy. Although the evidence must be considered preliminary, one study suggests that cyclic administration of low doses of estrogen may carry less risk than continuous administration, it therefore appears prudent to utilize such a regimen.

Close clinical surveillance of all women taking estrogens is important. In all cases of undiagnosed persistent of recurring abnormal vaginal bleeding, adequate diagnostic measures should be undertaken to rule out malignancy.

There is no evidence at present that "natural" estrogens are more or less hazardous than "synthetic" estrogens at equiestrogenic doses.

2. ESTROGENS SHOULD NOT BE USED DURING PREGNANCY.

The use of estrogens during early pregnancy may seriously damage the offspring. It has been reported that females exposed in utero to diethylstilbestrol, a nonsteroidal estrogen, may have an increased risk of developing in later life a form of vaginal or cervical cancer that is ordinarily extremely rare. This risk has been estimated statistically as not greater than 4 per 1000 exposures. In certain studies, a high percentage of such exposed women (from 30% to 90%) have been found to have vaginal adenosis, epithelial changes of the vagina and cervix. Although these changes are histologically benign, it is not known whether they are precursors of malignancy. Although similar data are not available with the use of other estrogens, it cannot be presumed they would not induce similar changes. Exposure to diethylstilbestrol has also been associated with adverse effects on reproductive performance, including increased rates of spontaneous abortion, ectopic pregnancy, premature deliveries, and perinatal deaths.

Several reports suggest an association between intrauterine fetal exposure to female sex hormones and congenital anomalies, including congenital heart defects and limb reduction defects. One case control study estimated a 4.7-fold increased risk of limb reduction defects in infants exposed in utero to sex hormones (oral contraceptives, hormone withdrawal tests for pregnancy, or attempted treatment for threatened abortion). Some of these exposures were very short and involved only a few days of treatment. The data suggests that the risk of limb reduction defects in exposed fetuses is somewhat less than 1 per 1000.

In the past, estrogens have been used during pregnancy in an attempt to treat threatened or habitual abortion. There is considerable evidence that estrogens are ineffective for these indications.

If ethinyl estradiol is used during pregnancy, or if the patient becomes pregnant while taking this drug, she should be apprised of the potential risks to the fetus, and the advisability of pregnancy continuation.

DESCRIPTION

Estinyl contains ethinyl estradiol, a potent synthetic estrogen, having the chemical name 19-Nor-17α-pregna-1,3,5(10)-trien-20-yne-3,17-diol; the chemical formula $C_{20}H_{24}O_2$; a molecular weight of 296.41.

Ethinyl estradiol is a white to creamy white, odorless, crystalline powder. It is insoluble in water, soluble in alcohol, chloroform, either, and vegetable oils.

Biologically, estrogens may be defined as compounds capable of stimulating, female secondary sex characteristics. Chemically, there are different groups of estrogens, depending on whether they are natural or synthetic, steroidal or non-steroidal. Natural human estrogens are ultimately formed from either androstenedione of testosterone as immediate precursors. Ethinyl estradiol is a synthetic, steroidal estrogen.

Ethinyl estradiol, for oral administration, is available in tablets containing 0.02, 0.05, or 0.5 mg ethinyl estradiol.

The inactive ingredients for ethinyl estradiol 0.02 mg include: acacia, butylparaben, calcium phosphate, calcium sulfate, carnauba wax, corn starch, FD&C blue no. 2 Al Lake, FD&C yellow no. 5, FD&C yellow no. 5 Al Lake, FD&C yellow no. 6 aluminum lake, gelatin, lactose, magnesium stearate, potato starch, sodium phosphate, sugar, and white wax. May contain talc.

The inactive ingredients for ethinyl estradiol 0.05 mg include, acacia, butylparaben, calcium phosphate, calcium sulfate, carnauba wax, corn starch, FD&C blue no. 1, FD&C red no. 3, gelatin, lactose, magnesium stearate, potato starch, sodium phosphate, and white wax. May also contain talc.

The inactive ingredients for ethinyl estradiol 0.5 mg include: corn starch, FD&C yellow no. 6, lactose, magnesium stearate and sodium phosphate.

Storage: Store between 2° and 30°C (36° and 86°F).

CLINICAL PHARMACOLOGY

Ethinyl estradiol is synthetic derivative of the natural estrogen, estradiol.

Ethinyl estradiol, like estradiol, promotes growth of the endometrium and thickening, stratification and cornification of the vagina. It causes growth of the ducts of the mammary glands, but inhibits lactation. It also inhibits the anterior pituitary and causes capillary dilatation, fluid retention, and protein anabolism.

Estradiol is the major estrogen in premenopausal women, with up to 100- 600 µg being secreted daily by the ovary. Natural estrogens are poorly effective when given by mouth. Apparently this is due to rapid clearance of the endogenous hormone from blood, along with a "first-pass-effect" after oral administration. The addition of a 17-alpha-ethinyl group to estradiol increases potency and enhances oral activity by impeding hepatic degradation. The oral efficacy of ethinyl estradiol is related to slower elimination than estradiol from the circulation. A part of ingested ethinyl estradiol is excreted in glucuronide form via urine in animals and in man, but also extensive metabolism of the steroid nucleus occurs. The major metabolism takes place mainly in the liver. Large amounts of ethinyl estradiol metabolites are excreted via human bite, much similar to what has been reported for estradiol. However, unlike, ethinyl estradiol metabolites do not exclusively leave via urine. Urinary recovery is much less than that of estradiol and substantial amounts of ethinyl estradiol metabolites appear in human feces. Quantitatively, the major metabolic pathway for ethinyl estradiol, both in rats and in humans, is aromatic hydroxylation, as it is for the natural estrogens.

Rapid and complete absorption follows oral intake of ethinyl estradiol. Elimination of ethinyl estradiol from plasma proceeds slower than that of estradiol. After oral administration, an initial peak occurs in plasma at 2-3 hours, with a secondary peak at about 12 hours after dosing; the second peak is interpreted as evidence for extensive enterohepatic circulation of ethinyl estradiol.

INDICATIONS AND USAGE

Ethinyl estradiol are indicated in the treatment of: (1) Moderate to severe *vasomotor* symptoms associated with the menopause. (There is no evidence that estrogens are effective for nervous symptoms or depression which might occur during menopause, and they should not be used to treat these conditions.) (2) Female hypogonadism. (3) Prostatic carcinoma-palliative therapy of advanced disease. (4) Breast cancer (for palliation only) in appropriately selected women; such as those who are more than 5 years postmenopausal with progressing inoperable or radiation-resistant disease.

ETHINYL ESTRADIOL HAS NOT BEEN SHOWN TO BE EFFECTIVE FOR ANY PURPOSE DURING PREGNANCY AND ITS USE MAY CAUSE SEVERE HARM TO THE FETUS (SEE BOXED WARNING.)

The lowest effective dose appropriate for the specific indication should be used. Studies of the addition of a progestin for 7 or more days or a cycle of estrogen administration have reported a lowered incidence of endometrial hyperplasia. Morphological and biochemical studies of endometrium suggest that 10-13 days or progestin are needed to provide maximal maturation of the endometrium and to eliminate any hyperplastic changes. Whether this will provide protection from endometrial carcinoma has not been clearly established. There are possible additional risks which may be associated with the inclusion of progestin in estrogen replacement regimens. The potential risks include adverse effects on carbohydrate and lipid metabolism. The choice of progestin and dosage may be important in minimizing these adverse effects.

NON-FDA APPROVED INDICATIONS

Other estrogens have been used for treatment of atrophic vaginitis, vulvular atrophy (kraurosis vulvae) and atrophic urethritis, for the prevention of osteoporosis in postmenopausal women, abnormal uterine bleeding, gastrointestinal bleeding in patients with renal failure, and gastrointestinal bleeding related to arteriovenous malformations.

CONTRAINDICATIONS

Estrogens should not be used in women (or men) with any of the following conditions:

1. Known or suspected cancer of the breast except in appropriately selected patients being treated for metastatic disease.
2. Known or suspected estrogen-dependent neoplasia.
3. Known or suspected pregnancy (see BOXED WARNING).
4. Undiagnosed abnormal genital bleeding.
5. Active thrombophlebitis or thromboembolic disorders.
6. A past history of thrombophlebitis, thrombosis, or thromboembolic disorders associated with previous estrogen use (except when used in treatment of breast or prostatic malignancy).

WARNINGS

INDUCTION OF MALIGNANT NEOPLASMS

Long-term continuous administration of natural and synthetic estrogens in certain animal species increases the frequency of carcinomas of the breast, cervix, vagina, and liver. There is now evidence that estrogens increase the risk of carcinoma of the endometrium in humans. (See BOXED WARNING.)

At the present time there is no satisfactory evidence that estrogens given to postmenopausal women increase the risk of cancer of the breast, although a recent long-term follow-up of a single physician's practice has raised this possibility. Because of the animal data, there is a need for caution in prescribing estrogens for women with a strong family history of breast cancer or who have breast nodules, fibrocystic disease, or abnormal mammograms.

Estrogens have been reported to be associated with carcinoma of the male breast and suspicious lesions in males receiving estrogen therapy should be investigated accordingly.

GALLBLADDER DISEASE

A recent study has reported a 2- to 3-fold increase in the risk of surgically confirmed gallbladder disease in women receiving postmenopausal estrogens, similar to the 2-fold increase previously noted in users of oral contraceptives. In the case of oral contraceptives, the increased risk appeared after 2 years of use.

EFFECTS SIMILAR TO THOSE CAUSED BY ESTROGEN-PROGESTOGEN ORAL CONTRACEPTIVES

There are several serious adverse effects of oral contraceptives, most of which have not, up to now, been documented as consequences of postmenopausal estrogen therapy. This may reflect the comparatively low doses of estrogen used in postmenopausal women. It would be expected that the larger doses of estrogen used to treat prostatic or breast cancer are more likely to result in these adverse effects, and, in fact, it has been shown that there is an increased risk of thrombosis in men receiving estrogens for prostatic cancer.

Thromboembolic Disease

It is now well established that users of oral contraceptives have an increased risk of various thromboembolic and thrombotic vascular diseases, such as thrombophlebitis, pulmonary embolism, stroke, and myocardial infarction. Cases of retinal thrombosis, mesenteric thrombosis, and optic neuritis have been reported in oral contraceptive users. There is evidence that the risk of several of these adverse reactions is related to the dose of the drug. An increased risk of postsurgery thromboembolic complications has also been reported in users of oral contraceptives. If feasible, estrogen should be discontinued at least 4 weeks before surgery of the type associated with an increased risk of thromboembolism, or during periods of immobilization.

While an increased rate of thromboembolic and thrombotic disease in postmenopausal users of estrogen has not been found, this does not rule out the possibility that such an increase may be present or that subgroups of women who have underlying risk factors or who are receiving relatively large doses of estrogens may have increased risk. Therefore, estrogens should not be used in persons with active thrombophlebitis or thromboembolic disorders, and they should not be used (except in treatment of malignancy) in persons with a history of such disorders in association with estrogen use. They should be used with caution in patients with cerebral vascular or coronary artery disease and only for those in whom estrogens are clearly needed.

Large doses of estrogen (5 mg conjugated estrogens per day), comparable to those used to treat cancer of the prostate and breast, have been shown in a large prospective clinical trial in men to increase the risk of nonfatal myocardial infarction, pulmonary embolism and thrombophlebitis. When estrogen doses of this size are used, any of the thromboembolic and thrombotic adverse effects associated with oral contraceptive use should be considered a clear risk.

Hepatic Adenoma

Benign hepatic adenomas appear to be associated with the use of oral contraceptives. Although benign, and rate, these may rupture and may cause death through intra-abdominal hemorrhage. Such lesions have not yet been reported in association with other estrogen or progestogen preparations, but should be considered in estrogen users having abdominal pain and tenderness, abdominal mass, or hypovolemic shock. Hepatocellular carcinoma has also been reported in women taking estrogen-containing oral contraceptives. The relationship of this malignancy to these drugs is not known at this time.

Elevated Blood Pressure

Increased blood pressure is not uncommon in women using oral contraceptives. There is now a report that this may occur with use of estrogens in the menopause and blood pressure should be monitored with estrogen use, especially if high doses are used.

Glucose Tolerance

A worsening or glucose tolerance has been observed in a significant percentage of patients on estrogen-containing oral contraceptives. For this reason, diabetic patients should be carefully observed while receiving estrogen.

HYPERCALCEMIA

Administration of estrogens may lead to severe hypercalcemia in patients with breast cancer and bone metastases. If this occurs, the drug should be stooped and appropriate measures taken to reduce the serum calcium level.

PRECAUTIONS

GENERAL

1. A complete medical and family history should be taken prior to the initiation of any estrogen therapy. The pretreatment and periodic physical examinations should include special reference to blood pressure, breasts, abdomen, and pelvic organs, and should include a Papanicolaou smear. As a general rule, estrogen should not be prescribed for longer than 1 year without another physical examination being performed.
2. Fluid retention-Because estrogens may cause some degree of fluid retention, conditions which might be influenced by this factor, such as epilepsy, migraine, and cardiac or renal dysfunction, require careful observation.
3. Certain patients may develop undesirable manifestations of excessive estrogenic stimulation, such as abnormal or excessive uterine bleeding, mastodynia, etc.
4. Oral contraceptives appear to be associated with an increased incidence of mental depression. Although it is not clear whether this is due to the estrogenic or progestogenic component of the contraceptive, patients with a history of depression should be carefully observed.
5. Preexisting uterine leiomyomata may increase in size during estrogen use.
6. The pathologist should be advised of estrogen therapy when relevant specimens are submitted.
7. Patients with a past history of jaundice during pregnancy have an increased risk of recurrence of jaundice while receiving estrogen-containing oral contraceptive therapy. If jaundice develops in any patient receiving estrogen, the medication should be discontinued while the cause is investigated.
8. Estrogens may be poorly metabolized in patients with impaired liver function and they should be administered with caution in such patients.
9. Because estrogens influence the metabolism or calcium an phosphorus, they should be used with caution in patients with metabolic bone diseases that are associated with hypercalcemia or in patients with renal insufficiency.
10. Because of the effects of estrogens on epiphyseal closure, they should be used judiciously in young patients in whom bone growth is not complete.
11. Ethinyl estradiol, 0.02 mg, contain FD&C Yellow No. 5 (tartrazine) which may cause allergic-type reactions (including bronchial asthma) in certain susceptible individuals. Although the overall incidence of FD&C Yellow No. 5 (tartrazine) sensitivity in the general population is low, it is frequently seen in patients who also have aspirin hypersensitivity.

CARCINOGENESIS, MUTAGENESIS, AND IMPAIRMENT OF FERTILITY

See BOXED WARNING.

PREGNANCY CATEGORY X

See CONTRAINDICATIONS and BOXED WARNING.

NURSING MOTHERS

Because of the potential for tumorigenicity shown for ethinyl estradiol in animal and human studies, a decision should be made whether to discontinue nursing or to discontinue the drug, taking into account the importance of the drug to the mother.

PEDIATRIC USE

Safety and effectiveness in children have not been established.

DRUG INTERACTIONS

Certain endocrine and liver function tests may be affected by estrogen-containing oral contraceptives. The following similar changes may be expected with large doses of estrogen:

Increased sulfobromophthalein retention; increased prothrombin and factors VII, VIII, IX, and X; decreased antithrombin 3; increased norepinephrine-induced platelet aggregation; increased thyroid binding globulin (TBG) leading to increased circulating total thyroid hormone, as measured by PBI, T_4 by column, or T_4 by radioimmunoassay. Free T_3 resin uptake is decrease, reflecting the elevated TBG; free T_4 concentration is unaltered; impaired glucose tolerance; decreased pregnanetriol excretion; reduced response to metyrapone test; reduced serum folate concentration; increased serum triglyceride and phospholipid concentration.

ADVERSE REACTIONS

See WARNINGS regarding induction of neoplasia, adverse effects on the fetus, increased incidence of gallbladder disease, and adverse effects similar to those oral contraceptives, including thromboembolism.

The following additional adverse reactions have been reported with estrogenic therapy, including oral contraceptives:

Genitourinary System: Breakthrough bleeding, spotting, change in menstrual flow; dysmenorrhea; premenstrual-lie syndrome; amenorrhea during and after treatment; increase in sizes of uterine fibromyomata; vaginal candidiasis; change in cervical eversion and in degree of cervical secretion; cystitis-like syndrome.

Breasts: Tenderness, enlargement, secretion.

Gastrointestinal: Nausea, vomiting; abdominal cramps, bloating; cholestatic jaundice.

Skin: Chloasma or melasma which may persist when drug is discontinued; erythema multiforme; erythema nodosum; hemorrhagic eruption; loss of scalp hair; hirsutism.

Eyes: Steeping of corneal curvature; intolerance to contact lenses.

CNS: Headache, migraine, dizziness; mental depression; chorea.

Miscellaneous: Increase or decrease in weight; reduced carbohydrate tolerance; aggravation of porphyria; edema; changes in libido.

DOSAGE AND ADMINISTRATION

1. ***Given cyclically for short-term use only:*** For treatment of moderate to severe vasomotor symptoms associated with the menopause. The lowest dose that will control symptoms should be chosen and medication should be discontinued as promptly as possible. Administration should be cyclic (*e.g.,* 3 weeks on a 1 week off). Attempts to discontinue or taper medication should be made at 3- to 6-month intervals. The usual dosage range is one 0.02 mg or 0.05 mg tablet daily. In some instances, the effective dose may be as low as one 0.02 mg tablet every other day. A useful dosage schedule for early menopause, while spontaneous menstruation continues, is 0.05 mg once a day for 21 days and then a rest period for 7 days. For the initial treatment of the late menopause, the same regimen is indicated with the 0.02 mg Estinyl Tablet for the first few cycles, after which the 0.05 mg dosage may be substituted. In more severe cases, such as those due to surgical and roentgenologic castration, one 0.05 mg tablet may be administered 3 times daily at the start of treatment. With adequate clinical improvement, usually obtainable in a few weeks, the dosage may be reduced to one 0.05 mg tablet daily and the patient continued thereafter on a maintenance dosage as in the average case.
2. ***Given cyclically, female hypogonadism:*** One 0.05 mg tablet is given 1-3 times daily during the first 2 weeks of a theoretical menstrual cycle. This is followed by progesterone during the last half of the arbitrary cycle. This regimen is continued for 3-6 months. The patients is then allowed to go untreated for 2 months to determine whether or not she can maintain the cycle without hormonal therapy. If not, additional courses of therapy may be prescribed.
3. ***Given chronically, inoperable progressing prostatic cancer:*** From three 0.05 mg to four 0.05 mg tablets may be administered daily for palliation.

Inoperable progressing breast cancer in appropriately selected postmenopausal women: (see INDICATIONS AND USAGE) Two 0.05 mg tablets 3 times daily for palliation.

Treated patients with an intact uterus should be monitored closely for signs of endometrial cancer and appropriate diagnostic measures should be taken to rule out malignancy in the event of persistent or recurring abnormal vaginal bleeding.

PRODUCT LISTING - EQUIVALENTS NOT AVAILABLE

Tablet - Oral - 0.02 mg

7's	$6.32	ESTINYL, Pd-Rx Pharmaceuticals	55289-0503-07
21's	$14.25	ESTINYL, Pd-Rx Pharmaceuticals	55289-0503-21
100's	$40.96	ESTINYL, Schering Corporation	00085-0298-03
250's	$96.26	ESTINYL, Schering Corporation	00085-0298-06

Tablet - Oral - 0.05 mg

100's	$68.98	ESTINYL, Schering Corporation	00085-0070-03
250's	$161.00	ESTINYL, Schering Corporation	00085-0070-06

Tablet - Oral - 0.5 mg

100's	$118.54	ESTINYL, Schering Corporation	00085-0150-03

Ethinyl Estradiol; Ethynodiol Diacetate *(001217)*

Categories: Contraception; Pregnancy Category X; FDA Approval Pre 1982
Drug Classes: Contraceptives; Estrogens; Hormones/hormone modifiers; Progestins
Brand Names: Conova; **Demulen**; Metrulen; Ovulen; Zovia
Foreign Brand Availability: Demulen 50 (Canada); Neovulen (Denmark); Ovulen 1 50 (Taiwan); Ovulen 50 (Belgium; Netherlands; Switzerland)
Cost of Therapy: $24.89 (Contraceptive; Demulen; 35 µg; 1 mg; 1 tablet/day; 21 day supply)
$29.61 (Contraceptive; Demulen; 35 µg; 1 mg; 1 tablet/day; 28 day supply)

DESCRIPTION

The chemical name for ethyndiol diacetate is 19-nor-17α-pregn-4-en-20-yne-3β,17-diol diacetate, and for ethinyl estradiol it is 19-nor-17α-pregna-1,3,5 (10)-trien-20-yne-3,17-diol.

DEMULEN 1/35-21 AND DEMULEN 1/35-28

Each white tablet contains 1 mg of ethynodiol diacetate and 35 µg of ethinyl estradiol. *Inactive Ingredients:* Calcium acetate, calcium phosphate, corn starch, hydrogenated castor oil, and povidone.

Each blue tablet in the Demulen 1/35-28 package is a placebo containing no active ingredients. *Inactive Ingredients:* Calcium sulfate, corn starch, FD&C blue no. 1 lake, magnesium stearate, and sucrose.

DEMULEN 1/50-21 AND DEMULEN 1/50-28

Each white tablet contains 1 mg of ethynodiol diacetate and 50 µg of ethinyl estradiol. *Inactive Ingredients:* Calcium acetate, calcium phosphate, corn starch, hydrogenated castor oil, and povidone.

Each pink tablet in the Demulen 1/50-28 package is a placebo containing no active ingredients. *Inactive Ingredients:* Calcium sulfate, corn starch, FD&C red no. 3, FD&C yellow no. 6, magnesium stearate, and sucrose.

For prescribing information refer to Ethinyl Estradiol; Norethindrone.

HOW SUPPLIED

DEMULEN 1/35

Each white Demulen 1/35 tablet is round in shape, with a debossed "SEARLE" on one side and "151" and design on the other side, and contains 1 mg of ethynodiol diacetate and 35 µg of ethinyl estradiol.

Blue placebo tablets have a debossed "SEARLE" on one side and a "P" on the other side.

DEMULEN 1/50

Each white Demulen 1/50 tablet is round in shape, with a debossed "SEARLE" on one side and "71" on the other side, and contains 1 mg of ethynodiol diacetate and 50 µg of ethinyl estradiol.

Blue placebo tablets have a debossed "SEARLE" on one side and a "P" on the other side.

PRODUCT LISTING - RATED THERAPEUTICALLY EQUIVALENT

Tablet - Oral - 35 mcg;1 mg

21 x 6	$174.00	GENERIC, Watson Laboratories Inc	52544-0532-21
28 x 6	$179.28	GENERIC, Watson Laboratories Inc	52544-0383-28
28's	$26.59	GENERIC, Allscripts Pharmaceutical Company	54569-4817-00

Tablet - Oral - 50 mcg;1 mg

21 x 6	$194.01	GENERIC, Watson Laboratories Inc	52544-0533-21
28 x 6	$199.74	GENERIC, Watson Laboratories Inc	52544-0384-28

PRODUCT LISTING - EQUIVALENTS NOT AVAILABLE

Tablet - Oral - 35 mcg;1 mg

21 x 6	$197.82	DEMULEN 1/35, Searle	00025-0151-07
21 x 24	$597.39	DEMULEN 1/35, Searle	00025-0151-24
28 x 6	$199.86	DEMULEN 1/35, Searle	00025-0161-09
28 x 24	$761.04	DEMULEN 1/35, Searle	00025-0161-24

Tablet - Oral - 50 mcg;1 mg

21 x 6	$220.62	DEMULEN 1/50, Searle	00025-0071-07
21 x 24	$608.38	DEMULEN 1/50, Searle	00025-0071-24
28 x 6	$222.60	DEMULEN 1/50, Searle	00025-0081-09
28 x 24	$786.48	DEMULEN 1/50, Searle	00025-0081-24

Ethinyl Estradiol; Ferrous Fumarate; Norethindrone Acetate *(001221)*

Categories: Contraception; Pregnancy Category X; FDA Approval Pre 1982
Drug Classes: Contraceptives; Estrogens; Hormones/hormone modifiers; Progestins
Brand Names: Estrostep Fe; **Loestrin Fe**; Loestrin Fe 1.5/30; Loestrin Fe 1/20; Norlestrin Fe; Norquest Fe
Foreign Brand Availability: Perlas (Philippines)
Cost of Therapy: $26.50 (Contraceptive; Loestrin Fe; 30 µg; 1.5 µg; 1 tablet/day; 28 day supply)
$27.69 (Contraceptive; Loestrin Fe 1/20; 20 µg; 1 µg; 1 tablet/day; 28 day supply)

DESCRIPTION

The name for norethindrone is [(17 alpha)-17 (acetylox)-19-norpregna-4-en-20-yn-3-one] and the name for ethinyl estradiol is [(17 alpha)-19-norpregna-1,3,5(10)-trien-20-yne-3,17-dio].

LOESTRIN FE

Each white tablet contains norethindrone acetate (17 alpha-ethinyl-19-nortestosterone acetate), 1 mg; ethinyl estradiol (17 alpha-ethinyl-1,3,5(10)-estratriene-3, 17 beta-diol), 20 µg. Also contains acacia, lactose, magnesium stearate, starch, confectioner's sugar, talc.

Each green tablet contains norethindrone acetate (17 alpha-ethinyl-19-nortestosterone acetate), 1.5 mg; ethinyl estradiol (17 alpha-ethinyl-1,3,5(10)-estratriene-3, 17 beta-diol), 30 µg. Also contains acacia, lactose, magnesium stearate, starch, confectioner's sugar, talc; D&C yellow no. 10; FD&C yellow no. 6; FD&C blue no. 1.

Each brown tablet contains microcrystalline cellulose, ferrous fumarate; magnesium stearate, povidone; sodium starch glycolate, sucrose with modified dextrins.

Loestrin Fe is a progestogen-estrogen combination.

Loestrin Fe 1/20 and 1.5/30: Each provides a continuous dosage regimen consisting of 21 oral contraceptive tablets and 7 ferrous fumarate tablets. The ferrous fumarate tablets are present to facilitate ease of drug administration via a 28 day regimen and do not serve any therapeutic purpose.

ESTROSTEP FE

Each triangular tablet contains 1 mg norethindrone acetate and 20 µg ethinyl estradiol; each white square tablet contains 1 mg norethindrone acetate and 30 µg ethinyl estradiol; each white round tablets contains 1 mg norethindrone acetate and 35 µg ethinyl estradiol; each brown tablet contains 75 mg ferrous fumarate.

Each Estrostep Fe tablet dispenser contains 5 white triangular tablets, 7 white square tablets, 9 white round tablets and 7 brown tablets. These tablets are to be taken in the following order: 1 triangular tablet each day for 5 days, then 1 square tablet each day for 7 days; followed by 1 round tablet each day for 9 days, and then 1 brown tablet each day for 7 days.

CLINICAL PHARMACOLOGY

Combination oral contraceptives act by suppression of gonadotropins. Although the primary mechanism of this action is inhibition of ovulation, other alterations include changes in the cervical mucus (which increase the difficulty of sperm entry into the uterus) and the endometrium (which reduce the likelihood of implantation).

In vitro and animal studies have shown that norethindrone combines high progestational activity with low intrinsic androgenicity. In humans, norethindrone acetate in combination with ethinyl estradiol does not counteract estrogen-induced increases in sex hormone binding globulin (SHBG). Following multiple-dose administration of ethinyl estradiol; ferrous fumarate; norethindrone acetate, serum SHBG concentrations increase 2- to 3-fold and free testosterone concentrations decrease by 47-64, indicating minimal androgenic activity.

PHARMACOKINETICS

Absorption

Norethindrone acetate appears to be completely and rapidly deacetylated to norethindrone after oral administration, since the disposition of norethindrone acetate is indistinguishable from that of orally administered norethindrone.[1] Norethindrone acetate and ethinyl estradiol are rapidly absorbed, with maximum plasma concentrations of norethindrone and ethinyl estradiol occurring 1-2 hours postdose. Both are subject to first-pass metabolism after oral dosing, resulting in an absolute bioavailability of approximately 64% for norethindrone and 43% for ethinyl estradiol.[1-3]

Administration of ethinyl estradiol; ferrous fumarate; norethindrone acetate tablets with a high fat meal decreases rate but not extent, of ethinyl estradiol absorption. The extent of norethindrone absorption is increased by 27% following administration with food.

Mean steady-state concentrations of norethindrone for the 20/1, 30/1, 35/1 tablet strengths increased as ethinyl estradiol dose increased over the 21 day dose regimen, due to dose-dependent effects of ethinyl estradiol on serum SHBG concentrations (TABLE 1). Mean steady-state plasma concentrations of ethinyl estradiol for the 20/1, 30/1, 35/1 tablet strengths were proportional to ethinyl estradiol dose (TABLE 1).

***TABLE 1** Mean (SD) Steady-State Pharmacokinetic Parameters* Following Chronic Administration of Ethinyl Estradiol; Ferrous Fumarate; Norethindrone Acetate*

Ethinyl Estradiol; Ferrous Fumarate; Norethindrone Acetate mg/µg	Cycle Day	C_{max} ng/ml	AUC ng·h/ml	CL/F ml/min	SHBG† nmol/L
		Norethindrone			
20/1	5	10.8 (3.9)	81.1 (28.5)	220 (137)	120 (33)
30/1	12	12.7 (4.1)	102 (32)	166 (85)	139 (42)
35/1	21	12.7 (4.1)	109 (32)	152 (73)	163 (40)
		Ethinyl Estradiol			
20/1	5	61.0 (16.8)	661 (190)	549 (171)	
30/1	12	92.4 (26.9)	973 (293)	546 (199)	
35/1	21	113 (44)	1149 (372)	568 (219)	

* C_{max}=Maximum plasma concentration; AUC (0-24)=Area under the plasma concentration-time curve over the dosing interval; CL/F=Apparent oral clearance.
† Mean (SD) baseline value=55 (29) nmol/L.

Distribution

Volume of distribution of norethindrone and ethinyl estradiol ranges from 2-4 L/kg.[1-3] Plasma protein binding of both steroids is extensive (>95%); norethindrone binds to both albumin and sex hormone binding globulin (SHBG), whereas ethinyl estradiol binds only to albumin.[4] Although ethinyl estradiol does not bind to SHBG, it induces SHBG synthesis. Ethinyl estradiol; ferrous fumarate; norethindrone acetate increases serum SHBG concentrations 2- to 3-fold (see TABLE 1).

Metabolism

Norethindrone undergoes extensive biotransformation, primarily via reduction, followed by sulfate and glucuronide conjugation. The majority of metabolites in the circulation are sulfates, with glucuronides accounting for most of the urinary metabolites.[5] A small amount of norethindrone acetate is metabolically converted to ethinyl estradiol. Ethinyl estradiol is also extensively metabolized, both by oxidation and by conjugation with sulfate and glucuronide. Sulfates are the major circulating conjugates of ethinyl estradiol and glucuronides predominate in urine. The primary oxidative metabolite is 2-hydroxy ethinyl estradiol, formed by the CYP3A4 isoform of cytochrome P450. Part of the first-pass metabolism of ethinyl estradiol is believed to occur in gastrointestinal mucosa. Ethinyl estradiol may undergo enterohepatic circulation.[6]

Excretion

Norethindrone and ethinyl estradiol are excreted in both urine and feces, primarily as metabolites.[5,6] Plasma clearance values for norethindrone and ethinyl estradiol are similar (approximately 0.4 L/h/kg).[1-3] Steady-state elimination half-lives of norethindrone and ethinyl estradiol following administration of ethinyl estradiol; ferrous fumarate; norenthindrone acetate tablets are approximately 13 hours and 19 hours, respectively.

SPECIAL POPULATIONS

Race: The effect of race on the disposition of ethinyl estradiol; ferrous fumarate; norenthindrone acetate has not been evaluated.

RENAL INSUFFICIENCY

The effect of renal disease on the disposition of ethinyl estradiol; ferrous fumarate; norenthindrone acetate has not been evaluated. In premenopausal women with chronic renal failure undergoing peritoneal dialysis who received multiple doses of an oral contraceptive containing ethinyl estradiol and norethindrone, plasma ethinyl estradiol concentrations were higher and norethindrone concentrations were unchanged compared to concentrations in premenopausal women with normal renal function.

HEPATIC INSUFFICIENCY

The effect of hepatic disease on the disposition of ethinyl estradiol; ferrous fumarate; norenthindrone acetate has not been evaluated. However, ethinyl estradiol and norethindrone may be poorly metabolized in patients with impaired liver function.

DRUG-DRUG INTERACTIONS

Numerous drug-drug interactions have been reported for oral contraceptives. A summary of these is found under DRUG INTERACTIONS

INDICATIONS AND USAGE

Ethinyl estradiol; norethindrone acetate is indicated for the prevention of pregnancy in women who elect to use oral contraceptives as a method of contraception.

Oral contraceptives are highly effective. TABLE 2 lists the typical accidental pregnancy rates for users of combination oral contraceptives and other methods of contraception. The efficacy of these contraceptive methods, except for sterilization, depends upon the reliability with which they are used. Correct and consistent use of methods can result in lower failure rates.

NON-CONTRACEPTIVE HEALTH BENEFITS

The following non-contraceptive health benefits related to the use of oral contraceptives are supported by epidemiological studies which largely utilized oral contraceptive formulations containing estrogen doses exceeding 0.035 mg of ethinyl estradiol or 0.05 mg of mestranol.[79-84]

Effects on Menses: Increased menstrual cycle regularity, decreased blood loss and decreased incidence of iron deficiency anemia, decreased incidence of dysmenorrhea.

Effects Related to Inhibition of Ovulation: Decreased incidence of functional ovarian cysts, decreased incidence of ectopic pregnancies.

Effects From Long-Term Use: Decreased incidence of fibroadenomas and fibrocystic disease of the breast, decreased incidence of acute pelvic inflammatory disease, decreased incidence of endometrial cancer, decreased incidence of ovarian cancer.

CONTRAINDICATIONS

Oral contraceptives should not be used in women who currently have the following conditions:

- Thrombophlebitis or thromboembolic disorders.
- A past history of deep vein thrombophlebitis or thromboembolic disorders.
- Cerebral vascular or coronary artery disease.
- Known or suspected carcinoma of the breast.
- Carcinoma of the endometrium or other known or suspected estrogen-dependent neoplasia.
- Undiagnosed abnormal genital bleeding.
- Cholestatic jaundice of pregnancy or jaundice with prior pill use.
- Hepatic adenomas or carcinomas.
- Known or suspected pregnancy.

WARNINGS

Cigarette smoking increases the risk of serious cardiovascular side effects from oral contraceptive use. This risk increases with age and with heavy smoking (15 or more cigarettes per day) and is quite marked in women over 35 years of age. Women who use oral contraceptives should be strongly advised not to smoke.

The use of oral contraceptives is associated with increased risks of several serious conditions including myocardial infarction, thromboembolism, stroke, hepatic neoplasia, and gallbladder disease, although the risk of serious morbidity or mortality is very small in healthy women without underlying risk factors. The risk of morbidity and mortality in-

TABLE 2 *Lowest Expected and Typical Failure Rates During the First Year of Continuous Use of a Method*[7]

% of Women Experiencing an Unintended Pregnancy in the First Year of Continuous Use		
Method	**Lowest Expected***	**Typical†**
(No Contraception)	(85%)	(85%)
Oral Contraceptives		
Combined	0.1%	N/A‡
Progestin Only	0.5%	N/A‡
Diaphragm With Spermicidal Cream or Jelly	6%	20%
Spermicides Alone (foam, creams, gels, vaginal suppositories and vaginal film)	6%	26%
Vaginal Sponge		
Nulliparous	9%	20%
Parous	20%	40%
Implant	0.05%	0.05%
Injection: Depot Medroxyprogesterone Acetate	0.3%	0.3%
IUD		
Progesterone T	1.5%	2.0%
Copper T 380A	0.6%	0.8%
LNg 20	0.1%	0.1%
Condom Without Spermicides		
Female	5%	21%
Male	3%	14%
Cervical Cap With Spermicidal Cream or Jelly		
Nulliparous	9%	20%
Parous	26%	40%
Periodic Abstinence (all methods)	1-9%	25%
Withdrawal	4%	19%
Female Sterilization	0.5%	0.5%
Male Sterilization	0.10%	0.15%

* The authors' best guess of the percentage of women expected to experience an accidental pregnancy among couples who initiate a method (not necessarily for the first time) and who use it consistently and correctly during the first year if they do not stop for any other reason.
† This term represents "typical" couples who initiate use of a method (not necessarily for the first time), who experience an accidental pregnancy during the first year if they do not stop use for any other reason.
‡ N/A=Data not available.

creases significantly in the presence of other underlying risk factors such as hypertension, hyperlipidemias, obesity, and diabetes.

Practitioners prescribing oral contraceptives should be familiar with the following information relating to these risks.

The information contained in this package insert is principally based on studies carried out in patients who used oral contraceptives with higher formulations of estrogens and progestogens than those in common use today. The effect of long-term use of the oral contraceptives with lower formulations of both estrogens and progestogens remains to be determined.

Throughout this labeling, epidemiological studies reported are of two types: retrospective or case control studies and prospective or cohort studies. Case control studies provide a measure of the relative risk of a disease, namely, a ratio of the incidence of a disease among oral contraceptive users to that among nonusers. The relative risk does not provide information on the actual clinical occurrence of a disease. Cohort studies provide a measure of attributable risk, which is the difference in the incidence of disease between oral contraceptive users and nonusers. The attributable risk does provide information about the actual occurrence of a disease in the population (adapted from References 8 and 9 with the author's permission). For further information, the reader is referred to a text on epidemiological methods.

THROMBOEMBOLIC DISORDERS AND OTHER VASCULAR PROBLEMS

Myocardial Infarction

An increased risk of myocardial infarction has been attributed to oral contraceptive use. This risk is primarily in smokers or women with other underlying risk factors for coronary artery disease such as hypertension, hypercholesterolemia, morbid obesity, and diabetes. The relative risk of heart attack for current oral contraceptive users has been estimated to be 2-6.[10-16] The risk is very low under the age of 30.

Smoking in combination with oral contraceptive use has been shown to contribute substantially to the incidence of myocardial infarctions in women in their mid-thirties or older with smoking accounting for the majority of excess cases.[17] Mortality rates associated with circulatory disease have been shown to increase substantially in smokers over the age of 35 and non-smokers over the age of 40 among women who use oral contraceptives.

Oral contraceptives may compound the effects of well-known risk factors, such as hypertension, diabetes, hyperlipidemias, age and obesity.[19] In particular, some progestogens are known to decrease HDL cholesterol and cause glucose intolerance, while estrogens may create a state of hyperinsulinism.[20-24] Oral contraceptives have been shown to increase blood pressure among users (see Elevated Blood Pressure). Similar effects on risk factors have been associated with an increased risk of heart disease. Oral contraceptives must be used with caution in women with cardiovascular disease risk factors.

Thromboembolism

An increased risk of thromboembolic and thrombotic disease associated with the use of oral contraceptives is well established. Case control studies have found the relative risk of users compared to nonusers to be 3 for the first episode of superficial venous thrombosis, 4-11 for deep vein thrombosis or pulmonary embolism, and 1.5-6 for women with predisposing conditions for venous thromboembolic disease.[9,10,25-30] Cohort studies have shown the relative risk to be somewhat lower, about 3 for new cases and about 4.5 for new cases requiring hospitalization.[31] The risk of thromboembolic disease due to oral contraceptives is not related to length of use and disappears after pill use is stopped.[8]

A 2- to 4-fold increase in relative risk of postoperative thromboembolic complications has been reported with the use of oral contraceptives.[15,32] The relative risk of venous thrombosis in women who have predisposing conditions is twice that of women without such medical conditions.[15,32] If feasible, oral contraceptives should be discontinued at least 4 weeks prior to and for 2 weeks after elective surgery of a type associated with an increase in risk of thromboembolism and during and following prolonged immobilization. Since the immediate postpartum period is also associated with an increased risk of thromboembolism, oral contraceptives should be started no earlier than 4-6 weeks after delivery in women who elect not to breastfeed.

Cerebrovascular Disease

Oral contraceptives have been shown to increase both the relative and attributable risks of cerebrovascular events (thrombotic and hemorrhagic strokes), although, in general, the risk is greatest among older (>35 years), hypertensive women who also smoke. Hypertension was found to be a risk factor for both users and nonusers, for both types of strokes, while smoking interacted to increase the risk for hemorrhagic strokes.[33-35]

In a large study, the relative risk of thrombotic strokes has been shown to range from 3 for normotensive users to 14 for users with severe hypertension.[36] The relative risk of hemorrhagic stroke is reported to be 1.2 for non-smokers who used oral contraceptives, 2.6 for smokers who did not use oral contraceptives, 7.6 for smokers who used oral contraceptives, 1.8 for normotensive users, and 25.7 for users with severe hypertension.[36] The attributable risk is also greater in older women.[9]

Dose-Related Risk of Vascular Disease From Oral Contraceptives

A positive association has been observed between the amount of estrogen and progestogen in oral contraceptives and the risk of vascular disease.[37-39] A decline in serum high-density lipoproteins (HDL) has been reported with many progestational agents.[20-22] A decline in serum high-density lipoproteins has been associated with an increased incidence of ischemic heart disease. Because estrogens increase HDL cholesterol, the net effect of an oral contraceptive depends on a balance achieved between doses of estrogen and progestin and the nature of the progestin used in the contraceptives. The amount and activity of both hormones should be considered in the choice of an oral contraceptive

Minimizing exposure to estrogen and progestogen is in keeping with good principles of therapeutics. For any particular oral contraceptive, the dosage regimen prescribed should be one which contains the least amount of estrogen and progestogen that is compatible with the needs of the individual patient. New acceptors of oral contraceptive agents should be started on preparations containing the lowest dose of estrogen which produces satisfactory results for the patient.

Persistence of Risk of Vascular Disease

There are two studies which have shown persistence of risk of vascular disease for ever-users of oral contraceptives. In a study in the United States, the risk of developing myocardial infarction after discontinuing oral contraceptives persists for at least 9 years for women 40-49 years who had used oral contraceptives for 5 or more years, but this increased risk was not demonstrated in other age groups.[14] In another study in Great Britain, the risk of developing cerebrovascular disease persisted for at least 6 years after discontinuation of oral contraceptives, although excess risk was very small.[40] However, both studies were performed with oral contraceptive formulations containing 50 µg or higher of estrogens.

ESTIMATES OF MORTALITY FROM CONTRACEPTIVE USE

One study gathered data from a variety of sources which have estimated the mortality rate associated with different methods of contraception at different ages (TABLE 3). These estimates include the combined risk of death associated with contraceptive methods plus the risk attributable to pregnancy in the event of method failure. Each method of contraception has its specific benefits and risks. The study concluded that with the exception of oral contraceptive users 35 and older who smoke and 40 and older who do not smoke, mortality associated with all methods of birth control is low and below that associated with childbirth. The observation of a possible increase in risk of mortality with age for oral contraceptive users is based on data gathered in the 1970s but not reported until 1983.[41] However, current clinical practice involves the use of lower estrogen dose formulations combined with careful restriction of oral contraceptive use to women who do not have the various risk factors listed in this labeling. Because of these changes in practice and, also, because of some limited new data which suggest that the risk of cardiovascular disease with the use of oral contraceptives may now be less than previously observed (Porter JB, Hunter J, Jick H, et al. Oral contraceptives and nonfatal vascular disease. Obstet Gynecol 1985; 66:1-4; and Porter JB, Hershel J, Walker AM. Mortality among oral contraceptive users. Obstet Gynecol 1987;70:29-32), the Fertility and Maternal Health Drugs Advisory Committee was asked to review the topic in 1989. The Committee concluded that although cardiovascular disease risks may be increased with oral contraceptive use after age 40 in healthy non-smoking women (even with the newer low-dose formulations), there are greater potential health risks associated with pregnancy in older women and with the alternative surgical and medical procedures which may be necessary if such women do not have access to effective and acceptable means of contraception.

Therefore, the Committee recommended that the benefits of oral contraceptive use by healthy non-smoking women over 40 may outweigh the possible risks. Of course, older women, as all women who take oral contraceptives, should take the lowest possible dose formulation that is effective.

CARCINOMA OF THE REPRODUCTIVE ORGANS

Numerous epidemiological studies have been performed on the incidence of breast, endometrial, ovarian, and cervical cancer in women using oral contraceptives. Most of the studies on breast cancer and oral contraceptive use report that the use of oral contraceptives is not associated with an increase in the risk of developing breast cancer.[42,44,89] Some studies have reported an increased risk of developing breast cancer in certain subgroups of oral contraceptive users, but the findings reported in these studies are not consistent.[43,45-49,85-88]

Some studies suggest that oral contraceptive use has been associated with an increase in the risk of cervical intraepithelial neoplasia in some populations of women.[51-54] However,

TABLE 3 *Annual Number of Birth-Related or Method-Related Deaths Associated With Control of Fertility per 100,000 Nonsterile Women by Fertility Control Method According to Age*[41]

Method of Control and Outcome	15-19	20-24	25-29	30-34	35-39	40-44
No fertility control methods*	7.0	7.4	9.1	14.8	25.7	28.2
Oral contraceptives non-smoker†	0.3	0.5	0.9	1.9	13.8	31.6
Oral contraceptives smoker†	2.2	3.4	6.6	13.5	51.1	117.2
IUD†	0.8	0.8	1.0	1.0	1.4	1.4
Condom*	1.1	1.6	0.7	0.2	0.3	0.4
Diaphragm/ spermicide*	1.9	1.2	1.2	1.3	2.2	2.8
Periodic abstinence*	2.5	1.6	1.6	1.7	2.9	3.6

* Deaths are birth related.
† Deaths are method related.

there continues to be controversy about the extent to which such findings may be due to differences in sexual behavior and other factors.

In spite of many studies of the relationship between oral contraceptive use and breast and cervical cancers, a cause and effect relationship has not been established.

HEPATIC NEOPLASIA

Benign hepatic adenomas are associated with oral contraceptive use, although the incidence of benign tumors is rare in the United States. Indirect calculations have estimated the attributable risk to be in the range of 3.3 cases/100,000 for users, a risk that increases after 4 or more years of use.[55] Rupture of rare, benign, hepatic adenomas may cause death through intraabdominal hemorrhage.[56,57]

Studies from Britain have shown an increased risk of developing hepatocellular carcinoma[58-60] in long-term (>8 years) oral contraceptive users. However, these cancers are extremely rare in the US, and the attributable risk (the excess incidence) of liver cancers in oral contraceptive users approaches less than one per million users.

OCULAR LESIONS

There have been clinical case reports of retinal thrombosis associated with the use of oral contraceptives. Oral contraceptives should be discontinued if there is unexplained partial or complete loss of vision; onset of proptosis or diplopia; papilledema; or retinal vascular lesions. Appropriate diagnostic and therapeutic measures should be undertaken immediately.

ORAL CONTRACEPTIVE USE BEFORE AND DURING EARLY PREGNANCY

Extensive epidemiological studies have revealed no increased risk of birth defects in women who have used oral contraceptives prior to pregnancy.[61-63] Studies also do not suggest a teratogenic effect, particularly insofar as cardiac anomalies and limb reduction defects are concerned,[61,62,64,65] when taken inadvertently during early pregnancy.

The administration of oral contraceptives to induce withdrawal bleeding should not be used as a test for pregnancy. Oral contraceptives should not be used during pregnancy to treat threatened or habitual abortion.

It is recommended that for any patient who has missed two consecutive periods, pregnancy should be ruled out before continuing oral contraceptive use. If the patient has not adhered to the prescribed schedule, the possibility of pregnancy should be considered at the time of the first missed period. Oral contraceptive use should be discontinued if pregnancy is confirmed.

GALLBLADDER DISEASE

Earlier studies have reported an increased lifetime relative risk of gallbladder surgery in users of oral contraceptives and estrogens.[66,67] More recent studies, however, have shown that the relative risk of developing gallbladder disease among oral contraceptive users may be minimal.[68-70] The recent findings of minimal risk may be related to the use of oral contraceptive formulations containing lower hormonal doses of estrogens and progestogens.

CARBOHYDRATE AND LIPID METABOLIC EFFECTS

Oral contraceptives have been shown to cause glucose intolerance in a significant percentage of users.[23] Oral contraceptives containing greater than 75 μg of estrogens cause hyperinsulinism, while lower doses of estrogen cause less glucose intolerance.[71] Progestogens increase insulin secretion and create insulin resistance, this effect varying with different progestational agents.[23,72] However, in the non-diabetic woman, oral contraceptives appear to have no effect on fasting blood glucose.[73] Because of these demonstrated effects, prediabetic and diabetic women should be carefully observed while taking oral contraceptives.

A small proportion of women will have persistent hypertriglyceridemia while on the pill. As discussed earlier (see Mycocardial Infarction and Dose-Related Risk of Vascular Disease From Oral Contraceptives), changes in serum triglycerides and lipoprotein levels have been reported in oral contraceptive users.

ELEVATED BLOOD PRESSURE

An increase in blood pressure has been reported in women taking oral contraceptives[74] and this increase is more likely in older oral contraceptive users[75] and with continued use.[74] Data from the Royal College of General Practitioners[18] and subsequent randomized trials have shown that the incidence of hypertension increases with increasing concentrations of progestogens.

Women with a history of hypertension or hypertension-related diseases or renal disease[76] should be encouraged to use another method of contraception. If women elect to use oral contraceptives, they should be monitored closely, and if significant elevation of blood pressure occurs, oral contraceptives should be discontinued. For most women, elevated blood pressure will return to normal after stopping oral contraceptives,[75] and there is no difference in the occurrence of hypertension among ever and never users.[74,76,77]

HEADACHE

The onset or exacerbation of migraine or development of headache with a new pattern which is recurrent, persistent, or severe requires discontinuation of oral contraceptives and evaluation of the cause.

BLEEDING IRREGULARITIES

Breakthrough bleeding and spotting are sometimes encountered in patients on oral contraceptives, especially during the first 3 months of use. Non-hormonal causes should be considered, and adequate diagnostic measures taken to rule out malignancy or pregnancy in the event of prolonged breakthrough bleeding, as in the case of any abnormal vaginal bleeding. If pathology has been excluded, time or a change to another formulation may solve the problem. In the event of amenorrhea, pregnancy should be ruled out.

Some women may encounter post-pill amenorrhea or oligomenorrhea, especially when such a condition was preexistent.

PRECAUTIONS

Patients should be counseled that this product does not protect against HIV infection (AIDS) and other sexually transmitted diseases.

PHYSICAL EXAMINATION AND FOLLOW-UP

It is good medical practice for all women to have annual history and physical examinations, including women using oral contraceptives. The physical examination, however, may be deferred until after initiation of oral contraceptives if requested by the woman and judged appropriate by the clinician. The physical examination should include special reference to blood pressure, breasts, abdomen and pelvic organs, including cervical cytology, and relevant laboratory tests. In case of undiagnosed, persistent or recurrent abnormal vaginal bleeding, appropriate measures should be conducted to rule out malignancy. Women with a strong family history of breast cancer or who have breast nodules should be monitored with particular care.

LIPID DISORDERS

Women who are being treated for hyperlipidemia should be followed closely if they elect to use oral contraceptives. Some progestogens may elevate LDL levels and may render the control of hyperlipidemias more difficult.

LIVER FUNCTION

If jaundice develops in any woman receiving such drugs, the medication should be discontinued. Steroid hormones may be poorly metabolized in patients with impaired liver function.

FLUID RETENTION

Oral contraceptives may cause some degree of fluid retention. They should be prescribed with caution, and only with careful monitoring, in patients with conditions which might be aggravated by fluid retention.

EMOTIONAL DISORDERS

Women with a history of depression should be carefully observed and the drug discontinued if depression recurs to a serious degree.

CONTACT LENSES

Contact lens wearers who develop visual changes or changes in lens tolerance should be assessed by an ophthalmologist.

INTERACTION WITH LABORATORY TESTS

Certain endocrine and liver function tests and blood components may be affected by oral contraceptives:

- Increased prothrombin and factors VII, VIII, IX, and X; decreased antithrombin 3; increased norepinephrine-induced platelet aggregability.
- Increased thyroid binding globulin (TBG) leading to increased circulating total thyroid hormone, as measured by protein-bound iodine (PBI), T4 by column or by radioimmunoassay. Free T3 resin uptake is decreased, reflecting the elevated TBG; free T4 concentration is unaltered.
- Other binding proteins may be elevated in serum.
- Sex-binding globulins are increased and result in elevated levels of total circulating sex steroids and corticoids; however, free or biologically active levels remain unchanged.
- Triglycerides may be increased.
- Glucose tolerance may be decreased.
- Serum folate levels may be depressed by oral contraceptive therapy. This may be of clinical significance if a woman becomes pregnant shortly after discontinuing oral contraceptives.

CARCINOGENESIS

See WARNINGS.

PREGNANCY CATEGORY X

See CONTRAINDICATIONS and WARNINGS.

NURSING MOTHERS

Small amounts of oral contraceptive steroids have been identified in the milk of nursing mothers, and a few adverse effects on the child have been reported, including jaundice and breast enlargement. In addition, oral contraceptives given in the postpartum period may interfere with lactation by decreasing the quantity and quality of breast milk. If possible, the nursing mother should be advised not to use oral contraceptives but to use other forms of contraception until she has completely weaned her child.

PEDIATRIC USE

Safety and efficacy of ethinyl estradiol; ferrous fumarate; norethindrone acetate have been established in women of reproductive age. Safety and efficacy are expected to be the same for postpubertal adolescents under the age of 16 and for users 16 years and older. Use of this product before menarche is not indicated.

DRUG INTERACTIONS

EFFECTS OF OTHER DRUGS ON ORAL CONTRACEPTIVES

Rifampin: Metabolism of both norethindrone and ethinyl estradiol is increased by rifampin. A reduction in contraceptive effectiveness and increased incidence of break-through bleeding and menstrual irregularities have been associated with concomitant use of rifampin.

Anticonvulsants: Anticonvulsants such as phenobarbital, phenytoin, and carbamazepine, have been shown to increase the metabolism of ethinyl estradiol and/or norethindrone, which could result in a reduction in contraceptive effectiveness.

Troglitazone: Administration of troglitazone with an oral contraceptive containing ethinyl estradiol and norethindrone reduced the plasma concentrations of both by approximately 30%, which could result in a reduction in contraceptive effectiveness.

Antibiotics: Pregnancy while taking oral contraceptives has been reported when the oral contraceptives were administered with antimicrobials such as ampicillin, tetracycline, and griseofulvin. However, clinical pharmacokinetic studies have not demonstrated any consistent effect of antibiotics (other than rifampin) on plasma concentrations of synthetic steroids.

Atorvastatin: Coadministration of atorvastatin and an oral contraceptive increased AUC values for norethindrone and ethinyl estradiol by approximately 30% and 20%, respectively.

Other: Ascorbic acid and acetaminophen may increase plasma ethinyl estradiol concentrations, possibly by inhibition of conjugation. A reduction in contraceptive effectiveness and increased incidence of breakthrough bleeding has been suggested with phenylbutazone.

EFFECTS OF ORAL CONTRACEPTIVES ON OTHER DRUGS

Oral contraceptive combinations containing ethinyl estradiol may inhibit the metabolism of other compounds. Increased plasma concentrations of cyclosporine, prednisolone, and theophylline have been reported with concomitant administration of oral contraceptives. In addition, oral contraceptives may induce the conjugation of other compounds. Decreased plasma concentrations of acetaminophen and increased clearance of temazepam, salicylic acid, morphine, and clofibric acid have been noted when these drugs were administered with oral contraceptives.

ADVERSE REACTIONS

An increased risk of the following serious adverse reactions has been associated with the use of oral contraceptives (see WARNINGS): Thrombophlebitis, cerebral hemorrhage, gallbladder disease, arterial thromboembolism, cerebral thrombosis, hepatic adenomas or benign liver tumors, pulmonary embolism, hypertension, myocardial infarction.

There is evidence of an association between the following conditions and the use of oral contraceptives, although additional confirmatory studies are needed: Mesenteric thrombosis and retinal thrombosis.

The following adverse reactions have been reported in patients receiving oral contraceptives and are believed to be drug-related: Nausea, change in weight (increase or decrease), vomiting, change in cervical erosion and secretion, gastrointestinal symptoms (such as abdominal cramps and bloating), diminution in lactation when given immediately postpartum, breakthrough bleeding, cholestatic jaundice, spotting, migraine, change in menstrual flow, rash (allergic), amenorrhea, mental depression, temporary infertility after discontinuation of treatment, reduced tolerance to carbohydrates, vaginal candidiasis, edema, change in corneal curvature (steepening), melasma which may persist, intolerance to contact lenses, breast changes: tenderness, enlargement, secretion.

The following adverse reactions have been reported in users of oral contraceptives and the association has been neither confirmed nor refuted: Pre-menstrual syndrome, hirsutism, impaired renal function, cataracts, loss of scalp hair, hemolytic uremic syndrome, changes in appetite, erythema multiforme, cystitis-like syndrome, erythema nodosum, Budd-Chiari syndrome, headache, hemorrhagic eruption, acne, nervousness, vaginitis, changes in libido, dizziness, porphyria, and colitis.

DOSAGE AND ADMINISTRATION

The tablet dispenser has been designed to make oral contraceptive dosing as easy and as convenient as possible. The tablets are arranged in either 3 or 4 rows of 7 tablets each, with the days of the week appearing on the tablet dispenser above the first row of tablets.

Note: Each tablet dispenser has been preprinted with the days of the week, starting with Sunday, to facilitate a Sunday-Start regimen. Six different day label strips have been provided with the Detailed Patient & Brief Summary Patient Package Insert in order to accomodate a Day-1 Start regimen. If the patient is using the Day-1 Start regimen, she should place the self-adhesive day label strip that corresponds to her starting day over the preprinted days.

Important: The patient should be instructed to use an additional method of protection until after the first week of administration in the initial cycle when utilizing the Sunday-Start regimen.

The possibility of ovulation and conception prior to initiation of use should be considered.

DOSAGE AND ADMINISTRATION FOR 28 DAY DOSAGE REGIMEN

To achieve maximum contraceptive effectiveness, Estrostep Fe should be taken exactly as directed and at intervals not exceeding 24 hours.

Estrostep Fe provides a continuous administration regimen consisting of 21 white tablets of Estrostep and 7 brown non-hormone containing tablets of ferrous fumarate. The ferrous fumarate tablets are present to facilitate ease of drug administration via a 28 day regimen and do not serve any therapeutic purpose. There is no need for the patient to count days between cycles because there are no "off-tablet days."

Sunday-Start Regimen

The patient begins taking the first white tablet from the top row of the dispenser (labeled Sunday) on the first Sunday after menstrual flow begins. When the menstrual flow begins on Sunday, the first white tablet is taken on the same day. The patient takes 1 white tablet daily for 21 days. The last white tablet in the dispenser will be taken on a Saturday. Upon completion of all 21 white tablets, and without interruption, the patient takes 1 brown tablet daily for 7 days. Upon completion of this first course of tablets, the patient begins a second course of 28 day tablets, without interruption, the next day (Sunday), starting with the Sunday white tablet in the top row. Adhering to this regimen of 1 white tablet daily for 21 days, followed without interruption by 1 brown tablet daily for 7 days, the patient will start all subsequent cycles on a Sunday.

Day-1 Start Regimen

The first day of menstrual flow is Day 1. The patient places the self-adhesive day label strip that corresponds to her starting day over the preprinted days on the tablet dispenser. She starts taking 1 white tablet daily, beginning with the first white tablet in the top row. After the last white tablet (at the end of the third row) has been taken, the patient will then take the brown tablets for a week (7 days). For all subsequent cycles, the patient begins a new 28 tablet regimen on the eighth day after taking her last white tablet, again starting with the first tablet in the top row after placing the appropriate day label strip over the preprinted days on the tablet dispenser. Following this regimen of 21 white tablets and 7 brown tablets, the patient will start all subsequent cycles on the same day of the week as the first course.

Tablets should be taken regularly at the same time each day and can be taken without regard to meals. It should be stressed that efficacy of medication depends on strict adherence to the dosage schedule.

Special Notes on Administration

Menstruation usually begins 2 or 3 days, but may begin as late as the 4th or 5th day, after the brown tablets have been started. In any event, the next course of tablets should be started without interruption. If spotting occurs while the patient is taking white tablets, continue medication without interruption.

If the patient forgets to take one or more white tablets, the following is suggested:

***One* tablet missed**

Take tablet as soon as remembered.
Take next tablet at the regular time.

***Two* Consecutive tablets are missed (Week 1 or Week 2)**

Take 2 tablets as soon as remembered.
Take 2 tablets the next day.
Use another birth control method for 7 days following the missed tablets.

***Two* consecutive tablets are missed (Week 3)**

Sunday-Start Regimen

Take 1 tablet daily until Sunday.
Discard remaining tablets.
Start new pack of tablets immediately (Sunday)
Use another birth control method for 7 days following the missed tablets.

Day-1 Start Regimen

Discard remaining tablets.
Start new pack of tablets that same day.
Use another birth control method for 7 days following the missed tablets.

***Three* (or more) consecutive tablets are missed**

Sunday-Start Regimen

Take 1 tablet daily until Sunday.
Discard remaining tablets.
Start new pack of tablets immediately (Sunday)
Use another birth control method for 7 days following the missed tablets.

Day-1 Start Regimen

Discard remaining tablets.
Start new pack of tablets that same day.
Use another birth control method for 7 days following the missed tablets.

The possibility of ovulation occurring increases with each successive day that scheduled white tablets are missed. While there is little likelihood of ovulation occurring if only 1 white tablet is missed, the possibility of spotting or bleeding is increased. This is particularly likely to occur if 2 or more consecutive white tablets are missed.

If the patient forgets to take any of the 7 brown tablets in week 4, those brown tablets that were missed are discarded and 1 brown tablet is taken each day until the pack is empty. A back-up birth control method is not required during this time. A new pack of tablets should be started no later than the eighth day after the last white tablet was taken.

In the rare case of bleeding which resembles menstruation, the patient should be advised to discontinue medication and then begin taking tablets from a new tablet dispenser on the next Sunday or the first day (Day 1), depending on her regimen. Persistent bleeding which is not controlled by this method indicates the need for reexamination of the patient, at which time nonfunctional causes should be considered.

USE OF ORAL CONTRACEPTIVES IN THE EVENT OF A MISSED MENSTRUAL PERIOD

(1) If the patient has not adhered to the prescribed dosage regimen, the possibility of pregnancy should be considered after the first missed period and oral contraceptives should be withheld until pregnancy has been ruled out.

(2) If the patient has adhered to the prescribed regimen and misses two consecutive periods, pregnancy should be ruled out before continuing the contraceptive regimen.

After several months on treatment, bleeding may be reduced to a point of virtual absence. This reduced flow may occur as a result of medication, in which event it is not indicative of pregnancy.

HOW SUPPLIED

Estrostep Fe is available in dispensers each containing 21 white tablets. The first 5 triangle tablets each contain 1 mg of norethindrone acetate and 20 µg of ethinyl estradiol; the next 7 square tablets each contain 1 mg of norethindrone acetate and 30 µg of ethinyl estradiol; the next 9 round tablets each contain 1 mg of norethindrone acetate and 35 µg of ethinyl estradiol; and the last 7 (brown) tablets each contain 75 mg ferrous fumarate.

Storage: Do not store above 25°C (77°F). Protect from light. Store tablets inside pouch when not in use.

Ethinyl Estradiol; Levonorgestrel *(001219)*

Categories: Contraception; Contraception, emergency; Pregnancy Category X; FDA Approved 1982 May; WHO Formulary

Drug Classes: Contraceptives; Estrogens; Hormones/hormone modifiers; Progestins

Brand Names: Alesse; Levlen; Levora-21; Levora-28; Minigynon; Tri-Levlen; Tri-Levlen 21; Triphasil; Trivora

Foreign Brand Availability: Adepal (France); Alesse 21 (Canada); Alesse 28 (Canada); Anna (Thailand); Anulette (Peru); Biphasil 28 (Australia); E-Gen-C (South-Africa); Gynatrol (Denmark); Klimonorm (Hong-Kong); Levlen ED (Australia; New-Zealand); Loette (New-Zealand; Singapore); Loette 21 (Singapore); Logynon (Bahrain; Benin; Burkina-Faso; Cyprus; Egypt; Ethiopia; Gambia; Ghana; Guinea; Iran; Iraq; Israel; Ivory-Coast; Jordan; Kenya; Kuwait; Lebanon; Liberia; Libya; Malawi; Mali; Mauritania; Mauritius; Morocco; Niger; Nigeria; Oman; Philippines; Qatar; Republic-of-Yemen; Saudi-Arabia; Senegal; Seychelles; Sierra-Leone; South-Africa; Sudan; Syria; Tanzania; Tunia; Uganda; United-Arab-Emirates; Zambia; Zimbabwe); Logynon ED (Australia; Bahamas; Barbados; Belize; Bermuda; Curacao; Guyana; Jamaica; Netherland-Antilles; New-Zealand; Puerto-Rico; South-Africa; Surinam; Trinidad); Microfemin (Colombia); Microfemin CD (Colombia); Microgest ED (Thailand); Microgyn (Denmark); Microgynon (Colombia; Costa-Rica; Czech-Republic; Denmark; Dominican-Republic; Ecuador; El-Salvador; Finland; Greece; Guatemala; Honduras; Indonesia; Israel; Italy; Mexico; Nicaragua; Norway; Panama; Peru; Philippines; Spain); Microgynon CD (Colombia; Costa-Rica; Dominican-Republic; Ecuador; El-Salvador; Guatemala; Honduras; Mexico; Nicaragua; Panama); Microgynon 20 ED (Australia; New-Zealand); Microgynon 21 (Germany); Microgynon 28 (Germany); Microgynon 30 (Australia; Austria; Bahamas; Bahrain; Barbados; Belgium; Belize; Benin; Bermuda; Burkina-Faso; Curacao; Cyprus; Egypt; England; Ethiopia; Gambia; Ghana; Guinea; Guyana; Hong-Kong; Iran; Iraq; Ireland; Israel; Ivory-Coast; Jamaica; Jordan; Kenya; Kuwait; Lebanon; Liberia; Libya; Malawi; Malaysia; Mali; Mauritania; Mauritius; Morocco; Netherland-Antilles; Netherlands; New-Zealand; Niger; Nigeria; Oman; Philippines; Puerto-Rico; Qatar; Republic-of-Yemen; Saudi-Arabia; Senegal; Seychelles; Sierra-Leone; South-Africa; Sudan; Surinam; Switzerland; Syria; Tanzania; Trinidad; Tunia; Uganda; United-Arab-Emirates; Zambia; Zimbabwe); Microgynon 30 ED (Australia; Hong-Kong; New-Zealand; Thailand); Minidril (France); Minisiston (Taiwan); Minivlar 30 (Korea); Min-Ovral 21 (Canada); Min-Ovral 28 (Canada); Monofeme 28 (Australia; New-Zealand); Neogynon 21 (Germany); Nordet (Mexico); Nordette (Argentina; Bahrain; Benin; Burkina-Faso; Costa-Rica; Cyprus; Dominican-Republic; Egypt; El-Salvador; Ethiopia; Gambia; Ghana; Greece; Guatemala; Guinea; Honduras; Hong-Kong; Iran; Iraq; Israel; Ivory-Coast; Jordan; Kenya; Kuwait; Lebanon; Liberia; Libya; Malawi; Malaysia; Mali; Mauritania; Mauritius; Morocco; Nicaragua; Niger; Nigeria; Oman; Panama; Peru; Philippines; Qatar; Republic-of-Yemen; Saudi-Arabia; Senegal; Seychelles; Sierra-Leone; South-Africa; Sudan; Syria; Taiwan; Tanzania; Tunia; Uganda; United-Arab-Emirates; Zambia; Zimbabwe); Nordette 21 (Australia; New-Zealand; Thailand); Nordette 28 (Australia; Colombia; Costa-Rica; Dominican-Republic; El-Salvador; Guatemala; Honduras; Indonesia; New-Zealand; Nicaragua; Panama; Thailand); Novastep (Germany); Ovoplex 30-150 (Spain); Ovranette (Austria; England); Preven (Canada); Rigevidon (Bahrain; Cyprus; Egypt; Iran; Iraq; Jordan; Kuwait; Lebanon; Libya; Oman; Qatar; Republic-of-Yemen; Saudi-Arabia; Syria; United-Arab-Emirates); Rigevidon 21+7 (Hong-Kong; Malaysia; Philippines); Sequilar ED (Australia); Stediril 30 (Belgium; Czech-Republic; Netherlands; Switzerland); Tetragynon (France); Triagynon (Spain); Triciclor (Spain); Trifeme 28 (Australia; New-Zealand); Trifeminal (Colombia); Trigoa (Germany); Trigynon (Austria; Belgium); Trinordiol (Austria; Bahrain; Belgium; Benin; Burkina-Faso; Costa-Rica; Cyprus; Czech-Republic; Denmark; Dominican-Republic; Ecuador; Egypt; El-Salvador; England; Ethiopia; France; Gambia; Germany; Ghana; Greece; Guatemala; Guinea; Honduras; Hong-Kong; Iran; Iraq; Ireland; Israel; Ivory-Coast; Jordan; Kenya; Kuwait; Lebanon; Liberia; Libya; Malawi; Malaysia; Mali; Mauritania; Mauritius; Mexico; Morocco; Netherlands; Nicaragua; Niger; Nigeria; Oman; Panama; Philippines; Qatar; Republic-of-Yemen; Russia; Saudi-Arabia; Senegal; Seychelles; Sierra-Leone; South-Africa; Sudan; Sweden; Syria; Taiwan; Tanzania; Tunia; Uganda; United-Arab-Emirates; Zambia; Zimbabwe); Trinordiol 21 (Germany; Indonesia); Trinordiol 28 (Indonesia); Triphasil 21 (Australia; Canada; New-Zealand); Triphasil 28 (Australia; Canada; New-Zealand); Triquilar (Australia; Bahrain; Canada; China; Costa-Rica; Cyprus; Czech-Republic; Dominican-Republic; Ecuador; Egypt; El-Salvador; Germany; Greece; Guatemala; Honduras; Hong-Kong; India; Iran; Iraq; Israel; Jordan; Korea; Kuwait; Lebanon; Libya; Malaysia; Mexico; New-Zealand; Nicaragua; Oman; Panama; Peru; Qatar; Republic-of-Yemen; Saudi-Arabia; Syria; United-Arab-Emirates); Triquilar ED (Australia; China; Hong-Kong; Indonesia; Malaysia; New-Zealand; Thailand); Tri-Regol (Philippines); Trolit (Peru)

Cost of Therapy: $16.40 (Contraceptive; Tri-Levlen; triphasic; 1 tablet/day; 21 day supply)
$16.40 (Contraceptive; Tri-Levlen; triphasic; 1 tablet/day; 28 day supply)
$30.86 (Contraceptive; Nordette; 30 µg; 0.15 mg; 1 tablet/day; 21 day supply)
$30.86 (Contraceptive; Nordette; 30 µg; 0.15 mg; 1 tablet/day; 28 day supply)

DESCRIPTION

TRIPHASIL

Each Triphasil cycle of 21 tablets consists of three different drug phases as follows: Phase 1 comprised of 6 brown tablets, each containing 0.050 mg of levonorgestrel, a totally synthetic progestogen, and 0.030 mg of ethinyl estradiol; phase 2 comprised of 5 white tablets, each containing 0.075 mg levongestrel and 0.040 mg ethinyl estradiol; phase 3 comprised of 10 light-yellow tablets, each containing 0.125 mg levongestrel and 0.030 mg ethinyl estradiol. *Inactive Ingredients:* Calcium carbonate, glycerin, iron oxides, lactose, magnesium stearate, methylparaben, polyethylene glycol, povidone, propylparaben, sodium benzoate, starch, sucrose, talc, and titanium dioxide.

NORDETTE

Each Nordette tablet contains 0.15 mg of levongestrel, a totally synthetic progestogen, and 0.03 mg of ethinyl estradiol. *Inactive Ingredients:* Cellulose, FD&C yellow 6, lactose, magnesium stearate, and polacrillin potassium. The tablets are round, light orange and marked with "WYETH" and "75".

FDA RECOMMENDED DOSAGE GUIDELINES FOR POSTCOITAL EMERGENCY CONTRACEPTION

The FDA has declared oral contraceptives safe and effective for emergency contraception. Vomiting, sometimes severe enough to prevent the pills from working, and nausea are potential side effects. The dosing regimens for ethinyl estradiol/levonorgestrel can be taken within 72 hours of unprotected intercourse with a follow-up dose of the same number of pills 12 hours after the first dose:

Levlen: Four light orange tablets.
Nordette: Four light orange tablets.
Triphasil: Four yellow tablets.
Tri-Levlen: Four yellow tablets.

The Preven Emergency Contraceptive Kit is intended to prevent pregnancy after known or suspected contraceptive failure or unprotected intercourse. Emergency contraceptive pills (like all oral contraceptives) do not protect against infection with HIV (the virus that causes AIDS) and other sexually transmitted diseases.

The Preven Emergency Contraceptive Kit consists of a patient information book, a urine pregnancy test and 4 emergency contraceptive pills (ECPs).

The pills in the Preven Emergency Contraceptive Kit are combination oral contraceptives (COCs) which are used to provide postcoital emergency contraception.

Each blue film-coated pill contains 0.25 mg levonorgestrel (18,19-Dinorpregn-4-en-20-yn-3-one, 13-Ethyl-17-hydroxy-, (17α)-(-), a totally synthetic progestogen, and 0.05 mg ethinyl estradiol (19-Nor-17α-pregna-1,3,5, (10)-trien-20-yne-3,17-diol). *Inactive Ingredients:* Polacrilin potassium, lactose, magnesium stearate, hydroxypropyl methylcellulose, titanium dioxide, polyethylene glycol, polysorbate 80 and FD&C blue no. 2 aluminum lake.

The Pregnancy Test uses monoclonal antibodies to detect the presence of hCG (Human Chorionic Gonadotropin) in the urine. It is sensitive to 20-25 mIU/ml.

E

CLINICAL PHARMACOLOGY

ECPs are not effective if the woman is pregnant; they act primarily by inhibiting ovulation. They may also act by altering tubal transport of sperm and/or ova (thereby inhibiting fertilization), and/or possibly altering the endometrium (thereby inhibiting implantation).

PHARMACOKINETICS

Absorption

No specific investigation of the absolute bioavailability of the ECPs in humans have been conducted. However, literature indicates that levonorgestrel is rapidly and completely absorbed after oral administration (bioavailability about 100%) and it is not subject to first-pass metabolism. Ethinyl estradiol is rapidly absorbed from the gastrointestinal tract but due to marked metabolism in the gut mucosa and during passage through the liver, ethinyl estradiol absolute bioavailability after oral administration is about 40-50%.

After a single oral dose of two ECPs to 35 postmenopausal women under fasting conditions, the bioavailabilities of levonorgestrel and ethinyl estradiol were about 94% and 97%, respectively, relative to the same two active drugs given in an oral reference tablet. The obtained pharmacokinetic parameters for levonorgestrel and ethinyl estradiol are presented in TABLE 1. The effect of food on the bioavailability of the ECPs following oral administration has not been evaluated.

TABLE 1 *Mean (SD) Pharmacokinetic Parameters After Oral Dose of 2 ECPs*

	C_{max}	T_{max}	AUC	$T_{½}$
Levonorgestrel (n=35)				
	10.9 ng/ml (4.0)	1.7 h (1.0)	167 ng/ml·h (92)	40.8 h (19.2)
Ethinyl Estradiol (n=35)				
	248.2 pg/ml (67)	1.7 h (0.4)	2747 pg/ml·h (701)	21.2 h (9.3)

Distribution

Levonorgestrel in serum is primarily bound to SHBG. Ethinyl estradiol is about 97% bound to plasma albumin. Ethinyl estradiol does not bind to SHBG but induces SHBG synthesis.

Metabolism

Levonorgestrel

The most important metabolic pathways occur in the reduction of the ≅e; 4-3-oxo group and hydroxylation at positions 2α, 10β, 16β, followed by conjugation. Most of the metabolites that circulate in the blood are sulfates of 3α, 5β-tetrahydro-levonorgestrel, while excretion occurs predominantly in the form of glucuronides. Some of the parent levonorgestrel also circulates as 17β-sulfate. Metabolic clearance rates may differ among individuals by several fold, and this may account in part for the high variability observed in levonorgestrel concentrations among users.

Ethinyl Estradiol

The cytochrome P450 enzyme (CYP3A4) is responsible for the 2-hydroxylation that is the major oxidative reaction. The 2-hydroxy metabolite is further transformed by methylation and glucuronidation prior to urinary and fecal excretion. Levels of Cytochrome P450 (CYP3A) vary widely among individuals and can explain the variation in rates of ethinyl estradiol 2-hydroxylation. Ethinyl estradiol is excreted in the urine and feces as glucoronides and sulfates and undergoes enterohepatic circulation.

Elimination

The elimination half-life for levonorgestrel after a single dose of two ECPs is 40.8 ± 19 hours. Levonorgestrel and its metabolites are primarily excreted in the urine. The elimination half-life of ethinyl estradiol is 21.2 ± 9.3 hours.

Special Populations

This product is not intended for use in geriatric (age 65 or older) or pediatric (premenarchal) populations and pharmacokinetic data are unavailable for these populations. Steroid hormones may be poorly metabolized in patients with impaired liver function.

Race, Hepatic Insuffiency, and Renal Insuffiency: No formal studies have evaluated the effect of race, hepatic disease and renal disease on the disposition of the ECPs.

INDICATIONS AND USAGE

INDICATIONS

Ethinyl estradiol, levonorgestrel is indicated for the prevention of pregnancy in women after known or suspected contraceptive failure or unprotected intercourse. To obtain optimal efficacy, use of these pills should begin as soon as possible but within 72 hours of intercourse.

EFFICACY

If 100 women used ECPs correctly in 1 month, about 2 women would become pregnant after a single act of intercourse. If no contraception is used about 8 women would become pregnant after a single act of intercourse. Therefore, the use of ECPs results in a 75% reduction in the number of pregnancies to be expected if no ECPs were used after unprotected intercourse. Notably, some clinical trials have shown that efficacy was greatest when ECPs were taken within 24 hours of unprotected intercourse, decreasing somewhat during each subsequent 24 hour period.

ECPs are not as effective as some other forms of contraception. For effectiveness rates of other contraceptive methods, refer to TABLE 2.

TABLE 2 *Percentage of Women Experiencing an Unintended Pregnancy During the First Year of Typical Use and the First Year of Contraception and the Percentage Continuing Use at the End of the First Year — United States.*

	% of Women Experiencing an Unintended Pregnancy within the First Year of Use		% of Women Continuing Use at 1 Year
Method (1)	**Typical Use* (2)**	**Perfect Use† (3)**	**(4)**
Chance‡	85%	85%	
Spermicides§	26%	6%	40%
Periodic abstinence	25%		63%
Calendar		9%	
Ovulation method		3%	
Symptom-thermal¤		2%	
Post-ovulation		1%	
Withdrawal	19%	4%	
Cap¶			
Parous women	40%	26%	42%
Nulliparous women	20%	9%	56%
Sponge			
Parous women	40%	20%	42%
Nulliparous women	20%	9%	56%
Diaphragm¶	20%	6%	56%
Condom**			
Female (Reality)	21%	5%	56%
Male	14%	3%	56%
Oral contraceptives	5%		71%
Progestin only		0.5%	
Combined		0.1%	
IUD			
Progestin T	2.0%	1.5%	81%
Copper T 380A	0.8%	0.6%	78%
LNG	0.1%	0.1%	81%
Depo-Provera	0.3%	0.3%	
Norplant and Norplant-2	0.05%	0.05%	88%
Female sterilization	0.5%	0.5%	100%
Male sterilization	0.15%	0.10%	100%

Emergency Contraceptive Pills: Treatment initiated within 72 hours after unprotected intercourse reduces the risk of pregnancy by at least 75%.

Lactational Amenorrhea Method: LAM is a highly effective temporary method of contraception.††

* Among typical couples who initiate use of a method (not necessarily for the first time) who experience an accidental pregnancy during the first year if they do not stop use for any other reason.

† Among couples who initiate use of a method (not necessarily for the first time) and who use it perfectly (both consistently and correctly) the percentage who experience an accidental pregnancy during the first year if they do not stop use for any other reason.

‡ The percent becoming pregnant in columns (2) and (3) are based on data from populations where contraception is not used and from women who cease using contraception in order to become pregnant. Among such populations, about 89% become pregnant within 1 year among women now relying on reversible methods of contraception if they abandoned contraception altogether.

§ Foams, creams, gels, vaginal suppositories, and vaginal film.

¤ Cervical mucus (ovulation) method supplemented by calendar in the pre-ovulatory and basal body temperature in the post-ovulatory phases.

¶ With spermicidal cream or jelly.

** Without spermicides.

†† However, to maintain an effective protection against pregnancy, another method of contraception must be used as soon as menstruation resumes, the frequency or duration of breastfeeds is reduced, bottle feeds are introduced, or the baby reaches 6 months of age.

Source: Trussell J. Contraceptive efficacy. In Hatcher RA, Trussell J, Stewart F, Cates W, Stewart GK, Guest F, Kowal D. Contraceptive Technology Seventeenth Revised Edition. New York NY: Irvington Publishers, 1998

CONTRAINDICATIONS

Ethinyl estradiol; levonorgestrel are combination oral contraceptive (COC) pills. The following are the known contraindications of daily cyclical combination oral contraceptive pill use (1 pill each day for 21 days of a 28 day cycle). It is not known whether these contraindications also apply to the ECP regimen of 4 oral contraceptive pills taken within a 12 hour period.

- Known or suspected pregnancy.
- Pulmonary embolism (current or history).
- Ischemic heart disease (current or history).
- History of cerebrovascular accidents.
- Valvular heart disease with complications.
- Severe hypertension.
- Diabetes with vascular involvement.
- Headaches with focal neurological symptoms.
- Major surgery with prolonged immobilization.
- Known or suspected carcinoma of the breast or personal history of breast cancer.
- Liver tumors (benign and malignant) active liver disease.
- Heavy smoking (>15 cigarettes per day) and over the age of 35.
- In addition, use is contraindicated in women who are known to be hypersensitive to any component of this product.

WARNINGS

Ethinyl estradiol; levonorgestrel are combination oral contraceptive (COC) pills. The following are the warnings given for daily cyclical combination oral contraceptive pill use (1 pill each day for 21 days of a 28 day cycle). It is not known whether these warnings also apply to the ECP regimen of four oral contraceptive pills taken within a 12 hour period.

Cigarette smoking increases the risk of serious cardiovascular side effects from COC use. This risk increases with age and heavy smoking (15 or more cigarettes per day) and is quite marked in women over 35 years of age. Women who use COCs should be strongly advised not to smoke.

CARDIOVASCULAR DISEASE (CVD)

COC use is associated with a small increase in the incidence of cardiovascular disease (CVD), primarily because of an increased risk of thrombosis rather than through an atherogenic mechanism. The degree of risk appears to be related primarily to the estrogen dosage. This increased risk is limited to the period during COC use and disappears upon cessation of use. Because the incidence of CVD is low during the reproductive years, the absolute risk attributable to COC use is quite small.

Deep Vein Thrombosis, Pulmonary Embolism

Use of COCs is associated with a low absolute risk of venous thromembolism which is nonetheless 3- to 6-fold higher than that among non-users. Smoking does not appear to be a risk factor.

The presence of factor V Leiden mutation and other hereditary coagulation disorders increases the risk of thromboembolic disease.

COC use is contraindicated for women who have deep vein thrombosis or pulmonary embolism and for those who have a history of these conditions.

Women who are immobilized for prolonged periods because of major surgery (or illness or injury) should not use COCs. For women undergoing major surgery without prolonged immobilization, the advantages of COC use generally outweigh the risk.

COC use should preferably not begin until two to three weeks postpartum, because of the risk of thrombosis.

Cerebrovascular Disease

In women who do not smoke and do not have hypertension, the risk of ischemic stroke in users of COCs is increased about 1.5 fold compared with non-users. The likelihood of hemorrhagic stroke is not increased among users of low-dose combined COCs who are under 35 years old and do not smoke or have hypertension. Women who have a history of stroke should not use COCs.

Ischemic Heart Disease

The likelihood of myocardial infarction is not increased among young women who use COCs and do not smoke or have hypertension or diabetes. Smokers older than 35 should not take COCs. Women who currently have ischemic heart disease, or who have a history of this disease, should not use COCs.

Valvular Heart Disease

COC use is contraindicated for women whose valvular heart disease is complicated by such factors as pulmonary hypertension, atrial fibrillation, or history of sub-acute bacterial endocarditis. COC use may be acceptable for women with uncomplicated valvular heart disease.

ELEVATED BLOOD PRESSURE

For women with an elevation in blood pressure (160+/100+ mm Hg), COC use would present an unacceptable health risk, and COCs should not be used. Similarly, hypertensive women with vascular disease should not use COCs.

OCULAR LESIONS

There have been clinical case reports of retinal thrombosis associated with the use of oral contraceptives. Oral contraceptives should be discontinued if there is unexplained partial or complete loss of vision; onset of proptosis or diplopia; papilledema; or retinal vascular lesions.

CARBOHYDRATE METABOLISM

For women with diabetes (both insulin-dependent and non-insulin dependent), who do not have vascular involvement, the advantages of COC use generally outweigh the risks, particularly the risks associated with pregnancy. The major concerns are vascular disease and added risk of thrombosis, although COC use by diabetic women appears to have only minimal effects on lipid metabolism and hemostasis. For diabetic women with nephropathy, retinopathy, neuropathy, or other vascular involvement, the risk-benefit ratio depends on the severity of the condition.

HEADACHES

For women with severe, recurrent headaches, including migraine headaches, the appropriateness of using COCs depends on the presence or absence of focal neurologic symptoms. These symptoms may reflect an increased risk of stroke and COC use is contraindicated in patients in whom they are present. The onset or exacerbation of migraines or the development of severe headache with focal neurological symptoms, which are recurrent or persistent, requires discontinuation of COC use and evaluation of the cause.

UNEXPLAINED VAGINAL BLEEDING

Women who have unexplained vaginal bleeding, suggestive of an underlying pathological condition or pregnancy, should be evaluated prior to initiation of COC use in order to avoid confusion of the pathological bleeding with COC side effects.

LIVER DISEASE

Because steroid hormones are metabolized by the liver, women taking COCs may experience adverse hepatobiliary effects. Although case-control studies have indicated that the risk of both benign and malignant liver tumors may be slightly increased by COC use, the incidence potentially attributable to COCs in the United States is minimal because the disease is very rare.

Women who currently have active liver disease should not use COCs.

ECTOPIC PREGNANCY

Ectopic as well as intrauterine pregnancy may occur in contraceptive failures.

PRECAUTIONS

SEXUALLY TRANSMITTED DISEASES

Women should be informed that this product does not protect against infection with HIV (the virus that causes AIDS) and other sexually transmitted diseases (STDs). If a woman is at high risk for STDs she should be encouraged to reduce risky behavior and to use condoms or other barrier methods (in addition to COCs).

PREGNANCY

Extensive research has found no significant effects on fetal development associated with long-term use of contraceptive doses of oral steroids before pregnancy or taken inadvertently during early pregnancy.

NURSING MOTHERS

Oral contraceptive steroids have been reported in the milk of breastfeeding mothers with no apparent clinical significance; long-term follow-up of breastfeeding mothers with no apparent clinical significance; long-term follow-up of children whose mothers used COCs while breastfeeding has shown no deleterious effects.

PEDIATRIC USE

The safety and efficacy of COCs have been established in women of reproductive age. Safety and efficacy are expected to be the same for postpubertal adolescents under 16 and users 16 and older. Use of this product before menarche is not indicated.

REPEATED USE OF EMERGENCY CONTRACEPTIVE PILLS

The effect of repeated use of ECPs (more than once in a menstrual cycle or in multiple cycles) is unknown.

See the Patient Instructions that are distributed with the prescription.

DRUG INTERACTIONS

No specific drug-drug interaction studies for the ECPs were conducted but there are many publications that indicate that interactions between ethinyl estradiol and other drugs may occur. Other drugs may decrease the effectiveness of ethinyl estradiol or other drugs may enhance ethinyl estradiol levels resulting in possible increased side-effects. Ethinyl estradiol may interfere with the metabolism of other compounds. In general, the effect of other drugs on ethinyl estradiol is due to interference with the absorption, metabolism or excretion of ethinyl estradiol, whereas the effect of ethinyl estradiol on other drugs is due to competition for metabolic pathways.

ABSORPTION INTERACTIONS

Infective diarrhea may induce failure of ethinyl estradiol by increasing gastrointestinal motility and reducing hormone absorption. Therefore, any drug which increases gastrointestinal transit and causes diarrhea is potentially likely to reduce concentrations of ethinyl estradiol.

INTERACTIONS WITH METABOLISM

Gastrointestinal Wall

The gastrointestinal wall has been shown to be a site for interaction for the sulfation of ethinyl estradiol. Inhibition of the sulfation in the gastrointestinal tract may increase the bioavailability of ethinyl estradiol and result in possible increased side-effects. (For example, ascorbic acid acts as competitive inhibitor for sulfation in the gastrointestinal wall increasing ethinyl estradiol bioavailability about 50%).

Hepatic Metabolism

The most clinically significant group of interactions occurs with other drugs that may induce ethinyl estradiol microsomal enzymes which may decrease ethinyl estradiol plasma levels below therapeutic level (for example, anticonvulsant agents; phenytoin, primidone, barbiturates, carbamazepine, ethosuximide, and methosuximide; antituberculous drugs such as rifampin; antifungal drugs such as griseofulvin).

INTERFERENCE WITH ENTEROHEPATIC CIRCULATION

Ethinyl estradiol conjugates are excreted in the bile and may be broken down by gut bacteria in the colon to liberate the active hormone which can then be reabsorbed. However, there are clinical reports that support the view that enterohepatic circulation of ethinyl estradiol decreases in women taking antibiotics such as ampicillin, tetracycline, etc.

INTERFERENCE IN THE METABOLISM OF OTHER DRUGS

Ethinyl estradiol can inhibit microsomal enzymes and therefore possibly interfere in the metabolism of other drugs. In this way it may slow the metabolism of other drugs, increasing their plasma and tissue concentrations and increasing the risk of side-effects (*i.e.,* analgesic anti-inflammatory drugs such as antipyrin, antidepressant agents, cyclosporin, theophylline, ethanol, etc.). In addition, estrogens appear to have the capacity to induce hepatic drug conjugation, particularly glucuronidation. This will have the opposite pharmacokinetic effect to the inhibitory action on hydroxylation.

ADVERSE REACTIONS

The pills provided in the Preven Emergency Contraceptive Kit are combination oral contraceptive (COC) pills. Based on clinical experience over several years of use of ECPs the most common side effects reported were as follows:

- Nausea.
- Vomiting.
- Menstrual irregularities.
- Breast tenderness.
- Headache.
- Abdominal pain/cramps.
- Dizziness.

DOSAGE AND ADMINISTRATION

The Preven Emergency Contraceptive Kit contains a pregnancy test. This test can be used to verify an existing pregnancy resulting from intercourse that occurred earlier in the current menstrual cycle or the previous cycle. If a positive pregnancy result is obtained, the patient should not take the pills in the Preven Kit.

The initial two pills must be taken as soon as possible but within **72 hours** of unprotected intercourse. This is followed by the second dose of two pills 12 hours later. The patient should be instructed that if she vomits within 1 hour of taking either dose of the medication, she should contact her healthcare professional to discuss whether to repeat that dose or to take an antinausea medication. ECPs are not indicated for ongoing pregnancy protection and should not be used as a woman's routine form of contraception.

HOW SUPPLIED

The Preven Emergency Contraceptive Kit is available in a carton which includes a patient information book, a pregnancy test in a sealed foil pack, four emergency contraceptive pills (ECPs) and detailed patient labeling.

Each pill contains 0.25 mg levonorgestrel and 0.05 mg ethinyl estradiol. The pills are marked with a "G" on one side and the numerals "891" on the other.

Storage: Store at 25°C (77°F); excursions permitted to 15-30°C (59-86°F).

PRODUCT LISTING - RATED THERAPEUTICALLY EQUIVALENT

Size	Price	Product	NDC
Tablet - Oral - Triphasic			
21 x 3	$97.35	TRIPHASIL, Wyeth-Ayerst Laboratories	00008-2535-01
21's	$31.69	TRIPHASIL, Wyeth-Ayerst Laboratories	00008-2535-05
28 x 3	$89.91	TRIPHASIL-28, Allscripts Pharmaceutical Company	54569-0695-01
28 x 3	$97.35	TRIPHASIL, Wyeth-Ayerst Laboratories	00008-2536-01
28 x 6	$164.92	GENERIC, Barr Laboratories Inc	51285-0514-28
28 x 6	$164.94	GENERIC, Watson Laboratories Inc	52544-0291-28
28's	$25.66	GENERIC, Allscripts Pharmaceutical Company	54569-5115-00
28's	$31.69	TRIPHASIL, Wyeth-Ayerst Laboratories	00008-2536-05
28's	$32.52	TRIPHASIL, Physicians Total Care	54868-0518-01
Tablet - Oral - 20 mcg;100 mcg			
21 x 3	$106.74	ALESSE, Lederle Laboratories	00008-0912-02
28 each	$32.95	ALESSE, Wyeth-Ayerst Laboratories	00008-2576-01
28 x 3	$106.74	ALESSE, Wyeth-Ayerst Laboratories	00008-2576-02
28 x 3	$106.77	LEVLITE, Berlex Laboratories	50419-0408-03
28 x 6	$177.90	AVIANE, Duramed Pharmaceuticals Inc	51285-0017-28
28's	$29.60	LEVLITE, Allscripts Pharmaceutical Company	54569-4710-00
Tablet - Oral - 30 mcg;0.15 mg			
21 x 6	$159.66	GENERIC, Watson/Rugby Laboratories Inc	52544-0277-21
21 x 6	$206.94	NORDETTE, Wyeth-Ayerst Laboratories	00008-0075-01
21's	$21.03	NORDETTE, Wyeth-Ayerst Laboratories	00008-0075-02
28 x 6	$185.58	GENERIC, Barr Laboratories Inc	00555-9020-58
28 x 6	$185.58	GENERIC, Watson/Rugby Laboratories Inc	52544-0279-28
28 x 6	$206.94	NORDETTE, Wyeth-Ayerst Laboratories	00008-2533-02
28's	$21.29	NORDETTE, Wyeth-Ayerst Laboratories	00008-2533-01
28's	$26.61	GENERIC, Allscripts Pharmaceutical Company	54569-4997-00

PRODUCT LISTING - RATED NOT THERAPEUTICALLY EQUIVALENT

Size	Price	Product	NDC
Tablet - Oral - 20 mcg;100 mcg			
28 x 6	$176.16	GENERIC, Barr Laboratories Inc	00555-9014-58
28 x 6	$191.94	GENERIC, Berlex Laboratories	00555-9045-58

PRODUCT LISTING - EQUIVALENTS NOT AVAILABLE

Size	Price	Product	NDC
Tablet - Oral - Triphasic			
21 x 3	$95.49	TRI-LEVLEN, Berlex Laboratories	50419-0432-03
21 x 6	$182.06	TRI-LEVLEN, Berlex Laboratories	50419-0432-06
28 x 3	$34.09	TRI-LEVLEN, Physicians Total Care	54868-3328-00
28 x 3	$98.37	TRI-LEVLEN, Berlex Laboratories	50419-0433-12
28 x 3	$98.38	TRI-LEVLEN, Berlex Laboratories	50419-0433-03
28 x 6	$187.56	TRI-LEVLEN, Berlex Laboratories	50419-0433-06
28's	$28.29	TRI-LEVLEN, Allscripts Pharmaceutical Company	54569-1439-00
Tablet - Oral - 0.05 mg;0.25 mg			
3's	$59.82	PREVEN EC, Gynetics Inc	63955-0010-01
4's	$12.50	PREVEN EC, Gynetics Inc	63955-0020-02
Tablet - Oral - 30 mcg;0.15 mg			
2's	$5.24	NORDETTE, Prescript Pharmaceuticals	00247-0247-02
5's	$8.05	NORDETTE, Prescript Pharmaceuticals	00247-0247-05
21 x 3	$102.99	GENERIC, Berlex Laboratories	50419-0410-21
28 x 3	$102.99	GENERIC, Berlex Laboratories	50419-0411-28
28 x 3	$103.00	GENERIC, Berlex Laboratories	50419-0411-12
28's	$29.67	NORDETTE, Prescript Pharmaceuticals	00247-0247-28
28's	$30.83	GENERIC, Allscripts Pharmaceutical Company	54569-3844-00

E

Ethinyl Estradiol; Norelgestromin *(003535)*

Categories: Contraception; FDA Approved 2001 Nov; Pregnancy Category X
Drug Classes: Contraceptives; Estrogens; Hormones/hormone modifiers; Progestins
Brand Names: **Ortho Evra**
Cost of Therapy: $35.13 (Contracepton; Ortho Evra Transdermal; 20 μg; 150 μg; 1 patch/week; 21 day supply)

DESCRIPTION

Note: The trade name has been used throughout this monograph for clarity.

Patients should be counseled that this product does not protect against HIV infection (AIDS) and other sexually transmitted diseases.

Ortho Evra is a combination transdermal contraceptive patch with a contact surface area of 20 cm^2. It contains 6.00 mg norelgestromin and 0.75 mg ethinyl estradiol (EE), and releases 150 μg of norelgestromin and 20 μg of EE to the bloodstream per 24 hours.

Ortho Evra is a thin, matrix-type transdermal contraceptive patch consisting of three layers. The backing layer is composed of a beige flexible film consisting of a low-density pigmented polyethylene outer layer and a polyester inner layer. It provides structural support and protects the middle adhesive layer from the environment. The middle layer contains polyisobutylene/polybutene adhesive, crospovidone, non-woven polyester fabric and lauryl lactate as inactive components. The active components in this layer are the hormones, norelgestromin and ethinyl estradiol. The third layer is the release liner, which protects the adhesive layer during storage and is removed just prior to application. It is a transparent polyethylene terephthalate (PET) film with a polydimethylsiloxane coating on the side that is in contact with the middle adhesive layer.

The outside of the backing layer is heat-stamped "ORTHO EVRA 150/20".

Molecular weight, norelgestromin: 327.47

Molecular weight, ethinyl estradiol: 296.41

Chemical name for norelgestromin: 18,19-dinorpregn-4-en-20-yn-3-one, 13-ethyl-17-hydroxy-, 3-oxime, (17α)

Chemical name for ethinyl estradiol: 19-norpregna-1,3,5 (10)-trien-20-yne-3,17-diol, (17α)

CLINICAL PHARMACOLOGY

PHARMACODYNAMICS

Norelgestromin is the active progestin largely responsible for the progestational activity that occurs in women following application of Ortho Evra. Norelgestromin is also the primary active metabolite produced following oral administration of norgestimate (NGM), the progestin component of the oral contraceptive products Ortho-Cyclen and Ortho Tri-Cyclen.

Combination oral contraceptives act by suppression of gonadotropins. Although the primary mechanism of this action is inhibition of ovulation, other alterations include changes in the cervical mucus (which increase the difficulty of sperm entry into the uterus) and the endometrium (which reduce the likelihood of implantation).

Receptor and human sex hormone-binding globulin (SHBG) binding studies, as well as studies in animals and humans, have shown that both norgestimate and norelgestromin exhibit high progestational activity with minimal intrinsic androgenicity.[90-93] Transdermally-administered norelgestromin, in combination with ethinyl estradiol, does not counteract the estrogen-induced increases in SHBG, resulting in lower levels of free testosterone in serum compared to baseline.

Pharmacokinetic studies with Ortho Evra demonstrated consistent elimination kinetics for norelgestromin and EE with half-life values of approximately 28 hours and 17 hours, respectively. One clinical trial assessed the return of hypothalamic-pituitary-ovarian axis function post-therapy and found that FSH, LH, and estradiol mean values, though suppressed during therapy, returned to near baseline values during the 6 weeks post therapy.

PHARMACOKINETICS

Absorption

Following application of Ortho Evra, both norelgestromin and EE rapidly appear in the serum, reach a plateau by approximately 48 hours, and are maintained at an approximate steady-state throughout the wear period. C^{SS} concentrations for norelgestromin and EE during 1 week of patch wear are approximately 0.6-0.8 ng/ml and 40-50 pg/ml, respectively, and are generally consistent from all studies and application sites. These C^{SS} concentrations are within the reference ranges for norelgestromin (0.6-1.2 ng/ml) and EE (25-75 pg/ml) established based upon the Cave concentrations observed with subjects taking Ortho-Cyclen.

Daily absorption of norelgestromin and EE from Ortho Evra was determined by comparison to an intravenous infusion of norelgestromin and EE. The results indicated that the average dose of norelgestromin and EE absorbed into the systemic circulation is 150 μg/day and 20 μg/day, respectively.

The absorption of norelgestromin and EE following application of Ortho Evra to the abdomen, buttock, upper outer arm and upper torso (excluding breast) was evaluated in a cross-over design study. The results of this study indicated that C^{SS} and AUC for the buttock, upper arm and torso for each analyte were equivalent. While C^{SS} values for the abdomen were within reference ranges for EE 35 μg/NGM 250 μg oral contraceptive users, exposure to the drugs was lower and strict bioequivalence requirements for AUC were not met in this study. However, in a separate parallel group multiple application pharmacokinetic study, C^{SS} and AUC for the buttock and abdomen were not statistically different. Therefore, all four sites may be considered therapeutically equivalent.

The absorption of norelgestromin and EE following application of Ortho Evra was studied under conditions encountered in a health club (sauna, whirlpool and treadmill) and in a cold water bath. The results indicated that for norelgestromin there were no significant treatment effects on C^{SS} or AUC when compared to normal wear. For EE, slight increases were observed due to sauna, whirlpool and treadmill, however, the C^{SS} values following these treatments were within the reference range. There was no significant effect of cold water on these parameters.

In multiple dose studies, C^{SS} and AUC for norelgestromin and EE were found to increase slightly over time when compared to Week 1 of Cycle 1. In a three-cycle study, these pharmacokinetic parameters reached steady-state conditions during all 3 weeks of Cycle 3. (See TABLE 1.)

***TABLE 1** Mean (SD) Pharmacokinetic Parameters of Norelgestromin and EE Following 3 Consecutive Cycles of Ortho Evra Wear on the Buttock*

	Cycle 1 Week 1	Cycle 3 Week 1	Cycle 3 Week 2	Cycle 3 Week 3
Norelgestromin				
C^{SS} (ng/ml)	0.70 (0.28)	0.70 (0.29)	0.80 (0.23)	0.70 (0.32)
AUC(0-168) (ng·h/ml)	107 (44.2)	105 (45.5)	132 (57.1)	120 (52.8)
T½ (h)	NC	NC	NC	32.1 (12.9
EE				
C^{SS} (pg/ml)	46.4 (17.9)	47.6 (17.3)	59.0 (25.1)	49.6 (27.0)
AUC (0-168) (pg·h/ml)	6796 (2673)	7160 (2893)	10054 (4205)	8840 (5176)
T½ (h)	NC	NC	NC	21.0 (9.07)

NC = Not calculated.

Results from a study of consecutive Ortho Evra wear for 7 and 10 days indicated that serum concentrations of norelgestromin and EE dropped slightly during the first 6 hours after the patch replacement, still stayed within the reference range, and recovered within 12 hours. Target C^{SS} of norelgestromin and EE were maintained during 2 days of extended wear of Ortho Evra.

Metabolism

Since Ortho Evra is applied transdermally, first-pass metabolism (via the gastrointestinal tract and/or liver) of norelgestromin and EE that would be expected with oral administration is avoided. Hepatic metabolism of norelgestromin occurs and metabolites include norgestrel, which is highly bound to SHBG, and various hydroxylated and conjugated metabolites. Ethinyl estradiol is also metabolized to various hydroxylated products and their glucuronide and sulfate conjugates.

Distribution

Norelgestromin and norgestrel (a serum metabolite of norelgestromin) are highly bound (>97%) to serum proteins. Norelgestromin is bound to albumin and not to SHBG, while norgestrel is bound primarily to SHBG, which limits its biological activity. Ethinyl estradiol is extensively bound to serum albumin.

Elimination

Following removal of patches, the elimination kinetics of norelgestromin and EE were consistent for all studies with half-life values of approximately 28 hours and 17 hours, respectively. The metabolites of norelgestromin and EE are eliminated by renal and fecal pathways.

SPECIAL POPULATIONS

Effects of Age, Body Weight, Body Surface Area and Race

The effects of age, body weight, body surface area and race on the pharmacokinetics of norelgestromin and EE were evaluated in 230 healthy women from nine pharmacokinetic studies of single 7 day applications of Ortho Evra. For both norelgestromin and EE, increasing age, body weight and body surface area each were associated with slight decreases in C^{SS} and AUC values. However, only a small fraction (10-25%) of the overall variability in the pharmacokinetics of norelgestromin and EE following application of Ortho Evra may be associated with any or all of the above demographic parameters. There was no significant effect of race with respect to Caucasians, Hispanics and Blacks.

RENAL AND HEPATIC IMPAIRMENT

No formal studies were conducted with Ortho Evra to evaluate the pharmacokinetics, safety, and efficacy in women with renal or hepatic impairment. Steroid hormones may be poorly metabolized in patients with impaired liver function (see PRECAUTIONS).

DRUG INTERACTIONS

The metabolism of hormonal contraceptives may be influenced by various drugs. Of potential clinical importance are drugs that cause the induction of enzymes that are responsible for the degradation of estrogens and progestins, and drugs that interrupt entero-hepatic recirculation of estrogen (*e.g.*, certain antibiotics).[72]

The proposed mechanism of interaction of antibiotics is different from that of liver enzyme-inducing drugs. Literature suggests possible interactions with the concomitant use of hormonal contraceptives and ampicillin or tetracycline. In a pharmacokinetic drug interaction study, oral administration of tetracycline HCl, 500 mg qid for 3 days prior to and 7 days during wear of Ortho Evra did not significantly affect the pharmacokinetics of norelgestromin or EE.

The major target for enzyme inducers is the hepatic microsomal estrogen-2-hydroxylase (cytochrome P450 3A4).[99] See also DRUG INTERACTIONS.

PATCH ADHESION

In the clinical trials with Ortho Evra, approximately 2% of the cumulative number of patches completely detached. The proportion of subjects with at least 1 patch that completely detached ranged from 2-6%, with a reduction from Cycle 1 (6%) to Cycle 13 (2%). For instructions on how to manage detachment of patches, refer to DOSAGE AND ADMINISTRATION.

INDICATIONS AND USAGE

Ortho Evra is indicated for the prevention of pregnancy.

Like oral contraceptives, Ortho Evra is highly effective if used as recommended in this label.

In 3 large clinical trials in North America, Europe and South Africa, 3330 women (ages 18-45) completed 22,155 cycles of Ortho Evra use, pregnancy rates were approximately 1 per 100 women-years of Ortho Evra use. The racial distribution was 91% Caucasian, 4.9% Black, 1.6% Asian, and 2.4% Other.

With respect to weight, 5 of the 15 pregnancies reported with Ortho Evra use were among women with a baseline body weight ≥198 lb (90 kg), which constituted <3% of the study population. The greater proportion of pregnancies among women at or above 198 lb was statistically significant and suggests that Ortho Evra may be less effective in these women.

Health Care Professionals who consider Ortho Evra for women at or above 198 lb should discuss the patient's individual needs in choosing the most appropriate contraceptive option.

TABLE 2 lists the accidental pregnancy rates for users of various methods of contraception. The efficacy of these contraceptive methods, except sterilization, IUD, and Norplant depends upon the reliability with which they are used. Correct and consistent use of methods can result in lower failure rates.

***TABLE 2** Percentage of Women Experiencing an Unintended Pregnancy During the First Year of Typical Use and the First Year of Perfect Use of Contraception and the Percentage Continuing Use at the End of the First Year — United States*

	% of Women Experiencing an Unintended Pregnancy Within the First Year of Use		% of Women Continuing
Method	**Typical Use***	**Perfect Use†**	**Use at 1 Year‡**
(1)	**(2)**	**(3)**	**(4)**
Chance§	85%	85%	
Spermicides¤	26%	6%	40%
Periodic abstinence	25%		63%
Calendar		9%	
Ovulation method		3%	
Sympto-thermal¶		2%	
Post-ovulation		1%	
Cap**			
Parous women	40%	26%	42%
Nulliparous women	20%	9%	56%
Sponge			
Parous women	40%	20%	42%
Nulliparous women	20%	9%	56%
Diaphragm**	20%	6%	56%
Withdrawal	19%	4%	
Condom††			
Female (Reality)	21%	5%	56%
Male	14%	3%	61%
Pill	5%		71%
Progestin only		0.5%	
Combined		0.1%	
IUD			
Progesterone T	2.0%	1.5%	81%
Copper T380A	0.8%	0.6%	78%
LNg 20	0.1%	0.1%	81%
Depo-Provera	0.3%	0.3%	70%
Norplant and Norplant-2	0.05%	0.05%	88%
Female sterilization	0.5%	0.5%	100%
Male sterilization	0.15%	0.10%	100%

Emergency Contraceptive Pills: Treatment initiated within 72 hours after unprotected intercourse reduces the risk of pregnancy by at least 75%.‡‡

Lactational Amenorrhea Method: LAM is highly effective, *temporary* method of contraception.§§

* Among *typical* couples who initiate use of a method (not necessarily for the first time), the percentage who experience an accidental pregnancy during the first year if they do not stop use for any other reason.

† Among couples who initiate use of a method (not necessarily for the first time) and who use it *perfectly* (both consistently and correctly), the percentage who experience an accidental pregnancy during the first year if they do not stop use for any other reason.

‡ Among couples attempting to avoid pregnancy, the percentage who continue to use a method for 1 year.

§ The percents becoming pregnant in columns (2) and (3) are based on data from populations where contraception is not used and from women who cease using contraception in order to become pregnant. Among such populations, about 89% become pregnant within 1 year. This estimate was lowered slightly (to 85%) to represent the percentage who would become pregnant within 1 year among women now relying on reversible methods of contraception if they abandoned contraception altogether.

¤ Foams, creams, gels, vaginal suppositories, and vaginal film.

¶ Cervical mucus (ovulation) method supplemented by calendar in the pre-ovulatory and basal body temperature in the post-ovulatory phases.

** With spermicidal cream or jelly.

†† Without spermicides.

‡‡ The treatment schedule is one dose within 72 hours after unprotected intercourse, and a second dose 12 hours after the first dose. The Food and Drug Administration has declared the following brands of oral contraceptives to be safe and effective for emergency contraception: Ovral (1 dose is 2 white pills), Alesse (1 dose is 5 pink pills), Nordette or Levlen (1 dose is 2 light-orange pills), Lo/Ovral (1 dose is 4 white pills), Triphasil or Tri-Levlen (1 dose is 4 yellow pills).

§§ However, to maintain effective protection against pregnancy, another method of contraception must be used as soon as menstruation resumes, the frequency or duration of breastfeeds is reduced, bottle feeds are introduced, or the baby reaches 6 months of age.

Source: Trussell J, Contraceptive efficacy. In Hatcher RA, Trussell J, Stewart F, Cates W, Stewart GK, Kowal D, Guest F, Contraceptive Technology: Seventeenth Revised Edition. New York NY: Irvington Publishers, 1998.

Ortho Evra has not been studied for and is not indicated for use in emergency contraception.

CONTRAINDICATIONS

Ortho Evra should not be used in women who currently have the following conditions:

Thrombophlebitis, thromboembolic disorders.
A past history of deep vein thrombophlebitis or thromboembolic disorders.
Cerebro-vascular or coronary artery disease (current or past history).
Valvular heart disease with complications.[103]
Severe hypertension.[103]
Diabetes with vascular involvement.[103]
Headaches with focal neurological symptoms.
Major surgery with prolonged immobilization.
Known or suspected carcinoma of the breast or personal history of breast cancer.
Carcinoma of the endometrium or other known or suspected estrogen-dependent neoplasia.
Undiagnosed abnormal genital bleeding.
Cholestatic jaundice of pregnancy or jaundice with prior hormonal contraceptive use.
Acute or chronic hepatocellular disease with abnormal liver function.[103]
Hepatic adenomas or carcinomas.
Known or suspected pregnancy.
Hypersensitivity to any component of this product.

WARNINGS

Cigarette smoking increases the risk of serious cardiovascular side effects from hormonal contraceptive use. This risk increases with age and with heavy smoking (15 or more cigarettes per day) and is quite marked in women over 35 years of age. Women who use hormonal contraceptives including Ortho Evra should be strongly advised not to smoke.

Ortho Evra and other contraceptives that contain both an estrogen and a progestin are called combination hormonal contraceptives. There is no epidemiologic data available to determine whether safety and efficacy with the transdermal route of administration would be different than the oral route. Practitioners prescribing Ortho Evra should be familiar with the following information relating to risks.

The use of combination hormonal contraceptives is associated with increased risks of several serious conditions including myocardial infarction, thromboembolism, stroke, hepatic neoplasia, and gallbladder disease, although the risk of serious morbidity or mortality is very small in healthy women without underlying risk factors. The risk of morbidity and mortality increases significantly in the presence of other underlying risk factors such as hypertension, hyperlipidemias, obesity and diabetes.

The information contained in this package insert is principally based on studies carried out in women who used combination oral contraceptives with higher formulations of estrogens and progestins than those in common use today. The effect of long-term use of combination hormonal contraceptives with lower doses of both estrogen and progestin administered by any route remains to be determined.

Throughout this labeling, epidemiological studies reported are of two types: retrospective or case control studies and prospective or cohort studies. Case control studies provide a measure of the relative risk of a disease, namely, a ratio of the incidence of a disease among oral contraceptive users to that among nonusers. The relative risk does not provide information on the actual clinical occurrence of a disease. Cohort studies provide a measure of attributable risk, which is the *difference* in the incidence of disease between hormonal contraceptive users and nonusers. The attributable risk does provide information about the actual occurrence of a disease in the population (adapted from refs. 2 and 3 with the author's permission). For further information, the reader is referred to a text on epidemiological methods.

THROMBOEMBOLIC DISORDERS AND OTHER VASCULAR PROBLEMS

Thromboembolism

An increased risk of thromboembolic and thrombotic disease associated with the use of hormonal contraceptives is well established. Case control studies have found the relative risk of users compared to nonusers to be 3 for the first episode of superficial venous thrombosis, 4 to 11 for deep vein thrombosis or pulmonary embolism, and 1.5 to 6 for women with predisposing conditions for venous thromboembolic disease.[2,3,19-24] Cohort studies have shown the relative risk to be somewhat lower, about 3 for new cases and about 4.5 for new cases requiring hospitalization.[25] The risk of thromboembolic disease associated with hormonal contraceptives is not related to length of use and disappears after hormonal contraceptive use is stopped.[2] A 2- to 4-fold increase in relative risk of post-operative thromboembolic complications has been reported with the use of hormonal contraceptives.[9,26] The relative risk of venous thrombosis in women who have predisposing conditions is twice that of women without such medical conditions.[9,26] If feasible, hormonal contraceptives should be discontinued at least 4 weeks prior to and for 2 weeks after elective surgery of a type associated with an increase in risk of thromboembolism and during and following prolonged immobilization. Since the immediate postpartum period is also associated with an increased risk of thromboembolism, hormonal contraceptives should be started no earlier than 4 weeks after delivery in women who elect not to breast-feed.

In the large clinical trials (n=3330 with 1704 women-years of exposure), 1 case of non-fatal pulmonary embolism occurred during Ortho Evra use, and 1 case of post-operative non-fatal pulmonary embolism was reported following Ortho Evra use. It is unknown if the risk of venous thromboembolism with Ortho Evra use is different than with use of combination oral contraceptives.

As with any combination hormonal contraceptives, the clinician should be alert to the earliest manifestations of thrombotic disorders (thrombophlebitis, pulmonary embolism, cerebrovascular disorders, and retinal thrombosis). Should any of these occur or be suspected, Ortho Evra should be discontinued immediately.

Myocardial Infarction

An increased risk of myocardial infarction has been attributed to hormonal contraceptive use. This risk is primarily in smokers or women with other underlying risk factors for coronary artery disease such as hypertension, hypercholesterolemia, morbid obesity, and diabetes. The relative risk of heart attack for current hormonal contraceptive users has been estimated to be two to six[4-10] compared to non-users. The risk is very low under the age of 30.

Smoking in combination with oral contraceptive use has been shown to contribute substantially to the incidence of myocardial infarctions in women in their mid-thirties or older with smoking accounting for the majority of excess cases.[11] Mortality rates associated with circulatory disease have been shown to increase substantially in smokers, especially in those 35 years of age and older among women who use oral contraceptives.

Hormonal contraceptives may compound the effects of well-known risk factors, such as hypertension, diabetes, hyperlipidemias, age and obesity.[13] In particular, some progestins are known to decrease HDL cholesterol and cause glucose intolerance, while estrogens may create a state of hyperinsulinism.[14-18] Hormonal contraceptives have been shown to increase blood pressure among some users (see WARNINGS, Elevated Blood Pressure). Similar effects on risk factors have been associated with an increased risk of heart disease. Hormonal contraceptives, including Ortho Evra, must be used with caution in women with cardiovascular disease risk factors.

Norgestimate and norelgestromin have minimal androgenic activity (see CLINICAL PHARMACOLOGY). There is some evidence that the risk of myocardial infarction associated with hormonal contraceptives is lower when the progestin has minimal androgenic activity than when the activity is greater.[97]

Cerebrovascular Diseases

Hormonal contraceptives have been shown to increase both the relative and attributable risks of cerebrovascular events (thrombotic and hemorrhagic strokes), although, in general, the risk is greatest among older (>35 years), hypertensive women who also smoke. Hypertension was found to be a risk factor for both users and nonusers, for both types of strokes, and smoking interacted to increase the risk of stroke.[27-29]

In a large study, the relative risk of thrombotic strokes has been shown to range from 3 for normotensive users to 14 for users with severe hypertension.[30] The relative risk of hemorrhagic stroke is reported to be 1.2 for non-smokers who used hormonal contraceptives, 2.6 for smokers who did not use hormonal contraceptives, 7.6 for smokers who used hormonal contraceptives, 1.8 for normotensive users and 25.7 for users with severe hypertension.[30] The attributable risk is also greater in older women.[3]

Dose-Related Risk of Vascular Disease From Hormonal Contraceptives

A positive association has been observed between the amount of estrogen and progestin in hormonal contraceptives and the risk of vascular disease.[31-33] A decline in serum high-density lipoproteins (HDL) has been reported with many progestational agents.[14-16] A decline in serum high-density lipoproteins has been associated with an increased incidence of ischemic heart disease. Because estrogens increase HDL cholesterol, the net effect of a hormonal contraceptive depends on a balance achieved between doses of estrogen and progestin and the activity of the progestin used in the contraceptives. The activity and amount of both hormones should be considered in the choice of a hormonal contraceptive.

Persistence of Risk of Vascular Disease

There are two studies that have shown persistence of risk of vascular disease for ever-users of combination hormonal contraceptives. In a study in the US, the risk of developing myocardial infarction after discontinuing combination hormonal contraceptives persists for at least 9 years for women 40-49 years who had used combination hormonal contraceptives for 5 or more years, but this increased risk was not demonstrated in other age groups.[8] In another study in Great Britain, the risk of developing cerebrovascular disease persisted for at least 6 years after discontinuation of combination hormonal contraceptives, although excess risk was very small.[34] However, both studies were performed with combination hormonal contraceptive formulations containing 50 µg or higher of estrogens.

It is unknown whether Ortho Evra is distinct from other combination hormonal contraceptives with regard to the occurrence of venous and arterial thrombosis.

ESTIMATES OF MORTALITY FROM COMBINATION HORMONAL CONTRACEPTIVE USE

One study gathered data from a variety of sources that have estimated the mortality rate associated with different methods of contraception at different ages (TABLE 3). These estimates include the combined risk of death associated with contraceptive methods plus the risk attributable to pregnancy in the event of method failure. Each method of contraception has its specific benefits and risks. The study concluded that with the exception of combination oral contraceptive users 35 and older who smoke, and 40 and older who do not smoke, mortality associated with all methods of birth control is low and below that associated with childbirth.

The observation of a possible increase in risk of mortality with age for combination oral contraceptive users is based on data gathered in the 1970's but not reported until 1983.[35] Current clinical recommendation involves the use of lower estrogen dose formulations and a careful consideration of risk factors. In 1989, the Fertility and Maternal Health Drugs Advisory Committee was asked to review the use of combination hormonal contraceptives in women 40 years of age and over. The Committee concluded that although cardiovascular disease risks may be increased with combination hormonal contraceptive use after age 40 in healthy non-smoking women (even with the newer low-dose formulations), there are also greater potential health risks associated with pregnancy in older women and with the alternative surgical and medical procedures that may be necessary if such women do not have access to effective and acceptable means of contraception. The Committee recommended that the benefits of low-dose combination hormonal contraceptive use by healthy non-smoking women over 40 may outweigh the possible risks.[36,37]

Although the data are mainly obtained with oral contraceptives, this is likely to apply to Ortho Evra as well. Women of all ages who use combination hormonal contraceptives, should use the lowest possible dose formulation that is effective and meets the individual patient needs.

CARCINOMA OF THE REPRODUCTIVE ORGANS AND BREASTS

Numerous epidemiological studies give conflicting reports on the relationship between breast cancer and COC use. The risk of having breast cancer diagnosed may be slightly increased among current and recent users of combination oral contraceptives. However, this excess risk appears to decrease over time after COC discontinuation and by 10 years after cessation the increased risk disappears. Some studies report an increased risk with duration of use while other studies do not and no consistent relationships have been found with dose or type of steroid. Some studies have found a small increase in risk for women who first use COCs before age 20. Most studies show a similar pattern of risk with COC use regardless of a woman's reproductive history or her family breast cancer history.

TABLE 3 *Annual Number of Birth-Related or Method-Related Deaths Associated With Control of Fertility per 100,000 Non-Sterile Women, by Fertility Control Method According to Age*

Method of Control and Outcome	15-19	20-24	25-29	30-34	35-39	40-44
No fertility control methods*	7.0	7.4	9.1	14.8	25.7	28.2
Oral contraceptives, non-smoker†	0.3	0.5	0.9	1.9	13.8	31.6
Oral contraceptives, smoker†	2.2	3.4	6.6	13.5	51.1	117.2
IUD†	0.8	0.8	1.0	1.0	1.4	1.4
Condom*	1.1	1.6	0.7	0.2	0.3	0.4
Diaphragm/spermicide*	1.9	1.2	1.2	1.3	2.2	2.8
Periodic abstinence*	2.5	1.6	1.6	1.7	2.9	3.6

* Deaths are birth-related.
† Deaths are method-related.
Adapted from H.W. Ory, *Family Planning Perspectives,* 15:57-63, 1983.

In addition, breast cancers diagnosed in current or ever oral contraceptive users may be less clinically advanced than in never-users.

Women who currently have or have had breast cancer should not use hormonal contraceptives because breast cancer is usually a hormonally sensitive tumor.

Some studies suggest that combination oral contraceptive use has been associated with an increase in the risk of cervical intraepithelial neoplasia in some populations of women.[45-48] However, there continues to be controversy about the extent to which such findings may be due to differences in sexual behavior and other factors.

In spite of many studies of the relationship between oral contraceptive use and breast and cervical cancers, a cause-and-effect relationship has not been established. It is not known whether Ortho Evra is distinct from oral contraceptives with regard to the above statements.

HEPATIC NEOPLASIA

Benign hepatic adenomas are associated with hormonal contraceptive use, although the incidence of benign tumors is rare in the US. Indirect calculations have estimated the attributable risk to be in the range of 3.3 cases/100,000 for users, a risk that increases after 4 or more years of use, especially with hormonal contraceptives containing 50 µg or more of estrogen.[49] Rupture of benign, hepatic adenomas may cause death through intra-abdominal hemorrhage.[50,51]

Studies from Britain and the US have shown an increased risk of developing hepatocellular carcinoma in long term (≥8 years)[52-54,96] oral contraceptive users. However, these cancers are extremely rare in the US and the attributable risk (the excess incidence) of liver cancers in oral contraceptive users approaches less than one per million users. It is unknown whether Ortho Evra is distinct from oral contraceptives in this regard.

OCULAR LESIONS

There have been clinical case reports of retinal thrombosis associated with the use of hormonal contraceptives. Ortho Evra should be discontinued if there is unexplained partial or complete loss of vision; onset of proptosis or diplopia; papilledema; or retinal vascular lesions. Appropriate diagnostic and therapeutic measures should be undertaken immediately.

HORMONAL CONTRACEPTIVE USE BEFORE OR DURING EARLY PREGNANCY

Extensive epidemiological studies have revealed no increased risk of birth defects in women who have used oral contraceptives prior to pregnancy.[56,57] Studies also do not indicate a teratogenic effect, particularly in so far as cardiac anomalies and limb reduction defects are concerned,[55,56,58,59] when oral contraceptives are taken inadvertently during early pregnancy.

Combination hormonal contraceptives such as Ortho Evra should not be used to induce withdrawal bleeding as a test for pregnancy. Ortho Evra should not be used during pregnancy to treat threatened or habitual abortion. It is recommended that for any patient who has missed two consecutive periods, pregnancy should be ruled out. If the patient has not adhered to the prescribed schedule for the use of Ortho Evra the possibility of pregnancy should be considered at the time of the first missed period. Hormonal contraceptive use should be discontinued if pregnancy is confirmed.

GALLBLADDER DISEASE

Earlier studies have reported an increased lifetime relative risk of gallbladder surgery in users of hormonal contraceptives and estrogens.[60,61] More recent studies, however, have shown that the relative risk of developing gallbladder disease among hormonal contraceptive users may be minimal.[62-64] The recent findings of minimal risk may be related to the use of hormonal contraceptive formulations containing lower hormonal doses of estrogens and progestins.

Combination hormonal contraceptives such as Ortho Evra may worsen existing gallbladder disease and may accelerate the development of this disease in previously asymptomatic women. Women with a history of combination hormonal contraceptive-related cholestasis are more likely to have the condition recur with subsequent combination hormonal contraceptive use.

CARBOHYDRATE AND LIPID METABOLIC EFFECTS

Hormonal contraceptives have been shown to cause a decrease in glucose tolerance in some users.[17] However, in the non-diabetic woman, combination hormonal contraceptives appear to have no effect on fasting blood glucose.[67]

Prediabetic and diabetic women in particular should be carefully monitored while taking combination hormonal contraceptives such as Ortho Evra.

In clinical trials with oral contraceptives containing ethinyl estradiol and norgestimate there were no clinically significant changes in fasting blood glucose levels. There were no clinically significant changes in glucose levels over 24 cycles of use. Moreover, glucose tolerance tests showed no clinically significant changes from baseline to cycles 3, 12 and 24. In a 6-cycle clinical trial with Ortho Evra there were no clinically significant changes in fasting blood glucose from baseline to end of treatment.

A small proportion of women will have persistent hypertriglyceridemia while taking hormonal contraceptives. As discussed earlier (see Thromboembolic Disorders and Other Vascular Problems: Thromboembolism and Dose-Related Risk of Vascular Disease From Hormonal Contraceptives), changes in serum triglycerides and lipoprotein levels have been reported in hormonal contraceptive users.

ELEVATED BLOOD PRESSURE

Women with significant hypertension should not be started on hormonal contraception.[103] Women with a history of hypertension or hypertension-related diseases, or renal disease[70] should be encouraged to use another method of contraception. If women elect to use Ortho Evra they should be monitored closely and if a clinically significant elevation of blood pressure occurs, Ortho Evra should be discontinued. For most women, elevated blood pressure will return to normal after stopping hormonal contraceptives, and there is no difference in the occurrence of hypertension between former and never users.[68-71]

An increase in blood pressure has been reported in women taking hormonal contraceptives[68] and this increase is more likely in older hormonal contraceptive users[69] and with extended duration of use.[61] Data from the Royal College of General Practitioners[12] and subsequent randomized trials have shown that the incidence of hypertension increases with increasing progestational activity.

HEADACHE

The onset or exacerbation of migraine headache or the development of headache with a new pattern that is recurrent, persistent or severe requires discontinuation of Ortho Evra and evaluation of the cause.

BLEEDING IRREGULARITIES

Breakthrough bleeding and spotting are sometimes encountered in women using Ortho Evra. Non-hormonal causes should be considered and adequate diagnostic measures taken to rule out malignancy, other pathology, or pregnancy in the event of breakthrough bleeding, as in the case of any abnormal vaginal bleeding. If pathology has been excluded, time or a change to another contraceptive product may resolve the bleeding. In the event of amenorrhea, pregnancy should be ruled out before initiating use of Ortho Evra.

Some women may encounter amenorrhea or oligomenorrhea after discontinuation of hormonal contraceptive use, especially when such a condition was pre-existent.

Bleeding Patterns

In the clinical trials most women started their withdrawal bleeding on the fourth day of the drug-free interval, and the median duration of withdrawal bleeding was 5-6 days. On average 26% of women per cycle had 7 or more total days of bleeding and/or spotting (this includes both withdrawal flow and breakthrough bleeding and/or spotting).

ECTOPIC PREGNANCY

Ectopic as well as intrauterine pregnancy may occur in contraceptive failures.

PRECAUTIONS

Women should be counseled that Ortho Evra does not protect against HIV infection (AIDS) and other sexually transmitted infections.

BODY WEIGHT ≥198 LB (90 KG)

Results of clinical trials suggest that Ortho Evra may be less effective in women with body weight ≥198 lb (90 kg) than in women with lower body weights.

PHYSICAL EXAMINATION AND FOLLOW-UP

It is good medical practice for women using Ortho Evra, as for all women, to have annual medical evaluation and physical examinations. The physical examination, however, may be deferred until after initiation of hormonal contraceptives if requested by the woman and judged appropriate by the clinician. The physical examination should include special reference to blood pressure, breasts, abdomen and pelvic organs, including cervical cytology, and relevant laboratory tests. In case of undiagnosed, persistent or recurrent abnormal vaginal bleeding, appropriate measures should be conducted to rule out malignancy or other pathology. Women with a strong family history of breast cancer or who have breast nodules should be monitored with particular care.

LIPID DISORDERS

Women who are being treated for hyperlipidemias should be followed closely if they elect to use Ortho Evra. Some progestins may elevate LDL levels and may render the control of hyperlipidemias more difficult.

LIVER FUNCTION

If jaundice develops in any woman using Ortho Evra, the medication should be discontinued. The hormones in Ortho Evra may be poorly metabolized in women with impaired liver function.

FLUID RETENTION

Steroid hormones like those in Ortho Evra may cause some degree of fluid retention. Ortho Evra should be prescribed with caution, and only with careful monitoring, in patients with conditions which might be aggravated by fluid retention.

EMOTIONAL DISORDERS

Women who become significantly depressed while using combination hormonal contraceptives such as Ortho Evra should stop the medication and use another method of contraception in an attempt to determine whether the symptom is drug related. Women with a history of depression should be carefully observed and Ortho Evra discontinued if significant depression occurs.

CONTACT LENSES

Contact lens wearers who develop visual changes or changes in lens tolerance should be assessed by an ophthalmologist.

INTERACTIONS WITH LABORATORY TESTS

Certain endocrine and liver function tests and blood components may be affected by hormonal contraceptives:

- Increased prothrombin and factors VII, VIII, IX, and X; decreased antithrombin 3; increased norepinephrine-induced platelet aggregability.
- Increased thyroid binding globulin (TBG) leading to increased circulating total thyroid hormone, as measured by protein-bound iodine (PBI), T4 by column or by radioimmunoassay. Free T3 resin uptake is decreased, reflecting the elevated TBG, free T4 concentration is unaltered.
- Other binding proteins may be elevated in serum.
- Sex hormone binding globulins are increased and result in elevated levels of total circulating endogenous sex steroids and corticoids; however, free or biologically active levels either decrease or remain unchanged.
- Triglycerides may be increased and levels of various other lipids and lipoproteins may be affected.
- Glucose tolerance may be decreased.
- Serum folate levels may be depressed by hormonal contraceptive therapy. This may be of clinical significance if a woman becomes pregnant shortly after discontinuing Ortho Evra.

CARCINOGENESIS, MUTAGENESIS, AND IMPAIRMENT OF FERTILITY

No carcinogenicity studies were conducted with norelgestromin. However, bridging PK studies were conducted using doses of NGM/EE which were used previously in the 2 year rat carcinogenicity study and 10 year monkey toxicity study to support the approval of Ortho-Cyclen and Ortho-Tri-Cyclen under NDAs 19-653 and 19-697, respectively. The PK studies demonstrated that rats and monkeys were exposed to 16 and 8 times the human exposure, respectively, with the proposed Ortho Evra transdermal contraceptive system.

Norelgestromin was tested in *in vitro* mutagenicity assays (bacterial plate incorporation mutation assay, CHO/HGPRT mutation assay, chromosomal aberration assay using cultured human peripheral lymphocytes) and in one *in vivo* test (rat micronucleus assay) and found to have no genotoxic potential.

See WARNINGS.

PREGNANCY CATEGORY X

See CONTRAINDICATIONS and WARNINGS.

Norelgestromin was tested for its reproductive toxicity in a rabbit developmental toxicity study by the SC route of administration. Doses of 0, 1, 2, 4 and 6 mg/kg body weight, which gave systemic exposure of approximately 25-125 times the human exposure with Ortho Evra, were administered daily on gestation days 7-19. Malformations reported were paw hyperflexion at 4 and 6 mg/kg and paw hyperextension and cleft palate at 6 mg/kg.

NURSING MOTHERS

The effects of Ortho Evra in nursing mothers have not been evaluated and are unknown. Small amounts of combination hormonal contraceptive steroids have been identified in the milk of nursing mothers and a few adverse effects on the child have been reported, including jaundice and breast enlargement. In addition, combination hormonal contraceptives given in the postpartum period may interfere with lactation by decreasing the quantity and quality of breast milk. Long-term follow-up of infants whose mothers used combination hormonal contraceptives while breast feeding has shown no deleterious effects. However, the nursing mother should be advised not to use Ortho Evra but to use other forms of contraception until she has completely weaned her child.

PEDIATRIC USE

Safety and efficacy of Ortho Evra have been established in women of reproductive age. Safety and efficacy are expected to be the same for post-pubertal adolescents under the age of 16 and for users 16 years and older. Use of this product before menarche is not indicated.

GERIATRIC USE

This product has not been studied in women over 65 years of age and is not indicated in this population.

SEXUALLY TRANSMITTED DISEASES

Patients should be counseled that this product does not protect against HIV infection (AIDS) and other sexually transmitted diseases.

PATCH ADHESION

Experience with more than 70,000 Ortho Evra patches worn for contraception for 6-13 cycles showed that 4.7% of patches were replaced because they either fell off (1.8%) or were partly detached (2.9%). Similarly, in a small study of patch wear under conditions of physical exertion and variable temperature and humidity, less than 2% of patches were replaced for complete or partial detachment.

If the Ortho Evra patch becomes partially or completely detached and remains detached, insufficient drug delivery occurs. A patch should not be re-applied if it is no longer sticky, if it has become stuck to itself or another surface, if it has other material stuck to it, or if it has become loose or fallen off before. If a patch cannot be reapplied, a new patch should be applied immediately. Supplemental adhesives or wraps should not be used to hold the Ortho Evra patch in place.

If a patch is partially or completely detached for more than 1 day (24 hours or more) OR if the woman is not sure how long the patch has been detached, she may not be protected from pregnancy. She should stop the current contraceptive cycle and start a new cycle immediately by applying a new patch. Back-up contraception, such as condoms, spermicide, or diaphragm, must be used for the first week of the new cycle.

INFORMATION FOR THE PATIENT

See Patient Labeling distributed with each prescription.

E

DRUG INTERACTIONS

CHANGES IN CONTRACEPTIVE EFFECTIVENESS ASSOCIATED WITH CO-ADMINISTRATION OF OTHER DRUGS

Contraceptive effectiveness may be reduced when hormonal contraceptives are co-administered with some antibiotics, antifungals, anticonvulsants, and other drugs that increase metabolism of contraceptive steroids. This could result in unintended pregnancy or breakthrough bleeding. Examples include barbiturates, griseofulvin, rifampin, phenylbutazone, phenytoin, carbamazepine, felbamate, oxcarbazepine, topiramate and possibly with ampicillin.

The proposed mechanism of interaction of antibiotics is different from that of liver enzyme-inducing drugs. Literature suggests possible interactions with the concomitant use of hormonal contraceptives and ampicillin or tetracycline. In a pharmacokinetic drug interaction study, oral administration of tetracycline HCl, 500 mg qid for 3 days prior to and 7 days during wear of Ortho Evra did not significantly affect the pharmacokinetics of norelgestromin or EE.

Several of the anti-HIV protease inhibitors have been studied with co-administration of oral combination hormonal contraceptives; significant changes (increase and decrease) in the mean AUC of the estrogen and progestin have been noted in some cases. The efficacy and safety of oral contraceptive products may be affected; it is unknown whether this applies to Ortho Evra. Healthcare professionals should refer to the label of the individual anti-HIV protease inhibitors for further drug-drug interaction information.

Herbal products containing St. John's Wort (hypericum perforatum) may induce hepatic enzymes (cytochrome P450) and p-glycoprotein transporter and may reduce the effectiveness of contraceptive steroids. This may also result in breakthrough bleeding.

INCREASE IN PLASMA HORMONE LEVELS ASSOCIATED WITH CO-ADMINISTERED DRUGS

Co-administration of atorvastatin and certain oral contraceptives containing ethinyl estradiol increase AUC values for ethinyl estradiol by approximately 20%. Ascorbic acid and acetaminophen may increase plasma ethinyl estradiol levels, possibly by inhibition of conjugation. CYP 3A4 inhibitors such as itraconazole or ketoconazole may increase plasma hormone levels.

CHANGES IN PLASMA LEVELS OF CO-ADMINISTERED DRUGS

Combination hormonal contraceptives containing some synthetic estrogens (*e.g.*, ethinyl estradiol) may inhibit the metabolism of other compounds. Increased plasma concentrations of cyclosporine, prednisolone, and theophylline have been reported with concomitant administration of oral contraceptives. In addition, oral contraceptives may induce the conjugation of other compounds. Decreased plasma concentrations of acetaminophen and increased clearance of temazepam, salicylic acid, morphine and clofibric acid have been noted when these drugs were administered with oral contraceptives.

Although norelgestromin and its metabolites inhibit a variety of P450 enzymes in human liver microsomes, the clinical consequence of such an interaction on the levels of other concomitant medications is likely to be insignificant. Under the recommended dosing regimen, the *in vivo* concentrations of norelgestromin and its metabolites, even at the peak serum levels, are relatively low compared to the inhibitory constant (Ki) (based on results of *in vitro* studies).

Health care professionals are advised to also refer to prescribing information of co-administered drugs for recommendations regarding management of concomitant therapy.

ADVERSE REACTIONS

The most common adverse events reported by 9-22% of women using Ortho Evra in clinical trials (n=3330) were the following, in order of decreasing incidence: Breast symptoms, headache, application site reaction, nausea, upper respiratory infection, menstrual cramps, and abdominal pain.

The most frequent adverse events leading to discontinuation in 1 to 2.4% of women using Ortho Evra in the trials included the following: Nausea and/or vomiting, application site reaction, breast symptoms, headache, and emotional lability.

Listed below are adverse events that have been associated with the use of combination hormonal contraceptives. These are also likely to apply to combination transdermal hormonal contraceptives such as Ortho Evra.

An increased risk of the following serious adverse reactions has been associated with the use of combination hormonal contraceptives (see WARNINGS).

Thrombophlebitis and venous thrombosis with or without embolism; arterial thromboembolism; pulmonary embolism; myocardial infarction; cerebral hemorrhage; cerebral thrombosis; hypertension; gallbladder disease; hepatic adenomas or benign liver tumors.

There is evidence of an association between the following conditions and the use of combination hormonal contraceptives:

Mesenteric thrombosis; retinal thrombosis.

The following adverse reactions have been reported in users of combination hormonal contraceptives and are believed to be drug-related:

Nausea; vomiting; gastrointestinal symptoms (such as abdominal cramps and bloating); breakthrough bleeding; spotting; change in menstrual flow; amenorrhea; temporary infertility after discontinuation of treatment; edema; melasma which may persist; breast changes: tenderness, enlargement, secretion; change in weight (increase or decrease); change in cervical erosion and secretion; diminution in lactation when given immediately postpartum; cholestatic jaundice; migraine; rash (allergic); mental depression; reduced tolerance to carbohydrates; vaginal candidiasis; change in corneal curvature (steepening); intolerance to contact lenses.

The following adverse reactions have been reported in users of combination hormonal contraceptives and a cause and effect association has been neither confirmed nor refuted:

Pre-menstrual syndrome; cataracts; changes in appetite; cystitis-like syndrome; headache; nervousness; dizziness; hirsutism; loss of scalp hair; erythema multiforme; erythema nodosum; hemorrhagic eruption; vaginitis; porphyria; impaired renal function; hemolytic uremic syndrome; acne; changes in libido; Colitis; Budd-Chiari syndrome.

DOSAGE AND ADMINISTRATION

To achieve maximum contraceptive effectiveness, Ortho Evra must be used exactly as directed.

Complete instructions to facilitate patient counseling on proper usage may be found in the Detailed Patient Labeling.

TRANSDERMAL CONTRACEPTIVE SYSTEM OVERVIEW

This system uses a 28 day (4 week) cycle. A new patch is applied each week for 3 weeks (21 total days). Week 4 is patch-free. Withdrawal bleeding is expected to begin during this time.

Every new patch should be applied on the same day of the week. This day is known as the "Patch Change Day". For example, if the first patch is applied on a Monday, all subsequent patches should be applied on a Monday. Only 1 patch should be worn at a time.

On the day after Week 4 ends a new 4 week cycle is started by applying a new patch. Under no circumstances should there be more than a 7 day patch-free interval between dosing cycles.

If the woman is starting Ortho Evra for the **first time,** she should **wait until the day she begins her menstrual period.** Either a First Day start or Sunday start may be chosen. The day she applies her first patch will be Day 1. Her "Patch Change Day" will be on this day every week.

- For **First Day Start:** The patient should apply her first patch during the first 24 hours of her menstrual period.

  If therapy starts after Day 1 of the menstrual cycle, a non-hormonal back-up contraceptive (such as condoms, spermicide or diaphragm) should be used concurrently for the first 7 consecutive days of the first treatment cycle.

OR

- For **Sunday Start:** The woman should apply her first patch on the first Sunday after her menstrual period starts. She must use back-up contraception for the first week of her first cycle.

If the menstrual period begins on a Sunday, the first patch should be applied on that day, and no back-up contraception is needed.

Where to apply the patch. The patch should be applied to clean, dry, intact healthy skin on the buttock, abdomen, upper outer arm or upper torso, in a place where it won't be rubbed by tight clothing. Ortho Evra should not be placed on skin that is red, irritated or cut, nor should it be placed on the breasts.

To prevent interference with the adhesive properties of Ortho Evra, no make-up, creams, lotions, powders or other topical products should be applied to the skin area where the Ortho Evra patch is or will be placed.

The patch is worn for 7 days (1 week). On the "Patch Change Day", Day 8, the used patch is removed and a new one is applied immediately. The used patch still contains some active hormones - it should be carefully folded in half so that it sticks to itself before throwing it away.

A new patch is applied for Week 2 (on Day 8) and again for Week 3 (on Day 15), on the usual "Patch Change Day". Patch changes may occur at any time on the Change Day. Each new Ortho Evra patch should be applied to a new spot on the skin to help avoid irritation, although they may be kept within the same anatomic area.

Week 4 is patch-free (Day 22 through Day 28), thus completing the 4 week contraceptive cycle. Bleeding is expected to begin during this time.

The next 4 week cycle is started by applying a new patch on the usual "Patch Change Day", the day after Day 28, no matter when the menstrual period begins or ends.

Under no circumstances should there be more than a 7 day patch-free interval between patch cycles.

If the Ortho Evra patch becomes partially or completely detached and remains detached, insufficient drug delivery occurs.

If a patch is partially or completely detached:

For less than 1 day (up to 24 hours), the woman should try to reapply it to the same place or replace it with a new patch immediately. No back-up contraception is needed. The woman's "Patch Change Day" will remain the same.

For more than 1 day (24 hours or more) **OR if the woman is not sure how long the patch has been detached,** SHE MAY NOT BE PROTECTED FROM PREGNANCY. She should stop the current contraceptive cycle and start a new cycle immediately by applying a new patch. There is now a new "Day 1" and a new "Patch Change Day." Back-up contraception, such as condoms, spermicide, or diaphragm, must be used for the first week of the new cycle.

A patch should not be re-applied if it is no longer sticky, if it has become stuck to itself or another surface, if it has other material stuck to it or if it has previously become loose or fallen off. If a patch cannot be re-applied, a new patch should be applied immediately. Supplemental adhesives or wraps should not be used to hold the Ortho Evra patch in place.

If the woman forgets to change her patch...

At the start of any patch cycle (Week 1 /Day 1): SHE MAY NOT BE PROTECTED FROM PREGNANCY. She should apply the first patch of her new cycle as soon as she remembers. There is now a new "Patch Change Day" and a new "Day 1". The woman must use back-up contraception, such as condoms, spermicide, or diaphragm, for the first week of the new cycle.

In the middle of the patch cycle (Week 2/Day 8 or Week 3/Day 15),

For **1 or 2 days** (up to 48 hours), she should apply a new patch immediately. The next patch should be applied on the usual "Patch Change Day". No back-up contraception is needed.

For **more than 2 days** (48 hours or more), SHE MAY NOT BE PROTECTED FROM PREGNANCY. She should stop the current contraceptive cycle and start a new 4 week cycle immediately by putting on a new patch. There is now a new "Patch Change Day" and a new "Day 1". The woman must use back-up contraception for 1 week.

At the end of the patch cycle (Week 4/Day 22), Week 4 (Day 22): If the woman forgets to remove her patch, she should take it off as soon as she remembers. The next cycle should be started on the usual "Patch Change Day", which is the day after Day 28. No back-up contraception is needed.

Under no circumstances should there be more than a 7 day patch-free interval between cycles. If there are more than 7 patch-free days, THE WOMAN MAY NOT BE PROTECTED FROM PREGNANCY and back-up contraception, such as condoms, spermicide, or diaphragm, must be used for 7 days. As with combined oral contraceptives, the risk of ovulation increases with each day beyond the recommended drug-free period. If coital exposure has occurred during such an extended patch-free interval, the possibility of fertilization should be considered.

CHANGE DAY ADJUSTMENT

If the woman wishes to change her Patch Change Day she should complete her current cycle, removing the third Ortho Evra patch on the correct day. During the patch-free week, she may select an earlier Patch Change Day by applying a new Ortho Evra patch on the desired day. In no case should there be more than 7 consecutive patch-free days.

SWITCHING FROM AN ORAL CONTRACEPTIVE

Treatment with Ortho Evra should begin on the first day of withdrawal bleeding. If there is no withdrawal bleeding within 5 days of the last active (hormone-containing) tablet, pregnancy must be ruled out. If therapy starts later than the first day of withdrawal bleeding, a non-hormonal contraceptive should be used concurrently for 7 days. If more than 7 days elapse after taking the last active oral contraceptive tablet, the possibility of ovulation and conception should be considered.

USE AFTER CHILDBIRTH

Women who elect not to breast-feed should start contraceptive therapy with Ortho Evra no sooner than 4 weeks after childbirth. If a woman begins using Ortho Evra postpartum, and has not yet had a period, the possibility of ovulation and conception occurring prior to use of Ortho Evra should be considered, and she should be instructed to use an additional method of contraception, such as condoms, spermicide, or diaphragm, for the first 7 days. (See PRECAUTIONS, Nursing Mothers; and WARNINGS, Thromboembolic and Other Vascular Problems.)

USE AFTER ABORTION OR MISCARRIAGE[106]

After an abortion or miscarriage that occurs in the first trimester, Ortho Evra may be started immediately. An additional method of contraception is not needed if Ortho Evra is started immediately. If use of Ortho Evra is not started within 5 days following a first trimester abortion, the woman should follow the instructions for a woman starting Ortho Evra for the first time. In the meantime she should be advised to use a nonhormonal contraceptive method. Ovulation may occur within 10 days of an abortion or miscarriage.

Ortho Evra should be started no earlier than 4 weeks after a second trimester abortion or miscarriage. When Ortho Evra is used postpartum or postabortion, the increased risk of thromboembolic disease must be considered. (See CONTRAINDICATIONS and WARNINGS concerning thromboembolic disease. See PRECAUTIONS, Nursing Mothers.)

BREAKTHROUGH BLEEDING OR SPOTTING

In the event of breakthrough bleeding or spotting (bleeding that occurs on the days that Ortho Evra is worn), treatment should be continued. If breakthrough bleeding persists longer than a few cycles, a cause other than Ortho Evra should be considered.

In the event of no withdrawal bleeding (bleeding that should occur during the patch-free week), treatment should be resumed on the next scheduled Change Day. If Ortho Evra has been used correctly, the absence of withdrawal bleeding is not necessarily an indication of pregnancy. Nevertheless, the possibility of pregnancy should be considered, especially if absence of withdrawal bleeding occurs in 2 consecutive cycles. Ortho Evra should be discontinued if pregnancy is confirmed.

IN CASE OF VOMITING OR DIARRHEA

Given the nature of transdermal application, dose delivery should be unaffected by vomiting.

IN CASE OF SKIN IRRITATION

If patch use results in uncomfortable irritation, the patch may be removed and a new patch may be applied to a different location until the next Change Day. Only 1 patch should be worn at a time.

ADDITIONAL INSTRUCTIONS FOR DOSING

Breakthrough bleeding, spotting, and amenorrhea are frequent reasons for patients discontinuing hormonal contraceptives. In case of breakthrough bleeding, as in all cases of irregular bleeding from the vagina, nonfunctional causes should be considered. In case of undiagnosed persistent or recurrent abnormal bleeding from the vagina, adequate diagnostic measures are indicated to rule out pregnancy or malignancy. If pathology has been excluded, time or a change to another method of contraception may solve the problem.

Use of hormonal contraceptives in the event of a missed menstrual period:

If the woman has not adhered to the prescribed schedule, the possibility of pregnancy should be considered at the time of the first missed period. Hormonal contraceptive use should be discontinued if pregnancy is confirmed.

If the woman has adhered to the prescribed regimen and misses one period, she should continue using her contraceptive patches.

If the woman has adhered to the prescribed regimen and misses two consecutive periods, pregnancy should be ruled out. Ortho Evra use should be discontinued if pregnancy is confirmed.

HOW SUPPLIED

Each beige Ortho Evra patch contains 6.0 mg norelgestromin and 0.75 mg EE, and releases 150 µg of norelgestromin and 20 µg of EE to the bloodstream per 24 hours. Each patch surface is heat stamped with Ortho Evra 150/20. Each patch is packaged in a protective pouch.

SPECIAL PRECAUTIONS FOR STORAGE AND DISPOSAL

Store at 25°C (77°F); excursions permitted to 15-30°C (59-86°F).

Store patches in their protective pouches. Apply immediately upon removal from the protective pouch.

Do not store in the refrigerator or freezer.

Used patches still contain some active hormones. Each patch should be carefully folded in half so that it sticks to itself before throwing it away.

PRODUCT LISTING - EQUIVALENTS NOT AVAILABLE

Film, Extended Release - Transdermal - 20 mcg;150 mcg/24 Hr

1 each	$12.29	ORTHO EVRA, Ortho Mcneil Pharmaceutical	00062-1920-01
3 x 6	$221.10	ORTHO EVRA, Ortho Mcneil Pharmaceutical	00062-1920-15

Ethinyl Estradiol; Norethindrone *(001220)*

Categories: Contraception; Pregnancy Category X; FDA Approval Pre 1982; WHO Formulary

Drug Classes: Contraceptives; Estrogens; Hormones/hormone modifiers; Progestins

Brand Names: Anovlar; Anovulatorio; Brevicon; Ciclovulan; Estrinor; Gencept; Genora; Jenest-28; Loestrin; Micronor; Milli; Minovlar; Modicon; N.E.E.; Nelova; Nodiol; Norcept-E; Norethin; Norinyl; Norlestrin; Orlest; **Ortho-Novum**; Ortho-Novum 7 7 7; Ovcon; Tri-Norinyl

Foreign Brand Availability: Brevinor (Australia; Benin; Burkina-Faso; Ethiopia; Gambia; Ghana; Guinea; Hong-Kong; Ivory-Coast; Kenya; Liberia; Malawi; Malaysia; Mali; Mauritania; Mauritius; Morocco; New-Zealand; Niger; Nigeria; Senegal; Seychelles; Sierra-Leone; Sudan; Tanzania; Tunia; Uganda; Zambia; Zimbabwe); Brevinor 21 (New-Zealand); Brevinor 28 (Australia; New-Zealand); Brevinor-1 21 (New-Zealand); Brevinor-1 28 (Australia; New-Zealand); Kliovance (New-Zealand); Neocon (Netherlands); Norimin (Australia; Bahrain; Benin; Burkina-Faso; Cyprus; Egypt; England; Ethiopia; Gambia; Ghana; Guinea; Hong-Kong; Iran; Iraq; Israel; Ivory-Coast; Jordan; Kenya; Kuwait; Lebanon; Liberia; Libya; Malawi; Mali; Mauritania; Mauritius; Morocco; New-Zealand; Niger; Nigeria; Oman; Qatar; Republic-of-Yemen; Saudi-Arabia; Senegal; Seychelles; Sierra-Leone; South-Africa; Sudan; Syria; Tanzania; Tunia; Uganda; United-Arab-Emirates; Zambia; Zimbabwe); Ortho 7 7 7 (Bahamas; Barbados; Belize; Bermuda; Canada; Curacao; Guyana; Jamaica; Netherland-Antilles; Puerto-Rico; Surinam; Trinidad); Ortho 1 35 (Canada); Ortho-Novum 1 35 (France; Mexico); Ortho-Novum 1 50 (Bahamas; Barbados; Belize; Bermuda; Curacao; Guyana; Jamaica; Netherland-Antilles; Puerto-Rico; Surinam; Trinidad); Ovysmen (Bahrain; Belgium; Benin; Burkina-Faso; Cyprus; Egypt; England; Ethiopia; Gambia; Ghana; Guinea; Iran; Iraq; Israel; Ivory-Coast; Jordan; Kenya; Kuwait; Lebanon; Liberia; Libya; Malawi; Mali; Mauritania; Mauritius; Morocco; Niger; Nigeria; Oman; Qatar; Republic-of-Yemen; Saudi-Arabia; Senegal; Seychelles; Sierra-Leone; South-Africa; Sudan; Syria; Tanzania; Tunia; Uganda; United-Arab-Emirates; Zambia; Zimbabwe); Ovysmen 0.5 35 (Austria; Germany; Switzerland); Ovysmen 1 35 (Austria; Germany; Switzerland); Synphase (Hong-Kong); Synphasic 28 (Australia; Canada; New-Zealand); Triella (France); Trinovum (Austria; Belgium; Benin; Burkina-Faso; Colombia; Denmark; England; Ethiopia; Gambia; Germany; Ghana; Guinea; Ireland; Israel; Italy; Ivory-Coast; Kenya; Liberia; Malawi; Mali; Mauritania; Mauritius; Mexico; Morocco; Netherlands; Niger; Nigeria; Russia; Senegal; Seychelles; Sierra-Leone; South-Africa; Sudan; Switzerland; Tanzania; Tunia; Uganda; Zambia; Zimbabwe); Trinovum 21 (Hong-Kong)

Cost of Therapy: $34.31 (Contraceptive; Ortho-Novum; biphasic; 1 tablet/day; 28 day supply)
$31.45 (Contraceptive; Ortho-Novum 7/7/7; 0.5 mg; 0.75 mg; 1 mg; 1 tablet/day; 28 day supply)
$29.98 (Contraceptive; Ortho-Novum 1/35; 35 µg; 1 mg; 1 tablet/day; 28 day supply)

WARNING

Patients should be counseled that this product does not protect against HIV infection (AIDS) and other sexually transmitted diseases.

DESCRIPTION

The chemical name for norethindrone is 17-hydroxy-19-nor-17α-pregn-4-en-20-yn-3-one, for ethinyl estradiol is 19-nor-17α-pregna-1,3,5(10)- trien -20-yne-3,17-diol, and for mestranol is 3-methoxy-19-nor-17α- pregna-1,3,5 (10)-trien-20-yn-17-ol.

Each of the following products is a combination oral contraceptive containing the progestational compound norethindrone and the estrogenic compound ethinyl estradiol:

ORTHO-NOVUM 7/7/7

Each white tablet contains 0.5 mg of norethindrone and 0.035 mg of ethinyl estradiol. *Inactive Ingredients:* Lactose, magnesium stearate and pregelatinized starch.

Each light peach tablet contains 0.75 mg of norethindrone and 0.035 mg of ethinyl estradiol. *Inactive Ingredients:* FD&C yellow no. 6 lactose, magnesium stearate and pregelatinized starch.

Each peach tablet contains 1 mg of norethindrone and 0.035 of ethinyl estradiol. *Inactive Ingredients:* FD&C yellow no. 6, lactose, magnesium stearate and pregelatinized starch.

Each green tablet in the Ortho-Novum 7/7/7 28 package contains only inert ingredients, as follows: D&C yellow no. 10 Aluminum Lake, FD&C blue no. 2 aluminum lake, lactose, magnesium stearate, microcrystalline cellulose and pregelatinized starch.

ORTHO-NOVUM 10/11
Each white tablet contains 0.5 mg of norethindrone and 0.035 mg of ethinyl estradiol. *Inactive Ingredients:* Lactose, magnesium stearate and pregelatinized starch.
 Each peach tablet contains 1 mg norethindrone and 0.035 ethinyl estradiol. *Inactive Ingredients:* FD&C yellow no. 6, lactose, magnesium stearate and pregelatinized starch.
 Each green tablet in the Ortho-Novum 10/11 28 package contains only inert ingredients, as listed under green tablets in Ortho-Novum 7/7/7 28.

ORTHO-NOVUM 1/35
Each peach tablet contains 1 mg of norethindrone and 0.035 mg of ethinyl estradiol. *Inactive Ingredients:* FD&C yellow no. 6, lactose, magnesium stearate and pregelatinized starch.
 Each green tablet in the Ortho-Novum 1/35 28 package contains only inert ingredients, as listed under green tablets in Ortho-Novum 7/7/7 28.

MODICON
Each white tablet contains 0.5 mg of norethindrone and 0.035 mg of ethinyl estradiol. *Inactive Ingredients:* Lactose, magnesium stearate and pregelatinized starch.
 Each green tablet in the Modicon 28 package contains only inert ingredients, as listed under green tablets in Ortho- Novum 7/7/7 28.

CLINICAL PHARMACOLOGY

COMBINATION ORAL CONTRACEPTIVES
Combination oral contraceptives act by suppression of gonadotropins. Although the primary mechanism of this action is inhibition of ovulation, other alterations include changes in the cervical mucus (which increase the difficulty of sperm entry into the uterus) and the endometrium (which may reduce the likelihood of implantation).

PROGESTIN-ONLY ORAL CONTRACEPTIVES
The primary mechanism through which norethindrone prevents conception is not known, but progestogen-only contraceptives are known to alter the cervical mucus, exert a progestational effect on the endometrium, interfering with implantation, and, in some patients, suppress ovulation.

INDICATIONS AND USAGE

Oral contraceptives are indicated for the prevention of pregnancy in women who elect to use the products as a method of contraception.
 Oral contraceptives are highly effective. TABLE 1 lists the typical accidental pregnancy rates for users of combination oral contraceptives and other methods of contraception. The efficacy of these contraceptive methods, except sterilization, depends upon the reliability upon the reliability with which they are used. Correct and consistent use of methods can result in lower failure rates.

***TABLE 1** Lowest Expected and Typical Failure Rates During the First Year of Continuous Use of a Method*

% of Women Experiencing an Accidental Pregnancy in the First Year of Continuous Use

Method	Lowest Expected*	Typical†
No contraception	(85)	(85)
Oral contraceptives		3
Combined	0.1	N/A‡
Progestin only	0.5	N/A‡
Diaphragm with spermicidal cream or jelly	6	18
Spermicides alone (foam, creams, gels, jellies, vaginal suppositories and vaginal film)	6	21
Vaginal sponge		
Nulliparous	9	18
Parous	20	36
Implant (6 capsules)	0.09	0.09
Injection: depot medroxyprogesterone acetate	0.3	0.3
IUD		
Progesterone T	1.5	2.0
Copper T 380 A	0.6	0.8
LN g 20	0.1	0.1
Condom without spermicides		
Female	5	21
Male	3	12
Cervical Cap with spermacidal cream or jelly	2	12
Nulliparous	9	18
Parous	26	36
Periodic abstinence (all methods)	1-9	20
Withdrawl	4	19
Female sterilization	0.4	0.4
Male sterilization	0.10	0.15

* The authors' best guess of the percentage of women expected to experience an accidental pregnancy among couples who initiate a method (not necessarily for the first time) and who use it consistently and correctly during first year if they do not stop for any other reason.
† This term represents "typical" couples who initiate a method (not necessarily for the first time), who experience an accidental pregnancy during the first year if they do not stop use for any other reason.
‡ N/A - Data not available.
Adapted from RA Hatcher *et al.,* Reference 7.

CONTRAINDICATIONS

Oral contraceptives should not be used in women who have the following combinations:

- Thrombophlebitis or thromboembolic disorders.
- A past history of deep vein thrombophlebitis or thromboembolic disorders.
- Cerebral vascular of coronary artery disease.
- Known or suspected carcinoma of the breast.
- Carcinoma of the endometrium or other known or suspected estrogen-dependent neoplasia.
- Undiagnosed abnormal genital bleeding.
- Cholestatic jaundice of pregnancy or jaundice with prior pill use.
- Hepatic adenomas or carcinomas.
- Known or suspected pregnancy.

WARNINGS

Cigarette smoking increases the risk of serious cardiovascular side effects from oral conceptive use. This risk increases with age and with heavy smoking (15 or more cigarettes per day) and is quite marked in women over 35 years of age. Women who use oral contraceptives should be strongly advised not to smoke.

The use of oral contraceptives is associated with increased risks of several serious conditions including myocardial infarction, thromboembolism, stroke, hepatic neoplasia and gallbladder disease, although the risk of serious morbidity or mortality is very small in healthy women with out underlying risk factors. The risk of morbidity and mortality increases significantly in the presence of other underlying risk factors such as hypertension, hyperlipidemias, hypercholesterolemia, obesity and diabetes.
 Practitioners prescribing oral should be familiar with the following information relating to these risks.
 The information contained in this package insert is principally based on studies carried out in patients who used oral contraceptives with higher formulations of estrogens and progestogens than those in common use today. The effect of long-term use of oral contraceptives with lower formulations of both estrogens and progestogens remains to be determined.
 Throughout this labeling, epidemiological studies reported are of two types: retrospective or case control studies and prospective or cohort studies. Case control studies provide a measure of the relative risk of a disease, namely, a *ratio* of the incidence of a disease among oral contraceptive users to that among non-users. The relative risk does not provide information on the actual clinical occurrence of a disease. Cohort studies provide a measure of attributable risk, which is the *difference* in the incidence of disease between oral contraceptive users and non-users. The attributable risk does provide information about the actual occurrence of a disease in the population (adapted from references 8 and 9 with the author's permission). For further information, the reader is referred to a text on epidemiological methods.

THROMBOEMBOLIC DISORDERS AND VASCULAR PROBLEMS

Myocardial Infarction

An increased risk of myocardial infarction has been attributed to oral contraceptive use. This risk is primarily in smokers or women with other underlying risk factors for coronary artery disease such as hypertension, hypercholesterolemia, morbid obesity and diabetes. The relative risk of heart attack for current oral contraceptive users has been estimated to be 2 to 6.[10-16] The risk is very low under the age of 30.
 Smoking in combination with oral contraceptive use has been shown to contribute substantially to the incidence of myocardial infarctions in women in their mid-thirties or older with smoking accounting for the majority of excess cases.[17] Mortality rates associated with circulatory disease have been shown to increase substantially in smokers over the age of 35 and non-smokers over the age of 40 among women who use oral contraceptives.
 Oral contraceptives may compound the effects of well-known risk factors such as hypertension, diabetes, hyperlipidemias, age and obesity.[19] In particular, some progestogens are known to decrease HDL cholesterol and cause glucose intolerance, while estrogens may create a state of hyperinsulinism.[20-24] Oral contraceptives have been shown to increase blood pressure among users (see Elevated Blood Pressure). Similar effects on risk factors have been associated with an increased risk of heart disease. Oral contraceptives must be used with caution in women with cardiovascular disease risk factors.

Thromboembolism

An increased risk of thromboembolic and thrombotic disease associated with the use of oral contraceptives is well established. Case control studies have found the relative risk of users compared to nonusers to be 3 for the first episode of superficial venous thrombosis, 4 to 11 for deep vein thrombosis or pulmonary embolism, and 1.5 to 6 for women with predisposing conditions for venous thromboembolic disease.[9,10,25-30] Cohort studies have shown the relative risk to be somewhat lower, about 3 for new cases and about 4.5 for new cases requiring hospitalization.[31] The risk of thromboembolic disease due to oral contraceptives is not related to length of use and disappears after pill use is stopped.[8]
 A 2- to 4-fold increase in relative risk of postoperative thromboembolic complications has been reported with the use of oral contraceptives.[15,32] The relative risk of venous thrombosis in women who have predisposing conditions is twice that of women without such medical conditions.[15,32] If feasible, oral contraceptives should be discontinued at least 4 weeks prior to and for 2 weeks after elective surgery of a type associated with an increase in risk of thromboembolism and during and following prolonged immobilization. Since the immediate postpartum period is also associated with an increased risk of thromboembolism, oral contraceptives should be started no earlier than 4-6 weeks after delivery in women who elect not to breast feed.

Cerebrovascular Diseases

Oral contraceptives have been shown to increase in both the relative and attributable risks of cerebrovascular events (thrombotic and hemorrhagic strokes) although, in general, the risk is greatest among older (>35 years), hypertensive women who also smoke. Hypertension was found to be a risk factor for both users and nonusers for both types of strokes while smoking interacted to increase the risk of stroke.[33-35]
 In a large study, the relative risk of thrombotic strokes has been shown to range from 3 for normotensive users to 14 for users with severe hypertension.[36] The relative risk of hemorrhagic stroke is reported to be 1.2 for non-smokers who used oral contraceptives, 2.6 for smokers who did not use oral contraceptives, 7.6 for smokers who used oral contraceptives, 1.8 for normotensive users and 25.7 for users with severe hypertension.[36] The attributable risk also is greater in older women.[9]

Dose-Related Risk of Vascular Disease From Oral Contraceptives

A positive association has been observed between the amount of estrogen and progestogen in oral contraceptives and the risk of vascular disease.[37-39] A decline in serum high density lipoproteins (HDL) has been reported with many progestational agents.[20-22] A decline in serum high density lipoproteins has been associated with an increased incidence of ischemic heart disease. Because estrogens increase HDL cholesterol, the net effect of an oral contraceptive depends on a balance achieved between doses of estrogen and progestogen and the nature of the progestin used in the contraceptives. The amount and activity of both hormones should be considered in the choice of an oral contraceptive.

Minimizing exposure to estrogen and progestogen is in keeping with good principles of therapeutics. For any particular oral contraceptive, the dosage regimen prescribed should be one which contains the least amount of estrogen and progestogen that is compatible with the needs of the individual patient. New acceptors of oral contraceptive agents should be started on preparations containing the lowest dose of estrogen which produces satisfactory results for the patient.

Persistence of Risk of Vascular Disease

There are two studies which have shown persistence of risk of vascular disease for ever-users of oral contraceptives. In a study in the United States, the risk of developing myocardial infarction after discontinuing oral contraceptives persists for at least 9 years for women 40-49 who had used oral contraceptives for 5 or more years, but this increased risk was not demonstrated in other age groups.[14] In another study in Great Britain, the risk of cerebrovascular disease persisted for at least 6 years after discontinuation of oral contraceptives, although excess risk was very small.[40] However, both studies were performed with oral contraceptive formulations containing 50 mcg or higher of estrogens.

ESTIMATES OF MORTALITY FROM CONTRACEPTIVE USE

One study gathered data from a variety of sources which have estimated the mortality rate associated with different methods of contraception at different ages (see TABLE 2). These estimates include the combined risk of death associated with contraceptive methods plus the risk attributable to pregnancy in the event of method failure. Each method of contraception has its specific benefits and risks. The study concluded that with the exception of oral contraceptive users 35 and older who smoke and 40 and older who do not smoke, mortality associated with all methods of birth control is low and below that associated with childbirth. The observation of an increase in risk of mortality with age for oral contraceptive users is based on data gathered in the 1970's but not reported until 1983.[41] However, current clinical practice involves the use of lower estrogen dose formulations combined with careful restriction of oral contraceptive use to women who do not have the various risk factors listed in this labeling.

Because of these changes in practice and, also, because of some limited new data which suggest that the risk of cardiovascular disease with the use of oral contraceptives may now be less than previously observed (Porter JB, Hunter J, Jick H, *et al.* Oral contraceptives and nonfatal vascular disease. Obset Gynecol 1985;66:1-4; and Porter JB, Hershel J, Walker AM. Mortality among oral contraceptive users. Obset Gunecol 1987;70:29-32), the Fertility and Maternal Health Drugs Advisory Committee was asked to review the topic in 1989. The Committee concluded that although cardiovascular disease risks may be increased with oral contraceptive use after age 40 in healthy non-smoking women (even with the newer low-dose formulations), there are greater potential health risks associated with pregnancy in older women and with the alternative surgical and medical procedures which may be necessary if such women do not have access to effective and acceptable means of contraception.

Therefore, the Committee recommended that the benefits of oral contraceptive use by healthy non-smoking women over 40 may outweigh the possible risks. Of course, older women, as all women who take oral contraceptives, should take an oral contraceptive which contains the least amount of estrogen and progestogen that is compatible with a low failure rate and individual patient needs.

TABLE 2 *Annual Number of Birth-Related or Method-Related Deaths Associated With Control of Fertility Per 100,000 Non-Sterile Women, by Fertility Control Method According to Age*

Method of control and outcome	15-19	20-24	25-29	30-34	35-39	40-44
No fertility controls methods*	7.0	7.4	9.1	14.8	25.7	28.2
Oral contraceptives non-smoker†	0.3	0.5	0.9	1.9	13.8	31.6
Oral contraceptives smoker†	2.2	3.4	6.6	13.5	51.1	117.2
IUD†	0.8	0.8	1.0	1.0	1.4	1.4
Condom*	1.1	1.6	0.7	0.2	0.3	0.4
Diaphragm/Spermicide*	1.9	1.2	1.2	1.3	2.2	2.8
Periodic abstinence*	2.5	1.6	1.6	1.7	2.9	3.6

* Deaths are birth-related
† Deaths are method-related
Adapted from H.W. Ory.[41]

CARCINOMA OF REPRODUCTIVE ORGANS

Numerous epidemiological studies have been performed or the incidence of breast, endometrial, ovarian and cervical cancer in women using oral contraceptives. Most of the studies on breast cancer and oral contraceptive use report that the use of oral contraceptives is not associated with an increase in the risk of developing breast cancer.[42,44,89] Some studies have reported an increased risk of developing breast cancer in certain subgroups of oral contraceptice users, but the findings reported in these studies are not consistent.[43,45-49,85-88]

Some studies suggest that oral contraceptive use has been associated with an increase in risk of cervical intraepithelial neoplasia in some populations of women.[51-54] However, there continues to be controversy about the extent to which such findings may be due to differences in sexual behavior and other factors.

In spite of many studies of the relationship between oral conraceptive use and breast and cervical cancers, a cause and effect relationship has not been established.

HEPATIC NEOPLASIA

Benign hepatic adenomas are associated with oral contraceptive use, although the incidence of benign tumors is rare in the United States. Indirect calculations have estimated the attributable risk to be in the range of 3.3 cases/100,000 for users, a risk that increases after 4 or more years of use.[55] Rupture of rare, benign, hepatic adenomas may cause death through intra-abdominal hemorrhage.[56,57]

Studies from Britain have shown an increased risk of developing hepatocellular carcinoma[58-60] in long-term (>8 years) oral contraceptive users. However, these cancers are extremely rare in the US and the attributable risk (the excess incidence) of liver cancers in oral contraceptive users approaches less than one per million users.

OCULAR LESIONS

There have been clinical case reports of retinal thrombosis associated with the use of oral contraceptives. Oral contraceptives should be discontinued if there is unexplained partial or complete loss of vision; onset of proptosis or diplopia; papilledema; or retinal vascular lesions. Appropriate diagnostic and therapeutic measures should be undertaken immediately.

E

ORAL CONTRACEPTIVE USE BEFORE OR DURING EARLY PREGNANCY

Extensive epidemiological studies have revealed no increased risk of birth defects in women who have used oral contraceptives prior to pregnancy.[61-63] Studies also do not suggest a teratogenic effect, particularly insofar as cardiac anomalies and limb reduction defects are concerned,[61,62,64,65] when taken inadvertently during early pregnancy.

The administration of oral contraceptives to induce withdrawal bleeding should not be used as a test for pregnancy. Oral contraceptives should not be used during pregnancy to treat threatened or habitual abortion.

It is recommended that for any patient who has missed 2 consecutive periods, (or after 45 days from the last menstrual period if the progestogen-only oral contraceptives are used) pregnancy should be ruled out before continuing oral contraceptive use. If the patient has not adhered to the prescribed schedule, the possibility of pregnancy should be considered at the time of the first missed period or upon missing 1 ethinyl estradiol; norethindrone tablet. Oral contraceptive use should be discontinued if pregnancy is confirmed.

GALLBLADDER DISEASE

Earlier studies have reported an increased lifetime relative risk of gallbladder surgery in users of oral contraceptives and estrogens.[66-67] More recent studies, however, have shown that the relative risk of developing gallbladder disease among oral contraceptive users may be minimal.[68-70] The recent findings of minimal risk may be related to the use of oral contraceptive formulations containing lower hormonal doses of estrogens and progestogens.

CARBOHYDRATE AND LIPID METABOLIC EFFECTS

Oral contraceptives have been shown to cause a glucose intolerance in a significant percentage of users.[23] Oral contraceptives containing greater than 75 μg of estrogens cause hyperinsulinism, while lower doses of estrogen cause less glucose intolerance.[71] Progestogens increase insulin secretion and create insulin resistance, this effect varying with different progestational agents.[23,72] However, in the non-diabetic woman, oral contraceptives appear to have no effect on fasting blood glucose.[73] Because of these demonstrated effects, prediabetic and diabetic women should be carefully observed while taking oral contraceptives.

A small proportion of women will have persistent hypertriglyceridemia while on the pill. As discussed earlier (see Myocardial Infarction and Dose Related Risk of Vascular Disease), changes in serum triglycerides and lipoprotein levels have been reported in oral contraceptive users.

ELEVATED BLOOD PRESSURE

An increase in blood pressure has been reported in women taking oral contraceptives[74] and this increase is more likely in older oral contraceptive users[75] and with extended duration of use.[74] Data from the Royal College of General Practitioners[18] and subsequent randomized trials have shown that the incidence of hypertension increases with increasing concentrations of progestogens.

Women with a history of hypertension or hypertension-related diseases, or renal disease[76] should be encouraged to use another method of contraception. If women elect to use oral contraceptives, they should be monitored closely and if significant elevation of blood pressure occurs, oral contraceptives should be discontinued. For most women, elevated blood pressure will return to normal after stopping oral contraceptives and there is no difference in the occurrence of hypertension between former and never users.[74,76,77]

HEADACHE

The onset or exacerbation of migraine or development of headache with a new pattern which is recurrent, persistent or severe requires discontinuation of oral contraceptives and evaluation of the cause.

BLEEDING IRREGULARITIES

Breakthrough bleeding and spotting are sometimes encountered in patients on oral contraceptives, especially during the first 3 months of use. Non-hormonal causes should be considered and adequate diagnostic measures taken to rule out malignancy or pregnancy in the event of breakthrough bleeding, as in the case of any abnormal vaginal bleeding. If pathology has been excluded, time or a change to another formulation may solve the problem. In the event of amenorrhea, pregnancy should be ruled out.

An alteration in menstrual patterns is likely to occur in women using progestogen-only contraceptives. The amount and duration of flow, cycle length, breakthrough bleeding, spotting and amenorrhea will probably be quite variable. Bleeding irregularities occur more frequently with the use of progestogen-only oral contraceptives than with the combinations and the dropout rate due to such conditions is higher.

Some women may encounter post-pill amenorrhea or oligomenorrhea, especially when such a condition was preexistent.

ECTOPIC PREGNANCY

Ectopic as well as intrauterine pregnancy may occur in contraceptive failures. However, in progestogen-only oral contraceptive failures, the ratio of ectopic to intrauterine pregnancies is higher than in women who are not receiving contraceptives, since the drugs are more effective in preventing intrauterine than ectopic pregnancies.

ADDITIONAL INFORMATION FOR PROGESTEN ONLY CONTRACEPTIVES

Masculinization of the female fetus has occurred who progestogens have been used in pregnant women.

Some beagle dogs treated with medroxyprogesterone acetate developed mammary nodules. Although nodules occasionally appeared in control animals they were intermittent in nature, whereas nodules in treated animals were larger and more numerous, and they persisted. There is no general agreement as to whether the nodules are benign or malignant. Their significance with respect to humans has not been estableised.

E

PRECAUTIONS

Patients should be counseled that this product does not protect against HIV infection (AIDS) and other sexually transmitted diseases.

PHYSICAL EXAMINATION AND FOLLOW-UP

It is good medical practice for all women to have annual history and physical examinations, including women using oral contraceptives. The physical examination, however, may be deferred until after initiation of oral contraceptives if requested by the women and judged appropriate by the clinician. The physical examination should include special reference to blood pressure, breasts, abdomen and pelvic organs, including cervical cytology, and relevant laboratory tests. In case of undiagnosed, persistent or recurrent abnormal vaginal bleeding, appropriate measures should be conducted to rule out malignancy. Women with a strong family history of breast cancer or who have breast nodules should be monitored with particular care.

LIPID DISORDERS

Women who are being treated for hyperlipidemia should be followed closely if they elect to use oral contraceptives. Some progestogens may elevate LDL levels and may render the control of hyperlipidemias more difficult.

LIVER FUNCTION

If jaundice develops in any woman receiving such drugs, the medication should be discontinued. Steroid hormones may be poorly metabolized in patients with impaired liver function.

FLUID RETENTION

Oral contraceptives may cause some degree of fluid retention. They should be prescribed with caution, and only with careful monitoring, in patients with conditions which might be aggravated by fluid retention.

EMOTIONAL DISORDERS

Women with a history of depression should be carefully observed and the drug discontinued if depression recurs to a serious degree.

CONTACT LENSES

Contact lens wearers who develop visual changes or changes in lens tolerance should be assessed by an ophthalmologist.

INTERACTIONS WITH LABORATORY TESTS

Certain endocrine and liver function tests and blood components may be affected by oral contraceptives:

a. Increased prothrombin and factors VII, VIII, IX, and X; decreased antithrombin 3; increased norepinephrine-induced platelet aggregability.

b. Increased thyroid binding globulins (TBG) leading to increased circulating total thyroid hormone, as measured by protein-bound iodine (PBI), T_4 by column or by radioimmunoassay. Free T_3 resin uptake is decreased, reflecting the elevated TBG. Free T_4 concentration is unaltered.

c. Other binding proteins may be elevated in serum.

d. Sex-binding globulins are increased and result in elevated levels of total circulating sex steroids and corticoids; however, free or biologically active levels remain unchanged.

e. Triglycerides may be increased.

f. Glucose tolerance may be decreased.

g. Serum folate levels may be depressed by oral contraceptive therapy. This may be of clinical significance if a woman becomes pregnant shortly after discontinuing oral contraceptives.

CARCINOGENESIS

See WARNINGS.

PREGNANCY CATEGORY X

See CONTRAINDICATIONS and WARNINGS.

NURSING MOTHERS

Small amounts of oral contraceptive steroids have been identified in the milk of nursing mothers, and a few adverse effects on the child have been reported, including jaundice and breast enlargement. In addition, oral contraceptives given in the postpartum period may interfere with lactation by decreasing the quantity and quality of breast milk. If possible, the nursing mother should be advised not to use oral contraceptives but to use other forms of contraception until she has completely weaned her child.

INFORMATION FOR THE PATIENT

See the Patient Instructions that are distributed with the prescription.

SEXUALLY TRANSMITTED DISEASES

Patients should be counseled that this product does not protect against HIV infection (AIDS) and other sexually transmitted diseases.

DRUG INTERACTIONS

Reduced efficacy and increased incidence of breakthrough bleeding and menstrual irregularities have been associated with concomitant use of rifampin. A similar association though less marked, has been suggested with barbiturates, phenylbutazone, phenytoin sodium, and possibly with griseofulvin, ampicillin and tetracyclines.[78]

ADVERSE REACTIONS

An increased risk of the following serious adverse reactions has been associated with the use of oral contraceptives: (See alsoWARNINGS.)Thrombophlebitis, arterial thromboembolism, pulmonary embolism, myocardial infarction, cerebral hemorrhage, cerebral thrombosis, hypertension, gallbladder disease, hepatic adenomas, carcinomas or benign liver tumors.

- ***There is evidence of an association between the following conditions and the use of oral contraceptives, although additional confirmatory studies are needed:*** Mesenteric thrombosis, retinal thrombosis.
- ***The following adverse reactions have been reported in patients receiving oral contraceptives and are believed to be drug-related:*** Nausea, vomiting, gastrointestinal symptoms (such as abdominal cramps and bloating), breakthrough bleeding, spotting, change in menstrual flow, amenorrhea, temporary infertility after discontinuation of treatment, edema, melasma which may persist, breast changes; tenderness, enlargement, secretion, change in weight (increase or decrease), change in cervical erosion and secretion, diminution in lactation when given immediately postpartum, cholestatic jaundice, migraine, rash (allergic), mental depression, reduced tolerance to carbohydrates, vaginal candidiasis, change in corneal curvature (steepening), intolerance to contact lenses.
- ***The following adverse reactions have been reported in users of oral contraceptives and the association has been neither confirmed nor refuted:*** Pre-menstrual syndrome, cataracts, changes in appetite, cystitis-like syndrome, headache, nervousness, dizziness, hirsutism, loss of scalp hair, erythema multiforme, erythema nodosum, hemorrhagic eruption, vaginitis, porphyria, impaired renal function, hemolytic uremic syndrome, budd chiari syndrome, acne, changes in libido, colitis.

DOSAGE AND ADMINISTRATION

To achieve maximum contraceptive effectiveness, tablets must be taken exactly as directed and at intervals not exceeding 24 hours.

The patient should be instructed to use an additional method of protection until after the first week of administration in the initial cycle when utilizing the Sunday-Start Regimen. Most dispensors are preset for Sunday Start. Day 1 Start is also available.

The possibility of ovulation and conception prior to initiation of use should be considered.

21-DAY REGIMEN (SUNDAY START)

The first tablet should be taken on the first Sunday after menstruation begins. If period begins on Sunday, the first tablet is taken on the same day. One (1) tablet is taken daily for 21 days. For subsequent cycles, no tablets are taken for 7 days, then a tablet is taken the next day (Sunday). For the first cycle of a Sunday Start regimen, another method of contraception should be used until after the first 7 consecutive days of administration.

21-DAY REGIMEN (DAY 1 START)

The initial cycle of therapy is 1 tablet administered daily from the 1st day through 21st day of the menstrual cycle, counting the first day of menstrual flow as "Day 1." For subsequent cycles, no tablets are taken for 7 days, then a new course is started of 1 tablet a day for 21 days. The dosage regimen then continues with 7 days of no medication, followed by 21 days of medication, instituting a 3-weeks-on, 1-week-off dosage regimen.

28-DAY REGIMEN (SUNDAY START)

The fist tablet should be taken on the first Sunday after menstruation begins. If period begins on Sunday, the first tablet should be taken that day. Take 1 active tablet daily for 21 days followed by 1 green placebo tablet daily for 7 days. After 28 tablets have been taken, a new course is started the next (Sunday). For the first cycle of a Sunday Start regimen, another method of contraception should be used until after the first 7 consecutive days of administration.

28-DAY REGIMEN (DAY 1 START)

The first initial cycle of therapy is 1 active tablet administered daily from the 1st through the 21st day of the menstrual cycle, counting the first day of menstrual flow as "Day 1" followed by 1 green tablet daily for 7 days. Tablets are taken without interruption for 28 days. After 28 tablets have been taken, a new course is started the next day.

The use of Ortho-Novum 7/7/7, Ortho-Novum 10/11, Ortho-Novum 1/35, Modicon and Ortho-Novum 1/50 for contraception may be initiated 4 weeks postpartum in women who elect not to breast feed. When the tablets are administered during the postpartum period, the increased risk of thromboembolic disease associated with the postpartum period must be considered. (See CONTRAINDICATIONS and WARNINGS, Thromboembolic diseases.) (See also PRECAUTIONS, Nursing Mothers.) The possibility of ovulation and conception prior to initiation of medication should considered.

See WARNINGS, Discussion of Dose, Related Risk of Vascular Disease from Oral Contraceptives.

NORETHINDRONE (CONTINUOUS REGIMEN)

Norethindrone is administered on a continuous daily dosage regimen starting on the first day of menstruation (*i.e.,* 1 tablet each day) every day of the year. Tablets should be taken at the same time each day and continued daily. The patient should be advised that if prolonged bleeding occurs she should consult her physician.

The use of norethindrone for contraception may be initiated postpartum (see WARNINGS). When norethindrone is administered during postpartum period, the increased risk of thromboembolic disease associated with the postpartum period must be considered. (See CONTRAINDICATIONS and WARNINGS) concerning thromboembolic disease.)

If the patient misses 1 tablet, norethindrone should be discontinued immediately and a method or nonhormonal contraception should be used until menses has appeared or pregnancy has been excluded.

Alternatively, if the patient has taken the tablets correctly, and if menses does not appear when expected, a nonhormonal method of contraception should be substituted until an appropriate diagnostic procedure is performed to rule out pregnancy.

ADDITIONAL INSTRUCTIONS FOR ALL DOSING REGIMENS

Breakthrough bleeding, spotting and amenorrhea are frequent reasons for patients discontinuing oral contraceptives. In breakthrough bleeding, as in all cases of irregular bleeding from the vagina, nonfunctional causes should be borne in mind. In undiagnosed persistent or recurrent abnormal bleeding from the vagina, adequate diagnostic measures are indicated to rule out pregnancy or malignancy. If pathology has been excluded, time or a change to another formulation may solve the problem. Changing to an oral contraceptive with a higher estrogen content, while potentially useful in minimizing menstrual irregularity, should be done only if necessary since this may increase the risk of thromboembolic disease.

SPECIAL NOTES ON ADMINISTRATION

Menstruation usually begins 2 or 3 days, but may begin as late as the fourth or fifth day, after discontinuing medication. If spotting occurs while on the usual regimen of one tablet daily, the patient should continue medication without interruption.

If the patient forgets to take 1 or more active tablets, the following is suggested:

One tablet missed:

- Take tablet as soon as remembered.
- Take next tablet at the regular time.

Two consecutive tablets are missed (week 1 or week 2):

- Take 2 tablets as soon as remembered.
- Take 2 tablets the next day.
- Use another birth control method for 7 days following the missed tablets.

Two consecutive tablets are missed (week 3):

- Take 1 tablet daily until Sunday.
- Discard remaining tablets.
- Start a new pack of tablets immediately (Sunday).
- Use another birth control method for 7 days following the missed tablets.

Three or more consecutive tablets are missed:

- Take 1 tablet daily until Sunday.
- Discard remaining tablets.
- Start a new pack of tablets immediately (Sunday).
- Use another birth control method for 7 days following the missed tablets.

The possibility of ovulation increases with each sucessive day that scheduled tablets are missed. While there is little likelihood of ovulation occurring if only 1 tablet is missed, the possibility of spotting or bleeding is increased. This is particularly likely if 2 or more consecutive tablets are missed.

In rare cases of bleeding which resembles menstruation, the patinet should be advised to discontinue medication and then begin taking tablets from a new tablet dispenser on the next Sunday. Persistent bleeding which is not controlled by this method indicates the need for reexaminstion of the patient, at which time nonfunctional causes should be considered.

Use of oral contraceptives in the event of a missed menstrual period:

1. If the patient has not adhered to the prescribed schedule, the possibility of pregnancy should be considered after the first missed period (or upon missing 1 Micronor Tablet) and oral contraceptive use should be withheld until pregnancy is ruled out.
2. If the patient has adhered to the prescribed regimen and misses two consecutive periods (or after 45 days from the last menstrual period if the progestogen-only oral contraceptives are used), pregnancy should be ruled out before continuing the contraceptive regimen.

NON-CONTRACEPTIVE HEALTH BENEFITS

The following non-contraceptive health benefits related to the use of oral contraceptives are supported by epidemiological studies which largely utilized oral contraceptive formulations containing estrogen doses exceeding 0.035 mg of ethinyl estradiol or 0.05 mg of mestranol.[79-84]

Effects on menses:

- Increased menstrual cycle regularity.
- Decreased blood loss and decreased incidence of iron deficiency anemia.
- Decreased incidence of dysmenorrhea.

Effects related to inhibition of ovulation:

- Decreased incidence of functional ovarian cysts.
- Decreased incidence of ectopic pregnancies.

Effects from long-term use:

- Decreased incidence of fibroadenomas and fibrocystic disease of the breast.
- Decreased incidence of acute pelvic inflammatory disease.
- Decreased incidence of endometrial cancer.
- Decreased incidence of ovarian cancer.

FDA RECOMMENDED DOSAGE GUIDELINES FOR POSTCOITAL EMERGENCY CONTRACEPTION

See Ethinyl Estradiol; Levonorgestrel and Ethinyl Estradiol; Norgestrel

PRODUCT LISTING - RATED THERAPEUTICALLY EQUIVALENT

Package	Price	Product, Manufacturer	NDC
Tablet - Oral - Biphasic			
21 x 6	$178.68	ORTHO-NOVUM 10/11, Janssen Pharmaceuticals	00062-1770-15
21 x 6	$192.84	GENERIC, Watson Laboratories Inc	52544-0553-21
28 x 6	$192.84	GENERIC, Watson Laboratories Inc	52544-0554-28
28 x 6	$248.28	ORTHO-NOVUM 10/11, Janssen Pharmaceuticals	00062-1771-15
Tablet - Oral - Triphasic 0.5 mg;0.75 mg;1 mg			
28 x 6	$193.38	GENERIC, Barr Laboratories Inc	00555-9012-58
Tablet - Oral - 35 mcg;0.5 mg			
21 x 6	$178.68	MODICON, Janssen Pharmaceuticals	00062-1712-15
21 x 6	$192.84	GENERIC, Watson Laboratories Inc	52544-0507-21
28 x 3	$101.22	BREVICON, Watson/Rugby Laboratories Inc	52544-0254-28
28 x 6	$192.84	GENERIC, Watson Laboratories Inc	52544-0550-28
28 x 6	$193.02	NORTREL, Barr Laboratories Inc	00555-9008-58
28 x 6	$248.28	MODICON, Janssen Pharmaceuticals	00062-1714-15
Tablet - Oral - 35 mcg;1 mg			
21 x 6	$90.30	NELOVA 1/35, Warner Chilcott Laboratories	00047-0930-11
21 x 6	$176.82	GENERIC, Watson Laboratories Inc	52544-0508-21
21 x 6	$177.00	NORTREL, Barr Laboratories Inc	00555-9009-57
28 each	$31.45	ORTHO-NOVUM 1/35, Allscripts Pharmaceutical Company	54569-0685-00
28 x 6	$23.27	ORTHO-NOVUM 1/35, Janssen Pharmaceuticals	00062-1761-20
28 x 6	$105.00	GENERIC, Watson/Rugby Laboratories Inc	00536-4055-48
28 x 6	$129.74	NELOVA 1/35, Allscripts Pharmaceutical Company	54569-2397-00
28 x 6	$176.82	GENERIC, Watson Laboratories Inc	52544-0552-28
28 x 6	$177.00	NORTREL, Barr Laboratories Inc	00555-9010-58
28 x 6	$219.72	NORINYL 1/35, Watson/Rugby Laboratories Inc	52544-0259-28
28 x 6	$227.58	ORTHO-NOVUM 1/35, Janssen Pharmaceuticals	00062-1761-15
28's	$12.13	GENERIC, Physicians Total Care	54868-4045-00
28's	$21.62	NELOVA 1/35, Allscripts Pharmaceutical Company	54569-2397-01
28's	$26.84	GENERIC, Allscripts Pharmaceutical Company	54569-4999-00

PRODUCT LISTING - EQUIVALENTS NOT AVAILABLE

Package	Price	Product, Manufacturer	NDC
Tablet - Oral - Biphasic			
28 x 6	$153.51	JENEST, Organon	00052-0269-06
Tablet - Oral - Triphasic 0.5 mg;0.75 mg;1 mg			
21's	$27.95	ORTHO-NOVUM 7/7/7, Physicians Total Care	54868-0508-00
28 x 6	$188.72	ORTHO-NOVUM 7/7/7, Allscripts Pharmaceutical Company	54569-0689-01
28 x 6	$193.20	GENERIC, Watson Laboratories Inc	52544-0936-28
28 x 6	$227.58	ORTHO-NOVUM 7/7/7, Janssen Pharmaceuticals	00062-1781-15
28 x 12	$451.68	ORTHO-NOVUM 7/7/7, Janssen Pharmaceuticals	00062-1781-22
28's	$23.23	ORTHO-NOVUM 7/7/7, Janssen Pharmaceuticals	00062-1781-20
28's	$31.45	ORTHO-NOVUM 7/7/7, Allscripts Pharmaceutical Company	54569-0689-00
Tablet - Oral - Triphasic 0.5 mg;1 mg;0.5 mg			
28 x 6	$213.36	TRI-NORINYL, Watson Laboratories Inc	52544-0274-28
28's	$32.95	TRI-NORINYL, Physicians Total Care	54868-0516-00
Tablet - Oral - Triphasic 20 mcg;30 mcg;35 mcg			
28 x 5	$171.30	ESTROSTEP FE, Parke-Davis	00071-0928-47
28 x 30	$1027.80	ESTROSTEP FE, Parke-Davis	00071-0928-15
Tablet - Oral - 5 mcg;1 mg			
28 x 5	$136.95	FEMHRT 1/5, Parke-Davis	00071-0144-45
90's	$88.01	FEMHRT 1/5, Parke-Davis	00071-0144-23
Tablet - Oral - 35 mcg;0.4 mg			
21 x 6	$189.78	OVCON 35, Warner Chilcott Laboratories	00430-0583-11
21 x 6	$190.56	OVCON 35, Bristol-Myers Squibb	00087-0583-42
28 x 6	$190.56	OVCON 35, Bristol-Myers Squibb	00087-0578-41
28 x 6	$210.60	OVCON 35, Warner Chilcott Laboratories	00430-0582-14
28's	$32.81	OVCON 35, Physicians Total Care	54868-0509-01
Tablet - Oral - 35 mcg;1 mg			
21 x 6	$75.23	NORETHIN 1/35 E, Roberts Pharmaceutical Corporation	54092-0087-21
28 x 6	$177.60	NORINYL 1/35, Watson/Rugby Laboratories Inc	52544-0259-88
Tablet - Oral - 50 mcg;1 mg			
28 x 6	$209.46	OVCON 50, Bristol-Myers Squibb	00087-0579-41
28 x 6	$232.44	OVCON 50, Warner Chilcott Laboratories	00430-0585-14
28's	$41.66	OVCON 50, Physicians Total Care	54868-3772-00

Ethinyl Estradiol; Norgestimate *(003270)*

Categories: Acne vulgaris; Contraception; Pregnancy Category X; FDA Approved 1989 Dec
Drug Classes: Contraceptives; Estrogens; Hormones/hormone modifiers; Progestins
Brand Names: **Ortho Cyclen**; Ortho Cyclen 21; Ortho Cyclen 28; Ortho Tri-Cyclen; Ortho Tri-Cyclen 21; Ortho Tri-Cyclen 28
Foreign Brand Availability: Cilest (Belgium; Bulgaria; Canada; Colombia; Costa-Rica; Czech-Republic; Denmark; Dominican-Republic; El-Salvador; England; Finland; France; Germany; Guatemala; Honduras; Hungary; Ireland; Mexico; Netherlands; Nicaragua; Panama; Peru; Switzerland); Cileste (Austria); Tricilest (Colombia; South-Africa); Tri-Cyclen (Canada)
Cost of Therapy: $31.15 (Contraception; Ortho Tri-Cyclen; triphasic; 1 tablet/day; 28 day supply)

DESCRIPTION

Note: The trade name has been used throughout this monograph for clarity.

Patients should be counseled that this product does not protect against HIV infection (AIDS) and other sexually transmitted diseases.

E

Each of the following products is a combination oral contraceptive containing the progestational compound norgestimate and the estrogenic compound ethinyl estradiol.

ORTHO TRI-CYCLEN 28 TABLETS

Each white tablet contains 0.180 mg of the progestational compound, norgestimate (18,19-Dinor-17-pregn-4-en-20-yn-3-one,17-(acetyloxy)-13-ethyl-,oxime,(17α)-(+)-) and 0.035 mg of the estrogenic compound, ethinyl estradiol (19-nor-17α-pregna,1,3,5(10)-trien-20-yne-3,17-diol). Inactive ingredients include lactose, magnesium stearate, and pregelatinized starch.

Each light blue tablet contains 0.215 mg of the progestational compound norgestimate (18,19-Dinor-17-pregn-4-en-20-yn-3-one,17-(acetyloxy)-13-ethyl-,oxime,(17α)-(+)-) and 0.035 mg of the estrogenic compound, ethinyl estradiol (19-nor-17α-pregna,1,3,5(10)-trien-20-yne-3,17-diol). Inactive ingredients include FD&C blue no. 2 aluminum lake, lactose, magnesium stearate, and pregelatinized starch.

Each blue tablet contains 0.250 mg of the progestational compound norgestimate (18,19-Dinor-17-pregn-4-en-20-yn-3-one,17-(acetyloxy)-13-ethyl-,oxime,(17α)-(+)-) and 0.035 mg of the estrogenic compound, ethinyl estradiol (19-nor-17α-pregna,1,3,5(10)-trien-20-yne-3,17-diol). Inactive ingredients include FD&C blue no. 2 aluminum lake, lactose, magnesium stearate, and pregelatinized starch.

Each green tablet contains only inert ingredients, as follows: D&C yellow no. 10 aluminum lake, FD&C blue no. 2 aluminum lake, lactose, magnesium stearate, microcrystalline cellulose and pregelatinized starch.

ORTHO-CYCLEN 28 TABLETS

Each blue tablet contains 0.250 mg of the progestational compound norgestimate (18,19-Dinor-17-pregn-4-en-20-yn-3-one,17-(acetyloxy)-13-ethyl-,oxime,(17α)-(+)-) and 0.035 mg of the estrogenic compound, ethinyl estradiol (19-nor-17α-pregna,1,3,5(10)-trien-20-yne-3,17-diol). Inactive ingredients include FD&C blue no. 2 aluminum lake, lactose, magnesium stearate, and pregelatinized starch.

Each green tablet contains only inert ingredients, as follows: D&C yellow no. 10 aluminum lake, FD&C blue no. 2 aluminum lake, lactose, magnesium stearate, microcrystalline cellulose and pregelatinized starch.

ORTHO TRI-CYCLEN LO TABLETS

Each white tablet contains 0.180 mg of the progestational compound, norgestimate (+)-13-Ethyl-17-hydroxy-18,19-dinor-17α-pregn-4-en-20-yn-3-one oxime acetate (ester) and 0.025 mg of the estrogenic compound, ethinyl estradiol (19-nor-17α-pregna,1,3,5(10)-trien-20-yne-3,17-diol). Inactive ingredients include lactose, magnesium stearate, croscarmellose sodium, microcrystalline cellulose, carnauba wax, hydroxypropylmethylcellulose, polyethylene glycol, titanium dioxide, and purified water.

Each light blue tablet contains 0.215 mg of the progestational compound norgestimate (+)-13-Ethyl-17-hydroxy-18,19-dinor-17α-pregn-4-en-20-yn-3-one oxime acetate (ester) and 0.025 mg of the estrogenic compound, ethinyl estradiol (19-nor-17α-pregna,1,3,5(10)-trien-20-yne-3,17-diol). Inactive ingredients include FD & C blue no. 2 aluminum lake, lactose, magnesium stearate, croscarmellose sodium, microcrystalline cellulose, carnauba wax, hydroxypropylmethylcellulose, polyethylene glycol, titanium dioxide, and purified water.

Each dark blue tablet contains 0.250 mg of the progestational compound norgestimate (+)-13-Ethyl-17-hydroxy-18,19-dinor-17α-pregn-4-en-20-yn-3-one oxime acetate (ester) and 0.025 mg of the estrogenic compound, ethinyl estradiol (19-nor-17α-pregna,1,3,5(10)-trien-20-yne-3,17-diol). Inactive ingredients include FD & C blue no. 2 aluminum lake, lactose, magnesium stearate, croscarmellose sodium, microcrystalline cellulose, polysorbate 80, carnauba wax, hydroxypropylmethylcellulose, polyethylene glycol, titanium dioxide, and purified water.

Each green tablet contains only inert ingredients, as follows: FD & C blue no. 1 aluminum lake, lactose, magnesium stearate, pregelatinized starch, ferric oxide, hydroxypropylmethylcellulose, polyethylene glycol, titanium dioxide, talc and purified water.

CLINICAL PHARMACOLOGY

ORTHO TRI-CYCLEN 28 TABLETS AND ORTHO-CYCLEN 28 TABLETS

Oral Contraception

Combination oral contraceptives act by suppression of gonadotropins. Although the primary mechanism of this action is inhibition of ovulation, other alterations include changes in the cervical mucus (which increase the difficulty of sperm entry into the uterus) and the endometrium (which reduce the likelihood of implantation).

Receptor binding studies, as well as studies in animals and humans, have shown that norgestimate and 17-deacetyl norgestimate, the major serum metabolite, combine high progestational activity with minimal intrinsic androgenicity.[90-93] Norgestimate, in combination with ethinyl estradiol, does not counteract the estrogen-induced increases in sex hormone binding globulin (SHBG), resulting in lower serum testosterone.[90,91,94]

Acne

Acne is a skin condition with a multifactorial etiology. The combination of ethinyl estradiol and norgestimate may increase sex hormone binding globulin (SHBG) and decrease free testosterone resulting in a decrease in the severity of facial acne in otherwise healthy women with this skin condition.

Norgestimate and ethinyl estradiol are well absorbed following oral administration of Ortho-Cyclen and Ortho Tri-Cyclen. On the average, peak serum concentrations of norgestimate and ethinyl estradiol are observed within 2 hours (0.5-2.0 hours for norgestimate and 0.75-3.0 hours for ethinyl estradiol) after administration followed by a rapid decline due to distribution and elimination. Although norgestimate serum concentrations following single or multiple dosing were generally below assay detection within 5 hours, a major norgestimate serum metabolite, 17-deacetyl norgestimate, (which exhibits a serum half-life ranging from 12-30 hours) appears rapidly in serum with concentrations greatly exceeding that of norgestimate. The 17-deacetylated metabolite is pharmacologically active and the pharmacologic profile is similar to that of norgestimate. The elimination half-life of ethinyl estradiol ranged from approximately 6-14 hours.

Both norgestimate and ethinyl estradiol are extensively metabolized and eliminated by renal and fecal pathways. Following administration of ^{14}C-norgestimate, 47% (45-49%) and 37% (16-49%) of the administered radioactivity was eliminated in the urine and feces, respectively. Unchanged norgestimate was not detected in the urine. In addition to 17-deacetyl norgestimate, a number of metabolites of norgestimate have been identified in human urine following administration of radiolabeled norgestimate. These include 18,19-Dinor-17-pregn-4-en-20-yn-3-one,17-hydroxy-13-ethyl,(17α)-(-);18,19-Dinor-5-17-pregnan-20-yn,3,17-dihy-droxy-13-ethyl,(17), various hydroxylated metabolites and conjugates of these metabolites. Ethinyl estradiol is metabolized to various hydroxylated products and their glucuronide and sulfate conjugates.

Non-Contraceptive Health Benefits

The following non-contraceptive health benefits related to the use of combination oral contraceptives are supported by epidemiological studies which largely utilized oral contraceptive formulations containing estrogen doses exceeding 0.035 mg of ethinyl estradiol or 0.05 mg mestranol.[73-78]

Effects on menses: Increased menstrual cycle regularity; decreased blood loss and decreased incidence of iron deficiency anemia; decreased incidence of dysmenorrhea.

Effects related to inhibition of ovulation: Decreased incidence of functional ovarian cysts; decreased incidence of ectopic pregnancies.

Other effects: Decreased incidence of fibroadenomas and fibrocystic disease of the breast; decreased incidence of acute pelvic inflammatory disease; decreased incidence of endometrial cancer; decreased incidence of ovarian cancer.

ORTHO TRI-CYCLEN LO TABLETS

Oral Contraception

Combination oral contraceptives act by suppression of gonadotropins. Although the primary mechanism of this action is inhibition of ovulation, other alterations include changes in the cervical mucus (which increase the difficulty of sperm entry into the uterus) and the endometrium (which reduce the likelihood of implantation).

Receptor binding studies, as well as studies in animals and humans, have shown that norgestimate and 17-deacetyl norgestimate, the major serum metabolite, combine high progestational activity with minimal intrinsic androgenicity.[90-93] Norgestimate, in combination with ethinyl estradiol, does not counteract the estrogen-induced increases in sex hormone binding globulin (SHBG), resulting in lower serum testosterone.[90,91,94]

Pharmacokinetics

Absorption

Norgestimate (NGM) and ethinyl estradiol (EE) are rapidly absorbed following oral administration. Norgestimate is rapidly and completely metabolized by first-pass (intestinal and/or hepatic) mechanisms to norelgestromin (NGMN) and norgestrel (NG), which are the major active metabolites of norgestimate. Mean pharmacokinetic parameters for NGMN, NG and EE during three cycles of administration of Ortho Tri-Cyclen LO are summarized in TABLE 1. These results indicate that: (1) Peak serum concentrations of NGMN and EE were generally reached by 2 hours after dosing; (2) Accumulation following multiple dosing of the 180 μg NGM/25 μg dose is approximately 1.5- to 2-fold for NGMN and approximately 1.5 fold for EE compared with single dose administration, in agreement with that predicted based on linear kinetics of NGMN and EE; (3) The kinetics of NGMN are dose proportional following NGM doses of 180-250 μg; (4) Steady-state conditions for NGMN following each NGM dose and for EE were achieved during the three cycle study; (5) Non-linear accumulation (4.5- to 14.5-fold) of norgestrel was observed as a result of high affinity binding to SHBG, which limits its biological activity. The effect of food on the pharmacokinetics of Ortho Tri-Cyclen LO has not been studied.

TABLE 1 provides a summary of norelgestromin, norgestrel and ethinyl estradiol pharmacokinetic parameters.

TABLE 1 *Mean (SD) Pharamacokinetic Parameters of Ortho Tri-Cyclen LO During a Three Cycle Study*

Analyte*	Cycle	Day	C_{max}	T_{max} (h)	AUC(0-24h)	T½ (h)
NGMN†‡§	1	1	0.91 (0.27)	1.8 (1.0)	5.86 (1.54)	NC
	3	7	1.42 (0.43)	1.8 (0.7)	11.3 (3.2)	NC
		14	1.57 (0.39)	1.8 (0.7)	13.9 (3.7)	NC
		21	1.82 (0.54)	1.5 (0.7)	16.1 (4.8)	28.1 (10.6)
NG†‡§	1	1	0.32 (0.14)	2.0 (1.1)	2.44 (2.04)	NC
	3	7	1.64 (0.89)	1.9 (0.9)	27.9 (18.1)	NC
		14	2.11 (1.13)	4.0 (6.3)	40.7 (24.8)	NC
		21	2.79 (1.42)	1.7 (1.2)	49.9 (27.6)	36.4 (10.2)
EE†‡¤	1	1	55.6 (18.1)	1.7 (0.5)	421 (118)	NC
	3	7	91.1 (36.7)	1.3 (0.3)	782 (329)	NC
		14	96.9 (38.5)	1.3 (0.3)	796 (273)	NC
		21	95.9 (38.9)	1.3 (0.6)	771 (303)	17.7 (4.4)

NC = not calculated.
* NGMN = Norelgestromin, NG = norgestrel, EE = ethinyl estradiol.
† C_{max} = peak serum concentration, T_{max} = time to reach peak serum concentration, AUC(0-24h) = area under serum concentration versus time curve from 0-24 hours, T½ = elimination half-life.
‡ Units for all analytes; h = hours.
§ Units for NGMN and NG — C_{max} = ng/ml, AUC(0-24) = h·ng/ml.
¤ Units for EE only — C_{max} = pg/ml, AUC(0-24h) = h·pg/ml.

Distribution

Norelgestromin and norgestrel (a serum metabolite of norelgestromin) are highly bound (>97%) to serum proteins. Norelgestromin is bound to albumin and not to SHBG, while norgestrel is bound primarily to SHBG. Ethinyl estradiol is extensively bound (>97%) to serum albumin.

Metabolism

Norgestimate is extensively metabolized by first-pass mechanisms in the gastrointestinal tract and/or liver. Norgestimate's primary active metabolite is norelgestromin. Subsequent hepatic metabolism of norelgestromin occurs and metabolites include norgestrel, which is also active and various hydroxylated and conjugated metabolites. Ethinyl estradiol is also metabolized to various hydroxylated products and their glucuronide and sulfate conjugates.

Excretion

Following 3 cycles of administration of Ortho Tri-Cyclen LO, the mean (±SD) elimination half-life values, at steady-state, for norelgestromin, norgestrel and ethinyl estradiol were 28.1 (±10.6) hours, 36.4 (±10.2) hours and 17.7 (±4.4) hours, respectively (TABLE 1). The metabolites of norelgestromin and ethinyl estradiol are eliminated by renal and fecal pathways.

Special Populations

Effects of Body Weight, Body Surface Area, and Age

The effects of body weight, body surface area, age and race on the pharmacokinetics of norelgestromin, norgestrel and ethinyl estradiol were evaluated in 79 healthy women using pooled data following single dose administration of NGM 180 or 250 µg/EE 25 µg tablets in four pharmacokinetic studies. Increasing body weight and body surface area were each associated with decreases in C_{max} and AUC(0-24h) values for norelgestromin and ethinyl estradiol and increases in CL/F (oral clearance) for ethinyl estradiol. Increasing body weight by 10 kg is predicted to reduce the following parameters: NGMN C_{max} by 9% and AUC(0-24h) by 19%, norgestrel C_{max} by 12% and AUC(0-24h) by 46%, EE C_{max} by 13% and AUC(0-24h) by 12%. These changes were statistically significant. Increasing age was associated with slight decreases (6% with increasing age by 5 years) in C_{max} and AUC(0-24h) for norelgestromin and were statistically significant, but there was no significant effect for norgestrel or ethinyl estradiol. Only a small to moderate fraction (5-40%) of the overall variability in the pharmacokinetics of norelgestromin and ethinyl estradiol following Ortho Tri-Cyclen LO tablets may be explained by any or all of the above demographic parameters.

In clinical studies involving 1673 subjects with a mean weight of 141 lb, there was no association between pregnancy and weight.

Renal and Hepatic Impairment

No studies with Ortho Tri-Cyclen LO have been conducted in women with renal or hepatic impairment.

Drug-Drug Interactions

Although norelgestromin and its metabolites inhibit a variety of P450 enzymes in human liver microsomes, under the recommended dosing regimen, the *in vivo* concentrations of norelgestromin and its metabolites, even at the peak serum levels, are relatively low compared to the inhibitory constant (K_i).

Interactions between oral contraceptives and other drugs have been reported in the literature. No formal drug-drug interaction studies were conducted with Ortho Tri-Cyclen LO (see PRECAUTIONS, Ortho Tri-Cyclen LO Tablets).

Non-Contraceptive Health Benefits

The following non-contraceptive health benefits related to the use of combination oral contraceptives are supported by epidemiological studies which largely utilized oral contraceptive formulations containing estrogen doses exceeding 0.035 mg of ethinyl estradiol or 0.05 mg mestranol.[73-78]

Effects on Menses:
- Increased menstrual cycle regularity.
- Decreased blood loss and decreased incidence of iron deficiency anemia.
- Decreased incidence of dysmenorrhea.

Effects Related to Inhibition of Ovulation:
- Decreased incidence of functional ovarian cysts.
- Decreased incidence of ectopic pregnancies.

Other Effects:
- Decreased incidence of fibroadenomas and fibrocystic disease of the breast.
- Decreased incidence of acute pelvic inflammatory disease.
- Decreased incidence of endometrial cancer.
- Decreased incidence of ovarian cancer.

INDICATIONS AND USAGE

ORTHO-TRI CYCLEN 28 TABLETS AND ORTHO-CYCLEN 28 TABLETS

Ortho-Cyclen and Ortho Tri-Cyclen tablets are indicated for the prevention of pregnancy in women who elect to use oral contraceptives as a method of contraception.

Ortho Tri-Cyclen is indicated for the treatment of moderate acne vulgaris in females, ≥15 years of age, who have no known contraindications to oral contraceptive therapy, desire contraception, have achieved menarche and are unresponsive to topical anti-acne medications.

Oral contraceptives are highly effective. TABLE 2 lists the typical accidental pregnancy rates for users of combination oral contraceptives and other methods of contraception. The efficacy of these contraceptive methods, except sterilization, depends upon the reliability with which they are used. Correct and consistent use of methods can result in lower failure rates.

In clinical trials with Ortho-Cyclen, 1,651 subjects completed 24,272 cycles and a total of 18 pregnancies were reported. This represents an overall use-efficacy (typical user efficacy) pregnancy rate of 0.96 per 100 women-years. This rate includes patients who did not take the drug correctly.

In four clinical trials with Ortho Tri-Cyclen, the use-efficacy pregnancy rate ranged from 0.68-1.47 per 100 women-years. In total, 4,756 subjects completed 45,244 cycles and a total of 42 pregnancies were reported. This represents an overall use-efficacy rate of 1.21 per 100 women-years. One of these 4 studies was a randomized comparative clinical trial in which 4,633 subjects completed 22,312 cycles. Of the 2312 patients on Ortho Tri-Cyclen, 8 pregnancies were reported. This represents an overall use-efficacy pregnancy rate of 0.94 per 100 women-years.

TABLE 2 *Percentage of Women Experiencing an Unintended Pregnancy During the First Year of Typical Use and the First Year of Perfect Use of Contraception and the Percentage Continuing Use at the End of the First Year; US*

Method (1)	% of Women Experiencing an Unintended Pregnancy* Typical Use‡ (2)	Perfect Use§ (3)	% of Women Continuing Use†¤ (4)
Chance¶	85%	85%	
Spermicides**	26%	6%	40%
Periodic Abstinence	25%		63%
Calendar		9%	
Ovulation method		3%	
Sympto-thermal††		2%	
Post-ovulation		1%	
Withdrawal	19%	4%	
Cap‡‡			
Parous women	40%	26%	42%
Nulliparous women	20%	9%	56%
Sponge			
Parous women	40%	20%	42%
Nulliparous women	20%	9%	56%
Diaphragm‡‡	20%	6%	56%
Condom§§			
Female (reality)	21%	5%	56%
Male	14%	3%	61%
Pill	5%		71%
Progestin only		0.5%	
Combined		0.1%	
IUD			
Progesterone T	2.0%	1.5%	81%
Copper T380A	0.8%	0.6%	78%
LNg 20	0.1%	0.1%	81%
Depo-Provera	0.3%	0.3%	70%
Norplant & Norplant-2	0.05%	0.05%	88%
Female Sterilization	0.5%	0.5%	100%
Male Sterilization	0.15%	0.10%	100%

Adapted from Hatcher *et al.*, 1998 reference no. 1.
* Within the first year of use.
† At 1 year.
‡ Among *typical* couples who initiate use of a method (not necessarily for the first time), the percentage who experience an accidental pregnancy during the first year if they do not stop use for any other reason.
§ Among couples who initiate use of a method (not necessarily for the first time) and who use it *perfectly* (both consistently and correctly), the percentage who experience an accidental pregnancy during the first year if they do not stop use for any other reason.
¤ Among couples attempting to avoid pregnancy, the percentage who continue to use a method for 1 year.
¶ The percents becoming pregnant in columns (2) and (3) are based on data from populations where contraception is not used and from women who cease using contraception in order to become pregnant. Among such populations, about 89% become pregnant within 1 year. This estimate was lowered slightly (to 85%) to represent the percent who would become pregnant within 1 year among women now relying on reversible methods of contraception if they abandoned contraception altogether.
** Foams, creams, gels, vaginal suppositories, and vaginal film.
†† Cervical mucus (ovulation) method supplemented by calendar in the pre-ovulatory and basal body temperature in the post-ovulatory phases.
‡‡ With spermicidal cream or jelly.
§§ Without spermicides.

In two double-blind, placebo-controlled, 6 month, multicenter clinical trials, Ortho Tri-Cyclen showed a statistically significant decrease in inflammatory lesion count and total lesion count (TABLE 3). The adverse reaction profile of Ortho Tri-Cyclen from these two controlled clinical trials is consistent with what has been noted from previous studies involving Ortho Tri-Cyclen and are the known risks associated with oral contraceptives.

TABLE 3 *Acne Vulgaris Indication — Combined Results: Two Multicenter, Placebo-Controlled Trials; Primary Efficacy Variables: Evaluable-for-Efficacy Population*

	Ortho-Tri-Cyclen n=163	Placebo n=161
Mean age at enrollment	27.3 years	28.0
Inflammatory lesions — Mean % reduction	56.6	36.6
Total lesions — Mean % reduction	49.6	30.3

ORTHO TRI-CYCLEN LO TABLETS

Ortho Tri-Cyclen LO Tablets are indicated for the prevention of pregnancy in women who elect to use oral contraceptives as a method of contraception.

In an active controlled clinical trial 1,673 subjects completed 11,003 cycles of Ortho Tri-Cyclen LO use and a total of 20 pregnancies were reported in Ortho Tri-Cyclen LO users.[99] This represents an overall use-efficacy (typical user efficacy) pregnancy rate of 2.36 per 100 women-years of use.

Oral contraceptives are highly effective for pregnancy prevention. TABLE 4 lists the typical accidental pregnancy rates for users of combination oral contraceptives and other methods of contraception. The efficacy of these contraceptive methods, except sterilization, the

IUD, and the Norplant system, depends upon the reliability with which they are used. Correct and consistent use of methods can result in lower failure rates.

TABLE 4 *Percentage of Women Experiencing an Unintended Pregnancy During the First Year of Typical Use and the First Year of Perfect Use of Contraception and the Percentage Continuing Use at the End of the First Year; US*

	Women Experiencing an Unintended Pregnancy Within the First Year of Use		Women Continuing Use at 1 Year‡
Method (1)	**Typical Use* (2)**	**Perfect Use† (3)**	**(4)**
Chance§	85%	85%	
Spermicides¤	26%	6%	40%
Periodic Abstinence	25%		63%
Calendar		9%	
Ovulation method		3%	
Sympto-thermal¶		2%	
Post-ovulation		1%	
Withdrawal	19%	4%	
Cap**			
Parous women	40%	26%	42%
Nulliparous women	20%	9%	56%
Sponge			
Parous women	40%	20%	42%
Nulliparous women	20%	9%	56%
Diaphragm**	20%	6%	56%
Condom††			
Female (Reality)	21%	5%	56%
Male	14%	3%	61%
Pill	5%		71%
Progestin only		0.5%	
Combined		0.1%	
IUD			
Progesterone T	2.0%	1.5%	81%
Copper T380A	0.8%	0.6%	78%
LNg 20	0.1%	0.1%	81%
	0.3%	0.3%	70%
	0.05%	0.05%	88%
Depo-Provera	0.3%	0.3%	70%
Norplant and Norplant-2	0.05%	0.05%	88%
Female Sterilization	0.5%	0.5%	100%
Male Sterilization	0.15%	0.10%	100%

Emergency Contraceptives Pills: Treatment initiated within 72 hours after unprotected intercourse reduces the risk of pregnancy by at least 75%. The treatment schedule is 1 dose within 72 hours after unprotected intercourse, and a second dose 12 hours after the first dose. The FDA has declared the following brands of oral contraceptives to be safe and effective for emergency contraception: Ovral (1 dose is 2 white pills), Alesse (1 dose is 5 pink pills), Nordette or Levlen (1 dose is 4 yellow pills).

Lactation Amenorrhea Method: LAM is a highly effective, temporary method of contraception. However, to maintain effective protection against pregnancy, another method of contraception must be used as soon as menstruation resumes, the frequency or duration of breastfeeds is reduced, bottle feeds are introduced, or the baby reaches 6 months of age.

Source: Trussell J. Contraceptive efficacy. In Hatcher RA, Trussell J, Stewart F, Cates W, Stewart GK, Kowel D, Guest F, Contraceptive Technology: Seventeenth Revised Edition. New York NY: Irvington Publishers, 1998.

* Among *typical* couples who initiate use of a method (not necessarily for the first time), the percentage who experience an accidental pregnancy during the first year if they do not stop use for any other reason.

† Among couples who initiate use of a method (not necessarily for the first time) and who use it *perfectly* (both consistently and correctly), the percentage who experience an accidental pregnancy during the first year if they do not stop use for any other reason.

‡ Among couples attempting to avoid pregnancy, the percentage who continue to use a method for 1 year.

§ The percents becoming pregnant in columns (2) and (3) are based on data from populations where contraception is not used and from women who cease using contraception in order to become pregnant. Among such populations, about 89% become pregnant within 1 year. This estimate was lowered slightly (to 85%) to represent the percent who would become pregnant within 1 year among women now relying on reversible methods of contraception if they abandoned contraception altogether.

¤ Foams, creams, gels, vaginal suppositories, and vaginal film.

¶ Cervical mucus (ovulation) method supplemented by calendar in the pre-ovulatory and basal body temperature in the post-ovulatory phases.

** With spermicidal cream or jelly.

†† Without spermicides.

Ortho Tri-Cyclen LO has not been studied for and is not indicated for use in emergency contraception.

CONTRAINDICATIONS

ORTHO TRI-CYCLEN 28 TABLETS AND ORTHO-CYCLEN 28 TABLETS

Oral contraceptives should not be used in women who currently have the following conditions:

- Thrombophlebitis or thromboembolic disorders.
- A past history of deep vein thrombophlebitis or thromboembolic disorders.
- Cerebral vascular or coronary artery disease.
- Migraine with focal aura.
- Known or suspected carcinoma of the breast.
- Carcinoma of the endometrium or other known or suspected estrogen dependent neoplasia.
- Undiagnosed abnormal genital bleeding.
- Cholestatic jaundice of pregnancy or jaundice with prior pill use.
- Acute or chronic hepatocellular disease with abnormal liver function.
- Hepatic adenomas or carcinomas.
- Known or suspected pregnancy.
- Hypersensitivity to any component of this product.

ORTHO TRI-CYCLEN LO TABLETS

Oral contraceptives should not be used in women who have any of the following conditions:

Thrombophlebitis or thromboembolic disorders.
A past history of deep vein thrombophlebitis or thromboembolic disorders.
Cerebral vascular or coronary artery disease (current or history).
Valvular heart disease with complications.
Severe hypertension.
Diabetes with vascular involvement.
Headaches with focal neurological symptoms.
Major surgery with prolonged immobilization.
Known or suspected carcinoma of the breast or personal history of breast cancer.
Carcinoma of the endometrium or other known or suspected estrogen-dependent neoplasia.
Undiagnosed abnormal genital bleeding.
Cholestatic jaundice of pregnancy or jaundice with prior pill use.
Hepatic adenomas or carcinomas.
Known or suspected pregnancy.
Hypersensitivity to any component of this product.

WARNINGS

ORTHO TRI-CYCLEN 28 TABLETS AND ORTHO-CYCLEN 28 TABLETS

Cigarette smoking increases the risk of serious cardiovascular side effects from oral contraceptive use. This risk increases with age and with heavy smoking (15 or more cigarettes per day) and is quite marked in women over 35 years of age. Women who use oral contraceptives should be strongly advised not to smoke.

The use of oral contraceptives is associated with increased risks of several serious conditions including myocardial infarction, thromboembolism, stroke, hepatic neoplasia, and gallbladder disease, although the risk of serious morbidity or mortality is very small in healthy women without underlying risk factors. The risk of morbidity and mortality increases significantly in the presence of other underlying risk factors such as hypertension, hyperlipidemias, obesity and diabetes.

Practitioners prescribing oral contraceptives should be familiar with the following information relating to these risks.

The information contained in prescribing information is principally based on studies carried out in patients who used oral contraceptives with higher formulations of estrogens and progestogens than those in common use today. The effect of long-term use of the oral contraceptives with lower formulations of both estrogens and progestogens remains to be determined.

Throughout this labeling, epidemiological studies reported are of two types: retrospective or case control studies and prospective or cohort studies. Case control studies provide a measure of the relative risk of a disease, namely, a *ratio* of the incidence of a disease among oral contraceptive users to that among nonusers. The relative risk does not provide information on the actual clinical occurrence of a disease. Cohort studies provide a measure of attributable risk, which is the *difference* in the incidence of disease between oral contraceptive users and nonusers. The attributable risk does provide information about the actual occurrence of a disease in the population (adapted from reference numbers 2 and 3 with the author's permission). For further information, the reader is referred to a text on epidemiological methods.

Thromboembolic Disorders and Other Vascular Problems

Myocardial Infarction

An increased risk of myocardial infarction has been attributed to oral contraceptive use. This risk is primarily in smokers or women with other underlying risk factors for coronary artery disease such as hypertension, hypercholesterolemia, morbid obesity, and diabetes. The relative risk of heart attack for current oral contraceptive users has been estimated to be 2-6.[4-10] The risk is very low under the age of 30.

Smoking in combination with oral contraceptive use has been shown to contribute substantially to the incidence of myocardial infarctions in women in their mid-thirties or older with smoking accounting for the majority of excess cases.[11] Mortality rates associated with circulatory disease have been shown to increase substantially in smokers, especially in those 35 years of age and older among women who use oral contraceptives.

Oral contraceptives may compound the effects of well-known risk factors, such as hypertension, diabetes, hyperlipidemias, age and obesity.[13] In particular, some progestogens are known to decrease HDL cholesterol and cause glucose intolerance, while estrogens may create a state of hyperinsulinism.[14-18] Oral contraceptives have been shown to increase blood pressure among users (see Ortho Tri-Cyclen 28 Tablets and Ortho-Cyclen 28 Tablets, Elevated Blood Pressure). Similar effects on risk factors have been associated with an increased risk of heart disease. Oral contraceptives must be used with caution in women with cardiovascular disease risk factors.

Norgestimate has minimal androgenic activity (see CLINICAL PHARMACOLOGY), and there is some evidence that the risk of myocardial infarction associated with oral contraceptives is lower when the progestogen has minimal androgenic activity than when the activity is greater.[97]

Thromboembolism

An increased risk of thromboembolic and thrombotic disease associated with the use of oral contraceptives is well established. Case control studies have found the relative risk of users compared to nonusers to be 3 for the first episode of superficial venous thrombosis, 4-11 for deep vein thrombosis or pulmonary embolism, and 1.5 to 6 for women with predisposing conditions for venous thromboembolic disease.[2,3,19-24] Cohort studies have shown the relative risk to be somewhat lower, about 3 for new cases and about 4.5 for new cases requiring hospitalization.[25] The risk of thromboembolic disease associated with oral contraceptives is not related to length of use and disappears after pill use is stopped.[2]

A 2- to 4-fold increase in relative risk of post-operative thromboembolic complications has been reported with the use of oral contraceptives.[9] The relative risk of venous thrombosis in women who have predisposing conditions is twice that of women without such medical conditions.[26] If feasible, oral contraceptives should be discontinued at least 4 weeks prior to and for 2 weeks after elective surgery of a type associated with an increase in risk of thromboembolism and during and following prolonged immobilization. Since the immediate postpartum period is also associated with an increased risk of thromboembolism, oral contraceptives should be started no earlier than 4 weeks after delivery in women who elect not to breast feed. After an induced or spontaneous abortion that occurs at or after 20 weeks gestation, hormonal contraceptives may be started either on day 21 post-abortion or on the first day of the first spontaneous menstruation, whichever comes first.[98]

Cerebrovascular Diseases

Oral contraceptives have been shown to increase both the relative and attributable risks of cerebrovascular events (thrombotic and hemorrhagic strokes), although, in general, the risk is greatest among older >35 years), hypertensive women who also smoke. Hypertension was found to be a risk factor for both users and nonusers, for both types of strokes, and smoking interacted to increase the risk of stroke.[27-29]

In a large study, the relative risk of thrombotic strokes has been shown to range from 3 for normotensive users to 14 for users with severe hypertension.[30] The relative risk of hemorrhagic stroke is reported to be 1.2 for non-smokers who used oral contraceptives, 2.6 for smokers who did not use oral contraceptives, 7.6 for smokers who used oral contraceptives, 1.8 for normotensive users and 25.7 for users with severe hypertension.[30] The attributable risk is also greater in older women.[3]

Dose-Related Risk of Vascular Disease From Oral Contraceptives

A positive association has been observed between the amount of estrogen and progestogen in oral contraceptives and the risk of vascular disease.[31-33] A decline in serum high density lipoproteins (HDL) has been reported with many progestational agents.[14-16] A decline in serum high density lipoproteins has been associated with an increased incidence of ischemic heart disease. Because estrogens increase HDL cholesterol, the net effect of an oral contraceptive depends on a balance achieved between doses of estrogen and progestogen and the activity of the progestogen used in the contraceptives. The activity and amount of both hormones should be considered in the choice of an oral contraceptive.

Minimizing exposure to estrogen and progestogen is in keeping with good principles of therapeutics. For any particular estrogen/progestogen combination, the dosage regimen prescribed should be one which contains the least amount of estrogen and progestogen that is compatible with a low failure rate and the needs of the individual patient. New acceptors of oral contraceptive agents should be started on preparations containing 0.035 mg or less of estrogen.

Persistence of Risk of Vascular Disease

There are two studies which have shown persistence of risk of vascular disease for ever-users of oral contraceptives. In a study in the US, the risk of developing myocardial infarction after discontinuing oral contraceptives persists for at least 9 years for women 40-49 years who had used oral contraceptives for 5 or more years, but this increased risk was not demonstrated in other age groups.[8] In another study in Great Britain, the risk of developing cerebrovascular disease persisted for at least 6 years after discontinuation of oral contraceptives, although excess risk was very small.[34] However, both studies were performed with oral contraceptive formulations containing 50 μg or higher of estrogens.

Estimates of Mortality From Contraceptive Use

One study gathered data from a variety of sources which have estimated the mortality rate associated with different methods of contraception at different ages (TABLE 5). These estimates include the combined risk of death associated with contraceptive methods plus the risk attributable to pregnancy in the event of method failure. Each method of contraception has its specific benefits and risks. The study concluded that with the exception of oral contraceptive users 35 and older who smoke, and 40 and older who do not smoke, mortality associated with all methods of birth control is low and below that associated with childbirth. The observation of an increase in risk of mortality with age for oral contraceptive users is based on data gathered in the 1970s.[35] Current clinical recommendation involves the use of lower estrogen dose formulations and a careful consideration of risk factors. In 1989, the Fertility and Maternal Health Drugs Advisory Committee was asked to review the use of oral contraceptives in women 40 years of age and over. The Committee concluded that although cardiovascular disease risks may be increased with oral contraceptive use after age 40 in healthy non-smoking women (even with the newer low-dose formulations), there are also greater potential health risks associated with pregnancy in older women and with the alternative surgical and medical procedures which may be necessary if such women do not have access to effective and acceptable means of contraception. The Committee recommended that the benefits of low-dose oral contraceptive use by healthy non-smoking women over 40 may outweigh the possible risks.

Of course, older women, as all women, who take oral contraceptives, should take an oral contraceptive which contains the least amount of estrogen and progestogen that is compatible with a low failure rate and individual patient needs.

Carcinoma of the Reproductive Organs and Breasts

Numerous epidemiological studies have been performed on the incidence of breast, endometrial, ovarian, and cervical cancer in women using oral contraceptives. While there are conflicting reports, most studies suggest that use of oral contraceptives is not associated with an overall increase in the risk of developing breast cancer. Some studies have reported an increased relative risk of developing breast cancer, particularly at a younger age. This increased relative risk has been reported to be related to duration of use.[36-44,79-89]

A meta-analysis of 54 studies found a small increase in the frequency of having breast cancer diagnosed for women who were currently using combined oral contraceptives or had used them within the past 10 years. This increase in the frequency of breast cancer diagnosis, within 10 years of stopping use, was generally accounted for by cancers localized to the breast. There was no increase in the frequency of having breast cancer diagnosed 10 or more years after cessation of use.[95]

Some studies suggest that oral contraceptive use has been associated with an increase in the risk of cervical intraepithelial neoplasia in some populations of women.[45-48] However,

TABLE 5 *Annual Number of Birth-Related or Method-Related Deaths Associated With Control of Fertility per 100,000 Non-Sterile Women, by Fertility Control Method According to Age*

Method of Control & Outcome	15-19	20-24	25-29	30-34	35-39	40-44
No fertility control methods*	7.0	7.4	9.1	14.8	25.7	28.2
Oral contraceptives non-smoker†	0.3	0.5	0.9	1.9	13.8	31.6
Oral contraceptives smoker†	2.2	3.4	6.6	13.5	51.1	117.2
IUD†	0.8	0.8	1.0	1.0	1.4	1.4
Condom*	1.1	1.6	0.7	0.2	0.3	0.4
Diaphragm/ spermicide*	1.9	1.2	1.2	1.3	2.2	2.8
Periodic abstinence*	2.5	1.6	1.6	1.7	2.9	3.6

* Deaths are birth-related.
† Deaths are method-related.
Adapted from H.W. Ory, reference no. 35.

there continues to be controversy about the extent to which such findings may be due to differences in sexual behavior and other factors.

Hepatic Neoplasia

Benign hepatic adenomas are associated with oral contraceptive use, although the incidence of benign tumors is rare in the US. Indirect calculations have estimated the attributable risk to be in the range of 3.3 cases/100,000 for users, a risk that increases after 4 or more years of use especially with oral contraceptives of higher dose.[49] Rupture of benign, hepatic adenomas may cause death through intra-abdominal hemorrhage.[50,51]

Studies have shown an increased risk of developing hepatocellular carcinoma [52-54,96] in oral contraceptive users. However, these cancers are rare in the US.

Ocular Lesions

There have been clinical case reports of retinal thrombosis associated with the use of oral contraceptives. Oral contraceptives should be discontinued if there is unexplained partial or complete loss of vision; onset of proptosis or diplopia; papilledema; or retinal vascular lesions. Appropriate diagnostic and therapeutic measures should be undertaken immediately.

Oral Contraceptive Use Before or During Early Pregnancy

Extensive epidemiological studies have revealed no increased risk of birth defects in women who have used oral contraceptives prior to pregnancy.[56,57] The majority of recent studies also do not indicate a teratogenic effect, particularly in so far as cardiac anomalies and limb reduction defects are concerned,[55,56,58,59] when taken inadvertently during early pregnancy.

The administration of oral contraceptives to induce withdrawal bleeding should not be used as a test for pregnancy. Oral contraceptives should not be used during pregnancy to treat threatened or habitual abortion.

It is recommended that for any patient who has missed 2 consecutive periods, pregnancy should be ruled out before continuing oral contraceptive use. If the patient has not adhered to the prescribed schedule, the possibility of pregnancy should be considered at the time of the first missed period. Oral contraceptive use should be discontinued until pregnancy is ruled out.

Gallbladder Disease

Earlier studies have reported an increased lifetime relative risk of gallbladder surgery in users of oral contraceptives and estrogens.[60,61] More recent studies, however, have shown that the relative risk of developing gallbladder disease among oral contraceptive users may be minimal.[62-64] The recent findings of minimal risk may be related to the use of oral contraceptive formulations containing lower hormonal doses of estrogens and progestogens.

Carbohydrate and Lipid Metabolic Effects

Oral contraceptives have been shown to cause a decrease in glucose tolerance in a significant percentage of users.[17] This effect has been shown to be directly related to estrogen dose.[65] Progestogens increase insulin secretion and create insulin resistance, this effect varying with different progestational agents.[17,66] However, in the non-diabetic woman, oral contraceptives appear to have no effect on fasting blood glucose.[67] Because of these demonstrated effects, prediabetic and diabetic women in particular should be carefully monitored while taking oral contraceptives.

A small proportion of women will have persistent hypertriglyceridemia while on the pill. As discussed earlier (see Myocardial Infarction and Thromboembolism), changes in serum triglycerides and lipoprotein levels have been reported in oral contraceptive users.

In clinical studies with Ortho-Cyclen there were no clinically significant changes in fasting blood glucose levels. No statistically significant changes in mean fasting blood glucose levels were observed over 24 cycles of use. Glucose tolerance tests showed minimal, clinically insignificant changes from baseline to cycles 3, 12, and 24.

In clinical studies with Ortho Tri-Cyclen there were no clinically significant changes in fasting blood glucose levels. Minimal statistically significant changes were noted in glucose levels over 24 cycles of use. Glucose tolerance tests showed no clinically significant changes from baseline to cycles 3, 12, and 24.

Elevated Blood Pressure

Women with significant hypertension should not be started on hormonal contraception.[98] An increase in blood pressure has been reported in women taking oral contraceptives[68] and this increase is more likely in older oral contraceptive users[69] and with extended duration of use.[61] Data from the Royal College of General Practitioners[12] and subsequent randomized trials have shown that the incidence of hypertension increases with increasing progestational activity.

Women with a history of hypertension or hypertension-related diseases, or renal disease[70] should be encouraged to use another method of contraception. If women elect to use oral contraceptives, they should be monitored closely and if significant elevation of blood pressure occurs, oral contraceptives should be discontinued. For most women, elevated blood pressure will return to normal after stopping oral contraceptives, and there is no difference in the occurrence of hypertension between former and never users.[68-71] It should be noted that in two separate large clinical trials (n=633 and n=911), no statistically significant changes in mean blood pressure were observed with Ortho-Cyclen.

Headache

The onset or exacerbation of migraine or development of headache with a new pattern which is recurrent, persistent or severe requires discontinuation of oral contraceptives and evaluation of the cause.

Bleeding Irregularities

Breakthrough bleeding and spotting are sometimes encountered in patients on oral contraceptives, especially during the first 3 months of use. Non-hormonal causes should be considered and adequate diagnostic measures taken to rule out malignancy or pregnancy in the event of breakthrough bleeding, as in the case of any abnormal vaginal bleeding. If pathology has been excluded, time or a change to another formulation may solve the problem. In the event of amenorrhea, pregnancy should be ruled out.

Some women may encounter post-pill amenorrhea or oligomenorrhea, especially when such a condition was preexistent.

Ectopic Pregnancy

Ectopic as well as intrauterine pregnancy may occur in contraceptive failures.

ORTHO TRI-CYCLEN LO TABLETS

Cigarette smoking increases the risk of serious cardiovascular side effects from oral contraceptive use. This risk increases with age and with heavy smoking (15 or more cigarettes per day) and is quite marked in women over 35 years of age. Women who use oral contraceptives should be strongly advised not to smoke.

The use of oral contraceptives is associated with increased risks of several serious conditions including myocardial infarction, thromboembolism, stroke, hepatic neoplasia, and gallbladder disease, although the risk of serious morbidity or mortality is very small in healthy women without underlying risk factors. The risk of morbidity and mortality increases significantly in the presence of other underlying risk factors such as hypertension, hyperlipidemias, obesity and diabetes.

Practitioners prescribing oral contraceptives should be familiar with the following information relating to these risks.

The information contained in this package insert is principally based on studies carried out in patients who used oral contraceptives with higher formulations of estrogens and progestogens than those in common use today. The effect of long-term use of the oral contraceptives with lower formulations of both estrogens and progestogens remains to be determined.

Throughout this labeling, epidemiological studies reported are of two types: retrospective or case control studies and prospective or cohort studies. Case control studies provide a measure of the relative risk of a disease, namely, a ratio of the incidence of a disease among oral contraceptive users to that among nonusers. The relative risk does not provide information on the actual clinical occurrence of a disease. Cohort studies provide a measure of attributable risk, which is the difference in the incidence of disease between oral contraceptive users and nonusers. The attributable risk does provide information about the actual occurrence of a disease in the population (adapted from 2 and 3 with the author's permission). For further information, the reader is referred to a text on epidemiological methods.

Thromboembolic Disorders and Other Vascular Problems

Myocardial Infarction

An increased risk of myocardial infarction has been attributed to oral contraceptive use. This risk is primarily in smokers or women with other underlying risk factors for coronary artery disease such as hypertension, hypercholesterolemia, morbid obesity, and diabetes. The relative risk of heart attack for current oral contraceptive users has been estimated to be 2-6.[4-10] The risk is very low under the age of 30.

Smoking in combination with oral contraceptive use has been shown to contribute substantially to the incidence of myocardial infarctions in women in their mid-thirties or older with smoking accounting for the majority of excess cases.[11] Mortality rates associated with circulatory disease have been shown to increase substantially in smokers, especially in those 35 years of age and older and in nonsmokers over the age of 40 among women who use oral contraceptives.

Oral contraceptives may compound the effects of well-known risk factors, such as hypertension, diabetes, hyperlipidemias, age and obesity.[13] In particular, some progestogens are known to decrease HDL cholesterol and cause glucose intolerance, while estrogens may create a state of hyperinsulinism.[14-18] Oral contraceptives have been shown to increase blood pressure among users (see Ortho Tri-Cyclen LO Tablets, Elevated Blood Pressure). Similar effects on risk factors have been associated with an increased risk of heart disease. Oral contraceptives must be used with caution in women with cardiovascular disease risk factors.

Norgestimate has minimal androgenic activity (see CLINICAL PHARMACOLOGY, Ortho Tri-Cyclen LO Tablets), and there is some evidence that the risk of myocardial infarction associated with oral contraceptives is lower when the progestogen has minimal androgenic activity than when the activity is greater.[97]

Thromboembolism

An increased risk of thromboembolic and thrombotic disease associated with the use of oral contraceptives is well established. Case control studies have found the relative risk of users compared to nonusers to be 3 for the first episode of superficial venous thrombosis, 4-11 for deep vein thrombosis or pulmonary embolism, and 1.5 to 6 for women with predisposing conditions for venous thromboembolic disease.[2,3,19-24] Cohort studies have shown the relative risk to be somewhat lower, about 3 for new cases and about 4.5 for new cases requiring hospitalization.[25] The risk of thromboembolic disease associated with oral contraceptives is not related to length of use and disappears after pill use is stopped.[2]

A 2- to 4-fold increase in relative risk of post-operative thromboembolic complications has been reported with the use of oral contraceptives.[9] The relative risk of venous thrombosis in women who have predisposing conditions is twice that of women without such medical conditions.[26] If feasible, oral contraceptives should be discontinued at least 4 weeks prior to and for 2 weeks after elective surgery of a type associated with an increase in risk of thromboembolism and during and following prolonged immobilization. Since the immediate postpartum period is also associated with an increased risk of thromboembolism, oral contraceptives should be started no earlier than 4 weeks after delivery in women who elect not to breast feed.

Cerebrovascular Diseases

Oral contraceptives have been shown to increase both the relative and attributable risks of cerebrovascular events (thrombotic and hemorrhagic strokes), although, in general, the risk is greatest among older (>35 years), hypertensive women who also smoke. Hypertension was found to be a risk factor for both users and nonusers, for both types of strokes, and smoking interacted to increase the risk of hemorrhagic stroke.[27-29]

In a large study, the relative risk of thrombotic strokes has been shown to range from 3 for normotensive users to 14 for users with severe hypertension.[30] The relative risk of hemorrhagic stroke is reported to be 1.2 for non-smokers who used oral contraceptives, 2.6 for smokers who did not use oral contraceptives, 7.6 for smokers who used oral contraceptives, 1.8 for normotensive users and 25.7 for users with severe hypertension.[30] The attributable risk is also greater in older women.[3]

Dose-Related Risk of Vascular Disease From Oral Contraceptives

A positive association has been observed between the amount of estrogen and progestogen in oral contraceptives and the risk of vascular disease.[31-33] A decline in serum high density lipoproteins (HDL) has been reported with many progestational agents.[14-16] A decline in serum high density lipoproteins has been associated with an increased incidence of ischemic heart disease. Because estrogens increase HDL cholesterol, the net effect of an oral contraceptive depends on a balance achieved between doses of estrogen and progestogen and the activity of the progestogen used in the contraceptives. The activity and amount of both hormones should be considered in the choice of an oral contraceptive.

Minimizing exposure to estrogen and progestogen is in keeping with good principles of therapeutics. For any particular estrogen/progestogen combination, the dosage regimen prescribed should be one which contains the least amount of estrogen and progestogen that is compatible with a low failure rate and the needs of the individual patient. New acceptors of oral contraceptive agents should be started on preparations containing the lowest estrogen content which is judged appropriate for an individual patient.

Persistence of Risk of Vascular Disease

There are two studies which have shown persistence of risk of vascular disease for ever-users of oral contraceptives. In a study in the US, the risk of developing myocardial infarction after discontinuing oral contraceptives persists for at least 9 years for women 40-49 years who had used oral contraceptives for 5 or more years, but this increased risk was not demonstrated in other age groups.[8] In another study in Great Britain, the risk of developing cerebrovascular disease persisted for at least 6 years after discontinuation of oral contraceptives, although excess risk was very small.[34] However, both studies were performed with oral contraceptive formulations containing 50 µg or higher of estrogens.

Estimates of Mortality From Contraceptive Use

One study gathered data from a variety of sources which have estimated the mortality rate associated with different methods of contraception at different ages (TABLE 6). These estimates include the combined risk of death associated with contraceptive methods plus the risk attributable to pregnancy in the event of method failure. Each method of contraception has its specific benefits and risks. The study concluded that with the exception of oral contraceptive users 35 and older who smoke, and 40 and older who do not smoke, mortality associated with all methods of birth control is low and below that associated with childbirth. The observation of an increase in risk of mortality with age for oral contraceptive users is based on data gathered in the 1970's.[35] Current clinical recommendation involves the use of lower estrogen dose formulations and a careful consideration of risk factors. In 1989, the Fertility and Maternal Health Drugs Advisory Committee was asked to review the use of oral contraceptives in women 40 years of age and over.

The Committee concluded that although cardiovascular disease risks may be increased with oral contraceptive use after age 40 in healthy non-smoking women (even with the newer low-dose formulations), there are also greater potential health risks associated with pregnancy in older women and with the alternative surgical and medical procedures which may be necessary if such women do not have access to effective and acceptable means of contraception. The Committee recommended that the benefits of low-dose oral contraceptive use by healthy non-smoking women over 40 may outweigh the possible risks.

Of course, older women, as all women, who take oral contraceptives, should take an oral contraceptive which contains the least amount of estrogen and progestogen that is compatible with a low failure rate and individual patient needs.

Carcinoma of the Reproductive Organs and Breasts

Numerous epidemiological studies have been performed on the incidence of breast, endometrial, ovarian, and cervical cancer in women using oral contraceptives.

The risk of having breast cancer diagnosed may be slightly increased among current and recent users of combination oral contraceptives. However, this excess risk appears to decrease over time after discontinuation of combination oral contraceptives and by 10 years after cessation the increased risk disappears. Some studies report an increased risk with duration of use while other studies do not and no consistent relationships have been found with dose or type of steroid. Some studies have found a small increase in risk for women who first use combination oral contraceptives before age 20. Most studies show a similar pattern of risk with combination oral contraceptive use regardless of a woman's reproductive history or her family breast cancer history.

TABLE 6 *Annual Number of Birth-Related or Method-Related Deaths Associated With Control of Fertility per 100,000 Non-Sterile Women, by Fertility Control Method According to Age*

Method of Control & Outcome	15-19	20-24	25-29	30-34	35-39	40-44
No fertility control methods*	7.0	7.4	9.1	14.8	25.7	28.2
Oral contraceptives non-smoker†	0.3	0.5	0.9	1.9	13.8	31.6
Oral contraceptives smoker†	2.2	3.4	6.6	13.5	51.1	117.2
IUD†	0.8	0.8	1.0	1.0	1.4	1.4
Condom*	1.1	1.6	0.7	0.2	0.3	0.4
Diaphragm/ spermicide*	1.9	1.2	1.2	1.3	2.2	2.8
Periodic abstinence*	2.5	1.6	1.6	1.7	2.9	3.6

* Deaths are birth-related.
† Deaths are method-related.
Adapted from H.W. Ory, Family Planning Perspectives, reference no. 35.

Breast cancers diagnosed in current or previous oral contraceptive users tend to be less clinically advanced than in nonusers.

Women who currently have or have had breast cancer should not use oral contraceptives because breast cancer is usually a hormonally-sensitive tumor.

Some studies suggest that oral contraceptive use has been associated with an increase in the risk of cervical intraepithelial neoplasia in some populations of women.[45-48] However, there continues to be controversy about the extent to which such findings may be due to differences in sexual behavior and other factors.

In spite of many studies of the relationship between oral contraceptive use and breast and cervical cancers, a cause-and-effect relationship has not been established.

Hepatic Neoplasia

Benign hepatic adenomas are associated with oral contraceptive use, although the incidence of benign tumors is rare in the US. Indirect calculations have estimated the attributable risk to be in the range of 3.3 cases/100,000 for users, a risk that increases after 4 or more years of use especially with oral contraceptives of higher dose.[49] Rupture of benign, hepatic adenomas may cause death through intra-abdominal hemorrhage.[50,51]

Studies from Britain have shown an increased risk of developing hepatocellular carcinoma in long-term (>8 years) oral contraceptive users. However, these cancers are extremely rare in the US and the attributable risk (the excess incidence) of liver cancers in oral contraceptive users approaches less than 1 per million users.

Ocular Lesions

There have been clinical case reports of retinal thrombosis associated with the use of oral contraceptives. Oral contraceptives should be discontinued if there is unexplained partial or complete loss of vision; onset of proptosis or diplopia; papilledema; or retinal vascular lesions. Appropriate diagnostic and therapeutic measures should be undertaken immediately.

Oral Contraceptive Use Before or During Early Pregnancy

Extensive epidemiological studies have revealed no increased risk of birth defects in women who have used oral contraceptives prior to pregnancy.[56,57] The majority of recent studies also do not indicate a teratogenic effect, particularly in so far as cardiac anomalies and limb reduction defects are concerned, when taken inadvertently during early pregnancy.

The administration of oral contraceptives to induce withdrawal bleeding should not be used as a test for pregnancy. Oral contraceptives should not be used during pregnancy to treat threatened or habitual abortion.

It is recommended that for any patient who has missed 2 consecutive periods, pregnancy should be ruled out. If the patient has not adhered to the prescribed schedule, the possibility of pregnancy should be considered at the time of the first missed period. Oral contraceptive use should be discontinued if pregnancy is confirmed.

Gallbladder Disease

Earlier studies have reported an increased lifetime relative risk of gallbladder surgery in users of oral contraceptives and estrogens.[60,61] More recent studies, however, have shown that the relative risk of developing gallbladder disease among oral contraceptive users may be minimal.[62-64] The recent findings of minimal risk may be related to the use of oral contraceptive formulations containing lower hormonal doses of estrogens and progestogens.

Carbohydrate and Lipid Metabolic Effects

Oral contraceptives have been shown to cause a decrease in glucose tolerance in a significant percentage of users.[17] This effect has been shown to be directly related to estrogen dose.[65] Progestogens increase insulin secretion and create insulin resistance, this effect varying with different progestational agents.[17,66] However, in the non-diabetic woman, oral contraceptives appear to have no effect on fasting blood glucose.[67] Because of these demonstrated effects, prediabetic and diabetic women in particular should be carefully monitored while taking oral contraceptives.

A small proportion of women will have persistent hypertriglyceridemia while on the pill. As discussed earlier (see Ortho Tri-Cyclen LO Tablets, Thromboembolic Disorders and Other Vascular Problems: Myocardial Infarction and Dose-Related Risk of Vascular Disease From Oral Contraceptives), changes in serum triglycerides and lipoprotein levels have been reported in oral contraceptive users.

Elevated Blood Pressure

Women with significant hypertension should not be started on hormonal contraception.[98] An increase in blood pressure has been reported in women taking oral contraceptives[68] and this increase is more likely in older oral contraceptive users[69] and with extended duration of use.[61] Data from the Royal College of General Practitioners[12] and subsequent randomized trials have shown that the incidence of hypertension increases with increasing progestational activity and concentrations of progestogens.

Women with a history of hypertension or hypertension-related diseases, or renal disease[70] should be encouraged to use another method of contraception. If women elect to use oral contraceptives, they should be monitored closely and if significant elevation of blood pressure occurs, oral contraceptives should be discontinued. For most women, elevated blood pressure will return to normal after stopping oral contraceptives, and there is no difference in the occurrence of hypertension between former and never users.[68-71]

Headache

The onset or exacerbation of migraine or development of headache with a new pattern which is recurrent, persistent or severe requires discontinuation of oral contraceptives and evaluation of the cause.

Bleeding Irregularities

Breakthrough bleeding and spotting are sometimes encountered in patients on oral contraceptives, especially during the first 3 months of use. Non-hormonal causes should be considered and adequate diagnostic measures taken to rule out malignancy or pregnancy in the event of breakthrough bleeding, as in the case of any abnormal vaginal bleeding. If pathology has been excluded, time or a change to another formulation may solve the problem. In the event of amenorrhea, pregnancy should be ruled out.

Some women may encounter post-pill amenorrhea or oligomenorrhea, especially when such a condition was preexistent.

Ectopic Pregnancy

Ectopic as well as intrauterine pregnancy may occur in contraceptive failures.

PRECAUTIONS

ORTHO TRI-CYCLEN 28 TABLETS AND ORTHO CYCLEN 28 TABLETS

Physical Examination and Follow Up

It is good medical practice for all women to have annual history and physical examinations, including women using oral contraceptives. The physical examination, however, may be deferred until after initiation of oral contraceptives if requested by the woman and judged appropriate by the clinician. The physical examination should include special reference to blood pressure, breasts, abdomen and pelvic organs, including cervical cytology, and relevant laboratory tests. In case of undiagnosed, persistent or recurrent abnormal vaginal bleeding, appropriate measures should be conducted to rule out malignancy. Women with a strong family history of breast cancer or who have breast nodules should be monitored with particular care.

Lipid Disorders

Women who are being treated for hyperlipidemias should be followed closely if they elect to use oral contraceptives. Some progestogens may elevate LDL levels and may render the control of hyperlipidemias more difficult.

Liver Function

If jaundice develops in any woman receiving such drugs, the medication should be discontinued. Steroid hormones may be poorly metabolized in patients with impaired liver function.

Fluid Retention

Oral contraceptives may cause some degree of fluid retention. They should be prescribed with caution, and only with careful monitoring, in patients with conditions which might be aggravated by fluid retention.

Emotional Disorders

Women with a history of depression should be carefully observed and the drug discontinued if depression recurs to a serious degree.

Contact Lenses

Contact lens wearers who develop visual changes or changes in lens tolerance should be assessed by an ophthalmologist.

Interactions With Laboratory Tests

Certain endocrine and liver function tests and blood components may be affected by oral contraceptives:

- Increased prothrombin and factors VII, VIII, IX, and X; decreased antithrombin 3; increased norepinephrine-induced platelet aggregability.
- Increased thyroid binding globulin (TBG) leading to increased circulating total thyroid hormone, as measured by protein-bound iodine (PBI), T4 by column or by radioimmunoassay. Free T3 resin uptake is decreased, reflecting the elevated TBG, free T4 concentration is unaltered.
- Other binding proteins may be elevated in serum.
- Sex hormone binding globulins are increased and result in elevated levels of total circulating sex steroids; however, free or biologically active levels either decrease or remain unchanged.
- High-density lipoprotein (HDL-C) and total cholesterol (Total-C) may be increased, low-density lipoprotein (LDL-C) may be increased or decreased, while LDL-C/HDL-C ratio may be decreased and triglycerides may be unchanged.
- Glucose tolerance may be decreased.
- Serum folate levels may be depressed by oral contraceptive therapy. This may be of clinical significance if a woman becomes pregnant shortly after discontinuing oral contraceptives.

Carcinogenesis

See WARNINGS, Ortho Tri-Cyclen 28 Tablets and Ortho-Cyclen 28 Tablets.

Pregnancy Category X
See CONTRAINDICATIONS, Ortho Tri-Cyclen 28 Tablets and Ortho-Cyclen 28 Tablets and WARNINGS, Ortho Tri-Cyclen 28 Tablets and Ortho-Cyclen 28 Tablets.

Nursing Mothers
Small amounts of oral contraceptive steroids have been identified in the milk of nursing mothers and a few adverse effects on the child have been reported, including jaundice and breast enlargement. In addition, combination oral contraceptives given in the postpartum period may interfere with lactation by decreasing the quantity and quality of breast milk. If possible, the nursing mother should be advised not to use combination oral contraceptives but to use other forms of contraception until she has completely weaned her child.

Pediatric Use
Safety and efficacy of Ortho-Cyclen tablets and Ortho Tri-Cyclen tablets have been established in women of reproductive age. Safety and efficacy are expected to be the same for postpubertal adolescents under the age of 16 and for users 16 years and older. Use of this product before menarche is not indicated.

E

Sexually Transmitted Diseases
Patients should be counseled that this product does not protect against HIV infection (AIDS) and other sexually transmitted diseases.

Information for the Patient
Refer to the Patient Instructions that are distributed with the prescription for complete instructions.

ORTHO TRI-CYCLEN LO TABLETS
General
Patients should be counseled that this product does not protect against HIV infection (AIDS) and other sexually transmitted diseases.

Physical Examination and Follow-Up
It is good medical practice for all women to have annual history and physical examinations, including women using oral contraceptives. The physical examination, however, may be deferred until after initiation of oral contraceptives if requested by the woman and judged appropriate by the clinician. The physical examination should include special reference to blood pressure, breasts, abdomen and pelvic organs, including cervical cytology, and relevant laboratory tests. In case of undiagnosed, persistent or recurrent abnormal vaginal bleeding, appropriate measures should be conducted to rule out malignancy. Women with a strong family history of breast cancer or who have breast nodules should be monitored with particular care.

Lipid Disorders
Women who are being treated for hyperlipidemias should be followed closely if they elect to use oral contraceptives. Some progestogens may elevate LDL levels and may render the control of hyperlipidemias more difficult.

Liver Function
If jaundice develops in any woman receiving oral contraceptives, the medication should be discontinued. Steroid hormones may be poorly metabolized in patients with impaired liver function.

Fluid Retention
Oral contraceptives may cause some degree of fluid retention. They should be prescribed with caution, and only with careful monitoring, in patients with conditions which might be aggravated by fluid retention.

Emotional Disorders
Women with a history of depression should be carefully observed and the drug discontinued if depression recurs to a serious degree.

Contact Lenses
Contact lens wearers who develop visual changes or changes in lens tolerance should be assessed by an ophthalmologist.

Interactions With Laboratory Tests
Certain endocrine and liver function tests and blood components may be affected by oral contraceptives:

- Increased prothrombin and factors VII, VIII, IX, and X; decreased antithrombin 3; increased norepinephrine-induced platelet aggregability.
- Increased thyroid binding globulin (TBG) leading to increased circulating total thyroid hormone, as measured by protein-bound iodine (PBI), T4 by column or by radioimmunoassay. Free T3 resin uptake is decreased, reflecting the elevated TBG, free T4 concentration is unaltered.
- Other binding proteins may be elevated in serum.
- Sex hormone binding globulins are increased and result in elevated levels of total circulating sex steroids; however, free or biologically active levels either decrease or remain unchanged.
- Triglycerides may be increased and levels of various other lipids and lipoproteins may be affected.
- Glucose tolerance may be decreased.
- Serum folate levels may be depressed by oral contraceptive therapy. This may be of clinical significance if a woman becomes pregnant shortly after discontinuing oral contraceptives.

Carcinogenesis
See WARNINGS, Ortho Tri-Cyclen LO Tablets.

Pregnancy Category X
See CONTRAINDICATIONS, Ortho Tri-Cyclen LO Tablets and WARNINGS, Ortho Tri-Cyclen LO Tablets.

Nursing Mothers
Small amounts of oral contraceptive steroids have been identified in the milk of nursing mothers and a few adverse effects on the child have been reported, including jaundice and breast enlargement. In addition, oral contraceptives given in the postpartum period may interfere with lactation by decreasing the quantity and quality of breast milk. If possible, the nursing mother should be advised not to use combination oral contraceptives but to use other forms of contraception until she has completely weaned her child.

Pediatric Use
Safety and efficacy of Ortho Tri-Cyclen LO Tablets have been established in women of reproductive age. Safety and efficacy are expected to be the same for postpubertal adolescents under the age of 16 and for users 16 years and older. Use of this product before menarche is not indicated.

Geriatric Use
This product has not been studied in women over 65 years of age and is not indicated in this population.

Information for the Patient
Refer to the Patient Instructions that are distributed with the prescription for complete instructions.

DRUG INTERACTIONS

ORTHO TRI-CYCLEN 28 TABLETS AND ORTHO CYCLEN 28 TABLETS
Reduced efficacy and increased incidence of breakthrough bleeding and menstrual irregularities have been associated with concomitant use of rifampin. A similar association, though less marked, has been suggested with barbiturates, phenylbutazone, phenytoin sodium, carbamazepine, griseofulvin, topiramate, and possibly with ampicillin and tetracyclines.[72] A possible interaction has been suggested with hormonal contraceptives and the herbal supplement St. John's Wort based on some reports of oral contraceptive users experiencing breakthrough bleeding shortly after starting St. John's Wort. Pregnancies have been reported by users of combined hormonal contraceptives who also used some form of St. John's Wort. Healthcare prescribers are advised to consult the package inserts of medication administered concomitantly with oral contraceptives.

ORTHO TRI-CYCLEN LO TABLETS
Changes in Contraceptive Effectiveness Associated With Co-Administration of Other Products
Contraceptive effectiveness may be reduced when hormonal contraceptives are coadministered with antibiotics, anticonvulsants, and other drugs that increase the metabolism of contraceptive steroids. This could result in unintended pregnancy or breakthrough bleeding. Examples include rifampin, barbiturates, phenylbutazone, phenytoin, carbamazepine, felbamate, oxcarbazepine, topiramate, and griseofulvin. Several cases of contraceptive failure and breakthrough bleeding have been reported in the literature with concomitant administration of antibiotics such as ampicillin and tetracyclines. However, clinical pharmacology studies investigating drug interaction between combined oral contraceptives and these antibiotics have reported inconsistent results.

Several of the anti-HIV protease inhibitors have been studied with co-administration of oral combination hormonal contraceptives; significant changes (increase and decrease) in the plasma levels of the estrogen and progestin have been noted in some cases. The safety and efficacy of oral contraceptive products may be affected with coadministration of anti-HIV protease inhibitors. Health care providers should refer to the label of the individual anti-HIV protease inhibitors for further drug-drug interaction information.

Herbal products containing St. John's Wort (hypericum perforatum) may induce hepatic enzymes (cytochrome P450) and p-glycoprotein transporter and may reduce the effectiveness of contraceptive steroids. This may also result in breakthrough bleeding.

Increase in Plasma Ethinyl Estradiol Levels Associated With Co-Administered Drugs
Co-administration of atorvastatin and certain oral contraceptives containing ethinyl estradiol increase AUC values for ethinyl estradiol by approximately 20%. Ascorbic acid and acetaminophen may increase plasma ethinyl estradiol levels, possibly by inhibition of conjugation. CYP 3A4 inhibitors such as itraconazole or ketoconazole may increase plasma hormone levels.

Changes in Plasma Levels of Co-Administered Drugs
Combination hormonal contraceptives containing some synthetic estrogens (*e.g.*, ethinyl estradiol) may inhibit the metabolism of other compounds. Increased plasma concentrations of cyclosporin, prednisolone, and theophylline have been reported with concomitant administration of oral contraceptives. Decreased plasma concentrations of acetaminophen and increased clearance of temazepam, salicylic acid, morphine and clofibric acid, due to induction of conjugation, have been noted when drugs were administered with oral contraceptives.

ADVERSE REACTIONS

ORTHO TRI-CYCLEN 28 TABLETS AND ORTHO CYCLEN 28 TABLETS
An increased risk of the following serious adverse reactions has been associated with the use of oral contraceptives (see WARNINGS, Ortho Tri-Cyclen 28 Tablets and Ortho-Cyclen 28 Tablets): Thrombophlebitis and venous thrombosis with or without embolism, arterial thromboembolism, pulmonary embolism, myocardial infarction, cerebral hemorrhage, cerebral thrombosis, hypertension, gallbladder disease, hepatic adenomas or benign liver tumors.

The following adverse reactions have been reported in patients receiving oral contraceptives and are believed to be drug-related: Nausea, vomiting, gastrointestinal symptoms (such as abdominal cramps and bloating), breakthrough bleeding, spotting, change in menstrual flow, amenorrhea, temporary infertility after discontinuation of treatment, edema, melasma which may persist, breast changes (tenderness, enlargement, secretion), change in weight (increase or decrease), change in cervical erosion and secretion, diminution in lactation when given immediately postpartum, cholestatic jaundice, migraine, rash (allergic), mental depression, reduced tolerance to carbohydrates, vaginal candidiasis, change in corneal curvature (steepening), intolerance to contact lenses.
The following adverse reactions have been reported in users of oral contraceptives and the association has been neither confirmed nor refuted: Pre-menstrual syndrome, cataracts, changes in appetite, cystitis-like syndrome, headache, nervousness, dizziness, hirsutism, loss of scalp hair, erythema multiforme, erythema nodosum, hemorrhagic eruption, vaginitis, porphyria, impaired renal function, hemolytic uremic syndrome, acne, changes in libido, colitis, Budd-Chiari Syndrome.

ORTHO TRI-CYCLEN LO TABLETS

An increased risk of the following serious adverse reactions has been associated with the use of oral contraceptives (see WARNINGS, Ortho Tri-Cyclen LO Tablets): Thrombophlebitis and venous thrombosis with or without embolism, arterial thromboembolism, pulmonary embolism, myocardial infarction, cerebral hemorrhage, cerebral thrombosis, hypertension, gallbladder disease, hepatic adenomas or benign liver tumors.
There is evidence of an association between the following conditions and the use of oral contraceptives: Mesenteric thrombosis, retinal thrombosis.
The following adverse reactions have been reported in patients receiving oral contraceptives and are believed to be drug-related: Nausea; vomiting; gastrointestinal symptoms (such as abdominal cramps and bloating); breakthrough bleeding; spotting; change in menstrual flow; amenorrhea; temporary infertility after discontinuation of treatment; edema; melasma which may persist; breast changes: tenderness, enlargement, secretion; change in weight (increase or decrease); change in cervical erosion and secretion; diminution in lactation when given immediately postpartum; cholestatic jaundice; migraine; rash (allergic); mental depression; reduced tolerance to carbohydrates; vaginal candidiasis; change in corneal curvature (steepening); intolerance to contact lenses.
The following adverse reactions have been reported in users of oral contraceptives and the association has been neither confirmed nor refuted: Pre-menstrual syndrome, cataracts, changes in appetite, cystitis-like syndrome, headache, nervousness, dizziness, hirsutism, loss of scalp hair, erythema multiforme, erythema nodosum, hemorrhagic eruption, vaginitis, porphyria, impaired renal function, hemolytic uremic syndrome, acne, changes in libido, colitis, Budd-Chiari syndrome.

DOSAGE AND ADMINISTRATION

ORTHO TRI-CYCLEN 28 TABLES AND ORTHO CYCLEN 28 TABLETS

Oral Contraception

To achieve maximum contraceptive effectiveness, Ortho Tri-Cyclen tablets and Ortho-Cyclen tablets must be taken exactly as directed and at intervals not exceeding 24 hours. Ortho Tri-Cyclen and Ortho-Cyclen are available in the Dialpak tablet dispenser which is preset for a Sunday start. Day 1 Start is also provided.

28 Day Regimen (Sunday start)

When taking Ortho Tri-Cyclen 28 and Ortho-Cyclen 28 the first tablet should be taken on the first Sunday after menstruation begins. If period begins on Sunday, the first tablet should be taken that day. Take 1 active tablet daily for 21 days followed by 1 green tablet daily for 7 days. After 28 tablets have been taken, a new course is started the next day (Sunday). For the first cycle of a Sunday Start regimen, another method of contraception should be used until after the first 7 consecutive days of administration.

If the patient misses 1 active tablet in weeks 1, 2, or 3, the tablet should be taken as soon as she remembers. If the patient misses 2 active tablets in week 1 or week 2, the patient should take 2 tablets the day she remembers and 2 tablets the next day; and then continue taking 1 tablet a day until she finishes the pack. The patient should be instructed to use a back-up method of birth control if she has sex in the 7 days after missing pills. If the patient misses 2 active tablets in the third week or misses 3 or more active tablets in a row, the patient should continue taking 1 tablet every day until Sunday. On Sunday the patient should throw out the rest of the pack and start a new pack that same day. The patient should be instructed to use a back-up method of birth control if she has sex in the 7 days after missing pills.

Complete instructions to facilitate patient counseling on proper pill usage may be found in the Detailed Patient Labeling ("How to Take the Pill") included with each prescription.

28 Day Regimen (day 1 start)

The dosage of Ortho Tri-Cyclen 28 and Ortho-Cyclen 28, for the initial cycle of therapy is 1 active tablet administered daily from the 1st day through the 21st day of the menstrual cycle, counting the first day of menstrual flow as "day 1" followed by 1 green tablet daily for 7 days. Tablets are taken without interruption for 28 days. After 28 tablets have been taken, a new course is started the next day.

If the patient misses 1 active tablet in weeks 1, 2, or 3, the tablet should be taken as soon as she remembers. If the patient misses 2 active tablets in week 1 or week 2, the patient should take 2 tablets the day she remembers and 2 tablets the next day; and then continue taking 1 tablet a day until she finishes the pack. The patient should be instructed to use a back-up method of birth control if she has sex in the 7 days after missing pills. If the patient misses 2 active tablets in the third week or misses 3 or more active tablets in a row, the patient should throw out the rest of the pack and start a new pack that same day. The patient should be instructed to use a back-up method of birth control if she has sex in the 7 days after missing pills.

Complete instructions to facilitate patient counseling on proper pill usage may be found in the Detailed Patient Labeling ("How to Take the Pill") included with each prescription.

The use of Ortho Tri-Cyclen and Ortho-Cyclen for contraception may be initiated 4 weeks postpartum in women who elect not to breast feed. When the tablets are administered during the postpartum period, the increased risk of thromboembolic disease associated with the postpartum period must be considered. (See CONTRAINDICATIONS, Ortho Tri-Cyclen 28 Tablets and Ortho-Cyclen 28 Tablets and WARNINGS, Ortho Tri-Cyclen 28 Tablets and Ortho-Cyclen 28 Tablets concerning thromboembolic disease. See also PRECAUTIONS, Ortho Tri-Cyclen 28 Tablets and Ortho-Cyclen 28 Tablets, Nursing Mothers.) The possibility of ovulation and conception prior to initiation of medication should be considered.

(See WARNINGS, Ortho Tri-Cyclen 28 Tablets and Ortho-Cyclen 28 Tablets, Thromboembolic Disorders and Other Vascular Problems, Dose-Related Risk of Vascular Disease From Oral Contraceptives.)

Additional Instructions for All Dosing Regimens

Breakthrough bleeding, spotting, and amenorrhea are frequent reasons for patients discontinuing oral contraceptives. In breakthrough bleeding, as in all cases of irregular bleeding from the vagina, nonfunctional causes should be borne in mind. In undiagnosed persistent or recurrent abnormal bleeding from the vagina, adequate diagnostic measures are indicated to rule out pregnancy or malignancy. If pathology has been excluded, time or a change to another formulation may solve the problem. Changing to an oral contraceptive with a higher estrogen content, while potentially useful in minimizing menstrual irregularity, should be done only if necessary since this may increase the risk of thromboembolic disease.

Use of oral contraceptives in the event of a missed menstrual period:

If the patient has not adhered to the prescribed schedule, the possibility of pregnancy should be considered at the time of the first missed period and oral contraceptive use should be discontinued and a non-hormonal method should be used until pregnancy is ruled out.

If the patient has adhered to the prescribed regimen and misses 2 consecutive periods, pregnancy should be ruled out before continuing oral contraceptive use.

Acne

The timing of initiation of dosing with Ortho Tri-Cyclen for acne should follow the guidelines for use of Ortho Tri-Cyclen as an oral contraceptive. **Consult DOSAGE AND ADMINISTRATION for oral contraceptives.** The dosage regimen for Ortho Tri-Cyclen for treatment of facial acne, as available in a Dialpak tablet dispenser, utilizes a 21 day active and a 7 day placebo schedule. Take 1 active tablet daily for 21 days followed by 1 green tablet for 7 days. After 28 tablets have been taken, a new course is started the next day.

ORTHO TRI-CYCLEN LO TABLETS

Oral Contraception

To achieve maximum contraceptive effectiveness, Ortho Tri-Cyclen LO Tablets must be taken exactly as directed and at intervals not exceeding 24 hours. The possibility of ovulation and conception prior to initiation of medication should be considered. Ortho Tri-Cyclen LO is available in the DIALPAK Tablet Dispenser which is preset for a Sunday Start. Day 1 Start is also provided.

Sunday Start

When taking Ortho Tri-Cyclen LO the first tablet should be taken on the first Sunday after menstruation begins. If the menstrual period begins on Sunday, the first tablet should be taken that day. Take 1 white, light blue or dark blue active tablet daily for 21 days followed by 1 green placebo tablet daily for 7 days. After 28 tablets have been taken, a new course is started the next day (Sunday). For the first cycle of a Sunday Start regimen, another method of contraception should be used until after the first 7 consecutive days of administration.

If the patient misses 1 active tablet in Weeks 1, 2, or 3, the tablet should be taken as soon as she remembers. If the patient misses 2 active tablets in Week 1 or Week 2, the patient should take 2 tablets the day she remembers and 2 tablets the next day; and then continue taking 1 tablet a day until she finishes the pack. The patient should be instructed to use a back-up method of birth control if she has sex in the 7 days after missing pills. If the patient misses 2 active tablets in the third week or misses 3 or more active tablets in a row, the patient should continue taking 1 tablet every day until Sunday. On Sunday the patient should throw out the rest of the pack and start a new pack that same day. The patient should be instructed to use a back-up method of birth control if she has sex in the 7 days after missing pills.

Complete instructions to facilitate patient counseling on proper pill usage may be found in the Detailed Patient Labeling ("How to Take the Pill" section).

Day 1 Start

The dosage of Ortho Tri-Cyclen LO for the initial cycle of therapy is 1 white, light blue or dark blue active tablet administered daily from the 1st day through the 21st day of the menstrual cycle, counting the first day of menstrual flow as "Day 1" followed by 1 green placebo tablet daily for 7 days. Tablets are taken without interruption for 28 days. After 28 tablets have been taken, a new course is started the next day.

If the patient misses 1 active tablet in Weeks 1, 2, or 3, the tablet should be taken as soon as she remembers. If the patient misses 2 active tablets in Week 1 or Week 2, the patient should take 2 tablets the day she remembers and 2 tablets the next day; and then continue taking 1 tablet a day until she finishes the pack. The patient should be instructed to use a back-up method of birth control if she has sex in the 7 days after missing pills. If the patient misses 2 active tablets in the third week or misses 3 or more active tablets in a row, the patient should throw out the rest of the pack and start a new pack that same day. The patient should be instructed to use a back-up method of birth control if she has sex in the 7 days after missing pills.

Complete instructions to facilitate patient counseling on proper pill usage may be found in the detailed patient labeling provided with the prescription.

When switching from another oral contraceptive, Ortho Tri-Cyclen LO should be started on the same day that a new pack of the previous oral contraceptive would have been started.

E

The use of Ortho Tri-Cyclen LO for contraception may be initiated 4 weeks postpartum in women who elect not to breast feed. When the tablets are administered during the postpartum period, the increased risk of thromboembolic disease associated with the postpartum period must be considered. (See CONTRAINDICATIONS, Ortho Tri-Cyclen LO Tablets and WARNINGS, Ortho Tri-Cyclen LO Tablets concerning thromboembolic disease. See also PRECAUTIONS, Ortho Tri-Cyclen LO Tablets, Nursing Mothers.) The possibility of ovulation and conception prior to initiation of medication should be considered. (See WARNINGS, Ortho Tri-Cyclen LO Tablets, Thromboembolic Disorders and Other Vascular Problems, Dose-Related Risk of Vascular Disease From Oral Contraceptives.)

Additional Instructions for All Dosing Regimens

Breakthrough bleeding, spotting, and amenorrhea are frequent reasons for patients discontinuing oral contraceptives. In breakthrough bleeding, as in all cases of irregular bleeding from the vagina, nonfunctional causes should be borne in mind. In undiagnosed persistent or recurrent abnormal bleeding from the vagina, adequate diagnostic measures are indicated to rule out pregnancy or malignancy. If pathology has been excluded, time or a change to another formulation may solve the problem. Changing to an oral contraceptive with a higher estrogen content, while potentially useful in minimizing menstrual irregularity, should be done only if necessary since this may increase the risk of thromboembolic disease.

Use of oral contraceptives in the event of a missed menstrual period:

If the patient has not adhered to the prescribed schedule, the possibility of pregnancy should be considered at the time of the first missed period and oral contraceptive use should be discontinued if pregnancy is confirmed.

If the patient has adhered to the prescribed regimen and misses 2 consecutive periods, pregnancy should be ruled out before continuing oral contraceptive use.

HOW SUPPLIED

ORTHO TRI-CYCLEN 28 TABLETS

Ortho Tri-Cyclen 28 tablets are available in a Dialpak tablet dispenser containing 28 tablets.

Each white tablet contains 0.180 mg of the progestational compound, norgestimate, together with 0.035 mg of the estrogenic compound, ethinyl estradiol. They are unscored, with "Ortho" and "180" debossed on each side.

Each light blue tablet contains 0.215 mg of the progestational compound, norgestimate, together with 0.035 mg of the estrogenic compound, ethinyl estradiol. They are unscored with "Ortho" and "215" debossed on each side.

Each blue tablet contains 0.250 mg of the progestational compound, norgestimate, together with 0.035 mg of the estrogenic compound, ethinyl estradiol. They are unscored with "Ortho" and "250" debossed on each side.

Each green tablet contains inert ingredients.

Ortho Tri-Cyclen 28 tablets are also available as refills.

Ortho Tri-Cyclen 28 tablets are available for clinic usage in a Veridate tablet dispenser (unfilled) and Veridate refills.

ORTHO-CYCLEN 28 TABLETS

Ortho-Cyclen 28 tablets are available in a Dialpak tablet dispenser containing 28 tablets as follows: 21 blue tablets and 7 green tablets.

Each blue tablet contains 0.250 mg of the progestational compound, norgestimate, together with 0.035 mg of the estrogenic compound, ethinyl estradiol which are unscored with "Ortho" and "250" debossed on each side.

Each green tablet contains inert ingredients.

Ortho-Cyclen 28 tablets are also available as refills.

Ortho-Cyclen 28 tablets are available for clinic usage in a Veridate tablet dispenser (unfilled) and Veridate refills.

ORTHO TRI-CYCLEN LO TABLETS

If the patient has adhered to the prescribed regimen and misses 2 consecutive periods, pregnancy should be ruled out before continuing oral contraceptive use.

Each of the 7 white tablets contains 0.180 mg of the progestational compound, norgestimate, together with 0.025 mg of the estrogenic compound, ethinyl estradiol. They are unscored, with "O-M" and "180" debossed on each side.

Each of the 7 light blue tablets contains 0.215 mg of the progestational compound, norgestimate, together with 0.025 mg of the estrogenic compound, ethinyl estradiol. They are unscored with "O-M" and "215" debossed on each side.

Each of the 7 dark blue tablets contains 0.250 mg of the progestational compound, norgestimate, together with 0.025 mg of the estrogenic compound, ethinyl estradiol. They are unscored with "O-M" and "250" debossed on each side.

Each of the 7 green tablets contains inert ingredients.

Ortho Tri-Cyclen LO Tablets are available for clinic usage in a Veridate Tablet Dispenser and Veridate Refills.

Storage: Protect from light.

PRODUCT LISTING - RATED THERAPEUTICALLY EQUIVALENT

Tablet - Oral - 35 mcg;0.25 mg

28 x 6	$193.38	GENERIC, Barr Laboratories Inc	00555-9016-58

PRODUCT LISTING - EQUIVALENTS NOT AVAILABLE

Tablet - Oral - Triphasic 25 mcg

28 x 6	$221.10	ORTHO TRI-CYCLEN LO, Ortho Mcneil Pharmaceutical	00062-1251-15

Tablet - Oral - Triphasic 35 mcg

28 x 6	$35.86	ORTHO TRI-CYCLEN, Physicians Total Care	54868-4093-00
28 x 6	$221.10	ORTHO TRI-CYCLEN, Janssen Pharmaceuticals	00062-1903-15
28 x 168	$4856.88	ORTHO TRI-CYCLEN, Janssen Pharmaceuticals	00062-1903-20

Tablet - Oral - 35 mcg;0.25 mg

28 x 6	$227.58	ORTHO CYCLEN, Janssen Pharmaceuticals	00062-1901-15
28 x 168	$4856.88	ORTHO CYCLEN, Janssen Pharmaceuticals	00062-1901-20
28's	$30.57	ORTHO CYCLEN, Physicians Total Care	54868-2606-00

Ethinyl Estradiol; Norgestrel (001222)

Categories: Contraception; Contraception, emergency; Pregnancy Category X; FDA Approval Pre 1982

Drug Classes: Contraceptives; Estrogens; Hormones/hormone modifiers; Progestins

Brand Names: Lo/Ovral; Low-Ogestrel; Ogestrel; Ovral

Foreign Brand Availability: Duoluton (Belgium; India; Japan; Mexico; Taiwan); Duoluton-L (India); Eugynon (Argentina; Hong-Kong; Mexico); Eugynon 21 (Spain); Eugynon 28 (Germany); Eugynon 30 (Ireland); Femenal (Philippines); Min-Ovral (Canada); Planovar (Japan); Stediril (Belgium; France)

Cost of Therapy: $30.61 (Contraceptive; Lo/Ovral; 30 µg; 0.3 mg; 1 tablet/day; 28 day supply)

DESCRIPTION

Note: The trade names have been used throughout this monograph for clarity.

LO/OVRAL

Patients should be counseled that this product does not protect against HIV infection (AIDS) and other sexually transmitted diseases.

Each Lo/Ovral tablet contains 0.3 mg of norgestrel (*dl*-13-beta-ethyl-17-alpha-ethinyl-17-beta-hydroxygon-4-en-3-one), a totally synthetic progestogen, and 0.03 mg of ethinyl estradiol (19-nor-17α-pregna-1,3,5 (10)-trien-20-yne-3,17-diol). The inactive ingredients present are cellulose, lactose, magnesium stearate, and polacrilin potassium.

LO/OVRAL-28

Patients should be counseled that this product does not protect against HIV infection (AIDS) and other sexually transmitted diseases.

21 white Lo/Ovral tablets, each containing 0.3 mg of norgestrel (*dl* -13-beta-ethyl-17-alpha-ethinyl-17-beta-hydroxygon-4-en-3-one), a totally synthetic progestogen, and 0.03 mg of ethinyl estradiol (19-nor-17α-pregna-1,3,5 (10)-trien-20-yne-3,17-diol), and 7 pink inert tablets. The inactive ingredients present are cellulose, D&C red 30, lactose, magnesium stearate, and polacrilin potassium.

CLINICAL PHARMACOLOGY

Combination oral contraceptives act by suppression of gonadotropins. Although the primary mechanism of this action is inhibition of ovulation, other alterations include changes in the cervical mucus (which increase the difficulty of sperm entry into the uterus) and the endometrium (which reduce the likelihood of implantation).

NONCONTRACEPTIVE HEALTH BENEFITS

The following noncontraceptive health benefits related to the use of oral contraceptives are supported by epidemiological studies which largely utilized oral-contraceptive formulations containing doses exceeding 0.035 mg of ethinyl estradiol or 0.05 mg of mestranol.

Effects on menses:

Increased menstrual cycle regularity.

Decreased blood loss and decreased incidence of iron-deficiency anemia.

Decreased incidence of dysmenorrhea.

Effects related to inhibition of ovulation:

Decreased incidence of functional ovarian cysts.

Decreased incidence of ectopic pregnancies.

Effects from long-term use:

Decreased incidence of fibroadenomas and fibrocystic disease of the breast.

Decreased incidence of acute pelvic inflammatory disease.

Decreased incidence of endometrial cancer.

Decreased incidence of ovarian cancer.

INDICATIONS AND USAGE

Oral contraceptives are indicated for the prevention of pregnancy in women who elect to use this product as a method of contraception.

Oral contraceptives are highly effective. TABLE 1 lists the typical accidental pregnancy rates for users of combination oral contraceptives and other methods of contraception. The efficacy of these contraceptive methods, except sterilization and the IUD, depends upon the reliability with which they are used. Correct and consistent use of methods can result in lower failure rates.

CONTRAINDICATIONS

Oral contraceptives should not be used in women with any of the following conditions:

Thrombophlebitis or thromboembolic disorders.

A past history of deep-vein thrombophlebitis or thromboembolic disorders.

Cerebral-vascular or coronary-artery disease.

Known or suspected carcinoma of the breast.

Carcinoma of the endometrium or other known or suspected estrogen-dependent neoplasia.

Undiagnosed abnormal genital bleeding.

Cholestatic jaundice of pregnancy or jaundice with prior pill use.

Hepatic adenomas or carcinomas.

Known or suspected pregnancy.

Hypersensitivity to any of the components of Lo/Ovral.

TABLE 1 *Percentage of Women Experiencing an Unintended Pregnancy During the First Year of Use of a Contraceptive Method*

Method	Perfect Use	Typical Use
Levonorgestrel implants	0.05%	0.05%
Male sterilization	0.1%	0.15%
Female sterilization	0.5%	0.5%
Depo-Provera (injectable progestogen)	0.3%	0.3%
Oral contraceptives		5%
Combined	0.1%	NA
Progestin only	0.5%	NA
IUD		
Progesterone	1.5%	2.0%
Copper T 380A	0.6%	0.8%
Condom		
(Male) without spermicide	3%	14%
(Female) without spermicide	5%	21%
Cervical cap		
Nulliparous women	9%	20%
Parous women	26%	40%
Vaginal sponge		
Nulliparous women	9%	20%
Parous women	20%	40%
Diaphragm with spermicidal cream or jelly	6%	20%
Spermicides alone (foam, creams, jellies, and vaginal suppositories)	6%	26%
Periodic abstinence (all methods)	1-9%*	25%
Withdrawal	4%	19%
No contraception (planned pregnancy)	85%	85%

NA Not Available.
* Depending on method (calendar, ovulation, symptothermal, post-ovulation) Adapted from Hatcher RA *et al., Contraceptive Technology: 17th Revised Edition.* NY, NY: Ardent Media, Inc., 1998.

WARNINGS

Cigarette smoking increases the risk of serious cardiovascular side effects from oral-contraceptive use. This risk increases with age and with heavy smoking (15 or more cigarettes per day) and is quite marked in women over 35 years of age. Women who use oral contraceptives should be strongly advised not to smoke.

The use of oral contraceptives is associated with increased risks of several serious conditions including myocardial infarction, thromboembolism, stroke, hepatic neoplasia, gallbladder disease, and hypertension, although the risk of serious morbidity or mortality is very small in healthy women without underlying risk factors. The risk of morbidity and mortality increases significantly in the presence of other underlying risk factors such as certain inherited thrombophilias, hypertension, hyperlipidemias, obesity, and diabetes.

Practitioners prescribing oral contraceptives should be familiar with the following information relating to these risks.

The information contained in this package insert is based principally on studies carried out in patients who used oral contraceptives with higher formulations of estrogens and progestogens than those in common use today. The effect of long-term use of the oral contraceptives with lower formulations of both estrogens and progestogens remains to be determined.

Throughout this labeling, epidemiological studies reported are of two types: retrospective or case control studies and prospective or cohort studies. Case control studies provide a measure of the relative risk of disease, namely, a ratio of the incidence of a disease among oral-contraceptive users to that among nonusers. The relative risk does not provide information on the actual clinical occurrence of a disease. Cohort studies provide a measure of attributable risk, which is the difference in the incidence of disease between oral-contraceptive users and nonusers. The attributable risk does provide information about the actual occurrence of a disease in the population. For further information, the reader is referred to a text on epidemiological methods.

THROMBOEMBOLIC DISORDERS AND OTHER VASCULAR PROBLEMS

Myocardial Infarction

An increased risk of myocardial infarction has been attributed to oral-contraceptive use. This risk is primarily in smokers or women with other underlying risk factors for coronary-artery disease such as hypertension, hypercholesterolemia, morbid obesity, and diabetes. The relative risk of heart attack for current oral-contraceptive users has been estimated to be 2-6. The risk is very low under the age of 30.

Smoking in combination with oral-contraceptive use has been shown to contribute substantially to the incidence of myocardial infarctions in women in their mid-thirties or older with smoking accounting for the majority of excess cases. Mortality rates associated with circulatory disease have been shown to increase substantially in smokers over the age of 35 and nonsmokers over the age of 40 among women who use oral contraceptives.

Oral contraceptives may compound the effects of well-known risk factors, such as hypertension, diabetes, hyperlipidemias, age, and obesity. In particular, some progestogens are known to decrease HDL cholesterol and cause glucose intolerance, while estrogens may create a state of hyperinsulinism. Oral contraceptives have been shown to increase blood pressure among users (see Elevated Blood Pressure). Similar effects on risk factors have been associated with an increased risk of heart disease. Oral contraceptives must be used with caution in women with cardiovascular disease risk factors.

Thromboembolism

An increased risk of thromboembolic and thrombotic disease associated with the use of oral contraceptives is well established. Case control studies have found the relative risk of users compared to nonusers to be 3 for the first episode of superficial venous thrombosis, 4-11 for deep-vein thrombosis or pulmonary embolism, and 1.5 to 6 for women with predisposing conditions for venous thromboembolic disease. Cohort studies have shown the relative risk to be somewhat lower, about 3 for new cases and about 4.5 for new cases requiring hospitalization. The risk of thromboembolic disease due to oral contraceptives is not related to length of use and disappears after pill use is stopped.

A 2- to 4-fold increase in relative risk of postoperative thromboembolic complications has been reported with the use of oral contraceptives. The relative risk of venous thrombosis in women who have predisposing conditions is twice that of women without such medical conditions. If feasible, oral contraceptives should be discontinued at least 4 weeks prior to and for 2 weeks after elective surgery of a type associated with an increase in risk of thromboembolism and during and following prolonged immobilization. Since the immediate postpartum period is also associated with an increased risk of thromboembolism, oral contraceptives should be started no earlier than 4-6 weeks after delivery in women who elect not to breast-feed, or a midtrimester pregnancy termination.

Cerebrovascular Diseases

Oral contraceptives have been shown to increase both the relative and attributable risks of cerebrovascular events (thrombotic and hemorrhagic strokes), although, in general, the risk is greatest among older (>35 years), hypertensive women who also smoke. Hypertension was found to be a risk factor for both users and nonusers, for both types of strokes, while smoking interacted to increase the risk for hemorrhagic strokes.

In a large study, the relative risk of thrombotic strokes has been shown to range from 3 for normotensive users to 14 for users with severe hypertension. The relative risk of hemorrhagic stroke is reported to be 1.2 for nonsmokers who used oral contraceptives, 2.6 for smokers who did not use oral contraceptives, 7.6 for smokers who used oral contraceptives, 1.8 for normotensive users, and 25.7 for users with severe hypertension. The attributable risk is also greater in older women.

Women with migraine (particularly migraine with aura) who take combination oral contraceptives may be at an increased risk of stroke.

Dose-Related Risk of Vascular Disease From Oral Contraceptives

A positive association has been observed between the amount of estrogen and progestogen in oral contraceptives and the risk of vascular disease. A decline in serum high-density lipoproteins (HDL) has been reported with many progestational agents. A decline in serum high-density lipoproteins has been associated with an increased incidence of ischemic heart disease. Because estrogens increase HDL cholesterol, the net effect of an oral contraceptive depends on a balance achieved between doses of estrogen and progestogen and the nature and absolute amount of progestogen used in the contraceptive. The amount of both hormones should be considered in the choice of an oral contraceptive.

Minimizing exposure to estrogen and progestogen is in keeping with good principles of therapeutics. For any particular estrogen/progestogen combination, the dosage regimen prescribed should be one which contains the least amount of estrogen and progestogen that is compatible with a low failure rate and the needs of the individual patient. New acceptors of oral-contraceptive agents should be started on preparations containing less than 50 μg of estrogen.

Persistence of Risk of Vascular Disease

There are two studies which have shown persistence of risk of vascular disease for ever-users of oral contraceptives. In a study in the US, the risk of developing myocardial infarction after discontinuing oral contraceptives persists for at least 9 years for women 40-49 years who had used oral contraceptives for 5 or more years, but this increased risk was not demonstrated in other age groups. In another study in Great Britain, the risk of developing cerebrovascular disease persisted for at least 6 years after discontinuation of oral contraceptives, although excess risk was very small. However, both studies were performed with oral-contraceptive formulations containing 50 μg or higher of estrogens.

ESTIMATES OF MORTALITY FROM CONTRACEPTIVE USE

One study gathered data from a variety of sources which have estimated the mortality rate associated with different methods of contraception at different ages (TABLE 2). These estimates include the combined risk of death associated with contraceptive methods plus the risk attributable to pregnancy in the event of method failure. Each method of contraception has its specific benefits and risks. The study concluded that with the exception of oral-contraceptive users 35 and older who smoke and 40 and older who do not smoke, mortality associated with all methods of birth control is less than that associated with childbirth. The observation of a possible increase in risk of mortality with age for oral-contraceptive users is based on data gathered in the 1970's — but not reported until 1983. However, current clinical practice involves the use of lower estrogen dose formulations combined with careful restriction of oral-contraceptive use to women who do not have the various risk factors listed in this labeling.

Because of these changes in practice and, also, because of some limited new data which suggest that the risk of cardiovascular disease with the use of oral contraceptives may now be less than previously observed, the Fertility and Maternal Health Drugs Advisory Committee was asked to review the topic in 1989. The Committee concluded that although cardiovascular disease risks may be increased with oral-contraceptive use after age 40 in healthy nonsmoking women (even with the newer low-dose formulations), there are greater potential health risks associated with pregnancy in older women and with the alternative surgical and medical procedures which may be necessary if such women do not have access to effective and acceptable means of contraception.

Therefore, the Committee recommended that the benefits of oral-contraceptive use by healthy nonsmoking women over 40 may outweigh the possible risks. Of course, older women, as all women who take oral contraceptives, should take the lowest possible dose formulation that is effective.

CARCINOMA OF THE REPRODUCTIVE ORGANS

A meta-analysis from 54 epidemiological studies reported that there is a slightly increased relative risk (RR=1.24) of having breast cancer diagnosed in women who are currently using combination oral contraceptives compared to never-users. The increased risk gradually disappears during the course of the 10 years after cessation of combination oral contraceptive use. These studies do not provide evidence for causation. The observed pattern of increased risk of breast cancer diagnosis may be due to earlier detection of breast cancer in combination oral contraceptive users, the biological effects of combination oral contracep-

TABLE 2 *Annual Number of Birth-Related or Method-Related Deaths Associated With Control of Fertility per 100,000 Nonsterile Women, By Fertility-Control Method and According to Age*

Method of control and outcome	15-19	20-24	25-29	30-34	35-39	40-44
No fertility-control methods*	7.0	7.4	9.1	14.8	25.7	28.2
Oral contraceptives - nonsmoker†	0.3	0.5	0.9	1.9	13.8	31.6
Oral contraceptives - smoker†	2.2	3.4	6.6	13.5	51.1	117.2
IUD†	0.8	0.8	1.0	1.0	1.4	1.4
Condom*	1.1	1.6	0.7	0.2	0.3	0.4
Diaphragm/spermicide*	1.9	1.2	1.2	1.3	2.2	2.8
Periodic abstinence*	2.5	1.6	1.6	1.7	2.9	3.6

* Deaths are birth related.
† Deaths are method related.
Adapted from H.W. Ory, Family Planning Perspectives, *15*:57-63, 1983.

tives, or a combination of both. Because breast cancer is rare in women under 40 years of age, the excess number of breast cancer diagnoses in current and recent combination oral contraceptive users is small in relation to the lifetime risk of breast cancer. Breast cancers diagnosed in ever-users tend to be less advanced clinically than the cancers diagnosed in never-users.

Some studies suggest that oral-contraceptive use has been associated with an increase in the risk of cervical intraepithelial neoplasia or cervical cancer in some populations of women. However, there continues to be controversy about the extent to which such findings may be due to differences in sexual behavior and other factors.

In spite of many studies of the relationship between oral-contraceptive use and breast and cervical cancers, a cause-and-effect relationship has not been established.

HEPATIC NEOPLASIA

Benign hepatic adenomas are associated with oral-contraceptive use, although the incidence of benign tumors is rare in the US. Indirect calculations have estimated the attributable risk to be in the range of 3.3 cases/100,000 for users, a risk that increases after 4 or more years of use. Rupture of rare, benign, hepatic adenomas may cause death through intra-abdominal hemorrhage.

Studies from Britain have shown an increased risk of developing hepatocellular carcinoma in long-term (>8 years) oral-contraceptive users. However, these cancers are extremely rare in the US, and the attributable risk (the excess incidence) of liver cancers in oral-contraceptive users approaches less than one per million users.

OCULAR LESIONS

There have been clinical case reports of retinal thrombosis associated with the use of oral contraceptives. Oral contraceptives should be discontinued if there is unexplained partial or complete loss of vision; onset of proptosis or diplopia; papilledema; or retinal vascular lesions. Appropriate diagnostic and therapeutic measures should be undertaken immediately.

ORAL-CONTRACEPTIVE USE BEFORE OR DURING EARLY PREGNANCY

Extensive epidemiological studies have revealed no increased risk of birth defects in women who have used oral contraceptives prior to pregnancy. Studies also do not suggest a teratogenic effect, particularly insofar as cardiac anomalies and limb-reduction defects are concerned, when taken inadvertently during early pregnancy.

The administration of oral contraceptives to induce withdrawal bleeding should not be used as a test for pregnancy. Oral contraceptives should not be used during pregnancy to treat threatened or habitual abortion.

It is recommended that for any patient who has missed two consecutive periods, pregnancy should be ruled out before continuing oral-contraceptive use. If the patient has not adhered to the prescribed schedule, the possibility of pregnancy should be considered at the time of the first missed period. Oral-contraceptive use should be discontinued if pregnancy is confirmed.

GALLBLADDER DISEASE

Earlier studies have reported an increased lifetime relative risk of gallbladder surgery in users of oral contraceptives and estrogens. More recent studies, however, have shown that the relative risk of developing gallbladder disease among oral-contraceptive users may be minimal.

The recent findings of minimal risk may be related to the use of oral-contraceptive formulations containing lower hormonal doses of estrogens and progestogens.

CARBOHYDRATE AND LIPID METABOLIC EFFECTS

Oral contraceptives have been shown to cause glucose intolerance in a significant percentage of users. Oral contraceptives containing greater than 75 μg of estrogens cause hyperinsulinism, while lower doses of estrogen cause less glucose intolerance. Progestogens increase insulin secretion and create insulin resistance, this effect varying with different progestational agents. However, in the nondiabetic woman, oral contraceptives appear to have no effect on fasting blood glucose. Because of these demonstrated effects, prediabetic and diabetic women should be carefully observed while taking oral contraceptives.

A small proportion of women will have persistent hypertriglyceridemia while on the pill. As discussed earlier (see Thromboembolic Disorders and Other Vascular Problems: Myocardial Infarction and Dose-Related Risk of Vascular Disease From Oral Contraceptives), changes in serum triglycerides and lipoprotein levels have been reported in oral-contraceptive users.

ELEVATED BLOOD PRESSURE

An increase in blood pressure has been reported in women taking oral contraceptives, and this increase is more likely in older oral-contraceptive users and with continued use. Data from the Royal College of General Practitioners and subsequent randomized trials have shown that the incidence of hypertension increases with increasing quantities of progestogens.

Women with a history of hypertension or hypertension-related diseases, or renal disease, should be encouraged to use another method of contraception. If women with hypertension elect to use oral contraceptives, they should be monitored closely, and if significant elevation of blood pressure occurs, oral contraceptives should be discontinued. For most women, elevated blood pressure will return to normal after stopping oral contraceptives, and there is no difference in the occurrence of hypertension among ever- and never-users.

HEADACHE

The onset or exacerbation of migraine or development of headache with a new pattern that is recurrent, persistent, or severe requires discontinuation of oral contraceptives and evaluation of the cause. (See Thromboembolic Disorders and Other Vascular Problems, Cerebrovascular Diseases.)

BLEEDING IRREGULARITIES

Breakthrough bleeding and spotting are sometimes encountered in patients on oral contraceptives, especially during the first 3 months of use. The type and dose of progestogen may be important. Nonhormonal causes should be considered and adequate diagnostic measures taken to rule out malignancy or pregnancy in the event of breakthrough bleeding, as in the case of any abnormal vaginal bleeding. If pathology has been excluded, time or a change to another formulation may solve the problem. In the event of amenorrhea, pregnancy should be ruled out.

Some women may encounter post-pill amenorrhea or oligomenorrhea, especially when such a condition was preexistent.

PRECAUTIONS

Patients should be counseled that this product does not protect against HIV infection (AIDS) and other sexually transmitted diseases.

PHYSICAL EXAMINATION AND FOLLOW-UP

A periodic history and physical examination is appropriate for all women, including women using oral contraceptives. The physical examination, however, may be deferred until after initiation of oral contraceptives if requested by the woman and judged appropriate by the clinician. The physical examination should include special reference to blood pressure, breasts, abdomen and pelvic organs, including cervical cytology, and relevant laboratory tests. In case of undiagnosed, persistent, or recurrent abnormal vaginal bleeding, appropriate measures should be conducted to rule out malignancy. Women with a strong family history of breast cancer or who have breast nodules should be monitored with particular care.

LIPID DISORDERS

Women who are being treated for hyperlipidemias should be followed closely if they elect to use oral contraceptives. Some progestogens may elevate LDL levels and may render the control of hyperlipidemias more difficult. (See WARNINGS, Thromboembolic Disorders and Other Vascular Problems, Dose-Related Risk of Vascular Disease From Oral Contraceptives.)

In patients with familial defects of lipoprotein metabolism receiving estrogen-containing preparations, there have been case reports of significant elevations of plasma triglycerides leading to pancreatitis.

LIVER FUNCTION

If jaundice develops in any woman receiving such drugs, the medication should be discontinued. Steroid hormones may be poorly metabolized in patients with impaired liver function.

FLUID RETENTION

Oral contraceptives may cause some degree of fluid retention. They should be prescribed with caution, and only with careful monitoring, in patients with conditions which might be aggravated by fluid retention.

EMOTIONAL DISORDERS

Patients becoming significantly depressed while taking oral contraceptives should stop the medication and use an alternate method of contraception in an attempt to determine whether the symptom is drug related. Women with a history of depression should be carefully observed and the drug discontinued if depression recurs to a serious degree.

CONTACT LENSES

Contact-lens wearers who develop visual changes or changes in lens tolerance should be assessed by an ophthalmologist.

INTERACTIONS WITH LABORATORY TESTS

Certain endocrine- and liver-function tests and blood components may be affected by oral contraceptives:

- Increased prothrombin and factors VII, VIII, IX, and X; decreased antithrombin 3; increased norepinephrine-induced platelet aggregability.
- Increased thyroid-binding globulin (TBG) leading to increased circulating total thyroid hormone, as measured by protein-bound iodine (PBI), T4 by column or by radioimmunoassay. Free T3 resin uptake is decreased, reflecting the elevated TBG; free T4 concentration is unaltered.
- Other binding proteins may be elevated in serum.
- Sex-binding globulins are increased and result in elevated levels of total circulating sex steroids and corticoids; however, free or biologically active levels remain unchanged.
- Triglycerides may be increased.

Glucose tolerance may be decreased.

Serum folate levels may be depressed by oral-contraceptive therapy. This may be of clinical significance if a woman becomes pregnant shortly after discontinuing oral contraceptives.

CARCINOGENESIS

See WARNINGS.

PREGNANCY CATEGORY X

See CONTRAINDICATIONS and WARNINGS.

NURSING MOTHERS

Small amounts of oral-contraceptive steroids have been identified in the milk of nursing mothers, and a few adverse effects on the child have been reported, including jaundice and breast enlargement. In addition, oral contraceptives given in the postpartum period may interfere with lactation by decreasing the quantity and quality of breast milk. If possible, the nursing mother should be advised not to use oral contraceptives but to use other forms of contraception until she has completely weaned her child.

PEDIATRIC USE

Safety and efficacy of Lo/Ovral have been established in women of reproductive age. Safety and efficacy are expected to be the same for postpubertal adolescents under the age of 16 and users 16 and older. Use of this product before menarche is not indicated.

INFORMATION FOR THE PATIENT

See the Patient Labeling that is distributed with the prescription.

DRUG INTERACTIONS

Reduced efficacy and increased incidence of breakthrough bleeding and menstrual irregularities have been associated with concomitant use of rifampin. A similar association, though less marked, has been suggested with barbiturates, phenylbutazone, phenytoin sodium, and possibly with griseofulvin, ampicillin, and tetracyclines.

Troleadomycin may increase the risk of intrahepatic cholestasis during coadministration with combination oral contraceptives.

ADVERSE REACTIONS

An increased risk of the following serious adverse reactions has been associated with the use of oral contraceptives (see WARNINGS): Thrombophlebitis, arterial thromboembolism, pulmonary embolism, myocardial infarction, cerebral hemorrhage, cerebral thrombosis, hypertension, gallbladder disease, hepatic adenomas or benign liver tumors.

There is evidence of an association between the following conditions and the use of oral contraceptives, although additional confirmatory studies are needed: Mesenteric thrombosis, retinal thrombosis.

The following adverse reactions have been reported in patients receiving oral contraceptives and are believed to be drug related: Nausea; vomiting; gastrointestinal symptoms (such as abdominal cramps and bloating); breakthrough bleeding; spotting; change in menstrual flow; amenorrhea; temporary infertility after discontinuation of treatment; edema; melasma which may persist; breast changes: tenderness, enlargement, secretion; change in weight (increase or decrease); change in cervical erosion and secretion; diminution in lactation when given immediately postpartum; cholestatic jaundice; migraine; rash (allergic); mental depression; reduced tolerance to carbohydrates; vaginal candidiasis; change in corneal curvature (steepening); intolerance to contact lenses.

The following adverse reactions have been reported in users of oral contraceptives, and the association has been neither confirmed nor refuted: Congenital anomalies; premenstrual syndrome; cataracts; optic neuritis; changes in appetite; cystitis-like syndrome; headache; nervousness; dizziness; hirsutism; loss of scalp hair; erythema multiforme; erythema nodosum; hemorrhagic eruption; vaginitis; porphyria; impaired renal function; hemolytic uremic syndrome; Budd-Chiari syndrome; acne; changes in libido; colitis; sickle-cell disease; cerebralvascular disease with mitral valve prolapse; lupus-like syndromes; pancreatitis.

DOSAGE AND ADMINISTRATION

LO/OVRAL

To achieve maximum contraceptive effectiveness, Lo/Ovral must be taken exactly as directed and at intervals not exceeding 24 hours.

The dosage of Lo/Ovral is 1 tablet daily for 21 consecutive days per menstrual cycle according to prescribed schedule. Tablets are then discontinued for 7 days (3 weeks on, 1 week off).

It is recommended that Lo/Ovral tablets be taken at the same time each day, preferably after the evening meal or at bedtime.

During the first cycle of medication, the patient is instructed to take 1 Lo/Ovral tablet daily for 21 consecutive days, beginning on the first day (Day 1 Start) of her menstrual cycle or on the Sunday after her period begins (Sunday Start). (The first day of menstruation is day 1.) The tablets are then discontinued for 1 week (7 days). Withdrawal bleeding should usually occur within 3 days following discontinuation of Lo/Ovral. (For Day 1 Start: If Lo/Ovral is first taken later than the first day of the first menstrual cycle of medication or postpartum, contraceptive reliance should not be placed on Lo/Ovral until after the first 7 consecutive days of administration. For Sunday Start: Contraceptive reliance should not be placed on Lo/Ovral until after the first 7 consecutive days of administration. The possibility of ovulation and conception prior to initiation of medication should be considered.)

The patient begins her next and all subsequent 21 day courses of Lo/Ovral tablets on the same day of the week that she began her first course, following the same schedule: 21 days on — 7 days off. She begins taking her tablets on the 8th day after discontinuance, regardless of whether or not a menstrual period has occurred or is still in progress. Any time a new cycle of Lo/Ovral is started later than the 8th day, the patient should be protected by another means of contraception until she has taken a tablet daily for 7 consecutive days.

If spotting or breakthrough bleeding occurs, the patient is instructed to continue on the same regimen. This type of bleeding is usually transient and without significance; however, if the bleeding is persistent or prolonged, the patient is advised to consult her physician. Although the occurrence of pregnancy is highly unlikely if Lo/Ovral is taken according to directions, if withdrawal bleeding does not occur, the possibility of pregnancy must be considered. If the patient has not adhered to the prescribed schedule (missed 1 or more tablets or started taking them on a day later than she should have), the probability of pregnancy should be considered at the time of the first missed period and appropriate diagnostic measures taken before the medication is resumed. If the patient has adhered to the prescribed regimen and misses two consecutive periods, pregnancy should be ruled out before continuing the contraceptive regimen.

For additional patient instructions regarding missed pills, see the Detailed Patient Labeling which is distributed with each prescription.

Any time the patient misses 2 or more tablets, she should also use another method of contraception until she has taken a tablet daily for 7 consecutive days. If breakthrough bleeding occurs following missed tablets, it will usually be transient and of no consequence. While there is little likelihood of ovulation occurring if only 1 or 2 tablets are missed, the possibility of ovulation increases with each successive day that scheduled tablets are missed.

In the nonlactating mother, Lo/Ovral may be initiated postpartum, for contraception. When the tablets are administered in the postpartum period, the increased risk of thromboembolic disease associated with the postpartum period must be considered (see CONTRAINDICATIONS, WARNINGS, and PRECAUTIONS concerning thromboembolic disease). It is to be noted that early resumption of ovulation may occur if Parlodel (bromocriptine mesylate) has been used for the prevention of lactation.

LO/OVRAL-28

To achieve maximum contraceptive effectiveness, Lo/Ovral-28 must be taken exactly as directed and at intervals not exceeding 24 hours.

The dosage of Lo/Ovral-28 is 1 white tablet daily for 21 consecutive days, followed by 1 pink inert tablet daily for 7 consecutive days, according to prescribed schedule. It is recommended that tablets be taken at the same time each day, preferably after the evening meal or at bedtime.

During the first cycle of medication, the patient is instructed to begin taking Lo/Ovral-28 on the first Sunday after the onset of menstruation. If menstruation begins on a Sunday, the first tablet (white) is taken that day. One (1) white tablet should be taken daily for 21 consecutive days followed by 1 pink inert tablet daily for 7 consecutive days. Withdrawal bleeding should usually occur within 3 days following discontinuation of white tablets. During the first cycle, contraceptive reliance should not be placed on Lo/Ovral-28 until a white tablet has been taken daily for 7 consecutive days. The possibility of ovulation and conception prior to initiation of medication should be considered.

The patient begins her next and all subsequent 28 day courses of tablets on the same day of the week (Sunday) on which she began her first course, following the same schedule: 21 days on white tablets — 7 days on pink inert tablets. If in any cycle the patient starts tablets later than the proper day, she should protect herself by using another method of birth control until she has taken a white tablet daily for 7 consecutive days.

If spotting or breakthrough bleeding occurs, the patient is instructed to continue on the same regimen. This type of bleeding is usually transient and without significance; however, if the bleeding is persistent or prolonged, the patient is advised to consult her physician. Although the occurrence of pregnancy is highly unlikely if Lo/Ovral-28 is taken according to directions, if withdrawal bleeding does not occur, the possibility of pregnancy must be considered. If the patient has not adhered to the prescribed schedule (missed 1 or more tablets or started taking them on a day later than she should have), the probability of pregnancy should be considered at the time of the first missed period and appropriate diagnostic measures taken before the medication is resumed. If the patient has adhered to the prescribed regimen and misses 2 consecutive periods, pregnancy should be ruled out before continuing the contraceptive regimen.

For additional patient instructions regarding missed pills, see the Detailed Patient Labeling which is distributed with each prescription.

Any time the patient misses 2 or more white tablets, she should also use another method of contraception until she has taken a white tablet daily for 7 consecutive days. If the patient misses 1 or more pink tablets, she is still protected against pregnancy **provided** she begins taking white tablets again on the proper day.

If breakthrough bleeding occurs following missed white tablets, it will usually be transient and of no consequence. While there is little likelihood of ovulation occurring if only 1 or 2 white tablets are missed, the possibility of ovulation increases with each successive day that scheduled white tablets are missed.

In the nonlactating mother, Lo/Ovral-28 may be initiated postpartum, for contraception. When the tablets are administered in the postpartum period, the increased risk of thromboembolic disease associated with the postpartum period must be considered (see CONTRAINDICATIONS, WARNINGS, and PRECAUTIONS concerning thromboembolic disease). It is to be noted that early resumption of ovulation may occur if Parlodel (bromocriptine mesylate) has been used for the prevention of lactation.

HOW SUPPLIED

LO/OVRAL

Lo/Ovral Tablets (0.3 mg norgestrel and 0.03 mg ethinyl estradiol) are available in packages of 6 PILPAK dispensers with 21 white, round tablets marked "WYETH" and "78" each.

Storage: Store at room temperature, approx. 25°C (77°F).

LO/OVRAL-28

Lo/Ovral-28 Tablets (0.3 mg norgestrel and 0.03 mg ethinyl estradiol) are available in packages of 12 PILPAK dispensers for clinic use only, each containing 28 tablets as follows:

21 active tablets, white, round tablet marked "WYETH" and "78".

7 inert tablets, pink, round tablet marked "WYETH" and "486".

Storage: Store at room temperature, approx. 25°C (77°F).

PRODUCT LISTING - RATED THERAPEUTICALLY EQUIVALENT

Tablet - Oral - 30 mcg;0.3 mg

1's	$31.96	LO/OVRAL-28, Allscripts Pharmaceutical Company	54569-0679-00
1's	$35.52	LO/OVRAL-28, Physicians Total Care	54868-0428-00
21 x 6	$216.24	LO/OVRAL, Wyeth-Ayerst Laboratories	00008-0078-01
28 each	$28.01	GENERIC, Allscripts Pharmaceutical Company	54569-4998-00
28 x 6	$183.12	GENERIC, Watson Laboratories Inc	52544-0847-28
28 x 6	$216.24	LO/OVRAL, Wyeth-Ayerst Laboratories	00008-2514-02

Tablet - Oral - 50 mcg;0.5 mg

21 x 6	$11.45	OVRAL, Pharma Pac	52959-0460-04
21 x 6	$318.30	OVRAL, Wyeth-Ayerst Laboratories	00008-0056-01
21's	$48.93	OVRAL, Allscripts Pharmaceutical Company	54569-0690-00
21's	$51.80	OVRAL, Wyeth-Ayerst Laboratories	00008-0056-02
28 x 6	$134.76	GENERIC, Watson Laboratories Inc	52544-0848-28
28 x 6	$318.30	OVRAL, Wyeth-Ayerst Laboratories	00008-2511-02
28's	$51.80	OVRAL, Wyeth-Ayerst Laboratories	00008-2511-01

PRODUCT LISTING - EQUIVALENTS NOT AVAILABLE

Tablet - Oral - 30 mcg;0.3 mg

28's	$22.30	LO/OVRAL, Wyeth-Ayerst Laboratories	00008-2514-01

Ethosuximide *(001226)*

Categories: Seizures, absence; FDA Approved 1960 Nov; Pregnancy Category C; WHO Formulary
Drug Classes: Anticonvulsants; Succinimides
Brand Names: Thosutin; **Zarontin**
Foreign Brand Availability: Emeside (England; Korea); Ethosuximide (India); Ethymal (Netherlands); Etosuximida (Spain); Petimid (Turkey); Petinimid (Austria; Czech-Republic); Petnidan (Germany); Suxilep (Bulgaria; Germany; Russia); Suximal (Portugal); Suxinutin (Austria; Bulgaria; Czech-Republic; Finland; Hungary; Sweden; Switzerland); Zarondan (Denmark; Norway)
Cost of Therapy: $62.99 (Epilepsy; Zarontin; 250 mg; 2 capsules/day; 30 day supply)

DESCRIPTION

Zarontin (ethosuximide) is an anticonvulsant succinimide, chemically designated as alpha-ethyl-alpha-methyl-succinimide.

Each Zarontin capsule contains 250 mg ethosuximide. Also contains: polyethylene glycol 400. The capsule contains D&C yellow no. 10; FD&C red no. 3; gelatin; glycerin; and sorbitol.

Storage: Store below 30°C (86°F).

CLINICAL PHARMACOLOGY

Ethosuximide suppresses the paroxysmal 3 cycle per second spike and wave activity associated with lapses of consciousness which is common in absence (petit mal) seizures. The frequency of epileptiform attacks is reduced, apparently by depression of the motor cortex and elevation of the threshold of the central nervous system to convulsive stimuli.

INDICATIONS AND USAGE

Zarontin is indicated for the control of absence (petit mal) epilepsy.

CONTRAINDICATIONS

Ethosuximide should not be used in patients with a history of hypersensitivity to succinimides.

WARNINGS

Blood dyscrasias, including some with fatal outcome, have been reported to be associated with the use of ethosuximide; therefore, periodic blood counts should be performed. Should signs and/or symptoms of infection (*e.g.*, sore throat, fever) develop, blood counts should be considered at that point.

Ethosuximide is capable of producing morphological and functional changes in the animal liver. In humans, abnormal liver and renal function studies have been reported.

Ethosuximide should be administered with extreme caution to patients with known liver or renal disease. Periodic urinalysis and liver function studies are advised for all patients receiving the drug.

Cases of systemic lupus erythematosus have been reported with the use of ethosuximide. The physician should be alert to this possibility.

USAGE IN PREGNANCY

Reports suggest an association between the use of anticonvulsant drugs by women with epilepsy and an elevated incidence of birth defects in children born to these women. Data are more extensive with respect to phenytoin and phenobarbital, but these are also the most commonly prescribed anticonvulsants; less systematic or anecdotal reports suggest a possible similar association with the use of all known anticonvulsant drugs.

The reports suggesting an elevated incidence of birth defects in children of drug-treated epileptic women cannot be regarded as adequate to prove a definite cause and effect relationship. There are intrinsic methodological problems in obtaining adequate data on drug teratogenicity in humans; the possibility also exists that other factors, *e.g.*, genetic factors or the epileptic condition itself, may be more important than drug therapy in leading to birth defects. The great majority of mothers on anticonvulsant medication deliver normal infants. It is important to note that anticonvulsant drugs should not be discontinued in patients in whom the drug is administered to prevent major seizures because of the strong possibility of precipitating status epilepticus with attendant hypoxia and threat to life. In individual cases where the severity and frequency of the seizure disorder are such that the removal of medication does not pose a serious threat to the patient, discontinuation of the drug may be considered prior to and during pregnancy, although it cannot be said with any confidence that even minor seizures do not pose some hazard to the developing embryo or fetus.

The prescribing physician will wish to weigh these considerations in treating or counseling epileptic women of childbearing potential.

PRECAUTIONS

GENERAL

Ethosuximide, when used alone in mixed types of epilepsy, may increase the frequency of grand mal seizures in some patients.

As with other anticonvulsants, it is important to proceed slowly when increasing or decreasing dosage, as well as when adding or eliminating other medication. Abrupt withdrawal of anticonvulsant medication may precipitate absence (petit mal) status.

INFORMATION FOR THE PATIENT

Ethosuximide may impair the mental and/or physical abilities required for the performance of potentially hazardous tasks, such as driving a motor vehicle or other such activity requiring alertness; therefore, the patient should be cautioned accordingly.

Patients taking ethosuximide should be advised of the importance of adhering strictly to the prescribed dosage regimen.

Patients should be instructed to promptly contact their physician if they develop signs and/or symptoms (*e.g.*, sore throat, fever) suggesting an infection.

PREGNANCY

See WARNINGS.

DRUG INTERACTIONS

Since ethosuximide may interact with concurrently administered antiepileptic drugs, periodic serum level determinations of these drugs may be necessary (*e.g.*, ethosuximide may elevate phenytoin serum levels and valproic acid has been reported to both increase and decrease ethosuximide levels).

ADVERSE REACTIONS

Gastrointestinal System: Gastrointestinal symptoms occur frequently and include anorexia, vague gastric upset, nausea and vomiting, cramps, epigastric and abdominal pain, weight loss, and diarrhea. There have been reports of gum hypertrophy and swelling of the tongue.

Hemopoietic System: Hemopoietic complications associated with the administration of ethosuximide have included leukopenia, agranulocytosis, pancytopenia, with or without bone marrow suppression, and eosinophilia.

Nervous System: Neurologic and sensory reactions reported during therapy with ethosuximide have included drowsiness, headache, dizziness, euphoria, hiccups, irritability, hyperactivity, lethargy, fatigue, and ataxia. Psychiatric or psychological aberrations associated with ethosuximide administration have included disturbances of sleep, night terrors, inability to concentrate, and aggressiveness. These effects may be noted particularly in patients who have previously exhibited psychological abnormalities. There have been rare reports of paranoid psychosis, increased libido, and increased state of depression with overt suicidal intentions.

Integumentary System: Dermatologic manifestations which have occurred with the administration of ethosuximide have included urticaria, Stevens-Johnson syndrome, systemic lupus erythematosus, pruritic erythematous rashes, and hirsutism.

Special Senses: Myopia.

Genitourinary System: Vaginal bleeding, microscopic hematuria.

DOSAGE AND ADMINISTRATION

Zarontin is administered by the oral route. The *initial* dose for patients 3-6 years of age is 1 capsule (250 mg) per day; for patients 6 years of age and older, 2 capsules (500 mg) per day. The dose thereafter must be individualized according to the patient's response. Dosage should be increased by small increments. One useful method is to increase the daily dose by 250 mg every four to seven days until control is achieved with minimal side effects. Dosages exceeding 1.5 g daily, in divided doses, should be administered only under the strictest supervision of the physician. The *optimal* dose for most children is 20 mg/kg/day. This dose has given average plasma levels within the accepted therapeutic range of 40-100 μg/ml. Subsequent dose schedules can be based on effectiveness and plasma level determinations.

Zarontin may be administered in combination with other anticonvulsants when other forms of epilepsy coexist with absence (petit mal). The *optimal* dose for most children is 20 mg/kg/day.

PRODUCT LISTING - RATED THERAPEUTICALLY EQUIVALENT

Syrup - Oral - 250 mg/5 ml

5 ml x 40	$76.00	GENERIC, Pharmaceutical Assoc Inc Div Beach Products	00121-0670-05
480 ml	$78.00	GENERIC, Pharmaceutical Assoc Inc Div Beach Products	00121-0670-16
480 ml	$80.95	GENERIC, Teva Pharmaceuticals Usa	00093-9660-16
480 ml	$80.95	GENERIC, Copley	38245-0660-07

PRODUCT LISTING - EQUIVALENTS NOT AVAILABLE

Capsule - Oral - 250 mg

100's	$90.70	GENERIC, Sidmak Laboratories Inc	50111-0901-01
100's	$104.99	ZARONTIN, Parke-Davis	00071-0237-24

Syrup - Oral - 250 mg/5 ml

480 ml	$110.44	ZARONTIN, Parke-Davis	00071-2418-23

Etidronate Disodium *(001234)*

Categories: Ossification, heterotopic; Paget's disease; Pregnancy Category B; FDA Approved 1977 Sep; Orphan Drugs
Drug Classes: Bisphosphonates
Brand Names: Didronel
Foreign Brand Availability: Didronat (Turkey); Didronate (Denmark; Norway; Sweden); Difosfen (Colombia; Costa-Rica; Dominican-Republic; El-Salvador; Guatemala; Panama; Peru; Singapore; Spain); Dinol (Korea); Dronate-OS (India); Etibon (Taiwan); Osteotop (Peru)
Cost of Therapy: $189.99 (Paget's Disease; Didronel; 400 mg; 1 tablet/day; 30 day supply)
HCFA JCODE(S): J1436 per 300 mg IV

INTRAVENOUS

DESCRIPTION

Note: The trade name has been used throughout this monograph for clarity.
Didronel IV infusion is a clear, colorless, sterile solution of etidronate disodium, the disodium salt of (1-hydroxyethylidene) diphosphonic acid. Each 6 ml ampule contains a 5% solution of 300 mg etidronate disodium in water for injection for slow intravenous infusion.

Etidronate disodium is a white powder, highly soluble in water, with a molecular weight of 250.

CLINICAL PHARMACOLOGY

Didronel acts primarily on bone. Its major pharmacologic action is the reduction of normal and abnormal bone resorption. Secondarily, it reduces bone formation since formation is coupled to resorption. This reduces bone turnover, but the reduction of bone turnover, *per se,* is not the important action in the reduction of hypercalcemia. Didronel's reduction of abnormal bone resorption is responsible for its therapeutic benefit in hypercalcemia. The antiresorptive action of Didronel has been demonstrated under a variety of conditions, although the exact mechanism(s) is not fully understood. It may be related to the drug's inhibition of hydroxyapatite crystal dissolution and/or its action on bone resorbing cells. The number of osteoclasts in active bone turnover sites is substantially reduced after Didronel therapy is administered. Didronel also can inhibit the formation and growth of hydroxyapatite crystals and their amorphous precursors at concentrations in excess of those required to inhibit crystal dissolution.

Etidronate disodium is not metabolized. A large fraction of the infused dose is excreted rapidly and unchanged in the urine. The mean residence time in the exchangeable pool is approximately 8.7 ± 1.0 hours. The mean volume of distribution at steady-state in normal humans is 1370 ± 203 ml/kg while the plasma half-life ($T_{1/2}$) is 6.0 ± 0.7 hours. In these same subjects, nonrenal clearance from the exchangeable pool amounts to 30-50% of the infused dose. This nonrenal clearance is considered to be due to uptake of the drug by bone; subsequently the drug is slowly eliminated through bone turnover. The half-life of the dose on bone is in excess of 90 days.

Hyperphosphatemia, which is often observed in association with oral Didronel medication at doses of 10-20 mg/kg/day, occurs less frequently, in association with intravenous medication of patients with hypercalcemia of malignancy.

Hyperphosphatemia is apparently due to increased tubular reabsorption of phosphate by the kidney. No adverse effects have been associated with Didronel-related hyperphosphatemia and its occurrence is not a contraindication to therapy. Serum phosphate elevations usually return to normal 2-4 weeks after medication is discontinued.

The responsiveness of animal tumors susceptible to four commonly employed classes or subclasses of chemotherapeutic agents, antitumor antibiotics (doxorubicin), a classic alkylating agent (cyclophosphamide), a nitrosourea (carmustine), and a pyrimidine antagonist (5-fluorouracil), were not adversely altered by the concurrent administration of intravenous Didronel.

HYPERCALCEMIA OF MALIGNANCY

Hypercalcemia of malignancy is usually related to increased bone resorption associated with the presence of neoplastic tissue. It occurs in 8-20% of patients with malignant disease. Whereas hypercalcemia is more often seen in patients with demonstrable osteolytic, osteoblastic, or mixed metastatic tumors in bone, discrete skeletal lesions cannot be demonstrated in at least 30% of patients.

Patients with certain types of neoplasms, such as carcinoma of the breast, bronchogenic carcinoma, renal cell carcinoma, cancers of the head and neck, lymphomas, and multiple myeloma, are especially prone to developing hypercalcemia.

As hypercalcemia of malignancy evolves, the renal tubules develop a diminished capacity to concentrate urine. The resultant polyuria and nocturia decrease the extracellular fluid volume. This decrease may be aggravated by vomiting and reduced fluid intake. Thus, the ability of the kidney to eliminate excess calcium is compromised. Renal impairment can eventually cause nitrogen retention, acidosis, renal failure, and further decrease in excretion of calcium. Didronel IV infusion, by inhibiting excessive bone resorption, interrupts this process. Salt loading and use of "high ceiling" or "loop" diuretics may be used to promote calcium excretion, because the rate of renal calcium excretion is directly related to the rate of sodium excretion.

The physiologic derangements induced by excessive serum calcium are due to increased levels of ionized calcium. The pathophysiologic effects of excessive serum calcium are heightened by reductions in serum albumin which normally binds a fraction (about 40%) of the total serum calcium. In patients with hypercalcemia of malignancy, serum albumin is often reduced and this tends to mask the magnitude of the increase in the level of ionized calcium. By reducing the flow of calcium from resorbing bone, Didronel IV infusion effectively reduces total and ionized serum calcium.

In the principal clinical study of Didronel for hypercalcemia of malignancy, patients with elevated calcium levels (10.1-17.4 mg/dl) were treated simultaneously with daily administrations of intravenous Didronel over a 3 day period and up to 3000 ml of saline and 80 mg of loop diuretic. The response to treatment for these patients was compared with that from patients treated with saline and loop diuretics alone. In terms of total serum calcium changes, 88% of patients treated with Didronel IV infusion as described, had reductions of serum calcium of 1 mg/dl or more. Total serum calcium returned to normal in 63% of patients within 7 days compared to 33% of patients treated with hydration alone.

Reductions in urinary calcium excretion, which accompany reductions in excessive bone resorption, became apparent after 24 hours. This was accompanied or followed by maximum decreases in serum calcium which were observed, most frequently, 72 hours after the first infusion.

The physiologically important component of serum calcium is the ionized portion. In most institutions, this cannot be measured directly. It is important to recognize that factors influencing the ratio of free and bound calcium such as serum proteins, particularly albumin, may complicate the interpretation of total serum calcium measurements. If indicated, a corrected serum calcium value should be calculated using an established algorithm.

When the total serum calcium values are adjusted for serum albumin levels, there was a return to normocalcemia in 24% of Didronel-treated patients and in 7% of patients treated with saline infusion. Eighty-seven percent (87%) of patients receiving Didronel and 67% of patients on saline had albumin-adjusted serum calcium levels returned to normal or reduced by at least 1 mg/dl.

In the above mentioned study, a second course of Didronel IV infusion was tried in a small number of patients who had a recurrence of hypercalcemia following an initial response to a 3 day infusion of the drug. All patients who received a second 3 day course of Didronel IV infusion showed a decrease of total serum calcium of at least 1 mg/dl. Normalization of total serum calcium occurred in 11 out of 14 patients.

Didronel IV infusion does not appear to alter renal tubular reabsorption of calcium, and does not affect hypercalcemia in patients with hyperparathyroidism where increased calcium reabsorption may be a factor in the hypercalcemia.

Limited clinical study results suggest that continuation of Didronel therapy with oral tablets may maintain clinically acceptable serum calcium levels and prolong normocalcemia.

INDICATIONS AND USAGE

Didronel IV infusion, together with achievement and maintenance of adequate hydration, is indicated for the treatment of hypercalcemia of malignancy inadequately managed by dietary modification and/or oral hydration.

In the treatment of hypercalcemia of malignancy, it is important to initiate rehydration with saline together with "high ceiling" or "loop" diuretics if indicated to restore urine output. This also is intended to increase the renal excretion of calcium and initiate a reduction in serum calcium. Since increased bone resorption is usually the underlying cause of an increased flux of calcium into the vascular compartment, concurrent therapy with Didronel IV infusion is recommended as soon as there is a restoration of urine output. Since Didronel is excreted by the kidney, it is important to know that renal function is adequate to handle not only the increased fluid load but also the excretion of the drug itself. (See WARNINGS.)

Didronel IV infusion is also indicated for the treatment of hypercalcemia of malignancy which persists after adequate hydration has been restored. Patients with and without metastases and with a variety of tumors have been responsive to treatment with Didronel IV infusion. Adequate hydration of patients should be maintained, but in aged patients and in those with cardiac failure, care must be taken to avoid overhydration.

NON-FDA APPROVED INDICATIONS

Although not an FDA approved indication, etidronate is also used in the management of postmenopausal and steroid-induced osteoporosis.

CONTRAINDICATIONS

In patients with Class Dc and higher renal functional impairment (serum creatinine greater than 5.0 mg/dl) Didronel IV infusion should be withheld.

WARNINGS

Occasional mild to moderate abnormalities in renal function (elevated BUN and/or serum creatinine) have been observed when Didronel IV infusion was given as directed to patients with hypercalcemia of malignancy. These changes were reversible or remained stable, without worsening, after completion of the course of Didronel IV infusion. In some patients with pre-existing renal impairment or in those who had received potentially nephrotoxic drugs, further depression of renal function was sometimes seen. This suggests that Didronel IV infusion may produce or aggravate the depression of renal function in approximately 8 of 203 treatment courses when used to treat hypercalcemia of malignancy. Therefore, it is recommended that appropriate monitoring of renal function with serum creatinine and/or BUN be carried out with Didronel IV infusion treatment.

The effects of Didronel IV infusion administration on renal function in patients with serum creatinine greater than 2.5 mg/dl (Class Cc and higher, Classification of Renal Functional Impairment, Council on the Kidney in Cardiovascular Disease, American Heart Association, Ann. Int. Med. 75:251-52, 1971) has not been systematically examined in controlled trials.

Since Didronel is excreted by the kidney, it is important to know that renal function is adequate to handle not only the increased fluid load but also the excretion of the drug itself. Since these capacities are impaired in patients with underlying renal disease and since experience with Didronel IV infusion in patients with serum creatinine >2.5 mg/dl is limited, the use of Didronel IV infusion in such patients should occur only after a careful assessment of renal status or potential risks and potential benefits. (See WARNINGS.)

Reduction of the dose of Didronel IV infusion, if used at all, may be advisable in Class Cc renal functional impairment (serum creatinine 2.5-4.9 mg/dl); and, Didronel IV infusion be used only if the potential benefit of hypercalcemia correction will substantially exceed the potential for worsening of renal function. In patients with Class Dc and higher renal functional impairment (serum creatinine greater than 5.0 mg/dl) Didronel IV infusion should be withheld.

PRECAUTIONS

GENERAL

Hypercalcemia may cause or exacerbate impaired renal function. In clinical trials, while elevations of serum creatinine or blood urea nitrogen were seen in patients with hypercalcemia of malignancy prior to treatment with Didronel IV infusion, these measurements improved in some patients or remained unchanged in most patients. Nevertheless, elevations in serum creatinine during treatment with Didronel IV infusion have been observed in approximately 10% of patients.

Rare cases of acute renal failure have been reported in association with the use of Didronel IV infusion (see also WARNINGS). Concomitant use of non-steroidal anti-inflammatory drugs and diuretics in these patients may have contributed to the renal failure.

In animal preclinical studies, administration of Didronel IV infusion in amounts or at rates in excess of those recommended produced transient hypocalcemia or induced proximal renal tubular damage.

In the principal clinical trial of Didronel IV infusion, 33 of 185 patients (18%) treated one or more times with Didronel IV infusion had serum calcium values below the lower limits of normal. When adjusted for levels of reduced serum albumin, less than 1% of the 185 patients are estimated to have hypocalcemic ionized serum calcium levels. No adverse effects have been traced to hypocalcemia.

The hypercalcemia of hyperparathyroidism is refractory to Didronel IV infusion. It is possible for this disease to coexist in patients with malignancy.

E

CARCINOGENESIS, MUTAGENESIS, AND IMPAIRMENT OF FERTILITY

Long-term studies in rats indicate that Didronel is not carcinogenic.

PREGNANCY, TERATOGENIC EFFECTS, PREGNANCY CATEGORY C

Animal reproduction studies have not been conducted with Didronel IV infusion. It is also not known whether Didronel IV infusion can cause fetal harm when administered to a pregnant woman or can affect reproduction capacity. Didronel IV infusion should be given to a pregnant woman only if clearly needed.

NURSING MOTHERS

It is not known whether this drug is excreted in human milk. Because many drugs are excreted in human milk, caution should be exercised when Didronel IV infusion is administered to a nursing woman.

PEDIATRIC USE

Safety and effectiveness in children have not been established.

ADVERSE REACTIONS

Hypercalcemia of malignancy is frequently associated with abnormal elevations of serum creatinine and BUN. One-third of the patients participating in multiclinic trials had such elevations before receiving Didronel IV infusion. In these trials, the elevations of BUN or serum creatinine improved in some patients, or remained unchanged in most patients; however, in approximately 10% of patients, occasional mild to moderate abnormalities in renal function (increases of >0.5 mg/dl serum creatinine) were observed during or immediately after treatment. The possibility that Didronel IV infusion contributed to these changes can not be excluded (see WARNINGS).

Of patients who participated in the controlled hypercalcemia trials, 10 of 221 (5%) treatment courses reported a metallic or altered taste, or loss of taste, which usually disappeared within hours, during and/or shortly after Didronel IV infusion. A few patients with Paget's Disease of bone have reported allergic skin rashes in association with oral Didronel medication.

DOSAGE AND ADMINISTRATION

DIDRONEL IV INFUSION

The recommended dose of Didronel IV infusion is 7.5 mg/kg body weight/day on 3 successive days. **This daily dose must be diluted in at least 250 ml of sterile normal saline.** Stability studies show that diluted solution stored at controlled room temperature (59-86°F or 15-30°C) shows no loss of drug for a 48 hour period.

THE DILUTED DOSE OF DIDRONEL IV INFUSION SHOULD BE ADMINISTERED INTRAVENOUSLY OVER A PERIOD OF AT LEAST 2 HOURS. Didronel IV infusion may be added to volumes of sterile, normal saline greater than 250 ml when this is convenient.

REGARDLESS OF THE VOLUME OF SOLUTION IN WHICH DIDRONEL IV INFUSION IS DILUTED, SLOW INFUSION IS IMPORTANT TO SAFETY. The minimum infusion time of 2 hours at the recommended dose or smaller doses, should be observed. The usual course of treatment is one infusion of 7.5 mg/kg body weight/day on each of 3 consecutive days but some patients have been treated for up to 7 days. When patients are treated for more than 3 days, there may be an increased possibility of producing hypocalcemia.

Retreatment with Didronel IV infusion may be appropriate if hypercalcemia recurs. There should be at least a 7 day interval between courses of treatment with Didronel IV infusion. The dose and manner of retreatment is the same as that for initial treatment. Retreatment for more than 3 days has not been adequately studied. The safety and efficacy of more than two courses of therapy with Didronel IV infusion have not been studied. In the presence of renal impairment, reduction of the dose may be advisable.

Parenteral drug products should be inspected visually for particulate matter and discoloration prior to administration whenever solution and container permit.

DIDRONEL ORAL TABLETS

Didronel (etidronate disodium) tablets may be started on the day following the last dose of Didronel IV infusion. The recommended oral dose of Didronel for patients who have had hypercalcemia is 20 mg/kg body for 30 days. If serum calcium levels remain normal or at clinically acceptable levels, treatment may be extended. Treatment for more than 90 days has not been adequately studied and is not recommended. Please consult the package insert pertaining to oral Didronel tablets for additional prescribing information.

HOW SUPPLIED

Didronel IV infusion is supplied in 6 ml ampules as a 5% solution containing 300 mg etidronate disodium.

Storage: Avoid excessive heat (over 40°C or 104°F) for undiluted product.

ORAL

DESCRIPTION

Note: The trade name has been used throughout this monograph for clarity.

Didronel tablets contain either 200 or 400 mg of etidronate disodium, the disodium salt of (1-hydroxyethylidene) diphosphonic acid, for oral administration. This compound, also known as EHDP, regulates bone metabolism. It is a white powder, highly soluble in water, with a molecular weight of 250.

Inactive Ingredients: Each tablet contains magnesium stearate, microcrystalline cellulose, and starch.

CLINICAL PHARMACOLOGY

Etidronate disodium acts primarily on bone. It can inhibit the formation, growth, and dissolution of hydroxyapatite crystals and their amorphous precursors by chemisorption to calcium phosphate surfaces. Inhibition of crystal resorption occurs at lower doses than are required to inhibit crystal growth. Both effects increase as the dose increases.

Etidronate disodium is not metabolized. The amount of drug absorbed after an oral dose is approximately 3%. In normal subjects, plasma half-life ($T_{1/2}$) of etidronate, based on non-compartmental pharmacokinetics is 1-6 hours. Within 24 hours, approximately half the absorbed dose is excreted in urine; the remainder is distributed to bone compartments from which it is slowly eliminated. Animal studies have yielded bone clearance estimates up to 165 days. In humans, the residence time on bone may vary due to such factors as specific metabolic condition and bone type. Unabsorbed drug is excreted intact in the feces. Preclinical studies indicate etidronate disodium does not cross the blood-brain barrier.

Etidronate disodium therapy does not adversely affect serum levels of parathyroid hormone or calcium.

PAGET'S DISEASE

Paget's disease of bone (osteitis deformans) is an idiopathic, progressive disease characterized by abnormal and accelerated bone metabolism in one or more bones. Signs and symptoms may include bone pain and/or deformity, neurologic disorders, elevated cardiac output and other vascular disorders, and increased serum alkaline phosphatase and/or urinary hydroxyproline levels. Bone fractures are common in patients with Paget's disease.

Etidronate disodium slows accelerated bone turnover (resorption and accretion) in pagetic lesions and, to a lesser extent, in normal bone. This has been demonstrated histologically, scintigraphically, biochemically, and through calcium kinetic and balance studies. Reduced bone turnover is often accompanied by symptomatic improvement, including reduced bone pain. Also, the incidence of pagetic fractures may be reduced, and elevated cardiac output and other vascular disorders may be improved by etidronate disodium therapy.

HETEROTOPIC OSSIFICATION

Heterotopic ossification, also referred to as myositis ossificans (circumscripta, progressiva or traumatica), ectopic calcification, periarticular ossification, or paraosteoarthropathy, is characterized by metaplastic osteogenesis. It usually presents with signs of localized inflammation or pain, elevated skin temperature, and redness. When tissues near joints are involved, functional loss may also be present.

Heterotopic ossification may occur for no known reason as in myositis ossificans progressiva or may follow a wide variety of surgical, occupational, and sports trauma (*e.g.*, hip arthroplasty, spinal cord injury, head injury, burns, and severe thigh bruises). Heterotopic ossification has also been observed in non-traumatic conditions (*e.g.*, infections of the central nervous system, peripheral neuropathy, tetanus, biliary cirrhosis, Peyronie's disease, as well as in association with a variety of benign and malignant neoplasms).

Clinical trials have demonstrated the efficacy of etidronate disodium in heterotopic ossification following total hip replacement, or due to spinal cord injury.

Heterotopic ossification complicating total hip replacement typically develops radiographically 3-8 weeks postoperatively in the pericapsular area of the affected hip joint. The overall incidence is about 50%; about one-third of these cases are clinically significant.

Heterotopic ossification due to spinal cord injury typically develops radiographically 1-4 months after injury. It occurs below the level of injury, usually at major joints. The overall incidence is about 40%; about one-half of these cases are clinically significant.

Etidronate disodium chemisorbs to calcium hydroxyapatite crystals and their amorphous precursors, blocking the aggregation, growth, and mineralization of these crystals. This is thought to be the mechanism by which etidronate disodium prevents or retards heterotopic ossification. There is no evidence etidronate disodium affects mature heterotopic bone.

INDICATIONS AND USAGE

Etidronate disodium is indicated for the treatment of symptomatic Paget's disease of bone and in the prevention and treatment of heterotopic ossification following total hip replacement or due to spinal cord injury. Etidronate disodium is not approved for the treatment of osteoporosis.

PAGET'S DISEASE

Etidronate disodium is indicated for the treatment of symptomatic Paget's disease of bone. Etidronate disodium therapy usually arrests or significantly impedes the disease process as evidenced by:

- Symptomatic relief, including decreased pain and/or increased mobility (experienced by 3 out of 5 patients).
- Reductions in serum alkaline phosphatase and urinary hydroxyproline levels (30% or more in 4 out of 5 patients).
- Histomorphometry showing reduced numbers of osteoclasts and osteoblasts, and more lamellar bone formation.
- Bone scans showing reduced radionuclide uptake at pagetic lesions.

In addition, reductions in pagetically elevated cardiac output and skin temperature have been observed in some patients.

In many patients, the disease process will be suppressed for a period of at least 1 year following cessation of therapy. The upper limit of this period has not been determined.

The effects of the etidronate disodium treatment in patients with asymptomatic Paget's disease have not been studied. However, etidronate disodium treatment of such patients may be warranted if extensive involvement threatens irreversible neurologic damage, major joints, or major weight-bearing bones.

HETEROTOPIC OSSIFICATION

Etidronate disodium is indicated in the prevention and treatment of heterotopic ossification following total hip replacement or due to spinal cord injury.

Etidronate disodium reduces the incidence of clinically important heterotopic bone by about two-thirds. Among those patients who form heterotopic bone, etidronate disodium retards the progression of immature lesions and reduces the severity by at least half. Follow-up data (at least 9 months posttherapy) suggest these benefits persist.

In total hip replacement patients, etidronate disodium does not promote loosening of the prosthesis or impede trochanteric reattachment.

In spinal cord injury patients, etidronate disodium does not inhibit fracture healing or stabilization of the spine.

NON-FDA APPROVED INDICATIONS

Although not an FDA approved indication, etidronate is also used in the management of postmenopausal and steroid-induced osteoporosis.

CONTRAINDICATIONS

Etidronate disodium tablets are contraindicated in patients with known hypersensitivity to etidronate disodium or in patients with clinically overt osteomalacia.

WARNINGS

PAGET'S DISEASE

In Paget's patients the response to therapy may be of slow onset and continue for months after etidronate disodium therapy is discontinued. Dosage should not be increased prematurely. A 90 day drug-free interval should be provided between courses of therapy.

HETEROTOPIC OSSIFICATION

No specific warnings.

PRECAUTIONS

GENERAL

Patients should maintain an adequate nutritional status, particularly an adequate intake of calcium and vitamin D.

Therapy has been withheld from some patients with enterocolitis since diarrhea may be experienced, particularly at higher doses.

Etidronate disodium is not metabolized and is excreted intact via the kidney. Hyperphosphatemia may occur at doses of 10-20 mg/kg/day, apparently as a result of drug-related increases in tubular reabsorption of phosphate. Serum phosphate levels generally return to normal 2-4 weeks posttherapy. There is no experience to specifically guide treatment in patients with impaired renal function. Etidronate disodium dosage should be reduced when reductions in glomerular filtration rates are present. Patients with renal impairment should be closely monitored. In approximately 10% of patients in clinical trials of etidronate disodium IV infusion for hypercalcemia of malignancy, occasional, mild-to-moderate abnormalities in renal function (increases of >0.5 mg/dl serum creatinine) were observed during or immediately after treatment.

Etidronate disodium suppresses bone turnover, and may retard mineralization of osteoid laid down during the bone accretion process. These effects are dose and time dependent. Osteoid, which may accumulate noticeably at doses of 10-20 mg/kg/day, mineralizes normally posttherapy. In patients with fractures, especially of long bones, it may be advisable to delay or interrupt treatment until callus is evident.

Paget's Disease

In Paget's patients, treatment regimens exceeding the recommended (see DOSAGE AND ADMINISTRATION) daily maximum dose of 20 mg/kg or continuous administration of medication for periods greater than 6 months may be associated with osteomalacia and an increased risk of fracture.

Long bones predominantly affected by lytic lesions, particularly in those patients unresponsive to etidronate disodium therapy, may be especially prone to fracture.

Patients with predominantly lytic lesions should be monitored radiographically and biochemically to permit termination of etidronate disodium in those patients unresponsive to treatment.

CARCINOGENESIS

Long-term studies in rats have indicated that etidronate disodium is not carcinogenic.

PREGNANCY, TERATOGENIC EFFECTS, PREGNANCY CATEGORY C

In teratology and developmental toxicity studies conducted in rats and rabbits treated with dosages of up to 100 mg/kg (5-20 times the clinical dose), no adverse or teratogenic effects have been observed in the offspring. Etidronate disodium has been shown to cause skeletal abnormalities in rats when given at oral dose levels of 300 mg/kg (15-60 times the human dose). Other effects on the offspring (including decreased live births) are at dosages that cause significant toxicity in the parent generation and are 25-200 times the human dose. The skeletal effects are thought to be the result of the pharmacological effects of the drug on bone.

There are no adequate and well-controlled studies in pregnant women. Etidronate disodium should be used during pregnancy only if the potential benefit justifies the potential risk to the fetus.

NURSING MOTHERS

It is not known whether this drug is excreted in human milk. Because many drugs are excreted in human milk, caution should be exercised when etidronate disodium is administered to a nursing woman.

PEDIATRIC USE

Safety and effectiveness in pediatric patients have not been established. Pediatric patients have been treated with etidronate disodium, at doses recommended for adults, to prevent heterotopic ossifications or soft tissue calcifications. A rachitic syndrome has been reported infrequently at doses of 10 mg/kg/day and more for prolonged periods approaching or exceeding a year. The epiphyseal radiologic changes associated with retarded mineralization of new osteoid and cartilage, and occasional symptoms reported, have been reversible when medication is discontinued.

GERIATRIC USE

Clinical studies of etidronate disodium did not include sufficient numbers of subjects aged 65 and over to determine whether they respond differently from younger subjects. Other reported clinical experience has not identified differences in responses between elderly and younger patients. In general, dose selection for an elderly patient should be cautious reflecting the greater frequency of decreased hepatic, renal, or cardiac function, and of concomitant disease or other drug therapy. This drug is known to be substantially excreted by the kidney, and the risk of toxic reactions to this drug may be greater in patients with impaired renal function. Because elderly patients are more likely to have decreased renal function, care should be taken when prescribing this drug therapy. As stated in PRECAUTIONS, etidronate disodium dosage should be reduced when reductions in glomerular filtration rates are present. In addition, patients with renal impairment should be closely monitored.

DRUG INTERACTIONS

There have been isolated reports of patients experiencing increases in their prothrombin times when etidronate was added to warfarin therapy. The majority of these reports concerned variable elevations in prothrombin times without clinically significant sequelae. Although the relevance of these reports and any mechanism of coagulation alterations is unclear, patients on warfarin should have their prothrombin time monitored.

ADVERSE REACTIONS

The incidence of gastrointestinal complaints (diarrhea, nausea) is the same for etidronate disodium at 5 mg/kg/day as for placebo, about 1 patient in 15. At 10-20 mg/kg/day the incidence may increase to 2 or 3 in 10. These complaints are often alleviated by dividing the total daily dose.

PAGET'S DISEASE

In Paget's patients, increased or recurrent bone pain at pagetic sites, and/or the onset of pain at previously asymptomatic sites has been reported. At 5 mg/kg/day about 1 patient in 10 (vs 1 in 15 in the placebo group) report these phenomena. At higher doses the incidence rises to about 2 in 10. When therapy continues, pain resolves in some patients but persists in others.

HETEROTOPIC OSSIFICATION

No specific adverse reactions.

WORLDWIDE POSTMARKETING EXPERIENCE

The worldwide postmarketing experience for etidronate disodium reflects its use in the following approved indications: Paget's disease, heterotopic ossification, and hypercalcemia of malignancy. It also reflects the use of etidronate disodium for osteoporosis where approved in countries outside the US. Other adverse events that have been reported and were thought to be possibly related to etidronate disodium include the following: alopecia; arthropathies, including arthralgia and arthritis; bone fracture; esophagitis; glossitis; hypersensitivity reactions, including angioedema, follicular eruption, macular rash, maculopapular rash, pruritus, a single case of Stevens-Johnson syndrome, and urticaria; osteomalacia; neuropsychiatric events, including amnesia, confusion, depression, and hallucination; and paresthesias.

In patients receiving etidronate disodium, there have been rare reports of agranulocytosis, pancytopenia, and a report of leukopenia with recurrence on rechallenge. In addition, there have been rare reports of exacerbation of asthma. Exacerbation of existing peptic ulcer disease has been reported in a few patients. In 1 patient, perforation also occurred.

In osteoporosis clinical trials, headache, gastritis, leg cramps, and arthralgia occurred at a significantly greater incidence in patients who received etidronate as compared with those who received placebo.

DOSAGE AND ADMINISTRATION

Etidronate disodium should be taken as a single, oral dose. However, should gastrointestinal discomfort occur, the dose may be divided. To maximize absorption, patients should avoid taking the following items within 2 hours of dosing:

Food, especially food high in calcium, such as milk or milk products.

Vitamins with mineral supplements or antacids which are high in metals such as calcium, iron, magnesium, or aluminum.

PAGET'S DISEASE

Initial Treatment Regimens

5-10 mg/kg/day, not to exceed 6 months, or 11-20 mg/kg/day, not to exceed 3 months.

The recommended initial dose is 5 mg/kg/day for a period not to exceed 6 months. Doses above 10 mg/kg/day should be reserved for when (1) lower doses are ineffective or (2) there is an overriding need to suppress rapid bone turnover (especially when irreversible neurologic damage is possible) or reduce elevated cardiac output. Doses in excess of 20 mg/kg/day are not recommended.

Retreatment Guidelines
Retreatment should be initiated only after (1) a etidronate disodium-free period of at least 90 days and (2) there is biochemical, symptomatic or other evidence of active disease process. It is advisable to monitor patients every 3-6 months although some patients may go drug free for extended periods. Retreatment regimens are the same as for initial treatment. For most patients the original dose will be adequate for retreatment. If not, consideration should be given to increasing the dose within the recommended guidelines.

HETEROTOPIC OSSIFICATION
The following treatment regimens have been shown to be effective:
Total Hip Replacement Patients: 20 mg/kg/day for 1 month before and 3 months after surgery (4 months total).
Spinal Cord Injured Patients: 20 mg/kg/day for 2 weeks followed by 10 mg/kg/day for 10 weeks (12 weeks total). Etidronate disodium therapy should begin as soon as medically feasible following the injury, preferably prior to evidence of heterotopic ossification.

Retreatment has not been studied.

HOW SUPPLIED

Didronel is available in:
200 mg: White, rectangular tablets with "P & G" on one face and "402" on the other.
400 mg: White, scored, capsule-shaped tablets with "N E" on one face and "406" on the other.
Storage: Avoid excessive heat (over 40°C or 104°F).

PRODUCT LISTING - EQUIVALENTS NOT AVAILABLE

Solution - Intravenous - 50 mg/ml
6 ml x 6 $402.00 DIDRONEL I.V., Mgi Pharma Inc 58063-0457-01
Tablet - Oral - 200 mg
60's $190.03 DIDRONEL, Procter and Gamble Pharmaceuticals 00149-0405-60
Tablet - Oral - 400 mg
60's $379.98 DIDRONEL, Procter and Gamble Pharmaceuticals 00149-0406-60

Etodolac *(003029)*

For related information, see the comparative table section in Appendix A.

Categories: Arthritis, osteoarthritis; Pain; Pregnancy Category C; FDA Approved 1991 Jan
Drug Classes: Analgesics, non-narcotic; Nonsteroidal anti-inflammatory drugs
Brand Names: Lodine
Foreign Brand Availability: Ecridoxan (Greece); Entrang (Korea); Etodin (Korea); Etonox (Thailand); Etopan (Israel); Etopan XL (Israel); Hypen (Japan); Lodine LP (France); Lodine Retard (Mexico); Lodine SR (Hong-Kong); Lonene (Indonesia); Lonine (Greece; Taiwan); Osteluc (Japan); Tedolan (Denmark); Toselac (Korea); Ultradol (Canada)
Cost of Therapy: $93.33 (Osteoarthritis; Lodine; 300 mg; 2 capsules/day; 30 day supply)
$75.14 (Osteoarthritis; Generic Capsules; 300 mg; 2 capsules/day; 30 day supply)

DESCRIPTION

Lodine is a pyranocarboxylic acid chemically designated as (±) 1,8-diethyl-1,3,4,9-tetrahydropyrano-[3,4-b]indole-1-acetic acid. Lodine is a racemic mixture of R- and S-etodolac.

The molecular formula for etodolac is $C_{17}H_{21}NO_3$. The molecular weight of the base is 287.37. It has a pKa of 4.65 and an n-octanol:water partition coefficient of 11.4 at pH 7.4. Etodolac is a white crystalline compound, insoluble in water but soluble in alcohols, chloroform, dimethyl sulfoxide, and aqueous polyethylene glycol.

The inactive ingredients present in the capsules are cellulose, gelatin, iron oxides, lactose, magnesium stearate, povidone, sodium lauryl sulfate, sodium starch glycolate, and titanium dioxide.

The inactive ingredients present in the tablets are cellulose, FD&C yellow no. 10, FD&C blue no. 2, FD&C yellow no. 6, hydroxypropyl methylcellulose, lactose, magnesium stearate, polyethylene glycol, polysorbate 80, povidone, sodium starch glycolate, and titanium dioxide.

Lodine is available in 200 and 300 mg capsules and 400 mg tablets for oral administration.

CLINICAL PHARMACOLOGY

Etodolac is a nonsteroidal anti-inflammatory drug (NSAID) that exhibits anti-inflammatory, analgesic, and antipyretic activities in animal models. The mechanism of action of etodolac, like that of other NSAIDs, is not known but is believed to be associated with the inhibition of prostaglandin biosynthesis.

Etodolac is a racemic mixture of [−]R- and [+]S-etodolac. As with other NSAIDs, it has been demonstrated in animals that the [+]S-form is biologically active. Both enantiomers are stable and there is no [−]R to [+]S conversion *in vivo*.

PHARMACODYNAMICS
Analgesia was demonstrable by ½ hour following single doses of 200-400 mg etodolac, with the peak effect occurring in 1-2 hours. The analgesic effect generally lasted for 4-6 hours.

PHARMACOKINETICS
The pharmacokinetics of etodolac have been evaluated in 267 normal subjects, 44 elderly patients (>65 years old), 19 patients with renal failure (creatinine clearance 37-88 ml/min), 9 patients on hemodialysis, and 10 patients with compensated hepatic cirrhosis.

Etodolac, when administered orally, exhibits kinetics that are well described by a two-compartment model with first-order absorption.

Etodolac has no apparent pharmacokinetic interaction when administered with phenytoin, glyburide, furosemide or hydrochlorothiazide.

ABSORPTION
Etodolac is well absorbed and had a relative bioavailability of 100% when 200 mg capsules were compared with a solution of etodolac. Based on mass balance studies, the systemic availability of etodolac from either the tablet or capsule formulation, is at least 80%. Etodolac does not undergo significant first-pass metabolism following oral administration. Mean (±1 SD) peak plasma concentrations range from approximately 14 ± 4 to 37 ± 9 µg/ml after 200-600 mg single doses and are reached in 80 ± 30 minutes (see TABLE 1 for summary of pharmacokinetic parameters). The dose-proportionality based on AUC (the area under the plasma concentration-time curve) is linear following doses up to 600 mg every 12 hours. Peak concentrations are dose-proportional for both total and free etodolac following doses up to 400 mg every 12 hours, but following a 600 mg dose, the peak is about 20% higher than predicted on the basis of lower doses.

***TABLE 1** Etodolac Steady-State Pharmacokinetic Parameters (N=267)*

Kinetic Parameters	Mean ± SD
Extent of oral absorption (bioavailability) [F]	≥80%
Oral-dose clearance [CL/F]	47 ± 16 ml/h/kg
Steady-state volume [V_{ss}/F]	362 ± 129 ml/kg
Distribution half-life [$T_{1/2}$, α]	0.71 ± 0.50 h
Terminal half-life [$T_{1/2}$, β]	7.3 ± 4.0 h

Antacid Effects
The extent of absorption of etodolac is not affected when etodolac is administered with an antacid. Coadministration with an antacid decreases the peak concentration reached by about 15-20%, with no measurable effect on time-to-peak.

Food Effect on Absorption
The extent of absorption of etodolac is not affected when etodolac is administered after a meal. Food intake, however, reduces the peak concentration reached by approximately one half and increases the time-to-peak concentration by 1.4-3.8 hours.

DISTRIBUTION
Etodolac has an apparent steady-state volume of distribution about 0.362 L/kg. Within the therapeutic dose range, etodolac is more than 99% bound to plasma proteins. The free fraction is less than 1% and is independent of etodolac total concentration over the dose range studied.

METABOLISM
Etodolac is extensively metabolized in the liver, with renal elimination of etodolac and its metabolites being the primary route of excretion. The intersubject variability of etodolac plasma levels, achieved after recommended doses, is substantial.

PROTEIN BINDING
Data from *in vitro* studies, using peak serum concentrations at reported therapeutic doses in humans, show that the etodolac free fraction is not significantly altered by acetaminophen, ibuprofen, indomethacin, naproxen, piroxicam, chlorpropamide, glipizide, glyburide, phenytoin, and probenecid.

ELIMINATION
The mean plasma clearance of etodolac, is 47 (± 16) ml/h/kg, and terminal disposition half-life is 7.3 (± 4.0) hours. Approximately 72% of the administered dose is recovered in the urine as the following, indicated as % of the administered dose.
- Etodolac, unchanged: 1%.
- Etodolac glucuronide: 13%.
- Hydroxylated metabolite (6-, 7-, and 8-OH): 5%.
- Hydroxylated metabolite glucuronides: 20%.
- Unidentified metabolites: 33%.

Fecal excretion accounted for 16% of the dose.

SPECIAL POPULATIONS
Elderly Patients
In clinical studies, etodolac clearance was reduced by about 15% in older patients (>65 years of age). In these studies, age was shown not to have any effect on etodolac half-life or protein binding, and there was no change in expected drug accumulation. No dosage adjustment is generally necessary in the elderly on the basis of pharmacokinetics. The elderly may need dosage adjustment, however, on the basis of body size (see PRECAUTIONS, Geriatric Use), as they may be more sensitive to antiprostaglandin effects than younger patients (see PRECAUTIONS, Geriatric Use).

Renal Impairment
Studies in patients with mild-to-moderate renal impairment (creatinine clearance 37-88 ml/min) showed no significant differences in the disposition of total and free etodolac. In patients undergoing hemodialysis, there was a 50% greater apparent clearance of total etodolac, due to a 50% greater unbound fraction. Free etodolac clearance was not altered, indicating the importance of protein binding in etodolac's disposition. Nevertheless, etodolac is not dialyzable.

Hepatic Impairment
In patients with compensated hepatic cirrhosis, the disposition of total and free etodolac is not altered. Although no dosage adjustment is generally required in this patient population, etodolac clearance is dependent on hepatic function and could be reduced in patients with severe hepatic failure.

INDICATIONS AND USAGE

Etodolac is indicated for acute and long-term use in the management of signs and symptoms of osteoarthritis. Etodolac is also indicated for the management of pain.

NON-FDA APPROVED INDICATIONS

While etodolac has also been used for the treatment of rheumatoid arthritis, it has generally been found to be less effective than other nonsteroidal anti-inflammatory agents. Etodolac is not FDA approved for the management of rheumatoid arthritis.

CONTRAINDICATIONS

Etodolac is contraindicated in patients with known hypersensitivity to etodolac. Etodolac should not be given to patients who have experienced asthma, urticaria, or other allergic-type reactions after taking aspirin or other NSAIDs. Severe, rarely fatal, anaphylactic-like reactions to etodolac have been reported in such patients (see WARNINGS, Anaphylactic Reactions).

WARNINGS

RISK OF GASTROINTESTINAL (GI) ULCERATION, BLEEDING, AND PERFORATION WITH NONSTEROIDAL ANTI-INFLAMMATORY DRUG (NSAID) THERAPY

Serious GI toxicity, such as bleeding, ulceration, and perforation, can occur at any time, with or without warning symptoms, in patients treated chronically with NSAIDs. Although minor upper GI problems, such as dyspepsia, are common, usually developing early in therapy, physicians should remain alert for ulceration and bleeding in patients treated chronically with NSAIDs, even in the absence of previous GI-tract symptoms. In patients observed in clinical trials of such agents for several months' to 2 years' duration, symptomatic upper GI ulcers, gross bleeding, or perforation appears to occur in approximately 1% of patients treated for 3-6 months and in about 2-4% of patients treated for 1 year. Physicians should inform patients about the signs and/or symptoms of serious GI toxicity and what steps to take if they occur.

Studies to date have not identified any subset of patients not at risk of developing peptic ulceration and bleeding. Except for a prior history of serious GI events and other risk factors known to be associated with peptic ulcer disease, such as alcoholism, smoking, etc., no risk factors (*e.g.*, age, sex) have been associated with increased risk. Elderly or debilitated patients seem to tolerate ulceration or bleeding less well than other individuals, and most spontaneous reports of fatal GI events are in this population. Studies to date are inconclusive concerning the relative risk of various NSAIDs in causing such reactions. High doses of any NSAID probably carry a greater risk of these reactions, although controlled clinical trials showing this do not exist in most cases. In considering the use of relatively large doses (within the recommended dosage range), sufficient benefit should be anticipated to offset the potential increased risk of GI toxicity.

ANAPHYLACTIC REACTIONS

Anaphylactoid reactions may occur in patients without prior exposure to etodolac. Etodolac should not be given to patients with the aspirin triad. The triad typically occurs in asthmatic patients who experience rhinitis with or without nasal polyps, or who exhibit severe, potentially fatal bronchospasm after taking aspirin or other nonsteroidal anti-inflammatory drugs. Fatal reactions have been reported in such patients (see CONTRAINDICATIONS and PRECAUTIONS, Pre-Existing Asthma). Emergency help should be sought in cases where an anaphylactoid reaction occurs.

ADVANCED RENAL DISEASE

In cases with advanced kidney disease, as with other NSAIDs, treatment with etodolac should only be initiated with close monitoring of the patient's kidney function (see PRECAUTIONS, Renal Effects).

USE IN PREGNANCY

In late pregnancy, as with other NSAIDs, etodolac should be avoided because it may cause premature closure of the ductus arteriosus (see PRECAUTIONS, Pregnancy, Teratogenic Effects, Pregnancy Category C).

PRECAUTIONS

GENERAL

Renal Effects

As with other NSAIDs, long-term administration of etodolac to rats has resulted in renal papillary necrosis and other renal medullary changes. Renal pelvic transitional epithelial hyperplasia, a spontaneous change occurring with variable frequency, was observed with increased frequency in treated male rats in a 2 year chronic study.

A second form of renal toxicity encountered with etodolac, as with other NSAIDs, is seen in patients with conditions in which renal prostaglandins have a supportive role in the maintenance of renal perfusion. In these patients, administration of a nonsteroidal anti-inflammatory drug may cause a dose-dependent reduction in prostaglandin formation and, secondarily, in renal blood flow, which may precipitate overt renal decompensation. Patients at greatest risk of this reaction are those with impaired renal function, heart failure, or liver dysfunction; those taking diuretics; and the elderly. Discontinuation of nonsteroidal anti-inflammatory drug therapy is usually followed by recovery to the pretreatment state.

Etodolac metabolites are eliminated primarily by the kidneys. The extent to which the inactive glucuronide metabolites may accumulate in patients with renal failure has not been studied. As with other drugs whose metabolites are excreted by the kidney, the possibility that adverse reactions (not listed in ADVERSE REACTIONS) may be attributable to these metabolites should be considered.

Hepatic Effects

Borderline elevations of one or more liver tests may occur in up to 15% of patients taking NSAIDs, including etodolac. These abnormalities may disappear, remain essentially unchanged, or progress with continued therapy. Meaningful elevations of ALT or AST (approximately three or more times the upper limit of normal) have been reported in approximately 1% of patients in clinical trials with etodolac. A patient with symptoms and/or signs suggesting liver dysfunction, or in whom an abnormal liver test has occurred, should be evaluated for evidence of the development of a more severe hepatic reaction while on therapy with etodolac. Rare cases of liver necrosis and hepatic failure, some of them with fatal outcomes have been reported. If clinical signs and symptoms consistent with liver disease develop, or if systemic manifestations occur (*e.g.*, eosinophilia, rash, etc.), etodolac should be discontinued.

Hematological Effects

Anemia is sometimes seen in patients receiving NSAIDs including etodolac. This may be due to fluid retention, GI blood loss, or an incompletely described effect upon erythropoiesis. Patients on long-term treatment with NSAIDs, including etodolac, should have their hemoglobin or hematocrit checked if they exhibit any signs or symptoms of anemia.

All drugs which inhibit the biosynthesis of prostaglandins may interfere to some extent with platelet function and vascular responses to bleeding.

Fluid Retention and Edema

Fluid retention and edema have been observed in some patients taking NSAIDs, including etodolac. Therefore, etodolac should be used with caution in patients with fluid retention, hypertension, or heart failure.

Pre-Existing Asthma

About 10% of patients with asthma may have aspirin-sensitive asthma. The use of aspirin in patients with aspirin-sensitive asthmas has been associated with severe bronchospasm which can be fatal. Since cross reactivity, including bronchospasm, between aspirin and other nonsteroidal anti-inflammatory drugs has been reported in such aspirin-sensitive patients, etodolac should not be administered to patients with this form of aspirin sensitivity and should be used with caution in all patients with pre-existing asthma.

INFORMATION FOR THE PATIENT

Etodolac, like other drugs of its class, can cause discomfort and, rarely, more serious side effects, such as gastrointestinal bleeding, which may result in hospitalization and even fatal outcomes.

Physicians may wish to discuss with their patients the potential risks (see WARNINGS, PRECAUTIONS, ADVERSE REACTIONS) and likely benefits of nonsteroidal anti-inflammatory drug treatment.

Patients on etodolac should report to their physicians signs or symptoms of gastrointestinal ulceration or bleeding, blurred vision or other eye symptoms, skin rash, weight gain, or edema.

Because serious gastrointestinal tract ulcerations and bleeding can occur without warning symptoms, physicians should follow chronically treated patients for the signs and symptoms of ulcerations and bleeding and should inform them of the importance of this follow-up (see WARNINGS, Risk of Gastrointestinal (GI) Ulceration, Bleeding and Perforation With Nonsteroidal Anti-Inflammatory Drug (NSAID) Therapy).

Patients should also be instructed to seek medical emergency help in case of an occurrence of anaphylactoid reactions (see WARNINGS).

LABORATORY TESTS

Patients on long-term treatment with etodolac, as with other NSAIDs, should have their hemoglobin or hematocrit checked periodically for signs or symptoms of anemia. Appropriate measures should be taken in case such signs of anemia occur.

If clinical signs and symptoms consistent with liver disease develop or if systemic manifestations occur (*e.g.*, eosinophilia, rash, etc.) and if abnormal liver tests are detected, persist or worsen, etodolac should be discontinued.

DRUG/LABORATORY TEST INTERACTIONS

The urine of patients who take etodolac can give a false-positive reaction for urinary bilirubin (urobilin) due to the presence of phenolic metabolites of etodolac. Diagnostic dipstick methodology, used to detect ketone bodies in urine, has resulted in false-positive findings in some patients treated with etodolac. Generally, this phenomenon has not been associated with other clinically significant events. No dose-relationship has been observed.

Etodolac treatment is associated with a small decrease in serum uric acid levels. In clinical trials, mean decreases of 1-2 mg/dl were observed in arthritic patients receiving etodolac (600-1000 mg/day) after 4 weeks of therapy. These levels then remained stable for up to 1 year of therapy.

CARCINOGENESIS, MUTAGENESIS, AND IMPAIRMENT OF FERTILITY

No carcinogenic effect of etodolac was observed in mice or rats receiving oral doses of 15 mg/kg/day (45-89 mg/m^2, respectively) or less for periods of 2 years or 18 months, respectively. Etodolac was not mutagenic in *in vitro* tests performed with *S. typhimurium* and mouse lymphoma cells as well as in an *in vivo* mouse micronucleus test. However, data from the *in vitro* human peripheral lymphocyte test showed an increase in the number of gaps (3.0-5.3% unstained regions in the chromatid without dislocation) among the etodolac-treated cultures (50-200 μg/ml) compared to negative controls (2.0%); no other difference was noted between the controls and drug-treated groups. Etodolac showed no impairment of fertility in male and female rats up to oral doses of 16 mg/kg (94 mg/m^2). However, reduced implantation of fertilized eggs occurred in the 8 mg/kg group.

PREGNANCY, TERATOGENIC EFFECTS, PREGNANCY CATEGORY C

In teratology studies, isolated occurrences of alterations in limb development were found and included polydactyly, oligodactyly, syndactyly, and unossified phalanges in rats and oligodactyly and synostosis of metatarsals in rabbits. These were observed at dose levels (2-14 mg/kg/day) close to human clinical doses. However, the frequency and the dosage group distribution of these findings in initial or repeated studies did not establish a clear drug or dose-response relationship.

There are no adequate or well-controlled studies in pregnant women. Etodolac should be used during pregnancy only if the potential benefits justify the potential risk to the fetus. Because of the known effects of NSAIDs on parturition and on the human fetal cardiovascular system with respect to closure of the ductus arteriosus, use during late pregnancy should be avoided.

LABOR AND DELIVERY

In rat studies with etodolac, as with other drugs known to inhibit prostaglandin synthesis, an increased incidence of dystocia, delayed parturition, and decreased pup survival occurred. The effects of etodolac on labor and delivery in pregnant women are unknown.

NURSING MOTHERS

It is not known whether etodolac is excreted in human milk. Because many drugs are excreted in human milk and because of the potential for serious adverse reactions in nursing infants from etodolac, a decision should be made whether to discontinue nursing or to discontinue the drug taking into account the importance of the drug to the mother.

PEDIATRIC USE

Safety and effectiveness in pediatric patients have not been established.

GERIATRIC USE

As with any NSAID, however, caution should be exercised in treating the elderly, and when individualizing their dosage, extra care should be taken when increasing the dose because the elderly seem to tolerate NSAID side effects less well than younger patients. In patients 65 years and older, no substantial differences in the side effect profile of etodolac were seen compared with the general population (see CLINICAL PHARMACOLOGY, Pharmacokinetics).

DRUG INTERACTIONS

Antacids: The concomitant administration of antacids has no apparent effect on the extent of absorption of etodolac. However, antacids can decrease the peak concentration reached by 15-20% but have no detectable effect on the time-to-peak.

Aspirin: When etodolac is administered with aspirin, its protein binding is reduced, although the clearance of free etodolac is not altered. The clinical significance of this interaction is not known; however, as with other NSAIDs, concomitant administration of etodolac and aspirin is not generally recommended because of the potential of increased adverse effects.

Warfarin: Short-term pharmacokinetic studies have demonstrated that concomitant administration of warfarin and etodolac results in reduced protein binding of warfarin, but there was no change in the clearance of free warfarin. There was no significant difference in the pharmacodynamic effect of warfarin administered alone and warfarin administered with etodolac as measured by prothrombin time. Thus, concomitant therapy with warfarin and etodolac should not require dosage adjustment of either drug. However, there have been a few spontaneous reports of prolonged prothrombin times in etodolac-treated patients receiving concomitant warfarin therapy. Caution should be exercised because interactions have been seen with other NSAIDs.

Cyclosporine, Digoxin, Lithium, Methotrexate: Etodolac, like other NSAIDs, through effects on renal prostaglandins, may cause changes in the elimination of these drugs leading to elevated serum levels of digoxin, lithium, and methotrexate and increased toxicity. Nephrotoxicity associated with cyclosporine may also be enhanced. Patients receiving these drugs who are given etodolac, or any other NSAID, and particularly those patients with altered renal function, should be observed for the development of the specific toxicities of these drugs.

Phenylbutazone: Phenylbutazone causes increase (by about 80%) in the free fraction of etodolac. Although *in vivo* studies have not been done to see if etodolac clearance is changed by coadministration of phenylbutazone, it is not recommended that they be coadministered.

ADVERSE REACTIONS

Adverse-reaction information for etodolac was derived from 2629 arthritic patients treated with etodolac in double-blind and open-label clinical trials of 4-320 weeks in duration and worldwide postmarketing surveillance studies. In clinical trials, most adverse reactions were mild and transient. The discontinuation rate in controlled clinical trials, because of adverse events, was up to 10% for patients treated with etodolac.

New patient complaints (with an incidence greater than or equal to 1%) are listed below by body system. The incidences were determined from clinical trials involving 465 patients with osteoarthritis treated with 300-500 mg of etodolac bid (*i.e.*, 600-1000 mg/day).

Incidence Greater Than or Equal To 1%—Probably Causally Related:

Body as a Whole: Chills and fever.

Digestive System: Dyspepsia (10%), abdominal pain*, diarrhea*, flatulence*, nausea*, constipation, gastritis, melena, vomiting.

Nervous System: Asthenia/malaise*, dizziness*, depression, nervousness.

Skin and Appendages: Pruritus, rash.

Special Senses: Blurred vision, tinnitus.

Urogenital System: Dysuria, urinary frequency.

*Drug-related patient complaints occurring in 3-9% of patients treated with etodolac.

Drug-related patient complaints occurring in fewer than 3%, but more than 1%, are unmarked.

Incidence Less Than 1%—Probably Causally Related :

Adverse reactions reported only in worldwide postmarketing experience, not seen in clinical trials, are considered rarer and are italicized.

Body as a Whole: *Allergic reactions, anaphylactoid reaction.*

Cardiovascular System: Hypertension, congestive heart failure, flushing, palpitations, syncope, *vasculitis (including necrotizing and allergic).*

Digestive System: Thirst, dry mouth, ulcerative stomatitis, anorexia, eructation, elevated liver enzymes, *cholestatic hepatitis,* hepatitis, *cholestatic jaundice, duodenitis, jaundice, hepatic failure, liver necrosis,* peptic ulcer with or without bleeding and/or perforation, *intestinal ulceration, pancreatitis.*

Hemic and Lymphatic System: Ecchymosis, anemia, thrombocytopenia, bleeding time increased, *agranulocytosis, hemolytic anemia, leukopenia, neutropenia, pancytopenia.*

Metabolic and Nutritional: Edema, serum creatinine increase, *hyperglycemia in previously controlled diabetic patients.*

Nervous System: Insomnia, somnolence.

Respiratory System: Asthma.

Skin and Appendages: Angioedema, sweating, urticaria, vesiculobullous rash, *cutaneous vasculitis with purpura, Stevens-Johnson syndrome,* hyperpigmentation, *erythema multiforme.*

Special Senses: Photophobia, transient visual disturbances.

Urogenital System: *Elevated BUN, renal failure, renal insufficiency, renal papillary necrosis.*

Incidence Less Than 1%—Causal Relationship Unknown :

Medical events occurring under circumstances where causal relationship to etodolac is uncertain. These reactions are listed as alerting information for physicians.

Body as a Whole: Infection, headache.

Cardiovascular System: Arrhythmias, myocardial infarction, cerebrovascular accident.

Digestive System: Esophagitis with or without stricture or cardiospasm, colitis.

Metabolic and Nutritional: Change in weight.

Nervous System: Paresthesia, confusion.

Respiratory System: Bronchitis, dyspnea, pharyngitis, rhinitis, sinusitis.

Skin and Appendages: Alopecia, maculopapular rash, photosensitivity, skin peeling.

Special Senses: Conjunctivitis, deafness, taste perversion.

Urogenital System: Cystitis, hematuria, leukorrhea, renal calculus, interstitial nephritis, uterine bleeding irregularities.

DOSAGE AND ADMINISTRATION

As with other NSAIDs, the lowest dose and longest dosing interval should be sought for each patient. Therefore, after observing the response to initial therapy with etodolac, the dose and frequency should be adjusted to suit an individual patient's needs.

Dosage adjustment of etodolac is generally not required in patients with mild to moderate renal impairment. Etodolac should be used with caution in such patients, because, as with other NSAIDs, it may further decrease renal function in some patients with impaired renal function. (See PRECAUTIONS, Renal Effects.)

ANALGESIA

The recommended total daily dose of etodolac for acute pain is up to 1000 mg, given as 200-400 mg every 6-8 hours. In some patients, if the potential benefits outweigh the risks; the dose may be increased to 1200 mg/day in order to achieve a therapeutic benefit that might not have been achieved with 1000 mg/day. Doses of etodolac greater than 1000 mg/day have not been adequately evaluated in well-controlled clinical trials.

OSTEOARTHRITIS

The recommended starting dose of etodolac for the management of the signs and symptoms of osteoarthritis is: 300 mg bid, tid, or 400 mg bid, or 500 mg bid. During long-term administration, the dose of etodolac may be adjusted up or down depending on the clinical response of the patient. A lower dose of 600 mg/day may suffice for long-term administration. In patients who tolerate 1000 mg/day, the dose may be increased to 1200 mg/day when a higher level of therapeutic activity is required. When treating patients with higher doses, the physician should observe sufficient increased clinical benefit to justify the higher dose. Physicians should be aware that doses above 1000 mg/day have not been adequately evaluated in well-controlled clinical trials.

In chronic conditions, a therapeutic response to therapy with etodolac is sometimes seen within one week of therapy, but most often is observed by two weeks. After a satisfactory response has been achieved, the patient's dose should be reviewed and adjusted as required.

HOW SUPPLIED

LODINE CAPSULES

Lodine capsules are available as: *200 mg Capsules:* Light gray with one wide red band with Lodine 200/white with two narrow red bands. *300 mg Capsules:* Light gray with one wide red band with Lodine 300/light gray with two narrow red bands.

Storage: Store at controlled room temperature, 15-30°C (59-86°F). Protect from moisture. Dispense in a tight, light-resistant container using a child-resistant closure.

LODINE TABLETS

Lodine 400 mg tablets: Are yellow-orange, oval, film-coated tablet, debossed Lodine 400 on one side.

Storage: Store at controlled room temperature, 15-30°C (59-86°F). Protect from moisture. Store tablets in original container until ready to use. Dispense in a tight, light-resistant container using a child-resistant closure.

PRODUCT LISTING - RATED THERAPEUTICALLY EQUIVALENT

Capsule - Oral - 200 mg

6 x 5	$32.98	GENERIC, Vangard Labs	00615-1329-65
31 x 10	$340.79	GENERIC, Vangard Labs	00615-1329-53
31 x 10	$340.79	GENERIC, Vangard Labs	00615-1329-63
100's	$48.00	FEDERAL UPPER LIMIT, H.C.F.A. F F P	99999-3029-01
100's	$110.56	GENERIC, Teva Pharmaceuticals Usa	00093-8399-01
100's	$114.15	GENERIC, Mylan Pharmaceuticals Inc	00378-7200-01
100's	$125.62	GENERIC, Taro Pharmaceuticals U.S.A. Inc	51672-4016-01
100's	$150.14	LODINE, Wyeth-Ayerst Laboratories	00046-0738-81

Capsule - Oral - 300 mg

14's	$24.66	LODINE, Prescript Pharmaceuticals	00247-0060-14
15's	$24.09	LODINE, Allscripts Pharmaceutical Company	54569-3264-02
15's	$26.19	LODINE, Prescript Pharmaceuticals	00247-0060-15

20's	$27.99	GENERIC, Pharma Pac	52959-0483-20
20's	$33.80	LODINE, Prescript Pharmaceuticals	00247-0060-20
20's	$43.63	LODINE, Pharma Pac	52959-0211-20
20's	$45.02	LODINE, Pd-Rx Pharmaceuticals	55289-0992-20
21's	$26.29	GENERIC, Allscripts Pharmaceutical Company	54569-4545-01
21's	$28.98	GENERIC, Pharma Pac	52959-0483-21
21's	$33.72	LODINE, Allscripts Pharmaceutical Company	54569-3264-01
21's	$35.32	LODINE, Prescript Pharmaceuticals	00247-0060-21
21's	$45.61	LODINE, Pharma Pac	52959-0211-21
21's	$46.28	LODINE, Pd-Rx Pharmaceuticals	55289-0992-21
30's	$35.85	GENERIC, Vangard Labs	00615-1330-65
30's	$41.04	GENERIC, Pharma Pac	52959-0483-30
30's	$48.18	LODINE, Allscripts Pharmaceutical Company	54569-3264-00
30's	$49.01	LODINE, Prescript Pharmaceuticals	00247-0060-30
30's	$55.59	LODINE, Physicians Total Care	54868-2018-01
30's	$64.28	LODINE, Pharma Pac	52959-0211-30
30's	$68.16	LODINE, Pd-Rx Pharmaceuticals	55289-0992-30
31 x 10	$340.79	GENERIC, Vangard Labs	00615-1330-53
31 x 10	$340.79	GENERIC, Vangard Labs	00615-1330-63
40's	$64.24	LODINE, Prescript Pharmaceuticals	00247-0060-40
40's	$64.24	LODINE, Allscripts Pharmaceutical Company	54569-3264-04
40's	$69.69	LODINE, Physicians Total Care	54868-2018-03
42's	$67.28	LODINE, Prescript Pharmaceuticals	00247-0060-42
42's	$67.45	LODINE, Allscripts Pharmaceutical Company	54569-3264-03
42's	$84.40	LODINE, Pharma Pac	52959-0211-42
42's	$89.28	LODINE, Pd-Rx Pharmaceuticals	55289-0992-42
60's	$94.67	LODINE, Prescript Pharmaceuticals	00247-0060-60
60's	$110.00	LODINE, Physicians Total Care	54868-2018-04
60's	$115.89	LODINE, Pd-Rx Pharmaceuticals	55289-0992-60
100's	$125.75	GENERIC, Ivax Corporation	00172-4177-60
100's	$126.38	GENERIC, Teva Pharmaceuticals Usa	00093-8397-01
100's	$129.25	GENERIC, Mylan Pharmaceuticals Inc	00378-7233-01
100's	$142.53	GENERIC, Taro Pharmaceuticals U.S.A. Inc	51672-4017-01
100's	$155.55	LODINE, Prescript Pharmaceuticals	00247-0060-00
100's	$170.03	LODINE, Wyeth-Ayerst Laboratories	00046-0739-81
180's	$221.20	LODINE, Allscripts Pharmaceutical Company	54569-8581-00

Tablet - Oral - 400 mg

12's	$13.50	GENERIC, Pd-Rx Pharmaceuticals	55289-0239-12
12's	$24.18	LODINE, Physicians Total Care	54868-2987-01
12's	$26.58	LODINE, Pd-Rx Pharmaceuticals	55289-0644-12
14's	$17.72	GENERIC, Allscripts Pharmaceutical Company	54569-4468-00
14's	$23.77	LODINE, Allscripts Pharmaceutical Company	54569-3764-02
14's	$31.05	LODINE, Pharma Pac	52959-0281-14
14's	$58.14	GENERIC, Pharma Pac	52959-0471-14
15's	$60.95	GENERIC, Pharma Pac	52959-0471-15
20's	$25.31	GENERIC, Allscripts Pharmaceutical Company	54569-4468-01
20's	$33.95	LODINE, Allscripts Pharmaceutical Company	54569-3764-00
20's	$43.44	LODINE, Pd-Rx Pharmaceuticals	55289-0644-20
20's	$77.91	GENERIC, Pharma Pac	52959-0471-20
21's	$23.77	GENERIC, Pd-Rx Pharmaceuticals	55289-0239-21
21's	$35.65	LODINE, Allscripts Pharmaceutical Company	54569-3764-03
28's	$105.97	GENERIC, Pharma Pac	52959-0471-28
30's	$30.40	GENERIC, Compumed Pharmaceuticals	00403-0694-30
30's	$34.05	GENERIC, Pd-Rx Pharmaceuticals	55289-0239-30
30's	$37.71	GENERIC, Vangard Labs	00615-4525-65
30's	$37.96	GENERIC, Allscripts Pharmaceutical Company	54569-4468-02
30's	$44.12	GENERIC, St. Mary'S Mpp	60760-0552-30
30's	$50.93	LODINE, Allscripts Pharmaceutical Company	54569-3764-01
30's	$63.19	LODINE, Pharma Pac	52959-0281-30
30's	$113.55	GENERIC, Pharma Pac	52959-0471-30
31 x 10	$389.70	GENERIC, Vangard Labs	00615-4525-53
31 x 10	$389.70	GENERIC, Vangard Labs	00615-4525-63
60's	$88.36	GENERIC, St. Mary'S Mpp	60760-0552-60
60's	$101.82	LODINE, Pharma Pac	52959-0281-60
60's	$194.04	GENERIC, Pharma Pac	52959-0471-60
62's	$44.10	LODINE, Pharma Pac	52959-0281-20
100's	$34.50	FEDERAL UPPER LIMIT, H.C.F.A. F F P	99999-3029-02
100's	$117.66	GENERIC, Mutual/United Research Laboratories	00677-1623-01
100's	$125.59	GENERIC, Major Pharmaceuticals Inc	00904-5246-60
100's	$129.50	GENERIC, Qualitest Products Inc	00603-3570-21
100's	$132.22	GENERIC, Geneva Pharmaceuticals	00781-1234-01
100's	$132.37	GENERIC, Eon Labs Manufacturing Inc	00185-0140-01
100's	$132.37	GENERIC, Esi Lederle Generics	59911-3608-01
100's	$133.02	GENERIC, Mova Pharmaceutical Corporation	55370-0552-07
100's	$138.93	GENERIC, Ranbaxy Laboratories	63304-0701-01
100's	$139.00	GENERIC, Mylan Pharmaceuticals Inc	00378-0237-01
100's	$146.70	GENERIC, Purepac Pharmaceutical Company	00228-2599-11
100's	$146.75	GENERIC, Ivax Corporation	00172-4175-60
100's	$146.78	GENERIC, Taro Pharmaceuticals U.S.A. Inc	51672-4018-01
100's	$146.80	GENERIC, Teva Pharmaceuticals Usa	00093-0892-01
100's	$146.80	GENERIC, Teva Pharmaceuticals Usa	55953-0393-40
100's	$179.75	LODINE, Wyeth-Ayerst Laboratories	00046-0761-81

Tablet - Oral - 500 mg

10's	$20.47	LODINE, Physicians Total Care	54868-3856-00
10's	$25.79	LODINE, Pd-Rx Pharmaceuticals	55289-0197-10
14's	$15.87	GENERIC, Pd-Rx Pharmaceuticals	55289-0418-14
20's	$22.70	GENERIC, Pd-Rx Pharmaceuticals	55289-0418-20
20's	$34.17	LODINE, Allscripts Pharmaceutical Company	54569-4416-00
20's	$48.40	LODINE, Pharma Pac	52959-0445-20
20's	$48.59	LODINE, Pd-Rx Pharmaceuticals	55289-0197-20
28's	$55.25	GENERIC, Pharma Pac	52959-0530-28
30's	$57.56	LODINE, Pharma Pac	52959-0445-30
60's	$95.20	GENERIC, St. Mary'S Mpp	60760-0714-60
100's	$100.32	FEDERAL UPPER LIMIT, H.C.F.A. F F P	99999-3029-03
100's	$139.09	GENERIC, Purepac Pharmaceutical Company	00228-2632-11
100's	$139.10	GENERIC, Esi Lederle Generics	59911-3787-01
100's	$140.62	GENERIC, Eon Labs Manufacturing Inc	00185-0139-01
100's	$146.50	GENERIC, Ivax Corporation	00172-4174-60
100's	$146.50	GENERIC, Mylan Pharmaceuticals Inc	00378-1242-01
100's	$146.50	GENERIC, Par Pharmaceutical Inc	49884-0596-01
100's	$150.14	GENERIC, Taro Pharmaceuticals U.S.A. Inc	51672-4036-01
100's	$150.15	GENERIC, Teva Pharmaceuticals Usa	55953-0392-40
100's	$180.90	LODINE, Wyeth-Ayerst Laboratories	00046-0787-81

Tablet, Extended Release - Oral - 400 mg

14's	$30.29	LODINE XL, Pharma Pac	52959-0467-14
20's	$25.22	LODINE XL, Allscripts Pharmaceutical Company	54569-4464-00
20's	$36.36	LODINE XL, Physicians Total Care	54868-3901-00
20's	$40.85	LODINE XL, Pd-Rx Pharmaceuticals	55289-0237-20
30's	$53.95	LODINE XL, Physicians Total Care	54868-3901-01
30's	$61.82	LODINE XL, Pharma Pac	52959-0467-30
60's	$106.72	LODINE XL, Physicians Total Care	54868-3901-02
100's	$140.17	GENERIC, Teva Pharmaceuticals Usa	00093-1122-01
100's	$140.17	GENERIC, Purepac Pharmaceutical Company	00228-2671-11
100's	$164.91	LODINE XL, Wyeth-Ayerst Laboratories	00046-0829-81

Tablet, Extended Release - Oral - 500 mg

28's	$45.36	LODINE XL, Pharma Pac	52959-0095-28
100's	$146.48	GENERIC, Teva Pharmaceuticals Usa	00093-7172-01
100's	$172.34	LODINE XL, Wyeth-Ayerst Laboratories	00046-0839-81

Tablet, Extended Release - Oral - 600 mg

14's	$52.56	LODINE XL, Pd-Rx Pharmaceuticals	55289-0220-14
100's	$265.21	GENERIC, Teva Pharmaceuticals Usa	00093-1118-01
100's	$312.01	LODINE XL, Wyeth-Ayerst Laboratories	00046-0831-81

PRODUCT LISTING - EQUIVALENTS NOT AVAILABLE

Capsule - Oral - 200 mg

14's	$17.95	GENERIC, Southwood Pharmaceuticals Inc	58016-0206-14
15's	$19.23	GENERIC, Southwood Pharmaceuticals Inc	58016-0206-15
20's	$25.64	GENERIC, Southwood Pharmaceuticals Inc	58016-0206-20
21's	$26.92	GENERIC, Southwood Pharmaceuticals Inc	58016-0206-21
30's	$38.46	GENERIC, Southwood Pharmaceuticals Inc	58016-0206-30
42's	$53.84	GENERIC, Southwood Pharmaceuticals Inc	58016-0206-42
100's	$40.00	GENERIC, Esi Lederle Generics	59911-3606-01
100's	$128.20	GENERIC, Southwood Pharmaceuticals Inc	58016-0206-00

Capsule - Oral - 300 mg

14's	$18.03	GENERIC, Allscripts Pharmaceutical Company	54569-4545-02
14's	$22.47	GENERIC, Southwood Pharmaceuticals Inc	58016-0209-14
15's	$24.08	GENERIC, Southwood Pharmaceuticals Inc	58016-0209-15
20's	$32.10	GENERIC, Southwood Pharmaceuticals Inc	58016-0209-20
21's	$33.71	GENERIC, Southwood Pharmaceuticals Inc	58016-0209-21
30's	$42.77	GENERIC, Allscripts Pharmaceutical Company	54569-4545-00
30's	$48.15	GENERIC, Southwood Pharmaceuticals Inc	58016-0209-30
42's	$67.41	GENERIC, Southwood Pharmaceuticals Inc	58016-0209-42
60's	$96.30	GENERIC, Southwood Pharmaceuticals Inc	58016-0209-60
100's	$125.23	GENERIC, Esi Lederle Generics	59911-3607-01
100's	$145.19	GENERIC, Southwood Pharmaceuticals Inc	58016-0209-00

Tablet - Oral - 400 mg

2's	$2.78	GENERIC, Allscripts Pharmaceutical Company	54569-4468-04
12's	$52.31	GENERIC, Pharma Pac	52959-0471-12
14's	$23.76	GENERIC, Southwood Pharmaceuticals Inc	58016-0208-14
15's	$25.46	GENERIC, Southwood Pharmaceuticals Inc	58016-0208-15
20's	$33.94	GENERIC, Southwood Pharmaceuticals Inc	58016-0208-20
21's	$35.64	GENERIC, Southwood Pharmaceuticals Inc	58016-0208-21
30's	$50.91	GENERIC, Southwood Pharmaceuticals Inc	58016-0208-30
42's	$71.27	GENERIC, Southwood Pharmaceuticals Inc	58016-0208-42
45's	$62.55	GENERIC, Allscripts Pharmaceutical Company	54569-4468-03
60's	$88.08	GENERIC, Allscripts Pharmaceutical Company	54569-4468-05
60's	$101.82	GENERIC, Southwood Pharmaceuticals Inc	58016-0208-60
90's	$152.73	GENERIC, Southwood Pharmaceuticals Inc	58016-0208-90
100's	$169.70	GENERIC, Southwood Pharmaceuticals Inc	58016-0208-00

Tablet - Oral - 500 mg

14's	$23.91	GENERIC, Southwood Pharmaceuticals Inc	58016-0375-14
14's	$27.01	GENERIC, Pharma Pac	52959-0530-14
20's	$30.03	GENERIC, Allscripts Pharmaceutical Company	54569-4630-00

20's	$34.16	GENERIC, Southwood Pharmaceuticals Inc	58016-0375-20
20's	$38.99	GENERIC, Pharma Pac	52959-0530-20
21's	$35.87	GENERIC, Southwood Pharmaceuticals Inc	58016-0375-21
28's	$47.82	GENERIC, Southwood Pharmaceuticals Inc	58016-0375-28
30's	$51.24	GENERIC, Southwood Pharmaceuticals Inc	58016-0375-30
30's	$56.70	GENERIC, Pharma Pac	52959-0530-30
40's	$68.32	GENERIC, Southwood Pharmaceuticals Inc	58016-0375-40
60's	$102.48	GENERIC, Southwood Pharmaceuticals Inc	58016-0375-60
100's	$139.00	GENERIC, Par Pharmaceutical Inc	49884-0596-10
100's	$170.80	GENERIC, Southwood Pharmaceuticals Inc	58016-0375-00
Tablet, Extended Release - Oral - 500 mg			
30's	$57.00	GENERIC, Pharma Pac	52959-0649-30

Etomidate *(001235)*

For complete prescribing information, refer to the CD-ROM included with the book.

Categories: Anesthesia, adjunct; Anesthesia, general; Pregnancy Category C; FDA Approved 1982 Sep
Drug Classes: Anesthetics, general
Brand Names: Amidate
Foreign Brand Availability: Hypnomidate (Austria; Belgium; Bulgaria; Czech-Republic; England; France; Germany; Greece; Mexico; Netherlands; Portugal; Russia; South-Africa; Spain; Switzerland; Taiwan; Turkey)

DESCRIPTION

Etomidate is a sterile, nonpyrogenic solution. Each milliliter contains etomidate, 2 mg, propylene glycol 35% v/v.

It is intended for the induction of general anesthesia by intravenous injection.

The drug etomidate is chemically identified as (R)-(+)-ethyl-1-(1- phenylethyl) -1H-imidazole-5-carboxylate.

Storage: Exposure of pharmaceutical products to heat should be minimized. Avoid excessive heat. Protect from freezing. It is recommended that the product be stored at room temperature (25°C); however, brief exposure up to 40°C does not adversely affect the product.

INDICATIONS AND USAGE

Etomidate is indicated by intravenous injection for the induction of general anesthesia. When considering use of etomidate, the usefulness of its hemodynamic properties should be weighed against the high frequency of transient skeletal muscle movements.

Intravenous etomidate is also indicated for the supplementation of subpotent anesthetic agents, such as nitrous oxide in oxygen, during maintenance of anesthesia for short operative procedures such as dilation and curettage or cervical conization.

CONTRAINDICATIONS

Etomidate is contraindicated in patients who have shown hypersensitivity to it.

WARNINGS

INTRAVENOUS ETOMIDATE SHOULD BE ADMINISTERED ONLY BY PERSONS TRAINED IN THE ADMINISTRATION OF GENERAL ANESTHETICS AND IN THE MANAGEMENT OF COMPLICATIONS ENCOUNTERED DURING THE CONDUCT OF GENERAL ANESTHESIA.

BECAUSE OF THE HAZARDS OF PROLONGED SUPPRESSION OF ENDOGENOUS CORTISOL AND ALDOSTERONE PRODUCTION, THIS FORMULATION IS NOT INTENDED FOR ADMINISTRATION BY PROLONGED INFUSION.

DOSAGE AND ADMINISTRATION

Etomidate injection is intended for administration only by the intravenous route. The dose for induction of anesthesia in adult patients and in children above the age of 10 years will vary between 0.2 and 0.6 mg/kg of body weight, and it must be individualized in each case. The usual dose for induction in these patients 0.3 mg/kg, injected over a period of 30-60 seconds. There are inadequate data to make dosage recommendations for induction of anesthesia in patients below the age of 10 years; therefore, such use is not recommended.

Smaller increments of intravenous etomidate may be administered to adult patients during short operative procedures to supplement subpotent anesthetic agents, such as nitrous oxide. The dosage employed under these circumstances, although usually smaller than the original induction dose, must be individualized. There are insufficient data to support this use of etomidate for longer adult procedures or for any procedures in children; therefore, such use is not recommended. The use of intravenous fentanyl and other neuroactive drugs employed during the conduct of anesthesia may alter the etomidate dosage requirements. Consult the prescribing information for all other such drugs before using.

Premedication: Etomidate injection is compatible with commonly administered preanesthetic medications, which may be employed as indicated. (See also and dosage recommendations for maintenance of anesthesia.)

Etomidate hypnosis does not significantly alter the usual dosage requirements of neuromuscular blocking agents employed for endotracheal intubation or other purposes shortly after induction of anesthesia.

Parenteral drug products should be inspected visually for particulate matter and discoloration prior to administration, whenever solution and container permit.

To prevent needle-stick injuries, needles should not be recapped, purposely bent, or broken by hand.

PRODUCT LISTING - RATED THERAPEUTICALLY EQUIVALENT

Solution - Intravenous - 2 mg/ml			
10 ml x 10	$162.69	AMIDATE, Abbott Pharmaceutical	00074-6695-01
10 ml x 10	$231.30	GENERIC, Bedford Laboratories	55390-0762-10
20 ml x 10	$236.91	AMIDATE, Abbott Pharmaceutical	00074-6695-02
20 ml x 10	$268.80	GENERIC, Bedford Laboratories	55390-0763-20
20 ml x 10	$288.00	AMIDATE, Abbott Pharmaceutical	00074-8060-03
20 ml x 10	$290.94	AMIDATE, Abbott Pharmaceutical	00074-8060-19
20 ml x 10	$307.68	AMIDATE, Abbott Pharmaceutical	00074-8060-29

PRODUCT LISTING - EQUIVALENTS NOT AVAILABLE

Solution - Intravenous - 2 mg/ml			
10 ml x 5	$74.87	AMIDATE, Abbott Pharmaceutical	00074-8062-01
20 ml x 5	$140.78	AMIDATE, Abbott Pharmaceutical	00074-8061-01
20 ml x 5	$274.08	AMIDATE, Abbott Pharmaceutical	00074-8060-01
20 ml x 10	$258.00	GENERIC, Bedford Laboratories	55390-0763-10

Etoposide *(001236)*

Categories: Carcinoma, lung; Carcinoma, testicular; Pregnancy Category D; FDA Approved 1983 Nov; WHO Formulary
Drug Classes: Antineoplastics, epipodophyllotoxins
Brand Names: Toposar; **Vepesid**
Foreign Brand Availability: Aside (Korea); Celltop (France); Eposin (Thailand); Etomedec (Germany); Etophos (Germany); Etopos (Mexico); Etoposide (Australia; Israel; New-Zealand); Etoposido (Colombia; Peru); Etosid (India); Lastet (China; India; Indonesia; Japan; Malaysia; Mexico; Philippines; Taiwan); Posid (Philippines); Vepeside (France); VP-TEC (Mexico)
HCFA JCODE(S): J9181 10 mg IV; J8560 50 mg ORAL

WARNING

Etoposide should be administered under the supervision of a qualified physician experienced in the use of cancer chemotherapeutic agents. Severe myelosuppression with resulting infection or bleeding may occur.

DESCRIPTION

Etoposide (also commonly known as VP-16) is a semisynthetic derivative of podophyllotoxin used in the treatment of certain neoplastic diseases. It is 4′-demethylepipodophyllotoxin 9-[4,6-0-(R)-ethylidene-β-D-glucopyranoside]. It is very soluble in methanol and chloroform, slightly soluble in ethanol, and sparingly soluble in water and ether. It is made more miscible with water by means of organic solvents. It has a molecular weight of 588.58 and a molecular formula of $C_{29}H_{32}O_{13}$.

VePesid may be administered either intravenously or orally. VePesid for injection is available in 100 mg (5 ml), 150 mg (7.5 ml), 500 mg (25 ml), or 1 g (50 ml), sterile, multiple dose vials. Toposar is available for intravenous use as a 20 mg/ml solution in 100 mg (5 ml), 200 mg (10 ml) and 500 mg (25 ml) sterile, multiple dose vials. The pH of the clear, nearly colorless to yellow solution is 3-4. Each ml contains 20 mg etoposide, 2 mg citric acid, 30 mg benzyl alcohol, 80 mg (modified) polysorbate 80/Tween 80, 650 mg polyethylene glycol 300, and 30.5% (v/v) alcohol. Vial headspace contains nitrogen.

VePesid is also available as 50 mg pink capsules. Each liquid filled, soft gelatin capsule contains 50 mg of etoposide in a vehicle consisting of citric acid, glycerin, purified water, and polyethylene glycol 400. The soft gelatin capsules contain gelatin, glycerin, sorbitol, purified water, and parabens (ethyl and propyl) with the following dye system: iron oxide (red) and titanium dioxide; the capsules are printed with edible ink.

CLINICAL PHARMACOLOGY

Etoposide has been shown to cause metaphase arrest in chick fibroblasts. Its main effect, however, appears to be at the G_2 portion of the cell cycle in mammalian cells. Two different dose-dependent responses are seen. At high concentrations (10 μg/ml or more), lysis of cells entering mitosis is observed. At low concentrations (0.3-10 μg/ml), cells are inhibited from entering prophase. It does not interfere with microtubular assembly. The predominant macromolecular effect of etoposide appears to be the induction of DNA strand breaks by an interaction with DNA topoisomerase II or the formation of free radicals.

PHARMACOKINETICS

On intravenous administration, the disposition of etoposide is best described as a biphasic process with a distribution half-life of about 1.5 hours and terminal elimination half-life ranging from 4-11 hours. Total body clearance values range from 33-48 ml/min or 16-36 ml/min/m^2 and, like the terminal elimination half-life, are independent of dose over a range 100-600 mg/m^2. Over the same dose range, the areas under the plasma concentration vs time curves (AUC) and the maximum plasma concentration (C_{max}) values increase linearly with dose. Etoposide does not accumulate in the plasma following daily administration of 100 mg/m^2 for 4-5 days.

The mean volumes of distribution at steady state fall in the range of 18-29 liters or 7-17 L/m^2. Etoposide enters the CSF poorly. Although it is detectable in CSF and intracerebral tumors, the concentrations are lower than in extracerebral tumors and in plasma. Etoposide concentrations are higher in normal lung than in lung metastases and are similar in primary tumors and normal tissues of the myometrium. *In vitro*, etoposide is highly protein bound (97%) to human plasma proteins. An inverse relationship between plasma albumin levels and etoposide renal clearance is found in children. In a study determining the effect of other therapeutic agents on the *in vitro* binding of carbon-14 labeled etoposide to human serum proteins, only phenylbutazone, sodium salicylate and aspirin displaced protein-bound etoposide at concentrations achieved *in vivo*.[1]

Etoposide binding ratio correlates directly with serum albumin in patients with cancer and in normal volunteers. The unbound fraction of etoposide significantly correlated with bilirubin in a population of cancer patients.[2,3] Data have suggested a significant inverse correlation between serum albumin concentration and free fraction of etoposide (see PRECAUTIONS).

After intravenous administration of ^3H-etoposide (70-290 mg/m^2), mean recoveries of radioactivity in the urine range from 42-67%, and fecal recoveries range from 0-16% of the dose. Less than 50% of an intravenous dose is excreted in the urine as etoposide with mean recoveries of 8% to 35% within 24 hours.

In children, approximately 55% of the dose is excreted in the urine as etoposide in 24 hours. The mean renal clearance of etoposide is 7-10 ml/min/m^2 or about 35% of the total body clearance over a dose range of 80-600 mg/m^2. Etoposide, therefore, is cleared by both renal and nonrenal processes, *i.e.,* metabolism and biliary excretion. The effect of renal disease on plasma etoposide clearance is not known.

Biliary excretion appears to be a minor route of etoposide elimination. Only 6% or less of an intravenous dose is recovered in the bile as etoposide. Metabolism accounts for most of the nonrenal clearance of etoposide. The major urinary metabolite of etoposide in adults and children is the hydroxy acid [4′-demethylepipodophyllic acid-9-(4,6-0-(R)-ethylidene-β-D-glucopyranoside)], formed by opening of the lactone ring. It is also present in human plasma, presumably as the **trans** isomer. Glucuronide and/or sulfate conjugates of etoposide are excreted in human urine and represent 5-22% of the dose. In addition, O-demethylation of the dimethoxyphenol ring occurs through the CYP450 3A4 isoenzyme pathway to produce the corresponding catechol.

After either intravenous infusion or oral capsule administration, the C_{max} and AUC values exhibit marked intra- and inter-subject variability. This results in variability in the estimates of the absolute oral bioavailability of etoposide oral capsules.

C_{max} and AUC values for orally administered etoposide capsules consistently fall in the same range as the C_{max} and AUC values for an intravenous dose of one-half the size of the oral dose. The overall mean value of oral capsule bioavailability is approximately 50% (range 25-75%). The bioavailability of etoposide capsules appears to be linear up to a dose of at least 250 mg/m^2.

There is no evidence of a first-pass effect for etoposide. For example, no correlation exists between the absolute oral bioavailability of etoposide capsules and nonrenal clearance. No evidence exists for any other differences in etoposide metabolism and excretion after administration of oral capsules as compared to intravenous infusion.

In adults, the total body clearance of etoposide is correlated with creatinine clearance, serum albumin concentration, and nonrenal clearance. Patients with impaired renal function receiving etoposide have exhibited reduced total body clearance, increased AUC and a lower volume of distribution at steady state (see PRECAUTIONS). Use of cisplatin therapy is associated with reduced total body clearance. In children, elevated serum SGPT levels are associated with reduced drug total body clearance. Prior use of cisplatin may also result in a decrease of etoposide total body clearance in children.

Although some minor differences in pharmacokinetic parameters between age and gender have been observed, these differences were not considered clinically significant.

INDICATIONS AND USAGE

Etoposide is indicated in the management of the following neoplasms:

Refractory testicular tumors: Etoposide injection in combination therapy with other approved chemotherapeutic agents in patients with refractory testicular tumors who have already received appropriate surgical, chemotherapeutic, and radiotherapeutic therapy.

Adequate data on the use of etoposide capsules in the treatment of testicular cancer are not available.

Small cell lung cancer: Etoposide injection and/or capsules in combination with other approved chemotherapeutic agents as first line treatment in patients with small cell lung cancer.

NON-FDA APPROVED INDICATIONS

Etoposide has been used without FDA approval for the treatment of Kaposi's sarcoma, non-Hodgkin's lymphoma, acute myelomonocytic leukemia, acute myelocytic leukemia, and neuroblastoma. It has also been used in the treatment of Ewing's sarcoma, brain tumors, Hodgkin's disease, choriocarcinoma, rhabdomyosarcoma, hepatocellular carcinoma, epithelial ovarian cancer, non-small-cell lung cancer, Wilms' tumor and refractory myeloma.

CONTRAINDICATIONS

Etoposide is contraindicated in patients who have demonstrated a previous hypersensitivity to etoposide or any component of the formulation.

WARNINGS

Patients being treated with etoposide must be frequently observed for myelosuppression both during and after therapy. Myelosuppression resulting in death has been reported. Dose-limiting bone marrow suppression is the most significant toxicity associated with etoposide therapy. Therefore, the following studies should be obtained at the start of therapy and prior to each subsequent dose of etoposide: platelet count, hemoglobin, white blood cell count, and differential. The occurrence of a platelet count below 50,000/mm^3 or an absolute neutrophil count below 500/mm^3 is an indication to withhold further therapy until the blood counts have sufficiently recovered.

Physicians should be aware of the possible occurrence of an anaphylactic reaction manifested by chills, fever, tachycardia, bronchospasm, dyspnea, and hypotension. Higher rates of anaphylactic-like reactions have been reported in children who received infusions at concentrations higher than those recommended. The role that concentration of infusion (or rate of infusion) plays in the development of anaphylactic-like reactions is uncertain. (See ADVERSE REACTIONS.) Treatment is symptomatic. The infusion should be terminated immediately, followed by the administration of pressor agents, corticosteroids, antihistamines, or volume expanders at the discretion of the physician.

For parenteral administration, etoposide should be given only by slow intravenous infusion (usually over a 30-60 minute period) since hypotension has been reported as a possible side effect of rapid intravenous injection.

PREGNANCY

Etoposide can cause fetal harm when administered to a pregnant woman. Etoposide has been shown to be teratogenic in mice and rats.

In rats, an intravenous etoposide dose of 0.4 mg/kg/day (about 1/20th of the human dose on a mg/m^2 basis) during organogenesis caused maternal toxicity, embryotoxicity, and teratogenicity (skeletal abnormalities, exencephaly, encephalocele, and anophthalmia); higher doses of 1.2 and 3.6 mg/kg/day (about 1/7th and 1/2 of human dose on a mg/m^2 basis) resulted in 90 and 100% embryonic resorptions. In mice, a single 1.0 mg/kg (1/16th of human dose on a mg/m^2 basis) dose of etoposide administered intraperitoneally on days 6, 7, 8 of gestation caused embryotoxicity, cranial abnormalities, and major skeletal malformations. An i.p. dose of 1.5 mg/kg (about 1/10th of human dose on a mg/m^2 basis) on day 7 of gestation caused an increase in the incidence of intrauterine death and fetal malformations and a significant decrease in the average fetal body weight.

Women of childbearing potential should be advised to avoid becoming pregnant. If this drug is used during pregnancy, or if the patient becomes pregnant while receiving this drug, the patient should be warned of the potential hazard to the fetus.

Etoposide should be considered a potential carcinogen in humans. The occurrence of acute leukemia with or without a preleukemic phase has been reported in rare instances in patients treated with etoposide alone or in association with other neo-plastic agents. The risk of development of a preleukemic or leukemic syndrome is unclear. Carcinogenicity tests with etoposide have not been conducted in laboratory animals.

PRECAUTIONS

GENERAL

In all instances where the use of etoposide is considered for chemotherapy, the physician must evaluate the need and usefulness of the drug against the risk of adverse reactions. Most such adverse reactions are reversible if detected early. If severe reactions occur, the drug should be reduced in dosage or discontinued and appropriate corrective measures should be taken according to the clinical judgment of the physician. Reinstitution of etoposide therapy should be carried out with caution, and with adequate consideration of the further need for the drug and alertness as to possible recurrence of toxicity.

Patients with low serum albumin may be at an increased risk of etoposide-associated toxicities.

LABORATORY TESTS

Periodic complete blood counts should be done during the course of etoposide treatment. They should be performed prior to each cycle of therapy and at appropriate intervals during and after therapy. At least one determination should be done prior to each dose of etoposide.

RENAL IMPAIRMENT

In patients with impaired renal function, the initial dose modification found in TABLE 1 should be considered based on measured creatinine clearance.

TABLE 1

Measured Creatinine Clearance	>50 ml/min	15-50 ml/min
Etoposide	100% of dose	75% of dose

Subsequent etoposide dosing should be based on patient tolerance and clinical effect.

Data are not available in patients with creatinine clearances <15 ml/min and further dose reduction should be considered in these patients.

CARCINOGENESIS, MUTAGENESIS, AND IMPAIRMENT OF FERTILITY

See WARNINGS for more information on carcinogenesis.

Etoposide has been shown to be mutagenic in Ames assay.

Treatment of Swiss-Albino mice with 1.5 mg/kg IP of etoposide on day 7 of gestation increased the incidence of intrauterine death and fetal malformations as well as significantly decreased the average fetal body weight. Maternal weight gain was not affected.

Irreversible testicular atrophy was present in rats treated with etoposide intravenously for 30 days at 0.5 mg/kg/day (about 1/16th of the human dose on a mg/m^2 basis).

PREGNANCY CATEGORY D

See WARNINGS.

NURSING MOTHERS

It is not known whether this drug is excreted in human milk. Because many drugs are excreted in human milk and because of the potential for serious adverse reactions in nursing infants from etoposide, a decision should be made whether to discontinue nursing or to discontinue the drug, taking into account the importance of the drug to the mother.

PEDIATRIC USE

Safety and effectiveness in pediatric patients have not been established.

Etoposide injection contains polysorbate 80. In premature infants, a life-threatening syndrome consisting of liver and renal failure, pulmonary deterioration, thrombocytopenia, and ascites has been associated with an injectable vitamin E product containing polysorbate 80. Anaphylactic reactions have been reported in children (see WARNINGS).

ADVERSE REACTIONS

The following data on adverse reactions are based on both oral and intravenous administration of etoposide as a single agent, using several different dose schedules for treatment of a wide variety of malignancies.

HEMATOLOGIC TOXICITY

Myelosuppression is dose related and dose limiting, with granulocyte nadirs occurring 7-14 days after drug administration and platelet nadirs occurring 9-16 days after drug administration. Bone marrow recovery is usually complete by day 20, and no cumulative toxicity has been reported. Fever and infection have also been reported in patients with neutropenia. Death associated with myelosuppression has been reported.

The occurrence of acute leukemia with or without a preleukemic phase has been reported rarely in patients treated with etoposide in association with other antineoplastic agents. (See WARNINGS.)

GASTROINTESTINAL TOXICITY

Nausea and vomiting are the major gastrointestinal toxicities. The severity of such nausea and vomiting is generally mild to moderate with treatment discontinuation required in 1% of patients. Nausea and vomiting can usually be controlled with standard antiemetic therapy. Gastrointestinal toxicities are slightly more frequent after oral administration than after intravenous infusion.

HYPOTENSION

Transient hypotension following rapid intravenous administration has been reported in 1-2% of patients. It has not been associated with cardiac toxicity or electrocardiographic changes. No delayed hypotension has been noted. To prevent this rare occurrence, it is recommended that etoposide be administered by slow intravenous infusion over a 30-60 minute period. If hypotension occurs, it usually responds to cessation of the infusion and administration of fluids or other supportive therapy as appropriate. When restarting the infusion, a slower administration rate should be used.

ALLERGIC REACTIONS

Anaphylactic-like reactions characterized by chills, fever, tachycardia, bronchospasm, dyspnea, and/or hypotension have been reported to occur in 0.7-2% of patients receiving intravenous etoposide and in less than 1% of the patients treated with the oral capsules. These reactions have usually responded promptly to the cessation of the infusion and administration of pressor agents, corticosteroids, antihistamines, or volume expanders as appropriate; however, the reactions can be fatal. Hypertension and/or flushing have also been reported. Blood pressure usually normalizes within a few hours after cessation of the infusion. Anaphylactic-like reactions have occurred during the initial infusion of etoposide.

Facial/tongue swelling, coughing, diaphoresis, cyanosis, tightness in throat, laryngospasm, back pain, and/or loss of consciousness have sometimes occurred in association with the above reactions. In addition, an apparent hypersensitivity-associated apnea has been reported rarely.

Rash, urticaria, and/or pruritus have infrequently been reported at recommended doses. At investigational doses, a generalized pruritic erythematous maculopapular rash, consistent with perivasculitis, has been reported.

ALOPECIA

Reversible alopecia, sometimes progressing to total baldness were observed in up to 66% of patients.

OTHER TOXICITIES

The following adverse reactions have been infrequently reported: abdominal pain, aftertaste, constipation, dysphagia, fever, transient cortical blindness, interstitial pneumonitis/pulmonary fibrosis, optic neuritis, pigmentation, seizure (occasionally associated with allergic reactions), and a single report of radiation recall dermatitis.

Hepatic toxicity, generally in patients receiving higher doses of the drug than those recommended, has been reported with etoposide. Metabolic acidosis has also been reported in patients receiving these higher doses.

The incidences of adverse reactions in TABLE 2 are derived from multiple data bases from studies in 2081 patients when etoposide was used either orally or by injection as a single agent.

TABLE 2

Adverse Drug Effect	Percent Range of Reported Incidence
Hematologic Toxicity	
Leukopenia (less than 1000 WBC/mm^3)	3-17%
Leukopenia (less than 4000 WBC/mm^3)	60-91%
Thrombocytopenia (less than 50,000 platelets/mm^3)	1-20%
Thrombocytopenia (less than 100,000 platelets/mm^3)	22-41%
Anemia	0-33%
Gastrointestinal Toxicity	
Nausea and vomiting	31-43%
Abdominal pain	0-2%
Anorexia	10-13%
Diarrhea	1-13%
Stomatitis	1-6%
Hepatic	0-3%
Alopecia	8-66%
Peripheral neurotoxicity	1-2%
Hypotension	1-2%
Allergic reaction	1-2%

DOSAGE AND ADMINISTRATION

Note: Plastic devices made of acrylic or ABS (a polymer composed of acrylonitrile, butadiene, and styrene) have been reported to crack and leak when used with *undiluted* etoposide injection.

Etoposide Injection: The usual dose of etoposide for injection in testicular cancer in combination with other approved chemotherapeutic agents ranges from 50-100 mg/m^2/day on days 1 through 5 to 100 mg/m^2/day on days 1, 3, and 5.

In small cell lung cancer, the etoposide for injection dose in combination with other approved chemotherapeutic drugs ranges from 35 mg/m^2/day for 4 days to 50 mg/m^2/day for 5 days.

For recommended dosing adjustments in patients with renal impairment, see PRECAUTIONS, Renal Impairment.

Chemotherapy courses are repeated at 3-4 week intervals after adequate recovery from any toxicity.

Etoposide Capsules: In small cell lung cancer, the recommended dose of etoposide capsules is 2 times the IV dose rounded to the nearest 50 mg.

The dosage, by either route, should be modified to take into account the myelosuppressive effects of other drugs in the combination or the effects of prior x-ray therapy or chemotherapy which may have compromised bone marrow reserve.

ADMINISTRATION PRECAUTIONS

As with other potentially toxic compounds, caution should be exercised in handling and preparing the solution of etoposide. Skin reactions associated with accidental exposure to etoposide may occur. The use of gloves is recommended. If etoposide solution contacts the skin or mucosa, immediately and thoroughly wash the skin with soap and water and flush the mucosa with water.

PREPARATION FOR INTRAVENOUS ADMINISTRATION

Etoposide for injection must be diluted prior to use with either 5% dextrose injection, or 0.9% sodium chloride injection, to give a final concentration of 0.2-0.4 mg/ml. If solutions are prepared at concentrations above 0.4 mg/ml, precipitation may occur. Hypotension following rapid intravenous administration has been reported, hence, it is recommended that the etoposide solution be administered over a 30-60 minute period. A longer duration of administration may be used if the volume of fluid to be infused is a concern. **Etoposide should not be given by rapid intravenous injection.**

Parenteral drug products should be inspected visually for particulate matter and discoloration prior to administration whenever solution and container permit.

STABILITY

Unopened vials of etoposide are stable for 24 months at room temperature (25°C). Vials diluted as recommended to a concentration of 0.2-0.4 mg/ml are stable for 96 and 24 hours, respectively, at room temperature (25°C) under normal room fluorescent lights in both glass and plastic containers.

Etoposide capsules must be stored under refrigeration 2-8°C (36-46°F). The capsules are stable for 24 months under such refrigeration conditions.

HANDLING AND DISPOSAL

Procedures for proper handling and disposal of anticancer drugs should be considered. Several guidelines on this subject have been published[4-10]. There is no general agreement that all of the procedures recommended in the guidelines are necessary or appropriate.

HOW SUPPLIED

VePesid is supplied in vials for injection and 50 mg pink capsules with "Bristol 3091" printed in black.

Storage: Capsules are to be stored under refrigeration 2-8°C (36-46°F). DO NOT FREEZE.

PRODUCT LISTING - RATED THERAPEUTICALLY EQUIVALENT

Capsule - Oral - 50 mg

Size	Price	Product	NDC
20's	$952.75	GENERIC, Mylan Pharmaceuticals Inc	00378-3266-94
20's	$952.75	GENERIC, Udl Laboratories Inc	51079-0965-05

Solution - Intravenous - 20 mg/ml

Size	Price	Product	NDC
5 ml	$42.75	GENERIC, Gensia Sicor Pharmaceuticals Inc	00703-5643-01
5 ml	$43.94	GENERIC, Gensia Sicor Pharmaceuticals Inc	00703-5653-01
5 ml	$110.00	GENERIC, Bedford Laboratories	55390-0291-01
5 ml	$131.00	GENERIC, Immunex Corporation	58406-0711-12
5 ml	$131.05	VEPESID, Bristol-Myers Squibb	00015-3095-20
5 ml	$142.95	GENERIC, Abbott Pharmaceutical	00074-1485-01
5 ml x 10	$157.60	GENERIC, American Pharmaceutical Partners	63323-0104-05
7.50 ml	$204.74	VEPESID, Bristol-Myers Squibb	00015-3084-20
25 ml	$69.69	GENERIC, Abbott Pharmaceutical	00074-1485-02
25 ml	$209.00	GENERIC, Gensia Sicor Pharmaceuticals Inc	00703-5646-01
25 ml	$214.94	GENERIC, Gensia Sicor Pharmaceuticals Inc	00703-5656-01
25 ml	$327.50	GENERIC, Immunex Corporation	58406-0714-18
25 ml	$550.00	GENERIC, Bedford Laboratories	55390-0292-01
25 ml	$638.87	VEPESID, Bristol-Myers Squibb	00015-3061-20
25 ml	$665.38	GENERIC, Pharmacia and Upjohn	00013-7356-88
25 ml x 1	$665.30	GENERIC, American Pharmaceutical Partners	63323-0104-25
50 ml	$127.75	GENERIC, Abbott Pharmaceutical	00074-1485-03
50 ml	$136.49	GENERIC, Pharmacia and Upjohn	00013-7336-91
50 ml	$272.98	GENERIC, Pharmacia and Upjohn	00013-7346-94
50 ml	$418.00	GENERIC, Abbott Pharmaceutical	00703-5667-01
50 ml	$429.88	GENERIC, Gensia Sicor Pharmaceuticals Inc	00703-5657-01
50 ml	$1100.00	GENERIC, Bedford Laboratories	55390-0293-01
50 ml	$1244.98	VEPESID, Bristol-Myers Squibb	00015-3062-20
50 ml	$1338.13	GENERIC, Gensia Sicor Pharmaceuticals Inc	00703-5668-01
50 ml	$1620.80	GENERIC, Pharmacia and Upjohn	00013-7366-73
50 ml x 1	$1393.40	GENERIC, American Pharmaceutical Partners	63323-0104-50
100 ml	$154.50	GENERIC, Baxter Pharmaceutical Products, Inc	10019-0930-01
500 ml	$650.00	GENERIC, Baxter Pharmaceutical Products, Inc	10019-0930-02

PRODUCT LISTING - EQUIVALENTS NOT AVAILABLE

Capsule - Oral - 50 mg

Size	Price	Product	NDC
20's	$1275.45	VEPESID, Bristol-Myers Squibb	00015-3091-45

Solution - Intravenous - 20 mg/ml

Size	Price	Product	NDC
5 ml	$131.05	VEPESID, Bristol-Myers Squibb	00015-3095-30
5 ml	$131.05	VEPESID, Bristol-Myers Squibb	00015-3095-95

5 ml	$141.50	GENERIC, Watson/Schein Pharmaceuticals Inc	00364-3028-53
5 ml	$141.97	GENERIC, Gensia Sicor Pharmaceuticals Inc	00703-5658-01
25 ml	$638.87	VEPESID, Bristol-Myers Squibb	00015-3061-24
50 ml	$1244.98	VEPESID, Bristol-Myers Squibb	00015-3062-24

Etoposide Phosphate *(003488)*

Categories: Carcinoma, lung; Carcinoma, testicular; FDA Approved 1998 Feb; Pregnancy Category D
Drug Classes: Antineoplastics, epipodophyllotoxins
Brand Names: Etopophos
Foreign Brand Availability: Exitop (Germany); Fytosid (Thailand); Posyd (Indonesia)

WARNING

Etoposide phosphate for injection should be administered under the supervision of a qualified physician experienced in the use of cancer chemotherapeutic agents. Severe myelosuppression with resulting infection or bleeding may occur.

DESCRIPTION

Etopophos (etoposide phosphate) for injection is an antineoplastic agent which is available for intravenous infusion as a sterile lyophile in single-dose vials containing etoposide phosphate equivalent to 100 mg etoposide, 32.7 mg sodium citrate, and 300 mg dextran 40.

Etoposide phosphate is a water soluble ester of etoposide (commonly known as VP-16), a semi-synthetic derivative of podophyllotoxin. The water solubility of etoposide phosphate lessens the potential for precipitation following dilution and during intravenous administration.

The chemical name for etoposide phosphate is: 4′-demethylepipodophyllotoxin 9-[4,6-O-(R)-ethylidene-β-D-glucopyranoside], 4′-(dihydrogen phosphate).

CLINICAL PHARMACOLOGY

The *in vitro* cytotoxicity observed for etoposide phosphate is significantly less than that seen with etoposide which is believed due to the necessity for conversion *in vivo* to the active moiety, etoposide, by dephosphorylation. The mechanism of action is believed to be the same as that of etoposide. Etoposide has been shown to cause metaphase arrest in chick fibroblasts. Its main effect, however, appears to be at the G_2 portion of the cell cycle in mammalian cells. Two different dose-dependent responses are seen. At high concentrations (10 μg/ml or more), lysis of cells entering mitosis is observed. At low concentrations (0.3-10 μg/ml), cells are inhibited from entering prophase. It does not interfere with microtubular assembly. The predominant macromolecular effect of etoposide appears to be the induction of DNA strand breaks by an interaction with DNA-topoisomerase II or the formation of free radicals.

ETOPOSIDE PHOSPHATE BIOEQUIVALENCE

Following intravenous administration of etoposide phosphate, etoposide phosphate is rapidly and completely converted to etoposide in plasma. A direct comparison of the pharmacokinetic parameters [area under the concentration time curve (AUC) and the maximum plasma concentration (C_{max})] of etoposide following intravenous administration of molar equivalent doses of etoposide phosphate and VePesid (etoposide) was made in 2 randomized cross-over studies in patients with a variety of malignancies. In the first study of 41 evaluable patients, the etoposide mean ±SD AUC values were 168.3 ± 48.2 μg·h/ml and 156.7 ± 43.4 μg·h/ml following administration of molar equivalent doses of 150 mg/m² etoposide phosphate or VePesid with a 3.5 hour infusion time; the corresponding mean ±SD C_{max} values were 20.0 ± 3.7 μg/ml and 19.6 ± 4.2 μg/ml, respectively. The point estimate (90% confidence interval) for the bioavailability of etoposide from etoposide phosphate, relative to VePesid, was 107% (105%, 110%) for AUC and 103% (99%, 106%) for C_{max}. In the second study of 29 evaluable patients following intravenous administration of 90, 100 and 110 mg/m² molar equivalents of etoposide phosphate or VePesid with a 60 minute infusion time, the etoposide mean ±SD AUC values (normalized to the 100 mg/m² dose) were 96.1 ± 22.6 μg·h/ml and 86.5 ± 25.8 μg·h/ml, respectively; the corresponding mean ±SD C_{max} values (normalized to the 100 mg/m² dose) were 20.1 ± 4.1 μg/ml and 19.0 ± 5.1 μg/ml, respectively. The point estimate (90% confidence interval) for the bioavailability of etoposide from etoposide phosphate, relative to VePesid, was 113% (107%, 119%) for AUC and 107% (101%, 113%) for C_{max} indicating bioequivalence. Results from both studies demonstrated no statistically significant differences in the AUC and C_{max} parameters for etoposide when administered as etoposide phosphate or VePesid. In addition, in the latter study, there were no statistically significant differences in the pharmacodynamic parameters (hematologic toxicity) after administration of etoposide phosphate or VePesid. Following VePesid administration, the mean nadir values (expressed as percent decrease from baseline) for leukocytes, granulocytes, hemoglobin and thrombocytes were 67.2 ± 17.0%, 84.1 ± 14.6%, 22.6 ± 9.8% and 46.4 ± 21.9%, respectively; the corresponding values after administration of etoposide phosphate were 67.3 ± 14.2%, 81.0 ± 16.5%, 21.4 ± 9.9% and 44.1 ± 20.7%, respectively.

Because of the similarity of pharmacokinetics and pharmacodynamics of etoposide after administration of either etoposide phosphate or VePesid, the following information on VePesid should be considered:

ETOPOSIDE PHOSPHATE PHARMACOKINETICS

On intravenous administration, the disposition of etoposide is best described as a biphasic process with a distribution half-life of about 1.5 hours and terminal elimination half-life ranging from 4-11 hours. Total body clearance values range from 33-48 ml/min or 16-36 ml/min/m² and, like the terminal elimination half-life, are independent of dose over a range 100-600 mg/m². Over the same dose range, the AUC and the C_{max} values increase linearly with dose. Etoposide does not accumulate in the plasma following daily administration of 100 mg/m² for 4-5 days. After intravenous infusion the C_{max} and AUC values exhibit marked intra- and inter-subject variability.

The mean volumes of distribution at steady state fall in the range of 18-29 liters or 7-17 L/m². Etoposide enters the CSF poorly. Although it is detectable in CSF and intracerebral tumors, the concentrations are lower than in extracerebral tumors and in plasma. Etoposide concentrations are higher in normal lung than in lung metastases and are similar in primary tumors and normal tissues of the myometrium. *In vitro,* etoposide is highly protein bound (97%) to human plasma proteins. An inverse relationship between plasma albumin levels and etoposide renal clearance is found in children. In a study determining the effect of other therapeutic agents on the *in vitro* binding of carbon-14 labeled etoposide to human serum proteins, only phenylbutazone, sodium salicylate, and aspirin displaced protein-bound etoposide at concentrations achieved *in vivo.*

Etoposide binding ratio correlates directly with serum albumin in patients with cancer and in normal volunteers. The unbound fraction of etoposide significantly correlated with bilirubin in a population of cancer patients. Data have suggested a significant inverse correlation between serum albumin concentration and free fraction of etoposide (see PRECAUTIONS).

After intravenous administration of ^{3}H-etoposide (70-290 mg/m²), mean recoveries of radioactivity in the urine range from 42-67%, and fecal recoveries range from 0-16% of the dose. Less than 50% of an intravenous dose is excreted in the urine as etoposide with mean recoveries of 8-35% within 24 hours.

In children, approximately 55% of the dose of VePesid (etoposide) is excreted in the urine as etoposide in 24 hours. The mean renal clearance of etoposide is 7-10 ml/min/m² or 35% of the total body clearance over a dose of 80-600 mg/m². Etoposide, therefore, is cleared by both renal and non-renal processes, *i.e.,* metabolism and biliary excretion. The effect of renal disease on plasma etoposide clearance is not known in children.

Biliary excretion appears to be a minor route of etoposide elimination. Only 6% or less of an intravenous dose is recovered in the bile as etoposide. Metabolism accounts for most of the nonrenal clearance of etoposide. The major urinary metabolite of etoposide in adults and children is the hydroxy acid [4′-demethylepipodophyllic acid-9-(4,6-O-(R)-ethylidene-β-D-glucopyra-noside)], formed by opening of the lactone ring. It is also present in human plasma, presumably as the trans isomer. Glucuronide and/or sulfate conjugates of etoposide are excreted in human urine and represent 5-22% of the dose. In addition, O-demethylation of the dimethoxyphenol ring occurs through the CYP450 3A4 isoenzyme pathway to produce the corresponding catechol.

In adults, the total body clearance of etoposide is correlated with creatinine clearance, serum albumin concentration, and nonrenal clearance. Patients with impaired renal function receiving etoposide have exhibited reduced total body clearance, increased AUC and a lower volume of distribution at steady state (see PRECAUTIONS). Use of cisplatin therapy is associated with reduced total body clearance. In children, elevated serum SGPT levels are associated with reduced drug total body clearance. Prior use of cisplatin may also result in a decrease of etoposide total body clearance in children.

Although some minor differences in pharmacokinetic parameters between age and gender have been observed, these differences were not considered clinically significant.

INDICATIONS AND USAGE

Etoposide phosphate for injection is indicated in the management of the following neoplasms:

Refractory Testicular Tumors: Etoposide phosphate for injection in combination therapy with other approved chemotherapeutic agents in patients with refractory testicular tumors who have already received appropriate surgical, chemotherapeutic, and radiotherapeutic therapy.

Small Cell Lung Cancer: Etoposide phosphate for injection in combination with other approved chemotherapeutic agents as first line treatment in patients with small cell lung cancer.

NON-FDA APPROVED INDICATIONS

Etoposide has been used without FDA approval for the treatment of Kaposi's sarcoma, non-Hodgkin's lymphoma, acute myelomonocytic leukemia, acute myelocytic leukemia, and neuroblastoma. It has also been used in the treatment of Ewing's sarcoma, brain tumors, Hodgkin's disease, choriocarcinoma, rhabdomyosarcoma, hepatocellular carcinoma, epithelial ovarian cancer, non-small-cell lung cancer, Wilms' tumor and refractory myeloma.

CONTRAINDICATIONS

Etoposide phosphate for injection is contraindicated in patients who have demonstrated a previous hypersensitivity to etoposide, etoposide phosphate, or any other component of the formulations.

WARNINGS

Patients being treated with etoposide phosphate must be frequently observed for myelosuppression both during and after therapy. Myelosuppression resulting in death has been reported following etoposide administration. Dose-limiting bone marrow suppression is the most significant toxicity associated with etoposide phosphate therapy. Therefore, the following studies should be obtained at the start of therapy and prior to each subsequent cycle of etoposide phosphate: platelet count, hemoglobin, white blood cell count, and differential. The occurrence of a platelet count below 50,000/mm³ or an absolute neutrophil count below 500/mm³ is an indication to withhold further therapy until the blood counts have sufficiently recovered. The toxicity of rapidly infused etoposide phosphate in patients with impaired renal or hepatic function has not been adequately evaluated. The toxicity profile of etoposide phosphate when infused at doses >175 mg/m² has not been delineated.

Physicians should be aware of the possible occurrence of an anaphylactic reaction manifested by chills, fever, tachycardia, bronchospasm, dyspnea and hypotension. Higher rates of anaphylactic-like reactions have been reported in children who received infusions of etoposide at concentrations higher than those recommended. The role that concentration of infusion (or rate of infusion) plays in the development of anaphylactic-like reactions is uncertain. (See ADVERSE REACTIONS.) Treatment is symptomatic. The infusion should be terminated immediately, followed by the administration of pressor agents, corticosteroids, antihistamines, or volume expanders at the discretion of the physician.

Etoposide phosphate can cause fetal harm when administered to a pregnant woman. Etoposide has been shown to be teratogenic in mice and rats, and it is therefore likely that etoposide phosphate is also teratogenic.

In rats, an intravenous etoposide dose of 0.4 mg/kg/day (about 1/20 of the human dose on a mg/m^2 basis) during organogenesis caused maternal toxicity, embryotoxicity, and teratogenicity (skeletal abnormalities, exencephaly, encephalocele, and anophthalmia); higher doses of 1.2 and 3.6 mg/kg/day (about 1/7 and 1/2 of the human dose on a mg/m^2 basis) resulted in 90% and 100% embryonic resorptions. In mice, a single 1.0 mg/kg (1/16 of the human dose on a mg/m^2 basis) dose of etoposide administered intraperitoneally on days 6, 7, or 8 of gestation caused embryotoxicity, cranial abnormalities, and major skeletal malformations. An i.p. dose of 1.5 mg/kg (about 1/10 of the human dose on a mg/m^2 basis) on day 7 of gestation caused an increase in the incidence of intrauterine death and fetal malformations and a significant decrease in the average fetal body weight.

If this drug is used during pregnancy, or if the patient becomes pregnant while receiving this drug, the patient should be warned of the potential hazard to the fetus. Women of childbearing potential should be advised to avoid becoming pregnant.

Etoposide phosphate should be considered a potential carcinogen in humans. The occurrence of acute leukemia with or without a preleukemic phase has been reported in rare instances in patients treated with etoposide alone or in association with other neoplastic agents. The risk of development of a preleukemic or leukemic syndrome is unclear. Carcinogenicity tests with etoposide phosphate have not been conducted in laboratory animals.

PRECAUTIONS

GENERAL

In all instances where the use of etoposide phosphate is considered for chemotherapy, the physician must evaluate the need and usefulness of the drug against the risk of adverse reactions. Most such adverse reactions are reversible if detected early. If severe reactions occur, the drug should be reduced in dosage or discontinued and appropriate corrective measures should be taken according to the clinical judgement of the physician. Reinstitution of etoposide phosphate therapy should be carried out with caution, and with adequate consideration of the further need for the drug and alertness as to possible recurrence of toxicity.

Patients with low serum albumin may be at an increased risk for etoposide associated toxicities.

LABORATORY TESTS

Periodic complete blood counts should be done during the course of etoposide phosphate treatment. They should be performed prior to each cycle of therapy and at appropriate intervals during and after therapy.

CARCINOGENESIS, MUTAGENESIS, AND IMPAIRMENT OF FERTILITY

See WARNINGS.

Etoposide phosphate was nonmutagenic in *in vitro* Ames microbial mutagenicity assay and the *E. coli* WP2 uvrA reverse mutation assay. Since etoposide phosphate is rapidly and completely converted to etoposide *in vivo* and etoposide has been shown to be mutagenic in Ames assay, etoposide phosphate should be considered as a potential mutagen *in vivo.*

In rats, an oral dose of etoposide phosphate at 86.0 mg/kg/day (about 10 times the human dose on a mg/m^2 basis) or above administered for 5 consecutive days resulted in irreversible testicular atrophy. Irreversible testicular atrophy was also present in rats treated with etoposide phosphate intravenously for 30 days at 5.11 mg/kg/day (about ½ of the human dose on a mg/m^2 basis).

PREGNANCY CATEGORY D

See WARNINGS.

NURSING MOTHERS

It is not known whether this drug is excreted in human milk. Because many drugs are excreted in human milk and because of the potential for serious adverse reactions in nursing infants from etoposide phosphate, a decision should be made whether to discontinue nursing or to discontinue the drug, taking into account the importance of the drug to the mother.

PEDIATRIC USE

Safety and effectiveness in pediatric patients have not been established. Anaphylactic reactions have been reported in pediatric patients who received etoposide (see WARNINGS).

RENAL IMPAIRMENT

In patients with impaired renal function, the following initial dose modification should be considered based on measured creatinine clearance:

TABLE 3

Measured Creatine Clearance	>50 ml/min	15-50 ml/min
Etoposide	100% of dose	75% of dose

Subsequent etoposide dosing should be based on patient tolerance and clinical effect. Equivalent dose adjustments of etoposide phosphate should be used.

Data are not available in patients with creatinine clearances <15 ml/min and further dose reduction should be considered in these patients.

DRUG INTERACTIONS

Caution should be exercised when administering etoposide phosphate with drugs that are known to inhibit phosphatase activities (*e.g.,* levamisole hydrochloride). High-dose cyclosporin A resulting in concentrations above 2000 ng/ml administered with oral etoposide has led to an 80% increase in etoposide exposure with a 38% decrease in total body clearance of etoposide compared to etoposide alone.

ADVERSE REACTIONS

Etoposide phosphate has been found to be well tolerated as a single agent in clinical studies involving 206 patients with a wide variety of malignancies, and in combination with cisplatin in 60 patients with small cell lung cancer. The most frequent clinically significant adverse experiences were leukopenia and neutropenia.

The incidences of adverse experiences in TABLE 4 that follows are derived from studies in which etoposide phosphate for injection was administered as a single agent. A total of 98 patients received total doses at or above 450 mg/m^2 on a 5 consecutive days or days 1, 3 and 5 schedule during the first course of therapy.

***TABLE 4** Summary of Adverse Events Reported With Single Agent Etoposide Phosphate Following Course 1 at Total Five Day Doses of ≥450 mg/m^2*

		Percent of Patients
Hematologic Toxicity		
Leukopenia	<4000 /mm^3	91%
	<1000 /mm^3	17%
Neutropenia	<2000 /mm^3	88%
	<500 /mm^3	37%
Thrombocytopenia	<100,000 /mm^3	23%
	<50,000 /mm^3	9%
Anemia	<11 g/dl	72%
	<8 g/dl	19%
Gastrointestinal Toxicity		
Nausea and/or vomiting		37%
Anorexia		16%
Mucositis		11%
Constipation		8%
Abdominal pain		7%
Diarrhea		6%
Taste alteration		6%
Asthenia/malaise		39%
Alopecia		33%
Chills and/or fever		24%
Dizziness		5%
Extravasation/phlebitis		5%

Since etoposide phosphate is converted to etoposide, those adverse experiences that are associated with etoposide can be expected to occur with etoposide phosphate.

HEMATOLOGIC TOXICITY

Myelosuppression after etoposide phosphate administration is dose related and dose limiting with the leukocyte nadir counts occurring from day 15 to day 22 after initiation of drug therapy, granulocyte nadir counts occurring day 12-19 after initiation of drug therapy, and platelet nadirs occurring from day 10-15. Bone marrow recovery usually occurs by day 21 but may be delayed, and no cumulative toxicity has been reported. Fever and infection have also been reported in patients with neutropenia. Death associated with myelosuppression has been reported following etoposide administration.

GASTROINTESTINAL TOXICITY

Nausea and vomiting are the major gastrointestinal toxicities. The severity of such nausea and vomiting is generally mild to moderate with treatment discontinuation required in 1% of patients. Nausea and vomiting can usually be controlled with standard antiemetic therapy.

BLOOD PRESSURE CHANGES

In clinical studies, 151 patients were treated with etoposide phosphate with infusion times ranging from 30 minutes to 3.5 hours. Sixty-three (63) patients received etoposide phosphate as a 5 minute bolus infusion. Four (4) patients experienced 1 or more episodes of hypertension and 8 patients experienced 1 or more episodes of hypotension, which may or may not be drug related. One episode of hypotension was reported among those patients who received a 5 minute bolus infusion. If clinically significant hypotension or hypertension occurs with etoposide phosphate, appropriate supportive therapy should be initiated.

ALLERGIC REACTIONS

Anaphylactic type reactions characterized by chills, rigors, tachycardia, bronchospasm, dyspnea, diaphoresis, fever, pruritus, hypertension or hypotension, loss of consciousness, nausea, and vomiting have been reported to occur in 3% (7/245) of all patients treated with etoposide phosphate. Facial flushing was reported in 2% and skin rashes in 3% of patients receiving etoposide phosphate. These reactions have usually responded promptly to the cessation of the infusion and administration of pressor agents, corticosteroids, antihistamines, or volume expanders as appropriate; however, the reactions can be fatal. Hypertension and/or flushing have also been reported. Blood pressure usually normalizes within a few hours after cessation of the initial infusion.

Anaphylactic-like reactions have occurred during the initial infusion of etoposide phosphate (see WARNINGS). Facial/tongue swelling, coughing, diaphoresis, cyanosis, tightness in throat, laryngospasm, back pain, and/or loss of consciousness have sometimes occurred in association with the above reactions. In addition, an apparent hypersensitivity-associated apnea has been reported rarely.

Rash, urticaria, and/or pruritus have infrequently been reported at recommended doses. At investigational doses, a generalized pruritic erythematous maculopapular rash, consistent with perivasculitis, has been reported.

ALOPECIA

Reversible alopecia, sometimes progressing to total baldness, was observed in up to 44% of patients.

OTHER TOXICITIES

The following adverse reactions have been infrequently reported: abdominal pain, aftertaste, constipation, dysphagia, fever, transient cortical blindness, interstitial pneumonitis/pulmonary fibrosis, optic neuritis, pigmentation, seizure (occasionally associated with allergic reactions), Stevens-Johnson Syndrome, toxic epidermal necrolysis, and a single report of radiation recall dermatitis. Rarely, hepatic toxicity may be seen.

The incidences of adverse reactions in TABLE 5 are derived from multiple data bases from studies in 2081 patients when etoposide was used either orally or by injection as a single agent.

TABLE 5

Adverse Drug Effects Observed With Single Agent VePesid		Percent Range of Reported Incidence
Hematologic Toxicity		
Leukopenia	$<1000\ /mm^3$	3-17%
	$<4000\ /mm^3$	60-91%
Thrombocytopenia	$<50{,}000/mm^3$	1-20%
	$<100{,}000/mm^3$	22-41%
Anemia		0-33%
Gastrointestinal Toxicity		
Nausea and vomiting		31-43%
Abdominal pain		0-2%
Anorexia		10-13%
Diarrhea		1-13%
Stomatitis		1-6%
Hepatic		0-3%
Alopecia		8-66%
Peripheral Neurotoxicity		1-2%
Hypotension		1-2%
Allergic Reaction		1-2%

DOSAGE AND ADMINISTRATION

The usual dose of etoposide for injection in testicular cancer in combination with other approved chemotherapeutic agents ranges from 50 to 100 mg/m^2/day on days 1 through 5 to 100 mg/m^2/day on days 1, 3, and 5. Equivalent doses of etoposide phosphate should be used.

In small cell lung cancer, the etoposide for injection dose in combination with other approved chemotherapeutic drugs ranges from 35 mg/m^2/day for 4 days to 50 mg/m^2/day for 5 days. Equivalent doses of etoposide phosphate should be used.

For recommended dosing adjustments in patients with renal impairment, see PRECAUTIONS.

Etoposide phosphate solutions may be administered at infusion rates from 5-210 minutes. Chemotherapy courses are repeated at 3-4 week intervals after adequate recovery from any toxicity.

The dosage should be modified to take into account the myelosuppressive effect of other drugs in the combination or the effects of prior x-ray therapy or chemotherapy which may have compromised bone marrow reserve.

ADMINISTRATION PRECAUTIONS

As with other potentially toxic compounds, caution should be exercised in handling and preparing the solution of etoposide phosphate. Skin reactions associated with accidental exposure to etoposide phosphate may occur. The use of gloves is recommended. If etoposide phosphate solution contacts the skin or mucosa, immediately and thoroughly wash the skin with soap and water and flush the mucosa with water.

PREPARATION FOR INTRAVENOUS ADMINISTRATION

Prior to use, the content of each vial must be reconstituted with either 5 ml or 10 ml sterile water for injection; 5% dextrose injection; 0.9% sodium chloride injection; sterile bacteriostactic water for injection with benzyl alcohol; or bacteriostatic sodium chloride for injection with benzyl alcohol to a concentration equivalent to 20 mg/ml or 10 mg/ml etoposide (22.7 mg/ml or 11.4 mg/ml etoposide phosphate), respectively. Following reconstitution the solution may be administered without further dilution or it can be further diluted to concentrations as low as 0.1 mg/ml etoposide with either 5% dextrose injection, or 0.9% sodium chloride injection.

Solutions of etoposide phosphate should be prepared in an aseptic manner. Parenteral drug products should be inspected visually for particulate matter and discoloration prior to administration whenever solution and container permit.

STABILITY

Unopened vials of etoposide phosphate for injection are stable until the date indicated on the package when stored under refrigeration 2-8°C (36-46°F) in the original package. When reconstituted and/or diluted as directed, etoposide phosphate solutions can be stored in glass or plastic containers at controlled room temperature 20-25°C (68-77°F) or under refrigeration 2-8°C (36-46°F) for 24 hours. Refrigerated solutions of etoposide phosphate should be used immediately upon return to room temperature.

HOW SUPPLIED

Individually cartoned single-dose vials with white flip-off seals containing etoposide phosphate equivalent to 100 mg etoposide.

Storage: Store the unopened vials under refrigeration 2-8°C (36-46°F). Retain in original package to protect from light.

HANDLING AND DISPOSAL

Procedures for proper handling and disposal of anticancer drugs should be considered. Several guidelines on this subject have been published.[1-7] There is no general agreement that all of the procedures recommended in the guidelines are necessary or appropriate.

PRODUCT LISTING - EQUIVALENTS NOT AVAILABLE

Powder For Injection - Intravenous - 100 mg

1's $124.14 ETOPOPHOS, Bristol-Myers Squibb 00015-3404-20

Exemestane *(003455)*

Categories: Carcinoma, breast; FDA Approved 1999 Oct; Pregnancy Category D; Orphan Drugs
Drug Classes: Antineoplastics, hormones/hormone modifiers; Antineoplastics, aromatase inhibitors; Hormones/hormone modifiers
Foreign Brand Availability: Aromasin (Australia; Bahrain; Canada; Colombia; Cyprus; Egypt; England; Germany; Hong-Kong; Iran; Iraq; Ireland; Israel; Jordan; Korea; Kuwait; Lebanon; Libya; Oman; Qatar; Republic-of-Yemen; Saudi-Arabia; Singapore; Syria; Thailand; United-Arab-Emirates); Aromasine (France)
Cost of Therapy: $245.41 (Breast Cancer; Aromasin; 25 mg; 1 tablet/day; 30 day supply)

DESCRIPTION

Aromasin tablets for oral administration contain 25 mg of exemestane, an irreversible, steroidal aromatase inactivator. Exemestane is chemically described as 6-methylenandrosta-1,4-diene-3,17 -dione. Its molecular formula is $C_{20}H_{24}O_2$.

The active ingredient is a white to slightly yellow crystalline powder with a molecular weight of 296.41. Exemestane is freely soluble in N, N-dimethylformamide, soluble in methanol, and practically insoluble in water.

Each Aromasin tablet contains the following inactive ingredients: Mannitol, crospovidone, polysorbate 80, hydroxypropyl methylcellulose, colloidal silicon dioxide, microcrystalline cellulose, sodium starch glycolate, magnesium stearate, simethicone, polyethylene glycol 6000, sucrose, magnesium carbonate, titanium dioxide, methylparaben, and polyvinyl alcohol.

CLINICAL PHARMACOLOGY

MECHANISM OF ACTION

Breast cancer cell growth may be estrogen-dependent. Exemestane is the principal enzyme that converts androgens to estrogens both in pre- and postmenopausal women. While the main source of estrogen (primarily estradiol) is the ovary in premenopausal women, the principal source of circulating estrogens in postmenopausal women is from conversion of adrenal and ovarian androgens (androstenedione and testosterone) to estrogens (estrone and estradiol) by the aromatase enzyme in peripheral tissues. Estrogen deprivation through aromatase inhibition is an effective and selective treatment for some postmenopausal patients with hormone-dependent breast cancer.

Exemestane is an irreversible, steroidal aromatase inactivator, structurally related to the natural substrate androstenedione. It acts as a false substrate for the aromatase enzyme, and is processed to an intermediate that binds irreversibly to the active site of the enzyme causing its inactivation, an effect also known as "suicide inhibition". Exemestane significantly lowers circulating estrogen concentrations in postmenopausal women, but has no detectable effect on adrenal biosynthesis of corticosteroids or aldosterone. Exemestane has no effect on other enzymes involved in the steroidogenic pathway up to a concentration at least 600 times higher than that inhibiting the aromatase enzyme.

PHARMACOKINETICS

Following oral administration to healthy postmenopausal women, exemestane is rapidly absorbed. After maximum plasma concentration is reached, levels decline polyexponentially with a mean terminal half-life of about 24 hours. Exemestane is extensively distributed and is cleared from the systemic circulation primarily by metabolism. The pharmacokinetics of exemestane are dose proportional after single (10-200 mg) or repeated oral doses (0.5 to 50 mg). Following repeated daily doses of exemestane 25 mg, plasma concentrations of unchanged drug are similar to levels measured after a single dose.

Pharmacokinetic parameters in postmenopausal women with advanced breast cancer following single or repeated doses have been compared with those in healthy, postmenopausal women. Exemestane appeared to be more rapidly absorbed in the women with breast cancer than in the healthy women, with a mean T_{max} of 1.2 hours in the women with breast cancer and 2.9 hours in the healthy women. After repeated dosing, the average oral clearance in women with advanced breast cancer was 45% lower than the oral clearance in healthy postmenopausal women, with corresponding higher systemic exposure. Mean AUC values following repeated doses in women with breast cancer (75.4 ng·h/ml) were about twice those in healthy women (41.4 ng·h/ml).

Absorption

Following oral administration of radiolabeled exemestane, at least 42% of radioactivity was absorbed from the gastrointestinal tract. Exemestane plasma levels increased by approximately 40% after a high-fat breakfast.

Distribution

Exemestane is distributed extensively into tissues. Exemestane is 90% bound to plasma proteins and the fraction bound is independent of the total concentration. Albumin and α_1-acid glycoprotein both contribute to the binding. The distribution of exemestane and its metabolites into blood cells is negligible.

Metabolism and Excretion

Following administration of radiolabeled exemestane to healthy postmenopausal women, the cumulative amounts of radioactivity excreted in urine and feces were similar (42 ± 3% in urine and 42 ± 6% in feces over a 1-week collection period). The amount of drug excreted unchanged in urine was less than 1% of the dose. Exemestane is extensively metabolized, with levels of the unchanged drug in plasma accounting for less than 10% of the total radioactivity. The initial steps in the metabolism of exemestane are oxidation of the methylene group in position 6 and reduction of the 17-keto group with subsequent formation of many secondary metabolites. Each metabolite accounts only for a limited amount of drug-related material. The metabolites are inactive or inhibit aromatase with decreased potency compared with the parent drug. One metabolite may have androgenic activity (see Pharmacodynamics, Other Endocrine Effects). Studies using human liver preparations indicate that cytochrome P-450 3A4 (CYP 3A4) is the principal isoenzyme involved in the oxidation of exemestane.

SPECIAL POPULATIONS

Geriatric

Healthy postmenopausal women aged 43-68 years were studied in the pharmacokinetic trials. Age-related alterations in exemestane pharmacokinetics were not seen over this age range.

Gender

The pharmacokinetics of exemestane following administration of a single, 25 mg tablet to fasted healthy males (mean age 32 years) were similar to the pharmacokinetics of exemestane in fasted healthy postmenopausal women (mean age 55 years).

Race

The influence of race on exemestane pharmacokinetics has not been evaluated.

Hepatic Insufficiency

The pharmacokinetics of exemestane have been investigated in subjects with moderate or severe hepatic insufficiency (Childs-Pugh B or C). Following a single 25 mg oral dose, the AUC of exemestane was approximately 3 times higher than that observed in healthy volunteers. (See PRECAUTIONS.)

Renal Insufficiency

The AUC of exemestane after a single 25 mg dose was approximately 3 times higher in subjects with moderate or severe renal insufficiency (creatinine clearance <35 ml/min/1.73 m^2) compared with the AUC in healthy volunteers (see PRECAUTIONS).

Pediatric

The pharmacokinetics of exemestane have not been studied in pediatric patients.

DRUG-DRUG INTERACTIONS

Exemestane is metabolized by cytochrome P-450 3A4 (CYP 3A4) and aldoketoreductases. It does not inhibit any of the major CYP isoenzymes, including CYP 1A2, 2C9, 2D6, 2E1, and 3A4. In a clinical pharmacokinetic study, ketoconazole showed no significant influence on the pharmacokinetics of exemestane. Although no other formal drug-drug interaction studies have been conducted, significant effects on exemestane clearance by CYP isoenzymes inhibitors appear unlikely. However, a possible decrease of exemestane plasma levels by known inducers of CYP 3A4 cannot be excluded.

PHARMACODYNAMICS

Effect on Estrogens

Multiple doses of exemestane ranging from 0.5 to 600 mg/day were administered to postmenopausal women with advanced breast cancer. Plasma estrogen (estradiol, estrone, and estrone sulfate) suppression was seen starting at a 5 mg daily dose of exemestane, with a maximum suppression of at least 85-95% achieved at a 25 mg dose. Exemestane 25 mg daily reduced whole body aromatization (as measured by injecting radiolabeled androstenedione) by 98% in postmenopausal women with breast cancer. After a single dose of exemestane 25 mg, the maximal suppression of circulating estrogens occurred 2-3 days after dosing and persisted for 4-5 days.

Effect on Corticosteroids

In multiple-dose trials of doses up to 200 mg daily, exemestane selectivity was assessed by examining its effect on adrenal steroids. Exemestane did not affect cortisol or aldosterone secretion at baseline or in response to ACTH at any dose. Thus, no glucocorticoid or mineralocorticoid replacement therapy is necessary with exemestane treatment.

Other Endocrine Effects

Exemestane does not bind significantly to steroidal receptors, except for a slightly affinity for the androgen receptor (0.28% relative to dihydrotestosterone). The binding affinity of its 17-dihydrometabolite for the androgen receptor, however, is 100-times that of the parent compound. Daily doses of exemestane up to 25 mg had no significant effect on circulating levels of testosterone, androstenedione, dehydroepiandrosterone sulfate, or 17-hydroxyprogesterone. Increases in testosterone and androstenedione levels have been observed at daily doses of 200 mg or more. A dose-dependent decrease in sex hormone binding globulin (SHBG) has been observed with daily exemestane doses of 2.5 mg or higher. Slight, nondose-dependent increases in serum lutenizing hormone (LH) and follicle-stimulating hormone (FSH) levels have been observed even at low doses as a consequence of feedback at the pituitary level.

INDICATIONS AND USAGE

Exemestane tablets are indicated for the treatment of advanced breast cancer in postmenopausal women whose disease has progressed following tamoxifen therapy.

CONTRAINDICATIONS

Exemestane tablets are contraindicated in patients with a known hypersensitivity to the drug or to any of the excipients.

WARNINGS

Exemestane tablets may cause fetal harm when administered to a pregnant woman. Radioactivity related to ^{14}C-exemestane crossed the placenta of rats following oral administration of 1 mg/kg exemestane. The concentration of exemestane and its metabolites was approximately equivalent in maternal and fetal blood. When rats were administered exemestane from 14 days prior to mating until either days 15 or 20 of gestation, and resuming for the 21 days of lactation, an increase in placental weight was seen at 4 mg/kg/d (approximately 1.5 times the recommended human daily dose on a mg/m^2 basis). Prolonged gestation and abnormal or difficult labor was observed at doses equal to or greater than 20 mg/kg/d. Increased resorption, reduced number of live fetuses, decreased fetal weight, and retarded ossification were also observed at these doses. No malformations were noted when exemestane was administered to pregnant rats during the organogenesis period at doses up to 810 mg/kg/day (approximately 320 times the recommended human dose on a mg/m^2 basis). Daily doses of exemestane, given to rabbits during organogenesis caused a decrease in placental weight at 90 mg/kg/day (approximately 70 times the recommended human daily dose on a mg/m^2 basis). Abortions, an increase in resorptions, and a reduction in fetal body weight were seen at 270 mg/kg/day. There was no increase in the incidence of malformations in rabbits at doses up to 270 mg/kg/day (approximately 210 times the recommended human dose on a mg/m^2 basis).

There are no studies in pregnant women using exemestane. Exemestane is indicated for postmenopausal women. If there is exposure to exemestane during pregnancy, the patient should be apprised of the potential hazard to the fetus and potential risk for loss of the pregnancy.

PRECAUTIONS

GENERAL

Exemestane tablets should not be administered to premenopausal women. Exemestane should not be coadministered with estrogen-containing agents as these could interfere with its pharmacologic action.

HEPATIC INSUFFICIENCY

The pharmacokinetics of exemestane have been investigated in subjects with moderate or severe hepatic insufficiency (Childs-Pugh B or C). Following a single 25 mg oral dose, the AUC of exemestane was approximately 3 times higher than that observed in healthy volunteers. The safety of chronic dosing in patients with moderate or severe hepatic impairment has not been studied. Based on experience with exemestane at repeated doses up to 200 mg daily that demonstrated a moderate increase in non-life threatening adverse events, dosage adjustment does not appear to be necessary.

RENAL INSUFFICIENCY

The AUC of exemestane after a single 25 mg dose was approximately 3 times higher in subjects with moderate or severe renal insufficiency (creatinine clearance <35 ml/min/1.73 m^2) compared with the AUC in healthy volunteers. The safety of chronic dosing in patients with moderate or severe renal impairment has not been studied. Based on experience with exemestane at repeated doses up to 200 mg daily that demonstrated a moderate increase in non-life threatening adverse events, dosage adjustment does not appear to be necessary.

LABORATORY TESTS

Approximately 20% of patients receiving exemestane in clinical studies, experienced Common Toxicity Criteria (CTC) grade 3 or 4 lymphocytopenia. Of these patients, 89% had a pre-existing lower grade lymphopenia. Forty percent (40%) of patients either recovered or improved to a lesser severity while on treatment. Patients did not have a significant increase in viral infections, and no opportunistic infections were observed. Elevations of serum levels of AST, ALT, alkaline phosphatase, and gamma glutamyl transferase >5 times the upper value of the normal range (*i.e.*, ≥ CTC grade 3) have been rarely reported but appear mostly attributable to the underlying presence of liver and/or bone metastases. In the comparative study, CTC grade 3 or 4 elevation of gamma glutamyl transferase without documented evidence of liver metastasis was reported in 2.7% of patients treated with exemestane and in 1.8% of patients treated with megestrol acetate.

DRUG/LABORATORY TEST INTERACTIONS

No clinically relevant changes in the results of clinical laboratory tests have been observed.

CARCINOGENESIS, MUTAGENESIS, AND IMPAIRMENT OF FERTILITY

Carcinogenicity studies have not been conducted with exemestane. Exemestane was not mutagenic in bacteria (Ames test) or mammalian cells (V79 Chinese hamster lung cells). Exemestane was clastogenic in human lymphocytes *in vitro* without metabolic activation but was not clastogenic *in vivo* (micronucleus assay in mouse bone marrow). Exemestane did not increase unscheduled DNA synthesis in rat hepatocytes.

Untreated female rats showed reduced fertility when mated to males treated with 500 mg/kg/day exemestane (approximately 200 times the recommended human dose on a mg/m^2 basis) for 63 days prior to and during cohabitation. Exemestane given to female rats 14 days prior to mating and through day 15 or 20 of gestation increased the placental weights at 4 mg/kg/day (approximately 1.5 times the human dose on a mg/m^2 basis). Exemestane showed no effects on female fertility parameters (*e.g.*, ovarian function, mating behavior, conception rate) in rats given doses up to 20 mg/kg/day (approximately 8 times the human dose on a mg/m^2 basis), but mean litter size was decreased at this dose. In general toxicology studies, changes in the ovary, including hyperplasia, an increase in ovarian cysts and a decrease in corpora lutea were observed with variable frequency in mice, rats, and dogs at doses that ranged from 3-20 times the human dose on a mg/m^2 basis.

PREGNANCY CATEGORY D

See WARNINGS.

NURSING MOTHERS

Exemestane is only indicated in postmenopausal women. However, radioactivity related to exemestane appeared in rat milk within 15 minutes of oral administration of radiolabeled exemestane. Concentrations of exemestane and its metabolites were approximately equivalent in the milk and plasma of rats for 24 hours after a single oral dose of 1 mg/kg ^{14}C-exemestane. It is not known whether exemestane is excreted in human milk. Because many drugs are excreted in human milk, caution should be exercised if a nursing woman is inadvertently exposed to exemestane (see WARNINGS).

PEDIATRIC USE

The safety and effectiveness of exemestane in pediatric patients have not been established.

GERIATRIC USE

The use of exemestane in geriatric patients does not require special precautions.

DRUG INTERACTIONS

Exemestane is extensively metabolized by CYP3A4, but coadministration of ketoconazole, a potent inhibitor of CYP 3A4, has no significant effect on exemestane pharmacokinetics. Significant pharmacokinetic interactions mediated by inhibition of CYP isoenzymes therefore appear unlikely; however, a possible decrease of exemestane plasma levels by known inducers of CYP 3A4 cannot be excluded (see CLINICAL PHARMACOLOGY, Pharmacokinetics).

ADVERSE REACTIONS

A total of 1058 patients were treated with exemestane 25 mg once daily in the clinical trials program. Exemestane was generally well tolerated, and adverse events were usually mild to moderate. Only 1 death was considered possibly related to treatment with exemestane; an 80-year-old women with known coronary artery disease had a myocardial infarction with multiple organ failure after 9 weeks on study treatment. In the clinical trials program, only 3% of the patients discontinued treatment with exemestane because of adverse events, mainly within the first 10 weeks of treatment; late discontinuations because of adverse events were uncommon (0.3%).

In the comparative study, adverse reactions were assessed for 358 patients treated with exemestane and 400 patients treated with megestrol acetate. Fewer patients receiving exemestane discontinued treatment because of adverse events than those treated with megestrol acetate (2% versus 5%). Adverse events that were considered drug related or of indeterminate cause included hot flashes (13% vs 5%), nausea (9% vs 5%), fatigue (8% vs 10%), increased sweating (4% vs 8%), and increased appetite (3% vs 6%). The proportion of patients experiencing an excessive weight gain (>10% of their baseline weight) was significantly higher with megestrol acetate than with exemestane (17% versus 8%). TABLE 3 shows the adverse events of all CTC grades, regardless of causality, reported in 5% or greater of patients in the study treated either with exemestane or megestrol acetate.

***TABLE 3** Incidence (%) of Adverse Events of all Grades* and Causes Occurring in ≥5% of Patients in Each Treatment Arm in the Comparative Study*

Event	Exemestane 25 mg once daily (n=358)	Megestrol Acetate 40 mg qid (n=400)
Autonomic Nervous		
Increased sweating	6%	9%
Body as a Whole		
Fatigue	22%	29%
Hot flashes	13%	6%
Pain	13%	13%
Influenza-like symptoms	6%	5%
Edema (includes edema, peripheral edema, leg edema)	7%	6%
Cardiovascular		
Hypertension	5%	6%
Nervous		
Depression	13%	9%
Insomnia	11%	9%
Anxiety	10%	11%
Dizziness	8%	6%
Headache	8%	7%
Gastrointestinal		
Nausea	18%	12%
Vomiting	7%	4%
Abdominal pain	6%	11%
Anorexia	6%	5%
Constipation	5%	8%
Diarrhea	4%	5%
Increased appetite	3%	6%
Respiratory		
Dyspnea	10%	15%
Coughing	6%	7%

* Graded according to Common Toxicity Criteria.

Less frequent adverse events of any cause (from 2-5%) reported in the comparative study for patients receiving exemestane 25 mg once daily were fever, generalized weakness, paresthesia, pathological fracture; bronchitis, sinusitis, rash, itching, urinary tract infection, and lymphedema.

Additional adverse events of any cause observed in the overall clinical trials program (n=1058) in 5% or greater of patients treated with exemestane 25 mg once daily but not in the comparative study included pain at tumor sites (8%), asthenia (6%), and fever (5%). Adverse events of any cause reported in 2-5% of all patients treated with exemestane 25 mg in the overall clinical trials program but not in the comparative study included chest pain, hypoesthesia, confusion, dyspepsia, arthralgia, back pain, skeletal pain, infection, upper respiratory tract infection, pharyngitis, rhinitis, and alopecia.

DOSAGE AND ADMINISTRATION

The recommended dose of exemestane tablets is 25 mg once daily after a meal. Treatment with exemestane should continue until tumor progression is evident.

The safety of chronic dosing in patients with moderate or severe hepatic or renal impairment has not been studied. Based on experience with exemestane at repeated doses up to 200 mg daily that demonstrated a moderate increase in non-life threatening adverse events, dosage adjustment does not appear to be necessary (see CLINICAL PHARMACOLOGY, Special Populations and PRECAUTIONS).

HOW SUPPLIED

Aromasin tablets are round, biconvex, and off-white to slightly gray. Each tablet contains 25 mg of exemestane. The tablets are printed on one side with the number "7663" in black.
Storage: Store at 25°C (77°F); excursions permitted to 15-30°C (59-86°F).

PRODUCT LISTING - EQUIVALENTS NOT AVAILABLE

Tablet - Oral - 25 mg
30's $245.41 AROMASIN, Pharmacia and Upjohn 00009-7663-04

Ezetimibe *(003574)*

For related information, see the comparative table section in Appendix A.

Categories: Hypercholesterolemia; Hyperlipidemia; Sitosterolemia; Pregnancy Category C; FDA Approved 2002 Oct
Drug Classes: Antihyperlipidemics
Brand Names: **Zetia**
Cost of Therapy: $72.38 (Hypercholesterolemia; Zetia; 10 mg; 1 tablet/day; 30 day supply)

E

DESCRIPTION

Ezetimibe is in a class of lipid-lowering compounds that selectively inhibits the intestinal absorption of cholesterol and related phytosterols. The chemical name of ezetimibe is 1-(4-fluorophenyl)-3(R)-[3-(4-fluorophenyl)-3(S)-hydroxypropyl]-4(S)-(4-hydroxyphenyl)-2-azetidinone. The empirical formula is $C_{24}H_{21}F_2NO_3$. Its molecular weight is 409.4.

Ezetimibe is a white, crystalline powder that is freely to very soluble in ethanol, methanol, and acetone and practically insoluble in water. Ezetimibe has a melting point of about 163°C and is stable at ambient temperature. Zetia is available as a tablet for oral administration containing 10 mg of ezetimibe and the following inactive ingredients: croscarmellose sodium, lactose monohydrate, magnesium stearate, microcrystalline cellulose, povidone, and sodium lauryl sulfate.

CLINICAL PHARMACOLOGY

BACKGROUND

Clinical studies have demonstrated that elevated levels of total cholesterol (total-C), low density lipoprotein cholesterol (LDL-C) and apolipoprotein B (Apo B), the major protein constituent of LDL, promote human atherosclerosis. In addition, decreased levels of high density lipoprotein cholesterol (HDL-C) are associated with the development of atherosclerosis. Epidemiologic studies have established that cardiovascular morbidity and mortality vary directly with the level of total-C and LDL-C and inversely with the level of HDL-C. Like LDL, cholesterol-enriched triglyceride-rich lipoproteins, including very-low-density lipoproteins (VLDL), intermediate-density lipoproteins (IDL), and remnants, can also promote atherosclerosis. The independent effect of raising HDL-C or lowering triglycerides (TG) on the risk of coronary and cardiovascular morbidity and mortality has not been determined.

Ezetimibe reduces total-C, LDL-C, Apo B, and TG, and increases HDL-C in patients with hypercholesterolemia. Administration of ezetimibe with an HMG-CoA reductase inhibitor is effective in improving serum total-C, LDL-C, Apo B, TG, and HDL-C beyond either treatment alone. The effects of ezetimibe given either alone or in addition to an HMG-CoA reductase inhibitor on cardiovascular morbidity and mortality have not been established.

MODE OF ACTION

Ezetimibe reduces blood cholesterol by inhibiting the absorption of cholesterol by the small intestine. In a 2 week clinical study in 18 hypercholesterolemic patients, ezetimibe inhibited intestinal cholesterol absorption by 54%, compared with placebo. Ezetimibe had no clinically meaningful effect on the plasma concentrations of the fat-soluble vitamins A, D, and E (in a study of 113 patients), and did not impair adrenocortical steroid hormone production (in a study of 118 patients).

The cholesterol content of the liver is derived predominantly from 3 sources. The liver can synthesize cholesterol, take up cholesterol from the blood from circulating lipoproteins, or take up cholesterol absorbed by the small intestine. Intestinal cholesterol is derived primarily from cholesterol secreted in the bile and from dietary cholesterol.

Ezetimibe has a mechanism of action that differs from those of other classes of cholesterol-reducing compounds (HMG-CoA reductase inhibitors, bile acid sequestrants [resins], fibric acid derivatives, and plant stanols).

Ezetimibe does not inhibit cholesterol synthesis in the liver, or increase bile acid excretion. Instead, ezetimibe localizes and appears to act at the brush border of the small intestine and inhibits the absorption of cholesterol, leading to a decrease in the delivery of intestinal cholesterol to the liver. This causes a reduction of hepatic cholesterol stores and an increase in clearance of cholesterol from the blood; this distinct mechanism is complementary to that of HMG-CoA reductase inhibitors.

PHARMACOKINETICS

Absorption

After oral administration, ezetimibe is absorbed and extensively conjugated to a pharmacologically active phenolic glucuronide (ezetimibe-glucuronide). After a single 10 mg dose of ezetimibe to fasted adults, mean ezetimibe peak plasma concentrations (C_{max}) of 3.4-5.5 ng/ml were attained within 4-12 hours (T_{max}). Ezetimibe-glucuronide mean C_{max} values of 45-71 ng/ml were achieved between 1 and 2 hours (T_{max}). There was no substantial deviation from dose proportionality between 5 and 20 mg. The absolute bioavailability of ezetimibe cannot be determined, as the compound is virtually insoluble in aqueous media suitable for injection. Ezetimibe has variable bioavailability; the coefficient of variation, based on intersubject variability, was 35-60% for AUC values.

Effect of Food on Oral Absorption

Concomitant food administration (high fat or non-fat meals) had no effect on the extent of absorption of ezetimibe when administered as ezetimibe 10 mg tablets. The C_{max} value of ezetimibe was increased by 38% with consumption of high fat meals. Ezetimibe can be administered with or without food.

Distribution
Ezetimibe and ezetimibe-glucuronide are highly bound (>90%) to human plasma proteins.

Metabolism and Excretion
Ezetimibe is primarily metabolized in the small intestine and liver via glucuronide conjugation (a phase II reaction) with subsequent biliary and renal excretion. Minimal oxidative metabolism (a phase I reaction) has been observed in all species evaluated.

In humans, ezetimibe is rapidly metabolized to ezetimibe-glucuronide. Ezetimibe and ezetimibe-glucuronide are the major drug-derived compounds detected in plasma, constituting approximately 10-20% and 80-90% of the total drug in plasma, respectively. Both ezetimibe and ezetimibe-glucuronide are slowly eliminated from plasma with a half-life of approximately 22 hours for both ezetimibe and ezetimibe-glucuronide. Plasma concentration-time profiles exhibit multiple peaks, suggesting enterohepatic recycling.

Following oral administration of ^{14}C-ezetimibe (20 mg) to human subjects, total ezetimibe (ezetimibe + ezetimibe-glucuronide) accounted for approximately 93% of the total radioactivity in plasma. After 48 hours, there were no detectable levels of radioactivity in the plasma.

Approximately 78% and 11% of the administered radioactivity were recovered in the feces and urine, respectively, over a 10 day collection period. Ezetimibe was the major component in feces and accounted for 69% of the administered dose, while ezetimibe-glucuronide was the major component in urine and accounted for 9% of the administered dose.

Special Populations

Geriatric Patients
In a multiple dose study with ezetimibe given 10 mg once daily for 10 days, plasma concentrations for total ezetimibe were about 2-fold higher in older (≥65 years) healthy subjects compared to younger subjects.

Pediatric Patients
In a multiple dose study with ezetimibe given 10 mg once daily for 7 days, the absorption and metabolism of ezetimibe were similar in adolescents (10-18 years) and adults. Based on total ezetimibe, there are no pharmacokinetic differences between adolescents and adults. Pharmacokinetic data in the pediatric population <10 years of age are not available.

Gender
In a multiple dose study with ezetimibe given 10 mg once daily for 10 days, plasma concentrations for total ezetimibe were slightly higher (<20%) in women than in men.

Race
Based on a meta-analysis of multiple-dose pharmacokinetic studies, there were no pharmacokinetic differences between Blacks and Caucasians. There were too few patients in other racial or ethnic groups to permit further pharmacokinetic comparisons.

Hepatic Insufficiency
After a single 10 mg dose of ezetimibe, the mean area under the curve (AUC) for total ezetimibe was increased approximately 1.7-fold in patients with mild hepatic insufficiency (Child-Pugh score 5-6), compared to healthy subjects. The mean AUC values for total ezetimibe and ezetimibe were increased approximately 3- to 4-fold and 5- 6-fold, respectively, in patients with moderate (Child-Pugh score 7-9) or severe hepatic impairment (Child-Pugh score 10-15). In a 14 day, multiple-dose study (10 mg daily) in patients with moderate hepatic insufficiency, the mean AUC values for total ezetimibe and ezetimibe were increased approximately 4-fold on Day 1 and Day 14 compared to healthy subjects. Due to the unknown effects of the increased exposure to ezetimibe in patients with moderate or severe hepatic insufficiency, ezetimibe is not recommended in these patients (see CONTRAINDICATIONS and PRECAUTIONS, Hepatic Insufficiency).

Renal Insufficiency
After a single 10 mg dose of ezetimibe in patients with severe renal disease (n=8; mean CRCL ≤30 ml/min/1.73 m^2), the mean AUC values for total ezetimibe, ezetimibe-glucuronide, and ezetimibe were increased approximately 1.5-fold, compared to healthy subjects (n=9).

DRUG INTERACTIONS
See also DRUG INTERACTIONS.

Ezetimibe had no significant effect on a series of probe drugs (caffeine, dextromethorphan, tolbutamide, and IV midazolam) known to be metabolized by cytochrome P450 (1A2, 2D6, 2C8/9 and 3A4) in a "cocktail" study of 12 healthy adult males. This indicates that ezetimibe is neither an inhibitor nor an inducer of these cytochrome P450 isozymes, and it is unlikely that ezetimibe will affect the metabolism of drugs that are metabolized by these enzymes.

Warfarin: Concomitant administration of ezetimibe (10 mg once daily) had no significant effect on bioavailability of warfarin and prothrombin time in a study of 12 healthy adult males.

Digoxin: Concomitant administration of ezetimibe (10 mg once daily) had no significant effect on the bioavailability of digoxin and the ECG parameters (HR, PR, QT, and QTc intervals) in a study of 12 healthy adult males.

Gemfibrozil: In a study of 12 healthy adult males, concomitant administration of gemfibrozil (600 mg twice daily) significantly increased the oral bioavailability of total ezetimibe by a factor of 1.7. Ezetimibe (10 mg once daily) did not significantly affect the bioavailability of gemfibrozil.

Oral Contraceptives: Coadministration of ezetimibe (10 mg once daily) with oral contraceptives had no significant effect on the bioavailability of ethinyl estradiol or levonorgestrel in a study of 18 healthy adult females.

Cimetidine: Multiple doses of cimetidine (400 mg twice daily) had no significant effect on the oral bioavailability of ezetimibe and total ezetimibe in a study of 12 healthy adults.

Antacids: In a study of 12 healthy adults, a single dose of antacid (Supralox 20 ml) administration had no significant effect on the oral bioavailability of total ezetimibe, ezetimibe-glucuronide, or ezetimibe based on AUC values. The C_{max} value of total ezetimibe was decreased by 30%.

Glipizide: In a study of 12 healthy adult males, steady-state levels of ezetimibe (10 mg once daily) had no significant effect on the pharmacokinetics and pharmacodynamics of glipizide. A single dose of glipizide (10 mg) had no significant effect on the exposure to total ezetimibe or ezetimibe.

HMG-CoA Reductase Inhibitors: In studies of healthy hypercholesterolemic (LDL-C ≥130 mg/dl) adult subjects, concomitant administration of ezetimibe (10 mg once daily) had no significant effect on the bioavailability of either lovastatin, simvastatin, pravastatin, atorvastatin, or fluvastatin. No significant effect on the bioavailability of total ezetimibe and ezetimibe was demonstrated by either lovastatin (20 mg once daily), pravastatin (20 mg once daily), atorvastatin (10 mg once daily), or fluvastatin (20 mg once daily).

Fenofibrate: In a study of 32 healthy hypercholesterolemic (LDL-C ≥130 mg/dl) adult subjects, concomitant fenofibrate (200 mg once daily) administration increased the mean C_{max} and AUC values of total ezetimibe approximately 64% and 48%, respectively. Pharmacokinetics of fenofibrate were not significantly affected by ezetimibe (10 mg once daily).

Cholestyramine: In a study of 40 healthy hypercholesterolemic (LDL-C ≥130 mg/dl) adult subjects, concomitant cholestyramine (4 g twice daily) administration decreased the mean AUC values of total ezetimibe and ezetimibe approximately 55% and 80%, respectively.

INDICATIONS AND USAGE

PRIMARY HYPERCHOLESTEROLEMIA

Monotherapy
Ezetimibe, administered alone is indicated as adjunctive therapy to diet for the reduction of elevated total-C, LDL-C, and Apo B in patients with primary (heterozygous familial and non-familial) hypercholesterolemia.

Combination Therapy With HMG-CoA Reductase Inhibitors
Ezetimibe, administered in combination with an HMG-CoA reductase inhibitor, is indicated as adjunctive therapy to diet for the reduction of elevated total-C, LDL-C, and Apo B in patients with primary (heterozygous familial and non-familial) hypercholesterolemia.

HOMOZYGOUS FAMILIAL HYPERCHOLESTEROLEMIA (HOFH)
The combination of ezetimibe and atorvastatin or simvastatin, is indicated for the reduction of elevated total-C and LDL-C levels in patients with HoFH, as an adjunct to other lipid-lowering treatments (*e.g.*, LDL apheresis) or if such treatments are unavailable.

HOMOZYGOUS SITOSTEROLEMIA
Ezetimibe is indicated as adjunctive therapy to diet for the reduction of elevated sitosterol and campesterol levels in patients with homozygous familial sitosterolemia.

Therapy with lipid-altering agents should be a component of multiple risk-factor intervention in individuals at increased risk for atherosclerotic vascular disease due to hypercholesterolemia. Lipid-altering agents should be used in addition to an appropriate diet (including restriction of saturated fat and cholesterol) and when the response to diet and other non-pharmacological measures has been inadequate. (See TABLE 7.)

Prior to initiating therapy with ezetimibe, secondary causes for dyslipidemia (*i.e.*, diabetes, hypothyroidism, obstructive liver disease, chronic renal failure, and drugs that increase LDL-C and decrease HDL-C [progestins, anabolic steroids, and corticosteroids]), should be excluded or, if appropriate, treated. A lipid profile should be performed to measure total-C, LDL-C, HDL-C and TG. For TG levels >400 mg/dl (>4.5 mmol/L), LDL-C concentrations should be determined by ultracentrifugation.

At the time of hospitalization for an acute coronary event, lipid measures should be taken on admission or within 24 hours. These values can guide the physician on initiation of LDL-lowering therapy before or at discharge.

CONTRAINDICATIONS

Hypersensitivity to any component of this medication.

The combination of ezetimibe with an HMG-CoA reductase inhibitor is contraindicated in patients with active liver disease or unexplained persistent elevations in serum transaminases.

All HMG-CoA reductase inhibitors are contraindicated in pregnant and nursing women. When ezetimibe is administered with an HMG-CoA reductase inhibitor in a woman of childbearing potential, refer to the pregnancy category and product labeling for the HMG-CoA reductase inhibitor. (See PRECAUTIONS, Pregnancy Category C.)

PRECAUTIONS

Concurrent administration of ezetimibe with a specific HMG-CoA reductase inhibitor should be in accordance with the product labeling for that HMG-CoA reductase inhibitor.

LIVER ENZYMES
In controlled clinical monotherapy studies, the incidence of consecutive elevations (≥3 × the upper limit of normal [ULN]) in serum transaminases was similar between ezetimibe (0.5%) and placebo (0.3%).

In controlled clinical combination studies of ezetimibe initiated concurrently with an HMG-CoA reductase inhibitor, the incidence of consecutive elevations (≥3 × ULN) in serum transaminases was 1.3% for patients treated with ezetimibe administered with HMG-CoA reductase inhibitors and 0.4% for patients treated with HMG-CoA reductase inhibitors alone. These elevations in transaminases were generally asymptomatic, not associated with cholestasis, and returned to baseline after discontinuation of therapy or with continued treatment. When ezetimibe is co-administered with an HMG-CoA reductase inhibitor, liver function tests should be performed at initiation of therapy and according to the recommendations of the HMG-CoA reductase inhibitor.

TABLE 7 *Summary of NCEP ATP III Guidelines*

Risk Category	LDL Goal (mg/dl)	LDL Level at Which to Initiate Therapeutic Lifestyle Changes* (mg/dl)	LDL Level at Which to Consider Drug Therapy (mg/dl)
CHD or CHD risk equivalents† (10 year risk >20%)‡	<100	≥100	≥130 (100-129: drug optional)§
2+ Risk factors¤ (10 year risk ≤20%)‡	<130	≥130	10 year risk 10-20%: ≥130‡ 10 year risk <10%: ≥160‡
0-1 Risk factor¶	<160	≥160	≥190 (160-189: LDL-lowering drug optional)

* Therapeutic lifestyle changes include: (1) dietary changes: reduced intake of saturated fats (<7% of total calories) and cholesterol (<200 mg/day), and enhancing LDL lowering with plant stanols/sterols (2 g/d) and increased viscous (soluble) fiber (10-25 g/d), (2) weight reduction, and (3) increased physical activity.
† CHD risk equivalents comprise: diabetes, multiple risk factors that confer a 10 year risk for CHD >20%, and other clinical forms of atherosclerotic disease (peripheral arterial disease, abdominal aortic aneurysm and symptomatic carotid artery disease).
‡ Risk assessment for determining the 10 year risk for developing CHD is carried out using the Framingham risk scoring. Refer to JAMA, May 16, 2001; 285 (19): 2486-2497, or the NCEP website (http://www.nhlbi.nih.gov) for more details.
§ Some authorities recommend use of LDL-lowering drugs in this category if an LDL cholesterol <100 mg/dl cannot be achieved by therapeutic lifestyle changes. Others prefer use of drugs that primarily modify triglycerides and HDL, *e.g.,* nicotinic acid or fibrate. Clinical judgment also may call for deferring drug therapy in this subcategory.
¤ Major risk factors (exclusive of LDL cholesterol) that modify LDL goals include cigarette smoking, hypertension (BP ≥140/90 mm Hg or on antihypertensive medication), low HDL cholesterol (<40 mg/dl), family history of premature CHD (CHD in male first-degree relative <55 years; CHD in female first-degree relative <65 years), age (men ≥45 years; women ≥55 years). HDL cholesterol ≥60 mg/dl counts as a "negative" risk factor; its presence removes 1 risk factor from the total count.
¶ Almost all people with 0-1 risk factor have a 10 year risk <10%; thus, 10 year risk assessment in people with 0-1 risk factor is not necessary.

SKELETAL MUSCLE

In clinical trials, there was no excess of myopathy or rhabdomyolysis associated with ezetimibe compared with the relevant control arm (placebo or HMG-CoA reductase inhibitor alone). However, myopathy and rhabdomyolysis are known adverse reactions to HMG-CoA reductase inhibitors and other lipid-lowering drugs. In clinical trials, the incidence of CPK >10 × ULN was 0.2% for ezetimibe versus 0.1% for placebo, and 0.1% for ezetimibe co-administered with an HMG-CoA reductase inhibitor versus 0.4% for HMG-CoA reductase inhibitors alone.

HEPATIC INSUFFICIENCY

Due to the unknown effects of the increased exposure to ezetimibe in patients with moderate or severe hepatic insufficiency, ezetimibe is not recommended in these patients. (See CLINICAL PHARMACOLOGY, Pharmacokinetics, Special Populations.)

CARCINOGENESIS, MUTAGENESIS, AND IMPAIRMENT OF FERTILITY

A 104 week dietary carcinogenicity study with ezetimibe was conducted in rats at doses up to 1500 mg/kg/day (males) and 500 mg/kg/day (females) [~20 times the human exposure at 10 mg daily based on AUC(0-24h) for total ezetimibe]. A 104 week dietary carcinogenicity study with ezetimibe was also conducted in mice at doses up to 500 mg/kg/day [>150 times the human exposure at 10 mg daily based on AUC(0-24h) for total ezetimibe]. There were no statistically significant increases in tumor incidences in drug-treated rats or mice.

No evidence of mutagenicity was observed *in vitro* in a microbial mutagenicity (Ames) test with *Salmonella typhimurium* and *Escherichia coli* with or without metabolic activation. No evidence of clastogenicity was observed *in vitro* in a chromosomal aberration assay in human peripheral blood lymphocytes with or without metabolic activation. In addition, there was no evidence of genotoxicity in the *in vivo* mouse micronucleus test.

In oral (gavage) fertility studies of ezetimibe conducted in rats, there was no evidence of reproductive toxicity at doses up to 1000 mg/kg/day in male or female rats [~7 times the human exposure at 10 mg daily based on AUC(0-24h) for total ezetimibe].

PREGNANCY CATEGORY C

There are no adequate and well-controlled studies of ezetimibe in pregnant women. Ezetimibe should be used during pregnancy only if the potential benefit justifies the risk to the fetus.

In oral (gavage) embryo-fetal development studies of ezetimibe conducted in rats and rabbits during organogenesis, there was no evidence of embryolethal effects at the doses tested (250, 500, 1000 mg/kg/day). In rats, increased incidences of common fetal skeletal findings (extra pair of thoracic ribs, unossified cervical vertebral centra, shortened ribs) were observed at 1000 mg/kg/day [~10 times the human exposure at 10 mg daily based on AUC(0-24h) for total ezetimibe]. In rabbits treated with ezetimibe, an increased incidence of extra thoracic ribs was observed at 1000 mg/kg/day [150 times the human exposure at 10 mg daily based on AUC(0-24h) for total ezetimibe]. Ezetimibe crossed the placenta when pregnant rats and rabbits were given multiple oral doses.

Multiple dose studies of ezetimibe given in combination with HMG-CoA reductase inhibitors (statins) in rats and rabbits during organogenesis result in higher ezetimibe and statin exposures. Reproductive findings occur at lower doses in combination therapy compared to monotherapy.

All HMG-CoA reductase inhibitors are contraindicated in pregnant and nursing women. When ezetimibe is administered with an HMG-CoA reductase inhibitor in a woman of childbearing potential, refer to the pregnancy category and package labeling for the HMG-CoA reductase inhibitor. (See CONTRAINDICATIONS.)

LABOR AND DELIVERY

The effects of ezetimibe on labor and delivery in pregnant women are unknown.

NURSING MOTHERS

In rat studies, exposure to total ezetimibe in nursing pups was up to half of that observed in maternal plasma. It is not known whether ezetimibe is excreted into human breast milk; therefore, ezetimibe should not be used in nursing mothers unless the potential benefit justifies the potential risk to the infant.

PEDIATRIC USE

The pharmacokinetics of ezetimibe in adolescents (10-18 years) have been shown to be similar to that in adults. Treatment experience with ezetimibe in the pediatric population is limited to 4 patients (9-17 years) in the sitosterolemia study and 5 patients (11-17 years) in the HoFH study. Treatment with ezetimibe in children (<10 years) is not recommended. (See CLINICAL PHARMACOLOGY, Pharmacokinetics, Special Populations.)

E

GERIATRIC USE

Of the patients who received ezetimibe in clinical studies, 948 were 65 and older (this included 206 who were 75 and older). The effectiveness and safety of ezetimibe were similar between these patients and younger subjects. Greater sensitivity of some older individuals cannot be ruled out. (See CLINICAL PHARMACOLOGY, Pharmacokinetics, Special Populations; and ADVERSE REACTIONS.)

DRUG INTERACTIONS

See also CLINICAL PHARMACOLOGY, Drug Interactions.

Cholestyramine: Concomitant cholestyramine administration decreased the mean AUC of total ezetimibe approximately 55%. The incremental LDL-C reduction due to adding ezetimibe to cholestyramine may be reduced by this interaction.

Fibrates: The safety and effectiveness of ezetimibe administered with fibrates have not been established.

Fibrates may increase cholesterol excretion into the bile, leading to cholelithiasis. In a preclinical study in dogs, ezetimibe increased cholesterol in the gallbladder bile (see ANIMAL PHARMACOLOGY). Coadministration of ezetimibe with fibrates is not recommended until use in patients is studied.

Fenofibrate: In a pharmacokinetic study, concomitant fenofibrate administration increased total ezetimibe concentrations approximately 1.5-fold.

Gemfibrozil: In a pharmacokinetic study, concomitant gemfibrozil administration increased total ezetimibe concentrations approximately 1.7-fold.

HMG-CoA Reductase Inhibitors: No clinically significant pharmacokinetic interactions were seen when ezetimibe was co-administered with atorvastatin, simvastatin, pravastatin, lovastatin, or fluvastatin.

Cyclosporine: The total ezetimibe level increased 12-fold in 1 renal transplant patient receiving multiple medications, including cyclosporine. Patients who take both ezetimibe and cyclosporine should be carefully monitored.

ADVERSE REACTIONS

Ezetimibe has been evaluated for safety in more than 4700 patients in clinical trials. Clinical studies of ezetimibe (administered alone or with an HMG-CoA reductase inhibitor) demonstrated that ezetimibe was generally well tolerated. The overall incidence of adverse events reported with ezetimibe was similar to that reported with placebo, and the discontinuation rate due to adverse events was also similar for ezetimibe and placebo.

MONOTHERAPY

Adverse experiences reported in ≥2% of patients treated with ezetimibe and at an incidence greater than placebo in placebo-controlled studies of ezetimibe, regardless of causality assessment, are shown in TABLE 8.

TABLE 8* *Clinical Adverse Events Occurring in ≥2% of Patients Treated With Ezetimibe and at an Incidence Greater Than Placebo, Regardless of Causality*

Body Sytem/Organ Class Adverse Event	Placebo n=795	Ezetimibe 10 mg n=1691
Body as a Whole — General Disorders		
Fatigue	1.8%	2.2%
Gastrointestinal System Disorders		
Abdominal pain	2.8%	3.0%
Diarrhea	3.0%	3.7%
Infection and Infestations		
Infection viral	1.8%	2.2%
Pharyngitis	2.1%	2.3%
Sinusitis	2.8%	3.6%
Musculoskeletal System Disorders		
Arthralgia	3.4%	3.8%
Back pain	3.9%	4.1%
Respiratory System Disorders		
Coughing	2.1%	2.3%

* Includes patients who received placebo or ezetimibe alone reported in TABLE 9.

The frequency of less common adverse events was comparable between ezetimibe and placebo.

COMBINATION WITH AN HMG-COA REDUCTASE INHIBITOR

Ezetimibe has been evaluated for safety in combination studies in more than 2000 patients.

In general, adverse experiences were similar between ezetimibe administered with HMG-CoA reductase inhibitors and HMG-CoA reductase inhibitors alone. However, the frequency of increased transaminases was slightly higher in patients receiving ezetimibe administered with HMG-CoA reductase inhibitors than in patients treated with HMG-CoA reductase inhibitors alone. (See PRECAUTIONS, Liver Enzymes.)

Clinical adverse experiences reported in ≥2% of patients and at an incidence greater than placebo in four placebo-controlled trials where ezetimibe was administered alone or initiated concurrently with various HMG-CoA reductase inhibitors, regardless of causality assessment, are shown in TABLE 9.

TABLE 9* *Clinical Adverse Events Occurring in ≥2% of Patients and at an Incidence Greater Than Placebo, Regardless of Causality, in Ezetimibe/Statin Combination Studies*

Body System/Organ Class Adverse Event	Placebo n=259	Ezetimibe 10 mg n=262	All Statins† n=936	Ezetimibe + All Statins† n=925
Body as a Whole — General Disorders				
Chest pain	1.2%	3.4%	2.0%	1.8%
Dizziness	1.2%	2.7%	1.4%	1.8%
Fatigue	1.9%	1.9%	1.4%	2.8%
Headache	5.4%	8.0%	7.3%	6.3%
Gastrointestinal System Disorders				
Abdominal pain	2.3%	2.7%	3.1%	3.5%
Diarrhea	1.5%	3.4%	2.9%	2.8%
Infection and Infestations				
Pharyngitis	1.9%	3.1%	2.5%	2.3%
Sinusitis	1.9%	4.6%	3.6%	3.5%
Upper respiratory tract infection	10.8%	13.0%	13.6%	11.8%
Musculoskeletal System Disorders				
Arthralgia	2.3%	3.8%	4.3%	3.4%
Back pain	3.5%	3.4%	3.7%	4.3%
Myalgia	4.6%	5.0%	4.1%	4.5%

* Includes four placebo-controlled combination studies in which ezetimibe was initiated concurrently with an HMG-CoA reductase inhibitor.
† All statins = all doses of all HMG-CoA reductase inhibitors.

DOSAGE AND ADMINISTRATION

The patient should be placed on a standard cholesterol-lowering diet before receiving ezetimibe and should continue on this diet during treatment with ezetimibe.

The recommended dose of ezetimibe is 10 mg once daily. Ezetimibe can be administered with or without food.

Ezetimibe may be administered with an HMG-CoA reductase inhibitor for incremental effect. For convenience, the daily dose of ezetimibe may be taken at the same time as the HMG-CoA reductase inhibitor, according to the dosing recommendations for the HMG-CoA reductase inhibitor.

PATIENTS WITH HEPATIC INSUFFICIENCY

No dosage adjustment is necessary in patients with mild hepatic insufficiency (see PRECAUTIONS, Hepatic Insufficiency).

PATIENTS WITH RENAL INSUFFICIENCY

No dosage adjustment is necessary in patients with renal insufficiency (see CLINICAL PHARMACOLOGY, Pharmacokinetics, Special Populations).

GERIATRIC PATIENTS

No dosage adjustment is necessary in geriatric patients (see CLINICAL PHARMACOLOGY, Pharmacokinetics, Special Populations).

COADMINISTRATION WITH BILE ACID SEQUESTRANTS

Dosing of ezetimibe should occur either ≥2 hours before or ≥4 hours after administration of a bile acid sequestrant (see DRUG INTERACTIONS).

ANIMAL PHARMACOLOGY

The hypocholesterolemic effect of ezetimibe was evaluated in cholesterol-fed Rhesus monkeys, dogs, rats, and mouse models of human cholesterol metabolism. Ezetimibe was found to have an ED_{50} value of 0.5 µg/kg/day for inhibiting the rise in plasma cholesterol levels in monkeys. The ED_{50} values in dogs, rats, and mice were 7, 30, and 700 µg/kg/day, respectively. These results are consistent with ezetimibe being a potent cholesterol absorption inhibitor.

In a rat model, where the glucuronide metabolite of ezetimibe (SCH 60663) was administered intraduodenally, the metabolite was as potent as the parent compound (SCH 58235) in inhibiting the absorption of cholesterol, suggesting that the glucuronide metabolite had activity similar to the parent drug.

In 1 month studies in dogs given ezetimibe (0.03-300 mg/kg/day), the concentration of cholesterol in gallbladder bile increased ~2- to 4-fold. However, a dose of 300 mg/kg/day administered to dogs for 1 year did not result in gallstone formation or any other adverse hepatobiliary effects. In a 14 day study in mice given ezetimibe (0.3-5 mg/kg/day) and fed a low-fat or cholesterol-rich diet, the concentration of cholesterol in gallbladder bile was either unaffected or reduced to normal levels, respectively.

A series of acute preclinical studies was performed to determine the selectivity of ezetimibe for inhibiting cholesterol absorption. Ezetimibe inhibited the absorption of C14 cholesterol with no effect on the absorption of triglycerides, fatty acids, bile acids, progesterone, ethyl estradiol, or the fat-soluble vitamins A and D.

In 4-12 week toxicity studies in mice, ezetimibe did not induce cytochrome P450 drug metabolizing enzymes. In toxicity studies, a pharmacokinetic interaction of ezetimibe with HMG-CoA reductase inhibitors (parents or their active hydroxy acid metabolites) was seen in rats, dogs, and rabbits.

HOW SUPPLIED

Zetia tablets, 10 mg, are white to off-white, capsule-shaped tablets debossed with "414" on one side.

Storage: Store at 25°C (77°F); excursions permitted to 15-30°C (59-86°F). Protect from moisture.

PRODUCT LISTING - EQUIVALENTS NOT AVAILABLE

Tablet - Oral - 10 mg

30's	$72.38	ZETIA, Schering Corporation	66582-0414-31
90's	$217.13	ZETIA, Schering Corporation	66582-0414-54
100's	$235.46	ZETIA, Schering Corporation	66582-0414-28

Famciclovir *(003213)*

Categories: Herpes genitalis; Herpes zoster; Infection, herpes simplex virus; Infection, varicella-zoster virus; FDA Approved 1994 Jun; Pregnancy Category B
Drug Classes: Antivirals
Brand Names: Famvir
Foreign Brand Availability: Oravir (France)
Cost of Therapy: $171.28 (Herpes Zoster; Famvir ; 500 mg; 3 tablets/day; 7 day supply)
$34.48 (Herpes Simplex; Famvir ; 125 mg; 2 tablets/day; 5 day supply)
$220.50 (Herpes Simplex Supression; Famvir ; 250 mg; 2 tablets/day; 30 day supply)

DESCRIPTION

Famciclovir is an orally administered prodrug of the antiviral agent penciclovir. Chemically, famciclovir is known as 2-[2-(2-amino-9*H*-purin-9-yl)ethyl]-1,3-propanediol diacetate. Its molecular formula is $C_{14}H_{19}N_5O_4$; its molecular weight is 321.3. It is a synthetic acyclic guanine derivative.

Famciclovir is a white to pale yellow solid. It is freely soluble in acetone and methanol, and sparingly soluble in ethanol and isopropanol. At 25°C famciclovir is freely soluble (>25% w/v) in water initially, but rapidly precipitates as the sparingly soluble (2-3% w/v) monohydrate. Famciclovir is not hygroscopic below 85% relative humidity. Partition coefficients are: octanol/water (pH 4.8) P=1.09 and octanol/phosphate buffer (pH 7.4) P=2.08.

Tablets for Oral Administration: Each white, film-coated tablet contains famciclovir. The 125 mg and 250 mg tablets are round; the 500 mg tablets are oval. Inactive ingredients consist of hydroxypropyl cellulose, hydroxypropyl methylcellulose, lactose, magnesium stearate, polyethylene glycols, sodium starch glycolate and titanium dioxide.

CLINICAL PHARMACOLOGY

MICROBIOLOGY

Mechanism of Antiviral Activity

Famciclovir undergoes rapid biotransformation to the active antiviral compound penciclovir, which has inhibitory activity against herpes simplex virus types 1 (HSV-1) and 2 (HSV-2) and varicella zoster virus (VZV). In cells infected with HSV-1, HSV-2 or VZV, viral thymidine kinase phosphorylates penciclovir to a monophosphate form that, in turn, is converted to penciclovir triphosphate by cellular kinases. *In vitro* studies demonstrate that penciclovir triphosphate inhibits HSV-2 DNA polymerase competitively with deoxyguanosine triphosphate. Consequently, herpes viral DNA synthesis and, therefore, replication are selectively inhibited.

Penciclovir triphosphate has an intracellular half-life of 10 hours in HSV-1-, 20 hours in HSV-2- and 7 hours in VZV-infected cells cultured *in vitro;* however, the clinical significance is unknown.

Antiviral Activity In Vitro and In Vivo

In cell culture studies, penciclovir has antiviral activity against the following herpesviruses (listed in decreasing order of potency): HSV-1, HSV-2, and VZV. Sensitivity test results, expressed as the concentration of the drug required to inhibit the growth of the virus by 50% (IC_{50}) or 99% (IC_{99}) in cell culture, vary greatly depending upon a number of factors, including the assay protocols, and in particular the cell type used. (See TABLE 1.)

TABLE 1

Method of Assay	Virus Type	Cell Type	IC_{50} (µg/ml)	IC_{99} (µg/ml)
Plaque reduction	VZV (c.i.)	MRC-5	5.0 ± 3.0	
	VZV (c.i.)	Hs68	0.9 ± 0.4	
	HSV-1 (c.i.)	MRC-5	0.2-0.6	
	HSV-1 (c.i.)	WISH	0.04-0.5	
	HSV-2 (c.i.)	MRC-5	0.9-2.1	
	HSV-2 (c.i.)	WISH	0.1-0.8	
Virus yield reduction	HSV-1 (c.i.)	MRC-5		0.4-0.5
	HSV-2 (c.i.)	MRC-5		0.6-0.7
DNA synthesis inhibition	VZV (Ellen)	MRC-5	0.1	
	HSV-1 (SC16)	MRC-5	0.04	
	HSV-2 (MS)	MRC-5	0.05	

(c.i.) = Clinical isolates.

Drug Resistance

Penciclovir-resistant mutants of HSV and VZV can result from mutations in the viral thymidine kinase (TK) and DNA polymerase genes. Mutations in the viral TK gene may lead to complete loss of viral TK activity (TK negative), reduced levels of TK activity (TK partial) or alteration in the ability of viral TK to phosphorylate the drug without an equivalent loss in the ability to phosphorylate thymidine (TK altered). The most commonly encountered acyclovir-resistant mutants are TK negative and they are also resistant to penciclovir. The possibility of viral resistance to penciclovir should be considered in patients who fail to respond or experience recurrent viral infections during therapy.

PHARMACOKINETICS

Absorption and Bioavailability

Famciclovir is the diacetyl 6-deoxy analog of the active antiviral compound penciclovir. Following oral administration, little or no famciclovir is detected in plasma or urine.

The absolute bioavailability of famciclovir is 77 ± 8% as determined following the administration of a 500 mg famciclovir oral dose and a 400 mg penciclovir IV dose to 12 healthy male subjects.

Penciclovir concentrations increased in proportion to dose over a famciclovir dose range of 125-750 mg administered as a single dose. Single oral dose administration of 125, 250 or 500 mg famciclovir to healthy male volunteers across 17 studies gave the following pharmacokinetic parameters (see TABLE 2).

TABLE 2

Dose	AUC(0-∞)*	C_{max}†	T_{max}‡
125 mg	2.24 μg·h/ml	0.8 μg/ml	0.9 hours
250 mg	4.48 μg·h/ml	1.6 μg/ml	0.9 hours
500 mg	8.95 μg·h/ml	3.3 μg/ml	0.9 hours

* AUC(0-∞) (μg·h/ml) = area under the plasma concentration-time profile extrapolated to infinity.
† C_{max} (μg/ml) = maximum observed plasma concentration.
‡ T_{max}(hours) = time to C_{max}.

Following single oral-dose administration of 500 mg famciclovir to 7 patients with herpes zoster, the mean ±SD AUC, C_{max}, and T_{max} were 12.1 ± 1.7 μg·h/ml, 4.0 ± 0.7 μg/ml, and 0.7 ± 0.2 hours, respectively. The AUC of penciclovir was approximately 35% greater in patients with herpes zoster as compared to healthy volunteers. Some of this difference may be due to differences in renal function between the two groups.

There is no accumulation of penciclovir after the administration of 500 mg famciclovir tid for 7 days.

Penciclovir C_{max} decreased approximately 50% and T_{max} was delayed by 1.5 hours when a capsule formulation of famciclovir was administered with food (nutritional content was approximately 910 Kcal and 26% fat). There was no effect on the extent of availability (AUC) of penciclovir. There was an 18% decrease in C_{max} and a delay in T_{max} of about 1 hour when famciclovir was given 2 hours after a meal as compared to its administration 2 hours before a meal. Because there was no effect on the extent of systemic availability of penciclovir, it appears that famciclovir can be taken without regard to meals.

Distribution

The volume of distribution (Vd_β) was 1.08 ± 0.17 L/kg in 12 healthy male subjects following a single IV dose of penciclovir at 400 mg administered as a 1 hour IV infusion.

Penciclovir is <20% bound to plasma proteins over the concentration range of 0.1 to 20 μg/ml. The blood/plasma ratio of penciclovir is approximately 1.

Metabolism

Following oral administration, famciclovir is deacetylated and oxidized to form penciclovir. Metabolites that are inactive include 6-deoxy penciclovir, monoacetylated penciclovir, and 6-deoxy monoacetylated penciclovir (5%, <0.5% and <0.5% of the dose in the urine, respectively). Little or no famciclovir is detected in plasma or urine.

An *in vitro* study using human liver microsomes demonstrated that cytochrome P450 does not play an important role in famciclovir metabolism. The conversion of 6-deoxy penciclovir to penciclovir is catalyzed by aldehyde oxidase.

Elimination

Approximately 94% of administered radioactivity was recovered in urine over 24 hours (83% of the dose was excreted in the first 6 hours) after the administration of 5 mg/kg radiolabeled penciclovir as a 1 hour infusion to 3 healthy male volunteers. Penciclovir accounted for 91% of the radioactivity excreted in the urine.

Following the oral administration of a single 500 mg dose of radiolabeled famciclovir to 3 healthy male volunteers, 73% and 27% of administered radioactivity were recovered in urine and feces over 72 hours, respectively. Penciclovir accounted for 82% and 6-deoxy penciclovir accounted for 7% of the radioactivity excreted in the urine. Approximately 60% of the administered radiolabeled dose was collected in urine in the first 6 hours.

After IV administration of penciclovir in 48 healthy male volunteers, mean ±SD total plasma clearance of penciclovir was 36.6 ± 6.3 L/h (0.48 ± 0.09 L/h/kg). Penciclovir renal clearance accounted for 74.5 ± 8.8% of total plasma clearance.

Renal clearance of penciclovir following the oral administration of a single 500 mg dose of famciclovir to 109 healthy male volunteers was 27.7 ± 7.6 L/h. The plasma elimination half-life of penciclovir was 2.0 ± 0.3 hours after IV administration of penciclovir to 48 healthy male volunteers and 2.3 ± 0.4 hours after oral administration of 500 mg famciclovir to 124 healthy male volunteers. The half-life in 7 patients with herpes zoster was 3.0 ± 1.1 hours.

HIV-Infected Patients

Following oral administration of a single dose of 500 mg famciclovir (the oral prodrug of penciclovir) to HIV-positive patients, the pharmacokinetic parameters of penciclovir were comparable to those observed in healthy subjects.

Renal Insufficiency

Apparent plasma clearance, renal clearance, and the plasma-elimination rate constant of penciclovir decreased linearly with reductions in renal function. After the administration of a single 500 mg famciclovir oral dose (n=27) to healthy volunteers and to volunteers with varying degrees of renal insufficiency (CLCR ranged from 6.4 to 138.8 ml/min), the results found in TABLE 3 were obtained.

TABLE 3

Parameter (mean ±SD)	CLCR* ≥60 (ml/min)	CLCR 40-59 (ml/min)	CLCR 20-39 (ml/min)	CLCR <20 (ml/min)
CLCR(ml/min)	88.1 ± 20.6	49.3 ± 5.9	26.5 ± 5.3	12.7 ± 5.9
CLR(L/h)	30.1 ± 10.6	13.0 ± 1.3†	4.2 ± 0.9	1.6 ± 1.0
CL/F‡(L/h)	66.9 ± 27.5	27.3 ± 2.8	12.8 ± 1.3	5.8 ± 2.8
Half-life (h)	2.3 ± 0.5	3.4 ± 0.7	6.2 ± 1.6	13.4 ± 10.2
n	15	5	4	3

* CLCR is measured creatinine clearance.
† n=4.
‡ CL/F consists of bioavailability factor and famciclovir to penciclovir conversion factor.

In a multiple dose study of famciclovir conducted in subjects with varying degrees of renal impairment (n=18), the pharmacokinetics of penciclovir were comparable to those after single doses.

A dosage adjustment is recommended for patients with renal insufficiency (see DOSAGE AND ADMINISTRATION).

Hepatic Insufficiency

Well-compensated chronic liver disease (chronic hepatitis [n=6], chronic ethanol abuse [n=8], or primary biliary cirrhosis [n=1]) had no effect on the extent of availability (AUC) of penciclovir following a single dose of 500 mg famciclovir. However, there was a 44% decrease in penciclovir mean maximum plasma concentration and the time to maximum plasma concentration was increased by 0.75 hours in patients with hepatic insufficiency compared to normal volunteers. No dosage adjustment is recommended for patients with well-compensated hepatic impairment. The pharmacokinetics of penciclovir have not been evaluated in patients with severe uncompensated hepatic impairment.

Elderly Subjects

Based on cross-study comparisons, mean penciclovir AUC was 40% larger and penciclovir renal clearance was 22% lower after the oral administration of famciclovir in elderly volunteers (n=18, age 65-79 years) compared to younger volunteers. Some of this difference may be due to differences in renal function between the two groups.

Gender

The pharmacokinetics of penciclovir was evaluated in 18 healthy male and 18 healthy female volunteers after single-dose oral administration of 500 mg famciclovir. AUC of penciclovir was 9.3 ± 1.9 μg·h/ml and 11.1 ± 2.1 μg·h/ml in males and females, respectively. Penciclovir renal clearance was 28.5 ± 8.9 L/h and 21.8 ± 4.3 L/h, respectively. These differences were attributed to differences in renal function between the two groups. No famciclovir dosage adjustment based on gender is recommended.

Pediatric Patients

The pharmacokinetics of famciclovir or penciclovir have not been evaluated in patients <18 years of age.

Race

The pharmacokinetics of famciclovir or penciclovir with respect to race have not been evaluated.

DRUG INTERACTIONS

Effects on Penciclovir

No clinically significant alterations in penciclovir pharmacokinetics were observed following single-dose administrtion of 500 mg famciclovir after pre-treatment with multiple doses of allopurinol, cimetidine, theophylline, or zidovudine. No clinically significant effect on penciclovir pharmacokinetics was observed following multiple-dose (tid) administration of famciclovir (500 mg) with multiple doses of digoxin.

Effects of Famciclovir on Coadministered Drugs

The steady-state pharmacokinetics of digoxin were not altered by concomitant administration of multiple doses of famciclovir (500 mg tid). No clinically significant effect on the pharmacokinetics of zidovudine or zidovudine glucuronide was observed following a single oral dose of 500 mg famciclovir.

INDICATIONS AND USAGE

HERPES ZOSTER

Famciclovir is indicated for the treatment of acute herpes zoster (shingles).

HERPES SIMPLEX INFECTIONS

Famciclovir is indicated for:

- Treatment or suppression of recurrent genital herpes in immunocompetent patients.
- Treatment of recurrent mucocutaneous herpes simplex infections in HIV-infected patients.

NON-FDA APPROVED INDICATIONS

Preliminary clinical data have also indicated efficacy in the treatment of first-episode herpes infection, although this use is not approved by the FDA.

CONTRAINDICATIONS

Famciclovir is contraindicated in patients with known hypersensitivity to the product, its components, and penciclovir cream.

PRECAUTIONS

GENERAL

The efficacy of famciclovir has not been established for initial episode genital herpes infection, ophthalmic zoster, disseminated zoster or in immunocompromised patients with herpes zoster.

Dosage adjustment is recommended when administering famciclovir to patients with creatinine clearance values <60 ml/min (see DOSAGE AND ADMINISTRATION). In patients with underlying renal disease who have received inappropriately high doses of famciclovir for their level of renal function, acute renal failure has been reported.

INFORMATION FOR THE PATIENT

Patients should be informed that famciclovir is not a cure for genital herpes. There are no data evaluating whether famciclovir will prevent transmission of infection to others. As genital herpes is a sexually transmitted disease, patients should avoid contact with lesions or intercourse when lesions and/or symptoms are present to avoid infecting partners. Genital herpes can also be transmitted in the absence of symptoms through asymptomatic viral shedding. If medical management of recurrent episodes is indicated, patients should be advised to initiate therapy at the first sign or symptom.

F

CARCINOGENESIS, MUTAGENESIS, AND IMPAIRMENT OF FERTILITY

Famciclovir was administered orally unless otherwise stated.

Carcinogenesis

Two (2) year dietary carcinogenicity studies with famciclovir were conducted in rats and mice. An increase in the incidence of mammary adenocarcinoma (a common tumor in animals of this strain) was seen in female rats receiving the high dose of 600 mg/kg/day (1.5-9.0× the human systemic exposure at the recommended daily oral doses of 500 mg tid, 250 mg bid, or 125 mg bid based on area under the plasma concentration curve comparisons [24 hour AUC] for penciclovir). No increases in tumor incidence were reported for male rats treated at doses up to 240 mg/kg/day (0.9-5.4× the human AUC), or in male and female mice at doses up to 600 mg/kg/day (0.4-2.4× the human AUC).

Mutagenesis

Famciclovir and penciclovir (the active metabolite of famciclovir) were tested for genotoxic potential in a battery of *in vitro* and *in vivo* assays. Famciclovir and penciclovir were negative in *in vitro* tests for gene mutation in bacteria (*S. typhimurium* and *E. coli*) and unscheduled DNA synthesis in mammalian HeLa 83 cells (at doses up to 10,000 and 5000 μg/plate, respectively). Famciclovir was also negative in the L5178Y mouse lymphoma assay (5000 μg/ml), the *in vivo* mouse micronucleus test (4800 mg/kg), and rat dominant lethal study (5000 mg/kg). Famciclovir induced increases in polyploidy in human lymphocytes *in vitro* in the absence of chromosomal damage (1200 μg/ml). Penciclovir was positive in the L5178Y mouse lymphoma assay for gene mutation/chromosomal aberrations, with and without metabolic activation (1000 μg/ml). In human lymphocytes, penciclovir caused chromosomal aberrations in the absence of metabolic activation (250 μg/ml). Penciclovir caused an increased incidence of micronuclei in mouse bone marrow *in vivo* when administered intravenously at doses highly toxic to bone marrow (500 mg/kg), but not when administered orally.

Impairment of Fertility

Testicular toxicity was observed in rats, mice, and dogs following repeated administration of famciclovir or penciclovir. Testicular changes included atrophy of the seminiferous tubules, reduction in sperm count, and/or increased incidence of sperm with abnormal morphology or reduced motility. The degree of toxicity to male reproduction was related to dose and duration of exposure. In male rats, decreased fertility was observed after 10 weeks of dosing at 500 mg/kg/day (1.9-11.4× the human AUC). The no observable effect level for sperm and testicular toxicity in rats following chronic administration (26 weeks) was 50 mg/kg/day (0.2-1.2× the human systemic exposure based on AUC comparisons). Testicular toxicity was observed following chronic administration to mice (104 weeks) and dogs (26 weeks) at doses of 600 mg/kg/day (0.4-2.4× the human AUC) and 150 mg/kg/day (1.7-10.2× the human AUC), respectively.

Famciclovir had no effect on general reproductive performance or fertility in female rats at doses up to 1000 mg/kg/day (3.6-21.6× the human AUC).

Two placebo-controlled studies in a total of 130 otherwise healthy men with a normal sperm profile over an 8 week baseline period and recurrent genital herpes receiving oral famciclovir (250 mg bid) (n=66) or placebo (n=64) therapy for 18 weeks showed no evidence of significant effects on sperm count, motility or morphology during treatment or during an 8 week follow-up.

PREGNANCY, TERATOGENIC EFFECTS, PREGNANCY CATEGORY B

Famciclovir was tested for effects on embryo-fetal development in rats and rabbits at oral doses up to 1000 mg/kg/day (approximately 3.6-21.6× and 1.8-10.8× the human systemic exposure to penciclovir based on AUC comparisons for the rat and the rabbit, respectively) and IV doses of 360 mg/kg/day in rats (2-12× the human dose based on body surface area [BSA] comparisons) or 120 mg/kg/day in rabbits (1.5-9.0× the human dose [BSA]). No adverse effects were observed on embryo-fetal development. Similarly, no adverse effects were observed following IV administration of penciclovir to rats (80 mg/kg/day, 0.4-2.6× the human dose [BSA]) or rabbits (60 mg/kg/day, 0.7-4.2× the human dose [BSA]). There are, however, no adequate and well-controlled studies in pregnant women. Because animal reproduction studies are not always predictive of human response, famciclovir should be used during pregnancy only if the benefit to the patient clearly exceeds the potential risk to the fetus.

Pregnancy Exposure Registry: To monitor maternal-fetal outcomes of pregnant women exposed to famciclovir, Novartis Pharmaceuticals Corporation maintains a Famciclovir Pregnancy Registry. Physicians are encouraged to register their patients by calling 888-669-6682.

NURSING MOTHERS

Following oral administration of famciclovir to lactating rats, penciclovir was excreted in breast milk at concentrations higher than those seen in the plasma. It is not known whether it is excreted in human milk. There are no data on the safety of famciclovir in infants.

USAGE IN CHILDREN

Safety and efficacy in children under the age of 18 years have not been established.

GERIATRIC USE

Of 816 patients with herpes zoster in clinical studies who were treated with famciclovir, 248 (30.4%) were ≥65 years of age and 103 (13%) were ≥75 years of age. No overall differences were observed in the incidence or types of adverse events between younger and older patients.

DRUG INTERACTIONS

Concurrent use with probenecid or other drugs significantly eliminated by active renal tubular secretion may result in increased plasma concentrations of penciclovir.

The conversion of 6-deoxy penciclovir to penciclovir is catalyzed by aldehyde oxidase. Interactions with other drugs metabolized by this enzyme could potentially occur.

ADVERSE REACTIONS

IMMUNOCOMPETENT PATIENTS

The safety of famciclovir has been evaluated in clinical studies involving 816 famciclovir-treated patients with herpes zoster (famciclovir, 250 mg tid to 750 mg tid); 528 famciclovir-treated patients with recurrent genital herpes (famciclovir, 125 mg bid to 500 mg tid); and 1197 patients with recurrent genital herpes treated with famciclovir as suppressive therapy (125 mg qd to 250 mg tid) of which 570 patients received famciclovir (open-labeled and/or double-blind) for at least 10 months. TABLE 5 lists selected adverse events.

TABLE 5 *Selected Adverse Events Reported by ≥2% of Patients in Placebo-Controlled Famciclovir Trials**

	Incidence					
	Herpes Zoster		Recurrent Genital Herpes		Genital Herpes-Suppression	
Event	Famciclovir (n=273)	Placebo (n=146)	Famciclovir (n=640)	Placebo (n=225)	Famciclovir (n=458)	Placebo (n=63)
Nervous System						
Headache	22.7%	17.8%	23.6%	16.4%	39.3%	42.9%
Paresthesia	2.6%	0.0%	1.3%	0.0%	0.9%	0.0%
Migraine	0.7%	0.7%	1.3%	0.4%	3.1%	0.0%
Gastrointestinal						
Nausea	12.5%	11.6%	10.0%	8.0%	7.2%	9.5%
Diarrhea	7.7%	4.8%	4.5%	7.6%	9.0%	9.5%
Vomiting	4.8%	3.4%	1.3%	0.9%	3.1%	1.6%
Flatulence	1.5%	0.7%	1.9%	2.2%	4.8%	1.6%
Abdominal pain	1.1%	3.4%	3.9%	5.8%	7.9%	7.9%
Body as a Whole						
Fatigue	4.4%	3.4%	6.3%	4.4%	4.8%	3.2%
Skin and Appendages						
Pruritus	3.7%	2.7%	0.9%	0.0%	2.2%	0.0%
Rash	0.4%	0.7%	0.6%	0.4%	3.3%	1.6%
Reproductive (Female)						
Dysmenorrhea	0.0%	0.7%	2.2%	1.3%	7.6%	6.3%

* Patients may have entered into more than one clinical trial.

The following adverse events have been reported during post-approval use of famciclovir: urticaria, hallucinations and confusion (including delirium, disorientation, confusional state, occurring predominantly in the elderly). Because these adverse events are reported voluntarily from a population of unknown size, estimates of frequency cannot be made.

TABLE 6 lists selected laboratory abnormalities in genital herpes suppression trials.

TABLE 6 *Selected Laboratory Abnormalities in Genital Herpes Supression Studies**

Parameter	Famciclovir (n=660)†	Placebo (n=210)†
Anemia (<0.8 × NRL)	0.1%	0.0%
Leukopenia (<0.75 × NRL)	1.3%	0.9%
Neutropenia (<0.8 × NRL)	3.2%	1.5%
AST (SGOT) (>2 × NRH)	2.3%	1.2%
ALT (SGPT) (>2 × NRH)	3.2%	1.5%
Total bilirubin (>1.5 × NRH)	1.9%	1.2%
Serum creatinine (>1.5 × NRH)	0.2%	0.3%
Amylase (>1.5 × NRH)	1.5%	1.9%
Lipase (>1.5 × NRH)	4.9%	4.7%

* Percentage of patients with laboratory abnormalities that were increased or decreased from baseline and were outside of specified ranges.
† n values represent the minimum number of patients assessed for each laboratory parameter.
NRH = Normal Range High.
NRL = Normal Range Low.

HIV-INFECTED PATIENTS

In HIV-infected patients, the most frequently reported adverse events for famciclovir (500 mg twice daily; n=150) and acyclovir (400 mg, 5×/day; n=143), respectively, were headache (16.0 vs 15.4%), nausea (10.7 vs 12.6%), diarrhea (6.7 vs 10.5%), vomiting (4.7 vs 3.5%), fatigue (4.0 vs 2.1%), and abdominal pain (3.3 vs 5.6%).

DOSAGE AND ADMINISTRATION

HERPES ZOSTER

The recommended dosage is 500 mg every 8 hours for 7 days. Therapy should be initiated promptly as soon as herpes zoster is diagnosed. No data are available on efficacy of treatment started greater than 72 hours after rash onset.

HERPES SIMPLEX INFECTIONS

Recurrent Genital Herpes

The recommended dosage is 125 mg twice daily for 5 days. Initiate therapy at the first sign or symptom if medical management of a genital herpes recurrence is indicated. The efficacy of famciclovir has not been established when treatment is initiated more than 6 hours after onset of symptoms or lesions.

Suppression of Recurrent Genital Herpes

The recommended dosage is 250 mg twice daily for up to 1 year. The safety and efficacy of famciclovir therapy beyond 1 year of treatment have not been established.

HIV-INFECTED PATIENTS

For recurrent orolabial or genital herpes simplex infection, the recommended dosage is 500 mg twice daily for 7 days.

In patients with reduced renal function, dosage reduction is recommended (see PRECAUTIONS, General). (See TABLE 7.)

TABLE 7

Indication and Normal Dosage Regimen	Creatinine Clearance (ml/min)	Adjusted Dosage Regimen Dose (mg)	Dosing Interval
Herpes Zoster			
500 mg every 8 hours	>60	500	every 8 hours
	40-59	500	every 12 hours
	20-39	500	every 24 hours
	<20	250	every 24 hours
	HD*	250	following each dialysis
Recurrent Genital Herpes			
125 mg every 12 hours	≥40	125	every 12 hours
	20-39	125	every 24 hours
	<20	125	every 24 hours
	HD*	125	following each dialysis
Suppression of Recurrent Genital Herpes			
250 mg every 12 hours	≥40	250	every 12 hours
	20-39	125	every 12 hours
	<20	125	every 24 hours
	HD*	125	following each dialysis
Recurrent Orolabial and Genital Herpes Simplex Infection in HIV-Infected Patients			
500 mg every 12 hours	≥40	500	every 12 hours
	20-39	500	every 24 hours
	<20	250	every 24 hours
	HD*	250	following each dialysis

* Hemodialysis.

ADMINISTRATION WITH FOOD

When famciclovir was administered with food, penciclovir C_{max} decreased approximately 50%. Because the systemic availability of penciclovir (AUC) was not altered, it appears that famciclovir may be taken without regard to meals.

HOW SUPPLIED

Famvir is supplied as film-coated tablets.

125 mg: White, round, debossed with "FAMVIR" on one side and "125" on the other.

250 mg: White, round, debossed with "FAMVIR" on one side and "250" on the other.

500 mg: White, oval, debossed with "FAMVIR" on one side and "500" on the other.

Storage: Store between 15 and 30°C (59 and 86°F).

PRODUCT LISTING - EQUIVALENTS NOT AVAILABLE

Tablet - Oral - 125 mg			
10's	$33.80	FAMVIR, Allscripts Pharmaceutical Company	54569-4533-00
30's	$101.40	FAMVIR, Glaxosmithkline	00007-4115-13
30's	$103.43	FAMVIR, Novartis Pharmaceuticals	00078-0366-15
100's	$245.15	FAMVIR, Glaxosmithkline	00007-4115-21
Tablet - Oral - 250 mg			
30's	$110.25	FAMVIR, Glaxosmithkline	00007-4116-13
30's	$112.45	FAMVIR, Novartis Pharmaceuticals	00078-0367-15
Tablet - Oral - 500 mg			
21's	$171.28	FAMVIR, Allscripts Pharmaceutical Company	54569-4534-00
30's	$221.30	FAMVIR, Glaxosmithkline	00007-4117-13
30's	$236.79	FAMVIR, Novartis Pharmaceuticals	00078-0368-15
50's	$407.80	FAMVIR, Glaxosmithkline	00007-4117-19
50's	$436.35	FAMVIR, Novartis Pharmaceuticals	00078-0368-64

Famotidine

(001246)

For related information, see the comparative table section in Appendix A.

Categories: Adenoma, multiple endocrine; Esophagitis, erosive; Gastroesophageal Reflux Disease; Ulcer, duodenal; Ulcer, gastric; Zollinger-Ellison syndrome; Esophagitis, erosive; Pregnancy Category B; FDA Approved 1986 Oct

Drug Classes: Antihistamines, H2; Gastrointestinals

Brand Names: **Pepcid**

Foreign Brand Availability: Agufam (Thailand); Antodine (Bahrain; Cyprus; Egypt; Iran; Iraq; Israel; Jordan; Kuwait; Lebanon; Libya; Oman; Qatar; Republic-of-Yemen; Saudi-Arabia; Syria; United-Arab-Emirates); Apo-Famotidine (New-Zealand); Apogastine (Israel); Bestidine (Korea); Blocacid (Singapore); Brolin (Spain); Cepal (Greece); Durater (Mexico); Facid (Indonesia); Fadin (Taiwan); Fadine (Malaysia; Thailand); Fafotin (Korea); Famo (Germany; Israel); FamoABZ (Germany); Famoc (Singapore); Famocid (Benin; Burkina-Faso; Ethiopia; Gambia; Ghana; Guinea; India; Ivory-Coast; Kenya; Liberia; Malawi; Mali; Mauritania; Mauritius; Morocco; Niger; Nigeria; Senegal; Seychelles; Sierra-Leone; South-Africa; Sudan; Tanzania; Tunia; Uganda; Zambia; Zimbabwe); Famodar (Bahrain; Cyprus; Egypt; Iran; Iraq; Israel; Jordan; Kuwait; Lebanon; Libya; Oman; Qatar; Republic-of-Yemen; Saudi-Arabia; Syria; United-Arab-Emirates); Famodil (Italy); Famodin (Bulgaria); Famodine (Bahrain; Cyprus; Egypt; Iran; Iraq; Israel; Jordan; Kuwait; Lebanon; Libya; Oman; Qatar; Republic-of-Yemen; Saudi-Arabia; Syria; United-Arab-Emirates); Famogal (Colombia); Famogard (Russia); Famolta (Hong-Kong); Famonerton (Germany); Famopril (Singapore); Famopsin (Hong-Kong; Malaysia; Thailand); Famos (Indonesia); Famosan (Bulgaria); Famotal (Norway); Famotep (Portugal); Famotin (Ecuador; Singapore); Famotine (Peru); Famowal (India); Famox (Hong-Kong; New-Zealand; Taiwan); Famoxal (Mexico); Fanox (Spain); Farmotex (Mexico); Farotin (Korea); Fenox (Colombia); Fibonel (Ecuador); Fudone (Benin; Burkina-Faso; Ethiopia; Gambia; Ghana; Guinea; Ivory-Coast; Kenya; Liberia; Malawi; Mali; Mauritania; Mauritius; Morocco; Niger; Nigeria; Senegal; Seychelles; Sierra-Leone; Sudan; Tanzania; Tunia; Uganda; Zambia; Zimbabwe); Fuweidin (Taiwan); Gardin (Korea); Gaster (China; Indonesia; Japan; Taiwan); Gastridin (Italy); Gastrion (Spain); Gastro (Israel); Gastrodomina (Benin; Burkina-Faso; Ethiopia; Gambia; Ghana; Guinea; Ivory-Coast; Kenya; Liberia; Malawi; Mali; Mauritania; Mauritius; Morocco; Niger; Nigeria; Senegal; Seychelles; Sierra-Leone; South-Africa; Sudan; Tanzania; Tunia; Uganda; Zambia; Zimbabwe); H2 Bloc (Philippines); Kemofam (Indonesia); Kimodin (Taiwan); Logos (South-Africa); Motiax (Italy); Motidine (Singapore); Pepcid AC (Canada; New-Zealand); Pepcidac (France); Pepcidin (Denmark; Finland; Netherlands; Norway; Sweden; Turkey); Pepcidin Rapitab (Norway); Pepcidina (Portugal); Pepcidine (Australia; Austria; Belgium; Costa-Rica; Ecuador; El-Salvador; Guatemala; Honduras; Hong-Kong; Malaysia; Mexico; New-Zealand; Nicaragua; Panama; Philippines; Russia; Switzerland); Pepdif (Turkey); Pepdine (Benin; Burkina-Faso; Ethiopia; France; Gambia; Ghana; Guinea; Ivory-Coast; Kenya; Liberia; Malawi; Mali; Mauritania; Mauritius; Morocco; Niger; Nigeria; Senegal; Seychelles; Sierra-Leone; South-Africa; Sudan; Tanzania; Tunia; Uganda; Zambia; Zimbabwe); Pepdul (Germany); Pepfamin (Thailand); Peptan (Greece); Pepticon (Korea); Peptifam (Bahrain; Cyprus; Egypt; Iran; Iraq; Israel; Jordan; Kuwait; Lebanon; Libya; Oman; Qatar; Republic-of-Yemen; Saudi-Arabia; Syria; United-Arab-Emirates); Pepzan (Hong-Kong; New-Zealand; Thailand); Purifam (Indonesia); Quamatel (China; Hong-Kong); Quamtel (Bahamas; Barbados; Belize; Bermuda; Curacao; Guyana; Jamaica; Netherland-Antilles; Puerto-Rico; Surinam; Trinidad); Restadin (Indonesia); Rogasti (Israel); Sedanium-R (Greece); Stomax (Bahrain; Cyprus; Egypt; Iran; Iraq; Jordan; Kuwait; Lebanon; Libya; Oman; Qatar; Republic-of-Yemen; Saudi-Arabia; Syria; United-Arab-Emirates); Supertidine (Taiwan); Tamin (Spain); Topcid (India); Ulcatif (Bahrain; Cyprus; Egypt; Iran; Iraq; Jordan; Kuwait; Lebanon; Libya; Oman; Qatar; Republic-of-Yemen; Saudi-Arabia; Syria; United-Arab-Emirates); Ulcedine (Hong-Kong); Ulceran (Bahrain; Cyprus; Egypt; Hong-Kong; Iran; Iraq; Israel; Jordan; Kuwait; Lebanon; Libya; Malaysia; Oman; Qatar; Republic-of-Yemen; Saudi-Arabia; Syria; United-Arab-Emirates); Ulcidine (Canada); Ulcofam (Thailand); Ulfadin (Colombia); Ulfagel (Ecuador); Ulfam (Indonesia); Ulped (Costa-Rica; Dominican-Republic; El-Salvador; Guatemala; Honduras; Nicaragua; Panama); Ulped AR (Costa-Rica; Dominican-Republic; El-Salvador; Guatemala; Honduras; Nicaragua; Panama); Weimok (Taiwan); Wiretin (Korea); Yamarin (Benin; Burkina-Faso; Ethiopia; Gambia; Ghana; Guinea; Ivory-Coast; Kenya; Liberia; Malawi; Mali; Mauritania; Mauritius; Morocco; Niger; Nigeria; Senegal; Seychelles; Sierra-Leone; Sudan; Tanzania; Tunia; Uganda; Zambia; Zimbabwe)

Cost of Therapy: $117.59 (Duodenal Ulcer; Pepcid; 40 mg; 1 tablet/day; 30 day supply)
$121.67 (GERD; Pepcid; 20 mg; 2 tablets/day; 30 day supply)

INTRAVENOUS

DESCRIPTION

The active ingredient in Pepcid (famotidine) injection premixed and injection is a histamine H_2-receptor antagonist. Famotidine is *N'*-(aminosulfonyl)-3-[[[2-[(diaminomethylene) amino]-4-thiazolyl]methyl]thio]propanimidamide. The empirical formula of famotidine is $C_8H_{15}N_7O_2S_3$ and its molecular weight is 337.43.

Famotidine is a white to pale yellow crystalline compound that is freely soluble in glacial acetic acid, slightly soluble in methanol, very slightly soluble in water, and practically insoluble in ethanol.

PEPCID INJECTION PREMIXED

Pepcid injection premixed is supplied as a sterile solution, for intravenous use only, in plastic single dose containers. Each 50 ml of the premixed, iso-osmotic intravenous injection contains 20 mg famotidine, and the following inactive ingredients: L-aspartic acid 6.8 mg, sodium chloride, 450 mg, and water for injection. The pH ranges from 5.7-6.4 and may have been adjusted with additional L-aspartic acid or with sodium hydroxide.

The plastic container is fabricated from a specially designed multilayer plastic (PL 2501). Solutions are in contact with the polyethylene layer of the container and can leach out certain chemical components of the plastic in very small amounts within the expiration period. The suitability and safety of the plastic have been confirmed in tests in animals according to the USP biological tests for plastic containers, as well as by tissue culture toxicity studies.

PEPCID INJECTION

Pepcid injection is supplied as a sterile concentrated solution for intravenous injection.

Each ml of the solution contains 10 mg of famotidine and the following inactive ingredients: L-aspartic acid 4 mg, mannitol 20 mg, and water for injection qs 1 ml. The multidose injection also contains benzyl alcohol 0.9% added as preservative.

CLINICAL PHARMACOLOGY

ADULTS

GI Effects

Famotidine is a competitive inhibitor of histamine H_2-receptors. The primary clinically important pharmacologic activity of famotidine is inhibition of gastric secretion. Both the acid concentration and volume of gastric secretion are suppressed by famotidine, while changes in pepsin secretion are proportional to volume output.

In normal volunteers and hypersecretors, famotidine inhibited basal and nocturnal gastric secretion, as well as secretion stimulated by food and pentagastrin. After oral administration, the onset of the antisecretory effect occurred within 1 hour; the maximum effect was dose-dependent, occurring within 1-3 hours. Duration of inhibition of secretion by doses of 20 and 40 mg was 10-12 hours.

After intravenous administration, the maximum effect was achieved within 30 minutes. Single intravenous doses of 10 and 20 mg inhibited nocturnal secretion for a period of 10-12 hours. The 20 mg dose was associated with the longest duration of action in most subjects.

Single evening oral doses of 20 and 40 mg inhibited basal and nocturnal acid secretion in all subjects; mean nocturnal gastric acid secretion was inhibited by 86% and 94%, respectively, for a period of at least 10 hours. The same doses given in the morning suppressed food-stimulated acid secretion in all subjects. The mean suppression was 76% and 84%, respectively, 3-5 hours after administration, and 25% and 30%, respectively, 8-10 hours after administration. In some subjects who received the 20 mg dose, however, the antisecretory effect was dissipated within 6-8 hours. There was no cumulative effect with repeated doses. The nocturnal intragastric pH was raised by evening doses of 20 and 40 mg of famotidine to mean values of 5.0 and 6.4, respectively. When famotidine was given after breakfast, the basal daytime interdigestive pH at 3 and 8 hours after 20 or 40 mg of famotidine was raised to about 5.

Famotidine had little or no effect on fasting or postprandial serum gastrin levels. Gastric emptying and exocrine pancreatic function were not affected by famotidine.

Other Effects

Systemic effects of famotidine in the CNS, cardiovascular, respiratory or endocrine systems were not noted in clinical pharmacology studies. Also, no antiandrogenic effects were noted. (See ADVERSE REACTIONS.) Serum hormone levels, including prolactin, cortisol, thyroxine (T_4), and testosterone, were not altered after treatment with famotidine.

Pharmacokinetics

Orally administered famotidine is incompletely absorbed and its bioavailability is 40-45%. Famotidine undergoes minimal first-pass metabolism. After oral doses, peak plasma levels occur in 1-3 hours. Plasma levels after multiple doses are similar to those after single doses. Fifteen (15) to 20% of famotidine in plasma is protein bound. Famotidine has an elimination half-life of 2.5-3.5 hours. Famotidine is eliminated by renal (65-70%) and metabolic (30-35%) routes. Renal clearance is 250-450 ml/min, indicating some tubular excretion. Twenty-five (25) to 30% of an oral dose and 65-70% of an intravenous dose are recovered in the urine as unchanged compound. The only metabolite identified in man is the S-oxide.

There is a close relationship between creatinine clearance values and the elimination half-life of famotidine. In patients with severe renal insufficiency, *i.e.*, creatinine clearance less than 10 ml/min, the elimination half-life of famotidine may exceed 20 hours and adjustment of dose or dosing intervals may be necessary (see PRECAUTIONS and DOSAGE AND ADMINISTRATION).

In elderly patients, there are no clinically significant age-related changes in the pharmacokinetics of famotidine. However, in elderly patients with decreased renal function, the clearance of the drug may be decreased (see PRECAUTIONS, Geriatric Use).

PEDIATRIC PATIENTS

Pharmacokinetics

TABLE 1 presents pharmacokinetic data from published studies of small numbers of pediatric patients given famotidine intravenously. Areas under the curve (AUCs) are normalized to a dose of 0.5 mg/kg IV for pediatric patients and compared with an extrapolated 40 mg intravenous dose in adults (extrapolation based on results obtained with a 20 mg IV adult dose).

TABLE 1 *Pharmacokinetic Parameters* of Intravenous Famotidine*

	Age		
	1-11 years (n=20)	11-15 years (n=6)	Adult (n=16)
Area under the curve (AUC) (ng·h/ml)	1089 ± 834	1140 ± 320	1726†
Total clearance (Cl) (L/h/kg)	0.54 ± 0.34	0.48 ± 0.14	0.39 ± 0.14
Volume of distribution (Vd) (L/kg)	2.07 ± 1.49	1.5 ± 0.4	1.3 ± 0.2
Elimination half-life ($T_{½}$) (hours)	3.38 ± 2.60	2.3 ± 0.4	2.83 ± 0.99

* Values are presented as means ±SD unless indicated otherwise.
† Mean value only.

Values of pharmacokinetic parameters for pediatric patients, ages 1-15 years, are comparable to those obtained for adults.

Bioavailability studies of 8 pediatric patients (11-15 years of age) showed a mean oral bioavailability of 0.5 compared to adult values of 0.42-0.49. Oral doses of 0.5 mg/kg achieved an AUC of 580 ± 60 ng·h/ml in pediatric patients 11-15 years of age compared to 482 ± 181 ng·h/ml in adults treated with 40 mg orally.

Pharmacodynamics

Pharmacodynamics of famotidine were evaluated in 5 pediatric patients 2-13 years of age using the sigmoid E_{max} model. These data suggest that the relationship between serum concentration of famotidine and gastric acid suppression is similar to that observed in one study of adults (TABLE 2).

TABLE 2 *Pharmacodynamics of Famotidine Using the Sigmoid E_{max} Model*

	EC_{50} (ng/ml)*
Pediatric patients	26 ± 13
Data from one study	
a) Healthy adult subjects	26.5 ± 10.3
b) Adult patients with upper GI bleeding	18.7 ± 10.8

* Serum concentration of famotidine associated with 50% maximum gastric acid reduction. Values are presented as means ±SD.

Four published studies (TABLE 3) examined the effect of famotidine on gastric pH and duration of acid suppression in pediatric patients. While each study had a different design, acid suppression data over time are summarized in TABLE 3.

TABLE 3

Dosage	Route	Effect*	
0.3 mg/kg, single dose	IV	gastric pH >3.5 for 8.7 ± 4.7† hours	n=6
0.4-0.8 mg/kg	IV	gastric pH >4 for 6-9 hours	n=18
0.5 mg/kg, single dose	IV	a >2 pH unit increase above baseline in gastric pH for >8 hours	n=9
0.5 mg/kg bid	IV	gastric pH >5 for 13.5 ± 1.8† hours	n=4
0.5 mg/kg bid	oral	gastric pH >5 for 5.0 ± 1.1† hours	n=4

* Values reported in published literature.
† Means ±SD.

INDICATIONS AND USAGE

Famotidine injection premixed, supplied as a premixed solution in plastic containers (PL 2501 Plastic), and famotidine injection, supplied as a concentrated solution for intravenous injection, are intended for intravenous use only. Famotidine injection premixed and injection are indicated in some hospitalized patients with pathological hypersecretory conditions or intractable ulcers, or as an alternative to the oral dosage forms for short term use in patients who are unable to take oral medication for the following conditions:

Short term treatment of active duodenal ulcer. Most adult patients heal within 4 weeks; there is rarely reason to use famotidine at full dosage for longer than 6-8 weeks. Studies have not assessed the safety of famotidine in uncomplicated active duodenal ulcer for periods of more than 8 weeks.

Maintenance therapy for duodenal ulcer patients at reduced dosage after healing of an active ulcer. Controlled studies in adults have not extended beyond 1 year.

Short term treatment of active benign gastric ulcer. Most adult patients heal within 6 weeks. Studies have not assessed the safety or efficacy of famotidine in uncomplicated active benign gastric ulcer for periods of more than 8 weeks.

Short term treatment of gastroesophageal reflux disease (GERD). Famotidine is indicated for short term treatment of patients with symptoms of GERD.

Famotidine is also indicated for the short term treatment of esophagitis due to GERD including erosive or ulcerative disease diagnosed by endoscopy.

Treatment of pathological hypersecretory conditions (*e.g.*, Zollinger-Ellison Syndrome, multiple endocrine adenomas).

NON-FDA APPROVED INDICATIONS

While not FDA approved indications, famotidine is also used in the management of upper gastrointestinal bleeding and for stress ulcer prophylaxis in the ICU, and to prevent NSAID-induced duodenal and gastric ulceration.

CONTRAINDICATIONS

Hypersensitivity to any component of these products. Cross sensitivity in this class of compounds has been observed. Therefore, famotidine should not be administered to patients with a history of hypersensitivity to other H_2-receptor antagonists.

PRECAUTIONS

GENERAL

Symptomatic response to therapy with famotidine does not preclude the presence of gastric malignancy.

PATIENTS WITH MODERATE OR SEVERE RENAL INSUFFICIENCY

Since CNS adverse effects have been reported in patients with moderate and severe renal insufficiency, longer intervals between doses or lower doses may need to be used in patients with moderate (creatinine clearance <50 ml/min) or severe (creatinine clearance <10 ml/min) renal insufficiency to adjust for the longer elimination half-life of famotidine (see CLINICAL PHARMACOLOGY, Adults, and DOSAGE AND ADMINISTRATION).

CARCINOGENESIS, MUTAGENESIS, AND IMPAIRMENT OF FERTILITY

In a 106 week study in rats and a 92 week study in mice given oral doses of up to 2000 mg/kg/day (approximately 2500 times the recommended human dose for active duodenal ulcer), there was no evidence of carcinogenic potential for famotidine.

Famotidine was negative in the microbial mutagen test (Ames test) using *Salmonella typhimurium* and *Escherichia coli* with or without rat liver enzyme activation at concentrations up to 10,000 µg/plate. In *in vivo* studies in mice, with a micronucleus test and a chromosomal aberration test, no evidence of a mutagenic effect was observed.

In studies with rats given oral doses of up to 2000 mg/kg/day or intravenous doses of up to 200 mg/kg/day, fertility and reproductive performance were not affected.

PREGNANCY CATEGORY B

Reproductive studies have been performed in rats and rabbits at oral doses of up to 2000 and 500 mg/kg/day, respectively, and in both species at IV doses of up to 200 mg/kg/day, and have revealed no significant evidence of impaired fertility or harm to the fetus due to famotidine. While no direct fetotoxic effects have been observed, sporadic abortions occurring only in mothers displaying marked decreased food intake were seen in some rabbits at oral doses of 200 mg/kg/day (250 times the usual human dose) or higher. There are, however, no adequate or well-controlled studies in pregnant women. Because animal reproductive studies are not always predictive of human response, this drug should be used during pregnancy only if clearly needed.

NURSING MOTHERS

Studies performed in lactating rats have shown that famotidine is secreted into breast milk. Transient growth depression was observed in young rats suckling from mothers treated with maternotoxic doses of at least 600 times the usual human dose. Famotidine is detectable in human milk. Because of the potential for serious adverse reactions in nursing infants from famotidine, a decision should be made whether to discontinue nursing or discontinue the drug, taking into account the importance of the drug to the mother.

PEDIATRIC USE

Use of famotidine in pediatric patients 1-16 years of age is supported by evidence from adequate and well-controlled studies of famotidine in adults, and by the following studies in pediatric patients: In published studies in small numbers of pediatric patients 1-15 years of age, clearance of famotidine was similar to that seen in adults. In pediatric patients 11-15 years of age, oral doses of 0.5 mg/kg were associated with a mean area under the curve (AUC) similar to that seen in adults treated orally with 40 mg. Similarly, in pediatric patients 1-15 years of age, intravenous doses of 0.5 mg/kg were associated with a mean AUC similar to that seen in adults treated intravenously with 40 mg. Limited published studies also suggest that the relationship between serum concentration and acid suppression is similar in pediatric patients 1-15 years of age as compared with adults. These studies suggest that the starting dose for pediatric patients 1-16 years of age is 0.25 mg/kg intravenously (injected over a period of not less than 2 minutes or as a 15 minute infusion) q12h up to 40 mg/day.

While published uncontrolled clinical studies suggest effectiveness of famotidine in the treatment of peptic ulcer, data in pediatric patients are insufficient to establish percent response with dose and duration of therapy. Therefore, treatment duration (initially based on adult duration recommendations) and dose should be individualized based on clinical response and/or gastric pH determination and endoscopy. Published uncontrolled studies in pediatric patients have demonstrated gastric acid suppression with doses up to 0.5 mg/kg intravenously q12h.

No pharmacokinetic or pharmacodynamic data are available on pediatric patients under 1 year of age.

GERIATRIC USE

Of the 4966 subjects in clinical studies who were treated with famotidine, 488 subjects (9.8%) were 65 and older, and 88 subjects (1.7%) were greater than 75 years of age. No overall differences in safety or effectiveness were observed between these subjects and younger subjects, and other reported clinical experience has not identified differences in responses between the elderly and younger patients, but greater sensitivity of some older individuals cannot be ruled out.

No dosage adjustment is required based on age (see CLINICAL PHARMACOLOGY, Adults, Pharmacokinetics). This drug is known to be substantially excreted by the kidney, and the risk of toxic reactions to this drug may be greater in patients with impaired renal function. Because elderly patients are more likely to have decreased renal function, care should be taken in dose selection, and it may be useful to monitor renal function. Dosage adjustment in the case of severe renal impairment is necessary (see Patients With Moderate or Severe Renal Insufficiency and DOSAGE AND ADMINISTRATION, Dosage Adjustments for Patients With Moderate or Severe Renal Insufficiency).

DRUG INTERACTIONS

No drug interactions have been identified. Studies with famotidine in man, in animal models, and *in vitro* have shown no significant interference with the disposition of compounds metabolized by the hepatic microsomal enzymes, *e.g.,* cytochrome P450 system. Compounds tested in man include warfarin, theophylline, phenytoin, diazepam, aminopyrine and antipyrine. Indocyanine green as an index of hepatic drug extraction has been tested and no significant effects have been found.

ADVERSE REACTIONS

The adverse reactions listed below have been reported during domestic and international clinical trials in approximately 2500 patients. In those controlled clinical trials in which famotidine tablets were compared to placebo, the incidence of adverse experiences in the group which received famotidine tablets, 40 mg at bedtime, was similar to that in the placebo group.

The following adverse reactions have been reported to occur in more than 1% of patients on therapy with famotidine in controlled clinical trials, and may be causally related to the drug: Headache (4.7%), dizziness (1.3%), constipation (1.2%), and diarrhea (1.7%).

The following other adverse reactions have been reported infrequently in clinical trials or since the drug was marketed. The relationship to therapy with famotidine has been unclear in many cases. Within each category the adverse reactions are listed in order of decreasing severity:

Body as a Whole: Fever, asthenia, fatigue.

Cardiovascular: Arrhythmia, AV block, palpitation.

Gastrointestinal: Cholestatic jaundice, liver enzyme abnormalities, vomiting, nausea, abdominal discomfort, anorexia, dry mouth.

Hematologic: Rare cases of agranulocytosis, pancytopenia, leukopenia, thrombocytopenia.

Hypersensitivity: Anaphylaxis, angioedema, orbital or facial edema, urticaria, rash, conjunctival injection.

Musculoskeletal: Musculoskeletal pain including muscle cramps, arthralgia.

Nervous System/Psychiatric: Grand mal seizure; psychic disturbances, which were reversible in cases for which follow-up was obtained, including hallucinations, confusion, agitation, depression, anxiety, decreased libido; paresthesia; insomnia; somnolence.

Respiratory: Bronchospasm.

Skin: Toxic epidermal necrolysis (very rare), alopecia, acne, pruritus, dry skin, flushing.

Special Senses: Tinnitus, taste disorder.

Other: Rare cases of impotence and rare cases of gynecomastia have been reported; however, in controlled clinical trials, the incidences were not greater than those seen with placebo.

The adverse reactions reported for famotidine tablets may also occur with famotidine for oral suspension, famotidine orally disintegrating tablets, injection premixed or injection. In addition, transient irritation at the injection site has been observed with famotidine injection.

DOSAGE AND ADMINISTRATION

In some hospitalized patients with pathological hypersecretory conditions or intractable ulcers, or in patients who are unable to take oral medication, famotidine injection premixed or famotidine injection may be administered until oral therapy can be instituted.

The recommended dosage for famotidine injection premixed and injection in adult patients is 20 mg intravenously q12h.

The doses and regimen for parenteral administration in patients with GERD have not been established.

DOSAGE FOR PEDIATRIC PATIENTS

See PRECAUTIONS, Pediatric Use.

The studies described in PRECAUTIONS, Pediatric Use suggest that the starting dose in pediatric patients 1-16 years of age is 0.25 mg/kg intravenously (injected over a period of not less than 2 minutes or as a 15 minute infusion) q12h up to 40 mg/day.

While published uncontrolled clinical studies suggest effectiveness of famotidine in the treatment of peptic ulcer, data in pediatric patients are insufficient to establish percent response with dose and duration of therapy. Therefore, treatment duration (initially based on adult duration recommendations) and dose should be individualized based on clinical response and/or gastric pH determination and endoscopy. Published uncontrolled studies in pediatric patients have demonstrated gastric acid suppression with doses up to 0.5 mg/kg intravenously q12h.

No pharmacokinetic or pharmacodynamic data are available on pediatric patients under 1 year of age.

DOSAGE ADJUSTMENTS FOR PATIENTS WITH MODERATE OR SEVERE RENAL INSUFFICIENCY

In adult patients with moderate (creatinine clearance <50 ml/min) or severe (creatinine clearance <10 ml/min) renal insufficiency, the elimination half-life of famotidine is increased. For patients with severe renal insufficiency, it may exceed 20 hours, reaching approximately 24 hours in anuric patients. Since CNS adverse effects have been reported in patients with moderate and severe renal insufficiency, to avoid excess accumulation of the drug in patients with moderate or severe renal insufficiency, the dose of famotidine injection premixed or injection may be reduced to half the dose, or the dosing interval may be prolonged to 36-48 hours as indicated by the patient's clinical response.

Based on the comparison of pharmacokinetic parameters for famotidine in adults and pediatric patients, dosage adjustment in pediatric patients with moderate or severe renal insufficiency should be considered.

PATHOLOGICAL HYPERSECRETORY CONDITIONS (E.G., ZOLLINGER-ELLISON SYNDROME, MULTIPLE ENDOCRINE ADENOMAS)

The dosage of famotidine in patients with pathological hypersecretory conditions varies with the individual patient. The recommended adult intravenous dose is 20 mg q12h. Doses should be adjusted to individual patient needs and should continue as long as clinically indicated. In some patients, a higher starting dose may be required. Oral doses up to 160 mg q6h have been administered to some adult patients with severe Zollinger-Ellison Syndrome.

CONCOMITANT USE OF ANTACIDS

Antacids may be given concomitantly if needed.

STABILITY

Parenteral drug products should be inspected visually for particulate matter and discoloration prior to administration whenever solution and container permit.

Pepcid Injection Premixed

Pepcid injection premixed, as supplied premixed in 0.9% sodium chloride in Galaxy containers (PL 2501 Plastic), is stable through the labeled expiration date when stored under the recommended conditions. (See HOW SUPPLIED, Storage.)

Pepcid Injection

When added to or diluted with most commonly used intravenous solutions, *e.g.,* water for injection, 0.9% sodium chloride injection, 5% and 10% dextrose injection, or lactated Ringer's injection, diluted famotidine injection is physically and chemically stable (*i.e.,* maintains at least 90% of initial potency) for 7 days at room temperature (see HOW SUPPLIED, Storage).

When added to or diluted with sodium bicarbonate injection, 5%, famotidine injection at a concentration of 0.2 mg/ml (the recommended concentration of famotidine intravenous infusion solutions) is physically and chemically stable (*i.e.,* maintains at least 90% of initial potency) for 7 days at room temperature (see HOW SUPPLIED, Storage). However, a precipitate may form at higher concentrations of famotidine injection (>0.2 mg/ml) in sodium bicarbonate injection, 5%.

HOW SUPPLIED

PEPCID INJECTION PREMIXED

Pepcid injection premixed 20 mg per 50 ml, is a clear, non-preserved, sterile solution premixed in a vehicle made iso-osmotic sodium chloride for administration as an infusion over a 15-30 minute period. *This premixed solution is for intravenous use only using sterile equipment.*

PEPCID INJECTION

Pepcid injection 10 mg per 1 ml, is a non-preserved, clear, colorless solution in a single dose vial.

Pepcid injection 10 mg per 1 ml, is a clear, colorless solution in a multidose vial.

STORAGE

Pepcid Injection Premixed

Store Pepcid injection premixed in Galaxy containers (PL 2501 Plastic) at room temperature (25°C, 77°F). Exposure of the premixed product to excessive heat should be avoided. Brief exposure to temperatures up to 35°C (95°F) does not adversely affect the product.

Pepcid Injection

Store Pepcid injection at 2-8°C (36-46°F). If solution freezes, bring to room temperature; allow sufficient time to solubilize all the components.

Although diluted Pepcid injection has been shown to be physically and chemically stable for 7 days at room temperature, there are no data on the maintenance of sterility after dilution. Therefore, it is recommended that if not used immediately after preparation, diluted solutions of Pepcid injection should be refrigerated and used within 48 hours (see DOSAGE AND ADMINISTRATION).

ORAL

DESCRIPTION

The active ingredient in Pepcid (famotidine) is a histamine H_2-receptor antagonist. Famotidine is N′-(aminosulfonyl)-3-[[[2-[(diaminomethylene)amino]-4-thiazolyl]methyl]thio] propanimidamide. The empirical formula of famotidine is $C_8H_{15}N_7O_2S_3$ and its molecular weight is 337.43.

Famotidine is a white to pale yellow crystalline compound that is freely soluble in glacial acetic acid, slightly soluble in methanol, very slightly soluble in water, and practically insoluble in ethanol.

PEPCID TABLETS

Each tablet for oral administration contains either 20 or 40 mg of famotidine and the following inactive ingredients: hydroxypropyl cellulose, hydroxypropyl methylcellulose, iron oxides, magnesium stearate, microcrystalline cellulose, corn starch, talc, and titanium dioxide.

PEPCID RPD ORALLY DISINTEGRATING TABLETS

Each orally disintegrating tablet for oral administration contains either 20 or 40 mg of famotidine and the following inactive ingredients: aspartame, mint flavor, gelatin, mannitol, red ferric oxide, and xanthan gum.

PEPCID FOR ORAL SUSPENSION

Each 5 ml of the oral suspension when prepared as directed contains 40 mg of famotidine and the following inactive ingredients: citric acid, flavors, microcrystalline cellulose and carboxymethylcellulose sodium, sucrose and xanthan gum. Added as preservatives are sodium benzoate 0.1%, sodium methylparaben 0.1%, and sodium propylparaben 0.02%.

CLINICAL PHARMACOLOGY

ADULTS

GI Effects

Famotidine is a competitive inhibitor of histamine H_2-receptors. The primary clinically important pharmacologic activity of famotidine is inhibition of gastric secretion. Both the acid concentration and volume of gastric secretion are suppressed by famotidine, while changes in pepsin secretion are proportional to volume output.

In normal volunteers and hypersecretors, famotidine inhibited basal and nocturnal gastric secretion, as well as secretion stimulated by food and pentagastrin. After oral administration, the onset of the antisecretory effect occurred within 1 hour; the maximum effect was dose-dependent, occurring within 1-3 hours. Duration of inhibition of secretion by doses of 20 and 40 mg was 10-12 hours.

Single evening oral doses of 20 and 40 mg inhibited basal and nocturnal acid secretion in all subjects; mean nocturnal gastric acid secretion was inhibited by 86% and 94%, respectively, for a period of at least 10 hours. The same doses given in the morning suppressed food-stimulated acid secretion in all subjects. The mean suppression was 76% and 84%, respectively, 3-5 hours after administration, and 25% and 30%, respectively, 8-10 hours after administration. In some subjects who received the 20 mg dose, however, the antisecretory effect was dissipated within 6-8 hours. There was no cumulative effect with repeated doses. The nocturnal intragastric pH was raised by evening doses of 20 and 40 mg of famotidine to mean values of 5.0 and 6.4, respectively. When famotidine was given after breakfast, the basal daytime interdigestive pH at 3 and 8 hours after 20 or 40 mg of famotidine was raised to about 5.

Famotidine had little or no effect on fasting or postprandial serum gastrin levels. Gastric emptying and exocrine pancreatic function were not affected by famotidine.

Other Effects

Systemic effects of famotidine in the CNS, cardiovascular, respiratory or endocrine systems were not noted in clinical pharmacology studies. Also, no antiandrogenic effects were noted. (See ADVERSE REACTIONS.) Serum hormone levels, including prolactin, cortisol, thyroxine (T_4), and testosterone, were not altered after treatment with famotidine.

Pharmacokinetics

Famotidine is incompletely absorbed. The bioavailability of oral doses is 40-45%. Famotidine tablets, famotidine for oral suspension and famotidine orally disintegrating tablets are bioequivalent. Bioavailability may be slightly increased by food, or slightly decreased by antacids; however, these effects are of no clinical consequence. Famotidine undergoes minimal first-pass metabolism. After oral doses, peak plasma levels occur in 1-3 hours. Plasma levels after multiple doses are similar to those after single doses. Fifteen (15) to 20% of famotidine in plasma is protein bound. Famotidine has an elimination half-life of 2.5-3.5 hours. Famotidine is eliminated by renal (65-70%) and metabolic (30-35%) routes. Renal clearance is 250-450 ml/min, indicating some tubular excretion. Twenty-five (25) to 30% of an oral dose and 65-70% of an intravenous dose are recovered in the urine as unchanged compound. The only metabolite identified in man is the S-oxide.

There is a close relationship between creatinine clearance values and the elimination half-life of famotidine. In patients with severe renal insufficiency, *i.e.*, creatinine clearance less than 10 ml/min, the elimination half-life of famotidine may exceed 20 hours and adjustment of dose or dosing intervals in moderate and severe renal insufficiency may be necessary (see PRECAUTIONS and DOSAGE AND ADMINISTRATION).

In elderly patients, there are no clinically significant age-related changes in the pharmacokinetics of famotidine. However, in elderly patients with decreased renal function, the clearance of the drug may be decreased (see PRECAUTIONS, Geriatric Use).

PEDIATRIC PATIENTS

Pharmacokinetics

TABLE 9 presents pharmacokinetic data from published studies of small numbers of pediatric patients given famotidine intravenously. Areas under the curve (AUCs) are normalized to a dose of 0.5 mg/kg IV for pediatric patients and compared with an extrapolated 40 mg intravenous dose in adults (extrapolation based on results obtained with a 20 mg IV adult dose).

TABLE 9 *Pharmacokinetic Parameters* of Intravenous Famotidine*

	Age		
	1-11 years (n=20)	**11-15 years (n=6)**	**Adult (n=16)**
Area under the curve (AUC) (ng·h/ml)	1089 ± 834	1140 ± 320	1726†
Total clearance (Cl) (L/h/kg)	0.54 ± 0.34	0.48 ± 0.14	0.39 ± 0.14
Volume of distribution (Vd) (L/kg)	2.07 ± 1.49	1.5 ± 0.4	1.3 ± 0.2
Elimination half-life (T½) (hours)	3.38 ± 2.60	2.3 ± 0.4	2.83 ± 0.99

* Values are presented as means ±SD unless indicated otherwise.
† Mean value only.

Values of pharmacokinetic parameters for pediatric patients, ages 1-15 years, are comparable to those obtained for adults.

Bioavailability studies of 8 pediatric patients (11-15 years of age) showed a mean oral bioavailability of 0.5 compared to adult values of 0.42-0.49. Oral doses of 0.5 mg/kg achieved an AUC of 580 ± 60 ng·h/ml in pediatric patients 11-15 years of age compared to 482 ± 181 ng·h/ml in adults treated with 40 mg orally.

Pharmacodynamics

Pharmacodynamics of famotidine were evaluated in 5 pediatric patients 2-13 years of age using the sigmoid E_{max} model. These data suggest that the relationship between serum concentration of famotidine and gastric acid suppression is similar to that observed in one study of adults (TABLE 10).

TABLE 10 *Pharmacodynamics of Famotidine Using the Sigmoid E_{max} Model*

	EC_{50} (ng/ml)*
Pediatric patients	26 ± 13
Data from one study	
a) Healthy adult subjects	26.5 ± 10.3
b) Adult patients with upper GI bleeding	18.7 ± 10.8

* Serum concentration of famotidine associated with 50% maximum gastric acid reduction. Values are presented as means ±SD.

Four published studies (TABLE 11) examined the effect of famotidine on gastric pH and duration of acid suppression in pediatric patients. While each study had a different design, acid suppression data over time are summarized in TABLE 11.

TABLE 11

Dosage	Route	Effect*	
0.3 mg/kg, single dose	IV	gastric pH >3.5 for 8.7 ± 4.7† hours	n=6
0.4-0.8 mg/kg	IV	gastric pH >4 for 6-9 hours	n=18
0.5 mg/kg, single dose	IV	a >2 pH unit increase above baseline in gastric pH for >8 hours	n=9
0.5 mg/kg bid	IV	gastric pH >5 for 13.5 ± 1.8† hours	n=4
0.5 mg/kg bid	oral	gastric pH >5 for 5.0 ± 1.1† hours	n=4

* Values reported in published literature.
† Means ±SD.

INDICATIONS AND USAGE

Famotidine is indicated in:

Short term treatment of active duodenal ulcer. Most adult patients heal within 4 weeks; there is rarely reason to use famotidine at full dosage for longer than 6-8 weeks. Studies have not assessed the safety of famotidine in uncomplicated active duodenal ulcer for periods of more than 8 weeks.

Maintenance therapy for duodenal ulcer patients at reduced dosage after healing of an active ulcer. Controlled studies in adults have not extended beyond 1 year.

Short term treatment of active benign gastric ulcer. Most adult patients heal within 6 weeks. Studies have not assessed the safety or efficacy of famotidine in uncomplicated active benign gastric ulcer for periods of more than 8 weeks.

Short term treatment of gastroesophageal reflux disease (GERD). Famotidine is indicated for short term treatment of patients with symptoms of GERD.

Famotidine is also indicated for the short term treatment of esophagitis due to GERD including erosive or ulcerative disease diagnosed by endoscopy.

Treatment of pathological hypersecretory conditions (*e.g.*, Zollinger-Ellison Syndrome, multiple endocrine adenomas).

NON-FDA APPROVED INDICATIONS

While not FDA approved indications, famotidine is also used in the management of upper gastrointestinal bleeding and for stress ulcer prophylaxis in the ICU, and to prevent NSAID-induced duodenal and gastric ulceration.

CONTRAINDICATIONS

Hypersensitivity to any component of these products. Cross sensitivity in this class of compounds has been observed. Therefore, famotidine should not be administered to patients with a history of hypersensitivity to other H_2-receptor antagonists.

PRECAUTIONS

GENERAL

Symptomatic response to therapy with famotidine does not preclude the presence of gastric malignancy.

PATIENTS WITH MODERATE OR SEVERE RENAL INSUFFICIENCY

Since CNS adverse effects have been reported in patients with moderate and severe renal insufficiency, longer intervals between doses or lower doses may need to be used in patients with moderate (creatinine clearance <50 ml/min) or severe (creatinine clearance <10 ml/min) renal insufficiency to adjust for the longer elimination half-life of famotidine (see CLINICAL PHARMACOLOGY, Adults and DOSAGE AND ADMINISTRATION).

INFORMATION FOR THE PATIENT

The patient should be instructed to shake the oral suspension vigorously for 5-10 seconds prior to each use. Unused constituted oral suspension should be discarded after 30 days.

Patients should be instructed to leave the famotidine orally disintegrating tablet in the unopened package until the time of use. Patients should then open the tablet blister pack with dry hands, place the tablet on the tongue to dissolve and be swallowed with saliva. No water is needed for taking the tablet.

Phenylketonurics: Phenylketonuric patients should be informed that famotidine contains phenylalanine 1.05 mg per 20 mg orally disintegrating tablet and 2.10 mg per 40 mg orally disintegrating tablet.

CARCINOGENESIS, MUTAGENESIS, AND IMPAIRMENT OF FERTILITY

In a 106 week study in rats and a 92 week study in mice given oral doses of up to 2000 mg/kg/day (approximately 2500 times the recommended human dose for active duodenal ulcer), there was no evidence of carcinogenic potential for famotidine.

Famotidine was negative in the microbial mutagen test (Ames test) using *Salmonella typhimurium* and *Escherichia coli* with or without rat liver enzyme activation at concentrations up to 10,000 µg/plate. In *in vivo* studies in mice, with a micronucleus test and a chromosomal aberration test, no evidence of a mutagenic effect was observed.

In studies with rats given oral doses of up to 2000 mg/kg/day or intravenous doses of up to 200 mg/kg/day, fertility and reproductive performance were not affected.

PREGNANCY CATEGORY B

Reproductive studies have been performed in rats and rabbits at oral doses of up to 2000 and 500 mg/kg/day, respectively, and in both species at IV doses of up to 200 mg/kg/day, and have revealed no significant evidence of impaired fertility or harm to the fetus due to famotidine. While no direct fetotoxic effects have been observed, sporadic abortions occurring only in mothers displaying marked decreased food intake were seen in some rabbits at oral doses of 200 mg/kg/day (250 times the usual human dose) or higher. There are, however, no adequate or well-controlled studies in pregnant women. Because animal reproductive studies are not always predictive of human response, this drug should be used during pregnancy only if clearly needed.

NURSING MOTHERS

Studies performed in lactating rats have shown that famotidine is secreted into breast milk. Transient growth depression was observed in young rats suckling from mothers treated with maternotoxic doses of at least 600 times the usual human dose. Famotidine is detectable in human milk. Because of the potential for serious adverse reactions in nursing infants from famotidine, a decision should be made whether to discontinue nursing or discontinue the drug, taking into account the importance of the drug to the mother.

PEDIATRIC USE

Use of famotidine in pediatric patients 1-16 years of age is supported by evidence from adequate and well-controlled studies of famotidine in adults, and by the following studies in pediatric patients: In published studies in small numbers of pediatric patients 1-15 years of age, clearance of famotidine was similar to that seen in adults. In pediatric patients 11-15 years of age, oral doses of 0.5 mg/kg were associated with a mean area under the curve (AUC) similar to that seen in adults treated orally with 40 mg. Similarly, in pediatric patients 1-15 years of age, intravenous doses of 0.5 mg/kg were associated with a mean AUC similar to that seen in adults treated intravenously with 40 mg. Limited published studies also suggest that the relationship between serum concentration and acid suppression is similar in pediatric patients 1-15 years of age as compared with adults. These studies suggest a starting dose for pediatric patients 1-16 years of age as follows:

Peptic ulcer: 0.5 mg/kg/day po at bedtime or divided bid up to 40 mg/day.

Gastroesophageal Reflux Disease with or without esophagitis including erosions and ulcerations: 1.0 mg/kg/day po divided bid up to 40 mg bid.

While published uncontrolled studies suggest effectiveness of famotidine in the treatment of gastroesophageal reflux disease and peptic ulcer, data in pediatric patients are insufficient to establish percent response with dose and duration of therapy. Therefore, treatment duration (initially based on adult duration recommendations) and dose should be individualized based on clinical response and/or pH determination (gastric or esophageal) and endoscopy. Published uncontrolled clinical studies in pediatric patients have employed doses up to 1 mg/kg/day for peptic ulcer and 2 mg/kg/day for GERD with or without esophagitis including erosions and ulcerations.

No pharmacokinetic or pharmacodynamic data are available on pediatric patients under 1 year of age.

GERIATRIC USE

Of the 4966 subjects in clinical studies who were treated with famotidine, 488 subjects (9.8%) were 65 and older, and 88 subjects (1.7%) were greater than 75 years of age. No overall differences in safety or effectiveness were observed between these subjects and younger subjects. However, greater sensitivity of some older individuals cannot be ruled out.

No dosage adjustment is required based on age (see CLINICAL PHARMACOLOGY, Adults, Pharmacokinetics). This drug is known to be substantially excreted by the kidney, and the risk of toxic reactions to this drug may be greater in patients with impaired renal function. Because elderly patients are more likely to have decreased renal function, care should be taken in dose selection, and it may be useful to monitor renal function. Dosage adjustment in the case of moderate or severe renal impairment is necessary (see Patients With Moderate or Severe Renal Insufficiency and DOSAGE AND ADMINISTRATION, Dosage Adjustment for Patients With Moderate or Severe Renal Insufficiency).

DRUG INTERACTIONS

No drug interactions have been identified. Studies with famotidine in man, in animal models, and *in vitro* have shown no significant interference with the disposition of compounds metabolized by the hepatic microsomal enzymes, *e.g.*, cytochrome P450 system. Compounds tested in man include warfarin, theophylline, phenytoin, diazepam, aminopyrine and antipyrine. Indocyanine green as an index of hepatic drug extraction has been tested and no significant effects have been found.

ADVERSE REACTIONS

The adverse reactions listed below have been reported during domestic and international clinical trials in approximately 2500 patients. In those controlled clinical trials in which famotidine tablets were compared to placebo, the incidence of adverse experiences in the group which received famotidine tablets, 40 mg at bedtime, was similar to that in the placebo group.

The following adverse reactions have been reported to occur in more than 1% of patients on therapy with famotidine in controlled clinical trials, and may be causally related to the drug: headache (4.7%), dizziness (1.3%), constipation (1.2%) and diarrhea (1.7%).

The following other adverse reactions have been reported infrequently in clinical trials or since the drug was marketed. The relationship to therapy with famotidine has been unclear in many cases. Within each category the adverse reactions are listed in order of decreasing severity:

Body as a Whole: Fever, asthenia, fatigue.

Cardiovascular: Arrhythmia, AV block, palpitation.

Gastrointestinal: Cholestatic jaundice, liver enzyme abnormalities, vomiting, nausea, abdominal discomfort, anorexia, dry mouth.

Hematologic: Rare cases of agranulocytosis, pancytopenia, leukopenia, thrombocytopenia.

Hypersensitivity: Anaphylaxis, angioedema, orbital or facial edema, urticaria, rash, conjunctival injection.

Musculoskeletal: Musculoskeletal pain including muscle cramps, arthralgia.

Nervous System/Psychiatric: Grand mal seizure; psychic disturbances, which were reversible in cases for which follow-up was obtained, including hallucinations, confusion, agitation, depression, anxiety, decreased libido; paresthesia; insomnia; somnolence.

Respiratory: Bronchospasm.

Skin: Toxic epidermal necrolysis (very rare), alopecia, acne, pruritus, dry skin, flushing.

Special Senses: Tinnitus, taste disorder.

Other: Rare cases of impotence and rare cases of gynecomastia have been reported; however, in controlled clinical trials, the incidences were not greater than those seen with placebo.

The adverse reactions reported for famotidine tablets may also occur with famotidine for oral suspension and orally disintegrating tablets.

DOSAGE AND ADMINISTRATION

DUODENAL ULCER

Acute Therapy: The recommended adult oral dosage for active duodenal ulcer is 40 mg once a day at bedtime. Most patients heal within 4 weeks; there is rarely reason to use famotidine at full dosage for longer than 6-8 weeks. A regimen of 20 mg bid is also effective.

Maintenance Therapy: The recommended adult oral dose is 20 mg once a day at bedtime.

BENIGN GASTRIC ULCER

Acute Therapy: The recommended adult oral dosage for active benign gastric ulcer is 40 mg once a day at bedtime.

GASTROESOPHAGEAL REFLUX DISEASE (GERD)

The recommended oral dosage for treatment of adult patients with symptoms of GERD is 20 mg bid for up to 6 weeks. The recommended oral dosage for the treatment of adult patients with esophagitis including erosions and ulcerations and accompanying symptoms due to GERD is 20 or 40 mg bid for up to 12 weeks.

DOSAGE FOR PEDIATRIC PATIENTS

See PRECAUTIONS, Pediatric Use.

The studies described in PRECAUTIONS, Pediatric Use suggest the following starting doses in pediatric patients 1-16 years of age:

Peptic ulcer: 0.5 mg/kg/day po at bedtime or divided bid up to 40 mg/day.

Gastroesophageal Reflux Disease with or without esophagitis including erosions and ulcerations: 1.0 mg/kg/day po divided bid up to 40 mg bid.

While published uncontrolled studies suggest effectiveness of famotidine in the treatment of gastroesophageal reflux disease and peptic ulcer, data in pediatric patients are insufficient to establish percent response with dose and duration of therapy. Therefore, treatment duration (initially based on adult duration recommendations) and dose should be individualized based on clinical response and/or pH determination (gastric or esophageal) and endoscopy. Published uncontrolled clinical studies in pediatric patients have employed doses up to 1 mg/kg/day for peptic ulcer and 2 mg/kg/day for GERD with or without esophagitis including erosions and ulcerations.

No pharmacokinetic or pharmacodynamic data are available on pediatric patients under 1 year of age.

PATHOLOGICAL HYPERSECRETORY CONDITIONS (E.G., ZOLLINGER-ELLISON SYNDROME, MULTIPLE ENDOCRINE ADENOMAS)

The dosage of famotidine in patients with pathological hypersecretory conditions varies with the individual patient. The recommended adult oral starting dose for pathological hypersecretory conditions is 20 mg q6h. In some patients, a higher starting dose may be required. Doses should be adjusted to individual patient needs and should continue as long as clinically indicated. Doses up to 160 mg q6h have been administered to some adult patients with severe Zollinger-Ellison Syndrome.

F

ORAL SUSPENSION

Famotidine for oral suspension may be substituted for famotidine tablets in any of the above indications. Each 5 ml contains 40 mg of famotidine after constitution of the powder with 46 ml of purified water as directed.

Stability of Famotidine for Oral Suspension

Unused constituted oral suspension should be discarded after 30 days.

ORALLY DISINTEGRATING TABLETS

Famotidine orally disintegrating tablets may be substituted for famotidine tablets in any of the above indications at the same recommended dosages.

Famotidine orally disintegrating tablets rapidly disintegrate on the tongue. No water is needed for taking the tablet. Patients should be instructed to open the tablet blister pack with dry hands, place the tablet on the tongue to disintegrate and be swallowed with saliva.

CONCOMITANT USE OF ANTACIDS

Antacids may be given concomitantly if needed.

DOSAGE ADJUSTMENT FOR PATIENTS WITH MODERATE OR SEVERE RENAL INSUFFICIENCY

In adult patients with moderate (creatinine clearance <50 ml/min) or severe (creatinine clearance <10 ml/min) renal insufficiency, the elimination half-life of famotidine is increased. For patients with severe renal insufficiency, it may exceed 20 hours, reaching approximately 24 hours in anuric patients. Since CNS adverse effects have been reported in patients with moderate and severe renal insufficiency, to avoid excess accumulation of the drug in patients with moderate or severe renal insufficiency, the dose of famotidine may be reduced to half the dose or the dosing interval may be prolonged to 36-48 hours as indicated by the patient's clinical response.

Based on the comparison of pharmacokinetic parameters for famotidine in adults and pediatric patients, dosage adjustment in pediatric patients with moderate or severe renal insufficiency should be considered.

HOW SUPPLIED

PEPCID TABLETS

20 mg: Beige colored, U-shaped, film-coated tablets coded "MSD 963" on one side and "PEPCID" on the other.

40 mg: Light brownish-orange, U-shaped, film-coated tablets coded "MSD 964" on one side and "PEPCID" on the other.

Storage

Store at 25°C (77°F); excursions permitted to 15-30°C (59-86°F).

PEPCID RPD ORALLY DISINTEGRATING TABLETS

20 mg: Pale rose colored, hexagonal-shaped, lyophilized tablets measuring 13.1 mm (side to side) and 15.2 mm (point to point), with a mint flavor.

40 mg: Pale rose colored, hexagonal-shaped, lyophilized tablets measuring 15.9 mm (side to side) and 18.4 mm (point to point), with a mint flavor.

Storage

Store at 25°C (77°F); excursions permitted to 15-30°C (59-86°F).

PEPCID FOR ORAL SUSPENSION

Pepcid for oral suspension is a white to off-white powder containing 400 mg of famotidine for constitution. When constituted as directed, Pepcid for oral suspension is a smooth, mobile, off-white, homogeneous suspension with a cherry-banana-mint flavor, containing 40 mg of famotidine per 5 ml.

Storage

Store Pepcid for oral suspension dry powder and suspension at 25°C (77°F); excursions permitted to 15-30°C (59-86°F). Protect the suspension from freezing.

Discard unused suspension after 30 days.

PRODUCT LISTING - RATED THERAPEUTICALLY EQUIVALENT

Solution - Intravenous - 10 mg/ml

2 ml	$11.30	GENERIC, American Pharmaceutical Partners	63323-0739-02
2 ml	$45.10	GENERIC, Faulding Pharmaceutical Company	61703-0238-07
2 ml x 10	$14.90	GENERIC, Bedford Laboratories	55390-0029-10
2 ml x 10	$22.56	GENERIC, Abbott Pharmaceutical	00074-2364-02
2 ml x 10	$47.30	PEPCID, Merck & Company Inc	00006-3539-04
2 ml x 25	$28.25	GENERIC, American Pharmaceutical Partners	63323-0739-12
4 ml	$2.25	GENERIC, American Pharmaceutical Partners	63323-0738-04
4 ml	$4.37	GENERIC, Abbott Pharmaceutical	00074-2362-04
4 ml	$8.99	GENERIC, Faulding Pharmaceutical Company	61703-0239-26
4 ml	$9.43	PEPCID, Merck & Company Inc	00006-3541-14
4 ml x 10	$27.80	GENERIC, Baxter Healthcare Corporation	10019-0046-02
4 ml x 10	$29.70	GENERIC, Bedford Laboratories	55390-0028-10
4 ml x 25	$93.75	GENERIC, Esi Lederle Generics	59911-5950-02
4 ml x 25	$183.00	GENERIC, Esi Lederle Generics	59911-5951-02
20 ml	$14.88	GENERIC, Bedford Laboratories	55390-0027-01
20 ml	$47.26	PEPCID, Merck & Company Inc	00006-3541-20
20 ml	$473.06	PEPCID, Merck & Company Inc	00006-3541-49
20 ml x 10	$112.50	GENERIC, American Pharmaceutical Partners	63323-0738-20
20 ml x 10	$217.91	GENERIC, Abbott Pharmaceutical	00074-2362-20
20 ml x 10	$365.00	GENERIC, Esi Lederle Generics	59911-5952-02
20 ml x 10	$451.00	GENERIC, Faulding Pharmaceutical Company	61703-0239-21
50 ml	$37.19	GENERIC, Bedford Laboratories	55390-0026-01

Solution - Intravenous - 20 mg/50 ml

50 ml x 24	$163.44	GENERIC, Baxter Healthcare Corporation	00338-5197-41

Tablet - Oral - 20 mg

2's	$3.69	PEPCID, Allscripts Pharmaceutical Company	54569-2352-04
6's	$19.80	PEPCID, Pd-Rx Pharmaceuticals	55289-0473-06
30's	$51.00	PEPCID, Southwood Pharmaceuticals Inc	58016-0635-30
30's	$52.14	GENERIC, Geneva Pharmaceuticals	00781-1736-31
30's	$52.15	GENERIC, Purepac Pharmaceutical Company	00228-2679-03
30's	$52.15	GENERIC, Mylan Pharmaceuticals Inc	00378-3020-93
30's	$52.20	GENERIC, Par Pharmaceutical Inc	49884-0608-11
30's	$60.68	PEPCID, Pharma Pac	52959-0465-30
30's	$60.84	PEPCID, Merck & Company Inc	00006-0963-31
31's	$1571.63	PEPCID, Merck & Company Inc	00006-0963-72
60's	$102.00	PEPCID, Southwood Pharmaceuticals Inc	58016-0635-60
90 x 12	$2190.15	PEPCID, Merck & Company Inc	00006-0963-94
90's	$153.00	PEPCID, Southwood Pharmaceuticals Inc	58016-0635-90
100's	$62.10	FEDERAL UPPER LIMIT, H.C.F.A. F F P	99999-1246-01
100's	$170.00	PEPCID, Southwood Pharmaceuticals Inc	58016-0635-00
100's	$173.00	GENERIC, Imx Pharmaceuticals	00172-5728-10
100's	$173.00	GENERIC, Imx Pharmaceuticals	00172-5728-60
100's	$173.50	GENERIC, Par Pharmaceutical Inc	49884-0608-01
100's	$173.80	GENERIC, Geneva Pharmaceuticals	00781-1736-01
100's	$173.90	GENERIC, Mylan Pharmaceuticals Inc	00378-3020-01
100's	$173.90	GENERIC, Udl Laboratories Inc	51079-0966-20
100's	$173.95	GENERIC, Purepac Pharmaceutical Company	00228-2679-11
100's	$173.99	GENERIC, Teva Pharmaceuticals Usa	00093-0896-01
100's	$174.00	GENERIC, Andrx Pharmaceuticals	62037-0955-01
100's	$191.32	GENERIC, Major Pharmaceuticals Inc	00904-5553-61
100's	$202.79	PEPCID, Merck & Company Inc	00006-0963-28
100's	$202.79	PEPCID, Merck & Company Inc	00006-0963-58

Tablet - Oral - 40 mg

30's	$100.75	GENERIC, Purepac Pharmaceutical Company	00228-2641-03
30's	$100.80	GENERIC, Mylan Pharmaceuticals Inc	00378-3040-93
30's	$100.89	GENERIC, Par Pharmaceutical Inc	49884-0609-11
30's	$117.59	PEPCID, Merck & Company Inc	00006-0964-31
30's	$173.00	GENERIC, Geneva Pharmaceuticals	00781-1746-31
100's	$120.00	FEDERAL UPPER LIMIT, H.C.F.A. F F P	99999-1246-02
100's	$332.64	GENERIC, Major Pharmaceuticals Inc	00904-5554-60
100's	$334.40	GENERIC, Ivax Corporation	00172-5729-10
100's	$334.40	GENERIC, Ivax Corporation	00172-5729-60
100's	$335.00	GENERIC, Par Pharmaceutical Inc	49884-0609-01
100's	$335.90	GENERIC, Purepac Pharmaceutical Company	00228-2641-11
100's	$335.92	GENERIC, Geneva Pharmaceuticals	00781-1746-01
100's	$336.10	GENERIC, Mylan Pharmaceuticals Inc	00378-3040-01
100's	$336.29	GENERIC, Andrx Pharmaceuticals	62037-0956-01
100's	$336.30	GENERIC, Teva Pharmaceuticals Usa	00093-0897-01
100's	$373.66	PEPCID, Merck & Company Inc	00006-0964-28
100's	$391.95	PEPCID, Merck & Company Inc	00006-0964-58

PRODUCT LISTING - RATED NOT THERAPEUTICALLY EQUIVALENT

Tablet - Oral - 20 mg

100's	$173.03	GENERIC, Watson Laboratories Inc	00591-3123-01

Tablet - Oral - 40 mg

100's	$334.43	GENERIC, Watson Laboratories Inc	00591-3124-01

PRODUCT LISTING - EQUIVALENTS NOT AVAILABLE

Powder For Reconstitution - Oral - 40 mg/5 ml

50 ml	$107.71	PEPCID, Merck & Company Inc	00006-3538-92

Solution - Intravenous - 10 mg/ml

2 ml x 10	$11.10	GENERIC, Baxter Healthcare Corporation	10019-0045-01
20 ml	$45.08	GENERIC, Faulding Pharmaceutical Company	61703-0239-22
20 ml x 10	$111.30	GENERIC, Baxter Healthcare Corporation	10019-0046-03

Solution - Intravenous - 20 mg/50 ml

50 ml x 24	$200.88	PEPCID, Merck & Company Inc	00006-3537-50

Tablet - Oral - 20 mg

4's	$6.16	PEPCID, Allscripts Pharmaceutical Company	54569-2352-01
4's	$14.64	PEPCID, Quality Care Pharmaceuticals Inc	60346-0355-44
6's	$9.92	PEPCID, Allscripts Pharmaceutical Company	54569-2352-02
7's	$11.57	PEPCID, Allscripts Pharmaceutical Company	54569-2352-03
20's	$56.60	PEPCID, Physicians Total Care	54868-0303-02
25's	$53.74	PEPCID, Quality Care Pharmaceuticals Inc	60346-0355-25
25's	$66.57	PEPCID, Pd-Rx Pharmaceuticals	55289-0162-97
30's	$49.60	PEPCID, Allscripts Pharmaceutical Company	54569-2352-00
40's	$74.84	PEPCID, Quality Care Pharmaceuticals Inc	60346-0355-40
60's	$113.20	PEPCID, Physicians Total Care	54868-0303-01

Tablet - Oral - 40 mg

4's	$14.70	PEPCID, Southwood Pharmaceuticals Inc	58016-0715-04
4's	$18.75	PEPCID, Pd-Rx Pharmaceuticals	55289-0146-04
4's	$90.48	PEPCID, Quality Care Pharmaceuticals Inc	60346-0152-44
12's	$35.73	PEPCID, Southwood Pharmaceuticals Inc	58016-0715-12
15's	$44.67	PEPCID, Southwood Pharmaceuticals Inc	58016-0715-15
25's	$95.48	PEPCID, Quality Care Pharmaceuticals Inc	60346-0152-25
25's	$105.32	PEPCID, Pd-Rx Pharmaceuticals	55289-0146-97
30's	$89.33	PEPCID, Southwood Pharmaceuticals Inc	58016-0715-30
30's	$95.87	PEPCID, Allscripts Pharmaceutical Company	54569-0431-00
30's	$105.78	PEPCID, Physicians Total Care	54868-0304-01
30's	$108.21	PEPCID, Cheshire Drugs	55175-2918-03
60's	$178.66	PEPCID, Allscripts Pharmaceutical Company	54569-0431-04
60's	$229.62	PEPCID, Quality Care Pharmaceuticals Inc	60346-0152-60
100's	$297.78	PEPCID, Southwood Pharmaceuticals Inc	58016-0715-00

Tablet, Disintegrating - Oral - 40 mg

30's	$108.75	PEPCID RPD, Merck & Company Inc	00006-3554-31
100's	$362.50	PEPCID RPD, Merck & Company Inc	00006-3554-48

Felbamate *(003077)*

Categories: Lennox-Gastaut syndrome; Seizures, partial; Pregnancy Category C; FDA Approved 1993 Jul; Orphan Drugs
Drug Classes: Anticonvulsants
Brand Names: Felbatol
Foreign Brand Availability: Taloxa (France; Netherlands; Sweden)
Cost of Therapy: $336.87 (Epilepsy; Felbatol; 600 mg; 6 tablets/day; 30 day supply)

WARNING

1. ***APLASTIC ANEMIA:*** **THE USE OF FELBAMATE IS ASSOCIATED WITH A MARKED INCREASE IN THE INCIDENCE OF APLASTIC ANEMIA, ACCORDINGLY, FELBAMATE SHOULD ONLY BE USED IN PATIENTS WHOSE EPILEPSY IS SO SEVERE THAT THE RISK OF APLASTIC ANEMIA IS DEEMED ACCEPTABLE IN LIGHT OF THE BENEFITS CONFERRED BY ITS USE (SEE INDICATIONS AND USAGE). ORDINARILY, A PATIENT SHOULD NOT BE PLACED ON AND/OR CONTINUED ON FELBATOL WITHOUT CONSIDERATION OF APPROPRIATE EXPERT HEMATOLOGIC CONSULTATION.**

AMONG FELBAMATE TREATED PATIENTS, APLASTIC ANEMIA (PANCYTOPENIA IN THE PRESENCE OF A BONE MARROW LARGELY DEPLETED OF HEMATOPOIETIC PRECURSORS) OCCURS AT AN INCIDENCE THAT MAY BE MORE THAN A 100 FOLD GREATER THAN THAT SEEN IN THE UNTREATED POPULATION (*I.E.,* 2-5 PER MILLION PERSONS PER YEAR). THE RISK OF DEATH IN PATIENTS WITH APLASTIC ANEMIA GENERALLY VARIES AS A FUNCTION OF ITS SEVERITY AND ETIOLOGY; CURRENT ESTIMATES OF THE OVERALL CASE FATALITY RATE ARE IN THE RANGE OF 20-30%, BUT RATES AS HIGH AS 70% HAVE BEEN REPORTED IN THE PAST.

THERE ARE TOO FEW FELBAMATE ASSOCIATED CASES, AND TOO LITTLE KNOWN ABOUT THEM TO PROVIDE A RELIABLE ESTIMATE OF THE SYNDROME'S INCIDENCE OR ITS CASE FATALITY RATE OR TO IDENTIFY THE FACTORS, IF ANY, THAT MIGHT CONCEIVABLY BE USED TO PREDICT WHO IS AT GREATER OR LESSER RISK.

IN MANAGING PATIENTS ON FELBAMATE, IT SHOULD BE BORNE IN MIND THAT THE CLINICAL MANIFESTATION OF APLASTIC ANEMIA MAY NOT BE SEEN UNTIL AFTER A PATIENT HAS BEEN ON FELBAMATE FOR SEVERAL MONTHS (*E.G.,* ONSET OF APLASTIC ANEMIA AMONG FELBAMATE EXPOSED PATIENTS FOR WHOM DATA ARE AVAILABLE HAS RANGED FROM 5-30 WEEKS). HOWEVER, THE INJURY TO BONE MARROW STEM CELLS THAT IS HELD TO BE ULTIMATELY RESPONSIBLE FOR THE ANEMIA MAY OCCUR WEEKS TO MONTHS EARLIER. ACCORDINGLY, PATIENTS WHO ARE DISCONTINUED FROM FELBAMATE REMAIN AT RISK FOR DEVELOPING ANEMIA FOR A VARIABLE, AND UNKNOWN, PERIOD AFTERWARDS.

IT IS NOT KNOWN WHETHER OR NOT THE RISK OF DEVELOPING APLASTIC ANEMIA CHANGES WITH DURATION OF EXPOSURE CONSEQUENTLY, IT IS NOT SAFE TO ASSUME THAT A PATIENT WHO HAS BEEN ON FELBAMATE WITHOUT SIGNS OF HEMATOLOGIC ABNORMALITY FOR LONG PERIODS OF TIME IS WITHOUT RISK.

IT IS NOT KNOWN WHETHER OR NOT THE DOSE OF FELBATOL AFFECTS THE INCIDENCE OF APLASTIC ANEMIA.

IT IS NOT KNOWN WHETHER OR NOT CONCOMITANT USE OF ANTIEPILEPTIC DRUGS AND/OR OTHER DRUGS AFFECTS THE INCIDENCE OF APLASTIC ANEMIA.

APLASTIC ANEMIA TYPICALLY DEVELOPS WITHOUT PREMONITORY CLINICAL OR LABORATORY SIGNS, THE FULL BLOWN SYNDROME PRESENTING WITH SIGNS OF INFECTION, BLEEDING, OR ANEMIA. ACCORDINGLY, ROUTINE BLOOD TESTING CANNOT BE RELIABLY USED TO REDUCE THE INCIDENCE OF APLASTIC ANEMIA, BUT, IT WILL, IN SOME CASES, ALLOW THE DETECTION OF THE HEMATOLOGIC CHANGES BEFORE THE SYNDROME DECLARES ITSELF CLINICALLY. FELBATOL SHOULD BE DISCONTINUED IF ANY EVIDENCE OF BONE MARROW DEPRESSION OCCURS.

WARNING — *Cont'd*

2. ***HEPATIC FAILURE:*** **HEPATIC FAILURE RESULTING IN FATALITIES HAS BEEN REPORTED WITH A MARKED INCREASE IN THE FREQUENCY IN PATIENTS RECEIVING FELBAMATE. ACCORDINGLY, FELBATOL SHOULD ONLY BE USED IN PATIENTS WHOSE EPILEPSY IS SO SEVERE THAT THE RISK OF LIVER FAILURE IS OUTWEIGHED BY THE POTENTIAL BENEFITS OF SEIZURE CONTROL.**

ALTHOUGH FULL INFORMATION IS NOT YET AVAILABLE, THE NUMBER OF CASES REPORTED GREATLY EXCEEDS THE NUMBER THAT IS EXPECTED BASED ON THE ANNUAL INCIDENCE OF ACUTE LIVER FAILURE IN THE UNITED STATES (I.E., ABOUT 2,000 CASES PER YEAR).

THERE ARE TOO FEW FELBAMATE ASSOCIATED CASES OF HEPATIC FAILURE AND TOO LITTLE KNOWN ABOUT THEM TO PROVIDE EITHER A RELIABLE ESTIMATE OF ITS INCIDENCE OR TO IDENTIFY THE FACTORS, IF ANY, THAT MIGHT BE USED TO PREDICT WHICH PATIENT IS AT GREATER OR LESSER RISK.

IT IS NOT KNOWN WHETHER OR NOT THE RISK OF DEVELOPING HEPATIC FAILURE CHANGES WITH DURATION OF EXPOSURE.

IT IS NOT KNOWN WHETHER OR NOT THE DOSAGE OF FELBATOL AFFECTS THE INCIDENCE OF HEPATIC FAILURE.

IT IS NOT KNOWN WHETHER CONCOMITANT USE OF OTHER ANTIEPILEPTIC DRUGS AND/OR OTHER DRUGS AFFECT THE INCIDENCE OF HEPATIC FAILURE.

FELBATOL SHOULD NOT BE PRESCRIBED FOR ANYONE WITH A HISTORY OF HEPATIC DYSFUNCTION.

PATIENTS PRESCRIBED FELBAMATE SHOULD HAVE LIVER FUNCTION TESTS (AST, ALT, BILIRUBIN) PERFORMED BEFORE INITIATING FELBATOL AND AT 1-2 WEEK INTERVALS WHILE TREATMENT CONTINUES. A PATIENT WHO DEVELOPS ABNORMAL LIVER FUNCTION TESTS SHOULD BE IMMEDIATELY WITHDRAWN FROM FELBAMATE TREATMENT.

DESCRIPTION

Before prescribing felbamate, the physician should be thoroughly familiar with the details of this prescribing information.

FELBAMATE SHOULD NOT BE USED BY PATIENTS UNTIL THERE HAS BEEN A COMPLETE DISCUSSION OF THE RISKS AND THE PATIENT, PARENT, OR GUARDIAN HAS PROVIDED WRITTEN INFORMED CONSENT.

Felbatol (felbamate) is an antiepileptic available as 400 mg and 600 mg tablets and as a 600 mg/5 ml suspension for oral administration. Its chemical name is 2-phenyl-1,3-propanediol dicarbamate.

Felbamate is a white to off-white crystalline powder with a characteristic odor. It is very slightly soluble in water, slightly soluble in ethanol, sparingly soluble in methanol, and freely soluble in dimethyl sulfoxide. The molecular weight is 238.24; felbamate's molecular formula is $C_{11}H_{14}N_2O_4$.

The inactive ingredients for Felbatol (felbamate) tablets 400 and 600 mg are starch, microcrystalline cellulose, croscarmellose sodium, lactose, magnesium stearate, FD&C yellow no. 6, D&C yellow no. 10, and FD&C red no. 40 (600 mg tablets only). The inactive ingredients for felbamate suspension 600 mg/5 ml are sorbitol, glycerin, microcrystalline cellulose, carboxymethylcellulose sodium, simethicone, polysorbate 80, methylparaben, saccharin sodium, propylparaben, FD&C yellow no. 6, FD&C red no. 40, flavorings, and purified water.

CLINICAL PHARMACOLOGY

MECHANISM OF ACTION

The mechanism by which felbamate exerts its anticonvulsant activity is unknown, but in animal test systems designed to detect anticonvulsant activity, felbamate has properties in common with other marketed anticonvulsants. Felbamate is effective in mice and rats in the maximal electroshock test, the subcutaneous pentylenetetrazol seizure test, and the subcutaneous picrotoxin seizure test. Felbamate also exhibits anticonvulsant activity against seizures induced by intracerebroventricular administration of glutamate in rats and N-methyl-D,L-aspartic acid in mice. Protection against maximal electroshock- induced seizures suggests that felbamate may reduce seizure spread, an effect possibly predictive of efficacy in generalized tonic-clonic or partial seizures. Protection against pentylenetetrazol-induced seizures suggests that felbamate may increase seizure threshold, an effect considered to be predictive of potential efficacy in absence seizures.

Receptor-binding studies *in vitro* indicate that felbamate has weak inhibitory effects on GABA-receptor binding, benzodiazepine receptor binding, and is devoid of activity at the MK-801 receptor binding site of the NMDA receptor-ionophore complex. However, felbamate does interact as an antagonist at the strychnine-insensitive glycine recognition site of the NMDA receptor-ionophore complex. Felbamate is not effective in protecting chick embryo retina tissue against the neurotoxic effects of the excitatory amino acid agonists NMDA, kainate, or quisqualate *in vitro*.

The monocarbamate, p-hydroxy, and 2-hydroxy metabolites were inactive in the maximal electroshock-induced seizure test in mice. The monocarbamate and p-hydroxy metabolites had only weak (0.2-0.6) activity compared with felbamate in the subcutaneous pentylenetetrazol seizure test. These metabolites did not contribute significantly to the anticonvulsant action of felbamate.

PHARMACOKINETICS

The numbers in the pharmacokinetic section are mean ± standard deviation.

Felbamate is well-absorbed after oral administration. Over 90% of the radioactivity after a dose of 100 mg ^{14}C felbamate was found in the urine. Absolute bioavailability (oral versus parenteral) has not been measured. The tablet and suspension were each shown to be bioequivalent to the capsule used in clinical trials, and pharmacokinetic parameters of the tablet and suspension are similar. There was no effect of food on absorption of the tablet; the effect of food on absorption of the suspension has not been evaluated.

Following oral administration, felbamate is the predominant plasma species (about 90% of plasma radioactivity). About 40-50% of absorbed dose appears unchanged in urine, and

F

an additional 40% is present as unidentified metabolites and conjugates. About 15% is present as parahydroxyfelbamate, 2-hydroxyfelbamate, and felbamate monocarbamate, none of which have significant anticonvulsant activity.

Binding of felbamate to human plasma protein was independent of felbamate concentrations between 10 and 310 micrograms/ml. Binding ranged from 22-25%, mostly to albumin, and was dependent on the albumin concentration.

Felbamate is excreted with a terminal half-life of 20-23 hours, which is unaltered after multiple doses. Clearance after a single 1200 mg dose is 26 ± 3 ml/h/kg, and after multiple daily doses of 3600 mg is 30 ± 8 ml/h/kg. The apparent volume of distribution was 756 ± 82 ml/kg after a 1200 mg dose. Felbamate C_{max} and AUC are proportionate to dose after single and multiple doses over a range of 100-800 mg single doses and 1200-3600 mg daily doses. C_{min} (trough) blood levels are also dose proportional. Multiple daily doses of 1200, 2400, and 3600 mg gave C_{min} values of 30 ± 5, 55 ± 8, and 83 ± 21 micrograms/ml (n=10 patients). Felbamate gave dose proportional steady-state peak plasma concentrations in children age 4-12 over a range of 15, 30, and 45 mg/kg/day with peak concentrations of 17, 32, and 49 micrograms/ml.

The effects of race and gender on felbamate pharmacokinetics have not been systematically evaluated, but plasma concentrations in males (n=5) and females (n=4) given felbamate have been similar. The effects of felbamate kinetics on renal and hepatic functional impairment have not been evaluated.

F

PHARMACODYNAMICS

Typical Physiologic Responses:

1. ***Cardiovascular:*** In adults, there is no effect of felbamate on blood pressure. Small but statistically significant mean increases in heart rate were seen during adjunctive therapy and monotherapy; however, these mean increases of up to 5 bpm were not clinically significant. In children, no clinically relevant changes in blood pressure or heart rate were seen during adjunctive therapy or monotherapy with felbamate.
2. ***Other Physiologic Effects:*** The only other change in vital signs was a mean decrease of approximately 1 respiration per minute in respiratory rate during adjunctive therapy in children. In adults, statistically significant mean reductions in body weight were observed during felbamate monotherapy and adjunctive therapy. In children, there were mean decreases in body weight during adjunctive therapy and monotherapy; however, these mean changes were not statistically significant. These mean reductions in adults and children were approximately 5% of the mean weights at baseline.

INDICATIONS AND USAGE

Felbamate is not indicated as a first line antiepileptic treatment (see WARNINGS). Felbamate is recommended for use only in those patients who respond inadequately to alternative treatments and whose epilepsy is so severe that a substantial risk of aplastic anemia and/or liver failure is deemed acceptable in light of the benefits conferred by its use.

If these criteria are met and the patient has been fully advised of the risk and has provided written, informed consent, felbamate can be considered for either monotherapy or adjunctive therapy in the treatment of partial seizures, with and without generalization, in adults with epilepsy and as adjunctive therapy in the treatment of partial and generalized seizures associated with Lennox-Gastaut syndrome in children.

CONTRAINDICATIONS

Felbamate is contraindicated in patients with known hypersensitivity to felbamate, its ingredients, or known sensitivity to other carbamates. It should not be used in patients with a history of any blood dyscrasia or hepatic dysfunction.

WARNINGS

See BOXED WARNING regarding aplastic anemia and hepatic failure.

Antiepileptic drugs should not be suddenly discontinued because of the possibility of increasing seizure frequency.

PRECAUTIONS

INFORMATION FOR THE PATIENT

Patients should be informed that the use of felbamate is associated with aplastic anemia and hepatic failure, potentially fatal conditions acutely or over a long term.

The physician should obtain written, informed consent prior to initiation of felbamate therapy.

APLASTIC ANEMIA

in the general population is relatively rare. The absolute risk for the individual patient is not known with any degree of reliability, but patients on felbamate may be at more than a 100 fold greater risk for developing the syndrome than the general population.

The long term outlook for patients with aplastic anemia is variable. Although many patients are apparently cured, others require repeated transfusions and other treatments for relapses, and some, although surviving for years, ultimately develop serious complications that sometimes prove fatal (*e.g.*, leukemia).

At present there is no way to predict who is likely to get aplastic anemia, nor is there a documented effective means to monitor the patient so as to avoid and/or reduce the risk. Patients with a history of any blood dyscrasia should not receive felbamate.

Patients should be advised to be alert for signs of infection, bleeding, easy bruising, or signs of anemia (fatigue, weakness, lassitude, etc.) and should be advised to report to the physician immediately if any such signs or symptoms appear.

HEPATIC FAILURE

Hepatic failure in the general population is relatively rare. The absolute risk for an individual patient is not known with any degree of reliability but patients on felbamate are at a greater risk for developing hepatic failure than the general population.

At present, there is no way to predict who is likely to develop hepatic failure, however, patients with a history of hepatic dysfunction should not be started on felbamate.

Patients should be advised to follow their physician's directives for liver function testing both before starting felbamate and at frequent intervals while taking felbamate.

LABORATORY TESTS

Full hematologic evaluations should be performed before felbamate therapy, frequently during therapy, and for a significant period of time after discontinuation of felbamate therapy. While it might appear prudent to perform frequent CBCs in patients continuing on felbamate, there is no evidence that such monitoring will allow early detection of marrow suppression before aplastic anemia occurs. (See BOXED WARNING.) Complete pretreatment blood counts, including platelets and reticulocytes should be obtained as a baseline. If any hematologic abnormalities are detected during the course of treatment, immediate consultation with a hematologist is advised. Felbamate should be discontinued if any evidence of bone marrow depression occurs.

Liver Function Testing

(AST, ALT, bilirubin) should be done before felbamate is started and at 1-2 week intervals while the patient is taking felbamate. If any liver abnormalities are detected during the course of treatment, felbamate should be discontinued immediately.

DRUG/LABORATORY TEST INTERACTIONS

There are no known interactions of felbamate with commonly used laboratory tests.

CARCINOGENESIS, MUTAGENESIS, AND IMPAIRMENT OF FERTILITY

Carcinogenicity studies were conducted in mice and rats. Mice received felbamate as a feed admixture for 92 weeks at doses of 300, 600, and 1200 mg/kg and rats were also dosed by feed admixture for 104 weeks at doses of 30, 100, and 300 (males) or 10, 30, and 100 (females) mg/kg. The maximum doses in these studies produced steady-state plasma concentrations that were equal to or less than the steady-state plasma concentrations in epileptic patients receiving 3600 mg/day. There was a statistically significant increase in hepatic cell adenomas in high-dose male and female mice and in high-dose female rats. Hepatic hypertrophy was significantly increased in a dose-related manner in mice, primarily males, but also in females. Hepatic hypertrophy was not found in female rats. The relationship between the occurrence of benign hepatocellular adenomas and the finding of liver hypertrophy resulting from liver enzyme induction has not been examined. There was a statistically significant increase in benign interstitial cell tumors of the testes in high-dose male rats receiving felbamate. The relevance of these findings to humans is unknown.

As a result of the synthesis process, felbamate could contain small amounts of two known animal carcinogens, the genotoxic compound ethyl carbamate (urethane) and the nongenotoxic compound methyl carbamate. It is theoretically possible that a 50 kg patient receiving 3600 mg of felbamate could be exposed to up to 0.72 micrograms of urethane and 1800 micrograms of methyl carbamate. These daily doses are approximately 1/35,000 (urethane) and 1/5500 (methyl carbamate) on a mg/kg basis, and 1/10,000 (urethane) and 1/1600 (methyl carbamate) on a mg/m^2 basis, of the dose levels shown to be carcinogenic in rodents. Any presence of these 2 compounds in felbamate used in the lifetime carcinogenicity studies was inadequate to cause tumors.

Microbial and mammalian cell assays revealed no evidence of mutagenesis in the Ames *Salmonella* microsome plate test, CHO/HGPRT mammalian cell forward gene mutation assay, sister chromatid exchange assay in CHO cells, and bone marrow cytogenetics assay.

Reproduction and fertility studies in rats showed no effects on male or female fertility at oral doses of up to 13.9 times the human total daily dose of 3600 mg on a mg/kg basis, or up to 3 times the human total daily dose on a mg/m^2 basis.

PREGNANCY CATEGORY C

The incidence of malformations was not increased compared to control in offspring of rats or rabbits given doses up to 13.9 times (rat) and 4.2 times (rabbit) the human daily dose on a mg/kg basis, or 3 times (rat) and less than 2 times (rabbit) the human daily dose on a mg/m^2 basis. However, in rats, there was a decrease in pup weight and an increase in pup deaths during lactation. The cause for these deaths is not known. The no effect dose for rat pup mortality was 6.9 times the human dose on a mg/kg basis or 1.5 times the human dose on a mg/m^2 basis.

Placental transfer of felbamate occurs in rat pups. There are, however, no studies in pregnant women. Because animal reproduction studies are not always predictive of human response, this drug should be used during pregnancy only if clearly needed.

LABOR AND DELIVERY

The effect of felbamate on labor and delivery in humans is unknown.

NURSING MOTHERS

Felbamate has been detected in human milk. The effect on the nursing infant is unknown (see Pregnancy).

PEDIATRIC USE

The safety and effectiveness of felbamate in children other than those with Lennox-Gastaut syndrome has not been established.

GERIATRIC USE

No systemic studies in geriatric patients have been conducted. Clinical studies of felbamate did not include sufficient numbers of patients aged 65 and over to determine whether they respond differently from younger patients. Other reported clinical experience has not identified differences in responses between the elderly and younger patients. In general, dosage selection for an elderly patient should be cautious, usually starting at the low end of the dosing range, reflecting the greater frequency of decreased hepatic, renal, or cardiac function, and of concomitant disease or other drug therapy.

DRUG INTERACTIONS

The drug interaction data described in this section were obtained from controlled clinical trials and studies involving otherwise health adults with epilepsy.

USED IN CONJUNCTION WITH OTHER ANTIEPILEPTIC DRUGS

(See DOSAGE AND ADMINISTRATION): The addition of felbamate to antiepileptic drugs (AEDs) affects the steady-state plasma concentrations of AEDs.The net effect of these interactions is summarized in TABLE 1.

TABLE 1 *Felbamate, Drug Interactions*

AED Coadministered	AED Concentration	Felbamate Concentration
Phenytoin	Increases	Decreases
Valproate	Increases	†
Carbamazepine (CBZ)	Decreases	Decreases
*CBZ epoxide	Increases	

* Not administered, but an active metabolite of carbamazepine.
† No significant effect.

SPECIAL EFFECTS OF FELBAMATE ON OTHER ANTIEPILEPTIC DRUGS

Phenytoin

Felbamate causes an increase in steady-state phenytoin plasma concentrations. In 10 otherwise healthy subjects with epilepsy ingesting phenytoin, the steady-state trough (C_{min}) phenytoin plasma concentration was 17 ± 5 micrograms/ml. The steady-state C_{min} increased to 21 ± 5 micrograms/ml when 1200 mg/day of felbamate was coadministered. Increasing the felbamate dose to 1800 mg/day in 6 of these subjects increased the steady-state phenytoin C_{min} to 25 ± 7 micrograms/ml. In order to maintain phenytoin levels, limit adverse experiences, and achieve the felbamate dose of 3600 mg/day, a phenytoin dose reduction of approximately 40% was necessary for 8 of these 10 subjects.

In a controlled clinical trial, a 20% reduction of the phenytoin dose at the initiation of felbamate therapy resulted in phenytoin levels comparable to those prior to felbamate administration.

Carbamazepine

Felbamate causes a decrease in the steady-state carbamazepine plasma concentration and an increase in the steady- state carbamazepine epoxide plasma concentration. In 9 otherwise healthy subjects with epilepsy ingesting carbamazepine, the steady-state trough (Cmin) carbamazepine concentration was 8 ± 2 micrograms/ml. The carbamazepine steady-state Cmin decreased 31% to 5 ± 1 micrograms/ml when felbamate (3000 mg/day, divided into three doses) was coadministered. Carbamazepine epoxide steady-state Cmin concentrations increased 57% from 1.0 ± 0.3 to 1.6 ± 0.4 micrograms/ml with the addition of felbamate.

In clinical trials, similar changes in carbamazepine and carbamazepine epoxide were seen.

Valproate

Felbamate causes an increase in steady-state valproate concentrations. In 4 subjects with epilepsy ingesting valproate, the steady-state trough (C_{min}) valproate plasma concentration was 63 ± 16 micrograms/ml. The steady-state C_{min} increased to 78 ± 14 micrograms/ml when 1200 mg/day of felbamate was coadministered. Increasing the felbamate dose to 2400 mg/day increased the steady-state valproate C_{min} to 96 ± 25 micrograms/ml. Corresponding values for free valproate C_{min} concentrations were 7 ± 3, 9 ± 4, and 11 ± 6 micrograms/ml for 0, 1200, and 2400 mg/day felbamate, respectively. The ratios of the AUCs of unbound valproate to the AUCs of the total valproate were 11.1%, 13.0%, and 11.5%, with coadministration of 0, 1200, and 2400 mg/day of felbamate, respectively. This indicates that the protein binding of valproate did not change appreciably with increasing doses of felbamate.

EFFECTS OF OTHER ANTIEPILEPTIC DRUGS ON FELBAMATE

Phenytoin

Phenytoin causes an approximate doubling of the clearance of felbamate at steady state and, therefore, the addition of phenytoin causes an approximate 45% decrease in the steady- state trough concentrations of felbamate as compared to the same dose of felbamate given as monotherapy.

Carbamazepine

Carbamazepine causes an approximate 50% increase in the clearance of felbamate at steady state and, therefore, the addition of carbamazepine results in an approximate 40% decrease in the steady-state trough concentrations of felbamate as compared to the same dose of felbamate given as monotherapy.

Valproate

Available data suggest that there is no significant effect of valproate on the clearance of felbamate at steady state. Therefore, the addition of valproate is not expected to cause a clinically important effect on felbamate plasma concentrations.

EFFECTS OF ANTACIDS ON FELBAMATE

The rate and extent of absorption of a 2400 mg dose of felbamate as monotherapy given as tablets was not affected when coadministered with antacids.

ADVERSE REACTIONS

The most common adverse reactions seen in association with felbamate in adults during monotherapy are anorexia, vomiting, insomnia, nausea, and headache. The most common adverse reactions seen in association with felbamate in adults during adjunctive therapy are anorexia, vomiting, insomnia, nausea, dizziness, somnolence, and headache.

The most common adverse reactions seen in association with felbamate in children during adjunctive therapy are anorexia, vomiting, insomnia, headache, and somnolence.

The dropout rate because of adverse experiences or intercurrent illnesses among adult felbamate patients was 12% (120/977). The dropout rate because of adverse experiences or intercurrent illnesses among pediatric felbamate patients was 6% (23/357). In adults, the body systems associated with causing these withdrawals in order of frequency were: digestive (4.3%), psychological (2.2%), whole body (1.7%), neurological (1.5%), and dermatological (1.5%). In children, the body systems associated with causing these withdrawals in order of frequency were: digestive (1.7%), neurological (1.4%), dermatological (1.4%), psychological (1.1%), and whole body (1.0%). In adults, specific events with an incidence of 1% or greater associated with causing these withdrawals, in order of frequency were: anorexia (1.6%), nausea (1.4%), rash (1.2%), and weight decrease (1.1%). In children, specific events with an incidence of 1% or greater associated with causing these withdrawals, in order of frequency was rash (1.1%).

INCIDENCE IN CLINICAL TRIALS

The prescriber should be aware that the figures cited in TABLE 2 cannot be used to predict the incidence of side effects in the course of usual medical practice where patient characteristics and other factors differ from those which prevailed in the clinical trials. Similarly, the cited frequencies cannot be compared with figures obtained from other clinical investigations involving different investigators, treatments, and uses including the use of felbamate as adjunctive therapy where the incidence of adverse events may be higher due to drug interactions. The cited figures, however, do provide the prescribing physician with some basis for estimating the relative contribution of drug and nondrug factors to the side effect incidence rate in the population studied.

INCIDENCE IN CONTROLLED CLINICAL TRIALS-MONOTHERAPY STUDIES IN ADULTS

TABLE 2 enumerates adverse events that occurred at an incidence of 2% or more among 58 adult patients who received felbamate monotherapy at dosages of 3600 mg/day in double-blind controlled trials. Reported adverse events were classified using standard WHO-based dictionary terminology.

TABLE 2 *Felbamate, Adverse Reactions*

Adults Treatment-Emergent Adverse Event Incidence in Controlled Monotherapy Trials

Body System/Event	Felbamate* (n=58)	Low-Dose Valproate† (n=50)
Body as a Whole		
Fatigue	6.9%	4.0%
Weight decrease	3.4%	0%
Face edema	3.4%	0%
Central Nervous System		
Insomnia	8.6%	4.0%
Headache	6.9%	18.0%
Anxiety	5.2%	2.0%
Dermatologic		
Acne	3.4%	0%
Rash	3.4%	0%
Digestive		
Dyspepsia	8.6%	2.0%
Vomiting	8.6%	2.0%
Constipation	6.9%	2.0%
Diarrhea	5.2%	0%
SGPT increased	5.2%	2.0%
Metabolic/Nutritional		
Hypophosphatemia	3.4%	0%
Respiratory		
Upper respiratory tract infection	8.6%	4.0%
Rhinitis	6.9%	0%
Special Senses		
Diplopia	3.4%	4.0%
Otitis media	3.4%	0%
Urogenital		
Intramenstrual bleeding	3.4%	0%
Urinary tract infection	3.4%	2.0%

* 3600 mg/day
† 15 mg/kg/day

INCIDENCE IN CONTROLLED ADD-ON CLINICAL STUDIES IN ADULTS

TABLE 3 enumerates adverse events that occurred at an incidence of 2% or more among 114 adult patients who received felbamate adjunctive therapy in add-on controlled trials at dosages up to 3600 mg/day. Reported adverse events were classified using standard WHO-based dictionary terminology.

Many adverse experiences that occurred during adjunctive therapy may be a result of drug interactions. Adverse experiences during adjunctive therapy typically resolved with conversion to monotherapy, or with adjustment of the dosage of other antiepileptic drugs.

INCIDENCE IN A CONTROLLED ADD-ON TRIAL IN CHILDREN WITH LENNOX-GASTAUT SYNDROME

TABLE 4 enumerates adverse events that occurred more than once among 31 pediatric patients who received felbamate up to 45 mg/kg/day or a maximum of 3600 mg/day. Reported adverse events were classified using standard WHO-based dictionary terminology.

OTHER EVENTS OBSERVED IN ASSOCIATION WITH THE ADMINISTRATION OF FELBAMATE

In the paragraphs that follow, the adverse clinical events, other than those in the preceding tables, that occurred in a total of 977 adults and 357 children exposed to felbamate and that are reasonably associated with its use are presented. They are listed in order of decreasing frequency. Because the reports cite events observed in open-label and uncontrolled studies, the role of felbamate in their causation cannot be reliably determined.

Events are classified within body system categories and enumerated in order of decreasing frequency using the following definitions: *frequent* adverse events are defined as those occurring on one or more occasions in at least 1/100 patients; *infrequent* adverse events are those occurring in 1/100-1/1000 patients; and *rare* events are those occurring in fewer than 1/1000 patients.

TABLE 3 *Felbamate, Adverse Reactions*

Adults Treatment-Emergent Adverse Event Incidence in Controlled Add-On Trials

Body System/Event	Felbamate (n=114)	Placebo (n=43)
Body as a Whole		
Fatigue	16.8%	7.0%
Fever	2.6%	4.7%
Chest pain	2.6%	0%
Central Nervous System		
Headache	36.8%	9.3%
Somnolence	19.3%	7.0%
Dizziness	18.4%	14.0%
Insomnia	17.5%	7.0%
Nervousness	7.0%	2.3%
Tremor	6.1%	2.3%
Anxiety	5.3%	4.7%
Gait abnormal	5.3%	0%
Depression	5.3%	0%
Paresthesia	3.5%	2.3%
Ataxia	3.5%	0%
Mouth dry	2.6%	0%
Stupor	2.6%	0%
Dermatologic		
Rash	3.5%	4.7%
Digestive		
Nausea	34.2%	2.3%
Anorexia	19.3%	2.3%
Vomiting	16.7%	4.7%
Dyspepsia	12.3%	7.0%
Constipation	11.4%	2.3%
Diarrhea	5.3%	2.33%
Abdominal pain	5.3%	0%
SGPT increased	3.5%	0%
Musculoskeletal		
Myalgia	2.6%	0%
Respiratory		
Upper respiratory tract infection	5.3%	7.0%
Sinusitis	3.5%	0%
Pharyngitis	2.6%	0%
Special Senses		
Diplopia	6.1%	0%
Taste perversion	6.1%	0%
Vision abnormal	5.3%	2.3%

TABLE 4 *Felbamate, Adverse Reactions*

Children Treatment-Emergent Adverse Event Incidence in a Controlled Add-On Lennox-Gastaut Trial

Body System/Event	Felbamate (n=31)	Placebo (n=27)
Body as a Whole		
Fever	22.6%	11.1%
Fatigue	9.7%	3.7%
Weight decrease	6.5%	0%
Pain	6.5%	0%
Central Nervous System		
Somnolence	48.4%	11.1%
Insomnia	16.1%	14.8%
Nervousness	16.1%	18.5%
Gait abnormal	9.7%	0%
Headache	6.5%	18.5%
Thinking abnormal	6.5%	3.7%
Ataxia	6.5%	3.7%
Urinary incontinence	6.5%	7.4%
Emotional lability	6.5%	0%
Miosis	6.5%	0%
Dermatologic		
Rash	9.7%	7.4%
Digestive		
Anorexia	54.8%	14.8%
Vomiting	38.7%	14.8%
Constipation	12.9%	
Hiccup	9.7%	3.7%
Nausea	6.5%	0%
Dyspepsia	6.5%	3.7%
Hematologic		
Purpura	12.9v	7.4%
Leukopenia	6.5%	0%
Respiratory		
Upper respiratory tract infection	45.2%	25.9%
Pharyngitis	9.7%	3.7%
Coughing	6.5%	0%
Special Senses		
Otitis media	9.7%	0%

Event frequencies are calculated as the number of patients reporting an event divided by the total number of patients (n=1334) exposed to felbamate.

Body as a Whole: *Frequent:* Weight increase, asthenia, malaise, influenza-like symptoms; *Rare:* Anaphylactoid reaction, chest pain substernal.

Cardiovascular: *Frequent:* Palpitation, tachycardia; *Rare:* Supraventricular tachycardia.

Central Nervous System: *Frequent:* Agitation, psychological disturbance, aggressive reaction; *Infrequent:* Hallucination, euphoria, suicide attempt, migraine.

Digestive: *Frequent:* SGOT increased;*Infrequent:*Esophagitis, appetite increased; *Rare:* GGT elevated.

Hematologic: *Infrequent:* Lymphadenopathy, leukopenia, leukocytosis, thrombocytopenia, granulocytopenia;*Rare:* Antinuclear factor test positive, qualitative platelet disorder, agranulocytosis.

Metabolic/Nutritional: *Infrequent:* Hypokalemia, hyponatremia, LDH increased, alkaline phosphatase increased, hypophosphatemia; *Rare:* Creatinine phosphokinase increased.

Musculoskeletal: *Infrequent:* Dystonia.

Dermatologic: *Frequent:* Pruritus;*Infrequent:* Urticaria, bullous eruption; *Rare:* Buccal mucous membrane swelling, Stevens-Johnson Syndrome.

Special Senses: *Rare:* Photosensitivity allergic reaction.

POSTMARKETING ADVERSE EVENT REPORTS

Voluntary reports of adverse events in patients taking felbamate (usually in conjunction with other drugs) have been received since market introduction and may have no causal relationship with the drug(s).

These include the following by body system:

Body as a Whole: Neoplasm, sepsis, placental disorder, L.E. syndrome, SIDS, sudden death, fetal death, edema, hypothermia, rigors, microcephaly.

Cardiovascular: Atrial fibrillation, atrial arrhythmia, cardiac arrest, torsade de pointes, cardiac failure, hypotension, hypertension, flushing, thrombophlebitis, ischemic necrosis, gangrene, peripheral ischemia.

Central & Peripheral Nervous System: Delusion, paralysis, mononeuritis, cerebrovascular disorder, cerebral edema, coma, manic reaction, encephalopathy, paranoid reaction, nystagmus, choreoathetosis, extrapyramidal disorder, confusion, psychosis, status epilepticus, dyskinesia, dysarthria, respiratory depression.

Dermatologic: Abnormal body odor, sweating, lichen planus, livedo reticularis, alopecia, toxic epidermal necrolysis.

Digestive: (See WARNINGS.) Hepatitis, hepatic failure, G.I. hemorrhage, hyperammonemia, pancreatitis, hematemesis, gastritis, esophagitis, rectal hemorrhage, flatulence, gingival bleeding, acquired megacolon, ileus, intestinal obstruction, enteritis, ulcerative stomatitis, glossitis, dysphagia, jaundice.

Hematologic: (See WARNINGS.) Increased and decreased prothrombin time, anemia, hypochromic anemia, aplastic anemia, pancytopenia, hemolytic uremic syndrome.

Metabolic/Nutritional: Hypernatremia, hypoglycemia, SIADH, hypomagnesemia, dehydration.

Musculoskeletal: Arthralgia, muscle weakness, involuntary muscle contraction, rhabdomyolysis.

Respiratory: Dyspnea, pneumonia, pneumonitis, hypoxia, epistaxis, pleural effusion, respiratory insufficiency, pulmonary hemorrhage.

Special Senses: Hemianopsia, decreased hearing, conjunctivitis.

Urogenital: Genital malformation, menstrual disorder, acute renal failure, hepatorenal syndrome, hematuria, urinary retention, nephrosis, vaginal hemorrhage.

DOSAGE AND ADMINISTRATION

Felbamate has been studied as monotherapy and adjunctive therapy in adults and as adjunctive therapy in children with seizures associated with Lennox-Gastaut syndrome. As felbamate is added to or substituted for existing AEDs, it is strongly recommended to reduce the dosage of those AEDs in the range of 20-33% to minimize side effects (see DRUG INTERACTIONS).

ADULTS (14 YEARS OF AGE AND OVER)

The majority of patients received 3600 mg/day in clinical trials evaluating its use as both monotherapy and adjunctive therapy.

MONOTHERAPY (INITIAL THERAPY)

Felbamate has not been systematically evaluated as initial monotherapy. Initiate felbamate at 1200 mg/day in divided doses 3 or 4 times daily. The prescriber is advised to titrate previously untreated patients under close clinical supervision, increasing the dosage in 600 mg increments every 2 weeks to 2400 mg/day based on clinical response and thereafter to 3600 mg/day if clinically indicated.

CONVERSION TO MONOTHERAPY

Initiate felbamate at 1200 mg/day in divided doses 3 or 4 times daily. Reduce the dosage of concomitant AEDs by one-third at initiation of felbamate therapy. At week 2, increase the felbamate dosage to 2400 mg/day while reducing the dosage of other AEDs up to an additional one-third of their original dosage. At week 3, increase the felbamate dosage up to 3600 mg/day and continue to reduce the dosage of other AEDs as clinically indicated.

ADJUNCTIVE THERAPY

Felbamate should be added at 1200 mg/day in divided doses 3-4 times daily while reducing present AEDs by 20% in order-control plasma concentrations of concurrent phenytoin, valproic acid, and carbamazepine and its metabolites. Further reductions of the concomitant AEDs dosage may be necessary to minimize side effects due to drug interactions. Increase the dosage of felbamate by 1200 mg/day increments at weekly intervals to 3600 mg/day. Most side effects seen during felbamate adjunctive therapy resolve as the dosage of concomitant AEDs is decreased. (See TABLE 5.)

TABLE 5 *Felbamate, Dosage Table (Adults)*

	WEEK 1	WEEK 2	WEEK 3
Dosage reduction of concomitant AEDs	REDUCE original dose by 20-33%*	REDUCE original dose by up to an additional 1/3*	REDUCE as clinically indicated
Felbamate dosage	1200 mg/day Initial dose	2400 mg/day Therapeutic dosage range	3600 mg/day Therapeutic dosage range

* See ***Conversion to Monotherapy***.

While the above felbamate conversion guidelines may result in a felbamate 3600 mg/day dose within 3 weeks, in some patients titration to a 3600 mg/day felbamate dose has been achieved in as little as 3 days with appropriate adjustment of other AEDs.

CHILDREN WITH LENNOX-GASTAUT SYNDROME (AGES 2-14 YEARS)

Adjunctive Therapy

Felbamate should be added at 15 mg/kg/day in divided doses 3 or 4 times daily while reducing present AEDs by 20% in order to control plasma levels of concurrent phenytoin, valproic acid, and carbamazepine and its metabolites. Further reductions of the concomitant AED dosage may be necessary to minimize side effects due to drug interactions. Increase the dosage of felbamate by 15 mg/kg/day increments at weekly intervals to 45 mg/kg/day. Most side effects seen during felbamate adjunctive therapy resolve as the dosage of concomitant AEDs is decreased.

HOW SUPPLIED

Felbatol Tablets, 400 mg Yellow, scored, capsule-shaped tablets, debossed "0430" on one side and "Wallace" on the other.

Felbatol Tablets, 600 mg, Peach-colored, scored, capsule- shaped tablets, debossed "0431" on one side and "Wallace" on the other.

Felbatol Oral Suspension, 600 mg/5 ml Peach-colored.

Shake suspension well before using.

Storage: Store at controlled room temperature 15°-30°C (59°-86°F). Dispense in tight container.

PRODUCT LISTING - EQUIVALENTS NOT AVAILABLE

Suspension - Oral - 600 mg/ 5 ml			
240 ml	$200.72	FELBATOL, Wallace Laboratories	00037-0442-67
960 ml	$514.99	FELBATOL, Wallace Laboratories	00037-0442-17
Tablet - Oral - 400 mg			
30's	$37.73	FELBATOL, Allscripts Pharmaceutical Company	54569-4749-00
100's	$135.85	FELBATOL, Wallace Laboratories	00037-0430-11
100's	$163.30	FELBATOL, Wallace Laboratories	00037-0430-01
Tablet - Oral - 600 mg			
90's	$129.74	FELBATOL, Allscripts Pharmaceutical Company	54569-4750-00
100's	$168.14	FELBATOL, Wallace Laboratories	00037-0431-11
100's	$187.15	FELBATOL, Wallace Laboratories	00037-0431-01

Felodipine *(003059)*

For related information, see the comparative table section in Appendix A.

Categories: Hypertension, essential; Pregnancy Category C; FDA Approved 1991 Jul
Drug Classes: Calcium channel blockers
Brand Names: **Plendil**
Foreign Brand Availability: AGON SR (Australia; New-Zealand); Dilopin (Korea); Felo-BASF (Germany); Felo-BASF Retardtab (Germany); Felo ER (New-Zealand); Felocor (Germany); Felocor Retardtab (Germany); Felodur ER (Australia); Felogard (India); Flodil LP (France); Hydac (Denmark; Finland; Sweden); Modip (Germany); Munobal (Germany; Japan; Mexico; Philippines); Munobal Retard (Austria; Germany; Switzerland); Nirmadil (Indonesia); Penedil (Israel); Plendil Depottab (Norway); Plendil ER (Australia; New-Zealand; Philippines); Plendil Retard (Austria); Renedil (Belgium; Canada); Splendil (Japan); Splendil ER (Korea)
Cost of Therapy: $36.56 (Hypertension; Plendil; 5 mg; 1 tablet/day; 30 day supply)

DESCRIPTION

Felodipine is a calcium antagonist (calcium channel blocker). Felodipine is a dihydropyridine derivative that is chemically described as ± ethyl methyl 4-(2,3-dichlorophenyl)-1,4-dihydro-2,6-dimethyl-3,5-pyridinedicarboxylate. Its empirical formula is $C_{18}H_{19}Cl_2NO_4$.

Felodipine is a slightly yellowish, crystalline powder with a molecular weight of 384.26. It is insoluble in water and is freely soluble in dichloromethane and ethanol. Felodipine is a racemic mixture.

Plendil tablets provide extended release of felodipine. They are available as tablets containing 2.5, 5, or 10 mg of felodipine for oral administration. In addition to the active ingredient felodipine, the tablets contain the following inactive ingredients:

Plendil tablets 2.5 mg: Hydroxypropyl cellulose, lactose, FD&C blue 2, sodium stearyl fumarate, titanium dioxide, yellow iron oxide, and other ingredients.

Plendil tablets 5 and 10 mg: Cellulose, red and yellow oxide, lactose, polyethylene glycol, sodium stearyl fumarate, titanium dioxide, and other ingredients.

CLINICAL PHARMACOLOGY

MECHANISM OF ACTION

Felodipine is a member of the dihydropyridine class of calcium channel antagonists (calcium channel blockers). It reversibly competes with nitrendipine and/or other calcium channel blockers for dihydropyridine binding sites, blocks voltage-dependent Ca^{++} currents in vascular smooth muscle and cultured rabbit atrial cells, and blocks potassium-induced contracture of the rat portal vein.

In vitro studies show that the effects of felodipine on contractile processes are selective, with greater effects on vascular smooth muscle than cardiac muscle. Negative inotropic effects can be detected *in vitro,* but such effects have not been seen in intact animals.

The effect of felodipine on blood pressure is principally a consequence of a dose-related decrease of peripheral vascular resistance in man, with a modest reflex increase in heart rate (see Cardiovascular Effects). With the exception of a mild diuretic effect seen in several animal species and man, the effects of felodipine are accounted for by its effects on peripheral vascular resistance.

PHARMACOKINETICS AND METABOLISM

Following oral administration, felodipine is almost completely absorbed and undergoes extensive first-pass metabolism. The systemic bioavailability of felodipine is approximately 20%. Mean peak concentrations following the administration of felodipine are reached in 2.5 to 5 hours. Both peak plasma concentration and the area under the plasma concentration time curve (AUC) increase linearly with doses up to 20 mg. Felodipine is greater than 99% bound to plasma proteins.

Following intravenous administration, the plasma concentration of felodipine declined triexponentially with mean disposition half-lives of 4.8 minutes, 1.5 hours, and 9.1 hours. The mean contributions of the three individual phases to the overall AUC were 15, 40, and 45%, respectively, in the order of increasing $T_{½}$.

Following oral administration of the immediate-release formulation, the plasma level of felodipine also declined polyexponentially with a mean terminal $T_{½}$ of 11-16 hours. The mean peak and trough steady-state plasma concentrations achieved after 10 mg of the immediate-release formulation given once a day to normal volunteers, were 20 and 0.5 nmol/L, respectively. The trough plasma concentration of felodipine in most individuals was substantially below the concentration needed to effect a half-maximal decline in blood pressure (EC_{50}) [4-6 nmol/L for felodipine], thus precluding once-a-day dosing with the immediate-release formulation.

Following administration of a 10 mg dose of felodipine, the extended-release formulation, to young, healthy volunteers, mean peak and trough steady-state plasma concentrations of felodipine were 7 and 2 nmol/L, respectively. Corresponding values in hypertensive patients (mean age 64) after a 20 mg dose of felodipine were 23 and 7 nmol/L. Since the EC_{50} for felodipine is 4-6 nmol/L, a 5-10 mg dose of felodipine in some patients, and a 20 mg dose in others, would be expected to provide an antihypertensive effect that persists for 24 hours (see Cardiovascular Effects and DOSAGE AND ADMINISTRATION).

The systemic plasma clearance of felodipine in young healthy subjects is about 0.8 L/min, and the apparent volume of distribution is about 10 L/kg.

Following an oral or intravenous dose of ^{14}C-labeled felodipine in man, about 70% of the dose of radioactivity was recovered in urine and 10% in the feces. A negligible amount of intact felodipine is recovered in the urine and feces (<0.5%). Six metabolites, which account for 23% of the oral dose, have been identified; none has significant vasodilating activity.

Following administration of felodipine to hypertensive patients, mean peak plasma concentrations at steady state are about 20% higher than after a single dose. Blood pressure response is correlated with plasma concentrations of felodipine.

The bioavailability of felodipine is influenced by the presence of food. When administered either with a high fat or carbohydrate diet, C_{max} is increased by approximately 60%; AUC is unchanged. When felodipine was administered after a light meal (orange juice, toast, and cereal), however, there is no effect on felodipine's pharmacokinetics. The bioavailability of felodipine was increased approximately 2-fold when taken with grapefruit juice. Orange juice does not appear to modify the kinetics of felodipine. A similar finding has been seen with other dihydropyridine calcium antagonists, but to a lesser extent than that seen with felodipine.

Geriatric Use

Plasma concentrations of felodipine, after a single dose and at steady state, increase with age. Mean clearance of felodipine in elderly hypertensives (mean age 74) was only 45% of that of young volunteers (mean age 26). At steady state mean AUC for young patients was 39% of that for the elderly. Data for intermediate age ranges suggest that the AUCs fall between the extremes of the young and the elderly.

Hepatic Dysfunction

In patients with hepatic disease, the clearance of felodipine was reduced to about 60% of that seen in normal young volunteers.

Renal impairment does not alter the plasma concentration profile of felodipine; although higher concentrations of the metabolites are present in the plasma due to decreased urinary excretion, these are inactive.

Animal studies have demonstrated that felodipine crosses the blood-brain barrier and the placenta.

CARDIOVASCULAR EFFECTS

Following administration of felodipine, a reduction in blood pressure generally occurs within 2-5 hours. During chronic administration, substantial blood pressure control lasts for 24 hours, with trough reductions in diastolic blood pressure approximately 40-50% of peak reductions. The antihypertensive effect is dose dependent and correlates with the plasma concentration of felodipine.

A reflex increase in heart rate frequently occurs during the first week of therapy; this increase attenuates over time. Heart rate increases of 5-10 beats per minute may be seen during chronic dosing. The increase is inhibited by beta-blocking agents.

The P-R interval of the ECG is not affected by felodipine when administered alone or in combination with a beta-blocking agent. Felodipine alone or in combination with a beta-blocking agent has been shown, in clinical and electrophysiologic studies, to have no significant effect on cardiac conduction (P-R, P-Q, and H-V intervals).

In clinical trials in hypertensive patients without clinical evidence of left ventricular dysfunction, no symptoms suggestive of a negative inotropic effect were noted; however, none would be expected in this population (see PRECAUTIONS).

RENAL/ENDOCRINE EFFECTS

Renal vascular resistance is decreased by felodipine while glomerular filtration rate remains unchanged. Mild diuresis, natriuresis, and kaliuresis have been observed during the first week of therapy. No significant effects on serum electrolytes were observed during short- and long-term therapy.

In clinical trials in patients with hypertension, increases in plasma noradrenaline levels have been observed.

F

INDICATIONS AND USAGE

Felodipine is indicated for the treatment of hypertension.

Felodipine may be used alone or concomitantly with other antihypertensive agents.

CONTRAINDICATIONS

Felodipine is contraindicated in patients who are hypersensitive to this product.

PRECAUTIONS

GENERAL

Hypotension

Felodipine, like other calcium antagonists, may occasionally precipitate significant hypotension and, rarely, syncope. It may lead to reflex tachycardia which in susceptible individuals may precipitate angina pectoris. (See ADVERSE REACTIONS.)

Heart Failure

Although acute hemodynamic studies in a small number of patients with NYHA Class II or III heart failure treated with felodipine have not demonstrated negative inotropic effects, safety in patients with heart failure has not been established. Caution, therefore, should be exercised when using felodipine in patients with heart failure or compromised ventricular function, particularly in combination with a beta blocker.

Patients With Impaired Liver Function

Patients with impaired liver function may have elevated plasma concentrations of felodipine and may respond to lower doses of felodipine; therefore, a starting dose of 2.5 mg once a day is recommended. These patients should have their blood pressure monitored closely during dosage adjustment of felodipine. (See CLINICAL PHARMACOLOGY and DOSAGE AND ADMINISTRATION.)

Peripheral Edema

Peripheral edema, generally mild and not associated with generalized fluid retention, was the most common adverse event in the clinical trials. The incidence of peripheral edema was both dose and age dependent. Frequency of peripheral edema ranged from about 10% in patients under 50 years of age taking 5 mg daily to about 30% in those over 60 years of age taking 20 mg daily. This adverse effect generally occurs within 2-3 weeks of the initiation of treatment.

INFORMATION FOR THE PATIENT

Patients should be instructed to take felodipine whole and not to crush or chew the tablets. They should be told that mild gingival hyperplasia (gum swelling) has been reported. Good dental hygiene decreases its incidence and severity.

Note: As with many other drugs, certain advice to patients being treated with felodipine is warranted. This information is intended to aid in the safe and effective use of this medication. It is not a disclosure of all possible adverse or intended effects.

CARCINOGENESIS, MUTAGENESIS, AND IMPAIRMENT OF FERTILITY

In a 2 year carcinogenicity study in rats fed felodipine at doses of 7.7, 23.1 or 69.3 mg/kg/day (up to 61 times* the maximum recommended human dose on a mg/m^2 basis), a dose-related increase in the incidence of benign interstitial cell tumors of the testes (Leydig cell tumors) was observed in treated male rats. These tumors were not observed in a similar study in mice at doses up to 138.6 mg/kg/day (61 times* the maximum recommended human dose on a mg/m^2 basis). Felodipine, at the doses employed in the 2 year rat study, has been shown to lower testicular testosterone and to produce a corresponding increase in serum luteinizing hormone in rats. The Leydig cell tumor development is possibly secondary to these hormonal effects which have not been observed in man.

In this same rat study a dose-related increase in the incidence of focal squamous cell hyperplasia compared to control was observed in the esophageal groove of male and female rats in all dose groups. No other drug-related esophageal or gastric pathology was observed in the rats or with chronic administration in mice and dogs. The latter species, like man, has no anatomical structure comparable to the esophageal groove.

Felodipine was not carcinogenic when fed to mice at doses up to 138.6 mg/kg/day (61 times* the maximum recommended human dose on a mg/m^2 basis) for periods of up to 80 weeks in males and 99 weeks in females.

Felodipine did not display any mutagenic activity *in vitro* in the Ames microbial mutagenicity test or in the mouse lymphoma forward mutation assay. No clastogenic potential was seen *in vivo* in the mouse micronucleus test at oral doses up to 2500 mg/kg (1100 times* the maximum recommended human dose on a mg/m^2 basis) or *in vitro* in a human lymphocyte chromosome aberration assay.

A fertility study in which male and female rats were administered doses of 3.8, 9.6 or 26.9 mg/kg/day (up to 24 times* the maximum recommended human dose on a mg/m^2 basis) showed no significant effect of felodipine on reproductive performance.

*Based on patient weight of 50 kg.

PREGNANCY CATEGORY C

Teratogenic Effects

Studies in pregnant rabbits administered doses of 0.46, 1.2, 2.3, and 4.6 mg/kg/day (from 0.8 to 8 times* the maximum recommended human dose on a mg/m^2 basis) showed digital anomalies consisting of reduction in size and degree of ossification of the terminal phalanges in the fetuses. The frequency and severity of the changes appeared dose related and were noted even at the lowest dose. These changes have been shown to occur with other members of the dihydropyridine class and are possibly a result of compromised uterine blood flow. Similar fetal anomalies were not observed in rats given felodipine.

In a teratology study in cynomolgus monkeys, no reduction in the size of the terminal phalanges was observed, but an abnormal position of the distal phalanges was noted in about 40% of the fetuses.

*Based on patient weight of 50 kg.

Nonteratogenic Effects

A prolongation of parturition with difficult labor and an increased frequency of fetal and early postnatal deaths were observed in rats administered doses of 9.6 mg/kg/day (8 times* the maximum human dose on a mg/m^2 basis) and above.

Significant enlargement of the mammary glands, in excess of the normal enlargement for pregnant rabbits, was found with doses greater than or equal to 1.2 mg/kg/day (2.1 times the maximum human dose on a mg/m^2 basis). This effect occurred only in pregnant rabbits and regressed during lactation. Similar changes in the mammary glands were not observed in rats or monkeys.

There are no adequate and well-controlled studies in pregnant women. If felodipine is used during pregnancy, or if the patient becomes pregnant while taking this drug, she should be apprised of the potential hazard to the fetus, possible digital anomalies of the infant, and the potential effects of felodipine on labor and delivery and on the mammary glands of pregnant females.

*Based on patient weight of 50 kg.

NURSING MOTHERS

It is not known whether this drug is secreted in human milk and because of the potential for serious adverse reactions from felodipine in the infant, a decision should be made whether to discontinue nursing or to discontinue the drug, taking into account the importance of the drug to the mother.

PEDIATRIC USE

Safety and effectiveness in pediatric patients have not been established.

GERIATRIC USE

Clinical studies of felodipine did not include sufficient numbers of subjects aged 65 and over to determine whether they respond differently from younger subjects. Other reported clinical experience has not identified differences in responses between the elderly and younger patients. Pharmacokinetics, however, indicate that the availability of felodipine is increased in older patients (see CLINICAL PHARMACOLOGY, Pharmacokinetics and Metabolism, Geriatric Use). In general, dose selection for an elderly patient should be cautious, usually starting at the low end of the dosing range, reflecting the greater frequency of decreased hepatic, renal, or cardiac function, and of concomitant disease or other drug therapy.

DRUG INTERACTIONS

CYP3A4 INHIBITORS

Felodipine is metabolized by CYP3A4. Coadministration of CYP3A4 inhibitors (*e.g.*, ketoconazole, itraconazole, erythromycin, grapefruit juice, cimetidine) with felodipine may lead to several-fold increases in the plasma levels of felodipine, either due to an increase in bioavailability or due to a decrease in metabolism. These increases in concentration may lead to increased effects, (lower blood pressure and increased heart rate). These effects have been observed with coadministration of itraconazole (a potent CYP3A4 inhibitor). Caution should be used when CYP3A4 inhibitors are coadministered with felodipine. A conservative approach to dosing felodipine should be taken. The following specific interactions have been reported:

Itraconazole: Coadministration of another extended-release formulation of felodipine with itraconazole resulted in approximately 8-fold increase in the AUC, more than 6-fold increase in the C_{max}, and 2-fold prolongation in the half-life of felodipine.

Erythromycin: Coadministration of felodipine with erythromycin resulted in approximately 2.5-fold increase in the AUC and C_{max}, and about 2-fold prolongation in the half-life of felodipine.

Grapefruit Juice: Coadministration of felodipine with grapefruit juice resulted in more than 2-fold increase in the AUC and C_{max}, but no prolongation in the half-life of felodipine.

Cimetidine: Coadministration of felodipine with cimetidine (a non-specific CYP-450 inhibitor) resulted in an increase of approximately 50% in the AUC and the C_{max}, of felodipine.

Beta-Blocking Agents: A pharmacokinetic study of felodipine in conjunction with metoprolol demonstrated no significant effects on the pharmacokinetics of felodipine. The AUC and C_{max} of metoprolol, however, were increased approximately 31 and 38%, respectively. In controlled clinical trials, however, beta blockers including metoprolol were concurrently administered with felodipine and were well tolerated.

Digoxin: When given concomitantly with felodipine the pharmacokinetics of digoxin in patients with heart failure were not significantly altered.

Anticonvulsants: In a pharmacokinetic study, maximum plasma concentrations of felodipine were considerably lower in epileptic patients on long-term anticonvulsant therapy (*e.g.*, phenytoin, carbamazepine, or phenobarbital) than in healthy volunteers. In such patients, the mean area under the felodipine plasma concentration-time curve was also reduced to approximately 6% of that observed in healthy volunteers. Since a clinically significant interaction may be anticipated, alternative antihypertensive therapy should be considered in these patients.

Other Concomitant Therapy: In healthy subjects there were no clinically significant interactions when felodipine was given concomitantly with indomethacin or spironolactone.

Interaction With Food: See CLINICAL PHARMACOLOGY, Pharmacokinetics and Metabolism.

ADVERSE REACTIONS

In controlled studies in the US and overseas, approximately 3000 patients were treated with felodipine as either the extended-release or the immediate-release formulation.

The most common clinical adverse events reported with felodipine administered as monotherapy at the recommended dosage range of 2.5 to 10 mg once a day were peripheral edema and headache. Peripheral edema was generally mild, but it was age and dose related and resulted in discontinuation of therapy in about 3% of the enrolled patients. Discontinuation of therapy due to any clinical adverse event occurred in about 6% of the patients receiving felodipine, principally for peripheral edema, headache, or flushing.

Adverse events that occurred with an incidence of 1.5% or greater at any of the recommended doses of 2.5 to 10 mg once a day (felodipine, n=861; placebo, n=334), without regard to causality, are compared to placebo and are listed by dose in TABLE 2. These events are reported from controlled clinical trials with patients who were randomized to a fixed dose of felodipine or titrated from an initial dose of 2.5 or 5 mg once a day. A dose of 20 mg once a day has been evaluated in some clinical studies. Although the antihypertensive effect of felodipine is increased at 20 mg once a day, there is a disproportionate increase in adverse events, especially those associated with vasodilatory effects (see DOSAGE AND ADMINISTRATION).

TABLE 2 *Percent of Patients With Adverse Events in Controlled Trials* of Felodipine (n=861) as Monotherapy Without Regard to Causality — Incidence of Discontinuations Shown in Parentheses*

Body System / Adverse Events	Placebo n=334	2.5 mg n=255	5 mg n=581	10 mg n=408
Body as a Whole				
Peripheral edema	3.3% (0.0%)	2.0% (0.0%)	8.8% (2.2%)	17.4% (2.5%)
Asthenia	3.3% (0.0%)	3.9% (0.0%)	3.3% (0.0%)	2.2% (0.0%)
Warm sensation	0.0% (0.0%)	0.0% (0.0%)	0.9% (0.2%)	1.5% (0.0%)
Cardiovascular				
Palpitation	2.4% (0.0%)	0.4% (0.0%)	1.4% (0.3%)	2.5% (0.5%)
Digestive				
Nausea	1.5% (0.9%)	1.2% (0.0%)	1.7% (0.3%)	1.0% (0.7%)
Dyspepsia	1.2% (0.0%)	3.9% (0.0%)	0.7% (0.0%)	0.5% (0.0%)
Constipation	0.9% (0.0%)	1.2% (0.0%)	0.3% (0.0%)	1.5% (0.2%)
Nervous				
Headache	10.2% (0.9%)	10.6% (0.4%)	11.0% (1.7%)	14.7% (2.0%)
Dizziness	2.7% (0.3%)	2.7% (0.0%)	3.6% (0.5%)	3.7% (0.5%)
Paresthesia	1.5% (0.3%)	1.6% (0.0%)	1.2% (0.0%)	1.2% (0.2%)
Respiratory				
Upper respiratory infection	1.8% (0.0%)	3.9% (0.0%)	1.9% (0.0%)	0.7% (0.0%)
Cough	0.3% (0.0%)	0.8% (0.0%)	1.2% (0.0%)	1.7% (0.0%)
Rhinorrhea	0.0% (0.0%)	1.6% (0.0%)	0.2% (0.0%)	0.2% (0.0%)
Sneezing	0.0% (0.0%)	1.6% (0.0%)	0.0% (0.0%)	0.0% (0.0%)
Skin				
Rash	0.9% (0.0%)	2.0% (0.0%)	0.2% (0.0%)	0.2% (0.0%)
Flushing	0.9% (0.3%)	3.9% (0.0%)	5.3% (0.7%)	6.9% (1.2%)

* Patients in titration studies may have been exposed to more than 1 dose level of felodipine.

Adverse events that occurred in 0.5 up to 1.5% of patients who received felodipine in all controlled clinical trials at the recommended dosage range of 2.5 to 10 mg once a day, and serious adverse events that occurred at a lower rate, or events reported during marketing experience (those lower rate events are in italics) are listed below. These events are listed in order of decreasing severity within each category, and the relationship of these events to administration of felodipine is uncertain:

Body as a Whole: Chest pain, facial edema, flu-like illness.

Cardiovascular: *Myocardial infarction, hypotension, syncope, angina pectoris, arrhythmia,* tachycardia, premature beats.

Digestive: Abdominal pain, diarrhea, vomiting, dry mouth, flatulence, acid regurgitation.

Endocrine: Gynecomastia.

Hematologic: *Anemia.*

Metabolic: ALT (SGPT) increased.

Musculoskeletal: Arthralgia, back pain, leg pain, foot pain, muscle cramps, myalgia, arm pain, knee pain, hip pain.

Nervous/Psychiatric: Insomnia, depression, anxiety disorders, irritability, nervousness, somnolence, decreased libido.

Respiratory: Dyspnea, pharyngitis, bronchitis, influenza, sinusitis, epistaxis, respiratory infection.

Skin: *Angioedema,* contusion, erythema, urticaria, *leukocytoclastic vasculitis.*

Special Senses: Visual disturbances.

Urogenital: Impotence, urinary frequency, urinary urgency, dysuria, polyuria.

Gingival Hyperplasia: Gingival hyperplasia, usually mild, occurred in <0.5% of patients in controlled studies. This condition may be avoided or may regress with improved dental hygiene. (See PRECAUTIONS, Information for the Patient.)

CLINICAL LABORATORY TEST FINDINGS

Serum Electrolytes: No significant effects on serum electrolytes were observed during short- and long-term therapy (see CLINICAL PHARMACOLOGY, Renal/Endocrine Effects).

Serum Glucose: No significant effects on fasting serum glucose were observed in patients treated with felodipine in the US controlled study.

Liver Enzymes: 1 of 2 episodes of elevated serum transaminases decreased once drug was discontinued in clinical studies; no follow-up was available for the other patient.

DOSAGE AND ADMINISTRATION

The recommended starting dose is 5 mg once a day. Depending on the patient's response, the dosage can be decreased to 2.5 mg or increased to 10 mg once a day. These adjustments should occur generally at intervals of not less than 2 weeks. The recommended dosage range is 2.5-10 mg once daily. In clinical trials, doses above 10 mg daily showed an increased blood pressure response but a large increase in the rate of peripheral edema and other vasodilatory adverse events (see ADVERSE REACTIONS). Modification of the recommended dosage is usually not required in patients with renal impairment.

Felodipine should regularly be taken either without food or with a light meal (see CLINICAL PHARMACOLOGY, Pharmacokinetics and Metabolism). Felodipine should be swallowed whole and not crushed or chewed.

GERIATRIC USE

Patients over 65 years of age are likely to develop higher plasma concentrations of felodipine (see CLINICAL PHARMACOLOGY). In general, dose selection for an elderly patient should be cautious, usually starting at the low end of the dosing range (2.5 mg daily). Elderly patients should have their blood pressure closely monitored during any dosage adjustment.

PATIENTS WITH IMPAIRED LIVER FUNCTION

Patients with impaired liver function may have elevated plasma concentrations of felodipine and may respond to lower doses of felodipine; therefore, patients should have their blood pressure monitored closely during dosage adjustment of felodipine (see CLINICAL PHARMACOLOGY).

HOW SUPPLIED

Plendil tablets are available as follows:

2.5 mg: Sage green, round convex tablets, with code "450" on one side and "PLENDIL" on the other.

5 mg: Light red-brown, round convex tablets, with code "451" on one side and "PLENDIL" on the other.

10 mg: Red-brown, round convex tablets, with code "452" on one side and "PLENDIL" on the other.

Storage: Store below 30°C (86°F). Keep container tightly closed. Protect from light.

PRODUCT LISTING - EQUIVALENTS NOT AVAILABLE

Tablet, Extended Release - Oral - 2.5 mg

30's	$36.55	PLENDIL, Astra-Zeneca Pharmaceuticals	00186-0450-31
100's	$121.85	PLENDIL, Astra-Zeneca Pharmaceuticals	00186-0450-58
100's	$127.94	PLENDIL, Astra-Zeneca Pharmaceuticals	00186-0450-28

Tablet, Extended Release - Oral - 5 mg

7's	$7.22	PLENDIL, Allscripts Pharmaceutical Company	54569-3718-03
30's	$30.96	PLENDIL, Allscripts Pharmaceutical Company	54569-3718-00
30's	$35.22	PLENDIL, Physicians Total Care	54868-2167-02
30's	$36.55	PLENDIL, Astra-Zeneca Pharmaceuticals	00186-0451-31
100's	$121.85	PLENDIL, Astra-Zeneca Pharmaceuticals	00186-0451-58
100's	$127.94	PLENDIL, Astra-Zeneca Pharmaceuticals	00186-0451-28

Tablet, Extended Release - Oral - 10 mg

30's	$55.63	PLENDIL, Allscripts Pharmaceutical Company	54569-3719-00
100's	$229.90	PLENDIL, Astra-Zeneca Pharmaceuticals	00186-0452-28

Fenofibrate *(003194)*

For related information, see the comparative table section in Appendix A.

Categories: Hypercholesterolemia; Hyperlipidemia; Hypertriglyceridemia; FDA Approved 1993 Dec; Pregnancy Category C
Drug Classes: Antihyperlipidemics; Fibric acid derivatives
Brand Names: **Lipidil**; Tricor
Foreign Brand Availability: Apo-Feno-Micro (Hong-Kong); Climage (Greece); Controlip (Mexico); Durafenat (Germany); Durafenat Micro (Germany); Evothyl (Indonesia); Fenofanton (Germany); Fenogal Lidose (Singapore); Hyperchol (Indonesia); Lexemin (Singapore; Thailand); Lipanthyl (Belgium; Bulgaria; China; Cyprus; Czech-Republic; France; Germany; Greece; Hong-Kong; Hungary; Indonesia; Italy; Kuwait; Malaysia; Philippines; Russia; Switzerland; Taiwan; Thailand); Lipantil (England; Portugal); Liparison (Spain); Lipidax (Italy); Lipilo (China); Lipofen (Portugal); Lipolin (Taiwan); Lipovas (Spain); Lipsin (Austria; South-Africa); Livesan Ge (France); Normalip (Germany); Normolip (Colombia); Secalip (France); Trichol (Indonesia); Trolip (Hong-Kong); Zerlubron (Greece); Zumafib (Indonesia)
Cost of Therapy: $29.58 (Hypertriglyceridemia; Tricor; 54 mg; 1 tablet/day; 30 day supply)
$88.74 (Hypercholesterolemia; Tricor; 160 mg; 1 tablet/day; 30 day supply)

DESCRIPTION

Tricor (fenofibrate tablets), is a lipid regulating agent available as tablets or capsules for oral administration. Each tablet contains 54 or 160 mg of fenofibrate. Each capsule contains 67, 134 or 200 mg of micronized fenofibrate. The chemical name for fenofibrate is 2-[4-(4-chlorobenzoyl)phenoxy]-2-methyl-propanoic acid,1-methylethyl ester.

The empirical formula is $C_{20}H_{21}O_4Cl$ and the molecular weight is 360.83; fenofibrate is insoluble in water. The melting point is 79-82°C. Fenofibrate is a white solid which is stable under ordinary conditions.

Inactive Ingredients: Each tablet contains colloidal silicon dioxide, crospovidone, lactose monohydrate, lecithin, microcrystalline cellulose, polyvinyl alcohol, povidone, sodium lauryl sulfate, sodium stearyl fumarate, talc, titanium dioxide, and xanthan gum. In addition, individual tablets contain: *54 mg tablets:* D&C yellow no. 10, FD&C yellow no. 6, FD&C blue no. 2. Each capsule also contains crospovidone, iron oxide, lactose, magnesium stearate, pregelatinized starch, sodium lauryl sulfate, and titanium dioxide.

CLINICAL PHARMACOLOGY

A variety of clinical studies have demonstrated that elevated levels of total cholesterol (total-C), low density lipoprotein cholesterol (LDL-C), and apolipoprotein B (apo B), and LDL membrane complex, are associated with human artherosclerosis. Similarly, decreased levels of high density lipoprotein cholesterol (HDL-C), and its transport complex apolipoprotein A (apo AI and apo AII) are associated with the development of artherosclerosis. Epidemiologic investigations have established that cardiovascular morbidity and mortality vary directly with the level of total-C, LDL-C, and triglycerides, and inversely with the level of HDL-C. The independent effect of raising HDL-C or lowering triglycerides (TG) on the risk of cardiovascular morbidity and mortality has not been determined.

Fenofibric acid, the active metabolite of fenofibrate, produces reductions in total cholesterol, LDL cholesterol, apoprotein B, total triglycerides and triglyceride rich lipoprotein

F

(VLDL) in treated patients. In addition, treatment with fenofibrate results in increases in high density lipoprotein (HDL), and apolipoproteins apo AI and apo AII.

The effects of fenofibric acid as seen in clinical practice have been explained *in vivo* in transgenic mice and *in vitro* in human hepaStocyte cultures by the activation of peroxisome proliferator activated receptor α (PPARα). Through this mechanism, fenofibrate increases lipolysis and elimination of triglyceride-rich particles from plasma by activating lipoprotein lipase and reducing production of apoprotein C-III (an inhibitor of lipoprotein lipase activity). The resulting fall in triglycerides produces an alteration in the size and composition of LDL from small, dense particles (which are thought to be atherogenic due to their susceptibility to oxidation), to large buoyant particles. These larger particles have a greater affinity for cholesterol receptors and are catabolized rapidly. Activation of PPARα also induces an increase in the systhesis of apoproteins A-I, A-II, and HDL-cholesterol.

Fenofibrate also reduces serum uric acid levels in hyperuricemic and normal individuals by increasing the urinary excretions of uric acid.

PHARMACOKINETICS AND METABOLISM

Plasma concentrations of fenofibric acid after administration of 54 and 160 mg tablets are equivalent under fed conditions to 67 and 200 mg capsules, respectively.

Clinical experience has been obtained with 2 different formulations of fenofibrate: a "micronized" and "non-micronized" formulation, which have been demonstrated to be bioequivalent. Comparisons of blood levels following oral administration of both formulations in healthy volunteers demonstrate that a single capsule containing 67 mg of the "micronized" formulation is bioequivalent to 100 mg of the "non-micronized" formulation. Three capsules containing 67 mg fenofibrate are bioequivalent to a single 200 mg fenofibrate capsule.

Absorption

The absolute bioavailability of fenofibrate cannot be determined as the compound is virtually insoluble in aqueous media suitable for injection. However, fenofibrate is well absorbed from the gastrointestinal tract. Following oral administration in healthy volunteers, approximately 60% of a single dose of radiolabelled fenofibrate appeared in urine, primarily as fenofibric acid and its glucuronate conjugate, and 25% was excreted in the feces. Peak plasma levels of fenofibric acid occur within 6-8 hours after administration.

The absorption of fenofibrate is increased when administered with food. With fenofibrate tablets and capsules, the extent of absorption is increased by approximately 35% under fed as compared to fasting conditions.

Distribution

In healthy volunteers, steady-state plasma levels of fenofibric acid were shown to be achieved within 5 days of dosing and did not demonstrate accumulation across time following multiple dose administration. Serum protein binding was approximately 99% in normal and hyperlipidemic subjects.

Metabolism

Following oral administration, fenofibrate is rapidly hydrolyzed by esterases to the active metabolite, fenofibric acid; no unchanged fenofibrate is detected in plasma.

Fenofibric acid is primarily conjugated with glucuronic acid and then excreted in urine. A small amount of fenofibric acid is reduced at the carbonyl moiety to a benzhydrol metabolite which is, in turn, conjugated with glucuronic acid and excreted in urine.

In vivo metabolism data indicate that neither fenofibrate nor fenofibric acid undergo oxidative metabolism (*e.g.,* cytochrome P450) to a significant event.

Excretion

After absorption, fenofibrate is mainly excreted in the urine in the form of metabolites, primarily fenofibric acid and fenofibric acid glucuronide. After administration of radiolabelled fenofibrate, approximately 60% of the dose appeared in the urine and 25% was excreted in the feces.

Fenofibric acid is eliminated with a half-life of 20 hours, allowing once daily administration in a clinical setting.

Special Populations

Geriatrics

In elderly volunteers 77-87 years of age, the oral clearance of fenofibric acid following a single oral dose of fenofibrate was 1.2 L/h, which compares to 1.1 L/h in young adults. This indicates that a similar dosage regimen can be used in the elderly, without increasing accumulation of the drug or metabolites.

Pediatrics

Fenofibrate has not been investigated in adequate and well-controlled trials in pediatric patients.

Gender

No pharmacokinetic difference between males and females has been observed for fenofibrate.

Race

The influence of race on the pharmacokinetics of fenofibrate has not been studied, however fenofibrate is not metabolized by enzymes known for exhibiting inter-ethnic variability. Therefore, inter-ethnic pharmacokinetic differences are very unlikely.

Renal Insufficiency

In a study in patients with severe renal impairment (creatinine clearance <50 ml/min), the rate of clearance of fenofibric acid was greatly reduced, and the compound accumulated during chronic dosage. However, in patients having moderate renal impairment (creatinine clearance of 50-90 ml/min), the oral clearance and the oral volume of distribution of fenofibric acid are increased compared to healthy adults (2.1 L/h and 95 L versus 1.1 L/h and 30 L, respectively). Therefore, the dosage of fenofibrate should be minimized in patients who have severe renal impairment, while no modification of dosage is required in patients having moderate renal impairment.

Hepatic Insufficiency

No pharmacokinetic studies have been conducted in patients having hepatic insufficiency.

Drug-Drug Interactions

In vitro studies using human liver microsomes indicate that fenofibrate and fenofibric acid are not inhibitors of cytochrome (CYP) P450 isoforms CYP3A4, CYP2D6, CYP2E1, or CYP1A2. They are weak inhibitors of CYP2C19 and CYP2A6, and mild-to-moderate inhibitors of CYP2C9 at therapeutic concentrations.

Potentiation of coumarin-type anticoagulants has been observed with prolongation of the prothrombin time/INR.

Bile acid sequestrants have been shown to bind other drugs given concurrently. Therefore, fenofibrate should be taken at least 1 hour before or 4-6 hours after a bile acid binding resin to avoid impeding its absorption (see WARNINGS and PRECAUTIONS).

INDICATIONS AND USAGE

TREATMENT OF HYPERCHOLESTEROLEMIA

Fenofibrate is indicated as adjunctive therapy to diet to reduce elevated LDL-C, Total-C, Triglycerides and Apo B, and to increase HDL-C in adult patients with primary hypercholesterolemia or mixed dyslipidemia (Fredricksons Types IIa and IIb). Lipid-altering agents should be used in addition to a diet restricted in saturated fat and cholesterol when response to diet and non-pharmacological interventions alone has been inadequate (see TABLE 4).

TREATMENT OF HYPERTRIGLYCERIDEMIA

Fenofibrate is also indicated as adjunctive therapy to diet for treatment of adult patients with hypertriglyceridemia (Fredrickson Types IV and V hyperlipidemia). Improving glycemic control in diabetic patients showing fasting chylomicronemia will usually reduce fasting triglycerides and eliminate chylomicronemia thereby obviating the need for pharmacologic intervention.

Markedly elevated levels of serum triglycerides (*e.g.,* >2000 mg/dl) may increase the risk of developing pancreatitis. The effect of fenofibrate therapy on reducing this risk has not been adequately studied.

Drug therapy is not indicated for patients with Type I hyperlipoproteinemia, who have elevations of chylomicrons and plasma triglycerides, but who have normal levels of very low density lipoprotein (VLDL). Inspection of plasma refrigerated for 14 hours is helpful in distinguishing Types I, IV and V hyperlipoproteinemia.[2]

The initial treatment for dyslipidemia is dietary therapy specific for the type of lipoprotein abnormality. Excess body weight and excess alcoholic intake may be important factors in hypertriglyceridemia and should be addressed prior to any drug therapy. Physical exercise can be an important ancillary measure. Diseases contributory to hyperlipidemia, such as hypothyroidism or diabetes mellitus should be looked for and adequately treated. Estrogen therapy, like thiazide diuretics and beta-blockers, is sometimes associated with massive rises in plasma triglycerides, especially in subjects with familial hypertriglyceridemia. In such cases, discontinuation of the specific etiologic agent may obviate the need for specific drug therapy of hypertriglyceridemia.

The use of drugs should be considered only when reasonable attempts have been made to obtain satisfactory results with non-drug methods. If the decision is made to use drugs, the patient should be instructed that this does not reduce the importance of adhering to diet. (See WARNINGS and PRECAUTIONS.)

TABLE 3 *Fredrickson Classification of Hyperlipoproteinemias*

Type	Lipoprotein Elevated	Lipid Elevation Major	Minor
I (rare)	chylomicrons	TG	C*
IIa	LDL	C	
IIb	LDL, VLDL	C	TG
III (rare)	IDL	C, TG	
IV	VLDL	TG	C*
V (rare)	chylomicrons, VLDL	TG	C*

* Increases or no change.

After the LDL-C goal has been achieved, if the TG is still >200 mg/dl, non HDL-C (total-C minus HDL-C) becomes a secondary target of therapy. Non-HDL-C goals are set 30 mg/dl higher than LDL-C goals for each risk category.

NON-FDA APPROVED INDICATIONS

Although not FDA approved, fenofibrate has been used as adjunct treatment of Fredrickson Type III hyperlipoproteinemia and for diabetic hyperlipoproteinemia.

CONTRAINDICATIONS

Fenofibrate is contraindicated in patients who exhibit hypersensitivity to fenofibrate.

Fenofibrate is contraindicated in patients with hepatic or severe renal dysfunction, including primary biliary cirrhosis, and patients with unexplained persistent liver function abnormality.

Fenofibrate is contraindicated in patients with preexisting gallbladder disease (see WARNINGS).

WARNINGS

LIVER FUNCTION

Fenofibrate use at doses equivalent to 107-160 mg fenofibrate per day has been associated with increases in serum transaminases [AST (SGOT) or ALT (SGPT)]. In a pooled analysis of 10 placebo-controlled trials, increases to >3 times the upper limit of normal occurred in 5.3% of patients taking fenofibrate versus 1.1% of patients taking placebo.

TABLE 4 *NCEP Treatment Guidelines: LDL-C Goals and Cutpoints for Therapeutic Lifestyle Changes and Drug Therapy in Different Risk Categories*

Risk Category	LDL Goal (mg/dl)	LDL Level at Which to Initiate Therapeutic Lifestyle Changes (mg/dl)	LDL Level at Which to Consider Drug Therapy (mg/dl)
CHD or CHD risk equivalents (10 year risk >20%)	<100	≥100	≥130 (100-129: drug optional)*
2+ Risk factors (10 year risk ≤20%)	<130	≥130	10 year risk 10-20%: ≥130 10 year risk <10%: ≥160
0-1 Risk factors†	<160	≥160	≥190 (160-189: LDL-lowering drug optional)

* Some authorities recommend use of LDL-lowering drugs in the category if an LDL-C level of <100 mg/dl cannot be acheived by therapeutic lifestyle changes. Others prefer use of drugs that primarily modify triglycerides and HDL-C, *e.g.*, nicotinic acid or fibrate. Clinical judgement also may call for deferring drug therapy in this subcategory.
† Almost all people with 0-1 risk factor have 10 year risk <10%; thus, 10 year risk assessment in people with 0-1 risk factor is not necessary.
CHD Coronary heart disease.

When transaminase determinations were followed either after discontinuation of treatment or during continued treatment, a return to normal limits was usually observed. The incidence of increases in transaminases related to fenofibrate therapy appear to be dose related. In an 8 week dose-ranging study, the incidence of ALT or AST elevations to at least 3 times the upper limit of normal was 13% in patients receiving dosages equivalent to 107-160 mg fenofibrate per day and was 0% in those receiving dosages equivalent to 54 mg or less fenofibrate per day, or placebo. Hepatocellular, chronic active and cholestatic hepatitis associated with fenofibrate therapy have been reported after exposures of weeks to several years. In extremely rare cases, cirrhosis has been reported in association with chronic hepatitis.

Regular periodic monitoring of liver function, including serum ALT (SGPT) should be performed for the duration of therapy with fenofibrate, and therapy discontinued if enzyme levels persist above 3 times the normal limit.

CHOLELITHIASIS

Fenofibrate, like clofibrate and gemfibrozil, may increase cholesterol excretion into the bile, leading to cholelithiasis. If cholelithiasis is suspected, gallbladder studies are indicated. Fenofibrate therapy should be discontinued if gallstones are found.

CONCOMITANT ORAL ANTICOAGULANTS

Caution should be exercised when anticoagulants are given in conjunction with fenofibrate because of the potentiation of coumarin-type anticoagulants in prolonging the prothrombin time/INR. The dosage of the anticoagulant should be reduced to maintain the prothrombin time/INR at the desired level to prevent bleeding complications. Frequent prothrombin time/INR determinations are advisable until it has been definitely determined that the prothrombin time/INR level has stabilized.

CONCOMITANT HMG-COA REDUCTASE INHIBITORS

The combined use of fenofibrate and HMG-CoA reductase inhibitors should be avoided unless the benefit of further alterations in lipid levels is likely to outweigh the increased risk of this drug combination.

In a single-dose drug interaction study in 23 healthy adults the concomitant administration of fenofibrate and pravastatin resulted in no clinically important difference in the pharmacokinetics of fenofibric acid, pravastatin or its active metabolite 3α-hydroxy iso-pravastatin when compared to either drug given alone.

The combined use of fibric acid derivatives and HMG-CoA reductase inhibitors has been associated, in the absence of a marked pharmacokinetic interaction, in numerous case reports, with rhabdomyolysis, markedly elevated creatine kinase (CK) levels and myoglobinuria, leading in a high proportion of cases to acute renal failure.

The use of fibrates alone, including fenofibrate, may occasionally be associated with myositis, myopathy, or rhabdomyolysis. Patients receiving fenofibrate and complaining of muscle pain, tenderness, or weakness should have prompt medical evaluation for myopathy, including serum creatine kinase level determination. If myopathy/myositis is suspected or diagnosed, fenofibrate therapy should be stopped.

MORTALITY

The effect of fenofibrate on coronary heart disease morbidity and mortality and non-cardiovascular mortality has not been established.

OTHER CONSIDERATIONS

In the Coronary Drug Project, a large study of post myocardial infarction of patients treated for 5 years with clofibrate, there was no difference in mortality seen between the clofibrate group and the placebo group. There was however, a difference in the rate of cholelithiasis and cholecystitis requiring surgery between the two groups (3.0% vs 1.8%).

Because of chemical, pharmacological, and clinical similarities between fenofibrate tablets, clofibrate, and gemfibrozil, the adverse findings in 4 large randomized, placebo-controlled clinical studies with these other fibrate drugs may also apply to fenofibrate.

In a study, conducted by the World Health Organization (WHO), 5000 subjects without known coronary heart disease were treated with placebo or clofibrate for 5 years and followed for an additional 1 year. There was a statistically significant, higher age-adjusted all-cause mortality in the clofibrate group compared with the placebo group (5.70% vs 3.96%, p ≤0.01). Excess mortality was due to a 33% increase in non-cardiovascular causes, including malignancy, post-cholecystectomy complications, and pancreatitis. This appeared to confirm the higher risk of gallbladder disease seen in clofibrate-treated patients studied in the Coronary Drug Project.

The Helsinki Heart Study was a large (n=4081) study of middle-aged men without a history of coronary artery disease. Subjects received either gemfibrozil or placebo for 5 years, with a 3.5 year open extension afterward. Total mortality was numerically higher in the gemfibrozil randomization group but did not achieve statistical significance (p=0.19, 95% confidence interval for relative risk G:P=0.91-1.64). Although cancer deaths trended higher in the gemfibrozil group (p=0.11), cancers (excluding basal cell carcinoma) were diagnosed with equal frequency in both study groups. Due to the limited size of the study, the relative risk of death from any cause was not shown to be different than that seen in the 9 year follow-up data from World Health Organization study (RR=1.29). Similarly, the numerical excess of gallbladder surgeries in the gemfibrozil group did not differ statistically from that observed in the WHO study.

The secondary prevention component of the Helsinki Heart Study enrolled middle-aged men excluded from the primary prevention study because of known or suspected coronary heart disease. Subjects received gemfibrozil or placebo for 5 years. Although cardiac deaths trended higher in the gemfibrozil group, this was not statistically significant (hazard ratio 2.2, 95% confidence interval: 0.94-5.05). The rate of gallbladder surgery was not statistically significant between the study groups, but did trend higher in the gemfibrozil group (1.9% vs 0.3%, p=0.07). There was a statistically significant difference in the number of appendectomies in the gemfibrozil group (6/311 vs 0/317, p=0.029).

F

PRECAUTIONS

INITIAL THERAPY

Laboratory studies should be done to ascertain that the lipid levels are consistently abnormal before instituting fenofibrate therapy. Every attempt should be made to control serum lipids with appropriate diet, exercise, weight loss in obese patients, and control of any medical problems such as diabetes mellitus and hypothyroidism that are contributing to the lipid abnormalities. Medications known to exacerbate hypertriglyceridemia (beta-blockers, thiazides, estrogens) should be discontinued or changed if possible prior to consideration of triglyceride-lowering drug therapy.

CONTINUED THERAPY

Periodic determination of serum lipids should be obtained during initial therapy in order to establish the lowest effective dose of fenofibrate. Therapy should be withdrawn in patients who do not have an adequate response after 2 months of treatment with the maximum recommended dose.

PANCREATITIS

Pancreatitis has been reported in patients taking fenofibrate, gemfibrozil, and clofibrate. This occurrence may represent a failure of efficacy in patients with hypertriglyceridemia, a direct drug effect, or a secondary phenomenon mediated through biliary tract stone or sludge formation and obstruction of the common bile duct.

HYPERSENSITIVITY REACTIONS

Acute hypersensitivity reactions including severe skin rashes requiring patient hospitalization and treatment with steroids have occurred very rarely during treatment with fenofibrate, including rare spontaneous reports of Stevens-Johnson syndrome, and toxic epidermal necrolysis. Urticaria was seen in 1.1 vs 0%, and rash in 1.4 vs 0.8% of fenofibrate and placebo patients respectively in controlled trials.

HEMATOLOGIC CHANGES

Mild to moderate hemoglobin, hematocrit, and white blood cell decreases have been observed in patients following initiation of fenofibrate therapy. However, these levels stabilize during long-term administration. Extremely rare spontaneous reports of thrombocytopenia and agranulocytosis have been received during post-marketing surveillance outside of the US. Periodic blood counts are recommended during the first 12 months of fenofibrate administration.

SKELETAL MUSCLE

The use of fibrates alone, including fenofibrate, may occasionally be associated with myopathy. Treatment with drugs of the fibrate class has been associated on rare occasions with rhabdomyolysis, usually in patients with impaired renal function. Myopathy should be considered in any patient with diffuse myalgias, muscle tenderness or weakness, and/or marked elevations of creatinine phosphokinase levels.

Patients should be advised to report promptly unexplained muscle pain, tenderness or weakness, particularly if accompanied by malaise or fever. CPK levels should be assessed in patients reporting these symptoms, and fenofibrate therapy should be discontinued if markedly elevated CPK levels occur or myopathy is diagnosed.

CARCINOGENESIS, MUTAGENESIS, AND IMPAIRMENT OF FERTILITY

In a 24 month study in rats (10, 45, and 200 mg/kg; 0.3, 1, and 6 times the maximum recommended human dose on the basis of mg/m^2 of surface area), the incidence of liver carcinoma was significantly increased at 6 times the maximum recommended human dose in males and females. A statistically significant increase in pancreatic carcinomas occurred in males at 1 and 6 times the maximum recommended human dose; there were also increases in pancreatic adenomas and benign testicular interstitial cell tumors at 6 times the maximum recommended human dose in males. In a second 24 month study in a different strain of rats (doses of 10 and 60 mg/kg; 0.3 and 2 times the maximum recommended human dose based on mg/m^2 surface area), there were significant increases in the incidence of pancreatic acinar adenomas in both sexes and increases in interstitial cell tumors of the testes at 2 times the maximum recommended human dose.

A comparative carcinogenicity study was done in rats comparing 3 drugs: fenofibrate (10 and 70 mg/kg; 0.3 and 1.6 times the maximum recommended human dose), clofibrate (400 mg/kg; 1.6 times the human dose), and gemfibrozil (250 mg/kg; 1.7 times the human dose) (multiples based on mg/m^2 surface area). Pancreatic acinar adenomas were increased in males and females on fenofibrate; hepatocellular carcinoma and pancreatic acinar adenomas were increased in males and hepatic neoplastic nodules in females treated with clofibrate; hepatic neoplastic nodules were increased in males and females treated with gemfibrozil while testicular interstitial cell tumors were increased in males on all 3 drugs.

In a 21 month study in mice at doses of 10, 45, and 200 mg/kg (approximately 0.2, 0.7 and 3 times the maximum recommended human dose on the basis of mg/m 2 surface area), there were statistically significant increases in liver carcinoma at 3 times the maximum recommended human dose in both males and females. In a second 18 month study at the same doses, there was a significant increase in liver carcinoma in male mice and liver adenoma in female mice at 3 times the maximum recommended human dose.

Electron microscopy studies have demonstrated peroxisomal proliferation following fenofibrate administration to the rat. An adequate study to test for peroxisome proliferation in humans has not been done, but changes in peroxisome morphology and numbers have been observed in humans after treatment with other members of the fibrate class when liver biopsies were compared before and after treatment in the same individual.

Fenofibrate has been demonstrated to be devoid of mutagenic potential in the following tests: Ames, mouse lymphoma, chromosomal aberration and unscheduled DNA synthesis.

F

PREGNANCY CATEGORY C

Fenofibrate has been shown to be embryocidal and teratogenic in rats when given in doses 7-10 times the maximum recommended human dose and embryocidal in rabbits when given at 9 times the maximum recommended human dose (on the basis of mg/m^2 surface area). There are no adequate and well-controlled studies in pregnant women. Fenofibrate should be used during pregnancy only if the potential benefit justifies the potential risk to the fetus.

Administration of 9 times the maximum recommended human dose of fenofibrate to female rats before and throughout gestation caused 100% of dams to delay delivery and resulted in a 60% increase in post-implantation loss, a decrease in litter size, a decrease in birth weight, a 40% survival of pups at birth, a 4% survival of pups as neonates, and a 0% survival of pups to weaning, and an increase in spina bifida.

Administration of 10 times the maximum recommended human dose to female rats on days 6-15 of gestation caused an increase in gross, visceral and skeletal findings in fetuses (domed head/hunched shoulders/rounded body/abnormal chest, kyphosis, stunted fetuses, elongated sternal ribs, malformed sternebrae, extra foramen in palatine, misshapen vertebrae, supernumerary ribs).

Administration of 7 times the maximum recommended human dose to female rats from day 15 of gestation through weaning caused a delay in delivery, a 40% decrease in live births, a 75% decrease in neonatal survival, and decreases in pup weight, at birth as well as on days 4 and 21 post-partum.

Administration of 9 and 18 times the maximum recommended human dose to female rabbits caused abortions in 10% of dams at 9 times and 25% of dams at 18 times the maximum recommended human dose and death of 7% of fetuses at 18 times the maximum recommended human dose.

NURSING MOTHERS

Fenofibrate should not be used in nursing mothers. Because of the potential for tumorigenicity seen in animal studies, a decision should be made whether to discontinue nursing or to discontinue the drug.

PEDIATRIC USE

Safety and efficacy in pediatric patients have not been established.

GERIATRIC USE

Fenofibric acid is known to be substantially excreted by the kidney, and the risk of adverse reactions to this drug may be greater in patients with impaired renal function. Because elderly patients are more likely to have decreased renal function, care should be taken in dose selection.

DRUG INTERACTIONS

ORAL ANTICOAGULANTS

CAUTION SHOULD BE EXERCISED WHEN COUMARIN ANTICOAGULANTS ARE GIVEN IN CONJUNCTION WITH FENOFIBRATE. THE DOSAGE OF THE ANTICOAGULANTS SHOULD BE REDUCED TO MAINTAIN THE PROTHROMBIN TIME/INR AT THE DESIRED LEVEL TO PREVENT BLEEDING COMPLICATIONS. FREQUENT PROTHROMBIN TIME/INR DETERMINATIONS ARE ADVISABLE UNTIL IT HAS BEEN DEFINITELY DETERMINED THAT THE PROTHROMBIN TIME/INR HAS STABILIZED.

HMG-COA REDUCTASE INHIBITORS

The combined use of fenofibrate and HMG-CoA reductase inhibitors should be avoided unless the benefit of further alterations in lipid levels is likely to outweigh the increased risk of this drug combination (see WARNINGS).

RESINS

Since bile acid sequestrants may bind other drugs given concurrently, patients should take fenofibrate at least 1 hour before or 4-6 hours after a bile acid binding resin to avoid impeding its absorption.

CYCLOSPORINE

Because cyclosporine can produce nephrotoxicity with decreases in creatinine clearance and rises in serum creatinine, and because renal excretion is the primary elimination route of fibrate drugs including fenofibrate, there is a risk that an interaction will lead to deterioration. The benefits and risks of using fenofibrate with immunosuppressants and other potentially nephrotoxic agents should be carefully considered, and the lowest effective dose employed.

ADVERSE REACTIONS

CLINICAL

Adverse events reported by 2% or more of patients treated with fenofibrate during the double-blind, placebo-controlled trials, regardless of causality, are listed in TABLE 5. Adverse events led to discontinuation of treatment in 5.0% of patients treated with fenofibrate and in 3.0% treated with placebo. Increases in liver function tests were the most frequent events, causing discontinuation of fenofibrate treatment in 1.6% of patients in double-blind trials.

TABLE 5

Body System Adverse Event	Fenofibrate* (n=439)	Placebo (n=365)
Body as a Whole		
Abdominal pain	4.6%	4.4%
Back pain	3.4%	2.5%
Headache	3.2%	2.7%
Asthenia	2.1%	3.0%
Flu syndrome	2.1%	2.7%
Digestive		
Liver function tests abnormal	7.5%†	1.4%
Diarrhea	2.3%	4.1%
Nausea	2.3%	1.9%
Constipation	2.1%	1.4%
Metabolic and Nutritional Disorders		
SGPT increased	3.0%	1.6%
Creatine phosphokinase increased	3.0%	1.4%
SGOT increased	3.4%†	0.5%
Respiratory		
Respiratory disorder	6.2%	5.5%
Rhinitis	2.3%	1.1%

* Dosage equivalent to 200 mg fenofibrate.
† Significantly different from placebo.

Additional adverse events reported by 3 or more patients in placebo-controlled trials or reported in other controlled or open trials, regardless of causality are listed below.

Body as a Whole: Chest pain, pain (unspecified), infection, malaise, allergic reaction, cyst, hernia, fever, photosensitivity reaction, accidental injury.

Cardiovascular System: Angina pectoris, hypertension, vasodilatation, coronary artery disorder, electrocardiogram abnormal, ventricular extrasystoles, myocardial infarct, peripheral vascular disorder, migraine, varicose vein, cardiovascular disorder, hypotension, palpitation, vascular disorder, arrhythmia, phlebitis, tachycardia, extrasystoles, and atrial fibrillation.

Digestive System: Dyspepsia, flatulence, nausea, increased appetite, gastroenteritis, cholelithiasis, rectal disorder, esophagitis, gastritis, colitis, tooth disorder, vomiting, anorexia, gastrointestinal disorder, duodenal ulcer, nausea and vomiting, peptic ulcer, rectal hemorrhage, liver fatty deposit, cholecystitis, eructation, gamma glutamyl transpeptidase, and diarrhea.

Endocrine System: Diabetes mellitus.

Hemic and Lymphatic System: Anemia, leukopenia, ecchymosis, eosinophilia, lymphadenopathy, and thrombocytopenia.

Metabolic and Nutritional Disorders: Creatinine increased, weight gain, hypoglycemia, gout, weight loss, edema, hyperuricemia, and peripheral edema.

Musculoskeletal System: Myositis, myalgia, arthralgia, arthritis, tenosynovitis, joint disorder, arthrosis, leg cramps, bursitis, and myasthenia.

Nervous System: Dizziness, insomnia, depression, vertigo, libido decreased, anxiety, paresthesia, dry mouth, hypertonia, nervousness, neuralgia, and somnolence.

Respiratory System: Pharyngitis, bronchitis, cough increased, dyspnea, asthma, pneumonia, laryngitis, and sinusitis.

Skin and Appendages: Rash, pruritus, eczema, herpes zoster, urticaria, acne, sweating, fungal dermatitis, skin disorder, alopecia, contact dermatitis, herpes simplex, maculopapular rash, nail disorder, and skin ulcer.

Special Senses: Conjuctivitis, eye disorder, amblyopia, ear pain, otitis media, abnormal vision, cataract specified, and refraction disorder.

Urogenital System: Urinary frequency, prostatic disorder, dysuria, kidney function abnormal, urolithiasis, gynecomastia, unintended pregnancy, vaginal moniliasis, and cystitis.

DOSAGE AND ADMINISTRATION

Patients should be placed on an appropriate lipid-lowering diet before receiving fenofibrate, and should continue this diet during treatment with fenofibrate. Fenofibrate tablets should be given with meals, thereby optimizing the bioavailability of the medication.

For the treatment of adult patients with primary hypercholesterolemia or mixed hyperlipidemia, the initial dose of fenofibrate is 160 mg/day (tablets) or 200 mg/day (capsules).

For adult patients with hypertriglyceridemia, the initial dose is 54-160 mg/day (tablets) or 67-200 mg/day (capsules). Dosage should be individualized according to patient response, and should be adjusted if necessary following repeat lipid determinations at 4-8 week intervals. The maximum dose is 160 mg/day (tablets) or 200 mg/day (capsules).

Treatment with fenofibrate should be initiated at a dose of 54 mg/day (tablets) or 67 mg/day (capsules) in patients having impaired renal function, and increased only after evaluation of the effects on renal function and lipid levels at this dose. In the elderly, the initial dose should likewise be limited to 54 mg/day (tablets) or 67 mg/day (capsules).

Lipid levels should be monitored periodically and consideration should be given to reducing the dosage of fenofibrate if lipid levels fall significantly below the targeted range.

HOW SUPPLIED

Tricor (fenofibrate tablets) are available in 2 strengths:

54 mg: Yellow tablets imprinted with the Abbott corporate logo and the Abbo-Code identification letters "TA".

160 mg: White tablets imprinted with the Abbott corporate logo and the Abbo-Code identification letters "TC".

Tricor (fenofibrate capsules), micronized, are available as hard gelatin capsules in 3 strengths:

67 mg: Yellow capsules, imprinted with the Abbott corporate logo and the Abbo-Code identification letters "FR".

134 mg: White capsules, imprinted with the Abbott corporate logo and the Abbo-Code identification letters "AR".

200 mg: Orange capsules, imprinted with the Abbott corporate logo and the Abbo-Code identification letters "SR".

Storage: Store at controlled room temperature, 15-30°C (59-86°F). Keep out of the reach of children. Protect from moisture.

PRODUCT LISTING - RATED THERAPEUTICALLY EQUIVALENT

Capsule - Oral - 134 mg

100's	$155.07	GENERIC, Teva Pharmaceuticals Usa	00093-8011-01

Capsule - Oral - 200 mg

100's	$232.60	GENERIC, Teva Pharmaceuticals Usa	00093-8012-01

PRODUCT LISTING - EQUIVALENTS NOT AVAILABLE

Capsule - Oral - 67 mg

90's	$77.54	TRICOR, Abbott Pharmaceutical	00074-4342-90
100's	$81.65	GENERIC, Gate Pharmaceuticals	57844-0322-01

Capsule - Oral - 134 mg

100's	$157.28	GENERIC, Gate Pharmaceuticals	57844-0323-01

Capsule - Oral - 200 mg

90's	$232.60	TRICOR, Abbott Pharmaceutical	00074-6415-90
100's	$244.96	GENERIC, Gate Pharmaceuticals	57844-0324-01

Tablet - Oral - 54 mg

90's	$88.74	TRICOR, Abbott Pharmaceutical	00074-4009-90

Tablet - Oral - 160 mg

90's	$266.21	TRICOR, Abbott Pharmaceutical	00074-4013-90

Fenoldopam Mesylate *(003506)*

For complete prescribing information, refer to the CD-ROM included with the book.

Categories: Hypertension, severe; Hypertension, malignant; FDA Approved 1997 Sep; Pregnancy Category B
Drug Classes: Vasodilators
Brand Names: Corlopam

DESCRIPTION

Corlopam (fenoldopam mesylate) is a dopamine D_1-like receptor agonist. The product is formulated as a solution to be diluted for intravenous infusion. Chemically it is 6-chloro-2,3,4,5-tetrahydro-1-(4-hydroxyphenyl)-[1*H*]-3-benzazepine-7,8-diol methanesulfonate.

Fenoldopam mesylate is a white to off-white powder with a molecular weight of 401.87 and a molecular formula of $C_{16}H_{16}ClNO_3 \cdot CH_3SO_3H$. It is sparingly soluble in water, ethanol and methanol, and is soluble in propylene glycol.

AMPULES

Each 1 ml contains, in sterile aqueous solution, citric acid 3.44 mg; fenoldopam mesylate equivalent to fenoldopam 10 mg; propylene glycol 518 mg; sodium citrate dihydrate 0.61 mg; sodium metabisulfite 1 mg.

Storage: Store at 2-30°C.

INDICATIONS AND USAGE

Fenoldopam mesylate is indicated for the in-hospital, short-term (up to 48 hours) management of severe hypertension when rapid, but quickly reversible, emergency reduction of blood pressure is clinically indicated, including malignant hypertension with deteriorating end-organ function. Transition to oral therapy with another agent can begin at any time after blood pressure is stable during fenoldopam mesylate infusion.

NON-FDA APPROVED INDICATIONS

Unapproved and investigational uses of fenoldopam have included treatment of chronic renal failure, peri-surgical hypertension, and congestive heart failure. Low doses have been used as an adjunct to saline hydration for prevention of contrast media-induced renal failure during angiography and percutaneous coronary intervention.

CONTRAINDICATIONS

None known.

WARNINGS

Contains sodium metabisulfite, a sulfite that may cause allergic-type reactions including anaphylactic symptoms and life-threatening or less severe asthmatic episodes in certain susceptible people. The overall prevalence of sulfite sensitivity in the general population is unknown and probably low. Sulfite sensitivity is seen more frequently in asthmatic than in nonasthmatic people.

DOSAGE AND ADMINISTRATION

The optimal magnitude and rate of blood pressure reduction in acutely hypertensive patients have not been rigorously determined, but, in general, both delay and too rapid decreases appear undesirable in sick patients. An initial fenoldopam mesylate dose may be chosen that produces the desired magnitude and rate of blood pressure reduction in a given clinical situation. Doses below 0.1 μg/kg/min have very modest effects and appear only marginally useful in this population. In general, as the initial dose increases, there is a greater and more rapid blood pressure reduction. However, lower initial doses (0.03-0.1 μg/kg/min) titrated slowly have been associated with less reflex tachycardia than have higher initial doses (≥0.3 μg/kg/min). In clinical trials, doses from 0.01-1.6 μg/kg/min have been studied. Most of the effect of a given infusion rate is attained in 15 minutes.

Fenoldopam mesylate should be administered by continuous intravenous infusion. **A bolus dose should not be used.** Hypotension and rapid decreases of blood pressure should be avoided. The initial dose should be titrated upward or downward, no more frequently than every 15 minutes (and less frequently as goal pressure is approached) to achieve the desired therapeutic effect. The recommended increments for titration are 0.05-0.1 μg/kg/min.

Use of a calibrated, mechanical infusion pump is recommended for proper control of infusion rate during fenoldopam mesylate infusion. In clinical trials, fenoldopam mesylate treatment was safely performed **without** the need for intra-arterial blood pressure monitoring; blood pressure and heart rate were monitored at frequent intervals, typically every 15 minutes. Frequent blood pressure monitoring is recommended.

Use of beta-blockers in conjunction with fenoldopam mesylate has not been studied in hypertensive patients and, if possible, concomitant use should be avoided. If the drugs are used together, caution should be exercised because unexpected hypotension could result from beta-blocker inhibition of the reflex response to fenoldopam.

The fenoldopam mesylate infusion can be abruptly discontinued or gradually tapered prior to discontinuation. Oral antihypertensive agents can be added during fenoldopam mesylate infusion or following its discontinuation. Patients in controlled clinical trials have received intravenous fenoldopam mesylate for as long as 48 hours.

PREPARATION OF INFUSION SOLUTION

WARNING: CONTENTS OF AMPULES MUST BE DILUTED BEFORE INFUSION. EACH AMPULE IS FOR SINGLE USE ONLY.

Dilution

The fenoldopam mesylate injection ampule concentrate must be diluted in 0.9% sodium chloride injection or 5% dextrose injection using the dilution schedule in TABLE 5.

TABLE 5

Milliliter of Concentrate (mg of drug)	Added to	Final Concentration
4 ml (40 mg)	1000 ml	40 μg/ml
2 ml (20 mg)	500 ml	40 μg/ml
1 ml (10 mg)	250 ml	40 μg/ml

The drug dose rate must be individualized according to body weight and according to the desired rapidity and extent of pharmacodynamic effect. TABLE 6 provides the calculated infusion volume in ml/min for a range of drug doses and body weights. The infusion should be administered using a calibrated mechanical infusion pump that can accurately and reliably deliver the desired infusion rate.

TABLE 6 *Infusion Rates (ml/min) to Achieve a Given Drug Dose Rate (μg/kg/min)*

	Drug Dose Rate (μg/kg/min)				
Body	0.025	0.05	0.1	0.2	0.3
Weight	Infusion Rates (ml/min)				
40 kg	0.025	0.05	0.10	0.20	0.30
50 kg	0.031	0.06	0.13	0.25	0.38
60 kg	0.038	0.08	0.15	0.30	0.45
70 kg	0.044	0.09	0.18	0.35	0.53
80 kg	0.050	0.10	0.20	0.40	0.60
90 kg	0.056	0.11	0.23	0.45	0.68
100 kg	0.063	0.13	0.25	0.50	0.75
110 kg	0.069	0.14	0.28	0.55	0.83
120 kg	0.075	0.15	0.30	0.60	0.90
130 kg	0.081	0.16	0.33	0.65	0.98
140 kg	0.088	0.18	0.35	0.70	1.05
150 kg	0.094	0.19	0.38	0.75	1.13

The diluted solution is stable under normal ambient light and temperature conditions for at least 24 hours. Diluted solution that is not used within 24 hours of preparation should be discarded. Parenteral products should be inspected visually. If particulate matter or cloudiness is observed, the drug should be discarded.

PRODUCT LISTING - RATED THERAPEUTICALLY EQUIVALENT

Solution - Intravenous - 10 mg/ml

1 ml	$260.00	CORLOPAM, Abbott Pharmaceutical	00074-2304-01
2 ml	$500.50	CORLOPAM, Abbott Pharmaceutical	00074-2304-02

PRODUCT LISTING - EQUIVALENTS NOT AVAILABLE

Solution - Intravenous - 10 mg/ml

1 ml	$240.00	CORLOPAM, Neurex	62860-0004-01
2 ml	$462.00	CORLOPAM, Neurex	62860-0002-02
5 ml	$1155.00	CORLOPAM, Neurex	62860-0003-01

Fenoprofen Calcium *(001253)*

For related information, see the comparative table section in Appendix A.

Categories: Arthritis, osteoarthritis; Arthritis, rheumatoid; Pain, mild to moderate; FDA Approved 1976 Mar; Pregnancy Category B; Pregnancy Category D, 3rd Trimester
Drug Classes: Analgesics, non-narcotic; Nonsteroidal anti-inflammatory drugs
Brand Names: **Nalfon**
Foreign Brand Availability: Fenoprex (Argentina); Fenopron (England; Hong-Kong; Ireland; Japan; Korea; South-Africa); Fepron (Italy; Netherlands); Nalgesic (France); Progesic (England)
Cost of Therapy: $24.63 (Osteoarthritis; Generic Capsules; 300 mg; 3 capsules/day; 30 day supply)
$34.88 (Osteoarthritis; Nalfon; 300 mg; 3 capsules/day; 30 day supply)

DESCRIPTION

Fenoprofen calcium is a nonsteroidal, anti-inflammatory, antiarthritic drug.

Chemically, fenoprofen calcium is an arylacetic acid derivative. Fenoprofen calcium is a benzeneacetic acid, α-methyl-3-phenoxy-, calcium salt dihydrate, (±)-, and has the empirical formula $C_{30}H_{26}CaO_6 \cdot 2\ H_2O$ representing a molecular weight of 558.65.

Fenoprofen calcium is a white crystalline powder that at 25°C, dissolves to a 15 mg/ml solution in alcohol (95%). It is slightly soluble in water and insoluble in benzene.

The pKa of fenoprofen calcium is 4.5 at 25°C.

Nalfon Pulvules contain fenoprofen calcium as the dihydrate in an amount equivalent to 200 mg (0.826 mmol) or 300 mg (1.24 mmol) of fenoprofen. The pulvules also contain cellulose, gelatin, iron oxides, silicone, titanium dioxide, and other inactive ingredients. The 300 mg pulvules also contain D&C yellow no. 10 and FD&C yellow no. 6.

Nalfon Tablets contain fenoprofen calcium as the dihydrate in an amount equivalent to 600 mg (2.48 mmol) of fenoprofen. The tablets also contain amberlite, benzyl alcohol, calcium phosphate, corn starch, D&C yellow no. 10, FD&C yellow no. 6, hydroxypropyl methylcellulose, magnesium stearate, polyethylene glycol, stearic acid, titanium dioxide, and other inactive ingredients.

Storage: Store at controlled room temperature, 15-30°C (59-86°F).

CLINICAL PHARMACOLOGY

Fenoprofen calcium is a nonsteroidal, anti-inflammatory, antiarthritic drug that also possesses analgesic and antipyretic activities. Its exact mode of action is unknown, but it is thought that prostaglandin synthetase inhibition is involved. Fenoprofen calcium has been shown to inhibit prostaglandin synthetase isolated from bovine seminal vesicles. Reproduction studies in rats have shown fenoprofen calcium to be associated with prolonged labor and difficult parturition when given during late pregnancy. Evidence suggests that this may be due to decreased uterine contractility resulting from the inhibition of prostaglandin synthesis. Its action is not mediated through the adrenal gland.

Fenoprofen shows anti-inflammatory effects in rodents by inhibiting the development of redness and edema in acute inflammatory conditions and by reducing soft-tissue swelling and bone damage associated with chronic inflammation. It exhibits analgesic activity in rodents by inhibiting the writhing response caused by the introduction of an irritant into the peritoneal cavities of mice and by elevating pain thresholds that are related to pressure in edematous hindpaws of rats. In rats made febrile by the subcutaneous administration of brewer's yeast, fenoprofen produces antipyretic action. These effects are characteristic of nonsteroidal, anti-inflammatory, antipyretic, analgesic drugs.

The results in humans confirmed the anti-inflammatory and analgesic actions found in animals. The emergence and degree of erythremic response were measured in adult male volunteers exposed to ultraviolet irradiation. The effects of fenoprofen calcium, aspirin, and indomethacin were each compared with those of a placebo. All 3 drugs demonstrated antierythemic activity.

In patients with rheumatoid arthritis, the anti-inflammatory action of fenoprofen calcium has been evidenced by relief of pain, increase in grip strength, and reductions in joint swelling, duration of morning stiffness, and disease activity (as assessed by both the investigator and the patient). The anti-inflammatory action of fenoprofen calcium has also been evidenced by increased mobility (*i.e.*, a decrease in the number of joints having limited motion).

The use of fenoprofen calcium in combination with gold salts or corticosteroids has been studied in patients with rheumatoid arthritis. The studies, however, were inadequate in demonstrating whether further improvement is obtained by adding fenoprofen calcium to maintenance therapy with gold salts or steroids. Whether or not fenoprofen calcium used in conjunction with partially effective doses of a corticosteroid has a "steroid-sparing" effect is unknown.

In patients with osteoarthritis, the anti-inflammatory and analgesic effects of fenoprofen calcium have been demonstrated by reduction in tenderness as a response to pressure and reductions in night pain, stiffness, swelling, and overall disease activity (as assessed by both the patient and the investigator). These effects have also been demonstrated by relief of pain with motion and at rest and increased range of motion in involved joints.

In patients with rheumatoid arthritis and osteoarthritis, clinical studies have shown fenoprofen calcium to be comparable to aspirin in controlling the aforementioned measures of disease activity, but mild gastrointestinal reactions (nausea, dyspepsia) and tinnitus occurred less frequently in patients treated with fenoprofen calcium than in aspirin-treated patients. It is not known whether fenoprofen calcium causes less peptic ulceration than does aspirin.

In patients with pain, the analgesic action of fenoprofen calcium has produced a reduction in pain intensity, an increase in pain relief, improvement in total analgesia scores, and a sustained analgesic effect.

Under fasting conditions, fenoprofen calcium is rapidly absorbed, and peak plasma levels of 50 μg/ml are achieved within 2 hours after oral administration of 600 mg doses. Good dose proportionality was observed between 200 mg and 600 mg doses in fasting male volunteers. The plasma half-life is approximately 3 hours. About 90% of a single oral dose is eliminated within 24 hours as fenoprofen glucuronide and 4'- hydroxyfenoprofen glucuronide, the major urinary metabolites of fenoprofen. Fenoprofen is highly bound (99%) to albumin.

The concomitant administration of antacid (containing both aluminum and magnesium hydroxide) does not interfere with absorption of fenoprofen calcium.

There is less suppression of collagen-induced platelet aggregation with single doses of fenoprofen calcium than there is with aspirin.

INDICATIONS AND USAGE

Fenoprofen calcium is indicated for relief of the signs and symptoms of rheumatoid arthritis and osteoarthritis. It is recommended for the treatment of acute flare-ups and exacerbations and for the long-term management of these diseases.

Fenoprofen calcium is also indicated for the relief of mild to moderate pain.

CONTRAINDICATIONS

Fenoprofen calcium is contraindicated in patients who have shown hypersensitivity to it.

The drug should not be administered to patients with a history of significantly impaired renal function.

Fenoprofen calcium should not be given to patients in whom aspirin and other nonsteroidal anti-inflammatory drugs induce the symptoms of asthma, rhinitis, or urticaria, because cross-sensitivity to these drugs occurs in a high proportion of such patients.

WARNINGS

RISK OF GI ULCERATION, BLEEDING AND PERFORATION WITH NSAID THERAPY

Serious gastrointestinal toxicity such as bleeding, ulceration, and perforation, can occur at any time, with or without warning symptoms, in patients treated chronically with NSAID therapy. Although minor upper gastrointestinal problems, such as dyspepsia, are common, usually developing early in therapy, physicians should remain alert for ulceration and bleeding in patients treated chronically with NSAIDs, even in the absence of previous GI tract symptoms. In patients observed in clinical trials of several months to 2 years duration, symptomatic upper GI ulcers, gross bleeding or perforation appear to occur in approximately 1% of patients treated for 3-6 months, and in about 2-4% of patients treated for 1 year. Physicians should inform patients about the signs and/or symptoms of serious GI toxicity and what steps to take if they occur.

Studies to date have not identified any subset of patients not at risk of developing peptic ulceration and bleeding. Except for a prior history of serious GI events and other risk factors known to be associated with peptic ulcer disease, such as alcoholism, smoking, etc., no risk factors (*e.g.*, age, sex) have been associated with increased risk. Elderly or debilitated patients seem to tolerate ulceration or bleeding less well than other individuals and most spontaneous reports of fatal GI events are in this population. Studies to date are inconclusive concerning the relative risk of various NSAIDs in causing such reactions. High doses of any NSAID probably carry a greater risk of these reactions, although controlled clinical trials showing this do not exist in most cases. In considering the use of relatively large doses (within the recommended dosage range), sufficient benefit should be anticipated to offset the potential increased risk of GI toxicity.

Since fenoprofen calcium has been marketed, there have been reports of genitourinary tract problems in patients taking it. The most frequently reported problems have been episodes of dysuria, cystitis, hematuria, interstitial nephritis, and nephrotic syndrome. This syndrome may be preceded by the appearance of fever, rash, arthralgia, oliguria, and azotemia and may progress to anuria. There may also be substantial proteinuria, and, on renal biopsy, electron microscopy has shown foot process fusion and T-lymphocyte infiltration in the renal interstitium. Early recognition of the syndrome and withdrawal of the drug have been followed by rapid recovery. Administration of steroids and the use of dialysis have also been included in the treatment. Because a syndrome with some of these characteristics has also been reported with other nonsteroidal anti-inflammatory drugs, it is recommended that patients who have had these reactions with other such drugs not be treated with fenoprofen calcium. In patients with possibly compromised renal function, periodic renal function examinations should be done.

PRECAUTIONS

GENERAL

Renal Effects

There have been reports of acute interstitial nephritis and nephrotic syndrome (see CONTRAINDICATIONS and WARNINGS).

A second form of renal toxicity has been seen in patients with prerenal conditions leading to a reduction in renal blood flow or blood volume, in which renal prostaglandins play a supportive role in the maintenance of renal perfusion. In these patients, administration of an NSAID may cause a dose-dependent reduction in prostaglandin formation and may precipitate overt renal decompensation at any time. Patients at greatest risk for this reaction are those with impaired renal function, heart failure, liver dysfunction, those taking diuretics, and the elderly. Discontinuation of NSAID therapy is typically followed by recovery to the pretreatment state.

Since fenoprofen calcium is primarily eliminated by the kidneys, patients with possibly compromised renal function (such as the elderly) should be monitored periodically, especially during long-term therapy. For such patients, it may be anticipated that a lower daily dosage will avoid excessive drug accumulation.

Miscellaneous

Peripheral edema has been observed in some patients taking fenoprofen calcium; therefore, fenoprofen calcium should be used with caution in patients with compromised cardiac function or hypertension. The possibility of renal involvement should be considered.

Studies to date have not shown changes in the eyes attributable to the administration of fenoprofen calcium. However, adverse ocular effects have been observed with other anti-inflammatory drugs. Eye examinations, therefore, should be performed if visual disturbances occur in patients taking fenoprofen calcium.

Caution should be exercised by patients whose activities require alertness if they experience CNS side effects while taking fenoprofen calcium.

Since the safety of fenoprofen calcium has not been established in patients with impaired hearing, these patients should have periodic tests of auditory function during prolonged therapy with fenoprofen calcium.

INFORMATION FOR THE PATIENT

Fenoprofen calcium, like other drugs of its class, is not free of side effects. The side effects of these drugs can cause discomfort and, rarely, there are more serious side effects, such as gastrointestinal bleeding, which may result in hospitalization and even fatal outcomes.

NSAIDs (Nonsteroidal Anti-Inflammatory Drugs) are often essential agents in the management of arthritis and have a major role in the treatment of pain, but they also may be commonly employed for conditions which are less serious.

Physicians may wish to discuss with their patients the potential risks (see WARNINGS, PRECAUTIONS, and ADVERSE REACTIONS) and likely benefits of NSAID treatment, particularly when the drugs are used for less serious conditions where treatment without NSAIDs may represent an acceptable alternative to both the patient and physician.

LABORATORY TESTS

In chronic studies in rats, high doses of fenoprofen calcium caused elevation of serum transaminase and hepatocellular hypertrophy. In clinical trials, some patients developed elevation of serum transaminase, LDH, and alkaline phosphatase that persisted for some months and usually, but not always, declined despite continuation of the drug. The significance of this is unknown. It is recommended, therefore, that fenoprofen calcium be discontinued if any significant liver abnormality occurs.

As with other nonsteroidal anti-inflammatory drugs, borderline elevations in 1 or more liver tests may occur in up to 15% of patients. These abnormalities may progress, may remain essentially unchanged, or may be transient with continued therapy. The SGPT (ALT) test is probably the most sensitive indicator of liver dysfunction. Meaningful (*i.e.,* 3 times the upper limit of normal) elevations of SGPT or SGOT (AST) occurred in controlled clinical trials in less than 1% of patients. A patient with symptoms and/or signs suggesting liver dysfunction, or in whom an abnormal liver test has occurred, should be evaluated for evidence of the development of more severe hepatic reactions while using fenoprofen calcium.

Severe hepatic reactions, including jaundice and cases of fatal hepatitis, have been reported with fenoprofen calcium, as with other nonsteroidal anti-inflammatory drugs. As a result, during long-term therapy, liver function tests should be monitored periodically. Although such reactions are rare, if liver tests continue to be abnormal or worsen, if clinical signs and symptoms consistent with liver disease develop, or if systemic manifestations occur (*e.g.,* eosinophilia and rash), fenoprofen calcium should be discontinued. If this drug is to be used in the presence of impaired liver function, it must be done under strict observation.

Patients with initial low hemoglobin values who are receiving long-term therapy with fenoprofen calcium should have a hemoglobin determination made at reasonable intervals.

Fenoprofen calcium decreases platelet aggregation and may prolong bleeding time. Patients who may be adversely affected by prolongation of the bleeding time should be carefully observed when fenoprofen calcium is administered.

Because serious GI tract ulceration and bleeding can occur without warning symptoms, physicians should follow chronically treated patients for the signs and symptoms of ulceration and bleeding and should inform them of the importance of this follow-up (see WARNINGS, Risk of GI Ulcerations, Bleeding and Perforation With NSAID Therapy).

LABORATORY TEST INTERACTIONS

Amerlex-M kit assay values of total and free triiodothyronine in patients receiving fenoprofen calcium have been reported as falsely elevated on the basis of a chemical cross-reaction that directly interferes with the assay. Thyroid-stimulating hormone, total thyroxine, and thyrotropin-releasing hormone response are not affected.

USAGE IN PREGNANCY

Safe use of fenoprofen calcium during pregnancy and lactation has not been established; therefore, administration to pregnant patients and nursing mothers is not recommended. Reproduction studies have been performed in rats and rabbits. When fenoprofen was given to rats during pregnancy and continued until the time of labor, parturition was prolonged. Similar results have been found with other nonsteroidal anti-inflammatory drugs that inhibit prostaglandin synthetase.

PEDIATRIC USE

Safety and effectiveness in pediatric patients have not been established.

DRUG INTERACTIONS

The coadministration of aspirin decreases the biologic half-life of fenoprofen because of an increase in metabolic clearance that results in a greater amount of hydroxylated fenoprofen in the urine. Although the mechanism of interaction between fenoprofen and aspirin is not totally known, enzyme induction and displacement of fenoprofen from plasma albumin binding sites are possibilities. Because fenoprofen calcium has not been shown to produce any additional effect beyond that obtained with aspirin alone and because aspirin increases the rate of excretion of fenoprofen calcium, the concomitant use of fenoprofen calcium and salicylates is not recommended.

Chronic administration of phenobarbital, a known enzyme inducer, may be associated with a decrease in the plasma half-life of fenoprofen. When phenobarbital is added to or withdrawn from treatment, dosage adjustment of fenoprofen calcium may be required.

In vitro studies have shown that fenoprofen, because of its affinity for albumin, may displace from their binding sites other drugs that are also albumin bound, and this may lead to drug interaction. Theoretically, fenoprofen could likewise be displaced. Patients receiving hydantoin, sulfonamides, or sulfonylureas should be observed for increased activity of these drugs and, therefore, signs of toxicity from these drugs. In patients receiving coumarin-type anticoagulants, the addition of fenoprofen calcium to therapy could prolong the prothrombin time. Patients receiving both drugs should be under careful observation. Patients treated with fenoprofen calcium may be resistant to the effects of loop diuretics.

In patients receiving fenoprofen calcium and a steroid concomitantly, any reduction in steroid dosage should be gradual in order to avoid the possible complications of sudden steroid withdrawal.

ADVERSE REACTIONS

During clinical studies for rheumatoid arthritis, osteoarthritis, or mild to moderate pain and studies of pharmacokinetics, complaints were compiled from a checklist of potential adverse reactions, and the following data emerged. These encompass observations in 6786 patients, including 188 observed for at least 52 weeks. For comparison, data are also presented from complaints received from the 266 patients who received placebo in these same trials. During short-term studies for analgesia, the incidence of adverse reactions was markedly lower than that seen in longer-term studies.

INCIDENCE GREATER THAN 1% — PROBABLE CAUSAL RELATIONSHIP

Digestive System: During clinical trials with fenoprofen calcium, the most common adverse reactions were gastrointestinal in nature and occurred in 20.8% of patients receiving fenoprofen calcium as compared to 16.9% of patients receiving placebo. In descending order of frequency, these reactions included dyspepsia (10.3%, fenoprofen calcium, vs 2.3%, placebo), nausea (7.7% vs 7.1%), constipation (7% vs 1.5%), vomiting (2.6% vs 1.9%), abdominal pain (2% vs 1.1%), and diarrhea (1.8% vs 4.1%).

The drug was discontinued because of adverse gastrointestinal reactions in less than 2% of patients during premarketing studies.

Nervous System: The most frequent adverse neurologic reactions were headache (8.7% treated vs 7.5% placebo) and somnolence (8.5% vs 6.4%). Dizziness (6.5% vs 5.6%), tremor (2.2% vs 0.4%), and confusion (1.4% vs none) were noted less frequently.

Fenoprofen calcium was discontinued in less than 0.5% of patients because of these side effects during premarketing studies.

Skin and Appendages: Increased sweating (4.6% vs 0.4%), pruritus (4.2% vs 0.8%), and rash (3.7% vs 0.4%) were reported.

Fenoprofen calcium was discontinued in about 1% of patients because of an adverse effect related to the skin during premarketing studies.

Special Senses: Tinnitus (4.5% vs 0.4%), blurred vision (2.2% vs none), and decreased hearing (1.6% vs none) were reported.

Fenoprofen calcium was discontinued in less than 0.5% of patients because of adverse effects related to the special senses during premarketing studies.

Cardiovascular: Palpitations (2.5% vs 0.4%).

Fenoprofen calcium was discontinued in about 0.5% of patients because of adverse cardiovascular reactions during premarketing studies.

Miscellaneous: Nervousness (5.7% vs 1.5%), asthenia (5.4% vs 0.4%), peripheral edema (5.0% vs 0.4%), dyspnea (2.8% vs none), fatigue (1.7% vs 1.5%), upper respiratory infection (1.5% vs 5.6%), and nasopharyngitis (1.2% vs none).

INCIDENCE LESS THAN 1% — PROBABLE CAUSAL RELATIONSHIP

The following adverse reactions, occurring in less than 1% of patients, were reported in controlled clinical trials and voluntary reports made since fenoprofen calcium was initially marketed. The probability of a causal relationship exists between fenoprofen calcium and these adverse reactions:

Digestive System: Gastritis, peptic ulcer with/without perforation, gastrointestinal hemorrhage, anorexia, flatulence, dry mouth, and blood in the stool. Increases in alkaline phosphatase, LDH, and SGOT, jaundice, and cholestatic hepatitis were observed (see PRECAUTIONS).

Genitourinary Tract: Renal failure, dysuria, cystitis, hematuria, oliguria, azotemia, anuria, interstitial nephritis, nephrosis, and papillary necrosis (see WARNINGS).

Hypersensitivity: Angioedema (angioneurotic edema).

Hematologic: Purpura, bruising, hemorrhage, thrombocytopenia, hemolytic anemia, aplastic anemia, agranulocytosis, and pancytopenia.

Miscellaneous: Anaphylaxis, urticaria, malaise, insomnia, and tachycardia.

INCIDENCE LESS THAN 1% — CAUSAL RELATIONSHIP UNKNOWN

Other reactions reported either in clinical trials or spontaneously, occurred in circumstances in which a causal relationship could not be established. However, with these rarely reported reactions, the possibility of such a relationship cannot be excluded. Therefore, these observations are listed to alert the physician.

Skin and Appendages: Exfoliative dermatitis, toxic epidermal necrolysis, Stevens-Johnson syndrome, and alopecia.

Digestive System: Aphthous ulcerations of the buccal mucosa, metallic taste, and pancreatitis.

Cardiovascular: Atrial fibrillation, pulmonary edema, electrocardiographic changes, and supraventricular tachycardia.

Nervous System: Depression, disorientation, seizures, and trigeminal neuralgia.

Special Senses: Burning tongue, diplopia, and optic neuritis.

Miscellaneous: Personality change, lymphadenopathy, mastodynia, and fever.

DOSAGE AND ADMINISTRATION

ANALGESIA

For the treatment of mild to moderate pain, the recommended dosage is 200 mg every 4-6 hours, as needed.

RHEUMATOID ARTHRITIS AND OSTEOARTHRITIS

The suggested dosage is 300-600 mg, 3 or 4 times a day. The dose should be tailored to the needs of the patient and may be increased or decreased depending on the severity of the symptoms. Dosage adjustments may be made after initiation of drug therapy or during exacerbations of the disease. Total daily dosage should not exceed 3200 mg.

If gastrointestinal complaints occur, fenoprofen calcium may be administered with meals or with milk. Although the total amount absorbed is not affected, peak blood levels are delayed and diminished.

Patients with rheumatoid arthritis generally seem to require larger doses of fenoprofen calcium than do those with osteoarthritis. The smallest dose that yields acceptable control should be employed.

Although improvement may be seen in a few days in many patients, an additional 2-3 weeks may be required to gauge the full benefits of therapy.

PRODUCT LISTING - RATED THERAPEUTICALLY EQUIVALENT

Package	Price	Product, Manufacturer	NDC
Capsule - Oral - 200 mg			
100's	$23.60	GENERIC, Watson Laboratories Inc	52544-0367-01
100's	$29.15	GENERIC, Major Pharmaceuticals Inc	00904-3778-60
100's	$29.21	GENERIC, Major Pharmaceuticals Inc	00904-3778-61
100's	$29.21	GENERIC, Major Pharmaceuticals Inc	00904-3784-61
100's	$30.63	GENERIC, Moore, H.L. Drug Exchange Inc	00839-7511-06
100's	$30.66	GENERIC, Geneva Pharmaceuticals	00781-2861-01
100's	$68.69	NALFON, Ranbaxy Laboratories	63304-0681-01
Capsule - Oral - 300 mg			
60's	$30.33	NALFON, Physicians Total Care	54868-0856-00
100's	$27.37	GENERIC, Watson Laboratories Inc	52544-0368-01
100's	$33.85	GENERIC, Major Pharmaceuticals Inc	00904-3785-60
100's	$34.69	GENERIC, Major Pharmaceuticals Inc	00904-3785-61
100's	$34.88	GENERIC, Geneva Pharmaceuticals	00781-2862-01
100's	$35.49	GENERIC, Moore, H.L. Drug Exchange Inc	00839-7512-06
100's	$38.76	NALFON, Dista Products Company	00777-0877-02
100's	$49.77	NALFON, Physicians Total Care	54868-0856-01
100's	$53.79	NALFON, Ranbaxy Laboratories	63304-0682-01
Tablet - Oral - 600 mg			
20's	$13.49	GENERIC, Pd-Rx Pharmaceuticals	55289-0334-20
30's	$10.85	GENERIC, Pd-Rx Pharmaceuticals	55289-0334-30
30's	$20.15	GENERIC, St. Mary'S Mpp	60760-0471-30
30's	$35.34	NALFON, Pd-Rx Pharmaceuticals	55289-0178-30
40's	$13.20	GENERIC, Pd-Rx Pharmaceuticals	55289-0334-40
100's	$24.00	FEDERAL UPPER LIMIT, H.C.F.A. F F P	99999-1253-05
100's	$26.00	GENERIC, Raway Pharmacal Inc	00686-0477-20
100's	$37.80	GENERIC, Watson Laboratories Inc	52544-0366-01
100's	$46.00	GENERIC, Major Pharmaceuticals Inc	00904-3786-60
100's	$46.29	GENERIC, Moore, H.L. Drug Exchange Inc	00839-7513-06
100's	$46.70	GENERIC, Martec Pharmaceuticals Inc	52555-0473-01
100's	$47.00	GENERIC, Watson/Schein Pharmaceuticals Inc	00364-2316-01
100's	$47.19	GENERIC, Esi Lederle Generics	00005-3559-43
100's	$47.80	GENERIC, Aligen Independent Laboratories Inc	00405-4424-01
100's	$48.10	GENERIC, Ivax Corporation	00182-1902-01
100's	$48.10	GENERIC, Geneva Pharmaceuticals	00781-1863-01
100's	$50.50	GENERIC, Ivax Corporation	00172-4141-60
100's	$50.50	GENERIC, Mylan Pharmaceuticals Inc	00378-0471-01
100's	$50.75	GENERIC, Purepac Pharmaceutical Company	00228-2317-10
100's	$56.15	GENERIC, Auro Pharmaceutical	55829-0252-10
100's	$63.64	GENERIC, Ivax Corporation	00182-1902-89
100's	$63.64	GENERIC, Vangard Labs	00615-3507-13

PRODUCT LISTING - EQUIVALENTS NOT AVAILABLE

Package	Price	Product, Manufacturer	NDC
Tablet - Oral - 600 mg			
4's	$2.03	GENERIC, Allscripts Pharmaceutical Company	54569-2105-06
6's	$4.81	GENERIC, Prescript Pharmaceuticals	00247-0365-06
6's	$5.13	GENERIC, Southwood Pharmaceuticals Inc	58016-0244-06
20's	$8.22	GENERIC, Prescript Pharmaceuticals	00247-0365-20
20's	$10.16	GENERIC, Allscripts Pharmaceutical Company	54569-2105-01
20's	$14.04	GENERIC, Southwood Pharmaceuticals Inc	58016-0244-20
20's	$14.20	GENERIC, Pharma Pac	52959-0067-20
20's	$15.76	GENERIC, Cardinal Pharmaceuticals	63874-0416-20
21's	$8.47	GENERIC, Prescript Pharmaceuticals	00247-0365-21
21's	$14.63	GENERIC, Southwood Pharmaceuticals Inc	58016-0244-21
28's	$10.18	GENERIC, Prescript Pharmaceuticals	00247-0365-28
28's	$18.53	GENERIC, Cardinal Pharmaceuticals	63874-0416-28
30's	$10.66	GENERIC, Prescript Pharmaceuticals	00247-0365-30
30's	$15.38	GENERIC, Allscripts Pharmaceutical Company	54569-2105-00
30's	$19.11	GENERIC, Southwood Pharmaceuticals Inc	58016-0244-30
30's	$19.15	GENERIC, Pharma Pac	52959-0067-30
30's	$21.28	GENERIC, Cardinal Pharmaceuticals	63874-0416-30
60's	$25.49	GENERIC, Southwood Pharmaceuticals Inc	58016-0244-60
100's	$70.66	GENERIC, Cardinal Pharmaceuticals	63874-0416-01

Fentanyl Citrate *(001254)*

For related information, see the comparative table section in Appendix A.

Categories: Anesthesia, adjunct; Anesthesia, general; Anesthesia, induction; Pain, cancer; Pain, chronic; Pregnancy Category C; DEA Class CII; FDA Approved 1968 Feb

Drug Classes: Analgesics, narcotic; Anesthetics, general

Brand Names: Actiq; Duragesic; **Sublimaze**

Foreign Brand Availability: Beatryl (Israel); Fenodid (Mexico); Fentanest (Italy; Mexico; Spain); Leptanal (Norway; Sweden); Trofentyl (India)

HCFA JCODE(S): J3010 up to 2 ml IM, IV

IM-IV

DESCRIPTION

Note: The trade names have been used throughout this monograph for clarity.

Sublimaze (fentanyl citrate) injection is a potent narcotic analgesic. Each ml contains fentanyl citrate equivalent to 50 µg of fentanyl base, adjusted to pH 4.0-7.5 with sodium hydroxide. Fentanyl citrate is chemically identified as N-(1-phenethyl-4- piperidyl) propionanilide citrate (1:1) with a molecular weight of 528.60. The empirical formula is $C_{22}H_{28}N_2O{\cdot}C_6H_8O_7$.

Sublimaze is a sterile, non-pyogenic, preservative free aqueous solution for intravenous or intramuscular injection.

CLINICAL PHARMACOLOGY

Fentanyl citrate is a narcotic analgesic. A dose of 100 µg (0.1 mg) (2.0 ml) is approximately equivalent in analgesic activity to 10 mg of morphine or 75 mg of meperidine. The principal actions of therapeutic value are analgesia and sedation. Alterations in respiratory rate and alveolar ventilation, associated with narcotic analgesics, may last longer than the analgesic effect. As the dose of narcotic is increased, the decrease in pulmonary exchange becomes greater. Large doses may produce apnea. Fentanyl appears to have less emetic activity than either morphine or meperidine. Histamine assays and skin wheal testing in man indicate that clinically significant histamine release rarely occurs with fentanyl. Recent assays in man show no clinically significant histamine release in dosages up to 50 µg/kg (0.05 mg/kg) (1 ml/kg). Fentanyl preserves cardiac stability and blunts stress-related hormonal changes at higher doses.

The pharmacokinetics of fentanyl can be described as a three-compartment model, with a distribution time of 1.7 minutes, redistribution of 13 minutes and a terminal elimination half-life of 219 minutes. The volume of distribution for fentanyl is 4 L/kg.

Sublimaze plasma protein binding capacity increases with increasing ionization of the drug. Alterations in pH may affect its distribution between plasma and the central nervous system. It accumulates in skeletal muscle and fat and is released slowly into the blood. Fentanyl, which is primarily transformed in the liver, demonstrates a high first pass clearance and releases approximately 75% of an IV dose in urine, mostly as metabolites with less than 10% representing the unchanged drug. Approximately 9% of the dose is recovered in the feces, primarily as metabolites. The onset of action of fentanyl is almost immediate when the drug is given intravenously; however, the maximal analgesic and respiratory depressant effect may not be noted for several minutes. The usual duration of action of the analgesic effect is 30-60 minutes after a single IV dose of up to 100 µg (0.1 mg) (2.2 ml). Following intramuscular administration, the onset of action is from 7-8 minutes, and the duration of action is 1-2 hours. As with longer acting narcotic analgesics, the duration of the respiratory depressant effect of fentanyl may be longer than the analgesic effect. The following observations have been reported concerning altered respiratory response to CO_2 stimulation following administration of fentanyl citrate to man:

DIMINISHED SENSITIVITY TO CO_2 STIMULATION MAY PERSIST LONGER THAN DEPRESSION OF RESPIRATORY RATE. (Altered sensitivity to CO_2 stimulation has been demonstrated for up to 4 hours following a single dose of 600 µg [0.6 mg] [12 ml] Sublimaze to healthy volunteers.) Sublimaze frequently slows the respiratory rate, duration and degree of respiratory depression being dose related.

The peak respiratory depressant effect of a single IV dose of fentanyl citrate is noted 5-15 minutes following injection. See also WARNINGS and PRECAUTIONS concerning respiratory depression.

INDICATIONS AND USAGE

Sublimaze (fentanyl citrate) injection is indicated for:

- Analgesic action of short duration during the anesthetic periods, premedication, induction and maintenance, and in the immediate postoperative period (recovery room) as the need arises.
- Use as a narcotic analgesic supplement in general or regional anesthesia.
- Administration with a neuroleptic such as droperidol injection as an anesthetic premedication, for the induction of anesthesia and as an adjunct in the maintenance of general and regional anesthesia.
- Use as an anesthetic agent with oxygen in selected high risk patients, such as those undergoing open heart surgery or certain complicated neurological or orthopedic procedures.

CONTRAINDICATIONS

Sublimaze (fentanyl citrate) injection is contraindicated in patients with known intolerance to the drug or other opioid agonists.

WARNINGS

SUBLIMAZE SHOULD BE ADMINISTERED ONLY BY PERSONS SPECIFICALLY TRAINED IN THE USE OF INTRAVENOUS ANESTHETICS AND MANAGEMENT OF THE RESPIRATORY EFFECTS OF POTENT OPIOIDS.

AN OPIOID ANTAGONIST, RESUSCITATIVE AND INTUBATION EQUIPMENT AND OXYGEN SHOULD BE READILY AVAILABLE.

See also discussion of narcotic antagonists in PRECAUTIONS.

If Sublimaze is administered with a tranquilizer such as droperidol, the user should become familiar with the special properties of each drug, particularly the widely differing durations of action. In addition, when such a combination is used, fluids and other countermeasures to manage hypotension should be available.

As with other potent narcotics, the respiratory depressant effect of Sublimaze may persist longer than the measured analgesic effect. The total dose of all narcotic analgesics administered should be considered by the practitioner before ordering narcotic analgesics during recovery from anesthesia. It is recommended that narcotics, when required, should be used in reduced doses initially, as low as 1/4 to 1/3 those usually recommended.

Sublimaze may cause muscle rigidity, particularly involving the muscles of respiration. This rigidity has been reported to occur or recur infrequently in the extended postoperative period usually following high dose administration. In addition, skeletal muscle movements of various groups in the extremities, neck and external eye have been reported during induction of anesthesia with fentanyl; these reported movements have, on rare occasions, been strong enough to pose patient management problems. This effect is related to the dose and speed of injection and its incidence can be reduced by: (1) administration of up to ¼ of the full paralyzing dose of a non-depolarizing neuromuscular blocking agent just prior to administration of Sublimaze; (2) administration of a full paralyzing dose of a neuromuscular blocking agent following loss of eyelash reflex when Sublimaze is used in anesthetic doses titrated by slow IV infusion; or, (3) simultaneous administration of Sublimaze and a full paralyzing dose of neuromuscular blocking agent when Sublimaze is used in rapidly administered anesthetic dosages. The neuromuscular blocking agent used should be compatible with the patient's cardiovascular status.

Adequate facilities should be available for postoperative monitoring and ventilation of patients administered anesthetic doses of Sublimaze. Where moderate or high doses are used (above 10 μg/kg), there must be adequate facilities for postoperative observation, and ventilation if necessary, of patients who have received Sublimaze. It is essential that these facilities be fully equipped to handle all degrees of respiratory depression.

Sublimaze may also produce other signs and symptoms characteristic of narcotic analgesics including euphoria, miosis, bradycardia and bronchoconstriction.

Severe and unpredictable potentiation by MAO inhibitors has been reported for other narcotic analgesics. Although this has not been reported for fentanyl, there are insufficient data to establish that this does not occur with fentanyl. Therefore, when fentanyl is administered to patients who have received MAO inhibitors within 14 days, appropriate monitoring and ready availability of vasodilators and beta-blockers for the treatment of hypertension is indicated.

HEAD INJURIES AND INCREASED INTRACRANIAL PRESSURE

Sublimaze should be used with caution in patients who may be particularly susceptible to respiratory depression, such as comatose patients who may have a head injury or brain tumor. In addition, fentanyl may obscure the clinical course of patients with head injury.

PRECAUTIONS

GENERAL

The initial dose of Sublimaze should be appropriately reduced in elderly and debilitated patients. The effect of the initial dose should be considered in determining incremental doses.

Nitrous oxide has been reported to produce cardiovascular depression when given with higher doses of IV fentanyl citrate.

Certain forms of conduction anesthesia, such as spinal anesthesia and some peridural anesthetics can alter respiration by blocking intercostal nerves. Through other mechanisms (see CLINICAL PHARMACOLOGY) Sublimaze can also alter respiration. Therefore, when Sublimaze is used to supplement these forms of anesthesia, the anesthetist should be familiar with the physicological alterations involved, and be prepared to manage them in the patients selected for these forms of anesthesia.

When a tranquilizer such as droperidol is used with Sublimaze, pulmonary arterial pressure may be decreased. This fact should be considered by those who conduct diagnostic and surgical procedures where interpretation of pulmonary arterial pressure measurements might determine final management of the patient. When high dose or anesthetic dosages of fentanyl are employed, even relatively small dosages of diazepam may cause cardiovascular depression.

When Sublimaze is used with a tranquilizer such as droperidol, hypotension can occur. If it occurs, the possibility of hypovolemia should also be considered and managed with appropriate parenteral fluid therapy.

Repositioning the patient to improve venous return to the heart should be considered when operative conditions permit. Care should be exercised in moving and positioning of patients because of the possiblility of orthostatic hypotension. If volume expansion with fluids plus other countermeasures do not correct hypotension, the administration of pressor agents other than epinephrine should be considered. Because of the alpha-adrenergic blocking action of droperidol, epinephrine may paradoxically decrease the blood pressure in patients treated with droperidol.

Elevated blood pressure, with and without pre-existing hypertension, has been reported following administration of fentanyl citrate combined with droperidol. This might be due to unexplained alterations in sympathetic activity following large doses; however, it is also frequently attributed to anesthetic and surgical stimulation during light anesthesia.

When droperidol is used with fentanyl and the EEG is used for postoperative monitoring, it may be found that the EEG pattern returns to normal slowly.

Vital signs should be monitored routinely.

Respiratory depression caused by opioid analgesics can be reversed by opioid antagonists such as naloxone. Because the duration of respiratory depression produced by Sublimaze may last longer than the duration of the opioid antagonist action, appropriate surveillance should be maintained. As with all potent opioids, profound analgesia is accompanied by respiratory depression and diminished sensitivity to CO_2 stimulation which may persist into or recur in the postoperative period. Respiratory depression secondary to chest wall rigidity has been reported in the postoperative period. Intraoperative hyperventilation may further alter postoperative response to CO_2. Appropriate postoperative monitoring should be employed to ensure that adequate spontaneous breathing is established and maintained in the absence of stimulation prior to discharging the patient from the recovery area.

IMPAIRED RESPIRATION

Sublimaze should be used with caution in patients with chronic obstructive pulmonary disease, patients with decreased respiratory reserve, and others with potentially compromised respiration. In such patients, narcotics may additionally decrease respiratory drive and increase airway resistance. During anesthesia, this can be managed by assisted or controlled respiration.

IMAPIRED HEPATIC OR RENAL FUNCTION

Sublimaze should be administered with caution to patients with liver and kidney dysfunction because of the importance of these organs in the metabolism and excretion of drugs.

CARDIOVASCULAR EFFECTS

Sublimaze may produce bradycardia, which may be treated with atropine. Sublimaze should be used with caution in patients with cardiac bradycardias.

CARCINOGENESIS, MUTAGENESIS, AND IMPAIRMENT OF FERTILITY

No carcinogenicity or mutagenicity studies have been conducted with Sublimaze. Reproduction studies in rats revealed a significant decrease in the pregnancy rate of all experimental groups. This decrease was most pronounced in the high dosed group (1.25 mg/kg — 12.5× human dose) in which 1 of 20 animals became pregnant.

PREGNANCY CATEGORY C

Sublimaze has been shown to impair fertility and to have an embryocidal effect in rats when given in doses 0.3 times the upper human dose for a period of 12 days. No evidence of teratogenic effects have been observed after administration of Sublimaze to rats. There are no adequate and well-controlled studies in pregnant women. Sublimaze should be used during pregnancy only if the potential benefit justifies the potential risk to the fetus.

LABOR AND DELIVERY

There are insufficient data to support the use of Sublimaze in labor and delivery. Therefore, such use is not recommended.

NURSING MOTHERS

It is not known whether this drug is excreted in human milk. Because many drugs are excreted in human milk, caution should be exercised when Sublimaze is administered to a nursing woman.

PEDIATRIC USE

The safety and efficacy of Sublimaze in children under 2 years of age have not been established. Rare cases of unexplained clinically significant methemoglobinemia have been reported in premature neonates undergoing emergency anesthesia and surgery which included combined use of fentanyl, pancuronium and atropine. A direct cause and effect relationship between the combined use of these drugs and the reported cases of methemoglobinemia has not been established.

DRUG INTERACTIONS

Other CNS depressant drugs (*e.g.*, barbiturates, tranquilizers, narcotics and general anesthetics) will have additive or potentiating effects with Sublimaze. When patients have received such drugs, the dose of Sublimaze required will be less than usual. Following the administration of Sublimaze, the dose of other CNS depressant drugs should be reduced.

ADVERSE REACTIONS

As with other narcotic analgesics, the most common serious adverse reactions reported to occur with Sublimaze are respiratory depression, apnea, rigidity, and bradycardia; if these remain untreated, respiratory arrest, circulatory depression or cardiac arrest could occur. Other adverse reactions that have been reported are hypertension, hypotension, dizziness, blurred vision, nausea, emesis, diaphoresis, pruritus, urticaria, laryngospasm and anaphylaxis. It has been reported that secondary rebound respiratory depression may occasionally occur postoperatively. Patients should be monitored for this possibility and appropriate countermeasures taken as necessary.

When a tranquilizer such as droperidol is used with Sublimaze, the following adverse reactions can occur: chills and/or shivering, restlessness, and postoperative hallucinatory episodes (sometimes associated with transient periods of mental depression); extrapyramidal symptoms (dystonia, akathisia and oculogyric crisis) have been observed up to 24 hours postoperatively. When they occur, extrapyramidal symptoms can usually be controlled with anti-parkinson agents. Postoperative drowsiness is also frequently reported following the use of droperidol.

DOSAGE AND ADMINISTRATION

50 μg = 0.05 mg = 1 ml

Dosage should be individualized. Some of the factors to be considered in determining the dose are age, body weight, physical status, underlying pathological condition, use of other drugs, type of anesthesia to be used and the surgical procedure involved. Dosage should be reduced in elderly or debilitated patients (see PRECAUTIONS).

Vital signs should be monitored routinely.

Premedication: Premedication (to be appropriately modified in the elderly, debilitated and those who have received other depressant drugs) 50-100 μg (0.05-0.1 mg) (1-2 ml) may be administered intramuscularly 30-60 minutes prior to surgery.

Adjunct to General Anesthesia: See Dosage Range Chart.

Adjunct to Regional Anesthesia: 50-100 μg (0.05-0.1 mg) (1-2 ml) may be administered intramuscularly or slowly intravenously, over 1-2 minutes, when additional analgesia is required.

Postoperatively (recovery room): 50-100 μg (0.05-0.1 mg) (1-2 ml) may be administered intramuscularly for the control of pain, tachypnea and emergence delirium. The dose may be repeated in 1-2 hours as needed.

Usage in Children: For induction and maintenance in children 2-12 years of age, a reduced dose as low as 2-3 µg/kg is recommended.

DOSAGE RANGE CHART
Total Dosage

Low Dose: 2 µg/kg (0.002 mg/kg) (0.04 ml/kg) Sublimaze. Sublimaze in small doses is most useful for minor, but painful, surgical procedures. In addition to the analgesia during surgery, Sublimaze may also provide some pain relief in the immediate postoperative period.

Moderate Dose: 2-20 µg/kg (0.002-0.02 mg/kg) (0.04-0.4 ml/kg) Sublimaze. Where surgery becomes more major, a larger dose is required. With this dose, in addition to adequate analgesia, one would expect to see some abolition of the stress response. However, respiratory depression will be such that artificial ventilation during anesthesia is necessary, and careful observation of ventilation postoperatively is essential.

High Dose: 20-50 µg/kg (0.02-0.05 mg/kg) (0.4-1 ml/kg) Sublimaze. During open heart surgery and certain more complicated neurosurgical and orthopedic procedures where surgery is more prolonged, and in the opinion of the anesthesiologist, the stress response to surgery would be detrimental to the well being of the patient, dosages of 20-50 µg/kg (0.02-0.05 mg/kg) (0.4-1 ml/kg) of Sublimaze with nitrous oxide/oxygen have been shown to attenuate the stress response as defined by increased levels of circulating growth hormone, catecholamine, ADH and prolactin. When dosages in this range have been used during surgery, postoperative ventilation and observation are essential due to extended postoperative respiratory depression. The main objective of this technique would be to produce "stress free" anesthesia.

Maintenance Dosage

Low Dose: 2 µg/kg (0.002 mg/kg) (0.04 ml/kg) Sublimaze. Additional dosages of Sublimaze are infrequently needed in these minor procedures.

Moderate Dose: 2-20 µg/kg (0.002-0.02 mg/kg) (0.04-0.4 ml/kg) Sublimaze. 25-100 µg (0.025-0.1 mg) (0.5-2 ml) may be administered intravenously or intramuscularly when movement and/or changes in vital signs indicate surgical stress or lightening of analgesia.

High Dose: 20-50 µg/kg (0.02-0.05 mg/kg) (0.4-1 ml/kg) Sublimaze. Maintenance dosage (ranging from 25 µg [0.025 mg] [0.5 ml] to one-half the initial loading dose) will be dictated by the changes in vital signs which indicate stress and lightening of analgesia. However, the additional dosage selected must be individualized especially if the anticipated remaining operative time is short.

AS A GENERAL ANESTHETIC

When attenuation of the responses to surgical stress is especially important, doses of 50-100 µg/kg (0.05-0.1 mg/kg) (1-2 ml/kg) may be administered with oxygen and a muscle relaxant. This technique has been reported to provide anesthesia without the use of additional anesthetic agents. In certain cases, doses up to 150 µg/kg (0.15 mg/kg) (3 ml/kg) may be necessary to produce this anesthetic effect. It has been used for open heart surgery and certain other major surgical procedures in patients for whom protection of the myocardium from excess oxygen demand is particularly indicated, and for certain complicated neurological and orthopedic procedures.

As noted above, it is essential that qualified personnel and adequate facilities be available for the management of respiratory depression.

See WARNINGS and PRECAUTIONS for use of Sublimaze (fentanyl citrate) with other CNS depressants, and in patients with altered response.

Parenteral drug products should be inspected visually for particulate matter and discoloration prior to administration, whenever solution and container permit.

Protect from light. Store at room temperature 15-30°C (59-86°F).

HOW SUPPLIED

Sublimaze is available in 2, 5, 10 and 20 ml ampoules containing 50 µg/ml of fentanyl base. **Storage:** PROTECT FROM LIGHT. STORE AT CONTROLLED ROOM TEMPERATURE 15-25°C (59-77°F).

ORAL

WARNING

Note: The trade names have been used throughout this monograph for clarity.

PHYSICIANS AND OTHER HEALTHCARE PROVIDERS MUST BECOME FAMILIAR WITH THE IMPORTANT WARNINGS IN THIS LABEL.

Actiq is indicated only for the management of breakthrough cancer pain in patients with malignancies who are already receiving and who are tolerant to opioid therapy for their underlying persistent cancer pain. Patients considered opioid tolerant are those who are taking at least 60 mg morphine/day, 50 µg transdermal fentanyl/hour, or an equianalgesic dose of another opioid for a week or longer.

Because life-threatening hypoventilation could occur at any dose in patients not taking chronic opiates, Actiq is contraindicated in the management of acute or postoperative pain. This product must not be used in opioid non-tolerant patients.

Actiq is intended to be used only in the care of cancer patients and only by oncologists and pain specialists who are knowledgeable of and skilled in the use of Schedule II opioids to treat cancer pain.

Patients and their caregivers must be instructed that Actiq contains a medicine in an amount which can be fatal to a child. Patients and their caregivers must be instructed to keep all units out of the reach of children and to discard open units properly. (See PRECAUTIONS, Information for Patients and Their Caregivers for disposal instructions.)

WARNING: May be habit forming.

DESCRIPTION

Actiq (oral transmucosal fentanyl citrate) is a solid formulation of fentanyl citrate, a potent opioid analgesic, intended for oral transmucosal administration. Actiq is formulated as a white to off-white solid drug matrix on a handle that is radiopaque and is fracture resistant (ABS plastic) under normal conditions when used as directed.

Actiq is designed to be dissolved slowly in the mouth in a manner to facilitate transmucosal absorption. The handle allows the Actiq unit to be removed from the mouth if signs of excessive opioid effects appear during administration.

Active Ingredient: Fentanyl citrate is N-(1-Phenethyl-4-piperidyl) propionanilide citrate (1:1). Fentanyl is a highly lipophilic compound (octanol-water partition coefficient at pH 7.4 is 816:1) that is freely soluble in organic solvents and sparingly soluble in water (1:40). The molecular weight of the free base is 336.5 (the citrate salt is 528.6). The pKa of the tertiary nitrogens are 7.3 and 8.4.

Actiq is available in 6 strengths equivalent to 200, 400, 600, 800, 1200, or 1600 µg fentanyl base that is identified by the text on the foil pouch, the shelf carton, and the dosage unit handle.

Inactive Ingredients: Sucrose, liquid glucose, artificial raspberry flavor, and white dispersion G.B. dye.

CLINICAL PHARMACOLOGY

Fentanyl, a pure opioid agonist, acts primarily through interaction with opioid mu-receptors located in the brain, spinal cord and smooth muscle. The primary site of therapeutic action is the central nervous system (CNS). The most clinically useful pharmacologic effects of the interaction of fentanyl with mu-receptors are analgesia and sedation.

Other opioid effects may include somnolence, hypoventilation, bradycardia, postural hypotension, pruritus, dizziness, nausea, diaphoresis, flushing, euphoria and confusion or difficulty in concentrating at clinically relevant doses.

ANALGESIA

The analgesic effects of fentanyl are related to the blood level of the drug, if proper allowance is made for the delay into and out of the CNS (a process with a 3-5 minute half-life). In opioid non-tolerant individuals, fentanyl provides effects ranging from analgesia at blood levels of 1-2 ng/ml, all the way to surgical anesthesia and profound respiratory depression at levels of 10-20 ng/ml.

In general, the minimum effective concentration and the concentration at which toxicity occurs rise with increasing tolerance to any and all opioids. The rate of development of tolerance varies widely among individuals. As a result, the dose of Actiq should be individually titrated to achieve the desired effect (see DOSAGE AND ADMINISTRATION).

GASTROINTESTINAL (GI) TRACT AND OTHER SMOOTH MUSCLE

Opioids increase the tone and decrease contractions of the smooth muscle of the gastrointestinal (GI) tract. This results in prolongation in GI transit time and may be responsible for the constipating effect of opioids. Because opioids may increase biliary tract pressure, some patients with biliary colic may experience worsening of pain.

While opioids generally increase the tone of urinary tract smooth muscle, the overall effect tends to vary, in some cases producing urinary urgency, in others, difficulty in urination.

RESPIRATORY SYSTEM

All opioid mu-receptor agonists, including fentanyl, produce dose dependent respiratory depression. The risk of respiratory depression is less in patients receiving chronic opioid therapy who develop tolerance to respiratory depression and other opioid effects. During the titration phase of the clinical trials, somnolence, which may be a precursor to respiratory depression, did increase in patients who were treated with higher doses of Actiq. In studies of opioid non-tolerant subjects, respiratory rate and oxygen saturation typically decrease as fentanyl blood concentration increases. Typically, peak respiratory depressive effects (decrease in respiratory rate) are seen 15-30 minutes from the start of oral transmucosal fentanyl citrate (OTFC) administration and may persist for several hours.

Serious or fatal respiratory depression can occur, even at recommended doses, in vulnerable individuals. As with other potent opioids, fentanyl has been associated with cases of serious and fatal respiratory depression in opioid non-tolerant individuals.

Fentanyl depresses the cough reflex as a result of its CNS activity. Although not observed with Actiq in clinical trials, fentanyl given rapidly by IV injection in large doses may interfere with respiration by causing rigidity in the muscles of respiration. Therefore, physicians and other healthcare providers should be aware of this potential complication.

(See BOXED WARNING, CONTRAINDICATIONS, WARNINGS, PRECAUTIONS and ADVERSE REACTIONS for additional information on hypoventilation.)

CLINICAL PHARMACOLOGY
PHARMACOKINETICS
Absorption

The absorption pharmacokinetics of fentanyl from the oral transmucosal dosage form is a combination of an initial rapid absorption from the buccal mucosa and a more prolonged absorption of swallowed fentanyl from the GI tract. Both the blood fentanyl profile and the bioavailability of fentanyl will vary depending on the fraction of the dose that is absorbed through the oral mucosa and the fraction swallowed.

Absolute bioavailability, as determined by area under the concentration-time curve, of 15 µg/kg in 12 adult males was 50% compared to intravenous fentanyl.

Normally, approximately 25% of the total dose of Actiq is rapidly absorbed from the buccal mucosa and becomes systemically available. The remaining 75% of the total dose is swallowed with the saliva and then is slowly absorbed from the GI tract. About 1/3 of this amount (25% of the total dose) escapes hepatic and intestinal first-pass elimination and becomes systemically available. Thus, the generally observed 50% bioavailability of Actiq is divided equally between rapid transmucosal and slower GI absorption. Therefore, a unit dose of Actiq, if chewed and swallowed, might result in lower peak concentrations and lower bioavailability than when consumed as directed.

Dose proportionality among 4 of the available strengths of Actiq (200, 400, 800, and 1600 µg) has been demonstrated in a balanced crossover design in adult subjects.

The pharmacokinetic parameters of the 4 strengths of Actiq tested in the dose-proportionality study are shown in TABLE 1. The mean C_{max} ranged from 0.39-2.51 ng/ml. The median time of maximum plasma concentration (T_{max}) across these 4 doses of Actiq varied from 20-40 minutes (range of 20-480 minutes) after a standardized consumption time of 15 minutes.

TABLE 1 *Pharmacokinetic Parameters in Adult Subjects Receiving 200, 400, 800, and 1600 µg Units of Actiq*

Pharmacokinetic Parameters	200 µg	400 µg	800 µg	1600 µg
T_{max}, min				
median (range)	40 (20-120)	25 (20-240)	25 (20-120)	20 (20-480)
C_{max}, ng/ml				
mean (%CV)	0.39 (23)	0.75 (33)	1.55 (30)	2.51 (23)
AUC(0-1440), ng/ml·min				
mean (%CV)	102 (65)	243 (67)	573 (64)	1026 (67)
T½, min				
mean (%CV)	193 (48)	386 (115)	381 (55)	358 (45)

Distribution

Fentanyl is highly lipophilic. Animal data showed that following absorption, fentanyl is rapidly distributed to the brain, heart, lungs, kidneys and spleen followed by a slower redistribution to muscles and fat. The plasma protein binding of fentanyl is 80-85%. The main binding protein is alpha-1-acid glycoprotein, but both albumin and lipoproteins contribute to some extent. The free fraction of fentanyl increases with acidosis. The mean volume of distribution at steady state (Vss) was 4 L/kg.

Metabolism

Fentanyl is metabolized in the liver and in the intestinal mucosa to norfentanyl by cytochrome P450 3A4 isoform. Norfentanyl was not found to be pharmacologically active in animal studies (see DRUG INTERACTIONS for additional information).

Elimination

Fentanyl is primarily (more than 90%) eliminated by biotransformation to N-dealkylated and hydroxylated inactive metabolites. Less than 7% of the dose is excreted unchanged in the urine, and only about 1% is excreted unchanged in the feces. The metabolites are mainly excreted in the urine, while fecal excretion is less important. The total plasma clearance of fentanyl was 0.5 L/h/kg (range 0.3-0.7 L/h/kg). The terminal elimination half-life after OTFC administration is about 7 hours.

Special Populations

Elderly Patients

Elderly patients have been shown to be twice as sensitive to the effects of fentanyl when administered intravenously, compared with the younger population. While a formal study evaluating the safety profile of Actiq in the elderly population has not been performed, in the 257 opioid tolerant cancer patients studied with Actiq, approximately 20% were over age 65 years. No difference was noted in the safety profile in this group compared to those aged less than 65 years, though they did titrate to lower doses than younger patients (see PRECAUTIONS).

Patients With Renal or Hepatic Impairment

Actiq should be administered with caution to patients with liver or kidney dysfunction because of the importance of these organs in the metabolism and excretion of drugs and effects on plasma-binding proteins (see PRECAUTIONS).

Although fentanyl kinetics are known to be altered in both hepatic and renal disease due to alterations in metabolic clearance and plasma proteins, individualized doses of Actiq have been used successfully for breakthrough cancer pain in patients with hepatic and renal disorders. The duration of effect for the initial dose of fentanyl is determined by redistribution of the drug, such that diminished metabolic clearance may only become significant with repeated dosing or with excessively large single doses. For these reasons, while doses titrated to clinical effect are recommended for all patients, special care should be taken in patients with severe hepatic or renal disease.

Gender

Both male and female opioid-tolerant cancer patients were studied for the treatment of breakthrough cancer pain. No clinically relevant gender differences were noted either in dosage requirement or in observed adverse events.

INDICATIONS AND USAGE

See BOXED WARNING and CONTRAINDICATIONS.

Actiq is indicated only for the management of breakthrough cancer pain in patients with malignancies who are **already receiving and who are tolerant to opioid therapy for their underlying persistent cancer pain.** Patients considered opioid tolerant are those who are taking at least 60 mg morphine/day, 50 µg transdermal fentanyl/hour, or an equianalgesic dose of another opioid for a week or longer.

Because life-threatening hypoventilation could occur at any dose in patients not taking chronic opiates, Actiq is contraindicated in the management of acute or postoperative pain. This product **must not** be used in opioid non-tolerant patients.

Actiq is intended to be used only in the care of cancer patients only by oncologists and pain specialists who are knowledgeable of and skilled in the use of Schedule II opioids to treat cancer pain.

Actiq should be individually titrated to a dose that provides adequate analgesia and minimizes side effects. If signs of excessive opioid effects appear before the unit is consumed, the dosage unit should be removed from the patient's mouth immediately, disposed of properly, and subsequent doses should be decreased (see DOSAGE AND ADMINISTRATION).

Patients and their caregivers must be instructed that Actiq contains a medicine in an amount that can be fatal to a child. Patients and their caregivers must be instructed to keep all units out of the reach of children and to discard opened units properly in a secured container.

CONTRAINDICATIONS

Because life-threatening hypoventilation could occur at any dose in patients not taking chronic opiates, Actiq is contraindicated in the management of acute or postoperative pain. The risk of respiratory depression begins to increase with fentanyl plasma levels of 2.0 ng/ml in opioid non-tolerant individuals (see CLINICAL PHARMACOLOGY, Pharmacokinetics). This product **must not** be used in opioid non-tolerant patients.

Patients considered opioid tolerant are those who are taking at least 60 mg morphine/day, 50 µg transdermal fentanyl/hour, or an equianalgesic dose of another opioid for a week or longer.

Actiq is contraindicated in patients with known intolerance or hypersensitivity to any of its components or the drug fentanyl.

WARNINGS

See BOXED WARNING.

The concomitant use of other CNS depressants, including other opioids, sedatives or hypnotics, general anesthetics, phenothiazines, tranquilizers, skeletal muscle relaxants, sedating antihistamines, potent inhibitors of cytochrome P450 3A4 isoform (*e.g.,* erythromycin, ketoconazole, and certain protease inhibitors), and alcoholic beverages may produce increased depressant effects. Hypoventilation, hypotension, and profound sedation may occur.

Actiq is not recommended for use in patients who have received MAO inhibitors within 14 days, because severe and unpredictable potentiation by MAO inhibitors has been reported with opioid analgesics.

PEDIATRIC USE

The appropriate dosing and safety of Actiq in opioid tolerant children with breakthrough cancer pain have not been established below the age of 16 years.

Patients and their caregivers must be instructed that Actiq contains a medicine in an amount which can be fatal to a child. Patients and their caregivers must be instructed to keep both used and unused dosage units out of the reach of children. While all units should be disposed of immediately after use, partially consumed units represent a special risk to children. In the event that a unit is not completely consumed it must be properly disposed as soon as possible. (See HOW SUPPLIED, Safety and Handling, PRECAUTIONS, and the Patient Leaflet distributed with the prescription for specific patient instructions.)

Physicians and dispensing pharmacists must specifically question patients or caregivers about the presence of children in the home on a full time or visiting basis and counsel them regarding the dangers to children from inadvertent exposure.

PRECAUTIONS

GENERAL

The initial dose of Actiq to treat episodes of breakthrough cancer pain should be 200 µg. Each patient should be individually titrated to provide adequate analgesia while minimizing side effects.

Opioid analgesics impair the mental and/or physical ability required for the performance of potentially dangerous tasks (*e.g.,* driving a car or operating machinery). Patients taking Actiq should be warned of these dangers and should be counseled accordingly.

The use of concomitant CNS active drugs requires special patient care and observation. (See WARNINGS.)

HYPOVENTILATION (RESPIRATORY DEPRESSION)

As with all opioids, there is a risk of clinically significant hypoventilation in patients using Actiq. Accordingly, all patients should be followed for symptoms of respiratory depression. Hypoventilation may occur more readily when opioids are given in conjunction with other agents that depress respiration.

CHRONIC PULMONARY DISEASE

Because potent opioids can cause hypoventilation, Actiq should be titrated with caution in patients with chronic obstructive pulmonary disease or pre-existing medical conditions predisposing them to hypoventilation. In such patients, even normal therapeutic doses of Actiq may further decrease respiratory drive to the point of respiratory failure.

HEAD INJURIES AND INCREASED INTRACRANIAL PRESSURE

Actiq should only be administered with extreme caution in patients who may be particularly susceptible to the intracranial effects of CO_2 retention such as those with evidence of increased intracranial pressure or impaired consciousness. Opioids may obscure the clinical course of a patient with a head injury and should be used only if clinically warranted.

CARDIAC DISEASE

Intravenous fentanyl may produce bradycardia. Therefore, Actiq should be used with caution in patients with bradyarrhythmias.

HEPATIC OR RENAL DISEASE

Actiq should be administered with caution to patients with liver or kidney dysfunction because of the importance of these organs in the metabolism and excretion of drugs and effects on plasma binding proteins (see CLINICAL PHARMACOLOGY, Pharmacokinetics).

INFORMATION FOR PATIENTS AND THEIR CAREGIVERS

Patients and their caregivers must be instructed that Actiq contains medicine in an amount that could be fatal to a child. Patients and their caregivers must be instructed to keep both used and unused dosage units out of the reach of children. Partially consumed units represent a special risk to children. In the event that a unit is not completely consumed it must be properly disposed as soon as possible. (See HOW SUPPLIED, Safety and Handling, WARNINGS, and the Patient Leaflet distributed with the prescription for specific patient instructions.)

Frequent consumption of sugar-containing products may increase the risk of dental caries (each Acquid unit contains approximately 2 g of sugar [sucrose, liquid glucose]). The occurrence of dry mouth associated with the use of opioid medications (such as fentanyl) may add to this risk. Therefore, patients using Actiq should consult their dentist to ensure appropriate oral hygiene.

Diabetic patients should be advised that Actiq contains approximately 2 g of sugar per unit.

Patients and their caregivers should be provided with an Actiq Welcome Kit, which contains educational materials and safe storage containers to help patients store Actiq and other medicines out of the reach of children. Patients and their caregivers should also have an opportunity to watch the patient safety video, which provides proper product use, storage, handling and disposal directions. Patients should also have an opportunity to discuss the video with their health care providers. Health care professionals should call 1-800-896-5855 to obtain a supply of welcome kits or videos for patient viewing.

DISPOSAL OF USED ACTIQ UNITS

Patients must be instructed to dispose of completely used and partially used Actiq units.

1. After consumption of the unit is complete and the matrix is totally dissolved, throw away the handle in a trash container that is out of the reach of children.
2. If any of the drug matrix remains on the handle, place the handle under hot running tap water until all of the drug matrix is dissolved, and then dispose of the handle in a place that is out of the reach of children.
3. Handles in the child-resistant container should be disposed of (as described in steps 1 and 2) at least once a day.

If the patient does not entirely consume the unit and the remaining drug cannot be immediately dissolved under hot running water, the patient or caregiver must temporarily store the Actiq unit in the specially provided child-resistant container out of the reach of children until proper disposal is possible.

DISPOSAL OF UNOPENED ACTIQ UNITS WHEN NO LONGER NEEDED

Patients and members of their household must be advised to dispose of any unopened units remaining from a prescription as soon as they are no longer needed.

To dispose of the unused Actiq units:

1. Remove the Actiq unit from its pouch using scissors, and hold the Actiq by its handle over the toilet bowl.
2. Using wire-cutting pliers cut off the drug matrix end so that it falls into the toilet.
3. Dispose of the handle in a place that is out of the reach of children.
4. Repeat steps 1, 2, and 3 for each Actiq unit. Flush the toilet twice after 5 units have been cut and deposited into the toilet.

Do not flush the entire Actiq units, Actiq handles, foil pouches, or cartons down the toilet. The handle should be disposed of where children cannot reach it (see HOW SUPPLIED, Safety and Handling).

Detailed instructions for the proper storage, administration, disposal, and important instructions for managing an overdose of Actiq are provided in the Actiq Patient Leaflet. Patients should be encouraged to read this information in its entirety and be given an opportunity to have their questions answered.

In the event that a caregiver requires additional assistance in disposing of excess unusable units that remain in the home after a patient has expired, they should be instructed to call the toll-free number (1-800-896-5855) or seek assistance from their local DEA office.

LABORATORY TESTS

The effects of Actiq on laboratory tests have not been evaluated.

CARCINOGENESIS, MUTAGENESIS, AND IMPAIRMENT OF FERTILITY

Because animal carcinogenicity studies have not been conducted with fentanyl citrate, the potential carcinogenic effect of Actiq is unknown.

Standard mutagenicity testing of fentanyl citrate has been conducted. There was no evidence of mutagenicity in the Ames *Salmonella* or *Escherichia* mutagenicity assay, the *in vitro* mouse lymphoma mutagenesis assay, and the *in vivo* micronucleus cytogenetic assay in the mouse.

Reproduction studies in rats revealed a significant decrease in the pregnancy rate of all experimental groups. This decrease was most pronounced in the high dose group (1.25 mg/kg subcutaneously) in which 1 of 20 animals became pregnant.

PREGNANCY CATEGORY C

Fentanyl has been shown to impair fertility and to have an embryocidal effect with an increase in resorptions in rats when given for a period of 12-21 days in doses of 30 µg/kg IV or 160 µg/kg subcutaneously.

No evidence of teratogenic effects has been observed after administration of fentanyl citrate to rats. There are no adequate and well-controlled studies in pregnant women. Actiq should be used during pregnancy only if the potential benefit justifies the potential risk to the fetus.

LABOR AND DELIVERY

Actiq is not indicated for use in labor and delivery.

NURSING MOTHERS

Fentanyl is excreted in human milk; therefore Actiq should not be used in nursing women because of the possibility of sedation and/or respiratory depression in their infants.

PEDIATRIC USE

See WARNINGS.

GERIATRIC USE

Of the 257 patients in clinical studies of Actiq in breakthrough cancer pain, 61 (24%) were 65 and over, while 15 (6%) were 75 and over.

Those patients over the age of 65 titrated to a mean dose that was about 200 µg less than the mean dose titrated to by younger patients. Previous studies with intravenous fentanyl showed that elderly patients are twice as sensitive to the effects of fentanyl as the younger population.

No difference was noted in the safety profile of the group over 65 as compared to younger patients in Actiq clinical trials. However, greater sensitivity in older individuals cannot be ruled out. Therefore, caution should be exercised in individually titrating Actiq in elderly patients to provide adequate efficacy while minimizing risk.

DRUG INTERACTIONS

See WARNINGS.

Fentanyl is metabolized in the liver and intestinal mucosa to norfentanyl by the cytochrome P450 3A4 isoform. Drugs that inhibit P450 3A4 activity may increase the bioavailability of swallowed fentanyl (by decreasing intestinal and hepatic first pass metabolism) and may decrease the systemic clearance of fentanyl. The expected clinical results would be increased or prolonged opioid effects. Drugs that induce cytochrome P450 3A4 activity may have the opposite effects. However, no *in vitro* or *in vivo* studies have been performed to assess the impact of those potential interactions on the administration of Actiq. Thus patients who begin or end therapy with potent inhibitors of CYP450 3A4 such as macrolide antibiotics (*e.g.,* erythromycin), azole antifungal agents (*e.g.,* ketoconazole and itraconazole), and protease inhibitors (*e.g.,* ritanovir) while receiving Actiq should be monitored for a change in opioid effects and, if warranted, the dose of Actiq should be adjusted.

ADVERSE REACTIONS

PRE-MARKETING CLINICAL TRIAL EXPERIENCE

The safety of Actiq has been evaluated in 257 opioid tolerant chronic cancer pain patients. The duration of Actiq use varied during the open-label study. Some patients were followed for over 21 months. The average duration of therapy in the open-label study was 129 days.

The adverse events seen with Actiq are typical opioid side effects. Frequently, these adverse events will cease or decrease in intensity with continued use of Actiq, as the patient is titrated to the proper dose. Opioid side effects should be expected and managed accordingly.

The most serious adverse effects associated with all opioids are respiratory depression (potentially leading to apnea or respiratory arrest), circulatory depression, hypotension, and shock. All patients should be followed for symptoms of respiratory depression.

Because the clinical trials of Actiq were designed to evaluate safety and efficacy in treating breakthrough cancer pain, all patients were also taking concomitant opioids, such as sustained-release morphine or transdermal fentanyl, for their persistent cancer pain. The adverse event data presented here reflect the actual percentage of patients experiencing each adverse effect among patients who received Actiq for breakthrough cancer pain along with a concomitant opioid for persistent cancer pain. There has been no attempt to correct for concomitant use of other opioids, duration of Actiq therapy, or cancer-related symptoms. Adverse events are included regardless of causality or severity.

Three short-term clinical trials with similar titration schemes were conducted in 257 patients with malignancy and breakthrough cancer pain. Data are available for 254 of these patients. The goal of titration in these trials was to find the dose of Actiq that provided adequate analgesia with acceptable side effects (successful dose). Patients were titrated from a low dose to a successful dose in a manner similar to current titration dosing guidelines. TABLE 3 lists by dose groups, adverse events with an overall frequency of 1% or greater that occurred during titration and are commonly associated with opioid administration or are of particular clinical interest. The ability to assign a dose-response relationship to these adverse events is limited by the titration schemes used in these studies. Adverse events are listed in descending order of frequency within each body system.

The following adverse events not reflected in TABLE 3 occurred during titration with an overall frequency of 1% or greater and are listed in descending order of frequency within each body system:

Body as a Whole: Pain, fever, abdominal pain, chills, back pain, chest pain, infection.
Cardiovascular: Migraine.
Digestive: Diarrhea, dyspepsia, flatulence.
Metabolic and Nutritional: Peripheral edema, dehydration.
Nervous: Hypesthesia.
Respiratory: Pharyngitis, cough increased.

The following events occurred during titration with an overall frequency of less than 1% and are listed in descending order of frequency within each body system:

Body as a Whole: Flu syndrome, abscess, bone pain.
Cardiovascular: Deep thrombophlebitis, hypertension, hypotension.
Digestive: Anorexia, eructation, esophageal stenosis, fecal impaction, gum hemorrhage, mouth ulceration, oral moniliasis.
Hemic and Lymphatic: Anemia, leukopenia.
Metabolic and Nutritional: Edema, hypercalcemia, weight loss.
Musculoskeletal: Myalgia, pathological fracture, myasthenia.
Nervous: Abnormal dreams, urinary retention, agitation, amnesia, emotional lability, euphoria, incoordination, libido decreased, neuropathy, paresthesia, speech disorder.
Respiratory: Hemoptysis, pleural effusion, rhinitis, asthma, hiccup, pneumonia, respiratory insufficiency, sputum increased.
Skin and Appendages: Alopecia, exfoliative dermatitis.
Special Senses: Taste perversion.
Urogenital: Vaginal hemorrhage, dysuria, hematuria, urinary incontinence, urinary tract infection.

A long-term extension study was conducted in 156 patients with malignancy and breakthrough cancer pain who were treated for an average of 129 days. Data are available for 152 of these patients. TABLE 4 lists by dose groups, adverse events with an overall frequency of 1% or greater that occurred during the long-term extension study and are commonly

TABLE 3 *Percent of Patients With Specific Adverse Events Commonly Associated With Opioid Administration or of Particular Clinical Interest Which Occurred During Titration — Events in 1% or More of Patients*

	Dose Group (μg)				
	200-600	800-1400	1600	>1600	Any
	n=230	n=138	n=54	n=41	n=254
Body as a Whole					
Asthenia	6%	4%	0%	7%	9%
Headache	3%	4%	6%	5%	6%
Accidental injury	1%	1%	4%	0%	2%
Digestive					
Nausea	14%	15%	11%	22%	23%
Vomiting	7%	6%	6%	15%	12%
Constipation	1%	4%	2%	0%	4%
Nervous					
Dizziness	10%	16%	6%	15%	17%
Somnolence	9%	9%	11%	20%	17%
Confusion	1%	6%	2%	0%	4%
Anxiety	3%	0%	2%	0%	3%
Abnormal gait	0%	1%	4%	0%	2%
Dry mouth	1%	1%	2%	0%	2%
Nervousness	1%	1%	0%	0%	2%
Vasodilatation	2%	0%	2%	0%	2%
Hallucinations	0%	1%	2%	2%	1%
Insomnia	0%	1%	2%	0%	1%
Thinking abnormal	0%	1%	2%	0%	1%
Vertigo	1%	0%	0%	0%	1%
Respiratory					
Dyspnea	2%	3%	6%	5%	4%
Skin					
Pruritus	1%	0%	0%	5%	2%
Rash	1%	1%	0%	2%	2%
Sweating	1%	1%	2%	2%	2%
Special Senses					
Abnormal vision	1%	0%	2%	0%	2%

associated with opioid administration or are of particular clinical interest. Adverse events are listed in descending order of frequency within each body system.

TABLE 4 *Percent of Patients With Adverse Events Commonly Associated With Opioid Administration or of Particular Clinical Interest Which Occurred During Long-Term Treatment — Events in 1% or More of Patients*

	Dose Group (μg)				
	200-600	800-1400	1600	>1600	Any
	n=98	n=83	n=53	n=27	n=152
Body as a Whole					
Asthenia	25%	30%	17%	15%	38%
Headache	12%	17%	13%	4%	20%
Accidental injury	4%	6%	4%	7%	9%
Hypertonia	2%	2%	2%	0%	3%
Digestive					
Nausea	31%	36%	25%	26%	45%
Vomiting	21%	28%	15%	7%	31%
Constipation	14%	11%	13%	4%	20%
Intestinal obstruction	0%	2%	4%	0%	3%
Cardiovascular					
Hypertension	1%	1%	0%	0%	1%
Nervous					
Dizziness	12%	10%	9%	0%	16%
Anxiety	9%	8%	8%	7%	15%
Somnolence	8%	13%	8%	7%	15%
Confusion	2%	5%	13%	7%	10%
Depression	9%	4%	2%	7%	9%
Insomnia	5%	1%	8%	4%	7%
Abnormal gait	5%	1%	0%	0%	4%
Dry mouth	3%	1%	2%	4%	4%
Nervousness	2%	2%	0%	4%	3%
Stupor	4%	1%	0%	0%	3%
Vasodilatation	1%	1%	4%	0%	3%
Thinking abnormal	2%	1%	0%	0%	2%
Abnormal dreams	1%	1%	0%	0%	1%
Convulsion	0%	1%	2%	0%	1%
Myoclonus	0%	0%	4%	0%	1%
Tremor	0%	1%	2%	0%	1%
Vertigo	0%	0%	4%	0%	1%
Respiratory					
Dyspnea	15%	16%	8%	7%	22%
Skin					
Rash	3%	5%	8%	4%	8%
Sweating	3%	2%	2%	0%	4%
Pruritus	2%	0%	2%	0%	2%
Special Senses					
Abnormal vision	2%	2%	0%	0%	3%
Urogenital					
Urinary retention	1%	2%	0%	0%	2%

The following events not reflected in TABLE 4 occurred with an overall frequency of 1% or greater in the long-term extension study and are listed in descending order of frequency within each body system:

Body as a Whole: Pain, fever, back pain, abdominal pain, chest pain, flu syndrome, chills, infection, abdomen enlarged, bone pain, ascites, sepsis, neck pain, viral infection, fungal infection, cachexia, cellulitis, malaise, pelvic pain.

Cardiovascular: Deep thrombophlebitis, migraine, palpitation, vascular disorder.

Digestive: Diarrhea, anorexia, dyspepsia, dysphagia, oral moniliasis, mouth ulceration, rectal disorder, stomatitis, flatulence, gastrointestinal hemorrhage, gingivitis, jaundice, periodontal abscess, eructation, glossitis, rectal hemorrhage.

Hemic and Lymphatic: Anemia, leukopenia, thrombocytopenia, ecchymosis, lymphadenopathy, lymphedema, pancytopenia.

Metabolic and Nutritional: Peripheral edema, edema, dehydration, weight loss, hyperglycemia, hypokalemia, hypercalcemia, hypomagnesemia.

Musculoskeletal: Myalgia, pathological fracture, joint disorder, leg cramps, arthralgia, bone disorder.

Nervous: Hypesthesia, paresthesia, hypokinesia, neuropathy, speech disorder.

Respiratory: Cough increased, pharyngitis, pneumonia, rhinitis, sinusitis, bronchitis, epistaxis, asthma, hemoptysis, sputum increased.

Skin and Appendages: Skin ulcer, alopecia.

Special Senses: Tinnitus, conjunctivitis, ear disorder, taste perversion.

Urogenital: Urinary tract infection, urinary incontinence, breast pain, dysuria, hematuria, scrotal edema, hydronephrosis, kidney failure, urinary urgency, urination impaired, breast neoplasm, vaginal hemorrhage, vaginitis.

The following events occurred with a frequency of less than 1% in the long-term extension study and are listed in descending order of frequency within each body system:

Body as a Whole: Allergic reaction, cyst, face edema, flank pain, granuloma, bacterial infection, injection site pain, mucous membrane disorder, neck rigidity.

Cardiovascular: Angina pectoris, hemorrhage, hypotension, peripheral vascular disorder, postural hypotension, tachycardia.

Digestive: Cheilitis, esophagitis, fecal incontinence, gastroenteritis, gastrointestinal disorder, gum hemorrhage, hemorrhage of colon, hepatorenal syndrome, liver tenderness, tooth caries, tooth disorder.

Hemic and Lymphatic: Bleeding time increased.

Metabolic and Nutritional: Acidosis, generalized edema, hypocalcemia, hypoglycemia, hyponatremia, hypoproteinemia, thirst.

Musculoskeletal: Arthritis, muscle atrophy, myopathy, synovitis, tendon disorder.

Nervous: Acute brain syndrome, agitation, cerebral ischemia, facial paralysis, foot drop, hallucinations, hemiplegia, miosis, subdural hematoma.

Respiratory: Hiccup, hyperventilation, lung disorder, pneumothorax, respiratory failure, voice alteration.

Skin and Appendages: Herpes zoster, maculopapular rash, skin discoloration, urticaria, vesiculobullous rash.

Special Senses: Ear pain, eye hemorrhage, lacrimation disorder, partial permanent deafness, partial transitory deafness.

Urogenital: Kidney pain, nocturia, oliguria, polyuria, pyelonephritis.

DOSAGE AND ADMINISTRATION

Actiq is contraindicated in non-opioid tolerant individuals.

Actiq should be individually titrated to a dose that provides adequate analgesia and minimizes side effects (see Dose Titration).

As with all opioids, the safety of patients using such products is dependent on health care professionals prescribing them in strict conformity with their approved labeling with respect to patient selection, dosing, and proper conditions for use.

Physicians and dispensing pharmacists must specifically question patients and caregivers about the presence of children in the home on a full time or visiting basis and counsel accordingly regarding the dangers to children of inadvertent exposure to Actiq.

ADMINISTRATION OF ACTIQ

The foil package should be opened with scissors immediately prior to product use. The patient should place the Actiq unit in his or her mouth between the cheek and lower gum, occasionally moving the drug matrix from one side to the other using the handle. The Actiq unit should be sucked, not chewed. A unit dose of Actiq, if chewed and swallowed, might result in lower peak concentrations and lower bioavailability than when consumed as directed.

The Actiq unit should be consumed over a 15 minute period. Longer or shorter consumption times may produce less efficacy than reported in Actiq clinical trials. If signs of excessive opioid effects appear before the unit is consumed, the drug matrix should be removed from the patient's mouth immediately and future doses should be decreased.

Patients and caregivers must be instructed that Actiq contains medicine in an amount that could be fatal to a child. While all units should be disposed of immediately after use, partially used units represent a special risk and must be disposed of as soon as they are consumed and/or no longer needed. Patients and caregivers should be advised to dispose of any units remaining from a prescription as soon as they are no longer needed (see Disposal of Actiq).

DOSE TITRATION

Starting Dose

The initial dose of Actiq to treat episodes of breakthrough cancer pain should be 200 μg. Patients should be prescribed an initial titration supply of six 200 μg Actiq units, thus limiting the number of units in the home during titration. Patients should use up all units before increasing to a higher dose.

From this initial dose, patients should be closely followed and the dosage level changed until the patient reaches a dose that provides adequate analgesia using a single Actiq dosage unit per breakthrough cancer pain episode.

Patients should record their use of Actiq over several episodes of breakthrough cancer pain and review their experience with their physicians to determine if a dosage adjustment is warranted.

Redosing Within a Single Episode
Until the appropriate dose is reached, patients may find it necessary to use an additional Actiq unit during a single episode. Redosing may start 15 minutes after the previous unit has been completed (30 minutes after the start of the previous unit). While patients are in the titration phase and consuming units which individually may be subtherapeutic, no more than 2 units should be taken for each individual breakthrough cancer pain episode.

Increasing the Dose
If treatment of several consecutive breakthrough cancer pain episodes requires more than one Actiq per episode, an increase in dose to the next higher available strength should be considered. At each new dose of Actiq during titration, it is recommended that 6 units of the titration dose be prescribed. Each new dose of Actiq used in the titration period should be evaluated over several episodes of breakthrough cancer pain (generally 1-2 days) to determine whether it provides adequate efficacy with acceptable side effects. The incidence of side effects is likely to be greater during this initial titration period compared to later, after the effective dose is determined.

Daily Limit
Once a successful dose has been found (*i.e.*, an average episode is treated with a single unit), patients should limit consumption to 4 or fewer units per day. If consumption increases above 4 units/day, the dose of the long-acting opioid used for persistent cancer pain should be re-evaluated.

ACTIQ TITRATION PROCESS
See BOXED WARNING.
I. Start at 200 μg (dispense no more than 6 units initially).
1. Consume Actiq unit over 15 minutes.
2. Wait 15 more minutes.
3. If needed, consume second unit over 15 minutes.
4. Try the Actiq dose for several episodes of breakthrough pain.

II. Adequate relief with one unit?
If **yes**, then a successful dose was determined.
If **no**, then increase dose to next highest strength* (dispense no more than 6 units initially), and return to Step I.
*Available dosage strengths include: 200, 400, 600, 800, 1200, and 1600 μg.

DOSE ADJUSTMENT
Experience in a long-term study of Actiq used in the treatment of breakthrough cancer pain suggests that dosage adjustment of both Actiq and the maintenance (around-the-clock) opioid analgesic may be required in some patients to continue to provide adequate relief of breakthrough cancer pain.

Generally, the Actiq dose should be increased when patients require more than one dosage unit per breakthrough cancer pain episode for several consecutive episodes. When titrating to an appropriate dose, small quantities (6 units) should be prescribed at each titration step. Physicians should consider increasing the around-the-clock opioid dose used for persistent cancer pain in patients experiencing more than 4 breakthrough cancer pain episodes daily.

DISCONTINUATION OF ACTIQ
For patients requiring discontinuation of opioids, a gradual downward titration is recommended because it is not known at what dose level the opioid may be discontinued without producing the signs and symptoms of abrupt withdrawal.

DISPOSAL OF ACTIQ
Patients must be advised to dispose of any units remaining from a prescription as soon as they are no longer needed. While all units should be disposed of immediately after use, partially consumed units represent a special risk because they are no longer protected by the child resistant pouch, yet may contain enough medicine to be fatal to a child (see PRECAUTIONS, Information for Patients and Their Caregivers).

A temporary storage bottle is provided as part of the Actiq Welcome Kit (see PRECAUTIONS, Information for Patients and Their Caregivers). This container is to be used by patients or their caregivers in the event that a partially consumed unit cannot be disposed of promptly. Instructions for usage of this container are included in the patient leaflet.

Patients and members of their household must be advised to dispose of any units remaining from a prescription as soon as they are no longer needed. Instructions are included in PRECAUTIONS, Information for Patients and Their Caregivers and in the patient leaflet. If additional assistance is required, referral to the Actiq 800 number (1–800–896–5855) should be made.

HOW SUPPLIED

Actiq is supplied in 6 dosage strengths. Each unit is individually wrapped in a child-resistant, protective foil pouch. These foil pouches are packed 24 per shelf carton for use when patients have been titrated to the appropriate dose.

Patients should be prescribed an initial titration supply of six 200 μg Actiq units. At each new dose of Actiq during titration, it is recommended that only 6 units of the next higher dose be prescribed.

Each dosage unit has a white to off-white color. The dosage strength of each unit is marked on the handle, the foil pouch and the carton.

SAFETY AND HANDLING
Actiq is supplied in individually sealed child-resistant foil pouches. The amount of fentanyl contained in Actiq can be fatal to a child. Patients and their caregivers must be instructed to keep Actiq out of the reach of children (see BOXED WARNING, WARNINGS, PRECAUTIONS and the Patient Leaflet distributed with the prescription).

Storage
Store at 25°C (77°F) with excursions permitted between 15° and 30°C (59-86°F) until ready to use.

TABLE 5

Dosage Strength (fentanyl base)	Carton/Foil Pouch Color
200 μg	Gray
400 μg	Blue
600 μg	Orange
800 μg	Purple
1200 μg	Green
1600 μg	Burgundy

Note: Colors are a secondary aid in product identification. Please be sure to confirm the printed dosage before dispensing.

Actiq should be protected from freezing and moisture. Do not store above 25°C. Do not use if the foil pouch has been opened.

TRANSDERMAL

WARNING

Note: The trade names have been used throughout this monograph for clarity.

BECAUSE SERIOUS OR LIFE-THREATENING HYPOVENTILATION COULD OCCUR, DURAGESIC IS CONTRAINDICATED:
- **In the management of acute or postoperative pain, including use in out-patient surgeries.**
- **In the management of mild or intermittent pain responsive to prn or non-opioid therapy.**
- **In doses exceeding 25 μg/h at the initiation of opioid therapy.**

(See CONTRAINDICATIONS for further information.)

DURAGESIC SHOULD NOT BE ADMINISTERED TO CHILDREN UNDER 12 YEARS OF AGE OR PATIENTS UNDER 18 YEARS OF AGE WHO WEIGH LESS THAN 50 KG (110 LB) EXCEPT IN AN AUTHORIZED INVESTIGATIONAL RESEARCH SETTING. (See PRECAUTIONS, Pediatric Use.)

Duragesic is indicated for treatment of chronic pain (such as that of malignancy) that:
- **Cannot be managed by lesser means such as acetaminophen-opioid combinations, non-steroidal analgesics, or prn dosing with short-acting opioids and**
- **Requires continuous opioid administration.**

The 50, 75, and 100 μg/h dosages should ONLY be used in patients who are already on and are tolerant to opioid therapy.

DESCRIPTION

Duragesic is a transdermal system providing continuous systemic delivery of fentanyl, a potent opioid analgesic, for 72 hours. The chemical name is N-Phenyl-N-(1-2-phenylethyl-4-piperidyl) propanamide.

The molecular weight of fentanyl base is 336.5, and the empirical formula is $C_{22}H_{28}N_2O$. The n-octanol:water partition coefficient is 860:1. The pKa is 8.4.

SYSTEM COMPONENTS AND STRUCTURE
The amount of fentanyl released from each system per hour is proportional to the surface area (25 μg/h/10 cm^2). The composition per unit area of all system sizes is identical. Each system also contains 0.1 ml of alcohol per 10 cm^2.

TABLE 6

Dose*	Size	Fentanyl Content
25 μg/h	10 cm^2	2.5 mg
50 μg/h†	20 cm^2	5 mg
75 μg/h†	30 cm^2	7.5 mg
100 μg/h†	40 cm^2	10 mg

* Nominal delivery rate per hour.
† FOR USE ONLY IN OPIOID TOLERANT PATIENTS.

Duragesic is a rectangular transparent unit comprising a protective liner and 4 functional layers. Proceeding from the outer surface toward the surface adhering to skin, these layers are:
1. A backing layer of polyester film;
2. A drug reservoir of fentanyl and alcohol gelled with hydroxyethyl cellulose;
3. An ethylene-vinyl acetate copolymer membrane that controls the rate of fentanyl delivery to the skin surface; and
4. A fentanyl containing silicone adhesive. Before use, a protective liner covering the adhesive layer is removed and discarded.

The active component of the system is fentanyl. The remaining components are pharmacologically inactive. Less than 0.2 ml of alcohol is also released from the system during use.

Do not cut or damage Duragesic. If the Duragesic system is cut or damaged, controlled drug delivery will not be possible.

CLINICAL PHARMACOLOGY

Fentanyl is an opioid analgesic. Fentanyl interacts predominately with the opioid μ-receptor. These μ-binding sites are discretely distributed in the human brain, spinal cord, and other tissues.

In clinical settings, fentanyl exerts its principal pharmacologic effects on the central nervous system. Its primary actions of therapeutic value are analgesia and sedation. Fentanyl may increase the patient's tolerance for pain and decrease the perception of suffering, although the presence of the pain itself may still be recognized.

In addition to analgesia, alterations in mood, euphoria and dysphoria, and drowsiness commonly occur. Fentanyl depresses the respiratory centers, depresses the cough reflex, and constricts the pupils. Analgesic blood levels of fentanyl may cause nausea and vomiting directly by stimulating the chemoreceptor trigger zone, but nausea and vomiting are significantly more common in ambulatory than in recumbent patients, as is postural syncope.

Opioids increase the tone and decrease the propulsive contractions of the smooth muscle of the gastrointestinal tract. The resultant prolongation in gastrointestinal transit time may be responsible for the constipating effect of fentanyl. Because opioids may increase biliary tract pressure, some patients with biliary colic may experience worsening rather than relief of pain.

While opioids generally increase the tone of urinary tract smooth muscle, the net effect tends to be variable, in some cases producing urinary urgency, in others, difficulty in urination.

At therapeutic dosages, fentanyl usually does not exert major effects on the cardiovascular system. However, some patients may exhibit orthostatic hypotension and fainting.

Histamine assays and skin wheal testing in man indicate that clinically significant histamine release rarely occurs with fentanyl administration. Assays in man show no clinically significant histamine release in dosages up to 50 μg/kg.

PHARMACOKINETICS

See TABLE 7 and TABLE 8.

Duragesic releases fentanyl from the reservoir at a nearly constant amount per unit time. The concentration gradient existing between the saturated solution of drug in the reservoir and the lower concentration in the skin drives drug release. Fentanyl moves in the direction of the lower concentration at a rate determined by the copolymer release membrane and the diffusion of fentanyl through the skin layers. While the actual rate of fentanyl delivery to the skin varies over the 72 hour application period, each system is labeled with a nominal flux which represents the average amount of drug delivered to the systemic circulation per hour across average skin.

While there is variation in dose delivered among patients, the nominal flux of the systems (25, 50, 75, and 100 μg of fentanyl per hour) are sufficiently accurate as to allow individual titration of dosage for a given patient. The small amount of alcohol which has been incorporated into the system enhances the rate of drug flux through the rate-limiting copolymer membrane and increases the permeability of the skin to fentanyl.

Following Duragesic application, the skin under the system absorbs fentanyl, and a depot of fentanyl concentrates in the upper skin layers. Fentanyl then becomes available to the systemic circulation. Serum fentanyl concentrations increase gradually following initial Duragesic application, generally leveling off between 12 and 24 hours and remaining relatively constant, with some fluctuation, for the remainder of the 72 hour application period. Peak serum concentrations of fentanyl generally occurred between 24 and 72 hours after initial application (see TABLE 7). Serum fentanyl concentrations achieved are proportional to the Duragesic delivery rate. With continuous use, serum fentanyl concentrations continue to rise for the first few system applications. After several sequential 72 hour applications, patients reach and maintain a steady state serum concentration that is determined by individual variation in skin permeability and body clearance of fentanyl (see TABLE 8).

After system removal, serum fentanyl concentrations decline gradually, falling about 50% in approximately 17 (range 13-22) hours. Continued absorption of fentanyl from the skin accounts for a slower disappearance of the drug from the serum than is seen after an IV infusion, where the apparent half-life is approximately 7 (range 3-12) hours.

TABLE 7 *Fentanyl Pharmacokinetic Parameters Following First 72 Hour Application of Duragesic*

Dose	T_{max}* (h) Mean (SD)	C_{max}† (ng/ml) Mean (SD)
Duragesic 25 μg/h	38.1 (18.0)	0.6 (0.3)
Duragesic 50 μg/h	34.8 (15.4)	1.4 (0.5)
Duragesic 75 μg/h	33.5 (14.5)	1.7 (0.7)
Duragesic 100 μg/h	36.8 (15.7)	2.5 (1.2)

* Time to maximal concentration.
† Maximal concentration.

Note: After system removal there is continued systemic absorption from residual fentanyl in the skin so that serum concentrations fall 50%, on average, in 17 hours.

TABLE 8 *Range of Pharmacokinetic Parameters of Intravenous Fentanyl in Patients*

	Clearance (L/h) Range [70 kg]	Vol. of Distribution Vss (L/kg) Range	Half-Life T½ (hours) Range
Surgical patients	27-75	3-8	3-12
Hepatically impaired patients	3-80*	0.8-8*	4-12*
Renally impaired patients	30-78	—	—

* Estimated.

Note: Information on volume of distribution and half-life not available for renally impaired patients.

Fentanyl plasma protein binding capacity decreases with increasing ionization of the drug. Alterations in pH may affect its distribution between plasma and the central nervous system. Fentanyl accumulates in the skeletal muscle and fat and is released slowly into the blood.

The average volume of distribution for fentanyl is 6 L/kg (range 3-8, n=8). The average clearance in patients undergoing various surgical procedures is 46 L/h (range 27-75, n=8). The kinetics of fentanyl in geriatric patients has not been well studied, but in geriatric patients the clearance of IV fentanyl may be reduced and the terminal half-life greatly prolonged (see PRECAUTIONS).

Fentanyl is metabolized primarily via human cytochrome P450 3A4 isoenzyme system. In humans the drug appears to be metabolized primarily by oxidative N-dealkylation to norfentanyl and other inactive metabolites that do not contribute materially to the observed activity of the drug. Within 72 hours of IV fentanyl administration, approximately 75% of the dose is excreted in urine, mostly as metabolites with less than 10% representing unchanged drug. Approximately 9% of the dose is recovered in the feces, primarily as metabolites. Mean values for unbound fractions of fentanyl in plasma are estimated to be between 13 and 21%.

Skin does not appear to metabolize fentanyl delivered transdermally. This was determined in a human keratinocyte cell assay and in clinical studies in which 92% of the dose delivered from the system was accounted for as unchanged fentanyl that appeared in the systemic circulation.

PHARMACODYNAMICS

Analgesia

Duragesic is a strong opioid analgesic. In controlled clinical trials in non-opioid-tolerant patients, 60 mg/day IM morphine was considered to provide analgesia approximately equivalent to Duragesic 100 μg/h in an acute pain model.

Minimum effective analgesic serum concentrations of fentanyl in opioid naive patients range from 0.2-1.2 ng/ml; side effects increase in frequency at serum levels above 2 ng/ml. Both the minimum effective concentration and the concentration at which toxicity occurs rise with increasing tolerance. The rate of development of tolerance varies widely among individuals.

Ventilatory Effects

At equivalent analgesic serum concentrations, fentanyl and morphine produce a similar degree of hypoventilation. A small number of patients have experienced clinically significant hypoventilation with Duragesic. Hypoventilation was manifest by respiratory rates of less than 8 breaths/minute or a pCO_2 greater than 55 mm Hg. In clinical trials of 357 postoperative (acute pain) patients treated with Duragesic, 13 patients experienced hypoventilation. In these studies the incidence of hypoventilation was higher in nontolerant women (10) than in men (3) and in patients weighing less than 63 kg (9 of 13). Although patients with impaired respiration were not common in the trials, they had higher rates of hypoventilation. In addition, post-marketing reports have been received of opioid-naive postoperative patients who have experienced clinically significant hypoventilation with Duragesic. Duragesic is contraindicated in the treatment of postoperative and acute pain.

While most patients using Duragesic chronically develop tolerance to fentanyl induced hypoventilation, episodes of slowed respirations may occur at any time during therapy; medical intervention generally was not required in these instances.

Hypoventilation can occur throughout the therapeutic range of fentanyl serum concentrations. However, in non-opioid-tolerant patients the risk of hypoventilation increases at serum fentanyl concentrations greater than 2 ng/ml, especially for patients who have an underlying pulmonary condition or who receive usual doses of opioids or other CNS drugs associated with hypoventilation in addition to Duragesic. The use of initial doses exceeding 25 μg/h is contraindicated in patients who are not tolerant to opioid therapy. The use of Duragesic should be monitored by clinical evaluation. As with other drug level measurements, serum fentanyl concentrations may be useful clinically, although they do not reflect patient sensitivity to fentanyl and should not be used by physicians as a sole indicator of effectiveness or toxicity.

See BOXED WARNING, CONTRAINDICATIONS, WARNINGS, PRECAUTIONS and ADVERSE REACTIONS for additional information on hypoventilation.

Cardiovascular Effects

Fentanyl may infrequently produce bradycardia. The incidence of bradycardia in clinical trials with Duragesic was less than 1%.

CNS Effects

In opioid naive patients, central nervous system effects increase when serum fentanyl concentrations are greater than 3 ng/ml.

INDICATIONS AND USAGE

Duragesic is indicated in the management of chronic pain in patients who require continuous opioid analgesia for pain that cannot be managed by lesser means such as acetaminophen-opioid combinations, non-steroidal analgesics, or prn dosing with short-acting opioids.

Duragesic should not be used in the management of acute or postoperative pain because serious or life-threatening hypoventilation could result. (See BOXED WARNING and CONTRAINDICATIONS.)

In patients with chronic pain, it is possible to individually titrate the dose of the transdermal system to minimize the risk of adverse effects while providing analgesia. In properly selected patients, Duragesic is a safe and effective alternative to other opioid regimens. (See DOSAGE AND ADMINISTRATION.)

CONTRAINDICATIONS

BECAUSE SERIOUS OR LIFE-THREATENING HYPOVENTILATION COULD OCCUR, DURAGESIC IS CONTRAINDICATED:

- **In the management of acute or postoperative pain, including use in out-patient surgeries because there is no opportunity for proper dose titration (see CLINICAL PHARMACOLOGY and DOSAGE AND ADMINISTRATION),**
- **In the management of mild or intermittent pain that can otherwise be managed by lesser means such as acetaminophen-opioid combinations, non-steriodal analgesics, or prn dosing with short-acting opioids, and**
- **In doses exceeding 25 μg/h at the initiation of opioid therapy because of the need to individualize dosing by titrating to the desired analgesic effect.**

Duragesic is also contraindicated in patients with known hypersensitivity to fentanyl or adhesives.

WARNINGS

DURAGESIC SHOULD NOT BE ADMINISTERED TO CHILDREN UNDER 12 YEARS OF AGE OR PATIENTS UNDER 18 YEARS OF AGE WHO WEIGH LESS THAN 50 KG (110 LB) EXCEPT IN AN AUTHORIZED INVESTIGATIONAL RESEARCH SETTING. (See PRECAUTIONS, Pediatric Use.)

PATIENTS WHO HAVE EXPERIENCED ADVERSE EVENTS SHOULD BE MONITORED FOR AT LEAST 12 HOURS AFTER DURAGESIC REMOVAL SINCE SERUM FENTANYL CONCENTRATIONS DECLINE GRADUALLY AND REACH AN APPROXIMATE 50% REDUCTION IN SERUM CONCENTRATIONS 17 HOURS AFTER SYSTEM REMOVAL.

DURAGESIC SHOULD BE PRESCRIBED ONLY BY PERSONS KNOWLEDGEABLE IN THE CONTINUOUS ADMINISTRATION OF POTENT OPIOIDS, IN THE MANAGEMENT OF PATIENTS RECEIVING POTENT OPIOIDS FOR TREATMENT OF PAIN, AND IN THE DETECTION AND MANAGEMENT OF HYPOVENTILATION INCLUDING THE USE OF OPIOID ANTAGONISTS.

THE CONCOMITANT USE OF OTHER CENTRAL NERVOUS SYSTEM DEPRESSANTS, INCLUDING OTHER OPIOIDS, SEDATIVES OR HYPNOTICS, GENERAL ANESTHETICS, PHENOTHIAZINES, TRANQUILIZERS, SKELETAL MUSCLE RELAXANTS, SEDATING ANTIHISTAMINES, AND ALCOHOLIC BEVERAGES MAY PRODUCE ADDITIVE DEPRESSANT EFFECTS. HYPOVENTILATION, HYPOTENSION AND PROFOUND SEDATION OR COMA MAY OCCUR. WHEN SUCH COMBINED THERAPY IS CONTEMPLATED, THE DOSE OF ONE OR BOTH AGENTS SHOULD BE REDUCED BY AT LEAST 50%.

F

ALL PATIENTS SHOULD BE ADVISED TO AVOID EXPOSING THE DURAGESIC APPLICATION SITE TO DIRECT EXTERNAL HEAT SOURCES, SUCH AS HEATING PADS OR ELECTRIC BLANKETS, HEAT LAMPS, SAUNAS, HOT TUBS, AND HEATED WATER BEDS, ETC., WHILE WEARING THE SYSTEM. THERE IS A POTENTIAL FOR TEMPERATURE-DEPENDENT INCREASES IN FENTANYL RELEASE FROM THE SYSTEM. (See PRECAUTIONS, Patients With Fever/External Heat.)

PRECAUTIONS

GENERAL

Duragesic doses greater than 25 μg/h are too high for initiation of therapy in non-opioid-tolerant patients and should not be used to begin Duragesic therapy in these patients. (See BOXED WARNING.)

Duragesic may impair mental and/or physical ability required for the performance of potentially hazardous tasks (*e.g.,* driving, operating machinery). Patients who have been given Duragesic should not drive or operate dangerous machinery unless they are tolerant to the side effects of the drug.

Patients should be instructed to keep both used and unused systems out of the reach of children. Used systems should be folded so that the adhesive side of the system adheres to itself and flushed down the toilet immediately upon removal. Patients should be advised to dispose of any systems remaining from a prescription as soon as they are no longer needed. Unused systems should be removed from their pouch and flushed down the toilet.

HYPOVENTILATION (RESPIRATORY DEPRESSION)

Hypoventilation may occur at any time during the use of Duragesic.

Because significant amounts of fentanyl are absorbed from the skin for 17 hours or more after the system is removed, hypoventilation may persist beyond the removal of Duragesic. Consequently, patients with hypoventilation should be carefully observed for degree of sedation and their respiratory rate monitored until respiration has stabilized.

The use of concomitant CNS active drugs requires special patient care and observation. (See WARNINGS.)

CHRONIC PULMONARY DISEASE

Because potent opioids can cause hypoventilation, Duragesic should be administered with caution to patients with preexisting medical conditions predisposing them to hypoventilation. In such patients, normal analgesic doses of opioids may further decrease respiratory drive to the point of respiratory failure.

HEAD INJURIES AND INCREASED INTRACRANIAL PRESSURE

Duragesic should not be used in patients who may be particularly susceptible to the intracranial effects of CO_2 retention such as those with evidence of increased intracranial pressure, impaired consciousness, or coma. Opioids may obscure the clinical course of patients with head injury. Duragesic should be used with caution in patients with brain tumors.

CARDIAC DISEASE

Fentanyl may produce bradycardia. Fentanyl should be administered with caution to patients with bradyarrhythmias.

HEPATIC OR RENAL DISEASE

At the present time insufficient information exists to make recommendations regarding the use of Duragesic in patients with impaired renal or hepatic function. If the drug is used in these patients, it should be used with caution because of the hepatic metabolism and renal excretion of fentanyl.

PATIENTS WITH FEVER/EXTERNAL HEAT

Based on a pharmacokinetic model, serum fentanyl concentrations could theoretically increase by approximately one-third for patients with a body temperature of 40°C (104°F) due to temperature-dependent increases in fentanyl release from the system and increased skin permeability. Therefore, patients wearing Duragesic systems who develop fever should be monitored for opioid side effects and the Duragesic dose should be adjusted if necessary.

ALL PATIENTS SHOULD BE ADVISED TO AVOID EXPOSING THE DURAGESIC APPLICATION SITE TO DIRECT EXTERNAL HEAT SOURCES, SUCH AS HEATING PADS OR ELECTRIC BLANKETS, HEAT LAMPS, SAUNAS, HOT TUBS, AND HEATED WATER BEDS, ETC., WHILE WEARING THE SYSTEM. THERE IS A POTENTIAL FOR TEMPERATURE-DEPENDENT INCREASES IN FENTANYL RELEASE FROM THE SYSTEM.

CARCINOGENESIS, MUTAGENESIS, AND IMPAIRMENT OF FERTILITY

Because long-term animal studies have not been conducted, the potential carcinogenic effects of Duragesic are unknown. There was no evidence of mutagenicity in the Ames *Salmonella typhimurium* mutagenicity assay, the primary rat hepatocyte unscheduled DNA synthesis assay, the BALB/c-3T3 transformation test, the mouse lymphoma assay, the human lymphocyte and CHO chromosomal aberration *in vitro* assays, or the *in vivo* micronucleus test.

PREGNANCY CATEGORY C

Fentanyl has been shown to impair fertility and to have an embryocidal effect in rats when given in IV doses 0.3 times the human dose for a period of 12 days. No evidence of teratogenic effects has been observed after administration of fentanyl to rats. There are no adequate and well-controlled studies in pregnant women. Duragesic should be used during pregnancy only if the potential benefit justifies the potential risk to the fetus.

LABOR AND DELIVERY

Duragesic is not recommended for analgesia during labor and delivery.

NURSING MOTHERS

Fentanyl is excreted in human milk; therefore Duragesic is not recommended for use in nursing women because of the possibility of effects in their infants.

PEDIATRIC USE

The safety and efficacy of Duragesic in pediatric patients have not been established. (See BOXED WARNING and CONTRAINDICATIONS.)

DURAGESIC SHOULD NOT BE ADMINISTERED TO CHILDREN UNDER 12 YEARS OF AGE OR PATIENTS UNDER 18 YEARS OF AGE WHO WEIGH LESS THAN 50 KG (110 LB) EXCEPT IN AN AUTHORIZED INVESTIGATIONAL RESEARCH SETTING.

GERIATRIC USE

Information from a pilot study of the pharmacokinetics of IV fentanyl in geriatric patients indicates that the clearance of fentanyl may be greatly decreased in the population above the age of 60. The relevance of these findings to transdermal fentanyl is unknown at this time.

Since elderly, cachectic, or debilitated patients may have altered pharmacokinetics due to poor fat stores, muscle wasting, or altered clearance, they should not be started on Duragesic doses higher than 25 μg/h unless they are already taking more than 135 mg of oral morphine a day or an equivalent dose of another opioid (see DOSAGE AND ADMINISTRATION).

INFORMATION FOR THE PATIENT

A patient instruction sheet is included in the package of Duragesic systems dispensed to the patient.

Disposal of Duragesic

Duragesic should be kept out of the reach of children. Duragesic systems should be folded so that the adhesive side of the system adheres to itself, then the system should be flushed down the toilet immediately upon removal. Patients should dispose of any systems remaining from a prescription as soon as they are no longer needed. Unused systems should be removed from their pouches and flushed down the toilet.

If the gel from the drug reservoir accidentally contacts the skin, the area should be washed with clear water.

DRUG INTERACTIONS

CENTRAL NERVOUS SYSTEM DEPRESSANTS

When patients are receiving Duragesic, the dose of additional opioids or other CNS depressant drugs (including benzodiazepines) should be reduced by at least 50%. With the concomitant use of CNS depressants, hypotension may occur.

AGENTS AFFECTING CYTOCHROME P450 3A4 ISOENZYME SYSTEM

CYP3A4 Inhibitors

Since the metabolism of fentanyl is mediated by the CYP3A4 isozyme, coadministration of drugs that inhibit CYP3A4 activity may cause decreased clearance of fentanyl. The expected clinical results would be increased or prolonged opioid effects. Thus patients coadministered with inhibitors of CYP3A4 such as macrolide antibiotics (*e.g.,* erythromycin), azole antifungal agents (*e.g.,* ketoconazole), and protease inhibitors (*e.g.,* ritanovir) while receiving Duragesic should be carefully monitored and dosage adjustment made if warranted.

CYP3A4 Inducers

Cytochrome P450 inducers, such as rifampin, carbamazepine, and phenytoin, induce metabolism and as such may cause increased clearance of fentanyl. Caution is advised when administering Duragesic to patients receiving these medications and if necessary dose adjustments should be considered.

DRUG OR ALCOHOL DEPENDENCE

Use of Duragesic in combination with alcoholic beverages and/or other CNS depressants can result in increased risk to the patient. Duragesic should be used with caution in individuals who have a history of drug or alcohol abuse, especially if they are outside a medically controlled environment.

AMBULATORY PATIENTS

Strong opioid analgesics impair the mental or physical abilities required for the performance of potentially dangerous tasks such as driving a car or operating machinery. Patients who have been given Duragesic should not drive or operate dangerous machinery unless they are tolerant to the effects of the drug.

ADVERSE REACTIONS

In post-marketing experience, deaths from hypoventilation due to inappropriate use of Duragesic have been reported. (See BOXED WARNING and CONTRAINDICATIONS.)

PRE-MARKETING CLINICAL TRIAL EXPERIENCE

The safety of Duragesic has been evaluated in 357 postoperative patients and 153 cancer patients for a total of 510 patients. Patients with acute pain used Duragesic for 1-3 days. The duration of Duragesic use varied in cancer patients; 56% of patients used Duragesic for over 30 days, 28% continued treatment for more than 4 months, and 10% used Duragesic for more than 1 year.

Hypoventilation was the most serious adverse reaction observed in 13 (4%) postoperative patients and in 3 (2%) of the cancer patients. Hypotension and hypertension were observed in 11 (3%) and 4 (1%) of the opioid-naive patients.

Various adverse events were reported; a causal relationship to Duragesic was not always determined. The frequencies presented here reflect the actual frequency of each adverse effect in patients who received Duragesic. There has been no attempt to correct for a placebo effect, concomitant use of other opioids, or to subtract the frequencies reported by placebo-treated patients in controlled trials.

The following adverse reactions were reported in 153 cancer patients at a frequency of 1% or greater; similar reactions were seen in the 357 postoperative patients studied.

Body as a Whole: Abdominal pain*, headache*.
Cardiovascular: Arrhythmia, chest pain.
Digestive: Nausea†, vomiting†, constipation†, dry mouth†, anorexia*, diarrhea*, dyspepsia*, flatulence.
Nervous: Somnolence†, confusion†, asthenia†, dizziness*, nervousness*, hallucinations*, anxiety*, depression*, euphoria*, tremor, abnormal coordination, speech disorder, abnormal thinking, abnormal gait, abnormal dreams, agitation, paresthesia, amnesia, syncope, paranoid reaction.
Respiratory: Dyspnea*, hypoventilation*, apnea*, hemoptysis, pharyngitis, hiccups.
Skin and Appendages: Sweating†, pruritus*, rash, application site reaction — erythema, papules, itching, edema.
Urogenital: Urinary retention*.

* Reactions occurring in 3-10% of Duragesic patients.
† Reactions occurring in 10% or more of Duragesic patients.

The following adverse effects have been reported in less than 1% of the 510 postoperative and cancer patients studied; the association between these events and Duragesic administration is unknown. This information is listed to serve as alerting information for the physician.

Cardiovascular: Bradycardia.
Digestive: Abdominal distention.
Nervous: Aphasia, hypertonia, vertigo, stupor, hypotonia, depersonalization, hostility.
Respiratory: Stertorous breathing, asthma, respiratory disorder.
Skin and Appendages, General: Exfoliative dermatitis, pustules.
Special Senses: Amblyopia.
Urogenital: Bladder pain, oliguria, urinary frequency.

POST-MARKETING EXPERIENCE

The following adverse reactions reported to have been observed in association with the use of Duragesic and not reported in the pre-marketing adverse reactions section above include:

Body as a Whole: Edema.
Cardiovascular: Tachycardia.
Metabolic and Nutritional: Weight loss.
Special Senses: Blurred vision.

DOSAGE AND ADMINISTRATION

With all opioids, the safety of patients using the products is dependent on health care practitioners prescribing them in strict conformity with their approved labeling with respect to patient selection, dosing, and proper conditions for use.

As with all opioids, dosage should be individualized. The most important factor to be considered in determining the appropriate dose is the extent of preexisting opioid tolerance. (See BOXED WARNING and CONTRAINDICATIONS.) Initial doses should be reduced in elderly or debilitated patients (see PRECAUTIONS).

Duragesic should be applied to non-irritated and non-irradiated skin on a flat surface such as chest, back, flank or upper arm. Hair at the application site should be clipped (not shaved) prior to system application. If the site of Duragesic application must be cleansed prior to application of the system, do so with clear water. Do not use soaps, oils, lotions, alcohol, or any other agents that might irritate the skin or alter its characteristics. Allow the skin to dry completely prior to system application.

Duragesic should be applied immediately upon removal from the sealed package. Do not alter the system (*e.g.,* cut) in any way prior to application.

The transdermal system should be pressed firmly in place with the palm of the hand for 30 seconds, making sure the contact is complete, especially around the edges.

Each Duragesic may be worn continuously for 72 hours. If analgesia for more than 72 hours is required, a new system should be applied to a different skin site after removal of the previous transdermal system.

Duragesic should be kept out of the reach of children. Used systems should be folded so that the adhesive side of the system adheres to itself, then the system should be flushed down the toilet immediately upon removal. Patients should dispose of any systems remaining from a prescription as soon as they are no longer needed. Unused systems should be removed from their pouches and flushed down the toilet.

DOSE SELECTION

DOSES MUST BE INDIVIDUALIZED BASED UPON THE STATUS OF EACH PATIENT AND SHOULD BE ASSESSED AT REGULAR INTERVALS AFTER DURAGESIC APPLICATION. REDUCED DOSES OF DURAGESIC ARE SUGGESTED FOR THE ELDERLY AND OTHER GROUPS DISCUSSED IN PRECAUTIONS.

DURAGESIC DOSES GREATER THAN 25 μg/h SHOULD NOT BE USED FOR INITIATION OF DURAGESIC THERAPY IN NON-OPIOID-TOLERANT PATIENTS.

In selecting an initial Duragesic dose, attention should be given to (1) the daily dose, potency, and characteristics of the opioid the patient has been taking previously (*e.g.,* whether it is a pure agonist or mixed agonist-antagonist), (2) the reliability of the relative potency estimates used to calculate the Duragesic dose needed (potency estimates may vary with the route of administration), (3) the degree of opioid tolerance, if any, and (4) the general condition and medical status of the patient. Each patient should be maintained at the lowest dose providing acceptable pain control.

INITIAL DURAGESIC DOSE SELECTION

There has been no systematic evaluation of Duragesic as an initial opioid analgesic in the management of chronic pain, since most patients in the clinical trials were converted to Duragesic from other narcotics. Therefore, unless the patient has pre-existing opioid tolerance, the lowest Duragesic dose, 25 μg/h, should be used as the initial dose.

To convert patients from oral or parenteral opioids to Duragesic use the following methodology:

1. Calculate the previous 24 hour analgesic requirement.
2. Convert this amount to the equianalgesic oral morphine dose using TABLE 9.
3. TABLE 10 displays the range of 24 hour oral morphine doses that are recommended for conversion to each Duragesic dose. Use TABLE 10 to find the calculated 24 hour morphine dose and the corresponding Duragesic dose. Initiate Duragesic treatment using the recommended dose and titrate patients upwards (no more frequently than every 3 days after the initial dose or than every 6 days thereafter) until analgesic efficacy is attained. The recommended starting dose when converting from other opioids to Duragesic is likely too low for 50% of patients. This starting dose is recommended to minimize the potential for overdosing patients with the first dose. For delivery rates in excess of 100 μg/h, multiple systems may be used.

TABLE 9* *Equianalgesic Potency Conversion*

Name	Equianalgesic Dose (mg) IM†‡	PO
Morphine	10	60 (30)§
Hydromorphone	1.5	7.5
Methadone	10	20
Oxycodone	15	30
Levorphanol	2	4
Oxymorphone	1	10 (PR)
Heroin	5	60
Meperidine	75	—
Codeine	130	200

* All IM and PO doses in this chart are considered equivalent to 10 mg of IM morphine in analgesic effect. IM denotes intramuscular, PO oral, and PR rectal.
† Based on single-dose studies in which an intramuscular dose of each drug listed was compared with morphine to establish the relative potency. Oral doses are those recommended when changing from parenteral to an oral route. Reference: Foley, K.M. (1985) The treatment of cancer pain. NEJM 313(2):84-95.
‡ Although controlled studies are not available, in clinical practice it is customary to consider the doses of opioid given IM, IV or subcutaneously to be equivalent. There may be some differences in pharmacokinetic parameters such as C_{max} and T_{max}.
§ The conversion ratio of 10 mg parenteral morphine = 30 mg oral morphine is based on clinical experience in patients with chronic pain. The conversion ratio of 10 mg parenteral morphine = 60 mg oral morphine is based on a potency study in acute pain. Reference: Ashburn and Lipman (1993) Management of pain in the cancer patient. Anesth Analg 76:402-416.

TABLE 10* *Recommended Initial Duragesic Dose Based Upon Daily Oral Morphine Dose*

Oral 24 hour Morphine	Duragesic Dose
45-134 mg/day	25 μg/h
135-224 mg/day	50 μg/h
225-314 mg/day	75 μg/h
315-404 mg/day	100 μg/h
405-494 mg/day	125 μg/h
495-584 mg/day	150 μg/h
585-674 mg/day	175 μg/h
675-764 mg/day	200 μg/h
765-854 mg/day	225 μg/h
855-944 mg/day	250 μg/h
945-1034 mg/day	275 μg/h
1035-1124 mg/day	300 μg/h

Note: In clinical trials these ranges of daily oral morphine doses were used as a basis for conversion to Duragesic.
* THIS TABLE SHOULD NOT BE USED TO CONVERT FROM DURAGESIC TO OTHER THERAPIES, BECAUSE THIS CONVERSION TO DURAGESIC IS CONSERVATIVE. USE OF THIS TABLE FOR CONVERSION TO OTHER ANALGESIC THERAPIES CAN OVERESTIMATE THE DOSE OF THE NEW AGENT. OVERDOSAGE OF THE NEW ANALGESIC AGENT IS POSSIBLE. (See Discontinuation of Duragesic.)

The majority of patients are adequately maintained with Duragesic administered every 72 hours. A small number of patients may not achieve adequate analgesia using this dosing interval and may require systems to be applied every 48 hours rather than every 72 hours. An increase in the Duragesic dose should be evaluated before changing dosing intervals in order to maintain patients on a 72 hour regimen. Because of the increase in serum fentanyl concentration over the first 24 hours following initial system application, the initial evaluation of the maximum analgesic effect of Duragesic cannot be made before 24 hours of wearing. The initial Duragesic dosage may be increased after 3 days (see Dose Titration).

During the initial application of Duragesic, patients should use short-acting analgesics as needed until analgesic efficacy with Duragesic is attained. Thereafter, some patients still may require periodic supplemental doses of other short-acting analgesics for "breakthrough" pain.

DOSE TITRATION

The recommended initial Duragesic dose based upon the daily oral morphine dose is conservative, and 50% of patients are likely to require a dose increase after initial application of Duragesic. The initial Duragesic dosage may be increased after 3 days based on the daily dose of supplemental analgesics required by the patient in the second or third day of the initial application.

Physicians are advised that it may take up to 6 days after increasing the dose of Duragesic for the patient to reach equilibrium on the new dose. Therefore, patients should wear a higher dose through two applications before any further increase in dosage is made on the basis of the average daily use of a supplemental analgesic.

Appropriate dosage increments should be based on the daily dose of supplementary opioids, using the ratio of 90 mg/24 hours of oral morphine to a 25 µg/h increase in Duragesic dose.

DISCONTINUATION OF DURAGESIC

To convert patients to another opioid, remove Duragesic and titrate the dose of the new analgesic based upon the patient's report of pain until adequate analgesia has been attained. Upon system removal, 17 hours or more are required for a 50% decrease in serum fentanyl concentrations. Opioid withdrawal symptoms (such as nausea, vomiting, diarrhea, anxiety, and shivering) are possible in some patients after conversion or dose adjustment. For patients requiring discontinuation of opioids, a gradual downward titration is recommended since it is not known what dose level the opioid may be discontinued without producing the signs and symptoms of abrupt withdrawal.

TABLE 10 SHOULD NOT BE USED TO CONVERT FROM DURAGESIC TO OTHER THERAPIES. BECAUSE THE CONVERSION TO DURAGESIC IS CONSERVATIVE, USE OF TABLE 10 FOR CONVERSION TO OTHER ANALGESIC THERAPIES CAN OVERESTIMATE THE DOSE OF THE NEW AGENT. OVERDOSAGE OF THE NEW ANALGESIC AGENT IS POSSIBLE.

HOW SUPPLIED

Duragesic is supplied in the following strengths and sizes (see TABLE 11).

TABLE 11

Duragesic Dose	Size	Fentanyl Content
Duragesic 25 µg/h	10 cm^2	2.5 mg
Duragesic 50* µg/h	20 cm^2	5 mg
Duragesic 75* µg/h	30 cm^2	7.5 mg
Duragesic 100* µg/h	40 cm^2	10 mg

* FOR USE ONLY IN OPIOID TOLERANT PATIENTS.

SAFETY AND HANDLING

Duragesic is supplied in sealed transdermal systems which pose little risk of exposure to health care workers. If the gel from the drug reservoir accidentally contacts the skin, the area should be washed with copious amounts of water. Do not use soap, alcohol, or other solvents to remove the gel because they may enhance the drug's ability to penetrate the skin. Do not cut or damage Duragesic. If the Duragesic system is cut or damaged, controlled drug delivery will not be possible.

KEEP DURAGESIC OUT OF THE REACH OF CHILDREN.

Storage: Do not store above 25°C (77°F). Apply immediately after removal from individually sealed package. Do not use if the seal is broken. **For transdermal use only.**

PRODUCT LISTING - RATED THERAPEUTICALLY EQUIVALENT

Device - Oral Transmucosal - 200 mcg
24's $188.00 ACTIQ, Abbott Pharmaceutical 00074-2460-24
Device - Oral Transmucosal - 600 mcg
24's $281.25 ACTIQ, Abbott Pharmaceutical 00074-2462-24
Device - Oral Transmucosal - 800 mcg
24's $349.00 ACTIQ, Abbott Pharmaceutical 00074-2463-24
Device - Oral Transmucosal - 1200 mcg
24's $433.75 ACTIQ, Abbott Pharmaceutical 00074-2464-24
Solution - Injectable - 0.05 mg/ml
2 ml x 10 $6.50 GENERIC, Abbott Pharmaceutical 00074-9093-32
2 ml x 10 $9.40 GENERIC, Abbott Pharmaceutical 00074-1276-02
2 ml x 10 $12.50 GENERIC, Abbott Pharmaceutical 00074-1276-32
2 ml x 10 $20.60 GENERIC, Esi Lederle Generics 00641-1116-33
2 ml x 10 $22.50 GENERIC, Baxter Pharmaceutical Products, Inc 10019-0038-67
2 ml x 10 $27.90 SUBLIMAZE, Taylor Pharmaceuticals 11098-0030-02
2 ml x 25 $23.45 GENERIC, Abbott Pharmaceutical 00074-9094-22
2 ml x 25 $196.88 GENERIC, Abbott Pharmaceutical 00074-9095-12
2 ml x 50 $46.32 GENERIC, Abbott Pharmaceutical 00074-9095-02
5 ml x 10 $8.60 GENERIC, Abbott Pharmaceutical 00074-9093-35
5 ml x 10 $17.80 GENERIC, Abbott Pharmaceutical 00074-1276-05
5 ml x 10 $25.60 GENERIC, Abbott Pharmaceutical 00074-1276-35
5 ml x 10 $34.40 GENERIC, Baxter Pharmaceutical Products, Inc 10019-0033-72
5 ml x 10 $37.90 GENERIC, Esi Lederle Generics 00641-1117-33
5 ml x 10 $50.70 SUBLIMAZE, Taylor Pharmaceuticals 11098-0030-05
5 ml x 25 $29.00 GENERIC, Abbott Pharmaceutical 00074-9094-25
10 ml x 5 $15.70 GENERIC, Abbott Pharmaceutical 00074-9093-36
10 ml x 5 $34.40 GENERIC, Baxter Pharmaceutical Products, Inc 10019-0034-73
10 ml x 5 $35.50 GENERIC, Esi Lederle Generics 00641-1118-34
10 ml x 5 $44.58 SUBLIMAZE, Taylor Pharmaceuticals 11098-0030-10
10 ml x 10 $194.28 GENERIC, Abbott Pharmaceutical 00074-9096-10
10 ml x 25 $90.75 GENERIC, Abbott Pharmaceutical 00074-9094-28
20 ml x 5 $16.45 GENERIC, Abbott Pharmaceutical 00074-9093-38
20 ml x 5 $69.90 GENERIC, Esi Lederle Generics 00641-1119-34
20 ml x 5 $93.60 SUBLIMAZE, Taylor Pharmaceuticals 11098-0030-20
20 ml x 10 $68.75 GENERIC, Baxter Pharmaceutical Products, Inc 10019-0035-74
20 ml x 10 $388.08 GENERIC, Abbott Pharmaceutical 00074-9096-20
20 ml x 25 $145.17 GENERIC, Abbott Pharmaceutical 00074-9094-31
30 ml $5.01 GENERIC, Baxter Pharmaceutical Products, Inc 10019-0036-82
50 ml $24.69 GENERIC, Abbott Pharmaceutical 10019-0037-83
50 ml x 25 $228.89 GENERIC, Abbott Pharmaceutical 00074-9094-61
Solution - Injectable - 1.5 mg/ml
30 ml $20.00 GENERIC, Esi Lederle Generics 00641-2402-41
Solution - Injectable - 2.5 mg/ml
50 ml $25.00 GENERIC, Esi Lederle Generics 00641-2403-41

PRODUCT LISTING - EQUIVALENTS NOT AVAILABLE

Device - Oral Transmucosal - 200 mcg
24's $194.00 ACTIQ, Cephalon, Inc 63459-0302-24
Device - Oral Transmucosal - 400 mcg
24's $230.00 ACTIQ, Abbott Pharmaceutical 00074-2461-24
24's $249.00 ACTIQ, Cephalon, Inc 63459-0304-24
Device - Oral Transmucosal - 600 mcg
24's $304.00 ACTIQ, Cephalon, Inc 63459-0306-24
Device - Oral Transmucosal - 800 mcg
24's $360.00 ACTIQ, Cephalon, Inc 63459-0308-24
Device - Oral Transmucosal - 1200 mcg
24's $469.00 ACTIQ, Cephalon, Inc 63459-0312-24
Device - Oral Transmucosal - 1600 mcg
24 x 1 $536.25 ACTIQ, Abbott Pharmaceutical 00074-2465-24
24 x 1 $580.00 ACTIQ, Cephalon, Inc 63459-0316-24
Film, Extended Release - Transdermal - 25 mcg/Hr
5's $72.74 DURAGESIC, Janssen Pharmaceuticals 50458-0033-05
Film, Extended Release - Transdermal - 50 mcg/Hr
5's $123.61 DURAGESIC, Janssen Pharmaceuticals 50458-0034-05
Film, Extended Release - Transdermal - 75 mcg/Hr
5's $194.31 DURAGESIC, Janssen Pharmaceuticals 50458-0035-05
Film, Extended Release - Transdermal - 100 mcg/Hr
5's $251.41 DURAGESIC, Janssen Pharmaceuticals 50458-0036-05

Ferrous Sulfate *(001275)*

Categories: Anemia, iron-deficiency; Deficiency, iron; WHO Formulary
Drug Classes: Hematinics; Vitamins/minerals
Brand Names: Chem-Sol; Fe-Mar; Fe-Max; Feosol; Fer-Gen-Sol; Fer-in-Sol; Fero-Gradumet Filmtab; Fersul; Ferra-Tab; Ferra-TD; Ferro-Time; Ironmar; Iron Sol; Siderol; Slow Fe
Foreign Brand Availability: Brofesol (Philippines); Com-Femic (Philippines); Duroferon (Finland; Norway; Sweden); Feospan (Bahrain; Benin; Burkina-Faso; Cyprus; Egypt; Ethiopia; Gambia; Ghana; Guinea; Hong-Kong; Iran; Iraq; Ivory-Coast; Jordan; Kenya; Kuwait; Lebanon; Liberia; Libya; Malawi; Mali; Mauritania; Mauritius; Morocco; Niger; Nigeria; Oman; Qatar; Republic-of-Yemen; Saudi-Arabia; Senegal; Seychelles; Sierra-Leone; Sudan; Syria; Tanzania; Tunia; Uganda; United-Arab-Emirates; Zambia; Zimbabwe); Ferro-Gradumet (Australia; Austria; Bahrain; Bulgaria; Cyprus; Egypt; Indonesia; Iran; Iraq; Israel; Jordan; Kuwait; Lebanon; Libya; New-Zealand; Oman; Portugal; Qatar; Republic-of-Yemen; Saudi-Arabia; Syria; United-Arab-Emirates); Ferro-grad (Italy); Ferrograd (England; Ireland); Ferrolent (Costa-Rica; Dominican-Republic; El-Salvador; Guatemala; Honduras; Nicaragua; Panama); Ferronemia (Peru); Ferrophor (Germany); Fespan (Taiwan); Haemoprotect (Germany); Hemobion (Mexico); Iberol Goths (Costa-Rica; Dominican-Republic; El-Salvador; Guatemala; Honduras; Nicaragua; Panama); Liquifer (Netherlands); Microfer (Finland; Greece); Mol-Iron (Colombia); Orafer (Mexico); Plastufer (Germany); Plexafer (Benin; Burkina-Faso; Ethiopia; Gambia; Ghana; Guinea; Ivory-Coast; Kenya; Liberia; Malawi; Mali; Mauritania; Mauritius; Morocco; Niger; Nigeria; Senegal; Seychelles; Sierra-Leone; Sudan; Tanzania; Tunia; Uganda; Zambia; Zimbabwe); Retafer (Bulgaria; Finland; Singapore)

DESCRIPTION

Slow Fe supplies ferrous sulfate, for the treatment of iron deficiency and iron deficiency anemia with a significant reduction in the incidence of the common side effects associated with taking oral iron preparations. The wax matrix delivery system of Slow Fe is designed to maximize the release of ferrous sulfate in the duodenum and the jejunum where it is best tolerated and absorbed. Slow Fe has been clinically shown to be associated with a lower incidence of constipation, diarrhea and abdominal discomfort when compared to an immediate release iron tablet[1] and a leading sustained-release iron capsule.[2]

FORMULA

Each tablet contains:

Active Ingredient: 160 mg dried ferrous sulfate, equivalent to 50 mg elemental iron.

Inactive Ingredients: Cetostearyl alcohol, hydroxypropyl methylcellulose, lactose, magnesium stearate, polysorbate 80, talc, titanium dioxide, yellow iron oxide, FD&C blue no. 2 aluminum lake.

INDICATIONS AND USAGE

NON-FDA APPROVED INDICATIONS

Ferrous sulfate is also used for anemia of chronic renal failure in patients receiving epoetin alfa therapy, although this use is not FDA approved.

WARNINGS

The treatment of any anemic condition should be under the advice and supervision of a physician. As oral iron products interfere with absorption of oral tetracycline antibiotics, these products should not be taken within 2 hours of each other. As with any drug, if you are pregnant or nursing a baby, seek the advice of a health professional before using this product.

Accidental overdose of iron-containing products is a leading cause of fatal poisoning in children under 6. KEEP THIS PRODUCT OUT OF REACH OF CHILDREN. In case of accidental overdose, call a doctor or poison control center immediately.

DOSAGE AND ADMINISTRATION

ADULTS

One (1) or 2 tablets daily or as recommended by a physician. A maximum of 4 tablets daily may be taken.

CHILDREN

One (1) tablet daily. Tablets must be swallowed whole.

Fexofenadine Hydrochloride *(003294)*

For related information, see the comparative table section in Appendix A.

Categories: Rhinitis, allergic; Urticaria, chronic idiopathic; Pregnancy Category C; FDA Approved 1996 Jul
Drug Classes: Antihistamines, H1
Brand Names: Allegra
Foreign Brand Availability: Telfast (Australia; Benin; Burkina-Faso; Ethiopia; France; Gambia; Germany; Ghana; Guinea; Hong-Kong; Israel; Ivory-Coast; Kenya; Liberia; Malawi; Mali; Mauritania; Mauritius; Morocco; New-Zealand; Niger; Nigeria; Senegal; Seychelles; Sierra-Leone; Sudan; Tanzania; Thailand; Tunia; Uganda; Zambia; Zimbabwe); Telfast BD (Indonesia)
Cost of Therapy: $64.60 (Allergic Rhinitis; Allegra; 60 mg; 2 capsules/day; 30 day supply)
$73.37 (Allergic Rhinitis; Allegra Extended Release; 180 mg; 1 tablet/day; 30 day supply)

DESCRIPTION

Fexofenadine hydrochloride is a histamine H_1-receptor antagonist with the chemical name (±)-4-[1 hydroxy-4-[4-(hydroxydiphenylmethyl)-l-piperidinyl]-butyl]-α,α-dimethyl benzeneacetic acid hydrochloride.

The molecular weight is 538.13 and the empirical formula is $C_{32}H_{39}NO_4 \cdot HCl$.

Fexofenadine hydrochloride is a white to off-white crystalline powder. It is freely soluble in methanol and ethanol, slightly soluble in chloroform and water, and insoluble in hexane. Fexofenadine hydrochloride is a racemate and exists as a zwitterion in aqueous media at a physiological pH.

Allegra is formulated as a capsule or tablet for oral administration. The manufacturer is no longer distributing the 60 mg capsules to avoid potential confusion between the 60 mg tablets and capsules.

TABLETS

Each tablet contains 30, 60, or 180 mg fexofenadine hydrochloride (depending on the dosage strength) and the following excipients: croscarmellose sodium, magnesium stearate, microcrystalline cellulose, and pregelatinized starch. The aqueous tablet film-coating is made from hydroxypropyl methylcellulose, iron oxide blends, polyethylene glycol, povidone, silicone dioxide, and titanium dioxide.

CLINICAL PHARMACOLOGY

MECHANISM OF ACTION

Fexofenadine HCl is an antihistamine with selective peripheral H_1-receptor antagonist activity. Both enantiomers of fexofenadine HCl displayed approximately equipotent antihistaminic effects. Fexofenadine inhibited histamine release from peritoneal mast cells in rats. In laboratory animals, no anticholinergic, alpha$_1$-adrenergic or beta-adrenergic-receptor blocking effects were observed. No sedative or other central nervous system effects were observed. Radiolabeled tissue distribution studies in rats indicated that fexofenadine does not cross the blood-brain barrier.

PHARMACOKINETICS

Absorption

Fexofenadine HCl was rapidly absorbed following oral administration of a single dose of two 60 mg capsules to healthy male volunteers with a mean time to maximum plasma concentration occurring at 2.6 hours postdose. After administration of a single 60 mg capsule to healthy subjects, the mean maximum plasma concentration was 131 ng/ml. Following single dose oral administrations of either the 60 and 180 mg tablet to healthy, adult male volunteers, mean maximum plasma concentrations were 142 and 494 ng/ml, respectively. The tablet formulations are bioequivalent to the capsule when administered at equal doses. Fexofenadine HCl pharmacokinetics are linear for oral doses up to a total daily dose of 240 mg (120 mg twice daily).

Distribution

Fexofenadine HCl is 60-70% bound to plasma proteins, primarily albumin and α_1-acid glycoprotein.

Elimination

The mean elimination half-life of fexofenadine was 14.4 hours following administration of 60 mg, twice daily, in normal volunteers.

Human mass balance studies documented a recovery of approximately 80% and 11% of the [^{14}C] fexofenadine HCl dose in the feces and urine, respectively. Because the absolute bioavailability of fexofenadine HCl has not been established, it is unknown if the fecal component represents unabsorbed drug or the result of biliary excretion.

Metabolism

Approximately 5% of the total oral dose was metabolized.

Special Populations

Special population pharmacokinetics (for geriatric subjects, renal and hepatic impairment), obtained after a single dose of 80 mg fexofenadine HCl, were compared to those for normal subjects from a separate study of similar design. While subject weights were relatively uniform between studies, these adult special population patients were substantially older than the healthy, young volunteers. Thus, an age effect may be confounding the pharmacokinetic differences observed in some of the special populations.

Seasonal Allergic Rhinitis (SAR) and Chronic Idiopathic Urticaria (CIU) Patients: The pharmacokinetics of fexofenadine HCl in seasonal allergic rhinitis and chronic idiopathic urticaria patients were similar to those in healthy subjects.

Geriatric Subjects: In older subjects (≥65 years old), peak plasma levels of fexofenadine were 99% greater than those observed in normal volunteers (<65 years old). Mean elimination half-lives were similar to those observed in normal volunteers.

Pediatric Patients: Cross study comparisons indicated that fexofenadine HCl area under the curve (AUC) following oral administration of a 60 mg dose to 7-12 year old pediatric allergic rhinitis patients was 56% greater compared to healthy adult subjects given the same dose. Plasma exposure in pediatric patients given 30 mg fexofenadine HCl is comparable to adults given 60 mg.

Renal Impairment: In patients with mild to moderate (creatinine clearance 41-80 ml/min) and severe (creatinine clearance 11-40 ml/min) renal impairment, peak plasma levels of fexofenadine were 87% and 111% greater, respectively, and mean elimination half-lives were 59% and 72% longer, respectively, than observed in normal volunteers. Peak plasma levels in patients on dialysis (creatinine clearance ≤10 ml/min) were 82% greater and half-life was 31% longer than observed in normal volunteers. Based on increases in bioavailability and half-life, a dose of 60 mg once daily is recommended as the starting dose in patients with decreased renal function. (See DOSAGE AND ADMINISTRATION.)

Hepatic Impairment: The pharmacokinetics of fexofenadine HCl in patients with hepatic disease did not differ substantially from that observed in healthy patients.

Effect of Gender: Across several trials, no clinically significant gender-related differences were observed in the pharmacokinetics of fexofenadine HCl.

PHARMACODYNAMICS

Wheal and Flare

Human histamine skin wheal and flare studies following single and twice daily doses of 20 and 40 mg fexofenadine HCl demonstrated that the drug exhibits an antihistamine effect by 1 hour, achieves maximum effect at 2-3 hours, and an effect is still seen at 12 hours. There was no evidence of tolerance to these effects after 28 days of dosing.

Histamine skin wheal and flare studies in 7-12 year old patients showed that following a single dose of 30 or 60 mg, antihistamine effect was observed at 1 hour and reached a maximum by 3 hours. Greater than 49% inhibition of wheal area, and 74% inhibition of flare area were maintained for 8 hours following the 30 and 60 mg dose.

Effects on QTc

In dogs (30 mg/kg orally twice a day), and in rabbits (10 mg/kg infused intravenously over 1 hour), fexofenadine HCl did not prolong QTc. In dogs the plasma fexofenadine concentration was approximately 9 times the therapeutic plasma concentrations in adults receiving the maximum recommended daily oral dose. In rabbits, the plasma fexofenadine concentration was approximately 20 times the therapeutic plasma concentration in adults receiving the maximum recommended daily oral dose. No effect was observed on calcium channel current, delayed potassium channel current, or action potential duration in guinea pig myocytes, sodium current in rat neonatal myocytes, or on several delayed rectifier potassium channels cloned from human heart at concentrations up to 1×10^{-5} M of fexofenadine HCl.

No statistically significant increase in mean QTc interval compared to placebo was observed in 714 seasonal allergic rhinitis patients given fexofenadine HCl capsules in doses of 60-240 mg twice daily for 2 weeks. Pediatric patients from two placebo-controlled trials (n=855) treated with up to 60 mg fexofenadine HCl twice daily demonstrated no significant treatment or dose-related increases in QTc. In addition, no statistically significant increase in mean QTc interval compared to placebo was observed in 40 healthy volunteers given fexofenadine HCl as an oral solution at doses up to 400 mg twice daily for 6 days, or in 231 healthy volunteers given fexofenadine HCl 240 mg once daily for 1 year.

INDICATIONS AND USAGE

Seasonal Allergic Rhinitis: Fexofenadine HCl is indicated for the relief of symptoms associated with seasonal allergic rhinitis in adults and children 6 years of age and older. Symptoms treated effectively include sneezing, rhinorrhea, and itchy nose/palate/throat, itchy/watery/red eyes.

Chronic Idiopathic Urticaria: Fexofenadine HCl is indicated for treatment of uncomplicated skin manifestations of chronic idiopathic urticaria in adults and children 6 years of age and older. It significantly reduces pruritus and the number of wheals.

CONTRAINDICATIONS

Fexofenadine HCl is contraindicated in patients with known hypersensitivity to any of its ingredients.

PRECAUTIONS

CARCINOGENESIS, MUTAGENESIS, AND IMPAIRMENT OF FERTILITY

The carcinogenic potential and reproductive toxicity of fexofenadine HCl were assessed using terfenadine studies with adequate fexofenadine HCl exposure (based on plasma area-under-the-concentration versus time [AUC] values). No evidence of carcinogenicity was observed in an 18 month study in mice and in a 24 month study in rats at oral doses of 150 mg/kg of terfenadine (which led to fexofenadine exposures that were respectively approximately 3 and 5 times the exposure from the maximum recommended daily oral dose of fexofenadine HCl in adults and children).

In *in vitro* (Bacterial Reverse Mutation, CHO/HGPRT Forward Mutation, and Rat Lymphocyte Chromosomal Aberration assays) and *in vivo* (Mouse Bone Marrow Micronucleus assay) tests, fexofenadine HCl revealed no evidence of mutagenicity.

In rat fertility studies, dose-related reductions in implants and increases in postimplantation losses were observed at an oral dose of 150 mg/kg of terfenadine (which led to fexofenadine HCl exposures that were approximately 3 times the exposure of the maximum recommended daily oral dose of fexofenadine HCl in adults).

PREGNANCY CATEGORY C

Teratogenic Effects

There was no evidence of teratogenicity in rats or rabbits at oral doses of terfenadine up to 300 mg/kg (which led to fexofenadine exposures that were approximately 4 and 31 times, respectively, the exposure from the maximum recommended daily oral dose of fexofenadine in adults).

There are no adequate and well controlled studies in pregnant women. Fexofenadine should be used during pregnancy only if the potential benefit justifies the potential risk to the fetus.

Nonteratogenic Effects

Dose-related decreases in pup weight gain and survival were observed in rats exposed to an oral dose of 150 mg/kg of terfenadine (approximately 3 times the maximum recommended daily oral dose of fexofenadine HCl in adults based on comparison of fexofenadine HCl AUCs).

NURSING MOTHERS

There are no adequate and well-controlled studies in women during lactation. Because many drugs are excreted in human milk, caution should be exercised when fexofenadine HCl is administered to a nursing woman.

PEDIATRIC USE

The recommended dose in patients 6-11 years of age is based on cross-study comparison of the pharmacokinetics of fexofenadine HCl in adults and pediatric patients and on the safety profile of fexofenadine HCl in both adult and pediatric patients at doses equal to or higher than the recommended doses.

The safety of fexofenadine HCl tablets at a dose of 30 mg twice daily has been demonstrated in 438 pediatric patients 6-11 years of age in two placebo-controlled, 2 week seasonal allergic rhinitis trials. The safety of fexofenadine HCl for the treatment of chronic idiopathic urticaria in patients 6-11 years of age is based on cross-study comparison of the pharmacokinetics of fexofenadine HCl in adult and pediatric patients and on the safety profile of fexofenadine in both adult and pediatric patients at doses equal to or higher than the recommended dose.

The effectiveness of fexofenadine HCl for the treatment of seasonal allergic rhinitis in patients 6-11 years of age was demonstrated in one trial (n=411) in which fexofenadine HCl tablets 30 mg twice daily significantly reduced total symptom scores compared to placebo, along with extrapolation of demonstrated efficacy in patients 12 years and above, and the pharmacokinetic comparisons in adults and children. The effectiveness of fexofenadine HCl for the treatment of chronic idiopathic urticaria in patients 6-11 years of age is based on an extrapolation of the demonstrated efficacy of fexofenadine HCl in adults with this condition and the likelihood that the disease course, pathophysiology and the drug's effect are substantially similar in children to that of adult patients.

The safety and effectiveness of fexofenadine HCl in pediatric patients under 6 years of age have not been established.

GERIATRIC USE

Clinical studies of fexofenadine HCl tablets and capsules did not include sufficient numbers of subjects aged 65 years and over to determine whether this population responds differently from younger patients. Other reported clinical experience has not identified differences in responses between the geriatric and younger patients. This drug is known to be substantially excreted by the kidney, and the risk of toxic reactions to this drug may be greater in patients with impaired renal function. Because elderly patients are more likely to have decreased renal function, care should be taken in dose selection, and may be useful to monitor renal function. (See CLINICAL PHARMACOLOGY.)

DRUG INTERACTIONS

DRUG INTERACTION WITH ERYTHROMYCIN AND KETOCONAZOLE

Fexofenadine HCl has been shown to exhibit minimal (ca. 5%) metabolism. However, coadministration of fexofenadine HCl with ketoconazole and erythromycin led to increased plasma levels of fexofenadine HCl. Fexofenadine HCl had no effect on the pharmacokinetics of erythromycin and ketoconazole. In two separate studies, fexofenadine HCl 120 mg twice daily (2 times the recommended twice daily dose) was coadministered with erythromycin 500 mg every 8 hours or ketoconazole 400 mg once daily under steady-state conditions to normal, healthy volunteers (n=24, each study). No differences in adverse events or QTc interval were observed when patients were administered fexofenadine HCl alone or in combination with erythromycin or ketoconazole. The findings of these studies are summarized in TABLE 1.

TABLE 1 *Effects on Steady-State Fexofenadine HCl Pharmacokinetics After 7 Days of Coadministration With Fexofenadine HCl 120 mg Every 12 Hours* in Normal Volunteers (n=24)*

Concomitant Drug	$C_{max,ss}$†	AUC_{ss}(0-12h)‡
Erythromycin (500 mg q8h)	+82%	+109%
Ketoconazole (400 mg once daily)	+135%	+164%

* Two times the recommended twice daily dose.
† Peak plasma concentration.
‡ Extent of systemic exposure.

The changes in plasma levels were within the range of plasma levels achieved in adequate and well-controlled clinical trials.

The mechanism of these interactions has been evaluated in *in vitro, in situ,* and *in vivo* animal models. These studies indicate that ketoconazole or erythromycin coadministration enhances fexofenadine gastrointestinal absorption. *In vivo* animal studies also suggest that in addition to increasing absorption, ketoconazole decreases fexofenadine HCl gastrointestinal secretion, while erythromycin may also decrease biliary excretion.

DRUG INTERACTIONS WITH ANTACIDS

Administration of 120 mg of fexofenadine HCl within 15 minutes of an aluminum and magnesium containing antacid decreased fexofenadine AUC by 41% and C_{max} by 43%. Fexofenadine HCl should not be taken closely in time with aluminum and magnesium containing antacids.

ADVERSE REACTIONS

SEASONAL ALLERGIC RHINITIS

Adults

In placebo-controlled seasonal allergic rhinitis clinical trials in patients 12 years of age and older, which included 2461 patients receiving fexofenadine HCl at doses of 20-240 mg twice daily, adverse events were similar in fexofenadine HCl and placebo-treated patients. All adverse events that were reported by greater than 1% of patients who received the recommended daily dose of fexofenadine HCl (60 mg twice daily), and that were more common with fexofenadine HCl than placebo, are listed in TABLE 2.

In a placebo-controlled clinical study in the US, which included 570 patients aged 12 years and older receiving fexofenadine HCl tablets at doses of 120 or 180 mg once daily, adverse events were similar in fexofenadine HCl and placebo-treated patients. TABLE 3 also lists adverse experiences that were reported by greater than 2% of patients treated with fexofenadine HCl tablets at doses of 180 mg once daily and that were more common with fexofenadine HCl than placebo.

The incidence of adverse events, including drowsiness, was not dose-related and was similar across subgroups defined by age, gender, and race.

TABLE 2 *Adverse Experiences in Patients Ages 12 Years and Older Reported in Placebo-Controlled Seasonal Allergic Rhinitis Clinical Trials in the US**

Adverse Experience	Fexofenadine 60 mg† (n=679)	Placebo† (n=671)
Viral infection (cold, flu)	2.5%	1.5%
Nausea	1.6%	1.5%
Dysmenorrhea	1.5%	0.3%
Drowsiness	1.3%	0.9%
Dyspepsia	1.3%	0.6%
Fatigue	1.3%	0.9%

* Twice daily dosing with fexofenadine at rates of greater than 1%.
† Twice daily.

TABLE 3 *Adverse Experiences in Patients Ages 12 Years and Older Reported in Placebo-Controlled Seasonal Allergic Rhinitis Clinical Trials in the US**

Adverse Experience	Fexofenadine 180 mg† (n=283)	Placebo (n=293)
Headache	10.6%	7.5%
Upper respiratory tract infection	3.2%	3.1%
Back pain	2.8%	1.4%

* Once daily dosing with fexofenadine HCl tablets at rates of greater than 2%.
† Once daily.

The frequency and magnitude of laboratory abnormalities were similar in fexofenadine HCl and placebo-treated patients.

Pediatric

TABLE 4 lists adverse experiences in patients aged 6-11 years of age which were reported by greater than 2% of patients treated with fexofenadine HCl tablets at a dose of 30 mg twice daily in placebo-controlled seasonal allergic rhinitis studies in the US and Canada that were more common with fexofenadine HCl than placebo.

TABLE 4 *Adverse Experiences Reported in Placebo-Controlled Seasonal Allergic Rhinitis Studies in Pediatric Patients Ages 6-11 in the US and Canada at Rates of Greater Than 2%*

Adverse Experience	Fexofenadine 30 mg* (n=209)	Placebo (n=229)
Headache	7.2%	6.6%
Accidental injury	2.9%	1.3%
Coughing	3.8%	1.3%
Fever	2.4%	0.9%
Pain	2.4%	0.4%
Otitis media	2.4%	0.0%
Upper respiratory tract infection	4.3%	1.7%

* Twice daily.

CHRONIC IDIOPATHIC URTICARIA

Adverse events reported by patients 12 years of age and older in placebo-controlled chronic idiopathic urticaria studies were similar to those reported in placebo-controlled seasonal allergic rhinitis studies. In placebo-controlled chronic idiopathic urticaria clinical trials, which included 726 patients 12 years of age and older receiving fexofenadine HCl tablets at doses of 20-240 mg twice daily, adverse events were similar in fexofenadine HCl and placebo-treated patients. TABLE 5 lists adverse experiences in patients aged 12 years and older that were reported by greater than 2% of patients treated with fexofenadine HCl 60 mg tablets twice daily in controlled clinical studies in the US and Canada and that were more common with fexofenadine HCl than placebo. The safety of fexofenadine HCl in the treatment of chronic idiopathic urticaria in pediatric patients 6-11 years of age is based on the safety profile of fexofenadine HCl in adults and adolescent patients at doses equal to or higher than the recommended dose (see PRECAUTIONS, Pediatric Use).

***TABLE 5** Adverse Experiences Reported in Patients 12 Years and Older in Placebo-Controlled Chronic Idiopathic Urticaria Studies in the US and Canada at Rates of Greater Than 2%*

Adverse Experience	Fexofenadine 60 mg* (n=186)	Placebo (n=178)
Back pain	2.2%	1.1%
Sinusitis	2.2%	1.1%
Dizziness	2.2%	0.6%
Drowsiness	2.2%	0.0%

* Twice daily.

Events that have been reported during controlled clinical trials involving seasonal allergic rhinitis and chronic idiopathic urticaria patients with incidences less than 1% and similar to placebo and have been rarely reported during postmarketing surveillance include: insomnia, nervousness, and sleep disorders or paroniria. In rare cases, rash, urticaria, pruritus and hypersensitivity reactions with manifestations such as angioedema, chest tightness, dyspnea, flushing and systemic anaphylaxis have been reported.

DOSAGE AND ADMINISTRATION

SEASONAL ALLERGIC RHINITIS

Adults and Children 12 Years and Older: The recommended dose of fexofenadine HCl is 60 mg twice daily, or 180 mg once daily. A dose of 60 mg once daily is recommended as the starting dose in patients with decreased renal function (see CLINICAL PHARMACOLOGY).

Children 6-11 Years: The recommended dose of fexofenadine HCl is 30 mg twice daily. A dose of 30 mg once daily is recommended as the starting dose in pediatric patients with decreased renal function (see CLINICAL PHARMACOLOGY).

CHRONIC IDIOPATHIC URTICARIA

Adults and Children 12 Years and Older: The recommended dose of fexofenadine HCl is 60 mg twice daily. A dose of 60 mg once daily is recommended as the starting dose in patients with decreased renal function (see CLINICAL PHARMACOLOGY).

Children 6-11 Years: The recommended dose of fexofenadine HCl is 30 mg twice daily. A dose of 30 mg once daily is recommended as the starting dose in pediatric patients with decreased renal function (see CLINICAL PHARMACOLOGY).

HOW SUPPLIED

Allegra Tablets are available in:

30 mg: Peach-colored film coated tablets with "03" on one side and either "0088" or scripted "E" on the other.

60 mg: Peach-colored film coated tablets with "06" on one side and either "0088" or scripted "E" on the other.

180 mg: Peach-colored film coated tablets with "018" on one side and either "0088" or scripted "E" on the other.

Storage: Store at controlled room temperature 20-25°C (68-77°F). Protect from excessive moisture.

PRODUCT LISTING - EQUIVALENTS NOT AVAILABLE

Capsule - Oral - 60 mg

Qty	Price	Product	NDC
1's	$1.03	ALLEGRA, Allscripts Pharmaceutical Company	54569-4388-06
6's	$16.47	ALLEGRA, Pd-Rx Pharmaceuticals	55289-0456-06
10's	$10.34	ALLEGRA, Allscripts Pharmaceutical Company	54569-4388-03
10's	$10.77	ALLEGRA, Southwood Pharmaceuticals Inc	58016-0131-10
10's	$13.34	ALLEGRA, Physicians Total Care	54868-3898-01
10's	$15.40	ALLEGRA, Pharma Pac	52959-0543-10
12's	$12.92	ALLEGRA, Southwood Pharmaceuticals Inc	58016-0131-12
14's	$14.48	ALLEGRA, Allscripts Pharmaceutical Company	54569-4388-01
14's	$21.42	ALLEGRA, Pharma Pac	52959-0543-14
15's	$16.15	ALLEGRA, Southwood Pharmaceuticals Inc	58016-0131-15
20's	$20.68	ALLEGRA, Allscripts Pharmaceutical Company	54569-4388-04
20's	$21.53	ALLEGRA, Southwood Pharmaceuticals Inc	58016-0131-20
20's	$24.88	ALLEGRA, St. Mary'S Mpp	60760-0102-20
20's	$25.50	ALLEGRA, Physicians Total Care	54868-3898-03
20's	$30.38	ALLEGRA, Pharma Pac	52959-0543-20
28's	$42.71	ALLEGRA, Pd-Rx Pharmaceuticals	55289-0456-28
30's	$31.02	ALLEGRA, Allscripts Pharmaceutical Company	54569-4388-05
30's	$32.30	ALLEGRA, Southwood Pharmaceuticals Inc	58016-0131-30
30's	$37.66	ALLEGRA, Physicians Total Care	54868-3898-00
30's	$43.56	ALLEGRA, Pharma Pac	52959-0543-30
60's	$61.74	ALLEGRA, Southwood Pharmaceuticals Inc	58016-0131-60
60's	$62.04	ALLEGRA, Allscripts Pharmaceutical Company	54569-4388-00
60's	$74.15	ALLEGRA, Physicians Total Care	54868-3898-02
100's	$107.67	ALLEGRA, Southwood Pharmaceuticals Inc	58016-0131-00
100's	$118.36	ALLEGRA, Aventis Pharmaceuticals	00088-1102-49
100's	$123.29	ALLEGRA, Aventis Pharmaceuticals	00088-1102-47

Tablet - Oral - 30 mg

Qty	Price	Product	NDC
100's	$70.58	ALLEGRA, Aventis Pharmaceuticals	00088-1106-47

Tablet - Oral - 60 mg

Qty	Price	Product	NDC
10's	$17.25	ALLEGRA, Pharma Pac	52959-0698-10
14's	$23.99	ALLEGRA, Pharma Pac	52959-0698-14
20's	$34.03	ALLEGRA, Pharma Pac	52959-0698-20
28's	$46.48	ALLEGRA, Pharma Pac	52959-0698-28
30's	$48.79	ALLEGRA, Pharma Pac	52959-0698-30
40's	$64.51	ALLEGRA, Pharma Pac	52959-0698-40
60's	$95.42	ALLEGRA, Pharma Pac	52959-0698-60
100's	$141.04	ALLEGRA, Aventis Pharmaceuticals	00088-1107-47
100's	$141.04	ALLEGRA, Aventis Pharmaceuticals	00088-1107-49
100's	$156.80	ALLEGRA, Pharma Pac	52959-0698-00

Tablet - Oral - 180 mg

Qty	Price	Product	NDC
30's	$62.03	ALLEGRA, Allscripts Pharmaceutical Company	54569-4938-00
100's	$244.55	ALLEGRA, Aventis Pharmaceuticals	00088-1109-47

F

Fexofenadine Hydrochloride; Pseudoephedrine Hydrochloride *(003388)*

For complete prescribing information, refer to the CD-ROM included with the book.

Categories: Rhinitis, seasonal allergic; FDA Approved 1997 Dec; Pregnancy Category C
Drug Classes: Antihistamines, H1; Decongestants, nasal
Brand Names: **Allegra-D**
Foreign Brand Availability: Telfast (Philippines); Telfast BD 60 (Indonesia); Telfast-D (Hong-Kong; Singapore); Telfast OD 120 (Indonesia); Telfast HD 180 (Indonesia); Telfast Decongestant (Australia); Telfast Plus (Indonesia)
Cost of Therapy: $86.03 (Allergic Rhinitis; Allegra-D, Extended Release; 60 mg; 120 mg; 2 tablets/day; 30 day supply)

DESCRIPTION

Allegra-D (fexofenadine hydrochloride and pseudoephedrine hydrochloride) extended-release tablets for oral administration contain 60 mg fexofenadine hydrochloride for immediate-release and 120 mg pseudoephedrine hydrochloride for extended-release. Tablets also contain as excipients: microcrystalline cellulose, pregelatinized starch, croscarmellose sodium, magnesium stearate, carnauba wax, stearic acid, silicon dioxide, hydroxypropyl methylcellulose and polyethylene glycol.

Fexofenadine hydrochloride is a histamine H_1-receptor antagonist with the chemical name (±)-4-[1-hydroxy-4-[4-(hydroxydiphenylmethyl)-1-piperidinyl]-butyl]-α, α-dimethyl benzeneacetic acid hydrochloride.

The molecular weight is 538.13 and the empirical formula is $C_{32}H_{39}NO_4 \cdot HCl$. Fexofenadine hydrochloride is a white to off-white crystalline powder. It is freely soluble in methanol and ethanol, slightly soluble in chloroform and water, and insoluble in hexane. Fexofenadine hydrochloride is a racemate and exists as a zwitterion in aqueous media at physiological pH.

Pseudoephedrine hydrochloride is an adrenergic (vasoconstrictor) agent with the chemical name [S-(R*,R*)]-α-[1-(methylamino)ethyl]-benzenemethanol hydrochloride.

The molecular weight is 201.70. The molecular formula is $C_{10}H_{15}NO \cdot HCl$. Pseudoephedrine hydrochloride occurs as fine, white to off-white crystals or powder, having a faint characteristic odor. It is very soluble in water, freely soluble in alcohol, and sparingly soluble in chloroform.

INDICATIONS AND USAGE

Fexofenadine HCl; pseudoephedrine HCl is indicated for the relief of symptoms associated with seasonal allergic rhinitis in adults and children 12 years of age and older. Symptoms treated effectively include sneezing, rhinorrhea, itchy nose/palate/ and/or throat, itchy/watery/red eyes, and nasal congestion.

Fexofenadine HCl; pseudoephedrine HCl should be administered when both the antihistaminic properties of fexofenadine HCl and the nasal decongestant properties of pseudoephedrine HCl are desired.

CONTRAINDICATIONS

Fexofenadine HCl; pseudoephedrine HCl is contraindicated in patients with known hypersensitivity to any of its ingredients.

Due to its pseudoephedrine component, fexofenadine HCl; pseudoephedrine HCl is contraindicated in patients with narrow-angle glaucoma or urinary retention, and in patients receiving monoamine oxidase (MAO) inhibitor therapy or within 14 days of stopping such treatment. It is also contraindicated in patients with severe hypertension, or severe coronary artery disease, and in those who have shown hypersensitivity or idiosyncrasy to its components, to adrenergic agents, or to other drugs of similar chemical structures. Manifestations of patient idiosyncrasy to adrenergic agents include: insomnia, dizziness, weakness, tremor, or arrhythmias.

WARNINGS

Sympathomimetic amines should be used judiciously and sparingly in patients with hypertension, diabetes mellitus, ischemic heart disease, increased intraocular pressure, hyperthyroidism, renal impairment, or prostatic hypertrophy (see CONTRAINDICATIONS). Sympathomimetic amines may produce central nervous system stimulation with convulsions or cardiovascular collapse with accompanying hypotension.

DOSAGE AND ADMINISTRATION

The recommended dose of fexofenadine HCl; pseudoephedrine HCl is 1 tablet twice daily for adults and children 12 years of age and older. It is recommended that the administration of fexofenadine HCl; pseudoephedrine HCl with food should be avoided. A dose of 1 tablet once daily is recommended as the starting dose in patients with decreased renal function.

PRODUCT LISTING - EQUIVALENTS NOT AVAILABLE

Tablet, Extended Release - Oral - 60 mg;120 mg

30's	$41.98	ALLEGRA-D, Physicians Total Care	54868-4258-00
60's	$54.45	ALLEGRA-D, Aventis Pharmaceuticals	00088-1090-41
100's	$111.18	ALLEGRA-D, Aventis Pharmaceuticals	00088-1090-49
100's	$143.39	ALLEGRA-D, Aventis Pharmaceuticals	00088-1090-47

Filgrastim *(003046)*

Categories: Leukemia, acute myelogenous, adjunct; Leukapheresis; Neutropenia; Transplant, bone marrow; Pregnancy Category C; Recombinant DNA Origin; FDA Approved 1991 Feb; Orphan Drugs
Drug Classes: Hematopoietic agents
Brand Names: **Neupogen**
Foreign Brand Availability: Biofigran (Colombia); Gran (Japan); Granulokine (Philippines); Grasin (Korea); Grimatin (Japan); Neotromax (Peru); Neutromax (Peru)
HCFA JCODE(S): J1440 300 μg SC, IV; J1441 480 μg SC, IV

DESCRIPTION

Filgrastim is a human granulocyte colony stimulating factor (G-CSF), produced by recombinant DNA technology. Neupogen is the Amgen Inc. trademark for filgrastim, which has been selected as the name for recombinant methionyl human granulocyte colony stimulating factor (r-metHuG-CSF).

Neupogen is a 175 amino acid protein manufactured by recombinant DNA technology.[1] Filgrastim is produced by *Escherichia coli* (*E. coli*) bacteria into which has been inserted the human granulocyte colony stimulating factor gene. Neupogen has a molecular weight of 18,800 daltons. The protein has an amino acid sequence that is identical to the natural sequence predicted from human DNA sequence analysis, except for the addition of an N-terminal methionine necessary for expression in *E. coli*. Because filgrastim is produced in *E. coli*, the product is nonglycosylated and thus differs from G-CSF isolated from a human cell.

Neupogen is a sterile, clear, colorless, preservative-free liquid for parenteral administration. Each single-use vial of Neupogen contains 300 μg/ml of filgrastim at a specific activity of $1.0 \pm 0.6 \times 10^8$U/mg, (as measured by a cell mitogenesis assay). The product is formulated in a 10 mM sodium acetate buffer at pH 4.0, containing 5% sorbitol, and 0.004% Tween 80.

The Quantitative Composition (per ml) of Neupogen is:

Filgrastim: 300 μg.
Acetate: 0.59 mg.
Sorbitol: 50.0 mg.
Tween 80: 0.004%.
Sodium: 0.035 mg.
Water for injection qs ad: 1.0 ml.

CLINICAL PHARMACOLOGY

COLONY STIMULATING FACTORS

Colony stimulating factors are glycoproteins which act on hematopoietic cells by binding to specific cell surface receptors and stimulating proliferation, differentiation commitment, and some end-cell functional activation.

Endogenous G-CSF is a lineage specific colony stimulating factor which is produced by monocytes, fibroblasts and endothelial cells. G-CSF regulates the production of neutrophils within the bone marrow and affects neutrophil progenitor proliferation,[2,3] differentiation[2,4] and selected end-cell functional activation (including enhanced phagocytic ability,[5] priming of the cellular metabolism associated with respiratory burst,[6] antibody dependent killing,[7] and the increased expression of some functions associated with cell surface antigens.[8] G-CSF is not species specific and has been shown to have minimal direct *in vivo* or *in vitro* effects on the production of hematopoietic cell types other than the neutrophil lineage.

PRECLINICAL EXPERIENCE

Filgrastim was administered to monkeys, dogs, hamsters, rats, and mice as part of a preclinical toxicology program which included both single-dose acute, repeated-dose subacute, subchronic, and chronic studies. Single-dose administration of filgrastim by the oral, intravenous (IV), subcutaneous (SC), or intraperitoneal (IP) routes resulted in no significant toxicity in mice, rats, hamsters, or monkeys. Although no deaths were observed in mice, rats, or monkeys at dose levels up to 3450 μg/kg and in hamsters using single doses up to approximately 860 μg/kg, deaths were observed in a subchronic (13 week) study in monkeys. In this study, evidence of neurological symptoms was seen in monkeys treated with doses of filgrastim greater than 1150 μg/kg/day for up to 18 days. Deaths were seen in 5 of the 8 treated animals and were associated with 15- to 28-fold increases in peripheral leukocyte counts, and neutrophil-infiltrated hemorrhagic foci were seen in both the cerebrum and cerebellum. In contrast, no monkeys died following 13 weeks of daily IV administration of filgrastim at a dose level of 115 μg/kg. In an ensuing 52 week study, one 115 μg/kg dose female monkey died after 18 weeks of daily IV administration of filgrastim. Death was attributed to cardiopulmonary insufficiency.

In subacute, repeated-dose studies, changes observed were attributable to the expected pharmacological actions of filgrastim (*i.e.,* dose-dependent increases in white cell counts, increased circulating segmented neutrophils, and increased myeloid:erythroid ratio in bone marrow). In all species, histopathologic examination of the liver and spleen revealed evidence of ongoing extramedullary granulopoiesis; increased spleen weights were seen in all species and appeared to be dose-related. A dose-dependent increase in serum alkaline phosphatase was observed in rats, and may reflect increased activity of osteoblasts and osteoclasts. Changes in serum chemistry values were reversible following discontinuation of treatment.

In rats treated at doses of 1150 μg/kg/day for 4 weeks (5 of 32 animals) and for 13 weeks at doses of 100 μg/kg/day (4 of 32 animals) and 500 μg/kg/day (6 of 32 animals) articular swelling of the hind legs was observed. Some degree of hind leg dysfunction was also observed; however, symptoms reversed following cessation of dosing. In rats, osteoclasis and osteoanagenesis were found in the femur, humerus, coccyx, and hind legs (where they were accompanied by synovitis) after IV treatment for four weeks (115-1150 μg/kg/day), and in the sternum after IV treatment for 13 weeks (115-575 μg/kg/day). These effects reversed to normal within 4-5 weeks following cessation of treatment.

In the 52 week chronic, repeated-dose studies performed in rats (IP injection up to 57.5 μg/kg/day), and cynomolgus monkeys (IV injection of up to 115 μg/kg/day), changes observed were similar to those noted in the subacute studies. Expected pharmacological actions of filgrastim included dose-dependent increases in white cell counts, increased circulating segmented neutrophils and alkaline phosphate levels, and increased myeloid: erythroid ratios in the bone marrow. Decreases in platelet counts were also noted in primates. In no animals tested were hemorrhagic complications observed. Rats displayed dose-related swelling of the hind limb, accompanied by some degree of hind limb dysfunction; osteopathy was noted microscopically. Enlarged spleens (both species) and livers (monkeys), reflective of ongoing extramedullary granulopoiesis, as well as myeloid hyperplasia of the bone marrow, were observed in a dose-dependent manner.

PHARMACOLOGIC EFFECTS OF FILGRASTIM

In Phase 1 studies involving 96 patients with various non-myeloid malignancies, filgrastim administration resulted in a dose-dependent increase in circulating neutrophil counts over the dose range of 1-70 μg/kg/day.[9-11] This increase in neutrophil counts was observed whether filgrastim was administered intravenously (1-70 μg/kg twice daily),[9] subcutaneously (1-3 μg/kg/daily),[11] or by continuous SC infusion (3-11 μg/kg/day).[10] With discontinuation of filgrastim therapy, neutrophil counts returned to baseline, in most cases within 4 days. Isolated neutrophils displayed normal phagocytic (measured by zymosan-stimulated chemoluminescence) and chemotactic [measured by migration under agarose using N-formyl-methionyl-leucyl-phenylamine (fMLP) as the chemotaxin] activity *in vitro*.

The absolute monocyte count was reported to increase in a dose-dependent manner in most patients receiving filgrastim, however, the percentage of monocytes in the differential count remained within the normal range. In all studies to date, absolute counts of both eosinophils and basophils did not change and were within the normal range following administration of filgrastim. Increases in lymphocyte counts following filgrastim administration have been reported in some normal subjects and cancer patients.

White blood cell (WBC) differentials obtained during clinical trials have demonstrated a shift towards earlier granulocyte progenitor cells (left shift) including the appearance of promyelocytes and myeloblasts, usually during neutrophil recovery following the chemotherapy-induced nadir. In addition, Dohle bodies, increased granulocyte granulation, as well as hypersegmented neutrophils have been observed. Such changes were transient, and were not associated with clinical sequelae nor were they necessarily associated with infection.

PHARMACOKINETICS

Absorption and clearance of filgrastim follows first-order pharmacokinetic modeling without apparent concentration dependence. A positive linear correlation occurred between the parenteral dose and both the serum concentration and area under the concentration-time curves. Continuous IV infusion of 20 μg/kg of filgrastim over 24 hours resulted in mean and median serum concentrations of approximately 48 and 56 ng/ml, respectively. SC administration of 3.45 μg/kg and 11.5 μg/kg resulted in maximum serum concentrations of 4 and 49 ng/ml, respectively, within 2-8 hours. The volume of distribution averaged 150 ml/kg in both normal subjects and cancer patients. The elimination half-life, in both normal subjects and cancer patients, was approximately 3.5 hours. Clearance rates of filgrastim were approximately 0.5-0.7 ml/min/kg. Single parenteral doses or daily IV doses, over a 14 day period, resulted in comparable half-lives. The half-lives were similar for IV administration (231 minutes, following doses of 34.5 μg/kg) and for SC administration (210 minutes, following filgrastim doses of 3.45 μg/kg). Continuous 24 hour IV infusions at 20 μg/kg over an 11-20 day period produced steady-state serum concentrations of filgrastim with no evidence of drug accumulation over the time period investigated.

INDICATIONS AND USAGE

CANCER PATIENTS RECEIVING MYELOSUPPRESSIVE CHEMOTHERAPY

Filgrastim is indicated to decrease the incidence of infection, as manifested by febrile neutropenia, in patients with non-myeloid malignancies receiving myelosuppressive anticancer drugs associated with a significant incidence of severe neutropenia with fever. A complete blood count (CBC) and platelet count should be obtained prior to chemotherapy, and twice per week (see PRECAUTIONS, Laboratory Monitoring) during filgrastim therapy to avoid leukocytosis and to monitor the neutrophil count. In phase 3 clinical studies, filgrastim therapy was discontinued when the absolute neutrophil count (ANC) was $\geq$10,000/mm^3 after the expected chemotherapy-induced nadir.

PATIENTS WITH ACUTE MYELOID LEUKEMIA RECEIVING INDUCTION OR CONSOLIDATION CHEMOTHERAPY

Filgrastim is indicated for reducing the time to neutrophil recovery and the duration of fever, following induction or consolidation chemotherapy treatment of adults with AML.

CANCER PATIENTS RECEIVING BONE MARROW TRANSPLANT (BMT)

Filgrastim is indicated to reduce the duration of neutropenia and neutropenia-related clinical sequelae (*e.g.,* febrile neutropenia, in patients with nonmyeloid malignancies undergoing myeloablative chemotherapy followed by marrow transplantation. It is recommended that CBCs and platelet counts be obtained at a minimum of three times per week (see PRECAUTIONS, Laboratory Monitoring) following marrow infusion to monitor the recovery of marrow reconstitution.

PATIENTS UNDERGOING PERIPHERAL BLOOD PROGENITOR CELL COLLECTION AND THERAPY

Filgrastim is indicated for the mobilization of hematopoietic progenitor cells into the peripheral blood for collection by leukapheresis. Mobilization allows for the collection of increased numbers of progenitor cells capable of engraftment compared with collection by leukapheresis without mobilization or bone marrow harvest. After myeloablative chemotherapy, the transplantation of an increased number of progenitor cells can lead to more rapid engraftment, which may result in a decreased need for supportive care.

PATIENTS WITH SEVERE CHRONIC NEUTROPENIA

Filgrastim is indicated for chronic administration to reduce the incidence and duration of sequelae of neutropenia (*e.g.*, fever, infections, oropharyngeal ulcers) in symptomatic patients with congenital neutropenia, cyclic neutropenia, or idiopathic neutropenia. It is essential that serial CBCs with differential and platelet counts, and an evaluation of bone marrow morphology and karyotype be performed prior to initiation of filgrastim therapy. The use of filgrastim prior to confirmation of SCN may impair diagnostic efforts and may thus impair or delay evaluation and treatment of an underlying condition, other than SCN, causing the neutropenia.

NON-FDA APPROVED INDICATIONS

Although not FDA approved, filgrastim has been used in myelodysplastic syndromes, AIDS or zidovudine-associated neutropenia, agranulocytosis, and drug- or radiation-induced neutropenia.

CONTRAINDICATIONS

Filgrastim is contraindicated in patients with known hypersensitivity to *E. coli*-derived proteins, filgrastim, or any component of the product.

WARNINGS

Allergic-type reactions occurring on initial or subsequent treatment have been reported in <1 in 4000 patients treated with filgrastim. These have generally been characterized by systemic symptoms involving at least two body systems, most often skin (rash, urticaria, facial edema), respiratory (wheezing, dyspnea), and cardiovascular (hypotension, tachycardia). Some reactions occurred on initial exposure. Reactions tended to occur within the first 30 minutes after administration and appeared to occur more frequently in patients receiving filgrastim IV. Rapid resolution of symptoms occurred in most cases after administration of antihistamines, steroids, bronchodilators, and/or epinephrine. Symptoms recurred in more than half the patients who were rechallenged.

PATIENTS WITH SEVERE CHRONIC NEUTROPENIA

The safety and efficacy of filgrastim in the treatment of neutropenia due to other hematopoietic disorders (*e.g.*, myelodysplastic disorders or myeloid leukopenia) have not been established. Care should be taken to confirm the diagnosis of SCN before initiating filgrastim therapy.

While 9 of 325 patients developed myelodysplasia or myeloid leukemia while receiving filgrastim during clinical trials, acute myeloid leukemia (AML) or abnormal cytogenetics have been reported to occur in the natural history of SCN without cytokine therapy.[16] Abnormal cytogenetics have been associated with the eventual development of myeloid leukemia. The effect of filgrastim on the development of abnormal cytogenetics and the effect of continued filgrastim administration in patients with abnormal cytogenetics are unknown. If a patient with SCN develops abnormal cytogenetics, the risks and benefits of continuing filgrastim should be carefully considered (see ADVERSE REACTIONS).

PRECAUTIONS

GENERAL

Simultaneous Use With Chemotherapy and Radiation Therapy

The safety and efficacy of filgrastim given simultaneously with cytotoxic chemotherapy have not been established. Because of the potential sensitivity of rapidly dividing myeloid cells to cytotoxic chemotherapy, do not use filgrastim in the period 24 hours before to 24 hours after the administration of cytotoxic chemotherapy (see DOSAGE AND ADMINISTRATION).

The efficacy of filgrastim has not been evaluated in patients receiving chemotherapy associated with delayed myelosuppression (*e.g.*, nitrosoureas) or with mitomycin C or with myelosuppressive doses of anti-metabolites such as 5-fluorouracil.

The safety and efficacy of filgrastim have not been evaluated in patients receiving concurrent radiation therapy. Simultaneous use of filgrastim with chemotherapy and radiation therapy should be avoided.

Potential Effect on Malignant Cells

Filgrastim is a growth factor that primarily stimulates neutrophils. However, the possibility that filgrastim can act as a growth factor for any tumor type, cannot be excluded. In a randomized study evaluating the effects of filgrastim versus placebo in patients undergoing remission induction for AML, there was no significant difference in remission rate, disease free or overall survival.

The safety of filgrastim in chronic myeloid leukemia (CML) and myelodysplasia (MDS) has not been established.

When filgrastim is used to mobilize PBPC, tumor cells may be released from the marrow and subsequently collected in the leukapheresis product. The effect of reinfusion of tumor cells has not been well-studied, and the limited data available are inconclusive.

Leukocytosis

Cancer Patients Receiving Myelosuppressive Chemotherapy

White blood cell counts of 100,000/mm³ or greater were observed in approximately 2% of patients receiving Filgrastim at doses above 5 μg/kg/day. There were no reports of adverse events associated with this degree of leukocytosis. In order to avoid the potential complications of excessive leukocytosis, a complete blood count (CBC) is recommended twice per week during filgrastim therapy (see PRECAUTIONS, Laboratory Monitoring).

Premature Discontinuation of Filgrastim Therapy: Cancer Patients Receiving Myelosuppressive Chemotherapy

A transient increase in neutrophil counts is typically seen 1-2 days after initiation of filgrastim therapy. However, for a sustained therapeutic response, filgrastim therapy should be continued following chemotherapy until the post nadir ANC reaches 10,000/mm³. Therefore, the premature discontinuation of filgrastim therapy, prior to the time of recovery from the expected neutrophil nadir, is generally not recommended (see DOSAGE AND ADMINISTRATION).

Other

In studies of filgrastim administration following chemotherapy, most reported side effects were consistent with those usually seen as a result of cytotoxic chemotherapy (see ADVERSE REACTIONS). Because of the potential of receiving higher doses of chemotherapy (*i.e.*, full doses on the prescribed schedule), the patient may be at greater risk of thrombocytopenia, anemia, and non-hematologic consequences of increased chemotherapy doses (please refer to the prescribing information of the specific chemotherapy agents used). Regular monitoring of the hematocrit and platelet count is recommended. Furthermore, care should be exercised in the administration of filgrastim in conjunction with other drugs known to lower the platelet count. In septic patients receiving filgrastim, the physician should be alert to the theoretical possibility of adult respiratory distress syndrome, due to the possible influx of neutrophils at the site of inflammation.

There have been rare reports (<1 in 7000 patients) of cutaneous vasculitis in patients treated with filgrastim. In most cases, the severity of cutaneous vasculitis was moderate or severe. Most of the reports involved patients with SCN receiving long-term filgrastim therapy. Symptoms of vasculitis generally developed simultaneously with an increase in the ANC and abated when the ANC decreased. Many patients were able to continue filgrastim at a reduced dose.

INFORMATION FOR THE PATIENT

In those situations in which the physician determines that the patient can safely and effectively self-administer filgrastim, the patient should be instructed as to the proper dosage and administration. Patients should be referred to the information included with the prescription. This patient information, however, is not intended to be a disclosure of all known or possible effects. If home use is prescribed, patients should be thoroughly instructed in the importance of proper disposal and cautioned against the reuse of needles, syringes, or drug product. A puncture-resistant container for the disposal of used syringes and needles should be available to the patient. The full container should be disposed of according to the directions provided by the physician.

LABORATORY MONITORING

Cancer Patients Receiving Myelosuppressive Chemotherapy

A CBC and platelet count should be obtained prior to chemotherapy, and at regular intervals (twice per week) during filgrastim therapy. Following cytotoxic chemotherapy, the neutrophil nadir occurred earlier during cycles when filgrastim was administered, and WBC differentials demonstrated a left shift, including the appearance of promyelocytes and myeloblasts. In addition, the duration of severe neutropenia was reduced, and was followed by an accelerated recovery in the neutrophil counts. Therefore, regular monitoring of WBC counts, particularly at the time of the recovery from the post chemotherapy nadir, is recommended in order to avoid excessive leukocytosis.

Cancer Patients Receiving Bone Marrow Transplant

Frequent CBCs and platelet counts are recommended (at least three times per week) following marrow transplantation.

Patients With Severe Chronic Neutropenia

During the initial 4 weeks of filgrastim therapy and during the 2 weeks following any dose adjustment, a CBC with differential and platelet count should be performed twice weekly. Once a patient is clinically stable, a CBC with differential and platelet count should be performed monthly.

In Clinical Trials, the Following Laboratory Results Were Observed:

- Cyclic fluctuations in the neutrophil counts were frequently observed in patients with congenital or idiopathic neutropenia after initiation of filgrastim therapy.
- Platelet counts were generally at the upper limits of normal prior to filgrastim therapy, platelet counts decreased but usually remained within normal limits (see ADVERSE REACTIONS).
- Early myeloid forms were noted in peripheral blood in most patients, including the appearance of metamyelocytes and myelocytes. Promyelocytes and myeloblasts were noted in some patients.
- Relative increases were occasionally noted in the number of circulating eosinophils and basophils. No consistent increases were observed with filgrastim therapy.
- As in other trials, increases were observed in serum uric acid, lactic dehydrogenase, and serum alkaline phosphatase.

CARCINOGENESIS, MUTAGENESIS, AND IMPAIRMENT OF FERTILITY

The carcinogenic potential of filgrastim has not been studied. Filgrastim failed to induce bacterial gene mutations in either the presence or absence of a drug metabolizing enzyme system. Filgrastim had no observed effect on the fertility of male or female rats, or on gestation doses up to 500 μg/kg.

PREGNANCY CATEGORY C

Filgrastim has been shown to have adverse effects in pregnant rabbits when given in doses 2-10 times the human dose. There are no adequate and well-controlled studies in pregnant women. Filgrastim should be used during pregnancy only if the potential benefit justifies the potential risk to the fetus.

In rabbits, increased abortion and embryolethality were observed in animals treated with filgrastim at 80 μg/kg/day. Filgrastim administered to pregnant rabbits at doses of 80 μg/kg/day during the period of organogenesis was associated with increased fetal resorption, genitourinary bleeding, developmental abnormalities, decreased body weight, live births, and food consumption. External abnormalities were not observed in the fetuses of dams treated at 80 µg/kg/day. Reproductive studies in pregnant rats have shown that filgrastim was not associated with lethal, teratogenic, or behavioral effects on fetuses when administered by daily IV injection during the period of organogenesis at dose levels up to 575 µg/kg/day.

In Segment III studies in rats, offspring of dams treated at >20 µg/kg/day exhibited a delay in external differentiation (detachment of auricles and descent of testes) and slight growth retardation, possibly due to lower body weight of females during rearing and nursing. Offspring of dams treated at 100 µg/kg/day exhibited decreased body weights at birth, and a slightly reduced 4 day survival rate.

NURSING MOTHERS

It is not known whether filgrastim is excreted in human milk. Because many drugs are excreted in human milk, caution should be exercised if filgrastim is administered to a nursing woman.

PEDIATRIC USE

Serious long-term risks associated with daily administration of filgrastim have not been identified in pediatric patients (ages 4 months to 17 years) with SCN. Limited data from patients who were followed in the phase 3 study for 1.5 years did not suggest alterations in growth and development, sexual maturation, or endocrine function.

The safety and efficacy in neonates and patients with autoimmune neutropenia of infancy have not been established.

In the cancer setting, 12 pediatric patients with neuroblastoma have received up to 6 cycles of cyclophosphamide, cisplatin, doxorubicin, and etoposide chemotherapy concurrently with filgrastim; in this population, filgrastim was well tolerated. There was one report of palpable splenomegaly associated with filgrastim therapy, however, the only consistently reported adverse event was musculoskeletal pain, which is no different from the experience in the adult population.

DRUG INTERACTIONS

Drug interactions between filgrastim and other drugs have not been fully evaluated. Drugs which may potentiate the release of neutrophils, such as lithium, should be used with caution.

ADVERSE REACTIONS

CANCER PATIENTS RECEIVING MYELOSUPPRESSIVE CHEMOTHERAPY

In clinical trials including over 350 patients receiving filgrastim following nonmyeloablative cytotoxic chemotherapy, most adverse experiences were the sequelae of the underlying malignancy or cytotoxic chemotherapy. In all phase 2 and 3 trials, medullary bone pain, reported in 24% of patients, was the only consistently observed adverse reaction attributed to filgrastim therapy. This bone pain was generally reported to be of mild-to-moderate severity, and could be controlled in most patients with non-narcotic analgesics; infrequently, bone pain was severe enough to require narcotic analgesics. Bone pain was reported more frequently in patients treated with higher doses (20-100 µg/kg/day) administered IV, and less frequently in patients treated with lower SC doses of filgrastim (3-10 µg/kg/day).

In the randomized, double-blind, placebo-controlled trial of filgrastim therapy following combination chemotherapy in patients (n=207) with small cell lung cancer, the adverse events shown in TABLE 5 were reported during blinded cycles of study medication (placebo or filgrastim at 4-8 µg/kg/day). Events are reported as exposure adjusted since patients remained on double-blind filgrastim a median of 3 cycles versus 1 cycle for placebo (see TABLE 5).

TABLE 5 *% of Blinded Cycles With Events*

Event	Filgrastim n=384 Patient Cycles	Placebo n=257 Patient Cycles
Nausea/vomiting	57%	64%
Skeletal pain	22%	11%
Alopecia	18%	27%
Diarrhea	14%	23%
Neutropenic fever	13%	35%
Mucositis	12%	20%
Fever	12%	11%
Fatigue	11%	16%
Anorexia	9%	11%
Dyspnea	9%	11%
Headache	7%	9%
Cough	6%	8%
Skin rash	6%	9%
Chest pain	5%	6%
Generalized weakness	4%	7%
Sore throat	4%	9%
Stomatitis	5%	10%
Constipation	5%	10%
Pain (unspecified)	2%	7%

In this study, there were no serious, life-threatening, or fatal adverse reactions attributed to filgrastim therapy. Specifically, there were no reports of flu-like symptoms, pleuritis, pericarditis, or other major systemic reactions to filgrastim.

Spontaneously reversible elevations in uric acid, lactate dehydrogenase, and alkaline phosphatase occurred in 27-58% of 98 patients receiving blinded filgrastim therapy following cytotoxic chemotherapy; increases were generally mild to moderate. Transient decreases in blood pressure (<90/60 mmHg), which did not require clinical treatment, were reported in 7 of 176 patients in phase 3 clinical studies following administration of filgrastim. Cardiac events (myocardial infarctions, arrhythmias) have been reported in 11 of 375 cancer patients receiving filgrastim in clinical studies; the relationship to filgrastim therapy is unknown. No evidence of interaction of filgrastim with other drugs was observed in the course of clinical trials (see PRECAUTIONS).

There has been no evidence for the development of antibodies or of a blunted or diminished response to filgrastim in treated patients, including those receiving filgrastim daily for almost 2 years.

PATIENTS WITH ACUTE MYELOID LEUKEMIA

In a randomized phase 3 clinical trial, 259 patients received filgrastim and 262 patients received placebo postchemotherapy. Overall, the frequency of all reported adverse events was similar in both the filgrastim and placebo groups (83% vs 82% in Induction 1, 61% vs 64% in Cosolidation 1). Adverse events reported more frequently in the filgrastim-treated group included: perechiae (17% vs 14%), epistaxis (9% vs 5%), and transfusion reactions (10% vs 5%). There were no significant differences in the frequency of these events.

There were a similar number of deaths in each treatment group during induction (25 filgrastim vs 27 placebo). The primary causes of death included infection (9 vs 18), persistent leukemia (7 vs 5), and hemorrhage (6 vs 3). Of the hemorrhagic deaths, 5 cerebral hemorrhages were reported in the filgrastim group and 1 in the placebo group. Other serious nonfatal hemorrhagic events were reported in the respiratory tract (4 vs 1), skin (4 vs 4), gastrointestinal tract (2 vs 2), urinary tract (1 vs 1), ocular (1 vs 0), and other nonspecific sites (2 vs 1). While 19 (7%) patients in the filgrastim group and 5 (2%) patients in the placebo group experienced severe or fatal hemorrhagic events, overall, hemorrhagic adverse events were reported at a similar frequency in both groups (40% vs 38%). The time to transfusion-independent platelet recovery and the number of days of platelet transfusions were similar in both groups.

CANCER PATIENTS RECEIVING BONE MARROW TRANSPLANT

In clinical trials, the reported adverse effects were those typically seen in patients receiving intensive chemotherapy followed by bone marrow transplantation (BMT). The most common events reported in both control and treatment groups included stomatitis, nausea, and vomiting, generally of mild-to-moderate severity and were considered unrelated to filgrastim. In the randomized studies of BMT involving 167 patients who received study drug, the following events occurred more frequently in patients treated with filgrastim than in controls: nausea (10% vs 4%), vomiting (7% vs 3%), hypertension (4% vs 0%), rash (12% vs 10%), and peritonitis (2% vs 0%). None of these events were reported by the Investigator to be related to filgrastim. One event of erythema nodosum was reported moderate in severity and possibly related to filgrastim.

Generally, adverse events observed in non-randomized studies were similar to those seen in randomized studies, occurred in a minority of patients, and were of mild-to-moderate severity. In one study (n=45), three serious adverse events reported by the Investigator were considered possibly related to filgrastim. These included two events of renal insufficiency and one event of capillary leak syndrome. The relationship of these events to filgrastim remains unclear since they occurred in patients with culture-proven infection with clinical sepsis who were receiving potentially nephrotoxic antibacterial and antifungal therapy.

CANCER PATIENTS UNDERGOING PERIPHERAL BLOOD PROGENITOR CELL COLLECTION AND THERAPY

In clinical trials, 126 patients received filgrastim for PBPC mobilization. In this setting, filgrastim was generally well tolerated. Adverse events related to filgrastim consisted primarily of mild-to-moderate musculoskeletal symptoms, reported in 44% of patients. These symptoms were predominantly events of medullary bone pain (33%). Headache was reported related to filgrastim in 7% of patients. Transient increases in alkaline phosphatase related to filgrastim were reported in 21% of the patients who had serum chemistries measured; most were mild-to-moderate.

All patients had increases in neutrophil counts during mobilization, consistent with the biological effects of filgrastim. Two patients had a WBC count >100,000 mm^3. No sequelae were associated with any grade of leukocytosis.

Sixty-five percent of patients had mild-to-moderate anemia and 97% of patients had decreases in platelet counts; five patients (out of 126) had decreased platelet counts to <50,000/mm^3. Anemia and thrombocytopenia have been reported to be related to leukapheresis; however, the possibility that filgrastim mobilization may contribute to anemia or thrombocytopenia has not been ruled out.

PATIENTS WITH SEVERE CHRONIC NEUTROPENIA

Mild-to-moderate bone pain was reported in approximately 33% of patients in clinical trials. This symptom was readily controlled with non-narcotic analgesics. Generalized musculoskeletal pain was also noted in higher frequency in patients treated with filgrastim. Palpable splenomegaly was observed in approximately 30% of patients. Abdominal or flank pain was seen infrequently and thrombocytopenia (<50,000/mm^3) was noted in 12% of patients with palpable spleens. Fewer than 3% of all patients underwent splenectomy, and most of these had a prestudy history of splenomegaly. Fewer than 6% of patients had thrombocytopenia (<50,000/mm^3) during filgrastim therapy, most of whom had a pre-existing history of thrombocytopenia. In most cases, thrombocytopenia was managed by filgrastim dose reduction or interruption. An additional 5% of patients had platelet counts between 50,000-100,000/mm^3. There were no associated serious hemorrhagic sequelae in these patients. Epistaxis was noted in 15% of patients treated with filgrastim, but was associated with thrombocytopenia in 2% of patients. Anemia was reported in approximately 10% of patients, but in most cases appeared to be related to frequent diagnostic phlebotomy, chronic illness, or concomitant medications. In clinical trials, myelodysplasia or myeloid leukemia was reported to have developed during filgrastim threrapy in approximately 3% of patients (9 of 3250) (see WARNINGS). Twelve (12) patients from a subset of 102 who had normal cytogenetic evaluations at baseline were subsequently found to have abnormalities, including monosomy 7, on routine repeat evaluation conducted after 18-52 months of filgrastim therapy. It is unknown whether the development of these findings is related to chronic daily filgrastim administration or reflects the natural history of SCN. Other adverse events infrequently observed and possibly related to filgrastim therapy were: injection site reaction, rash, hepatomegaly, arthralgia, osteoporosis, cutaneous vasculitis, hematuria/proteinuria, alopecia, and exacerbation of some pre-existing skin disorders (*e.g.,* psoriasis).

DOSAGE AND ADMINISTRATION

CANCER PATIENTS RECEIVING MYELOSUPPRESSIVE CHEMOTHERAPY

The recommended starting dose of filgrastim is 5 μg/kg/day, administered as a single daily injection by SC bolus injection, by short IV infusion (15-30 minutes), or by continuous SC or continuous IV infusion. A CBC platelet count should be obtained before instituting filgrastim therapy, and monitored twice weekly during therapy. Doses may be increased in increments of 5 μg/kg for each chemotherapy cycle, according to the duration and severity of the ANC nadir.

Filgrastim should be administered no earlier than 24 hours after the administration of cytotoxic chemotherapy. Filgrastim should not be administered in the period 24 hours before the administration of chemotherapy (see PRECAUTIONS). Filgrastim should be administered daily for up to 2 weeks, until the ANC has reached 10,000/mm³ following the expected chemotherapy-induced neutrophil nadir. The duration of filgrastim therapy needed to attenuate chemotherapy-induced neutropenia may be dependent on the myelosuppressive potential of the chemotherapy regimen employed. Filgrastim therapy should be discontinued if the ANC surpasses 10,000/mm³ after the expected chemotherapy-induced neutrophil nadir (see PRECAUTIONS). In phase 3 trials, efficacy was observed at doses of 4-8 μg/kg/day.

CANCER PATIENTS RECEIVING BONE MARROW TRANSPLANT

The recommended dose of filgrastim following BMT is 10 μg/kg/day given as an IV infusion of 4 or 24 hours, or as a continuous 24 hour SC infusion. For patients receiving BMT, the first dose of filgrastim should be administered at least 24 hours after cytotoxic chemotherapy and at least 24 hours after bone marrow infusion.

During the period of neutrophil recovery, the daily dose of filgrastim should be titrated against the neutrophil response as found in TABLE 6.

TABLE 6

Absolute Neutrophil Count	Filgrastim Dose Adjustment
When ANC >1000/mm³ for 3 consecutive days then:	Reduce to 5 μg/kg/day*
If ANC remains >1000/mm³ for 3 more consecutive days then:	Discontinue filgrastim
If ANC decreases to <1000/mm³	Resume at 5 μg/kg/day

* If ANC decreases to <1000/mm³ at any time during the 5 μg/kg/day administration, filgrastim should be increased to 10 μg/kg/day, and the above steps should then be followed.

Peripheral Blood Progenitor Cell Collection and Therapy in Cancer Patients

The recommended dose of filgrastim for the mobilization of PBPC is 10 μg/kg/day subcutaneously, either as a bolus or a continuous infusion. It is recommended that filgrastim be given for at least 4 days before the first leukapheresis procedure and continued until the last leukapheresis. Although the optimal duration of filgrastim administration and leukapheresis schedule have not been established, administration of filgrastim for 6-7 days with leukaphereses on days 5, 6 and 7 was found to be safe and effective. Neutrophil counts should be monitored after 4 days of filgrastim, and filgrastim dose-modification should be considered for those patients who develop a WBC count >100,000/mm³.

In all clinical trials of filgrastim for the mobilization of PBPC, filgrastim was also administered after reinfusion of the collected cells.

PATIENTS WITH SEVERE CHRONIC NEUTROPENIA

Filgrastim should be administered to those patients in whom a diagnosis of congenital, cyclic, or idiopathic neutropenia has been definitively confirmed. Other diseases associated with neutropenia should be ruled out.

Starting Dose:

Congenital Neutropenia: The recommended daily starting dose is 6 μg/kg bid subcutaneously every day.

Idiopathic or Cyclic Neutropenia: The recommended daily starting dose is 5 μg/kg as a single injection subcutaneously every day.

Dose Adjustments

Chronic daily administration is required to maintain clinical benefit. ANC should not be used as the sole indication of efficacy. The dose should be individually adjusted based on the patients' clinical course as well as ANC. In the phase 3 study, the target absolute neutrophil count was 1500/mm³. However, patients may experience clinical benefit with absolute neutrophil counts below this target range. The dose should be reduced if the absolute neutrophil count is persistently greater than 10,000/mm³.

Dilution

If required, filgrastim may be diluted in 5% dextrose. Filgrastim diluted to concentrations between 5 and 15 μg/ml should be protected from adsorption to plastic materials by addition of Albumin (Human) to a final concentration of 2 mg/ml. When diluted in 5% dextrose or 5% dextrose plus Albumin (Human), filgrastim is compatible with glass bottles, PVC and polyolefin IV bags, and polypropylene syringes.

Dilution of filgrastim to a final concentration of less than 5 μg/ml is not recommended at any time. **Do not dilute with saline at any time; product may precipitate.**

HOW SUPPLIED

Neupogen: Use only one dose per vial; do not reenter the vial. Discard unused portions. Do not save unused drug for later administration.

Single-dose, preservative-free vials containing 300 μg (1 ml) of filgrastim (300 μg/ml).

Single-dose, preservative-free vials containing 480 ml (1.6 ml) of filgrastim (300 μg/ml).

Storage: Neupogen should be stored at 2°-8° C (36°-46° F). Do not freeze. Avoid shaking. Prior to injection, filgrastim may be allowed to reach room temperature for a maximum of 24 hours. Any vial left at room temperature for greater than 24 hours should be discarded. Parenteral drug products should be inspected visually for particulate matter and discoloration prior to administration, whenever solution and container permit, if particulates or discoloration are observed, the container should not be used.

PRODUCT LISTING - EQUIVALENTS NOT AVAILABLE

Solution - Injectable - 300 mcg/ml

1 ml	$156.10	NEUPOGEN, Amgen	55513-0347-01
1 ml	$172.59	NEUPOGEN, Physicians Total Care	54868-2522-00
1 ml	$197.80	NEUPOGEN, Amgen	55513-0530-01
1 ml x 10	$1548.00	NEUPOGEN, Amgen	55513-0347-10
1 ml x 10	$1885.00	NEUPOGEN, Allscripts Pharmaceutical Company	54569-4824-00
1 ml x 10	$2075.00	NEUPOGEN, Amgen	55513-0530-10
1.60 ml	$242.50	NEUPOGEN, Amgen	55513-0348-01
1.60 ml	$315.10	NEUPOGEN, Amgen	55513-0546-01
1.60 ml x 10	$2466.00	NEUPOGEN, Amgen	55513-0348-10
1.60 ml x 10	$3306.30	NEUPOGEN, Amgen	55513-0546-10

Solution - Injectable - 600 mcg/ml

0.50 ml	$197.90	NEUPOGEN, Amgen	55513-0924-01
0.50 ml x 10	$2276.30	NEUPOGEN, Amgen	55513-0924-10
0.80 ml	$345.60	NEUPOGEN, Amgen	55513-0209-01
0.80 ml x 10	$3626.30	NEUPOGEN, Amgen	55513-0209-10

F

Finasteride (003078)

Categories: Alopecia, androgenetic; Hyperplasia, benign prostatic; Pregnancy Category X; FDA Approved 1992 Jun
Drug Classes: 5-alpha-reductase inhibitors; Antiandrogens; Hormones/hormone modifiers
Brand Names: Propecia; **Proscar**
Foreign Brand Availability: Chibro-Proscar (France); Fincar (India); Finired (Indonesia); Finpro (Indonesia); Fistrin (Colombia); Nasterol (Colombia); Pro-Cure (Israel); Prohair (Bahrain; Cyprus; Egypt; Iran; Iraq; Jordan; Kuwait; Lebanon; Libya; Oman; Qatar; Republic-of-Yemen; Saudi-Arabia; Syria; United-Arab-Emirates); Propeshia (Mexico); Proscar 5 (South-Africa); Prosh (Indonesia); Prostacare (Bahrain; Cyprus; Egypt; Iran; Iraq; Jordan; Kuwait; Lebanon; Libya; Oman; Qatar; Republic-of-Yemen; Saudi-Arabia; Syria; United-Arab-Emirates); Prostacom (Indonesia); Reprostom (Indonesia); Tensen (Taiwan)
Cost of Therapy: $75.88 (BPH; Proscar; 5 mg; 1 tablet/day; 30 day supply)
$49.35 (Male Pattern Hair Loss; Proscar; 1 mg; 1 tablet/day; 30 day supply)

DESCRIPTION

Note: The trade names have been used throughout this monograph for clarity.

PROPECIA

Propecia (finasteride), a synthetic 4-azasteroid compound, is a specific inhibitor of steroid Type II 5α-reductase, an intracellular enzyme that converts the androgen testosterone into 5α-dihydrotestosterone (DHT).

Finasteride is 4-azaandrost-1-ene-17-carboxamide,*N*-(1,1-dimethylethyl)-3-oxo-,(5α,17β)-. The empirical formula of finasteride is $C_{23}H_{36}N_2O_2$ and its molecular weight is 372.55.

Finasteride is a white crystalline powder with a melting point near 250°C. It is freely soluble in chloroform and in lower alcohol solvents but is practically insoluble in water.

Propecia tablets for oral administration are film-coated tablets that contain 1 mg of finasteride and the following inactive ingredients: lactose monohydrate, microcrystalline cellulose, pregelatinized starch, sodium starch glycolate, docusate sodium, magnesium stearate, hydroxypropyl methylcellulose 2910, hydroxypropyl cellulose, titanium dioxide, talc, yellow ferric oxide, and red ferric oxide.

PROSCAR

Proscar (finasteride), a synthetic 4-azasteroid compound, is a specific inhibitor of steroid Type II 5α-reductase, an intracellular enzyme that converts the androgen testosterone into 5α-dihydrotestosterone (DHT).

Finasteride is 4-azaandrost-1-ene-17-carboxamide,*N*-(1,1-dimethylethyl)-3-oxo-,(5α,17β)-. The empirical formula of finasteride is $C_{23}H_{36}N_2O_2$ and its molecular weight is 372.55.

Finasteride is a white crystalline powder with a melting point near 250°C. It is freely soluble in chloroform and in lower alcohol solvents, but is practically insoluble in water.

Proscar (finasteride) tablets for oral administration are film-coated tablets that contain 5 mg of finasteride and the following inactive ingredients: hydrous lactose, microcrystalline cellulose, pregelatinized starch, sodium starch glycolate, hydroxypropyl cellulose LF, hydroxypropylmethyl cellulose, titanium dioxide, magnesium stearate, talc, docusate sodium, FD&C blue 2 aluminum lake and yellow iron oxide.

CLINICAL PHARMACOLOGY

PROPECIA

Finasteride is a competitive and specific inhibitor of Type II 5α-reductase, an intracellular enzyme that converts the androgen testosterone into DHT. Two distinct isozymes are found in mice, rats, monkeys, and humans: Type I and II. Each of these isozymes is differentially expressed in tissues and developmental stages. In humans, Type I 5α-reductase is predominant in the sebaceous glands of most regions of skin, including scalp, and liver. Type I 5α-reductase is responsible for approximately one-third of circulating DHT. The Type II 5α-reductase isozyme is primarily found in prostate, seminal vesicles, epididymides, and hair follicles as well as liver, and is responsible for two-thirds of circulating DHT.

In humans, the mechanism of action of finasteride is based on its preferential inhibition of the Type II isozyme. Using native tissues (scalp and prostate), *in vitro* binding studies examining the potential of finasteride to inhibit either isozyme revealed a 100-fold selectivity for the human Type II 5α-reductase over Type I isozyme (IC_{50} = 500 and 4.2 nM for Type I and II, respectively). For both isozymes, the inhibition by finasteride is accompanied by reduction of the inhibitor to dihydrofinasteride and adduct formation with NADP+. The turnover for the enzyme complex is slow ($T_{1/2}$ approximately 30 days for the Type II enzyme complex and 14 days for the Type I complex).

Finasteride has no affinity for the androgen receptor and has no androgenic, antiandrogenic, estrogenic, antiestrogenic, or progestational effects. Inhibition of Type II 5α-reductase blocks the peripheral conversion of testosterone to DHT, resulting in significant decreases in serum and tissue DHT concentrations. Finasteride produces a rapid reduction in serum DHT concentration, reaching 65% suppression within 24 hours of oral dosing with a 1 mg tablet.

In men with male pattern hair loss (androgenetic alopecia), the balding scalp contains miniaturized hair follicles and increased amounts of DHT compared with hairy scalp. Administration of finasteride decreases scalp and serum DHT concentrations in these men. The relative contributions of these reductions to the treatment effect of finasteride have not been defined. By this mechanism, finasteride appears to interrupt a key factor in the development of androgenetic alopecia in those patients genetically predisposed.

A 48 week, placebo-controlled study designed to assess by phototrichogram the effect of Propecia on total and actively growing (anagen) scalp hairs in vertex baldness enrolled 212 men with androgenetic alopecia. At baseline and 48 weeks, total and anagen hair counts were obtained in a 1 cm_2 target area of the scalp. Men treated with Propecia showed increases from baseline in total and anagen hair counts of 7 hairs and 18 hairs, respectively, whereas men treated with placebo had decreases of 10 hairs and 9 hairs, respectively. These changes in hair counts resulted in a between-group difference of 17 hairs in total hair count ($p < 0.001$) and 27 hairs in anagen hair count ($p < 0.001$), and an improvement in the proportion of anagen hairs from 62% at baseline to 68% for men treated with Propecia.

F

Finasteride had no effect on circulating levels of cortisol, thyroid-stimulating hormone, or thyroxine, nor did it affect the plasma lipid profile (*e.g.*, total cholesterol, low-density lipoproteins, high-density lipoproteins and triglycerides) or bone mineral density. In studies with finasteride, no clinically meaningful changes in luteinizing hormone (LH) or follicle-stimulating hormone (FSH) were detected. In healthy volunteers, treatment with finasteride did not alter the response of LH and FSH to gonadotropin-releasing hormone, indicating that the hypothalamic-pituitary-testicular axis was not affected. Mean circulating levels of testosterone and estradiol were increased by approximately 15% as compared to baseline in the first year of treatment, but these levels were within the physiologic range.

Pharmacokinetics

Following an oral dose of ^{14}C-finasteride in man, a mean of 39% (range, 32-46%) of the dose was excreted in the urine in the form of metabolites; 57% (range, 51-64%) was excreted in the feces. The major compound isolated from urine was the monocarboxylic acid metabolite; virtually no unchanged drug was recovered. The t-butyl side chain monohydroxylated metabolite has been isolated from plasma. These metabolites possessed no more than 20% of the 5α-reductase inhibitory activity of finasteride.

In a study in 15 healthy male subjects, the mean bioavailability of finasteride 1 mg tablets was 65% (range 26-170%), based on the ratio of AUC relative to a 5 mg IV dose infused over 60 minutes. Following IV infusion, mean plasma clearance was 165 ml/min (range, 70-279 ml/min) and mean steady-state volume of distribution was 76 L (range, 44-96 L). In a separate study, the bioavailability of finasteride was not affected by food.

Approximately 90% of circulating finasteride is bound to plasma proteins. Finasteride has been found to cross the blood-brain barrier.

There is a slow accumulation phase for finasteride after multiple dosing. At steady state following dosing with 1 mg/day, maximum finasteride plasma concentration averaged 9.2 ng/ml (range, 4.9-13.7 ng/ml) and was reached 1-2 hours postdose; AUC(0-24h) was 53 ng·h/ml (range, 20-154 ng·h/ml) and mean terminal half-life of elimination was 4.8 hours (range, 3.3-13.4 hours).

Semen levels have been measured in 35 men taking finasteride 1 mg daily for 6 weeks. In 60% (21 of 35) of the samples, finasteride levels were undetectable. The mean finasteride level was 0.26 ng/ml and the highest level measured was 1.52 ng/ml. Using this highest semen level measured and assuming 100% absorption from a 5 ml ejaculate per day, human exposure through vaginal absorption would be up to 7.6 ng/day, which is 750 times lower than the exposure from the no-effect dose for developmental abnormalities in Rhesus monkeys (see PRECAUTIONS, Propecia, Pregnancy, Teratogenic Effects, Pregnancy Category X).

The elimination rate of finasteride decreases somewhat with age. Mean terminal half-life is approximately 5-6 hours in men 18-60 years of age and 8 hours in men more than 70 years of age. These findings are of no clinical significance, and a reduction in dosage in the elderly is not warranted.

No dosage adjustment is necessary in patients with renal insufficiency. In patients with chronic renal impairment (creatinine clearance ranging from 9.0 to 55 ml/min), the values for AUC, maximum plasma concentration, half-life, and protein binding after a single dose of ^{14}C-finasteride were similar to those obtained in healthy volunteers. Urinary excretion of metabolites was decreased in patients with renal impairment. This decrease was associated with an increase in fecal excretion of metabolites. Plasma concentrations of metabolites were significantly higher in patients with renal impairment (based on a 60% increase in total radioactivity AUC). Furthermore, finasteride has been well tolerated in men with normal renal function receiving up to 80 mg/day for 12 weeks where exposure of these patients to metabolites would presumably be much greater.

PROSCAR

The development and enlargement of the prostate gland is dependent on the potent androgen, 5α-dihydrotestosterone (DHT). Type II 5α-reductase metabolizes testosterone to DHT in the prostate gland, liver and skin. DHT induces androgenic effects by binding to androgen receptors in the cell nuclei of these organs.

Finasteride is a competitive and specific inhibitor of Type II 5α-reductase with which it slowly forms a stable enzyme complex. Turnover from this complex is extremely slow ($T_{1/2}$ ~30 days). This has been demonstrated both *in vivo* and *in vitro*. Finasteride has no affinity for the androgen receptor. In man, the 5α-reduced steroid metabolites in blood and urine are decreased after administration of finasteride.

In man, a single 5 mg oral dose of Proscar produces a rapid reduction in serum DHT concentration, with the maximum effect observed 8 hours after the first dose. The suppression of DHT is maintained throughout the 24 hour dosing interval and with continued treatment. Daily dosing of Proscar at 5 mg/day for up to 4 years has been shown to reduce the serum DHT concentration by approximately 70%. The median circulating level of testosterone increased by approximately 10-20% but remained within the physiologic range.

Adult males with genetically inherited Type II 5α-reductase deficiency also have decreased levels of DHT. Except for the associated urogenital defects present at birth, no other clinical abnormalities related to Type II 5α-reductase deficiency have been observed in these individuals. These individuals have a small prostate gland throughout life and do not develop BPH.

In patients with BPH treated with finasteride (1-100 mg/day) for 7-10 days prior to prostatectomy, an approximate 80% lower DHT content was measured in prostatic tissue removed at surgery, compared to placebo; testosterone tissue concentration was increased up to 10 times over pretreatment levels, relative to placebo. Intraprostatic content of prostate-specific antigen (PSA) was also decreased.

In healthy male volunteers treated with Proscar for 14 days, discontinuation of therapy resulted in a return of DHT levels to pretreatment levels in approximately 2 weeks. In patients treated for 3 months, prostate volume, which declined by approximately 20%, returned to close to baseline value after approximately 3 months of discontinuation of therapy.

Pharmacokinetics

Absorption

In a study of 15 healthy young subjects, the mean bioavailability of finasteride 5 mg tablets was 63% (range 34-108%), based on the ratio of area under the curve (AUC) relative to an intravenous (IV) reference dose. Maximum finasteride plasma concentration averaged 37 ng/ml (range, 27-49 ng/ml) and was reached 1-2 hours postdose.

Bioavailability of finasteride was not affected by food.

Distribution

Mean steady-state volume of distribution was 76 L (range, 44-96 L). Approximately 90% of circulating finasteride is bound to plasma proteins. There is a slow accumulation phase for finasteride after multiple dosing. After dosing with 5 mg/day of finasteride for 17 days, plasma concentrations of finasteride were 47 and 54% higher than after the first dose in men 45-60 years old (n=12) and ≥70 years old (n=12), respectively. Mean trough concentrations after 17 days of dosing were 6.2 ng/ml (range, 2.4-9.8 ng/ml) and 8.1 ng/ml (range, 1.8-19.7 ng/ml), respectively, in the two age groups. Although steady state was not reached in this study, mean trough plasma concentration in another study in patients with BPH (mean age, 65 years) receiving 5 mg/day was 9.4 ng/ml (range, 7.1-13.3 ng/ml; n=22) after over a year of dosing.

Finasteride has been shown to cross the blood brain barrier but does not appear to distribute preferentially to the CSF.

In 2 studies of healthy subjects (n=69) receiving Proscar 5 mg/day for 6-24 weeks, finasteride concentrations in semen ranged from undetectable (<0.1 ng/ml) to 10.54 ng/ml. In an earlier study using a less sensitive assay, finasteride concentrations in the semen of 16 subjects receiving Proscar 5 mg/day ranged from undetectable (<1.0 ng/ml) to 21 ng/ml. Thus, based on a 5 ml ejaculate volume, the amount of finasteride in semen was estimated to be 50- to 100-fold less than the dose of finasteride (5 μg) that had no effect on circulating DHT levels in men (see also PRECAUTIONS, Proscar, Pregnancy Category X).

Metabolism

Finasteride is extensively metabolized in the liver, primarily via the cytochrome P450 3A4 enzyme subfamily. Two metabolites, the t-butyl side chain monohydroxylated and monocarboxylic acid metabolites, have been identified that possess no more than 20% of the 5α-reductase inhibitory activity of finasteride.

Excretion

In healthy young subjects (n=15), mean plasma clearance of finasteride was 165 ml/min (range, 70-279 ml/min) and mean elimination half-life in plasma was 6 hours (range, 3-16 hours). Following an oral dose of ^{14}C-finasteride in man (n=6), a mean of 39% (range, 32-46%) of the dose was excreted in the urine in the form of metabolites; 57% (range, 51-64%) was excreted in the feces.

The mean terminal half-life of finasteride in subjects ≥70 years of age was approximately 8 hours (range, 6-15 hours; n=12), compared with 6 hours (range, 4-12 hours; n=12) in subjects 45-60 years of age. As a result, mean AUC (0-24h) after 17 days of dosing was 15% higher in subjects ≥70 years of age than in subjects 45-60 years of age (p=0.02).

Special Populations

Pediatric

Finasteride pharmacokinetics have not been investigated in patients <18 years of age.

Gender

Finasteride pharmacokinetics in women are not available.

Geriatric

No dosage adjustment is necessary in the elderly. Although the elimination rate of finasteride is decreased in the elderly, these findings are of no clinical significance. See also Pharmacokinetics, Excretion; PRECAUTIONS, Proscar, Geriatric Use; and DOSAGE AND ADMINISTRATION, Proscar.

Race

The effect of race on finasteride pharmacokinetics has not been studied.

Renal Insufficiency

No dosage adjustment is necessary in patients with renal insufficiency. In patients with chronic renal impairment, with creatinine clearances ranging from 9.0 to 55 ml/min, AUC, maximum plasma concentration, half-life, and protein binding after a single dose of ^{14}C-finasteride were similar to values obtained in healthy volunteers. Urinary excretion of metabolites was decreased in patients with renal impairment. This decrease was associated with an increase in fecal excretion of metabolites. Plasma concentrations of metabolites were significantly higher in patients with renal impairment (based on a 60% increase in total radioactivity AUC). However, finasteride has been well tolerated in BPH patients with normal renal function receiving up to 80 mg/day for 12 weeks, where exposure of these patients to metabolites would presumably be much greater.

Hepatic Insufficiency

The effect of hepatic insufficiency on finasteride pharmacokinetics has not been studied. Caution should be used in the administration of Proscar in those patients with liver function abnormalities, as finasteride is metabolized extensively in the liver.

Drug Interactions

Also see DRUG INTERACTIONS, Proscar.

No drug interactions of clinical importance have been identified. Finasteride does not appear to affect the cytochrome P450-linked drug metabolism enzyme system. Compounds that have been tested in man have included antipyrine, digoxin, propranolol, theophylline, and warfarin, and no clinically meaningful interactions were found.

TABLE 1 *Mean (SD) Pharmacokinetic Parameters in Healthy Young Subjects (n=15)*

	Mean (±SD)
Bioavailability	63% (34-108%)*
Clearance (ml/min)	165 (55)
Volume of distribution (L)	76 (14)
Half-life (hours)	6.2 (2.1)

* Range.

TABLE 2 *Mean (SD) Noncompartmental Pharmacokinetic Parameters After Multiple Doses of 5 mg/day in Older Men*

	Mean (±SD)	
	45-60 years old (n=12)	≥70 years old (n=12)
AUC (ng·h/ml)	389 (98)	463 (186)
Peak concentration (ng/ml)	46.2 (8.7)	48.4 (14.7)
Time to peak (hours)	1.8 (0.7)	1.8 (0.6)
Half-life (hours)*	6.0 (1.5)	8.2 (2.5)

* First-dose values; all other parameters are last-dose values.

INDICATIONS AND USAGE

PROPECIA

Propecia is indicated for the treatment of male pattern hair loss (androgenetic alopecia) in **MEN ONLY.** Safety and efficacy were demonstrated in men between 18-41 years of age with mild to moderate hair loss of the vertex and anterior mid-scalp area.

Efficacy in bitemporal recession has not been established.

Propecia is not indicated in women (see CONTRAINDICATIONS, Propecia).

Propecia is not indicated in children (see PRECAUTIONS, Propecia, Pediatric Use).

PROSCAR

Proscar is indicated for the treatment of symptomatic benign prostatic hyperplasia (BPH) in men with an enlarged prostate to:

Improve symptoms.

Reduce the risk of acute urinary retention.

Reduce the risk of the need for surgery including transurethral resection of the prostate (TURP) and prostatectomy.

NON-FDA APPROVED INDICATIONS

Finasteride has been used experimentally for the treatment of prostate cancer, hirsutism, and acne. However, further study is needed to fully assess the utility of finasteride in the management of these conditions.

CONTRAINDICATIONS

PROPECIA

Propecia is contraindicated in the following:

Pregnancy: Finasteride use is contraindicated in women when they are or may potentially be pregnant. Because of the ability of 5α-reductase inhibitors to inhibit the conversion of testosterone to DHT, finasteride may cause abnormalities of the external genitalia of a male fetus of a pregnant woman who receives finasteride. If this drug is used during pregnancy, or if pregnancy occurs while taking this drug, the pregnant woman should be apprised of the potential hazard to the male fetus. (See also WARNINGS, Propecia, Exposure of Women — Risk to Male Fetus; PRECAUTIONS, Propecia: Information for the Patient and Pregnancy, Teratogenic Effects, Pregnancy Category X.) In female rats, low doses of finasteride administered during pregnancy have produced abnormalities of the external genitalia in male offspring.

Hypersensitivity to any component of this medication.

PROSCAR

Proscar is contraindicated in the following:

Hypersensitivity to any component of this medication.

Pregnancy: Finasteride use is contraindicated in women when they are or may potentially be pregnant. Because of the ability of Type II 5α-reductase inhibitors to inhibit the conversion of testosterone to DHT, finasteride may cause abnormalities of the external genitalia of a male fetus of a pregnant woman who receives finasteride. If this drug is used during pregnancy, or if pregnancy occurs while taking this drug, the pregnant woman should be apprised of the potential hazard to the male fetus. (See also WARNINGS, Proscar, Exposure of Women — Risk to Male Fetus; PRECAUTIONS, Proscar: Information for the Patient and Pregnancy Category X.) In female rats, low doses of finasteride administered during pregnancy have produced abnormalities of the external genitalia in male offspring.

WARNINGS

PROPECIA

Propecia is not indicated for use in pediatric patients (see INDICATIONS AND USAGE, Propecia; and PRECAUTIONS, Propecia, Pediatric Use) or women (see alsoPRECAUTIONS, Propecia: Information for the Patient and Pregnancy, Teratogenic Effects, Pregnancy Category X; and HOW SUPPLIED, Propecia, Storage and Handling).

Exposure of Women — Risk to Male Fetus

Women should not handle crushed or broken Propecia tablets when they are pregnant or may potentially be pregnant because of the possibility of absorption of finasteride and the subsequent potential risk to a male fetus. Propecia tablets are coated and will prevent contact with the active ingredient during normal handling, provided that the tablets have not been broken or crushed. (See also CONTRAINDICATIONS, Propecia; PRECAUTIONS, Propecia: Information for the Patient and Pregnancy, Teratogenic Effects, Pregnancy Category X; and HOW SUPPLIED, Propecia, Storage and Handling.)

PROSCAR

Proscar is not indicated for use in pediatric patients (see PRECAUTIONS, Proscar, Pediatric Use) or women (see also WARNINGS, Proscar, Exposure of Women — Risk to Male Fetus; PRECAUTIONS, Proscar, Information for the Patient; PRECAUTIONS, Proscar, Pregnancy Category X; and HOW SUPPLIED, Proscar).

Exposure of Women — Risk to Male Fetus

Women should not handle crushed or broken Proscar tablets when they are pregnant or may potentially be pregnant because of the possibility of absorption of finasteride and the subsequent potential risk to a male fetus.

Proscar tablets are coated and will prevent contact with the active ingredient during normal handling, provided that the tablets have not been broken or crushed. (See CONTRAINDICATIONS, Proscar; PRECAUTIONS, Proscar: Information for the Patient and Pregnancy Category X; and HOW SUPPLIED, Proscar.)

PRECAUTIONS

PROPECIA

General

Caution should be used in the administration of Propecia in patients with liver function abnormalities, as finasteride is metabolized extensively in the liver.

Information for the Patient

Women should not handle crushed or broken Propecia tablets when they are pregnant or may potentially be pregnant because of the possibility of absorption of finasteride and the subsequent potential risk to a male fetus. Propecia tablets are coated and will prevent contact with the active ingredient during normal handling, provided that the tablets have not been broken or crushed. (See also CONTRAINDICATIONS, Propecia; WARNINGS, Propecia, Exposure of Women — Risk to Male Fetus; PRECAUTIONS, Propecia, Pregnancy, Teratogenic Effects, Pregnancy Category X; and HOW SUPPLIED, Propecia, Storage and Handling.) See also the Patient Package Insert included with the prescription.

Drug/Laboratory Test Interactions

In clinical studies with Propecia in men 18-41 years of age, the mean value of serum prostate-specific antigen (PSA) decreased from 0.7 ng/ml at baseline to 0.5 ng/ml at month 12. When finasteride is used in older men who have benign prostatic hyperplasia (BPH), PSA levels are decreased by approximately 50%. Until further information is gathered in men >41 years of age without BPH, consideration should be given to doubling the PSA level in men undergoing this test while taking Propecia.

Carcinogenesis, Mutagenesis, and Impairment of Fertility

No evidence of a tumorigenic effect was observed in a 24 month study in Sprague-Dawley rats receiving doses of finasteride up to 160 mg/kg/day in males and 320 mg/kg/day in females. These doses produced respective systemic exposure in rats of 888 and 2192 times those observed in man receiving the recommended human dose of 1 mg/day. All exposure calculations were based on calculated AUC(0-24h) for animals and mean AUC(0-24h) for man (0.05 μg·h/ml).

In a 19 month carcinogenicity study in CD-1 mice, a statistically significant ($p \leq 0.05$) increase in the incidence of testicular Leydig cell adenomas was observed at a dose of 250 mg/kg/day (1824 times the human exposure). In mice at a dose of 25 mg/kg/day (184 times the human exposure, estimated) and in rats at a dose of ≥40 mg/kg/day (312 times the human exposure) an increase in the incidence of Leydig cell hyperplasia was observed. A positive correlation between the proliferative changes in the Leydig cells and an increase in serum LH levels (2- to 3-fold above control) has been demonstrated in both rodent species treated with high doses of finasteride. No drug-related Leydig cell changes were seen in either rats or dogs treated with finasteride for 1 year at doses of 20 mg/kg/day and 45 mg/kg/day (240 and 2800 times, respectively, the human exposure) or in mice treated for 19 months at a dose of 2.5 mg/kg/day (18.4 times the human exposure).

No evidence of mutagenicity was observed in an *in vitro* bacterial mutagenesis assay, a mammalian cell mutagenesis assay, or in an *in vitro* alkaline elution assay. In an *in vitro* chromosome aberration assay, when Chinese hamster ovary cells were treated with high concentrations (450-550 μmol) of finasteride, there was a slight increase in chromosome aberrations. These concentrations correspond to 18,000-22,000 times the peak plasma levels in man given a total dose of 1 mg. Further, the concentrations (450-550 μmol) used in *in vitro* studies are not achievable in a biological system. In an *in vivo* chromosome aberration assay in mice, no treatment-related increase in chromosome aberration was observed with finasteride at the maximum tolerated dose of 250 mg/kg/day (1824 times the human exposure, estimated) as determined in the carcinogenicity studies.

In sexually mature male rabbits treated with finasteride at 80 mg/kg/day (4344 times the estimated human exposure) for up to 12 weeks, no effect on fertility, sperm count, or ejaculate volume was seen. In sexually mature male rats treated with 80 mg/kg/day of finasteride (488 times the estimated human exposure), there were no significant effects on fertility after 6 or 12 weeks of treatment; however, when treatment was continued for up to 24 or 30 weeks, there was an apparent decrease in fertility, fecundity, and an associated significant decrease in the weights of the seminal vesicles and prostate. All these effects were reversible within 6 weeks of discontinuation of treatment. No drug-related effect on testes or on mating performance has been seen in rats or rabbits. This decrease in fertility in finasteride-treated rats is secondary to its effect on accessory sex organs (prostate and seminal vesicles) resulting in failure to form a seminal plug. The seminal plug is essential for normal fertility in rats but is not relevant in man.

Pregnancy, Teratogenic Effects, Pregnancy Category X

See CONTRAINDICATIONS, Propecia.

Propecia is not indicated for use in women.

Administration of finasteride to pregnant rats at doses ranging from 100 μg/kg/day to 100 mg/kg/day (5-5000 times the recommended human dose of 1 mg/day) resulted in dose-dependent development of hypospadias in 3.6 to 100% of male offspring. Pregnant rats produced male offspring with decreased prostatic and seminal vesicular weights, delayed preputial separation, and transient nipple development when given finasteride at ≥30 μg/kg/day (≥1.5 times the recommended human dose of 1 mg/day) and decreased anogenital distance when given finasteride at ≥3 μg/kg/day (one-fifth the recommended human dose of 1 mg/day). The critical period during which these effects can be induced in male rats has been defined to be days 16-17 of gestation. The changes described above are expected pharmacological effects of drugs belonging to the class of Type II 5α-reductase inhibitors and are similar to those reported in male infants with a genetic deficiency of Type II 5α-reductase. No abnormalities were observed in female offspring exposed to any dose of finasteride *in utero*.

No developmental abnormalities have been observed in first filial generation (F_1) male or female offspring resulting from mating finasteride-treated male rats (80 mg/kg/day; 488 times the human exposure) with untreated females. Administration of finasteride at 3 mg/kg/day (150 times the recommended human dose of 1 mg/day) during the late gestation and lactation period resulted in slightly decreased fertility in F_1 male offspring. No effects were seen in female offspring. No evidence of malformations has been observed in rabbit fetuses exposed to finasteride *in utero* from days 6-18 of gestation at doses up to 100 mg/kg/day (5000 times the recommended human dose of 1 mg/day). However, effects on male genitalia would not be expected since the rabbits were not exposed during the critical period of genital system development.

The *in utero* effects of finasteride exposure during the period of embryonic and fetal development were evaluated in the rhesus monkey (gestation days 20-100), a species more predictive of human development than rats or rabbits. Intravenous administration of finasteride to pregnant monkeys at doses as high as 800 ng/day (at least 750 times the highest estimated exposure of pregnant women to finasteride from semen of men taking 1 mg/day) resulted in no abnormalities in male fetuses. In confirmation of the relevance of the rhesus model for human fetal development, oral administration of a very high dose of finasteride (2 mg/kg/day; 100 times the recommended human dose of 1 mg/day or approximately 12 million times the highest estimated exposure to finasteride from semen of men taking 1 mg/day) to pregnant monkeys resulted in external genital abnormalities in male fetuses. No other abnormalities were observed in male fetuses and no finasteride-related abnormalities were observed in female fetuses at any dose.

Nursing Mothers

Propecia is not indicated for use in women.

It is not known whether finasteride is excreted in human milk.

Pediatric Use

Propecia is not indicated for use in pediatric patients.

Safety and effectiveness in pediatric patients have not been established.

Geriatric Use

Clinical efficacy studies with Propecia did not include subjects aged 65 and over. Based on the pharmacokinetics of finasteride 5 mg, no dosage adjustment is necessary in the elderly for Propecia (see CLINICAL PHARMACOLOGY, Propecia, Pharmacokinetics). However the efficacy of Propecia in the elderly has not been established.

PROSCAR

General

Prior to initiating therapy with Proscar, appropriate evaluation should be performed to identify other conditions such as infection, prostate cancer, stricture disease, hypotonic bladder or other neurogenic disorders that might mimic BPH.

Patients with large residual urinary volume and/or severely diminished urinary flow should be carefully monitored for obstructive uropathy. These patients may not be candidates for finasteride therapy.

Caution should be used in the administration of Proscar in those patients with liver function abnormalities, as finasteride is metabolized extensively in the liver.

Effects on PSA and Prostate Cancer Detection

No clinical benefit has been demonstrated in patients with prostate cancer treated with Proscar. Patients with BPH and elevated PSA were monitored in controlled clinical studies with serial PSAs and prostate biopsies. In these studies, Proscar did not appear to alter the rate of prostate cancer detection. The overall incidence of prostate cancer was not significantly different in patients treated with Proscar or placebo.

Proscar causes a decrease in serum PSA levels by approximately 50% in patients with BPH, even in the presence of prostate cancer. This decrease is predictable over the entire range of PSA values, although it may vary in individual patients. Analysis of PSA data from over 3000 patients in PLESS confirmed that in typical patients treated with Proscar for 6 months or more, PSA values should be doubled for comparison with normal ranges in untreated men. This adjustment preserves the sensitivity and specificity of the PSA assay and maintains its ability to detect prostate cancer.

Any sustained increases in PSA levels while on Proscar should be carefully evaluated, including consideration of non-compliance to therapy with Proscar.

Percent free PSA (free to total PSA ratio) is not significantly decreased by Proscar. The ratio of free to total PSA remains constant even under the influence of Proscar. If clinicians elect to use percent free PSA as an aid in the detection of prostate cancer in men undergoing finasteride therapy, no adjustment to its value appears necessary.

Information for the Patient

Women should not handle crushed or broken Proscar tablets when they are pregnant or may potentially be pregnant because of the possibility of absorption of finasteride and the subsequent potential risk to the male fetus (see CONTRAINDICATIONS, Proscar; WARNINGS, Proscar, Exposure of Women — Risk to Male Fetus; PRECAUTIONS, Proscar, Pregnancy Category X; and HOW SUPPLIED, Proscar).

Physicians should inform patients that the volume of ejaculate may be decreased in some patients during treatment with Proscar. This decrease does not appear to interfere with normal sexual function. However, impotence and decreased libido may occur in patients treated with Proscar (see ADVERSE REACTIONS, Proscar).

Physicians should instruct their patients to read the patient package insert before starting therapy with Proscar and to reread it each time the prescription is renewed so that they are aware of current information for patients regarding Proscar.

Drug/Laboratory Test Interactions

In patients with BPH, Proscar has no effect on circulating levels of cortisol, estradiol, prolactin, thyroid-stimulating hormone, or thyroxine. No clinically meaningful effect was observed on the plasma lipid profile (*i.e.*, total cholesterol, low density lipoproteins, high density lipoproteins and triglycerides) or bone mineral density. Increases of about 10% were observed in luteinizing hormone (LH) and follicle-stimulating hormone (FSH) in patients receiving Proscar, but levels remained within the normal range. In healthy volunteers, treatment with Proscar did not alter the response of LH and FSH to gonadotropin-releasing hormone indicating that the hypothalamic-pituitary-testicular axis was not affected.

Treatment with Proscar for 24 weeks to evaluate semen parameters in healthy male volunteers revealed no clinically meaningful effects on sperm concentration, mobility, morphology, or pH. A 0.6 ml (22.1%) median decrease in ejaculate volume with a concomitant reduction in total sperm per ejaculate, was observed. These parameters remained within the normal range and were reversible upon discontinuation of therapy with an average time to return to baseline of 84 weeks.

Carcinogenesis, Mutagenesis, and Impairment of Fertility

No evidence of a tumorigenic effect was observed in a 24 month study in Sprague-Dawley rats receiving doses of finasteride up to 160 mg/kg/day in males and 320 mg/kg/day in females. These doses produced respective systemic exposure in rats of 111 and 274 times those observed in man receiving the recommended human dose of 5 mg/day. All exposure calculations were based on calculated AUC(0-24h) for animals and mean AUC (0-24h) for man (0.4 μg·h/ml).

In a 19 month carcinogenicity study in CD-1 mice, a statistically significant ($p \leq 0.05$) increase in the incidence of testicular Leydig cell adenomas was observed at a dose of 250 mg/kg/day (228 times the human exposure). In mice at a dose of 25 mg/kg/day (23 times the human exposure, estimated) and in rats at a dose of ≥40 mg/kg/day (39 times the human exposure) an increase in the incidence of Leydig cell hyperplasia was observed. A positive correlation between the proliferative changes in the Leydig cells and an increase in serum LH levels (2- to 3-fold above control) has been demonstrated in both rodent species treated with high doses of finasteride. No drug-related Leydig cell changes were seen in either rats or dogs treated with finasteride for 1 year at doses of 20 mg/kg/day and 45 mg/kg/day (30 and 350 times, respectively, the human exposure) or in mice treated for 19 months at a dose of 2.5 mg/kg/day (2.3 times the human exposure, estimated).

No evidence of mutagenicity was observed in an *in vitro* bacterial mutagenesis assay, a mammalian cell mutagenesis assay, or in an *in vitro* alkaline elution assay. In an *in vitro* chromosome aberration assay, using Chinese hamster ovary cells, there was a slight increase in chromosome aberrations. These concentrations correspond to 4000-5000 times the peak plasma levels in man given a total dose of 5 mg. In an *in vivo* chromosome aberration assay in mice, no treatment-related increase in chromosome aberration was observed with finasteride at the maximum tolerated dose of 250 mg/kg/day (228 times the human exposure) as determined in the carcinogenicity studies.

In sexually mature male rabbits treated with finasteride at 80 mg/kg/day (543 times the human exposure) for up to 12 weeks, no effect on fertility, sperm count, or ejaculate volume was seen. In sexually mature male rats treated with 80 mg/kg/day of finasteride (61 times the human exposure), there were no significant effects on fertility after 6 or 12 weeks of treatment; however, when treatment was continued for up to 24 or 30 weeks, there was an apparent decrease in fertility, fecundity and an associated significant decrease in the weights of the seminal vesicles and prostate. All these effects were reversible within 6 weeks of discontinuation of treatment. No drug-related effect on testes or on mating performance has been seen in rats or rabbits. This decrease in fertility in finasteride-treated rats is secondary to its effect on accessory sex organs (prostate and seminal vesicles) resulting in failure to form a seminal plug. The seminal plug is essential for normal fertility in rats and is not relevant in man.

Pregnancy Category X

See CONTRAINDICATIONS, Proscar.

Proscar is not indicated for use in women.

Administration of finasteride to pregnant rats at doses ranging from 100 μg/kg/day to 100 mg/kg/day (1-1000 times the recommended human dose of 5 mg/day) resulted in dose-dependent development of hypospadias in 3.6 to 100% of male offspring. Pregnant rats produced male offspring with decreased prostatic and seminal vesicular weights, delayed preputial separation and transient nipple development when given finasteride at ≥30 μg/kg/day ≥3/10 of the recommended human dose of 5 mg/day) and decreased anogenital distance when given finasteride at ≥3 μg/kg/day ≥3/100 of the recommended human dose of 5 mg/day). The critical period during which these effects can be induced in male rats has been defined to be days 16-17 of gestation. The changes described above are expected pharmacological effects of drugs belonging to the class of Type II 5α-reductase inhibitors and are similar to those reported in male infants with a genetic deficiency of Type II 5α-reductase. No abnormalities were observed in female offspring exposed to any dose of finasteride *in utero*.

No developmental abnormalities have been observed in first filial generation (F_1) male or female offspring resulting from mating finasteride-treated male rats (80 mg/kg/day; 61 times the human exposure) with untreated females. Administration of finasteride at 3 mg/kg/day (30 times the recommended human dose of 5 mg/day) during the late gestation and lactation period resulted in slightly decreased fertility in F_1 male offspring. No effects were seen in female offspring. No evidence of malformations has been observed in rabbit fetuses exposed to finasteride *in utero* from days 6-18 of gestation at doses up to 100 mg/kg/day (1000 times the recommended human dose of 5 mg/day). However, effects on male genitalia would not be expected since the rabbits were not exposed during the critical period of genital system development.

The *in utero* effects of finasteride exposure during the period of embryonic and fetal development were evaluated in the rhesus monkey (gestation days 20-100), a species more predictive of human development than rats or rabbits. Intravenous administration of finasteride to pregnant monkeys at doses as high as 800 ng/day (at least 60-120 times the highest estimated exposure of pregnant women to finasteride from semen of men taking 5 mg/day) resulted in no abnormalities in male fetuses. In confirmation of the relevance of the rhesus model for human fetal development, oral administration of a dose of finasteride (2 mg/kg/day; 20 times the recommended human dose of 5 mg/day or approximately 1-2 million times the highest estimated exposure to finasteride from semen of men taking 5 mg/day) to pregnant monkeys resulted in external genital abnormalities in male fetuses. No other abnormalities were observed in male fetuses and no finasteride-related abnormalities were observed in female fetuses at any dose.

Nursing Mothers

Proscar is not indicated for use in women.

It is not known whether finasteride is excreted in human milk.

Pediatric Use

Proscar is not indicated for use in pediatric patients.

Safety and effectiveness in pediatric patients have not been established.

Geriatric Use

Of the total number of subjects included in PLESS, 1480 and 105 subjects were 65 and over and 75 and over, respectively. No overall differences in safety or effectiveness were observed between these subjects and younger subjects, and other reported clinical experience has not identified differences in responses between the elderly and younger patients. No dosage adjustment is necessary in the elderly (see CLINICAL PHARMACOLOGY, Proscar, Pharmacokinetics).

DRUG INTERACTIONS

PROPECIA

No drug interactions of clinical importance have been identified. Finasteride does not appear to affect the cytochrome P450-linked drug metabolizing enzyme system. Compounds that have been tested in man include antipyrine, digoxin, propranolol, theophylline, and warfarin and no interactions were found.

Other Concomitant Therapy

Although specific interaction studies were not performed, finasteride doses of 1 mg or more were concomitantly used in clinical studies with acetaminophen, α-blockers, analgesics, angiotensin-converting enzyme (ACE) inhibitors, anticonvulsants, benzodiazepines, beta blockers, calcium-channel blockers, cardiac nitrates, diuretics, H_2 antagonists, HMG-CoA reductase inhibitors, prostaglandin synthetase inhibitors (NSAIDs), and quinolone anti-infectives without evidence of clinically significant adverse interactions.

PROSCAR

No drug interactions of clinical importance have been identified. Finasteride does not appear to affect the cytochrome P450-linked drug metabolizing enzyme system. Compounds that have been tested in man have included antipyrine, digoxin, propranolol, theophylline, and warfarin and no clinically meaningful interactions were found.

Other Concomitant Therapy

Although specific interaction studies were not performed, Proscar was concomitantly used in clinical studies with acetaminophen, acetylsalicylic acid, α-blockers, angiotensin-converting enzyme (ACE) inhibitors, analgesics, anti-convulsants, beta-adrenergic blocking agents, diuretics, calcium channel blockers, cardiac nitrates, HMG-CoA reductase inhibitors, nonsteroidal anti-inflammatory drugs (NSAIDs), benzodiazepines, H^2 antagonists and quinolone anti-infectives without evidence of clinically significant adverse interactions.

ADVERSE REACTIONS

PROPECIA

Clinical Studies for Propecia (finasteride 1 mg) in the Treatment of Male Pattern Hair Loss

In controlled clinical trials for Propecia of 12 month duration, 1.4% of the patients were discontinued due to adverse experiences that were considered to be possibly, probably or definitely drug-related (1.6% for placebo); 1.2% of patients on Propecia and 0.9% of patients on placebo discontinued therapy because of a drug-related sexual adverse experience. The following clinical adverse reactions were reported as possibly, probably or definitely drug-related in ≥1% of patients treated for 12 months with Propecia or placebo, respectively: decreased libido (1.8%, 1.3%), erectile dysfunction (1.3%, 0.7%) and ejaculation disorder (1.2%, 0.7%; primarily decreased volume of ejaculate: [0.8%, 0.4%]). Integrated analysis of clinical adverse experiences showed that during treatment with Propecia, 36 (3.8%) of 945 men had reported one or more of these adverse experiences as compared to 20 (2.1%) of 934 men treated with placebo (p=0.04). Resolution occurred in all men who discontinued therapy with Propecia due to these side effects and in most of those who continued therapy. The incidence of each of the above side effects decreased to ≤0.3% by the fifth year of treatment with Propecia.

In a study of finasteride 1 mg daily in healthy men, a median decrease in ejaculate volume of 0.3 ml (-11%) compared with 0.2 ml (-8%) for placebo was observed after 48 weeks of treatment. Two other studies showed that finasteride at 5 times the dosage of Propecia (5 mg daily) produced significant median decreases of approximately 0.5 ml (-25%) compared to placebo in ejaculate volume but this was reversible after discontinuation of treatment.

In the clinical studies with Propecia, the incidences for breast tenderness and enlargement, hypersensitivity reactions, and testicular pain in finasteride-treated patients were not different from those in patients treated with placebo.

Postmarketing Experience for Propecia (finasteride 1 mg)

Breast tenderness and enlargement; hypersensitivity reactions including rash, pruritus, urticaria, and swelling of the lips and face; and testicular pain.

Controlled Clinical Trials and Long-Term Open Extension Studies for Proscar (finasteride 5 mg) in the Treatment of Benign Prostatic Hyperplasia

In controlled clinical trials for Proscar of 12 month duration, 1.3% of the patients were discontinued due to adverse experiences that were considered to be possibly, probably or definitely drug-related (0.9% for placebo); only 1 patient on Proscar (0.2%) and 1 patient on placebo (0.2%) discontinued therapy because of a drug-related sexual adverse experience. The following clinical adverse reactions were reported as possibly, probably or definitely drug-related in ≥1% of patients treated for 12 months with Proscar or placebo, respectively: erectile dysfunction (3.7%, 1.1%), decreased libido (3.3%, 1.6%) and decreased volume of ejaculate (2.8%, 0.9%). The adverse experience profiles for patients treated with finasteride 1 mg/day for 12 months and those maintained on Proscar for 24-48 months were similar to that observed in the 12 month controlled studies with Proscar. Sexual adverse experiences resolved with continued treatment in over 60% of patients who reported them.

PROSCAR

Proscar is generally well tolerated; adverse reactions usually have been mild and transient.

4 Year Placebo-Controlled Study

In PLESS, 1524 patients treated with Proscar and 1516 patients treated with placebo were evaluated for safety over a period of 4 years. The most frequently reported adverse reactions were related to sexual function. 3.7% (57 patients) treated with Proscar and 2.1% (32 patients) treated with placebo discontinued therapy as a result of adverse reactions related to sexual function, which are the most frequently reported adverse reactions.

TABLE 4 presents the only clinical adverse reactions considered possibly, probably or definitely drug related by the investigator, for which the incidence on Proscar was ≥1% and greater than placebo over the 4 years of the study. In years 2-4 of the study, there was no significant difference between treatment groups in the incidences of impotence, decreased libido and ejaculation disorder.

TABLE 4 *Drug-Related Adverse Experiences*

	Year 1		Years 2, 3 and 4*	
	Finasteride	Placebo	Finasteride	Placebo
Impotence	8.1%	3.7%	5.1%	5.1%
Decreased libido	6.4%	3.4%	2.6%	2.6%
Decreased volume of ejaculate	3.7%	0.8%	1.5%	0.5%
Ejaculation disorder	0.8%	0.1%	0.2%	0.1%
Breast enlargement	0.5%	0.1%	1.8%	1.1%
Breast tenderness	0.4%	0.1%	0.7%	0.3%
Rash	0.5%	0.2%	0.5%	0.1%

* Combined years 2-4.
n=1524 and 1516, finasteride versus placebo, respectively.

Phase 3 Studies and 5 Year Open Extensions

The adverse experience profile in the 1 year, placebo-controlled, Phase 3 studies, the 5 year open extensions, and PLESS were similar.

There is no evidence of increased adverse experiences with increased duration of treatment with Proscar. New reports of drug-related sexual adverse experiences decreased with duration of therapy.

The following additional adverse effects have been reported in post-marketing experience:

Hypersensitivity reactions, including pruritus, urticaria, and swelling of the lips and face.

Testicular pain.

DOSAGE AND ADMINISTRATION

PROPECIA

The recommended dosage is 1 mg once a day.

Propecia may be administered with or without meals.

In general, daily use for 3 months or more is necessary before benefit is observed. Continued use is recommended to sustain benefit which should be re-evaluated periodically. Withdrawal of treatment leads to reversal of effect within 12 months.

PROSCAR

The recommended dose is 5 mg orally once a day.

Proscar may be administered with or without meals.

No dosage adjustment is necessary for patients with renal impairment or for the elderly (see CLINICAL PHARMACOLOGY, Proscar, Pharmacokinetics).

HOW SUPPLIED

PROPECIA

Propecia tablets, 1 mg, are tan, octagonal, film-coated convex tablets with "stylized P" logo on one side and "PROPECIA" on the other.

Storage and Handling

Store at room temperature, 15-30°C (59-86°F). Keep container closed and protect from moisture.

Women should not handle crushed or broken Propecia tablets when they are pregnant or may potentially be pregnant because of the possibility of absorption of finasteride and the subsequent potential risk to a male fetus. Propecia tablets are coated and will prevent contact with the active ingredient during normal handling, provided that the tablets are not broken or crushed. (See WARNINGS, Propecia, Exposure of Women — Risk to Male Fetus and PRECAUTIONS, Propecia:Information for the Patient and Pregnancy, Teratogenic Effects, Pregnancy Category X.)

PROSCAR

Proscar tablets 5 mg are blue, modified apple-shaped, film-coated tablets, with the code "MSD 72" on one side and "PROSCAR" on the other.

Storage and Handling

Store at room temperatures below 30°C (86°F). Protect from light and keep container tightly closed.

Women should not handle crushed or broken Proscar tablets when they are pregnant or may potentially be pregnant because of the possibility of absorption of finasteride and the subsequent potential risk to a male fetus (see WARNINGS, Proscar, Exposure of Women — Risk to Male Fetus; PRECAUTIONS, Proscar: Information for the Patient and Pregnancy Category X).

PRODUCT LISTING - EQUIVALENTS NOT AVAILABLE

Tablet - Oral - 1 mg

30 x 3	$156.41	PROPECIA, Merck & Company Inc	00006-0071-61
30's	$49.35	PROPECIA, Allscripts Pharmaceutical Company	54569-4544-00
30's	$52.14	PROPECIA, Merck & Company Inc	00006-0071-31
30's	$56.32	PROPECIA, Physicians Total Care	54868-4120-00

Tablet - Oral - 5 mg

30's	$70.97	PROSCAR, Allscripts Pharmaceutical Company	54569-8597-01
30's	$80.76	PROSCAR, Physicians Total Care	54868-2719-01
30's	$81.46	PROSCAR, Merck & Company Inc	00006-0072-31
90's	$175.92	PROSCAR, Allscripts Pharmaceutical Company	54569-8597-00
100's	$252.94	PROSCAR, Physicians Total Care	54868-2719-02
100's	$271.54	PROSCAR, Merck & Company Inc	00006-0072-28
100's	$271.54	PROSCAR, Merck & Company Inc	00006-0072-58

Flecainide Acetate (001299)

For complete prescribing information, refer to the CD-ROM included with the book.

Categories: Arrhythmia, ventricular; Fibrillation, paroxysmal atrial; Flutter, paroxysmal atrial; Tachycardia, paroxysmal supraventricular; Tachycardia, ventricular; Pregnancy Category C; FDA Approved 1985 Oct
Drug Classes: Antiarrhythmics, class IC
Brand Names: Tambocor
Foreign Brand Availability: Almarytm (Italy); Apocard (Spain); Flecaine (France)
Cost of Therapy: $116.06 (Arrhythmia; Tambocor; 50 mg; 2 tablets/day; 30 day supply)
$104.37 (Arrhythmia; Generic Tablets; 50 mg; 2 tablets/day; 30 day supply)

DESCRIPTION

Tambocor is an antiarrhythmic drug available in tablets of 50, 100, or 150 mg for oral administration.

Flecainide acetate is benzamide, N-(2-piperidinyl-methyl)-2, 5-bis(2,2,2-trifluoroethoxy)-monoacetate.

Flecainide acetate is a white crystalline substance with a pKa of 9.3. It has an aqueous solubility of 48.4 mg/ml at 37°C.

Tambocor tablets also contain: Croscarmellose sodium, hydrogenated vegetable oil, magnesium stearate, microcrystalline cellulose and starch.

INDICATIONS AND USAGE

In patients without structural heart disease, flecainide acetate is indicated for the prevention of:

- Paroxysmal supraventricular tachycardias (PSVT), including atrioventricular nodal reentrant tachycardia, atrioventricular reentrant tachycardia and other supraventricular tachycardias of unspecified mechanism associated with disabling symptoms
- Paroxysmal atrial fibrillation/flutter (PAF) associated with disabling symptoms

Flecainide acetate is also indicated for the prevention of:

- Documented ventricular arrhythmias, such as sustained ventricular tachycardia (sustained VT), that in the judgment of the physician, are life-threatening.

Use of flecainide acetate for the treatment of sustained VT, like other antiarrhythmics, should be initiated in the hospital. The use of flecainide acetate is not recommended in patients with less severe ventricular arrhythmias even if the patients are symptomatic.

Because of the proarrhythmic effects of flecainide acetate, its use should be reserved for patients in whom, in the opinion of the physician, the benefits of treatment outweigh the risks.

Flecainide acetate should not be used in patients with recent myocardial infarction. (See WARNINGS.)

Use of flecainide acetate in chronic atrial fibrillation has not been adequately studied and is not recommended. (See WARNINGS.)

As is the case for other antiarrhythmic agents, there is no evidence from controlled trials that the use of flecainide acetate favorably affects survival or the incidence of sudden death.

CONTRAINDICATIONS

Flecainide acetate is contraindicated in patients with preexisting second- or third-degree AV block, or with right bundle branch block when associated with a left hemiblock (bifascicular block), unless a pacemaker is present to sustain the cardiac rhythm should complete heart block occur. Flecainide acetate is also contraindicated in the presence of cardiogenic shock or known hypersensitivity to the drug.

WARNINGS

MORTALITY

Flecainide acetate was included in the National Heart Lung and Blood Institute's Cardiac Arrhythmia Suppression Trial (CAST), a long-term, multicenter, randomized, double-blind study in patients with asymptomatic non-life-threatening ventricular arrhythmias who had a myocardial infarction more than 6 days but less than 2 years previously. An excessive mortality or non-fatal cardiac arrest rate was seen in patients assigned to a carefully matched placebo-treated group. This rate was 16/315 (5.1%) for flecainide acetate and 7/309 (2.3%) for its matched placebo. The average duration of treatment with flecainide acetate in this study was 10 months.

The applicability of the CAST results to other populations (*e.g.*, those without recent myocardial infarction) is uncertain, but at present it is prudent to consider the risks of Class IC agents (including flecainide acetate), coupled with the lack of any evidence of improved survival, generally unacceptable in patients without life-threatening ventricular arrhythmias, even if the patients are experiencing unpleasant, but not life-threatening, symptoms or signs.

VENTRICULAR PRO-ARRHYTHMIC EFFECTS IN PATIENTS WITH ATRIAL FIBRILLATION/FLUTTER

A review of the world literature revealed reports of 568 patients treated with oral flecainide acetate for paroxysmal atrial fibrillation/flutter (PAF). Ventricular tachycardia was experienced in 0.4% (2/568) of these patients. Of 19 patients in the literature with chronic atrial fibrillation (CAF), 10.5% (2) experienced VT or VF. FLECAINIDE IS NOT RECOMMENDED FOR USE IN PATIENTS WITH CHRONIC ATRIAL FIBRILLATION. Case reports of ventricular proarrhythmic effects in patients treated with flecainide acetate for atrial fibrillation/flutter have included increased PVCs, VT, ventricular fibrillation (VF), and death.

As with other Class I agents, patients treated with flecainide acetate for atrial flutter have been reported with 1:1 atrioventricular conduction due to slowing the atrial rate. A paradoxical increase in the ventricular rate also may occur in patients with atrial fibrillation who receive flecainide acetate. Concomitant negative chronotropic therapy such as digoxin or beta-blockers may lower the risk of this complication.

PROARRHYTHMIC EFFECTS

Flecainide acetate, like other antiarrhythmic agents, can cause new or worsened supraventricular or ventricular arrhythmias. Ventricular proarrhythmic effects range from an increase in frequency of PVCs to the development of more severe ventricular tachycardia, *e.g.*, tachycardia that is more sustained or more resistant to conversion to sinus rhythm, with potentially fatal consequences. In studies of ventricular arrhythmia patients treated with flecainide acetate, three-fourths of proarrhythmic events were new or worsened ventricular tachyarrhythmias, the remainder being increased frequency of PVCs or new supraventricular arrhythmias. In patients treated with flecainide for sustained ventricular tachycardia, 80% (51/64) of proarrhythmic events occurred within 14 days of the onset of therapy. In studies of 225 patients with supraventricular arrhythmia (108 with paroxysmal supraventricular tachycardia and 117 with paroxysmal atrial fibrillation), there were 9 (4%) proarrhythmic events, 8 of them in patients with paroxysmal atrial fibrillation. Of the 9, 7 (including the 1 in a PSVT patient) were exacerbations of supraventricular arrhythmias (longer duration, more rapid rate, harder to reverse) while 2 were ventricular arrhythmias, including 1 fatal case of VT/VF and 1 wide complex VT (the patient showed inducible VT, however, after withdrawal of flecainide), both in patients with paroxysmal atrial fibrillation and known coronary artery disease.

It is uncertain if flecainide acetate's risk of proarrhythmia is exaggerated in patients with chronic atrial fibrillation (CAF), high ventricular rate, and/or exercise. Wide complex tachycardia and ventricular fibrillation have been reported in 2 of 12 CAF patients undergoing maximal exercise tolerance testing.

In patients with complex ventricular arrhythmias, it is often difficult to distinguish a spontaneous variation in the patient's underlying rhythm disorder from drug-induced worsening, so that the following occurrence rates must be considered approximations. Their frequency appears to be related to dose and to the underlying cardiac disease.

Among patients treated for sustained VT (who frequently also had CHF, a low ejection fraction, a history of myocardial infarction and/or an episode of cardiac arrest), the incidence of proarrhythmic events was 13% when dosage was initiated at 200 mg/day with slow upward titration, and did not exceed 300 mg/day in most patients. In early studies in patients with sustained VT utilizing a higher initial dose (400 mg/day) the incidence of proarrhythmic events was 26%; moreover, in about 10% of the patients treated proarrhythmic events resulted in death, despite prompt medical attention. With lower initial doses, the incidence of proarrhythmic events resulting in death decreased to 0.5% of these patients. Accordingly, it is extremely important to follow the recommended dosage schedule. (See DOSAGE AND ADMINISTRATION.)

The relatively high frequency of proarrhythmic events in patients with sustained VT and serious underlying heart disease, and the need for careful titration and monitor-

ing, requires that therapy of patients with sustained VT be started in the hospital. (See DOSAGE AND ADMINISTRATION.)

HEART FAILURE

Flecainide acetate has a negative inotropic effect and may cause or worsen CHF, particularly in patients with cardiomyopathy, preexisting severe heart failure (NYHA functional class III or IV) or low ejection fractions (less than 30%). In patients with supraventricular arrhythmias new or worsened CHF developed in 0.4% (1/225) of patients. In patients with sustained ventricular tachycardia during a mean duration of 7.9 months of flecainide acetate therapy, 6.3% (20/317) developed new CHF. In patients with sustained ventricular tachycardia and a history of CHF, during a mean duration of 5.4 months of flecainide acetate therapy, 25.7% (78/304) developed worsened CHF. Exacerbation of preexisting CHF occurred more commonly in studies which included patients with class III or IV failure than in studies which excluded such patients. Flecainide acetate should be used cautiously in patients who are known to have a history of CHF or myocardial dysfunction. The initial dosage in such patients should be no more than 100 mg bid (see DOSAGE AND ADMINISTRATION) and patients should be monitored carefully. Close attention must be given to maintenance of cardiac function, including optimization of digitalis, diuretic, or other therapy. In cases where CHF has developed or worsened during treatment with flecainide acetate, the time of onset has ranged from a few hours to several months after starting therapy. Some patients who develop evidence of reduced myocardial function while on flecainide acetate can continue on flecainide acetate with adjustment of digitalis or diuretics, others may require dosage reduction or discontinuation of flecainide acetate. When feasible, it is recommended that plasma flecainide levels be monitored. Attempts should be made to keep trough plasma levels below 0.7-1.0 μg/ml.

Effects on Cardiac Conduction

Flecainide acetate slows cardiac conduction in most patients to produce dose-related increases in PR, QRS, and QT intervals. PR interval increases on average about 25% (0.04 seconds) and as much as 118% in some patients. Approximately one-third of patients may develop new first-degree AV heart block (PR interval ≥0.20 seconds). The QRS complex increases on average about 25% (0.02 seconds) and as much as 150% in some patients. Many patients develop QRS complexes with a duration of 0.12 seconds or more. In one study, 4% of patients developed new bundle branch block while on flecainide acetate. The degree of lengthening of PR and QRS intervals does not predict either efficacy or the development of cardiac adverse effects. In clinical trials, it was unusual for PR intervals to increase to 0.30 seconds or more, or for QRS intervals to increase to 0.18 seconds or more. Thus, caution should be used when such intervals occur, and dose reductions may be considered. The QT interval widens about 8%, but most of this widening (about 60-90%) is due to widening of the QRS duration. The JT interval (QT minus QRS) only widens about 4% on the average. Significant JT prolongation occurs in less than 2% of patients. There have been rare cases of Torsade de Pointes-type arrhythmia associated with flecainide acetate therapy.

Clinically significant conduction changes have been observed at these rates: sinus node dysfunction such as sinus pause, sinus arrest and symptomatic bradycardia (1.2%), second-degree AV block (0.5%) and third-degree AV block (0.4%). An attempt should be made to manage the patient on the lowest effective dose in an effort to minimize these effects. (See DOSAGE AND ADMINISTRATION.) If second- or third-degree AV block, or right bundle branch block associated with a left hemiblock occur, flecainide acetate therapy should be discontinued unless a temporary or implanted ventricular pacemaker is in place to ensure an adequate ventricular rate.

Sick Sinus Syndrome (Bradycardia-Tachycardia Syndrome)

Flecainide acetate should be used only with extreme caution in patients with sick sinus syndrome because it may cause sinus bradycardia, sinus pause, or sinus arrest.

Effects on Pacemaker Thresholds

Flecainide acetate is known to increase endocardial pacing thresholds and may suppress ventricular escape rhythms. These effects are reversible if flecainide is discontinued. It should be used with caution in patients with permanent pacemakers or temporary pacing electrodes and should not be administered to patients with existing poor thresholds or non-programmable pacemakers unless suitable pacing rescue is available.

The pacing threshold in patients with pacemakers should be determined prior to instituting therapy with flecainide acetate, again after 1 week of administration and at regular intervals thereafter. Generally threshold changes are within the range of multiprogrammable pacemakers and, when these occur, a doubling of either voltage or pulse width is usually sufficient to regain capture.

Electrolyte Disturbances

Hypokalemia or hyperkalemia may alter the effects of Class I antiarrhythmic drugs. Preexisting hypokalemia or hyperkalemia should be corrected before administration of flecainide acetate.

Pediatric Use

The safety and efficacy of flecainide acetate in the fetus, infant, or child have not been established in double-blind, randomized, placebo-controlled trials. The proarrhythmic effects of flecainide acetate, as described previously, apply also to children. In pediatric patients with structural heart disease, flecainide acetate has been associated with cardiac arrest and sudden death. Flecainide acetate should be started in the hospital with rhythm monitoring. Any use of flecainide acetate in children should be directly supervised by a cardiologist skilled in the treatment of arrhythmias in children.

DOSAGE AND ADMINISTRATION

For patients with sustained VT, no matter what their cardiac status, flecainide acetate, like other antiarrhythmics, should be initiated in-hospital with rhythm monitoring.

Flecainide has a long half-life (12-27 hours in patients). Steady-state plasma levels, in patients with normal renal and hepatic function, may not be achieved until the patient has received 3-5 days of therapy at a given dose. Therefore, **increases in dosage should be made no more frequently than once every 4 days,** since during the first 2-3 days of therapy the optimal effect of a given dose may not be achieved.

For patients with PSVT and patients with PAF the recommended starting dose is 50 mg every 12 hours. Flecainide acetate doses may be increased in increments of 50 mg bid every 4 days until efficacy is achieved. For PAF patients, a substantial increase in efficacy without a substantial increase in discontinuations for adverse experiences may be achieved by increasing the flecainide acetate dose from 50-100 mg bid. The maximum recommended dose for patients with paroxysmal supraventricular arrhythmias is 300 mg/day.

For sustained VT the recommended starting dose is 100 mg every 12 hours. This dose may be increased in increments of 50 mg bid every 4 days until efficacy is achieved. Most patients with sustained VT do not require more than 150 mg every 12 hours (300 mg/day), and the maximum dose recommended is 400 mg/day.

In patients with sustained VT, use of higher initial doses and more rapid dosage adjustments have resulted in an increased incidence of proarrhythmic events and CHF, particularly during the first few days of dosing (see WARNINGS). Therefore, a loading dose is not recommended.

Intravenous lidocaine has been used occasionally with flecainide acetate while awaiting the therapeutic effect of flecainide acetate. No adverse drug interactions were apparent. However, no formal studies have been performed to demonstrate the usefulness of this regimen.

An occasional patient not adequately controlled by (or intolerant to) a dose given at 12 hour intervals may be dosed at 8 hour intervals.

Once adequate control of the arrhythmia has been achieved, it may be possible in some patients to reduce the dose as necessary to minimize side effects or effects on conduction. In such patients, efficacy at the lower dose should be evaluated.

Flecainide acetate should be used cautiously in patients with a history of CHF or myocardial dysfunction (see WARNINGS).

Any use of flecainide acetate in children should be directly supervised by a cardiologist skilled in the treatment of arrhythmias in children. Because of the evolving nature of information in this area, specialized literature should be consulted. Under 6 months of age, the initial starting dose of flecainide acetate in children is approximately 50 mg/m^2 body surrface area daily, divided into 2 or 3 equally spaced doses. Over 6 months of age, the initial starting dose may be increased to 100 mg/m^2/day. The maximum recommended dose is 200 mg/m^2/day. This dose should not be exceeded. In some children on higher doses, despite previously low plasma levels, the level has increased rapidly to far above therapeutic values while taking the same dose. Small changes in dose may also lead to disproportionate increases in plasma levels. Plasma trough (less than 1 hour pre-dose) flecainide levels and electrocardiograms should be obtained at presumed steady state (after at least 5 doses) either after initiation or change in flecainide acetate dose, whether the dose was increased for lack of effectiveness, or increased growth of the patient. For the first year on therapy, whenever the patient is seen for reasons of clinical follow-up, it is suggested that a 12-lead electrocardiogram and plasma trough flecainide level are obtained. The usual therapeutic level of flecainide in children is 200-500 ng/ml. In some cases, levels as high as 800 ng/ml may be required for control.

In patients with severe renal impairment (creatinine clearance of 35 ml/min/1.73 m^2 or less), the initial dosage should be 100 mg once daily (or 50 mg bid); when used in such patients, frequent plasma level monitoring is required to guide dosage adjustments (see Plasma Level Monitoring). In patients with less severe renal disease, the initial dosage should be 100 mg every 12 hours; plasma level monitoring may also be useful in these patients during dosage adjustment. In both groups of patients, dosage increases should be made very cautiously when plasma levels have plateaued (after more than 4 days), observing the patient closely for signs of adverse cardiac effects or other toxicity. It should be borne in mind that in these patients it may take longer than 4 days before a new steady-state plasma level is reached following a dosage change.

Based on theoretical considerations, rather than experimental data, the following suggestion is made: When transferring patients from another antiarrhythmic drug to flecainide acetate allow at least 2 to 4 plasma half-lives to elapse for the drug being discontinued before starting flecainide acetate at the usual dosage. In patients where withdrawal of a previous anti-arrhythmic agent is likely to produce life-threatening arrhythmias, the physician should consider hospitalizing the patient.

When flecainide is given in the presence of amiodarone, reduce the usual flecainide dose by 50% and monitor the patient closely for adverse effects. Plasma level monitoring is strongly recommended to guide dosage with such combination therapy (see Plasma Level Monitoring).

PLASMA LEVEL MONITORING

The large majority of patients successfully treated with flecainide acetate were found to have trough plasma levels between 0.2 and 1.0 μg/ml. The probability of adverse experiences, especially cardiac, may increase with higher trough plasma levels, especially when these exceed 1.0 μg/ml. Periodic monitoring of trough plasma levels may be useful in patient management. Plasma level monitoring is required in patients with severe renal failure or severe hepatic disease, since elimination of flecainide from plasma may be markedly slower. Monitoring of plasma levels is strongly recommended in patients on concurrent amiodarone therapy and may also be helpful in patients with CHF and in patients with moderate renal disease.

PRODUCT LISTING - RATED THERAPEUTICALLY EQUIVALENT

Tablet - Oral - 50 mg

24's	$174.09	GENERIC, Geneva Pharmaceuticals	00781-5062-01
100's	$173.95	GENERIC, Mylan Pharmaceuticals Inc	00378-8505-01
100's	$174.08	GENERIC, Barr Laboratories Inc	00555-0859-02
100's	$174.08	GENERIC, Par Pharmaceutical Inc	49884-0694-01

Tablet - Oral - 100 mg

24's	$273.07	GENERIC, Geneva Pharmaceuticals	00781-5063-01
100's	$272.80	GENERIC, Mylan Pharmaceuticals Inc	00378-8510-01
100's	$273.06	GENERIC, Par Pharmaceutical Inc	49884-0695-01

Tablet - Oral - 150 mg

24's	$375.84	GENERIC, Geneva Pharmaceuticals	00781-5064-01
100's	$375.45	GENERIC, Mylan Pharmaceuticals Inc	00378-8515-01
100's	$375.81	GENERIC, Forest Pharmaceuticals	00555-0861-02
100's	$375.81	GENERIC, Par Pharmaceutical Inc	49884-0696-01

PRODUCT LISTING - EQUIVALENTS NOT AVAILABLE

Tablet - Oral - 50 mg

60's	$104.46	GENERIC, Roxane Laboratories Inc	00054-0010-21
100's	$70.68	TAMBOCOR, 3M Pharmaceuticals	00089-0305-16
100's	$193.44	TAMBOCOR, 3M Pharmaceuticals	00089-0305-10

Tablet - Oral - 100 mg

60's	$163.85	GENERIC, Roxane Laboratories Inc	00054-0011-21
100's	$134.34	TAMBOCOR, 3M Pharmaceuticals	00089-0307-16
100's	$303.42	TAMBOCOR, 3M Pharmaceuticals	00089-0307-10

Tablet - Oral - 150 mg

60's	$225.50	GENERIC, Roxane Laboratories Inc	00054-0012-21
100's	$417.60	TAMBOCOR, 3M Pharmaceuticals	00089-0314-10

F

Floxuridine (001300)

For complete prescribing information, refer to the CD-ROM included with the book.

Categories: Carcinoma, gastrointestinal; Pregnancy Category D; FDA Approved 1970 Dec
Drug Classes: Antineoplastics, antimetabolites
Brand Names: FUDR
HCFA JCODE(S): J9200 500 mg IV

WARNING

FOR INTRA-ARTERIAL INFUSION ONLY.

It is recommended that Floxuridine be given only by or under the supervision of a qualified physician who is experienced in cancer chemotherapy and intra-arterial drug therapy and is well versed in the use of potent antimetabolites.

Because of the possibility of severe toxic reactions, all patients should be hospitalized for initiation of the first course of therapy.

DESCRIPTION

Floxuridine, an antineoplastic antimetabolite, is available as a sterile, nonpyrogenic, lyophilized powder for reconstitution. Each vial contains 500 mg of floxuridine which is to be reconstituted with 5 ml of sterile water for injection. An appropriate amount of reconstituted solution is then diluted with a parenteral solution for intra-arterial infusion (see DOSAGE AND ADMINISTRATION).

Floxuridine is a fluorinated pyrimidine. Chemically, floxuridine is 2′-deoxy-5-fluorouridine with an empirical formula of $C_9H_{11}FN_2O_5$. It is a white to off-white odorless solid which is freely soluble in water.

The 2% aqueous solution has a pH of between 4.0 and 5.5. The molecular weight of floxuridine is 246.19.

Storage: The sterile powder should be stored at 15-30°C (59- 86°F). Reconstituted vials should be stored under refrigeration (2-8°C, 36-46°F) for not more than 2 weeks.

INDICATIONS AND USAGE

Floxuridine is effective in the palliative management of gastrointestinal adenocarcinoma metastatic to the liver, when given by continuous regional intra-arterial infusion in carefully selected patients who are considered incurable by surgery or other means. Patients with known disease extending beyond an area capable of infusion via a single artery should, except in unusual circumstances, be considered for systemic therapy with other chemotherapeutic agents.

CONTRAINDICATIONS

Floxuridine therapy is contraindicated for patients in a poor nutritional state, those with depressed bone marrow function or those with potentially serious infections.

WARNINGS

BECAUSE OF THE POSSIBILITY OF SEVERE TOXIC REACTIONS, ALL PATIENTS SHOULD BE HOSPITALIZED FOR THE FIRST COURSE OF THERAPY.

Floxuridine should be used with extreme caution in poor risk patients with impaired hepatic or renal function or a history of high-dose pelvic irradiation or previous use of alkylating agents. The drug is not intended as an adjuvant to surgery.

Floxuridine may cause fetal harm when administered to a pregnant woman. It has been shown to be teratogenic in the chick embryo, mouse (at doses of 2.5 to 100 mg/kg) and rat (at doses of 75-150 mg/kg). Malformations included cleft palates; skeletal defects; and deformed appendages, paws and tails. The dosages which were teratogenic in animals are 4.2 to 125 times the recommended human therapeutic dose.

There are no adequate and well-controlled studies with floxuridine in pregnant women. If this drug is used during pregnancy or if the patient becomes pregnant while taking (receiving) this drug, the patient should be apprised of the potential hazard to the fetus. Women of childbearing potential should be advised to avoid becoming pregnant.

Combination Therapy: Any form of therapy which adds to the stress of the patient, interferes with nutrition or depresses bone marrow function will increase the toxicity of floxuridine.

DOSAGE AND ADMINISTRATION

Each vial must be reconstituted with 5 ml of sterile water for injection to yield a solution containing approximately 100 mg of floxuridine/ml. The calculated daily dose(s) of the drug is then diluted with 5% dextrose or 0.9% sodium chloride injection to a volume appropriate for the infusion apparatus to be used. The administration of FUDR is best achieved with the use of an appropriate pump to overcome pressure in large arteries and to ensure a uniform rate of infusion.

Parenteral drug products should be inspected visually for particulate matter and discoloration prior to administration whenever solution and container permit.

The recommended therapeutic dosage schedule of floxuridine by continuous arterial infusion is 0.1 to 0.6 mg/kg/day. The higher dosage ranges (0.4-0.6 mg) are usually employed for hepatic artery infusion because the liver metabolizes the drug, thus reducing the potential for systemic toxicity. Therapy can be given until adverse reactions appear. When these side effects have subsided, therapy may be resumed. The patient should be maintained on therapy as long as response to floxuridine continues.

Procedures for proper handling and disposal of anticancer drugs should be considered. Several guidelines on this subject have been published.[1-6] There is no general agreement that all of the procedures recommended in the guidelines are necessary or appropriate.

PRODUCT LISTING - RATED THERAPEUTICALLY EQUIVALENT

Powder For Injection - Injectable - 0.5 Gm

1's	$136.38	FUDR, Roche Laboratories	00004-1935-08
1's	$136.39	GENERIC, Bedford Laboratories	55390-0435-01
1's	$148.75	GENERIC, American Pharmaceutical Partners	63323-0141-07
1's	$150.00	GENERIC, Bedford Laboratories	55390-0135-01
1's	$155.00	FUDR, Faulding Pharmaceutical Company	61703-0331-09

Fluconazole (001301)

For related information, see the comparative table section in Appendix A.

Categories: Candidiasis; Candidiasis, prophylaxis; Meningitis, cryptococcal; Transplantation, bone marrow, adjunct; Pregnancy Category C; FDA Approved 1990 Jan; WHO Formulary
Drug Classes: Antifungals
Brand Names: Diflucan
Foreign Brand Availability: Baten (Colombia); Biozolene (Italy); Cancid (Indonesia); Cryptal (Indonesia); Flucand (Bahrain; Cyprus; Egypt; Iran; Iraq; Jordan; Kuwait; Lebanon; Libya; Oman; Qatar; Republic-of-Yemen; Saudi-Arabia; Syria; United-Arab-Emirates); Flucazol (Bahrain; Cyprus; Egypt; Iran; Iraq; Israel; Jordan; Kuwait; Lebanon; Libya; Oman; Qatar; Republic-of-Yemen; Saudi-Arabia; Syria; United-Arab-Emirates); Flucoral (Indonesia); Flucozal (Hong-Kong); Fludizol (Thailand); Flukezol (Mexico); Flunco (Thailand); Flunizol (Peru); Fluzone (Benin; Burkina-Faso; Ethiopia; Gambia; Ghana; Guinea; Ivory-Coast; Kenya; Liberia; Malawi; Mali; Mauritania; Mauritius; Morocco; Niger; Nigeria; Senegal; Seychelles; Sierra-Leone; South-Africa; Sudan; Tanzania; Tunia; Uganda; Zambia; Zimbabwe); Forcan (India); Fumay (Taiwan); Funazol (Korea); Fungata (Austria; Germany); Govazol (Indonesia); Medoflucon (China); Mutum (Peru); Mycocyst (Bahamas; Barbados; Belize; Bermuda; Curacao; Guyana; Jamaica; Netherland-Antilles; Puerto-Rico; Surinam; Trinidad); Mycorest (Singapore); Nobzol-1 (Colombia); Nobzol-2 (Colombia); Oneflu (Korea); Oxifugol (Mexico); Plunazol (Korea); Stalene (Thailand); Syscan (India); Tavor (Colombia); Treflucan (Bahrain; Cyprus; Egypt; Iran; Iraq; Jordan; Kuwait; Lebanon; Libya; Oman; Qatar; Republic-of-Yemen; Saudi-Arabia; Syria; United-Arab-Emirates); Triflucan (France; Israel; Turkey); Zemyc (Indonesia)
Cost of Therapy: $13.60 (Candidiasis, Vaginal; Diflucan; 150 mg; 1 tablet/day; 1 day supply)
$104.56 (Candidiasis, Oropharyngeal; Diflucan; 100 mg; 1 tablet/day; 14 day supply)

DESCRIPTION

Fluconazole is designated chemically as 2,4-difluoro-α,α′-bis(1H-1,2,4-triazol-1-ylmethyl) benzyl alcohol with an empirical formula of $C_{13}H_{12}F_2N_6O$ and molecular weight 306.3.

Fluconazole is a white crystalline solid which is slightly soluble in water and saline.

Diflucan (fluconazole), the first of a new subclass of synthetic triazole antifungal agents, is available as tablets for oral administration, as a powder for oral suspension and as a sterile solution for intravenous use in glass and in Viaflex Plus plastic containers.

DIFLUCAN TABLETS

Contain 50, 100, or 200 mg of fluconazole. *Inactive Ingredients:* Microcrystalline cellulose, dibasic calcium phosphate anhydrous, povidone, croscarmellose sodium, FD&C red no. 40 aluminum lake dye, and magnesium stearate.

DIFLUCAN FOR ORAL SUSPENSION

Contains 350 or 1400 mg of fluconazole. *Inactive Ingredients:* Sucrose, sodium citrate dihydrate, citric acid anhydrous, sodium benzoate, titanium dioxide, colloidal silicon dioxide, xanthan gum and natural orange flavor. After reconstitution with 24 ml of distilled water or purified water, each ml of reconstituted suspension contains 10 or 40 mg of fluconazole.

DIFLUCAN INJECTION

An iso-osmotic, sterile, nonpyrogenic solution of fluconazole in a sodium chloride or dextrose diluent. Each ml contains 2 mg of fluconazole and 9 mg of sodium chloride or 56 mg of dextrose, hydrous. The pH ranges from 4.0-8.0 in the sodium chloride diluent and from 3.5-6.5 in the dextrose diluent. Injection volumes of 100 ml and 200 ml are packaged in glass and in Viaflex Plus plastic containers.

The Viaflex Plus plastic container is fabricated from a specially formulated polyvinyl chloride (PL 146 Plastic). The amount of water that can permeate from inside the container into the overwrap is insufficient to affect the solution significantly. Solutions in contact with the plastic container can leach out certain of its chemical components in very small amounts within the expiration period, *e.g.*, di-2-ethylhexylphthalate (DEHP), up to 5 parts per million. However, the suitability of the plastic has been confirmed in tests in animals according to USP biological tests for plastic containers as well as by tissue culture toxicity studies.

CLINICAL PHARMACOLOGY

MODE OF ACTION

Fluconazole is a highly selective inhibitor of fungal cytochrome P-450 sterol C-14 alpha-demethylation. Mammalian cell demethylation is much less sensitive to fluconazole inhibition. The subsequent loss of normal sterols correlates with the accumulation of 14 alpha-methyl sterols in fungi and may be responsible for the fungistatic activity of fluconazole.

PHARMACOKINETICS AND METABOLISM

The pharmacokinetic properties of fluconazole are similar following administration by the intravenous or oral routes. In normal volunteers, the bioavailability of orally administered fluconazole is over 90% compared with intravenous administration. Bioequivalence was established between the 100 mg tablet and both suspension strengths when administered as a single 200 mg dose.

Peak plasma concentrations (C_{max}) in fasted normal volunteers occur between 1 and 2 hours with a terminal plasma elimination half-life of approximately 30 hours (range 20-50 hours) after oral administration.

In fasted normal volunteers, administration of a single oral 400 mg dose of fluconazole leads to a mean C_{max} of 6.72 µg/ml (range: 4.12-8.08 µg/ml) and after single oral doses of 50-400 mg, fluconazole plasma concentrations and AUC (area under the plasma concentration-time curve) are dose proportional.

Administration of a single oral 150 mg tablet of fluconazole to 10 lactating women resulted in a mean C_{max} of 2.61 µg/ml (range: 1.57-3.65 µg/ml).

Steady-state concentrations are reached within 5-10 days following oral doses of 50-400 mg given once daily. Administration of a loading dose (on day 1) of twice the usual daily dose results in plasma concentrations close to steady-state by the second day. The apparent volume of distribution of fluconazole approximates that of total body water. Plasma protein binding is low (11-12%). Following either single- or multiple-oral doses for up to 14 days, fluconazole penetrates into all body fluids studied (see TABLE 1). In normal volunteers, saliva concentrations of fluconazole were equal to or slightly greater than plasma concentrations regardless of dose, route, or duration of dosing. In patients with bronchiectasis, sputum concentrations of fluconazole following a single 150 mg oral dose were equal to plasma concentrations at both 4 and 24 hours post dose. In patients with fungal meningitis, fluconazole concentrations in the CSF are approximately 80% of the corresponding plasma concentrations.

A single oral 150 mg dose of fluconazole administered to 27 patients penetrated into vaginal tissue, resulting in tissue:plasma ratios ranging from 0.94-1.14 over the first 48 hours following dosing.

A single oral 150 mg dose of fluconazole administered to 14 patients penetrated into vaginal fluid, resulting in fluid:plasma ratios ranging from 0.36-0.71 over the first 72 hours following dosing (see TABLE 1).

TABLE 1

Tissue or Fluid	Ratio of Fluconazole Tissue (Fluid)/Plasma Concentration*
Cerebrospinal fluid†	0.5-0.9
Saliva	1
Sputum	1
Blister fluid	1
Urine	10
Normal skin	10
Nails	1
Blister skin	2
Vaginal tissue	1
Vaginal fluid	0.4-0.7

* Relative to concurrent concentrations in plasma in subjects with normal renal function.
† Independent of degree of meningeal inflammation.

In normal volunteers, fluconazole is cleared primarily by renal excretion, with approximately 80% of the administered dose appearing in the urine as unchanged drug. About 11% of the dose is excreted in the urine as metabolites.

The pharmacokinetics of fluconazole are markedly affected by reduction in renal function. There is an inverse relationship between the elimination half-life and creatinine clearance. The dose of fluconazole may need to be reduced in patients with impaired renal function (see DOSAGE AND ADMINISTRATION). A 3 hour hemodialysis session decreases plasma concentrations by approximately 50%.

In normal volunteers, fluconazole administration (doses ranging from 200- 400 mg once daily for up to 14 days) was associated with small and inconsistent effects on testosterone concentrations, endogenous corticosteroid concentrations, and the ACTH-stimulated cortisol response.

Pharmacokinetics in Children: In children, the following pharmacokinetic data [MEAN (%CV)] have been reported (see TABLE 2A and TABLE 2B).

TABLE 2A

Age Studied	Dose (mg/kg)	Clearance (ml/min/kg)
9 Months-13 Years	Single-Oral 2 mg/kg	0.40 (38%) n=14
9 Months-13 Years	Single-Oral 8 mg/kg	0.51 (60%) n=15
5-15 years	Multiple IV 2 mg/kg	0.49 (40%) n=4
5-15 years	Multiple IV 4 mg/kg	0.59 (64%) n=5
5-15 years	Multiple IV 8 mg/kg	0.66 (31%) n=5

Clearance corrected for body weight was not affected by age in these studies. Mean body clearance in adults is reported to be 0.23 (17%) ml/min/kg.

TABLE 2B

Half-life (hours)	C_{max} (µg/ml)	Vdss (l/kg)
25.0	2.9 (22%) n=16	—
19.5	9.8 (20%) n=15	—
17.4	5.5 (25%) n=5	0.722 (36%) n=4
15.2	11.4 (44%) n=6	0.729 (33%) n=5
17.6	14.1 (22%) n=8	1.069 (37%) n=7

In premature newborns (gestational age 26-29 weeks), the mean (% cv) clearance within 36 hours of birth was 0.180 (35%, n=7) ml/min/kg, which increased with time to a mean of 0.218 (31%, n=9) ml/min/kg 6 days later and 0.333 (56%, n=4) ml/min/kg 12 days later. Similarly, the half- life was 73.6 hours, which decreased with time to a mean of 53.2 hours 6 days later and 46.6 hours 12 days later.

MICROBIOLOGY

Fluconazole exhibits *in vitro* activity against *Cryptococcus neoformans* and *Candida* spp. Fungistatic activity has also been demonstrated in normal and immunocompromised animal models for systemic and intracranial fungal infections due to *Cryptococcus neoformans* and for systemic infections due to *Candida albicans.*

In common with other azole antifungal agents, most fungi show a higher apparent sensitivity to fluconazole *in vivo* than *in vitro.* Fluconazole administered orally and/or intravenously was active in a variety of animal models of fungal infection using standard laboratory strains of fungi. Activity has been demonstrated against fungal infections caused by *Aspergillus flavus* and *Aspergillus fumigatus* in normal mice. Fluconazole has also been shown to be active in animal models of endemic mycoses, including one model of *Blastomyces dermatitidis* pulmonary infections in normal mice; one model of *Coccidioides immitis* intracranial infections in normal mice; and several models of *Histoplasma capsulatum* pulmonary infection in normal and immunosuppressed mice. The clinical significance of results obtained in these studies is unknown.

Concurrent administration of fluconazole and amphotericin B in infected normal and immunosuppressed mice showed the following results: a small additive antifungal effect in systemic infection with *C. albicans,* no interaction in intracranial infection with *Cr. neoformans,* and antagonism of the two drugs in systemic infection with *Asp. fumigatus.* The clinical significance of results obtained in these studies is unknown.

There have been reports of cases of superinfection with Candida species other than *C. albicans,* which are often inherently not susceptible to Diflucan (*e.g., Candida krusei*). Such cases may require alternative antifungal therapy.

INDICATIONS AND USAGE

Fluconazole is indicated for the treatment of:

1. Vaginal Candidiasis (vaginal yeast infections due to *Candida*).
2. Oropharyngeal and esophageal candidiasis. In open noncomparative studies of relatively small numbers of patients, fluconazole was also effective for the treatment of *Candida* urinary tract infections, peritonitis, and systemic *Candida* infections including candidemia, disseminated candidiasis, and pneumonia.
3. Cryptococcal meningitis. Studies comparing fluconazole to amphotericin B in non-HIV infected patients have not been conducted.

PROPHYLAXIS

Fluconazole is also indicated to decrease the incidence of candidiasis in patients undergoing bone marrow transplantation who receive cytotoxic chemotherapy and/or radiation therapy.

Specimens for fungal culture and other relevant laboratory studies (serology, histopathology) should be obtained prior to therapy to isolate and identify causative organisms. Therapy may be instituted before the results of the cultures and other laboratory studies are known; however, once these results become available, anti-infective therapy should be adjusted accordingly.

CONTRAINDICATIONS

Fluconazole is contraindicated in patients who have shown hypersensitivity to fluconazole or to any of its excipients. There is no information regarding cross hypersensitivity between fluconazole and other azole antifungal agents. Caution should be used in prescribing fluconazole to patients with hypersensitivity to other azoles.

WARNINGS

1. ***Hepatic Injury:*** Fluconazole has been associated with rare cases of serious hepatic toxicity, including fatalities primarily in patients with serious underlying medical conditions. In cases of fluconazole associated hepatotoxicity, no obvious relationship to total daily dose, duration of therapy, sex or age of the patient has been observed. Fluconazole hepatotoxicity has usually, but not always, been reversible on discontinuation of therapy. Patients who develop abnormal liver function tests during fluconazole therapy should be monitored for the development of more severe hepatic injury. Fluconazole should be discontinued if clinical signs and symptoms consistent with liver disease develop that may be attributable to fluconazole.
2. ***Anaphylaxis:*** In rare cases, anaphylaxis has been reported.
3. ***Dermatologic:*** Patients have rarely developed exfoliative skin disorders during treatment with fluconazole. In patients with serious underlying diseases (predominantly AIDS and malignancy), these have rarely resulted in a fatal outcome. Patients who develop rashes during treatment with fluconazole should be monitored closely and the drug discontinued if lesions progress.

PRECAUTIONS

GENERAL

Single Dose

The convenience and efficacy of the single dose oral tablet of fluconazole regimen for the treatment of vaginal yeast infections should be weighed against the acceptability of a higher incidence of drug related adverse events with fluconazole (26%) versus intravaginal agents (16%) in US comparative clinical studies. (See ADVERSE REACTIONS.)

CARCINOGENESIS, MUTAGENESIS, AND IMPAIRMENT OF FERTILITY

Fluconazole showed no evidence of carcinogenic potential in mice and rats treated orally for 24 months at doses of 2.5, 5 or 10 mg/kg/day (approximately 2-7× the recommended human dose). Male rats treated with 5 and 10 mg/kg/day had an increased incidence of hepatocellular adenomas.

Fluconazole, with or without metabolic activation, was negative in tests for mutagenicity in 4 strains of *S. typhimurium,* and in the mouse lymphoma L5178Y system. Cytogenetic studies *in vivo* (murine bone marrow cells, following oral administration of fluconazole) and *in vitro* (human lymphocytes exposed to fluconazole at 1000 µg/ml) showed no evidence of chromosomal mutations.

Fluconazole did not affect the fertility of male or female rats treated orally with daily doses of 5, 10, or 20 mg/kg or with parenteral doses of 5, 25, or 75 mg/kg, although the onset of parturition was slightly delayed at 20 mg/kg p.o. In an intravenous perinatal study in rats at 5, 20, and 40 mg, dystocia and prolongation of parturition were observed in a few dams at 20 mg/kg (approximately 5-15× the recommended human dose) and 40 mg/kg, but not at 5 mg/kg. The disturbances in parturition were reflected by a slight increase in the number of still-born pups and decrease of neonatal survival at these dose levels. The effects on parturition in rats are consistent with the species specific estrogen-lowering property produced by high doses of fluconazole. Such a hormone change has not been observed in women treated with fluconazole. (See CLINICAL PHARMACOLOGY.)

PREGNANCY, TERATOGENIC EFFECTS, PREGNANCY CATEGORY C

Fluconazole was administered orally to pregnant rabbits during organogenesis in two studies, at 5, 10, and 20 mg/kg and at 5, 25, and 75 mg/kg, respectively. Maternal weight gain was impaired at all dose levels, and abortions occurred at 75 mg/kg (approximately 20-60× the recommended human dose); no adverse fetal effects were detected. In several studies in which pregnant rats were treated orally with fluconazole during organogenesis, maternal weight gain was impaired and placental weights were increased at 25 mg/kg. There were no fetal effects at 5 or 10 mg/kg; increases in fetal anatomical variants (supernumerary ribs, renal pelvis dilation) and delays in ossification were observed at 25 and 50 mg/kg and higher doses. At doses ranging from 80 mg/kg (approximately 20-60× the recommended human dose) to 320 mg/kg embryolethality in rats was increased and fetal abnormalities included wavy ribs, cleft palate and abnormal cranio-facial ossification. These effects are consistent with the inhibition of estrogen synthesis in rats and may be a result of known effects of lowered estrogen on pregnancy, organogenesis and parturition.

There are no adequate and well controlled studies in pregnant women. Fluconazole should be used in pregnancy only if the potential benefit justifies the possible risk to the fetus.

NURSING MOTHERS

Fluconazole is secreted in human milk at concentrations similar to plasma. Therefore, the use of fluconazole in nursing mothers is not recommended.

PEDIATRIC USE

An open-label, randomized, controlled trial has shown Diflucan to be effective in the treatment of oropharyngeal candidiasis in children 6 months to 13 years of age.

The use of fluconazole in children with cryptococcal meningitis, *Candida* esophagitis, or systemic *Candida* infections is supported by the efficacy shown for these indications in adults and by the results from several small noncomparative pediatric clinical studies. In addition, pharmacokinetic studies in children (see CLINICAL PHARMACOLOGY), have established a dose proportionality between children and adults. (See DOSAGE AND ADMINISTRATION.)

In a noncomparative study of children with serious systemic fungal infections, most of which were candidemia, the effectiveness of fluconazole was similar to that reported for the treatment of candidemia in adults. Of 17 subjects with culture-confirmed candidemia, 11 of 14 (79%) with baseline symptoms (3 were asymptomatic) had a clinical cure: 13/15 (87%) of evaluable patients had a mycologic cure at the end of treatment but 2 of these patients relapsed at 10 and 18 days, respectively, following cessation of therapy.

The efficacy of fluconazole for the suppression of cryptococcal meningitis was successful in 4 of 5 children treated in a compassionate-use study of fluconazole for the treatment of life-threatening or serious mycosis. There is no information regarding the efficacy of fluconazole for primary treatment of cryptococcal meningitis in children.

The safety profile of fluconazole in children has been studied in 577 children ages 1 day to 17 years who received doses ranging from 1-15 mg/kg/day for 1-1616 days. (See ADVERSE REACTIONS.)

Efficacy of fluconazole has not been established in infants less than 6 months of age. (See CLINICAL PHARMACOLOGY.) A small number of patients (29) ranging in age from 1 day to 6 months have been treated safely with fluconazole.

DRUG INTERACTIONS

See PRECAUTIONS, General.

Clinically or potentially significant drug interactions between fluconazole and the following agents/classes have been observed. These are described in greater detail below:

Oral Hypoglycemics: Clinically significant hypoglycemia may be precipitated by the use of fluconazole with oral hypoglycemic agents: 1 fatality has been reported from hypoglycemia in association with combined fluconazole and glyburide use. Fluconazole reduces the metabolism of tolbutamide, glyburide, and glipizide and increases the plasma concentration of these agents. When fluconazole is used concomitantly with these or other sulfonylurea oral hypoglycemic agents, blood glucose concentrations should be carefully monitored and the dose of the sulfonylurea should be adjusted as necessary.

Coumarin-Type Anticoagulants: Prothrombin time may be increased in patients receiving concomitant fluconazole and coumarin-type anticoagulants. Careful monitoring of prothrombin time in patients receiving fluconazole and coumarin-type anticoagulants is recommended.

Phenytoin: Fluconazole increases the plasma concentrations of phenytoin. Careful monitoring of phenytoin concentrations in patients receiving fluconazole and phenytoin is recommended.

Cyclosporine: Fluconazole may significantly increase cyclosporine levels in renal transplant patients with or without renal impairment. Careful monitoring of cyclosporine concentrations and serum creatinine is recommended in patients receiving fluconazole and cyclosporine.

Rifampin: Rifampin enhances the metabolism of concurrently administered fluconazole. Depending on clinical circumstances, consideration should be given to increasing the dose of fluconazole when it is administered with rifampin.

Theophylline: Fluconazole increases the serum concentrations of theophylline. Careful monitoring of serum theophylline concentrations in patients receiving fluconazole and theophylline is recommended.

Terfenadine: Because of the occurrence of serious cardiac dysrhythmias in patients receiving other azole antifungals in conjunction with terfenadine, an interaction study has been performed (see Drug Interaction Studies), and failed to demonstrate a clinically significant drug interaction. Although these events have not been observed in patients receiving fluconazole, the co-administration of fluconazole and terfenadine should be carefully monitored.

Fluconazole tablets coadministered with ethinyl estradiol- and levonorgestrel -containing oral contraceptives produced an overall mean increase in ethinyl estradiol and levonorgestrel levels; however, in some patients there were decreases up to 47% and 33% of ethinyl estradiol and levonorgestrel levels (see Drug Interaction Studies). The data presently available indicate that the decreases in some individual ethinyl estradiol and levonorgestrel AUC values with fluconazole treatment are likely the result of random variation. While there is evidence that fluconazole can inhibit the metabolism of ethinyl estradiol and levonorgestrel, there is no evidence that fluconazole is a net inducer of ethinyl estradiol or levonorgestrel metabolism. The clinical significance of these effects is presently unknown.

Physicians should be aware that interaction studies with medications other than those listed in CLINICAL PHARMACOLOGY have not been conducted, but such interactions may occur.

DRUG INTERACTION STUDIES

Oral Contraceptives

Oral contraceptives were administered as a single dose both before and after the oral administration of fluconazole 50 mg once daily for 10 days in 10 healthy women. There was no significant difference in ethinyl estradiol or levonorgestrel AUC after the administration of 50 mg of fluconazole. The mean increase in ethinyl estradiol AUC was 6% (range: -47 to 108%) and levonorgestrel AUC increased 17% (range: -33 to 141%).

Twenty-five (25) normal females received daily doses of both 200 mg of fluconazole tablets or placebo for two, 10 day periods. The treatment cycles were 1 month apart with all subjects receiving fluconazole during one cycle and placebo during the other. The order of study treatment was random. Single doses of an oral contraceptive tablet containing levonorgestrel and ethinyl estradiol were administered on the final treatment day (day 10) of both cycles. Following administration of 200 mg of fluconazole, the mean percentage increase of AUC for levonorgestrel compared to placebo was 25% (range: -12 to 82%) and the mean percentage increase for ethinyl estradiol compared to placebo was 38% (range: -11 to 101%). Both of these increases were statistically significantly different from placebo.

Cimetidine

Fluconazole 100 mg was administered as a single oral dose alone and 2 hours after a single dose of cimetidine 400 mg to 6 healthy male volunteers. After the administration of cimetidine, there was a significant decrease in fluconazole AUC and C_{max}. There was a mean ±SD decrease in fluconazole AUC of 13% ± 11% (range: -3.4 to -31%) and C_{max} decreased 19% ± 14% (range: -5 to -40%). However, the administration of cimetidine 600-900 mg intravenously over a 4 hour period (from 1 hour before to 3 hours after a single oral dose of fluconazole 200 mg) did not affect the bioavailability or pharmacokinetics of fluconazole in 24 healthy male volunteers.

Antacid

Administration of Maalox (20 ml) to 14 normal male volunteers immediately prior to a single dose of fluconazole 100 mg had no effect on the absorption or elimination of fluconazole.

Hydrochlorothiazide

Concomitant oral administration of 100 mg Diflucan and 50 mg hydrochlorothiazide for 10 days in 13 normal volunteers resulted in a significant increase in fluconazole AUC and C_{max} compared to Diflucan given alone. There was a mean ±SD increase in fluconazole AUC and C_{max} 45% ± 31% (range: 19-114%) and 43% ± 31% (range: 19-122%), respectively. These changes are attributable to a mean ±SD reduction in renal clearance of 30% ± 12% (range: -10 to -50%).

Rifampin

Administration of a single oral 200 mg dose of fluconazole after 15 days of rifampin administration as 600 mg daily in 8 healthy male volunteers resulted in a significant decrease in fluconazole AUC and a significant increase in apparent oral clearance of fluconazole. There was a mean ±SD reduction in fluconazole AUC of 23% ± 9% (range: - 13 to -42%). Apparent oral clearance of fluconazole increased 32% ± 17% (range: 16-72%). Fluconazole half-life decreased from 33.4 ± 4.4 hours to 26.8 ± 3.9 hours. (See PRECAUTIONS.)

Warfarin

There was a significant increase in prothrombin time response (area under the prothrombin time-time curve) following a single dose of warfarin (15 mg) administered to 13 normal male volunteers following oral fluconazole 200 mg administered daily for 14 days as compared to the administration of warfarin alone. There was a mean ±SD increase in the prothrombin time response (area under the prothrombin time-time curve) of 7% ± 4% (range: -2 to 13%). (See PRECAUTIONS.) Mean is based on data from 12 subjects as 1 of 13 subjects experienced a 2-fold increase in his prothrombin time response.

Phenytoin

Phenytoin AUC was determined after 4 days of phenytoin dosing (200 mg daily, orally for 3 days followed by 250 mg intravenously for 1 dose) both with and without the administration of fluconazole (oral fluconazole 200 mg daily for 16 days) in 10 normal male volunteers. There was a significant increase in phenytoin AUC. The mean ±SD increase in phenytoin AUC was 88% ± 68% (range: 16-247%). The absolute magnitude of this interaction is unknown because of the intrinsically nonlinear disposition of phenytoin. (See PRECAUTIONS.)

Cyclosporine

Cyclosporine AUC and C_{max} were determined before and after the administration of fluconazole 200 mg daily for 14 days in 8 renal transplant patients who had been on cyclosporine therapy for at least 6 months and on a stable cyclosporine dose for at least 6 weeks. There was a significant increase in cyclosporine AUC, C_{max}, C_{min} (24 hour concentration), and a significant reduction in apparent oral clearance following the administration of fluconazole. The mean ±SD increase in AUC was 92% ± 43% (range: 18-147%). The C_{max} increased 60% ± 48% (range: -5 to 133%). The C_{min} increased 157% ± 96% (range: 33-360%). The apparent oral clearance decreased 45% ± 15% (range: -15 to -60%). (See PRECAUTIONS.)

Zidovudine

Plasma zidovudine concentrations were determined on two occasions (before and following fluconazole 200 mg daily for 15 days) in 13 volunteers with AIDS or ARC who were on a stable zidovudine dose for at least 2 weeks. There was a significant increase in zidovudine AUC following the administration of fluconazole. The mean ±SD increase in AUC was 20% ± 32% (range: -27 to 104%). The metabolite, GZDV to parent drug ratio significantly decreased after the administration of fluconazole, from 7.6 ± 3.6 to 5.7 ± 2.2.

Theophylline

The pharmacokinetics of theophylline were determined from a single intravenous dose of aminophylline (6 mg/kg) before and after the oral administration of fluconazole 200 mg daily for 14 days in 16 normal male volunteers. There were significant increases in theophylline AUC, C_{max}, and half-life with a corresponding decrease in clearance. The mean ±SD theophylline AUC increased 21% ± 16% (range: -5 to 48%). The C_{max} increased 13% ± 17% (range: -13 to 40%). Theophylline clearance decreased 16% ± 11% (range: -32 to 5%). The half-life of theophylline increased from 6.6 ± 1.7 hours to 7.9 ± 1.5 hours.

Terfenadine

Six (6) healthy volunteers received terfenadine 60 mg bid for 15 days. Fluconazole 200 mg was administered daily from days 9 through 15. Fluconazole did not affect terfenadine plasma concentrations. Terfenadine acid metabolite AUC increased 36% ± 36% (range: 7 to 102%) from day 8 to 15 with the concomitant administration of fluconazole. There was no change in cardiac repolarization as a measure by Holter QTc intervals.

Oral Hypoglycemics

The effects of fluconazole on the pharmacokinetics of the sulfonylurea oral hypoglycemic agents tolbutamide, glipizide, and glyburide were evaluated in three placebo-controlled studies in normal volunteers. All subjects received the sulfonylurea alone as a single dose and again as a single dose following the administration of fluconazole 100 mg daily for 7 days. In these three studies 22/46 (47.8%) of fluconazole treated patients and 9/22 (40.1%) of placebo treated patients experienced symptoms consistent with hypoglycemia. (See PRECAUTIONS.)

Tolbutamide

In 13 normal male volunteers, there was significant increase in tolbutamide (500 mg single dose) AUC and C_{max} following the administration of fluconazole. There was a mean ±SD increase in tolbutamide AUC of 26% ± 9% (range: 12 to 39%). Tolbutamide C_{max} increased 11% ± 9% (range: -6 to 27%). (See PRECAUTIONS.)

Glipizide

The AUC and C_{max} of glipizide (2.5 mg single dose) were significantly increased following the administration of fluconazole in 13 normal male volunteers. There was mean ±SD increase in AUC of 49% ± 13% (range: 27 to 73%) and an increase in C_{max} of 19% ± 23% (range: -11 to 79%). (See PRECAUTIONS.)

Glyburide

The AUC and C_{max} of glyburide (5 mg single dose) were significantly increased following the administration of fluconazole in 20 normal male volunteers. There was a mean ±SD increase in AUC of 44% ± 29% (range: -13 to 115%) and C_{max} increased 19% ± 19% (range: -23 to 62%). Five (5) subjects required oral glucose following the ingestion of glyburide after 7 days of fluconazole administration. (See PRECAUTIONS.)

ADVERSE REACTIONS

IN PATIENTS RECEIVING A SINGLE DOSE FOR VAGINAL CANDIDIASIS

During comparative clinical studies conducted in the US, 448 patients with vaginal candidiasis were treated with Diflucan, 150 mg single dose. The overall incidence of side effects possibly related to Diflucan was 26%. In 422 patients receiving active comparative agents, the incidence was 16%. The most common treatment-related adverse events reported in the patients who received 150 mg single dose fluconazole for vaginitis were headache (13%), nausea (7%), and abdominal pain (6%). Other side effects reported with an incidence equal to or greater than 1% included diarrhea (3%), dyspepsia (1%), dizziness (1%), and taste perversion (1%). Most of the reported side effects were mild to moderate in severity. Rarely, angioedema and anaphylactic reaction have been reported in marketing experience.

IN PATIENTS RECEIVING MULTIPLE DOSES FOR OTHER INFECTIONS

Sixteen percent (16%) of over 4000 patients treated with fluconazole in clinical trials of 7 days or more experienced adverse events. Treatment was discontinued in 1.5% of patients due to adverse clinical events and in 1.3% of patients due to laboratory test abnormalities.

Clinical adverse events were reported more frequently in HIV infected patients (21%) than in non-HIV infected patients (13%); however, the patterns in HIV infected and non-HIV infected patients were similar. The proportions of patients discontinuing therapy due to clinical adverse events were similar in the two groups (1.5%).

The following treatment-related clinical adverse events occurred at an incidence of 1% or greater in 4048 patients receiving Diflucan for 7 or more days in clinical trials: nausea 3.7%, headache 1.9%, skin rash 1.8%, vomiting 1.7%, abdominal pain 1.7%, and diarrhea 1.5%.

The following adverse events have occurred under conditions where a casual association is probable:

Hepatobiliary: In combined clinical trials and marketing experience, there have been rare cases of serious hepatic reactions during treatment with fluconazole. (See WARNINGS.) The spectrum of these hepatic reactions has ranged from mild transient elevations in transaminases to clinical hepatitis, cholestasis and fulminant hepatic failure, including fatalities. Instances of fatal hepatic reactions were noted to occur primarily in patients with serious underlying medical conditions (predominantly AIDS or malignancy) and often while taking multiple concomitant medications. Transient hepatic reactions, including hepatitis and jaundice, have occurred among patients with no other identifiable risk factors. In each of these cases, liver function returned to baseline on discontinuation of fluconazole.

In two comparative trials evaluating the efficacy of fluconazole for the suppression of relapse of cryptococcal meningitis, a statistically significant increase was observed in median AST (SGOT) levels from a baseline value of 30 IU/l to 41 IU/l in one trial and 34 IU/l to 66 IU/l in the other. The overall rate of serum transaminase elevations of more than 8 times the upper limit of normal was approximately 1% in fluconazole-treated patients in clinical trials. These elevations occurred in patients with severe underlying disease, predominantly AIDS or malignancies, most of whom were receiving multiple concomitant medications, including many known to be hepatotoxic. The incidence of abnormally elevated serum transaminases was greater in patients taking fluconazole concomitantly with one or more of the following medications: rifampin, phenytoin, isoniazid, valproic acid, or oral sulfonylurea hypoglycemic agents.

Immunological: In rare cases, anaphylaxis has been reported.

The following adverse events have occurred under conditions where a casual association is uncertain:

Central Nervous System: Seizures.

Dermatologic: Exfoliative skin disorders including Stevens-Johnson Syndrome and toxic epidermal necroivsis (See WARNINGS, alopecia).

Hematopoietic and Lymphatic: Leukopenia, thrombocytopenia.

Metabolic: Hypercholesterolemia, hypertriglyceridemia, hypokalemia.

ADVERSE REACTIONS IN CHILDREN

In Phase 2/3 clinical trials conducted in the US and in Europe, 577 pediatric patients, ages 1 day to 17 years were treated with fluconazole at doses up to 15 mg/kg/day for up to 1616 days. Thirteen percent of children experienced treatment related adverse events. The most commonly reported events were vomiting (5%), abdominal pain (3%), nausea (2%), and diarrhea (2%). Treatment was discontinued inn 2.3% of patients due to adverse clinical events and in 1.4% of patients due to laboratory test abnormalities. The majority of treatment-related laboratory abnormalities were elevations of transaminases or alkaline phosphatase (see TABLE 6).

TABLE 6 *Percentage of Patients With Treatment-Related Side Effects*

	Fluconazole (n=577)	Comparative Agents (n=451)
With any side effect	13.0%	9.3%
Vomiting	5.4%	5.1%
Abdominal pain	2.8%	1.6%
Nausea	2.3%	1.6%
Diarrhea	2.1%	2.2%

DOSAGE AND ADMINISTRATION

DOSAGE AND ADMINISTRATION IN ADULTS

Single Dose

Vaginal candidiasis: The recommended dosage of fluconazole for vaginal candidiasis is 150 mg as a single oral dose.

Multiple Dose

SINCE ORAL ABSORPTION IS RAPID AND ALMOST COMPLETE, THE DAILY DOSE OF FLUCONAZOLE IS THE SAME FOR ORAL (TABLETS AND SUSPENSION) AND INTRAVENOUS ADMINISTRATION. In general, a leading dose of twice the daily dose is recommended on the first day of therapy to result in plasma concentrations close to steady-state by the second day of therapy.

The daily dose of fluconazole for the treatment of infections other than vaginal candidiasis should be based on the infecting organism and the patient's response to therapy. Treatment should be continued until clinical parameters or laboratory tests indicate that active fungal infection has subsided. An inadequate period of treatment may lead to recurrence of active infection. Patients with AIDS and cryptococcal meningitis or recurrent oropharyngeal candidiasis usually require maintenance therapy to prevent relapse.

Oropharyngeal Candidiasis: The recommended dosage of fluconazole for oropharyngeal candidiasis is 200 mg on the first day, followed by 100 mg once daily. Clinical evidence of oropharyngeal candidiasis generally resolves within several days, but treatment should be continued for at least 2 weeks to decrease the likelihood of relapse.

Esophageal Candidiasis: The recommended dosage of fluconazole for esophageal candidiasis is 200 mg on the first day, followed by 100 mg once daily. Doses up to 400 mg/day may be used, based on medical judgment of the patient's response to therapy. Patients with esophageal candidiasis should be treated for a minimum of 3 weeks and for at least 2 weeks following resolution of symptoms.

Systemic Candida Infections: For systemic Candida infections including candidemia, disseminated candidiasis, and pneumonia, optimal therapeutic dosage and duration of therapy have not been established. In open, noncomparative studies of small numbers of patients, doses of up to 400 mg daily have been used.

Urinary Tract Infection and Peritonitis: For the treatment of Candida urinary tract infections and peritonitis, daily doses of 50-200 mg have been used in open, non-comparative studies of small numbers of patients.

Cryptococcal Meningitis: The recommended dosage for treatment of acute cryptococcal meningitis is 400 mg on the first day, followed by 200 mg once daily. A dosage of 400 mg once daily may be used, based on medical judgment of the patient's response to therapy. The recommended duration of treatment for initial therapy of cryptococcal meningitis is 10-12 weeks after the cerebrospinal fluid becomes culture negative. The recommended dosage of fluconazole for suppression of relapse of cryptococcal meningitis in patients with AIDS is 200 mg once daily.

Prophylaxis in Patients Undergoing Bone Marrow Transplantation: The recommended fluconazole daily dosage for the prevention of candidiasis of patients undergoing bone marrow transplantation is 400 mg once daily. Patients who are anticipated to have severe granulocytopenia (less than 500 neutrophils/mm^3) should start fluconazole prophylaxis several days before the anticipated onset of neutropenia, and continue for 7 days after the neutrophil count rises above 1000 cells/mm^3.

DOSAGE AND ADMINISTRATION IN CHILDREN

The following dose equivalency scheme should generally provide equivalent exposure in pediatric and adult patients (see TABLE 7).

TABLE 7

Pediatric Patients	Adults
3 mg/kg	100 mg
6 mg/kg	200 mg
12* mg/kg	400 mg

* Some older children may have clearances similar to that of adults. Absolute doses exceeding 600 mg/day are not recommended.

Experience with fluconazole in neonates is limited to pharmacokinetic studies in premature newborns. (See CLINICAL PHARMACOLOGY.) Based on the prolonged half-life seen in premature newborns (gestational age 26-29 weeks), these children, in the first 2 weeks of life, should receive the same dosage (mg/kg) as in older children, but administered every 72 hours. After the first 2 weeks, these children should be dosed once daily. No information regarding fluconazole pharmacokinetics in full-term newborns is available.

Oropharyngeal Candidiasis: The recommended dosage of fluconazole for oropharyngeal candidiasis in children is 6 mg/kg on the first day, followed by 3 mg/kg once daily. Treatment should be administered for at least 2 weeks to decrease the likelihood of relapse.

Esophageal Candidiasis: For the treatment of esophageal candidiasis, the recommended dosage of fluconazole in children is 6 mg/kg on the first day, followed by 3 mg/kg once daily. Doses up to 12 mg/kg/day may be used based on medical judgment of the patient's response to therapy. Patients with esophageal candidiasis should be treated for a minimum of 3 weeks for at least 2 weeks following the resolution of symptoms.

Systemic Candida Infections: For the treatment of candidemia and disseminated Candida infections, daily doses of 6-12 mg/kg/day have been used in an open, noncomparative study of a small number of children.

Cryptococcal Meningitis: For the treatment of acute cryptococcal meningitis, the recommended dosage is 12 mg/kg on the first day, followed by 6 mg/kg once daily. A dosage of 12 mg/kg once daily may be used, based on medical judgment of the patient's response to therapy. The recommended duration of treatment for initial therapy of cryptococcal meningitis is 10-12 weeks after the cerebrospinal fluid becomes culture negative. For suppression of relapse of cryptococcal meningitis in children with AIDS, the recommended dose of fluconazole is 6 mg/kg once daily.

DOSAGE IN PATIENTS WITH IMPAIRED RENAL FUNCTION

Fluconazole is cleared primarily by renal excretion as unchanged drug. There is no need to adjust single dose therapy for vaginal candidiasis because of impaired renal function. In patients with impaired renal function who will receive multiple doses of fluconazole, an initial loading dose of 50-400 mg should be given. After the loading dose, the daily dose (according to indication) should be based on TABLE 8.

TABLE 8

Creatinine Clearance (ml/min)	Percent of Recommended Dose
>50	100%
11-50	50%
Patients receiving regular hemodialysis.	One recommended dose after each dialysis.

These are suggested dose adjustments based on pharmacokinetics following administration of multiple doses. Further adjustment may be needed depending upon clinical condition.

When serum creatinine is the only measure of renal function available, the formula below (based on sex, weight, and age of the patient) should be used to estimate the creatinine clearance:

Males: [Weight (kg) × (140-Age)] ÷ [72 × Serum Creatnine (mg/100ml]

Females: 0.85 × the above value

Although the pharmacokinetics of fluconazole has not been studied in children with renal insufficiency, dosage reduction in children with renal insufficiency should parallel that recommended for adults. The formula below may be used to estimate creatinine clearance in children:

[K × Linear Length or Height (cm)] ÷ [Serum Creatnine (mg/100 ml)]

K=0.55 for children older than 1 year and 0.45 for infants.

ADMINISTRATION

Fluconazole may be administered either orally or by intravenous infusion. Diflucan injection has been used safely for up to fourteen days of intravenous therapy. The intravenous infusion of fluconazole should be administered at a maximum rate of approximately 200 mg/hour, given as a continuous infusion.

Fluconazole injections in glass and Viaflex Plus plastic containers are intended only for intravenous administration using sterile equipment.

Parenteral drug products should be inspected visually for particulate matter and discoloration prior to administration whenever solution and container permit.

Do not use if the solution is cloudy or precipitated or if the seal is not intact.

HOW SUPPLIED

DIFLUCAN TABLETS:

Pink trapezoidal tablets containing 50, 100, or 200 mg of fluconazole are packaged in bottles or unit dose blisters. The 150 mg fluconazole tablets are pink and oval shaped, packaged in a single dose unit blister.

Storage: Store tablets below 30°C (86°F).

DIFLUCAN FOR ORAL SUSPENSION

Diflucan for oral suspension is supplied as an orange-flavored powder to provide 35 ml per bottle.

Storage: Store dry powder below 30°C (86°F). Store reconstituted suspension between 30°C (86°F) and 5°C (41°F) and discard unused portion after 2 weeks. Protect from freezing.

DIFLUCAN INJECTIONS

Diflucan injections for intravenous infusion administration are formulated as sterile iso-osmotic solutions containing 2 mg/ml of fluconazole. They are supplied in glass bottles or in Viaflex Plus plastic containers containing volumes of 100 or 200 ml affording doses of 200 and 400 mg of fluconazole, respectively.

Storage: Store between 30°C (86°F) and 5°C (41°F). Protect from freezing.

Diflucan injections in Viaflex Plus plastic containers are available in both sodium chloride and dextrose diluents.

Storage: Store between 25°C (77°F) and 5°C (41°F). Brief exposure up to 40°C (104°F) does not adversely affect the product. Protect from freezing.

PRODUCT LISTING - EQUIVALENTS NOT AVAILABLE

Powder For Reconstitution - Oral - 10 mg/ml

35 ml	$34.94	DIFLUCAN, Pfizer U.S. Pharmaceuticals	00049-3440-19

Powder For Reconstitution - Oral - 40 mg/ml

35 ml	$126.91	DIFLUCAN, Pfizer U.S. Pharmaceuticals	00049-3450-19

Solution - Intravenous - 200 mg/100 ml

100 ml x 6	$605.88	DIFLUCAN, Pfizer U.S. Pharmaceuticals	00049-3371-26
100 ml x 6	$605.88	DIFLUCAN, Pfizer U.S. Pharmaceuticals	00049-3435-26
100 ml x 6	$605.88	DIFLUCAN, Pfizer U.S. Pharmaceuticals	00049-3437-26

Solution - Intravenous - 400 mg/200 ml

200 ml x 6	$838.74	DIFLUCAN, Pfizer U.S. Pharmaceuticals	00049-3438-26
200 ml x 6	$885.48	DIFLUCAN, Pfizer U.S. Pharmaceuticals	00049-3372-26
200 ml x 6	$885.48	DIFLUCAN, Pfizer U.S. Pharmaceuticals	00049-3436-26

Tablet - Oral - 50 mg

30's	$163.11	DIFLUCAN, Pfizer U.S. Pharmaceuticals	00049-3410-30

Tablet - Oral - 100 mg

7's	$55.27	DIFLUCAN, Physicians Total Care	54868-1863-02
10's	$78.45	DIFLUCAN, Physicians Total Care	54868-1863-01
15's	$112.03	DIFLUCAN, Pharma Pac	54569-3926-01
30's	$224.06	DIFLUCAN, Pharma Pac	54569-3926-00
30's	$224.06	DIFLUCAN, Physicians Total Care	54868-1863-03
30's	$256.31	DIFLUCAN, Pfizer U.S. Pharmaceuticals	00049-3420-30
100's	$854.38	DIFLUCAN, Pfizer U.S. Pharmaceuticals	00049-3420-41

Tablet - Oral - 150 mg

1's	$11.89	DIFLUCAN, Allscripts Pharmaceutical Company	54569-3954-00
1's	$18.71	DIFLUCAN, Pharma Pac	52959-0455-01
12's	$163.20	DIFLUCAN, Pfizer U.S. Pharmaceuticals	00049-3500-79

Tablet - Oral - 200 mg

1's	$12.22	DIFLUCAN, Allscripts Pharmaceutical Company	54569-3269-00
1's	$21.68	DIFLUCAN, Pd-Rx Pharmaceuticals	55289-0148-01
30's	$392.26	DIFLUCAN, Physicians Total Care	54868-1034-01
30's	$419.44	DIFLUCAN, Pfizer U.S. Pharmaceuticals	00049-3430-30
100's	$1398.13	DIFLUCAN, Pfizer U.S. Pharmaceuticals	00049-3430-41

Flucytosine (001302)

For related information, see the comparative table section in Appendix A.

Categories: Endocarditis, candidal; Infection, respiratory tract, due to Candida; Infection, respiratory tract, due to Cryptococcus; Infection, urinary tract, due to Candida; Meningitis, due to Cryptococcus; Septicemia, due to Candida; Pregnancy Category C; FDA Approved 1971 Nov; WHO Formulary
Drug Classes: Antifungals
Brand Names: Ancobon
Foreign Brand Availability: Alcobon (Bahrain; Cyprus; Egypt; England; Iran; Iraq; Ireland; Jordan; Kuwait; Lebanon; Libya; New-Zealand; Oman; Qatar; Republic-of-Yemen; Saudi-Arabia; South-Africa; Syria; United-Arab-Emirates); Ancotil (Austria; Bulgaria; Czech-Republic; Denmark; France; Hong-Kong; Italy; Japan; Netherlands; Norway; Sweden; Switzerland)
Cost of Therapy: $899.42 (Candidiasis, systemic; Ancobon; 500 mg; 8 capsules/day; 14 day supply)

WARNING

Use with extreme caution in patients with impaired renal function. Close monitoring of hematologic, renal and hepatic status of all patients is essential. These instructions should be thoroughly reviewed before administration of flucytosine.

DESCRIPTION

Flucytosine, an antifungal agent, is available as 250 mg and 500 mg capsules for oral administration. Each capsule also contains corn starch, lactose and talc. Ancobon gelatin capsule shells contain parabens (butyl, methyl, propyl) and sodium propionate, with the following dye systems: 250 mg capsules — black iron oxide, FD&C blue no. 1, FD&C yellow no. 6, D&C yellow no. 10 and titanium dioxide; 500 mg capsules — black iron oxide and titanium dioxide. Chemically, flucytosine is 5-fluorocytosine, a fluorinated pyrimidine which is related to fluorouracil and floxuridine. It is a white to off-white crystalline powder with a molecular weight of 129.09.

CLINICAL PHARMACOLOGY

Flucytosine is rapidly and virtually completely absorbed following oral administration. Bioavailability estimated by comparing the area under the curve of serum concentrations after oral and intravenous administration showed 78-89% absorption of the oral dose. Peak blood concentrations of 30-40 μg/ml were reached within 2 hours of administration of a 2 g oral dose to normal subjects. The mean blood concentrations were approximately 70-80 μg/ml 1-2 hours after a dose in patients with normal renal function who received a 6 week regimen of flucytosine (150 mg/kg/day given in divided doses every 6 hours) in combination with amphotericin B. The half-life in the majority of normal subjects ranged between 2.4 and 4.8 hours. Flucytosine is excreted via the kidneys by means of glomerular filtration without significant tubular reabsorption. More than 90% of the total radioactivity after oral administration was recovered in the urine as intact drug. Approximately 1% of the dose is present in the urine as the α-fluoro-β-ureido-propionic acid metabolite. A small portion of the dose is excreted in the feces.

The half-life of flucytosine is prolonged in patients with renal insufficiency; the average half-life in nephrectomized or anuric patients was 85 hours (range: 29.9-250 hours). A linear correlation was found between the elimination rate constant of flucytosine and creatinine clearance.

In vitro studies have shown that 2.9-4% of flucytosine is protein-bound over the range of therapeutic concentrations found in the blood. Flucytosine readily penetrates the blood-brain barrier, achieving clinically significant concentrations in cerebrospinal fluid. Studies in pregnant rats have shown that flucytosine injected intraperitoneally crosses the placental barrier (see PRECAUTIONS).

METABOLISM

Flucytosine has *in vitro* and *in vivo* activity against *Candida* and *Cryptococcus*. Although the exact mode of action is unknown, it has been proposed that flucytosine acts directly on fungal organisms by competitive inhibition of purine and pyrimidine uptake and indirectly by intracellular metabolism to 5-fluorouracil. Flucytosine enters the fungal cell via cytosine permease; thus, flucytosine is metabolized to 5-fluorouracil within fungal organisms. The 5-fluorouracil is extensively incorporated into fungal RNA and inhibits synthesis of both DNA and RNA. The result is unbalanced growth and death of the fungal organism. Antifungal synergism between flucytosine and polyene antibiotics, particularly amphotericin B, has been reported.

Flucytosine has *in vitro* and *in vivo* activity against *Candida* and *Cryptococcus*. The exact mode of action against these fungi is not known. Flucytosine is not metabolized significantly when given orally to man.

SUSCEPTIBILITY

Cryptococcus

Most strains initially isolated from clinical material have shown flucytosine minimal inhibitory concentrations (MICs) ranging from 0.46 to 7.8 μg/ml. Any isolate with an MIC greater than 12.5 μg/ml is considered resistant. *In vitro* resistance has developed in originally susceptible strains during therapy. It is recommended that clinical cultures for susceptibility testing be taken initially and at weekly intervals during therapy. The initial culture should be reserved as a reference in susceptibility testing of subsequent isolates.

Candida

As high as 40-50% of the pretreatment clinical isolates of *Candida* have been reported to be resistant to flucytosine. It is recommended that susceptibility studies be performed as early as possible and be repeated during therapy. An MIC value greater than 100 μg/ml is considered resistant.

Interference with *in vitro* activity of flucytosine occurs in complex or semisynthetic media. In order to rely upon the recommended *in vitro* interpretations of susceptibility, it is essential that the broth medium and the testing procedure used be that described by Shadomy.[1]

INDICATIONS AND USAGE

Flucytosine is indicated only in the treatment of serious infections caused by susceptible strains of *Candida* and/or *Cryptococcus.*

Candida: Septicemia, endocarditis and urinary system infections have been effectively treated with flucytosine. Limited trials in pulmonary infections justify the use of flucytosine.

Cryptococcus: *Meningitis and pulmonary infections have been treated effectively. Studies in septicemias and urinary tract infections are limited, but good responses have been reported.*

CONTRAINDICATIONS

Flucytosine should not be used in patients with a known hypersensitivity to the drug.

WARNINGS

Flucytosine must be given with extreme caution to patients with impaired renal function. Since flucytosine is excreted primarily by the kidneys, renal impairment may lead to accumulation of the drug. Flucytosine blood concentrations should be monitored to determine the adequacy of renal excretion in such patients.[1] Dosage adjustments should be made in patients with renal insufficiency to prevent progressive accumulation of active drug.

Flucytosine must be given with extreme caution to patients with bone marrow depression. Patients may be more prone to depression of bone marrow function if they: (1) have a hematologic disease, (2) are being treated with radiation or drugs which depress bone marrow, or (3) have a history of treatment with such drugs or radiation. Frequent monitoring of hepatic function and of the hematopoietic system is indicated during therapy.

PRECAUTIONS

GENERAL

Before therapy with flucytosine is instituted, electrolytes (because of hypokalemia) and the hematologic and renal status of the patient should be determined (see WARNINGS). Close monitoring of the patient during therapy is essential.

LABORATORY TESTS

Since renal impairment can cause progressive accumulation of the drug, blood concentrations and kidney function should be monitored during therapy. Hematologic status (leucocyte and thrombocyte count) and liver function (alkaline phosphatase, SGOT and SGPT) should be determined at frequent intervals during treatment as indicated.

DRUG/LABORATORY TEST INTERACTIONS

Measurement of serum creatinine levels should be determined by the Jaffe method, since flucytosine does not interfere with the determination of creatinine values by this method, as it does when the dry-slide enzymatic method with the Kodak Ektachem analyzer is used.

CARCINOGENESIS, MUTAGENESIS, AND IMPAIRMENT OF FERTILITY

Flucytosine has not undergone adequate animal testing to evaluate carcinogenic potential. The mutagenic potential of flucytosine was evaluated in Ames-type studies with five different mutants of *S. typhimurium* and no mutagenicity was detected in the presence or absence of activating enzymes. Flucytosine was nonmutagenic in three different repair assay systems.

There have been no adequate trials in animals on the effects of flucytosine on fertility or reproductive performance. The fertility and reproductive performance of the offspring (F_1 generation) of mice treated with 100, 200, or 400 mg/kg/day of flucytosine on days 7-13 of gestation was studied; the *in utero* treatment had no adverse effect on the fertility or reproductive performance of the offspring.

PREGNANCY, TERATOGENIC EFFECTS, PREGNANCY CATEGORY C

Flucytosine has been shown to be teratogenic in the rat and mouse at doses of 40 mg/kg/day (*i.e.,* 0.27 times the maximum recommended human dose). There are no adequate and well-controlled studies in pregnant women. Flucytosine should be used during pregnancy only if the potential benefit justifies the potential risk to the fetus.

The teratogenicity of flucytosine is apparently species-related. Although there is confirmation of rat teratogenicity in the published literature, three studies in the mouse and studies in the rabbit and monkey have failed to reveal a teratogenic liability.

NURSING MOTHERS

It is not known whether this drug is excreted in human milk. Because many drugs are excreted in human milk and because of the potential for serious adverse reactions in nursing infants from flucytosine, a decision should be made whether to discontinue nursing or to discontinue the drug, taking into account the importance of the drug to the mother.

PEDIATRIC USE

Safety and effectiveness in children have not been established.

DRUG INTERACTIONS

Cytosine arabinoside, a cytostatic agent, has been reported to inactivate the antifungal activity of flucytosine by competitive inhibition. Drugs which impair glomerular filtration may prolong the biological half-life of flucytosine. Antifungal synergism between flucytosine and polyene antibiotics, particularly amphotericin B, has been reported.

ADVERSE REACTIONS

The adverse reactions which have occurred during treatment with flucytosine are grouped according to organ system affected.

Cardiovascular: Cardiac arrest.

Respiratory: Respiratory arrest, chest pain, dyspnea.

Dermatologic: Rash, pruritus, urticaria, photosensitivity.

Gastrointestinal: Nausea, emesis, abdominal pain, diarrhea, anorexia, dry mouth, duodenal ulcer, gastrointestinal hemorrhage, hepatic dysfunction, jaundice, ulcerative colitis, bilirubin elevation.

Genitourinary: Azotemia, creatinine and BUN elevation, crystalluria, renal failure.

Hematologic: Anemia, agranulocytosis, aplastic anemia, eosinophilia, leukopenia, pancytopenia, thrombocytopenia.

Neurologic: Ataxia, hearing loss, headache, paresthesia, parkinsonism, peripheral neuropathy, pyrexia, vertigo, sedation.

Psychiatric: Confusion, hallucinations, psychosis.

Miscellaneous: Fatigue, hypoglycemia, hypokalemia, weakness.

DOSAGE AND ADMINISTRATION

The usual dosage of flucytosine is 50-150 mg/kg/day administered in divided doses at 6 hour intervals. Nausea or vomiting may be reduced or avoided if the capsules are given a few at a time over a 15 minute period. If the BUN or the serum creatinine is elevated, or if there are other signs of renal impairment, the initial dose should be at the lower level (see WARNINGS).

F

PRODUCT LISTING - RATED THERAPEUTICALLY EQUIVALENT

Capsule - Oral - 250 mg
100's $403.69 ANCOBON, Icn Pharmaceuticals Inc 00187-3554-10
Capsule - Oral - 500 mg
100's $803.05 ANCOBON, Icn Pharmaceuticals Inc 00187-3555-10

Fludarabine Phosphate *(003047)*

Categories: Leukemia, chronic lymphocytic; Pregnancy Category D; FDA Approved 1991 Apr; Orphan Drugs
Drug Classes: Antineoplastics, antimetabolites
Brand Names: Fludara
Foreign Brand Availability: Beneflur (Spain)
HCFA JCODE(S): J9185 50 mg IV

WARNING

FOR INJECTION.

FOR INTRAVENOUS USE ONLY.

Fludarabine phosphate for injection should be administered under the supervision of a qualified physician experienced in the use of antineoplastic therapy. Fludarabine phosphate for injection can severely suppress bone marrow function. When used at high doses in dose-ranging studies in patients with acute leukemia, fludarabine phosphate for injection was associated with severe neurologic effects, including blindness, coma, and death. This severe central nervous system toxicity occurred in 36% of patients treated with doses approximately four times greater (96 mg/m²/day for 5-7 days) than the recommended dose. Similar severe central nervous system toxicity has been rarely (≤0.2%) reported in patients treated at doses in the range of the dose recommended for chronic lymphocytic leukemia.

Instances of life-threatening and sometimes fatal autoimmune hemolytic anemia have been reported to occur after one or more cycles of treatment with fludarabine phosphate for injection. Patients undergoing treatment with fludarabine phosphate for injection should be evaluated and closely monitored for hemolysis.

In a clinical investigation using fludarabine phosphate for injection in combination with pentostatin (deoxycoformycin) for the treatment of refractory chronic lymphocytic leukemia (CLL), there was an unacceptably high incidence of fatal pulmonary toxicity. Therefore, the use of fludarabine phosphate for injection in combination with pentostatin is not recommended.

DESCRIPTION

Fludara for injection contains fludarabine phosphate, a fluorinated nucleotide analog of the antiviral agent vidarabine, 9-β-D-arabinofuranosyladenine (ara-A) that is relatively resistant to deamination by adenosine deaminase. Each vial of sterile lyophilized solid cake contains 50 mg of the active ingredient fludarabine phosphate, 50 mg of mannitol, and sodium hydroxide to adjust pH to 7.7. The pH range for the final product is 7.2-8.2. Reconstitution with 2 ml of sterile water for injection results in a solution containing 25 mg/ml of fludarabine phosphate intended for intravenous administration.

The chemical name for fludarabine phosphate is 9*H*-Purin-6-amine, 2-fluoro-9-(5-*O*-phosphono-β-D-arabinofuranosyl) (2-fluoro-ara-AMP).

The molecular formula of fludarabine phosphate is $C_{10}H_{13}FN_5O_7P$. The molecular weight is 365.2.

CLINICAL PHARMACOLOGY

Fludarabine phosphate is rapidly dephosphorylated to 2-fluoro-ara-A and then phosphorylated intracellularly by deoxycytidine kinase to the active triphosphate, 2-fluoro-ara-ATP. This metabolite appears to act by inhibiting DNA polymerase alpha, ribonucleotide reductase and DNA primase, thus inhibiting DNA synthesis. The mechanism of action of this antimetabolite is not completely characterized and may be multi-faceted.

Phase 1 studies in humans have demonstrated that fludarabine phosphate is rapidly converted to the active metabolite, 2-fluoro-ara-A, within minutes after intravenous infusion. Consequently, clinical pharmacology studies have focused on 2-fluoro-ara-A pharmacokinetics. After the five daily doses of 25 mg 2-fluoro-ara-AMP/m² to cancer patients infused over 30 minutes, 2-fluoro-ara-A concentrations show a moderate accumulation. During a 5 day treatment schedule, 2-fluoro-ara-A plasma trough levels increased by a factor of about 2. The terminal half-life of 2-fluoro-ara-A was estimated as approximately 20 hours. *In vitro,* plasma protein binding of fludarabine ranged between 19 and 29%.

A correlation was noted between the degree of absolute granulocyte count nadir and increased area under the concentration × time curve (AUC).

SPECIAL POPULATIONS

Patients With Renal Impairment

The total body clearance of the principal metabolite 2-fluoro-ara-A correlated with the creatinine clearance, indicating the importance of the renal excretion pathway for the elimination of the drug. Renal clearance represents approximately 40% of the total body clearance. Patients with moderate renal impairment (17-41 ml/min/m²) receiving 20% reduced fludarabine phosphate dose had a similar exposure (AUC; 21 versus 20 nM·h/ml) compared to patients with normal renal function receiving recommended dose. The mean total body clearance was 172 ml/min for normal and 124 ml/min for patients with moderately impaired renal function.

INDICATIONS AND USAGE

Fludarabine phosphate for injection is indicated for the treatment of patients with B-cell chronic lymphocytic leukemia (CLL) who have not responded to or whose disease has progressed during treatment with at least one standard alkylating-agent containing regimen. The safety and effectiveness of fludarabine phosphate for injection in previously untreated or non-refractory patients with CLL have not been established.

NON-FDA APPROVED INDICATIONS

Fludarabine has been used without approval for the treatment of non-Hodgkin's lymphoma, Waldenstrom's macroglobulinemia, prolymphocytic leukemia or prolymphocytoid variant of CLL, mycosis fungoides, hairy cell leukemia, some types of acute leukemia, and Hodgkin's disease.

CONTRAINDICATIONS

Fludarabine phosphate for injection is contraindicated in those patients who are hypersensitive to this drug or its components.

WARNINGS

See BOXED WARNING.

There are clear dose dependent toxic effects seen with fludarabine phosphate for injection. Dose levels approximately 4 times greater (96 mg/m²/day for 5-7 days) than that recommended for CLL (25 mg/m²/day for 5 days) were associated with a syndrome characterized by delayed blindness, coma and death. Symptoms appeared from 21-60 days following the last dose. Thirteen (13) of 36 patients (36%) who received fludarabine phosphate for injection at high doses (96 mg/m²/day for 5-7 days) developed this severe neurotoxicity. This syndrome has been reported rarely in patients treated with doses in the range of the recommended CLL dose of 25 mg/m²/day for 5 days every 28 days. The effect of chronic administration of fludarabine phosphate for injection on the central nervous system is unknown, however, patients have received the recommended dose for up to 15 courses of therapy.

Severe bone marrow suppression, notably anemia, thrombocytopenia and neutropenia, has been reported in patients treated with fludarabine phosphate for injection. In a Phase I study in solid tumor patients, the median time to nadir counts was 13 days (range, 3-25 days) for granulocytes and 16 days (range, 2-32) for platelets. Most patients had hematologic impairment at baseline either as a result of disease or as a result of prior myelosuppressive therapy. Cumulative myelosuppression may be seen. While chemotherapy-induced myelosuppression is often reversible, administration of fludarabine phosphate for injection requires careful hematologic monitoring.

Several instances of trilineage bone marrow hypoplasia or aplasia resulting in pancytopenia, sometimes resulting in death, have been reported. The duration of clinically significant cytopenia in the reported cases has ranged from approximately 2 months to approximately 1 year. These episodes have occurred both in previously treated or untreated patients.

Instances of life-threatening and sometimes fatal autoimmune hemolytic anemia have been reported to occur after one or more cycles of treatment with fludarabine phosphate for injection in patients with or without a previous history of autoimmune hemolytic anemia or a positive Coombs' test and who may or may not be in remission for their disease. Steroids may or may not be effective in controlling these hemolytic episodes. The majority of patients rechallenged with fludarabine phosphate for injection developed a recurrence in the hemolytic process. The mechanism(s) which predispose patients to the development of this complication has not been identified. Patients undergoing treatment with fludarabine phosphate for injection should be evaluated and closely monitored for hemolysis.

Transfusion-associated graft-versus-host disease has been observed rarely after transfusion of non-irradiated blood in fludarabine phosphate for injection treated patients. Consideration should, therefore, be given to the use of irradiated blood products in those patients requiring transfusions while undergoing treatment with fludarabine phosphatefor injection.

In a clinical investigation using fludarabine phosphate for injection in combination with pentostatin (deoxycoformycin) for the treatment of refractory chronic lymphocytic leukemia (CLL), there was an unacceptably high incidence of fatal pulmonary toxicity. Therefore, the use of fludarabine phosphate for injection in combination with pentostatin is not recommended.

Of the 133 CLL patients in the two trials, there were 29 fatalities during study. Approximately 50% of the fatalities were due to infection and 25% due to progressive disease.

PREGNANCY CATEGORY D

Fludarabine phosphate for injection may cause fetal harm when administered to a pregnant woman. Fludarabine phosphate was teratogenic in rats and in rabbits. Fludarabine phosphate was administered intravenously at doses of 0, 1, 10 or 30 mg/kg/day to pregnant rats on days 6-15 of gestation. At 10 and 30 mg/kg/day in rats, there was an increased incidence of various skeletal malformations. Fludarabine phosphate was administered intravenously at doses of 0, 1, 5 or 8 mg/kg/day to pregnant rabbits on days 6-15 of gestation. Dose-related teratogenic effects manifested by external deformities and skeletal malformations were observed in the rabbits at 5 and 8 mg/kg/day. Drug-related deaths or toxic effects on maternal and fetal weights were not observed. There are no adequate and well-controlled studies in pregnant women.

If fludarabine phosphate for injection is used during pregnancy, or if the patient becomes pregnant while taking this drug, the patient should be apprised of the potential hazard to the fetus. Women of childbearing potential should be advised to avoid becoming pregnant.

PRECAUTIONS

GENERAL

Fludarabine phosphate for injection is a potent antineoplastic agent with potentially significant toxic side effects. Patients undergoing therapy should be closely observed for signs of hematologic and nonhematologic toxicity. Periodic assessment of peripheral blood counts is recommended to detect the development of anemia, neutropenia and thrombocytopenia.

Tumor lysis syndrome associated with fludarabine phosphate for injection treatment has been reported in CLL patients with large tumor burdens. Since fludarabine phosphate for injection can induce a response as early as the first week of treatment, precautions should be taken in those patients at risk of developing this complication.

There are inadequate data on dosing of patients with renal insufficiency. Fludarabine phosphate for injection must be administered cautiously in patients with renal insufficiency. The total body clearance of 2-fluoro-ara-A has been shown to be directly correlated with creatinine clearance. Patients with moderate impairment of renal function (creatinine clearance 30-70 ml/min/1.73 m^2) should have fludarabine phosphate dose reduced by 20% and be monitored closely. Fludarabine phosphate is not recommended for patients with severely impaired renal function (creatinine clearance less than 30 ml/min/1.73 m^2).

LABORATORY TESTS

During treatment, the patient's hematologic profile (particularly neutrophils and platelets) should be monitored regularly to determine the degree of hematopoietic suppression.

CARCINOGENESIS

No animal carcinogenicity studies with fludarabine phosphate for injection have been conducted.

MUTAGENESIS

Fludarabine phosphate was not mutagenic to bacteria (Ames test) or mammalian cells (HGRPT assay in Chinese hamster ovary cells) either in the presence or absence of metabolic activation. Fludarabine phosphate was clostogenic *in vitro* to Chinese hamster ovary cells (chromosome aberrations in the presence of metabolic activation) and induced sister chromatid exchanges both with and without metabolic activation. In addition, fludarabine phosphate was clastogenic *in vivo* (mouse micronucleus assay) but was not mutagenic to germ cells (dominant lethal test in male mice).

IMPAIRMENT OF FERTILITY

Studies in mice, rats and dogs have demonstrated dose-related adverse effects on the male reproductive system. Observations consisted of a decrease in mean testicular weights in mice and rats with a trend toward decreased testicular weights in dogs and degeneration and necrosis of spermatogenic epithelium of the testes in mice, rats and dogs. The possible adverse effects on fertility in humans have not been adequately evaluated.

PREGNANCY CATEGORY D

See WARNINGS.

NURSING MOTHERS

It is not known whether this drug is excreted in human milk. Because many drugs are excreted in human milk and because of the potential for serious adverse reactions in nursing infants from fludarabine phosphate for injection, a decision should be made to discontinue nursing or discontinue the drug, taking into account the importance of the drug for the mother.

PEDIATRIC USE

The safety and effectiveness of fludarabine phosphate for injection in children have not been established.

DRUG INTERACTIONS

The use of fludarabine phosphate for injection in combination with pentostatin is not recommended due to the risk of severe pulmonary toxicity (see WARNINGS).

ADVERSE REACTIONS

The most common adverse events include myelosuppression (neutropenia, thrombocytopenia and anemia), fever and chills, infection, and nausea and vomiting. Other commonly reported events include malaise, fatigue, anorexia, and weakness. Serious opportunistic infections have occurred in CLL patients treated with fludarabine phosphate. The most frequently reported adverse events and those reactions which are more clearly related to the drug are arranged below according to body system.

Hematopoietic Systems: Hematologic events (neutropenia, thrombocytopenia, and/or anemia) were reported in the majority of CLL patients treated with fludarabine phosphate for injection. During fludarabine phosphate for injection treatment of 133 patients with CLL, the absolute neutrophil count decreased to less than 500/mm^3 in 59% of patients, hemoglobin decreased from pretreatment values by at least 2 g percent in 60%, and platelet count decreased from pretreatment values by at least 50% in 55%. Myelosuppression may be severe, cumulative, and may affect multiple cell lines. Bone marrow fibrosis occurred in 1 CLL patient treated with fludarabine phosphate for injection.

Several instances of trilineage bone marrow hypoplasia or aplasia resulting in pancytopenia, sometimes resulting in death, have been reported in postmarketing surveillance. The duration of clinically significant cytopenia in the reported cases has ranged from approximately 2 months to approximately 1 year. These episodes have occurred both in previously treated or untreated patients.

Life-threatening and sometimes fatal autoimmune hemolytic anemia have been reported to occur in patients receiving fludarabine phosphate for injection (see WARNINGS). The majority of patients rechallenged with fludarabine phosphate for injection developed a recurrence in the hemolytic process.

Metabolic: Tumor lysis syndrome has been reported in CLL patients treated with fludarabine phosphate for injection. This complication may include hyperuricemia, hyperphosphatemia, hypocalcemia, metabolic acidosis, hyperkalemia, hematuria, urate crystalluria, and renal failure. The onset of this syndrome may be heralded by flank pain and hematuria.

Nervous System: See WARNINGS. Objective weakness, agitation, confusion, visual disturbances, and coma have occurred in CLL patients treated with fludarabine phosphate for injection at the recommended dose. Peripheral neuropathy has been observed in patients treated with fludarabine phosphate for injection and one case of wrist-drop was reported.

Pulmonary System: Pneumonia, a frequent manifestation of infection in CLL patients, occurred in 16%, and 22% of those treated with fludarabine phosphate for injection in the MDAH and SWOG studies, respectively. Pulmonary hypersensitivity reactions to fludarabine phosphate for injection characterized by dyspnea, cough and interstitial pulmonary infiltrate have been observed.

In post-marketing experience, cases of severe pulmonary toxicity have been observed with fludarabine phosphate use which resulted in ARDS, respiratory distress, pulmonary hemorrhage, pulmonary fibrosis, and respiratory failure. After an infectious origin has been excluded, some patients experienced symptom improvement with corticosteroids.

Gastrointestinal System: Gastrointestinal disturbances such as nausea and vomiting, anorexia, diarrhea, stomatitis and gastrointestinal bleeding have been reported in patients treated with fludarabine phosphate for injection.

Cardiovascular: Edema has been frequently reported. One patient developed a pericardial effusion possibly related to treatment with fludarabine phosphate. No other severe cardiovascular events were considered to be drug related.

Genitourinary System: Rare cases of hemorrhagic cystitis have been reported in patients treated with fludarabine phosphate for injection.

Skin: Skin toxicity, consisting primarily of skin rashes, has been reported in patients treated with fludarabine phosphate for injection.

Data in TABLE 1 are derived from the 133 patients with CLL who received fludarabine phosphate for injection in the MDAH and SWOG studies.

More than 3000 patients received fludarabine phosphate for injection in studies of other leukemias, lymphomas, and other solid tumors. The spectrum of adverse effects reported in these studies was consistent with the data presented in TABLE 1.

DOSAGE AND ADMINISTRATION

USUAL DOSE

The recommended dose of fludarabine phosphate for injection is 25 mg/m^2 administered intravenously over a period of approximately 30 minutes daily for 5 consecutive days. Each 5 day course of treatment should commence every 28 days. Dosage may be decreased or delayed based on evidence of hematologic or nonhematologic toxicity. Physicians should consider delaying or discontinuing the drug if neurotoxicity occurs.

A number of clinical settings may predispose to increased toxicity from fludarabine phosphate for injection. These include advanced age, renal insufficiency, and bone marrow impairment. Such patients should be monitored closely for excessive toxicity and the dose modified accordingly.

The optimal duration of treatment has not been clearly established. It is recommended that three additional cycles of fludarabine phosphate for injection be administered following the achievement of a maximal response and then the drug should be discontinued.

RENAL INSUFFICIENCY

Patients with moderate impairment of renal function (creatinine clearance 30-70 ml/min/1.73 m^2) should have a 20% dose reduction of fludarabine phosphate for injection. Fludarabine phosphate for injection should not be administered to patients with severely impaired renal function (creatinine clearance less than 30 ml/min/1.73 m^2).

PREPARATION OF SOLUTIONS

Fludarabine phosphate for injection should be prepared for parenteral use by aseptically adding sterile water for injection. When reconstituted with 2 ml of sterile water for injection, the solid cake should fully dissolve in 15 seconds or less; each ml of the resulting solution will contain 25 mg of fludarabine phosphate, 25 mg of mannitol, and sodium hydroxide to adjust the pH to 7.7. The pH range for the final product is 7.2-8.2. In clinical studies, the product has been diluted to 100 or 125 cc of 5% dextrose injection or 0.9% sodium chloride.

Reconstituted fludarabine phosphate for injection contains no antimicrobial preservative and thus should be used within 8 hours of reconstitution. Care must be taken to assure the sterility of prepared solutions. Parenteral drug products should be inspected visually for particulate matter and discoloration prior to administration.

HANDLING AND DISPOSAL

Procedures for proper handling and disposal should be considered. Consideration should be given to handling and disposal according to guidelines issued for cytotoxic drugs. Several guidelines on this subject have been published.[2-9] There is no general agreement that all of the procedures recommended in the guidelines are necessary or appropriate.

Caution should be exercised in the handling and preparation of fludarabine phosphate for injection solution. The use of latex gloves and safety glasses is recommended to avoid exposure in case of breakage of the vial or other accidental spillage. If the solution contacts the skin or mucous membranes, wash thoroughly with soap and water; rinse eyes thoroughly with plain water. Avoid exposure by inhalation or by direct contact of the skin or mucous membranes.

TABLE 1 *Percent of CLL Patients Reporting Non-Hematologic Adverse Events*

Adverse Events	MDAH (n=101)	SWOG (n=32)
Any Adverse Event	88%	91%
Body as a Whole	72%	84%
Fever	60%	69%
Chills	11%	19%
Fatigue	10%	38%
Infection	33%	44%
Pain	20%	22%
Malaise	8%	6%
Diaphoresis	1%	13%
Alopecia	0%	3%
Anaphylaxis	1%	0%
Hemorrhage	1%	0%
Hyperglycemia	1%	6%
Dehydration	1%	0%
Neurological	21%	69%
Weakness	9%	65%
Paresthesia	4%	12%
Headache	3%	0%
Visual disturbance	3%	15%
Hearing loss	2%	6%
Sleep disorder	1%	3%
Depression	1%	0%
Cerebellar syndrome	1%	0%
Impaired mentation	1%	0%
Pulmonary	35%	69%
Cough	10%	44%
Pneumonia	16%	22%
Dyspnea	9%	22%
Sinusitis	5%	0%
Pharyngitis	0%	9%
Upper respiratory infection	2%	16%
Allergic pneumonitis	0%	6%
Epistaxis	1%	0%
Hemoptysis	1%	6%
Bronchitis	1%	0%
Hypoxia	1%	0%
Gastrointestinal	46%	63%
Nausea/vomiting	36%	31%
Diarrhea	15%	13%
Anorexia	7%	34%
Stomatitis	9%	0%
GI bleeding	3%	13%
Esophagitis	3%	0%
Mucositis	2%	0%
Liver failure	1%	0%
Abnormal liver function test	1%	3%
Cholelithiasis	0%	3%
Constipation	1%	3%
Dysphagia	1%	0%
Cutaneous	17%	18%
Rash	15%	15%
Pruritus	1%	3%
Seborrhea	1%	0%
Genitourinary	12%	22%
Dysuria	4%	3%
Urinary infection	2%	15%
Hematuria	2%	3%
Renal failure	1%	0%
Abnormal renal function test	1%	0%
Proteinuria	1%	0%
Hesitancy	0%	3%
Cardiovascular	12%	38%
Edema	8%	19%
Angina	0%	6%
Congestive heart failure	0%	3%
Arrhythmia	0%	3%
Supraventricular tachycardia	0%	3%
Myocardial infarction	0%	3%
Deep venous thrombosis	1%	3%
Phlebitis	1%	3%
Transient ischemic attack	1%	0%
Aneurysm	1%	0%
Cerebrovascular accident	0%	3%
Musculoskeletal	7%	16%
Myalgia	4%	16%
Osteoporosis	2%	0%
Arthralgia	1%	0%
Tumor Lysis Syndrome	1%	0%

HOW SUPPLIED

FLUDARA FOR INJECTION

Fludara for injection is supplied as a white, lyophilized solid cake. Each vial contains 50 mg of fludarabine phosphate, 50 mg of mannitol and sodium hydroxide to adjust pH to 7.7. The pH range for the final product is 7.2-8.2.

Storage: Store under refrigeration, between 2-8°C (36-46°F).

PRODUCT LISTING - EQUIVALENTS NOT AVAILABLE

Powder For Injection - Intravenous - 50 mg

1's $374.81 FLUDARA, Berlex Laboratories 50419-0511-06

Fludrocortisone Acetate (001303)

Categories: Addison's disease; Pregnancy Category C; FDA Approved 1955 Aug; WHO Formulary
Drug Classes: Corticosteroids
Brand Names: **Florinef**
Foreign Brand Availability: Astonin (Spain); Astonin H (Austria; Czech-Republic; Germany; Hungary)
Cost of Therapy: $26.48 (Addison's Disease; Florinef; 0.1 mg; 1 tablet/day; 30 day supply)
$22.43 (Addison's Disease; Generic Tablets; 0.1 mg; 1 tablet/day; 30 day supply)

DESCRIPTION

Fludrocortisone acetate is a synthetic adrenocortical steroid possessing very potent mineralocorticoid properties and high glucocorticoid activity; it is used only for its mineralocorticoid effects. The chemical name for fludrocortisone acetate is 9-fluoro-11β,17,21-trihydroxypregn-4-ene-3,20-dione 21-acetate.

The molecular formula is $C_{23}H_{31}FO_6$, and the molecular weight is 422.49.

Florinef Acetate is available for oral administration as scored tablets providing 0.1 mg fludrocortisone acetate per tablet. *Inactive Ingredients:* Calcium phosphate, color additive (D&C red no. 27), corn starch, lactose, magnesium stearate, sodium benzoate, and talc.

Storage: Store at room temperature; avoid excessive heat.

CLINICAL PHARMACOLOGY

Corticosteroids are thought to act, at least in part, by controlling the rate of synthesis of proteins. Although there are a number of instances in which the synthesis of specific proteins is known to be induced by corticosteroids, the links between the initial actions of the hormones and final metabolic effects have not been completely elucidated.

The physiologic action of fludrocortisone acetate is similar to that of hydrocortisone. However, the effects of fludrocortisone acetate, particularly on electrolyte balance, but also on carbohydrate metabolism, are considerably heightened and prolonged. Mineralocorticoids act on the distal tubules of the kidney to enhance the reabsorption of sodium ions from the tubular fluid into the plasma; they increase the urinary excretion of both potassium and hydrogen ions. The consequence of these three primary effects together with similar actions on cation transport in other tissues appear to account for the entire spectrum of physiological activities that are characteristic of mineralocorticoids. In small oral doses, fludrocortisone acetate produces marked sodium retention and increased urinary potassium excretion. It also causes a rise in blood pressure, apparently because of these effects on electrolyte levels.

In larger doses, fludrocortisone acetate inhibits endogenous adrenal cortical secretion, thymic activity, and pituitary corticotropin excretion; promotes the deposition of liver glycogen; and, unless protein intake is adequate, induces negative nitrogen balance.

The approximate plasma half-life of fludrocortisone (fluorohydrocortisone) is 3.5 hours or more and the biological half-life is 18-36 hours.

INDICATIONS AND USAGE

Fludrocortisone acetate is indicated as partial replacement therapy for primary and secondary adrenocortical insufficiency in Addison's disease and for the treatment of salt-losing adrenogenital syndrome.

NON-FDA APPROVED INDICATIONS

Although not FDA approved, fludrocortisone has been used as a diagnostic aid for and treatment of Type IV renal tubular acidosis and in conjunction with increased sodium intake as treatment of idiopathic orthostatic hypotension.

CONTRAINDICATIONS

Corticosteroids are contraindicated in patients with systemic fungal infections and in those with a history of possible or known hypersensitivity to these agents.

WARNINGS

BECAUSE OF ITS MARKED EFFECT ON SODIUM RETENTION, THE USE OF FLUDROCORTISONE ACETATE IN THE TREATMENT OF CONDITIONS OTHER THAN THOSE INDICATED HEREIN IS NOT ADVISED.

Corticosteroids may mask some signs of infection, and new infections may appear during their use. There may be decreased resistance and inability to localize infection when corticosteroids are used. If an infection occurs during fludrocortisone acetate therapy, it should be promptly controlled by suitable antimicrobial therapy.

Prolonged use of corticosteroids may produce posterior subcapsular cataracts, glaucoma with possible damage to the optic nerves, and may enhance the establishment of secondary ocular infections due to fungi or viruses.

Average and large doses of hydrocortisone or cortisone can cause elevation of blood pressure, salt and water retention, and increased excretion of potassium. These effects are less likely to occur with the synthetic derivatives except when used in large doses. However, since fludrocortisone acetate is a potent mineralocorticoid, both the dosage and salt intake should be carefully monitored in order to avoid the development of hypertension, edema, or weight gain. **Periodic checking of serum electrolyte levels is advisable during prolonged therapy; dietary salt restriction and potassium supplementation may be necessary.** All corticosteroids increase calcium excretion.

Patients should not be vaccinated against smallpox while on corticosteroid therapy. Other immunization procedures should not be undertaken in patients who are on corticosteroids, especially on high dose, because of possible hazards of neurological complications and a lack of antibody response.

The use of fludrocortisone acetate tablets in active tuberculosis should be restricted to those cases of fulminating or disseminated tuberculosis in which the corticosteroid is used for the management of the disease in conjunction with an appropriate antituberculous regimen. If corticosteroids are indicated in patients with latent tuberculosis or tuberculin reactivity, close observation is necessary since reactivation of the disease may occur. During prolonged corticosteroid therapy these patients should receive chemoprophylaxis.

Children who are on immunosuppressant drugs are more susceptible to infections than healthy children. Chicken pox and measles, for example, can have a more serious or even fatal course in children on immunosuppressant corticosteroids. In such children, or in adults who have not had these diseases, particular care should be taken to avoid exposure. If exposed, therapy with varicella zoster immune globulin (VZIG) or pooled intravenous immunoglobulin (IVIG), as appropriate, may be indicated. If chicken pox develops, treatment with antiviral agents may be considered.

PRECAUTIONS

GENERAL

Adverse reactions to corticosteroids may be produced by too rapid withdrawal or by continued use of large doses.

To avoid drug-induced adrenal insufficiency, supportive dosage may be required in times of stress (such as trauma, surgery, or severe illness) both during treatment with fludrocortisone acetate and for a year afterwards.

There is an enhanced corticosteroid effect in patients with hypothyroidism and in those with cirrhosis.

Corticosteroids should be used cautiously in patients with ocular herpes simplex because of possible corneal perforation.

The lowest possible dose of corticosteroid should be used to control the condition being treated. A gradual reduction in dosage should be made when possible.

Psychic derangements may appear when corticosteroids are used. These may range from euphoria, insomnia, mood swings, personality changes, and severe depression to frank psychotic manifestations. Existing emotional instability or psychotic tendencies may also be aggravated by corticosteroids.

Aspirin should be used cautiously in conjunction with corticosteroids in patients with hypoprothrombinemia.

Corticosteroids should be used with caution in patients with nonspecific ulcerative colitis if there is a probability of impending perforation, abscess or other pyrogenic infection. Corticosteroids should also be used cautiously in patients with diverticulitis, fresh intestinal anastomoses, active or latent peptic ulcer, renal insufficiency, hypertension, osteoporosis, and myasthenia gravis.

INFORMATION FOR THE PATIENT

The physician should advise the patient to report any medical history of heart disease, high blood pressure, or kidney or liver disease and to report current use of any medicines to determine if these medicines might interact adversely with fludrocortisone acetate (see DRUG INTERACTIONS).

Patients who are on immunosuppressant doses of corticosteroids should be warned to avoid exposure to chicken pox or measles, and, if exposed, to obtain medical advice.

The patient's understanding of his steroid-dependent status and increased dosage requirement under widely variable conditions of stress is vital. Advise the patient to carry medical identification indicating his dependence on steroid medication and, if necessary, instruct him to carry an adequate supply of medication for use in emergencies.

Stress to the patient the importance of regular follow-up visits to check his progress and the need to promptly notify the physician of dizziness, severe or continuing headaches, swelling of feet or lower legs, or unusual weight gain.

Advise the patient to use the medicine only as directed, to take a missed dose as soon as possible, unless it is almost time for the next dose, and not to double the next dose.

Inform the patient to keep this medication and all drugs out of the reach of children.

LABORATORY TESTS

Patients should be monitored regularly for blood pressure determinations and serum electrolyte determinations (see WARNINGS).

DRUG/LABORATORY TEST INTERACTIONS

Corticosteroids may affect the nitrobluetetrazolium test for bacterial infection and produce false-negative results.

CARCINOGENESIS, MUTAGENESIS, AND IMPAIRMENT OF FERTILITY

Adequate studies have not been performed in animals to determine whether fludrocortisone acetate has carcinogenic or mutagenic activity or whether it affects fertility in males or females.

PREGNANCY CATEGORY C

Adequate animal reproduction studies have not been conducted with fludrocortisone acetate. However, many corticosteroids have been shown to be teratogenic in laboratory animals at low doses. Teratogenicity of these agents in man has not been demonstrated. It is not known whether fludrocortisone acetate can cause fetal harm when administered to a pregnant woman or can affect reproduction capacity. Fludrocortisone acetate should be given to a pregnant woman only if clearly needed.

Nonteratogenic Effects

Infants born of mothers who have received substantial doses of fludrocortisone acetate during pregnancy should be carefully observed for signs of hypoadrenalism.

Maternal treatment with corticosteroids should be carefully documented in the infant's medical records to assist in follow up.

NURSING MOTHERS

Corticosteroids are found in the breast milk of lactating women receiving systemic therapy with these agents. Caution should be exercised when fludrocortisone acetate is administered to a nursing woman.

PEDIATRIC USE

Safety and effectiveness in children have not been established.

Growth and development of infants and children on prolonged corticosteroid therapy should be carefully observed.

DRUG INTERACTIONS

When administered concurrently, the following drugs may interact with adrenal corticosteroids:

Amphotericin B or Potassium-Depleting Diuretics: (Benzothiadiazines and related drugs, ethacrynic acid and furosemide-enhanced hypokalemia. Check serum potassium levels at frequent intervals; use potassium supplements if necessary (see WARNINGS).

Digitalis Glycosides: Enhanced possibility of arrhythmias of digitalis toxicity associated with hypokalemia. Monitor serum potassium levels; use potassium supplements if necessary.

Oral Anticoagulants: Decreased prothrombin time response. Monitor prothrombin levels and adjust anticoagulant dosage accordingly.

Antidiabetic Drugs: (Oral agents and insulin) — diminished antidiabetic effect. Monitor for symptoms of hyperglycemia; adjust dosage of antidiabetic drug upward if necessary.

Aspirin: Increased ulcerogenic effect; decreased pharmacologic effect of aspirin. Rarely salicylate toxicity may occur in patients who discontinue steroids after concurrent high-dose aspirin therapy. Monitor salicylate levels or the therapeutic effect for which aspirin is given; adjust salicylate dosage accordingly if effect is altered (see PRECAUTIONS, General).

Barbiturates, Phenytoin, or Rifampin: Increased metabolic clearance of fludrocortisone acetate because of the induction of hepatic enzymes. Observe the patient for possible diminished effect of steroid and increase the steroid dosage accordingly.

Anabolic Steroids (Particularly C-17 alkylated androgens such as oxymetholone, methandrostenolone, norethandrolone, and similar compounds) — enhanced tendency toward edema. Use caution when giving these drugs together, especially in patients with hepatic or cardiac disease.

Vaccines: Neurological complications and lack of antibody response (see WARNINGS).

Estrogen: increased levels of corticosteroid-binding globulin, thereby increasing the bound (inactive) fraction; this effect is at least balanced by decreased metabolism of corticosteroids. When estrogen therapy is initiated, a reduction in corticosteroid dosage may be required, and increased amounts may be required when estrogen is terminated.

ADVERSE REACTIONS

Most adverse reactions are caused by the drug's mineralocorticoid activity (retention of sodium and water) and include hypertension, edema, cardiac enlargement, congestive heart failure, potassium loss, and hypokalemic alkalosis.

When fludrocortisone is used in the small dosages recommended, the glucocorticoid side effects often seen with cortisone and its derivatives are not usually a problem; however the following untoward effects should be kept in mind, particularly when fludrocortisone is used over a prolonged period of time or in conjunction with cortisone or a similar glucocorticoid.

Musculoskeletal: Muscle weakness, steroid myopathy, loss of muscle mass, osteoporosis, vertebral compression fractures, aseptic necrosis of femoral and humeral heads, pathologic fracture of long bones, and spontaneous fractures.

Gastrointestinal: Peptic ulcer with possible perforation and hemorrhage, pancreatitis, abdominal distention, and ulcerative esophagitis.

Dermatologic: Impaired wound healing, thin fragile skin, bruising, petechiae and ecchymoses, facial erythema, increased sweating, subcutaneous fat atrophy, purpura, striae, hyperpigmentation of the skin and nails, hirsutism, acneiform eruptions, and hives and/or allergic skin rash; reactions to skin tests may be suppressed.

Neurological: Convulsions, increased intracranial pressure with papilledema (pseudotumor cerebri) usually after treatment, vertigo, headache, and severe mental disturbances.

Endocrine: Menstrual irregularities; development of the cushingoid state; suppression of growth in children; secondary adrenocortical and pituitary unresponsiveness, particularly in times of stress (*e.g.*, trauma, surgery, or illness); decreased carbohydrate tolerance; manifestations of latent diabetes mellitus; and increased requirements for insulin or oral hypoglycemic agents in diabetics.

Ophthalmic: Posterior subcapsular cataracts, increased intraocular pressure, glaucoma, and exophthalmos.

Metabolic: Hyperglycemia, glycosuria, and negative nitrogen balance due to protein catabolism.

Other adverse reactions that may occur following the administration of a corticosteroid are necrotizing angitis, thrombophlebitis, aggravation or masking of infections, insomnia, syncopal episodes, and anaphylactoid reactions.

DOSAGE AND ADMINISTRATION

Dosage depends on the severity of the disease and the response of the patient. Patients should be continually monitored for signs that indicate dosage adjustment is necessary, such as remissions or exacerbations of the disease and stress (surgery, infection, trauma) (see WARNINGS and PRECAUTIONS, General).

ADDISON'S DISEASE

In Addison's disease, the combination of fludrocortisone acetate tablets with a glucocorticoid such as hydrocortisone or cortisone provides substitution therapy approximating normal adrenal activity with minimal risks of unwanted effects.

The usual dose is 0.1 mg of fludrocortisone acetate daily, although dosage ranging from 0.1 mg three times a week to 0.2 mg daily has been employed. In the event transient hypertension develops as a consequence of therapy, the dose should be reduced to 0.05 mg daily. Fludrocortisone acetate is preferably administered in conjunction with cortisone (10-37.5 mg daily in divided doses) or hydrocortisone (10-30 mg daily in divided doses).

SALT-LOSING ADRENOGENITAL SYNDROME

The recommended dosage for treating the salt-losing adrenogenital syndrome is 0.1-0.2 mg of fludrocortisone acetate daily.

PRODUCT LISTING - EQUIVALENTS NOT AVAILABLE

Tablet - Oral - 0.1 mg

30's	$21.35	FLORINEF ACETATE, Allscripts Pharmaceutical Company	54569-3170-00
100's	$74.77	GENERIC, Global Pharmaceutical Corporation	00115-7033-01
100's	$79.35	GENERIC, Barr Laboratories Inc	00555-0997-02
100's	$88.26	FLORINEF ACETATE, Bristol-Myers Squibb	00003-0429-50

Flumazenil *(003104)*

Categories: Antidote, benzodiazepine; Pregnancy Category C; FDA Approved 1991 Dec
Drug Classes: Antidotes
Brand Names: **Mazicon**; Romazicon
Foreign Brand Availability: Anexate (Australia; Austria; Bahrain; Belgium; Benin; Bulgaria; Burkina-Faso; Canada; China; Cyprus; Czech-Republic; Egypt; England; Ethiopia; France; Gambia; Germany; Ghana; Greece; Guinea; Hong-Kong; Hungary; Indonesia; Iran; Iraq; Ireland; Israel; Italy; Ivory-Coast; Japan; Jordan; Kenya; Korea; Kuwait; Lebanon; Liberia; Libya; Malawi; Malaysia; Mali; Mauritania; Mauritius; Morocco; Netherlands; New-Zealand; Niger; Nigeria; Norway; Oman; Portugal; Qatar; Republic-of-Yemen; Saudi-Arabia; Senegal; Seychelles; Sierra-Leone; South-Africa; Spain; Sudan; Switzerland; Syria; Taiwan; Tanzania; Thailand; Tunia; Turkey; Uganda; United-Arab-Emirates; Zambia; Zimbabwe); Lanexat (Bahamas; Barbados; Belize; Bermuda; Colombia; Curacao; Denmark; Finland; Guyana; Jamaica; Mexico; Netherland-Antilles; Peru; Puerto-Rico; Surinam; Sweden; Trinidad)

DESCRIPTION

Romazicon (flumazenil) is a benzodiazepine receptor antagonist. Chemically, flumazenil is ethyl 8-fluoro-5,6-dihydro- 5-methyl-6-oxo-4H-imidazo[1,5-a](1,4) benzodiazepine-3-carboxylate. Flumazenil has an imidazobenzodiazepine structure and a calculated molecular weight of 303.3.

Flumazenil is a white to off-white crystalline compound with an octanol:buffer partition coefficient of 14 to 1 at pH 7.4. It is insoluble in water but slightly soluble in acidic aqueous solutions. Flumazenil is available as a sterile parenteral dosage form for intravenous administration. Each ml contains 0.1 mg of flumazenil compounded with 1.8 mg of methylparaben, 0.2 mg of propylparaben, 0.9% sodium chloride, 0.01% edetate disodium, and 0.01% acetic acid; the pH is adjusted to approximately 4 with hydrochloric acid and/or, if necessary, sodium hydroxide.

Storage: Store at 59-86°F (15-30°C).

CLINICAL PHARMACOLOGY

Flumazenil, an imidazobenzodiazepine derivative, antagonizes the actions of benzodiazepines on the central nervous system. Flumazenil competitively inhibits the activity at the benzodiazepine recognition site on the GABA/benzodiazepine receptor complex. Flumazenil is a weak partial agonist in some animal models of activity, but has little or no agonist activity in man.

Flumazenil does not antagonize the central nervous system effects of drugs affecting GABA-ergic neurons by means other than the benzodiazepine receptor (including ethanol, barbiturates, or general anesthetics) and does not reverse the effects of opioids.

PHARMACODYNAMICS

Intravenous flumazenil has been shown to antagonize sedation, impairment of recall and psychomotor impairment produced by benzodiazepines in healthy human volunteers.

The duration and degree of reversal of benzodiazepine effects are related to the dose and plasma concentrations of flumazenil.

Generally, doses of approximately 0.1-0.2 mg (corresponding to peak plasma levels of 3-6 ng/ml) produce partial antagonism, whereas higher doses of 0.4-1.0 mg (peak plasma levels of 12-28 ng/ml) usually produce complete antagonism in patients who have received the usual sedating doses of benzodiazepines. The onset of reversal is usually evident within 1-2 minutes after the injection is completed. Eighty percent response will be reached within 3 minutes, with the peak effect occurring at 6-10 minutes. The duration and degree of reversal are related to the plasma concentration of the sedating benzodiazepine as well as the dose of flumazenil given.

In healthy volunteers, flumazenil did not alter intraocular pressure when given alone and reversed the decrease in intraocular pressure seen after administration of midazolam.

PHARMACOKINETICS

After IV administration, plasma concentrations of flumazenil follow a two compartment open pharmacokinetic model with an initial distribution half-life of 7-15 minutes and a terminal half-life of 41-79 minutes. Peak concentrations of flumazenil are proportional to dose, with an apparent initial volume of distribution of 0.5 L/kg. After redistribution the apparent volume of distribution (V_{ss}) ranges from 0.77-1.60 L/kg. Protein binding is approximately 50% and the drug shows no preferential partitioning into red blood cells.

Flumazenil is a highly extracted drug. Clearance of flumazenil occurs primarily by hepatic metabolism and is dependent on hepatic blood flow. In pharmacokinetic studies of normal volunteers, total clearance ranges from 0.7-1.3 L/h/kg, with less than 1% of the administered dose eliminated unchanged in the urine. The major metabolites of flumazenil identified in urine are the de-ethylated free acid and its glucuronide conjugate. In preclinical studies there was no evidence of pharmacologic activity exhibited by the de-ethylated free acid. Elimination of radiolabeled drug is essentially complete within 72 hours, with 90-95% of the radioactivity appearing in urine and 5-10% in the feces.

Pharmacokinetic Parameters Following a 5 minute infusion of a total of 1 mg of flumazenil Mean (Coefficient of variation, Range) (see TABLE 1).

The pharmacokinetics of flumazenil are not significantly affected by gender, age, renal failure (creatinine clearance <10 ml/min), or hemodialysis beginning 1 hour after drug administration. Mean total clearance is decreased to 40-60% of normal in patients with moderate liver dysfunction and to 25% of normal in patients with severe liver dysfunction compared with age-matched healthy subjects. This results in a prolongation of the half-life

TABLE 1

C_{max} (ng/ml)	24 (38%, 11-43)
AUC (ng · h/ml)	15 (22%, 10-22)
V_{ss} (L/kg)	1 (24%, 0.8-1.6)
Cl (L/h/kg)	1 (20%, 0.7-1.4)
Half-life (min)	54 (21%, 41-79)

from 0.8 hours in healthy subjects to 1.3 hours in patients with moderate hepatic impairment and 2.4 hours in severely impaired patients. Ingestion of food during an intravenous infusion of the drug results in a 50% increase in clearance, most likely due to the increased hepatic blood flow that accompanies a meal. The pharmacokinetic profile of flumazenil is unaltered in the presence of benzodiazepine agonists and the kinetic profiles of those benzodiazepines are unaltered by flumazenil.

INDIVIDUALIZATION OF DOSAGES

General Principles

The serious adverse effects of flumazenil are related to the reversal of benzodiazepine effects. Using more than the minimally effective dose of flumazenil is tolerated by most patients but may complicate the management of patients who are physically dependent on benzodiazepines or patients who are depending on benzodiazepines for therapeutic effect (such as suppression of seizures in cyclic antidepressant overdose).

In high-risk patients, it is important to administer the smallest amount of flumazenil that is effective. The 1 minute wait between individual doses in the dose-titration recommended for general clinical populations may be too short for high risk patients. This is because it takes 6-10 minutes for any single dose of flumazenil to reach full effects. Practitioners should slow the rate of administration of flumazenil administered to high risk patients as recommended below.

ANESTHESIA AND CONSCIOUS SEDATION

Flumazenil is well tolerated at the recommended doses in individuals who have no tolerance to (or dependence on) benzodiazepines. The recommended dosages and titration rates in anesthesia and conscious sedation (0.2 to 1 mg given at 0.2 mg/min) are well tolerated in patients receiving the drug for reversal of a single benzodiazepine exposure in most clinical settings (see ADVERSE REACTIONS). The major risk will be resedation because the duration of effect of a long-acting (or large dose of a short-acting) benzodiazepine may exceed that of flumazenil. Resedation may be treated by giving a repeat dose at no less than 20 minute intervals. For repeat treatment, no more than 1 mg (at 0.2 mg/min doses) should be given at any one time and no more than 3 mg should be given in any one hour.

OVERDOSE PATIENTS

The risk of confusion, agitation, emotional lability and perceptual distortion with the doses recommended in patients with benzodiazepine overdose (3-5 mg administered as 0.5 mg/min) may be greater than that expected with lower doses and slower administration. The recommended doses represent a compromise between a desirable slow awakening and the need for prompt response and a persistent effect in the overdose situation. If circumstances permit, the physician may elect to use the 0.2 mg/minute titration rate to slowly awaken the patient over 5-10 minutes, which may help to reduce signs and symptoms on emergence.

Flumazenil has no effect in cases where benzodiazepines are not responsible for sedation. Once doses of 3-5 mg have been reached without clinical response, additional flumazenil is likely to have no effect.

PATIENTS TOLERANT TO BENZODIAZEPINES

Flumazenil may cause benzodiazepine withdrawal symptoms in individuals who have been taking benzodiazepines long enough to have some degree of tolerance. Patients who had been taking benzodiazepines prior to entry into the flumazenil trials who were given flumazenil in doses over 1 mg experienced withdrawal-like events 2-5 times more frequently than patients who received less than 1 mg.

In patients who may have tolerance to benzodiazepines, as indicated by clinical history or by the need for larger than usual doses of benzodiazepine, slower titration rates of 0.1 mg/min and lower total doses may help reduce the frequency of emergent confusion and agitation. In such cases special care must be taken to monitor the patients for resedation because of the lower doses of flumazenil used.

PATIENTS PHYSICALLY DEPENDENT ON BENZODIAZEPINES

Flumazenil is known to precipitate withdrawal seizures in patients who are physically dependent on benzodiazepines, even if such dependence was established in a relatively few days of high dose sedation in Intensive Care Unit environments. The risk of either seizures or resedation in such cases is high and patients have experienced seizures before regaining consciousness. Flumazenil should be used in such settings with extreme caution, since the use of flumazenil in this situation has not been studied and no information as to dose and rate of titration is available. Flumazenil should be used in such patients only if the potential benefits of using the drug outweigh the risks of precipitated seizures. Physicians are directed to the scientific literature for the most current information in this area.

INDICATIONS AND USAGE

Flumazenil is indicated for the complete or partial reversal of the sedative effects of benzodiazepines in cases where general anesthesia has been induced and/or maintained with benzodiazepines, where sedation has been produced with benzodiazepines for diagnostic and therapeutic procedures, and for the management of benzodiazepine overdose.

NON-FDA APPROVED INDICATIONS

Flumazenil has been used anecdotally in the acute treatment of overdose from other drugs (like zolpidem, carbamazepine, choral hydrate and baclofen) some of whose pharmacologic effects may be, in part, mediated by benzodiazepine receptors. This use is not FDA approved. Additionally some investigators have suggested that flumazenil may be useful in the treatment of hepatic encephalopathy and in the diagnosis of coma of unknown etiology. These applications are currently controversial and are not approved by the FDA.

CONTRAINDICATIONS

Flumazenil is Contraindicated:

- In patients with a known hypersensitivity to flumazenil or to benzodiazepines.
- In patients who have been given a benzodiazepine for control of a potentially life-threatening condition (*e.g.,* control of intracranial pressure or status epilepticus).
- In patients who are showing signs of serious cyclic antidepressant overdose. (See WARNINGS.)

WARNINGS

THE USE OF FLUMAZENIL HAS BEEN ASSOCIATED WITH THE OCCURRENCE OF SEIZURES.

THESE ARE MOST FREQUENT IN PATIENTS WHO HAVE BEEN ON BENZODIAZEPINES FOR LONG-TERM SEDATION OR IN OVERDOSE CASES WHERE PATIENTS ARE SHOWING SIGNS OF SERIOUS CYCLIC ANTIDEPRESSANT OVERDOSE.

PRACTITIONERS SHOULD INDIVIDUALIZE THE DOSAGE OF FLUMAZENIL AND BE PREPARED TO MANAGE SEIZURES.

RISK OF SEIZURES

The reversal of benzodiazepine effects may be associated with the onset of seizures in certain high-risk populations. Possible risk factors for seizures include: concurrent major sedative-hypnotic drug withdrawal, recent therapy with repeated doses of parenteral benzodiazepines, myoclonic jerking or seizure activity prior to flumazenil administration in overdose cases, or concurrent cyclic anti-depressant poisoning.

Flumazenil is not recommended in cases of serious cyclic antidepressant poisoning, as manifested by motor abnormalities (twitching, rigidity, focal seizure), dysrhythmia (wide QRS, ventricular dysrhythmia, heart block), anticholinergic signs (mydriasis, dry mucosa, hypo-peristalsis), and cardiovascular collapse at presentation. In such cases flumazenil should be withheld and the patient should be allowed to remain sedated (with ventilatory and circulatory support as needed) until the signs of antidepressant toxicity have subsided. Treatment with flumazenil has no known benefit to the seriously ill mixed-overdose patient other than reversing sedation and should not be used in cases where seizures (from any cause) are likely.

Most convulsions associated with flumazenil administration require treatment and have been successfully managed with benzodiazepines, phenytoin or barbiturates. Because of the presence of flumazenil, higher than usual doses of benzodiazepines may be required.

HYPOVENTILATION

Patients who have received flumazenil for the reversal of benzodiazepine effects (after conscious sedation or general anesthesia) should be monitored for resedation, respiratory depression, or other residual benzodiazepine effects for an appropriate period (up to 120 minutes) based on the dose and duration of effect of the benzodiazepine employed.

This is because flumazenil has not been established as an effective treatment for hypoventilation due to benzodiazepine administration. In healthy male volunteers, flumazenil is capable of reversing benzodiazepine induced depression of the ventilatory responses to hypercapnia and hypoxia after a benzodiazepine alone. However, such depression may recur because the ventilatory effects of typical doses of flumazenil (1 mg or less) may wear off before the effects of many benzodiazepines. The effects of flumazenil on ventilatory response following sedation with a benzodiazepine in combination with an opioid are inconsistent and have not been adequately studied. The availability of flumazenil does not diminish the need for prompt detection of hypoventilation and the ability to effectively intervene by establishing an airway and assisting ventilation.

Overdose cases should always be monitored for resedation until the patients are stable and resedation is unlikely.

PRECAUTIONS

RETURN OF SEDATION

Flumazenil may be expected to improve the alertness of patients recovering from a procedure involving sedation or anesthesia with benzodiazepines, but should not be substituted for an adequate period of post-procedure monitoring. The availability of flumazenil does not reduce the risks associated with the use of large doses of benzodiazepines for sedation.

Patients should be monitored for resedation, respiratory depression (see WARNINGS), or other persistent or recurrent agonist effects for an adequate period of time after administration of flumazenil.

Resedation is least likely in cases where flumazenil is administered to reverse a low dose of a short-acting benzodiazepine (<10 mg midazolam). It is most likely in cases where a large single or cumulative dose of a benzodiazepine has been given in the course of a long procedure along with neuromuscular blocking agents and multiple anesthetic agents.

Profound resedation was observed in 1-3% of patients in the clinical studies. In clinical situations where resedation must be prevented, physicians may wish to repeat the initial dose (up to 1 mg of flumazenil given at 0.2 mg/min) at 30 minutes and possibly again at 60 minutes. This dosage schedule, although not studied in clinical trials, was effective in preventing resedation in a pharmacologic study in normal volunteers.

USE IN THE ICU

Flumazenil should be used with caution in the Intensive Care Unit because of the increased risk of unrecognized benzodiazepine dependence in such settings. Flumazenil may produce convulsions in patients physically dependent on benzodiazepines. (See WARNINGS and CLINICAL PHARMACOLOGY, Individualization of Dosage.)

Administration of flumazenil to diagnose benzodiazepine-induced sedation in the Intensive Care Unit is not recommended due to the risk of adverse events as described above. In addition, the prognostic significance of a patient's failure to respond to flumazenil in cases confounded by metabolic disorder, traumatic injury, drugs other than benzodiazepines, or any other reasons not associated with benzodiazepine receptor occupancy is not known.

USE IN OVERDOSE

Flumazenil is intended as an adjunct to, not as a substitute for proper management of airway, assisted breathing, circulatory access and support, internal decontamination by lavage and charcoal, and adequate clinical evaluation.

Necessary measures should be instituted to secure airway, ventilation and intravenous access prior to administering flumazenil. Upon arousal patients may attempt to withdraw endotracheal tubes and/or intravenous lines as the result of confusion and agitation following awakening.

HEAD INJURY

Flumazenil should be used with caution in patients with head injury as it may be capable of precipitating convulsions or altering cerebral blood flow in patients receiving benzodiazepines. It should be used only by practitioners prepared to manage such complications should they occur.

USE WITH NEUROMUSCULAR BLOCKING AGENTS

Flumazenil should not be used until the effects of neuromuscular blockade have been fully reversed.

USE IN PSYCHIATRIC PATIENTS

Flumazenil has been reported to provoke panic attacks in patients with a history of panic disorder.

PAIN ON INJECTION

To minimize the likelihood of pain or inflammation at the injection site, flumazenil should be administered through a freely flowing intravenous infusion into a large vein. Local irritation may occur following extravasation into perivascular tissues.

USE IN RESPIRATORY DISEASE:

The primary treatment of patients with serious lung disease who experience serious respiratory depression due to benzodiazepines should be appropriate ventilatory support (see PRECAUTIONS) rather than the administration of flumazenil. Flumazenil is capable of partially reversing benzodiazepine-induced alterations in ventilatory drive in healthy volunteers, but has not been shown to be clinically effective.

USE IN CARDIOVASCULAR DISEASE

Flumazenil did not increase the work of the heart when used to reverse benzodiazepines in cardiac patients when given at a rate of 0.1 mg/min in total doses of less than 0.5 mg in studies reported in the clinical literature. Flumazenil alone had no significant effects on cardiovascular parameters when administered to patients with stable ischemic heart disease.

USE IN LIVER DISEASE

The clearance of flumazenil is reduced to 40-60% of normal in patients with mild to moderate hepatic disease and to 25% of normal in patients with severe hepatic dysfunction (see CLINICAL PHARMACOLOGY, Pharmacokinetics). While the dose of flumazenil used for initial reversal of benzodiazepine effects is not affected, repeat doses of the drug in liver disease should be reduced in size or frequency.

USE IN DRUG AND ALCOHOL DEPENDENT PATIENTS

Flumazenil should be used with caution in patients with alcoholism and other drug dependencies due to the increased frequency of benzodiazepine tolerance and dependence observed in these patient populations.

Flumazenil is not recommended either as a treatment for benzodiazepine dependence or for the management of protracted benzodiazepine abstinence syndromes, as such use has not been studied.

The administration of flumazenil can precipitate benzodiazepine withdrawal in animals and man. This has been seen in healthy volunteers treated with therapeutic doses of oral lorazepam for up to 2 weeks who exhibited effects such as hot flushes, agitation and tremor when treated with cumulative doses of up to 3 mg doses of flumazenil.

Similar adverse experiences suggestive of flumazenil precipitation of benzodiazepine withdrawal have occurred in some patients in clinical trials. Such patients had a short-lived syndrome characterized by dizziness, mild confusion, emotional lability, agitation (with signs and symptoms of anxiety), and mild sensory distortions. This response was dose-related, most common at doses above 1 mg, rarely required treatment other than reassurance and was usually short lived. When required (5-10 cases), these patients were successfully treated with usual doses of a barbiturate, a benzodiazepine, or other sedative drug.

Practitioners should assume that flumazenil administration may trigger dose-dependent withdrawal syndromes in patients with established physical dependence on benzodiazepines and may complicate the management of withdrawal syndrome for alcohol, barbiturates and cross-tolerant sedatives.

USE IN AMBULATORY PATIENTS

The effects of flumazenil may wear off before a long-acting benzodiazepine is completely cleared from the body. In general, if a patient shows no signs of sedation within 2 hours after a 1 mg dose of flumazenil, serious resedation at a later time is unlikely. An adequate period of observation must be provided for any patient in whom either long-acting benzodiazepines (such as diazepam) or large doses of short-acting benzodiazepines (such as >10 mg of midazolam) have been used. See CLINICAL PHARMACOLOGY, Individualization of Dosage.

Because of the increased risk of adverse reactions in patients who have been taking benzodiazepines on a regular basis, it is particularly important that physicians query carefully about benzodiazepine, alcohol and sedative use as part of the history prior to any procedure in which the use of flumazenil is planned. See PRECAUTIONS, Drug And Alcohol Dependent Patients.

INFORMATION FOR THE PATIENT

Flumazenil does not consistently reverse amnesia. Patients cannot be expected to remember information told to them in the post-procedure period and instructions given to patients should be reinforced in writing or given to a responsible family member. Physicians are advised to discuss with their patients, both before surgery and at discharge, that although the patient may feel alert at the time of discharge, the effects of the benzodiazepine may recur. As a result, the patient should be instructed, preferably in writing, that their memory and judgement may be impaired and specifically advised:

1. Not to engage in any activities requiring complete alertness, and not to operate hazardous machinery or a motor vehicle until at least 18-24 hours after discharge, and it is certain no residual sedative effects of the benzodiazepine remain.
2. Not to take any alcohol or non-prescription drugs for 18-24 hours after flumazenil administration or if the effects of the benzodiazepine persist.

LABORATORY TESTS

No specific laboratory tests are recommended to follow the patient's response or to identify possible adverse reactions.

DRUG/LABORATORY TEST INTERACTIONS

The possible interaction of flumazenil with commonly used laboratory tests has not been evaluated.

F

CARCINOGENESIS, MUTAGENESIS, AND IMPAIRMENT OF FERTILITY

Carcinogenesis

No studies in animals to evaluate the carcinogenic potential of flumazenil have been conducted.

Mutagenesis

No evidence for mutagenicity was noted in the Ames test using five different tester strains. Assays for mutagenic potential in *S. cerevisiae* D7 and in Chinese hamster cells were considered to be negative as were blastogenesis assays *in vitro* in peripheral human lymphocytes and *in vivo* in a mouse micronucleus assay. Flumazenil caused a slight increase in unscheduled DNA synthesis in rat hepatocyte culture at concentrations which were also cytotoxic; no increase in DNA repair was observed in male mouse germ cells in an *in vivo* DNA repair assay.

Impairment of Fertility

A reproduction study in male and female rats did not show any impairment of fertility at oral dosages of 125 mg/kg/day. From the available data on the area under the curve (AUC) in animals and man the dose represented 120 × the human exposure from a maximum recommended intravenous dose of 5 mg.

PREGNANCY CATEGORY C

There are no adequate and well-controlled studies of the use of flumazenil in pregnant women. Flumazenil should be used during pregnancy only if the potential benefit justifies the potential risk to the fetus.

Teratogenic Effects

Flumazenil has been studied for teratogenicity in rats and rabbits following oral treatments of up to 150 mg/kg/day. The treatments during the major organogenesis were on days 6-15 of gestation in the rat and days 6-18 of gestation in the rabbit. No teratogenic effects were observed in rats or rabbits at 150 mg/kg; the dose, based on the available data on the area under the plasma concentration-time curve (AUC) represented 120 x to 600 x the human exposure from a maximum recommended intravenous dose of 5 mg in humans. In rabbits, embryocidal effects (as evidenced by increased pre-implantation and post-implantation losses) were observed at 50 mg/kg or 200 x the human exposure from a maximum recommended intravenous dose of 5 mg. The no-effect dose of 15 mg/kg in rabbits represents 60 x the human exposure.

Nonteratogenic Effects

An animal reproduction study was conducted in rats at oral dosages of 5, 25 and 125 mg/kg/day of flumazenil. Pup survival was decreased during the lactating period, pup liver weight at weaning was increased for the high-dose group (125 mg/kg/day) and incisor eruption and ear opening in the offspring were delayed; the delay in ear opening was associated with a delay in the appearance of the auditory startle response. No treatment-related adverse effects were noted for the other dose groups. Based on the available data from AUC, the effect level (125 mg/kg), represents 120 × the human exposure from 5 mg, the maximum recommended intravenous dose in humans. The no-effect level represents 24 × the human exposure from an intravenous dose of 5 mg.

LABOR AND DELIVERY

The use of flumazenil to reverse the effects of benzodiazepines used during labor and delivery is not recommended because the effects of the drug in the newborn are unknown.

NURSING MOTHERS

Caution should be exercised when deciding to administer flumazenil to a nursing woman because it is not known whether flumazenil is excreted in human milk.

PEDIATRIC USE

Flumazenil is not recommended for use in children (either for the reversal of sedation, the management of overdose or the resuscitation of the newborn), as no clinical studies have been performed to determine the risks, benefits and dosages to be used.

GERIATRIC USE

The pharmacokinetics of flumazenil have been studied in the elderly and are not significantly different from younger patients. Several studies of flumazenil in patients over the age of 65 and one study in patients over the age of 80 suggest that while the doses of benzodiazepine used to induce sedation should be reduced, ordinary doses of flumazenil may be used for reversal.

DRUG INTERACTIONS

Interaction with central nervous system depressants other than benzodiazepines has not been specifically studied; however, no deleterious interactions were seen when flumazenil was administered after narcotics, inhalational anesthetics, muscle relaxants and muscle relaxant antagonists administered in conjunction with sedation or anesthesia.

Particular caution is necessary when using flumazenil in cases of mixed drug overdosage since the toxic effects (such as convulsions and cardiac dysrhythmias) of other drugs taken in overdose (especially cyclic antidepressants) may emerge with the reversal of the benzodiazepine effect by flumazenil. (See WARNINGS.)

The pharmacokinetics of benzodiazepines are unaltered in the presence of flumazenil.

ADVERSE REACTIONS

SERIOUS ADVERSE REACTIONS

Deaths have occurred in patients who received flumazenil in a variety of clinical settings. The majority of deaths occurred in patients with serious underlying disease or in patients who had ingested large amounts of non-benzodiazepine drugs, (usually cyclic antidepressants) as part of an overdose.

Serious adverse events have occurred in all clinical settings, and convulsions are the most common serious adverse event-reported. Flumazenil administration has been associated with the onset of convulsions in patients who are relying on benzodiazepine effects to control seizures, are physically dependent on benzodiazepines, or who have ingested large doses of other drugs. (See WARNINGS.)

Two (2) of the 446 patients who received flumazenil in controlled clinical trials for the management of a benzodiazepine overdosage had cardiac dysrhythmias (1 ventricular tachycardia, 1 junctional tachycardia).

ADVERSE EVENTS IN CLINICAL STUDIES

The following adverse reactions were considered to be related to flumazenil administration (both alone and for the reversal of benzodiazepine effects) and were reported in studies involving 1875 individuals who received flumazenil in controlled trials. Adverse events most frequently associated with flumazenil alone were limited to dizziness, injection site pain, increased sweating, headache and abnormal or blurred vision (3-9%).

Body as a Whole: Fatigue (asthenia, malaise), Headache, Injection Site Pain*, Injection Site Reaction (thrombophlebitis, skin abnormality, rash).
Cardiovascular System: Cutaneous vasodilation (sweating, flushing, hot flushes).
Digestive System: Nausea and Vomiting (11%).
Nervous System: Agitation (anxiety, nervousness, dry mouth, tremor, palpitations, insomnia, dyspnea, hyperventilation)*, Dizziness (vertigo, ataxia) (10%), Emotional lability (crying abnormal, depersonalization, euphoria, increased tears, depression, dysphoria, paranoia).
Special Senses: Abnormal Vision (visual field defect, diplopia), Paresthesia (sensation abnormal, hypoesthesia).
(All adverse reactions occurred in 1-3% of cases unless otherwise marked.)
*Indicates reaction in 3-9% of cases.
Observed percentage reported if greater than 9%.

The following adverse events were observed infrequently (less than 1%) in the clinical studies, but were judged as probably related to flumazenil administration and/or reversal of benzodiazepine effects:

Nervous System: Confusion (difficulty concentrating, delirium), Convulsions (See WARNINGS), Somnolence (stupor).
Special Senses: Abnormal Hearing (transient hearing impairment, hyperacusis, tinnitus).

The following adverse events occurred with frequencies less than 1% in the clinical trials. Their relationship to flumazenil administration is unknown, but they are included as alerting information for the physician.

Body as a Whole: Rigors, shivering.
Cardiovascular: Arrhythmia (atrial, nodal, ventricular extrasystoles), bradycardia, tachycardia, hypertension, chest pain.
Digestive System: Hiccup.
Nervous System: Speech disorder (dysphoria, thick tongue).

Not included in this list is operative site pain that occurred with the same frequency in patients receiving placebo as in patients receiving flumazenil for reversal of sedation following a surgical procedure.

DOSAGE AND ADMINISTRATION

Flumazenil is recommended for intravenous use only. It is compatible with 5% dextrose in water, lactated Ringer's and normal saline solutions. If flumazenil is drawn into a syringe or mixed with any of these solutions, it should be discarded after 24 hours. For optimum sterility, flumazenil should remain in the vial until just before use. As with all parenteral drug products, flumazenil should be inspected visually for particulate matter and discoloration prior to administration, whenever solution and container permit.

To minimize the likelihood of pain at the injection site, flumazenil should be administered through a freely running intravenous infusion into a large vein.

REVERSAL OF CONSCIOUS SEDATION OR IN GENERAL ANESTHESIA

For the reversal of the sedative effects of benzodiazepines administered for conscious sedation or general anesthesia, the recommended initial dose of flumazenil is 0.2 mg (2 ml) administered intravenously over 15 seconds. If the desired level of consciousness is not obtained after waiting an additional 45 seconds, a further dose of 0.2 mg (2 ml) can be injected and repeated at 60-second intervals where necessary (up to a maximum of 4 additional times) to a maximum total dose of 1 mg (10 ml). The dose should be individualized based on the patient's response, with most patients responding to doses of 0.6 to 1 mg. (See CLINICAL PHARMACOLOGY, Individualization Of Dosage.)

In the event of resedation, repeated doses may be administered at 20 minute intervals as needed. For repeat treatment, no more than 1 mg (given as 0.2 mg/min) should be administered at any one time, and no more than 3 mg should be given in any one hour.

It is recommended that flumazenil be administered as the series of small injections described (not as a single bolus injection) to allow the practitioner to control the reversal of sedation to the approximate endpoint desired and to minimize the possibility of adverse effects. See CLINICAL PHARMACOLOGY, Individualization of Dosage.

MANAGEMENT OF SUSPECTED BENZODIAZEPINE OVERDOSE

For initial management of a known or suspected benzodiazepine overdose, the recommended initial dose of flumazenil is 0.2 mg (2 ml) administered intravenously over 30 seconds. If the desired level of consciousness is not obtained after waiting 30 seconds, a further dose of 0.3 mg (3 ml) can be administered over another 30 seconds. Further doses of 0.5 mg (5 ml) can be administered over 30 seconds at 1 minute intervals up to a cumulative dose of 3 mg.

Do not rush the administration of flumazenil. Patients should have a secure airway and intravenous access before administration of the drug and be awakened gradually. (See PRECAUTIONS.)

Most patients with benzodiazepine overdose will respond to a cumulative dose of 1-3 mg of flumazenil, and doses beyond 3 mg do not reliably produce additional effects. On rare occasions, patients with a partial response at 3 mg may require additional titration up to a total dose of 5 mg (administered slowly in the same manner).

If a patient has not responded 5 minutes after receiving a cumulative dose of 5 mg flumazenil, the major cause of sedation is likely not to be due to benzodiazepines, and additional flumazenil is likely to have no effect.

In the event of resedation, repeated doses may be given at 20 minute intervals if needed. For repeat treatment, no more than 1 mg (given as 0.5 mg/min) should be given at any one time and no more than 3 mg should be given in any one hour.

SAFETY AND HANDLING

Flumazenil is supplied in sealed dosage forms and poses no known risk to the health care provider. Routine care should be taken to avoid aerosol generation when preparing syringes for injection, and spilled medication should be rinsed from the skin with cool water.

PRODUCT LISTING - EQUIVALENTS NOT AVAILABLE

Solution - Intravenous - 0.1 mg/ml

5 ml x 5	$50.40	ROMAZICON, Allscripts Pharmaceutical Company	54569-3956-01
5 ml x 10	$628.40	ROMAZICON, Roche Laboratories	00004-6911-06
10 ml x 10	$999.80	ROMAZICON, Roche Laboratories	00004-6912-06

Flunisolide *(001305)*

For related information, see the comparative table section in Appendix A.

Categories: Asthma; Rhinitis, perennial allergic; Rhinitis, seasonal allergic; Pregnancy Category C; FDA Approved 1981 Sep
Drug Classes: Corticosteroids, inhalation
Brand Names: Aerobid; Aerobid-M; **Nasalide**; Nasarel
Foreign Brand Availability: Bronalide (Bahamas; Barbados; Belize; Bermuda; Canada; Curacao; Guyana; Jamaica; Netherland-Antilles; Puerto-Rico; Surinam; Trinidad); Bronilide (France); Flunase (Israel); Flunitec (Peru); Gibiflu (Italy); Inhacort (Germany); Locasyn (Denmark); Lokilan (Norway); Lokilan Nasal (Finland; Sweden); Lunibron-A (Italy); Lunis (Italy); Rhinalar (Canada); Sanergal (Slovenia); Synaclyn (Japan); Syntaris (Austria; Bahamas; Bahrain; Barbados; Belgium; Belize; Bermuda; Bulgaria; Curacao; Czech-Republic; England; Germany; Guyana; Hungary; Italy; Jamaica; Kuwait; Netherland-Antilles; Netherlands; Portugal; South-Africa; Surinam; Switzerland; Trinidad); Syntaris Nasal Spray (Benin; Burkina-Faso; Ethiopia; Gambia; Ghana; Guinea; Ivory-Coast; Kenya; Liberia; Malawi; Mali; Mauritania; Mauritius; Morocco; Niger; Nigeria; Senegal; Seychelles; Sierra-Leone; Sudan; Tanzania; Tunia; Uganda; Zambia; Zimbabwe)
Cost of Therapy: $52.24 (Allergic Rhinitis; Nasalide Spray; 25 µg/inhalation; 25 ml; 8 sprays/day; 25 day supply)
$54.61 (Asthma; Aerobid Aerosol; 250 µg/inhalation; 7 g; 4 inhalations/day; 25 day supply)
$46.49 (Asthma; Generic Nasal Spray; 25 µg/inhalation; 25 ml; 8 sprays/day; 25 day supply)

DESCRIPTION

NASAL SOLUTION

Flunisolide nasal solution is intended for administration as a spray to the nasal mucosa. Flunisolide, the active component of Flunisolide nasal solution, is an anti-inflammatory steroid with the chemical name: 6α-fluoro-11β,16α,17,21-tetrahydroxypregna-1,4-diene-3,20-dione cyclic 16,17-acetal with acetone (USAN).

Flunisolide is a white to creamy white crystalline powder with a molecular weight of 434.49. It is insoluble in acetone, sparingly soluble in chloroform, slightly soluble in methanol, and practically insoluble in water. It has a melting point of about 245°C.

Each 25 ml spray bottle contains flunisolide 6.25 mg (0.25 mg/ml) in a solution of propylene glycol, polyethylene glycol 3350, citric acid, sodium citrate, butylated hydroxyanisole, edetate disodium, benzalkonium chloride, and purified water, with NaOH and/or HCl added to adjust the pH to approximately 5.3. It contains no fluorocarbons.

After priming the delivery system for Flunisolide, each actuation of the unit delivers a metered droplet spray containing approximately 25 µg of flunisolide. The size of the droplets produced by the unit is in excess of 8 microns to facilitate deposition on the nasal mucosa. The contents of one nasal spray bottle deliver at least 200 sprays.

ORAL INHALER

Flunisolide, the active component of Aerobid inhaler system, is an anti-inflammatory steroid having the chemical name 6α-fluoro-11β,16α,17,21-tetrahydroxypregna-1,4-diene-3,20-dione cyclic-16,17-acetal with acetone.

Flunisolide is a white to creamy white crystalline powder with a molecular weight of 434.49. It is soluble in acetone, sparingly soluble in chloroform, slightly soluble in methanol, and practically insoluble in water. It has a melting point of about 245°C.

Aerobid inhaler is delivered in a metered-dose aerosol system containing a microcrystalline suspension of flunisolide as the hemihydrate in propellants (trichloromonofluoromethane, dichlorodifluoromethane and dichlorotetrafluoroethane) with sorbitan trioleate as a dispersing agent. Aerobid-M also contains menthol as a flavoring agent. Each activation delivers approximately 250 µg of flunisolide to the patient. One Aerobid inhaler system is designed to deliver at least 100 metered inhalations.

CLINICAL PHARMACOLOGY

NASAL SOLUTION

Flunisolide has demonstrated potent glucocorticoid and weak mineralocorticoid activity in classical animal test systems. As a glucocorticoid it is several hundred times more potent than the cortisol standard. Clinical studies with flunisolide have shown therapeutic activity on nasal mucous membranes with minimal evidence of systemic activity at the recommended doses.

A study in approximately 100 patients which compared the recommended dose of flunisolide nasal solution with an oral dose providing equivalent systemic amounts of flunisolide has shown that the clinical effectiveness of Flunisolide, when used topically as recommended, is due to its direct local effect and not to an indirect effect through systemic absorption.

Following administration to flunisolide to man, approximately half of the administered dose is recovered in the urine and half in the stool; 65-70% of the dose recovered in urine is the primary metabolite, which has undergone loss of the 6α fluorine and addition of a 6β hydroxy group. Flunisolide is well absorbed but is rapidly converted by the liver to the much less active primary metabolite and to glucuronate and/or sulfate conjugates. Because of first-pass liver metabolism, only 20% of the flunisolide reaches the systemic circulation when it is given orally whereas 50% of the flunisolide administered intranasally reaches the systemic circulation unmetabolized. The plasma half-life of flunisolide is 1-2 hours.

The effects of flunisolide on hypothalamic-pituitary-adrenal (HPA) axis function has been studied in volunteers. Flunisolide was administered intranasally as a spray in total doses over 7 times the recommended dose (2200 µg equivalent to 88 sprays/days) in 2 subjects for 4 days, about 3 times the recommended dose (800 µg, equivalent to 32 sprays/day) in 4 subjects for 10 days. Early morning plasma cortisol concentrations and 24 hour urinary 17-ketogenic steroids were measured daily. There was evidence of decreased endogenous cortisol production at all three doses.

In controlled studies, Flunisolide was found to be effective in reducing symptoms of stuffy nose, runny nose and sneezing in most patients. These controlled clinical studies have been conducted in 488 adult patients at doses ranging from 8 to 16 sprays (200-400 µg) per day and 127 children at doses ranging from 6-8 sprays (150-200 µg) per day for periods as long as 3 months. In 170 patients who had cortisol levels evaluated at baseline and after 3 months or more of flunisolide treatment, there was no unequivocal flunisolide-related depression of plasma cortisol levels.

The mechanisms responsible for the anti-inflammatory action of corticosteroids and for the activity of the aerosolized drug on the nasal mucosa are unknown.

ORAL INHALER

Flunisolide has demonstrated marked anti-inflammatory and anti-allergic activity in classical test systems. It is a corticosteroid that is several hundred times more potent in animal anti-inflammatory assays than the cortisol standard. The molar dose of each activation of flunisolide in this preparation is approximately 2.5 to 7 times that of comparable inhaled corticosteroid products marketed for the same indication. The dose of flunisolide delivered per activation in this preparation is 10 times that per activation of flunisolide nasal solution. Clinical studies have shown therapeutic activity on bronchial mucosa with minimal evidence of systemic activity at recommended doses.

After oral inhalation of 1 mg flunisolide, total systemic availability was 40%. The flunisolide that is swallowed is rapidly and extensively converted to the 6β-OH metabolite and to water-soluble conjugates during the first pass through the liver. This offers a metabolic explanation for the low systemic activity of oral flunisolide itself since the metabolite has the low corticosteroid potency (on the order of the cortisol standard). The inhaled flunisolide absorbed through the bronchial tree is converted to the same metabolites. Repeated inhalation of 2.0 mg of flunisolide per day (the maximum recommended dose) of 14 days did not show accumulation of the drug in plasma. The plasma half-life of flunisolide is approximately 1.8 hours.

The following observations relevant to systemic absorption were made in clinical studies. In one uncontrolled study a statistically significant decrease in responsiveness to metyrapone was noted in 15 adult steroid-independent patients treated with 2.0 mg of flunisolide per day (the maximum recommended dose) for 3 months. A small but statistically significant drop in eosinophils from 11.5% to 7.4% of total circulating leukocytes was noted in another study in children who were not taking oral corticosteroids simultaneously. A 5% incidence of menstrual disturbances was reported during open studies, in which there were no control groups for comparison.

Aerosol administration of flunisolide 2.0 mg twice daily for 1 week to 6 healthy male subjects revealed neither suppression of adrenal function as measured by early morning cortisol levels nor impairment of HPA axis function as determined by insulin hypoglycemia tests.

Controlled clinical studies have included over 500 patients with asthma, among them 150 children age 6 and over. More than 120 patients have been treated in open trials for 2 years or more. No significant adrenal suppression attributed to flunisolide was seen in these studies.

Significant decreases of systemic steroid dosages have been possible in flunisolide-treated patients. Recommended doses of flunisolide appear to be the therapeutic equivalent of an average of 10 mg/day of oral prednisone. Asthma patients have had further symptomatic improvement with flunisolide treatment even while reducing concomitant medication.

INDICATIONS AND USAGE

NASAL SOLUTION

Flunisolide is indicated for the topical treatment of the symptoms of seasonal or perennial or perennial rhinitis when effectiveness of or tolerance to conventional treatment is unsatisfactory.

Clinical studies have shown that improvement is based on a local effect rather than systemic absorption, and is usually apparent within a few days starting Flunisolide. However, symptomatic relief may not occur in some patients for as long as 2 weeks. Although systemic effects are minimal at recommended doses, Flunisolide should not be continued beyond 3 weeks in the absence of significant symptomatic improvement.

Flunisolide should not be used in the presence of untreated localized infection involving nasal mucosa.

ORAL INHALER

Flunisolide inhaler is indicated in the maintenance treatment of asthma as prophylactic therapy. Flunisolide is also indicated for asthma patients who require systemic corticosteroid administration, where adding flunisolide may reduce or eliminate the need for the systemic corticosteroids.

Flunisolide inhaler is NOT indicated for the relief of acute bronchospasm.

CONTRAINDICATIONS

NASAL SOLUTION

Hypersensitivity to any of the ingredients.

ORAL INHALER

Flunisolide inhaler is contraindicated in the primary treatment of status asthmaticus or other acute episodes of asthma where intensive measures are required.

Hypersensitivity to any of the ingredients of this preparation contraindicates its use.

WARNINGS

NASAL SOLUTION

The replacement of a systemic corticosteroid with a topical corticoid can be accompanied by signs of adrenal insufficiency, and in addition some patients may experience symptoms of withdrawal *e.g.,* joint and/or muscular pain, lassitude and depression. Patients previously treated for prolonged periods with systemic corticosteroids and transferred to flunisolide should be carefully monitored to avoid acute adrenal insufficiency in response to stress.

When transferred to Flunisolide, careful attention must be given to patients previously treated for prolonged periods with systemic corticosteroids. This is particularly important in those patients who have associated asthma or other clinical conditions, where too rapid a decrease in systemic corticosteroids may cause a severe exacerbation of their symptoms.

The use of Flunisolide with alternate-day prednisone systemic treatment could increase the likelihood of HPA suppression compared to a therapeutic dose of either one alone. Therefore, Flunisolide treatment should be used with caution in patients already on alternate-day prednisone regimens for any disease.

ORAL INHALER

Particular care is needed in patients who are transferred from systemically active corticosteroids to flunisolide inhaler because deaths due to adrenal insufficiency have occurred in asthmatic patients during and after transfer from systemic corticosteroids to aerosol corticosteroids. After withdrawal from systemic corticosteroids, a number of months are required for recovery of hypothalamic-pituitary-adrenal (HPA) function. During this period of HPA suppression, patients may exhibit signs and symptoms of adrenal insufficiency when exposed to trauma, surgery, or infections, particularly gastroenteritis. Although flunisolide Inhaler may provide control of asthmatic symptoms during these episodes, it does NOT provide the systemic steroid that is necessary for coping with emergencies.

During periods of stress or a severe asthmatic attack, patients who have been withdrawn from systemic corticosteroids should be instructed to resume systemic steroids (in larger doses) immediately and to contact their physician for further instruction. These patients should also be instructed to carry a warning card indicating that they may need supplementary systemic steroids during periods of stress or a severe asthma attack. To assess the risk of adrenal insufficiency in emergency situations, routine tests of adrenal cortical function, including measurement of early morning cortisol levels, should be performed periodically in all patients. An early morning resting cortisol level may be accepted as normal if it falls at or near the normal mean level.

Localized infections with *Candida albicans* or *Aspergillus niger* have occurred in the mouth and pharynx and occasionally in the larynx. Positive cultures for oral *Candida* may be present in up to 34% of patients. Although the frequency of clinically apparent infection is considerably lower, these infections may require treatment with appropriate antifungal therapy or discontinuance of treatment with flunisolide inhaler.

Flunisolide inhaler is not to be regarded as a bronchodilator and is not indicated for rapid relief of bronchospasm.

Patients should be instructed to contact their physician immediately when episodes of asthma that are not responsive to bronchodilators occur during the course of treatment. During such episodes, patients may require therapy with systemic corticosteroids. Theoretically, the use of inhaled corticosteroids with alternate day prednisone systemic treatment should be accompanied by more HPA suppression than a therapeutically equivalent regimen of either alone.

Transfer of patients from systemic steroid therapy to flunisolide inhaler may unmask allergic conditions previously suppressed by the systemic steroid therapy, *e.g.,* rhinitis, conjunctivitis, and eczema.

Persons who are on drugs which suppress the immune system are more susceptible to infections than healthy individuals. Chicken pox and measles, for example, can have a more serious or even fatal course in non-immune children or adults on corticosteroids. In such children or adults who have not had these diseases, particular care should be taken to avoid exposure. How the dose, route and duration of corticosteroid administration affects the risk of developing a disseminated infection is not known. The contribution of the underlying disease and/or prior corticosteroid treatment to the risk is also not known. If exposed to chicken pox, prophylaxis with varicella zoster immune globulin (VZIG) may be indicated. If exposed to measles, prophylaxis with pooled intramuscular immunoglobulin (IG) may be indicated. (See the respective monographs for complete VZIG and IG prescribing information.) If chicken pox develops, treatment with antiviral agents may be considered.

PRECAUTIONS

NASAL SOLUTION

General

In clinical studies with flunisolide administered intranasally, the development of localized infections of the nose and pharynx with *Candida albicans* has occurred only rarely. When such an infection develops it may require treatment with appropriate local therapy or discontinuance of treatment with flunisolide.

Flunisolide is absorbed into the circulation. Use of excessive doses of Flunisolide may suppress hypothalamic-pituitary-adrenal function.

Flunisolide should be used with caution, if at all in patients with active quiescent tuberculosis infections of the respiratory tract or in treated fungal, bacterial or systemic viral infections or ocular herpes simplex.

Because of the inhibitory effect of corticosteroids on wound healing, in patients who have experienced recent nasal septal ulcers, recurrent epistaxis, nasal surgery or trauma, a nasal corticosteroid should be used with caution until healing has occurred.

Although systemic effects have been minimal with recommended doses, this potential increases with excessive dosages. Therefore, larger than recommended doses should be avoided.

Information for the Patient

Patients should use Flunisolide at regular intervals since its effectiveness depends on its regular use. The patient should take the medication as directed. It is not acutely effective and the prescribed dosage should not be increased. Instead, nasal vasoconstrictors or oral antihistamines may be needed until the effects of Flunisolide are fully manifested. One (1) or 2 weeks may pass before full relief is obtained. The patient should contact the physician if symptoms do not improve, or if the condition worsens, or if sneezing or nasal irritation occurs.

For the proper use of this unit and to attain maximum improvement, the patient should read and follow the accompanying Patient Instructions carefully. (Contact the manufacturer for this information).

ORAL INHALER

General

Because of the relatively high molar dose of flunisolide per activation in this preparation, and because of the evidence suggesting higher levels of systemic absorption with flunisolide than with other comparable inhaled corticosteroids (see CLINICAL PHARMACOLOGY), patients treated with flunisolide should be observed carefully for any evidence of systemic corticosteroid effect, including suppression of bone growth in children. Particular care should be taken in observing patients post-operatively or during periods of stress for evidence of a decrease in adrenal function. During withdrawal from oral steroids, some patients may experience symptoms of systemically active steroid withdrawal, *e.g.,* joint and/or muscular pain, lassitude and depression, despite maintenance of even improvement of respiratory function (see DOSAGE AND ADMINISTRATION for details).

In responsive patients, flunisolide may permit control of asthmatic symptoms without suppression of HPA function. Since flunisolide is absorbed into the circulation and can be systemically active, the beneficial effects of flunisolide inhaler in minimizing or preventing HPA dysfunction may be expected only when recommended dosages are not exceeded.

The long-term local and systemic effects of flunisolide in human subjects are still not fully known. In particular, the effects resulting from chronic use of flunisolide on developmental or immunologic processes in the mouth, pharynx, trachea, and lung are unknown.

Inhaled corticosteroids should be used with caution, if at all, in patients with active or quiescent tuberculosis infection of the respiratory tract; untreated systemic fungal, bacterial, parasitic or viral infections; or ocular herpes simplex.

Pulmonary infiltrates with eosinophilia may occur in patients on flunisolide inhaler therapy. Although it is possible that in some patients this state may become manifest because of systemic steroid withdrawal when inhalational steroids are administered, a causative role for the drug and/or its vehicle cannot be ruled out.

Information for the Patient

Since the relief from flunisolide inhaler depends on its regular use and on proper inhalation technique, patients must be instructed to take inhalations at regular intervals. They should also be instructed in the correct method of use (refer to the Patient Instructions that are distributed with the prescription for complete instructions).

Patients whose systemic corticosteroids have been reduced or withdrawn should be instructed to carry a warning card indicating that they may need supplemental systemic steroids during periods of stress or a severe asthmatic attack that is not responsive to bronchodilators.

Persons who are on immunosuppressant doses of corticosteroids should be warned to avoid exposure to chicken pox or measles. Patients should also be advised that if they are exposed, medical advice should be sought without delay.

CONTENTS UNDER PRESSURE.

Do not puncture. Do not use or store near heat or open flame. Exposure to temperatures above 120°F (49°C) may cause container to explode. Never throw container into fire or incinerator. Keep out of reach of children.

Pediatric Use

Safety and effectiveness have not been established in children below the age of 6. Oral corticoids have been shown to cause growth suppression in children and adolescents, particularly with higher doses over extended periods. If a child or adolescent on any corticoid appears to have growth suppression, the possibility that they are particularly sensitive to this effect of steroids should be considered.

NASAL SOLUTION AND ORAL INHALER

Carcinogenesis

Long-term studies were conducted in mice and rats using oral administration to evaluate the carcinogenic potential of the drug. There was an increase in the incidence of pulmonary adenomas in mice, but not in rats.

Female rats receiving the highest oral dose had an increased incidence of mammary adenocarcinoma compared to control rats. An increased incidence of this tumor type has been reported for other corticosteroids.

Impairment of Fertility

Female rats receiving high doses of flunisolide (200 μg/kg/day) showed some evidence of impaired fertility. Reproductive performance in low (8 μg/kg/day) and mid-dose (40 μg/kg/day) groups was comparable to controls.

Pregnancy, Teratogenic Effects, Pregnancy Category C

As with other corticosteroids, flunisolide has been shown to be teratogenic in rabbits and rats at doses of 40 and 200 μg/kg/day respectively. It was also fetotoxic in these animal reproductive studies. There are no adequate and well-controlled studies in pregnant women. Flunisolide should be used during pregnancy only if the potential benefit justifies the potential risk to the fetus.

Nursing Mothers

It not known whether this drug is excreted in human milk. Because other corticosteroids are excreted in human milk, caution should be exercised when flunisolide is administered to nursing women.

ADVERSE REACTIONS

NASAL SOLUTION

Adverse reactions reported in controlled clinical trials and long-term open studies in 595 patients treated with Flunisolide are described below. Of these patients, 409 were treated for 3 months or longer, 323 for 6 months or longer, 259 for 1 year or longer, and 91 for 2 years or longer.

In general, side effects elicited in the clinical studies have been primarily associated with the nasal mucous membranes. The most frequent complaints were those of mild transient nasal burning and stinging, which were reported in approximately 45% of the patients treated with Flunisolide in placebo-controlled and long-term studies. These complaints do not usually interfere with treatment; in only 3% of patients was it necessary to decrease dosage or stop treatment because of these symptoms. Approximately the same incidence of mild transient nasal burning and stinging was reported in patients on placebo as was reported in patients treated with Flunisolide in controlled studies, implying that these complaints may be related to the vehicle or the delivery system.

The incidence of complaints of nasal burning and stinging decreased with increasing duration of treatment.

Other side effects reported at frequency of 5% or less were: nasal congestion, sneezing, epistaxis and/or bloody mucus, nasal irritation, watery eyes, sore throat, nausea and/or vomiting, headache and loss of sense of smell and taste. As is the case with other nasally inhaled corticosteroids, nasal septal perforations have been observed in rare instances.

Systemic corticosteroid side effects were not reported during the controlled clinical trials. If recommended doses are exceeded or if individuals are particularly sensitive, symptoms of hypercorticism, *i.e.,* Cushing's syndrome, could occur.

ORAL INHALER

Adverse events reported in controlled clinical trials and long-term open studies in 514 patients treated with flunisolide are described below. Of those patients, 463 were treated for 3 months or longer, 407 for 6 months or longer, 287 for 1 year or longer, and 122 for 2 years or longer.

Musculoskeletal reactions were reported in 35% of steroid-dependent patients in whom the dose of oral steroid was being tapered. This is a well-known effect of steroid withdrawal.

Incidence 10% or Greater:

Gastrointestinal: Diarrhea (10%), nausea and/or vomiting (25%), upset stomach (10%).

General: Flu (10%).

Mouth and Throat: Sore throat (20%).

Nervous system: Headache (25%).

Respiratory: Cold symptoms (15%), nasal congestion (15%), upper respiratory infection (25%).

Special Senses: Unpleasant tastes (10%).

Incidence 3-9%:

Cardiovascular: Palpitations.

Gastrointestinal: Abdominal pain, heartburn.

General: Chest pain, decreased appetite, edema, fever.

Mouth and Throat: *Candida* infection.

Nervous System: Dizziness, irritability, nervousness, shakiness.

Reproductive: Menstrual disturbances.

Respiratory: Chest congestion, cough*, hoarseness, rhinitis, runny nose, sinus congestion, sinus drainage, sinus infection, sinusitis, sneezing, sputum, wheezing*.

Skin: Eczema, itching (pruritus), rash.

Special Senses: Ear infection, loss of smell or taste.

Incidence 1-3%:

General: Chills, increased appetite and weight gain, malaise, peripheral edema, sweating, weakness.

Cardiovascular: Hypertension, tachycardia.

Gastrointestinal: Constipation, dyspepsia, gas.

Hemic/Lymph: Capillary fragility, enlarged lymph nodes.

Mouth and Throat: Dry throat, glossitis, mouth irritation, pharyngitis, phlegm, throat irritation.

Nervous System: Anxiety, depression, faintness, fatigue, hyperactivity, hypoactivity, insomnia, moodiness, numbness, vertigo.

Respiratory: Bronchitis, chest tightness*, dyspnea, epistaxis, head stuffiness, laryngitis, nasal irritation, pleurisy, pneumonia, sinus discomfort.

Skin: Acne, hives, or urticaria.

Special Senses: Blurred vision, earache, eye discomfort, eye infection.

Incidence Less Than 1%: *Judged by investigators as possibly or probably drug related:* Abdominal fullness, shortness of breath.

*The incidences as shown of cough, wheezing, and chest tightness were judged by investigators to be possibly or probably drug-related. In placebo-controlled trials, the *overall* incidences of these adverse events (regardless of investigators' judgement of drug relationship) were similar for drug and placebo-treated groups. They may be related to the vehicle or delivery system.

DOSAGE AND ADMINISTRATION

NASAL SOLUTION

The therapeutic effects of corticosteroids, unlike those of decongestants, are not immediate. This should be explained to the patient in advance in order to ensure cooperation and continuation of treatment with the prescribed dosage regimen. Full therapeutic benefit requires regular use, and is usually evident within a few days. However, a longer period of therapy may be required may be required for some patients to achieve maximum benefit (up to 3 weeks). If no improvement is evidence by that time, flunisolide should not be continued.

Patients with blocked nasal passages should be encouraged to use a decongestant just before Flunisolide administration to ensure adequate penetration of the spray. Patients should also be advised to clear nasal passages of secretions prior to use.

Adults: The recommended starting dose of Flunisolide is 2 sprays (50 μg) in each nostril 2 times a day (total dose 200 μg/day). If needed, this dose may be increased to 2 sprays in each nostril 3 times a day (total dose 300 μg/day).

Children: 6-14 years: The recommended starting dose of Flunisolide is one spray (25 μg) in each nostril 3 times a day or 2 sprays (50 μg) in each nostril 2 times a day (total dose 150-200 μg/day). Flunisolide is not recommended for use for children less than 6 years of age as safety and efficacy studies, including possible adverse effects on growth, have not been conducted.

Maximum total daily doses should not exceed 8 sprays in each nostril for adults (total dose 400 μg/day) and 4 sprays in each nostril for children under 14 years of age (total dose 200 μg/day). Since there is no evidence that exceeding the maximum recommended dosage is more effective and increased systemic absorption would occur, higher doses should be avoided.

After the desired clinical effect is obtained, the maintenance dose should be reduced to the smallest amount necessary to control the symptoms. Approximately 15% of the patients with perennial rhinitis may be maintained on as little as 1 spray in each nostril per day.

Store at controlled room temperature, 15°-30°C (59°-86°F).

ORAL INHALER

The flunisolide inhaler system is for oral inhalation only.

Adults: The recommended starting dose is 2 inhalations twice daily, morning and evening, for a total daily dose of 1 mg. The maximum daily dose should not exceed 4 inhalations twice a day for a total daily dose of 2 mg. When the drug is used chronically at 2 mg/day, patients should be monitored periodically for effects on the hypothalamic-pituitary-adrenal (HPA) axis.

Pediatric Patients: For children and adolescents 6-15 years of age, two inhalations may be administered twice daily for a total daily dose of 1 mg. Higher doses have not been studied. Insufficient information is available to warrant use in pediatric patients under age 6. With chronic use, pediatric patients should be monitored for growth as well as for effects on the HPA axis.

Rinsing the mouth after inhalation is advised.

Different considerations must be given to the following groups of patients in order to obtain the full therapeutic benefit of flunisolide inhaler.

Patients Not Receiving Systemic Corticosteroids

Patients who require maintenance therapy of their asthma may benefit from treatment with flunisolide at the doses recommended above. In patients who respond to flunisolide, improvement in pulmonary function is usually apparent within 1-4 weeks after the start of therapy. Once the desired effect is achieved, consideration should be given to tapering to the lowest effective dose.

Patients Maintained on Systemic Corticosteroids

Clinical studies have shown that flunisolide may be effective in the management of asthmatics dependent or maintained on systemic corticosteroids and may permit replacement or significant reduction in the dosage of systemic corticosteroids.

The patient's asthma should be reasonably stable before treatment with flunisolide inhaler is started. Initially, flunisolide should be used concurrently with the patient's usual maintenance dose of systemic corticosteroid. After approximately 1 week, gradual withdrawal of the systemic corticosteroid is started by reducing the daily or alternate daily dose. Reductions may be made after an interval of 1 or 2 weeks, depending on the response of the patient. A slow rate of withdrawal is strongly recommended. Generally, these decrements should not exceed 2.5 mg of prednisone or its equivalent. During withdrawal, some patients may experience symptoms of systemic corticosteroid withdrawal, (*e.g.,* joint and/or muscular pain, lassitude and depression), despite maintenance or even improvement in pulmonary function. Such patients should be encouraged to continue with the inhaler but should be monitored for objective signs of adrenal insufficiency. If evidence of adrenal insufficiency occurs, the systemic corticosteroid doses should be increased temporarily and thereafter withdrawal should continue more slowly.

During periods of stress or severe asthma attack, transfer patients may require supplementary treatment with systemic corticosteroids.

HOW SUPPLIED

Note: The statement below is required by the Federal government's Clean Air Act for all products containing or manufactured with chlorofluorocarbons (CFC's).

WARNING: Contains trichloromonofluoromethane, dichlorodifluoromethane and dichlorotetrafluoroethane, substances which harm public health and enviornment by destryoing ozone in the upper atmosphere.

PRODUCT LISTING - RATED THERAPEUTICALLY EQUIVALENT

Spray - Nasal - 25 mcg/Inh

Size	Price	Product	NDC
25 ml	$31.22	NASALIDE, Physicians Total Care	54868-1015-01
25 ml	$46.49	GENERIC, Bausch and Lomb	24208-0344-25
25 ml	$52.24	NASALIDE, Ivax Corporation	51479-0038-25

PRODUCT LISTING - RATED NOT THERAPEUTICALLY EQUIVALENT

Spray - Nasal - 25 mcg/Inh

Size	Price	Product	NDC
25 ml	$43.51	NASAREL, Allscripts Pharmaceutical Company	54569-4735-00
25 ml	$48.44	NASAREL, Physicians Total Care	54868-4162-00
25 ml	$51.89	NASAREL, Ivax Corporation	59310-0037-25

PRODUCT LISTING - EQUIVALENTS NOT AVAILABLE

Size	Price	Product	NDC
Aerosol - Inhalation - 250 mcg/Inh			
7 gm	$54.61	AEROBID-M, Quality Care Pharmaceuticals Inc	60346-0282-74
7 gm	$67.01	AEROBID-M, Allscripts Pharmaceutical Company	54569-3976-00
7 gm	$73.87	AEROBID-M, Forest Pharmaceuticals	00456-0670-99
Aerosol with Adapter - Inhalation - 250 mcg/Inh			
7 gm	$67.01	AEROBID, Allscripts Pharmaceutical Company	54569-1013-00
7 gm	$73.87	AEROBID, Forest Pharmaceuticals	00456-0672-99
7 gm	$76.06	AEROBID, Pharma Pac	52959-0131-00
7 gm	$79.43	AEROBID, Physicians Total Care	54868-1883-01

Fluocinolone Acetonide *(001306)*

Categories: Dermatosis, corticosteroid-responsive; Pregnancy Category C; FDA Approved 1963 Jun
Drug Classes: Corticosteroids, topical; Dermatologics
Brand Names: Bio-Syn; Derma-Smoothe Fs; FS Shampoo; Fluocet; Fluonid; Flurosyn; Lidex; **Synalar**; Synalar-Hp; Synemol
Foreign Brand Availability: Alfabios (Italy); Alvadermo Fuerte (Spain); Aplosyn (Philippines); Cinolon (Indonesia); Clofeet (Japan); Cortilona (Mexico); Cremisona (Mexico); Dermalar (Israel); Dermoflam (Peru); Dermoran (Japan); Esacinone (Bahrain; Cyprus; Egypt; Iran; Iraq; Jordan; Kuwait; Lebanon; Libya; Oman; Qatar; Republic-of-Yemen; Saudi-Arabia; Syria; United-Arab-Emirates); Flozet (Philippines); Fluciderm (Thailand); Flucort (India; Japan; Taiwan); Flulone (Argentina); Flunolone-V (Hong-Kong; Singapore); Fluoderm (Canada); Fluzon (Japan); Fusalar (Mexico); Jellin (Germany); Luci (India); Radiocin (Bahrain; Benin; Burkina-Faso; Cyprus; Egypt; Ethiopia; Gambia; Ghana; Guinea; Iran; Iraq; Ivory-Coast; Jordan; Kenya; Kuwait; Lebanon; Liberia; Libya; Malawi; Mali; Mauritania; Mauritius; Morocco; Niger; Nigeria; Oman; Qatar; Republic-of-Yemen; Saudi-Arabia; Senegal; Seychelles; Sierra-Leone; Sudan; Syria; Tanzania; Tunia; Uganda; United-Arab-Emirates; Zambia; Zimbabwe); Supralan (Thailand); Synalar 25 (Philippines); Synalar Simple (Peru)

DESCRIPTION

Note: The trade names have been used throughout this monograph for clarity.

DERMA-SMOOTHE/FS

For Dermatologic Use Only - Not for Ophthalmic Use

Derma-Smoothe/FS contains fluocinolone acetonide {(6α,11β,16α)-6,9-difluoro-11,21-dihydroxy-16,17[(1-methylethylidene)bis(oxy)]-pregna-1,4-diene-3,20-dione, cyclic 16,17 acetal with acetone}, a synthetic corticosteroid for topical dermatologic use. Chemically, fluocinolone acetonide is $C_{24}H_{30}F_2O_6$.

Fluocinolone acetonide in Derma-Smoothe/FS has a molecular weight of 452.50. It is a white crystalline powder that is odorless, stable in light, and melts at 270°C with decomposition; soluble in alcohol, acetone and methanol; slightly soluble in chloroform; insoluble in water.

Each gram of Derma-Smoothe/FS contains approximately 0.11 mg of fluocinolone acetonide in a blend of oils, which contains isopropyl alcohol, isopropyl myristate, light mineral oil, oleth-2, refined peanut oil and fragrances.

LIDEX AND SYNALAR

These preparations are all intended for topical administration.

Lidex preparations have as their active component the corticosteroid fluocinonide, which is the 21-acetate ester of fluocinolone acetonide and has the chemical name pregna-1,4-diene-3,20-dione, 21-(acetyloxy)-6,9-difluoro-11-hydroxy-16,17-[(1-methylethylidene)bis(oxy)]-,(6(α),11(β), 16(α))-.

Lidex Cream contains fluocinonide 0.5 mg/g in FAPG cream, a specially formulated cream base consisting of citric acid, 1,2,6-hexanetriol, polyethylene glycol 8000, propylene glycol and stearyl alcohol. This white cream vehicle is greaseless, non-staining, anhydrous and completely water miscible. The base provides emollient and hydrophilic properties. In this formulation, the active ingredient is totally in solution.

Lidex Gel contains fluocinonide 0.5 mg/g in a specially formulated gel base consisting of carbomer 940, edetate disodium, propyl gallate, propylene glycol, sodium hydroxide and/or hydrochloric acid (to adjust the pH), and water (purified). This clear, colorless, thixotropic vehicle is greaseless, non-staining and completely water miscible. In this formulation, the active ingredient is totally in solution.

Lidex Ointment contains fluocinonide 0.5 mg/g in a specially formulated ointment base consisting of glyceryl monostearate, white petrolatum, propylene carbonate, propylene glycol and white wax. It provides the occlusive and emollient effects desirable in an ointment. In this formulation, the active ingredient is totally in solution.

Lidex Topical Solution contains fluocinonide 0.5 mg/ml in a solution of alcohol (35%), citric acid, diisopropyl adipate, and propylene glycol. In this formulation, the active ingredient is totally in solution.

Lidex-E Cream contains fluocinonide 0.5 mg/g in a water-washable aqueous emollient base of cetyl alcohol, citric acid, mineral oil, polysorbate 60, propylene glycol, sorbitan monostearate, stearyl alcohol and water (purified).

Synalar preparations have as their active component the corticosteroid fluocinolone acetonide, which has the chemical name pregna-1,4-diene-3,20-dione,6,9-difluoro-11,21-dihydroxy-16,17-[(1-methylethylidene)bis(oxy)]-,(6(α),11(β), 16(α))-.

Synalar Cream contains fluocinolone acetonide 0.25 mg/g in a water-washable aqueous base of butylated hydroxytoluene, cetyl alcohol, citric acid, edetate disodium, methylparaben and propylparaben (preservatives), mineral oil, polyoxyl 20 cetostearyl ether, propylene glycol, simethicone, stearyl alcohol, water (purified) and white wax.

Synalar Ointment contains fluocinolone acetonide 0.25 mg/g in a white petroleum vehicle.

Synalar Topical Solution contains fluocinolone acetonide 0.1 mg/ml in a water-washable base of citric acid and propylene glycol.

Synemol Cream contains fluocinolone acetonide 0.25 mg/g in a water-washable aqueous emollient base of cetyl alcohol, citric acid, mineral oil, polysorbate 60, propylene glycol, sorbitan monostearate, stearyl alcohol and water (purified).

CLINICAL PHARMACOLOGY

DERMA-SMOOTHE/FS

Like other topical corticosteroids, fluocinolone acetonide has anti-inflammatory, antipruritic, and vasoconstrictive properties. The mechanism of the anti-inflammatory activity of the topical steroids, in general, is unclear. However, corticosteroids are thought to act by the induction of phospholipase A_2 inhibitory proteins, collectively called lipocortins. It is postulated that these proteins control the biosynthesis of potent mediators of inflammation such as prostaglandins and leukotrienes by inhibiting the release of their common precursor arachidonic acid. Arachidonic acid is released from membrane phospholipids by phospholipase A_2.

Pharmacokinetics

The extent of percutaneous absorption of topical corticosteroids is determined by many factors including the vehicle and the integrity of the epidermal barrier. Occlusion of topical corticosteroids can enhance penetration. Topical corticosteroids can be absorbed from normal intact skin.

Also, inflammation and/or other disease processes in the skin can increase percutaneous absorption.

Derma-Smoothe/FS is in the low to medium range of potency as compared with other topical corticosteroids.

LIDEX AND SYNALAR

Topical corticosteroids share anti-inflammatory, anti-pruritic and vasoconstrictive actions.

The mechanism of anti-inflammatory activity of the topical corticosteroids is unclear. Various laboratory methods, including vasoconstrictor assays, are used to compare and predict potencies and/or clinical efficacies of the topical corticosteroids. There is some evidence to suggest that a recognizable correlation exists between vasoconstrictor potency and therapeutic efficacy in man.

Pharmacokinetics

The extent of percutaneous absorption of topical corticosteroids is determined by many factors including the vehicle, the integrity of the epidermal barrier, and the use of occlusive dressings. A significantly greater amount of fluocinonide is absorbed from the solution than from the cream or gel formulations.

Topical corticosteroids can be absorbed from normal intact skin. Inflammation and/or other disease processes in the skin increase percutaneous absorption. Occlusive dressings substantially increase the percutaneous absorption of topical corticosteroids. Thus, occlusive dressings may be a valuable therapeutic adjunct for treatment of resistant dermatoses. (See DOSAGE AND ADMINISTRATION, Lidex and Synalar.)

Once absorbed through the skin, topical corticosteroids are handled through pharmacokinetic pathways similar to systemically administered corticosteroids. Corticosteroids are bound to plasma proteins in varying degrees. Corticosteroids are metabolized primarily in the liver and are then excreted by the kidneys. Some of the topical corticosteroids and their metabolites are also excreted into the bile.

INDICATIONS AND USAGE

DERMA-SMOOTHE/FS

Derma-Smoothe/FS is a low to medium potency corticosteroid indicated:

In adult patients for the treatment of atopic dermatitis or psoriasis of the scalp.

In pediatric patients 2 years and older with moderate to severe atopic dermatitis. It may be used for up to 4 weeks.

LIDEX AND SYNALAR

These products are indicated for the relief of the inflammatory and pruritic manifestations of corticosteroid-responsive dermatoses.

CONTRAINDICATIONS

DERMA-SMOOTHE/FS

Derma-Smoothe/FS is contraindicated in those patients with a history of hypersensitivity to any of the components of the preparation.

This product contains refined peanut oil (see PRECAUTIONS, Derma-Smoothe/FS).

LIDEX AND SYNALAR

Topical corticosteroids are contraindicated in those patients with a history of hypersensitivity to any of the components of the preparation.

PRECAUTIONS

DERMA-SMOOTHE/FS

General

Systemic absorption of topical corticosteroids can produce reversible hypothalamic-pituitary-adrenal (HPA) axis suppression with the potential for glucocorticosteroid insufficiency after withdrawal of treatment. Manifestations of Cushing's syndrome, hyperglycemia, and glucosuria can also be produced in some patients by systemic absorption of topical corticosteroids while on treatment.

Patients applying a topical steroid to a large surface area or to areas under occlusion should be evaluated periodically for evidence of HPA axis suppression. This may be done by using the ACTH stimulation, AM plasma cortisol, and urinary free cortisol tests.

If HPA axis suppression is noted, an attempt should be made to withdraw the drug, to reduce the frequency of application, or to substitute a less potent corticosteroid. Infrequently, signs and symptoms of glucocorticoid insufficiency may occur requiring supplemental systemic corticosteroids. For information on systemic supplementation, see prescribing information for those products.

Children may be more susceptible to systemic toxicity from equivalent doses due to their larger skin surface to body mass ratios. (See Pediatric Use.)

Allergic contact dermatitis to any component of topical corticosteroids is usually diagnosed by a *failure to heal* rather than noting a clinical exacerbation, which may occur with most topical products not containing corticosteroids. Such an observation should be corroborated with appropriate diagnostic testing.

If concomitant skin infections are present or develop, an appropriate antifungal or antibacterial agent should be used. If a favorable response does not occur promptly, use of Derma-Smoothe/FS should be discontinued until the infection has been adequately controlled.

If wheal and flare type reactions (which may be limited to pruritus) or other manifestations of hypersensitivity develop, Derma-Smoothe/FS should be discontinued immediately and appropriate therapy instituted. One peanut sensitive child experienced a flare of his atopic dermatitis during 2 weeks of twice daily treatment with Derma-Smoothe/FS.

Derma-Smoothe/FS is formulated with 48% refined peanut oil. Peanut oil used in this product is routinely tested for peanut proteins using a sandwich enzyme-linked immunosorbent assay test (S-ELISA) kit, which can detect peanut proteins to as low as 2.5 parts per million (ppm).

Physicians should use caution in prescribing Derma-Smoothe/FS for peanut-sensitive children.

Information for the Patient

Patients using topical corticosteroids should receive the following information and instructions:

This medication is to be used as directed by the physician. It is for external use only. Avoid contact with the eyes. In case of contact, wash eyes liberally with water.

This medication should not be used for any disorder other than that for which it was prescribed.

Patients should promptly report to their physician any worsening of their skin condition.

Parents of pediatric patients should be advised not to use Derma-Smoothe/FS in the treatment of diaper dermatitis. Derma-Smoothe/FS should not be applied to the diaper area as diapers or plastic pants may constitute occlusive dressing.

This medication should not be used on the face, underarm, or groin unless directed by the physician.

As with other corticosteroids, therapy should be discontinued when control is achieved. If no improvement is seen within 2 weeks, contact the physician.

Laboratory Tests

The following tests may be helpful in evaluating patients for HPA axis suppression:

ACTH stimulation test
AM plasma cortisol test
Urinary free cortisol test

Carcinogenesis, Mutagenesis, and Impairment of Fertility

Long-term animal studies have not been performed to evaluate the carcinogenic potential or the effect on fertility of Derma-Smoothe/FS. Studies have not been performed to evaluate the mutagenic potential of fluocinolone acetonide, the active ingredient in Derma-Smoothe/FS. Some corticosteroids have been found to be genotoxic in various genotoxicity tests (*i.e.*, the *in vitro* human peripheral blood lymphocyte chromosome aberration assay with metabolic activation, the *in vivo* mouse bone marrow micronucleus assay, the Chinese hamster micronucleus test and the *in vitro* mouse lymphoma gene mutation assay).

Pregnancy, Teratogenic Effects, Pregnancy Category C

Corticosteroids have been shown to be teratogenic in laboratory animals when administered systemically at relatively low dosage levels. Some corticosteroids have been shown to be teratogenic after dermal application in laboratory animals.

There are no adequate and well-controlled studies in pregnant women on teratogenic effects from Derma-Smoothe/FS. Therefore, Derma-Smoothe/FS should be used during pregnancy only if the potential benefit justifies the potential risk to the fetus.

Nursing Mothers

Systemically administered corticosteroids appear in human milk and could suppress growth, interfere with endogenous corticosteroid production, or cause other untoward effects. It is not known whether topical administration of corticosteroids could result in sufficient systemic absorption to produce detectable quantities in human milk. Because many drugs are excreted in human milk, caution should be exercised when Derma-Smoothe/FS is administered to a nursing woman.

Pediatric Use

Derma-Smoothe/FS may be used in pediatric patients 2 years and older with moderate to severe atopic dermatitis when used twice daily for no longer than 4 weeks. Derma-Smoothe/FS should not be applied to the face or diaper area. Application to intertriginous areas should be avoided due to the increased possibility of local adverse events such as striae, atrophy, and telangiectasia, which may be irreversible. The smallest amount of drug needed to cover the affected areas should be applied. Long-term safety in the pediatric population has not been established.

Because of a higher ratio of skin surface area to body mass, children are at a greater risk than adults of HPA-axis-suppression when they are treated with topical corticosteroids. They are therefore also at greater risk of glucocorticosteroid insufficiency after withdrawal of treatment and of Cushing's syndrome while on treatment. Adverse effects including striae have been reported with inappropriate use of topical corticosteroids in infants and children. (See PRECAUTIONS, Derma-Smoothe/FS.)

HPA axis suppression, Cushing's syndrome, and intracranial hypertension have been reported in children receiving topical corticosteroids. Children may be more susceptible to systemic toxicity from equivalent doses due to their larger skin surface to body mass ratios. Manifestations of adrenal suppression in children include linear growth retardation, delayed weight gain, low plasma cortisol levels, and absence of response to ACTH stimulation. Manifestations of intracranial hypertension include bulging fontanelles, headaches, and bilateral papilledema.

Derma-Smoothe/FS is formulated with 48% refined peanut oil, in which peanut protein is not detectable at 2.5 ppm. Physicians should use caution in prescribing Derma-Smoothe/FS for peanut sensitive individuals.

LIDEX AND SYNALAR

General

Systemic absorption of topical corticosteroids has produced reversible hypothalamic-pituitary-adrenal (HPA) axis suppression, manifestations of Cushing's syndrome, hyperglycemia, and glucosuria in some patients.

Conditions which augment systemic absorption include the application of the more potent steroids, use over large surface areas, prolonged use, and the addition of occlusive dressings.

Therefore, patients receiving a large dose of a potent topical steroid applied to a large surface area or under an occlusive dressing should be evaluated periodically for evidence of HPA axis suppression by using the urinary free cortisol and ACTH stimulation tests. If HPA axis suppression is noted, an attempt should be made to withdraw the drug, to reduce the frequency of application, or to substitute a less potent steroid.

Recovery of HPA axis function is generally prompt and complete upon discontinuation of the drug. Infrequently, signs and symptoms of steroid withdrawal may occur, requiring supplemental systemic corticosteroids.

Children may absorb proportionally larger amounts of topical corticosteroids and thus be more susceptible to systemic toxicity. (See Pediatric Use.) These preparations are not for ophthalmic use. Severe irritation is possible if fluocinonide solution contacts the eye. If that should occur, immediate flushing of the eye with a large volume of water is recommended.

If irritation develops, topical corticosteroids should be discontinued and appropriate therapy instituted.

As with any topical corticosteroid product, prolonged use may produce atrophy of the skin and subcutaneous tissues. When used on intertriginous or flexor areas, or on the face, this may occur even with short-term use.

In the presence of dermatological infections, the use of an appropriate antifungal or antibacterial agent should be instituted. If a favorable response does not occur promptly, the corticosteroid should be discontinued until the infection has been adequately controlled.

Information for the Patient

Patients using topical corticosteroids should receive the following information and instructions:

This medication is to be used as directed by the physician. It is for external use only. Avoid contact with the eyes.

Patients should be advised not to use this medication for any disorder other than that for which it was prescribed.

The treated skin area should not be bandaged or otherwise covered or wrapped as to be occlusive unless directed by the physician.

Patients should report any signs of local adverse reactions especially under occlusive dressing.

Parents of pediatric patients should be advised not to use tight-fitting diapers or plastic pants on a child being treated in the diaper area as these garments may constitute occlusive dressings.

Laboratory Tests

The following tests may be helpful in evaluating HPA axis suppression: Urinary free cortisol test and ACTH stimulation test.

Carcinogenesis, Mutagenesis, and Impairment of Fertility

Long-term animal studies have not been performed to evaluate the carcinogenic potential or the effect on fertility of topical corticosteroids.

Studies to determine mutagenicity with prednisolone and hydrocortisone have revealed negative results.

Pregnancy Category C

Corticosteroids are generally teratogenic in laboratory animals when administered systemically at relatively low dosage levels. The more potent corticosteroids have been shown to be teratogenic after dermal application in laboratory animals. There are no adequate and well-controlled studies in pregnant women on teratogenic effects from topically applied corticosteroids. Therefore, topical corticosteroids should be used during pregnancy only if the potential benefit justifies the potential risk to the fetus. Drugs of this class should not be used extensively on pregnant patients, in large amounts, or for prolonged periods of time.

Nursing Mothers

It is not known whether topical administration of corticosteroids could result in sufficient systemic absorption to produce detectable quantities in breast milk. Systemically administered corticosteroids are secreted into breast milk in quantities not likely to have a deleterious effect on the infant. Nevertheless, caution should be exercised when topical corticosteroids are administered to a nursing woman.

Pediatric Use

Pediatric patients may demonstrate greater susceptibility to topical corticosteroid-induced hypothalamic-pituitary-adrenal (HPA) axis suppression and Cushing's syndrome than mature patients because of a larger skin surface area to body weight ratio. HPA axis suppression, Cushing's syndrome, and intracranial hypertension have been reported in children receiving topical corticosteroids. Manifestations of adrenal suppression in children include linear growth retardation, delayed weight gain, low plasma cortisol levels, and absence of response to ACTH stimulation. Manifestations of intracranial hypertension include bulging fontanelles, headaches, and bilateral papilledema.

Administration of topical corticosteroids to children should be limited to the least amount compatible with an effective therapeutic regimen. Chronic corticosteroid therapy may interfere with the growth and development of children.

ADVERSE REACTIONS

DERMA-SMOOTHE/FS

The following local adverse reactions have been reported infrequently with topical corticosteroids. They may occur more frequently with the use of occlusive dressings, especially with higher potency corticosteroids. These reactions are listed in an approximate decreasing order of occurrence: burning, itching, irritation, dryness, folliculitis, acneiform eruptions, hypopigmentation, perioral dermatitis, allergic contact dermatitis, secondary infection, skin atrophy, striae, and miliaria. One peanut sensitive child experienced a flare of his atopic dermatitis during 2 weeks of twice daily treatment with Derma-Smoothe/FS.

LIDEX AND SYNALAR

The following local adverse reactions are reported infrequently with topical corticosteroids, but may occur more frequently with the use of occlusive dressings. These reactions are listed in an approximate decreasing order of occurrence: burning, itching, irritation, dryness, folliculitis, hypertrichosis, acneiform eruptions, hypopigmentation, perioral dermatitis, allergic contact dermatitis, maceration of the skin, secondary infection, skin atrophy, striae, miliaria.

DOSAGE AND ADMINISTRATION

DERMA-SMOOTHE/FS

Atopic dermatitis in adults:

For the treatment of atopic dermatitis, Derma-Smoothe/FS should be applied as a thin film to the affected area 3 times daily.

Scalp psoriasis in adults:

For the treatment of scalp psoriasis, wet or dampen hair and scalp thoroughly. Apply a thin film of Derma-Smoothe/FS on the scalp, massage well and cover scalp with the supplied shower cap. Leave on overnight or for a minimum of 4 hours before washing off. Wash hair with regular shampoo and rinse thoroughly.

Atopic dermatitis in pediatric patients 2 years and older:

Moisten skin. Apply Derma-Smoothe/FS as a thin film to the affected areas twice daily for no longer than 4 weeks.

LIDEX AND SYNALAR

Topical corticosteroids are generally applied to the affected area as a thin film from 2-4 times daily depending on the severity of the condition. In hairy sites, the hair should be parted to allow direct contact with the lesion.

Occlusive dressings may be used for the management of psoriasis or recalcitrant conditions. Some plastic films may be flammable and due care should be exercised in their use. Similarly, caution should be employed when such films are used on children or left in their proximity, to avoid the possibility of accidental suffocation.

If an infection develops, the use of occlusive dressings should be discontinued and appropriate antimicrobial therapy instituted.

HOW SUPPLIED

DERMA-SMOOTHE/FS

Derma-Smoothe/FS is supplied in bottles containing 4 fluid ounces.
Storage: Store between 20-25°C (68-77°F) in tightly closed containers.

LIDEX AND SYNALAR

Lidex (fluocinonide) Topical Solution 0.05% — Plastic squeeze bottles: 20 or 60 cc. *Storage:* Store at room temperature. Avoid excessive heat, above 40°C (104°F).

Lidex (fluocinonide) Cream 0.05% — 15, 30, 60 or 120 g tube. *Storage:* Store at room temperature. Avoid excessive heat, above 40°C (104°F).

Lidex (fluocinonide) Gel 0.05% — 15, 30, or 60 g tube. *Storage:* Store at controlled room temperature: 15°-30°C (59°-86°F).

Lidex (fluocinonide) Ointment 0.05% — 15, 30, 60 or 120 g tube.*Storage:* Store at room temperature. Avoid temperature over 30°C (86°F).

Lidex-E (fluocinonide) Cream 0.05% — 15, 30, or 60 g tube. *Storage:* Store at room temperature. Avoid excessive heat, above 40°C (104°F).

Synalar (fluocinolone acetonide) Cream 0.025% — 15 or 60 g tube. *Storage:* Store at room temperature; avoid freezing and excessive heat, above 40°C (104°F).

Synalar (fluocinolone acetonide) Topical Solution 0.01% — 20 or 60 cc. *Storage:* Store at room temperature. Avoid freezing.

Synalar (fluocinolone acetonide) Ointment 0.025% — 15 or 60 g tube. *Storage:* Store at room temperature, avoid freezing and excessive heat, above 40°C (104°F).

Synemol (fluocinolone acetonide) Cream 0.025% — 60 g tube. *Storage:* Store at room temperature. Avoid excessive heat, above 40°C (104°F).

PRODUCT LISTING - RATED THERAPEUTICALLY EQUIVALENT

Size	Price	Product	NDC
Cream - Topical - 0.01%			
15 gm	$1.50	GENERIC, Thames Pharmacal Company Inc	49158-0142-20
15 gm	$1.60	GENERIC, Moore, H.L. Drug Exchange Inc	00839-6346-47
15 gm	$1.65	GENERIC, Geneva Pharmaceuticals	00781-7003-27
15 gm	$1.66	GENERIC, Qualitest Products Inc	00603-7747-74
15 gm	$1.80	GENERIC, Interstate Drug Exchange Inc	00814-3188-93
15 gm	$1.95	GENERIC, Watson/Rugby Laboratories Inc	00536-4431-20
15 gm	$2.00	GENERIC, Clay-Park Laboratories Inc	45802-0067-35
15 gm	$2.10	GENERIC, Major Pharmaceuticals Inc	00904-2660-36
15 gm	$2.22	GENERIC, Fougera	00168-0058-15
60 gm	$3.20	GENERIC, Thames Pharmacal Company Inc	49158-0142-24
60 gm	$3.36	GENERIC, Moore, H.L. Drug Exchange Inc	00839-6346-50
60 gm	$3.60	GENERIC, Geneva Pharmaceuticals	00781-7003-35
60 gm	$3.74	GENERIC, Qualitest Products Inc	00603-7747-88
60 gm	$4.10	GENERIC, Major Pharmaceuticals Inc	00904-2660-02
60 gm	$4.13	GENERIC, Interstate Drug Exchange Inc	00814-3188-91
60 gm	$4.20	GENERIC, Ivax Corporation	00182-1149-52
60 gm	$4.25	GENERIC, Cmc-Consolidated Midland Corporation	00223-4297-60
60 gm	$4.55	GENERIC, Fougera	00168-0058-60
60 gm	$4.70	GENERIC, Clay-Park Laboratories Inc	45802-0067-37
100 gm	$1.95	GENERIC, Cmc-Consolidated Midland Corporation	00223-4297-15
425 gm	$11.90	GENERIC, Clay-Park Laboratories Inc	45802-0067-38
425 gm	$13.98	GENERIC, Thames Pharmacal Company Inc	49158-0142-23
425 gm	$17.50	GENERIC, Cmc-Consolidated Midland Corporation	00223-4297-13
Cream - Topical - 0.025%			
15 gm	$1.67	GENERIC, Moore, H.L. Drug Exchange Inc	00839-6347-47
15 gm	$1.80	GENERIC, Thames Pharmacal Company Inc	49158-0143-20
15 gm	$2.00	GENERIC, Major Pharmaceuticals Inc	00904-2659-36
15 gm	$2.25	GENERIC, Interstate Drug Exchange Inc	00814-3190-93
15 gm	$2.35	GENERIC, Geneva Pharmaceuticals	00781-7001-27
15 gm	$2.50	GENERIC, Cmc-Consolidated Midland Corporation	00223-4296-15
15 gm	$2.70	GENERIC, Ivax Corporation	00182-1150-51
15 gm	$2.90	GENERIC, Qualitest Products Inc	00603-7748-74
15 gm	$2.90	GENERIC, Clay-Park Laboratories Inc	45802-0068-35
15 gm	$3.05	GENERIC, Fougera	00168-0060-15
15 gm	$14.44	SYNEMOL, Syntex Laboratories Inc	00033-2509-13
15 gm	$26.13	SYNALAR, Medicis Dermatologics Inc	99207-0501-13
60 gm	$3.81	GENERIC, Moore, H.L. Drug Exchange Inc	00839-6347-50
60 gm	$4.20	GENERIC, Thames Pharmacal Company Inc	49158-0143-24
60 gm	$4.41	GENERIC, Qualitest Products Inc	00603-7748-88
60 gm	$4.75	GENERIC, Ivax Corporation	00182-1150-52
60 gm	$4.90	GENERIC, Geneva Pharmaceuticals	00781-7001-35
60 gm	$5.40	GENERIC, Interstate Drug Exchange Inc	00814-3190-91
60 gm	$5.75	GENERIC, Clay-Park Laboratories Inc	45802-0068-37
60 gm	$6.58	GENERIC, Major Pharmaceuticals Inc	00904-2659-02
60 gm	$7.20	GENERIC, Fougera	00168-0060-60
60 gm	$7.25	GENERIC, Cmc-Consolidated Midland Corporation	00223-4296-60
60 gm	$61.41	SYNALAR, Medicis Dermatologics Inc	99207-0501-17
100 gm	$4.95	GENERIC, Cmc-Consolidated Midland Corporation	00223-4290-15
100 gm	$10.75	GENERIC, Cmc-Consolidated Midland Corporation	00223-4290-60
425 gm	$25.37	GENERIC, Clay-Park Laboratories Inc	45802-0068-38
425 gm	$26.56	GENERIC, Major Pharmaceuticals Inc	00904-2659-27
425 gm	$27.50	GENERIC, Thames Pharmacal Company Inc	49158-0143-23
425 gm	$45.00	GENERIC, Cmc-Consolidated Midland Corporation	00223-4296-13
Ointment - Topical - 0.025%			
15 gm	$4.00	GENERIC, Major Pharmaceuticals Inc	00904-2580-36
15 gm	$4.15	GENERIC, Watson/Rugby Laboratories Inc	00536-4462-20
15 gm	$4.20	GENERIC, Fougera	00168-0064-15
15 gm	$16.41	SYNALAR, Physicians Total Care	54868-2448-03
15 gm	$22.93	SYNALAR, Medicis Dermatologics Inc	99207-0504-13
30 gm	$22.04	SYNALAR, Physicians Total Care	54868-2448-01
60 gm	$9.95	GENERIC, Major Pharmaceuticals Inc	00904-2580-02
60 gm	$9.96	GENERIC, Fougera	00168-0064-60
60 gm	$39.27	SYNALAR, Physicians Total Care	54868-2448-02
60 gm	$61.42	SYNALAR, Medicis Dermatologics Inc	99207-0504-17
Solution - Topical - 0.01%			
20 ml	$3.95	GENERIC, Major Pharmaceuticals Inc	00904-2661-55
20 ml	$4.17	GENERIC, Moore, H.L. Drug Exchange Inc	00839-6660-97
20 ml	$4.60	GENERIC, Geneva Pharmaceuticals	00781-6304-80
20 ml	$32.74	SYNALAR, Medicis Dermatologics Inc	99207-0506-44
60 ml	$7.03	FEDERAL UPPER LIMIT, H.C.F.A. F F P	99999-1306-01
60 ml	$9.00	GENERIC, Watson/Schein Pharmaceuticals Inc	00364-7343-58
60 ml	$9.30	GENERIC, Interstate Drug Exchange Inc	00814-3195-74
60 ml	$9.93	GENERIC, Moore, H.L. Drug Exchange Inc	00839-6660-64
60 ml	$10.60	GENERIC, Geneva Pharmaceuticals	00781-6304-61
60 ml	$10.60	GENERIC, Major Pharmaceuticals Inc	00904-2661-03
60 ml	$10.60	GENERIC, Allscripts Pharmaceutical Company	54569-3393-00
60 ml	$10.80	GENERIC, Ivax Corporation	00182-1564-68
60 ml	$11.00	GENERIC, Fougera	00168-0059-60

60 ml	$40.04	FLUONID, Allergan Inc	00023-0878-60
60 ml	$64.78	SYNALAR, Medicis Dermatologics Inc	99207-0506-46
100 ml	$5.00	GENERIC, Cmc-Consolidated Midland Corporation	00223-6180-20
100 ml	$11.50	GENERIC, Cmc-Consolidated Midland Corporation	00223-6180-60
Solution - Topical - 0.025%			
60 ml	$12.30	GENERIC, Ivax Corporation	00182-5015-52

PRODUCT LISTING - RATED NOT THERAPEUTICALLY EQUIVALENT

Kit - Topical - 0.01%			
1's	$38.46	DERMA-SMOOTHE/FS ATOPIC PAK, Hill Dermaceuticals Inc	28105-0125-12
Shampoo - Topical - 0.01%			
120 ml	$34.75	CAPEX, Galderma Laboratories Inc	00299-5500-04

PRODUCT LISTING - EQUIVALENTS NOT AVAILABLE

Cream - Topical - 0.01%			
15 gm	$2.27	GENERIC, Allscripts Pharmaceutical Company	54569-1544-00
15 gm	$2.50	GENERIC, Raway Pharmacal Inc	00686-0142-20
15 gm	$4.78	GENERIC, Southwood Pharmaceuticals Inc	58016-3083-01
15 gm	$12.95	GENERIC, Pharma Pac	52959-0314-00
60 gm	$4.95	GENERIC, Raway Pharmacal Inc	00686-0142-24
Cream - Topical - 0.025%			
15 gm	$3.05	GENERIC, Allscripts Pharmaceutical Company	54569-3390-00
15 gm	$3.10	GENERIC, Raway Pharmacal Inc	00686-6838-35
15 gm	$4.40	GENERIC, Prescript Pharmaceuticals	00247-0394-15
15 gm	$4.64	GENERIC, Southwood Pharmaceuticals Inc	58016-3104-01
60 gm	$4.00	GENERIC, Raway Pharmacal Inc	00686-0068-37
Cream - Topical - 0.2%			
12 gm	$27.33	SYNALAR-HP, Syntex Laboratories Inc	00033-2503-12
Lotion - Topical - 0.01%			
60 ml	$2.98	GENERIC, Raway Pharmacal Inc	00686-0067-37
Oil - Topical - 0.01%			
120 ml	$25.00	DERMA-SMOOTH/FS, Hill Dermaceuticals Inc	28105-0149-04
120 ml	$33.60	DERMA-SMOOTH/FS, Hill Dermaceuticals Inc	28105-0150-04
Solution - Topical - 0.01%			
20 ml	$6.60	GENERIC, Thames Pharmacal Company Inc	49158-0209-40
60 ml	$13.20	GENERIC, Thames Pharmacal Company Inc	49158-0209-32

Fluocinolone Acetonide; Hydroquinone; Tretinoin *(003551)*

For complete prescribing information, refer to the CD-ROM included with the book.

Categories: Melasma; Pregnancy Category C; FDA Approved 2002 Jan
Drug Classes: Corticosteroids, topical; Depigmenting agents; Dermatologics; Keratolytics; Retinoids
Brand Names: Tri-Luma
Cost of Therapy: $86.40 (Melasma; Tri-Luma Cream; 0.01%; 4%; 0.05%; 1 application/day; variable day supply)

DESCRIPTION

Note: The trade name has been used throughout this monograph for clarity.

For External Use Only.

Not for Ophthalmic Use.

Tri-Luma cream (fluocinolone acetonide 0.01%, hydroquinone 4%, tretinoin 0.05%) contains fluocinolone acetonide, hydroquinone, and tretinoin, in a hydrophilic cream base for topical application.

FLUOCINOLONE ACETONIDE

Fluocinolone acetonide is a synthetic fluorinated corticosteroid for topical dermatological use and is classified therapeutically as an anti-inflammatory. It is a white crystalline powder that is odorless and stable in light.

The chemical name for fluocinolone acetonide is: (6α,11β,16α)-6,9-difluoro-11,21-dihydroxy-16,17-[(1-methylethylidene)bis(oxy)]-pregna-1,-4-diene-3,20-dione.

The molecular formula is $C_{24}H_{30}F_2O_6$ and molecular weight is 452.50.

HYDROQUINONE

Hydroquinone is classified therapeutically as a depigmenting agent. It is prepared from the reduction of *p*-benzoquinone with sodium bisulfite. It occurs as fine white needles that darken on exposure to air.

The chemical name for hydroquinone is: 1,4-benzenediol.

The molecular formula is $C_6H_6O_2$ and molecular weight is 110.11.

TRETINOIN

Tretinoin is all-*trans*-retinoic acid formed from the oxidation of the aldehyde group of retinene to a carboxyl group. It occurs as yellow to light-orange crystals or crystalline powder with a characteristic odor of ensilage. It is highly reactive to light and moisture.

Tretinoin is classified therapeutically as a keratolytic.

The chemical name for tretinoin is: *(all-E)*-3,7-dimethyl-9-(2,6,6-trimethyl-1-cyclohexen-1-yl)-2,4,6,8-nonatetraenoic acid.

The molecular formula is $C_{20}H_{28}O_2$ and molecular weight is 300.44.

TRI-LUMA

Each gram of Tri-Luma cream contains:

Active: Fluocinolone acetonide 0.01% (0.1 mg), hydroquinone 4% (40 mg), and tretinoin 0.05% (0.5 mg).

Inactive: Butylated hydroxytoluene, cetyl alcohol, citric acid, glycerin, glyceryl stearate, magnesium aluminum silicate, methyl gluceth-10, methylparaben, PEG-100 stearate, propylparaben, purified water, sodium metabisulfite, stearic acid, and stearyl alcohol.

INDICATIONS AND USAGE

Tri-Luma cream is indicated for the short-term treatment of moderate to severe melasma of the face, in the presence of measures for sun avoidance, including the use of sunscreens.

The following are important statements relating to the indication and usage of Tri-Luma cream:

Tri-Luma cream, a combination drug product containing corticosteroid, retinoid, and bleaching agent, is NOT indicated for the maintenance treatment of melasma. After achieving control with Tri-Luma cream, some patients may be managed with other treatments instead of triple therapy with Tri-Luma cream. Because melasma usually recurs upon discontinuation of Tri-Luma cream, patients need to avoid sunlight exposure, use sunscreen with appropriate SPF, wear protective clothing, and change to non-hormonal forms of birth control, if hormonal methods are used.

In clinical trials used to support the use of Tri-Luma cream in the treatment of melasma, patients were instructed to avoid sunlight exposure to the face, wear protective clothing and use a sunscreen with SPF 30 each day. They were to apply the study medication each night, after washing their face with a mild soapless cleanser.

The safety and efficacy of Tri-Luma cream in patients of skin types V and VI have not been studied. Excessive bleaching resulting in undesirable cosmetic effect in patients with darker skin cannot be excluded.

The safety and efficacy of Tri-Luma cream in the treatment of hyperpigmentation conditions other than melasma of the face have not been studied.

Because pregnant and lactating women were excluded from, and women of child-bearing potential had to use birth control measures in the clinical trials, the safety and efficacy of Tri-Luma cream in pregnant women and nursing mothers have not been established.

CONTRAINDICATIONS

Tri-Luma cream is contraindicated in individuals with a history of hypersensitivity, allergy, or intolerance to this product or any of its components.

WARNINGS

Tri-Luma cream contains sodium metabisulfite, a sulfite that may cause allergic-type reactions including anaphylactic symptoms and life-threatening asthmatic episodes in susceptible people.

Tri-Luma cream contains hydroquinone, which may produce exogenous ochronosis, a gradual blue-black darkening of the skin, whose occurrence should prompt discontinuation of therapy. The majority of patients developing this condition are Black, but it may also occur in Caucasians and Hispanics.

Cutaneous hypersensitivity to the active ingredients of Tri-Luma cream has been reported in the literature. In a patch test study to determine sensitization potential in 221 healthy volunteers, 3 volunteers developed sensitivity reactions to Tri-Luma cream or its components.

DOSAGE AND ADMINISTRATION

Tri-Luma cream should be applied once daily at night. It should be applied at least 30 minutes before bedtime.

Gently wash the face and neck with a mild cleanser. Rinse and pat the skin dry. Apply a thin film of the cream to the hyperpigmented areas of melasma including about ½ inch of normal appearing skin surrounding each lesion. Rub lightly and uniformly into the skin. Do not use occlusive dressing.

During the day, use a sunscreen of SPF 30, and wear protective clothing. Avoid sunlight exposure. Patients may use moisturizers and/or cosmetics during the day.

PRODUCT LISTING - EQUIVALENTS NOT AVAILABLE

Cream - Topical - 0.01%;4%;0.05%			
30 gm	$86.40	TRI-LUMA, Hill Dermaceuticals Inc	28105-0300-30
30 gm	$92.50	TRI-LUMA, Galderma Laboratories Inc	00299-5950-30

Fluocinonide (001310)

Categories: Dermatosis, corticosteroid-responsive; Pregnancy Category C; FDA Approved 1971 Jun
Drug Classes: Corticosteroids, topical; Dermatologics
Brand Names: **Lidex**; Lidex-E
Foreign Brand Availability: Bestasone (Japan); Biscosal (Japan); Cusigel (Spain); Flu-21 (Italy); Flubiol (Japan); Gelisyn (Mexico); Klariderm (Spain); Lidemol (Canada; Philippines); Lyderm (Canada); Metosyn (Bahamas; Barbados; Belize; Benin; Bermuda; Burkina-Faso; Curacao; Czech-Republic; Denmark; England; Ethiopia; Finland; Gambia; Ghana; Guinea; Guyana; Ireland; Ivory-Coast; Jamaica; Kenya; Liberia; Malawi; Malaysia; Mali; Mauritania; Mauritius; Morocco; Netherland-Antilles; Niger; Nigeria; Norway; Senegal; Seychelles; Sierra-Leone; Sudan; Surinam; Tanzania; Trinidad; Tunia; Uganda; Zambia; Zimbabwe); Novoter (Malaysia; Spain); Rawracid (Japan); Tohsino (Japan); Topsym (Austria; Bahrain; Cyprus; Ecuador; Egypt; Germany; Iran; Iraq; Japan; Jordan; Kuwait; Lebanon; Libya; Oman; Peru; Portugal; Qatar; Republic-of-Yemen; Saudi-Arabia; Switzerland; Syria; Taiwan; United-Arab-Emirates); Topsym F (Austria; Switzerland); Topsymin (Switzerland); Topsyn (Canada; Italy); Topsyne (Netherlands)

DESCRIPTION

For prescribing information, please see Fluocinolone Acetonide

PRODUCT LISTING - RATED THERAPEUTICALLY EQUIVALENT

Cream - Topical - 0.05%

Size	Price	Manufacturer	NDC
15 gm	$3.20	GENERIC, Thames Pharmacal Company Inc	49158-0212-20
15 gm	$5.93	GENERIC, Interstate Drug Exchange Inc	00814-3200-93
15 gm	$6.60	GENERIC, Moore, H.L. Drug Exchange Inc	00839-7698-47
15 gm	$6.89	GENERIC, Genetco Inc	00302-3010-15
15 gm	$7.30	GENERIC, Major Pharmaceuticals Inc	00904-0770-36
15 gm	$7.32	GENERIC, Qualitest Products Inc	00603-7759-74
15 gm	$7.88	GENERIC, Clay-Park Laboratories Inc	45802-0017-35
15 gm	$7.90	GENERIC, Moore, H.L. Drug Exchange Inc	00839-7013-47
15 gm	$8.85	GENERIC, Ivax Corporation	00182-1731-51
15 gm	$8.97	GENERIC, Teva Pharmaceuticals Usa	00093-0262-15
15 gm	$9.00	GENERIC, Fougera	00168-0139-15
15 gm	$10.00	GENERIC, Alpharma Uspd Makers Of Barre and Nmc	00472-3901-15
15 gm	$10.45	GENERIC, Major Pharmaceuticals Inc	00904-0773-36
15 gm	$11.95	GENERIC, Moore, H.L. Drug Exchange Inc	00839-7758-47
15 gm	$12.35	GENERIC, Qualitest Products Inc	00603-7763-74
15 gm	$13.55	GENERIC, Taro Pharmaceuticals U.S.A. Inc	51672-1253-01
15 gm	$16.36	GENERIC, Watson Laboratories Inc	52544-0449-73
15 gm	$19.90	GENERIC, Teva Pharmaceuticals Usa	00093-0263-15
15 gm	$19.90	GENERIC, Taro Pharmaceuticals U.S.A. Inc	51672-1254-01
15 gm	$21.04	GENERIC, Alpharma Uspd Makers Of Barre and Nmc	00472-0392-15
15 gm	$28.69	LIDEX-E, Medicis Dermatologics Inc	99207-0513-13
15 gm	$30.41	LIDEX, Medicis Dermatologics Inc	99207-0511-13
30 gm	$7.30	GENERIC, Thames Pharmacal Company Inc	49158-0212-68
30 gm	$9.68	GENERIC, Qualitest Products Inc	00603-7759-78
30 gm	$10.15	GENERIC, Major Pharmaceuticals Inc	00904-0770-31
30 gm	$10.25	GENERIC, Moore, H.L. Drug Exchange Inc	00839-7013-49
30 gm	$10.25	GENERIC, Moore, H.L. Drug Exchange Inc	00839-7698-49
30 gm	$12.40	GENERIC, Ivax Corporation	00182-1731-56
30 gm	$12.53	GENERIC, Fougera	00168-0139-30
30 gm	$12.67	GENERIC, Clay-Park Laboratories Inc	45802-0017-11
30 gm	$13.02	GENERIC, Teva Pharmaceuticals Usa	00093-0262-30
30 gm	$13.90	GENERIC, Taro Pharmaceuticals U.S.A. Inc	51672-1253-02
30 gm	$14.00	GENERIC, Alpharma Uspd Makers Of Barre and Nmc	00472-3901-30
30 gm	$14.00	GENERIC, Watson/Rugby Laboratories Inc	52544-0447-03
30 gm	$15.75	GENERIC, Major Pharmaceuticals Inc	00904-0773-31
30 gm	$16.60	GENERIC, Ivax Corporation	00182-5051-56
30 gm	$17.48	GENERIC, Moore, H.L. Drug Exchange Inc	00839-7758-49
30 gm	$27.50	GENERIC, Teva Pharmaceuticals Usa	00093-0263-30
30 gm	$27.50	GENERIC, Taro Pharmaceuticals U.S.A. Inc	51672-1254-02
30 gm	$29.17	GENERIC, Alpharma Uspd Makers Of Barre and Nmc	00472-0392-30
30 gm	$43.41	LIDEX-E, Medicis Dermatologics Inc	99207-0513-14
30 gm	$43.43	LIDEX, Medicis Dermatologics Inc	99207-0511-14
60 gm	$8.27	GENERIC, Thames Pharmacal Company Inc	49158-0212-24
60 gm	$10.73	FEDERAL UPPER LIMIT, H.C.F.A. F F P	99999-1310-03
60 gm	$13.37	GENERIC, Moore, H.L. Drug Exchange Inc	00839-7698-50
60 gm	$14.93	GENERIC, Interstate Drug Exchange Inc	00814-3200-91
60 gm	$16.05	GENERIC, Moore, H.L. Drug Exchange Inc	00839-7013-50
60 gm	$16.26	GENERIC, Qualitest Products Inc	00603-7759-88
60 gm	$16.50	GENERIC, Major Pharmaceuticals Inc	00904-0770-02
60 gm	$18.60	GENERIC, Clay-Park Laboratories Inc	45802-0017-37
60 gm	$19.25	GENERIC, Major Pharmaceuticals Inc	00904-0773-02
60 gm	$21.00	GENERIC, Fougera	00168-0139-60
60 gm	$21.84	GENERIC, Teva Pharmaceuticals Usa	00093-0262-92
60 gm	$23.50	GENERIC, Alpharma Uspd Makers Of Barre and Nmc	00472-3901-60
60 gm	$23.72	GENERIC, Taro Pharmaceuticals U.S.A. Inc	51672-1253-03
60 gm	$24.50	GENERIC, Watson/Rugby Laboratories Inc	52544-0447-06
60 gm	$25.68	GENERIC, Geneva Pharmaceuticals	00781-7103-35
60 gm	$25.91	GENERIC, Moore, H.L. Drug Exchange Inc	00839-7589-50
60 gm	$27.75	GENERIC, Qualitest Products Inc	00603-7763-88
60 gm	$46.00	GENERIC, Teva Pharmaceuticals Usa	00093-0263-92
60 gm	$46.00	GENERIC, Taro Pharmaceuticals U.S.A. Inc	51672-1254-03
60 gm	$48.93	GENERIC, Alpharma Uspd Makers Of Barre and Nmc	00472-0392-60
60 gm	$72.84	LIDEX, Medicis Dermatologics Inc	99207-0511-17
60 gm	$72.84	LIDEX-E, Medicis Dermatologics Inc	99207-0513-17
120 gm	$22.00	GENERIC, Moore, H.L. Drug Exchange Inc	00839-7698-53
120 gm	$26.95	GENERIC, Major Pharmaceuticals Inc	00904-0770-22
120 gm	$30.00	GENERIC, Clay-Park Laboratories Inc	45802-0017-13
120 gm	$35.05	GENERIC, Ivax Corporation	00182-1731-57
120 gm	$44.65	GENERIC, Major Pharmaceuticals Inc	00904-0773-22
120 gm	$77.00	GENERIC, Taro Pharmaceuticals U.S.A. Inc	51672-1253-04
120 gm	$103.82	LIDEX, Medicis Dermatologics Inc	99207-0511-22

Gel - Topical - 0.05%

Size	Price	Manufacturer	NDC
15 gm	$20.87	GENERIC, Taro Pharmaceuticals U.S.A. Inc	51672-1279-01
15 gm	$21.01	GENERIC, Fougera	00168-0135-15
15 gm	$31.33	LIDEX, Medicis Dermatologics Inc	99207-0507-13
30 gm	$27.40	GENERIC, Taro Pharmaceuticals U.S.A. Inc	51672-1279-02
30 gm	$43.41	LIDEX, Medicis Dermatologics Inc	99207-0507-14
60 gm	$29.79	FEDERAL UPPER LIMIT, H.C.F.A. F F P	99999-1310-08
60 gm	$41.46	GENERIC, Moore, H.L. Drug Exchange Inc	00839-7590-50
60 gm	$46.01	GENERIC, Teva Pharmaceuticals Usa	00093-0265-92
60 gm	$48.55	GENERIC, Taro Pharmaceuticals U.S.A. Inc	51672-1279-03
60 gm	$48.83	GENERIC, Fougera	00168-0135-60
60 gm	$72.84	LIDEX, Medicis Dermatologics Inc	99207-0507-17

Ointment - Topical - 0.05%

Size	Price	Manufacturer	NDC
15 gm	$15.00	GENERIC, Qualitest Products Inc	00603-7761-74
15 gm	$15.25	GENERIC, Major Pharmaceuticals Inc	00904-7677-36
15 gm	$18.43	GENERIC, Moore, H.L. Drug Exchange Inc	00839-7731-47
15 gm	$19.91	FLUOCINONIDE, Teva Pharmaceuticals Usa	00093-0264-15
15 gm	$20.85	GENERIC, Fougera	00168-0140-15
15 gm	$21.04	GENERIC, Taro Pharmaceuticals U.S.A. Inc	51672-1264-01
15 gm	$23.64	LIDEX, Allscripts Pharmaceutical Company	54569-0769-00
15 gm	$31.33	LIDEX, Medicis Dermatologics Inc	99207-0514-13
30 gm	$21.00	GENERIC, Qualitest Products Inc	00603-7761-78
30 gm	$25.64	GENERIC, Moore, H.L. Drug Exchange Inc	00839-7731-49
30 gm	$27.51	GENERIC, Teva Pharmaceuticals Usa	00093-0264-30
30 gm	$28.90	GENERIC, Fougera	00168-0140-30
30 gm	$29.19	GENERIC, Taro Pharmaceuticals U.S.A. Inc	51672-1264-02
30 gm	$43.41	LIDEX, Medicis Dermatologics Inc	99207-0514-14
60 gm	$21.85	GENERIC, Major Pharmaceuticals Inc	00904-7677-31
60 gm	$34.35	GENERIC, Qualitest Products Inc	00603-7761-88
60 gm	$35.00	GENERIC, Major Pharmaceuticals Inc	00904-7677-02
60 gm	$42.11	GENERIC, Moore, H.L. Drug Exchange Inc	00839-7731-50
60 gm	$46.01	GENERIC, Teva Pharmaceuticals Usa	00093-0264-92
60 gm	$48.49	GENERIC, Fougera	00168-0140-60
60 gm	$49.00	GENERIC, Taro Pharmaceuticals U.S.A. Inc	51672-1264-03
60 gm	$72.84	LIDEX, Medicis Dermatologics Inc	99207-0514-17

Solution - Topical - 0.05%

Size	Price	Manufacturer	NDC
20 ml	$8.70	GENERIC, Thames Pharmacal Company Inc	49158-0316-54
20 ml	$16.88	GENERIC, Taro Pharmaceuticals U.S.A. Inc	51672-1273-02
20 ml	$32.65	LIDEX, Medicis Dermatologics Inc	99207-0517-44
60 ml	$14.90	FEDERAL UPPER LIMIT, H.C.F.A. F F P	99999-1310-15
60 ml	$18.75	GENERIC, Thames Pharmacal Company Inc	49158-0316-48
60 ml	$20.48	GENERIC, Qualitest Products Inc	00603-1230-49
60 ml	$21.59	GENERIC, Moore, H.L. Drug Exchange Inc	00839-7583-64
60 ml	$23.58	GENERIC, Geneva Pharmaceuticals	00781-6308-61
60 ml	$24.15	GENERIC, Alpharma Uspd Makers Of Barre and Nmc	00472-0829-02
60 ml	$25.45	GENERIC, Major Pharmaceuticals Inc	00904-0769-03
60 ml	$26.08	GENERIC, Fougera	00168-0134-60
60 ml	$26.18	GENERIC, Teva Pharmaceuticals Usa	00093-0266-39
60 ml	$26.18	GENERIC, Ivax Corporation	00182-5050-68
60 ml	$27.00	GENERIC, Taro Pharmaceuticals U.S.A. Inc	51672-1273-04
60 ml	$70.59	LIDEX, Medicis Dermatologics Inc	99207-0517-46

PRODUCT LISTING - EQUIVALENTS NOT AVAILABLE

Size	Price	Product	NDC
Cream - Topical - 0.05%			
15 gm	$7.22	GENERIC, Prescript Pharmaceuticals	00247-0010-15
15 gm	$7.55	GENERIC, Allscripts Pharmaceutical Company	54569-2177-00
15 gm	$7.55	GENERIC, Allscripts Pharmaceutical Company	54569-7062-00
15 gm	$9.61	GENERIC, Prescript Pharmaceuticals	00247-0076-15
15 gm	$23.29	GENERIC, Southwood Pharmaceuticals Inc	58016-3042-01
15 gm	$25.36	GENERIC, Pharma Pac	52959-0093-01
30 gm	$11.09	GENERIC, Prescript Pharmaceuticals	00247-0010-30
30 gm	$12.00	GENERIC, Pedinol Pharmacal Inc	00884-5793-01
30 gm	$15.25	GENERIC, Allscripts Pharmaceutical Company	54569-3887-00
30 gm	$24.90	GENERIC, Southwood Pharmaceuticals Inc	58016-3121-01
30 gm	$30.35	GENERIC, Pharma Pac	52959-0093-03
60 gm	$25.39	GENERIC, Allscripts Pharmaceutical Company	54569-2275-00
60 gm	$48.98	GENERIC, Pharma Pac	52959-0093-02
Gel - Topical - 0.05%			
60 gm	$52.55	GENERIC, Southwood Pharmaceuticals Inc	58016-3274-01
Ointment - Topical - 0.05%			
15 gm	$19.91	GENERIC, Allscripts Pharmaceutical Company	54569-4210-00
15 gm	$22.15	GENERIC, Pharma Pac	52959-0315-01
30 gm	$30.50	GENERIC, Pharma Pac	52959-0315-03
Solution - Topical - 0.05%			
60 ml	$23.90	GENERIC, Alpharma Uspd Makers Of Barre and Nmc	23317-0393-60

Fluoride; Polyvitamin *(001314)*

Categories: Caries, dental, prevention; Nutrition, supplement; FDA Pre 1938 Drugs
Drug Classes: Vitamins/minerals
Brand Names: Bio-Poly-Flor; Florvite; Multi Vita-Bets; Multiple Vitamins W/Fluoride; Multivitamins W/Fluoride; Mulvidren-F; Poly-Flor; Poly-V; **Poly-Vi-Flor**; Poly-Vi-Tab W/Fluoride; Poly-Vites W/Fluoride; Polytab-F; Polyvite/Fluoride; Soluvite; Uni-Multi-Fluor; V-Fluorodex; Vi-Daylin/F; Vitastex-F

DESCRIPTION

CHEWABLE TABLETS

Active Ingredient for Caries Prophylaxis: Fluoride as sodium fluoride.

Other Ingredients: Ascorbic acid, cholecalciferol (0.25 and 0.5 mg only), colloidal silicon dioxide, cyanocobalamin (0.25 and 0.5 mg only), dextrates, FD&C blue no. 2 (aluminum lake), FD&C red no. 40 (aluminum lake), FD&C yellow no. 6 (aluminum lake), folic acid, fruit flavors (artificial), lactose (0.25 and 0.5 mg only), magnesium stearate, niacinamide, pyridoxine hydrochloride (0.25 and 0.5 mg only), riboflavin, silica gel, sodium ascorbate, sodium chloride, sucrose, thiamin mononitrate, dl-alpha-tocopheryl acetate (0.25 and 0.5 mg only), vitamin A acetate. *Additional Ingredients for the 1.0 mg Chewable Tablets:* Vitamin B_6 hydrochloride, vitamin B_{12}, vitamin D_3, and vitamin E acetate.

TABLE 1 *Nutrition Facts, Chewable Tablets*

Amount Per Tablet	% DV Adults & Children 4 Years or More
Vitamin A 2500 IU	50%
Vitamin C 60 mg	100%
Vitamin D 400 IU	100%
Vitamin E 15 IU	50%
Thiamin 1.05 mg	70%
Riboflavin 1.2 mg	70%
Niacin 13.5 mg	68%
Vitamin B_6 1.05 mg	53%
Folate 0.3 mg	75%
Vitamin B_{12} 4.5 µg	75%
Fluoride 0.25 mg (0.25 mg tablets); 0.5 mg (0.5 mg tablets); and 1 mg (1 mg tablets)	*

* Daily Value (DV) not established.

DROPS

Active Ingredient for Caries Prophylaxis: Fluoride as sodium fluoride.

Other Ingredients: Ascorbic acid, caramel color, cholecalciferol, cyanocobalamin, ferrous sulfate, fruit flavor (artificial), glycerin, niacinamide, polysorbate 80, pyridoxine hydrochloride, riboflavin-5-phosphate sodium, thiamin hydrochloride, d-alpha-tocopheryl acid succinate, vitamin A palmitate, water, and other ingredients.

CLINICAL PHARMACOLOGY

It is well established that fluoridation of the water supply (1 ppm fluoride) during the period of tooth development leads to a significant decrease in the incidence of dental caries.

Fluoride; polyvitamin 0.5 mg tablets provide sodium fluoride (0.5 mg fluoride) and ten essential vitamins in a chewable tablet. Because the tablets are chewable, they provide a *topical* as well as *systemic* source of fluoride.[1,2]

Hydroxyapatite is the principal crystal for all calcified tissue in the human body. The fluoride ion reacts with the *hydroxyapatite* in the tooth as it is formed to produce the more caries-resistant crystal, *fluorapatite.* The reaction may be expressed by the equation:[3]

$$Ca_{10}(PO_4)_6(OH)_2 + 2F^- \rightarrow Ca_{10}(PO_4)_6F_2 + 2\ OH^-$$

(Hydroxyapatite) → (Fluorapatite)

TABLE 2 *Nutrition Facts, Drops*

Amount Per 1 ml	% DV Infants (0.25 mg drops only)	% DV Adults & Children 4 Years or More
Vitamin A 1500 IU	100%	50%
Vitamin C 35 mg	100%	100%
Vitamin D 400 IU	100%	100%
Vitamin E 5 IU	100%	50%
Thiamin .05 mg	100%	70%
Riboflavin 0.6mg	100%	70%
Niacin 8 mg	100%	68%
Vitamin B_6 0.4 mg	100%	53%
Vitamin B_{12} 2 mcg	100%	75%
Fluoride 0.25 mg (0.25 mg drops) 0.5 mg (0.5 mg drops)	*	*

* Daily Value (DV) not established.

Three stages of fluoride deposition in tooth enamel can be distinguished:[3]

1. Small amounts (reflecting the low levels of fluoride in tissue fluids) are incorporated into the enamel crystals while they are being formed.
2. After enamel has been laid down, fluoride deposition continues in the surface enamel. Diffusion of fluoride from the surface inward is apparently restricted.
3. After eruption, the surface enamel acquires fluoride from water, food, supplementary fluoride, and smaller amounts from saliva.

INDICATIONS AND USAGE

CHEWABLE TABLETS AND DROPS

Supplementation of the diet with ten essential vitamins for the chewable tablets, nine for the drops.

Supplementation of the diet with fluoride for caries prophylaxis, *and with the 0.25 mg chewable tablets only:* for children 4-6 years of age where the drinking water contains 0.3-0.6 ppm of fluoride.[4]

Fluoride; polyvitamin supplies significant amounts of vitamins A, C, D, E, thiamin, riboflavin, niacin, vitamin B_6, vitamin B_{12}, and folate to supplement the diet, and to help assure that nutritional deficiencies of these vitamins will not develop. Thus, in a single easy-to-use preparation, children (and infants for the drops) obtain 10 essential vitamins (for the chewable tablets, 9 for the drops) and the important mineral, fluoride.

The American Academy of Pediatrics recommends that children up to age 16, in areas where drinking water contains less than optimal levels of fluoride, receive daily fluoride supplementation.

CHEWABLE TABLETS

Fluoride; polyvitamin 0.5 mg chewable tablets provide fluoride in tablet form for children 4 to 6 years of age where the drinking water has a fluoride content less than 0.3 ppm, and for children 6 years of age and above where the drinking water contains 0.3 through 0.6 ppm of fluoride.[4]

Fluoride; polyvitamin 1.0 mg chewable tablets were developed to provide fluoride in tablet form for children 6 to 16 years of age in areas where the water fluoride level is less than 0.3 ppm.[4]

Children using fluoride; polyvitamin chewable tablets regularly should receive semiannual dental examinations. The regular brushing of teeth and attention to good oral hygiene practices are also essential.

DROPS

Fluoride; polyvitamin drops provide fluoride in drop form for children ages 3-6 years in areas where the drinking water contains less than 0.3 ppm fluoride; and for children 6 years of age and older in areas where the drinking water contains 0.3 through 0.6 ppm of fluoride. Each 1.0 ml supplies sodium fluoride (0.5 mg fluoride) plus nine essential vitamins.

Additional Information for the 0.5 mg Drops Only

A comprehensive 5½ year series of studies of the effectiveness of fluoride; multivitamin and fluoride; polyvitamin products in caries protection has been published.[1,2,5,6] Children in this continuing study lived in an area where the water supply contained only 0.05 ppm fluoride. The subjects were divided into two groups, one which used only non-fluoridated Vi-Sol vitamin products, and the other fluoride; multivitamin and fluoride; polyvitamin products.

The 3 year interim report showed 63% fewer carious surfaces in primary teeth and 43% fewer carious surfaces in permanent teeth of the children taking fluoride; multivitamin products.

After 4 years the studies continued to support the effectiveness of fluoride; multivitamins and fluoride; polyvitamins, showing a reduction in carious surfaces of 68% in primary teeth and 46% in permanent teeth.[2]

Results at the end of 5½ years further confirmed the previous findings and indicated that significant reductions in dental caries are apparent with the continued use of fluoride; multivitamin products.[5]

WARNINGS

As in the case of all medications, keep out of the reach of children.

The chewable tablets should be chewed. The chewable tablets are not recommended for children under age 4 due to risk of choking.

PRECAUTIONS

The suggested dose *should not be exceeded,* since dental fluorosis may result from continued ingestion of large amounts of fluoride.

Before prescribing fluoride; polyvitamin:

1. Determine the fluoride content of the drinking water from all major sources.
2. Make sure the child is not receiving significant amounts of fluoride from other sources such as medications and swallowed toothpaste.

3. Periodically check to make sure that the child does not develop significant dental fluorosis.

Additional Information for Drops: Fluoride; polyvitamin drops should be dispensed in the original plastic container, since contact with glass leads to instability and precipitation. (The amount of sodium fluoride in the 50 ml size is well below the maximum to be dispensed at 1 time according to recommendations of the American Dental Association.

ADVERSE REACTIONS

Allergic rash and other idiosyncrasies have been rarely reported.

DOSAGE AND ADMINISTRATION

Chewable Tablets: One tablet daily or as prescribed.

Drops: 1.0 ml or as prescribed. May be dropped directly into mouth with "Safti-Dropper", or mixed with cereal, fruit juice, or other food. **USE FULL DOSAGE.**

F

Fluorouracil *(001319)*

Categories: Carcinoma, breast; Carcinoma, colorectal; Carcinoma, pancreatic; Carcinoma, basal cell; Carcinoma, gastric; Keratoses, actinic; Pregnancy Category D; FDA Approved 1962 Apr; WHO Formulary
Drug Classes: Antineoplastics, antimetabolites; Dermatologics
Brand Names: Adrucil; Efudex; Fluoroplex
Foreign Brand Availability: Actino-Hermal (Germany); Efudix (Australia; Bahamas; Bahrain; Barbados; Belgium; Belize; Bermuda; Bulgaria; Curacao; Cyprus; Czech-Republic; Egypt; England; France; Germany; Ghana; Guyana; Hong-Kong; Iran; Iraq; Ireland; Israel; Italy; Jamaica; Japan; Jordan; Kenya; Kuwait; Lebanon; Libya; Mexico; Netherland-Antilles; Netherlands; New-Zealand; Oman; Peru; Qatar; Republic-of-Yemen; Saudi-Arabia; Singapore; South-Africa; Spain; Surinam; Switzerland; Syria; Taiwan; Tanzania; Trinidad; Uganda; United-Arab-Emirates; Zambia)
HCFA JCODE(S): J9190 500 mg IV

WARNING

It is recommended that fluorouracil be given only by or under the supervision of a qualified physician who is experienced in cancer chemotherapy and who is well versed in the use of potent antimetabolites. Because of the possibility of severe toxic reactions, it is recommended that patients be hospitalized at least during the initial course of therapy.

These instructions should be thoroughly reviewed before administration of fluorouracil.

DESCRIPTION

INJECTION

Adrucil, an antineoplastic antimetabolite, is a colorless to faint yellow aqueous, sterile, nonpyrogenic injectable solution for intravenous administration. Each 10 ml contains 500 mg of fluorouracil; pH is adjusted to 8.6-9.2 with sodium hydroxide and hydrochloric acid if necessary.

Chemically, fluorouracil, a fluorinated pyrimidine, is 5-fluoro-2,4 (*1H,3H*)-pyrimidinedione. It is a white to practically white crystalline powder which is sparingly soluble in water. The molecular formula is $C_4H_3FN_2O_2$. The molecular weight of fluorouracil is 130.08.

TOPICAL SOLUTIONS AND CREAMS

Fluorouracil topical solutions and cream are chemotherapeutic agents for the treatment of solar keratoses and superficial basal cell carcinomas. They contain the fluorinated pyrimidine 5-fluorouracil, antineoplastic antimetabolite. Fluorouracil solution consists of 2% or 5% fluorouracil on a weight/weight basis, compounded with propylene glycol, tris (hydroxymethyl), aminomethane, hydroxypropyl cellulose, parabens (methyl and propyl) and disodium edetate.

Fluorouracil cream contains 5% fluorouracil in a vanishing cream base consisting of white petrolatum, stearyl alcohol, propylene glycol, polysorbate 60 and parabens (methyl and propyl).

Note: Although fluorouracil solution may discolor slightly during storage, the potency and safety are not adversely affected.

Storage: Store at room temperature 15-30°C (59-86°F). Protect from light. Retain in carton until time of use.

CLINICAL PHARMACOLOGY

There is evidence that the metabolism of fluorouracil in the anabolic pathway blocks the methylation reaction of deoxyuridylic acid to thymidylic acid. In this manner, fluorouracil interferes with the synthesis of deoxyribonucleic acid (DNA) and to a lesser extent inhibits the formation of ribonucleic acid (RNA). Since DNA and RNA are essential for cell division and growth, the effect of fluorouracil may be to create a thymine deficiency which provokes unbalanced growth and death of the cell. The effects of DNA and RNA deprivation are most marked on those cells which grow more rapidly and which take up fluorouracil at a more rapid rate.

Following intravenous injection, fluorouracil distributes into tumors, intestinal mucosa, bone marrow, liver and other tissues throughout the body. In spite of its limited lipid solubility, fluorouracil diffuses readily across the blood-brain barrier and distributes into cerebrospinal fluid and brain tissue.

Seven (7) to 20% of the parent drug is excreted unchanged in the urine in 6 hours; of this over 90% is excreted in the first hour. The remaining percentage of the administered dose is metabolized, primarily in the liver. The catabolic metabolism of fluorouracil results in degradation products (*e.g.*, CO_2 urea and α-fluoro-β-alanine) which are inactive. The inactive metabolites are excreted in the urine over the next 3 to 4 hours. When fluorouracil is labeled in the six carbon position, thus preventing the ^{14}C metabolism to CO_2, approximately 90% of the total radioactivity is excreted in the urine. When fluorouracil is labeled in the two carbon position approximately 90% of the total radioactivity is excreted in expired CO_2. Ninety percent (90%) of the dose is accounted for during the first 24 hours following intravenous administration.

Following intravenous administration of fluorouracil, the mean half-life of elimination from plasma is approximately 16 minutes, with a range of 8-20 minutes, and is dose dependent. No intact drug can be detected in the plasma 3 hours after an intravenous injection.

Additional Information for Topicals: Studies in man with topical application of ^{14}C-labeled fluorouracil demonstrated insignificant absorption as measured by ^{14}C content of plasma, urine, and respiratory CO_2.

INDICATIONS AND USAGE

INJECTION

Fluorouracil is effective in the palliative management of carcinoma of the colon, rectum, breast, stomach and pancreas.

TOPICAL SOLUTIONS AND CREAMS

Fluorouracil is recommended for the topical treatment of multiple actinic or solar keratoses. In the 5% strength it is also useful in the treatment of superficial basal cell carcinomas, when conventional methods are impractical, such as with multiple lesions or difficult treatment sites. The diagnosis should be established prior to treatment, since this new method has not been proven effective in other types of basal cell carcinomas. With isolated, easily accessible lesions, conventional techniques are preferred since success with such lesions is almost 100% with these methods. The success rate with fluorouracil topicals is approximately 93%. This 93% success rate is based on 113 lesions in 54 patients. Twenty-five (25) lesions treated with the solution produced 1 failure and 88 lesions treated with the cream produced 7 failures.

CONTRAINDICATIONS

INJECTION

Fluorouracil therapy is contraindicated for patients in a poor nutritional state, those with depressed bone marrow function, those with potentially serious infections or those with a known hypersensitivity to fluorouracil.

TOPICAL SOLUTIONS AND CREAMS

Contraindicated in patients with known hypersensitivity to any of its components.

WARNINGS

INJECTION

THE DAILY DOSE OF FLUOROURACIL IS NOT TO EXCEED 800 MG. IT IS RECOMMENDED THAT PATIENTS BE HOSPITALIZED DURING THEIR FIRST COURSE OF TREATMENT.

Fluorouracil should be used with extreme caution in poor risk patients with a history of high-dose pelvic irradiation or previous use of alkylating agents, those who have a widespread involvement of bone marrow by metastatic tumors or those with impaired hepatic or renal function.

Rarely, unexpected, severe toxicity (*e.g.*, stomatitis, diarrhea, neutropenia, and neurotoxicity) associated with 5-fluorouracil has been attributed to deficiency of dipyrimidine dehydrogenase activity. A few patients have been rechallenged with 5-fluorouracil and despite 5-fluorouracil dose lowering, toxicity recurred and progressed with worse morbidity. Absence of this catabolic enzyme appears to result in prolonged clearance of 5-fluorouracil.

Pregnancy, Teratogenic Effects, Pregnancy Category D

Fluorouracil may cause fetal harm when administered to a pregnant woman. Fluorouracil has been shown to be teratogenic in laboratory animals. Fluorouracil exhibited maximum teratogenicity when given to mice as single intraperitoneal injections of 10 to 40 mg/kg on day 10 or 12 of gestation. Similarly, intraperitoneal doses of 12-37 mg/kg given to rats between days 9 and 12 of gestation and intramuscular doses of 3-9 mg given to hamsters between days 8 and 11 of gestation were teratogenic. Malformations included cleft palates, skeletal defects and deformed appendages, paws and tails. The dosages which were teratogenic in animals are 1-3 times the maximum recommended human therapeutic dose. In monkeys, divided doses of 40 mg/kg given between days 20 and 24 of gestation were not teratogenic.

There are no adequate and well-controlled studies with fluorouracil in pregnant women. While there is no evidence of teratogenicity in humans due to fluorouracil, it should be kept in mind that other drugs which inhibit DNA synthesis (*e.g.*, methotrexate and aminopterin) have been reported to be teratogenic in humans. Women of childbearing potential should be advised to avoid becoming pregnant. If the drug is used during pregnancy, or if the patient becomes pregnant while taking the drug, the patient should be told of the potential hazard to the fetus. Fluorouracil should be used during pregnancy only if the potential benefit justifies the potential risk to the fetus.

Combination Therapy

Any form of therapy which adds to the stress of the patient, interferes with nutrition or depresses bone marrow function will increase the toxicity of fluorouracil.

TOPICAL SOLUTIONS AND CREAMS

If an occlusive dressing is used, there may be an increase in the incidence of inflammatory reactions in the adjacent normal skin. A porous gauze dressing may be applied for cosmetic reasons without an increase in reaction.

Prolonged exposure to ultraviolet rays should be avoided while under treatment with fluorouracil because the intensity of the reaction may be increased.

Use in Pregnancy: Safety for use in pregnancy has not been established.

PRECAUTIONS

INJECTION

General

Fluorouracil is a highly toxic drug with a narrow margin of safety. Therefore, patients should be carefully supervised, since therapeutic response is unlikely to occur without some evidence of toxicity. Severe hematological toxicity, gastrointestinal hemorrhage and even death may result from the use of fluorouracil despite meticulous selection of patients and careful adjustment of dosage. Although severe toxicity is more likely in poor risk patients, fatalities may be encountered occasionally even in patients in relatively good condition.

Therapy is to be discontinued promptly whenever one of the following signs of toxicity appears:

- Stomatitis or esophagopharyngitis, at the first visible sign.
- Leukopenia (WBC under 3500) or a rapidly falling white blood count.
- Vomiting, intractable.
- Diarrhea, frequent bowel movements or watery stools.
- Gastrointestinal ulceration and bleeding.
- Thrombocytopenia, (platelets under 100,000).
- Hemorrhage from any site.

The administration of 5-fluorouracil has been associated with the occurrence of palmar-plantar erythrodysesthesia syndrome, also known as hand-foot syndrome. This syndrome has been characterized as a tingling sensation of hands and feet which may progress over the next few days to pain when holding objects or walking. The palms and soles become symmetrically swollen and erythematous with tenderness of the distal phalanges, possibly accompanied by desquamation. Interruption of therapy is followed by gradual resolution over 5-7 days. Although pyridoxine has been reported to ameliorate the palmar-plantar erythrodysesthesia syndrome, its safety and effectiveness have not been established.

Information for the Patient

Patients should be informed of expected toxic effects, particularly oral manifestations. Patients should be alerted to the possibility of alopecia as a result of therapy and should be informed that it is usually a transient effect.

Laboratory Tests

White blood counts with differential are recommended before each dose.

Carcinogenesis, Mutagenesis, and Impairment of Fertility

Carcinogenesis

Long-term studies in animals to evaluate the carcinogenic potential of fluorouracil have not been conducted. However, there was no evidence of carcinogenicity in small groups of rats given fluorouracil orally at doses of 0.01, 0.3, 1 or 3 mg per rat 5 days per week for 52 weeks, followed by a 6 month observation period. Also, in other studies, 33 mg/kg of fluorouracil was administered intravenously to male rats once a week for 52 weeks followed by observation for the remainder of their lifetimes with no evidence of carcinogenicity. Female mice were given 1 mg of fluorouracil intravenously once a week for 16 weeks with no effect on the incidence of lung adenomas. On the basis of the available data, no evaluation can be made of the carcinogenic risk of fluorouracil to humans.

Mutagenesis

Oncogenic transformation of fibroblasts from mouse embryo has been induced *in vitro* by fluorouracil, but the relationship between oncogenicity and mutagenicity is not clear. Fluorouracil has been shown to be mutagenic to several strains of *Salmonella typhimurium,* including TA 1535, TA 1537 and TA 1538, and to *Saccharomyces cerevisiae,* although no evidence of mutagenicity was found with *Salmonella typhimurium* strains TA 92, TA 98 and TA 100. In addition, a positive effect was observed in the micronucleus test on bone marrow cells of the mouse, and fluorouracil at very high concentrations produced chromosomal breaks in hamster fibroblasts *in vitro.*

Impairment of Fertility

Fluorouracil has not been adequately studied in animals to permit an evaluation of its effects on fertility and general reproductive performance. However, doses of 125 or 250 mg/kg, administered intraperitoneally, have been shown to induce chromosomal aberrations and changes in chromosomal organization of spermatogonia in rats. Spermatogonial differentiation was also inhibited by fluorouracil, resulting in transient infertility. However, in studies with a strain of mouse which is sensitive to the induction of sperm head abnormalities after exposure to a range of chemical mutagens and carcinogens, fluorouracil did not produce any abnormalities at oral doses of up to 80 mg/kg/day. In female rats, fluorouracil, administered intraperitoneally at weekly doses of 25 or 50 mg/kg for 3 weeks during the pre-ovulatory phase of oogenesis, significantly reduced the incidence of fertile matings, delayed the development of pre- and post-implantation embryos, increased the incidence of pre-implantation lethality and induced chromosomal anomalies in these embryos. In a limited study in rabbits, a single 25 mg/kg dose of fluorouracil or 5 daily doses of 5 mg/kg had no effect on ovulation, appeared not to affect implantation and had only a limited effect in producing zygote destruction. Compounds such as fluorouracil, which interfere with DNA, RNA and protein synthesis, might be expected to have adverse effects on gametogenesis.

Pregnancy Category D

See WARNINGS, Pregnancy, Teratogenic Effects, Pregnancy Category D.

Pregnancy, Nonteratogenic Effects

Fluorouracil has not been studied in animals for its effects on peri- and postnatal development. However, fluorouracil has been shown to cross the placenta and enter into fetal circulation in the rat. Administration of fluorouracil has resulted in increased resorptions and embryolethality in rats. In monkeys, maternal doses higher than 40 mg/kg resulted in abortion of all embryos exposed to fluorouracil. Compounds which inhibit DNA, RNA and protein synthesis might be expected to have adverse effects on peri- and postnatal development.

Nursing Mothers

It is not known whether fluorouracil is excreted in human milk. Because fluorouracil inhibits DNA, RNA and protein synthesis, mothers should not nurse while receiving this drug.

Pediatric Use

Safety and effectiveness in pediatric patients have not been established.

TOPICAL SOLUTIONS AND CREAMS

If fluorouracil is applied with the fingers, the hands should be washed immediately afterward. Fluorouracil should be applied with care near the eyes, nose, and mouth. Solar keratoses which do no not respond should be biopsied to confirm the diagnosis. Patients should be forewarned that the reaction in the treated areas may be unsightly during therapy, and, in some cases, for several weeks following the cessation of therapy.

Follow-up biopsies should be performed as indicated in the management of superficial basal cell carcinoma.

DRUG INTERACTIONS

Leucovorin calcium may enhance the toxicity of fluorouracil.

Also see WARNINGS.

ADVERSE REACTIONS

INJECTION

Stomatitis and esophagopharyngitis (which may lead to sloughing and ulceration), diarrhea, anorexia, nausea and emesis are commonly seen during therapy.

Leukopenia usually follows every course of adequate therapy with fluorouracil. The lowest white blood cell counts are commonly observed between the 9th and 14th days after the first course of treatment, although uncommonly the maximal depression may be delayed for as long as 20 days. By the 30th day the count has usually returned to the normal range.

Alopecia and dermatitis may be seen in a substantial number of cases. The dermatitis most often seen is a pruritic maculopapular rash usually appearing on the extremities and less frequently on the trunk. It is generally reversible and usually responsive to symptomatic treatment.

Other adverse reactions are:

- ***Hematologic:*** Pancytopenia, thrombocytopenia, agranulocytosis, anemia.
- ***Cardiovascular:*** Myocardial ischemia, angina.
- ***Gastrointestinal:*** Gastrointestinal ulceration and bleeding.
- ***Allergic Reactions:*** Anaphylaxis and generalized allergic reactions.
- ***Neurologic:*** Acute cerebellar syndrome (which may persist following discontinuance of treatment), nystagmus, headache.
- ***Dermatologic:*** Dry skin, fissuring, photosensitivity, as manifested by erythema or increased pigmentation of the skin; vein pigmentation; palmar-plantar erythrodysesthesia syndrome, as manifested by tingling of the hands and feet followed by pain, erythema and swelling.
- ***Ophthalmic:*** Lacrimal duct stenosis, visual changes, lacrimation, photophobia.
- ***Psychiatric:*** Disorientation, confusion, euphoria.
- ***Miscellaneous:*** Thrombophlebitis, epistaxis, nail changes (including loss of nails).

TOPICAL SOLUTIONS AND CREAMS

The most frequently encountered local reactions are pain, pruritus, hyperpigmentation and burning at the site of the application. Other local reactions include allergic contact dermatitis, scarring, soreness, tenderness, suppuration, scaling, and swelling.

Also reported are alopecia, insomnia, stomatitis, irritability, medicinal taste, photosensitivity, lacrimation, telangiectasia and urticaria, although a causal relationship is remote.

Laboratory abnormalities reported are leukocytosis, thrombocytopenia, toxic granulation and eosinophilia.

DOSAGE AND ADMINISTRATION

INJECTION

General Instructions

Fluorouracil injection should be administered only intravenously, using care to avoid extravasation. No dilution is required.

All dosages are based on the patient's actual weight. However, the estimated lean body mass (dry weight) is used if the patient is obese or if there has been a spurious weight gain due to edema, ascites or other forms of abnormal fluid retention.

It is recommended that prior to treatment each patient be carefully evaluated in order to estimate as accurately as possible the optimum initial dosage of fluorouracil.

Dosage

Twelve (12) mg/kg are given intravenously once daily for 4 successive days. The daily dose should not exceed 800 mg.

If No Toxicity is Observed

6 mg/kg are given on the 6th, 8th, 10th and 12th days *unless toxicity occurs.* No therapy is given on the 5th, 7th, 9th or 11th days. *Therapy is to be discontinued at the end of the 12th day, even if no toxicity has become apparent.* (See WARNINGS and PRECAUTIONS.)

Poor risk patients or those who are not in an adequate nutritional state (see CONTRAINDICATIONS and WARNINGS) should receive 6 mg/kg/day for 3 days. *If no toxicity is observed,* 3 mg/kg may be given on the 5th, 7th and 9th days *unless toxicity occurs.* No therapy is given on the 4th, 6th or 8th days. The daily dose should not exceed 400 mg.

A sequence of injections on either schedule constitutes a "course of therapy".

Maintenance Therapy

In instances where toxicity has not been a problem, it is recommended that therapy be continued using either of the following schedules:

1. Repeat dosage of first course every 30 days after the last day of the previous course of treatment.
2. When toxic signs resulting from the initial course of therapy have subsided, administer a maintenance dosage of 10-15 mg/kg/week as a single dose. Do not exceed 1 g per week.

The patient's reaction to the previous course of therapy should be taken into account in determining the amount of the drug to be used, and the dosage should be adjusted accordingly. Some patients have received from 9-45 courses of treatment during periods which ranged from 12-60 months.

Handling and Disposal

Procedures for proper handling and disposal of anticancer drugs should be considered. Several guidelines on this subject have been published.[1-7] There is no general agreement that all of the procedures recommended in the guidelines are necessary or appropriate.

Note: Parenteral drug products should be inspected visually for particulate matter and discoloration prior to administration, whenever solution and container permit. If a precipitate occurs due to exposure to low temperatures, resolubilize by heating to 140°F and shaking vigorously; allow to cool to body temperature before using.

TOPICAL SOLUTIONS AND CREAMS

When fluorouracil is applied to a lesion, a response occurs with the following sequence: erythema, usually followed by vesiculation, erosion, ulceration, necrosis and epithelization.

Actinic or Solar Keratosis

Apply cream or solution twice daily in an amount sufficient to cover the lesions. Medication should be continued until the inflammatory response reaches the erosion, necrosis and the ulceration stage, at which time use of the drug should be terminated. The usual duration of therapy is from 2-4 weeks. Complete healing of the lesions may not be evident for 1-2 months following cessation of fluorouracil therapy.

Superficial Basal Cell Carcinomas

Only the 5% strength is recommended. Apply cream or solution twice daily in an amount sufficient to cover the lesions. Treatment should be continued for at least 3-6 weeks. Therapy may be required for as long as 10-12 weeks before the lesions are obliterated. As in any neoplastic condition, the patient should be followed for a reasonable period of time to determine if a cure has been obtained.

PRODUCT LISTING - RATED THERAPEUTICALLY EQUIVALENT

Size	Price	Product	NDC
Solution - Intravenous - 50 mg/ml			
10 ml	$2.60	GENERIC, Baxter Pharmaceutical Products, Inc	10019-0950-02
10 ml	$32.00	GENERIC, Pharmacia and Upjohn	00013-1036-91
10 ml x 10	$15.24	GENERIC, Solo Pak Medical Products Inc	39769-0012-10
10 ml x 10	$21.80	GENERIC, Icn Pharmaceuticals Inc	00187-3953-64
10 ml x 10	$37.45	GENERIC, Faulding Pharmaceutical Company	61703-0409-32
10 ml x 10	$37.50	GENERIC, American Pharmaceutical Partners	63323-0117-10
20 ml x 10	$75.00	GENERIC, American Pharmaceutical Partners	63323-0117-20
50 ml	$7.69	GENERIC, Pharmacia and Upjohn	00013-1046-94
50 ml x 1	$13.45	GENERIC, American Pharmaceutical Partners	63323-0117-51
100 ml	$15.50	GENERIC, Chiron Therapeutics	00702-1710-30
100 ml	$160.30	GENERIC, Pharmacia and Upjohn	00013-1056-94
100 ml x 1	$32.13	GENERIC, American Pharmaceutical Partners	63323-0117-61
100 ml x 10	$250.00	GENERIC, Solo Pak Medical Products Inc	39769-0012-90
Solution - Topical - 5%			
10 ml	$102.13	EFUDEX, Icn Pharmaceuticals Inc	00187-3203-10

PRODUCT LISTING - EQUIVALENTS NOT AVAILABLE

Size	Price	Product	NDC
Cream - Topical - 0.5%			
30 gm	$99.75	CARAC, Aventis Pharmaceuticals	00066-7150-30
Cream - Topical - 1%			
30 gm	$75.61	FLUOROPLEX, Allergan Inc	00023-0812-30
Cream - Topical - 5%			
25 gm	$58.44	EFUDEX, Roche Laboratories	00004-1506-03
25 gm	$105.19	EFUDEX, Icn Pharmaceuticals Inc	00187-3204-26
Solution - Topical - 1%			
30 ml	$75.61	FLUOROPLEX, Allergan Inc	00023-0810-30
Solution - Topical - 2%			
10 ml	$50.63	EFUDEX, Roche Laboratories	00004-1704-06

Fluoxetine Hydrochloride *(001320)*

For related information, see the comparative table section in Appendix A.

Categories: Bulimia nervosa; Depression; Obsessive-compulsive disorder; Panic disorder; Premenstrual dysphoric disorder; Pregnancy Category C; FDA Approved 1987 Dec

Drug Classes: Antidepressants, serotonin specific reuptake inhibitors

***Brand Names:* Prozac**

Foreign Brand Availability: Adofen (Spain); Alzac 20 (Guatemala); Andep (India); Ansilan (Colombia); Auroken (Mexico); Deprexin (Bahamas; Barbados; Belize; Bermuda; Curacao; Guyana; Jamaica; Netherland-Antilles; Puerto-Rico; Singapore; Surinam; Trinidad); Deproxin (Thailand); Fluctin (Germany); Fluctine (Austria; Switzerland); Fludac (Benin; Burkina-Faso; Ethiopia; Gambia; Ghana; Guinea; India; Ivory-Coast; Kenya; Liberia; Malawi; Mali; Mauritania; Mauritius; Morocco; Niger; Nigeria; Senegal; Seychelles; Sierra-Leone; South-Africa; Sudan; Tanzania; Tunia; Uganda; Zambia; Zimbabwe); Flufran (India); Flunil (India); Fluox (Germany); Fluoxac (Mexico); Fluoxeren (Italy); Fluoxil (Dominican-Republic); Fluox-Puren (Germany); Fluronin (Taiwan); Flusac (Thailand); Flutin (Colombia; Korea); Flutine (Israel; Thailand); Fluxen (Taiwan); Fluxetil (Singapore); Fluxetin (Singapore); Fluxil (Bahrain; Cyprus; Egypt; Hong-Kong; Iran; Iraq; Israel; Jordan; Kuwait; Lebanon; Libya; Oman; Qatar; Republic-of-Yemen; Saudi-Arabia; Syria; United-Arab-Emirates); Fontex (Denmark; Finland; Norway; Sweden); Foxetin (Korea); Landic (Korea); Lorien (South-Africa); Lovan (Australia); Magrilan (Singapore); Margrilan (Bahrain; Cyprus; Egypt; Hong-Kong; Iran; Iraq; Jordan; Kuwait; Lebanon; Libya; Oman; Qatar; Republic-of-Yemen; Saudi-Arabia; Syria; Thailand; United-Arab-Emirates); Modipran (Benin; Burkina-Faso; Ethiopia; Gambia; Ghana; Guinea; Ivory-Coast; Kenya; Liberia; Malawi; Mali; Mauritania; Mauritius; Morocco; Niger; Nigeria; Senegal; Seychelles; Sierra-Leone; Sudan; Tanzania; Tunia; Uganda; Zambia; Zimbabwe); Neupax (Peru); Nopres (Indonesia); Nuzak (South-Africa); Oxedep (China; India); Pragmaten (Ecuador); Prizma (Israel); Proctin (Korea); Prodep (Benin; Burkina-Faso; Ethiopia; Gambia; Ghana; Guinea; India; Ivory-Coast; Kenya; Liberia; Malawi; Mali; Mauritania; Mauritius; Morocco; Niger; Nigeria; Senegal; Seychelles; Sierra-Leone; South-Africa; Sudan; Tanzania; Tunia; Uganda; Zambia; Zimbabwe); Prozac 20 (Korea; Malaysia; Mexico; Philippines; Taiwan; Thailand); Rowexetina (Costa-Rica; Dominican-Republic; El-Salvador; Guatemala; Honduras; Nicaragua; Panama); Salipax (Bahamas; Barbados; Belize; Bermuda; Curacao; Guyana; Jamaica; Netherland-Antilles; Puerto-Rico; Surinam; Trinidad); Sanzur (South-Africa); Sinzac (Taiwan); ZAC (Indonesia); Zactin (Australia; Singapore; Taiwan); Zepax (Colombia)

Cost of Therapy: $99.10 (Depression; Prozac; 20 mg; 1 capsule/day; 30 day supply)
$79.59 (Depression; Generic Capsules; 20 mg; 1 capsule/day; 30 day supply)
$297.30 (Bulimia Nervosa; Prozac; 20 mg; 3 capsules/day; 30 day supply)
$93.28 (PMDD; Sarafem; 20 mg; 1 capsule/day; 28 day supply)

DESCRIPTION

Note: The trade names have been used throughout this monograph for clarity.

Prozac (fluoxetine hydrochloride), a selective serotonin reuptake inhibitor (SSRI), is a psychotropic drug for oral administration. It is also marketed for the treatment of premenstrual dysphoric disorder (Sarafem, fluoxetine hydrochloride). It is designated (±)-N-methyl-3-phenyl-3-[(α,α,α-trifluoro-*p*-tolyl)oxy]propylamine hydrochloride and has the empirical formula of $C_{17}H_{18}F_3NO{\cdot}HCl$. Its molecular weight is 345.79.

Fluoxetine hydrochloride is a white to off-white crystalline solid with a solubility of 14 mg/ml in water.

EACH PROZAC PULVULE CONTAINS

Fluoxetine hydrochloride equivalent to 10 mg (32.3 μmol), 20 mg (64.7 μmol), or 40 mg (129.3 μmol) of fluoxetine. The Pulvules also contain starch, gelatin, silicone, titanium dioxide, iron oxide, and other inactive ingredients. The 10 and 20 mg Pulvules also contain FD&C blue no. 1, and the 40 mg Pulvule also contains FD&C blue no. 1 and FD&C yellow no. 6.

EACH PROZAC TABLET CONTAINS

Fluoxetine hydrochloride equivalent to 10 mg (32.3 μmol) of fluoxetine. The tablets also contain microcrystalline cellulose, magnesium stearate, crospovidone, hydroxypropyl methylcellulose, titanium dioxide, polyethylene glycol, and yellow iron oxide. In addition to the above ingredients, the 10 mg tablet contains FD&C blue no. 1 aluminum lake, and polysorbate 80.

THE PROZAC ORAL SOLUTION CONTAINS

Fluoxetine hydrochloride equivalent to 20 mg/5 ml (64.7 μmol) of fluoxetine. It also contains alcohol 0.23%, benzoic acid, flavoring agent, glycerin, purified water, and sucrose.

EACH PROZAC WEEKLY CAPSULE (A DELAYED-RELEASE FORMULATION) CONTAINS

Enteric-coated pellets of fluoxetine hydrochloride equivalent to 90 mg (291 μmol) of fluoxetine. The capsules also contain D&C yellow no. 10, FD&C blue no. 2, gelatin, hydroxypropyl methylcellulose, hydroxypropyl methylcellulose acetate succinate, sodium lauryl sulfate, sucrose, sugar spheres, talc, titanium dioxide, triethyl citrate, and other inactive ingredients.

EACH SARAFEM PULVULE CONTAINS

Fluoxetine hydrochloride equivalent to 10 mg (32.3 μmol) or 20 mg (64.7 μmol) of fluoxetine. The Pulvules also contain dimethicone, FD&C blue no. 1, FD&C red no. 3, FD&C yellow no. 6, gelatin, sodium lauryl sulfate, starch, and titanium dioxide.

CLINICAL PHARMACOLOGY

PHARMACODYNAMICS

The antidepressant, antiobsessive-compulsive, and antibulimic actions of fluoxetine and the mechanism of action of fluoxetine in premenstrual dysphoric disorder (PMDD) are presumed to be linked to its inhibition of CNS neuronal uptake of serotonin. Studies at clinically relevant doses humans have demonstrated that fluoxetine blocks the uptake of serotonin into human platelets. Studies in animals also suggest that fluoxetine is a much more potent uptake inhibitor of serotonin than of norepinephrine.

Antagonism of muscarinic, histaminergic, and α_1-adrenergic receptors has been hypothesized to be associated with various anticholinergic, sedative, and cardiovascular effects of classical tricyclic antidepressant (TCA) drugs. Fluoxetine binds to these and other membrane receptors from brain tissue much less potently *in vitro* than do the tricyclic drugs.

ABSORPTION, DISTRIBUTION, METABOLISM, AND EXCRETION
Systemic Bioavailability
In humans, following a single oral 40 mg dose, peak plasma concentrations of fluoxetine from 15-55 ng/ml are observed after 6-8 hours.
The Pulvule, tablet, oral solution, and Prozac Weekly capsule dosage forms of fluoxetine are bioequivalent. Food does not appear to affect the systemic bioavailability of fluoxetine, although it may delay its absorption by 1-2 hours, which is probably not clinically significant. Thus, fluoxetine may be administered with or without food. Prozac Weekly capsules, a delayed-release formulation, contain enteric-coated pellets that resist dissolution until reaching a segment of the gastrointestinal tract where the pH exceeds 5.5. The enteric coating delays the onset of absorption of fluoxetine 1-2 hours relative to the immediate release formulations.

Protein Binding
Over the concentration range from 200-1000 ng/ml, approximately 94.5% of fluoxetine is bound *in vitro* to human serum proteins, including albumin and α_1-glycoprotein. The interaction between fluoxetine and other highly protein-bound drugs has not been fully evaluated, but may be important (see PRECAUTIONS).

Enantiomers
Fluoxetine is a racemic mixture (50/50) of *R*-fluoxetine and *S*-fluoxetine enantiomers. In animal models, both enantiomers are specific and potent serotonin uptake inhibitors with essentially equivalent pharmacologic activity. The *S*-fluoxetine enantiomer is eliminated more slowly and is the predominant enantiomer present in plasma at steady-state.

Metabolism
Fluoxetine is extensively metabolized in the liver to norfluoxetine and a number of other unidentified metabolites. The only identified active metabolite, norfluoxetine, is formed by demethylation of fluoxetine. In animal models, *S*-norfluoxetine is a potent and selective inhibitor of serotonin uptake and has activity essentially equivalent to *R*- or *S*-fluoxetine. *R*-norfluoxetine is significantly less potent than the parent drug in the inhibition of serotonin uptake. The primary route of elimination appears to be hepatic metabolism to inactive metabolites excreted by the kidney.

Clinical Issues Related to Metabolism/Elimination
The complexity of the metabolism of fluoxetine has several consequences that may potentially affect fluoxetine's clinical use.

Variability in Metabolism
A subset (about 7%) of the population has reduced activity of the drug metabolizing enzyme cytochrome P450IID6. Such individuals are referred to as "poor metabolizers" of drugs such as debrisoquin, dextromethorphan, and the TCAs. In a study involving labeled and unlabeled enantiomers administered as a racemate, these individuals metabolized *S*-fluoxetine at a slower rate and thus achieved higher concentrations of *S*-fluoxetine. Consequently, concentrations of *S*-norfluoxetine at steady-state were lower. The metabolism of *R*-fluoxetine in these poor metabolizers appears normal. When compared with normal metabolizers, the total sum at steady-state of the plasma concentrations of the 4 active enantiomers was not significantly greater among poor metabolizers. Thus, the net pharmacodynamic activities were essentially the same. Alternative, nonsaturable pathways (non-IID6) also contribute to the metabolism of fluoxetine. This explains how fluoxetine achieves a steady-state concentration rather than increasing without limit.
Because fluoxetine's metabolism, like that of a number of other compounds including TCAs and other selective serotonin reuptake inhibitors, involves the P450IID6 system, concomitant therapy with drugs also metabolized by this enzyme system (such as the TCAs) may lead to drug interactions (see DRUG INTERACTIONS).

Accumulation and Slow Elimination
The relatively slow elimination of fluoxetine (elimination half-life of 1-3 days after acute administration and 4-6 days after chronic administration) and its active metabolite, norfluoxetine (elimination half-life of 4-16 days after acute and chronic administration), leads to significant accumulation of these active species in chronic use and delayed attainment of steady-state, even when a fixed dose is used. After 30 days of dosing at 40 mg/day, plasma concentrations of fluoxetine in the range of 91-302 ng/ml and norfluoxetine in the range of 72-258 ng/ml have been observed. Plasma concentrations of fluoxetine were higher than those predicted by single-dose studies, because fluoxetine's metabolism is not proportional to dose. Norfluoxetine, however, appears to have linear pharmacokinetics. Its mean terminal half-life after a single-dose was 8.6 days and after multiple dosing was 9.3 days. Steady-state levels after prolonged dosing are similar to levels seen at 4-5 weeks.
The long elimination half-lives of fluoxetine and norfluoxetine assure that, even when dosing is stopped, active drug substance will persist in the body for weeks (primarily depending on individual patient characteristics, previous dosing regimen, and length of previous therapy at discontinuation). This is of potential consequence when drug discontinuation is required or when drugs are prescribed that might interact with fluoxetine and norfluoxetine following the discontinuation of Prozac or Sarafem.

Weekly Dosing
Administration of Prozac Weekly once-weekly results in increased fluctuation between peak and trough concentrations of fluoxetine and norfluoxetine compared to once-daily dosing (for fluoxetine: 24% [daily] to 164% [weekly] and for norfluoxetine: 17% [daily] to 43% [weekly]). Plasma concentrations may not necessarily be predictive of clinical response. Peak concentrations from once-weekly doses of Prozac Weekly capsules of fluoxetine are in the range of the average concentration for 20 mg once-daily dosing. Average trough concentrations are 76% lower for fluoxetine and 47% lower for norfluoxetine than the concentrations maintained by 20 mg once-daily dosing. Average steady-state concentrations of either once-daily or once-weekly dosing are in relative proportion to the total dose administered. Average steady-state fluoxetine concentrations are approximately 50% lower following the once-weekly regimen compared to a once-daily regimen.
C_{max} for fluoxetine following the 90 mg dose was approximately 1.7-fold higher than the C_{max} value for the established 20 mg once-daily regimen following transition the next day to the once-weekly regimen. In contrast, when the first 90 mg once-weekly dose and the last 20 mg once-daily dose were separated by 1 week, C_{max} values were similar. Also, there was a transient increase in the average steady-state concentrations of fluoxetine observed following transition the next day to the once-weekly regimen. From a pharmacokinetic perspective, it may be better to separate the first 90 mg weekly dose and the last 20 mg once-daily dose by 1 week (see DOSAGE AND ADMINISTRATION).

Liver Disease
As might be predicted from its primary site of metabolism, liver impairment can affect the elimination of fluoxetine. The elimination half-life of fluoxetine was prolonged in a study of cirrhotic patients, with a mean of 7.6 days compared to the range of 2-3 days seen in subjects without liver disease; norfluoxetine elimination was also delayed, with a mean duration of 12 days for cirrhotic patients compared to the range of 7-9 days in normal subjects. This suggests that the use of fluoxetine in patients with liver disease must be approached with caution. If fluoxetine is administered to patients with liver disease, a lower or less frequent dose should be used (see PRECAUTIONS, Use in Patients With Concomitant Illness and DOSAGE AND ADMINISTRATION).

F

Renal Disease
In depressed patients on dialysis (n=12), fluoxetine administered as 20 mg once-daily for 2 months produced steady-state fluoxetine and norfluoxetine plasma concentrations comparable to those seen in patients with normal renal function. While the possibility exists that renally excreted metabolites of fluoxetine may accumulate to higher levels in patients with severe renal dysfunction, use of a lower or less frequent dose is not routinely necessary in renally impaired patients (see PRECAUTIONS, Use in Patients With Concomitant Illness and DOSAGE AND ADMINISTRATION).

Age
Geriatric Pharmacokinetics
The disposition of single-doses of fluoxetine in healthy elderly subjects (greater than 65 years of age) did not differ significantly from that in younger normal subjects. However, given the long half-life and nonlinear disposition of the drug, a single-dose study is not adequate to rule out the possibility of altered pharmacokinetics in the elderly, particularly if they have systemic illness or are receiving multiple drugs for concomitant diseases. The effects of age upon the metabolism of fluoxetine have been investigated in 260 elderly but otherwise healthy depressed patients (≥60 years of age) who received 20 mg fluoxetine for 6 weeks. Combined fluoxetine plus norfluoxetine plasma concentrations were 209.3 ± 85.7 ng/ml at the end of 6 weeks. No unusual age-associated pattern of adverse events was observed in those elderly patients.

Pediatric Pharmacokinetics (children and adolescents)
Fluoxetine pharmacokinetics were evaluated in 21 pediatric patients (10 children ages 6 to <13, 11 adolescents ages 13 to <18) diagnosed with major depressive disorder or obsessive-compulsive disorder (OCD). Fluoxetine 20 mg/day was administered for up to 62 days. The average steady-state concentrations of fluoxetine in these children were 2-fold higher than in adolescents (171 ng/ml and 86 ng/ml, respectively). The average norfluoxetine steady-state concentrations in these children were 1.5-fold higher than in adolescents (195 ng/ml and 113 ng/ml, respectively). These differences can be almost entirely explained by differences in weight. No gender-associated difference in fluoxetine pharmacokinetics was observed. Similar ranges of fluoxetine and norfluoxetine plasma concentrations were observed in another study in 94 pediatric patients (ages 8 to <18) diagnosed with major depressive disorder.
Higher average steady-state fluoxetine and norfluoxetine concentrations were observed in children relative to adults; however, these concentrations were within the range of concentrations observed in the adult population. As in adults, fluoxetine and norfluoxetine accumulated extensively following multiple oral dosing; steady-state concentrations were achieved within 3-4 weeks of daily dosing.

INDICATIONS AND USAGE

MAJOR DEPRESSIVE DISORDER
Prozac is indicated for the treatment of major depressive disorder.

Adult
The efficacy of Prozac was established in 5 and 6 week trials with depressed adult and geriatric outpatients (≥18 years of age) whose diagnoses corresponded most closely to the DSM-III (currently DSM-IV) category of major depressive disorder.
A major depressive episode (DSM-IV) implies a prominent and relatively persistent (nearly every day for at least 2 weeks) depressed or dysphoric mood that usually interferes with daily functioning, and includes at least 5 of the following 9 symptoms: Depressed mood; loss of interest in usual activities; significant change in weight and/or appetite; insomnia or hypersomnia; psychomotor agitation or retardation; increased fatigue; feelings of guilt or worthlessness; slowed thinking or impaired concentration; a suicide attempt or suicidal ideation.
The effects of Prozac in hospitalized depressed patients have not been adequately studied.
The efficacy of Prozac 20 mg once-daily in maintaining a response in major depressive disorder for up to 38 weeks following 12 weeks of open-label acute treatment (50 weeks total) was demonstrated in a placebo-controlled trial.
The efficacy of Prozac Weekly once-weekly in maintaining a response in major depressive disorder has been demonstrated in a placebo-controlled trial for up to 25 weeks following open-label acute treatment of 13 weeks with Prozac 20 mg daily for a total treatment of 38 weeks. However, it is unknown whether or not Prozac Weekly given on a once-weekly basis provides the same level of protection from relapse as that provided by Prozac 20 mg daily.

Pediatric (children and adolescents)

The efficacy of Prozac in children and adolescents was established in two 8-9 week placebo-controlled clinical trials in depressed outpatients whose diagnosis corresponded most closely to the DSM-III-R or DSM-IV category of major depressive disorder.

The usefulness of the drug in adult and pediatric patients receiving fluoxetine for extended periods should be reevaluated periodically.

OBSESSIVE-COMPULSIVE DISORDER

Adult

Prozac is indicated for the treatment of obsessions and compulsions in patients with obsessive-compulsive disorder (OCD), as defined in the DSM-III-R; *i.e.,* the obsessions or compulsions cause marked distress, are time-consuming, or significantly interfere with social or occupational functioning.

The efficacy of Prozac was established in 13 week trials with obsessive-compulsive outpatients whose diagnoses corresponded most closely to the DSM-III-R category of obsessive-compulsive disorder.

Obsessive-compulsive disorder is characterized by recurrent and persistent ideas, thoughts, impulses, or images (obsessions) that are ego-dystonic and/or repetitive, purposeful, and intentional behaviors (compulsions) that are recognized by the person as excessive or unreasonable.

The effectiveness of Prozac in long-term use (*i.e.,* for more than 13 weeks) has not been systematically evaluated in placebo-controlled trials. Therefore, the physician who elects to use Prozac for extended periods should periodically reevaluate the long-term usefulness of the drug for the individual patient (see DOSAGE AND ADMINISTRATION).

Pediatric (children and adolescents)

The efficacy of Prozac in children and adolescents was established in a 13 week dose titration, clinical trial in patients with OCD, as defined in DSM-IV.

BULIMIA NERVOSA

Prozac is indicated for the treatment of binge-eating and vomiting behaviors in patients with moderate to severe bulimia nervosa.

The efficacy of Prozac was established in 8-16 week trials for adult outpatients with moderate to severe bulimia nervosa (*i.e.,* at least 3 bulimic episodes/week for 6 months).

The efficacy of Prozac 60 mg/day in maintaining a response, in patients with bulimia who responded during an 8 week acute treatment phase while taking Prozac 60 mg/day and were then observed for relapse during a period of up to 52 weeks, was demonstrated in a placebo-controlled trial. Nevertheless, the physician who elects to use Prozac for extended periods should periodically reevaluate the long-term usefulness of the drug for the individual patient (see DOSAGE AND ADMINISTRATION).

PANIC DISORDER

Prozac is indicated for the treatment of panic disorder, with or without agoraphobia, as defined in DSM-IV. Panic disorder is characterized by the occurrence of unexpected panic attacks, and associated concern about having additional attacks, worry about the implications or consequences of the attacks, and/or a significant change in behavior related to the attacks.

The efficacy of Prozac was established in two 12 week clinical trials in patients whose diagnoses corresponded to the DSM-IV category of panic disorder.

Panic disorder (DSM-IV) is characterized by recurrent, unexpected panic attacks, *i.e.,* a discrete period of intense fear or discomfort in which 4 or more of the following symptoms develop abruptly and reach a peak within 10 minutes: (1) palpitations, pounding heart, or accelerated heart rate; (2) sweating; (3) trembling or shaking; (4) sensations of shortness of breath or smothering; (5) feeling of choking; (6) chest pain or discomfort; (7) nausea or abdominal distress; (8) feeling dizzy, unsteady, lightheaded, or faint; (9) fear of losing control; (10) fear of dying; (11) paresthesias (numbness or tingling sensations); (12) chills or hot flashes.

The effectiveness of Prozac in long-term use, that is, for more than 12 weeks, has not been established in placebo-controlled trials. Therefore, the physician who elects to use Prozac for extended periods should periodically reevaluate the long-term usefulness of the drug for the individual patient (see DOSAGE AND ADMINISTRATION).

PREMENSTRUAL DYSPHORIC DISORDER (PMDD)

Sarafem is indicated for the treatment of premenstrual dysphoric disorder (PMDD).

The efficacy of fluoxetine in the treatment of PMDD was established in 3 placebo-controlled trials.

The essential features of PMDD, according to the DSM-IV, include markedly depressed mood, anxiety or tension, affective lability, and persistent anger or irritability. Other features include decreased interest in usual activities, difficulty concentrating, lack of energy, change in appetite or sleep, and feeling out of control. Physical symptoms associated with PMDD include breast tenderness, headache, joint and muscle pain, bloating, and weight gain. These symptoms occur regularly during the luteal phase and remit within a few days following onset of menses; the disturbance markedly interferes with work or school or with usual social activities and relationships with others. In making the diagnosis, care should be taken to rule out other cyclical mood disorders that may be exacerbated by treatment with an antidepressant.

The effectiveness of Sarafem in long-term use, that is, for more than 6 months, has not been systematically evaluated in controlled trials. Therefore, the physician who elects to use Sarafem for extended periods should periodically reevaluate the long-term usefulness of the drug for the individual patient.

NON-FDA APPROVED INDICATIONS

Fluoxetine and other SSRIs may also have clinical utility for the treatment of a number of other conditions including substance abuse, headaches, premature ejaculation, post-traumatic stress disorder, seasonal affective disorder, chronic pain, and bipolar II major depression, although none of these uses is approved by the FDA and comparative efficacy trials for many of these uses have not yet been performed.

CONTRAINDICATIONS

Fluoxetine is contraindicated in patients known to be hypersensitive to it.

MONOAMINE OXIDASE INHIBITORS

There have been reports of serious, sometimes fatal, reactions (including hyperthermia, rigidity, myoclonus, autonomic instability with possible rapid fluctuations of vital signs, and mental status changes that include extreme agitation progressing to delirium and coma) in patients receiving fluoxetine in combination with a monoamine oxidase inhibitor (MAOI), and in patients who have recently discontinued fluoxetine and are then started on an MAOI. Some cases presented with features resembling neuroleptic malignant syndrome. Therefore, fluoxetine should not be used in combination with an MAOI, or within a minimum of 14 days of discontinuing therapy with an MAOI. Since fluoxetine and its major metabolite have very long elimination half-lives, at least 5 weeks (perhaps longer, especially if fluoxetine has been prescribed chronically and/or at higher doses [see CLINICAL PHARMACOLOGY, Accumulation and Slow Elimination]) should be allowed after stopping Prozac before starting an MAOI.

THIORIDAZINE

Thioridazine should not be administered with Prozac or within a minimum of 5 weeks after Prozac has been discontinued (see WARNINGS).

WARNINGS

RASH AND POSSIBLY ALLERGIC EVENTS

In US fluoxetine clinical trials for conditions other than PMDD as of May 8, 1995, 7% of 10,782 patients developed various types of rashes and/or urticaria. Among the cases of rash and/or urticaria reported in premarketing clinical trials, almost a third were withdrawn from treatment because of the rash and/or systemic signs or symptoms associated with the rash. In 4 clinical trials for PMDD, 4% of 415 patients treated with Sarafem reported rash and/or urticaria. None of these cases were classified as serious and 2 of 415 patients (both receiving 60 mg) were withdrawn from treatment because of rash and/or urticaria. Clinical findings reported in association with rash include fever, leukocytosis, arthralgias, edema, carpal tunnel syndrome, respiratory distress, lymphadenopathy, proteinuria, and mild transaminase elevation. Most patients improved promptly with discontinuation of fluoxetine and/or adjunctive treatment with antihistamines or steroids, and all patients experiencing these events were reported to recover completely.

In premarketing clinical trials, 2 patients are known to have developed a serious cutaneous systemic illness. In neither patient was there an unequivocal diagnosis, but 1 was considered to have a leukocytoclastic vasculitis, and the other, a severe desquamating syndrome that was considered variously to be a vasculitis or erythema multiforme. Other patients have had systemic syndromes suggestive of serum sickness.

Since the introduction of Prozac, systemic events, possibly related to vasculitis and including lupus-like syndrome, have developed in patients with rash. Although these events are rare, they may be serious, involving the lung, kidney, or liver. Death has been reported to occur in association with these systemic events.

Anaphylactoid events, including bronchospasm, angioedema, laryngospasm, and urticaria alone and in combination, have been reported.

Pulmonary events, including inflammatory processes of varying histopathology and/or fibrosis, have been reported rarely. These events have occurred with dyspnea as the only preceding symptom.

Whether these systemic events and rash have a common underlying cause or are due to different etiologies or pathogenic processes is not known. Furthermore, a specific underlying immunologic basis for these events has not been identified. Upon the appearance of rash or of other possibly allergic phenomena for which an alternative etiology cannot be identified, fluoxetine should be discontinued.

POTENTIAL INTERACTION WITH THIORIDAZINE

In a study of 19 healthy male subjects, which included 6 slow and 13 rapid hydroxylators of debrisoquin, a single 25 mg oral dose of thioridazine produced a 2.4-fold higher C_{max} and a 4.5-fold higher AUC for thioridazine in the slow hydroxylators compared to the rapid hydroxylators. The rate of debrisoquin hydroxylation is felt to depend on the level of cytochrome P450IID6 isozyme activity. Thus, this study suggests that drugs which inhibit P450IID6, such as certain SSRIs, including fluoxetine, will produce elevated plasma levels of thioridazine (see PRECAUTIONS).

Thioridazine administration produces a dose-related prolongation of the QTc interval, which is associated with serious ventricular arrhythmias, such as torsades de pointes-type arrhythmias, and sudden death. This risk is expected to increase with fluoxetine-induced inhibition of thioridazine metabolism (see CONTRAINDICATIONS).

PRECAUTIONS

GENERAL

Anxiety and Insomnia

In US placebo-controlled clinical trials for major depressive disorder, 12-16% of patients treated with Prozac and 7-9% of patients treated with placebo reported anxiety, nervousness, or insomnia.

In US placebo-controlled clinical trials for OCD, insomnia was reported in 28% of patients treated with Prozac and in 22% of patients treated with placebo. Anxiety was reported in 14% of patients treated with Prozac and in 7% of patients treated with placebo.

In US placebo-controlled clinical trials for bulimia nervosa, insomnia was reported in 33% of patients treated with Prozac 60 mg, and 13% of patients treated with placebo. Anxiety and nervousness were reported respectively in 15% and 11% of patients treated with Prozac 60 mg, and in 9% and 5% of patients treated with placebo.

Among the most common adverse events associated with discontinuation (incidence at least twice that for placebo and at least 1% for Prozac in clinical trials collecting only a primary event associated with discontinuation) in US placebo-controlled fluoxetine clinical trials were anxiety (2% in OCD), insomnia (1% in combined indications and 2% in bulimia), and nervousness (1% in major depressive disorder) (see TABLE 5).

In 2 placebo-controlled trials of fluoxetine in PMDD, treatment-emergent adverse events were assessed. Rates were as follows for Sarafem 20 mg (the recommended dose) continuous and intermittent pooled, Sarafem 60 mg continuous, and pooled placebo, respectively: anxiety (3%, 9%, and 4%), nervousness (5%, 9%, and 3%), and insomnia (9%, 26%, and 7%). For individual rates for Sarafem 20 mg given as continuous and intermittent dosing, see TABLE 6 and accompanying footnote. Events associated with discontinuation for Sarafem 20 mg continuous and intermittent pooled, Sarafem 60 mg continuous, and pooled placebo, respectively, were: anxiety (0%, 6%, and 1%), nervousness (1%, 0%, and 0.5%), and insomnia (1%, 4%, and 0.5%). In US placebo-controlled clinical trials of fluoxetine for other approved indications, anxiety, nervousness, and insomnia have been among the most commonly reported adverse events (see TABLE 7).

Altered Appetite and Weight

Significant weight loss, especially in underweight depressed or bulimic patients may be an undesirable result of treatment with fluoxetine.

In US placebo-controlled clinical trials for major depressive disorder, 11% of patients treated with Prozac and 2% of patients treated with placebo reported anorexia (decreased appetite). Weight loss was reported in 1.4% of patients treated with Prozac and in 0.5% of patients treated with placebo. However, only rarely have patients discontinued treatment with Prozac because of anorexia or weight loss (see also Pediatric Use).

In US placebo-controlled clinical trials for OCD, 17% of patients treated with Prozac and 10% of patients treated with placebo reported anorexia (decreased appetite). One patient discontinued treatment with Prozac because of anorexia (see also Pediatric Use).

In US placebo-controlled clinical trials for bulimia nervosa, 8% of patients treated with Prozac, 60 mg, and 4% of patients treated with placebo reported anorexia (decreased appetite). Patients treated with Prozac, 60 mg, on average lost 0.45 kg compared with a gain of 0.16 kg by patients treated with placebo in the 16 week double-blind trial. Weight change should be monitored during therapy.

In 2 placebo-controlled trials of fluoxetine in PMDD, rates for anorexia were as follows for Sarafem 20 mg (the recommended dose) continuous and intermittent pooled, Sarafem 60 mg continuous, and pooled placebo, respectively: 4%, 13%, and 2%. For individual rates for Sarafem 20 mg continuous and intermittent, see footnote accompanying TABLE 6. In 2 placebo-controlled trials (only 1 of which included a dose of 60 mg/day), potentially clinically significant weight gain (≥7%) occurred in 8% of patients on Sarafem 20 mg, 6% of patients on Sarafem 60 mg, and 1% of patients on placebo. Potentially clinically significant weight loss (≥7%) occurred in 7% of patients on Sarafem 20 mg, 12% of patients on Sarafem 60 mg, and 3% of patients on placebo.

Activation of Mania/Hypomania

In US placebo-controlled clinical trials for major depressive disorder, mania/hypomania was reported in 0.1% of patients treated with Prozac and 0.1% of patients treated with placebo. Activation of mania/hypomania has also been reported in a small proportion of patients with Major Affective Disorder treated with other marketed drugs effective in the treatment of major depressive disorder (see also Pediatric Use).

In US placebo-controlled clinical trials for OCD, mania/hypomania was reported in 0.8% of patients treated with Prozac and no patients treated with placebo. No patients reported mania/hypomania in US placebo-controlled clinical trials for bulimia. In all US Prozac clinical trials as of May 8, 1995, 0.7% of 10,782 patients reported mania/hypomania (see also Pediatric Use).

No patients treated with Sarafem in 4 PMDD clinical trials (n=415) reported mania/hypomania.

Seizures

In US placebo-controlled clinical trials for major depressive disorder, convulsions (or events described as possibly having been seizures) were reported in 0.1% of patients treated with Prozac and 0.2% of patients treated with placebo. No patients reported convulsions in US placebo-controlled clinical trials for either OCD, bulimia, or PMDD. In all US Prozac clinical trials as of May 8, 1995, 0.2% of 10,782 patients reported convulsions. The percentage appears to be similar to that associated with other marketed drugs effective in the treatment of major depressive disorder. Fluoxetine should be introduced with care in patients with a history of seizures.

Suicide

The possibility of a suicide attempt is inherent in major depressive disorder and may persist until significant remission occurs. Close supervision of high risk patients should accompany initial drug therapy. Prescriptions for Prozac should be written for the smallest quantity of capsules consistent with good patient management, in order to reduce the risk of overdose.

Because of well-established comorbidity between both OCD and major depressive disorder and bulimia and major depressive disorder, the same precautions observed when treating patients with major depressive disorder should be observed when treating patients with OCD or bulimia.

No patients treated with Sarafem in 4 PMDD clinical trials (n=415) attempted suicide.

The Long Elimination Half-Lives of Fluoxetine and Its Metabolites

Because of the long elimination half-lives of the parent drug and its major active metabolite, changes in dose will not be fully reflected in plasma for several weeks, affecting both strategies for titration to final dose and withdrawal from treatment (see CLINICAL PHARMACOLOGY and DOSAGE AND ADMINISTRATION).

Use in Patients With Concomitant Illness

Clinical experience with fluoxetine in patients with concomitant systemic illness is limited. Caution is advisable in using fluoxetine in patients with diseases or conditions that could affect metabolism or hemodynamic responses.

Fluoxetine has not been evaluated or used to any appreciable extent in patients with a recent history of myocardial infarction or unstable heart disease. Patients with these diagnoses were systematically excluded from clinical studies during the product's premarket testing. However, the electrocardiograms of 312 patients who received fluoxetine in double-blind trials were retrospectively evaluated; no conduction abnormalities that resulted in heart block were observed. The mean heart rate was reduced by approximately 3 beats/min.

In subjects with cirrhosis of the liver, the clearances of fluoxetine and its active metabolite, norfluoxetine, were decreased, thus increasing the elimination half-lives of these substances. A lower or less frequent dose should be used in patients with cirrhosis.

Studies in depressed patients on dialysis did not reveal excessive accumulation of fluoxetine or norfluoxetine in plasma (see CLINICAL PHARMACOLOGY, Renal Disease). Use of a lower or less frequent dose for renally impaired patients is not routinely necessary (see DOSAGE AND ADMINISTRATION).

In patients with diabetes, fluoxetine may alter glycemic control. Hypoglycemia has occurred during therapy with fluoxetine, and hyperglycemia has developed following discontinuation of the drug. As is true with many other types of medication when taken concurrently by patients with diabetes, insulin and/or oral hypoglycemic dosage may need to be adjusted when therapy with fluoxetine is instituted or discontinued.

Interference With Cognitive and Motor Performance

Any psychoactive drug may impair judgment, thinking, or motor skills, and patients should be cautioned about operating hazardous machinery, including automobiles, until they are reasonably certain that the drug treatment does not affect them adversely.

INFORMATION FOR THE PATIENT

Physicians are advised to discuss the following issues with patients for whom they prescribe Prozac:

Because Prozac may impair judgment, thinking, or motor skills, patients should be advised to avoid driving a car or operating hazardous machinery until they are reasonably certain that their performance is not affected.

Patients should be advised to inform their physician if they are taking or plan to take any prescription or over-the-counter drugs, or alcohol.

Patients should be advised to notify their physician if they become pregnant or intend to become pregnant during therapy.

Patients should be advised to notify their physician if they are breastfeeding an infant.

Patients should be advised to notify their physician if they develop a rash or hives.

LABORATORY TESTS

There are no specific laboratory tests recommended.

CARCINOGENESIS, MUTAGENESIS, AND IMPAIRMENT OF FERTILITY

There is no evidence of carcinogenicity, mutagenicity, or impairment of fertility with fluoxetine.

Carcinogenesis

The dietary administration of fluoxetine to rats and mice for 2 years at doses of up to 10 and 12 mg/kg/day, respectively (approximately 1.2 and 0.7 times, respectively, the maximum recommended human dose [MRHD] of 80 mg on a mg/m^2 basis), produced no evidence of carcinogenicity.

Mutagenicity

Fluoxetine and norfluoxetine have been shown to have no genotoxic effects based on the following assays: bacterial mutation assay, DNA repair assay in cultured rat hepatocytes, mouse lymphoma assay, and *in vivo* sister chromatid exchange assay in Chinese hamster bone marrow cells.

Impairment of Fertility

Two fertility studies conducted in rats at doses of up to 7.5 and 12.5 mg/kg/day (approximately 0.9 and 1.5 times the MRHD on a mg/m^2 basis) indicated that fluoxetine had no adverse effects on fertility.

PREGNANCY CATEGORY C

In embryo-fetal development studies in rats and rabbits, there was no evidence of teratogenicity following administration of up to 12.5 and 15 mg/kg/day, respectively (1.5 and 3.6 times, respectively, the maximum recommended human dose [MRHD] of 80 mg on a mg/m^2 basis) throughout organogenesis. However, in rat reproduction studies, an increase in stillborn pups, a decrease in pup weight, and an increase in pup deaths during the first 7 days postpartum occurred following maternal exposure to 12 mg/kg/day (1.5 times the MRHD on a mg/m^2 basis) during gestation or 7.5 mg/kg/day (0.9 times the MRHD on a mg/m^2 basis) during gestation and lactation. There was no evidence of developmental neurotoxicity in the surviving offspring of rats treated with 12 mg/kg/day during gestation. The no-effect dose for rat pup mortality was 5 mg/kg/day (0.6 times the MRHD on a mg/m^2 basis). Fluoxetine should be used during pregnancy only if the potential benefit justifies the potential risk to the fetus.

LABOR AND DELIVERY

The effect of fluoxetine on labor and delivery in humans is unknown. However, because fluoxetine crosses the placenta and because of the possibility that fluoxetine may have adverse effects on the newborn, fluoxetine should be used during labor and delivery only if the potential benefit justifies the potential risk to the fetus.

NURSING MOTHERS

Because fluoxetine is excreted in human milk, nursing while on fluoxetine is not recommended. In 1 breast milk sample, the concentration of fluoxetine plus norfluoxetine was 70.4 ng/ml. The concentration in the mother's plasma was 295.0 ng/ml. No adverse effects on the infant were reported. In another case, an infant nursed by a mother on Prozac developed crying, sleep disturbance, vomiting, and watery stools. The infant's plasma drug levels were 340 ng/ml of fluoxetine and 208 ng/ml of norfluoxetine on the second day of feeding.

PEDIATRIC USE

The efficacy of fluoxetine for the treatment of major depressive disorder was demonstrated in two 8-9 week placebo-controlled clinical trials with 315 pediatric outpatients ages 8 to ≤18.

The efficacy of fluoxetine for the treatment of OCD was demonstrated in one 13 week placebo-controlled clinical trial with 103 pediatric outpatients ages 7 to <18.

Safety and effectiveness in pediatric patients less than 8 years of age in major depressive disorder and less than 7 years of age in OCD have not been established.

Fluoxetine pharmacokinetics were evaluated in 21 pediatric patients (ages 6 to ≤18) with major depressive disorder or OCD (see CLINICAL PHARMACOLOGY, Pediatric Pharmacokinetics (children and adolescents)).

The acute adverse event profiles in the three studies (n=418 randomized; 228 fluoxetine-treated, 190 placebo-treated) were generally similar to that observed in adult studies with fluoxetine. The longer-term adverse event profile observed in the 19 week major depressive disorder study (n=219 randomized; 109 fluoxetine-treated, 110 placebo-treated) was also similar to that observed in adult trials with fluoxetine (see ADVERSE REACTIONS).

Manic reaction, including mania and hypomania, was reported in 6 (1 mania, 5 hypomania) out of 228 (2.6%) fluoxetine-treated patients and in 0 out of 190 (0%) placebo-treated patients. Mania/hypomania led to the discontinuation of 4 (1.8%) fluoxetine-treated patients from the acute phases of the three studies combined. Consequently, regular monitoring for the occurrence of mania/hypomania is recommended.

As with other SSRIs, decreased weight gain has been observed in association with the use of fluoxetine in children and adolescent patients. After 19 weeks of treatment in a clinical trial, pediatric subjects treated with fluoxetine gained an average of 1.1 cm less in height (p=0.004) and 1.1 kg less in weight (p=0.008) than subjects treated with placebo. In addition, fluoxetine treatment was associated with a decrease in alkaline phosphatase levels. The safety of fluoxetine treatment for pediatric patients has not been systematically assessed for chronic treatment longer than several months in duration. In particular, there are no studies that directly evaluate the longer-term effects of fluoxetine on the growth, development, and maturation of children and adolescent patients. Therefore, height and weight should be monitored periodically in pediatric patients receiving fluoxetine.

GERIATRIC USE

US fluoxetine clinical trials as of May 8, 1995 (10,782 patients) included 687 patients ≥65 years of age and 93 patients ≥75 years of age. The efficacy in geriatric patients has been established. For pharmacokinetic information in geriatric patients see CLINICAL PHARMACOLOGY, Age. No overall differences in safety or effectiveness were observed between these subjects and younger subjects, and other reported clinical experience has not identified differences in responses between the elderly and younger patients, but greater sensitivity of some older individuals cannot be ruled out. As with other SSRIs, fluoxetine has been associated with cases of clinically significant hyponatremia in elderly patients (see Hyponatremia).

HYPONATREMIA

Cases of hyponatremia (some with serum sodium lower than 110 mmol/L) have been reported. The hyponatremia appeared to be reversible when Prozac was discontinued. Although these cases were complex with varying possible etiologies, some were possibly due to the syndrome of inappropriate antidiuretic hormone secretion (SIADH). The majority of these occurrences have been in older patients and in patients taking diuretics or who were otherwise volume depleted. In two 6 week controlled studies in patients ≥60 years of age, 10 of 323 fluoxetine patients and 6 of 327 placebo recipients had a lowering of serum sodium below the reference range; this difference was not statistically significant. The lowest observed concentration was 129 mmol/L. The observed decreases were not clinically significant.

PLATELET FUNCTION

There have been rare reports of altered platelet function and/or abnormal results from laboratory studies in patients taking fluoxetine. While there have been reports of abnormal bleeding in several patients taking fluoxetine, it is unclear whether fluoxetine had a causative role.

DRUG INTERACTIONS

As with all drugs, the potential for interaction by a variety of mechanisms (*e.g.,* pharmacodynamic, pharmacokinetic drug inhibition or enhancement, etc.) is a possibility (see CLINICAL PHARMACOLOGY, Accumulation and Slow Elimination).

DRUGS METABOLIZED BY P450IID6

Approximately 7% of the normal population has a genetic defect that leads to reduced levels of activity of the cytochrome P450 isoenzyme P450IID6. Such individuals have been referred to as "poor metabolizers" of drugs such as debrisoquin, dextromethorphan, and TCAs. Many drugs, such as most drugs effective in the treatment of major depressive disorder, including fluoxetine and other selective uptake inhibitors of serotonin, are metabolized by this isoenzyme; thus, both the pharmacokinetic properties and relative proportion of metabolites are altered in poor metabolizers. However, for fluoxetine and its metabolite the sum of the plasma concentrations of the four active enantiomers is comparable between poor and extensive metabolizers (see CLINICAL PHARMACOLOGY, Variability in Metabolism).

Fluoxetine, like other agents that are metabolized by P450IID6, inhibits the activity of this isoenzyme, and thus may make normal metabolizers resemble "poor metabolizers." Therapy with medications that are predominantly metabolized by the P450IID6 system and that have a relatively narrow therapeutic index (see CNS Active Drugs), should be initiated at the low end of the dose range if a patient is receiving fluoxetine concurrently or has taken it in the previous 5 weeks. Thus, his/her dosing requirements resemble those of "poor metabolizers." If fluoxetine is added to the treatment regimen of a patient already receiving a drug metabolized by P450IID6, the need for decreased dose of the original medication should be considered. Drugs with a narrow therapeutic index represent the greatest concern (*e.g.,* flecainide, vinblastine, and TCAs). Due to the risk of serious ventricular arrhythmias and sudden death potentially associated with elevated plasma levels of thioridazine, thioridazine should not be administered with fluoxetine or within a minimum of 5 weeks after fluoxetine has been discontinued (see CONTRAINDICATIONS and WARNINGS).

DRUGS METABOLIZED BY CYTOCHROME P450IIIA4

In an *in vivo* interaction study involving coadministration of fluoxetine with single-doses of terfenadine (a cytochrome P450IIIA4 substrate), no increase in plasma terfenadine concentrations occurred with concomitant fluoxetine. In addition, *in vitro* studies have shown ketoconazole, a potent inhibitor of P450IIIA4 activity, to be at least 100 times more potent than fluoxetine or norfluoxetine as an inhibitor of the metabolism of several substrates for this enzyme, including astemizole, cisapride, and midazolam. These data indicate that fluoxetine's extent of inhibition of cytochrome P450IIIA4 activity is not likely to be of clinical significance.

CNS ACTIVE DRUGS

The risk of using fluoxetine in combination with other CNS active drugs has not been systematically evaluated. Nonetheless, caution is advised if the concomitant administration of fluoxetine and such drugs is required. In evaluating individual cases, consideration should be given to using lower initial doses of the concomitantly administered drugs, using conservative titration schedules, and monitoring of clinical status (see CLINICAL PHARMACOLOGY, Accumulation and Slow Elimination).

Anticonvulsants

Patients on stable doses of phenytoin and carbamazepine have developed elevated plasma anticonvulsant concentrations and clinical anticonvulsant toxicity following initiation of concomitant fluoxetine treatment.

Antipsychotics

Some clinical data suggests a possible pharmacodynamic and/or pharmacokinetic interaction between serotonin specific reuptake inhibitors (SSRIs) and antipsychotics. Elevation of blood levels of haloperidol and clozapine has been observed in patients receiving concomitant fluoxetine. A single case report has suggested possible additive effects of pimozide and fluoxetine leading to bradycardia. For thioridazine, see CONTRAINDICATIONS and WARNINGS.

Benzodiazepines

The half-life of concurrently administered diazepam may be prolonged in some patients (see CLINICAL PHARMACOLOGY, Accumulation and Slow Elimination). Coadministration of alprazolam and fluoxetine has resulted in increased alprazolam plasma concentrations and in further psychomotor performance decrement due to increased alprazolam levels.

Lithium

There have been reports of both increased and decreased lithium levels when lithium was used concomitantly with fluoxetine. Cases of lithium toxicity and increased serotonergic effects have been reported. Lithium levels should be monitored when these drugs are administered concomitantly.

Tryptophan

Five patients receiving Prozac in combination with tryptophan experienced adverse reactions, including agitation, restlessness, and gastrointestinal distress.

Monoamine Oxidase Inhibitors

See CONTRAINDICATIONS.

Other Drugs Effective in the Treatment of Major Depressive Disorder

In two studies, previously stable plasma levels of imipramine and desipramine have increased greater than 2- to 10-fold when fluoxetine has been administered in combination. This influence may persist for 3 weeks or longer after fluoxetine is discontinued. Thus, the dose of TCA may need to be reduced and plasma TCA concentrations may need to be monitored temporarily when fluoxetine is coadministered or has been recently discontinued (see CLINICAL PHARMACOLOGY, Accumulation and Slow Elimination and DRUG INTERACTIONS, Drugs Metabolized by P450IID6).

Sumatriptan

There have been rare postmarketing reports describing patients with weakness, hyperreflexia, and incoordination following the use of an SSRI and sumatriptan. If concomitant treatment with sumatriptan and an SSRI (*e.g.,* fluoxetine, fluvoxamine, paroxetine, sertraline, or citalopram) is clinically warranted, appropriate observation of the patient is advised.

POTENTIAL EFFECTS OF COADMINISTRATION OF DRUGS TIGHTLY BOUND TO PLASMA PROTEINS

Because fluoxetine is tightly bound to plasma protein, the administration of fluoxetine to a patient taking another drug that is tightly bound to protein (*e.g.,* warfarin, digitoxin) may cause a shift in plasma concentrations potentially resulting in an adverse effect. Conversely, adverse effects may result from displacement of protein bound fluoxetine by other tightly bound drugs (see CLINICAL PHARMACOLOGY, Accumulation and Slow Elimination).

WARFARIN

Altered anti-coagulant effects, including increased bleeding, have been reported when fluoxetine is coadministered with warfarin. Patients receiving warfarin therapy should receive careful coagulation monitoring when fluoxetine is initiated or stopped.

ELECTROCONVULSIVE THERAPY

There are no clinical studies establishing the benefit of the combined use of ECT and fluoxetine. There have been rare reports of prolonged seizures in patients on fluoxetine receiving ECT treatment.

ADVERSE REACTIONS

Multiple doses of Prozac had been administered to 10,782 patients with various diagnoses in US clinical trials as of May 8, 1995. In addition, there have been 425 patients administered Prozac in panic clinical trials. Adverse events were recorded by clinical investigators using descriptive terminology of their own choosing. Consequently, it is not possible to provide a meaningful estimate of the proportion of individuals experiencing adverse events without first grouping similar types of events into a limited (*i.e.,* reduced) number of standardized event categories.

In TABLE 3A, TABLE 3B, TABLE 3C, TABLE 3D, TABLE 4, TABLE 5, and the tabulations that follow, COSTART Dictionary terminology has been used to classify reported adverse events. The stated frequencies represent the proportion of individuals who experienced, at least once, a treatment-emergent adverse event of the type listed. An event was considered treatment-emergent if it occurred for the first time or worsened while receiving therapy following baseline evaluation. It is important to emphasize that events reported during therapy were not necessarily caused by it.

The prescriber should be aware that the figures in TABLE 3A, TABLE 3B, TABLE 3C, TABLE 3D, TABLE 4, TABLE 5 and the tabulations cannot be used to predict the incidence of side effects in the course of usual medical practice where patient characteristics and other factors differ from those that prevailed in the clinical trials. Similarly, the cited frequencies cannot be compared with figures obtained from other clinical investigations involving different treatments, uses, and investigators. The cited figures, however, do provide the prescribing physician with some basis for estimating the relative contribution of drug and nondrug factors to the side effect incidence rate in the population studied.

INCIDENCE IN MAJOR DEPRESSIVE DISORDER, OCD, BULIMIA, AND PANIC DISORDER PLACEBO-CONTROLLED CLINICAL TRIALS (EXCLUDING DATA FROM EXTENSIONS OF TRIALS)

TABLE 3A, TABLE 3B, TABLE 3C, and TABLE 3D enumerate the most common treatment-emergent adverse events associated with the use of Prozac (incidence of at least 5% for Prozac and at least twice that for placebo within at least 1 of the indications) for the treatment of major depressive disorder, OCD, and bulimia in US controlled clinical trials and panic disorder in US plus non-US controlled trials. TABLE 4 enumerates treatment-emergent adverse events that occurred in 2% or more patients treated with Prozac and with incidence greater than placebo who participated in US major depressive disorder, OCD, and bulimia controlled clinical trials and US plus non-US panic disorder controlled clinical trials. TABLE 4 provides combined data for the pool of studies that are provided separately by indication in TABLE 3A, TABLE 3B, TABLE 3C, and TABLE 3D.

TABLE 3A *Most Common Treatment-Emergent Adverse Events: Incidence in Major Depressive Disorder Placebo-Controlled Clinical Trials*

Body System / Adverse Event	Prozac (n=1728)	Placebo (n=975)
Body as a Whole		
Asthenia	9%	5%
Flu syndrome	3%	4%
Cardiovascular System		
Vasodilatation	3%	2%
Digestive System		
Nausea	21%	9%
Diarrhea	12%	8%
Anorexia	11%	2%
Dry mouth	10%	7%
Dyspepsia	7%	5%
Nervous System		
Insomnia	16%	9%
Anxiety	12%	7%
Nervousness	14%	9%
Somnolence	13%	6%
Tremor	10%	3%
Libido decreased	3%	—
Abnormal dreams	1%	1%
Respiratory System		
Pharyngitis	3%	3%
Sinusitis	1%	4%
Yawn	—	—
Skin and Appendages		
Sweating	8%	3%
Rash	4%	3%
Urogenital System		
Impotence*	2%	—
Abnormal ejaculation*	—	—

* Denominator used was for males only (n=690 Prozac; n=410 placebo).
— Incidence less than 1%.

TABLE 3B *Most Common Treatment-Emergent Adverse Events: Incidence in OCD Placebo-Controlled Clinical Trials*

Body System / Adverse Event	Prozac (n=266)	Placebo (n=89)
Body as a Whole		
Asthenia	15%	11%
Flu syndrome	10%	7%
Cardiovascular System		
Vasodilatation	5%	—
Digestive System		
Nausea	26%	13%
Diarrhea	18%	13%
Anorexia	17%	10%
Dry mouth	12%	3%
Dyspepsia	10%	4%
Nervous System		
Insomnia	28%	22%
Anxiety	14%	7%
Nervousness	14%	15%
Somnolence	17%	7%
Tremor	9%	1%
Libido decreased	11%	2%
Abnormal dreams	5%	2%
Respiratory System		
Pharyngitis	11%	9%
Sinusitis	5%	2%
Yawn	7%	—
Skin and Appendages		
Sweating	7%	—
Rash	6%	3%
Urogenital System		
Impotence*	—	—
Abnormal ejaculation*	7%	—

* Denominator used was for males only (n=116 Prozac; n=43 placebo).
— Incidence less than 1%.

TABLE 3C *Most Common Treatment-Emergent Adverse Events: Incidence in Bulimia Placebo-Controlled Clinical Trials*

Body System / Adverse Event	Prozac (n=450)	Placebo (n=267)
Body as a Whole		
Asthenia	21%	9%
Flu syndrome	8%	3%
Cardiovascular System		
Vasodilatation	2%	1%
Digestive System		
Nausea	29%	11%
Diarrhea	8%	6%
Anorexia	8%	4%
Dry mouth	9%	6%
Dyspepsia	10%	6%
Nervous System		
Insomnia	33%	13%
Anxiety	15%	9%
Nervousness	11%	5%
Somnolence	13%	5%
Tremor	13%	1%
Libido decreased	5%	1%
Abnormal dreams	5%	3%
Respiratory System		
Pharyngitis	10%	5%
Sinusitis	6%	4%
Yawn	11%	—
Skin and Appendages		
Sweating	8%	3%
Rash	4%	4%
Urogenital System		
Impotence*	7%	—
Abnormal ejaculation*	7%	—

* Denominator used was for males only (n=14 Prozac; n=1 placebo).
— Incidence less than 1%.

ASSOCIATED WITH DISCONTINUATION IN MAJOR DEPRESSIVE DISORDER, OCD, BULIMIA, AND PANIC DISORDER PLACEBO-CONTROLLED CLINICAL TRIALS (EXCLUDING DATA FROM EXTENSIONS OF TRIALS)

TABLE 5 lists the adverse events associated with discontinuation of Prozac treatment (incidence at least twice that for placebo and at least 1% for Prozac in clinical trials collecting only a primary event associated with discontinuation) in major depressive disorder, OCD, bulimia, and panic disorder clinical trials, plus non-US panic disorder clinical trials.

OTHER ADVERSE EVENTS IN PEDIATRIC PATIENTS (CHILDREN AND ADOLESCENTS)

Treatment-emergent adverse events were collected in 322 pediatric patients (180 fluoxetine-treated, 142 placebo-treated). The overall profile of adverse events was generally similar to that seen in adult studies, as shown in TABLE 3A, TABLE 3B, TABLE 3C, TABLE 3D and TABLE 4. However, the following adverse events (excluding those which appear in the body or footnotes of TABLE 3A, TABLE 3B, TABLE 3C, TABLE 3D and TABLE 4 and those for which the COSTART terms were uninformative or misleading) were reported at an incidence of at least 2% for fluoxetine and greater than placebo: thirst, hyperkinesia, agitation, personality disorder, epistaxis, urinary frequency, and menorrhagia.

The most common adverse event (incidence at least 1% for fluoxetine and greater than placebo) associated with discontinuation in three pediatric placebo-controlled trials (n=418 randomized; 228 fluoxetine-treated; 190 placebo-treated) was mania/hypomania (1.8% for fluoxetine-treated, 0% for placebo-treated). In these clinical trials, only a primary event associated with discontinuation was collected.

EVENTS OBSERVED IN PROZAC WEEKLY CLINICAL TRIALS

Treatment-emergent adverse events in clinical trials with Prozac Weekly were similar to the adverse events reported by patients in clinical trials with Prozac daily. In a placebo-controlled clinical trial, more patients taking Prozac Weekly reported diarrhea than patients taking placebo (10% vs 3%, respectively) or taking Prozac 20 mg daily (10% vs 5%, respectively).

PMDD

In 1 of 3 placebo-controlled, continuous-dosing trials and 1 placebo-controlled, intermittent-dosing trial of fluoxetine in PMDD, treatment-emergent adverse events reporting rates were assessed. The information from TABLE 6 is based on data from the continuous-dosing trial at the recommended dose of Sarafem (Sarafem 20 mg, n=104; pla-

TABLE 3D *Most Common Treatment-Emergent Adverse Events: Incidence in Panic Disorder Placebo-Controlled Clinical Trials*

Body System Adverse Event	Prozac (n=425)	Placebo (n=342)
Body as a Whole		
Asthenia	7%	7%
Flu syndrome	5%	5%
Cardiovascular System		
Vasodilatation	1%	—
Digestive System		
Nausea	12%	7%
Diarrhea	9%	4%
Anorexia	4%	1%
Dry mouth	4%	4%
Dyspepsia	6%	2%
Nervous System		
Insomnia	10%	7%
Anxiety	6%	2%
Nervousness	8%	6%
Somnolence	5%	2%
Tremor	3%	1%
Libido decreased	1%	2%
Abnormal dreams	1%	1%
Respiratory System		
Pharyngitis	3%	3%
Sinusitis	2%	3%
Yawn	1%	—
Skin and Appendages		
Sweating	2%	2%
Rash	2%	2%
Urogenital System		
Impotence*	1%	—
Abnormal ejaculation*	2%	1%

* Denominator used was for males only (n=162 Prozac; n=121 placebo).
— Incidence less than 1%.

TABLE 4 *Treatment-Emergent Adverse Events: Incidence in Major Depressive Disorder, OCD, Bulimia, and Panic Disorder Placebo-Controlled Clinical Trials**

Body System Adverse Event†	Prozac (n=2869)	Placebo (n=1673)
Body as a Whole		
Headache	21%	19%
Asthenia	11%	6%
Flu syndrome	5%	4%
Fever	2%	1%
Cardiovascular System		
Vasodilatation	2%	1%
Digestive System		
Nausea	22%	9%
Diarrhea	11%	7%
Anorexia	10%	3%
Dry mouth	9%	6%
Dyspepsia	8%	4%
Constipation	5%	4%
Flatulence	3%	2%
Vomiting	3%	2%
Metabolic and Nutritional Disorders		
Weight loss	2%	1%
Nervous System		
Insomnia	19%	10%
Nervousness	13%	8%
Anxiety	12%	6%
Somnolence	12%	5%
Dizziness	9%	6%
Tremor	9%	2%
Libido decreased	4%	1%
Thinking abnormal	2%	1%
Respiratory System		
Yawn	3%	—
Skin and Appendages		
Sweating	7%	3%
Rash	4%	3%
Pruritus	3%	2%
Special Senses		
Abnormal vision	2%	1%

* Includes US data for major depressive disorder, OCD, bulimia, and panic disorder clinical trials, plus non-US data for panic disorder clinical trials.
† Included are events reported by at least 2% of patients taking fluoxetine, except the following events, which had an incidence on placebo ≥ fluoxetine (major depressive disorder, OCD, bulimia, and panic disorder combined): abdominal pain, abnormal dreams, accidental injury, back pain, cough increased, major depressive disorder (includes suicidal thoughts), dysmenorrhea, infection, myalgia, pain, paresthesia, pharyngitis, rhinitis, sinusitus.
— Incidence less than 1%.

cebo, n=108) and data from the intermittent-dosing trial of fluoxetine in PMDD (Sarafem 20 mg, n=86; placebo, n=88). In addition, a broader set of information on treatment-emergent adverse events in the population of female patients, 18-45 years of age, from the US placebo-controlled depression, OCD, and bulimia clinical trials, is presented for comparison (see TABLE 7).

Adverse events were recorded by clinical investigators using descriptive terminology of their own choosing. Consequently, it is not possible to provide a meaningful estimate of the proportion of individuals experiencing adverse events without first grouping similar types of events into a limited (*i.e.*, reduced) number of standardized event categories.

TABLE 5 *Most Common Adverse Events Associated With Discontinuation in Major Depressive Disorder, OCD, Bulimia, and Panic Disorder Placebo-Controlled Clinical Trials*

Major Depressive Disorder, OCD, Bulimia, and Panic Disorder Combined (n=1533)	Major Depressive Disorder (n=392)	OCD (n=266)	Bulimia (n=450)	Panic Disorder (n=425)
Anxiety (1%)	—	Anxiety (2%)	—	Anxiety (2%)
—	—	—	Insomnia (2%)	—
—	Nervousness (1%)	—	—	Nervousness (1%)
—	—	Rash (1%)	—	—

* Includes US major depressive disorder, OCD, bulimia, and panic disorder clinical trials, plus non-US panic disorder clinical trials.

In TABLE 6, TABLE 7, and the tabulations that follow, COSTART Dictionary terminology has been used to classify reported adverse events. The stated frequencies represent the proportion of individuals who experienced, at least once, a treatment-emergent adverse event of the type listed. An event was considered treatment-emergent if it occurred for the first time or worsened while receiving therapy following baseline evaluation. It is important to emphasize that events reported during therapy were not necessarily caused by it.

The prescriber should be aware that the figures in TABLE 6, TABLE 7, and tabulations that follow cannot be used to predict the incidence of side effects in the course of usual medical practice where patient characteristics and other factors differ from those that prevailed in the clinical trials. Similarly, the cited frequencies cannot be compared with figures obtained from other clinical investigations involving different treatments, uses, and investigators. The cited figures, however, do provide the prescribing physician with some basis for estimating the relative contribution of drug and nondrug factors to the side effect incidence rate in the population studied.

Incidence in Placebo-Controlled PMDD Clinical Trials

TABLE 6 enumerates the most common treatment-emergent adverse events associated with the use of Sarafem 20 mg (incidence of at least 5% for Sarafem 20 mg and greater than placebo) for the treatment of PMDD.

TABLE 6 *Most Common Treatment-Emergent Adverse Events: Incidence in a PMDD Placebo-Controlled Clinical Trial*

Body System Adverse Event*	Sarafem 20 mg/day Continuously (n=104)	 Intermittently (n=86)	Placebo (n=196)
Body as a Whole			
Headache	13%	15%	11%
Asthenia	12%	8%	4%
Pain	9%	3%	7%
Accidental injury	8%	1%	5%
Infection	7%	0%	3%
Flu syndrome	12%	3%	7%
Digestive System			
Nausea	13%	9%	6%
Diarrhea	6%	2%	6%
Nervous System			
Insomnia	9%	10%	7%
Dizziness	7%	2%	3%
Nervousness	7%	3%	3%
Thinking abnormal†	6%	5%	0%
Libido decreased	3%	9%	1%
Respiratory System			
Rhinitis	23%	16%	15%
Pharyngitis	10%	6%	5%

* Included in the table are events reported by at least 5% of patients taking Sarafem 20 mg either continuously or intermittently. For additional adverse event terms referenced in PRECAUTIONS, reporting rates for Sarafem 20 mg continuous and intermittent were, respectively: anxiety 4.8%, 1.2% and anorexia 3.8%, 3.5%.
† Thinking abnormal is the COSTART term that captures concentration difficulties.

Incidence in US Depression, OCD, and Bulimia Placebo-Controlled Clinical Trials (excluding data from extensions of trials)

TABLE 7 enumerates the most common treatment-emergent adverse events associated with the use of fluoxetine up to 80 mg (incidence of at least 2% for fluoxetine and greater than placebo) in female patients ages 18-45 years from US placebo-controlled clinical trials in the treatment of depression, OCD, and bulimia.

Associated With Discontinuation in Two Placebo-Controlled PMDD Clinical Trials

In a continuous-dosing PMDD placebo-controlled trial, the most common adverse event (incidence at least 2% for Sarafem 20 mg and greater than placebo) associated with discontinuation was nausea (3% for Sarafem 20 mg, n=104 and 1% for placebo, n=108). In an intermittent-dosing placebo-controlled trial, no events associated with discontinuation reached an incidence of 2% for Sarafem 20 mg. In these clinical trials, more than 1 event may have been recorded as the cause of discontinuation.

MALE AND FEMALE SEXUAL DYSFUNCTION WITH SSRIS

Although changes in sexual desire, sexual performance, and sexual satisfaction often occur as manifestations of a psychiatric disorder, they may also be a consequence of pharmacologic treatment. In particular, some evidence suggests that SSRIs can cause such untoward sexual experiences. Reliable estimates of the incidence and severity of untoward experiences involving sexual desire, performance, and satisfaction are difficult to obtain, however,

TABLE 7 *Treatment-Emergent Adverse Events: Incidence in Female Patients Ages 18-45 Years in US Depression, OCD, and Bulimia Placebo-Controlled Clinical Trials*

Body System / Adverse Event*	Fluoxetine (n=1145)	Placebo (n=553)
Body as a Whole		
Headache	24%	21%
Asthenia	14%	6%
Flu syndrome	7%	3%
Abdominal pain	6%	5%
Accidental injury	4%	3%
Fever	3%	2%
Cardiovascular System		
Palpitation	3%	2%
Vasodilatation	3%	1%
Digestive System		
Nausea	27%	11%
Anorexia	11%	4%
Dry mouth	11%	8%
Diarrhea	10%	7%
Dyspepsia	7%	5%
Constipation	5%	3%
Vomiting	3%	2%
Metabolic and Nutritional Disorders		
Weight loss	3%	1%
Nervous System		
Insomnia	24%	11%
Nervousness	14%	10%
Anxiety	13%	9%
Somnolence	13%	6%
Tremor	12%	1%
Dizziness	11%	5%
Libido decreased	4%	1%
Abnormal dreams	3%	2%
Thinking abnormal†	3%	2%
Respiratory System		
Pharyngitis	6%	5%
Yawn	5%	—
Skin and Appendages		
Sweating	8%	3%
Rash	5%	3%
Special Senses		
Abnormal vision	3%	1%
Urogenital System		
Urinary frequency	2%	1%

* Included are events reported by at least 2% of patients taking fluoxetine, except the following events, which had an incidence on placebo >fluoxetine (depression, OCD, and bulimia combined): back pain, cough increased, depression (includes suicidal thoughts), dysmenorrhea, flatulence, infection, myalgia, pain, puritus, rhinitis, sinusitus.
† Thinking abnormal is the COSTART term that captures concentration difficulties.
— Incidence less than 0.5%.

in part because patients and physicians may be reluctant to discuss them. Accordingly, estimates of the incidence of untoward sexual experience and performance, cited in product labeling, are likely to underestimate their actual incidence. In patients enrolled in US major depressive disorder, OCD, and bulimia placebo-controlled clinical trials, decreased libido was the only sexual side effect reported by at least 2% of patients taking fluoxetine (4% fluoxetine, <1% placebo). There have been spontaneous reports in women taking fluoxetine of orgasmic dysfunction, including anorgasmia.

There are no adequate and well-controlled studies examining sexual dysfunction with fluoxetine treatment.

Priapism has been reported with all SSRIs.

While it is difficult to know the precise risk of sexual dysfunction associated with the use of SSRIs, physicians should routinely inquire about such possible side effects.

OTHER EVENTS OBSERVED IN CLINICAL TRIALS

Following is a list of all treatment-emergent adverse events reported at anytime by individuals taking fluoxetine in US clinical trials as of May 8, 1995 (10,782 patients) except:

- Those listed in the body or footnotes of TABLE 3A, TABLE 3B, TABLE 3C, TABLE 3D, or TABLE 4 or elsewhere in the prescribing information.
- Those for which the COSTART terms were uninformative or misleading.
- Those events for which a causal relationship to Prozac use was considered remote.
- Events occurring in only 1 patient treated with Prozac and which did not have a substantial probability of being acutely life-threatening.

Events are classified within body system categories using the following definitions: *Frequent Adverse Events:* Defined as those occurring on one or more occasions in at least 1/100 patients. *Infrequent Adverse Events:* Those occurring in 1/100 to 1/1000 patients. *Rare Events:* Those occurring in less than 1/1000 patients.

Body as a Whole: *Frequent:* Chest pain, chills. *Infrequent:* Chills and fever, face edema, intentional overdose, malaise, pelvic pain, suicide attempt. *Rare:* Abdominal syndrome acute, hypothermia, intentional injury, neuroleptic malignant syndrome (the COSTART term which best captures serotonin syndrome), photosensitivity reaction.

Cardiovascular System: *Frequent:* Hemorrhage, hypertension, palpitation. *Infrequent:* Angina pectoris, arrhythmia, congestive heart failure, hypotension, migraine, myocardial infarct, postural hypotension, syncope, tachycardia, vascular headache. *Rare:* Atrial fibrillation, bradycardia, cerebral embolism, cerebral ischemia, cerebrovascular accident, extrasystoles, heart arrest, heart block, pallor, peripheral vascular disorder, phlebitis, shock, thrombophlebitis, thrombosis, vasospasm, ventricular arrhythmia, ventricular extrasystoles, ventricular fibrillation.

Digestive System: *Frequent:* Increased appetite, nausea and vomiting. *Infrequent:* Aphthous stomatitis, cholelithiasis, colitis, dysphagia, eructation, esophagitis, gastritis, gastroenteritis, glossitis, gum hemorrhage, hyperchlorhydria, increased salivation, liver function tests abnormal, melena, mouth ulceration, nausea/vomiting/diarrhea, stomach ulcer, stomatitis, thirst. *Rare:* Biliary pain, bloody diarrhea, cholecystitis, duodenal ulcer, enteritis, esophageal ulcer, fecal incontinence, gastrointestinal hemorrhage, hematemesis, hemorrhage of colon, hepatitis, intestinal obstruction, liver fatty deposit, pancreatitis, peptic ulcer, rectal hemorrhage, salivary gland enlargement, stomach ulcer hemorrhage, tongue edema.

Endocrine System: *Infrequent:* Hypothyroidism. *Rare:* Diabetic acidosis, diabetes mellitus.

Hemic and Lymphatic System: *Infrequent:* Anemia, ecchymosis. *Rare:* Blood dyscrasia, hypochromic anemia, leukopenia, lymphedema, lymphocytosis, petechia, purpura, thrombocythemia, thrombocytopenia.

Metabolic and Nutritional: *Frequent:* Weight gain. *Infrequent:* Dehydration, generalized edema, gout, hypercholesteremia, hyperlipemia, hypokalemia, peripheral edema. *Rare:* Alcohol intolerance, alkaline phosphatase increased, BUN increased, creatine phosphokinase increased, hyperkalemia, hyperuricemia, hypocalcemia, iron deficiency anemia, SGPT increased.

Musculoskeletal System: *Infrequent:* Arthritis, bone pain, bursitis, leg cramps, tenosynovitis. *Rare:* Arthrosis, chondrodystrophy, myasthenia, myopathy, myositis, osteomyelitis, osteoporosis, rheumatoid arthritis.

Nervous System: *Frequent:* Agitation, amnesia, confusion, emotional lability, sleep disorder. *Infrequent:* Abnormal gait, acute brain syndrome, akathisia, apathy, ataxia, buccoglossal syndrome, CNS depression, CNS stimulation, depersonalization, euphoria, hallucinations, hostility, hyperkinesia, hypertonia, hypesthesia, incoordination, libido increased, myoclonus, neuralgia, neuropathy, neurosis, paranoid reaction, personality disorder (the COSTART term for designating non-aggressive objectionable behavior), psychosis, vertigo. *Rare:* Abnormal electroencephalogram, antisocial reaction, circumoral paresthesia, coma, delusions, dysarthria, dystonia, extrapyramidal syndrome, foot drop, hyperesthesia, neuritis, paralysis, reflexes decreased, reflexes increased, stupor.

Respiratory System: *Infrequent:* Asthma, epistaxis, hiccup, hyperventilation. *Rare:* Apnea, atelectasis, cough decreased, emphysema, hemoptysis, hypoventilation, hypoxia, larynx edema, lung edema, pneumothorax, stridor.

Skin and Appendages: *Infrequent:* Acne, alopecia, contact dermatitis, eczema, maculopapular rash, skin discoloration, skin ulcer, vesiculobullous rash. *Rare:* Furunculosis, herpes zoster, hirsutism, petechial rash, psoriasis, purpuric rash, pustular rash, seborrhea.

Special Senses: *Frequent:* Ear pain, taste perversion, tinnitus. *Infrequent:* Conjunctivitis, dry eyes, mydriasis, photophobia. *Rare:* Blepharitis, deafness, diplopia, exophthalmos, eye hemorrhage, glaucoma, hyperacusis, iritis, parosmia, scleritis, strabismus, taste loss, visual field defect.

Urogenital System: *Frequent:* Urinary frequency. *Infrequent:* Abortion*, albuminuria, amenorrhea*, anorgasmia, breast enlargement, breast pain, cystitis, dysuria, female lactation*, fibrocystic breast*, hematuria, leukorrhea*, menorrhagia*, metrorrhagia*, nocturia, polyuria, urinary incontinence, urinary retention, urinary urgency, vaginal hemorrhage*. *Rare:* Breast engorgement, glycosuria, hypomenorrhea*, kidney pain, oliguria, priapism*, uterine hemorrhage*, uterine fibroids enlarged*.

* Adjusted for gender.

POSTINTRODUCTION REPORTS

Voluntary reports of adverse events temporally associated with fluoxetine that have been received since market introduction and that may have no causal relationship with the drug include the following: Aplastic anemia, atrial fibrillation, cataract, cerebral vascular accident, cholestatic jaundice, confusion, dyskinesia (including, for example, a case of buccal-lingual-masticatory syndrome with involuntary tongue protrusion reported to develop in a 77-year-old female after 5 weeks of fluoxetine therapy and which completely resolved over the next few months following drug discontinuation), eosinophilic pneumonia, epidermal necrolysis, erythema nodosum, exfoliative dermatitis, gynecomastia, heart arrest, hepatic failure/necrosis, hyperprolactinemia, hypoglycemia, immune-related hemolytic anemia, kidney failure, misuse/abuse, movement disorders developing in patients with risk factors including drugs associated with such events and worsening of preexisting movement disorders, neuroleptic malignant syndrome-like events, optic neuritis, pancreatitis, pancytopenia, priapism, pulmonary embolism, pulmonary hypertension, QT prolongation, serotonin syndrome (a range of signs and symptoms that can rarely, in its most severe form, resemble neuroleptic malignant syndrome), Stevens-Johnson syndrome, sudden unexpected death, suicidal ideation, thrombocytopenia, thrombocytopenic purpura, vaginal bleeding after drug withdrawal, ventricular tachycardia (including torsades de pointes-type arrhythmias), and violent behaviors.

DOSAGE AND ADMINISTRATION

MAJOR DEPRESSIVE DISORDER

Initial Treatment

Adult

In controlled trials used to support the efficacy of fluoxetine, patients were administered morning doses ranging from 20-80 mg/day. Studies comparing fluoxetine 20, 40, and 60 mg/day to placebo indicate that 20 mg/day is sufficient to obtain a satisfactory response in major depressive disorder in most cases. Consequently, a dose of 20 mg/day, administered in the morning, is recommended as the initial dose.

A dose increase may be considered after several weeks if insufficient clinical improvement is observed. Doses above 20 mg/day may be administered on a once a day (morning) or bid schedule (*i.e.*, morning and noon) and should not exceed a maximum dose of 80 mg/day.

Pediatric (children and adolescents)

In the short-term (8-9 weeks) controlled clinical trials of fluoxetine supporting its effectiveness in the treatment of major depressive disorder, patients were administered fluoxetine doses of 10-20 mg/day. Treatment should be initiated with a dose of 10 or 20 mg/day. After 1 week at 10 mg/day, the dose should be increased to 20 mg/day.

However, due to higher plasma levels in lower weight children, the starting and target dose in this group may be 10 mg/day. A dose increase to 20 mg/day may be considered after several weeks if insufficient clinical improvement is observed.

All Patients

As with other drugs effective in the treatment of major depressive disorder, the full effect may be delayed until 4 weeks of treatment or longer.

As with many other medications, a lower or less frequent dosage should be used in patients with hepatic impairment. A lower or less frequent dosage should also be considered for the elderly (see PRECAUTIONS, Geriatric Use), and for patients with concurrent disease or on multiple concomitant medications. Dosage adjustments for renal impairment are not routinely necessary (see CLINICAL PHARMACOLOGY: Liver Disease and Renal Disease; and PRECAUTIONS, Use in Patients With Concomitant Illness).

Maintenance/Continuation/Extended Treatment

It is generally agreed that acute episodes of major depressive disorder require several months or longer of sustained pharmacologic therapy. Whether the dose needed to induce remission is identical to the dose needed to maintain and/or sustain euthymia is unknown.

Daily Dosing

Systematic evaluation of Prozac has shown that its efficacy in major depressive disorder is maintained for periods of up to 38 weeks following 12 weeks of open-label acute treatment (50 weeks total) at a dose of 20 mg/day.

Weekly Dosing

Systematic evaluation of Prozac Weekly has shown that its efficacy in major depressive disorder is maintained for periods of up to 25 weeks with once-weekly dosing following 13 weeks of open-label treatment with Prozac 20 mg once-daily. However, therapeutic equivalence of Prozac Weekly given on a once-weekly basis with Prozac 20 mg given daily for delaying time to relapse has not been established.

Weekly dosing with Prozac Weekly capsules is recommended to be initiated 7 days after the last daily dose of Prozac 20 mg (see CLINICAL PHARMACOLOGY).

If satisfactory response is not maintained with Prozac Weekly, consider reestablishing a daily dosing regimen.

OBSESSIVE-COMPULSIVE DISORDER

Initial Treatment

Adult

In the controlled clinical trials of fluoxetine supporting its effectiveness in the treatment of obsessive-compulsive disorder, patients were administered fixed daily doses of 20, 40, or 60 mg of fluoxetine or placebo. In one of these studies, no dose response relationship for effectiveness was demonstrated. Consequently, a dose of 20 mg/day, administered in the morning, is recommended as the initial dose. Since there was a suggestion of a possible dose response relationship for effectiveness in the second study, a dose increase may be considered after several weeks if insufficient clinical improvement is observed. The full therapeutic effect may be delayed until 5 weeks of treatment or longer.

Doses above 20 mg/day may be administered on a once a day (*i.e.,* morning) or bid schedule (*i.e.,* morning and noon). A dose range of 20-60 mg/day is recommended, however, doses of up to 80 mg/day have been well tolerated in open studies of OCD. The maximum fluoxetine dose should not exceed 80 mg/day.

Pediatric (children and adolescents)

In the controlled clinical trial of fluoxetine supporting its effectiveness in the treatment of OCD, patients were administered fluoxetine doses in the range of 10-60 mg/day. In adolescents and higher weight children, treatment should be initiated with a dose of 10 mg/day. After 2 weeks, the dose should be increased to 20 mg/day. Additional dose increases may be considered after several more weeks if insufficient clinical improvement is observed. A dose range of 20-60 mg/day is recommended.

In lower weight children, treatment should be initiated with a dose of 10 mg/day. Additional dose increases may be considered after several more weeks if insufficient clinical improvement is observed. A dose range of 20-30 mg/day is recommended. Experience with daily doses greater than 20 mg is very minimal, and there is no experience with doses greater than 60 mg.

All Patients

As with the use of Prozac in the treatment of major depressive disorder, a lower or less frequent dosage should be used in patients with hepatic impairment. A lower or less frequent dosage should also be considered for the elderly (see PRECAUTIONS, Geriatric Use), and for patients with concurrent disease or on multiple concomitant medications. Dosage adjustments for renal impairment are not routinely necessary (see CLINICAL PHARMACOLOGY: Liver Disease and Renal Disease; and PRECAUTIONS, Use in Patients With Concomitant Illness).

Maintenance/Continuation Treatment

While there are no systematic studies that answer the question of how long to continue Prozac, OCD is a chronic condition and it is reasonable to consider continuation for a responding patient. Although the efficacy of Prozac after 13 weeks has not been documented in controlled trials, patients have been continued in therapy under double-blind conditions for up to an additional 6 months without loss of benefit. However, dosage adjustments should be made to maintain the patient on the lowest effective dosage, and patients should be periodically reassessed to determine the need for treatment.

BULIMIA NERVOSA

Initial Treatment

In the controlled clinical trials of fluoxetine supporting its effectiveness in the treatment of bulimia nervosa, patients were administered fixed daily fluoxetine doses of 20 or 60 mg, or placebo. Only the 60 mg dose was statistically significantly superior to placebo in reducing the frequency of binge-eating and vomiting. Consequently, the recommended dose is 60 mg/day, administered in the morning. For some patients it may be advisable to titrate up to this target dose over several days. Fluoxetine doses above 60 mg/day have not been systematically studied in patients with bulimia.

As with the use of Prozac in the treatment of major depressive disorder and OCD, a lower or less frequent dosage should be used in patients with hepatic impairment. A lower or less frequent dosage should also be considered for the elderly (see PRECAUTIONS, Geriatric Use), and for patients with concurrent disease or on multiple concomitant medications. Dosage adjustments for renal impairment are not routinely necessary (see CLINICAL PHARMACOLOGY: Liver Disease and Renal Disease; and PRECAUTIONS, Use in Patients With Concomitant Illness).

Maintenance/Continuation Treatment

Systematic evaluation of continuing Prozac 60 mg/day for periods of up to 52 weeks in patients with bulimia who have responded while taking Prozac 60 mg/day during an 8 week acute treatment phase has demonstrated a benefit of such maintenance treatment. Nevertheless, patients should be periodically reassessed to determine the need for maintenance treatment.

SWITCHING PATIENTS TO A TRICYCLIC ANTIDEPRESSANT (TCA)

Dosage of a TCA may need to be reduced, and plasma TCA concentrations may need to be monitored temporarily when fluoxetine is coadministered or has been recently discontinued (see DRUG INTERACTIONS, Other Drugs Effective in the Treatment of Major Depressive Disorder).

SWITCHING PATIENTS TO OR FROM A MONOAMINE OXIDASE INHIBITOR

At least 14 days should elapse between discontinuation of an MAOI and initiation of therapy with Prozac. In addition, at least 5 weeks, perhaps longer, should be allowed after stopping Prozac before starting an MAOI (see CONTRAINDICATIONS and PRECAUTIONS).

PANIC DISORDER

Initial Treatment

In the controlled clinical trials of fluoxetine supporting its effectiveness in the treatment of panic disorder, patients were administered fluoxetine doses in the range of 10-60 mg/day. Treatment should be initiated with a dose of 10 mg/day. After 1 week, the dose should be increased to 20 mg/day. The most frequently administered dose in the 2 flexible-dose clinical trials was 20 mg/day.

A dose increase may be considered after several weeks if no clinical improvement is observed. Fluoxetine doses above 60 mg/day have not been systematically evaluated in patients with panic disorder.

As with the use of Prozac in other indications, a lower or less frequent dosage should be used in patients with hepatic impairment. A lower or less frequent dosage should also be considered for the elderly (see PRECAUTIONS, Geriatric Use), and for patients with concurrent disease or on multiple concomitant medications. Dosage adjustments for renal impairment are not routinely necessary (see CLINICAL PHARMACOLOGY: Liver Disease and Renal Disease; and PRECAUTIONS, Use in Patients With Concomitant Illness).

Maintenance/Continuation Treatment

While there are no systematic studies that answer the question of how long to continue Prozac, panic disorder is a chronic condition and it is reasonable to consider continuation for a responding patient. Nevertheless, patients should be periodically reassessed to determine the need for continued treatment.

PREMENSTRUAL DYSPHORIC DISORDER

Initial Treatment

The recommended dose of Sarafem for the treatment of PMDD is 20 mg/day given continuously (every day of the menstrual cycle) or intermittently (defined as starting a daily dose 14 days prior to the anticipated onset of menstruation through the first full day of menses and repeating with each new cycle). The dosing regimen should be determined by the physician based on individual patient characteristics. In a study comparing continuous dosing of fluoxetine 20 and 60 mg/day to placebo, both doses were proven to be effective, but there was no statistically significant added benefit for the 60 mg/day compared with the 20 mg/day dose. Fluoxetine doses above 60 mg/day have not been systematically studied in patients with PMDD. The maximum fluoxetine dose should not exceed 80 mg/day.

As with many other medications, a lower or less frequent dosage should be considered in patients with hepatic impairment. A lower or less frequent dosage should also be considered for patients with concurrent disease or on multiple concomitant medications. Dosage adjustments for renal impairment are not routinely necessary (see CLINICAL PHARMACOLOGY: Liver Disease and Renal Disease; and PRECAUTIONS, Use in Patients With Concomitant Illness).

Maintenance/Continuation Treatment

Systematic evaluation of Sarafem has shown that its efficacy in PMDD is maintained for periods of up to 6 months at a dose of 20 mg/day given continuously and up to 3 month at a dose of 20 mg/day given intermittently. Patients should be periodically reassessed to determine the need for continued treatment.

ANIMAL PHARMACOLOGY

Phospholipids are increased in some tissues of mice, rats, and dogs given fluoxetine chronically. This effect is reversible after cessation of fluoxetine treatment. Phospholipid accumulation in animals has been observed with many cationic amphiphilic drugs, including fenfluramine, imipramine, and ranitidine. The significance of this effect in humans is unknown.

HOW SUPPLIED

PROZAC

Prozac is available in the following dosage forms (all strengths are fluoxetine base equivalent):

Pulvules

10 mg Pulvule: Opaque green and green, imprinted with "DISTA 3104" on the cap and "Prozac 10 mg" on the body.
20 mg Pulvule: Opaque green cap and off-white body, imprinted with "DISTA 3105" on the cap and "Prozac 20 mg" on the body.
40 mg Pulvule: Opaque green cap and opaque orange body, imprinted with "DISTA 3107" on the cap and "Prozac 40 mg" on the body.
Storage: Store at controlled room temperature, 15-30°C (59-86°F). Protect from light.

Oral Solution

Oral Solution: 20 mg/5 ml with mint flavor.
Storage: Store at controlled room temperature, 15-30°C (59-86°F). Dispense in a tight, light-resistant container.

Tablets

10 mg Tablet: Green, elliptical shaped, and scored with "PROZAC 10" debossed on opposite side of score.
Storage: Store at controlled room temperature, 15-30°C (59-86°F).

Weekly Capsules

90 mg Capsule: Opaque green cap and clear body containing discretely visible white pellets through the clear body of the capsule, imprinted with "Lilly" on the cap, and "3004" and "90 mg" on the body.
Storage: Store at controlled room temperature, 15-30°C (59-86°F).

SARAFEM

10 mg Pulvule: The 10 mg Pulvule has an opaque lavender body and cap, and is imprinted with "10 mg" on the body and "LILLY 3210" on the cap.
20 mg Pulvule: The 20 mg Pulvule has an opaque pink body with opaque lavender cap, and is imprinted with "20 mg" on the body and "LILLY 3220" on the cap.
Storage: Store at controlled room temperature, 15-30°C (59-86°F). Protect from light.

PRODUCT LISTING - RATED THERAPEUTICALLY EQUIVALENT

Capsule - Oral - 10 mg

1's	$2.38	PROZAC, Dista Products Company	00777-3104-01
3's	$12.55	PROZAC, Prescript Pharmaceuticals	00247-0644-03
7's	$24.81	PROZAC, Prescript Pharmaceuticals	00247-0644-07
7's	$26.37	PROZAC, Pd-Rx Pharmaceuticals	55289-0308-07
10's	$34.00	PROZAC, Prescript Pharmaceuticals	00247-0644-10
14's	$46.27	PROZAC, Prescript Pharmaceuticals	00247-0644-14
14's	$50.91	PROZAC, Pd-Rx Pharmaceuticals	55289-0308-14
28's	$89.18	PROZAC, Prescript Pharmaceuticals	00247-0644-28
30's	$61.10	PROZAC, Compumed Pharmaceuticals	00403-4807-30
30's	$64.44	PROZAC, Heartland Healthcare Services	61392-0234-30
30's	$77.86	GENERIC, Mutual Pharmaceutical Co Inc	53489-0373-07
30's	$80.40	PROZAC, Allscripts Pharmaceutical Company	54569-4129-00
30's	$94.26	PROZAC, Physicians Total Care	54868-3033-00
30's	$95.31	PROZAC, Prescript Pharmaceuticals	00247-0644-30
30's	$99.50	PROZAC, Pharma Pac	52959-0665-30
60's	$128.88	PROZAC, Heartland Healthcare Services	61392-0234-60
60's	$155.71	GENERIC, Mutual Pharmaceutical Co Inc	53489-0373-06
60's	$187.26	PROZAC, Prescript Pharmaceuticals	00247-0644-60
90's	$193.32	PROZAC, Heartland Healthcare Services	61392-0234-90
100's	$258.65	GENERIC, Ivax Corporation	00172-4363-60
100's	$259.52	GENERIC, Mutual/United Research Laboratories	00677-1766-01
100's	$259.52	GENERIC, Mutual Pharmaceutical Co Inc	53489-0373-01
100's	$259.83	GENERIC, Teva Pharmaceuticals Usa	00093-1042-01
100's	$259.83	GENERIC, Watson Laboratories Inc	00591-0826-01
100's	$259.83	GENERIC, Parke-Davis	49884-0732-01
100's	$259.83	GENERIC, Sidmak Laboratories Inc	50111-0647-01
100's	$259.85	GENERIC, Mylan Pharmaceuticals Inc	00378-4210-01
100's	$260.09	GENERIC, Mallinckrodt Medical Inc	00406-0661-01
100's	$260.09	GENERIC, Barr Laboratories Inc	00555-0876-02
100's	$260.12	GENERIC, Eon Labs Manufacturing Inc	00185-0080-01
100's	$272.82	GENERIC, Geneva Pharmaceuticals	00781-2823-01
100's	$309.87	PROZAC, Prescript Pharmaceuticals	00247-0644-00
100's	$324.71	PROZAC, Dista Products Company	00777-3104-02

Capsule - Oral - 20 mg

1's	$2.44	PROZAC, Dista Products Company	00777-3105-01
3's	$13.16	PROZAC, Prescript Pharmaceuticals	00247-0372-03
4's	$16.44	PROZAC, Prescript Pharmaceuticals	00247-0372-04
7's	$16.92	PROZAC, Allscripts Pharmaceutical Company	54569-1732-06
7's	$26.25	PROZAC, Prescript Pharmaceuticals	00247-0372-07
10 x 10	$274.00	GENERIC, Mallinckrodt Medical Inc	00406-0663-62
10's	$29.64	PROZAC, Southwood Pharmaceuticals Inc	58016-0828-10
10's	$36.05	PROZAC, Prescript Pharmaceuticals	00247-0372-10
10's	$40.20	PROZAC, Pharma Pac	52959-0233-10
14's	$34.50	PROZAC, Allscripts Pharmaceutical Company	54569-1732-04
14's	$49.13	PROZAC, Prescript Pharmaceuticals	00247-0372-14
14's	$54.32	PROZAC, Pharma Pac	52959-0233-14
15's	$33.03	PROZAC, Heartland Healthcare Services	61392-0235-15
15's	$52.40	PROZAC, Prescript Pharmaceuticals	00247-0372-15
20's	$59.29	PROZAC, Southwood Pharmaceuticals Inc	58016-0828-20
20's	$73.00	PROZAC, Pharma Pac	52959-0233-20
22's	$77.62	PROZAC, Pd-Rx Pharmaceuticals	55289-0215-22
25's	$66.74	GENERIC, Udl Laboratories Inc	51079-0971-19
28's	$94.91	PROZAC, Prescript Pharmaceuticals	00247-0372-28
30's	$66.06	PROZAC, Heartland Healthcare Services	61392-0235-30
30's	$73.92	PROZAC, Allscripts Pharmaceutical Company	54569-1732-00
30's	$79.59	GENERIC, Watson Laboratories Inc	00591-0827-30
30's	$79.96	GENERIC, Mutual Pharmaceutical Co Inc	53489-0374-07
30's	$79.99	GENERIC, Sidmak Laboratories Inc	50111-0648-10
30's	$88.93	PROZAC, Southwood Pharmaceuticals Inc	58016-0828-30
30's	$97.66	PROZAC, Physicians Total Care	54868-0511-01
30's	$99.92	PROZAC, Dista Products Company	00777-3105-30
30's	$101.45	PROZAC, Prescript Pharmaceuticals	00247-0372-30
30's	$103.94	PROZAC, Pharma Pac	52959-0233-30
30's	$105.87	PROZAC, Pd-Rx Pharmaceuticals	55289-0215-30
40's	$118.57	PROZAC, Southwood Pharmaceuticals Inc	58016-0828-40
40's	$133.60	PROZAC, Pharma Pac	52959-0233-40
45's	$99.09	PROZAC, Heartland Healthcare Services	61392-0235-45
50's	$116.76	PROZAC, Allscripts Pharmaceutical Company	54569-1732-02
50's	$162.50	PROZAC, Pharma Pac	52959-0233-50
60's	$132.12	PROZAC, Heartland Healthcare Services	61392-0235-60
60's	$135.00	PROZAC, Compumed Pharmaceuticals	00403-1781-71
60's	$145.01	PROZAC, Allscripts Pharmaceutical Company	54569-1732-05
60's	$159.91	GENERIC, Mutual Pharmaceutical Co Inc	53489-0374-06
60's	$177.86	PROZAC, Southwood Pharmaceuticals Inc	58016-0828-60
60's	$184.54	PROZAC, Physicians Total Care	54868-0511-05
60's	$199.54	PROZAC, Prescript Pharmaceuticals	00247-0372-60
90's	$198.18	PROZAC, Heartland Healthcare Services	61392-0235-90
90's	$202.09	PROZAC, Allscripts Pharmaceutical Company	54569-8013-00
90's	$202.09	PROZAC, Allscripts Pharmaceutical Company	54569-8522-00
90's	$266.79	PROZAC, Southwood Pharmaceuticals Inc	58016-0828-90
100's	$241.69	PROZAC, Allscripts Pharmaceutical Company	54569-1732-03
100's	$259.10	PROZAC, Pharma Pac	52959-0233-00
100's	$265.30	GENERIC, Ivax Corporation	00172-4356-60
100's	$266.40	GENERIC, Mallinckrodt Medical Inc	00406-0663-01
100's	$266.52	GENERIC, Mutual Pharmaceutical Co Inc	00677-1767-01
100's	$266.52	GENERIC, Geneva Pharmaceuticals	00781-2822-01
100's	$266.52	GENERIC, Mutual Pharmaceutical Co Inc	53489-0374-01
100's	$266.55	GENERIC, Mylan Pharmaceuticals Inc	00378-4220-01
100's	$266.81	GENERIC, Teva Pharmaceuticals Usa	00093-1043-01
100's	$266.81	GENERIC, Eon Labs Manufacturing Inc	00185-0085-01
100's	$266.81	GENERIC, Barr Laboratories Inc	00555-0877-02
100's	$266.81	GENERIC, Watson Laboratories Inc	00591-0827-01
100's	$266.81	GENERIC, Par Pharmaceutical Inc	49884-0733-01
100's	$266.81	GENERIC, Sidmak Laboratories Inc	50111-0648-01
100's	$266.95	GENERIC, Udl Laboratories Inc	51079-0971-20
100's	$306.16	PROZAC, Physicians Total Care	54868-0511-00
100's	$330.33	PROZAC, Prescript Pharmaceuticals	00247-0372-00
100's	$333.07	PROZAC, Dista Products Company	00777-3105-02
100's	$339.56	PROZAC, Dista Products Company	00777-3105-33
118's	$389.19	PROZAC, Prescript Pharmaceuticals	00247-0372-52
180's	$404.17	PROZAC, Allscripts Pharmaceutical Company	54569-8522-01

Capsule - Oral - 40 mg

30's	$160.09	GENERIC, Teva Pharmaceuticals Usa	00093-7198-56
30's	$160.09	GENERIC, Par Pharmaceutical Inc	49884-0743-11
100's	$533.05	GENERIC, Geneva Pharmaceuticals	00781-2824-01
100's	$533.56	GENERIC, Par Pharmaceutical Inc	49884-0743-01

Solution - Oral - 20 mg/5 ml

5 ml x 40	$234.00	GENERIC, Pharmaceutical Assoc Inc Div Beach Products	00121-0721-05
120 ml	$118.00	GENERIC, Mallinckrodt Medical Inc	00406-0667-01
120 ml	$118.30	GENERIC, Alpharma Uspd Makers Of Barre and Nmc	00472-0021-04
120 ml	$118.35	GENERIC, Apotex Usa Inc	60505-0352-01
120 ml	$118.49	GENERIC, Teva Pharmaceuticals Usa	00093-6108-12
120 ml	$123.03	GENERIC, Pharmaceutical Assoc Inc Div Beach Products	00121-0721-04
120 ml	$147.91	PROZAC, Dista Products Company	00777-5120-58

Tablet - Oral - 10 mg

30's	$78.03	GENERIC, Barr Laboratories Inc	00555-0201-01
30's	$78.04	GENERIC, Teva Pharmaceuticals Usa	00093-7188-56
30's	$81.93	GENERIC, Par Pharmaceutical Inc	49884-0734-11
30's	$97.42	PROZAC, Lilly, Eli and Company	00002-4006-30
100's	$258.65	GENERIC, Ivax Corporation	00172-4510-60
100's	$273.10	GENERIC, Par Pharmaceutical Inc	49884-0734-01
100's	$324.71	PROZAC, Lilly, Eli and Company	00002-4006-02

Tablet - Oral - 20 mg

30's	$84.02	GENERIC, Par Pharmaceutical Inc	49884-0735-11
100's	$280.06	GENERIC, Par Pharmaceutical Inc	49884-0735-01

PRODUCT LISTING - EQUIVALENTS NOT AVAILABLE

Capsule - Oral - 10 mg

28's	$90.92	SARAFEM, Lilly, Eli and Company	00002-3210-45
30's	$91.04	GENERIC, Southwood Pharmaceuticals Inc	58016-0906-30
60's	$182.08	GENERIC, Southwood Pharmaceuticals Inc	58016-0906-60
90's	$273.12	GENERIC, Southwood Pharmaceuticals Inc	58016-0906-90

F

100's	$259.80	GENERIC, Purepac Pharmaceutical Company	00008-2702-11
100's	$303.47	GENERIC, Southwood Pharmaceuticals Inc	58016-0906-00
Capsule - Oral - 20 mg			
28's	$93.28	SARAFEM, Lilly, Eli and Company	00002-3220-45
100's	$266.50	GENERIC, Purepac Pharmaceutical Company	00228-2703-11
Capsule - Oral - 40 mg			
30's	$165.00	GENERIC, Southwood Pharmaceuticals Inc	58016-0704-30
30's	$199.85	PROZAC, Lilly, Eli and Company	00777-3107-30
60's	$330.00	GENERIC, Southwood Pharmaceuticals Inc	58016-0704-60
90's	$495.00	GENERIC, Southwood Pharmaceuticals Inc	58016-0704-90
100's	$550.00	GENERIC, Southwood Pharmaceuticals Inc	58016-0704-00
Capsule, Extended Release - Oral - 90 mg			
4's	$77.75	PROZAC WEEKLY, Pharma Pac	52959-0638-04
4's	$88.48	PROZAC WEEKLY, Lilly, Eli and Company	00002-3004-75
Solution - Oral - 20 mg/5 ml			
5 ml x 50	$555.04	PROZAC, Xactdose Inc	50962-0500-60
Tablet - Oral - 20 mg			
100's	$311.21	GENERIC, Par Pharmaceutical Inc	49884-0759-01

F

Fluphenazine Decanoate *(001322)*

Categories: Psychosis; Schizophrenia; FDA Approved 1972 Jun; Pregnancy Category C; WHO Formulary
Drug Classes: Antipsychotics; Phenothiazines
Brand Names: Fluphenazine; **Prolixin Decanoate**
Foreign Brand Availability: Anatensol (India; Netherlands); Anatensol Decanoato (Peru); Dapotum d (Hungary); Dapotum D (Switzerland); Dapatum D25 (Germany); Dapotum Depot (Austria); Deca (China; Malaysia; Thailand); Decafen (South-Africa); Flucan (Taiwan); Fludecasine (Japan); Fludecate (Israel); Fludecate Multidose (South-Africa); Modecate (Australia; Bahamas; Barbados; Belize; Benin; Bermuda; Burkina-Faso; Canada; China; Curacao; England; Ethiopia; France; Gambia; Ghana; Guinea; Guyana; Hong-Kong; Indonesia; Ireland; Ivory-Coast; Jamaica; Kenya; Liberia; Malawi; Mali; Mauritania; Mauritius; Morocco; Netherland-Antilles; New-Zealand; Niger; Nigeria; Senegal; Seychelles; Sierra-Leone; Singapore; South-Africa; Spain; Sudan; Surinam; Tanzania; Trinidad; Tunia; Uganda; Zambia; Zimbabwe); Moditen (Czech-Republic); Moditen Depot (Hungary); Phenazine (Thailand); Phlufdek (Philippines); Prolixin-D (Colombia); Siqualone (Finland; Norway; Sweden); Sydepres (Philippines)
HCFA JCODE(S): J2680 up to 25 mg IM, SC

DESCRIPTION

Fluphenazine decanoate is the decanoate ester of a trifluoromethyl phenothiazine derivative. It is a highly potent behavior modifier with a markedly extended duration of effect. Fluphenazine decanoate is available for intramuscular or subcutaneous administration, providing 25 mg fluphenazine decanoate per ml in a sesame oil vehicle with 1.2% (w/v) benzyl alcohol as a preservative. At the time of manufacture, the air in the vials is replaced by nitrogen.

Storage: Store at room temperature; avoid freezing and excessive heat. Protect from light.

CLINICAL PHARMACOLOGY

The basic effects of fluphenazine decanoate appear to be no different from those of fluphenazine HCl, with the exception of duration of action. The esterification of fluphenazine markedly prolongs the drug's duration of effect without unduly attenuating the its beneficial action.

Fluphenazine decanoate has activity at all levels of the central nervous system as well as on multiple organ systems. The mechanism whereby its therapeutic action is exerted is unknown.

Fluphenazine differs from other phenothiazine derivatives in several respects: it is more potent on a milligram basis, it has less potentiating effect on central nervous system depressants and anesthetics than do some of the phenothiazines to produce hypotension (nevertheless, appropriate cautions should be observed — see PRECAUTIONS and ADVERSE REACTIONS).

INDICATIONS AND USAGE

Fluphenazine decanoate injection is a long-acting parenteral antipsychotic drug intended for use in the management of patients requiring prolonged parenteral neuroleptic therapy (*e.g.*, chronic schizophrenics).

Fluphenazine decanoate has not been shown effective in the management of behavioral complications in patients with mental retardation.

CONTRAINDICATIONS

Phenothiazines are contraindicated in patients with suspected or established or established subcortical brain damage.

Phenothiazine compounds should not be used in patients receiving large doses of hypnotics.

Fluphenazine decanoate injection is contraindicated in comatose or severely depressed states.

The presence of blood dyscrasia or liver damage precludes the use of fluphenazine decanoate.

Fluphenazine decanoate is not intended for use in children under 12 years of age.

Fluphenazine decanoate is contraindicated in patients who have shown hypersensitivity to fluphenazine; cross-sensitivity to phenothiazine derivatives may occur.

WARNINGS

TARDIVE DYSKINESIA

Tardive dyskinesia, a syndrome consisting of potentially irreversible, involuntary, dyskinetic movements may develop in patients treated with neuroleptic (antipsychotic) drugs. Although the prevalence of the syndrome appears to be highest among the elderly, especially elderly women, it is impossible to rely upon prevalence estimates to predict, at the inception of neuroleptic treatment, which patients are likely to develop the syndrome. Whether neuroleptic drug products differ in their potential to cause tardive dyskinesia is unknown.

Both the risk of developing the syndrome and the likelihood that it will become irreversible are believed to increase as the duration of treatment and the total cumulative dose of neuroleptic drugs administered to the patient increase. However, the syndrome can develop, although much less commonly, after relatively brief treatment periods at low doses.

There is no known treatment for established cases of tardive dyskinesia, although the syndrome may remit, partially or completely, if neuroleptic treatment is withdrawn. Neuroleptic treatment, itself, however, may suppress (or partially suppress) the signs and symptoms of the syndrome and thereby may possibly mask the underlying disease process. The effect that symptomatic suppression has upon the long-term course of the syndrome is unknown.

Given these considerations, neuroleptics should be prescribed in a manner that is most likely to minimize the occurrence of tardive dyskinesia. Chronic neuroleptic treatment should generally be reserved for patients who suffer from a chronic illness that, (1) is known to respond to neuroleptic drugs, and, (2) for whom alternative, equally effective, but potentially less harmful treatments are *not* available or appropriate. In patients who do require chronic treatment, the smallest dose and the shortest duration of treatment producing a satisfactory clinical response should be sought. The need for continued treatment should be reassessed periodically.

If signs and symptoms of tardive dyskinesia appear in a patient on neuroleptics, drug discontinuation should be considered. However, some patients may require treatment despite the presence of the syndrome. (For further information about the description of tardive dyskinesia and its clinical detention, please refer to PRECAUTIONS, Information for Patients and ADVERSE REACTIONS, Tardive Dyskinesia.)

NEUROLEPTIC MALIGNANT SYNDROME (NMS)

A potentially fatal symptom complex sometimes referred to as Neuroleptic Malignant Syndrome (NMS) has been reported in association with antipsychotic drugs. Clinical manifestations of NMS are hyperpyrexia, muscle rigidity, altered mental status and evidence of autonomic instability (irregular pulse or blood pressure, tachycardia, diaphoresis, and cardiac dysrhythmias).

The diagnostic evaluation of patients with this syndrome is complicated. In arriving at a diagnosis, it is important to identify cases where the clinical presentation includes both serious mental illness (*e.g.*, pneumonia, systemic infection, etc.) and untreated or inadequately treated extrapyramidal signs and symptoms (EPS). Other important considerations in the differential diagnosis include anticholinergic toxicity, heat stroke, drug fever and primary central nervous system (CNS) pathology.

The management of NMS should include (1) immediate discontinuation of antipsychotic drugs and other drugs not essential to concurrent therapy, (2) intensive symptomatic treatment and medical monitoring, and (3) treatment of any concomitant serious medical problems for which specific treatments are available. There is no general agreement about specific pharmacological treatment regimens for uncomplicated NMS.

If a patient requires antipsychotic drug treatment after recovery from NMS, the potential reintroduction of drug therapy should be carefully considered. The patient should be carefully monitored, since recurrences of NMS have been reported.

The use of this drug may impair the mental and physical abilities required for driving a car or operating heavy machinery.

Physicians should be alert to the possibility that severe reactions may which require immediate medical attention.

Potentiation of the effects of alcohol may occur with use of this drug.

Since there is no adequate experience in children who have received this drug, safety and efficacy in children have not been established.

USAGE IN PREGNANCY

The safety for the use of the drug during pregnancy has not been established; therefore, the possible hazards should be weighed against the potential benefits when administering this drug to pregnant patients.

PRECAUTIONS

GENERAL

Because of the possibility of cross-sensitivity, fluphenazine decanoate should be used cautiously in patients who have developed cholestatic jaundice, dermatoses, or other allergic reactions to phenothiazine derivatives.

Psychotic patients on large doses of a phenothiazine drug who are undergoing surgery should be watched carefully for possible hypotensive phenomena. Moreover, it should be remembered that reduced amounts of anesthetics or central nervous system depressants may be necessary.

The effects of atropine may be potentiated in some patients receiving fluphenazine because of added anticholinergic effects.

Fluphenazine decanoate should be used cautiously in patients exposed to extreme heat or phosphorus insecticides.

The preparation should be used with caution in patients with a history of convulsive disorders, since grand mal convulsions have been know to occur.

Use with caution in patients with special medical disorders such as mitral insufficiency or other cardiovascular diseases and pheochromocytoma.

The possibility of liver damage, pigmentary retinopathy, lenticular and corneal deposits, and development of irreversible dyskinesia should be remembered when patients are on prolonged therapy.

Outside state hospitals or psychiatric institutions, fluphenazine decanoate should be administered under the direction of a physician experienced in the clinical use of psychotropic drugs, particularly phenothiazine derivatives. Furthermore, facilities should be available for periodic checking of hepatic function, renal function, and the blood picture. Renal function of patients on long-term therapy should be monitored; If BUN (blood urea nitrogen) becomes abnormal, treatment should be discontinued.

As with any phenothiazine, the physician should be alert to the possible development of "silent pneumonias" in patients under treatment with fluphenazine decanoate.

Neuroleptic drugs elevate prolactin levels; the elevation persists during chronic administration. Tissue culture experiments indicate that approximately one-third of human breast cancers are prolactin dependent *in vitro,* a factor of potential importance if the prescription of these drugs is contemplated in a patient with previously detected breast cancer. Although disturbances such as galactorrhea, amenorrhea, gynecomastia, and impotence have been reported, the clinical significance of elevated serum prolactin levels is unknown for most patients. An increase in mammary neoplasms has been found in rodents after chronic administration of neuroleptic drugs. Neither clinical studies nor epidemiologic studies conducted to date, however, have shown an association between chronic administration of these drugs and mammary tumorigenesis; the available evidence is considered too limited to be conclusive at this time.

INFORMATION FOR THE PATIENT

Given the likelihood that a substantial proportion of patients exposed chronically to neuroleptics will develop tardive dyskinesia, it is advised that patients in whom chronic use is contemplated to be given, if possible, full information about this risk. The decision to inform patients and/or their guardians must obviously take into account the clinical circumstances and the competency of the patient to understand the information provided.

ADVERSE REACTIONS

CENTRAL NERVOUS SYSTEM

The side effects most frequently reported with phenothiazine compounds are extrapyramidal symptoms including pseudoparkinsonism, dystonia, dyskinesia, akathisia, oculogyric crises, opisthotonos, and hyperreflexia. Muscle rigidity sometimes accompanied by hyperthermia has been reported following use of fluphenazine decanoate. Most often these extrapyramidal symptoms are reversible; however, they may be persistent (see next paragraph). The frequency of such reactions is related in part to chemical structure: one can expect a higher incidence with fluphenazine decanoate than with less potent piperazine derivatives or with straight-chain phenothiazines such as chlorpromazine. With any given phenothiazine derivative, the incidence and severity of such reactions depend more on individual patient sensitivity than on other factors, but dosage level and patient age are also determinants.

Extrapyramidal reactions may be alarming, and the patient should be forewarned and reassured. These reactions can usually be controlled by administration of antiparkinsonism drugs such as Benztropine Mesylate or intravenous Caffeine and Sodium Benzoate Injection, and by subsequent reduction in dosage.

TARDIVE DYSKINESIA

See WARNINGS. The syndrome is characterized by involuntary choreoathetoid movements which variously involve the tongue, face, mouth, lips, or jaw (*e.g.,* protrusion of the tongue, puffing of cheeks, puckering of mouth, chewing movements), trunk and extremities. The severity of the syndrome and the degree of impairment produced may vary widely.

The syndrome may become clinically recognizable either during treatment, upon dosage reduction, or upon withdrawal of treatment. Early detection of tardive dyskinesia is important. To increase the likelihood of detecting the syndrome at the earliest possible time, the dosage of neuroleptic drug should be reduced periodically (if clinically possible) and the patient observed for signs of the disorder. This maneuver is critical, since neuroleptic drugs may mask the signs of the syndrome.

OTHER CNS EFFECTS

Occurrence of neuroleptic malignant syndrome (NMS) have been reported in patients on neuroleptic therapy (see WARNINGS, Neuroleptic Malignant Syndrome); leukocytosis, elevated CPK, liver function abnormalities, and acute renal failure may also occur with NMS.

Drowsiness or lethargy, if they occur, may necessitate a reduction in dosage; the induction of a catatonic-like state has been known to occur with dosages of fluphenazine far in excess of the recommended amounts. As with other phenothiazine compounds, reactivation or aggravation of psychotic processes may be encountered.

Phenothiazine derivatives have been known to cause, in some patients, restlessness, excitement, or bizarre dreams.

AUTONOMIC NERVOUS SYSTEM

Hypertension and fluctuations in blood pressure have been reported with fluphenazine.

Hypotension has rarely presented a problem with fluphenazine. However, patients with pheochromocytoma, cerebral vascular or renal insufficiency, or a severe cardiac reserve deficiency such as mitral insufficiency appear to be particularly prone to hypotensive reactions with phenothiazine compounds, and should therefore be observed closely when the drug is administered. If severe hypotension should occur, supportive measures including the use of intravenous vasopressor drugs should be instituted immediately. Levarterenol Bitartrate Injection is the most suitable drug for this purpose; *epinephrine should not be used* since phenothiazine derivatives have been found to reverse its action, resulting in a further lowering of blood pressure.

Autonomic reactions including nausea and loss of appetite, salivation, polyuria, perspiration, dry mouth, headache, and constipation may occur. Autonomic effects can usually be controlled by reducing or temporarily discontinuing dosage.

In some patients, phenothiazine derivatives have caused blurred vision, glaucoma, bladder paralysis, fecal impaction, paralytic ileus, tachycardia, or nasal congestion.

METABOLIC AND ENDOCRINE

Weight change, peripheral edema, abnormal lactation, gynecomastia, menstrual irregularities, false results on pregnancy tests, impotency in men and increased libido in women have all been known to occur in some patients on phenothiazine therapy.

ALLERGIC REACTIONS

Skin disorders such as itching, erythema, urticaria, seborrhea, photosensitivity, eczema and even exfoliative dermatitis have been reported with phenothiazine derivatives. The possibility of anaphylactoid reactions occurring in some patients should be borne in mind.

HEMATOLOGIC

Routine blood counts are advisable during therapy since blood dyscrasias including leukopenia, agranulocytosis, thrombocytopenic or nonthrombocytopenic purpura, eosinophilia, and pancytopenia have been observed with phenothiazine derivatives. Furthermore, if any soreness of the mouth, gums, or throat, or any symptoms of upper respiratory infection occur and confirmatory leukocyte count indicates cellular depression, therapy should be discontinued and other appropriate measures instituted immediately.

HEPATIC

Liver damage as manifested by cholestatic jaundice may be encountered, particularly during the first months of therapy; treatment should be discontinued if this occurs. An increase in cephalin flocculation, sometimes accompanied by alterations in other liver function tests, has been reported in patients receiving the enanthate ester of fluphenazine (a closely related compound) who have had no clinical evidence of liver damage.

OTHER

Sudden, unexpected and unexplained deaths have been reported in hospitalized psychotic patients receiving phenothiazines. Previous brain damage or seizures may be predisposing factors; high doses should be avoided in known seizure patients. Several patients have shown sudden flare-ups of psychotic behavior patterns shortly before death. Autopsy findings have usually revealed acute fulminating pneumonia or pneumonitis, aspiration of gastric contents, or intramyocardial lesions.

Although this is not a general feature of fluphenazine, potentiation of central nervous system depressants (opiates, analgesics, antihistamines, barbiturates, alcohol) may occur.

The following adverse reactions have also occurred with phenothiazine derivatives: Systemic lupus erythematosus-like syndrome, hypotension severe enough to cause fatal cardiac arrest, altered electrocardiographic and electroencephalographic tracings, altered cerebrospinal fluid proteins , cerebral edema, asthma, laryngeal edema, angioneurotic edema; with long-term use—skin pigmentation, and lenticular and corneal opacities.

Injections of fluphenazine decanoate are extremely well tolerated, local tissue reactions occurring only rarely.

DOSAGE AND ADMINISTRATION

Parenteral drug products should be inspected visually for particulate matter and discoloration prior to administration, whenever solution and container permit.

Fluphenazine decanoate injection may be given intramuscularly or subcutaneously. A dry syringe and needle of at least 21 gauge should be used. Use of a wet needle or syringe may cause the solution to become cloudy.

To begin therapy with fluphenazine decanoate the following regimens are suggested:

FOR MOST PATIENTS

A dose of 12.5-25 mg (0.5-1 ml) may be given to initiate therapy. The onset of action generally appears between 24 and 72 hours after injection and the effects of the drug on psychotic symptoms becomes significant within 48-96 hours. Subsequent injections and the dosage interval are determined in accordance with the patient's response. When administered as maintenance therapy, a single injection may be effective in controlling schizophrenic symptoms up to 4 weeks or longer. The response to a single dose has been found to last as long as 6 weeks in a few patients on maintenance therapy.

It may be advisable that patients who have no history of taking phenothiazines should be treated initially with a shorter-acting form of fluphenazine before administering the decanoate to determine the patient's response to fluphenazine and to establish appropriate dosage. For psychotic patients who have been stabilized on a fixed daily dosage of fluphenazine HCl tablets, fluphenazine hcl elixir, or fluphenazine HCL oral solution, conversion of therapy from these short-acting oral forms to the long-acting injectable fluphenazine decanoate may be indicated.

Appropriate dosage of fluphenazine decanoate injection should be individualized for each patient and responses carefully monitored. No precise formula can be given to convert to use of fluphenazine decanoate; however, a controlled multicenter study,[1] in patients receiving oral doses from 5-60 mg fluphenazine HCl daily, showed that 20 mg fluphenazine HCl daily was equivalent to 25 mg (1 ml) fluphenazine decanoate every 3 weeks. This represents an approximate conversion ratio of 0.5 ml (12.5 mg) of decanoate every 3 weeks for every 10 mg of fluphenazine HCl daily.

Once conversion to fluphenazine decanoate is made, careful clinical monitoring of the patient and appropriate dosage adjustment should be made at the time of each injection.

SEVERELY AGITATED PATIENTS

Severely agitated patients may be treated initially with a rapid- acting phenothiazine compound such as fluphenazine HCl Injection. When acute symptoms have subsided, 25 mg (1 ml) of fluphenazine decanoate may be administered; subsequent dosage is adjusted as necessary.

"POOR RISK" PATIENTS

(Those with known hypersensitivity to phenothiazines, or with disorders that predispose to undue reactions.) Therapy may be initiated cautiously with oral or parenteral fluphenazine HCl. When the pharmacologic effects and an appropriate dosage are apparent, an equivalent dose of fluphenazine decanoate may be administered. Subsequent dosage adjustments are made in accordance with the response of the patient.

The optimal amount of the drug and the frequency of administration must be determined for each patient, since dosage requirements have been found to vary with clinical circumstances as well as with individual response to the drug.

Dosage should not exceed 100 mg. If doses greater than 50 mg are deemed necessary, the next dose and succeeding doses should be increased cautiously in increments of 12.5 mg.

Fluphenazine Hydrochloride (001324)

Categories: Psychosis; FDA Approved 1959 Sep; Pregnancy Category C
Drug Classes: Antipsychotics; Phenothiazines
Brand Names: Flunazine; Fluphenazine Hcl; Fluzine; Permitil; **Prolixin**
Foreign Brand Availability: Anatensol (Australia; Belgium; Hong-Kong; Indonesia; Netherlands; New-Zealand); Apo-Fluphenazine (Malaysia); Cenilene (Portugal); Dapotum (Austria; Germany; Switzerland); Fluzine-P (Thailand); Lyogen (Germany); Lyogen Depot (Germany); Moditen (Bahrain; Benin; Burkina-Faso; Canada; England; Ethiopia; France; Gambia; Ghana; Guinea; Iraq; Ireland; Israel; Ivory-Coast; Kenya; Kuwait; Liberia; Malawi; Mali; Mauritania; Mauritius; Morocco; Niger; Nigeria; Senegal; Seychelles; Sierra-Leone; Sudan; Switzerland; Tanzania; Tunia; Uganda; Zambia; Zimbabwe); Omca (Germany); Pacinol (Denmark; Finland; Sweden); Pacinol Prolong (Norway); Potensone (Thailand); Siqualone (Finland; Sweden)
Cost of Therapy: \$37.57 (Schizophrenia; Prolixin; 1 mg; 1 tablet/day; 30 day supply)
\$9.33 (Schizophrenia; Generic Tablets; 1 mg; 1 tablet/day; 30 day supply)

DESCRIPTION

TABLETS AND ELIXIR

Fluphenazine Hydrochloride is a trifluoroethyl phenothiazine derivative intended for the management of schizophrenia.

Fluphenazine HCl tablets contain 1, 2.5, 5, and 10 mg Fluphenazine HCl per tablet. Inactive ingredients: acacia, carnauba wax for 1 and 2.5 only, castor oil; Aluminum lakes of the following colorants: (D&C red no. 27 for 1 and 10 mg only; D&C yellow no. 10 for 5 and 10 mg only; FD&C blue no. 1 for 5 and 10 mg only; FD&C blue no. 2 for 2.5 mg only; FD&C yellow no. 5 (tartrazine) for 2.5, 5 an 10 mg only; FC&C yellow no. 6 for 1 mg only); corn starch; ethylcellulose; gelatin; lactose; magnesium carbonate; magnesium stearate; pharmaceutical glaze; polyethylene glycol for 1 and 2.5 mg only; povidone for 1,2.5, and 10 mg only; precipitated calcium carbonate; sodium benzoate; sucrose; synthetic iron oxide; talc; titanium dioxide; white wax for 1 and 2.5 mg only; and other ingredients.

Fluphenazine HCl elixir contains 0.5 mg fluphenazine hydrochloride per ml. Inactive ingredients: alcohol (14% (v/v)) colorant (FD&C yellow no. 6), flavors, glycerin, polysorbate 40, purified water, sodium benzoate, and sucrose.

INJECTION

Fluphenazine HCl injection is available in multiple dose vials providing 2.5 mg fluphenazine HCl per ml. The preparation also includes sodium chloride for isotonicity, sodium hydroxide or hydrochloric acid to adjust the pH to 4.8-5.2, and 0.1% methylparaben and 0.01% propylparaben as preservatives. At the time of manufacture, the air in the vials is replaced by nitrogen.

CLINICAL PHARMACOLOGY

Fluphenazine HCl has activity at all levels of the central nervous system as well as on multiple organ systems. The mechanism whereby its therapeutic action is extended action exerted is unknown.

INDICATIONS AND USAGE

Fluphenazine HCl is indicated in the management of manifestations of psychotic disorders.

Fluphenazine HCl has not been shown effective in the management of behavioral complications in patients with mental retardation.

CONTRAINDICATIONS

Phenothiazines are contraindicated in patients with suspected or established subcortical brain damage, in patients receiving large doses of hypnotics, & in comatose or severely depressed states. The presence of blood dyscrasia or liver damage precludes the use of fluphenazine HCl. This drug is contraindicated in patients who have shown hypersensitivity to fluphenazine; cross-sensitivity to phenothiazine derivatives may occur.

WARNINGS

TARDIVE DYSKINESIA

Tardive Dyskinesia a syndrome consisting of potentially irreversible, involuntary, dyskinetic movements may develop in patients treated with neuroleptic (antipsychotic) drugs. Although the prevalence of the syndrome appears to be highest among the elderly, especially elderly women, it is impossible to rely upon prevalence estimates to predict, at the inception of neuroleptic treatment, which patients are likely to develop the syndrome. Whether neuroleptic drug products differ in their potential to cause tardive dyskinesia is unknown.

Both the risk of developing the syndrome and the likelihood that it will become irreversible are believed to increase as the duration of treatment and the total cumulative dose of neuroleptic drugs administered to the patient increase. However, the syndrome can develop, although much less commonly, after relatively brief treatment periods at low doses.

There is no known treatment for established cases of tardive dyskinesia, although the syndrome may remit, partially or completely, if neuroleptic treatment is withdrawn. Neuroleptic treatment, itself, however, amy suppress (or partially suppress) the signs and symptoms of the syndrome and thereby may possibly mask the underlying disease process. The effect that symptomatic suppression has upon the long-term course of the syndrome is unknown.

Given these considerations, neuroleptics should be prescribed in a manner that is most likely to minimize the occupance of tardive dyskinesia. Chronic neuroleptic treatment should generally be reserved for patients who suffer from a chronic illness that (1) is known to respond to neuroleptic drugs, and, (2) for whom alternative, equally effective, but potentially less harmful treatments are *not* available or appropriate. In patients who do require chronic treatment, the smallest dose and the shortest duration of treatment of treatment producing a satisfactory clinical response should be sought. The need for continued treatment should be reassessed periodically.

If signs and symptoms of tardive dyskinesia appear in a patient on neuroleptics, drug discontinuation should be considered. However, some patients may require treatment despite the presence of the syndrome.

(For further information about the description of tardive dyskinesia and its clinical detection, please refer to the sections on PRECAUTIONS, Information for the Patient, and ADVERSE REACTIONS, Tardive Dyskinesia).

NEUROLEPTIC MALIGNANT SYNDROME (NMS)

A potentially fatal symptom complex sometimes referred to as Neuroleptic Malignant Syndrome (NMS) has been reported in association with antipsychotic drugs. Clinical manifestations of NMS are hyperpyrexia, muscle rigidity, altered mental status and evidence of automatic instability (irregular pulse or blood pressure, tachycardia, diaphoresis, and cardiac dysrhythmias).

The diagnostic evaluation of patients with this syndrome is complicated. In arriving at a diagnosis, it is important to identify cases where the clinical presentation includes both serious medical illness (*e.g.,* pneumonia, systemic infection, etc.) and untreated or inadequately treated extrapyramidal signs and symptoms. Other important considerations in the differential diagnosis include central anticholinergic toxicity, heat stroke, drug fever and primary central nervous system pathology.

The management of NMS should include: (1) immediate discontinuation of antipsychotic and other drugs not essential to concurrent therapy; (2) intensive symptomatic treatment and medical monitoring; and (3) treatment of any concomitant serious medical problems for which specific treatments are available. There is no general agreement about specific pharmacologic treatment regimens for uncomplicated NMS.

If a patient requires antipsychotic drug treatment after recovery from NMS, the potential reintroduction of drug therapy should be carefully considered. The patient should be carefully monitored, since recurrences of NMS have been reported.

The use of this drug may impair the mental and physical abilities for driving or operating heavy machinery.

Potentiation of the effects of alcohol may occur with the use of this drug.

Since there is no adequate experience in children who have received this drug, safety and efficacy in children have not been established.

USAGE IN PREGNANCY

The safety for the use of this drug during pregnancy has not been established; therefore, the possible hazards should be weighed against the potential benefits when administering this drug to pregnant patients.

PRECAUTIONS

GENERAL

Because of the possibility of cross-sensitivity, fluphenazine HCl should be used cautiously in patients who have developed cholestatic jaundice, dermatoses, or other allergic reactions to phenothiazine derivatives.

Fluphenazine HCl tablets 2.5, 5. and 10 mg contain FD&C yellow no. 5 (tartrazine) which may cause allergic-type reactions (including bronchial asthma) in certain susceptible individuals. Although the overall incidence of FD&C yellow no. 5 (tartrazine) sensitivity in the general population is low, it is frequently seen in patients who also have aspirin hypersensitivity.

Psychotic patients on large doses of a phenothiazine drug who are undergoing surgery should be watched carefully for possible hypotensive phenomena. Moreover, it should be remembered that reduced amounts of anesthetics or central nervous system depressants may be necessary.

The effects of atropine may be potentiated in some patients receiving fluphenazine HCl because of added anticholinergic effects.

Fluphenazine HCl should be used cautiously in patients exposed to extreme heat or phosphorus insecticides; in patients with a history of convulsive disorders, since grand mal convulsions have been known to occur; and in patients with a special medical disorders, such as mitral insufficiency or other cardiovascular diseases and pheochromocytoma.

The possibility of liver damage, pigmentary retinopathy, lenticular and corneal deposits, and development of irreversible dyskinesia should be remembered when patients are on prolonged therapy.

Neuroleptic drugs elevate prolactin levels; the elevation persists during chronic administration. Tissue culture experiments indicate that approximately one-third of human breast cancers are prolactin dependent *in vitro,* a factor of potential importance if the prescription of these drugs is contemplated in a patient with previously detectable breast cancer. Although disturbances such as galactorrhea, amenorrhea, gynecomastia, and impotence have been reported, the clinical significance of elevated serum prolactin levels is unknown for most patients. An increase in mammary neoplasms have been found in rodents after chronic administration of neuroleptic drugs. Neither clinical studies nor epidemiologic studies conducted to date, however, have shown an association between chronic administration of these drugs and mammary tumorigenesis; the available evidence is considered too limited to be conclusive at this time.

INFORMATION FOR THE PATIENT

Given the likelihood that some patients exposed chronically to neuroleptics will develop tardive dyskinesia, it is advised that all patients in whom chronic use is contemplated be given, if possible, full information about this risk. The decision to inform patients and/or their guardians must obviously take into account the clinical circumstances and the competency of the patient to understand the information provided.

ABRUPT WITHDRAWAL

In general, phenothiazines do not produce psychic dependence; however, gastritis, nausea and vomiting, dizziness, and tremulousness have been reported following abrupt cessation of high dose therapy. Reports suggest that these symptoms can be reduced if concomitant antiparkinsonian agents are continued for several weeks after the phenothiazine is withdrawn.

Facilities should be available for periodic checking of the hepatic function, renal function and the blood picture. Renal function of the patient on long-term therapy should be monitored; if BUN (blood urea nitrogen) becomes abnormal, treatment should be discontinued.

As with any phenothiazines, the physicians should be alert to the possible development of "silent pneumonias" in patients under treatment with fluphenazine HCl.

ADVERSE REACTIONS

CENTRAL NERVOUS SYSTEM

The side effects most frequently reported with phenothiazine compounds are extrapyramidal symptoms, including pseudoparkinsonism, dystonia, dyskinesia, akathisia, oculogyric crises, opisthotonos, and hyperreflexia. Most often these extrapyramidal symptoms are reversible; however, they may be persistent see below. With any given phenothiazine derivative, the incidence and severity of such reactions depend more on the individual patient sensitivity than on other factors, but dosage level and patient age are also determinants.

Extrapyramidal reactions may be alarming, and the patient should be forewarned and reassured. These reactions can usually be controlled by administration of antiparkinsonian drugs such as benztropine mesylate or IV caffeine and sodium benzoate injection, and by subsequent reduction in dosage.

TARDIVE DYSKINESIA

See WARNINGS. The syndrome is characterized by involuntary choreoathetoid movements which variously involve the tongue, face, mouth, lips, or jaw (*e.g.,* protrusion of the tongue, puffing of cheeks, puckering of the mouth, chewing movements), trunk and extremities. The severity of the syndrome and the degree of impairment produced vary widely.

The syndrome may become clinically recognizable either during treatment, upon dosage reduction, or upon withdrawal of treatment. Early detection of tardive dyskinesia is important. To increase the likelihood of detecting the syndrome at the earliest possible time, the dosage of neuroleptic drug should be reduced periodically (if clinically possible) and the patient observed for signs of the disorder. This maneuver is critical, since neuroleptic drugs may mask the signs of the syndrome.

OTHER CNS EFFECTS

Occurrences of neuroleptic malignant syndrome (NMS) have been reported in patients on neuroleptic therapy (see WARNINGS, Neuroleptic Malignant Syndrome). Leukocytosis, elevated CPK, liver function abnormalities, and acute renal failure may also occur with NMS.

Drowsiness or lethargy, if they occur, may necessitate a reduction in dosage; the induction of a catatonic-like state has been known to occur with dosages of fluphenazine far in excess of the compounds, reactivation or aggravation of psychotic processes may be encountered.

Phenothiazine derivatives have been known to cause, in some patients, restlessness, excitement, or bizarre dreams.

Automatic Nervous System: Hypertension and fluctuation in blood pressure have been reported with fluphenazine HCl.

Hypotension has rarely presented a problem with fluphenazine HCl. However, patients with pheochromocytoma, cerebral vascular or renal insufficiency, or a severe cardiac reserve deficiency (such as mitral insufficiency) appear to be particularly prone to hypotensive reactions with phenothiazine compounds, and should therefore be observed closely when the drug is administered. If severe hypotension should occur, supportive measures including the use of IV vasopressor drugs should be instituted immediately. Levarterenol bitartrate injection is the most suitable drug for this purpose; *epinephrine should not be used* since phenothiazine derivatives have been found to reverse its action, resulting in a further lowering of blood pressure.

Autonomic reactions including nausea and loss of appetite, salivation, polyuria, perspiration, dry mouth, headache, and constipation may occur. Autonomic effects can usually be controlled by reducing or temporarily discontinuing dosage.

In some patients, phenothiazine derivatives have caused blurred vision, glaucoma, bladder paralysis, fecal impaction, paralytic ileus, tachycardia, or nasal congestion.

METABOLIC AND ENDOCRINE

Weight change, peripheral edema, abnormal lactation, gynecomastia, menstrual irregularities, false results on pregnancy tests, impotency in men and increased libido in women have all been known to occur in some patients on phenothiazine therapy.

ALLERGIC REACTIONS

Skin disorders such as itching, erythema, urticaria, seborrhea, photosensitivity, eczema and even exfoliative dermatitis have been reported with phenothiazine derivatives. The possibility of anaphylactoid reactions occurring in some patients should be borne in mind.

HEMATOLOGIC

Routine blood counts are advisable during therapy since blood dyscrasias including leukopenia, agranulocytosis, thrombocytopenic or nonthrombocytopenic purpura, eosinophilia, and pancytopenia have been observed with phenothiazine derivatives. Furthermore, if any soreness of the mouth, gums, or throat, or any symptoms of upper respiratory infection occur and confirmatory leukocyte indicates cellular depression, therapy should be discontinued and other appropriate measures instituted immediately.

HEPATIC

Liver damage as manifested by cholestatic jaundice may be encountered, particularly during the first months of therapy; treatment should be discontinued if this occurs. An increase in cephalin flocculation, sometimes accompanied by alterations in other liver function tests, has been reported in patients receiving fluphenazine HCl who have had no clinical evidence of liver damage.

OTHERS

Sudden, unexpected and unexplained deaths have been reported in hospitalized psychotic patients receiving phenothiazines. Previous brain damage or seizures may be predisposing factors; high doses should be avoided in known seizure patients. Several patients have shown sudden flare-ups of psychotic behavior patterns shortly before death. Autopsy findings have usually revealed acute fulminating pneumonia or pneumonitis, aspiration of gastric contents, or intramyocardial lesions.

Although this is not a general feature of fluphenazine HCl, potentiation of central nervous system depressants (opiates, analgesics, antihistamines, barbiturates, alcohol) may occur.

The following adverse reactions have also occurred with phenothiazine derivatives: Systemic lupus erythematosus-like syndrome, hypotension severe enough to cause fatal cardiac arrest, altered electrocardiographic and electroencephalographic tracings, altered cerebrospinal fluid proteins, cerebral edema, asthma, laryngeal edema, and angioneurotic edema; with long-term use - skin pigmentation, and lenticular and corneal opacities.

DOSAGE AND ADMINISTRATION

TABLETS AND ELIXIR

Fluphenazine HCl elixir should be inspected prior to use. Upon standing a slight wispy precipitate or globular material may develop due to the flavoring oils separating from the solution (potency is not affected). Gentle shaking redisperses the oils and the solution becomes clear. Solutions that do not clarify should not be used.

Depending on the severity and duration of symptoms, total dosage for *adult* psychotic patients may range initially from 2.5-10.0 mg and should be divided and given at 6-8 hour intervals.

The smallest amount that will produce the desired results must be carefully determined for each individual, since optimal dosage levels of the potent drug vary from patient to patient. In general, the oral dose has been found to be approximately 2-3 times the parenteral dose of fluphenazine HCl. Treatment is best instituted with a *low initial dosage,* which may be increased, if necessary, until the desired clinical effects are achieved. Therapeutic effect is often achieved with doses under 20 mg daily. Patients remaining severely distributed or inadequately controlled may require upward titration of dosage. Daily doses up to 40 mg may be necessary; controlled clinical studies have not been performed to demonstrate safety of prolonged administration of such doses.

When symptoms are controlled, dosage can generally be reduced gradually to daily maintenance doses of 1.0 or 5.0 mg, often given as a single daily dose. Continued treatment is needed to achieve maximum therapeutic benefits; further adjustments in dosage may be necessary during the course of therapy to meet the patient's requirements.

For psychotic patients who have been stabilized on a fixed daily dosage or orally administered fluphenazine HCl dosage forms, conversion to the long-acting injectable Fluphenazine Decanoate may be indicated (see package insert for fluphenazine decanoate Injection for conversion information).

For *geriatric* patients, the suggested starting dose is 1.0-2.5 mg daily, adjusted according to the response of the patient.

Fluphenazine HCl injection is useful when psychotic patients are unable or unwilling to take oral therapy.

STORAGE

Store tablets and elixir at room temperature. Protect from light. Keep tightly closed.

Tablets: Avoid excessive heat.

Elixir : Avoid freezing.

INJECTION

The average well-tolerated starting dose for adult psychotic patients is 1.25 mg (0.5 ml) intramuscularly. Depending on the severity and duration of symptoms, initial total daily dosage may range from 2.5-10.0 mg and should be divided and given at 6-8 hour intervals.

The smallest amount that will produce the desired results must be carefully determined for each individual, since optimal dosage levels of this potent drug very from patient to patient. In general, the parenteral dose for fluphenazine has been found to be approximately 1/3 to 1/2 the oral dose. Treatment may be instituted with a *low initial dosage,* which may be increased, if necessary, until the desired clinical effects are achieved. Dosages exceeding 10.0 mg daily should be used with caution.

When symptoms are controlled, oral maintenance therapy can generally be instituted, often with single daily doses. Continued treatment, by the oral route if possible, is needed to achieve maximum therapeutic benefits; further adjustments in dosage may be necessary during the course of therapy to meet the patient's requirements.

STORAGE

Solutions should be protected from exposure to light. Parenteral solutions may vary in color from essentially colorless to light amber. If a solution has become any darker than light amber or is discolored in any other way it should not be used.

Store at room temperature; avoid freezing.

PRODUCT LISTING - RATED THERAPEUTICALLY EQUIVALENT

Size	Price	Product	NDC
Concentrate - Oral - 5 mg/ml			
118 ml	$90.92	PERMITIL, Schering Corporation	00085-0296-05
120 ml	$57.50	GENERIC, Pharmaceutical Assoc Inc Div Beach Products	00121-0653-04
120 ml	$112.80	GENERIC, Teva Pharmaceuticals Usa	00093-9630-12
120 ml	$160.44	PROLIXIN, Bristol-Myers Squibb	00003-0801-10
Elixir - Oral - 2.5 mg/5 ml			
60 ml	$16.09	GENERIC, Pharmaceutical Assoc Inc Div Beach Products	00121-0654-02
473 ml	$128.70	GENERIC, Pharmaceutical Assoc Inc Div Beach Products	00121-0654-16
473 ml	$142.75	GENERIC, Teva Pharmaceuticals Usa	00093-9686-16
Solution - Injectable - Decanoate 25 mg/ml			
1 ml	$28.14	PROLIXIN DECANOATE, Bristol-Myers Squibb	00003-0569-02
5 ml	$14.29	GENERIC, Insource Inc	63252-1126-50
5 ml	$25.00	GENERIC, Gensia Sicor Pharmaceuticals Inc	00703-5003-01
5 ml	$25.00	GENERIC, Bedford Laboratories	55390-0465-05
5 ml	$25.00	GENERIC, Apotex Usa Inc	60505-0664-02
5 ml	$69.30	GENERIC, American Pharmaceutical Partners	63323-0272-05

5 ml	$74.18	GENERIC, American Pharmaceutical Partners	63323-0272-55
5 ml	$80.25	GENERIC, Able Laboratories Inc	53265-0301-01
5 ml	$87.00	GENERIC, Pasadena Research Laboratories Inc	00418-2720-10
5 ml	$125.45	PROLIXIN DECANOATE, Bristol-Myers Squibb	00003-0569-15
Solution - Injectable - 2.5 mg/ml			
10 ml	$65.13	GENERIC, American Pharmaceutical Partners	63323-0281-10
10 ml	$68.83	PROLIXIN, Bristol-Myers Squibb	00003-0586-30
Tablet - Oral - 1 mg			
30's	$24.71	GENERIC, Heartland Healthcare Services	61392-0057-30
30's	$24.71	GENERIC, Heartland Healthcare Services	61392-0057-39
31's	$25.53	GENERIC, Heartland Healthcare Services	61392-0057-31
32's	$26.35	GENERIC, Heartland Healthcare Services	61392-0057-32
45's	$37.06	GENERIC, Heartland Healthcare Services	61392-0057-45
50's	$26.10	GENERIC, Geneva Pharmaceuticals	00781-1436-50
60's	$49.41	GENERIC, Heartland Healthcare Services	61392-0057-60
90's	$74.12	GENERIC, Heartland Healthcare Services	61392-0057-90
100's	$22.73	FEDERAL UPPER LIMIT, H.C.F.A. F F P	99999-1324-03
100's	$31.09	GENERIC, Warner Chilcott Laboratories	00047-0796-24
100's	$45.90	GENERIC, Dixon-Shane Inc	17236-0489-01
100's	$47.05	GENERIC, Major Pharmaceuticals Inc	00904-3673-60
100's	$47.95	GENERIC, Parmed Pharmaceuticals Inc	00349-8983-01
100's	$48.18	GENERIC, Moore, H.L. Drug Exchange Inc	00839-6440-06
100's	$48.31	GENERIC, Aligen Independent Laboratories Inc	00405-4439-01
100's	$48.70	GENERIC, Ivax Corporation	00182-1365-01
100's	$49.75	GENERIC, Geneva Pharmaceuticals	00781-1436-01
100's	$54.90	GENERIC, Mylan Pharmaceuticals Inc	00378-6004-01
100's	$54.90	GENERIC, Par Pharmaceutical Inc	49884-0061-01
100's	$62.40	GENERIC, Dixon-Shane Inc	17236-0489-11
100's	$62.40	GENERIC, Udl Laboratories Inc	51079-0485-20
100's	$62.99	GENERIC, Geneva Pharmaceuticals	00781-1436-13
100's	$63.00	GENERIC, Ivax Corporation	00182-1365-89
100's	$74.43	GENERIC, Major Pharmaceuticals Inc	00904-3673-61
100's	$125.24	PROLIXIN, Bristol-Myers Squibb	00003-0863-50
Tablet - Oral - 2.5 mg			
30's	$34.93	GENERIC, Heartland Healthcare Services	61392-0058-30
30's	$34.93	GENERIC, Heartland Healthcare Services	61392-0058-39
31's	$36.09	GENERIC, Heartland Healthcare Services	61392-0058-31
32's	$37.26	GENERIC, Heartland Healthcare Services	61392-0058-32
45's	$52.39	GENERIC, Heartland Healthcare Services	61392-0058-45
50's	$40.57	GENERIC, Geneva Pharmaceuticals	00781-1437-50
60's	$69.86	GENERIC, Heartland Healthcare Services	61392-0058-60
90's	$104.79	GENERIC, Heartland Healthcare Services	61392-0058-90
100's	$27.75	FEDERAL UPPER LIMIT, H.C.F.A. F F P	99999-1324-07
100's	$44.10	GENERIC, Warner Chilcott Laboratories	00047-0797-24
100's	$64.98	GENERIC, Dixon-Shane Inc	17236-0490-01
100's	$67.25	GENERIC, Major Pharmaceuticals Inc	00904-3674-60
100's	$68.24	GENERIC, Moore, H.L. Drug Exchange Inc	00839-6441-06
100's	$68.95	GENERIC, Parmed Pharmaceuticals Inc	00349-8981-01
100's	$75.42	GENERIC, Aligen Independent Laboratories Inc	00405-4440-01
100's	$75.75	GENERIC, Ivax Corporation	00182-1366-01
100's	$75.75	GENERIC, Geneva Pharmaceuticals	00781-1437-01
100's	$83.50	GENERIC, Mylan Pharmaceuticals Inc	00378-6009-01
100's	$83.50	GENERIC, Par Pharmaceutical Inc	49884-0062-01
100's	$89.60	GENERIC, Dixon-Shane Inc	17236-0490-11
100's	$89.60	GENERIC, Udl Laboratories Inc	51079-0486-20
100's	$90.99	GENERIC, Geneva Pharmaceuticals	00781-1437-13
100's	$91.00	GENERIC, Ivax Corporation	00182-1366-89
100's	$101.67	GENERIC, Major Pharmaceuticals Inc	00904-3674-61
100's	$155.40	PROLIXIN, Bristol-Myers Squibb	00003-0864-50
Tablet - Oral - 5 mg			
25's	$9.34	GENERIC, Udl Laboratories Inc	51079-0487-19
30's	$45.19	GENERIC, Heartland Healthcare Services	61392-0059-30
30's	$45.19	GENERIC, Heartland Healthcare Services	61392-0059-39
31 x 10	$418.28	GENERIC, Vangard Labs	00615-1501-53
31's	$46.70	GENERIC, Heartland Healthcare Services	61392-0059-31
32 x 10	$418.28	GENERIC, Vangard Labs	00615-1501-63
32's	$48.20	GENERIC, Heartland Healthcare Services	61392-0059-32
45's	$67.79	GENERIC, Heartland Healthcare Services	61392-0059-45
50's	$47.17	GENERIC, Geneva Pharmaceuticals	00781-1438-50
60's	$90.38	GENERIC, Heartland Healthcare Services	61392-0059-60
90's	$135.57	GENERIC, Heartland Healthcare Services	61392-0059-90
100's	$35.46	FEDERAL UPPER LIMIT, H.C.F.A. F F P	99999-1324-11
100's	$56.88	GENERIC, Warner Chilcott Laboratories	00047-0798-24
100's	$83.75	GENERIC, Dixon-Shane Inc	17236-0491-01
100's	$83.88	GENERIC, Aligen Independent Laboratories Inc	00405-4441-01
100's	$84.25	GENERIC, Major Pharmaceuticals Inc	00904-3675-60
100's	$87.95	GENERIC, Moore, H.L. Drug Exchange Inc	00839-6442-06
100's	$89.95	GENERIC, Geneva Pharmaceuticals	00781-1438-01
100's	$97.10	GENERIC, Mylan Pharmaceuticals Inc	00378-6074-01
100's	$97.10	GENERIC, Par Pharmaceutical Inc	49884-0076-01
100's	$132.74	GENERIC, Dixon-Shane Inc	17236-0491-11
100's	$132.74	GENERIC, Udl Laboratories Inc	51079-0487-20
100's	$134.99	GENERIC, Geneva Pharmaceuticals	00781-1438-13
100's	$135.00	GENERIC, Ivax Corporation	00182-1367-89
100's	$136.49	GENERIC, Major Pharmaceuticals Inc	00904-3675-61
100's	$167.38	PROLIXIN, Bristol-Myers Squibb	00003-0877-52
100's	$229.06	PROLIXIN, Bristol-Myers Squibb	00003-0877-50
Tablet - Oral - 10 mg			
30's	$58.84	GENERIC, Heartland Healthcare Services	61392-0060-30
30's	$58.84	GENERIC, Heartland Healthcare Services	61392-0060-39
31 x 10	$527.62	GENERIC, Vangard Labs	00615-3574-53
31's	$60.80	GENERIC, Heartland Healthcare Services	61392-0060-31
32 x 10	$527.62	GENERIC, Vangard Labs	00615-3574-63
32's	$62.77	GENERIC, Heartland Healthcare Services	61392-0060-32
45's	$88.26	GENERIC, Heartland Healthcare Services	61392-0060-45
50's	$60.24	GENERIC, Geneva Pharmaceuticals	00781-1439-50
60's	$117.69	GENERIC, Heartland Healthcare Services	61392-0060-60
90's	$176.53	GENERIC, Heartland Healthcare Services	61392-0060-90
100's	$50.99	FEDERAL UPPER LIMIT, H.C.F.A. F F P	99999-1324-15
100's	$74.03	GENERIC, Warner Chilcott Laboratories	00047-0799-24
100's	$109.05	GENERIC, Aligen Independent Laboratories Inc	00405-4442-01
100's	$109.05	GENERIC, Dixon-Shane Inc	17236-0492-01
100's	$111.40	GENERIC, Major Pharmaceuticals Inc	00904-3676-60
100's	$114.48	GENERIC, Moore, H.L. Drug Exchange Inc	00839-7452-06
100's	$114.75	GENERIC, Ivax Corporation	00182-1368-01
100's	$114.75	GENERIC, Geneva Pharmaceuticals	00781-1439-01
100's	$125.00	GENERIC, Mylan Pharmaceuticals Inc	00378-6097-01
100's	$125.00	GENERIC, Par Pharmaceutical Inc	49884-0064-01
100's	$168.50	GENERIC, Dixon-Shane Inc	17236-0492-11
100's	$168.50	GENERIC, Udl Laboratories Inc	51079-0488-20
100's	$170.30	GENERIC, Ivax Corporation	00182-1368-89
100's	$170.30	GENERIC, Geneva Pharmaceuticals	00781-1439-13
100's	$179.57	GENERIC, Major Pharmaceuticals Inc	00904-3676-61
100's	$278.90	PROLIXIN, Bristol-Myers Squibb	00003-0956-50

PRODUCT LISTING - RATED NOT THERAPEUTICALLY EQUIVALENT

Tablet - Oral - 2.5 mg			
100's	$127.19	PERMITIL, Schering Corporation	00085-0442-04
Tablet - Oral - 5 mg			
100's	$152.42	PERMITIL, Schering Corporation	00085-0550-04

PRODUCT LISTING - EQUIVALENTS NOT AVAILABLE

Elixir - Oral - 2.5 mg/5 ml			
60 ml	$25.51	PROLIXIN, Bristol-Myers Squibb	00003-0820-30

Flurandrenolide *(001325)*

For complete prescribing information, refer to the CD-ROM included with the book.

Categories: Dermatosis, corticosteroid-responsive; Pregnancy Category C; FDA Approved 1961 Jul
Drug Classes: Corticosteroids, topical; Dermatologics
Brand Names: **Cordran**; Cordran Tape Patch; Haelan
Foreign Brand Availability: Drenison (Canada; Spain); Drenison 1 4 (Canada)

DESCRIPTION

Flurandrenolide is a potent corticosteroid intended for topical use. It occurs as white to off-white, fluffy, crystalline powder and is odorless. Flurandrenolide is practically insoluble in water and in ether. One (1) gram dissolves in 72 ml of alcohol and in 10 ml of chloroform. The molecular weight of flurandrenolide is 436.52.

The chemical name of flurandrenolide is pregn-4-ene-3,20-dione, 6-fluro-11,21-dihydroxy-16,17-[(1-methylethylidene)bis (oxy)]-, (6α-11β, 16α)-; its empirical formula is $C_{24}H_{33}FO_6$.

CORDRAN SP CREAM

Each gram of Cordran SP cream contains 0.5 mg (1.145 μmol; 0.05%) or 0.25 mg (0.57 μmol; 0.025%) flurandrenolide in an emulsified base composed of cetyl alcohol, citric acid, mineral oil, polyoxyl 40 stearate, propylene glycol, sodium citrate, stearic acid, and purified water.

CORDRAN OINTMENT

Each gram of Cordran ointment contains 0.5 mg (1.145 μmol; 0.05%) or 0.25 mg (0.57 μmol; 0.25%) flurandrenolide in a base composed of white wax, cetyl alcohol, sorbitan sesquioleate, and white petrolatum.

CORDRAN LOTION

Each ml of Cordran lotion contains 0.5 mg (1.145 μmol) (0.05%) flurandrenolide in an oil-in-water emulsion base composed of glycerin, cetyl alcohol, stearic acid, glyceryl monostearate, mineral oil, polyoxyl 40 stearate, menthol, benzyl alcohol, and purified water.

CORDRAN TAPE

Cordran tape is a transparent, inconspicuous plastic surgical tape, impervious to moisture.

Each square centimeter contains 4 μg (0.00916 μmol) flurandrenolide uniformly distributed in the adhesive layer. The tape is made of a thin, matte-finish poly-ethylene film that is slightly elastic and highly flexible.

The adhesive is a synthetic copolymer of acrylate ester and acrylic acid that is free from substances of plant origin. The pressure-sensitive adhesive surface is covered with a protective paper liner to permit handling and trimming before application.

INDICATIONS AND USAGE

Flurandrenolide is indicated for the relief of the inflammatory and pruritic manifestations of corticosteroid-responsive dermatoses, (particularly dry, scale localized lesions —Tape only).

CONTRAINDICATIONS

Topical corticosteroids are contraindicated in patients with a history of hypersensitivity to any of the components of these preparations.

Tape: Use of flurandrenolide tape is not recommended for lesions exuding serum or in intertriginous areas.

DOSAGE AND ADMINISTRATION

CREAM, OINTMENT, AND LOTION

Topical corticosteroids are generally applied to the affected area as a thin film from 1 to 4 times daily, depending on the severity of the condition.

A small quantity of flurandrenolide cream or lotion should be rubbed gently into the affected area 2 or 3 times daily.

Occlusive dressings may be used for the management of psoriasis or recalcitrant conditions.

If an infection develops, the use of occlusive dressings should be discontinued and appropriate antimicrobial therapy instituted.

Use With Occlusive Dressings

The technique of occlusive dressings (for management of psoriasis and other persistent dermatoses) is as follows:

1. Remove as much as possible of the superficial scaling before applying flurandrenolide cream, ointment or lotion. Soaking in a bath will help soften the scales and permit easier removal by brushing, picking, or rubbing.
2. Rub the lotion thoroughly into the affected areas.
3. Cover with an occlusive plastic film, such as polyethylene, Saran Wrap, or Handi-Wrap. (Added moisture may be provided by placing a slightly dampened cloth or gauze over the lesion before the plastic film is applied.)
4. Seal the edges to adjacent normal skin with tape or hold in place by a gauze wrapping.
5. For convenience, the patient may remove the dressing during the day. The dressing should then be reapplied each night.
6. For daytime therapy, the condition may be treated by rubbing flurandrenolide cream, ointment or lotion sparingly into the affected areas.
7. In more resistant cases, leaving the dressing in place for 3-4 days at a time may result in a better response.
8. Thin polyethylene gloves are suitable for treatment of the hands and fingers; plastic garment bags may be utilized for treating lesions on the trunk or buttocks. A tight shower cap is useful in treating lesions on the scalp.

Occlusive Dressings Have the Following Advantages

1. Percutaneous penetration of the corticosteroid is enhanced.
2. Medication is concentrated on the areas of skin where it is most needed.
3. This method of administration frequently is more effective in very resistant dermatoses than is the conventional application of Flurandrenolide.

Precautions to Be Observed in Therapy With Occlusive Dressings

Treatment should be continued for at least a few days after clearing of the lesions. If it is stopped too soon, a relapse may occur. Reinstitution of treatment frequently will cause remission.

Because of the increased hazard of secondary infection from resistant strains of staphylococci among hospitalized patients, it is suggested that the use of occlusive plastic films for corticosteroid therapy in such cases be restricted.

Generally, occlusive dressings should not be used on weeping, or exudative, lesions.

When large areas of the body are covered, thermal homeostasis may be impaired. If elevation of body temperature occurs, use of the occlusive dressing should be discontinued.

Rarely, a patient may develop miliaria, folliculitis, or a sensitivity to either the particular dressing material or a combination of Flurandrenolide and the occlusive dressing. If miliaria or folliculitis occurs, use of the occlusive dressing should be discontinued. Treatment by inunction with Flurandrenolide may be continued. If the sensitivity is caused by the particular material of the dressing, substitution of a different material may be tried.

Warnings

Some plastic films are readily flammable. Patients should be cautioned against the use of any such material.

When plastic films are used on infants and children, the persons caring for the patients must be reminded of the danger of suffocation if the plastic material accidentally covers the face.

TAPE

Occlusive dressings may be used for the management of psoriasis or recalcitrant conditions.

If an infection develops, the use of flurandrenolide tape and other occlusive dressings should be discontinued and appropriate antimicrobial therapy instituted.

Replacement of the tape every 12 hours produces the lowest incidence of adverse reactions, but it may be left in place for 24 hours it is well tolerated and adheres satisfactorily. When necessary, the tape may be used at night only and removed during the day.

If ends of the tape loosen prematurely, they may be trimmed off and replaced with fresh tape.

The directions given below are included on a separate package insert for the patient to follow unless otherwise instructed by the physician.

PRODUCT LISTING - EQUIVALENTS NOT AVAILABLE

Cream - Topical - 0.025%			
30 gm	$22.33	CORDRAN SP, Oclassen Pharmaceuticals Inc	55515-0034-30
60 gm	$31.54	CORDRAN SP, Oclassen Pharmaceuticals Inc	55515-0034-60
Cream - Topical - 0.05%			
15 gm	$20.16	CORDRAN SP, Oclassen Pharmaceuticals Inc	55515-0035-15
30 gm	$28.50	CORDRAN SP, Oclassen Pharmaceuticals Inc	55515-0035-30
60 gm	$52.94	CORDRAN SP, Oclassen Pharmaceuticals Inc	55515-0035-60
Lotion - Topical - 0.05%			
15 ml	$15.73	CORDRAN, Oclassen Pharmaceuticals Inc	55515-0052-15
60 ml	$41.33	CORDRAN, Oclassen Pharmaceuticals Inc	55515-0052-60
Ointment - Topical - 0.025%			
30 gm	$22.33	CORDRAN, Oclassen Pharmaceuticals Inc	55515-0024-30
60 gm	$31.54	CORDRAN, Oclassen Pharmaceuticals Inc	55515-0024-60
Ointment - Topical - 0.05%			
15 gm	$20.16	CORDRAN, Oclassen Pharmaceuticals Inc	55515-0026-15
30 gm	$28.50	CORDRAN, Oclassen Pharmaceuticals Inc	55515-0026-30
60 gm	$47.65	CORDRAN, Oclassen Pharmaceuticals Inc	55515-0026-60
Tape - Topical - 4 mcg/Cm2			
1's	$20.93	CORDRAN TAPE, Oclassen Pharmaceuticals Inc	55515-0014-24
1's	$44.94	CORDRAN TAPE, Oclassen Pharmaceuticals Inc	55515-0014-80
12's	$20.93	CORDRAN TAPE, Oclassen Pharmaceuticals Inc	55515-0014-12

F

Flurazepam Hydrochloride *(001327)*

Categories: Insomnia; DEA Class CIV; FDA Approved 1970 Apr; Pregnancy Category X
Drug Classes: Benzodiazepines; Sedatives/hypnotics
Brand Names: **Dalmane**; Fluleep; Midorm; Niotal; Paxane
Foreign Brand Availability: Apo-Flurazepam (Canada); Benozil (Japan); Dalmadorm (Denmark; Germany; Ghana; Guatemala; Hong-Kong; Italy; Kenya; Korea; Malaysia; Netherlands; Portugal; South-Africa; Switzerland; Taiwan; Tanzania; Uganda; Zambia); Dalmate (Japan); Dormodor (South-Africa; Spain); Felison (Italy); Flunox (Italy); Fluzepam (Slovenia); Fordrim (Argentina); Insumin (Japan); Irdal (Ireland); Manlsum (Taiwan); Midorm AR (Italy); Natam (Argentina); Nergart (Japan); Nindral (India); Remdue (Italy); Somlan (Argentina); Staurodorm (Austria; Bahrain; Belgium; Cyprus; Czech-Republic; Egypt; Germany; Iran; Iraq; Jordan; Kuwait; Lebanon; Libya; Oman; Qatar; Republic-of-Yemen; Saudi-Arabia; Syria; Taiwan; United-Arab-Emirates); Valdorm (Italy)
Cost of Therapy: $16.55 (Insomnia; Dalmane; 30 mg; 1 capsule/day; 10 day supply)
$1.00 (Insomnia; Generic Capsules; 30 mg; 1 capsule/day; 10 day supply)

DESCRIPTION

Dalmane is available as capsules containing 15 or 30 mg flurazepam hydrochloride. Each 15 mg capsule also contains corn starch, lactose, magnesium stearate and talc; gelatin capsule shells may contain methyl and propyl parabens and potassium sorbate, with the following dye systems: FD&C red no. 3, FD&C yellow no. 6 and D&C yellow no. 10. Each 30 mg capsule also contains corn starch, lactose and magnesium stearate; gelatin capsule shells may contain methyl and propyl parabens and potassium sorbate, with the following dye systems: FD&C blue no. 1, FD&C yellow no. 6, D&C yellow no. 10 and either FD&C red no. 3 or FD&C red no. 40.

Flurazepam hydrochloride is chemically 7-chloro-1-[2-(diethylamino)ethyl]-5-(*o*-fluorophenyl)-1,3-dihydro-2*H*-1,4-benzodiazepin-2-one dihydrochloride. It is a pale yellow, crystalline compound, freely soluble in alcohol and very soluble in water. It has a molecular weight of 460.826.

CLINICAL PHARMACOLOGY

Flurazepam HCl is rapidly absorbed from the GI tract. Flurazepam is rapidly metabolized and is excreted primarily in the urine. Following a single oral dose, peak flurazepam plasma concentrations ranging from 0.5-4.0 ng/ml occur at 30-60 minutes post-dosing. The harmonic mean apparent half-life of flurazepam is 2.3 hours. The blood level profile of flurazepam and its major metabolites was determined in man following the oral administration of 30 mg daily for 2 weeks. The N_1-hydroxyethyl-flurazepam was measurable only during the early hours after a 30 mg dose and was not detectable after 24 hours. The major metabolite in blood was N_1-desalkyl-flurazepam, which reached steady-state (plateau) levels after 7-10 days of dosing, at levels approximately 5- to 6-fold greater than the 24 hour levels observed on day 1. The half-life of elimination of N_1-desalkyl-flurazepam ranged from 47-100 hours. The major urinary metabolite is conjugated N_1-hydroxyethyl-flurazepam which accounts for 22-55% of the dose. Less than 1% of the dose is excreted in the urine as N_1-desalkyl-flurazepam.

This pharmacokinetic profile may be responsible for the clinical observation that flurazepam is increasingly effective on the second or third night of consecutive use and that for 1 or 2 nights after the drug is discontinued both sleep latency and total wake time may still be decreased.

GERIATRIC PHARMACOKINETICS

The single dose pharmacokinetics of flurazepam were studied in 12 healthy geriatric subjects (aged 61-85 years). The mean elimination half-life of desalkyl-flurazepam was longer in elderly male subjects (160 hours) compared with younger male subjects (74 hours), while mean elimination half-life was similar in geriatric female subjects (120 hours) and younger female subjects (90 hours). After multiple dosing, mean steady state plasma levels of desalkyl-flurazepam were higher in elderly male subjects (81 ng/ml) compared with younger male subjects (53 ng/ml), while values were similar between elderly female subjects (85 ng/ml) and younger female subjects (86 ng/ml). The mean washout half-life of desalkyl-flurazepam was longer in elderly male and female subjects (126 and 158 hours, respectively) compared with younger male and female subjects (111 and 113 hours, respectively).[1]

INDICATIONS AND USAGE

Flurazepam HCl is a hypnotic agent useful for the treatment of insomnia characterized by difficulty in falling asleep, frequent nocturnal awakenings, and/or early morning awakening. Flurazepam HCl can be used effectively in patients with recurring insomnia or poor sleeping habits, and in acute or chronic medical situations requiring restful sleep. Sleep laboratory studies have objectively determined that flurazepam HCl is effective for at least 28 consecutive nights of drug administration. Since insomnia is often transient and intermittent, short-term use is usually sufficient. Prolonged use of hypnotics is usually not indicated and should only be undertaken concomitantly with appropriate evaluation of the patient.

CONTRAINDICATIONS

Flurazepam HCl is contraindicated in patients with known hypersensitivity to the drug.

USAGE IN PREGNANCY

Benzodiazepines may cause fetal damage when administered during pregnancy. An increased risk of congenital malformations associated with the use of diazepam and chlordiazepoxide during the first trimester of pregnancy has been suggested in several studies.

Flurazepam HCl is contraindicated in pregnant women. Symptoms of neonatal depression have been reported; a neonate whose mother received 30 mg of flurazepam HCl nightly for insomnia during the 10 days prior to delivery appeared hypotonic and inactive during the first 4 days of life. Serum levels of N_1-desalkyl-flurazepam in the infant indicated transplacental circulation and implicate this long-acting metabolite in this case. If there is a likelihood of the patient becoming pregnant while receiving flurazepam, she should be warned of the potential risks to the fetus. Patients should be instructed to discontinue the drug prior to becoming pregnant. The possibility that a woman of childbearing potential may be pregnant at the time of institution of therapy should be considered.

WARNINGS

Patients receiving flurazepam HCl should be cautioned about possible combined effects with alcohol and other CNS depressants. Also, caution patients that an additive effect may occur if alcoholic beverages are consumed during the day following the use of flurazepam HCl for nighttime sedation. The potential for this interaction continues for several days following discontinuance of flurazepam, until serum levels of psychoactive metabolites have declined.

Patients should also be cautioned about engaging in hazardous occupations requiring complete mental alertness such as operating machinery or driving a motor vehicle after ingesting the drug, including potential impairment of the performance of such activities which may occur the day following ingestion of flurazepam HCl.

Usage in Children: Clinical investigations of flurazepam HCl have not been carried out in children. Therefore, the drug is not currently recommended for use in persons under 15 years of age.

Withdrawal symptoms of the barbiturate type have occurred after the discontinuation of benzodiazepines.

PRECAUTIONS

Since the risk of the development of oversedation, dizziness, confusion and/or ataxia increases substantially with larger doses in elderly and debilitated patients, it is recommended that in such patients the dosage be limited to 15 mg. If flurazepam HCl is to be combined with other drugs having known hypnotic properties or CNS-depressant effects, due consideration should be given to potential additive effects.

The usual precautions are indicated for severely depressed patients or those in whom there is any evidence of latent depression; particularly the recognition that suicidal tendencies may be present and protective measures may be necessary.

The usual precautions should be observed in patients with impaired renal or hepatic function and chronic pulmonary insufficiency.

INFORMATION FOR THE PATIENT

To assure the safe and effective use of benzodiazepines, patients should be informed that since benzodiazepines may produce psychological and physical dependence, it is advisable that they consult with their physician before either increasing the dose or abruptly discontinuing this drug.

GERIATRIC USE

Since the risk of the development of oversedation, dizziness, confusion and/or ataxia increases substantially with larger doses in elderly and debilitated patients, it is recommended that in such patients the dosage be limited to 15 mg. Staggering and falling have also been reported, particularly in geriatric patients.

After multiple dosing, elimination half-life of desalkyl-flurazepam was longer in all elderly subjects compared with younger subjects, and mean steady-state serum concentrations were higher only in elderly male subjects relative to younger subjects (see CLINICAL PHARMACOLOGY, Geriatric Pharmacokinetics).

ADVERSE REACTIONS

Dizziness, drowsiness, light-headedness, staggering, ataxia and falling have occurred, particularly in elderly or debilitated persons. Severe sedation, lethargy, disorientation and coma, probably indicative of drug intolerance or overdosage, have been reported.

Also reported were headache, heartburn, upset stomach, nausea, vomiting, diarrhea, constipation, gastrointestinal pain, nervousness, talkativeness, apprehension, irritability, weakness, palpitations, chest pains, body and joint pains and genitourinary complaints. There have also been rare occurrences of leukopenia, granulocytopenia, sweating flushes, difficulty in focusing, blurred vision, burning eyes, faintness, hypotension, shortness of breath, pruritus, skin rash, dry mouth, bitter taste, excessive salivation, anorexia, euphoria, depression, slurred speech, confusion, restlessness, hallucinations, and elevated SGOT, SGPT, total and direct bilirubins, and alkaline phosphatase. Paradoxical reactions, *e.g.*, excitement, stimulation and hyperactivity, have also been reported in rare instances.

DOSAGE AND ADMINISTRATION

Dosage should be individualized for maximal beneficial effects. The usual adult dosage is 30 mg before retiring. In some patients, 15 mg may suffice. In elderly and/or debilitated patients, 15 mg is usually sufficient for a therapeutic response and it is therefore recommended that therapy be initiated with this dosage.

HOW SUPPLIED

Dalmane capsules are supplied as:

15 mg: Orange and ivory.

30 mg: Red and ivory.

PRODUCT LISTING - RATED THERAPEUTICALLY EQUIVALENT

Capsule - Oral - 15 mg

Size	Price	Supplier	NDC
100's	$7.50	FEDERAL UPPER LIMIT, H.C.F.A. F F P	99999-1327-02
100's	$8.93	GENERIC, Interstate Drug Exchange Inc	00814-3244-14
100's	$22.10	GENERIC, Aligen Independent Laboratories Inc	00405-0085-01
100's	$23.50	GENERIC, Ivax Corporation	00182-1817-01
100's	$23.63	GENERIC, Qualitest Products Inc	00603-3691-21
100's	$28.25	GENERIC, West Ward Pharmaceutical Corporation	00143-3367-01
100's	$28.25	GENERIC, Auro Pharmaceutical	55829-0836-10
100's	$28.50	GENERIC, Mylan Pharmaceuticals Inc	00378-4415-01
100's	$29.36	GENERIC, Udl Laboratories Inc	51079-0302-20
100's	$29.75	GENERIC, Major Pharmaceuticals Inc	00904-2800-60
100's	$31.97	GENERIC, Udl Laboratories Inc	51079-0302-21
100's	$34.46	GENERIC, Major Pharmaceuticals Inc	00904-2800-61
100's	$152.13	DALMANE, Icn Pharmaceuticals Inc	00187-4051-10

Capsule - Oral - 30 mg

Size	Price	Supplier	NDC
100's	$9.22	FEDERAL UPPER LIMIT, H.C.F.A. F F P	99999-1327-05
100's	$11.40	GENERIC, Interstate Drug Exchange Inc	00814-3245-14
100's	$24.55	GENERIC, Aligen Independent Laboratories Inc	00405-0086-01
100's	$26.70	GENERIC, Ivax Corporation	00182-1818-01
100's	$26.70	GENERIC, Watson/Rugby Laboratories Inc	00536-3796-01
100's	$28.39	GENERIC, Major Pharmaceuticals Inc	00904-2801-60
100's	$29.92	GENERIC, Vangard Labs	00615-0461-47
100's	$30.95	GENERIC, Auro Pharmaceutical	55829-0837-10
100's	$34.25	GENERIC, West Ward Pharmaceutical Corporation	00143-3370-01
100's	$34.40	GENERIC, Mylan Pharmaceuticals Inc	00378-4430-01
100's	$34.87	GENERIC, Major Pharmaceuticals Inc	00904-2801-61
100's	$35.43	GENERIC, Udl Laboratories Inc	51079-0303-20
100's	$38.26	GENERIC, Udl Laboratories Inc	51079-0303-21
100's	$165.48	DALMANE, Icn Pharmaceuticals Inc	00187-4052-10

PRODUCT LISTING - EQUIVALENTS NOT AVAILABLE

Capsule - Oral - 15 mg

Size	Price	Supplier	NDC
5's	$3.75	GENERIC, Southwood Pharmaceuticals Inc	58016-0811-05
15's	$11.25	GENERIC, Southwood Pharmaceuticals Inc	58016-0811-15
30's	$22.50	GENERIC, Southwood Pharmaceuticals Inc	58016-0811-30
40's	$30.00	GENERIC, Southwood Pharmaceuticals Inc	58016-0811-40

Capsule - Oral - 30 mg

Size	Price	Supplier	NDC
2's	$3.48	GENERIC, Prescript Pharmaceuticals	00247-0345-02
3's	$3.55	GENERIC, Prescript Pharmaceuticals	00247-0345-03
6's	$4.99	GENERIC, Southwood Pharmaceuticals Inc	58016-0812-06
7's	$3.81	GENERIC, Prescript Pharmaceuticals	00247-0345-07
9's	$7.49	GENERIC, Southwood Pharmaceuticals Inc	58016-0812-09
10's	$4.01	GENERIC, Prescript Pharmaceuticals	00247-0345-10
10's	$8.32	GENERIC, Southwood Pharmaceuticals Inc	58016-0812-10
12's	$9.98	GENERIC, Southwood Pharmaceuticals Inc	58016-0812-12
14's	$11.64	GENERIC, Southwood Pharmaceuticals Inc	58016-0812-14
15's	$4.34	GENERIC, Prescript Pharmaceuticals	00247-0345-15
15's	$12.48	GENERIC, Southwood Pharmaceuticals Inc	58016-0812-15
20's	$4.68	GENERIC, Prescript Pharmaceuticals	00247-0345-20
20's	$16.63	GENERIC, Southwood Pharmaceuticals Inc	58016-0812-20
21's	$17.47	GENERIC, Southwood Pharmaceuticals Inc	58016-0812-21
24's	$19.96	GENERIC, Southwood Pharmaceuticals Inc	58016-0812-24
30's	$5.34	GENERIC, Prescript Pharmaceuticals	00247-0345-30
30's	$24.95	GENERIC, Southwood Pharmaceuticals Inc	58016-0812-30
60's	$49.90	GENERIC, Southwood Pharmaceuticals Inc	58016-0812-60
100's	$9.98	GENERIC, Prescript Pharmaceuticals	00247-0345-00
100's	$83.17	GENERIC, Southwood Pharmaceuticals Inc	58016-0812-00

Flurbiprofen (001328)

For related information, see the comparative table section in Appendix A.

Categories: Arthritis, osteoarthritis; Arthritis, rheumatoid; Miosis, inhibition; Pregnancy Category B; FDA Approved 1988 Oct
Drug Classes: Analgesics, non-narcotic; Nonsteroidal anti-inflammatory drugs; Ophthalmics
Brand Names: Ansaid; Ocufen
Foreign Brand Availability: Apo-Flurbiprofen (Canada); Arflur (India); Bifen Cataplasma (Korea); Cebutid (France); Florphen (Taiwan); Flupen (Taiwan); Flurofen (Denmark; Greece); Flurozin (Bahamas; Barbados; Belize; Bermuda; Curacao; Guyana; Jamaica; Netherland-Antilles; Surinam; Thailand; Trinidad); Froben (Austria; Bahrain; Belgium; Canada; Cyprus; Egypt; England; Germany; India; Iran; Iraq; Ireland; Italy; Japan; Jordan; Kuwait; Lebanon; Libya; Malaysia; Netherlands; New-Zealand; Oman; Portugal; Qatar; Republic-of-Yemen; Saudi-Arabia; South-Africa; Spain; Switzerland; Syria; United-Arab-Emirates); Froben SR (Canada; New-Zealand); Lapole (Japan); Mirafen (Colombia); Ocuflur (Austria; Belgium; Bulgaria; Czech-Republic; Greece; Hungary; India; Portugal; Russia; Spain; Switzerland); Strepfen (Australia)
Cost of Therapy: $116.15 (Osteoarthritis; Ansaid; 100 mg; 2 tablets/day; 30 day supply)
$63.83 (Osteoarthritis; Generic Tablets; 100 mg; 2 tablets/day; 30 day supply)

OPHTHALMIC

DESCRIPTION

Flurbiprofen sodium ophthalmic solution 0.03% is a sterile topical nonsteroidal anti-inflammatory product for ophthalmic use.
Chemical name: Sodium (±)-2-(2-fluoro-4-biphenyl)-propionate dihydrate.
Ocufen contains:
Active: Flurbiprofen sodium 0.03%.
Preservative: Thimerosal 0.005%.
Inactives: Polyvinyl alcohol 1.4%; edetate disodium; potassium chloride; sodium chloride; sodium citrate; citric acid; hydrochloric acid and/or sodium hydroxide to adjust the pH; and purified water.
Note: Store at room temperature.

CLINICAL PHARMACOLOGY

Flurbiprofen sodium is one of a series of phenylalkanoic acids that have shown analgesic, antipyretic, and anti-inflammatory activity in animal inflammatory diseases. Its mechanism of action is believed to be through inhibition of the cyclo-oxygenase enzyme that is essential in the biosynthesis of prostaglandins.

Prostaglandins have been shown in many animal models to be mediators of certain kinds of intraocular inflammation. In studies performed on animal eyes, prostaglandins have been shown to produce disruption of the blood-aqueous humor barrier, vasodilation, increased vascular permeability, leukocytosis, and increased intraocular pressure.

Prostaglandins also appear to play a role in the miotic response produced during ocular surgery by constricting the iris sphincter independently of cholinergic mechanisms. In clinical studies, flurbiprofen sodium has been shown to inhibit the miosis induced during the course of cataract surgery.

Results from clinical studies indicate that flurbiprofen sodium has no significant effect upon intraocular pressure.

INDICATIONS AND USAGE

Flurbiprofen sodium ophthalmic solution is indicated for the inhibition of intraoperative miosis.

CONTRAINDICATIONS

Flurbiprofen sodium is contraindicated in individuals who are hypersensitive to any components of the medication.

WARNINGS

With nonsteroidal anti-inflammatory drugs, there exists the potential for increased bleeding due to interference with thrombocyte aggregation. There have been reports that flurbiprofen sodium solution may cause increased bleeding of ocular tissues in conjunction with ocular surgery.

There exists the potential for cross-sensitivity to acetylsalicylic acid and other nonsteroidal anti-inflammatory drugs. Therefore, caution should be used when treating individuals who have previously exhibited sensitivities to these drugs.

PRECAUTIONS

GENERAL

Wound healing may be delayed with the use of flurbiprofen sodium. It is recommended that flurbiprofen sodium ophthalmic solution 0.03% be used with caution in surgical patients with known bleeding tendencies or who are receiving other medications which may prolong bleeding time.

CARCINOGENESIS, MUTAGENESIS, AND IMPAIRMENT OF FERTILITY

Long-term studies in mice and/or rats have shown no evidence of carcinogenicity or impairment of fertility with flurbiprofen.

Long-term mutagenicity studies in animals have not been performed.

PREGNANCY CATEGORY C

Flurbiprofen has been shown to be embryocidal, delay parturition, prolong gestation, reduce weight, and/or slightly retard growth of fetuses when given to rats in daily oral doses of 0.4 mg/kg (approximately 67 times the human daily topical dose) and above. There are no adequate and well-controlled studies in pregnant women. Flurbiprofen sodium solution should be used during pregnancy only if the potential benefit justifies the potential risk to the fetus.

NURSING MOTHERS

It is not known whether this drug is excreted in human milk. Because many drugs are excreted in human milk and because of the potential for serious adverse reactions in nursing infants from flurbiprofen sodium, a decision should be made whether to discontinue nursing or to discontinue the drug, taking into account the importance of the drug to the mother.

PEDIATRIC USE

Safety and effectiveness in pediatric patients have not been established.

GERIATRIC USE

No overall differences in safety or effectiveness have been observed between elderly and younger patients.

DRUG INTERACTIONS

Interaction of flurbiprofen sodium ophthalmic solution with other topical ophthalmic medications has not been fully investigated.

Although clinical studies with acetylcholine chloride and animal studies with acetylcholine chloride or carbachol revealed no interference, and there is no known pharmacological basis for an interaction, there have been reports that acetylcholine chloride and carbachol have been ineffective when used in patients treated with flurbiprofen sodium.

ADVERSE REACTIONS

Transient burning and stinging upon instillation and other minor symptoms of ocular irritation have been reported with the use of flurbiprofen sodium ophthalmic solution. Other adverse reactions reported with the use of flurbiprofen sodium include: fibrosis, miosis, and mydriasis.

Increased bleeding tendency of ocular tissues in conjunction with ocular surgery has also been reported.

DOSAGE AND ADMINISTRATION

A total of 4 drops of flurbiprofen sodium solution should be administered by instilling 1 drop approximately every ½ hour beginning 2 hours before surgery.

ORAL

DESCRIPTION

Ansaid tablets contain flurbiprofen, which is a member of the phenylalkanoic acid derivative group of nonsteroidal anti-inflammatory drugs. Ansaid tablets are white, oval, film-coated tablets for oral administration. Flurbiprofen is a racemic mixture of (+)S- and (-)R-enantiomers. Flurbiprofen is a white or slightly yellow crystalline powder. It is slightly soluble in water at pH 7.0 and readily soluble in most polar solvents. The chemical name is [1,1′-biphenyl]-4-acetic acid, 2-fluoro-alpha-methyl-, (±)-. The molecular weight is 244.26. Its molecular formula is $C_{15}H_{13}FO_2$.

The inactive ingredients in Ansaid (both strengths) include carnauba wax, colloidal silicon dioxide, croscarmellose sodium, hydroxypropyl methylcellulose, lactose, magnesium stearate, microcrystalline cellulose, propylene glycol, and titanium dioxide. In addition, the 100 mg tablet contains FD&C blue no. 2.

CLINICAL PHARMACOLOGY

PHARMACODYNAMICS

Flurbiprofen tablets contain flurbiprofen, a nonsteroidal anti-inflammatory drug that exhibits anti-inflammatory, analgesic, and antipyretic activities in animal models. The mechanism of action of flurbiprofen tablets, like that of other nonsteroidal anti-inflammatory drugs, is not completely understood but may be related to prostaglandin synthetase inhibition.

PHARMACOKINETICS

Absorption

The mean oral bioavailability of flurbiprofen from flurbiprofen tablets 100 mg is 96% relative to an oral solution. Flurbiprofen is rapidly and non-stereoselectively absorbed from flurbiprofen tablets, with peak plasma concentrations occurring at about 2 hours (see TABLE 1). Administration of flurbiprofen tablets with either food or antacids may alter the rate but not the extent of flurbiprofen absorption. Ranitidine has been shown to have no effect on either the rate or extent of flurbiprofen absorption from flurbiprofen tablets.

Distribution

The apparent volume of distribution (Vz/F) of both R- and S-flurbiprofen is approximately 0.12 L/kg. Both flurbiprofen enantiomers are more than 99% bound to plasma proteins, primarily albumin. Plasma protein binding is relatively constant for the typical average steady-state concentrations (≤10 μg/ml) achieved with recommended doses. Flurbiprofen is poorly excreted into human milk. The nursing infant dose is predicted to be approximately 0.1 mg/day in the established milk of a woman taking flurbiprofen tablets 200 mg/day (see PRECAUTIONS, Nursing Mothers).

Metabolism

Several flurbiprofen metabolites have been identified in human plasma and urine. These metabolites include 4′-hydroxy-flurbiprofen, 3′,4′-dihydroxy-flurbiprofen, 3′-hydroxy-4′-methoxy-flurbiprofen, their conjugates, and conjugated flurbiprofen. Unlike other arylpropionic acid derivatives (*e.g.,* ibuprofen), metabolism of R-flurbiprofen to S-flurbiprofen is minimal. *In vitro* studies have demonstrated that cytochrome P450 2C9 plays an important role in the metabolism of flurbiprofen to its major metabolite, 4′-hydroxy-flurbiprofen. The 4′-hydroxy-flurbiprofen metabolite showed little anti-inflammatory activity in animal models of inflammation. Flurbiprofen does not induce enzymes that alter its metabolism.

The total plasma clearance of unbound flurbiprofen is not stereoselective, and clearance of flurbiprofen is independent of dose when used within the therapeutic range.

Excretion

Following dosing with flurbiprofen tablets, less than 3% of flurbiprofen is excreted unchanged in the urine, with about 70% of the dose eliminated in the urine as parent drug and metabolites. Because renal elimination is a significant pathway of elimination of flurbiprofen metabolites, dosing adjustment in patients with moderate or severe renal dysfunction may be necessary to avoid accumulation of flurbiprofen metabolites. The mean terminal disposition half-lives (T½) of R- and S-flurbiprofen are similar, about 4.7 and 5.7 hours, respectively. There is little accumulation of flurbiprofen following multiple doses of flurbiprofen tablets.

TABLE 1 *Mean (SD) R,S-Flurbiprofen Pharmacokinetic Parameters Normalized to a 100 mg Dose of Flurbiprofen Tablets*

Pharmacokinetic Parameter	Normal Healthy Adults* (18-40 years) n=15	Geriatric Arthritis Patients† (65-83 years) n=13	End Stage Renal Disease Patients* (23-42 years) n=8	Alcoholic Cirrhosis Patients‡ (31-61 years) n=8
Peak concentration (Tg/ml)	14 (4)	16 (5)	9§	9§
Time of peak concentration (h)	1.9 (1.5)	2.2 (3)	2.3§	1.2§
Urinary recovery of unchanged flurbiprofen (% of dose)	2.9 (1.3)	0.6 (0.6)	0.02 (0.02)	NA¤
Area under the curve (AUC)¶ (Tg h/ml)	83 (20)	77 (24)	44§	50§
Apparent volume of distribution (Vz/F, L)	14 (3)	12 (5)	10§	14§
Terminal disposition half-life (T½, h)	7.5 (0.8)	5.8 (1.9)	3.3**	5.4**

* 100 mg single-dose.
† Steady-state evaluation of 100 mg every 12 hours.
‡ 200 mg single-dose.
§ Calculated from mean parameter values of both flurbiprofen enantiomers.
¤ Not available.
¶ AUC from 0 to infinity for single doses and from 0 to the end of the dosing interval for multiple-doses.
** Value for S-flurbiprofen.

SPECIAL POPULATIONS

Pediatric

The pharmacokinetics of flurbiprofen have not been investigated in pediatric patients.

Race

No pharmacokinetic differences due to race have been identified.

Geriatric

Flurbiprofen pharmacokinetics were similar in geriatric arthritis patients, younger arthritis patients, and young healthy volunteers receiving flurbiprofen tablets 100 mg as either single or multiple doses.

Hepatic Insufficiency

Hepatic metabolism may account for >90% of flurbiprofen elimination, so patients with hepatic disease may require reduced doses of flurbiprofen tablets compared to patients with normal hepatic function. The pharmacokinetics of R- and S-flurbiprofen were similar, however, in alcoholic cirrhosis patients (n=8) and young healthy volunteers (n=8) following administration of a single 200 mg dose of flurbiprofen tablets.

Flurbiprofen plasma protein binding may be decreased in patients with liver disease and serum albumin concentrations below 3.1 g/dl (see PRECAUTIONS, General, Hepatic Effects).

Renal Insufficiency

Renal clearance is an important route of elimination for flurbiprofen metabolites, but a minor route of elimination for unchanged flurbiprofen (≤3% of total clearance). The unbound clearances of R- and S-flurbiprofen did not differ significantly between normal healthy volunteers (n=6, 50 mg single dose) and patients with renal impairment (n=8, insulin clearances ranging from 11-43 ml/min, 50 mg multiple doses). Flurbiprofen plasma protein binding may be decreased in patients with renal impairment and serum albumin concentrations below 3.9 g/dl. Elimination of flurbiprofen metabolites may be reduced in patients with renal impairment (see PRECAUTIONS, General, Renal Effects).

Flurbiprofen is not significantly removed from the blood into dialysate in patients undergoing continuous ambulatory peritoneal dialysis.

DRUG-DRUG INTERACTIONS

See also DRUG INTERACTIONS.

Antacids

Administration of flurbiprofen tablets to volunteers under fasting conditions or with antacid suspension yielded similar serum flurbiprofen-time profiles in young adult subjects (n=12). In geriatric subjects (n=7), there was a reduction in the rate but not the extent of flurbiprofen absorption.

Aspirin

Concurrent administration of flurbiprofen tablets and aspirin resulted in 50% lower serum flurbiprofen concentrations. This effect of aspirin (which is also seen with other nonsteroidal anti-inflammatory drugs) has been demonstrated in patients with rheumatoid arthritis (n=15) and in healthy volunteers (n=16) (see DRUG INTERACTIONS).

Beta-Adrenergic Blocking Agents

The effect of flurbiprofen on blood pressure response to propranolol and atenolol was evaluated in men with mild uncomplicated hypertension (n=10). Flurbiprofen pretreatment attenuated the hypotensive effect of a single dose of propranolol but not atenolol. Flurbiprofen did not appear to affect the beta-blocker-mediated reduction in heart rate. Flurbiprofen did not affect the pharmacokinetic profile of either drug (see DRUG INTERACTIONS).

Cimetidine, Ranitidine

In normal volunteers (n=9), pretreatment with cimetidine or ranitidine did not affect flurbiprofen pharmacokinetics, except for a small (13%) but statistically significant increase in the area under the serum concentration curve of flurbiprofen in subjects who received cimetidine.

Digoxin

In studies of healthy males (n=14), concomitant administration of flurbiprofen and digoxin did not change the steady state serum levels of either drug.

Diuretics

Studies in healthy volunteers have shown that, like other nonsteroidal anti-inflammatory drugs, flurbiprofen can interfere with the effects of furosemide. Although results have varied from study to study, effects have been shown on furosemide-stimulated diuresis, natriuresis, and kaliuresis. Other nonsteroidal anti-inflammatory drugs that inhibit prostaglandin synthesis have been shown to interfere with thiazide and potassium-sparing diuretics (see DRUG INTERACTIONS).

Lithium

In a study of 11 women with bipolar disorder receiving lithium carbonate at a dosage of 600-1200 mg/day, administration of 100 mg flurbiprofen tablets every 12 hours increased plasma lithium concentrations by 19%. Four (4) of 11 patients experienced a clinically important increase (>25% or >0.2 mmol/L). Nonsteroidal anti-inflammatory drugs have also been reported to decrease the renal clearance of lithium by about 20% (see DRUG INTERACTIONS).

Methotrexate

In a study of 6 adult arthritis patients, coadministration of methotrexate (10-25 mg/dose) and flurbiprofen tablets (300 mg/day) resulted in no observable interaction between these 2 drugs.

Oral Hypoglycemic Agents

In a clinical study, flurbiprofen was administered to adult diabetics who were already receiving glyburide (n=4), metformin (n=2), chlorpropamide with phenformin (n=3), or glyburide with phenformin (n=6). Although there was a slight reduction in blood sugar concentrations during concomitant administration of flurbiprofen and hypoglycemic agents, there were no signs or symptoms of hypoglycemia.

INDICATIONS AND USAGE

Flurbiprofen tablets are indicated for relief of the signs and symptoms of rheumatoid arthritis and osteoarthritis.

NON-FDA APPROVED INDICATIONS

While not FDA approved indications, flurbiprofen has also been used in the management of pain and other nonrheumatic inflammatory conditions.

CONTRAINDICATIONS

Flurbiprofen tablets are contraindicated in patients with known hypersensitivity to flurbiprofen. Flurbiprofen tablets should not be given to patients who have experienced asthma, urticaria, or allergic-type reactions after taking aspirin or other nonsteroidal anti-inflammatory drugs. Severe, rarely fatal, anaphylactic-like reactions to nonsteroidal anti-inflammatory drugs have been reported in such patients (see WARNINGS, Anaphylactoid Reactions, and PRECAUTIONS, General, Preexisting Asthma). Flurbiprofen tablets should not be given to patients with the aspirin triad. This symptom complex typically occurs in asthmatic patients who experience rhinitis, with or without nasal polyps, or severe, potentially fatal bronchospasm after taking aspirin or other nonsteroidal anti-inflammatory drugs.

WARNINGS

GASTROINTESTINAL (GI) EFFECTS — RISK OF GI ULCERATION, BLEEDING, AND PERFORATION

Serious GI toxicity, such as inflammation, bleeding, ulceration, or perforation of the stomach, small intestine, or large intestine, can occur at any time, with or without warning symptoms, in patients treated with nonsteroidal anti-inflammatory drugs. Minor upper GI problems, such as dyspepsia, are common and may also occur at any time during therapy. Therefore, physicians and patients should remain alert for ulceration and bleeding, even in the absence of previous GI tract symptoms. Patients should be informed about the signs and/or symptoms of serious GI toxicity and the steps to take if they occur. The utility of periodic laboratory monitoring has not been demonstrated, nor has it been adequately assessed. Only 1 in 5 patients who develop a serious upper GI adverse event during therapy with a nonsteroidal anti-inflammatory drug is symptomatic. Upper GI ulcers, gross bleeding, or perforation caused by nonsteroidal anti-inflammatory drugs appear to occur in approximately 1% of patients treated for 3-6 months, and in about 2-4% of patients treated for 1 year. These trends continue over time, thus increasing the likelihood of a patient developing a serious GI event at some time during the course of therapy. However, even short-term therapy is not without risk.

Nonsteroidal anti-inflammatory drugs should be prescribed with extreme caution to patients with a prior history of ulcer disease or GI bleeding. Most spontaneous reports of fatal GI events are in elderly or debilitated patients; therefore, special care should be taken in treating this population. **To minimize the potential risk for an adverse GI event, the lowest effective dose should be used for the shortest possible duration.** For high risk patients, alternate therapies that do not involve nonsteroidal anti-inflammatory drugs should be considered.

Studies have shown that patients with a prior history of peptic ulcer disease and/or GI bleeding who use nonsteroidal anti-inflammatory drugs have a greater than 10-fold risk for developing a GI bleed as compared with patients with neither of these risk factors. In addition to a past history of ulcer disease, pharmacoepidemiological studies have identified several other co-therapies or comorbid conditions that may increase the risk for GI bleeding, such as the following: treatment with oral corticosteroids, treatment with anticoagulants, longer duration of therapy with nonsteroidal anti-inflammatory drugs, smoking, alcoholism, older age, and poor general health status.

ANAPHYLACTOID REACTIONS

As with other nonsteroidal anti-inflammatory drugs, anaphylactoid reactions may occur in patients without known prior exposure to flurbiprofen tablets (see CONTRAINDICATIONS; WARNINGS; and PRECAUTIONS, General, Preexisting Asthma). If an anaphylactoid reaction occurs, the patient should immediately seek emergency help.

ADVANCED RENAL DISEASE

Treatment with flurbiprofen tablets is not recommended in patients with advanced kidney disease. However, if therapy with a nonsteroidal anti-inflammatory drug must be initiated, close monitoring of the patient's kidney function is advisable (see PRECAUTIONS, General, Renal Effects).

PREGNANCY

As with other nonsteroidal anti-inflammatory drugs, treatment with flurbiprofen tablets should be avoided in late pregnancy because it may cause premature closure of the ductus arteriosus in the neonate.

PRECAUTIONS

GENERAL

Hepatic Effects

Borderline elevations of 1 or more liver tests may occur in up to 15% of patients taking nonsteroidal anti-inflammatory drugs, including flurbiprofen tablets. These laboratory abnormalities may progress, may remain unchanged, or may be transient with continuing therapy. Notable elevations of ALT or AST (approximately 3 or more times the upper limit of normal) have been reported in approximately 1% of patients in clinical trials with nonsteroidal anti-inflammatory drugs. In addition, rare cases of severe hepatic reactions have been reported, including jaundice, fulminant hepatitis, liver necrosis, and hepatic failure, some of them with fatal outcomes.

A patient with symptoms and/or signs suggesting liver dysfunction, or with abnormal liver test values, should be evaluated for evidence of the development of a more severe hepatic reaction while on therapy with flurbiprofen tablets. If clinical signs and symptoms consistent with liver disease develop, or if systemic manifestations occur (*e.g.*, eosinophilia, rash, etc.), flurbiprofen tablets should be discontinued.

Renal Effects

Caution should be used when initiating treatment with flurbiprofen tablets in patients with considerable dehydration. It is advisable to rehydrate patients first and then start therapy with flurbiprofen tablets. Caution is also recommended in patients with preexisting kidney disease (see WARNINGS, Advanced Renal Disease).

As with other nonsteroidal anti-inflammatory drugs, long-term administration of flurbiprofen tablets has resulted in renal papillary necrosis and other renal medullary changes. A second form of renal toxicity has been seen in patients in whom renal prostaglandins have a compensatory role in the maintenance of renal perfusion. In these patients, administration of a nonsteroidal anti-inflammatory drug may cause a dose-dependent reduction in prostaglandin formation and, secondarily, in renal blood flow, which may precipitate overt renal decompensation. Patients at greatest risk of this reaction are those with impaired renal function, heart failure, or liver dysfunction, as well as those taking diuretics or ACE inhibitors, and the elderly. Discontinuation of nonsteroidal anti-inflammatory drug therapy is usually followed by recovery to the pretreatment state.

In clinical studies, the elimination half-life of flurbiprofen was unchanged in patients with renal impairment. Flurbiprofen metabolites are eliminated primarily by the kidneys. Elimination of 4′-hydroxy-flurbiprofen was reduced in patients with moderate to severe renal impairment. Therefore, patients with significantly impaired renal function may require a reduction of dosage to avoid accumulation of flurbiprofen metabolites. Such patients should be closely monitored (see CLINICAL PHARMACOLOGY).

Hematological Effects

Anemia is sometimes seen in patients receiving nonsteroidal anti-inflammatory drugs, including flurbiprofen tablets. This may be due to fluid retention, GI blood loss, or an incompletely described effect upon erythropoiesis. Patients on long-term treatment with nonsteroidal anti-inflammatory drugs, including flurbiprofen tablets, should have their hemoglobin or hematocrit checked periodically even if they do not exhibit any signs or symptoms of anemia.

All drugs that inhibit the biosynthesis of prostaglandins may interfere to some extent with platelet function and vascular responses to bleeding.

Nonsteroidal anti-inflammatory drugs inhibit platelet aggregation and have been shown to prolong bleeding time in some patients. Unlike aspirin, their effect on platelet function is quantitatively less, of shorter duration, and reversible. Flurbiprofen tablets does not generally affect platelet counts, prothrombin time (PT), or partial thromboplastin time (PTT). Patients receiving flurbiprofen tablets who may be adversely affected by alterations in platelet function, such as those with coagulation disorders or patients receiving anticoagulants, should be carefully monitored.

Fluid Retention and Edema

Fluid retention and edema have been observed in some patients taking nonsteroidal anti-inflammatory drugs. Therefore, as with other nonsteroidal anti-inflammatory drugs, flurbiprofen tablets should be used with caution in patients with fluid retention, hypertension, or heart failure.

Preexisting Asthma

About 10% of patients with asthma have aspirin-sensitive asthma. The use of aspirin in patients with aspirin-sensitive asthma has been associated with severe bronchospasm that can be fatal. Since cross reactivity, including bronchospasm, between aspirin and other nonsteroidal anti-inflammatory drugs has been reported in such aspirin-sensitive patients, flurbiprofen tablets should not be administered to patients with this form of aspirin sensitivity and should be used with caution in patients with preexisting asthma.

Vision Changes

Blurred and/or diminished vision has been reported with the use of flurbiprofen tablets and other nonsteroidal anti-inflammatory drugs. Patients experiencing eye complaints should have ophthalmologic examinations.

INFORMATION FOR THE PATIENT

Flurbiprofen tablets, like other drugs of its class, can cause discomfort and, rarely, more serious side effects, such as GI bleeding, which may result in hospitalization and even fatal outcomes. Although serious GI tract ulceration and bleeding can occur without warning symptoms, patients should be alert for the signs and symptoms of ulceration and bleeding, and should ask for medical advice when observing any indicative sign or symptoms. Patients should be apprised of the importance of this follow-up [see WARNINGS, Gastrointestinal (GI) Effects — Risk of GI Ulceration, Bleeding, and Perforation].

Patients should report to their physicians any signs or symptoms of GI ulceration or bleeding, skin rash, weight gain, or edema.

Patients should be informed of the warning signs and symptoms of hepatotoxicity (*e.g.*, nausea, fatigue, lethargy, pruritus, jaundice, right upper quadrant tenderness, and "flu-like" symptoms). If these occur, patients should be instructed to stop therapy with flurbiprofen tablets and seek immediate medical therapy.

Patients should also be instructed to seek immediate emergency help in the case of an anaphylactoid reaction (see WARNINGS, Anaphylactoid Reactions).

As with other nonsteroidal anti-inflammatory drugs, flurbiprofen tablets should be avoided in late pregnancy because it may cause premature closure of the ductus arteriosus.

LABORATORY TESTS

Patients on long-term treatment with nonsteroidal anti-inflammatory drugs should have their complete blood count and chemistry profile checked periodically. If clinical signs and symptoms consistent with liver or renal disease develop, systemic manifestations occur (*e.g.*, eosinophilia, rash, etc.), or abnormal liver tests persist or worsen, flurbiprofen tablets should be discontinued.

PREGNANCY, TERATOGENIC EFFECTS, PREGNANCY CATEGORY C

No developmental abnormalities were seen in reproductive studies conducted in mice and rabbits. However, animal reproduction studies are not always predictive of human response. There are no adequate and well-controlled studies in pregnant women.

NONTERATOGENIC EFFECTS

Because of the known effects of nonsteroidal anti-inflammatory drugs on the fetal cardiovascular system (closure of ductus arteriosus), use during late pregnancy should be avoided.

LABOR AND DELIVERY

In rat studies with nonsteroidal anti-inflammatory drugs, as with other drugs known to inhibit prostaglandin synthesis, an increased incidence of dystocia, delayed parturition, and decreased pup survival occurred. The effects of flurbiprofen tablets on labor and delivery in pregnant women are unknown.

NURSING MOTHERS

Concentrations of flurbiprofen in breast milk and plasma of nursing mothers suggest that a nursing infant could receive approximately 0.10 mg flurbiprofen/day in the established milk of a woman taking flurbiprofen tablets 200 mg/day. Because of possible adverse effects of prostaglandin-inhibiting drugs on neonates, a decision should be made whether to discontinue nursing or to discontinue the drug, taking into account the importance of the drug to the mother.

PEDIATRIC USE

Safety and effectiveness in pediatric patients have not been established.

GERIATRIC USE

Clinical experience with flurbiprofen tablets suggests that elderly patients may have a higher incidence of gastrointestinal complaints than younger patients, including ulceration, bleeding, flatulence, bloating, and abdominal pain. **To minimize the potential risk for gastrointestinal events, the lowest effective dose should be used for the shortest possible duration** [see WARNINGS, Gastrointestinal (GI) Effects — Risk of GI Ulceration, Bleeding, and Perforation]. Likewise, elderly patients are at greater risk of developing renal decompensation (see PRECAUTIONS, General, Renal Effects).

The pharmacokinetics of flurbiprofen do not seem to differ in elderly patients from those in younger individuals (see CLINICAL PHARMACOLOGY, Special Populations). The rate of absorption of flurbiprofen tablets was reduced in elderly patients who also received antacids, although the extent of absorption was not affected (see CLINICAL PHARMACOLOGY, Drug-Drug Interactions).

DRUG INTERACTIONS

ACE-Inhibitors: Reports suggest that nonsteroidal anti-inflammatory drugs may diminish the antihypertensive effect of ACE-inhibitors. This interaction should be given consideration in patients taking nonsteroidal anti-inflammatory drugs concomitantly with ACE-inhibitors.

Anticoagulants: Patients who take warfarin concomitantly with nonsteroidal anti-inflammatory drugs have a risk of serious clinical bleeding greater than that in users of either drug alone. The physician should be cautious when administering flurbiprofen tablets to patients taking warfarin or other anticoagulants.

Aspirin: Concurrent administration of aspirin lowers serum flurbiprofen concentrations (see CLINICAL PHARMACOLOGY, Drug-Drug Interactions). The clinical significance of this interaction is not known; however, as with other nonsteroidal anti-inflammatory drugs, concomitant administration of flurbiprofen tablets and aspirin is not recommended.

Beta-Adrenergic Blocking Agents: Flurbiprofen attenuated the hypotensive effect of propranolol but not atenolol (see CLINICAL PHARMACOLOGY, Drug-Drug Interactions). The mechanism underlying this interference is unknown. Patients taking both flurbiprofen and a beta-blocker should be monitored to ensure that a satisfactory hypotensive effect is achieved.

Diuretics: Nonsteroidal anti-inflammatory drugs can reduce the natriuretic effect of furosemide and thiazides in some patients (see CLINICAL PHARMACOLOGY, Drug-Drug Interactions). This effect has been attributed to inhibition of renal prostaglandin synthesis. Patients receiving diuretics concomitantly with flurbiprofen tablets should be observed closely for signs of renal failure (see PRECAUTIONS, General, Renal Effects) and to assure that the desired diuretic effect is obtained.

Lithium: Nonsteroidal anti-inflammatory drugs have produced an elevation of plasma lithium levels and a reduction in renal lithium clearance (see CLINICAL PHARMACOLOGY, Drug-Drug Interactions). These effects have been attributed to inhibition of renal prostaglandin synthesis by the nonsteroidal anti-inflammatory drug. Thus, when nonsteroidal anti-inflammatory drugs and lithium are administered concurrently, subjects should be observed carefully for signs of lithium toxicity.

Methotrexate: Nonsteroidal anti-inflammatory drugs have been reported to competitively inhibit methotrexate accumulation in rabbit kidney slices. This may indicate that they could enhance the toxicity of methotrexate. Caution should be used when nonsteroidal anti-inflammatory drugs are administered concomitantly with methotrexate.

ADVERSE REACTIONS

REPORTED ADVERSE EVENTS IN PATIENTS RECEIVING FLURBIPROFEN TABLETS OR OTHER NONSTEROIDAL ANTI-INFLAMMATORY DRUGS

Reported in Patients Treated With Flurbiprofen Tablets

Incidence of 1% or greater from clinical trials:

Body as a Whole: Edema.

Digestive System: Abdominal pain, constipation, diarrhea, dyspepsia/heartburn, elevated liver enzymes, flatulence, GI bleeding, nausea, vomiting.

Metabolic and Nutritional System: Body weight changes.

Nervous System: Headache; nervousness and other manifestations of central nervous system (CNS) stimulation (*e.g.,* anxiety, insomnia, increased reflexes, tremor).

Respiratory System: Rhinitis.

Skin and Appendages: Rash.

Special Senses: Changes in vision, dizziness/vertigo, tinnitus.

Urogenital System: Signs and symptoms suggesting urinary tract infection.

Incidence less than 1% (causal relationship probable) from clinical trials, post-marketing surveillance, or literature:

Body as a Whole: Anaphylactic reaction, chills, fever.

Cardiovascular System: Congestive heart failure, hypertension, vascular diseases, vasodilation.

Digestive System: Bloody diarrhea, esophageal disease, gastric/peptic ulcer disease, gastritis, jaundice (cholestatic and noncholestatic), hematemesis, hepatitis, stomatitis/glossitis.

Hemic and Lymphatic System: Aplastic anemia (including agranulocytosis or pancytopenia), decrease in hemoglobin and hematocrit, ecchymosis/purpura, eosinophilia, hemolytic anemia, iron deficiency anemia, leukopenia, thrombocytopenia.

Metabolic and Nutritional System: Hyperuricemia.

Nervous System: Ataxia, cerebrovascular ischemia, confusion, paresthesia, twitching.

Respiratory System: Asthma, epistaxis.

Skin and Appendages: Angioedema, eczema, exfoliative dermatitis, photosensitivity, pruritus, toxic epidermal necrolysis, urticaria.

Special Senses: Conjunctivitis, parosmia.

Urogenital System: Hematuria, interstitial nephritis, renal failure.

Incidence less than 1% (causal relationship unknown) from clinical trials, post-marketing surveillance, or literature:

Cardiovascular System: Angina pectoris, arrhythmias, myocardial infarction.

Digestive System: Appetite changes, cholecystitis, colitis, dry mouth, exacerbation of inflammatory bowel disease, periodontal abscess, small intestine inflammation with loss of blood and protein.

Hemic and Lymphatic System: Lymphadenopathy.

Metabolic and Nutritional System: Hyperkalemia.

Nervous System: Convulsion, cerebrovascular accident, emotional lability, hypertonia, meningitis, myasthenia, subarachnoid hemorrhage.

Respiratory System: Bronchitis, dyspnea, hyperventilation, laryngitis, pulmonary embolism, pulmonary infarct.

Skin and Appendages: Alopecia, dry skin, herpes simplex/zoster, nail disorder, sweating.

Special Senses: Changes in taste, corneal opacity, ear disease, glaucoma, retinal hemorrhage, retrobulbar neuritis, transient hearing loss.

Urogenital System: Menstrual disturbances, prostate disease, vaginal and uterine hemorrhage, vuvlovaginitis.

Reported in Patients Treated With Other Products but not Flurbiprofen Tablets

Body as a Whole: ***<1%:*** Death, infection, sepsis.

Cardiovascular System: ***<1%:*** Hypotension, palpitations, syncope, tachycardia, vasculitis.

Digestive System: ***>1%:*** GI perforation, GI ulcers (gastic/duodenal); ***<1%:*** Eructation, liver failure, pancreatitis.

Hemic and Lymphatic System: ***>1%:*** Anemia, increased bleeding time; ***<1%:*** Melena, rectal bleeding.

Metabolic and Nutritional System: ***<1%:*** Hyperglycemia.

Nervous System: ***<1%:*** Coma, dream abnormalities, drowsiness, hallucinations.

Respiratory System: ***<1%:*** Pneumonia, respiratory depression.

Skin and Appendages: ***<1%:*** Erythema multiforme, Stevens Johnson syndrome.

Special Senses: ***>1%:*** Pruritus; ***<1%:*** Hearing impairment.

Urogenital System: ***>1%:*** Abnormal renal function; ***<1%:*** Dysuria, oliguria, polyuria, proteinuria.

DOSAGE AND ADMINISTRATION

As with other nonsteroidal anti-inflammatory drugs, the lowest dose should be sought for each patient. Therefore, after observing the response to initial therapy with flurbiprofen tablets, the physician should adjust the dose and frequency to suit an individual patient's needs.

For relief of the signs and symptoms of rheumatoid arthritis or osteoarthritis, the recommended starting dose of flurbiprofen tablets is 200-300 mg/day, divided for administration 2, 3, or 4 times a day. The largest recommended single dose in a multiple-dose daily regimen is 100 mg.

HOW SUPPLIED

Ansaid tablets are available as follows:

50 mg: White, oval, film-coated, imprinted "ANSAID 50 mg".

100 mg: Blue, oval, film-coated, imprinted "ANSAID 100 mg".

Storage: Store at controlled room temperature 20-25°C (68-77°F).

PRODUCT LISTING - RATED THERAPEUTICALLY EQUIVALENT

Solution - Ophthalmic - 0.03%			
2 ml	$8.14	FEDERAL UPPER LIMIT, H.C.F.A. F F P	99999-1328-03
2.50 ml	$8.73	GENERIC, Bausch and Lomb	24208-0314-25
2.50 ml	$9.48	GENERIC, Pacific Pharma	60758-0910-03
2.50 ml	$16.64	OCUFEN, Southwood Pharmaceuticals Inc	58016-1131-01
2.50 ml	$17.89	OCUFEN, Allscripts Pharmaceutical Company	54569-2514-00
2.50 ml	$20.48	OCUFEN, Allergan Inc	11980-0801-03
3 ml	$20.80	OCUFEN, Physicians Total Care	54868-1158-00
Tablet - Oral - 50 mg			
30's	$21.57	GENERIC, Allscripts Pharmaceutical Company	54569-3857-00
100's	$68.02	GENERIC, Warrick Pharmaceuticals Corporation	59930-1771-01
100's	$68.15	GENERIC, Moore, H.L. Drug Exchange Inc	00839-8003-06
100's	$71.34	GENERIC, Aligen Independent Laboratories Inc	00405-4443-01
100's	$72.00	GENERIC, Geneva Pharmaceuticals	00781-1031-01
100's	$73.97	GENERIC, Novopharm Usa Inc	55953-0573-41
100's	$76.80	GENERIC, Ivax Corporation	00172-4361-60
100's	$78.80	GENERIC, Mylan Pharmaceuticals Inc	00378-0076-01
100's	$146.44	ANSAID, Pharmacia Corporation	00009-0170-07
Tablet - Oral - 100 mg			
9's	$61.02	ANSAID, Pd-Rx Pharmaceuticals	55289-0647-09
12's	$25.62	ANSAID, Physicians Total Care	54868-1113-01
14's	$27.02	ANSAID, Allscripts Pharmaceutical Company	54569-2413-01
14's	$68.07	ANSAID, Pd-Rx Pharmaceuticals	55289-0647-14
20's	$25.66	GENERIC, St. Mary'S Mpp	60760-0711-20
20's	$38.60	ANSAID, Allscripts Pharmaceutical Company	54569-2413-05
20's	$97.23	ANSAID, Pd-Rx Pharmaceuticals	55289-0647-20
21's	$23.36	GENERIC, Allscripts Pharmaceutical Company	54569-3858-01
30's	$13.01	GENERIC, Pd-Rx Pharmaceuticals	55289-0561-30
30's	$33.68	GENERIC, Allscripts Pharmaceutical Company	54569-3858-00
30's	$35.33	GENERIC, Heartland Healthcare Services	61392-0062-30
30's	$35.33	GENERIC, Heartland Healthcare Services	61392-0062-39
30's	$57.90	ANSAID, Allscripts Pharmaceutical Company	54569-2413-00
30's	$66.61	ANSAID, Pharma Pac	52959-0017-30
30's	$144.42	ANSAID, Pd-Rx Pharmaceuticals	55289-0647-30
31's	$36.51	GENERIC, Heartland Healthcare Services	61392-0062-31
32's	$37.69	GENERIC, Heartland Healthcare Services	61392-0062-32
45's	$53.00	GENERIC, Heartland Healthcare Services	61392-0062-45
60's	$70.66	GENERIC, Heartland Healthcare Services	61392-0062-60
60's	$123.41	ANSAID, Physicians Total Care	54868-1113-03
90's	$105.99	GENERIC, Heartland Healthcare Services	61392-0062-90
100's	$36.00	FEDERAL UPPER LIMIT, H.C.F.A. F F P	99999-1328-02
100's	$106.38	GENERIC, Moore, H.L. Drug Exchange Inc	00839-8004-06
100's	$106.95	GENERIC, Qualitest Products Inc	00603-3700-21
100's	$107.58	GENERIC, Warrick Pharmaceuticals Corporation	59930-1772-01
100's	$108.25	GENERIC, Teva Pharmaceuticals Usa	00093-0711-01

100's	$111.23	GENERIC, Allscripts Pharmaceutical Company	54569-3858-02
100's	$111.98	GENERIC, Aligen Independent Laboratories Inc	00405-4444-01
100's	$115.70	GENERIC, Ivax Corporation	00172-4362-60
100's	$117.60	GENERIC, Ivax Corporation	00182-2621-89
100's	$118.70	GENERIC, Mylan Pharmaceuticals Inc	00378-0093-01
100's	$123.10	GENERIC, Vangard Labs	00615-3575-13
100's	$193.58	ANSAID, Physicians Total Care	54868-1113-02
100's	$228.89	ANSAID, Pharmacia Corporation	00009-0305-03

PRODUCT LISTING - EQUIVALENTS NOT AVAILABLE

Tablet - Oral - 50 mg

10's	$8.25	GENERIC, Southwood Pharmaceuticals Inc	58016-0340-10
15's	$12.38	GENERIC, Southwood Pharmaceuticals Inc	58016-0340-15
20's	$16.50	GENERIC, Southwood Pharmaceuticals Inc	58016-0340-20
28's	$23.10	GENERIC, Southwood Pharmaceuticals Inc	58016-0340-28
30's	$24.75	GENERIC, Southwood Pharmaceuticals Inc	58016-0340-30
40's	$33.00	GENERIC, Southwood Pharmaceuticals Inc	58016-0340-40
100's	$82.50	GENERIC, Southwood Pharmaceuticals Inc	58016-0340-00
100's	$89.41	ANSAID, Pharmacia and Upjohn	00009-0170-08

Tablet - Oral - 100 mg

2's	$3.72	GENERIC, Prescript Pharmaceuticals	00247-0091-02
10's	$5.15	GENERIC, Prescript Pharmaceuticals	00247-0091-10
10's	$14.49	GENERIC, Southwood Pharmaceuticals Inc	58016-0750-10
12's	$17.08	GENERIC, Southwood Pharmaceuticals Inc	58016-0750-12
14's	$5.88	GENERIC, Prescript Pharmaceuticals	00247-0091-14
14's	$19.74	GENERIC, Pharma Pac	52959-0346-14
14's	$19.92	GENERIC, Southwood Pharmaceuticals Inc	58016-0750-14
15's	$21.35	GENERIC, Southwood Pharmaceuticals Inc	58016-0750-15
20's	$6.95	GENERIC, Prescript Pharmaceuticals	00247-0091-20
20's	$12.48	GENERIC, Alpharma Uspd Makers Of Barre and Nmc	63874-0340-20
20's	$27.76	GENERIC, Pharma Pac	52959-0346-20
20's	$28.47	GENERIC, Southwood Pharmaceuticals Inc	58016-0750-20
21's	$7.14	GENERIC, Prescript Pharmaceuticals	00247-0091-21
21's	$29.13	GENERIC, Pharma Pac	52959-0346-21
28's	$39.85	GENERIC, Southwood Pharmaceuticals Inc	58016-0750-28
30's	$8.76	GENERIC, Prescript Pharmaceuticals	00247-0091-30
30's	$13.52	GENERIC, Alpharma Uspd Makers Of Barre and Nmc	63874-0340-30
30's	$37.65	GENERIC, Pharma Pac	52959-0346-30
30's	$42.70	GENERIC, Southwood Pharmaceuticals Inc	58016-0750-30
40's	$10.56	GENERIC, Prescript Pharmaceuticals	00247-0091-40
40's	$56.93	GENERIC, Southwood Pharmaceuticals Inc	58016-0750-40
100's	$109.95	GENERIC, Major Pharmaceuticals Inc	00904-5019-60
100's	$112.25	GENERIC, Greenstone Limited	59762-3724-01
100's	$117.40	GENERIC, Udl Laboratories Inc	51079-0815-20
100's	$142.33	GENERIC, Southwood Pharmaceuticals Inc	58016-0750-00
180's	$191.48	GENERIC, Greenstone Limited	59762-3724-05

Flutamide *(001330)*

For complete prescribing information, refer to the CD-ROM included with the book.

Categories: Carcinoma, prostate; Pregnancy Category D; FDA Approved 1989 Jan
Drug Classes: Antineoplastics, antiandrogens; Hormones/hormone modifiers
Brand Names: Etaconil; **Eulexin**; Flucinome
Foreign Brand Availability: Apimid (Germany); Cytamid (Germany); Drogenil (Ecuador; England; Ireland); Euflex (Canada); Eulexine (France); Flucinom (Czech-Republic; Greece; Russia; Switzerland); Flugerel (Australia; Taiwan); Fluken (Mexico); Flulem (Mexico); Flutamex (Germany); Flutan (Hong-Kong; Thailand); Flutol (New-Zealand); Fugerel (Austria; Hong-Kong; Hungary; Indonesia; Malaysia; Philippines; Thailand); Odyne (Japan); Prostamid (India); Prostogenat (Germany); Testac (Germany)
Cost of Therapy: $462.41 (Prostatic Carcinoma; Eulexin; 125 mg; 6 capsules/day; 30 day supply)
$374.50 (Prostatic Carcinoma; Generic capsule; 125 mg; 6 capsules/day; 30 day supply)

WARNING

Hepatic Injury

There have been post-marketing reports of hospitalization and rarely death due to liver failure in patients taking flutamide. Evidence of hepatic injury included elevated serum transaminase levels, jaundice, hepatic encephalopathy and death related to acute hepatic failure. The hepatic injury was reversible after discontinuation of therapy in some patients. Approximately half of the reported oases occurred within the initial 3 months of treatment with flutamide.

Serum transaminase levels should be measured prior to starting treatment with flutamide. Flutamide is not recommended in patients whose ALT values exceed twice the upper limit of normal. Serum transaminase levels should then be measured monthly for the first 4 months of therapy, and periodically thereafter. Liver function tests also should be obtained at the first signs and symptoms suggestive of liver dysfunction, *e.g.,* nausea, vomiting, abdominal pain, fatigue, anorexia, "flu-like" symptoms, hyperbilirubinuria, jaundice or right upper quadrant tenderness. If at any time, a patient has jaundice, or their ALT rises above 2 times the upper limit of normal, flutamide should be immediately discontinued with close follow-up of liver function tests until resolution.

DESCRIPTION

Eulexin capsules contain flutamide, an acetanilid, nonsteroidal, orally active antiandrogen having the chemical name, 2-methyl-*N*-[4-nitro-3-(trifluoromethyl)phenyl] propanamide.

Each capsule contains 125 mg flutamide. The compound is a buff to yellow powder with a molecular weight of 276.2.

The inactive ingredients for Eulexin capsules include: Corn starch, lactose, magnesium stearate, povidone, and sodium lauryl sulfate. Gelatin capsule shells may contain methylparaben, propylparaben, butylparaben and the following dye systems: FD&C blue 1, FD&C yellow 6 and either FD&C red 3 or FD&C red 40 plus D&C yellow 10, with titanium dioxide and other inactive ingredients.

INDICATIONS AND USAGE

Flutamide is indicated for use in combination with LHRH agonists for the management of locally confined Stage B_2-C and Stage D_2 metastatic carcinoma of the prostate.

STAGE B_2-C PROSTATIC CARCINOMA

Treatment with flutamide and the LHRH agonist should start 8 weeks prior to initiating radiation therapy and continue during radiation therapy.

STAGE D_2 METASTATIC CARCINOMA

To achieve benefit from treatment, flutamide should be initiated with the LHRH agonist and continued until progression.

NON-FDA APPROVED INDICATIONS

Flutamide has also been used experimentally in the treatment of benign prostatic hyperplasia and in combination with oral contraceptives in the treatment of hirsutism in females. However, these uses have not been approved by the FDA.

CONTRAINDICATIONS

Flutamide is contraindicated in patients who are hypersensitive to flutamide or any component of this preparation.

Flutamide capsules are contraindicated in patients with severe hepatic impairment (baseline hepatic enzymes should be evaluated prior to treatment).

WARNINGS

HEPATIC INJURY

SEE BOXED WARNING.

USE IN WOMEN

Flutamide capsules are for use **only** in men. This product has no indication for women and should not be used in this population, particularly for nonserious or nonlife-threatening conditions.

FETAL TOXICITY

Flutamide may cause fetal harm when administered to a pregnant woman.

ANILINE TOXICITY

One metabolite of flutamide is 4-nitro-3-flouro-methylaniline. Several toxicities consistent with aniline exposure, including methmoglobinemia, hemolytic anemia and cholestatic jaundice have been observed in both animals and humans after flutamide administration. In patients susceptible to aniline toxicity (*e.g.,* persons with glucose-6-phosphate dehydrogenase deficiency, hemoglobin M disease and smokers), monitoring of methomoglobin levels should be considered.

DOSAGE AND ADMINISTRATION

The recommended dosage is 2 capsules three times a day at 8 hour intervals for a total daily dose of 750 mg.

PRODUCT LISTING - RATED THERAPEUTICALLY EQUIVALENT

Capsule - Oral - 125 mg

100's	$209.22	GENERIC, Eon Labs Manufacturing Inc	00185-1125-88
180's	$374.50	GENERIC, Ivax Corporation	00172-4960-58
180's	$376.18	GENERIC, Barr Laboratories Inc	00555-0870-63
180's	$376.60	GENERIC, Teva Pharmaceuticals Usa	00093-7120-86
180's	$376.60	GENERIC, Eon Labs Manufacturing Inc	00185-1125-18
180's	$462.41	EULEXIN, Schering Corporation	00085-0525-06

PRODUCT LISTING - EQUIVALENTS NOT AVAILABLE

Capsule - Oral - 125 mg

100's	$272.35	EULEXIN, Schering Corporation	00085-0525-03

F

Fluticasone Propionate (003011)

For related information, see the comparative table section in Appendix A.

Categories: Asthma; Dermatitis; Pruritus; Rhinitis, allergic; Pregnancy Category C; FDA Approved 1990 Dec
Drug Classes: Corticosteroids, inhalation; Corticosteroids, topical; Dermatologics
Brand Names: **Cutivate**; Flonase; Flonase Aq; Flovent
Foreign Brand Availability: Allegro (Israel); Atemur Mite (Germany); Flixonase (Austria; Bahamas; Barbados; Belize; Bermuda; Bulgaria; Colombia; Costa-Rica; Curacao; Czech-Republic; Denmark; Dominican-Republic; El-Salvador; England; Finland; France; Guatemala; Guyana; Honduras; Hong-Kong; Hungary; Indonesia; Ireland; Israel; Italy; Jamaica; Korea; Malaysia; Mexico; Netherland-Antilles; Netherlands; Nicaragua; Panama; Peru; Puerto-Rico; Russia; Singapore; Surinam; Taiwan; Thailand; Trinidad; Turkey); Flixonase Nasal Spray (New-Zealand); Flixonase 24 hour (New-Zealand); Flixotide (Austria; Bahamas; Barbados; Belize; Bermuda; Bulgaria; China; Curacao; Czech-Republic; Denmark; England; Finland; France; Guyana; Hong-Kong; Hungary; Indonesia; Ireland; Israel; Italy; Jamaica; Korea; Mexico; Netherland-Antilles; Netherlands; Peru; Philippines; Puerto-Rico; Russia; Singapore; South-Africa; Surinam; Taiwan; Thailand; Trinidad; Turkey); Flixotide Disk (China; New-Zealand); Flixotide Disks (Australia); Flixotide Inhaler (Australia); Flixovate (France); Flunase (Japan); Flutide (Germany; Japan); Flutivate (Germany; Norway); Zoflut (India)
Cost of Therapy: $53.36 (Allergic Rhinitis; Flonase Spray; 0.05 mg/inh;16 g; 4 sprays/day; 30 day supply)
$64.64 (Asthma; Flovent Aerosol; 110 µg/inh;13 g; 2 inhalations/day; variable day supply)

F

INHALATION

DESCRIPTION

Note: The trade names have been used throughout this monograph for clarity.

FLOVENT INHALATION AEROSOL

For Oral Inhalation Only

The active component of Flovent 44 µg, 110 µg, and 220 µg inhalation aerosol is fluticasone propionate, a glucocorticoid having the chemical name S-(fluoromethyl)6α,9-difluoro-11β,17-dihydroxy-16α-methyl-3-oxoandrosta-1,4-diene-17β-carbothioate, 17-propionate.

Fluticasone propionate is a white to off-white powder with a molecular weight of 500.6. It is practically insoluble in water, freely soluble in dimethyl sulfoxide and dimethylformamide, and slightly soluble in methanol and 95% ethanol.

Flovent 44 µg, 110 µg, and 220 µg inhalation aerosol are pressurized, metered-dose aerosol units intended for oral inhalation only. Each unit contains a microcrystalline suspension of fluticasone propionate (micronized) in a mixture of two chlorofluorocarbon propellants (trichlorofluoromethane and dichlorodifluoromethane) with lecithin. Each actuation of the inhaler delivers 50, 125, or 250 µg of fluticasone propionate from the valve, and 44, 110, or 220 µg, respectively, of fluticasone propionate from the actuator.

FLOVENT DISKUS

For Oral Inhalation Only

The active component of Flovent Diskus 50 µg, Flovent Diskus 100 µg, and Flovent Diskus 250 µg is fluticasone propionate, a corticosteroid having the chemical name S-(fluoromethyl)6α,9-difluoro-11β,17-dihydroxy-16α-methyl-3-oxoandrosta-1,4-diene-17β-carbothioate, 17-propionate.

Fluticasone propionate is a white to off-white powder with a molecular weight of 500.6, and the empirical formula is $C_{25}H_{31}F_3O_5S$. It is practically insoluble in water, freely soluble in dimethyl sulfoxide and dimethylformamide, and slightly soluble in methanol and 95% ethanol.

Flovent Diskus 50 µg, 100 µg, and 250 µg are specially designed plastic devices containing a double-foil blister strip of a powder formulation of fluticasone propionate intended for oral inhalation only. Each blister on the double-foil strip within the device contains 50, 100, or 250 µg of microfine fluticasone propionate in 12.5 mg of formulation containing lactose. After a blister containing medication is opened by activating the device, the medication is dispersed into the airstream created by the patient inhaling through the mouthpiece.

Under standardized *in vitro* test conditions, Flovent Diskus delivers 47, 94, or 235 µg of fluticasone propionate from Flovent Diskus 50 µg, 100 µg, or 250 µg, respectively, when tested at a flow rate of 60 L/min for 2 seconds. In adult patients with obstructive lung disease and severely compromised lung function (mean forced expiratory volume in 1 second [FEV_1] 20-30% of predicted), mean peak inspiratory flow (PIF) through a Diskus device was 82.4 L/min (range, 46.1-115.3 L/min). In children with asthma 4 and 8 years old, mean PIF through Flovent Diskus was 70 and 104 L/min, respectively (range, 48-123 L/min).

The actual amount of drug delivered to the lung will depend on patient factors, such as inspiratory flow profile.

FLOVENT ROTADISK

For Oral Inhalation Only

For Use With the Diskhaler Inhalation Device

The active component of Flovent Rotadisk 50 µg, Flovent Rotadisk 100 µg, and Flovent Rotadisk 250 µg is fluticasone propionate, a corticosteroid having the chemical name S-(fluoromethyl)6α,9-difluoro-11β,17-dihydroxy-16α-methyl-3-oxoandrosta-1,4-diene-17β-carbothioate, 17-propionate.

Fluticasone propionate is a white to off-white powder with a molecular weight of 500.6, and the empirical formula is $C_{25}H_{31}F_3O_5S$. It is practically insoluble in water, freely soluble in dimethyl sulfoxide and dimethylformamide, and slightly soluble in methanol and 95% ethanol.

Flovent Rotadisk 50 µg, 100 µg, and 250 µg contain a dry powder presentation of fluticasone propionate intended for oral inhalation only. Each double-foil Rotadisk contains 4 blisters. Each blister contains a mixture of 50, 100, or 250 µg of microfine fluticasone propionate blended with lactose to a total weight of 25 mg. The contents of each blister are inhaled using a specially designed plastic device for inhaling powder called the Diskhaler. After a fluticasone propionate Rotadisk is loaded into the Diskhaler, a blister containing medication is pierced and the fluticasone propionate is dispersed into the air stream created when the patient inhales through the mouthpiece.

The amount of drug delivered to the lung will depend on patient factors such as inspiratory flow. Under standardized *in vitro* testing, Flovent Rotadisk delivers 44, 88, or 220 µg of fluticasone propionate from Flovent Rotadisk 50 µg, 100 µg, or 250 µg, respectively, when tested at a flow rate of 60 L/min for 3 seconds. In adult and adolescent patients with asthma, mean peak inspiratory flow (PIF) through the Diskhaler was 123 L/min (range, 88-159 L/min), and in pediatric patients 4-11 years of age with asthma, mean PIF was 110 L/min (range, 43-175 L/min).

CLINICAL PHARMACOLOGY

FLOVENT INHALATION AEROSOL

Fluticasone propionate is a synthetic, trifluorinated glucocorticoid with potent anti-inflammatory activity. *In vitro* assays using human lung cytosol preparations have established fluticasone propionate as a human glucocorticoid receptor agonist with an affinity 18 times greater than dexamethasone, almost twice that of beclomethasone-17-monopropionate (BMP), the active metabolite of beclomethasone dipropionate, and over 3 times that of budesonide. Data from the McKenzie vasoconstrictor assay in man are consistent with these results.

The precise mechanisms of glucocorticoid action in asthma are unknown. Inflammation is recognized as an important component in the pathogenesis of asthma. Glucocorticoids have been shown to inhibit multiple cell types (*e.g.*, mast cells, eosinophils, basophils, lymphocytes, macrophages, and neutrophils) and mediator production or secretion (*e.g.*, histamine, eicosanoids, leukotrienes, and cytokines) involved in the asthmatic response. These anti-inflammatory actions of glucocorticoids may contribute to their efficacy in asthma.

Though highly effective for the treatment of asthma, glucocorticoids do not affect asthma symptoms immediately. However, improvement following inhaled administration of fluticasone propionate can occur within 24 hours of beginning treatment, although maximum benefit may not be achieved for 1-2 weeks or longer after starting treatment. When glucocorticoids are discontinued, asthma stability may persist for several days or longer.

Pharmacokinetics

Absorption

The activity of Flovent inhalation aerosol is due to the parent drug, fluticasone propionate. Studies using oral dosing of labeled and unlabeled drug have demonstrated that the oral systemic bioavailability of fluticasone propionate is negligible (<1%), primarily due to incomplete absorption and pre-systemic metabolism in the gut and liver. In contrast, the majority of the fluticasone propionate delivered to the lung is systemically absorbed. The systemic bioavailability of fluticasone propionate inhalation aerosol in healthy volunteers averaged about 30% of the dose delivered from the actuator.

Peak plasma concentrations after an 880 µg inhaled dose ranged from 0.1-1.0 ng/ml.

Distribution

Following intravenous administration, the initial disposition phase for fluticasone propionate was rapid and consistent with its high lipid solubility and tissue binding. The volume of distribution averaged 4.2 L/kg. The percentage of fluticasone propionate bound to human plasma proteins averaged 91%. Fluticasone propionate is weakly and reversibly bound to erythrocytes. Fluticasone propionate is not significantly bound to human transcortin.

Metabolism

The total clearance of fluticasone propionate is high (average, 1093 ml/min), with renal clearance accounting for less than 0.02% of the total. The only circulating metabolite detected in man is the 17β-carboxylic acid derivative of fluticasone propionate, which is formed through the cytochrome P450 3A4 pathway. This metabolite had approximately 2000 times less affinity than the parent drug for the glucocorticoid receptor of human lung cytosol *in vitro* and negligible pharmacological activity in animal studies. Other metabolites detected *in vitro* using cultured human hepatoma cells have not been detected in man.

Excretion

Following intravenous dosing, fluticasone propionate showed polyexponential kinetics and had a terminal elimination half-life of approximately 7.8 hours. Less than 5% of a radiolabeled oral dose was excreted in the urine as metabolites, with the remainder excreted in the feces as parent drug and metabolites.

Special Populations

Formal pharmacokinetic studies using fluticasone propionate were not carried out in any special populations. In a clinical study using fluticasone propionate inhalation powder, trough fluticasone propionate plasma concentrations were collected in 76 males and 74 females after inhaled administration of 100 and 500 µg twice daily. Full pharmacokinetic profiles were obtained from 7 female patients and 13 male patients at these doses, and no overall differences in pharmacokinetic behavior were found.

Pharmacodynamics

To confirm that systemic absorption does not play a role in the clinical response to inhaled fluticasone propionate, a double-blind clinical study comparing inhaled and oral fluticasone propionate was conducted. Doses of 100 and 500 µg twice daily of fluticasone propionate inhalation powder were compared to oral fluticasone propionate, 20,000 µg given once daily, and placebo for 6 weeks. Plasma levels of fluticasone propionate were detectable in all 3 active groups, but the mean values were highest in the oral group. Both doses of inhaled fluticasone propionate were effective in maintaining asthma stability and improving lung function while oral fluticasone propionate and placebo were ineffective. This demonstrates that the clinical effectiveness of inhaled fluticasone propionate is due to its direct local effect and not to an indirect effect through systemic absorption.

The potential systemic effects of inhaled fluticasone propionate on the hypothalamic-pituitary-adrenal (HPA) axis were also studied in asthma patients. Fluticasone propionate given by inhalation aerosol at doses of 220, 440, 660, or 880 µg twice daily was compared with placebo or oral prednisone 10 mg given once daily for 4 weeks. For most patients, the ability to increase cortisol production in response to stress, as assessed by 6 hour cosyntropin stimulation, remained intact with inhaled fluticasone propionate treatment. No patient had an abnormal response (peak less than 18 µg/dl) after dosing with placebo or 220 µg twice daily. Ten percent (10%) to 16% of patients treated with fluticasone propionate at doses of 440 μg or more twice daily had an abnormal response as compared to 29% of patients treated with prednisone.

FLOVENT DISKUS

Mechanism of Action

Fluticasone propionate is a synthetic, trifluorinated corticosteroid with potent anti-inflammatory activity. *In vitro* assays using human lung cytosol preparations have established fluticasone propionate as a human glucocorticoid receptor agonist with an affinity 18 times greater than dexamethasone, almost twice that of beclomethasone-17-monopropionate (BMP), the active metabolite of beclomethasone dipropionate, and over 3 times that of budesonide. Data from the McKenzie vasoconstrictor assay in man are consistent with these results.

The precise mechanisms of fluticasone propionate action in asthma are unknown. Inflammation is recognized as an important component in the pathogenesis of asthma. Corticosteroids have been shown to inhibit multiple cell types (*e.g.,* mast cells, eosinophils, basophils, lymphocytes, macrophages, and neutrophils) and mediator production or secretion (*e.g.,* histamine, eicosanoids, leukotrienes, and cytokines) involved in the asthmatic response. These anti-inflammatory actions of corticosteroids may contribute to their efficacy in asthma.

Though highly effective for the treatment of asthma, corticosteroids do not affect asthma symptoms immediately. However, improvement following inhaled administration of fluticasone propionate can occur within 24 hours of beginning treatment, although maximum benefit may not be achieved for 1-2 weeks or longer after starting treatment. When corticosteroids are discontinued, asthma stability may persist for several days or longer.

Studies in asthmatic patients have shown a favorable ratio between topical anti-inflammatory activity and systemic corticosteroid effects over recommended doses of Flovent Diskus. This is explained by a combination of a relatively high local anti-inflammatory effect, negligible oral systemic bioavailability (<1%), and the minimal pharmacological activity of the only metabolite detected in man. Lung absorption does occur (see below).

Pharmacokinetics

Absorption

The activity of Flovent Diskus is due to the parent drug, fluticasone propionate. Studies using oral dosing of labeled and unlabeled drug have demonstrated that the oral systemic bioavailability of fluticasone propionate is negligible (<1%), primarily due to incomplete absorption and presystemic metabolism in the gut and liver. In contrast, the majority of the fluticasone propionate delivered to the lung is systemically absorbed. The systemic bioavailability of fluticasone propionate from the Diskus device in healthy adult volunteers averages about 18%.

Peak steady-state fluticasone propionate plasma concentrations in adult patients with asthma (n=11) ranged from undetectable to 266 pg/ml after a 500 μg twice-daily dose of fluticasone propionate inhalation powder using the Diskus device. The mean fluticasone propionate plasma concentration was 110 pg/ml.

Distribution

Following intravenous administration, the initial disposition phase for fluticasone propionate was rapid and consistent with its high lipid solubility and tissue binding. The volume of distribution averaged 4.2 L/kg.

The percentage of fluticasone propionate bound to human plasma proteins averages 91%. Fluticasone propionate is weakly and reversibly bound to erythrocytes. Fluticasone propionate is not significantly bound to human transcortin.

Metabolism

The total clearance of fluticasone propionate is high (average, 1093 ml/min), with renal clearance accounting for less than 0.02% of the total. The only circulating metabolite detected in man is the 17β-carboxylic acid derivative of fluticasone propionate, which is formed through the cytochrome P450 3A4 pathway. This metabolite had less affinity (approximately 1/2000) than the parent drug for the glucocorticoid receptor of human lung cytosol *in vitro* and negligible pharmacological activity in animal studies. Other metabolites detected *in vitro* using cultured human hepatoma cells have not been detected in man.

Elimination

Following intravenous dosing, fluticasone propionate showed polyexponential kinetics and had a terminal elimination half-life of approximately 7.8 hours. Less than 5% of a radiolabeled oral dose was excreted in the urine as metabolites, with the remainder excreted in the feces as parent drug and metabolites.

Hepatic Impairment

Since fluticasone propionate is predominantly cleared by hepatic metabolism, impairment of liver function may lead to accumulation of fluticasone propionate in plasma. Therefore, patients with hepatic disease should be closely monitored.

Gender

Full pharmacokinetic profiles were obtained from 9 female and 16 male patients given 500 μg twice daily. No overall differences in fluticasone propionate pharmacokinetics were observed.

Pediatrics

In a clinical study conducted in patients 4-11 years of age with mild to moderate asthma, fluticasone propionate concentrations were obtained in 61 patients at 20 and 40 minutes after dosing with 50 and 100 μg twice daily of fluticasone propionate inhalation powder using the Diskus. Plasma concentrations were low and ranged from undetectable (about 80% of the plasma samples) to 88 pg/ml. Mean fluticasone propionate plasma concentrations at the 2 dose levels were 5 and 8 pg/ml, respectively.

Special Populations

Formal pharmacokinetic studies using fluticasone propionate were not carried out in other special populations.

Drug-Drug Interactions

In a multiple-dose drug interaction study, coadministration of fluticasone propionate (500 μg twice daily) and erythromycin (333 mg 3 times daily) did not affect fluticasone propionate pharmacokinetics. In another drug interaction study, coadministration of fluticasone propionate (1000 μg) and ketoconazole (200 mg once daily) resulted in increased fluticasone propionate concentrations and reduced plasma cortisol area under the plasma concentration versus time curve (AUC), but had no effect on urinary excretion of cortisol. Since fluticasone propionate is a substrate of cytochrome P450 3A4, caution should be exercised when cytochrome P450 3A4 inhibitors (*e.g.,* ritonavir, ketoconazole) are coadministered with fluticasone propionate as this could result in increased plasma concentrations of fluticasone propionate.

Pharmacodynamics

To confirm that systemic absorption does not play a role in the clinical response to inhaled fluticasone propionate, a double-blind clinical study comparing inhaled and oral fluticasone propionate was conducted. Doses of 100 and 500 μg twice daily of fluticasone propionate inhalation powder were compared to oral fluticasone propionate, 20,000 μg given once daily, and placebo for 6 weeks. Plasma levels of fluticasone propionate were detectable in all 3 active groups, but the mean values were highest in the oral group. Both doses of inhaled fluticasone propionate were effective in maintaining asthma stability and improving lung function while oral fluticasone propionate and placebo were ineffective. This demonstrates that the clinical effectiveness of inhaled fluticasone propionate is due to its direct local effect and not to an indirect effect through systemic absorption.

The potential systemic effects of inhaled fluticasone propionate on the hypothalamic-pituitary-adrenal (HPA) axis were also studied in asthma patients. Fluticasone propionate given by inhalation aerosol at doses of 220, 440, 660, or 880 μg twice daily was compared with placebo or oral prednisone 10 mg given once daily for 4 weeks. For most patients, the ability to increase cortisol production in response to stress, as assessed by 6 hour cosyntropin stimulation, remained intact with inhaled fluticasone propionate treatment. No patient had an abnormal response (peak serum cortisol <18 μg/dl) after dosing with placebo or fluticasone propionate 220 μg twice daily. For patients treated with 440, 660, and 880 μg twice daily, 10%, 16%, and 12%, respectively, had an abnormal response as compared to 29% of patients treated with prednisone.

In clinical trials with fluticasone propionate inhalation powder using doses up to and including 250 μg twice daily, occasional abnormal short cosyntropin tests (peak serum cortisol <18 μg/dl) were noted both in patients receiving fluticasone propionate and in patients receiving placebo. The incidence of abnormal tests at 500 μg twice daily was greater than placebo. In a 2 year study carried out with the Diskhaler inhalation device in 64 patients with mild, persistent asthma (mean FEV_1 91% of predicted) randomized to fluticasone propionate 500 μg twice daily or placebo, no patient receiving fluticasone propionate had an abnormal response to 6 hour cosyntropin infusion (peak serum cortisol <18 μg/dl). With a peak cortisol threshold <35 μg/dl, 1 patient receiving fluticasone propionate (4%) had an abnormal response at 1 year; repeat testing at 18 months and 2 years was normal. Another patient receiving fluticasone propionate (5%) had an abnormal response at 2 years. No patient on placebo had an abnormal response at 1 or 2 years.

In a placebo-controlled clinical study conducted in patients 4-11 years of age, a 30 minute cosyntropin stimulation test was performed in 41 patients after 12 weeks of dosing with 50 or 100 μg twice daily of fluticasone propionate via the Diskus device. One patient receiving fluticasone propionate via Diskus had a prestimulation plasma cortisol concentration <5 μg/dl, and 2 patients had a rise in cortisol of <7 μg/dl. However, all poststimulation values were >18 μg/dl.

FLOVENT ROTADISK

Fluticasone propionate is a synthetic, trifluorinated corticosteroid with potent anti-inflammatory activity. *In vitro* assays using human lung cytosol preparations have established fluticasone propionate as a human glucocorticoid receptor agonist with an affinity 18 times greater than dexamethasone, almost twice that of beclomethasone-17-monopropionate (BMP), the active metabolite of beclomethasone dipropionate, and over 3 times that of budesonide. Data from the McKenzie vasoconstrictor assay in man are consistent with these results.

The precise mechanisms of fluticasone propionate action in asthma are unknown. Inflammation is recognized as an important component in the pathogenesis of asthma. Corticosteroids have been shown to inhibit multiple cell types (*e.g.,* mast cells, eosinophils, basophils, lymphocytes, macrophages, and neutrophils) and mediator production or secretion (*e.g.,* histamine, eicosanoids, leukotrienes, and cytokines) involved in the asthmatic response. These anti-inflammatory actions of corticosteroids may contribute to their efficacy in asthma.

Though highly effective for the treatment of asthma, corticosteroids do not affect asthma symptoms immediately. However, improvement following inhaled administration of fluticasone propionate can occur within 24 hours of beginning treatment, although maximum benefit may not be achieved for 1-2 weeks or longer after starting treatment. When corticosteroids are discontinued, asthma stability may persist for several days or longer.

Pharmacokinetics

Absorption

The activity of Flovent Rotadisk inhalation powder is due to the parent drug, fluticasone propionate. Studies using oral dosing of labeled and unlabeled drug have demonstrated that the oral systemic bioavailability of fluticasone propionate is negligible (<1%), primarily due to incomplete absorption and pre-systemic metabolism in the gut and liver. In contrast, the majority of the fluticasone propionate delivered to the lung is systemically absorbed. The systemic bioavailability of fluticasone propionate inhalation powder in healthy volunteers averaged about 13.5% of the nominal dose.

Peak plasma concentrations after a 1000 μg dose of fluticasone propionate inhalation powder ranged from 0.1-1.0 ng/ml.

Distribution

Following intravenous administration, the initial disposition phase for fluticasone propionate was rapid and consistent with its high lipid solubility and tissue binding. The volume of distribution averaged 4.2 L/kg. The percentage of fluticasone propionate bound to human plasma proteins averaged 91%.

Fluticasone propionate is weakly and reversibly bound to erythrocytes. Fluticasone propionate is not significantly bound to human transcortin.

Metabolism

The total clearance of fluticasone propionate is high (average, 1093 ml/min), with renal clearance accounting for less than 0.02% of the total. The only circulating metabolite detected in man is the 17β-carboxylic acid derivative of fluticasone propionate, which is formed through the cytochrome P450 3A4 pathway. This metabolite had approximately 2000 times less affinity than the parent drug for the glucocorticoid receptor of human lung cytosol *in vitro* and negligible pharmacological activity in animal studies. Other metabolites detected *in vitro* using cultured human hepatoma cells have not been detected in man.

In a multiple-dose drug interaction study, coadministration of fluticasone propionate (500 µg twice daily) and erythromycin (333 mg three times daily) did not affect fluticasone propionate pharmacokinetics.

In a drug interaction study, coadministration of fluticasone propionate (1000 µg) and ketoconazole (200 mg once daily) resulted in increased fluticasone propionate concentrations, a reduction in plasma cortisol AUC, and no effect on urinary excretion of cortisol.

Excretion

Following intravenous dosing, fluticasone propionate showed polyexponential kinetics and had a terminal elimination half-life of approximately 7.8 hours. Less than 5% of a radiolabeled oral dose was excreted in the urine as metabolites, with the remainder excreted in the feces as parent drug and metabolites.

Special Populations

Formal pharmacokinetic studies using fluticasone propionate were not carried out in any special populations. In a clinical study using fluticasone propionate inhalation powder, trough fluticasone propionate plasma concentrations were collected in 76 males and 74 females after inhaled administration of 100 and 500 µg twice daily. Full pharmacokinetic profiles were obtained from 7 female patients and 13 male patients at these doses, and no overall differences in pharmacokinetic behavior were found.

Plasma concentrations of fluticasone propionate were measured 20 and 40 minutes after dosing from 29 children aged 4-11 years who were taking either 50 or 100 µg twice daily of fluticasone propionate inhalation powder. Plasma concentration values ranged from below the limit of quantitation (25 pg/ml) to 117 pg/ml (50 µg dose) or 154 pg/ml (100 µg dose). In a study with adults taking the 100 µg twice-daily dose, the plasma concentrations observed ranged from below the limit of quantitation to 73.1 pg/ml. The median fluticasone propionate plasma concentrations for the 100 µg dose in children was 58.7 pg/ml; in adults the median plasma concentration was 39.5 pg/ml.

Pharmacodynamics

To confirm that systemic absorption does not play a role in the clinical response to inhaled fluticasone propionate, a double-blind clinical study comparing inhaled and oral fluticasone propionate was conducted. Doses of 100 and 500 µg twice daily of fluticasone propionate inhalation powder were compared to oral fluticasone propionate, 20,000 µg given once daily, and placebo for 6 weeks. Plasma levels of fluticasone propionate were detectable in all 3 active groups, but the mean values were highest in the oral group. Both doses of inhaled fluticasone propionate were effective in maintaining asthma stability and improving lung function while oral fluticasone propionate and placebo were ineffective. This demonstrates that the clinical effectiveness of inhaled fluticasone propionate is due to its direct local effect and not to an indirect effect through systemic absorption.

The potential systemic effects of inhaled fluticasone propionate on the hypothalamic-pituitary-adrenal (HPA) axis were also studied in asthma patients. Fluticasone propionate given by inhalation aerosol at doses of 220, 440, 660, or 880 µg twice daily was compared with placebo or oral prednisone 10 mg given once daily for 4 weeks. For most patients, the ability to increase cortisol production in response to stress, as assessed by 6 hour cosyntropin stimulation, remained intact with inhaled fluticasone propionate treatment. No patient had an abnormal response (peak serum cortisol <18 µg/dl) after dosing with placebo or fluticasone propionate 220 µg twice daily. For patients treated with 440, 660, and 880 µg twice daily, 10%, 16%, and 12%, respectively, had an abnormal response as compared to 29% of patients treated with prednisone.

In clinical trials with fluticasone propionate inhalation powder, using doses up to and including 250 µg twice daily, occasional abnormal short cosyntropin tests (peak serum cortisol <18 µg/dl) were noted in patients receiving fluticasone propionate or placebo. The incidence of abnormal tests at 500 µg twice daily was greater than placebo. In a 2 year study carried out in 64 patients randomized to fluticasone propionate 500 µg twice daily or placebo, 1 patient receiving fluticasone propionate (4%) had an abnormal response to 6 hour cosyntropin infusion at 1 year; repeat testing at 18 months and 2 years was normal. Another patient receiving fluticasone propionate (5%) had an abnormal response at 2 years. No patient on placebo had an abnormal response at 1 or 2 years.

INDICATIONS AND USAGE

FLOVENT INHALATION AEROSOL

Flovent inhalation aerosol is indicated for the maintenance treatment of asthma as prophylactic therapy. It is also indicated for patients requiring oral corticosteroid therapy for asthma. Many of these patients may be able to reduce or eliminate their requirement for oral corticosteroids over time.

Flovent inhalation aerosol is NOT indicated for the relief of acute bronchospasm.

FLOVENT DISKUS

Flovent Diskus is indicated for the maintenance treatment of asthma as prophylactic therapy in adult and pediatric patients 4 years of age and older. It is also indicated for patients requiring oral corticosteroid therapy for asthma. Many of these patients may be able to reduce or eliminate their requirement for oral corticosteroids over time.

Flovent Diskus is NOT indicated for the relief of acute bronchospasm.

FLOVENT ROTADISK

Flovent Rotadisk is indicated for the maintenance treatment of asthma as prophylactic therapy in patients 4 years of age and older. It is also indicated for patients requiring oral corticosteroid therapy for asthma. Many of these patients may be able to reduce or eliminate their requirement for oral corticosteroids over time.

Flovent Rotadisk is NOT indicated for the relief of acute bronchospasm.

CONTRAINDICATIONS

FLOVENT INHALATION AEROSOL

Flovent inhalation aerosol is contraindicated in the primary treatment of status asthmaticus or other acute episodes of asthma where intensive measures are required.

Hypersensitivity to any of the ingredients of these preparations contraindicates their use.

FLOVENT DISKUS

Flovent Diskus is contraindicated in the primary treatment of status asthmaticus or other acute episodes of asthma where intensive measures are required.

Hypersensitivity to any of the ingredients of these preparations contraindicates their use.

FLOVENT ROTADISK

Flovent Rotadisk is contraindicated in the primary treatment of status asthmaticus or other acute episodes of asthma where intensive measures are required.

Hypersensitivity to any of the ingredients of these preparations contraindicates their use.

WARNINGS

FLOVENT INHALATION AEROSOL

Particular care is needed for patients who are transferred from systemically active corticosteroids to Flovent inhalation aerosol because deaths due to adrenal insufficiency have occurred in patients with asthma during and after transfer from systemic corticosteroids to less systemically available inhaled corticosteroids. After withdrawal from systemic corticosteroids, a number of months are required for recovery of HPA function.

Patients who have been previously maintained on 20 mg or more per day of prednisone (or its equivalent) may be most susceptible, particularly when their systemic corticosteroids have been almost completely withdrawn. During this period of HPA suppression, patients may exhibit signs and symptoms of adrenal insufficiency when exposed to trauma, surgery, or infection (particularly gastroenteritis) or other conditions associated with severe electrolyte loss. Although fluticasone propionate inhalation aerosol may provide control of asthma symptoms during these episodes, in recommended doses it supplies less than normal physiological amounts of glucocorticoid systemically and does NOT provide the mineralocorticoid activity that is necessary for coping with these emergencies.

During periods of stress or a severe asthma attack, patients who have been withdrawn from systemic corticosteroids should be instructed to resume oral corticosteroids (in large doses) immediately and to contact their physicians for further instruction. These patients should also be instructed to carry a warning card indicating that they may need supplementary systemic corticosteroids during periods of stress or a severe asthma attack.

Patients requiring oral corticosteroids should be weaned slowly from systemic corticosteroid use after transferring to fluticasone propionate inhalation aerosol. In a trial of 96 patients, prednisone reduction was successfully accomplished by reducing the daily prednisone dose by 2.5 mg on a weekly basis during transfer to inhaled fluticasone propionate. Successive reduction of prednisone dose was allowed only when lung function, symptoms, and as-needed beta-agonist use were better than or comparable to that seen before initiation of prednisone dose reduction. Lung function (FEV_1 or AM PEFR), beta-agonist use, and asthma symptoms should be carefully monitored during withdrawal of oral corticosteroids. In addition to monitoring asthma signs and symptoms, patients should be observed for signs and symptoms of adrenal insufficiency such as fatigue, lassitude, weakness, nausea and vomiting, and hypotension.

Transfer of patients from systemic corticosteroid therapy to fluticasone propionate inhalation aerosol may unmask conditions previously suppressed by the systemic corticosteroid therapy, *e.g.*, rhinitis, conjunctivitis, eczema, and arthritis.

Persons who are on drugs that suppress the immune system are more susceptible to infections than healthy individuals. Chickenpox and measles, for example, can have a more serious or even fatal course in susceptible children or adults on corticosteroids. In such children or adults who have not had these diseases, particular care should be taken to avoid exposure. How the dose, route, and duration of corticosteroid administration affects the risk of developing a disseminated infection is not known. The contribution of the underlying disease and/or prior corticosteroid treatment to the risk is also not known. If exposed to chickenpox, prophylaxis with varicella zoster immune globulin (VZIG) may be indicated. If exposed to measles, prophylaxis with pooled intramuscular immunoglobulin (IG) may be indicated. (See the respective package inserts for complete VZIG and IG prescribing information.) If chickenpox develops, treatment with antiviral agents may be considered.

Fluticasone propionate inhalation aerosol is not to be regarded as a bronchodilator and is not indicated for rapid relief of bronchospasm.

As with other inhaled asthma medications, bronchospasm may occur with an immediate increase in wheezing after dosing. If bronchospasm occurs following dosing with Flovent inhalation aerosol, it should be treated immediately with a fast-acting inhaled bronchodilator. Treatment with Flovent inhalation aerosol should be discontinued and alternative therapy instituted.

Patients should be instructed to contact their physicians immediately when episodes of asthma that are not responsive to bronchodilators occur during the course of treatment with fluticasone propionate inhalation aerosol. During such episodes, patients may require therapy with oral corticosteroids.

FLOVENT DISKUS

Particular care is needed for patients who are transferred from systemically active corticosteroids to Flovent Diskus because deaths due to adrenal insufficiency have occurred in patients with asthma during and after transfer

Cont'd

from systemic corticosteroids to less systemically available inhaled corticosteroids. After withdrawal from systemic corticosteroids, a number of months are required for recovery of HPA function.

Patients who have been previously maintained on 20 mg or more per day of prednisone (or its equivalent) may be most susceptible, particularly when their systemic corticosteroids have been almost completely withdrawn. During this period of HPA suppression, patients may exhibit signs and symptoms of adrenal insufficiency when exposed to trauma, surgery, or infection (particularly gastroenteritis) or other conditions associated with severe electrolyte loss. Although fluticasone propionate inhalation powder may provide control of asthma symptoms during these episodes, in recommended doses it supplies less than normal physiological amounts of glucocorticoid systemically and does NOT provide the mineralocorticoid activity that is necessary for coping with these emergencies.

During periods of stress or a severe asthma attack, patients who have been withdrawn from systemic corticosteroids should be instructed to resume oral corticosteroids (in large doses) immediately and to contact their physicians for further instruction. These patients should also be instructed to carry a warning card indicating that they may need supplementary systemic corticosteroids during periods of stress or a severe asthma attack.

Patients requiring oral corticosteroids should be weaned slowly from systemic corticosteroid use after transferring to fluticasone propionate inhalation powder. In a clinical trial of 111 patients, prednisone reduction was successfully accomplished by reducing the daily prednisone dose by 2.5 mg on a weekly basis during transfer to inhaled fluticasone propionate. Successive reduction of prednisone dose was allowed only when lung function, symptoms, and as-needed beta-agonist use were better than or comparable to that seen before initiation of prednisone dose reduction. Lung function (FEV_1 or AM PEFR), beta-agonist use, and asthma symptoms should be carefully monitored during withdrawal of oral corticosteroids. In addition to monitoring asthma signs and symptoms, patients should be observed for signs and symptoms of adrenal insufficiency such as fatigue, lassitude, weakness, nausea and vomiting, and hypotension.

Transfer of patients from systemic corticosteroid therapy to fluticasone propionate inhalation powder may unmask conditions previously suppressed by the systemic corticosteroid therapy, *e.g.*, rhinitis, conjunctivitis, eczema, arthritis, and eosinophilic conditions.

Persons who are using drugs that suppress the immune system are more susceptible to infections than healthy individuals. Chickenpox and measles, for example, can have a more serious or even fatal course in susceptible children or adults using corticosteroids. In such children or adults who have not had these diseases or been properly immunized, particular care should be taken to avoid exposure. How the dose, route, and duration of corticosteroid administration affect the risk of developing a disseminated infection is not known. The contribution of the underlying disease and/or prior corticosteroid treatment to the risk is also not known. If exposed to chickenpox, prophylaxis with varicella zoster immune globulin (VZIG) may be indicated. If exposed to measles, prophylaxis with pooled intramuscular immunoglobulin (IG) may be indicated. (See the respective package inserts for complete VZIG and IG prescribing information.) If chickenpox develops, treatment with antiviral agents may be considered.

Fluticasone propionate inhalation powder is not to be regarded as a bronchodilator and is not indicated for rapid relief of bronchospasm.

As with other inhaled asthma medications, bronchospasm may occur with an immediate increase in wheezing after dosing. If bronchospasm occurs following dosing with Flovent Diskus, it should be treated immediately with a fast-acting inhaled bronchodilator. Treatment with Flovent Diskus should be discontinued and alternative therapy instituted.

Patients should be instructed to contact their physicians immediately when episodes of asthma that are not responsive to bronchodilators occur during the course of treatment with fluticasone propionate inhalation powder. During such episodes, patients may require therapy with oral corticosteroids.

FLOVENT ROTADISK

Particular care is needed for patients who are transferred from systemically active corticosteroids to Flovent Rotadisk because deaths due to adrenal insufficiency have occurred in asthmatic patients during and after transfer from systemic corticosteroids to less systemically available inhaled corticosteroids. After withdrawal from systemic corticosteroids, a number of months are required for recovery of HPA function.

Patients who have been previously maintained on 20 mg or more per day of prednisone (or its equivalent) may be most susceptible, particularly when their systemic corticosteroids have been almost completely withdrawn. During this period of HPA suppression, patients may exhibit signs and symptoms of adrenal insufficiency when exposed to trauma, surgery, or infection (particularly gastroenteritis) or other conditions associated with severe electrolyte loss. Although fluticasone propionate inhalation powder may provide control of asthma symptoms during these episodes, in recommended doses it supplies less than normal physiological amounts of corticosteroid systemically and does NOT provide the mineralocorticoid activity that is necessary for coping with these emergencies.

During periods of stress or a severe asthma attack, patients who have been withdrawn from systemic corticosteroids should be instructed to resume oral corticosteroids (in large doses) immediately and to contact their physicians for further instruction. These patients should also be instructed to carry a warning card indicating that they may need supplementary systemic corticosteroids during periods of stress or a severe asthma attack.

Patients requiring oral corticosteroids should be weaned slowly from systemic corticosteroid use after transferring to fluticasone propionate inhalation powder. In a clinical trial of 96 patients, prednisone reduction was successfully accomplished by reducing the daily prednisone dose by 2.5 mg on a weekly basis during transfer to inhaled fluticasone propionate. Successive reduction of prednisone dose was allowed only when lung function, symptoms, and as-needed beta-agonist use were better than or comparable to that seen before initiation of prednisone dose reduction. Lung function (FEV_1 or AM PEFR), beta-agonist use, and asthma symptoms should be carefully monitored during withdrawal of oral corticosteroids. In addition to monitoring asthma signs and symptoms, patients should be observed for signs and symptoms of adrenal insufficiency such as fatigue, lassitude, weakness, nausea and vomiting, and hypotension.

Transfer of patients from systemic corticosteroid therapy to fluticasone propionate inhalation powder may unmask conditions previously suppressed by the systemic corticosteroid therapy, *e.g.*, rhinitis, conjunctivitis, eczema, and arthritis.

Persons who are on drugs that suppress the immune system are more susceptible to infections than healthy individuals. Chickenpox and measles, for example, can have a more serious or even fatal course in susceptible children or adults on corticosteroids. In such children or adults who have not had these diseases, particular care should be taken to avoid exposure. How the dose, route, and duration of corticosteroid administration affects the risk of developing a disseminated infection is not known. The contribution of the underlying disease and/or prior corticosteroid treatment to the risk is also not known. If exposed to chickenpox, prophylaxis with varicella zoster immune globulin (VZIG) may be indicated. If exposed to measles, prophylaxis with pooled intramuscular immunoglobulin (IG) may be indicated. (See the respective package inserts for complete VZIG and IG prescribing information.) If chickenpox develops, treatment with antiviral agents may be considered.

Fluticasone propionate inhalation powder is not to be regarded as a bronchodilator and is not indicated for rapid relief of bronchospasm.

As with other inhaled asthma medications, bronchospasm may occur with an immediate increase in wheezing after dosing. If bronchospasm occurs following dosing with Flovent Rotadisk, it should be treated immediately with a fast-acting inhaled bronchodilator. Treatment with inhaled fluticasone propionate should be discontinued and alternative therapy instituted.

Patients should be instructed to contact their physicians immediately when episodes of asthma that are not responsive to bronchodilators occur during the course of treatment with fluticasone propionate inhalation powder. During such episodes, patients may require therapy with oral corticosteroids.

F

PRECAUTIONS

FLOVENT INHALATION AEROSOL

General

During withdrawal from oral corticosteroids, some patients may experience symptoms of systemically active corticosteroid withdrawal, *e.g.*, joint and/or muscular pain, lassitude, and depression, despite maintenance or even improvement of respiratory function.

Fluticasone propionate will often permit control of asthma symptoms with less suppression of HPA function than therapeutically equivalent oral doses of prednisone. Since fluticasone propionate is absorbed into the circulation and can be systemically active at higher doses, the beneficial effects of fluticasone propionate inhalation aerosol in minimizing HPA dysfunction may be expected only when recommended dosages are not exceeded and individual patients are titrated to the lowest effective dose. A relationship between plasma levels of fluticasone propionate and inhibitory effects on stimulated cortisol production has been shown after 4 weeks of treatment with fluticasone propionate inhalation aerosol. Since individual sensitivity to effects on cortisol production exists, physicians should consider this information when prescribing fluticasone propionate inhalation aerosol.

Because of the possibility of systemic absorption of inhaled corticosteroids, patients treated with these drugs should be observed carefully for any evidence of systemic corticosteroid effects. Particular care should be taken in observing patients postoperatively or during periods of stress for evidence of inadequate adrenal response.

It is possible that systemic corticosteroid effects such as hypercorticism and adrenal suppression may appear in a small number of patients, particularly at higher doses. If such changes occur, fluticasone propionate inhalation aerosol should be reduced slowly, consistent with accepted procedures for reducing systemic corticosteroids and for management of asthma symptoms.

A reduction of growth velocity in children or teenagers may occur as a result of inadequate control of chronic diseases such as asthma or from use of corticosteroids for treatment. Physicians should closely follow the growth of adolescents taking corticosteroids by any route and weigh the benefits of corticosteroid therapy and asthma control against the possibility of growth suppression if an adolescent's growth appears slowed.

The long-term effects of fluticasone propionate in human subjects are not fully known. In particular, the effects resulting from chronic use of fluticasone propionate on developmental or immunologic processes in the mouth, pharynx, trachea, and lung are unknown. Some patients have received fluticasone propionate inhalation aerosol on a continuous basis for periods of 3 years or longer. In clinical studies with patients treated for nearly 2 years with inhaled fluticasone propionate, no apparent differences in the type or severity of adverse reactions were observed after long- versus short-term treatment.

Rare instances of glaucoma, increased intraocular pressure, and cataracts have been reported following the inhaled administration of corticosteroids, including fluticasone propionate.

In clinical studies with inhaled fluticasone propionate, the development of localized infections of the pharynx with *Candida albicans* has occurred. When such an infection develops, it should be treated with appropriate local or systemic (*i.e.*, oral antifungal) therapy while remaining on treatment with fluticasone propionate inhalation aerosol, but at times therapy with fluticasone propionate may need to be interrupted.

Inhaled corticosteroids should be used with caution, if at all, in patients with active or quiescent tuberculosis infection of the respiratory tract; untreated systemic fungal, bacterial, viral or parasitic infections; or ocular herpes simplex.

Eosinophilic Conditions

In rare cases, patients on inhaled fluticasone propionate may present with systemic eosinophilic conditions, with some patients presenting with clinical features of vasculitis consistent with Churg-Strauss syndrome, a condition that is often treated with systemic corticosteroid therapy. These events usually, but not always, have been associated with the reduction and/or withdrawal of oral corticosteroid therapy following the introduction of fluticasone propionate. Cases of serious eosinophilic conditions have also been reported with other inhaled corticosteroids in this clinical setting. Physicians should be alert to eosinophilia, vasculitic rash, worsening pulmonary symptoms, cardiac complications, and/or neuropathy presenting in their patients. A causal relationship between fluticasone propionate and these underlying conditions has not been established (see ADVERSE REACTIONS, Flovent Inhalation Aerosol).

Information for the Patient

Patients being treated with Flovent inhalation aerosol should receive the following information and instructions. This information is intended to aid them in the safe and effective use of this medication. It is not a disclosure of all possible adverse or intended effects.

Patients should use Flovent inhalation aerosol at regular intervals as directed. Results of clinical trials indicated significant improvement may occur within the first day or 2 of treatment; however, the full benefit may not be achieved until treatment has been administered for 1-2 weeks or longer. The patient should not increase the prescribed dosage but should contact the physician if symptoms do not improve or if the condition worsens.

After inhalation, rinse the mouth with water without swallowing.

Patients should be warned to avoid exposure to chickenpox or measles and, if they are exposed, to consult their physicians without delay.

For the proper use of Flovent inhalation aerosol and to attain maximum improvement, the patient should read and follow carefully the accompanying Patient's Instructions for Use.

Carcinogenesis, Mutagenesis, and Impairment of Fertility

Fluticasone propionate demonstrated no tumorigenic potential in studies of oral doses up to 1000 μg/kg (approximately 2 times the maximum human daily inhalation dose based on μg/m^2) for 78 weeks in the mouse or inhalation of up to 57 μg/kg (approximately ¼ the maximum human daily inhalation dose based on μg/m^2) for 104 weeks in the rat.

Fluticasone propionate did not induce gene mutation in prokaryotic or eukaryotic cells *in vitro*. No significant clastogenic effect was seen in cultured human peripheral lymphocytes *in vitro* or in the mouse micronucleus test when administered at high doses by the oral or subcutaneous routes. Furthermore, the compound did not delay erythroblast division in bone marrow.

No evidence of impairment of fertility was observed in reproductive studies conducted in rats dosed subcutaneously with doses up to 50 μg/kg (approximately ¼ the maximum human daily inhalation dose based on μg/m^2) in males and females. However, prostate weight was significantly reduced in rats.

Pregnancy, Teratogenic Effects, Pregnancy Category C

Subcutaneous studies in the mouse and rat at 45 and 100 μg/kg, respectively (approximately 1/10 and 1/2 the maximum human daily inhalation dose based on μg/m^2, respectively), revealed fetal toxicity characteristic of potent glucocorticoid compounds, including embryonic growth retardation, omphalocele, cleft palate, and retarded cranial ossification.

In the rabbit, fetal weight reduction and cleft palate were observed following subcutaneous doses of 4 μg/kg (approximately 1/25 the maximum human daily inhalation dose based on μg/m^2). However, following oral administration of up to 300 μg/kg (approximately 3 times the maximum human daily inhalation dose based on μg/m^2) of fluticasone propionate to the rabbit, there were no maternal effects nor increased incidence of external, visceral, or skeletal fetal defects. No fluticasone propionate was detected in the plasma in this study, consistent with the established low bioavailability following oral administration (see CLINICAL PHARMACOLOGY, Flovent Inhalation Aerosol).

Less than 0.008% of the administered dose crossed the placenta following oral administration of 100 μg/kg to rats or 300 μg/kg to rabbits (approximately ½ and 3 times the maximum human daily inhalation dose based on μg/m^2, respectively).

There are no adequate and well-controlled studies in pregnant women. Fluticasone propionate should be used during pregnancy only if the potential benefit justifies the potential risk to the fetus.

Experience with oral glucocorticoids since their introduction in pharmacologic, as opposed to physiologic, doses suggests that rodents are more prone to teratogenic effects from glucocorticoids than humans. In addition, because there is a natural increase in glucocorticoid production during pregnancy, most women will require a lower exogenous glucocorticoid dose and many will not need glucocorticoid treatment during pregnancy.

Nursing Mothers

It is not known whether fluticasone propionate is excreted in human breast milk. Subcutaneous administration of 10 μg/kg tritiated drug to lactating rats (approximately 1/20 the maximum human daily inhalation dose based on μg/m^2) resulted in measurable radioactivity in both plasma and milk. Because glucocorticoids are excreted in human milk, caution should be exercised when fluticasone propionate inhalation aerosol is administered to a nursing woman.

Pediatric Use

One hundred thirty-seven (137) patients between the ages of 12 and 16 years were treated with fluticasone propionate inhalation aerosol in the US pivotal clinical trials. The safety and effectiveness of Flovent inhalation aerosol in children below 12 years of age have not been established. Oral corticosteroids have been shown to cause a reduction in growth velocity in children and teenagers with extended use. If a child or teenager on any corticosteroid appears to have growth suppression, the possibility that they are particularly sensitive to this effect of corticosteroids should be considered (see PRECAUTIONS, Flovent Inhalation Aerosol).

Geriatric Use

Five hundred seventy-four (574) patients 65 years of age or older have been treated with fluticasone propionate inhalation aerosol in US and non-US clinical trials. There were no differences in adverse reactions compared to those reported by younger patients.

FLOVENT DISKUS

General

Orally inhaled corticosteroids may cause a reduction in growth velocity when administered to pediatric patients (see Pediatric Use).

During withdrawal from oral corticosteroids, some patients may experience symptoms of systemically active corticosteroid withdrawal, *e.g.*, joint and/or muscular pain, lassitude, and depression, despite maintenance or even improvement of respiratory function.

Fluticasone propionate will often permit control of asthma symptoms with less suppression of HPA function than therapeutically equivalent oral doses of prednisone. Since fluticasone propionate is absorbed into the circulation and can be systemically active at higher doses, the beneficial effects of fluticasone propionate inhalation powder in minimizing HPA dysfunction may be expected only when recommended dosages are not exceeded and individual patients are titrated to the lowest effective dose. A relationship between plasma levels of fluticasone propionate and inhibitory effects on stimulated cortisol production has been shown after 4 weeks of treatment with fluticasone propionate inhalation aerosol. Since individual sensitivity to effects on cortisol production exists, physicians should consider this information when prescribing fluticasone propionate inhalation powder.

Because of the possibility of systemic absorption of inhaled corticosteroids, patients treated with these drugs should be observed carefully for any evidence of systemic corticosteroid effects. Particular care should be taken in observing patients postoperatively or during periods of stress for evidence of inadequate adrenal response.

It is possible that systemic corticosteroid effects such as hypercorticism and adrenal suppression may appear in a small number of patients, particularly at higher doses. If such changes occur, fluticasone propionate inhalation powder should be reduced slowly, consistent with accepted procedures for reducing systemic corticosteroids and for management of asthma symptoms.

The long-term effects of fluticasone propionate in human subjects are not fully known. In particular, the effects resulting from chronic use of fluticasone propionate on developmental or immunologic processes in the mouth, pharynx, trachea, and lung are unknown. Some patients have received inhaled fluticasone propionate on a continuous basis for periods of 3 years or longer. In clinical studies with patients treated for 2 years with inhaled fluticasone propionate, no apparent differences in the type or severity of adverse reactions were observed after long- versus short-term treatment.

Rare instances of glaucoma, increased intraocular pressure, and cataracts have been reported following the inhaled administration of corticosteroids, including fluticasone propionate.

In clinical studies with inhaled fluticasone propionate, the development of localized infections of the pharynx with *Candida albicans* has occurred. When such an infection develops, it should be treated with appropriate local or systemic (*i.e.*, oral antifungal) therapy while remaining on treatment with fluticasone propionate inhalation powder, but at times therapy with fluticasone propionate may need to be interrupted.

Inhaled corticosteroids should be used with caution, if at all, in patients with active or quiescent tuberculosis infections of the respiratory tract; untreated systemic fungal, bacterial, viral, or parasitic infections; or ocular herpes simplex.

Eosinophilic Conditions

In rare cases, patients on inhaled fluticasone propionate may present with systemic eosinophilic conditions, with some patients presenting with clinical features of vasculitis consistent with Churg-Strauss syndrome, a condition that is often treated with systemic corticosteroid therapy. These events usually, but not always, have been associated with the reduction and/or withdrawal of oral corticosteroid therapy following the introduction of fluticasone propionate. Cases of serious eosinophilic conditions have also been reported with other inhaled corticosteroids in this clinical setting. Physicians should be alert to eosinophilia, vasculitic rash, worsening pulmonary symptoms, cardiac complications, and/or neuropathy presenting in their patients. A causal relationship between fluticasone propionate and these underlying conditions has not been established (see ADVERSE REACTIONS, Flovent Diskus).

Information for the Patient

Patients being treated with Flovent Diskus should receive the following information and instructions. This information is intended to aid them in the safe and effective use of this medication. It is not a disclosure of all possible adverse or intended effects.

It is important that patients understand how to use the Diskus inhalation device appropriately and how it should be used in relation to other asthma medications they are taking.

Patients should be given the following information:

Patients should use Flovent Diskus at regular intervals as directed. Results of clinical trials indicated significant improvement may occur within the first day or 2 of treatment; however, the full benefit may not be achieved until treatment has been administered for 1-2 weeks or longer. The patient should not increase the prescribed dosage but should contact the physician if symptoms do not improve or if the condition worsens.

Flovent Diskus should not be used with a spacer device.

If you are pregnant or nursing, contact your physician about the use of Flovent Diskus.

Effective and safe use of Flovent Diskus includes an understanding of the way that it should be used:

Never exhale into the Diskus.

Never attempt to take the Diskus apart.

Always activate and use the Diskus in a level, horizontal position.

Never wash the mouthpiece or any part of the Diskus. KEEP IT DRY.

Always keep the Diskus in a dry place.

Discard **6 weeks (50 μg strength) or 2 months (100 and 250 μg strengths)** after removal from the moisture-protective foil overwrap pouch or after all blisters have been used (when the dose indicator reads "0"), whichever comes first.

Patients should be warned to avoid exposure to chickenpox or measles and, if they are exposed, to consult their physicians without delay.

For the proper use of Flovent Diskus and to attain maximum improvement, the patient should read and follow carefully the Patient's Instructions for Use accompanying the product.

Carcinogenesis, Mutagenesis, and Impairment of Fertility

Fluticasone propionate demonstrated no tumorigenic potential in mice at oral doses up to 1000 μg/kg (approximately 2 times the maximum recommended daily inhalation dose in adults and approximately 10 times the maximum recommended daily inhalation dose in children on a μg/m^2 basis) for 78 weeks or in rats at inhalation doses up to 57 μg/kg (less than the maximum recommended daily inhalation dose in adults and approximately equal to the maximum recommended daily inhalation dose in children on a μg/m^2 basis) for 104 weeks.

Fluticasone propionate did not induce gene mutation in prokaryotic or eukaryotic cells *in vitro*. No significant clastogenic effect was seen in cultured human peripheral lymphocytes *in vitro* or in the mouse micronucleus test.

No evidence of impairment of fertility was observed in reproductive studies conducted in male and female rats at subcutaneous doses up to 50 μg/kg (less than the maximum recommended daily inhalation dose in adults on a μg/m^2 basis). Prostate weight was significantly reduced at a subcutaneous dose of 50 μg/kg.

Pregnancy, Teratogenic Effects, Pregnancy Category C

Subcutaneous studies in the mouse and rat at 45 and 100 μg/kg, respectively, (less than the maximum recommended daily inhalation dose in adults on a μg/m^2 basis) revealed fetal toxicity characteristic of potent corticosteroid compounds, including embryonic growth retardation, omphalocele, cleft palate, and retarded cranial ossification.

In the rabbit, fetal weight reduction and cleft palate were observed at a subcutaneous dose of 4 μg/kg (less than the maximum recommended daily inhalation dose in adults on a μg/m^2 basis). However, no teratogenic effects were reported at oral doses up to 300 μg/kg (approximately 3 times the maximum recommended daily inhalation dose in adults on a μg/m^2 basis) of fluticasone propionate. No fluticasone propionate was detected in the plasma in this study, consistent with the established low bioavailability following oral administration (see CLINICAL PHARMACOLOGY, Flovent Diskus).

Fluticasone propionate crossed the placenta following administration of a subcutaneous dose of 100 μg/kg to mice (less than the maximum recommended daily inhalation dose in adults on a μg/m^2 basis), a subcutaneous or an oral dose of 100 μg/kg to rats (less than the maximum recommended daily inhalation dose in adults on a μg/m^2 basis), and an oral dose of 300 μg/kg to rabbits (approximately 3 times the maximum recommended daily inhalation dose in adults on a μg/m^2 basis).

There are no adequate and well-controlled studies in pregnant women. Fluticasone propionate should be used during pregnancy only if the potential benefit justifies the potential risk to the fetus.

Experience with oral corticosteroids since their introduction in pharmacologic, as opposed to physiologic, doses suggests that rodents are more prone to teratogenic effects from corticosteroids than humans. In addition, because there is a natural increase in corticosteroid production during pregnancy, most women will require a lower exogenous corticosteroid dose and many will not need corticosteroid treatment during pregnancy.

Nursing Mothers

It is not known whether fluticasone propionate is excreted in human breast milk. However, other corticosteroids have been detected in human milk. Subcutaneous administration to lactating rats of 10 μg/kg of tritiated fluticasone propionate (less than the maximum recommended daily inhalation dose in adults on a μg/m^2 basis) resulted in measurable radioactivity in the milk. Since there are no data from controlled trials on the use of Flovent Diskus by nursing mothers, a decision should be made whether to discontinue nursing or to discontinue Flovent Diskus, taking into account the importance of Flovent Diskus to the mother.

Pediatric Use

Five hundred twenty (520) patients 4-11 years of age and 66 patients 12-16 years of age were treated with Flovent Diskus in US pivotal clinical trials. The safety and effectiveness of Flovent Diskus in children below 4 years of age have not been established.

Controlled clinical studies have shown that inhaled corticosteroids may cause a reduction in growth in pediatric patients. In these studies, the mean reduction in growth velocity was approximately 1 cm/year (range, 0.3-1.8 cm/year) and appears to depend upon the dose and duration of exposure. The specific growth effects of inhaled fluticasone propionate have also been studied in a controlled clinical trial (see data below). This effect was observed in the absence of laboratory evidence of HPA axis suppression, suggesting that growth velocity is a more sensitive indicator of systemic corticosteroid exposure in pediatric patients than some commonly used tests of HPA axis function. The long-term effects of this reduction in growth velocity associated with orally inhaled corticosteroids, including the impact on final adult height, are unknown. The potential for "catch-up" growth following discontinuation of treatment with orally inhaled corticosteroids has not been adequately studied. The growth of children and adolescents receiving orally inhaled corticosteroids, including Flovent Diskus, should be monitored routinely (*e.g.*, via stadiometry). The potential growth effects of prolonged treatment should be weighed against the clinical benefits obtained and the risks associated with alternative therapies. To minimize the systemic effects of orally inhaled corticosteroids, including Flovent Diskus, each patient should be titrated to the lowest dose that effectively controls his/her symptoms.

A 52 week, placebo-controlled study to assess the potential growth effects of fluticasone propionate inhalation powder at 50 and 100 μg twice daily was conducted in the US in 325 prepubescent children (244 males and 81 females) 4-11 years of age. The mean growth velocities at 52 weeks observed in the intent-to-treat population were 6.32 cm/year in the placebo group (n=76), 6.07 cm/year in the 50 μg group (n=98), and 5.66 cm/year in the 100 μg group (n=89). An imbalance in the proportion of children entering puberty between groups and a higher dropout rate in the placebo group due to poorly controlled asthma may be confounding factors in interpreting these data. A separate subset analysis of children who remained prepubertal during the study revealed growth rates at 52 weeks of 6.10 cm/year in the placebo group (n=57), 5.91 cm/year in the 50 μg group (n=74), and 5.67 cm/year in the 100 μg group (n=79). The clinical significance of these growth data is not certain. In children 8.5 years of age, the mean age of children in this study, the range for expected growth velocity is: *Boys:* 3rd percentile = 3.8 cm/year, 50th percentile = 5.4 cm/year, and 97th percentile = 7.0 cm/year; *Girls:* 3rd percentile = 4.2 cm/year, 50th percentile = 5.7 cm/year, and 97th percentile = 7.3 cm/year.

Geriatric Use

Of the total number of patients in clinical studies of Flovent Diskus, 152 were 65 years of age or older and 4 were 75 years of age or older. No overall differences in safety were observed between these patients and younger patients, and other reported clinical experience has not identified differences in responses between the elderly and younger patients, but greater sensitivity of some older individuals cannot be ruled out. Based on available data for Flovent Diskus, no adjustment of dosage of Flovent Diskus in geriatric patients is warranted.

FLOVENT ROTADISK

General

During withdrawal from oral corticosteroids, some patients may experience symptoms of systemically active corticosteroid withdrawal, *e.g.*, joint and/or muscular pain, lassitude, and depression, despite maintenance or even improvement of respiratory function.

Fluticasone propionate will often permit control of asthma symptoms with less suppression of HPA function than therapeutically equivalent oral doses of prednisone. Since fluticasone propionate is absorbed into the circulation and can be systemically active at higher doses, the beneficial effects of fluticasone propionate inhalation powder in minimizing HPA dysfunction may be expected only when recommended dosages are not exceeded and individual patients are titrated to the lowest effective dose. A relationship between plasma levels of fluticasone propionate and inhibitory effects on stimulated cortisol production has been shown after 4 weeks of treatment with fluticasone propionate inhalation aerosol. Since individual sensitivity to effects on cortisol production exists, physicians should consider this information when prescribing fluticasone propionate inhalation powder.

Because of the possibility of systemic absorption of inhaled corticosteroids, patients treated with these drugs should be observed carefully for any evidence of systemic corticosteroid effects. Particular care should be taken in observing patients postoperatively or during periods of stress for evidence of inadequate adrenal response.

It is possible that systemic corticosteroid effects such as hypercorticism and adrenal suppression may appear in a small number of patients, particularly at higher doses. If such changes occur, fluticasone propionate inhalation powder should be reduced slowly, consistent with accepted procedures for reducing systemic corticosteroids and for management of asthma symptoms.

A reduction of growth velocity in children or adolescents may occur as a result of poorly controlled asthma or from the therapeutic use of corticosteroids, including inhaled corticosteroids. A 52 week placebo-controlled study to assess the potential growth effects of fluticasone propionate inhalation powder at 50 and 100 μg twice daily was conducted in the US in 325 prepubescent children (244 males and 81 females), 4-11 years of age. The mean growth velocities at 52 weeks observed in the intent-to-treat population were 6.32 cm/year in the placebo group (n=76), 6.07 cm/year in the 50 μg group (n=98), and 5.66 cm/year in the 100 μg group (n=89). An imbalance in the proportion of children entering puberty between groups and a higher dropout rate in the placebo group due to poorly controlled asthma may be confounding factors in interpreting these data. A separate subset analysis of children who remained prepubertal during the study revealed growth rates at 52 weeks of 6.10 cm/year in the placebo group (n=57), 5.91 cm/year in the 50 μg group (n=74), and 5.67 cm/year in the 100 μg group (n=79). The clinical significance of these growth data is not certain. In children 8.5 years of age, the mean age of children in this study, the range for expected growth velocity is: *Boys:* 3rd percentile = 3.8 cm/year, 50th percentile = 5.4 cm/year, and 97th percentile = 7.0 cm/year; *Girls:* 3rd percentile = 4.2 cm/year, 50th percentile = 5.7 cm/year, and 97th percentile = 7.3 cm/year. The effects of long-term treatment of children with inhaled corticosteroids, including fluticasone propionate, on final adult height are not known. Physicians should closely follow the growth of children and adolescents taking corticosteroids by any route, and weigh the benefits of corticosteroid therapy against the possibility of growth suppression if growth appears slowed. Patients should be maintained on the lowest dose of inhaled corticosteroid that effectively controls their asthma.

The long-term effects of fluticasone propionate in human subjects are not fully known. In particular, the effects resulting from chronic use of fluticasone propionate on developmental or immunologic processes in the mouth, pharynx, trachea, and lung are unknown. Some patients have received inhaled fluticasone propionate on a continuous basis for periods of 3 years or longer. In clinical studies with patients treated for 2 years with inhaled fluticasone propionate, no apparent differences in the type or severity of adverse reactions were observed after long- versus short-term treatment.

Rare instances of glaucoma, increased intraocular pressure, and cataracts have been reported following the inhaled administration of corticosteroids, including fluticasone propionate.

In clinical studies with inhaled fluticasone propionate, the development of localized infections of the pharynx with *Candida albicans* has occurred. When such an infection develops, it should be treated with appropriate local or systemic (*i.e.*, oral antifungal) therapy while remaining on treatment with fluticasone propionate inhalation powder, but at times therapy with fluticasone propionate may need to be interrupted.

Inhaled corticosteroids should be used with caution, if at all, in patients with active or quiescent tuberculous infections of the respiratory tract; untreated systemic fungal, bacterial, viral, or parasitic infections; or ocular herpes simplex.

Eosinophilic Conditions

In rare cases, patients on inhaled fluticasone propionate may present with systemic eosinophilic conditions, with some patients presenting with clinical features of vasculitis consistent with Churg-Strauss syndrome, a condition that is often treated with systemic corticosteroid therapy. These events usually, but not always, have been associated with the reduction and/or withdrawal of oral corticosteroid therapy following the introduction of fluticasone propionate. Cases of serious eosinophilic conditions have also been reported with other inhaled corticosteroids in this clinical setting. Physicians should be alert to eosinophilia, vasculitic rash, worsening pulmonary symptoms, cardiac complications, and/or neuropathy presenting in their patients. A causal relationship between fluticasone propionate and these underlying conditions has not been established (see ADVERSE REACTIONS, Flovent Rotadisk).

Information for the Patient

Patients being treated with Flovent Rotadisk should receive the following information and instructions. This information is intended to aid them in the safe and effective use of this medication. It is not a disclosure of all possible adverse or intended effects.

Patients should use Flovent Rotadisk at regular intervals as directed. Results of clinical trials indicated significant improvement may occur within the first day or 2 of treatment; however, the full benefit may not be achieved until treatment has been administered for 1-2 weeks or longer. The patient should not increase the prescribed dosage but should contact the physician if symptoms do not improve or if the condition worsens.

Patients should be warned to avoid exposure to chickenpox or measles and, if they are exposed, to consult their physicians without delay.

For the proper use of Flovent Rotadisk inhalation powder and to attain maximum improvement, the patient should read and follow carefully the accompanying Patient's Instructions for Use.

Carcinogenesis, Mutagenesis, and Impairment of Fertility

Fluticasone propionate demonstrated no tumorigenic potential in mice at oral doses up to 1000 μg/kg (approximately 2 times the maximum recommended daily inhalation dose in adults and approximately 10 times the maximum recommended daily inhalation dose in children on a μg/m^2 basis) for 78 weeks or in rats at inhalation doses up to 57 μg/kg (approximately ¼ the maximum recommended daily inhalation dose in adults and comparable to the maximum recommended daily inhalation dose in children on a μg/m^2 basis) for 104 weeks.

Fluticasone propionate did not induce gene mutation in prokaryotic or eukaryotic cells *in vitro*. No significant clastogenic effect was seen in cultured human peripheral lymphocytes *in vitro* or in the mouse micronucleus test when administered at high doses by the oral or subcutaneous routes. Furthermore, the compound did not delay erythroblast division in bone marrow.

F

No evidence of impairment of fertility was observed in reproductive studies conducted in male and female rats at subcutaneous doses up to 50 μg/kg (approximately 1/5 the maximum recommended daily inhalation dose in adults on a μg/m^2 basis). Prostate weight was significantly reduced at a subcutaneous dose of 50 μg/kg.

Pregnancy, Teratogenic Effects, Pregnancy Category C

Subcutaneous studies in the mouse and rat at 45 and 100 μg/kg, respectively, (approximately 1/10 and 1/3, respectively, the maximum recommended daily inhalation dose in adults on a μg/m^2 basis) revealed fetal toxicity characteristic of potent corticosteroid compounds, including embryonic growth retardation, omphalocele, cleft palate, and retarded cranial ossification.

In the rabbit, fetal weight reduction and cleft palate were observed at a subcutaneous dose of 4 μg/kg (approximately 1/30 the maximum recommended daily inhalation dose in adults on a μg/m^2 basis). However, no teratogenic effects were reported at oral doses up to 300 μg/kg (approximately 2 times the maximum recommended daily inhalation dose in adults on a μg/m^2 basis) of fluticasone propionate. No fluticasone propionate was detected in the plasma in this study, consistent with the established low bioavailability following oral administration (see CLINICAL PHARMACOLOGY, Flovent Rotadisk).

Fluticasone propionate crossed the placenta following oral administration of 100 μg/kg to rats or 300 μg/kg to rabbits (approximately 1/3 and 2 times, respectively, the maximum recommended daily inhalation dose in adults on a μg/m^2 basis).

There are no adequate and well-controlled studies in pregnant women. Fluticasone propionate should be used during pregnancy only if the potential benefit justifies the potential risk to the fetus.

Experience with oral corticosteroids since their introduction in pharmacologic, as opposed to physiologic, doses suggests that rodents are more prone to teratogenic effects from corticosteroids than humans. In addition, because there is a natural increase in corticosteroid production during pregnancy, most women will require a lower exogenous corticosteroid dose and many will not need corticosteroid treatment during pregnancy.

Nursing Mothers

It is not known whether fluticasone propionate is excreted in human breast milk. Subcutaneous administration to lactating rats of 10 μg/kg tritiated fluticasone propionate (approximately 1/25 the maximum recommended daily inhalation dose in adults on a μg/m^2 basis) resulted in measurable radioactivity in milk. Because other corticosteroids are excreted in human milk, caution should be exercised when fluticasone propionate inhalation powder is administered to a nursing woman.

Pediatric Use

Two hundred fourteen (214) patients 4-11 years of age and 142 patients 12-16 years of age were treated with fluticasone propionate inhalation powder in US clinical trials. The safety and effectiveness of Flovent Rotadisk inhalation powder in children below 4 years of age have not been established.

Inhaled corticosteroids, including fluticasone propionate, may cause a reduction in growth in children and adolescents (see PRECAUTIONS, Flovent Rotadisk). If a child or adolescent on any corticosteroid appears to have growth suppression, the possibility that they are particularly sensitive to this effect of corticosteroids should be considered. Patients should be maintained on the lowest dose of inhaled corticosteroid that effectively controls their asthma.

Geriatric Use

Safety data have been collected on 280 patients (Flovent Diskus n=83, Flovent Rotadisk n=197) 65 years of age or older and 33 patients (Flovent Diskus n=14, Flovent Rotadisk n=19) 75 years of age or older who have been treated with fluticasone propionate inhalation powder in US and non-US clinical trials. There were no differences in adverse reactions compared to those reported by younger patients. In addition, there were no apparent differences in efficacy between patients 65 years of age or older and younger patients. Fifteen (15) patients 65 years of age or older and 1 patient 75 years of age or older were included in the efficacy evaluation of US clinical studies.

DRUG INTERACTIONS

FLOVENT DISKUS

In a placebo-controlled, crossover study in 8 healthy volunteers, coadministration of a single dose of fluticasone propionate (1000 μg) with multiple doses of ketoconazole (200 mg) to steady state resulted in increased mean fluticasone propionate concentrations, a reduction in plasma cortisol AUC, and no effect on urinary excretion of cortisol. This interaction may be due to an inhibition of cytochrome P450 3A4 by ketoconazole, which is also the route of metabolism of fluticasone propionate. Care should be exercised when Flovent is coadministered with long-term ketoconazole and other known cytochrome P450 3A4 inhibitors.

FLOVENT ROTADISK

In a placebo-controlled, crossover study in 8 healthy volunteers, coadministration of a single dose of fluticasone propionate (1000 μg) with multiple doses of ketoconazole (200 mg) to steady state resulted in increased mean fluticasone propionate concentrations, a reduction in plasma cortisol AUC, and no effect on urinary excretion of cortisol. This interaction may be due to an inhibition of the cytochrome P450 3A4 isoenzyme system by ketoconazole, which is also the route of metabolism of fluticasone propionate. Care should be exercised when Flovent is coadministered with long-term ketoconazole and other known cytochrome P450 3A4 inhibitors.

ADVERSE REACTIONS

FLOVENT INHALATION AEROSOL

The incidence of common adverse experiences in TABLE 1 is based upon 7 placebo-controlled US clinical trials in which 1243 patients (509 female and 734 male adolescents and adults previously treated with as-needed bronchodilators and/or inhaled corticosteroids) were treated with fluticasone propionate inhalation aerosol (doses of 88-440 μg twice daily for up to 12 weeks) or placebo.

TABLE 1 *Overall Adverse Experiences With >3% Incidence on Fluticasone Propionate in US Controlled Clinical Trials With MDI in Patients Previously Receiving Bronchodilators and/or Inhaled Corticosteroids*

		Flovent Twice Daily		
Adverse Event	Placebo (n=475)	88 μg (n=488)	220 μg (n=95)	440 μg (n=185)
Ear, Nose, and Throat				
Pharyngitis	7%	10%	14%	14%
Nasal congestion	8%	8%	16%	10%
Sinusitis	4%	3%	6%	5%
Nasal discharge	3%	5%	4%	4%
Dysphonia	1%	4%	3%	8%
Allergic rhinitis	4%	5%	3%	3%
Oral candidiasis	1%	2%	3%	5%
Respiratory				
Upper respiratory infection	12%	15%	22%	16%
Influenza	2%	3%	8%	5%
Neurological				
Headache	14%	17%	22%	17%
Average Duration of Exposure (days)	44	66	64	59

TABLE 1 includes all events (whether considered drug-related or nondrug-related by the investigator) that occurred at a rate of over 3% in the combined fluticasone propionate inhalation aerosol groups and were more common than in the placebo group. In considering these data, differences in average duration of exposure should be taken into account.

These adverse reactions were mostly mild to moderate in severity, with ≤2% of patients discontinuing the studies because of adverse events. Rare cases of immediate and delayed hypersensitivity reactions, including urticaria and rash and other rare events of angioedema and bronchospasm, have been reported.

Systemic glucocorticoid side effects were not reported during controlled clinical trials with fluticasone propionate inhalation aerosol. If recommended doses are exceeded, however, or if individuals are particularly sensitive, symptoms of hypercorticism, *e.g.*, Cushing's syndrome, could occur.

Other adverse events that occurred in these clinical trials using fluticasone propionate inhalation aerosol with an incidence of 1-3% and which occurred at a greater incidence than with placebo were:

Ear, Nose, and Throat: Pain in nasal sinus(es), rhinitis.
Eye: Irritation of the eye(s).
Gastrointestinal: Nausea and vomiting, diarrhea, dyspepsia and stomach disorder.
Miscellaneous: Fever.
Mouth and Teeth: Dental problem.
Musculoskeletal: Pain in joint, sprain/strain, aches and pains, pain in limb.
Neurological: Dizziness/giddiness.
Respiratory: Bronchitis, chest congestion.
Skin: Dermatitis, rash/skin eruption.
Urogenital: Dysmenorrhea.

In a 16 week study in patients with asthma requiring oral corticosteroids, the effects of fluticasone propionate inhalation aerosol, 660 μg twice daily (n=32) and 880 μg twice daily (n=32), were compared with placebo.

Adverse events (whether considered drug-related or nondrug-related by the investigator) reported by more than 3 patients in either fluticasone propionate group and which were more common with fluticasone propionate than placebo are:

Ear, Nose, and Throat: Pharyngitis (9% and 25%), nasal congestion (19% and 22%), sinusitis (19% and 22%), nasal discharge (16% and 16%), dysphonia (19% and 9%), pain in nasal sinus(es) (13% and 0%), Candida-like oral lesions (16% and 9%), oropharyngeal candidiasis (25% and 19%).

Respiratory: Upper respiratory infection (31% and 19%), influenza (0% and 13%).

Other: Headache (28% and 34%), pain in joint (19% and 13%), nausea and vomiting (22% and 16%), muscular soreness (22% and 13%), malaise/fatigue (22% and 28%), insomnia (3% and 13%).

Observed During Clinical Practice

In addition to adverse experiences reported from clinical trials, the following experiences have been identified during postapproval use of fluticasone propionate. Because they are reported voluntarily from a population of unknown size, estimates of frequency cannot be made. These experiences have been chosen for inclusion due to either their seriousness, frequency of reporting, causal connection to fluticasone propionate, or a combination of these factors.

Ear, Nose, and Throat: Aphonia, facial and oropharyngeal edema, hoarseness, laryngitis, and throat soreness and irritation.

Endocrine and Metabolic: Cushingoid features, growth velocity reduction in children/adolescents, hyperglycemia, osteoporosis, and weight gain.

Eye: Cataracts.

Psychiatry: Agitation, aggression, depression, and restlessness.

Respiratory: Asthma exacerbation, bronchospasm, chest tightness, cough, dyspnea, immediate bronchospasm, parodoxical bronchospasm, pneumonia, and wheeze.

Skin: Contusions, ecchymoses, and pruritus.

Eosinophilic Conditions

In rare cases, patients on inhaled fluticasone propionate may present with systemic eosinophilic conditions, with some patients presenting with clinical features of vasculitis consistent with Churg-Strauss syndrome, a condition that is often treated with systemic corticosteroid therapy. These events usually, but not always, have been associated with the reduction and/or withdrawal of oral corticosteroid therapy following the introduction of fluticasone propionate. Cases of serious eosinophilic conditions have also been reported with other inhaled corticosteroids in this clinical setting. Physicians should be alert to eosinophilia, vasculitic rash, worsening pulmonary symptoms, cardiac complications, and/or neuropathy presenting in their patients. A causal relationship between fluticasone propionate and these underlying conditions has not been established (see PRECAUTIONS, Flovent Inhalation Aerosol, Eosinophilic Conditions).

FLOVENT DISKUS

The incidence of common adverse experiences in TABLE 2 is based upon 7 placebo-controlled US clinical trials in which 1176 pediatric, adolescent, and adult patients (466 females and 710 males) previously treated with as-needed bronchodilators and/or inhaled corticosteroids were treated with fluticasone propionate inhalation powder (doses of 50-500 μg twice daily for up to 12 weeks) or placebo.

TABLE 2 *Overall Adverse Experiences With >3% Incidence on Fluticasone Propionate in US Controlled Clinical Trials With Flovent Diskus in Patients Previously Receiving Bronchodilators and/or Inhaled Corticosteroids*

		Flovent Diskus Twice Daily			
Adverse Event	**Placebo (n=543)**	**50 μg (n=178)**	**100 μg (n=305)**	**250 μg (n=86)**	**500 μg (n=64)**
Ear, Nose, and Throat					
Upper respiratory tract infection	16%	20%	18%	21%	14%
Throat irritation	8%	13%	13%	3%	22%
Sinusitis/sinus infection	6%	9%	10%	6%	6%
Upper respiratory inflammation	3%	5%	5%	0%	5%
Rhinitis	2%	4%	3%	1%	2%
Oral candidiasis	7%	<1%	9%	6%	5%
Gastrointestinal					
Nausea and vomiting	4%	8%	4%	1%	2%
Gastrointestinal discomfort and pain	3%	4%	3%	2%	2%
Viral gastrointestinal infection	1%	4%	3%	3%	5%
Non-Site Specific					
Fever	4%	7%	7%	1%	2%
Viral infection	2%	2%	2%	0%	5%
Lower Respiratory					
Viral respiratory infection	4%	4%	5%	1%	2%
Cough	4%	3%	5%	1%	5%
Bronchitis	1%	2%	3%	0%	8%
Neurological					
Headache	7%	12%	12%	2%	14%
Musculoskeletal and Trauma					
Muscle injury	1%	2%	0%	1%	5%
Musculoskeletal pain	2%	4%	3%	2%	5%
Injury	<1%	2%	<1%	0%	5%
Average Duration of Exposure (days)	56	76	73	79	78

TABLE 2 includes all events (whether considered drug-related or nondrug-related by the investigator) that occurred at a rate of over 3% in any of the fluticasone propionate inhalation powder groups and were more common than in the placebo group. In considering these data, differences in average duration of exposure should be taken into account.

These adverse reactions were mostly mild to moderate in severity, with <2% of patients discontinuing the studies because of adverse events. Rare cases of immediate and delayed hypersensitivity reactions, including rash and other rare events of angioedema and bronchospasm, have been reported.

Other adverse events that occurred in these clinical trials using fluticasone propionate inhalation powder with an incidence of 1-3% and that occurred at a greater incidence than with placebo were:

Cardiovascular: Palpitations.

Drug Interaction, Overdose, and Trauma: Soft tissue injuries; contusions and hematomas; wounds and lacerations; postoperative complications; burns; poisoning and toxicity; pressure-induced disorders.

Ear, Nose, and Throat: Ear signs and symptoms; rhinorrhea/postnasal drip; hoarseness/dysphonia; epistaxis; tonsillitis; nasal signs and symptoms; laryngitis; unspecified oropharyngeal plaques; otitis; ear, nose, throat, and tonsil signs and symptoms; ear, nose, and throat polyps; allergic ear, nose, and throat disorders; throat constriction.

Endocrine and Metabolic: Fluid disturbances; weight gain; goiter; disorders of uric acid metabolism; appetite disturbances.

Eye: Keratitis and conjunctivitis; blepharoconjunctivitis.

Gastrointestinal: Diarrhea; gastrointestinal signs and symptoms; oral ulcerations; dental discomfort and pain; gastroenteritis; gastrointestinal infections; abdominal discomfort and pain; oral erythema and rashes; mouth and tongue disorders; oral discomfort and pain; tooth decay.

Hepatobiliary Tract and Pancreas: Cholecystitis.

Lower Respiratory: Lower respiratory infections.

Musculoskeletal: Muscle pain; arthralgia and articular rheumatism; muscle cramps and spasms; musculoskeletal inflammation.

Neurological: Dizziness; sleep disorders; migraines; paralysis of cranial nerves.

Non-Site Specific: Chest symptoms; malaise and fatigue; pain; edema and swelling; bacterial infections; fungal infections; mobility disorders; cysts, lumps, and masses.

Psychiatry: Mood disorders.

Reproduction: Bacterial reproductive infections.

Skin: Skin rashes; urticaria; photodermatitis; dermatitis and dermatosis; viral skin infections; eczema; fungal skin infections; pruritus; acne and folliculitis.

Urology: Urinary infections.

Three (3) of the 7 placebo-controlled US clinical trials were pediatric studies. A total of 592 patients 4-11 years were treated with Flovent Diskus (doses of 50 or 100 μg twice daily) or placebo; an additional 174 patients 4-11 years received Flovent Rotadisk at the same doses. There were no clinically relevant differences in the pattern or severity of adverse events in children compared with those reported in adults.

In the first 16 weeks of a 52 week clinical trial in adult asthma patients who previously required oral corticosteroids (daily doses of 5-40 mg oral prednisone), the effects of Flovent Diskus 500 μg twice daily (n=41) and 1000 μg twice daily (n=36) were compared with placebo (n=34) for the frequency of reported adverse events. Adverse events, whether or not considered drug related by the investigators, reported in more than 5 patients in the group taking Flovent Diskus and that occurred more frequently with Flovent Diskus than with placebo are shown below (percent Flovent Diskus and percent placebo). In considering these data, the increased average duration of exposure for patients taking Flovent Diskus (105 days for Flovent Diskus versus 75 days for placebo) should be taken into account.

Ear, Nose, and Throat: Hoarseness/dysphonia (9% and 0%), nasal congestion/blockage (16% and 0%), oral candidiasis (31% and 21%), rhinitis (13% and 9%), sinusitis/sinus infection (33% and 12%), throat irritation (10% and 9%), and upper respiratory tract infection (31% and 24%).

Gastrointestinal: Nausea and vomiting (9% and 0%).

Lower Respiratory: Cough (9% and 3%) and viral respiratory infections (9% and 6%).

Musculoskeletal: Arthralgia and articular rheumatism (17% and 3%) and muscle pain (12% and 0%).

Non-Site Specific: Malaise and fatigue (16% and 9%) and pain (10% and 3%).

Skin: Pruritus (6% and 0%) and skin rashes (8% and 3%).

Observed During Clinical Practice

In addition to adverse events reported from clinical trials, the following events have been identified during postapproval use of fluticasone propionate in clinical practice. Because they are reported voluntarily from a population of unknown size, estimates of frequency cannot be made. These events have been chosen for inclusion due to either their seriousness, frequency of reporting, or causal connection to fluticasone propionate or a combination of these factors.

Ear, Nose, and Throat: Aphonia and throat soreness.

Endocrine and Metabolic: Cushingoid features, growth velocity reduction in children/adolescents, hyperglycemia, weight gain, and osteoporosis.

Eye: Cataracts.

Psychiatry: Agitation, aggression, depression, and restlessness.

Respiratory: Asthma exacerbation, bronchospasm, chest tightness, cough, dyspnea, immediate bronchospasm, wheeze, and pneumonia.

Skin: Contusions and ecchymoses.

Eosinophilic Conditions

In rare cases, patients on inhaled fluticasone propionate may present with systemic eosinophilic conditions, with some patients presenting with clinical features of vasculitis consistent with Churg-Strauss syndrome, a condition that is often treated with systemic corticosteroid therapy. These events usually, but not always, have been associated with the reduction and/or withdrawal of oral corticosteroid therapy following the introduction of fluticasone propionate. Cases of serious eosinophilic conditions have also been reported with other inhaled corticosteroids in this clinical setting. Physicians should be alert to eosinophilia, vasculitic rash, worsening pulmonary symptoms, cardiac complications, and/or neuropathy presenting in their patients. A causal relationship between fluticasone propionate and these underlying conditions has not been established (see PRECAUTIONS, Flovent Diskus, Eosinophilic Conditions).

FLOVENT ROTADISK

The incidence of common adverse experiences in TABLE 3 is based upon 6 placebo-controlled clinical trials in which 1384 patients ≥4 years of age (520 females and 864 males) previously treated with as-needed bronchodilators and/or inhaled corticosteroids were treated with fluticasone propionate inhalation powder (doses of 50-500 μg twice daily for up to 12 weeks) or placebo.

TABLE 3 includes all events (whether considered drug-related or nondrug-related by the investigator) that occurred at a rate of over 3% in any of the fluticasone propionate inha-

TABLE 3 *Overall Adverse Experiences With >3% Incidence on Fluticasone Propionate in Controlled Clinical Trials With Flovent Rotadisk in Patients ≥4 Years Previously Receiving Bronchodilators and/or Inhaled Corticosteroids*

		Flovent Rotadisk Twice Daily			
	Placebo	50 µg	100 µg	250 µg	500 µg
Adverse Event	**(n=438)**	**(n=255)**	**(n=331)**	**(n=176)**	**(n=184)**
Ear, Nose, and Throat					
Pharyngitis	7%	6%	8%	8%	13%
Nasal congestion	5%	4%	4%	7%	7%
Sinusitis	4%	5%	4%	6%	4%
Rhinitis	4%	4%	9%	2%	3%
Dysphonia	0%	<1%	4%	6%	4%
Oral candidiasis	1%	3%	3%	4%	11%
Respiratory					
Upper respiratory infection	13%	16%	17%	22%	16%
Influenza	2%	3%	3%	3%	4%
Bronchitis	2%	4%	2%	1%	2%
Other					
Headache	11%	11%	9%	14%	15%
Diarrhea	1%	2%	2%	0%	4%
Back problems	<1%	<1%	1%	1%	4%
Fever	3%	4%	4%	2%	2%
Average duration of exposure (days)	53	77	68	78	60

lation powder groups and were more common than in the placebo group. In considering these data, differences in average duration of exposure should be taken into account.

These adverse reactions were mostly mild to moderate in severity, with <2% of patients discontinuing the studies because of adverse events. Rare cases of immediate and delayed hypersensitivity reactions, including rash and other rare events of angioedema and bronchospasm, have been reported.

Other adverse events that occurred in these clinical trials using fluticasone propionate inhalation powder with an incidence of 1-3% and which occurred at a greater incidence than with placebo were:

Ear, Nose, and Throat: Otitis media, tonsillitis, nasal discharge, earache, laryngitis, epistaxis, sneezing.

Eye: Conjunctivitis.

Gastrointestinal: Abdominal pain, viral gastroenteritis, gastroenteritis/colitis, abdominal discomfort.

Miscellaneous: Injury.

Mouth and Teeth: Mouth irritation.

Musculoskeletal: Sprain/strain, pain in joint, disorder/symptoms of neck, muscular soreness, aches and pains.

Neurological: Migraine, nervousness.

Respiratory: Chest congestion, acute nasopharyngitis, dyspnea, irritation due to inhalant.

Skin: Dermatitis, urticaria.

Urogenital: Dysmenorrhea, candidiasis of vagina, pelvic inflammatory disease, vaginitis/vulvovaginitis, irregular menstrual cycle.

There were no clinically relevant differences in the pattern or severity of adverse events in children compared with those reported in adults.

Fluticasone propionate inhalation aerosol (660 or 880 µg twice daily) was administered for 16 weeks to asthmatics requiring oral corticosteroids. Adverse events reported more frequently in these patients compared to patients not on oral corticosteroids included sinusitis, nasal discharge, oropharyngeal candidiasis, headache, joint pain, nausea and vomiting, muscular soreness, malaise/fatigue, and insomnia.

Observed During Clinical Practice

In addition to adverse experiences reported from clinical trials, the following experiences have been identified during postapproval use of fluticasone propionate in clinical practice. Because they are reported voluntarily from a population of unknown size, estimates of frequency cannot be made. These events have been chosen for inclusion due to either their seriousness, frequency of reporting, causal connection to fluticasone propionate or a combination of these factors.

Ear, Nose, and Throat: Aphonia, facial and oropharyngeal edema, hoarseness, and throat soreness and irritation.

Endocrine and Metabolic: Cushingoid features, growth velocity reduction in children/adolescents, hyperglycemia, and weight gain.

Eye: Cataracts.

Psychiatry: Agitation, aggression, depression, and restlessness.

Respiratory: Asthma exacerbation, bronchospasm, chest tightness, cough, immediate bronchospasm, paradoxical bronchospasm, pneumonia, and wheeze.

Skin: Contusions, ecchymoses, and pruritus.

Eosinophilic Conditions

In rare cases, patients on inhaled fluticasone propionate may present with systemic eosinophilic conditions, with some patients presenting with clinical features of vasculitis consistent with Churg-Strauss syndrome, a condition that is often treated with systemic corticosteroid therapy. These events usually, but not always, have been associated with the reduction and/or withdrawal of oral corticosteroid therapy following the introduction of fluticasone propionate. Cases of serious eosinophilic conditions have also been reported with other inhaled corticosteroids in this clinical setting. Physicians should be alert to eosinophilia, vasculitic rash, worsening pulmonary symptoms, cardiac complications, and/or neuropathy presenting in their patients. A causal relationship between fluticasone propionate and these underlying conditions has not been established (see PRECAUTIONS, Flovent Rotadisk, Eosinophilic Conditions).

DOSAGE AND ADMINISTRATION

FLOVENT INHALATION AEROSOL

Flovent inhalation aerosol should be administered by the orally inhaled route in patients 12 years of age and older. Individual patients will experience a variable time to onset and degree of symptom relief. Generally, fluticasone propionate inhalation aerosol has a relatively rapid onset of action for an inhaled glucocorticoid. Improvement in asthma control following inhaled administration of fluticasone propionate can occur within 24 hours of beginning treatment, although maximum benefit may not be achieved for 1-2 weeks or longer after starting treatment.

After asthma stability has been achieved (see below), it is always desirable to titrate to the lowest effective dose to reduce the possibility of side effects. For patients who do not respond adequately to the starting dose after 2 weeks of therapy, higher doses may provide additional asthma control. The safety and efficacy of Flovent inhalation aerosol when administered in excess of recommended doses has not been established.

The recommended starting dose and the highest recommended dose of fluticasone propionate inhalation aerosol, based on prior antiasthma therapy, are listed in TABLE 4.

TABLE 4

Previous Therapy	Recommended Starting Dose	Highest Recommended Dose
Bronchodilators alone	88 µg twice daily	440 µg twice daily
Inhaled corticosteroids	88-220 µg twice daily*	440 µg twice daily
Oral corticosteroids†	880 µg twice daily	880 µg twice daily

* Starting doses above 88 µg twice daily may be considered for patients with poorer asthma control or those who have previously required doses of inhaled corticosteroids that are in the higher range for that specific agent.

NOTE: In all patients, it is desirable to titrate to the lowest effective dose once asthma stability is achieved.

† **For patients currently receiving chronic oral corticosteroid therapy:** Prednisone should be reduced no faster than 2.5 mg/day on a weekly basis, beginning after at least 1 week of therapy with Flovent inhalation aerosol. Patients should be carefully monitored for signs of asthma instability, including serial objective measures of airflow, and for signs of adrenal insufficiency (see WARNINGS, Flovent Inhalation Aerosol). Once prednisone reduction is complete, the dosage of fluticasone propionate should be reduced to the lowest effective dosage.

Geriatric Use

In studies where geriatric patients (65 years of age or older, see PRECAUTIONS, Flovent Inhalation Aerosol) have been treated with fluticasone propionate inhalation aerosol, efficacy and safety did not differ from that in younger patients. Consequently, no dosage adjustment is recommended.

Directions for Use

Illustrated Patient's Instructions for Use accompany each package of Flovent inhalation aerosol.

FLOVENT DISKUS

Flovent Diskus should be administered by the orally inhaled route in patients 4 years of age and older. Individual patients will experience a variable time to onset and degree of symptom relief. Generally, fluticasone propionate inhalation powder has a relatively rapid onset of action for an inhaled corticosteroid. Improvement in asthma control following inhaled administration of fluticasone propionate can occur within 24 hours of beginning treatment, although maximum benefit may not be achieved for 1-2 weeks or longer after starting treatment.

After asthma stability has been achieved, it is always desirable to titrate to the lowest effective dose to reduce the possibility of side effects. For patients who do not respond adequately to the starting dose after 2 weeks of therapy, higher doses may provide additional asthma control. The safety and efficacy of Flovent Diskus when administered in excess of recommended doses have not been established.

Rinsing the mouth after inhalation is advised.

The recommended starting dose and the highest recommended dose of fluticasone propionate inhalation powder, based on prior asthma therapy, are listed in TABLE 5.

Pediatric Use

Because individual responses may vary, children previously maintained on Flovent Rotadisk 50 or 100 µg twice daily may require dosage adjustments upon transfer to Flovent Diskus.

Geriatric Use

In studies where geriatric patients (65 years of age or older, see PRECAUTIONS, Flovent Diskus) have been treated with fluticasone propionate inhalation powder, efficacy and safety did not differ from that in younger patients. Based on available data for Flovent Diskus, no dosage adjustment is recommended.

Directions for Use

Illustrated Patient's Instructions for Use accompany each package of Flovent Diskus.

FLOVENT ROTADISK

Flovent Rotadisk should be administered by the orally inhaled route in patients 4 years of age and older. Individual patients will experience a variable time to onset and degree of symptom relief. Generally, fluticasone propionate inhalation powder has a relatively rapid onset of action for an inhaled corticosteroid. Improvement in asthma control following inhaled administration of fluticasone propionate can occur within 24 hours of beginning treatment, although maximum benefit may not be achieved for 1-2 weeks or longer after starting treatment.

After asthma stability has been achieved, it is always desirable to titrate to the lowest effective dose to reduce the possibility of side effects. Doses as low as 50 µg twice daily have been shown to be effective in some patients. For patients who do not respond ad-

TABLE 5

Previous Therapy	Recommended Starting Dose	Highest Recommended Dose
Adults and Adolescents		
Bronchodilators alone	100 µg twice daily	500 µg twice daily
Inhaled corticosteroids	100-250 µg twice daily*	500 µg twice daily
Oral corticosteroids†	500-1000 µg twice daily‡	1000 µg twice daily
Children 4-11 Years		
Bronchodilators alone	50 µg twice daily	100 µg twice daily
Inhaled corticosteroids	50 µg twice daily	100 µg twice daily

NOTE: In all patients, it is desirable to titrate to the lowest effective dose once asthma stability is achieved.

* Starting doses above 100 µg twice daily for adults and adolescents and 50 µg twice daily for children 4-11 years of age may be considered for patients with poorer asthma control or those who have previously required doses of inhaled corticosteroids that are in the higher range for that specific agent.

† **For patients currently receiving chronic oral corticosteroid therapy:** Prednisone should be reduced no faster than 2.5 mg/day on a weekly basis, beginning after at least 1 week of therapy with Flovent Diskus. Patients should be carefully monitored for signs of asthma instability, including serial objective measures of airflow, and for signs of adrenal insufficiency (see WARNINGS, Flovent Diskus). Once prednisone reduction is complete, the dosage of fluticasone propionate should be reduced to the lowest effective dosage.

‡ The choice of starting dose should be made on the basis of individual patient assessment. A controlled clinical study of 111 oral corticosteroid-dependent patients with asthma showed few significant differences between the 2 doses of Flovent Diskus on safety and efficacy endpoints. However, inability to decrease the dose of oral corticosteroids further during corticosteroid reduction may be indicative of the need to increase the dose of fluticasone propionate up to the maximum of 1000 µg twice daily.

equately to the starting dose after 2 weeks of therapy, higher doses may provide additional asthma control. The safety and efficacy of Flovent Rotadisk when administered in excess of recommended doses have not been established.

Rinsing the mouth after inhalation is advised.

The recommended starting dose and the highest recommended dose of fluticasone propionate inhalation powder, based on prior anti-asthma therapy, are listed in TABLE 6.

TABLE 6

Previous Therapy	Recommended Starting Dose	Highest Recommended Dose
Adults and Adolescents		
Bronchodilators alone	100 µg twice daily	500 µg twice daily
Inhaled corticosteroids	100-250 µg twice daily*	500 µg twice daily
Oral corticosteroids†	1000 µg twice daily‡	1000 µg twice daily‡
Children 4-11 Years		
Bronchodilators alone	50 µg twice daily	100 µg twice daily
Inhaled corticosteroids	50 µg twice daily	100 µg twice daily

* Starting doses above 100 µg twice daily for adults and adolescents and 50 µg twice daily for children 4-11 years of age may be considered for patients with poorer asthma control or those who have previously required doses of inhaled corticosteroids that are in the higher range for that specific agent.

NOTE: In all patients, it is desirable to titrate to the lowest effective dose once asthma stability is achieved.

† **For patients currently receiving chronic oral corticosteroid therapy:** Prednisone should be reduced no faster than 2.5 mg/day on a weekly basis, beginning after at least 1 week of therapy with Flovent. Patients should be carefully monitored for signs of asthma instability, including serial objective measures of airflow, and for signs of adrenal insufficiency (see WARNINGS, Flovent Rotadisk). Once prednisone reduction is complete, the dosage of fluticasone propionate should be reduced to the lowest effective dosage.

‡ This dosing recommendation is based on clinical data from a study conducted using Flovent inhalation aerosol. No clinical trials have been conducted in patients on oral corticosteroids using the Rotadisk formulation; no direct assessment of the clinical comparability of equal nominal doses for the Flovent Rotadisk and Flovent inhalation aerosol formulations in this population has been conducted.

Geriatric Use

In studies where geriatric patients (65 years of age or older, see PRECAUTIONS, Flovent Rotadisk) have been treated with fluticasone propionate inhalation powder, efficacy and safety did not differ from that in younger patients. Consequently, no dosage adjustment is recommended.

Directions for Use

Illustrated Patient's Instructions for Use accompany each package of Flovent Rotadisk.

HOW SUPPLIED

FLOVENT INHALATION AEROSOL

Flovent 44 µg inhalation aerosol is supplied in 7.9 g canisters containing 60 metered inhalations and in 13 g canisters containing 120 metered inhalations. Each canister is supplied with a dark orange-colored oral actuator with a peach-colored strapcap and patient's instructions. Each actuation of the inhaler delivers 44 µg of fluticasone propionate from the actuator.

Flovent 110 µg inhalation aerosol is supplied in 7.9 g canisters containing 60 metered inhalations and in 13 g canisters containing 120 metered inhalations. Each canister is supplied with a dark orange-colored oral actuator with a peach-colored strapcap and patient's instructions. Each actuation of the inhaler delivers 110 µg of fluticasone propionate from the actuator.

Flovent 220 µg inhalation aerosol is supplied in 7.9 g canisters containing 60 metered inhalations and in 13 g canisters containing 120 metered inhalations. Each canister is supplied with a dark orange-colored oral actuator with a peach-colored strapcap and patient's instructions. Each actuation of the inhaler delivers 220 µg of fluticasone propionate from the actuator.

Flovent canisters are for use with Flovent inhalation aerosol actuators only. The actuators should not be used with other aerosol medications.

The correct amount of medication in each inhalation cannot be assured after 60 inhalations from the 7.9 g canister or 120 inhalations from the 13 g canister even though the canister is not completely empty. The canister should be discarded when the labeled number of actuations has been used.

Storage

Store between 2 and 30°C (36 and 86°F). Store canister with mouthpiece down. Protect from freezing temperatures and direct sunlight.

Avoid spraying in eyes. Contents under pressure. Do not puncture or incinerate. Do not store at temperatures above 120°F. Keep out of reach of children. For best results, the canister should be at room temperature before use. Shake well before using.

Note: The statement below is required by the Federal Government's Clean Air Act for all products containing or manufactured with chlorofluorocarbons (CFCs).

WARNING: Contains trichlorofluoromethane and dichlorodifluoromethane, substances which harm public health and environment by destroying ozone in the upper atmosphere.

A notice similar to the above WARNING has been placed in the patient information leaflet of this product pursuant to EPA regulations.

F

FLOVENT DISKUS

Flovent Diskus 50 µg is supplied as a disposable, orange-colored device containing 60 blisters. The Diskus inhalation device is packaged within an orange-colored, plastic-coated, moisture-protective foil pouch. Flovent Diskus 50 µg is also supplied in an institutional pack of 1 orange-colored, disposable Diskus inhalation device containing 28 blisters. The Diskus inhalation device is packaged within an orange-colored, plastic-coated foil pouch.

Flovent Diskus 100 µg is supplied as a disposable, orange-colored device containing 60 blisters. The Diskus inhalation device is packaged within an orange-colored, plastic-coated, moisture-protective foil pouch. Flovent Diskus 100 µg is also supplied in an institutional pack of 1 orange-colored, disposable Diskus inhalation device containing 28 blisters. The Diskus inhalation device is packaged within an orange-colored, plastic-coated foil pouch.

Flovent Diskus 250 µg is supplied as a disposable, orange-colored device containing 60 blisters. The Diskus inhalation device is packaged within an orange-colored, plastic-coated, moisture-protective foil pouch. Flovent Diskus 250 µg is also supplied in an institutional pack of 1 orange-colored, disposable Diskus inhalation device containing 28 blisters. The Diskus inhalation device is packaged within an orange-colored, plastic-coated foil pouch.

Storage

Store at controlled room temperature, 20-25°C (68-77°F) in a dry place away from direct heat or sunlight. Keep out of reach of children. The Diskus inhalation device is not reusable. The device should be discarded 6 weeks (50 µg strength) or 2 months (100 and 250 µg strengths) after removal from the moisture-protective foil overwrap pouch or after all blisters have been used (when the dose indicator reads "0"), whichever comes first. Do not attempt to take the device apart.

FLOVENT ROTADISK

Flovent Rotadisk 50 µg is a circular double-foil pack containing 4 blisters of the drug and 1 dark orange- and peach-colored Diskhaler inhalation device.

Flovent Rotadisk 100 µg is a circular double-foil pack containing 4 blisters of the drug and 1 dark orange- and peach-colored Diskhaler inhalation device.

Flovent Rotadisk 250 µg is a circular double-foil pack containing 4 blisters of the drug and 1 dark orange- and peach-colored Diskhaler inhalation device.

Storage

Store at controlled room temperature, 20-25°C (68-77°F) in a dry place. Keep out of reach of children. Do not puncture any fluticasone propionate Rotadisk blister until taking a dose using the Diskhaler.

Use the Rotadisk blisters within 2 months after opening of the moisture-protective foil overwrap or before the expiration date, whichever comes first. Place the sticker provided with the product on the tube and enter the date the foil overwrap is opened and the 2 month use date.

INTRANASAL

DESCRIPTION

Note: The trade names have been used throughout this monograph for clarity.

For Intranasal Use Only.

SHAKE GENTLY BEFORE USE.

Fluticasone propionate, the active ingredient of Flonase nasal spray, is a synthetic corticosteroid with the chemical name of S-(fluoromethyl)6α,9-difluoro-11β-17-dihydroxy-16α-methyl-3-oxoandrosta-1,4-diene-17β-carbothioate, 17-propionate.

Fluticasone propionate is a white to off-white powder with a molecular weight of 500.6, and the empirical formula is $C_{25}H_{31}F_3O_5S$. It is practically insoluble in water, freely soluble in dimethyl sulfoxide and dimethylformamide, and slightly soluble in methanol and 95% ethanol.

Flonase nasal spray 50 µg is an aqueous suspension of microfine fluticasone propionate for topical administration to the nasal mucosa by means of a metering, atomizing spray pump. Flonase nasal spray also contains microcrystalline cellulose and carboxymethylcellulose sodium, dextrose, 0.02% w/w benzalkonium chloride, polysorbate 80, and 0.25% w/w phenylethyl alcohol, and has a pH between 5 and 7.

It is necessary to prime the pump before first use or after a period of non-use (1 week or more). After initial priming (6 actuations), each actuation delivers 50 µg of fluticasone propionate in 100 mg of formulation through the nasal adapter. Each 16 g bottle of Flonase nasal spray provides 120 metered sprays. After 120 metered sprays, the amount of fluticasone propionate delivered per actuation may not be consistent and the unit should be discarded.

CLINICAL PHARMACOLOGY

MECHANISM OF ACTION

Fluticasone propionate is a synthetic, trifluorinated corticosteroid with anti-inflammatory activity. *In vitro* dose response studies on a cloned human glucocorticoid receptor system involving binding and gene expression afforded 50% responses at 1.25 and 0.17 nM concentrations, respectively. Fluticasone propionate was 3- to 5-fold more potent than dexamethasone in these assays. Data from the McKenzie vasoconstrictor assay in man also support its potent glucocorticoid activity.

In preclinical studies, fluticasone propionate revealed progesterone-like activity similar to the natural hormone. However, the clinical significance of these findings in relation to the low plasma levels (see Pharmacokinetics) is not known.

F

The precise mechanism through which fluticasone propionate affects allergic rhinitis symptoms is not known. Corticosteroids have been shown to have a wide range of effects on multiple cell types (*e.g.*, mast cells, eosinophils, neutrophils, macrophages, and lymphocytes) and mediators (*e.g.*, histamine, eicosanoids, leukotrienes, and cytokines) involved in inflammation. In 7 trials in adults, fluticasone propionate nasal spray has decreased nasal mucosal eosinophils in 66% (35% for placebo) of patients and basophils in 39% (28% for placebo) of patients. The direct relationship of these findings to long-term symptom relief is not known.

Flonase nasal spray, like other corticosteroids, is an agent that does not have an immediate effect on allergic symptoms. A decrease in nasal symptoms has been noted in some patients 12 hours after initial treatment with Flonase nasal spray. Maximum benefit may not be reached for several days. Similarly, when corticosteroids are discontinued, symptoms may not return for several days.

PHARMACOKINETICS

Absorption

The activity of Flonase nasal spray is due to the parent drug, fluticasone propionate. Indirect calculations indicate that fluticasone propionate delivered by the intranasal route has an absolute bioavailability averaging less than 2%. After intranasal treatment of patients with allergic rhinitis for 3 weeks, fluticasone propionate plasma concentrations were above the level of detection (50 pg/ml) only when recommended doses were exceeded and then only in occasional samples at low plasma levels. Due to the low bioavailability by the intranasal route, the majority of the pharmacokinetic data was obtained via other routes of administration. Studies using oral dosing of radiolabeled drug have demonstrated that fluticasone propionate is highly extracted from plasma and absorption is low. Oral bioavailability is negligible, and the majority of the circulating radioactivity is due to an inactive metabolite.

Distribution

Following intravenous administration, the initial dispostion phase for fluticasone propionate was rapid and consistent with its high lipid solubility and tissue binding. The volume of distribution averaged 4.2 L/kg.

The percentage of fluticasone propionate bound to human plasma proteins averaged 91% with no obvious concentration relationship. Fluticasone propionate is weakly and reversibly bound to erythrocytes and freely equilibrates between erythrocytes and plasma. Fluticasone propionate is not significantly bound to human transcortin.

Metabolism

The total blood clearance of fluticasone propionate is high (average, 1093 ml/min), with renal clearance accounting for less than 0.02% of the total. The only circulating metabolite detected in man is the 17β-carboxylic acid derivative of fluticasone propionate, which is formed through the cytochrome P450 3A4 pathway. This inactive metabolite had less affinity (approximately 1/2000) than the parent drug for the glucocorticoid receptor of human lung cytosol *in vitro* and negligible pharmacological activity in animal studies. Other metabolites detected *in vitro* using cultured human hepatoma cells have not been detected in man.

Elimination

Following intravenous dosing, fluticasone propionate showed polyexponential kinetics and had a terminal elimination half-life of approximately 7.8 hours. Less than 5% of a radiolabeled oral dose was excreted in the urine as metabolites, with the remainder excreted in the feces as parent drug and metabolites.

SPECIAL POPULATIONS

Fluticasone propionate nasal spray was not studied in any special populations, and no gender-specific pharmacokinetic data have been obtained.

DRUG-DRUG INTERACTIONS

In a multiple-dose drug interaction study, coadministration of orally inhaled fluticasone propionate (500 µg twice daily) and erythromycin (333 mg three times daily) did not affect fluticasone propionate pharmacokinetics. In another drug interaction study, coadministration of orally inhaled fluticasone propionate (1000 µg, 5 times the maximum daily intranasal dose) and ketoconazole (200 mg once daily) resulted in increased fluticasone propionate concentrations and reduced plasma cortisol area under the plasma concentration versus time curve (AUC), but had no effect on urinary excretion of cortisol. Due to very low plasma concentrations achieved after intranasal dosing, clinically significant drug interactions are unlikely; however, since fluticasone propionate is a substrate of cytochrome P450 3A4, caution should be exercised when known strong cytochrome P450 3A4 inhibitors (*e.g.*, ritonavir, ketoconazole) are coadministered with fluticasone propionate as this could result in increased plasma concentrations of fluticasone propionate.

PHARMACODYNAMICS

In a trial to evaluate the potential systemic and topical effects of Flonase nasal spray on allergic rhinitis symptoms, the benefits of comparable drug blood levels produced by Flonase nasal spray and oral fluticasone propionate were compared. The doses used were 200 µg of Flonase nasal spray, the nasal spray vehicle (plus oral placebo), and 5 and 10 mg of oral fluticasone propionate (plus nasal spray vehicle) per day for 14 days. Plasma levels were undetectable in the majority of patients after intranasal dosing, but present at low levels in the majority after oral dosing. Flonase nasal spray was significantly more effective in reducing symptoms of allergic rhinitis than either the oral fluticasone propionate or the nasal vehicle. This trial demonstrated that the therapeutic effect of Flonase nasal spray can be attributed to the topical effects of fluticasone propionate.

In another trial, the potential systemic effects of Flonase nasal spray on the hypothalamic-pituitary-adrenal (HPA) axis were also studied in allergic patients. Flonase nasal spray given as 200 µg once daily or 400 µg twice daily was compared with placebo or oral prednisone 7.5 or 15 mg given in the morning. Flonase nasal spray at either dose for 4 weeks did not affect the adrenal response to 6 hour cosyntropin stimulation, while both doses of oral prednisone significantly reduced the response to cosyntropin.

INDICATIONS AND USAGE

Flonase nasal spray is indicated for the management of the nasal symptoms of seasonal and perennial allergic and nonallergic rhinitis in adults and pediatric patients 4 years of age and older.

Safety and effectiveness of Flonase nasal spray in children below 4 years of age have not been adequately established.

CONTRAINDICATIONS

Flonase nasal spray is contraindicated in patients with a hypersensitivity to any of its ingredients.

WARNINGS

The replacement of a systemic corticosteroid with a topical corticosteroid can be accompanied by signs of adrenal insufficiency, and in addition some patients may experience symptoms of withdrawal, *e.g.*, joint and/or muscular pain, lassitude, and depression. Patients previously treated for prolonged periods with systemic corticosteroids and transferred to topical corticosteroids should be carefully monitored for acute adrenal insufficiency in response to stress. In those patients who have asthma or other clinical conditions requiring long-term systemic corticosteroid treatment, too rapid a decrease in systemic corticosteroids may cause a severe exacerbation of their symptoms.

The concomitant use of intranasal corticosteroids with other inhaled corticosteroids could increase the risk of signs or symptoms of hypercorticism and/or suppression of the HPA axis.

Patients who are using drugs that suppress the immune system are more susceptible to infections than healthy individuals. Chickenpox and measles, for example, can have a more serious or even fatal course in susceptible children or adults using corticosteroids. In children or adults who have not had these diseases or been properly immunized, particular care should be taken to avoid exposure. How the dose, route, and duration of corticosteroid administration affect the risk of developing a disseminated infection is not known. The contribution of the underlying disease and/or prior corticosteroid treatment to the risk is also not known. If exposed to chickenpox, prophylaxis with varicella zoster immune globulin (VZIG) may be indicated. If exposed to measles, prophylaxis with pooled intramuscular immunoglobulin (IG) may be indicated. (See the respective package inserts for complete VZIG and IG prescribing information.) If chickenpox develops, treatment with antiviral agents may be considered.

Avoid spraying in eyes.

PRECAUTIONS

GENERAL

Intranasal corticosteroids may cause a reduction in growth velocity when administered to pediatric patients (see Pediatric Use).

Rarely, immediate hypersensitivity reactions or contact dermatitis may occur after the administration of Flonase nasal spray. Rare instances of wheezing, nasal septum perforation, cataracts, glaucoma and increased intraocular pressure have been reported following the intranasal application of corticosteroids, including fluticasone propionate.

Use of excessive doses of corticosteroids may lead to signs or symptoms of hypercorticism and/or suppression of HPA function.

Although systemic effects have been minimal with recommended doses of Flonase nasal spray, potential risk increases with larger doses. Therefore, larger than recommended doses of Flonase nasal spray should be avoided.

When used at higher than recommended doses or in rare individuals at recommended doses, systemic corticosteroid effects such as hypercorticism and adrenal suppression may appear. If such changes occur, the dosage of Flonase nasal spray should be discontinued slowly consistent with accepted procedures for discontinuing oral corticosteroid therapy.

In clinical studies with fluticasone propionate administered intranasally, the development of localized infections of the nose and pharynx with *Candida albicans* has occurred only rarely. When such an infection develops, it may require treatment with appropriate local therapy and discontinuation of treatment with Flonase nasal spray. Patients using Flonase nasal spray over several months or longer should be examined periodically for evidence of *Candida* infection or other signs of adverse effects on the nasal mucosa.

Intranasal corticosteroids should be used with caution, if at all, in patients with active or quiescent tuberculous infections of the respiratory tract; untreated local or systemic fungal or bacterial infections; systemic viral or parasitic infections; or ocular herpes simplex.

Because of the inhibitory effect of corticosteroids on wound healing, patients who have experienced recent nasal septal ulcers, nasal surgery, or nasal trauma should not use a nasal corticosteroid until healing has occurred.

INFORMATION FOR THE PATIENT

Patients being treated with Flonase nasal spray should receive the following information and instructions. This information is intended to aid them in the safe and effective use of this medication. It is not a disclosure of all possible adverse or intended effects.

Patients should be warned to avoid exposure to chickenpox or measles and, if exposed, to consult their physician without delay.

Patients should use Flonase nasal spray at regular intervals for optimal effect. Some patients (12 years of age and older) with seasonal allergic rhinitis may find as-needed use of 200 μg once daily effective for symptom control.

A decrease in nasal symptoms may occur as soon as 12 hours after starting therapy with Flonase nasal spray. Results in several clinical trials indicate statistically significant improvement within the first day or 2 of treatment; however, the full benefit of Flonase nasal spray may not be achieved until treatment has been administered for several days. The patient should not increase the prescribed dosage but should contact the physician if symptoms do not improve or if the condition worsens.

For the proper use of Flonase nasal spray and to attain maximum improvement, the patient should read and follow carefully the patient's instructions that accompany the product.

CARCINOGENESIS, MUTAGENESIS, AND IMPAIRMENT OF FERTILITY

Fluticasone propionate demonstrated no tumorigenic potential in mice at oral doses up to 1000 μg/kg (approximately 20 times the maximum recommended daily intranasal dose in adults and approximately 10 times the maximum recommended daily intranasal dose in children on a μg/m^2 basis) for 78 weeks or in rats at inhalation doses up to 57 μg/kg (approximately 2 times the maximum recommended daily intranasal dose in adults and approximately equivalent to the maximum recommended daily intranasal dose in children on a μg/m^2 basis) for 104 weeks.

Fluticasone propionate did not induce gene mutation in prokaryotic or eukaryotic cells *in vitro*. No significant clastogenic effect was seen in cultured human peripheral lymphocytes *in vitro* or in the mouse micronucleus test.

No evidence of impairment of fertility was observed in reproductive studies conducted in male and female rats at subcutaneous doses up to 50 μg/kg (approximately 2 times the maximum recommended daily intranasal dose in adults on a μg/m^2 basis). Prostate weight was significantly reduced at a subcutaneous dose of 50 μg/kg.

PREGNANCY, TERATOGENIC EFFECTS, PREGNANCY CATEGORY C

Subcutaneous studies in the mouse and rat at 45 and 100 μg/kg, respectively (approximately equivalent to and 4 times the maximum recommended daily intranasal dose in adults on a μg/m^2 basis, respectively) revealed fetal toxicity characteristic of potent corticosteroid compounds, including embryonic growth retardation, omphalocele, cleft palate, and retarded cranial ossification.

In the rabbit, fetal weight reduction and cleft palate were observed at a subcutaneous dose of 4 μg/kg (less than the maximum recommended daily intranasal dose in adults on a μg/m^2 basis). However, no teratogenic effects were reported at oral doses up to 300 μg/kg (approximately 25 times the maximum recommended daily intranasal dose in adults on a μg/m^2 basis) of fluticasone propionate to the rabbit. No fluticasone propionate was detected in the plasma in this study, consistent with the established low bioavailability following oral administration (see CLINICAL PHARMACOLOGY).

Fluticasone propionate crossed the placenta following oral administration of 100 μg/kg to rats or 300 μg/kg to rabbits (approximately 4 and 25 times, respectively, the maximum recommended daily intranasal dose in adults on a μg/m^2 basis).

There are no adequate and well-controlled studies in pregnant women. Fluticasone propionate should be used during pregnancy only if the potential benefit justifies the potential risk to the fetus.

Experience with oral corticosteroids since their introduction in pharmacologic, as opposed to physiologic, doses suggests that rodents are more prone to teratogenic effects from corticosteroids than humans. In addition, because there is a natural increase in corticosteroid production during pregnancy, most women will require a lower exogenous corticosteroid dose and many will not need corticosteroid treatment during pregnancy.

NURSING MOTHERS

It is not known whether fluticasone propionate is excreted in human breast milk. However, other corticosteroids have been detected in human milk. Subcutaneous administration to lactating rats of 10 μg/kg of tritiated fluticasone propionate (less than the maximum recommended daily intranasal dose in adults on a μg/m_2 basis) resulted in measurable radioactivity in the milk. Since there are no data from controlled trials on the use of intranasal fluticasone propionate by nursing mothers, caution should be exercised when Flonase nasal spray is administered to a nursing woman.

PEDIATRIC USE

Five hundred (500) patients aged 4-11 years of age and 440 patients aged 12-17 years were studied in US clinical trials with fluticasone propionate nasal spray. The safety and effectiveness of Flonase nasal spray in children below 4 years of age have not been established.

Controlled clinical studies have shown that intranasal corticosteroids may cause a reduction in growth velocity in pediatric patients. This effect has been observed in the absence of laboratory evidence of HPA axis suppression, suggesting that growth velocity is a more sensitive indicator of systemic corticosteroid exposure in pediatric patients than some commonly used tests of HPA axis function. The long-term effects of this reduction in growth velocity associated with intranasal corticosteroids, including the impact on final adult height, are unknown. The potential for "catch-up" growth following discontinuation of treatment with intranasal corticosteroids has not been adequately studied. The growth of pediatric patients receiving intranasal corticosteroids, including Flonase nasal spray, should be monitored routinely (*e.g.*, via stadiometry). The potential growth effects of prolonged treatment should be weighed against the clinical benefits obtained and the risks/benefits of treatment alternatives. To minimize the systemic effects of intranasal corticosteroids, including Flonase nasal spray, each patient should be titrated to the lowest dose that effectively controls his/her symptoms.

GERIATRIC USE

A limited number of patients 65 years of age and older (n=129) or 75 years of age and older (n=11) have been treated with Flonase nasal spray in US and non-US clinical trials. While the number of patients is too small to permit separate analysis of efficacy and safety, the adverse reactions reported in this population were similar to those reported by younger patients.

DRUG INTERACTIONS

In a placebo-controlled, crossover study in 8 healthy volunteers, coadministration of a single dose of orally inhaled fluticasone propionate (1000 μg, 5 times the maximum daily intranasal dose) with multiple doses of ketoconazole (200 mg) to steady state resulted in increased mean fluticasone propionate concentrations, a reduction in plasma cortisol AUC, and no effect on urinary excretion of cortisol. This interaction may be due to an inhibition of the cytochrome P450 3A4 by ketoconazole, which is also the route of metabolism of fluticasone propionate. No drug interaction studies have been conducted with Flonase nasal spray; however, care should be exercised when fluticasone propionate is coadministered with long-term ketoconazole and other known cytochrome P450 3A4 inhibitors.

ADVERSE REACTIONS

In controlled US studies, more than 3300 patients with seasonal allergic, perennial allergic, or perennial nonallergic rhinitis received treatment with intranasal fluticasone propionate. In general, adverse reactions in clinical studies have been primarily associated with irritation of the nasal mucous membranes, and the adverse reactions were reported with approximately the same frequency by patients treated with the vehicle itself. The complaints did not usually interfere with treatment. Less than 2% of patients in clinical trials discontinued because of adverse events; this rate was similar for vehicle placebo and active comparators.

Systemic corticosteroid side effects were not reported during controlled clinical studies up to 6 months' duration with Flonase nasal spray. If recommended doses are exceeded, however, or if individuals are particularly sensitive or taking Flonase nasal spray in conjunction with administration of other corticosteroids, symptoms of hypercorticism, *e.g.*, Cushing's syndrome, could occur.

The following incidence of common adverse reactions (>3%, where incidence in fluticasone propionate-treated subjects exceeded placebo) is based upon 7 controlled clinical trials in which 536 patients (57 girls and 108 boys aged 4-11 years, 137 female and 234 male adolescents and adults) were treated with Flonase nasal spray 200 μg once daily over 2-4 weeks and 2 controlled clinical trials in which 246 patients (119 female and 127 male adolescents and adults) were treated with Flonase nasal spray 200 μg once daily over 6 months (see TABLE 7). Also included in TABLE 7 are adverse events from 2 studies in which 167 children (45 girls and 122 boys aged 4-11 years) were treated with Flonase nasal spray 100 μg once daily for 2-4 weeks.

TABLE 7 *Overall Adverse Experiences With >3% Incidence on Fluticasone Propionate in Controlled Clinical Trials With Flonase Nasal Spray in Patients ≥4 Years With Seasonal or Perennial Allergic Rhinitis*

		Flonase Once Daily	
Adverse Experience	**Vehicle Placebo (n=758)**	**100 μg (n=167)**	**200 μg (n=782)**
Headache	14.6%	6.6%	16.1%
Pharyngitis	7.2%	6.0%	7.8%
Epistaxis	5.4%	6.0%	6.9%
Nasal burning/nasal irritation	2.6%	2.4%	3.2%
Nausea/vomiting	2.0%	4.8%	2.6%
Asthma symptoms	2.9%	7.2%	3.3%
Cough	2.8%	3.6%	3.8%

Other adverse events that occurred in ≤3% but ≥1% of patients and that were more common with fluticasone propionate (with uncertain relationship to treatment) included: Blood in nasal mucus, runny nose, abdominal pain, diarrhea, fever, flu-like symptoms, aches and pains, dizziness, bronchitis.

OBSERVED DURING CLINICAL PRACTICE

In addition to adverse events reported from clinical trials, the following events have been identified during postapproval use of fluticasone propionate in clinical practice. Because they are reported voluntarily from a population of unknown size, estimates of frequency cannot be made. These events have been chosen for inclusion due to either their seriousness, frequency of reporting, or causal connection to fluticasone propionate or a combination of these factors.

General: Hypersensitivity reactions, including angioedema, skin rash, edema of the face and tongue, pruritus, urticaria, bronchospasm, wheezing, dyspnea, and anaphylaxis/anaphylactoid reactions, which in rare instances were severe.

Ear, Nose, and Throat: Alteration or loss of sense of taste and/or smell and, rarely, nasal septal perforation, nasal ulcer, sore throat, throat irritation and dryness, cough, hoarseness, and voice changes.

Eye: Dryness and irritation, conjunctivitis, blurred vision, glaucoma, increased intraocular pressure, and cataracts.

Cases of growth suppression have been reported for intranasal corticosteroids, including Flonase (see PRECAUTIONS, Pediatric Use).

DOSAGE AND ADMINISTRATION

Patients should use Flonase nasal spray at regular intervals for optimal effect.

ADULTS

The recommended starting dosage in **adults** is 2 sprays (50 μg of fluticasone propionate each) in each nostril once daily (total daily dose, 200 μg). The same dosage divided into 100 μg given twice daily (*e.g.*, 8 AM and 8 PM) is also effective. After the first few days, patients may be able to reduce their dosage to 100 µg (1 spray in each nostril) once daily for maintenance therapy. Some patients (12 years of age and older) with seasonal allergic rhinitis may find as-needed use of 200 µg once daily effective for symptom control. Greater symptom control may be achieved with scheduled regular use.

ADOLESCENTS AND CHILDREN (4 YEARS OF AGE AND OLDER)

Patients should be started with 100 µg (1 spray in each nostril once daily). Patients not adequately responding to 100 µg may use 200 µg (2 sprays in each nostril). Once adequate control is achieved, the dosage should be decreased to 100 µg (1 spray in each nostril) daily.

The maximum total daily dosage should not exceed 2 sprays in each nostril (200 µg/day). Flonase nasal spray is not recommended for children under 4 years of age.

DIRECTIONS FOR USE

Illustrated patient's instructions for proper use accompany each package of Flonase nasal spray.

HOW SUPPLIED

Flonase nasal spray 50 µg is supplied in an amber glass bottle fitted with a white metering atomizing pump, white nasal adapter, and green dust cover in a box of 1 with patient's instructions for use. Each bottle contains a net fill weight of 16 g and will provide 120 actuations. Each actuation delivers 50 µg of fluticasone propionate in 100 mg of formulation through the nasal adapter. The correct amount of medication in each spray cannot be assured after 120 sprays even though the bottle is not completely empty. The bottle should be discarded when the labeled number of actuations has been used.

Storage: Store between 4 and 30°C (39 and 86°F).

TOPICAL

DESCRIPTION

Note: The trade names have been used throughout this monograph for clarity.

CUTIVATE CREAM, 0.05%

For Dermatologic Use Only — Not for Ophthalmic Use.

Cutivate (fluticasone propionate cream) cream, 0.05% contains fluticasone propionate [(6α,11β,16α,17α)-6,9,-difluoro-11-hydroxy-16-methyl-3-oxo-17-(1-oxopropoxy)androsta-1,4-diene-17-carbothioic acid,S-fluoromethyl ester], a synthetic fluorinated corticosteroid, for topical dermatologic use. The topical corticosteroids constitute a class of primarily synthetic steroids used as anti-inflammatory and antipruritic agents.

Chemically, fluticasone propionate is $C_{25}H_{31}F_3O_5S$.

Fluticasone propionate has a molecular weight of 500.6. It is a white to off-white powder and is insoluble in water.

Each gram of Cutivate Cream contains fluticasone propionate 0.5 mg in a base of propylene glycol, mineral oil, cetostearyl alcohol, Ceteth-20, isopropyl myristate, dibasic sodium phosphate, citric acid, purified water, and imidurea as preservative.

CUTIVATE OINTMENT, 0.005%

For Dermatologic Use Only — Not for Ophthalmic Use.

Cutivate ointment, 0.005% contains fluticasone propionate [(6α,11β,16α,17α)-6,9,-difluoro-11-hydroxy-16-methyl-3-oxo-17-(1-oxopropoxy)androsta-1,4-diene-17-carbothioic acid,S-fluoromethyl ester], a synthetic fluorinated corticosteroid, for topical dermatologic use. The topical corticosteroids constitute a class of primarily synthetic steroids used as anti-inflammatory and antipruritic agents.

Chemically, fluticasone propionate is $C_{25}H_{31}F_3O_5S$.

Fluticasone propionate has a molecular weight of 500.6. It is a white to off-white powder and is insoluble in water.

Each gram of Cutivate ointment contains fluticasone propionate 0.05 mg in a base of liquid paraffin, microcrystalline wax, propylene glycol, and sorbitan sesquioleate.

CLINICAL PHARMACOLOGY

CUTIVATE CREAM, 0.05%

Like other topical corticosteroids, fluticasone propionate has anti-inflammatory, antipruritic, and vasoconstrictive properties. The mechanism of the anti-inflammatory activity of the topical steroids, in general, is unclear. However, corticosteroids are thought to act by the induction of phospholipase A_2 inhibitory proteins, collectively called lipocortins. It is postulated that these proteins control the biosynthesis of potent mediators of inflammation such as prostaglandins and leukotrienes by inhibiting the release of their common precursor, arachidonic acid. Arachidonic acid is released from membrane phospholipids by phospholipase A_2.

Fluticasone propionate is lipophilic and has a strong affinity for the glucocorticoid receptor. It has weak affinity for the progesterone receptor, and virtually no affinity for the mineralocorticoid, estrogen, or androgen receptors. The therapeutic potency of glucocorticoids is related to the half-life of the glucocorticoid-receptor complex. The half-life of the fluticasone propionate-glucocorticoid receptor complex is approximately 10 hours.

Studies performed with Cutivate cream indicate that it is in the medium range of potency as compared with other topical corticosteroids.

Pharmacokinetics

Absorption

The activity of Cutivate is due to the parent drug, fluticasone propionate. The extent of percutaneous absorption of topical corticosteroids is determined by many factors, including the vehicle and the integrity of the epidermal barrier. Occlusive dressing enhances penetration. Topical corticosteroids can be absorbed from normal intact skin. Inflammation and/or other disease processes in the skin increase percutaneous absorption.

In a human study of 12 healthy males receiving 12.5 g of 0.05% fluticasone propionate cream twice daily for 3 weeks, plasma levels were generally below the level of quantification (0.05 ng/ml). In another study of 6 healthy males administered 25 g of 0.05% fluticasone propionate cream under occlusion for 5 days, plasma levels of fluticasone ranged from 0.07-0.39 ng/ml.

In an animal study using radiolabeled 0.05% fluticasone propionate cream and ointment preparations, rats received a topical dose of 1 g/kg for a 24 hour period. Total recovery of radioactivity was approximately 80% at the end of 7 days. The majority of the dose (73%) was recovered from the surface of the application site. Less than 1% of the dose was recovered in the skin at the application site. Approximately 5% of the dose was absorbed systemically through the skin. Absorption from the skin continued for the duration of the study (7 days), indicating a long retention time at the application site.

Distribution

Following intravenous administration of 1 mg fluticasone propionate in healthy volunteers, the initial disposition phase for fluticasone propionate was rapid and consistent with its high lipid solubility and tissue binding. The apparent volume of distribution averaged 4.2 L/kg (range, 2.3-16.7 L/kg). The percentage of fluticasone propionate bound to human plasma proteins averaged 91%. Fluticasone propionate is weakly and reversibly bound to erythrocytes. Fluticasone propionate is not significantly bound to human transcortin.

Metabolism

No metabolites of fluticasone propionate were detected in an *in vitro* study of radiolabeled fluticasone propionate incubated in a human skin homogenate. The total blood clearance of systemically absorbed fluticasone propionate averages 1093 ml/min (range, 618-1702 ml/min) after a 1 mg intravenous dose, with renal clearance accounting for less than 0.02% of the total. Fluticasone propionate is metabolized in the liver by cytochrome P450 3A4-mediated hydrolysis of the 5-fluoromethyl carbothioate grouping. This transformation occurs in 1 metabolic step to produce the inactive 17-β-carboxylic acid metabolite, the only known metabolite detected in man. This metabolite has approximately 2000 times less affinity than the parent drug for the glucocorticoid receptor of human lung cytosol *in vitro* and negligible pharmacological activity in animal studies. Other metabolites detected *in vitro* using cultured human hepatoma cells have not been detected in man.

Excretion

Following intravenous dose of 1 mg in healthy volunteers, fluticasone propionate showed polyexponential kinetics and had an average terminal half-life of 7.2 hours (range, 3.2-11.2 hours).

CUTIVATE OINTMENT, 0.005%

Like other topical corticosteroids, fluticasone propionate has anti-inflammatory, antipruritic, and vasoconstrictive properties. The mechanism of the anti-inflammatory activity of the topical steroids, in general, is unclear. However, corticosteroids are thought to act by the induction of phospholipase A_2 inhibitory proteins, collectively called lipocortins. It is postulated that these proteins control the biosynthesis of potent mediators of inflammation such as prostaglandins and leukotrienes by inhibiting the release of their common precursor, arachidonic acid. Arachidonic acid is released from membrane phospholipids by phospholipase A_2.

Fluticasone propionate is lipophilic and has a strong affinity for the glucocorticoid receptor. It has weak affinity for the progesterone receptor, and virtually no affinity for the mineralocorticoid, estrogen, or androgen receptors. The therapeutic potency of glucocorticoids is related to the half-life of the glucocorticoid-receptor complex. The half-life of the fluticasone propionate-glucocorticoid receptor complex is approximately 10 hours.

Studies performed with Cutivate ointment indicate that it is in the medium range of potency as compared with other topical corticosteroids.

Pharmacokinetics

Absorption

The activity of Cutivate is due to the parent drug, fluticasone propionate. The extent of percutaneous absorption of topical corticosteroids is determined by many factors, including the vehicle and the integrity of the epidermal barrier. Occlusive dressing enhances penetration. Topical corticosteroids can be absorbed from normal intact skin. Inflammation and/or other disease processes in the skin increase percutaneous absorption.

In a study of 6 healthy volunteers applying 25 g of fluticasone propionate ointment 0.005% twice daily to the trunk and legs for up to 5 days under occlusion, plasma levels of fluticasone ranged from 0.08-0.22 ng/ml.

In an animal study using radiolabeled 0.05% fluticasone propionate cream and ointment preparations, rats received a topical dose of 1 g/kg for a 24 hour period. Total recovery of radioactivity was approximately 80% at the end of 7 days. The majority of the dose (73%) was recovered from the surface of the application site. Less than 1% of the dose was recovered in the skin at the application site. Approximately 5% of the dose was absorbed systemically through the skin. Absorption from the skin continued for the duration of the study (7 days), indicating a long retention time at the application site.

Distribution

Following intravenous administration of 1 mg of fluticasone propionate in healthy volunteers, the initial disposition phase for fluticasone propionate was rapid and consistent with its high lipid solubility and tissue binding. The apparent volume of distribution averaged 4.2 L/kg (range, 2.3-16.7 L/kg). The percentage of fluticasone propionate bound to human plasma proteins averaged 91%. Fluticasone propionate is weakly and reversibly bound to erythrocytes. Fluticasone propionate is not significantly bound to human transcortin.

Metabolism

No metabolites of fluticasone propionate were detected in an *in vitro* study of radiolabeled fluticasone propionate incubated in a human skin homogenate. The total blood clearance of systemically absorbed fluticasone propionate averages 1093 ml/min (range, 618-1702 ml/min) after a 1 mg intravenous dose, with renal clearance accounting for less than 0.02% of the total.

Fluticasone propionate is metabolized in the liver by cytochrome P450 3A4-mediated hydrolysis of the 5-fluoromethyl carbothioate grouping. This transformation occurs in 1 metabolic step to produce the inactive 17-β-carboxylic acid metabolite, the only known metabolite detected in man. This metabolite has approximately 2000 times less affinity than the parent drug for the glucocorticoid receptor of human lung cytosol *in vitro* and negligible pharmacological activity in animal studies. Other metabolites detected *in vitro* using cultured human hepatoma cells have not been detected in man.

Excretion

Following an intravenous dose of 1 mg in healthy volunteers, fluticasone propionate showed polyexponential kinetics and had an average terminal half-life of 7.2 hours (range, 3.2-11.2 hours).

INDICATIONS AND USAGE

CUTIVATE CREAM, 0.05%

Cutivate cream is a medium potency corticosteroid indicated for the relief of the inflammatory and pruritic manifestations of corticosteroid-responsive dermatoses. Cutivate cream may be used with caution in pediatric patients 3 months of age or older. The safety and efficacy of drug use for longer than 4 weeks in this population have not been established. The safety and efficacy of Cutivate cream in pediatric patients below 3 months of age have not been established.

CUTIVATE OINTMENT, 0.005%

Cutivate ointment is a medium potency corticosteroid indicated for the relief of the inflammatory and pruritic manifestations of corticosteroid-responsive dermatoses in adult patients.

CONTRAINDICATIONS

CUTIVATE CREAM, 0.05%

Cutivate cream is contraindicated in those patients with a history of hypersensitivity to any of the components in the preparation.

CUTIVATE OINTMENT, 0.005%

Cutivate ointment is contraindicated in those patients with a history of hypersensitivity to any of the components in the preparation.

PRECAUTIONS

CUTIVATE CREAM, 0.05%

General

Systemic absorption of topical corticosteroids can produce reversible hypothalamic-pituitary-adrenal (HPA) axis suppression with the potential for glucocorticosteroid insufficiency after withdrawal from treatment. Manifestations of Cushing's syndrome, hyperglycemia, and glucosuria can also be produced in some patients by systemic absorption of topical corticosteroids while on treatment.

Patients applying a potent topical steroid to a large surface area or to areas under occlusion should be evaluated periodically for evidence of HPA axis suppression. This may be done by using the ACTH stimulation, AM plasma cortisol, and urinary free cortisol tests.

If HPA axis suppression is noted, an attempt should be made to withdraw the drug, to reduce the frequency of application, or to substitute a less potent steroid. Recovery of HPA axis function is generally prompt upon discontinuation of topical corticosteroids. Infrequently, signs and symptoms of glucocorticosteroid insufficiency may occur requiring supplemental systemic corticosteroids. For information on systemic supplementation, see prescribing information for those products.

Fluticasone propionate cream, 0.05% caused depression of AM plasma cortisol levels in 1 of 6 adult patients when used daily for 7 days in patients with psoriasis or eczema involving at least 30% of the body surface. After 2 days of treatment, this patient developed a 60% decrease from pretreatment values in the AM plasma cortisol level.

There was some evidence of corresponding decrease in the 24 hour urinary free cortisol levels. The AM plasma cortisol level remained slightly depressed for 48 hours but recovered by day 6 of treatment.

Fluticasone propionate cream, 0.05%, caused HPA axis suppression in 2 of 43 pediatric patients, ages 2 and 5 years old, who were treated for 4 weeks covering at least 35% of the body surface area. Follow-up testing 12 days after treatment discontinuation, available for 1 of the 2 subjects, demonstrated a normally responsive HPA axis (see Pediatric Use).

Pediatric patients may be more susceptible to systemic toxicity from equivalent doses due to their larger skin surface to body mass ratios (see Pediatric Use).

Fluticasone propionate cream, 0.05% may cause local cutaneous adverse reactions (see ADVERSE REACTIONS, Cutivate Cream, 0.05%).

If irritation develops, Cutivate cream should be discontinued and appropriate therapy instituted. Allergic contact dermatitis with corticosteroids is usually diagnosed by observing failure to heal rather than noting a clinical exacerbation as with most topical products not containing corticosteroids. Such an observation should be corroborated with appropriate diagnostic patch testing.

If concomitant skin infections are present or develop, an appropriate antifungal or antibacterial agent should be used. If a favorable response does not occur promptly, use of Cutivate cream should be discontinued until the infection has been adequately controlled.

Cutivate cream should not be used in the presence of preexisting skin atrophy and should not be used where infection is present at the treatment site. Cutivate cream should not be used in the treatment of rosacea and perioral dermatitis.

Information for the Patient

Patients using topical corticosteroids should receive the following information and instructions:

This medication is to be used as directed by the physician. It is for external use only. Avoid contact with the eyes.

This medication should not be used for any disorder other than that for which it was prescribed.

The treated skin area should not be bandaged or otherwise covered or wrapped so as to be occlusive unless directed by the physician.

Patients should report to their physician any signs of local adverse reactions.

Parents of pediatric patients should be advised not to use this medication in the treatment of diaper dermatitis. Cutivate cream should not be applied in the diaper areas as diapers or plastic pants may constitute occlusive dressing (see DOSAGE AND ADMINISTRATION, Cutivate Cream, 0.05%).

This medication should not be used on the face, underarms, or groin areas unless directed by a physician.

As with other corticosteroids, therapy should be discontinued when control is achieved. If no improvement is seen within 2 weeks, contact the physician.

Laboratory Tests

The following tests may be helpful in evaluating patients for HPA axis suppression:

ACTH stimulation test
AM plasma cortisol test
Urinary free cortisol test

Carcinogenesis, Mutagenesis, and Impairment of Fertility

Two 18 month studies were performed in mice to evaluate the carcinogenic potential of fluticasone propionate when given topically (as an 0.05% ointment) and orally. No evidence of carcinogenicity was found in either study.

Fluticasone propionate was not mutagenic in the standard Ames test, *E. coli* luctuation test, *S. cerevisiae* gene conversion test, or Chinese Hamster ovarian cell assay. It was not clastogenic in mouse micronucleus or cultured human lymphocyte tests.

In a fertility and general reproductive performance study in rats, fluticasone propionate administered subcutaneously to females at up to 50 μg/kg/day and to males at up to 100 μg/kg/day (later reduced to 50 μg/kg/day) had no effect upon mating performance or fertility. These doses are approximately 15 and 30 times, respectively, the human systemic exposure following use of the recommended human topical dose of fluticasone propionate cream, 0.05%, assuming human percutaneous absorption of approximately 3% and the use in a 70 kg person of 15 g/day.

Pregnancy, Teratogenic Effects, Pregnancy Category C

Corticosteroids have been shown to be teratogenic in laboratory animals when administered systemically at relatively low dosage levels. Some corticosteroids have been shown to be teratogenic after dermal application in laboratory animals. Teratology studies in the mouse demonstrated fluticasone propionate to be teratogenic (cleft palate) when administered subcutaneously in doses of 45 μg/kg/day and 150 μg/kg/day. This dose is approximately 14 and 45 times, respectively, the human topical dose of fluticasone propionate cream, 0.05%. There are no adequate and well-controlled studies in pregnant women. Cutivate cream should be used during pregnancy only if the potential benefit justifies the potential risk to the fetus.

Nursing Mothers

Systemically administered corticosteroids appear in human milk and could suppress growth, interfere with endogenous corticosteroid production, or cause other untoward effects. It is not known whether topical administration of corticosteroids could result in sufficient systemic absorption to produce detectable quantities in human milk. Because many drugs are excreted in human milk, caution should be exercised when Cutivate cream is administered to a nursing woman.

Pediatric Use

Cutivate cream may be used with caution in pediatric patients as young as 3 months of age. The safety and efficacy of drug use for longer than 4 weeks in this population have not been established. The safety and efficacy of Cutivate cream in pediatric patients below 3 months of age have not been established.

Fluticasone propionate cream, 0.05%, caused HPA axis suppression in 2 of 43 pediatric patients, ages 2 and 5 years old, who were treated for 4 weeks covering at least 35% of the body surface area. Follow-up testing 12 days after treatment discontinuation, available for 1 of the 2 subjects, demonstrated a normally responsive HPA axis (see ADVERSE REACTIONS, Cutivate Cream, 0.05%). Adverse effects including striae have been reported with use of topical corticosteroids in pediatric patients.

HPA axis suppression, Cushing's syndrome, linear growth retardation, delayed weight gain, and intracranial hypertension have been reported in pediatric patients receiving topical corticosteroids. Manifestations of adrenal suppression in pediatric patients include low plasma cortisol levels to an absence of response to ACTH stimulation. Manifestations of intracranial hypertension include bulging fontanelles, headaches, and bilateral papilledema.

Geriatric Use

A limited number of patients above 65 years of age (n=133) have been treated with Cutivate cream in US and non-US clinical trials. While the number of patients is too small to permit separate analysis of efficacy and safety, the adverse reactions reported in this population were similar to those reported by younger patients. Based on available data, no adjustment of dosage of Cutivate in geriatric patients is warranted.

CUTIVATE OINTMENT, 0.005%

General

Systemic absorption of topical corticosteroids can produce reversible hypothalamic-pituitary-adrenal (HPA) axis suppression with the potential for glucocorticosteroid insufficiency after withdrawal from treatment. Manifestations of Cushing's syndrome, hyperglycemia, and glucosuria can also be produced in some patients by systemic absorption of topical corticosteroids while on treatment.

Patients applying a topical steroid to a large surface area or to areas under occlusion should be evaluated periodically for evidence of HPA axis suppression. This may be done by using the ACTH stimulation, AM plasma cortisol, and urinary free cortisol tests.

If HPA axis suppression is noted, an attempt should be made to withdraw the drug, to reduce the frequency of application, or to substitute a less potent corticosteroid. Recovery of HPA axis function is generally prompt upon discontinuation of topical corticosteroids. Infrequently, signs and symptoms of glucocorticosteroid insufficiency may occur, requiring supplemental systemic corticosteroids. For information on systemic supplementation, see prescribing information for those products.

Pediatric patients may be more susceptible to systemic toxicity from equivalent doses due to their larger skin surface to body mass ratios (see Pediatric Use).

Fluticasone propionate ointment, 0.005% may cause local cutaneous adverse reactions (see ADVERSE REACTIONS, Cutivate Ointment 0.005%).

If irritation develops, Cutivate ointment should be discontinued and appropriate therapy instituted. Allergic contact dermatitis with corticosteroids is usually diagnosed by observing failure to heal rather than noting a clinical exacerbation as with most topical products not containing corticosteroids. Such an observation should be corroborated with appropriate diagnostic patch testing.

If concomitant skin infections are present or develop, an appropriate antifungal or antibacterial agent should be used. If a favorable response does not occur promptly, use of Cutivate ointment should be discontinued until the infection has been adequately controlled.

Cutivate ointment should not be used in the presence of preexisting skin atrophy and should not be used where infection is present at the treatment site. Cutivate ointment should not be used in the treatment of rosacea and perioral dermatitis.

Information for the Patient

Patients using topical corticosteroids should receive the following information and instructions:

This medication is to be used as directed by the physician. It is for external use only. Avoid contact with the eyes.

This medication should not be used for any disorder other than that for which it was prescribed.

The treated skin area should not be bandaged or otherwise covered or wrapped so as to be occlusive unless directed by the physician.

Patients should report to their physician any signs of local adverse reactions.

This medication should not be used on the face, underarms, or groin areas unless directed by a physician.

As with other corticosteroids, therapy should be discontinued when control is achieved. If no improvement is seen within 2 weeks, contact the physician.

Laboratory Tests

The following tests may be helpful in evaluating patients for HPA axis suppression:

ACTH stimulation test

AM plasma cortisol test

Urinary free cortisol test

A concentrated fluticasone propionate ointment, 0.05% (10 times that of the marketed fluticasone propionate ointment, 0.005%) suppressed 24 hour urinary free cortisol levels in 2 of 6 patients when used at a dose of 30 g/day for a week in patients with psoriasis or atopic eczema. No suppression of AM plasma cortisol was observed. In a second study of the same concentrated formulation of fluticasone propionate ointment, 0.05%, depression of AM plasma cortisol levels was noted in 2 of 8 normal volunteers when applied at doses of 50 g/day for 21 days. Morning plasma levels returned to normal levels within 4 days upon discontinuation of fluticasone propionate. In this study there was no corresponding decrease in 24 hour urinary free cortisol levels.

In a study of 35 pediatric patients treated with fluticasone propionate ointment 0.005% for atopic dermatitis over at least 35% of body surface area, subnormal adrenal function was observed with cosyntropin stimulation testing at the end of 3-4 weeks of treatment in 4 patients who had normal testing prior to treatment. It is not known if these patients had recovery of adrenal function because follow-up testing was not performed (see Pediatric Use and ADVERSE REACTIONS, Cutivate Ointment 0.005%). Adrenal suppression was indicated by either a ≤5 μg/dl pre-stimulation cortisol, or a cosyntropin post-stimulation cortisol ≤18 μg/dl, and/or an increase of <7 μg/dl from the baseline cortisol level.

Carcinogenesis, Mutagenesis, and Impairment of Fertility

Two 18 month studies were performed in mice to evaluate the carcinogenic potential of fluticasone propionate when given topically (as an 0.05% ointment) and orally. No evidence of carcinogenicity was found in either study.

Fluticasone propionate was not mutagenic in the standard Ames test, *E. coli* fluctuation test, *S. cerevisiae* gene conversion test, or Chinese Hamster ovarian cell assay. It was not clastogenic in mouse micronucleus or cultured human lymphocyte tests.

In a fertility and general reproductive performance study in rats, fluticasone propionate administered subcutaneously to females at up to 50 μg/kg/day and to males at up to 100 μg/kg/day (later reduced to 50 μg/kg/day) had no effect upon mating performance or fertility. These doses are approximately 150 and 300 times, respectively, the human systemic exposure following use of the recommended human topical dose of fluticasone propionate ointment, 0.005%, assuming human percutaneous absorption of approximately 3% and the use in a 70 kg person of 15 g/day.

Pregnancy, Teratogenic Effects, Pregnancy Category C

Corticosteroids have been shown to be teratogenic in laboratory animals when administered systemically at relatively low dosage levels. Some corticosteroids have been shown to be teratogenic after dermal application in laboratory animals. Teratology studies in the mouse demonstrated fluticasone propionate to be teratogenic (cleft palate) when administered subcutaneously in doses of 45 μg/kg/day and 150 μg/kg/day. This dose is approximately 140 and 450 times, respectively, the human topical dose of fluticasone propionate ointment, 0.005%. There are no adequate and well-controlled studies in pregnant women. Cutivate ointment should be used during pregnancy only if the potential benefit justifies the potential risk to the fetus.

Nursing Mothers

Systemically administered corticosteroids appear in human milk and could suppress growth, interfere with endogenous corticosteroid production, or cause other untoward effects. It is not known whether topical administration of corticosteroids could result in sufficient systemic absorption to produce detectable quantities in human milk. Because many drugs are excreted in human milk, caution should be exercised when Cutivate ointment is administered to a nursing woman.

Pediatric Use

Use of Cutivate ointment in pediatric patients is not recommended.

In a study of 35 pediatric patients treated with fluticasone propionate ointment 0.005% for atopic dermatitis over at least 35% of body surface area, subnormal adrenal function was observed with cosyntropin stimulation testing at the end of 3-4 weeks of treatment in 4 patients who had normal testing prior to treatment. It is not known if these patients had recovery of adrenal function because follow-up testing was not performed (see Pediatric Use and ADVERSE REACTIONS Cutivate Ointment 0.005%). The decreased responsiveness to cosyntropin testing was not correlated to age of patient, amount of fluticasone propionate ointment used, or serum levels of fluticasone propionate. Plasma fluticasone propionate were not performed in a 6 month old patient who demonstrated an abnormal response to cosyntropin stimulation testing.

Pediatric patients may demonstrate greater susceptibility to topical corticosteroid-induced HPA axis suppression and Cushing's syndrome than mature patients because of a larger skin surface to body weight ratio.

HPA axis suppression, Cushing's syndrome, linear growth retardation, delayed weight gain, and intracranial hypertension have been reported in pediatric patients receiving topical corticosteroids. Manifestations of adrenal suppression in pediatric patients include low plasma cortisol levels and an absence of response to ACTH stimulation.

Manifestations of intracranial hypertension include bulging fontanelles, headaches, and bilateral papilledema.

Geriatric Use

A limited number of patients above 65 years of age (n=203) have been treated with Cutivate ointment in US and non-US clinical trials. While the number of patients is too small to permit separate analysis of efficacy and safety, the adverse reactions reported in this population were similar to those reported by younger patients. Based on available data, no adjustment of dosage of Cutivate in geriatric patients is warranted.

ADVERSE REACTIONS

CUTIVATE CREAM, 0.05%

In controlled clinical trials of twice-daily administration, the total incidence of adverse reactions associated with the use of Cutivate cream was approximately 4%. These adverse reactions were usually mild; self-limiting; and consisted primarily of pruritus, dryness, numbness of fingers, and burning. These events occurred in 2.9%, 1.2%, 1.0%, and 0.6% of patients, respectively.

Two clinical studies compared once- to twice-daily administration of Cutivate cream for the treatment of moderate to severe eczema. The local drug-related adverse events for the 491 patients enrolled in both studies are shown in TABLE 12. In the study enrolling both adult and pediatric patients, the incidence of local adverse events in the 119 pediatric patients ages 1-12 years was comparable to the 140 patients ages 13-62 years.

Fifty-one (51) pediatric patients ages 3 months to 5 years, with moderate to severe eczema, were enrolled in an open-label HPA axis safety study. Cutivate cream was applied twice daily for 3-4 weeks over an arithmetic mean body surface area of 64% (range, 35-95%). The mean morning cortisol levels with standard deviations before treatment (prestimulation mean value = 13.76 ± 6.94 μg/dl, poststimulation mean value = 30.53 ± 7.23 μg/dl) and at end treatment (prestimulation mean value = 12.32 ± 6.92 μg/dl, poststimulation mean value = 28.84 ± 7.16 μg/dl) showed little change. In 2 of 43 (4.7%) patients with end-treatment results, peak cortisol levels following cosyntropin stimulation testing were ≤18 μg/dl, indicating adrenal suppression. Follow-up testing after treatment discontinuation, available for 1 of the 2 subjects, demonstrated a normally responsive HPA axis. Local drug-related adverse events were transient burning, resolving the same day it was reported; transient urticaria, resolving the same day it was reported; erythematous rash; dusky erythema, resolving within 1 month after cessation of Cutivate cream; and telangiectasia, resolving within 3 months after stopping Cutivate cream.

***TABLE 12** Drug-Related Adverse Events — Skin*

	Fluticasone		
Adverse Events	Once Daily (n=210)	Twice Daily (n=203)	Vehicle Twice Daily (n=78)
Skin infection	1 (0.5%)	0	0
Infected eczema	1 (0.5%)	2 (1.0%)	0
Viral warts	0	1 (0.5%)	0
Herpes simplex	0	1 (0.5%)	0
Impetigo	1 (0.5%)	0	0
Atopic dermatitis	1 (0.5%)	0	0
Eczema	1 (0.5%)	0	0
Exacerbation of eczema	4 (1.9%)	1 (0.5%)	1 (1.3%)
Erythema	0	2 (1.0%)	0
Burning	2 (1.0%)	2 (1.0%)	2 (2.6%)
Stinging	0	2 (1.0%)	1 (1.3%)
Skin irritation	6 (2.9%)	2 (1.0%)	0
Pruritus	2 (1.0%)	4 (1.9%)	4 (5.1%)
Exacerbation of pruritus	4 (1.9%)	1 (0.5%)	1 (1.3%)
Folliculitis	1 (0.5%)	1 (0.5%)	0
Blisters	0	1 (0.5%)	0
Dryness of skin	3 (1.4%)	1 (0.5%)	0

The following local adverse reactions have been reported infrequently with topical corticosteroids, and they may occur more frequently with the use of occlusive dressings and higher potency corticosteroids. These reactions are listed in an approximately decreasing order of occurrence: irritation, folliculitis, acneiform eruptions, hypopigmentation, perioral dermatitis, allergic contact dermatitis, secondary infection, skin atrophy, striae, and miliaria.

TABLE 13 *Adverse Events* From Pediatric Open-Label Trial (n=51)*

Adverse Events	Fluticasone Twice Daily
Burning	1 (2.0%)
Dusky erythema	1 (2.0%)
Erythematous rash	1 (2.0%)
Facial telangiectasia†	2 (4.9%)
Non-facial telangiectasia	1 (2.0%)
Uticaria	1 (2.0%)

* See text for additional detail.
† n=41.

Also, there are reports of the development of pustular psoriasis from chronic plaque psoriasis following reduction or discontinuation of potent topical corticosteroid products.

CUTIVATE OINTMENT, 0.005%

In controlled clinical trials, the total incidence of adverse reactions associated with the use of Cutivate ointment was approximately 4%. These adverse reactions were usually mild, self-limiting, and consisted primarily of pruritus, burning, hypertrichosis, increased erythema, hives, irritation, and lightheadedness. Each of these events occurred individually in less than 1% of patients.

In a study of 35 pediatric patients treated with fluticasone propionate ointment 0.005% for atopic dermatitis over at least 35% of body surface area, subnormal adrenal function was observed with cosyntropin stimulation testing at the end of 3-4 weeks of treatment in 4 patients who had normal testing prior to treatment. It is not known if these patients had recovery of adrenal function because follow-up testing was not performed (see PRECAUTIONS, Cutivate Ointment 0.005%, Pediatric Use and ADVERSE REACTIONS, Cutivate Ointment 0.005%). Telangiectasia on the face was noted 1 patient on the eighth day of a 4 week treatment period. Facial use was discontinued and the telangiectasia resolved.

The following additional local adverse reactions have been reported infrequently with topical corticosteroids, including fluticasone propionate, and they may occur more frequently with the use of occlusive dressings and higher potency corticosteroids. These reactions are listed in an approximately decreasing order of occurrence: dryness, folliculitis, acneiform eruptions, hypopigmentation, perioral dermatitis, allergic contact dermatitis, secondary infection, skin atrophy, striae, and miliaria. Also, there are reports of the development of pustular psoriasis from chronic plaque psoriasis following reduction or discontinuation of potent topical corticosteroid products.

DOSAGE AND ADMINISTRATION

CUTIVATE CREAM, 0.05%

Cutivate cream may be used in adult and pediatric patients 3 months of age or older. Safety and efficacy of Cutivate cream in pediatric patients for more than 4 weeks of use have not been established (see PRECAUTIONS, Cutivate Cream, 0.05%, Pediatric Use). The safety and efficacy of Cutivate cream in pediatric patients below 3 months of age have not been established.

Atopic Dermatitis: Apply a thin film of Cutivate cream to the affected skin areas once or twice daily. Rub in gently.

Other Corticosteroid-Responsive Dermatoses: Apply a thin film of Cutivate cream to the affected skin areas twice daily. Rub in gently.

As with other corticosteroids, therapy should be discontinued when control is achieved. If no improvement is seen within 2 weeks, reassessment of diagnosis may be necessary.

Cutivate cream should not be used with occlusive dressings. Cutivate cream should not be applied in the diaper area, as diapers or plastic pants may constitute occlusive dressings.

Geriatric Use

In studies where geriatric patients (65 years of age or older, see PRECAUTIONS, Cutivate Cream, 0.05%) have been treated with Cutivate cream, safety did not differ from that in younger patients; therefore, no dosage adjustment is recommended.

CUTIVATE OINTMENT, 0.005%

Apply a thin film of Cutivate ointment to the affected skin areas twice daily. Rub in gently.

Cutivate ointment should not be used with occlusive dressings.

Geriatric Use

In studies where geriatric patients (65 years of age or older, see PRECAUTIONS, Cutivate Ointment, 0.005%) have been treated with Cutivate ointment, safety did not differ from that in younger patients; therefore, no dosage adjustment is recommended.

HOW SUPPLIED

CUTIVATE CREAM, 0.05%

Cutivate Cream is supplied in 15, 30, and 60 g tubes.
Storage: Store between 2 and 30°C (36 and 86°F).

CUTIVATE OINTMENT, 0.005%

Cutivate Ointment, 0.005% is supplied in 15, 30, and 60 g tubes.
Storage: Store between 2 and 30°C (36 and 86°F).

PRODUCT LISTING - EQUIVALENTS NOT AVAILABLE

Aerosol with Adapter - Inhalation - 44 mcg/Inh

7.90 gm	$41.66	FLOVENT, Glaxosmithkline	00173-0497-00
13 gm	$46.94	FLOVENT, Allscripts Pharmaceutical Company	54569-4863-00
13 gm	$55.54	FLOVENT, Glaxosmithkline	00173-0491-00

Aerosol with Adapter - Inhalation - 110 mcg/Inh

7.90 gm	$53.61	FLOVENT, Glaxosmithkline	00173-0498-00
13 gm	$64.64	FLOVENT, Allscripts Pharmaceutical Company	54569-4602-00
13 gm	$77.20	FLOVENT, Glaxosmithkline	00173-0494-00

Aerosol with Adapter - Inhalation - 220 mcg/Inh

7.90 gm	$84.85	FLOVENT, Glaxosmithkline	00173-0499-00
13 gm	$99.44	FLOVENT, Allscripts Pharmaceutical Company	54569-4603-00
13 gm	$119.91	FLOVENT, Glaxosmithkline	00173-0495-00

Cream - Topical - 0.05%

15 gm	$17.17	CUTIVATE, Dura Pharmaceuticals	51479-0430-00
15 gm	$17.17	CUTIVATE, Allscripts Pharmaceutical Company	54569-4169-00
30 gm	$26.46	CUTIVATE, Dura Pharmaceuticals	51479-0430-01
60 gm	$41.71	CUTIVATE, Dura Pharmaceuticals	51479-0430-02

Ointment - Topical - 0.005%

15 gm	$17.17	CUTIVATE, Dura Pharmaceuticals	51479-0431-00
30 gm	$26.46	CUTIVATE, Dura Pharmaceuticals	51479-0431-01
60 gm	$41.71	CUTIVATE, Dura Pharmaceuticals	51479-0431-02

Powder - Inhalation - 50 mcg

4 x 15	$35.05	FLOVENT ROTADISK, Allscripts Pharmaceutical Company	54569-4896-00
4 x 15	$41.46	FLOVENT ROTADISK, Glaxosmithkline	00173-0511-00

Powder - Inhalation - 100 mcg

4 x 15	$58.30	FLOVENT ROTADISK, Glaxosmithkline	00173-0509-00

Powder - Inhalation - 250 mcg

4 x 15	$81.09	FLOVENT ROTADISK, Glaxosmithkline	00173-0504-00

Spray - Nasal - 0.05 mg/Inh

16 gm	$53.36	FLONASE, Allscripts Pharmaceutical Company	54569-4120-00
16 gm	$57.00	FLONASE, Southwood Pharmaceuticals Inc	58016-6533-01
16 gm	$65.01	FLONASE, Glaxosmithkline	00173-0453-01

F

Fluticasone Propionate; Salmeterol Xinafoate *(003503)*

For complete prescribing information, refer to the CD-ROM included with the book.

Categories: Asthma; FDA Approved 2000 Aug; Pregnancy Category C
Drug Classes: Adrenergic agonists; Bronchodilators; Corticosteroids, inhalation
Brand Names: Advair Diskus
Foreign Brand Availability: Seretide (Bahamas; Barbados; Belize; Bermuda; Colombia; Curacao; England; France; Guyana; Hong-Kong; Indonesia; Ireland; Jamaica; Korea; Netherland-Antilles; Philippines; Puerto-Rico; Singapore; South-Africa; Surinam; Thailand; Trinidad); Seretide Accuhaler (Australia; Mexico)
Cost of Therapy: $117.10 (Asthma; Advair Diskus; 100 µg; 50 µg; 2 inhalations/day; 30 day supply)

DESCRIPTION

Note: The trade name has been used throughout this monograph for clarity.

Advair Diskus 100/50, Advair Diskus 250/50, and Advair Diskus 500/50 are combinations of fluticasone propionate and salmeterol xinafoate.

One active component of Advair Diskus is fluticasone propionate, a corticosteroid having the chemical name S-(fluoromethyl) 6α,9-difluoro-11β,17-dihydroxy-16α-methyl-3-oxoandrosta-1,4-diene-17β-carbothioate, 17-propionate.

Fluticasone propionate is a white to off-white powder with a molecular weight of 500.6, and the empirical formula is $C_{25}H_{31}F_3O_5S$. It is practically insoluble in water, freely soluble in dimethyl sulfoxide and dimethylformamide, and slightly soluble in methanol and 95% ethanol.

The other active component of Advair Diskus is salmeterol xinafoate, a highly selective beta$_2$-adrenergic bronchodilator. Salmeterol xinafoate is the racemic form of the 1-hydroxy-2-naphthoic acid salt of salmeterol. The chemical name of salmeterol xinafoate is 4-hydroxy-α^1-[[[6-(4-phenylbutoxy)hexyl]amino]methyl]-1,3-benzenedimethanol, 1-hydroxy-2-naphthalenecarboxylate.

Salmeterol xinafoate is a white to off-white powder with a molecular weight of 603.8, and the empirical formula is $C_{25}H_{37}NO_4 \cdot C_{11}H_8O_3$. It is freely soluble in methanol; slightly soluble in ethanol, chloroform, and isopropanol; and sparingly soluble in water.

Advair Diskus 100/50, Advair Diskus 250/50, and Advair Diskus 500/50 are specially designed plastic devices containing a double-foil blister strip of a powder formulation of fluticasone propionate and salmeterol xinafoate intended for oral inhalation only. Each blister on the double-foil strip within the device contains 100, 250, or 500 µg of microfine fluticasone propionate and 72.5 µg of microfine salmeterol xinafoate salt, equivalent to 50 µg of salmeterol base, in 12.5 mg of formulation containing lactose. Each blister contains 1 complete dose of both medications. After a blister containing medication is opened by activating the device, the medication is dispersed into the airstream created by the patient inhaling through the mouthpiece.

Under standardized *in vitro* test conditions, Advair Diskus delivers 93, 233, and 465 µg of fluticasone propionate and 45 µg of salmeterol base/blister from Advair Diskus 100/50, 250/50, and 500/50, respectively, when tested at a flow rate of 60 L/min for 2 seconds. In adult patients (n=9) with obstructive lung disease and severely compromised lung function (mean forced expiratory volume in 1 second [FEV$_1$] 20-30% of predicted), mean peak inspiratory flow (PIF) through a Diskus device was 80.0 L/min (range, 46.1-115.3 L/min).

Inhalation profiles for adolescent (n=13, aged 12-17 years) and adult (n=17, aged 18-50 years) patients with asthma inhaling maximally through the Diskus device show mean PIF of 122.2 L/min (range, 81.6-152.1 L/min).

The actual amount of drug delivered to the lung will depend on patient factors, such as inspiratory flow profile.

INDICATIONS AND USAGE

Advair Diskus is indicated for the long-term, twice-daily, maintenance treatment of asthma in patients 12 years of age and older.

Advair Diskus is NOT indicated for the relief of acute bronchospasm.

CONTRAINDICATIONS

Advair Diskus is contraindicated in the primary treatment of status asthmaticus or other acute episodes of asthma where intensive measures are required.

Hypersensitivity to any of the ingredients of these preparations contraindicates their use.

WARNINGS

Advair Diskus should not be used for transferring patients from systemic corticosteroid therapy. Particular care is needed for patients who have been transferred from systemically active corticosteroids to inhaled corticosteroids because deaths due to adrenal insufficiency have occurred in patients with asthma during and after transfer from systemic corticosteroids to less systemically available inhaled corticosteroids. After withdrawal from systemic corticosteroids, a number of months are required for recovery of HPA function.

F

Patients who have been previously maintained on 20 mg or more/day of prednisone (or its equivalent) may be most susceptible, particularly when their systemic corticosteroids have been almost completely withdrawn. During this period of HPA suppression, patients may exhibit signs and symptoms of adrenal insufficiency when exposed to trauma, surgery, or infection (particularly gastroenteritis) or other conditions associated with severe electrolyte loss. Although inhaled corticosteroids may provide control of asthma symptoms during these episodes, in recommended doses they supply less than normal physiological amounts of glucocorticoid systemically and do NOT provide the mineralocorticoid activity that is necessary for coping with these emergencies.

During periods of stress or a severe asthma attack, patients who have been withdrawn from systemic corticosteroids should be instructed to resume oral corticosteroids (in large doses) immediately and to contact their physicians for further instruction. These patients should also be instructed to carry a warning card indicating that they may need supplementary systemic corticosteroids during periods of stress or a severe asthma attack.

ADVAIR DISKUS SHOULD NOT BE INITIATED IN PATIENTS DURING RAPIDLY DETERIORATING OR POTENTIALLY LIFE-THREATENING EPISODES OF ASTHMA. Serious acute respiratory events, including fatalities, have been reported both in the US and worldwide when salmeterol, a component of Advair Diskus, has been initiated in patients with significantly worsening or acutely deteriorating asthma. In most cases, these have occurred in patients with severe asthma (*e.g.,* patients with a history of corticosteroid dependence, low pulmonary function, intubation, mechanical ventilation, frequent hospitalizations, or previous life-threatening acute asthma exacerbations) and/or in some patients in whom asthma has been acutely deteriorating (*e.g.,* unresponsive to usual medications; increasing need for inhaled, short-acting beta$_2$-agonists; increasing need for systemic corticosteroids; significant increase in symptoms; recent emergency room visits; sudden or progressive deterioration in pulmonary function). However, they have occurred in a few patients with less severe asthma as well. It was not possible from these reports to determine whether salmeterol contributed to these events or simply failed to relieve the deteriorating asthma.

Do not use Advair Diskus to treat acute symptoms: An inhaled, short-acting beta$_2$-agonist, not Advair Diskus, should be used to relieve acute asthma symptoms. When prescribing Advair Diskus, the physician must also provide the patient with an inhaled, short-acting beta$_2$-agonist (*e.g.,* albuterol) for treatment of symptoms that occur acutely, despite regular twice daily (morning and evening) use of Advair Diskus.

When beginning treatment with Advair Diskus, patients who have been taking oral or inhaled, short-acting beta$_2$-agonists on a regular basis (*e.g.,* 4 times a day) should be instructed to discontinue the regular use of these drugs. For patients on Advair Diskus, short-acting, inhaled beta$_2$-agonists should only be used for symptomatic relief of acute asthma symptoms.

Watch for increasing use of inhaled, short-acting beta$_2$-agonists, which is a marker of deteriorating asthma: Asthma may deteriorate acutely over a period of hours or chronically over several days or longer. If the patient's inhaled, short-acting beta$_2$-agonist becomes less effective, the patient needs more inhalations than usual, or the patient develops a significant decrease in PEF, these may be a marker of destabilization of asthma. In this setting, the patient requires immediate reevaluation with reassessment of the treatment regimen, giving special consideration to the possible need for replacing the current strength of Advair Diskus with a higher strength, adding additional inhaled corticosteroid, or initiating systemic corticosteroids. Patients should not use more than 1 inhalation twice daily (morning and evening) of Advair Diskus.

Do not use an inhaled, long-acting beta$_2$-agonist in conjunction with Advair Diskus: Patients who are receiving Advair Diskus twice daily should not use salmeterol or other long-acting inhaled beta$_2$-agonists for prevention of exercise-induced bronchospasm or the maintenance treatment of asthma. Additional benefit would not be gained from using supplemental salmeterol for prevention of exercise-induced bronchospasm since Advair Diskus already contains salmeterol.

Do not exceed recommended dosage: Advair Diskus should not be used more often or at higher doses than recommended. Fatalities have been reported in association with excessive use of inhaled sympathomimetic drugs. Large doses of inhaled or oral salmeterol (12-20 times the recommended dose) have been associated with clinically significant prolongation of the QTc interval, which has the potential for producing ventricular arrhythmias.

Paradoxical bronchospasm: As with other inhaled asthma medications, Advair Diskus can produce paradoxical bronchospasm, which may be life threatening. If paradoxical bronchospasm occurs following dosing with Advair Diskus, it should be treated immediately with a short-acting, inhaled bronchodilator, Advair Diskus should be discontinued immediately, and alternative therapy should be instituted.

Immediate hypersensitivity reactions: Immediate hypersensitivity reactions may occur after administration of Advair Diskus, as demonstrated by cases of urticaria, angioedema, rash, and bronchospasm.

Upper airway symptoms: Symptoms of laryngeal spasm, irritation, or swelling, such as stridor and choking, have been reported in patients receiving fluticasone propionate and salmeterol, components of Advair Diskus.

Cardiovascular disorders: Advair Diskus, like all products containing sympathomimetic amines, should be used with caution in patients with cardiovascular disorders, especially coronary insufficiency, cardiac arrhythmias, and hypertension. Salmeterol, a component of Advair Diskus, can produce a clinically significant cardiovascular effect in some patients as measured by pulse rate, blood pressure, and/or symptoms. Although such effects are uncommon after administration of salmeterol at recommended doses, if they occur, the drug may need to be discontinued. In addition, beta-agonists have been reported to produce electrocardiogram (ECG) changes, such as flattening of the T wave, prolongation of the QTc interval, and ST segment depression. The clinical significance of these findings is unknown.

Discontinuation of systemic corticosteroids: Transfer of patients from systemic corticosteroid therapy to Advair Diskus may unmask conditions previously suppressed by the systemic corticosteroid therapy, *e.g.,* rhinitis, conjunctivitis, eczema, and arthritis.

Immunosuppression: Persons who are using drugs that suppress the immune system are more susceptible to infections than healthy individuals. Chickenpox and measles, for example, can have a more serious or even fatal course in susceptible children or adults using corticosteroids. In such children or adults who have not had these diseases or been properly immunized, particular care should be taken to avoid exposure. How the dose, route, and duration of corticosteroid administration affect the risk of developing a disseminated infection is not known. The contribution of the underlying disease and/or prior corticosteroid treatment to the risk is also not known. If exposed to chickenpox, prophylaxis with varicella zoster immune globulin (VZIG) may be indicated. If exposed to measles, prophylaxis with pooled intramuscular immunoglobulin (IG) may be indicated. (See the respective package inserts for complete VZIG and IG prescribing information.) If chickenpox develops, treatment with antiviral agents may be considered.

DOSAGE AND ADMINISTRATION

Advair Diskus is available in 3 strengths, Advair Diskus 100/50, Advair Diskus 250/50, and Advair Diskus 500/50, containing 100, 250, and 500 μg of fluticasone propionate, respectively, and 50 μg of salmeterol/inhalation. Advair Diskus should be administered by the orally inhaled route only (see Patient's Instructions for Use).

For patients 12 years of age and older, the dosage is 1 inhalation twice daily (morning and evening, approximately 12 hours apart).

The recommended starting dosages for Advair Diskus are based upon patients' current asthma therapy.

- For patients who are not currently on an inhaled corticosteroid, whose disease severity warrants treatment with 2 maintenance therapies, including patients on non-corticosteroid maintenance therapy, the recommended starting dosage is Advair Diskus 100/50 twice daily.
- For patients on an inhaled corticosteroid, TABLE 4 provides the recommended starting dosage.

The maximum recommended dosage is Advair Diskus 500/50 twice daily.

For all patients it is desirable to titrate to the lowest effective strength after adequate asthma stability is achieved.

TABLE 4 *Recommended Doses of Advair Diskus for Patients Taking Inhaled Corticosteroids*

Current *Daily Dose* of Inhaled Corticosteroid	Recommended Strength and Dosing Schedule of Advair Diskus
Beclomethasone Dipropionate	
≤420 μg	100/50 twice daily
462-840 μg	250/50 twice daily
Budesonide	
≤400 μg	100/50 twice daily
800-1200 μg	250/50 twice daily
1600 μg*	500/50 twice daily
Flunisolide	
≤1000 μg	100/50 twice daily
1250-2000 μg	250/50 twice daily
Fluticasone Propionate Inhalation Aerosol	
≤176 μg	100/50 twice daily
440 μg	250/50 twice daily
660-880 μg*	500/50 twice daily
Fluticasone Propionate Inhalation Powder	
≤200 μg	100/50 twice daily
500 μg	250/50 twice daily
1000 μg*	500/50 twice daily
Triamcinolone Acetonide	
≤1000 μg	100/50 twice daily
1100-1600 μg	250/50 twice daily

* Advair Diskus should not be used for transferring patients from systemic corticosteroid therapy.

Advair Diskus should be administered twice daily every day. More frequent administration (more than twice daily) or a higher number of inhalations (more than 1 inhalation twice daily) of the prescribed strength of Advair Diskus is not recommended as some patients are more likely to experience adverse effects with higher doses of salmeterol. The safety and efficacy of Advair Diskus when administered in excess of recommended doses have not been established.

If symptoms arise in the period between doses, an inhaled, short-acting beta$_2$-agonist should be taken for immediate relief.

Patients who are receiving Advair Diskus twice daily should not use salmeterol for prevention of exercise-induced bronchospasm, or for any other reason.

Improvement in asthma control following inhaled administration of Advair Diskus can occur within 30 minutes of beginning treatment, although maximum benefit may not be achieved for 1 week or longer after starting treatment. Individual patients will experience a variable time to onset and degree of symptom relief.

For patients who do not respond adequately to the starting dosage after 2 weeks of therapy, replacing the current strength of Advair Diskus with a higher strength may provide additional asthma control.

If a previously effective dosage regimen of Advair Diskus fails to provide adequate control of asthma, the therapeutic regimen should be reevaluated and additional therapeutic options, *e.g.*, replacing the current strength of Advair Diskus with a higher strength, adding additional inhaled corticosteroid, or initiating oral corticosteroids, should be considered.

GERIATRIC USE

In studies where geriatric patients (65 years of age or older) have been treated with Advair Diskus, efficacy and safety did not differ from that in younger patients. Based on available data for Advair Diskus and its active components, no dosage adjustment is recommended.

DIRECTIONS FOR USE

Illustrated Patient's Instructions for Use accompany each package of Advair Diskus.

PRODUCT LISTING - EQUIVALENTS NOT AVAILABLE

Powder - Inhalation - 100 mcg;50 mcg

28's	$79.04	ADVAIR DISKUS, Glaxosmithkline	00173-0695-02
60's	$117.10	ADVAIR DISKUS, Glaxosmithkline	00173-0695-00

Powder - Inhalation - 250 mcg;50 mcg

28's	$97.54	ADVAIR DISKUS, Glaxosmithkline	00173-0696-02
60's	$148.23	ADVAIR DISKUS, Glaxosmithkline	00173-0696-00

Powder - Inhalation - 500 mcg;50 mcg

28's	$137.19	ADVAIR DISKUS, Glaxosmithkline	00173-0697-02
60's	$203.74	ADVAIR DISKUS, Glaxosmithkline	00173-0697-00

Fluvastatin Sodium *(003193)*

For related information, see the comparative table section in Appendix A.

Categories: Atherosclerosis; Coronary heart disease, prevention; Hypercholesterolemia; Hyperlipidemia; Pregnancy Category X; FDA Approved 1993 Dec
Drug Classes: Antihyperlipidemics; HMG CoA reductase inhibitors
Brand Names: **Lescol**; Lescol XR
Foreign Brand Availability: Canef (Mexico); Cranoc (Germany); Fractal (France); Fractal LP (France); Lescol LP (France); Lescol XL (England; Philippines; Singapore; Thailand); Locol (Germany); Vastin (Australia; New-Zealand)
Cost of Therapy: $55.56 (Hypercholesterolemia; Lescol; 20 mg; 1 capsule/day; 30 day supply)
$71.27 (Hypercholesterolemia; Lescol XL; 80 mg; 1 capsule/day; 30 day supply)

DESCRIPTION

Note: The trade names have been used throughout this monograph for clarity.

Lescol (fluvastatin sodium), is a water-soluble cholesterol lowering agent which acts through the inhibition of 3-hydroxy-3-methylglutaryl-coenzyme A (HMG-CoA) reductase.

Fluvastatin sodium is [*R**,*S**-(*E*)]-(±)-7-[3-(4-fluorophenyl)-1-(1-methylethyl)-1*H*-indol-2-yl]-3,5-dihydroxy-6-heptenoic acid, monosodium salt. The empirical formula of fluvastatin sodium is $C_{24}H_{25}FNO_4{\cdot}Na$, and its molecular weight is 433.46.

This molecular entity is the first entirely synthetic HMG-CoA reductase inhibitor, and is in part structurally distinct from the fungal derivatives of this therapeutic class.

Fluvastatin sodium is a white to pale yellow, hygroscopic powder soluble in water, ethanol and methanol. Lescol is supplied as capsules containing fluvastatin sodium, equivalent to 20 or 40 mg of fluvastatin, for oral administration. Lescol XL is supplied as extended-release tablets containing fluvastatin sodium, equivalent to 80 mg of fluvastatin, for oral administration.

Active ingredient: Fluvastatin sodium.

Inactive ingredients in capsules: Gelatin, magnesium stearate, microcrystalline cellulose, pregelatinized starch (corn), red iron oxide, sodium lauryl sulfate, talc, titanium dioxide, yellow iron oxide, and other ingredients.

Capsules may also include: Benzyl alcohol, black iron oxide, butylparaben, carboxymethylcellulose sodium, edetate calcium disodium, methylparaben, propylparaben, silicon dioxide and sodium propionate.

Inactive ingredients in extended-release tablets: Microcrystalline cellulose, hydroxypropyl cellulose, hydroxypropyl methyl cellulose, potassium bicarbonate, povidone, magnesium stearate, iron oxide yellow, titanium dioxide and polyethylene glycol 8000.

CLINICAL PHARMACOLOGY

A variety of clinical studies have demonstrated that elevated levels of total cholesterol (Total-C), low density lipoprotein cholesterol (LDL-C), triglycerides (TG), and apolipoprotein B (a membrane transport complex for LDL-C) promote human atherosclerosis. Similarly, decreased levels of HDL-cholesterol (HDL-C) and its transport complex, apolipoprotein A, are associated with the development of atherosclerosis. Epidemiologic investigations have established that cardiovascular morbidity and mortality vary directly with the level of Total-C and LDL-C and inversely with the level of HDL-C.

Like LDL, cholesterol-enriched triglyceride-rich lipoproteins, including VLDL, IDL and remnants, can also promote atherosclerosis. Elevated plasma triglycerides are frequently found in a triad with low HDL-C levels and small LDL particles, as well as in association with non-lipid metabolic risk factors for coronary heart disease. As such, total plasma TG has not consistently been shown to be an independent risk factor for CHD. Furthermore, the independent effect of raising HDL or lowering TG on the risk of coronary and cardiovascular morbidity and mortality has not been determined.

In patients with hypercholesterolemia and mixed dyslipidemia, treatment with Lescol or Lescol XL reduced Total-C, LDL-C, apolipoprotein B, and triglycerides while producing an increase in HDL-C. Increases in HDL-C are greater in patients with low HDL-C (<35 mg/dl). Neither agent had a consistent effect on either Lp(a) or fibrinogen. The effect of Lescol or Lescol XL induced changes in lipoprotein levels, including reduction of serum cholesterol, on cardiovascular morbidity or mortality has not been determined.

MECHANISM OF ACTION

Lescol is a competitive inhibitor of HMG-CoA reductase, which is responsible for the conversion of 3-hydroxy-3-methylglutaryl-coenzyme A (HMG-CoA) to mevalonate, a precursor of sterols, including cholesterol. The inhibition of cholesterol biosynthesis reduces the cholesterol in hepatic cells, which stimulates the synthesis of LDL receptors and thereby increases the uptake of LDL particles. The end result of these biochemical processes is a reduction of the plasma cholesterol concentration.

PHARMACOKINETICS AND METABOLISM

Oral Absorption

Fluvastatin is absorbed rapidly and completely following oral administration of the capsule, with peak concentrations reached in less than 1 hour. Following administration of a 10 mg dose, the absolute bioavailability is 24% (range 9-50%). Administration with food reduces the rate but not the extent of absorption. At steady-state, administration of fluvastatin with the evening meal results in a 2-fold decrease in C_{max} and more than 2-fold increase in T_{max} as compared to administration 4 hours after the evening meal. No significant differences in extent of absorption or in the lipid-lowering effects were observed between the 2 administrations. After single or multiple doses above 20 mg, fluvastatin exhibits saturable first-pass metabolism resulting in higher-than-expected plasma fluvastatin concentrations.

Fluvastatin has 2 optical enantiomers, an active 3R,5S and an inactive 3S,5R form. *In vivo* studies showed that stereo-selective hepatic binding of the active form occurs during the first pass resulting in a difference in the peak levels of the 2 enantiomers, with the active to inactive peak concentration ratio being about 0.7. The approximate ratio of the active to inactive approaches unity after the peak is seen and thereafter the 2 enantiomers decline with the same half-life. After an IV administration, bypassing the first-pass metabolism, the ratios of the enantiomers in plasma were similar throughout the concentration-time profiles.

Fluvastatin administered as Lescol XL 80 mg tablets reaches peak concentration in approximately 3 hours under fasting conditions, after a low-fat meal, or 2.5 hours after a low-fat meal. The mean relative bioavailability of the XL tablet is approximately 29% (range: 9-66%) compared to that of the Lescol immediate-release capsule administered under fasting conditions. Administration of a high fat meal delayed the absorption (T_{max}: 6H) and increased the bioavailability of the XL tablet by approximately 50%. Once Lescol XL begins to be absorbed, fluvastatin concentrations rise rapidly. The maximum concentration seen after a high fat meal is much less than the peak concentration following a single dose or twice daily dose of the 40 mg Lescol capsule. Overall variability in the pharmacokinetics of Lescol XL is large (42-64% CV for C_{max} and AUC), and especially so after a high fat meal (63-89% for C_{max} and AUC). Intrasubject variability in the pharmacokinetics of Lescol XL under fasting conditions (about 25% for C_{max} and AUC) tends to be much smaller as compared to the overall variability. Multiple peaks in plasma fluvastatin concentrations have been observed after Lescol XL administration.

Distribution

Fluvastatin is 98% bound to plasma proteins. The mean volume of distribution (VDss) is estimated at 0.35 L/kg. The parent drug is targeted to the liver and no active metabolites are present systemically. At therapeutic concentrations, the protein binding of fluvastatin is not affected by warfarin, salicylic acid and glyburide.

Metabolism

Fluvastatin is metabolized in the liver, primarily via hydroxylation of the indole ring at the 5- and 6-positions. N-dealkylation and beta-oxidation of the side-chain also occurs. The hydroxy metabolites have some pharmacologic activity, but do not circulate in the blood. Both enantiomers of fluvastatin are metabolized in a similar manner.

In vitro studies demonstrated that fluvastatin undergoes oxidative metabolism, predominantly via 2C9 isozyme systems (75%). Other isozymes that contribute to fluvastatin metabolism are 2C8 (~5%) and 3A4 (~20%). (See DRUG INTERACTIONS.)

Elimination

Fluvastatin is primarily (about 90%) eliminated in the feces as metabolites, with less than 2% present as unchanged drug. Urinary recovery is about 5%. After a radiolabeled dose of fluvastatin, the clearance was 0.8 L/h/kg. Following multiple oral doses of radiolabeled compound, there was no accumulation of fluvastatin; however, there was a 2.3-fold accumulation of total radioactivity.

Steady-state plasma concentrations show no evidence of accumulation of fluvastatin following immediate release capsule administration of up to 80 mg daily, as evidenced by a beta-elimination half-life of less than 3 hours. However, under conditions of maximum rate of absorption (*i.e.*, fasting) systemic exposure to fluvastatin is increased 33-53% compared to a single 20 or 40 mg dose of the immediate release capsule. Following once daily administration of the 80 mg Lescol XL tablet for 7 days, systemic exposure to fluvastatin is increased (20-30%) compared to a single dose of the 80 mg Lescol XL tablet. Terminal half-life of Lescol XL was about 9 hours as a result of the slow-release formulation.

Single-dose and steady-state pharmacokinetic parameters in 33 subjects with hypercholesterolemia for the capsules and in 35 healthy subjects for the extended-release tablets are summarized in TABLE 1.

SPECIAL POPULATIONS

Renal Insufficiency

No significant (<6%) renal excretion of fluvastatin occurs in humans.

Hepatic Insufficiency

Fluvastatin is subject to saturable first-pass metabolism/sequestration by the liver and is eliminated primarily via the biliary route. Therefore, the potential exists for drug accumulation in patients with hepatic insufficiency. Caution should therefore be exercised when fluvastatin sodium is administered to patients with a history of liver disease or heavy alcohol ingestion (see WARNINGS).

Fluvastatin AUC and C_{max} values increased by about 2.5-fold in hepatic insufficiency patients. This result was attributed to the decreased presystemic metabolism due to hepatic dysfunction. The enantiomer ratios of the 2 isomers of fluvastatin in hepatic insufficiency patients were comparable to those observed in healthy subjects.

TABLE 1 *Single-Dose and Steady-State Pharmacokinetic Parameters*

	Mean ±SD (range)				
	C_{max} (ng/ml)	AUC (ng·h/ml)	T_{max} (h)	CL/F (L/h)	T½ (h)
Capsules					
20 mg single dose (n=17)	166 ± 106 (48.9-517)	207 ± 65 (111-288)	0.9 ± 0.4 (0.5-2.0)	107 ± 38.1 (69.5-181)	2.5 ± 1.7 (0.5-6.6)
20 mg bid (n=17)	200 ± 86 (71.8-366)	275 ± 111 (91.6-467)	1.2 ± 0.9 (0.5-4.0)	87.8 ± 45 (42.8-218)	2.8 ± 1.7 (0.9-6.0)
40 mg single dose (n=16)	273 ± 189 (72.8-812)	456 ± 259 (207-1221)	1.2 ± 0.7 (0.75-3.0)	108 ± 44.7 (32.8-193)	2.7 ± 1.3 (0.8-5.9)
40 mg bid (n=16)	432 ± 236 (119-990)	697 ± 275 (359-1559)	1.2 ± 0.6 (0.5-2.5)	64.2 ± 21.1 (25.7-111)	2.7 ± 1.3 (0.7-5.0)
Extended-Release Tablets 80 mg Single Dose (n=24)					
Fasting	126 ± 53 (37-242)	579 ± 341 (144-1760)	3.2 ± 2.6 (1-12)	-	-
Fed state — high fat meal	183 ± 163 (21-733)	861 ± 632 (199-3132)	6 (2-24)	-	-
Extended-Release Tablets 80 mg Following 7 Days Dosing (steady-state) (n=11)					
80 mg once daily, fasting (n=11)	102 ± 42 (43.9-181)	630 ± 326 (247-1406)	2.6 ± 0.91 (1.5-4)	-	-

Age

Plasma levels of fluvastatin are not affected by age.

Gender

Women tend to have slightly higher (but statistically insignificant) fluvastatin concentrations than men for the immediate-release capsule. This is most likely due to body weight differences, as adjusting for body weight decreases the magnitude of the differences seen. For Lescol XL, there are 67% and 77% increases in systemic availability for women over men under fasted and high fat meal conditions.

Pediatric

No data are available. Fluvastatin is not indicated for use in the pediatric population.

INDICATIONS AND USAGE

Therapy with lipid-altering agents should be a component of multiple risk factor intervention in those individuals at significantly increased risk for atherosclerosis vascular disease due to hypercholesterolemia.

HYPERCHOLESTEROLEMIA (HETEROZYGOUS FAMILIAL AND NON FAMILIAL) AND MIXED DYSLIPIDEMIA

Lescol and Lescol XL are indicated as an adjunct to diet to reduce elevated total cholesterol (Total-C), LDL-C, TG and Apo B levels, and to increase HDL-C in patients with primary hypercholesterolemia and mixed dyslipidemia (Fredrickson Type IIa and IIb) whose response to dietary restriction of saturated fat and cholesterol and other nonpharmacological measures has not been adequate.

ATHEROSCLEROSIS

Lescol and Lescol XL are also indicated to slow the progression of coronary atherosclerosis in patients with coronary heart disease as part of a treatment strategy to lower total and LDL cholesterol to target levels.

Therapy with lipid-altering agents should be considered only after secondary causes for hyperlipidemia such as poorly controlled diabetes mellitus, hypothyroidism, nephrotic syndrome, dysproteinemias, obstructive liver disease, other medication, or alcoholism, have been excluded. Prior to initiation of fluvastatin sodium, a lipid profile should be performed to measure Total-C, HDL-C and TG. For patients with TG <400 mg/dl (<4.5 mmol/L), LDL-C can be estimated using the following equation:

LDL-C = (Total-C) - (HDL-C) - 1/5 TG

For TG levels >400 mg/dl (>4.5 mmol/L), this equation is less accurate and LDL-C concentrations should be determined by ultracentrifugation. In many hypertriglyceridemic patients LDL-C may be low or normal despite elevated Total-C. In such cases, Lescol is not indicated.

Lipid determinations should be performed at intervals of no less than 4 weeks and dosage adjusted according to the patient's response to therapy.

The Natural Cholesterol Education Program (NCEP) Treatment Guidelines are summarized in TABLE 3.

After the LDL-C goal has been achieved, if the TG is still ≥200 mg/dl, non-HDL-C (total-C minus HDL-C) becomes a secondary target of therapy. Non-HDL-C goals are set 30 mg/dl higher than LDL-C goals for each risk category.

At the time of hospitalization for an acute coronary event, consideration can be given to initiating drug therapy at discharge if the LDL-C level is ≥130 mg/dl (NCEP-ATP II).

Since the goal of treatment is to lower LDL-C, the NCEP recommends that the LDL-C levels be used to initiate and assess treatment response. Only if LDL-C levels are not available, should the Total-C be used to monitor therapy.

Neither the Lescol nor Lescol XL have been studied in conditions where the major abnormality is elevation of chylomicrons, VLDL, or IDL (*i.e.,* hypolipoproteinemia Types I, III, IV, or V).

TABLE 3 *NCEP Treatment Guidelines: LDL-C Goals and Cutpoints for Therapeutic Lifestyle Changes and Drug Therapy in Different Risk Categories*

		LDL Level at Which To:	
Risk Category	LDL Goal (mg/dl)	Initiate Therapeutic Lifestyle Changes (mg/dl)	Consider Drug Therapy (mg/dl)
CHD* or CHD risk equivalents†	<100	≥100	≥130 (100-129: drug optional)‡
2+ Risk factors§	<130	≥130	10 year risk 10-20%: ≥130 10 year risk <10%: ≥160
0-1 Risk factor¤	<160	≥160	≥190 (160-189: LDL-lowering drug optional)

* CHD, coronary heart disease.
† 10 year risk >20%.
‡ Some authorities recommend use of LDL-lowering drugs in this category if an LDL-C level of <100 mg/dl cannot be achieved by therapeutic lifestyle changes. Others prefer use of drugs that primarily modify triglycerides and HDL-C, *e.g.,* nicotinic acid or fibrate. Clinical judgement also may call for deferring drug therapy in this subcategory.
§ 10 year risk ≤20%.
¤ Almost all people with 0-1 risk factor have 10 year risk <10%; thus, 10 year risk assessment in people with 0-1 risk factor is not necessary.

TABLE 4 *Classification of Hyperlipoproteinemias*

		Lipid Elevations	
Type	Lipoproteins Elevated	Major	Minor
I (rare)	Chylomicrons	TG	C*
IIa	LDL	C	—
IIb	LDL, VLDL	C	TG
III (rare)	IDL	C/TG	—
IV	VLDL	TG	C*
V (rare)	Chylomicrons, VLDL	TG	C*

C = cholesterol, TG = triglycerides, LDL = low density lipoprotein, VLDL = very low density lipoprotein, IDL = intermediate density lipoprotein.
* Increases or no change.

CONTRAINDICATIONS

Hypersensitivity to any component of this medication. Lescol and Lescol XL are contraindicated in patients with active liver disease or unexplained, persistent elevations in serum transaminases (see WARNINGS).

PREGNANCY AND LACTATION

Atherosclerosis is a chronic process and discontinuation of lipid-lowering drugs during pregnancy should have little impact on the outcome of long-term therapy of primary hypercholesterolemia. Cholesterol and other products of cholesterol biosynthesis are essential components for fetal development (including synthesis of steroids and cell membranes). Since HMG-CoA reductase inhibitors decrease cholesterol synthesis and possibly the synthesis of other biologically active substances derived from cholesterol, they may cause fetal harm when administered to pregnant women. Therefore, HMG-CoA reductase inhibitors are contraindicated during pregnancy and in nursing mothers. **Fluvastatin sodium should be administered to women of childbearing age only when such patients are highly unlikely to conceive and have been informed of the potential hazards.** If the patient becomes pregnant while taking this class of drug, therapy should be discontinued and the patient apprised of the potential hazard to the fetus.

WARNINGS

LIVER ENZYMES

Biochemical abnormalities of liver function have been associated with HMG-CoA reductase inhibitors and other lipid-lowering agents. Approximately 1.1% of patients treated with Lescol capsules in worldwide trials developed dose-related, persistent elevations of transaminase levels to more than 3 times the upper limit of normal. Fourteen (14) of these patients (0.6%) were discontinued from therapy. In all clinical trials, a total of 33/2969 patients (1.1%) had persistent transaminase elevations with an average fluvastatin exposure of approximately 71.2 weeks; 19 of these patients (0.6%) were discontinued. The majority of patients with these abnormal biochemical findings were asymptomatic.

In a pooled analysis of all placebo-controlled studies in which Lescol capsules were used, persistent transaminase elevations (>3 times the upper limit of normal [ULN] on 2 consecutive weekly measurements) occurred in 0.2%, 1.5%, and 2.7% of patients treated with 20, 40, and 80 mg (titrated to 40 mg twice daily) Lescol capsules, respectively. Ninety-one percent (91%) of the cases of persistent liver function test abnormalities (20 of 22 patients) occurred within 12 weeks of therapy and in all patients with persistent liver function test abnormalities there was an abnormal liver function test present at baseline or by Week 8.

In the pooled analysis of the 24 week controlled trials, persistent transaminase elevation occurred in 1.9%, 1.8%, and 4.9% of patients treated with Lescol XL 80 mg, Lescol 40 mg and Lescol 40 mg twice daily, respectively. In 13 of 16 patients treated with Lescol XL the abnormality occurred within 12 weeks of initiation of treatment with Lescol XL 80 mg.

It is recommended that liver function tests be performed before the initiation of therapy and at 12 weeks following initiation of treatment or elevation in dose. Patients who develop transaminase elevations or signs and symptoms of liver disease should be monitored to confirm the finding and should be followed thereafter with frequent liver function tests until the levels return to normal. Should an increase in AST or ALT of 3 times the upper limit of normal or greater persist (found on 2 consecutive occasions) withdrawal of fluvastatin sodium therapy is recommended.

Active liver disease or unexplained transaminase elevations are contraindications to the use of Lescol and Lescol XL (see CONTRAINDICATIONS). Caution should be exercised when fluvastatin sodium is administered to patients with a history of liver disease or heavy alcohol ingestion (see CLINICAL PHARMACOLOGY, Pharmacokinetics and Metabolism). Such patients should be closely monitored.

SKELETAL MUSCLE

Rhabdomyolysis with renal dysfunction secondary to myoglobinuria has been reported with fluvastatin and with other drugs in this class. Myopathy, defined as muscle aching or muscle weakness in conjunction with increases in creatine phosphokinase (CPK) values to greater than 10 times the upper limit of normal, has been reported.

Myopathy should be considered in any patients with diffuse myalgias, muscle tenderness or weakness, and/or marked elevation of CPK. Patients should be advised to report promptly unexplained muscle pain, tenderness or weakness, particularly if accompanied by malaise or fever. Fluvastatin sodium therapy should be discontinued if markedly elevated CPK levels occur or myopathy is diagnosed or suspected. Fluvastatin sodium therapy should also be temporarily withheld in any patient experiencing an acute or serious condition predisposing to the development of renal failure secondary to rhabdomyolysis, *e.g.*, sepsis; hypotension; major surgery; trauma; severe metabolic, endocrine, or electrolyte disorders; or uncontrolled epilepsy.

The risk of myopathy and/or rhabdomyolysis during treatment with HMG-CoA reductase inhibitors has been reported to be increased if therapy with either cyclosporine, gemfibrozil, erythromycin, or niacin is administered concurrently. Myopathy was not observed in a clinical trial in 74 patients involving patients who were treated with fluvastatin sodium together with niacin.

Uncomplicated myalgia has been observed infrequently in patients treated with Lescol at rates indistinguishable from placebo.

The use of fibrates alone may occasionally be associated with myopathy. The combined use of HMG-CoA reductase inhibitors and fibrates should generally be avoided.

PRECAUTIONS

GENERAL

Before instituting therapy with Lescol or Lescol XL, an attempt should be made to control hypercholesterolemia with appropriate diet, exercise, and weight reduction in obese patients, and to treat other underlying medical problems (see INDICATIONS AND USAGE).

The HMG-CoA reductase inhibitors may cause elevation of creatine phosphokinase and transaminase levels (see WARNINGS and ADVERSE REACTIONS). This should be considered in the differential diagnosis of chest pain in a patient on therapy with fluvastatin sodium.

HOMOZYGOUS FAMILIAL HYPERCHOLESTEROLEMIA

HMG-CoA reductase inhibitors are reported to be less effective in patients with rare homozygous familial hypercholesterolemia, possibly because these patients have few functional LDL receptors.

INFORMATION FOR THE PATIENT

Patients should be advised to report promptly unexplained muscle pain, tenderness or weakness, particularly if accompanied by malaise or fever.

Women should be informed that if they become pregnant while receiving Lescol or Lescol XL the drug should be discontinued immediately to avoid possible harmful effects on a developing fetus from a relative deficit of cholesterol and biological products derived from cholesterol. In addition, Lescol or Lescol XL should not be taken during nursing. (See CONTRAINDICATIONS.)

ENDOCRINE FUNCTION

HMG-CoA reductase inhibitors interfere with cholesterol synthesis and lower circulating cholesterol levels and, as such, might theoretically blunt adrenal or gonadal steroid hormone production.

Fluvastatin exhibited no effect upon non-stimulated cortisol levels and demonstrated no effect upon thyroid metabolism as assessed by TSH. Small declines in total testosterone have been noted in treated groups, but no commensurate elevation in LH occurred, suggesting that the observation was not due to a direct effect upon testosterone production. No effect upon FSH in males was noted. Due to the limited number of premenopausal females studied to date, no conclusions regarding the effect of fluvastatin upon female sex hormones may be made.

Two clinical studies in patients receiving fluvastatin at doses up to 80 mg daily for periods of 24-28 weeks demonstrated no effect of treatment upon the adrenal response to ACTH stimulation. A clinical study evaluated the effect of fluvastatin at doses up to 80 mg daily for 28 weeks upon the gonadal response to HCG stimulation. Although the mean total testosterone response was significantly reduced ($p < 0.05$) relative to baseline in the 80 mg group, it was not significant in comparison to the changes noted in groups receiving either 40 mg of fluvastatin or placebo.

Patients treated with fluvastatin sodium who develop clinical evidence of endocrine dysfunction should be evaluated appropriately. Caution should be exercised if an HMG-CoA reductase inhibitor or other agent used to lower cholesterol levels is administered to patients receiving other drugs (*e.g.*, ketoconazole, spironolactone, or cimetidine) that may decrease the levels of endogenous steroid hormones.

CNS TOXICITY

CNS effects, as evidenced by decreased activity, ataxia, loss of righting reflex, and ptosis were seen in the following animal studies: the 18 month mouse carcinogenicity study at 50 mg/kg/day, the 6 month dog study at 36 mg/kg/day, the 6 month hamster study at 40 mg/kg/day, and in acute, high-dose studies in rats and hamsters (50 mg/kg), rabbits (300 mg/kg) and mice (1500 mg/kg). CNS toxicity in the acute high-dose studies was characterized (in mice) by conspicuous vacuolation in the ventral white columns of the spinal cord at a dose of 5000 mg/kg and (in rat) by edema with separation of myelinated fibers of the ventral spinal tracts and sciatic nerve at a dose of 1500 mg/kg. CNS toxicity, characterized by periaxonal vacuolation, was observed in the medulla of dogs that died after treatment for 5 weeks with 48 mg/kg/day; this finding was not observed in the remaining dogs when the dose level was lowered to 36 mg/kg/day. CNS vascular lesions, characterized by perivascular hemorrhages, edema, and mononuclear cell infiltration of perivascular spaces, have been observed in dogs treated with other members of this class. No CNS lesions have been observed after chronic treatment for up to 2 years with fluvastatin in the mouse (at doses up to 350 mg/kg/day), rat (up to 24 mg/kg/day), or dog (up to 16 mg/kg/day).

Prominent bilateral posterior Y suture lines in the ocular lens were seen in dogs after treatment with 1, 8, and 16 mg/kg/day for 2 years.

CARCINOGENESIS, MUTAGENESIS, AND IMPAIRMENT OF FERTILITY

A 2 year study was performed in rats at dose levels of 6, 9, and 18-24 (escalated after 1 year) mg/kg/day. These treatment levels represented plasma drug levels of approximately 9, 13, and 26-35 times the mean human plasma drug concentration after a 40 mg oral dose. A low incidence of forestomach squamous papillomas and 1 carcinoma of the forestomach at the 24 mg/kg/day dose level was considered to reflect the prolonged hyperplasia induced by direct contact exposure to fluvastatin sodium rather than to a systemic effect of the drug. In addition, an increased incidence of thyroid follicular cell adenomas and carcinomas was recorded for males treated with 18-24 mg/kg/day. The increased incidence of thyroid follicular cell neoplasm in male rats with fluvastatin sodium appears to be consistent with findings from other HMG-CoA reductase inhibitors. In contrast to other HMG-CoA reductase inhibitors, no hepatic adenomas or carcinomas were observed.

The carcinogenicity study conducted in mice at dose levels of 0.3, 15 and 30 mg/kg/day revealed, as in rats, a statistically significant increase in forestomach squamous cell papillomas in males and females at 30 mg/kg/day and in females at 15 mg/kg/day. These treatment levels represented plasma drug levels of approximately 0.05, 2, and 7 times the mean human plasma drug concentration after a 40 mg oral dose.

No evidence of mutagenicity was observed *in vitro,* with or without rat-liver metabolic activation, in the following studies: microbial mutagen tests using mutant strains of *Salmonella typhimurium* or *Escherichia coli;* malignant transformation assay in BALB/3T3 cells; unscheduled DNA synthesis in rat primary hepatocytes; chromosomal aberrations in V79 Chinese Hamster cells; HGPRT V79 Chinese Hamster cells. In addition, there was no evidence of mutagenicity *in vivo* in either a rat or mouse micronucleus test.

In a study in rats at dose levels for females of 0.6, 2 and 6 mg/kg/day and at dose levels for males of 2, 10 and 20 mg/kg/day, fluvastatin sodium had no adverse effects on the fertility or reproductive performance.

Seminal vesicles and testes were small in hamsters treated for 3 months at 20 mg/kg/day (approximately 3 times the 40 mg human daily dose based on surface area, mg/m^2). There was tubular degeneration and aspermatogenesis in testes as well as vesiculitis of seminal vesicles. Vesiculitis of seminal vesicles and edema of the testes were also seen in rats treated for 2 years at 18 mg/kg/day (approximately 4 times the human C_{max} achieved with a 40 mg daily dose).

PREGNANCY CATEGORY X

See CONTRAINDICATIONS.

Fluvastatin sodium produced delays in skeletal development in rats at doses of 12 mg/kg/day and in rabbits at doses of 10 mg/kg/day. Malaligned thoracic vertebrae were seen in rats at 36 mg/kg, a dose that produced maternal toxicity. These doses resulted in 2 times (rat at 12 mg/kg) or 5 times (rabbit at 10 mg/kg) the 40 mg human exposure based on mg/m^2 surface area. A study in which female rats were dosed during the third trimester at 12 and 24 mg/kg/day resulted in maternal mortality at or near term and postpartum. In addition, fetal and neonatal lethality were apparent. No effects on the dam or fetus occurred at 2 mg/kg/day. A second study at levels of 2, 6, 12 and 24 mg/kg/day confirmed the findings in the first study with neonatal mortality beginning at 6 mg/kg. A modified Segment III study was performed at dose levels of 12 or 24 mg/kg/day with or without the presence of concurrent supplementation with mevalonic acid, a product of HMG-CoA reductase which is essential for cholesterol biosynthesis. The concurrent administration of mevalonic acid completely prevented the maternal and neonatal mortality but did not prevent low body weights in pups at 24 mg/kg on Days 0 and 7 postpartum. Therefore, the maternal and neonatal lethality observed with fluvastatin sodium reflect its exaggerated pharmacologic effect during pregnancy. There are no data with fluvastatin sodium in pregnant women. However, rare reports of congenital anomalies have been received following intrauterine exposure to other HMG-CoA reductase inhibitors. There has been 1 report of severe congenital bony deformity, tracheo-esophageal fistula, and anal atresia (VATER association) in a baby born to a woman who took another HMG-CoA reductase inhibitor with dextroamphetamine sulfate during the first trimester of pregnancy. **Lescol or Lescol XL should be administered to women of child-bearing potential only when such patients are highly unlikely to conceive and have been informed of the potential hazards.** If a woman becomes pregnant while taking Lescol or Lescol XL, the drug should be discontinued and the patient advised again as to the potential hazards to the fetus.

NURSING MOTHERS

Based on preclinical data, drug is present in breast milk in a 2:1 ratio (milk:plasma). Because of the potential for serious adverse reactions in nursing infants, nursing women should not take Lescol or Lescol XL (see CONTRAINDICATIONS).

PEDIATRIC USE

Safety and effectiveness in individuals less than 18 years old have not been established. Treatment in patients less than 18 years of age is not recommended at this time.

GERIATRIC USE

The effect of age on the pharmacokinetics of immediate-release fluvastatin sodium was evaluated. Results indicate that for the general patient population plasma concentrations of fluvastatin sodium do not vary as a function of age. (See also CLINICAL PHARMACOLOGY, Pharmacokinetics and Metabolism.) Elderly patients ($\geq$65 years of age) demonstrated a greater treatment response in respect to LDL-C, Total-C and LDL/HDL ratio than patients $<$65 years of age.

F

DRUG INTERACTIONS

The drug interaction information listed below is derived from studies using immediate-release fluvastatin. Similar studies have not been conducted using the Lescol XL tablet.

IMMUNOSUPPRESSIVE DRUGS, GEMFIBROZIL, NIACIN (NICOTINIC ACID), ERYTHROMYCIN

See WARNINGS, Skeletal Muscle.

In vitro data indicate that fluvastatin metabolism involves multiple Cytochrome P450 (CYP) isozymes. CYP2C9 isoenzyme is primarily involved in the metabolism of fluvastatin (~75%), while CYP2C8 and CYP3A4 isoenzymes are involved to a much less extent, *i.e.*, ~5% and ~20%, respectively. If 1 pathway is inhibited in the elimination process of fluvastatin, other pathways may compensate.

In vivo drug interaction studies with CYP3A4 inhibitors/substrates such as cyclosporine, erythromycin, and itraconazole result in minimal changes in the pharmacokinetics of fluvastatin, confirming less involvement of CYP3A4 isozyme. Concomitant administration of fluvastatin and phenytoin increased the levels of phenytoin and fluvastatin, suggesting predominant involvement of CYP2C9 in fluvastatin metabolism.

Niacin/Propranolol: Concomitant administration of immediate-release fluvastatin sodium with niacin or propranolol has no effect on the bioavailability of fluvastatin sodium.

Cholestyramine: Administration of immediate-release fluvastatin sodium concomitantly with, or up to 4 hours after cholestyramine, results in fluvastatin decreases of more than 50% for AUC and 50-80% for C_{max}. However, administration of immediate-release fluvastatin sodium 4 hours after cholestyramine resulted in a clinically significant additive effect compared with that achieved with either component drug.

Cyclosporine: Plasma cyclosporine levels remain unchanged when fluvastatin (20 mg daily) was administered concurrently in renal transplant recipients on stable cyclosporine regimens. Fluvastatin AUC increased 1.9-fold, and C_{max} increased 1.3-fold compared to historical controls.

Digoxin: In a crossover study involving 18 patients chronically receiving digoxin, a single 40 mg dose of immediate-release fluvastatin had no effect on digoxin AUC, but had an 11% increase in digoxin C_{max} and small increase in digoxin urinary clearance.

Erythromycin: Erythromycin (500 mg, single dose) did not affect steady-state plasma levels of fluvastatin (40 mg daily).

Itraconazole: Concomitant administration of fluvastatin (40 mg) and itraconazole (100 mg daily × 4 days) does not affect plasma itraconazole or fluvastatin levels.

Gemfibrozil: There is no change in either fluvastatin (20 mg twice daily) or gemfibrozil (600 mg twice daily) plasma levels when these drugs are coadministered.

Phenytoin: Single morning dose administration of phenytoin (300 mg extended-release) increased mean steady-state fluvastatin (40 mg) C_{max} by 27% and AUC by 40% whereas fluvastatin increased the mean phenytoin C_{max} by 5% and AUC by 20%. Patients on phenytoin should continue to be monitored appropriately when fluvastatin therapy is initiated or when the fluvastatin dosage is changed.

Diclofenac: Concurrent administration of fluvastatin (40 mg) increased the mean C_{max} and AUC of diclofenac by 60% and 25%, respectively.

Tolbutamide: In healthy volunteers, concurrent administration of either single or multiple daily doses of fluvastatin sodium (40 mg) with tolbutamide (1 g) did not affect the plasma levels of either drug to a clinically significant extent.

Glibenclamide (glyburide): In glibenclamide-treated NIDDM patients (n=32), administration of fluvastatin (40 mg twice daily for 14 days) increased the mean C_{max}, AUC, and $T_{1/2}$ of glibenclamide approximately 50%, 69% and 121%, respectively. Glibenclamide (5-20 mg daily) increased the mean C_{max} and AUC of fluvastatin by 44% and 51%, respectively. In this study there were no changes in glucose, insulin and C-peptide levels. However, patients on concomitant therapy with glibenclamide (glyburide) and fluvastatin should continue to be monitored appropriately when their fluvastatin dose is increased to 40 mg twice daily.

Losartan: Concomitant administration of fluvastatin with losartan has no effect on the bioavailability of either losartan or its active metabolite.

Cimetidine/Ranitidine/Omeprazole: Concomitant administration of immediate-release fluvastatin sodium with cimetidine, ranitidine and omeprazole results in a significant increase in the fluvastatin C_{max} (43%, 70% and 50%, respectively) and AUC (24-33%), with an 18-23% decrease in plasma clearance.

Rifampicin: Administration of immediate-release fluvastatin sodium to subjects pretreated with rifampicin results in significant reduction in C_{max} (59%) and AUC (51%), with a large increase (95%) in plasma clearance.

Warfarin: *In vitro* protein binding studies demonstrated no interaction at therapeutic concentrations. Concomitant administration of a single dose of warfarin (30 mg) in young healthy males receiving immediate-release fluvastatin sodium (40 mg/day × 8 days) resulted in no elevation of racemic warfarin concentration. There was also no effect on prothrombin complex activity when compared to concomitant administration of placebo and warfarin. However, bleeding and/or increased prothrombin times have been reported in patients taking coumarin anticoagulants concomitantly with other HMG-CoA reductase inhibitors. Therefore, patients receiving warfarin-type anticoagulants should have their prothrombin times closely monitored when fluvastatin sodium is initiated or the dosage of fluvastatin sodium is changed.

ADVERSE REACTIONS

In all clinical studies of Lescol, 1.0% (32/2969) of fluvastatin-treated patients were discontinued due to adverse experiences attributed to study drug (mean exposure approximately 16 months ranging in duration from 1 to >36 months). This results in an exposure adjusted rate of 0.8% (32/4051) per patient year in fluvastatin patients in controlled studies compared to an incidence of 1.1% (4/355) in placebo patients. Adverse reactions have usually been of mild to moderate severity.

In controlled clinical studies, 3.9% (36/912) of patients treated with Lescol XL 80 mg discontinued due to adverse events (causality not determined).

Adverse experiences occurring in the Lescol and Lescol XL controlled studies with a frequency >2%, regardless of causality, are shown in TABLE 5.

TABLE 5 *Adverse Experiences Occurring in >2% of Patients in Lescol and Lescol XL Controlled Studies*

Adverse Event	Lescol* (n=2326)	Placebo* (n=960)	Lescol XL† (n=912)
Integumentary			
Rash	2.3%	2.4%	1.6%
Musculoskeletal			
Back pain	5.7%	6.6%	4.7%
Myalgia	5.0%	4.5%	3.8%
Arthralgia	4.0%	4.1%	1.3%
Arthritis	2.1%	2.0%	1.3%
Arthropathy	NA	NA	3.2%
Respiratory			
Upper respiratory tract infection	16.2%	16.5%	12.5%
Pharyngitis	3.8%	3.8%	2.4%
Rhinitis	4.7%	4.9%	1.5%
Sinusitis	2.6%	1.9%	3.5%
Coughing	2.4%	2.9%	1.9%
Bronchitis	1.8%	1.0%	2.6%
Gastrointestinal			
Dyspepsia	7.9%	3.2%	3.5%
Diarrhea	4.9%	4.2%	3.3%
Abdominal pain	4.9%	3.8%	3.7%
Nausea	3.2%	2.0%	2.5%
Constipation	3.1%	3.3%	2.3%
Flatulence	2.6%	2.5%	1.4%
Misc. tooth disorder	2.1%	1.7%	1.4%
Central Nervous System			
Dizziness	2.2%	2.5%	1.9%
Psychiatric Disorders			
Insomnia	2.7%	1.4%	0.8%
Genitourinary			
Urinary tract infection	1.6%	1.1%	2.7%
Miscellaneous			
Headache	8.9%	7.8%	4.7%
Influenza-like symptoms	5.1%	5.7%	7.1%
Accidental trauma	5.1%	4.8%	4.2%
Fatigue	2.7%	2.3%	1.6%
Allergy	2.3%	2.2%	1.0%

* Controlled trials with Lescol capsules (20 and 40 mg daily and 40 mg twice daily).
† Controlled trials with Lescol XL 80 mg tablets.

The following effects have been reported with drugs in this class. Not all the effects listed below have necessarily been associated with fluvastatin sodium therapy.

Skeletal: Muscle cramps, myalgia, myopathy, rhabdomyolysis, arthralgias.

Neurological: Dysfunction of certain cranial nerves (including alteration of taste, impairment of extraocular movement, facial paresis), tremor, dizziness, vertigo, memory loss, paresthesia, peripheral neuropathy, peripheral nerve palsy, psychic disturbances, anxiety, insomnia, depression.

Hypersensitivity Reactions: ***An apparent hypersensitivity syndrome has been reported rarely which has included 1 or more of the following features:*** Anaphylaxis, angioedema, lupus erythematosus-like syndrome, polymyalgia rheumatica, vasculitis, purpura, thrombocytopenia, leukopenia, hemolytic anemia, positive ANA, ESR increase, eosinophilia, arthritis, arthralgia, urticaria, asthenia, photosensitivity, fever, chills, flushing, malaise, dyspnea, toxic epidermal necrolysis, erythema multiforme, including Stevens-Johnson syndrome.

Gastrointestinal: Pancreatitis, hepatis, including chronic active hepatitis, cholestatic jaundice, fatty change in liver, and, rarely, cirrhosis, fulminant hepatic necrosis, and hepatoma; anorexia, vomiting.

Skin: Alopecia, pruritus. A variety of skin changes (*e.g.*, nodules, discoloration, dryness of skin/mucous membranes, changes to hair/nails) have been reported.

Reproductive: Gynecomastia, loss of libido, erectile dysfunction.

Eye: Progression of cataracts (lens opacities), ophthalmoplegia.

Laboratory Abnormalities: Elevated transaminases, alkaline phosphatase, γ-glutamyl transpeptidase, and bilirubin; thyroid function abnormalities.

CONCOMITANT THERAPY

Fluvastatin sodium has been administered concurrently with cholestyramine and nicotinic acid. No adverse reactions unique to the combination or in addition to those previously reported for this class of drugs alone have been reported. Myopathy and rhabdomyolysis (with or without acute renal failure) have been reported when another HMG-CoA reductase inhibitor was used in combination with immunosuppressive drugs, gemfibrozil, erythromycin, or lipid-lowering doses of nicotinic acid. Concomitant therapy with HMG-CoA reductase inhibitors and these agents is generally not recommended (see WARNINGS, Skeletal Muscle).

DOSAGE AND ADMINISTRATION

The patient should be placed on a standard cholesterol-lowering diet before receiving Lescol or Lescol XL and should continue on this diet during treatment with Lescol or Lescol XL. (See NCEP Treatment Guidelines for details on dietary therapy.)

For patients requiring LDL-C reduction to a goal of ≥25%, the recommended starting dose is 40 mg as 1 capsule, 80 mg as 1 Lescol XL tablet administered as a single dose in the evening or 80 mg in divided doses of the 40 mg capsule given twice daily. For patients requiring LDL-C reduction to a goal of <25%, a starting dose of 20 mg may be used. The recommended dosing range is 20-80 mg/day. Lescol or Lescol XL may be taken without regard to meals, since there are no apparent differences in the lipid-lowering effects of fluvastatin sodium administered with the evening meal or 4 hours after the evening meal. Since the maximal reductions in LDL-C of a given dose are seen within 4 weeks, periodic lipid determinations should be performed and dosage adjustment made according to the patient's response to therapy and established treatment guidelines. The therapeutic effect of Lescol or Lescol XL is maintained with prolonged administration.

CONCOMITANT THERAPY

Lipid-lowering effects on total cholesterol and LDL cholesterol are additive when immediate-release Lescol is combined with a bile-acid binding resin or niacin. When administering a bile-acid resin (*e.g.*, cholestyramine) and fluvastatin sodium, Lescol should be administered at bedtime, at least 2 hours following the resin to avoid a significant interaction due to drug binding to resin. (See ADVERSE REACTIONS, Concomitant Therapy.)

DOSAGE IN PATIENTS WITH RENAL INSUFFICIENCY

Since fluvastatin sodium is cleared hepatically with less than 6% of the administered dose excreted into the urine, dose adjustments for mild to moderate renal impairment are not necessary. Fluvastatin has not been studied at doses greater than 40 mg in patients with severe renal impairment; therefore caution should be exercised when treating such patients at higher doses.

HOW SUPPLIED

LESCOL CAPSULES

20 mg: Brown and light brown imprinted twice with "S" (surrounded by a triangle) and "20" on 1 half and "LESCOL" and the Lescol logo twice on the other half of the capsule.
40 mg: Brown and gold imprinted twice with "S" (surrounded by a triangle) and "40" on 1 half and "LESCOL" and the Lescol logo twice on the other half of the capsule.

LESCOL XL EXTENDED-RELEASE TABLETS

80 mg: Yellow, round, slightly biconvex film-coated tablet with beveled edges debossed with "Lescol XL" on 1 side and "80" on the other.

STORE AND DISPENSE

Store at 25°C (77°F); excursions permitted to 15-30°C (59-86°F). Dispense in a tight container. Protect from light.

PRODUCT LISTING - EQUIVALENTS NOT AVAILABLE

Qty	Price	Product	NDC
Capsule - Oral - 20 mg			
30's	$42.28	LESCOL, Allscripts Pharmaceutical Company	54569-3821-00
30's	$45.46	LESCOL, Physicians Total Care	54868-3329-00
30's	$55.65	LESCOL, Novartis Pharmaceuticals	00078-0176-15
60's	$79.84	LESCOL, Allscripts Pharmaceutical Company	54569-3821-01
60's	$111.30	LESCOL, Pd-Rx Pharmaceuticals	55289-0740-60
100's	$185.19	LESCOL, Novartis Pharmaceuticals	00078-0176-05
Capsule - Oral - 40 mg			
30's	$42.21	LESCOL, Allscripts Pharmaceutical Company	54569-4761-00
30's	$55.65	LESCOL, Novartis Pharmaceuticals	00078-0234-15
30's	$62.31	LESCOL, Pd-Rx Pharmaceuticals	55289-0476-30
100's	$185.19	LESCOL, Novartis Pharmaceuticals	00078-0234-05
Tablet, Extended Release - Oral - 80 mg			
30's	$71.28	LESCOL XL, Novartis Pharmaceuticals	00078-0354-15
100's	$237.58	LESCOL XL, Novartis Pharmaceuticals	00078-0354-05

Fluvoxamine Maleate *(003080)*

For related information, see the comparative table section in Appendix A.

Categories: Obsessive compulsive disorder; Pregnancy Category C; FDA Approved 1994 Dec
Drug Classes: Antidepressants, serotonin specific reuptake inhibitors
Brand Names: Floxyfral; **Luvox**
Foreign Brand Availability: Dumirox (Korea; Spain); Dumyrox (Greece; Portugal); Faverin (Australia; Bahrain; Cyprus; Egypt; England; Hong-Kong; Iran; Iraq; Ireland; Jordan; Kuwait; Lebanon; Libya; Oman; Philippines; Qatar; Republic-of-Yemen; Saudi-Arabia; Singapore; Syria; Thailand; United-Arab-Emirates); Favoxil (Israel); Fevarin (Bulgaria; Denmark; Finland; Germany; Hungary; Italy; Netherlands; Norway; Sweden; Turkey); Fluvohexal (Germany); Fluvoxin (India); Voxamin (Colombia)
Cost of Therapy: $79.19 (Obsessive-Compulsive Disorder; Luvox; 100 mg; 1 tablet/day; 30 day supply)
$78.80 (Obsessive-Compulsive Disorder; Generic Tablets; 100 mg; 1 tablet/day; 30 day supply)

DESCRIPTION

Fluvoxamine maleate is a selective serotonin (5-HT) reuptake inhibitor (SSRI) belonging to a new chemical series, the 2-aminoethyl oxime ethers of aralkylketones. It is chemically unrelated to other SSRIs and clomipramine. It is chemically designated as 5-methoxy-4'-(trifluoromethyl)valerophenone-(E)-O-(2-aminoethyl)oxime maleate (1:1) and has the empirical formula $C_{15}H_{21}O_2N_2F_3 \cdot C_4H_4O_4$. Its molecular weight is 434.4.

Fluvoxamine maleate is a white or off white, odorless, crystalline powder which is sparingly soluble in water, freely soluble in ethanol and chloroform and practically insoluble in diethyl ether.

Luvox (fluvoxamine maleate) tablets are available in 25, 50 and 100 mg strengths for oral administration. In addition to the active ingredient, fluvoxamine maleate, each tablet contains the following inactive ingredients: carnauba wax, hydroxypropyl methylcellulose, mannitol, polyethylene glycol, polysorbate 80, pregelatinized starch (potato), silicon dioxide, sodium stearyl fumarate, starch (corn), and titanium dioxide. The 50 and 100 mg tablets also contain synthetic iron oxides.

CLINICAL PHARMACOLOGY

PHARMACODYNAMICS

The mechanism of action of fluvoxamine maleate in Obsessive Compulsive Disorder is presumed to be linked to its specific serotonin reuptake inhibition in brain neurons. In preclinical studies, it was found that fluvoxamine inhibited neuronal uptake of serotonin.

In *in vitro* studies fluvoxamine maleate had no significant affinity for histaminergic, alpha or beta adrenergic, muscarinic, or dopaminergic receptors. Antagonism of some of these receptors is thought to be associated with various sedative, cardiovascular, anticholinergic, and extrapyramidal effects of some psychotropic drugs.

PHARMACOKINETICS

Bioavailability

The absolute bioavailability of fluvoxamine maleate is 53%. Oral bioavailability is not significantly affected by food.

In a dose proportionality study involving fluvoxamine maleate at 100, 200, and 300 mg/day for 10 consecutive days in 30 normal volunteers, steady-state was achieved after about a week of dosing. Maximum plasma concentrations at steady-state occurred within 3-8 hours of dosing and reached concentrations averaging 88, 283, and 546 ng/ml, respectively. Thus, fluvoxamine had nonlinear pharmacokinetics over this dose range, *i.e.*, higher doses of fluvoxamine maleate produced disproportionately higher concentrations than predicted from the lower dose.

Distribution/Protein Binding

The mean apparent volume of distribution for fluvoxamine is approximately 25 L/kg, suggesting extensive tissue distribution.

Approximately 80% of fluvoxamine is bound to plasma protein, mostly albumin, over a concentration range of 20-2000 ng/ml.

Metabolism

Fluvoxamine maleate is extensively metabolized by the liver; the main metabolic routes are oxidative demethylation and deamination. Nine metabolites were identified following a 5 mg radiolabeled dose of fluvoxamine maleate, constituting approximately 85% of the urinary excretion products of fluvoxamine. The main human metabolite was fluvoxamine acid which, together with its N-acetylated analog, accounted for about 60% of the urinary excretion products. A third metabolite, fluvoxethanol, formed by oxidative deamination, accounted for about 10%. Fluvoxamine acid and fluvoxethanol were tested in an *in vitro* assay of serotonin and norepinephrine reuptake inhibition in rats; they were inactive except for a weak effect of the former metabolite on inhibition of serotonin uptake (1-2 orders of magnitude less potent than the parent compound). Approximately 2% of fluvoxamine was excreted in urine unchanged. (See DRUG INTERACTIONS.)

Elimination

Following a ^{14}C-labeled oral dose of fluvoxamine maleate (5 mg), an average of 94% of drug-related products was recovered in the urine within 71 hours.

The mean plasma half-life of fluvoxamine at steady-state after multiple oral doses of 100 mg/day in healthy, young volunteers was 15.6 hours.

Elderly Subjects

In a study of fluvoxamine maleate tablets at 50 and 100 mg comparing elderly (aged 66-73) and young subjects (ages 19-35), mean maximum plasma concentrations in the elderly were 40% higher. The multiple dose elimination half-life of fluvoxamine was 17.4 and 25.9 hours in the elderly compared to 13.6 and 15.6 hours in the young subjects at steady-state for 50 and 100 mg doses, respectively.

In elderly patients, the clearance of fluvoxamine was reduced by about 50% and, therefore, fluvoxamine maleate tablets should be slowly titrated during initiation of therapy.

Hepatic and Renal Disease

A cross study comparison (healthy subjects versus patients with hepatic dysfunction) suggested a 30% decrease in fluvoxamine clearance in association with hepatic dysfunction. The mean minimum plasma concentrations in renally impaired patients (creatinine clearance of 5-45 ml/min) after 4 and 6 weeks of treatment (50 mg bid, n=13) were comparable to each other, suggesting no accumulation of fluvoxamine in these patients. (See PRECAUTIONS, Use in Patients With Concomitant Illness.)

INDICATIONS AND USAGE

Fluvoxamine maleate tablets are indicated for the treatment of obsessions and compulsions in patients with Obsessive Compulsive Disorder (OCD), as defined in the DSM-III-R. The obsessions or compulsions cause marked distress, are time-consuming, or significantly interfere with social or occupational functioning.

The efficacy of fluvoxamine maleate tablets was established in three 10 week trials with obsessive compulsive outpatients with the diagnosis of Obsessive Compulsive Disorder as defined in DSM-III-R.

Obsessive Compulsive Disorder is characterized by recurrent and persistent ideas, thoughts, impulses or images (obsessions) that are ego-dystonic and/or repetitive, purposeful, and intentional behaviors (compulsions) that are recognized by the person as excessive or unreasonable.

The effectiveness of fluvoxamine maleate tablets for long-term use, *i.e.*, for more than 10 weeks, has not been systematically evaluated in placebo-controlled trials. Therefore, the physician who elects to use fluvoxamine maleate tablets for extended periods should periodically re-evaluate the long-term usefulness of the drug for the individual patient. (See DOSAGE AND ADMINISTRATION.)

NON-FDA APPROVED INDICATIONS

Fluvoxamine has been reported to improve symptoms of social anxiety disorder, post-traumatic stress disorder, depression, panic disorder, pathological gambling, compulsive buying, trichotillomania, kleptomania, body dysmorphic disorder, eating disorders, and autistic disorders. However, these uses have not been approved by the FDA and further clinical trials are needed.

CONTRAINDICATIONS

Co-administration of thioridazine, terfenadine, astemizole, cisapride, or pimozide with fluvoxamine maleate tablets is contraindicated (see WARNINGS and PRECAUTIONS).

Fluvoxamine maleate tablets are contraindicated in patients with a history of hypersensitivity to fluvoxamine maleate.

WARNINGS

POTENTIAL FOR INTERACTION WITH MONOAMINE OXIDASE INHIBITORS

In patients receiving another serotonin reuptake inhibitor drug in combination with monoamine oxidase inhibitors (MAOI), there have been reports of serious, sometimes fatal, reactions including hyperthermia, rigidity, myoclonus, autonomic instability with possible rapid fluctuations of vital signs, and mental status changes that include extreme agitation progressing to delirium and coma. These reactions have also been reported in patients who have discontinued that drug and have been started on a MAOI. Some cases presented with features resembling neuroleptic malignant syndrome. Therefore, it is recommended that fluvoxamine maleate tablets not be used in combination with a MAOI, or within 14 days of discontinuing treatment with a MAOI. After stopping fluvoxamine maleate tablets, at least 2 weeks should be allowed before starting a MAOI.

F

POTENTIAL INTERACTION WITH THIORIDAZINE

The effect of fluvoxamine (25 mg bid for 1 week) on thioridazine steady-state concentrations was evaluated in 10 male inpatients with schizophrenia. Concentrations of thioridazine and its two active metabolites, mesoridazine and sulforidazine, increased 3-fold following co-administration of fluvoxamine.

Thioridazine administration produces a dose-related prolongation of the QTc interval, which is associated with serious ventricular arrhythmias, such as torsade de pointes-type arrhythmias, and sudden death. It is likely that this experience underestimates the degree of risk that might occur with higher doses of thioridazine. Moreover, the effect of fluvoxamine may be even more pronounced when it is administered at higher doses.

Therefore, fluvoxamine and thioridazine should not be co-administered (see CONTRAINDICATIONS and PRECAUTIONS).

POTENTIAL TERFENADINE, ASTEMIZOLE, CISAPRIDE, AND PIMOZIDE INTERACTIONS

Terfenadine, astemizole, cisapride, and pimozide are all metabolized by the cytochrome P450IIIA4 isozyme, and it has been demonstrated that ketoconazole, a potent inhibitor of IIIA4, blocks the metabolism of these drugs, resulting in increased plasma concentrations of parent drug. Increased plasma concentrations of terfenadine, astemizole, cisapride, and pimozide cause QT prolongation and have been associated with torsades de pointes-type ventricular tachycardia, sometimes fatal. As noted below, a substantial pharmacokinetic interaction has been observed for fluvoxamine in combination with alprazolam, a drug that is known to be metabolized by the IIIA4 isozyme. Although it has not been definitively demonstrated that fluvoxamine is a potent IIIA4 inhibitor, it is likely to be, given the substantial interaction of fluvoxamine with alprazolam. Consequently, it is recommended that fluvoxamine not be used in combination with either terfenadine, astemizole, cisapride, or pimozide (see CONTRAINDICATIONS and PRECAUTIONS).

OTHER POTENTIALLY IMPORTANT DRUG INTERACTIONS

Also see DRUG INTERACTIONS.

Benzodiazepines

Benzodiazepines metabolized by hepatic oxidation (*e.g.,* alprazolam, midazolam, triazolam, etc.) should be used with caution because the clearance of these drugs is likely to be reduced by fluvoxamine. The clearance of benzodiazepines metabolized by glucuronidation (*e.g.,* lorazepam, oxazepam, temazepam) is unlikely to be affected by fluvoxamine.

Alprazolam

When fluvoxamine maleate (100 mg qd) and alprazolam (1 mg qid) were co-administered to steady-state, plasma concentrations and other pharmacokinetic parameters (AUC, C_{max}, $T_{1/2}$) of alprazolam were approximately twice those observed when alprazolam was administered alone; oral clearance was reduced by about 50%. The elevated plasma alprazolam concentrations resulted in decreased psychomotor performance and memory. This interaction, which has not been investigated using higher doses of fluvoxamine, may be more pronounced if a 300 mg daily dose is co-administered, particularly since fluvoxamine exhibits non-linear pharmacokinetics over the dosage range 100-300 mg. If alprazolam is co-administered with fluvoxamine maleate tablets, the initial alprazolam dosage should be at least halved and titration to the lowest effective dose is recommended. No dosage adjustment is required for fluvoxamine maleate tablets.

Diazepam

The co-administration of fluvoxamine maleate tablets and diazepam is generally not advisable. Because fluvoxamine reduces the clearance of both diazepam and its active metabolite, N-desmethyldiazepam, there is a strong likelihood of substantial accumulation of both species during chronic co-administration.

Evidence supporting the conclusion that it is inadvisable to co-administer fluvoxamine and diazepam is derived from a study in which healthy volunteers taking 150 mg/day of fluvoxamine were administered a single oral dose of 10 mg of diazepam. In these subjects (n=8), the clearance of diazepam was reduced by 65% and that of N-desmethyldiazepam to a level that was too low to measure over the course of the 2 week long study.

It is likely that this experience significantly underestimates the degree of accumulation that might occur with repeated diazepam administration. Moreover, as noted with alprazolam, the effect of fluvoxamine may even be more pronounced when it is administered at higher doses.

Accordingly, diazepam and fluvoxamine should not ordinarily be co-administered.

Mexiletine

The effect of steady-state fluvoxamine (50 mg bid for 7 days) on the single dose pharmacokinetics of mexiletene (200 mg) was evaluated in 6 healthy Japanese males. The clearance of mexiletene was reduced by 38% following co-administration with fluvoxamine compared to mexiletene alone. If fluvoxamine and mexiletene are co-administered, serum mexiletene levels should be monitored.

Theophylline

The effect of steady-state fluvoxamine (50 mg bid) on the pharmacokinetics of a single dose of theophylline (375 mg as 442 mg aminophylline) was evaluated in 12 healthy non-smoking, male volunteers. The clearance of theophylline was decreased approximately 3-fold. Therefore, if theophylline is co-administered with fluvoxamine maleate, its dose should be reduced to one-third of the usual daily maintenance dose and plasma concentrations of theophylline should be monitored. No dosage adjustment is required for fluvoxamine maleate tablets.

Warfarin

When fluvoxamine maleate (50 mg tid) was administered concomitantly with warfarin for 2 weeks, warfarin plasma concentrations increased by 98% and prothrombin times were prolonged. Thus patients receiving oral anticoagulants and fluvoxamine maleate tablets should have their prothrombin time monitored and their anticoagulant dose adjusted accordingly. No dosage adjustment is required for fluvoxamine maleate tablets.

PRECAUTIONS

GENERAL

Activation of Mania/Hypomania

During premarketing studies involving primarily depressed patients, hypomania or mania occurred in approximately 1% of patients treated with fluvoxamine. In a 10 week pediatric OCD study, 2 out of 57 patients (4%) treated with fluvoxamine experienced manic reactions, compared to none of 63 placebo patients. Activation of mania/hypomania has also been reported in a small proportion of patients with major affective disorder who were treated with other marketed antidepressants. As with all antidepressants, fluvoxamine maleate tablets should be used cautiously in patients with a history of mania.

Seizures

During premarketing studies, seizures were reported in 0.2% of fluvoxamine-treated patients. Fluvoxamine maleate tablets should be used cautiously in patients with a history of seizures. It should be discontinued in any patient who develops seizures.

Suicide

The possibility of a suicide attempt is inherent in patients with depressive symptoms, whether these occur in primary depression or in association with another primary disorder such as OCD. Close supervision of high risk patients should accompany initial drug therapy. Prescriptions for fluvoxamine maleate tablets should be written for the smallest quantity of tablets consistent with good patient management in order to reduce the risk of overdose.

Hyponatremia

Several cases of hyponatremia have been reported. In cases where the outcome was known, the hyponatremia appeared to be reversible when fluvoxamine was discontinued. The majority of these occurrences have been in elderly individuals, some in patients taking diuretics or with concomitant conditions that might cause hyponatremia. In patients receiving fluvoxamine maleate tablets and suffering from Syndrome of Inappropriate Secretion of Antidiuretic Hormone (SIADH), displacement syndromes, edematous states, adrenal disease or conditions of fluid loss, it is recommended that serum electrolytes, especially sodium as well as BUN and plasma creatinine, be monitored regularly.

Use in Patients With Concomitant Illness

Closely monitored clinical experience with fluvoxamine maleate tablets in patients with concomitant systemic illness is limited. Caution is advised in administering fluvoxamine maleate tablets to patients with diseases or conditions that could affect hemodynamic responses or metabolism.

Fluvoxamine maleate tablets have not been evaluated or used to any appreciable extent in patients with a recent history of myocardial infarction or unstable heart disease. Patients with these diagnoses were systematically excluded from many clinical studies during the product's premarketing testing. Evaluation of the electrocardiograms for patients with depression or OCD who participated in premarketing studies revealed no differences between fluvoxamine and placebo in the emergence of clinically important ECG changes.

In patients with liver dysfunction, fluvoxamine clearance was decreased by approximately 30%. Fluvoxamine maleate tablets should be slowly titrated in patients with liver dysfunction during the initiation of treatment.

INFORMATION FOR THE PATIENT

Physicians are advised to discuss the following issues with patients for whom they prescribe fluvoxamine maleate tablets:

Interference with cognitive or motor performance: Since any psychoactive drug may impair judgement, thinking, or motor skills, patients should be cautioned about operating hazardous machinery, including automobiles, until they are certain that fluvoxamine maleate tablets therapy does not adversely affect their ability to engage in such activities.

Pregnancy: Patients should be advised to notify their physicians if they become pregnant or intend to become pregnant during therapy with fluvoxamine maleate tablets.

Nursing: Patients receiving fluvoxamine maleate tablets should be advised to notify their physicians if they are breast feeding an infant. (See Nursing Mothers.)

Concomitant medication: Patients should be advised to notify their physicians if they are taking, or plan to take, any prescription or over-the-counter drugs, since there is a potential for clinically important interactions with fluvoxamine maleate tablets.

Alcohol: As with other psychotropic medications, patients should be advised to avoid alcohol while taking fluvoxamine maleate tablets.

Allergic reactions: Patients should be advised to notify their physicians if they develop a rash, hives, or a related allergic phenomenon during therapy with fluvoxamine maleate tablets.

LABORATORY TESTS

There are no specific laboratory tests recommended.

CARCINOGENESIS, MUTAGENESIS, AND IMPAIRMENT OF FERTILITY

Carcinogenesis

There is no evidence of carcinogenicity, mutagenicity, or impairment of fertility with fluvoxamine maleate.

There was no evidence of carcinogenicity in rats treated orally with fluvoxamine maleate for 30 months or hamsters treated orally with fluvoxamine maleate for 20 (females) or 26 (males) months. The daily doses in the high dose groups in these studies were increased over the course of the study from a minimum of 160 mg/kg to a maximum of 240 mg/kg in rats, and from a minimum of 135 mg/kg to a maximum of 240 mg/kg in hamsters. The maximum dose of 240 mg/kg is approximately 6 times the maximum human daily dose on a mg/m^2 basis.

Mutagenesis

No evidence of mutagenic potential was observed in a mouse micronucleus test, an *in vitro* chromosome aberration test, or the Ames microbial mutagen test with or without metabolic activation.

Impairment of Fertility

In fertility studies of male and female rats, up to 80 mg/kg/day orally of fluvoxamine maleate, (approximately 2 times the maximum human daily dose on a mg/m^2 basis) had no effect on mating performance, duration of gestation, or pregnancy rate.

PREGNANCY, TERATOGENIC EFFECTS, PREGNANCY CATEGORY C

In teratology studies in rats and rabbits, daily oral doses of fluvoxamine maleate of up to 80 and 40 mg/kg, respectively (approximately 2 times the maximum human daily dose on a mg/m^2 basis) caused no fetal malformations. However, in other reproduction studies in which pregnant rats were dosed through weaning there was (1) an increase in pup mortality at birth (seen at 80 mg/kg and above but not at 20 mg/kg), and (2) decreases in postnatal pup weights (seen at 160 but not at 80 mg/kg) and survival (seen at all doses; lowest dose tested = 5 mg/kg). (Doses of 5, 20, 80, and 160 mg/kg are approximately 0.1, 0.5, 2, and 4 times the maximum human daily dose on a mg/m^2 basis.) While the results of a cross-fostering study implied that at least some of these results likely occurred secondarily to maternal toxicity, the role of a direct drug effect on the fetuses or pups could not be ruled out. There are no adequate and well-controlled studies in pregnant women. Fluvoxamine maleate should be used during pregnancy only if the potential benefit justifies the potential risk to the fetus.

LABOR AND DELIVERY

The effect of fluvoxamine on labor and delivery in humans is unknown.

NURSING MOTHERS

As for many other drugs, fluvoxamine is secreted in human breast milk. The decision of whether to discontinue nursing or to discontinue the drug should take into account the potential for serious adverse effects from exposure to fluvoxamine in the nursing infant as well as the potential benefits of fluvoxamine maleate tablets therapy to the mother.

PEDIATRIC USE

The efficacy of fluvoxamine maleate for the treatment of Obsessive Compulsive Disorder was demonstrated in a 10 week multicenter placebo controlled study with 120 outpatients ages 8-17. The adverse event profile observed in that study was generally similar to that observed in adult studies with fluvoxamine (see ADVERSE REACTIONS and DOSAGE AND ADMINISTRATION).

Decreased appetite and weight loss have been observed in association with the use of fluvoxamine as well as other SSRIs. Consequently, regular monitoring of weight and growth is recommended if treatment of a child with an SSRI is to be continued long term.

The risks, if any, that may be associated with fluvoxamine's extended use in children and adolescents with OCD have not been systematically assessed. The prescriber should be mindful that the evidence relied upon to conclude that fluvoxamine is safe for use in children and adolescents derives from relatively short term clinical studies and from extrapolation of experience gained with adult patients. In particular, there are no studies that directly evaluate the effects of long term fluvoxamine use on the growth, development, and maturation of children and adolescents. Although there is no affirmative finding to suggest that fluvoxamine possesses a capacity to adversely affect growth, development or maturation, the absence of such findings is not compelling evidence of the absence of the potential of fluvoxamine to have adverse effects in chronic use.

GERIATRIC USE

Approximately 230 patients participating in controlled premarketing studies with fluvoxamine maleate tablets were 65 years of age or over. No overall differences in safety were observed between these patients and younger patients. Other reported clinical experience has not identified differences in response between the elderly and younger patients. However, fluvoxamine has been associated with several cases of clinically significant hyponatremia in elderly patients (see General). Furthermore, the clearance of fluvoxamine is decreased by about 50% in elderly compared to younger patients (see CLINICAL PHARMACOLOGY, Pharmacokinetics), and greater sensitivity of some older individuals also cannot be ruled out. Consequently, fluvoxamine maleate tablets should be slowly titrated during initiation of therapy.

DRUG INTERACTIONS

POTENTIAL INTERACTIONS WITH DRUGS THAT INHIBIT OR ARE METABOLIZED BY CYTOCHROME P450 ISOZYMES

Multiple hepatic cytochrome P450 (CYP450) enzymes are involved in the oxidative biotransformation of a large number of structurally different drugs and endogenous compounds. The available knowledge concerning the relationship of fluvoxamine and the CYP450 enzyme system has been obtained mostly from pharmacokinetic interaction studies conducted in healthy volunteers, but some preliminary *in vitro* data are also available. Based on a finding of substantial interactions of fluvoxamine with certain of these drugs (see later parts of this section and also WARNINGS for details) and limited *in vitro* data for the IIIA4 isozyme, it appears that fluvoxamine inhibits the following isozymes that are known to be involved in the metabolism of the drugs listed below:

IA2: Warfarin, theophylline, and propranolol.

IIC9: Warfarin.

IIIA4: Alprazolam.

In vitro data suggest that fluvoxamine is a relatively weak inhibitor of the IID6 isozyme.

Approximately 7% of the normal population has a genetic defect that leads to reduced levels of activity of cytochrome P450IID6 isozyme. Such individuals have been referred to as "poor metabolizers" (PM) of drugs such as debrisoquin, dextromethorphan, and tricyclic antidepressants. While none of the drugs studied for drug interactions significantly affected the pharmacokinetics of fluvoxamine, an *in vivo* study of fluvoxamine single-dose pharmacokinetics in 13 PM subjects demonstrated altered pharmacokinetic properties compared to 16 "extensive metabolizers" (EM): mean C_{max}, AUC, and half-life were increased by 52%, 200%, and 62%, respectively, in the PM compared to the EM group. This suggests that fluvoxamine is metabolized, at least in part, by IID6 isozyme. Caution is indicated in patients known to have reduced levels of P450IID6 activity and those receiving concomitant drugs known to inhibit this isozyme (*e.g.*, quinidine).

The metabolism of fluvoxamine has not been fully characterized and the effects of potent P450 isozyme inhibition, such as the ketoconazole inhibition of IIIA4, on fluvoxamine metabolism have not been studied.

A clinically significant fluvoxamine interaction is possible with drugs having a narrow therapeutic ratio such as terfenadine, astemizole, cisapride, or pimozide, warfarin, theophylline, certain benzodiazepines and phenytoin. If fluvoxamine maleate tablets are to be administered together with a drug that is eliminated via oxidative metabolism and has a narrow therapeutic window, plasma levels and/or pharmacodynamic effects of the latter drug should be monitored closely, at least until steady-state conditions are reached (see CONTRAINDICATIONS and WARNINGS).

CNS ACTIVE DRUGS

Monoamine Oxidase Inhibitors: See WARNINGS.

Alprazolam: See WARNINGS.

Diazepam: See WARNINGS.

Alcohol: Studies involving single 40 g doses of ethanol (oral administration in one study and intravenous in the other) and multiple dosing with fluvoxamine maleate (50 mg bid) revealed no effect of either drug on the pharmacokinetics or pharmacodynamics of the other.

Carbamazepine: Elevated carbamazepine levels and symptoms of toxicity have been reported with the co-administration of fluvoxamine maleate and carbamazepine.

Clozapine: Elevated serum levels of clozapine have been reported in patients taking fluvoxamine maleate and clozapine. Since clozapine related seizures and orthostatic hypotension appear to be dose related, the risk of these adverse events may be higher when fluvoxamine and clozapine are co-administered. Patients should be closely monitored when fluvoxamine maleate and clozapine are used concurrently.

Lithium: As with other serotonergic drugs, lithium may enhance the serotonergic effects of fluvoxamine and, therefore, the combination should be used with caution. Seizures have been reported with the co-administration of fluvoxamine maleate and lithium.

Lorazepam: A study of multiple doses of fluvoxamine maleate (50 mg bid) in healthy male volunteers (n=12) and a single dose of lorazepam (4 mg single dose) indicated no significant pharmacokinetic interaction. On average, both lorazepam alone and lorazepam with fluvoxamine produced substantial decrements in cognitive functioning; however, the co-administration of fluvoxamine and lorazepam did not produce larger mean decrements compared to lorazepam alone.

Methadone: Significantly increased methadone (plasma level:dose) ratios have been reported when fluvoxamine maleate was administered to patients receiving maintenance methadone treatment, with symptoms of opioid intoxication in 1 patient. Opioid withdrawal symptoms were reported following fluvoxamine maleate discontinuation in another patient.

Sumatriptan: There have been rare postmarketing reports describing patients with weakness, hyperreflexia, and incoordination following the use of a selective serotonin reuptake inhibitor (SSRI) and sumatriptan. If concomitant treatment with sumatriptan and an SSRI (*e.g.*, fluoxetine, fluvoxamine, paroxetine, sertraline) is clinically warranted, appropriate observation of the patient is advised.

Tacrine: In a study of 13 healthy, male volunteers, a single 40 mg dose of tacrine added to fluvoxamine 100 mg/day administered at steady-state was associated with 5- and 8-fold increases in tacrine C_{max} and AUC, respectively, compared to the administration of tacrine alone. Five (5) subjects experienced nausea, vomiting, sweating, and diarrhea following co-administration, consistent with the cholinergic effects of tacrine.

Thioridazine: See CONTRAINDICATIONS and WARNINGS.

Tricyclic Antidepressants (TCAs): Significantly increased plasma TCA levels have been reported with the co-administration of fluvoxamine maleate tablets and amitriptyline, clomipramine or imipramine. Caution is indicated with the co-administration of fluvoxamine maleate tablets and TCAs; plasma TCA concentrations may need to be monitored, and the dose of TCA may need to be reduced.

Tryptophan: Tryptophan may enhance the serotonergic effects of fluvoxamine, and the combination should, therefore, be used with caution. Severe vomiting has been reported with the co-administration of fluvoxamine maleate and tryptophan.

OTHER DRUGS

Theophylline: See WARNINGS.

Warfarin: See WARNINGS.

Digoxin: Administration of fluvoxamine maleate 100 mg daily for 18 days (n=8) did not significantly affect the pharmacokinetics of a 1.25 mg single intravenous dose of digoxin.

Diltiazem: Bradycardia has been reported with the co-administration of fluvoxamine maleate and diltiazem.

Propranolol and Other Beta-Blockers: Co-administration of fluvoxamine maleate 100 mg/day and propranolol 160 mg/day in normal volunteers resulted in a mean 5-fold increase (range 2-17) in minimum propranolol plasma concentrations. In this study, there was a slight potentiation of the propranolol-induced reduction in heart rate and reduction in the exercise diastolic pressure.

One case of bradycardia and hypotension and a second case of orthostatic hypotension have been reported with the co-administration of fluvoxamine maleate and metoprolol.

If propranolol or metoprolol is co-administered with fluvoxamine maleate tablets, a reduction in the initial beta-blocker dose and more cautious dose titration is recommended. No dosage adjustment is required for fluvoxamine maleate tablets.

Co-administration of fluvoxamine maleate 100 mg/day with atenolol 100 mg/day (n=6) did not affect the plasma concentrations of atenolol. Unlike propranolol and metoprolol which undergo hepatic metabolism, atenolol is eliminated primarily by renal excretion.

EFFECTS OF SMOKING ON FLUVOXAMINE METABOLISM

Smokers had a 25% increase in the metabolism of fluvoxamine compared to nonsmokers.

ELECTROCONVULSIVE THERAPY (ECT)

There are no clinical studies establishing the benefits or risks of combined use of ECT and fluvoxamine maleate.

ADVERSE REACTIONS

ASSOCIATED WITH DISCONTINUATION OF TREATMENT

Of the 1087 OCD and depressed patients treated with fluvoxamine maleate in controlled clinical trials conducted in North America, 22% discontinued treatment due to an adverse event. The most common events (≥1%) associated with discontinuation and considered to be drug-related (*i.e.*, those events associated with dropout at a rate at least twice that of placebo) included those listed in TABLE 3.

TABLE 3 *Adverse Events Associated With Discontinuation of Treatment in OCD and Depression Populations*

Body System / Adverse Event	Fluvoxamine	Placebo
Body as a Whole		
Headache	3%	1%
Asthenia	2%	<1%
Abdominal pain	1%	0%
Digestive		
Nausea	9%	1%
Diarrhea	1%	<1%
Vomiting	2%	<1%
Anorexia	1%	<1%
Dyspepsia	1%	<1%
Nervous System		
Insomnia	4%	1%
Somnolence	4%	<1%
Nervousness	2%	<1%
Agitation	2%	<1%
Dizziness	2%	<1%
Anxiety	1%	<1%
Dry mouth	1%	<1%

INCIDENCE IN CONTROLLED TRIALS

Commonly Observed Adverse Events in Controlled Clinical Trials

Fluvoxamine maleate tablets have been studied in controlled trials of OCD (n=320) and depression (n=1350). In general, adverse event rates were similar in the two data sets as well as in the pediatric OCD study. The most commonly observed adverse events associated with the use of fluvoxamine maleate tablets and likely to be drug-related (incidence of 5% or greater and at least twice that for placebo) derived from TABLE 4 were: *somnolence, insomnia, nervousness, tremor, nausea, dyspepsia, anorexia, vomiting, abnormal ejaculation, asthenia, and sweating.* In a pool of two studies involving only patients with OCD, the following additional events were identified using the above rule: *dry mouth, decreased libido, urinary frequency, anorgasmia, rhinitis and taste perversion.* In a study of pediatric patients with OCD, the following additional events were identified using the above rule: *agitation, depression, dysmenorrhea, flatulence, hyperkinisia, and rash.*

Adverse Events Occurring at an Incidence of 1%

TABLE 4 enumerates adverse events that occurred in adults at a frequency of 1% or more, and were more frequent than in the placebo group, among patients treated with fluvoxamine maleate tablets in two short-term placebo controlled OCD trials (10 week) and depression trials (6 week) in which patients were dosed in a range of generally 100-300 mg/day. TABLE 4 shows the percentage of patients in each group who had at least one occurrence of an event at some time during their treatment. Reported adverse events were classified using a standard COSTART-based dictionary terminology.

The prescriber should be aware that these figures cannot be used to predict the incidence of side effects in the course of usual medical practice where patient characteristics and other factors may differ from those that prevailed in the clinical trials. Similarly, the cited frequencies cannot be compared with figures obtained from other clinical investigations involving different treatments, uses, and investigators. The cited figures, however, do provide the prescribing physician with some basis for estimating the relative contribution of drug and non-drug factors to the side-effect incidence rate in the population studied.

TABLE 4 *Treatment-Emergent Adverse Event Incidence Rates by Body System in Adult OCD and Depression Populations Combined**

Body System / Adverse Event	Fluvoxamine n=892	Placebo n=778
Body as Whole		
Headache	22%	20%
Asthenia	14%	6%
Flu syndrome	3%	2%
Chills	2%	1%
Cardiovascular		
Palpitations	3%	2%
Digestive System		
Nausea	40%	14%
Diarrhea	11%	7%
Constipation	10%	8%
Dyspepsia	10%	5%
Anorexia	6%	2%
Vomiting	5%	2%
Flatulence	4%	3%
Tooth disorder†	3%	1%
Dysphagia	2%	1%
Nervous System		
Somnolence	22%	8%
Insomnia	21%	10%
Dry mouth	14%	10%
Nervousness	12%	5%
Dizziness	11%	6%
Tremor	5%	1%
Anxiety	5%	3%
Vasodilatation‡	3%	1%
Hypertonia	2%	1%
Agitation	2%	1%
Decreased libido	2%	1%
Depression	2%	1%
CNS stimulation	2%	1%
Respiratory System		
Upper respiratory infection	9%	5%
Dyspnea	2%	1%
Yawn	2%	0%
Skin		
Sweating	7%	3%
Special Senses		
Taste perversion	3%	1%
Amblyopia§	3%	2%
Urogenital		
Abnormal ejaculation¤¶	8%	1%
Urinary frequency	3%	2%
Impotence¶	2%	1%
Anorgasmia	2%	0%
Urinary retention	1%	0%

* Events for which fluvoxamine maleate incidence was equal to or less than placebo are not listed in the table above, but include the following: abdominal pain, abnormal dreams, appetite increase, back pain, chest pain, confusion, dysmenorrhea, fever, infection, leg cramps, migraine, myalgia, pain, paresthesia, pharyngitis, postural hypotension, pruritus, rash, rhinitis, thirst and tinnitus.

† Includes "toothache," "tooth extraction and abscess," and "caries."

‡ Mostly feeling warm, hot, or flushed.

§ Mostly "blurred vision."

¤ Mostly "delayed ejaculation."

¶ Incidence based on number of male patients.

Adverse Events in OCD Placebo Controlled Studies Which Are Markedly Different (defined as at least a 2-fold difference) in Rate From the Pooled Event Rates in OCD and Depression Placebo Controlled Studies

The events in OCD studies with a 2-fold decrease in rate compared to event rates in OCD and depression studies were dysphagia and amblyopia (mostly blurred vision). Additionally, there was an approximate 25% decrease in nausea.

The events in OCD studies with a 2-fold increase in rate compared to event rates in OCD and depression studies were: *asthenia, abnormal ejaculation (mostly delayed ejaculation), anxiety, infection, rhinitis, anorgasmia (in males), depression, libido decreased, pharyngitis, agitation, impotence, myoclonus/twitch, thirst, weight loss, leg cramps, myalgia, and urinary retention.* These events are listed in order of decreasing rates in the OCD trials.

OTHER ADVERSE EVENTS IN OCD PEDIATRIC POPULATION

In pediatric patients (n=57) treated with fluvoxamine maleate tablets, the overall profile of adverse events was generally similar to that seen in adult studies, as shown in TABLE 4. However, the following adverse events, not appearing in TABLE 4, were reported in 2 or more of the pediatric patients and were more frequent with fluvoxamine maleate tablets than with placebo: abnormal thinking, cough increase, dysmenorrhea, ecchymosis, emotional lability, epistaxis, hyperkinesia, infection, manic reaction, rash, sinusitis, and weight decrease.

VITAL SIGN CHANGES

Comparisons of fluvoxamine maleate and placebo groups in separate pools of short-term OCD and depression trials on (1) median change from baseline on various vital signs variables and on (2) incidence of patients meeting criteria for potentially important changes from baseline on various vital signs variables revealed no important differences between fluvoxamine maleate and placebo.

LABORATORY CHANGES

Comparisons of fluvoxamine maleate and placebo groups in separate pools of short-term OCD and depression trials on (1) median change from baseline on various serum chemistry, hematology, and urinalysis variables and on (2) incidence of patients meeting criteria for potentially important changes from baseline on various serum chemistry, hematology, and urinalysis variables revealed no important differences between fluvoxamine maleate and placebo.

ECG CHANGES

Comparisons of fluvoxamine maleate and placebo groups in separate pools of short-term OCD and depression trials on (1) mean change from baseline on various ECG variables and on (2) incidence of patients meeting criteria for potentially important changes from baseline on various ECG variables revealed no important differences between fluvoxamine maleate and placebo.

OTHER EVENTS OBSERVED DURING THE PREMARKETING EVALUATION OF FLUVOXAMINE MALEATE TABLETS

During premarketing clinical trials conducted in North America and Europe, multiple doses of fluvoxamine maleate were administered for a combined total of 2737 patient exposures in patients suffering OCD or Major Depressive Disorder. Untoward events associated with this exposure were recorded by clinical investigators using descriptive terminology of their own choosing. Consequently, it is not possible to provide a meaningful estimate of the proportion of individuals experiencing adverse events without first grouping similar types of untoward events into a limited (*i.e.,* reduced) number of standard event categories.

In the tabulations which follow, a standard COSTART-based dictionary terminology has been used to classify reported adverse events. If the COSTART term for an event was so general as to be uninformative, it was replaced with a more informative term. The frequencies presented, therefore, represent the proportion of the 2737 patient exposures to multiple doses of fluvoxamine maleate who experienced an event of the type cited on at least 1 occasion while receiving fluvoxamine maleate. All reported events are included in the list below, with the following exceptions: (1) those events already listed in TABLE 4, which tabulates incidence rates of common adverse experiences in placebo-controlled OCD and depression clinical trials, are excluded; (2) those events for which a drug cause was considered remote (*i.e.,* neoplasia, gastrointestinal carcinoma, herpes simplex, herpes zoster, application site reaction, and unintended pregnancy) are omitted; and (3) events which were reported in only 1 patient and judged to not be potentially serious are not included. It is important to emphasize that, although the events reported did occur during treatment with fluvoxamine maleate, a causal relationship to fluvoxamine maleate has not been established. **Events are further classified within body system categories and enumerated in order of decreasing frequency using the following definitions:** *Frequent* adverse events are defined as those occurring on one or more occasions in at least 1/100 patients; *infrequent* adverse events are those occurring between 1/100 and 1/1000 patients; and *rare* adverse events are those occurring in less than 1/1000 patients.

Body as a Whole: *Frequent:* Accidental injury, malaise. *Infrequent:* Allergic reaction, neck pain, neck rigidity, overdose, photosensitivity reaction, suicide attempt. *Rare:* Cyst, pelvic pain, sudden death.

Cardiovascular System: *Frequent:* Hypertension, hypotension, syncope, tachycardia. *Infrequent:* Angina pectoris, bradycardia, cardiomyopathy, cardiovascular disease, cold extremities, conduction delay, heart failure, myocardial infarction, pallor, pulse irregular, ST segment changes. *Rare:* AV block, cerebrovascular accident, coronary artery disease, embolus, pericarditis, phlebitis, pulmonary infarction, supraventricular extrasystoles.

Digestive System: *Frequent:* Elevated liver transaminases. *Infrequent:* Colitis, eructation, esophagitis, gastritis, gastroenteritis, gastrointestinal hemorrhage, gastrointestinal ulcer, gingivitis, glossitis, hemorrhoids, melena, rectal hemorrhage, stomatitis. *Rare:* Biliary pain, cholecystitis, cholelithiasis, fecal incontinence, hematemesis, intestinal obstruction, jaundice.

Endocrine System: *Infrequent:* Hypothyroidism. *Rare:* Goiter.

Hemic and Lymphatic Systems: *Infrequent:* Anemia, ecchymosis, leukocytosis, lymphadenopathy, thrombocytopenia. *Rare:* Leukopenia, purpura.

Metabolic and Nutritional Systems: *Frequent:* Edema, weight gain, weight loss. *Infrequent:* Dehydration, hypercholesterolemia. *Rare:* Diabetes mellitus, hyperglycemia, hyperlipidemia, hypoglycemia, hypokalemia, lactate dehydrogenase increased.

Musculoskeletal System: *Infrequent:* Arthralgia, arthritis, bursitis, generalized muscle spasm, myasthenia, tendinous contracture, tenosynovitis. *Rare:* Arthrosis, myopathy, pathological fracture.

Nervous System: *Frequent:* Amnesia, apathy, hyperkinesia, hypokinesia, manic reaction, myoclonus, psychotic reaction. *Infrequent:* Agoraphobia, akathisia, ataxia, CNS depression, convulsion, delirium, delusion, depersonalization, drug dependence, dyskinesia, dystonia, emotional lability, euphoria, extrapyramidal syndrome, gait unsteady, hallucinations, hemiplegia, hostility, hypersomnia, hypochondriasis, hypotonia, hysteria, incoordination, increased salivation, increased libido, neuralgia, paralysis, paranoid reaction, phobia, psychosis, sleep disorder, stupor, twitching, vertigo. *Rare:* Akinesia, coma, fibrillations, mutism, obsessions, reflexes decreased, slurred speech, tardive dyskinesia, torticollis, trismus, withdrawal syndrome.

Respiratory System: *Frequent:* Cough increased, sinusitis. *Infrequent:* Asthma, bronchitis, epistaxis, hoarseness, hyperventilation. *Rare:* Apnea, congestion of upper airway, hemoptysis, hiccups, laryngismus, obstructive pulmonary disease, pneumonia.

Skin: *Infrequent:* Acne, alopecia, dry skin, eczema, exfoliative dermatitis, furunculosis, seborrhea, skin discoloration, urticaria.

Special Senses: *Infrequent:* Accommodation abnormal, conjunctivitis, deafness, diplopia, dry eyes, ear pain, eye pain, mydriasis, otitis media, parosmia, photophobia, taste loss, visual field defect. *Rare:* Corneal ulcer, retinal detachment.

Urogenital System: *Infrequent:* Anuria, breast pain, cystitis, delayed menstruation*, dysuria, female lactation*, hematuria, menopause*, menorrhagia*, metrorrhagia*, nocturia, polyuria, premenstrual syndrome*, urinary incontinence, urinary tract infection, urinary urgency, urination impaired, vaginal hemorrhage*, vaginitis*. *Rare:* Kidney calculus, hematospermia (based on the number of males), oliguria.

* Based on the number of females.

POSTMARKETING REPORTS

Voluntary reports of adverse events in patients taking fluvoxamine maleate tablets that have been received since market introduction and are of unknown causal relationship to fluvoxamine maleate tablets use include: ventricular tachycardia (including torsades de pointes), porphria, toxic epidermal necrolysis, Stevens-Johnson syndrome, Henoch-Schoenlein purpura, bullous eruption, priapism, agranulocytosis, neuropathy, aplastic anemia, anaphylactic reaction, angioedema, vasculitis, hyponatremia, acute renal failure, hepatitis, pancreatitis, ileus, serotonin syndrome, neuropathy, laryngismus, and severe akinesia with fever when fluvoxamine was co-administered with antipsychotic medication.

DOSAGE AND ADMINISTRATION

DOSAGE FOR ADULTS

The recommended starting dose for fluvoxamine maleate tablets in adult patients is 50 mg, administered as a single daily dose at bedtime. In the controlled clinical trials establishing the effectiveness of fluvoxamine maleate tablets in OCD, patients were titrated within a dose range of 100-300 mg/day. Consequently, the dose should be increased in 50 mg increments every 4-7 days, as tolerated, until maximum therapeutic benefit is achieved, not exceed 300 mg/day. It is advisable that a total daily dose of more than 100 mg should be given in 2 divided doses. If the doses are not equal, the larger dose should be given at bedtime.

DOSAGE FOR PEDIATRIC POPULATION (CHILDREN AND ADOLESCENTS)

The recommended starting dose for fluvoxamine maleate tablets in pediatric populations (ages 8-17 years) is 25 mg, administered as a single daily dose at bedtime. In a controlled clinical trial establishing the effectiveness of fluvoxamine maleate tablets in OCD, pediatric patients (ages 8-17) were titrated within a dose range of 50-200 mg/day. The dose should be increased in 25 mg increments every 4-7 days, as tolerated, until maximum therapeutic benefit is achieved, not to exceed 200 mg/day. It is advisable that a total daily dose of more than 50 mg should be given in 2 divided doses. If the 2 divided doses are not equal, the larger dose should be given at bedtime.

DOSAGE FOR ELDERLY OR HEPATICALLY IMPAIRED PATIENTS

Elderly patients and those with hepatic impairment have been observed to have a decreased clearance of fluvoxamine maleate. Consequently, it may be appropriate to modify the initial dose and the subsequent dose titration for these patient groups.

MAINTENANCE/CONTINUATION EXTENDED TREATMENT

Although the efficacy of fluvoxamine maleate tablets beyond 10 weeks of dosing for OCD has not been documented in controlled trials, OCD is a chronic condition, and it is reasonable to consider continuation for a responding patient. Dosage adjustments should be made to maintain the patient on the lowest effective dosage, and patients should be periodically reassessed to determine the need for continued treatment.

HOW SUPPLIED

Luvox Tablets

25 mg: Unscored, white, elliptical, film-coated (debossed "SOLVAY" and "4202" on one side).

50 mg: Scored, yellow, elliptical, film-coated (debossed "SOLVAY" and "4205" on one side and scored on the other).

100 mg: Scored, beige, elliptical, film-coated (debossed "SOLVAY" and "4210" on one side and scored on the other).

Storage: Luvox tablets should be protected from high humidity and stored at controlled room temperature, 15-30°C (59-86°F). Dispense in tight containers.

PRODUCT LISTING - RATED THERAPEUTICALLY EQUIVALENT

Tablet - Oral - 25 mg

100's	$229.18	GENERIC, Ivax Corporation	00172-4389-60
100's	$230.20	GENERIC, Apotex Usa Inc	60505-0164-01
100's	$230.21	GENERIC, Geneva Pharmaceuticals	00781-5040-01
100's	$230.30	GENERIC, Mylan Pharmaceuticals Inc	00378-0407-01
100's	$230.45	GENERIC, Purepac Pharmaceutical Company	00228-2704-11
100's	$264.74	GENERIC, Barr Laboratories Inc	00555-0967-02
100's	$265.03	GENERIC, Eon Labs Manufacturing Inc	00185-0017-01
100's	$294.48	LUVOX, Solvay Pharmaceuticals Inc	00032-4202-01
100's	$294.48	LUVOX, Solvay Pharmaceuticals Inc	00032-4202-11

Tablet - Oral - 50 mg

100's	$256.10	GENERIC, Ivax Corporation	00172-4391-60
100's	$257.20	GENERIC, Apotex Usa Inc	60505-0165-01
100's	$257.35	GENERIC, Mylan Pharmaceuticals Inc	00378-0412-01
100's	$257.35	GENERIC, Udl Laboratories Inc	51079-0992-20
100's	$257.50	GENERIC, Purepac Pharmaceutical Company	00228-2655-11
100's	$295.82	GENERIC, Barr Laboratories Inc	00555-0968-02
100's	$296.15	GENERIC, Eon Labs Manufacturing Inc	00185-0027-01

Tablet - Oral - 100 mg

100's	$262.67	GENERIC, Ivax Corporation	00172-4392-60
100's	$263.85	GENERIC, Apotex Usa Inc	60505-0166-01
100's	$263.95	GENERIC, Mylan Pharmaceuticals Inc	00378-0414-01
100's	$263.95	GENERIC, Udl Laboratories Inc	51079-0993-20
100's	$264.10	GENERIC, Purepac Pharmaceutical Company	00228-2656-11
100's	$303.42	GENERIC, Mylan Pharmaceuticals Inc	00555-0969-02
100's	$303.76	GENERIC, Eon Labs Manufacturing Inc	00185-0157-01

PRODUCT LISTING - EQUIVALENTS NOT AVAILABLE

Tablet - Oral - 50 mg

100's	$257.24	GENERIC, Geneva Pharmaceuticals	00781-5041-01
100's	$329.06	LUVOX, Solvay Pharmaceuticals Inc	00032-4205-01
100's	$332.88	LUVOX, Solvay Pharmaceuticals Inc	00032-4205-11

Tablet - Oral - 100 mg

100's	$263.85	GENERIC, Geneva Pharmaceuticals	00781-5042-01
100's	$337.51	LUVOX, Solvay Pharmaceuticals Inc	00032-4210-01
100's	$344.10	LUVOX, Solvay Pharmaceuticals Inc	00032-4210-11

Folic Acid (001331)

Categories: Anemia, megaloblastic; FDA Approved 1971 Dec; Pregnancy Category A; WHO Formulary
Drug Classes: Hematinics; Vitamins/minerals
Brand Names: Acido; Folasic; Folicet; Folico; **Folvite**; Nifolin; Renal Multivit Form Forte Zinc
Foreign Brand Availability: Acfol (Spain); Acide Folique CCD (France); Acido Folico (Colombia; Ecuador; Peru); Apo-Folic (Canada; New-Zealand); Filicine (Greece); Folacin (Sweden); Folart (Philippines); Foliamin (Hong-Kong; Thailand); Folic Acid DHA (Malaysia); Folicid (Korea); Folina (Italy); Folinsyre (Denmark; Norway); Folitab (Mexico); Folivit (Thailand); Folsan (Austria; Germany; Hungary); Folverlan (Germany); Ingafol (India); Lexpec (England); Megafol (Australia); RubieFol (Germany)

DESCRIPTION

Folic acid, N-(p(((2-amino-4-hydroxy-6-pteridinyl)-methyl)amino)benzoyl) glutamic acid, is a complex organic compound present in liver, yeast and other substances, and which may be prepared synthetically.

Tablets: 1 mg folic acid.

Parenteral: Each ml of folic acid-solution contains sodium folate equivalent to 5 mg of folic acid.

Inactive ingredients: Sequestrene sodium 0.2% and water for injection qs 100%. Sodium hydroxide to approx. pH 9.

Preservative: Benzyl alcohol 1.5%.

CLINICAL PHARMACOLOGY

In man, an exogenous source of folate is required for nucleoprotein synthesis and the maintenance of normal erythropoiesis. Folic acid, whether given by mouth or parenterally, stimulates specifically the production of red blood cells, white blood cells, and platelets in persons suffering from certain megaloblastic anemias.

INDICATIONS AND USAGE

Folic acid is effective in the treatment of megaloblastic anemias due to a deficiency of folic acid as may be seen in tropical or non-tropical sprue, in anemias of nutritional origin, pregnancy, infancy, or childhood.

NON-FDA APPROVED INDICATIONS

Studies have also shown that increased folic acid intake may play a role in the prevention of arteriosclerotic vascular disease (by decreasing total homocysteine levels). One large study (n=88,756), which reported that long term use of multivitamins may substantially reduce the risk of colon cancer, concluded that this effect may be related to the folic acid contained in the multivitamins. These uses are not FDA approved and require further study.

WARNINGS

Folic acid alone is improper therapy in the treatment of pernicious anemia and other megaloblastic anemias where vitamin B_{12} is deficient.

PRECAUTIONS

Folic acid in doses above 0.1 mg daily may obscure pernicious anemia in that hematologic remission can occur while neurological manifestations remain progressive.

ADVERSE REACTIONS

Allergic sensitization has been reported following both oral and parenteral administration of folic acid.

DOSAGE AND ADMINISTRATION

Oral Administration: Folic acid is well absorbed and may be administered orally with satisfactory results except in severe instances of intestinal malabsorption.

Parenteral Administration: Intramuscular, intravenous, and subcutaneous routes may be used if the disease is exceptionally severe, or if gastrointestinal absorption may be, or is known to be, impaired.

Usual Therapeutic Dosage: Adults and children regardless of age, up to 1.0 mg daily. Resistant cases may require larger doses.

Maintenance Level: When clinical symptoms have subsided and the blood picture has become normal, a maintenance level should be used, *i.e.,* 0.1 mg for infants and up to 0.3 mg for children under 4 years of age, 0.4 mg for adults and children 4 or more years of age, and 0.8 mg for pregnant and lactating women, per day, but never less than 0.1 mg/day. Patients should be kept under close supervision and adjustment of the maintenance level made if relapse appears imminent.

In the presence of alcoholism, hemolytic anemia, anticonvulsant therapy, or chronic infection, the maintenance level may need to be increased.

PRODUCT LISTING - RATED THERAPEUTICALLY EQUIVALENT

Solution - Injectable - 5 mg/ml

10 ml	$12.50	GENERIC, Bedford Laboratories	55390-0410-10
10 ml	$14.33	GENERIC, Lederle Laboratories	00205-4154-34
10 ml x 10	$12.33	GENERIC, American Pharmaceutical Partners	63323-0184-10

Tablet - Oral - 1 mg

20's	$2.40	GENERIC, Allscripts Pharmaceutical Company	54569-0958-03
25's	$2.63	GENERIC, Udl Laboratories Inc	51079-0041-19
30 x 25	$115.05	GENERIC, Sky Pharmaceuticals Packaging, Inc	63739-0110-03
30's	$1.85	GENERIC, Major Pharmaceuticals Inc	00904-0625-46
30's	$3.24	GENERIC, Pd-Rx Pharmaceuticals	55289-0492-30
30's	$3.60	GENERIC, Allscripts Pharmaceutical Company	54569-0958-02
30's	$4.17	GENERIC, Heartland Healthcare Services	61392-0244-30
30's	$4.17	GENERIC, Heartland Healthcare Services	61392-0244-39
31 x 10	$48.48	GENERIC, Vangard Labs	00615-0664-53
31 x 10	$48.48	GENERIC, Vangard Labs	00615-0664-63
31's	$4.31	GENERIC, Heartland Healthcare Services	61392-0244-31
32's	$4.45	GENERIC, Heartland Healthcare Services	61392-0244-32
60's	$8.34	GENERIC, Heartland Healthcare Services	61392-0244-60
90's	$3.34	GENERIC, Golden State Medical	60429-0212-90
90's	$12.51	GENERIC, Heartland Healthcare Services	61392-0244-90
100's	$0.66	GENERIC, Global Pharmaceutical Corporation	00115-3585-01
100's	$1.41	GENERIC, Allscripts Pharmaceutical Company	54569-0958-00
100's	$2.25	GENERIC, Halsey Drug Company Inc	00879-0081-01
100's	$2.63	GENERIC, Interstate Drug Exchange Inc	00814-3250-14
100's	$2.75	GENERIC, Cmc-Consolidated Midland Corporation	00223-1002-01
100's	$2.80	GENERIC, Major Pharmaceuticals Inc	00904-0625-60
100's	$4.56	FEDERAL UPPER LIMIT, H.C.F.A. F F P	99999-1331-01
100's	$5.00	GENERIC, Raway Pharmacal Inc	00686-0041-20
100's	$5.89	GENERIC, Major Pharmaceuticals Inc	00904-0625-61
100's	$6.85	GENERIC, Paddock Laboratories Inc	00574-0060-11
100's	$8.50	GENERIC, West Ward Pharmaceutical Corporation	00143-1248-25
100's	$12.00	GENERIC, Watson/Schein Pharmaceuticals Inc	00364-0137-01
100's	$15.90	GENERIC, American Health Packaging	62584-0708-01
100's	$15.95	GENERIC, Udl Laboratories Inc	51079-0041-20
100's	$22.67	GENERIC, Ivax Corporation	00182-0507-89
100's	$34.50	GENERIC, West Ward Pharmaceutical Corporation	00143-1248-01
100's	$36.00	GENERIC, Watson/Schein Pharmaceuticals Inc	00591-5216-01

PRODUCT LISTING - EQUIVALENTS NOT AVAILABLE

Solution - Injectable - 5 mg/ml

10 ml	$12.50	GENERIC, Raway Pharmacal Inc	00686-1840-30

Tablet - Oral - 1 mg

15's	$2.08	GENERIC, Heartland Healthcare Services	61392-0244-15
30's	$5.22	GENERIC, Marlex Pharmaceuticals	10135-0182-30
45's	$6.26	GENERIC, Heartland Healthcare Services	61392-0244-45
60's	$4.85	GENERIC, Marlex Pharmaceuticals	10135-0182-60
90's	$3.70	GENERIC, Pharmaceutical Corporation Of America	51655-0008-26
90's	$6.33	GENERIC, Marlex Pharmaceuticals	10135-0182-90
100's	$3.38	GENERIC, Vangard Labs	00615-0664-01
100's	$3.58	GENERIC, Moore, H.L. Drug Exchange Inc	00839-5066-06
100's	$12.32	GENERIC, Marlex Pharmaceuticals	10135-0182-01

Folic Acid; Nicotinamide; Zinc Oxide (003526)

Categories: Acne rosacea; Acne vulgaris; FDA Approved 2001 Mar
Drug Classes: Vitamins/minerals
Brand Names: Nicomide
Cost of Therapy: $10.97 (Acne; Nicomide; 500 mg; 750 mg; 25 mg; 1 tablet/day; 30 day supply)

DESCRIPTION

Note: The trade name has been left throughout this monograph for clarity.

Nicomide tablets for oral administration are peach colored, oval shaped tablets imprinted "Sirius" above and "726" below a score line in blue ink on one side.

Each tablet provides:

Nicotinamide; 750 mg
Zinc oxide; 25 mg
Folic acid; 500 μg

Inactive Ingrediants: Carnauba wax powder, FD&C blue no. 1, FD&C yellow no. 6 aluminum lake, hydroxypropyl methyl cellulose, magnesium stearate, microcrystalline cellulose, polyethlene glycol, polysorbate 80, stearic acid and titanium dioxide.

CLINICAL PHARMACOLOGY

Nicotinamide is a water-soluble component of the vitamin B complex group. *In vivo,* nicotinamide is incorporated into nicotinamide adenine dinucleotide (NAD) and nicotinamide adenine dinucleotide phosphate (NADP). NAD and NADP function as coenzymes in a wide variety of enzymatic oxidation-reduction reactions essential for tissue respiration, lipid metabolism, and glycogenolysis.

Nicotinamide has demonstrated anti-inflammatory actions which may be of benefit in patients with inflammatory acne vulgaris, including but not limited to, suppression of antigen induced-lymphocytic transformation and inhibition of 3′-5′ cyclic AMP phosphodiesterase. Nicotinamide has demonstrated the ability to block the inflammatory actions of iodides known to precipitate or exacerbate inflammatory acne.

Nicotinamide lacks the vasodilator, gastrointestinal, hepatic, and hypolipemic actions of nicotinic acid (niacin). As such nicotinamide has not been shown to produce the flushing, itching and burning skin sensations commonly observed when large doses of nicotinic acid are administered orally. (See ADVERSE REACTIONS.)

Zinc has been shown to inhibit inflammatory polymorphonuclear leukocyte chemotaxis in acne patients. Zinc has also been demonstrated to have an inhibitory effect on the lipase of the three *Propionibacterium* species found in human pilosebaceous follicles. Patients with inflammatory acne have been shown to have significantly lower serum zinc levels than matched healthy controls.

Folic acid serves as an essential cofactor for the biosynthesis of thymidine and purine nucleotides required for normal cellular DNA synthesis. Deficiencies of folic acid have been demonstrated to occur in some cutaneous inflammatory disorders.

INDICATIONS AND USAGE

Indicated for nonpregnant patients with acne vulgaris, acne rosacea, or other inflammatory skin disorders who are deficient in, or at risk of deficiency in, one or more of the components of Nicomide.

CONTRAINDICATIONS

Nicomide is contraindicated in patients with hypersensitivity to any of its components.

WARNINGS

Folic acid alone is improper treatment of pernicious anemia and other megaloblastic anemias where vitamin B_{12} is deficient.

PRECAUTIONS

GENERAL

Large doses of nicotinamide should be administered with caution in patients with a history of jaundice, liver disease, or diabetes mellitus.

Folic acid above 0.1 mg daily may obscure pernicious anemia (hematologic remission may occur while neurological manifestations remain progressive).

PREGNANCY

Large doses of nicotinamide or zinc should be avoided in pregnancy.

NURSING MOTHERS

Caution should be exercised when using Nicomide in nursing mothers.

PEDIATRICS

Safety and effectiveness of Nicomide in pediatric patients have not been established.

GERIATRICS

Clinical studies of Nicomide have not been performed to determine whether elderly subjects respond differently than younger subjects. In general, dose selection for an elderly patient should be cautious, usually starting at the low end of the dosing range, reflecting the greater frequency of decreased hepatic, renal, or cardiac function, and of concomitant disease or other drug therapy.

DRUG INTERACTIONS

Nicotinamide: The clearance of primidone and carbamazepine may be reduced with the concomitant use of nicotinamide.

Zinc Oxide: The absorption of quinolones or tetracycline may be decreased with the concomitant use of zinc.

ADVERSE REACTIONS

Allergic sensitization has been reported rarely following oral and parenteral administration of folic acid.

At recommended doses, Nicomide is expected to be well-tolerated. Gastrointestinal distress such as nausea or vomiting have been associated with the administration of nicotinamide or zinc at doses greater than the recommended dose of Nicomide. These effects usually resolved when nicotinamide or zinc was administered with food.

Although rare, transient elevations of liver functions tests have been reported when nicotinamide was administered in doses greater than the recommended dose of Nicomide.

DOSAGE AND ADMINISTRATION

Usual adult dose is one tablet taken once or twice a day or as prescribed by a physician.

HOW SUPPLIED

Nicomide tablets for oral administration are peach colored, oval shaped tablets imprinted "Sirius" above and "726" below a score line in blue ink on one side.

Each tablet provides:

Nicotinamide; 750 mg
Zinc oxide; 25 mg
Folic acid; 500 µg

Storage: Store at controlled room temperature, 15-30°C (59-86°F).

Fomepizole *(003373)*

For complete prescribing information, refer to the CD-ROM included with the book.

Categories: Poisoning, ethylene glycol; Poisoning, methanol; FDA Approved 1997 Dec; Pregnancy Category C; Orphan Drugs
Drug Classes: Antidotes
Brand Names: **Antizole**
Foreign Brand Availability: Antizol (Israel)

DESCRIPTION

Caution: Must be diluted prior to use.

Fomepizole injection is a competitive inhibitor of alcohol dehydrogenase.

The chemical name of fomepizole is 4-methylpyrazole. It has the molecular formula $C_4H_6N_2$ and a molecular weight of 82.1.

It is a clear to yellow liquid at room temperature. Its melting point is 25°C (77°F) and it may present in a solid form at room temperature. Fomepizole is soluble in water and very soluble in ethanol, diethyl ether, and chloroform. Each Antizol vial contains 1.5 ml (1 g/ml) of fomepizole.

F

INDICATIONS AND USAGE

Fomepizole is indicated as an antidote for ethylene glycol (such as antifreeze) or methanol poisoning, or for use in suspected ethylene glycol or methanol ingestion, either alone or in combination with hemodialysis (see DOSAGE AND ADMINISTRATION).

CONTRAINDICATIONS

Fomepizole should not be administered to patients with a documented serious hypersensitivity reaction to fomepizole or other pyrazoles.

DOSAGE AND ADMINISTRATION

TREATMENT GUIDELINES

If ethylene glycol or methanol poisoning is left untreated, the natural progression of the poisoning leads to accumulation of toxic metabolites, including glycolic and oxalic acids (ethylene glycol intoxication) and formic acid (methanol intoxication). These metabolites can induce metabolic acidosis, nausea/vomiting, seizures, stupor, coma, calcium oxaluria, acute tubular necrosis, blindness, and death. The diagnosis of these poisonings may be difficult because ethylene glycol and methanol concentrations diminish in the blood as they are metabolized to their respective metabolites. Hence, both ethylene glycol and methanol concentrations and acid base balance, as determined by serum electrolyte (anion gap) and/or arterial blood gas analysis, should be frequently monitored and used to guide treatment.

Treatment consists of blocking the formation of toxic metabolites using inhibitors of alcohol dehydrogenase, such as fomepizole, and correction of metabolic abnormalities. In patients with high ethylene glycol or methanol concentrations (≥50 mg/dl), significant metabolic acidosis, or renal failure, hemodialysis should be considered to remove ethylene glycol or methanol and the respective toxic metabolites of these alcohols.

Treatment With Fomepizole

Begin fomepizole treatment immediately upon suspicion of ethylene glycol or methanol ingestion based on patient history and/or anion gap metabolic acidosis, increased osmolar gap, visual disturbances, or oxalate crystals in the urine, **OR** a documented serum ethylene glycol or methanol concentration greater than 20 mg/dl.

Hemodialysis

Hemodialysis should be considered in addition to fomepizole in the case of renal failure, significant or worsening metabolic acidosis, or a measured ethylene glycol or methanol concentration of greater than or equal to 50 mg/dl. Patients should be dialyzed to correct metabolic abnormalities and to lower the ethylene glycol concentrations below 50 mg/dl.

Discontinuation of Fomepizole Treatment

Treatment with fomepizole may be discontinued when ethylene glycol or methanol concentrations are undetectable or have been reduced below 20 mg/dl, and the patient is asymptomatic with normal pH.

DOSING OF FOMEPIZOLE

A loading dose of 15 mg/kg should be administered, followed by doses of 10 mg/kg every 12 hours for 4 doses, then 15 mg/kg every 12 hours thereafter until ethylene glycol or methanol concentrations are undetectable or have been reduced below 20 mg/dl, and the patient is asymptomatic with normal pH. All doses should be administered as a slow intravenous infusion over 30 minutes (see Administration).

Dosage With Renal Dialysis

Fomepizole injection is dialyzable and the frequency of dosing should be increased to every 4 hours during hemodialysis (see TABLE 1).

Administration

Fomepizole solidifies at temperatures less than 25°C (77°F). If the fomepizole solution has become solid in the vial, the solution should be liquefied by running the vial under warm water or by holding in the hand. Solidification does not affect the efficacy, safety, or stability of fomepizole. Using sterile technique, the appropriate dose of fomepizole should be drawn from the vial with a syringe and injected into **at least 100 ml of sterile 0.9% sodium chloride injection or dextrose 5% injection.** Mix well. The entire contents of the resulting solution should be infused over 30 minutes. Fomepizole, like all parenteral products, should be inspected visually for particulate matter prior to administration.

TABLE 1 *Fomepizole Dosing in Patients Requiring Hemodialysis*

DOSE AT THE BEGINNING OF HEMODIALYSIS	
If <6 hours since last fomepizole dose: Do not administer dose.	**If ≥6 hours since last fomepizole dose:** Administer next scheduled dose.
DOSING DURING HEMODIALYSIS	
Dose every 4 hours.	
DOSING AT THE TIME HEMODIALYSIS IS COMPLETED	
Time between last dose and the end of hemodialysis:	
<1 hour	Do not administer dose at the end of hemodialysis.
1-3 hours	Administer ½ of next scheduled dose.
>3 hours	Administer next scheduled dose.
MAINTENANCE DOSING OFF HEMODIALYSIS	
Give next scheduled dose 12 hours from last dose administered.	

Stability

Fomepizole diluted in 0.9% sodium chloride injection or dextrose 5% injection remains stable and sterile for at least 24 hours when stored refrigerated or at room temperature. Fomepizole does not contain preservatives. Therefore, maintain sterile conditions, and after dilution do not use beyond 24 hours. Solutions showing haziness, particulate matter, precipitate, discoloration, or leakage should not be used.

PRODUCT LISTING - EQUIVALENTS NOT AVAILABLE

Solution - Intravenous - 1 Gm/ml

1.50 ml x 4 $4841.52 ANTIZOL, Orphan Medical 62161-0003-34

Fomivirsen Sodium *(003415)*

Categories: Retinitis, secondary to cytomegalovirus; FDA Approved 1998 Aug; Pregnancy Category C
Drug Classes: Antivirals; Ophthalmics
Brand Names: Vitravene

DESCRIPTION

Fomivirsen sodium intravitreal injectable is a sterile, aqueous, preservative-free, bicarbonate-buffered solution for intravitreal injection.

Fomivirsen sodium is a phosphorothioate oligonucleotide, twenty-one nucleotides in length, with the following sequence:

5′-GCG TTT GCT CTT CTT CTT GCG-3′.

The chemical name for fomivirsen sodium is as follows:

2′-Deoxyguanosylyl-(3′→5′ *O,O*-phosphorothioyl)-2′-deoxycytidylyl-(3′→5′ *O,O*-phosphorothioyl)-2′-deoxyguanosylyl-(3′→5′ *O,O*-phosphorothioyl)-thymidylyl-(3′→5′ *O,O*-phosphorothioyl)-thymidylyl-(3′→5′ *O,O*-phosphorothioyl)-thymidylyl-(3′→5′ *O,O*-phosphorothioyl)-2′-deoxyguanosylyl-(3′→5′ *O,O*-phosphorothioyl)-2′-deoxycytidylyl-(3′→5′ *O,O*-phosphorothioyl)-thymidylyl-(3′→5′ *O,O*-phosphorothioyl)-2′-deoxycytidylyl-(3′→5′ *O,O*-phosphorothioyl)-thymidylyl-(3′→5′ *O,O*-phosphorothioyl)-thymidylyl-(3′→5′ *O,O*-phosphorothioyl)-2′-deoxycytidylyl-(3′→5′ *O,O*-phosphorothioyl)-thymidylyl-(3′→5′ *O,O*-phosphorothioyl)-thymidylyl-(3′→5′ *O,O*-phosphorothioyl)-2′-deoxycytidylyl-(3′→5′ *O,O*-phosphorothioyl)-thymidylyl-(3′→5′ *O,O*-phosphorothioyl)-thymidylyl-(3′→5′ *O,O*-phosphorothioyl)-2′-deoxyguanosylyl-(3′→5′ *O,O*-phosphorothioyl)-2′-deoxycytidylyl-(3′→5′ *O,O*-phosphorothioyl)-2′-deoxyguanosine, 20-sodium salt.

Fomivirsen sodium is a white to off-white, hygroscopic, amorphous powder with a molecular formula of $C_{204}H_{243}N_{63}O_{114}P_{20}S_{20}Na_{20}$ and a molecular weight of 7122.

Each ml of Vitravene Contains: *Active:* Fomivirsen sodium 6.6 mg. *Inactive:* Sodium bicarbonate, sodium chloride, sodium carbonate, and water for injection. Sodium hydroxide and/or hydrochloric acid may be added to adjust pH. Vitravene injection is formulated to have an osmolality of 290 mOsm/kg, and a pH of 8.7.

Storage: Store Vitravene between 2 and 25°C (35 and 77°F). Protect from excessive heat and light.

CLINICAL PHARMACOLOGY

VIROLOGY

Mechanism of Action

Fomivirsen is a phosphorothioate oligonucleotide that inhibits human cytomegalovirus (HCMV) replication through an antisense mechanism. The nucleotide sequence of fomivirsen is complementary to a sequence in mRNA transcripts of the major immediate early region 2 (IE2) of HCMV. This region of mRNA encodes several proteins responsible for regulation of viral gene expression that are essential for production of infectious CMV. Binding of fomivirsen to the target mRNA results in inhibition of IE2 protein synthesis, subsequently inhibiting virus replication.

Resistance

Through persistent selection pressure *in vitro* it was possible to isolate a clone of HCMV that was 10-fold less sensitive to inhibition of replication than the parent strain. The molecular basis for the resistance has not been elucidated. It is possible that resistant strains may occur in clinical use.

Cross-Resistance

The antisense mechanism of action and molecular target of fomivirsen are different from that of other inhibitors of HCMV replication, which function by inhibiting the viral DNA polymerase. Fomivirsen was equally potent against 21 independent clinical HCMV isolates, including several that were resistant to ganciclovir, foscarnet and/or cidofovir. Isolates which are resistant to fomivirsen may be sensitive to ganciclovir, focarnet and/or cidofovir.

Pharmacokinetics

The assessment of ocular pharmacokinetic parameters in patients has been limited and is still ongoing.

INDICATIONS AND USAGE

Fomivirsen sodium is indicated for the local treatment of cytomegalovirus (CMV) retinitis in patients with acquired immunodeficiency syndrome (AIDS) who are intolerant of or have a contraindication to other treatment(s) for CMV retinitis or who were insufficiently responsive to previous treatment(s) for CMV retinitis.

The diagnosis and evaluation of CMV retinitis is ophthalmologic and should be made by comprehensive retinal examination including indirect ophthalmoscopy. Other conditions that should be considered in the differential diagnosis of CMV retinitis include ocular infections caused by syphilis, candidiasis, toxoplasmosis, histoplasmosis, herpes simplex virus and varicella-zoster virus as well as retinal scars, and cotton wool spots, any of which may produce a retinal appearance similar to CMV. For this reason, it is essential that a physician familiar with the retinal presentation of these conditions establish the diagnosis of CMV retinitis.

CONTRAINDICATIONS

Fomivirsen sodium is contraindicated in those persons who have a known hypersensitivity to any component of this preparation.

WARNINGS

Fomivirsen sodium is for intravitreal injection use only.

CMV retinitis may be associated with CMV disease elsewhere in the body. Fomivirsen sodium intravitreal injection provides localized therapy limited to the treated eye. The use of fomivirsen sodium does not provide treatment for systemic CMV disease. Patients should be monitored for extraocular CMV disease or disease in the contralateral eye.

Fomivirsen sodium is not recommended for use in patients who have recently (2-4 weeks) been treated with either intravenous or intravitreal cidofovir because of the risk of exaggerated ocular inflammation.

PRECAUTIONS

GENERAL

FOR OPHTHALMIC USE ONLY.

Ocular inflammation (uveitis) including iritis and vitritis has been reported to occur in approximately 1 in 4 patients. Inflammatory reactions are more common during induction dosing. Topical corticosteroids have been useful in the medical management of inflammatory changes, and with both medical management and time, patients may be able to continue to receive intraviteal injections of fomivirsen sodium after the inflammation has resolved.

Increased intraocular pressure has been commonly reported. The increase is usually a transient event and in most cases the pressure returns to the normal range without any treatment or with temporary use of topical medications. Intraocular pressure should be monitored at each visit and elevations of intraocular pressure, if sustained, should be managed with medications to lower intraocular pressure.

INFORMATION FOR THE PATIENT

Fomivirsen sodium intravitreal injection is not a cure for CMV retinitis, and some immunocompromised patients may continue to experience progression of retinitis during and following treatment. Patients receiving fomivirsen sodium should be advised to have regular ophthalmologic follow-up examinations. Patients may also experience other manifestations of CMV disease despite fomivirsen sodium therapy.

Fomivirsen sodium treats only the eye(s) in which it has been injected. CMV may exist as a systemic disease, in addition to CMV retinitis. Therefore, patients should be monitored for extraocular CMV infections (*e.g.*, pneumonitis, colitis) and retinitis in the opposite eye, if only one infected eye is being treated.

HIV-infected patients should continue taking antiretroviral therapy as otherwise indicated.

CARCINOGENESIS, MUTAGENESIS, AND IMPAIRMENT OF FERTILITY

No studies have been conducted to evaluate the carcinogenic potential of fomivirsen sodium.

Fomivirsen sodium was not mutagenic in Salmonella/Microsome (Ames) and mouse lymphoma tests or clastogenic in the *in vivo* mouse micronucleous assay. However, equivocal results were observed in the chromosome aberration test with Chinese hamster ovary cells.

No studies have been conducted to evaluate the potential of fomivirsen sodium to affect fertility.

PREGNANCY, TERATOGENIC EFFECTS, PREGNANCY CATEGORY C

Animal reproductive studies have not been conducted with fomivirsen sodium. It is also not known whether fomivirsen sodium can cause fetal harm when administered to a pregnant woman or can affect reproduction capacity.

There are no adequate and well-controlled studies in pregnant women. Fomivirsen sodium should be used during pregnancy only if the potential benefit justifies the potential risk to the fetus.

NURSING MOTHERS

It is not known whether fomivirsen sodium is excreted in human milk. Because many drugs are excreted in human milk and because of the potential for serious adverse reactions in nursing infants from fomivirsen sodium, a decision should be made whether to discontinue nursing or to discontinue the drug, taking into account the importance of the drug to the mother.

PEDIATRIC USE

Safety and effectiveness in pediatric patients have not been established.

GERIATRIC USE

Clinical studies of fomivirsen sodium did not include sufficient numbers of subjects aged 65 and over to determine whether they respond differently than younger subjects.

DRUG INTERACTIONS

The interaction in humans between fomivirsen sodium and other drugs has not been studied.

Results from *in vitro* tests demonstrated no inhibition of anti-HCMV activity of fomivirsen by AZT or ddC.

ADVERSE REACTIONS

The most frequently observed adverse experiences have been cases of ocular inflammation (uveitis) including iritis and vitritis. Ocular inflammation has been reported to occur in approximately 1 in 4 patients. Inflammatory reactions are more common during induction dosing. Delaying additional treatment with fomivirsen sodium and the use of topical corticosteroids have been useful in the medical management of inflammatory changes (see PRECAUTIONS, General).

Adverse experiences reported in approximately 5-20% of patients have included:

Ocular: Abnormal vision, anterior chamber inflammation, blurred vision, cataract, conjunctival hemorrhage, decreased visual acuity, desaturation of color vision, eye pain, floaters, increased intraocular pressure, photophobia, retinal detachment, retinal edema, retinal hemorrhage, retinal pigment changes, uveitis, vitritis.

Systemic: Abdominal pain, anemia, asthenia, diarrhea, fever, headache, infection, nausea, pnuemonia, rash, sepsis, sinusitis, systemic CMV, vomiting.

Adverse experiences reported in approximately 2-5% of patients have included:

Ocular: Application site reaction, conjunctival hyperemia, conjunctivitis, corneal edema, decreased peripheral vision, eye irritation, hypotony, keratic precipitates, optic neuritis, photopsia, retinal vascular disease, visual field defect, vitreous hemorrhage, vitreous opacity.

Systemic: Abnormal liver function, abnormal thinking, allergic reactions, anorexia, back pain, bronchitis, cachexia, catheter infection, chest pain, decreased weight, dehydration, depression, dizziness, dyspnea, flu syndrome, increased cough, increased GGTP, kidney failure, lymphoma-like reaction, neuropathy, neutropenia, oral monilia, pain, pancreatitis, sweating, thrombocytopenia.

DOSAGE AND ADMINISTRATION

Treatment with fomivirsen sodium involves an induction and a maintenance phase. The recommended dose of fomivirsen sodium is 330 µg (0.05 ml). The induction dose of fomivirsen sodium should be 1 injection every other week for 2 doses. Subsequent maintenance doses should be administered once every 4 weeks after induction.

For unacceptable inflammation in the face of controlled CMVR, it is worthwhile interrupting therapy until the level of inflammation decreases and therapy can resume.

For patients whose disease progresses on fomivirsen during maintenance, an attempt at reinduction at the same dose may result in resumed disease control.

INSTRUCTIONS FOR INTRAVITREAL INJECTION

Fomivirsen sodium is administered by intravitreal injection (0.05 ml/eye) into the affected eye following application of standard topical and/or local anesthetics and antimicrobials using a 30 gauge needle on a low-volume (*e.g.,* tuberculin) syringe.

INSTRUCTIONS FOR POST-INJECTION MONITORING

Monitor light perception and optic nerve head perfusion: if not completely perfused by 7-10 minutes, perform anterior chamber paracentesis with a 30 gauge needle on a plungerless tuberculin syringe at the slit lamp.

ANIMAL PHARMACOLOGY

OCULAR KINETICS

Fomivirsen is cleared from the vitreous in rabbits over the course of 7-10 days, by a combination of tissue distribution and metabolism. In the eye, fomivirsen concentrations were greatest in the retina and iris. Fomivirsen was detectable in retina within hours after injection, and concentrations increased over 3-5 days.

METABOLISM AND ELIMINATION

Metabolism is the primary route of elimination from the eye. Metabolites of fomivirsen are detected in the retina and vitreous in animals. Fomivirsen sodium is metabolized by exonucleases in a process that sequentially removes residues from the terminal ends of the oligonucleotide yielding shortened oligonucleotides and mononucleotide metabolites. Data with related compounds indicate that mononucleotide metabolites are further catabolized similar to endogenous nucleotides and are excreted as low molecular weight metabolites. In rabbits, a small amount of fomivirsen-derived radioactivity was eliminated in urine (16%) or feces (3%) as low molecular weight metabolites. Expired air has been shown to be a major route of excretion for CO_2 generated by catabolism of nucleotides after administration of phosphorothioate oligonucleotides.

SYSTEMIC EXPOSURE

Systemic exposure to fomivirsen following single or repeated intravitreal injections in monkeys was below limits of quantitation (70 ng/ml in plasma and 350 ng/g in tissue). In monkeys treated every other week for up to 3 months with fomivirsen there were isolated instances when fomivirsen's metabolites were observed in liver, kidney, and plasma at a concentration near the level of detection (14 ng/ml in plasma and 70 ng/g in tissue).

PROTEIN BINDING

Analysis of vitreous samples from treated rabbits and monkeys indicate that approximately 40% of fomivirsen is bound to proteins.

PRODUCT LISTING - EQUIVALENTS NOT AVAILABLE

Solution - Intraocular - 6.6 mg/ml

0.25 ml $1000.00 VITRAVENE, Ciba Vision Ophthalmics 58768-0902-35

Fondaparinux Sodium *(003552)*

Categories: Embolism, pulmonary, prophylaxis; Thrombosis, deep vein, prophylaxis; FDA Approved 2001 Dec; Pregnancy Category B

Drug Classes: Anticoagulants

Brand Names: **Arixtra**

Cost of Therapy: $217.50 (Deep Vein Thrombosis; Arixtra Injection; 2.5 mg/0.5 ml; 1 injection/day; 5 day supply)

WARNING

SPINAL/EPIDURAL HEMATOMAS

When neuraxial anesthesia (epidural/spinal anesthesia) or spinal puncture is employed, patients anticoagulated or scheduled to be anticoagulated with low molecular weight heparins, heparinoids or fondaparinux sodium for prevention of thromboembolic complications are at risk of developing an epidural or spinal hematoma which can result in long-term or permanent paralysis.

The risk of these events is increased by the use of indwelling epidural catheters for administration of analgesia or by the concomitant use of drugs affecting hemostasis such as non-steroidal anti-inflammatory drugs (NSAIDs), platelet inhibitors, or other anticoagulants. The risk also appears to be increased by traumatic or repeated epidural or spinal puncture.

Patients should be frequently monitored for signs and symptoms of neurological impairment. If neurologic compromise is noted, urgent treatment is necessary.

The physician should consider the potential benefit versus risk before neuraxial intervention in patients anticoagulated or to be anticoagulated for thromboprophylaxis (see also WARNINGS, Hemorrhage and DRUG INTERACTIONS).

DESCRIPTION

Arixtra injection is a sterile solution containing fondaparinux sodium. It is a synthetic and specific inhibitor of activated Factor X (Xa). Fondaparinux sodium is methyl O-2-deoxy-6-O-sulfo-2-(sulfoamino)-α-D-glucopyranosyl-(1→4)-O-β-D-glucopyra-nuronosyl-(1→4)-O-2-deoxy-3,6-di-O-sulfo-2-(sulfoamino)-α-D-glucopyranosyl-(1→4)-O-2-O-sulfo-α-L-idopyranuronosyl-(1→4)-2-deoxy-6-O-sulfo-2-(sulfoamino)-α-D-glucopyranoside, decasodium salt.

The molecular formula of fondaparinux sodium is $C_{31}H_{43}N_3Na_{10}O_{49}S_8$ and its molecular weight is 1728.

Arixtra is provided as a sterile, preservative-free injectable solution for subcutaneous use. Each single dose, prefilled syringe of Arixtra, affixed with an automatic needle protection system, contains 2.5 mg of fondaparinux sodium in 0.5 ml of an isotonic solution of sodium chloride and water for injection. The final drug product is a clear and colorless liquid with a pH between 5.0 and 8.0.

CLINICAL PHARMACOLOGY

PHARMACODYNAMICS

Mechanism of Action

The antithrombotic activity of fondaparinux sodium is the result of antithrombin III (ATIII)-mediated selective inhibition of Factor Xa. By selectively binding to ATIII, fondaparinux sodium potentiates (about 300 times) the innate neutralization of Factor Xa by ATIII. Neutralization of Factor Xa interrupts the blood coagulation cascade and thus inhibits thrombin formation and thrombus development.

Fondaparinux sodium does not inactivate thrombin (activated Factor II) and has no known effect on platelet function. At the recommended dose, fondaparinux sodium does not affect fibrinolytic activity or bleeding time.

Anti-Xa Activity

The pharmacodynamics/pharmacokinetics of fondaparinux sodium are derived from fondaparinux plasma concentrations quantified via anti-Factor Xa activity. Only fondaparinux can be used to calibrate the anti-Xa assay. (The international standards of heparin or LMWH are not appropriate for this use.) As a result, the activity of fondaparinux sodium is expressed as milligrams (mg) of the fondaparinux calibrator. The anti-Xa activity of the drug increases with increasing drug concentration, reaching maximum values in approximately 3 hours.

PHARMACOKINETICS

Absorption

Fondaparinux sodium administered by SC injection is rapidly and completely absorbed (absolute bioavailability is 100%). Following a single SC dose of fondaparinux sodium 2.5 mg in young male subjects, C_{max} of 0.34 mg/L is reached in approximately 2 hours. In patients undergoing treatment with fondaparinux sodium injection 2.5 mg, once daily, the peak steady-state plasma concentration is, on average, 0.39-0.50 mg/L and is reached approximately 3 hours post dose. In these patients, the minimum steady-state plasma concentration is 0.14-0.19 mg/L.

Distribution

In healthy adults, intravenously or subcutaneously administered fondaparinux sodium distributes mainly in blood and only to a minor extent in extravascular fluid as evidenced by steady-state and non-steady-state apparent volume of distribution of 7-11 L. Similar fondaparinux distribution occurs in patients undergoing elective hip surgery or hip fracture surgery. *In vitro,* fondaparinux sodium is highly (at least 94%) and specifically bound to antithrombin III (ATIII) and does not bind significantly to other plasma proteins (including platelet Factor 4 [PF4]) or red blood cells.

Metabolism

In vivo metabolism of fondaparinux has not been investigated since the majority of the administered dose is eliminated unchanged in urine in individuals with normal kidney function.

Elimination

In individuals with normal kidney function fondaparinux is eliminated in urine mainly as unchanged drug. In healthy individuals up to 75 years of age, up to 77% of a single SC or IV fondaparinux dose is eliminated in urine as unchanged drug in 72 hours. The elimination half-life is 17-21 hours.

SPECIAL POPULATIONS

Renal Impairment

Fondaparinux elimination is prolonged in patients with renal impairment since the major route of elimination is urinary excretion of unchanged drug. In patients undergoing elective hip surgery or hip fracture surgery, the total clearance of fondaparinux is approximately 25% lower in patients with mild renal impairment (creatinine clearance 50-80 ml/min), approximately 40% lower in patients with moderate renal impairment (creatinine clearance 30-50 ml/min) and approximately 55% lower in patients with severe renal impairment (<30 ml/min) compared to patients with normal renal function (see CONTRAINDICATIONS and WARNINGS, Renal Impairment).

F

Hepatic Impairment

The pharmacokinetic properties of fondaparinux have not been studied in patients with hepatic impairment.

Elderly Patients

Fondaparinux elimination is prolonged in patients over 75 years old. In studies evaluating fondaparinux sodium 2.5 mg in hip fracture surgery or elective hip surgery, the total clearance of fondaparinux was approximately 25% lower in patients over 75 years old as compared to patients less than 65 years old.

Patients Weighing Less Than 50 kg

Total clearance of fondaparinux sodium is decreased by approximately 30% in patients weighing less than 50 kg (see CONTRAINDICATIONS).

Gender

The pharmacokinetic properties of fondaparinux sodium are not significantly affected by gender.

Race

Pharmacokinetic differences due to race have not been studied prospectively. However, studies performed in Asian (Japanese) healthy subjects did not reveal a different pharmacokinetic profile compared to Caucasian healthy subjects. Similarly, no plasma clearance differences were observed between Black and Caucasian patients undergoing orthopedic surgery.

Drug Interactions

See DRUG INTERACTIONS.

INDICATIONS AND USAGE

Fondaparinux sodium injection is indicated for the prophylaxis of deep vein thrombosis, which may lead to pulmonary embolism:

- In patients undergoing hip fracture surgery.
- In patients undergoing hip replacement surgery.
- In patients undergoing knee replacement surgery.

CONTRAINDICATIONS

Fondaparinux sodium injection is contraindicated in patients with severe renal impairment (creatinine clearance <30 ml/min). Fondaparinux sodium is eliminated primarily by the kidneys, and such patients are at increased risk for major bleeding episodes (see WARNINGS, Renal Impairment).

Fondaparinux sodium is contraindicated in patients with body weight <50 kg. In clinical trials, occurrence of major bleeding was doubled in patients with body weight <50 kg compared to those with body weight ≥50 kg (5.4% vs 2.1%).

The use of fondaparinux sodium is contraindicated in patients with active major bleeding, bacterial endocarditis, in patients with thrombocytopenia associated with a positive *in vitro* test for anti-platelet antibody in the presence of fondaparinux sodium, or in patients with known hypersensitivity to fondaparinux sodium.

WARNINGS

Fondaparinux sodium injection is not intended for intramuscular administration.

Fondaparinux sodium cannot be used interchangeably (unit for unit) with heparin, low molecular weight heparins or heparinoids, as they differ in manufacturing process, anti-Xa and anti-IIa activity, units, and dosage. Each of these medicines has its own instructions for use.

RENAL IMPAIRMENT

The risk of hemorrhage increases with increasing renal impairment. Occurrences of major bleeding in patients with normal renal function, mild renal impairment, moderate renal impairment and severe renal impairment have been found to be 1.6% (25/1565), 2.4% (31/1288), 3.8% (19/504) and 4.8% (4/83), respectively (see CLINICAL PHARMACOLOGY, Special Populations, Renal Impairment and CONTRAINDICATIONS).

Therefore, fondaparinux sodium is contraindicated in patients with severe renal impairment (creatinine clearance <30 ml/min) and should be used with caution in patients with moderate renal impairment (creatinine clearance 30-50 ml/min).

Renal function should be assessed periodically in patients receiving the drug. Fondaparinux sodium should be discontinued immediately in patients who develop severe renal impairment or labile renal function while on therapy. After discontinuation of fondaparinux sodium, its anticoagulant effects may persist for 2-4 days in patients with normal renal function (*i.e.*, at least 3-5 half-lives). The anticoagulant effects of fondaparinux sodium may persist even longer in patients with renal impairment (see CLINICAL PHARMACOLOGY).

HEMORRHAGE

Fondaparinux sodium, like other anticoagulants, should be used with extreme caution in conditions with increased risk of hemorrhage, such as congenital or acquired bleeding disorders, active ulcerative and angiodysplastic gastrointestinal disease, hemorrhagic stroke, or shortly after brain, spinal, or ophthalmological surgery, or in patients treated concomitantly with platelet inhibitors.

LABORATORY TESTING

Because routine coagulation tests such as Prothrombin Time (PT) and Activated Partial Thromboplastin Time (aPTT) are relatively insensitive measures of fondaparinux sodium activity and international standards of heparin or LMWH are not calibrators to measure anti-Factor Xa activity of fondaparinux sodium, if during fondaparinux sodium therapy unexpected changes in coagulation parameters or major bleeding occurs, fondaparinux sodium should be discontinued (see PRECAUTIONS, Laboratory Tests).

NEURAXIAL ANESTHESIA AND POST-OPERATIVE INDWELLING EPIDURAL CATHETER USE

Spinal or epidural hematomas, which may result in long-term or permanent paralysis, can occur with the use of anticoagulants and neuraxial (spinal/epidural) anesthesia or spinal puncture. The risk of these events may be higher with post-operative use of indwelling epidural catheters or concomitant use of other drugs affecting hemostasis such as NSAIDs (see BOXED WARNING).

THROMBOCYTOPENIA

Thrombocytopenia can occur with the administration of fondaparinux sodium. Moderate thrombocytopenia (platelet counts between 100,000/mm^3 and 50,000/mm^3) occurred at a rate of 2.9% in patients given fondaparinux sodium 2.5 mg in clinical trials. Severe thrombocytopenia (platelet counts less than 50,000/mm^3) occurred at a rate of 0.2% in patients given fondaparinux sodium 2.5 mg in clinical trials.

Thrombocytopenia of any degree should be monitored closely. If the platelet count falls below 100,000/mm^3, fondaparinux sodium should be discontinued.

PRECAUTIONS

GENERAL

Fondaparinux sodium injection should be administered according to the recommended regimen, especially with respect to the timing of the first dose after surgery. In clinical studies, the administration of fondaparinux sodium before 6 hours after surgery has been associated with an increased risk of major bleeding (see ADVERSE REACTIONS, Hemorrhage and DOSAGE AND ADMINISTRATION).

Fondaparinux sodium injection should be used with care in patients with a bleeding diathesis, uncontrolled arterial hypertension or a history of recent gastrointestinal ulceration, diabetic retinopathy, and hemorrhage.

Fondaparinux sodium injection should be used with caution in elderly patients (see Geriatric Use).

Fondaparinux sodium should be used with caution in patients with a history of heparin-induced thrombocytopenia.

Fondaparinux sodium injection should not be mixed with other injections or infusions.

If thrombotic events occur despite fondaparinux sodium prophylaxis, appropriate therapy should be initiated.

LABORATORY TESTS

Periodic routine complete blood counts (including platelet count), serum creatinine level, and stool occult blood tests are recommended during the course of treatment with fondaparinux sodium injection.

When administered at the recommended prophylaxis dose, routine coagulation tests such as Prothrombin Time (PT) and Activated Partial Thromboplastin Time (aPTT) are relatively insensitive measures of fondaparinux sodium activity, and are therefore, unsuitable for monitoring.

The anti-factor Xa activity of fondaparinux sodium can be measured by anti-Xa assay using the appropriate calibrator (fondaparinux). Since the international standards of heparin or LMWH are not appropriate calibrators, the activity of fondaparinux sodium is expressed in milligrams (mg) of the fondaparinux and cannot be compared with activities of heparin or low molecular weight heparins. (See CLINICAL PHARMACOLOGY: Pharmacodynamics and Pharmacokinetics; and WARNINGS, Laboratory Testing.)

CARCINOGENESIS, MUTAGENESIS, AND IMPAIRMENT OF FERTILITY

No long-term studies in animals have been performed to evaluate the carcinogenic potential of fondaparinux sodium.

Fondaparinux sodium was not genotoxic in the Ames test, the mouse lymphoma cell (L5178Y/TK$^{+/-}$) forward mutation test, the human lymphocyte chromosome aberration test, the rat hepatocyte unscheduled DNA synthesis (UDS) test, or the rat micronucleus test.

At SC doses up to 10 mg/kg/day (about 32 times the recommended human dose based on body surface area) fondaparinux sodium found to have no effect on fertility and reproductive performance of male and female rats.

PREGNANCY, TERATOGENIC EFFECTS, PREGNANCY CATEGORY B

Reproduction studies have been performed in pregnant rats at SC doses up to 10 mg/kg/day (about 32 times the recommended human dose based on body surface area) and pregnant rabbits at SC doses up to 10 mg/kg/day (about 65 times the recommended human dose based on body surface area) and have revealed no evidence of impaired fertility or harm to the fetus due to fondaparinux sodium. There are, however, no adequate and well-controlled studies in pregnant women. Because animal reproduction studies are not always predictive of human response, this drug should be used during pregnancy only if clearly needed.

NURSING MOTHERS

Fondaparinux sodium was found to be excreted in the milk of lactating rats. However, it is not known whether this drug is excreted in human milk. Because many drugs are excreted in human milk, caution should be exercised when fondaparinux sodium is administered to a nursing mother.

PEDIATRIC USE

Safety and effectiveness of fondaparinux sodium in pediatric patients have not been established.

GERIATRIC USE

Fondaparinux sodium should be used with caution in elderly patients. Over 2300 patients, 65 years and older, have received fondaparinux sodium 2.5 mg in randomized clinical trials in the orthopedic surgery program. The efficacy of fondaparinux sodium in the elderly (equal or older than 65 years) was similar to that seen in younger patients (younger than 65 years). The risk of fondaparinux sodium-associated major bleeding increased with age: 1.8% (23/1253) in patients <65 years, 2.2% (24/1111) in those 65-74 years, and 2.7% (33/1227) in those ≥75 years. Serious adverse events increased with age for patients receiving fondaparinux sodium. Careful attention to dosing directions and concomitant medications (especially antiplatelet medication) is advised. (See CLINICAL PHARMACOLOGY and PRECAUTIONS, General.)

Fondaparinux sodium is substantially excreted by the kidney, and the risk of toxic reactions to fondaparinux sodium may be greater in patients with impaired renal function. Because elderly patients are more likely to have decreased renal function, it may be useful to monitor renal function. (See CONTRAINDICATIONS and WARNINGS, Renal Impairment.)

DRUG INTERACTIONS

In clinical studies performed with fondaparinux sodium, the concomitant use of oral anticoagulants (warfarin), platelet inhibitors (acetylsalicylic acid), NSAIDs (piroxicam) and digoxin did not significantly affect the pharmacokinetics/pharmacodynamics of fondaparinux sodium. In addition, fondarparinux sodium neither influenced the pharmacodynamics of warfarin, acetylsalicylic acid, piroxicam and digoxin, nor the pharmacokinetics of digoxin at steady-state.

Agents that may enhance the risk of hemorrhage should be discontinued prior to initiation of fondaparinux sodium therapy. If coadministration is essential, close monitoring may be appropriate.

In an *in vitro* study in human liver microsomes, inhibition of CYP2A6 hydroxylation of coumarin by fondaparinux (200 μM *i.e.,* 350 mg/L) was 17-28%. Inhibition of the other isozymes evaluated (CYPs 2A1, 2C9, 2C19, 2D6, 3A4, and 3E1) was 0-16%. Since fondaparinux does not markedly inhibit CYP450s (CYP1A2, CYP2A6, CYP2C9, CYP2C19, CYP2D6, CYP2E1 or CYP3A4) *in vitro,* fondaparinux sodium is not expected to significantly interact with other drugs *in vivo* by inhibition of metabolism mediated by these isozymes.

Since fondaparinux sodium does not bind significantly to plasma proteins other than ATIII, no drug interactions by protein-binding displacement are expected.

ADVERSE REACTIONS

Because clinical trials are conducted under widely varying conditions, adverse reaction rates observed in the clinical trials of a drug cannot be directly compared to rates in the clinical trials of another drug and may not reflect the rates observed in practice. The adverse reaction information from clinical trials does, however, provide a basis for identifying possible adverse events and for approximating rates.

The data described below reflect exposure to fondaparinux sodium injection in 4823 patients undergoing hip fracture, hip replacement, or major knee surgeries.

Fondaparinux sodium was studied primarily in two large dose-response (n=989) and four active-controlled trials with enoxaparin sodium (n=3616). The population ranged in age from 17-97 years and in body weight between 30 and 169 kg. The population included 58% females and 42% males, and 95% Caucasian, 3% Black, 1% Asian, 1% other races. Over 3500 patients received fondaparinux sodium 2.5 mg once daily with treatment ranging up to 11 days while over 90% of patients were treated between 5 and 9 days. Patients with serum creatinine >2.0 mg/dl were excluded from these clinical trials.

HEMORRHAGE

During fondaparinux sodium administration, the most common adverse reactions were bleeding complications (see WARNINGS).

The rates of major bleeding events reported during clinical trials with fondaparinux sodium 2.5 mg injection are provided in TABLE 4 and TABLE 5.

A separate analysis of major bleeding across all clinical studies according to the time of the first injection of fondaparinux sodium after surgical closure was performed in patients who received fondaparinux sodium only post-operatively. In this analysis the incidences of major bleeding were as follows: <4 hours was 4.8% (5/104), 4-6 hours was 2.3% (28/1196), 6-8 hours was 1.9% (38/1965).

THROMBOCYTOPENIA

See WARNINGS, Thrombocytopenia.

LOCAL REACTIONS

Mild local irritation (injection site bleeding, rash and pruritus) may occur following SC injection of fondaparinux sodium.

ELEVATIONS OF SERUM AMINOTRANSFERASES

Asymptomatic increases in aspartate (AST [SGOT]) and alanine (ALT [SGPT]) aminotransferase levels greater than 3 times the upper limit of normal of the laboratory reference range have been reported in 1.7% and 2.6% of patients, respectively, during treatment with fondaparinux sodium 2.5 mg injection versus 3.2% and 3.9% of patients, respectively, during treatment with enoxaparin sodium 30 mg every 12 hours or 40 mg once daily enoxaparin sodium. Such elevations are fully reversible and are rarely associated with increases in bilirubin.

Since aminotransferase determinations are important in the differential diagnosis of myocardial infarction, liver disease, and pulmonary emboli, elevations that might be caused by drugs like fondaparinux sodium should be interpreted with caution.

OTHER

Other adverse events that occurred during treatment with fondaparinux sodium or enoxaparin sodium in clinical trials with patients undergoing hip fracture surgery, hip replacement surgery, or knee replacement surgery and that occurred at a rate of at least 2% in either treatment group, are provided in TABLE 6.

TABLE 4 *Major Bleeding Episodes* in Hip Fracture, Hip Replacement, and Knee Replacement Surgery Studies*

Indications	Fondaparinux Sodium 2.5 mg SC Once Daily	Enoxaparin Sodium†‡
Hip fracture	18/831 (2.2%)	19/842 (2.3%)
Hip replacement	67/2268 (3.0%)	55/2597 (2.1%)
Knee replacement	11/517 (2.1%)§	1/517 (0.2%)

* Major bleeding was defined as clinically overt bleeding that was (1) fatal, (2) bleeding at critical site (*e.g.,* intracranial, retroperitoneal, intra-ocular, pericardial, spinal or into adrenal gland), (3) associated with reoperation at operative site, or (4) with a bleeding index (BI) ≥2 calculated as [number of whole blood or packed red blood cells units transfused - [(pre-bleeding) - (post-bleeding)] hemoglobin (g/dl) values].
† Enoxaparin sodium dosing regimen: 30 mg every 12 hours or 40 mg once daily.
‡ Not approved for use in patients undergoing hip fracture surgery.
§ p value versus enoxaparin sodium: <0.01, 95% confidence interval: [1.1%, 3.3%] in fondaparinux sodium group versus [0.0%, 1.1%] in enoxaparin sodium group.

TABLE 5 *Bleeding Across Hip Fracture, Hip Replacement, and Knee Replacement Surgery Studies*

Indications	Fondaparinux Sodium 2.5 mg SC Once Daily n=3616	Enoxaparin Sodium*† n=3956
Major Bleeding‡	96 (2.7%)	75 (1.9%)
Fatal bleeding	0 (0.0%)	1 (<0.1%)
Non-fatal bleeding at critical site	0 (0.0%)	1 (<0.1%)
Reoperation due to bleeding	12 (0.3%)	10 (0.3%)
BI ≥2§	84 (2.3%)	63 (1.6%)
Minor Bleeding¤	109 (3.0%)	116 (2.9%)

* Enoxaparin sodium dosing regimen: 30 mg every 12 hours or 40 mg once daily.
† Not approved for use in patients undergoing hip fracture surgery.
‡ Major bleeding was defined as clinically overt bleeding that was (1) fatal, (2) bleeding at critical site (*e.g.,* intracranial, retroperitoneal, intra-ocular, pericardial, spinal or into adrenal gland), (3) associated with reoperation at operative site, or (4) with a bleeding index (BI) ≥2.
§ BI ≥2: overt bleeding associated only with a bleeding index (BI) ≥2 calculated as [number of whole blood or packed red blood cell units transfused - [(pre-bleeding) - (post-bleeding)] hemoglobin (g/dl) values].
¤ Minor bleeding was defined as clinically overt bleeding that was not major.

TABLE 6 *Adverse Events Occurring in ≥2% of Fondaparinux Sodium or Enoxaparin Sodium Treated Patients Regardless of Relationship to Study Drug Across Hip Fracture Surgery, Hip Replacement Surgery, or Knee Replacement Surgery Studies*

Adverse Events	Fondaparinux Sodium 2.5 mg SC Once Daily n=3616	Enoxaparin Sodium*† n=3956
Anemia	707 (19.6%)	670 (16.9%)
Fever	491 (13.6%)	610 (15.4%)
Nausea	409 (11.3%)	484 (12.2%)
Edema	313 (8.7%)	348 (8.8%)
Constipation	309 (8.5%)	416 (10.5%)
Rash	273 (7.5%)	329 (8.3%)
Vomiting	212 (5.9%)	236 (6.0%)
Insomnia	179 (5.0%)	214 (5.4%)
Wound drainage increased	161 (4.5%)	184 (4.7%)
Hypokalemia	152 (4.2%)	164 (4.1%)
Urinary tract infection	136 (3.8%)	135 (3.4%)
Dizziness	131 (3.6%)	165 (4.2%)
Purpura	128 (3.5%)	137 (3.5%)
Hypotension	126 (3.5%)	125 (3.2%)
Confusion	113 (3.1%)	132 (3.3%)
Bullious eruption	112 (3.1%)	102 (2.6%)
Urinary retention	106 (2.9%)	117 (3.0%)
Hematoma	103 (2.8%)	109 (2.8%)
Diarrhea	90 (2.5%)	102 (2.6%)
Dyspepsia	87 (2.4%)	102 (2.6%)
Post-operative hemorrhage	85 (2.4%)	69 (1.7%)
Headache	72 (2.0%)	97 (2.5%)
Pain	62 (1.7%)	101 (2.6%)

* Enoxaparin sodium dosing regimen: 30 mg every 12 hours or 40 mg once daily.
† Not approved for use in patients undergoing hip fracture surgery.

In ongoing studies for other indications, major bleeding events include intracranial hemorrhage, cerebral hemorrhage, and retroperitoneal hemorrhage.

DOSAGE AND ADMINISTRATION

Fondaparinux sodium injection is administered by subcutaneous injection.

In patients undergoing hip fracture, hip replacement, or knee replacement surgery, the recommended dose of fondaparinux sodium is 2.5 mg administered by SC injection once daily. After hemostasis has been established, the initial dose should be given 6-8 hours after surgery. Administration before 6 hours after surgery has been associated with an increased risk of major bleeding. The usual duration of administration is 5-9 days; and up to 11 days administration has been tolerated. (See WARNINGS, Laboratory Testing and ADVERSE REACTIONS.)

INSTRUCTIONS FOR USE

Parenteral drug products should be inspected visually for particulate matter and discoloration prior to administration.

Fondaparinux sodium injection is provided in a single dose, prefilled syringe affixed with an automatic needle protection system. Fondaparinux sodium is administered by SC injection. It must not be administered by IM injections.

To avoid the loss of drug when using the pre-filled syringe do not expel the air bubble from the syringe before the injection. Administration should be made in the fatty tissue, alternating injection sites (*e.g.*, between the left and right anterolateral or the left and right posterolateral abdominal wall).

HOW SUPPLIED

Arixtra injection is available in 2.5 mg fondaparinux sodium in 0.5 ml single dose prefilled syringe, affixed with a 27-gauge × ½ inch needle with an automatic needle protection system.

Storage: Store at 25°C (77°F); excursions permitted to 15-30°C (59-86°F).

Keep out of the reach of children.

PRODUCT LISTING - EQUIVALENTS NOT AVAILABLE

Solution - Subcutaneous - 2.5 mg/0.5 ml
1 x 10 $435.00 ARIXTRA, Organon 66203-2300-01

Formoterol Fumarate (001329)

For related information, see the comparative table section in Appendix A.

Categories: Asthma; Bronchitis, chronic; Bronchospasm, exercise-induced; Chronic obstructive pulmonary disease; Emphysema; Pregnancy Category C; FDA Approved 2001 Feb
Drug Classes: Adrenergic agonists; Bronchodilators
Brand Names: **Foradil**
Foreign Brand Availability: Atock (China; Japan; Korea; Philippines; Taiwan); Foradile (Australia); Foradil P (Germany); Formoclean (Korea); Forterol (Korea); Newtock (Korea); Oxis (Australia; Bahamas; Barbados; Belize; Benin; Bermuda; Burkina-Faso; Curacao; Ethiopia; Gambia; Germany; Ghana; Guinea; Guyana; Indonesia; Ireland; Ivory-Coast; Jamaica; Kenya; Liberia; Malawi; Mali; Mauritania; Mauritius; Morocco; Netherland-Antilles; Netherlands; New-Zealand; Niger; Nigeria; Philippines; Puerto-Rico; Senegal; Seychelles; Sierra-Leone; Singapore; South-Africa; Sudan; Surinam; Sweden; Tanzania; Thailand; Trinidad; Tunia; Uganda; Zambia; Zimbabwe); Sortel (Korea)
Cost of Therapy: $83.15 (Asthma; Foradil; 12 µg; 2 inhalations/day; 30 day supply)

DESCRIPTION

Foradil Aerolizer consists of a capsule dosage form containing a dry powder formulation of Foradil (formoterol fumarate) intended for oral inhalation only with the Aerolizer Inhaler.

Each clear, hard gelatin capsule contains a dry powder blend of 12 µg of formoterol fumarate and 25 mg of lactose as a carrier.

The active component of Foradil is formoterol fumarate, a racemate. Formoterol fumarate is a selective beta$_2$-adrenergic bronchodilator. Its chemical name is (±)-2-hydroxy-5-[(1RS)-1-hydroxy-2-[[(1RS)-2-(4-methoxyphenyl)-1-methylethyl]-amino]ethyl]formanilide fumarate dihydrate.

Formoterol fumarate has a molecular weight of 840.9, and its empirical formula is $(C_{19}H_{24}N_2O_4)_2 \cdot C_4H_4O_4 \cdot 2H_2O$. Formoterol fumarate is a white to yellowish crystalline powder, which is freely soluble in glacial acetic acid, soluble in methanol, sparingly soluble in ethanol and isopropanol, slightly soluble in water, and practically insoluble in acetone, ethyl acetate, and diethyl ether.

The aerolizer inhaler is a plastic device used for inhaling formoterol fumarate. The amount of drug delivered to the lung will depend on patient factors, such as inspiratory flow rate and inspiratory time. Under standardized *in vitro* testing at a fixed flow rate of 60 L/min for 2 seconds, the aerolizer inhaler delivered 10 µg of formoterol fumarate from the mouthpiece. Peak inspiratory flow rates (PIFR) achievable through the aerolizer inhaler were evaluated in 33 adult and adolescent patients and 32 pediatric patients with mild-to-moderate asthma. Mean PIFR was 117.82 L/min (range 34-188 L/min) for adult and adolescent patients, and 99.66 L/min (range 43-187 L/min) for pediatric patients. Approximately 90% of each population studied generated a PIFR through the device exceeding 60 L/min.

To use the delivery system, a formoterol fumarate capsule is placed in the well of the aerolizer inhaler, and the capsule is pierced by pressing and releasing the buttons on the side of the device. The formoterol fumarate formulation is dispersed into the air stream when the patient inhales rapidly and deeply through the mouthpiece.

CLINICAL PHARMACOLOGY

MECHANISM OF ACTION

Formoterol fumarate is a long-acting selective beta$_2$-adrenergic receptor agonist (beta$_2$-agonist). Inhaled formoterol fumarate acts locally in the lung as a bronchodilator. *In vitro* studies have shown that formoterol has more than 200-fold greater agonist activity at beta$_2$-receptors than at beta$_1$-receptors. Although beta$_2$-receptors are the predominant adrenergic receptors in bronchial smooth muscle and beta$_1$-receptors are the predominant receptors in the heart, there are also beta$_2$-receptors in the human heart comprising 10-50% of the total beta-adrenergic receptors. The precise function of these receptors has not been established, but they raise the possibility that even highly selective beta$_2$-agonists may have cardiac effects.

The pharmacologic effects of beta$_2$-adrenoceptor agonist drugs, including formoterol, are at least in part attributable to stimulation of intracellular adenyl cyclase, the enzyme that catalyzes the conversion of adenosine triphosphate (ATP) to cyclic-3′,5′-adenosine monophosphate (cyclic AMP). Increased cyclic AMP levels cause relaxation of bronchial smooth muscle and inhibition of release of mediators of immediate hypersensitivity from cells, especially from mast cells.

In vitro tests show that formoterol is an inhibitor of the release of mast cell mediators, such as histamine and leukotrienes, from the human lung. Formoterol also inhibits histamine-induced plasma albumin extravasation in anesthetized guinea pigs and inhibits allergen-induced eosinophil influx in dogs with airway hyper-responsiveness. The relevance of these *in vitro* and animal findings to humans is unknown.

PHARMACOKINETICS

Information on the pharmacokinetics of formoterol in plasma has been obtained in healthy subjects by oral inhalation of doses higher than the recommended range and in Chronic Obstructive Pulmonary Disease (COPD) patients after oral inhalation of doses at and above the therapeutic dose. Urinary excretion of unchanged formoterol was used as an indirect measure of systemic exposure. Plasma drug disposition data parallel urinary excretion, and the elimination half-lives calculated for urine and plasma are similar.

Absorption

Following inhalation of a single 120 µg dose of formoterol fumarate by 12 healthy subjects, formoterol was rapidly absorbed into plasma, reaching a maximum drug concentration of 92 pg/ml within 5 minutes of dosing. In COPD patients treated for 12 weeks with formoterol fumarate 12 or 24 µg bid, the mean plasma concentrations of formoterol ranged between 4.0 and 8.8 pg/ml and 8.0 and 17.3 pg/ml, respectively, at 10 minutes, 2 hours and 6 hours post inhalation.

Following inhalation of 12-96 µg of formoterol fumarate by 10 healthy males, urinary excretion of both (R,R)- and (S,S)-enantiomers of formoterol increased proportionally to the dose. Thus, absorption of formoterol following inhalation appeared linear over the dose range studied.

In a study in patients with asthma, when formoterol 12 or 24 µg twice daily was given by oral inhalation for 4 or 12 weeks, the accumulation index, based on the urinary excretion of unchanged formoterol ranged from 1.63-2.08 in comparison with the first dose. For COPD patients, when formoterol 12 or 24 µg twice daily was given by oral inhalation for 12 weeks, the accumulation index, based on the urinary excretion of unchanged formoterol was 1.19-1.38. This suggests some accumulation of formoterol in plasma with multiple dosing. The excreted amounts of formoterol at steady-state were close to those predicted based on single-dose kinetics. As with many drug products for oral inhalation, it is likely that the majority of the inhaled formoterol fumarate delivered is swallowed and then absorbed from the gastrointestinal tract.

Distribution

The binding of formoterol to human plasma proteins *in vitro* was 61-64% at concentrations from 0.1 to 100 ng/ml. Binding to human serum albumin *in vitro* was 31-38% over a range of 5-500 ng/ml. The concentrations of formoterol used to assess the plasma protein binding were higher than those achieved in plasma following inhalation of a single 120 µg dose.

Metabolism

Formoterol is metabolized primarily by direct glucuronidation at either the phenolic or aliphatic hydroxyl group and O-demethylation followed by glucuronide conjugation at either phenolic hydroxyl groups. Minor pathways involve sulfate conjugation of formoterol and deformylation followed by sulfate conjugation. The most prominent pathway involves direct conjugation at the phenolic hydroxyl group. The second major pathway involves O-demethylation followed by conjugation at the phenolic 2′-hydroxyl group. Four cytochrome P450 isozymes (CYP2D6, CYP2C19, CYP2C9 and CYP2A6) are involved in the O-demethylation of formoterol. Formoterol did not inhibit CYP450 enzymes at therapeutically relevant concentrations. Some patients may be deficient in CYP2D6 or 2C19 or both. Whether a deficiency in one or both of these isozymes results in elevated systemic exposure to formoterol or systemic adverse effects has not been adequately explored.

Excretion

Following oral administration of 80 µg of radiolabeled formoterol fumarate to 2 healthy subjects, 59-62% of the radioactivity was eliminated in the urine and 32-34% in the feces over a period of 104 hours. Renal clearance of formoterol from blood in these subjects was about 150 ml/min. Following inhalation of a 12 or 24 µg dose by 16 patients with asthma, about 10% and 15-18% of the total dose was excreted in the urine as unchanged formoterol and direct conjugates of formoterol, respectively. Following inhalation of 12 or 24 µg dose by 18 patients with COPD the corresponding values were 7% and 6-9% of the dose, respectively.

Based on plasma concentrations measured following inhalation of a single 120 µg dose by 12 healthy subjects, the mean terminal elimination half-life was determined to be 10 hours. From urinary excretion rates measured in these subjects, the mean terminal elimination half-lives for the (R,R)- and (S,S)-enantiomers were determined to be 13.9 and 12.3 hours, respectively. The (R,R)- and (S,S)-enantiomers represented about 40% and 60% of unchanged drug excreted in the urine, respectively, following single inhaled doses between 12 and 120 µg in healthy volunteers and single and repeated doses of 12 and 24 µg in patients with asthma. Thus, the relative proportion of the two enantiomers remained constant over the dose range studied and there was no evidence of relative accumulation of one enantiomer over the other after repeated dosing.

Special Populations

Gender

After correction for body weight, formoterol pharmacokinetics did not differ significantly between males and females.

Geriatric and Pediatric

The pharmacokinetics of formoterol have not been studied in the elderly population, and limited data are available in pediatric patients.

In a study of children with asthma who were 5-12 years of age, when formoterol fumarate 12 or 24 µg was given twice daily by oral inhalation for 12 weeks, the accumulation index ranged from 1.18-1.84 based on urinary excretion of unchanged formoterol. Hence, the accumulation in children did not exceed that in adults, where the accumulation index ranged from 1.63-2.08 (see Absorption). Approximately 6% and 6.5 to 9% of the dose was recovered in the urine of the children as unchanged and conjugated formoterol, respectively.

Hepatic/Renal Impairment

The pharmacokinetics of formoterol have not been studied in subjects with hepatic or renal impairment.

PHARMACODYNAMICS

Systemic Safety and Pharmacokinetic/Pharmacodynamic Relationships

The major adverse effects of inhaled beta$_2$-agonists occur as a result of excessive activation of the systemic beta-adrenergic receptors. The most common adverse effects in adults and adolescents include skeletal muscle tremor and cramps, insomnia, tachycardia, decreases in plasma potassium, and increases in plasma glucose.

Pharmacokinetic/pharmacodynamic (PK/PD) relationships between heart rate, ECG parameters, and serum potassium levels and the urinary excretion of formoterol were evaluated in 10 healthy male volunteers (25-45 years of age) following inhalation of single doses containing 12, 24, 48, or 96 µg of formoterol fumarate. There was a linear relationship between urinary formoterol excretion and decreases in serum potassium, increases in plasma glucose, and increases in heart rate.

In a second study, PK/PD relationships between plasma formoterol levels and pulse rate, ECG parameters, and plasma potassium levels were evaluated in 12 healthy volunteers following inhalation of a single 120 µg dose of formoterol fumarate (10 times the recommended clinical dose). Reductions of plasma potassium concentration were observed in all subjects. Maximum reductions from baseline ranged from 0.55-1.52 mmol/L with a median maximum reduction of 1.01 mmol/L. The formoterol plasma concentration was highly correlated with the reduction in plasma potassium concentration. Generally, the maximum effect on plasma potassium was noted 1-3 hours after peak formoterol plasma concentrations were achieved. A mean maximum increase of pulse rate of 26 bpm was observed 6 hours post-dose. The maximum increase of mean corrected QT interval (QTc) was 25 milliseconds when calculated using Bazett's correction and was 8 milliseconds when calculated using Fredericia's correction. The QTc returned to baseline within 12-24 hours post-dose. Formoterol plasma concentrations were weakly correlated with pulse rate and increase of QTc duration. The effects on plasma potassium, pulse rate, and QTc interval are known pharmacological effects of this class of study drug and were not unexpected at the very high formoterol dose (120 µg single dose, 10 times the recommended single dose) tested in this study. These effects were well-tolerated by the healthy volunteers.

The electrocardiographic and cardiovascular effects of formoterol fumarate inhalation powder were compared with those of albuterol and placebo in two pivotal 12 week double-blind studies of patients with asthma. A subset of patients underwent continuous electrocardiographic monitoring during three 24 hour periods. No important differences in ventricular or supraventricular ectopy between treatment groups were observed. In these two studies, the total number of patients with asthma sexposed to any dose of formoterol fumarate inhalation powder who had continuous electrocardiographic monitoring was about 200.

Continuous electrocardiographic monitoring was not included in the clinical studies of formoterol fumarate inhalation powder that were performed in COPD patients. The electrocardiographic effects of formoterol fumarate inhalation powder were evaluated versus placebo in a 12 month pivotal double-blind study of patients with COPD. An analysis of ECG intervals was performed for patients who participated at study sites in the US, including 46 patients treated with formoterol fumarate inhalation powder 12 µg twice daily, and 50 patients treated with formoterol fumarate inhalation powder 24 µg twice daily. ECGs were performed pre-dose, and at 5-15 minutes and 2 hours post-dose at study baseline and after 3, 6 and 12 months of treatment. The results showed that there was no clinically meaningful acute or chronic effect on ECG intervals, including QTc, resulting from treatment with formoterol fumarate inhalation powder.

Tachyphylaxis/Tolerance

In a clinical study in 19 adult patients with mild asthma, the bronchoprotective effect of formoterol, as assessed by methacholine challenge, was studied following an initial dose of 24 µg (twice the recommended dose) and after 2 weeks of 24 µg twice daily. Tolerance to the bronchoprotective effects of formoterol was observed as evidenced by a diminished bronchoprotective effect on FEV$_1$ after 2 weeks of dosing, with loss of protection at the end of the 12 hour dosing period.

Rebound bronchial hyper-responsiveness after cessation of chronic formoterol therapy has not been observed.

In three large clinical trials in patients with asthma, while efficacy of formoterol versus placebo was maintained, a slightly reduced bronchodilatory response (as measured by 12 hour FEV$_1$ AUC) was observed within the formoterol arms over time, particularly with the 24 µg twice daily dose (twice the daily recommended dose). A similarly reduced FEV$_1$ AUC over time was also noted in the albuterol treatment arms (180 µg four times daily by metered-dose inhaler).

INDICATIONS AND USAGE

Formoterol fumarate inhalation powder is indicated for long-term, twice-daily (morning and evening) administration in the maintenance treatment of asthma and in the prevention of bronchospasm in adults and children 5 years of age and older with reversible obstructive airways disease, including patients with symptoms of nocturnal asthma, who require regular treatment with inhaled, short-acting, beta$_2$-agonists. It is not indicated for patients whose asthma can be managed by occasional use of inhaled, short-acting, beta$_2$-agonists.

Formoterol fumarate inhalation powder is also indicated for the acute prevention of exercise-induced bronchospasm (EIB) in adults and children 12 years of age and older, when administered on an occasional, as needed basis.

Formoterol fumarate inhalation powder can be used to treat asthma concomitantly with short-acting beta$_2$-agonists, inhaled or systemic corticosteroids, and theophylline therapy (see DRUG INTERACTIONS). A satisfactory clinical response to formoterol fumarate inhalation powder does not eliminate the need for continued treatment with an anti-inflammatory agent.

Formoterol fumarate inhalation powder is indicated for the long-term, twice daily (morning and evening) administration in the maintenance treatment of bronchoconstriction in patients with Chronic Obstructive Pulmonary Disease including chronic bronchitis and emphysema.

CONTRAINDICATIONS

Formoterol fumarate is contraindicated in patients with a history of hypersensitivity to formoterol fumarate or to any components of this product.

WARNINGS

IMPORTANT INFORMATION: FORMOTEROL FUMARATE INHALATION POWDER SHOULD NOT BE INITIATED IN PATIENTS WITH SIGNIFICANTLY WORSENING OR ACUTELY DETERIORATING ASTHMA, WHICH MAY BE A LIFE-THREATENING CONDITION. The use of formoterol fumarate inhalation powder in this setting is inappropriate.

FORMOTEROL FUMARATE INHALATION POWDER IS NOT A SUBSTITUTE FOR INHALED OR ORAL CORTICOSTEROIDS. Corticosteroids should not be stopped or reduced at the time formoterol fumarate inhalation powder is initiated. (See PRECAUTIONS, Information for the Patient and refer to the Patient Instructions for Use that are distributed with the prescription for complete instructions.)

When beginning treatment with formoterol fumarate inhalation powder, patients who have been taking inhaled, short-acting beta$_2$-agonists on a regular basis (*e.g.,* 4 times a day) should be instructed to discontinue the regular use of these drugs and use them only for symptomatic relief of acute asthma symptoms (see PRECAUTIONS, Information for the Patient).

PARADOXICAL BRONCHOSPASM

As with other inhaled beta$_2$-agonists, formoterol can produce paradoxical bronchospasm, that may be life-threatening. If paradoxical bronchospasm occurs, formoterol fumarate inhalation powder should be discontinued immediately and alternative therapy instituted.

DETERIORATION OF ASTHMA

Asthma may deteriorate acutely over a period of hours or chronically over several days or longer. If the usual dose of formoterol fumarate inhalation powder no longer controls the symptoms of bronchoconstriction, and the patient's inhaled, short-acting beta$_2$-agonist becomes less effective or the patient needs more inhalation of short-acting beta$_2$-agonist than usual, these may be markers of deterioration of asthma. In this setting, a re-evaluation of the patient and the asthma treatment regimen should be undertaken at once, giving special consideration to the possible need for anti-inflammatory treatment, *e.g.,* corticosteroids. Increasing the daily dosage of formoterol fumarate inhalation powder beyond the recommended dose in this situation is not appropriate. Formoterol fumarate inhalation powder should not be used more frequently than twice daily (morning and evening) at the recommended dose.

USE OF ANTI-INFLAMMATORY AGENTS

The use of beta$_2$-agonists alone may not be adequate to control asthma in many patients. Early consideration should be given to adding anti-inflammatory agents, *e.g.,* corticosteroids. There are no data demonstrating that formoterol fumarate has any clinical anti-inflammatory effect and therefore it cannot be expected to take the place of corticosteroids. Patients who already require oral or inhaled corticosteroids for treatment of asthma should be continued on this type of treatment even if they feel better as a result of initiating or increasing the dose of formoterol fumarate inhalation powder. Any change in corticosteroid dosage, in particular a reduction, should be made ONLY after clinical evaluation (see PRECAUTIONS, Information for the Patient).

CARDIOVASCULAR EFFECTS

Formoterol fumarate, like other beta$_2$-agonists, can produce a clinically significant cardiovascular effect in some patients as measured by increases in pulse rate, blood pressure, and/or symptoms. Although such effects are uncommon after administration of formoterol fumarate inhalation powder at recommended doses, if they occur, the drug may need to be discontinued. In addition, beta-agonists have been reported to produce ECG changes, such as flattening of the T wave, prolongation of the QTc interval, and ST segment depression. The clinical significance of these findings is unknown. Therefore, formoterol fumarate, like other sympathomimetic amines, should be used with caution in patients with cardiovascular disorders, especially coronary insufficiency, cardiac arrhythmias, and hypertension (see PRECAUTIONS, General).

IMMEDIATE HYPERSENSITIVITY REACTIONS

Immediate hypersensitivity reactions may occur after administration of formoterol fumarate inhalation powder, as demonstrated by cases of anaphylactic reactions, urticaria, angioedema, rash, and bronchospasm.

DO NOT EXCEED RECOMMENDED DOSE

Fatalities have been reported in association with excessive use of inhaled sympathomimetic drugs in patients with asthma. The exact cause of death is unknown, but cardiac arrest following an unexpected development of a severe acute asthmatic crisis and subsequent hypoxia is suspected.

PRECAUTIONS

GENERAL

Formoterol fumarate inhalation powder should not be used to treat acute symptoms of asthma. Formoterol fumarate inhalation powder has not been studied in the relief of acute asthma symptoms and extra doses should not be used for that purpose. When prescribing formoterol fumarate inhalation powder, the physician should also provide the patient with an inhaled, short-acting beta$_2$-agonist for treatment of symptoms that occur acutely, despite regular twice-daily (morning and evening) use of formoterol fumarate inhalation powder. Patients should also be cautioned that increasing inhaled beta$_2$-agonist use is a signal of deteriorating asthma. (See Information for the Patient and refer to the Patient Instructions for Use that are distributed with the prescription for complete instructions.)

Formoterol fumarate, like other sympathomimetic amines, should be used with caution in patients with cardiovascular disorders, especially coronary insufficiency, cardiac arrhythmias, and hypertension; in patients with convulsive disorders or thyrotoxicosis; and in patients who are unusually responsive to sympathomimetic amines. Clinically significant changes in systolic and/or diastolic blood pressure, pulse rate and electrocardiograms have been seen infrequently in individual patients in controlled clinical studies with formoterol. Doses of the related beta$_2$-agonist albuterol, when administered intravenously, have been reported to aggravate preexisting diabetes mellitus and ketoacidosis.

F

Beta-agonist medications may produce significant hypokalemia in some patients, possibly through intracellular shunting, which has the potential to produce adverse cardiovascular effects. The decrease in serum potassium is usually transient, not requiring supplementation.

Clinically significant changes in blood glucose and/or serum potassium were infrequent during clinical studies with long-term administration of formoterol fumarate inhalation powder at the recommended dose.

Formoterol fumarate capsules should ONLY be used with the aerolizer inhaler and SHOULD NOT be taken orally.

Formoterol fumarate capsules should always be stored in the blister, and only removed IMMEDIATELY before use.

INFORMATION FOR THE PATIENT

It is important that patients understand how to use the aerolizer inhaler appropriately and how it should be used in relation to other asthma medications they are taking (refer to the Patient Instructions for Use that are distributed with the prescription for complete instructions).

The active ingredient formoterol fumarate is a long-acting, bronchodilator used for the treatment of asthma, including nocturnal asthma, and for the prevention of exercise-induced bronchospasm. Formoterol fumarate inhalation powder provides bronchodilation for up to 12 hours. Patients should be advised not to increase the dose or frequency of formoterol fumarate inhalation powder without consulting the prescribing physician. Patients should be warned not to stop or reduce concomitant asthma therapy without medical advice.

Formoterol fumarate aerolizer is not indicated to relieve acute asthma symptoms and extra doses should not be used for that purpose. Acute symptoms should be treated with an inhaled, short-acting, beta$_2$-agonist (the health-care provider should prescribe the patient with such medication and instruct the patient in how it should be used). Patients should be instructed to seek medical attention if their symptoms worsen, if formoterol fumarate aerolizer treatment becomes less effective, or if they need more inhalations of a short-acting beta$_2$-agonist than usual. Patients should not inhale more than the contents of the prescribed number of capsules at any one time. The daily dosage of fomoterol fumarate aerolizer should not exceed 1 capsule twice daily (24 μg total daily dose).

When formoterol fumarate inhalation powder is used for the prevention of EIB, the contents of 1 capsule should be taken at least 15 minutes prior to exercise. Additional doses of formoterol fumarate inhalation powder should not be used for 12 hours. Prevention of EIB has not been studied in patients who are receiving chronic formoterol fumarate inhalation powder administration twice daily and these patients should not use additional formoterol fumarate inhalation powder for prevention of EIB.

Formoterol fumarate inhalation powder should not be used as a substitute for oral or inhaled corticosteroids. The dosage of these medications should not be changed and they should not be stopped without consulting the physician, even if the patient feels better after initiating treatment with formoterol fumarate inhalation powder.

Patients should be informed that treatment with beta$_2$-agonists may lead to adverse events which include palpitations, chest pain, rapid heart rate, tremor or nervousness. Patients should be informed never to use formoterol fumarate inhalation powder with a spacer and never to exhale into the device.

Patients should avoid exposing the formoterol fumarate capsules to moisture and should handle the capsules with dry hands. The aerolizer inhaler should never be washed and should be kept dry. The patient should always use the new aerolizer inhaler that comes with each refill.

Women should be advised to contact their physician if they become pregnant or if they are nursing.

Patients should be told that in rare cases, the gelatin capsule might break into small pieces. These pieces should be retained by the screen built into the aerolizer inhaler. However, it remains possible that rarely, tiny pieces of gelatin might reach the mouth or throat after inhalation. The capsule is less likely to shatter when pierced if: storage conditions are strictly followed, capsules are removed from the blister immediately before use, and the capsules are only pierced once.

CARCINOGENESIS, MUTAGENESIS, AND IMPAIRMENT OF FERTILITY

The carcinogenic potential of formoterol fumarate has been evaluated in 2 year drinking water and dietary studies in both rats and mice. In rats, the incidence of ovarian leiomyomas was increased at doses of 15 mg/kg and above in the drinking water study and at 20 mg/kg in the dietary study, but not at dietary doses up to 5 mg/kg (AUC exposure approximately 450 times human exposure at the maximum recommended daily inhalation dose). In the dietary study, the incidence of benign ovarian theca-cell tumors was increased at doses of 0.5 mg/kg and above (AUC exposure at the low dose of 0.5 mg/kg was approximately 45 times human exposure at the maximum recommended daily inhalation dose). This finding was not observed in the drinking water study, nor was it seen in mice.

In mice, the incidence of adrenal subcapsular adenomas and carcinomas was increased in males at doses of 69 mg/kg and above in the drinking water study, but not at doses up to 50 mg/kg (AUC exposure approximately 590 times human exposure at the maximum recommended daily inhalation dose) in the dietary study. The incidence of hepatocarcinomas was increased in the dietary study at doses of 20 and 50 mg/kg in females and 50 mg/kg in males, but not at doses up to 5 mg/kg in either males or females (AUC exposure approximately 60 times human exposure at the maximum recommended daily inhalation dose). Also in the dietary study, the incidence of uterine leiomyomas and leiomyosarcomas was increased at doses of 2 mg/kg and above (AUC exposure at the low dose of 2 mg/kg was approximately 25 times human exposure at the maximum recommended daily inhalation dose). Increases in leiomyomas of the rodent female genital tract have been similarly demonstrated with other beta-agonist drugs.

Formoterol fumarate was not mutagenic or clastogenic in the following tests: Mutagenicity tests in bacterial and mammalian cells, chromosomal analyses in mammalian cells, unscheduled DNA synthesis repair tests in rat hepatocytes and human fibroblasts, transformation assay in mammalian fibroblasts and micronucleus tests in mice and rats.

Reproduction studies in rats revealed no impairment of fertility at oral doses up to 3 mg/kg (approximately 1000 times the maximum recommended daily inhalation dose in humans on a mg/m^2 basis).

PREGNANCY, TERATOGENIC EFFECTS, PREGNANCY CATEGORY C

Formoterol fumarate has been shown to cause stillbirth and neonatal mortality at oral doses of 6 mg/kg (approximately 2000 times the maximum recommended daily inhalation dose in humans on a mg/m^2 basis) and above in rats receiving the drug during the late stage of pregnancy. These effects, however, were not produced at a dose of 0.2 mg/kg (approximately 70 times the maximum recommended daily inhalation dose in humans on a mg/m^2 basis). When given to rats throughout organogenesis, oral doses of 0.2 mg/kg and above delayed ossification of the fetus, and doses of 6 mg/kg and above decreased fetal weight. Formoterol fumarate did not cause malformations in rats or rabbits following oral administration. Because there are no adequate and well-controlled studies in pregnant women, formoterol fumarate inhalation powder should be used during pregnancy only if the potential benefit justifies the potential risk to the fetus.

USE IN LABOR AND DELIVERY

Formoterol fumarate has been shown to cause stillbirth and neonatal mortality at oral doses of 6 mg/kg (approximately 2000 times the maximum recommended daily inhalation dose in humans on a mg/m^2 basis) and above in rats receiving the drug for several days at the end of pregnancy. These effects were not produced at a dose of 0.2 mg/kg (approximately 70 times the maximum recommended daily inhalation dose in humans on a mg/m^2 basis). There are no adequate and well-controlled human studies that have investigated the effects of formoterol fumarate inhalation powder during labor and delivery.

Because beta-agonists may potentially interfere with uterine contractility, formoterol fumarate inhalation powder should be used during labor only if the potential benefit justifies the potential risk.

NURSING MOTHERS

In reproductive studies in rats, formoterol was excreted in the milk. It is not known whether formoterol is excreted in human milk, but because many drugs are excreted in human milk, caution should be exercised if formoterol fumarate inhalation powder is administered to nursing women. There are no well-controlled human studies of the use of formoterol fumarate inhalation powder in nursing mothers.

PEDIATRIC USE

Asthma

A total of 776 children 5 years of age and older with asthma were studied in three multiple-dose controlled clinical trials. Of the 512 children who received formoterol, 508 were 5-12 years of age, and approximately one-third were 5-8 years of age.

Exercise Induced Bronchoconstriction

A total of 20 adolescent patients, 12-16 years of age, were studied in three well-controlled single-dose clinical trials.

The safety and effectiveness of formoterol fumarate inhalation powder in pediatric patients below 5 years of age has not been established. (See ADVERSE REACTIONS, Experience in Pediatric, Adolescent and Adult Patients.)

GERIATRIC USE

Of the total number of patients who received formoterol fumarate inhalation powder in adolescent and adult chronic dosing asthma clinical trials, 318 were 65 years of age or older and 39 were 75 years of age and older. Of the 811 patients who received formoterol fumarate inhalation powder in two pivotal multiple-dose controlled clinical studies in patients with COPD, 395 (48.7%) were 65 years of age or older while 62 (7.6%) were 75 years of age or older. No overall differences in safety or effectiveness were observed between these subjects and younger subjects. A slightly higher frequency of chest infection was reported in the 39 asthma patients 75 years of age and older, although a causal relationship with formoterol fumarate has not been established. Other reported clinical experience has not identified differences in responses between the elderly and younger adult patients, but greater sensitivity of some older individuals cannot be ruled out. (See DRUG INTERACTIONS.)

DRUG INTERACTIONS

If additional adrenergic drugs are to be administered by any route, they should be used with caution because the pharmacologically predictable sympathetic effects of formoterol may be potentiated.

Concomitant treatment with xanthine derivatives, steroids, or diuretics may potentiate any hypokalemic effect of adrenergic agonists.

The ECG changes and/or hypokalemia that may result from the administration of non-potassium sparing diuretics (such as loop or thiazide diuretics) can be acutely worsened by beta-agonists, especially when the recommended dose of the beta-agonist is exceeded. Although the clinical significance of these effects is not known, caution is advised in the co-administration of beta-agonist with non-potassium sparing diuretics.

Formoterol, as with other $beta_2$-agonists, should be administered with extreme caution to patients being treated with monamine oxidase inhibitors, tricyclic antidepressants, or drugs known to prolong the QTc interval because the action of adrenergic agonists on the cardiovascular system may be potentiated by these agents. Drugs that are known to prolong the QTc interval have an increased risk of ventricular arrhythmias.

Beta-adrenergic receptor antagonists (beta-blockers) and formoterol may inhibit the effect of each other when administered concurrently. Beta-blockers not only block the therapeutic effects of beta-agonists, such as formoterol, but may produce severe bronchospasm in asthmatic patients. Therefore, patients with asthma should not normally be treated with beta-blockers. However, under certain circumstances, *e.g.*, as prophylaxis after myocardial infarction, there may be no acceptable alternatives to the use of beta-blockers in patients with asthma. In this setting, cardioselective beta-blockers could be considered, although they should be administered with caution.

ADVERSE REACTIONS

Adverse reactions to formoterol fumarate are similar in nature to other selective $beta_2$-adrenoceptor agonists; *e.g.*, angina, hypertension or hypotension, tachycardia, arrhythmias, nervousness, headache, tremor, dry mouth, palpitation, muscle cramps, nausea, dizziness, fatigue, malaise, hypokalemia, hyperglycemia, metabolic acidosis and insomnia.

EXPERIENCE IN PEDIATRIC, ADOLESCENT AND ADULT PATIENTS WITH ASTHMA

Of the 5824 patients in multiple-dose controlled clinical trials, 1985 were treated with formoterol fumarate inhalation powder at the recommended dose of 12 μg twice daily. TABLE 1 shows adverse events where the frequency was greater than or equal to 1% in the formoterol fumarate twice daily group and where the rates in the formoterol fumarate group exceeded placebo. Three adverse events showed dose ordering among tested doses of 6, 12 and 24 μg administered twice daily; tremor, dizziness and dysphonia.

***TABLE 1** Number and Frequency of Adverse Experiences in Patients 5 Years of Age and Older From Multiple-Dose Controlled Clinical Trials*

Adverse Event	Formoterol Fumarate Inhalation Powder* n	Placebo n
Total patients	1985 (100%)	969 (100%)
Infection viral	341 (17.2%)	166 (17.1%)
Bronchitis	92 (4.6%)	42 (4.3%)
Chest infection	54 (2.7%)	4 (0.4%)
Dyspnea	42 (2.1%)	16 (1.7%)
Chest pain	37 (1.9%)	13 (1.3%)
Tremor	37 (1.9%)	4 (0.4%)
Dizziness	31 (1.6%)	15 (1.5%)
Insomnia	29 (1.5%)	8 (0.8%)
Tonsillitis	23 (1.2%)	7 (0.7%)
Rash	22 (1.1%)	7 (0.7%)
Dysphonia	19 (1.0%)	9 (0.9%)

* 12 μg twice daily.

EXPERIENCE IN CHILDREN WITH ASTHMA

The safety of formoterol fumarate inhalation powder compared to placebo was investigated in one large, multicenter, randomized, double-blind clinical trial in 518 children with asthma (ages 5-12 years) in need of daily bronchodilators and anti-inflammatory treatment. The numbers and percent of patients who reported adverse events were comparable in the 12 μg twice daily and placebo groups. In general, the pattern of the adverse events observed in children differed from the usual pattern seen in adults. The adverse events that were more frequent in the formoterol group than in the placebo group reflected infection/inflammation (viral infection, rhinitis, tonsillitis, gastroenteritis) or abdominal complaints (abdominal pain, nausea, dyspepsia).

EXPERIENCE IN ADULT PATIENTS WITH COPD

Of the 1634 patients in two pivotal multiple-dose Chronic Obstructive Pulmonary Disease (COPD) controlled trials, 405 were treated with formoterol fumarate inhalation powder 12 μg twice daily. The numbers and percent of patients who reported adverse events were comparable in the 12 μg twice daily and placebo groups. Adverse events (AEs) experienced were similar to those seen in asthmatic patients, but with a higher incidence of COPD-related AEs in both placebo and formoterol treated patients.

TABLE 2 shows adverse events where the frequency was greater than or equal to 1% in the formoterol fumarate inhalation powder group and where the rates in the formoterol fumarate inhalation powder group exceeded placebo. The two clinical trials included doses of 12 and 24 μg, administered twice daily. Seven adverse events showed dose ordering among tested doses of 12 and 24 μg administered twice daily; pharyngitis, fever, muscle cramps, increased sputum, dysphonia, myalgia, and tremor.

Overall, the frequency of all cardiovascular adverse events in the two pivotal studies was low and comparable to placebo (6.4% for formoterol fumarate inhalation powder 12 μg twice daily, and 6.0% for placebo). There were no frequently-occurring specific cardiovascular adverse events for formoterol fumarate inhalation powder (frequency greater than or equal to 1% and greater than placebo).

***TABLE 2** Number and Frequency of Adverse Experiences in Adult COPD Patients Treated in Multiple-Dose Controlled Clinical Trials*

Adverse Event	Formoterol Fumarate Inhalation Powder* n	Placebo n
Total patients	405 (100%)	420 (100%)
Upper respiratory tract infection	30 (7.4%)	24 (5.7%)
Pain back	17 (4.2%)	17 (4.0%)
Pharyngitis	14 (3.5%)	10 (2.4%)
Pain chest	13 (3.2%)	9 (2.1%)
Sinusitis	11 (2.7%)	7 (1.7%)
Fever	9 (2.2%)	6 (1.4%)
Cramps leg	7 (1.7%)	2 (0.5%)
Cramps muscle	7 (1.7%)	0
Anxiety	6 (1.5%)	5 (1.2%)
Pruritus	6 (1.5%)	4 (1.0%)
Sputum increased	6 (1.5%)	5 (1.2%)
Mouth dry	5 (1.2%)	4 (1.0%)
Trauma	5 (1.2%)	0

* 12 μg twice daily.

POST MARKETING EXPERIENCE

In extensive worldwide marketing experience with formoterol fumarate, serious exacerbations of asthma, including some that have been fatal, have been reported. While most of these cases have been in patients with severe or acutely deteriorating asthma (see WARNINGS), a few have occurred in patients with less severe asthma. The contribution of formoterol fumarate to these cases could not be determined.

Rare reports of anaphylactic reactions, including severe hypotension and angioedema, have also been received in association with the use of formoterol fumarate inhalation powder.

DOSAGE AND ADMINISTRATION

Formoterol fumarate capsules should be administered only by the oral inhalation route (refer to the Patient Instructions for Use that are distributed with the prescription for complete instructions) and only using the aerolizer inhaler. Formoterol fumarate capsules should not be ingested (*i.e.*, swallowed) orally. Formoterol fumarate capsules should always be stored in the blister, and only removed IMMEDIATELY BEFORE USE.

FOR MAINTENANCE TREATMENT OF ASTHMA

For adults and children 5 years of age and older, the usual dosage is the inhalation of the contents of one 12 μg formoterol fumarate capsule every 12 hours using the aerolizer inhaler. The patient must not exhale into the device. The total daily dose of formoterol fumarate should not exceed 1 capsule twice daily (24 μg total daily dose). More frequent administration or administration of a larger number of inhalations is not recommended. If symptoms arise between doses, an inhaled short-acting $beta_2$-agonist should be taken for immediate relief.

If a previously effective dosage regimen fails to provide the usual response, medical advice should be sought immediately as this is often a sign of destabilization of asthma. Under these circumstances, the therapeutic regimen should be re-evaluated and additional therapeutic options, such as inhaled or systemic corticosteroids, should be considered.

FOR PREVENTION OF EXERCISE-INDUCED BRONCHOSPASM (EIB)

For adults and adolescents 12 years of age or older, the usual dosage is the inhalation of the contents of one 12 μg formoterol fumarate capsule at least 15 minutes before exercise administered on an occasional as-needed basis.

Additional doses of formoterol fumarate inhalation powder should not be used for 12 hours after the administration of this drug. Regular, twice-daily dosing has not been studied in preventing EIB. Patients who are receiving formoterol fumarate inhalation powder twice daily for maintenance treatment of their asthma should not use additional doses for prevention of EIB and may require a short-acting bronchodilator.

FOR MAINTENANCE TREATMENT OF CHRONIC OBSTRUCTIVE PULMONARY DISEASE (COPD)

The usual dosage is the inhalation of the contents of one 12 μg formoterol fumarate capsule every 12 hours using the aerolizer inhaler.

A total daily dose of greater than 24 μg is not recommended.

If a previously effective dosage regimen fails to provide the usual response, medical advice should be sought immediately as this is often a sign of destabilization of COPD. Under these circumstances, the therapeutic regimen should be re-evaluated and additional therapeutic options should be considered.

ANIMAL PHARMACOLOGY

Studies in laboratory animals (minipigs, rodents, and dogs) have demonstrated the occurrence of cardiac arrhythmias and sudden death (with histologic evidence of myocardial necrosis) when beta-agonists and methylxanthines are administered concurrently. The clinical significance of these findings is unknown.

HOW SUPPLIED

Foradil Aerolizer contains 12 μg Foradil (formoterol fumarate) clear gelatin capsules with "CG" printed on one end and "FXF" printed on the opposite end; one Aerolizer Inhaler; and Patient Instructions for Use.

Foradil capsules should be used with the Aerolizer Inhaler only. The Aerolizer Inhaler should not be used with any other capsules.

STORAGE

Prior to Dispensing: Store in a refrigerator, 2-8°C (36-46°F).

After Dispensing to Patient: Store at 20-25°C (68-77°F). Protect from heat and moisture. CAPSULES SHOULD ALWAYS BE STORED IN THE BLISTER AND ONLY REMOVED FROM THE BLISTER IMMEDIATELY BEFORE USE.

Always discard the Foradil capsules and Aerolizer Inhaler by the "Use by" date and always use the new Aerolizer Inhaler provided with each new prescription.

Keep out of the reach of children.

PRODUCT LISTING - EQUIVALENTS NOT AVAILABLE

Capsule - Inhalation - 12 mcg

12's	$26.35	FORADIL AEROLIZER, Novartis Pharmaceuticals	00083-0167-02
18's	$26.82	FORADIL AEROLIZER, Novartis Pharmaceuticals	00083-0167-11
60's	$83.15	FORADIL AEROLIZER, Novartis Pharmaceuticals	00083-0167-74

Foscarnet Sodium (003061)

F

Categories: Infection, herpes simplex virus; Retinitis, secondary to cytomegalovirus; Pregnancy Category C; FDA Approved 1991 Sep
Drug Classes: Antivirals
Brand Names: Foscavir
Foreign Brand Availability: Foscovir (Denmark)
HCFA JCODE(S): J1455 per 1,000 mg IV

WARNING

RENAL IMPAIRMENT IS THE MAJOR TOXICITY OF FOSCARNET SODIUM. FREQUENT MONITORING OF SERUM CREATININE, WITH DOSE ADJUSTMENT FOR CHANGES IN RENAL FUNCTION, AND ADEQUATE HYDRATION WITH ADMINISTRATION OF FOSCARNET SODIUM, IS IMPERATIVE. (See DOSAGE AND ADMINISTRATION, Hydration.)

SEIZURES, RELATED TO ALTERATIONS IN PLASMA MINERALS AND ELECTROLYTES, HAVE BEEN ASSOCIATED WITH FOSCARNET SODIUM TREATMENT. THEREFORE, PATIENTS MUST BE CAREFULLY MONITORED FOR SUCH CHANGES AND THEIR POTENTIAL SEQUELAE. MINERAL AND ELECTROLYTE SUPPLEMENTATION MAY BE REQUIRED.

FOSCARNET SODIUM IS INDICATED FOR USE ONLY IN IMMUNOCOMPROMISED PATIENTS WITH CMV RETINITIS AND MUCOCUTANEOUS ACYCLOVIR-RESISTANT HSV INFECTIONS. (See INDICATIONS AND USAGE.)

DESCRIPTION

Foscavir is the brand name for foscarnet sodium. The chemical name of foscarnet sodium is phosphonoformic acid, trisodium salt. Foscarnet sodium is a white, crystalline powder containing 6 equivalents of water of hydration with an empirical formula of $Na_3CO_5P \cdot 6H_2O$ and a molecular weight of 300.1.

Foscavir has the potential to chelate divalent metal ions, such as calcium and magnesium, to form stable coordination compounds. Foscavir injection is a sterile, isotonic aqueous solution for intravenous administration only. The solution is clear and colorless. Each milliliter of Foscavir contains 24 mg of foscarnet sodium hexahydrate in water for injection. Hydrochloric acid and/or sodium hydroxide may have been added to adjust the pH of the solution to 7.4. Foscavir injection contains no preservatives.

STORAGE

Foscavir Injection should be stored at controlled room temperature, 15-30°C (59-86°F), and should be protected from excessive heat (above 40°C) and from freezing. Foscavir Injection should be used only if the bottle and seal are intact, a vacuum is present, and the solution is clear and colorless.

CLINICAL PHARMACOLOGY

MECHANISM OF ACTION

Foscarnet sodium is an organic analogue of inorganic pyrophosphate that inhibits replication of herpesviruses *in vitro* including cytomegalovirus (CMV) and herpes simplex virus types 1 and 2 (HSV-1 and HSV-2).

Foscarnet sodium exerts its antiviral activity by a selective inhibition at the pyrophosphate binding site on virus-specific DNA polymerases at concentrations that do not affect cellular DNA polymerases. Foscarnet sodium does not require activation (phosphorylation) by thymidine kinase or other kinases and therefore is active *in vitro* against HSV TK deficient mutants and CMV UL97 mutants. Thus, HSV strains resistant to acyclovir or CMV strains resistant to ganciclovir may be sensitive to foscarnet sodium. However, acyclovir or ganciclovir resistant mutants with alterations in the viral DNA polymerase may be resistant to foscarnet sodium and may not respond to therapy with foscarnet sodium. The combination of foscarnet sodium and ganciclovir has been shown to have enhanced activity *in vitro*.

ANTIVIRAL ACTIVITY — IN VITRO AND IN VIVO

The quantitative relationship between the *in vitro* susceptibility of human cytomegalovirus (CMV) or herpes simplex virus 1 and 2 (HSV-1 and HSV-2) to foscarnet sodium and clinical response to therapy has not been established and virus sensitivity testing has not been standardized. Sensitivity test results, expressed as the concentration of drug required to inhibit by 50% the growth of virus in cell culture (IC_{50}), vary greatly depending on the assay method used, cell type employed and the laboratory performing the test. A number of sensitive viruses and their IC_{50} values are listed in TABLE 1.

Statistically significant decreases in positive CMV cultures from blood and urine have been demonstrated in two studies (FOS-03 and ACTG-015/915) of patients treated with foscarnet sodium. Although median time to progression of CMV retinitis was increased in patients treated with foscarnet sodium, reductions in positive blood or urine cultures have not been shown to correlate with clinical efficacy in individual patients.

TABLE 1 Foscarnet Inhibition of Virus Multiplication in Cell Culture

Virus	IC_{50} (μM)
CMV	50-800*
HSV-1, HSV-2	10-130
Ganciclovir resistant CMV	190
HSV-TK negative mutant	67
HSV-DNA polymerase mutants	5-443

* Mean = 269 μM.

*TABLE 2 Blood and Urine Culture Results From CMV Retinitis Patients**

Blood	+CMV	−CMV
Baseline	27	34
End of induction†	1	60
Urine	**+CMV**	**−CMV**
Baseline	52	6
End of induction†	21	37

* A total of 77 patients were treated with foscarnet sodium in two clinical trials (FOS-03 and ACTG-015/915). Not all patients had blood or urine cultures done and some patients had results from both cultures.
† (60 mg/kg foscarnet sodium tid for 2-3 weeks).

RESISTANCE

Strains of both HSV and CMV that are resistant to foscarnet sodium can be readily selected *in vitro* by passage of wild type virus in the presence of increasing concentrations of the drug. All foscarnet sodium resistant mutants are known to be generated through mutation in the viral DNA polymerase gene. CMV strains with double mutations conferring resistance to both foscarnet sodium and ganciclovir have been isolated from patients with AIDS. The possibility of viral resistance should be considered in patients who show poor clinical response or experience persistent viral excretion during therapy.

PHARMACOKINETICS

The pharmacokinetics of foscarnet have been determined after administration as an intermittent intravenous infusion during induction therapy in AIDS patients with CMV retinitis. Observed plasma foscarnet concentrations in four studies (FOS-01, ACTG-015, FP48PK, FP49PK) are summarized in TABLE 3.

*TABLE 3 Foscarnet Pharmacokinetic Characteristics**

Parameter	60 mg/kg q8h	90 mg/kg q12h
C_{max} at steady-state (μM)	589 ± 192 (24)	623 ± 132 (19)
C_{trough} at steady-state (μM)	114 ± 91 (24)	63 ± 57 (17)
Volume of distribution (L/kg)	0.41 ± 0.13 (12)	0.52 ± 0.20 (18)
Plasma half-life (h)	4.0 ± 2.0 (24)	3.3 ± 1.4 (18)
Systemic clearance (L/h)	6.2 ± 2.1 (24)	7.1 ± 2.7 (18)
Renal clearance (L/h)	5.6 ± 1.9 (5)	6.4 ± 2.5 (13)
CSF:plasma ratio	0.69 ± 0.19 (9)†	0.66 ± 0.11 (5)‡

* Values expressed as mean ± S.D. (number of subjects studied) for each parameter.
† 50 mg/kg Q8h for 28 days, samples taken 3 hours after end of 1 hour infusion (Astra Report 815-04 AC025-1).
‡ 90 mg/kg Q12h for 28 days, samples taken 1 hour after end of 2 hour infusion (Hengge *et al.*, 1993).

DISTRIBUTION

In vitro studies have shown that 14-17% of foscarnet is protein bound at plasma drug concentrations of 1-1000 μM.

The foscarnet terminal half-life determined by urinary excretion was 87.5 ± 41.8 hours, possibly due to release of foscarnet from bone. Postmortem data on several patients in European clinical trials provide evidence that foscarnet does accumulate in bone in humans; however, the extent to which this occurs has not been determined. In animal studies (mice), 40% of an intravenous dose of foscarnet sodium was deposited in bone in young animals and 7% was deposited in adult animals.

SPECIAL POPULATIONS

Adults With Impaired Renal Function

The pharmacokinetic properties of foscarnet have been determined in a small group of adult subjects with normal and impaired renal function, as summarized in TABLE 4.

TABLE 4 Pharmacokinetic Parameters (Mean ± SD) After a Single 60 mg/kg Dose of Foscarnet Sodium in 4 Groups of Adults With Varying Degrees of Renal Function*

Parameter	Group 1 (n=6)	Group 2 (n=6)	Group 3 (n=6)	Group 4 (n=4)
Creatinine clearance (ml/min)	108 ± 16	68 ± 8	34 ± 9	20 ± 4
Foscarnet CL (ml/min/kg)	2.13 ± 0.71	1.33 ± 0.43	0.46 ± 0.14	0.43 ± 0.26
Foscarnet half-life (h)	1.93 ± 0.12	3.35 ± 0.87	13.0 ± 4.05	25.3 ± 18.7

* Group 1 patients had normal renal function defined as a creatinine clearance (CrCl) of >80 ml/min, Group 2 CrCl was 50-80 ml/min, Group 3 CrCl was 25-49 ml/min and Group 4 CrCl was 10-24 ml/min.

Total systemic clearance (CL) of foscarnet decreased and half-life increased with diminishing renal function (as expressed by creatinine clearance). Based on these observations, it is necessary to modify the dosage of foscarnet in patients with renal impairment (see DOSAGE AND ADMINISTRATION).

INDICATIONS AND USAGE

CMV RETINITIS

Foscarnet sodium is indicated for the treatment of CMV retinitis in patients with acquired immunodeficiency syndrome (AIDS). Combination therapy with foscarnet sodium and ganciclovir is indicated for patients who have relapsed after monotherapy with either drug. SAFETY AND EFFICACY OF FOSCARNET SODIUM HAVE NOT BEEN ESTABLISHED FOR TREATMENT OF OTHER CMV INFECTIONS (*e.g.,* PNEUMONITIS, GASTROENTERITIS); CONGENITAL OR NEONATAL CMV DISEASE; OR NON-IMMUNOCOMPROMISED INDIVIDUALS.

MUCOCUTANEOUS ACYCLOVIR-RESISTANT HSV INFECTIONS

Foscarnet sodium is indicated for the treatment of acyclovir-resistant mucocutaneous HSV infections in immunocompromised patients. SAFETY AND EFFICACY OF FOSCARNET SODIUM HAVE NOT BEEN ESTABLISHED FOR TREATMENT OF OTHER HSV INFECTIONS (*e.g.,* RETINITIS, ENCEPHALITIS); CONGENITAL OR NEONATAL HSV DISEASE; OR HSV IN NON-IMMUNOCOMPROMISED INDIVIDUALS.

CONTRAINDICATIONS

Foscarnet sodium is contraindicated in patients with clinically significant hypersensitivity to foscarnet sodium.

WARNINGS

RENAL IMPAIRMENT

THE MAJOR TOXICITY OF FOSCARNET SODIUM IS RENAL IMPAIRMENT (see ADVERSE REACTIONS). Renal impairment is most likely to become clinically evident during the second week of induction therapy, but may occur at any time during foscarnet sodium treatment. Renal function should be monitored carefully during both induction and maintenance therapy (see DOSAGE AND ADMINISTRATION, Patient Monitoring). Elevations in serum creatinine are usually, but not always, reversible following discontinuation or dose adjustment of foscarnet sodium. Safety and efficacy data for patients with baseline serum creatinine levels greater than 2.8 mg/dl or measured 24 hour creatinine clearances <50 ml/min are limited.

BECAUSE OF FOSCARNET SODIUM'S POTENTIAL TO CAUSE RENAL IMPAIRMENT, DOSE ADJUSTMENT BASED ON SERUM CREATININE IS NECESSARY. Hydration may reduce the risk of nephrotoxicity. It is recommended that 750-1000 ml of normal saline or 5% dextrose solution should be given prior to the first infusion of foscarnet sodium to establish diuresis. With subsequent infusions, 750-1000 ml of hydration fluid should be given with 90-120 mg/kg of foscarnet sodium, and 500 ml with 40-60 mg/kg of foscarnet sodium. Hydration fluid may need to be decreased if clinically warranted.

After the first dose, the hydration fluid should be administered concurrently with each infusion of foscarnet sodium.

MINERAL AND ELECTROLYTE ABNORMALITIES

Foscarnet sodium has been associated with changes in serum electrolytes including hypocalcemia, hypophosphatemia, hyperphosphatemia, hypomagnesemia, and hypokalemia (see ADVERSE REACTIONS). Foscarnet sodium may also be associated with a dose-related decrease in ionized serum calcium which may not be reflected in total serum calcium. This effect is likely to be related to chelation of divalent metal ions such as calcium by foscarnet. Patients should be advised to report symptoms of low ionized calcium such as perioral tingling, numbness in the extremities and paresthesias. Particular caution and careful management of serum electrolytes is advised in patients with altered calcium or other electrolyte levels before treatment and especially in those with neurologic or cardiac abnormalities and those receiving other drugs known to influence minerals and electrolytes (see DOSAGE AND ADMINISTRATION, Patient Monitoring and DRUG INTERACTIONS). Physicians should be prepared to treat these abnormalities and their sequalae such as tetany, seizures or cardiac disturbances. The rate of foscarnet sodium infusion may also affect the decrease in ionized calcium. **Therefore, an infusion pump must be used for administration to prevent rapid intravenous infusion (see DOSAGE AND ADMINISTRATION).** Slowing the infusion rate may decrease or prevent symptoms.

SEIZURES

Seizures related to mineral and electrolyte abnormalities have been associated with foscarnet sodium treatment (see Mineral and Electrolyte Abnormalities). Several cases of seizures were associated with death. Risk factors associated with seizures included impaired baseline renal function, low total serum calcium, and underlying CNS conditions.

PRECAUTIONS

GENERAL

Care must be taken to infuse solutions containing foscarnet sodium only into veins with adequate blood flow to permit rapid dilution and distribution to avoid local irritation (see DOSAGE AND ADMINISTRATION). Local irritation and ulcerations of penile epithelium have been reported in male patients receiving foscarnet sodium, possibly related to the presence of drug in the urine. One case of vulvovaginal ulcerations in a female receiving foscarnet sodium has been reported. Adequate hydration with close attention to personal hygiene may minimize the occurrence of such events.

HEMOPOIETIC SYSTEM

Anemia has been reported in 33% of patients receiving foscarnet sodium in controlled studies. Granulocytopenia has been reported in 17% of patients receiving foscarnet sodium in controlled studies; however, only 1% (2/189) were terminated from these studies because of neutropenia.

INFORMATION FOR THE PATIENT

CMV Retinitis

Patients should be advised that foscarnet sodium is not a cure for CMV retinitis, and that they may continue to experience progression of retinitis during or following treatment. They should be advised to have regular ophthalmologic examinations.

Mucocutaneous Acyclovir-Resistant HSV Infections

Patients should be advised that foscarnet sodium is not a cure for HSV infections. While complete healing is possible, relapse occurs in most patients. Because relapse may be due to acyclovir-sensitive HSV, sensitivity testing of the viral isolate is advised. In addition, repeated treatment with foscarnet sodium has led to the development of resistance associated with poorer response. In the case of poor therapeutic response, sensitivity testing of the viral isolate also is advised.

General

Patients should be informed that the major toxicities of foscarnet are renal impairment, electrolyte disturbances, and seizures, and that dose modifications and possibly discontinuation may be required. The importance of close monitoring while on therapy must be emphasized. Patients should be advised of the importance of reporting to their physicians symptoms of perioral tingling, numbness in the extremities or paresthesias during or after infusion as possible symptoms of electrolyte abnormalities. Should such symptoms occur, the infusion of foscarnet sodium should be stopped, appropriate laboratory samples for assessment of electrolyte concentrations obtained, and a physician consulted before resuming treatment. The rate of infusion must be no more than 1 mg/kg/minute. The potential for renal impairment may be minimized by accompanying foscarnet sodium administration with hydration adequate to establish and maintain a diuresis during dosing.

F

CARCINOGENESIS, MUTAGENESIS, AND IMPAIRMENT OF FERTILITY

Carcinogenicity studies were conducted in rats and mice at oral doses of 500 and 250 mg/kg/day. Oral bioavailability in unfasted rodents is <20%. No evidence of oncogenicity was reported at plasma drug levels equal to 1/3 and 1/5, respectively, of those in humans (at the maximum recommended human daily dose) as measured by the area-under-the-time/concentration curve (AUC).

Foscarnet sodium showed genotoxic effects in the BALB/3T3 *in vitro* transformation assay at concentrations greater than 0.5 µg/ml and an increased frequency of chromosome aberrations in the sister chromatid exchange assay at 1000 µg/ml. A high dose of foscarnet (350 mg/kg) caused an increase in micronucleated polychromatic erythrocytes *in vivo* in mice at doses that produced exposures (area under curve) comparable to that anticipated clinically.

PREGNANCY, TERATOGENIC EFFECTS, PREGNANCY CATEGORY C

Foscarnet sodium did not adversely affect fertility and general reproductive performance in rats. The results of peri- and post-natal studies in rats were also negative. However, these studies used exposures that are inadequate to define the potential for impairment of fertility at human drug exposure levels.

Daily subcutaneous doses up to 75 mg/kg administered to female rats prior to and during mating, during gestation, and 21 days post-partum caused a slight increase (<5%) in the number of skeletal anomalies compared with the control group. Daily subcutaneous doses up to 75 mg/kg administered to rabbits and 150 mg/kg administered to rats during gestation caused an increase in the frequency of skeletal anomalies/variations. On the basis of estimated drug exposure (as measured by AUC), the 150 mg/kg dose in rats and 75 mg/kg dose in rabbits were approximately one-eighth (rat) and one-third (rabbit) the estimated maximal daily human exposure. These studies are inadequate to define the potential teratogenicity at levels to which women will be exposed.

There are no adequate and well controlled studies in pregnant women. Because animal reproductive studies are not always predictive of human response, foscarnet sodium should be used during pregnancy only if clearly needed.

NURSING MOTHERS

It is not known whether foscarnet sodium is excreted in human milk; however, in lactating rats administered 75 mg/kg, foscarnet sodium was excreted in maternal milk at concentrations 3 times higher than peak maternal blood concentrations.

PEDIATRIC USE

The safety and effectiveness of foscarnet sodium in children have not been established. Foscarnet sodium is deposited in teeth and bone and deposition is greater in young and growing animals. Foscarnet sodium has been demonstrated to adversely affect development of tooth enamel in mice and rats. The effects of this deposition on skeletal development have not been studied. Since deposition in human bone has also been shown to occur, it is likely that it does so to a greater degree in developing bone in children. Administration to children should be undertaken only after careful evaluation and only if the potential benefits for treatment outweigh the risks.

GERIATRIC USE

No studies of the efficacy or safety of foscarnet sodium in persons over age 65 have been conducted. Since these individuals frequently have reduced glomerular filtration, particular attention should be paid to assessing renal function before and during foscarnet sodium administration (see DOSAGE AND ADMINISTRATION).

DRUG INTERACTIONS

A possible drug interaction of foscarnet sodium and intravenous pentamidine has been described. Concomitant treatment of 4 patients in the United Kingdom with foscarnet sodium and intravenous pentamidine may have caused hypocalcemia; 1 patient died with severe hypocalcemia. Toxicity associated with concomitant use of aerosolized pentamidine has not been reported.

Because of foscarnet's tendency to cause renal impairment, the use of foscarnet sodium should be avoided in combination with potentially nephrotoxic drugs such as aminoglycosides, amphotericin B and intravenous pentamidine (see above) unless the potential benefits outweigh the risks to the patient.

Since foscarnet sodium decreases serum concentrations of ionized calcium, concurrent treatment with other drugs known to influence serum calcium concentrations should be used with particular caution.

Ganciclovir: The pharmacokinetics of foscarnet and ganciclovir were not altered in 13 patients receiving either concomitant therapy or daily alternating therapy for maintenance of CMV disease.

ADVERSE REACTIONS

THE MAJOR TOXICITY OF FOSCARNET SODIUM IS RENAL IMPAIRMENT (see WARNINGS). Approximately 33% of 189 patients with AIDS and CMV retinitis who received foscarnet sodium (60 mg/kg tid), without adequate hydration, developed significant impairment of renal function (serum creatinine ≥ 2.0 mg/dl). The incidence of renal impairment in subsequent clinical trials in which 1000 ml of normal saline or 5% dextrose solution was given with each infusion of foscarnet sodium was 12% (34/280).

Foscarnet sodium has been associated with changes in serum electrolytes including hypocalcemia (15-30%), hypophosphatemia (8-26%) and hyperphosphatemia (6%), hypomagnesemia (15-30%), and hypokalemia (16-48%) (see WARNINGS). The higher percentages were derived from those patients receiving hydration.

Foscarnet sodium treatment was associated with seizures in 18/189 (10%) AIDS patients in the initial five controlled studies (see WARNINGS). Risk factors associated with seizures included impaired baseline renal function, low total serum calcium, and underlying CNS conditions predisposing the patient to seizures. The rate of seizures did not increase with duration of treatment. Three cases were associated with overdoses of foscarnet sodium.

In five controlled US clinical trials the most frequently reported adverse events in patients with AIDS and CMV retinitis are shown in TABLE 5. These figures were calculated without reference to drug relationship or severity.

TABLE 5 *Adverse Events Reported in Five Controlled US Clinical Trials*

	n = 189
Fever	65%
Nausea	47%
Anemia	33%
Diarrhea	30%
Abnormal renal function	27%
Vomiting	26%
Headache	26%
Seizures	10%

From the same controlled studies, adverse events categorized by investigator as "severe" are shown in TABLE 6. Although death was specifically attributed to foscarnet sodium in only one case, other complications of foscarnet sodium (*i.e.*, renal impairment, electrolyte abnormalities, and seizures) may have contributed to patient deaths (see WARNINGS).

TABLE 6 *Severe Adverse Events*

	n = 189
Death	14%
Abnormal renal function	14%
Marrow suppression	10%
Anemia	9%
Seizures	7%

From the five initial US controlled trials of foscarnet sodium, the following list of adverse events has been compiled regardless of causal relationship to foscarnet sodium. Evaluation of these reports was difficult because of the diverse manifestations of the underlying disease and because most patients received numerous concomitant medications.

Incidence 5% or Greater:

Body as a Whole: Fever, fatigue, rigors, asthenia, malaise, pain, infection, sepsis, death.

Central and Peripheral Nervous System: Headache, paresthesia, dizziness, involuntary muscle contractions, hypoesthesia, neuropathy, seizures including grand mal seizures (see WARNINGS).

Gastrointestinal System: Anorexia, nausea, diarrhea, vomiting, abdominal pain.

Hematologic: Anemia, granulocytopenia, leukopenia (see PRECAUTIONS).

Metabolic and Nutritional: Mineral and electrolyte imbalances (see WARNINGS) including hypokalemia, hypocalcemia, hypomagnesemia, hypophosphatemia, hyperphosphatemia.

Psychiatric: Depression, confusion, anxiety.

Respiratory System: Coughing, dyspnea.

Skin and Appendages: Rash, increased sweating.

Urinary: Alterations in renal function including increased serum creatinine, decreased creatinine clearance, and abnormal renal function (see WARNINGS).

Special Senses: Vision abnormalities.

Incidence Between 1% and 5%:

Application Site: Injection site pain, injection site inflammation.

Body as a Whole: Back pain, chest pain, edema, influenza-like symptoms, bacterial infections, moniliasis, fungal infections, abscess.

Cardiovascular: Hypertension, palpitations, ECG abnormalities including sinus tachycardia, first degree AV block and non-specific ST-T segment changes, hypotension, flushing, cerebrovascular disorder (see WARNINGS).

Central and Peripheral Nervous System: Tremor, ataxia, dementia, stupor, generalized spasms, sensory disturbances, meningitis, aphasia, abnormal coordination, leg cramps, EEG abnormalities (see WARNINGS).

Gastrointestinal: Constipation, dysphagia, dyspepsia, rectal hemorrhage, dry mouth, melena, flatulence, ulcerative stomatitis, pancreatitis.

Hematologic: Thrombocytopenia, platelet abnormalities, thrombosis, white blood cell abnormalities, lymphadenopathy.

Liver and Biliary: Abnormal A-G ratio, abnormal hepatic function, increased SGPT, increased SGOT.

Metabolic and Nutritional: Hyponatremia, decreased weight, increased alkaline phosphatase, increased LDH, increased BUN, acidosis, cachexia, thirst, hypercalcemia (see WARNINGS).

Musculo-Skeletal: Arthralgia, myalgia.

Neoplasms: Lymphoma-like disorder, sarcoma.

Psychiatric: Insomnia, somnolence, nervousness, amnesia, agitation, aggressive reaction, hallucination.

Respiratory System: Pneumonia, sinusitis, pharyngitis, rhinitis, respiratory disorders, respiratory insufficiency, pulmonary infiltration, stridor, pneumothorax, hemoptysis, bronchospasm.

Skin and Appendages: Pruritus, skin ulceration, seborrhea, erythematous rash, maculopapular rash, skin discoloration.

Special Senses: Taste perversions, eye abnormalities, eye pain, conjunctivitis.

Urinary System: Albuminuria, dysuria, polyuria, urethral disorder, urinary retention, urinary tract infections, acute renal failure, nocturia, facial edema.

Selected adverse events occurring at a rate of less than 1% in the five initial US controlled clinical trials of foscarnet sodium include: syndrome of inappropriate antidiuretic hormone secretion, pancytopenia, hematuria, dehydration, hypoproteinemia, increases in amylase and creatinine phosphokinase, cardiac arrest, coma, and other cardiovascular and neurologic complications.

Selected adverse event data from the Foscarnet vs. Ganciclovir CMV Retinitis Trial (FGCRT), performed by the Studies of the Ocular Complications of AIDS (SOCA) Research Group, are shown in TABLE 7.

TABLE 7 *FGCRT: Selected Adverse Events**

Event	Ganciclovir No. of Events	Ganciclovir No. of Patients	Ganciclovir Rates†	Foscarnet No. of Events	Foscarnet No. of Patients	Foscarnet Rates†
Absolute neutrophil count decreasing to <0.50 × 10^9 per L	63	41	1.30	31	17	0.72
Serum creatinine increasing to >260 μmol/L (>2.9 mg/dl)	6	4	0.12	13	9	0.30
Seizure‡	21	13	0.37	19	13	0.37
Catheterization-related infection	49	27	1.26	51	28	1.46
Hospitalization	209	91	4.74	202	75	5.03

* Values for the treatment groups refer only to patients who completed at least one follow-up visit—*i.e.*, 113-119 patients in the ganciclovir group and 93-100 in the foscarnet group. "Events" denotes all events observed and "patients" the number of patients with one or more of the indicated events.

† Per person-year at risk.

‡ Final frozen SOCA I database dated October 1991.

Selected adverse events from ACTG Study 228 (CRRT) comparing combination therapy with foscarnet sodium or ganciclovir monotherapy are shown in TABLE 8A and TABLE 8B. The most common reason for a treatment change in patients assigned to either foscarnet sodium or ganciclovir was retinitis progression. The most frequent reason for a treatment change in the combination treatment group was toxicity.

TABLE 8A *CRRT: Selected Adverse Events*

	Foscarnet Sodium n=88 No. Events	No. pts.*	Rate†	Ganciclovir n=93 No. Events	No. pts.*	Rate†
Anemia (Hgb <70 g/L)	11	7	0.20	9	7	0.14
Neutropenia‡						
ANC <0.75 × 10^9 cells/L	86	32	1.53	95	41	1.51
ANC <0.50 × 10^9 cells/L	50	25	0.91	49	28	0.80
Thrombocytopenia						
Platelets <50 × 10^9/L	28	14	0.50	19	8	0.43
Platelets <20 × 10^9/L	1	1	0.01	6	2	0.05
Nephrotoxicity						
Creatinine > 260 μmol/L (>2.9 mg/dl)	9	7	0.15	10	7	0.17
Seizures	6	6	0.17	7	6	0.15
Hospitalizations	86	53	1.86	111	59	2.36

* Pts. = patients with event.

† Rate = events/person/year.

‡ ANC = absolute neutrophil count.

Adverse events that have been reported in post-marketing surveillance include: ventricular arrhythmia, prolongation of QT interval, diabetes insipidus (usually nephrogenic), and muscle disorders including myopathy, myositis, muscle weakness and rare cases of rhabdomyolysis. Cases of vesiculobullous eruptions including erythema multiforme, toxic epidermal necrolysis, and Stevens-Johnson Syndrome have been reported. In most cases, patients were taking other medications that have been associated with toxic epidermal necrolysis or Stevens-Johnson Syndrome.

DOSAGE AND ADMINISTRATION

CAUTION: DO NOT ADMINISTER FOSCARNET SODIUM BY RAPID OR BOLUS INTRAVENOUS INJECTION. THE TOXICITY OF FOSCAVIR MAY BE INCREASED AS A RESULT OF EXCESSIVE PLASMA LEVELS. CARE SHOULD BE TAKEN TO AVOID UNINTENTIONAL OVERDOSE BY CAREFULLY CONTROL-

TABLE 8B *CRRT: Selected Adverse Events*

	Combination n=93		
	No. Events	No. pts.*	Rate†
Anemia (Hgb <70 g/L)	19	15	0.33
Neutropenia‡			
ANC <0.75 × 10^9 cells/L	107	51	1.91
ANC <0.50 × 10^9 cells/L	50	28	0.85
Thrombocytopenia			
Platelets <50 × 10^9/L	40	15	0.56
Platelets <20 × 10^9/L	7	6	0.18
Nephrotoxicity			
Creatinine >260 μmol/L (>2.9 mg/dl)	11	10	0.20
Seizures	10	5	0.18
Hospitalizations	118	64	2.36

* Pts. = patients with event.
† Rate = events/person/year.
‡ ANC = absolute neutrophil count.

LING THE RATE OF INFUSION. THEREFORE, AN INFUSION PUMP MUST BE USED. IN SPITE OF THE USE OF AN INFUSION PUMP, OVERDOSES HAVE OCCURRED.

ADMINISTRATION

Foscarnet sodium is administered by controlled intravenous infusion, either by using a central venous line or by using a peripheral vein. The standard 24 mg/ml solution may be used with or without dilution when using a central venous catheter for infusion. When a peripheral vein catheter is used, the 24 mg/ml solution **must** be diluted to 12 mg/ml with 5% dextrose in water or with a normal saline solution prior to administration to avoid local irritation of peripheral veins. Since the dose of foscarnet sodium is calculated on the basis of body weight, it may be desirable to remove and discard any unneeded quantity from the bottle before starting with the infusion to avoid overdosage. Dilutions and/or removals of excess quantities should be accomplished under aseptic conditions. Solutions thus prepared should be used within 24 hours of first entry into a sealed bottle. *To reduce the risk of nephrotoxicity, creatinine clearance (ml/min/kg) should be calculated even if serum creatinine is within the normal range, and doses should be adjusted accordingly.*

Hydration

Hydration may reduce the risk of nephrotoxicity. It is recommended that 750-1000 ml of normal saline or 5% dextrose solution should be given prior to the first infusion of foscarnet sodium to establish diuresis. With subsequent infusions, 750-1000 ml of hydration fluid should be given with 90-120 mg/kg of foscarnet sodium, and 500 ml with 40-60 mg/kg of foscarnet sodium. Hydration fluid may need to be decreased if clinically warranted.

After the first dose, the hydration fluid should be administered concurrently with each infusion of foscarnet sodium.

Compatibility With Other Solutions/Drugs

Other drugs and supplements can be administered to a patient receiving foscarnet sodium. However, care must be taken to ensure that foscarnet sodium is only administered with normal saline or 5% dextrose solution and that no other drug or supplement is administered concurrently via the same catheter. Foscarnet has been reported to be chemically incompatible with 30% dextrose, amphotericin B, and solutions containing calcium such as Ringer's lactate and TPN. Physical incompatibility with other IV drugs has also been reported including acyclovir sodium, ganciclovir, trimetrexate glucuronate, pentamidine isethionate, vancomycin, trimethoprim/sulfamethoxazole, diazepam, midazolam, digoxin, phenytoin, leucovorin, and prochlorperazine. Because of foscarnet's chelating properties, a precipitate can potentially occur when divalent cations are administered concurrently in the same catheter.

Parenteral drug products must be inspected visually for particulate matter and discoloration prior to administration whenever the solution and container permit. Solutions that are discolored or contain particulate matter should not be used.

Accidental Exposure

Accidental skin and eye contact with foscarnet sodium solution may cause local irritation and burning sensation. If accidental contact occurs, the exposed area should be flushed with water.

THE RECOMMENDED DOSAGE, FREQUENCY, OR INFUSION RATES SHOULD NOT BE EXCEEDED. ALL DOSES MUST BE INDIVIDUALIZED FOR PATIENTS' RENAL FUNCTION.

Induction Treatment: The recommended initial dose of foscarnet sodium for patients with normal renal function is:

- For CMV retinitis patients, either 90 mg/kg (1½ to 2 hour infusion) every 12 hours or 60 mg/kg (minimum 1 hour infusion) every 8 hours over 2-3 weeks depending on clinical response.
- For acyclovir-resistant HSV patients, 40 mg/kg (minimum 1 hour infusion) either every 8 or 12 hours for 2-3 weeks or until healed.

An infusion pump must be used to control the rate of infusion. Adequate hydration is recommended to establish a diuresis (see Hydration for recommendation), both prior to and during treatment to minimize renal toxicity (see WARNINGS), provided there are no clinical contraindications.

MAINTENANCE TREATMENT

Following induction treatment the recommended maintenance dose of foscarnet sodium for CMV retinitis is 90-120 mg/kg/day (individualized for renal function) given as an intravenous infusion over 2 hours. Because the superiority of the 120 mg/kg/day has not been established in controlled trials, and given the likely relationship of higher plasma foscarnet levels to toxicity, it is recommended that most patients be started on maintenance treatment with a dose of 90 mg/kg/day. Escalation to 120 mg/kg/day may be considered should early reinduction be required because of retinitis progression. Some patients who show excellent tolerance to foscarnet sodium may benefit from initiation of maintenance treatment at 120 mg/kg/day earlier in their treatment.

An infusion pump must be used to control the rate of infusion with all doses. Again, hydration to establish diuresis both prior to and during treatment is recommended to minimize renal toxicity, provided there are no clinical contraindications (see WARNINGS).

Patients who experience progression of retinitis while receiving foscarnet sodium maintenance therapy may be retreated with the induction and maintenance regimens given above or with a combination of foscarnet sodium and ganciclovir. **Because of physical incompatibility, foscarnet sodium and ganciclovir must NOT be mixed.**

USE IN PATIENTS WITH ABNORMAL RENAL FUNCTION

Foscarnet sodium should be used with caution in patients with abnormal renal function because reduced plasma clearance of foscarnet will result in elevated plasma levels (see CLINICAL PHARMACOLOGY). In addition, foscarnet sodium has the potential to further impair renal function (see WARNINGS). Safety and efficacy data for patients with baseline serum creatinine levels greater than 2.8 mg/dl or measured 24 hour creatinine clearances <50 ml/min are limited.

Renal function must be monitored carefully at baseline and during induction and maintenance therapy with appropriate dose adjustments for foscarnet sodium as outlined in Dose Adjustment and Patient Monitoring. During foscarnet sodium therapy if creatinine clearance falls below the limits of the dosing nomograms (0.4 ml/min/kg), foscarnet sodium should be discontinued, the patient hydrated, and monitored daily until resolution of renal impairment is ensured.

DOSE ADJUSTMENT

Foscarnet sodium dosing must be individualized according to the patient's renal function status. Refer to TABLE 9A and TABLE 9B for recommended doses and adjust the dose as indicated. Even patients with serum creatinine in the normal range may require dose adjustment; therefore, the dose should be calculated at baseline and frequently thereafter.

To use this dosing guide, actual 24 hour creatinine clearance (ml/min) must be divided by body weight (kg), or the estimated creatinine clearance in ml/min/kg can be calculated from serum creatinine (mg/dl) using the following formula (modified Cockcroft and Gault equation):

For Males: [140-age] ÷ [serum creatinine × 72] (× 0.85 for females)=ml/min/kg

TABLE 9A *Foscarnet Sodium Dosing Guide Induction*

	HSV: Equivalent to		CMV: Equivalent to	
	80 mg/kg/day total	120 mg/kg/day total	180 mg/kg/day total	
CrCl (ml/min/kg)	(40 mg/kg q12h)	(40 mg/kg q8h)	(60 mg/kg q8h)	(90 mg/kg q12h)
> 1.4	40 q12h	40 q8h	60 q8h	90 q12h
>1.0-1.4	30 q12h	30 q8h	45 q8h	70 q12h
>0.8-1.0	20 q12h	**35 q12h**	**50 q12h**	50 q12h
>0.6-0.8	**35 q24h**	**25 q12h**	**40 q12h**	**80 q24h**
>0.5-0.6	**25 q24h**	40 q24h	60 q24h	**60 q24h**
≥0.4-0.5	**20 q24h**	35 q24h	50 q24h	**50 q24h**
<0.4	Not Recommended	Not Recommended	Not Recommended	Not Recommended

TABLE 9B *Maintenance*

	CMV: Equivalent to	
CrCl (ml/min/kg)	90 mg/kg/day (once daily)	120 mg/kg/day (once daily)
>1.4	90 q24h	120 q24h
>1.0-1.4	70 q24h	90 q24h
>0.8-1.0	50 q24h	65 q24h
>0.6-0.8	**80 q48h**	**105 q48h**
>0.5-0.6	**60 q48h**	**80 q48h**
≥0.4-0.5	**50 q48h**	**65 q48h**
<0.4	Not Recommended	Not Recommended

> Means "greater than."
≥ Means "greater than or equal to."
< Means "less than."

PATIENT MONITORING

The majority of patients will experience some decrease in renal function due to foscarnet sodium administration. Therefore it is recommended that creatinine clearance, either measured or estimated using the modified Cockcroft and Gault equation based on serum creatinine, be determined at baseline, 2-3 times per week during induction therapy and at least every 1-2 weeks during maintenance therapy, with foscarnet sodium dose adjusted accordingly (see Dose Adjustment). More frequent monitoring may be required for some patients. It is also recommended that a 24 hour creatinine clearance be determined at baseline and periodically thereafter to ensure correct dosing (assuming verification of an adequate collection using creatinine index). Foscarnet sodium should be discontinued if creatinine clearance drops below 0.4 ml/min/kg.

Due to foscarnet sodium's propensity to chelate divalent metal ions and alter levels of serum electrolytes, patients must be monitored closely for such changes. It is recommended that a schedule similar to that recommended for serum creatinine (see Dose Adjustment) be used to monitor serum calcium, magnesium, potassium and phosphorus. Particular caution is advised in patients with decreased total serum calcium or other electrolyte levels before treatment, as well as in patients with neurologic or cardiac abnormalities, and in patients receiving other drugs known to influence serum calcium levels. Any clinically significant metabolic changes should be corrected. Also, patients who experience mild (*e.g.*, perioral numbness or paresthesias) or severe (*e.g.*, seizures) symptoms of electrolyte abnormalities should have serum electrolyte and mineral levels assessed as close in time to the event as possible.

Careful monitoring and appropriate management of electrolytes, calcium, magnesium and creatinine are of particular importance in patients with conditions that may predispose them to seizures (see WARNINGS).

PRODUCT LISTING - EQUIVALENTS NOT AVAILABLE

Solution - Intravenous - 24 mg/ml

250 ml x 12	$995.28	FOSCAVIR, Astra-Zeneca Pharmaceuticals	00186-1905-01
500 ml x 12	$1982.16	FOSCAVIR, Astra-Zeneca Pharmaceuticals	00186-1906-01

F

Fosfomycin Tromethamine (003341)

For complete prescribing information, refer to the CD-ROM included with the book.

Categories: Infection, urinary tract; Pregnancy Category B; FDA Approved 1997 Jan
Drug Classes: Antibiotics, miscellaneous; Antiseptics, urinary tract
Brand Names: Monurol
Foreign Brand Availability: Monuril (Colombia; France; Germany); Monuril Pediatrico (Colombia); Uridoz (France)
Cost of Therapy: $36.49 (Urinary Tract Infection; Monurol Sachet; 3 g; 3 g; 1 day supply)

DESCRIPTION

Monurol (fosfomycin tromethamine) sachet contains fosfomycin tromethamine, a synthetic, broad-spectrum, bactericidal antibiotic for oral administration. It is available as a single-dose sachet which contains white granules consisting of 5.631 g of fosfomycin tromethamine (equivalent to 3 g of fosfomycin), and the following inactive ingredients: mandarin flavor, orange flavor, saccharin, and sucrose. The contents of the sachet must be dissolved in water. Fosfomycin tromethamine, a phosphoric acid derivative, is available as (1*R*,2*S*)-(1,2-epoxypropyl)phosphonic acid, compound with 2-amino-2-(hydroxymethyl)-1,3-propanediol (1:1) It is a white granular compound with a molecular weight of 259.2. Its empirical formula is $C_3H_7O_4P{\cdot}C_4H_{11}NO_3$.

INDICATIONS AND USAGE

Fosfomycin tromethamine is indicated only for the treatment of uncomplicated urinary tract infections (acute cystitis) in women due to susceptible strains of *Escherichia coli* and *Enterococcus faecalis.* Fosfomycin tromethamine is not indicated for the treatment of pyelonephritis or perinephric abscess.

If persistence or reappearance of bacteriuria occurs after treatment with fosfomycin tromethamine, other therapeutic agents should be selected.

NON-FDA APPROVED INDICATIONS

Although not approved by the FDA, fosfomycin has been used successfully to treat genitourinary tract infections in men. Fosfomycin has also been demonstrated to be effective in hospital-acquired urinary tract infections, bacteriuria of pregnancy and for prophylaxis during transurethral prostatic resection. Experimentally, fosfomycin is being investigated as a potential antidote for dose-limiting ototoxicity and nephrotoxicity associated with cisplatin chemotherapy.

CONTRAINDICATIONS

Fosfomycin tromethamine is contraindicated in patients with known hypersensitivity to the drug.

DOSAGE AND ADMINISTRATION

The recommended dosage for women 18 years of age and older for uncomplicated urinary tract infection (acute cystitis) is 1 sachet of fosfomycin tromethamine. Fosfomycin tromethamine may be taken with or without food.

Fosfomycin tromethamine should not be taken in its dry form. Always mix fosfomycin tromethamine with water before ingesting. (See Preparation.)

PREPARATION

Fosfomycin tromethamine should be taken orally. Pour the entire contents of a single-dose sachet of fosfomycin tromethamine into 3-4 ounces of water (½ cup) and stir to dissolve. Do not use hot water. Fosfomycin tromethamine should be taken immediately after dissolving in water.

PRODUCT LISTING - EQUIVALENTS NOT AVAILABLE

Powder For Reconstitution - Oral - 3 Gm

1's	$30.08	MONUROL, Allscripts Pharmaceutical Company	54569-4539-00
3's	$109.48	MONUROL, Forest Pharmaceuticals	00456-4300-08

Fosinopril Sodium (003052)

For related information, see the comparative table section in Appendix A.

Categories: Hypertension, essential; Pregnancy Category D; FDA Approved 1991 May
Drug Classes: Angiotensin converting enzyme inhibitors
Brand Names: Monopril
Foreign Brand Availability: Acenor-M (Indonesia); Dynacil (Germany); Fosinil (Belgium); Fosinorm (Germany); Fosipres (Italy); Fositen (Portugal; Switzerland); Fositens (Austria; Bahrain; Cyprus; Egypt; Iran; Iraq; Israel; Jordan; Kuwait; Lebanon; Libya; Oman; Qatar; Republic-of-Yemen; Saudi-Arabia; Spain; Syria; United-Arab-Emirates); Fovas (India); Fozitec (France); Sapril (Philippines); Staril (England); Vasopril (Israel)
Cost of Therapy: $33.12 (Hypertension; Monopril; 10 mg; 1 tablet/day; 30 day supply)
$37.07 (Hypertension; Monopril HCT; 10 mg; 12.5 mg; 1 tablet/day; 30 day supply)

WARNING

Use in Pregnancy: When used in pregnancy during the second and third trimesters, ACE inhibitors can cause injury and even death to the developing fetus. When pregnancy is detected, fosinopril sodium should be discontinued as soon as possible. (See WARNINGS, Fetal/Neonatal Morbidity and Mortality.)

DESCRIPTION

Monopril is the sodium salt of fosinopril, the ester prodrug of an angiotensin converting enzyme (ACE) inhibitor, fosinoprilat. It contains a phosphinate group capable of specific binding to the active site of angiotensin converting enzyme. Fosinopril sodium is designated chemically as: L-proline,4-cyclohexyl-1-[[[2-methyl-1-(1-oxopropoxy)propoxy](4-phenylbutyl)phosphinyl]acetyl]-, sodium salt, *trans*-.

Fosinopril sodium is a white to off-white crystalline powder. It is soluble in water (100 mg/ml), methanol, and ethanol and slightly soluble in hexane.

Its empirical formula is $C_{30}H_{45}NNaO_7P$, and its molecular weight is 585.65.

Monopril is available for oral administration as 10, 20, and 40 mg tablets. Inactive ingredients include: lactose, microcrystalline cellulose, crospovidone, povidone, and sodium stearyl fumarate.

CLINICAL PHARMACOLOGY

MECHANISM OF ACTION

In animals and humans, fosinopril sodium is hydrolyzed by esterases to the pharmacologically active form, fosinoprilat, a specific competitive inhibitor of angiotensin converting enzyme (ACE).

ACE is a peptidyl dipeptidase that catalyzes the conversion of angiotensin I to the vasoconstrictor substance, angiotensin II. Angiotensin II also stimulates aldosterone secretion by the adrenal cortex. Inhibition of ACE results in decreased plasma angiotensin II, which leads to decreased vasopressor activity and to decreased aldosterone secretion. The latter decrease may result in a small increase of serum potassium.

In 647 hypertensive patients treated with fosinopril alone for an average of 29 weeks, mean increases in serum potassium of 0.1 mEq/L were observed. Similar increases were observed among all patients treated with fosinopril, including those receiving concomitant diuretic therapy. Removal of angiotensin II negative feedback on renin secretion leads to increased plasma renin activity.

ACE is identical to kininase, an enzyme that degrades bradykinin. Whether increased levels of bradykinin, a potent vasopressor peptide, play a role in the therapeutic effects of fosinopril sodium remains to be elucidated.

While the mechanism through which fosinopril sodium lowers blood pressure is believed to be primarily suppression of the renin-angiotensin-aldosterone system, fosinopril sodium has an antihypertensive effect even in patients with low-renin hypertension. Although fosinopril sodium was antihypertensive in all races studied, black hypertensive patients (usually a low-renin hypertensive population) had a smaller average response to ACE inhibitor monotherapy than non-black patients.

In patients with heart failure, the beneficial effects of fosinopril sodium are thought to result primarily from suppression of the renin-angiotensin-aldosterone system; inhibition of the angiotensin converting enzyme produces decreases in both preload and afterload.

PHARMACOKINETICS AND METABOLISM

Following oral administration, fosinopril (the prodrug) is absorbed slowly. The absolute absorption of fosinopril averaged 36% of an oral dose. The primary site of absorption is the proximal small intestine (duodenum/jejunum). While the rate of absorption may be slowed by the presence of food in the gastrointestinal tract, the extent of absorption of fosinopril is essentially unaffected.

Fosinoprilat is highly protein-bound (approximately 99.4%), has a relatively small volume of distribution, and has negligible binding to cellular components in blood. After single and multiple oral doses, plasma levels, areas under plasma concentration-time curves (AUCs) and peak concentrations (C_{maxs}) are directly proportional to the dose of fosinopril. Times to peak concentrations are independent of dose and are achieved in approximately 3 hours.

After an oral dose of radiolabeled fosinopril, 75% of radioactivity in plasma was present as active fosinoprilat, 20-30% as a glucuronide conjugate of fosinoprilat, and 1-5% as a *p*-hydroxy metabolite of fosinoprilat. Since fosinoprilat is not biotransformed after intravenous (IV) administration, fosinopril, not fosinoprilat, appears to be the precursor for the glucuronide and *p*-hydroxy metabolites. In rats, the *p*- hydroxy metabolite of fosinoprilat is as potent an inhibitor of ACE as fosinoprilat; the glucuronide conjugate is devoid of ACE inhibitory activity.

After IV administration, fosinoprilat was eliminated approximately equally by the liver and kidney. After oral administration of radiolabeled fosinopril, approximately half of the absorbed dose is excreted in the urine and the remainder is excreted in the feces. In two studies involving healthy subjects, the mean body clearance of IV fosinoprilat was between 26 and 39 ml/min.

In healthy subjects, the terminal elimination half-life ($T_{1/2}$) of an IV dose of radiolabeled fosinoprilat is approximately 12 hours. In hypertensive patients with normal renal and hepatic function, who received repeated doses of fosinopril, the effective $T_{1/2}$ for accumulation of fosinoprilat averaged 11.5 hours. In patients with heart failure, the effective $T_{1/2}$ was 14 hours.

In Patients With Mild-to-Severe Renal Insufficiency (creatinine clearance 10-80 ml/min/1.73 m²)

The clearance of fosinoprilat does not differ appreciably from normal, because of the large contribution of hepatobiliary elimination. In patients with end-stage renal disease (creatinine clearance <10 ml/min/1.73 m²), the total body clearance of fosinoprilat is approximately one-half of that in patients with normal renal function. (See DOSAGE AND ADMINISTRATION.)

Fosinopril is not well dialyzed. Clearance of fosinoprilat by hemodialysis and peritoneal dialysis averages 2% and 7%, respectively, of urea clearances.

In Patients With Hepatic Insufficiency (alcoholic or biliary cirrhosis)

The extent of hydrolysis of fosinopril is not appreciably reduced, although the rate of hydrolysis may be slowed; the apparent total body clearance of fosinoprilat is approximately one-half of that in patients with normal hepatic function.

In Elderly (male) Subjects (65-74 years old) With Clinically Normal Renal and Hepatic Function

There appear to be no significant differences in pharmacokinetic parameters for fosinoprilat compared to those of younger subjects (20-35 years old).

Fosinoprilat was found to cross the placenta of pregnant animals.

Studies in animals indicate that fosinopril and fosinoprilat do not cross the blood-brain barrier.

PHARMACODYNAMICS AND CLINICAL EFFECTS

Serum ACE activity was inhibited ≥90% at 2-12 hours after single doses of 10-40 mg of fosinopril. At 24 hours, serum ACE activity remained suppressed by 85%, 93%, and 93% in the 10, 20 and 40 mg dose groups, respectively.

HYPERTENSION

Administration of fosinopril sodium tablets to patients with mild-to-moderate hypertension results in a reduction of both supine and standing blood pressure to about the same extent with no compensatory tachycardia. Symptomatic postural hypotension is infrequent, although it can occur in patients who are salt- and/or volume-depleted (see WARNINGS). Use of fosinopril sodium in combination with thiazide diuretics gives a blood pressure-lowering effect greater than that seen with either agent alone.

Following oral administration of single doses of 10-40 mg, fosinopril sodium lowered blood pressure within 1 hour, with peak reductions achieved 2-6 hours after dosing. The antihypertensive effect of a single dose persisted for 24 hours. Following 4 weeks of monotherapy in placebo-controlled trials in patients with mild-to-moderate hypertension, once-daily doses of 20-80 mg lowered supine or seated systolic and diastolic blood pressures at 24 hours after dosing by an average of 8-9/6-7 mm Hg more than placebo. The trough effect was about 50-60% of the peak diastolic response and about 80% of the peak systolic response.

In most trials, the antihypertensive effect of fosinopril sodium increased during the first several weeks of repeated measurements. The antihypertensive effect of fosinopril sodium has been shown to continue during long-term therapy for at least 2 years. Abrupt withdrawal of fosinopril sodium has not resulted in a rapid increase in blood pressure.

Limited experience in controlled and uncontrolled trials combining fosinopril with a calcium channel blocker or a loop diuretic has indicated no unusual drug-drug interactions. Other ACE inhibitors have had less than additive effects with beta-adrenergic blockers, presumably because both drugs lower blood pressure by inhibiting parts of the renin-angiotensin system.

ACE inhibitors are generally less effective in blacks than in non-blacks. The effectiveness of fosinopril sodium was not influenced by age, sex, or weight.

In hemodynamic studies in hypertensive patients, after 3 months of therapy, responses (changes in BP, heart rate, cardiac index, and PVR) to various stimuli (*e.g.*, isometric exercise, 45° head-up tilt, and mental challenge) were unchanged compared to baseline, suggesting that fosinopril sodium does not affect the activity of the sympathetic nervous system. Reduction in systemic blood pressure appears to have been mediated by a decrease in peripheral vascular resistance without reflex cardiac effects. Similarly, renal, splanchnic, cerebral, and skeletal muscle blood flow were unchanged compared to baseline, as was glomerular filtration rate.

HEART FAILURE

In a randomized, double-blind, placebo-controlled trial, 179 patients with heart failure, all receiving diuretics and some receiving digoxin, were administered single doses of 1, 20, or 40 mg of fosinopril sodium or placebo. Doses of 20 and 40 mg of fosinopril sodium resulted in acute decreases in pulmonary capillary wedge pressure (preload) and mean arterial blood pressure and systemic vascular resistance (afterload). One hundred fifty-five (155) patients were re-randomized to once-daily therapy with fosinopril sodium (1, 20, or 40 mg) for an additional 10 weeks. Hemodynamic measurements made 24 hours after dosing showed (relative to baseline) continued reduction in pulmonary capillary wedge pressure, mean arterial blood pressure, right atrial pressure and an increase in cardiac index and stroke volume for the 20 and 40 mg dose groups. No tachyphylaxis was seen.

Fosinopril sodium was studied in 3 double-blind, placebo-controlled, 12-24 week trials including a total of 734 patients with heart failure, with fosinopril sodium doses from 10-40 mg daily. Concomitant therapy in 2 of these 3 trials included diuretics and digitalis; in the third trial patients were receiving only diuretics. All 3 trials showed statistically significant benefits of fosinopril sodium therapy, compared to placebo, in 1 or more of the following: exercise tolerance (1 study), symptoms of dyspnea, orthopnea and paroxysmal nocturnal dyspnea (2 studies), NYHA classification (2 studies), hospitalization for heart failure (2 studies), study withdrawals for worsening heart failure (2 studies), and/or need for supplemental diuretics (2 studies). Favorable effects were maintained for up to 2 years. Effects of fosinopril sodium on long-term mortality in heart failure have not been evaluated. The once-daily dosage for the treatment of congestive heart failure was the only dosage regimen used during clinical trial development and was determined by the measurement of hemodynamic responses.

INDICATIONS AND USAGE

Fosinopril sodium is indicated for the treatment of hypertension. It may be used alone or in combination with thiazide diuretics.

Fosinopril sodium is indicated in the management of heart failure as adjunctive therapy when added to conventional therapy including diuretics with or without digitalis (see DOSAGE AND ADMINISTRATION).

In using fosinopril sodium, consideration should be given to the fact that another angiotensin converting enzyme inhibitor (captopril) has caused agranulocytosis, particularly in patients with renal impairment or collagen-vascular disease. Available data are insufficient to show that fosinopril sodium does not have a similar risk (see WARNINGS).

In considering use of fosinopril sodium, it should be noted that in controlled trials ACE inhibitors have an effect on blood pressure that is less in black patients than in non-blacks. In addition, ACE inhibitors (for which adequate data are available) cause a higher rate of angioedema in black than in non-black patients (see WARNINGS, Anaphylactic and Possible Related Reactions, Angioedema).

F

NON-FDA APPROVED INDICATIONS

Other ACE inhibitors have been approved for the treatment of diabetic nephropathy, left ventricular dysfunction, left ventricular hypertrophy, and acute myocardial infarction.

CONTRAINDICATIONS

Fosinopril sodium is contraindicated in patients who are hypersensitive to this product or to any other angiotensin converting enzyme inhibitor (*e.g.*, a patient who has experienced angioedema with any other ACE inhibitor therapy).

WARNINGS

ANAPHYLACTIC AND POSSIBLE RELATED REACTIONS

Presumably because angiotensin-converting enzyme inhibitors affect the metabolism of eicosanoids and polypeptides, including endogenous bradykinin, patients receiving ACE inhibitors (including fosinopril sodium) may be subject to a variety of adverse reactions, some of them serious.

Angioedema

Angioedema involving the extremities, face, lips, mucous membranes, tongue, glottis or larynx has been reported in patients treated with ACE inhibitors. If angioedema involves the tongue, glottis or larynx, airway obstruction may occur and be fatal. If laryngeal stridor or angioedema of the face, lips, mucous membranes, tongue, glottis or extremities occurs, treatment with fosinopril sodium should be discontinued and appropriate therapy instituted immediately. **Where there is involvement of the tongue, glottis, or larynx, likely to cause airway obstruction, appropriate therapy, *e.g.*, subcutaneous epinephrine solution 1:1000 (0.3-0.5 ml) should be promptly administered** (see PRECAUTIONS, Information for the Patient and ADVERSE REACTIONS).

Anaphylactic Reactions During Desensitization

Two patients undergoing desensitizing treatment with hymenoptera venom while receiving ACE inhibitors sustained life-threatening anaphylactic reactions. In the same patients, these reactions were avoided when ACE inhibitors were temporarily withheld, but they reappeared upon inadvertent rechallenge.

Anaphylactic Reactions During Membrane Exposure

Anaphylactic reactions have been reported in patients dialyzed with high-flux membranes and treated concomitantly with an ACE inhibitor. Anaphylactoid reactions have also been reported in patients undergoing low-density lipoprotein apheresis with dextran sulfate absorption.

HYPOTENSION

Fosinopril sodium can cause symptomatic hypotension. Like other ACE inhibitors, fosinopril has been only rarely associated with hypotension in uncomplicated hypertensive patients. Symptomatic hypotension is most likely to occur in patients who have been volume- and/or salt-depleted as a result of prolonged diuretic therapy, dietary salt restriction, dialysis, diarrhea, or vomiting. Volume and/or salt depletion should be corrected before initiating therapy with fosinopril sodium.

In patients with heart failure, with or without associated renal insufficiency, ACE inhibitor therapy may cause excessive hypotension, which may be associated with oliguria or azotemia and, rarely, with acute renal failure and death. In such patients, fosinopril sodium therapy should be started under close medical supervision; they should be followed closely for the first 2 weeks of treatment and whenever the dose of fosinopril or diuretic is increased. Consideration should be given to reducing the diuretic dose in patients with normal or low blood pressure who have been treated vigorously with diuretics or who are hyponatremic.

If hypotension occurs, the patient should be placed in a supine position, and, if necessary, treated with IV infusion of physiological saline. Fosinopril sodium treatment usually can be continued following restoration of blood pressure and volume.

NEUTROPENIA/AGRANULOCYTOSIS

Another angiotensin converting enzyme inhibitor, captopril, has been shown to cause agranulocytosis and bone marrow depression, rarely in uncomplicated patients but more frequently in patients with renal impairment, especially if they also have a collagen-vascular disease such as systemic lupus erythematosus or scleroderma. Available data from clinical trials of fosinopril are insufficient to show that fosinopril does not cause agranulocytosis at similar rates. Monitoring of white blood cell counts should be considered in patients with collagen-vascular disease, especially if the disease is associated with impaired renal function.

FETAL/NEONATAL MORBIDITY AND MORTALITY

ACE inhibitors can cause fetal and neonatal morbidity and death when administered to pregnant women. Several dozen cases have been reported in the world literature. When pregnancy is detected, ACE inhibitors should be discontinued as soon as possible.

The use of ACE inhibitors during the second and third trimesters of pregnancy has been associated with fetal and neonatal injury, including hypotension, neonatal skull hypoplasia, anuria, reversible or irreversible renal failure, and death. Oligohydramnios has also been reported, presumably resulting from decreased fetal renal function; oligohydramnios in this setting has been associated with fetal limb contractures, craniofacial deformation, and hypoplastic lung development. Prematurity, intrauterine growth retardation, and patent ductus arteriosus have also been reported, although it is not clear whether these occurrences were due to the ACE inhibitor exposure.

These adverse effects do not appear to have resulted from intrauterine ACE inhibitor exposure that has been limited to the first trimester. Mothers whose embryos and fetuses are exposed to ACE inhibitors only during the first trimester should be so informed. Nonetheless, when patients become pregnant, physicians should make every effort to discontinue the use of fosinopril as soon as possible.

F

Rarely (probably less often than once in every 1000 pregnancies), no alternative to ACE inhibitors will be found. In these rare cases, the mothers should be apprised of the potential hazards to their fetuses, and serial ultrasound examinations should be performed to assess the intraamniotic environment.

If oligohydramnios is observed, fosinopril should be discontinued unless it is considered life-saving for the mother. Contraction stress testing (CST), a non-stress test (NST), or biophysical profiling (BPP) may be appropriate, depending upon the week of pregnancy. Patients and physicians should be aware, however, that oligohydramnios may not appear until after the fetus has sustained irreversible injury.

Infants with histories of *in utero* exposure to ACE inhibitors should be closely observed for hypotension, oliguria, and hyperkalemia. If oliguria occurs, attention should be directed toward support of blood pressure and renal perfusion. Exchange transfusion or dialysis may be required as a means of reversing hypotension and/or substituting for disordered renal function. Fosinopril is poorly dialyzed from the circulation of adults by hemodialysis and peritoneal dialysis. There is no experience with any procedure for removing fosinopril from the neonatal circulation.

When fosinopril was given to pregnant rats at doses about 80-250 times (on a mg/kg basis) the maximum recommended human dose, 3 similar orofacial malformations and 1 fetus with *situs inversus* were observed among the offspring. No teratogenic effects of fosinopril were seen in studies in pregnant rabbits at doses up to 25 times (on a mg/kg basis) the maximum recommended human dose.

HEPATIC FAILURE

Rarely, ACE inhibitors have been associated with a syndrome that starts with cholestatic jaundice and progresses to fulminant hepatic necrosis and (sometimes) death. The mechanism of this syndrome is not understood. Patients receiving ACE inhibitors who develop jaundice or marked elevations of hepatic enzymes should discontinue the ACE inhibitor and receive appropriate medical follow-up.

PRECAUTIONS

GENERAL

Impaired Renal Function

As a consequence of inhibiting the renin-angiotensin-aldosterone system, changes in renal function may be anticipated in susceptible individuals. In patients with severe congestive heart failure whose renal function may depend on the activity of the renin-angiotensin-aldosterone system, treatment with angiotensin converting enzyme inhibitors, including fosinopril sodium, may be associated with oliguria and/or progressive azotemia, and (rarely) with acute renal failure and/or death.

In hypertensive patients with renal artery stenosis in a solitary kidney or bilateral renal artery stenosis, increases in blood urea nitrogen and serum creatinine may occur. Experience with another angiotensin converting enzyme inhibitor suggests that these increases are usually reversible upon discontinuation of ACE inhibitor and/or diuretic therapy. In such patients, renal function should be monitored during the first few weeks of therapy. Some hypertensive patients with no apparent preexisting renal vascular disease have developed increases in blood urea nitrogen and serum creatinine, usually minor and transient, especially when fosinopril sodium has been given concomitantly with a diuretic. This is more likely to occur in patients with preexisting renal impairment. Dosage reduction of fosinopril sodium and/or discontinuation of the diuretic may be required.

Evaluation of patients with hypertension or heart failure should always include assessment of renal function (see DOSAGE AND ADMINISTRATION).

Impaired renal function decreases total clearance of fosinoprilat and approximately doubles AUC. In general, no adjustment of dosing is needed. However, patients with heart failure and severely reduced renal function may be more sensitive to the hemodynamic effects (*e.g.*, hypotension) of ACE inhibition (see CLINICAL PHARMACOLOGY).

Hyperkalemia

In clinical trials, hyperkalemia (serum potassium greater than 10% above the upper limit of normal) has occurred in approximately 2.6% of hypertensive patients receiving fosinopril sodium. In most cases, these were isolated values which resolved despite continued therapy. In clinical trials, 0.1% of patients (2 patients) were discontinued from therapy due to an elevated serum potassium. Risk factors for the development of hyperkalemia include renal insufficiency, diabetes mellitus, and concomitant use of potassium-sparing diuretics, potassium supplements, and/or potassium-containing salt substitutes, which should be used cautiously, if at all, with fosinopril sodium (see DRUG INTERACTIONS).

Cough

Presumably due to the inhibition of the degradation of endogenous bradykinin, persistent nonproductive cough has been reported with all ACE inhibitors, always resolving after discontinuation of therapy. ACE inhibitor-induced cough should be considered in the differential diagnosis of cough.

Impaired Liver Function

Since fosinopril is primarily metabolized by hepatic and gut wall esterases to its active moiety, fosinoprilat, patients with impaired liver function could develop elevated plasma levels of unchanged fosinopril. In a study in patients with alcoholic or biliary cirrhosis, the extent of hydrolysis was unaffected, although the rate was slowed. In these patients, the apparent total body clearance of fosinoprilat was decreased and the plasma AUC approximately doubled.

Surgery/Anesthesia

In patients undergoing surgery or during anesthesia with agents that produce hypotension, fosinopril will block the angiotensin II formation that could otherwise occur secondary to compensatory renin release. Hypotension that occurs as a result of this mechanism can be corrected by volume expansion.

HEMODIALYSIS

Recent clinical observations have shown an association of hypersensitivity-like (anaphylactoid) reactions during hemodialysis with high-flux dialysis membranes (*e.g.*, AN69) in patients receiving ACE inhibitors as medication. In these patients, consideration should be given to using a different type of dialysis membrane or a different class of medication. (See WARNINGS, Anaphylactic and Possible Related Reactions, Anaphylactoid Reactions During Membrane Exposure.)

INFORMATION FOR THE PATIENT

Angioedema

Angioedema, including laryngeal edema, can occur with treatment with ACE inhibitors, especially following the first dose. Patients should be advised to immediately report to their physician any signs or symptoms suggesting angioedema (*e.g.*, swelling of face, eyes, lips, tongue, larynx, mucous membranes, and extremities; difficulty in swallowing or breathing; hoarseness) and to discontinue therapy. (See WARNINGS, Anaphylactic and Possible Related Reactions, Angioedema; and ADVERSE REACTIONS.)

Symptomatic Hypotension

Patients should be cautioned that lightheadedness can occur, especially during the first days of therapy, and it should be reported to a physician. Patients should be told that if syncope occurs, fosinopril sodium should be discontinued until the physician has been consulted.

All patients should be cautioned that inadequate fluid intake or excessive perspiration, diarrhea, or vomiting can lead to an excessive fall in blood pressure, with the same consequences of lightheadedness and possible syncope.

Hyperkalemia

Patients should be told to not use potassium supplements or salt substitutes containing potassium without consulting the physician.

Neutropenia

Patients should be told to promptly report any indication of infection (*e.g.*, sore throat, fever), which could be a sign of neutropenia.

PREGNANCY

Female patients of childbearing age should be told about the consequences of second- and third-trimester exposure to ACE inhibitors, and they should also be told that these consequences do not appear to have resulted from intrauterine ACE inhibitor exposure that has been limited to the first trimester. These patients should be asked to report pregnancies to their physicians as soon as possible.

DRUG/LABORATORY TEST INTERACTIONS

Fosinopril may cause a false low measurement of serum digoxin levels with the Digi-Tab RIA Kit for Digoxin. Other kits, such as the Coat-A-Count RIA Kit, may be used.

CARCINOGENESIS, MUTAGENESIS, AND IMPAIRMENT OF FERTILITY

No evidence of a carcinogenic effect was found when fosinopril was given in the diet to mice and rats for up to 24 months at doses up to 400 mg/kg/day. On a body weight basis, the highest dose in mice and rats is about 250 times the maximum recommended human dose of 80 mg, assuming a 50 kg subject. On a body surface area basis, in mice, this dose is 20 times maximum human dose; in rats, this dose is 40 times the maximum human dose. Male rats given the highest dose level had a slightly higher incidence of mesentery/omentum lipomas.

Neither fosinopril nor the active fosinoprilat was mutagenic in the Ames microbial mutagen test, the mouse lymphoma forward mutation assay, or a mitotic gene conversion assay. Fosinopril was also not genotoxic in a mouse micronucleus test *in vivo* and a mouse bone marrow cytogenic assay *in vivo*.

In the Chinese hamster ovary cell cytogenic assay, fosinopril increased the frequency of chromosomal aberrations when tested without metabolic activation at a concentration that was toxic to the cells. However, there was no increase in chromosomal aberrations at lower drug concentrations without metabolic activation or at any concentration with metabolic activation.

There were no adverse reproductive effects in male and female rats treated with 15 or 60 mg/kg daily. On a body weight basis, the high dose of 60 mg/kg is about 38 times the maximum recommended human dose. On a body surface area basis, this dose is 6 times the maximum recommended human dose. There was no effect on pairing time prior to mating in rats until a daily dose of 240 mg/kg, a toxic dose, was given; at this dose, a slight increase in pairing time was observed. On a body weight basis, this dose is 150 times the maximum recommended human dose. On a body surface area basis, this dose is 24 times the maximum recommended human dose.

PREGNANCY CATEGORY C (FIRST TRIMESTER) AND PREGNANCY CATEGORY D (SECOND AND THIRD TRIMESTERS)

See WARNINGS, Fetal/Neonatal Morbidity and Mortality.

NURSING MOTHERS

Ingestion of 20 mg daily for 3 days resulted in detectable levels of fosinoprilat in breast milk. Fosinopril sodium should not be administered to nursing mothers.

GERIATRIC USE

Clinical studies of fosinopril sodium did not include a sufficient number of subjects aged 65 and over to determine whether they respond differently from younger subjects. Other reported clinical experience has not identified differences in responses between the elderly and younger patients. In general, dose selection for an elderly patient should be cautious, usually starting at the low end of the dosing range, reflecting the greater frequency of decreased hepatic, renal, or cardiac function, and of concomitant disease or other drug therapy.

PEDIATRIC USE

Safety and effectiveness in pediatric patients have not been established.

DRUG INTERACTIONS

WITH DIURETICS

Patients on diuretics, especially those with intravascular volume depletion, may occasionally experience an excessive reduction of blood pressure after initiation of therapy with fosinopril sodium. The possibility of hypotensive effects with fosinopril sodium can be minimized by either discontinuing the diuretic or increasing salt intake prior to initiation of treatment with fosinopril sodium. If this is not possible, the starting dose should be reduced and the patient should be observed closely for several hours following an initial dose and until blood pressure has stabilized (see DOSAGE AND ADMINISTRATION).

WITH POTASSIUM SUPPLEMENTS AND POTASSIUM-SPARING DIURETICS

Fosinopril sodium can attenuate potassium loss caused by thiazide diuretics. Potassium-sparing diuretics (spironolactone, amiloride, triamterene, and others) or potassium supplements can increase the risk of hyperkalemia. Therefore, if concomitant use of such agents is indicated, they should be given with caution, and the patient's serum potassium should be monitored frequently.

WITH LITHIUM

Increased serum lithium levels and symptoms of lithium toxicity have been reported in patients receiving ACE inhibitors during therapy with lithium. These drugs should be coadministered with caution, and frequent monitoring of serum lithium levels is recommended. If a diuretic is also used, the risk of lithium toxicity may be increased.

WITH ANTACIDS

In a clinical pharmacology study, coadministration of an antacid (aluminum hydroxide, magnesium hydroxide, and simethicone) with fosinopril reduced serum levels and urinary excretion of fosinoprilat as compared with fosinopril administered alone, suggesting that antacids may impair absorption of fosinopril. Therefore, if concomitant administration of these agents is indicated, dosing should be separated by 2 hours.

OTHER

Neither fosinopril sodium nor its metabolites have been found to interact with food. In separate single or multiple dose pharmacokinetic interaction studies with chlorthalidone, nifedipine, propanolol, hydrochlorothiazide, cimetidine, metoclopramide, propantheline, digoxin, and warfarin, the bioavailability of fosinoprilat was not altered by coadministration of fosinopril with any one of these drugs. In a study with concomitant administration of aspirin and fosinopril sodium, the bioavailability of unbound fosinoprilat was not altered.

In a pharmacokinetic interaction study with warfarin, bioavailability parameters, the degree of protein binding, and the anticoagulant effect (measured by prothrombin time) of warfarin were not significantly changed.

ADVERSE REACTIONS

Fosinopril sodium has been evaluated for safety in more than 2100 individuals in hypertension and heart failure trials, including approximately 530 patients treated for a year or more. Generally adverse events were mild and transient, and their frequency was not prominently related to dose within the recommended daily dosage range.

HYPERTENSION

In placebo-controlled clinical trials (688 fosinopril sodium-treated patients), the usual duration of therapy was 2-3 months. Discontinuations due to any clinical or laboratory adverse event were 4.1 and 1.1% in fosinopril sodium-treated and placebo-treated patients, respectively. The most frequent reasons (0.4-0.9%) were headache, elevated transaminases, fatigue, cough (see PRECAUTIONS, General, Cough), diarrhea, and nausea and vomiting.

During clinical trials with any fosinopril sodium regimen, the incidence of adverse events in the elderly (≥65 years old) was similar to that seen in younger patients.

Clinical adverse events probably or possibly related or of uncertain relationship to therapy, occurring in at least 1% of patients treated with fosinopril sodium alone and at least as frequent on fosinopril sodium as on placebo in placebo-controlled clinical trials are shown in TABLE 1.

The following events were also seen at >1% on fosinopril sodium but occurred in the placebo group at a greater rate: Headache, diarrhea, fatigue, and sexual dysfunction.

Other clinical events probably or possibly related, or of uncertain relationship to therapy occurring in 0.2-1.0% of patients (except as noted) treated with fosinopril sodium in controlled or uncontrolled clinical trials (n=1479) and less frequent, clinically significant events include (listed by body system):

TABLE 1 *Clinical Adverse Events in Placebo-Controlled Trials (Hypertension)*

	Incidence (Discontinuation)	
	Fosinopril Sodium (n=688)	Placebo (n=184)
Cough	2.2 (0.4)	0.0 (0.0)
Dizziness	1.6 (0.0)	0.0 (0.0)
Nausea/vomiting	1.2 (0.4)	0.5 (0.0)

General: Chest pain, edema, weakness, excessive sweating.

Cardiovascular: Angina/myocardial infarction, cerebrovascular accident, hypertensive crisis, rhythm disturbances, palpitations, hypotension, syncope, flushing, claudication.

Orthostatic hypotension occurred in 1.4% of patients treated with fosinopril monotherapy. Hypotension or orthostatic hypotension was a cause for discontinuation of therapy in 0.1% of patients.

Dermatologic: Urticaria, rash, photosensitivity, pruritus.

Endocrine/Metabolic: Gout, decreased libido.

Gastrointestinal: Pancreatitis, hepatitis, dysphagia, abdominal distention, abdominal pain, flatulence, constipation, heartburn, appetite/weight change, dry mouth.

Hematologic: Lymphadenopathy.

Immunologic: Angioedema. (See WARNINGS, Anaphylactic and Possible Related Reactions, Angioedema.)

Musculoskeletal: Arthralgia, musculoskeletal pain, myalgia/muscle cramp.

Nervous/Psychiatric: Memory disturbance, tremor, confusion, mood change, paresthesia, sleep disturbance, drowsiness, vertigo.

Respiratory: Bronchospasm, pharyngitis, sinusitis/rhinitis, laryngitis/hoarseness, epistaxis. A symptom-complex of cough, bronchospasm, and eosinophilia has been observed in 2 patients treated with fosinopril.

Special Senses: Tinnitus, vision disturbance, taste disturbance, eye irritation.

Urogenital: Renal insufficiency, urinary frequency.

HEART FAILURE

In placebo-controlled clinical trials (361 fosinopril sodium-treated patients), the usual duration of therapy was 3-6 months. Discontinuations due to any clinical or laboratory adverse event, except for heart failure, were 8.0% and 7.5% in fosinopril sodium-treated and placebo-treated patients, respectively. The most frequent reason for discontinuation of fosinopril sodium was angina pectoris (1.1%). Significant hypotension after the first dose of fosinopril sodium occurred in 14/590 (2.4%) of patients; 5/590 (0.8%) patients discontinued due to first dose hypotension.

Clinical adverse events probably or possibly related or of uncertain relationship to therapy, occurring in at least 1% of patients treated with fosinopril sodium and at least as common as the placebo group, in placebo-controlled trials are shown in TABLE 2.

TABLE 2 *Clinical Adverse Events in Placebo-Controlled Trials (Heart Failure)*

	Incidence (Discontinuation)	
	Fosinopril Sodium (n=361)	Placebo (n=373)
Dizziness	11.9 (0.6)	5.4 (0.3)
Cough	9.7 (0.8)	5.1 (0.0)
Hypotension	4.4 (0.8)	0.8 (0.0)
Musculoskeletal pain	3.3 (0.0)	2.7 (0.0)
Nausea/vomiting	2.2 (0.6)	1.6 (0.3)
Diarrhea	2.2 (0.0)	1.3 (0.0)
Chest pain (non-cardiac)	2.2 (0.0)	1.6 (0.0)
Upper respiratory infection	2.2 (0.0)	1.3 (0.0)
Orthostatic hypotension	1.9 (0.0)	0.8 (0.0)
Subjective cardiac rhythm disturbance	1.4 (0.6)	0.8 (0.3)
Weakness	1.4 (0.3)	0.5 (0.0)

The following events also occurred at a rate of 1% or more on fosinopril sodium tablets but occurred on placebo more often: Fatigue, dyspnea, headache, rash, abdominal pain, muscle cramp, angina pectoris, edema, and insomnia.

The incidence of adverse events in the elderly (≥65 years old) was similar to that seen in younger patients.

Other clinical events probably or possibly related, or of uncertain relationship to therapy occurring in 0.4-1.0% of patients (except as noted) treated with fosinopril sodium in controlled clinical trials (n=516) and less frequent, clinically significant events include (listed by body system):

General: Fever, influenza, weight gain, hyperhidrosis, sensation of cold, fall, pain.

Cardiovascular: Sudden death, cardiorespiratory arrest, shock (0.2%), atrial rhythm disturbance, cardiac rhythm disturbances, non-anginal chest pain, edema lower extremity, hypertension, syncope, conduction disorder, bradycardia, tachycardia.

Dermatologic: Pruritus.

Endocrine/Metabolic: Gout, sexual dysfunction.

Gastrointestinal: Hepatomegaly, abdominal distension, decreased appetite, dry mouth, constipation, flatulence.

Immunologic: Angioedema (0.2%).

Musculoskeletal: Muscle ache, swelling of an extremity, weakness of an extremity.

Nervous/Psychiatric: Cerebral infarction, TIA, depression, numbness, paresthesia, vertigo, behavior change, tremor.

Respiratory: Abnormal vocalization, rhinitis, sinus abnormality, tracheobronchitis, abnormal breathing, pleuritic chest pain.

Special Senses: Vision disturbance, taste disturbance.

Urogenital: Abnormal urination, kidney pain.

FETAL/NEONATAL MORBIDITY AND MORTALITY
See WARNINGS, Fetal/Neonatal Morbidity and Mortality.

POTENTIAL ADVERSE EFFECTS REPORTED WITH ACE INHIBITORS

Body as a Whole: Anaphylactoid reactions (see WARNINGS, Anaphylactic and Possible Related Reactions and PRECAUTIONS, Hemodialysis).

Other medically important adverse effects reported with ACE inhibitors include: Cardiac arrest; eosinophilic pneumonitis; neutropenia/agranulocytosis; pancytopenia, anemia (including hemolytic and aplastic); thrombocytopenia; acute renal failure; hepatic failure, jaundice (hepatocellular or cholestatic); symptomatic hyponatremia; bullous pemphigus; exfoliative dermatitis; a syndrome which may include: arthralgia/arthritis, vasculitis, serositis, myalgia, fever, rash or other dermatologic manifestations, a positive ANA, leukocytosis, eosinophilia, or an elevated ESR.

LABORATORY TEST ABNORMALITIES

Serum Electrolytes

Hyperkalemia, (see PRECAUTIONS); hyponatremia, (see DRUG INTERACTIONS, With Diuretics).

BUN/Serum Creatinine

Elevations, usually transient and minor, of BUN or serum creatinine have been observed. In placebo-controlled clinical trials, there were no significant differences in the number of patients experiencing increases in serum creatinine (outside the normal range or 1.33 times the pretreatment value) between the fosinopril and placebo treatment groups. Rapid reduction of longstanding or markedly elevated blood pressure by any antihypertensive therapy can result in decreases in the glomerular filtration rate and, in turn, lead to increases in BUN or serum creatinine. (See PRECAUTIONS, General.)

Hematology

In controlled trials, a mean *hemoglobin* decrease of 0.1 g/dl was observed in fosinopril-treated patients. In individual patients, decreases in hemoglobin or hematocrit were usually transient, small, and not associated with symptoms. No patient was discontinued from therapy due to the development of anemia.

Other

Neutropenia (see WARNINGS), leukopenia and eosinophilia.

Liver Function Tests

Elevations of transaminases, LDH, alkaline phosphatase, and serum bilirubin have been reported. Fosinopril therapy was discontinued because of serum transaminase elevations in 0.7% of patients. In the majority of cases, the abnormalities were either present at baseline or were associated with other etiologic factors. In those cases that were possibly related to fosinopril therapy, the elevations were generally mild and transient and resolved after discontinuation of therapy.

DOSAGE AND ADMINISTRATION

HYPERTENSION

The recommended initial dose of fosinopril sodium is 10 mg once a day, both as monotherapy and when the drug is added to a diuretic. Dosage should then be adjusted according to blood pressure response at peak (2-6 hours) and trough (about 24 hours after dosing) blood levels. The usual dosage range needed to maintain a response at trough is 20-40 mg but some patients appear to have a further response to 80 mg. In some patients treated with once-daily dosing, the antihypertensive effect may diminish toward the end of the dosing interval. If trough response is inadequate, dividing the daily dose should be considered. If blood pressure is not adequately controlled with fosinopril sodium alone, a diuretic may be added.

Concomitant administration of fosinopril sodium with potassium supplements, potassium salt substitutes, or potassium-sparing diuretics can lead to increases of serum potassium (see PRECAUTIONS).

In patients who are currently being treated with a diuretic, symptomatic hypotension occasionally can occur following the initial dose of fosinopril sodium. To reduce the likelihood of hypotension, the diuretic should, if possible, be discontinued 2-3 days prior to beginning therapy with fosinopril sodium (see WARNINGS). Then, if blood pressure is not controlled with fosinopril sodium alone, diuretic therapy should be resumed. If diuretic therapy cannot be discontinued, an initial dose of 10 mg of fosinopril sodium should be used with careful medical supervision for several hours and until blood pressure has stabilized. (See WARNINGS; PRECAUTIONS, Information for the Patient; and DRUG INTERACTIONS.)

Since concomitant administration of fosinopril sodium with potassium supplements, or potassium-containing salt substitutes or potassium-sparing diuretics may lead to increases in serum potassium, they should be used with caution (see PRECAUTIONS).

HEART FAILURE

Digitalis is not required for fosinopril sodium to manifest improvements in exercise tolerance and symptoms. Most placebo-controlled clinical trial experience has been with both digitalis and diuretics present as background therapy.

The usual starting dose of fosinopril sodium should be 10 mg once daily. Following the initial dose of fosinopril sodium, the patient should be observed under medical supervision for at least 2 hours for the presence of hypotension or orthostasis and, if present, until blood pressure stabilizes. An initial dose of 5 mg is preferred in heart failure patients with moderate to severe renal failure or those who have been vigorously diuresed.

Dosage should be increased, over a several week period, to a dose that is maximal and tolerated but not exceeding 40 mg once daily. The usual effective dosage range is 20-40 mg once daily.

The appearance of hypotension, orthostasis, or azotemia early in dose titration should not preclude further careful dose titration. Consideration should be given to reducing the dose of concomitant diuretic.

For Hypertensive or Heart Failure Patients With Renal Impairment

In patients with impaired renal function, the total body clearance of fosinoprilat is approximately 50% slower than in patients with normal renal function. Since hepatobiliary elimination partially compensates for diminished renal elimination, the total body clearance of fosinoprilat does not differ appreciably with any degree of renal insufficiency (creatinine clearances <80 ml/min/1.73 m^2), including end-stage renal failure (creatinine clearance <10 ml/min/1.73 m^2). This relative constancy of body clearance of active fosinoprilat, resulting from the dual route of elimination, permits use of the usual dose in patients with any degree of renal impairment. (See WARNINGS, Anaphylactic and Possible Related Reactions, Anaphylactic Reactions During Membrane Exposure and PRECAUTIONS, Hemodialysis.)

HOW SUPPLIED

Monopril tablets are supplied as:

10 mg: White to off-white, biconvex flat-end diamond-shaped, compressed partially scored tablets with *"BMS"* on one side and *"Monopril 10"* on the other.

20 mg: White to off-white, oval-shaped, compressed tablets with "**BMS**" on one side and "**Monopril 20**" on the other.

40 mg: White to off-white, biconvex hexagonal-shaped, compressed tablets with "**BMS**" on one side and "**Monopril 40**" on the other.

Storage: Store at 25°C (77°F): excursions permitted to 15-30°C (59-86°F). Protect from moisture by keeping tightly closed.

PRODUCT LISTING - EQUIVALENTS NOT AVAILABLE

Tablet - Oral - 10 mg			
30's	$26.91	MONOPRIL, Allscripts Pharmaceutical Company	54569-3808-00
30's	$33.95	MONOPRIL, Physicians Total Care	54868-2368-01
90's	$65.69	MONOPRIL, Allscripts Pharmaceutical Company	54569-8592-00
90's	$98.90	MONOPRIL, Physicians Total Care	54868-2368-02
90's	$111.19	MONOPRIL, Bristol-Myers Squibb	00087-0158-46
100's	$110.41	MONOPRIL, Physicians Total Care	54868-2368-00
Tablet - Oral - 20 mg			
30's	$29.93	MONOPRIL, Allscripts Pharmaceutical Company	54569-3809-00
60's	$66.72	MONOPRIL, Physicians Total Care	54868-3279-00
90's	$111.19	MONOPRIL, Bristol-Myers Squibb	00087-0609-42
100's	$99.77	MONOPRIL, Bristol-Myers Squibb	00087-0609-45
100's	$109.82	MONOPRIL, Physicians Total Care	54868-3279-02
Tablet - Oral - 40 mg			
30's	$27.97	MONOPRIL, Allscripts Pharmaceutical Company	54569-4948-00
90's	$111.19	MONOPRIL, Bristol-Myers Squibb	00087-1202-13

Fosinopril Sodium; Hydrochlorothiazide *(003245)*

For complete prescribing information, refer to the CD-ROM included with the book.

Categories: Hypertension, essential; Pregnancy Category D; FDA Approved 1994 Nov
Drug Classes: Angiotensin converting enzyme inhibitors; Diuretics, thiazide and derivatives
Brand Names: **Monopril-HCT**
Foreign Brand Availability: Dynacil (Germany); Fosicomp (Switzerland); Fosinorm (Germany); Foziretic (France); Monoplus (Australia); Monozide (South-Africa); Vasopril Plus (Israel)
Cost of Therapy: $27.97 (Hypertension; Monopril HCT; 10 mg; 12.5 mg; 1 tablet/day; 30 day supply)

WARNING

USE IN PREGNANCY: When used in pregnancy during the second and third trimesters, ACE inhibitors can cause injury and even death to the developing fetus.When pregnancy is detected, fosinopril sodium; hydrochlorothiazide tablets should be discontinued as soon as possible. See WARNINGS, Fetal/Neonatal Morbidity and Mortality.

DESCRIPTION

Fosinopril sodium is a white to off-white crystalline powder, soluble (>100 mg/ml) in water, in ethanol, and in methanol, and slightly soluble in hexane. Fosinopril sodium's chemical name is L-proline, 4-cyclohexyl-1-[[[2-methyl-1-(1-oxopropoxy)-propoxy]-(4 phenylbutyl)-phosphinyl]acetyl]-, sodium salt, *trans*-.

Its empirical formula is $C_{30}H_{45}NNaO_7P$, and its molecular weight is 585.65.

Fosinoprilat, the active metabolite of fosinopril, is a non-sulfhydryl angiotensin-converting enzyme inhibitor. Fosinopril is converted to fosinoprilat by hepatic cleavage of the ester group.

Hydrochlorothiazide is a white, or practically white, practically odorless, crystalline powder. It is slightly soluble in water; freely soluble in sodium hydroxide solution, in n-butylamine, and in dimethylformamide; sparingly soluble in methanol; and insoluble in ether, in chloroform, and in dilute mineral acids. Hydrochlorothiazide's chemical name is 6-chloro-3,4-dihydro-2*H*-1,2,4-benzothiadiazine-7-sulfonamide 1,1-dioxide.

Its empirical formula is $C_7H_8ClN_3O_4S_2$, and its molecular weight is 297.73. Hydrochlorothiazide is a thiazide diuretic.

Monopril-HCT (fosinopril sodium; hydrochlorothiazide tablets) is a combination of fosinopril sodium and hydrochlorothiazide. *It is available for oral use in two tablet strengths:* Monopril-HCT 10/12.5, containing 10 mg of fosinopril sodium and 12.5 mg of hydrochlorothiazide; and Monopril-HCT 20/12.5, containing 20 mg of fosinopril sodium and 12.5 mg of hydrochlorothiazide. The inactive ingredients of the tablets include lactose, croscarmellose sodium, povidone, sodium stearyl fumarate, and iron oxide.

INDICATIONS AND USAGE

Fosinopril sodium; hydrochlorothiazide tablets are indicated for the treatment of hypertension.

These fixed dose combinations are not indicated for initial therapy. (See DOSAGE AND ADMINISTRATION.)

In using fosinopril sodium; hydrochlorothiazide tablets, consideration should be given to the fact that another angiotensin-converting enzyme inhibitor, captopril, has caused agranulocytosis, particularly in patients with renal impairment or collagen-vascular disease. Available data are insufficient to show that fosinopril does not have a similar risk (see WARNINGS, Neutropenia/Agranulocytosis).

ACE inhibitors (for which adequate data are available) cause a higher rate of angioedema in black than in non-black patients (see WARNINGS, Angioedema).

CONTRAINDICATIONS

Fosinopril sodium; hydrochlorothiazide tablets are contraindicated in patients who are anuric. Fosinopril sodium; hydrochlorothiazide tablets are also contraindicated in patients who are hypersensitive to fosinopril, to any other ACE inhibitor, to hydrochlorothiazide, or other sulfonamide-derived drugs, or any other ingredient or component in the formulation. Hypersensitivity reactions are more likely to occur in patients with a history of allergy or bronchial asthma.

WARNINGS

ANAPHYLACTOID AND POSSIBLY RELATED REACTIONS

Presumably because angiotensin-converting enzyme inhibitors affect the metabolism of eicosanoids and polypeptides, including endogenous bradykinin, patients receiving ACE inhibitors (including fosinopril sodium; hydrochlorothiazide tablets) may be subject to a variety of adverse reactions, some of them serious.

Angioedema

Angioedema of the face, extremities, lips, tongue, glottis and larynx has been reported in patients treated with angiotensin-converting enzyme inhibitors. Angioedema associated with laryngeal edema can be fatal. If laryngeal stridor or angioedema of the face, tongue, or glottis occurs, treatment with fosinopril sodium; hydrochlorothiazide tablets should be discontinued and appropriate therapy instituted immediately. *When involvement of the tongue, glottis, or larynx appears likely to cause airway obstruction, appropriate therapy, e.g., subcutaneous epinephrine injection 1:1000 (0.3-0.5 ml) should be promptly administered.*

Anaphylactoid Reactions During Desensitization

Two (2) patients undergoing desensitizing treatment with hymenoptera venom while receiving ACE inhibitors sustained life-threatening anaphylactoid reactions. In the same patients, these reactions were avoided when ACE inhibitors were temporarily withheld, but they reappeared upon inadvertent rechallenge.

Anaphylactoid Reactions During Membrane Exposure

Anaphylactoid reactions have been reported in patients dialyzed with high-flux membranes and treated concomitantly with an ACE inhibitor. Anaphylactoid reactions have also been reported in patients undergoing low-density lipoprotein apheresis with dextran sulfate absorption.

HYPOTENSION

Fosinopril sodium; hydrochlorothiazide tablets can cause symptomatic hypotension. Like other ACE inhibitors, fosinopril has been only rarely associated with hypotension in uncomplicated hypertensive patients. Symptomatic hypotension is most likely to occur in patients who have been volume- and/or salt-depleted as a result of prolonged diuretic therapy, dietary salt restriction, dialysis, diarrhea, or vomiting. Volume and/or salt depletion should be corrected before initiating therapy with fosinopril sodium; hydrochlorothiazide tablets.

Fosinopril sodium; hydrochlorothiazide tablets should be used cautiously in patients receiving concomitant therapy with other antihypertensives. The thiazide component of fosinopril sodium; hydrochlorothiazide tablets may potentiate the action of other antihypertensive drugs, especially ganglionic or peripheral adrenergic-blocking drugs. The antihypertensive effects of the thiazide component may also be enhanced in the postsympathectomy patient.

In patients with congestive heart failure, with or without associated renal insufficiency, ACE inhibitor therapy may cause excessive hypotension, which may be associated with oliguria, azotemia, and (rarely) with acute renal failure and death. In such patients, fosinopril sodium; hydrochlorothiazide tablets therapy should be started under close medical supervision; they should be followed closely for the first 2 weeks of treatment and whenever the dose of fosinopril or diuretic is increased.

If hypotension occurs, the patient should be placed in a supine position, and, if necessary, treated with intravenous infusion of physiological saline. Fosinopril sodium; hydrochlorothiazide treatment usually can be continued following restoration of blood pressure and volume.

IMPAIRED RENAL FUNCTION

Fosinopril sodium; hydrochlorothiazide tablets should be used with caution in patients with severe renal disease. Thiazides may precipitate azotemia in such patients, and the effects of repeated dosing may be cumulative.

When the renin-angiotensin-aldosterone system is inhibited by ACE inhibitors, changes in renal function may be anticipated in susceptible individuals. In patients with **severe congestive heart failure,** whose renal function may depend on the activity of the renin-angiotensin-aldosterone system, treatment with angiotensin-converting enzyme inhibitors (including fosinopril) may be associated with oliguria and/or progressive azotemia and (rarely) with acute renal failure and/or death.

In some studies of hypertensive patients with **unilateral or bilateral renal artery stenosis,** treatment with ACE inhibitors has been associated with increases in blood urea nitrogen and serum creatinine; these increases were reversible upon discontinuation of ACE inhibitor therapy, concomitant diuretic therapy, or both. When such patients are treated with fosinopril sodium; hydrochlorothiazide tablets, renal function should be monitored during the first few weeks of therapy.

Some ACE-inhibitor-treated hypertensive patients with **no apparent pre-existing renal vascular disease** have developed increases in blood urea nitrogen and serum creatinine, usually minor and transient, especially when the ACE-inhibitor has been given concomitantly with a diuretic. Dosage reduction of fosinopril sodium; hydrochlorothiazide tablets may be required. **Evaluation of the hypertensive patient should always include assessment of renal function** (see DOSAGE AND ADMINISTRATION).

NEUTROPENIA/AGRANULOCYTOSIS

Another angiotensin-converting enzyme inhibitor, captopril, has been shown to cause agranulocytosis and bone marrow depression, rarely in uncomplicated patients (incidence probably less than once per 10,000 exposures), but more frequently (incidence possibly as great as once per 1000 exposures) in patients with renal impairment, especially those who also have a collagen-vascular disease such as systemic lupus erythematosus or scleroderma. Available data from clinical trials of fosinopril are insufficient to show that fosinopril does not cause agranulocytosis at similar rates. Monitoring of white blood cell counts should be considered in patients with collagen-vascular disease, especially if the disease is associated with impaired renal function.

Neutropenia/agranulocytosis has also been associated with thiazide diuretics.

FETAL/NEONATAL MORBIDITY AND MORTALITY

ACE inhibitors can cause fetal and neonatal morbidity and death when administered to pregnant women. Several dozen cases have been reported in the world literature. When pregnancy is detected, fosinopril sodium; hydrochlorothiazide tablets should be discontinued as soon as possible.

The use of ACE inhibitors during the second and third trimesters of pregnancy has been associated with fetal and neonatal injury, including hypotension, neonatal skull hypoplasia, anuria, reversible or irreversible renal failure, and death. Oligohydramnios has also been reported, presumably resulting from decreased fetal renal function; oligohydramnios in this setting has been associated with fetal limb contractures, craniofacial deformation, and hypoplastic lung development. Prematurity, intrauterine growth retardation, and patent ductus arteriosus have also been reported, although it is not clear whether these occurrences were due to the ACE-inhibitor exposure.

These adverse effects do not appear to have resulted from intrauterine ACE-inhibitor exposure that has been limited to the first trimester. Mothers whose embryos and fetuses are exposed to ACE inhibitors only during the first trimester should be so informed. Nonetheless, when patients become pregnant, physicians should make every effort to discontinue the use of fosinopril as soon as possible.

Rarely (probably less often than once in every thousand pregnancies), no alternative to ACE inhibitors will be found. In these rare cases, the mothers should be apprised of the potential hazards to their fetuses, and serial ultrasound examinations should be performed to assess the intraamniotic environment.

If oligohydramnios is observed, fosinopril should be discontinued unless it is considered life-saving for the mother. Contraction stress testing (CST), a non-stress test (NST), or biophysical profiling (BPP) may be appropriate, depending upon the week of pregnancy. Patients and physicians should be aware, however, that oligohydramnios may not appear until after the fetus has sustained irreversible injury.

Infants with histories of *in utero* exposure to ACE inhibitors should be closely observed for hypotension, oliguria, and hyperkalemia. If oliguria occurs, attention should be directed toward support of blood pressure and renal perfusion. Exchange transfusion or peritoneal dialysis may be required as a means of reversing hypotension and/or substituting for disordered renal function. Fosinopril is poorly dialyzed from the circulation of adults, and indeed there is no experience with any procedure for removing fosinopril from the neonatal circulation, but limited experience with other ACE inhibitors has not shown that such removal is central to the treatment of these infants.

When fosinopril is given to pregnant rats at doses about 80-250 times (on a mg/kg basis) the maximum recommended human dose, 3 similar orofacial malformations and 1 fetus with *situs inversus* were observed among the offspring. In pregnant rabbits, no teratogenic effects of fosinopril were seen in studies at doses up to 25 times (on a mg/kg basis) the maximum recommended human dose.

IMPAIRED HEPATIC FUNCTION

Rarely, ACE inhibitors have been associated with a syndrome that begins with cholestatic jaundice and progresses to fulminant hepatic necrosis and (sometimes) death. The mechanism of this syndrome is not understood. A patient receiving fosinopril sodium; hydrochlorothiazide tablets who develops jaundice or marked elevation of hepatic enzymes should discontinue fosinopril sodium; hydrochlorothiazide tablets and receive appropriate medical follow-up.

Fosinopril sodium; hydrochlorothiazide tablets should be used with caution in patients with impaired hepatic function or progressive liver disease, since minor alterations of fluid and electrolyte balance may precipitate hepatic coma. Also, since the metabolism of fosinopril to fosinoprilat is normally dependent upon hepatic esterases, patients with impaired liver function could develop elevated plasma levels of fosinopril. In a study of patients with alcoholic or biliary cirrhosis the rate (but not the extent) of hydrolysis to fosinoprilat was reduced. In these patients the clearance of fosinoprilat was reduced, and the area under the fosinoprilat-time curve was approximately doubled.

SYSTEMIC LUPUS ERYTHEMATOSUS

Thiazide diuretics have been reported to cause exacerbation or activation of systemic lupus erythematosus.

DOSAGE AND ADMINISTRATION

Fosinopril is an effective treatment of hypertension in once-daily doses of 10-80 mg, while hydrochlorothiazide is effective in doses of 12.5-50 mg/day. In clinical trials of fosinopril; hydrochlorothiazide combination therapy using fosinopril doses of 2.5-40 mg and hydro-

F

chlorothiazide doses at 5-37.5 mg, the anti-hypertensive effects increased with increasing dose of either component.

The hazards (see WARNINGS) of fosinopril are generally rare and apparently independent of dose; those of hydrochlorothiazide are a mixture of dose-dependent phenomena (primarily hypokalemia) and dose-independent phenomena (*e.g.*, pancreatitis), the former much more common than the latter. Therapy with any combination of fosinopril and hydrochlorothiazide will be associated with both sets of dose-independent hazards. To minimize dose-independent hazards, it is usually appropriate to begin combination therapy only after a patient has failed to achieve the desired effect with monotherapy.

DOSE TITRATION BY CLINICAL EFFECT

A patient whose blood pressure is not adequately controlled with fosinopril or hydrochlorothiazide monotherapy may be switched to combination therapy with fosinopril sodium; hydrochlorothiazide tablets. Dosage must be guided by clinical response; controlled clinical trials showed that the addition of 12.5 mg of hydrochlorothiazide to 10-20 mg of fosinopril will typically be associated with additional reduction in seated diastolic blood pressure at 24 hours after dosing. On average, the effect of the combination of 10 mg of fosinopril with 12.5 mg of hydrochlorothiazide was similar to the effect seen with monotherapy using either 40 mg of fosinopril or 37.5 mg of hydrochlorothiazide.

F

USE IN RENAL IMPAIRMENT

In patients with severe renal impairment (creatinine clearance is <30 ml/min/1.73 m^2, serum creatine roughly ≥3 mg/dl or 265 μmol/L), loop diuretics are preferred to thiazides, so fosinopril sodium; hydrochlorothiazide tablets are not recommended. In patients with lesser degrees of renal impairment, fosinopril sodium; hydrochlorothiazide tablets may be used with no change in dosage.

PRODUCT LISTING - EQUIVALENTS NOT AVAILABLE

Tablet - Oral - 10 mg;12.5 mg
100's $123.55 MONOPRIL HCT, Bristol-Myers Squibb 00087-1492-01
Tablet - Oral - 20 mg;12.5 mg
100's $123.55 MONOPRIL HCT, Bristol-Myers Squibb 00087-1493-01

Fosphenytoin Sodium *(003298)*

Categories: Seizures, secondary to neurosurgery; Status epilepticus; Pregnancy Category D; FDA Approved 1996 Aug; Orphan Drugs
Drug Classes: Anticonvulsants; Hydantoins
Brand Names: Cerebyx
Foreign Brand Availability: Prodilantin (France)

DESCRIPTION

Fosphenytoin sodium injection is a prodrug intended for parenteral administration; its active metabolite is phenytoin. Each Cerebyx vial contains 75 mg/ml fosphenytoin sodium (hereafter referred to as fosphenytoin) **equivalent to 50 mg/ml phenytoin sodium** after administration. Cerebyx is supplied in vials as a ready-mixed solution in water for injection, and tromethamine (TRIS), buffer adjusted to pH 8.6-9.0 with either hydrochloric acid, or sodium hydroxide. Fosphenytoin is a clear, colorless to pale yellow sterile solution.

The chemical name of fosphenytoin is 5,5-diphenyl-3-[(phosphonooxy)methyl]-2,4-imidazolidinedione disodium salt. The molecular weight of fosphenytoin is 406.24.

IMPORTANT NOTE: Throughout all fosphenytoin product labeling, the amount and concentration of fosphenytoin is expressed in terms of phenytoin sodium equivalents (PE). Fosphenytoin's weight is expressed as phenytoin sodium equivalents to avoid the need to perform molecular weight-based adjustments when converting between fosphenytoin and phenytoin sodium doses. Fosphenytoin should always be prescribed and dispensed in phenytoin sodium equivalent units (PE) (see DOSAGE AND ADMINISTRATION).

CLINICAL PHARMACOLOGY

INTRODUCTION

Following parenteral administration of fosphenytoin, it is converted to the anticonvulsant phenytoin. For every mmol of fosphenytoin administered, 1 mmol of phenytoin is produced. The pharmacological and toxicological effects of fosphenytoin include those of phenytoin. However, the hydrolysis of fosphenytoin to phenytoin yields two metabolites, phosphate and formaldehyde. Formaldehyde is subsequently converted to formate, which is in turn metabolized via a folate dependent mechanism. Although phosphate and formaldehyde (formate) have potentially important biological effect, these effects typically occur at concentrations considerably in excess of those obtained when fosphenytoin is administered under conditions of use recommended in this labeling.

MECHANISM OF ACTION

Fosphenytoin is a prodrug of phenytoin and accordingly, its anticonvulsant effects are attributable to phenytoin.

After IV administration to mice, fosphenytoin blocked the tonic phase of maximal electroshock seizures at doses equivalent to those effective for phenytoin. In addition to its ability to suppress maximal electroshock seizures in mice and rats, phenytoin exhibits anticonvulsant activity against kindled seizures in rats, audiogenic seizures in mice, and seizures produced by electrical stimulation of the brainstem in rats. The cellular mechanisms of phenytoin thought to be responsible for its anticonvulsant actions include modulation of voltage-dependent sodium channels of neurons, inhibition of calcium flux across neuronal membranes, modulation of voltage-dependent calcium channels of neurons, and enhancement of the sodium-potassium ATPase activity of neurons and glial cells. The modulation of sodium channels may be a primary anticonvulsant mechanism because this property is shared with several other anticonvulsants in addition to phenytoin.

PHARMACOKINETICS AND DRUG METABOLISM

Fosphenytoin

Absorption/Bioavailability

Intravenous: When fosphenytoin is administered by IV infusion, maximum plasma fosphenytoin concentrations are achieved at the end of the infusion. Fosphenytoin has a half-life of approximately 15 minutes.

Intramuscular: Fosphenytoin is completely bioavailable following IM administration of fosphenytoin. Peak concentrations occur at approximately 30 minutes postdose. Plasma fosphenytoin concentrations following IM administration are lower but more sustained than those following IV administration due to the time required for absorption of fosphenytoin from the injection site.

Distribution

Fosphenytoin is extensively bound (95-99%) to human plasma proteins, primarily albumin. Binding to plasma proteins is saturable with the result that the percent bound decreases as total fosphenytoin concentrations increase. Fosphenytoin displaces phenytoin from protein binding sites. The volume of distribution of fosphenytoin increases with fosphenytoin dose and rate, and ranges from 4.3-10.8 liters.

Metabolism and Elimination

The conversion half-life of fosphenytoin to phenytoin is approximately 15 minutes. The mechanism of fosphenytoin conversion has not been determined, but photophatases probably play a major role. Fosphenytoin is not excreted in urine. Each mmol of fosphenytoin is metabolized to 1 mmol of phenytoin, phosphate, and formate (see Introduction and PRECAUTIONS, General, Fosphenytoin Specific, Phosphate Load).

Phenytoin (after fosphenytoin administration)

In general, IM administration of fosphenytoin generates systemic phenytoin concentrations that are similar enough to oral phenytoin sodium to allow essentially interchangeable use.

The pharmacokinetics of fosphenytoin following IV administration of fosphenytoin, however, are complex, and when used in an emergency setting (*e.g.*, status epilepticus), differences in rate of availability of phenytoin could be critical. Studies have therefore empirically determined an infusion rate for fosphenytoin that gives a rate and extent of phenytoin systemic availability similar to that of a 50 mg/min phenytoin sodium infusion.

A dose of 15-20 mg PE/kg of fosphenytoin infused at 100-150 mg PE/min yields plasma free phenytoin concentrations over time that approximate those achieved when an equivalent dose of phenytoin sodium (*e.g.*, parenteral phenytoin sodium) is administered at 50 mg/min (see DOSAGE AND ADMINISTRATION and WARNINGS).

Following administration of single IV fosphenytoin doses of 400-1200 mg PE, mean maximum total phenytoin concentrations increase in proportion to dose, but do not change appreciably with changes in infusion rate. In contrast, mean maximum unbound protein concentrations increase with both dose and rate.

Absorption/Bioavailability

Fosphenytoin is completely converted to phenytoin following IV administration, with a half-life of approximately 15 minutes. Fosphenytoin is also completely converted to phenytoin following IM administration and plasma total phenytoin concentrations peak in approximately 3 hours.

Distribution

Phenytoin is highly bound to plasma proteins, primarily albumin, although to a lesser extent than fosphenytoin. In the absence of fosphenytoin, approximately 12% of total plasma phenytoin is unbound over the clinically relevant concentration range. However, fosphenytoin displaces phenytoin from plasma protein binding sites. This increases the fraction of phenytoin unbound (up to 30% unbound) during the period required for conversion of fosphenytoin to phenytoin (approximately 0.5 to 1 hour postinfusion).

Metabolism and Elimination

Phenytoin derived from administration of fosphenytoin is extensively metabolised in the liver and excreted in urine primarily as 5-(p-hydroxyphenyl)-5-phenylhydantoin and its glucuronide; little unchanged phenytoin (1-5% of the fosphenytoin dose) is recovered in urine. Phenytoin hepatic metabolism is satuable, and following administration of single IV fosphenytoin doses of 400-1200 mg PE, total and unbound phenytoin AUC values increase disproportionately with dose. Mean total phenytoin half-life values (12.0-28.9 hours) following fosphenytoin administration at these doses are similar to those after equal doses of parenteral phenytoin sodium and tend to be greater at higher plasma phenytoin concentrations.

SPECIAL POPULATIONS

Patients With Renal or Hepatic Disease

Due to an increased fraction of unbound phenytoin in patients with renal or hepatic disease, or in those with hypoalbuminemia, the interpretation of total phenytoin plasma concentrations should be made with caution (see DOSAGE AND ADMINISTRATION). Unbound phenytoin concentration may be more useful in these patient populations. After IV administration of fosphenytoin to patients with renal and/or hepatic disease, or in those with hypoalbuminemia, fosphenytoin clearance to phenytoin may be increased without similar increase in phenytoin clearance. This has the potential to increase the frequency and severity of adverse events (see PRECAUTIONS).

Age

The effect of age was evaluated in patients 5-98 years of age. Patient age had no significant impact on fosphenytoin pharmacokinetics. Phenytoin clearance tends to decrease with increasing age (20% less in patients over 70 years of age relative to that in patients 20-30 years of age). Phenytoin dosing requirements are highly variable and must be individualized (see DOSAGE AND ADMINISTRATION).

Gender and Race

Gender and race have no significant impact on fosphenytoin or phenytoin pharmacokinetics.

Pediatrics

Only limited pharmacokinetic data are available in children (n=8; age 5-10 years). In these patients with status epilepticus who received loading doses of fosphenytoin, the plasma fosphenytoin, total phenytoin, and unbound phenytoin concentration-time profiles did not signal any major differences from those in adult patients with status epilepticus receiving comparable doses.

INDICATIONS AND USAGE

Fosphenytoin is indicated for short-term parenteral administration when other means of phenytoin administration are unavailable, inappropriate or deemed less advantageous. The safety and effectiveness of fosphenytoin in this use has not been systemically evaluated for more than 5 days.

Fosphenytoin can be used for the control of generalized convulsive status epilepticus and prevention and treatment of seizures occurring during neuosurgery. It can also be substituted, short-term, for oral phenytoin.

CONTRAINDICATIONS

Fosphenytoin is contraindicated in patients who have demonstrated hypersensitivity to fosphenytoin or its ingredients, or to phenytoin or other hydantoins.

Because of the effect of parenteral phenytoin on ventricular automaticity, fosphenytoin is contraindicated in patients with sinus bradycardia, sino-atrial block, second and third degree AV block, and Adams-Stokes syndrome.

WARNINGS

DOSES OF FOSPHENYTOIN ARE EXPRESSED AS THEIR PHENYTOIN SODIUM EQUIVALENTS IN THIS LABELING (PE = Phenytoin Sodium Equivalent).

DO NOT, THEREFORE, MAKE ANY ADJUSTMENT IN THE RECOMMENDED DOSES WHEN SUBSTITUTING FOSPHENYTOIN FOR PHENYTOIN SODIUM OR VICE VERSA.

The following warnings are based on experience with fosphenytoin or phenytoin.

STATUS EPILEPTICUS DOSING REGIMEN

Do not administer fosphenytoin at a rate greater than 150 mg PE/min.

The dose of IV fosphenytoin (15-20 mg PE/kg) that is used to treat status epilepticus is administered at a maximum rate of 150 mg PE/min. The typical fosphenytoin infusion administered to a 50 kg patient would take between 5 and 7 minutes. Note that the delivery of an identical molar dose of phenytoin using parenteral Dilantin or generic phenytoin sodium injection cannot be accomplished in less than 15-20 minutes because of the untoward cardiovascular effects that accompany the direct intravenous administration of phenytoin at rates greater than 50 mg/min.

If rapid phenytoin loading is a primary goal, IV administration of fosphenytoin is preferred because the time to achieve therapeutic plasma phenytoin concentrations is greater following IM than that following IV administration (see DOSAGE AND ADMINISTRATION).

WITHDRAWAL PRECIPITATED SEIZURE, STATUS EPILEPTICUS

Antiepileptic drugs should not be abruptly discontinued because of the possibility of increased seizure frequency, including status epilepticus. When, in the judgement of the clinician, the need for dosage reduction, discontinuation, or substitution of alternative antiepileptic medication arises, this should be done gradually. However, in the event of an allergic or hypersensitivity reaction, rapid substitution of alternative therapy may be necessary. In this case, alternative therapy should be an antiepileptic drug not belonging to the hydantoin chemical class.

CARDIOVASCULAR DEPRESSION

Hypotension may occur, especially after IV administration at high doses and high rates of administration. Following administration of phenytoin, severe cardiovascular reactions and fatalities have been reported with atrial and ventricular conduction depression and ventricular fibrillation. Severe complications are most commonly encountered in elderly or gravely ill patients. Therefore, careful cardiac monitoring is needed when administering IV loading doses of fosphenytoin. Reduction in rate of administration or discontinuation of dosing may be needed.

Fosphenytoin should be used with caution in patients with hypotension and severe myocardial insufficiency.

RASH

Fosphenytoin should be discontinued if a skin rash appears. If the rash is exfoliative purpuric, or bullous, or if lupus erythematosus, Stevens-Johnson syndrome or toxic epidermal necrolysis is suspected, use of this drug should not be resumed and alternative therapy should be considered. If the rash is of a milder type (measles-like or scarlatiniform), therapy may be resumed after the rash has completely disappeared. If the rash recurs upon reinstitution of therapy, further fosphenytoin or phenytoin administration is contraindicated.

HEPATIC INJURY

Cases of acute hepatotoxicity, including infrequent cases of acute hepatic failure, have been reported with phenytoin. These incidents have been associated with a hypersensitivity syndrome characterized by fever, skin eruptions, and lymphadenopathy, and usually occur within the first 2 months of treatment. Other common manifestations include jaundice, hepatomegaly, elevated serum transaminase levels, leukocytosis, and eosinophilia. The clinical course of acute phenytoin hepatotoxicity ranges from prompt recovery to fatal outcomes. In these patients with acute hepatotoxicity, fosphenytoin should be immediately discontinued and not readministered.

HEMOPOIETIC SYSTEM

Hemopoietic complications, some fatal, have occasionally been reported in association with administration of phenytoin. These have included thrombocytopenia, leukopenia, granulocytopenia, agranulocytosis, and pancytopenia with or without bone marrow suppression.

There have been a number of reports that have suggested a relationship between phenytoin and the development of lymphadenopathy (local or generalized), including benign lymph node hyperplasia, pseudolymphoma, lymphoma, and Hodgkin's disease. Although a cause and effect relationship has not been established, the occurrence of lymphadenopathy indicates the need to differentiate such a condition from other types of lymph node pathology. Lymph node involvement may occur with or without symptoms and signs resembling serum sickness *e.g.,* fever, rash and liver involvement. In all cases of lymphadenopathy, follow-up observation for an extended period is indicated and every effort should be made to achieve seizure control using alternative antiepileptic drugs.

ALCOHOL USE

Acute alcohol intake may increase plasma phenytoin concentrations while chronic alcohol use may decrease plasma concentrations.

USAGE IN PREGNANCY

Clinical

Risks to Mother: An increase in seizure frequency may occur during pregnancy because of altered phenytoin pharmacokinetics. Periodic measurement of plasma phenytoin concentrations may be valuable in the management of pregnant women as a guide to appropriate adjustment of dosage (see PRECAUTIONS, Laboratory Tests). However, postpartum restoration of the original dosage will probably be indicated.

Risks to the Fetus: If this drug is used during pregnancy, or if the patient becomes pregnant while taking the drug, the patient should be apprised of the potential harm to the fetus.

Prenatal exposure to phenytoin may increase the risks for congenital malformations and other adverse developmental outcomes. Increased frequencies of major malformations (such as orofacial clefts and cardiac defects), minor anomalies (dysmorphic facial features, nail and digit hypoplasia), growth abnormalities (including microcephaly), and mental deficiency have been reported among children born to epileptic women who took phenytoin alone or in combination with other antiepileptic drugs during pregnancy. There have also been several reported cases of malignancies, including neuroblastoma, in children whose mothers received phenytoin during pregnancy. The overall incidence of malformations for children of epileptic women treated with antiepileptic drugs (phenytoin and/or others) during pregnancy is about 10%, or 2- to 3-fold that in the general population. However, the relative contributions of antiepileptic drugs and other factors associated with epilepsy to this increased risk are uncertain and in most cases it has not been possible to attribute specific developmental abnormalities to particular antiepileptic drugs.

Patients should consult with their physicians to weigh the risks and benefits of phenytoin during pregnancy.

Postpartum Period: A potentially life-threatening bleeding disorder related to decreased levels of vitamin K-dependent clotting factors may occur in newborns exposed to phenytoin *in utero.* This drug-induced condition can be prevented with vitamin K administration to the mother before delivery and to the neonate after birth.

Preclinical

Increased frequencies of malformations (brain, cardiovascular, digit, and skeletal anomalies), death, growth retardation, and functional impairment (chromodacryorrhea, hyperactivity, circling) were observed among the offspring of rats receiving fosphenytoin during pregnancy. Most of the adverse effects on embryo-fetal development occurred at doses of 33 mg PE/kg or higher (approximately 30% of the maximum human loading dose or higher on a mg/m^2 basis), which produced peak maternal plasma phenytoin concentrations of approximately 20 µg/ml or greater. Maternal toxicity was often associated with these doses and plasma concentrations, however, there is no evidence to suggest that the developmental effects were secondary to the maternal effects. The single occurrence of a rare brain malformation at a non-maternotoxic dose of 17 mg PE/kg (approximately 10% of the maximum human loading dose on a mg/m^2 basis) was also considered drug-induced. The developmental effects of fosphenytoin in rats were similar to those which have been reported following administration of phenytoin to pregnant rats.

No effects on embryo-fetal development were observed when rabbits were given up to 33 mg PE/kg of fosphenytoin (approximately 50% of the maximum human loading dose on a mg/m^2 basis) during pregnancy. Increased resorption and malformation rates have been reported following administration of phenytoin doses of 75 mg/kg or higher (approximately 120% of the maximum human loading dose or higher on a mg/m^2 basis) to pregnant rabbits.

PRECAUTIONS

GENERAL

Fosphenytoin Specific

Sensory Disturbances

Severe burning, itching, and/or paresthesia were reported by 7 of 16 normal volunteers administered IV fosphenytoin at a dose of 1200 mg PE at the maximum rate of administration (150 mg PE/min). The severe sensory disturbance lasted from 3-50 minutes in 6 of these subjects and for 14 hours in the seventh subject. In some cases, milder sensory disturbances persisted for as long as 24 hours. The location of the discomfort varied among subjects with the groin mentioned most frequently as an area of discomfort. In a separate cohort of 16 normal volunteers (taken from 2 other studies) who were administered IV fosphenytoin at a dose of 1200 mg PE at the maximum rate of administration (150 mg PE/min), none experienced severe disturbances, but most experienced mild to moderate itching or tingling.

Patients administered fosphenytoin at doses of 20 mg PE/kg at 150 mg PE/min are expected to experience discomfort of some degree. The occurrence and intensity of the discomfort can be lessened by slowing or temporarily stopping the infusion.

The effect of continuing infusion unaltered in the presence of these sensations is unknown. No permanent sequelae have been reported thus far. The pharmacologic basis for these positive sensory phenomena is unknown, but other phosphate ester drugs, which de-

F

liver smaller phosphate loads, have been associated with burning, itching, and/or tingling predominantly in the groin area.

Phosphate Load

The phosphate load provided by fosphenytoin (0.0037 mmol phosphate/mg PE fosphenytoin) should be considered when treating patients who require phosphate restriction, such as those with severe renal impairment.

IV Loading in Renal and/or Hepatic Disease or in Those With Hypoalbuminemia

After IV administration to patients with renal and/or hepatic disease, or in those with hypoalbuminemia, fosphenytoin clearance to phenytoin may be increased without a similar increase in phenytoin clearance. This has the potential to increase the frequency and severity of adverse events (see CLINICAL PHARMACOLOGY, Special Populations and DOSAGE AND ADMINISTRATION, Dosing in Special Populations).

Phenytoin Associated

Fosphenytoin is *not* indicated for the treatment of *absence seizures.*

A small percentage of individuals who have been treated with phenytoin have been shown to metabolize the drug slowly. *Slow metabolism* may be due to limited enzyme availability and lack of induction; it appears to be genetically determined.

Phenytoin and other hydantoins are contraindicated in patients who have experienced phenytoin hypersensitivity. Additionally, caution should be exercised if using structurally similar (*e.g.* barbiturates, succinimides, oxazolidinediones, and other related compounds) in these same patients.

Phenytoin has been infrequently associated with the exacerbation of *porphyria.* Caution should be exercised when fosphenytoin is used in patients with this disease.

Hyperplycemia, resulting from phenytoin's inhibitory effect on insulin release has been reported. Phenytoin may also raise the serum glucose concentrations in diabetic patients. Plasma concentrations of phenytoin sustained above the optimal range may produce confusional states referred to as "delirium", "psychosis", or "encephalopathy", or rarely, irreversible cerebellar dysfunction. Accordingly, at the first sign of *acute toxicity,* determination of plasma phenytoin concentrations is recommended (see Laboratory Tests). Fosphenytoin dose reduction is indicated if phenytoin concentrations are excessive; if symptoms persist, administration of fosphenytoin should be discontinued.

The liver is the primary site of biotransformation of phenytoin; patients with impaired liver function, elderly patients, or those who are gravely ill may show early signs of toxicity.

Phenytoin and other hydantoins are not indicated for seizures due to hypoglycemic or other metabolic causes. Appropriate diagnostic procedures should be performed as indicated.

Phenytoin has the potential to lower serum folate levels.

LABORATORY TESTS

Phenytoin doses are usually selected to attain therapeutic plasma total phenytoin concentrations of 10-20 μg/ml, (unbound phenytoin concentrations of 1-2 μg/ml). Following fosphenytoin administration, it is recommended that phenytoin concentrations not be monitored until conversion to phenytoin is essentially complete. This occurs within approximately 2 hours after the end of IV infusion and 4 hours after IM injection.

Prior to complete conversion commonly used immunoanalytical techniques such as TDx/TDxFLx (fluorescence polarization) and Emit 2000 (enzyme multiplied), may significantly overestimate plasma phenytoin concentrations because of cross-reactivity with fosphenytoin. The error is dependent on plasma phenytoin and fosphenytoin concentration (influenced by fosphenytoin dose, route and rate of administration, and time of sampling relative to dosing), and analytical method. Chromatographic assay methods accurately quantitate phenytoin concentrations in biological fluids in the presence of fosphenytoin. Prior to complete conversion, blood samples for phenytoin monitoring should be collected in tubes containing EDTA as an anticoagulant to minimize *ex vivo* conversion of fosphenytoin to phenytoin. However, even with specific assay methods, phenytoin concentrations measured before conversion of fosphenytoin is complete will not reflect phenytoin concentrations ultimately achieved.

DRUG/LABORATORY TEST INTERACTIONS

Phenytoin may decrease serum concentrations of T_4. It may also produce artifactually low results in dexamethasone or metyrapone tests. Phenytoin may also cause increased serum concentrations of glucose, alkaline phosphatase, and gamma glutamyl transpeptidase (GGT).

Care should be taken when using immunoanalytical methods to measure plasma phenytoin concentrations following fosphenytoin administration (see Laboratory Tests).

CARCINOGENESIS, MUTAGENESIS, AND IMPAIRMENT OF FERTILITY

The carcinogenic potential of fosphenytoin has not been studied. Assessment of the carcinogenic potential of phenytoin in mice and rats is ongoing.

Structural chromosome aberration frequency in cultured V79 Chinese hamster lung cells was increased by exposure to fosphenytoin in the presence of metabolic activation. No evidence of mutagenicity was observed in bacteria (Ames test) or Chinese hamster lung cells *in vitro,* and no evidence for clastogenic activity was observed in an *in vivo* mouse bone marrow micronucleus test.

No effects on fertility were noted in rats of either sex given fosphenytoin. Maternal toxicity and altered estrous cycles, delayed mating, prolonged gestation length, and developmental toxicity were observed following administration of fosphenytoin during mating, gestation, and lactation at doses of 50 mg PE/kg or higher (approximately 40% of the maximum human loading dose or higher on a mg/m^2 basis).

PREGNANCY CATEGORY D

See WARNINGS.

USE IN NURSING MOTHERS

It is not known whether fosphenytoin is excreted in human milk.

Following administration of phenytoin sodium, phenytoin appears to be excreted in low concentrations in human milk. Therefore, breast-feeding is not recommended for women receiving fosphenytoin.

PEDIATRIC USE

The safety of fosphenytoin in pediatric patients has not been established.

GERIATRIC USE

No systematic studies in geriatric patients have been conducted. Phenytoin clearance tends to decrease with increasing age (see CLINICAL PHARMACOLOGY, Special Populations).

DRUG INTERACTIONS

No drugs are known to interfere with the conversion of fosphenytoin to phenytoin. Conversion could be affected by alterations in the level of phosphatase activity, but given the abundance and wide distribution of phosphatases in the body it is unlikely that drugs would affect this activity enough to affect conversion of fosphenytoin to phenytoin. Drugs highly bound to albumin could increase the unbound fraction of fosphenytoin. Although, it is unknown whether this could result in clinically significant effects, caution is advised when administering fosphenytoin with other drugs that significantly bind to serum albumin.

The pharmacokinetics and protein binding of fosphenytoin, phenytoin, and diazepam were not altered when diazepam and fosphenytoin were concurrently administered in single submaximal doses.

The most significant drug interactions following administration of fosphenytoin are expected to occur with drugs that interact with phenytoin. Phenytoin is extensively bound to serum plasma proteins and is prone to competitive displacement. Phenytoin is metabolized by hepatic cytochrome P450 enzymes and is particularly susceptible to inhibitory drug interactions because it is subject to saturable metabolism. Inhibition of metabolism may produce significant increases in circulating phenytoin concentrations and enhance the risk of drug toxicity. Phenytoin is a potent inducer of hepatic drug-metabolizing enzymes.

The most commonly occurring drug interactions are listed below:

Drugs that may increase plasma phenytoin concentrations include: Acute alcohol intake, amiodarone, chloramphenicol, chlordiazepoxide, cimetidine, diazepam, dicumarol, disulfiram, estrogens, ethosuximide, fluoxetine, H_2-antagonists, halothane, isoniazid, methylphenidate, phenothiazines, phenylbutazone, salicylates, succinimides, sulfonamides, tolbutamide, trazodone.

Drugs that may decrease plasma phenytoin concentrations include: Carbamazepine, chronic alcohol abuse, reserpine.

Drugs that may either increase or decrease plasma phenytoin concentrations include: Phenobarbital, valproic acid, and sodium valproate. Similarly, the effects of phenytoin on phenobarbital, valproic acid and sodium plasma valproate concentrations are unpredictable.

Although not a true drug interaction, tricyclic antidepressants may precipitate seizures in susceptible patients and fosphenytoin dosage may need to be adjusted.

Drugs whose efficacy is impaired by phenytoin include: Anticoagulants, corticosteroids, coumarin, digitoxin, doxycycline, estrogens, furosemide, oral contraceptives, rifampin, quinidine, theophylline, vitamin D.

Monitoring of plasma phenytoin concentrations may be helpful when possible drug interactions are suspected (see Laboratory Tests).

ADVERSE REACTIONS

The more important adverse clinical events caused by the IV use of fosphenytoin or phenytoin are cardiovascular collapse and/or central nervous system depression. Hypotension can occur when either drug is administered rapidly by the IV route. The rate of administration is very important; for fosphenytoin, it should not exceed 150 mg PE/min.

The adverse clinical events most commonly observed with the use of fosphenytoin in clinical trials were nystagmus, dizziness, pruritus, paresthesia, headache, somnolence, and ataxia. With two exceptions, these events are commonly associated with the administration of IV phenytoin. Paresthesia and pruritus, however, were seen much more often following fosphenytoin administration and occurred more often with IV fosphenytoin administration than with IM fosphenytoin administration. These events were dose and rate related; most alert patients (41 of 64; 64%) administered doses of ≥15 mg PE/kg at 150 mg PE/min experienced discomfort of some degree. These sensations, generally described as itching, burning or tingling, were usually not at the infusion site. The location of the discomfort varied with the groin mentioned most frequently as a site of involvement. The paresthesia and pruritus were transient events that occurred within several minutes of the start of infusion and generally resolved within 10 minutes after completion of fosphenytoin infusion. Some patients experienced symptoms for hours. These events did not increase in severity with repeated administration. Concurrent adverse events or clinical laboratory change suggesting an allergic process were not seen (see PRECAUTIONS,General, Fosphenytoin Specific, Sensory Disturbances).

Approximately 2% of the 859 individuals who received fosphenytoin in premarketing clinical trials discontinued treatment because of an adverse event. The adverse events most commonly associated with withdrawal were pruritus (0.5%), hypotension (0.3%), and bradycardia (0.2%).

DOSE AND RATE DEPENDENCY OF ADVERSE EVENTS FOLLOWING LV FOSPHENYTOIN

The incidence of adverse events tended to increase as both dose and infusion rate increased. In particular, at doses of ≥15 mg PE/kg and rates ≥150 mg PE/min, transient pruritus, tinnitus, nystagmus, somnolence, and ataxia occurred 2-3 times more often than at lower doses or rates.

INCIDENCE IN CONTROLLED CLINICAL TRIALS

All adverse events were recorded during the trials by the clinical investigators using terminology of their own choosing. Similar types of events were grouped into standardized categories using modified COSTART dictionary terminology. These categories are used in the tables and listings with the frequencies representing the proportion of individuals exposed to fosphenytoin or comparative therapy.

The prescriber should be aware that these figures cannot be used to predict the frequency of adverse events in the course of usual medical practice where patient characteristics and other factors may differ from those prevailing during clinical studies. Similarly, the cited frequencies cannot be directly compared with figures obtained from other clinical investigations involving different treatments, uses or investigators. An inspection of these frequencies, however, does provide the prescribing physician with one basis to estimate the relative contribution of drug and nondrug factors to the adverse event incidences in the population studied.

Incidence in Controlled Clinical Trials — IV Administration to Patients With Epilepsy or Neurosurgical Patients

TABLE 2 lists treatment-emergent adverse events that occurred in at least 2% of patients treated with IV fosphenytoin at the maximum dose and rate in a randomized, double blind, controlled clinical trial where the rates for phenytoin and fosphenytoin administration would have resulted in equivalent systemic exposure to phenytoin.

TABLE 2 *Treatment-Emergent Adverse Event Incidence Following IV Administration at the Maximum Dose and Rate to Patients With Epilepsy or Neurosurgical Patients (events in at least 2% of fosphenytoin-treated patients)*

Body System Adverse Event	IV Fosphenytoin n=90	IV Phenytoin n=22
Body as a Whole		
Pelvic pain	4.4%	0.0%
Asthenia	2.2%	0.0%
Back pain	2.2%	0.0%
Headache	2.2%	4.5%
Cardiovascular		
Hypotension	7.7%	9.1%
Vasodilatation	5.6%	4.5%
Tachycardia	2.2%	0.0%
Digestive		
Nausea	8.9%	13.6%
Tongue disorder	4.4%	0.0%
Dry mouth	4.4%	4.5%
Vomiting	2.2%	9.1%
Nervous		
Nystagmus	44.4%	59.1%
Dizziness	31.1%	27.3%
Somnolence	21.0%	27.3%
Ataxia	11.1%	18.2%
Stupor	7.7%	4.5%
Incoordination	4.4%	4.5%
Paresthesia	4.4%	0.0%
Extrapyramidal syndrome	4.4%	0.0%
Tremor	3.3%	9.1%
Agitation	3.3%	0.0%
Hypesthesia	2.2%	9.1%
Dysarthria	2.2%	0.0%
Vertigo	2.2%	0.0%
Brain edema	2.2%	4.5%
Skin and Appendages		
Pruritus	48.9%	4.5%
Special Senses		
Tinnitus	8.9%	9.1%
Diplopia	3.3%	0.0%
Taste perversion	3.3%	0.0%
Amblyopia	2.2%	9.1%
Deafness	2.2%	0.0%

Incidence in Controlled Trials — IM Administration to Patients With Epilepsy

TABLE 3 lists treatment-emergent adverse events that occurred in at least 2% of fosphenytoin-treated patients in a double-blind, randomized, controlled clinical trial of adult epilepsy patients receiving either IM fosphenytoin substituted for oral phenytoin sodium or continuing oral phenytoin sodium. Both treatments were administered for 5 days.

TABLE 3 *Treatment-Emergent Adverse Event Incidence Following Substitution of IM Fosphenytoin for Oral Phenytoin Sodium in Patients With Epilepsy (events in at least 2% of fosphenytoin-treated patients)*

Body System Adverse Event	IM Fosphenytoin n=179	Oral Phenytoin Sodium n=61
Body as a Whole		
Headache	8.9%	4.9%
Asthenia	3.9%	3.3%
Accidental injury	3.4%	6.6%
Digestive		
Nausea	4.5%	0.0%
Vomiting	2.8%	0.0%
Hematologic and Lymphatic		
Ecchymosis	7.3%	4.9%
Nervous		
Nystagmus	15.1%	8.2%
Tremor	9.5%	13.1%
Ataxia	8.4%	8.2%
Incoordination	7.8%	4.9%
Somnolence	6.7%	9.8%
Dizziness	5.0%	3.3%
Paresthesia	3.9%	3.3%
Reflexes decreased	2.8%	4.9%
Skin and Appendages		
Pruritus	2.8%	0.0%

ADVERSE EVENTS DURING ALL CLINICAL TRIALS

Fosphenytoin has been administered to 859 individuals during all clinical trials. All adverse events seen at least twice are listed in the following except those already included in previous tables and listings. Events are further classified within body system categories and enumerated in order of increasing frequency using the following definitions: *frequent* adverse events are defined as those occurring in greater than 1/100 individuals *infrequent* adverse events are those occurring in 1/100 to 1/1000 individuals.

Body as a Whole: *Frequent:* Fever, injection-site reaction, infection, chills, face edema, injection-site pain. *Infrequent:* Sepsis, injection-site inflammation, injection-site edema, injection-site hemorrhage, flu syndrome, malaise, generalized edema, shock, photosensitivity reaction, cachexia, cryptococcosis.

Cardiovascular: *Frequent:* Hypertension. *Infrequent:* Cardiac arrest, migraine, syncope cerebral hemorrhage, palpitation, sinus bradycardia, atrial flutter, bundle branch block, cardiomegaly, cerebral infarct, postural hypotension, pulmonary embolus, QT interval prolongation, thrombophlebitis, ventricular extrasystoles, congestive heart failure.

Digestive: *Frequent:* Constipation. *Infrequent:* Dyspepsia, diarrhea, anorexia, gastrointestinal hemorrhage, increased salivation, liver function tests abnormal, tenesmus, tongue edema, dysphagia, flatulence, gastritis, ileus.

Endocrine: *Infrequent:* Diabetes insipidus.

Hematologic and Lymphatic: *Infrequent:* Thrombocytopenia, anemia, leukocytosis, cyanosis, hypochromic anemia, leukopenia, lymphadenopathy, petechia.

Metabolic and Nutritional: *Frequent:* Hypokalemia. *Infrequent:* Hyperglycemia, hypophosphatemia, alkalosis, acidosis, dehydration, hyperkalemia, ketosis.

Musculoskeletal: *Frequent:* Myasthenia. *Infrequent:* Myopathy, leg cramps, arthralgia, myalgia.

Nervous: *Frequent:* Reflexes increased, speech disorder, dysarthria, intracranial hypertension, thinking abnormal, nervousness, hypesthesia. *Infrequent:* Confusion, twitching, Babinski sign positive, circumoral paresthesia, hemiplegia, hypotonia, convulsion, extrapyramidal syndrome, insomnia, meningitis, depersonalization, CNS depression, depression, hypokinesia, hyperkinesia, brain edema, paralysis, psychosis, aphasia, emotional lability, coma, hyperesthesia, myoclonus, personality disorder, acute brain syndrome, encephalitis, subdural hematoma, encephalopathy, hostility, akathisia, amnesia, neurosis.

Respiratory: *Frequent:* Pneumonia. *Infrequent:* Pharyngitis, sinusitis, hyperventilation, rhinitis, apnea, aspiration pneumonia, asthma, dyspnea, atelectasis, cough increased, sputum increased, epistaxis, hypoxia, pneumothorax, hemoptysis, bronchitis.

Skin and Appendages: *Frequent:* Rash. *Infrequent:* Maculopapular rash, urticaria, sweating, skin discoloration, contact dermatitis, pustular rash, skin nodule.

Special Senses: *Frequent:* Taste perversion. *Infrequent:* Deafness, visual field defect, eye pain, conjunctivitis, photophobia, hyperacusis, mydriasis, parosmia, ear pain, taste loss.

Urogenital: *Infrequent:* Urinary retention, oliguria, dysuria, vaginitis, albuminuria, genital edema, kidney failure, polyuria, urethral pain, urinary incontinence, vaginal moniliasis.

DOSAGE AND ADMINISTRATION

The dose, concentration in dosing solutions, and infusion rate of IV fosphenytoin is expressed as phenytoin sodium equivalents (PE) to avoid the need to perform molecular weight-based adjustments when converting between fosphenytoin and phenytoin sodium doses. Fosphenytoin should always be prescribed and dispensed in phenytoin sodium equivalent units (PE). Fosphenytoin has important differences in administration from those for parenteral phenytoin sodium (see below).

Products with particulate matter or discoloration should not be used. Prior to IV infusion, dilute fosphenytoin in 5% dextrose or 0.9% saline solution for injection to a concentration ranging from 1.5 to 25 mg PE/ml.

STATUS EPILEPTICUS

The loading dose of fosphenytoin is 15-20 mg PE/kg administered at 100-150 mg PE/min.

Because of the risk of hypotension, fosphenytoin should be administered no faster than 150 mg PE/min. Continuous monitoring of the electrocardiogram, blood pressure, and respiratory function is essential and the patient should be observed throughout the period where maximal serum phenytoin concentrations occur, approximately 10-20 minutes after the end of fosphenytoin infusions.

Because the full antiepileptic effect of phenytoin whether given as fosphenytoin or parenteral phenytoin, is not immediate, other measures, including concomitant administration of an IV benzodiazepine, will usually be necessary for the control of status epilepticus.

The loading dose should be followed by maintenance doses of fosphenytoin, or phenytoin either orally or parenterally.

If administration of fosphenytoin does not terminate seizures, the use of other anticonvulsants and other appropriate measures should be considered.

IM fosphenytoin should not be used in the treatment of status epilepticus because therapeutic phenytoin concentrations may not be reached as quickly as with IV administration. If IV access is impossible, loading doses of fosphenytoin have been given by the IM route for other indications.

NONEMERGENT LOADING AND MAINTENANCE DOSING

The loading dose of fosphenytoin is 10-20 mg PE/kg given IV or IM. The rate of administration for IV fosphenytoin should be no greater than 150 mg PE/min. Continuous monitoring of the electrocardiogram, blood pressure, and respiratory function is essential and the patient should be observed throughout the period where maximal serum phenytoin concentrations occur, approximately 10-20 minutes after the end of fosphenytoin infusions.

The initial daily maintenance dose of fosphenytoin is 4-6 mg PE/kg/day.

IM OR IV SUBSTITUTION FOR ORAL PHENYTOIN THERAPY

Fosphenytoin can be substituted for oral phenytoin sodium therapy at the same total daily dose.

Phenytoin sodium capsules are approximately 90% bioavailable by the oral route. Phenytoin, supplied as fosphenytoin, is 100% bioavailable by both the IM and IV routes. For this reason, plasma phenytoin concentrations may increase modestly when IM or IV fosphenytoin is substituted for oral phenytoin sodium therapy.

The rate of administration for IV fosphenytoin should be no greater than 150 mg PE/min.

In controlled trials, IM fosphenytoin was administered as a single daily dose utilizing either 1 or 2 injection sites. Some patients may require more frequent dosing.

DOSING IN SPECIAL POPULATIONS

Patients With Renal or Hepatic Disease

Due to an increased fraction of unbound phenytoin in patients with renal or hepatic disease, or in those with hypoalbuminemia, the interpretation of total phenytoin plasma concentrations should be made with caution (see CLINICAL PHARMACOLOGY, Special Populations). Unbound phenytoin concentrations may be more useful in these patient populations. After IV fosphenytoin administration to patients with renal and/or hepatic disease, or in those with hypoalbuminemia, fosphenytoin clearance to phenytoin may be increased without a similar increase in phenytoin clearance. This has the potential to increase the frequency and severity of adverse events (see PRECAUTIONS).

F

Elderly Patients

Age does not have a significant impact on the pharmacokinetics of fosphenytoin following fosphenytoin administration. Phenytoin clearance is decreased slightly in elderly patients and lower or less frequent dosing may be required.

Pediatric

The safety of fosphenytoin in pediatric patients has not been established.

HOW SUPPLIED

Cerebyx injection is supplied as follows:

Each 10 ml vial contains fosphenytoin sodium 750 mg equivalent to 500 mg of phenytoin sodium.

Each 2 ml vial contains fosphenytoin sodium 150 mg equivalent to 100 mg of phenytoin sodium.

Both sizes of vials contain tromethamine (TRIS), hydrochloric acid, or sodium hydroxide, and water for injection.

Fosphenytoin should always be prescribed in phenytoin sodium equivalent units (PE) (see DOSAGE AND ADMINISTRATION).

Storage: Store under refrigeration at 2-8°C (36-46°F). The product should not be stored at room temperature for more than 48 hours. Vials that develop particulate matter should not be used.

PRODUCT LISTING - EQUIVALENTS NOT AVAILABLE

Solution - Injectable - 50 mg/ml

2 ml x 25	$533.25	CEREBYX, Parke-Davis	00071-4007-05
10 ml x 10	$639.90	CEREBYX, Parke-Davis	00071-4008-10

Frovatriptan Succinate (003561)

For related information, see the comparative table section in Appendix A.

Categories: Headache, migraine; FDA Approved 2001 Nov; Pregnancy Category C
Drug Classes: Serotonin receptor agonists
Brand Names: Frova
Cost of Therapy: $15.41 (Migraine Headache; Frova; 2.5 mg; 1 tablet/day; 1 day supply)

DESCRIPTION

Frova (frovatriptan succinate) tablets contain frovatriptan succinate, a selective 5-hydroxytryptamine1 ($5\text{-}HT_{1B/1D}$) receptor subtype agonist, as the active ingredient.

Frovatriptan succinate is chemically designated as R-(+) 3-methylamino-6-carboxamido-1,2,3,4-tetrahydrocarbazole monosuccinate monohydrate.

The empirical formula is $C_{14}H_{17}N_3O{\cdot}C_4H_6O_4{\cdot}H_2O$, representing a molecular weight of 379.4.

Frovatriptan succinate is a white to off-white powder that is soluble in water. Each Frova tablet for oral administration contains 3.91 mg frovatriptan succinate, equivalent to 2.5 mg of frovatriptan base. Each tablet also contains the inactive ingredients lactose, microcrystalline cellulose, colloidal silicon dioxide, sodium starch glycolate, magnesium stearate, hydroxypropylmethylcellulose, polyethylene glycol 3000, triacetin, and titanium dioxide.

CLINICAL PHARMACOLOGY

MECHANISM OF ACTION

Frovatriptan is a 5-HT receptor agonist that binds with high affinity for $5\text{-}HT_{1B}$ and $5\text{-}HT_{1D}$ receptors. Frovatriptan has no significant effects on $GABA_A$ mediated channel activity and has no significant affinity for benzodiazepine binding sites.

Frovatriptan is believed to act on extracerebral, intracranial arteries and to inhibit excessive dilation of these vessels in migraine. In anesthetized dogs and cats, intravenous administration of frovatriptan produced selective constriction of the carotid vascular bed and had no effect on blood pressure (both species) or coronary resistance (in dogs).

PHARMACOKINETICS

Mean maximum blood concentrations (C_{max}) in patients are achieved approximately 2-4 hours after administration of a single oral dose of frovatriptan 2.5 mg. The absolute bioavailability of an oral dose of frovatriptan 2.5 mg in healthy subjects is about 20% in males and 30% in females. Food has no significant effect on the bioavailability of frovatriptan, but delays T_{max} by 1 hour.

Binding of frovatriptan to serum proteins is low (approximately 15%). Reversible binding to blood cells at equilibrium is approximately 60%, resulting in a blood:plasma ratio of about 2:1 in both males and females. The mean steady state volume of distribution of frovatriptan following intravenous administration of 0.8 mg is 4.2 L/kg in males and 3.0 L/kg in females.

In vitro, cytochrome P450 1A2 appears to be the principal enzyme involved in the metabolism of frovatriptan. Following administration of a single oral dose of radiolabeled frovatriptan 2.5 mg to healthy male and female subjects, 32% of the dose was recovered in urine and 62% in feces. Radiolabeled compounds excreted in urine were unchanged frovatriptan, hydroxylated frovatriptan, N-acetyl desmethyl frovatriptan, hydroxylated N-acetyl desmethyl frovatriptan and desmethyl frovatriptan, together with several other minor metabolites. Desmethyl frovatriptan has lower affinity for $5\text{-}HT_{1B/1D}$ receptors compared to the parent compound. The N-acetyl desmethyl metabolite has no significant affinity for 5-HT receptors. The activity of the other metabolites is unknown.

After an intravenous dose, mean clearance of frovatriptan was 220 and 130 ml/min in males and females, respectively. Renal clearance accounted for about 40% (82 ml/min) and 45% (60 ml/min) of total clearance in males and females, respectively. The mean terminal elimination half-life of frovatriptan in both males and females is approximately 26 hours.

The pharmacokinetics of frovatriptan are similar in migraine patients and healthy subjects.

SPECIAL POPULATIONS

Age

Mean AUC of frovatriptan was 1.5- to 2-fold higher in healthy elderly subjects (age 65-77 years) compared to those in healthy younger subjects (age 21-37 years). There was no difference in T_{max} or $T_{1/2}$ between the two populations.

Gender

There was no difference in the mean terminal elimination half-life of frovatriptan in males and females. Bioavailability was higher, and systemic exposure to frovatriptan was approximately 2-fold greater, in females than males, irrespective of age.

Renal Impairment

Since less than 10% of frovatriptan succinate is excreted in urine after an oral dose, it is unlikely that the exposure to frovatriptan will be affected by renal impairment. The pharmacokinetics of frovatriptan following a single oral dose of 2.5 mg was not different in patients with renal impairment (5 males and 6 females, creatinine clearance 16-73 ml/min) and in subjects with normal renal function.

Hepatic Impairment

There is no clinical or pharmacokinetic experience with frovatriptan succinate in patients with severe hepatic impairment. The AUC in subjects with mild (Child-Pugh 5-6) to moderate (Child-Pugh 7-9) hepatic impairment is about twice as high as the AUC in young, healthy subjects, but within the range found among normal elderly subjects.

Race

The effect of race on the pharmacokinetics of frovatriptan has not been examined.

DRUG INTERACTIONS

See also DRUG INTERACTIONS.

Frovatriptan is not an inhibitor of human monoamine oxidase (MAO) enzymes or cytochrome P450 (isozymes 1A2, 2C9, 2C19, 2D6, 2E1, 3A4) *in vitro* at concentrations up to 250- to 500-fold higher than the highest blood concentrations observed in man at a dose of 2.5 mg. No induction of drug metabolizing enzymes was observed following multiple dosing of frovatriptan to rats or on addition to human hepatocytes *in vitro*. Although no clinical studies have been performed, it is unlikely that frovatriptan will affect the metabolism of co-administered drugs metabolized by these mechanisms.

Oral Contraceptives: Retrospective analysis of pharmacokinetic data from females across trials indicated that the mean C_{max} and AUC of frovatriptan are 30% higher in those subjects taking oral contraceptives compared to those not taking oral contraceptives.

Ergotamine: The AUC and C_{max} of frovatriptan (2×2.5 mg dose) were reduced by approximately 25% when co-administered with ergotamine tartrate.

Propranolol: Propranolol increased the AUC of frovatriptan 2.5 mg in males by 60% and in females by 29%. The C_{max} of frovatriptan was increased 23% in males and 16% in females in the presence of propranolol. The T_{max} as well as half-life of frovatriptan, though slightly longer in the females, were not affected by concomitant administration of propranolol.

Moclobemide: The pharmacokinetic profile of frovatriptan was unaffected when a single oral dose of frovatriptan 2.5 mg was administered to healthy female subjects receiving the MAO-A inhibitor, moclobemide, at an oral dose of 150 mg bid for 8 days.

INDICATIONS AND USAGE

Frovatriptan succinate is indicated for the acute treatment of migraine attacks with or without aura in adults.

Frovatriptan succinate is not intended for the prophylactic therapy of migraine or for use in the management of hemiplegic or basilar migraine (see CONTRAINDICATIONS). The safety and effectiveness of frovatriptan succinate have not been established for cluster headache, which is present in an older, predominately male, population.

CONTRAINDICATIONS

Frovatriptan succinate should not be given to patients with ischemic heart disease (*e.g.*, angina pectoris, history of myocardial infarction, or documented silent ischemia), or to patients who have symptoms or findings consistent with ischemic heart disease, coronary artery vasospasm, including Prinzmetal's variant angina or other significant underlying cardiovascular disease (see WARNINGS).

Frovatriptan succinate should not be given to patients with cerebrovascular syndromes including (but not limited to) strokes of any type as well as transient ischemic attacks.

Frovatriptan succinate should not be given to patients with peripheral vascular disease including (but is not limited to) ischemic bowel disease (see WARNINGS).

Frovatriptan succinate should not be given to patients with uncontrolled hypertension (see WARNINGS).

Frovatriptan succinate should not be administered to patients with hemiplegic or basilar migraine.

Frovatriptan succinate should not be used within 24 hours of treatment with another 5-HT_1 agonist, an ergotamine containing or ergot-type medication such as dihydroergotamine (DHE) or methysergide.

Frovatriptan succinate is contraindicated in patients who are hypersensitive to frovatriptan or any of the inactive ingredients in the tablets.

WARNINGS

Frovatriptan succinate should only be used where a clear diagnosis of migraine has been established.

RISK OF MYOCARDIAL ISCHEMIA AND/OR INFARCTION AND OTHER ADVERSE CARDIAC EVENTS

Because of the potential of this class of compound (5-HT_1 agonists) to cause coronary vasospasm, frovatriptan should not be given to patients with documented ischemic or vasospastic coronary artery disease (CAD) (see CONTRAINDICATIONS). It is strongly recommended that frovatriptan not be given to patients in whom unrecognized CAD is predicted by the presence of risk factors (*e.g.*, hypertension, hypercholesterolemia, smoker, obesity, diabetes, strong family history of CAD, female with surgical or physiological menopause, or male over 40 years of age) unless a cardiovascular evaluation provides satisfactory clinical evidence that the patient is reasonably free of coronary artery and ischemic myocardial disease or other significant underlying cardiovascular disease. The sensitivity of cardiac diagnostic procedures to detect cardiovascular disease or predisposition to coronary artery vasospasm is modest, at best. If, during the cardiovascular evaluation, the patient's medical history, electrocardiographic, or other investigations reveal findings indicative of, or consistent with, coronary artery vasospasm or myocardial ischemia, frovatriptan should not be administered (see CONTRAINDICATIONS).

For patients with risk factors predictive of CAD, who are determined to have a satisfactory cardiovascular evaluation, it is strongly recommended that administration of the first dose of frovatriptan take place in the setting of a physician's office or similar medically staffed and equipped facility unless the patient has previously received frovatriptan.

Because cardiac ischemia can occur in the absence of clinical symptoms, consideration should be given to obtaining on the first occasion of use an electrocardiogram (ECG) during the interval immediately following administration of frovatriptan succinate in these patients with risk factors.

It is recommended that patients who are intermittent long-term users of 5-HT_1 agonists, including frovatriptan succinate, and who have or acquire risk factors predictive of CAD, as described above, undergo periodic cardiovascular evaluation as they continue to use frovatriptan succinate.

The systematic approach described above is intended to reduce the likelihood that patients with unrecognized cardiovascular disease would be inadvertently exposed to frovatriptan.

CARDIAC EVENTS AND FATALITIES WITH 5-HT_1 AGONISTS

Serious adverse cardiac events, including acute myocardial infarction, life-threatening disturbances of cardiac rhythm and death have been reported within a few hours of administration of 5-HT_1 agonists. Considering the extent of use of 5-HT_1 agonists in patients with migraine, the incidence of these events is extremely low.

Premarketing Experience With Frovatriptan: Among more than 3000 patients with migraine who participated in premarketing clinical trials of frovatriptan succinate, no deaths or serious cardiac events were reported which were related to the use of frovatriptan succinate.

CEREBROVASCULAR EVENTS AND FATALITIES WITH 5-HT_1 AGONISTS

Cerebral hemorrhage, subarachnoid hemorrhage, stroke and other cerebrovascular events have been reported in patients treated with 5-HT_1 agonists; and some have resulted in fatalities. In a number of cases, it appears possible that the cerebrovascular events were primary, the agonist having been administered in the incorrect belief that the symptoms experienced were a consequence of migraine, when they were not. It should be noted that patients with migraine may be at increased risk of certain cerebrovascular events (*e.g.*, stroke, hemorrhage, transient ischemic attack).

OTHER VASOSPASM-RELATED EVENTS

5-HT_1 agonists may cause vasospastic reactions other than coronary artery spasm. Both peripheral vascular ischemia and colonic ischemia with abdominal pain and bloody diarrhea have been reported with 5-HT_1 agonists.

EFFECTS ON BLOOD PRESSURE

In young healthy subjects, there were statistically significant increases in systolic and diastolic blood pressure after single doses of 80 mg frovatriptan (32 times the clinical dose) and above. These increases were transient, resolved spontaneously and were not clinically significant. At the recommended dose of 2.5 mg, transient changes in systolic blood pressure were recorded in some elderly subjects (65-77 years). Any increases were generally small, resolved spontaneously, and blood pressure remained within the normal range. Frovatriptan is contraindicated in patients with uncontrolled hypertension (see CONTRAINDICATIONS).

An 18% increase in mean pulmonary artery pressure was seen following dosing with another 5-HT_1 agonist in a study evaluating subjects undergoing cardiac catheterization.

PRECAUTIONS

GENERAL

As with other 5-HT_1 agonists, sensations of pain, tightness, pressure and heaviness have been reported in the chest, throat, neck and jaw after treatment with frovatriptan succinate. These events have not been associated with arrhythmias or ischemic ECG changes in clinical trials with frovatriptan succinate. Because 5-HT_1 agonists may cause coronary vasospasm, patients who experience signs or symptoms suggestive of angina following dosing should be evaluated for the presence of CAD. Patients shown to have CAD and those with Prinzmetal's variant angina should not receive 5-HT_1 agonists (see CONTRAINDICATIONS). Patients who experience other symptoms or signs suggestive of decreased arterial flow, such as ischemic bowel syndrome or Raynaud's syndrome following the use of any 5-HT_1 agonist are candidates for further evaluation. If a patient has no response for the first migraine attack treated with frovatriptan succinate, the diagnosis of migraine should be reconsidered before frovatriptan is administered to treat any subsequent attacks.

HEPATICALLY IMPAIRED PATIENTS

There is no clinical or pharmacokinetic experience with frovatriptan succinate in patients with severe hepatic impairment. The AUC of frovatriptan in patients with mild (Child-Pugh 5-6) to moderate (Child-Pugh 7-9) hepatic impairment was about twice that of young, healthy subjects, but within the range observed in healthy elderly subjects and was considerably lower than the values attained with higher doses of frovatriptan (up to 40 mg), which were not associated with any serious adverse effects. Therefore, no dosage adjustment is necessary when frovatriptan succinate is given to patients with mild to moderate hepatic impairment (see CLINICAL PHARMACOLOGY, Special Populations).

BINDING TO MELANIN-CONTAINING TISSUES

When pigmented rats were given a single oral dose of 5 mg/kg of radiolabeled frovatriptan, the radioactivity in the eye after 28 days was 87% of the value measured after 8 hours. This suggests that frovatriptan and/or its metabolites may bind to the melanin of the eye. Because there could be accumulation in melanin rich tissues over time, this raises the possibility that frovatriptan could cause toxicity in these tissues after extended use. However, no effects on the retina related to treatment with frovatriptan were noted in the toxicity studies. Although no systematic monitoring of ophthalmologic function was undertaken in clinical trials and no specific recommendations for ophthalmologic monitoring are made, prescribers should be aware of the possibility of long-term ophthalmologic effects.

INFORMATION FOR THE PATIENT

Physicians should instruct their patients to read the patient package insert that is distributed with the prescription before taking frovatriptan succinate.

LABORATORY TESTS

No specific laboratory tests are recommended for monitoring patients prior to and/or after treatment with frovatriptan succinate.

DRUG/LABORATORY TEST INTERACTIONS

Frovatriptan succinate is not known to interfere with commonly employed clinical laboratory tests.

CARCINOGENESIS, MUTAGENESIS, AND IMPAIRMENT OF FERTILITY

Carcinogenesis

The carcinogenic potential of frovatriptan was evaluated in an 84 week study in mice (4, 13, and 40 mg/kg/day), a 104 week study in rats (8.5, 27 and 85 mg/kg/day), and a 26 week study in p53(+/-) transgenic mice (20, 62.5, 200, and 400 mg/kg/day). Although the maximum tolerated dose (MTD) was not achieved in the 84 week mouse study and in female rats, exposures at the highest doses studied were many fold greater than those achieved at the maximum recommended daily human dose (MRHD) of 7.5 mg. There were no increases in tumor incidence in the 84 week mouse study at doses producing 140 times the exposure achieved at the MRHD based on blood AUC comparisons. In the rat study, there was a statistically significant increase in the incidence of pituitary adenomas in males only at 85 mg/kg/day, a dose that produced 250 times the exposure achieved at the MRHD based on AUC comparisons. In the 26 week p53(+/-) transgenic mouse study, there was an increased incidence of subcutaneous sarcomas in females dosed at 200 and 400 mg/kg/day, or 390 and 630 times the human exposure based on AUC comparisons. The incidence of sarcomas was not increased at lower doses that achieved exposures 180 and 60 times the human exposure. These sarcomas were physically associated with subcutaneously implanted animal identification transponders. There were no other increases in tumor incidence of any type in any dose group. These sarcomas are not considered to be relevant to humans.

Mutagenesis

Frovatriptan was clastogenic in human lymphocyte cultures, in the absence of metabolic activation. In the bacterial reverse mutation assay (Ames test), frovatriptan produced an equivocal response in the absence of metabolic activation. No mutagenic or clastogenic activities were seen in an *in vitro* mouse lymphoma assay, an *in vivo* mouse bone marrow micronucleus test, or an *ex vivo* assay for unscheduled DNA synthesis in rat liver.

Impairment of Fertility

Male and female rats were dosed prior to and during mating, and up to implantation, at doses of 100, 500, and 1000 mg/kg/day (equivalent to approximately 130, 650 and 1300 times the MRHD on a mg/m^2 basis). At all dose levels there was an increase in the number of females that mated on the first day of pairing compared to control animals. This occurred in conjunction with a prolongation of the estrous cycle. In addition females had a decreased mean number of corpora lutea, and consequently a lower number of live fetuses per litter, which suggested a partial impairment of ovulation. There were no other fertility-related effects.

PREGNANCY CATEGORY C

When pregnant rats were administered frovatriptan during the period of organogenesis at oral doses of 100, 500 and 1000 mg/kg/day (equivalent to 130, 650 and 1300 times the maximum recommended human dose [MRHD] on a mg/m^2 basis) there were dose related increases in incidences of both litters and total numbers of fetuses with dilated ureters, unilateral and bilateral pelvic cavitation, hydronephrosis, and hydroureters. A no-effect dose for renal effects was not established. This signifies a syndrome of related effects on a specific organ in the developing embryo in all treated groups, which is consistent with a slight delay in fetal maturation. This delay was also indicated by a treatment related increased incidence of incomplete ossification of the sternebrae, skull and nasal bones in all treated groups. Slightly lower fetal weights and an increased incidence of early embryonic deaths in treated rats were observed; although not statistically significant compared to control, the latter effect occurred in both the embryofetal developmental study and in the prenatal-postnatal developmental study. There was no evidence of this latter effect at the lowest dose level studied, 100 mg/kg/day (equivalent to 130 times the MRHD on a mg/m^2 basis). When pregnant rabbits were dosed throughout organogenesis at doses up to 80 mg/kg/day (equivalent to 210 times the MRHD on a mg/m^2 basis) no effects on fetal development were observed.

There are no adequate and well-controlled studies in pregnant women; therefore, frovatriptan should be used during pregnancy only if the potential benefit justifies the potential risk to the fetus.

NURSING MOTHERS

It is not known whether frovatriptan is excreted in human milk. Frovatriptan and/or its metabolites are excreted in the milk of lactating rats with the maximum concentration being 4-fold higher than that seen in blood. Therefore, caution should be exercised when considering the administration of frovatriptan succinate to a nursing woman.

PEDIATRIC USE

Safety and effectiveness of frovatriptan succinate in pediatric patients have not been established; therefore, frovatriptan succinate is not recommended for use in patients under 18 years of age. Postmarketing experience with other triptans includes a limited number of reports that describe pediatric patients who have experienced clinically serious adverse events that are similar in nature to those reported rarely in adults.

USE IN THE ELDERLY

Mean blood concentrations of frovatriptan in elderly subjects were 1.5- to 2-times higher than those seen in younger adults (see CLINICAL PHARMACOLOGY, Special Populations). Because migraine occurs infrequently in the elderly, clinical experience with frovatriptan succinate is limited in such patients.

DRUG INTERACTIONS

See also CLINICAL PHARMACOLOGY, Drug Interactions.

Ergot-containing drugs have been reported to cause prolonged vasospastic reactions. Due to a theoretical risk of a pharmacodynamic interaction, use of ergotamine-containing or ergot-type medications (like dihydroergotamine or methysergide) and frovatriptan succinate within 24 hours of each other should be avoided (see CONTRAINDICATIONS).

Concomitant use of other $5\text{-}HT_{1B/1D}$ agonists within 24 hours of frovatriptan succinate treatment is not recommended (see CONTRAINDICATIONS).

Selective serotonin reuptake inhibitors (SSRIs) (*e.g.*, fluoxetine, fluvoxamine, paroxetine, sertraline) have been reported, rarely, to cause weakness, hyperreflexia, and incoordination when coadministered with $5\text{-}HT_1$ agonists. If concomitant treatment with frovatriptan and an SSRI is clinically warranted, appropriate observation of the patient is advised.

ADVERSE REACTIONS

Serious cardiac events, including some that have been fatal, have occurred following use of $5\text{-}HT_1$ agonists. These events are extremely rare and most have been reported in patients with risk factors predictive of CAD. Events reported have included coronary artery vasospasm, transient myocardial ischemia, myocardial infarction, ventricular tachycardia and ventricular fibrillation (see CONTRAINDICATIONS, WARNINGS and PRECAUTIONS).

INCIDENCE IN CONTROLLED CLINICAL TRIALS

Among 1554 patients treated with frovatriptan succinate in four placebo-controlled trials (Trials 1, 3, 4 and 5), only 1% (16) patients withdrew because of treatment-emergent adverse events. In a long term, open-label study where patients were allowed to treat multiple migraine attacks with frovatriptan succinate for up to 1 year, 5% (26/496) patients discontinued due to treatment-emergent adverse events.

The treatment-emergent adverse events that occurred most frequently following administration of frovatriptan 2.5 mg (*i.e.*, in at least 2% of patients), and at an incidence ≥1% greater than with placebo, in the four placebo-controlled trials were dizziness, paresthesia, headache, dry mouth, fatigue, flushing, hot or cold sensation and chest pain.

TABLE 2 lists treatment-emergent adverse events reported within 48 hours of drug administration that occurred with frovatriptan 2.5 mg at an incidence of ≥2% and more often than on placebo, in the first attack in four placebo-controlled trials (Trials 1, 3, 4 and 5). These studies involved 2392 patients (1554 frovatriptan 2.5 mg and 838 placebo). The events cited reflect experience gained under closely monitored conditions of clinical trials in a highly selected patient population. In actual clinical practice or in other clinical trials, these incidence estimates may not apply, as the conditions of use, reporting behavior, and the kinds of patients treated may differ.

Other events that occurred at ≥2% on frovatriptan that were equally or more common in the placebo group were somnolence and nausea.

Frovatriptan succinate is generally well tolerated. The incidence of adverse events in clinical trials did not increase when up to 3 doses were used within 24 hours. The majority of adverse events were mild or moderate and transient. The incidence of adverse events in four placebo-controlled clinical trials was not affected by gender, age or concomitant medications commonly used by migraine patients. There were insufficient data to assess the impact of race on the incidence of adverse events.

OTHER EVENTS OBSERVED IN ASSOCIATION WITH FROVATRIPTAN SUCCINATE

In the paragraphs that follow, the incidence of less commonly reported adverse events in four placebo-controlled trials are presented. Variability associated with adverse event reporting, the terminology used to describe adverse events etc., limit the value of the incidence

***TABLE 2** Treatment-Emergent Adverse Events (Incidence ≥2% and Greater Than Placebo) of Patients in Four Placebo-Controlled Migraine Trials*

Adverse Events	Frovatriptan 2.5 mg (n=1554)	Placebo (n=838)
Central & Peripheral Nervous System		
Dizziness	8%	5%
Headache	4%	3%
Paresthesia	4%	2%
Gastrointestinal System		
Dry mouth	3%	1%
Dyspepsia	2%	1%
Body as a Whole - General Disorders		
Fatigue	5%	2%
Hot or cold sensation	3%	2%
Chest pain	2%	1%
Musculoskeletal System		
Skeletal pain	3%	2%
Vascular System		
Flushing	4%	2%

estimates provided. The incidence of each adverse event is calculated as the number of patients reporting the event at least once divided by the number of patients who used frovatriptan succinate. All adverse events reported within 48 hours of drug administration in the first attack in four placebo-controlled trials involving 2392 patients (1554 frovatriptan 2.5 mg and 838 placebo) are included, except those already listed in TABLE 2, those too general to be informative, those not reasonably associated with the use of the drug and those which occurred at the same or a greater incidence in the placebo group. Events are further classified within body system categories and enumerated in order of decreasing frequency using the following definitions: *frequent* adverse events are those occurring in at least 1/100 patients, *infrequent* adverse events are those occurring in between 1/100 and 1/1000 patients, and *rare* adverse events are those occurring in fewer than 1/1000 patients.

Central and peripheral nervous system: *Frequent:* Dysesthesia and hypoesthesia; *Infrequent:* Tremor, hyperesthesia, migraine aggravated, involuntary muscle contractions, vertigo, ataxia, abnormal gait and speech disorder; *Rare:* Hypertonia, hypotonia, abnormal reflexes and tongue paralysis.

Gastrointestinal: *Frequent:* Vomiting, abdominal pain and diarrhea; *Infrequent:* Dysphagia, flatulence, constipation, anorexia, esophagospasm and increased salivation; *Rare:* Change in bowel habits, cheilitis, eructation, gastroesophageal reflux, hiccup, peptic ulcer, salivary gland pain, stomatitis and toothache.

Body as a whole: *Frequent:* Pain; *Infrequent:* Asthenia, rigors, fever, hot flushes and malaise; *Rare:* Feeling of relaxation, leg pain and edema mouth.

Psychiatric: *Frequent:* Insomnia and anxiety; *Infrequent:* Confusion, nervousness, agitation, euphoria, impaired concentration, depression, emotional lability, amnesia, thinking abnormal and depersonalization; *Rare:* Depression aggravated, abnormal dreaming and personality disorder.

Musculoskeletal: *Infrequent:* Myalgia, back pain, arthralgia, arthrosis, leg cramps and muscle weakness.

Respiratory: *Frequent:* Sinusitis and rhinitis; *Infrequent:* Pharyngitis, dyspnea, hyperventilation and laryngitis.

Vision disorders: *Frequent:* Vision abnormal; *Infrequent:* Eye pain, conjunctivitis and abnormal lacrimation.

Skin and appendages: *Frequent:* Sweating increased; *Infrequent:* Pruritus, and bullous eruption.

Hearing and vestibular disorders: *Frequent:* Tinnitus; *Infrequent:* Ear ache, and hyperacusis.

Heart rate and rhythm: *Frequent:* Palpitation; *Infrequent:* Tachycardia; *Rare:* Bradycardia.

Metabolic and nutritional disorders: *Infrequent:* Thirst and dehydration; *Rare:* Hypocalcemia and hypoglycemia.

Special senses, other disorders: *Infrequent:* Taste perversion.

Urinary system disorders: *Infrequent:* Micturition frequency and polyuria; *Rare:* Nocturia, renal pain and abnormal urine.

Cardiovascular disorders, general: *Infrequent:* Abnormal ECG.

Platelet, bleeding and clotting disorders: *Infrequent:* Epistaxis; *Rare:* Purpura.

Autonomic nervous system: *Rare:* Syncope.

DOSAGE AND ADMINISTRATION

The recommended dose is a single tablet of frovatriptan 2.5 mg taken orally with fluids.

If the headache recurs after initial relief, a second tablet may be taken, providing there is an interval of at least 2 hours between doses. The total daily dose of frovatriptan should not exceed 3 tablets (3 × 2.5 mg/day).

There is no evidence that a second dose of frovatriptan is effective in patients who do not respond to a first dose of the drug for the same headache.

The safety of treating an average of more than 4 migraine attacks in a 30 day period has not been established.

HOW SUPPLIED

Frova tablets, containing 2.5 mg of frovatriptan (base) as the succinate, are available as round, white, film-coated tablets with "77" on one side and the "e" logo on the other side. **Storage:** Store at controlled room temperature, 25°C (77°F) excursions permitted to 15-30°C (59-86°F), protect from moisture and light.

PRODUCT LISTING - EQUIVALENTS NOT AVAILABLE

Tablet - Oral - 2.5 mg

9's	$138.71	GENERIC, Elan Pharmaceuticals	59075-0740-89

Fulvestrant (003553)

Categories: Carcinoma, breast; Pregnancy Category D; FDA Approved 2002 Apr
Drug Classes: Antineoplastics, antiestrogens; Estrogen receptor modulators, selective; Hormones/hormone modifiers
Brand Names: Faslodex
Cost of Therapy: $921.88 (Breast Cancer; Faslodex Injection; 50 mg/ml; 5 ml; 250 mg/month; 30 day supply)

DESCRIPTION

Faslodex (fulvestrant) injection for intramuscular administration is an estrogen receptor antagonist without known agonist effects. The chemical name is 7-alpha-[9-(4,4,5,5,5-penta fluoropentylsulphinyl) nonyl]estra-1,3,5-(10)-triene-3,17-beta-diol. The molecular formula is $C_{32}H_{47}F_5O_3S$.

Fulvestrant is a white powder with a molecular weight of 606.77. The solution for injection is a clear, colorless to yellow, viscous liquid.

Each injection contains as inactive ingredients: alcohol, benzyl alcohol, and benzyl benzoate, as co-solvents, and castor oil as a co-solvent and release rate modifier.

Faslodex is supplied in sterile single patient pre-filled syringes containing 50 mg/ml fulvestrant either as a single 5 ml or two concurrent 2.5 ml injections to deliver the required monthly dose. Faslodex is administered as an intramuscular injection of 250 mg once monthly.

CLINICAL PHARMACOLOGY

MECHANISM OF ACTION

Many breast cancers have estrogen receptors (ER), and the growth of these tumors can be stimulated by estrogen. Fulvestrant is an estrogen receptor antagonist that binds to the estrogen receptor in a competitive manner with affinity comparable to that of estradiol. Fulvestrant downregulates the ER protein in human breast cancer cells.

In a clinical study in postmenopausal women with primary breast cancer treated with single doses of fulvestrant 15-22 days prior to surgery, there was evidence of increasing down regulation of ER with increasing dose. This was associated with a dose-related decrease in the expression of the progesterone receptor, an estrogen-regulated protein. These effects on the ER pathway were also associated with a decrease in Ki67 labeling index, a marker of cell proliferation.

In vitro studies demonstrated that fulvestrant is a reversible inhibitor of the growth of tamoxifen-resistant, as well as estrogen-sensitive human breast cancer (MCF-7) cell lines. In *in vivo* tumor studies, fulvestrant delayed the establishment of tumors from xenografts of human breast cancer MCF-7 cells in nude mice. Fulvestrant inhibited the growth of established MCF-7 xenografts and of tamoxifen-resistant breast tumor xenografts. Fulvestrant resistant breast tumor xenografts may also be cross-resistant to tamoxifen.

Fulvestrant showed no agonist-type effects in *in vivo* uterotropic assays in immature or ovariectomized mice and rats. In *in vivo* studies in immature rats and ovariectomized monkeys, fulvestrant blocked the uterotrophic action of estradiol. In postmenopausal women, the absence of changes in plasma concentrations of FSH and LH in response to fulvestrant treatment (250 mg monthly) suggests no peripheral steroidal effects.

PHARMACOKINETICS

Following intravenous administration, fulvestrant is rapidly cleared at a rate approximating hepatic blood flow (about 10.5 ml plasma/min/kg). After an intramuscular injection plasma concentrations are maximal at about 7 days and are maintained over a period of at least 1 month, with trough concentration about one-third of C_{max}. The apparent half-life was about 40 days. After administration of 250 mg of fulvestrant intramuscularly every month, plasma levels approach steady-state after 3-6 doses, with an average 2.5-fold increase in plasma AUC compared to single dose AUC and trough levels about equal to the single dose C_{max} (see TABLE 1).

TABLE 1 *Summary of Fulvestrant Pharmacokinetic Parameters in Postmenopausal Advanced Breast Cancer Patients After Intramuscular Administration of a 250 mg Dose (mean ± SD)*

	C_{max} ng/ml	C_{min} ng/ml	AUC ng·d/ml	T½ days	CL ml/min
Single dose	8.5 ± 5.4	2.6 ± 1.1	131 ± 62	40 ± 11	690 ± 226
Multiple dose steady state	15.8 ± 2.4	7.4 ± 1.7	328 ± 48		

Fulvestrant was subject to extensive and rapid distribution. The apparent volume of distribution at steady state was approximately 3-5 L/kg. This suggests that distribution is largely extravascular. Fulvestrant was highly (99%) bound to plasma proteins; VLDL, LDL and HDL lipoprotein fractions appear to be the major binding components. The role of sex hormone-binding globulin, if any, could not be determined.

METABOLISM AND EXCRETION

Biotransformation and disposition of fulvestrant in humans have been determined following intramuscular and intravenous administration of ^{14}C-labeled fulvestrant. Metabolism of fulvestrant appears to involve combinations of a number of possible biotransformation pathways analogous to those of endogenous steroids, including oxidation, aromatic hydroxylation, conjugation with glucuronic acid and/or sulphate at the 2, 3 and 17 positions of the steroid nucleus, and oxidation of the side chain sulphoxide. Identified metabolites are either less active or exhibit similar activity to fulvestrant in antiestrogen models. Studies using human liver preparations and recombinant human enzymes indicate that cytochrome P-450 3A4 (CYP 3A4) is the only P-450 isoenzyme involved in the oxidation of fulvestrant; however, the relative contribution of P-450 and non-P-450 routes *in vivo* is unknown.

Fulvestrant was rapidly cleared by the hepatobiliary route with excretion primarily via the feces (approximately 90%). Renal elimination was negligible (less than 1%).

SPECIAL POPULATIONS

Geriatric

In patients with breast cancer, there was no difference in fulvestrant pharmacokinetic profile related to age (range 33-89 years).

Gender

Following administration of a single intravenous dose, there were no pharmacokinetic differences between men and women or between premenopausal and postmenopausal women. Similarly, there were no apparent differences between men and postmenopausal women after intramuscular administration.

Race

In the advanced breast cancer treatment trials, the potential for pharmacokinetic differences due to race have been evaluated in 294 women including 87.4% Caucasian, 7.8% Black, and 4.4% Hispanic. No differences in fulvestrant plasma pharmacokinetics were observed among these groups. In a separate trial, pharmacokinetic data from postmenopausal ethnic Japanese women were similar to those obtained in non-Japanese patients.

Renal Impairment

Negligible amounts of fulvestrant are eliminated in urine; therefore, a study in patients with renal impairment was not conducted. In the advanced breast cancer trials, fulvestrant concentrations in women with estimated creatinine clearance as low as 30 ml/min were similar to women with normal creatinine.

Hepatic Impairment

Fulvestrant is metabolized primarily in the liver. In clinical trials in patients with locally advanced or metastatic breast cancer, pharmacokinetic data were obtained following administration of a 250 mg dose of fulvestrant to 261 patients classified as having normal liver function and to 24 patient with mild impairment. Mild impairment was defined as an alanine aminotransferase concentration (at any visit) greater than the upper limit of the normal (ULN) reference range, but less than 2 times the ULN; or if any 2 of the following 3 parameters were between 1- and 2-times the ULN:aspartate aminotransferase, alkaline phosphatase, or total bilirubin.

There was no clear relationship between fulvestrant clearance and hepatic impairment and the safety profile in patients with mild hepatic impairment was similar to that seen in patients with no hepatic impairment. Safety and efficacy have not been evaluated in patients with moderate to severe hepatic impairment (see PRECAUTIONS, Hepatic Impairment and DOSAGE AND ADMINISTRATION, Patients With Hepatic Impairment).

Pediatric

The pharmacokinetics of fulvestrant have not been evaluated in pediatric patients.

DRUG-DRUG INTERACTIONS

There are no known drug-drug interactions. Fulvestrant does not significantly inhibit any of the major CYP isoenzymes, including CYP 1A2, 2C9, 2C19, 2D6, and 3A4 *in vitro*, and studies of co-administration of fulvestrant with midazolam indicate that therapeutic doses of fulvestrant have no inhibitory effects on CYP 3A4 or alter blood levels of drug metabolized by that enzyme. Also, although fulvestrant is partly metabolized by CYP 3A4, a clinical study with rifampin, an inducer of CYP 3A4, showed no effect on the pharmacokinetics of fulvestrant. Clinical studies of the effect of strong CYP 3A4 inhibitors on the pharmacokinetics of fulvestrant have not been performed.

INDICATIONS AND USAGE

Fulvestrant is indicated for the treatment of hormone receptor positive metastatic breast cancer in postmenopausal women with disease progression following antiestrogen therapy.

CONTRAINDICATIONS

Fulvestrant is contraindicated in pregnant women, and in patients with a known hypersensitivity to the drug or to any of its components.

WARNINGS

Women of childbearing potential should be advised not to become pregnant while receiving fulvestrant. Fulvestrant can cause fetal harm when administered to a pregnant woman and has been shown to cross the placenta following single intramuscular doses in rats and in rabbits. In studies in the pregnant rat, intramuscular doses of fulvestrant 100 times lower than the maximum recommended human dose (based on body surface area [BSA]), caused an increased incidence of fetal abnormalities and death. Similarly, rabbits failed to maintain pregnancy and the fetuses showed an increased incidence of skeletal variations when fulvestrant was administered at one-half the recommended human dose (based on BSA).

There are no studies in pregnant women using fulvestrant. If fulvestrant is used during pregnancy or if the patient becomes pregnant while receiving this drug, the patient should be apprised of the potential hazard to the fetus, or potential risk for loss of the pregnancy. See PRECAUTIONS, Pregnancy Category D.

Because fulvestrant is administered intramuscularly, it should not be used in patients with bleeding diatheses, thrombocytopenia or patients on anticoagulants.

PRECAUTIONS

GENERAL

Before starting treatment with fulvestrant, pregnancy must be excluded (see WARNINGS).

HEPATIC IMPAIRMENT

Safety and efficacy have not been evaluated in patients with moderate to severe hepatic impairment (see CLINICAL PHARMACOLOGY, Hepatic Impairment and DOSAGE AND ADMINISTRATION, Patients With Hepatic Impairment).

CARCINOGENESIS, MUTAGENESIS, AND IMPAIRMENT OF FERTILITY

A 2 year carcinogenesis study was conducted in female and male rats, at intramuscular doses of 15 mg/kg/30 days, 10 mg/rat/30 days and 10 mg/rat/15 days. These doses correspond to approximately 1-, 3-, and 5-fold (in females) and 1.3-, 1.3-, and 1.6-fold (in males) the systemic exposure [AUC(0-30 days)] achieved in women receiving the recommended dose of 250 mg/month. An increased incidence of benign ovarian granulosa cell tumors and testicular Leydig cell tumors was evident, in females dosed at 10 mg/rat/15 days and males dosed at 15 mg/rat/30 days, respectively. Induction of such tumors is consistent with the pharmacology-related endocrine feedback alterations in gonadotropin levels caused by an antiestrogen.

Fulvestrant was not mutagenic or clastogenic in multiple *in vitro* tests with and without the addition of a mammalian liver metabolic activation factor (bacterial mutation assay in strains of *Salmonella typhimurium* and *Escherichia coli*, *in vitro* cytogenetics study in human lymphocytes, mammalian cell mutation assay in mouse lymphoma cells and *in vivo* micronucleus test in rat.

In female rats, fulvestrant administered at doses ≥0.01 mg/kg/day (approximately one-hundredth of the human recommended dose based on body surface area [BSA], for 2 weeks prior to and for 1 week following mating, caused a reduction in fertility and embryonic survival. No adverse effects on female fertility and embryonic survival were evident in female animals dosed at 0.001 mg/kg/day (approximately one-thousandth of the human dose based on BSA). Restoration of female fertility to values similar to controls was evident following a 29 day withdrawal period after dosing at 2 mg/kg/day (twice the human dose based on BSA). The effects of fulvestrant on the fertility of female rats appear to be consistent with its anti-estrogenic activity. The potential effects of fulvestrant on the fertility of male animals were not studied but in a 6 month toxicology study, male rats treated with intramuscular doses of 15 mg/kg/30 days, 10 mg/rat/30 days, or 10 mg/rat/15 days fulvestrant showed a loss of spermatozoa from the seminiferous tubules, seminiferous tubular atrophy, and degenerative changes in the epididymides. Changes in the testes and epididymides had not recovered 20 weeks after cessation of dosing. These fulvestrant doses correspond to approximately 2-, 3-, and 3-fold the systemic exposure [AUC(0-30 days)] achieved in women.

PREGNANCY CATEGORY D

See WARNINGS.

In studies in female rats at doses ≥0.01 mg/kg/day (IM; approximately one-hundredth of the human recommended dose based on body surface area [BSA]), fulvestrant caused a reversible reduction in female fertility, as well as effects on embryo/fetal development consistent with its anti-estrogenic activity. Fulvestrant caused an increased incidence of fetal abnormalities in rats (tarsal flexure of the hind paw at 2 mg/kg/day IM; twice the human dose on BSA) and non-ossification of the odontoid and ventral tubercle of the first cervical vertebra at doses ≥0.1 mg/kg/day IM (approximately one-tenth of the human dose on BSA) when administered during the period of organogenesis. Rabbits failed to maintain pregnancy when dosed with 1 mg/kg/day fulvestrant IM (twice the human dose on BSA) during the period of organogenesis. Further, in rabbits dosed at 0.25 mg/kg/day (about one-half the human dose on BSA), increases in placental weight and post-implantation loss were observed but, there were no observed effects on fetal development. Fulvestrant was associated with an increased incidence of fetal variations in rabbits (backwards displacement of the pelvic girdle, and 27 pre-sacral vertebrae at 0.25 mg/kg/day IM; one-half the human dose on BSA) when administered during the period of organogenesis. Because pregnancy could not be maintained in the rabbit following doses of fulvestrant of 1 mg/kg/day and above, this study was inadequate to fully define the possible adverse effects on fetal development at clinically relevant exposures.

NURSING MOTHERS

Fulvestrant is found in rat milk at levels significantly higher (approximately 12-fold) than plasma after administration of 2 mg/kg. Drug exposure in rodent pups from fulvestrant-treated lactating dams was estimated as 10% of the administered dose. It is not known if fulvestrant is excreted in human milk. Because many drugs are excreted in human milk, and because of the potential for serious adverse reactions from fulvestrant in nursing infants, a decision should be made whether to discontinue nursing or to discontinue the drug taking into account the importance of the drug to the mother.

PEDIATRIC USE

The safety and efficacy of fulvestrant in pediatric patients have not been established.

GERIATRIC USE

When tumor response was considered by age, objective responses were seen in 24% and 22% of patients under 65 years of age and in 16% and 11% of patients 65 years of age and older, who were treated with fulvestrant in the European and North American trials, respectively.

DRUG INTERACTIONS

Fulvestrant is metabolized by CYP 3A4 *in vitro*. Clinical studies of the effect of strong CYP 3A4 inhibitors on the pharmacokinetics of fulvestrant have not been performed (see CLINICAL PHARMACOLOGY, Drug-Drug Interactions).

ADVERSE REACTIONS

The most commonly reported adverse experiences in the fulvestrant and anastrozole treatment groups, regardless of the investigator's assessment of causality, were gastrointestinal symptoms (including nausea, vomiting, constipation, diarrhea and abdominal pain), headache, back pain, vasodilatation (hot flushes), and pharyngitis.

Injection site reactions with mild transient pain and inflammation were seen with fulvestrant and occurred in 7% of patients (1% of treatments) given the single 5 ml injection (European Trial) and in 27% of patients (4.6% of treatments) given the 2 × 2.5 ml injections (North American Trial).

TABLE 4 lists adverse experiences reported with an incidence of 5% or greater, regardless of causality, from the two controlled clinical trials comparing the administration of fulvestrant 250 mg intramuscularly once a month with anastrozole 1 mg orally once a day.

TABLE 4 *Combined Trials Adverse Events ≥5%*

Body System Adverse Event*	Fulvestrant 250 mg n=423	Anastrozole 1 mg n=423
Body as a Whole	68.3%	67.6%
Asthenia	22.7%	27.0%
Pain	18.9%	20.3%
Headache	15.4%	16.8%
Back pain	14.4%	13.2%
Abdominal pain	11.8%	11.6%
Injection site pain†	10.9%	6.6%
Pelvic pain	9.9%	9.0%
Chest pain	7.1%	5.0%
Flu syndrome	7.1%	6.4%
Fever	6.4%	6.4%
Accidental injury	4.5%	5.7%
Cardiovascular System	30.3%	27.9%
Vasodilatation	17.7%	17.3%
Digestive System	51.5%	48.0%
Nausea	26.0%	25.3%
Vomiting	13.0%	11.8%
Constipation	12.5%	10.6%
Diarrhea	12.3%	12.8%
Anorexia	9.0%	10.9%
Hemic and Lymphatic Systems	13.7%	13.5%
Anemia	4.5%	5.0%
Metabolic and Nutritional Disorders	18.2%	17.7%
Peripheral edema	9.0%	10.2%
Musculoskeletal System	25.5%	27.9%
Bone pain	15.8%	13.7%
Arthritis	2.8%	6.1%
Nervous System	34.3%	33.8%
Dizziness	6.9%	6.6%
Insomnia	6.9%	8.5%
Paresthesia	6.4%	7.6%
Depression	5.7%	6.9%
Anxiety	5.0%	3.8%
Respiratory System	38.5%	33.6%
Pharyngitis	16.1%	11.6%
Dyspnea	14.9%	12.3%
Cough increased	10.4%	10.4%
Skin and Appendages	22.2%	23.4%
Rash	7.3%	8.0%
Sweating	5.0%	5.2%
Urogenital System	18.2%	14.9%
Urinary tract infection	6.1%	3.5%

* A patient may have more than one adverse event.
† All patients on fulvestrant received injections, but only those anastrozole patients who were in the North American study received placebo injections.

Other adverse events reported as drug-related and seen infrequently (<1%) include thromboembolic phenomena, myalgia, vertigo, and leukopenia.

Vaginal bleeding has been reported infrequently (<1%), mainly in patients during the first 6 weeks after changing from existing hormonal therapy to treatment with fulvestrant. If bleeding persists, further evaluation should be considered.

DOSAGE AND ADMINISTRATION

ADULTS (INCLUDING THE ELDERLY)

The recommended dose is 250 mg to be administered intramuscularly into the buttock at intervals of 1 month as either a single 5 ml injection or two concurrent 2.5 ml injections (see HOW SUPPLIED). The injection should be administered slowly.

PATIENTS WITH HEPATIC IMPAIRMENT

Fulvestrant has not been studied in patients with moderate or severe hepatic compromise. No dosage adjustment is recommended in patients with mild hepatic impairment (see CLINICAL PHARMACOLOGY, Hepatic Impairment and PRECAUTIONS, Hepatic Impairment).

HOW SUPPLIED

FASLODEX INJECTION

One 5 ml clear neutral glass (Type 1) barrel containing 5 ml (50 mg/ml) Faslodex injection for intramuscular injection and fitted with a tamper-evident closure.

Two 5 ml clear neutral glass (Type 1) barrels, each containing 2.5 ml (50 mg/ml) of Faslodex injection for intramuscular injection and fitted with a tamper-evident closure.

The syringes are presented in a tray with polystyrene plunger rod and a safety needle (Safety Glide) for connection to the barrel.

Storage: Store in a refrigerator, 2-8°C (36-46°F). Store in original container.

PRODUCT LISTING - EQUIVALENTS NOT AVAILABLE

Injection - Intramuscular - 50 mg/ml

2.50 ml x 2	$921.88	FASLODEX, Astra-Zeneca Pharmaceuticals	00310-0720-25
5 ml	$921.88	FASLODEX, Astra-Zeneca Pharmaceuticals	00310-0720-50

Furosemide (001342)

Categories: Edema; Edema, pulmonary; Hypertension, essential; Pregnancy Category C; FDA Approved 1968 Mar; WHO Formulary

Drug Classes: Diuretics, loop

Brand Names: Furocot; Furomide M.D.; **Lasix**

Foreign Brand Availability: Aldic (Thailand); Anfuramaide (Taiwan); Apo-Frusemide (New-Zealand); Apo-Furosemide (Canada); Aquarid (South-Africa); Arasemide (Japan); Cetasix (Indonesia); Dirine (Malaysia); Diural (Denmark; Norway; Sweden; Switzerland); Diuresal (Bahamas; Bahrain; Barbados; Belize; Benin; Bermuda; Burkina-Faso; Curacao; Cyprus; Egypt; Ethiopia; Gambia; Ghana; Guinea; Guyana; Iran; Iraq; Israel; Ivory-Coast; Jamaica; Jordan; Kenya; Kuwait; Lebanon; Liberia; Libya; Malawi; Mali; Mauritania; Mauritius; Morocco; Netherland-Antilles; Niger; Nigeria; Oman; Puerto-Rico; Qatar; Republic-of-Yemen; Saudi-Arabia; Senegal; Seychelles; Sierra-Leone; South-Africa; Sudan; Surinam; Syria; Taiwan; Tanzania; Trinidad; Tunia; Uganda; United-Arab-Emirates; Zambia; Zimbabwe); Diurin (New-Zealand); Diurolasa (Spain); Diusemide (Benin; Burkina-Faso; Ethiopia; Gambia; Ghana; Guinea; Ivory-Coast; Kenya; Liberia; Malawi; Mali; Mauritania; Mauritius; Morocco; Niger; Nigeria; Senegal; Seychelles; Sierra-Leone; Sudan; Tanzania; Tunia; Uganda; Zambia; Zimbabwe); Dryptal (England; Ireland); Durafurid (Germany); Edenol (Mexico); Errolon (Argentina); Eutensin (Japan); Franyl (Japan); Furmid (Malaysia); Frusedan (Benin; Burkina-Faso; Ethiopia; Gambia; Ghana; Guinea; Ivory-Coast; Kenya; Liberia; Malawi; Mali; Mauritania; Mauritius; Morocco; Niger; Nigeria; Senegal; Seychelles; Sierra-Leone; South-Africa; Sudan; Tanzania; Tunia; Uganda; Zambia; Zimbabwe); Frusema (Philippines); Furanthril (Czech-Republic); Furanturil (Bulgaria); Furetic (Thailand); Furix (Norway; Sweden); Furo-Basan (Switzerland); Furomen (Finland); Furomex (Czech-Republic); Furo-Puren (Germany); Furorese (Germany); Furoscan (Philippines); Furosix (Indonesia); Furovite (Israel); Fusid (Germany; Israel); Hissuflux (Colombia); Hydrex (South-Africa); Impugan (Denmark; Indonesia; Sweden; Switzerland; Thailand); Kofuzon (Taiwan); Kutrix (Japan); Lasiletten (Netherlands); Lasilix (France; Morocco); Lasix Retard (Denmark; Netherlands; Norway; Portugal; Sweden); Laxur (Chile); Marsemide (Philippines); Naclex (Indonesia); Nephron (Argentina); Odemex (Costa-Rica; Dominican-Republic; Ecuador; El-Salvador; Guatemala; Honduras; Nicaragua; Panama); Oedemex (Bahrain; Cyprus; Egypt; Iran; Iraq; Israel; Jordan; Kuwait; Lebanon; Libya; Oman; Qatar; Republic-of-Yemen; Saudi-Arabia; Switzerland; Syria; United-Arab-Emirates); Promedes (Japan); Radisemide (Bahrain; Benin; Burkina-Faso; Cyprus; Egypt; Ethiopia; Gambia; Ghana; Guinea; Iran; Iraq; Israel; Ivory-Coast; Jordan; Kenya; Kuwait; Lebanon; Liberia; Libya; Malawi; Mali; Mauritania; Mauritius; Morocco; Niger; Nigeria; Oman; Qatar; Republic-of-Yemen; Saudi-Arabia; Senegal; Seychelles; Sierra-Leone; South-Africa; Sudan; Syria; Tanzania; Tunia; Uganda; United-Arab-Emirates; Zambia; Zimbabwe); Retep (Argentina); Seguril (Spain); Selectofur (Mexico); Uremide (Australia; New-Zealand); Urenil (Japan); Uresix (Indonesia); Urex (Australia; Hong-Kong; Japan; New-Zealand); Urex-M (Australia; New-Zealand); Zafurida (Mexico)

Cost of Therapy: $19.04 (Hypertension; Lasix; 40 mg; 2 tablets/day; 30 day supply)
$1.50 (Hypertension; Generic Tablets; 40 mg; 2 tablets/day; 30 day supply)

HCFA JCODE(S): J1940 up to 20 mg IM, IV

WARNING

Furosemide is a potent diuretic which, if given in excessive amounts, can lead to a profound diuresis with water and electrolyte depletion. Therefore, careful medical supervision is required and dose and dose schedule must be adjusted to the individual patient's needs. (See DOSAGE AND ADMINISTRATION.)

DESCRIPTION

TABLETS

Lasix is a diuretic which is an anthranilic acid derivative. Lasix for oral administration contains furosemide as the active ingredient and the following inactive ingredients: lactose, magnesium stearate, starch, and talc. Chemically, it is 4-chloro-N-furfuryl-5-sulfamoylanthranilic acid. Furosemide is available as white tablets for oral administration in dosage strengths of 20, 40 and 80 mg.

Furosemide is a white to off-white odorless crystalline powder. It is practically insoluble in water, sparingly soluble in alcohol, freely soluble in dilute alkali solutions and insoluble in dilute acids.

The CAS Registry Number is 54-31-9.

INJECTION

Lasix injection is composed of 4-chloro-N-furfuryl-5- sulfamoylanthranilic acid, sodium chloride for isotonicity and sodium hydroxide to adjust pH.

Lasix injection 10 mg/ml is a sterile, non-pyrogenic solution in ampules, disposable syringes and single dose vials for intravenous and intramuscular injection.

ORAL SOLUTION

Lasix oral solution contains furosemide as the active ingredient and the following inactive ingredients: alcohol 11.5%, D&C yellow no. 10, FD&C yellow no. 6 as color additives, flavors, glycerin, parabens, purified water, sorbitol; sodium hydroxide added to adjust pH. Lasix oral solution 10 mg/ml is an orange flavored liquid for oral administration.

CLINICAL PHARMACOLOGY

Investigations into the mode of action of furosemide have utilized micropuncture studies in rats, stop flow experiments in dogs and various clearance studies in both humans and experimental animals. It has been demonstrated that furosemide inhibits primarily the absorption of sodium and chloride not only in the proximal and distal tubules but also in the loop of Henle. The high degree of efficacy is largely due to this unique site of action. The action on the distal tubule is independent of any inhibitory effect on carbonic anhydrase and aldosterone.

Recent evidence suggests that furosemide glucuronide is the only or at least the major biotransformation product of furosemide in man. Furosemide is extensively bound to plasma proteins, mainly to albumin. Plasma concentrations ranging from 1 to 400 μg/ml are 91-99% bound in healthy individuals. The unbound fraction averages 2.3-4.1% at therapeutic concentrations.

The onset of diuresis following oral administration is within 1 hour. The peak effect occurs within the first or second hour. The duration of diuretic effect is 6-8 hours.

The onset of diuresis following intravenous administration is within 5 minutes and somewhat later after intramuscular administration. The peak effect occurs within the first half hour. The duration of diuretic effect is approximately 2 hours.

In fasted normal men, the mean bioavailability of furosemide from tablets and oral solution is 64% and 60%, respectively, of that from an intravenous injection of the drug. Although furosemide is more rapidly absorbed from the oral solution (50 minutes) than from the tablet (87 minutes), peak plasma levels and area under the plasma concentration-time curves do not differ significantly. Peak plasma concentrations increase with increasing dose but times-to-peak do not differ among doses. The terminal half-life of furosemide is approximately 2 hours.

Significantly more furosemide is excreted in urine following the IV injection than after the tablet or oral solution. There are no significant differences between the two oral formulations in the amount of unchanged drug excreted in urine.

INDICATIONS AND USAGE

Parenteral therapy should be reserved for patients unable to take oral medication or for patients in emergency clinical situations.

TABLETS, INJECTION, AND ORAL SOLUTION

Edema: Furosemide is indicated in adults and pediatric patients for the treatment of edema associated with congestive heart failure, cirrhosis of the liver, and renal disease, including the nephrotic syndrome. Furosemide is particularly useful when an agent with greater diuretic potential is desired.

TABLETS AND ORAL SOLUTION

Hypertension: Oral furosemide may be used in adults for the treatment of hypertension alone or in combination with other antihypertensive agents. Hypertensive patients who cannot be adequately controlled with thiazides will probably also not be adequately controlled with furosemide alone.

INJECTION

Furosemide is indicated as adjunctive therapy in acute pulmonary edema. The intravenous administration of furosemide is indicated when a rapid onset of diuresis is desired, *e.g.*, in acute pulmonary edema.

If gastrointestinal absorption is impaired or oral medication is not practical for any reason, furosemide is indicated by the intravenous or intramuscular route. Parenteral use should be replaced with oral furosemide as soon as practical.

NON-FDA APPROVED INDICATIONS

Because inhaled furosemide has been shown to protect the asthmatic airways against various bronchoconstrictor stimuli, some respiratory medicine experts are evaluating its therapeutic role in reactive airways disease. Use of furosemide to treat reactive airways disease is not approved by the FDA.

CONTRAINDICATIONS

Furosemide is contraindicated in patients with anuria and in patients with a history of hypersensitivity to furosemide.

WARNINGS

TABLETS, INJECTION, AND ORAL SOLUTION

In patients with hepatic cirrhosis and ascites, furosemide therapy is best initiated in the hospital. In hepatic coma and in states of electrolyte depletion, therapy should not be instituted until the basic condition is improved. Sudden alterations of fluid and electrolyte balance in patients with cirrhosis may precipitate hepatic coma; therefore, strict observation is necessary during the period of diuresis. Supplemental potassium chloride and, if required, an aldosterone antagonist are helpful in preventing hypokalemia and metabolic alkalosis.

If increasing azotemia and oliguria occur during treatment of severe progressive renal disease, furosemide should be discontinued.

Cases of tinnitus and reversible or irreversible hearing impairment have been reported. Usually, reports indicate that furosemide ototoxicity is associated with rapid injection, severe renal impairment, doses exceeding several times the usual recommended dose, or concomitant therapy with aminoglycoside antibiotics, ethacrynic acid, or other ototoxic drugs. If the physician elects to use high dose parenteral therapy, controlled intravenous infusion is advisable (for adults, an infusion rate not exceeding 4 mg furosemide per minute has been used).

INJECTION

Pediatric Use: In premature neonates with respiratory distress syndrome, diuretic treatment with furosemide in the first few weeks of life may increase the risk of persistent patent ductus arteriosus (PDA), possibly through a prostaglandin-E-mediated process.

Hearing loss in neonates has been associated with the use of furosemide injection (see WARNINGS).

PRECAUTIONS

TABLETS, INJECTION, AND ORAL SOLUTION

General

Excessive diuresis may cause dehydration and blood volume reduction with circulatory collapse and possibly vascular thrombosis and embolism, particularly in elderly patients. As with any effective diuretic, electrolyte depletion may occur during furosemide therapy, especially in patients receiving higher doses and a restricted salt intake. Hypokalemia may develop with furosemide, especially with brisk diuresis, inadequate oral electrolyte intake, when cirrhosis is present, or during concomitant use of corticosteroids or ACTH. Digitalis therapy may exaggerate metabolic effects of hypokalemia, especially myocardial effects.

All patients receiving furosemide therapy should be observed for these signs or symptoms of fluid or electrolyte imbalance (hyponatremia, hypochloremic alkalosis, hypokalemia, hypomagnesemia or hypocalcemia): dryness of mouth, thirst, weakness, lethargy, drowsiness, restlessness, muscle pains or cramps, muscular fatigue, hypotension, oliguria, tachycardia, arrhythmia, or gastrointestinal disturbances such as nausea and vomiting. Increases in blood glucose and alterations in glucose tolerance tests (with abnormalities of the fasting and 2 hour postprandial sugar) have been observed, and rarely, precipitation of diabetes mellitus has been reported.

Asymptomatic hyperuricemia can occur and gout may rarely be precipitated.

F

ORAL SOLUTION
The sorbitol present in the vehicle may cause diarrhea (especially in children) when higher doses of furosemide oral solution are given.

TABLETS, INJECTION, AND ORAL SOLUTION
Patients allergic to sulfonamides may also be allergic to furosemide. The possibility exists of exacerbation or activation of systemic lupus erythematosus.

As with many other drugs, patients should be observed regularly for the possible occurrence of blood dyscrasias, liver or kidney damage, or other idiosyncratic reactions.

Information for the Patient
Patients receiving furosemide should be advised that they may experience symptoms from excessive fluid and/or electrolyte losses. The postural hypotension that sometimes occurs can usually be managed by getting up slowly. Potassium supplements and/or dietary measures may be needed to control or avoid hypokalemia.

Patients with diabetes mellitus should be told that furosemide may increase blood glucose levels and thereby affect urine glucose tests. The skin of some patients may be more sensitive to the effects of sunlight while taking furosemide.

Hypertensive patients should avoid medications that may increase blood pressure, including over-the-counter products for appetite suppression and cold symptoms.

Laboratory Tests
Serum electrolytes (particularly potassium), CO_2, creatinine and BUN should be determined frequently during the first few months of furosemide therapy and periodically thereafter. Serum and urine electrolyte determinations are particularly important when the patient is vomiting profusely or receiving parenteral fluids. Abnormalities should be corrected or the drug temporarily withdrawn. Other medications may also influence serum electrolytes.

Reversible elevations of BUN may occur and are associated with dehydration, which should be avoided, particularly in patients with renal insufficiency.

Urine and blood glucose should be checked periodically in diabetics receiving furosemide, even in those suspected of latent diabetes.

Furosemide may lower serum levels of calcium (rarely cases of tetany have been reported) and magnesium. Accordingly, serum levels of these electrolytes should be determined periodically.

Carcinogenesis, Mutagenesis, and Impairment of Fertility
Furosemide was tested for carcinogenicity by oral administration in one strain of mice and one strain of rats. A small but significantly increased incidence of mammary gland carcinomas occurred in female mice at a dose 17.5 times the maximum human dose of 600 mg. There were marginal increases in uncommon tumors in male rats at a dose of 15 mg/kg (slightly greater than the maximum human dose) but not at 30 mg/kg.

Furosemide was devoid of mutagenic activity in various strains of *Salmonella typhimurium* when tested in the presence or absence of an *in vitro* metabolic activation system, and questionably positive for gene mutation in mouse lymphoma cells in the presence of rat liver S9 at the highest dose tested. Furosemide did not induce sister chromatid exchange in human cells *in vitro*, but other studies on chromosomal aberrations in human cells *in vitro* gave conflicting results. In Chinese hamster cells it induced chromosomal damage but was questionably positive for sister chromatid exchange. Studies on the induction by furosemide of chromosomal aberrations in mice were inconclusive. The urine of rats treated with this drug did not induce gene conversion in *Saccharomyces cerevisiae*.

Furosemide produced no impairment of fertility in male or female rats, at 100 mg/kg/day (the maximum effective diuretic dose in the rat and 8 times the maximal human dose of 600 mg/day).

Pregnancy Category C
Furosemide has been shown to cause unexplained maternal deaths and abortions in rabbits at 2, 4 and 8 times the maximal recommended human dose. There are no adequate and well-controlled studies in pregnant women. Furosemide should be used during pregnancy only if the potential benefit justifies the potential risk to the fetus.

The effects of furosemide on embryonic and fetal development and on pregnant dams were studied in mice, rats and rabbits.

Furosemide caused unexplained maternal deaths and abortions in the rabbit at the lowest dose of 25 mg/kg (2 times the maximal recommended human dose of 600 mg/day). In another study, a dose of 50 mg/kg (4 times the maximal recommended human dose of 600 mg/day) also caused maternal deaths and abortions when administered to rabbits between Days 12 and 17 of gestation. In a third study, none of the pregnant rabbits survived a dose of 100 mg/kg. Data from the above studies indicate fetal lethality that can precede maternal deaths.

The results of the mouse study and one of the three rabbit studies also showed an increased incidence and severity of hydronephrosis (distention of the renal pelvis and, in some cases, of the ureters) in fetuses derived from the treated dams as compared with the incidence in fetuses from the control group.

Nursing Mothers
Because it appears in breast milk, caution should be exercised when furosemide is administered to a nursing mother.

INJECTION
Pediatric Use: Renal calcifications (from barely visible on x-ray to staghorn) have occurred in some severely premature infants treated with intravenous furosemide for edema due to patent ductus arteriosus and hyaline membrane disease. The concurrent use of chlorothiazide has been reported to decrease hypercalciuria and dissolve some calculi.

DRUG INTERACTIONS

Furosemide may increase the ototoxic potential of aminoglycoside antibiotics, especially in the presence of impaired renal function. Except in life-threatening situations, avoid this combination.

Furosemide should not be used concomitantly with ethacrynic acid because of the possibility of ototoxicity. Patients receiving high doses of salicylates concomitantly with furosemide, as in rheumatic disease, may experience salicylate toxicity at lower doses because of competitive renal excretory sites.

Furosemide has a tendency to antagonize the skeletal muscle relaxing effect of tubocurarine and may potentiate the action of succinylcholine.

Lithium generally should not be given with diuretics because they reduce lithium's renal clearance and add a high risk of lithium toxicity.

Furosemide may add to or potentiate the therapeutic effect of other antihypertensive drugs. Potentiation occurs with ganglionic or peripheral adrenergic blocking drugs.

Furosemide may decrease arterial responsiveness to norepinephrine. However, norepinephrine may still be used effectively.

TABLETS
Simultaneous administration of sucralfate and furosemide tablets may reduce the natriuretic and antihypertensive effects of furosemide. Patients receiving both drugs should be observed closely to determine if the desired diuretic and/or antihypertensive effect of furosemide is achieved. The intake of furosemide and sucralfate should be separated by at least 2 hours.

TABLETS, INJECTION, AND ORAL SOLUTION
One study in 6 subjects demonstrated that the combination of furosemide and acetylsalicylic acid temporarily reduced creatinine clearance in patients with chronic renal insufficiency. There are case reports of patients who developed increased BUN, serum creatinine and serum potassium levels, and weight gain when furosemide was used in conjunction with NSAIDs.

Literature reports indicate that coadministration of indomethacin may reduce the natriuretic and antihypertensive effects of furosemide in some patients by inhibiting prostaglandin synthesis. Indomethacin may also affect plasma renin levels, aldosterone excretion, and renin profile evaluation. Patients receiving both indomethacin and furosemide should be observed closely to determine if the desired diuretic and/or antihypertensive effect of furosemide is achieved.

ADVERSE REACTIONS

Adverse reactions are categorized below by organ system and listed by decreasing severity:

Gastrointestinal System Reactions: Pancreatitis, jaundice (intrahepatic cholestatic jaundice), anorexia, oral and gastric irritation, cramping, diarrhea, constipation, nausea, and vomiting.

Systemic Hypersensitivity Reactions: Systemic vasculitis, interstitial nephritis, and necrotizing angiitis.

Central Nervous System Reactions: Tinnitus and hearing loss, paresthesias, vertigo, dizziness, headache, blurred vision, and xanthopsia.

Hematologic Reactions: Aplastic anemia (rare), thrombocytopenia, agranulocytosis (rare), hemolytic anemia, leukopenia, and anemia.

Dermatologic-Hypersensitivity Reactions: Exfoliative dermatitis, erythema multiforme, purpura, photosensitivity, urticaria, rash, and pruritus.

Cardiovascular Reaction: Orthostatic hypotension may occur and be aggravated by alcohol, barbiturates or narcotics.

Other Reactions: Hyperglycemia, glycosuria, hyperuricemia, muscle spasm, weaknesses, restlessness, urinary bladder spasm, thrombophlebitis, and fever.

Whenever adverse reactions are moderate or severe, furosemide dosage should be reduced or therapy withdrawn.

DOSAGE AND ADMINISTRATION

TABLETS AND ORAL SOLUTION
Edema
Therapy should be individualized according to patient response to gain maximal therapeutic response and to determine the minimal dose needed to maintain that response.

Adults
The usual initial dose of furosemide is 20-80 mg given as a single dose. Ordinarily a prompt diuresis ensues. If needed, the same dose can be administered 6-8 hours later or the dose may be increased. The dose may be raised by 20 or 40 mg and given not sooner than 6 to 8 hours after the previous dose until the desired diuretic effect has been obtained. This individually determined single dose should then be given once or twice daily (*e.g.*, at 8 am and 2 pm). The dose of furosemide may be carefully titrated up to 600 mg/day in patients with clinically severe edematous states.

Edema may be most efficiently and safely mobilized by giving furosemide on 2-4 consecutive days each week.

When doses exceeding 80 mg/day are given for prolonged periods, careful clinical observation and laboratory monitoring are particularly advisable. (See PRECAUTIONS, Laboratory Tests.)

Pediatric Patients
The usual initial dose of oral furosemide in pediatric patients is 2 mg/kg body weight, given as a single dose. If the diuretic response is not satisfactory after the initial dose, dosage may be increased by 1 or 2 mg/kg no sooner than 6-8 hours after the previous dose. Doses greater than 6 mg/kg body weight are not recommended. For maintenance therapy in pediatric patients, the dose should be adjusted to the minimum effective level.

Hypertension
Therapy should be individualized according to the patient's response to gain maximal therapeutic response and to determine the minimal dose needed to maintain the therapeutic response.

Adults

The usual initial dose of furosemide for hypertension is 80 mg, usually divided into 40 mg twice a day. Dosage should then be adjusted according to response. If response is not satisfactory, add other antihypertensive agents.

Changes in blood pressure must be carefully monitored when furosemide is used with other antihypertensive drugs, especially during initial therapy. To prevent excessive drop in blood pressure, the dosage of other agents should be reduced by at least 50% when furosemide is added to the regimen. As the blood pressure falls under the potentiating effect of furosemide, a further reduction in dosage or even discontinuation of other antihypertensive drugs may be necessary.

INJECTION

Adults

Parenteral therapy with furosemide injection should be used only in patients unable to take oral medication or in emergency situations and should be replaced with oral therapy as soon as practical.

Edema

The usual initial dose of furosemide is 20-40 mg given as a single dose, injected intramuscularly or intravenously. The intravenous dose should be given slowly (1-2 minutes). Ordinarily a prompt diuresis ensues. If needed, another dose may be administered in the same manner 2 hours later or the dose may be increased. The dose may be raised by 20 mg and given not sooner than 2 hours after the previous dose until the desired diuretic effect has been obtained. This individually determined single dose should then be given once or twice daily.

Therapy should be individualized according to patient response to gain maximal therapeutic response to determine the minimal dose needed to maintain that response. Close medical supervision is necessary.

If the physician elects to use high dose parenteral therapy, add the furosemide to either sodium chloride injection, lactated ringer's injection, or dextrose (5%) injection after pH has been adjusted to above 5.5, and administer as a controlled intravenous infusion at a rate not greater than 4 mg/min. Furosemide injection is a buffered alkaline solution with a pH of about 9 and the drug may precipitate at pH values below 7. Care must be taken to ensure that the pH of the prepared infusion solution is in the weakly alkaline to neutral range. Acid solutions, including other parenteral medications (*e.g.,* labetalol, ciprofloxacin, amrinone, and milrinone) must not be administered concurrently in the same infusion because they may cause precipitation of the furosemide. In addition, furosemide injection should not be added to a running intravenous line containing any of these acidic products.

Acute Pulmonary Edema

The usual initial dose of furosemide is 40 mg injected slowly intravenously (over 1-2 minutes). If a satisfactory response does not occur within 1 hour, the dose may be increased to 80 mg injected slowly intravenously (over 1-2 minutes).

If necessary, additional therapy (*e.g.,* digitalis, oxygen) may be administered concomitantly.

Pediatric Patients

Parenteral therapy should be used only in patients unable to take oral medication or in emergency situations and should be replaced with oral therapy as soon as practical.

The usual initial dose of furosemide injection (intravenously or intramuscularly) in pediatric patients is 1 mg/kg body weight and should be given slowly under close medical supervision. If the diuretic response to the initial dose is not satisfactory, dosage may be increased by 1 mg/kg not sooner than 2 hours after the previous dose, until the desired diuretic effect has been obtained. Doses greater than 6 mg/kg body weight are not recommended.

Furosemide injection should be inspected visually for particulate matter and discoloration before administration. Do not use if solution is discolored.

To insure patient safety, this needle should be handled with care and should be destroyed and discarded if damaged in any manner. If cannula is bent, no attempt should be made to straighten.

To prevent needle-stick injuries, needles should not be recapped, purposely bent, or broken by hand.

HOW SUPPLIED

TABLETS

Dispense in well-closed, light-resistant containers. Exposure to light might cause a slight discoloration. Discolored tablets should not be dispensed.

20 mg Tablets: Lasix tablets 20 mg are supplied as white, oval, monogrammed tablets. They are imprinted with "Lasix" on one side and "Hoechst" on the other.

40 mg Tablets: Lasix tablets 40 mg are supplied as white, round, monogrammed, scored tablets. They are imprinted with "Lasix" on one side and the Hoechst logo on the other.

80 mg Tablets: Lasix tablets 80 mg are supplied as white, round, monogrammed, facetted edge tablets. They are imprinted with "Lasix 80" on one side and the Hoechst logo on the other.

ORAL SOLUTION

Store at controlled room temperature (59-86°F). Dispense in light-resistant containers. Discard opened bottle after 60 days.

INJECTION

Storage: Store at controlled room temperature (59-86°F).

Do not use if solution is discolored.

Protect syringes from light. Do not remove syringe from individual package until time of use.

PRODUCT LISTING - RATED THERAPEUTICALLY EQUIVALENT

Size	Price	Product	NDC
Liquid - Oral - 10 mg/ml			
60 ml	$7.14	GENERIC, Moore, H.L. Drug Exchange Inc	00839-7431-64
60 ml	$9.05	GENERIC, Aligen Independent Laboratories Inc	00405-2832-56
60 ml	$9.10	GENERIC, Roxane Laboratories Inc	00054-3294-46
60 ml	$10.40	GENERIC, Qualitest Products Inc	00603-1250-52
60 ml	$10.40	GENERIC, Morton Grove Pharmaceuticals Inc	60432-0613-60
60 ml	$10.50	GENERIC, Major Pharmaceuticals Inc	00904-1477-03
60 ml	$12.00	LASIX, Aventis Pharmaceuticals	00039-0063-06
120 ml	$12.90	GENERIC, Ivax Corporation	00182-6053-37
120 ml	$13.96	GENERIC, Major Pharmaceuticals Inc	00904-1477-20
120 ml	$14.28	GENERIC, Morton Grove Pharmaceuticals Inc	60432-0613-04
120 ml	$17.67	GENERIC, Roxane Laboratories Inc	00054-3294-50
120 ml	$19.98	LASIX, Aventis Pharmaceuticals	00039-0063-40
Solution - Injectable - 10 mg/ml			
2 ml	$0.98	GENERIC, Hauser, A.F. Inc	52637-0010-10
2 ml	$2.10	GENERIC, Interstate Drug Exchange Inc	00814-3306-35
2 ml x 5	$5.94	LASIX, Aventis Pharmaceuticals	00039-0061-15
2 ml x 5	$8.94	LASIX, Aventis Pharmaceuticals	00039-0062-08
2 ml x 10	$7.10	GENERIC, Sanofi Winthrop Pharmaceuticals	00024-0611-03
2 ml x 10	$7.50	GENERIC, Abbott Pharmaceutical	00074-1275-02
2 ml x 10	$12.35	GENERIC, Abbott Pharmaceutical	00074-1275-22
2 ml x 10	$23.75	GENERIC, Abbott Pharmaceutical	00074-1275-12
2 ml x 25	$18.70	GENERIC, Abbott Pharmaceutical	00074-6102-02
2 ml x 25	$19.30	GENERIC, Abbott Pharmaceutical	00074-6101-02
2 ml x 25	$19.76	GENERIC, Esi Lederle Generics	00641-0382-25
2 ml x 25	$22.25	GENERIC, American Regent Laboratories Inc	00517-5702-25
2 ml x 25	$25.75	GENERIC, American Pharmaceutical Partners	63323-0280-02
2 ml x 25	$36.66	LASIX, Aventis Pharmaceuticals	00039-0162-25
2 ml x 50	$56.10	LASIX, Aventis Pharmaceuticals	00039-0061-05
4 ml x 5	$10.02	LASIX, Aventis Pharmaceuticals	00039-0061-45
4 ml x 5	$11.94	LASIX, Aventis Pharmaceuticals	00039-0064-08
4 ml x 10	$13.68	GENERIC, Abbott Pharmaceutical	00074-1274-04
4 ml x 10	$14.25	GENERIC, Abbott Pharmaceutical	00074-1274-14
4 ml x 10	$16.86	GENERIC, Abbott Pharmaceutical	00074-1274-34
4 ml x 10	$25.90	GENERIC, Astra-Zeneca Pharmaceuticals	00186-0635-01
4 ml x 10	$27.31	GENERIC, Abbott Pharmaceutical	00074-9631-04
4 ml x 10	$59.00	GENERIC, Abbott Pharmaceutical	00074-6055-14
4 ml x 25	$19.75	GENERIC, Baxter Pharmaceutical Products, Inc	10019-0010-76
4 ml x 25	$22.27	GENERIC, Abbott Pharmaceutical	00074-6102-04
4 ml x 25	$26.42	GENERIC, Abbott Pharmaceutical	00074-6101-04
4 ml x 25	$31.00	GENERIC, American Pharmaceutical Partners	63323-0280-04
4 ml x 25	$36.00	GENERIC, American Regent Laboratories Inc	00517-5704-25
4 ml x 25	$49.02	LASIX, Aventis Pharmaceuticals	00039-0061-65
4 ml x 25	$56.10	LASIX, Aventis Pharmaceuticals	00039-0163-25
5 ml x 10	$14.30	GENERIC, Abbott Pharmaceutical	00074-1274-24
8 ml x 10	$45.60	GENERIC, Abbott Pharmaceutical	00074-6056-17
10 ml	$2.36	GENERIC, Moore, H.L. Drug Exchange Inc	00839-6677-30
10 ml	$6.95	GENERIC, Roberts/Hauck Pharmaceutical Corporation	43797-0028-12
10 ml x 5	$28.44	LASIX, Aventis Pharmaceuticals	00039-0061-08
10 ml x 5	$29.94	LASIX, Aventis Pharmaceuticals	00039-0065-08
10 ml x 10	$45.80	GENERIC, Abbott Pharmaceutical	00074-1639-10
10 ml x 10	$48.20	GENERIC, Astra-Zeneca Pharmaceuticals	00186-0636-01
10 ml x 10	$124.44	GENERIC, Abbott Pharmaceutical	00074-6056-10
10 ml x 10	$149.60	GENERIC, Abbott Pharmaceutical	00074-6056-18
10 ml x 25	$12.25	GENERIC, Abbott Pharmaceutical	00074-6102-10
10 ml x 25	$16.25	GENERIC, Abbott Pharmaceutical	00074-6101-10
10 ml x 25	$49.08	GENERIC, Abbott Pharmaceutical	00074-6055-04
10 ml x 25	$54.50	GENERIC, American Pharmaceutical Partners	63323-0280-10
10 ml x 25	$57.25	GENERIC, American Regent Laboratories Inc	00517-5710-25
10 ml x 25	$73.50	GENERIC, Astra-Zeneca Pharmaceuticals	00186-1117-12
10 ml x 25	$137.88	LASIX, Aventis Pharmaceuticals	00039-0061-25
10 ml x 25	$143.88	LASIX, Aventis Pharmaceuticals	00039-0164-25
50 ml	$11.50	GENERIC, Pasadena Research Laboratories Inc	00418-0361-02
50 ml	$27.25	GENERIC, Cmc-Consolidated Midland Corporation	00223-7700-02
60 ml	$7.00	GENERIC, Major Pharmaceuticals Inc	00904-1485-10
80 ml	$71.04	GENERIC, Abbott Pharmaceutical	00074-6056-20
100 ml	$37.50	GENERIC, Cmc-Consolidated Midland Corporation	00223-7704-04
Solution - Oral - 10 mg/ml			
60 ml	$7.80	FEDERAL UPPER LIMIT, H.C.F.A. F F P	99999-1342-14
Tablet - Oral - 20 mg			
6's	$3.12	GENERIC, Pd-Rx Pharmaceuticals	55289-0593-06
15's	$1.59	GENERIC, Heartland Healthcare Services	61392-0256-15
25's	$2.81	GENERIC, Udl Laboratories Inc	51079-0072-19
25's	$5.49	GENERIC, Pd-Rx Pharmaceuticals	55289-0593-97
30 x 25	$96.30	GENERIC, Sky Pharmaceuticals Packaging, Inc	63739-0111-03
30 x 25	$115.11	GENERIC, Sky Pharmaceuticals Packaging, Inc	63739-0111-01

30's	$1.85	GENERIC, Major Pharmaceuticals Inc	00904-1580-46
30's	$2.60	GENERIC, Circle Pharmaceuticals Inc	00659-1304-30
30's	$3.18	GENERIC, Heartland Healthcare Services	61392-0256-30
30's	$3.18	GENERIC, Heartland Healthcare Services	61392-0256-39
30's	$3.66	GENERIC, Pd-Rx Pharmaceuticals	55289-0593-30
31 x 10	$39.99	GENERIC, Vangard Labs	00615-1569-53
31 x 10	$39.99	GENERIC, Vangard Labs	00615-1569-63
32's	$3.39	GENERIC, Heartland Healthcare Services	61392-0256-32
45's	$4.77	GENERIC, Heartland Healthcare Services	61392-0256-45
60's	$6.35	GENERIC, Heartland Healthcare Services	61392-0256-60
90's	$2.80	GENERIC, Major Pharmaceuticals Inc	00904-1580-89
90's	$4.25	GENERIC, Allscripts Pharmaceutical Company	54569-8557-00
90's	$9.53	GENERIC, Heartland Healthcare Services	61392-0256-90
100's	$2.93	GENERIC, Interstate Drug Exchange Inc	00814-3300-14
100's	$4.25	GENERIC, Moore, H.L. Drug Exchange Inc	00839-6345-06
100's	$4.98	GENERIC, Aligen Independent Laboratories Inc	00405-4452-01
100's	$5.00	GENERIC, Raway Pharmacal Inc	00686-0072-20
100's	$5.10	GENERIC, Creighton Products Corporation	50752-0286-05
100's	$5.18	GENERIC, Pd-Rx Pharmaceuticals	55289-0593-01
100's	$5.25	GENERIC, Roxane Laboratories Inc	00054-4297-25
100's	$5.63	FEDERAL UPPER LIMIT, H.C.F.A. F F P	99999-1342-02
100's	$6.06	GENERIC, Moore, H.L. Drug Exchange Inc	00839-7782-06
100's	$6.39	GENERIC, Major Pharmaceuticals Inc	00904-1480-61
100's	$7.57	GENERIC, Roxane Laboratories Inc	00054-8297-25
100's	$8.75	GENERIC, Watson/Schein Pharmaceuticals Inc	00364-0568-90
100's	$11.30	GENERIC, Auro Pharmaceutical	55829-0265-10
100's	$11.36	GENERIC, Esi Lederle Generics	00005-3708-23
100's	$12.44	GENERIC, Geneva Pharmaceuticals	00781-1818-13
100's	$12.52	GENERIC, American Health Packaging	62584-0709-01
100's	$12.78	GENERIC, Major Pharmaceuticals Inc	00904-1580-61
100's	$13.25	GENERIC, Medirex Inc	57480-0328-01
100's	$13.45	GENERIC, Major Pharmaceuticals Inc	00904-1580-60
100's	$14.30	GENERIC, Mylan Pharmaceuticals Inc	00378-0208-01
100's	$14.73	GENERIC, Udl Laboratories Inc	51079-0072-20
100's	$15.38	GENERIC, Ivax Corporation	00172-2908-60
100's	$16.27	GENERIC, Ivax Corporation	00182-1170-89
100's	$22.66	LASIX, Aventis Pharmaceuticals	00039-0067-10

Tablet - Oral - 40 mg

4's	$1.34	GENERIC, Pd-Rx Pharmaceuticals	55289-0118-04
10's	$2.84	GENERIC, Pd-Rx Pharmaceuticals	55289-0118-10
12's	$3.21	GENERIC, Pd-Rx Pharmaceuticals	55289-0118-12
15's	$2.17	GENERIC, Heartland Healthcare Services	61392-0253-15
25's	$3.60	GENERIC, Udl Laboratories Inc	51079-0073-19
25's	$5.30	GENERIC, Pd-Rx Pharmaceuticals	55289-0118-97
30 x 25	$132.90	GENERIC, Sky Pharmaceuticals Packaging, Inc	63739-0112-01
30 x 25	$132.90	GENERIC, Sky Pharmaceuticals Packaging, Inc	63739-0112-03
30's	$1.90	GENERIC, Major Pharmaceuticals Inc	00904-1481-46
30's	$3.75	GENERIC, Pd-Rx Pharmaceuticals	55289-0118-30
30's	$4.35	GENERIC, Heartland Healthcare Services	61392-0253-30
30's	$4.35	GENERIC, Heartland Healthcare Services	61392-0253-39
30's	$8.71	LASIX, Allscripts Pharmaceutical Company	54569-0573-00
30's	$10.64	LASIX, Physicians Total Care	54868-0788-01
31 x 10	$56.42	GENERIC, Vangard Labs	00615-0446-53
31 x 10	$56.42	GENERIC, Vangard Labs	00615-0446-63
31's	$3.28	GENERIC, Heartland Healthcare Services	61392-0256-31
31's	$4.49	GENERIC, Heartland Healthcare Services	61392-0253-31
32's	$4.64	GENERIC, Heartland Healthcare Services	61392-0253-32
45's	$6.52	GENERIC, Heartland Healthcare Services	61392-0253-45
60's	$8.69	GENERIC, Heartland Healthcare Services	61392-0253-60
90's	$2.95	GENERIC, Major Pharmaceuticals Inc	00904-1481-89
90's	$4.86	GENERIC, Pd-Rx Pharmaceuticals	55289-0118-90
90's	$5.34	GENERIC, Allscripts Pharmaceutical Company	54569-8523-00
90's	$13.04	GENERIC, Heartland Healthcare Services	61392-0253-90
100's	$3.50	GENERIC, Mova Pharmaceutical Corporation	55370-0515-07
100's	$3.53	GENERIC, Interstate Drug Exchange Inc	00814-3301-14
100's	$5.25	GENERIC, Raway Pharmacal Inc	00686-0073-20
100's	$5.32	GENERIC, Aligen Independent Laboratories Inc	00405-4453-01
100's	$5.66	GENERIC, Moore, H.L. Drug Exchange Inc	00839-6323-06
100's	$5.85	GENERIC, Creighton Products Corporation	50752-0287-05
100's	$5.99	FEDERAL UPPER LIMIT, H.C.F.A. F F P	99999-1342-08
100's	$6.28	GENERIC, Moore, H.L. Drug Exchange Inc	00839-7783-06
100's	$6.70	GENERIC, Pd-Rx Pharmaceuticals	55289-0118-01
100's	$8.49	GENERIC, Roxane Laboratories Inc	00054-8299-25
100's	$12.10	GENERIC, Watson/Schein Pharmaceuticals Inc	00364-0514-90
100's	$13.56	GENERIC, Esi Lederle Generics	00005-3709-23
100's	$14.10	GENERIC, Auro Pharmaceutical	55829-0266-10
100's	$14.31	GENERIC, American Health Packaging	62584-0710-01
100's	$15.35	GENERIC, Major Pharmaceuticals Inc	00904-1481-60
100's	$15.50	GENERIC, Geneva Pharmaceuticals	00781-1966-01
100's	$16.30	GENERIC, Roxane Laboratories Inc	00054-4299-25
100's	$16.30	GENERIC, Mylan Pharmaceuticals Inc	00378-0216-01
100's	$16.79	GENERIC, Udl Laboratories Inc	51079-0073-20
100's	$17.49	GENERIC, Ivax Corporation	00172-2907-60
100's	$18.46	GENERIC, Geneva Pharmaceuticals	00781-1966-13
100's	$19.05	GENERIC, Major Pharmaceuticals Inc	00904-1481-61
100's	$21.67	GENERIC, Ivax Corporation	00182-1161-89
100's	$29.04	LASIX, Aventis Pharmaceuticals	00039-0060-11
100's	$31.74	LASIX, Aventis Pharmaceuticals	00039-0060-13
100's	$33.42	LASIX, Physicians Total Care	54868-0788-00
100's	$47.60	GENERIC, Creighton Products Corporation	50752-0287-09

Tablet - Oral - 80 mg

25's	$5.48	GENERIC, Udl Laboratories Inc	51079-0527-19
30 x 25	$164.03	GENERIC, Sky Pharmaceuticals Packaging, Inc	63739-0113-03
30's	$8.50	GENERIC, Heartland Healthcare Services	61392-0254-30
30's	$8.50	GENERIC, Heartland Healthcare Services	61392-0254-39
30's	$133.40	GENERIC, Medirex Inc	57480-0330-06
31 x 10	$77.35	GENERIC, Vangard Labs	00615-1571-53
31 x 10	$77.35	GENERIC, Vangard Labs	00615-1571-63
31's	$8.79	GENERIC, Heartland Healthcare Services	61392-0254-31
32's	$9.07	GENERIC, Heartland Healthcare Services	61392-0254-32
45's	$12.75	GENERIC, Heartland Healthcare Services	61392-0254-45
50's	$25.66	LASIX, Aventis Pharmaceuticals	00039-0066-05
60's	$17.01	GENERIC, Heartland Healthcare Services	61392-0254-60
90's	$25.51	GENERIC, Heartland Healthcare Services	61392-0254-90
100's	$7.75	GENERIC, Raway Pharmacal Inc	00686-0527-20
100's	$7.80	GENERIC, Interstate Drug Exchange Inc	00814-3303-14
100's	$9.15	FEDERAL UPPER LIMIT, H.C.F.A. F F P	99999-1342-12
100's	$13.05	GENERIC, Creighton Products Corporation	50752-0288-05
100's	$13.07	GENERIC, Moore, H.L. Drug Exchange Inc	00839-6777-06
100's	$19.25	GENERIC, Ivax Corporation	00182-1736-01
100's	$19.98	GENERIC, Aligen Independent Laboratories Inc	00405-4454-01
100's	$20.69	GENERIC, Esi Lederle Generics	00005-3100-23
100's	$21.50	GENERIC, Auro Pharmaceutical	55829-0267-10
100's	$29.75	GENERIC, Geneva Pharmaceuticals	00781-1446-13
100's	$29.75	GENERIC, Major Pharmaceuticals Inc	00904-1482-61
100's	$41.19	GENERIC, Major Pharmaceuticals Inc	00904-1482-60
100's	$41.60	GENERIC, Geneva Pharmaceuticals	00781-1446-01
100's	$43.70	GENERIC, Roxane Laboratories Inc	00054-4301-25
100's	$43.70	GENERIC, Mylan Pharmaceuticals Inc	00378-0232-01
100's	$44.28	LASIX, Aventis Pharmaceuticals	00039-0066-11
100's	$45.01	GENERIC, Udl Laboratories Inc	51079-0527-20
100's	$52.44	GENERIC, Roxane Laboratories Inc	00054-8301-25

PRODUCT LISTING - EQUIVALENTS NOT AVAILABLE

Solution - Injectable - 10 mg/ml

2 ml x 25	$37.79	GENERIC, Allscripts Pharmaceutical Company	54569-2306-00
2 ml x 25	$40.00	GENERIC, Cmc-Consolidated Midland Corporation	00223-7701-02
4 ml x 25	$19.76	GENERIC, Allscripts Pharmaceutical Company	54569-3590-00
4 ml x 25	$55.00	GENERIC, Consolidated Midland Corporation	00223-7705-04
10 ml	$6.25	GENERIC, Cmc-Consolidated Midland Corporation	00223-7708-20
10 ml	$8.90	GENERIC, Hyrex Pharmaceuticals	00314-0510-70
10 ml x 25	$125.00	GENERIC, Cmc-Consolidated Midland Corporation	00223-7707-10

Solution - Oral - 40 mg/5 ml

5 ml x 40	$60.00	GENERIC, Roxane Laboratories Inc	00054-8298-16
10 ml x 40	$68.11	GENERIC, Roxane Laboratories Inc	00054-8300-16
500 ml	$36.74	GENERIC, Roxane Laboratories Inc	00054-3298-63

Tablet - Oral - 20 mg

4's	$0.76	GENERIC, Southwood Pharmaceuticals Inc	58016-0538-04
12's	$2.28	GENERIC, Southwood Pharmaceuticals Inc	58016-0538-12
15's	$2.85	GENERIC, Southwood Pharmaceuticals Inc	58016-0538-15
20's	$3.80	GENERIC, Southwood Pharmaceuticals Inc	58016-0538-20
30's	$3.87	GENERIC, Allscripts Pharmaceutical Company	54569-0572-00
30's	$5.70	GENERIC, Southwood Pharmaceuticals Inc	58016-0538-30
50's	$9.50	GENERIC, Southwood Pharmaceuticals Inc	58016-0538-50
60's	$2.16	GENERIC, Circle Pharmaceuticals Inc	00659-1304-60
60's	$7.74	GENERIC, Allscripts Pharmaceutical Company	54569-0572-02
90's	$12.05	GENERIC, Pharmaceutical Corporation Of America	51655-0193-26
100's	$2.00	GENERIC, Cmc-Consolidated Midland Corporation	00223-1012-01
100's	$12.90	GENERIC, Allscripts Pharmaceutical Company	54569-0572-01
100's	$19.00	GENERIC, Southwood Pharmaceuticals Inc	58016-0538-00

Tablet - Oral - 40 mg

2's	$0.28	GENERIC, Allscripts Pharmaceutical Company	54569-0574-06
3's	$3.44	GENERIC, Prescript Pharmaceuticals	00247-0199-03
4's	$3.46	GENERIC, Prescript Pharmaceuticals	00247-0199-04
10's	$2.65	GENERIC, Southwood Pharmaceuticals Inc	58016-0539-10
12's	$3.18	GENERIC, Southwood Pharmaceuticals Inc	58016-0539-12
14's	$3.71	GENERIC, Southwood Pharmaceuticals Inc	58016-0539-14
15's	$2.12	GENERIC, Allscripts Pharmaceutical Company	54569-0574-02
15's	$3.75	GENERIC, Prescript Pharmaceuticals	00247-0199-15
15's	$3.98	GENERIC, Southwood Pharmaceuticals Inc	58016-0539-15
20's	$5.30	GENERIC, Southwood Pharmaceuticals Inc	58016-0539-20
21's	$5.57	GENERIC, Southwood Pharmaceuticals Inc	58016-0539-21
24's	$6.36	GENERIC, Southwood Pharmaceuticals Inc	58016-0539-24
25's	$6.63	GENERIC, Southwood Pharmaceuticals Inc	58016-0539-25

F

28's	$7.42	GENERIC, Southwood Pharmaceuticals Inc	58016-0539-28
30's	$4.15	GENERIC, Prescript Pharmaceuticals	00247-0199-30
30's	$4.24	GENERIC, Allscripts Pharmaceutical Company	54569-0574-00
30's	$5.20	GENERIC, Pharmaceutical Corporation Of America	51655-0081-24
30's	$7.95	GENERIC, Southwood Pharmaceuticals Inc	58016-0539-30
40's	$10.60	GENERIC, Southwood Pharmaceuticals Inc	58016-0539-40
60's	$8.48	GENERIC, Allscripts Pharmaceutical Company	54569-0574-03
60's	$9.40	GENERIC, Pharmaceutical Corporation Of America	51655-0081-25
60's	$15.90	GENERIC, Southwood Pharmaceuticals Inc	58016-0539-60
90's	$13.60	GENERIC, Pharmaceutical Corporation Of America	51655-0081-26
100's	$2.50	GENERIC, Cmc-Consolidated Midland Corporation	00223-1013-01
100's	$6.00	GENERIC, Prescript Pharmaceuticals	00247-0199-00
100's	$14.14	GENERIC, Allscripts Pharmaceutical Company	54569-0574-01
100's	$15.05	GENERIC, Pharmaceutical Corporation Of America	51655-0081-21
100's	$26.50	GENERIC, Southwood Pharmaceuticals Inc	58016-0539-00
180's	$10.80	GENERIC, Allscripts Pharmaceutical Company	54569-8523-01
180's	$26.40	GENERIC, Pharmaceutical Corporation Of America	51655-0081-83

Tablet - Oral - 80 mg

10's	$3.60	GENERIC, Southwood Pharmaceuticals Inc	58016-0576-10
12's	$4.32	GENERIC, Southwood Pharmaceuticals Inc	58016-0576-12
14's	$5.04	GENERIC, Southwood Pharmaceuticals Inc	58016-0576-14
15's	$5.40	GENERIC, Southwood Pharmaceuticals Inc	58016-0576-15
18's	$6.48	GENERIC, Southwood Pharmaceuticals Inc	58016-0576-18
20's	$7.20	GENERIC, Southwood Pharmaceuticals Inc	58016-0576-20
21's	$7.56	GENERIC, Southwood Pharmaceuticals Inc	58016-0576-21
24's	$8.64	GENERIC, Southwood Pharmaceuticals Inc	58016-0576-24
25's	$9.00	GENERIC, Southwood Pharmaceuticals Inc	58016-0576-25
28's	$10.08	GENERIC, Southwood Pharmaceuticals Inc	58016-0576-28
30's	$10.80	GENERIC, Southwood Pharmaceuticals Inc	58016-0576-30
30's	$11.15	GENERIC, Allscripts Pharmaceutical Company	54569-0570-01
40's	$14.40	GENERIC, Southwood Pharmaceuticals Inc	58016-0576-40
50's	$17.95	GENERIC, Southwood Pharmaceuticals Inc	58016-0576-50
60's	$21.60	GENERIC, Southwood Pharmaceuticals Inc	58016-0576-60
100's	$35.90	GENERIC, Southwood Pharmaceuticals Inc	58016-0576-00

Gabapentin *(003175)*

Categories: Neuralgia, postherpetic; Seizures, partial; Pregnancy Category C; FDA Approved 1993 Dec
Drug Classes: Anticonvulsants
Brand Names: **Neurontin**
Foreign Brand Availability: Gantin (Australia); Kaptin (Colombia)
Cost of Therapy: $119.13 (Epilepsy; Neurontin; 300 mg; 3 capsules/day; 30 day supply)

DESCRIPTION

Neurontin (gabapentin) capsules, tablets, and oral solution are supplied as imprinted hard shell capsules containing 100, 300, and 400 mg of gabapentin, elliptical film-coated tablets containing 600 and 800 mg of gabapentin or an oral solution containing 250 mg/5 ml of gabapentin.

Gabapentin is described as 1-(aminomethyl)cyclohexanacetic acid with a molecular formula of $C_9H_{17}NO_2$ and a molecular weight of 171.24.

Gabapentin is a white to off-white crystalline solid with a pK_{a1} of 3.7 and a pK_{a2} of 10.7. It is freely soluble in water and both basic and acidic aqueous solutions. The log of the partition coefficient (n-octanol/0.05M phosphate buffer) at pH 7.4 is -1.25.

CAPSULES

The inactive ingredients for the capsules are lactose, cornstarch, and talc. The 100 mg capsule shell contains gelatin and titanium dioxide. The 300 mg capsule shell contains gelatin, titanium dioxide, and yellow iron oxide. The 400 mg capsule shell contains gelatin, red iron oxide, titanium dioxide, and yellow iron oxide. The imprinting ink contains FD&C blue no. 2 and titanium dioxide.

TABLETS

The inactive ingredients for the tablets are poloxamer 407, copolyvidonum, cornstarch, magnesium stearate, hydroxypropyl cellulose, talc, candelilla wax and purified water. The imprinting ink for the 600 mg tablets contains synthetic black iron oxide, pharmaceutical shellac, pharmaceutical glaze, propylene glycol, ammonium hydroxide, isopropyl alcohol and n-butyl alcohol. The imprinting ink for the 800 mg tablets contains synthetic yellow iron oxide, synthetic red iron oxide, hydroxypropyl methylcellulose, propylene glycol, methanol, isopropyl alcohol and deionized water.

ORAL SOLUTION

The inactive ingredients for the oral solution are glycerin, xylitol, purified water and artificial cool strawberry anise flavor.

CLINICAL PHARMACOLOGY

MECHANISM OF ACTION

The mechanism by which gabapentin exerts its analgesic action is unknown, but in animal models of analgesia, gabapentin prevents allodynia (pain-related behavior in response to a normally innocuous stimulus) and hyperalgesia (exaggerated response to painful stimuli). In particular, gabapentin prevents pain-related responses in several models of neuropathic pain in rats or mice (*e.g.,* spinal nerve ligation models, streptozocin-induced diabetes model, spinal cord injury model, acute herpes zoster infection model). Gabapentin also decreases pain-related responses after peripheral inflammation (carrageenan footpad test, late phase of formalin test). Gabapentin did not alter immediate pain-related behaviors (rat tail flick test, formalin footpad acute phase, acetic acid abdominal constriction test, footpad heat irradiation test). The relevance of these models to human pain is not known.

The mechanism by which gabapentin exerts its anticonvulsant action is unknown, but in animal test systems designed to detect anticonvulsant activity, gabapentin prevents seizures as do other marketed anticonvulsants. Gabapentin exhibits antiseizure activity in mice and rats in both the maximal electroshock and pentylenetetrazole seizure models and other preclinical models (*e.g.,* strains with genetic epilepsy, etc.). The relevance of these models to human epilepsy is not known.

Gabapentin is structurally related to the neurotransmitter GABA (gamma-aminobutyric acid) but it does not modify $GABA_A$ or $GABA_B$ radioligand binding, it is not converted metabolically into GABA or a GABA agonist, and it is not an inhibitor of GABA uptake or degradation. Gabapentin was tested in radioligand binding assays at concentrations up to 100 μM and did not exhibit affinity for a number of other common receptor sites, including benzodiazepine, glutamate, N-methyl-D-aspartate (NMDA), quisqualate, kainate, strychnine-insensitive or strychnine-sensitive glycine, alpha 1, alpha 2, or beta adrenergic, adenosine A1 or A2, cholinergic muscarinic or nicotinic, dopamine D1 or D2, histamine H1, serotonin S1 or S2, opiate mu, delta or kappa, cannabinoid 1, voltage-sensitive calcium channel sites labeled with nitrendipine or diltiazem, or at voltage-sensitive sodium channel sites labeled with batrachotoxinin A 20-alpha-benzoate. Furthermore, gabapentin did not alter the cellular uptake of dopamine, noradrenaline, or serotonin.

In vitro studies with radiolabeled gabapentin have revealed a gabapentin binding site in areas of rat brain including neocortex and hippocampus. A high-affinity binding protein in animal brain tissue has been identified as an auxiliary subunit of voltage-activated calcium channels. However, functional correlates of gabapentin binding, if any, remain to be elucidated.

PHARMACOKINETICS AND DRUG METABOLISM

All pharmacological actions following gabapentin administration are due to the activity of the parent compound; gabapentin is not appreciably metabolized in humans.

Oral Bioavailability

Gabapentin bioavailability is not dose proportional; *i.e.,* as dose is increased, bioavailability decreases. Bioavailability of gabapentin is approximately 60%, 47%, 34%, 33%, and 27% following 900, 1200, 2400, 3600, and 4800 mg/day given in 3 divided doses, respectively. Food has only a slight effect on the rate and extent of absorption of gabapentin (14% increase in AUC and C_{max}).

Distribution

Less than 3% of gabapentin circulates bound to plasma protein. The apparent volume of distribution of gabapentin after 150 mg intravenous administration is 58 ± 6 L (mean ±SD). In patients with epilepsy, steady-state predose (C_{min}) concentrations of gabapentin in cerebrospinal fluid were approximately 20% of the corresponding plasma concentrations.

Elimination

Gabapentin is eliminated from the systemic circulation by renal excretion as unchanged drug. Gabapentin is not appreciably metabolized in humans.

Gabapentin elimination half-life is 5-7 hours and is unaltered by dose or following multiple dosing. Gabapentin elimination rate constant, plasma clearance, and renal clearance are directly proportional to creatinine clearance (see Special Populations, Adult Patients With Renal Insufficiency). In elderly patients, and in patients with impaired renal function, gabapentin plasma clearance is reduced. Gabapentin can be removed from plasma by hemodialysis.

Dosage adjustment in patients with compromised renal function or undergoing hemodialysis is recommended (see TABLE 5).

SPECIAL POPULATIONS

Adult Patients With Renal Insufficiency

Subjects (n=60) with renal insufficiency (mean creatinine clearance ranging from 13-114 ml/min) were administered single 400 mg oral doses of gabapentin. The mean gabapentin half-life ranged from about 6.5 hours (patients with creatinine clearance >60 ml/min) to 52 hours (creatinine clearance <30 ml/min) and gabapentin renal clearance from about 90 ml/min (>60 ml/min group) to about 10 ml/min (<30 ml/min). Mean plasma clearance (CL/F) decreased from approximately 190 ml/min to 20 ml/min.

Dosage adjustment in adult patients with compromised renal function is necessary (see DOSAGE AND ADMINISTRATION). Pediatric patients with renal insufficiency have not been studied.

Hemodialysis

In a study in anuric subjects (n=11), the apparent elimination half-life of gabapentin on nondialysis days was about 132 hours; during dialysis the apparent half-life of gabapentin was reduced to 3.8 hours. Hemodialysis thus has a significant effect on gabapentin elimination in anuric subjects.

Dosage adjustment in patients undergoing hemodialysis is necessary (see DOSAGE AND ADMINISTRATION).

Hepatic Disease

Because gabapentin is not metabolized, no study was performed in patients with hepatic impairment.

Age

The effect of age was studied in subjects 20-80 years of age. Apparent oral clearance (CL/F) of gabapentin decreased as age increased, from about 225 ml/min in those under 30 years of age to about 125 ml/min in those over 70 years of age. Renal clearance (CLR) and CLR adjusted for body surface area also declined with age; however, the decline in the renal clearance of gabapentin with age can largely be explained by the decline in renal function. Reduction of gabapentin dose may be required in patients who have age related compromised renal function. (See PRECAUTIONS, Geriatric Use, and DOSAGE AND ADMINISTRATION.)

Pediatric

Gabapentin pharmacokinetics were determined in 48 pediatric subjects between the ages of 1 month and 12 years following a dose of approximately 10 mg/kg. Peak plasma concentrations were similar across the entire age group and occurred 2-3 hours postdose. In general, pediatric subjects between 1 month and <5 years of age achieved approximately 30% lower exposure (AUC) than that observed in those 5 years of age and older. Accordingly, oral clearance normalized per body weight was higher in the younger children. Apparent oral clearance of gabapentin was directly proportional to creatinine clearance. Gabapentin elimination half-life averaged 4.7 hours and was similar across the age groups studied.

A population pharmacokinetic analysis was performed in 253 pediatric subjects between 1 month and 13 years of age. Patients received 10-65 mg/kg/day given tid. Apparent oral clearance (CL/F) was directly proportional to creatinine clearance and this relationship was similar following a single dose and at steady state. Higher oral clearance values were observed in children <5 years of age compared to those observed in children 5 years of age and older, when normalized per body weight. The clearance was highly variable in infants <1 year of age. The normalized CL/F values observed in pediatric patients 5 years of age and older were consistent with values observed in adults after a single dose. The oral volume of distribution normalized per body weight was constant across the age range.

These pharmacokinetic data indicate that the effective daily dose in pediatric patients with epilepsy ages 3 and 4 years should be 40 mg/kg/day to achieve average plasma concentrations similar to those achieved in patients 5 years of age and older receiving gabapentin at 30 mg/kg/day. (See DOSAGE AND ADMINISTRATION.)

Gender

Although no formal study has been conducted to compare the pharmacokinetics of gabapentin in men and women, it appears that the pharmacokinetic parameters for males and females are similar and there are no significant gender differences.

Race

Pharmacokinetic differences due to race have not been studied. Because gabapentin is primarily renally excreted and there are no important racial differences in creatinine clearance, pharmacokinetic differences due to race are not expected.

INDICATIONS AND USAGE

POSTHERPETIC NEURALGIA

Gabapentin is indicated for the management of postherpetic neuralgia in adults.

EPILEPSY

Gabapentin is indicated as adjunctive therapy in the treatment of partial seizures with and without secondary generalization in patients over 12 years of age with epilepsy. Gabapentin is also indicated as adjunctive therapy in the treatment of partial seizures in pediatric patients age 3-12 years.

NON-FDA APPROVED INDICATIONS

Gabapentin has been reported to be effective in the treatment of cocaine dependence, multiple sclerosis, neuropathic pain (including trigeminal neuralgia), cancer pain, diabetic neuropathy, panic disorder, bipolar disorder, restless legs syndrome, somatization disorder, and other disorders. While preliminary results are promising, additional confirmatory trials are needed. These uses have not been approved by the FDA.

CONTRAINDICATIONS

Gabapentin is contraindicated in patients who have demonstrated hypersensitivity to the drug or its ingredients.

WARNINGS

NEUROPSYCHIATRIC ADVERSE EVENTS — PEDIATRIC PATIENTS 3-12 YEARS OF AGE

Gabapentin use in pediatric patients with epilepsy 3-12 years of age is associated with the occurrence of central nervous system related adverse events. The most significant of these can be classified into the following categories: (1) emotional lability (primarily behavioral problems); (2) hostility, including aggressive behaviors; (3) thought disorder, including concentration problems and change in school performance; and (4) hyperkinesia (primarily restlessness and hyperactivity). Among the gabapentin-treated patients, most of the events were mild to moderate in intensity.

In controlled trials in pediatric patients 3-12 years of age, the incidence of these adverse events was: Emotional lability 6% (gabapentin-treated patients) vs 1.3% (placebo-treated patients); hostility 5.2% vs 1.3%; hyperkinesia 4.7% vs 2.9%; and thought disorder 1.7% vs 0%. One of these events, a report of hostility, was considered serious. Discontinuation of gabapentin treatment occurred in 1.3% of patients reporting emotional lability and hyperkinesia and 0.9% of gabapentin-treated patients reporting hostility and thought disorder. One placebo-treated patient (0.4%) withdrew due to emotional lability.

WITHDRAWAL PRECIPITATED SEIZURE, STATUS EPILEPTICUS

Antiepileptic drugs should not be abruptly discontinued because of the possibility of increasing seizure frequency.

In the placebo-controlled studies in patients >12 years of age, the incidence of status epilepticus in patients receiving gabapentin was 0.6% (3 of 543) vs 0.5% in patients receiving placebo (2 of 378). Among the 2074 patients >12 years of age treated with gabapentin across all studies (controlled and uncontrolled) 31 (1.5%) had status epilepticus. Of these, 14 patients had no prior history of status epilepticus either before treatment or while on other medications. Because adequate historical data are not available, it is impossible to say whether or not treatment with gabapentin is associated with a higher or lower rate of status epilepticus than would be expected to occur in a similar population not treated with gabapentin.

TUMORIGENIC POTENTIAL

In standard preclinical *in vivo* lifetime carcinogenicity studies, an unexpectedly high incidence of pancreatic acinar adenocarcinomas was identified in male, but not female, rats. (See PRECAUTIONS, Carcinogenesis, Mutagenesis, and Impairment of Fertility.) The clinical significance of this finding is unknown. Clinical experience during gabapentin's premarketing development provides no direct means to assess its potential for inducing tumors in humans.

In clinical studies in adjunctive therapy in epilepsy comprising 2085 patient-years of exposure in patients >12 years of age, new tumors were reported in 10 patients (2 breast, 3 brain, 2 lung, 1 adrenal, 1 non-Hodgkin's lymphoma, 1 endometrial carcinoma *in situ*), and pre-existing tumors worsened in 11 patients (9 brain, 1 breast, 1 prostate) during or up to 2 years following discontinuation of gabapentin. Without knowledge of the background incidence and recurrence in a similar population not treated with gabapentin, it is impossible to know whether the incidence seen in this cohort is or is not affected by treatment.

SUDDEN AND UNEXPLAINED DEATH IN PATIENTS WITH EPILEPSY

During the course of premarketing development of gabapentin, 8 sudden and unexplained deaths were recorded among a cohort of 2203 patients treated (2103 patient-years of exposure).

Some of these could represent seizure-related deaths in which the seizure was not observed, *e.g.,* at night. This represents an incidence of 0.0038 deaths per patient-year. Although this rate exceeds that expected in a healthy population matched for age and sex, it is within the range of estimates for the incidence of sudden unexplained deaths in patients with epilepsy not receiving gabapentin (ranging from 0.0005 for the general population of epileptics to 0.003 for a clinical trial population similar to that in the gabapentin program, to 0.005 for patients with refractory epilepsy). Consequently, whether these figures are reassuring or raise further concern depends on comparability of the populations reported upon to the gabapentin cohort and the accuracy of the estimates provided.

PRECAUTIONS

INFORMATION FOR THE PATIENT

Patients should be instructed to take gabapentin only as prescribed.

Patients should be advised that gabapentin may cause dizziness, somnolence and other symptoms and signs of CNS depression. Accordingly, they should be advised neither to drive a car nor to operate other complex machinery until they have gained sufficient experience on gabapentin to gauge whether or not it affects their mental and/or motor performance adversely.

Patients who require concomitant treatment with morphine may experience increases in gabapentin concentrations. Patients should be carefully observed for signs of CNS depression, such as somnolence, and the dose of gabapentin or morphine should be reduced appropriately (see DRUG INTERACTIONS).

LABORATORY TESTS

Clinical trials data do not indicate that routine monitoring of clinical laboratory parameters is necessary for the safe use of gabapentin. The value of monitoring gabapentin blood concentrations has not been established. Gabapentin may be used in combination with other antiepileptic drugs without concern for alteration of the blood concentrations of gabapentin or of other antiepileptic drugs.

DRUG/LABORATORY TEST INTERACTIONS

Because false positive readings were reported with the Ames N-Multistix SG dipstick test for urinary protein when gabapentin was added to other antiepileptic drugs, the more specific sulfosalicylic acid precipitation procedure is recommended to determine the presence of urine protein.

CARCINOGENESIS, MUTAGENESIS, AND IMPAIRMENT OF FERTILITY

Gabapentin was given in the diet to mice at 200, 600, and 2000 mg/kg/day and to rats at 250, 1000, and 2000 mg/kg/day for 2 years. A statistically significant increase in the incidence of pancreatic acinar cell adenomas and carcinomas was found in male rats receiving the high dose; the no-effect dose for the occurrence of carcinomas was 1000 mg/kg/day. Peak plasma concentrations of gabapentin in rats receiving the high dose of 2000 mg/kg were 10 times higher than plasma concentrations in humans receiving 3600 mg/day and in rats receiving 1000 mg/kg/day peak plasma concentrations were 6.5 times higher than in humans receiving 3600 mg/day. The pancreatic acinar cell carcinomas did not affect survival, did not metastasize and were not locally invasive. The relevance of this finding to carcinogenic risk in humans is unclear.

Studies designed to investigate the mechanism of gabapentin-induced pancreatic carcinogenesis in rats indicate that gabapentin stimulates DNA synthesis in rat pancreatic acinar cells *in vitro* and, thus, may be acting as a tumor promoter by enhancing mitogenic activity. It is not known whether gabapentin has the ability to increase cell proliferation in other cell types or in other species, including humans.

Gabapentin did not demonstrate mutagenic or genotoxic potential in three *in vitro* and four *in vivo* assays. It was negative in the Ames test and the *in vitro* HGPRT forward mutation assay in Chinese hamster lung cells; it did not produce significant increases in chromosomal aberrations in the *in vitro* Chinese hamster lung cell assay; it was negative in the *in vivo* chromosomal aberration assay and in the *in vivo* micronucleus test in Chinese hamster bone marrow; it was negative in the *in vivo* mouse micronucleus assay; and it did not induce unscheduled DNA synthesis in hepatocytes from rats given gabapentin.

No adverse effects on fertility or reproduction were observed in rats at doses up to 2000 mg/kg (approximately 5 times the maximum recommended human dose on a mg/m^2 basis).

PREGNANCY CATEGORY C

Gabapentin has been shown to be fetotoxic in rodents, causing delayed ossification of several bones in the skull, vertebrae, forelimbs and hindlimbs. These effects occurred when pregnant mice received oral doses of 1000 or 3000 mg/kg/day during the period of organogenesis, or approximately 1-4 times the maximum dose of 3600 mg/day given to epileptic patients on a mg/m^2 basis. The no-effect level was 500 mg/kg/day or approximately ½ of the human dose on a mg/m^2 basis.

When rats were dosed prior to and during mating, and throughout gestation, pups from all dose groups (500, 1000 and 2000 mg/kg/day) were affected. These doses are equivalent to less than approximately 1-5 times the maximum human dose on a mg/m^2 basis. There was an increased incidence of hydroureter and/or hydronephrosis in rats in a study of fertility and general reproductive performance at 2000 mg/kg/day with no effect at 1000 mg/kg/day, in a teratology study at 1500 mg/kg/day with no effect at 300 mg/kg/day, and in a perinatal and postnatal study at all doses studied (500, 1000 and 2000 mg/kg/day). The doses at which the effects occurred are approximately 1-5 times the maximum human dose of 3600 mg/day on a mg/m^2 basis; the no-effect doses were approximately 3 times (Fertility and General Reproductive Performance study) and approximately equal to (Teratogenicity study) the maximum human dose on a mg/m^2 basis. Other than hydroureter and hydronephrosis, the etiologies of which are unclear, the incidence of malformations was not increased compared to controls in offspring of mice, rats, or rabbits given doses up to 50 times (mice), 30 times (rats), and 25 times (rabbits) the human daily dose on a mg/kg basis, or 4 times (mice), 5 times (rats), or 8 times (rabbits) the human daily dose on a mg/m^2 basis.

In a teratology study in rabbits, an increased incidence of postimplantation fetal loss occurred in dams exposed to 60, 300 and 1500 mg/kg/day, or less than approximately ¼ to 8 times the maximum human dose on a mg/m^2 basis. There are no adequate and well-controlled studies in pregnant women. This drug should be used during pregnancy only if the potential benefit justifies the potential risk to the fetus.

USE IN NURSING MOTHERS

Gabapentin is secreted into human milk following oral administration. A nursed infant could be exposed to a maximum dose of approximately 1 mg/kg/day of gabapentin. Because the effect on the nursing infant is unknown, gabapentin should be used in women who are nursing only if the benefits clearly outweigh the risks.

PEDIATRIC USE

Safety and effectiveness of gabapentin in the management of postherpetic neuralgia in pediatric patients have not been established.

Effectiveness as adjunctive therapy in the treatment of partial seizures in pediatric patients below the age of 3 years has not been established.

GERIATRIC USE

The total number of patients treated with gabapentin in controlled clinical trials in patients with postherpetic neuralgia was 336, of which 102 (30%) were 65-74 years of age, and 168 (50%) were 75 years of age and older. There was a larger treatment effect in patients 75 years of age and older compared with younger patients who received the same dosage. Since gabapentin is almost exclusively eliminated by renal excretion, the larger treatment effect observed in patients ≥75 years may be a consequence of increased gabapentin exposure for a given dose that results from an age-related decrease in renal function. However, other factors cannot be excluded. The types and incidence of adverse events were similar across age groups except for peripheral edema and ataxia, which tended to increase in incidence with age.

Clinical studies of gabapentin in epilepsy did not include sufficient numbers of subjects aged 65 and over to determine whether they responded differently from younger subjects. Other reported clinical experience has not identified differences in responses between the elderly and younger patients. In general, dose selection for an elderly patient should be cautious, usually starting at the low end of the dosing range, reflecting the greater frequency of decreased hepatic, renal, or cardiac function, and of concomitant disease or other drug therapy.

This drug is known to be substantially excreted by the kidney, and the risk of toxic reactions to this drug may be greater in patients with impaired renal function. Because elderly patients are more likely to have decreased renal function, care should be taken in dose selection, and dose should be adjusted based on creatinine clearance values in these patients (see CLINICAL PHARMACOLOGY, ADVERSE REACTIONS, and DOSAGE AND ADMINISTRATION).

DRUG INTERACTIONS

In vitro studies were conducted to investigate the potential of gabapentin to inhibit the major cytochrome P450 enzymes (CYP1A2, CYP2A6, CYP2C9, CYP2C19, CYP2D6, CYP2E1, and CYP3A4) that mediate drug and xenobiotic metabolism using isoform selective marker substrates and human liver microsomal preparations. Only at the highest concentration tested (171 μg/ml; 1 mM) was a slight degree of inhibition (14-30%) of isoform CYP2A6 observed. No inhibition of any of the other isoforms tested was observed at gabapentin concentrations up to 171 μg/ml (approximately 15 times the C_{max} at 3600 mg/day).

Gabapentin is not appreciably metabolized nor does it interfere with the metabolism of commonly coadministered antiepileptic drugs.

The drug interaction data described in this section were obtained from studies involving healthy adults and adult patients with epilepsy.

Phenytoin: In a single (400 mg) and multiple dose (400 mg tid) study of gabapentin in epileptic patients (n=8) maintained on phenytoin monotherapy for at least 2 months, gabapentin had no effect on the steady-state trough plasma concentrations of phenytoin and phenytoin had no effect on gabapentin pharmacokinetics.

Carbamazepine: Steady-state trough plasma carbamazepine and carbamazepine 10, 11 epoxide concentrations were not affected by concomitant gabapentin (400 mg tid; n=12) administration. Likewise, gabapentin pharmacokinetics were unaltered by carbamazepine administration.

Valproic Acid: The mean steady-state trough serum valproic acid concentrations prior to and during concomitant gabapentin administration (400 mg tid; n=17) were not different and neither were gabapentin pharmacokinetic parameters affected by valproic acid.

Phenobarbital: Estimates of steady-state pharmacokinetic parameters for phenobarbital or gabapentin (300 mg tid; n=12) are identical whether the drugs are administered alone or together.

Naproxen: Coadministration (n=18) of naproxen sodium capsules (250 mg) with gabapentin (125 mg) appears to increase the amount of gabapentin absorbed by 12-15%. Gabapentin had no effect on naproxen pharmacokinetic parameters. These doses are lower than the therapeutic doses for both drugs. The magnitude of interaction within the recommended dose ranges of either drug is not known.

Hydrocodone: Coadministration of gabapentin (125-500 mg; n=48) decreases hydrocodone (10 mg; n=50) C_{max} and AUC values in a dose-dependent manner relative to administration of hydrocodone alone; C_{max} and AUC values are 3-4% lower, respectively, after administration of 125 mg gabapentin and 21-22% lower, respectively, after administration of 500 mg gabapentin. The mechanism for this interaction is unknown. Hydrocodone increases gabapentin AUC values by 14%. The magnitude of interaction at other doses is not known.

Morphine: A literature article reported that when a 60 mg controlled release morphine capsule was administered 2 hours prior to a 600 mg gabapentin capsule (n=12), mean gabapentin AUC increased by 44% compared to gabapentin administered without morphine (see PRECAUTIONS). Morphine pharmacokinetic parameter values were not affected by administration of gabapentin 2 hours after morphine. The magnitude of interaction at other doses is not known.

Cimetidine: In the presence of cimetidine at 300 mg qid (n=12) the mean apparent oral clearance of gabapentin fell by 14% and creatinine clearance fell by 10%. Thus cimetidine appeared to alter the renal excretion of both gabapentin and creatinine, an endogenous marker of renal function. This small decrease in excretion of gabapentin by cimetidine is not expected to be of clinical importance. The effect of gabapentin on cimetidine was not evaluated.

Oral Contraceptives: Based on AUC and half-life, multiple-dose pharmacokinetic profiles of norethindrone and ethinyl estradiol following administration of tablets containing 2.5 mg of norethindrone acetate and 50 μg of ethinyl estradiol were similar with and without coadministration of gabapentin (400 mg tid; n=13). The C_{max} of norethindrone was 13% higher when it was coadministered with gabapentin; this interaction is not expected to be of clinical importance.

Antacid (Maalox): Maalox reduced the bioavailability of gabapentin (n=16) by about 20%. This decrease in bioavailability was about 5% when gabapentin was administered 2 hours after Maalox. It is recommended that gabapentin be taken at least 2 hours following Maalox administration.

Effect of Probenecid: Probenecid is a blocker of renal tubular secretion. Gabapentin pharmacokinetic parameters without and with probenecid were comparable. This indicates that gabapentin does not undergo renal tubular secretion by the pathway that is blocked by probenecid.

ADVERSE REACTIONS

POSTHERPETIC NEURALGIA

The most commonly observed adverse events associated with the use of gabapentin in adults, not seen at an equivalent frequency among placebo-treated patients, were dizziness, somnolence, and peripheral edema.

In the 2 controlled studies in postherpetic neuralgia, 16% of the 336 patients who received gabapentin and 9% of the 227 patients who received placebo discontinued treatment because of an adverse event. The adverse events that most frequently led to withdrawal in gabapentin-treated patients were dizziness, somnolence, and nausea.

INCIDENCE IN CONTROLLED CLINICAL TRIALS

TABLE 2 lists treatment-emergent signs and symptoms that occurred in at least 1% of gabapentin-treated patients with postherpetic neuralgia participating in placebo-controlled trials and that were numerically more frequent in the gabapentin group than in the placebo group. Adverse events were usually mild to moderate in intensity.

Other events in more than 1% of patients but equally or more frequent in the placebo group included pain, tremor, neuralgia, back pain, dyspepsia, dyspnea, and flu syndrome.

There were no clinically important differences between men and women in the types and incidence of adverse events. Because there were few patients whose race was reported as other than white, there are insufficient data to support a statement regarding the distribution of adverse events by race.

EPILEPSY

The most commonly observed adverse events associated with the use of gabapentin in combination with other antiepileptic drugs in patients >12 years of age, not seen at an equivalent frequency among placebo-treated patients, were somnolence, dizziness, ataxia, fatigue, and nystagmus. The most commonly observed adverse events reported with the use of gabapentin in combination with other antiepileptic drugs in pediatric patients 3-12 years of age, not seen at an equal frequency among placebo-treated patients, were viral infection, fever, nausea and/or vomiting, somnolence, and hostility (see WARNINGS, Neuropsychiatric Adverse Events).

Approximately 7% of the 2074 patients >12 years of age and approximately 7% of the 449 pediatric patients 3-12 years of age who received gabapentin in premarketing clinical trials discontinued treatment because of an adverse event. The adverse events most commonly associated with withdrawal in patients >12 years of age were somnolence (1.2%), ataxia (0.8%), fatigue (0.6%), nausea and/or vomiting (0.6%), and dizziness (0.6%). The adverse events most commonly associated with withdrawal in pediatric patients were emotional lability (1.6%), hostility (1.3%), and hyperkinesia (1.1%).

INCIDENCE IN CONTROLLED CLINICAL TRIALS

TABLE 3 lists treatment-emergent signs and symptoms that occurred in at least 1% of gabapentin-treated patients >12 years of age with epilepsy participating in placebo-controlled trials and were numerically more common in the gabapentin group. In these stud-

G

TABLE 2 *Treatment-Emergent Adverse Event Incidence in Controlled Trials in Postherpetic Neuralgia**

Body System/ Preferred Term	Gabapentin n=336	Placebo n=227
Body as a Whole		
Asthenia	5.7%	4.8%
Infection	5.1%	3.5%
Headache	3.3%	3.1%
Accidental injury	3.3%	1.3%
Abdominal pain	2.7%	2.6%
Digestive System		
Diarrhea	5.7%	3.1%
Dry mouth	4.8%	1.3%
Constipation	3.9%	1.8%
Nausea	3.9%	3.1%
Vomiting	3.3%	1.8%
Flatulence	2.1%	1.8%
Metabolic and Nutritional Disorders		
Peripheral edema	8.3%	2.2%
Weight gain	1.8%	0.0%
Hyperglycemia	1.2%	0.4%
Nervous System		
Dizziness	28.0%	7.5%
Somnolence	21.4%	5.3%
Ataxia	3.3%	0.0%
Thinking abnormal	2.7%	0.0%
Abnormal gait	1.5%	0.0%
Incoordination	1.5%	0.0%
Amnesia	1.2%	0.9%
Hypesthesia	1.2%	0.9%
Respiratory System		
Pharyngitis	1.2%	0.4%
Skin and Appendages		
Rash	1.2%	0.9%
Special Senses		
Amblyopia†	2.7%	0.9%
Conjunctivitis	1.2%	0.0%
Diplopia	1.2%	0.0%
Otitis media	1.2%	0.0%

* Events in at least 1% of gabapentin-treated patients and numerically more frequent than in the placebo group.
† Reported as blurred vision.

ies, either gabapentin or placebo was added to the patient's current antiepileptic drug therapy. Adverse events were usually mild to moderate in intensity.

The prescriber should be aware that these figures, obtained when gabapentin was added to concurrent antiepileptic drug therapy, cannot be used to predict the frequency of adverse events in the course of usual medical practice where patient characteristics and other factors may differ from those prevailing during clinical studies. Similarly, the cited frequencies cannot be directly compared with figures obtained from other clinical investigations involving different treatments, uses, or investigators. An inspection of these frequencies, however, does provide the prescribing physician with one basis to estimate the relative contribution of drug and nondrug factors to the adverse event incidences in the population studied.

Other events in more than 1% of patients >12 years of age but equally or more frequent in the placebo group included: Headache, viral infection, fever, nausea and/or vomiting, abdominal pain, diarrhea, convulsions, confusion, insomnia, emotional lability, rash, acne.

Among the treatment-emergent adverse events occurring at an incidence of at least 10% of gabapentin-treated patients, somnolence and ataxia appeared to exhibit a positive dose-response relationship.

The overall incidence of adverse events and the types of adverse events seen were similar among men and women treated with gabapentin. The incidence of adverse events increased slightly with increasing age in patients treated with either gabapentin or placebo. Because only 3% of patients (28/921) in placebo-controlled studies were identified as nonwhite (black or other), there are insufficient data to support a statement regarding the distribution of adverse events by race.

TABLE 4 lists treatment-emergent signs and symptoms that occurred in at least 2% of gabapentin-treated patients age 3-12 years of age with epilepsy participating in placebo-controlled trials and were numerically more common in the gabapentin group. Adverse events were usually mild to moderate in intensity.

Other events in more than 2% of pediatric patients 3-12 years of age but equally or more frequent in the placebo group included: Pharyngitis, upper respiratory infection, headache, rhinitis, convulsions, diarrhea, anorexia, coughing, and otitis media.

OTHER ADVERSE EVENTS OBSERVED DURING ALL CLINICAL TRIALS

Clinical Trials in Adults and Adolescents With Epilepsy

Gabapentin has been administered to 2074 patients >12 years of age during all adjunctive therapy clinical trials in epilepsy, only some of which were placebo-controlled. During these trials, all adverse events were recorded by the clinical investigators using terminology of their own choosing. To provide a meaningful estimate of the proportion of individuals having adverse events, similar types of events were grouped into a smaller number of standardized categories using modified COSTART dictionary terminology. These categories are used in the listing below. The frequencies presented represent the proportion of the 2074 patients >12 years of age exposed to gabapentin who experienced an event of the type cited on at least one occasion while receiving gabapentin. All reported events are included except those already listed in TABLE 3, those too general to be informative, and those not reasonably associated with the use of the drug.

Events are further classified within body system categories and enumerated in order of decreasing frequency using the following definitions: *frequent* adverse events are defined as those occurring in at least 1/100 patients; *infrequent* adverse events are those occuring in 1/100 to 1/1000 patients; *rare* events are those occurring in fewer than 1/1000 patients.

TABLE 3 *Treatment-Emergent Adverse Event Incidence in Controlled Add-On Trials in Patients >12 Years of Age**

Body System Adverse Event	Gabapentin† n=543	Placebo† n=378
Body as a Whole		
Fatigue	11.0%	5.0%
Weight increase	2.9%	1.6%
Back pain	1.8%	0.5%
Peripheral edema	1.7%	0.5%
Cardiovascular		
Vasodilation	1.1%	0.3%
Digestive System		
Dyspepsia	2.2%	0.5%
Mouth or throat dry	1.7%	0.5%
Constipation	1.5%	0.8%
Dental abnormalities	1.5%	0.3%
Increased appetite	1.1%	0.8%
Hematologic and Lymphatic Systems		
Leukopenia	1.1%	0.5%
Musculoskeletal System		
Myalgia	2.0%	1.9%
Fracture	1.1%	0.8%
Nervous System		
Somnolence	19.3%	8.7%
Dizziness	17.1%	6.9%
Ataxia	12.5%	5.6%
Nystagmus	8.3%	4.0%
Tremor	6.8%	3.2%
Nervousness	2.4%	1.9%
Dysarthria	2.4%	0.5%
Amnesia	2.2%	0.0%
Depression	1.8%	1.1%
Thinking abnormal	1.7%	1.3%
Twitching	1.3%	0.5%
Coordination abnormal	1.1%	0.3%
Respiratory System		
Rhinitis	4.1%	3.7%
Pharyngitis	2.8%	1.6%
Coughing	1.8%	1.3%
Skin and Appendages		
Abrasion	1.3%	0.0%
Pruritus	1.3%	0.5%
Urogenital System		
Impotence	1.5%	1.1%
Special Senses		
Diplopia	5.9%	1.9%
Amblyopia‡	4.2%	1.1%
Laboratory Deviations		
WBC decreased	1.1%	0.5%

* Events in at least 1% of gabapentin patients and numerically more frequent than in the placebo group.
† Plus background antiepileptic drug therapy.
‡ Amblyopia was often described as blurred vision.

TABLE 4 *Treatment-Emergent Adverse Event Incidence in Pediatric Patients Age 3-12 Years in a Controlled Add-On Trial*

Body System Adverse Event	Gabapentin† n=119	Placebo† n=128
Body as a Whole		
Viral infection	10.9%	3.1%
Fever	10.1%	3.1%
Weight increase	3.4%	0.8%
Fatigue	3.4%	1.6%
Digestive System		
Nausea and/or vomiting	8.4%	7.0%
Nervous System		
Somnolence	8.4%	4.7%
Hostility	7.6%	2.3%
Emotional lability	4.2%	1.6%
Dizziness	2.5%	1.6%
Hyperkinesia	2.5%	0.8%
Respiratory System		
Bronchitis	3.4%	0.8%
Respiratory infection	2.5%	0.8%

* Events in at least 2% of gabapentin patients and numerically more frequent than in the placebo group.
† Plus background antiepileptic drug therapy.

Body as a Whole: *Frequent:* Asthenia, malaise, face edema; *Infrequent:* Allergy, generalized edema, weight decrease, chill; *Rare:* Strange feelings, lassitude, alcohol intolerance, hangover effect.

Cardiovascular System: *Frequent:* Hypertension; *Infrequent:* Hypotension, angina pectoris, peripheral vascular disorder, palpitation, tachycardia, migraine, murmur; *Rare:* Atrial fibrillation, heart failure, thrombophlebitis, deep thrombophlebitis, myocardial infarction, cerebrovascular accident, pulmonary thrombosis, ventricular extrasystoles, bradycardia, premature atrial contraction, pericardial rub, heart block, pulmonary embolus, hyperlipidemia, hypercholesterolemia, pericardial effusion, pericarditis.

Digestive System: *Frequent:* Anorexia, flatulence, gingivitis; *Infrequent:* Glossitis, gum hemorrhage, thirst, stomatitis, increased salivation, gastroenteritis, hemorrhoids, bloody stools, fecal incontinence, hepatomegaly; *Rare:* Dysphagia, eructation, pancreatitis, peptic ulcer, colitis, blisters in mouth, tooth discolor, perlèche, salivary gland enlarged, lip hemorrhage, esophagitis, hiatal hernia, hematemesis, proctitis, irritable bowel syndrome, rectal hemorrhage, esophageal spasm.

Endocrine System: *Rare:* Hyperthyroid, hypothyroid, goiter, hypoestrogen, ovarian failure, epididymitis, swollen testicle, cushingoid appearance.

Hematologic and Lymphatic System: *Frequent:* Purpura most often described as bruises resulting from physical trauma; *Infrequent:* Anemia, thrombocytopenia, lymphadenopathy; *Rare:* WBC count increased, lymphocytosis, non-Hodgkin's lymphoma, bleeding time increased.

Musculoskeletal System: *Frequent:* Arthralgia; *Infrequent:* Tendinitis, arthritis, joint stiffness, joint swelling, positive Romberg test; *Rare:* Costochondritis, osteoporosis, bursitis, contracture.

Nervous System: *Frequent:* Vertigo, hyperkinesia, paresthesia, decreased or absent reflexes, increased reflexes, anxiety, hostility; *Infrequent:* CNS tumors, syncope, dreaming abnormal, aphasia, hypesthesia, intracranial hemorrhage, hypotonia, dysesthesia, paresis, dystonia, hemiplegia, facial paralysis, stupor, cerebellar dysfunction, positive Babinski sign, decreased position sense, subdural hematoma, apathy, hallucination, decrease or loss of libido, agitation, paranoia, depersonalization, euphoria, feeling high, doped-up sensation, suicidal, psychosis; *Rare:* Choreoathetosis, orofacial dyskinesia, encephalopathy, nerve palsy, personality disorder, increased libido, subdued temperament, apraxia, fine motor control disorder, meningismus, local myoclonus, hyperesthesia, hypokinesia, mania, neurosis, hysteria, antisocial reaction, suicide gesture.

Respiratory System: *Frequent:* Pneumonia; *Infrequent:* Epistaxis, dyspnea, apnea; *Rare:* Mucositis, aspiration pneumonia, hyperventilation, hiccup, laryngitis, nasal obstruction, snoring, bronchospasm, hypoventilation, lung edema.

Dermatologic: *Infrequent:* Alopecia, eczema, dry skin, increased sweating, urticaria, hirsutism, seborrhea, cyst, herpes simplex; *Rare:* Herpes zoster, skin discolor, skin papules, photosensitive reaction, leg ulcer, scalp seborrhea, psoriasis, desquamation, maceration, skin nodules, subcutaneous nodule, melanosis, skin necrosis, local swelling.

Urogenital System: *Infrequent:* Hematuria, dysuria, urination frequency, cystitis, urinary retention, urinary incontinence, vaginal hemorrhage, amenorrhea, dysmenorrhea, menorrhagia, breast cancer, unable to climax, ejaculation abnormal; *Rare:* Kidney pain, leukorrhea, pruritus genital, renal stone, acute renal failure, anuria, glycosuria, nephrosis, nocturia, pyuria, urination urgency, vaginal pain, breast pain, testicle pain.

Special Senses: *Frequent:* Abnormal vision; *Infrequent:* Cataract, conjunctivitis, eyes dry, eye pain, visual field defect, photophobia, bilateral or unilateral ptosis, eye hemorrhage, hordeolum, hearing loss, earache, tinnitus, inner ear infection, otitis, taste loss, unusual taste, eye twitching, ear fullness; *Rare:* Eye itching, abnormal accommodation, perforated ear drum, sensitivity to noise, eye focusing problem, watery eyes, retinopathy, glaucoma, iritis, corneal disorders, lacrimal dysfunction, degenerative eye changes, blindness, retinal degeneration, miosis, chorioretinitis, strabismus, eustachian tube dysfunction, labyrinthitis, otitis externa, odd smell.

CLINICAL TRIALS IN PEDIATRIC PATIENTS WITH EPILEPSY

Adverse events occurring during clinical trials in 449 pediatric patients 3-12 years of age treated with gabapentin that were not reported in adjunctive trials in adults are:

Body as a Whole: Dehydration, infectious mononucleosis.

Digestive System: Hepatitis.

Hemic and Lymphatic System: Coagulation defect.

Nervous System: Aura disappeared, occipital neuralgia.

Psychobiologic Function: Sleepwalking.

Respiratory System: Pseudocroup, hoarseness.

CLINICAL TRIALS IN ADULTS WITH NEUROPATHIC PAIN OF VARIOUS ETIOLOGIES

Safety information was obtained in 1173 patients during double-blind and open-label clinical trials including neuropathic pain conditions for which efficacy has not been demonstrated. Adverse events reported by investigators were grouped into standardized categories using modified COSTART IV terminology. Listed below are all reported events except those already listed in TABLE 2 and those not reasonably associated with the use of the drug. **Events are further classified within body system categories and enumerated in order of decreasing frequency using the following definitions:** *Frequent* adverse events are defined as those occurring in at least 1/100 patients; *Infrequent* adverse events are those occurring in 1/100 to 1/1000 patients; *Rare* events are those occurring in fewer than 1/1000 patients.

Body as a Whole: *Infrequent:* Chest pain, cellulitis, malaise, neck pain, face edema, allergic reaction, abscess, chills, chills and fever, mucous membrane disorder; *Rare:* Body odor, cyst, fever, hernia, abnormal BUN value, lump in neck, pelvic pain, sepsis, viral infection.

Cardiovascular System: *Infrequent:* Hypertension, syncope, palpitation, migraine, hypotension, peripheral vascular disorder, cardiovascular disorder, cerebrovascular accident, congestive heart failure, myocardial infarction, vasodilatation; *Rare:* Angina pectoris, heart failure, increased capillary fragility, phlebitis, thrombophlebitis, varicose vein.

Digestive System: *Infrequent:* Gastroenteritis, increased appetite, gastrointestinal disorder, oral moniliasis, gastritis, tongue disorder, thirst, tooth disorder, abnormal stools, anorexia, liver function tests abnormal, periodontal abscess; *Rare:* Cholecystitis, cholelithiasis, duodenal ulcer, fecal incontinence, gamma glutamyl transpeptidase increased, gingivitis, intestinal obstruction, intestinal ulcer, melena, mouth ulceration, rectal disorder, rectal hemorrhage, stomatitis.

Endocrine System: *Infrequent:* Diabetes mellitus.

Hemic and Lymphatic System: *Infrequent:* Ecchymosis, anemia; *Rare:* Lymphadenopathy, lymphoma-like reaction, prothrombin decreased.

Metabolic and Nutritional: *Infrequent:* Edema, gout, hypoglycemia, weight loss; *Rare:* Alkaline phosphatase increased, diabetic ketoacidosis, lactic dehydrogenase increased.

Musculoskeletal: *Infrequent:* Arthritis, arthralgia, myalgia, arthrosis, leg cramps, myasthenia; *Rare:* Shin bone pain, joint disorder, tendon disorder.

Nervous System: *Frequent:* Confusion, depression; *Infrequent:* Vertigo, nervousness, paresthesia, insomnia, neuropathy, libido decreased, anxiety, depersonalization, reflexes decreased, speech disorder, abnormal dreams, dysarthria, emotional lability, nystagmus, stupor, circumoral paresthesia, euphoria, hyperesthesia, hypokinesia; *Rare:* Agitation, hypertonia, libido increased, movement disorder, myoclonus, vestibular disorder.

Respiratory System: *Infrequent:* Cough increased, bronchitis, rhinitis, sinusitis, pneumonia, asthma, lung disorder, epistaxis; *Rare:* Hemoptysis, voice alteration.

Skin and Appendages: *Infrequent:* Pruritus, skin ulcer, dry skin, herpes zoster, skin disorder, fungal dermatitis, furunculosis, herpes simplex, psoriasis, sweating, urticaria, vesiculobullous rash; *Rare:* Acne, hair disorder, maculopapular rash, nail disorder, skin carcinoma, skin discoloration, skin hypertrophy.

Special Senses: *Infrequent:* Abnormal vision, ear pain, eye disorder, taste perversion, deafness; *Rare:* Conjunctival hyperemia, diabetic retinopathy, eye pain, fundi with microhemorrhage, retinal vein thrombosis, taste loss.

Urogenital System: *Infrequent:* Urinary tract infection, dysuria, impotence, urinary incontinence, vaginal moniliasis, breast pain, menstrual disorder, polyuria, urinary retention; *Rare:* Cystitis, ejaculation abnormal, swollen penis, gynecomastia, nocturia, pyelonephritis, swollen scrotum, urinary frequency, urinary urgency, urine abnormality.

G

POSTMARKETING AND OTHER EXPERIENCE

In addition to the adverse experiences reported during clinical testing of gabapentin, the following adverse experiences have been reported in patients receiving marketed gabapentin. These adverse experiences have not been listed above and data are insufficient to support an estimate of their incidence or to establish causation. The listing is alphabetized: angioedema, blood glucose fluctuation, erythema multiforme, elevated liver function tests, fever, hyponatremia, jaundice, Stevens-Johnson syndrome.

DOSAGE AND ADMINISTRATION

Gabapentin is given orally with or without food.

POSTHERPETIC NEURALGIA

In adults with postherpetic neuralgia, gabapentin therapy may be initiated as a single 300 mg dose on Day 1, 600 mg/day on Day 2 (divided bid), and 900 mg/day on Day 3 (divided tid). The dose can subsequently be titrated up as needed for pain relief to a daily dose of 1800 mg (divided tid). In clinical studies, efficacy was demonstrated over a range of doses from 1800-3600 mg/day with comparable effects across the dose range. Additional benefit of using doses greater than 1800 mg/day was not demonstrated.

EPILEPSY

Gabapentin is recommended for add-on therapy in patients 3 years of age and older. Effectiveness in pediatric patients below the age of 3 years has not been established.

Patients >12 Years of Age: The effective dose of gabapentin is 900-1800 mg/day and given in divided doses (3 times a day) using 300 or 400 mg capsules, or 600 or 800 mg tablets. The starting dose is 300 mg three times a day. If necessary, the dose may be increased using 300 or 400 mg capsules, or 600 or 800 mg tablets three times a day up to 1800 mg/day. Dosages up to 2400 mg/day have been well tolerated in long-term clinical studies. Doses of 3600 mg/day have also been administered to a small number of patients for a relatively short duration, and have been well tolerated. The maximum time between doses in the tid schedule should not exceed 12 hours.

Pediatric Patients Age 3-12 Years: The starting dose should range from 10-15 mg/kg/day in 3 divided doses, and the effective dose reached by upward titration over a period of approximately 3 days. The effective dose of gabapentin in patients 5 years of age and older is 25-35 mg/kg/day and given in divided doses (3 times a day). The effective dose in pediatric patients ages 3 and 4 years is 40 mg/kg/day and given in divided doses (3 times a day). (See CLINICAL PHARMACOLOGY, Special Populations, Pediatric.) Gabapentin may be administered as the oral solution, capsule, or tablet, or using combinations of these formulations. Dosages up to 50 mg/kg/day have been well-tolerated in a long-term clinical study. The maximum time interval between doses should not exceed 12 hours.

It is not necessary to monitor gabapentin plasma concentrations to optimize gabapentin therapy. Further, because there are no significant pharmacokinetic interactions among gabapentin and other commonly used antiepileptic drugs, the addition of gabapentin does not alter the plasma levels of these drugs appreciably.

If gabapentin is discontinued and/or an alternate anticonvulsant medication is added to the therapy, this should be done gradually over a minimum of 1 week.

DOSAGE IN RENAL IMPAIRMENT

Creatinine clearance is difficult to measure in outpatients. In patients with stable renal function, creatinine clearance (CCR) can be reasonably well estimated using the equation of Cockcroft and Gault:

For Females: CCR = [(0.85)(140-age)(weight)] ÷ [(72)(SCR)]

For Males: CCR = [(140-age)(weight)] ÷ [(72)(SCR)]

Where age is in years, weight is in kilograms and SCR is serum creatinine in mg/dl.

Dosage adjustment in patients ≥12 years of age with compromised renal function or undergoing hemodialysis is recommended as found in TABLE 5.

The use of gabapentin in patients <12 years of age with compromised renal function has not been studied.

DOSAGE IN ELDERLY

Because elderly patients are more likely to have decreased renal function, care should be taken in dose selection, and dose should be adjusted based on creatinine clearance values in these patients.

TABLE 5 *Gabapentin Dosage Based on Renal Function*

Renal Function Creatinine Clearance	Total Daily Dose Range	Dose Regimen				
≥60 (ml/min)	900-3600 (mg/day)	300 mg tid	400 mg tid	600 mg tid	800 mg tid	1200 mg tid
>30-59 (ml/min)	400-1400 (mg/day)	200 mg bid	300 mg bid	400 mg bid	500 mg bid	700 mg bid
>15-29 (ml/min)	200-700 (mg/day)	200 mg qd	300 mg qd	400 mg qd	500 mg qd	700 mg qd
15* (ml/min)	100-300 (mg/day)	100 mg qd	125 mg qd	150 mg qd	200 mg qd	300 mg qd
		Post-Hemodialysis Supplemental Dose (mg)†				
Hemodialysis	—	125†	150†	200†	250†	350†

* For patients with creatinine clearance <15 ml/min, reduce daily dose in proportion to creatinine clearance (*e.g.*, patients with a creatinine clearance of 7.5 ml/min should receive one-half the daily dose that patients with a creatinine clearance of 15 ml/min receive).

† Patients on hemodialysis should receive maintenance doses based on estimates of creatinine clearance as indicated in the upper portion of the table and a supplemental post-hemodialysis dose administered after each 4 hours of hemodialysis as indicated in the lower portion of the table.

HOW SUPPLIED

CAPSULES

Neurontin capsules are supplied as follows:

100 mg: White hard gelatin capsules printed with "PD" on one side and "Neurontin/100 mg" on the other.

300 mg: Yellow hard gelatin capsules printed with "PD" on one side and "Neurontin/300 mg" on the other.

400 mg: Orange hard gelatin capsules printed with "PD" on one side and "Neurontin/400 mg" on the other.

Storage: Store at 25°C (77°F); excursions permitted to 15-30°C (59-86°F).

TABLETS

Neurontin tablets are supplied as follows:

600 mg: White elliptical film-coated tablets printed in black ink with "Neurontin 600" on one side.

800 mg: White elliptical film-coated tablets printed in orange with "Neurontin 800" on one side.

Storage: Store at 25°C (77°F); excursions permitted to 15-30°C (59-86°F).

ORAL SOLUTION

Neurontin oral solution is supplied as follows:

250 mg/5 ml: Clear colorless to slightly yellow solution; each 5 ml of oral solution contains 250 mg of gabapentin.

Storage: Store refrigerated, 2-8°C (36-46°F).

PRODUCT LISTING - EQUIVALENTS NOT AVAILABLE

Capsule - Oral - 100 mg

10's	$5.29	NEURONTIN, Southwood Pharmaceuticals Inc	58016-0427-10
14's	$7.41	NEURONTIN, Southwood Pharmaceuticals Inc	58016-0427-14
15's	$7.94	NEURONTIN, Southwood Pharmaceuticals Inc	58016-0427-15
20's	$10.59	NEURONTIN, Southwood Pharmaceuticals Inc	58016-0427-20
21's	$11.12	NEURONTIN, Southwood Pharmaceuticals Inc	58016-0427-21
21's	$23.68	NEURONTIN, Pharma Pac	52959-0506-21
28's	$14.82	NEURONTIN, Southwood Pharmaceuticals Inc	58016-0427-28
30's	$13.93	NEURONTIN, Allscripts Pharmaceutical Company	54569-4576-01
30's	$15.88	NEURONTIN, Southwood Pharmaceuticals Inc	58016-0427-30
30's	$32.26	NEURONTIN, Pharma Pac	52959-0506-30
40's	$21.17	NEURONTIN, Southwood Pharmaceuticals Inc	58016-0427-40
45's	$47.30	NEURONTIN, Pharma Pac	52959-0506-45
50's	$26.47	NEURONTIN, Southwood Pharmaceuticals Inc	58016-0427-50
50's	$32.33	NEURONTIN, Parke-Davis	00071-0803-40
60's	$31.76	NEURONTIN, Southwood Pharmaceuticals Inc	58016-0427-60
60's	$73.87	NEURONTIN, Pharma Pac	52959-0506-60
90's	$47.64	NEURONTIN, Southwood Pharmaceuticals Inc	58016-0427-90
100's	$51.09	NEURONTIN, Physicians Total Care	54868-3529-00
100's	$52.93	NEURONTIN, Southwood Pharmaceuticals Inc	58016-0427-00
100's	$55.60	NEURONTIN, Parke-Davis	00071-0803-24
120's	$88.64	NEURONTIN, Pharma Pac	52959-0506-02

Capsule - Oral - 300 mg

10's	$13.24	NEURONTIN, Southwood Pharmaceuticals Inc	58016-0481-10
14's	$18.53	NEURONTIN, Southwood Pharmaceuticals Inc	58016-0481-14
15's	$19.86	NEURONTIN, Southwood Pharmaceuticals Inc	58016-0481-15
20's	$26.47	NEURONTIN, Southwood Pharmaceuticals Inc	58016-0481-20
20's	$44.68	NEURONTIN, Pharma Pac	52959-0434-20
21's	$27.80	NEURONTIN, Southwood Pharmaceuticals Inc	58016-0481-21
28's	$37.06	NEURONTIN, Southwood Pharmaceuticals Inc	58016-0481-28
30's	$34.82	NEURONTIN, Allscripts Pharmaceutical Company	54569-4577-01
30's	$39.71	NEURONTIN, Southwood Pharmaceuticals Inc	58016-0481-30
30's	$42.14	NEURONTIN, Physicians Total Care	54868-3768-01
30's	$62.11	NEURONTIN, Pharma Pac	52959-0434-30
40's	$52.95	NEURONTIN, Southwood Pharmaceuticals Inc	58016-0481-40
45's	$67.96	NEURONTIN, Pharma Pac	52959-0434-45
50's	$66.18	NEURONTIN, Southwood Pharmaceuticals Inc	58016-0481-50
50's	$76.01	NEURONTIN, Parke-Davis	00071-0805-40
60's	$79.42	NEURONTIN, Southwood Pharmaceuticals Inc	58016-0481-60
60's	$89.70	NEURONTIN, Pharma Pac	52959-0434-60
90's	$119.13	NEURONTIN, Southwood Pharmaceuticals Inc	58016-0481-90
90's	$132.03	NEURONTIN, Pharma Pac	52959-0434-90
100's	$132.37	NEURONTIN, Southwood Pharmaceuticals Inc	58016-0481-00
100's	$139.00	NEURONTIN, Parke-Davis	00071-0805-24
100's	$141.14	NEURONTIN, Pharma Pac	52959-0434-00

Capsule - Oral - 400 mg

10's	$15.88	NEURONTIN, Southwood Pharmaceuticals Inc	58016-0433-10
14's	$22.24	NEURONTIN, Southwood Pharmaceuticals Inc	58016-0433-14
15's	$23.83	NEURONTIN, Southwood Pharmaceuticals Inc	58016-0433-15
20's	$31.77	NEURONTIN, Southwood Pharmaceuticals Inc	58016-0433-20
21's	$33.36	NEURONTIN, Southwood Pharmaceuticals Inc	58016-0433-21
28's	$44.47	NEURONTIN, Southwood Pharmaceuticals Inc	58016-0433-28
30's	$46.63	NEURONTIN, Physicians Total Care	54868-3931-00
30's	$47.65	NEURONTIN, Southwood Pharmaceuticals Inc	58016-0433-30
40's	$63.53	NEURONTIN, Southwood Pharmaceuticals Inc	58016-0433-40
50's	$79.42	NEURONTIN, Southwood Pharmaceuticals Inc	58016-0433-50
50's	$88.26	NEURONTIN, Parke-Davis	00071-0806-40
60's	$95.30	NEURONTIN, Southwood Pharmaceuticals Inc	58016-0433-60
90's	$142.95	NEURONTIN, Southwood Pharmaceuticals Inc	58016-0433-90
100's	$158.83	NEURONTIN, Southwood Pharmaceuticals Inc	58016-0433-00
100's	$166.78	NEURONTIN, Parke-Davis	00071-0806-24

Solution - Oral - 250 mg/5 ml

480 ml	$103.71	NEURONTIN, Parke-Davis	00071-2012-23

Tablet - Oral - 600 mg

10's	$21.85	NEURONTIN, Southwood Pharmaceuticals Inc	58016-0482-10
14's	$30.59	NEURONTIN, Southwood Pharmaceuticals Inc	58016-0482-14
15's	$32.77	NEURONTIN, Southwood Pharmaceuticals Inc	58016-0482-15
20's	$43.69	NEURONTIN, Southwood Pharmaceuticals Inc	58016-0482-20
21's	$45.88	NEURONTIN, Southwood Pharmaceuticals Inc	58016-0482-21
28's	$61.17	NEURONTIN, Southwood Pharmaceuticals Inc	58016-0482-28
30's	$65.54	NEURONTIN, Southwood Pharmaceuticals Inc	58016-0482-30
40's	$87.39	NEURONTIN, Southwood Pharmaceuticals Inc	58016-0482-40
50's	$109.23	NEURONTIN, Southwood Pharmaceuticals Inc	58016-0482-50
60's	$131.08	NEURONTIN, Southwood Pharmaceuticals Inc	58016-0482-60
90's	$196.62	NEURONTIN, Southwood Pharmaceuticals Inc	58016-0482-90
100's	$218.47	NEURONTIN, Southwood Pharmaceuticals Inc	58016-0482-00
100's	$218.49	NEURONTIN, Parke-Davis	00071-0416-24

Tablet - Oral - 800 mg

10's	$26.22	NEURONTIN, Southwood Pharmaceuticals Inc	58016-0483-10
20's	$52.43	NEURONTIN, Southwood Pharmaceuticals Inc	58016-0483-20
30's	$78.65	NEURONTIN, Southwood Pharmaceuticals Inc	58016-0483-30

40's	$104.87	NEURONTIN, Southwood Pharmaceuticals Inc	58016-0483-40
50's	$131.08	NEURONTIN, Southwood Pharmaceuticals Inc	58016-0483-50
60's	$157.30	NEURONTIN, Southwood Pharmaceuticals Inc	58016-0483-60
90's	$235.95	NEURONTIN, Southwood Pharmaceuticals Inc	58016-0483-90
100's	$262.17	NEURONTIN, Southwood Pharmaceuticals Inc	58016-0483-00
100's	$262.18	NEURONTIN, Parke-Davis	00071-0426-24

Galantamine Hydrobromide *(001844)*

Categories: Alzheimer's disease; FDA Approved 2001 Feb; Pregnancy Category B
Drug Classes: Cholinesterase inhibitors
Brand Names: **Reminyl**
Foreign Brand Availability: Nivalin (Austria; Bulgaria; Germany; Hungary; Russia)
Cost of Therapy: $149.96 (Alzheimer's Disease; Reminyl; 8 mg; 2 tablets/day; 30 day supply)

DESCRIPTION

Reminyl (galantamine hydrobromide) is a reversible, competitive acetylcholinesterase inhibitor. It is known chemically as (4a*S*,6*R*,8a*S*)-4a,5,9,10,11,12-hexahydro-3-methoxy-11-methyl-6*H*-benzofuro[3a,3,2*ef*][2]benzazepin-6-ol hydrobromide. It has an empirical formula of $C_{17}H_{21}NO_3$·HBr and a molecular weight of 368.27. Galantamine hydrobromide is a white to almost white powder and is sparingly soluble in water.

Reminyl for oral use is available in circular biconvex film-coated tablets of 4 mg (off-white), 8 mg (pink), and 12 mg (orange-brown). Each 4, 8, and 12 mg (base equivalent) tablet contains 5.126, 10.253, and 15.379 mg of galantamine hydrobromide, respectively. Inactive ingredients include colloidal silicon dioxide, crospovidone, hydroxypropyl methylcellulose, lactose monohydrate, magnesium stearate, microcrystalline cellulose, propylene glycol, talc, and titanium dioxide. The 4 mg tablets contain yellow ferric oxide. The 8 mg tablets contain red ferric oxide. The 12 mg tablets contain red ferric oxide and FD&C yellow no. 6 aluminum lake.

Reminyl is also available as a 4 mg/ml oral solution. The inactive ingredients for this solution are methyl parahydroxybenzoate, propyl parahydroxybenzoate, sodium saccharin, sodium hydroxide and purified water.

CLINICAL PHARMACOLOGY

MECHANISM OF ACTION

Although the etiology of cognitive impairment in Alzheimer's disease (AD) is not fully understood, it has been reported that acetylcholine-producing neurons degenerate in the brains of patients with Alzheimer's disease. The degree of this cholinergic loss has been correlated with degree of cognitive impairment and density of amyloid plaques (a neuropathological hallmark of Alzheimer's disease).

Galantamine, a tertiary alkaloid, is a competitive and reversible inhibitor of acetylcholinesterase. While the precise mechanism of galantamine's action is unknown, it is postulated to exert its therapeutic effect by enhancing cholinergic function. This is accomplished by increasing the concentration of acetylcholine through reversible inhibition of its hydrolysis by cholinesterase. If this mechanism is correct, galantamine's effect may lessen as the disease process advances and fewer cholinergic neurons remain functionally intact. There is no evidence that galantamine alters the course of the underlying dementing process.

PHARMACOKINETICS

Galantamine is well absorbed with absolute oral bioavailability of about 90%. It has a terminal elimination half-life of about 7 hours and pharmacokinetics are linear over the range of 8-32 mg/day.

The maximum inhibition of anticholinesterase activity of about 40% was achieved about 1 hour after a single oral dose of 8 mg galantamine in healthy male subjects.

Absorption and Distribution

Galantamine is rapidly and completely absorbed with time to peak concentration about 1 hour. Bioavailability of the tablet was the same as the bioavailability of an oral solution. Food did not affect the AUC of galantamine but C_{max} decreased by 25% and T_{max} was delayed by 1.5 hours. The mean volume of distribution of galantamine is 175 L.

The plasma protein binding of galantamine is 18% at therapeutically relevant concentrations. In whole blood, galantamine is mainly distributed to blood cells (52.7%). The blood to plasma concentration ratio of galantamine is 1.2.

Metabolism and Elimination

Galantamine is metabolized by hepatic cytochrome P450 enzymes, glucuronidated, and excreted unchanged in the urine. *In vitro* studies indicate that cytochrome CYP2D6 and CYP3A4 were the major cytochrome P450 isoenzymes involved in the metabolism of galantamine, and inhibitors of both pathways increase oral bioavailability of galantamine modestly (see Drug-Drug Interactions). O-demethylation, mediated by CYP2D6 was greater in extensive metabolizers of CYP2D6 than in poor metabolizers. In plasma from both poor and extensive metabolizers, however, unchanged galantamine and its glucuronide accounted for most of the sample radioactivity.

In studies of oral ^{3}H-galantamine, unchanged galantamine and its glucuronide, accounted for most plasma radioactivity in poor and extensive CYP2D6 metabolizers. Up to 8 hours post-dose, unchanged galantamine accounted for 39-77% of the total radioactivity in the plasma, and galantamine glucuronide for 14-24%. By 7 days, 93-99% of the radioactivity had been recovered, with about 95% in urine and about 5% in the feces. Total urinary recovery of unchanged galantamine accounted for, on average, 32% of the dose and that of galantamine glucuronide for another 12% on average.

After IV or oral administration, about 20% of the dose was excreted as unchanged galantamine in the urine in 24 hours, representing a renal clearance of about 65 ml/min, about 20-25% of the total plasma clearance of about 300 ml/min.

SPECIAL POPULATIONS

CYP2D6 Poor Metabolizers

Approximately 7% of the normal population has a genetic variation that leads to reduced levels of activity of CYP2D6 isozyme. Such individuals have been referred to as poor metabolizers. After a single oral dose of 4 or 8 mg galantamine, CYP2D6 poor metabolizers demonstrated a similar C_{max} and about 35% AUC(∞) increase of unchanged galantamine compared to extensive metabolizers.

A total of 356 patients with Alzheimer's disease enrolled in two Phase 3 studies were genotyped with respect to CYP2D6 (n=210 hetero-extensive metabolizers, 126 homo-extensive metabolizers, and 20 poor metabolizers). Population pharmacokinetic analysis indicated that there was a 25% decrease in median clearance in poor metabolizers compared to extensive metabolizers. Dosage adjustment is not necessary in patients identified as poor metabolizers as the dose of drug is individually titrated to tolerability.

Hepatic Impairment

Following a single 4 mg dose of galantamine, the pharmacokinetics of galantamine in subjects with mild hepatic impairment (n=8; Child-Pugh score of 5-6) were similar to those in healthy subjects. In patients with moderate hepatic impairment (n=8; Child-Pugh score of 7-9), galantamine clearance was decreased by about 25% compared to normal volunteers. Exposure would be expected to increase further with increasing degree of hepatic impairment (see PRECAUTIONS and DOSAGE AND ADMINISTRATION).

G

Renal Impairment

Following a single 8 mg dose of galantamine, AUC increased by 37% and 67% in moderate and severely renal-impaired patients compared to normal volunteers. (See PRECAUTIONS and DOSAGE AND ADMINISTRATION.)

Elderly

Data from clinical trials in patients with Alzheimer's disease indicate that galantamine concentrations are 30-40% higher than in healthy young subjects.

Gender and Race

No specific pharmacokinetic study was conducted to investigate the effect of gender and race on the disposition of galantamine hydrobromide, but a population pharmacokinetic analysis indicates (n=539 males and 550 females) that galantamine clearance is about 20% lower in females than in males (explained by lower body weight in females) and race (n=1029 White, 24 Black, 13 Asian and 23 other) did not affect the clearance of galantamine hydrobromide.

DRUG-DRUG INTERACTIONS

Multiple metabolic pathways and renal excretion are involved in the elimination of galantamine so no single pathway appears predominant. Based on *in vitro* studies, CYP2D6 and CYP3A4 were the major enzymes involved in the metabolism of galantamine. CYP2D6 was involved in the formation of O-desmethyl-galantamine, whereas CYP3A4 mediated the formation of galantamine-N-oxide. Galantamine is also glucuronidated and excreted unchanged in urine.

Effect of Other Drugs on the Metabolism of Galantamine Hydrobromide

Drugs that are potent inhibitors for CYP2D6 or CYP3A4 may increase the AUC of galantamine. Multiple dose pharmacokinetic studies demonstrated that the AUC of galantamine increased 30% and 40%, respectively, during coadministration of ketoconazole and paroxetine. As coadministered with erythromycin, another CYP3A4 inhibitor, the galantamine AUC increased only 10%. Population PK analysis with a database of 852 patients with Alzheimer's disease showed that the clearance of galantamine was decreased about 25-33% by concurrent administration of amitriptyline (n=17), fluoxetine (n=48), fluvoxamine (n=14), and quinidine (n=7), known inhibitors of CYP2D6.

Concurrent administration of H2-antagonists demonstrated that ranitidine did not affect the pharmacokinetics of galantamine, and cimetidine increased the galantamine AUC by approximately 16%.

Effect of Galantamine Hydrobromide on the Metabolism of Other Drugs

In vitro studies show that galantamine did not inhibit the metabolic pathways catalyzed by CYP1A2, CYP2A6, CYP3A4, CYP4A, CYP2C, CYP2D6 and CYP2E1. This indicated that the inhibitory potential of galantamine towards the major forms of cytochrome P450 is very low. Multiple doses of galantamine (24 mg/day) had no effect on the pharmacokinetics of digoxin and warfarin (R- and S-forms). Galantamine had no effect on the increased prothrombin time induced by warfarin.

INDICATIONS AND USAGE

Galantamine hydrobromide is indicated for the treatment of mild to moderate dementia of the Alzheimer's type.

CONTRAINDICATIONS

Galantamine hydrobromide is contraindicated in patients with known hypersensitivity to galantamine hydrobromide or to any excipients used in the formulation.

WARNINGS

ANESTHESIA

Galantamine, as a cholinesterase inhibitor, is likely to exaggerate the neuromuscular blockade effects of succinylcholine-type and similar neuromuscular blocking agents during anesthesia.

CARDIOVASCULAR CONDITIONS

Because of their pharmacological action, cholinesterase inhibitors have vagotonic effects on the sinoatrial and atrioventricular nodes, leading to bradycardia and AV block. These actions may be particularly important to patients with supraventricular cardiac conduction disorders or to patients taking other drugs concomitantly that significantly slow heart rate. Postmarketing surveillance of marketed anticholinesterase inhibitors has shown, however, that bradycardia and all types of heart block have been reported in patients both with and without known underlying cardiac conduction abnormalities. Therefore all patients should be considered at risk for adverse effects on cardiac conduction.

In randomized controlled trials, bradycardia was reported more frequently in galantamine-treated patients than in placebo-treated patients, but rarely led to treatment discontinuation. The overall frequency of this event was 2-3% for galantamine doses up to 24 mg/day compared with <1% for placebo. No increased incidence of heart block was observed at the recommended doses.

Patients treated with galantamine up to 24 mg/day using the recommended dosing schedule showed a dose-related increase in risk of syncope (placebo 0.7% [2/286]; 4 mg bid 0.4% [3/692]; 8 mg bid 1.3% [7/552]; 12 mg bid 2.2% [6/273]).

GASTROINTESTINAL CONDITIONS

Through their primary action, cholinomimetics may be expected to increase gastric acid secretion due to increased cholinergic activity. Therefore, patients should be monitored closely for symptoms of active or occult gastrointestinal bleeding, especially those with an increased risk for developing ulcers, *e.g.*, those with a history of ulcer disease or patients using concurrent nonsteroidal anti-inflammatory drugs (NSAIDS). Clinical studies of galantamine hydrobromide have shown no increase, relative to placebo, in the incidence of either peptic ulcer disease or gastrointestinal bleeding.

Galantamine hydrobromide, as a predictable consequence of its pharmacological properties, has been shown to produce nausea, vomiting, diarrhea, anorexia, and weight loss. (See ADVERSE REACTIONS.)

GENITOURINARY

Although this was not observed in clinical trials with galantamine hydrobromide, cholinomimetics may cause bladder outflow obstruction.

NEUROLOGICAL CONDITIONS

Seizures: Cholinesterase inhibitors are believed to have some potential to cause generalized convulsions. However, seizure activity may also be a manifestation of Alzheimer's disease. In clinical trials, there was no increase in the incidence of convulsions with galantamine hydrobromide compared to placebo.

PULMONARY CONDITIONS

Because of its cholinomimetic action, galantamine should be prescribed with care to patients with a history of severe asthma or obstructive pulmonary disease.

PRECAUTIONS

INFORMATION FOR THE PATIENT AND CAREGIVERS

Caregivers should be instructed in the recommended administration (twice/day, preferably with morning and evening meal) and dose escalation (dose increases should follow minimum of 4 weeks at prior dose).

Patients and caregivers should be advised that the most frequent adverse events associated with use of the drug can be minimized by following the recommended dosage and administration.

Patients and caregivers should be informed that if therapy has been interrupted for several days or longer, the patient should be restarted at the lowest dose and the dose escalated to the current dose.

Caregivers should be instructed in the correct procedure for administering galantamine hydrobromide oral solution. In addition, they should be informed of the existence of an Instruction Sheet (included with the product) describing how the solution is to be administered. They should be urged to read this sheet prior to administering galantamine hydrobromide oral solution. Caregivers should direct questions about the administration of the solution to either their physician or pharmacist.

SPECIAL POPULATIONS

Hepatic Impairment

In patients with moderately impaired hepatic function, dose titration should proceed cautiously (see CLINICAL PHARMACOLOGY and DOSAGE AND ADMINISTRATION). The use of galantamine hydrobromide in patients with severe hepatic impairment is not recommended.

Renal Impairment

In patients with moderately impaired renal function, dose titration should proceed cautiously (see CLINICAL PHARMACOLOGY and DOSAGE AND ADMINISTRATION). In patients with severely impaired renal function (CLCR <9 ml/min) the use of galantamine hydrobromide is not recommended.

CARCINOGENESIS, MUTAGENESIS, AND IMPAIRMENT OF FERTILITY

In a 24 month oral carcinogenicity study in rats, a slight increase in endometrial adenocarcinomas was observed at 10 mg/kg/day (4 times the Maximum Recommended Human Dose [MRHD] on a mg/m^2 basis or 6 times on an exposure [AUC] basis and 30 mg/kg/day [12 times MRHD on a mg/m^2 basis] or 19 times on an AUC basis). No increase in neoplastic changes was observed in females at 2.5 mg/kg/day (equivalent to the MRHD on a mg/m^2 basis or 2 times on an AUC basis) or in males up to the highest dose tested of 30 mg/kg/day (12 times the MRHD on a mg/m^2 and AUC basis).

Galantamine was not carcinogenic in a 6 month oral carcinogenicity study in transgenic (P 53-deficient) mice up to 20 mg/kg/day, or in a 24 month oral carcinogenicity study in male and female mice up to 10 mg/kg/day (2 times the MRHD on a mg/m^2 basis and equivalent on an AUC basis).

Galantamine produced no evidence of genotoxic potential when evaluated in the *in vitro* Ames *S. typhimurium* or *E. coli* reverse mutation assay, *in vitro* mouse lymphoma assay, *in vivo* micronucleus test in mice, or *in vitro* chromosome aberration assay in Chinese hamster ovary cells.

No impairment of fertility was seen in rats given up to 16 mg/kg/day (7 times the MRHD on a mg/m^2 basis) for 14 days prior to mating in females and for 60 days prior to mating in males.

PREGNANCY CATEGORY B

In a study in which rats were dosed from day 14 (females) or day 60 (males) prior to mating through the period of organogenesis, a slightly increased incidence of skeletal variations was observed at doses of 8 mg/kg/day (3 times the Maximum Recommended Human Dose [MRHD] on a mg/m^2 basis) and 16 mg/kg/day. In a study in which pregnant rats were dosed from the beginning of organogenesis through day 21 post-partum, pup weights were decreased at 8 and 16 mg/kg/day, but no adverse effects on other postnatal developmental parameters were seen. The doses causing the above effects in rats produced slight maternal toxicity. No major malformations were caused in rats given up to 16 mg/kg/day. No drug related teratogenic effects were observed in rabbits given up to 40 mg/kg/day (32 times the MRHD on a mg/m^2 basis) during the period of organogenesis.

There are no adequate and well-controlled studies of galantamine hydrobromide in pregnant women. Galantamine hydrobromide should be used during pregnancy only if the potential benefit justifies the potential risk to the fetus.

NURSING MOTHERS

It is not known whether galantamine is excreted in human breast milk. Galantamine hydrobromide has no indication for use in nursing mothers.

PEDIATRIC USE

There are no adequate and well-controlled trials documenting the safety and efficacy of galantamine in any illness occurring in children. Therefore, use of galantamine hydrobromide in children is not recommended.

DRUG INTERACTIONS

USE WITH ANTICHOLINERGICS

Galantamine hydrobromide has the potential to interfere with the activity of anticholinergic medications.

USE WITH CHOLINOMIMETICS AND OTHER CHOLINESTERASE INHIBITORS

A synergistic effect is expected when cholinesterase inhibitors are given concurrently with succinylcholine, other cholinesterase inhibitors, similar neuromuscular blocking agents or cholinergic agonists such as bethanechol.

Effect of Other Drugs on Galantamine

In Vitro

CYP3A4 and CYP2D6 are the major enzymes involved in the metabolism of galantamine. CYP3A4 mediates the formation of galantamine-N-oxide; CYP2D6 leads to the formation of O-desmethyl-galantamine. Because galantamine is also glucuronidated and excreted unchanged, no single pathway appears predominant.

In Vivo

Cimetidine and Ranitidine: Galantamine was administered as a single dose of 4 mg on day 2 of a 3 day treatment with either cimetidine (800 mg daily) or ranitidine (300 mg daily). Cimetidine increased the bioavailability of galantamine by approximately 16%. Ranitidine had no effect on the PK of galantamine.

Ketoconazole: Ketoconazole, a strong inhibitor of CYP3A4 and an inhibitor of CYP2D6, at a dose of 200 mg bid for 4 days, increased the AUC of galantamine by 30%.

Erythromycin: Erythromycin, a moderate inhibitor of CYP3A4, at a dose of 500 mg qid for 4 days, affected the AUC of galantamine minimally (10% increase).

Paroxetine: Paroxetine, a strong inhibitor of CYP2D6, at 20 mg/day for 16 days, increased the oral bioavailability of galantamine by about 40%.

Effect of Galantamine on Other Drugs

In Vitro

Galantamine did not inhibit the metabolic pathways catalyzed by CYP1A2, CYP2A6, CYP3A4, CYP4A, CYP2C, CYP2D6 or CYP2E1. This indicates that the inhibitory potential of galantamine towards the major forms of cytochrome P450 is very low.

In Vivo

Warfarin: Galantamine at 24 mg/day had no effect on the pharmacokinetics of R-and-S-warfarin (25 mg single dose) or on the prothrombin time. The protein binding of warfarin was unaffected by galantamine.

Digoxin: Galantamine at 24 mg/day had no effect on the steady-state pharmacokinetics of digoxin (0.375 mg once daily) when they were coadministered. In this study, however, one healthy subject was hospitalized for 2nd and 3rd degree heart block and bradycardia.

ADVERSE REACTIONS

ADVERSE EVENTS LEADING TO DISCONTINUATION

In two large scale, placebo-controlled trials of 6 months duration, in which patients were titrated weekly from 8 to 16 to 24, and to 32 mg/day, the risk of discontinuation because of an adverse event in the galantamine group exceeded that in the placebo group by about 3-fold. In contrast, in a 5 month trial with escalation of the dose by 8 mg/day every 4 weeks, the overall risk of discontinuation because of an adverse event was 7%, 7%, and 10% for the placebo, galantamine 16 mg/day, and galantamine 24 mg/day groups, respectively, with gastrointestinal adverse effects the principle reason for discontinuing galantamine. TABLE 5 shows the most frequent adverse events leading to discontinuation in this study.

TABLE 5 *Most Frequent Adverse Events Leading to Discontinuation in a Placebo-Controlled, Double-Blind Trial With a 4 Week Dose-Escalation Schedule*

		4 Week Escalation	
	Placebo	16 mg/day	24 mg/day
Adverse Event	n=286	n=279	n=273
Nausea	<1%	2%	4%
Vomiting	0%	1%	3%
Anorexia	<1%	1%	<1%
Dizziness	<1%	2%	1%
Syncope	0%	0%	1%

ADVERSE EVENTS REPORTED IN CONTROLLED TRIALS

The reported adverse events in galantamine hydrobromide trials reflect experience gained under closely monitored conditions in a highly selected patient population. In actual practice or in other clinical trials, these frequency estimates may not apply, as the conditions of use, reporting behavior and the types of patients treated may differ.

The majority of these adverse events occurred during the dose-escalation period. In those patients who experienced the most frequent adverse event, nausea, the median duration of the nausea was 5-7 days.

Administration of galantamine hydrobromide with food, the use of anti-emetic medication, and ensuring adequate fluid intake may reduce the impact of these events.

The most frequent adverse events, defined as those occurring at a frequency of at least 5% and at least twice the rate on placebo with the recommended maintenance dose of either 16 or 24 mg/day of galantamine hydrobromide under conditions of every 4 week dose-escalation for each dose increment of 8 mg/day, are shown in TABLE 6. These events were primarily gastrointestinal and tended to be less frequent with the 16 mg/day recommended initial maintenance dose.

TABLE 6 *The Most Frequent Adverse Events in the Placebo-Controlled Trial With Dose-Escalation Every 4 Weeks Occurring in at Least 5% of Patients Receiving Galantamine Hydrobromide and at Least Twice the Rate on Placebo*

		Galantamine Hydrobromide	
	Placebo	16 mg/day	24 mg/day
Adverse Event	n=286	n=279	n=273
Nausea	5%	13%	17%
Vomiting	1%	6%	10%
Diarrhea	6%	12%	6%
Anorexia	3%	7%	9%
Weight decrease	1%	5%	5%

The most common adverse events (adverse events occurring with an incidence of at least 2% with galantamine hydrobromide treatment and in which the incidence was greater than with placebo treatment) are listed in TABLE 7 for four placebo-controlled trials for patients treated with 16 or 24 mg/day of galantamine hydrobromide.

TABLE 7 *Adverse Events Reported in at Least 2% of Patients With Alzheimer's Disease Administered Galantamine Hydrobromide and at a Frequency Greater Than With Placebo*

Body System	Placebo	Galantamine Hydrobromide*
Adverse Event	n=801	n=1040
Body as a Whole — General Disorders		
Fatigue	3%	5%
Syncope	1%	2%
Central & Peripheral Nervous System Disorders		
Dizziness	6%	9%
Headache	5%	8%
Tremor	2%	3%
Gastrointestinal System Disorders		
Nausea	9%	24%
Vomiting	4%	13%
Diarrhea	7%	9%
Abdominal pain	4%	5%
Dyspepsia	2%	5%
Heart Rate and Rhythm Disorders		
Bradycardia	1%	2%
Metabolic and Nuritional Disorders		
Weight decrease	2%	7%
Psychiatric Disorders		
Anorexia	3%	9%
Depression	5%	7%
Insomnia	4%	5%
Somnolence	3%	4%
Red Blood Cell Disorders		
Anemia	2%	3%
Respiratory System Disorders		
Rhinitis	3%	4%
Urinary System Disorders		
Urinary tract infection	7%	8%
Hematuria	2%	3%

* Adverse events in patients treated with 16 or 24 mg/day of galantamine hydrobromide in 4 placebo-controlled trials are included.

Adverse events occurring with an incidence of at least 2% in placebo-treated patients that was either equal to or greater than with galantamine hydrobromide treatment were constipation, agitation, confusion, anxiety, hallucination, injury, back pain, peripheral edema, asthenia, chest pain, urinary incontinence, upper respiratory tract infection, bronchitis, coughing, hypertension, fall, and purpura.

There were no important differences in adverse event rate related to dose or sex. There were too few non-Caucasian patients to assess the effects of race on adverse event rates.

No clinically relevant abnormalities in laboratory values were observed.

OTHER ADVERSE EVENTS OBSERVED DURING CLINICAL TRIALS

Galantamine hydrobromide was administered to 3055 patients with Alzheimer's disease. A total of 2357 patients received galantamine in placebo-controlled trials and 761 patients with Alzheimer's disease received galantamine 24 mg/day, the maximum recommended maintenance dose. About 1000 patients received galantamine for at least 1 year and approximately 200 patients received galantamine for 2 years.

To establish the rate of adverse events, data from all patients receiving any dose of galantamine in 8 placebo-controlled trials and 6 open-label extension trials were pooled. The methodology to gather and codify these adverse events was standardized across trials, using WHO terminology. All adverse events occurring in approximately 0.1% are included, except for those already listed elsewhere in labeling, WHO terms too general to be informative, or events unlikely to be drug caused. Events are classified by body system and listed using the following definitions: frequent adverse events — those occurring in at least 1/100 patients; infrequent adverse events — those occurring in 1/100 to 1/1000 patients; rare adverse events — those occurring in fewer than 1/1000 patients. These adverse events are not necessarily related to galantamine hydrobromide treatment and in most cases were observed at a similar frequency in placebo-treated patients in the controlled studies.

Body as a Whole — General Disorders: *Frequent:* Chest pain.

Cardiovascular System Disorders: *Infrequent:* Postural hypotension, hypotension, dependent edema, cardiac failure.

Central & Peripheral Nervous System Disorders: *Infrequent:* Vertigo, hypertonia, convulsions, involuntary muscle contractions, paresthesia, ataxia, hypokinesia, hyperkinesia, apraxia, aphasia.

Gastrointestinal System Disorders: *Frequent:* Flatulence; *Infrequent:* Gastritis, melena, dysphagia, rectal hemorrhage, dry mouth, saliva increased, diverticulitis, gastroenteritis, hiccup; *Rare:* Esophageal perforation.

Heart Rate & Rhythm Disorders: *Infrequent:* AV block, palpitation, atrial fibrillation, QT prolonged, bundle branch block, supraventricular tachycardia, T-wave inversion, ventricular tachycardia.

Metabolic & Nutritional Disorders: *Infrequent:* Hyperglycemia, alkaline phosphatase increased.

Platelet, Bleeding & Clotting Disorders: *Infrequent:* Purpura, epistaxis, thrombocytopenia.

Psychiatric Disorders: *Infrequent:* Apathy, paroniria, paranoid reaction, libido increased, delirium.

Urinary System Disorders: *Frequent:* Incontinence; *Infrequent:* Hematuria, micturition frequency, cystitis, urinary retention, nocturia, renal calculi.

DOSAGE AND ADMINISTRATION

The dosage of galantamine hydrobromide shown to be effective in controlled clinical trials is 16-32 mg/day given as twice daily dosing. As the dose of 32 mg/day is less well tolerated than lower doses and does not provide increased effectiveness, the recommended dose range is 16-24 mg/day given in a bid regimen. The dose of 24 mg/day did not provide a statistically significant greater clinical benefit than 16 mg/day. It is possible, however, that a daily dose of 24 mg of galantamine hydrobromide might provide additional benefit for some patients.

The recommended starting dose of galantamine hydrobromide is 4 mg twice a day (8 mg/day). After a minimum of 4 weeks of treatment, if this dose is well tolerated, the dose should be increased to 8 mg twice a day (16 mg/day). A further increase to 12 mg twice a day (24 mg/day) should be attempted only after a minimum of 4 weeks at the previous dose.

Galantamine hydrobromide should be administered twice a day, preferably with morning and evening meals.

Patients and caregivers should be informed that if therapy has been interrupted for several days or longer, the patient should be restarted at the lowest dose and the dose escalated to the current dose.

Caregivers should be instructed in the correct procedure for administering galantamine hydrobromide oral solution. In addition, they should be informed of the existence of an Instruction Sheet (included with the product) describing how the solution is to be administered. They should be urged to read this sheet prior to administering galantamine hydrobromide oral solution. Caregivers should direct questions about the administration of the solution to either their physician or pharmacist.

The abrupt withdrawal of galantamine hydrobromide in those patients who had been receiving doses in the effective range was not associated with an increased frequency of adverse events in comparison with those continuing to receive the same doses of that drug. The beneficial effects of galantamine hydrobromide are lost, however, when the drug is discontinued.

DOSING IN SPECIAL POPULATIONS

Galantamine plasma concentrations may be increased in patients with moderate to severe hepatic impairment. In patients with moderately impaired hepatic function (Child-Pugh score of 7-9), the dose should generally not exceed 16 mg/day. The use of galantamine hydrobromide in patients with severe hepatic impairment (Child-Pugh score of 10-15) is not recommended.

For patients with moderate renal impairment the dose should generally not exceed 16 mg/day. In patients with severe renal impairment (creatinine clearance <9 ml/min), the use of galantamine hydrobromide is not recommended.

HOW SUPPLIED

Reminyl tablets are available in 4, 8 and 12 mg strengths.

4 mg: Off-white tablet imprinted "JANSSEN" on one side, and "G" and "4" on the other.

8 mg: Pink tablet imprinted "JANSSEN" on one side, and "G" and "8" on the other.

12 mg: Orange-brown tablet imprinted "JANSSEN" on one side, and "G" and "12" on the other.

Reminyl 4 mg/ml oral solution is a clear colorless solution supplied in 100 ml bottles with a calibrated (in milligrams and milliliters) pipette. The minimum calibrated volume is 0.5 ml, while the maximum calibrated volume is 4 ml.

STORAGE AND HANDLING

Reminyl tablets should be stored at 25°C (77°F); excursions permitted to 15-30°C (59-86°F).

Reminyl oral solution should be stored at 25°C (77°F); excursions permitted to 15-30°C (59-86°F). DO NOT FREEZE.

Keep out of reach of children.

PRODUCT LISTING - EQUIVALENTS NOT AVAILABLE

Solution - Oral - 4 mg/ml
100 ml $157.35 REMINYL, Janssen Pharmaceuticals 50458-0399-10

Tablet - Oral - 4 mg
60's $149.96 REMINYL, Janssen Pharmaceuticals 50458-0390-60

Tablet - Oral - 8 mg
60's $149.96 REMINYL, Janssen Pharmaceuticals 50458-0391-60

Tablet - Oral - 12 mg
60's $149.96 REMINYL, Janssen Pharmaceuticals 50458-0392-60

G

Ganciclovir Sodium *(001343)*

Categories: Retinitis, cytomegalovirus; Pregnancy Category C; FDA Approved 1989 Jun; Orphan Drugs
Drug Classes: Antivirals
Brand Names: Cytovene
Foreign Brand Availability: Cymevan (France); Cymeven (Germany); Cymevene (Australia; Austria; Bahamas; Bahrain; Barbados; Belgium; Belize; Benin; Bermuda; Bulgaria; Burkina-Faso; Colombia; Curacao; Cyprus; Czech-Republic; Denmark; Egypt; England; Ethiopia; Finland; Gambia; Ghana; Greece; Guinea; Guyana; Hong-Kong; Hungary; Indonesia; Iran; Iraq; Israel; Italy; Ivory-Coast; Jamaica; Jordan; Kenya; Korea; Kuwait; Lebanon; Liberia; Libya; Malawi; Malaysia; Mali; Mauritania; Mauritius; Mexico; Morocco; Netherland-Antilles; Netherlands; New-Zealand; Niger; Nigeria; Norway; Oman; Peru; Philippines; Portugal; Qatar; Republic-of-Yemen; Saudi-Arabia; Senegal; Seychelles; Sierra-Leone; South-Africa; Spain; Sudan; Surinam; Sweden; Switzerland; Syria; Taiwan; Tanzania; Thailand; Trinidad; Tunia; Turkey; Uganda; United-Arab-Emirates; Zambia; Zimbabwe); Denosine (Japan); Virgan (Philippines); Vitrasert Implant (Austria; Belgium; Bulgaria; Czech-Republic; Denmark; England; Finland; France; Germany; Greece; Hungary; Ireland; Italy; Netherlands; Norway; Poland; Portugal; Slovenia; Spain; Sweden; Switzerland; Turkey)
Cost of Therapy: $780.90 (CMV Retinitis; Cytovene; 500 mg; 6 capsules/day; 30 day supply)
HCFA JCODE(S): J1570 500 mg IV

WARNING

THE CLINICAL TOXICITY OF GANCICLOVIR SODIUM CAPSULES AND GANCICLOVIR SODIUM IV INCLUDES GRANULOCYTOPENIA, ANEMIA, AND THROMBOCYTOPENIA. IN ANIMAL STUDIES GANCICLOVIR WAS CARCINOGENIC, TERATOGENIC, AND CAUSED ASPERMATOGENESIS.

GANCICLOVIR SODIUM IV IS INDICATED FOR USE *ONLY* IN THE TREATMENT OF CYTOMEGALOVIRUS (CMV) RETINITIS IN IMMUNOCOMPROMISED PATIENTS AND FOR THE PREVENTION OF CMV DISEASE IN TRANSPLANT PATIENTS AT RISK FOR CMV DISEASE.

GANCICLOVIR SODIUM CAPSULES ARE INDICATED *ONLY* FOR PREVENTION OF CMV DISEASE IN PATIENTS WITH ADVANCED HIV INFECTION AT RISK FOR CMV DISEASE, FOR MAINTENANCE TREATMENT OF CMV RETINITIS IN IMMUNOCOMPROMISED PATIENTS, AND FOR PREVENTION OF CMV DISEASE IN SOLID ORGAN TRANSPLANT RECIPIENTS (See INDICATIONS AND USAGE).

BECAUSE GANCICLOVIR SODIUM CAPSULES ARE ASSOCIATED WITH A RISK OF MORE RAPID RATE OF CMV RETINITIS PROGRESSION, THEY SHOULD BE USED AS MAINTENANCE TREATMENT ONLY IN THOSE PATIENTS FOR WHOM THIS RISK IS BALANCED BY THE BENEFIT ASSOCIATED WITH AVOIDING DAILY IV INFUSIONS.

DESCRIPTION

Ganciclovir is a synthetic guanine derivative active against cytomegalovirus (CMV). Cytovene-IV and Cytovene are the brand names for ganciclovir sodium for injection and ganciclovir capsules, respectively.

Cytovene-IV: Available as sterile lyophilized powder in strength of 500 mg per vial for IV administration only. Each vial of Cytovene-IV contains the equivalent of 500 mg ganciclovir as the sodium salt (46 mg sodium). Reconstitution with 10 ml of sterile water for injection yields a solution with pH 11 and a ganciclovir concentration of approximately 50 mg/ml. Further dilution in an appropriate IV solution must be performed before infusion (see DOSAGE AND ADMINISTRATION).

Cytovene: Available as 250 and 500 mg capsules. Each capsule contains 250 or 500 mg ganciclovir, respectively, and inactive ingredients croscarmellose sodium, magnesium stearate, and povidone. The hard gelatin shells consist of gelatin, titanium dioxide, yellow iron oxide, and FD&C blue no. 2.

Ganciclovir is a white to off-white crystalline powder with a molecular formula of $C_9H_{13}N_5O_4$ and a molecular weight of 255.23. The chemical name for ganciclovir is 9-[[2-hydroxy-1- (hydroxymethyl)ethoxy]methyl]guanine. Ganciclovir is a polar hydrophilic compound with a solubility of 2.6 mg/ml in water at 25°C and an n-octanol/water partition coefficient of 0.022. The pKas for ganciclovir are 2.2 and 9.4.

Ganciclovir, when formulated as monosodium salt in the IV dosage form, is a white to off-white lyophilized powder with a molecular formula of $C_9H_{12}N_5NaO_4$, and molecular weight of 277.22. The chemical name for ganciclovir sodium is 9-[[2-hydroxy-1-(hydroxymethyl)ethoxy]methyl]guanine, monosodium salt. The lyophilized powder has an aqueous solubility of greater than 50 mg/ml at 25°C. At physiological pH, ganciclovir sodium exists as the un-ionized form with a solubility of approximately 6 mg/ml at 37°C.

All doses in this insert are specified in terms of ganciclovir.

CLINICAL PHARMACOLOGY

VIROLOGY

Mechanism of Action

Ganciclovir is an acyclic nucleoside analogue of 2′-deoxyguanosine that inhibits replication of herpes viruses. Ganciclovir has been shown to be active against cytomegalovirus (CMV) and herpes simplex virus (HSV) in human clinical studies.

To achieve anti-CMV activity, ganciclovir is phosphorylated first to the monophosphate form by a CMV-encoded (UL97 gene) protein kinase homologue, then to the di- and triphosphate forms by cellular kinases. Ganciclovir triphosphate concentrations may be 100-fold greater in CMV-infected than in uninfected cells, indicating preferential phosphorylation in infected cells. Ganciclovir triphosphate, once formed, persists for days in the CMV-infected cell. Ganciclovir triphosphate is believed to inhibit viral DNA synthesis by (1) competitive inhibition of viral DNA polymerases; and (2) incorporation into viral DNA, resulting in eventual termination of viral DNA elongation.

Antiviral Activity

The median concentration of ganciclovir that inhibits CMV replication (IC_{50}) *in vitro* (laboratory strains or clinical isolates) has ranged from 0.02-3.48 μg/ml. Ganciclovir inhibits mammalian cell proliferation (CIC_{50}) *in vitro* at higher concentrations ranging from 30-725 μg/ml. Bone marrow-derived colony-forming cells are more sensitive (CIC_{50} 0.028-0.7 μg/ml). The relationship of *in vitro* sensitivity of CMV to ganciclovir and clinical response has not been established.

Clinical Antiviral Effect Of Ganciclovir Sodium IV and Capsules

Ganciclovir Sodium IV

In a study of ganciclovir sodium IV treatment of life- or sight-threatening CMV disease in immunocompromised patients, 121 of 314 patients had CMV cultured within 7 days prior to treatment and sequential posttreatment viral cultures of urine, blood, throat and/or semen. As judged by conversion to culture negativity, or a greater than 100-fold decrease in *in vitro* CMV titer, at least 83% of patients had a virologic response with a median response time of 7-15 days.

Antiviral activity of ganciclovir sodium IV was demonstrated in two randomized studies for the prevention of CMV disease in transplant recipients (see TABLE 1).

TABLE 1 *Patients With Positive CMV Cultures*

Time	Heart Allograft* (n=147) Ganciclovir Sodium IV†	Heart Allograft* (n=147) Placebo	Bone Marrow Allograft (n=72) Ganciclovir Sodium IV‡	Bone Marrow Allograft (n=72) Placebo
Pretreatment	1/67 (2%)	5/64 (8%)	37/37 (100%)	35/35 (100%)
Week 2	2/75 (3%)	11/67 (16%)	2/31 (6%)	19/28 (68%)
Week 4	3/66 (5%)	28/66 (43%)	0/24 (0%)	16/20 (80%)

* CMV seropositive or receiving graft from seropostitive donor.
† 5 mg/kg bid for 14 days followed by 6 mg/kg qd for 5 days/week for 14 days.
‡ 5 mg/kg bid for 7 days followed by 5 mg/kg qd until day 100 post-transplant.

Ganciclovir Sodium Capsules

In trials comparing ganciclovir sodium IV with ganciclovir sodium capsules for the maintenance treatment of CMV retinitis in patients with AIDS, serial urine cultures and other available cultures (semen, biopsy specimens, blood and others) showed that a small proportion of patients remained culture-positive during maintenance therapy with no statistically significant differences in CMV isolation rates between treatment groups.

A study of ganciclovir sodium capsules (1000 mg q8h) for prevention of CMV disease in individuals with advanced HIV infection (ICM 1654) evaluated antiviral activity as measured by CMV isolation in culture; most cultures were from urine. At baseline, 40% (176/436) and 44% (92/210) of ganciclovir and placebo recipients, respectively, had positive cultures (urine or blood). After 2 months on treatment, 10% vs 44% of ganciclovir versus placebo recipients had positive cultures.

Viral Resistance

The current working definition of CMV resistance to ganciclovir in *in vitro* assays is IC_{50} >3.0 μg/ml (12.0 μM). CMV resistance to ganciclovir has been observed in individuals with AIDS and CMV retinitis who have never received ganciclovir therapy. Viral resistance has also been observed in patients receiving prolonged treatment for CMV retinitis with ganciclovir sodium IV. In a controlled study of oral ganciclovir for prevention of AIDS-associated CMV disease, 364 individuals had one or more cultures performed after at least 90 days of ganciclovir treatment. Of these, 113 had at least one positive culture. The last available isolate from each subject was tested for reduced sensitivity, and 2 of 40 were found to be resistant to ganciclovir. These resistant isolates were associated with subsequent treatment failure for retinitis.

The possibility of viral resistance should be considered in patients who show poor clinical response or experience persistent viral excretion during therapy. The principal mechanism of resistance to ganciclovir in CMV is the decreased ability to form the active triphosphate moiety; resistant viruses have been described that contain mutations in the UL97 gene of CMV that controls phosphorylation of ganciclovir. Mutations in the viral DNA polymerase have also been reported to confer viral resistance to ganciclovir.

PHARMACOKINETICS

BECAUSE THE MAJOR ELIMINATION PATHWAY FOR GANCICLOVIR IS RENAL, DOSAGE REDUCTIONS ACCORDING TO CREATININE CLEARANCE ARE REQUIRED FOR GANCICLOVIR SODIUM IV AND SHOULD BE CONSIDERED FOR GANCICLOVIR SODIUM CAPSULES. FOR DOSING INSTRUCTIONS IN PATIENTS WITH RENAL IMPAIRMENT, REFER TO DOSAGE AND ADMINISTRATION.

Absorption

The absolute bioavailability of oral ganciclovir under fasting conditions was approximately 5% (n=6) and following food was 6-9% (n=32). When ganciclovir was administered orally with food at a total daily dose of 3 g/day (500 mg q3h, 6 times daily and 1000 mg tid), the steady-state absorption as measured by area under the serum concentration versus time curve (AUC) over 24 hours and maximum serum concentrations (C_{max}) were similar following both regimens with an AUC(0-24) of 15.9 ± 4.2 (mean ±SD) and 15.4 ± 4.3 µg·h/ml and C_{max} of 1.02 ± 0.24 and 1.18 ± 0.36 µg/ml, respectively (n=16).

At the end of a 1 hour IV infusion of 5 mg/kg ganciclovir, total AUC ranged between 22.1 ± 3.2 (n=16) and 26.8 ± 6.1 µg·h/ml (n=16) and C_{max} ranged between 8.27 ± 1.02 (n=16) and 9.0 ± 1.4 µg/ml (n=16).

Food Effects

When ganciclovir sodium capsules were given with a meal containing 602 calories and 46.5% fat at a dosage of 1000 mg every 8 hours to 20 HIV-positive subjects, the steady-state AUC increased by 22 ± 22% (range: -6 to 68%) and there was a significant prolongation of time to peak serum concentrations (T_{max}) from 1.8 ± 0.8 to 3.0 ± 0.6 hours and a higher C_{max} (0.85 ± 0.25 vs 0.96 ± 0.27 µg/ml) (n=20).

Distribution

The steady-state volume of distribution of ganciclovir after IV administration was 0.74 ± 0.15 L/kg (n=98). For ganciclovir sodium capsules, no correlation was observed between AUC and reciprocal weight (range: 55-128 kg); oral dosing according to weight is not required. Cerebrospinal fluid concentrations obtained 0.25-5.67 hours postdose in 3 patients who received 2.5 mg/kg ganciclovir intravenously q8h or q12h ranged from 0.31-0.68 µg/ml representing 24-70% of the respective plasma concentrations. Binding to plasma proteins was 1-2% over ganciclovir concentrations of 0.5 and 51 µg/ml.

Metabolism

Following oral administration of a single 1000 mg dose of ^{14}C-labeled ganciclovir, 86 ± 3% of the administered dose was recovered in the feces and 5 ± 1% was recovered in the urine (n=4). No metabolite accounted for more than 1-2% of the radioactivity recovered in urine or feces.

Elimination

When administered intravenously, ganciclovir exhibits linear pharmacokinetics over the range of 1.6-5.0 mg/kg and when administered orally, it exhibits linear kinetics up to a total daily dose of 4 g/day. Renal excretion of unchanged drug by glomerular filtration and active tubular secretion is the major route of elimination of ganciclovir. In patients with normal renal function, 91.3 ± 5.0% (n=4) of intravenously administered ganciclovir was recovered unmetabolized in the urine. Systemic clearance of intravenously administered ganciclovir was 3.52 ± 0.80 ml/min/kg (n=98) while renal clearance was 3.20 ± 0.80 ml/min/kg (n=47), accounting for 91 ± 11% of the systemic clearance (n=47). After oral administration of ganciclovir, steady-state is achieved within 24 hours. Renal clearance following oral administration was 3.1 ± 1.2 ml/min/kg (n=22). Half-life was 3.5 ± 0.9 hours (n=98) following IV administration and 4.8 ± 0.9 hours (n=39) following oral administration.

SPECIAL POPULATIONS

Renal Impairment

The pharmacokinetics following IV administration of ganciclovir sodium IV solution were evaluated in 10 immunocompromised patients with renal impairment who received doses ranging from 1.25 to 5 mg/kg (see TABLE 2).

TABLE 2

Estimated Creatinine Clearance (ml/min)	n	Dose	Mean ± SD Clearance (ml/min)	Half-Life (hours)
50-79	4	3.2-5 mg/kg	128 ± 63	4.6 ± 1.4
25-49	3	3-5 mg/kg	57 ± 8	4.4 ± 0.4
<25	3	1.25-5 mg/kg	30 ± 13	10.7 ± 5.7

The pharmacokineticsof ganciclovir following oral administration of ganciclovir sodium capsules were evaluated in 44 patients, who were either solid organ transplant recipients or HIV positive. Apparent oral clearance of ganciclovir decreased and AUC(0-24h) increased with diminishing renal function (as expressed by creatinine clearance).

Based on these observations, it is necessary to modify the dosage of ganciclovir in patients with renal impairment (see DOSAGE AND ADMINISTRATION).

Hemodialysis reduces plasma concentrations of ganciclovir by about 50% after both IV and oral administration.

Race/Ethnicity and Gender

The effects of race/ethnicity and gender were studied in subjects receiving a dose regimen of 1000 mg every 8 hours. Although the numbers of blacks (16%) and Hispanics (20%) were small, there appeared to be a trend towards a lower steady-state C_{max} and AUC(0-8) in these subpopulations as compared to Caucasians. No definitive conclusions regarding gender differences could be made because of the small number of females (12%); however, no differences between males and females were observed.

Pediatrics

Ganciclovir pharmacokinetics were studied in 27 neonates, aged 2-49 days. At an IV dose of 4 mg/kg (n=14) or 6 mg/kg (n=13), the pharmacokinetic parameters were, respectively, C_{max} of 5.5 ± 1.6 and 7.0 ± 1.6 µg/ml, systemic clearance of 3.14 ± 1.75 and 3.56 ± 1.27 ml/min/kg, and T½ of 2.4 hours (harmonic mean) for both.

Ganciclovir pharmacokinetics were also studied in 10 pediatric patients, aged 9 months to 12 years. The pharmacokinetic characteristics of ganciclovir were the same after single and multiple (q12h) IV doses (5 mg/kg). The steady-state volume of distribution was 0.64 ± 0.22 L/kg, C_{max} was 7.9 ± 3.9 µg/ml, systemic clearance was 4.7 ± 2.2 ml/min/kg, and T½ was 2.4 ± 0.7 hours. The pharmacokinetics of IV ganciclovir in pediatric patients are similar to those observed in adults.

Elderly

No studies have been conducted in adults older than 65 years of age.

INDICATIONS AND USAGE

Ganciclovir sodium IV is indicated for the treatment of CMV retinitis in immunocompromised patients, including patients with acquired immunodeficiency syndrome (AIDS). Ganciclovir sodium IV is also indicated for the prevention of CMV disease in transplant recipients at risk for CMV disease.

Ganciclovir sodium capsules are indicated for the prevention of CMV disease in solid organ transplant recipients and in individuals with advanced HIV infection at risk for developing CMV disease. Ganciclovir sodium capsules are also indicated as an alternative to the IV formulation for maintenance treatment of CMV retinitis in immunocompromised patients, including patients with AIDS, in whom retinitis is stable following appropriate induction therapy and for whom the risk of more rapid progression is balanced by the benefit associated with avoiding daily IV infusions.

SAFETY AND EFFICACY OF **GANCICLOVIR SODIUM IV** AND **CAPSULES** HAVE NOT BEEN ESTABLISHED FOR CONGENITAL OR NEONATAL CMV DISEASE; NOR FOR THE TREATMENT OF ESTABLISHED CMV DISEASE OTHER THAN RETINITIS; NOR FOR USE IN NON-IMMUNOCOMPROMISED INDIVIDUALS. THE SAFETY AND EFFICACY OF **GANCICLOVIR SODIUM** CAPSULES HAVE NOT BEEN ESTABLISHED FOR TREATING ANY MANIFESTATION OF CMV DISEASE OTHER THAN MAINTENANCE TREATMENT OF CMV RETINITIS.

NON-FDA APPROVED INDICATIONS

Intravenous ganciclovir is also commonly given to treat other manifestations of CMV, including pneumonitis, central nervous system infections, gastroenteritis, and hepatitis, although such uses are not approved by the FDA.

CONTRAINDICATIONS

Ganciclovir sodium IV and capsules are contraindicated in patients with hypersensitivity to ganciclovir or acyclovir.

WARNINGS

HEMATOLOGIC

Ganciclovir sodium IV and capsules should not be administered if the absolute neutrophil count is less than 500 cells/µl or the platelet count is less than 25,000 cells/µl. Granulocytopenia (neutropenia), anemia and thrombocytopenia have been observed in patients treated with ganciclovir sodium IV and capsules. The frequency and severity of these events vary widely in different patient populations (see ADVERSE REACTIONS).

Ganciclovir sodium IV and capsules should, therefore, be used with caution in patients with pre-existing cytopenias or with a history of cytopenic reactions to other drugs, chemicals, or irradiation. Granulocytopenia usually occurs during the first or second week of treatment but may occur at any time during treatment. Cell counts usually begin to recover within 3-7 days of discontinuing drug. Colony-stimulating factors have been shown to increase neutrophil and white blood cell counts in patients receiving ganciclovir sodium IV solution for treatment of CMV retinitis.

IMPAIRMENT OF FERTILITY

Animal data indicate that administration of ganciclovir causes inhibition of spermatogenesis and subsequent infertility. These effects were reversible at lower doses and irreversible at higher doses (see PRECAUTIONS: Carcinogenesis, Mutagenesis and Impairment of Fertility). Although data in humans have not been obtained regarding this effect, it is considered probable that ganciclovir at the recommended doses causes temporary or permanent inhibition of spermatogenesis. Animal data also indicate that suppression of fertility in females may occur.

TERATOGENESIS

Because of the mutagenic and teratogenic potential of ganciclovir, women of childbearing potential should be advised to use effective contraception during treatment. Similarly, men should be advised to practice barrier contraception during and for at least 90 days following treatment with ganciclovir sodium IV or ganciclovir sodium capsules (see PRECAUTIONS, Pregnancy Category C).

PRECAUTIONS

GENERAL

In clinical studies with ganciclovir sodium IV, the maximum single dose administered was 6 mg/kg by IV infusion over 1 hour. Larger doses have resulted in increased toxicity. It is likely that more rapid infusions would result in increased toxicity. Administration of ganciclovir sodium IV solution should be accompanied by adequate hydration.

Initially, reconstituted solutions of ganciclovir sodium IV have a high pH (pH 11). Despite further dilution in IV fluids, phlebitis and/or pain may occur at the site of IV infusion. Care must be taken to infuse solutions containing ganciclovir sodium IV only into veins with adequate blood flow to permit rapid dilution and distribution (see DOSAGE AND ADMINISTRATION).

Since ganciclovir is excreted by the kidneys, normal clearance depends on adequate renal function. IF RENAL FUNCTION IS IMPAIRED, DOSAGE ADJUSTMENTS ARE REQUIRED FOR GANCICLOVIR SODIUM IVAND SHOULD BE CONSIDERED FOR GANCICLOVIR SODIUM CAPSULES. Such adjustments should be based on measured or estimated creatinine clearance values. (see DOSAGE AND ADMINISTRATION).

G

INFORMATION FOR THE PATIENT

All patients should be informed that the major toxicities of ganciclovir are granulocytopenia (neutropenia), anemia, and thrombocytopenia and that dose modifications may be required, including discontinuation. The importance of close monitoring of blood counts while on therapy should be emphasized. Patients should be informed that ganciclovir has been associated with elevations in serum creatinine.

Patients should be instructed to take ganciclovir sodium capsules with food to maximize bioavailability.

Patients should be advised that ganciclovir has caused decreased sperm production in animals and may cause infertility in humans. Women of childbearing potential should be advised that ganciclovir causes birth defects in animals and should not be used during pregnancy. Women of childbearing potential should be advised to use effective contraception during treatment with ganciclovir sodium IV or ganciclovir sodium capsules. Similarly, men should be advised to practice barrier contraception during and for at least 90 days following treatment with ganciclovir sodium IV or ganciclovir sodium capsules.

Patients should be advised that ganciclovir causes tumors in animals. Although there is no information from human studies, ganciclovir should be considered a potential carcinogen.

All HIV+ Patients

These patients may be receiving zidovudine. Patients should be counseled that treatment with both ganciclovir and zidovudine simultaneously may not be tolerated by some patients and may result in severe granulocytopenia (neutropenia). Patients with AIDS may be receiving didanosine. Patients should be counseled that concomitant treatment with both ganciclovir and didanosine can cause didanosine serum concentrations to be significantly increased.

HIV+ Patients With CMV Retinitis

Ganciclovir is not a cure for CMV retinitis, and immunocompromised patients may continue to experience progression of retinitis during or following treatment. Patients should be advised to have ophthalmologic follow-up examinations at a minimum of every 4-6 weeks while being treated with ganciclovir sodium IV or ganciclovir sodium capsules. Some patients will require more frequent follow-up.

Transplant Recipients

Transplant recipients should be counseled regarding the high frequency of impaired renal function in transplant recipients who received ganciclovir sodium IV solution in controlled clinical trials, particularly in patients receiving concomitant administration of nephrotoxic agents such as cyclosporine and amphotericin B. Although the specific mechanism of this toxicity, which in most cases was reversible, has not been determined, the higher rate of renal impairment in patients receiving ganciclovir sodium IV solution compared with those who received placebo in the same trials may indicate that ganciclovir sodium IV played a significant role.

LABORATORY TESTS

Due to the frequency of neutropenia, anemia and thrombocytopenia in patients receiving ganciclovir sodium IV and capsules (see ADVERSE REACTIONS), it is recommended that complete blood counts and platelet counts be performed frequently, especially in patients in whom ganciclovir or other nucleoside analogues have previously resulted in leukopenia, or in whom neutrophil counts are less than 1000 cells/μl at the beginning of treatment. Increased serum creatinine levels have been observed in trials evaluating both ganciclovir sodium IV and capsules. Patients should have serum creatinine or creatinine clearance values monitored carefully to allow for dosage adjustments in renally impaired patients (see DOSAGE AND ADMINISTRATION).

CARCINOGENESIS, MUTAGENESIS*

Ganciclovir was carcinogenic in the mouse at oral doses of 20 and 1000 mg/kg/day (approximately 0.1× and 1.4×, respectively, the mean drug exposure in humans following the recommended IV dose of 5 mg/kg, based on area under the plasma concentration curve [AUC] comparisons). At the dose of 1000 mg/kg/day there was a significant increase in the incidence of tumors of the preputial gland in males, forestomach (nonglandular mucosa) in males and females, and reproductive tissues (ovaries, uterus, mammary gland, clitoral gland, and vagina) and liver in females. At the dose of 20 mg/kg/day, a slightly increased incidence of tumors was noted in the preputial and harderian glands in males, forestomach in males and females, and liver in females. No carcinogenic effect was observed in mice administered ganciclovir at 1 mg/kg/day (estimated as 0.01× the human dose based on AUC comparison). Except for histiocytic sarcoma of the liver, ganciclovir-induced tumors were generally of epithelial or vascular origin. Although the preputial and clitoral glands, forestomach, and harderian glands of mice do not have human counterparts, ganciclovir should be considered a potential carcinogen in humans.

Ganciclovir increased mutations in mouse lymphoma cells and DNA damage in human lymphocytes *in vitro* at concentrations between 50-500 and 250-2000 μg/ml, respectively. In the mouse micronucleus assay, ganciclovir was clastogenic at doses of 150 and 500 mg/kg (IV) (2.8-10× human exposure based on AUC) but not 50 mg/kg (exposure approximately comparable to the human based on AUC). Ganciclovir was not mutagenic in the Ames *Salmonella* assay at concentrations of 500-5000 μg/ml.

IMPAIRMENT OF FERTILITY*

Ganciclovir caused decreased mating behavior, decreased fertility, and an increased incidence of embryolethality in female mice following IV doses of 90 mg/kg/day (approximately 1.7× the mean drug exposure in humans following the dose of 5 mg/kg, based on AUC comparisons). Ganciclovir caused decreased fertility in male mice and hypospermatogenesis in mice and dogs following daily oral or IV administration of doses ranging from 0.2 to 10 mg/kg. Systemic drug exposure (AUC) at the lowest dose showing toxicity in each species ranged from 0.03 to 0.1× the AUC of the recommended human IV dose.

PREGNANCY CATEGORY C*

Ganciclovir has been shown to be embryotoxic in rabbits and mice following IV administration and teratogenic in rabbits. Fetal resorptions were present in at least 85% of rabbits and mice administered 60 and 108 mg/kg/day (2× the human exposure based on AUC comparisons), respectively. Effects observed in rabbits included: fetal growth retardation, embryolethality, teratogenicity, and/or maternal toxicity. Teratogenic changes included cleft palate, anophthalmia/microphthalmia, aplastic organs (kidney and pancreas), hydrocephaly, and brachygnathia. In mice, effects observed were maternal/fetal toxicity and embryolethality.

Daily IV doses of 90 mg/kg administered to female mice prior to mating, during gestation, and during lactation caused hypoplasia of the testes and seminal vesicles in the month-old male offspring, as well as pathologic changes in the nonglandular region of the stomach (see Carcinogenesis, Mutagenesis, and Impairment of Fertility). The drug exposure in mice as estimated by the AUC was approximately 1.7× the human AUC.

Ganciclovir may be teratogenic or embryotoxic at dose levels recommended for human use. There are no adequate and well-controlled studies in pregnant women. Ganciclovir sodium IV or ganciclovir sodium capsules should be used during pregnancy only if the potential benefits justify the potential risk to the fetus.

*All dose comparisons presented in Carcinogenesis, Mutagenesis, Impairment of Fertility, andPregnancy Category C are based on the human AUC following administration of a single 5 mg/kg IV infusion of ganciclovir sodium IV as used during the maintenance phase of treatment. Compared with the single 5 mg/kg IV infusion, human exposure is doubled during the IV induction phase (5 mg/kg bid) and approximately halved during maintenance treatment with ganciclovir sodium capsules (1000 mg tid). The cross-species dose comparisons should be divided by 2 for IV induction treatment with ganciclovir sodium IV and multiplied by 2 for ganciclovir sodium capsules.

NURSING MOTHERS

It is not known whether ganciclovir is excreted in human milk. However, many drugs are excreted in human milk and, because carcinogenic and teratogenic effects occurred in animals treated with ganciclovir, the possibility of serious adverse reactions from ganciclovir in nursing infants is considered likely (see Pregnancy Category C). Mothers should be instructed to discontinue nursing if they are receiving ganciclovir sodium IV or capsules. The minimum interval before nursing can safely be resumed after the last dose of ganciclovir sodium IV or capsules is unknown.

PEDIATRIC USE

SAFETY AND EFFICACY OF GANCICLOVIR SODIUM IV AND CAPSULES IN PEDIATRIC PATIENTS HAVE NOT BEEN ESTABLISHED. THE USE OF GANCICLOVIR SODIUM IV OR CAPSULES IN THE PEDIATRIC POPULATION WARRANTS EXTREME CAUTION DUE TO THE PROBABILITY OF LONG-TERM CARCINOGENICITY AND REPRODUCTIVE TOXICITY. ADMINISTRATION TO PEDIATRIC PATIENTS SHOULD BE UNDERTAKEN ONLY AFTER CAREFUL EVALUATION AND ONLY IF THE POTENTIAL BENEFITS OF TREATMENT OUTWEIGH THE RISKS.

The spectrum of adverse events reported in 120 immunocompromised pediatric clinical trial participants with serious CMV infections receiving ganciclovir sodium IV solution were similar to those reported in adults. Granulocytopenia (17%) and thrombocytopenia (10%) were the most common adverse events reported.

Sixteen (16) pediatric patients (8 months to 15 years of age) with life- or sight-threatening CMV infections were evaluated in an open-label, ganciclovir sodium IV solution, pharmacokinetics study. Adverse events reported for more than 1 pediatric patient were as follows: hypokalemia (4/16, 25%), abnormal kidney function (3/16, 19%), sepsis (3/16, 19%), thrombocytopenia (3/16, 19%), leukopenia (2/16, 13%), coagulation disorder (2/16, 13%), hypertension (2/16, 13%), pneumonia (2/16, 13%), and immune system disorder (2/16, 13%).

There has been very limited clinical experience using ganciclovir sodium IV for the treatment of CMV retinitis in patients under the age of 12 years. Two (2) pediatric patients (ages 9 and 5 years) showed improvement or stabilization of retinitis for 23 and 9 months, respectively. These pediatric patients received induction treatment with 2.5 mg/kg tid followed by maintenance therapy with 6 to 6.5 mg/kg once per day, 5-7 days/week. When retinitis progressed during once-daily maintenance therapy, both pediatric patients were treated with the 5 mg/kg bid regimen. Two (2) other pediatric patients (ages 2.5 and 4 years) who received similar induction regimens showed only partial or no response to treatment. Another pediatric patient, a 6-year-old with T-cell dysfunction, showed stabilization of retinitis for 3 months while receiving continuous infusions of ganciclovir sodium IV at doses of 2-5 mg/kg/24 hours. Continuous infusion treatment was discontinued due to granulocytopenia.

Eleven (11) of the 72 patients in the placebo-controlled trial in bone marrow transplant recipients were pediatric patients, ranging in age from 3-10 years (5 treated with ganciclovir sodium IV and 6 with placebo). Five (5) of the pediatric patients treated with ganciclovir sodium IV received 5 mg/kg intravenously bid for up to 7 days; 4 patients went on to receive 5 mg/kg qd up to day 100 posttransplant. Results were similar to those observed in adult transplant recipients treated with ganciclovir sodium IV. Two (2) of the 6 placebo-treated pediatric patients developed CMV pneumonia versus none of the 5 patients treated with ganciclovir sodium IV. The spectrum of adverse events in the pediatric group was similar to that observed in the adult patients.

Ganciclovir sodium capsules have not been studied in children under age 13.

GERIATRIC USE

The pharmacokinetic profiles of ganciclovir sodium IV and capsules in elderly patients have not been established. Since elderly individuals frequently have a reduced glomerular filtration rate, particular attention should be paid to assessing renal function before and during administration of ganciclovir sodium IV or capsules (see DOSAGE AND ADMINISTRATION).

Clinical studies of ganciclovir sodium IV and capsules did not include sufficient numbers of subjects aged 65 and over to determine whether they respond differently from younger subjects. In general, dose selection for an elderly patient should be cautious, reflecting the greater frequency of decreased hepatic, renal, or cardiac function, and of concomitant disease or other drug therapy. Ganciclovir sodium IV and capsules are known to be substantially excreted by the kidney, and the risk of toxic reactions to this drug may be greater in patients with impaired renal function. Because elderly patients are more likely to have decreased renal function, care should be taken in dose selection. In addition, renal function should be monitored and dosage adjustments should be made accordingly (see Use in Patients With Renal Impairment and DOSAGE AND ADMINISTRATION).

USE IN PATIENTS WITH RENAL IMPAIRMENT

Ganciclovir sodium IV and capsules should be used with caution in patients with impaired renal function because the half-life and plasma/serum concentrations of ganciclovir will be increased due to reduced renal clearance (see DOSAGE AND ADMINISTRATION and ADVERSE REACTIONS).

Hemodialysis has been shown to reduce plasma levels of ganciclovir by approximately 50%.

DRUG INTERACTIONS

DIDANOSINE

At an oral dose of 1000 mg of ganciclovir sodium capsules every 8 hours and didanosine, 200 mg every 12 hours, the steady-state didanosine AUC(0-12) increased 111 ± 114% (range: 10-493%) when didanosine was administered either 2 hours prior to or concurrent with administration of ganciclovir sodium capsules (n=12 patients, 23 observations). A decrease in steady-state ganciclovir AUC of 21 ± 17% (range: -44 to 5%) was observed when didanosine was administered 2 hours prior to administration of ganciclovir sodium capsules, but ganciclovir AUC was not affected by the presence of didanosine when the 2 drugs were administered simultaneously (n=12). There were no significant changes in renal clearance for either drug.

When the standard IV ganciclovir induction dose (5 mg/kg infused over 1 hour every 12 hours) was coadministered with didanosine at a dose of 200 mg orally every 12 hours, the steady-state didanosine AUC(0-12) increased 70 ± 40% (range: 3-121%, n=11) and C_{max} increased 49 ± 48% (range: -28 to 125%). In a separate study, when the standard IV ganciclovir maintenance dose (5 mg/kg infused over 1 hour every 24 hours) was coadministered with didanosine at a dose of 200 mg orally every 12 hours, didanosine AUC(0-12) increased 50 ± 26% (range: 22-110%, n=11) and C_{max} increased 36 ± 36% (range: -27 to 94%) over the first didanosine dosing interval. Didanosine plasma concentrations [AUC(12-24)] were unchanged during the dosing intervals when ganciclovir was not coadministered. Ganciclovir pharmacokinetics were not affected by didanosine. In neither study were there significant changes in the renal clearance of either drug.

ZIDOVUDINE

At an oral dose of 1000 mg of ganciclovir sodium every 8 hours, mean steady-state ganciclovir AUC(0-8) decreased 17 ± 25% (range: -52 to 23%) in the presence of zidovudine, 100 mg every 4 hours (n=12). Steady-state zidovudine AUC(0-4) increased 19 ± 27% (range: -11 to 74%) in the presence of ganciclovir.

Since both zidovudine and ganciclovir have the potential to cause neutropenia and anemia, some patients may not tolerate concomitant therapy with these drugs at full dosage.

PROBENECID

At an oral dose of 1000 mg of ganciclovir sodium capsules every 8 hours (n=10), ganciclovir AUC(0-8) increased 53 ± 91% (range: -14 to 299%) in the presence of probenecid, 500 mg every 6 hours. Renal clearance of ganciclovir decreased 22 ± 20% (range: -54 to -4%), which is consistent with an interaction involving competition for renal tubular secretion.

IMIPENEM-CILASTATIN

Generalized seizures have been reported in patients who received ganciclovir and imipenem-cilastatin. These drugs should not be used concomitantly unless the potential benefits outweigh the risks.

OTHER MEDICATIONS

It is possible that drugs that inhibit replication of rapidly dividing cell populations such as bone marrow, spermatogonia, and germinal layers of skin and gastrointestinal mucosa may have additive toxicity when administered concomitantly with ganciclovir. Therefore, drugs such as dapsone, pentamidine, flucytosine, vincristine, vinblastine, adriamycin, amphotericin B, trimethoprim/sulfamethoxazole combinations or other nucleoside analogues, should be considered for concomitant use with ganciclovir only if the potential benefits are judged to outweigh the risks.

No formal drug interaction studies of ganciclovir sodium IV solution or capsules and drugs commonly used in transplant recipients have been conducted. Increases in serum creatinine were observed in patients treated with ganciclovir sodium IV plus either cyclosporine or amphotericin B, drugs with known potential for nephrotoxicity (see ADVERSE REACTIONS). In a retrospective analysis of 93 liver allograft recipients receiving ganciclovir (5 mg/kg infused over 1 hour every 12 hours) and oral cyclosporine (at therapeutic doses), there was no evidence of an effect on cyclosporine whole blood concentrations.

ADVERSE REACTIONS

Adverse events that occurred during clinical trials of ganciclovir sodium IV solution and ganciclovir sodium capsules are summarized below, according to the participating study subject population.

SUBJECTS WITH AIDS

Three controlled, randomized, Phase 3 trials comparing ganciclovir sodium IV solution and ganciclovir sodium capsules for maintenance treatment of CMV retinitis have been completed. During these trials, ganciclovir sodium IV or capsules were prematurely discontinued in 9% of subjects because of adverse events. In a placebo-controlled, randomized, Phase 3 trial of ganciclovir sodium capsules for prevention of CMV disease in AIDS, treatment was prematurely discontinued because of adverse events, new or worsening intercurrent illness, or laboratory abnormalities in 19.5% of subjects treated with ganciclovir sodium capsules and 16% of subjects receiving placebo. Laboratory data and adverse events reported during the conduct of these controlled trials are summarized in TABLE 6A and TABLE 6B.

Laboratory Data

See TABLE 6A and TABLE 6B.

TABLE 6A *Selected Laboratory Abnormalities in Trials for Treatment of CMV Retinitis**

	Ganciclovir Sodium	
	Capsules†	IV‡
Treatment	3000 mg/day	mg/kg/day
Subjects, number	320	175
Neutropenia		
<500 ANC/µl	18%	25%
500 - <749	17%	14%
750 - <1000	19%	26%
Anemia		
Hemoglobin:		
<6.5 g/dl	2%	5%
6.5 - <8.0	10%	16%
8.0 - <9.5	25%	26%
Maximum Serum Creatinine		
≥2.5 mg/dl	1%	2%
≥1.5 - <2.5	12%	14%

* Pooled data from Treatment Studies, ICM 1653, Study ICM 1774, and Study AVI 034.
† Mean time on therapy = 91 days, including allowed reinduction treatment period.
‡ Mean time on therapy = 103 days, including allowed reinduction treatment period.

TABLE 6B *Selected Laboratory Abnormalities in Trials for Prevention of CMV Disease**

	Ganciclovir Sodium Capsules†	
Treatment	3000 mg/day	Placebo‡
Subjects, number	478	234
Neutropenia		
<500 ANC/µl	10%	6%
500 - <749	16%	7%
750 - <1000	22%	16%
Anemia		
Hemoglobin:		
<6.5 g/dl	1%	<1%
6.5 - <8.0	5%	3%
8.0 - <9.5	15%	16%
Maximum Serum Creatinine		
≥2.5 mg/dl	1%	2%
≥1.5 - <2.5	19%	11%

* Data from Prevention Study, ICM 1654.
† Mean time on ganciclovir = 269 days.
‡ Mean time on placebo = 240 days.

Adverse Events

TABLE 7A and TABLE 7B show selected adverse events reported in 5% or more of the subjects in three controlled clinical trials during treatment with either ganciclovir sodium IV solution (5 mg/kg/day) or capsules (3000 mg/day), and in one controlled clinical trial in which ganciclovir sodium capsules (3000 mg/day) were compared to placebo for the prevention of CMV disease.

TABLE 7A *Selected Adverse Events Reported ≥5% of Subjects in Three Randomized Phase 3 Studies Comparing Ganciclovir Sodium Capsules to Ganciclovir Sodium IV Solution for Maintenance Treatment of CMV Retinitis*

	Maintenance Treatment Studies	
	Capsules	IV
Body System/Adverse Event	(n=326)	(n=179)
Body as a Whole		
Fever	38%	48%
Infection	9%	13%
Chills	7%	10%
Sepsis	4%	15%
Digestive System		
Diarrhea	41%	44%
Anorexia	15%	14%
Vomiting	13%	13%
Hemic and Lymphatic System		
Leukopenia	29%	41%
Anemia	19%	25%
Thrombocytopenia	6%	6%
Nervous System		
Neuropathy	8%	9%
Other		
Sweating	11%	12%
Pruritus	6%	5%
Catheter Related*		
Total catheter events	6%	22%
Catheter infection	4%	9%
Catheter sepsis	1%	8%

* Some of these events also appear under other body systems.

TABLE 7B *Selected Adverse Events Reported in ≥5% of Subjects in One Phase 3 Randomized Study Comparing Ganciclovir Sodium Capsules to Placebo for Prevention of CMV Disease*

	Prevention Study	
Body System/Adverse Event	**Capsules (n=478)**	**Placebo (n=234)**
Body as a Whole		
Fever	35%	33%
Infection	8%	4%
Chills	7%	4%
Sepsis	3%	2%
Digestive System		
Diarrhea	48%	42%
Anorexia	19%	16%
Vomiting	14%	11%
Hemic and Lymphatic System		
Leukopenia	17%	9%
Anemia	9%	7%
Thrombocytopenia	3%	1%
Nervous System		
Neuropathy	21%	15%
Other		
Sweating	14%	12%
Pruritus	10%	9%
Catheter Related*		
Total catheter events	—	—
Catheter infection	—	—
Catheter sepsis	—	—

* Some of these events also appear under other body systems.

The following events were frequently observed in clinical trials but occurred with equal or greater frequency in placebo-treated subjects: Abdominal pain, nausea, flatulence, pneumonia, paresthesia, rash.

Retinal Detachment

Retinal detachment has been observed in subjects with CMV retinitis both before and after initiation of therapy with ganciclovir. Its relationship to therapy with ganciclovir is unknown. Retinal detachment occurred in 11% of patients treated with ganciclovir sodium IV solution and in 8% of patients treated with ganciclovir sodium capsules. Patients with CMV retinitis should have frequent ophthalmologic evaluations to monitor the status of their retinitis and to detect any other retinal pathology.

TRANSPLANT RECIPIENTS

There have been three controlled clinical trials of ganciclovir sodium IV solution and one controlled clinical trial of ganciclovir sodium capsules for the prevention of CMV disease in transplant recipients. Laboratory data and adverse events reported during these trials are summarized in TABLE 8A and TABLE 8B.

Laboratory Data

TABLE 8A and TABLE 8B show the frequency of granulocytopenia (neutropenia) and thrombocytopenia observed.

TABLE 8A *Controlled Trials*

Transplant Recipients

	Heart Allograft*		Bone Marrow Allograft†	
	Ganciclovir Sodium IV (n=76)	**Placebo (n=73)**	**Ganciclovir Sodium IV (n=57)**	**Control (n=55)**
Neutropenia				
Minumum ANC <500/μl	4%	3%	12%	6%
Minimum ANC 500-1000/μl	3%	8%	29%	17%
Total ANC ≤1000/μl	7%	11%	41%	23%
Thrombocytopenia				
Platelet count <25,000/μl	3%	1%	32%	28%
Platelet count 25,000-50,000/μl	5%	3%	25%	37%
Total Platelet ≤50,000/μl	8%	4%	57%	65%

* Study ICM 1496. Mean duration of treatment = 28 dyas.
† Study ICM 1570 and ICM 1689. Mean duration of treatment = 45 days.

TABLE 9 shows the frequency of elevated serum creatinine values in these controlled clinical trials.

In 3 out of 4 trials, patients receiving either ganciclovir sodium IV solution or ganciclovir sodium capsules had elevated serum creatinine levels when compared to those receiving placebo. Most patients in these studies also received cyclosporine. The mechanism of impairment of renal function is not known. However, careful monitoring of renal function during therapy with ganciclovir sodium IV solution or capsules is essential, especially for those patients receiving concomitant agents that may cause nephrotoxicity.

TABLE 8B *Controlled Trials*

Transplant Recipients

	Live Allograft*	
	Ganciclovir Capsules (n=150)	**Placebo (n=154)**
Neutropenia		
Minumum ANC <500/μl	3%	1%
Minimum ANC 500-1000/μl	3%	2%
Total ANC ≤1000/μl	6%	3%
Thrombocytopenia		
Platelet count <25,000/μl	0%	3%
Platelet count 25,000-50,000/μl	5%	3%
Total Platelet ≤50,000/μl	5%	6%

* Study GAN040. Mean duration of ganciclovir treatment = 82 days.

TABLE 9 *Controlled Trials*

Transplant Recipients

		Maximum Serum Creatinine Levels	
	n	**Serum Creatinine ≥2.5 mg/dl**	**Serum Creatinine ≥1.5 - <2.5 mg/dl**
		Ganciclovir Sodium IV	
Heart Allograft (ICM 1496)			
Ganciclovir sodium IV	76	18%	58%
Placebo	73	4%	69%
Bone Marrow Allograft (ICM 1570)			
Ganciclovir sodium IV	20	20%	50%
Control	20	0%	35%
Bone Marrrow Allograft (ICM 1689)			
Ganciclovir sodium IV	37	0%	43%
Control	35	0%	44%
		Ganciclovir Sodium Capsules	
Liver Allograft (Study 040)			
Ganciclovir sodium capsules	150	16%	39%
Placebo	154	10%	42%

GENERAL

Other adverse events that were thought to be "probably" or "possibly" related to ganciclovir sodium IV solution or capsules in clinical studies in either subjects with AIDS or transplant recipients are listed below. These events all occurred in at least 3 subjects.

Body as a Whole: Abdomen enlarged, asthenia, chest pain, edema, headache, injection site inflammation, malaise, pain.

Digestive System: Abnormal liver function test, aphthous stomatitis, constipation, dyspepsia, eructation.

Hemic and Lymphatic System: Pancytopenia.

Respiratory System: Cough increased, dyspnea.

Nervous System: Abnormal dreams, anxiety, confusion, depression, dizziness, dry mouth, insomnia, seizures, somnolence, thinking abnormal, tremor.

Skin and Appendages: Alopecia, dry skin.

Special Senses: Abnormal vision, taste perversion, tinnitus, vitreous disorder.

Metabolic and Nutritional Disorders: Creatinine increased, SGOT increased, SGPT increased, weight loss.

Cardiovascular System: Hypertension, phlebitis, vasodilatation.

Urogenital System: Creatinine clearance decreased, kidney failure, kidney function abnormal, urinary frequency.

Musculoskeletal System: Arthralgia, leg cramps, myalgia, myasthenia.

The following adverse events reported in patients receiving ganciclovir may be potentially fatal: gastrointestinal perforation, multiple organ failure, pancreatitis and sepsis.

ADVERSE EVENTS REPORTED DURING POSTMARKETING EXPERIENCE WITH GANCICLOVIR SODIUM IV AND CAPSULES

The following events have been identified during postapproval use of the drug. Because they are reported voluntarily from a population of unknown size, estimates of frequency cannot be made. These events have been chosen for inclusion due to either the seriousness, frequency of reporting, the apparent causal connection or a combination of these factors: acidosis, allergic reaction, anaphylactic reaction, arthritis, bronchospasm, cardiac arrest, cardiac conduction abnormality, cataracts, cholelithiasis, cholestasis, congenital anomaly, dry eyes, dysesthesia, dysphasia, elevated triglyceride levels, encephalopathy, exfoliative dermatitis, extrapyramidal reaction, facial palsy, hallucinations, hemolytic anemia, hemolytic uremic syndrome, hepatic failure, hepatitis, hypercalcemia, hyponatremia, inappropriate serum ADH, infertility, intestinal ulceration, intracranial hypertension, irritability, loss of memory, loss of sense of smell, myelopathy, oculomotor nerve paralysis, peripheral ischemia, pulmonary fibrosis, renal tubular disorder, rhabdomyolysis, Stevens-Johnson syndrome, stroke, testicular hypotrophy, torsades de pointes, vasculitis, ventricular tachycardia.

DOSAGE AND ADMINISTRATION

CAUTION — DO NOT ADMINISTER GANCICLOVIR SODIUM IV SOLUTION BY RAPID OR BOLUS INTRAVENOUS INJECTION. THE TOXICITY OF GANCICLOVIR SODIUM IV MAY BE INCREASED AS A RESULT OF EXCESSIVE PLASMA LEVELS.

CAUTION — INTRAMUSCULAR OR SUBCUTANEOUS INJECTION OF RECONSTITUTED GANCICLOVIR SODIUM IV SOLUTION MAY RESULT IN SEVERE TISSUE IRRITATION DUE TO HIGH pH (11).

DOSAGE

THE RECOMMENDED DOSE FOR GANCICLOVIR SODIUM IV SOLUTION AND GANCICLOVIR SODIUM CAPSULES SHOULD NOT BE EXCEEDED. THE RECOMMENDED INFUSION RATE FOR GANCICLOVIR SODIUM IV SOLUTION SHOULD NOT BE EXCEEDED.

For Treatment of CMV Retinitis in Patients With Normal Renal Function

Induction Treatment

The recommended initial dosage for patients with normal renal function is 5 mg/kg (given intravenously at a constant rate over 1 hour) every 12 hours for 14-21 days. Ganciclovir sodium capsules should not be used for induction treatment.

Maintenance Treatment

Ganciclovir Sodium IV: Following induction treatment, the recommended maintenance dose of ganciclovir sodium IV solution is 5 mg/kg given as a constant-rate IV infusion over 1 hour once daily, 7 days/week, or 6 mg/kg once daily, 5 days/week.

Ganciclovir Sodium Capsules: Following induction treatment, the recommended maintenance dosage of ganciclovir sodium capsules is 1000 mg tid with food. Alternatively, the dosing regimen of 500 mg six times daily every 3 hours with food, during waking hours, may be used.

For patients who experience progression of CMV retinitis while receiving maintenance treatment with either formulation of ganciclovir, reinduction treatment is recommended.

For the Prevention of CMV Disease in Patients With Advanced HIV Infection and Normal Renal Function

Ganciclovir Sodium Capsules: The recommended prophylactic dose of ganciclovir sodium capsules is 1000 mg tid with food.

For the Prevention of CMV Disease in Transplant Recipients With Normal Renal Function

Ganciclovir Sodium IV: The recommended initial dosage of ganciclovir sodium IV solution for patients with normal renal function is 5 mg/kg (given intravenously at a constant rate over 1 hour) every 12 hours for 7-14 days, followed by 5 mg/kg once daily 7 days/week, or 6 mg/kg once daily 5 days/week.

Ganciclovir Sodium Capsules: The recommended prophylactic dosage of ganciclovir sodium capsules is 1000 mg tid with food.

The duration of treatment with ganciclovir sodium IV solution and capsules in transplant recipients is dependent upon the duration and degree of immunosuppression. In controlled clinical trials in bone marrow allograft recipients, treatment with ganciclovir sodium IV was continued until day 100-120 posttransplantation. CMV disease occurred in several patients who discontinued treatment with ganciclovir sodium IV solution prematurely. In heart allograft recipients, the onset of newly diagnosed CMV disease occurred after treatment with ganciclovir sodium IV was stopped at day 28 posttransplant, suggesting that continued dosing may be necessary to prevent late occurrence of CMV disease in this patient population. In a controlled clinical trial of liver allograft recipients, treatment with ganciclovir sodium capsules was continued through week 14 posttransplantation (see INDICATIONS AND USAGE for a more detailed discussion).

Renal Impairment

Ganciclovir Sodium IV

For patients with impairment of renal function, refer to TABLE 10 for recommended doses of ganciclovir sodium IV solution and adjust the dosing interval as indicated.

TABLE 10

Creatinine Clearance* (ml/min)	Ganciclovir Sodium IV Induction Dose (mg/kg)	Dosing Interval (hours)	Ganciclovir Sodium IV Maintenance Dose (mg/kg)	Dosing Interval (hours)
≥70	5.0	12	5.0	24
50-69	2.5	12	2.5	24
25-49	2.5	24	1.25	24
10-24	1.25	24	0.625	24
<10	1.25	†	0.625	†

* Creatinine clearance can be related to serum creatinine by the formulas given below.
† 3 times/week, following hemodialysis.

Dosing for patients undergoing hemodialysis should not exceed 1.25 mg/kg three times/week, following each hemodialysis session. Ganciclovir sodium IV should be given shortly after completion of the hemodialysis session, since hemodialysis has been shown to reduce plasma levels by approximately 50%.

Ganciclovir Sodium Capsules

In patients with renal impairment, the dose of ganciclovir sodium capsules should be modified as shown in TABLE 11.

PATIENT MONITORING

Due to the frequency of granulocytopenia, anemia, and thrombocytopenia in patients receiving ganciclovir (see ADVERSE REACTIONS), it is recommended that complete blood counts and platelet counts be performed frequently, especially in patients in whom ganciclovir or other nucleoside analogues have previously resulted in cytopenia, or in whom neutrophil counts are less than 1000 cells/µl at the beginning of treatment. Patients should have serum creatinine or creatinine clearance values followed carefully to allow for dosage adjustments in renally impaired patients (see DOSAGE AND ADMINISTRATION).

TABLE 11

Creatinine Clearance* ml/min	Ganciclovir Sodium Capsule Doses
≥70	1000 mg tid or 500 mg q3h, 6×/day
50-69	1500 mg qd or 500 mg tid
25-49	1000 mg qd or 500 mg bid
10-24	500 mg qd
<10	500 mg three times/week, following hemodialysis

* Creatinine clearance can be related to serum creatinine by the following formulae:
Creatinine clearance for males = [(140 - age [yrs]) (body wt [kg])] ÷ [(72) (serum creatinine [mg/dl])]
Creatinine clearance for females = 0.85 × male value.

REDUCTION OF DOSE

Dosage reductions in renally impaired patients are required for ganciclovir sodium IV and should be considered for ganciclovir sodium capsules (see Renal Impairment). Dosage reductions should also be considered for those with neutropenia, anemia and/or thrombocytopenia (see ADVERSE REACTIONS). Ganciclovir should not be administered in patients with severe neutropenia (ANC less than 500/µl) or severe thrombocytopenia (platelets less than 25,000/µl).

HANDLING AND DISPOSAL

Caution should be exercised in the handling and preparation of solutions of ganciclovir sodium IV and in the handling of ganciclovir sodium capsules. Solutions of ganciclovir sodium IV are alkaline (pH 11). Avoid direct contact with the skin or mucous membranes of the powder contained in ganciclovir sodium capsules or IV solutions. If such contact occurs, wash thoroughly with soap and water; rinse eyes thoroughly with plain water. Ganciclovir sodium capsules should not be opened or crushed.

Because ganciclovir shares some of the properties of antitumor agents (*i.e.*, carcinogenicity and mutagenicity), consideration should be given to handling and disposal according to guidelines issued for antineoplastic drugs. Several guidelines on this subject have been published.[8-10]

There is no general agreement that all of the procedures recommended in the guidelines are necessary or appropriate.

HOW SUPPLIED

CYTOVENE IV

Cytovene IV is supplied in 10 ml sterile vials, each containing ganciclovir sodium equivalent to 500 mg of ganciclovir.

Storage: Store vials at temperatures below 40°C (104°F).

CYTOVENE CAPSULES

250 mg: Two-pieced, size no. 1, opaque green hard gelatin capsules with "ROCHE" and "CYTOVENE 250 mg" imprinted on the capsules in dark blue ink and with 2 blue lines partially encircling the capsule body. Each capsule contains 250 mg of ganciclovir as a white to off-white powder.

500 mg: Two-pieced, size no. 0 elongated, opaque yellow/opaque green hard gelatin capsules with "ROCHE" and "CYTOVENE 500 mg" imprinted on the capsules in dark blue ink and with 2 blue lines partially encircling the capsule body. Each capsule contains 500 mg of ganciclovir as a white to off-white powder.

Storage: Store between 5 and 25°C (41 and 77°F).

PRODUCT LISTING - EQUIVALENTS NOT AVAILABLE

Capsule - Oral - 250 mg

180's	$780.90	CYTOVENE, Physicians Total Care	54868-3507-00
180's	$867.15	CYTOVENE, Roche Laboratories	00004-0269-48

Capsule - Oral - 500 mg

180's	$1734.29	CYTOVENE, Roche Laboratories	00004-0278-48

Implant - Ophthalmic - 4.5 mg

1's	$5000.00	VITRASERT, Chiron Therapeutics	61772-0002-01

Powder For Injection - Intravenous - 500 mg

25's	$891.76	CYTOVENE, Allscripts Pharmaceutical Company	54569-4738-00
25's	$966.08	CYTOVENE, Roche Laboratories	00004-6940-03

Gatifloxacin (003463)

For related information, see the comparative table section in Appendix A.

Categories: Bronchitis, chronic, acute exacerbation; Conjunctivitis, bacterial; Gonorrhea; Infection, lower respiratory tract; Infection, rectal; Infection, sexually transmitted; Infection, sinus; Infection, skin and skin structures; Infection, upper respiratory tract; Infection, urinary tract; Pneumonia, community-acquired; Pyelonephritis; FDA Approved 1999 Dec; Pregnancy Category C
Drug Classes: Antibiotics, quinolones
Brand Names: Tequin; Zymar
Cost of Therapy: $65.82 (Infection; Tequin; 400 mg; 1 tablet/day; 7 day supply)

DESCRIPTION

Tequin contains gatifloxacin, a synthetic broad-spectrum 8-methoxyfluoroquinolone antibacterial agent for oral or intravenous (IV) administration. Chemically, gatifloxacin is (±)-1-cyclopropyl-6-fluoro-1,4-dihydro-8-methoxy-7-(3-methyl-1-piperazinyl)-4-oxo-3-quinolinecarboxylic acid sesquihydrate.

Its empirical formula is $C_{19}H_{22}FN_3O_4 \cdot 1.5\ H_2O$ and its molecular weight is 402.42. Gatifloxacin is a sesquihydrate crystalline powder and is white to pale yellow in color. It exists as a racemate, with no net optical rotation. The solubility of the compound is pH dependent. The maximum aqueous solubility (40-60 mg/ml) occurs at a pH range of 2-5.

TEQUIN TABLETS FOR ORAL ADMINISTRATION

Tequin tablets are available as 200 and 400 mg white, film-coated tablets and contain the following inactive ingredients: hydroxypropyl methylcellulose, magnesium stearate, methylcellulose, microcrystalline cellulose, polyethylene glycol, polysorbate 80, simethicone, sodium starch glycolate, sorbic acid, and titanium dioxide.

TEQUIN INJECTION FOR IV ADMINISTRATION

Tequin injection is available in 40 ml (400 mg) single-use vials as a sterile, preservative-free aqueous solution of gatifloxacin with pH ranging from 3.5-5.5. Tequin injection is also available in ready-to-use 100 ml (200 mg) and 200 ml (400 mg) flexible bags as a sterile, preservative-free aqueous solution of gatifloxacin with pH ranging from 3.5-5.5. The appearance of the IV solution may range from light yellow to greenish-yellow in color. The color does not affect nor is it indicative of product stability.

The IV formulation contains dextrose, anhydrous or dextrose, monohydrate, and water for injection, and may contain hydrochloric acid and/or sodium hydroxide for pH adjustment.

G

ZYMAR OPHTHALMIC SOLUTION

ZYMAR is a sterile, clear, pale yellow colored isotonic unbuffered solution. It has an osmolality of 260-330 mOsm/kg.

Zymar Ophthalmic Solution Contains:

- ***Active:*** Gatifloxacin 0.3% (3 mg/ml).
- ***Preservative:*** Benzalkonium chloride 0.005%.
- ***Inactives:*** Edetate disodium; purified water and sodium chloride. May contain hydrochloric acid and/or sodium hydroxide to adjust pH to approximately 6.

CLINICAL PHARMACOLOGY

Gatifloxacin is administered as a racemate, with the disposition and antibacterial activity of the R- and S-enantiomers virtually identical.

ABSORPTION

Gatifloxacin is well absorbed from the gastrointestinal tract after oral administration and can be given without regard to food. The absolute bioavailability of gatifloxacin is 96%. Peak plasma concentrations of gatifloxacin usually occur 1-2 hours after oral dosing.

The oral and IV routes of administration for gatifloxacin can be considered interchangeable, since the pharmacokinetics of gatifloxacin after 1 hour IV administration are similar to those observed for orally administered gatifloxacin when equal doses are administered (see DOSAGE AND ADMINISTRATION).

PHARMACOKINETICS

The mean (SD) pharmacokinetic parameters of gatifloxacin following oral administration to healthy subjects with bacterial infections and subjects with renal insufficiency are listed in TABLE 1. The mean (SD) pharmacokinetic parameters of gatifloxacin following IV administration to healthy subjects are listed in TABLE 2.

TABLE 1 *Gatifloxacin Pharmacokinetic Parameters — Oral Administration*

	C_{max} (µg/ml)	T_{max}* (h)	AUC† (µg·h/ml)	T½ (h)	CL/F (ml/min)	CLR (ml/min)	UR (%)
200 mg — Healthy Volunteers							
Single dose (n=12)	2.0 ± 0.4	1.00 (0.50, 2.50)	14.2 ± 0.4	—	241 ± 40	—	73.8 ± 10.9
400 mg — Healthy Volunteers							
Single dose (n=202)‡	3.8 ± 1.0	1.00 (0.50, 6.00)	33.0 ± 6.2	7.8 ± 1.3	210 ± 44	151 ± 46	72.4 ± 18.1
Multiple dose (n=18)	4.2 ± 1.3	1.50 (0.50, 4.00)	34.4 ± 5.7	7.1 ± 0.6	199 ± 31	159 ± 34	80.2 ± 12.1
400 mg — Patients With Infection							
Multiple dose (n=140)§	4.2 ± 1.9	—	51.3 ± 20.4	—	147 ± 48	—	—
400 mg — Single Dose Subjects With Renal Insufficiency							
CLCR 50-89 ml/min (n=8)	4.4 ± 1.1	1.13 (0.75-2.00)	48.0 ± 12.7	11.2 ± 2.8	148 ± 41	124 ± 38	83.7 ± 7.8
CLCR 30-49 ml/min (n=8)	5.1 ± 1.8	0.75 (0.50, 6.00)	74.9 ± 12.6	17.2 ± 8.5	92 ± 17	67 ± 24	71.1 ± 17.4
CLCR <30 ml/min (n=8)	4.5 ± 1.2	1.50 (0.50, 6.00)	149.3 ± 35.6	30.7 ± 8.4	48 ± 16	23 ± 13	44.7 ± 13.0
Hemodialysis (n=8)	4.7 ± 1.0	1.50 (1.00, 3.00)	180.3 ± 34.4	35.7 ± 7.0	38 ± 8	—	—
CAPD (n=8)	4.7 ± 1.3	1.75 (0.50, 3.00)	227.0 ± 60.0	40.3 ± 8.3	31 ± 8	—	—

* Median (minimum, maximum).
† Single dose: AUC(0-∞), Multiple dose: AUC(0-24).
‡ n=184 for CL/F, n=134 for CLR, and n=132 for UR.
§ Based on the patient population pharmacokinetic modeling, n=103 for C_{max}.
C_{max}: Maximum serum concentration; T_{max}: Time to C_{max}; AUC: Area under concentration versus time curve; T½: Serum half-life; CL/F: Apparent total clearance; CLR: Renal clearance; UR: Urinary recovery.

TABLE 2 *Gatifloxacin Pharmacokinetic Parameters — IV Administration*

	C_{max} (µg/ml)	T_{max}* (h)	AUC† (µg·h/ml)	T½ (h)	Vdss (L/kg)	CL (ml/min)	CLR (ml/min)	UR (%)
200 mg — Healthy Volunteers								
Single dose (n=12)	2.2 ± 0.3	1.00 (0.67, 1.50)	15.9 ± 2.6	11.1 ± 4.1	1.9 ± 0.1	214 ± 36	155 ± 32	71.7 ± 6.8
Multiple dose (n=8)‡	2.4 ± 0.4	1.00 (0.67, 1.00)	16.8 ± 3.6	12.3 ± 4.6	2.0 ± 0.3	207 ± 44	155 ± 55	72.4 ± 16.4
400 mg — Healthy Volunteers								
Single dose (n=30)	5.5 ± 1.0	1.00 (0.50, 1.00)	35.1 ± 6.7	7.4 ± 1.6	1.5 ± 0.2	196 ± 33	124 ± 41	62.3 ± 16.7
Multiple dose (n=5)	4.6 ± 0.6	1.00 (1.00, 1.00)	35.4 ± 4.6	13.9 ± 3.9	1.6 ± 0.5	190 ± 24	161 ± 43	83.5 ± 13.8

* Median (minimum, maximum).
† Single dose: AUC(0-∞), Multiple dose: AUC(0-24).
‡ n=7 for CLR and UR.
C_{max}: Maximum serum concentration; T_{max}: Time to C_{max}; AUC: Area under concentration versus time curve; T½: Serum half-life; Vdss: Volume of distribution; CL: Total clearance; CLR: Renal clearance; UR: Urinary recovery.

Gatifloxacin pharmacokinetics are linear and time-independent at doses ranging from 200-800 mg administered over a period of up to 14 days. Steady-state concentrations are achieved by the third daily oral or IV dose of gatifloxacin. The mean steady-state peak and trough plasma concentrations attained following a dosing regimen of 400 mg once daily are approximately 4.2 µg/ml and 0.4 µg/ml, respectively, for oral administration and 4.6 µg/ml and 0.4 µg/ml, respectively, for IV administration.

Gatifloxacin ophthalmic solution 0.3 or 0.5% was administered to one eye of 6 healthy male subjects each in an escalated dosing regimen starting with a single 2 drop dose, then 2 drops 4 times daily for 7 days and finally 2 drops 8 times daily for 3 days. At all time points, serum gatifloxacin levels were below the lower limit of quantification (5 ng/ml) in all subjects.

Distribution

Serum protein binding of gatifloxacin is approximately 20% in volunteers and is concentration independent. Consistent with the low protein binding, concentrations of gatifloxacin in saliva were approximately equal to those in plasma [mean (range) saliva:plasma ratio was 0.88 (0.46-1.57)]. The mean volume of distribution of gatifloxacin at steady-state (Vdss) ranged from 1.5-2.0 L/kg. Gatifloxacin is widely distributed throughout the body into many body tissues and fluids. Rapid distribution of gatifloxacin into tissues results in higher gatifloxacin concentrations in most target tissues than in serum (see TABLE 3).

TABLE 3 *Gatifloxacin Tissue — Fluid/Serum Ratio (Range)**

Fluid or Tissue	Tissue-Fluid/Serum Ratio (range)*
Respiratory	
Alveolar macrophages	26.5 (10.9-61.1)
Bronchial mucosa	1.65 (1.12-2.22)
Lung epithelial lining fluid	1.67 (0.81-4.46)
Lung parenchyma	4.09 (0.50-9.22)
Sinus mucosa	1.78 (1.17-2.49)
Sputum (multiple dose)	1.28 (0.49-2.38)
Skin	
Skin blister fluid	1.00 (0.50-1.47)
Reproductive	
Ejaculate	1.07 (0.86-1.32)
Seminal fluid	1.01 (0.81-1.21)
Vagina	1.22 (0.57-1.63)
Cervix	1.45 (0.56-2.64)

* Mean of individual ratios collected over 24 hours following single (100, 150, 200, 300, or 400 mg) or multiple (150 or 200 mg bid) doses of gatifloxacin except for the skin blister fluid, where mean AUC ratio is presented.

Metabolism

Gatifloxacin undergoes limited biotransformation in humans with less than 1% of the dose excreted in the urine as ethylenediamine and methylethylenediamine metabolites.

In vitro studies with cytochrome P450 isoenzymes (CYP) indicate that gatifloxacin does not inhibit CYP3A4, CYP2D6, CYP2C9, CYP2C19, or CYP1A2, suggesting that gatifloxacin is unlikely to alter the pharmacokinetics of drugs metabolized by these enzymes (*e.g.*, midazolam, cyclosporine, warfarin, theophylline).

In vivo studies in animals and humans indicate that gatifloxacin is not an enzyme inducer; therefore, gatifloxacin is unlikely to alter the metabolic elimination of itself or other coadministered drugs.

Excretion

Gatifloxacin is excreted as unchanged drug primarily by the kidney. More than 70% of an administered gatifloxacin dose was recovered as unchanged drug in the urine within 48 hours following oral and IV administration, and 5% was recovered in the feces. Less than 1% of the dose is recovered in the urine as two metabolites. Crystals of gatifloxacin have not been observed in the urine of normal, healthy human subjects following administration of IV or oral doses up to 800 mg.

The mean elimination half-life of gatifloxacin ranges from 7-14 hours and is independent of dose and route of administration. Renal clearance is independent of dose with mean value ranging from 124-161 ml/min. The magnitude of this value, coupled with the significant decrease in the elimination of gatifloxacin seen with concomitant probenecid administration, indicates that gatifloxacin undergoes both glomerular filtration and tubular secretion. Gatifloxacin may also undergo minimal biliary and/or intestinal elimination, since 5% of dose was recovered in the feces as unchanged drug. This finding is supported by the 5-fold higher concentration of gatifloxacin in the bile compared to the plasma [mean bile: plasma ratio (range) 5.34 (0.33-14.0)].

Special Populations

Patients With Bacterial Infections

The pharmacokinetics of gatifloxacin were similar between healthy volunteers and patients with infection, when underlying renal function was taken into account (see TABLE 1).

Geriatric

Following a single oral 400 mg dose of gatifloxacin in young (18-40 years) and elderly (≥65 years) male and female subjects, there were only modest differences in the pharmacokinetics of gatifloxacin noted in female subjects; elderly females had a 21% increase in C_{max} and a 32% increase in AUC(0-∞) compared to young females. These differences were mainly due to decreasing renal function with increasing age and are not thought to be clinically important. No dosage adjustment based on age alone is necessary for elderly subjects when administering gatifloxacin.

Pediatric

The pharmacokinetics of gatifloxacin in pediatric populations (<18 years of age) have not been established.

Gender

Following a single oral 400 mg dose of gatifloxacin in male and female subjects, there were only modest differences in the pharmacokinetics of gatifloxacin, mainly confined to elderly subjects. Elderly females had a 21% increase in C_{max} and a 33% increase in AUC(0-∞) compared to elderly males. Both results were accounted for by gender-related differences in body weight and are not thought to be clinically important. Dosage adjustment of gatifloxacin is not necessary based on gender.

Chronic Hepatic Disease

Following a single oral 400 mg dose of gatifloxacin in healthy subjects and in subjects with moderate hepatic impairment (Child-Pugh B classification of cirrhosis), C_{max}, and AUC(0-∞) values for gatifloxacin were modestly higher (32% and 23% respectively). Due to the concentration-dependent antimicrobial activity associated with quinolones, the modestly higher C_{max} values in the subjects with moderate hepatic impairment are not expected to negatively impact the outcome of gatifloxacin therapy in this population. Dosage adjustment of gatifloxacin is not necessary in patients with moderate hepatic impairment. The effect of severe hepatic impairment on the pharmacokinetics of gatifloxacin is unknown.

Renal Insufficiency

Following administration of a single oral 400 mg dose of gatifloxacin to subjects with varying degrees of renal impairment, apparent total clearance of gatifloxacin (CL/F) was reduced and systemic exposure (AUC) was increased commensurate with the decrease in renal function (see TABLE 1). Total gatifloxacin clearance was reduced 57% in moderate renal insufficiency (CLCR 30-49 ml/min) and 77% in severe renal insufficiency (CLCR <30 ml/min). Systemic exposure to gatifloxacin was approximately 2 times higher in moderate renal insufficiency and approximately 4 times higher in severe renal insufficiency, compared to subjects with normal renal function. Mean C_{max} values were modestly increased. A reduced dosage of gatifloxacin is recommended in patients with creatinine clearance <40 ml/min, including patients requiring hemodialysis or continuous ambulatory peritoneal dialysis (CAPD) (see PRECAUTIONS, General and DOSAGE AND ADMINISTRATION, Impaired Renal Function).

Diabetes Mellitus

The pharmacokinetics of gatifloxacin in patients with Type 2 diabetes (non-insulin-dependent diabetes mellitus), following gatifloxacin 400 mg orally for 10 days, were comparable to those in healthy subjects.

GLUCOSE HOMEOSTASIS

Disturbances of blood glucose, including symptomatic hyper- and hypoglycemia, have been reported with gatifloxacin, usually in diabetic patients. Therefore, careful monitoring of blood glucose is recommended when gatifloxacin is administered to patients with diabetes (see WARNINGS; PRECAUTIONS, Information for the Patient; DRUG INTERACTIONS; and ANIMAL PHARMACOLOGY).

In a postmarketing study conducted in non-infected patients (n=70) with Type 2 diabetes mellitus controlled primarily with either the combination of glyburide and metformin or metformin alone, daily administration of gatifloxacin 400 mg orally for 14 days was associated with initial hypoglycemia followed by hyperglycemia. Upon initiation of gatifloxacin dosing (*i.e.*, first 2 days of treatment), there were increases in serum insulin concentrations and resulting decreases in serum glucose, as compared to baseline glucose values, despite ingestion of dietary restricted meals. In some patients, the reductions in glucose produced signs and symptoms of hypoglycemia (asthenia, sweating, dizziness) and necessitated administration of additional food. With continued gatifloxacin dosing (*i.e.*, from the third day of treatment and throughout the dosing period), fasting serum glucose concentrations were increased compared to baseline. The serum glucose concentrations returned to baseline in most of these uninfected patients by 28 days after the cessation of gatifloxacin treatment. Single doses of insulin were administered to 3 patients in this study to correct the hyperglycemia during continued gatifloxacin administration.

In two premarketing studies, no clinically significant changes in glucose tolerance (via measurement of oral glucose challenge) and glucose homeostasis (via measurement of fasting serum glucose, serum insulin and c-peptide) were observed following single or multiple IV infusion doses of 200-800 mg gatifloxacin in healthy volunteers (n=30), or 400 mg oral doses of gatifloxacin for 10 days in patients (n=16) with type 2 (non-insulin-dependent) diabetes mellitus controlled on diet and exercise. Compared to placebo, transient modest increases in serum insulin of approximately 20-40% and decreases in glucose concentrations of approximately 30% were noted with the first dose of IV or oral gatifloxacin.

In another premarketing study, following administration of single oral 400 mg doses of gatifloxacin for 10 days in patients (n=16) with Type 2 diabetes mellitus controlled with glyburide, decreases in serum insulin concentrations of approximately 30-40%, as compared to placebo, were noted following oral glucose challenge; however, these decreases were not accompanied by statistically significant changes in serum glucose levels. In this study, modest increases in fasting glucose (average increases of 40 mg/dl) were also noted by Day 4 of continued gatifloxacin administration, although these changes did not reach statistical significance.

PHOTOSENSITIVITY POTENTIAL

In a study of the skin response to ultraviolet and visible radiation conducted in 48 healthy, male Caucasian volunteers (12/group), the minimum erythematous dose was measured for ciprofloxacin (500 mg bid), lomefloxacin (400 mg qd), gatifloxacin (400 mg qd), and placebo before and after drug administration for 7 days. In this study, gatifloxacin was comparable to placebo at all wavelengths tested and had a lower potential for producing delayed photosensitivity skin reactions than ciprofloxacin or lomefloxacin.

ELECTROCARDIOGRAM

In premarketing studies of volunteer subjects with pre- and post-dose ECGs obtained in 55 male volunteers receiving oral or IV gatifloxacin doses of 200-800 mg, the mean change in the post-dose QTc interval was <10 msec and there were no subjects with prolonged post-dose QTc intervals of >450 msec. In a postmarketing study of 34 healthy male and female volunteers receiving single oral doses of gatifloxacin 400, 800, and 1200 mg and placebo, an association between increases in post-dose QTc interval changes from baseline and increases in gatifloxacin plasma concentrations were observed. At the therapeutic dose of 400 mg, the mean change in the post-dose QTc interval from baseline was <10 msec. There were no subjects with prolonged post-dose QTc intervals of >450 msec for males and >470 msec for females.

In a postmarketing clinical trial of 262 patients with respiratory tract infections receiving repeated 400 mg oral doses of gatifloxacin who were studied with pre- and post-dose ECGs, the mean change in the post-dose QTc interval was <10 msec following the first 400 mg dose. In another postmarketing study of patients with an acute coronary syndrome occurring within 4 weeks prior to gatifloxacin administration, pre- and post-dose ECGs were obtained in patients who were administered gatifloxacin 400 mg orally after single (n=372) and repeated (steady-state; n=36) dosing. The mean changes in the post-dose QTc interval in these patients were <10 msec after both single and repeated dosing.

There is limited information available on the potential for a pharmacodynamic interaction in humans between gatifloxacin and drugs that prolong the QTc interval of an electrocardiogram. Therefore, gatifloxacin should not be used with Class IA and Class III antiarrhythmics (see WARNINGS and PRECAUTIONS, Information for the Patient).

SPIROMETRY

No clinically significant changes in spirometry were observed following single or multiple 200, 400, 600, and 800 mg IV infusion doses of gatifloxacin in healthy volunteers.

DRUG-DRUG INTERACTIONS

Systemic exposure to gatifloxacin is increased following concomitant administration of gatifloxacin and probenecid, and is reduced by concomitant administration of gatifloxacin and ferrous sulfate or antacids containing aluminum or magnesium salts. Gatifloxacin can be administered 4 hours before the administration of dietary supplements containing zinc, magnesium, or iron (such as multivitamins).

Probenecid: Concomitant administration of gatifloxacin (single oral 200 mg dose) with probenecid (500 mg bid × 1 day) resulted in a 42% increase in AUC and a 44% longer half-life of gatifloxacin.

Iron: When gatifloxacin (single oral 400 mg dose) was administered concomitantly with ferrous sulfate (single oral 325 mg dose), bioavailability of gatifloxacin was reduced (54% reduction in mean C_{max} and 35% reduction in mean AUC). Administration of gatifloxacin (single oral 400 mg dose) 2 hours after or 2 hours before ferrous sulfate (single oral 325 mg dose) did not significantly alter the oral bioavailability of gatifloxacin (see DOSAGE AND ADMINISTRATION).

Antacids: When gatifloxacin (single oral 400 mg dose) was administered 2 hours before, concomitantly, or 2 hours after an aluminum/magnesium-containing antacid (1800 mg of aluminum oxide and 1200 mg of magnesium hydroxide single oral dose), there was a 15%, 69%, and 47% reduction in C_{max} and a 17%, 64%, and 40% reduction in AUC of gatifloxacin, respectively. An aluminum/magnesium-containing antacid did not have a clinically significant effect on the pharmacokinetics of gatifloxacin when administered 4 hours after gatifloxacin administration (single oral 400 mg dose) (see DOSAGE AND ADMINISTRATION).

Milk, calcium, and calcium-containing antacids: No significant pharmacokinetic interactions occur when milk or calcium carbonate is administered concomitantly with gatifloxacin. Concomitant administration of 200 ml of milk or 1000 mg of calcium carbonate with gatifloxacin (200 mg gatifloxacin dose for the milk study and 400 mg gatifloxacin dose for the calcium carbonate study) had no significant effect on the pharmacokinetics of gatifloxacin. Gatifloxacin can be administered 4 hours before the administration of dietary supplements containing zinc, magnesium, or iron (such as multivitamins).

Minor pharmacokinetic interactions occur following concomitant administration of gatifloxacin and digoxin; a priori dosage adjustments of either drug are not warranted.

Digoxin: Overall, only modest increases in C_{max} and AUC of digoxin were noted (12% and 19% respectively) in 8 of 11 healthy volunteers who received concomitant administration of gatifloxacin (400 mg oral tablet, once daily for 7 days) and digoxin (0.25 mg orally, once daily for 7 days). In 3 of 11 subjects, however, a significant increase in digoxin concentrations was observed. In these 3 subjects, digoxin C_{max} increased by 18, 29, and 58% while digoxin AUC increased by 66, 104, and 79%, and digoxin clearance decreased by 40, 51, and 45%. Although dose adjustments for digoxin are not warranted with initiation of gatifloxacin treatment, patients taking

G

digoxin should be monitored for signs and/or symptoms of toxicity. In patients who display signs and/or symptoms of digoxin intoxication, serum digoxin concentrations should be determined, and digoxin dosage should be adjusted as appropriate. The pharmacokinetics of gatifloxacin was not altered by digoxin.

No significant pharmacokinetic interactions occur when cimetidine, midazolam, theophylline, warfarin, or glyburide is administered concomitantly with gatifloxacin. These results and the data from *in vitro* studies suggest that gatifloxacin is unlikely to significantly alter the metabolic clearance of drugs metabolized by CYP3A, CYP1A2, CYP2C9, CYP2C19, and CYP2D6 isoenzymes.

Cimetidine: Administration of gatifloxacin (single oral dose of 200 mg) 1 hour after cimetidine (single oral dose of 200 mg) had no significant effect on the pharmacokinetics of gatifloxacin. These results suggest that absorption of gatifloxacin is expected to be unaffected by H_2-receptor antagonists like cimetidine.

Midazolam: Gatifloxacin administration had no significant effect on the systemic clearance of IV midazolam. A single IV dose of midazolam (0.0145 mg/kg) had no effect on the steady-state pharmacokinetics of gatifloxacin (once daily oral doses of 400 mg for 5 days). These results are consistent with the lack of effect of gatifloxacin in *in vitro* studies with the human CYP3A4 isoenzyme.

Theophylline: Concomitant administration of gatifloxacin (once daily oral doses of 400 mg for 5 days) and theophylline (300 mg bid oral dose for 10 days) had no significant effect on the pharmacokinetics of either drug. These results are consistent with the lack of effect of gatifloxacin in *in vitro* studies with the human CYP1A2 isoenzyme.

Warfarin: Concomitant administration of gatifloxacin (once daily oral doses of 400 mg for 11 days) and warfarin (single oral dose of 25 mg) had no significant effect on the pharmacokinetics of either drug nor was the prothrombin time significantly altered. These results are consistent with the lack of effect of gatifloxacin in *in vitro* studies with the human CYP2C9, CYP1A2, CYP3A4 and CYP2C19 isoenzymes (see DRUG INTERACTIONS).

Glyburide: Pharmacodynamic changes in glucose homeostasis were seen with concomitant administration of gatifloxacin (once daily oral doses of 400 mg for 10 days) and glyburide (steady-state once daily regimen) in patients with Type 2 diabetes mellitus. This was not associated with significant effects on the pharmacokinetic disposition of either drug. These latter results are consistent with the lack of effect of gatifloxacin in *in vitro* studies with the human CYP3A4 isoenzyme (see CLINICAL PHARMACOLOGY, Glucose Homeostasis and WARNINGS).

MICROBIOLOGY

Gatifloxacin is an 8-methoxyfluoroquinolone with *in vitro* activity against a wide range of gram-negative and gram-positive microorganisms. The antibacterial action of gatifloxacin results from inhibition of DNA gyrase and topoisomerase IV. DNA gyrase is an essential enzyme that is involved in the replication, transcription and repair of bacterial DNA. Topoisomerase IV is an enzyme known to play a key role in the partitioning of the chromosomal DNA during bacterial cell division. It appears that the C-8-methoxy moiety contributes to enhanced activity and lower selection of resistant mutants of gram-positive bacteria compared to the non-methoxy C-8 moiety.

The mechanism of action of fluoroquinolones including gatifloxacin is different from that of penicillins, cephalosporins, aminoglycosides, macrolides, and tetracyclines. Therefore, fluoroquinolones may be active against pathogens that are resistant to these antibiotics. There is no cross-resistance between gatifloxacin and the mentioned classes of antibiotics.

From *in vitro* synergy tests, gatifloxacin, as with other fluoroquinolones, is antagonistic with rifampin against enterococci.

Resistance to gatifloxacin *in vitro* develops slowly via multiple-step mutations. Resistance to gatifloxacin *in vitro* occurs at a general frequency of between 1×10^{-7} to 10^{-10}. Although cross-resistance has been observed between gatifloxacin and some other fluoroquinolones, some microorganisms resistant to other fluoroquinolones may be susceptible to gatifloxacin.

Gatifloxacin Oral and IV

Gatifloxacin has been shown to be active against most strains of the following microorganisms, both *in vitro* and in clinical infections as described in INDICATIONS AND USAGE.

Aerobic Gram-Positive Microorganisms:
Staphylococcus aureus (methicillin-susceptible strains only)
Streptococcus pneumoniae (penicillin-susceptible strains)
Streptococcus pyogenes

Aerobic Gram-Negative Microorganisms:
Escherichia coli
Haemophilus influenzae
Haemophilus parainfluenzae
Klebsiella pneumoniae
Moraxella catarrhalis
Neisseria gonorrhoeae
Proteus mirabilis

Other Microorganisms:
Chlamydia pneumoniae
Legionella pneumophila
Mycoplasma pneumoniae

The following *in vitro* data are available, **but their clinical significance is unknown.**

Gatifloxacin exhibits *in vitro* minimum inhibitory concentrations (MICs) of ≤2 μg/ml (≤1 μg/ml for *Streptococcus pneumoniae*) against most (≥90%) strains of the following microorganisms; however, the safety and effectiveness of gatifloxacin in treating clinical infections due to these microorganisms have not been established in adequate and well-controlled clinical trials.

Aerobic Gram-Positive Microorganisms:
Staphylococcus epidermidis (methicillin-susceptible strains only)
Staphylococcus saprophyticus
Streptococcus (Group C/G/F)
Streptococcus agalactiae
Streptococcus pneumoniae (penicillin-resistant strains)
Streptococcus (viridans group)

Aerobic Gram-Negative Microorganisms:
Acinetobacter lwoffii
Citrobacter freundii
Citrobacter koseri
Enterobacter aerogenes
Enterobacter cloacae
Klebsiella oxytoca
Morganella morganii
Proteus vulgaris

Anaerobic Microorganisms:
Peptostreptococcus species

NOTE: The activity of gatifloxacin against *Treponema pallidum* has not been evaluated; however, other quinolones are not active against *Treponema pallidum* (see WARNINGS).

NOTE: Extended-spectrum β-lactamase producing gram-negative microorganisms may have reduced susceptibility to quinolones.

Susceptibility Testing

Dilution Techniques

Quantitative methods are used to determine antimicrobial minimum inhibitory concentrations (MICs). These MICs provide estimates of the susceptibility of bacteria to antimicrobial compounds. The MICs should be determined using a standardized procedure. Standardized procedures are based on a dilution method[1] (broth or agar) or equivalent with standardized inoculum concentrations and standardized concentrations of gatifloxacin powder. The MIC values should be interpreted according to the following criteria:

For testing *Enterobacteriaceae, Staphylococcus* species, *Haemophilus influenzae* and *Haemophilus parainfluenzae** see TABLE 4.

TABLE 4

MIC	Interpretation
***Enterobacteriaceae* and *Staphylococcus* species**	
≤2.0 μg/ml	Susceptible (S)
4.0 μg/ml	Intermediate (I)
≥8.0 μg/ml	Resistant (R)
Haemophilus influenzae* and *Haemophilus parainfluenzae*	
≤1.0 μg/ml	Susceptible (S)

* This interpretive standard is applicable only to broth microdilution susceptibility tests with *Haemophilus influenzae* and *Haemophilus parainfluenzae* using *Haemophilus* Test Medium (HTM)[1].

The current absence of data on resistant strains precludes defining any results other than "Susceptible".

Strains yielding MIC results suggestive of a "nonsusceptible" category should be submitted to a reference laboratory for further testing.

For testing *Streptococcus pneumoniae**, *Streptococcus* species other than *Streptococcus pneumoniae**, and *Neisseria gonorrhoeae*† see TABLE 5.

TABLE 5

MIC	Interpretation
Streptococcus pneumoniae*	
≤1.0 μg/ml	Susceptible (S)
2.0 μg/ml	Intermediate (I)
≥4.0 μg/ml	Resistant (R)
Streptococcus* species other than *Streptococcus pneumoniae*	
≤2.0 μg/ml	Susceptible (S)
4.0 μg/ml	Intermediate (I)
≥8.0 μg/ml	Resistant (R)
***Neisseria gonorrhoeae*†**	
≤0.125 μg/ml	Susceptible (S)
0.25 μg/ml	Intermediate (I)
≥0.5 μg/ml	Resistant (R)

* These interpretive standards are applicable only to broth microdilution susceptibility tests using cation-adjusted Mueller-Hinton broth with 2-5% lysed horse blood.
† These interpretive standards are applicable to agar dilution tests with GC agar base and 1% defined growth supplement.

A report of "Susceptible" indicates that the pathogen is likely to be inhibited if the antimicrobial compound in the blood reaches the concentration usually achievable. A report of "Intermediate" indicates that the result should be considered equivocal, and if the microorganism is not fully susceptible to alternative, clinically feasible drugs, the test should be repeated. This category implies possible clinical applicability in body sites where the drug is physiologically concentrated or in situations where high dosage of drug can be used. This category also provides a buffer zone, which prevents small uncontrolled technical factors from causing major discrepancies in interpretation. A report of "Resistant" indicates that the pathogen is not likely to be inhibited if the antimicrobial compound in the blood reaches the concentration usually achievable; other therapy should be selected.

Standardized susceptibility test procedures require the use of laboratory control microorganisms to control the technical aspects of the laboratory procedures. Standard gatifloxacin powder should provide the MIC values shown in TABLE 6.

Diffusion Techniques

Quantitative methods that require measurement of zone diameters also provide reproducible estimates of the susceptibility of bacteria to antimicrobial compounds. One such standardized procedure[2] requires the use of standardized inoculum concentrations. This procedure

TABLE 6

Microorganism	MIC Range
Enterococcus faecalis ATCC 29212	0.12-1.0 µg/ml
Escherichia coli ATCC 25922	0.008-0.03 µg/ml
Haemophilus influenzae ATCC 49247*	0.004-0.03 µg/ml
Neisseria gonorrhoeae ATCC 49226†	0.002-0.016 µg/ml
Pseudomonas aeruginosa ATCC 27853	0.5-2.0 µg/ml
Staphylococcus aureus ATCC 29213	0.03-0.12 µg/ml
Streptococcus pneumoniae ATCC 49619‡	0.12-0.5 µg/ml

* This quality control range is applicable to only *H. influenzae* ATCC 49247 tested by a broth microdilution procedure using HTM.[1]
† This quality control range is applicable to only *N. gonorrhoeae* ATCC 49226 tested by an agar dilution procedure using GC agar base with 1% defined growth supplement.[1]
‡ This quality control range is applicable to only *S. pneumoniae* ATCC 49619 tested by a microdilution procedure using cation-adjusted Mueller-Hinton broth with 2-5% lysed horse blood.[1]

uses paper disks impregnated with 5 µg gatifloxacin to test the susceptibility of microorganisms to gatifloxacin.

Reports from the laboratory providing results of the standard single-disk susceptibility test with a 5 µg gatifloxacin disk should be interpreted according to the following criteria:

The following zone diameter interpretive criteria should be used for testing *Enterobacteriaceae, Staphylococcus* species, *Haemophilus influenzae* and *Hemophilus parainfluenzae** (see TABLE 7).

TABLE 7

Zone Diameter	Interpretation
***Enterobacteriaceae* and *Staphylococcus* species**	
≥18 mm	Susceptible (S)
15-17 mm	Intermediate (I)
≤14 mm	Resistant (R)
***Haemophilus influenzae* and *Hemophilus parainfluenzae*†**	
≥18 mm	Susceptible (S)

* This zone diameter standard is applicable only to tests with *Haemophilus influenzae* and *Haemophilus parainfluenzae* using *Haemophilus* Test Medium (HTM).[2]

The current absence of data on resistant strains precludes defining any results other than "Susceptible". Strains yielding MIC results suggestive of a "nonsusceptible" category should be submitted to a reference laboratory for further testing.

For testing *Streptococcus pneumoniae**, *Streptococcus* species other than *Streptococcus pneumoniae** and *Neisseria gonorrhoeae*† see TABLE 8.

TABLE 8

Zone Diameter	Interpretation
Streptococcus pneumoniae*	
≥21 mm	Susceptible (S)
18-20 mm	Intermediate (I)
≤17 mm	Resistant (R)
Streptococcus* species other than *Streptococcus pneumoniae*	
≥18 mm	Susceptible (S)
15-17 mm	Intermediate (I)
≤14 mm	Resistant (R)
***Neisseria gonorrhoeae*†**	
≥38 mm	Susceptible (S)
34-37 mm	Intermediate (I)
≤33 mm	Resistant (R)

* These zone diameter standards only apply to tests performed using Mueller-Hinton agar supplemented with 5% sheep blood incubated in 5% CO_2.[2]
† These interpretive standards are applicable to disk diffusion tests with GC agar base and 1% defined growth supplement incubated in 5% CO_2.

Interpretation should be as stated above for results using dilution techniques. Interpretation involves correlation of the diameter obtained in the disk test with the MIC for gatifloxacin.[2]

As with standardized dilution techniques, methods require the use of laboratory control microorganisms that are used to control the technical aspects of the laboratory procedures. For the diffusion technique, the 5 µg gatifloxacin disk should provide the following zone diameters in these laboratory quality control strains (see TABLE 9).

TABLE 9

Microorganism	Zone Diameter Range
Escherichia coli ATCC 25922	30-37 mm
Haemophilus influenzae ATCC 49247*	33-41 mm
Neisseria gonorrhoeae ATCC 49226†	45-56 mm
Pseudomonas aeruginosa ATCC 27853	20-28 mm
Staphylococcus aureus ATCC 25923	27-33 mm
Streptococcus pneumoniae ATCC 49619‡	24-31 mm

* This quality control range applies to tests conducted with *Haemophilus influenzae* ATCC 49247 using *Haemophilus* Test Medium (HTM).[2]
† This quality control range is only applicable to tests conducted with *N. gonorrhoeae* ATCC 49226 performed by disk diffusion using GC agar base and 1% defined growth supplement.[2]
‡ This quality control range is applicable only to tests conducted with *S. pneumoniae* ATCC 49619 performed by disk diffusion using Mueller-Hinton agar supplemented with 5% defibrinated sheep blood.

Gatifloxacin Ophthalmic Solution

Gatifloxacin has been shown to be active against most strains of the following organisms both *in vitro* and clinically, in conjunctival infections as described in INDICATIONS AND USAGE.

Aerobes, Gram-Positive:
Cornyebacterium propinquum, Staphylococcus aureus, Staphylococcus epidermidis, Streptococcus mitis,* Streptococcus pneumoniae.*

Aerobes, Gram-Negative:
Haemophilus influenzae.

* Efficacy for this organism was studied in fewer than 10 infections.

The following *in vitro* data are available, **but their clinical significance in ophthalmic infections is unknown.** The safety and effectiveness of gatifloxacin in treating ophthalmic infections due to the following organisms have not been established in adequate and well-controlled clinical trials.

The following organisms are considered susceptible when evaluated using systemic breakpoints. However, a correlation between the *in vitro* systemic breakpoint and ophthalmological efficacy has not been established. The following list of organisms is provided as guidance only in assessing the potential treatment of conjunctival infections. Gatifloxacin exhibits *in vitro* minimal inhibitory concentrations (MICs) of 2 µg/ml or less (systemic susceptible breakpoint) against most (≥90%) strains of the following ocular pathogens.

Aerobes, Gram-Positive:
Listeria monocytogenes, Staphylococcus saprophyticus, Streptococcus agalactiae, Streptococcus pyogenes, Streptococcus viridans Group, *Streptococcus* Groups C, F, G.

Aerobes, Gram-Negative:
Acinetobacter lwoffii, Enterobacter aerogenes, Enterobacter cloacae, Escherichia coli, Citrobacter freundii, Citrobacter koseri, Haemophilus parainfluenzae, Klebsiella oxytoca, Klebsiella pneumoniae, Moraxella catarrhalis, Morganella morganii, Neisseria gonorrhoeae, Neisseria meningitides, Proteus mirabilis, Proteus vulgaris, Serratia marcescens, Vibrio cholerae, Yersinia enterocolitica.

Other Microorganisms:
Chlamydia pneumoniae, Legionella pneumophila, Mycobacterium marinum, Mycobacterium fortuitum, Mycoplasma pneumoniae.

Anaerobic Microorganisms:
Bacteroides fragilis, Clostridium perfringens.

INDICATIONS AND USAGE

Gatifloxacin is indicated for the treatment of infections due to susceptible strains of the designated microorganisms in the conditions listed below (see DOSAGE AND ADMINISTRATION).

Acute bacterial exacerbation of chronic bronchitis due to *Streptococcus pneumoniae, Haemophilus influenzae, Haemophilus parainfluenzae, Moraxella catarrhalis,* or *Staphylococcus aureus.*

Acute sinusitis due to *Streptococcus pneumoniae* or *Haemophilus influenzae.*

Community-acquired pneumonia due to *Streptococcus pneumoniae, Haemophilus influenzae, Haemophilus parainfluenzae, Moraxella catarrhalis, Staphylococcus aureus, Mycoplasma pneumoniae, Chlamydia pneumoniae,* or *Legionella pneumophila.*

Uncomplicated skin and skin structure infections (*i.e.,* simple abscesses, furuncles, folliculitis, wound infections, and cellulitis) due to *Staphylococcus aureus* (methicillin-susceptible strains only) or *Streptococcus pyogenes.*

NOTE: An insufficient number of patients with the diagnosis of impetiginous lesions were available for evaluation.

Uncomplicated urinary tract infections (cystitis) due to *Escherichia coli, Klebsiella pneumoniae,* or *Proteus mirabilis.*

Complicated urinary tract infections due to *Escherichia coli, Klebsiella pneumoniae,* or *Proteus mirabilis.*

Pyelonephritis due to *Escherichia coli.*

Uncomplicated urethral and cervical gonorrhea due to *Neisseria gonorrhoeae.* **Acute, uncomplicated rectal infections in women** due to *Neisseria gonorrhoeae* (see WARNINGS).

Appropriate culture and susceptibility tests should be performed before treatment in order to isolate and identify organisms causing infection and to determine their susceptibility to gatifloxacin. Therapy with gatifloxacin may be initiated before results of these tests are known; once results become available, appropriate therapy should be continued.

Gatifloxacin ophthalmic solution is indicated for the treatment of bacterial conjunctivitis caused by susceptible strains of the following organisms:

Aerobic Gram-Positive Bacteria: *Cornyebacterium propinquum,* Staphylococcus aureus, Staphylococcus epidermidis, Streptococcus mitis,* Streptococcus pneumoniae.*

Aerobic Gram-Negative Bacteria: *Haemophilus influenzae.*

* Efficacy for this organism was studied in fewer than 10 infections.

NON-FDA APPROVED INDICATIONS

Although not FDA approved, additional uses of gatifloxacin have included the treatment of atypical pneumonia and chronic prostatitis.

CONTRAINDICATIONS

Gatifloxacin is contraindicated in persons with a history of hypersensitivity to gatifloxacin or any member of the quinolone class of antimicrobial agents.

WARNINGS

THE SAFETY AND EFFECTIVENESS OF GATIFLOXACIN IN PEDIATRIC PATIENTS, ADOLESCENTS (LESS THAN 18 YEARS OF AGE), PREGNANT WOMEN, AND LACTATING WOMEN HAVE NOT BEEN ESTABLISHED (see PRECAUTIONS: Pediatric Use, Pregnancy Category C, and Nursing Mothers).

PROLONGATION OF THE QTC INTERVAL

GATIFLOXACIN HAS THE POTENTIAL TO PROLONG THE QTc INTERVAL OF THE ELECTROCARDIOGRAM IN SOME PATIENTS. DUE TO THE LACK OF CLINICAL EXPERIENCE IN PATIENTS WITH KNOWN PROLONGATION OF THE QTc INTERVAL, PATIENTS WITH UNCORRECTED HYPOKALEMIA, AND PATIENTS RECEIVING CLASS IA (*e.g.,* QUINIDINE, PROCAINAMIDE) OR CLASS III (*e.g.,* AMIODARONE, SOTALOL) ANTIARRHYTHMIC AGENTS GATIFLOXACIN SHOULD BE AVOIDED IN THESE PATIENT POPULATIONS.

Pharmacokinetic and pharmacodynamic studies between gatifloxacin and drugs that prolong the QTc interval such as cisapride, erythromycin, antipsychotics, and tricyclic antidepressants have not been performed. Gatifloxacin should be used with caution when given concurrently with these drugs, as well as in patients with ongoing proarrhythmic conditions, such as clinically significant bradycardia or acute myocardial ischemia.

The magnitude of QTc prolongation increases with increasing concentrations of the drug; therefore, the recommended dose and the recommended IV infusion rate should not be exceeded (see DOSAGE AND ADMINISTRATION for dosing recommendations for patients with or without renal impairment). QTc prolongation may lead to an increased risk for ventricular arrhythmias including torsades de pointes (see CLINICAL PHARMACOLOGY, Electrocardiogram).

No cardiovascular morbidity or mortality attributable to QTc prolongation has occurred in over 44,000 patients treated with gatifloxacin in clinical trials; these include 118 patients concurrently receiving drugs known to prolong the QTc internal and 139 patients known to have uncorrected hypokalemia (ECG monitoring was not performed). During postmarketing surveillance, rare cases of torsades de pointes have been reported in patients taking gatifloxacin. These cases have occurred primarily in elderly patients with underlying medical problems for which they were receiving concomitant medications known to prolong the QTc interval; the contribution, if any, of gatifloxacin to the development of torsades de pointes in these patients is unknown.

DISTURBANCES IN BLOOD GLUCOSE

Disturbances of blood glucose, including symptomatic hyper- and hypoglycemia, have been reported with gatifloxacin, usually in diabetic patients. Therefore, careful monitoring of blood glucose is recommended when gatifloxacin is administered to patients with diabetes (see CLINICAL PHARMACOLOGY; PRECAUTIONS,Information for the Patient; DRUG INTERACTIONS; and ANIMAL PHARMACOLOGY).

Studies conducted in non-infected patients with Type 2 diabetes mellitus controlled on oral hypoglycemic agents have demonstrated that gatifloxacin is associated with disturbances in glucose homeostasis including an increase in serum insulin and decrease in serum glucose usually following administration of initial doses (*i.e.,* first 2 days of treatment), and sometimes associated with symptomatic hypoglycemia. Increases in fasting serum glucose were also observed, usually after the third day of gatifloxacin administration, continuing throughout the duration of treatment, and returning to baseline by 28 days after the cessation of gatifloxacin treatment in most patients.

During the postmarketing period, there have been reports of serious disturbances of glucose homeostasis in patients being treated with gatifloxacin. Hypoglycemic episodes, in some cases severe, have been reported in patients with diabetes mellitus treated with either sulfonylurea or non-sulfonylurea oral hypoglycemic medications. These events frequently occurred on the first day of therapy and usually within 3 days following the initiation of gatifloxacin. Hyperglycemic episodes, in some cases severe and associated with hyperosmolar non-ketotic hyperglycemic coma, were reported in diabetic patients, mostly between 4 and 10 days following the initiation of gatifloxacin therapy. Some of the hyperglycemic and hypoglycemic events were life-threatening and many required hospitalization, although these events were reversible when appropriately managed. Many of these patients had other underlying medical problems and were receiving concomitant medications that may have contributed to the glucose abnormality. Episodes of hyperglycemia, including hyperosmolar non-ketotic hyperglycemic coma, also occurred in patients not previously diagnosed with diabetes mellitus. Elderly patients who may have unrecognized diabetes, age-related decrease in renal function, underlying medical problems and/or are taking concomitant medications associated with hyperglycemia may be at particular risk of serious hyperglycemia.

The dose of gatifloxacin should be adjusted based on underlying renal function (see DOSAGE AND ADMINISTRATION). When gatifloxacin is used in diabetic patients, blood glucose should be closely monitored. Signs and symptom of hypoglycemia should be monitored, especially during the first 3 days of therapy, and signs and symptoms of hyperglycemia should be monitored in diabetics and patients who may be at risk for hyperglycemia, especially with continued treatment with gatifloxacin beyond 3 days. If signs and symptoms of either hypoglycemia or hyperglycemia occur in any patient being treated with gatifloxacin, appropriate therapy must be initiated immediately and gatifloxacin should be discontinued.

OTHER

As with other members of the quinolone class, gatifloxacin has caused arthropathy and/or chondrodysplasia in immature dogs. The relevance of these findings to the clinical use of gatifloxacin is unknown (see ANIMAL PHARMACOLOGY).

Convulsions, increased intracranial pressure, and psychosis have been reported in patients receiving quinolones. Quinolones may also cause central nervous system (CNS) stimulation, which may lead to tremors, restlessness, lightheadedness, confusion, hallucinations, paranoia, depression, nightmares and insomnia. These reactions may occur following the first dose. If these reactions occur in patients receiving gatifloxacin, the drug should be discontinued and appropriate measures instituted (see ADVERSE REACTIONS).

As with other quinolones, gatifloxacin should be used with caution in patients with known or suspected CNS disorders, such as severe cerebral atherosclerosis, epilepsy, and other factors that predispose to seizures.

Serious and occasionally fatal hypersensitivity and/or anaphylactic reactions have been reported in patients receiving therapy with quinolones. These reactions may occur following the first dose. Some reactions have been accompanied by cardiovascular collapse, hypotension/shock, seizure, loss of consciousness, tingling, angioedema (including tongue, laryngeal, throat or facial edema/swelling), airway obstruction (including bronchospasm, shortness of breath, and acute respiratory distress), dyspnea, urticaria, itching, and other serious skin reactions.

Gatifloxacin should be discontinued at the first appearance of a skin rash or any other sign of hypersensitivity. Serious acute hypersensitivity reactions may require treatment with epinephrine and other resuscitative measures, including oxygen, IV fluids, antihistamines, corticosteroids, pressor amines, and airway management, as clinically indicated (see PRECAUTIONS).

Serious and sometimes fatal events, some due to hypersensitivity and some due to uncertain etiology, have been reported in patients receiving antibacterial therapy. These events may be severe and generally occur following the administration of multiple doses. Clinical manifestations may include 1 or more of the following: fever, rash or severe dermatologic reactions (*e.g.,* toxic epidermal necrolysis, Stevens-Johnson syndrome); vasculitis, arthralgia, myalgia, serum sickness; allergic pneumonitis, interstitial nephritis; acute renal insufficiency or failure; hepatitis, jaundice, acute hepatic necrosis or failure; anemia, including hemolytic and aplastic; thrombocytopenia, including thrombotic thrombocytopenic purpura; leukopenia; agranulocytosis; pancytopenia; and/or other hematologic abnormalities.

Pseudomembranous colitis has been reported with nearly all antibacterial agents, including gatifloxacin, and may range in severity from mild to life-threatening. It is important, therefore, to consider this diagnosis in patients who present with diarrhea subsequent to the administration of any antibacterial agent.

Treatment with antibacterial agents alters the flora of the colon and may permit overgrowth of clostridia. Studies indicate that a toxin produced by *Clostridium difficile* is the primary cause of "antibiotic-associated colitis".

After the diagnosis of pseudomembranous colitis has been established, therapeutic measures should be initiated. Mild cases of pseudomembranous colitis usually respond to drug discontinuation alone. In moderate to severe cases, consideration should be given to management with fluids and electrolytes, protein supplementation, and treatment with an antibacterial drug clinically effective against *C. difficile* colitis.

Ruptures of the shoulder, hand, and Achilles tendons that required surgical repair or resulted in prolonged disability have been reported in patients receiving quinolones. Gatifloxacin should be discontinued if the patient experiences pain, inflammation or rupture of a tendon. Patients should rest and refrain from exercise until the diagnosis of tendonitis or tendon rupture has been confidently excluded. Tendon rupture can occur during or after therapy with quinolones.

Gatifloxacin has not been shown to be effective in the treatment of syphilis. Antimicrobial agents used in high doses for short periods of time to treat gonorrhea may mask or delay the symptoms of incubating syphilis. All patients with gonorrhea should have a serologic test for syphilis at the time of diagnosis.

Gatifloxacin ophthalmic solution should not be injected subconjunctivally, nor should it be introduced directly into the anterior chamber of the eye.

PRECAUTIONS

GENERAL

Gatifloxacin Oral and IV

Quinolones may cause central nervous system (CNS) events including nervousness, agitation, insomnia, anxiety, nightmares, or paranoia (see WARNINGS and PRECAUTIONS, Information for the Patient).

Administer gatifloxacin with caution in the presence of renal insufficiency. Careful clinical observation and appropriate laboratory studies should be performed prior to and during therapy since elimination of gatifloxacin may be reduced. In patients with impaired renal function (creatinine clearance <40 ml/min), adjustment of the dosage regimen is necessary to avoid the accumulation of gatifloxacin due to decreased clearance (see CLINICAL PHARMACOLOGY and DOSAGE AND ADMINISTRATION).

Because a hypotonic solution results, water for injection should not be used as a diluent when preparing a 2 mg/ml solution from the concentrated solution of gatifloxacin (10 mg/ml) (see DOSAGE AND ADMINISTRATION).

Disturbances of blood glucose homeostasis have been reported during the postmarketing period (see CLINICAL PHARMACOLOGY, WARNINGS, and ANIMAL PHARMACOLOGY).

Gatifloxacin Ophthalmic Solution

As with other anti-infectives, prolonged use may result in overgrowth of nonsusceptible organisms, including fungi. If superinfection occurs discontinue use and institute alternative therapy. Whenever clinical judgment dictates, the patient should be examined with the aid of magnification, such as slit lamp biomicroscopy and, where appropriate, fluorescein staining.

Patients should be advised not to wear contact lenses if they have signs and symptoms of bacterial conjunctivitis.

INFORMATION FOR THE PATIENT

Gatifloxacin Oral and IV

See the Patient Information that is distributed with the prescription.

To assure safe and effective use of gatifloxacin, the following information and instructions should be communicated to the patient when appropriate.

Patients Should Be Advised:

- That gatifloxacin may produce changes in the electrocardiogram (QTc interval prolongation).
- That gatifloxacin should be avoided in patients receiving Class IA (*e.g.,* quinidine, procainamide) or Class III (*e.g.,* amiodarone, sotalol) antiarrhythmic agents.
- That gatifloxacin should be used with caution in patients receiving drugs that may effect the QTc interval such as cisapride, erythromycin, antipsychotics, and tricyclic antidepressants.
- To inform their physician of any personal or family history of QTc prolongation or proarrhythmic conditions such as recent hypokalemia, significant bradycardia, or recent myocardial ischemia.
- That disturbances of blood glucose, including symptomatic hyper- and hypoglycemia, have been reported with gatifloxacin, usually in diabetic patients or in patients at risk for

hyperglycemia. If a hypoglycemic reaction or symptoms of hyperglycemia occur, patients should initiate appropriate therapy immediately, discontinue gatifloxacin, and contact their physician (see CLINICAL PHARMACOLOGY and WARNINGS).

- To inform their physician of any other medications when taken concurrently with gatifloxacin, including over-the-counter medications.
- To contact their physician if they experience palpitations or fainting spells while taking gatifloxacin.
- That gatifloxacin tablets may be taken with or without meals.
- That gatifloxacin tablets should be taken 4 hours before any aluminum- or magnesium-based antacids (see DRUG INTERACTIONS).
- That gatifloxacin tablets should be taken at least 4 hours before the administration of ferrous sulfate or dietary supplements containing zinc, magnesium, or iron (such as multivitamins) (see DRUG INTERACTIONS).
- That gatifloxacin should be taken 4 hours before didanosine (Videx) buffered tablets, buffered solution, or buffered powder for oral suspension.
- That gatifloxacin may be associated with hypersensitivity reactions, even following the first dose, and to discontinue the drug at the first sign of a skin rash, hives or other skin reactions, difficulty in swallowing or breathing, any swelling suggesting angioedema (*e.g.*, swelling of the lips, tongue, face, tightness of the throat, hoarseness), or other symptoms of an allergic reaction (see WARNINGS and ADVERSE REACTIONS).
- To discontinue treatment; rest and refrain from exercise; and inform their physician if they experience pain, inflammation, or rupture of a tendon.
- That gatifloxacin may cause dizziness and lightheadedness; therefore, patients should know how they react to this drug before they operate an automobile or machinery or engage in activities requiring mental alertness or coordination.
- That phototoxicity has been reported in patients receiving certain quinolones. There was no phototoxicity seen with gatifloxacin at the recommended dose. In keeping with good medical practice, avoid excessive sunlight or artificial ultraviolet light (*e.g.,* tanning beds). If sunburn-like reaction or skin eruptions occur, contact their physician (see CLINICAL PHARMACOLOGY, Photosensitivity Potential).
- That convulsions have been reported in patients receiving quinolones, and they should notify their physician before taking this drug if there is a history of this condition.

Gatifloxacin Ophthalmic Solution

Avoid contaminating the applicator tip with material from the eye, fingers or other source.

Systemic quinolones, including gatifloxacin, have been associated with hypersensitivity reactions, even following a single dose. Discontinue use immediately and contact your physician at the first sign of a rash or allergic reaction.

LABORATORY TEST INTERACTIONS

There are no reported laboratory test interactions.

CARCINOGENESIS, MUTAGENESIS, AND IMPAIRMENT OF FERTILITY

B6C3F1 mice given gatifloxacin in the diet for 18 months at doses with an average intake up to 81 mg/kg/day in males and 90 mg/kg/day in females showed no increases in neoplasms. These doses are approximately 0.13 and 0.18 times the maximum recommended human dose based upon daily systemic exposure (AUC).

In a 2 year dietary carcinogenicity study in Fischer 344 rats, no increases in neoplasms were seen in males given doses up to 47 mg/kg/day and females given up to 139 mg/kg/day. These doses are approximately 0.36 (males) and 0.81 (females) times the maximum recommended human dose based upon daily systemic exposure. A statistically significant increase in the incidence of large granular lymphocyte (LGL) leukemia was seen in males treated with a high dose of 100 mg/kg/day (approximately 0.74 times the maximum recommended human dose based upon daily systemic exposure) versus controls. Although Fischer 344 rats have a high spontaneous background rate of LGL leukemia, the incidence in high-dose males slightly exceeded the historical control range established for this strain. The findings in high-dose males are not considered a concern with regard to the safe use of gatifloxacin in humans.

In genetic toxicity tests, gatifloxacin was not mutagenic in several strains of bacteria used in the Ames test; however, it was mutagenic to *Salmonella* strain TA102. Gatifloxacin was negative in four *in vivo* assays that included oral and IV micronucleus tests in mice, an oral cytogenetics test in rats, and an oral DNA repair test in rats. Gatifloxacin was positive in *in vitro* gene-mutation assays in Chinese hamster V-79 cells and *in vitro* cytogenetics assays in Chinese hamster CHL/IU cells. These findings were not unexpected; similar findings have been seen with other quinolones and may be due to the inhibitory effects of high concentrations on eukaryotic type II DNA topoisomerase.

There were no adverse effects on fertility or reproduction in rats given gatifloxacin orally at doses up to 200 mg/kg/day [approximately equivalent to the maximum human dose based on systemic exposure (AUC)].

PREGNANCY CATEGORY C

There were no teratogenic effects observed in rats or rabbits at oral gatifloxacin doses up to 150 or 50 mg/kg, respectively (approximately 0.7 and 1.9 times the maximum human dose based on systemic exposure). However, skeletal malformations were observed in fetuses from rats given 200 mg/kg/day orally or 60 mg/kg/day intravenously during organogenesis. Developmental delays in skeletal ossification, including wavy ribs, were observed in fetuses from rats given oral doses of ≥150 mg/kg or IV doses of ≥30 mg/kg daily during organogenesis, suggesting that gatifloxacin is slightly fetotoxic at these doses. Similar findings have been seen with other quinolones. These changes were not seen in rats or rabbits given oral doses of gatifloxacin up to 50 mg/kg (approximately 0.2 and 1.9 times the maximum human dose, respectively, based on systemic exposure).

When rats were given oral doses of 200 mg/kg of gatifloxacin beginning in late pregnancy and continuing throughout lactation, late postimplantation loss increased, as did neonatal and perinatal mortalities. These observations also suggest fetotoxicity. Similar findings have been seen with other quinolones.

Because there are no adequate and well-controlled studies in pregnant women, gatifloxacin should be used during pregnancy only if the potential benefit outweighs the potential risk to the fetus.

NURSING MOTHERS

Gatifloxacin is excreted in the breast milk of rats. It is not known whether this drug is excreted in human milk. Because many drugs are excreted in human milk, caution should be exercised when gatifloxacin is administered to a nursing woman.

PEDIATRIC USE

The safety and effectiveness of gatifloxacin in pediatric populations (<18 years of age) have not been established. Quinolones, including gatifloxacin, cause arthropathy and osteochondrotoxicity in juvenile animals (rats and dogs).

GERIATRIC USE

During the postmarketing period, serious disturbances of glucose homeostasis have been reported in elderly patients being treated with gatifloxacin (see WARNINGS, DRUG INTERACTIONS, and ANIMAL PHARMACOLOGY).

In multiple-dose clinical trials of gatifloxacin (n=2891), 22% of patients were ≥65 years of age and 10% were ≥75 years of age. No overall differences in safety or efficacy were observed in clinical trials between these subjects and younger subjects, and other reported clinical experience has not identified differences in responses between the elderly and younger patients, but greater sensitivity of some older individuals cannot be ruled out.

This drug is known to be substantially excreted by the kidney, and the risk of toxic reactions to this drug may be greater in patients with impaired renal function. Because elderly patients are more likely to have decreased renal function, care should be taken in dose selection, and it may be useful to monitor renal function (see DOSAGE AND ADMINISTRATION).

G

DRUG INTERACTIONS

Gatifloxacin can be taken 4 hours before ferrous sulfate, dietary supplements containing zinc, magnesium, or iron (such as multivitamins), or aluminum/magnesium-containing antacids without any significant pharmacokinetic interactions (see CLINICAL PHARMACOLOGY).

Milk, calcium carbonate, cimetidine, theophylline, warfarin, or midazolam: No significant interactions have been observed when administered concomitantly with gatifloxacin. No dosage adjustments are necessary when these drugs are administered concomitantly with gatifloxacin (see CLINICAL PHARMACOLOGY).

Antidiabetic agents: Pharmacodynamic changes in glucose homeostasis have been seen with concomitant glyburide use. However, no significant pharmacokinetic interactions have been observed when glyburide was administered concomitantly with gatifloxacin (see CLINICAL PHARMACOLOGY, Glucose Homeostasis and WARNINGS).

Digoxin: Concomitant administration of gatifloxacin and digoxin did not produce significant alteration of the pharmacokinetics of gatifloxacin; however, an increase in digoxin concentrations was observed for 3 of 11 subjects. Patients taking digoxin should therefore be monitored for signs and/or symptoms of toxicity. In patients who display signs and/or symptoms of digoxin intoxication, serum digoxin concentrations should be determined, and digoxin dosage should be adjusted as appropriate (see CLINICAL PHARMACOLOGY).

Probenecid: The systemic exposure of gatifloxacin is significantly increased following the concomitant administration of gatifloxacin and probenecid (see CLINICAL PHARMACOLOGY).

Warfarin: In subjects receiving warfarin, no significant change in clotting time was observed when gatifloxacin was coadministered. However, because some quinolones have been reported to enhance the effects of warfarin or its derivatives, prothrombin time or other suitable anticoagulation test should be monitored closely if a quinolone antimicrobial is administered with warfarin or its derivatives.

Nonsteroidal anti-inflammatory drugs (NSAIDs): Although not observed with gatifloxacin in preclinical and clinical trials, the concomitant administration of nonsteroidal anti-inflammatory drugs with a quinolone may increase the risks of CNS stimulation and convulsions (see WARNINGS).

ADVERSE REACTIONS

Over 5000 patients have been treated with gatifloxacin in single- and multiple-dose clinical efficacy trials worldwide.

In gatifloxacin studies, the majority of adverse reactions were described as mild in nature. Gatifloxacin was discontinued for adverse events thought related to drug in 2.7% of patients.

Drug-related adverse events classified as possibly, probably, or definitely related with a frequency of ≥3% in patients receiving gatifloxacin in single- and multiple-dose clinical trials are as follows: nausea 8%, vaginitis 6%, diarrhea 4%, headache 3%, dizziness 3%.

In patients who were treated with either IV gatifloxacin or with IV followed by oral therapy, the incidence of adverse events was similar to those who received oral therapy alone. Local injection site reactions (redness at injection site) were noted in 5% of patients.

Additional drug-related adverse events (possibly, probably, or definitely related) considered clinically relevant that occurred in ≥0.1% to <3% of patients receiving gatifloxacin in single- and multiple-dose clinical trials are as follows:

Body as a Whole: Allergic reaction, asthenia, back pain, chest pain, chills, face edema, fever.

Cardiovascular System: Hypertension, palpitation.

Digestive System: Abdominal pain, anorexia, constipation, dyspepsia, flatulence, gastritis, glossitis, mouth ulcer, oral moniliasis, stomatitis, vomiting.

Metabolic/Nutritional System: Hyperglycemia, peripheral edema, thirst.

Musculoskeletal System: Arthralgia, leg cramp.

Nervous System: Abnormal dream, agitation, anxiety, confusion, insomnia, nervousness, paresthesia, somnolence, tremor, vasodilatation, vertigo.

Respiratory System: Dyspnea, pharyngitis.

Skin/Appendages: Dry skin, pruritus, rash, sweating.

Special Senses: Abnormal vision, taste perversion, tinnitus.

Urogenital System: Dysuria.

Additional drug-related adverse events considered clinically relevant that occurred in <0.1% (rare adverse events) of patients receiving gatifloxacin in single- and multiple-

dose clinical trials are as follows: Abnormal thinking, alcohol intolerance, arthritis, asthma (bronchospasm), ataxia, bone pain, bradycardia, breast pain, cheilitis, colitis, convulsion, cyanosis, depersonalization, depression, diabetes mellitus, dysphagia, ear pain, ecchymosis, edema, epistaxis, euphoria, eye pain, eye photosensitivity, gastrointestinal hemorrhage, generalized edema, gingivitis, halitosis, hallucination, hematemesis, hematuria, hostility, hyperesthesia, hypertonia, hyperventilation, hypoglycemia, lymphadenopathy, maculopapular rash, metrorrhagia, migraine, mouth edema, myalgia, myasthenia, neck pain, panic attack, paranoia, parosmia, photophobia, pseudomembranous colitis, psychosis, ptosis, rectal hemorrhage, stress, substernal chest pain, tachycardia, taste loss, tongue edema, and vesiculobullous rash.

LABORATORY CHANGES

Clinically relevant changes in laboratory parameters, without regard to drug relationship, occurred in fewer than 1% of gatifloxacin-treated patients. These included the following: neutropenia, increased ALT or AST levels, alkaline phosphatase, bilirubin, serum amylase, and electrolytes abnormalities. It is not known whether these abnormalities were caused by the drug or the underlying condition being treated.

POSTMARKETING ADVERSE EVENT REPORTS

The following events have been reported during postapproval use of gatifloxacin. Because these events are reported voluntarily from a population of uncertain size, it is not always possible to reliably estimate their frequency or establish a causal relationship to drug exposure.

G

Acute allergic reaction including anaphylactic reaction and angioneurotic edema, hepatitis, increased International Normalized Ratio (INR)/prothrombin time, severe hyperglycemia (including hyperosmolar nonketotic hyperglycemia), severe hypoglycemia, tendon rupture, thrombocytopenia, and torsades de pointes.

OPHTHALMIC USE

The most frequently reported adverse events in the overall study population were conjunctival irritation, increased lacrimation, keratitis, and papillary conjunctivitis. These events occurred in approximately 5-10% of patients. Other reported reactions occurring in 1-4% of patients were chemosis, conjunctival hemorrhage, dry eye, eye discharge, eye irritation, eye pain, eyelid edema, headache, red eye, reduced visual acuity and taste disturbance.

DOSAGE AND ADMINISTRATION

GATIFLOXACIN ORAL AND IV

The recommended dosage for gatifloxacin tablets or injection is described in TABLE 10. Doses of gatifloxacin are administered once every 24 hours. These recommendations apply to all patients with a creatinine clearance ≥40 ml/min. For patients with a creatinine clearance <40 ml/min, see Impaired Renal Function.

Gatifloxacin can be administered without regard to food, including milk and dietary supplements containing calcium.

Oral doses of gatifloxacin should be administered at least 4 hours before the administration of ferrous sulfate, dietary supplements containing zinc, magnesium, or iron (such as multivitamins), aluminum/magnesium-containing antacids, or didanosine buffered tablets, buffered solution, or buffered powder for oral suspension.

Gatifloxacin can be administered without regard to gender or age (≥18 years). Consideration should be given to the possibility that the elderly may have impaired renal function (see PRECAUTIONS, Geriatric Use).

When switching from IV to oral dosage administration, no dosage adjustment is necessary. Patients whose therapy is started with gatifloxacin injection may be switched to gatifloxacin tablets when clinically indicated at the discretion of the physician.

Gatifloxacin injection should be administered by IV infusion only. It is not intended for intramuscular, intrathecal, intraperitoneal, or subcutaneous administration.

Single-use vials require dilution prior to administration.

Gatifloxacin injection should be administered by IV infusion over a period of 60 minutes. *CAUTION:* RAPID OR BOLUS IV INFUSION SHOULD BE AVOIDED.

TABLE 10 *Gatifloxacin — Dosage Guidelines*

Infection*	Daily Dose†	Duration
Acute bacterial exacerbation of chronic bronchitis	400 mg	5 days
Acute sinusitis	400 mg	10 days
Community-acquired pneumonia	400 mg	7-14 days
Uncomplicated skin and skin structure infections	400 mg	7-10 days
Uncomplicated urinary tract infections (cystitis)	400 mg or 200 mg	Single dose 3 days
Complicated urinary tract infections	400 mg	7-10 days
Acute pyelonephritis	400 mg	7-10 days
Uncomplicated urethral gonorrhea in men; endocervical and rectal gonorrhea in women	400 mg	Single dose

* Due to the designated pathogens (see INDICATIONS AND USAGE).
† For either the oral or IV routes of administration for gatifloxacin (see CLINICAL PHARMACOLOGY).

Impaired Renal Function

Since gatifloxacin is eliminated primarily by renal excretion, a dosage modification of gatifloxacin is recommended for patients with creatinine clearance <40 ml/min, including patients on hemodialysis and on CAPD. The recommended dosage of gatifloxacin is shown in TABLE 11.

Administer gatifloxacin after a dialysis session for patients on hemodialysis.

Single 400 mg dose gatifloxacin regimen (for the treatment of uncomplicated urinary tract infections and gonorrhea) and 200 mg once daily for 3 days gatifloxacin regimen (for the treatment of uncomplicated urinary tract infections) require no dosage adjustment in patients with impaired renal function.

TABLE 11 *Recommended Dosage of Gatifloxacin in Adult Patients With Renal Impairment*

Creatinine Clearance	Initial Dose	Subsequent Dose*
≥40 ml/min	400 mg	400 mg every day
<40 ml/min	400 mg	200 mg every day
Hemodialysis	400 mg	200 mg every day
Continuous peritoneal dialysis	400 mg	200 mg every day

* Start subsequent dose on Day 2 of dosing.

Chronic Hepatic Disease

No adjustment in the dosage of gatifloxacin is necessary in patients with moderate hepatic impairment (Child-Pugh Class B). There are no data in patients with severe hepatic impairment (Child-Pugh Class C). (See CLINICAL PHARMACOLOGY.)

GATIFLOXACIN OPHTHALMIC SOLUTION

The recommended dosage regimen for the treatment of bacterial conjunctivitis is: *Days 1 and 2:* Instill 1 drop every 2 hours in the affected eye(s) while awake, up to 8 times daily. *Days 3-7:* Instill 1 drop up to 4 times daily while awake.

ANIMAL PHARMACOLOGY

In 3 animal species (rats, beagle dogs, and cynomolgus monkeys) given oral gatifloxacin doses approximately 1.0 to 19 times the approved human dose (based on body surface area) from 1-6 months, electron microscopy showed vesiculation of rough endoplasmic reticulum and decreased secretory granules in pancreatic β-cells of all 3 species. These ultrastructural changes correlated with vacuolation of pancreatic β-cells seen by light microscopy in dogs given a dose level for 1 or 6 months that was approximately equivalent to the human dose (based upon body surface area and plasma AUC). Following a 4 week recovery period without gatifloxacin, partial recovery from these pancreatic changes was seen in the rat, and complete recovery was evident in beagle dogs and cynomolgus monkeys (see WARNINGS and CLINICAL PHARMACOLOGY).

In contrast to some other quinolone antibacterials, there was no evidence of phototoxicity when gatifloxacin was evaluated in the hairless mouse or guinea pig models using simulated sunlight or UVA radiation, respectively.

Unlike some other members of the quinolone class, crystalluria, ocular toxicity, and testicular degeneration were not observed in 6 month repeat dose studies with rats or dogs given gatifloxacin.

While some quinolone antibacterials have proconvulsant activity that is exacerbated with concomitant use of nonsteroidal anti-inflammatory drugs (NSAIDs), gatifloxacin did not produce an increase in seizure activity when administered intravenously to mice at doses up to 100 mg/kg in combination with the NSAID fenbufen.

Quinolone antibacterials have been shown to cause arthropathy in immature animals. There is no evidence of arthropathy in fully mature rats and dogs given gatifloxacin for 6 months at doses of 240 or 24 mg/kg, respectively (approximately 1.5 times the maximum human dose in both species based on systemic exposure). Arthropathy and chondrodysplasia were observed in immature dogs given 10 mg/kg gatifloxacin orally for 7 days (approximately equal to the maximum human dose based upon systemic exposure) [see WARNINGS]. The relevance of these findings to the clinical use of gatifloxacin is unknown.

Some other members of the quinolone class have been shown to cause prolongation of the QT interval in dogs. Intravenous 10 mg/kg bolus doses of gatifloxacin had no effect on QT interval in anesthetized dogs.

HOW SUPPLIED

TABLETS

Tequin tablets are available as 200 and 400 mg white, film-coated tablets. The tablets are almond shaped and biconvex and contain gatifloxacin sesquihydrate equivalent to either 200 or 400 mg gatifloxacin.

200 mg: White, biconvex, debossed with "BMS" on one side and "TEQUIN" and "200" on the other.

400 mg: White, biconvex, debossed with "BMS" on one side and "TEQUIN" and "400" on the other.

Storage: Store at 25°C (77°F); excursions permitted to 15-30°C (59-86°F).

IV SOLUTION — SINGLE-USE VIALS

Tequin (gatifloxacin) injection is available for IV administration in single-use vials containing a clear, light yellow to greenish-yellow solution at a concentration of 10 mg/ml gatifloxacin.

Storage: Store at 25°C (77°F); excursions permitted to 15-30°C (59-86°F).

IV SOLUTION — PREMIX BAGS

Tequin (gatifloxacin in 5% dextrose) injection is also available in ready-to-use flexible bags containing a dilute solution of 200 or 400 mg of gatifloxacin in 5% dextrose.

Storage: Store at 25°C (77°F); excursions permitted to 15-30°C (59-86°F). Do not freeze.

OPHTHALMIC SOLUTION

Zymar (gatifloxacin ophthalmic solution) 0.3% is supplied sterile (2.5 or 5 ml) in a white, low density polyethylene (LDPE) (6 or 8 ml) bottle with a controlled dropper tip and a tan, high impact polystyrene (HIPS) cap.

Storage: Store between 15-25°C (59-77°F). Protect from freezing.

PRODUCT LISTING - EQUIVALENTS NOT AVAILABLE

Solution - Intravenous - 2 mg/ml
100 ml x 10 $180.00 TEQUIN, Bristol-Myers Squibb 00015-1180-80

200 ml x 10	$380.50	TEQUIN, Bristol-Myers Squibb	00015-1181-80
Solution - Intravenous - 10 mg/ml			
40 ml	$38.05	TEQUIN, Bristol-Myers Squibb	00015-1179-80
Tablet - Oral - 200 mg			
30's	$282.08	TEQUIN, Bristol-Myers Squibb	00015-1117-50
100's	$940.25	TEQUIN, Bristol-Myers Squibb	00015-1117-80
Tablet - Oral - 400 mg			
7's	$48.97	TEQUIN, Allscripts Pharmaceutical Company	54569-4921-00
10's	$69.96	TEQUIN, Allscripts Pharmaceutical Company	54569-4921-01
14's	$114.41	TEQUIN TEQPAQ, Bristol-Myers Squibb	00015-1177-19
15's	$141.03	TEQUIN TEQPAQ, Bristol-Myers Squibb	00015-1177-21
50's	$470.13	TEQUIN, Bristol-Myers Squibb	00015-1177-60
100's	$940.25	TEQUIN, Bristol-Myers Squibb	00015-1177-80

Gefitinib *(003596)*

Categories: Carcinoma, lung; Pregnancy Category D; FDA Approved 2003 May
Drug Classes: Antineoplastics, signal transduction inhibitors
Brand Names: Iressa
Cost of Therapy: $1,950.00 (Lung Cancer; Iressa; 250 mg; 1 tablet/day; 30 day supply)

DESCRIPTION

FOR ONCOLOGY USE ONLY.

Iressa tablets contain 250 mg of gefitinib and are available as brown film-coated tablets for daily oral administration.

Gefitinib is an anilinoquinazoline with the chemical name 4-Quinazolinamine, *N*-(3-chloro-4-fluorophenyl)-7-methoxy-6-[3-4-morpholin) propoxy].

It has the molecular formula $C_{22}H_{24}ClFN_4O_3$, a relative molecular mass of 446.9 and is a white-colored powder. Gefitinib is a free base. The molecule has pK_as of 5.4 and 7.2 and therefore ionizes progressively in solution as the pH falls. Gefitinib can be defined as sparingly soluble at pH 1, but is practically insoluble above pH 7, with the solubility dropping sharply between pH 4 and pH 6. In non-aqueous solvents, gefitinib is freely soluble in glacial acetic acid and dimethylsulphoxide, soluble in pyridine, sparingly soluble in tetrahydrofuran, and slightly soluble in methanol, ethanol (99.5%), ethyl acetate, propan-2-ol and acetonitrile.

The inactive ingredients of Iressa tablets are: *Tablet core:* Lactose monohydrate, microcrystalline cellulose, croscarmellose sodium, povidone, sodium lauryl sulfate and magnesium stearate. *Coating:* Hydroxypropyl methylcellulose, polyethylene glycol 300, titanium dioxide, red ferric oxide and yellow ferric oxide.

CLINICAL PHARMACOLOGY

MECHANISM OF ACTION

The mechanism of the clinical antitumor action of gefitinib is not fully characterized. Gefitinib inhibits the intracellular phosphorylation of numerous tyrosine kinases associated with transmembrane cell surface receptors, including the tyrosine kinases associated with the epidermal growth factor receptor (EGFR-TK). EGFR is expressed on the cell surface of many normal cells and cancer cells. No clinical studies have been performed that demonstrate a correlation between EGFR receptor expression and response to gefitinib.

PHARMACOKINETICS

Gefitinib is absorbed slowly after oral administration with mean bioavailability of 60%. Elimination is by metabolism (primarily CYP 3A4) and excretion in feces. The elimination half-life is about 48 hours. Daily oral administration of gefitinib to cancer patients resulted in a 2-fold accumulation compared to single dose administration. Steady state plasma concentrations are achieved within 10 days.

Absorption and Distribution

Gefitinib is slowly absorbed, with peak plasma levels occurring 3-7 hours after dosing and mean oral bioavailability of 60%. Bioavailability is not significantly altered by food. Gefitinib is extensively distributed throughout the body with a mean steady state volume of distribution of 1400 L following intravenous administration. *In vitro* binding of gefitinib to human plasma proteins (serum albumin and α1-acid glycoprotein) is 90% and is independent of drug concentrations.

Metabolism and Elimination

Gefitinib undergoes extensive hepatic metabolism in humans, predominantly by CYP3A4. Three sites of biotransformation have been identified: metabolism of the N-propoxymorpholino-group, demethylation of the methoxy-substituent on the quinazoline, and oxidative defluorination of the halogenated phenyl group.

Five metabolites were identified in human plasma. Only O-desmethyl gefitinib has exposure comparable to gefitinib. Although this metabolite has similar EGFR-TK activity to gefitinib in the isolated enzyme assay, it had only 1/14 of the potency of gefitinib in one of the cell-based assays.

Gefitinib is cleared primarily by the liver, with total plasma clearance and elimination half-life values of 595 ml/min and 48 hours, respectively, after intravenous administration. Excretion is predominantly via the feces (86%), with renal elimination of drug and metabolites accounting for less than 4% of the administered dose.

Special Populations

In population based data analyses, no relationships were identified between predicted steady state trough concentration and patient age, body weight, gender, ethnicity or creatinine clearance.

Pediatric

There are no pharmacokinetic data in pediatric patients.

Hepatic Impairment

The influence of hepatic metastases with elevation of serum aspartate aminotransferase (AST/SGOT), alkaline phosphatase, and bilirubin has been evaluated in patients with normal (14 patients), moderately elevated (13 patients) and severely elevated (4 patients) levels of one or more of these biochemical parameters. Patients with moderately and severely elevated biochemical liver abnormalities had gefitinib pharmacokinetics similar to individuals without liver abnormalities (see PRECAUTIONS).

Renal Impairment

No clinical studies were conducted with gefitinib in patients with severely compromised renal function (see PRECAUTIONS). Gefitinib and its metabolites are not significantly excreted via the kidney (<4%).

Drug-Drug Interactions

In human liver microsome studies, gefitinib had no inhibitory effect on CYP1A2, CYP2C9, and CYP3A4 activities at concentrations ranging from 2-5000 ng/ml. At the highest concentration studied (5000 ng/ml), gefitinib inhibited CYP2C19 by 24% and CYP2D6 by 43%. Exposure to metoprolol, a substrate of CYP2D6, was increased by 30% when it was given in combination with gefitinib (500 mg daily for 28 days) in patients with solid tumors.

Rifampicin, an inducer of CYP3A4, reduced mean AUC of gefitinib by 85% in healthy male volunteers (see DRUG INTERACTIONS and DOSAGE AND ADMINISTRATION, Dose Adjustment).

Concomitant administration of itraconazole (200 mg qd for 12 days), an inhibitor of CYP3A4, with gefitinib (250 mg single dose) to healthy male volunteers, increased mean gefitinib AUC by 88% (see DRUG INTERACTIONS).

Co-administration of high doses of ranitidine with sodium bicarbonate (to maintain the gastric pH above pH 5.0) reduced mean gefitinib AUC by 44% (see DRUG INTERACTIONS).

International Normalized Ratio (INR) elevations and/or bleeding events have been reported in some patients taking warfarin while on gefitinib therapy. Patients taking warfarin should be monitored regularly for changes in prothrombin time or INR (see DRUG INTERACTIONS and ADVERSE REACTIONS).

INDICATIONS AND USAGE

Gefitinib is indicated as monotherapy for the treatment of patients with locally advanced or metastatic non-small cell lung cancer after failure of both platinum-based and docetaxel chemotherapies.

The effectiveness of gefitinib is based on objective response rates. There are no controlled trials demonstrating a clinical benefit, such as improvement in disease-related symptoms or increased survival.

Results from two large, controlled, randomized trials in first-line treatment of non-small cell lung cancer showed no benefit from adding gefitinib to doublet, platinum-based chemotherapy. Therefore, gefitinib is not indicated for use in this setting.

CONTRAINDICATIONS

Gefitinib is contraindicated in patients with severe hypersensitivity to gefitinib or to any other component of gefitinib.

WARNINGS

PULMONARY TOXICITY

Cases of interstitial lung disease (ILD) have been observed in patients receiving gefitinib at an overall incidence of about 1%. Approximately 1/3 of the cases have been fatal. The reported incidence of ILD was about 2% in the Japanese post-marketing experience, about 0.3% in approximately 23,000 patients treated with gefitinib in a US expanded access program and about 1% in the studies of first-line use in NSCLC (but with similar rates in both treatment and placebo groups). Reports have described the adverse event as interstitial pneumonia, pneumonitis and alveolitis. Patients often present with the acute onset of dyspnea, sometimes associated with cough or low-grade fever, often becoming severe within a short time and requiring hospitalization. ILD has occurred in patients who have received prior radiation therapy (31% of reported cases), prior chemotherapy (57% of reported patients), and no previous therapy (12% of reported cases). Patients with concurrent idiopathic pulmonary fibrosis whose condition worsens while receiving gefitinib have been observed to have an increased mortality compared to those without concurrent idiopathic pulmonary fibrosis.

In the event of acute onset or worsening of pulmonary symptoms (dyspnea, cough, fever), gefitinib therapy should be interrupted and a prompt investigation of these symptoms should occur. If interstitial lung disease is confirmed, gefitinib should be discontinued and the patient treated appropriately (see PRECAUTIONS, Information for the Patient; ADVERSE REACTIONS; and DOSAGE AND ADMINISTRATION, Dose Adjustment).

PREGNANCY CATEGORY D

Gefitinib may cause fetal harm when administered to a pregnant woman. A single dose study in rats showed that gefitinib crosses the placenta after an oral dose of 5 mg/kg (30 mg/m^2, about 1/5 the recommended human dose on a mg/m^2 basis). When pregnant rats were treated with 5 mg/kg from the beginning of organogenesis to the end of weaning gave birth, there was a reduction in the number of offspring born alive. This effect was more severe at 20 mg/kg and was accompanied by high neonatal mortality soon after parturition. In this study a dose of 1 mg/kg caused no adverse effects.

In rabbits, a dose of 20 mg/kg/day (240 mg/m^2, about twice the recommended dose in humans on a mg/m^2 basis) caused reduced fetal weight.

There are no adequate and well-controlled studies in pregnant women using gefitinib. If gefitinib is used during pregnancy or if the patient becomes pregnant while receiving this drug, she should be apprised of the potential hazard to the fetus or potential risk for loss of the pregnancy.

PRECAUTIONS

HEPATOTOXICITY

Asymptomatic increases in liver transaminases have been observed in gefitinib treated patients; therefore, periodic liver function (transaminases, bilirubin, and alkaline phosphatase) testing should be considered. Discontinuation of gefitinib should be considered if changes are severe.

PATIENTS WITH HEPATIC IMPAIRMENT

In vitro and *in vivo* evidence suggest that gefitinib is cleared primarily by the liver. Therefore, gefitinib exposure may be increased in patients with hepatic dysfunction. In patients with liver metastases and moderately to severely elevated biochemical liver abnormalities, however, gefitinib pharmacokinetics were similar to the pharmacokinetics of individuals without liver abnormalities (see CLINICAL PHARMACOLOGY, Pharmacokinetics, Special Populations). The influence of non-cancer related hepatic impairment on the pharmacokinetics of gefitinib has not been evaluated.

INFORMATION FOR THE PATIENT

Patients should be advised to seek medical advice promptly if they develop (1) severe or persistent diarrhea, nausea, anorexia, or vomiting, as these have sometimes been associated with dehydration; (2) an onset or worsening of pulmonary symptoms, *i.e.*, shortness of breath or cough; (3) an eye irritation; or, (4) any other new symptom (see WARNINGS, Pulmonary Toxicity; ADVERSE REACTIONS; and DOSAGE AND ADMINISTRATION, Dose Adjustment).

Women of childbearing potential must be advised to avoid becoming pregnant (see WARNINGS, Pregnancy Category D).

CARCINOGENESIS, MUTAGENESIS, AND IMPAIRMENT OF FERTILITY

Gefitinib has been tested for genotoxicity in a series of *in vitro* (bacterial mutation, mouse lymphoma, and human lymphocyte) assays and an *in vivo* rat micronucleus test. Under the conditions of these assays, gefitinib did not cause genetic damage.

Carcinogenicity studies have not been conducted with gefitinib.

PREGNANCY CATEGORY D

See WARNINGS and PRECAUTIONS, Information for the Patient.

NURSING MOTHERS

It is not known whether gefitinib is excreted in human milk. Following oral administration of carbon-14 labeled gefitinib to rats 14 days postpartum, concentrations of radioactivity in milk were higher than in blood. Levels of gefitinib and its metabolites were 11- to 19-fold higher in milk than in blood, after oral exposure of lactating rats to a dose of 5 mg/kg. Because many drugs are excreted in human milk and because of the potential for serious adverse reactions in nursing infants, women should be advised against breast-feeding while receiving gefitinib therapy.

PEDIATRIC USE

Safety and effectiveness of gefitinib in pediatric patients have not been studied.

GERIATRIC USE

Of the total number of patients participating in trials of second- and third-line gefitinib treatment of NSCLC, 65% were aged 64 years or less, 30.5% were aged 65-74 years, and 5% of patients were aged 75 years or older. No differences in safety or efficacy were observed between younger and older patients.

PATIENTS WITH SEVERE RENAL IMPAIRMENT

The effect of severe renal impairment on the pharmacokinetics of gefitinib is not known. Patients with severe renal impairment should be treated with caution when given gefitinib.

DRUG INTERACTIONS

Substances that are inducers of CYP3A4 activity increase the metabolism of gefitinib and decrease its plasma concentrations. In patients receiving a potent CYP3A4 inducer such as rifampicin or phenytoin, a dose increase to 500 mg daily should be considered in the absence of severe adverse drug reaction, and clinical response and adverse events should be carefully monitored (see CLINICAL PHARMACOLOGY, Pharmacokinetics, Drug-Drug Interactions and DOSAGE AND ADMINISTRATION, Dose Adjustment).

International Normalized Ratio (INR) elevations and/or bleeding events have been reported in some patients taking warfarin while on gefitinib therapy. Patients taking warfarin should be monitored regularly for changes in prothrombin time or INR (see CLINICAL PHARMACOLOGY, Pharmacokinetics, Drug-Drug Interactions and ADVERSE REACTIONS).

Substances that are potent inhibitors of CYP3A4 activity (*e.g.*, ketoconazole and itraconazole) decrease gefitinib metabolism and increase gefitinib plasma concentrations. This increase may be clinically relevant as adverse experiences are related to dose and exposure; therefore, caution should be used when administering CYP3A4 inhibitors with gefitinib (see CLINICAL PHARMACOLOGY, Pharmacokinetics, Drug-Drug Interactions and ADVERSE REACTIONS).

Drugs that cause significant sustained elevation in gastric pH (histamine H^2-receptor antagonists such as ranitidine or cimetidine) may reduce plasma concentrations of gefitinib and therefore potentially may reduce efficacy (see CLINICAL PHARMACOLOGY, Pharmacokinetics, Drug-Drug Interactions).

ADVERSE REACTIONS

The safety database includes 941 patients from clinical trials and approximately 23,000 patients in the Expanded Access Program.

TABLE 3 includes drug-related adverse events with an incidence of ≥5% for the 216 patients who received either 250 mg or 500 mg of gefitinib monotherapy for treatment of NSCLC. The most common adverse events reported at the recommended 250 mg daily dose were diarrhea, rash, acne, dry skin, nausea, and vomiting (see PRECAUTIONS, Information for the Patient and DOSAGE AND ADMINISTRATION, Dose Adjustment). The 500 mg dose showed a higher rate for most of these adverse events.

TABLE 4 provides drug-related adverse events with an incidence of ≥5% by CTC grade for the patients who received the 250 mg/day dose of gefitinib monotherapy for treatment of NSCLC. Only 2% of patients stopped therapy due to an adverse drug reaction (ADR). The onset of these ADRs occurred within the first month of therapy.

TABLE 3 *Drug-Related Adverse Events With an Incidence of ≥5% in Either 250 mg or 500 mg Dose Group*

Drug-Related Adverse Event*	250 mg/day (n=102)	500 mg/day (n=114)
Diarrhea	49 (48%)	76 (67%)
Rash	44 (43%)	61 (54%)
Acne	25 (25%)	37 (33%)
Dry skin	13 (13%)	30 (26%)
Nausea	13 (13%)	20 (18%)
Vomiting	12 (12%)	10 (9%)
Pruritus	8 (8%)	10 (9%)
Anorexia	7 (7%)	11 (10%)
Asthenia	6 (6%)	5 (4%)
Weight loss	3 (3%)	6 (5%)

* A patient may have had more than 1 drug-related adverse event.

TABLE 4 *Drug Related Adverse Events ≥5% at 250 mg Dose by Worst CTC Grade (n=102)*

		CTC Grade			
Adverse Event	All Grades	1	2	3	4
Diarrhea	48%	41%	6%	1%	0%
Rash	43%	39%	4%	0%	0%
Acne	25%	19%	6%	0%	0%
Dry skin	13%	12%	1%	0%	0%
Nausea	13%	7%	5%	1%	0%
Vomiting	12%	9%	2%	1%	0%
Pruritus	8%	7%	1%	0%	0%
Anorexia	7%	3%	4%	0%	0%
Asthenia	6%	2%	2%	1%	1%

Other adverse events reported at an incidence of <5% in patients who received either 250 mg or 500 mg as monotherapy for treatment of NSCLC (along with their frequency at the 250 mg recommended dose) include the following: peripheral edema (2%), amblyopia (2%), dyspnea (2%), conjunctivitis (1%), vesiculobullous rash (1%), and mouth ulceration (1%).

INTERSTITIAL LUNG DISEASE

Cases of interstitial lung disease (ILD) have been observed in patients receiving gefitinib at an overall incidence of about 1%. Approximately 1/3 of the cases have been fatal. The reported incidence of ILD was about 2% in the Japanese postmarketing experience, about 0.3% in approximately 23,000 patients treated with gefitinib in a US expanded access program and about 1% in the studies of first-line use in NSCLC (but with similar rates in both treatment and placebo groups). Reports have described the adverse event as interstitial pneumonia, pneumonitis and alveolitis. Patients often present with the acute onset of dyspnea, sometimes associated with cough or low-grade fever, often becoming severe within a short time and requiring hospitalization. ILD has occurred in patients who have received prior radiation therapy (31% of reported cases), prior chemotherapy (57% of reported patients), and no previous therapy (12% of reported cases). Patients with concurrent idiopathic pulmonary fibrosis whose condition worsens while receiving gefitinib have been observed to have an increased mortality compared to those without concurrent idiopathic pulmonary fibrosis.

In the event of acute onset or worsening of pulmonary symptoms (dyspnea, cough, fever), gefitinib therapy should be interrupted and a prompt investigation of these symptoms should occur. If interstitial lung disease is confirmed, gefitinib should be discontinued and the patient treated appropriately (see WARNINGS, Pulmonary Toxicity; PRECAUTIONS, Information for the Patient; and DOSAGE AND ADMINISTRATION, Dose Adjustment).

In patients receiving gefitinib therapy, there were reports of eye pain and corneal erosion/ulcer, sometimes in association with aberrant eyelash growth (see PRECAUTIONS, Information for the Patient). There were also rare reports of pancreatitis and very rare reports of corneal membrane sloughing, ocular ischemia/hemorrhage, toxic epidermal necrolysis, erythema multiforme, and allergic reactions, including angioedema and urticaria.

International Normalized Ratio (INR) elevations and/or bleeding events have been reported in some patients taking warfarin while on gefitinib therapy. Patients taking warfarin should be monitored regularly for changes in prothrombin time or INR (see CLINICAL PHARMACOLOGY, Pharmacokinetics, Drug-Drug Interactions and DRUG INTERACTIONS).

Data from non-clinical (*in vitro* and *in vivo*) studies indicate that gefitinib has the potential to inhibit the cardiac action potential repolarization process (*e.g.*, QT interval). The clinical relevance of these findings is unknown.

DOSAGE AND ADMINISTRATION

The recommended daily dose of gefitinib is one 250 mg tablet with or without food. Higher doses do not give a better response and cause increased toxicity.

DOSE ADJUSTMENT

Patients with poorly tolerated diarrhea (sometimes associated with dehydration) or skin adverse drug reactions may be successfully managed by providing a brief (up to 14 days) therapy interruption followed by reinstatement of the 250 mg daily dose.

In the event of acute onset or worsening of pulmonary symptoms (dyspnea, cough, fever), gefitinib therapy should be interrupted and a prompt investigation of these symptoms should occur and appropriate treatment initiated. If interstitial lung disease is confirmed, gefitinib should be discontinued and the patient treated appropriately (see WARNINGS, Pulmonary Toxicity; PRECAUTIONS, Information for the Patient; and ADVERSE REACTIONS).

Patients who develop onset of new eye symptoms such as pain should be medically evaluated and managed appropriately, including gefitinib therapy interruption and removal of an aberrant eyelash if present. After symptoms and eye changes have resolved, the decision should be made concerning reinstatement of the 250 mg daily dose (see PRECAUTIONS, Information for the Patient and ADVERSE REACTIONS).

In patients receiving a potent CYP3A4 inducer such as rifampicin or phenytoin, a dose increase to 500 mg daily should be considered in the absence of severe adverse drug reaction, and clinical response and adverse events should be carefully monitored (see CLINICAL PHARMACOLOGY, Pharmacokinetics, Drug-Drug Interactions and DRUG INTERACTIONS).

No dosage adjustment is required on the basis of patient age, body weight, gender, ethnicity, or renal function; or in patients with moderate to severe hepatic impairment due to liver metastases (see CLINICAL PHARMACOLOGY, Pharmacokinetics, Special Populations).

HOW SUPPLIED

Iressa tablets are supplied as round, biconvex, brown film-coated tablets intagliated with "IRESSA 250" on one side and plain on the other side, each containing 250 mg of gefitinib.
Storage: Store at controlled room temperature 20-25°C (68-77°F).

Gemcitabine Hydrochloride *(003266)*

Categories: Carcinoma, lung; Carcinoma, pancreatic; FDA Approved 1996 May; Pregnancy Category D
Drug Classes: Antineoplastics, antimetabolites
Brand Names: Gemzar
Foreign Brand Availability: Gemcite (India)
HCFA JCODE(S): J9201 200 mg IV

DESCRIPTION

Gemzar (gemcitabine hydrochloride) is a nucleoside analogue that exhibits antitumor activity. Gemcitabine hydrochloride is 2′-deoxy-2′,2′-difluorocytidine monohydrochloride (β-isomer).

The empirical formula for gemcitabine hydrochloride is $C_9H_{11}F_2N_3O_4 \cdot HCl$. It has a molecular weight of 299.66.

Gemcitabine hydrochloride is a white to off-white solid. It is soluble in water, slightly soluble in methanol, and practically insoluble in ethanol and polar organic solvents.

The clinical formulation is supplied in a sterile form for intravenous (IV) use only. Vials of gemcitabine hydrochloride contain either 200 mg or 1 g of gemcitabine hydrochloride (expressed as free base) formulated with mannitol (200 mg or 1 g, respectively) and sodium acetate (12.5 mg or 62.5 mg, respectively) as a sterile lyophilized powder. Hydrochloric acid and/or sodium hydroxide may have been added for pH adjustment.

CLINICAL PHARMACOLOGY

Gemcitabine exhibits cell phase specificity, primarily killing cells undergoing DNA synthesis (S-phase) and also blocking the progression of cells through the G1/S-phase boundary. Gemcitabine is metabolized intracellularly by nucleoside kinases to the active diphosphate (dFdCDP) and triphosphate (dFdCTP) nucleosides. The cytotoxic effect of gemcitabine is attributed to a combination of 2 actions of the diphosphate and the triphosphate nucleosides, which leads to inhibition of DNA synthesis. First, gemcitabine diphosphate inhibits ribonucleotide reductase, which is responsible for catalyzing the reactions that generate the deoxynucleoside triphosphates for DNA synthesis. Inhibition of this enzyme by the diphosphate nucleoside causes a reduction in the concentrations of deoxynucleotides, including dCTP. Second, gemcitabine triphosphate competes with dCTP for incorporation into DNA. The reduction in the intracellular concentration of dCTP (by the action of the diphosphate) enhances the incorporation of gemcitabine triphosphate into DNA (self-potentiation). After the gemcitabine nucleotide is incorporated into DNA, only 1 additional nucleotide is added to the growing DNA strands. After this addition, there is inhibition of further DNA synthesis. DNA polymerase epsilon is unable to remove the gemcitabine nucleotide and repair the growing DNA strands (masked chain termination). In CEM T lymphoblastoid cells, gemcitabine induces internucleosomal DNA fragmentation, one of the characteristics of programmed cell death.

Gemcitabine demonstrated dose-dependent synergistic activity with cisplatin *in vitro*. No effect of cisplatin on gemcitabine triphosphate accumulation or DNA double-strand breaks was observed. *In vivo*, gemcitabine showed activity in combination with cisplatin against the LX-1 and CALU-6 human lung xenografts, but minimal activity was seen with the NCI-H460 or NCI-H520 xenografts. Gemcitabine was synergistic with cisplatin in the Lewis lung murine xenograft. Sequential exposure to gemcitabine 4 hours before cisplatin produced the greatest interaction.

HUMAN PHARMACOKINETICS

Gemcitabine disposition was studied in 5 patients who received a single 1000 mg/m²/30 min infusion of radiolabeled drug. Within 1 week, 92-98% of the dose was recovered, almost entirely in the urine. Gemcitabine (<10%) and the inactive uracil metabolite, 2′-deoxy-2′,2′-difluorouridine (dFdU), accounted for 99% of the excreted dose. The metabolite dFdU is also found in plasma. Gemcitabine plasma protein binding is negligible.

The pharmacokinetics of gemcitabine were examined in 353 patients, about 2/3 men, with various solid tumors. Pharmacokinetic parameters were derived using data from patients treated for varying durations of therapy given weekly with periodic rest weeks and using both short infusions (<70 minutes) and long infusions (70-285 minutes). The total gemcitabine HCl dose varied from 500-3600 mg/m².

Gemcitabine pharmacokinetics are linear and are described by a 2-compartment model. Population pharmacokinetic analyses of combined single and multiple dose studies showed that the volume of distribution of gemcitabine was significantly influenced by duration of infusion and gender. Clearance was affected by age and gender. Differences in either clearance or volume of distribution based on patient characteristics or the duration of infusion result in changes in half-life and plasma concentrations. TABLE 1 shows plasma clearance and half-life of gemcitabine following short infusions for typical patients by age and gender.

Gemcitabine half-life for short infusions ranged from 32-94 minutes, and the value for long infusions varied from 245-638 minutes, depending on age and gender, reflecting a greatly increased volume of distribution with longer infusions. The lower clearance in women and the elderly results in higher concentrations of gemcitabine for any given dose.

TABLE 1 *Gemcitabine Clearance and Half-Life for the "Typical" Patient*

	Clearance		Half-Life*	
Age	Men (L/h/m²)	Women (L/h/m²)	Men (min)	Women (min)
29	92.2	69.4	42	49
45	75.7	57.0	48	57
65	55.1	41.5	61	73
79	40.7	30.7	79	94

* Half-life for patients receiving a short infusion (<70min).

The volume of distribution was increased with infusion length. Volume of distribution of gemcitabine was 50 L/m² following infusions lasting <70 minutes, indicating that gemcitabine, after short infusions, is not extensively distributed into tissues. For long infusions, the volume of distribution rose to 370 L/m², reflecting slow equilibration of gemcitabine within the tissue compartment.

The maximum plasma concentrations of dFdU (inactive metabolite) were achieved up to 30 minutes after discontinuation of the infusions and the metabolite is excreted in urine without undergoing further biotransformation. The metabolite did not accumulate with weekly dosing, but its elimination is dependent on renal excretion, and could accumulate with decreased renal function.

The effects of significant renal or hepatic insufficiency on the disposition of gemcitabine have not been assessed.

The active metabolite, gemcitabine triphosphate, can be extracted from peripheral blood mononuclear cells. The half-life of the terminal phase for gemcitabine triphosphate from mononuclear cells ranges from 1.7-19.4 hours.

DRUG INTERACTIONS

When gemcitabine (1250 mg/m² on Days 1 and 8) and cisplatin (75 mg/m² on Day 1) was administered in NSCLC patients, the clearance of gemcitabine on Day 1 was 128 L/hr/m² and on Day 8 was 107 L/hr/m². The clearance of cisplatin in the same study was reported to be 3.94 mL/min/m² with a corresponding half-life of 134 hours (see DRUG INTERACTIONS).

INDICATIONS AND USAGE

THERAPEUTIC INDICATIONS

Non-Small Cell Lung Cancer

Gemcitabine HCl is indicated in combination with cisplatin for the first-line treatment of patients with inoperable, locally advanced (Stage IIIA or IIIB) or metastatic (Stage IV) non-small cell lung cancer.

Pancreatic Cancer

Gemcitabine HCl is indicated as first-line treatment for patients with locally advanced (non-resectable Stage II or Stage III) or metastatic (Stage IV) adenocarcinoma of the pancreas. Gemcitabine HCl is indicated for patients previously treated with 5-FU.

NON-FDA APPROVED INDICATIONS

Gemcitabine has been used without FDA approval in breast cancer, bladder cancer (with a response rate of 56%), advanced ovarian cancer (20%), squamous cell carcinoma of the head and neck (13%), and renal cell carcinoma (6%). When administered to patients with carcinoma of unknown primary cite, 8% of patients had a partial response and 25% had minor responses or stable disease with improved symptoms. Gemcitabine has been reported to show marginal activity in patients with advanced hepatocellular carcinoma, although the response duration was short lived.

CONTRAINDICATIONS

Gemcitabine HCl is contraindicated in those patients with a known hypersensitivity to the drug (see ADVERSE REACTIONS, Allergic).

WARNINGS

Caution: Prolongation of the infusion time beyond 60 minutes and more frequent than weekly dosing have been shown to increase toxicity.

HEMATOLOGY

Gemcitabine HCl can suppress bone marrow function as manifested by leukopenia, thrombocytopenia and anemia (see ADVERSE REACTIONS), and myelosuppression is usually the dose-limiting toxicity. Patients should be monitored for myelosuppression during therapy. See DOSAGE AND ADMINISTRATION for recommended dose adjustments.

PULMONARY

Pulmonary toxicity has been reported with the use of gemcitabine HCl. In cases of severe lung toxicity, gemcitabine HCl therapy should be discontinued immediately and appropriate supportive care measures instituted (see ADVERSE REACTIONS: Pulmonary and , Post-Marketing Experience).

RENAL

HUS and or renal failure have been reported following 1 or more doses of gemcitabine HCl. Renal failure leading to death or requiring dialysis, despite discontinuation of therapy, has been rarely reported. The majority of the cases of renal failure leading to death were due to HUS (see ADVERSE REACTIONS: Renal and Post-Marketing Experience).

HEPATIC

Serious hepatotoxicity, including liver failure and death has been reported very rarely in patients receiving gemcitabine HCl alone or in combination with other potentially heaptotoxic drugs (see ADVERSE REACTIONS: Hepatic and Post-Marketing Experience).

PREGNANCY CATEGORY D

Gemcitabine HCl can cause fetal harm when administered to a pregnant woman. Gemcitabine is embryotoxic causing fetal malformations (cleft palate, incomplete ossification) at doses of 1.5 mg/kg/day in mice (about 1/200 the recommended human dose on a mg/m^2 basis). Gemcitabine is fetotoxic causing fetal malformations (fused pulmonary artery, absence of gall bladder) at doses of 0.1 mg/kg/day in rabbits (about 1/600 the recommended human dose on a mg/m^2 basis). Embryotoxicity was characterized by decreased fetal viability, reduced live litter sizes, and developmental delays. There are no studies of gemcitabine HCl in pregnant women. If gemcitabine HCl is used during pregnancy, or if the patient becomes pregnant while taking gemcitabine HCl, the patient should be apprised of the potential hazard to the fetus.

G

PRECAUTIONS

GENERAL

Patients receiving therapy with gemcitabine HCl should be monitored closely by a physician experienced in the use of cancer chemotherapeutic agents. Most adverse events are reversible and do not need to result in discontinuation, although doses may need to be withheld or reduced. There was a greater tendency in women, especially older women, not to proceed to the next cycle.

LABORATORY TESTS

Patients receiving gemcitabine HCl should be monitored prior to each dose with a complete blood count (CBC), including differential and platelet count. Suspension or modification of therapy should be considered when marrow suppression is detected (see DOSAGE AND ADMINISTRATION).

Laboratory evaluation of renal and hepatic function should be performed prior to initiation of therapy and periodically thereafter (see WARNINGS).

CARCINOGENESIS, MUTAGENESIS, AND IMPAIRMENT OF FERTILITY

Long-term animal studies to evaluate the carcinogenic potential of gemcitabine HCl have not been conducted. Gemcitabine induced forward mutations *in vitro* in a mouse lymphoma (L5178Y) assay and was clastogenic in an *in vivo* mouse micronucleus assay. Gemcitabine was negative when tested using the Ames, *in vivo* sister chromatid exchange, and *in vitro* chromosomal aberration assays, and did not cause unscheduled DNA synthesis *in vitro*. Gemcitabine IP doses of 0.5 mg/kg/day (about 1/700 the human dose on a mg/m^2 basis) in male mice had an effect on fertility with moderate to severe hypospermatogenesis, decreased fertility, and decreased implantations. In female mice fertility was not affected but maternal toxicities were observed at 1.5 mg/kg/day IV (about 1/200 the human dose on a mg/m^2 basis) and fetotoxicity or embryolethality was observed at 0.25 mg/kg/day IV (about 1/1300 the human dose on a mg/m^2 basis).

PREGNANCY CATEGORY D

See WARNINGS.

NURSING MOTHERS

It is not known whether gemcitabine HCl or its metabolites are excreted in human milk. Because many drugs are excreted in human milk and because of the potential for serious adverse reactions from gemcitabine HCl in nursing infants, the mother should be warned and a decision should be made whether to discontinue nursing or to discontinue the drug, taking into account the importance of the drug to the mother and the potential risk to the infant.

GERIATRIC USE

Gemcitabine HCl clearance is affected by age (see CLINICAL PHARMACOLOGY). There is no evidence, however, that unusual dose adjustments, (*i.e.*, other than those already recommended in DOSAGE AND ADMINISTRATION) are necessary in patients over 65, and, in general adverse reaction rates in the single-agent safety database of 979 patients were similar in patients above and below 65. Grade 3/4 thrombocytopenia was more common in the elderly.

GENDER

Gemcitabine HCl clearance is affected by gender (see CLINICAL PHARMACOLOGY). In the single agent safety database (n=979 patients), however, there is no evidence that unusual dose adjustments (*i.e.*, other than those already recommended in DOSAGE AND ADMINISTRATION) are necessary in women. In general, in single agent studies of gemcitabine adverse reaction rates were similar in men and women, but women, especially older women, were more likely not to proceed to a subsequent cycle and to experience Grade 3/4 neutropenia and thrombocytopenia.

PEDIATRIC USE

Gemcitabine HCl has not been studied in pediatric patients. Safety and effectiveness in pediatric patients have not been established.

PATIENTS WITH RENAL AND HEPATIC IMPAIRMENT

Gemcitabine HCl should be used with caution in patients with preexisting renal impairment or hepatic insufficiency. Gemcitabine HCl has not been studied in patients with significant renal or hepatic impairment.

RADIATION THERAPY

Safe and effective regimens for the administration of gemcitabine HCl with therapeutic doses of radiation have not yet been determined.

DRUG INTERACTIONS

No specific drug interaction studies have been conducted. For information on the pharmacokinetics of gemcitabine HCl and cisplatin in combination, see CLINICAL PHARMACOLOGY, Drug Interactions.

ADVERSE REACTIONS

Gemcitabine HCl has been used in a wide variety of malignancies, both as a single agent and in combination with other cytotoxic drugs. The following discussion focuses on single agent use where the effects of gemcitabine HCl can be most readily determined and on the specific combination use that is the basis for its use in NSCLC.

SINGLE-AGENT USE

Myelosuppression is the principal dose-limiting toxicity with gemcitabine HCl therapy. Dosage adjustments for hematologic toxicity are frequently needed and are described in DOSAGE AND ADMINISTRATION.

The data in TABLE 4 are based on 979 patients receiving gemcitabine HCl as a single-agent administered weekly as a 30 minute infusion for treatment of a wide variety of malignancies. The gemcitabine HCl starting doses ranged from 800-1250 mg/m^2. Data are also shown for the subset of patients with pancreatic cancer treated in five clinical studies. The frequency of all grades and severe (WHO Grade 3/4) adverse events were generally similar in the single-agent safety database of 979 patients and the subset of patients with pancreatic cancer. Adverse reactions reported in the single-agent safety database resulted in discontinuation of gemcitabine HCl therapy in about 10% of patients. In the comparative trial in pancreatic cancer, the discontinuation rate for adverse reactions was 14.3% for the gemcitabine arm and 4.8% for the 5-FU arm.

All WHO-graded laboratory events are listed in TABLE 4, regardless of causality. Non-laboratory adverse events listed in TABLE 4 or discussed below were those reported, regardless of causality, for at least 10% of all patients, except the categories of Extravasation, Allergic, and Cardiovascular and certain specific events under the Renal, Pulmonary, and Infection categories. TABLE 5 presents the data from the comparative trial of gemcitabine HCl and 5-FU in pancreatic cancer for the same adverse events as those in TABLE 4, regardless of incidence.

Hematologic: In studies in pancreatic cancer myelosuppression is the dose-limiting toxicity with gemcitabine, but <1% of patients discontinued therapy for either anemia, leukopenia, or thrombocytopenia. Red blood cell transfusions was required by 19% of patients. The incidence of sepsis was less than 1%. Petechiae or mild blood loss (hemorrhage), from any cause, were reported in 16% of patients; less than 1% of patients required platelet transfusions. Patients should be monitored for myelosuppression during gemcitabine therapy and dosage modified or suspended according to the degree of hematologic toxicity (see DOSAGE AND ADMINISTRATION).

Gastrointestinal: Nausea and vomiting were commonly reported (69%) but were usually of mild to moderate severity. Severe nausea and vomiting (WHO Grade 3/4) occurred in <15% of patients. Diarrhea was reported by 19% of patients, and stomatitis by 11% of patients.

Hepatic: In clinical trials, gemcitabine HCl was associated with transient elevations of 1 or both serum transaminases in approximately 70% of patients, but there was no evidence of increasing hepatic toxicity with either longer duration of exposure to gemcitabine HCl or with greater total cumulative dose. Serious hepatotoxicity, including liver failure and death, has been reported very rarely in patients receiving gemcitabine HCl alone or in combination with other potentially hepatotoxic drugs (see Post-Marketing Experience, Hepatic).

Renal: In clinical trials, mild proteinuria and hematuria were commonly reported. Clinical findings consistent with the hemolytic uremic syndrome (HUS) were reported in 6 of 2429 patients (0.25%) receiving gemcitabine HCl in clinical trials. Four patients developed HUS on gemcitabine HCl therapy, 2 immediately post-therapy. The diagnosis of HUS should be considered if the patient develops anemia with evidence of microangiopathic hemolysis, elevation of bilirubin or LDH, reticulocytosis, severe thrombocytopenia, and/or evidence of renal failure (elevation of serum creatinine or BUN). Gemcitabine HCl therapy should be discontinued immediately. Renal failure may not be reversible even with discontinuation of therapy and dialysis may be required (see Post-Marketing Experience, Renal).

Fever: The overall incidence of fever was 41%. This is in contrast to the incidence of infection (16%) and indicates that gemcitabine HCl may cause fever in the absence of clinical infection. Fever was frequently associated with other flu-like symptoms and was usually mild and clinically manageable.

Rash: Rash was reported in 30% of patients. The rash was typically a macular or finely granular maculopapular pruritic eruption of mild to moderate severity involving the trunk and extremities. Pruritus was reported for 13% of patients.

Pulmonary: In clinical trials, dyspnea, unrelated to underlying disease, has been reported in association with gemcitabine HCl therapy. Dyspnea was occasionally accompanied by bronchospasm. Pulmonary lung toxicity has been reported with the use of gemcitabine HCl (see Post-Marketing Experience, Pulmonary). The etiology of these effects is unknown. If such effects develop, gemcitabine HCl should be discontinued. Early use of supportive care measures may help ameliorate these conditions.

Edema: Edema (13%), peripheral edema (20%) and generalized edema (<1%) were reported. Less than 1% of patients discontinued due to edema.

Flu-Like Symptoms: "Flu syndrome" was reported for 19% of patients. Individual symptoms of fever, asthenia, anorexia, headache, cough, chills, and myalgia were commonly reported. Fever and asthenia were also reported frequently as isolated symptoms. Insomnia, rhinitis, sweating, and malaise were reported infrequently. Less than 1% of patients discontinued due to flu-like symptoms.

Infection: Infections were reported for 16% of patients. Sepsis was rarely reported (<1%).

Alopecia: Hair loss, usually minimal, was reported by 15% of patients.

Neurotoxicity: There was a 10% incidence of mild paresthesias and a <1% rate of severe paresthesias.

Extravasation: Injection-site related events were reported for 4% of patients. There were no reports of injection site necrosis. Gemcitabine HCl is not a vesicant.

Allergic: Bronchospasm was reported for less than 2% of patients. Anaphylactoid reaction has been reported rarely. Gemcitabine HCl should not be administered to patients with a known hypersensitivity to this drug (see CONTRAINDICATIONS).

Cardiovascular: During clinical trials, 2% of patients discontinued therapy with gemcitabine HCl due to cardiovascular events such as myocardial infarction, cerebrovascular accident, arrhythmia, and hypertension. Many of these patients had a prior history of cardiovascular disease (see Post-Marketing Experience, Cardiovascular).

TABLE 5 *Selected WHO-Graded Adverse Events From Comparative Trial of Gemcitabine HCl and 5-FU in Pancreatic Cancer — WHO Grades (% incidence)**

	Gemcitabine HCl†			5-FU‡		
	All Grades	Grade 3	Grade 4	All Grades	Grade 3	Grade 4
Laboratory§						
Hematologic						
Anemia	65	7	3	45	0	0
Leukopenia	71	10	0	15	2	0
Neutropenia	62	19	7	18	2	3
Thrombocytopenia	47	10	0	15	2	0
Hepatic						
ALT	72	8	2	38	0	0
AST	72	10	2	52	2	0
Alkaline phosphatase	71	16	0	64	10	3
Bilirubin	16	2	2	25	6	3
Renal						
Proteinuria	10	0	0	2	0	0
Hematuria	13	0	0	0	0	0
BUN	8	0	0	10	0	0
Creatinine	2	0	0	0	0	0
Non-Laboratory¤						
Nausea and vomiting	64	10	3	58	5	0
Pain	10	2	0	7	0	0
Fever	30	0	0	16	0	0
Rash	24	0	0	13	0	0
Dyspnea	6	0	0	3	0	0
Constipation	10	3	0	11	2	0
Diarrhea	24	2	0	31	5	0
Hemorrhage	0	0	0	2	0	0
Infection	8	0	0	3	2	0
Alopecia	18	0	0	16	0	0
Stomatitis	14	0	0	15	0	0
Somnolence	5	2	0	7	2	0
Paresthesias	2	0	0	2	0	0

* Grade based on criteria from the World Health Organization (WHO)
† n=58-63; all gemcitabine patients with laboratory or non-laboratory data.
‡ n=61-63; all 5-FU patients with laboratory or non-laboratory data.
§ Regardless of causality.
¤ Non-laboratory events were graded only if assessed to be possibly drug-related.

COMBINATION USE IN NON-SMALL CELL LUNG CANCER

TABLE 4 *Selected WHO-Graded Adverse Events in Patients Receiving Single Agent Gemcitabine HCl — WHO Grades (% incidence)**

	All Patients†			Pancreatic Cancer Patients‡			Discontinuations (%)§
	All Grades	Grade 3	Grade 4	All Grades	Grade 3	Grade 4	All Patients
Laboratory¤							
Hematologic							
Anemia	68	7	1	73	8	2	<1
Leukopenia	62	9	<1	64	8	1	<1
Neutropenia	63	19	6	61	17	7	—
Thrombocytopenia	24	4	1	36	7	<1	<1
Hepatic							<1
ALT	68	8	2	72	10	1	
AST	67	6	2	78	12	5	
Alkaline phosphatase	55	7	2	77	16	4	
Bilirubin	13	2	<1	26	6	2	
Renal							<1
Proteinuria	45	<1	0	32	<1	0	
Hematuria	35	<1	0	23	0	0	
BUN	16	0	0	15	0	0	
Creatinine	8	<1	0	6	0	0	
Non-Laboratory¶							
Nausea and vomiting	69	13	1	71	10	2	<1
Pain	48	9	<1	42	6	<1	<1
Fever	41	2	0	38	2	0	<1
Rash	30	<1	0	28	<1	0	<1
Dyspnea	23	3	<1	10	0	<1	<1
Constipation	23	1	<1	31	3	<1	0
Diarrhea	19	1	0	30	3	0	0
Hemorrhage	17	<1	<1	4	2	<1	<1
Infection	16	1	<1	10	2	<1	<1
Alopecia	15	<1	0	16	0	0	0
Stomatitis	11	<1	0	10	<1	0	<1
Somnolence	11	<1	<1	11	2	<1	<1
Paresthesias	10	<1	0	10	<1	0	0

* Grade based on criteria from the World Health Organization (WHO).
† n=699-974; all patients with laboratory or non-laboratory data.
‡ n=161-241; all pancreatic cancer patients with laboratory or non-laboratory data.
§ n=979.
¤ Regardless of causality.
¶ Table includes non-laboratory data with incidence for all patients ≥10%. For approximately 60% of the patients, non-laboratory events were graded only if assessed to be possibly drug-related.

In the gemcitabine HCl plus cisplatin versus cisplatin study, dose adjustments occurred with 35% of gemcitabine HCl injections and 17% of cisplatin injections on the combination arm, versus 6% on the cisplatin only arm. Dose adjustments were required in greater than 90% of patients on the combination, versus 16% on cisplatin. Study discontinuations for possibly drug-related adverse events occurred in 15% of patients on the combination arm and 8% of patients on the cisplatin arm. With a median of 4 cycles of gemcitabine HCl plus cisplatin treatment, 94 of 262 patients (36%) experienced a total of 149 hospitalizations due to possibly treatment-related adverse events. With a median of 2 cycles of cisplatin treatment, 61 of 260 patients (23%) experienced 78 hospitalizations due to possibly treatment-related adverse events.

In the gemcitabine HCl plus cisplatin versus etoposide plus cisplatin study, dose adjustments occurred with 20% of gemcitabine HCl injections and 16% of cisplatin injections in the gemcitabine HCl plus cisplatin arm compared with 20% of etoposide injections and 15% of cisplatin injections in the etoposide plus cisplatin arm. With a median of 5 cycles of gemcitabine HCl plus cisplatin treatment, 15 of 69 patients (22%) experienced 15 hospitalizations due to possibly treatment-related adverse events. With a median of 4 cycles of etoposide plus cisplatin treatment, 18 of 66 patients (27%) experienced 22 hospitalizations due to possibly treatment related adverse events. In patients who completed more than 1 cycle, dose adjustments were reported in 81% of the gemcitabine HCl plus cisplatin patients, compared with 68% on the etoposide plus cisplatin arm. Study discontinuations for possibly drug-related adverse events occurred in 14% of patients on the gemcitabine plus cisplatin arm and in 8% of patients on the etoposide plus cisplatin arm. The incidence of myelosuppression was increased in frequency with gemcitabine HCl plus cisplatin treatment (~90%) compared to that with the gemcitabine HCl monotherapy (~60%). With combination therapy gemcitabine HCl dosage adjustments for hematologic toxicity were required more often while cisplatin dose adjustments were less frequently required.

TABLE 6 presents the safety data from the gemcitabine HCl plus cisplatin versus cisplatin study in non-small cell lung cancer. The NCI Common Toxicity Criteria (CTC) were used. The 2 drug combination was more myelosuppressive with four (1.5%) possibly treatment-related deaths, including 3 resulting from myelosuppression with infection and 1 case of renal failure associated with pancytopenia and infection. No deaths due to treatment were reported on the cisplatin arm. Nine cases of febrile neutropenia were reported on the combination therapy arm compared to 2 on the cisplatin arm. More patients required RBC and platelet transfusions on the gemcitabine HCl plus cisplatin arm.

Myelosuppression occurred more frequently on the combination arm, and in 4 possibly treatment-related deaths myelosuppression was observed. Sepsis was reported in 4% of patients on the gemcitabine HCl plus cisplatin arm compared to 1% on the cisplatin arm. Platelet transfusions were required in 21% of patients on the combination arm and <1% of patients on the cisplatin arm. Hemorrhagic events occurred in 14% of patients on the combination arm and 4% on the cisplatin arm. However, severe hemorrhagic events were rare. Red blood cell transfusions were required in 39% of the patients on the gemcitabine HCl plus cisplatin arm, versus 13% on the cisplatin arm. The data suggest cumulative anemia with continued gemcitabine HCl plus cisplatin use.

Nausea and vomiting despite the use of antiemetics occurred slightly more often with gemcitabine HCl plus cisplatin therapy (78%) than with cisplatin alone (71%). In studies with single-agent gemcitabine HCl, a lower incidence of nausea and vomiting (58-69%) was reported. Renal function abnormalities, hypomagnesemia, neuromotor, neurocortical, and neurocerebellar toxicity occurred more often with gemcitabine HCl plus cisplatin than with cisplatin monotherapy. Neurohearing toxicity was similar on both arms.

Cardiac dysrrhythmias of Grade 3 or greater were reported in 7 (3%) patients treated with gemcitabine HCl plus cisplatin compared to one (<1%) Grade 3 dysrrhythmia reported with cisplatin therapy. Hypomagnesemia and hypokalemia were associated with one Grade 4 arrhythmia on the gemcitabine HCl plus cisplatin combination arm.

TABLE 7 presents data from the randomized study of gemcitabine HCl plus cisplatin versus etoposide plus cisplatin in 135 patients with NSCLC for the same WHO-graded adverse events as those in TABLE 5. One death (1.5%) was reported on the gemcitabine HCl plus cisplatin arm due to febrile neutropenia associated with renal failure which was possibly treatment-related. No deaths related to treatment occurred on the etoposide plus cisplatin arm. The overall incidence of Grade 4 neutropenia on the gemcitabine HCl plus cisplatin arm was less than on the etoposide plus cisplatin arm (28% vs 56%). Sepsis was experienced by 2% of patients on both treatment arms. Grade 3 anemia and Grade 3/4 thrombocytopenia were more common on the gemcitabine HCl plus cisplatin arm. RBC transfusions were given to 29% of the patients who received gemcitabine HCl plus cisplatin versus 21% of patients who received etoposide plus cisplatin. Platelet transfusions were given to 3% of the patients who received gemcitabine HCl plus cisplatin versus 8% of patients who received etoposide plus cisplatin. Grade 3/4 nausea and vomiting were also more common on the gemcitabine HCl plus cisplatin arm. On the gemcitabine HCl plus cisplatin arm, 7% of participants were hospitalized due to febrile neutropenia compared to 12% on the etoposide plus cisplatin arm. More than twice as many patients had dose reductions or omissions of a scheduled dose of gemcitabine HCl as compared to etoposide, which may explain the differences in the incidence of neutropenia and febrile neutropenia between treatment arms. Flu syndrome was reported by 3% of patients on the gemcitabine HCl plus cisplatin arm with none reported on the comparator arm. Eight (8) patients (12%) on the gemcitabine HCl plus cisplatin arm reported edema compared to 1 patient (2%) on the etoposide plus cisplatin arm.

***TABLE 6** Selected CTC-Graded Adverse Events From Comparative Trial of Gemcitabine Plus Cisplatin Versus Single-Agent Cisplatin in NSCLC — CTC Grades (% incidence)**

	Gemcitabine HCl plus Cisplatin†			Cisplatin‡		
	All Grades	**Grade 3**	**Grade 4**	**All Grades**	**Grade 3**	**Grade 4**
Laboratory§						
Hematologic						
Anemia	89	22	3	67	6	1
RBC Transfusions¤	39			13		
Leukopenia	82	35	11	25	2	1
Neutropenia	79	22	35	20	3	1
Thrombocytopenia	85	25	25	13	3	1
Platelet Transfusions¤	21			<1		
Lymphocytes	75	25	18	51	12	5
Hepatic						
Transaminase	22	2	1	10	1	0
Alkaline phosphatase	19	1	0	13	0	0
Renal						
Proteinuria	23	0	0	18	0	0
Hematuria	15	0	0	13	0	0
Creatinine	38	4	<1	31	2	<1
Other Laboratory						
Hyperglycemia	30	4	0	23	3	0
Hypomagnesemia	30	4	3	17	2	0
Hypocalcemia	18	2	0	7	0	<1
Non-Laboratory¶						
Nausea	93	25	2	87	20	<1
Vomiting	78	11	12	71	10	9
Alopecia	53	1	0	33	0	0
Neuro motor	35	12	0	15	3	0
Constipation	28	3	0	21	0	0
Neuro hearing	25	6	0	21	6	0
Diarrhea	24	2	2	13	0	0
Neuro sensory	23	1	0	18	1	0
Infection	18	3	2	12	1	0
Fever	16	0	0	5	0	0
Neuro cortical	16	3	1	9	1	0
Neuro mood	16	1	0	10	1	0
Local	15	0	0	6	0	0
Neuro headache	14	0	0	7	0	0
Stomatitis	14	1	0	5	0	0
Hemorrhage	14	1	0	4	0	0
Dyspnea	12	4	3	11	3	2
Hypotension	12	1	0	7	1	0
Rash	11	0	0	3	0	0

* Grade based on Common Toxicity Criteria (CTC). Table includes data for adverse events with incidence ≥10% in either arm.
† n=217-253; all gemcitabine HCl plus cisplatin patients with laboratory or non-laboratory data. Gemcitabine HCl at 1000 mg/m^2 on Days 1, 8, and 15 and cisplatin at 100 mg/m^2 on Day 1 every 28 days.
‡ n=213-248; all cisplatin patients with laboratory data. Cisplatin at 100 mg/m^2 on Day 1 every 28 days.
§ Regardless of causality.
¤ Percent of patients receiving transfusions. Percent transfusions are not CTC-graded events.
¶ Non-laboratory events were graded only if assessed to be possibly drug-related.

POST-MARKETING EXPERIENCE

The following adverse events have been identified during post-approval use of gemcitabine HCl. These events have occurred after gemcitabine HCl single-agent use and gemcitabine HCl in combination with other cytotoxic agents. Decisions to include these events are based on the seriousness of the event, frequency of reporting, or potential causal connection to gemcitabine HCl.

Cardiovascular

Congestive heart failure and myocardial infarction have been reported very rarely with the use of gemcitabine HCl. Arrhythmias, predominantly supraventricular in nature, have been reported very rarely.

Vascular Disorders

Vascular toxicity reported with gemcitabine HCl includes clinical signs of vasculitis which has been reported very rarely. Gangrene has also been reported very rarely.

Skin

Cellulitis and non-serious injection site reactions in the absence of extravasation have been rarely reported.

Hepatic

Serious hepatotoxicity, including liver failure and death has been reported very rarely in patients receiving gemcitabine HCl alone or in combination with other potentially hepatotoxic drugs.

***TABLE 7** Selected WHO-Graded Adverse Events from Comparative Trial of Gemcitabine HCl Plus Cisplatin Versus Etoposide Plus Cisplatin in NSCLC — WHO Grades (% Incidence)**

	Gemcitabine HCl Plus Cisplatin†			Etoposide Plus Cisplatin‡		
	All Grades	**Grade 3**	**Grade 4**	**All Grades**	**Grade 3**	**Grade 4**
Laboratory§						
Hematologic						
Anemia	88	22	0	77	13	2
RBC Transfusions¤	29			21		
Leukopenia	86	26	3	87	36	7
Neutropenia	88	36	28	87	20	56
Thrombocytopenia	81	39	16	45	8	5
Platelet Transfusions¤	3			8		
Hepatic						
ALT	6	0	0	12	0	0
AST	3	0	0	11	0	0
Alkaline phosphatase	16	0	0	11	0	0
Bilirubin	0	0	0	0	0	0
Renal						
Proteinuria	12	0	0	5	0	0
Hematuria	22	0	0	10	0	0
BUN	6	0	0	4	0	0
Creatinine	2	0	0	2	0	0
Non-Laboratory¶**						
Nausea and Vomiting	96	35	4	86	19	7
Fever	6	0	0	3	0	0
Rash	10	0	0	3	0	0
Dyspnea	1	0	1	3	0	0
Constipation	17	0	0	15	0	0
Diarrhea	14	1	1	13	0	2
Hemorrhage	9	0	3	3	0	3
Infection	28	3	1	21	8	0
Alopecia	77	13	0	92	51	0
Stomatitis	20	4	0	18	2	0
Somnolence	3	0	0	3	2	0
Paresthesias	38	0	0	16	2	0

* Grade based on criteria from the World Health Organization (WHO).
† n=67-69; all gemcitabine HCl plus cisplatin patients with laboratory or non-laboratory data. Gemcitabine HCl at 1250 mg/m^2 on Days 1 and 8 and cisplatin at 100 mg/m^2 on Day 1 every 21 days.
‡ n=57-63; all cisplatin plus etoposide patients with laboratory data. Cisplatin at 100 mg/m^2 on Day 1 and IV etoposide at 100 mg/m^2 on Days 1, 2, and 3 every 21 days.
§ Regardless of causality.
¤ Percent of patients receiving transfusions. Percent transfusions are not CTC-graded events.
¶ Non-laboratory events were graded only if assessed to be possibly drug-related.
** Pain data were not collected.

Pulmonary

Parenchymal toxicity, including interstitial pneumonitis, pulmonary fibrosis, pulmonary edema, and adult respiratory distress syndrome (ARDS) has been reported rarely following 1 or more doses of gemcitabine HCl administered to patients with various malignancies. Some patients experienced the onset of pulmonary symptoms up to 2 weeks after the last gemcitabine HCl dose. Respiratory failure and death occurred very rarely in some patients despite discontinuation of therapy.

Renal

HUS and or renal failure have been reported following 1 or more doses of gemcitabine HCl. Renal failure leading to death or requiring dialysis, despite discontinuation of therapy, has been rarely reported. The majority of the cases of renal failure leading to death were due to HUS.

DOSAGE AND ADMINISTRATION

Gemcitabine HCl is for intravenous use only.

Adults

SINGLE-AGENT USE

Pancreatic Cancer

Gemcitabine HCl should be administered by IV infusion at a dose of 1000 mg/m^2 over 30 minutes once weekly for up to 7 weeks (or until toxicity necessitates reducing or holding a dose), followed by a week of rest from treatment. Subsequent cycles should consist of infusions once weekly for 3 consecutive weeks out of every 4 weeks.

Dose Modifications

Dosage adjustment is based upon the degree of hematologic toxicity experienced by the patient (see WARNINGS). Clearance in women and the elderly is reduced and women were somewhat less able to progress to subsequent cycles (see CLINICAL PHARMACOLOGY, Human Pharmacokinetics and PRECAUTIONS).

Patients receiving gemcitabine HCl should be monitored prior to each dose with a complete blood count (CBC), including differential and platelet count. If marrow suppression is detected, therapy should be modified or suspended according to the guidelines in TABLE 8.

Laboratory evaluation of renal and hepatic function, including transaminases and serum creatinine, should be performed prior to initiation of therapy and periodically thereafter.

TABLE 8 *Dosage Reduction Guidelines*

Absolute Granulocyte Count (× 10⁶/L)		Platelet Count (× 10⁶/L)	% of Full Dose
≥1000	and	≥100,000	100
500-999	or	50,000-99,000	75
<500	or	<50,000	Hold

Gemcitabine HCl should be administered with caution in patients with evidence of significant renal or hepatic impairment.

Patients treated with gemcitabine HCl who complete an entire cycle of therapy may have the dose for subsequent cycles increased by 25%, provided that the absolute granulocyte count (AGC) and platelet nadirs exceed 1500 × 10^6/L and 100,000 × 10^6/L, respectively, and if non-hematologic toxicity has not been greater than WHO Grade 1. If patients tolerate the subsequent course of gemcitabine HCl at the increased dose, the dose for the next cycle can be further increased by 20%, provided again that the AGC and platelet nadirs exceed 1500 × 10^6/L and 100,000 × 10^6/L, respectively, and that non-hematologic toxicity has not been greater than WHO Grade 1.

COMBINATION USE

Non-Small Cell Lung Cancer

Two schedules have been investigated and the optimum schedule has not been determined. With the 4 week schedule, gemcitabine HCl should be administered intravenously at 1000 mg/m² over 30 minutes on Days 1, 8, and 15 of each 28 day cycle. Cisplatin should be administered intravenously at 100 mg/m² on Day 1 after the infusion of gemcitabine HCl. With the 3 week schedule, gemcitabine HCl should be administered intravenously at 1250 mg/m² over 30 minutes on Days 1 and 8 of each 21 day cycle. Cisplatin at a dose of 100 mg/m² should be administered intravenously after the infusion of gemcitabine HCl on Day 1. For cisplatin administration and hydration guidelines see manufacturer's prescribing information.

Dose Modifications

Dosage adjustments for hematologic toxicity may be required for gemcitabine HCl and for cisplatin. Gemcitabine HCl dosage adjustment for hematological toxicity is based on the granulocyte and platelet counts taken on the day of therapy. Patients receiving gemcitabine HCl should be monitored prior to each dose with a complete blood count (CBC), including differential and platelet counts. If marrow suppression is detected, therapy should be modified or suspended according to the guidelines in TABLE 8. For cisplatin dosage adjustment, see the prescribing information that accompany drug.

In general, for severe (Grade 3/4) non-hematological toxicity, except alopecia and nausea/vomiting, therapy with gemcitabine HCl plus cisplatin should be held or decreased by 50% depending on the judgement of the treating physician. During combination therapy with cisplatin, serum creatinine, serum potassium, serum calcium, and serum magnesium should be carefully monitored (Grade 3/4; serum creatinine toxicity for gemcitabine HCl plus cisplatin was 5% vs 2% for cisplatin alone).

Gemcitabine HCl may be administered on an outpatient basis.

INSTRUCTIONS FOR USE/HANDLING

The recommended diluent for reconstitution of gemcitabine HCl is 0.9% sodium chloride injection without preservatives. Due to solubility considerations, the maximum concentration for gemcitabine HCl upon reconstitution is 40 mg/ml. Reconstitution at concentrations greater than 40 mg/ml may result in incomplete dissolution, and should be avoided.

To reconstitute, add 5 ml of 0.9% sodium chloride injection to the 200 mg vial or 25 ml of 0.9% sodium chloride injection to the 1 g vial. Shake to dissolve. These dilutions each yield a gemcitabine concentration of 38 mg/ml which includes accounting for the displacement volume of the lyophilized powder (0.26 ml for the 200 mg vial or 1.3 ml for the 1 g vial). The total volume upon reconstitution will be 5.26 ml or 26.3 ml, respectively. Complete withdrawal of the vial contents will provide 200 mg or 1 g of gemcitabine, respectively. The appropriate amount of drug may be administered as prepared or further diluted with 0.9% sodium chloride injection to concentrations as low as 0.1 mg/ml.

Reconstituted gemcitabine HCl is a clear, colorless to light straw-colored solution. After reconstitution with 0.9% sodium chloride injection, the pH of the resulting solution lies in the range of 2.7-3.3. The solution should be inspected visually for particulate matter and discoloration, prior to administration, whenever solution or container permit. If particulate matter or discoloration is found, do not administer.

When prepared as directed, gemcitabine HCl solutions are stable for 24 hours at controlled room temperature 20-25°C (68-77°F). Discard unused portion. Solutions of reconstituted gemcitabine HCl should not be refrigerated, as crystallization may occur.

The compatibility of gemcitabine HCl with other drugs has not been studied. No incompatibilities have been observed with infusion bottles or polyvinyl chloride bags and administration sets.

Unopened vials of gemcitabine HCl are stable until the expiration date indicated on the package when stored at controlled room temperature 20-25°C (68-77°F).

Caution should be exercised in handling and preparing gemcitabine HCl solutions. The use of gloves is recommended. If gemcitabine HCl solution contacts the skin or mucosa, immediately wash the skin thoroughly with soap and water or rinse the mucosa with copious amounts of water. Although acute dermal irritation has not been observed in animal studies, 2 of 3 rabbits exhibited drug-related systemic toxicities (death, hypoactivity, nasal discharge, shallow breathing) due to dermal absorption.

Procedures for proper handling and disposal of anti-cancer drugs should be considered. Several guidelines on this subject have been published.[1-8] There is no general agreement that all of the procedures recommended in the guidelines are necessary or appropriate.

HOW SUPPLIED

Gemzar is supplied as:

200 mg: White, lyophilized powder in a 10 ml size sterile single use vial.

1 g: White, lyophilized powder in a 50 ml size sterile single use vial.

Storage: Store at controlled room temperature (20-25°C) (68-77°F). The USP has defined controlled room temperature as "A temperature maintained thermostatically that encompasses the usual and customary working environment of 20-25°C (68-77°F); that results in a mean kinetic temperature calculated to be not more than 25°C; and that allows for excursions between 15 and 30°C (59 and 86°F) that are experienced in pharmacies, hospitals, and warehouses."

PRODUCT LISTING - EQUIVALENTS NOT AVAILABLE

Powder For Injection - Intravenous - 1 Gm
1's $636.90 GEMZAR, Lilly, Eli and Company 00002-7502-01

Powder For Injection - Intravenous - 200 mg
1's $127.38 GEMZAR, Lilly, Eli and Company 00002-7501-01

Gemfibrozil *(001351)*

For related information, see the comparative table section in Appendix A.

Categories: Hypercholesterolemia; Hyperlipidemia; Hyperlipoproteinemia; Hypertriglyceridemia; Pregnancy Category C; FDA Approved 1986 Nov

Drug Classes: Antihyperlipidemics; Fibric acid derivatives

Brand Names: **Lopid**; Tripid

Foreign Brand Availability: Apo-Gemfibrozil (New-Zealand); Ausgem (Australia); Bolutol (Spain); Brozil (Malaysia); Chlorestrol (Thailand); Cholespid (Philippines); Clearol (Taiwan); Decrelip (Spain); Elmogan (Hong-Kong); Fetinor (Indonesia); Fibralip (Indonesia); Fibrocit (Italy); Gemd (Taiwan); Gemfi (Germany); Gemfibril (Thailand); Gemfibromax (Australia); Gemizol (New-Zealand); Gemlipid (Italy; Turkey); Gemnpid (Taiwan); Gemzil (Hong-Kong); Gevilon (Czech-Republic; Finland; Germany; Hungary; Poland; Switzerland); Gevilon Uno (Germany); Gozid (Thailand); Grifogemzilo (Peru); Hidil (Thailand); Hipolixan (Ecuador); Ipolipid (Bahrain; Benin; Burkina-Faso; Cyprus; Egypt; Ethiopia; Gambia; Ghana; Guinea; Hong-Kong; Iran; Iraq; Israel; Ivory-Coast; Jordan; Kenya; Kuwait; Lebanon; Liberia; Libya; Malawi; Malaysia; Mali; Mauritania; Mauritius; Morocco; Niger; Nigeria; Oman; Qatar; Republic-of-Yemen; Saudi-Arabia; Senegal; Seychelles; Sierra-Leone; South-Africa; Sudan; Syria; Tanzania; Tunia; Uganda; United-Arab-Emirates; Zambia; Zimbabwe); Jezil (Australia; New-Zealand); Lanaterom (Indonesia); Lifibron (Indonesia); Lipazil (Australia); Lipidys (Thailand); Lipigem (India; Philippines); Lipira (Indonesia); Lipison (Hong-Kong); Lipistorol (Hong-Kong); Lipizyl (India); Lipofor (Hong-Kong); Lipolo (Thailand); Lipur (France); Lowin (Hong-Kong); Low-Lip (Bahrain; Cyprus; Egypt; Iran; Iraq; Israel; Jordan; Kuwait; Lebanon; Libya; Oman; Qatar; Republic-of-Yemen; Saudi-Arabia; Syria; United-Arab-Emirates); Manobrozil (Thailand); Normolip (Benin; Burkina-Faso; Ethiopia; Gambia; Ghana; Guinea; India; Ivory-Coast; Kenya; Liberia; Malawi; Mali; Mauritania; Mauritius; Morocco; Niger; Nigeria; Senegal; Seychelles; Sierra-Leone; South-Africa; Sudan; Tanzania; Tunia; Uganda; Zambia; Zimbabwe); Panazil (Taiwan); Polyxit (Thailand); Progemzal (Indonesia); Reducel (Philippines); Regulip (Bahrain; Benin; Burkina-Faso; Cyprus; Egypt; Ethiopia; Gambia; Ghana; Guinea; Iran; Iraq; Israel; Ivory-Coast; Jordan; Kenya; Kuwait; Lebanon; Liberia; Libya; Malawi; Mali; Mauritania; Mauritius; Morocco; Niger; Nigeria; Oman; Qatar; Republic-of-Yemen; Saudi-Arabia; Senegal; Seychelles; Sierra-Leone; South-Africa; Sudan; Syria; Tanzania; Tunia; Uganda; United-Arab-Emirates; Zambia; Zimbabwe); Synbrozil (Hong-Kong); Triglizil (Colombia); Zilop (Colombia; Indonesia)

Cost of Therapy: $99.88 (Hypertriglyceridemia; Lopid; 600 mg; 2 tablets/day; 30 day supply)
$53.50 (Hypertriglyceridemia; Generic Tablets; 600 mg; 2 tablets/day; 30 day supply)

DESCRIPTION

Lopid (gemfibrozil tablets) is a lipid regulating agent. It is available as tablets for oral administration. Each tablet contains 600 mg gemfibrozil. Each also contains calcium stearate, candelilla wax, microcrystalline cellulose, hydroxypropyl cellulose, hydroxypropylmethylcellulose, methylparaben, Opaspray white; polyethylene glycol, polysorbate 80, propylparaben, colloidal silicon dioxide, pregelatinized starch. The chemical name is 5-(2,5-dimethylphenoxy)-2,2-dimethylpentanoic acid.

The empirical formula is $C_{15}H_{22}O_3$ and the molecular weight is 250.35; the solubility in water and acid is 0.0019% and in dilute base it is greater than 1%. The melting point is 58-61°C.

Gemfibrozil is a white solid which is stable under ordinary conditions.

CLINICAL PHARMACOLOGY

Gemfibrozil is a lipid regulating agent which decreases serum triglycerides and very low density lipoprotein (VLDL) cholesterol, and increases high density lipoprotein (HDL) cholesterol. While modest decreases in total and low density lipoprotein (LDL) cholesterol may be observed with gemfibrozil therapy, treatment of patients with elevated triglycerides due to Type IV hyperlipoproteinemia often results in a rise in LDL-cholesterol. LDL-cholesterol levels in Type IIb patients with elevations of both serum LDL-cholesterol and triglycerides are, in general, minimally affected by gemfibrozil treatment; however, gemfibrozil usually raises HDL-cholesterol significantly in this group. Gemfibrozil increases levels of high density lipoprotein (HDL) subfractions HDL_2 and HDL_3, as well as apolipoproteins AI and AII. Epidemiological studies have shown that both low HDL-cholesterol and high LDL-cholesterol are independent risk factors for coronary heart disease.

In the primary prevention component of the Helsinki Heart Study,[1,2] in which 4081 male patients between the ages of 40 and 55 were studied in a randomized, double-blind, placebo-controlled fashion, gemfibrozil therapy was associated with significant reductions in total plasma triglycerides and a significant increase in high density lipoprotein cholesterol. Moderate reductions in total plasma cholesterol and low density lipoprotein cholesterol were observed for the gemfibrozil treatment group as a whole, but the lipid response was heterogeneous, especially among different Fredrickson types. The study involved subjects with serum non-HDL-cholesterol of over 200 mg/dl and no previous history of coronary heart disease. Over the 5 year study period, the gemfibrozil group experienced a 1.4% absolute (34% relative) reduction in the rate of serious coronary events (sudden cardiac deaths plus fatal and nonfatal myocardial infarctions) compared to placebo, p=0.04 (see TABLE 1). There was a 37% relative reduction in the rate of nonfatal myocardial infarction compared to placebo, equivalent to a treatment-related difference of 13.1 events per 1000 persons. Deaths from any cause during the double-blind portion of the study totaled 44 (2.2%) in the gemfibrozil randomization group and 43 (2.1%) in the placebo group.

Among Fredrickson types, during the 5 year double-blind portion of the primary prevention component of the Helsinki Heart Study, the greatest reduction in the incidence of serious coronary events occurred in Type IIb patients who had elevations of both LDL-cholesterol and total plasma triglycerides. This subgroup of Type IIb gemfibrozil group patients had a lower mean HDL-cholesterol level at baseline than the Type IIa subgroup that

TABLE 1 *Reduction in CHD Rates (events per 1000 patients) by Baseline Lipids* in the Helsinki Heart Study, Years 0-5†*

	Incidence of Events
All Patients	
Placebo	41
Gemfibrozil	27
Difference‡	14
LDL-C >175; HDL-C >46.4	
Placebo	32
Gemfibrozil	29
Difference‡	3
LDL-C >175; TG >177	
Placebo	71
Gemfibrozil	44
Difference‡	27
LDL-C >175; TG >200; HDL-C <35	
Placebo	149
Gemfibrozil	64
Difference‡	85

* Lipid values in mg/dl at baseline.
† Difference in rates between placebo and gemfibrozil groups.
‡ Fatal and nonfatal myocardial infarctions plus sudden cardiac deaths (events per 1000 patients over 5 years).

had elevations of LDL-cholesterol and normal plasma triglycerides. The mean increase in HDL-cholesterol among the Type IIb patients in this study was 12.6% compared to placebo. The mean change in LDL-cholesterol among Type IIb patients was -4.1% with gemfibrozil compared to a rise of 3.9% in the placebo subgroup. The Type IIb subjects in the Helsinki Heart Study had 26 fewer coronary events per 1000 persons over 5 years in the gemfibrozil group compared to placebo. The difference in coronary events was substantially greater between gemfibrozil and placebo for that subgroup of patients with the triad of LDL-cholesterol >175 mg/dl (>4.5 mmol), triglycerides >200 mg/dl (>2.2 mmol), and HDL-cholesterol <35 mg/dl (<0.90 mmol) (see TABLE 1).

Further information is available from a 3.5 year (8.5 year cumulative) follow-up of all subjects who had participated in the Helsinki Heart Study. At the completion of the Helsinki Heart Study, subjects could choose to start, stop, or continue to receive gemfibrozil; without knowledge of their own lipid values or double-blind treatment, 60% of patients originally randomized to placebo began therapy with gemfibrozil and 60% of patients originally randomized to gemfibrozil continued medication. After approximately 6.5 years following randomization, all patients were informed of their original treatment group and lipid values during the 5 years of the doubleblind treatment. After further elective changes in gemfibrozil treatment status, 61% of patients in the group originally randomized to gemfibrozil were taking drug; in the group originally randomized to placebo, 65% were taking gemfibrozil. The event rate per 1000 occurring during the open-label follow-up period is detailed in TABLE 2.

TABLE 2 *Cardiac Events and All-Cause Mortality (events per 1000 patients) Occurring During the 3.5 Year Open-Label Follow-Up to the Helsinki Heart Study**

		Cardiac Events	All-Cause Mortality
PDrop	(n=215)	38.8	41.9
PN	(n=494)	22.9	22.3
PG	(n=1283)	22.5	15.6
GDrop	(n=221)	37.2	72.3
GN	(n=574)	28.3	19.2
GG	(n=1207)	25.4	24.9

* The six open-label groups are designated first by the original randomization (P = Placebo, G = Gemfibrozil) and then by the drug taken in the follow-up period (N = Attend clinic but took no drug, G= Gemfibrozil, Drop = No attendance at clinic during open-label).

Cumulative mortality through 8.5 years showed a 20% relative excess of deaths in the group originally randomized to gemfibrozil versus the originally randomized placebo group and a 20% relative decrease in cardiac events in the group originally randomized to gemfibrozil versus the originally randomized placebo group (see TABLE 3). This analysis of the originally randomized "intent-to-treat" population neglects the possible complicating effects of treatment switching during the open-label phase. Adjustment of hazard ratios taking into account open-label treatment status from years 6.5-8.5 could change the reported hazard ratios for mortality toward unity.

TABLE 3 *Cardiac Events, Cardiac Deaths, Non-Cardiac Deaths and All-Cause Mortality in the Helsinki Heart Study, Years 0-8.5**

	Study Start		Hazard Ratio	
Event	Gemfibrozil	Placebo	G:P†	CI‡
Cardiac events§	110	131	0.80	0.62-1.03
Cardiac deaths	36	38	0.98	0.63-1.54
Non-cardiac deaths	65	45	1.40	0.95-2.05
All-cause mortality	101	83	1.20	0.90-1.61

* Intention-to-Treat Analysis of originally randomized patients neglecting the open-label treatment switches and exposure to study conditions.
† Hazard ratio for risk of event in the group originally randomized to gemfibrozil compared to the group originally randomized to placebo neglecting open-label treatment switch and exposure to study condition.
‡ 95% confidence intervals of gemfibrozil:placebo group hazard ratio.
§ Fatal and non-fatal myocardial infarctions plus sudden cardiac deaths over the 8.5 year period.

It is not clear to what extent the findings of the primary prevention component of the Helsinki Heart Study can be extrapolated to other segments of the dyslipidemic population not studied (such as women, younger or older males, or those with lipid abnormalities limited solely to HDL-cholesterol) or to other lipid-altering drugs.

The secondary prevention component of the Helsinki Heart Study was conducted over 5 years in parallel and at the same centers in Finland in 628 middle-aged males excluded from the primary prevention component of the Helsinki Heart Study because of a history of angina, myocardial infarction or unexplained ECG changes.[3] The primary efficacy endpoint of the study was cardiac events (the sum of fatal and non-fatal myocardial infarctions and sudden cardiac deaths). The hazard ratio (gemfibrozil:placebo) for cardiac events was 1.47 (95% confidence limits 0.88-2.48, p=0.14). Of the 35 patients in the gemfibrozil group who experienced cardiac events, 12 patients suffered events after discontinuation from the study. Of the 24 patients in the placebo group with cardiac events, 4 patients suffered events after discontinuation from the study. There were 17 cardiac deaths in the gemfibrozil group and 8 in the placebo group (hazard ratio 2.18; 95% confidence limits 0.94-5.05, p=0.06). Ten (10) of these deaths in the gemfibrozil group and 3 in the placebo group occurred after discontinuation from therapy. In this study of patients with known or suspected coronary heart disease, no benefit from gemfibrozil treatment was observed in reducing cardiac events or cardiac deaths. Thus, gemfibrozil has shown benefit only in selected dyslipidemic patients without suspected or established coronary heart disease. Even in patients with coronary heart disease and the triad of elevated LDL-cholesterol, elevated triglycerides, plus low HDL-cholesterol, the possible effect of gemfibrozil on coronary events has not been adequately studied.

No efficacy in the patients with established coronary heart disease was observed during the Coronary Drug Project with the chemically and pharmacologically related drug, clofibrate. The Coronary Drug Project was a 6 year randomized, double-blind study involving 1000 clofibrate, 1000 nicotinic acid, and 3000 placebo patients with known coronary heart disease. A clinically and statistically significant reduction in myocardial infarctions was seen in the concurrent nicotinic acid group compared to placebo; no reduction was seen with clofibrate.

The mechanism of action of gemfibrozil has not been definitely established. In man, gemfibrozil has been shown to inhibit peripheral lipolysis and to decrease the hepatic extraction of free fatty acids, thus reducing hepatic triglyceride production. Gemfibrozil inhibits synthesis and increases clearance of VLDL carrier apolipoprotein B, leading to a decrease in VLDL production.

Animal studies suggest that gemfibrozil may, in addition to elevating HDL-cholesterol, reduce incorporation of long-chain fatty acids into newly formed triglycerides, accelerate turnover and removal of cholesterol from the liver, and increase excretion of cholesterol in the feces. Gemfibrozil is well absorbed from the gastrointestinal tract after oral administration. Peak plasma levels occur in 1-2 hours with a plasma half-life of 1.5 hours following multiple doses.

Gemfibrozil is completely absorbed after oral administration of gemfibrozil tablets, reaching peak plasma concentrations 1-2 hours after dosing. Gemfibrozil pharmacokinetics are affected by the timing of meals relative to time of dosing. In one study,[4] both the rate and extent of absorption of the drug were significantly increased when administered 0.5 hour before meals. Average AUC was reduced by 14-44% when gemfibrozil was administered after meals compared to 0.5 hour before meals. In a subsequent study,[4] rate of absorption of gemfibrozil was maximum when administered 0.5 hour before meals with the C_{max} 50-60% greater than when given either with meals or fasting. In this study, there were no significant effects on AUC of timing of dose relative to meals (see DOSAGE AND ADMINISTRATION).

Gemfibrozil mainly undergoes oxidation of a ring methyl group to successively form a hydroxymethyl and a carboxyl metabolite. Approximately 70% of the administered human dose is excreted in the urine, mostly as the glucuronide conjugate, with less than 2% excreted as unchanged gemfibrozil. Six percent (6%) of the dose is accounted for in the feces. Gemfibrozil is highly bound to plasma proteins and there is potential for displacement interactions with other drugs (see PRECAUTIONS).

INDICATIONS AND USAGE

Gemfibrozil is indicated as adjunctive therapy to diet for:

Treatment of adult patients with very high elevations of serum triglyceride levels (Types IV and V hyperlipidemia) who present a risk of pancreatitis and who do not respond adequately to a determined dietary effort to control them. Patients who present such risk typically have serum triglycerides over 2000 mg/dl and have elevations of VLDL-cholesterol as well as fasting chylomicrons (Type V hyperlipidemia). Subjects who consistently have total serum or plasma triglycerides below 1000 mg/dl are unlikely to present a risk of pancreatitis. Gemfibrozil therapy may be considered for those subjects with triglyceride elevations between 1000 and 2000 mg/dl who have a history of pancreatitis or of recurrent abdominal pain typical of pancreatitis. It is recognized that some Type IV patients with triglycerides under 1000 mg/dl may, through dietary or alcoholic indiscretion, convert to a Type V pattern with massive triglyceride elevations accompanying fasting chylomicronemia, but the influence of gemfibrozil therapy on the risk of pancreatitis in such situations has not been adequately studied. Drug therapy is not indicated for patients with Type I hyperlipoproteinemia, who have elevations of chylomicrons and plasma triglycerides, but who have normal levels of very low density lipoprotein (VLDL). Inspection of plasma refrigerated for 14 hours is helpful in distinguishing Types I, IV, and V hyperlipoproteinemia.[5]

Reducing the risk of developing coronary heart disease **only** in Type IIb patients without history of or symptoms of existing coronary heart disease who have had an inadequate response to weight loss, dietary therapy, exercise, and other pharmacologic agents (such as bile acid sequestrants and nicotinic acid, known to reduce LDL- and raise HDL-cholesterol) **and** who have the following triad of lipid abnormalities: low HDL-cholesterol levels in addition to elevated LDL-cholesterol and elevated triglycerides (see WARNINGS, PRECAUTIONS, and CLINICAL PHARMACOLOGY). The National Cholesterol Education Program has defined a serum HDL-cholesterol value that is consistently below 35 mg/dl as constituting an independent risk factor for coronary heart disease.[6] Patients with significantly elevated triglycerides should be closely observed when treated with gemfibrozil. In some patients with high triglyceride levels, treatment with gemfibrozil is associated with a significant increase in LDL-cholesterol. BECAUSE OF POTENTIAL TOXICITY SUCH AS MALIGNANCY, GALLBLADDER DISEASE, ABDOMINAL PAIN LEADING TO APPENDECTOMY AND OTHER ABDOMINAL SURGERIES, AN INCREASED INCIDENCE IN NON-CORONARY MORTALITY, AND THE 44% RELATIVE INCREASE DURING THE TRIAL PERIOD IN AGE-ADJUSTED ALL-CAUSE MORTALITY SEEN WITH THE CHEMICALLY AND PHARMACOLOGICALLY RELATED DRUG, CLOFIBRATE, THE POTENTIAL BENEFIT OF GEMFIBROZIL IN TREATING TYPE IIA PATIENTS WITH ELEVATIONS OF LDL-CHOLESTEROL ONLY IS NOT LIKELY TO OUTWEIGH THE RISKS. GEMFIBROZIL IS ALSO NOT INDICATED FOR THE TREATMENT OF PATIENTS WITH LOW HDL-CHOLESTEROL AS THEIR ONLY LIPID ABNORMALITY.

In a subgroup analysis of patients in the Helsinki Heart Study with above-median HDL-cholesterol values at baseline (greater than 46.4 mg/dl), the incidence of serious coronary events was similar for gemfibrozil and placebo subgroups (see TABLE 1).

The initial treatment for dyslipidemia is dietary therapy specific for the type of lipoprotein abnormality. Excess body weight and excess alcohol intake may be important factors in hypertriglyceridemia and should be managed prior to any drug therapy. Physical exercise can be an important ancillary measure, and has been associated with rises in HDL-cholesterol. Diseases contributory to hyperlipidemia such as hypothyroidism or diabetes mellitus should be looked for and adequately treated. Estrogen therapy is sometimes associated with massive rises in plasma triglycerides, especially in subjects with familial hypertriglyceridemia. In such cases, discontinuation of estrogen therapy may obviate the need for specific drug therapy of hypertriglyceridemia. The use of drugs should be considered only when reasonable attempts have been made to obtain satisfactory results with nondrug methods. If the decision is made to use drugs, the patient should be instructed that this does not reduce the importance of adhering to diet.

CONTRAINDICATIONS

Combination therapy of gemfibrozil with cerivastatin due to the increased risk of myopathy and rhabdomyolysis (see WARNINGS).

Hepatic or severe renal dysfunction, including primary biliary cirrhosis.

Preexisting gallbladder disease (see WARNINGS).

Hypersensitivity to gemfibrozil.

WARNINGS

Because of chemical, pharmacological, and clinical similarities between gemfibrozil and clofibrate, the adverse findings with clofibrate in two large clinical studies may also apply to gemfibrozil. In the first of those studies, the Coronary Drug Project, 1000 subjects with previous myocardial infarction were treated for 5 years with clofibrate. There was no difference in mortality between the clofibrate-treated subjects and 3000 placebo-treated subjects, but twice as many clofibrate-treated subjects developed cholelithiasis and cholecystitis requiring surgery. In the other study, conducted by the World Health Organization (WHO), 5000 subjects without known coronary heart disease were treated with clofibrate for 5 years and followed 1 year beyond. There was a statistically significant, 44%, higher age-adjusted total mortality in the clofibrate-treated than in a comparable placebo-treated control group during the trial period. The excess mortality was due to a 33% increase in non-cardiovascular causes, including malignancy, post-cholecystectomy complications, and pancreatitis. The higher risk of clofibrate-treated subjects for gallbladder disease was confirmed.

Because of the more limited size of the Helsinki Heart Study, the observed difference in mortality from any cause between the gemfibrozil and placebo group is not statistically significantly different from the 29% excess mortality reported in the clofibrate group in the separate WHO study at the 9 year follow-up (see CLINICAL PHARMACOLOGY). Noncoronary heart disease related mortality showed an excess in the group originally randomized to gemfibrozil primarily due to cancer deaths observed during the open-label extension.

During the 5 year primary prevention component of the Helsinki Heart Study, mortality from any cause was 44 (2.2%) in the gemfibrozil group and 43 (2.1%) in the placebo group; including the 3.5 year follow-up period since the trial was completed, cumulative mortality from any cause was 101 (4.9%) in the gemfibrozil group and 83 (4.1%) in the group originally randomized to placebo (hazard ratio 1:20 in favor of placebo). Because of the more limited size of the Helsinki Heart Study, the observed difference in mortality from any cause between the gemfibrozil and placebo groups at Year 5 or at Year 8.5 is not statistically significantly different from the 29% excess mortality reported in the clofibrate group in the separate WHO study at the 9 year follow-up. Noncoronary heart disease related mortality showed an excess in the group originally randomized to gemfibrozil at the 8.5 year follow-up (65 gemfibrozil versus 45 placebo noncoronary deaths).

The incidence of cancer (excluding basal cell carcinoma) discovered during the trial and in the 3.5 years after the trial was completed was 51 (2.5%) in both originally randomized groups. In addition, there were 16 basal cell carcinomas in the group originally randomized to gemfibrozil and 9 in the group randomized to placebo (p=0.22). There were 30 (1.5%) deaths attributed to cancer in the group originally randomized to gemfibrozil and 18 (0.9%) in the group originally randomized to placebo (p=0.11). Adverse outcomes, including coronary events, were higher in gemfibrozil patients in a corresponding study in men with a history of known or suspected coronary heart disease in the secondary prevention component of the Helsinki Heart Study. (See CLINICAL PHARMACOLOGY.)

A comparative carcinogenicity study was also done in rats comparing three drugs in this class: fenofibrate (10 and 60 mg/kg; 0.3 and 1.6 times the human dose), clofibrate (400 mg/kg; 1.6 times the human dose), and gemfibrozil (250 mg/kg; 1.7 times the human dose). Pancreatic acinar adenomas were increased in males and females on fenofibrate; hepatocellular carcinoma and pancreatic acinar adenomas were increased in males and hepatic neoplastic nodules in females treated with clofibrate; hepatic neoplastic nodules were increased in males and females treated with clofibrate; hepatic neoplastic nodules were increased in males and females treated with gemfibrozil while testicular interstitial cell (Leydig cell) tumors were increased in males on all three drugs.

A gallstone prevalence substudy of 450 Helsinki Heart Study participants showed a trend toward a greater prevalence of gallstones during the study within the gemfibrozil treatment group (7.5% vs 4.9% for the placebo group, a 55% excess for the gemfibrozil group). A trend toward a greater incidence of gallbladder surgery was observed for the gemfibrozil group (17 vs 11 subjects, a 54% excess). This result did not differ statistically from the increased incidence of cholecystectomy observed in the WHO study in the group treated with clofibrate. Both clofibrate and gemfibrozil may increase cholesterol excretion into the bile leading to cholelithiasis. If cholelithiasis is suspected, gallbladder studies are indicated. Gemfibrozil therapy should be discontinued if gallstones are found.

Since a reduction of mortality from coronary heart disease has not been demonstrated and because liver and interstitial cell testicular tumors were increased in rats, gemfibrozil should be administered only to those patients described in INDICATIONS AND USAGE. If a significant serum lipid response is not obtained, gemfibrozil should be discontinued.

Concomitant Anticoagulants: Caution should be exercised when anticoagulants are given in conjunction with gemfibrozil. The dosage of the anticoagulant should be reduced to maintain the prothrombin time at the desired level to prevent bleeding complications. Frequent prothrombin determinations are advisable until it has been definitely determined that the prothrombin level has stabilized.

Concomitant therapy with gemfibrozil and an HMG-CoA reductase inhibitor is associated with an increased risk of skeletal muscle toxicity manifested as rhabdomyolysis, markedly elevated creatine kinase (CPK) levels and myoglobinuria, leading in a high proportion of cases to acute renal failure and death. **Because of an observed marked increased risk of myopathy and rhabdomyolysis, the specific combination of gemfibrozil and cerivastatin is absolutely contraindicated (see CONTRAINDICATIONS).** IN PATIENTS WHO HAVE HAD AN UNSATISFACTORY LIPID RESPONSE TO EITHER DRUG ALONE, THE BENEFIT OF COMBINED THERAPY WITH GEMFIBROZIL AND HMG-CoA REDUCTASE INHIBITORS OTHER THAN CERIVASTATIN DOES NOT OUTWEIGH THE RISKS OF SEVERE MYOPATHY, RHABDOMYOLYSIS, AND ACUTE RENAL FAILURE[7-10] (see DRUG INTERACTIONS). The use of fibrates alone, including gemfibrozil may occasionally be associated with myositis. Patients receiving gemfibrozil and complaining of muscle pain, tenderness, or weakness should have prompt medical evaluation for myositis, including serum creatine-kinase level determination. If myositis is suspected or diagnosed, gemfibrozil therapy should be withdrawn.

Cataracts: Subcapsular bilateral cataracts occurred in 10% and unilateral in 6.3% of male rats treated with gemfibrozil at 10 times the human dose.

PRECAUTIONS

INITIAL THERAPY

Laboratory studies should be done to ascertain that the lipid levels are consistently abnormal. Before instituting gemfibrozil therapy, every attempt should be made to control serum lipids with appropriate diet, exercise, weight loss in obese patients, and control of any medical problems such as diabetes mellitus and hypothyroidism that are contributing to the lipid abnormalities.

CONTINUED THERAPY

Periodic determination of serum lipids should be obtained, and the drug withdrawn if lipid response is inadequate after 3 months of therapy.

CARCINOGENESIS, MUTAGENESIS, AND IMPAIRMENT OF FERTILITY

Long-term studies have been conducted in rats at 0.2 and 1.3 times the human exposure (based on AUC). The incidence of benign liver nodules and liver carcinomas was significantly increased in high dose male rats. The incidence of liver carcinomas increased also in low dose males, but this increase was not statistically significant (p=0.1). Male rats had a dose-related and statistically significant increase of benign Leydig cell tumors. The higher dose female rats had a significant increase in the combined incidence of benign and malignant liver neoplasms.

Long-term studies have been conducted in mice at 0.1 and 0.7 times the human exposure (based on AUC). There were no statistically significant differences from controls in the incidence of liver tumors, but the doses tested were lower than those shown to be carcinogenic with other fibrates.

Electron microscopy studies have demonstrated a florid hepatic peroxisome proliferation following gemfibrozil administration to the male rat. An adequate study to test for peroxisome proliferation has not been done in humans but changes in peroxisome morphology have been observed. Peroxisome proliferation has been shown to occur in humans with either of two other drugs of the fibrate class when liver biopsies were compared before and after treatment in the same individual.

Administration of approximately 2 times the human dose (based on surface area) to male rats for 10 weeks resulted in a dose-related decrease of fertility. Subsequent studies demonstrated that this effect was reversed after a drug-free period of about 8 weeks, and it was not transmitted to the offspring.

PREGNANCY CATEGORY C

Gemfibrozil has been shown to produce adverse effects in rats and rabbits at doses between 0.5 and 3 times the human dose (based on surface area). There are no adequate and well-controlled studies in pregnant women. Gemfibrozil should be used during pregnancy only if the potential benefit justifies the potential risk to the fetus.

Administration of gemfibrozil to female rats 2 times the human dose (based on surface area) before and throughout gestation caused a dose-related decrease in conception rate and an increase in stillborns and a slight reduction in pup weight during lactation. There were also dose-related increased skeletal variations. Anophthalmia occurred, but rarely.

G

Administration of 0.6 and 2 times the human dose (based on surface area) of gemfibrozil to female rats from gestation day 15 through weaning caused dose-related decreases in birth weight and suppressions of pup growth during lactation.

Administration of 1 and 3 times the human dose (based on surface area) of gemfibrozil to female rabbits during organogenesis caused a dose-related decrease in litter size and, at the high dose, an increased incidence of parietal bone variations.

NURSING MOTHERS

It is not known whether this drug is excreted in human milk. Because many drugs are excreted in human milk and because of the potential for tumorigenicity shown for gemfibrozil in animal studies, a decision should be made whether to discontinue nursing or to discontinue the drug, taking into account the importance of the drug to the mother.

HEMATOLOGIC CHANGES

Mild hemoglobin, hematocrit and white blood cell decreases have been observed in occasional patients following initiation of gemfibrozil therapy. However, these levels stabilize during long-term administration. Rarely, severe anemia, leukopenia, thrombocytopenia, and bone marrow hypoplasia have been reported. Therefore, periodic blood counts are recommended during the first 12 months of gemfibrozil administration.

LIVER FUNCTION

Abnormal liver function tests have been observed occasionally during gemfibrozil administration, including elevations of AST (SGOT), ALT (SGPT), LDH, bilirubin, and alkaline phosphatase. These are usually reversible when gemfibrozil is discontinued. Therefore, periodic liver function studies are recommended and gemfibrozil therapy should be terminated if abnormalities persist.

KIDNEY FUNCTION

There have been reports of worsening renal insufficiency upon the addition of gemfibrozil therapy in individuals with baseline plasma creatinine >2.0 mg/dl. In such patients, the use of alternative therapy should be considered against the risks and benefits of a lower dose of gemfibrozil.

PEDIATRIC USE

Safety and efficacy in pediatric patients have not been established.

DRUG INTERACTIONS

HMG-COA REDUCTASE INHIBITORS

The risk of myopathy and rhabdomyolysis is increased with combined gemfibrozil and HMG-CoA reductase inhibitor therapy (see CONTRAINDICATIONS). Myopathy or rhabdomyolysis with or without acute renal failure have been reported as early as 3 weeks after initiation of combined therapy or after several months.[7-10] (See WARNINGS.) There is no assurance that periodic monitoring of creatine kinase will prevent the occurrence of severe myopathy and kidney damage.

ANTICOAGULANTS

CAUTION SHOULD BE EXERCISED WHEN ANTI-COAGULANTS ARE GIVEN IN CONJUNCTION WITH GEMFIBROZIL. THE DOSAGE OF THE ANTICOAGULANT SHOULD BE REDUCED TO MAINTAIN THE PROTHROMBIN TIME AT THE DESIRED LEVEL TO PREVENT BLEEDING COMPLICATIONS. FREQUENT PROTHROMBIN DETERMINATIONS ARE ADVISABLE UNTIL IT HAS BEEN DEFINITELY DETERMINED THAT THE PROTHROMBIN LEVEL HAS STABILIZED.

ADVERSE REACTIONS

In the double-blind controlled phase of the primary prevention component of the Helsinki Heart Study, 2046 patients received gemfibrozil for up to 5 years. In that study, the following adverse reactions were statistically more frequent in subjects in the gemfibrozil group (see TABLE 4).

TABLE 4

	Gemfibrozil (n=2046)	Placebo (n=2035)
Gastrointestinal reactions	34.2%	23.8%
Dyspepsia	19.6%	11.9%
Abdominal pain	9.8%	5.6%
Acute appendicitis*	1.2%	0.6%
Atrial fibrillation	0.7%	0.1%
Adverse events reported by more than 1% of subjects, but without a significant difference between groups		
Diarrhea	7.2%	6.5%
Fatigue	3.8%	3.5%
Nausea/vomiting	2.5%	2.1%
Eczema	1.9%	1.2%
Rash	1.7%	1.3%
Vertigo	1.5%	1.3%
Constipation	1.4%	1.3%
Headache	1.2%	1.1%

* Histologically confirmed in most cases where data were available.

Gallbladder surgery was performed in 0.9% of gemfibrozil and 0.5% of placebo subjects in the primary prevention component, a 64% excess, which is not statistically different from the excess of gallbladder surgery observed in the clofibrate compared to the placebo group of the WHO study. Gallbladder surgery was also performed more frequently in the gemfibrozil group compared to placebo (1.9% vs 0.3%, p=0.07) in the secondary prevention component. A statistically significant increase in appendectomy in the gemfibrozil group was seen also in the secondary prevention component (6 on gemfibrozil vs 0 on placebo, p=0.014).

Nervous system and special senses adverse reactions were more common in the gemfibrozil group. These included hypesthesia, paresthesias, and taste perversion. Other adverse reactions that were more common among gemfibrozil treatment group subjects but where a causal relationship was not established include cataracts, peripheral vascular disease, and intracerebral hemorrhage.

From other studies it seems probable that gemfibrozil is causally related to the occurrence of MUSCULOSKELETAL SYMPTOMS (see WARNINGS), and to ABNORMAL LIVER FUNCTION TESTS and HEMATOLOGIC CHANGES (see PRECAUTIONS).

Reports of viral and bacterial infections (common cold, cough, urinary tract infections) were more common in gemfibrozil treated patients in other controlled clinical trials of 805 patients. Additional adverse reactions that have been reported for gemfibrozil are listed below by system. These are categorized according to whether a causal relationship to treatment with gemfibrozil is probable or not established (see TABLE 5).

TABLE 5

	Causal Relationship Probable	Causal Relationship Not Established
General:		Weight loss.
Cardiac:		Extrasystoles.
Gastrointestinal:	Cholestatic jaundice.	Pancreatitis, hepatoma, colitis.
Central Nervous System:	Dizziness, somnolence, paresthesia, peripheral neuritis, decreased libido, depression, headache.	Confusion, convulsions, syncope.
Eye:	Blurred vision.	Retinal edema.
Genitourinary:	Impotence.	Decreased male fertility, renal dysfunction.
Musculoskeletal:	Myopathy, myasthenia, myalgia, painful extremities, arthralgia, synovitis, rhabdomyolysis*.	
Clinical Laboratory:	Increased creatinine phosphokinase, increased bilirubin, increased liver transaminases (AST [SGOT], ALT [SGPT]), increased alkaline phosphatase.	Positive antinuclear antibody.
Hematopoietic:	Anemia, leukopenia, bone marrow hypoplasia, eosinophilia.	Thrombocytopenia.
Immunologic:	Angioedema, laryngeal edema, urticaria.	Anaphylaxis, Lupus-like syndrome, vasculitis.
Integumentary:	Exfoliative dermatitis, rash, dermatitis, pruritus.	Alopecia, photosensitivity.

* See WARNINGS and DRUG INTERACTIONS.

DOSAGE AND ADMINISTRATION

The recommended dose for adults is 1200 mg administered in two divided doses 30 minutes before the morning and evening meal (see CLINICAL PHARMACOLOGY).

HOW SUPPLIED

Lopid is available as white, elliptical, film-coated, scored tablets, each containing 600 mg gemfibrozil.

Storage: Store at controlled room temperature 20-25°C (68-77°F). Protect from light and humidity.

PRODUCT LISTING - RATED THERAPEUTICALLY EQUIVALENT

Tablet - Oral - 600 mg

6's	$5.73	GENERIC, Allscripts Pharmaceutical Company	54569-3695-01
25's	$25.95	GENERIC, Udl Laboratories Inc	51079-0787-19
30's	$35.32	GENERIC, Heartland Healthcare Services	61392-0116-30
30's	$35.32	GENERIC, Heartland Healthcare Services	61392-0116-39
30's	$52.65	LOPID, Physicians Total Care	54868-1418-00
31 x 10	$321.80	GENERIC, Vangard Labs	00615-3559-53
31 x 10	$321.80	GENERIC, Vangard Labs	00615-3559-63
31's	$36.50	GENERIC, Heartland Healthcare Services	61392-0116-31
32's	$37.68	GENERIC, Heartland Healthcare Services	61392-0116-32
45's	$52.98	GENERIC, Heartland Healthcare Services	61392-0116-45
60's	$53.50	GENERIC, Aligen Independent Laboratories Inc	00405-4456-31
60's	$54.05	GENERIC, Purepac Pharmaceutical Company	00228-2552-06
60's	$54.92	GENERIC, Qualitest Products Inc	00603-3750-20
60's	$55.65	GENERIC, West Point Pharma	59591-0017-68
60's	$55.89	GENERIC, Watson Laboratories Inc	52544-0454-60
60's	$56.63	GENERIC, Moore, H.L. Drug Exchange Inc	00839-7787-05
60's	$57.10	GENERIC, Creighton Products Corporation	50752-0310-80
60's	$57.35	GENERIC, Allscripts Pharmaceutical Company	54569-3695-00
60's	$59.60	GENERIC, Watson/Rugby Laboratories Inc	00536-3854-08
60's	$59.60	GENERIC, Martec Pharmaceuticals Inc	52555-0634-60
60's	$64.70	GENERIC, Mylan Pharmaceuticals Inc	00378-0517-91
60's	$64.72	GENERIC, Geneva Pharmaceuticals	00781-1056-60
60's	$70.65	GENERIC, Heartland Healthcare Services	61392-0116-60
60's	$74.75	GENERIC, Major Pharmaceuticals Inc	00904-5379-52
60's	$74.75	GENERIC, Apotex Usa Inc	60505-0034-04
60's	$74.80	GENERIC, Teva Pharmaceuticals Usa	00093-0670-06
60's	$99.88	LOPID, Parke-Davis	00071-0737-20
60's	$103.54	LOPID, Physicians Total Care	54868-1418-01
90's	$86.02	GENERIC, Allscripts Pharmaceutical Company	54569-8511-01
90's	$105.97	GENERIC, Heartland Healthcare Services	61392-0116-90

100's	$89.50	GENERIC, Purepac Pharmaceutical Company	00228-2552-10
100's	$103.82	GENERIC, Udl Laboratories Inc	51079-0787-20
100's	$115.50	GENERIC, Ivax Corporation	00182-1956-89
100's	$121.65	GENERIC, Major Pharmaceuticals Inc	00904-5379-61
180's	$172.05	GENERIC, Allscripts Pharmaceutical Company	54569-8016-00
180's	$172.05	GENERIC, Allscripts Pharmaceutical Company	54569-8511-00

PRODUCT LISTING - EQUIVALENTS NOT AVAILABLE

Tablet - Oral - 600 mg

60's	$59.95	GENERIC, Watson/Rugby Laboratories Inc	00536-5554-08
60's	$87.75	GENERIC, Southwood Pharmaceuticals Inc	58016-0540-60
100's	$138.66	GENERIC, Southwood Pharmaceuticals Inc	58016-0540-00

Gemifloxacin Mesylate *(003592)*

Categories: Bronchitis, chronic, acute exacerbation; Infection, respiratory tract, lower; Pneumonia; Pregnancy Category C; FDA Approved 2003 Apr
Drug Classes: Antibiotics, quinolones
Brand Names: Factive

DESCRIPTION

To reduce the development of drug-resistant bacteria and maintain the effectiveness of gemifloxacin mesylate and other antibacterial drugs, gemifloxacin mesylate should be used only to treat infections that are proven or strongly suspected to be caused by bacteria.

Factive (gemifloxacin mesylate) is a synthetic broad-spectrum antibacterial agent for oral administration. Gemifloxacin, a compound related to the fluoroquinolone class of antibiotics, is available as the mesylate salt in the sesquihydrate form. Chemically, gemifloxacin is (*R,S*)-7-[(4Z)-3-(aminomethyl)-4-(methoxyimino)-1-pyrrolidinyl]-1-cyclopropyl-6-fluoro-1,4-dihydro-4-oxo-1,8-naphthyridine-3-carboxylic acid. The mesylate salt is a white to light brown solid with a molecular weight of 485.49. Gemifloxacin is considered freely soluble at neutral pH (350 µg/ml at 37°C, pH 7.0). Its empirical formula is $C_{18}H_{20}FN_5O_4{\cdot}CH_4O_3S$.

Each white to off-white, oval, film-coated Factive tablet has breaklines and "GE 320" debossed on both faces and contains gemifloxacin mesylate equivalent to 320 mg gemifloxacin. The inactive ingredients are crospovidone, hydroxypropyl methylcellulose, magnesium stearate, microcrystalline cellulose, polyethylene glycol, povidone, and titanium dioxide.

CLINICAL PHARMACOLOGY

PHARMACOKINETICS

The pharmacokinetics of gemifloxacin are approximately linear over the dose range from 40-640 mg. There was minimal accumulation of gemifloxacin following multiple oral doses up to 640 mg/day for 7 days (mean accumulation <20%). Following repeat oral administration of 320 mg gemifloxacin once daily, steady-state is achieved by the third day of dosing.

Absorption and Bioavailability

Gemifloxacin given as an oral tablet, is rapidly absorbed from the gastrointestinal tract. Peak plasma concentrations of gemifloxacin were observed between 0.5 and 2 hours following oral tablet administration and the absolute bioavailability of the 320 mg tablet averaged approximately 71% (95% CI 60-84%). Following repeat oral doses of 320 mg to healthy subjects, the mean ±SD maximal gemifloxacin plasma concentrations (C_{max}) and systemic drug exposure [AUC(0-24)] were 1.61 ± 0.51 µg/ml (range 0.70-2.62 µg/ml) and 9.93 ± 3.07 µg·h/ml (range 4.71-20.1 µg·h/ml), respectively. In patients with respiratory and urinary tract infections (n=1423), similar estimates of systemic drug exposure were determined using a population pharmacokinetics analysis (geometric mean AUC(0-24), 8.36 µg·h/ml; range 3.2-47.7 µg·h/ml).

The pharmacokinetics of gemifloxacin were not significantly altered when a 320 mg dose was administered with a high-fat meal. Therefore gemifloxacin mesylate tablets may be administered without regard to meals.

Distribution

In vitro binding of gemifloxacin to plasma proteins in healthy subjects is approximately 60-70% and is concentration independent. After repeated doses, the *in vivo* plasma protein binding in healthy elderly and young subjects ranged from 55-73% and was unaffected by age. Renal impairment does not significantly affect the protein binding of gemifloxacin. The blood-to-plasma concentration ratio of gemifloxacin was 1.2:1. The geometric mean for Vdss/F is 4.18 L/kg (range, 1.66-12.12 L/kg).

Gemifloxacin is widely distributed throughout the body after oral administration. Concentrations of gemifloxacin in bronchoalveolar lavage fluid exceed those in the plasma. Gemifloxacin penetrates well into lung tissue and fluids. After 5 daily doses of 320 mg gemifloxacin, concentrations in plasma, bronchoalveolar macrophages, epithelial lining fluid and bronchial mucosa at approximately 2 hours were as in TABLE 1.

Metabolism

Gemifloxacin its metabolized to a limited extent by the liver. The unchanged compound is the predominant drug-related component detected in plasma (approximately 65%) up to 4 hours after dosing. All metabolites formed are minor (<10% of the administered oral dose); the principal ones are N-acetyl gemifloxacin, the E-isomer of gemifloxacin and the carbamyl glucuronide of gemifloxacin. Cytochrome P450 enzymes do not play an important role in gemifloxacin metabolism, and the metabolic activity of these enzymes is not significantly inhibited by gemifloxacin.

TABLE 1

Tissue	Concentration (mean ±SD)	Ratio Compared With Plasma (mean ±SD)
Plasma	1.40 (0.442) µg/ml	—
Bronchoalveolar macrophages	107 (77) µg/g	90.5 (106.3)
Epithelial lining fluid	2.69 (1.96) µg/ml	1.99 (1.32)
Bronchial mucosa	9.52 (5.15) µg/g	7.21 (4.03)

Excretion

Gemifloxacin and it metabolites are excreted via dual routes of excretion. Following oral administration of gemifloxacin to healthy subjects, a mean (±SD) of 61 ± 9.5% of the dose was excreted in the feces and 36 ± 9.3% in the urine as unchanged drug and metabolites. The mean (±SD) renal clearance following repeat doses of 320 mg was approximately 11.6 ± 3.9 L/h (range 4.6-17.6 L/h), which indicates active secretion is involved in the renal excretion of gemifloxacin. The mean (±SD) plasma elimination half-life at steady-state following 320 mg to healthy subjects was approximately 7 ± 2 hours (range 4-12 hours).

Special Populations

Pediatric

The pharmacokinetics of gemifloxacin in pediatric subjects have not been studied.

Geriatric

In adult subjects, the pharmacokinetics of gemifloxacin are not affected by age.

Gender

There are no significant differences between gemifloxacin pharmacokinetics in males and females when differences in body weight are taken into account. Population pharmacokinetic studies indicated that following administration of 320 mg gemifloxacin, AUC values were approximately 10% higher in healthy female patients compared to males. Males and females had mean AUC values of 7.98 µg·h/ml (range, 3.21-42.71 µg·h/ml) and 8.80 µg·h/ml (range, 3.33-47.73 µg·h/ml), respectively. No gemifloxacin dosage adjustment based on gender is necessary.

Hepatic Insufficiency

The pharmacokinetics following a single 320 mg dose of gemifloxacin were studied in patients with mild (Child-Pugh Class A) to moderate (Child-Pugh Class B) liver disease. There was a mean increase in AUC(0-inf) of 34% and a mean increase in C_{max} of 25% in these patients with hepatic impairment compared to healthy volunteers.

The pharmacokinetics of a single 320 mg dose of gemifloxacin were also studied in patients with severe hepatic impairment (Child-Pugh Class C). There was a mean increase in AUC(0-inf) of 45% and a mean increase in C_{max} of 41% in these subjects with hepatic impairment compared to healthy volunteers.

These average pharmacokinetic increases are not considered to be clinically significant. There was no significant change in plasma elimination half-life in the mild, moderate or severe hepatic impairment patients. No dosage adjustment is recommended in patients with mild (Child-Pugh Class A), moderate (Child-Pugh Class B) or severe (Child-Pugh Class C) hepatic impairment. (See DOSAGE AND ADMINISTRATION.)

Renal Insufficiency

Results from population pharmacokinetic and clinical pharmacology studies with repeated 320 mg doses indicate the clearance of gemifloxacin is reduced and the plasma elimination is prolonged, leading to an average increase in AUC values of approximately 70% in patients with renal insufficiency. In the pharmacokinetic studies, gemifloxacin C_{max} was not significantly altered in subjects with renal insufficiency. Dose adjustment in patients with creatinine clearance >40 ml/min is not required. Modification of the dosage is recommended for patients with creatinine clearance ≤40 ml/min. (See DOSAGE AND ADMINISTRATION.)

Hemodialysis removes approximately 20-30% of an oral dose of gemifloxacin from plasma.

Photosensitivity Potential

In a study of the skin response to ultraviolet and visible radiation conducted in 40 healthy volunteers, the minimum erythematous dose (MED) was assessed following administration of either gemifloxacin 160 mg once daily, gemifloxacin 320 mg once daily, ciprofloxacin 500 mg bid, or placebo for 7 days. At 5 of the 6 wavelengths tested (295-430 nm), the photosensitivity potential of gemifloxacin was not statistically different from placebo. At 365 nm (UVA region), gemifloxacin showed a photosensitivity potential similar to that of ciprofloxacin 500 mg bid and the photosensitivity potential for both drugs were statistically greater than that of placebo. Photosensitivity reactions were reported rarely in clinical trials with gemifloxacin (0.039%). (See ADVERSE REACTIONS.)

DRUG-DRUG INTERACTIONS

Antacids/Di- and Trivalent Cations

The systemic availability of gemifloxacin is significantly reduced when an aluminum- and magnesium-containing antacid is concomitantly administered (AUC decreased 85%; C_{max} decreased 87%. Administration of an aluminum- and magnesium-containing antacid or ferrous sulfate (325 mg) at 3 hours before or at 2 hours after gemifloxacin did not significantly alter the systemic availability of gemifloxacin. Therefore, aluminum- and/or magnesium-containing antacids, ferrous sulfate (iron), multivitamin preparations containing zinc or other metal cations, or Videx (didanosine) chewable/buffered tablets or the pediatric powder for oral solution should not be taken within 3 hours before or 2 hours after taking gemifloxacin mesylate tablets.

Calcium carbonate (1000 mg) given either 2 hours before or 2 hours after gemifloxacin administration showed no notable reduction in gemifloxacin systemic availability. Calcium carbonate administered simultaneously with gemifloxacin resulted in a small, not clinically

G

significant, decrease in gemifloxacin exposure [AUC(0-inf) decreased 21% and C_{max} decreased].

Sucralfate

When sucralfate (2 g) was administered 3 hours prior to gemifloxacin, the oral bioavailability of gemifloxacin was significantly reduced (53% decrease in AUC; 69% decrease in C_{max}). When sucralfate (2 g) was administered 2 hours after gemifloxacin, the oral bioavailability of gemifloxacin was not significantly affected; therefore gemifloxacin mesylate should be taken at least 2 hours before sucralfate. (See PRECAUTIONS.)

In Vitro Metabolism

Results of *in vitro* inhibition studies indicate that hepatic cytochrome P450 (CYP450) enzymes do not play an important role in gemifloxacin metabolism. Therefore gemifloxacin should not cause significant *in vivo* pharmacokinetic interactions with other drugs that are metabolized by CYP450 enzymes.

Theophylline

Gemifloxacin 320 mg at steady-state did not affect the repeat dose pharmacokinetics of theophylline (300-400 mg bid to healthy male subjects).

Digoxin

Gemifloxacin 320 mg at steady-state did not affect the repeat dose pharmacokinetics of digoxin (0.25 mg once daily to healthy elderly subjects).

Oral Contraceptives

The effect of an oral estrogen/progesterone contraceptive product (once daily for 21 days) on the pharmacokinetics of gemifloxacin (320 mg once daily for 6 days) in healthy female subjects indicates that concomitant administration caused an average reduction in gemifloxacin AUC and C_{max} of 19% and 12%. These changes are not considered clinically significant. Gemifloxacin 320 mg at steady-state did not affect the repeat dose pharmacokinetics of an ethinylestradiol/levonorgestrol oral contraceptive product (30 µg/150 µg once daily for 21 days to healthy female subjects).

Cimetidine

Co-administration of a single dose of 320 mg gemifloxacin with cimetidine 400 mg four times daily for 7 days resulted in slight average increases in gemifloxacin AUC(0-inf) and C_{max} of 10% and 6%, respectively. These increases are not considered clinically significant.

Omeprazole

Co-administration of a single dose of 320 mg gemifloxacin with omeprazole 40 mg once daily for 4 days resulted in slight average increases in gemifloxacin AUC(0-inf) and C_{max} of 10% and 11%, respectively. These increases are not considered clinically significant.

Warfarin

Administration of repeated doses of gemifloxacin (320 mg once daily for 7 days) to healthy subjects on stable warfarin therapy had no significant effect on warfarin-induced anticoagulant activity (*i.e.*, International Normalized Ratios for Prothrombin Time). (See DRUG INTERACTIONS.)

Probenecid

Administration of a single dose of 320 mg gemifloxacin to healthy subjects who also received repeat doses of probenecid (total dose = 4.5 g) reduced the mean renal clearance of gemifloxacin by approximately 50%, resulting in a mean increase of 45% in gemifloxacin AUC(0-inf) and a prolongation of mean half-life by 1.6 hours. Mean gemifloxacin C_{max} increased 8%.

MICROBIOLOGY

Gemifloxacin has *in vitro* activity against a wide range of Gram-negative and Gram-positive microorganisms. Gemifloxacin is bactericidal with minimum bactericidal concentrations (MBCs) generally within one dilution of the minimum inhibitory concentrations (MICs). Gemifloxacin acts by inhibiting DNA synthesis through the inhibition of both DNA gyrase and topoisomerase IV (TOPO IV), which are essential for bacterial growth. *Streptococcus pneumoniae* showing mutations in both DNA gyrase and TOPO IV (double mutants) are resistant to most fluoroquinolones. Gemifloxacin has the ability to inhibit both enzyme systems at therapeutically relevant drug levels in *S. pneumoniae* (dual targeting), and has MIC values that are still in the susceptible range for some of these double mutants. The mechanism of action of quinolones, including gemifloxacin, is different from that of macrolides, beta-lactams, aminoglycosides, or tetracyclines; therefore, microorganisms resistant to these classes of drugs may be susceptible to gemifloxacin and other quinolones.

There is no known cross-resistance between gemifloxacin and the above mentioned classes of antimicrobials.

The main mechanism of fluoroquinolone resistance is due to mutations in DNA gyrase and/or TOPO IV. Resistance to gemifloxacin develops slowly via multistep mutations and efflux in a manner similar to other fluoroquinolones. The frequency of spontaneous mutation is low (10^{-7} to $<10^{-10}$). Although cross-resistance has been observed between gemifloxacin and other fluoroquinolones, some microorganisms resistant to other fluoroquinolones may be susceptible to gemifloxacin.

Gemifloxacin has been shown to be active against most strains of the following microorganisms, both *in vitro* and in clinical infections as described in INDICATIONS AND USAGE.

Aerobic Gram-Positive Microorganisms:

Streptococcus pneumoniae (including penicillin-resistant strains, MIC value for penicillin ≥2 µg/ml).

Aerobic Gram-Negative Microorganisms:

Haemophilus influenzae, Haemophilus parainfluenzae, Klebsiella pneumoniae (many strains are only moderately susceptible), and *Moraxella catarrhalis.*

Other Microorganisms:

Chlamydia pneumoniae and *Mycoplasma pneumoniae.*

The following data are available, **but their clinical significance is unknown.**

Gemifloxacin exhibits *in vitro* minimal inhibitory concentrations (MICs) of (0.25 µg/ml) or less against most (≥90%) strains of the following microorganisms; however, the safety and effectiveness of gemifloxacin in treating clinical infections due to these microorganisms has not been established in adequate and well-controlled clinical trials:

Aerobic Gram-Positive Microorganisms:

Staphylococcus aureus (methicillin-susceptible strains only), and *Streptococcus pyogenes.*

Aerobic Gram-Negative Microorganisms:

Acinetobacter lwoffi, Klebsiella oxytoca, Legionella pneumophila, and *Proteus vulgaris.*

Susceptibility Testing

Dilution Techniques

Quantitative methods are used to determine antimicrobial minimum inhibitory concentrations (MICs). These MICs provide estimates of the susceptibility of bacteria to antimicrobial compounds. The MICs should be determined using a standardized procedure. Standardized procedures are based on a dilution method[1] (broth or agar) or equivalent with standardized inoculum concentrations and standardized concentrations of gemifloxacin powder. The MICs should be interpreted according to the following criteria:

For testing *Enterobacteriaceae, Haemophilus influenzae,* and *Haemophilus parainfluenzae** see TABLE 2.

TABLE 2

MIC	Interpretation
Enterobacteriaceae	
≤0.25 µg/ml	Susceptible (S)
0.5 µg/ml	Intermediate (I)
≥1.0 µg/ml	Resistant (R)
Haemophilus influenzae and *Haemophilus parainfluenzae**	
≤0.12 µg/ml	Susceptible (S)

* This interpretive standard is applicable only to broth microdilution susceptibility testing with *Haemophilus influenzae* and *Haemophilus parainfluenzae* using *Haemophilus* Test Medium (HTM).[1]

The current absence of data on resistant strains precludes defining any results other than "Susceptible". Strains yielding MIC results suggestive of a "nonsusceptible" category should be submitted to a reference laboratory for further testing.

For testing *Streptococcus pneumoniae** see TABLE 3.

TABLE 3

MIC	Interpretation
≤0.12 µg/ml	Susceptible (S)
0.25 µg/ml	Intermediate (I)
≥0.5 µg/ml	Resistant (R)

* These interpretive standards are applicable only to broth microdilution susceptibility tests using cation-adjusted Muller-Hinton broth with 2-5% lysed horse blood.

A report of "Susceptible" indicates that the pathogen is likely to be inhibited if the antimicrobial compound in the blood reaches the concentration usually achievable. A report of "Intermediate" indicates that the result should be considered equivocal, and if the microorganism is not fully susceptible to alternative, clinically feasible drugs, the test should be repeated. This category implies possible clinical applicability in body sites where the drug is physiologically concentrated or in situations where high dosage of drug can be used. This category also provides a buffer zone, which prevents small uncontrolled technical factors from causing major discrepancies in interpretation. A report of "Resistant" indicates that the pathogen is not likely to be inhibited if the antimicrobial compound in the blood reaches the concentration usually achievable; other therapy should be selected.

Standardized susceptibility test procedures require the use of laboratory control microorganisms to control the technical aspects of the laboratory procedures. Standard gemifloxacin powder should provide the following MIC values (see TABLE 4).

TABLE 4

Microorganism	MIC Range
Enterococcus faecalis ATCC 29212	0.016-0.12 µg/ml
Escherichia coli ATCC 25922	0.004-0.016 µg/ml
Haemophilus influenzae ATCC 49247*	0.002-0.008 µg/ml
Streptococcus pneumoniae ATCC 49619†	0.008-0.03 µg/ml

* This quality control range is applicable to only *H. influenzae* ATCC 49247 tested by a broth microdilution procedure using *Haemophilus* Test Medium (HTM).[1]

† This quality control range is applicable to only *S. pneumoniae* ATCC 49619 tested by a broth microdilution procedure using cation-adjusted Mueller-Hinton broth with 2-5% lysed horse blood.

Diffusion Techniques

Quantitative methods that require measurement of zone diameters also provide reproducible estimates of the susceptibility of bacteria to antimicrobial compounds. One such standardized procedure[2] requires the use of standardized inoculum concentrations. This procedure uses paper disks impregnated with 5 µg gemifloxacin to test the susceptibility of microorganisms to gemifloxacin.

Reports from the laboratory providing results of the standard single-disk susceptibility test with a 5 µg gemifloxacin disk should be interpreted according to the following criteria:

For testing *Enterobacteriaceae, Haemophilus influenzae,* and *Haemophilus parainfluenzae** see TABLE 5.

TABLE 5

Zone Diameter	Interpretation
Enterobacteriaceae	
≥20 mm	Susceptible (S)
16-19 mm	Intermediate (I)
≤15 mm	Resistant (R)
Haemophilus influenzae and *Haemophilus parainfluenzae**	
≥18 mm	Susceptible (S)

* This interpretive standard is applicable only to disk diffusion susceptibility testing with *Haemophilus influenzae* and *Haemophilus parainfluenzae* using *Haemophilus* Test Medium (HTM).[2]

The current absence of data on resistant strains precludes defining any results other than "Susceptible". Strains yielding zone diameter results suggestive of a "nonsusceptible" category should be submitted to a reference laboratory for further testing.

For testing *Streptococcus pneumoniae** see TABLE 6.

TABLE 6

Zone Diameter	Interpretation
≥23 mm	Susceptible (S)
20-22 mm	Intermediate (I)
≤19 mm	Resistant (R)

* These zone diameter standards apply only to tests performed using Mueller-Hinton agar supplemented with 5% defibrinated sheep blood incubated in 5% CO_2.

Interpretation should be as stated above for results using dilution techniques. Interpretation involves correlation of the diameter obtained in the disk test with the MIC for gemifloxacin.

As with standardized dilution techniques, diffusion methods require the use of laboratory control microorganisms that are used to control the technical aspects of the laboratory procedures. For the diffusion technique, the 5 μg gemifloxacin disk should provide the following zone diameters in these laboratory quality control strains (see TABLE 7).

TABLE 7

Microorganism	Zone Diameter
Escherichia coli ATCC 25922	29-36 mm
Haemophilus influenzae ATCC 49247*	30-37 mm
Streptococcus pneumoniae ATCC 49619†	28-34 mm

* This quality control range is applicable to only *H. influenzae* ATCC 49247 tested by a disk diffusion procedure using *Haemophilus* Test Medium (HTM).[2]

† This quality control range is applicable to only *S. pneumoniae* ATCC 49619 tested by a disk diffusion procedure using Mueller-Hinton agar supplemented with 5% defibrinated sheep blood and incubated in 5% CO_2.

INDICATIONS AND USAGE

Gemifloxacin mesylate is indicated for the treatment of infections caused by susceptible strains of the designated microorganisms in the conditions listed below. (See DOSAGE AND ADMINISTRATION.)

Acute bacterial exacerbation of chronic bronchitis caused by *Streptococcus pneumoniae, Haemophilus influenzae, Haemophilus parainfluenzae,* or *Moraxella catarrhalis.*

Community-acquired pneumonia (of mild to moderate severity) caused by *Streptococcus pneumoniae* (including penicillin-resistant strains, MIC value for penicillin ≥2 μg/ml), *Haemophilus influenzae, Moraxella catarrhalis, Mycoplasma pneumoniae, Chlamydia pneumoniae,* or *Klebsiella pneumoniae**.

* In the clinical trials, there were 13 subjects with *Klebsiella pneumoniae,* primarily from non-comparative studies. Ten (10) subjects had mild disease, 2 had moderate disease, and 1 had severe disease. There were 2 clinical failures in subjects with mild disease (1 of these had a bacteriologic recurrence).

To reduce the development of drug-resistant bacteria and maintain the effectiveness of gemifloxacin mesylate and other antibacterial drugs, gemifloxacin mesylate should be used only to treat infections that are proven or strongly suspected to be caused by susceptible bacteria. When culture and susceptibility information are available, they should be considered in selecting or modifying antibacterial therapy. In the absence of such data, local epidemiology and susceptibility patterns may contribute to the empiric selection of therapy.

CONTRAINDICATIONS

Gemifloxacin is contraindicated in patients with a history of hypersensitivity to gemifloxacin, fluoroquinolone antibiotic agents, or any of the product components.

WARNINGS

THE SAFETY AND EFFECTIVENESS OF GEMIFLOXACIN MESYLATE IN CHILDREN, ADOLESCENTS (LESS THAN 18 YEARS OF AGE), PREGNANT WOMEN, AND LACTATING WOMEN HAVE NOT BEEN ESTABLISHED. (See PRECAUTIONS: Pediatric Use, Pregnancy, Teratogenic Effects, Pregnancy Category C, and Nursing Mothers.)

QT EFFECTS

GEMIFLOXACIN MAY PROLONG THE QT INTERVAL IN SOME PATIENTS. GEMIFLOXACIN SHOULD BE AVOIDED IN PATIENTS WITH A HISTORY OF PROLONGATION OF THE QTc INTERVAL, PATIENTS WITH UNCORRECTED ELECTROLYTE DISORDERS (HYPOKALEMIA OR HYPOMAGNESEMIA), AND PATIENTS RECEIVING CLASS IA (*e.g.,* QUINIDINE, PROCAINAMIDE) OR CLASS III (*e.g.,* AMIODARONE, SOTALOL) ANTIARRHYTHMIC AGENTS.

Pharmacokinetic studies between gemifloxacin and drugs that prolong the QTc interval such as erythromycin, antipsychotics, and tricyclic antidepressants have not been performed. Gemifloxacin should be used with caution when given concurrently with these drugs, as well as in patients with ongoing proarrhythmic conditions, such as clinically significant bradycardia or acute myocardial ischemia. No cardiovascular morbidity or mortality attributable to QTc prolongation occurred with gemifloxacin treatment in over 6775 patients, including 653 patients concurrently receiving drugs known to prolong the QTc interval and 5 patients with hypokalemia.

The likelihood of QTc prolongation may increase with increasing dose of the drug; therefore, the recommended dose should not be exceeded especially in patients with renal or hepatic impairment where the C_{max} and AUC are slightly higher. QTc prolongation may lead to an increased risk for ventricular arrhythmias including torsades de pointes. The maximal change in the QTc interval occurs approximately 5-10 hours following oral administration of gemifloxacin.

HYPERSENSITIVITY REACTIONS

Serious and occasionally fatal hypersensitivity and/or anaphylactic reactions have been reported in patients receiving fluoroquinolone therapy. These reactions may occur following the first dose. Some reactions have been accompanied by cardiovascular collapse, hypotension/shock, seizure, loss of consciousness, tingling, angioedema (including tongue, laryngeal, throat or facial edema/swelling), airway obstruction (including bronchospasm, shortness of breath and acute respiratory distress), dyspnea, urticaria, itching and other serious skin reactions.

Gemifloxacin should be discontinued immediately at the appearance of any sign of an immediate type I hypersensitivity skin rash or any other manifestation of a hypersensitivity reaction; the need for continued fluoroquinolone therapy should be evaluated. As with other drugs, serious acute hypersensitivity reactions may require treatment with epinephrine and other resuscitative measures, including oxygen, intravenous fluids, antihistamines, corticosteroids, pressor amines and airway management as clinically indicated. (See PRECAUTIONS and ADVERSE REACTIONS.)

Serious and occasionally fatal events, some due to hypersensitivity and/or some of uncertain etiology, have been reported in patients receiving fluoroquinolones. These events may be severe and generally occur following the administration of multiple doses. Clinical manifestations usually include new onset fever and 1 or more of the following: rash or severe dermatologic reactions (*e.g.,* toxic epidermal necrolysis, Stevens-Johnson Syndrome); vasculitis, arthralgia, myalgia, serum sickness; allergic pneumonitis, interstitial nephritis; acute renal insufficiency or failure; hepatitis, jaundice, acute hepatic necrosis or failure; anemia, including hemolytic and aplastic; thrombocytopenia, including thrombotic thrombocytopenic purpura; leukopenia; agranulocytosis; pancytopenia; and/or other hematologic abnormalities.

TENDON AND CARTILAGE EFFECTS

Fluoroquinolones as a class have been shown to cause arthropathy and osteochondrosis in immature rats and dogs. The relevance of these findings to humans is unknown.

Tendonitis and rupture of the shoulder, hand, and Achilles tendons that required surgical repair or resulted in prolonged disability have been reported in patients receiving fluoroquinolones. Gemifloxacin should be discontinued if the patient experiences pain, inflammation, or rupture of a tendon. Patients should rest and refrain from exercise until the diagnosis of tendonitis or tendon rupture has been confidently excluded. Tendon rupture can occur either during or after treatment. Elderly patients, athletes, and patients taking corticosteroids are more prone to tendonitis.

CNS EFFECTS

In clinical studies with gemifloxacin, Central nervous system (CNS) effects have been reported infrequently. As with other fluoroquinolones, gemifloxacin should be used with caution in patients with CNS diseases such as epilepsy or patients predisposed to convulsions. Although not seen in gemifloxacin clinical trials, convulsions, increased intracranial pressure, and toxic psychosis have been reported in patients receiving other fluoroquinolones. CNS stimulation which may lead to tremors, restlessness, anxiety, lightheadedness, confusion, hallucinations, paranoia, depression, insomnia, and rarely suicidal thoughts or acts may also be caused by other fluoroquinolones. If these reactions occur in patients receiving gemifloxacin, the drug should be discontinued and appropriate measures instituted.

ANTIBIOTIC ASSOCIATED COLITIS

Pseudomembranous colitis has been reported with nearly all antibacterial agents, including gemifloxacin, and may range in severity from mild to life-threatening. Therefore, it is important to consider this diagnosis in patients who present with diarrhea subsequent to the administration of any antibacterial agent.

Treatment with antibacterial agents alters the normal flora of the colon and may permit overgrowth of clostridia. Studies indicate that a toxin produced by *Clostridium difficile* is the primary cause of "antibiotic-associated colitis."

After the diagnosis of pseudomembranous colitis has been established, therapeutic measures should be initiated. Mild cases of pseudomembranous colitis usually respond to drug discontinuation alone. In moderate to severe cases, consideration should be given to management with fluids and electrolytes, protein supplementation, and treatment with an antibacterial drug clinically effective against *Clostridium difficile* colitis. (See ADVERSE REACTIONS.)

PRECAUTIONS

GENERAL

Prescribing gemifloxacin mesylate tablets in the absence of a proven or strongly suspected bacterial infection is unlikely to provide benefit to the patient and increase the risk of the development of drug-resistant bacteria.

RASH

In clinical studies, the overall rate of drug-related rash was 2.8%. The most common form of rash associated with gemifloxacin was described as maculopapular and mild to moderate in severity; 0.3% were described as urticarial in appearance. Rash usually appeared 8-10 days after start of therapy; 60% of the rashes resolved within 7 days, and 80% resolved within 14 days. Approximately 10% of those patients developing rash had a rash described as of severe intensity. Histology was evaluated in a clinical pharmacology study and was consistent with an uncomplicated exanthematous skin reaction and showed no evidence of phototoxicity, vasculitis, or necrosis. There were no documented cases in the clinical trials of more serious skin reactions known to be associated with significant morbidity or mortality.

Rash was more commonly observed in patients <40 years of age, especially females and post-menopausal females taking hormone replacement therapy. The incidence of rash also correlated with longer treatment duration (>7 days). Prolonging duration of therapy beyond 7 days causes the incidence of rash to increase significantly in all subgroups except men over the age of 40 (see TABLE 11). Gemifloxacin therapy should be discontinued in patients developing a rash while on treatment (see ADVERSE REACTIONS).

TABLE 11 *Rash Incidence in Gemifloxacin Mesylate Treated Patients From the Clinical Studies Population* by Gender, Age, and Duration of Therapy*

Gender & Age (years)	Duration of Gemifloxacin Therapy			
Category	5 Days	7 Days	10 Days†	14 Days†
Female <40	5/242 (2.1%)	39/324 (12.0%)	20/131 (15.3%)	7/31 (22.6%)
Female ≥40	19/1210 (1.6%)	30/695 (4.3%)	19/308 (6.2%)	10/126 (7.9%)
Male <40	4/218 (1.8%)	20/318 (6.3%)	7/74 (9.5%)	3/39 (7.7%)
Male ≥40	9/1321 (0.7%)	23/776 (3.0%)	9/345 (2.6%)	3/116 (2.6%)
Totals	37/2991 (1.2%)	112/2113 (5.3%)	55/858 (6.4%)	23/312 (7.4%)

* Includes patients from studies of community-acquired pneumonia, acute bacterial exacerbation of chronic bronchitis, and other indications.

† Exceeds the recommended duration of therapy (see DOSAGE AND ADMINISTRATION).

Photosensitivity reactions have been reported very rarely in clinical trials with gemifloxacin mesylate tablets. (See CLINICAL PHARMACOLOGY.) However, as with all drugs of this class, it is recommended that patients avoid unnecessary exposure to strong sunlight or artificial UV rays (*e.g.*, sunlamps, solariums), and should be advised of the appropriate use of broad spectrum sun block if in bright sunlight. Treatment should be discontinued if a photosensitivity reaction is suspected.

HEPATIC EFFECTS

Liver enzyme elevations (increased ALT and/or AST) occurred at similar rates in patients receiving gemifloxacin 320 mg daily relative to comparator antimicrobial agents (ciprofloxacin, levofloxacin, clarithromycin/cefuroxime axetil, amoxicillin/clavulanate potassium, and ofloxacin). In patients who received gemifloxacin at doses of 480 mg/day or greater there was an increased incidence of elevations in liver enzymes. (See ADVERSE REACTIONS.)

There were no clinical symptoms associated with these liver enzyme elevations. The liver enzyme elevations resolved following cessation of therapy. The recommended dose of gemifloxacin 320 mg daily should not be exceeded and the recommended length of therapy should not be exceeded. (See DOSAGE AND ADMINISTRATION.)

Alteration of the dosage regimen is necessary for patients with impairment of renal function (creatinine clearance ≤40 ml/min). (See DOSAGE AND ADMINISTRATION.)

Adequate hydration of patients receiving gemifloxacin should be maintained to prevent the formation of a highly concentrated urine.

INFORMATION FOR THE PATIENT

Patients Should Be Advised:

- That antibacterial drugs including gemifloxacin mesylate should only be used to treat bacterial infections. They do not treat viral infections (*e.g.*, common cold). When gemifloxacin mesylate is prescribed to treat a bacterial infection, patients should be told that although it is common to feel better early in the course of therapy, the medication should be taken exactly as directed. Skipping doses or not completing the full course of therapy may (1) decrease effectiveness of the immediate treatment and (2) increase the likelihood that bacteria will develop resistance.
- That gemifloxacin mesylate has been associated with rash. Patients should discontinue drug and call their healthcare provider if they develop a rash.
- That gemifloxacin mesylate may be associated with hypersensitivity reactions, including anaphylactic reactions, even following a single dose; patients should immediately discontinue the drug at the sign of a rash or other allergic reaction and seek medical care.
- That gemifloxacin mesylate may produce changes in the electrocardiogram (QTc interval prolongation).
- That gemifloxacin mesylate should be avoided in patients receiving Class IA (*e.g.*, quinidine, procainamide) or Class III (*e.g.*, amiodarone, sotalol) antiarrhythmic agents.
- That gemifloxacin mesylate should be used with caution in patients receiving drugs that may affect the QTc interval such as erythromycin, antipsychotics, and tricyclic antidepressants.
- To inform their physician of any personal or family history of QTc prolongation or proarrhythmic conditions such as recent hypokalemia, significant bradycardia, or recent myocardial ischemia.
- To inform their physician of any other medications when taken concurrently with gemifloxacin mesylate, including over-the-counter medications and dietary supplements.
- To contact their physician if they experience palpitations or fainting spells while taking gemifloxacin mesylate.
- That gemifloxacin mesylate may be taken with or without meals.
- To drink fluids liberally.
- Not to take antacids containing magnesium and/or aluminum or products containing ferrous sulfate (iron), multivitamin preparations containing zinc or other metal cations, or Videx (didanosine) chewable/buffered tablets or the pediatric powder for oral solution within 3 hours before or 2 hours after taking gemifloxacin mesylate.
- That gemifloxacin mesylate should be taken at least 2 hours before sucralfate.
- That phototoxicity has been reported with certain quinolones. The potential for gemifloxacin mesylate to cause phototoxicity was low (3/7659) at the recommended dose in clinical studies. In keeping with good clinical practice, avoid excessive sunlight or artificial ultraviolet light (*e.g.*, tanning beds). If a sunburn-like reaction or skin eruption occurs, contact your physician; (see CLINICAL PHARMACOLOGY, Special Populations, Photosensitivity Potential).
- That gemifloxacin mesylate may cause dizziness; if this occurs, patients should not operate an automobile or machinery or engage in activities requiring mental alertness or coordination.
- That they should discontinue gemifloxacin mesylate therapy and inform their physician if they feel pain, tenderness or rupture of a tendon. Patients should rest and avoid exercise until the diagnosis of tendonitis or tendon rupture has been excluded.
- That convulsions have been reported in patients receiving quinolones; and they should notify their physician before taking this drug if there is a history of this condition.

CARCINOGENESIS, MUTAGENESIS, AND IMPAIRMENT OF FERTILITY

Carcinogenesis

Long term studies in animals to determine the carcinogenic potential of gemifloxacin have not been conducted.

Photocarcinogenesis

Gemifloxacin did not shorten the time to development of UVR-induced skin tumors in hairless albino (Skh-1) mice; thus, it was not photocarcinogenic in this model. These mice received oral gemifloxacin and concurrent irradiation with simulated sunlight 5 days/week for 40 weeks followed by a 12 week treatment-free observation period. The daily dose of UV radiation used in this study was approximately 1/3 of the minimal dose of UV radiation that would induce erythema in Caucasian humans. The median time to the development of skin tumors in the hairless mice was similar in the vehicle control group (36 weeks) and those given up to 100 mg/kg gemifloxacin daily (39 weeks). Following repeat doses of 100 mg/kg gemifloxacin per day, the mice had skin gemifloxacin concentrations of approximately 7.4 µg/g. Plasma levels following this dose were approximately1.4 µg/ml in the mice around the time of irradiation. There are no data on gemifloxacin skin levels in humans, but the mouse plasma gemifloxacin levels are in the expected range of human plasma C_{max} levels (0.7-2.6 µg/ml, with an overall mean of about 1.6 µg/ml) following multiple 320 mg oral doses.

Mutagenesis

Gemifloxacin was not mutagenic in 4 bacterial strains (TA 98, TA 100, TA 1535, TA 1537) used in an Ames *Salmonella* reversion assay. It did not induce micronuclei in the bone marrow of mice following intraperitoneal doses of up to 40 mg/kg and it did not induce unscheduled DNA synthesis in hepatocytes from rats which received oral doses of up to 1600 mg/kg. Gemifloxacin was clastogenic *in vitro* in the mouse lymphoma and human lymphocyte chromosome aberration assays. It was clastogenic *in vivo* in the rat micronucleus assay at oral and intravenous dose levels (≥800 mg/kg and ≥40 mg/kg, respectively) that produced bone marrow toxicity. Fluoroquinolone clastogenicity is apparently due to inhibition of mammalian topoisomerase activity which has threshold implications.

Impairment of Fertility

Gemifloxacin did not affect the fertility of male or female rats at AUC levels following oral administration (216 and 600 mg/kg/day) that were approximately 3- to 4-fold higher than the AUC levels at the clinically recommended dose.

PREGNANCY, TERATOGENIC EFFECTS, PREGNANCY CATEGORY C

Gemifloxacin treatment during organogenesis caused fetal growth retardation in mice (oral dosing at 450 mg/kg/day), rats (oral dosing at 600 mg/kg/day) and rabbits (IV dosing at 40 mg/kg/day) at AUC levels which were 2-, 4- and 3-fold those in women given oral doses of 320 mg. In rats, this growth retardation appeared to be reversible in a pre- and postnatal development study (mice and rabbits were not studied for the reversibility of this effect). Treatment of pregnant rats at 8-fold clinical exposure (based upon AUC comparisons) caused fetal brain and ocular malformations in the presence of maternal toxicity. The overall no-effect exposure level in pregnant animals was approximately 0.8- to 3-fold clinical exposure.

The safety of gemifloxacin in pregnant women has not been established. Gemifloxacin should not be used in pregnant women unless the potential benefit to the mother outweighs the risk to the fetus. There are no adequate and well-controlled studies in pregnant women.

NURSING MOTHERS

Gemifloxacin is excreted in the breast milk of rats. There is no information on excretion of gemifloxacin into human milk. Therefore, gemifloxacin should not be used in lactating women unless the potential benefit to the mother outweighs the risk.

PEDIATRIC USE

Safety and effectiveness in children and adolescents less than 18 years of age have not been established. Fluoroquinolones, including gemifloxacin, cause arthropathy and osteochondrosis in immature animals. (See WARNINGS.)

GERIATRIC USE

Of the total number of subjects in clinical studies of gemifloxacin, 30% (2064) were 65 and over, while 12% (779) were 75 and over. No overall difference in effectiveness was observed between these subjects and younger subjects; the adverse event rates for this group was similar to or lower than that for younger subjects with the exception that the incidence of rash was lower in geriatric patients compared to patients less than 40 years of age.

DRUG INTERACTIONS

Administration of repeat doses of gemifloxacin mesylate had no effect on the repeat dose pharmacokinetics of theophylline, digoxin or an ethinylestradiol/levonorgestrol oral contraceptive product in healthy subjects. (See CLINICAL PHARMACOLOGY, Drug-Drug Interactions.)

Concomitant administration of gemifloxacin mesylate and calcium carbonate, cimetidine, omeprazole, or an estrogen/progesterone oral contraceptive produced minor changes in the pharmacokinetics of gemifloxacin, which were considered to be without clinical significance. (See CLINICAL PHARMACOLOGY.)

Concomitant administration of gemifloxacin mesylate with probenecid resulted in a 45% increase in systemic exposure to gemifloxacin. (See CLINICAL PHARMACOLOGY.)

Gemifloxacin mesylate had no significant effect on the anticoagulant effect of warfarin in healthy subjects on stable warfarin therapy. However, because some quinolones have been reported to enhance the anticoagulant effects of warfarin or its derivatives in patients, the prothrombin time or other suitable coagulation test should be closely monitored if a quinolone antimicrobial is administered concomitantly with warfarin or its derivatives.

Quinolones form chelates with alkaline earth and transition metals. The absorption of oral gemifloxacin is significantly reduced by the concomitant administration of an antacid containing aluminum and magnesium. Magnesium- and/or aluminum-containing antacids, products containing ferrous sulfate (iron), multivitamin preparations containing zinc or other metal cations, or Videx (didanosine) chewable/buffered tablets or the pediatric powder for oral solution should not be taken within 3 hours before or 2 hours after gemifloxacin mesylate. Sucralfate should not be taken within 2 hours of gemifloxacin mesylate. (See CLINICAL PHARMACOLOGY.)

ADVERSE REACTIONS

In clinical studies, 6775 patients received daily oral doses of 320 mg gemifloxacin. In addition, 1797 healthy volunteers and 81 patients with renal or hepatic impairment received single or repeat doses of gemifloxacin in clinical pharmacology studies. The majority of adverse reactions experienced by patients in clinical trials were considered to be of mild to moderate severity.

Gemifloxacin was discontinued because of an adverse event (possibly or probably related) in 2.2% of patients, primarily due to rash (0.9%), nausea (0.3%), diarrhea (0.3%), urticaria (0.3%) and vomiting (0.2%). Comparator antibiotics were discontinued because of an adverse event at an overall comparable rate of 2.1%, primarily due to diarrhea (0.5%), nausea (0.3%), vomiting (0.3%) and rash (0.3%).

Drug-related adverse events, classified as possibly or probably related with a frequency of ≥1% for patients receiving 320 mg of gemifloxacin or comparator drug are presented in TABLE 12.

TABLE 12

	Gemifloxacin 320 mg n=6775	All Oral Comparators* n=5248
Diarrhea	3.6%	4.6%
Rash	2.8%	0.6%
Nausea	2.7%	3.2%
Headache	1.2%	1.5%
Abdominal pain	0.9%	1.1%
Vomiting	0.9%	1.1%
Dizziness	0.8%	1.5%
Taste perversion	0.3%	1.9%

* Beta-lactam antibiotics, macrolides, and other fluoroquinolones.

Gemifloxacin appears to have a low potential for photosensitivity. In clinical trials, treatment-related photosensitivity occurred in only 0.039% (3/7659) of patients.

Additional drug-related adverse events (possibly or probably related) in >0.1 to 1% of patients who received 320 mg of gemifloxacin were: abdominal pain, anorexia, arthralgia, constipation, dermatitis, dizziness, dry mouth, dyspepsia, fatigue, flatulence, fungal infection, gastritis, genital moniliasis, hyperglycemia, insomnia, leukopenia, moniliasis, pruritus, somnolence, taste perversion, thrombocythemia, urticaria, vaginitis, and vomiting.

Other adverse events reported from clinical trials which have potential clinical significance and which were considered to have a suspected relationship to the drug, that occurred in ≤0.1% of patients were: abnormal urine, anemia, asthenia, back pain, bilirubinemia, dyspnea, eczema, eosinophilia, flushing, gastroenteritis, granulocytopenia, hot flashes, increase GGT, leg cramps, myalgia, nervousness, non-specified gastrointestinal disorder, pain, pharyngitis, pneumonia, thrombocytopenia, tremor, vertigo, and vision abnormality.

In clinical trials of acute bacterial exacerbation of chronic bronchitis (ABECB) and community acquired pneumonia (CAP), the incidences of rash are shown in TABLE 13.

See PRECAUTIONS.

TABLE 13

	ABECB (5 days) n=2284		CAP (7 days) n=643	
Totals	27/2284	1.2%	26/643	4.0%
Females <40 years	NA*		8/88	9.1%
Females ≥40 years	16/1040	1.5%	5/214	2.3%
Males <40 years	NA*		5/101	5.0%
Males ≥40 years	11/1203	0.9%	8/240	3.3%

* Insufficient number of patients in this category for a meaningful analysis.

LABORATORY CHANGES

The percentages of patients who received multiple doses of gemifloxacin and had a laboratory abnormality are listed below. It is not known whether these abnormalities were related to gemifloxacin or an underlying condition.

Clinical Chemistry: Increased ALT (1.5%), increased AST (1.1%), increased creatine phosphokinase (0.6%), increased potassium (0.5%), decreased sodium (0.3%), increased gammaglutamyl transferase (0.5%), increased alkaline phosphatase (0.3%), increased total bilirubin (0.3%), increased blood urea nitrogen (0.3%), decreased calcium (0.2%), decreased albumin (0.3%), increased serum creatinine (0.2%), decreased total protein (0.1%) and increased calcium (<0.1%).

CPK Elevations Were Noted Infrequently: 0.8% in gemifloxacin patients versus 0.4% in the comparator patients.

Hematology: Increased platelets (0.9%), decreased neutrophils (0.5%), increased neutrophils (0.5%), decreased hematocrit (0.3%), decreased hemoglobin (0.2%), decreased platelets (0.2%), decreased red blood cells (0.1%), increased hematocrit (0.1%), increased hemoglobin (0.1%), and increased red blood cells (0.1%).

In clinical studies, approximately 7% of the gemifloxacin treated patients had elevated ALT values immediately prior to entry into the study. Of these patients, approximately 10% showed a further elevation of their ALT at the on-therapy visit and 5% showed a further elevation at the end of therapy visit. None of these patients demonstrated evidence of hepatocellular jaundice. For the pooled comparators, approximately 6% of patients had elevated ALT values immediately prior to entry into the study. Of these patients, approximately 7% showed a further elevation of their ALT at the on-therapy visit and 4% showed a further elevation at the end of therapy visit.

In a clinical trial where 638 patients received either a single 640 mg dose of gemifloxacin or 250 mg bid of ciprofloxacin for 3 days, there was an increased incidence of ALT elevations in the gemifloxacin arm (3.9%) versus the comparator arm (1.0%). In this study, 2 patients experienced ALT elevations of 8-10 times the upper limit of normal. These elevations were asymptomatic and reversible.

DOSAGE AND ADMINISTRATION

Gemifloxacin mesylate tablets can be taken with or without food and should be swallowed whole with a liberal amount of liquid. The recommended dose of gemifloxacin mesylate tablets is 320 mg daily, according to TABLE 14.

TABLE 14

Indication	Dose	Duration
Acute bacterial exacerbation of chronic bronchitis	One 320 mg tablet daily	5 days
Community-acquired pneumonia (of mild to moderate severity)	One 320 mg tablet daily	7 days

The recommended dose and duration of gemifloxacin mesylate tablets should not be exceeded (see TABLE 11).

RENALLY IMPAIRED PATIENTS

Dose adjustment in patients with creatinine clearance >40 ml/min is not required. Modification of the dosage is recommended for patients with creatinine clearance ≤40 ml/min. TABLE 15 provides dosage guidelines for use in patients with renal impairment.

TABLE 15 *Recommended Starting and Maintenance Doses for Patients With Impaired Renal Function*

Creatinine Clearance	Dose
>40 ml/min	See usual dosage
≤40 ml/min	160 mg q24h

Patients requiring routine hemodialysis or continuous ambulatory peritoneal dialysis (CAPD) should receive 160 mg q24h.

When only the serum creatinine concentration is known, the following formula may be used to estimate creatinine clearance.

Men: Creatinine clearance (ml/min) = [weight (kg) × (140 - age)] ÷ [72 × serum creatinine (mg/dl)]

Women: 0.85 × the value calculated for men

USE IN HEPATICALLY IMPAIRED PATIENTS

No dosage adjustment is recommended in patients with mild (Child-Pugh Class A), moderate (Child-Pugh Class B) or severe (Child-Pugh Class C) hepatic impairment.

USE IN ELDERLY

No dosage adjustment is recommended.

ANIMAL PHARMACOLOGY

Quinolones have been shown to cause arthropathy in immature animals. Degeneration of articular cartilage occurred in juvenile dogs given at least 192 mg/kg/day gemifloxacin in a 28 day study (producing about 6 times the systemic exposure at the clinical dose), but not in mature dogs. There was no damage to the articular surfaces of joints in immature rats given repeated doses of up to 800 mg/kg/day.

Some quinolones have been reported to have proconvulsant properties that are potentiated by the concomitant administration of non-steroidal anti-inflammatory drugs (NSAIDs). Gemifloxacin alone had effects in tests of behaviour or CNS interaction typically at doses of at least 160 mg/kg. No convulsions occurred in mice given the active metabolite of the NSAID, fenbufen, followed by 80 mg/kg gemifloxacin.

Dogs given 192 mg/kg/day (about 6 times the systemic exposure at the clinical dose) for 28 days, or 24 mg/kg/day (approximately equivalent to the systemic exposure at the clinical dose) for 13 weeks showed reversible increases in plasma ALT activities and local periportal liver changes associated with blockage of small bile ducts by crystals containing gemifloxacin.

Quinolones have been associated with prolongation of the electrocardiographic QT interval in dogs. Gemifloxacin produced no effect on the QT interval in dogs dosed orally to provide about 4 times human therapeutic plasma concentrations at C_{max}, and transient prolongation after intravenous administration at more than 4 times human plasma levels at C_{max}. Gemifloxacin exhibited weak activity in the cardiac I_{Kr} (hERG) channel inhibition assay, having an IC_{50} of approximately 270 μM.

Gemifloxacin, like many other quinolones, tends to crystallise at the alkaline pH of rodent urine, resulting in a nephropathy in rats that is reversible on drug withdrawal (oral no-effect dose 24 mg/kg/day).

Gemifloxacin was weakly phototoxic to hairless mice given a single 200 mg/kg oral dose and exposed to UVA radiation, however, no evidence of phototoxicity was observed at 100 mg/kg/day dosed orally for 13 weeks in a standard hairless mouse model, using simulated sunlight.

HOW SUPPLIED

Factive is available as white to off-white, oval, film-coated tablets with breaklines and "GE 320" debossed on both faces. Each tablet contains gemifloxacin mesylate equivalent to 320 mg of gemifloxacin.

Storage: Store at 25°C (77°F); excursions permitted to 15-30°C (59-86°F). Protect from light.

G

Gemtuzumab Ozogamicin *(003492)*

For complete prescribing information, refer to the CD-ROM included with the book.

Categories: Leukemia, acute myeloid; FDA Approved 2000 May; Pregnancy Category D; Orphan Drugs
Drug Classes: Antineoplastics, monoclonal antibodies; Monoclonal antibodies
Brand Names: Mylotarg

WARNING

FOR INTRAVENOUS USE ONLY.

Gemtuzumab ozogamicin should be administered under the supervision of physicians experienced in the treatment of acute leukemia and in facilities equipped to monitor and treat leukemia patients.

There are no controlled trials demonstrating efficacy and safety using gemtuzumab ozogamicin in combination with other chemotherapeutic agents. Therefore, gemtuzumab ozogamicin should only be used as single agent chemotherapy and not in combination chemotherapy regimens outside clinical trials.

Severe myelosuppression occurs when gemtuzumab ozogamicin is used at recommended doses.

HYPERSENSITIVITY REACTIONS INCLUDING ANAPHYLAXIS, INFUSION REACTIONS, PULMONARY EVENTS

Gemtuzumab ozogamicin administration can result in severe hypersensitivity reactions (including anaphylaxis), and other infusion-related reactions which may include severe pulmonary events. Infrequently, hypersensitivity reactions and pulmonary events have been fatal. In most cases, infusion-related symptoms occurred during the infusion or within 24 hours of administration of gemtuzumab ozogamicin and resolved. Gemtuzumab ozogamicin infusion should be interrupted for patients experiencing dyspnea or clinically significant hypotension. Patients should be monitored until signs and symptoms completely resolve. Discontinuation of gemtuzumab ozogamicin treatment should be strongly considered for patients who develop anaphylaxis, pulmonary edema, or acute respiratory distress syndrome. Since patients with high peripheral blast counts may be at greater risk for pulmonary events and tumor lysis syndrome, physicians should consider leukoreduction with hydroxyurea or leukapheresis to reduce the peripheral white count to below 30,000/µl prior to administration of gemtuzumab ozogamicin. (See WARNINGS.)

HEPATOTOXICITY

Hepatotoxicity, including severe hepatic veno-occlusive disease (VOD), has been reported in association with the use of gemtuzumab ozogamicin as a single agent, as part of a combination chemotherapy regimen, and in patients without a history of liver disease or hematopoietic stem-cell transplant (HSCT). (See WARNINGS.)

Patients who receive gemtuzumab ozogamicin either before or after HSCT, patients with underlying hepatic disease or abnormal liver function, and patients receiving gemtuzumab ozogamicin in combinations with other chemotherapy may be at increased risk for developing severe VOD. Death from liver failure and from VOD has been reported in patients who received gemtuzumab ozogamicin.

Physicians should monitor their patients carefully for symptoms of hepatotoxicity, particularly VOD. These symptoms can include: rapid weight gain, right upper quadrant pain, hepatomegaly, ascites, elevations in bilirubin and/or liver enzymes. However, careful monitoring may not identify all patients at risk or prevent the complications of hepatotoxicity.

DESCRIPTION

Mylotarg (gemtuzumab ozogamicin for injection) is a chemotherapy agent composed of a recombinant humanized IgG_4, kappa antibody conjugated with a cytotoxic antitumor antibiotic, calicheamicin, isolated from fermentation of a bacterium, *Micromonospora echinospora* ssp. *calichensis.* The antibody portion of gemtuzumab ozogamicin binds specifically to the CD33 antigen, a sialic acid-dependent adhesion protein found on the surface of leukemic myeloblasts and immature normal cells of myelomonocytic lineage, but not on normal hematopoetic stem cells. The anti-CD33 hP67.6 antibody is produced by mammalian cell suspension culture using a myeloma NS0 cell line and is purified under conditions which remove or inactivate viruses. Three separate and independent steps in the hP67.6 antibody purification process achieve retrovirus inactivation and removal. These include low pH treatment, DEAE-Sepharose chromatography, and viral filtration. Mylotarg contains amino acid sequences of which approximately 98.3% are of human origin. The constant region and framework regions contain human sequences while the complementarity-determining regions are derived from amurine antibody (p67.6) that binds CD33. This antibody is linked to N-acetyl-gamma calicheamicin via a bifunctional linker. Gemtuzumab ozogamicin has approximately 50% of the antibody loaded with 4-6 moles calicheamicin per mole of antibody. The remaining 50% of the antibody is not linked to the calicheamicin derivative. Gemtuzumab ozogamicin has a molecular weight of 151-153 kDa.

Mylotarg is a sterile, white, preservative-free lyophilized powder containing 5 mg of drug conjugate (protein equivalent) in a 20 ml amber vial. The drug product is light sensitive and must be protected from direct and indirect sunlight and unshielded fluorescent light during the preparation and administration of the infusion. The inactive ingredients are: dextran 40; sucrose; sodium chloride; monobasic and dibasic sodium phosphate.

INDICATIONS AND USAGE

Gemtuzumab ozogamicin is indicated for the treatment of patients with CD33 positive acute myeloid leukemia in first relapse who are 60 years of age or older and who are not considered candidates for cytotoxic chemotherapy. The safety and efficacy of gemtuzumab ozogamicin in patients with poor performance status and organ dysfunction has not been established.

The effectiveness of gemtuzumab ozogamicin is based on OR rates. There are no controlled trials demonstrating a clinical benefit, such as improvement in disease-related symptoms or increased survival, compared to any other treatment.

CONTRAINDICATIONS

Gemtuzumab ozogamicin is contraindicated in patients with a known hypersensitivity to gemtuzumab ozogamicin or any of its components: anti-CD33 antibody (hP67.6), calicheamicin derivatives, or inactive ingredients.

WARNINGS

Gemtuzumab ozogamicin should be administered under the supervision of physicians experienced in the treatment of acute leukemia and in facilities equipped to monitor and treat leukemia patients.

There are no controlled trials demonstrating efficacy and safety using gemtuzumab ozogamicin in combination with other chemotherapeutic agents. Therefore, gemtuzumab ozogamicin should only be used as single agent chemotherapy and not in combination chemotherapy regimens outside clinical trials.

MYELOSUPPRESSION

Severe myelosuppression will occur in all patients given the recommended dose of this agent. Careful hematologic monitoring is required. Systemic infections should be treated.

HYPERSENSITIVITY REACTIONS INCLUDING ANAPHYLAXIS, INFUSION REACTIONS, PULMONARY EVENTS

Gemtuzumab ozogamicin administration can result in severe hypersensitivity reactions (including anaphylaxis), and other infusion-related reactions which may include severe pulmonary events. Infrequently, hypersensitivity reactions and pulmonary events have been fatal. In most cases, infusion-related symptoms occurred during the infusion or within 24 hours of administration of gemtuzumab ozogamicin and resolved.

Gemtuzumab ozogamicin infusion should be interrupted for patients experiencing dyspnea or clinically significant hypotension. Patients should be monitored until signs and symptoms completely resolve. Discontinuation of further gemtuzumab ozogamicin treatment should be strongly considered for patients who develop anaphylaxis, pulmonary edema, or acute respiratory distress syndrome. Since patients with high peripheral blast counts may be at greater risk for such reactions, physicians should consider leukoreduction with hydroxyurea or leukapheresis to reduce the peripheral white count to below 30,000/µl prior to administration of gemtuzumab ozogamicin.

INFUSION REACTIONS

Gemtuzumab ozogamicin can produce a post-infusion symptom complex of fever and chills, and less commonly hypotension and dyspnea that may occur during the first 24 hours after administration. Grade 3 or 4 non-hematologic infusion-related adverse events included chills, fever, hypotension, hypertension, hyperglycemia, hypoxia, and dyspnea. Most patients received the following prophylactic medications before administration: diphenhydramine 50 mg po and acetaminophen 650-1000 mg po; thereafter, two additional doses of acetaminophen 650-1000 mg po, one every 4 hours as needed. Vital signs should be monitored during infusion and for the 4 hours following infusion.

In clinical studies, these symptoms generally occurred after the end of the 2 hour intravenous infusion and resolved after 2-4 hours with a supportive therapy of acetaminophen, diphenhydramine, and IV fluids. Fewer infusion-related events were observed after the second dose.

PULMONARY EVENTS

Severe pulmonary events leading to death have been reported infrequently with the use of gemtuzumab ozogamicin in the postmarketing setting. Signs, symptoms and clinical findings include dyspnea, pulmonary infiltrates, pleural effusions, non-cardiogenic pulmonary edema, pulmonary insufficiency and hypoxia, and acute respiratory distress syndrome. These events occur as sequelae of infusion reactions; patients with WBC counts >30,000/µl may be at increased risk. (See Infusion Reactions.) Physicians should consider leukoreduction with hydroxyurea or leukapheresis to reduce the peripheral white count to below 30,000 µl prior to administration of gemtuzumab ozogamicin. Patients with symptomatic intrinsic lung disease may also be at greater risk of severe pulmonary reactions.

HEPATOTOXICITY

Hepatotoxicity, including severe VOD, has been reported in association with the use of gemtuzumab ozogamicin as a single agent, as part of a combination chemotherapy regimen, and in patients without a history of liver disease or HSCT. Patients who receive gemtuzumab ozogamicin either before or after HSCT, patients with underlying hepatic disease or abnormal liver function, and patients receiving gemtuzumab ozogamicin in combinations with other chemotherapy may be at increased risk for developing severe VOD. Death from liver failure and from VOD has been reported in patients who received gemtuzumab ozogamicin. Physicians should monitor their patients carefully for symptoms of hepatotoxicity, particularly VOD. These symptoms can include: rapid weight gain, right upper quadrant pain, hepatomegaly, ascites, elevations in bilirubin and/or liver enzymes. However, careful monitoring may not identify all patients at risk or prevent the complications of hepatotoxicity.

USE IN PATIENTS WITH HEPATIC IMPAIRMENT

Gemtuzumab ozogamicin has not been studied in patients with bilirubin >2 mg/dl. Extra caution should be exercised when administering gemtuzumab ozogamicin in patients with hepatic impairment.

TUMOR LYSIS SYNDROME (TLS)

TLS may be a consequence of leukemia treatment with any chemotherapeutic agent including gemtuzumab ozogamicin. Renal failure secondary to TLS has been reported in association with the use of gemtuzumab ozogamicin. Appropriate measures, (*e.g.*, hydration and allopurinol), must be taken to prevent hyperuricemia. Physicians should consider leukoreduction with hydroxyurea or leukapheresis to reduce the peripheral white blood count to <30,000/μl prior to administration of gemtuzumab ozogamicin.

PREGNANCY

Gemtuzumab ozogamicin may cause fetal harm when administered to a pregnant woman. Daily treatment of pregnant rats with gemtuzumab ozogamicin during organogenesis caused dose-related decreases in fetal weight in association with dose-related decreases in fetal skeletal ossification beginning at 0.025 mg/kg/day. Doses of 0.060 mg/kg/day (approximately 0.04 times the recommended human single dose on a mg/m^2 basis) produced increased embryo-fetal mortality (increased numbers of resorptions and decreased numbers of live fetuses per litter). Gross external, visceral, and skeletal alterations at the 0.060 mg/kg/day dose level included digital malformations (ectrodactyly, brachydactyly) in one or both hind feet, absence of the aortic arch, wavy ribs, anomalies of the long bones in the forelimb(s) (short/thick humerus, misshapen radius and ulna, and short/thick ulna), misshapen scapula, absence of vertebral centrum, and fused sternebrae. This dose was also associated with maternal toxicity (decreased weight gain, decreased food consumption). There are no adequate and well-controlled studies in pregnant women. If gemtuzumab ozogamicin is used in pregnancy, or if the patient becomes pregnant while taking it, the patient should be apprised of the potential hazard to the fetus. Women of childbearing potential should be advised to avoid becoming pregnant while receiving treatment with gemtuzumab ozogamicin.

DOSAGE AND ADMINISTRATION

The recommended dose of gemtuzumab ozogamicin is 9 mg/m^2, administered as a 2 hour intravenous infusion. Physicians should consider leukoreduction with hydroxyurea or leukapheresis to reduce the peripheral white blood count to below 30,000/μl prior to administration of gemtuzumab ozogamicin. Appropriate measures (*e.g.*, hydration and allopurinol) must be taken to prevent hyperuricemia. Patients should receive the following prophylactic medications 1 hour before gemtuzumab ozogamicin administration: diphenhydramine 50 mg po and acetaminophen 650-1000 mg po; thereafter, two additional doses of acetaminophen 650-1000 mg po, one every 4 hours as needed. Vital signs should be monitored during infusion and for 4 hours following infusion. The recommended treatment course with gemtuzumab ozogamicin is a total of 2 doses with 14 days between the doses. Full recovery from hematologic toxicities is not a requirement for administration of the second dose.

HEPATIC INSUFFICIENCY

Patients with hepatic impairment were not included in the clinical studies. See WARNINGS.

RENAL INSUFFICIENCY

Patients with renal impairment were not included in the clinical studies.

INSTRUCTIONS FOR RECONSTITUTION

The drug product is light sensitive and must be protected from direct and indirect sunlight and unshielded fluorescent light during the preparation and administration of the infusion. **All preparation should take place in a biologic safety hood with the fluorescent light off.** Prior to reconstitution, allow drug vials to come to room temperature. Reconstitute the contents of each vial with 5 ml sterile water for injection, using sterile syringes. Gently swirl each vial. Each vial should be inspected for complete solution and for particulate. The final concentration of drug in the vial is 1 mg/ml. While in the vial, the reconstituted drug may be stored refrigerated (2-8°C) and protected from light for up to 8 hours.

INSTRUCTIONS FOR DILUTION

Withdraw the desired volume from each vial and inject into a 100 ml IV bag of 0.9% sodium chloride injection. Place the 100 ml IV bag into an UV protectant bag. The resulting drug solution in the IV bag should be used immediately.

ADMINISTRATION

DO NOT ADMINISTER AS AN INTRAVENOUS PUSH OR BOLUS.

Once the reconstituted gemtuzumab ozogamicin is diluted into the IV bag containing normal saline, the resulting solution should be infused over a 2 hour period. A separate IV line equipped with a low protein-binding 1.2 micron terminal filter must be used for administration of the drug. Gemtuzumab ozogamicin may be given peripherally or through a central line. Premedication, consisting of acetaminophen and diphenhydramine, should be given before each infusion to reduce the incidence of a post-infusion symptom complex.

Instructions for Use, Handling and for Disposal

Gemtuzumab ozogamicin should be inspected visually for particulate matter and discoloration, following reconstitution and prior to administration. Protect from light and use an UV protective bag over the IV bag during infusion. Procedures for handling and disposal of anticancer drugs should be considered. Several guidelines on this subject have been published.1-3

PRODUCT LISTING - EQUIVALENTS NOT AVAILABLE

Powder For Injection - Intravenous - 5 mg

1's $2298.75 MYLOTARG, Wyeth-Ayerst Laboratories 00008-4510-01

Gentamicin Sulfate *(001352)*

Categories: Blepharitis; Blepharoconjunctivitis; Burns; Conjunctivitis, infectious; Dacryocystitis; Infection, bone; Infection, central nervous system; Infection, gastrointestinal tract; Infection, intra-abdominal; Infection, ophthalmic; Infection, respiratory tract; Infection, skin and skin structures; Infection, urinary tract; Keratitis; Keratoconjunctivitis; Meibomianitis; Meningitis; Peritonitis; Septicemia; Ulcer, corneal; Pregnancy Category C; FDA Approved 1966 Mar; WHO Formulary

Drug Classes: Antibiotics, aminoglycosides; Anti-infectives, ophthalmic; Anti-infectives, otic; Anti-infectives, topical; Dermatologics; Ophthalmics; Otics

Brand Names: Apogen; Bristagen; Ed-Mycin; G-Mycin; G-Myticin; **Garamycin**; Garasone; Genoptic; Gentacidin; Gentafair; Gentak; Gentasol; Isotonic Gentamicin; Ocu-Mycin; Oftalmogenta; U-Gencin

Foreign Brand Availability: Adelanin (Philippines); Alcomicin (Bahrain; Belgium; Benin; Burkina-Faso; Cyprus; Egypt; Ethiopia; Gambia; Ghana; Guinea; Indonesia; Iran; Iraq; Ivory-Coast; Jordan; Kenya; Kuwait; Lebanon; Liberia; Libya; Malawi; Mali; Mauritania; Mauritius; Morocco; Niger; Nigeria; Oman; Qatar; Republic-of-Yemen; Saudi-Arabia; Senegal; Seychelles; Sierra-Leone; Sudan; Syria; Tanzania; Thailand; Tunia; Uganda; United-Arab-Emirates; Zambia; Zimbabwe); Apigent (Bahrain; Cyprus; Egypt; Iran; Iraq; Jordan; Kuwait; Lebanon; Libya; Oman; Qatar; Republic-of-Yemen; Saudi-Arabia; Syria; United-Arab-Emirates); Bactiderm (Philippines); Biogaracin (India); Cidomycin (Bahamas; Bahrain; Barbados; Belize; Bermuda; Curacao; Cyprus; Egypt; England; Guyana; Iran; Iraq; Ireland; Jamaica; Jordan; Kuwait; Lebanon; Libya; Malaysia; Netherland-Antilles; Oman; Qatar; Republic-of-Yemen; Saudi-Arabia; South-Africa; Surinam; Syria; Trinidad; United-Arab-Emirates); Danigen (Indonesia); Dermogen (Malaysia); Diakarmon (Bahrain; Benin; Burkina-Faso; Cyprus; Egypt; Ethiopia; Gambia; Ghana; Greece; Guinea; Iran; Iraq; Ivory-Coast; Jordan; Kenya; Kuwait; Lebanon; Liberia; Libya; Malawi; Mali; Mauritania; Mauritius; Morocco; Niger; Nigeria; Oman; Qatar; Republic-of-Yemen; Saudi-Arabia; Senegal; Seychelles; Sierra-Leone; Sudan; Syria; Tanzania; Tunia; Uganda; United-Arab-Emirates; Zambia; Zimbabwe); Epigent (Bahrain; Cyprus; Egypt; Iran; Iraq; Jordan; Kuwait; Lebanon; Libya; Oman; Qatar; Republic-of-Yemen; Saudi-Arabia; Syria; United-Arab-Emirates); Fermentmycin (South-Africa); Garabiotic (Indonesia); Garamicin (Thailand); Garamicina (Colombia; Costa-Rica; Dominican-Republic; Ecuador; El-Salvador; Guatemala; Honduras; Mexico; Nicaragua; Panama); Garamicina Cream (Colombia); Garamicina Crema (Ecuador; Mexico); Garamicina Oftalmica (Colombia; Ecuador; Mexico); Garalone (Portugal); Garbilocin (Greece); Gencin (South-Africa); Genrex (Mexico); Gensumycin (Denmark; Finland; Norway; Sweden); Genta Grin (Mexico); Gentabiotic (Costa-Rica; Dominican-Republic; El-Salvador; Guatemala; Honduras; Nicaragua; Panama; Peru); Gentabiox (Peru); Gentacin (Hong-Kong; Japan; Korea); Gentacor (Philippines); Gentacyl (Indonesia); Gentagram (Peru); Gental (Thailand); Gentalline (France); Gentalol (Japan); Gentalyn (Italy; Peru); Gentalyn Oftalmico-Otico (Peru); Gentamax (Ecuador); Gentamedical (Spain); Gentamen (Bahrain; Cyprus; Egypt; Iran; Iraq; Jordan; Kuwait; Lebanon; Libya; Oman; Qatar; Republic-of-Yemen; Saudi-Arabia; Syria; United-Arab-Emirates); Gentamerck (Indonesia); Gentamina (Argentina); Gentamytrex (Germany; Hungary; Netherlands; Philippines); Gentamytrex Ophthiole (Malaysia); Gentarad (Bahrain; Cyprus; Egypt; Iran; Iraq; Jordan; Kuwait; Lebanon; Libya; Oman; Qatar; Republic-of-Yemen; Saudi-Arabia; Syria; United-Arab-Emirates); Gentasil (Peru); Gentasporin (India); Gentatrim (Israel); Genticin (Bahrain; Benin; Burkina-Faso; Cyprus; Egypt; England; Ethiopia; Gambia; Ghana; Guinea; Iran; Iraq; Ireland; Ivory-Coast; Jordan; Kenya; Kuwait; Lebanon; Liberia; Libya; Malawi; Mali; Mauritania; Mauritius; Morocco; Niger; Nigeria; Oman; Qatar; Republic-of-Yemen; Saudi-Arabia; Senegal; Seychelles; Sierra-Leone; Sudan; Syria; Tanzania; Tunia; Uganda; United-Arab-Emirates; Zambia; Zimbabwe); Genticina (Spain); Genticyn (India); Gentiderm (Indonesia); Genum (Philippines); Geomycine (Belgium); Gevramycin (Spain); Grammicin (Thailand); Hexamycin (Denmark); Konigen (Indonesia); Lacromycin (Israel); Lisagent (Taiwan); Miragenta (Colombia); Miramycin (Hong-Kong; Malaysia; Singapore; Taiwan; Thailand); Nichogencin (Indonesia); Obogen (Philippines); Ocugenta (Korea); Oftagen (Peru); Ophtagram (Belgium; Germany; Philippines; Switzerland); Optigen (Hong-Kong; Malaysia); Opti-Genta (Israel); Optimycin (Benin; Burkina-Faso; Ethiopia; Gambia; Ghana; Guinea; Ivory-Coast; Kenya; Liberia; Malawi; Mali; Mauritania; Mauritius; Morocco; Niger; Nigeria; Senegal; Seychelles; Sierra-Leone; Sudan; Tanzania; Tunia; Uganda; Zambia; Zimbabwe); Ottogenta (Indonesia); Pyogenta (Indonesia); Refobacin (Austria; Germany); Rigaminol (Peru); Rocy Gen (Philippines); Rovixida (Argentina); Sagestam eye drops (Indonesia); Sedanazin (Japan); Servigenta (Malaysia); Skinfect (Thailand); Sulmycin (Germany); Terramycin N Augensalbe (Germany); Terramycin N Augentropfen (Germany); Versigen (Thailand); Yectamicina (Mexico)

HCFA JCODE(S): J1580 up to 80 mg IM, IV

IM-IV

WARNING

Patients treated with aminoglycosides should be under close clinical observation because of the potential toxicity associated with their use.

As with other aminoglycosides, gentamicin sulfate pediatric injectable is potentially nephrotoxic. The risk of nephrotoxicity is greater in patients with impaired renal function and in those who receive high dosage or prolonged therapy.

Neurotoxicity manifested by ototoxicity, both vestibular and auditory, can occur in patients treated with gentamicin sulfate pediatric injectable, primarily in those with pre-existing renal damage and in patients with normal renal function treated with higher doses and/or for longer periods than recommended. Aminoglycoside-induced ototoxicity is usually irreversible. Other manifestations of neurotoxicity may include numbness, skin tingling, muscle twitching, and convulsions.

Renal and eighth cranial nerve functions should be closely monitored, especially in patients with known or suspected reduced renal function at onset of therapy, and also in those whose renal function is initially normal but who develop signs of renal dysfunction during therapy. Urine should be examined for decreased specific gravity, increased excretion of protein, and the presence of cells or casts. Blood urea nitrogen, serum creatinine, or creatinine clearance should be determined periodically. When feasible, it is recommended that serial audiograms be obtained in patients old enough to be tested, particularly high-risk patients. Evidence of ototoxicity (dizziness, vertigo, ataxia, tinnitus, roaring in the ears, or hearing loss) or nephrotoxicity requires dosage adjustment or discontinuance of the drug. As with the other aminoglycosides, on rare occasions changes in renal and eighth cranial nerve function may not become manifest until soon after completion of therapy.

WARNING — Cont'd

Serum concentrations of aminoglycosides should be monitored when feasible to assure adequate levels and to avoid potentially toxic levels. When monitoring gentamicin peak concentrations, dosage should be adjusted so that prolonged levels above 12 μg/ml are avoided. When monitoring gentamicin trough concentrations, dosage should be adjusted so that levels above 2 μg/ml are avoided. Excessive peak and/or trough serum concentrations of aminoglycosides may increase the risk of renal and eighth cranial nerve toxicity. In the event of overdose or toxic reactions, hemodialysis may aid in the removal of gentamicin from the blood, especially if renal function is, or becomes, compromised. The rate of removal of gentamicin is considerably less by peritoneal dialysis than by hemodialysis. In the newborn infant, exchange transfusions may also be considered.

Concurrent and/or sequential systemic or topical use of other potentially neurotoxic and/or nephrotoxic drugs, such as cisplatin, cephaloridine, kanamycin, amikacin, neomycin, polymyxin B, colistin, paromomycin, streptomycin, tobramycin, vancomycin, and viomycin, should be avoided. Another factor which may increase patient risk of toxicity is dehydration.

The concurrent use of gentamicin with potent diuretics, such as ethacrynic acid or furosemide, should be avoided, since certain diuretics by themselves may cause ototoxicity. In addition, when administered intravenously, diuretics may enhance aminoglycoside toxicity by altering the antibiotic concentration in serum and tissue.

DESCRIPTION

Gentamicin sulfate, a water-soluble antibiotic of the aminoglycoside group, is derived from *Micromonospora purpurea*, an actinomycete. Garamycin pediatric injectable and Garamycin adult injectable is a sterile, aqueous solution for parenteral administration.

Pediatric Injection: Each ml contains gentamicin sulfate equivalent to 10 mg gentamicin base; 1.3 mg methylparaben and 0.2 mg propylparaben as preservatives; 3.2 mg sodium bisulfite; and 0.1 mg edetate disodium.

Adult Injection: Each ml contains gentamicin sulfate equivalent to 40 mg gentamicin base; 1.8 mg methylparaben and 0.2 mg propylparaben as preservatives; 3.2 mg sodium bisulfite; and 0.1 mg edetate disodium.

CLINICAL PHARMACOLOGY

PEDIATRIC INJECTION

After intramuscular administration of gentamicin sulfate pediatric injectable, peak serum concentrations usually occur between 30 and 60 minutes and serum levels are measurable for 6-12 hours. In infants, a single dose of 2.5 mg/kg usually provides a peak serum level in the range of 3-5 μg/ml. When gentamicin is administered by intravenous infusion over a 2 hour period, the serum concentrations are similar to those obtained by intramuscular administration. Age markedly affects the peak concentrations: in one report, a 1 mg/kg dose produced mean peak concentrations of 1.58, 2.03, and 2.81 μg/ml in patients 6 months to 5 years old, 5-10 years old, and over 10 years old, respectively.

In infants 1 week to 6 months of age, the half-life is 3 to 3½ hours. In full-term and large premature infants less than 1 week old, the approximate serum half-life of gentamicin is 5½ hours. In small premature infants, the half-life is inversely related to birth weight. In premature infants weighing less than 1500 g, the half-life is 11½ hours; in those weighing 1500-2000 g, the half-life is 8 hours; in those weighing over 2000 g, the half-life is approximately 5 hours. While some variation is to be expected due to a number of variables such as age, body temperature, surface area, and physiologic differences, the individual patient given the same dose tends to have similar levels in repeated determinations.

ADULT INJECTION

After intramuscular administration of gentamicin sulfate injectable, peak serum concentrations usually occur between 30 and 60 minutes and serum levels are measurable for 6-8 hours. When gentamicin is administered by intravenous infusion over a 2 hour period, the serum concentrations are similar to those obtained by intramuscular administration.

In patients with normal renal functions, peak serum concentrations of gentamicin (μg/ml) are usually up to 4 times the single intramuscular dose (mg/kg); for example, a 1.0 mg/kg injection in adults may be expected to result in a peak serum concentration up to 4 μg/ml; a 1.5 mg/kg dose may produce levels up to 6 μg/ml. While some variation is to be expected due to a number of variables such as age, body temperature, surface area, and physiologic differences, the individual patient given the same dose tends to have similar levels in repeated determinations. Gentamicin administered at 1.0 mg/kg every 8 hours for the usual 7-10 day treatment period to patients with normal renal function does not accumulate in the serum.

PEDIATRIC AND ADULT INJECTION

Gentamicin, like all aminoglycosides, may accumulate in the serum and tissues of patients treated with higher doses and/or for prolonged periods, particularly in the presence of impaired or immature renal function. In patients with immature or impaired renal function, gentamicin is cleared from the body more slowly than in patients with normal renal function. The more severe the impairment, the slower the clearance. (Dosage must be adjusted.)

Since gentamicin is distributed in extracellular fluid, peak serum concentrations may be lower than usual in patients who have a large volume of this fluid. Serum concentrations of gentamicin in febrile patients may be lower than those in afebrile patients given the same dose. When body temperature returns to normal, serum concentrations of the drug may rise. Febrile and anemic states may be associated with a shorter than usual serum half-life. (Dosage adjustment is usually not necessary.) In severely burned patients, the half-life may be significantly decreased and resulting serum concentrations may be lower than anticipated from the mg/kg dose.

Protein-binding studies have indicated that the degree of gentamicin binding is low; depending upon the methods used for testing, this may be between 0 and 30%.

PEDIATRIC INJECTION

In neonates less than 3 days old, approximately 10% of the administered dose is excreted in 12 hours; in infants 5-40 days old, approximately 40% is excreted over the same period. Excretion of gentamicin correlates with postnatal age and creatinine clearance. Thus, with increasing postnatal age and concomitant increase in renal maturity, gentamicin is excreted more rapidly. Little, if any, metabolic transformation occurs; the drug is excreted principally by glomerular filtration. After several days of treatment, the amount of gentamicin excreted in the urine approaches, but does not equal, the daily dose administered. As with other aminoglycosides, a small amount of the gentamicin dose may be retained in the tissues, especially in the kidneys. Minute quantities of aminoglycosides have been detected in the urine of some patients weeks after drug administration was discontinued. Renal clearance of gentamicin is similar to that of endogenous creatinine.

ADULT INJECTION

After initial administration to patients with normal renal function, generally 70% or more of the gentamicin dose is recoverable in the urine in 24 hours; concentrations in urine above 100 μg/ml may be achieved. Little, if any, metabolic transformation occurs; the drug is excreted principally by glomerular filtration. After several days of treatment, the amount of gentamicin excreted in the urine approaches the daily dose administered. As with other aminoglycosides, a small amount of the gentamicin dose may be retained in the tissues, especially in the kidneys. Minute quantities of aminoglycosides have been detected in the urine weeks after drug administration was discontinued. Renal clearance of gentamicin is similar to that of endogenous creatinine.

PEDIATRIC AND ADULT INJECTION

In patients with marked impairment of renal function, there is a decrease in the concentration of aminoglycosides in urine and in their penetration into defective renal parenchyma. This decreased drug excretion, together with the potential nephrotoxicity of aminoglycosides, should be considered when treating such patients who have urinary tract infections.

Probenecid does not affect renal tubular transport of gentamicin.

The endogenous creatinine clearance rate and the serum creatinine level have a high correlation with the half-life of gentamicin in serum. Results of these tests may serve as guides for adjusting dosage in patients with renal impairment (see DOSAGE AND ADMINISTRATION).

Following parenteral administration, gentamicin can be detected in serum, lymph, tissues, sputum, and in pleural, synovial, and peritoneal fluids. Concentrations in renal cortex sometimes may be 8 times higher than the usual serum levels. Concentrations in bile, in general, have been low and have suggested minimal biliary excretion. Gentamicin crosses the peritoneal as well as the placental membranes. Since aminoglycosides diffuse poorly into the subarachnoid space after parenteral administration, concentrations of gentamicin in cerebrospinal fluid are often low and dependent upon dose, rate of penetration, and degree of meningeal inflammation. There is minimal penetration of gentamicin into ocular tissues following intramuscular or intravenous administration.

Microbiology

In vitro tests have demonstrated that gentamicin is a bactericidal antibiotic which acts by inhibiting normal protein synthesis in susceptible microorganisms. It is active against a wide variety of pathogenic bacteria including *Escherichia coli, Proteus* species (indole-positive and indole-negative), *Pseudomonas aeruginosa,* species of the *Klebsiella-Enterobacter-Serratia* group, *Citrobacter* species, and *Staphylococcus* species (including penicillin- and methicillin-resistant strains). Gentamicin is also active *in vitro* against species of *Salmonella* and *Shigella.* The following bacteria are usually resistant to aminoglycosides: *Streptococcus pneumoniae,* most species of streptococci, particularly group D and anaerobic organisms, such as *Bacteroides* species or *Clostridium* species.

In vitro studies have shown that an aminoglycoside combined with an antibiotic that interferes with cell wall synthesis may act synergistically against some group D streptococcal strains. The combination of gentamicin and penicillin G has a synergistic bactericidal effect against virtually all strains of *Streptococcus faecalis* and its varieties (*S. faecalis* var. *liquifaciens, S. faecalis* var. *zymogenes*), *S. faecium* and *S. durans.* An enhanced killing effect against many of these strains has also been shown *in vitro* with combinations of gentamicin and ampicillin, carbenicillin, nafcillin, or oxacillin.

The combined effect of gentamicin and carbenicillin is synergistic for many strains of *Pseudomonas aeruginosa. In vitro* synergism against other gram-negative organisms has been shown with combinations of gentamicin and cephalosporins.

Gentamicin may be active against clinical isolates of bacteria resistant to other aminoglycosides. Bacteria resistant to one aminoglycoside may be resistant to one or more other aminoglycosides. Bacterial resistance to gentamicin is generally developed slowly.

Susceptibility Testing

If the disc method of susceptibility testing used is that described by Bauer *et al.* (*Am J Clin Path* 45:493, 1966; *Federal Register* 37:20525-20529, 1972), a disc containing 10 μg of gentamicin should give a zone of inhibition of 15 mm or more to indicate susceptibility of the infecting organism. A zone of 12 mm or less indicates that the infecting organism is likely to be resistant. Zones greater than 12 mm and less than 15 mm indicate intermediate susceptibility. In certain conditions it may be desirable to do additional susceptibility testing by the tube or agar dilution method; gentamicin substance is available for this purpose.

INDICATIONS AND USAGE

Gentamicin sulfate injectable is indicated in the treatment of serious infections caused by susceptible strains of the following microorganisms: *Pseudomonas aeruginosa, Proteus* species (indole-positive and indole-negative), *Escherichia coli, Klebsiella-Enterobacter-Serratia* species, *Citrobacter* species, and *Staphylococcus* species (coagulase-positive and coagulase-negative).

Clinical studies have shown gentamicin sulfate pediatric injectable to be effective in bacterial neonatal sepsis; bacterial septicemia; and serious bacterial infections of the central nervous system (meningitis), urinary tract, respiratory tract, gastrointestinal tract (including peritonitis), skin, bone and soft tissue (including burns).

Aminoglycosides, including gentamicin, are not indicated in uncomplicated initial episodes of urinary tract infections unless the causative organisms are susceptible to these antibiotics and are not susceptible to antibiotics having less potential for toxicity.

Specimens for bacterial culture should be obtained to isolate and identify causative organisms and to determine their susceptibility to gentamicin.

Gentamicin sulfate may be considered as initial therapy in suspected or confirmed gram-negative infections, and therapy may be instituted before obtaining results of susceptibility testing. The decision to continue therapy with this drug should be based on the results of susceptibility tests, the severity of the infection, and the important additional concepts contained in BOXED WARNING. If the causative organisms are resistant to gentamicin, other appropriate therapy should be instituted.

In serious infections when the causative organisms are unknown, gentamicin sulfate may be administered as initial therapy in conjunction with a penicillin-type or cephalosporin-type drug before obtaining results of susceptibility testing. If anaerobic organisms are suspected as etiologic agents, consideration should be given to using other suitable antimicrobial therapy in conjunction with gentamicin. Following identification of the organism and its susceptibility, appropriate antibiotic therapy should then be continued.

Gentamicin sulfate has been used effectively in combination with carbenicillin for the treatment of life-threatening infections caused by *Pseudomonas aeruginosa.* It has also been found effective when used in conjunction with a penicillin-type drug for the treatment of endocarditis caused by group D streptococci.

Gentamicin sulfate pediatric and adult injectables have also been shown to be effective in the treatment of serious staphylococcal infections. While not the antibiotic of first choice, gentamicin sulfate pediatric and adult injectables may be considered when penicillins or other less potentially toxic drugs are contraindicated and bacterial susceptibility tests and clinical judgment indicate its use. It may also be considered in mixed infections caused by susceptible strains of staphylococci and gram-negative organisms.

In the neonate with suspected bacterial sepsis or staphylococcal pneumonia, a penicillin-type drug is also usually indicated as concomitant therapy with gentamicin.

CONTRAINDICATIONS

Hypersensitivity to gentamicin is a contraindication to its use. A history of hypersensitivity or serious toxic reactions to other aminoglycosides may contraindicate use of gentamicin because of the known cross-sensitivity of patients to drugs in this class.

WARNINGS

See BOXED WARNING.

Aminoglycosides can cause fetal harm when administered to a pregnant woman. Aminoglycoside antibiotics cross the placenta, and there have been several reports of total irreversible bilateral congenital deafness in children whose mothers received streptomycin during pregnancy. Serious side effects to mother, fetus, or newborn have not been reported in the treatment of pregnant women with other aminoglycosides. Animal reproduction studies conducted on rats and rabbits did not reveal evidence of impaired fertility or harm to the fetus due to gentamicin sulfate.

It is not known whether gentamicin sulfate can cause fetal harm when administered to a pregnant woman or can affect reproduction capacity. If gentamicin is used during pregnancy or if the patient becomes pregnant while taking gentamicin, she should be apprised of the potential hazard to the fetus.

Gentamicin sulfate injectable contains sodium bisulfite, a sulfite that may cause allergic-type reactions including anaphylactic symptoms and life-threatening or less severe asthmatic episodes in certain susceptible people. The overall prevalence of sulfite sensitivity in the general population is unknown and probably low. Sulfite sensitivity is seen more frequently in asthmatic than in nonasthmatic people.

PRECAUTIONS

Neurotoxic and nephrotoxic antibiotics may be absorbed in significant quantities from body surfaces after local irrigation or application. The potential toxic effect of antibiotics administered in this fashion should be considered.

Increased nephrotoxicity has been reported following concomitant administration of aminoglycoside antibiotics and cephalosporins.

Neuromuscular blockade and respiratory paralysis have been reported in the cat receiving high doses (40 mg/kg) of gentamicin. The possibility of these phenomena occurring in man should be considered if aminoglycosides are administered by any route to patients receiving anesthetics, or to patients receiving neuromuscular blocking agents, such as succinylcholine, tubocurarine, or decamethonium, or in patients receiving massive transfusions of citrate-anticoagulated blood. If neuromuscular blockade occurs, calcium salts may reverse it.

Aminoglycosides should be used with caution in patients with neuromuscular disorders, such as myasthenia gravis, since these drugs may aggravate muscle weakness because of their potential curare-like effects on the neuromuscular junction. During or following gentamicin therapy, paresthesias, tetany, positive Chvostek and Trousseau signs, and mental confusion have been described in patients with hypomagnesemia, hypocalcemia, and hypokalemia. When this has occurred in infants, tetany and muscle weakness has been described. Both adults and infants required appropriate corrective electrolyte therapy.

Elderly patients may have reduced renal function which may not be evident in the results of routine screening tests, such as BUN or serum creatinine. A creatinine clearance determination may be more useful. Monitoring of renal function during treatment with gentamicin, as with other aminoglycosides, is particularly important in such patients.

A Fanconi-like syndrome, with aminoaciduria and metabolic acidosis, has been reported in some adults and infants being given gentamicin injections.

Cross-allergenicity among aminoglycosides has been demonstrated.

Patients should be well hydrated during treatment.

Although the *in vitro* mixing of gentamicin and carbenicillin results in a rapid and significant inactivation of gentamicin, this interaction has not been demonstrated in patients with normal renal function who received both drugs by different routes of administration. A reduction in gentamicin serum half-life has been reported in patients with severe renal impairment receiving carbenicillin concomitantly with gentamicin.

Treatment with gentamicin may result in overgrowth of nonsusceptible organisms. If this occurs, appropriate therapy is indicated.

See BOXED WARNING regarding concurrent use of potent diuretics and regarding concurrent and/or sequential use of other neurotoxic and/or nephrotoxic antibiotics and for other essential information.

USAGE IN PREGNANCY

Safety for use in pregnancy has not been established.

ADVERSE REACTIONS

NEPHROTOXICITY

Adverse renal effects, as demonstrated by the presence of casts, cells, or protein in the urine or by rising BUN, NPN, serum creatinine or oliguria, have been reported. They occur more frequently in patients treated for longer periods or with larger dosages than recommended.

NEUROTOXICITY

Serious adverse effects on both vestibular and auditory branches of the eighth cranial nerves have been reported, primarily in patients with renal impairment (especially if dialysis is required) and in patients on high doses and/or prolonged therapy. Symptoms include dizziness, vertigo, ataxia, tinnitus, roaring in the ears and hearing loss, which, as with the other aminoglycosides, may be irreversible. Hearing loss is usually manifested initially by diminution of high-tone acuity. Other factors which may increase the risk of toxicity include excessive dosage, dehydration, and previous exposure to other ototoxic drugs.

Peripheral neuropathy or encephalopathy, including numbness, skin tingling, muscle twitching, convulsions, and a myasthenia gravis-like syndrome, have been reported.

Note: The risk of toxic reactions is low in neonates, infants, children, and adults with normal renal function who do not receive gentamicin sulfate injectable at higher doses or for longer periods of time than recommended.

Other reported adverse reactions possibly related to gentamicin include: Respiratory depression, lethargy, confusion, depression, visual disturbances, decreased appetite, weight loss, and hypotension and hypertension; rash, itching, urticaria, generalized burning, laryngeal edema, anaphylactoid reactions, fever, and headache; nausea, vomiting, increased salivation, and stomatitis; purpura, pseudotumor cerebri, acute organic brain syndrome, pulmonary fibrosis, alopecia, joint pain, transient hepatomegaly, and splenomegaly.

Laboratory abnormalities possibly related to gentamicin include: Increased levels of serum transaminase (SGOT, SGPT), serum LDH, and bilirubin; decreased serum calcium, magnesium, sodium, and potassium; anemia, leukopenia, granulocytopenia, transient agranulocytosis, eosinophilia, increased and decreased reticulocyte counts, and thrombocytopenia.

While clinical laboratory test abnormalities may be isolated findings, they may also be associated with clinically related signs and symptoms. For example, tetany and muscle weakness may be associated with hypomagnesemia, hypocalcemia, and hypokalemia.

While local tolerance of gentamicin sulfate pediatric injectable is generally excellent, there has been an occasional report of pain at the injection site. Subcutaneous atrophy or fat necrosis suggesting local irritation has been reported rarely.

DOSAGE AND ADMINISTRATION

Gentamicin sulfate pediatric injectable may be given intramuscularly or intravenously. The patient's pretreatment body weight should be obtained for calculation of correct dosage. The dosage of aminoglycosides in obese patients should be based on an estimate of the lean body mass. It is desirable to limit the duration of treatment with aminoglycosides to short term.

DOSAGE FOR PATIENTS WITH NORMAL RENAL FUNCTION

Children: 6 to 7.5 mg/kg/day. (2.0-2.5 mg/kg administered every 8 hours.)

Infants and neonates: 7.5 mg/kg/day. (2.5 mg/kg administered every 8 hours.)

Premature or full-term neonates 1 week of age or less: 5 mg/kg/day. (2.5 mg/kg administered every 12 hours.)

Adults: The recommended dosage of gentamicin sulfate injectable for patients with serious infections and normal renal function is 3 mg/kg/day, administered in 3 equal doses every 8 hours (TABLE 1).

For patients with life-threatening infections, dosages up to 5 mg/kg/day may be administered in 3 or 4 equal doses. This dosage should be reduced to 3 mg/kg/day as soon as clinically indicated (TABLE 1).

It is desirable to measure periodically both peak and trough serum concentrations of gentamicin when feasible during therapy to assure adequate but not excessive drug levels. For example, the peak concentration (at 30-60 minutes after intramuscular injection) is expected to be in the range of 3-5 μg/ml for pediatric patients, and 4-6 μg/ml for adult patients. When monitoring peak concentrations after intramuscular or intravenous administration, dosage should be adjusted so that prolonged levels above 12 μg/ml are avoided. When monitoring trough concentrations (just prior to the next dose), dosage should be adjusted so that levels above 2 μg/ml are avoided. Determination of the adequacy of a serum level for a particular patient must take into consideration the susceptibility of the causative organism, the severity of the infection, and the status of the patient's host-defense mechanisms.

In patients with extensive burns, altered pharmacokinetics may result in reduced serum concentrations of aminoglycosides. In such patients treated with gentamicin, measurement of serum concentrations is recommended as a basis for dosage adjustment.

The usual duration of treatment is 7-10 days. In difficult and complicated infections, a longer course of therapy may be necessary. In such cases monitoring of renal, auditory, and vestibular functions is recommended, since toxicity is more apt to occur with treatment extended for more than 10 days. Dosage should be reduced if clinically indicated.

FOR INTRAVENOUS ADMINISTRATION

The intravenous administration of gentamicin may be particularly useful for treating patients with bacterial septicemia or those in shock. It may also be the preferred route of administration for some patients with congestive heart failure, hematologic disorders, severe burns, or those with reduced muscle mass.

For intermittent intravenous administration, a single dose of gentamicin sulfate injectable may be diluted in sterile isotonic saline solution (50-200 ml in adults) or in a sterile solution of dextrose 5% in water. In infants and children, the volume of diluent should be less. The solution may be infused over a period of ½ to 2 hours.

The recommended dosage for intravenous and intramuscular administration is identical.

Gentamicin sulfate injectable should not be physically premixed with other drugs, but should be administered separately in accordance with the recommended route of administration and dosage schedule.

TABLE 1 *Dosage Schedule Guide For Adults With Normal Renal Function (Dosage at 8 hour Intervals) 40 mg/ml*

Patient's Weight*		Usual Dose for Serious Infections		Dose For Life-Threatening Infections (reduce as soon as clinically indicated)	
		1 mg/kg q8h		1.7 mg/kg q8h†	
kg	(lb)	(3 mg/kg/day)		(5 mg/kg/day)	
		mg/dose q8h	ml/dose	mg/dose q8h	ml/dose
40	(88)	40	1.0	66	1.6
45	(99)	45	1.1	75	1.9
50	(110)	50	1.25	83	2.1
55	(121)	55	1.4	91	2.25
60	(132)	60	1.5	100	2.5
65	(143)	65	1.6	108	2.7
70	(154)	70	1.75	116	2.9
75	(165)	75	1.9	125	3.1
80	(176)	80	2.0	133	3.3
85	(187)	85	2.1	141	3.5
90	(198)	90	2.25	150	3.75
95	(209)	95	2.4	158	4.0
100	(220)	100	2.5	166	4.2

* The dosage of aminoglycosides in obese patients should be based on an estimate of the lean body mass.

† For q6h schedules, dosage should be recalculated.

DOSAGE FOR PATIENTS WITH IMPAIRED RENAL FUNCTION

Dosage must be adjusted in patients with impaired renal function to assure therapeutically adequate, but not excessive, blood levels. Whenever possible, serum concentrations of gentamicin should be monitored. One method of dosage adjustment is to increase the interval between administration of the usual doses. Since the serum creatinine concentration has a high correlation with the serum half-life of gentamicin, this laboratory test may provide guidance for adjustment of the interval between doses. In adults, the interval between doses (in hours) may be approximately by multiplying the serum creatinine level (mg/100 ml) by 8. For example, a patient weighing 60 kg with a serum creatinine level of 2.0 mg/100 ml could be given 60 mg (1 mg/kg) every 16 hours (2 × 8). These guidelines may be considered when treating patients with serious renal impairment.

In patients with serious systemic infections and renal impairment, it may be desirable to administer the antibiotic more frequently but in reduced dosage. In such patients, serum concentrations of gentamicin should be measured so that adequate but not excessive levels result. A peak and trough concentration measured intermittently during therapy will provide optimal guidance for adjusting dosage. After the usual initial dose, a rough guide for determining reduced dosage at 8 hour intervals is to divide the normally recommended dose by the serum creatinine level (TABLE 2). For example, after an initial dose of 20 mg (2.0 mg/kg), a child weighing 10 kg with a serum creatinine level of 2.0 mg/100 ml could be given 10 mg every 8 hours (20 ÷ 2). It should be noted that the status of renal function may be changing over the course of the infectious process. It is important to recognize that deteriorating renal function may require a greater reduction in dosage than that specified in the above guidelines for patients with stable renal impairment.

TABLE 2 *Dosage Adjustment Guide for Patients With Renal Impairment (Dosage at 8 hour Intervals After the Usual Initial Dose)*

Serum Creatinine (mg %)	Approximate Creatinine Clearance Rate (ml/min/1.73 m^2)	Percent of Usual Doses Shown Above
≤1.0	>100	100%
1.1-1.3	70-100	80%
1.4-1.6	55-70	65%
1.7-1.9	45-55	55%
2.0-2.2	40-45	50%
2.3-2.5	35-40	40%
2.6-3.0	30-35	35%
3.1-3.5	25-30	30%
3.6-4.0	20-25	25%
4.1-5.1	15-20	20%
5.2-6.6	10-15	15%
6.7-8.0	<10	10%

In patients with renal failure undergoing hemodialysis, the amount of gentamicin removed from the blood may vary depending upon several factors including the dialysis method used. An 8 hour hemodialysis may reduce serum concentrations of gentamicin by approximately 50%. In children the recommended dose at the end of each dialysis period is 2.0-2.5 mg/kg depending upon the severity of infection. The recommended dosage at the end of each adult dialysis period is 1-1.7 mg/kg depending upon the severity of infection.

The above dosage schedules are not intended as rigid recommendations but are provided as guides to dosage when the measurement of gentamicin serum levels is not feasible.

A variety of methods are available to measure gentamicin concentrations in body fluids; these include microbiologic, enzymatic, and radioimmunoassay techniques.

HOW SUPPLIED

Garamycin pediatric injectable and adult injectable are clear, stable solutions that requires no refrigeration.

Storage: Store between 2-30°C (36-86°F).

TOPICAL

DESCRIPTION

Each gram of Garamycin cream 0.1% contains 1.7 mg gentamicin sulfate, equivalent to 1.0 mg gentamicin base, with 1.0 mg methylparaben and 4.0 mg butylparaben as preservatives, in a bland, emulsion-type vehicle composed of stearic acid, propylene glycol stearate, isopropyl myristate, propylene glycol, polysorbate 40, sorbitol solution and purified water.

Each gram of Garamycin ointment 0.1% contains 1.7 mg gentamicin sulfate, equivalent to 1.0 mg gentamicin base, with 0.5 mg methylparaben and 0.1 mg propylparaben as preservatives in a bland, unctuous petrolatum base.

CLINICAL PHARMACOLOGY

Gentamicin sulfate, a wide-spectrum antibiotic, provides highly effective topical treatment in primary and secondary bacterial infections of the skin. Gentamicin sulfate may clear infections that have not responded to other topical antibiotic agents. In impetigo contagiosa and other primary skin infections, treatment 3 or 4 times daily with gentamicin sulfate usually clears the lesions promptly. In secondary skin infections, gentamicin sulfate facilitates the treatment of the underlying dermatosis by controlling the infection. Bacteria susceptible to the action of gentamicin sulfate include sensitive strains of streptococci (group A beta-hemolytic, alpha-hemolytic), *Staphylococcus aureus* (coagulase-positive, coagulase-negative, and some penicillinase-producing strains), and the gram-negative bacteria, *Pseudomonas aeruginosa, Aerobacter aerogenes, Escherichia coli, Proteus vulgaris,* and *Klebsiella pneumoniae*.

INDICATIONS AND USAGE

Primary Skin Infections: Impetigo contagiosa, superficial folliculitis, ecthyma, furunculosis, sycosis barbae, and pyoderma gangrenosum.

Secondary Skin Infections: Infectious eczematoid dermatitis, pustular acne, pustular psoriasis, infected seborrheic dermatitis, infected contact dermatitis (including poison ivy), infected excoriations, and bacterial superinfections of fungal or viral infections.

Note: Gentamicin sulfate is a bactericidal agent that is not effective against viruses or fungi in skin infections. Gentamicin sulfate is useful in the treatment of infected skin cysts and certain other skin abscesses when preceded by incision and drainage to permit adequate contact between the antibiotic and the infecting bacteria. Good results have been obtained in the treatment of infected stasis and other skin ulcers, infected superficial burns, paronychia, infected insect bites and stings, infected lacerations and abrasions, and wounds from minor surgery. Patients sensitive to neomycin can be treated with gentamicin, although regular observation of patients sensitive to topical antibiotics is advisable when such patients are treated with any topical antibiotic. Gentamicin sulfate ointment helps retain moisture and has been useful in infection on dry eczematous or psoriatic skin. Gentamicin sulfate cream is recommended for wet, oozing primary infections and greasy, secondary infections, such as pustular acne or infected seborrheic dermatitis. If a water-washable preparation is desired, gentamicin sulfate cream is preferable. Gentamicin sulfate ointment and cream have been used successfully in infants over 1 year of age, as well as in adults and children.

CONTRAINDICATIONS

This drug is contraindicated in individuals with a history of sensitivity reactions to any of its components.

PRECAUTIONS

Use of topical antibiotics occasionally allows overgrowth of nonsusceptible organisms, including fungi. If this occurs, or if irritation, sensitization, or superinfection develops, treatment with gentamicin should be discontinued and appropriate therapy instituted.

ADVERSE REACTIONS

In patients with dermatoses treated with gentamicin, irritation (erythema and pruritus) that did not usually require discontinuance of treatment has been reported in a small percentage of cases. There was no evidence of irritation or sensitization, however, in any of these patients patch-tested subsequently with gentamicin on normal skin. Possible photosensitization has been reported in several patients but could not be elicited in these patients by reapplication of gentamicin followed by exposure to ultraviolet radiation.

DOSAGE AND ADMINISTRATION

A small amount of gentamicin sulfate cream or ointment should be applied gently to the lesions 3 or 4 times daily. The area treated may be covered with a gauze dressing, if desired. In impetigo contagiosa, the crusts should be removed before application of gentamicin sulfate to permit maximum contact between the antibiotic and the infection. Care should be exercised to avoid further contamination of the infected skin. Infected stasis ulcers have responded well to gentamicin sulfate under gelatin packing.

HOW SUPPLIED

Storage: Store between 2-30°C (36-86°F).

OPHTHALMIC

DESCRIPTION

Gentamicin sulfate is a water-soluble antibiotic of the aminoglycoside group.

Gentamicin sulfate ophthalmic solution is a sterile, aqueous solution buffered to approximately pH 7 for ophthalmic use. Each ml contains gentamicin sulfate (equivalent to 3.0 mg gentamicin), disodium phosphate, monosodium phosphate, sodium chloride, and benzalkonium chloride (0.1 mg) as a preservative.

Gentamicin sulfate ophthalmic ointment is a sterile ointment, each gram containing gentamicin sulfate (equivalent to 3.0 mg gentamicin) in a base of white petrolatum, with methylparaben (0.5 mg) and propylparaben (0.1 mg) as preservatives.

Gentamicin is obtained from cultures of *Micromonospora purpurea.* It is a mixture of the sulfate salts of gentamicin C_1, C_2 and C_{1A}. All three components appear to have similar antimicrobial activities. Gentamicin sulfate occurs as a white powder and is soluble in water and insoluble in alcohol.

Storage: Store Garamycin Ophthalmic Ointment and Solution between 2-30°C (36-86°F).

CLINICAL PHARMACOLOGY

MICROBIOLOGY

Gentamicin sulfate is active *in vitro* against many strains of the following microorganisms:

Staphylococcus aureus Staphylococcus epidermidis, Streptococcus pyogenes, Streptococcus pneumoniae, Enterobacter aerogenes, Escherichia coli, Haemophilus influenzae, Klebsiella pneumoniae, Neisseria gonorrhoeae, Pseudomonas aeruginosa, and *Serratia marcescens.*

INDICATIONS AND USAGE

Gentamicin sulfate sterile ophthalmic solution and ointment are indicated in the topical treatment of ocular bacterial infections, including conjunctivitis, keratitis, keratoconjunctivitis, corneal ulcers, blepharitis, blepharoconjunctivitis, acute meibomianitis, and dacryocystitis caused by susceptible strains of the following microorganisms:

Staphylococcus aureus, Staphylococcus epidermidis, Streptococcus pyogenes, Streptococcus pneumoniae, Enterobacter aerogenes, Escherichia coli, Haemophilus influenzae, Klebsiella pneumoniae, Neisseria gonorrhoeae, Pseudomonas aeruginosa, and *Serratia marcescens.*

CONTRAINDICATIONS

Gentamicin sulfate ophthalmic solution and ointment are contraindicated in patients with known hypersensitivity to any of the components.

WARNINGS

NOT FOR INJECTION INTO THE EYE. Gentamicin sulfate ophthalmic solution and ointment are not for injection. They should never be injected subconjunctivally, nor should they be directly introduced into the anterior chamber of the eye.

PRECAUTIONS

GENERAL

Prolonged use of topical antibiotics may give rise to overgrowth of nonsusceptible organisms including fungi. Bacterial resistance to gentamicin may also develop. If purulent discharge, inflammation or pain becomes aggravated, the patient should discontinue use of the medication and consult a physician.

If irritation or hypersensitivity to any component of the drug develops, the patient should discontinue use of this preparation, and appropriate therapy should be instituted.

Ophthalmic ointments may retard corneal healing.

INFORMATION FOR THE PATIENT

To avoid contamination, do not touch tip of container to the eye, eyelid, or any surface.

CARCINOGENESIS, MUTAGENESIS, AND IMPAIRMENT OF FERTILITY

There are no published carcinogenicity or impairment of fertility studies on gentamicin. Aminoglycoside antibiotics have been found to be non-mutagenic.

PREGNANCY CATEGORY C

Gentamicin has been shown to depress body weights, kidney weights, and median glomerular counts in newborn rats when administered systemically to pregnant rats in daily doses approximately 500 times the maximum recommended ophthalmic human dose. There are no adequate and well-controlled studies in pregnant women. Gentamicin should be used during pregnancy only if the potential benefit justifies the potential risk to the fetus.

ADVERSE REACTIONS

Bacterial and fungal corneal ulcers have developed during treatment with gentamicin ophthalmic preparations.

The most frequently reported adverse reactions are ocular burning and irritation upon drug instillation, non-specific conjunctivitis, conjunctival epithelial defects, and conjunctival hyperemia.

Other adverse reactions which have occurred rarely are allergic reactions, thrombocytopenic purpura, and hallucinations.

DOSAGE AND ADMINISTRATION

Gentamicin Sulfate Ophthalmic Solution: Instill 1 or 2 drops into the affected eye every 4 hours. In severe infections, dosage may be increased to as much as 2 drops once every hour.

Gentamicin Sulfate Ophthalmic Ointment: Apply a small amount (about ½ inch) to the affected eye 2-3 times a day.

PRODUCT LISTING - RATED THERAPEUTICALLY EQUIVALENT

Cream - Topical - 0.1%

Size	Price	Product	NDC
15 gm	$2.90	GENERIC, Qualitest Products Inc	00603-7769-74
15 gm	$3.00	GENERIC, Interstate Drug Exchange Inc	00814-3446-93
15 gm	$3.00	GENERIC, Interstate Drug Exchange Inc	00814-3447-93
15 gm	$3.00	GENERIC, Clay-Park Laboratories Inc	45802-0056-35
15 gm	$3.10	GENERIC, Major Pharmaceuticals Inc	00904-2663-36
15 gm	$3.10	GENERIC, Major Pharmaceuticals Inc	00904-2664-36
15 gm	$3.23	GENERIC, Ivax Corporation	00182-1403-51
15 gm	$3.23	GENERIC, Moore, H.L. Drug Exchange Inc	00839-6492-47
15 gm	$3.25	GENERIC, Cmc-Consolidated Midland Corporation	00223-4304-15
15 gm	$3.25	GENERIC, Cmc-Consolidated Midland Corporation	00223-4306-15
15 gm	$3.56	GENERIC, Thames Pharmacal Company Inc	49158-0162-20
15 gm	$3.60	GENERIC, Fougera	00168-0071-15
30 gm	$4.75	GENERIC, Watson/Schein Pharmaceuticals Inc	00364-7305-56
30 gm	$4.80	GENERIC, Thames Pharmacal Company Inc	49158-0162-68
30 gm	$4.90	GENERIC, Clay-Park Laboratories Inc	45802-0056-11
454 gm	$86.40	GENERIC, Clay-Park Laboratories Inc	00414-0056-05
454 gm	$86.40	GENERIC, Clay-Park Laboratories Inc	45802-0056-05

Ointment - Ophthalmic - 0.3%

Size	Price	Product	NDC
3.50 gm	$12.96	GENERIC, Ciba Vision Ophthalmics	58768-0251-05
3.50 gm	$14.56	GENERIC, Alpharma Uspd Makers Of Barre and Nmc	63874-0173-04
3.50 gm	$19.67	GENERIC, Akorn Inc	17478-0284-35
3.50 gm	$19.98	GARAMYCIN OPHTHALMIC, Allscripts Pharmaceutical Company	54569-4029-00
3.50 gm	$20.50	GARAMYCIN OPHTHALMIC, Southwood Pharmaceuticals Inc	58016-6433-01
3.50 gm	$21.64	GARAMYCIN OPHTHALMIC, Southwood Pharmaceuticals Inc	58016-6433-00
3.50 gm	$21.84	GARAMYCIN OPHTHALMIC, Schering Corporation	00085-0151-05
3.50 gm	$23.82	GARAMYCIN OPHTHALMIC, Pharma Pac	52959-0327-00

Ointment - Topical - 0.1%

Size	Price	Product	NDC
15 gm	$2.90	GENERIC, Qualitest Products Inc	00603-7770-74
15 gm	$3.00	GENERIC, Clay-Park Laboratories Inc	45802-0046-35
15 gm	$3.23	GENERIC, Moore, H.L. Drug Exchange Inc	00839-6599-47
15 gm	$3.60	GENERIC, Fougera	00168-0078-15
15 gm	$3.75	GENERIC, Ivax Corporation	00182-1474-51
15 gm	$4.00	GENERIC, Thames Pharmacal Company Inc	49158-0191-20
30 gm	$4.50	GENERIC, Ivax Corporation	00182-1474-56
30 gm	$4.80	GENERIC, Thames Pharmacal Company Inc	49158-0191-68
30 gm	$4.90	GENERIC, Clay-Park Laboratories Inc	45802-0046-11
454 gm	$86.40	GENERIC, Clay-Park Laboratories Inc	00414-0046-05
454 gm	$86.40	GENERIC, Clay-Park Laboratories Inc	45802-0046-05

Solution - Injectable - 10 mg/ml

Size	Price	Product	NDC
2 ml x 10	$22.49	GARAMYCIN, Schering Corporation	00085-0013-06
2 ml x 25	$19.50	GENERIC, Esi Lederle Generics	00641-0394-25
2 ml x 25	$29.50	GENERIC, American Pharmaceutical Partners	63323-0513-02
2 ml x 25	$31.00	GENERIC, American Pharmaceutical Partners	63323-0173-02
6 ml x 25	$59.67	GENERIC, Abbott Pharmaceutical	00074-3400-01
8 ml x 25	$61.45	GENERIC, Abbott Pharmaceutical	00074-3401-01
10 ml x 25	$64.72	GENERIC, Abbott Pharmaceutical	00074-3402-01

Solution - Injectable - 40 mg/ml

Size	Price	Product	NDC
2 ml	$2.15	GENERIC, Moore, H.L. Drug Exchange Inc	00839-6503-23
2 ml x 25	$21.00	GENERIC, Abbott Pharmaceutical	00074-1207-03
2 ml x 25	$39.89	GENERIC, Esi Lederle Generics	00641-0395-25
2 ml x 25	$64.50	GENERIC, American Pharmaceutical Partners	63323-0010-02
2 ml x 25	$157.68	GARAMYCIN, Schering Corporation	00085-0069-04
20 ml	$7.74	GENERIC, Major Pharmaceuticals Inc	00904-0799-55
20 ml	$9.95	GENERIC, Roberts/Hauck Pharmaceutical Corporation	43797-0144-26
20 ml	$11.25	GENERIC, Watson/Rugby Laboratories Inc	00536-4690-73
20 ml x 10	$159.47	GENERIC, Esi Lederle Generics	00641-2331-43
20 ml x 25	$140.75	GENERIC, American Pharmaceutical Partners	63323-0010-20
50 ml x 10	$325.90	GENERIC, American Pharmaceutical Partners	63323-0010-50

Solution - Intravenous - 40 mg/50 ml;0.9%

Size	Price	Product	NDC
50 ml x 24	$93.90	GENERIC, Baxter I.V. Systems Division	00338-0503-41

Solution - Intravenous - 60 mg/50 ml;0.9%

Size	Price	Product	NDC
50 ml x 24	$86.40	GENERIC, B. Braun/Mcgaw Inc	00264-5812-38
50 ml x 24	$106.32	GENERIC, Abbott Pharmaceutical	00074-7879-13
50 ml x 24	$222.91	GENERIC, Baxter I.V. Systems Division	00338-0507-41

Solution - Intravenous - 60 mg/100 ml;0.9%

Size	Price	Product	NDC
100 ml x 24	$112.08	GENERIC, Baxter I.V. Systems Division	00338-0501-48
100 ml x 24	$115.85	GENERIC, Baxter I.V. Systems Division	00338-0507-48
100 ml x 24	$258.24	GENERIC, B. Braun/Mcgaw Inc	00264-5806-32

Solution - Intravenous - 70 mg/50 ml;0.9%

Size	Price	Product	NDC
50 ml x 24	$110.01	GENERIC, Abbott Pharmaceutical	00074-7881-13

Solution - Intravenous - 80 mg/50 ml;0.9%

Size	Price	Product	NDC
50 ml x 24	$104.00	GENERIC, B. Braun/Mcgaw Inc	00264-5816-38
50 ml x 24	$114.00	GENERIC, Abbott Pharmaceutical	00074-7883-13
50 ml x 24	$237.84	GENERIC, Baxter I.V. Systems Division	00338-0509-41

Solution - Intravenous - 80 mg/100 ml;0.9%

Size	Price	Product	NDC
100 ml x 24	$97.50	GENERIC, B. Braun/Mcgaw Inc	00264-5808-32
100 ml x 24	$138.72	GENERIC, Abbott Pharmaceutical	00074-7884-23
100 ml x 24	$237.84	GENERIC, Baxter Healthcare Corporation	00338-0503-48

Solution - Intravenous - 90 mg/100 ml;0.9%

Size	Price	Product	NDC
100 ml x 24	$142.22	GENERIC, Abbott Pharmaceutical	00074-7886-23

Solution - Intravenous - 100 mg/50 ml;0.9%

Size	Price	Product	NDC
50 ml x 24	$258.60	GENERIC, Baxter I.V. Systems Division	00338-0511-41

Solution - Intravenous - 100 mg/100 ml;0.9%

100 ml x 24	$105.00	GENERIC, B. Braun/Mcgaw Inc	00264-5810-32
100 ml x 24	$146.40	GENERIC, Abbott Pharmaceutical	00074-7889-23
100 ml x 24	$258.72	GENERIC, Baxter I.V. Systems Division	00338-0505-48

Solution - Ophthalmic - 0.3%

1 ml	$3.76	GENOPTIC, Allergan Inc	11980-0117-01
5 ml	$2.95	GENERIC, Paco Pharmaceutical Services, Inc	52967-0505-35
5 ml	$3.27	FEDERAL UPPER LIMIT, H.C.F.A. F F P	99999-1352-14
5 ml	$4.85	GENERIC, Major Pharmaceuticals Inc	00904-1908-38
5 ml	$5.10	GENERIC, Interstate Drug Exchange Inc	00814-3448-38
5 ml	$5.52	GENERIC, Moore, H.L. Drug Exchange Inc	00839-6745-25
5 ml	$5.89	GENERIC, Parmed Pharmaceuticals Inc	00349-8579-75
5 ml	$6.00	GENERIC, Fougera	00168-0248-03
5 ml	$6.10	GENERIC, Geneva Pharmaceuticals	00781-7110-75
5 ml	$6.14	GENERIC, Aligen Independent Laboratories Inc	00405-6060-05
5 ml	$6.38	GENERIC, Ocusoft	54799-0510-05
5 ml	$8.00	GENERIC, Ivax Corporation	00182-1695-62
5 ml	$8.17	GENERIC, Bausch and Lomb	24208-0419-05
5 ml	$8.75	GENERIC, Pacific Pharma	60758-0188-05
5 ml	$9.44	GENERIC, Major Pharmaceuticals Inc	00904-1907-05
5 ml	$9.54	GENERIC, Akorn Inc	17478-0283-10
5 ml	$9.62	GENERIC, Ciba Vision Ophthalmics	58768-0365-05
5 ml	$11.82	GENERIC, Ciba Vision Ophthalmics	00058-0151-05
5 ml	$14.86	GARAMYCIN OPHTHALMIC, Southwood Pharmaceuticals Inc	58016-6441-01
5 ml	$17.93	GENOPTIC, Allergan Inc	11980-0117-05
5 ml	$18.25	GENERIC, Qualitest Products Inc	00603-7158-37
5 ml	$19.98	GARAMYCIN OPHTHALMIC, Allscripts Pharmaceutical Company	54569-0866-00
5 ml	$21.20	GARAMYCIN OPHTHALMIC, Schering Corporation	00085-0899-05
5 ml	$21.64	GARAMYCIN OPHTHALMIC, Southwood Pharmaceuticals Inc	58016-6441-05
5 ml	$22.03	GARAMYCIN OPHTHALMIC, Pharma Pac	52959-0320-00
15 ml	$3.45	GENERIC, Paco Pharmaceutical Services, Inc	52967-0505-45
15 ml	$6.38	GENERIC, Interstate Drug Exchange Inc	00814-3448-42
15 ml	$7.35	GENERIC, Major Pharmaceuticals Inc	00904-1907-35
15 ml	$7.52	GENERIC, Aligen Independent Laboratories Inc	00405-6060-15
15 ml	$8.95	GENERIC, Geneva Pharmaceuticals	00781-7110-85
15 ml	$10.78	GENERIC, Bausch and Lomb	24208-0419-15
15 ml	$11.91	GENERIC, Akorn Inc	17478-0283-12

PRODUCT LISTING - EQUIVALENTS NOT AVAILABLE

Cream - Topical - 0.1%

15 gm	$2.55	GENERIC, Raway Pharmacal Inc	00686-0056-35
15 gm	$3.60	GENERIC, Allscripts Pharmaceutical Company	54569-1117-00
15 gm	$13.07	GENERIC, Alpharma Uspd Makers Of Barre and Nmc	63874-0132-15
15 gm	$24.13	GARAMYCIN TOPICAL, Schering Corporation	00085-0008-05
30 gm	$26.10	GENERIC, Alpharma Uspd Makers Of Barre and Nmc	63874-0132-30

Ointment - Ophthalmic - 0.3%

3.50 gm	$4.10	OCU-MYCIN, Ocumed Inc	51944-3335-00
3.50 gm	$4.75	GENERIC, Raway Pharmacal Inc	00686-0575-55
3.50 gm	$9.55	GENERIC, Sidmak Laboratories Inc	50111-0819-20
3.50 gm	$14.88	GENERIC, Allscripts Pharmaceutical Company	54569-1229-00
3.50 gm	$18.60	GENERIC, Southwood Pharmaceuticals Inc	58016-6026-01
3.50 gm	$21.12	GENERIC, Pharma Pac	52959-0078-03

Ointment - Topical - 0.1%

15 gm	$2.10	GENERIC, Raway Pharmacal Inc	00686-0046-35
15 gm	$3.60	GENERIC, Allscripts Pharmaceutical Company	54569-1144-00
15 gm	$17.47	GENERIC, Alpharma Uspd Makers Of Barre and Nmc	63874-0172-15
15 gm	$18.60	GENERIC, Southwood Pharmaceuticals Inc	58016-3027-01
30 gm	$33.54	GENERIC, Alpharma Uspd Makers Of Barre and Nmc	63874-0172-30

Solution - Injectable - 10 mg/ml

2 ml	$1.75	GENERIC, Cmc-Consolidated Midland Corporation	00223-7715-02
2 ml x 25	$37.50	GENERIC, Cmc-Consolidated Midland Corporation	00223-7714-02

Solution - Injectable - 40 mg/ml

2 ml	$2.25	GENERIC, Cmc-Consolidated Midland Corporation	00223-7719-02
2 ml	$2.93	GENERIC, Interstate Drug Exchange Inc	00814-3446-35
2 ml	$4.00	GENERIC, Bolan Pharmaceutical Inc	44437-0559-02
2 ml x 25	$50.00	GENERIC, Cmc-Consolidated Midland Corporation	00223-7721-02
2 ml x 25	$52.50	GENERIC, Cmc-Consolidated Midland Corporation	00223-7719-25
2 ml x 25	$65.10	GENERIC, Allscripts Pharmaceutical Company	54569-3149-00
20 ml	$7.43	GENERIC, Interstate Drug Exchange Inc	00814-3446-44
20 ml	$8.25	GENERIC, Cmc-Consolidated Midland Corporation	00223-7717-20

Solution - Ophthalmic - 0.3%

5 ml	$3.75	GENERIC, Logen	00820-0105-22
5 ml	$4.10	OCU-MYCIN, Ocumed Inc	51944-4335-05
5 ml	$4.75	GENERIC, Cmc-Consolidated Midland Corporation	00223-6651-05
5 ml	$4.76	GENERIC, Prescript Pharmaceuticals	00247-0011-05
5 ml	$5.10	GENERIC, Raway Pharmacal Inc	00686-0580-60
5 ml	$9.50	GENERIC, Falcon Pharmaceuticals, Ltd.	61314-0633-05
5 ml	$11.44	GENERIC, Alpharma Uspd Makers Of Barre and Nmc	63874-0133-05
5 ml	$18.60	GENERIC, Southwood Pharmaceuticals Inc	58016-6027-01
5 ml	$20.49	GENERIC, Pharma Pac	52959-0103-00
15 ml	$4.65	OCU-MYCIN, Ocumed Inc	51944-4335-02
15 ml	$5.50	GENERIC, Cmc-Consolidated Midland Corporation	00223-6651-45
15 ml	$6.00	GENERIC, Raway Pharmacal Inc	00686-0580-64
15 ml	$7.59	GENERIC, Prescript Pharmaceuticals	00247-0011-15
15 ml	$11.91	GENERIC, Allscripts Pharmaceutical Company	54569-1218-00
15 ml	$37.71	GENERIC, Pharma Pac	52959-0103-01

Glatiramer Acetate (003332)

Categories: Multiple sclerosis; Pregnancy Category B; FDA Approved 1997 Feb; Orphan Drugs
Drug Classes: Immunosuppressives
Brand Names: **Copaxone**
Cost of Therapy: $1/038.46 (Multiple Sclerosis; Capaxone Injection; 20 mg; 20 mg/day; 30 day supply)

DESCRIPTION

Copaxone is the brand name for glatiramer acetate (formerly known as copolymer-1). Glatiramer acetate, the active ingredient of Copaxone, consists of the acetate salts of synthetic polypeptides, containing four naturally occurring amino acids: L-glutamic acid, L-alanine, L-tyrosine, and L-lysine with an average molar fraction of 0.141, 0.427, 0.095, and 0.338, respectively. The average molecular weight of glatiramer acetate is 4,700-11,000 daltons.

Chemically, glatiramer acetate is designated L-glutamic acid polymer with L-alanine, L-lysine and L-tyrosine, acetate (salt).

Copaxone injection is a clear, colorless to slightly yellow, sterile, non-pyrogenic solution for subcutaneous injection. Each 1.0 ml of solution contains 20 mg of glatiramer acetate and 40 mg of mannitol. The pH range of the solution is approximately 5.5 to 8.5.

CLINICAL PHARMACOLOGY

MECHANISM OF ACTION

The mechanism(s) by which glatiramer acetate exerts its effects in patients with Multiple Sclerosis (MS) is (are) not fully elucidated. However, it is thought to act by modifying immune processes that are currently believed to be responsible for the pathogenesis of MS. This hypothesis is supported by findings of studies that have been carried out to explore the pathogenesis of experimental allergic encephalomyelitis (EAE), a condition induced in several animal species through immunization against central nervous system derived material containing myelin and often used as an experimental animal model of MS. Studies in animals and *in vitro* systems suggest that upon its administration, glatiramer acetate-specific suppressor T-cells are induced and activated in the periphery.

Because glatiramer acetate can modify immune functions, concerns exist about its potential to alter naturally occurring immune responses. Results of a limited battery of tests designed to evaluate this risk produced no finding of concern; nevertheless, there is no logical way to absolutely exclude this possibility (see PRECAUTIONS).

PHARMACOKINETICS

Results obtained in pharmacokinetic studies performed in humans (healthy volunteers) and animals support the assumption that a substantial fraction of the therapeutic dose delivered to patients subcutaneously is hydrolyzed locally. Nevertheless, larger fragments of glatiramer acetate can be recognized by glatiramer acetate-reactive antibodies. Some fraction of the injected material, either intact or partially hydrolyzed, is presumed to enter the lymphatic circulation, enabling it to reach regional lymph nodes, and some may enter the systemic circulation intact.

INDICATIONS AND USAGE

Glatiramer acetate for injection is indicated for reduction of the frequency of relapses in patients with Relapsing-Remitting Multiple Sclerosis.

CONTRAINDICATIONS

Glatiramer acetate for injection is contraindicated in patients with known hypersensitivity to glatiramer acetate or mannitol.

WARNINGS

The only recommended route of administration of glatiramer acetate injection is the subcutaneous route. Glatiramer acetate for injection should not be administered by the intravenous route.

PRECAUTIONS

GENERAL

Patients should be instructed in self-injection techniques to assure the safe administration of glatiramer acetate for injection (see Information for the Patient and the glatiramer acetate for injection Patient Information Leaflet that is distributed with the prescription). Current data indicate that no special caution is required for patients operating an automobile or using complex machinery.

CONSIDERATIONS REGARDING THE USE OF A PRODUCT CAPABLE OF MODIFYING IMMUNE RESPONSES

Because glatiramer acetate can modify immune response, it could possibly interfere with useful immune functions. For example, treatment with glatiramer acetate might, in theory, interfere with the recognition of foreign antigens in a way that would undermine the body's tumor surveillance and its defenses against infection. There is no evidence that glatiramer acetate does this, but there has as yet been no systematic evaluation of this risk. Because glatiramer acetate is an antigenic material, it is possible that its use may lead to the induction of host responses that are untoward, but systematic surveillance for these effects has not been undertaken.

Although glatiramer acetate is intended to minimize the autoimmune response to myelin, there is the possibility that continued alteration of cellular immunity due to chronic treatment with glatiramer acetate might result in untoward effects.

Glatiramer acetate-reactive antibodies are formed in practically all patients exposed to daily treatment with the recommended dose. Studies in both the rat and monkey have suggested that immune complexes are deposited in the renal glomeruli. Furthermore, in a controlled trial of 125 RR MS patients given glatiramer acetate, 20 mg, subcutaneously every day for 2 years, serum IgG levels reached at least 3 times baseline values in 80% of patients by 3 months of initiation of treatment. By 12 months of treatment, however, 30% of patients still had IgG levels at least 3 times baseline values, and 90% had levels above baseline by 12 months. The antibodies are exclusively of the IgG subtype- and predominantly of the IgG-1 subtype. No IgE type antibodies could be detected in any of the 94 sera tested; nevertheless, anaphylaxis can be associated with the administration of most any foreign substance, and therefore, this risk cannot be excluded.

INFORMATION FOR THE PATIENT

To assure safe and effective use of glatiramer acetate for injection, the following information and instructions should be given to patients:

Inform your physician if you are pregnant, if you are planning to have a child, or if you become pregnant while taking this medication.

Inform your physician if you are nursing.

Do not change the dose or dosing schedule without consulting your physician.

Do not stop taking the drug without consulting your physician.

Patients should be instructed in the use of aseptic techniques when administering glatiramer acetate for injection. Appropriate instructions for the self-injection of glatiramer acetate should be given, including a careful review of the glatiramer acetate injection Patient Information Leaflet that is distributed with the prescription. The first injection should be performed under the supervision of an appropriately qualified health care professional. Patient understanding and use of aseptic self-injection techniques and procedures should be periodically reevaluated. Patients should be cautioned against the reuse of needles or syringes and instructed in safe disposal procedures. They should use a puncture-resistant container for disposal of used needles and syringes. Patients should be instructed on the safe disposal of full containers according to local laws.

Awareness of Adverse Reactions

Physicians are advised to counsel patients about adverse reactions associated with the use of glatiramer acetate for injection (see ADVERSE REACTIONS). In addition, patients should be advised to read the glatiramer acetate for injection Patient Information Leaflet that is distributed with the prescription and resolve any questions regarding it prior to beginning glatiramer acetate injection therapy.

LABORATORY TESTS

Data collected during premarketing development do not suggest the need for routine laboratory monitoring.

DRUG/LABORATORY TEST INTERACTIONS

None are known.

CARCINOGENESIS, MUTAGENESIS, AND IMPAIRMENT OF FERTILITY

Carcinogenesis

In a 2 year carcinogenicity study, mice were administered up to 60 mg/kg/day glatiramer acetate by subcutaneous injection (up to 15 times the human therapeutic dose on a mg/m^2 basis). No increase in systemic neoplasms was observed. In males of the high dose group (60 mg/kg/day), but not in females, there was an increased incidence of fibrosarcomas at the injection sites. These sarcomas were associated with skin damage precipitated by repetitive injections of an irritant over a limited skin area.

In a 2 year carcinogenicity study, rats were administered up to 30 mg/kg/day glatiramer acetate by subcutaneous injection (up to 15 times the human therapeutic dose on a mg/m^2 basis). No increase in systemic neoplasms was observed.

Mutagenesis

Glatiramer acetate was not mutagenic in four strains of *Salmonella typhimurium* and two strains of *Escherichia coli* (Ames test) or in the *in vitro* mouse lymphoma assay in L5178Y cells. Glatiramer acetate was clastogenic in two separate *in vitro* chromosomal aberration assays in cultured human lymphocytes; it was not clastogenic in an *in vivo* mouse bone marrow micronucleus assay.

Impairment of Fertility

In a multigeneration reproduction and fertility study in rats, glatiramer acetate at subcutaneous doses of up to 36 mg/kg (18 times the human therapeutic dose on a mg/m^2 basis) had no adverse effects on reproductive parameters.

PREGNANCY CATEGORY B

No adverse effects on embryofetal development occurred in reproduction studies in rats and rabbits receiving subcutaneous doses of up to 37.5 mg/kg of glatiramer acetate during the period of organogenesis (18 and 36 times the therapeutic human dose on a mg/m^2 basis, respectively). In a prenatal and postnatal study in which rats received subcutaneous glatiramer acetate at doses of up to 36 mg/kg from day 15 of pregnancy throughout lactation, no significant effects on delivery or on offspring growth and development were observed.

There are no adequate and well-controlled studies in pregnant women. Because animal reproduction studies are not always predictive of human response, glatiramer acetate should be used during pregnancy only if clearly needed.

LABOR AND DELIVERY

In a prenatal and postnatal study, in which rats received subcutaneous glatiramer acetate at doses of up to 36 mg/kg from day 15 of pregnancy throughout lactation, no significant effects on delivery were observed. The relevance of these findings to humans is unknown.

NURSING MOTHERS

It is not known whether glatiramer acetate is excreted in human milk. Because many drugs are excreted in human milk, caution should be exercised when glatiramer acetate for injection is administered to a nursing woman.

PEDIATRIC USE

The safety and efficacy of glatiramer acetate for injection have not been established in individuals under 18 years of age.

USE IN THE ELDERLY

Glatiramer acetate for injection has not been studied specifically in elderly patients.

USE IN PATIENTS WITH IMPAIRED RENAL FUNCTION

The pharmacokinetics of glatiramer acetate in patients with impaired renal function have not been determined.

DRUG INTERACTIONS

Interactions between glatiramer acetate injection and other drugs have not been fully evaluated. Results from existing clinical trials do not suggest any significant interactions of glatiramer acetate injection with therapies commonly used in MS patients, including the concurrent use of corticosteroids for up to 28 days. Glatiramer acetate injection has not been formally evaluated in combination with Interferon beta.

ADVERSE REACTIONS

During premarketing clinical trials approximately 900 individuals received at least 1 dose of glatiramer acetate.

In controlled clinical trials the most commonly observed adverse experiences associated with the use of glatiramer acetate and not seen at an equivalent frequency among placebo-treated patients were: injection site reactions, vasodilatation, chest pain, asthenia, infection, pain, nausea, arthralgia, anxiety, and hypertonia.

Approximately 8% of the 893 subjects receiving glatiramer acetate discontinued treatment because of an adverse reaction. The adverse reactions most commonly associated with discontinuation were: injection site reaction (6.5%), vasodilatation, unintended pregnancy, depression, dyspnea, urticaria, tachycardia, dizziness, and tremor.

IMMEDIATE POST-INJECTION REACTION

Approximately 10% of MS patients exposed to glatiramer acetate in premarketing studies experienced a constellation of symptoms immediately after injection that included flushing, chest pain, palpitations, anxiety, dyspnea, constriction of the throat, and urticaria. In clinical trials, the symptoms were generally transient and self-limited and did not require specific treatment. In general, these symptoms have their onset several months after the initiation of treatment, although they may occur earlier, and a given patient may experience one or several episodes of these symptoms. Whether or not any of these symptoms actually represent a specific syndrome is uncertain. During the postmarketing period, there have been reports of patients with similar symptoms who received emergency medical care.

Whether an immunologic or non-immunologic mechanism mediates these episodes, or whether several similar episodes seen in a given patient have identical mechanisms, is unknown.

CHEST PAIN

Approximately 21% of glatiramer acetate patients in the pre-marketing controlled studies (compared to 11% of placebo patients) experienced at least one episode of what was described as transient chest pain. While some of these episodes occurred in the context of the Immediate Post-Injection Reaction described above, many did not. The temporal relationship of this chest pain to an injection of glatiramer acetate was not always known. The pain was transient (usually lasting only a few minutes), often unassociated with other symptoms, and appeared to have no important clinical sequelae. There has been only one episode of chest pain during which a full EKG was performed; that EKG showed no evidence of ischemia. Some patients experienced more than one such episode, and episodes usually began at least 1 month after the initiation of treatment. The pathogenesis of this symptom is unknown.

INCIDENCE IN CONTROLLED CLINICAL STUDIES

TABLE 4A and TABLE 4B list treatment-emergent signs and symptoms that occurred in at least 2% of MS patients treated with glatiramer acetate in the pre-marketing placebo-controlled trials. These signs and symptoms were numerically more common in patients treated with glatiramer acetate than in patients treated with placebo. These trials include the first two controlled trials in RR MS patients and a controlled trial in patients with Chronic-Progressive MS. Adverse reactions were usually mild in intensity.

The prescriber should be aware that these figures cannot be used to predict the frequency of adverse experiences in the course of usual medical practice where patient characteristics and other factors may differ from those prevailing during clinical studies. Similarly, the cited frequencies cannot be directly compared with figures obtained from other clinical investigations involving different treatments, uses, or investigators. An inspection of these frequencies, however, does provide the prescriber with one basis on which to estimate the relative contribution of drug and nondrug factors to the adverse reaction incidences in the population studied.

TABLE 4A *Controlled Trials in Patients With Multiple Sclerosis: Incidence of Glatiramer Acetate Adverse Reactions ≥2% and More Frequent Than Placebo*

Preferred Term	Glatiramer Acetate (n=201)	Placebo (n=206)
Body as Whole		
Asthenia	83 (41%)	78 (38%)
Back pain	33 (16%)	30 (15%)
Bacterial infection	11 (5%)	9 (4%)
Chest pain	43 (21%)	22 (11%)
Chills	8 (4%)	2 (1%)
Cyst	5 (2%)	1 (0%)
Face edema	12 (6%)	2 (1%)
Fever	17 (8%)	15 (7%)
Flu syndrome	38 (19%)	35 (17%)
Infection	101 (50%)	99 (48%)
Injection site erythema	132 (66%)	40 (19%)
Injection site hemorrhage	11 (5%)	6 (3%)
Injection site induration	26 (13%)	1 (0%)
Injection site inflammation	98 (49%)	22 (11%)
Injection site mass	54 (27%)	21 (10%)
Injection site pain	147 (73%)	78 (38%)
Injection site pruritus	80 (40%)	12 (6%)
Injection site urticaria	10 (5%)	0 (0%)
Injection site welt	22 (11%)	5 (2%)
Neck pain	16 (8%)	9 (4%)
Pain	56 (28%)	52 (25%)
Cardiovascular System		
Migraine	10 (5%)	5 (2%)
Palpitations	35 (17%)	16 (8%)
Syncope	10 (5%)	5 (2%)
Tachycardia	11 (5%)	8 (4%)
Vasodilatation	55 (27%)	21 (10%)
Digestive System		
Anorexia	17 (8%)	15 (7%)
Diarrhea	25 (12%)	23 (11%)
Gastroenteritis	6 (3%)	2 (1%)
Gastrointestinal disorder	10 (5%)	8 (4%)
Nausea	44 (22%)	34 (17%)
Vomiting	13 (6%)	8 (4%)
Hemic and Lymphatic System		
Ecchymosis	16 (8%)	13 (6%)
Lymphadenopathy	25 (12%)	12 (6%)

TABLE 4B *Controlled Trials in Patients With Multiple Sclerosis: Incidence of Glatiramer Acetate Adverse Reactions ≥2% and More Frequent Than Placebo*

Preferred Term	Glatiramer Acetate (n=201)	Placebo (n=206)
Metabolic and Nutritional		
Edema	5 (3%)	1 (0%)
Peripheral edema	14 (7%)	8 (4%)
Weight gain	7 (3%)	0 (0%)
Musculoskeletal System		
Arthralgia	49 (24%)	39 (19%)
Nervous System		
Agitation	8 (4%)	4 (2%)
Anxiety	46 (23%)	40 (19%)
Confusion	5 (2%)	1 (0%)
Foot drop	6 (3%)	4 (2%)
Hypertonia	44 (22%)	37 (18%)
Nervousness	4 (2%)	2 (1%)
Nystagmus	5 (2%)	2 (1%)
Speech disorder	5 (2%)	3 (1%)
Tremor	14 (7%)	7 (3%)
Vertigo	12 (6%)	11 (5%)
Respiratory System		
Bronchitis	18 (9%)	12 (6%)
Dyspnea	38 (19%)	15 (7%)
Laryngismus	10 (5%)	7 (3%)
Rhinitis	29 (14%)	27 (13%)
Skin and Appendages		
Erythema	8 (4%)	4 (2%)
Herpes simplex	8 (4%)	6 (3%)
Pruritus	36 (18%)	26 (13%)
Rash	37 (18%)	30 (15%)
Skin nodule	4 (2%)	1 (0%)
Sweating	31 (15%)	21 (10%)
Urticaria	9 (4%)	5 (2%)
Special Senses		
Ear pain	15 (7%)	12 (6%)
Eye disorder	8 (4%)	1 (0%)
Urogenital System		
Dysmenorrhea	12 (6%)	10 (5%)
Urinary urgency	20 (10%)	17 (8%)
Vaginal moniliasis	16 (8%)	9 (4%)

Other events which occurred in at least 2% of glatiramer acetate patients but were present at equal or greater rates in the placebo group included:

Body as a Whole: Headache, injection site ecchymosis, accidental injury, abdominal pain, allergic rhinitis, neck rigidity, and malaise.

Digestive System: Dyspepsia, constipation, dysphagia, fecal incontinence, flatulence, nausea and vomiting, gastritis, gingivitis, periodontal abscess, and dry mouth.

Musculoskeletal: Myasthenia and myalgia.

Nervous System: Dizziness, hypesthesia, paresthesia, insomnia, depression, dysesthesia, incoordination, somnolence, abnormal gait, amnesia, emotional lability, Lhermitte's sign, abnormal thinking, twitching, euphoria, and sleep disorder.

Respiratory System: Pharyngitis, sinusitis, increased cough, and laryngitis.

Skin and Appendages: Acne, alopecia, and nail disorder.

Special Senses: Abnormal vision, diplopia, amblyopia, eye pain, conjunctivitis, tinnitus, taste perversion, and deafness.

Urogenital System: Urinary tract infection, urinary frequency, urinary incontinence, urinary retention, dysuria, cystitis, metrorrhagia, breast pain, and vaginitis.

Data on adverse reactions occurring in the controlled clinical trials were analyzed to evaluate differences based on sex. No clinically significant differences were identified. Ninety-two percent (92%) of patients in these clinical trials were Caucasian. This percentage reflects the racial composition of the MS population. In addition, the vast majority of patients treated with glatiramer acetate for injection were between the ages of 18 and 45. Consequently, data are inadequate to perform an analysis of the adverse reaction incidence related to clinically relevant age subgroups.

Laboratory analyses were performed on all patients participating in the clinical program for glatiramer acetate. Clinically significant laboratory values for hematology, chemistry, and urinalysis were similar for both glatiramer acetate and placebo groups in blinded clinical trials. No patient receiving glatiramer acetate withdrew from any trial because of abnormal laboratory findings.

OTHER ADVERSE EVENTS OBSERVED DURING CLINICAL TRIALS

Glatiramer acetate was administered to 979 individuals during premarketing clinical trials, only some of which were placebo-controlled. During these trials, all adverse events were recorded by the clinical investigators, using terminology of their own choosing. To provide a meaningful estimate of the proportion of individuals having adverse events, similar types of events were grouped into standardized categories using COSTART dictionary terminology. All reported events occurring at least twice and potentially important events occurring once are listed below, except those already listed in TABLE 4A and TABLE 4B, those too general to be informative, trivial events, and other reactions which occurred in at least 2% of treated patients and were present at equal or greater rates in the placebo group. Additional adverse reactions reported during the post-marketing period are included.

Events are further classified within body system categories and listed in order of decreasing frequency using the following definitions: *Frequent* adverse events are defined as those occurring in at least 1/100 patients; *Infrequent* adverse events are those occurring in 1/100 to 1/1000 patients; *Rare* adverse events are those occurring in less than 1/1000 patients.

Body as a Whole: *Frequent:* Injection site edema, injection site atrophy, abscess, injection site hypersensitivity. *Infrequent:* Injection site hematoma, injection site fibrosis, moon face, cellulitis, generalized edema, hernia, injection site abscess, serum sickness, suicide attempt, injection site hypertrophy, injection site melanosis, lipoma, and photosensitivity reaction.

Cardiovascular: *Frequent:* Hypertension. *Infrequent:* Hypotension, midsystolic click, systolic murmur, atrial fibrillation, bradycardia, fourth heart sound, postural hypotension, and varicose veins.

Digestive: *Infrequent:* Dry mouth, stomatitis, burning sensation on tongue, cholecystitis, colitis, esophageal ulcer, esophagitis, gastrointestinal carcinoma, gum hemorrhage, hepatomegaly, increased appetite, melena, mouth ulceration, pancreas disorder, pancreatitis, rectal hemorrhage, tenesmus, tongue discoloration, and duodenal ulcer.

Endocrine: *Infrequent:* Goiter, hyperthyroidism, and hypothyroidism.

Gastrointestinal: *Frequent:* Bowel urgency, oral moniliasis, salivary gland enlargement, tooth caries, and ulcerative stomatitis.

Hemic and Lymphatic: *Infrequent:* Leukopenia, anemia, cyanosis, eosinophilia, hematemesis, lymphedema, pancytopenia, and splenomegaly.

Metabolic and Nutritional: *Infrequent:* Weight loss, alcohol intolerance, Cushing's syndrome, gout, abnormal healing, and xanthoma.

Musculoskeletal: *Infrequent:* Arthritis, muscle atrophy, bone pain, bursitis, kidney pain, muscle disorder, myopathy, osteomyelitis, tendon pain, and tenosynovitis.

Nervous: *Frequent:* Abnormal dreams, emotional lability, and stupor. *Infrequent:* Aphasia, ataxia, convulsion, circumoral paresthesia, depersonalization, hallucinations, hostility, hypokinesia, coma, concentration disorder, facial paralysis, decreased libido, manic reaction, memory impairment, myoclonus, neuralgia, paranoid reaction, paraplegia, psychotic depression, and transient stupor.

Respiratory: *Frequent:* Hyperventilation, hay-fever. *Infrequent:* Asthma, pneumonia, epistaxis, hypoventilation, and voice alteration.

Skin and Appendages: *Frequent:* Eczema, herpes zoster, pustular rash, skin atrophy, and warts. *Infrequent:* Dry skin, skin hypertrophy, dermatitis, furunculosis, psoriasis, angioedema, contact dermatitis, erythema nodosum, fungal dermatitis, maculopapular rash, pigmentation, benign skin neoplasm, skin carcinoma, skin striae, and vesiculobullous rash.

Special Senses: *Frequent:* Visual field defect. *Infrequent:* Dry eyes, otitis externa, ptosis, cataract, corneal ulcer, mydriasis, optic neuritis, photophobia, and taste loss.

Urogenital: *Frequent:* Amenorrhea, hematuria, impotence, menorrhagia, suspicious papanicolaou smear, urinary frequency and vaginal hemorrhage. *Infrequent:* Vaginitis, flank pain (kidney), abortion, breast engorgement, breast enlargement, carcinoma *in situ* cervix, fibrocystic breast, kidney calculus, nocturia, ovarian cyst, priapism, pyelonephritis, abnormal sexual function, and urethritis.

POSTMARKETING CLINICAL EXPERIENCE

Postmarketing experience has shown an adverse event profile similar to that presented above. Reports of adverse reactions occurring under treatment with glatiramer acetate not mentioned above that have been received since market introduction and that may have or not have causal relationship to the drug include the following:

Body as a Whole: Sepsis; LE syndrome; hydrocephalus; enlarged abdomen; injection site hypersensitivity; allergic reaction; anaphylactoid reaction.

Cardiovascular System: Thrombosis; peripheral vascular disease; pericardial effusion; myocardial infarct; deep thrombophlebitis; coronary occlusion; congestive heart failure; cardiomyopathy; cardiomegaly; arrhythmia; angina pectoris.

Digestive System: Tongue edema; stomach ulcer, hemorrhage; liver function abnormality; liver damage; hepatitis; eructation; cirrhosis of the liver; cholelithiasis.

Hemic and Lymphatic System: Thrombocytopenia; lymphoma-like reaction; acute leukemia.
Metabolic and Nutritional Disorders: Hypercholesterolemia.
Musculoskeletal System: Rheumatoid arthritis; generalized spasm.
Nervous System: Myelitis; meningitis; CNS neoplasm; cerebrovascular accident; brain edema; abnormal dreams; aphasia; convulsion; neuralgia.
Respiratory System: Pulmonary embolus; pleural effusion; carcinoma of lung; hay fever.
Special Senses: Glaucoma; blindness; visual field defect.
Urogenital System: Urogenital neoplasm; urine abnormality; ovarian carcinoma; nephrosis; kidney failure; breast carcinoma; bladder carcinoma; urinary frequency.

DOSAGE AND ADMINISTRATION

The recommended dose of glatiramer acetate injection for the treatment of RR MS is 20 mg/day injected subcutaneously.

INSTRUCTIONS FOR USE

Remove one blister with the syringe inside from the glatiramer acetate injection pre-filled syringes package from the refrigerator. Let the pre-filled syringe package stand at room temperature 20 minutes to allow the solution to warm up to room temperature. Store all unused syringes in the refrigerator. Inspect the product visually and discard or return the product to the pharmacist before use if it contains any particulate matter.

Sites for self-injection include arms, abdomen, hips, and thighs. The pre-filled syringe is suitable for single use only; unused portions should be discarded. (See the glatiramer acetate injection Patient Information Leaflet that is distributed with the prescription for instructions for injecting glatiramer acetate.)

HOW SUPPLIED

Copaxone injection is supplied as a single-use pre-filled syringe containing 1.0 ml of a clear, colorless to slightly yellow, sterile, non-pyrogenic solution containing 20 mg of glatiramer acetate and 40 mg mannitol.

STORAGE

The recommended storage condition for Copaxone injection is refrigeration (2-8°C/36-46°F). However, excursions from recommended storage conditions to room temperature conditions (15-30°C/59-86°F) for up to 1 week have been shown to have no adverse impact on the product. Exposure to higher temperatures or intense light should be avoided.

Copaxone injection contains no preservative. Do not use if the solution contain any particulate matter.

PRODUCT LISTING - EQUIVALENTS NOT AVAILABLE

Powder For Injection - Subcutaneous - 20 mg
1's $1107.69 COPAXONE, Aventis Pharmaceuticals 00088-1150-03
Solution - Subcutaneous - 20 mg
1's $1107.69 COPAXONE, Aventis Pharmaceuticals 00088-1153-30

Glimepiride (003279)

For related information, see the comparative table section in Appendix A.

Categories: Diabetes mellitus; FDA Approved 1995 Nov; Pregnancy Category C
Drug Classes: Antidiabetic agents; Sulfonylureas, second generation
Brand Names: Amaryl
Foreign Brand Availability: Euglim (India); Glimerid (Colombia); Solosa (Philippines)
Cost of Therapy: $10.04 (Diabetes mellitus; Amaryl; 1 mg; 1 tablet/day; 30 day supply)

DESCRIPTION

Glimepiride tablets are an oral blood-glucose-lowering drug of the sulfonylurea class. Glimepiride is a white to yellowish-white, crystalline, odorless to practically odorless powder formulated into tablets of 1, 2, and 4 mg strengths for oral administration. Amaryl tablets contain the active ingredient glimepiride and the following inactive ingredients: lactose (hydrous), sodium starch glycolate, povidone, microcrystalline cellulose, and magnesium stearate. In addition, Amaryl 1 mg tablets contain ferric oxide red, Amaryl 2 mg tablets contain ferric oxide yellow and FD&C blue no. 2 aluminum lake, and Amaryl 4 mg tablets contain FD&C blue no. 2 aluminum lake.

Chemically, glimepiride is identified as 1-[[p-[2-(3-ethyl-4-methyl-2-oxo-3-pyrroline-1-carboxamido)ethyl]phenyl]sulfonyl]-3-(trans-4-methylcyclohexyl)urea.

The molecular formula for glimepiride is $C_{24}H_{34}N_4O_5S$. The molecular weight is 490.62. Glimepiride is practically insoluble in water.

CLINICAL PHARMACOLOGY

MECHANISM OF ACTION

The primary mechanism of action of glimepiride in lowering blood glucose appears to be dependent on stimulating the release of insulin from functioning pancreatic beta cells. In addition, extrapancreatic effects may also play a role in the activity of sulfonylureas such as glimepiride. This is supported by both preclinical and clinical studies demonstrating that glimepiride administration can lead to increased sensitivity of peripheral tissues to insulin. These findings are consistent with the results of a long-term, randomized, placebo-controlled trial in which glimepiride therapy improved postprandial insulin/C-peptide responses and overall glycemic control without producing clinically meaningful increases in fasting insulin/C-peptide levels. However, as with other sulfonylureas, the mechanism by which glimepiride lowers blood glucose during long-term administration has not been clearly established.

Glimepiride is effective as initial drug therapy. In patients where monotherapy with glimepiride or metformin has not produced adequate glycemic control, the combination of glimepiride and metformin may have a synergistic effect, since both agents act to improve glucose tolerance by different primary mechanisms of action. This complementary effect has been observed with metformin and other sulfonylureas, in multiple studies.

PHARMACODYNAMICS

A mild glucose-lowering effect first appeared following single oral doses as low as 0.5-0.6 mg in healthy subjects. The time required to reach the maximum effect (*i.e.*, minimum blood glucose level [T_{min}]) was about 2-3 hours. In noninsulin-dependent (Type 2) diabetes mellitus (NIDDM) patients, both fasting and 2 hour postprandial glucose levels were significantly lower with glimepiride (1, 2, 4, and 8 mg once daily) than with placebo after 14 days of oral dosing. The glucose-lowering effect in all active treatment groups was maintained over 24 hours.

In larger dose-ranging studies, blood glucose and HbA1c were found to respond in a dose-dependent manner over the range of 1-4 mg/day of gilmepiride. Some patients, particularly those with higher fasting plasma glucose (FPG) levels, may benefit from doses of glimepiride up to 8 mg once daily. No difference in response was found when glimepiride was administered once or twice daily.

In two 14 week, placebo-controlled studies in 720 subjects, the average net reduction in HbA1c for glimepiride tablet patients treated with 8 mg once daily was 2.0% in absolute units compared with placebo-treated patients. In a long-term, randomized, placebo-controlled study of NIDDM patients unresponsive to dietary management, glimepiride therapy improved postprandial insulin/C-peptide responses, and 75% of patients achieved and maintained control of blood glucose and HbA1c. Efficacy results were not affected by age, gender, weight, or race.

In long-term extension trials with previously-treated patients, no meaningful deterioration in mean fasting blood glucose (FBG) or HbA1c levels was seen after 2½ years of glimepiride therapy.

Combination therapy with glimepiride and insulin (70% NPH/30% regular) was compared to placebo/insulin in secondary failure patients whose body weight was >130% of their ideal body weight. Initially, 5-10 units of insulin were administered with the main evening meal and titrated upward weekly to achieve predefined FPG values. Both groups in this double-blind study achieved similar reductions in FPG levels but the glimepiride/insulin therapy group used approximately 38% less insulin.

Glimepiride therapy is effective in controlling blood glucose without deleterious changes in the plasma lipoprotein profiles of patients treated for NIDDM.

PHARMACOKINETICS

Absorption

After oral administration, glimepiride is completely (100%) absorbed from the GI tract. Studies with single oral doses in normal subjects and with multiple oral doses in patients with NIDDM have shown significant absorption of glimepiride within 1 hour after administration and peak drug levels (C_{max}) at 2-3 hours. When glimepiride was given with meals, the mean T_{max} (time to reach C_{max}) was slightly increased (12%) and the mean C_{max} and AUC (area under the curve) were slightly decreased (8% and 9%, respectively).

Distribution

After intravenous (IV) dosing in normal subjects, the volume of distribution (Vd) was 8.8 L (113 ml/kg), and the total body clearance (CL) was 47.8 ml/min. Protein binding was greater than 99.5%.

Metabolism

Glimepiride is completely metabolized by oxidative biotransformation after either an IV or oral dose. The major metabolites are the cyclohexyl hydroxy methyl derivative (M1) and the carboxyl derivative (M2). Cytochrome P450 II C9 has been shown to be involved in the biotransformation of glimepiride to M1. M1 is further metabolized to M2 by one or several cytosolic enzymes. M1, but not M2, possesses about 1/3 of the pharmacological activity as compared to its parent in an animal model; however, whether the glucose-lowering effect of M1 is clinically meaningful is not clear.

Excretion

When ^{14}C-glimepiride was given orally, approximately 60% of the total radioactivity was recovered in the urine in 7 days and M1 (predominant) and M2 accounted for 80-90% of that recovered in the urine. Approximately 40% of the total radioactivity was recovered in the feces and M1 and M2 (predominant) accounted for about 70% of that recovered in feces. No parent drug was recovered from urine or feces. After IV dosing in patients, no significant biliary excretion of glimepiride or its M1 metabolite has been observed.

Pharmacokinetic Parameters

The pharmacokinetic parameters of glimepiride obtained from a single-dose, crossover, dose-proportionality (1, 2, 4, and 8 mg) study in normal subjects and from a single- and multiple-dose, parallel, dose-proportionality (4 and 8 mg) study in patients with NIDDM are summarized in TABLE 1.

These data indicate that glimepiride did not accumulate in serum, and the pharmacokinetics of glimepiride were not different in healthy volunteers and in NIDDM patients. Oral clearance of glimepiride did not change over the 1-8 mg dose range, indicating linear pharmacokinetics.

Variability

In normal healthy volunteers, the intra-individual variabilities of C_{max}, AUC, and CL/f for glimepiride were 23%, 17%, and 15%, respectively, and the inter-individual variabilities were 25%, 29%, and 24%, respectively.

SPECIAL POPULATIONS

Geriatric

Comparison of glimepiride pharmacokinetics in NIDDM patients ≤65 years and those >65 years was performed in a study using a dosing regimen of 6 mg daily. There were no significant differences in glimepiride pharmacokinetics between the two age groups. The mean AUC at steady state for the older patients was about 13% lower than that for the younger

TABLE 1

	Volunteers	Patients with NIDDM	
	Single Dose	Single Dose (Day 1)	Multiple Dose (Day 10)
	Mean ±SD	Mean ±SD	Mean ±SD
C_{max} (ng/ml)			
1 mg	103 ± 34 (12)	—	—
2 mg	177 ± 44 (12)	—	—
4 mg	308 ± 69 (12)	352 ± 222 (12)	309 ± 134 (12)
8 mg	557± 152 (12)	591 ± 232 (14)	578 ± 265 (11)
T_{max}(h)	2.4 ± 0.8 (48)	2.5 ± 1.2 (26)	2.8 ± 2.2 (23)
CL/f (ml/min)	52.1 ± 16.0 (48)	48.5 ± 29.3 (26)	52.7 ± 40.3 (23)
Vd/f (L)	21.8 ± 13.9 (48)	19.8 ± 12.7 (26)	37.1 ± 18.2 (23)
T½ (h)	5.3 ± 4.1 (48)	5.0 ± 2.5 (26)	9.2 ± 3.6 (23)

() = Number of subjects.
CL/f = Total body clearance after oral dosing.
Vd/f = Volume of distribution calculated after oral dosing.

patients; the mean weight-adjusted clearance for the older patients was about 11% higher than that for the younger patients.

Pediatric

No studies were performed in pediatric patients.

Gender

There were no differences between males and females in the pharmcokinetics of glimepiride when adjustment was made for differences in body weight.

Race

No pharmacokinetic studies to assess the effects of race have been performed, but in placebo-controlled studies of glimepiride tablets in patients with NIDDM, the antihyperglycemic effect was comparable in whites (n=536), blacks (n=63), and Hispanics (n=63).

Renal Insufficiency

A single-dose, open-label study was conducted in 15 patients with renal impairment. Glimepiride (3 mg) was administered to 3 groups of patients with different levels of mean creatinine clearance (CLCR); (Group I, CLCR = 77.7 ml/min, n=5), (Group II, CLCR = 27.7 ml/min, n=3), and (Group III, CLCR = 9.4 ml/min, n=7). Glimepiride was found to be well tolerated in all 3 groups. The results showed that glimepiride serum levels decreased as renal function decreased. However, M1 and M2 serum levels (mean AUC values) increased 2.3 and 8.6 times from Group I to Group III. The apparent terminal half-life (T½) for glimepiride did not change, while the half-lives for M1 and M2 increased as renal function decreased. Mean urinary excretion of M1 plus M2 as percent of dose, however, decreased (44.4%, 21.9%, and 9.3% for Groups I to III).

A multiple-dose titration study was also conducted in 16 NIDDM patients with renal impairment using doses ranging from 1-8 mg daily for 3 months. The results were consistent with those observed after single doses. All patients with a CLCR less than 22 ml/min had adequate control of their glucose levels with a dosage regimen of only 1 mg daily. The results from this study suggested that a starting dose of 1 mg glimepiride may be given to NIDDM patients with kidney disease, and the dose may be titrated based on fasting blood glucose levels.

Hepatic Insufficiency

No studies were performed in patients with hepatic insufficiency.

Other Populations

There were no important differences in glimepiride metabolism in subjects identified as phenotypically different drug-metabolizers by their metabolism of sparteine.

The pharmacokinetics of glimepiride in morbidly obese patients were similar to those in the normal weight group, except for a lower C_{max} and AUC. However, since neither C_{max} nor AUC values were normalized for body surface area, the lower values of C_{max} and AUC for the obese patients were likely the result of their excess weight and not due to a difference in the kinetics of glimepiride.

Drug Interactions

The hypoglycemic action of sulfonylureas may be potentiated by certain drugs, including nonsteroidal anti-inflammatory drugs and other drugs that are highly protein bound, such as salicylates, sulfonamides, chloramphenicol, coumarins, probenecid, monamine oxidase inhibitors, and beta adrenergic blocking agents. When these drugs are administered to a patient receiving glimepiride, the patient should be observed closely for hypoglycemia. When these drugs are withdrawn from a patient receiving glimepiride, the patient should be observed closely for loss of glycemic control.

Certain drugs tend to produce hyperglycemia and may lead to loss of control. These drugs include the thiazides and other diurectics, corticosteroids, phenothiazines, thyroid products, estrogens, oral contraceptives, phenytoin, nicotinic acid, sympathomimetics, and isoniazid. When these drugs are administered to a patient receiving glimepiride, the patient should be closely observed for loss of control. When these drugs are withdrawn from a patient receiving glimepiride, the patient should be observed closely for hypoglycemia.

Coadministration of aspirin (1 g tid) and glimepiride led to a 34% decrease in the mean glimepiride AUC and, therefore, a 34% increase in the mean CL/f. The mean C_{max} had a decrease of 4%. Blood glucose and serum C-peptide concentrations were unaffected and no hypoglycemic symptoms were reported. Pooled data from clinical trials showed no evidence of clinically significant adverse interactions with uncontrolled concurrent administration of aspirin and other salicylates.

Coadministration of either cimetidine (800 mg once daily) or ranitidine (150 mg bid) with a single 4 mg oral dose of glimepiride did not significantly alter the absorption and disposition of glimepiride, and no differences were seen in hypoglycemic symptomatology. Pooled data from clinical trials showed no evidence of clinically significant adverse interactions with uncontrolled concurrent administration of H2-receptor antagonists.

Concomitant administration of propranolol (40 mg tid) and glimepiride significantly increased C_{max}, AUC, and T½ of glimepiride by 23%, 22%, and 15%, respectively, and it decreased CL/f by 18%. The recovery of M1 and M2 from urine, however, did not change. The pharmacodynamic responses to glimepiride were nearly identical in normal subjects receiving propranolol and placebo. Pooled data from clinical trials in patients with NIDDM showed no evidence of clinically significant adverse interactions with uncontrolled concurrent administration of beta-blockers. However, if beta-blockers are used, caution should be exercised and patients should be warned about the potential for hypoglycemia.

Concomitant administration of glimepiride tablets (4 mg once daily) did not alter the pharmacokinetic characteristics of R- and S-warfarin enantiomers following administration of a single dose (25 mg) of racemic warfarin to healthy subjects. No changes were observed in warfarin plasma protein binding. Glimepiride treatment did result in a slight, but statistically significant, decrease in the pharmacodyhamic response to warfarin. The reductions in mean area under the prothrombin time (PT) curve and maximum PT values during glimepiride treatment were very small (3.3% and 9.9%, respectively) and are unlikely to be clinically important.

The responses of serum glucose, insulin, C-peptide, and plasma glucagon to 2 mg glimepiride were unaffected by coadministration of ramipril (an ACE inhibitor) 5 mg once daily in normal subjects. No hypoglycemic symptoms were reported. Pooled data from clinical trials in patients with NIDDM showed no evidence of clinically significant adverse interactions with uncontrolled concurrent administration of ACE inhibitors.

A potential interaction between oral miconazole and oral hypoglycemic agents leading to severe hypoglycemia has been reported. Whether this interaction also occurs with the intravenous, topical, or vaginal preparations of miconazole is not known. Potential interactions of glimepiride with other drugs metabolized by cytochrome P450 II C9 also include phenytoin, diclofenac, ibuprofen, naproxen, and mefenamic acid.

Although no specific interaction studies were performed, pooled data from clinical trials showed no evidence of clinically significant adverse interactions with uncontrolled concurrent administration of calcium-channel blockers, estrogens, fibrates, NSAIDS, HMG CoA reductase inhibitors, sulfonamides, or thyroid hormone.

INDICATIONS AND USAGE

Glimepiride is indicated as an adjunct to diet and exercise to lower the blood glucose in patients with noninsulin-dependent (Type 2) diabetes mellitus (NIDDM) whose hyperglycemia cannot be controlled by diet and exercise alone. Glimepiride may be used concomitantly with metformin when diet, exercise, and glimepiride or metformin alone do not result in adequeate glycemic control.

Glimepiride is also indicated for use in combination with insulin to lower blood glucose in patients whose hyperglycemia cannot be controlled by diet and exercise in conjunction with an oral hypoglycemic agent. Combined use of glimepiride and insulin may increase the potential for hypoglycemia.

In initiating treatment for noninsulin-dependent diabetes, diet and exercise should be emphasized as the primary form of treatment. Caloric restriction, weight loss, and exercise are essential in the obese diabetic patient. Proper dietary management and exercise alone may be effective in controlling the blood glucose and symptoms of hyperglycemia. In addition to regular physical activity, cardiovascular risk factors should be identified and corrective measures taken where possible.

If this treatment program fails to reduce symptoms and/or blood glucose, the use of an oral sulfonylurea or insulin should be considered. Use of glimepiride must be viewed by both the physician and patient as a treatment in addition to diet and exercise and not as substitute for diet and exercise or as a convenient mechanism for avoiding dietary restraint. Furthermore, loss of blood glucose control on diet and exercise alone may be transient, thus requiring only short-term administration of glimepiride.

During maintenance programs, glimepiride monotherapy should be discontinued if satisfactory lowering of blood glucose is no longer achieved. Judgements should be based on regular clinical and laboratory evaluations. Secondary failures to glimepiride monotherapy can be treated with glimepiride-insulin combination therapy.

In considering the use of glimepiride in asymptomatic patients, it should be recognized that blood glucose control in NIDDM has not definitely been established to be effective in preventing the long-term cardiovascular and neural complications of diabetes. However, the Diabetes Control and Complications Trial (DCCT) demonstrated that control of HbA1c and glucose was associated with a decrease in retinopathy, neuropathy, and nephropathy for insulin-dependent diabetic (IDDM) patients.

CONTRAINDICATIONS

Glimepiride is contraindicated in patients with:

1. Known hypersensitivity to the drug.
2. Diabetic ketoacidosis, with or without coma. This condition should be treated with insulin.

WARNINGS

SPECIAL WARNING ON INCREASED RISK OF CARDIOVASCULAR MORTALITY

The administration of oral hypoglycemic drugs has been reported to be associated with increased cardiovascular mortality as compared to treatment with diet alone or diet plus insulin. This warning is based on the study conducted by the University Group Diabetes Program (UGDP), a long-term, prospective clinical trial designed to evaluate the effectiveness of glucose-lowering drugs in preventing or delaying vascular complications in patients with non-insulin-dependent diabetes. The study involved 823 patients who were randomly assigned to one of four treatment groups.[1]

UGDP reported that patients treated for 5-8 years with diet plus a fixed dose of tolbutamide (1.5 g/day) had a rate of cardiovascular mortality approximately 2½ times that of patients treated with diet alone. A significant increase in total mortality was not observed, but the use of tolbutamide was discontinued based on the increase in cardiovascular mortality, thus limiting the opportunity for the study to show an increase in overall mortality. Despite controversy regarding the interpretation of these

results, the findings of the UGDP study provide an adequate basis for this warning. The patient should be informed of the potential risks and advantages of glimepiride tablets and of alternative modes of therapy.

Although only one drug in the sulfonylurea class (tolbutamide) was included in this study, it is prudent from a safety standpoint to consider that this warning may also apply to other oral hypoglycemic drugs in this class, in view of their close similarities in mode of action and chemical structure.

PRECAUTIONS

GENERAL

Hypoglycemia

All sulfonylurea drugs are capable of producing severe hypoglycemia. Proper patient selection, dosage, and instructions are important to avoid hypoglycemic episodes. Patients with impaired renal function may be more sensitive to the glucose-lowering effect of glimepiride. A starting dose of 1 mg once daily followed by appropriate dose titration is recommended in those patients. Debilitated or malnourished patients, and those with adrenal, pituitary, or hepatic insufficiency are particularly susceptible to the hypoglycemic action of glucose-lowering drugs. Hypoglycemia may be difficult to recognize in the elderly and in people who are taking beta-adrenergic blocking drugs or other sympatholytic agents. Hypoglycemia is more likely to occur when caloric intake is deficient, after severe or prolonged exercise, when alcohol is ingested, or when more than one glucose-lowering drug is used. Combined use of glimepiride with insulin or metformin may increase the potential for hypoglycemia.

Loss of Control of Blood Glucose

When a patient stabilized on any diabetic regimen is exposed to stress such as fever, trauma, infection, or surgery, a loss of control may occur. At such times, it may be necessary to add insulin in combination with glimepiride or even use insulin monotherapy. The effectiveness of any oral hypoglycemic drug, including glimepiride, in lowering blood glucose to a desired level decreases in many patients over a period of time, which may be due to progression of the severity of the diabetes or to diminished responsiveness to the drug. This phenomenon is known as secondary failure, to distinguish it from primary failure in which the drug is ineffective in an individual patient when first given. Should secondary failure occur with glimepiride or metformin monotherapy, combined therapy with glimepiride and metformin or glimepiride and insulin may result in a response. Should secondary failure occur with combined glimepiride/metformin therapy, it may be necessary to initiate insulin therapy.

INFORMATION FOR THE PATIENT

Patients should be informed of the potential risks and advantages of glimepiride and of alternative modes of therapy. They should also be informed about the importance of adherence to dietary instructions, of a regular exercise program, and of regular testing of blood glucose.

The risks of hypoglycemia, its symptoms and treatment, and conditions that predispose to its development should be explained to patients and responsible family members. The potential for primary and secondary failure should also be explained.

LABORATORY TESTS

Fasting blood glucose should be monitored periodically to determine therapeutic response. Glycosylated hemoglobin should also be monitored, usually every 3-6 months, to more precisely assess long-term glycemic control.

CARCINOGENESIS, MUTAGENESIS, AND IMPAIRMENT OF FERTILITY

Studies in rats at doses of up to 5000 ppm in complete feed (approximately 340 times the maximum recommended human dose, based on surface area) for 30 months showed no evidence of carcinogenesis. In mice, administration of glimepiride for 24 months resulted in an increase in benign pancreatic adenoma formation which was dose related and is thought to be the result of chronic pancreatic stimulation. The no-effect dose for adenoma formation in mice in this study was 320 ppm in complete feed, or 46-54 mg/kg body weight/day. This is about 35 times the maximum human recommended dose of 8 mg once daily based on surface area.

Glimepiride was non-mutagenic in a battery of *in vitro* and *in vivo* mutagenicity studies (Ames test, somatic cell mutation, chromosomal aberration, unscheduled DNA synthesis, mouse micronucleus test).

There was no effect of glimepiride on male mouse fertility in animals exposed up to 2500 mg/kg body weight (>1700 times the maximum recommended human dose based on surface area). Glimepiride had no effect on the fertility of male and female rats administered up to 4000 mg/kg body weight (approximately 4000 times the maximum recommended human dose based on surface area).

PREGNANCY

Teratogenic Effects, Pregnancy Category C

Glimepiride did not produce teratogenic effects in rats exposed orally up to 4000 mg/kg body weight (approximately 4000 times the maximum recommended human dose based on surface area) or in rabbits exposed up to 32 mg/kg body weight (approximately 60 times the maximum recommended human dose based on surface area). Glimepiride has been shown to be associated with intrauterine fetal death in rats when given in doses as low as 50 times the human dose based on surface area and in rabbits when given in doses as low as 0.1 times the human dose based on surface area. This fetotoxicity, observed only at dose inducing maternal hypoglycemia, has been similarly noted with other sulfonylureas, and is believed to be directly related to the pharmacologic (hypoglycemic) action of glimepiride.

There are no adequate and well-controlled studies in pregnant women. On the basis of results from animal studies, glimepiride tablets should not be used during pregnancy. Because recent information suggests that abnormal blood glucose levels during pregnancy are associated with a higher incidence of congenital abnormalities, many experts recommend that insulin be used during pregnancy to maintain glucose levels as close to normal as possible.

Nonteratogenic Effects

In some studies in rats, offspring of dams exposed to high levels of glimepiride during pregnancy and lactation developed skeletal deformities consisting of shortening, thickening, and bending of the humerus during the postnatal period. Significant concentrations of glimepiride were observed in the serum and breast milk of the dams as well as in the serum of the pups. These skeletal deformations were determined to be the result of nursing from mothers exposed to glimepiride.

Prolonged severe hypoglycemia (4-10 days) has been reported in neonates born to mothers who were receiving a sulfonylurea drug at the time of delivery. This has been reported more frequently with the use of agents with prolonged half-lives. Patients who are planning a pregnancy should consult their physician, and it is recommended that they change over to insulin for the entire course of pregnancy and lactation.

NURSING MOTHERS

In rat reproduction studies, significant concentrations of glimpiride were observed in the serum and breast milk of the dams, as well as in the serum of the pups. Although it is not known whether glimepiride is excreted in human milk, other sulfonylureas are excreted in human milk. Because the potential for hypoglycemia in nursing infants may exist, and because of the effects on nursing animals, glimepiride should be discontinued in nursing mothers. If glimepiride is discontinued, and if diet and exercise alone are inadequate for controlling blood glucose, insulin therapy should be considered. (See Pregnancy, Nonteratogenic Effects.)

PEDIATRIC USE

Safety and effectiveness in pediatric patients have not been established.

DRUG INTERACTIONS

See CLINICAL PHARMACOLOGY, Special Populations, Drug Interactions.

ADVERSE REACTIONS

The incidence of hypoglycemia with glimepiride, as documented by blood glucose values <60 mg/dl, ranged from 0.9-1.7% in two large, well-controlled, 1 year studies. (See WARNINGS and PRECAUTIONS.)

Glimepiride has been evaluated for safety in 2013 patients in US controlled trials, and in 1551 patients in foreign controlled trials. More than 1650 of these patients were treated for at least 1 year.

Adverse events, other than hypoglycemia, considered to be possibly or probably related to study drug that occurred in US placebo-controlled trials in more than 1% of patients treated with glimepiride are shown in TABLE 2.

TABLE 2 *Adverse Events Occurring in ≥1% Glimepiride Patients*

	Glimepiride		Placebo	
	No.	%	No.	%
Total treated	746	100	294	100
Dizziness	13	1.7	1	0.3
Asthenia	12	1.6	3	1.0
Headache	11	1.5	4	1.4
Nausea	8	1.1	0	0.0

GASTROINTESTINAL REACTIONS

Vomiting, gastrointestinal pain, and diarrhea have been reported, but the incidence in placebo-controlled trials was less than 1%. In rare cases, there may be an elevation of liver enzyme levels. In isolated instances, impairment of liver function (*e.g.*, with cholestasis and jaundice), as well as hepatitis, which may also lead to liver failure have been reported with sulfonylureas, including glimepiride.

DERMATOLOGIC REACTIONS

Allergic skin reactions, *e.g.*, pruritus, erythema, urticaria, and morbilliform or maculopapular eruptions, occur in less than 1% of treated patients. These may be transient and may disappear despite continued use of glimepiride. If those hypersensitivity reactions persist or worsen, the drug should be discontinued. Porphyria cutanea tarda, photosensitivity reactions, and allergic vasculitis have been reported with sulfonylureas.

HEMATOLOGIC REACTIONS

Leukopenia, agranulocytosis, thrombocytopenia, hemolytic anemia, aplastic anemia, and pancytopenia have been reported with sulfonylureas.

METABOLIC REACTIONS

Hepatic porphyria reactions and disulfiram-like reactions have been reported with sulfonylureas; however, no cases have yet been reported with glimepiride tablets. Cases of hyponatremia have been reported with glimepiride and all other sulfonylureas, most often in patients who are on other medications or have medical conditions known to cause hyponatremia or increase release of antidiuretic hormone. The syndrome of inappropriate antidiuretic hormone (SIADH) secretion has been reported with certain other sulfonylureas, and it has been suggested that these sulfonylureas may augment the peripheral (antidiuretic) action of ADH and/or increase release of ADH.

OTHER REACTIONS

Changes in accommodation and/or blurred vision may occur with the use of glimepiride. This is thought to be due to changes in blood glucose, and may be more pronounced when treatment is initiated. This condition is also seen in untreated diabetic patients, and may actually be reduced by treatment. In placebo-controlled trials of glimepiride, the incidence of blurred vision was placebo, 0.7%, and glimepiride, 0.4%.

HUMAN OPHTHALMOLOGY DATA

Ophthalmic examinations were carried out in over 500 subjects during long-term studies using the methodology of Taylor and West and Laties *et al.* No significant differences were seen between glimepiride and glyburide in the number of subjects with clinically important changes in visual acuity, intra-ocular tension, or in any of the five lens-related variables examined.

Ophthalmic examinations were carried out during long-term studies using the method of Chylack *et al.* No significant or clinically meaningful differences were seen between glimepiride and glipizide with respect to cataract progression by subjective LOCS II grading and objective image analysis systems, visual acuity, intraocular pressure, and general ophthalmic examination.

DOSAGE AND ADMINISTRATION

There is no fixed dosage regimen for the management of diabetes mellitus with glimepiride or any other hypoglycemic agent. The patient's fasting blood glucose and HbA1c must be measured periodically to determine the minimum effective dose for the patient; to detect primary failure, *i.e.*, inadequate lowering of blood glucose at the maximum recommended dose of medication; and to detect secondary failure, *i.e.*, loss of adequate blood glucose lowering response after an initial period of effectiveness. Glycosylated hemoglobin levels should be performed to monitor the patient's response to therapy.

Short-term administration of glimepiride may be sufficient during periods of transient loss of control in patients usually controlled well on diet and exercise.

G

USUAL STARTING DOSE

The usual starting dose of glimepiride as initial therapy is 1-2 mg once daily, administered with breakfast or the first main meal. Those patients who may be more sensitive to hypoglycemic drugs should be started at 1 mg once daily, and should be titrated carefully. (See PRECAUTIONS for patients at increased risk.)

No exact dosage relationship exists between glimepiride and the other oral hypoglycemic agents. The maximum starting dose of glimepiride should be no more than 2 mg.

Failure to follow an appropriate dosage regimen may precipitate hypoglycemia. Patients who do not adhere to their prescribed dietary and drug regimen are more prone to exhibit unsatisfactory response to therapy.

USUAL MAINTENANCE DOSE

The usual maintenance dose is 1-4 mg once daily. The maximum recommended dose is 8 mg once daily. After reaching a dose of 2 mg, dosage increases should be made in increments of no more than 2 mg at 1-2 week intervals based upon the patient's blood glucose response. Long-term efficacy should be monitored by measurement of HbA1c levels, for example, every 3-6 months.

GLIMEPIRIDE-METFORMIN COMBINATION THERAPY

If patients do not respond adequately to the maixmal dose of glimepiride monotherapy, addition of metformin may be considered. Published clinical information exists for the use of other sulfonylureas including glyburide, glipizide, chlorpropamide, and tolbutamide in combination with metformin.

With concomitant glimepiride and metformin therapy, the desired control of blood glucose may be obtained by adjusting the dose of each drug. However, attempts should be made to identify the minimum effective dose of each drug to achieve this goal. With concomitant glimepiride and metformin therapy, the risk of hypoglycemia associated with glimepiride therapy continues and may be increased. Appropriate precautions should be taken.

GLIMEPIRIDE-INSULIN COMBINATION THERAPY

Combination therapy with glimepiride and insulin may be used in secondary failure patients. The fasting glucose level for instituting combination therapy is in the range of >150 mg/dl in plasma or serum depending on the patient. The recommended glimepiride dose is 8 mg once daily administered with the first main meal. After starting with low-dose insulin, upward adjustments of insulin can be done approximately weekly as guided by frequent measurements of fasting blood glucose. Once stable, combination-therapy patients should monitor their capillary blood glucose on an ongoing basis, preferably daily. Periodic adjustments of insulin may also be necessary during maintenance as guided by glucose and HbA1c levels.

SPECIFIC PATIENT POPULATIONS

Glimepiride tablets are not recommended for use in pregnancy, nursing mothers, or children. In elderly, debilitated, or malnourished patients, or in patients with renal or hepatic insufficiency, the initial dosing, dose increments, and maintenance dosage should be conservative to avoid hypoglycemic reactions. (See CLINICAL PHARMACOLOGY, Special Populations and PRECAUTIONS, General.)

PATIENTS RECEIVING OTHER ORAL HYPOGLYCEMIC AGENTS

As with other sulfonylurea hypoglycemic agents, no transition period is necessary when transferring patients to glimepiride. Patients should be observed carefully (1-2 weeks) for hypoglycemia when being transferred from longer half-life sulfonylureas (*e.g.*, chlorpropamide) to glimepiride due to potential overlapping of drug effect.

ANIMAL PHARMACOLOGY

Reduced serum glucose values and degranulation of the pancreatic beta cells were observed in beagle dogs exposed to 320 mg glimepiride/kg/day for 12 months (approximately 1000 times the recommended human dose based on surface area). No evidence of tumor formation was observed in any organ. One female and one male dog developed bilateral subscapsular cataracts. Non-GLP studies indicated that glimepiride was unlikely to exacerbate cataract formation. Evaluation of the co-cataractogenic potential of glimepiride in several diabetic and cataract rat models was negative and there was no adverse effect of glimepiride on bovine ocular lens metabolism in organ culture.

HOW SUPPLIED

Amaryl tablets are available in:

- *1 mg:* Pink, flat-faced, oblong with notched sides at double bisect, imprinted with "AMA RYL" on one side and the Hoechst logo on both sides of the bisect on the other side.
- *2 mg:* Green, flat-faced, oblong with notched sides at double bisect, imprinted with "AMA RYL" on one side and the Hoechst logo on both sides of the bisect on the other side.
- *4 mg:* Blue, flat-faced, oblong with notched sides at double bisect, imprinted with "AMA RYL" on one side and the Hoechst logo on both sides of the bisect on the other side.

Storage: Store between 15-30°C (59-86°F). Dispense in well-closed containers with safety closures.

PRODUCT LISTING - EQUIVALENTS NOT AVAILABLE

Tablet - Oral - 1 mg			
100's	$33.48	AMARYL, Aventis Pharmaceuticals	00039-0221-10
Tablet - Oral - 2 mg			
30's	$15.73	AMARYL, Physicians Total Care	54868-4205-00
100's	$54.26	AMARYL, Aventis Pharmaceuticals	00039-0222-10
100's	$54.26	AMARYL, Aventis Pharmaceuticals	00039-0222-11
Tablet - Oral - 4 mg			
30's	$74.76	AMARYL, Allscripts Pharmaceutical Company	54569-4453-01
100's	$77.76	AMARYL, Allscripts Pharmaceutical Company	54569-4453-00
100's	$102.34	AMARYL, Aventis Pharmaceuticals	00039-0223-10
100's	$102.34	AMARYL, Aventis Pharmaceuticals	00039-0223-11

Glipizide *(001357)*

For related information, see the comparative table section in Appendix A.

Categories: Diabetes mellitus; Pregnancy Category C; FDA Approved 1984 May

Drug Classes: Antidiabetic agents; Sulfonylureas, second generation

Brand Names: **Glucotrol**; Glucotrol Xl

Foreign Brand Availability: Aldiab (Indonesia); Apamid (Thailand); Beapizide (Singapore); Decose (Taiwan); Depizide (Thailand); Diabes (Taiwan); Diasef (Hong-Kong; Singapore); Digrin (Korea); Dipazide (Thailand); Gipzide (Thailand); Glibenese (Bahrain; Belgium; Benin; Burkina-Faso; Cyprus; Denmark; Egypt; Ethiopia; Finland; France; Gambia; Germany; Ghana; Guinea; Iran; Iraq; Israel; Ivory-Coast; Jordan; Kenya; Kuwait; Lebanon; Liberia; Libya; Malawi; Mali; Mauritania; Mauritius; Morocco; Netherlands; Niger; Nigeria; Oman; Qatar; Republic-of-Yemen; Russia; Saudi-Arabia; Senegal; Seychelles; Sierra-Leone; South-Africa; Spain; Sudan; Sweden; Switzerland; Syria; Tanzania; Tunia; Uganda; United-Arab-Emirates; Zambia; Zimbabwe); Glibetin (Taiwan); Glican (El-Salvador); Glidiab (China; Taiwan); Glipicontin (India); Glipid (New-Zealand); Glizide (Thailand); Glucodiab (Thailand); Glucolip (India); Gluconil (Philippines); Gluco-Rite (Israel); Glucozide (Taiwan); Glupitel (Mexico); Glupizide (Taiwan); Glutrol (China); Glyde (India); Glygen (Thailand); Glynase (India); Glyzid (Indonesia); Glyzip (India); Melizide (Australia; Finland; New-Zealand; Singapore); Mindiab (Finland; Hong-Kong; Norway; Russia; Sweden); Minidiab (Australia; Austria; Bahrain; Belgium; Benin; Bulgaria; Burkina-Faso; China; Cyprus; Czech-Republic; Denmark; Egypt; Ethiopia; France; Gambia; Ghana; Guinea; Hong-Kong; Hungary; Indonesia; Iran; Iraq; Israel; Italy; Ivory-Coast; Jordan; Kenya; Kuwait; Lebanon; Liberia; Libya; Malawi; Malaysia; Mali; Mauritania; Mauritius; Morocco; New-Zealand; Niger; Nigeria; Oman; Philippines; Portugal; Qatar; Republic-of-Yemen; Saudi-Arabia; Senegal; Seychelles; Sierra-Leone; South-Africa; Sudan; Syria; Taiwan; Tanzania; Thailand; Tunia; Turkey; Uganda; United-Arab-Emirates; Zambia; Zimbabwe); Minodiab (Argentina; Costa-Rica; Dominican-Republic; El-Salvador; England; Greece; Honduras; Ireland; Mexico; Nicaragua; Panama; Spain); Napizide (Taiwan); Ozidia (France); Sucrazide (Bahrain; Cyprus; Egypt; Iran; Iraq; Israel; Jordan; Kuwait; Lebanon; Libya; Oman; Qatar; Republic-of-Yemen; Saudi-Arabia; Syria; United-Arab-Emirates)

Cost of Therapy: $12.93 (Diabetes Mellitus; Glucotrol; 5 mg; 1 tablet/day; 30 day supply)
$9.33 (Diabetes Mellitus; Generic Tablets; 5 mg; 1 tablet/day; 30 day supply)
$12.80 (Diabetes Mellitus; Glucotrol XL Extended-Release; 5 mg; 1 tablet/day; 30 day supply)

DESCRIPTION

IMMEDIATE- AND EXTENDED-RELEASE TABLETS

Glipizide is an oral blood-glucose-lowering drug of the sulfonylurea class.

The chemical abstracts name of glipizide is 1-cyclohexyl-3-[[p-(2-(5-methylpyrazinecarboxamido)ethyl]phenyl]sulfonyl]urea. The molecular formula is $C_{21}H_{27}N_5O_4S$; the molecular weight is 445.55.

Glipizide is a whitish, odorless powder with a pKa of 5.9. It is insoluble in water and alcohols, but soluble in 0.1 *N* NaOH; it is freely soluble in dimethylformamide.

Immediate-Release Tablets: Each immediate-release tablet, for oral administration contains glipizide, 5 or 10 mg and the following inactive ingredients: corn starch, anhydrous lactose, microcrystalline cellulose, colloidal silicon dioxide and stearic acid.

Extended-Release Tablets: Inert ingredients in the formulations are: polyethylene oxide, hydroxypropyl methylcellulose, magnesium stearate, sodium chloride, red ferric oxide, cellulose acetate, polyethylene glycol, opadry white and black ink.

EXTENDED-RELEASE TABLETS

Glucotrol XL extended-release tablets are similar in appearance to a conventional tablet. It consists, however, of an osmotically active drug core surrounded by a semipermeable membrane. The core itself is divided into two layers: an "active" layer containing the drug, and a "push" layer containing pharmacologically insert (but osmotically active) components. The membrane surrounding the tablet is permeable to water but not to drug or osmotic excipients. As water from the gastrointestinal tract enters the tablet pressure increases in the osmotic layer and "pushes" against the drug layer, resulting in the release of through a small, laser-drilled orifice in the membrane on the drug side of the tablet.

The Glucotrol XL extended-release tablet is designed to provide a controlled rate of delivery of glipizide into the gastrointestinal lumen which is independent of pH or gastrointestinal motility. The function of the Glucotrol XL extended-release tablet depends upon the existence of an osmotic gradient between the contents of the bi-layer core and fluid in the GI tract. Drug delivery is essentially constant as long as the osmotic gradient remains constant, and then gradually falls to zero. The biologically inert components of the tablet remain intact during GI transit and are eliminated in the feces as an insoluble shell.

CLINICAL PHARMACOLOGY

IMMEDIATE-RELEASE TABLETS

Mechanism of Action

The primary mode of action of glipizide in experimental animals appears to be the stimulation of insulin secretion from the beta cells of pancreatic islet tissue and is thus dependent on functioning beta cells in the pancreatic islets. In humans glipizide appears to lower the blood glucose acutely by stimulating the release of insulin from the pancreas, an effect dependent upon functioning beta cells in the pancreatic islets. The mechanism by which glipizide lowers blood glucose during long-term administration has not been clearly established. In man, stimulation of insulin secretion by glipizide in response to a meal is undoubtedly of major importance. Fasting insulin levels are not elevated even on long-term glipizide administration, but the postprandial insulin response continues to be enhanced after at least 6 months of treatment. The insulinotropic response to a meal occurs within 30 minutes after an oral dose of glipizide in diabetic patients, but elevated insulin levels do not persist beyond the time of the meal challenge. Extrapancreatic effects may play a part in the mechanism of action of oral sulfonylurea hypoglycemic drugs.

Blood sugar control persists in some patients for up to 24 hours after a single dose of glipizide, even though plasma levels have declined to a small fraction of peak levels by that time (see Pharmacokinetics).

Some patients fail to respond initially, or gradually lose their responsiveness to sulfonylurea drugs, including glipizide. Alternatively, glipizide may be effective in some patients who have not responded or have ceased to respond to other sulfonylureas.

Pharmacokinetics

Gastrointestinal absorption of glipizide in man is uniform, rapid, and essentially complete. Peak plasma concentrations occur 1-3 hours after a single oral dose. The half-life of elimination ranges from 2-4 hours in normal subjects, whether given intravenously or orally. The metabolic and excretory patterns are similar with the two routes of administration, indicating that first-pass metabolism is not significant. Glipizide does not accumulate in plasma on repeated oral administration. It has been reported that total absorption and disposition of an oral dose was unaffected by food in normal volunteers, but absorption was delayed by about 40 minutes. Thus glipizide was more effective when administered about 30 minutes before, rather than with, a test meal in diabetic patients. Protein binding was studied in serum from volunteers who received either oral or intravenous glipizide and found to be 98-99% one hour after either route of administration. The apparent volume of distribution of glipizide after intravenous administration was 11 L, indicative of localization within the extracellular fluid compartment. In mice no glipizide or metabolites were detectable autoradiographically in the brain or spinal cord of males or females, nor in the fetuses of pregnant females. In another study, however, very small amounts of radioactivity were detected in the fetuses of rats given labelled drug.

The metabolism of glipizide is extensive and occurs mainly in the liver. The primary metabolites are inactive hydroxylation products and polar conjugates and are excreted mainly in the urine. Less than 10% unchanged glipizide is found in the urine.

EXTENDED-RELEASE TABLETS

Mechanism of Action

Glipizide appears to lower blood glucose acutely by stimulating the release of insulin from the pancreas, an effect dependent upon functioning beta cells in the pancreatic islets. Extrapancreatic effects also may play a part in the mechanism of action of oral sulfonylurea hypoglycemic drugs. Two extrapancreatic effects shown to be important in the action of glipizide are an increase in insulin sensitivity and a decrease in hepatic glucose production. However, the mechanism by which glipizide lowers blood glucose during long-term administration has not been clearly established. Stimulation of insulin secretion by glipizide in response to a meal is of major importance. The insulinotropic response to a meal is enhanced with glipizide extended-release tablets administration in diabetic patients. The postprandial insulin and C-peptide responses continue to be enhanced after at least 6 months of treatment. In 2 randomized, double blind, dose-response studies comprising a total of 347 patients, there was no significant increase in fasting insulin in all glipizide extended-release tablets-treated patients combined compared to placebo, although minor elevations were observed at some doses. There was no increase in fasting insulin over the long-term.

Some patients fail to respond initially, or gradually lose their responsiveness to sulfonylurea drugs, including glipizide. Alternatively, glipizide may be effective in some patients who have not responded or have ceased to respond to other sulfonylureas.

Effects on Blood Glucose

The effectiveness of glipizide extended-release tablets in NIDDM at doses from 5-60 mg once daily has been evaluated in 4 therapeutic clinical trials each with long-term open extensions involving a total of 598 patients. Once daily administration of 5, 10, and 20 mg produced statistically significant reductions from placebo in hemoglobin A_{1C}, fasting plasma glucose and postprandial glucose in mild to severe NIDDM patients. In a pooled analysis of the patients treated with 5 mg and 20 mg, the relationship between dose and glipizide extended-release tablets's effect of reducing hemoglobin A_{1C} was not established. However, in the case of fasting plasma glucose patients treated with 20 mg, a statistically significant reduction of fasting plasma glucose compared to the 5 mg-treated group was found.

The reductions in hemoglobin A_{1C} and fasting plasma glucose were similar in younger and older patients. Efficacy of glipizide extended-release tablets was not affected by gender, race, or weight (as assessed by body mass index). In long term extension trials, efficacy of glipizide extended-release tablets was maintained in 81% of patients for up to 12 months.

In an open, two-way crossover study 132 patients were randomly assigned to either glipizide extended-release tablets or glipizide for 8 weeks and then crossed over to the other drug for an additional 8 weeks. Glipizide extended-release tablet administration resulted in significantly lower fasting plasma glucose levels and equivalent hemoglobin A_{1C} levels, as compared to glipizide.

Pharmacokinetics and Metabolism

Glipizide is rapidly and completely absorbed following oral administration in an immediate-release dosage form. The absolute bioavailability of glipizide was 100% after single doses in patients with NIDDM. Beginning 2-3 hours after administration of glipizide extended-release tablets, plasma drug concentrations gradually rise reaching maximum concentrations within 6-12 hours after dosing. With subsequent once daily dosing of glipizide extended-release tablets, effective plasma glipizide concentrations are maintained throughout the 24 hour dosing interval with less peak to through fluctuation than that observed with twice daily dosing of immediate-release glipizide. The mean relative bioavailability of glipizide in 21 males with NIDDM after administration of 20 mg glipizide extended-release tablets, compared to immediate-release glipizide (10 mg given twice daily), was 90% at steady state. Steady state plasma concentrations were achieved by at least the fifth day of dosing with glipizide extended-release tablets in 21 male with NIDDM and patients younger than 65 years. Approximately 1-2 days longer were required to reach steady state in 24 elderly (≥65 years) males and females with NIDDM. No accumulation of drug was observed in patients with NIDDM during chronic dosing with glipizide extended-release tablets. Administration of glipizide extended-release tablets with food has no effect on the 2 to 3 hour lag time in drug absorption. In a single dose, food effect study in 21 healthy males subjects, the administration of glipizide extended-release tablets immediately before a high fat breakfast resulted in a 40% increase in the glipizide mean C_{max} value, which was significant, but the effect on the AUC was not significant. There was no change in glucose response between the fed and fasting state. Markedly reduced GI retention times of the glipizide extended-release tablets over prolonged periods (*e.g.*, short bowel syndrome) may influence the pharmacokinetic profile of the drug and potentially result in lower plasma concentrations. In a multiple dose study in 26 males with NIDDM, the pharmacokinetics of glipizide were linear over the dose range of 5-60 mg of glipizide extended-release tablets in that the plasma drug concentrations increased proportionately with dose. In a single dose study in 24 healthy subjects, four 5 mg, two 10 mg, and one 20 mg glipizide extended-release tablets were bioequivalent.

Glipizide is eliminated primarily by hepatic biotransformation: less than 10% of a dose is excreted as unchanged drug in urine and feces; approximately 90% of a dose is excreted as biotransformation products in urine (80%) and feces (10%). The major metabolites of glipizide are products of aromatic hydroxylation and have no hypoglycemic activity. A minor metabolite which accounts for less than 2% of a dose, an acetylaminoethyl benzine derivatives, is reported to have 1/10 to 1/3 as much hypoglycemic activity as the parent compound. The mean total body clearance of glipizide was approximately 3 L/h after single intravenous doses in patients with NIDDM. The mean apparent volume of distribution was approximately 10 L. Glipizide is 98-99% bound to serum proteins, primarily to albumin. The mean terminal elimination half-life of glipizide ranged from 2-5 hours after single or multiple doses in patients with NIDDM. There were no significant differences in the pharmacokinetics of glipizide after single dose administration to older diabetic subjects compared to younger healthy subjects. There is only limited information regarding the effects of renal impairment on the disposition of glipizide and no information regarding the effects of hepatic disease. However, since glipizide is highly protein bound and hepatic biotransformation is the predominant route of elimination the pharmacokinetics and/or pharmacodynamics of glipizide may be altered in patients with renal or hepatic impairment.

In mice no glipizide or metabolites were detectable autoradiographically in the brain or spinal cord of males or females, nor in the fetuses of pregnant females. In another study, however, very small amounts of radioactivity were detected in the fetuses of rats given labeled drug.

IMMEDIATE- AND EXTENDED-RELEASE TABLETS

Other Effects: It has been shown that glipizide therapy was effective in controlling blood sugar without deleterious changes in the plasma lipoprotein profiles of patients treated for NIDDM.

In a placebo-controlled, crossover study in normal volunteers, glipizide had no anti-diuretic activity, and, in fact, led to a slight increase in free water clearance.

INDICATIONS AND USAGE

IMMEDIATE- AND EXTENDED-RELEASE TABLETS

Glipizide is indicated as an adjunct to diet for the control of hyperglycemia and its associated symptomatology in patients with non-insulin-dependent diabetes mellitus (NIDDM; Type II), formerly known as maturity-onset diabetes, after an adequate trial of dietary therapy has proved unsatisfactory.

In initiating treatment for non-insulin-dependent diabetes, diet should be emphasized as the primary form of treatment. Caloric restriction and weight loss are essential in the obese diabetic patient. Proper dietary management alone may be effective in controlling the blood glucose and symptoms of hyperglycemia. The importance of regular physical activity should also be stressed, cardiovascular risk factors should be identified, and corrective measures taken where possible.

If this treatment program fails to reduce symptoms and/or blood glucose, the use of an oral sulfonylurea should be considered. If additional reduction of symptoms and/or blood glucose is required, the addition of insulin to the treatment regimen should be considered. Use of glipizide must be viewed by both the physician and patient as a treatment in addition to diet, and not as a substitute for diet or as a convenient mechanism for avoiding dietary restraint. Furthermore, loss of blood glucose control on diet alone also may be transient, thus requiring only short-term administration of glipizide.

During maintenance programs, glipizide should be discontinued if satisfactory lowering of blood glucose is no longer achieved. Judgments should be based on regular clinical and laboratory evaluations.

In considering the use of glipizide in asymptomatic patients, it should be recognized that controlling blood glucose in non-insulin-dependent diabetes has not been definitely established to be effective in preventing the long-term cardiovascular or neural complications of diabetes. In insulin-dependent diabetes mellitus controlling blood glucose has been effective in slowing the progression of diabetic retinopathy, nephropathy, and neuropathy.

EXTENDED-RELEASE TABLETS

In 12 week, well-controlled studies there was a maximal average net reduction in hemoglobin A_{1C} of 1.7% in absolute units between placebo-treated and glipizide extended-release tablets-treated patients.

CONTRAINDICATIONS

Glipizide is contraindicated in patients with:

1. Known hypersensitivity to the drug.
2. Diabetic ketoacidosis, with or without coma. This condition should be treated with insulin.

WARNINGS

IMMEDIATE- AND EXTENDED-RELEASE TABLETS

SPECIAL WARNING ON INCREASED RISK OF CARDIOVASCULAR MORTALITY: The administration of oral hypoglycemic drugs has been reported to be associated with increased cardiovascular mortality as compared to treatment with diet alone or diet plus insulin. This warning is based on the study conducted by the University Group Diabetes Program (UGDP), a long-term prospective clinical trial designed to evaluate the effectiveness of glucose-lowering drugs in preventing or delaying vascular complications in patients with non-insulin-dependent diabetes. The study involved 823 patients who were randomly assigned to one of four treatment groups.[1]

UGDP reported that patients treated for 5-8 years with diet plus a fixed dose of tolbutamide (1.5 g/day) had a rate of cardiovascular mortality approximately 2½ times that of patients treated with diet alone. A significant increase in total mortality was not observed, but the use of tolbutamide was discontinued based on the increase in cardiovascular mortality, thus limiting the opportunity for the study to show an increase in overall mortality. Despite controversy regarding the interpretation of these results, the findings of the UGDP study provide an adequate basis for this warning. The patient should be informed of the potential risks and advantages of glipizide and of alternative modes of therapy.

Although only one drug in the sulfonylurea class (tolbutamide) was included in this study, it is prudent from a safety standpoint to consider that this warning may also apply to other oral hypoglycemic drugs in this class, in view of their close similarities in mode of action and chemical structure.

As with any other non-deformable material, caution should be used when administering glipizide extended-release tablets in patients with preexisting severe gastrointestinal narrowing (pathologic or iatrogenic). There have been rare reports of obstructive symptoms in patients with known structures in association with the ingestion of another drug in this non-deformable sustained release formulation.

PRECAUTIONS

GENERAL

Renal and Hepatic Disease

The metabolism and excretion of glipizide may be slowed in patients with impaired renal and/or hepatic function. If hypoglycemia should occur in such patients, it may be prolonged and appropriate management should be instituted.

Hypoglycemia

All sulfonylurea drugs are capable of producing severe hypoglycemia. Proper patient selection, dosage, and instructions are important to avoid hypoglycemic episodes. Renal or hepatic insufficiency may cause elevated blood levels of glipizide and the latter may also diminish gluconeogenic capacity, both of which increase the risk of serious hypoglycemic reactions. Elderly, debilitated or malnourished patients, and those with adrenal or pituitary insufficiency are particularly susceptible to the hypoglycemic action of glucose-lowering drugs. Hypoglycemia may be difficult to recognize in the elderly, and in people who are taking beta-adrenergic blocking drugs. Hypoglycemia is more likely to occur when caloric intake is deficient, after severe or prolonged exercise, when alcohol is ingested, or when more than one glucose-lowering drug is used. Therapy with a combination of glucose-lowering agents may increase the potential for hypoglycemia.

Loss of Control of Blood Glucose

When a patient stabilized on any diabetic regimen is exposed to stress such as fever, trauma, infection, or surgery, a loss of control may occur. At such times, it may be necessary to discontinue glipizide and administer insulin.

The effectiveness of any oral hypoglycemic drug, including glipizide, in lowering blood glucose to a desired level decreases in many patients over a period of time, which may be due to progression of the severity of the diabetes or to diminished responsiveness to the drug. This phenomenon is known as secondary failure, to distinguish it from primary failure in which the drug is ineffective in an individual patient when first given. Adequate adjustment of dose and adherence to diet should be assessed before classifying a patient as a secondary failure.

LABORATORY TESTS

Blood and urine glucose should be monitored periodically. Measurement of glycosylated hemoglobin may be useful.

CARCINOGENESIS, MUTAGENESIS, AND IMPAIRMENT OF FERTILITY

A 20 month study in rats and an eighteen month study in mice at doses up to 75 times the maximum human dose revealed no evidence of drug-related carcinogenicity. Bacterial and *in vivo* mutagenicity tests were uniformly negative. Studies in rats of both sexes at doses up to 75 times the human dose showed no effects on fertility.

PREGNANCY, TERATOGENIC EFFECTS, PREGNANCY CATEGORY C

Glipizide was found to be mildly fetotoxic in rat reproductive studies at all dose levels (5-50 mg/kg). This fetotoxicity has been similarly noted with other sulfonylureas, such as tolbutamide and tolazamide. The effect is perinatal and believed to be directly related to the pharmacologic (hypoglycemic) action of glipizide. In studies in rats and rabbits no teratogenic effects were found. There are no adequate and well controlled studies in pregnant women. Glipizide should be used during pregnancy only if the potential benefit justifies the potential risk to the fetus.

Because recent information suggests that abnormal blood glucose levels during pregnancy are associated with a higher incidence of congenital abnormalities, many experts recommend that insulin be used during pregnancy to maintain blood glucose levels as close to normal as possible.

Nonteratogenic Effects

Prolonged severe hypoglycemia (4-10 days) has been reported in neonates born to mothers who were receiving a sulfonylurea drug at the time of delivery. This has been reported more frequently with the use of agents with prolonged half-lives. If glipizide is used during pregnancy, it should be discontinued at least 1 month before the expected delivery date.

NURSING MOTHERS

Although it is not known whether glipizide is excreted in human milk, some sulfonylurea drugs are known to be excreted in human milk. Because the potential for hypoglycemia in nursing infants may exist, a decision should be made whether to discontinue nursing or to discontinue the drug, taking into account the importance of the drug to the mother. If the drug is discontinued and if diet alone is inadequate for controlling blood glucose, insulin therapy should be considered.

PEDIATRIC USE

Safety and effectiveness in pediatric patients have not been established.

IMMEDIATE-RELEASE TABLETS

Information for the Patient

Patients should be informed of the potential risks and advantages of glipizide and of alternative modes of therapy. They should also be informed about the importance of adhering to dietary instructions, of a regular exercise program, and of regular testing of urine and/or blood glucose.

The risks of hypoglycemia, its symptoms and treatment, and conditions that predispose to its development should be explained to patients and responsible family members. Primary and secondary failure should also be explained.

EXTENDED-RELEASE TABLETS

GI Disease

Markedly reduced GI retention times of the glipizide extended-release tablets may influence the pharmacokinetic profile and hence the clinical efficacy of the drug.

Adequate adjustment of dose and adherence to diet should be assessed before classifying a patient as a secondary failure.

Information for the Patient

Patients should be informed that glipizide extended-release tablets should be swallowed whole. Patients should not chew, divide or crush tablets. Patients should not be concerned if they occasionally notice in their stool something that looks like a tablet. In the glipizide extended-release tablet, the medication is contained within a shell that has been specially designed to slowly release the drug so the body can absorb it. When this process is completed, the empty tablet is eliminated from the body.

Patients should be informed of the potential risks and advantages of glipizide extended-release tablets and of alternative modes of therapy. They should also be informed about the importance of adhering to dietary instructions, of a regular exercise program, and of regular testing of urine and/or blood glucose.

The risk of hypoglycemia, its symptoms and treatment, and conditions that predispose to its development should be explained to patients and responsible family members. Primary and secondary failure also should be explained.

Geriatric Use

Of the total number of patients in clinical studies of glipizide extended-release tablets 33% were 65 and over. No overall differences in effectiveness or safety were observed between these patients and younger patients, but greater sensitivity of some individuals cannot be ruled out. Approximately 1-2 days longer were required to reach steady state in the elderly. (See CLINICAL PHARMACOLOGY and DOSAGE AND ADMINISTRATION.)

DRUG INTERACTIONS

The hypoglycemic action of sulfonylureas may be potentiated by certain drugs including nonsteroidal anti-inflammatory agents, some azoles and other drugs that are highly protein bound, salicylates, sulfonamides, chloramphenicol, probenecid, coumarins, monoamine oxidase inhibitors, and beta adrenergic blocking agents. When such drugs are administered to a patient receiving glipizide, the patient should be observed closely for hypoglycemia. When such drugs are withdrawn from a patient receiving glipizide, the patient should be observed closely for loss of control. *In vitro* binding studies with human serum proteins indicate that glipizide binds differently than tolbutamide and does not interact with salicylate or dicumarol. However, caution must be exercised in extrapolating these findings to the clinical situation and in the use of glipizide with these drugs.

Certain drugs tend to produce hyperglycemia and may lead to loss of control. These drugs include the thiazides and other diuretics, corticosteroids, phenothiazines, thyroid products, estrogens, oral contraceptives, phenytoin, nicotinic acid, sympathomimetics, calcium channel blocking drugs, and isoniazid. When such drugs are administered to a patient receiving glipizide, the patient should be closely observed for loss of control. When such drugs are withdrawn from a patient receiving glipizide, the patient should be observed closely for hypoglycemia.

A potential interaction between oral miconazole and oral hypoglycemic agents leading to severe hypoglycemia has been reported. Whether this interaction also occurs with the intravenous, topical, or vaginal preparations of miconazole is not known. The effect of concomitant administration of fluconazole and glipizide has been demonstrated in a placebo-controlled crossover study in normal volunteers. All subjects received glipizide alone and following treatment with 100 mg of fluconazole as a single daily oral dose for 7 days. The mean percentage increase in the glipizide AUC after fluconazole administration was 56.9% (range: 35-81).

ADVERSE REACTIONS

IMMEDIATE-RELEASE TABLETS

In US and foreign controlled studies, the frequency of serious adverse reactions reported was very low. Of 702 patients, 11.8% reported adverse reactions and in only 1.5% was glipizide discontinued.

Hypoglycemia: See PRECAUTIONS.

Gastrointestinal: Gastrointestinal disturbances are the most common reactions. Gastrointestinal complaints were reported with the following approximate incidence: nausea and diarrhea, 1 in 70; constipation and gastralgia, 1 in 100. They appear to be dose-related and may disappear on division or reduction of dosage. Cholestatic jaundice may occur rarely with sulfonylureas; glipizide should be discontinued if this occurs.

Dermatologic: Allergic skin reactions including erythema, morbilliform or maculopapular eruptions, urticaria, pruritus, and eczema have been reported in about 1 in 70 patients. These may be transient and may disappear despite continued use of glipizide; if skin reactions persist, the drug should be discontinued. Porphyria cutanea tarda and photosensitivity reactions have been reported with sulfonylureas.

Miscellaneous: Dizziness, drowsiness, and headache have each been reported in about 1 in 50 patients treated with glipizide. They are usually transient and seldom require discontinuance of therapy.

EXTENDED-RELEASE TABLETS

In US controlled studies the frequency of serious adverse experiences reported was very low and causal relationship has not been established. The 580 patients from 31-87 years of age who recieved glipizide extended-release tablets in doses from 5-60 mg in both controlled and open trials were included in the evaluation of adverse experiences. All adverse experiences reported were tabulated independently of their possible causal relation to medication.

Hypoglycemia: See PRECAUTIONS.

Only 3.4% of patients receiving glipizide extended-release tablets had hypoglycemia documented by/ a blood glucose measurement <60 mg/dl and or symptoms believed to be associated with hypoglycemia. In a comparative efficacy study of glipizide extended-release tablets and glipizide, hypoglycemia occurred rarely with an incidence of less than 1% with both drugs.

In double-blind, placebo-controlled studies the adverse experiences reported with an incidence of 3% or more in glipizide extended-release tablets-treated patients include:

TABLE 1

Adverse Effect	Glipizide Extended-Release Tablets (n=278)	Placebo (n=69)
Asthenia	10.1%	13.0%
Headache	8.6%	8.7%
Dizziness	6.8%	5.8%
Nervousness	3.6%	2.9%
Tremor	3.6%	0.0%
Diarrhea	5.4%	0.0%
Flatulence	3.2%	1.4%

The following adverse experiences occurred with an incidence of less than 3% in glipizide extended-release tablets-treated patients:

Body as a Whole: Pain.

Nervous System: Insomnia, paresthesia, anxiety, depression and hypesthesia.

Gastrointestinal: Nausea, dyspepsia, constipation and vomiting.

Metabolic: Hypoglycemia.

Musculoskeletal: Arthralgia, leg cramps and myalgia.

Cardiovascular: Syncope.

Skin: Sweating and pruritus.

Respiratory: Rhinitis.

Special Senses: Blurred vision.

Urogenital: Polyuria.

Other adverse experiences occurred with an incidence of less than 1% in glipizide extended-release tablets-treated patients:

Body as a Whole: Chills.

Nervous System: Hypertonia, confusion, vertigo, somnolence, gait abnormality and decreases libido.

Gastrointestinal: Anorexia and trace blood in stool.

Metabolic: Thirst and edema.

Cardiovascular: Arrhythmia, migraine, flushing and hypertension.

Skin: Rash and urticaria.

Respiratory: Pharyngitis and dyspnea.

Special Senses: Pain in the eye, conjunctivitis and retinal hemorrhage.

Urogenital: Dysuria.

Although these adverse experiences occurred in patients treated with glipizide extended-release tablets, a causal relationship to the medication has not been established in all cases.

There have been rare reports of gastrointestinal irritation and gastrointestinal bleeding with use of another drug in this non-deformable sustained release formulation, although causal relationship to the drug is uncertain.

IMMEDIATE-RELEASE TABLETS

The following are adverse experiences reported with immediate-release glipizide and other sulfonylureas, but have not been observed with glipizide extended-release tablets:

Hematologic: Leukopenia, agranulocytosis, thrombocytopenia, hemolytic anemia, aplastic anemia, and pancytopenia have been reported with sulfonylureas.

Metabolic: Hepatic porphyria and disulfiram-like reactions have been reported with sulfonylureas. In the mouse, glipizide pretreatment did not cause an accumulation of acetaldehyde after ethanol administration. Clinical experience to date has shown that glipizide has an extremely low incidence of disulfiram-like alcohol reactions.

Endocrine Reactions: Cases of hyponatremia and the syndrome of inappropriate antidiuretic hormone (SIADH) secretion have been reported with this and other sulfonylureas.

LABORATORY TESTS

The pattern of laboratory test abnormalities observed with glipizide was similar to that for other sulfonylureas. Occasional mild to moderate elevations of SGOT, LDH, alkaline phosphatase, BUN and creatinine were noted. One case of jaundice was reported. The relationship of these abnormalities to glipizide is uncertain, and they have rarely been associated with clinical symptoms.

DOSAGE AND ADMINISTRATION

IMMEDIATE- AND EXTENDED-RELEASE TABLETS

There is no fixed dosage regimen for the management of diabetes mellitus with glipizide or any other hypoglycemic agent. In addition to the usual monitoring of urinary glucose, the patient's blood glucose must also be monitored periodically to determine the minimum effective dose for the patient; to detect primary failure, *i.e.*, inadequate lowering of blood glucose at the maximum recommended dose of medication; and to detect secondary failure, *i.e.*, loss of an adequate blood-glucose-lowering response after an initial period of effectiveness. Glycosylated hemoglobin levels may also be of value in monitoring the patient's response to therapy.

Short-term administration of glipizide may be sufficient during periods of transient loss of control in patients usually controlled well on diet.

Patients Receiving Insulin

As with other sulfonylurea-class hypoglycemics, many stable non-insulin-dependent diabetic patients receiving insulin may be safely placed on glipizide. When transferring patients from insulin to glipizide, the following general guidelines should be considered:

For patients whose daily insulin requirement is 20 units or less, insulin may be discontinued and glipizide therapy may begin at usual dosages. Several days should elapse between glipizide titration steps.

For patients whose daily insulin requirement is greater than 20 units, the insulin dose should be reduced by 50% and glipizide therapy may begin at usual dosages. Subsequent reductions in insulin dosage should depend on individual patient response. Several days should elapse between glipizide titration steps.

During the insulin withdrawal period, the patient should test urine samples for sugar and ketone bodies at least 3 times daily. Patients should be instructed to contact the prescriber immediately if these tests are abnormal. In some cases, especially when patient has been receiving greater than 40 units of insulin daily, it may be advisable to consider hospitalization during the transition period.

Patients Receiving Other Oral Hypoglycemic Agents

As with other sulfonylurea-class hypoglycemics, no transition period is necessary when transferring patients to glipizide. Patients should be observed carefully (1-2 weeks) for hypoglycemia when being transferred from longer half-life sulfonylureas (*e.g.*, chlorpropamide) to glipizide due to potential over-lapping of drug effect.

EXTENDED-RELEASE TABLETS

Recommended Dosing

The recommended stating dose of glipizide extended-release tablets is 5 mg/day, given with breakfast. The recommended dose for geriatric patients is also 5 mg/day.

Dosage adjustment should be based on laboratory measures of glycemic control. While fasting blood glucose levels generally reach steady state following initiation of change in glipizide XL dosage, a single fasting glucose determination may not accurately reflect the response to therapy. In most cases, hemoglobin A_{1C} level measured at 3 month intervals is the preferred means of monitoring response to therapy.

Hemoglobin A_{1C} should be measured as glipizide extended-release tablet therapy is initiated at the 5 mg dose and repeated approximately 3 months later. If the result of this test suggests that glycemic control over the preceding 3 months was inadequate, the glipizide extended-release tablet dose may be increased to 10 mg. Subsequent dosage adjustments should be made on the basis of hemoglobin A_{1C} levels measured at 3 month intervals. If no improvement is seen after 3 months of therapy with a higher dose, the previous dose should be resumed. Decisions which utilize fasting blood glucose to adjust glipizide extended-release tablet therapy should be based on at least two or more similar, consecutive values obtained 7 days or more after the previous dose adjustment.

Most patients will be controlled with 5 mg or 10 mg taken once daily. However, some patients may require up to the maximum recommended daily dose of 20 mg. While the glycemic control of selected patients may improve with doses which exceed 10 mg, clinical studies conducted to date have not demonstrated an additional group average reduction of hemoglobin A_{1C} beyond what was achieved with the 10 mg dose.

Based on the results of a randomized crossover study patients receiving immediate-release glipizide may be switched safely to glipizide extended-release tablets once-a-day at the nearest equivalent total daily dose. Patients receiving immediate-release glipizide also may be titrated to the appropriate dose of glipizide extended-release tablets starting with 5 mg once daily. The decision to switch to the nearest equivalent dose or to titrate should be based on clinical judgement.

In elderly patients, debilitated or malnourished patients, and patients with impaired renal or hepatic function, the initial and maintenance dosing should be conservative to avoid hypoglycemic reactions (see PRECAUTIONS.)

When glipizide extended-release tablets are used in combination with other oral blood glucose-lowering agents, the second agent should be added at the lowest recommended dose and patients should be observed carefully. Titration of the added oral agent should be based on clinical judgment.

IMMEDIATE-RELEASE TABLETS

In general, glipizide should be given approximately 30 minutes before a meal to achieve the greatest reduction in postprandial hyperglycemia.

Initial Dose

The recommended starting dose is 5 mg, given before breakfast. Geriatric patients or those with liver disease may be started on 2.5 mg.

Titration

Dosage adjustments should ordinarily be in increments of 2.5-5 mg, as determined by blood glucose response. At least several days should elapse between titration steps. If response to a single dose is not satisfactory, dividing that dose may prove effective. The maximum recommended once daily dose is 15 mg. Doses above 15 mg should ordinarily be divided and given before meals of adequate caloric content. The maximum recommended total daily dose is 40 mg.

Maintenance

Some patients may be effectively controlled on a once-a-day regimen, while others show better response with divided dosing. Total daily doses above 15 mg should ordinarily be divided. Total daily doses above 30 mg have been safely given on a bid basis to long-term patients.

In elderly patients, debilitated or malnourished patients, and patients with impaired renal or hepatic function, the initial and maintenance dosing should be conservative to avoid hypoglycemic reactions (see PRECAUTIONS).

HOW SUPPLIED

IMMEDIATE-RELEASE TABLETS

Glucotrol tablets are supplied as follows:

- *5 mg:* White, dye-free, scored, diamond-shaped, and imprinted "Pfizer 411".
- *10 mg:* White, dye-free, scored, diamond-shaped, and imprinted "Pfizer 412".

Storage: Store below 30°C (86°F).

EXTENDED-RELEASE TABLETS

Glucotrol XL extended-release tablets are supplied as follows:

5 mg: White, round, biconvex tablet imprinted with "GLUCOTROL XL 5" in black ink on one side.

10 mg: White, round, biconvex tablet imprinted with "GLUCOTROL XL 10" in black ink on one side.

Storage: The tablets should be protected from moisture and humidity and stored at controlled room temperature, 15-30°C (59-86°F).

PRODUCT LISTING - RATED THERAPEUTICALLY EQUIVALENT

Tablet - Oral - 5 mg

Size	Price	Product	NDC
25 x 30	$255.68	GENERIC, Sky Pharmaceuticals Packaging, Inc	63739-0116-03
25's	$3.89	GENERIC, Udl Laboratories Inc	51079-0810-19
30's	$7.57	GENERIC, Pd-Rx Pharmaceuticals	55289-0806-30
30's	$10.38	GENERIC, Heartland Healthcare Services	61392-0063-30
30's	$10.38	GENERIC, Heartland Healthcare Services	61392-0063-39
30's	$12.93	GLUCOTROL, Allscripts Pharmaceutical Company	54569-0206-01
30's	$20.13	GENERIC, Golden State Medical	60429-0082-30
31 x 10	$117.74	GENERIC, Vangard Labs	00615-3595-53
31 x 10	$117.74	GENERIC, Vangard Labs	00615-3595-63
31's	$10.73	GENERIC, Heartland Healthcare Services	61392-0063-31
32's	$11.07	GENERIC, Heartland Healthcare Services	61392-0063-32
45's	$15.57	GENERIC, Heartland Healthcare Services	61392-0063-45
60's	$20.76	GENERIC, Heartland Healthcare Services	61392-0063-60
60's	$25.86	GLUCOTROL, Allscripts Pharmaceutical Company	54569-0206-03
60's	$28.75	GENERIC, Golden State Medical	60429-0082-60
90's	$31.14	GENERIC, Heartland Healthcare Services	61392-0063-90
90's	$31.91	GLUCOTROL, Allscripts Pharmaceutical Company	54569-8565-00
100's	$6.99	FEDERAL UPPER LIMIT, H.C.F.A. F F P	99999-1357-01
100's	$31.09	GENERIC, Par Pharmaceutical Inc	49884-0451-01
100's	$31.50	GENERIC, Mutual/United Research Laboratories	00677-1544-01
100's	$31.70	GENERIC, Dixon-Shane Inc	17236-0441-01
100's	$31.90	GENERIC, Watson/Rugby Laboratories Inc	00536-5702-01
100's	$31.94	GENERIC, Duramed Pharmaceuticals Inc	51285-0598-02
100's	$33.60	GENERIC, Geneva Pharmaceuticals	00781-1452-01
100's	$34.75	GENERIC, Mylan Pharmaceuticals Inc	00378-1105-01
100's	$35.00	GENERIC, Ivax Corporation	00172-3649-60
100's	$36.35	GENERIC, Ivax Corporation	00182-1994-89
100's	$37.70	GENERIC, Watson Laboratories Inc	00591-0460-01
100's	$37.70	GENERIC, Watson Laboratories Inc	52544-0460-01
100's	$43.10	GLUCOTROL, Allscripts Pharmaceutical Company	54569-0206-02
100's	$45.21	GLUCOTROL, Pfizer U.S. Pharmaceuticals	00049-4110-66

Tablet - Oral - 10 mg

Size	Price	Product	NDC
14's	$4.20	GENERIC, Pd-Rx Pharmaceuticals	55289-0976-14
25 x 30	$464.78	GENERIC, Sky Pharmaceuticals Packaging, Inc	63739-0117-03
25's	$15.60	GENERIC, Udl Laboratories Inc	51079-0811-19
30's	$11.52	GENERIC, Pd-Rx Pharmaceuticals	55289-0976-30
30's	$18.72	GENERIC, Heartland Healthcare Services	61392-0064-30
30's	$18.72	GENERIC, Heartland Healthcare Services	61392-0064-39
30's	$27.25	GENERIC, Golden State Medical	60429-0083-30
31 x 10	$117.74	GENERIC, Vangard Labs	00615-3596-63
31 x 10	$215.05	GENERIC, Vangard Labs	00615-3596-53
31's	$19.34	GENERIC, Heartland Healthcare Services	61392-0064-31
32's	$19.97	GENERIC, Heartland Healthcare Services	61392-0064-32
45's	$28.08	GENERIC, Heartland Healthcare Services	61392-0064-45
60's	$37.44	GENERIC, Heartland Healthcare Services	61392-0064-60
60's	$43.00	GENERIC, Golden State Medical	60429-0083-60
90's	$56.16	GENERIC, Heartland Healthcare Services	61392-0064-90
100's	$9.44	FEDERAL UPPER LIMIT, H.C.F.A. F F P	99999-1357-02
100's	$57.09	GENERIC, Par Pharmaceutical Inc	49884-0452-01
100's	$58.40	GENERIC, Dixon-Shane Inc	17236-0442-01
100's	$58.50	GENERIC, Geneva Pharmaceuticals	00781-1453-01
100's	$58.87	GENERIC, Duramed Pharmaceuticals Inc	51285-0599-02
100's	$59.75	GENERIC, Watson Laboratories Inc	00591-0461-01
100's	$63.00	GENERIC, Ivax Corporation	00172-3650-60
100's	$63.77	GENERIC, Endo Laboratories Llc	60951-0714-70
100's	$66.90	GENERIC, Ivax Corporation	00182-1995-89
100's	$67.00	GENERIC, Mylan Pharmaceuticals Inc	00378-1110-01
100's	$67.00	GENERIC, Watson Laboratories Inc	52544-0461-01
100's	$73.15	GLUCOTROL, Southwood Pharmaceuticals Inc	58016-0961-00
100's	$83.01	GLUCOTROL, Pfizer U.S. Pharmaceuticals	00049-4120-66
120's	$70.86	GENERIC, Golden State Medical	60429-0083-12

PRODUCT LISTING - EQUIVALENTS NOT AVAILABLE

Tablet - Oral - 5 mg

Size	Price	Product	NDC
10's	$3.07	GENERIC, Southwood Pharmaceuticals Inc	58016-0876-10
12's	$3.68	GENERIC, Southwood Pharmaceuticals Inc	58016-0876-12
14's	$4.30	GENERIC, Southwood Pharmaceuticals Inc	58016-0876-14
15's	$4.60	GENERIC, Southwood Pharmaceuticals Inc	58016-0876-15
20's	$6.14	GENERIC, Southwood Pharmaceuticals Inc	58016-0876-20
21's	$6.44	GENERIC, Southwood Pharmaceuticals Inc	58016-0876-21
24's	$7.36	GENERIC, Southwood Pharmaceuticals Inc	58016-0876-24
28's	$8.59	GENERIC, Southwood Pharmaceuticals Inc	58016-0876-28
30's	$9.20	GENERIC, Southwood Pharmaceuticals Inc	58016-0876-30
30's	$9.98	GENERIC, Allscripts Pharmaceutical Company	54569-3841-00
40's	$12.27	GENERIC, Southwood Pharmaceuticals Inc	58016-0876-40
50's	$15.34	GENERIC, Southwood Pharmaceuticals Inc	58016-0876-50
60's	$18.41	GENERIC, Southwood Pharmaceuticals Inc	58016-0876-60
60's	$19.87	GENERIC, Allscripts Pharmaceutical Company	54569-3841-01
100's	$31.50	GENERIC, Major Pharmaceuticals Inc	00904-7924-60
100's	$31.90	GENERIC, Warner Chilcott Laboratories	00047-0463-24
100's	$33.12	GENERIC, Allscripts Pharmaceutical Company	54569-3841-02
100's	$37.49	GENERIC, Udl Laboratories Inc	51079-0810-20

Tablet - Oral - 10 mg

Size	Price	Product	NDC
30's	$18.23	GENERIC, Allscripts Pharmaceutical Company	54569-3842-00
60's	$36.70	GENERIC, Allscripts Pharmaceutical Company	54569-3842-01
100's	$57.95	GENERIC, Major Pharmaceuticals Inc	00904-7925-60
100's	$58.54	GENERIC, Warner Chilcott Laboratories	00047-0464-24
100's	$61.16	GENERIC, Allscripts Pharmaceutical Company	54569-3842-02
100's	$69.01	GENERIC, Udl Laboratories Inc	51079-0811-20

Tablet, Extended Release - Oral - 2.5 mg

Size	Price	Product	NDC
30's	$12.80	GLUCOTROL XL, Pfizer U.S. Pharmaceuticals	00049-1620-30

Tablet, Extended Release - Oral - 5 mg

Size	Price	Product	NDC
30's	$10.66	GLUCOTROL XL, Allscripts Pharmaceutical Company	54569-3937-00
100's	$42.66	GLUCOTROL XL, Pfizer U.S. Pharmaceuticals	00049-1550-66

Tablet, Extended Release - Oral - 10 mg

Size	Price	Product	NDC
30's	$21.09	GLUCOTROL XL, Allscripts Pharmaceutical Company	54569-3938-00
60's	$42.17	GLUCOTROL XL, Allscripts Pharmaceutical Company	54569-3938-01
100's	$84.50	GLUCOTROL XL, Pfizer U.S. Pharmaceuticals	00049-1560-66

Glipizide; Metformin Hydrochloride (003575)

For complete prescribing information, refer to the CD-ROM included with the book.

For related information, see the comparative table section in Appendix A.

Categories: Diabetes mellitus; Pregnancy Category C; FDA Approved 2002 Oct
Drug Classes: Antidiabetic agents; Biguanides; Sulfonylureas, second generation
Brand Names: **Metaglip**
Cost of Therapy: $24.64 (Diabetes Mellitus; Metaglip; 2.5 mg/250 mg; 1 tablet/day; 30 day supply)

DESCRIPTION

Note: The trade name was used throughout this monograph for clarity.

Metaglip (glipizide; metformin hydrochloride) tablets contains 2 oral antihyperglycemic drugs used in the management of Type 2 diabetes, glipizide and metformin hydrochloride.

Glipizide is an oral antihyperglycemic drug of the sulfonylurea class. The chemical name for glipizide is 1-cyclohexyl-3-[[*p*-[2-(5-methylpyrazinecarboxamido)ethyl]phenyl] sulfonyl]urea. Glipizide is a whitish, odorless powder with a molecular formula of

$C_{21}H_{27}N_5O_4S$, a molecular weight of 445.55 and a pK_a of 5.9. It is insoluble in water and alcohols, but soluble in 0.1 *N* NaOH; it is freely soluble in dimethylformamide.

Metformin hydrochloride is an oral antihyperglycemic drug used in the management of Type 2 diabetes. Metformin hydrochloride (*N,N*-dimethylimidodicarbonimidic diamide mono-hydrochloride) is not chemically or pharmacologically related to sulfonylureas, thiazolidinediones, or a-glucosidase inhibitors. It is a white to off-white crystalline compound with a molecular formula of $C_4H_{12}ClN_5$ (mono-hydrochloride) and a molecular weight of 165.63. Metformin hydrochloride is freely soluble in water and is practically insoluble in acetone, ether, and chloroform. The pK_a of metformin is 12.4. The pH of a 1% aqueous solution of metformin hydrochloride is 6.68.

Metaglip is available for oral administration in tablets containing 2.5 mg glipizide with 250 mg metformin hydrochloride, 2.5 mg glipizide with 500 mg metformin hydrochloride, and 5 mg glipizide with 500 mg metformin hydrochloride. In addition, each tablet contains the following inactive ingredients: microcrystalline cellulose, povidone, croscarmellose sodium, and magnesium stearate. The tablets are film coated, which provides color differentiation.

INDICATIONS AND USAGE

Metaglip (glipizide; metformin HCl) tablets are indicated as initial therapy, as an adjunct to diet and exercise, to improve glycemic control in patients with Type 2 diabetes whose hyperglycemia cannot be satisfactorily managed with diet and exercise alone.

Metaglip is indicated as second-line therapy when diet, exercise, and initial treatment with a sulfonylurea or metformin do not result in adequate glycemic control in patients with Type 2 diabetes.

CONTRAINDICATIONS

Metaglip is contraindicated in patients with:

- Renal disease or renal dysfunction (*e.g.*, as suggested by serum creatinine levels ≥1.5 mg/dl [males], ≥1.4 mg/dl [females], or abnormal creatinine clearance) which may also result from conditions such as cardiovascular collapse (shock), acute myocardial infarction, and septicemia (see WARNINGS).
- Congestive heart failure requiring pharmacologic treatment.
- Known hypersensitivity to glipizde or metformin HCl.
- Acute or chronic metabolic acidosis, including diabetic ketoacidosis, with or without coma. Diabetic ketoacidosis should be treated with insulin.

Metaglip should be temporarily discontinued in patients undergoing radiologic studies involving intravascular administration of iodinated contrast materials, because use of such products may result in acute alteration of renal function.

WARNINGS

METFORMIN HCl

Lactic Acidosis:

Lactic acidosis is a rare, but serious, metabolic complication that can occur due to metformin accumulation during treatment with Metaglip; when it occurs, it is fatal in approximately 50% of cases. Lactic acidosis may also occur in association with a number of pathophysiologic conditions, including diabetes mellitus, and whenever there is significant tissue hypoperfusion and hypoxemia. Lactic acidosis is characterized by elevated blood lactate levels (>5 mmol/L), decreased blood pH, electrolyte disturbances with an increased anion gap, and an increased lactate/pyruvate ratio. When metformin is implicated as the cause of lactic acidosis, metformin plasma levels >5 µg/ml are generally found.

The reported incidence of lactic acidosis in patients receiving metformin HCl is very low (approximately 0.03 cases/1000 patient-years, with approximately 0.015 fatal cases/1000 patient-years). Reported cases have occurred primarily in diabetic patients with significant renal insufficiency, including both intrinsic renal disease and renal hypoperfusion, often in the setting of multiple concomitant medical/surgical problems and multiple concomitant medications. Patients with congestive heart failure requiring pharmacologic management, in particular those with unstable or acute congestive heart failure who are at risk of hypoperfusion and hypoxemia, are at increased risk of lactic acidosis. The risk of lactic acidosis increases with the degree of renal dysfunction and the patient's age. The risk of lactic acidosis may, therefore, be significantly decreased by regular monitoring of renal function in patients taking metformin and by use of the minimum effective dose of metformin. In particular, treatment of the elderly should be accompanied by careful monitoring of renal function. Metaglip treatment should not be initiated in patients ≥80 years of age unless measurement of creatinine clearance demonstrates that renal function is not reduced, as these patients are more susceptible to developing lactic acidosis. In addition, Metaglip should be promptly withheld in the presence of any condition associated with hypoxemia, dehydration, or sepsis. Because impaired hepatic function may significantly limit the ability to clear lactate, Metaglip should generally be avoided in patients with clinical or laboratory evidence of hepatic disease. Patients should be cautioned against excessive alcohol intake, either acute or chronic, when taking Metaglip, since alcohol potentiates the effects of metformin HCl on lactate metabolism. In addition, Metaglip should be temporarily discontinued prior to any intravascular radiocontrast study and for any surgical procedure.

The onset of lactic acidosis often is subtle, and accompanied only by nonspecific symptoms such as malaise, myalgias, respiratory distress, increasing somnolence, and nonspecific abdominal distress. There may be associated hypothermia, hypotension, and resistant bradyarrhythmias with more marked acidosis. The patient and the patient's physician must be aware of the possible importance of such symptoms and the patient should be instructed to notify the physician immediately if they occur. Metaglip should be withdrawn until the situation is clarified. Serum electrolytes, ketones, blood glucose, and if indicated, blood pH, lactate levels, and even blood metformin levels may be useful. Once a patient is stabilized on any dose level of Metaglip, gastrointestinal symptoms, which are common during initiation of therapy with metformin, are unlikely to be drug related. Later occurrence of gastrointestinal symptoms could be due to lactic acidosis or other serious disease.

Levels of fasting venous plasma lactate above the upper limit of normal but less than 5 mmol/L in patients taking Metaglip do not necessarily indicate impending lactic acidosis and may be explainable by other mechanisms, such as poorly controlled diabetes or obesity, vigorous physical activity, or technical problems in sample handling.

Lactic acidosis should be suspected in any diabetic patient with metabolic acidosis lacking evidence of ketoacidosis (ketonuria and ketonemia).

Lactic acidosis is a medical emergency that must be treated in a hospital setting. In a patient with lactic acidosis who is taking Metaglip, the drug should be discontinued immediately and general supportive measures promptly instituted. Because metformin HCl is dialyzable (with a clearance of up to 170 ml/min under good hemodynamic conditions), prompt hemodialysis is recommended to correct the acidosis and remove the accumulated metformin. Such management often results in prompt reversal of symptoms and recovery. (See also CONTRAINDICATIONS.)

SPECIAL WARNING ON INCREASED RISK OF CARDIOVASCULAR MORTALITY

The administration of oral hypoglycemic drugs has been reported to be associated with increased cardiovascular mortality as compared to treatment with diet alone or diet plus insulin. This warning is based on the study conducted by the University Group Diabetes Program (UGDP), a long-term prospective clinical trial designed to evaluate the effectiveness of glucose-lowering drugs in preventing or delaying vascular complications in patients with non-insulin-dependent diabetes. The study involved 823 patients who were randomly assigned to 1 of 4 treatment groups (*Diabetes* 19 (Suppl. 2):747-830, 1970).

UGDP reported that patients treated for 5-8 years with diet plus a fixed dose of tolbutamide (1.5 g/day) had a rate of cardiovascular mortality approximately 2½ times that of patients treated with diet alone. A significant increase in total mortality was not observed, but the use of tolbutamide was discontinued based on the increase in cardiovascular mortality, thus limiting the opportunity for the study to show an increase in overall mortality. Despite controversy regarding the interpretation of these results, the findings of the UGDP study provide an adequate basis for this warning. The patient should be informed of the potential risks and benefits of glipizide and of alternative modes of therapy.

Although only one drug in the sulfonylurea class (tolbutamide) was included in this study, it is prudent from a safety standpoint to consider that this warning may also apply to other hypoglycemic drugs in this class, in view of their close similarities in mode of action and chemical structure.

DOSAGE AND ADMINISTRATION

GENERAL CONSIDERATIONS

Dosage of Metaglip must be individualized on the basis of both effectiveness and tolerance while not exceeding the maximum recommended daily dose of 20 mg glipizide/2000 mg metformin. Metaglip should be given with meals and should be initiated at a low dose, with gradual dose escalation as described below, in order to avoid hypoglycemia (largely due to glipizide), to reduce GI side effects (largely due to metformin), and to permit determination of the minimum effective dose for adequate control of blood glucose for the individual patient.

With initial treatment and during dose titration, appropriate blood glucose monitoring should be used to determine the therapeutic response to Metaglip and to identify the minimum effective dose for the patient. Thereafter, HbA_{1c} should be measured at intervals of approximately 3 months to assess the effectiveness of therapy. The therapeutic goal in all patients with Type 2 diabetes is to decrease FPG, PPG, and HbA_{1c} to normal or as near normal as possible. Ideally, the response to therapy should be evaluated using HbA_{1c} (glycosylated hemoglobin), which is a better indicator of long-term glycemic control than FPG alone.

No studies have been performed specifically examining the safety and efficacy of switching to Metaglip therapy in patients taking concomitant glipizide (or other sulfonylurea) plus metformin. Changes in glycemic control may occur in such patients, with either hyperglycemia or hypoglycemia possible. Any change in therapy of Type 2 diabetes should be undertaken with care and appropriate monitoring.

METAGLIP AS INITIAL THERAPY

For patients with Type 2 diabetes whose hyperglycemia cannot be satisfactorily managed with diet and exercise alone, the recommended starting dose of Metaglip is 2.5 mg/250 mg once a day with a meal. For patients whose FPG is 280-320 mg/dl a starting dose of Metaglip 2.5 mg/500 mg twice daily should be considered. The efficacy of Metaglip (glipizide; metformin HCl) tablets in patients whose FPG exceeds 320 mg/dl has not been established. Dosage increases to achieve adequate glycemic control should be made in increments of 1 tablet/day every 2 weeks up to maximum of 10 mg/1000 mg or 10 mg/2000 mg Metaglip per day given in divided doses. In clinical trials of Metaglip as initial therapy, there was no experience with total daily doses greater than 10 mg/2000 mg per/day.

METAGLIP AS SECOND-LINE THERAPY

For patients not adequately controlled on either glipizide (or another sulfonylurea) or metformin alone, the recommended starting dose of Metaglip is 2.5 mg/500 mg or 5 mg/500 mg twice daily with the morning and evening meals. In order to avoid hypoglycemia, the starting dose of Metaglip should not exceed the daily doses of glipizide or metformin already being taken. The daily dose should be titrated in increments of no more than 5 mg/500 mg up to the minimum effective dose to achieve adequate control of blood glucose or to a maximum dose of 20 mg/2000 mg/day.

Patients previously treated with combination therapy of glipizide (or another sulfonylurea) plus metformin may be switched to Metaglip 2.5 mg/500 mg or 5 mg/500 mg; the starting dose should not exceed the daily dose of glipizide (or equivalent dose of another sulfonylurea) and metformin already being taken. The decision to switch to the nearest equivalent dose or to titrate should be based on clinical judgment. Patients should be monitored closely for signs and symptoms of hypoglycemia following such a switch and the dose of Metaglip should be titrated as described above to achieve adequate control of blood glucose.

SPECIFIC PATIENT POPULATIONS

Metaglip is not recommended for use during pregnancy or for use in pediatric patients. The initial and maintenance dosing of Metaglip should be conservative in patients with advanced age, due to the potential for decreased renal function in this population. Any dosage adjustment requires a careful assessment of renal function. Generally, elderly, debilitated, and malnourished patients should not be titrated to the maximum dose of Metaglip to avoid the risk of hypoglycemia. Monitoring of renal function is necessary to aid in prevention of metformin-associated lactic acidosis, particularly in the elderly. (See WARNINGS.)

PRODUCT LISTING - EQUIVALENTS NOT AVAILABLE

Tablet - Oral - 2.5 mg;250 mg
100's $82.13 METAGLIP, Bristol-Myers Squibb 00087-6081-31
Tablet - Oral - 2.5 mg;500 mg
100's $97.96 METAGLIP, Bristol-Myers Squibb 00087-6077-31
Tablet - Oral - 5 mg;500 mg
100's $97.96 METAGLIP, Bristol-Myers Squibb 00087-6078-31

Glucagon (rDNA origin) (003432)

For complete prescribing information, refer to the CD-ROM included with the book.

Categories: Hypoglycemia; Imaging, colon, adjunct; Imaging, duodenum, adjunct; Imaging, small bowel, adjunct; Imaging, stomach, adjunct; Pregnancy Category B
Drug Classes: Antihypoglycemics; Hormones/hormone modifiers
Brand Names: Glucagon
Foreign Brand Availability: Glucagen (Australia; China; Colombia; Denmark; Greece; New-Zealand; Switzerland); Glucagen Novo (Hong-Kong); GlucaGen (Israel; Singapore)

G

DESCRIPTION

Glucagon for injection (rDNA origin) is a polypeptide hormone identical to human glucagon that increases blood glucose and relaxes smooth muscle of the gastrointestinal tract. Glucagon is synthesized in a special non-pathogenic laboratory strain of *Escherichia coli* bacteria that has been genetically altered by the addition of the gene for glucagon.

Glucagon is a single-chain polypeptide that contains 29 amino acid residues and has a molecular weight of 3483.

The empirical formula is $C_{153}H_{225}N_{43}O_{49}S$.

Crystalline glucagon is a white to off-white powder. It is relatively insoluble in water but is soluble at a pH of less than 3 or more than 9.5.

Glucagon is available for use intravenously, intramuscularly, or subcutaneously in a kit that contains a vial of sterile glucagon and a syringe of sterile diluent. The vial contains 1 mg (1 unit) of glucagon and 49 mg of lactose. Hydrochloric acid may have been added during manufacture to adjust the pH of the glucagon. One International Unit of glucagon is equivalent to 1 mg of glucagon.[1] The diluent syringe contains 12 mg/ml of glycerin, water for injection, and hydrochloric acid.

INDICATIONS AND USAGE

FOR THE TREATMENT OF HYPOGLYCEMIA

Glucagon is indicated as a treatment for severe hypoglycemia.

Because patients with Type 1 diabetes may have less of an increase in blood glucose levels compared with a stable Type 2 patient, supplementary carbohydrate should be given as soon as possible, especially to a pediatric patient.

FOR USE AS A DIAGNOSTIC AID

Glucagon is indicated as a diagnostic aid in the radiologic examination of the stomach, duodenum, small bowel, and colon when diminished intestinal motility would be advantageous.

Glucagon is as effective for this examination as are the anticholinergic drugs. However, the addition of the anticholinergic agent may result in increased side effects.

CONTRAINDICATIONS

Glucagon is contraindicated in patients with known hypersensitivity to it or in patients with known pheochromocytoma.

WARNINGS

Glucagon should be administered cautiously to patients with a history suggestive of insulinoma, pheochromocytoma, or both. In patients with insulinoma, intravenous administration of glucagon may produce an initial increase in blood glucose; however, because of glucagon's hyperglycemic effect the insulinoma may release insulin and cause subsequent hypoglycemia. A patient developing symptoms of hypoglycemia after a dose of glucagon should be given glucose orally, intravenously, or by gavage, whichever is most appropriate.

Exogenous glucagon also stimulates the release of catecholamines. In the presence of pheochromocytoma, glucagon can cause the tumor to release catecholamines, which may result in a sudden and marked increase in blood pressure. If a patient develops a sudden increase in blood pressure, 5-10 mg of phentolamine mesylate may be administered intravenously in an attempt to control the blood pressure.

Generalized allergic reactions, including urticaria, respiratory distress, and hypotension, have been reported in patients who received glucagon by injection.

DOSAGE AND ADMINISTRATION

GENERAL INSTRUCTIONS FOR USE

- The diluent is provided for use only in the preparation of glucagon for parenteral injection and for no other use.
- Glucagon should not be used at concentrations greater than 1 mg/ml (1 unit/ml).
- Reconstituted glucagon should be used immediately. **Discard any unused portion.**
- Reconstituted glucagon solutions should be used only if they are clear and of a water-like consistency.
- Parenteral drug products should be inspected visually for particulate matter and discoloration prior to administration.

DIRECTIONS FOR TREATMENT OF SEVERE HYPOGLYCEMIA

Severe hypoglycemia should be treated initially with intravenous glucose, if possible.

- If parenteral glucose can not be used, dissolve the lyophilized glucagon using the accompanying diluting solution and use immediately.
- For adults and for pediatric patients weighing more than 44 lb (20 kg), give 1 mg (1 unit) by subcutaneous, intramuscular, or intravenous injection.
- For pediatric patients weighing less than 44 lb (20 kg), give 0.5 mg (0.5 unit) or a dose equivalent to 20-30 μg/kg.[2-6]
- **Discard any unused portion.**
- An unconscious patient will usually awaken within 15 minutes following the glucagon injection. If the response is delayed, there is no contraindication to the administration of an additional dose of glucagon; however, in view of the deleterious effects of cerebral hypoglycemia, emergency aid should be sought so that parenteral glucose can be given.
- After the patient responds, supplemental carbohydrate should be given to restore liver glycogen and to prevent secondary hypoglycemia.

DIRECTIONS FOR USE AS A DIAGNOSTIC AID

Dissolve the lyophilized glucagon using the accompanying diluting solution and use immediately. **Discard any unused portion.**

The doses in TABLE 1 may be administered for relaxation of the stomach, duodenum, and small bowel, depending on the onset and duration of effect required for the examination. Since the stomach is less sensitive to the effect of glucagon, 0.5 mg (0.5 units) IV or 2 mg (2 units) IM are recommended.

TABLE 1

Dose	Route of Administration	Time of Onset of Action	Approximate Duration of Effect
0.25-0.5 mg (0.25-0.5 units)	IV	1 minute	9-17 minutes
1 mg (1 unit)	IM	8-10 minutes	12-27 minutes
2 mg*(2 units)	IV	1 minute	22-25 minutes
2 mg*(2 units)	IM	4-7 minutes	21-32 minutes

* Administration of 2 mg (2 units) doses produces a higher incidence of nausea and vomiting than do lower doses.

For examination of the colon, it is recommended that a 2 mg (2 units) dose be administered intramuscularly approximately 10 minutes prior to the procedure. Colon relaxation and reduction of patient discomfort may allow the radiologist to perform a more satisfactory examination.

PRODUCT LISTING - RATED THERAPEUTICALLY EQUIVALENT

Powder For Injection - Injectable - Recombinant 1 mg
1's $78.13 GENERIC, Lilly, Eli and Company 00002-8031-01
1's $78.13 GENERIC, Lilly, Eli and Company 00002-8085-01

PRODUCT LISTING - EQUIVALENTS NOT AVAILABLE

Powder For Injection - Injectable - Recombinant 1 mg
1's $71.39 GENERIC, Bedford Laboratories 55390-0004-01
10's $743.63 GENERIC, Bedford Laboratories 55390-0004-10

Glyburide

(001368)

For related information, see the comparative table section in Appendix A.

Categories: Diabetes mellitus; Pregnancy Category C; FDA Approved 1984 May; WHO Formulary
Drug Classes: Antidiabetic agents; Sulfonylureas, second generation
Brand Names: Diabeta; Glynase; **Micronase**
Foreign Brand Availability: Apo-Glibenclamide (New-Zealand); Benclamin (Thailand); Betanase (Bahrain; Cyprus; Egypt; Iran; Iraq; Israel; Jordan; Kuwait; Lebanon; Libya; Oman; Qatar; Republic-of-Yemen; Saudi-Arabia; Syria; United-Arab-Emirates); Betanese 5 (Benin; Burkina-Faso; Ethiopia; Gambia; Ghana; Guinea; Ivory-Coast; Kenya; Liberia; Malawi; Mali; Mauritania; Mauritius; Morocco; Niger; Nigeria; Senegal; Seychelles; Sierra-Leone; South-Africa; Sudan; Tanzania; Tunia; Uganda; Zambia; Zimbabwe); Calabren (Czech-Republic); Clamide (Hong-Kong); Cytagon (Thailand); Daonil (Argentina; Australia; Bahamas; Bahrain; Barbados; Belgium; Belize; Benin; Bermuda; Burkina-Faso; CIS; Costa-Rica; Curacao; Cyprus; Dominican-Republic; Ecuador; Egypt; El-Salvador; England; Ethiopia; France; Gambia; Ghana; Greece; Guatemala; Guinea; Guyana; Honduras; Hong-Kong; India; Indonesia; Iran; Iraq; Israel; Italy; Ivory-Coast; Jamaica; Japan; Jordan; Kenya; Korea; Kuwait; Lebanon; Liberia; Libya; Malawi; Malaysia; Mali; Mauritania; Mauritius; Mexico; Morocco; Netherland-Antilles; Netherlands; New-Zealand; Nicaragua; Niger; Nigeria; Oman; Panama; Peru; Philippines; Puerto-Rico; Qatar; Republic-of-Yemen; Russia; Saudi-Arabia; Senegal; Seychelles; Sierra-Leone; South-Africa; Spain; Sudan; Surinam; Switzerland; Syria; Taiwan; Tanzania; Thailand; Trinidad; Tunia; Uganda; United-Arab-Emirates; Zambia; Zimbabwe); Daono (Thailand); Debtan (Thailand); Diaben (Bahrain; Cyprus; Egypt; Iran; Iraq; Israel; Jordan; Kuwait; Lebanon; Libya; Oman; Qatar; Republic-of-Yemen; Saudi-Arabia; Syria; United-Arab-Emirates); Diabet (Korea); Dibelet (Malaysia; Thailand); Euglucan (France); Euglucon (Argentina; Australia; Austria; Bahamas; Bahrain; Barbados; Belgium; Belize; Benin; Bermuda; Burkina-Faso; Canada; CIS; Colombia; Curacao; Cyprus; Czech-Republic; Ecuador; Egypt; England; Ethiopia; Gambia; Germany; Ghana; Greece; Guinea; Guyana; Hong-Kong; India; Indonesia; Iran; Iraq; Israel; Italy; Ivory-Coast; Jamaica; Japan; Jordan; Kenya; Korea; Kuwait; Lebanon; Liberia; Libya; Malawi; Malaysia; Mali; Mauritania; Mauritius; Mexico; Morocco; Netherland-Antilles; Netherlands; New-Zealand; Niger; Nigeria; Oman; Peru; Philippines; Puerto-Rico; Qatar; Republic-of-Yemen; Russia; Saudi-Arabia; Senegal; Seychelles; Sierra-Leone; South-Africa; Spain; Sudan; Surinam; Switzerland; Syria; Taiwan; Tanzania; Thailand; Trinidad; Tunia; Uganda; United-Arab-Emirates; Zambia; Zimbabwe); G.B.N. (Singapore); Gilemal (Austria; Bulgaria; China; Hungary); Glencamide (Thailand); Gliban (Bahrain; Cyprus; Egypt; Iran; Iraq; Israel; Jordan; Kuwait; Lebanon; Libya; Oman; Qatar; Republic-of-Yemen; Saudi-Arabia; Syria; United-Arab-Emirates); Glibemid (Singapore); Gliben (Hong-Kong; Italy; New-Zealand; Taiwan); Glibenhexal (China); Glibenil (Mexico); Glibens (Colombia); Glibesyn (Malaysia); Glibet (India); Glibetic (Israel); Glibil (Bahrain; Cyprus; Egypt; Iran; Iraq; Israel; Jordan; Kuwait; Lebanon; Libya; Oman; Qatar; Republic-of-Yemen; Saudi-Arabia; Syria; United-Arab-Emirates); Gliboral (Benin; Burkina-Faso; Ethiopia; Gambia; Ghana; Guinea; Ivory-Coast; Kenya; Liberia; Malawi; Mali; Mauritania; Mauritius; Morocco; Niger; Nigeria; Senegal; Seychelles; Sierra-Leone; South-Africa; Sudan; Tanzania; Tunia; Uganda; Zambia; Zimbabwe); Glicem (Ecuador); Glidiabet (Peru); Glikeyer (Mexico); Glimel (Australia; Hong-Kong; New-Zealand); Glimide (Malaysia); Glisulin (Korea); Glitisol (Bahamas; Barbados; Belize; Bermuda; Curacao; Guyana; Jamaica; Netherland-Antilles; Puerto-Rico; Surinam; Taiwan; Trinidad); Gluben (Israel); Glucal (Mexico); Glucolon (Spain); Glucomid (Benin; Burkina-Faso; Ethiopia; Gambia; Ghana; Guinea; Ivory-Coast; Kenya; Liberia; Malawi; Mali; Mauritania; Mauritius; Morocco; Niger; Nigeria; Senegal; Seychelles; Sierra-Leone; Sudan; Tanzania; Tunia; Uganda; Zambia; Zimbabwe); Gluconic (Indonesia); Glyben (South-Africa); Glycomin (South-Africa); Hemi-Daonil (Argentina; France; Morocco; Netherlands); Humedia (Germany); Locose (Thailand); Lodulce (Philippines); Manoglucon (Thailand); Med-Glionil (Thailand); Melix (Bahamas; Bahrain; Barbados; Belize; Benin; Bermuda; Burkina-Faso; Curacao; Cyprus; Egypt; Ethiopia; Gambia; Ghana; Guinea; Guyana; Iran; Iraq; Israel; Ivory-Coast; Jamaica; Jordan; Kenya; Kuwait; Lebanon; Liberia; Libya; Malawi; Mali; Mauritania; Mauritius; Morocco; Netherland-Antilles; Niger; Nigeria; Oman; Puerto-Rico; Qatar; Republic-of-Yemen; Saudi-Arabia; Senegal; Seychelles; Sierra-Leone; South-Africa; Sudan; Surinam; Syria; Tanzania; Trinidad; Tunia; Uganda; United-Arab-Emirates; Zambia; Zimbabwe); Miglucan (France); Norboral (Mexico); Orabetic (Philippines); Pira (Argentina); Prodiabet (Indonesia); Renabetic (Indonesia); Semi-Daonil (Argentina; Australia; Bahrain; Cyprus; Egypt; England; Hong-Kong; Indonesia; Iran; Iraq; Ireland; Israel; Jordan; Kuwait; Lebanon; Libya; Morocco; Oman; Qatar; Republic-of-Yemen; Saudi-Arabia; Switzerland; Syria; United-Arab-Emirates); Semi-Euglucon (Argentina; Australia; Austria; Hong-Kong; India; Indonesia; Netherlands; New-Zealand; Philippines; Switzerland; Thailand); Sugril (Thailand); Suraben (Korea); Tiabet (Indonesia); Xeltic (Hong-Kong)
Cost of Therapy: $30.27 (Diabetes Mellitus; Micronase; 5 mg; 1 tablet/day; 30 day supply)
$23.29 (Diabetes Mellitus; DiaBeta; 5 mg; 1 tablet/day; 30 day supply)
$10.32 (Diabetes Mellitus; Generic Tablets; 5 mg; 1 tablet/day; 30 day supply)
$29.50 (Diabetes Mellitus; Glynase Pres-Tab Micronized; 3 mg; 1 tablet/day; 30 day supply)
$18.06 (Diabetes Mellitus; Generic Micronized; 3 mg; 1 tablet/day; 30 day supply)

DESCRIPTION

MICRONASE TABLETS (STANDARD GLYBURIDE)

Micronase tablets contain glyburide, which is an oral blood-glucose-lowering drug of the sulfonylurea class. Glyburide is a white, crystalline compound, formulated as Micronase tablets of 1.25, 2.5, and 5 mg strengths for oral administration. *Inactive Ingredients:* Colloidal silicon dioxide, dibasic calcium phosphate, magnesium stearate, microcrystalline cellulose, sodium alginate, talc. In addition, the **2.5 mg** contains aluminum oxide and FD&C red no. 40 and the **5 mg** contains aluminum oxide and FD&C blue no. 1. The chemical name for glyburide is 1-[[p-[2-(5-chloro-o-anisamido)-ethyl]phenyl]-sulfonyl]-3-cyclohexylurea and the molecular weight is 493.99.

GLYNASE PRESTAB TABLETS (MICRONIZED GLYBURIDE)

Glynase PresTab tablets contain micronized (smaller particle size) glyburide, which is an oral blood-glucose-lowering drug of the sulfonylurea class. Glyburide is a white, crystalline compound, formulated as Glynase Prestab tablets of 1.5, 3, and 6 mg strengths for oral administration. *Inactive Ingredients:* Colloidal silicon dioxide, corn starch, lactose, magnesium stearate. In addition the **3 mg** strength contains FD&C blue no. 1 aluminum lake, and the **6 mg** tablet contains D&C yellow no. 10 aluminum lake. The chemical name for glyburide is 1-[[p-[2-(5-chloro-o-anisamido)ethyl]phenyl]-sulfonyl]-3-cyclohexylurea and the molecular weight is 493.99.

CLINICAL PHARMACOLOGY

MECHANISM OF ACTION

Glyburide appears to lower the blood glucose acutely by stimulating the release of insulin from the pancreas, an effect dependent upon functioning beta cells in the pancreatic islets. The mechanism by which glyburide lowers blood glucose during long-term administration has not been clearly established. With chronic administration in Type II diabetic patients, the blood glucose lowering effect persists despite a gradual decline in the insulin secretory response to the drug. Extrapancreatic effects may be involved in the mechanism of action of oral sulfonylurea hypoglycemic drugs. The combination of glyburide and metformin may have a synergistic effect, since both agents act to improve glucose tolerance by different but complementary mechanisms.

Some patients who are initially responsive to oral hypoglycemic drugs, including glyburide, may become unresponsive or poorly responsive over time. Alternatively, glyburide may be effective in some patients who have become unresponsive to one or more other sulfonylurea drugs.

In addition to its blood glucose lowering actions, glyburide produces a mild diuresis by enhancement of renal free water clearance. Disulfiram-like reactions have very rarely been reported in patients treated with glyburide.

PHARMACOKINETICS

Single dose studies with glyburide tablets in normal subjects demonstrate significant absorption of glyburide within 1 hour, peak drug levels at about 4 hours (2-3 hours for micronized glyburide), and low but detectable levels at 24 hours. Mean serum levels of glyburide, as reflected by areas under the serum concentration-time curve, increase in proportion to corresponding increases in dose. Multiple dose studies with glyburide in diabetic patients demonstrate drug level concentration-time curves similar to single dose studies, indicating no buildup of drug in tissue depots. The decrease of standard glyburide in the serum of normal healthy individuals is biphasic; the terminal half-life is about 10 hours. In single dose studies in fasting normal subjects who were administered standard glyburide, the degree and duration of blood glucose lowering is proportional to the dose administered and to the area under the drug level concentration-time curve. The blood glucose lowering effect persists for 24 hours following single morning doses in nonfasting diabetic patients. Under conditions of repeated administration in diabetic patients, however, there is no reliable correlation between blood drug levels and fasting blood glucose levels. A 1 year study of diabetic patients treated with glyburide showed no reliable correlation between administered dose and serum drug level.

The major metabolite of glyburide is the 4-trans-hydroxy derivative. A second metabolite, the 3-cis-hydroxy derivative, also occurs. These metabolites probably contribute no significant hypoglycemic action in humans since they are only weakly active (1/400th and 1/40th as active, respectively, as glyburide) in rabbits.

Glyburide is excreted as metabolites in the bile and urine, approximately 50% by each route. This dual excretory pathway is qualitatively different from that of other sulfonylureas, which are excreted primarily in the urine.

Sulfonylurea drugs are extensively bound to serum proteins. Displacement from protein binding sites by other drugs may lead to enhanced hypoglycemic action. *In vitro*, the protein binding exhibited by glyburide is predominantly non-ionic, whereas that of other sulfonylureas (chlorpropamide, tolbutamide, tolazamide) is predominantly ionic. Acidic drugs such as phenylbutazone, warfarin, and salicylates displace the ionic-binding sulfonylureas from serum proteins to a far greater extent than the non-ionic binding glyburide. It has not been shown that this difference in protein binding will result in fewer drug-drug interactions with glyburide tablets in clinical use.

Additional Information for Micronized Glyburide Tablets

Bioavailability studies have demonstrated that micronized glyburide tablets 3 mg provide serum glyburide concentrations that are not bioequivalent to those from standard glyburide tablets 5 mg. Therefore, the patient should be retitrated.

In a single-dose bioavailability study in which subjects received micronized glyburide tablets 3 mg and standard glyburide tablets 5 mg with breakfast, the peak of the mean serum glyburide concentration-time curve was 97.2 ng/ml for micronized glyburide tablets 3 mg and 87.5 ng/ml for standard glyburide tablets 5 mg. The mean of the individual maximum serum concentration values of glyburide (C_{max}) from micronized glyburide tablets 3 mg was 106 ng/ml and that from standard glyburide tablets 5 mg was 104 ng/ml. The mean glyburide area under the serum concentration time curve (AUC) for this study was 568 ng × hr/ml for micronized glyburide tablets 3 mg and 746 ng × hr/ml for standard glyburide tablets 5 mg.

In a steady-state study in diabetic patients receiving micronized glyburide tablets 6 mg once daily or micronized glyburide tablets 3 mg twice daily, no difference was seen between the two dosage regimens in average 24 hour glyburide concentrations following 2 weeks of dosing. The once-daily and twice-daily regimens provided equivalent glucose control as measured by fasting plasma glucose levels, 4 hour postprandial glucose AUC values, and 24 hour glucose AUC values. Insulin AUC response over the 24 hour period was not different for the two regimens. There were differences in insulin response between the regimens for the breakfast and supper 4 hour postprandial periods, but these did not translate into differences in glucose control.

The serum concentration of glyburide in normal subjects decreased with a half-life of about 4 hours.

INDICATIONS AND USAGE

Glyburide tablets are indicated as an adjunct to diet to lower the blood glucose in patients with non-insulin-dependent diabetes mellitus (Type II) whose hyperglycemia cannot be satisfactorily controlled by diet alone.

Glyburide may be used concomitantly with metformin when diet and glyburide or diet and metformin alone do not result in adequate glycemic control (see the metformin prescribing information).

In initiating treatment for non-insulin-dependent diabetes, diet should be emphasized as the primary form of treatment. Caloric restriction and weight loss are essential in the obese diabetic patient. Proper dietary management alone may be effective in controlling the blood glucose and symptoms of hyperglycemia. The importance of regular physical activity should also be stressed, and cardiovascular risk factors should be identified and corrective measures taken where possible. If this treatment program fails to reduce symptoms and/or blood glucose, the use of an oral sulfonylurea or insulin should be considered. Use of glyburide must be viewed by both the physician and patient as a treatment in addition to diet and not as a substitution or as a convenient mechanism for avoiding dietary restraint. Furthermore, loss of blood glucose control on diet alone may be transient, thus requiring only short-term administration of glyburide.

During maintenance programs, glyburide should be discontinued if satisfactory lowering of blood glucose is no longer achieved. Judgment should be based on regular clinical and laboratory evaluations.

In considering the use of glyburide in asymptomatic patients, it should be recognized that controlling blood glucose in non-insulin-dependent diabetes has not been definitely established to be effective in preventing the long-term cardiovascular or neural complications of diabetes.

G

CONTRAINDICATIONS

Glyburide tablets are contraindicated in patients with:

1. Known hypersensitivity or allergy to the drug.
2. Diabetic ketoacidosis, with or without coma. This condition should be treated with insulin.
3. Type I diabetes mellitus, as sole therapy.

WARNINGS

SPECIAL WARNING ON INCREASED RISK OF CARDIOVASCULAR MORTALITY: The administration of oral hypoglycemic drugs has been reported to be associated with increased cardiovascular mortality as compared to treatment with diet alone or diet plus insulin. This warning is based on the study conducted by the University Group Diabetes Program (UGDP), a long-term prospective clinical trial designed to evaluate the effectiveness of glucose-lowering drugs in preventing or delaying vascular complications in patients with non-insulin-dependent diabetes. The study involved 823 patients who were randomly assigned to one of four treatment groups.[1]

UGDP reported that patients treated for 5-8 years with diet plus a fixed dose of tolbutamide (1.5 g/day) had a rate of cardiovascular mortality approximately 2½ times that of patients treated with diet alone. A significant increase in total mortality was not observed, but the use of tolbutamide was discontinued based on the increase in cardiovascular mortality, thus limiting the opportunity for the study to show an increase in overall mortality. Despite controversy regarding the interpretation of these results, the findings of the UGDP study provide an adequate basis for this warning. The patient should be informed of the potential risks and advantages of glyburide and of alternative modes of therapy.

Although only one drug in the sulfonylurea class (tolbutamide) was included in this study, it is prudent from a safety standpoint to consider that this warning may also apply to other oral hypoglycemic drugs in this class, in view of their close similarities in mode of action and chemical structure.

G

PRECAUTIONS

GENERAL

Hypoglycemia

All sulfonylureas are capable of producing severe hypoglycemia. Proper patient selection and dosage and instructions are important to avoid hypoglycemic episodes. Renal or hepatic insufficiency may cause elevated drug levels of glyburide and the latter may also diminish gluconeogenic capacity, both of which increase the risk of serious hypoglycemic reactions. Elderly, debilitated or malnourished patients, and those with adrenal or pituitary insufficiency, are particularly susceptible to the hypoglycemic action of glucose-lowering drugs. Hypoglycemia may be difficult to recognize in the elderly and in people who are taking beta-adrenergic blocking drugs. Hypoglycemia is more likely to occur when caloric intake is deficient, after severe or prolonged exercise, when alcohol is ingested, or when more than one glucose lowering drug is used. The risk of hypoglycemia may be increased with combination therapy.

Loss of Control of Blood Glucose

When a patient stabilized on any diabetic regimen is exposed to stress such as fever, trauma, infection or surgery, a loss of control may occur. At such times it may be necessary to discontinue glyburide and administer insulin.

The effectiveness of any hypoglycemic drug, including glyburide, in lowering blood glucose to a desired level decreases in many patients over a period of time which may be due to progression of the severity of diabetes or to diminished responsiveness to the drug. This phenomenon is known as secondary failure, to distinguish it from primary failure in which the drug is ineffective in an individual patient when glyburide is first given. Adequate adjustment of dose and adherence to diet should be assessed before classifying a patient as a secondary failure.

INFORMATION FOR THE PATIENT

Patients should be informed of the potential risks and advantages of glyburide and of alternative modes of therapy. They also should be informed about the importance of adherence to dietary instructions, of a regular exercise program, and of regular testing of urine and/or blood glucose.

The risks of hypoglycemia, its symptoms and treatment, and conditions that predispose to its development should be explained to patients and responsible family members. Primary and secondary failure also should be explained.

LABORATORY TESTS

Therapeutic response to glyburide tablets should be monitored by frequent urine glucose tests and periodic blood glucose tests. Measurement of glycosylated hemoglobin levels may be helpful in some patients.

CARCINOGENESIS, MUTAGENESIS, AND IMPAIRMENT OF FERTILITY

Studies in rats at doses up to 300 mg/kg/day for 18 months showed no carcinogenic effects. Glyburide is nonmutagenic when studied in the Salmonella microsome test (Ames test) and in the DNA damage/alkaline elution assay. No drug related effects were noted in any of the criteria evaluated in the 2 year oncogenicity study of glyburide in mice.

PREGNANCY, TERATOGENIC EFFECTS, PREGNANCY CATEGORY B

Reproduction studies have been performed in rats and rabbits at doses up to 500 times the human dose and have revealed no evidence of impaired fertility or harm to the fetus due to glyburide. There are, however, no adequate and well-controlled studies in pregnant women. Because animal reproduction studies are not always predictive of human response, this drug should be used during pregnancy only if clearly needed.

Because recent information suggests that abnormal blood glucose levels during pregnancy are associated with a higher incidence of congenital abnormalities, many experts recommend that insulin be used during pregnancy to maintain blood glucose as close to normal as possible.

Nonteratogenic Effects: Prolonged severe hypoglycemia (4-10 days) has been reported in neonates born to mothers who were receiving a sulfonylurea drug at the time of delivery. This has been reported more frequently with the use of agents with prolonged half-lives. If glyburide is used during pregnancy, it should be discontinued at least 2 weeks before the expected delivery date.

NURSING MOTHERS

Although it is not known whether glyburide is excreted in human milk, some sulfonylurea drugs are known to be excreted in human milk. Because the potential for hypoglycemia in nursing infants may exist, a decision should be made whether to discontinue nursing or to discontinue the drug, taking into account the importance of the drug to the mother. If the drug is discontinued, and if diet alone is inadequate for controlling blood glucose, insulin therapy should be considered.

PEDIATRIC USE

Safety and effectiveness in pediatric patients have not been established.

ADDITIONAL INFORMATION FOR MICRONIZED GLYBURIDE

Bioavailability studies have demonstrated that micronized glyburide tablets 3 mg provide serum glyburide concentrations that are not bioequivalent to those from glyburide tablets 5 mg. Therefore, patients should be retitrated when transferred from glyburide or other oral hypoglycemic agents.

DRUG INTERACTIONS

The hypoglycemic action of sulfonylureas may be potentiated by certain drugs including nonsteroidal anti-inflammatory agents and other drugs that are highly protein bound, salicylates, sulfonamides, chloramphenicol, probenecid, coumarins, monoamine oxidase inhibitors, and beta adrenergic blocking agents. When such drugs are administered to a patient receiving glyburide, the patient should be observed closely for hypoglycemia. When such drugs are withdrawn from a patient receiving glyburide, the patient should be observed closely for loss of control.

Certain drugs tend to produce hyperglycemia and may lead to loss of control. These drugs include the thiazides and other diuretics, corticosteroids, phenothiazines, thyroid products, estrogens, oral contraceptives, phenytoin, nicotinic acid, sympathomimetics, calcium channel blocking drugs, and isoniazid. When such drugs are administered to a patient receiving glyburide, the patient should be closely observed for loss of control. When such drugs are withdrawn from a patient receiving glyburide, the patient should be observed closely for hypoglycemia.

A possible interaction between glyburide and ciprofloxacin, a fluoroquinolone antibiotic, has been reported, resulting in a potentiation of the hypoglycemic action of glyburide. The mechanism of action for this interaction is not known.

A potential interaction between oral miconazole and oral hypoglycemic agents leading to severe hypoglycemia has been reported. Whether this interaction also occurs with the intravenous, topical or vaginal preparations of miconazole is not known.

Metformin: In a single-dose interaction study in NIDDM subjects, decreases in glyburide AUC and C_{max} were observed, but were highly variable. The single-dose nature of this study and the lack of correlation between glyburide blood levels and pharmacodynamic effects, makes the clinical significance of this interaction uncertain. Coadministration of glyburide and metformin did not result in any changes in either metformin pharmacokinetics or pharmacodynamics.

ADVERSE REACTIONS

HYPOGLYCEMIA

See PRECAUTIONS.

GASTROINTESTINAL REACTIONS

Cholestatic jaundice and hepatitis may occur rarely; glyburide should be discontinued if this occurs.

Liver function abnormalities, including isolated transaminase elevations, have been reported.

Gastrointestinal disturbances (*e.g.*, nausea, epigastric fullness, and heartburn) are the most common reactions, having occurred in 1.8% of treated patients during clinical trials. They tend to be dose related and may disappear when dosage is reduced.

DERMATOLOGIC REACTIONS

Allergic skin reactions (*e.g.*, pruritus, erythema, urticaria, and morbilliform or maculopapular eruptions) occurred in 1.5% of treated patients during clinical trials. These may be transient and may disappear despite continued use of glyburide: If skin reactions persist, the drug should be discontinued.

Porphyria cutanea tarda and photosensitivity reactions have been reported with sulfonylureas.

HEMATOLOGIC REACTIONS

Leukopenia, agranulocytosis, thrombocytopenia, hemolytic anemia, aplastic anemia, and pancytopenia have been reported with sulfonylureas.

METABOLIC REACTIONS

Hepatic porphyria and disulfiram-like reactions have been reported with sulfonylureas; however, hepatic porphyria has not been reported with glyburide and disulfiram-like reactions have been reported very rarely.

Cases of hyponatremia have been reported with glyburide and all other sulfonylureas, most often in patients who are on other medications or have medical conditions known to cause hyponatremia or increase release of antidiuretic hormone. The syndrome of inappropriate antidiuretic hormone (SIADH) secretion has been reported with certain other sulfonylureas, and it has been suggested that these sulfonylureas may augment the peripheral (antidiuretic) action of ADH and/or increase release of ADH.

OTHER REACTIONS
Changes in accommodation and/or blurred vision have been reported with glyburide and other sulfonylureas. These are thought to be related to fluctuation in glucose levels.
In addition to dermatologic reactions, allergic reactions such as angioedema, arthralgia, myalgia, and vasculitis have been reported.

DOSAGE AND ADMINISTRATION

Patients should be retitrated when transferred from standard glyburide tablets or other oral hypoglycemic agents to glyburide micronized tablets.
There is no fixed dosage regimen for the management of diabetes mellitus with glyburide or any other hypoglycemic agent. In addition to the usual monitoring of urinary glucose, the patient's blood glucose must also be monitored periodically to determine the minimum effective dose for the patient; to detect primary failure (*i.e.,* inadequate lowering of blood glucose at the maximum recommended dose of medication); and to detect secondary failure (*i.e.,* loss of adequate blood glucose lowering response after an initial period of effectiveness). Glycosylated hemoglobin levels may also be of value in monitoring the patient's response to therapy.
Short-term administration of glyburide may be sufficient during periods of transient loss of control in patients usually controlled well on diet.

USUAL STARTING DOSE
The usual starting dose of standard glyburide tablets is 2.5-5 mg daily (micronized glyburide tablets: 1.5-3 mg daily), administered with breakfast or the first main meal. Those patients who may be more sensitive to hypoglycemic drugs should be started at 1.25 mg of standard glyburide daily (0.75 mg for micronized glyburide daily). (See PRECAUTIONS for patients at increased risk.) Failure to follow an appropriate dosage regimen may precipitate hypoglycemia. Patients who do not adhere to their prescribed dietary and drug regimen are more prone to exhibit unsatisfactory response to therapy.

TRANSFER FROM OTHER HYPOGLYCEMIC THERAPY; PATIENTS RECEIVING OTHER ORAL ANTIDIABETIC THERAPY
Standard Glyburide
Transfer of patients from other oral antidiabetic regimens to standard glyburide should be done conservatively and the initial daily dose should be 2.5-5 mg. When transferring patients from oral hypoglycemic agents other than chlorpropamide to standard glyburide, no transition period and no initial or priming dose are necessary. When transferring patients from chlorpropamide, particular care should be exercised during the first 2 weeks because the prolonged retention of chlorpropamide in the body and subsequent overlapping drug effects may provoke hypoglycemia.

Micronized Glyburide
Patients should be re-titrated when transferring from standard glyburide or other oral hypoglycemic agents. The initial daily dose should be 1.5-3 mg. When transferring patients from oral hypoglycemic agents other than chlorpropamide to micronized glyburide, no transition period and no initial or priming dose are necessary. When transferring patients from chlorpropamide, particular care should be exercised during the first 2 weeks because the prolonged retention of chlorpropamide in the body and subsequent overlapping drug effects may provoke hypoglycemia.

PATIENTS RECEIVING INSULIN
Some Type II diabetic patients being treated with insulin may respond satisfactorily to glyburide. If the insulin dose is less than 20 units daily, substitution of standard glyburide tablets 2.5-5 mg (micronized glyburide tablets 1.5-3 mg) as a single daily dose may be tried. If the insulin dose is between 20 and 40 units daily, the patient may be placed directly on standard glyburide tablets 5 mg (micronized glyburide tablets 3 mg) daily as a single dose. If the insulin dose is more than 40 units daily, a transition period is required for conversion to glyburide. In these patients, insulin dosage is decreased by 50% and standard glyburide tablets 5 mg daily (micronized glyburide tablets 3 mg daily) is started. Please refer to Titration to Maintenance Dose for further explanation.

TITRATION TO MAINTENANCE DOSE
Standard Glyburide
The usual maintenance dose is in the range of 1.25-20 mg daily, which may be given as a single dose or in divided doses (see Dosage Interval). Dosage increases should be made in increments of no more than 2.5 mg at weekly intervals based upon the patient's blood glucose response.
No exact dosage relationship exists between standard glyburide and the other oral hypoglycemic agents. Although patients may be transferred from the maximum dose of other sulfonylureas, the maximum starting dose of 5 mg of standard glyburide tablets should be observed. A maintenance dose of 5 mg of standard glyburide tablets provides approximately the same degree of blood glucose control as 250-375 mg chlorpropamide, 250-375 mg tolazamide, 500-750 mg acetohexamide, or 1000-1500 mg tolbutamide.
When transferring patients receiving more than 40 units of insulin daily, they may be started on a daily dose of standard glyburide tablets 5 mg concomitantly with a 50% reduction in insulin dose. Progressive withdrawal of insulin and increase of standard glyburide in increments of 1.25-2.5 mg every 2-10 days is then carried out. During this conversion period when both insulin and standard glyburide are being used, hypoglycemia may rarely occur. During insulin withdrawal, patients should test their urine for glucose and acetone at least 3 times daily and report results to their physician. The appearance of persistent acetonuria with glycosuria indicates that the patient is a Type I diabetic who requires insulin therapy.

Micronized Glyburide
The usual maintenance dose is in the range of 0.75-12 mg daily, which may be given as a single dose or in divided doses (see Dosage Interval). Dosage increases should be made in increments of no more than 1.5 mg at weekly intervals based upon the patient's blood glucose response.
No exact dosage relationship exists between micronized glyburide and the other oral hypoglycemic agents, including standard glyburide. Although patients may be transferred from the maximum dose of other sulfonylureas, the maximum starting dose of 3 mg of micronized glyburide tablets should be observed. A maintenance dose of 3 mg of micronized glyburide tablets provides approximately the same degree of blood glucose control as 250-375 mg chlorpropamide, 250-375 mg tolazamide, 5 mg of glyburide (nonmicronized tablets), 500-750 mg acetohexamide, or 1000-1500 mg tolbutamide.
When transferring patients receiving more than 40 units of insulin daily, they may be started on a daily dose of micronized glyburide tablets 3 mg concomitantly with a 50% reduction in insulin dose. Progressive withdrawal of insulin and increase of micronized glyburide in increments of 0.75-1.5 mg every 2-10 days is then carried out. During this conversion period when both insulin and micronized glyburide are being used, hypoglycemia may rarely occur. During insulin withdrawal, patients should test their urine for glucose and acetone at least 3 times daily and report results to their physician. The appearance of persistent acetonuria with glycosuria indicates that the patient is a Type I diabetic who requires insulin therapy.

CONCOMITANT GLYBURIDE AND METFORMIN THERAPY
Glyburide should be added gradually to the dosing regimen of patients who have not responded to the maximum dose of metformin monotherapy after 4 weeks (see Usual Starting Dose and Titration to Maintenance Dose). Refer to the metformin prescribing information.
With concomitant glyburide and metformin therapy, the desired control of blood glucose may be obtained by adjusting the dose of each drug. However, attempts should be made to identify the optimal dose of each drug needed to achieve this goal. With concomitant glyburide and metformin therapy, the risk of hypoglycemia associated with sulfonylurea therapy continues and may be increased. Appropriate precautions should be taken (see PRECAUTIONS).

G

MAXIMUM DOSE
Standard Glyburide: Daily doses of more than 20 mg are not recommended.
Micronized Glyburide: Daily doses of more than 12 mg are not recommended.

DOSAGE INTERVAL
Standard Glyburide: Once-a-day therapy is usually satisfactory. Some patients, particularly those receiving more than 10 mg daily, may have a more satisfactory response with twice-a-day dosage.
Micronized Glyburide: Once-a-day therapy is usually satisfactory. Some patients, particularly those receiving more than 6 mg daily, may have a more satisfactory response with twice-a-day dosage.

SPECIFIC PATIENT POPULATIONS
Glyburide is not recommended for use in pregnancy or for use in pediatric patients.
In elderly patients, debilitated or malnourished patients, and patients with impaired renal or hepatic function, the initial and maintenance dosing should be conservative to avoid hypoglycemic reactions (see PRECAUTIONS).

HOW SUPPLIED

MICRONASE
Micronase tablets are supplied in:
1.25 mg: White, round, scored and imprinted "MICRONASE 1.25".
2.5 mg: Dark pink, round, scored and imprinted "MICRONASE 2.5"
5 mg: Blue, round, scored and imprinted "MICRONASE 5"
Storage: Store at controlled room temperature 20-25°C (68-77°F). Keep container tightly closed. Dispensed in well-closed containers with safety closures.

GLYNASE PRESTAB
Glynase PresTab tablets are supplied in:
1.5 mg: White, ovoid, imprinted "GLYNASE 1.5/PT" Score PT, contour, scored.
3 mg: Blue, ovoid, imprinted "GLYNASE 3/PT" Score Pt, contour, scored.
6 mg: Yellow, ovoid, imprinted "GLYNASE 6/PT" Score PT, contour, scored.
The PresTab tablet can be easily divided in half for a more flexible dosing regimen. Press gently on the score and the PresTab tablet will split in even halves.
Storage: Store at controlled room temperature 20-25°C (68-77°F). Dispensed in well-closed containers with safety closures. Keep container tightly closed.

PRODUCT LISTING - RATED THERAPEUTICALLY EQUIVALENT

Tablet - Oral - Micronized 1.5 mg			
100's	$35.65	GENERIC, Teva Pharmaceuticals Usa	00093-8034-01
100's	$37.40	GENERIC, Mylan Pharmaceuticals Inc	00378-1113-01
100's	$37.77	GENERIC, Greenstone Limited	59762-3781-01
100's	$37.78	GENERIC, Watson Laboratories Inc	52544-0558-01
100's	$37.78	GENERIC, Mova Pharmaceutical Corporation	55370-0146-07
100's	$45.26	GENERIC, Zoetica Pharmaceutical	64909-0101-07
100's	$51.25	GLYNASE PRES-TAB, Pharmacia and Upjohn	00009-0341-02
100's	$58.16	GLYNASE PRES-TAB, Pharmacia Corporation	00009-0341-01
Tablet - Oral - Micronized 3 mg			
30's	$23.21	GLYNASE PRES-TAB, Allscripts Pharmaceutical Company	54569-3690-00
60's	$46.41	GLYNASE PRES-TAB, Allscripts Pharmaceutical Company	54569-3690-01
100's	$60.20	GENERIC, Teva Pharmaceuticals Usa	00093-8035-01
100's	$63.20	GENERIC, Mylan Pharmaceuticals Inc	00378-1125-01
100's	$63.87	GENERIC, Greenstone Limited	59762-3782-01
100's	$63.88	GENERIC, Watson Laboratories Inc	52544-0559-01
100's	$63.88	GENERIC, Mova Pharmaceutical Corporation	55370-0147-07

100's	$72.36	GLYNASE PRES-TAB, Pharmacia and Upjohn	00009-0352-14
100's	$76.85	GENERIC, Zoetica Pharmaceutical	64909-0102-07
100's	$86.60	GLYNASE PRES-TAB, Pharmacia and Upjohn	00009-0352-02
100's	$98.33	GLYNASE PRES-TAB, Pharmacia Corporation	00009-0352-01
Tablet - Oral - Micronized 4.5 mg			
100's	$98.50	GENERIC, Zoetica Pharmaceutical	64909-0104-07
Tablet - Oral - Micronized 6 mg			
100's	$84.09	GENERIC, Teva Pharmaceuticals Usa	00093-8036-01
100's	$106.70	GENERIC, Mylan Pharmaceuticals Inc	00378-1142-01
100's	$107.30	GENERIC, Watson Laboratories Inc	52544-0560-01
100's	$107.30	GENERIC, Greenstone Limited	59762-3783-01
100's	$107.32	GENERIC, Mova Pharmaceutical Corporation	55370-0506-07
100's	$121.46	GENERIC, Zoetica Pharmaceutical	64909-0105-07
100's	$155.05	GLYNASE PRES-TAB, Pharmacia Corporation	00009-3449-01
Tablet - Oral - 1.25 mg			
60's	$22.42	MICRONASE, Physicians Total Care	54868-1688-01
100's	$18.34	GENERIC, Qualitest Products Inc	00603-3762-21
100's	$19.03	GENERIC, Brightstone Pharma	62939-3211-01
100's	$27.56	GENERIC, Teva Pharmaceuticals Usa	00093-8342-01
100's	$37.53	MICRONASE, Pharmacia and Upjohn	00009-0131-01
Tablet - Oral - 1.5 mg			
100's	$25.49	FEDERAL UPPER LIMIT, H.C.F.A. F F P	99999-1368-01
Tablet - Oral - 2.5 mg			
3's	$1.33	GENERIC, Allscripts Pharmaceutical Company	54569-3830-01
25's	$7.60	GENERIC, Udl Laboratories Inc	51079-0872-19
30's	$18.68	MICRONASE, Physicians Total Care	54868-1244-01
60's	$36.19	MICRONASE, Physicians Total Care	54868-1244-03
100's	$30.55	GENERIC, Qualitest Products Inc	00603-3763-21
100's	$30.60	GENERIC, Udl Laboratories Inc	51079-0872-20
100's	$30.96	GENERIC, Brightstone Pharma	62939-3221-01
100's	$45.93	GENERIC, Teva Pharmaceuticals Usa	00093-8343-01
100's	$52.54	MICRONASE, Physicians Total Care	54868-1244-02
100's	$58.50	MICRONASE, Pharmacia and Upjohn	00009-0141-02
100's	$62.51	MICRONASE, Pharmacia and Upjohn	00009-0141-01
240's	$133.44	MICRONASE, Physicians Total Care	54868-1244-00
Tablet - Oral - 3 mg			
100's	$32.02	FEDERAL UPPER LIMIT, H.C.F.A. F F P	99999-1368-02
Tablet - Oral - 5 mg			
15's	$6.89	GENERIC, Pd-Rx Pharmaceuticals	55289-0892-15
25's	$13.15	GENERIC, Udl Laboratories Inc	51079-0873-19
25's	$20.87	GENERIC, Pd-Rx Pharmaceuticals	55289-0892-97
30's	$13.80	GENERIC, Pd-Rx Pharmaceuticals	55289-0892-30
30's	$24.20	MICRONASE, Pharma Pac	52959-0177-30
30's	$24.20	MICRONASE, Pd-Rx Pharmaceuticals	55289-0173-30
30's	$26.46	MICRONASE, Pharmacia and Upjohn	00009-0171-11
30's	$28.25	GENERIC, Pharma Pac	52959-0449-30
30's	$31.09	MICRONASE, Physicians Total Care	54868-1245-01
60's	$12.93	GENERIC, Pd-Rx Pharmaceuticals	55289-0892-60
60's	$60.42	MICRONASE, Physicians Total Care	54868-1245-05
60's	$63.39	MICRONASE, Pharmacia Corporation	00009-0171-12
90's	$46.42	GENERIC, Greenstone Limited	59762-3727-03
90's	$46.87	GENERIC, Allscripts Pharmaceutical Company	54569-8601-03
100's	$34.40	GENERIC, Pd-Rx Pharmaceuticals	55289-0892-01
100's	$51.95	GENERIC, Brightstone Pharma	62939-3231-01
100's	$52.60	GENERIC, Udl Laboratories Inc	51079-0873-20
100's	$52.95	GENERIC, Watson/Rugby Laboratories Inc	00536-5752-01
100's	$58.35	GENERIC, Pharma Pac	52959-0449-01
100's	$77.70	GENERIC, Teva Pharmaceuticals Usa	00093-8344-01
100's	$100.90	MICRONASE, Physicians Total Care	54868-1245-02
100's	$105.68	MICRONASE, Pharmacia Corporation	00009-0171-05
100's	$118.35	MICRONASE, Pharmacia Corporation	00009-0171-03
120's	$81.73	GENERIC, Allscripts Pharmaceutical Company	54569-3831-04
120's	$120.81	MICRONASE, Physicians Total Care	54868-1245-03
180's	$93.74	GENERIC, Allscripts Pharmaceutical Company	54569-8601-02
270's	$140.62	GENERIC, Allscripts Pharmaceutical Company	54569-8601-01

PRODUCT LISTING - RATED NOT THERAPEUTICALLY EQUIVALENT

Tablet - Oral - 1.25 mg			
30's	$4.48	GENERIC, Allscripts Pharmaceutical Company	54569-3832-00
30's	$5.78	GENERIC, Heartland Healthcare Services	61392-0117-30
30's	$5.78	GENERIC, Heartland Healthcare Services	61392-0117-39
31's	$5.98	GENERIC, Heartland Healthcare Services	61392-0117-31
32's	$6.17	GENERIC, Heartland Healthcare Services	61392-0117-32
45's	$8.68	GENERIC, Heartland Healthcare Services	61392-0117-45
50's	$11.66	DIABETA, Aventis Pharmaceuticals	00039-0053-05
50's	$13.78	GENERIC, Teva Pharmaceuticals Usa	00093-9477-53
60's	$11.57	GENERIC, Heartland Healthcare Services	61392-0117-60
90's	$17.35	GENERIC, Heartland Healthcare Services	61392-0117-90
100's	$18.35	GENERIC, Warrick Pharmaceuticals Corporation	59930-1592-01
100's	$27.56	GENERIC, Greenstone Limited	59762-3725-01
Tablet - Oral - 2.5 mg			
30's	$8.38	GENERIC, Allscripts Pharmaceutical Company	54569-3830-00
30's	$9.21	GENERIC, Heartland Healthcare Services	61392-0119-30
30's	$9.21	GENERIC, Heartland Healthcare Services	61392-0119-39
31's	$9.52	GENERIC, Heartland Healthcare Services	61392-0119-31
32's	$9.82	GENERIC, Heartland Healthcare Services	61392-0119-32
45's	$13.82	GENERIC, Heartland Healthcare Services	61392-0119-45
60's	$18.42	GENERIC, Heartland Healthcare Services	61392-0119-60
90's	$27.63	GENERIC, Heartland Healthcare Services	61392-0119-90
100's	$30.60	GENERIC, Warrick Pharmaceuticals Corporation	59930-1622-01
100's	$34.62	DIABETA, Aventis Pharmaceuticals	00039-0051-11
100's	$45.65	DIABETA, Aventis Pharmaceuticals	00039-0051-10
100's	$45.93	GENERIC, Teva Pharmaceuticals Usa	00093-9433-01
100's	$45.93	GENERIC, Copley	38245-0433-10
100's	$45.93	GENERIC, Greenstone Limited	59762-3726-03
Tablet - Oral - 5 mg			
30's	$15.64	GENERIC, Allscripts Pharmaceutical Company	54569-3831-00
30's	$16.40	GENERIC, Heartland Healthcare Services	61392-0120-30
30's	$16.40	GENERIC, Heartland Healthcare Services	61392-0120-39
30's	$22.09	DIABETA, Allscripts Pharmaceutical Company	54569-0200-00
31's	$16.94	GENERIC, Heartland Healthcare Services	61392-0120-31
32's	$17.49	GENERIC, Heartland Healthcare Services	61392-0120-32
45's	$24.60	GENERIC, Heartland Healthcare Services	61392-0120-45
60's	$31.28	GENERIC, Allscripts Pharmaceutical Company	54569-3831-02
60's	$32.80	GENERIC, Heartland Healthcare Services	61392-0120-60
60's	$54.17	DIABETA, Pd-Rx Pharmaceuticals	55289-0614-60
90's	$49.19	GENERIC, Heartland Healthcare Services	61392-0120-90
90's	$53.01	DIABETA, Allscripts Pharmaceutical Company	54569-8556-01
100's	$52.13	GENERIC, Allscripts Pharmaceutical Company	54569-3831-01
100's	$53.00	GENERIC, Warrick Pharmaceuticals Corporation	59930-1639-01
100's	$77.63	DIABETA, Pd-Rx Pharmaceuticals	55289-0614-01
100's	$77.68	GENERIC, Greenstone Limited	59762-3727-04
100's	$77.70	GENERIC, Teva Pharmaceuticals Usa	00093-9364-01
100's	$77.70	GENERIC, Copley	38245-0364-10
100's	$78.04	DIABETA, Aventis Pharmaceuticals	00039-0052-11
100's	$83.73	DIABETA, Aventis Pharmaceuticals	00039-0052-10
180's	$84.96	GENERIC, Golden State Medical	60429-0085-18
180's	$106.02	DIABETA, Allscripts Pharmaceutical Company	54569-8556-00
270's	$159.03	DIABETA, Allscripts Pharmaceutical Company	54569-8556-03

PRODUCT LISTING - EQUIVALENTS NOT AVAILABLE

Tablet - Oral - 1.25 mg			
50's	$1086.00	GENERIC, Pharmaceutical Corporation Of America	51655-0758-77
Tablet - Oral - 2.5 mg			
30's	$8.55	GENERIC, Pharmaceutical Corporation Of America	51655-0753-24
100's	$31.00	GENERIC, Watson/Rugby Laboratories Inc	00536-5751-01
Tablet - Oral - 5 mg			
30's	$14.21	GENERIC, Pharmaceutical Corporation Of America	51655-0904-24
60's	$27.43	GENERIC, Pharmaceutical Corporation Of America	51655-0904-25

Glyburide; Metformin Hydrochloride *(003501)*

For complete prescribing information, refer to the CD-ROM included with the book.

For related information, see the comparative table section in Appendix A.

Categories: Diabetes mellitus; FDA Approved 2000 Jul; Pregnancy Category B
Drug Classes: Antidiabetic agents; Biguanides; Sulfonylureas, second generation
Brand Names: **Glucovance**
Foreign Brand Availability: Bi-Euglucon (Colombia); Bi-Euglucon M "5" (Mexico); Glibomet (Italy; Korea)
Cost of Therapy: $24.64 (Diabetes mellitus; Glucovance; 1.25 mg; 250 mg; 1 tablet/day; 30 day supply)

DESCRIPTION

Note: The trade name has been used throughout this monograph for clarity.

Glucovance contains 2 oral antihyperglycemic drugs used in the management of Type 2 diabetes, glyburide and metformin hydrochloride.

Glyburide is an oral antihyperglycemic drug of the sulfonylurea class. The chemical name for glyburide is 1-[[*p*-[2-(5-chloro-*o*-anisamido)ethyl]phenyl]sulfonyl]-3-cyclohexylurea. Glyburide is a white to off-white crystalline compound with a molecular formula of $C_{23}H_{28}ClN_3O_5S$ and a molecular weight of 494.01. The glyburide used in Glucovance has a particle size distribution of 25% undersize value not more than 6 μm, 50% undersize value not more than 7-10 μm, and 75% undersize value not more than 21 μm.

Metformin HCl is an oral antihyperglycemic drug used in the management of Type 2 diabetes. Metformin HCl (*N,N*-dimethylimidodicarbonimidic diamide monohydrochloride) is not chemically or pharmacologically related to sulfonylureas, thiazolidinediones, or α-glucosidase inhibitors. It is a white to off-white crystalline compound with a molecular formula of $C_4H_{12}ClN_5$ (monohydrochloride) and a molecular weight of 165.63. Metformin HCl is freely soluble in water and is practically insoluble in acetone, ether, and chloroform. The pKa of metformin is 12.4. The pH of a 1% aqueous solution of metformin HCl is 6.68.

Glucovance is available for oral administration in tablets containing 1.25 mg glyburide with 250 mg metformin HCl, 2.5 mg glyburide with 500 mg metformin HCl, and 5 mg glyburide with 500 mg metformin HCl. In addition, each tablet contains the following inactive ingredients: microcrystalline cellulose, povidone, croscarmellose sodium, and magnesium stearate. The tablets are film coated, which provides color differentiation.

INDICATIONS AND USAGE

Glucovance is indicated as initial therapy, as an adjunct to diet and exercise, to improve glycemic control in patients with Type 2 diabetes whose hyperglycemia cannot be satisfactorily managed with diet and exercise alone.

Glucovance is indicated as second-line therapy when diet, exercise, and initial treatment with a sulfonylurea or metformin do not result in adequate glycemic control in patients with Type 2 diabetes. For patients requiring additional therapy, a thiazolidinedione may be added to Glucovance to achieve additional glycemic control.

CONTRAINDICATIONS

Glucovance is contraindicated in patients with:

Renal disease or renal dysfunction (*e.g.*, as suggested by serum creatinine levels ≥1.5 mg/dl [males], ≥1.4 mg/dl [females], or abnormal creatinine clearance) which may also result from conditions such as cardiovascular collapse (shock), acute myocardial infarction, and septicemia (see WARNINGS).

Congestive heart failure requiring pharmacologic treatment.

Known hypersensitivity to metformin HCl or glyburide.

Acute or chronic metabolic acidosis, including diabetic ketoacidosis, with or without coma. Diabetic ketoacidosis should be treated with insulin.

Glucovance should be temporarily discontinued in patients undergoing radiologic studies involving intravascular administration of iodinated contrast materials, because use of such products may result in acute alteration of renal function.

WARNINGS

METFORMIN HCl

Lactic Acidosis

Lactic acidosis is a rare, but serious, metabolic complication that can occur due to metformin accumulation during treatment with Glucovance; when it occurs, it is fatal in approximately 50% of cases. Lactic acidosis may also occur in association with a number of pathophysiologic conditions, including diabetes mellitus, and whenever there is significant tissue hypoperfusion and hypoxemia. Lactic acidosis is characterized by elevated blood lactate levels (>5 mmol/L), decreased blood pH, electrolyte disturbances with an increased anion gap, and an increased lactate/pyruvate ratio. When metformin is implicated as the cause of lactic acidosis, metformin plasma levels >5 µg/ml are generally found.

The reported incidence of lactic acidosis in patients receiving metformin HCl is very low (approximately 0.03 cases/1000 patient years, with approximately 0.015 fatal cases/1000 patient-years). Reported cases have occurred primarily in diabetic patients with significant renal insufficiency, including both intrinsic renal disease and renal hypoperfusion, often in the setting of multiple concomitant medical/surgical problems and multiple concomitant medications. Patients with congestive heart failure requiring pharmacologic management, in particular those with unstable or acute congestive heart failure who are at risk of hypoperfusion and hypoxemia, are at increased risk of lactic acidosis. The risk of lactic acidosis increases with the degree of renal dysfunction and the patient's age. The risk of lactic acidosis may, therefore, be significantly decreased by regular monitoring of renal function in patients taking metformin and by use of the minimum effective dose of metformin. In particular, treatment of the elderly should be accompanied by careful monitoring of renal function. Glucovance treatment should not be initiated in patients ≥80 years of age unless measurement of creatinine clearance demonstrates that renal function is not reduced, as these patients are more susceptible to developing lactic acidosis. In addition, Glucovance should be promptly withheld in the presence of any condition associated with hypoxemia, dehydration, or sepsis. Because impaired hepatic function may significantly limit the ability to clear lactate, Glucovance should generally be avoided in patients with clinical or laboratory evidence of hepatic disease. Patients should be cautioned against excessive alcohol intake, either acute or chronic, when taking Glucovance, since alcohol potentiates the effects of metformin HCl on lactate metabolism. In addition, Glucovance should be temporarily discontinued prior to any intravascular radiocontrast study and for any surgical procedure.

The onset of lactic acidosis often is subtle, and accompanied only by nonspecific symptoms such as malaise, myalgias, respiratory distress, increasing somnolence, and nonspecific abdominal distress. There may be associated hypothermia, hypotension, and resistant bradyarrhythmias with more marked acidosis. The patient and the patient's physician must be aware of the possible importance of such symptoms and the patient should be instructed to notify the physician immediately if they occur. Glucovance should be withdrawn until the situation is clarified. Serum electrolytes, ketones, blood glucose, and if indicated, blood pH, lactate levels, and even blood metformin levels may be useful. Once a patient is stabilized on any dose level of Glucovance, gastrointestinal symptoms, which are common during initiation of therapy with metformin, are unlikely to be drug related. Later occurrence of gastrointestinal symptoms could be due to lactic acidosis or other serious disease.

Levels of fasting venous plasma lactate above the upper limit of normal but less than 5 mmol/L in patients taking Glucovance do not necessarily indicate impending lactic acidosis and may be explainable by other mechanisms, such as poorly controlled diabetes or obesity, vigorous physical activity, or technical problems in sample handling.

Lactic acidosis should be suspected in any diabetic patient with metabolic acidosis lacking evidence of ketoacidosis (ketonuria and ketonemia).

Lactic acidosis is a medical emergency that must be treated in a hospital setting. In a patient with lactic acidosis who is taking Glucovance, the drug should be discontinued immediately and general supportive measures promptly instituted. Because metformin HCl is dialyzable (with a clearance of up to 170 ml/min under good hemodynamic conditions), prompt hemodialysis is recommended to correct the acidosis and remove the accumulated metformin. Such management often results in prompt reversal of symptoms and recovery. (See also CONTRAINDICATIONS.)

SPECIAL WARNING ON INCREASED RISK OF CARDIOVASCULAR MORTALITY

The administration of oral hypoglycemic drugs has been reported to be associated with increased cardiovascular mortality as compared to treatment with diet alone or diet plus insulin. This warning is based on the study conducted by the University Group Diabetes Program (UGDP), a long-term prospective clinical trial designed to evaluate the effectiveness of glucose-lowering drugs in preventing or delaying vascular complications in patients with non-insulin-dependent diabetes. The study involved 823 patients who were randomly assigned to 1 of 4 treatment groups [*Diabetes* 19 (Suppl 2):747-830, 1970].

UGDP reported that patients treated for 5-8 years with diet plus a fixed dose of tolbutamide (1.5 g/day) had a rate of cardiovascular mortality approximately 2½ times that of patients treated with diet alone. A significant increase in total mortality was not observed, but the use of tolbutamide was discontinued based on the increase in cardiovascular mortality, thus limiting the opportunity for the study to show an increase in overall mortality. Despite controversy regarding the interpretation of these results, the findings of the UGDP study provide an adequate basis for this warning. The patient should be informed of the potential risks and benefits of glyburide and of alternative modes of therapy.

Although only 1 drug in the sulfonylurea class (tolbutamide) was included in this study, it is prudent from a safety standpoint to consider that this warning may also apply to other hypoglycemic drugs in this class, in view of their close similarities in mode of action and chemical structure.

DOSAGE AND ADMINISTRATION

GENERAL CONSIDERATIONS

Dosage of Glucovance must be individualized on the basis of both effectiveness and tolerance while not exceeding the maximum recommended daily dose of 20 mg glyburide/2000 mg metformin. Glucovance should be given with meals and should be initiated at a low dose, with gradual dose escalation as described below, in order to avoid hypoglycemia (largely due to glyburide), to reduce GI side effects (largely due to metformin), and to permit determination of the minimum effective dose for adequate control of blood glucose for the individual patient.

With initial treatment and during dose titration, appropriate blood glucose monitoring should be used to determine the therapeutic response to Glucovance and to identify the minimum effective dose for the patient. Thereafter, HbA_{1c} should be measured at intervals of approximately 3 months to assess the effectiveness of therapy. The therapeutic goal in all patients with Type 2 diabetes is to decrease FPG, PPG, and HbA_{1c} to normal or as near normal as possible. Ideally, the response to therapy should be evaluated using HbA_{1c} (glycosylated hemoglobin), which is a better indicator of long-term glycemic control than FPG alone.

No studies have been performed specifically examining the safety and efficacy of switching to Glucovance therapy in patients taking concomitant glyburide (or other sulfonylurea) plus metformin. Changes in glycemic control may occur in such patients, with either hyperglycemia or hypoglycemia possible. Any change in therapy of Type 2 diabetes should be undertaken with care and appropriate monitoring.

GLUCOVANCE AS INITIAL THERAPY

Recommended starting dose: 1.25 mg/250 mg once or twice daily with meals.

For patients with Type 2 diabetes whose hyperglycemia cannot be satisfactorily managed with diet and exercise alone, the recommended starting dose of Glucovance is 1.25 mg/250 mg once a day with a meal. As initial therapy in patients with baseline HbA_{1c} >9% or an FPG >200 mg/dl, a starting dose of Glucovance 1.25 mg/250 mg twice daily with the morning and evening meals may be used. Dosage increases should be made in increments of 1.25 mg/250 mg/day every 2 weeks up to the minimum effective dose necessary to achieve adequate control of blood glucose. In clinical trials of Glucovance as initial therapy, there was no experience with total daily doses greater than 10 mg/2000 mg/day. **Glucovance 5 mg/500 mg should not be used as initial therapy due to an increased risk of hypoglycemia.**

GLUCOVANCE USE IN PREVIOUSLY TREATED PATIENTS (SECOND-LINE THERAPY)

Recommended starting dose: 2.5 mg/500 mg or 5 mg/500 mg twice daily with meals.

For patients not adequately controlled on either glyburide (or another sulfonylurea) or metformin alone, the recommended starting dose of Glucovance is 2.5 mg/500 mg or 5 mg/500 mg twice daily with the morning and evening meals. In order to avoid hypoglycemia, the starting dose of Glucovance should not exceed the daily doses of glyburide or metformin already being taken. The daily dose should be titrated in increments of no more than 5 mg/500 mg up to the minimum effective dose to achieve adequate control of blood glucose or to a maximum dose of 20 mg/2000 mg/day.

For patients previously treated with combination therapy of glyburide (or another sulfonylurea) plus metformin, if switched to Glucovance, the starting dose should not exceed the daily dose of glyburide (or equivalent dose of another sulfonylurea) and metformin already being taken. Patients should be monitored closely for signs and symptoms of hypoglycemia following such a switch and the dose of Glucovance should be titrated as described above to achieve adequate control of blood glucose.

ADDITION OF THIAZOLIDINEDIONES TO GLUCOVANCE THERAPY

For patients not adequately controlled on Glucovance, a thiazolidinedione can be added to Glucovance therapy. When a thiazolidinedione is added to Glucovance therapy, the current dose of Glucovance can be continued and the thiazolidinedione initiated at its recommended starting dose. For patients needing additional glycemic control, the dose of the thiazolidenedione can be increased based on its recommended titration schedule. The increased glycemic control attainable with Glucovance plus a thiazolidinedione may increase the potential for hypoglycemia at any time of day. In patients who develop hypoglycemia when receiving Glucovance and a thiazolidinedione, consideration should be given to reducing the dose of the glyburide component of Glucovance. As clinically warranted, adjustment of the dosages of the other components of the antidiabetic regimen should also be considered.

SPECIFIC PATIENT POPULATIONS

Glucovance is not recommended for use during pregnancy or for use in pediatric patients. The initial and maintenance dosing of Glucovance should be conservative in patients with advanced age, due to the potential for decreased renal function in this population. Any dosage adjustment requires a careful assessment of renal function. Generally, elderly, debilitated, and malnourished patients should not be titrated to the maximum dose of Glucovance to avoid the risk of hypoglycemia. Monitoring of renal function is necessary to aid in prevention of metformin-associated lactic acidosis, particularly in the elderly. (See WARNINGS.)

PRODUCT LISTING - EQUIVALENTS NOT AVAILABLE

Tablet - Oral - 1.25 mg;250 mg
100's $82.13 GLUCOVANCE, Bristol-Myers Squibb 00087-6072-11
Tablet - Oral - 2.5 mg;500 mg
100's $97.96 GLUCOVANCE, Bristol-Myers Squibb 00087-6073-11
Tablet - Oral - 5 mg;500 mg
100's $97.96 GLUCOVANCE, Bristol-Myers Squibb 00087-6074-11

Glycopyrrolate *(001377)*

Categories: Anesthesia, adjunct; Ulcer, peptic; Pregnancy Category B; FDA Approved 1961 Aug
Drug Classes: Anticholinergics; Gastrointestinals
Brand Names: Robinul
Foreign Brand Availability: Gastrodyn Inj (Finland); Glycopyrrolate Inj (India); Robinul Forte (Canada); Robinul Inj. (Australia; Austria; Denmark; England; Finland; Germany; Netherlands; New-Zealand; Norway; Sweden; Switzerland); Sroton (Japan); Strodin (Korea)
Cost of Therapy: $59.42 (Peptic Ulcer; Robinul; 1 mg; 3 tablets/day; 30 day supply)
$66.35 (Peptic Ulcer; Robinul Forte; 2 mg; 2 tablets/day; 30 day supply)

DESCRIPTION

Glycopyrrolate is a quaternary ammonium compound with the following chemical name: 3-((cyclopentylhydroxyphenylacetyl)oxy)-1, 1-dimethylpyrrolidinium bromide.

TABLETS

Glycopyrrolate and glycopyrrolate extra strength tablets contain the synthetic anticholinergic, glycopyrrolate.

Robinul tablets are scored, compressed white tablets engraved AHR. Each tablet contains 1 mg glycopyrrolate.

Robinul Forte tablets are scored, compressed white tablets engraved AHR. Each tablet contains 2 mg glycopyrrolate.

Inactive Ingredients: Dibasic calcium phosphate, lactose, magnesium stearate, povidone, sodium starch glycolate.

INJECTION

Glycopyrrolate is a synthetic anticholinergic agent. Each 1 ml contains: Glycopyrrolate 0.2 mg; water for injection, qs; benzyl alcohol, 0.9% (preservative); pH adjusted, when necessary, with hydrochloric acid and/or sodium hydroxide.

For intramuscular or intravenous administration.

Unlike atropine, glycopyrrolate is completely ionized at physiological pH values.

Glycopyrrolate injectable is a clear, colorless, sterile liquid; pH 2.0- 3.0.

Storage: Store at controlled room temperature between 15-30°C (59-86°F).

CLINICAL PHARMACOLOGY

Glycopyrrolate, like other anticholinergic (antimuscarinic) agents, inhibits the action of acetylcholine on structures innervated by postganglionic cholinergic nerves and on smooth muscles that respond to acetylcholine but lack cholinergic innervation. These peripheral cholinergic receptors are present in the autonomic effector cells of smooth muscle, cardiac muscle, the sino-atrial node, the atrioventricular node, exocrine glands, and, to a limited degree, in the autonomic ganglia. Thus, it diminishes the volume and free acidity of gastric secretions and controls excessive pharyngeal, tracheal, and bronchial secretions.

Glycopyrrolate antagonizes muscarinic symptoms (*e.g.,* bronchorrhea, bronchospasm, bradycardia, and intestinal hypermotility) induced by cholinergic drugs such as the anticholinesterases.

The highly polar quaternary ammonium group of glycopyrrolate limits its passage across lipid membranes, such as the blood-brain barrier, in contrast to atropine sulfate and scopolamine hydrobromide, which are non-polar tertiary amines which penetrate lipid barriers easily.

INJECTION

Peak effects occur approximately 30-45 minutes after intramuscular administration. The vagal blocking effects persist for 2-3 hours and the antisialagogue effects persist up to 7 hours, periods longer than for atropine. With intravenous injection, the onset of action is generally evident within 1 minute.

INDICATIONS AND USAGE

TABLETS

For use as adjunctive therapy in the treatment of peptic ulcer.

INJECTION

In Anesthesia

Glycopyrrolate injectable is indicated for use as a preoperative antimuscarinic to reduce salivary, tracheobronchial, and pharyngeal secretions; to reduce the volume and free acidity of gastric secretions; and, to block cardiac vagal inhibitory reflexes during induction of anesthesia and intubation. When indicated, glycopyrrolate injectable may be used intraoperatively to counteract drug-induced or vagal traction reflexes with the associated arrhythmias. Glycopyrrolate protects against the peripheral muscarinic effects (*e.g.,* bradycardia and excessive secretions) of cholinergic agents such as neostigmine and pyridostigmine given to reverse the neuromuscular blockade due to nondepolarizing muscle relaxants.

In Peptic Ulcer

For use in adults as adjunctive therapy for the treatment of peptic ulcer when rapid anticholinergic effect is desired or when oral medication is not tolerated.

CONTRAINDICATIONS

Glaucoma; obstructive uropathy (for example, bladder neck obstruction due to prostatic hypertrophy); obstructive disease of the gastrointestinal tract (as in achalasia, pyloroduodenal stenosis, etc.); paralytic ileus; intestinal atony of the elderly or debilitated patient; unstable cardiovascular status in acute hemorrhage; severe ulcerative colitis; toxic megacolon complicating ulcerative colitis; myasthenia gravis.

Glycopyrrolate tablets are contraindicated in those patients with a hypersensitivity to glycopyrrolate.

INJECTION

Due to its benzyl alcohol content, glycopyrrolate injectable should not be used in newborns (children less than 1 month of age).

WARNINGS

In the presence of a high environmental temperature, heat prostration (fever and heat stroke due to decreased sweating) can occur with use of glycopyrrolate.

Diarrhea may be an early symptom of incomplete intestinal obstruction, especially in patients with ileostomy or colostomy. In this instance treatment with this drug would be inappropriate and possibly harmful.

Glycopyrrolate may produce drowsiness or blurred vision. In this event, the patient should be warned not to engage in activities requiring mental alertness such as operating a motor vehicle or other machinery, or performing hazardous work while taking this drug.

TABLETS

Theoretically, with overdosage, a curare-like action may occur, *i.e.,* neuromuscular blockade leading to muscular weakness and possible paralysis.

INJECTION

This drug should be used with great caution, if at all, in patients with glaucoma or asthma.

PRECAUTIONS

TABLETS

Use glycopyrrolate with caution in the elderly and in all patients with:

- Autonomic neuropathy.
- Hepatic or renal disease.
- Ulcerative colitis-large doses may suppress intestinal motility to the point of producing a paralytic ileus and for this reason may precipitate or aggravate "toxic megacolon," a serious complication of the disease.
- Hyperthyroidism, coronary heart disease, congestive heart failure,cardiac tachyarrhythmias, tachycardia, hypertension and prostatic hypertrophy.
- Hiatal hernia associated with reflux esophagitis, since anticholinergic drugs may aggravate this condition.

Pregnancy

The safety of this drug during pregnancy has not been established. The use of any drug during pregnancy requires that the potential benefits of the drug be weighed against possible hazards to mother and child. Reproduction studies in rats revealed no teratogenic effects from glycopyrrolate; however, the potent anticholinergic action of this agent resulted in diminished rates of conception and of survival at weaning, in a dose-related manner. Other studies in dogs suggest that this may be due to diminished seminal secretion which is evident at high doses of glycopyrrolate. Information on possible adverse effects in the pregnant female is limited to uncontrolled data derived from marketing experience. Such experience has revealed no reports of teratogenic or other fetus- damaging potential. No controlled studies to establish the safety of the drug in pregnancy have been performed.

Nursing Mothers

It is not known whether this drug is excreted in human milk. As a general rule, nursing should not be undertaken while a patient is on a drug since many drugs are excreted in human milk.

Pediatric Use

Since there is no adequate experience in children who have received this drug, safety and efficacy in children have not been established.

INJECTION

General

Investigate any tachycardia before giving glycopyrrolate since an increase in the heart rate may occur.

Use with caution in patients with: coronary artery disease; congestive heart failure; cardiac arrhythmias; hypertension; hyperthyroidism.

In managing ulcer patients, use glycopyrrolate with caution in the elderly and in all patients with autonomic neuropathy, hepatic or renal disease, ulcerative colitis or hiatal hernia, since anticholinergic drugs may aggravate these conditions.

With overdosage, a curare-like action may occur.

Carcinogenesis, Mutagenesis, and Impairment of Fertility

Long-term studies in animals have not been performed to evaluate carcinogenic potential. In the teratology studies, diminished rates of conception and of survival at weaning were observed in rats, in a dose-related manner. Studies in dogs suggest that this may be due to diminished seminal secretion which is evident at high doses of glycopyrrolate.

Pregnancy Category B

Reproduction studies have been performed in rats and rabbits up to 1000 times the human dose and have revealed no teratogenic effects from glycopyrrolate. There are, however, no adequate and well-controlled studies in pregnant women. Because animal reproduction studies are not always predictive of human response, this drug should be used during pregnancy only if clearly needed.

Nursing Mothers

It is not known whether this drug is excreted in human milk. Because many drugs are excreted in human milk, caution should be exercised when glycopyrrolate is administered to a nursing woman.

Pediatric Use

Safety and effectiveness in children below the age of 12 years have not been established for the management of peptic ulcer.

DRUG INTERACTIONS

TABLETS

There are no known drug interactions.

INJECTION

The intravenous administration of any anticholinergic in the presence of cyclopropane anesthesia can result in ventricular arrhythmias; therefore, caution should be observed if glycopyrrolate injectable is used during cyclopropane anesthesia. If the drug is given in small incremental doses of 0.1 mg or less, the likelihood of producing ventricular arrhythmias is reduced.

ADVERSE REACTIONS

Anticholinergics produce certain effects, most of which are extensions of their fundamental pharmacological actions. Adverse reactions to anticholinergics in general may include xerostomia; decreased sweating; urinary hesitancy and retention; blurred vision; tachycardia; palpitations; dilatation of the pupil; cycloplegia; increased ocular tension; loss of taste; headaches; nervousness; mental confusion; drowsiness; weakness; dizziness; insomnia; nausea; vomiting; constipation; bloated feeling; impotence; suppression of lactation; severe allergic reaction or drug idiosyncrasies including anaphylaxis, urticaria and other dermal manifestations.

Glycopyrrolate is chemically a quaternary ammonium compound; hence, its passage across lipid membranes, such as the blood-brain barrier, is limited in contrast to atropine sulfate and scopolamine hydrobromide. For this reason the occurrence of CNS related side effects is lower, in comparison to their incidence following administration of anticholinergics which are chemically tertiary amines that can cross this barrier readily.

DOSAGE AND ADMINISTRATION

TABLETS

The dosage of glycopyrrolate or glycopyrrolate extra strength should be adjusted to the needs of the individual patient to assure symptomatic control with a minimum of adverse reactions. The presently recommended maximum daily dosage of glycopyrrolate is 8 mg.

Glycopyrrolate: *1 mg Tablets:* The recommended initial dosage of glycopyrrolate for adults is 1 tablet 3 times daily (in the morning, early afternoon, and at bedtime). Some patients may require 2 tablets at bedtime to assure overnight control of symptoms. For maintenance, a dosage of 1 tablet twice a day is frequently adequate.

Glycopyrrolate Extra Strength: *2 mg Tablets:* The recommended dosage of glycopyrrolate extra strength for adults is 1 tablet 2 or 3 times daily at equally spaced intervals.

Glycopyrrolate tablets are not recommended for use in children under the age of 12 years.

INJECTION

Glycopyrrolate injectable may be administered intramuscularly, or intravenously, without dilution, in the following indications:

Adults:

Preanesthetic Medication: The recommended dose of glycopyrrolate injectable is 0.002 mg (0.01 ml) per pound of body weight by intramuscular injection, given 30 to 60 minutes prior to the anticipated time of induction of anesthesia or at the time the preanesthetic narcotic and/or sedative are administered.

Intraoperative Medication: Glycopyrrolate injectable may be used during surgery to counteract drug induced or vagal taction reflexes with the associated arrhythmias (*e.g.*, bradycardia). It should be administered intravenously as single doses of 0.1 mg (0.5 ml) and repeated, as needed, at intervals of 2-3 minutes. The usual attempts should be made to determine the etiology of the arrhythmia, and the surgical or anesthetic manipulations necessary to correct parasympathetic imbalance should be performed.

Reversal of Neuromuscular Blockade: The recommended dose of glycopyrrolate injectable is 0.2 mg (1.0 ml) for each 1.0 mg of neostigmine or 5.0 mg of pyridostigmine. In order to minimize the appearance of cardiac side effects, the drugs may be administered simultaneously by intravenous injection and may be mixed in the same syringe.

Peptic Ulcer: The usual recommended dose of glycopyrrolate injectable is 0.1 mg (0.5 ml) administered at 4-hour intervals. 3 or 4 times daily intravenously or intramuscularly. Where more profound effect is required, 0.2 mg (1.0 ml) may be given. Some patients may be given. Some patients may need only a single dose, and frequency of administration should be dictated by patient response up to a maximum of 4 times daily.

Children:

(Read CONTRAINDICATIONS.)

Preanesthetic Medication: The recommended dose of glycopyrrolate injectable in children 1 month to 12 years of age is 0.002 mg (0.01 ml) per pound of body weight intramuscularly, given 30 to 60 minutes prior to the anticipated time of induction of anesthesia or at the time the preanesthetic narcotic and/or sedative are administered.

Children 1 month to 2 years of age may require up to 0.004 mg (0.02 ml) per pound of body weight.

Intraoperative Medication: Because of the long duration of action of glycopyrrolate if used as preanesthetic medication, additional glycopyrrolate injectable for anticholinergic effect intraoperatively is rarely needed; in the event it is required the recommended pediatric dose 0.002 mg (0.01 ml) per pound of body weight intravenously, not to exceed 0.1 mg (0.5 ml) in a single dose which may be repeated, as needed, at intervals of 2-3 minutes. The usual attempts should be made to determine the etiology of the arrhythmia, and the surgical or anesthetic manipulations necessary to correct parasympathetic imbalance should be performed.

Reversal of Neuromuscular Blockade: The recommended pediatric dose of glycopyrrolate injectable is 0.2 mg (1.0 ml) for each 1.0 mg of neostigmine or 5.0 mg of pyridostigmine. In order to minimize the appearance of cardiac side effects, the drugs may be administered simultaneously by intravenous injection and may be mixed in the same syringe.

Glycopyrrolate injectable is not recommended for peptic ulcer in children under 12 years of age. (See PRECAUTIONS.)

Note: Parenteral drug products should be inspected visually for particulate matter and discoloration prior to administration whenever solution and container permit.

Admixture Compatibilities: Glycopyrrolate injectable is compatible for mixing and injection with the following injectable dosage forms: 5% and 10% glucose in water or saline; atropine sulfate; physostigmine salicylate; diphenhydramine HCl; codeine phosphate; benzquinamide HCl; hydromorphone HCl; droperidol; droperidol and fentabyl citrate; propiomazine HCl; levorphanol tartrate); lidocaine; meperidine and promethazine HCls; meperidine HCl; pyridostigmine bromide; morphine sulfate; alphaprodine HCl; nalbuphine HCl; oxymorphone HCl; opium alkaloids HCls; procaine HCl; promethazine HCl; neostigmine methylsulfate; scopolamine HBr; promazine HCl; butorphanol tartrate; fentanyl citrate; pentazocine lactate; tri-methobenzamide HCl; tri-flupromazine HCl; hydroxyzine HCl. Glycopyrrolate injectable may be administered via the tubing of a running infusion of physiological saline or lactated Ringer's solution.

Since the stability of glycopyrrolate is questionable above a pH of 6.0 do *not* combine glycopyrrolate injectable in the same syringe with methohexital Na; chloramphenicol Na succinate; dimenhydrinate; pentobarbital Na; thiopental Na; secobarbital Na; sodium bicarbonate; or diazepam. A gas will evolve or precipitate may form. Mixing with dexamethazone Na phosphate or a buffered solution of lactated Ringer's solution will result in a pH higher than 6.0. Mixing chlorpromazine HCl , or prochlorperazine with other agents in a syringe is not recommended by the manufacturer, although the mixture with glycopyrrolate is physically compatible.

PRODUCT LISTING - RATED THERAPEUTICALLY EQUIVALENT

Solution - Injectable - 0.2 mg/ml

Size	Price	Product	NDC
1 ml x 25	$22.00	ROBINUL, Baxter Pharmaceutical Products, Inc	10019-0016-81
1 ml x 25	$22.25	GENERIC, American Regent Laboratories Inc	00517-4601-25
1 ml x 25	$30.71	ROBINUL, Physicians Total Care	54868-3231-01
2 ml x 25	$26.75	ROBINUL, Baxter Pharmaceutical Products, Inc	10019-0016-17
2 ml x 25	$36.00	GENERIC, American Regent Laboratories Inc	00517-4602-25
5 ml	$3.30	GENERIC, Watson/Schein Pharmaceuticals Inc	00364-3013-53
5 ml x 25	$32.75	ROBINUL, Baxter Pharmaceutical Products, Inc	10019-0016-54
5 ml x 25	$78.50	GENERIC, American Regent Laboratories Inc	00517-4605-25
20 ml	$7.63	ROBINUL, Allscripts Pharmaceutical Company	54569-3519-00
20 ml	$14.64	ROBINUL, Baxter Pharmaceutical Products, Inc	10019-0016-63
20 ml x 25	$156.00	GENERIC, American Regent Laboratories Inc	00517-4620-25
25 ml	$17.65	GENERIC, Watson/Schein Pharmaceuticals Inc	00364-3013-46

Tablet - Oral - 1 mg

Size	Price	Product	NDC
100's	$66.02	ROBINUL, First Horizon Pharmaceutical Corporation	59630-0200-10

Tablet - Oral - 2 mg

Size	Price	Product	NDC
100's	$110.58	ROBINUL FORTE, First Horizon Pharmaceutical Corporation	59630-0205-10

PRODUCT LISTING - EQUIVALENTS NOT AVAILABLE

Solution - Injectable - 0.2 mg/ml

Size	Price	Product	NDC
5 ml x 25	$125.00	GENERIC, Cmc-Consolidated Midland Corporation	00223-7722-05
20 ml	$6.00	GENERIC, Cmc-Consolidated Midland Corporation	00223-7723-20

G

Gold Sodium Thiomalate (001379)

For complete prescribing information, refer to the CD-ROM included with the book.

Categories: Arthritis, rheumatoid; Pregnancy Category C; FDA Pre 1938 Drugs
Drug Classes: Disease modifying antirheumatic drugs; Gold compounds
Brand Names: Aurolate; **Myochrysine**
Foreign Brand Availability: Aurothio (Korea); Miocrin (Colombia; Costa-Rica; Dominican-Republic; El-Salvador; Panama; Singapore; Spain); Myocrisin (Australia; Bahamas; Bahrain; Barbados; Belize; Bermuda; Curacao; Cyprus; Denmark; Egypt; England; Finland; Guyana; Hong-Kong; Hungary; Iran; Iraq; Ireland; Jamaica; Jordan; Kuwait; Lebanon; Libya; Netherland-Antilles; New-Zealand; Norway; Oman; Qatar; Republic-of-Yemen; Saudi-Arabia; South-Africa; Surinam; Sweden; Syria; Thailand; Trinidad; United-Arab-Emirates); Shiosol (Japan); Tauredon (Austria; Czech-Republic; Germany; Hungary; Portugal; Russia; Switzerland)
Cost of Therapy: $236.22 (Rheumatoid Arthritis; Myochrisine Injection; 50 mg/ml; 10 ml; 25 mg/week; variable day supply)
$217.00 (Rheumatoid Arthritis; Generic injection; 50 mg/ml; 10 ml; 25 mg/week; variable day supply)
HCFA JCODE(S): J1600 up to 50 mg IM

WARNING

Physicians planning to use gold sodium thiomalate should thoroughly familiarize themselves with its toxicity and its benefits. The possibility of toxic reactions should always be explained to the patient before starting therapy. Patients should be warned to report promptly any symptoms suggesting toxicity. Before each injection of gold sodium thiomalate the physician should review the results of laboratory work, and see the patient to determine the presence or absence of adverse reactions since some of these can be severe or even fatal.

DESCRIPTION

Gold sodium thiomalate is a sterile aqueous solution of gold sodium thiomalate. It contains 0.5% benzyl alcohol added as a preservative. The pH of the product is 5.8-6.5.

Gold sodium thiomalate is a mixture of the mono- and di-sodium salts of gold thiomalic acid.

The molecular weight for $C_4H_3AuNa_2O_4S$ (the disodium salt) is 390.07. The molecular weight for $C_4H_4AuNaO_4S$ (the mono-sodium salt) is 368.09.

Gold sodium thiomalate is supplied as a solution for intramuscular injection containing 25 or 50 mg of gold sodium thiomalate per ml.

Storage: Protect from light. Store container in carton until contents have been used.

INDICATIONS AND USAGE

Gold sodium thiomalate is indicated in the treatment of selected cases of active rheumatoid arthritis — both adult and juvenile type. The greatest benefit occurs in the early active stage. In late stages of the illness when cartilage and bone damage have occurred, gold can only check the progression of rheumatoid arthritis and prevent further structural damage to joints. It cannot repair damage caused by previously active disease.

Gold sodium thiomalate should be used only as *one part* of a complete program of therapy; alone it is not a complete treatment.

CONTRAINDICATIONS

The following are contraindications for using gold sodium thiomalate:

- Hypersensitivity to any component of this product.
- Severe toxicity resulting from previous exposure to gold or other heavy metals.
- Severe debilitation.
- Systemic lupus erythematosus.

WARNINGS

Before treatment is started, the patient's hemoglobin, erythrocyte, white blood cell, differential and platelet counts should be determined, and urinalysis should be done to serve as basic reference. Urine should be analyzed for protein and sediment changes prior to each injection. Complete blood counts including platelet estimation should be made before every second injection throughout treatment. The occurrence of purpura or ecchymoses at any time always requires a platelet count.

Danger signals of possible gold toxicity include: rapid reduction of hemoglobin, leukopenia below 4000 WBC/mm^3, eosinophilia above 5%, platelet decrease below 100,000/mm^3, albuminuria, hematuria, pruritus, skin eruption, stomatitis, or persistent diarrhea. No additional injections of gold sodium thiomalate should be given unless further studies show these abnormalities to be caused by conditions other than gold toxicity.

DOSAGE AND ADMINISTRATION

Gold sodium thiomalate should be administered only by intramuscular injection, preferably intragluteally. It should be given with the patient lying down. He should remain recumbent for approximately 10 minutes after the injection.

Therapeutic effects from gold sodium thiomalate occur slowly. Early improvement, often limited to a reduction in morning stiffness, may begin after 6-8 weeks of treatment, but beneficial effects may not be observed until after months of therapy.

Parenteral drug products should be inspected visually for particulate matter and discoloration prior to administration. Do not use if material has darkened. Color should not exceed pale yellow.

For the adult of average size the following dosage schedule is suggested:

Weekly Injections:

1st Injection: 10 mg.

2nd Injection: 25 mg.

3rd and Subsequent Injections: 25 to 50 mg until there is toxicity or major clinical improvement, or, in the absence of either of these, the cumulative dose of gold sodium thiomalate reaches 1 g.

Gold sodium thiomalate is continued until the cumulative dose reaches 1 g unless toxicity or major clinical improvement occurs. If significant clinical improvement occurs before a cumulative dose of 1 g has been administered, the dose may be decreased or the interval between injections increased as with maintenance therapy. Maintenance doses of 25 to 50 mg every other week for 2-20 weeks are recommended. If the clinical course remains stable, injections of 25 to 50 mg may be given every third and subsequently every fourth week indefinitely. Some patients may require maintenance treatment at intervals of 1-3 weeks. Should the arthritis exacerbate during maintenance therapy, weekly injections may be resumed temporarily until disease activity is suppressed.

Should a patient fail to improve during initial therapy (cumulative dose of 1 g), several options are available:

1. The patient may be considered to be unresponsive and gold sodium thiomalate is discontinued
2. The same dose (25-50 mg) of gold sodium thiomalate may be continued for approximately 10 additional weeks
3. The dose of gold sodium thiomalate may be increased by increments of 10 mg every 1-4 weeks, not to exceed 100 mg in a single injection.

If significant clinical improvement occurs using option 2 or 3, the maintenance schedule described above should be initiated. If there is no significant improvement or if toxicity occurs, therapy with gold sodium thiomalate should be stopped. The higher the individual dose of gold sodium thiomalate, the greater the risk of gold toxicity. Selection of one of these options for chrysotherapy should be based upon a number of factors including the physician's experience with gold salt therapy, the course of the patient's condition, the choice of alternative treatments, and the availability of the patient for the close supervision required.

JUVENILE RHEUMATOID ARTHRITIS

The pediatric dose of gold sodium thiomalate is proportional to the adult dose on a weight basis. After the initial test dose of 10 mg, the recommended dose for children is 1 mg/kg body weight, not to exceed 50 mg for a single in injection. Otherwise, the guidelines given above for administration to adults also apply to children.

Concomitant Drug Therapy

Gold salts should not be used concomitantly with penicillamine.

The safety of coadministration with cytotoxic drugs has not been established. Other measures, such as salicylates, other non-steroidal anti-inflammatory drugs, or systemic corticosteroids, may be continued when gold sodium thiomalate is initiated. After improvement commences, analgesic and anti-inflammatory drugs may be discontinued slowly as symptoms permit.

PRODUCT LISTING - EQUIVALENTS NOT AVAILABLE

Suspension - Intramuscular - 50 mg/ml

Size	Price	Product	NDC
1 ml	$16.75	GENERIC, Apotex Usa Inc	61147-8006-00
1 ml x 6	$57.26	GENERIC, Pasadena Research Laboratories Inc	00418-4450-01
1 ml x 6	$85.38	MYOCHRYSINE, Taylor Pharmaceuticals	11098-0533-01
6 ml	$74.78	GENERIC, Pasadena Research Laboratories Inc	00418-4450-21
10 ml	$108.50	GENERIC, Pasadena Research Laboratories Inc	00418-4450-10
10 ml	$118.11	MYOCHRYSINE, Taylor Pharmaceuticals	11098-0533-10
10 ml	$156.86	GENERIC, Apotex Usa Inc	61147-8006-03

Goserelin Acetate (001382)

Categories: Carcinoma, breast; Carcinoma, prostate; Endometriosis; Pregnancy Category X; FDA Approved 1989 Dec
Drug Classes: Antineoplastics, hormones/hormone modifiers; Hormones/hormone modifiers
Brand Names: Zoladex
Foreign Brand Availability: Prozoladex (Mexico); Zoladex Depot (South-Africa); Zoladex Implant (Australia; Austria; Belgium; Bulgaria; Czech-Republic; Denmark; England; Finland; France; Germany; Greece; Hungary; Ireland; Italy; Netherlands; Norway; Poland; Portugal; Slovenia; Spain; Sweden; Switzerland; Turkey); Zoladex Inj. (New-Zealand); Zoladex LA (Canada; Indonesia; Philippines; Singapore)
Cost of Therapy: $469.99 (Prostate Cancer; Zoladex Injection; 3.6 mg; 3.6 mg/month; 28 day supply)
HCFA JCODE(S): J9202 per 3.6 mg SC

DESCRIPTION

Goserelin acetate implant contains a potent synthetic decapeptide analogue of luteinizing hormone-releasing hormone (LHRH), also known as a gonadotropin releasing hormone (GnRH) agonist analogue. Goserelin acetate is chemically described as an acetate salt of [D-Ser(Bu^t)^6, Azgly^{10}]LHRH. Its chemical structure is pyro-Glu-His-Trp-Ser-Tyr-D-Ser(Bu^t)-Leu-Arg-Pro-Azgly-NH_2 acetate [$C_{59}H_{84}N_{18}O_{14}\cdot(C_2H_4O_2)_x$ where x = 1 to 2.4].

Goserelin acetate is an off-white powder with a molecular weight of 1269 Daltons (free base). It is freely soluble in glacial acetic acid. It is soluble in water, 0.1 M hydrochloric acid, 0.1 M sodium hydroxide, dimethylformamide and dimethyl sulfoxide. Goserelin acetate is practically insoluble in acetone, chloroform and ether.

Zoladex is supplied as a sterile, biodegradable product containing goserelin acetate equivalent to 3.6 mg (or 10.8 mg) of goserelin. Zoladex is designed for subcutaneous injection with continuous release over a 28-day (or 12-week) period. Goserelin acetate is dispersed in a matrix of D,L-lactic and glycolic acids copolymer (13.3-14.3 mg/dose) or (12.82–14.76 mg/dose) containing less than 2.5% (2%) acetic acid and up to 12% (10%) goserelin-related substances and presented as a sterile, white to cream colored 1-mm (1.5 mm) diameter cylinder, preloaded in a special single use syringe with a 16 gauge (14 gauge) needle and overwrapped in a sealed, light- and moisture-proof, aluminum foil laminate pouch containing a desiccant capsule.

Studies of the D,L-lactic and glycolic acids copolymer have indicated that it is completely biodegradable and has no demonstrable antigenic potential.

CLINICAL PHARMACOLOGY

MECHANISM OF ACTION

Goserelin acetate is a synthetic decapeptide analogue of LHRH. Goserelin acetate acts as a potent inhibitor of pituitary gonadotropin secretion when administered in the biodegradable formulation.

Following initial administration in males, goserelin acetate causes an initial increase in serum luteinizing hormone (LH) and follicle stimulating hormone (FSH) levels with subsequent increases in serum levels of testosterone. Chronic administration of goserelin acetate leads to sustained suppression of pituitary gonadotropins, and serum levels of testosterone consequently fall into the range normally seen in surgically castrated men approximately 21 days after initiation of therapy. This leads to accessory sex organ regression.

In animal and in *in vitro* studies, administration of goserelin resulted in the regression or inhibition of growth of the hormonally sensitive dimethylbenzanthracene (DMBA)-induced rat mammary tumor and Dunning R3327 prostate tumor.

In clinical trials using goserelin 3.6 mg with follow-up of more than 2 years, suppression of serum testosterone to castrate levels has been maintained for the duration of therapy.

In females (3.6 mg only), a similar down-regulation of the pituitary gland by chronic exposure to goserelin acetate leads to suppression of gonadotropin secretion, a decrease in serum estradiol to levels consistent with the postmenopausal state, and would be expected to lead to a reduction of ovarian size and function, reduction in the size of the uterus and mammary gland, as well as a regression of sex hormone-responsive tumors, if present. Serum estradiol is suppressed to levels similar to those observed in postmenopausal women within 3 weeks following initial administration; however, after supression was attained, isolated elevations of estradiol were seen in 10% of the patients enrolled in clinical trials. Serum LH and FSH are suppressed to follicular phase levels within 4 weeks after initial administration of the drug and are usually maintained in that range with continued use of goserelin acetate. In 5% or less of women treated with goserelin, FSH and LH levels may not be suppressed to follicular phase levels on day 28 post treatment with use of a single 3.6 mg depot injection. In certain individuals, suppression of any of these hormones to such levels may not be achieved with goserelin. Estradiol, LH and FSH levels return to pretreatment values within 12 weeks following the last implant administration in all but rare cases.

3.6 MG IMPLANT

Pharmacokinetics: The pharamcokinetics of goserelin have been determined in both male and female healthy volunteers and patients. In these studies, goserelin was administered as a single 250 mcg (aqueous solution) dose and as a single or multiple 3.6 mg depot dose by subcutaneous route. The absorption of radiolabeled drug was rapid, and the peak blood radioactivity levels occurred between 0.5 and 1.0 hour after dosing. The pharamcokinetic parameter estimates of goserelin after administration of 3.6 mg depot for 2 months in males and females are presented in TABLE 1.

TABLE 1 *Pharmacokinetic Parameters of 3.6 mg Implant*

Parameters (Units)	Males (n=7)	Females (n=9)
Peak Plasma Concentration (ng/ml)	2.84±1.81	1.46±0.82
Time to Peak Concentration (days)	12-15	8-22
Area Under the Curve (0-28 days)(ng.h/ml)	27.8±15.3	18.5±10.3
Systemic Clearance (ml/min)	110.5±47.5	163.9±71.0
*Apparent Volume of Distribution (L)	44.1±13.6	20.3±4.1
*Elimination Half-life (h)	4.2±1.1	2.3±0.6

* The apparent volume of distribution and the elimination half-life were determined after subcutaneous administration of 250 mcg aqueous solution of goserelin.

Pharmacokinetic data were obtained using a nonspecific RIA method.

Goserelin is released from the depot at a much slower rate initially for the first 8 days, and then there is more rapid and continuous release for the remainder of the 28–day dosing period. Despite the change in the releasing rate of goserelin, administration of goserelin every 28 days resulted in testosterone levels that were suppressed to and maintained in the range normally seen in surgically castrated men.

When goserelin 3.6 mg depot was used for treating male and female patients with normal renal and hepatic function, there was no significant evidence of drug accumulation. However, in clinical trials the minimum serum levels of a few patients were increased. These levels can be attributed to interpatient variation.

Distribution: The apparent volumes of distribution determined after subcutaneous administration of 250 mcg aqueous solution of goserelin were 44.1 and 20.3 liters for males and females, respectively. The plasma protein binding of goserelin obtained from one sample was found to be 27.3%.

Metabolism: Metabolism of goserelin, by hydrolysis of the C-terminal amino acids, is the major clearance mechanism. The major circulating component in serum appeared to be 1-7 fragment, and the major component presented in urine of one healthy male volunteer was 5-10 fragment. The metabolism of goserelin in humans yields a similar but narrow profile of metabolites to that found in other species. All metabolites found in humans have also been found in toxicology species.

Excretion: Clearance of goserelin following subcutaneous administration of the solution formulation of goserelin is very rapid and occurs via a combination of hepatic metabolism and urinary excretion. More than 90% of a subcutaneous, radiolabeled solution formulation dose of goserelin is excreted in urine. Approximately 20% of the dose in urine is accounted for by unchanged goserelin. The total body clearance of goserelin (administered subcutaneously as 3.6 mg depot) was significantly ($p<0.05$) greater (163.9 versus 110.5 ml/min) in females compared to males.

Special Populations: In clinical trials with the solution formulation of goserelin, male patients with impaired renal function (creatinine clearance <20 ml/min) had a total body clearance and serum elimination half-life of 31.5 ml/min and 12.1 hours, respectively, compared to 133 ml/min and 4.2 hours for subjects with normal renal function (creatinine clearance >70 ml/min). In females, the effects of reduced goserelin clearance due to impaired renal function on drug efficacy and toxicity are unknown. The total body clearances and serum elimination half-lives were similar between normal and hepatic impaired patients receiving 250 mcg solution formulation of goserelin. Pharmacokinetic studies using the aqueous formulation of goserelin in patients with renal and hepatic impairment do not indicate a need for dose adjustment with the use of the depot formulation.

10.8 MG IMPLANT

Pharmacokinetics: The pharmacokinetics of goserelin have been determined in healthy male volunteers and prostate cancer patients using an RIA method, which has been shown to be specific for goserelin in the presence of its metabolites.

The profiles for serum goserelin concentrations in prostate cancer patients administered three 3.6 mg depots followed by one 10.8 are primarily dependent upon the rate of drug release from the depots. For the 3.6 mg depot, mean concentrations gradually rise to reach a peak of about 3 ng/ml at around 15 days after administration and then decline to approximately 0.5 ng/ml by the end of the treatment period. For the 10.8 mg depot, mean concentrations increase to reach a peak of about 8 ng/ml within the first 24 hours and then decline rapidly up to Day 4. Thereafter, mean concentrations remain relatively stable in the range of about 0.3 to 1 ng/ml up to the end of the treatment period.

Absorption: The absorption of radiolabelled drug was rapid following administration as a single 250 mcg (aqueous solution) dose to volunteers by the subcutaneous route. The pharmacokinetics of goserelin following administration of goserelin acetate 10.8 mg depot to patients with prostate cancer are determined by the release of drug from the depot; representative data are summarized in TABLE 2.

G

Release of goserelin from the depot was relatively rapid shortly after administration resulting in peak concentration being observed 2 hours after dosing. Sustained release of goserelin produced a reasonably stable systemic exposure from Day 4 until the end of the 12-week dosing interval. This overall profile resulted in testosterone levels that were suppressed to and maintained within the range normally observed in surgically castrated men (0-1.73 nmol/L or 0-50 ng/dl), over the dosing interval in approximately 91% (145/160) of patients studied. In 6 of 15 patients that escaped from castrate range, serum testosterone levels were maintained below 2.0 nmol/L (58 ng/dl) and in only one of the 15 patients did the depot completely fail to maintain serum testosterone levels to within the recognized castrate range over a 336-day period (4 depot injections). In the 8 additional patients, a transient escape was followed 14 days later by a level within the castrate range. There is no clinically significant accumulation of goserelin following administration of four depots administered at 12-week intervals.

Distribution: The plasma protein-binding of goserelin is low (<30%).

Metabolism/Elimination: Clearance of goserelin following subcutaneous administration of the solution formulation of goserelin is very rapid and occurs via a combination of hepatic metabolism and urinary excretion. The metabolism of goserelin in humans yields a similar but narrow profile of metabolites to that found in other species. All the human metabolites have also been found in the toxicology species. The major component in serum was the 1-7 fragment formed by hydrolysis of the C-terminal amino acid.

Excretion: More than 90% of a subcutaneous radiolabelled solution formulation dose of goserelin is excreted in urine. Approximately 20% of the dose recovered in urine is accounted for by unchanged goserelin.

Special Populations

Renal Insufficiency: In clinical trials with the solution formulation of goserelin, subjects with impaired renal function (creatinine clearance less than 20 ml/min) had a serum elimination half-life of 12.1 hours compared to 4.2 hours for subjects with normal renal function (creatinine clearance greater than 70 ml/min). However, there was no evidence for any accumulation of goserelin on multiple dosing of the goserelin acetate 10.8 mg depot to subjects with impaired renal function. There was no evidence for any increase in incidence of adverse events in renally impaired patients administered the 10.8 mg depot. These data indicate that there is no need for any dosage adjustment when administering goserelin 10.8 mg to subjects with impaired renal function.

Hepatic Insufficiency: The clearance and half-life of goserelin administered as an aqueous solution are not affected by hepatic impairment. These data indicate that there is no need for any dosage adjustment when administering goserelin acetate 10.8 mg to subjects with impaired hepatic function.

Geriatric: There is no need for any dosage adjustment when administering goserelin acetate 10.8 mg to geriatric patients.

Body Weight: A decline of approximately 1 to 2.5% in the AUC after administration of a 10.8 mg depot was observed with a kilogram increase in body weight. In obese patients who have not responded clinically, testosterone levels should be monitored closely.

TABLE 2 *Goserelin Pharmacokinetic Parameters for the 10.8 mg Depot*

Parameter	n	Mean	SE	95% CI Lower	95% CI Upper
Systemic clearance (ml/min)	41	121	6.6	108	134
C_{max} (ng/ml)	41	8.85	0.44	7.96	9.74
T_{max} (h)	41	1.80	0.05	1.70	1.92
C_{min} (ng/ml)	44	0.37	0.03	0.30	0.43
Elimination Half-life (h)*	7	4.16	0.40	3.12	5.20

* determined after subcutaneous administration of 250 mcg aqueous soltion of goserelin.
SE =standard error of the mean
95% CI =95% confidence interval

INDICATIONS AND USAGE

Prostatic Carcinoma: Goserelin acetate is indicated in the palliative treatment of advanced carcinoma of the prostate. Goserelin offers an alternative treatment of prostatic cancer when orchiectomy or estrogen administration are either not indicated or unacceptable to the patient.

In controlled studies of patients with advanced prostatic cancer comparing goserelin 3.6 mg to orchiectomy, the long-term endocrine responses and objective responses were similar between the two treatment arms. Additionally, duration of survival was similar between the two treatment arms in a major comparative trial.

In controlled studies of patients with advanced prostatic cancer comparing goserelin acetate 10.8 mg implant produced pharmacodynamically similar effect in terms of supression of serum testosterone to that achieved with goserelin 3.6 mg implant. Clinical outcome similar to that produced with the use of the goserelin acetate 3.6 mg implant administered every 28 days is predicted with the goserelin acetate 10.8 mg implant administered every 12 weeks.

Endometriosis: Goserelin is indicated for the management of endometriosis; including pain relief and reduction of endometriotic lesions for the duration of therapy. Experience with goserelin for the management of endometriosis has been limited to women 18 years of age and older treated for 6 months.

Advanced Breast Cancer: Goserelin is indicated for use in the palliative treatment of advanced breast cancer in pre- and perimenopausal women.

The estrogen and progesterone receptor values may help to predict whether goserelin therapy is likely to be beneficial. (See CLINICAL PHARMACOLOGY.)

NON-FDA APPROVED INDICATIONS

G

Several studies on the use of goserelin in the treatment of uterine fibroids have demonstrated considerable reductions in fibroid size. One study which included 185 women concluded that in patients with uterine leiomyomata and anemia, goserelin acetate 3.6 mg once monthly in combination with iron therapy showed significant advantages over iron therapy alone in restoring hematologic normality, decreasing uterine and fibroid volumes and reducing operative blood loss. These uses are not approved by the FDA.

CONTRAINDICATIONS

A report of anaphylactic reaction to synthetic GnRH (Factrel) has been reported in medical literature. Goserelin is contraindicated in those patients who have a known hypersensitivity to LHRH, LHRH agonist analogues or any of the components in goserelin acetate.

Goserelin acetate 10.8 mg implant is not indicated in women as the data are insufficient to support reliable suppression of serum estradiol. (See INDICATIONS AND USAGE for female patients requiring treatment with goserelin.)

Goserelin is contraindicated in women being treated for endometriosis who are or may become pregnant while receiving the drug. In studies in rats and rabbits, goserelin increased preimplantation loss, resorptions, and abortions (see Pregnancy, Teratogenic Effects, Pregnancy Category X). In rats and dogs, goserelin suppressed ovarian function, decreased ovarian weight and size, and led to atropic changes in secondary sex organs. Further evidence suggests that fertility was reduced in female rats that became pregnant after goserelin was stopped. These effects are an expected consequence of the hormonal alterations produced by goserelin in humans. If a patient becomes pregnant during treatment, the drug must be discontinued and the patient must be apprised of the potential risk for loss of the pregnancy due to possible hormonal imbalance as a result of the expected pharmacologic action of goserelin treatment. In animal studies, there was no evidence that goserelin possessed the potential to cause teratogenicity in rabbits; however, in rats the incidence of umbilical hernia was significantly increased with treatment. (See Pregnancy, Teratogenic Effects, Pregnancy Category X)

Goserelin can cause fetal harm when administered to a pregnant woman. Effects on reproductive function, as a result of antigonadotrophic properties of the drug, are expected to occur on chronic administration.

Effective nonhormonal contraception must be used by all premenopausal women during goserelin therapy and for 12 weeks following discontinuation of therapy. There are no adequate and well-controlled studies in pregnant women using goserelin. If this drug is used during pregnancy, or the patient being treated for endometriosis becomes pregnant while taking this drug, the patient should be apprised of the potential hazard to the fetus or potential risk for loss of the pregnancy. Women of childbearing potential should be advised to avoid becoming pregnant.

For a description of findings in animal reproductive toxicity studies, (see WARNINGS).

Goserelin is contraindicated in women who are breast feeding (see Nursing Mothers).

WARNINGS

Before starting treatment with goserelin, pregnancy must be excluded. Safe use of goserelin in pregnancy has not been established. Goserelin can cause fetal harm when administered to a pregnant woman. Goserelin has been found to cross the placenta following subcutaneous administration of 50 and 1000 mcg/kg in rats and rabbits, respectively. Studies in both rats and rabbits at doses equal to or greater than 2 and 20 mcg/kg/day, respectively (about 1/10 and 2 times the daily maximum recommended dose, respectively, on a mg/m^2 basis), administered during the period of organogenesis, have confirmed that goserelin will increase pregnancy loss, and is embryotoxic/fetotoxic (characterized by increased preimplantation loss, increased resorption and an increase in umbilical hernia in rats at a dose of ≥10 mcg/kg/day [about 1/2 the recommended human dose on a mg/m^2 basis]; effects were dose-related. In additional reproduction studies in rats, goserelin was found to decrease fetus and pup survival.

There are no adequate and well-controlled studies in pregnant women using goserelin. Women of childbearing potential should be advised to avoid becoming pregnant.

When used every 28 days, goserelin usually inhibits ovulation and stops menstruation. Contraception is not ensured, however, by taking goserelin. During treatment, pregnancy must be avoided by the use of nonhormonal methods of contraception. If goserelin is used during pregnancy in a patient with advanced breast cancer or the patient becomes pregnant while receiving this drug, the patient must be apprised of the potential risk for loss of the pregnancy due to possible hormonal imbalance as a result of the expected pharmacologic action of goserelin treatment.

Following the last goserelin injection, nonhormonal methods of contraception must be continued until the return of menses or for at least 12 weeks. (See CONTRAINDICATIONS.)

Prostate and Breast Cancer: Initially, goserelin, like other LHRH agonists, causes transient increases in serum levels of testosterone in men with prostate cancer, and estrogen in women with breast cancer. Transient worsening of symptoms, or the occurrence of additional signs and symptoms of prostate or breast cancer, may occasionally develop during the first few weeks of goserelin treatment. A small number of patients may experience a temporary increase in bone pain, which can be managed symptomatically. As with other LHRH agonists, isolated cases of ureteral obstruction and spinal cord compression have been observed in patients with prostate cancer. If spinal cord compression or renal impairment develops, standard treatment of these complications should be instituted. For extreme cases in prostate cancer patients, an immediate orchiectomy should be considered.

As with other LHRH agonists or hormonal therapies (antiestrogens, estrogens, etc.), hypercalcemia has been reported in some prostate and breast cancer patients with bone metastases after starting treatment with goserelin. If hypercalcemia does occur, appropriate treatment measures should be initiated.

PRECAUTIONS

GENERAL

Hypersensitivity, antibody formation and anaphylactic reactions have been reported with LHRH agonist analogues.

Of 115 women worldwide treated with goserelin and tested for development of binding to goserelin following treatment with goserelin, one patient showed low-titer binding to goserelin. On further testing of this patient's plasma obtained following treatment, her goserelin binding component was found not to be precipitated with rabbit antihuman immunoglobulin polyvalent sera. These findings suggest the possibility of antibody formation.

INFORMATION FOR THE PATIENT

Males: The use of goserelin in patients at particular risk of developing ureteral obstruction or spinal cord compression should be considered carefully and the patients monitored closely during the first month of therapy. Patients with ureteral obstruction or spinal cord compression should have appropriate treatment prior to initiation of goserelin therapy.

Females: Patients must be made aware of the following information

1. Since menstruation should stop with effective doses of goserelin the patient should notify her physician if regular menstruation persists. Patients missing one or more successive doses of goserelin may experience breakthrough menstrual bleeding.
2. Goserelin should not be prescribed if the patient is pregnant, breast feeding, lactating, has nondiagnosed abnormal vaginal bleeding, or is allergic to any of the components of goserelin.
3. Use of goserelin in pregnancy is contraindicated in women being treated for endometriosis. Therefore, a nonhormonal method of contraception should be used during treatment. Patients should be advised that if they miss one or more successive doses of goserelin, breakthrough menstrual bleeding or ovulation may occur with the potential for conception. If a patient becomes pregnant during treatment for endometriosis, goserelin treatment should be discontinued and the patient should be advised of the possible risks to the pregnancy and fetus. (See CONTRAINDICATIONS.) For patients being treated for advanced breast cancer (see WARNINGS).
4. Those adverse events occurring most frequently in clinical studies with goserelin are associated with hypoestrogenism; of these the most frequently reported are hot flashes (flushes), headaches, vaginal dryness, emotional lability, change in libido, depression, sweating and change in breast size.
5. As with other LHRH agonist analogues, treatment with goserelin induces a hypoestrogenic state which results in a loss of bone mineral density (BMD) over the course of treatment, some of which may not be reversible. In patients with a history of prior treatment that may have resulted in bone mineral density loss and/or in patients with major risk factors for decreased bone mineral density such as chronic alcohol abuse and/or tobacco abuse, significant family history of osteoporosis, or chronic use of drugs that can reduce bone density such as anticonvulsants or corticosteroids, goserelin therapy may pose an additional risk. In these patients the risks and benefits must be weighed carefully before therapy with goserelin is instituted.
6. Currently, there are no clinical data on the effects of retreatment or treatment of benign gynecological conditions with goserelin for periods in excess of 6 months.
7. As with other hormonal interventions that disrupt the pituitary-gonadal axis, some patients may have delayed return to menses. The rare patient, however, may experience persistent amenorrhea.

DRUG/LABORATORY TEST INTERACTIONS

Administration of goserelin in therapeutic doses results in suppression of the pituitary-gonadal system. Because of this suppression, diagnostic tests of pituitary-gonadotropic and gonadal functions conducted during treatment and until the resumption of menses may show results which are misleading. Normal function is usually restored within 12 weeks after treatment is discontinued.

CARCINOGENESIS, MUTAGENESIS, AND IMPAIRMENT OF FERTILITY

The subcutaneous implant of goserelin in male and female rats once every 4 weeks for 1 year and recovery for 23 weeks at doses of about 80 and 150 mcg/kg (males) and 50 and 100 mcg/kg (females) daily (about 3 to 9 times the recommended human dose on a mg/m^2 basis) resulted in an incresed incidence of pituitary adenomas. An increased incidence of pituitary adenomas was also observed following subcutaneous implant of goserelin in rats at similar dose levels for a period of 72 weeks in males and 101 weeks in females. The relevance of the rat pituitary adenomas to humans has not been established. Subcutaneous implants of goserelin every 3 weeks for 2 years delivered to mice at doses of up to 2400 mcg/kg/day (about 70 times the recommended human dose on a mg/m^2 basis) resulted in an increased incidence of histiocytic sarcoma of the vertebral column and femur.

Mutagenicity tests using bacterial and mammalian systems for point mutations and cytogenetic effects have provided no evidence for mutagenic potential.

Administration of goserelin led to changes that were consistent with gonadal suppression in both male and female rats as a result of its endocrine action. In male rats administered 500-1000 mcg/kg/day (about 30-60 times the recommended human dose on a mg/m^2 basis), a decrease in weight and atrophic histological changes were observed in the testes, epididymis, seminal vesicle, and prostate gland with complete suppression of spermatogenesis. In female rats administered 50-1000 mcg/kg/day (about 3-60 times the recommended human dose on a mg/m^2 basis), suppression of ovarian function led to decreased size and weight of ovaries and secondary sex organs; follicular development was arrested at the antral stage and the corpora lutea were reduced in size and number. Except for the testes, almost complete histologic reversal of these effects in males and females was observed several weeks after dosing was stopped; however, fertility and general reproductive performance were reduced in those that became pregnant after goserelin was discontinued. Fertile matings occurred within 2 weeks after cessation of dosing, even though total recovery of reproductive function may not have occurred before mating took place; and, the ovulation rate, the corresponding implantation rate, and number of live fetuses were reduced.

Based on histological examination, drug effects on reproductive organs were reversible in male and female dogs administered 107-214 mcg/kg/day (about 20-40 times the recommended human dose on a mg/m^2 basis) when drug treatment was stopped after continuous administration for 1 year.

PREGNANCY, TERATOGENIC EFFECTS, PREGNANCY CATEGORY X

(See CONTRAINDICATIONS.) Goselerin 10.8 mg is not indicated in women as the data are insufficient to support reliable suppression of serum estradiol. Studies in both rats and rabbits at doses of 2, 10, 20 and 50 mcg/kg/day and 20, 250, and 1,000 mcg/kg/day, respectively (up to 1/10 to 3 times and 2 to 100 times the maximum recommended human dose, respectively, on a mg/m^2 basis) administered during the period of organogenesis, have confirmed that goserelin will increase pregnancy loss in a dose-related manner. While there was no evidence that goserelin possessed the potential to cause teratogenicity in rabbits, in rats the incidence of umbilical hernia was significantly increased at doses greater than 10 mcg/kg/day (about 1/2 the recommended dose on a mg/m^2 basis).

Nursing Mothers: Goserelin has been shown to be excreted in the milk of lactating rats. It is not known if this drug is excreted in human milk. Because many drugs are excreted in human milk and because of the potential for serious adverse reactions from goserelin in nursing infants, mothers receiving goserelin should discontinue nursing prior to taking the drug. (See CONTRAINDICATIONS.)

Pediatric Use: The safety and efficacy of goserelin in pediatric patients have not been established.

DRUG INTERACTIONS

No formal drug interaction studies with other drugs have been conducted with goserelin. No confirmed interactions have been reported between goserelin and other drugs.

ADVERSE REACTIONS

General: Rarely, hypersensitivity reactions (including urticaria and anaphylaxis) have been reported in patients receiving goserelin.

MALES

As with other endocrine therapies, hypercalcemia (increased calcium) has rarely been reported in cancer patients with bone metastases following initiation of treatment with goserelin or other LHRH agonists.

Goserelin has been found to be generally well tolerated in clinical trials. Adverse reactions reported in these trials were rarely severe enough to result in the patients' withdrawal from goserelin treatment. As seen with other hormonal therapies, the most commonly observed adverse events during goserelin therapy were due to the expected physiological effects from decreased testosterone levels. These included hot flashes, sexual dysfunction and decreased erections.

Initially, goserelin, like other LHRH agonists, causes transient increases in serum levels of testosterone. A small percentage of patients experienced a temporary worsening of signs and symptoms (see WARNINGS), usually manifested by an increase in cancer-related pain which was managed symptomatically. Isolated cases of exacerbation of disease symptoms, either ureteral obstruction or spinal cord compression, occurred at similar rates in controlled clinical trials with both goserelin and orchiectomy. The relationship of these events to therapy is uncertain.

In the controlled clinical trails of goserelin versus orchiectomy, the following events were reported as adverse reactions in greater than 5% of the patients.

TABLE 4 *Treatment Received*

Adverse Event	Goserelin (n=242) %	Orchiectomy (n=254) %
Hot Flashes	62	53
Sexual Dysfunction	21	15
Decreased Erections	18	16
Lower Urinary Tract Symptoms	13	8
Lethargy	8	4
Pain (worsened in the first 30 days)	8	3
Edema	7	8
Upper Respiratory Infection	7	2
Rash	6	1
Sweating	6	4
Anorexia	5	2
Chronic Obstructive Pulmonary Disease	5	3
Congestive Heart Failure	5	1
Dizziness	5	4
Insomnia	5	1
Nausea	5	2
Complications of Surgery	0	18†

† Complications related to surgery were reported in 18% of the orchiectomy patients, while only 3% of goserelin patients reported adverse reactions at the injection site. The surgical complications included scrotal infection (5.9%), groin pain (4.7%), wound seepage (3.1%), scrotal hematoma (2.8%), incisional discomfort (1.6%), and skin necrosis (1.2%).

The following additional adverse reactions were reported in greater than 1% but less than 5% of the patients treated with goserelin:

Cardiovascular: arrhythmia, cerebrovascular accident, hypertension, myocardial infarction, peripheral vascular disorder, chest pain;
Central Nervous System: anxiety, depression, headache;
Gastrointestinal: constipation, diarrhea, ulcer, vomiting;
Hematologic: anemia;
Metabolic/ Nutritional: gout, hyperglycemia, weight increase;
Miscellaneous: chills, fever;
Urogenital: renal insufficiency, urinary tract obstruction, urinary tract infection, breast swelling and tenderness.

FEMALES

As would be expected with a drug that results in hypoestrogenism, the most frequently reported adverse reactions were those related to this effect.

Endometriosis: In controlled clinical trials comparing goserelin every 28 days and danazol daily for the treatment of endometriosis, the events in TABLE 5 were reported at a frequency of 5% or greater.

TABLE 5 *Treatment Received*

Adverse Event	Goserelin (n=411) %	Danazol (n=207) %
Hot Flushes	96	67
Vaginitis	75	43
Headache	75	63
Emotional Lability	60	56
Libido Decreased	61	44
Sweating	45	30
Depression	54	48
Acne	42	55
Breast Atrophy	33	42
Seborrhea	26	52
Peripheral Edema	21	34
Breast Enlargement	18	15
Pelvic Symptoms	18	23
Pain	17	16
Dyspareunia	14	5
Libido Increased	12	19
Infection	13	11
Asthenia	11	13
Nausea	8	14
Hirsutism	7	15
Insomnia	11	4
Breast Pain	7	4
Abdominal Pain	7	7
Back Pain	7	13
Flu Syndrome	5	5
Dizziness	6	4
Application Site Reaction	6	-
Voice Alterations	3	8
Pharyngitis	5	2
Hair Disorders	4	11
Myalgia	3	11
Nervousness	3	5
Weight Gain	3	23
Leg Cramps	2	6
Increased Appetite	2	5
Pruritus	2	6
Hypertonia	1	10

The following adverse events not already listed above were reported at a frequency of 1% or greater, regardless of causality, in goserelin-treated women from all clinical trials:

Whole Body: allergic reaction, chest pain, fever, malaise;
Cardiovascular: hemorrhage, hypertension, migraine, palpitations, tachycardia;
Digestive: anorexia, constipation, diarrhea, dry mouth, dyspepsia, flatulence;
Hematologic: ecchymosis;
Metabolic and Nutritional: edema;
Musculoskeletal: arthralgia, joint disorder;
CNS: anxiety, paresthesia, somnolence, thinking abnormal;
Respiratory: bronchitis, cough increased, epistaxis, rhinitis, sinusitis;
Skin: alopecia, dry skin, rash, skin discoloration;
Special Senses: amblyopia, dry eyes;
Urogenital: dysmenorrhea, urinary frequency, urinary tract infection, vaginal hemorrhage.

Changes in Bone Mineral Density: After 6 months of goserelin treatment, 109 female patients treated with goserelin showed an average 4.3% decrease of vertebral trabecular bone mineral density (BMD) as compared to pretreatment values. BMD was measured by dual-photon absorptiometry or dual energy x-ray absorptiometry. Sixty-six of these patients were assessed for BMD loss 6 months after the completion (posttherapy) of the 6-month therapy period. Data from these patients showed an average 2.4% BMD loss compared to pretreatment values. Twenty-eight of the 109 patients were assessed for BMD at 12 months posttherapy. Data from these patients showed an average decrease of 2.5% in BMD compared to pretreatment values. These data suggest a possibility of partial reversibility.

CHANGES IN LABORATORY VALUES DURING TREATMENT

Plasma Enzymes: Elevation of liver enzymes (AST, ALT) have been reported in female patients exposed to goserelin 3.6 mg (representing less than 1% of all patients). There was no other evidence of abnormal liver function. Causality between these changes and goserelin have not been established.

Lipids: In a controlled trial, goserelin 3.6 mg therapy resulted in a minor, but statistically significant effect on serum lipids. In patients treated for endometriosis at 6 months following initiation of therapy, danazol treatment resulted in a mean increase in LDL cholesterol of 33.3 mg/dl and a decrease in HDL cholesterol of 21.3 mg/dl compared to increases of 21.3 and 2.7 mg/dl in LDL cholesterol and HDL cholesterol, respectively, for goserelin-treated patients. Triglycerides increased by 8.0 mg/dl in goserelin-treated patients compared to a decrease of 8.9 mg/dl in danazol-treated patients.

In patients treated for endometriosis, goserelin increased total cholesterol and LDL cholesterol during 6 months of treatment. However, goserelin therapy resulted in HDL cholesterol levels which were significantly higher relative to danazol therapy. At the end of 6 months of treatment, HDL cholesterol fractions (HDL_2 and HDL_3) were decreased by 13.5 and 7.7 mg/dl, respectively, for danazol-treated patients compared to treatment increases of 1.9 and 0.8 mg/dl, respectively, for goserelin treated patients.

Breast Cancer: The adverse event profile for women with advanced breast cancer treated with goserelin is consistent with the profile described above for women treated with goserelin for endometriosis. In a controlled clinical trial (SWOG-8692) comparing goserelin with oophorectomy in premenopausal and perimenopausal women with advanced breast cancer, the following events were reported at a frequency of 5% or greater in either treatment group regardless of causality.

G

TABLE 6 *Treatment Received*

Adverse Event	Goserelin (n=57) %	Oophorectomy (n=55) %
Hot Flashes	70	47
Tumor Flare	23	4
Nausea	11	7
Edema	5	0
Malaise/Fatigue/Lethargy	5	2
Vomiting	4	7

In the Phase II clinical trial program in 333 pre- and perimenopausal women with advanced breast cancer, hot flashes were reported in 75.9% of patients and decreased libido was noted in 47.7% of patients. These two adverse events reflect the pharmacological actions of goserelin.

Injection site reactions were reported in less than 1% of patients.

DOSAGE AND ADMINISTRATION

Goserelin, at a dosage of 3.6 mg, should be administered subcutaneously every 28 days into the upper abdominal wall using an aseptic technique under the supervision of a physician.

Goserelin, at a dosage of 10.8 mg, should be administered subcutaneously every 12 weeks into the upper abdominal wall using an aseptic technique under the supervision of a physician.

While a delay of a few days is permissible, every effort should be made to adhere to the 28-day or 12 week schedule.

For the management of advanced prostate cancer, goserelin is intended for long-term administration unless clinically inappropriate.

For the management of endometriosis, the recommended duration of administration is 6 months.

Currently, there are no clinical data on the effect of treatment of benign gynecological conditions with goserelin for periods in excess of 6 months.

Retreatment cannot be recommended for the management of endometriosis since safety data for retreatment are not available. If the symptoms of endometriosis recur after a course of therapy, and further treatment with goserelin is contemplated, consideration should be given to monitoring bone mineral density.

No dosage adjustment in necessary for patients with renal or hepatic impairment.

Administration Technique: The proper method of administration of goserelin is described in the instructions that follow.

1. The package should be inspected for damage prior to opening. If the package is damaged, the syringe should not be used. Do not remove the sterile syringe from the package until immediately before use. Examine the syringe for damage, and check that goserelin is visible in the translucent chamber.
2. Clean an area of skin of the upper abdominal wall with an alcohol swab. (A local anesthetic may be used in the normal fashion at the option of the administrator or patient.)
3. Grasp red (blue for 10.8 mg) plastic safety clip tab, pull out and away from needle, and discard immediately. Then remove needle cover.
4. Using an aseptic technique, stretch or pinch the patient's skin with one hand, and grip the syringe barrel. Insert the hypodermic needle into the subcutaneous tissue. *Note:* The goserelin syringe cannot be used for aspiration. If the hypodermic needle penetrates a large vessel, blood will be seen instantly in the syringe chamber. If a vessel is penetrated, withdraw the needle and inject with a new syringe elsewhere.
5. Change the direction of the needle so it parallels the abdominal wall. Push the needle in until the barrel hub touches the patient's skin. Withdraw the needle one centimeter to create a space to discharge goserelin. Fully depress the plunger to discharge goserelin.
6. Withdraw the needle. Then bandage the site. Confirm discharge of goserelin by ensuring tip of the plunger is visible within the tip of the needle. Dispose of the used needle and syringe in a safe manner. *Note:* In the unlikely event of the need to surgically remove goserelin, it may be localized by ultrasound.

HOW SUPPLIED

Zoladex is supplied as a sterile and totally biodegradable D,L-lactic and glycolic acids copolymer (13.3-14.3 mg/dose) impregnated with goserelin acetate equivalent to 3.6 mg or 10.8 mg of goserelin in a disposable syringe device fitted with a 16 gauge or 14 gauge hypodermic needle. The unit is sterile and comes in a sealed, light and moisture proof, aluminum foil laminate pouch containing a desiccant capsule.

Storage: Store at room temperature (do not exceed 25°C).

PRODUCT LISTING - EQUIVALENTS NOT AVAILABLE

Implant - Subcutaneous - 3.6 mg
1's $469.99 ZOLADEX, Astra-Zeneca Pharmaceuticals 00310-0960-36

Implant - Subcutaneous - 10.8 mg
1's $1409.98 ZOLADEX, Astra-Zeneca Pharmaceuticals 00310-0961-30

Granisetron Hydrochloride *(003157)*

Categories: Nausea, postoperative; Nausea, secondary to cancer chemotherapy; Vomiting, postoperative; Vomiting, secondary to cancer chemotherapy; FDA Approved 1993 Dec; Pregnancy Category B
Drug Classes: Antiemetics/antivertigo; Serotonin receptor antagonists
Brand Names: Kytril
Foreign Brand Availability: Granicip (India); Setron (Israel)
Cost of Therapy: $136.64 (Nausea; Kytril Injection; 1 mg/ml;4 ml; 0.7 ml/dose; variable day supply)
$94.09 (Nausea; Kytril; 1 mg; 2 tablets/day; 1 day supply)
HCFA JCODE(S): J1625 per 1 mg IV; J1626 100 µg IV

INTRAVENOUS

DESCRIPTION

Note: The trade names have been used throughout this monograph for clarity.

Kytril (granisetron hydrochloride) injection is an antinauseant and antiemetic agent. Chemically it is endo-N-(9-methyl-9-azabicyclo [3.3.1] non-3-yl)-1-methyl-1H-indazole-3-carboxamide hydrochloride with a molecular weight of 348.9 (312.4 free base). Its empirical formula is $C_{18}H_{24}N_4O{\cdot}HCl$.

Granisetron hydrochloride is a white to off-white solid that is readily soluble in water and normal saline at 20°C. Kytril injection is a clear, colorless, sterile, nonpyrogenic, aqueous solution for intravenous (IV) administration.

Kytril is available in 1 ml single-dose and 4 ml multi-dose vials:

Single-Dose Vials: Each 1 ml of preservative-free aqueous solution contains 1.12 mg granisetron hydrochloride equivalent to granisetron, 1 mg and sodium chloride, 9 mg. The solution's pH ranges from 4.7-7.3.

Multi-Dose Vials: Each 1 ml contains 1.12 mg granisetron hydrochloride equivalent to granisetron, 1 mg; sodium chloride, 9 mg; citric acid, 2 mg; benzyl alcohol, 10 mg, as a preservative. The solution's pH ranges from 4.0-6.0.

CLINICAL PHARMACOLOGY

Granisetron is a selective 5-hydroxytryptamine$_3$ (5-HT_3) receptor antagonist with little or no affinity for other serotonin receptors, including 5-HT_1; 5-HT_{1A}; 5-$HT_{1B/C}$; 5-HT_2; for alpha$_1$-, alpha$_2$- or beta-adrenoreceptors; for dopamine-D_2; or for histamine-H_1; benzodiazepine; picrotoxin, or opioid receptors.

Serotonin receptors of the 5-HT_3 type are located peripherally on vagal nerve terminals and centrally in the chemoreceptor trigger zone of the area postrema. During chemotherapy-induced vomiting, mucosal enterochromaffin cells release serotonin, which stimulates 5-HT_3 receptors. This evokes vagal afferent discharge, inducing vomiting. Animal studies demonstrate that, in binding to 5-HT_3 receptors, granisetron blocks serotonin stimulation and subsequent vomiting after emetogenic stimuli such as cisplatin. In the ferret animal model, a single granisetron injection prevented vomiting due to high-dose cisplatin or arrested vomiting within 5-30 seconds.

In most human studies, granisetron has had little effect on blood pressure, heart rate or ECG. No evidence of an effect on plasma prolactin or aldosterone concentrations has been found in other studies.

Kytril injection exhibited no effect on oro-cecal transit time in normal volunteers given a single IV infusion of 50 or 200 µg/kg. Single and multiple oral doses slowed colonic transit in normal volunteers.

PHARMACOKINETICS

Chemotherapy-Induced Nausea and Vomiting

In adult cancer patients undergoing chemotherapy and in volunteers, mean pharmacokinetic data obtained from an infusion of a single 40 µg/kg dose of Kytril Injection are shown in TABLE 1.

TABLE 1 *Pharmacokinetic Parameters in Adult Cancer Patients Undergoing Chemotherapy and in Volunteers, Following a Single IV 40 µg/kg Dose of Kytril Injection*

	Peak Plasma Concentration	Terminal Phase Plasma Half-Life	Total Clearance	Volume of Distribution
Cancer Patients				
Mean	63.8 ng/ml*	8.95 h*	0.38 L/h/kg*	3.07 L/kg*
Range	18.0-176 ng/ml	0.90-31.1 h	0.14-1.54 L/h/kg	0.85-10.4 L/kg
Volunteers				
21-42 years				
Mean	64.3 ng/ml†	4.91 h†	0.79 L/h/kg†	3.04 L/kg†
Range	11.2-182 ng/ml	0.88-15.2 h	0.20-2.56 L/h/kg	1.68-6.13 L/kg
65-81 years				
Mean	57.0 ng/ml†	7.69 h†	0.44 L/h/kg†	3.97 L/kg†
Range	14.6-153 ng/ml	2.65-17.7 h	0.17-1.06 L/h/kg	1.75-7.01 L/kg

* 5 minute infusion.
† 3 minute infusion.

Distribution: Plasma protein binding is approximately 65% and granisetron distributes freely between plasma and red blood cells.

Metabolism: Granisetron metabolism involves N-demethylation and aromatic ring oxidation followed by conjugation. *In vitro* liver microsomal studies show that granisetron's major route of metabolism is inhibited by ketoconazole, suggestive of metabolism mediated by the cytochrome P-450 3A subfamily. Animal studies suggest that some of the metabolites may also have 5-HT_3 receptor antagonist activity.
Elimination: Clearance is predominantly by hepatic metabolism. In normal volunteers, approximately 12% of the administered dose is eliminated unchanged in the urine in 48 hours. The remainder of the dose is excreted as metabolites, 49% in the urine, and 34% in the feces.

SUBPOPULATIONS

Gender

There was high inter- and intra-subject variability noted in these studies. No difference in mean AUC was found between males and females, although males had a higher C_{max} generally.

There was high inter- and intrasubject variability noted in these studies. No difference in mean AUC was found between males and females, although males had a higher C_{max} generally.

Geriatrics

The ranges of the pharmacokinetic parameters in geriatric volunteers (mean age 71 years), given a single 40 µg/kg intravenous dose of Kytril injection, were generally similar to those in younger healthy volunteers; mean values were lower for clearance and longer for half-life in the geriatric patients (see TABLE 1).

Pediatric Patients

A pharmacokinetic study in pediatric cancer patients (2-16 years of age), given a single 40 µg/kg intravenous dose of Kytril injection, showed that volume of distribution and total clearance increased with age. No relationship with age was observed for peak plasma concentration or terminal phase plasma half-life. When volume of distribution and total clearance are adjusted for body weight, the pharmacokinetics of granisetron are similar in pediatric and adult cancer patients.

Renal Failure Patients

Total clearance of granisetron was not affected in patients with severe renal failure who received a single 40 µg/kg intravenous dose of granisetron HCl injection.

Hepatically Impaired Patients

A pharmacokinetic study in patients with hepatic impairment due to neoplastic liver involvement showed that total clearance was approximately halved compared to patients without hepatic impairment. Given the wide variability in pharmacokinetic parameters noted in patients and the good tolerance of doses well above the recommended 10 µg/kg dose, dosage adjustment in patients with possible hepatic functional impairment is not necessary.

Postoperative Nausea and Vomiting

In adult patients (age range, 18-64 years) recovering from elective surgery and receiving general balanced anesthesia, mean pharmacokinetic data obtained from a single 1 mg dose of Kytril injection administered intravenously over 30 seconds are shown in TABLE 2.

TABLE 2 *Pharmacokinetic Parameters in 16 Adult Surgical Patients Following a Single Intravenous 1 mg Dose of Kytril injection Injection*

	Terminal Phase Plasma Half-life	Total Clearance	Volume of Distribution
Mean	8.63 h	0.28 L/h/kg	2.42 L/kg
Range	1.77-17.73 h	0.07-0.71 L/h/kg	0.71-4.13 L/kg

The pharmacokinetics of granisetron in patients undergoing surgery were similar to those seen in cancer patients undergoing chemotherapy.

INDICATIONS AND USAGE

Kytril Injection Is Indicated for:

- The prevention of nausea and vomiting associated with initial and repeat courses of emetogenic cancer therapy, including high-dose cisplatin.
- The prevention and treatment of postoperative nausea and vomiting. As with other antiemetics, routine prophylaxis is not recommended in patients in whom there is little expectation that nausea and/or vomiting will occur postoperatively. In patients where nausea and/or vomiting must be avoided during the postoperative period, Kytril injection is recommended even where the incidence of postoperative nausea and/or vomiting is low.

NON-FDA APPROVED INDICATIONS

Granisetron has also been used for the treatment of acute migraine headache.

CONTRAINDICATIONS

Kytril injection is contraindicated in patients with known hypersensitivity to the drug or to any of its components.

WARNINGS

Hypersensitivity reactions may occur in patients who have exhibited hypersensitivity to other selective 5-HT_3 receptor antagonists.

PRECAUTIONS

Kytril is not a drug that stimulates gastric or intestinal peristalsis. It should not be used instead of nasogastric suction. The use of Kytril in patients following abdominal surgery or in patients with chemotherapy-induced nausea and vomiting may mask a progressive ileus and/or gastric distention.

CARCINOGENESIS, MUTAGENESIS, AND IMPAIRMENT OF FERTILITY

In a 24 month carcinogenicity study, rats were treated orally with granisetron 1, 5 or 50 mg/kg/day (6, 30 or 300 mg/m^2/day). The 50 mg/kg/day dose was reduced to 25 mg/kg/day (150 mg/m^2/day) during week 59 due to toxicity. For a 50 kg person of average height (1.46 m^2 body surface area), these doses represent 16, 81 and 405 times the recommended clinical dose (0.37 mg/m^2, IV) on a body surface area basis. There was a statistically significant increase in the incidence of hepatocellular carcinomas and adenomas in males treated with 5 mg/kg/day (30 mg/m^2/day, 81 times the recommended human dose based on body surface area) and above, and in females treated with 25 mg/kg/day (150 mg/m^2/day, 405 times the recommended human dose based on body surface area). No increase in liver tumors was observed at a dose of 1 mg/kg/day (6 mg/m^2/day, 16 times the recommended human dose based on body surface area) in males and 5 mg/kg/day (30 mg/m^2/day, 81 times the recommended human dose based on body surface area) in females. In a 12 month oral toxicity study, treatment with granisetron 100 mg/kg/day (600 mg/m^2/day, 1622 times the recommended human dose based on body surface area) produced hepatocellular adenomas in male and female rats while no such tumors were found in the control rats. A 24 month mouse carcinogenicity study of granisetron did not show a statistically significant increase in tumor incidence, but the study was not conclusive.

Because of the tumor findings in rat studies, Kytril injection should be prescribed only at the dose and for the indication recommended (see INDICATIONS AND USAGE and DOSAGE AND ADMINISTRATION).

Granisetron was not mutagenic in *in vitro* Ames test and mouse lymphoma cell forward mutation assay, and *in vivo* mouse micronucleus test and *in vitro* and *ex vivo* rat hepatocyte UDS assays. It, however, produced a significant increase in UDS in HeLa cells *in vitro* and a significant increased incidence of cells with polyploidy in an *in vitro* human lymphocyte chromosomal aberration test.

Granisetron at subcutaneous doses up to 6 mg/kg/day (36 mg/m^2/day, 97 times the recommended human dose based on body surface area) was found to have no effect on fertility and reproductive performance of male and female rats.

PREGNANCY, TERATOGENIC EFFECTS, PREGNANCY CATEGORY B

Reproduction studies have been performed in pregnant rats at intravenous doses up to 9 mg/kg/day (54 mg/m^2/day, 146 times the recommended human dose based on body surface area) and pregnant rabbits at intravenous doses up to 3 mg/kg/day (35.4 mg/m^2/day, 96 times the recommended human dose based on body surface area) and have revealed no evidence of impaired fertility or harm to the fetus due to granisetron. There are, however, no adequate and well-controlled studies in pregnant women. Because animal reproduction studies are not always predictive of human response, this drug should be used during pregnancy only if clearly needed.

NURSING MOTHERS

It is not known whether granisetron is excreted in human milk. Because many drugs are excreted in human milk, caution should be exercised when Kytril injection is administered to a nursing woman.

PEDIATRIC USE

See DOSAGE AND ADMINISTRATION for use in chemotherapy-induced nausea and vomiting in children 2-16 years of age. Safety and effectiveness in children under 2 years of age have not been established. Safety and effectiveness of Kytril injection have not been established in children for the prevention or treatment of postoperative nausea or vomiting.

GERIATRIC USE

During chemotherapy clinical trials, 713 patients 65 years of age or older received Kytril injection. Effectiveness and safety were similar in patients of various ages.

During postoperative nausea and vomiting clinical trials , 168 patients 65 years of age or older, of which 47 were 75 years of age or older, received Kytril injection. Clinical studies of Kytril injection did not include sufficient numbers of subjects aged 65 years and over to determine whether they respond differently from younger subjects. Other reported clinical experience has not identified differences in responses between the elderly and younger patients.

DRUG INTERACTIONS

Granisetron does not induce or inhibit the cytochrome P-450 drug-metabolizing enzyme system. There have been no definitive drug-drug interaction studies to examine pharmacokinetic or pharmacodynamic interaction with other drugs, but in humans, Kytril injection has been safely administered with drugs representing benzodiazepines, neuroleptics and anti-ulcer medications commonly prescribed with antiemetic treatments. Kytril injection also does not appear to interact with emetogenic cancer chemotherapies. Because granisetron is metabolized by hepatic cytochrome P-450 drug-metabolizing enzymes, inducers or inhibitors of these enzymes may change the clearance and, hence, the half-life of granisetron.

ADVERSE REACTIONS

CHEMOTHERAPY-INDUCED NAUSEA AND VOMITING

The following have been reported during controlled clinical trials or in the routine management of patients. The percentage figures are based on clinical trial experience only. TABLE 10 gives the comparative frequencies of the 5 most commonly reported adverse events ($\geq$3%) in patients receiving Kytril injection, in single-day chemotherapy trials. These patients received chemotherapy, primarily cisplatin, and intravenous fluids during the 24 hour period following Kytril injection administration. Events were generally recorded over 7 days post-Kytril injection administration. In the absence of a placebo group, there is uncertainty as to how many of these events should be attributed to Kytril, except for headache, which was clearly more frequent than in comparison groups.

In over 3000 patients receiving Kytril injection (2-160 µg/kg) in single-day and multiple-day clinical trials with emetogenic cancer therapies, adverse events, other than those in TABLE 10, were observed; attribution of many of these events to Kytril is uncertain.

TABLE 10 *Principal Adverse Events in Clinical Trials — Single-Day Chemotherapy*

	Percent of Patients With Event	
	Kytril Injection 40 µg/kg (n=1268)	Comparator* (n=422)
Headache	14%	6%
Asthenia	5%	6%
Somnolence	4%	15%
Diarrhea	4%	6%
Constipation	3%	3%

* Metoclopramide/dexamethasone and phenothiazines/dexamethasone.

Hepatic: In comparative trials, mainly with cisplatin regimens, elevations of AST and ALT (>2 times the upper limit of normal) following administration of Kytril injection occurred in 2.8% and 3.3% of patients, respectively. These frequencies were not significantly different from those seen with comparators (AST: 2.1%; ALT: 2.4%).

Cardiovascular: Hypertension (2%); hypotension, arrhythmias such as sinus bradycardia, atrial fibrillation, varying degrees of A-V block, ventricular ectopy including non-sustained tachycardia, and ECG abnormalities have been observed rarely.

Central Nervous System: Agitation, anxiety, CNS stimulation and insomnia were seen in less than 2% of patients. Extrapyramidal syndrome occurred rarely and only in the presence of other drugs associated with this syndrome.

Hypersensitivity: Rare cases of hypersensitivity reactions, sometimes severe (*e.g.*, anaphylaxis, shortness of breath, hypotension, urticaria) have been reported.

Other: Fever (3%), taste disorder (2%), skin rashes (1%). In multiple-day comparative studies, fever occurred more frequently with Kytril injection (8.6%) than with comparative drugs (3.4%, P <0.014), which usually included dexamethasone.

POSTOPERATIVE NAUSEA AND VOMITING

The adverse events listed in TABLE 11 were reported in ≥2% of adults receiving Kytril injection 1 mg during controlled clinical trials.

TABLE 11 *Adverse Events ≥2%*

	Kytril injection (1 mg) (n=267)	Placebo (n=266)
Pain	10.1%	8.3%
Constipation	9.4%	12.0%
Anemia	9.4%	10.2%
Headache	8.6%	7.1%
Fever	7.9%	4.5%
Abdominal pain	6.0%	6.0%
Hepatic enzymes increased	5.6%	4.1%
Insomnia	4.9%	6.0%
Bradycardia	4.5%	5.3%
Dizziness	4.1%	3.4%
Leukocytosis	3.7%	4.1%
Anxiety	3.4%	3.8%
Hypotension	3.4%	3.8%
Diarrhea	3.4%	1.1%
Flatulence	3.0%	3.0%
Infection	3.0%	2.3%
Dyspepsia	3.0%	1.9%
Hypertension	2.6%	4.1%
Urinary tract infection	2.6%	3.4%
Oliguria	2.2%	1.5%
Coughing	2.2%	1.1%

In a clinical study conducted in Japan, the types of adverse events differed notably from those reported in TABLE 11. The adverse events in the Japanese study that occurred in ≥2% of patients and were more frequent with Kytril 1 mg than with placebo were: fever (56% to 50%), sputum increased (2.7% to 1.7%), and dermatitis (2.7% to 0%).

DOSAGE AND ADMINISTRATION

PREVENTION OF CHEMOTHERAPY-INDUCED NAUSEA AND VOMITING

The recommended dosage for Kytril injection is 10 µg/kg administered intravenously within 30 minutes before initiation of chemotherapy, and only on the day(s) chemotherapy is given.

Infusion Preparation

Kytril injection may be administered intravenously either undiluted over 30 seconds, or diluted with 0.9% sodium chloride or 5% dextrose and infused over 5 minutes.

Stability

Intravenous infusion of Kytril injection should be prepared at the time of administration. However, Kytril injection has been shown to be stable for at least 24 hours when diluted in 0.9% Sodium Chloride or 5% Dextrose and stored at room temperature under normal lighting conditions.

As a general precaution, Kytril injection should not be mixed in solution with other drugs. Parenteral drug products should be inspected visually for particulate matter and discoloration before administration whenever solution and container permit.

Pediatric Use

The recommended dose in pediatric patients 2-16 years of age is 10 µg/kg. Pediatric patients under 2 years of age have not been studied.

Geriatric Patients, Renal Failure Patients or Hepatically Impaired Patients

No dosage adjustment is recommended (see CLINICAL PHARMACOLOGY, Pharmacokinetics).

PREVENTION AND TREATMENT OF POSTOPERATIVE NAUSEA AND VOMITING

The recommended dosage for prevention of postoperative nausea and vomiting is 1 mg of Kytril, undiluted, administered intravenously over 30 seconds, before induction of anesthesia or immediately before reversal of anesthesia.

The recommended dosage for the treatment of nausea and/or vomiting after surgery is 1 mg of Kytril, undiluted, administered intravenously over 30 seconds.

Pediatric Use

Safety and effectiveness of Kytril injection injection have not been established in children for the prevention or treatment of postoperative nausea or vomiting.

Geriatric, Renal Failure or Hepatically Impaired Patients

No dosage adjustment is recommended (see CLINICAL PHARMACOLOGY, Pharmacokinetics).

HOW SUPPLIED

Kytril injection, 1 mg/ml (free base), is supplied in 1 ml Single-Use Vials and 4 ml Multi-Dose Vials.

STORAGE

Store single-dose vials and multi-dose vials at 25°C (77°F); excursions permitted to 15-30°C (59-86°F).

Once the multi-dose vial is penetrated, its contents should be used within 30 days.

Do not freeze. Protect from light.

ORAL

DESCRIPTION

Note: The trade names have been used throughout this monograph for clarity.

Kytril tablets and oral solution contain granisetron hydrochloride, an antinauseant and antiemetic agent. Chemically it is *endo*-N-(9-methyl-9-azabicyclo [3.3.1] non-3-yl)-1-methyl-1H-indazole-3-carboxamide hydrochloride with a molecular weight of 348.9 (312.4 free base). Its empirical formula is $C_{18}H_{24}N_4O·HCl$.

Granisetron hydrochloride is a white to off-white solid that is readily soluble in water and normal saline at 20°C.

TABLETS FOR ORAL ADMINISTRATION

Each white, triangular, biconvex, film-coated Kytril tablet contains 1.12 mg granisetron hydrochloride equivalent to granisetron, 1 mg. Inactive ingredients are: hydroxypropyl methylcellulose, lactose, magnesium stearate, microcrystalline cellulose, polyethylene glycol, polysorbate 80, sodium starch glycolate and titanium dioxide.

ORAL SOLUTION

Each 10 ml of clear, orange-colored, orange-flavored Kytril oral solution contains 2.24 mg of granisetron hydrochloride equivalent to 2 mg granisetron. Inactive ingredients: citric acid anhydrous, FD&C yellow no. 6, orange flavor, purified water, sodium benzoate, and sorbitol.

CLINICAL PHARMACOLOGY

Granisetron is a selective 5-hydroxytryptamine$_3$ (5-HT$_3$) receptor antagonist with little or no affinity for other serotonin receptors, including 5-HT$_1$; 5-HT$_{1A}$; 5-HT$_{1B/C}$; 5-HT$_2$; for alpha$_1$-, alpha$_2$- or beta-adrenoreceptors; for dopamine-D$_2$; or for histamine-H$_1$; benzodiazepine; picrotoxin, or opioid receptors.

Serotonin receptors of the 5-HT$_3$ type are located peripherally on vagal nerve terminals and centrally in the chemoreceptor trigger zone of the area postrema. During chemotherapy that induces vomiting, mucosal enterochromaffin cells release serotonin, which stimulates 5-HT$_3$ receptors. This evokes vagal afferent discharge, inducing vomiting. Animal studies demonstrate that, in binding to 5-HT$_3$ receptors, granisetron blocks serotonin stimulation and subsequent vomiting after emetogenic stimuli such as cisplatin. In the ferret animal model, a single granisetron injection prevented vomiting due to high-dose cisplatin or arrested vomiting within 5-30 seconds.

In most human studies, granisetron has had little effect on blood pressure, heart rate or ECG. No evidence of an effect on plasma prolactin or aldosterone concentrations has been found in other studies.

Following single and multiple oral doses, Kytril tablets slowed colonic transit in normal volunteers. However, Kytril had no effect on oro-cecal transit time in normal volunteers when given as a single IV infusion of 50 or 200 µg/kg.

PHARMACOKINETICS

In healthy volunteers and adult cancer patients undergoing chemotherapy, administration of Kytril tablets produced the following mean pharmacokinetic data (see TABLE 12).

The effects of gender on the pharmacokinetics of Kytril tablets have not been studied. However, after IV infusion of Kytril, no difference in mean AUC was found between males and females, although males had a higher C_{max} generally.

When Kytril tablets were administered with food, AUC was decreased by 5% and C_{max} increased by 30% in non-fasted healthy volunteers who received a single dose of 10 mg.

Granisetron metabolism involves N-demethylation and aromatic ring oxidation followed by conjugation. Animal studies suggest that some of the metabolites may also have 5-HT$_3$ receptor antagonist activity.

Clearance is predominantly by hepatic metabolism. In normal volunteers, approximately 11% of the orally administered dose is eliminated unchanged in the urine in 48 hours. The remainder of the dose is excreted as metabolites, 48% in the urine and 38% in the feces.

TABLE 12 *Pharmacokinetic Parameters (median [range]) Following Kytril Tablets*

	Peak Plasma Concentration (ng/ml)	Terminal Phase Plasma Half-Life (h)	Volume of Distribution (L/kg)	Total Clearance (L/h/kg)
Cancer Patients 1 mg bid, 7 days (n=27)	5.99 [0.63–30.9]	ND*	ND	0.52 [0.09-7.37]
Volunteers single 1 mg dose (n=39)	3.63 [0.27–9.14	6.23 [0.96-19.9]	3.94 [1.89-39.4]	0.41 [0.11-24.6]

* Not determined after oral administration; following a single IV dose of 40 μg/kg, terminal phase half-life was determined to be 8.95 hours.
ND = Not determined.

In vitro liver microsomal studies show that granisetron's major route of metabolism is inhibited by ketoconazole, suggestive of metabolism mediated by the cytochrome P-450 3A subfamily.

Plasma protein binding is approximately 65% and granisetron distributes freely between plasma and red blood cells.

A 2 mg dose of Kytril oral solution is bioequivalent to the corresponding dose of Kytril tablets (1 mg × 2) and may be used interchangeably.

In elderly and pediatric patients and in patients with renal failure or hepatic impairment, the pharmacokinetics of granisetron was determined following administration of IV Kytril:

Elderly: The ranges of the pharmacokinetic parameters in elderly volunteers (mean age 71 years), given a single 40 μg/kg IV dose of Kytril injection, were generally similar to those in younger healthy volunteers; mean values were lower for clearance and longer for half-life in the elderly.

Renal Failure Patients: Total clearance of granisetron was not affected in patients with severe renal failure who received a single 40 μg/kg IV dose of Kytril.

Hepatically Impaired Patients: A pharmacokinetic study with intravenous Kytril in patients with hepatic impairment due to neoplastic liver involvement showed that total clearance was approximately halved compared to patients without hepatic impairment. Given the wide variability in pharmacokinetic parameters noted in patients and the good tolerance of doses well above the recommended dose, dosage adjustment in patients with possible hepatic functional impairment is not necessary.

Pediatric Patients: A pharmacokinetic study in pediatric cancer patients (2-16 years of age), given a single 40 μg/kg IV dose of Kytril injection, showed that volume of distribution and total clearance increased with age. No relationship with age was observed for peak plasma concentration or terminal phase plasma half-life. When volume of distribution and total clearance are adjusted for body weight, the pharmacokinetics of granisetron are similar in pediatric and adult cancer patients.

INDICATIONS AND USAGE

Kytril Is Indicated for the Prevention of:

Nausea and vomiting associated with initial and repeat courses of emetogenic cancer therapy, including high-dose cisplatin.

Nausea and vomiting associated with radiation, including total body irradiation and fractionated abdominal radiation.

NON-FDA APPROVED INDICATIONS

Granisetron has also been used to prevent post-operative nausea and vomiting, and for the treatment of acute migraine headache.

CONTRAINDICATIONS

Kytril is contraindicated in patients with known hypersensitivity to the drug or any of its components.

PRECAUTIONS

CARCINOGENESIS, MUTAGENESIS, AND IMPAIRMENT OF FERTILITY

In a 24 month carcinogenicity study, rats were treated orally with granisetron 1, 5 or 50 mg/kg/day (6, 30 or 300 mg/m^2/day). The 50 mg/kg/day dose was reduced to 25 mg/kg/day (150 mg/m^2/day) during week 59 due to toxicity. For a 50 kg person of average height (1.46 m^2 body surface area), these doses represent 4, 20 and 101 times the recommended clinical dose (1.48 mg/m^2, oral) on a body surface area basis. There was a statistically significant increase in the incidence of hepatocellular carcinomas and adenomas in males treated with 5 mg/kg/day (30 mg/m^2/day, 20 times the recommended human dose based on body surface area) and above, and in females treated with 25 mg/kg/day (150 mg/m^2/day, 101 times the recommended human dose based on body surface area). No increase in liver tumors was observed at a dose of 1 mg/kg/day (6 mg/m^2/day, 4 times the recommended human dose based on body surface area) in males and 5 mg/kg/day (30 mg/m^2/day, 20 times the recommended human dose based on body surface area) in females. In a 12 month oral toxicity study, treatment with granisetron 100 mg/kg/day (600 mg/m^2/day, 405 times the recommended human dose based on body surface area) produced hepatocellular adenomas in male and female rats while no such tumors were found in the control rats. A 24 month mouse carcinogenicity study of granisetron did not show a statistically significant increase in tumor incidence, but the study was not conclusive.

Because of the tumor findings in rat studies, Kytril should be prescribed only at the dose and for the indication recommended (see INDICATIONS AND USAGE, and DOSAGE AND ADMINISTRATION).

Granisetron was not mutagenic in *in vitro* Ames test and mouse lymphoma cell forward mutation assay, and *in vivo* mouse micronucleus test and *in vitro* and *ex vivo* rat hepatocyte UDS assays. It, however, produced a significant increase in UDS in HeLa cells *in vitro* and a significant increased incidence of cells with polyploidy in an *in vitro* human lymphocyte chromosomal aberration test.

Granisetron at oral doses up to 100 mg/kg/day (600 mg/m^2/day, 405 times the recommended human dose based on body surface area) was found to have no effect on fertility and reproductive performance of male and female rats.

PREGNANCY, TERATOGENIC EFFECTS, PREGNANCY CATEGORY B

Reproduction studies have been performed in pregnant rats at oral doses up to 125 mg/kg/day (750 mg/m^2/day, 507 times the recommended human dose based on body surface area) and pregnant rabbits at oral doses up to 32 mg/kg/day (378 mg/m^2/day, 255 times the recommended human dose based on body surface area) and have revealed no evidence of impaired fertility or harm to the fetus due to granisetron. There are, however, no adequate and well-controlled studies in pregnant women. Because animal reproduction studies are not always predictive of human response, this drug should be used during pregnancy only if clearly needed.

NURSING MOTHERS

It is not known whether granisetron is excreted in human milk. Because many drugs are excreted in human milk, caution should be exercised when Kytril is administered to a nursing woman.

PEDIATRIC USE

Safety and effectiveness in pediatric patients have not been established.

GERIATRIC USE

During clinical trials, 325 patients 65 years of age or older received Kytril tablets; 298 were 65-74 years of age and 27 were 75 years of age or older. Efficacy and safety were maintained with increasing age.

DRUG INTERACTIONS

Granisetron does not induce or inhibit the cytochrome P-450 drug-metabolizing enzyme system. There have been no definitive drug-drug interaction studies to examine pharmacokinetic or pharmacodynamic interaction with other drugs but, in humans, Kytril injection has been safely administered with drugs representing benzodiazepines, neuroleptics and anti-ulcer medications commonly prescribed with antiemetic treatments. Kytril injection also does not appear to interact with emetogenic cancer chemotherapies. Because granisetron is metabolized by hepatic cytochrome P-450 drug-metabolizing enzymes, inducers or inhibitors of these enzymes may change the clearance and, hence, the half-life of granisetron.

ADVERSE REACTIONS

CHEMOTHERAPY-INDUCED NAUSEA AND VOMITING

Over 3700 patients have received Kytril tablets in clinical trials with emetogenic cancer therapies consisting primarily of cyclophosphamide or cisplatin regimens.

In patients receiving Kytril tablets 1 mg bid for 1, 7 or 14 days, or 2 mg qd for 1 day, TABLE 15 lists adverse experiences reported in more than 5% of the patients with comparator and placebo incidences.

TABLE 15 *Principal Adverse Events in Clinical Trials*

	Kytril Tablets*			
	1 mg bid (n=978)	2 mg qd (n=1450)	Comparator† (n=599)	Placebo (n=185)
Headache‡	21%	20%	13%	12%
Constipation	18%	14%	16%	8%
Asthenia	14%	18%	10%	4%
Diarrhea	8%	9%	10%	4%
Abdominal pain	6%	4%	6%	3%
Dyspepsia	4%	6%	5%	4%

* Adverse events were recorded for 7 days when Kytril tablets were given on a single day and for up to 28 days when Kytril tablets were administered for 7 or 14 days.
† Metoclopramide/dexamethasone; phenothiazines/dexamethasone; dexamethasone alone; prochlorperazine.
‡ Usually mild to moderate in severity.

Other adverse events reported in clinical trials were:

Gastrointestinal: In single-day dosing studies in which adverse events were collected for 7 days, nausea (20%) and vomiting (12%) were recorded as adverse events after the 24 hour efficacy assessment period.

Hepatic: In comparative trials, elevation of AST and ALT (>2 times the upper limit of normal) following the administration of Kytril tablets occurred in 5% and 6% of patients, respectively. These frequencies were not significantly different from those seen with comparators (AST: 2%; ALT: 9%).

Cardiovascular: Hypertension (1%); hypotension, angina pectoris, atrial fibrillation and syncope have been observed rarely.

Central Nervous System: Dizziness (5%), insomnia (5%), anxiety (2%), somnolence (1%). One case compatible with but not diagnostic of extrapyramidal symptoms has been reported in a patient treated with Kytril tablets.

Hypersensitivity: Rare cases of hypersensitivity reactions, sometimes severe (*e.g.*, anaphylaxis, shortness of breath, hypotension, urticaria) have been reported.

Other: Fever (5%). Events often associated with chemotherapy also have been reported: leukopenia (9%), decreased appetite (6%), anemia (4%), alopecia (3%), thrombocytopenia (2%).

Over 5000 patients have received injectable Kytril in clinical trials.

TABLE 16 gives the comparative frequencies of the 5 commonly reported adverse events (≥3%) in patients receiving Kytril injection, 40 μg/kg, in single-day chemotherapy trials. These patients received chemotherapy, primarily cisplatin, and intravenous fluids during the 24 hour period following Kytril injection administration.

TABLE 16 *Principal Adverse Events in Clinical Trials — Single-Day Chemotherapy*

	Kytril Injection* 40 µg/kg (n=1268)	Comparator (n=422)
Headache	14%	6%
Asthenia	5%	6%
Somnolence	4%	15%
Diarrhea	4%	6%
Constipation	3%	3%

* Adverse events were generally recorded over 7 days post-Kytril injection administration.
† Metoclopramide/dexamethasone and phenothiazines/dexamethasone.

In the absence of a placebo group, there is uncertainty as to how many of these events should be attributed to Kytril, except for headache, which was clearly more frequent than in comparison groups.

G

RADIATION-INDUCED NAUSEA AND VOMITING

In controlled clinical trials, the adverse events reported by patients receiving Kytril tablets and concurrent radiation were similar to those reported by patients receiving Kytril tablets prior to chemotherapy. The most frequently reported adverse events were diarrhea, asthenia and constipation. Headache, however, was less prevalent in this patient population.

DOSAGE AND ADMINISTRATION

EMETOGENIC CHEMOTHERAPY

The recommended adult dosage of oral Kytril is 2 mg once daily or 1 mg twice daily. In the 2 mg once-daily regimen, two 1 mg tablets or 10 ml of Kytril oral solution (2 teaspoonfuls, equivalent to 2 mg of granisetron) are given up to 1 hour before chemotherapy. In the 1 mg twice-daily regimen, the first 1 mg tablet or 1 teaspoonful (5 ml) of Kytril oral solution is given up to 1 hour before chemotherapy, and the second tablet or second teaspoonful (5 ml) of Kytril oral solution, 12 hours after the first. Either regimen is administered only on the day(s) chemotherapy is given. Continued treatment, while not on chemotherapy, has not been found to be useful.

Use in the elderly, pediatric patients, renal failure patients or hepatically impaired patients: No dosage adjustment is recommended (see CLINICAL PHARMACOLOGY, Pharmacokinetics).

RADIATION (EITHER TOTAL BODY IRRADIATION OR FRACTIONATED ABDOMINAL RADIATION)

The recommended adult dosage of oral Kytril is 2 mg once daily. Two 1 mg tablets or 10 ml of Kytril oral solution (2 teaspoonfuls, equivalent to 2 mg of granisetron) are taken within 1 hour of radiation.

Pediatric Use: There is no experience with oral Kytril in the prevention of radiation-induced nausea and vomiting in pediatric patients.

Use in the Elderly: No dosage adjustment is recommended.

HOW SUPPLIED

TABLETS

White, triangular, biconvex, film-coated tablets; tablets are debossed "K1" on one face.

Storage: Store between 15 and 30°C (59 and 86°F). Protect from light.

ORAL SOLUTION

Clear, orange-colored, orange-flavored, 2 mg/10 ml, in 30 ml amber glass bottles with child-resistant closures.

Storage: Store at 25°C (77°F); excursions permitted to 15-30°C (59-86°F). Keep bottle closed tightly and stored in an upright position. Protect from light.

PRODUCT LISTING - EQUIVALENTS NOT AVAILABLE

Solution - Intravenous - 1 mg/ml			
1 ml	$195.20	KYTRIL, Roche Laboratories	00004-0239-09
1 ml	$195.20	KYTRIL, Glaxosmithkline	00029-4149-01
4 ml	$780.80	KYTRIL, Roche Laboratories	00004-0240-09
4 ml	$780.80	KYTRIL, Glaxosmithkline	00029-4152-01
Solution - Oral - 2 mg/10 ml			
30 ml	$282.30	KYTRIL, Roche Laboratories	00004-0237-09
Tablet - Oral - 1 mg			
2's	$94.10	KYTRIL, Roche Laboratories	00004-0241-33
2's	$94.10	KYTRIL, Glaxosmithkline	00029-4151-39
6's	$282.30	KYTRIL, Allscripts Pharmaceutical Company	54569-4871-00
20's	$940.85	KYTRIL, Roche Laboratories	00004-0241-26
20's	$940.85	KYTRIL, Glaxosmithkline	00029-4151-05

Griseofulvin, Microcrystalline *(001388)*

For related information, see the comparative table section in Appendix A.

Categories: Tinea barbae; Tinea capitis; Tinea corporis; Tinea cruris; Tinea pedis; Tinea unguium; FDA Approved 1962 Aug; Pregnancy Category C; WHO Formulary
Drug Classes: Antifungals
Brand Names: Brofulin; Fulvicin U F; Grifulin; Grifulvin V; **Grisactin**; Microfulvin; Microgris
Foreign Brand Availability: Fulcin (Bulgaria; Ecuador; Peru); Fulcin Forte (Mexico); Fungin (Thailand); Grisefuline (France); Grisenova (Greece); Griseofulvin (England; Hungary); Griseofulvin Prafa (Indonesia); Griseofulvine (Netherlands); Grisflavin (Thailand); Grisfulvin V (Philippines); Grisovin (Australia; Bahrain; Cyprus; Egypt; Iran; Iraq; Jordan; Kuwait; Lebanon; Libya; Oman; Peru; Qatar; Republic-of-Yemen; Saudi-Arabia; Syria; United-Arab-Emirates); Grisovin-FP (India; Malaysia; Mexico); Grisuvin (Malaysia); Grivin (Malaysia); Krisovin (Malaysia); Likuden M (Germany); Microfulvin-500 (Indonesia); Mycostop (Indonesia)
Cost of Therapy: $105.41 (Tinea Pedis; Grifulvin V; 500 mg; 2 tablets/day; 28 day supply)
$52.70 (Tinea Corporis; Grifulvin V; 500 mg; 1 tablet/day; 28 day supply)

DESCRIPTION

Griseofulvin is an antibiotic derived from a species of *Penicillium.* Each Grifulvin V tablet contains either 250 or 500 mg of griseofulvin microsize, and also contains calcium stearate, colloidal silicon dioxide, starch, and wheat gluten. Additionally, the 250 mg tablet also contains dibasic calcium phosphate. Each 5 ml of Grifulvin V suspension contains 125 mg of griseofulvin microsize and also contains alcohol 0.2%, docusate sodium, FD&C red no. 40, FD&C yellow no. 6, flavors, magnesium aluminum silicate, menthol, methylparaben, propylene glycol, propylparaben, saccharin sodium, simethicone emulsion, sodium alginate, sucrose, and purified water.

CLINICAL PHARMACOLOGY

Griseofulvin acts systemically to inhibit the growth of *Trichophyton, Microsporum,* and *Epidermophyton* genera of fungi. Fungistatic amounts are deposited in the keratin, which is gradually exfoliated and replaced by noninfected tissue.

Griseofulvin absorption from the gastrointestinal tract varies considerably among individuals, mainly because of insolubility of the drug in aqueous media of the upper GI tract. The peak serum level found in fasting adults given 0.5 g occurs at about 4 hours and ranges between 0.5 and 2.0 µg/ml.

It should be noted that some individuals are consistently "poor absorbers" and tend to attain lower blood levels at all times. This may explain unsatisfactory therapeutic results in some patients. Better blood levels can probably be attained in most patients if the tablets are administered after a meal with a high fat content.

INDICATIONS AND USAGE

Major indications for griseofulvin are:

- Tinea capitis (ringworm of the scalp), Tinea corporis (ringworm of the body), Tinea pedis (athlete's foot), Tinea unguium (onychomycosis; ringworm of the nails), Tinea cruris (ringworm of the thigh), and Tinea barbae (barber's itch).

Griseofulvin inhibits the growth of those genera of fungi that commonly cause ringworm infections of the hair, skin, and nails, such as:

- *Trichophyton rubrum, Trichophyton tonsurans, Trichophyton mentagrophytes, Trichophyton interdigitalis, Trichophyton verrucosum, Trichophyton sulphureum, Trichophyton schoenleini, Microsporum audouini, Microsporum canis, Microsporum gypseum, Epidermophyton floccosum, Trichophyton megnini, Trichophyton gallinae,* and *Trichophyton crateriform.*

Note: Prior to therapy, the type of fungi responsible for the infection should be identified. The use of the drug is not justified in minor or trivial infections which will respond to topical anti-fungal agents alone.

It is *not* effective in:

- Bacterial infections, Candidiasis (Moniliasis), Histoplasmosis, Actinomycosis, Sporotrichosis, Chromoblastomycosis, Coccidioidomycosis, North American Blastomycosis, Cryptococcosis (Torulosis), Tinea versicolor, and Nocardiosis.

CONTRAINDICATIONS

This drug is contraindicated in patients with porphyria, hepatocellular failure, and in individuals with a history of hypersensitivity to griseofulvin.

Two (2) cases of conjoined twins have been reported in patients taking griseofulvin during the first trimester of pregnancy. Griseofulvin should not be prescribed to pregnant patients.

WARNINGS

Prophylactic Usage: Safety and efficacy of prophylactic use of this drug has not been established.

Chronic feeding of griseofulvin, at levels ranging from 0.5-2.5% of the diet, resulted in the development of liver tumors in several strains of mice, particularly in males. Smaller particle sizes result in an enhanced effect. Lower oral dosage levels have not been tested. Subcutaneous administration of relatively small doses of griseofulvin once a week during the first 3 weeks of life has also been reported to induce hepatomata in mice. Although studies in other animal species have not yielded evidence of tumorigenicity, these studies were not of adequate design to form a basis for conclusions in this regard.

In subacute toxicity studies, orally administered griseofulvin produced hepatocellular necrosis in mice, but this has not been seen in other species. Disturbances in porphyrin metabolism have been reported in griseofulvin-treated laboratory animals. Griseofulvin has been reported to have a colchicine-like effect on mitosis and cocarcinogenicity with methylcholanthrene in cutaneous tumor induction in laboratory animals.

Reports of animal studies in the Soviet literature state that a griseofulvin preparation was found to be embryotoxic and teratogenic on oral administration to pregnant Wistar rats. Rat reproduction studies done in the US and Great Britain were inconclusive in this regard. Pups with abnormalities have been reported in the litters of a few bitches treated with griseofulvin. Because the potential for adverse effects on the human fetus cannot be ruled out, additional contraceptive precautions should be taken during treatment with griseofulvin and for a month after termination of treatment. Griseofulvin should not be prescribed to women intending to become pregnant within 1 month following cessation of therapy.

Suppression of spermatogenesis has been reported to occur in rats but investigation in man failed to confirm this. Griseofulvin interferes with chromosomal distribution during cell division, causing aneuploidy in plant and mammalian cells. These effects have been demonstrated *in vitro* at concentrations that may be achieved in the serum with the recommended therapeutic dosage.

Since griseofulvin has demonstrated harmful effects *in vitro* on the genotype in bacteria, plants, and fungi, males should wait at least 6 months after completing griseofulvin therapy before fathering a child.

PRECAUTIONS

Patients on prolonged therapy with any potent medication should be under close observation. Periodic monitoring of organ system function, including renal, hepatic and hemopoietic, should be done.

Since griseofulvin is derived from species of penicillin, the possibility of cross sensitivity with penicillin exists; however, known penicillin-sensitive patients have been treated without difficulty.

Since a photosensitivity reaction is occasionally associated with griseofulvin therapy, patients should be warned to avoid exposure to intense natural or artificial sunlight. Should a photosensitivity reaction occur, lupus erythematosus may be aggravated.

DRUG INTERACTIONS

Patients on warfarin-type anticoagulant therapy may require dosage adjustment of the anticoagulant during and after griseofulvin therapy. Concomitant use of barbiturates usually depresses griseofulvin activity and may necessitate raising the dosage.

The concomitant administration of griseofulvin has been reported to reduce the efficacy of oral contraceptives and to increase the incidence of breakthrough bleeding.

ADVERSE REACTIONS

When adverse reactions occur, they are most commonly of the hypersensitivity type such as skin rashes, urticaria and rarely, angioneurotic edema or erythema multiforme-like drug reaction, and may necessitate withdrawal of therapy and appropriate countermeasures. Paresthesias of the hands and feet have been reported rarely after extended therapy. Other side effects reported occasionally are oral thrush, nausea, vomiting, epigastric distress, diarrhea, headache, fatigue, dizziness, insomnia, mental confusion and impairment of performance of routine activities.

Proteinuria and leukopenia have been reported rarely. Administration of the drug should be discontinued if granulocytopenia occurs.

When rare, serious reactions occur with griseofulvin, they are usually associated with high dosages, long periods of therapy, or both.

DOSAGE AND ADMINISTRATION

Accurate diagnosis of the infecting organism is essential. Identification should be made either by direct microscopic examination of a mounting of infected tissue in a solution of potassium hydroxide or by culture on an appropriate medium.

Medication must be continued until the infecting organism is completely eradicated as indicated by appropriate clinical or laboratory examination. Representative treatment periods are tinea capitis, 4-6 weeks; tinea corporis, 2-4 weeks; tinea pedis, 4-8 weeks; tinea unguium — depending on rate of growth — fingernails, at least 4 months; toenails, at least 6 months.

General measures in regard to hygiene should be observed to control sources of infection or reinfection. Concomitant use of appropriate topical agents is usually required, particularly in treatment of tinea pedis since in some forms of athlete's foot, yeasts and bacteria may be involved. Griseofulvin will not eradicate the bacterial or monilial infection.

Adults: A daily dose of 500 mg will give a satisfactory response in most patients with tinea corporis, tinea cruris, and tinea capitis.

For those fungus infections more difficult to eradicate such as tinea pedis and tinea unguium, a daily dose of 1.0 g is recommended.

Children: Approximately 5 mg/lb of body weight per day is an effective dose for most children. On this basis the following dosage schedule for children is suggested:

Children weighing 30-50 pounds: 125-250 mg daily.

Children weighing over 50 pounds: 250-500 mg daily.

HOW SUPPLIED

GRISEOFULVIN V TABLETS

250 mg: White, scored, imprinted "ORTHO 211".

500 mg: White, scored, imprinted "ORTHO 214".

Storage: STORE AT ROOM TEMPERATURE.

GRISEOFULVIN V SUSPENSION

Griseofulvin V Suspension 125 mg per 5 ml.

Storage: STORE AT ROOM TEMPERATURE.

PRODUCT LISTING - RATED THERAPEUTICALLY EQUIVALENT

Tablet - Oral - Microcrystalline 250 mg			
60's	$60.40	FULVICIN U/F, Schering Corporation	00085-0948-03
250's	$202.54	FULVICIN U/F, Schering Corporation	00085-0948-06
Tablet - Oral - Microcrystalline 500 mg			
60's	$62.59	GENERIC, Esi Lederle Generics	59911-5808-01
60's	$92.61	GRISACTIN 500, Wyeth-Ayerst Laboratories	00046-0444-60
60's	$103.50	FULVICIN U/F, Schering Corporation	00085-0496-03
100's	$188.23	GRIFULVIN V, Janssen Pharmaceuticals	00062-0214-60
250's	$391.90	FULVICIN U/F, Schering Corporation	00085-0496-06
Tablet - Oral - Ultramicrocrystalline 125 mg			
100's	$33.11	GENERIC, Warrick Pharmaceuticals Corporation	59930-1620-01
100's	$34.10	GENERIC, Martec Pharmaceuticals Inc	52555-0583-01
100's	$60.77	FULVICIN P/G, Schering Corporation	00085-0228-03
100's	$69.00	GRIS-PEG, Pedinol Pharmacal Inc	00884-0763-04
Tablet - Oral - Ultramicrocrystalline 165 mg			
100's	$47.65	GENERIC, Major Pharmaceuticals Inc	00904-0723-60
100's	$53.15	GENERIC, Sidmak Laboratories Inc	50111-0415-01
100's	$85.19	FULVICIN P/G, Schering Corporation	00085-0654-03
Tablet - Oral - Ultramicrocrystalline 250 mg			
100's	$64.96	GENERIC, Warrick Pharmaceuticals Corporation	59930-1621-01
100's	$73.40	GENERIC, Martec Pharmaceuticals Inc	52555-0584-01
100's	$79.00	GENERIC, Ivax Corporation	00182-1490-01
100's	$119.23	FULVICIN P/G, Schering Corporation	00085-0507-03
100's	$138.00	GRIS-PEG, Pedinol Pharmacal Inc	00884-0773-04
Tablet - Oral - Ultramicrocrystalline 330 mg			
100's	$82.25	GENERIC, Major Pharmaceuticals Inc	00904-0724-60
100's	$82.47	GENERIC, Warrick Pharmaceuticals Corporation	59930-1624-01
100's	$82.48	GENERIC, Qualitest Products Inc	00603-3771-21
100's	$84.50	GENERIC, Sidmak Laboratories Inc	50111-0416-01
100's	$87.85	GENERIC, Ivax Corporation	00182-1500-01
100's	$89.70	GENERIC, Martec Pharmaceuticals Inc	52555-0585-01
100's	$151.42	FULVICIN P/G, Schering Corporation	00085-0352-03

PRODUCT LISTING - EQUIVALENTS NOT AVAILABLE

Suspension - Oral - Microcrystalline 125 mg/5 ml			
120 ml	$31.10	GRIFULVIN V, Allscripts Pharmaceutical Company	54569-1739-01
120 ml	$39.28	GRIFULVIN V, Janssen Pharmaceuticals	00062-0206-04

Griseofulvin, Ultramicrocrystalline *(001389)*

For related information, see the comparative table section in Appendix A.

Categories: Tinea barbae; Tinea capitis; Tinea corporis; Tinea cruris; Tinea pedis; Tinea unguium; FDA Approved 1978 Feb; Pregnancy Category C; WHO Formulary
Drug Classes: Antifungals
Brand Names: Fulvicin P G; **Gris-Peg**; Grisactin Ultra; Griseofulvin Ultramicrosize; Ultragris; Ultramicrosize Griseofulvin
Foreign Brand Availability: Fulvina P G (Mexico); Griseofort (Indonesia); Griseostatin (Australia; Taiwan); Polygris (Germany); Sporostatin P G (Peru); Sporostatin U F (Ecuador; Philippines)
Cost of Therapy: $84.80 (Tinea Pedis; Fulvicin P/G; 330 mg; 2 tablets/day; 28 day supply)
$46.06 (Tinea Pedis; Generic tablets; 330 mg; 2 tablets/day; 28 day supply)
$42.40 (Tinea Corporis; Fulvicin P/G; 330 mg; 1 tablet/day; 28 day supply)
$23.03 (Tinea Corporis; Generic tablets; 330 mg; 1 tablet/day; 28 day supply)

DESCRIPTION

Griseofulvin tablets contain ultramicrosize crystals of griseofulvin, an antibiotic derived from a species of *Penicillium.* Griseofulvin crystals are partly dissolved in polyethylene glycol 6000 and partly dispersed throughout the tablet matrix.

Each griseofulvin tablet contains 125, 165, 250, or 330 mg griseofulvin ultramicrosize.

The inactive ingredients for griseofulvin tablets, 125 or 250 mg, include: corn starch, lactose, magnesium stearate, PEG, and sodium lauryl sulfate.

Storage: Store between 2-30°C (36-86°F).

CLINICAL PHARMACOLOGY

MICROBIOLOGY

Griseofulvin is fungistatic with *in vitro* activity against various species of *Microsporum, Epidermophyton,* and *Trichophyton.* It has no effect on bacteria or on the other genera of fungi.

HUMAN PHARMACOLOGY

Following oral administration, griseofulvin is deposited in the keratin precursor cells and has a greater affinity for diseased tissue. The drug is tightly bound to the new keratin which becomes highly resistant to fungal invasions.

The efficiency of gastrointestinal absorption of ultramicrocrystalline griseofulvin is approximately one and one-half times that of the conventional microsize griseofulvin. This factor permits the oral intake of two-thirds as much ultramicrocrystalline griseofulvin as the microsize form. However, there is currently no evidence that this lower dose confers any significant clinical difference with regard to safety and/or efficacy.

INDICATIONS AND USAGE

Griseofulvin tablets are indicated for the treatment of ringworm infections of the skin, hair, nails, namely: tinea corporis, tinea pedis, tinea cruris, tinea barbae, tinea capitis, tinea unguium (onychomycosis) when caused by one or more of the following genera of fungi: *trichophyton rubrum, trichophyton tonsurans, trichophyton mentagrophytes, trichophyton interdigitale, trichophyton verrucosum, trichophyton megninii, trichophyton gallinae, trichophyton craterifome, trichophyton sulphureum, trichophyton schoenleinii, microsporum audouini, microsporum canis, microsporum gypseum, and epidermophyton floccosum.*

Note: Prior to therapy, the type of fungi responsible for the infection should be identified. The use of this drug is not justified in minor or trivial infections which will respond to topical agents alone.

Griseofulvin is not effective in the following: bacterial infections, candidiasis (moniliasis), histoplasmosis, actinomycosis, sporotrichosis, chromoblastomycosis, coccidioidomycosis, North American blastomycosis, cryptococcosis, (torulosis), tinea versicolor, and nocardiosis.

CONTRAINDICATIONS

This drug is contraindicated in patients with porphyria, hepatocellular failure, and in individuals with a history of hypersensitivity to griseofulvin.

Rare cases of conjoined twins have been reported in patients taking griseofulvin during the first trimester of pregnancy. Griseofulvin should not be prescribed to pregnant patients or women contemplating pregnancy.

WARNINGS

PROPHYLACTIC USAGE

Safety and efficacy of griseofulvin for prophylaxis of fungal infections has not been established.

ANIMAL TOXICOLOGY

Chronic feeding of griseofulvin, at levels ranging from 0.5-2.5% of the diet, resulted in the development of liver tumors in several strains of mice, particularly in males. Smaller particle sizes result in an enhanced effect. Lower oral dosage levels have not been tested. Subcutaneous administration of relatively small doses of griseofulvin, once a week during the first 3 weeks of life has also been reported to induce hepatomata in mice. Thyroid tumors, mostly adenomas but some carcinomas, have been reported in male rats receiving griseofulvin at levels of 2.0%, 1.0%, and 0.2% of the diet, and in female rats receiving the two higher dose levels. Although studies in other animal species have not yielded evidence of tumorigenicity, these studies were not of adequate design to form a basis for conclusions in this regard.

In subacute toxicity studies, orally administered griseofulvin produced hepatocellular necrosis in mice, but this has not been seen in other species. Disturbances in porphyrin metabolism have been reported in griseofulvin-treated laboratory animals. Griseofulvin has been reported to have a colchicine-like effect on mitosis and cocarcinogenicity with methylcholanthrene in cutaneous tumor induction in laboratory animals.

USAGE IN PREGNANCY

The safety of this drug during pregnancy has not been established.

ANIMAL REPRODUCTION STUDIES

It has been reported in the literature that griseofulvin was found to be embryotoxic and teratogenic on oral administration to pregnant rats. Pups with abnormalities have been reported in the litters of a few bitches treated with griseofulvin. Additional animal reproduction studies are in progress.

Suppression of spermatogenesis has been reported to occur in rats, but investigation in man failed to confirm this.

PRECAUTIONS

Patients on prolonged therapy with any potent medication should be under close observation. Periodic monitoring of organ system function, including renal, hepatic, and hematopoietic, should be done.

Since griseofulvin is derived from species of *Penicillium,* the possibility of cross-sensitivity with penicillin exists; however, known penicillin sensitive patients have been treated without difficulty.

Since a photosensitivity reaction is occasionally associated with griseofulvin therapy, patients should be warned to avoid exposure to intense natural or artificial sunlight.

Lupus erythematosus, lupus-like syndromes, or exacerbation of existing lupus erythematosus have been reported in patients receiving griseofulvin.

DRUG INTERACTIONS

Griseofulvin decreases the activity of warfarin-type anticoagulants so that patients receiving these drugs concomitantly may require dosage adjustment of the anticoagulant during and after griseofulvin therapy.

Barbiturates usually depress griseofulvin activity and concomitant administration may require a dosage adjustment of the antifungal agent.

The effect of alcohol may be potentiated by griseofulvin, producing such effects as tachycardia and flush.

Griseofulvin may potentiate an increase in hepatic enzymes that metabolize estrogens at an increased rate, including the estrogen components of oral contraceptive effects and menstrual irregularities.

ADVERSE REACTIONS

When adverse reactions occur, they are most commonly of the hypersensitivity type such as skin rashes, urticaria, and rarely, angioneurotic edema, and may necessitate withdrawal of therapy and appropriate countermeasures. Paresthesias of the hands and feet have been reported rarely after extended therapy. Other side effects reported occasionally are oral thrush, nausea, vomiting, epigastric distress, diarrhea, headache, fatigue, dizziness, insomnia, mental confusion, and impairment of performance of routine activities.

Proteinuria and leukopenia have been reported rarely. Administration of the drug should be discontinued if granulocytopenia occurs.

When rare, serious reactions occur with griseofulvin, they are usually associated with high dosages, long periods of therapy, or both.

DOSAGE AND ADMINISTRATION

Accurate diagnosis of the infecting organism is essential. Identification should be made either by direct microscopic examination of a mounting of infected tissue in a solution of potassium hydroxide or by culture on an appropriate medium.

Medication must be continued until the infecting organism is completely eradicated as indicated by appropriate clinical or laboratory examination. Representative treatment periods are — *tinea capitis,* 4-6 weeks; *tinea corporis,* 2-4 weeks; *tinea pedis,* 4-8 weeks; *tinea unguium* — depending on rate of growth — fingernails, at least 4 months; toenails, at least 6 months.

General measures in regard to hygiene should be observed to control sources of infection or reinfection. Concomitant use of appropriate topical agents is usually required, particularly in treatment of *tinea pedis.* In some forms of athlete's foot, yeasts and bacteria may be involved as well as fungi. Griseofulvin will not eradicate the bacterial or monilial infection.

ADULTS

Daily administration of 330 mg (as a single dose or in divided doses) will give a satisfactory response in most patients with tinea corporis, tinea cruris, and tinea capitis. For those fungal infections more difficult to eradicate such as tinea pedis and tinea unguium, a divided dose of 660 mg is recommended.

CHILDREN

Approximately 3.3 mg/lb of body weight per day of ultramicrosize griseofulvin is an effective dose for most children. On this basis, the following dosage schedules are suggested:

Children weighing 35-50 pounds: 82.5 mg to 165 mg daily. Children weighing over 50 pounds: 165 mg to 330 mg daily.

Children 2 years of age and younger: dosage has not been established.

Clinical experience with griseofulvin in children with tinea capitis indicates that a single daily dose is effective. Clinical relapse will occur if the medication is not continued until the infecting organism is eradicated.

Guaifenesin *(001391)*

Categories: Cough; Pregnancy Category C; FDA Pre 1938 Drugs
Drug Classes: Expectorants
Brand Names: Fenex La; Fenesin; **Humibid L.A.**; Muco-Fen-La; Mucobid-L.A.; Organidin Nr; Pneumomist; Prolex; Touro Ex; Tussin
Foreign Brand Availability: 44 Exp (Mexico); Balminil Expectorant (Canada); Bronchocol (Israel); Codimal (Philippines); Desbly (France); Dextricyl (Philippines); Ecolate (Thailand); Excaugh 100 (Hong-Kong); Expectorin Cough (Philippines); Fagusan N Losung (Germany); Flemonex (Philippines); Pharmachem (Philippines); Probat (Indonesia); Resyl (Ecuador; Switzerland); Resyl S (Finland; Sweden); Robitussin (Australia; Bahamas; Bahrain; Barbados; Belize; Bermuda; Canada; Colombia; Curacao; Cyprus; Egypt; England; Finland; Guyana; Hong-Kong; Iran; Iraq; Ireland; Israel; Italy; Jamaica; Jordan; Kuwait; Lebanon; Libya; Malaysia; Netherland-Antilles; Oman; Philippines; Qatar; Republic-of-Yemen; Saudi-Arabia; Spain; Surinam; Sweden; Syria; Taiwan; Thailand; Trinidad; United-Arab-Emirates); Robitussin jarabe (Ecuador); Sipla (Indonesia); Suprekof (Philippines); Tintus (Finland); Transpulmin G (Philippines)
Cost of Therapy: $8.12 (Cough; Humibid L.A.; 600 mg; 2 tablets/day; 7 day supply)
$2.40 (Cough; Generic Tablets; 600 mg; 2 tablets/day; 7 day supply)

DESCRIPTION

Each Humibid L.A. light green scored, sustained-release tablet provides 600 mg guaifenesin. *Inactive ingredients:* Dicalcium phosphate, methocel, magnesium stearate, silicon dioxide, stearic acid, FD&C blue no. 1 lake, D&C yellow no. 10 lake. Chemically, guaifenesin is 3-(2-methoxyphenoxy)-1, 2-propanediol.

Storage: Store at controlled room temperature between 15-30°C (59-86°F). Dispense in tight containers.

CLINICAL PHARMACOLOGY

Guaifenesin is an expectorant which increases respiratory tract fluid secretions and helps to loosen phlegm and bronchial secretions. By reducing the viscosity of secretions, guaifenesin increases the efficiency of the cough reflex and of ciliary action in removing accumulated secretions from the trachea and bronchi. Guaifenesin is readily absorbed from the gastrointestinal tract and is rapidly metabolized and excreted in the urine. Guaifenesin has a plasma half-life of 1 hour. The major urinary metabolite is B-(2-methoxyphenoxy) lactic acid.

INDICATIONS AND USAGE

Guaifenesin tablets are indicated for the temporary relief of coughs associated with respiratory tract infections and related conditions such as sinusitis, pharyngitis, bronchitis, and asthma, when these conditions are complicated by tenacious mucus and/or mucus plugs and congestion. The drug is effective in productive as well as non-productive cough, but is of particular value in dry, non-productive cough which tends to injure the mucous membrane of the air passages.

CONTRAINDICATIONS

This drug is contraindicated in patients with hypersensitivity to guaifenesin.

PRECAUTIONS

GENERAL

Before prescribing medication to suppress or modify cough, it is important to ascertain that the underlying cause of cough is identified, that modification of cough does not increase the risk of clinical or physiological complications, and that appropriate therapy for the primary disease is instituted.

DRUG/LABORATORY TEST INTERACTIONS

Guaifenesin may increase renal clearance for urate and thereby lower serum uric acid levels. Guaifenesin may produce an increase in urinary 5-hydroxy-indoleacetic acid and may therefore interfere with the interpretation of this test for the diagnosis of carcinoid syndrome. It may also falsely elevate the VMA test for catechols. Administration of this drug should be discontinued 48 hours prior to the collection of urine specimens for such tests.

CARCINOGENESIS, MUTAGENESIS, AND IMPAIRMENT OF FERTILITY

No data are available on the long-term potential for carcinogenesis, mutagenesis, or impairment of fertility in animals or humans.

PREGNANCY CATEGORY C

Animal reproduction studies have not been conducted with guaifenesin. It is also not known whether guaifenesin can cause fetal harm when administered to a pregnant woman or can affect reproduction capacity. Guaifenesin should be given to a pregnant woman only if clearly needed.

NURSING MOTHERS

It is not known whether guaifenesin is excreted in human milk. Because many drugs are excreted in human milk, caution should be exercised when guaifenesin is administered to a nursing woman and a decision should be made whether to discontinue nursing or to discontinue the drug, taking into account the importance of the drug to the mother.

ADVERSE REACTIONS

No serious side effects from guaifenesin have been reported.

DOSAGE AND ADMINISTRATION

Adults and children over 12 years of age: One or two tablets every 12 hours not to exceed 4 tablets (2400 mg) in 24 hours.

Children 6-12 years: One tablet every 12 hours not to exceed 2 tablets (1200 mg) in 24 hours.

Children 2-6 years: ½ tablet every 12 hours not to exceed 1 tablet (600 mg) in 24 hours.

PRODUCT LISTING - RATED THERAPEUTICALLY EQUIVALENT

Tablet, Extended Release - Oral - 600 mg

100's	$25.62	GENERIC, Ecr Pharmaceuticals	00095-0600-01

PRODUCT LISTING - EQUIVALENTS NOT AVAILABLE

Capsule, Extended Release - Oral - 300 mg

100's	$55.73	HUMIBID PEDIATRIC, Celltech Pharmacuetica ls Inc	53014-0402-10

Liquid - Oral - 100 mg/5 ml

480 ml	$36.95	GENERIC, Cypress Pharmaceutical Inc	60258-0256-16
480 ml	$37.15	GENERIC, Qualitest Products Inc	00603-1328-58

Tablet - Oral - 200 mg

100's	$10.94	GENERIC, Moore, H.L. Drug Exchange Inc	00839-7977-06
100's	$19.95	GENERIC, Qualitest Products Inc	00603-4885-21
100's	$20.15	GENERIC, Trinity Technologies Corporation	61355-0502-10
100's	$23.95	GENERIC, Major Pharmaceuticals Inc	00904-5154-60
100's	$23.95	GENERIC, Econolab	55053-0270-01
100's	$24.92	GENERIC, Alphagen Laboratories Inc	59743-0019-01
100's	$24.95	IOFEN, Superior Pharmaceutical Company	00144-1645-01
100's	$26.26	GENERIC, Aligen Independent Laboratories Inc	00405-4455-01
100's	$26.50	GENERIC, Integrity Pharmaceutical Corporation	64731-0275-01
100's	$31.49	GENERIC, Ivax Corporation	00182-2614-01
100's	$31.49	GENERIC, Mutual/United Research Laboratories	00677-1661-01
100's	$53.24	ORGANIDIN NR, Wallace Laboratories	00037-4312-01

Tablet, Extended Release - Oral - 575 mg

100's	$43.00	TOURO EX, Dartmouth Pharmaceuticals Inc	58869-0421-01

Tablet, Extended Release - Oral - 600 mg

2's	$3.41	GENERIC, Prescript Pharmaceuticals	00247-0266-02
3's	$3.44	GENERIC, Prescript Pharmaceuticals	00247-0266-03
8's	$4.58	GENERIC, Southwood Pharmaceuticals Inc	58016-0150-08
10's	$3.62	GENERIC, Prescript Pharmaceuticals	00247-0266-10
10's	$3.87	GENERIC, Pharmaceutical Corporation Of America	51655-0948-53
12's	$3.67	GENERIC, Prescript Pharmaceuticals	00247-0266-12
14's	$3.73	GENERIC, Prescript Pharmaceuticals	00247-0266-14
14's	$4.42	GENERIC, Allscripts Pharmaceutical Company	54569-4392-03
14's	$5.84	GENERIC, Pharma Pac	52959-0438-14
14's	$6.92	GENERIC, Cheshire Drugs	55175-2696-01
14's	$7.07	HUMIBID L.A., Allscripts Pharmaceutical Company	54569-1489-05
15's	$3.75	GENERIC, Prescript Pharmaceuticals	00247-0266-15
20's	$3.88	GENERIC, Prescript Pharmaceuticals	00247-0266-20
20's	$3.98	GENERIC, Pd-Rx Pharmaceuticals	55289-0598-20
20's	$6.31	GENERIC, Allscripts Pharmaceutical Company	54569-4392-01
20's	$6.69	GENERIC, Pharmaceutical Corporation Of America	51655-0948-52
20's	$8.25	GENERIC, Cheshire Drugs	55175-2696-02
20's	$10.50	GENERIC, Pharma Pac	52959-0438-20
20's	$11.27	GENERIC, Adams Laboratories	63824-0008-20
20's	$17.18	HUMIBID L.A., Pd-Rx Pharmaceuticals	55289-0461-20
24's	$3.99	GENERIC, Prescript Pharmaceuticals	00247-0266-24
28's	$9.44	GENERIC, Pharma Pac	52959-0438-28
30's	$4.15	GENERIC, Prescript Pharmaceuticals	00247-0266-30
30's	$4.88	GENERIC, Pd-Rx Pharmaceuticals	55289-0598-30
30's	$9.62	GENERIC, Allscripts Pharmaceutical Company	54569-4392-00
30's	$10.43	GENERIC, Allscripts Pharmaceutical Company	54569-3928-00
30's	$15.14	HUMIBID L.A., Allscripts Pharmaceutical Company	54569-1489-01
30's	$16.75	GENERIC, Southwood Pharmaceuticals Inc	58016-0792-30
30's	$24.69	HUMIBID L.A., Pd-Rx Pharmaceuticals	55289-0461-30
31 x 10	$93.75	GENERIC, Vangard Labs	00615-4524-53
31 x 10	$93.75	GENERIC, Vangard Labs	00615-4524-63
40's	$12.60	GENERIC, Allscripts Pharmaceutical Company	54569-4392-02
40's	$13.20	GENERIC, Cheshire Drugs	55175-2696-04
40's	$18.46	GENERIC, Pharma Pac	52959-0438-40
40's	$20.19	HUMIBID L.A., Allscripts Pharmaceutical Company	54569-1489-03
40's	$23.79	GENERIC, Adams Laboratories	63824-0008-40
40's	$30.85	HUMIBID L.A., Pharma Pac	52959-0189-40
50's	$42.86	HUMIBID L.A., Pd-Rx Pharmaceuticals	55289-0461-50
60's	$30.41	GENERIC, Southwood Pharmaceuticals Inc	58016-0792-60
100's	$12.80	GENERIC, Htd Pharmaceutical	60354-0004-01
100's	$17.15	GENERIC, Alphagen Laboratories Inc	59743-0018-01
100's	$18.56	GENERIC, Moore, H.L. Drug Exchange Inc	00839-7655-06
100's	$21.95	GENERIC, Iomed Laboratories Inc	61646-0125-01
100's	$22.50	GENERIC, Vintage Pharmaceuticals Inc	00254-5312-28
100's	$23.95	GENERIC, Major Pharmaceuticals Inc	00904-7759-60
100's	$24.92	GENERIC, Tmk Pharmaceuticals	59582-0001-01
100's	$25.00	GENERIC, We Pharmaceuticals Inc	59196-0008-01
100's	$25.00	GENERIC, Trinity Technologies Corporation	61355-0501-10
100's	$25.65	GENERIC, Respa Pharmaceuticals Inc	60575-0786-19
100's	$26.00	GENERIC, Caraco Pharmaceutical Laboratories	57664-0152-08
100's	$26.20	GENERIC, Aligen Independent Laboratories Inc	00405-4457-01
100's	$26.45	GENERIC, Md Pharmaceutical Inc	43567-0501-07
100's	$26.80	GENERIC, Martec Pharmaceuticals Inc	52555-0628-01
100's	$29.00	GENERIC, King Pharmaceuticals Inc	60793-0049-01
100's	$29.17	GENERIC, Roberts/Hauck Pharmaceutical Corporation	43797-0048-03
100's	$29.17	GENERIC, Roberts/Hauck Pharmaceutical Corporation	59441-0152-01
100's	$30.96	GENERIC, Marnel Pharmaceuticals Inc	00682-0006-01
100's	$31.00	GENERIC, Ion Laboratories Inc	11808-0300-01
100's	$31.93	GENERIC, Capellon Pharmaceuticals	64543-0131-01
100's	$31.95	GENERIC, Monarch Pharmaceuticals Inc	61570-0026-01
100's	$32.50	GENERIC, Dura Pharmaceuticals	51479-0009-01
100's	$34.73	GENERIC, Ethex Corporation	58177-0205-04
100's	$34.76	GENERIC, Dj Pharma Inc	64455-0009-01
100's	$36.35	GENERIC, Ivax Corporation	00182-1188-01
100's	$36.35	GENERIC, Duramed Pharmaceuticals Inc	51285-0417-02
100's	$40.37	GENERIC, Qualitest Products Inc	00603-5543-21
100's	$40.37	GENERIC, Mutual/United Research Laboratories	00677-1475-01
100's	$40.37	GENERIC, Amide Pharmaceutical Inc	52152-0106-02
100's	$40.37	GENERIC, Mutual Pharmaceutical Co Inc	53489-0423-01
100's	$43.49	GENERIC, Seatrace Pharmaceuticals	00551-0189-01
100's	$49.00	GENERIC, Southwood Pharmaceuticals Inc	58016-0792-00
100's	$58.03	HUMIBID L.A., Celltech Pharmacuetica ls Inc	53014-0012-10
150's	$37.95	GENERIC, Sky Pharmaceuticals Packaging, Inc	63739-0292-15
250's	$53.40	GENERIC, Vintage Pharmaceuticals Inc	00254-5312-33
250's	$53.40	GENERIC, Qualitest Products Inc	00603-5543-24
250's	$54.90	GENERIC, Alphagen Laboratories Inc	59743-0018-25
250's	$55.45	GENERIC, Major Pharmaceuticals Inc	00904-7759-70
250's	$56.80	GENERIC, Aligen Independent Laboratories Inc	00405-4457-04
250's	$64.95	GENERIC, Trinity Technologies Corporation	61355-0501-25
250's	$79.95	GENERIC, Amide Pharmaceutical Inc	52152-0106-03

Tablet, Extended Release - Oral - 800 mg

100's	$26.29	GENERIC, Mutual/United Research Laboratories	00677-1772-01
100's	$35.38	GENERIC, Ivax Corporation	59310-0109-10

Tablet, Extended Release - Oral - 1000 mg

100's	$29.99	GENERIC, Mutual/United Research Laboratories	00677-1811-01
100's	$35.04	GENERIC, Prasco Laboratories	66993-0322-02
100's	$40.88	MUCO-FEN, Ivax Corporation	59310-0118-10
100's	$60.70	ALLFEN, Mcr/American Pharmaceuticals Inc	58605-0513-01

Tablet, Extended Release - Oral - 1200 mg

100's	$32.25	GENERIC, Qualitest Products Inc	00603-3773-21
100's	$32.25	GENERIC, Alphagen Laboratories Inc	59743-0028-01
100's	$33.75	GENERIC, Iomed Laboratories Inc	61646-0172-01
100's	$34.11	GENERIC, Mutual/United Research Laboratories	00677-1643-01
100's	$43.55	GENERIC, Major Pharmaceuticals Inc	00904-5453-60
100's	$43.95	GENERIC, Breckenridge Inc	51991-0204-01
100's	$48.87	GENERIC, Qualitest Products Inc	00603-3503-21
100's	$48.87	GENERIC, Amide Pharmaceutical Inc	52152-0245-02
100's	$49.46	GUAIFENEX G, Ethex Corporation	58177-0308-04
100's	$54.29	GENERIC, Ivax Corporation	59310-0120-10
100's	$54.34	GENERIC, Duramed Pharmaceuticals Inc	51285-0857-02
100's	$56.00	GENERIC, Capellon Pharmaceuticals	64543-0121-01
100's	$61.99	GENERIC, Cypress Pharmaceutical Inc	60258-0258-01
100's	$73.70	GENERIC, Ucb Pharma Inc	50474-0620-01

Guaifenesin; Pseudoephedrine Hydrochloride (001405)

Categories: Congestion, nasal; Cough; Pregnancy Category C; FDA Pre 1938 Drugs
Drug Classes: Decongestants, nasal; Expectorants
Brand Names: Anatuss La; Congess Jr.; Congess Sr.; Decongestant Ii; **Deconsal**; Deconsal Ii; Defen-L.A.; Demibid Ii; Entex Pse; Eudal Sr; Eudal-Sr; Fenex-Pse; G-Phed; G-Phed-Pd; G-Tuss; Gp 500; Guai-Sudo; Guaibid D; Guaifed; Guaifed-Pd; Guaifen Pse; Guaimax-D; Guiadrine Ii; Guiafed; Guiatex Ii; Guiatex Pse; Histalet X; Iotex Pse; K-Gest, S.A.; Maxifed; Maxifed-G; Medent; Nalex; Nasabid; Nasatab La; Pan-Mist La; Pseudo G/Psi; Pseudo-G/Psi; Pseudocot-G; Pseudofen; Pseudofen-Pd; Respaire-120; Respaire-120 Sr; Respaire-60; Respaire-60 Sr; Respinol La; Ru-Tuss De; Rymed; Sinumist-Sr; Stamoist E; Syn-Rx; Touro La; Tuss-La; V-Dec-M; Zaptec Pse; Zephrex; Zephrex La; Zephrex-La
Foreign Brand Availability: Actifed Chesty Syrup (New-Zealand); Guaifenex PSE 60 (Hong-Kong)

G

DESCRIPTION

Note: The trade names have been used throughout this monograph for clarity.

Deconsal II: Each scored, dark blue Deconsal II tablet provides 60 mg pseudoephedrine HCl and 600 mg guaifenesin in a sustained-release formulation intended for oral administration. *Inactive ingredients:* Stearic acid, dibasic calcium phosphate, FD&C blue #1 lake, sodium lauryl sulfate, ethylcellulose, magnesium stearate.

Deconsal LA: Each scored, light blue Deconsal LA tablet provides 120 mg pseudoephedrine HCl and 400 mg guaifenesin in a sustained-release formulation intended for oral administration.

Pseudoephedrine HCl is a nasal decongestant and is an adrenergic (vasoconstrictor) which exists as fine, white to off-white crystals or powder, having a faint, characteristic odor. It is very soluble in water, freely soluble in alcohol and sparingly soluble in chloroform. Chemically, it is [S-(R*,R*)]-α-[1-(methylamino)ethyl]-, benzenemethanol HCl and has the following formula: $C_{10}H_{15}NO{\cdot}HCl$ and a molecular weight of 201.70.

Guaifenesin is an expectorant. It occurs as a white to slightly gray, crystalline powder having a bitter taste. It may have a slight characteristic odor. It is soluble in water, alcohol, chloroform, glycerine, and propylene glycol. Chemically it is, 3-(2-methoxyphenoxy)-1,2-propanediol and has the following chemical formula: $C_{10}H_{14}O_4$ and a molecular weight of 198.22.

Storage: Store at controlled room temperature between 15-30°C (59-86°F). Dispense in tight, light-resistant container with a child-resistant closure.

CLINICAL PHARMACOLOGY

Pseudoephedrine HCl is an orally indirect acting sympathomimetic amine and exerts a decongestant action on the nasal mucosa. It does this by vasoconstriction which results in reduction of tissue hyperemia, edema, nasal congestion, and an increase in nasal airway patency. The vasoconstriction action of pseudoephedrine is similar to that of ephedrine. In the usual dose it has minimal vasopressor effects. Pseudoephedrine is rapidly and almost completely absorbed from the gastrointestinal tract. It has a plasma half-life of 6-8 hours. Acid urine is associated with faster elimination of the drug (acidic urine is associated with faster elimination). The drug is distributed to body tissues and fluids, including fetal tissue, breast milk and the central nervous system (CNS). Approximately 50-75% of the administered dose is excreted unchanged in the urine; the remainder is apparently metabolized in the liver to inactive compounds by N-demethylation, parahydroxylation and oxidative deamination.

Guaifenesin is an expectorant which increases respiratory tract fluid secretions and helps loosen phlegm and bronchial secretions. By reducing the viscosity of secretions, guaifenesin increases the efficiency of the cough relfex and of ciliary action in removing accumulated secretions from trachea and bronchi. Guaifenesin is readily absorbed from the gastrointestinal tract and is rapidly metabolized and excreted in the urine. Guaifenesin has a plasma half-life of 1 hour. The major urinary metabolite is β-(2-methoxyphenoxy) lactic acid.

INDICATIONS AND USAGE

Guaifenesin; pseudoephedrine HCl tablets are indicated for the temporary relief of nasal congestion and cough associated with respiratory tract infections and related conditions such as sinusitis, pharyngitis, bronchitis, and asthma, when these conditions are complicated by tenacious mucus and/or mucus plugs and congestion. The product is effective in productive as well as non-productive cough which tends to injure the mucus membrane of the air passages.

CONTRAINDICATIONS

Guaifenesin; pseudoephedrine HCl tablets are contraindicated in patients with hypersensitivity to guaifenesin, or with hypersensitivity or idiosyncrasy to sympathomimetic amines which may be manifested by insomnia, dizziness, weakness and tremor or arrhythmias. Patients known to be hypersensitive to other sympathomimetic amines may exhibit cross sensitivity with pseudoephedrine.

Sympathomimetic amines are contraindicated in patients with severe hypertension, severe coronary artery disease and patients on monoamine oxidase inhibitor (MAO inhibitor) therapy and for 14 days after stopping MAO inhibitor therapy. (See DRUG INTERACTIONS.)

WARNINGS

Sympathomimetic amines should be used with caution in patients with hypertension, ischemic heart disease, diabetes mellitus, increased intraocular pressure, hyperthyroidism, or prostatic hypertrophy. Sympathomimetics may produce central nervous system stimulation with convulsions or cardiovascular collapse with accompanying hypotension.

Do not exceed recommended dosage.

Hypertensive crises can occur with concurrent use of pseudoephedrine or phenylephrine and MAO inhibitors, and for 14 days after stopping MAO inhibitor therapy, indomethacin, or with beta-blockers and methyldopa. If a hypertensive crisis occurs, these drugs should be discontinued immediately and therapy to lower blood pressure should be instituted. Fever should be managed by means of external cooling.

PRECAUTIONS

GENERAL

Use with caution in patients with diabetes, hypertension, cardiovascular disease and intolerance to ephedrine.

Before prescribing medication to suppress or modify cough, it is important too ascertain that the underlying cause of cough is identified, that modification of cough does not increase the risk of clinical or physiologic complications, and that appropriate therapy for the primary disease is instituted.

INFORMATION FOR THE PATIENT

Patients should be instructed to check with physician if symptoms do not improve within 5 days or if fever is present.

PEDIATRIC USE

This product is not recommended for use in pediatric patients under 2 years of age.

GERIATRIC USE

The elderly (60 years and older) are more likely to experience adverse reactions to sympathomimetics. Overdosage of sympathomimetics in this age group may cause hallucinations, convulsions, CNS depression, and death.

DRUG/LABORATORY TEST INTERACTIONS

Guaifenesin may increase renal clearance for urate and thereby lower serum uric acid levels. Guaifenesin may produce an increase in urinary 5-hydroxy-indoleacetic acid and may therefore interfere with the interpretation of this test for the diagnosis of carcinoid syndrome. It may also falsely elevate the VMA test for catechols. Administration of this drug should be discontinued 48 hours prior to the collection of urine specimens for such tests.

CARCINOGENESIS, MUTAGENESIS, AND IMPAIRMENT OF FERTILITY

No data are available on the long-term potential of the components of this product for carcinogenesis, mutagenesis, or impairment of fertility in animals or or humans.

Pregnancy Category C: Animal reproduction studies have not been conducted with guaifenesin; pseudoephedrine HCl tablets. It is also not known whether guaifenesin; pseudoephedrine HCl tablets can cause fetal harm when administered to a pregnant woman or can affect reproduction capacity. Guaifenesin; pseudoephedrine HCl should be given to a pregnant woman only if clearly needed.

NURSING MOTHERS

Pseudoephedrine is excreted in breast milk. Use of this product by nursing mothers is not recommended because of the higher than usual risk for infants from sympathomimetic amines.

DRUG INTERACTIONS

Do not prescribe this product for use in patients that are now taking a prescription MAO inhibitor (certain drugs for depression, psychiatric or emotional conditions, or Parkinson's disease), or for 14 days after stopping the MAO inhibitor drug therapy. Beta-adrenergic blockers and MAO inhibitor may potentiate the pressor effect of pseudoephedrine. (see WARNINGS.) Concurrent use of digitalis glycosides may increase the possibility of cardiac arrhythmias. Sympathomimetics may reduce the hypotensive effects of guanethidine, mecamylamine, methyldopa, reserpine and veratrum alkaloids. Concurrent use of tricyclic antidepressants may antagonize the effects of pseudoephedrine.

ADVERSE REACTIONS

Hyperreactive individuals may display ephedrine-like reactions such as tachycardia, palpitations, headache, dizziness, or nausea. Sympathomimetics have been associated with certain untoward reactions including fear, anxiety, nervousness, restlessness, tremor, weakness, pallor, respiratory difficulty, dysuria, insomnia, hallucinations, convulsions, CNS depression, arrhythmias, and cardiovascular collapse with hypotension. No serious side effects have been reported with the use of guaifenesin.

DOSAGE AND ADMINISTRATION

Adults and adolescents over 12 years of age: One or two tablets every 12 hours not to exceed 4 tablets in 24 hours.

Children 6 to under 12 years: ½-1 tablet every 12 hours not to exceed 2 tablets in 24 hours.

Children 2-6 years: ½ tablet every 12 hours not to exceed 1 tablet in 24 hours.

PRODUCT LISTING - EQUIVALENTS NOT AVAILABLE

Capsule, Extended Release - Oral - 125 mg;60 mg

100's	$31.00	GENERIC, Fleming and Company	00256-0174-01

Capsule, Extended Release - Oral - 200 mg;60 mg

20's	$8.15	RESPAIRE-60 SR, Allscripts Pharmaceutical Company	54569-0708-01
30's	$12.23	RESPAIRE-60 SR, Allscripts Pharmaceutical Company	54569-0708-00
100's	$39.58	RESPAIRE-60 SR, Laser Inc	00277-0174-01

Capsule, Extended Release - Oral - 250 mg;120 mg

12's	$14.27	GUAIFED, Allscripts Pharmaceutical Company	54569-3244-00
30's	$27.35	GENERIC, Southwood Pharmaceuticals Inc	58016-0790-30
60's	$52.65	GENERIC, Southwood Pharmaceuticals Inc	58016-0790-60
100's	$29.76	GENERIC, Qualitest Products Inc	00603-3776-21
100's	$30.50	GENERIC, Duramed Pharmaceuticals Inc	51285-0894-02
100's	$35.03	GENERIC, Moore, H.L. Drug Exchange Inc	00839-7925-06
100's	$39.00	GENERIC, Alphagen Laboratories Inc	59743-0002-01
100's	$47.77	GENERIC, Laser Inc	00277-0169-01
100's	$56.80	GENERIC, Ethex Corporation	58177-0045-04
100's	$56.95	GENERIC, Ivax Corporation	00182-2601-01

100's	$58.42	GENERIC, Econolab	55053-0860-01
100's	$61.50	GENERIC, Aligen Independent Laboratories Inc	00405-4466-01
100's	$84.92	GENERIC, Southwood Pharmaceuticals Inc	58016-0790-00
100's	$142.21	GUAIFED SR, Muro Pharmaceuticals Inc	00451-4002-50

Capsule, Extended Release - Oral - 300 mg;60 mg

20's	$18.97	GUAIFED-PD, Allscripts Pharmaceutical Company	54569-2191-00
30's	$22.34	GENERIC, Southwood Pharmaceuticals Inc	58016-0791-30
60's	$41.97	GENERIC, Southwood Pharmaceuticals Inc	58016-0791-60
100's	$27.82	GENERIC, Qualitest Products Inc	00603-3777-21
100's	$28.25	GENERIC, Duramed Pharmaceuticals Inc	51285-0895-02
100's	$30.80	GENERIC, Moore, H.L. Drug Exchange Inc	00839-7924-06
100's	$35.00	GENERIC, Alphagen Laboratories Inc	59743-0003-01
100's	$37.24	GENERIC, Roberts/Hauck Pharmaceutical Corporation	59441-0151-01
100's	$43.35	GENERIC, Ivax Corporation	00182-2602-01
100's	$45.28	GENERIC, Ethex Corporation	58177-0046-04
100's	$47.29	GENERIC, Seatrace Pharmaceuticals	00551-0173-01
100's	$48.94	GENERIC, Aligen Independent Laboratories Inc	00405-4465-01
100's	$67.70	GENERIC, Southwood Pharmaceuticals Inc	58016-0791-00
100's	$113.38	GUAIFED-PD, Muro Pharmaceuticals Inc	00451-4003-50

Syrup - Oral - 50 mg;15 mg/5 ml

120 ml	$4.81	TRIAMINIC CHEST CONGESTION, Novartis Consumer Health	00043-0568-04
240 ml	$7.79	TRIAMINIC CHEST CONGESTION, Novartis Consumer Health	00043-0568-08

Syrup - Oral - 200 mg;40 mg/5 ml

480 ml	$39.64	PANMIST-S, Pan American Laboratories	00525-0798-16

Tablet - Oral - 400 mg;60 mg

100's	$85.34	GENERIC, Sanofi Winthrop Pharmaceuticals	00024-2624-01

Tablet, Chewable - Oral - 50 mg;15 mg

18's	$4.71	TRIAMINIC SOFTCHEWS CHEST CONGESTION, Novartis Consumer Health	00067-0353-18

Tablet, Extended Release - Oral - 100 mg;60 mg

100's	$7.00	GENERIC, C.O. Truxton Inc	00463-7014-01

Tablet, Extended Release - Oral - 400 mg;120 mg

20's	$12.21	EUDAL SR, Pd-Rx Pharmaceuticals	55289-0366-20
100's	$34.50	NASATAB LA, Ecr Pharmaceuticals	00095-0225-01
100's	$44.48	EUDAL SR, Forest Pharmaceuticals	00785-6301-01
100's	$59.70	ANATUSS LA, Merz Pharmaceuticals	00259-0379-01

Tablet, Extended Release - Oral - 500 mg;60 mg

100's	$31.20	GENERIC, United Research Laboratories, Inc.	00677-1851-01
100's	$36.70	GENERIC, Atley Pharmaceuticals	59702-0060-01
100's	$42.80	GENERIC, Mcr/American Pharmaceuticals Inc	58605-0506-01

Tablet, Extended Release - Oral - 500 mg;120 mg

100's	$25.81	GENERIC, Hyrex Pharmaceuticals	00314-8050-01
100's	$32.00	GENERIC, Huckaby Pharmacal Inc	58407-0375-01
100's	$55.98	GENERIC, Seatrace Pharmaceuticals	00551-0170-01
100's	$63.00	TOURO LA, Dartmouth Pharmaceuticals Inc	58869-0536-01

Tablet, Extended Release - Oral - 525 mg;120 mg

100's	$63.96	GENERIC, Dartmouth Pharmaceuticals Inc	58869-0636-01

Tablet, Extended Release - Oral - 550 mg;60 mg

100's	$60.81	GENERIC, Mcr/American Pharmaceuticals Inc	58605-0514-01

Tablet, Extended Release - Oral - 600 mg;45 mg

100's	$44.98	GENERIC, Breckenridge Inc	51991-0068-01
100's	$45.00	GENERIC, Mutual/United Research Laboratories	00677-1830-01
100's	$47.93	GENERIC, Pan American Laboratories	00525-0762-01

Tablet, Extended Release - Oral - 600 mg;60 mg

10's	$35.85	GENERIC, Mutual/United Research Laboratories	53489-0425-01
14's	$5.81	GENERIC, Allscripts Pharmaceutical Company	54569-4727-00
30's	$18.98	GENERIC, Southwood Pharmaceuticals Inc	58016-0788-30
56's	$23.32	GENERIC, Allscripts Pharmaceutical Company	54569-4727-01
56's	$24.05	GENERIC, Iomed Laboratories Inc	61646-0700-56
56's	$25.45	GENERIC, Ethex Corporation	58177-0276-17
56's	$27.00	GENERIC, Duramed Pharmaceuticals Inc	51285-0588-88
56's	$31.20	SYN-RX, Allscripts Pharmaceutical Company	54569-4445-00
60's	$35.66	GENERIC, Southwood Pharmaceuticals Inc	58016-0788-60
100's	$32.50	GENERIC, Md Pharmaceutical Inc	43567-0500-07
100's	$34.21	GENERIC, Aligen Independent Laboratories Inc	00405-4467-01
100's	$34.25	GENERIC, Iomed Laboratories Inc	61646-0122-01
100's	$35.85	GENERIC, Mutual/United Research Laboratories	00677-1487-01
100's	$35.90	GENERIC, Ethex Corporation	58177-0214-04
100's	$38.80	GENERIC, Ivax Corporation	00182-1037-01
100's	$38.90	GENERIC, Qualitest Products Inc	00603-3116-21
100's	$38.90	GENERIC, Alphagen Laboratories Inc	59743-0050-01
100's	$39.80	GUIATEX II SR, Watson Laboratories Inc	52544-0435-01
100's	$39.95	GENERIC, Pecos Pharmaceutical	59879-0116-01
100's	$40.00	GENERIC, Respa Pharmaceuticals Inc	60575-0108-19
100's	$40.61	GENERIC, Respa Pharmaceuticals Inc	60575-0087-19
100's	$42.60	GENERIC, Major Pharmaceuticals Inc	00904-5150-60
100's	$42.60	GENERIC, Trinity Technologies Corporation	61355-0201-10
100's	$42.65	GENERIC, Moore, H.L. Drug Exchange Inc	00839-7898-06
100's	$49.80	GENERIC, We Pharmaceuticals Inc	59196-0005-01
100's	$53.80	DEFEN-LA, First Horizon Pharmaceutical Corporation	59630-0110-10
100's	$57.52	GENERIC, Southwood Pharmaceuticals Inc	58016-0788-00
100's	$71.28	GENERIC, Celltech PharmacuetICALS Inc	53014-0017-10

Tablet, Extended Release - Oral - 600 mg;90 mg

100's	$24.99	GENERIC, Hawthorn Pharmaceuticals	63717-0301-01
100's	$48.29	GENERIC, We Pharmaceuticals Inc	59196-0060-01
100's	$79.20	NASABID SR, Jones Pharma Inc	52604-0600-01

Tablet, Extended Release - Oral - 600 mg;120 mg

2's	$5.45	ENTEX PSE, Prescript Pharmaceuticals	00247-0176-02
10's	$11.32	GENERIC, Pd-Rx Pharmaceuticals	55289-0391-10
10's	$13.81	ENTEX PSE, Prescript Pharmaceuticals	00247-0176-10
14's	$8.31	GENERIC, Allscripts Pharmaceutical Company	54569-3949-01
15's	$10.91	RU TUSS DE, Allscripts Pharmaceutical Company	54569-3534-00
15's	$21.38	GENERIC, Pd-Rx Pharmaceuticals	55289-0423-15
20's	$11.87	GENERIC, Allscripts Pharmaceutical Company	54569-3949-00
20's	$18.25	GENERIC, Pharma Pac	52959-0397-20
20's	$19.71	GENERIC, Physicians Total Care	54868-0523-02
20's	$22.62	ENTEX PSE, Allscripts Pharmaceutical Company	54569-3440-00
20's	$24.27	ENTEX PSE, Prescript Pharmaceuticals	00247-0176-20
20's	$24.90	RU TUSS DE, Pd-Rx Pharmaceuticals	55289-0797-20
20's	$27.96	GENERIC, Pd-Rx Pharmaceuticals	55289-0423-20
30's	$17.80	GENERIC, Allscripts Pharmaceutical Company	54569-3949-02
30's	$26.15	GENERIC, Pharma Pac	52959-0397-30
30's	$26.30	GENERIC, Pd-Rx Pharmaceuticals	55289-0391-30
30's	$28.98	GENERIC, Physicians Total Care	54868-0523-03
30's	$29.32	GENERIC, Southwood Pharmaceuticals Inc	58016-0789-30
30's	$35.67	GENERIC, Pd-Rx Pharmaceuticals	55289-0423-30
30's	$38.78	RU TUSS DE, Pd-Rx Pharmaceuticals	55289-0797-30
60's	$55.08	GENERIC, Southwood Pharmaceuticals Inc	58016-0789-60
100's	$15.63	GENERIC, American Generics Inc	58634-0033-01
100's	$26.04	GENERIC, Marnel Pharmaceuticals Inc	00682-0500-01
100's	$39.98	FENEX-PSE, Tmk Pharmaceuticals	59582-0003-01
100's	$44.35	GENERIC, Md Pharmaceutical Inc	43567-0451-07
100's	$45.16	GENERIC, Aligen Independent Laboratories Inc	00405-4040-01
100's	$46.75	GENERIC, Martec Pharmaceuticals Inc	52555-0635-01
100's	$47.75	GENERIC, Breckenridge Inc	51991-0245-01
100's	$48.20	GENERIC, Duramed Pharmaceuticals Inc	51285-0401-02
100's	$49.90	GENERIC, Major Pharmaceuticals Inc	00904-5404-60
100's	$49.94	GENERIC, Moore, H.L. Drug Exchange Inc	00839-7754-06
100's	$49.95	GENERIC, Caraco Pharmaceutical Laboratories	57664-0222-08
100's	$52.00	GENERIC, Ivax Corporation	00182-1740-01
100's	$52.90	GENERIC, Trinity Technologies Corporation	61355-0202-10
100's	$53.15	GENERIC, Ethex Corporation	58177-0208-04
100's	$53.30	GENERIC, Watson Laboratories Inc	52544-0436-01
100's	$55.95	GENERIC, Iomed Laboratories Inc	61646-0121-01
100's	$55.99	GENERIC, Vintage Pharmaceuticals Inc	00254-6211-28
100's	$55.99	GENERIC, Qualitest Products Inc	00603-3767-21
100's	$55.99	GENERIC, Qualitest Products Inc	00603-5668-21
100's	$56.00	GENERIC, Amide Pharmaceutical Inc	52152-0130-02
100's	$56.05	GENERIC, Alphagen Laboratories Inc	59743-0059-01
100's	$56.70	GENERIC, Major Pharmaceuticals Inc	00904-7689-60
100's	$56.99	GENERIC, Mutual/United Research Laboratories	00677-1476-01
100's	$56.99	GENERIC, Mutual/United Research Laboratories	53489-0424-01
100's	$59.90	GENERIC, Major Pharmaceuticals Inc	00904-7861-60
100's	$60.98	GENERIC, Eon Labs Manufacturing Inc	00185-0784-01
100's	$67.58	GUAI-VENT/PSE, Dj Pharma Inc	64455-0015-01
100's	$67.85	GENERIC, Duramed Pharmaceuticals Inc	51285-0402-02
100's	$72.61	GUAIMAX-D, Schwarz Pharma	00131-2055-37
100's	$80.58	ENTEX PSE, Procter and Gamble Pharmaceuticals	00149-0427-02
100's	$80.93	GENERIC, Able Laboratories Inc	53265-0248-10
100's	$84.92	GENERIC, Southwood Pharmaceuticals Inc	58016-0789-00
100's	$97.76	GENERIC, Ucb Pharma Inc	50474-0612-01
100's	$101.21	GENERIC, Cypress Pharmaceutical Inc	60258-0275-01
100's	$101.60	GENERIC, Sanofi Winthrop Pharmaceuticals	00024-2627-01
100's	$124.40	ENTEX PSE, Dura Pharmaceuticals	51479-0032-01
100's	$141.22	ENTEX PSE, Andrx Pharmaceuticals	62022-0032-01
250's	$113.40	GENERIC, Major Pharmaceuticals Inc	00904-7689-70
250's	$113.40	GENERIC, Major Pharmaceuticals Inc	00904-7861-70
250's	$124.74	GENERIC, Eon Labs Manufacturing Inc	00185-0784-52

Tablet, Extended Release - Oral - 700 mg;80 mg

100's	$61.13	MAXIFED, Mcr/American Pharmaceuticals Inc	58605-0520-01

Tablet, Extended Release - Oral - 800 mg;45 mg

100's	$54.01	GENERIC, Ivax Corporation	59310-0307-10

Tablet, Extended Release - Oral - 800 mg;60 mg

100's	$40.85	MEDENT LD, Stewart-Jackson Pharmaceutical Inc	45985-0642-01

Tablet, Extended Release - Oral - 800 mg;80 mg

100's	$33.75	GENERIC, We Pharmaceuticals Inc	59196-0065-01
100's	$45.78	GENERIC, Mutual/United Research Laboratories	00677-1787-01
100's	$49.00	PANMIST LA, Pan American Laboratories	00525-0742-01
100's	$50.47	GENERIC, Mutual/United Research Laboratories	00677-1789-01
100's	$51.03	GENERIC, Ethex Corporation	58177-0413-04

Tablet, Extended Release - Oral - 800 mg;90 mg

100's	$69.26	PROFEN FORTE, Ivax Corporation	59310-0315-10

Tablet, Extended Release - Oral - 1200 mg;60 mg

100's	$78.18	GENERIC, Cypress Pharmaceutical Inc	60258-0272-01
100's	$101.95	GENERIC, United Research Laboratories, Inc.	00677-1841-01

Tablet, Extended Release - Oral - 1200 mg;75 mg

100's	$96.32	AQUATAB D, Adams Laboratories	63824-0068-10

Tablet, Extended Release - Oral - 1200 mg;90 mg

100's	$87.71	GUAIFENESIN-PSEUDOEPHEDRINE HYDROCHLORIDE SR, United Research Laboratories, Inc.	00677-1850-01
100's	$103.19	DYNEX, Andrx Pharmaceuticals	62022-0033-01

Tablet, Extended Release - Oral - 1200 mg;120 mg

20 x 5	$156.95	DURATUSS AM/PM, Ucb Pharma Inc	50474-0650-40
100's	$69.99	GUAIFENESIN-PSEUDOEPHEDRINE HYDROCHLORIDE SR, Cypress Pharmaceutical Inc	60258-0266-01
100's	$77.02	GENERIC, Ethex Corporation	58177-0373-04
100's	$81.06	GENERIC, Qualitest Products Inc	00603-3506-21
100's	$81.10	GUAIFENESIN-PSEUDOEPHEDRINE HYDROCHLORIDE SR, Mutual/United Research Laboratories	00677-1785-01
100's	$107.51	DURATUSS GP, Ucb Pharma Inc	50474-0640-01

Guanabenz Acetate *(001408)*

Categories: Hypertension, essential; Pregnancy Category C; FDA Approved 1982 Sep
Drug Classes: Antiadrenergics, central
Brand Names: **Wytensin**
Foreign Brand Availability: Rexitene (Austria); Wytens (Japan)
Cost of Therapy: $35.60 (Hypertension; Generic Tablets; 4 mg; 2 tablets/day; 30 day supply)

DESCRIPTION

Guanabenz acetate, an antihypertensive agent for oral administration, is an aminoguanidine derivative, 2,6-dichlorobenzylideneaminoguanidine acetate.

It is an odorless, white to off-white, crystalline substance, sparingly soluble in water and soluble in alcohol, with a molecular weight of 291.14. Each tablet of Wytensin is equivalent to 4 or 8 mg of free guanabenz base. The inactive ingredients present are cellulose, iron oxide, lactose, and magnesium stearate. The 8 mg dosage strength also contains FD&C blue no. 2.

Wytensin is available as 4 or 8 mg tablets for oral administration.

CLINICAL PHARMACOLOGY

Guanabenz acetate is an orally active central alpha-2 adrenergic agonist. Its antihypertensive action appears to be mediated via stimulation of central alpha adrenergic receptors, resulting in a decrease of sympathetic outflow from the brain at the bulbar level to the peripheral circulatory system.

PHARMACOKINETICS

In human studies, about 75% of an orally administered dose of guanabenz acetate is absorbed and metabolized with less than 1% of unchanged drug recovered from the urine. Peak plasma concentrations of unchanged drug occur between 2 and 5 hours after a single oral dose. The average half-life for guanabenz acetate is about 6 hours. The site or sites of metabolism of guanabenz acetate have not been determined. The effect of meals on the absorption of guanabenz acetate has not been studied.

PHARMACODYNAMICS

The onset of the antihypertensive action of guanabenz acetate begins within 60 minutes after a single oral dose and reaches a peak effect within 2-4 hours. The effect of an acute single dose is reduced appreciably 6-8 hours after administration, and blood pressure approaches baseline values within 12 hours of administration.

The acute antihypertensive effect of guanabenz acetate occurs without major changes in peripheral resistance, but its chronic effect appears to be a decrease in peripheral resistance. A decrease in blood pressure is seen in both the supine and standing positions without alterations of normal postural mechanisms, so that postural hypotension has not been observed. Guanabenz acetate decreases pulse rate by about 5 beats per minute. Cardiac output and left ventricular ejection fraction are unchanged during long-term therapy.

In clinical trials, guanabenz acetate, given orally to hypertensive patients, effectively controlled blood pressure without any significant effect on glomerular filtration rate, renal blood flow, body fluid volume or body weight. Guanabenz acetate given parenterally to dogs has produced a natriuresis. Similarly, hypertensive subjects, 24 hours after salt loading, have shown a decrease in blood pressure and a natriuresis (5-240% increase in sodium excretion) following a single oral dose of guanabenz acetate. After 7 consecutive days of administration and effective blood-pressure control, no significant change on glomerular filtration rate, renal blood flow, or body weight was observed. However, in clinical trials of 6-30 months duration, hypertensive patients with effective blood-pressure control by guanabenz acetate lost 1-4 pounds of body weight. The mechanism of this weight loss has not been established. Tolerance to the antihypertensive effect of guanabenz acetate has not been observed.

During long-term administration of guanabenz acetate, there is a small decrease in serum cholesterol and total triglycerides without any change in the high-density lipoprotein fraction. Plasma norepinephrine, serum dopamine beta-hydroxylase, and plasma renin activity are decreased during chronic administration of guanabenz acetate. No changes in serum electrolytes, uric acid, blood urea nitrogen, calcium, or glucose have been observed.

Guanabenz acetate and hydrochlorothiazide have been shown to have at least partially additive effects in patients not responding adequately to either drug alone.

INDICATIONS AND USAGE

Guanabenz acetate is indicated in the treatment of hypertension. It may be employed alone or in combination with a thiazide diuretic.

CONTRAINDICATIONS

Guanabenz acetate is contraindicated in patients with a known sensitivity to the drug or any of the tablet ingredients.

PRECAUTIONS

GENERAL

Sedation

Guanabenz acetate causes sedation or drowsiness in a large fraction of patients. When guanabenz acetate is used with centrally active depressants, such as phenothiazines, barbiturates, and benzodiazepines, the potential for additive sedative effects should be considered.

Patients With Vascular Insufficiency

Guanabenz acetate, like other antihypertensive agents, should be used with caution in patients with severe coronary insufficiency, recent myocardial infarction, cerebrovascular disease, or severe hepatic or renal failure.

Rebound

Sudden cessation of therapy with central alpha agonists like guanabenz acetate may rarely result in "overshoot" hypertension and more commonly produces an increase in serum catecholamines and subjective symptomatology.

Patients With Hepatic Impairment

The disposition of orally administered guanabenz acetate is altered in patients with alcohol-induced liver disease. Mean plasma concentrations of guanabenz acetate were higher in these patients than in healthy subjects. The clinical significance of this finding is unknown. However, careful monitoring of blood pressure is suggested when guanabenz acetate is administered to patients with hypertension and coexisting chronic hepatic dysfunction.

Patients With Renal Impairment:

The disposition of orally administered guanabenz acetate is altered modestly in patients with renal impairment. Guanabenz acetate's half-life is prolonged and clearance decreased, more so in patients on hemodialysis. The clinical significance of these findings is unknown. Careful monitoring of blood pressure during guanabenz acetate dose titration is suggested in patients with coexisting hypertension and renal impairment.

INFORMATION FOR THE PATIENT

Patients who receive guanabenz acetate should be advised to exercise caution when operating dangerous machinery or driving motor vehicles until it is determined that they do not become drowsy or dizzy from the medication. Patients should be warned that their tolerance for alcohol and other CNS depressants may be diminished. Patients should be advised not to discontinue therapy abruptly.

LABORATORY TESTS

In clinical trials, no clinically significant laboratory-test abnormalities were identified during either acute or chronic therapy with guanabenz acetate. Tests carried out included CBC, urinalysis, electrolytes, SGOT, bilirubin, alkaline phosphatase, uric acid, BUN, creatinine, glucose, calcium, phosphorus, total protein, and Coombs' test. During long-term administration of guanabenz acetate, there was a small decrease in serum cholesterol and total triglycerides without any change in the high-density lipoprotein fraction. In rare instances an occasional nonprogressive increase in liver enzymes has been observed. However, no clinical evidence of hepatic disease has been found.

DRUG/LABORATORY TEST INTERACTIONS

No laboratory-test abnormalities were identified with the use of guanabenz acetate.

CARCINOGENESIS, MUTAGENESIS, AND IMPAIRMENT OF FERTILITY

Two year studies were conducted with oral guanabenz acetate administered in the diet to mice and rats. No evidence of carcinogenic potential was seen in mice given doses of up to 11.5 mg/kg/day (41.4 mg/m^2/day) or in rats given doses of up to 9.5 mg/kg/day (83.8 mg/m^2/day). On a body-weight basis, these doses are 9× and 7×, respectively, the maximum recommended human daily dose (MRHDD) of 64 mg (based on a 50 kg individual). On a body-surface-area basis, these doses are 1× (mice) and 2× (rats) the MRHDD. In the Salmonella microsome mutagenicity (Ames) test system, guanabenz acetate at 200-500 μg per plate or at 30-50 μg/ml in suspension gave dose-related increases in the number of mutants in one (TA 1537) of five *Salmonella typhimurium* strains with or without inclusion of rat liver microsomes. No mutagenic activity was seen at doses up to those which inhibit growth in the eukaryotic microorganisms, *Schizosaccharomyces pombe,* or in Chinese hamster ovary cells at doses up to those which were lethal to the cells in culture. In another eukaryotic system, *Saccharomyces cerevisiae,* guanabenz acetate produced no activity in an assay measuring induction of repairable DNA damage. Reproductive studies showed a decreased pregnancy rate in rats administered high oral doses (9.6 mg/kg) of guanabenz acetate, suggesting an impairment of fertility. The fertility of treated males (9.6 mg/kg) may also have been affected, as suggested by the decreased pregnancy rate of their mates, even though the females received guanabenz acetate only during the last third of pregnancy.

PREGNANCY CATEGORY C

GUANABENZ ACETATE MAY HAVE ADVERSE EFFECTS ON THE FETUS WHEN ADMINISTERED TO PREGNANT WOMEN. A teratology study in mice has indicated a possible increase in skeletal abnormalities when guanabenz acetate is given orally at doses of 3-6 times the maximum recommended human dose of 1.0 mg/kg. These abnormalities, principally costal and vertebral, were not noted in similar studies in rats and rabbits. However, increased fetal loss has been observed after oral guanabenz acetate administration to pregnant rats (14 mg/kg) and rabbits (20 mg/kg). Reproductive studies of guanabenz acetate in rats have shown slightly decreased live-birth indices, decreased fetal survival rate, and decreased pup body weight at oral doses of 6.4 and 9.6 mg/kg. There are no adequate, well controlled studies in pregnant women. Guanabenz acetate should be used during pregnancy only if the potential benefit justifies the potential risk to the fetus.

NURSING MOTHERS

It is not known whether this drug is excreted in human milk. Because many drugs are excreted in human milk, caution should be exercised when guanabenz acetate is administered to a nursing woman.

PEDIATRIC USE

The safety and effectiveness of guanabenz acetate in pediatric patients have not been established.

DRUG INTERACTIONS

Guanabenz acetate has not been demonstrated to cause any drug interactions when administered with other drugs, such as digitalis, diuretics, analgesics, anxiolytics, and anti-inflammatory or anti-infective agents, in clinical trials. However, the potential for increased sedation when guanabenz acetate is administered concomitantly with CNS-depressant drugs should be noted.

ADVERSE REACTIONS

The incidence of adverse effects has been ascertained from controlled clinical studies conducted in the US and is based on data from 859 patients who received guanabenz acetate for up to 3 years. There is some evidence that the side effects are dose-related.

TABLE 1 shows the incidence of adverse effects, occurring in at least 5% of patients in a study comparing guanabenz acetate to placebo, at a starting dose of 8 mg bid.

TABLE 1

Adverse Effect	Placebo n=102	Guanabenz Acetate n=109
Dry mouth	7%	28%
Drowsiness or sedation	12%	39%
Dizziness	7%	17%
Weakness	7%	10%
Headache	6%	5%

In other controlled clinical trials at the starting dose of 16 mg/day in 476 patients, the incidence of dry mouth was slightly higher (38%) and that of dizziness was slightly lower (12%), but the incidence of the most frequent adverse effects was similar to the placebo-controlled trial. Although these side effects were not serious, they led to discontinuation of treatment about 15% of the time. In more recent studies using an initial dose of 8 mg/day in 274 patients, the incidence of drowsiness or sedation was lower, about 20%.

Other adverse effects were reported during clinical trials with guanabenz acetate but are not clearly distinguishable from placebo effects and occurred with a frequency of 3% or less:

Cardiovascular: Chest pain, edema, arrhythmias, palpitations.

Gastrointestinal: Nausea, epigastric pain, diarrhea, vomiting, constipation, abdominal discomfort.

Central Nervous System: Anxiety, ataxia, depression, sleep disturbances.

ENT Disorders: Nasal congestion.

Eye Disorders: Blurring of vision.

Musculoskeletal: Aches in extremities, muscle aches.

Respiratory: Dyspnea.

Dermatologic: Rash, pruritus.

Urogenital: Urinary frequency, disturbances of sexual function (decreased libido, impotence).

Other: Gynecomastia, taste disorders.

In very rare instances atrioventricular dysfunction, up to and including complete AV block, has been caused by guanabenz acetate.

DOSAGE AND ADMINISTRATION

Dosage with guanabenz acetate should be individualized. A starting dose of 4 mg twice a day is recommended, whether guanabenz acetate is used alone or with a thiazide diuretic. Dosage may be increased in increments of 4-8 mg per day every 1-2 weeks, depending on the patients's response. The maximum dose studied to date has been 32 mg twice daily, but doses as high as this are rarely needed.

HOW SUPPLIED

Wytensin tablets are available in:

4 mg: Orange, five-sided tablet with a raised "W" and a "4" under the "W" on one side and "WYETH 73" on reverse side.

8 mg: Gray, five-sided tablet with a raised "W" and a "8" under the "W" on one side and "WYETH 74" on scored reverse side.

STORAGE

Keep tightly closed.

Store at room temperature, approximately 25°C (77°F).

Protect from light.

Dispense in a light-resistant, tight container.

PRODUCT LISTING - RATED THERAPEUTICALLY EQUIVALENT

Tablet - Oral - 4 mg

100's	$59.33	GENERIC, Moore, H.L. Drug Exchange Inc	00839-7932-06
100's	$59.45	GENERIC, Martec Pharmaceuticals Inc	52555-0555-01
100's	$66.20	GENERIC, Watson Laboratories Inc	52544-0451-01
100's	$71.00	GENERIC, Ivax Corporation	00172-4226-60

Tablet - Oral - 8 mg

100's	$89.10	GENERIC, Moore, H.L. Drug Exchange Inc	00839-7933-06
100's	$89.25	GENERIC, Martec Pharmaceuticals Inc	52555-0556-01
100's	$99.40	GENERIC, Watson Laboratories Inc	52544-0452-01
100's	$125.00	GENERIC, Ivax Corporation	00172-4227-60

Guanadrel Sulfate *(001409)*

G

Categories: Hypertension, essential; Pregnancy Category B; FDA Approved 1982 Dec
Drug Classes: Antiadrenergics, peripheral
Brand Names: Hylorel
Cost of Therapy: $22.46 (Hypertension; Hylorel; 10 mg; 1 tablet/day; 30 day supply)

DESCRIPTION

Hylorel tablets for oral administration contain guanadrel sulfate, an antihypertensive agent belonging to the class of adrenergic neuron blocking drugs. Guanadrel sulfate is (1,4-Dioxaspiro[4.5] dec-2-ylmethyl) guanidine sulfate with a molecular weight of 524.63. The empirical formula is $(C_{10}H_{19}N_3O_2)_2{\cdot}H_2SO_4$. It is a white to off-white crystalline powder, which melts with decomposition at about 235°C. It is soluble in water to the extent of 76 mg/ml.

Hylorel tablets are available in two strengths: 10 and 25 mg. Inactive ingredients: colloidal silicon dioxide, corn starch, lactose monohydrate, magnesium stearate, microcrystalline cellulose and talc. The 10 mg tablet also contains FD&C Yellow No. 6.

CLINICAL PHARMACOLOGY

Guanadrel sulfate is an orally effective antihypertensive agent that lowers both systolic and diastolic arterial blood pressures. Guanadrel sulfate inhibits sympathetic vasoconstriction by inhibiting norepinephrine release from neuronal storage sites in response to stimulation of the nerve and also causes depletion of norepinephrine from the nerve ending. This results in relaxation of vascular smooth muscle which decreases total peripheral resistance, and decreases venous return, both of which reduce the ability to maintain blood pressure in the upright position. The result is a hypotensive effect that is greater in the standing than in the supine position by about 10 mm Hg systolic and 3.5 mm Hg diastolic, on the average. Heart rate is also decreased usually by about 5 beats/minute. Fluid retention occurs during treatment with guanadrel, particularly when it is not accompanied by a diuretic. The drug does not inhibit parasympathetic nerve function nor does it enter the central nervous system.

Guanadrel sulfate is rapidly absorbed after oral administration. Plasma concentrations generally peak 1½ to 2 hours after ingestion. The half-life is about 10 hours, but individual variability is great. Approximately 85% of the drug is eliminated in the urine. Urinary excretion is approximately 85% complete within 24 hours after administration; about 40% of the dose is excreted as unchanged drug. The disposition of guanadrel sulfate is significantly altered in patients with impaired renal function. A study in such patients has shown that as renal function (measured as creatinine clearance) declines, apparent total body clearance, renal and apparent nonrenal clearances decrease, and the terminal elimination half-life is prolonged. Dosage adjustments may be necessary, especially in patients with creatinine clearances of less than 60 ml/min (see DOSAGE AND ADMINISTRATION.)

Guanadrel sulfate begins to decrease blood pressure within 2 hours and produces maximal decreases in 4-6 hours. No significant change in cardiac output accompanies the blood pressure decline in normal individuals.

Because drugs of the adrenergic neuron blocking class are transported into the neuron by the "norepinephrine pump", drugs that compete for the pump may block their effects. Tricyclic antidepressants have been shown to block the norepinephrine-depleting effect of guanadrel sulfate in rats and monkeys, and the blood pressure lowering effect of guanadrel sulfate in monkeys. Similar effects have been seen with guanethidine and inhibition of the antihypertensive effects of guanadrel sulfate by tricyclic antidepressants in humans should be presumed.

Therefore caution is recommended if guanadrel sulfate and a tricyclic antidepressant are used concomitantly. Should patients be on both a tricyclic antidepressant and guanadrel sulfate, caution is advised upon discontinuation of the tricyclic antidepressant, especially if discontinued abruptly, as an enhanced effect of guanadrel sulfate may occur.

Chlorpromazine seems to have a similar effect on guanethidine and may affect guanadrel as well. Indirectly acting adrenergic amines are transported into the neuron by the "norepinephrine pump" and may interfere with uptake or may displace blocking agents. Ephedrine rapidly reverses the effects of guanadrel but other agents have not been studied.

Agents of the guanethidine class cause increased sensitivity to circulating norepinephrine, probably by preventing uptake of norepinephrine by adrenergic neurons, the usual mechanism for terminating norepinephrine effects. Agents of this class are thus dangerous in the presence of excess norepinephrine, e.g., in the presence of a pheochromocytoma.

In controlled clinical studies comparing guanadrel to guanethidine and methyldopa, involving about 2000 patients exposed to guanadrel, patients with initial supine blood pressures averaging 160-170/105-110 mm Hg had decreases in blood pressure of 20-25/15-20 mm Hg in the standing position. The decreases in supine blood pressure were less than the decreases in standing blood pressure by 6-10/2-7 mm Hg in different studies. Guanethidine and guanadrel were very similar in effectiveness while methyldopa had a larger effect on supine systolic pressure. Side effects of guanadrel and guanethidine were generally similar in type (see ADVERSE REACTIONS) while methyldopa had more central nervous system effects (depression, drowsiness) but fewer orthostatic effects and less diarrhea.

INDICATIONS AND USAGE

Guanadrel sulfate tablets are indicated for the treatment of hypertension in patients not responding adequately to a thiazide type diuretic. Guanadrel sulfate should be added to a diuretic regimen for optimum blood pressure control.

NON-FDA APPROVED INDICATIONS

Guanadrel has also been used alone or as an adjunct in the treatment of cardiovascular and neuromuscular complications of thyrotoxicosis; however, this use is not approved by the FDA.

CONTRAINDICATIONS

Guanadrel sulfate tablets are contraindicated in known or suspected pheochromocytoma.

Guanadrel sulfate should not be used concurrently with, or within 1 week of, monoamine oxidase inhibitors.

Guanadrel sulfate should not be used in patients hypersensitive to the drug.

Guanadrel sulfate should not be used in patients with frank congestive heart failure.

G

WARNINGS

ORTHOSTATIC HYPOTENSION

Orthostatic hypotension and its consequences (dizziness and weakness) are frequent in people treated with guanadrel sulfate tablets. Rarely, fainting upon standing or exercise is seen. Careful instructions to the patient can minimize these symptoms, as can recognition by the physician that the supine blood pressure does not constitute an adequate assessment of the effects of this drug. Patients with known regional vascular disease (cerebral, coronary) are at particular risk from marked orthostatic hypotension and guanadrel sulfate should be avoided in them unless drugs with lesser degrees of orthostatic hypotension are ineffective or unacceptable. In such patients hypotensive episodes should be avoided, even if this requires accepting a poorer degree of blood pressure control.

Instructions to Patients

Patients should be advised about the risk of orthostatic hypotension and told to sit or lie down immediately at the onset of dizziness or weakness so that they can prevent loss of consciousness. They should be told that postural hypotension is worst in the morning and upon arising, and may be exaggerated by alcohol, fever, hot weather, prolonged standing, or exercise.

SURGERY

To reduce the possibility of vascular collapse during anesthesia, guanadrel should be discontinued 48-72 hours before elective surgery. If emergency surgery is required, the anesthesiologist should be made aware that the patient has been taking guanadrel sulfate and that preanesthetic and anesthetic agents should be administered cautiously in reduced dosage. If vasopressors are needed they must be used cautiously, as guanadrel can enhance the pressor response to such agents and increase their arrhythmogenicity.

ASTHMATIC PATIENTS

Special care is needed in patients with bronchial asthma, as their condition may be aggravated by catecholamine depletion and sympathomimetic amines may interfere with the hypotensive effect of guanadrel.

PRECAUTIONS

GENERAL

Salt and water retention may occur with the use of guanadrel sulfate tablets. In clinical studies major problems did not arise because of concomitant diuretic use. Patients with heart failure have not been studied on guanadrel sulfate, but guanadrel could interfere with the adrenergic mechanisms that maintain compensation.

In patients with a history of peptic ulcer, which could be aggravated by a relative increase in parasympathetic tone, guanadrel sulfate should be used cautiously.

In patients with compromised renal function, decreases in renal and nonrenal clearances and an increase in the elimination half-life of guanadrel sulfate have been found. This could possibly lead to an increased incidence of side effects if standard doses are used in these patients. Titration of dose based on the blood pressure response is necessary because of marked interpatient variability (see DOSAGE AND ADMINISTRATION.)

A transient increase in blood pressure has been observed in some patients.

INFORMATION FOR THE PATIENT

See WARNINGS section.

CARCINOGENESIS, MUTAGENESIS, AND IMPAIRMENT OF FERTILITY

No evidence of carcinogenic potential appeared in a 2 year mouse study of guanadrel sulfate. In a 2 year rat study, an increased number of benign testicular interstitial cell tumors was observed at dosages of 100 mg/kg/day and 400 mg/kg/day. These are common spontaneous tumors in aged rats and their significance to therapy with guanadrel sulfate in man is unknown. *Salmonella* testing (Ames test) showed no evidence of mutagenic activity.

A reproduction study was performed in male and female rats at dosages of 0, 10, 30, and 100 mg/kg/day. Suppressed libido and reduced fertility were noted at 100 mg/kg/day (12 times the maximum human dose in a 50 kg subject) and libido was suppressed to a lesser extent at 30 mg/kg/day.

PREGNANCY CATEGORY B

Teratology studies performed in rats and rabbits at doses up to 12 times the maximum recommended human dose (in a 50 kg subject) revealed no significant harm to the fetus due to guanadrel sulfate. There are, however, no adequate and well-controlled studies in pregnant women. Because animal reproduction studies are not always predictive, guanadrel sulfate should be used in pregnant women only when the potential benefit outweighs the potential risk to mother and infant.

NURSING MOTHERS

Whether guanadrel sulfate is excreted in human milk is not known, but because many drugs are excreted in human milk and because of the potential for serious adverse reactions in nursing infants from guanadrel, a decision should be made whether to discontinue nursing or discontinue the drug, taking into account the importance of the drug to the mother.

PEDIATRIC USE

Safety and effectiveness in children have not been established.

DRUG INTERACTIONS

As discussed in CLINICAL PHARMACOLOGY, tricyclic antidepressants and indirect-acting sympathomimetics such as ephedrine or phenylpropanolamine, and possibly phenothiazines, can reverse the effects of neuronal blocking agents. IN VIEW OF THE PRESENCE OF SYMPATHOMIMETIC AMINES IN MANY NON-PRESCRIPTION DRUGS FOR THE TREATMENT OF COLDS, ALLERGY, OR ASTHMA, PATIENTS GIVEN GUANADREL SHOULD BE SPECIFICALLY WARNED NOT TO USE SUCH PREPARATIONS WITHOUT THEIR PHYSICIAN'S ADVICE.

Guanadrel enhances the activity of direct-acting sympathomimetics, like norepinephrine, by blocking neuronal uptake.

Drugs that affect the adrenergic response by the same or other mechanisms would be expected to potentiate the effects of guanadrel, causing excessive postural hypotension and bradycardia. These include alpha- or beta-adrenergic blocking agents and reserpine. There is no clinical experience with the combination of guanadrel sulfate with alpha-adrenergic blocking agents or reserpine.

When guanadrel sulfate was added to the treatment regimen in hypertensive patients inadequately controlled with a diuretic and propranolol, no significant adverse effects, including bradycardia, were reported in the 26 patients treated concomitantly with the three drugs.

The use of guanadrel sulfate with vasodilators has not been adequately studied and is not generally recommended because concomitant use may increase the potential for symptomatic orthostatic hypotension.

ADVERSE REACTIONS

The adverse reaction data for guanadrel is derived principally from comparative long-term (6 months to 3 years) studies with methyldopa and guanethidine in which side effects were assessed through use of periodic questionnaires, a method that tends to give high adverse reaction rates. In the tables that follow, some of the adverse effects reported may not be drug-related, but in the absence of a placebo-treated group, these cannot be readily distinguished. Comparative results with two well-known drugs, methyldopa and guanethidine should aid in interpretation of these adverse reaction rates.

TABLE 1A, TABLE 1B, and TABLE 1C display the frequency of side effects which are believed to be related to sympathetic blocking agents: orthostatic faintness, increased bowel movements and ejaculation disturbances for peripherally acting drugs such as guanadrel and drowsiness for centrally acting drugs such as methyldopa. The frequencies observed were generally higher during the first 8 weeks of therapy. Week 0 frequencies, which were recorded just prior to administration of the antihypertensive drugs while the patients were receiving diuretics, serve as a reference point. Frequency while on therapy are shown for the first 8 weeks and for weeks 9-52.

TABLE 1A *Frequency of Side Effects*

Percent of clinic visits in which side effect was reported

Week	Guanadrel Pre-Drug 0	1-8	9-52
Number of clinic visits analyzed	470	3003	4260
Side Effect			
Morning orthostatic faintness	6.6%	9.4%	6.8%
Orthostatic faintness during the day	7.5%	10.8%	8.5%
Other faintness	7.8%	4.8%	4.5%
Increased bowel movements	4.9%	7.9%	6.1%
Drowsiness	15.3%	14.4%	8.7%
Fatigue	25.7%	26.6%	23.7%
Ejaculation disturbance	7.0%	17.5%	12.0%

TABLE 1B *Frequency of Side Effects*

Percent of clinic visits in which side effect was reported

Week	Methyldopa Pre-Drug 0	1-8	9-52
Number of clinic visits analyzed	266	1610	2216
Side Effect			
Morning orthostatic faintness	6.8%	8.1%	7.4%
Orthostatic faintness during the day	7.5%	8.0%	7.8%
Other faintness	6.2%	3.7%	3.8%
Increased bowel movements	4.9%	5.9%	3.8%
Drowsiness	13.2%	21.2%	18.6%
Fatigue	32.9%	22.6%	27.6%
Ejaculation disturbance	10.3%	13.4%	11.5%

The frequency of side effects over time may be reduced by the discontinuation of drugs in patients who experience intolerable side effects. Reasons for discontinuation of therapy with guanadrel are shown in TABLE 2.

TABLE 1C *Frequency of Side Effects*

Percent of clinic visits in which side effect was reported

Week	Guanethidine Pre-Drug 0	1-8	9-52
Number of clinic visits analyzed	215	1421	2009
Side Effect			
Morning orthostatic faintness	4.6%	10.7%	7.9%
Orthostatic faintness during the day	5.6%	8.9%	6.3%
Other faintness	5.9%	2.7%	2.0%
Increased bowel movements	3.7%	7.9%	9.4%
Drowsiness	10.2%	10.3%	6.4%
Fatigue	21.4%	20.5%	17.5%
Ejaculation disturbance	6.9%	16.6%	18.2%

TABLE 2 *Percent of Patients Who Discontinued*

	Guanadrel	Methyldopa	Guanethidine
Orthostatic faintness	0.6%	0.7%	6.0%*
Syncope	0.4%	0.3%	2.0%
Other faintness	1.2%	0.0%	0.0%
Increased bowel movements	0.8%	0.7%	1.4%
Drowsiness	0.0%	1.9%*	0.0%
Fatigue	0.2%	2.6%*	0.0%
Ejaculation disturbances	0.4%	0.0%	0.0%

* significantly greater than guanadrel sulfate, p <0.003

The following paragraph shows the incidence of reactions often associated with adrenergic neuron blockers as the percent of patients who reported the event at least once over the treatment periods of 6 months to 3 years. For such long-term studies these incidence rates of side effects, which are found often in untreated patients, tend to be high and accumulate with time. The incidence rates for two well-known comparison drugs, methyldopa and guanethidine should aid in interpreting the high rates. It can be seen that the serious consequences of the orthostatic effect of guanadrel, such as syncope, were very uncommon.

1544 guanadrel, 743 methyldopa and 330 guanethidine patients were evaluated in comparison studies. The observed incidence rates of major drug related side effects for guanadrel, methyldopa and guanethidine, respectively, are as follows: orthostatic faintness: 49%, 41%, 48%; other faintness: 47%, 46%, 45%; increased bowel movements: 31%, 28%, 36%; ejaculation disturbances: 18%, 21%, 22%; impotence: 5.1%, 12.2%, 7.2%; syncope: 0.4%, 0.3%, 2%; urine retention: 0.2%, 0%, 0%.

Apart from these adverse effects, many others were reported. Relationship to therapy is less clear, although some (such as peripheral edema with all three drugs, depression with methyldopa) are in part drug related. All adverse effects reported in at least 1% of guanadrel patients are listed in TABLE 3.

TABLE 3

Event	Guanadrel n=1544	Methyldopa n=743	Guanethidine n=330
Cardiovascular - Respiratory			
Chest pain	27.9%	37.4%	27.3%
Coughing	26.9%	36.2%	21.5%
Palpitations	29.5%	35.0%	24.5%
Shortness of breath at rest	18.3%	22.3%	17.0%
Shortness of breath on exertion	45.9%	53.2%	48.8%
Central Nervous System - Special Senses			
Confusion	14.8%	22.6%	10.9%
Depression	1.9%	3.9%	1.8%
Drowsiness	44.6%	64.1%	28.5%
Headache	58.1%	69.0%	49.7%
Paresthesias	25.1%	35.1%	16.4%
Psychological problems	3.8%	4.8%	3.9%
Sleep disorders	2.1%	2.3%	2.7%
Visual disturbances	29.2%	35.3%	26.1%
Gastrointestinal			
Abdominal distress or pain	1.7%	1.9%	1.5%
Anorexia	18.7%	23.0%	17.6%
Constipation	21.0%	29.1%	20.3%
Dry mouth, dry throat	1.7%	4.0%	0.6%
Gas pain	32.0%	39.7%	29.4%
Glossitis	8.4%	10.8%	4.8%
Indigestion	23.7%	30.8%	18.5%
Nausea and/or vomiting	3.9%	4.8%	3.6%
Genitourinary			
Hematuria	2.3%	4.2%	2.1%
Nocturia	48.4%	52.4%	41.5%
Peripheral edema	28.6%	37.4%	22.7%
Urination urgency or frequency	33.6%	39.8%	27.6%
Miscellaneous			
Excessive weight gain	44.3%	53.7%	42.4%
Excessive weight loss	42.2%	51.1%	41.5%
Fatigue	63.6%	76.2%	57.0%
Musculoskeletal			
Aching limbs	42.9%	51.7%	33.9%
Backache or neckache	1.5%	1.1%	1.8%
Joint pain or inflammation	1.7%	2.0%	2.4%
Leg cramps during the day	21.1%	26.0%	20.0%
Leg cramps during the night	25.6%	32.6%	21.2%

DOSAGE AND ADMINISTRATION

As with other sympathetic suppressant drugs, the dose response to guanadrel sulfate tablets varies widely and must be adjusted for each patient until the therapeutic goal is achieved. With long-term therapy, some tolerance may occur and the dosage may have to be increased.

Because guanadrel sulfate has a substantial orthostatic effect, monitoring both supine and standing pressures is essential, especially while dosage is being adjusted.

Guanadrel sulfate should be administered in divided doses. The usual starting dosage for treating hypertension is 10 mg/day, which can be given as 5 mg bid by breaking the 10 mg tablet. The dosage should be adjusted weekly or monthly until blood pressure is controlled. Most patients will require daily dosage in the range of 20-75 mg usually in twice daily doses. For larger doses 3 or 4 times daily dosing may be needed. A dosage of more than 400 mg/day is rarely required.

Dosage should be adjusted for patients with impaired renal function (see CLINICAL PHARMACOLOGY and PRECAUTIONS). As a general guideline, it is recommended that initial therapy with guanadrel sulfate in patients with creatinine clearances of 30-60 ml/min be reduced to 5 mg every 24 hours. In patients with creatinine clearances less than 30 ml/min, the dosing interval should be increased to 48 hours. The time to achieve steady state will be increased. Dosage increases should be made cautiously at intervals not less than 7 days in patients with moderate renal insufficiency and not less than 14 days in patients with severe renal insufficiency. These recommendations are based upon human pharmacokinetic data and not clinical experience.

HOW SUPPLIED

Hylorel tablets are available as follows:

10 mg: Scored elliptical tablets (light orange).

25 mg: Scored elliptical tablets (white).

Storage: Store at controlled room temperature 15-30°C (59-86°F). Keep out of the reach of children.

PRODUCT LISTING - EQUIVALENTS NOT AVAILABLE

Tablet - Oral - 10 mg

100's	$74.87	HYLOREL, Celltech Pharmacueticals Inc	00585-0787-71
100's	$181.58	HYLOREL, Celltech Pharmacueticals Inc	53014-0787-71

Tablet - Oral - 25 mg

100's	$108.36	HYLOREL, Celltech Pharmacueticals Inc	00585-0788-71
100's	$108.36	HYLOREL, Celltech Pharmacueticals Inc	53014-0788-71

Guanethidine Monosulfate *(001410)*

Categories: Hypertension, essential; Pregnancy Category C; FDA Approved 1960 Jul
Drug Classes: Antiadrenergics, peripheral
Brand Names: Antipres; Declindin; Ingadine; **Ismelin**; Normalin; Sanotensin
Foreign Brand Availability: Ismeline (Belgium)
Cost of Therapy: $32.31 (Hypertension; Ismelin; 25 mg; 1 tablet/day; 30 day supply)

DESCRIPTION

Ismelin, guanethidine monosulfate, is an antihypertensive, available as tablets of 10 and 25 mg for oral administration. Each 10 and 25 mg tablet contains guanethidine monosulfate equivalent to 10 and 25 mg of guanethidine sulfate. Its chemical name is (2-(hexahydro-1(*2H*)-azocinyl)ethyl) guanidine sulfate 1:1.

Guanethidine monosulfate is a white to off-white crystalline powder with a molecular weight of 296.38. It is very soluble in water, sparingly soluble in alcohol, and practically insoluble in chloroform.

Ismelin inactive ingredients: Calcium stearate, colloidal silicon dioxide, D&C yellow no. 10 (10 mg tablets), lactose, starch, stearic acid, and sucrose.

Storage: Do not store above 30°C (86°F). *Dispense in tight container.*

CLINICAL PHARMACOLOGY

Guanethidine monosulfate acts at the sympathetic neuroeffector junction by inhibiting or interfering with the release and/or distribution of the chemical mediator (presumably the catecholamine norepinephrine), rather than acting at the effector cell by inhibiting the association of the transmitter with its receptors. In contrast to ganglionic blocking agents, guanethidine monosulfate suppresses equally the responses mediated by alpha-and beta-adrenergic receptors but does not produce parasympathetic blockade. Since sympathetic blockade results in modest decreases in peripheral resistance and cardiac output, guanethidine monosulfate lowers blood pressure in the supine position. It further reduces blood pressure by decreasing the degree of vasoconstriction that normally results from reflex sympathetic nervous activity upon assumption of the upright posture, thus reducing venous return and cardiac output more. The inhibition of sympathetic venoconstrictive mechanisms results in venous pooling of blood. Therefore, the effect of guanethidine monosulfate is especially pronounced when the patient is standing. Both the systolic and diastolic pressures are reduced.

Other actions at the sympathetic nerve terminal include depletion of norepinephrine. Once it gains access to the neuron, guanethidine monosulfate accumulates within the intraneuronal storage vesicles and causes depletion of norepinephrine stores within the nerve terminal. Prolonged oral administration of guanethidine monosulfate produces a denervation sensitivity of the neuroeffector junction, probably resulting from the chronic reduction in norepinephrine released by the sympathetic nerve endings. Systemic responses to catecholamines released from the adrenal medulla are not prevented and may even be augmented as a result of this denervation sensitivity. A paradoxical hypertensive crisis may occur if guanethidine monosulfate is given to patients with pheochromocytoma or if norepinephrine is given to a patient receiving the drug.

Due to its poor lipid solubility, guanethidine monosulfate does not readily cross the blood-brain barrier. In contrast to most neural blocking agents, guanethidine monosulfate does not appear to suppress plasma renin activity in many patients.

PHARMACOKINETICS

The pharmacokinetics of guanethidine monosulfate are complex. The amount of drug in plasma and in urine is linearly related to dose, although large differences occur between individuals because of variation in absorption and metabolism. Adrenergic blockade occurs with a minimum concentration in plasma of 8 ng/ml; this concentration is achieved in different individuals with dosages of 10-50 mg/day at steady state. Guanethidine monosulfate is eliminated slowly because of extensive tissue binding. After chronic oral administration, the initial phase of elimination with a half-life of 1.5 days is followed by a second phase of elimination with a half-life of 4-8 days. The renal clearance of guanethidine monosulfate is 56 ml/min. Guanethidine monosulfate is converted by the liver to three metabolites, which are excreted in the urine. The metabolites are pharmacologically less active than guanethidine monosulfate.

INDICATIONS AND USAGE

Guanethidine monosulfate is indicated for the treatment of moderate and severe hypertension, either alone or as an adjunct, and for the treatment of renal hypertension, including that secondary to pyelonephritis, renal amyloidosis, and renal artery stenosis.

NON-FDA APPROVED INDICATIONS

Guanethidine injection has been used in the treatment of reflex sympathetic dystrophy and Raynaud's disease; however, these uses are not approved by the FDA.

G

CONTRAINDICATIONS

Known or suspected pheochromocytoma; hypersensitivity; frank congestive heart failure not due to hypertension; use of monoamine oxidase (MAO) inhibitors.

WARNINGS

Guanethidine monosulfate is a potent drug and its use can lead to disturbing and serious clinical problems. Before prescribing, physicians should familiarize themselves with the details of its use and warn patients not to deviate from instructions.

Orthostatic hypotension can occur frequently, and patients should be properly instructed about this potential hazard. Fainting spells may occur unless the patient is forewarned to sit or lie down with the onset of dizziness or weakness. Postural hypotension is most marked in the morning and is accentuated by hot weather, alcohol, or exercise. Dizziness or weakness may be particularly bothersome during the initial period of dosage adjustment and with postural changes, such as arising the morning. The potential occurrence of these symptoms may require alteration of previous daily activity. The patient should be cautioned to avoid sudden or prolonged standing or exercise while taking the drug.

Inhibition of ejaculation has been reported in animals (see PRECAUTIONS, Carcinogenesis, Mutagenesis, and Impairment of Fertility) as well as in men given guanethidine monosulfate. This effect, which result from the sympathetic blockade caused by the drug's action, is reversible after guanethidine monosulfate has been discontinued for several weeks. The drug does not cause parasympathetic blockade, and erectile potency is usually retained during administration of guanethidine monosulfate. The possible occurrence of inhibition of ejaculation should be kept in mind when considering the use of guanethidine in men or reproductive age.

If possible, therapy should be withdrawn 2 weeks prior to surgery to reduce the possibility of vascular collapse and cardiac arrest during anesthesia. If emergency surgery is indicated, preanesthetic and anesthetic agents should be administered cautiously in reduced dosage. Oxygen, atropine, vasopressors, and adequate solutions for volume replacement should be ready for immediate use to counteract vascular collapse in the surgical patient. Vasopressors should be used only with extreme caution, since guanethidine monosulfate augments responsiveness to exogenously administered norepinephrine and vasopressors; specially; blood pressure may rise and cardiac arrhythmias may be produced.

PRECAUTIONS

GENERAL

Dosage requirements may be reduced in the presence of fever.

Special care should be exercised when treating patients with a history of bronchial asthma; asthmatic patients are more apt to be hypersensitive to catecholamine depletion, and their condition may be aggravated.

The effects of guanethidine monosulfate are cumulative over long periods; initial doses should be small and increased gradually in small increments.

Guanethidine monosulfate should be used very cautiously in hypertensive patients with: renal disease and nitrogen retention or rising BUN levels, since decreased blood pressure may further compromise renal function; coronary insufficiency or recent myocardial infarction; and cerebrovascular disease, especially with encephalopathy.

Guanethidine monosulfate should not be given to patients with severe cardiac failure except with extreme caution, since guanethidine monosulfate may interfere with the compensatory role of the adrenergic system in producing circulatory adjustment in patients with congestive heart failure.

Patients with incipient cardiac decompensation should be watched for weight gain or edema, which may be averted by the concomitant administration of a thiazide.

Guanethidine monosulfate should be used cautiously in patients with a history of peptic ulcer or other chronic disorders that may be aggravated by a relative increase in parasympathetic tone.

INFORMATION FOR THE PATIENT

The patient should be advised to take guanethidine monosulfate exactly as directed. If the patient misses a dose, he or she should be told to take only the next scheduled dose (without doubling it).

The patient should be advised to avoid sudden or prolonged standing or exercise and to arise slowly, especially in the morning, to reduce the orthostatic hypotensive effects of dizziness, lightheadedness, or fainting.

The patient should be cautioned about ingesting alcohol, since it aggravates the orthostatic hypotensive effects of guanethidine monosulfate.

Male patients should be advised that guanethidine may interfere with ejaculation.

CARCINOGENESIS, MUTAGENESIS, AND IMPAIRMENT OF FERTILITY

Long-term carcinogenicity studies in animals have not been conducted with guanethidine monosulfate.

While inhibition of sperm passage and accumulation of sperm debris have been reported in rats and rabbits after several weeks of administration of guanethidine monosulfate, 5 or 10 mg/kg/day, subcutaneously or intraperitoneally, recovery of ejaculatory function and fertility has been demonstrated in rats given guanethidine monosulfate intramuscularly, 25 mg/kg/day, for 8 weeks. Inhibition of ejaculation has also been reported in men (see WARNINGS and ADVERSE REACTIONS). This effect, which is attributable to the sympathetic blockade caused by the drug, is reversible several weeks after discontinuance of the drug.

PREGNANCY CATEGORY C

Animal reproduction studies have not been conducted with guanethidine monosulfate. It is also not known whether guanethidine monosulfate can cause fetal harm when administered to a pregnant woman or can affect reproduction capacity. Guanethidine monosulfate should be given to a pregnant woman only if clearly needed.

NURSING MOTHERS

Guanethidine monosulfate is excreted in breast milk in very small quantity. Caution should be exercised when guanethidine monosulfate is administered to a nursing woman.

PEDIATRIC USE

Safety and effectiveness in children have not been established.

DRUG INTERACTIONS

Concurrent use of guanethidine monosulfate and rauwolfia derivatives may cause excessive postural hypotension, bradycardia, and mental depression.

Both digitalis and guanethidine monosulfate slow the heart rate.

Thiazide diuretics enhance the antihypertensive action of guanethidine monosulfate (see DOSAGE AND ADMINISTRATION).

Amphetamine-like compounds, stimulants (*e.g.*, ephedrine, methylphenidate), tricyclic antidepressants (*e.g.*, amitriptyline, imipramine, desipramine) and other psychopharmacologic agents (*e.g.*, phenothiazines and related compounds), as well as oral contraceptives, may reduce the hypotensive effect of guanethidine monosulfate.

MAO inhibitors should be discontinued for at least 1 week before starting therapy with guanethidine monosulfate.

ADVERSE REACTIONS

The following adverse reactions have been observed, but there are not enough data to support an estimate of their frequency. Consequently the reactions are categorized by organ system and are listed in decreasing order of severity and not frequency.

Digestive: Diarrhea, which may be severe at times and necessitate discontinuance of medication; vomiting; nausea; increased bowel movements; dry mouth; parotid tenderness.

Cardiovascular: Chest pains (angina); bradycardia; a tendency toward fluid retention and edema with occasional development of congestive heart failure.

Respiratory: Dyspnea; asthma in susceptible individuals; nasal congestion.

Neurologic: Syncope resulting from either postural or exertional hypotension; dizziness; blurred vision; muscle tremor; ptosis of the lids; mental depression; chest paresthesias; weakness; lassitude; fatigue.

Muscular: Myalgia.

Genitourinary: Rise in BUN; urinary incontinence; inhibition of ejaculation; nocturia.

Metabolic: Weight gain.

Skin and Appendages: Dermatitis; scalp hair loss.

Although a causal relationship has not been established, a few instances of blood dyscrasias (anemia, thrombocytopenia, and leukopenia) and of priapism or impotence have been reported.

DOSAGE AND ADMINISTRATION

Better control may be obtained, especially in the initial phases of treatment, if the patient can have his blood pressure recorded regularly at home.

AMBULATORY PATIENTS

Initial doses should be small (10 mg) and increased gradually, depending upon the patient's response. Guanethidine monosulfate has a long duration of action; therefore, dosage increases should not be made more often than every 5-7 days, unless the patient is hospitalized.

Blood pressure should be measured in the supine position, after standing for 10 minutes, and immediately after exercise if feasible. Dosage may be increased only if there has been no decrease in the standing blood pressure from previous levels. The average daily dose is 25-50 mg; only one dose a day is usually required (TABLE 1).

TABLE 1 *Dosage Chart for Ambulatory Patients*

Visits (intervals of 5- 7 days)	Daily Dose
Visit 1 (Patient may be started on 10 mg tablets)	10 mg
Visit 2	20 mg
Visit 3 (Patient may be changed to 25 mg tablets whenever convenient)	30 mg (three 10 mg tablets) or 37.5 mg (one and one-half 25 mg tablets)
Visit 4	50 mg
Visit 5 and subsequent	Dosage may be increased by 12.5 mg or 25 mg if necessary.

The dosage should be reduced in any of the following situations: (1) normal supine pressure; (2) excessive orthostatic fall in pressure; (3) severe diarrhea.

HOSPITALIZED PATIENTS

Initial oral dose is 25-50 mg, increased by 25 or 50 mg daily or every other day, as indicated. This higher dosage is possible because hospitalized patients can be watched carefully. Unless absolutely impossible, the standing blood pressure should be measured regularly. Patients should not be discharged from the hospital until the effect of the drug on the standing blood pressure is known. Patients should be told about the possibility of orthostatic hypotension and warned not to get out of bed without help during the period of dosage adjustment.

COMBINATION THERAPY

Guanethidine monosulfate may be added gradually to thiazides and/or hydralazine. Thiazide diuretics enhance the effectiveness of guanethidine monosulfate and may reduce the incidence of edema. When thiazide diuretics are added to the regimen in patients taking guanethidine monosulfate, it is usually necessary to reduce the dosage of guanethidine monosulfate. After control is established, the dosage of all drugs should be reduced to the lowest effective level.

Note: When guanethidine monosulfate is replacing MAO inhibitors, at least 1 week should elapse before commencing treatment with guanethidine monosulfate (see CONTRAINDICATIONS). If ganglionic blockers have not been discontinued before guanethidine monosulfate is started, they should be gradually withdrawn to prevent a spiking blood pressure response during the transfer period.

Guanfacine Hydrochloride *(001412)*

Categories: Hypertension, essential; Pregnancy Category B; FDA Approved 1986 Oct
Drug Classes: Antiadrenergics, central
Brand Names: Entulic; **Tenex**
Foreign Brand Availability: Estulic (Belgium; Benin; Burkina-Faso; Czech-Republic; Ecuador; Ethiopia; France; Gambia; Germany; Ghana; Guinea; Hungary; Indonesia; Ivory-Coast; Japan; Kenya; Liberia; Malawi; Mali; Mauritania; Mauritius; Morocco; Netherlands; Niger; Nigeria; Philippines; Russia; Senegal; Seychelles; Sierra-Leone; Spain; Sudan; Tanzania; Tunia; Turkey; Uganda; Zambia; Zimbabwe)
Cost of Therapy: $54.27 (Hypertension; Tenex; 1 mg; 1 tablet/day; 30 day supply)
$21.17 (Hypertension; Generic Tablets; 1 mg; 1 tablet/day; 30 day supply)

DESCRIPTION

Guanfacine hydrochloride is a centrally acting antihypertensive with α_2-adrenoceptor agonist properties in tablet form for oral administration.

The chemical name of guanfacine hydrochloride is N-amidino-2-(2,6-dichlorophenyl) acetamide hydrochloride and its molecular weight is 282.56.

Guanfacine hydrochloride is a white to off-white powder; sparingly soluble in water and alcohol and slightly soluble in acetone.

Tenex tablets contain the following inactive ingredients:

Tenex 1 mg: FD&C red 40 aluminum lake, lactose, microcrystalline cellulose, povidone, stearic acid.

Tenex 2 mg: D&C yellow 10 aluminum lake, lactose, microcrystalline cellulose, povidone, stearic acid.

CLINICAL PHARMACOLOGY

Guanfacine HCl is an orally active antihypertensive agent whose principal mechanism of action appears to be stimulation of central α_2-adrenergic receptors. By stimulating these receptors, guanfacine reduces sympathetic nerve impulses from the vasomotor center to the heart and blood vessels. This results in a decrease in peripheral vascular resistance and a reduction in heart rate.

Controlled clinical trials in patients with mild to moderate hypertension who were receiving a thiazide-type diuretic have defined the dose- response relationship for blood pressure response and adverse reactions of guanfacine given at bedtime and have shown that the blood pressure response to guanfacine can persist for 24 hours after a single dose. In the dose-response study, patients were randomized to placebo or to doses of 0.5, 1, 2, and 3 mg of guanfacine, each given at bedtime. The observed mean changes from baseline, tabulated in TABLE 1, indicate the similarity of response for placebo and the 0.5 mg dose. Doses of 1, 2, and 3 mg resulted in decreased blood pressure in the sitting position with no real differences among the three doses. In the standing position there was some increase in response with dose.

TABLE 1 *Mean Decrease in Seated and Standing Blood Pressure (BP) by guanfacine dosage group*

Vital Sign		Placebo	0.5 mg	1 mg	2 mg	3 mg
	n =	63	63	64	58	59
Change in systolic (seated)	BP	-5	-5	-14	-12	-16
Change in diastolic (seated)	BP	-7	-6	-13	-13	-13
Change in systolic (standing)	BP	-3	-5	-11	- 9	-15
Change in diastolic (standing)	BP	-5	-4	- 9	-10	-12

While most of the effectiveness of guanfacine was present at 1 mg, adverse reactions at this dose were not clearly distinguishable from those associated with placebo. Adverse reactions were clearly present at 2 and 3 mg (see ADVERSE REACTIONS).

In a placebo-controlled study of guanfacine HCl a significant decrease in blood pressure was maintained for a full 24 hours after dosing. While there was no significant difference between the 12 and 24 hour blood pressure readings, the fall in blood pressure at 24 hours was numerically smaller, suggesting possible escape of blood pressure in some patients and the need for individualization of therapy.

In a double-blind, randomized trial, either guanfacine or clonidine was given at recommended doses with 25 mg chlorthalidone for 24 weeks and then abruptly discontinued. Results showed equal degrees of blood pressure reduction with the two drugs and there was no tendency for blood pressures to increase despite maintenance of the same daily dose of the two drugs. Signs and symptoms of rebound phenomena were infrequent upon discontinuation of either drug. Abrupt withdrawal of clonidine produced a rapid return of diastolic and especially, systolic blood pressure to approximately pre-treatment levels, with occasional values significantly greater than baseline, whereas guanfacine withdrawal produced a more gradual increase to pre-treatment levels, but also with occasional values significantly greater than baseline.

PHARMACODYNAMICS

Hemodynamic studies in man showed that the decrease in blood pressure observed after single-dose or long-term oral treatment with guanfacine was accompanied by a significant decrease in peripheral resistance and a slight reduction in heart rate (5 beats/min). Cardiac output under conditions of rest or exercise was not altered by guanfacine.

Guanfacine HCl lowered elevated plasma renin activity and plasma catecholamine levels in hypertensive patients, but this does not correlate with individual blood-pressure responses.

Growth hormone secretion was stimulated with single oral doses of 2 and 4 mg of guanfacine. Long-term use of guanfacine HCl had no effect on growth hormone levels.

Guanfacine had no effect on plasma aldosterone. A slight but insignificant decrease in plasma volume occurred after 1 month of guanfacine therapy. There were no changes in mean body weight or electrolytes.

PHARMACOKINETICS

Relative to an intravenous dose of 3 mg, the absolute oral bioavailability of guanfacine is about 80%. Peak plasma concentrations occur from 1-4 hours with an average of 2.6 hours after single oral doses or at steady state.

The area under the concentration-time curve (AUC) increases linearly with the dose.

In individuals with normal renal function, the average elimination half-life is approximately 17 hours (range 10-30 hours). Younger patients tend to have shorter elimination half-lives (13-14 hours) while older patients tend to have half-lives at the upper end of the range. Steady state blood levels were attained within 4 days in most subjects.

In individuals with normal renal function, guanfacine and its metabolites are excreted primarily in the urine. Approximately 50% (40-75%) of the dose is eliminated in the urine as unchanged drug; the remainder is eliminated mostly as conjugates of metabolites produced by oxidative metabolism of the aromatic ring.

The guanfacine-to-creatinine clearance ratio is greater than 1.0, which would suggest that tubular secretion of drug occurs.

The drug is approximately 70% bound to plasma proteins, independent of drug concentration.

The whole body volume of distribution is high (a mean of 6.3 L/kg), which suggests a high distribution of drug to the tissues.

The clearance of guanfacine in patients with varying degrees of renal insufficiency is reduced, but plasma levels of drug are only slightly increased compared to patients with normal renal function. When prescribing for patients with renal impairment, the low end of the dosing range should be used. Patients on dialysis also can be given usual doses of guanfacine hydrochloride as the drug is poorly dialyzed.

INDICATIONS AND USAGE

Guanfacine HCl is indicated in the management of hypertension. Since dosing information (see DOSAGE AND ADMINISTRATION) has been established in the presence of a thiazide-type diuretic; guanfacine HCl should, therefore, be used in patients who are already receiving a thiazide-type diuretic.

NON-FDA APPROVED INDICATIONS

Guanfacine has been used for the treatment of heroin withdrawal symptoms and hypertension in pregnancy; however, this use is not approved by the FDA.

CONTRAINDICATIONS

Guanfacine HCl is contraindicated in patients with known hypersensitivity to guanfacine hydrochloride.

PRECAUTIONS

GENERAL

Like other antihypertensive agents, guanfacine HCl should be used with caution in patients with severe coronary insufficiency, recent myocardial infarction, cerebrovascular disease or chronic renal or hepatic failure.

Sedation

Guanfacine HCl, like other orally active central alpha-2 adrenergic agonists, causes sedation or drowsiness, especially when beginning therapy. These symptoms are dose-related (see ADVERSE REACTIONS). When guanfacine HCl is used with other centrally active depressants (such as phenothiazines, barbiturates, or benzodiazepines), the potential for additive sedative effects should be considered.

Rebound

Abrupt cessation of therapy with orally active central alpha-2 adrenergic agonists may be associated with increases (from depressed on-therapy levels) in plasma and urinary catecholamines, symptoms of "nervousness and anxiety" and, less commonly, increases in blood pressure to levels significantly greater than those prior to therapy.

INFORMATION FOR THE PATIENT

Patients who receive guanfacine HCl should be advised to exercise caution when operating dangerous machinery or driving motor vehicles until it is determined that they do not become drowsy or dizzy from the medication. Patients should be warned that their tolerance for alcohol and other CNS depressants may be diminished. Patients should be advised not to discontinue therapy abruptly.

LABORATORY TESTS

In clinical trials, no clinically relevant laboratory test abnormalities were identified as causally related to drug during short-term treatment with guanfacine HCl.

DRUG/LABORATORY TEST INTERACTIONS

No laboratory test abnormalities related to the use of guanfacine HCl have been identified.

CARCINOGENESIS, MUTAGENESIS, AND IMPAIRMENT OF FERTILITY

No carcinogenic effect was observed in studies of 78 weeks in mice at doses more than 150 times the maximum recommended human dose and 102 weeks in rats at doses more than 100 times the maximum recommended human dose. In a variety of test models guanfacine was not mutagenic.

No adverse effects were observed in fertility studies in male and female rats.

G

PREGNANCY CATEGORY B

Administration of guanfacine to rats at 70 times the maximum recommended human dose and rabbits at 20 times the maximum recommended human dose resulted in no evidence of impaired fertility or harm to the fetus. Higher doses (100 and 200 times the maximum recommended human dose in rabbits and rats respectively) were associated with reduced fetal survival and maternal toxicity. Rat experiments have shown that guanfacine crosses the placenta.

There are, however, no adequate and well-controlled studies in pregnant women. Because animal reproduction studies are not always predictive of human response, this drug should be used during pregnancy only if clearly needed.

LABOR AND DELIVERY

Guanfacine HCl is not recommended in the treatment of acute hypertension associated with toxemia of pregnancy. There is no information available on the effects of guanfacine on the course of labor and delivery.

NURSING MOTHERS

It is not known whether guanfacine HCl is excreted in human milk. Because many drugs are excreted in human milk, caution should be exercised when guanfacine HCl is administered to a nursing woman. Experiments with rats have shown that guanfacine is excreted in the milk.

PEDIATRIC USE

Safety and effectiveness in children under 12 years of age have not been demonstrated. Therefore, the use of guanfacine HCl in this age group is not recommended.

DRUG INTERACTIONS

The potential for increased sedation when guanfacine HCl is given with other CNS-depressant drugs should be appreciated.

The administration of guanfacine concomitantly with a known microsomal enzyme inducer (phenobarbital or phenytoin) to 2 patients with renal impairment reportedly resulted in significant reductions in elimination half-life and plasma concentration. In such cases, therefore, more frequent dosing may be required to achieve or maintain the desired hypotensive response. Further, if guanfacine is to be discontinued in such patients, careful tapering of the dosage may be necessary in order to avoid rebound phenomena (see PRECAUTIONS, General, Rebound.)

Anticoagulants: Ten (10) patients who were stabilized on oral anticoagulants were given guanfacine, 1-2 mg/day, for 4 weeks. No changes were observed in the degree of anticoagulation.

In several well-controlled studies, guanfacine was administered together with diuretics with no drug interactions reported. In the long-term safety studies, guanfacine HCl was given concomitantly with many drugs without evidence of any interactions. The principal drugs given (number of patients in parentheses) were: cardiac glycosides (115), sedatives and hypnotics (103), coronary vasodilators (52), oral hypoglycemics (45), cough and cold preparations (45), NSAIDs (38), anti-hyperlipidemics (29), antigout drugs (24), oral contraceptives (18), bronchodilators (13), insulin (10), and beta blockers (10).

ADVERSE REACTIONS

Adverse reactions noted with guanfacine HCl are similar to those of other drugs of the central alpha-2 adrenoreceptor agonist class: dry mouth, sedation (somnolence), weakness (asthenia), dizziness, constipation, and impotence. While the reactions are common, most are mild and tend to disappear on continued dosing.

Skin rash with exfoliation has been reported in a few cases; although clear cause and effect relationships to guanfacine HCl could not be established, should a rash occur, guanfacine HCl should be discontinued and the patient monitored appropriately.

In a 12 week placebo-controlled, dose-response study the frequency of the most commonly observed adverse reactions showed a clear dose relationship from 0.5 to 3 mg (seeTABLE 2).

There were 41 premature terminations because of adverse reactions in this study. The percent of patients who terminated and the dose at which they terminated are shown in TABLE 3.

Reasons for dropouts among patients who received guanfacine were: somnolence, headache, weakness, dry mouth, dizziness, impotence, insomnia, constipation, syncope, urinary incontinence, conjunctivitis, paresthesia, and dermatitis. In a second placebo-controlled study in which the dose should be adjusted upward to 3 mg per day in 1 mg increments at 3 week intervals, *i.e.,* a setting more similar to ordinary clinical use, the most commonly recorded reactions were: dry mouth 47%, constipation 16%, fatigue 12%, somnolence 10%, asthenia 6%, dizziness 6%, headache 4%, and insomnia 4%.

TABLE 2

		Assigned Treatment Group			
	Placebo	0.5 mg	1.0 mg	2.0 mg	3.0 mg
Adverse Reaction	n=73	n=72	n=72	n=72	n=72
Dry mouth	5 (7%)	4 (5%)	6 (8%)	8 (11%)	20 (28%)
Somnolence	1 (1%)	3 (4%)	0 (0%)	1 (1%)	10 (14%)
Asthenia	0 (0%)	2 (3%)	0 (0%)	2 (2%)	7 (10%)
Dizziness	2 (2%)	1 (1%)	3 (4%)	6 (8%)	3 (4%)
Headache	3 (4%)	4 (3%)	3 (4%)	1 (1%)	2 (2%)
Impotence	1 (1%)	1 (0%)	0 (0%)	1 (1%)	3 (4%)
Constipation	0 (0%)	0 (0%)	0 (0%)	1 (1%)	1 (1%)
Fatigue	3 (3%)	2 (3%)	2 (3%)	5 (6%)	3 (4%)

TABLE 3

Dose	Placebo	0.5 mg	1 mg	2 mg	3 mg
Terminated	6.9%	4.2%	3.2%	6.9%	8.3%

Reasons for dropouts among patients who received guanfacine were: somnolence, dry mouth, dizziness, impotence, constipation, confusion, depression, and palpitations.

In the clonidine/guanfacine comparison described in Clinical Pharmacology, the most common adverse reactions noted are shown in TABLE 4.

TABLE 4

	Guanfacine (n=279)	Clonidine (n=278)
Dry mouth	30%	37%
Somnolence	21%	35%
Dizziness	11%	8%
Constipation	10%	5%
Fatigue	9%	8%
Headache	4%	4%
Insomnia	4%	3%

Adverse reactions occurring in 3% or less of patients in the three controlled trials were:

Cardiovascular: Bradycardia, palpitations, substernal pain.
Gastrointestinal: Abdominal pain, diarrhea, dyspepsia, dysphagia, nausea.
CNS: Amnesia, confusion, depression, insomnia, libido decrease.
ENT disorders: Rhinitis, taste perversion, tinnitus.
Eye disorders: Conjunctivitis, iritis, vision disturbance.
Musculoskeletal: Leg cramps, hypokinesia.
Respiratory: Dyspnea.
Dermatologic: Dermatitis, pruritus, purpura, sweating.
Urogenital: Testicular disorder, urinary incontinence.
Other: Malaise, paresthesia, paresis.

Adverse reaction reports tend to decrease over time. In an open-label trial of 1 year's duration, 580 hypertensive subjects were given guanfacine, titrated to achieve goal blood pressure, alone (51%), with diuretic (38%), with beta blocker (3%), with diuretic plus beta blocker (6%), or with diuretic plus vasodilator (2%). The mean daily dose of guanfacine reached was 4.7 mg (see TABLE 5).

TABLE 5

Adverse Reaction	Incidence of adverse reactions at any time during the study (n=580)	Incidence of adverse at end of 1 year (n=580)
Dry mouth	60%	15%
Drowsiness	33%	6%
Dizziness	15%	1%
Constipation	14%	3%
Weakness	5%	1%
Headache	4%	0.2%
Insomnia	5%	0%

There were 52 (8.9%) dropouts due to adverse effects in this 1-year trial. The causes were: dry mouth (n=20), weakness (n=12), constipation (n=7), somnolence (n=3), nausea (n=3), orthostatic hypotension (n=2), insomnia (n=1), rash (n=1), nightmares (n=1), headache (n=1), and depression (n=1).

POSTMARKETING EXPERIENCE

An open-label postmarketing study involving 21,718 patients was conducted to assess the safety of guanfacine HCl 1 mg/day given at bedtime for 28 days. Guanfacine HCl was administered with or without other antihypertensive agents. Adverse events reported in the postmarketing study at an incidence greater than 1% included dry mouth, dizziness, somnolence, fatigue, headache and nausea. The most commonly reported adverse events in this study were the same as those observed in controlled clinical trials.

Less frequent, possibly guanfacine HCl-related events observed in the postmarketing study and/or reported spontaneously include:

Body as a Whole: Asthenia, chest pain, edema, malaise, tremor.
Cardiovascular: Bradycardia, palpitations, syncope, tachycardia.
Central Nervous System: Paresthesias, vertigo.

Eye Disorders: Blurred vision.
Gastrointestinal System: Abdominal pain, constipation, diarrhea, dyspepsia.
Liver And Biliary System: Abnormal liver function tests.
Musculo-Skeletal System: Arthralgia, leg cramps, leg pain, myalgia.
Psychiatric: Agitation, anxiety, confusion, depression, insomnia, nervousness.
Reproductive System, Male: Impotence.
Respiratory System: Dyspnea.
Skin And Appendages: Alopecia, dermatitis, exfoliative pruritus, rash, dermatitis.
Special Senses: Alterations in taste.
Urinary System: Nocturia, urinary frequency.

Rare, serious disorders with no definitive cause and effect relationship to guanfacine HCl have been reported spontaneously and/or in the postmarketing study. These events include acute renal failure, cardiac fibrillation, cerebrovascular accident, congestive heart failure, heart block, and myocardial infarction.

DOSAGE AND ADMINISTRATION

The recommended dose of guanfacine HCl is 1 mg daily given at bedtime to minimize somnolence. Patients should already be receiving a thiazide type diuretic.

If after 3-4 weeks of therapy, 1 mg does not give a satisfactory result, doses of 2 and then subsequently 3 mg may be given, although most of the effect of guanfacine HCl is seen at 1 mg (see CLINICAL PHARMACOLOGY). Some patients may show a rise in pressure toward the end of the dosing interval; in this event a divided dose may be utilized.

Higher daily doses (rarely up to 40 mg/day, in divided doses) have been used, but adverse reactions increase significantly with doses above 3 mg/day and there is no evidence of increased efficacy. No studies have established an appropriate dose or dosing interval when guanfacine HCl is given as the sole antihypertensive agent.

The frequency of rebound hypertension is low, but rebound can occur. When rebound occurs, it does so after 2-4 days, which is delayed compared with clonidine hydrochloride. This is consistent with the longer half-life of guanfacine. In most cases, after abrupt withdrawal of guanfacine, blood pressure returns to pretreatment levels slowly (within 2-4 days) without ill effects.

Store at controlled room temperature, between 15-30°C (59-86°F).

PRODUCT LISTING - RATED THERAPEUTICALLY EQUIVALENT

Package	Price	Supplier	NDC
Tablet - Oral - 1 mg			
90's	$78.40	TENEX, Allscripts Pharmaceutical Company	54569-8563-00
100's	$52.50	FEDERAL UPPER LIMIT, H.C.F.A. F F P	99999-1412-03
100's	$70.55	GENERIC, Qualitest Products Inc	00603-3774-21
100's	$70.58	GENERIC, Major Pharmaceuticals Inc	00904-5133-60
100's	$74.99	GENERIC, Amide Pharmaceutical Inc	52152-0118-02
100's	$78.99	GENERIC, Ivax Corporation	00182-2641-01
100's	$80.26	GENERIC, Moore, H.L. Drug Exchange Inc	00839-8046-06
100's	$81.07	GENERIC, Watson/Rugby Laboratories Inc	00536-5756-01
100's	$83.00	GENERIC, Watson Laboratories Inc	52544-0444-01
100's	$87.20	GENERIC, Mylan Pharmaceuticals Inc	00378-1160-01
100's	$87.20	GENERIC, Watson Laboratories Inc	00591-0444-01
100's	$87.20	GENERIC, Par Pharmaceutical Inc	49884-0572-01
100's	$180.90	TENEX, Wyeth-Ayerst Laboratories	00031-8901-63
Tablet - Oral - 2 mg			
100's	$72.00	FEDERAL UPPER LIMIT, H.C.F.A. F F P	99999-1412-04
100's	$96.75	GENERIC, Qualitest Products Inc	00603-3775-21
100's	$96.77	GENERIC, Major Pharmaceuticals Inc	00904-5134-60
100's	$102.99	GENERIC, Amide Pharmaceutical Inc	52152-0119-02
100's	$107.36	GENERIC, Ivax Corporation	00182-2642-01
100's	$110.09	GENERIC, Moore, H.L. Drug Exchange Inc	00839-8047-06
100's	$111.14	GENERIC, Watson/Rugby Laboratories Inc	00536-5757-01
100's	$117.60	GENERIC, Mylan Pharmaceuticals Inc	00378-1190-01
100's	$117.60	GENERIC, Watson Laboratories Inc	00591-0453-01
100's	$117.60	GENERIC, Par Pharmaceutical Inc	49884-0573-01
100's	$117.60	GENERIC, Watson Laboratories Inc	52544-0453-01
100's	$136.87	GENERIC, Major Pharmaceuticals Inc	00904-5580-60
100's	$268.66	TENEX, Wyeth-Ayerst Laboratories	00031-8903-63

Haemophilus B Conjugate Vaccine *(001414)*

For complete prescribing information, refer to the CD-ROM included with the book.

Categories: Immunization, Haemophilus B; Pregnancy Category C; FDA Approved 1988 Dec
Drug Classes: Vaccines
Brand Names: ActHIB; HibTITER; **PedvaxHIB**; ProHIBIT
Foreign Brand Availability: Act-HIB (Korea); HIBest (France)

DESCRIPTION

PEDVAXHIB

PedvaxHIB (Haemophilus b Conjugate Vaccine (Meningococcal Protein Conjugate)) is a highly purified capsular polysaccharide (polyribosylribitol phosphate or PRP) of *Haemophilus influenzae* type b (Haemophilus b, Ross strain) that is covalently bound to an outer membrane protein complex (OMPC) of the B11 strain of *Neisseria meningitidis* serogroup B. The covalent bonding of the PRP to the OMPC which is necessary for enhanced immunogenicity of the PRP is confirmed by analysis of the conjugate's components by chemical treatment which yields a unique amino acid. This PRP-OMPC conjugate vaccine is a lyophilized preparation containing lactose as a stabilizer.

PedvaxHIB, when reconstituted as directed, is a sterile suspension for intramuscular use formulated to contain: 15 μg of Haemophilus b PRP, 250 μg of *Neisseria meningitidis* OMPC, 225 μg of aluminum as aluminum hydroxide, thimerosal (a mercury derivative) at 1:20,000 as a preservative, and 2.0 mg of lactose, in 0.9% sodium chloride.

Storage

Before reconstitution, store at 2-8°C (36-46°F).

Store reconstituted vaccine in the vaccine vial at 2-8°C (36-46°F) and discard if not used within 24 hours.

DO NOT FREEZE the aluminum hydroxide diluent or the reconstituted vaccine.

HIBTITER

HibTITER Haemophilus b Conjugate Vaccine (Diphtheria CRM_{197} Protein Conjugate) is a sterile solution of a conjugate of oligosaccharides of the capsular antigen of *Haemophilus influenzae* type b (Haemophilus b) and diphtheria CRM_{197} protein (CRM_{197}) dissolved in 0.9% sodium chloride. The oligosaccharides are derived from highly purified capsular polysaccharide, polyribosylribitol phosphate, isolated from Haemophilus b strain Eagan grown in a chemically defined medium (a mixture of mineral salts, amino acids, and cofactors). The oligosaccharides are purified and sized by diafiltrations through a series of ultrafiltration membranes, and coupled by reductive amination directly to highly purified CRM_{197}.[1,2] CRM_{197} is a nontoxic variant of diphtheria toxin isolated from cultures of *Corynebacterium diphtheriae* C7 (β197) grown in a casamino acids and yeast extract-based medium that is ultrafiltered before use. CRM_{197} is purified through ultrafiltration, ammonium sulfate precipitation and ion-exchange chromatography to high purity. The conjugate is purified to remove unreacted protein, oligosaccharides, and reagents; sterilized by filtration; and filled into vials. HibTITER is intended for intramuscular use.

The vaccine is a clear, colorless solution. Each single dose of 0.5 ml is formulated to contain 10 μg of purified Haemophilus b saccharide and approximately 25 μg of CRM_{197} protein. Multidose vials contain thimerosal (mercurial derivative) 1:10,000 as a preservative.

INDICATIONS AND USAGE

PEDVAXHIB

PedvaxHIB is indicated for routine immunization against invasive disease caused by *Haemophilus influenzae* type b in infants and children 2-71 months of age.

PedvaxHIB will not protect against disease caused by *Haemophilus influenzae* other than type b or against other microorganisms that cause invasive disease such as meningitis or sepsis.

Revaccination

Infants completing the primary two dose regimen before 12 months of age should receive a booster dose (see DOSAGE AND ADMINISTRATION).

Use With Other Vaccines

Studies have been conducted in which PedvaxHIB has been administered concomitantly with the primary vaccination series of DTP and OPV, or concomitantly with M-M-R II (Measles, Mumps, and Rubella Virus Vaccine Live,) (using separate sites and syringes) or with a booster dose of OPV plus DTP (using separate sites and syringes for PedvaxHIB and DTP). No impairment of immune response to individual tested vaccine antigens was demonstrated. The type, frequency and severity of adverse experiences observed in these studies with PedvaxHIB were similar to those seen when the other vaccines were given alone.

PedvaxHIB IS NOT RECOMMENDED FOR USE IN INFANTS YOUNGER THAN 2 MONTHS OF AGE.

HIBTITER

HibTITER Haemophilus b Conjugate Vaccine (Diphtheria CRM_{197} Protein Conjugate) is indicated for the immunization of children 2 months to 71 months of age against invasive diseases caused by *H. influenzae* type b.

As with any vaccine, HibTITER may not protect 100% of individuals receiving the vaccine.

HibTITER may be administered simultaneously but at different sites from other routine pediatric vaccines, *e.g.*, Diphtheria and Tetanus Toxoids and Pertussis Vaccine Adsorbed (DTP), Oral Poliovirus Vaccine (OPV), and Measles-Mumps-Rubella Vaccine (MMR).[31,32]

CONTRAINDICATIONS

PEDVAXHIB

Hypersensitivity to any component of the vaccine or the diluent.

HIBTITER

Hypersensitivity to any component of the vaccine, including diphtheria toxoid, or thimerosal in the multidose presentation, is a contraindication to use of HibTITER.

WARNINGS

PEDVAXHIB

USE ONLY THE ALUMINUM HYDROXIDE DILUENT SUPPLIED.

If PedvaxHIB is used in persons with malignancies or those receiving immunosuppressive therapy or who are otherwise immunocompromised, the expected immune response may not be obtained.

HIBTITER

HibTITER WILL NOT PROTECT AGAINST *H. INFLUENZAE* OTHER THAN TYPE b STRAINS, NOR WILL HibTITER PROTECT AGAINST OTHER MICROORGANISMS THAT CAUSE MENINGITIS OR SEPTIC DISEASE.

AS WITH ANY INTRAMUSCULAR INJECTION, HibTITER SHOULD BE GIVEN WITH CAUTION TO INFANTS OR CHILDREN WITH THROMBOCYTOPENIA OR ANY COAGULATION DISORDER THAT WOULD CONTRAINDICATE INTRAMUSCULAR INJECTION.

ANTIGENURIA HAS BEEN DETECTED FOLLOWING RECEIPT OF HAEMOPHILUS b CONJUGATE VACCINE[33] AND THEREFORE ANTIGEN DETECTION IN

URINE MAY NOT HAVE DIAGNOSTIC VALUE IN SUSPECTED HAEMOPHILUS b DISEASE WITHIN 2 WEEKS OF IMMUNIZATION.

DOSAGE AND ADMINISTRATION

PEDVAXHIB

2-14 Months of Age

FOR INTRAMUSCULAR ADMINISTRATION. DO NOT INJECT INTRAVENOUSLY. Infants 2-14 months of age should receive a 0.5 ml dose of vaccine ideally beginning at 2 months of age followed by a 0.5 ml dose 2 months later (or as soon as possible thereafter). When the primary two dose regimen is completed before 12 months of age, a booster dose is required (see Booster Dose.

15 Months of Age and Older

Children 15 months of age and older previously unvaccinated against Haemophilus b disease should receive a single 0.5 ml dose of vaccine.

Booster Dose

In infants completing the primary two dose regimen before 12 months of age, a booster dose (0.5 ml) should be administered at 12-15 months of age but not earlier than 2 months after the second dose. DATA ARE NOT AVAILABLE REGARDING THE INTERCHANGEABILITY OF OTHER HAEMOPHILUS b CONJUGATE VACCINES AND PedvaxHIB.

Vaccination regimens by age group are outlined in TABLE 7.

TABLE 7

Age (Months) at First Dose	Primary	Age (Months) at Booster Dose
2-10	2 doses, 2 mo. apart	12-15
11-14	2 doses, 2 mo. apart	—
15-71	1 dose	—

TO RECONSTITUTE, USE ONLY THE ALUMINUM HYDROXIDE DILUENT SUPPLIED.

It is recommended that the vaccine be used as soon as possible after reconstitution. Store reconstituted vaccine in the vaccine vial at 2-8°C (36-46°F) and discard if not used within 24 hours. Agitate prior to injection.

Parenteral drug products should be inspected visually for extraneous particulate matter and discoloration prior to administration whenever solution and container permit. Aluminum hydroxide diluent and PedvaxHIB when reconstituted are slightly opaque white suspensions.

Special care should be taken to ensure that the injection does not enter a blood vessel.

It is important to use a separate sterile syringe and needle for each patient to prevent transmission of hepatitis B or other infectious agents from one person to another.

HIBTITER

HibTITER is for Intramuscular Use Only.

Any parenteral drug product should be inspected visually for extraneous particulate matter and/or discoloration prior to administration whenever solution and container permit. If these conditions exist, HibTITER should not be administered.

Before injection, the skin over the site to be injected should be cleansed with a suitable germicide. After insertion of the needle, aspirate to help avoid inadvertent injection into a blood vessel.

The vaccine should be injected intramuscularly, preferably into the midlateral muscles of the thigh or deltoid, with care to avoid major peripheral nerve trunks.

HibTITER is indicated for children 2 months to 71 months of age for the prevention of invasive Haemophilus b disease. For infants 2-6 months of age, the immunizing dose is three separate injections of 0.5 ml given at approximately 2 months apart. Children from 12 through 14 months of age who have not been vaccinated previously receive 1 injection. All vaccinated children receive a single booster dose at 15 months of age or older, but not less than 2 months after the previous dose. Previously unvaccinated children 15-71 months of age receive a single injection of HibTITER.[31,32] Preterm infants should be vaccinated with HibTITER according to their chronological birth [31] (see TABLE 8).

TABLE 8 *Recommended Immunization Schedule*

Age at First Immunization	No. of Doses	Booster
2-6 months	3	Yes
7-11 months	2	Yes
12-14 months	1	Yes
15 months and over	1	No

Interruption of the recommended schedules with a delay between doses does not interfere with the final immunity achieved nor does it necessitate starting the series over again, regardless of the length of time elapsed between doses.[31, 32]

NO DATA ARE AVAILABLE TO SUPPORT THE INTERCHANGEABILITY OF HibTITER OR OTHER HAEMOPHILUS b CONJUGATE VACCINES WITH ONE ANOTHER FOR THE PRIMARY IMMUNIZATION SERIES. THEREFORE, IT IS RECOMMENDED THAT THE SAME CONJUGATE VACCINE BE USED THROUGHOUT EACH IMMUNIZATION SCHEDULE, CONSISTENT WITH THE DATA SUPPORTING APPROVAL AND LICENSURE OF THE VACCINE.

Each dose of 0.5 ml is formulated to contain 10 µg of purified Haemophilus b saccharide and approximately 25 µg of CRM_{197} protein.

PRODUCT LISTING - EQUIVALENTS NOT AVAILABLE

Powder For Injection - Intramuscular - 10 mcg;24 mcg/0.5 ml

5's	$93.75	OMNIHIB, Glaxosmithkline	00007-4408-05
5's	$135.20	ACTHIB, Aventis Pharmaceuticals	49281-0545-05

Powder For Injection - Intramuscular - 15 mcg;250 mcg/0.5 ml

1's	$20.78	PEDVAX HIB, Merck & Company Inc	00006-4792-00
5's	$103.88	PEDVAX HIB, Merck & Company Inc	00006-4797-00

Solution - Intramuscular - 7.5 mcg;125 mcg/0.5 ml

1 ml	$25.34	PEDVAX HIB, Merck & Company Inc	00006-4877-00
1 ml x 10	$255.99	PEDVAX HIB, Merck & Company Inc	00006-4897-00

Solution - Intramuscular - 18 mcg;25 mcg/ 0.5 ml

0.50 ml x 5	$105.75	PROHIBIT, Aventis Pharmaceuticals	49281-0541-05
0.50 ml x 5	$120.25	PROHIBIT, Aventis Pharmaceuticals	49281-0541-01
5 ml	$211.50	PROHIBIT, Aventis Pharmaceuticals	49281-0541-10

Solution - Intramuscular - 25 mcg;10 mcg/0.5 ml

0.50 ml x 4	$93.40	HIBTITER, Lederle Laboratories	53124-0104-41
0.50 ml x 5	$113.52	HIBTITER, Wyeth-Ayerst Laboratories	00005-0104-41
5 ml	$141.90	HIBTITER, Wyeth-Ayerst Laboratories	00005-0104-32
5 ml	$188.20	HIBTITER, Compumed Pharmaceuticals	00403-4911-18
5 ml	$210.70	HIBTITER, Lederle Laboratories	53124-0201-10
5 ml	$229.35	HIBTITER, Allscripts Pharmaceutical Company	54569-3350-00
5 ml	$256.84	HIBTITER, Wyeth-Ayerst Laboratories	00005-0201-10
5 ml x 5	$141.09	HIBTITER, Wyeth-Ayerst Laboratories	53124-0104-32

Haemophilus B Conjugate Vaccine; Hepatitis B Vaccine *(003514)*

For complete prescribing information, refer to the CD-ROM included with the book.

Categories: Immunization, Haemophilus B; Immunization, hepatitis B; FDA Approved 1996 Oct; Pregnancy Category C

Drug Classes: Vaccines

Brand Names: Comvax

DESCRIPTION

Note: The trade names have been left in this monograph for clarity.

Comvax [Haemophilus b Conjugate (Meningococcal Protein Conjugate) and Hepatitis B (Recombinant) Vaccine] is a sterile bivalent vaccine made of the antigenic components used in producing PedvaxHIB [Haemophilus b Conjugate Vaccine (Meningococcal Protein Conjugate)] and Recombivax HB [Hepatitis B Vaccine (Recombinant)]. These components are the *Haemophilus influenzae* type b capsular polysaccharide (PRP) that is covalently bound to an outer membrane protein complex (OMPC) of *Neisseria meningitidis* and hepatitis B surface antigen (HBsAg) from recombinant yeast cultures.

Haemophilus influenzae type b and *Neisseria meningitidis* serogroup B are grown in complex fermentation media. The PRP is purified from the culture broth by purification procedures which include ethanol fractionation, enzyme digestion, phenol extraction and diafiltration. The OMPC from *Neisseria meningitidis* is purified by detergent extraction, ultracentrifugation, diafiltration and sterile filtration.

The PRP-OMPC conjugate is prepared by the chemical coupling of the highly purified PRP (polyribosylribitol phosphate) of *Haemophilus influenzae* type b (Haemophilus b, Ross strain) to an OMPC of the B11 strain of *Neisseria meningitidis* serogroup B. The coupling of the PRP to the OMPC, which is necessary for enhanced immunogenicity of the PRP, is confirmed by analysis of the conjugate's components following chemical treatment which yields a unique amino acid. After conjugation, the aqueous bulk is then adsorbed onto an aluminum hydroxide adjuvant.

HBsAg is produced in recombinant yeast cells. A portion of the hepatitis B virus gene, coding for HBsAg, is cloned into yeast, and the vaccine for hepatitis B is produced from cultures of this recombinant yeast strain according to methods developed in the Merck Research Laboratories. The antigen is harvested and purified from fermentation cultures of a recombinant strain of the yeast *Saccharomyces cerevisiae* containing the gene for the *adw* subtype of HBsAg. The HBsAg protein is released from the yeast cells by cell disruption and purified by a series of physical and chemical methods. The vaccine contains no detectable yeast DNA but may contain not more than 1% yeast protein. The aqueous bulk is treated with formaldehyde and then adsorbed onto an aluminum hydroxide adjuvant.

After each PRP-OMPC and HBsAg aqueous bulk is adsorbed onto the aluminum hydroxide adjuvant, they are then combined to produce Comvax. Each 0.5 ml dose of Comvax is formulated to contain 7.5 µg of Haemophilus b PRP, 125 µg of *Neisseria meningitidis* OMPC, 5 µg of HBsAg, approximately 225 µg of aluminum as aluminum hydroxide, and 35 µg sodium borate (decahydrate) as a pH stabilizer, in 0.9% sodium chloride.

The product contains no preservative.

Comvax is a sterile suspension for intramuscular injection.

INDICATIONS AND USAGE

Comvax is indicated for vaccination against invasive disease caused by *Haemophilus influenzae* type b and against infection caused by all known subtypes of hepatitis B virus in infants 6 weeks to 15 months of age born of HBsAg negative mothers. Infants born of HBsAg positive mothers should receive Hepatitis B Immune Globulin and Hepatitis B Vaccine (Recombinant) at birth and should complete the hepatitis B vaccination series given according to a particular schedule (see the prescribing information for Hepatitis B Vaccine [Recombinant]).

Infants born of mothers of unknown HBsAg status should receive Hepatitis B Vaccine (Recombinant) at birth and should complete the hepatitis B vaccination series given according to a particular schedule (see the prescribing information for Hepatitis B Vaccine [Recombinant]).

Vaccination with Comvax should ideally begin at approximately 2 months of age or as soon thereafter as possible. In order to complete the 3 dose regimen of Comvax, vaccination should be initiated no later than 10 months of age. Infants in whom vaccination with a PRP-OMPC-containing product (*i.e.*, PedvaxHIB, Comvax) is not initiated until 11 months of age do not require 3 doses of PRP-OMPC; however, 3 doses of an HBsAg-containing product are required for complete vaccination against hepatitis B, regardless of age. For infants and children not vaccinated according to the recommended schedule see DOSAGE AND ADMINISTRATION.

USE WITH OTHER VACCINES

Results from clinical studies indicate that Comvax can be administered concomitantly with DTP, OPV, eIPV (enhanced inactivated poliovirus vaccine), VARIVAX [Varicella Virus Vaccine Live (Oka/Merck)], and M-M-R II, and with a booster dose of DTaP at approximately 15 months of age, using separate sites and syringes for injectable vaccines. No impairment of immune response to these individually tested vaccine antigens was demonstrated.

Comvax has been administered concomitantly with the primary series of DTaP to a limited number of infants. No serious vaccine-related adverse events were reported. Immune response data are satisfactory for Comvax but are currently unavailable for DTaP.

COMVAX SHOULD NOT BE USED IN INFANTS YOUNGER THAN 6 WEEKS OF AGE.

CONTRAINDICATIONS

Hypersensitivity to any component of the vaccine.

WARNINGS

If Comvax is used in persons with malignancies or those receiving immunosuppressive therapy or who are otherwise immunocompromised, the expected immune response may not be obtained.

Patients who develop symptoms suggestive of hypersensitivity after an injection should not receive further injections of the vaccine (see CONTRAINDICATIONS).

DOSAGE AND ADMINISTRATION

FOR INTRAMUSCULAR ADMINISTRATION.

Do not inject intravenously, intradermally, or subcutaneously.

RECOMMENDED SCHEDULE

Infants born of HBsAg negative mothers should be vaccinated with three 0.5 ml doses of Comvax, ideally at 2, 4, and 12-15 months of age. If the recommended schedule cannot be followed exactly, the interval between the first 2 doses should be at least 2 months and the interval between the second and third dose should be as close as possible to 8-11 months.

Infants born of HBsAg-positive mothers should receive Hepatitis B Immune Globulin and Hepatitis B Vaccine (Recombinant) at birth and should complete the hepatitis B vaccination series given according to a particular schedule (see the prescribing information for Hepatitis B Vaccine [Recombinant]).

Infants born of mothers of unknown HBsAg status should receive Hepatitis B Vaccine (Recombinant) at birth and should complete the hepatitis B vaccination series given according to a particular schedule (see the prescribing information for Hepatitis B Vaccine [Recombinant]).

The subsequent administration of Comvax for completion of the hepatitis B vaccination series in infants who were born of HBsAg positive mothers and received HBIG or infants born of mothers of unknown status has not been studied.

Comvax should not be administered to any infant before the age of 6 weeks.

MODIFIED SCHEDULES

Children previously vaccinated with one or more doses of either hepatitis B vaccine or Haemophilus b conjugate vaccine: Children who receive 1 dose of hepatitis B vaccine at or shortly after birth may be administered Comvax on the schedule of 2, 4, and 12-15 months of age. There are no data to support the use of a 3 dose series of Comvax in infants who have previously received more than 1 dose of hepatitis B vaccine. However, Comvax may be administered to children otherwise scheduled to receive concurrent Recombivax HB and PedvaxHIB.

Children not vaccinated according to recommended schedule: Vaccination schedules for children not vaccinated according to the recommended schedule should be considered on an individual basis. The number of doses of a PRP-OMPC-containing product (*i.e.,* Comvax, PedvaxHIB) depends on the age that vaccination is begun. An infant 2-10 months of age should receive 3 doses of a product containing PRP-OMPC. An infant 11-14 months of age should receive 2 doses of a product containing PRP-OMPC. A child 15-71 months of age should receive 1 dose of a product containing PRP-OMPC. Infants and children, regardless of age, should receive 3 doses of an HBsAg-containing product.

Comvax is for intramuscular injection. The *anterolateral thigh* is the recommended site for intramuscular injection in infants. Data suggests that injections given in the buttocks frequently are given into fatty tissue instead of into muscle. Such injections have resulted in a lower seroconversion rate (for hepatitis B vaccine) than was expected.

Injection must be accomplished with a needle long enough to ensure intramuscular deposition of the vaccine. The ACIP has recommended that for intramuscular injections, the needle should be of sufficient length to reach the muscle mass itself. In a clinical trial with Comvax vaccination was accomplished with a needle length of 5/8 inches in accordance with ACIP recommendations in effect at that time.[64] ACIP currently recommends that needles of longer length (7/8 to 1 inch) be used.[65]

The vaccine should be used as supplied; no reconstitution is necessary.

Shake well before withdrawal and use. Thorough agitation is necessary to maintain suspension of the vaccine.

Parenteral drug products should be inspected visually for extraneous particulate matter and discoloration prior to administration whenever solution and container permit. After thorough agitation, Comvax is a slightly opaque, white suspension.

It is important to use a separate sterile syringe and needle for each patient to prevent transmission of infectious agents from one person to another.

PRODUCT LISTING - EQUIVALENTS NOT AVAILABLE

Suspension - Intramuscular - Strength n/a

0.50 ml	$51.51	COMVAX, Merck & Company Inc	00006-4843-00
0.50 ml x 10	$533.20	COMVAX, Merck & Company Inc	00006-4898-00

Haemophilus B; Tetanus Toxoid *(001415)*

For complete prescribing information, refer to the CD-ROM included with the book.

Categories: Immunization, Haemophilus B; Immunization, tetanus; FDA Pre 1938 Drugs; Pregnancy Category C
Drug Classes: Vaccines
Brand Names: Acthib; OmniHib

DESCRIPTION

OmniHIB, Haemophilus b Conjugate Vaccine (Tetanus Toxoid Conjugate), produced by Pasteur Merieux Serums & Vaccins, S.A., for intramuscular use, is a sterile, lyophilized powder which is reconstituted at the time of use with saline diluent (0.4% Sodium Chloride). The vaccine consists of the Haemophilus b polysaccharide, a high molecular weight polymer prepared from the *Haemophilus influenzae* type b strain 1482 grown in a semi-synthetic medium, covalently bound to tetanus toxoid.[1] The lyophilized powder and saline diluent contain no preservatives. Each single dose of 0.5 ml is formulated to contain 10 mcg of purified capsular polysaccharide, 24 mcg of tetanus toxoid and 8.5% of sucrose. The tetanus toxoid is prepared by extraction, ammonium sulfate purification, and formalin inactivation of the toxin from cultures of *Clostridium tetani* (Harvard strain) grown in a modified Mueller and Miller medium.[2] The toxoid is filter sterilized prior to the conjugation process. Potency of OmniHIB is specified on each lot by limits on the content of PRP polysaccharide and protein in each dose and the proportion of polysaccharide and protein in the vaccine which is characterized as high molecular weight conjugate. The reconstituted vaccine is clear and colorless.

INDICATIONS AND USAGE

OmniHIB is indicated for the active immunization of infants and children 2 months through 5 years of age for the prevention of invasive disease caused by *H. influenzae* type b.

Antibody levels associated with protection may not be achieved earlier than two weeks following the last recommended dose.

CONTRAINDICATIONS

As with Any Vaccine, Vaccination with OmniHIB May not Protect 100% of Susceptible Individuals: OmniHIB IS CONTRAINDICATED IN CHILDREN WITH A HISTORY OF HYPERSENSITIVITY TO ANY COMPONENT OF THIS VACCINE, INCLUDING TETANUS TOXOID.

WARNINGS

If OmniHIB is administered to immunosuppressed persons or persons receiving immunosuppressive therapy, the expected antibody response may not be obtained. This includes patients with asymptomatic or symptomatic HIV-infection,[20] severe combined immunodeficiency, hypogammaglobulinemia, or agammaglobulinemia; altered immune states due to diseases such as leukemia, lymphoma, or generalized malignancy; or an immune system compromised by treatment with corticosteroids, alkylating drugs, antimetabolites or radiation.[21]

IMMUNIZATION WITH OmniHIB ALONE DOES NOT SUBSTITUTE FOR ROUTINE TETANUS IMMUNIZATION.

DOSAGE AND ADMINISTRATION

Parenteral drug products should be inspected visually for particulate matter and/or discoloration prior to administration, whenever solution and container permit. If these conditions exist, the vaccine should not be administered.

Reconstitution with Supplied Diluent: Prior to reconstitution, cleanse the vaccine vial rubber barrier with a suitable germicide and inject the entire volume of diluent contained in the syringe into the vial of lyophilized vaccine. Thorough agitation is advised to ensure complete rehydration. The entire volume of reconstituted vaccine is then drawn back into a new syringe before injection of one 0.5 ml dose. The vaccine will appear clear and colorless.

Reconstitution instructions for diluent supplied:

Administer OmniHIB intramuscularly after reconstitution with diluent supplied. (In the event of coagulation disorders, OmniHIB may be given subcutaneously in the mid-lateral aspect of the thigh.[14]) **Vaccine should be used immediately after reconstitution.**

1. Insert syringe needle through the rubber barrier into the OmniHIB vial and inject 0.6 ml of diluent supplied.
2. Agitate vial thoroughly to ensure complete reconstitution.
3. After reconstitution, discard syringe and withdraw total volume of reconstituted vaccine in a new syringe and administer 0.5 ml intramuscularly (or subcutaneously if coagulation disorders exist).

Each 0.5 ml dose is formulated to contain 10 mcg of purified capsular polysaccharide conjugated to 24 mcg of inactivated tetanus toxoid and 8.5% of sucrose.

Before injection, the skin over the site to be injected should be cleansed with a suitable germicide. After insertion of the needle, aspirate to ensure that the needle has not entered a blood vessel.

DO NOT INJECT INTRAVENOUSLY.

Each dose of OmniHIB is administered intramuscularly in the outer aspect of the vastus lateralis (mid-thigh) or deltoid. The vaccine should not be injected into the gluteal area or areas where there may be a nerve trunk. During the course of primary immunizations, injections should not be made more than once at the same site.

H

OmniHIB is indicated for infants and children 2 months through 5 years of age for intramuscular administration in accordance with the schedule indicated in (see TABLE 6).[14,16]

Infants between 2 and 6 months of age should receive three 0.5 ml doses at eight week intervals, followed by a booster dose at 15 to 18 months of age. Infants 7 to 11 months of age who have not been previously immunized should receive two 0.5 ml doses at eight week intervals, followed by a booster dose at 15 to 18 months of age; children 12 to 14 months of age who have not been previously immunized should receive one 0.5 ml dose, followed by a booster dose at 15 to 18 months of age; and children 15 to 60 months of age who have not been previously immunized should receive a single 0.5 ml dose.

TABLE 6

Age At First Dose	Primary Series	Booster
2 to 6 months	3 Doses, 8 weeks apart	1 Dose, 15 to 18 months
7 to 11 months	2 Doses, 8 weeks apart	1 Dose, 15 to 18 months
12 to 14 months	1 Dose	1 Dose, 15 to 18 months*
15 to 60 months	1 Dose	None

* Administer vaccine not earlier than 2 months after the previous dose.

Preterm infants should be vaccinated according to their chronological age from birth.[33]

Interruption of the recommended schedule with a delay between doses should not interfere with the final immunity achieved with OmniHIB. There is no need to start the series over again, regardless of the time elapsed between doses.

No data are available to support the interchangeability of OmniHIB and ActHIB with other Haemophilus b conjugate vaccines. Therefore, it is recommended that the same conjugate vaccine be used throughout each immunization schedule, consistent with the data supporting approval and licensure of the vaccine. Since OmniHIB and ActHIB are the same vaccine these may be used interchangeably.

Haloperidol (001418)

Categories: Conduct disorders in children; Psychosis; Tourette's syndrome; FDA Approved 1974 Apr; Pregnancy Category C; WHO Formulary

Drug Classes: Antipsychotics

Brand Names: **Haldol**; Haloperidol Lactate; Pacedol; Pericate; Seranase

Foreign Brand Availability: Alased (Greece); Aloperidin (Greece); Apo-Haloperidol (Canada; Malaysia); Avant (Taiwan); Binison (Taiwan); Brotopon (Japan); Cereen (South-Africa); Cizoren (India); Depidol (India); Dozic (England); Duraperidol (Germany); Einalon S (Japan); Govotil (Indonesia); Halidol (India; Israel); Halojust (Japan); Halomed (Thailand); Halo-P (Thailand); Haloper (Czech-Republic; Germany; Russia); Haloperil (Mexico); Haloperin (Finland); Halopidol (Argentina; Colombia); Halopol (Thailand); Halosten (Japan); Haricon (Thailand); Haridol-D (China); Inin (Taiwan); Linton (Japan); Mixidol (Japan); Motivan (Malaysia); Novoperidol (Canada); Peluces (Japan); Perida (Thailand); Peridol (Canada; China; Korea); Peridor (Israel); Selezyme (Japan); Seranace (England; South-Africa); Serenace (Australia; Benin; Burkina-Faso; Ethiopia; Gambia; Ghana; Guinea; Hong-Kong; India; Ireland; Ivory-Coast; Japan; Kenya; Liberia; Malawi; Malaysia; Mali; Mauritania; Mauritius; Morocco; New-Zealand; Niger; Nigeria; Philippines; Senegal; Seychelles; Sierra-Leone; Sudan; Taiwan; Tanzania; Tunia; Uganda; Zambia; Zimbabwe); Serenase (Belgium; Denmark; Finland; Italy); Serenelfi (Portugal); Sigaperidol (Germany; Switzerland); Trancodol-5 (India); Trancodol-10 (India)

Cost of Therapy: $2.45 (Schizophrenia; Generic Tablets; 0.5 mg; 2 tablets/day; 30 day supply)
$9.90 (Schizophrenia; Haldol Injection; 5 mg/ml; 1 ml; 1 injection; variable day supply)
$1.78 (Schizophrenia; Generic Injection; 5 mg/ml; 1 ml; 1 injection; variable day supply)

HCFA JCODE(S): J1630 up to 5 mg IM, IV

DESCRIPTION

Haloperidol is the first of the butyrophenone series of major tranquilizers. The chemical designation is 4-[4-(p-chlorophenyl)-4-hydroxypiperidino]-4′-fluorobutyrophenone.

Haloperidol dosage forms include: tablets (½, 1, 2, 5, 10, and 20 mg); a concentrate with 2 mg/ml haloperidol (as the lactate); and a sterile parenteral form for intramuscular injection. The injection provides 5 mg haloperidol (as the lactate) with 1.8 mg methylparaben and 0.2 mg propylparaben per ml, and lactic acid for pH adjustment between 3.0-3.6.

Inactive Ingredients: *Tablets:* Calcium phosphate, calcium stearate, corn starch and flavor; *1 mg contains:* FD&C yellow no. 10 and FD&C red no. 40; *2 mg contains:* D&C red no. 33 and FD&C blue no. 2; *5 mg contains:* FD&C blue no. 1 and D&C yellow no. 10 and D&C red no. 30; *10 mg contains:* FD&C blue no. 1, FD&C yellow no. 10, and D&C red no. 30; *20 mg contains:* FD&C red no. 40. *Concentrate:* Lactic acid and methylparaben.

CLINICAL PHARMACOLOGY

The precise mechanism of action has not been clearly established.

INDICATIONS AND USAGE

Haloperidol is indicated for use in the management of manifestations of psychotic disorders.

Haloperidol is indicated for the control of tics and vocal utterances of Tourette's Disorder in children and adults.

Haloperidol is effective for the treatment of severe behavior problems in children of combative, explosive hyperexcitability (which cannot be accounted for by immediate provocation). Haloperidol is also effective in the short-term treatment of hyperactive children who show excessive motor activity with accompanying conduct disorders consisting of some or all of the following symptoms: impulsivity, difficulty sustaining attention, aggressivity, mood lability and poor frustration tolerance. Haloperidol should be reserved for these two groups of children only after failure to respond to psychotherapy or medications other than antipsychotics.

NON-FDA APPROVED INDICATIONS

Haloperidol has also been used for the treatment of the acute manic phase of bipolar disorder, for the symptomatic treatment of non-psychotic behavior associated with dementia, and for the treatment of nausea and vomiting due to emetogenic chemotherapy, although these uses are not approved by the FDA.

CONTRAINDICATIONS

Haloperidol is contraindicated in severe toxic central nervous system depression or comatose states from any cause and in individuals who are hypersensitive to this drug or have Parkinson's disease.

WARNINGS

TARDIVE DYSKINESIA

A syndrome consisting of potentially irreversible, involuntary, dyskinetic movements may develop in patients treated with antipsychotic drugs. Although the prevalence of the syndrome appears to be highest among the elderly, especially elderly women, it is impossible to rely upon prevalence estimates to predict, at the inception of antipsychotic treatment, which patients are likely to develop the syndrome. Whether antipsychotic drug products differ in their potential to cause tardive dyskinesia is unknown.

Both the risk of developing tardive dyskinesia and the likelihood that it will become irreversible are believed to increase as the duration of treatment and the total cumulative dose of antipsychotic drugs administered to the patient increase. However, the syndrome can develop, although much less commonly, after relatively brief treatment periods at low doses.

There is no known treatment for established cases of tardive dyskinesia, although the syndrome may remit, partially or completely, if antipsychotic treatment is withdrawn. Antipsychotic treatment, itself, however, may suppress (or partially suppress) the signs and symptoms of the syndrome and thereby may possibly mask the underlying process. The effect that symptomatic suppression has upon the long-term course of the syndrome is unknown.

Given these considerations, antipsychotic drugs should be prescribed in a manner that is most likely to minimize the occurrence of tardive dyskinesia. Chronic antipsychotic treatment should generally be reserved for patients who suffer from a chronic illness that, 1) is known to respond to antipsychotic drugs, and 2) for whom alternative, equally effective, but potentially less harmful treatments are **not** available or appropriate. In patients who do require chronic treatment, the smallest dose and the shortest duration of treatment producing a satisfactory clinical response should be sought. The need for continued treatment should be reassessed periodically.

If signs and symptoms of tardive dyskinesia appear in a patient on antipsychotics, drug discontinuation should be considered. However, some patients may require treatment despite the presence of the syndrome.

(For further information about the description of tardive dyskinesia and its clinical detection, please refer to ADVERSE REACTIONS.)

NEUROLEPTIC MALIGNANT SYNDROME (NMS)

A potentially fatal symptom complex sometimes referred to as Neuroleptic Malignant Syndrome (NMS) has been reported in association with antipsychotic drugs. Clinical manifestations of NMS are hyperpyrexia, muscle rigidity, altered mental status (including catatonic signs) and evidence of autonomic instability (irregular pulse or blood pressure, tachycardia, diaphoresis, and cardiac dysrhythmias). Additional signs may include elevated creatine phosphokinase, myoglobinuria (rhabdomyolysis) and acute renal failure.

The diagnostic evaluation of patients with this syndrome is complicated. In arriving at a diagnosis, it is important to identify cases where the clinical presentation includes both serious medical illness (*e.g.*, pneumonia, systemic infection, etc.) and untreated or inadequately treated extrapyramidal signs and symptoms (EPS). Other important considerations in the differential diagnosis include central anticholinergic toxicity, heat stroke, drug fever and primary central nervous system (CNS) pathology.

The management of NMS should include (1) immediate discontinuation of antipsychotic drugs and other drugs not essential to concurrent therapy, (2) intensive symptomatic treatment and medical monitoring, and (3) treatment of any concomitant serious medical problems for which specific treatments are available. There is no general agreement about specific pharmacological treatment regimens for uncomplicated NMS.

If a patient requires antipsychotic drug treatment after recovery from NMS, the potential reintroduction of drug therapy should be carefully considered. The patient should be carefully monitored, since recurrences of NMS have been reported.

Hyperpyrexia and heat stroke, not associated with the above symptom complex, have also been reported with haloperidol.

USE IN PREGNANCY

Rodents given 2-20 times the usual maximum human dose of haloperidol by oral or parenteral routes showed an increase in incidence of resorption, reduced fertility, delayed delivery and pup mortality. No teratogenic effect has been reported in rats, rabbits or dogs at dosages within this range, but cleft palate has been observed in mice given 15 times the usual maximum human dose. Cleft palate in mice appears to be a nonspecific response to stress or nutritional imbalance as well as to a variety of drugs, and there is no evidence to relate this phenomenon to predictable human risk for most of these agents.

There are no well controlled studies with haloperidol in pregnant women. There are reports, however, of cases of limb malformations observed following maternal use of haloperidol along with other drugs which have suspected teratogenic potential during the first trimester of pregnancy. Causal relationships were not established in these cases. Since such experience does not exclude the possibility of fetal damage due to haloperidol, this drug should be used during pregnancy or in women likely to become pregnant only if the benefit clearly justifies a potential risk to the fetus. Infants should not be nursed during drug treatment.

GENERAL

A number of cases of bronchopneumonia, some fatal, have followed the use of antipsychotic drugs, including haloperidol. It has been postulated that lethargy and decreased sensation of thirst due to central inhibition may lead to dehydration, hemoconcentration and reduced pulmonary ventilation. Therefore, if the above signs and symptoms appear, especially in the elderly, the physician should institute remedial therapy promptly.

Although not reported with haloperidol, decreased serum cholesterol and/or cutaneous and ocular changes have been reported in patients receiving chemically-related drugs.

Haloperidol may impair the mental and/or physical abilities required for the performance of hazardous tasks such as operating machinery or driving a motor vehicle. The ambulatory patient should be warned accordingly.

The use of alcohol with this drug should be avoided due to possible additive effects and hypotension.

PRECAUTIONS

Haloperidol should be administered cautiously to patients:

- With severe cardiovascular disorders, because of the possibility of transient hypotension and/or precipitation of anginal pain. Should hypotension occur and a vasopressor be required, epinephrine should not be used since haloperidol may block its vasopressor activity and paradoxical further lowering of the blood pressure may occur. Instead, metaraminol, phenylephrine or norepinephrine should be used.
- Receiving anticonvulsant medications, with a history of seizures, or with EEG abnormalities, because haloperidol may lower the convulsive threshold. If indicated, adequate anticonvulsant therapy should be concomitantly maintained.
- With known allergies, or with a history of allergic reactions to drugs.
- Receiving anticoagulants, since an isolated instance of interference occurred with the effects of one anticoagulant (phenindione).

If concomitant antiparkinson medication is required, it may have to be continued after haloperidol is discontinued because of the difference in excretion rates. If both are discontinued simultaneously, extrapyramidal symptoms may occur. The physician should keep in mind the possible increase in intraocular pressure when anticholinergic drugs, including antiparkinson agents, are administered concomitantly with haloperidol.

As with other antipsychotic agents, it should be noted that haloperidol may be capable of potentiating CNS depressants such as anesthetics, opiates, and alcohol.

When haloperidol is used to control mania in cyclic disorders, there may be a rapid mood swing to depression.

Severe neurotoxicity (rigidity, inability to walk or talk) may occur in patients with thyrotoxicosis who are also receiving antipsychotic medication, including haloperidol.

No mutagenic potential of haloperidol was found in the Ames *Salmonella* microsomal activation assay. Negative or inconsistent positive findings have been obtained in *in vitro* and *in vivo* studies of effects of haloperidol on chromosome structure and number. The available cytogenetic evidence is considered too inconsistent to be conclusive at this time.

Carcinogenicity studies using oral haloperidol were conducted in Wistar rats (dosed at up to 5 mg/kg daily for 24 months) and in Albino Swiss mice (dosed at up to 5 mg/kg daily for 18 months). In the rat study survival was less than optimal in all dose groups, reducing the number of rats at risk for developing tumors. However, although a relatively greater number of rats survived to the end of the study in high-dose male and female groups, these animals did not have a greater incidence of tumors than control animals. Therefore, although not optimal, this study does suggest the absence of a haloperidol related increase in the incidence of neoplasia in rats at doses up to 20 times the usual daily human dose for chronic or resistant patients.

In female mice at 5 and 20 times the highest initial daily dose for chronic or resistant patients, there was a statistically significant increase in mammary gland neoplasia and total tumor incidence; at 20 times the same daily dose there was a statistically significant increase in pituitary gland neoplasia. In male mice, no statistically significant differences in incidences of total tumors or specific tumor types were noted.

Antipsychotic drugs elevate prolactin levels; the elevation persists during chronic administration. Tissue culture experiments indicate that approximately one-third of human breast cancers are prolactin dependent *in vitro,* a factor of potential importance if the prescription of these drugs is contemplated in a patient with a previously detected breast cancer. Although disturbances such as galactorrhea, amenorrhea, gynecomastia, and impotence have been reported, the clinical significance of elevated serum prolactin levels is unknown for most patients. An increase in mammary neoplasms has been found in rodents after chronic administration of antipsychotic drugs. Neither clinical studies nor epidemiologic studies conducted to date, however, have shown an association between chronic administration of these drugs and mammary tumorigenesis; the available evidence is considered too limited to be conclusive at this time.

DRUG INTERACTIONS

COMBINED USE OF HALOPERIDOL AND LITHIUM

An encephalopathic syndrome (characterized by weakness, lethargy, fever, tremulousness and confusion, extrapyramidal symptoms, leukocytosis, elevated serum enzymes, BUN, and FBS) followed by irreversible brain damage has occurred in a few patients treated with lithium plus haloperidol. A causal relationship between these events and the concomitant administration of lithium and haloperidol has not been established; however, patients receiving such combined therapy should be monitored closely for early evidence of neurological toxicity and treatment discontinued promptly if such signs appear.

ADVERSE REACTIONS

CNS EFFECTS

Extrapyramidal Symptoms (EPS)

EPS during the administration of haloperidol have been reported frequently, often during the first few days of treatment. EPS can be categorized generally as Parkinson-like symptoms, akathisia, or dystonia (including opisthotonos and oculogyric crisis). While all can occur at relatively low doses, they occur more frequently and with greater severity at higher doses. The symptoms may be controlled with dose reductions or administration of antiparkinson drugs such as benztropine mesylate or trihexyphenidyl HCl. It should be noted that persistent EPS have been reported; the drug may have to be discontinued in such cases.

Withdrawal Emergent Neurological Signs

Generally, patients receiving short-term therapy experience no problems with abrupt discontinuation of antipsychotic drugs. However, some patients on maintenance treatment experience transient dyskinetic signs after abrupt withdrawal. In certain of these cases the dyskinetic movements are indistinguishable from the syndrome described in Tardive Dyskinesia except for duration. It is not known whether gradual withdrawal of antipsychotic drugs will reduce the rate of occurrence of withdrawal emergent neurological signs but until further evidence becomes available, it seems reasonable to gradually withdraw use of haloperidol.

Tardive Dyskinesia

As with all antipsychotic agents haloperidol has been associated with persistent dyskinesias. Tardive dyskinesia, a syndrome consisting of potentially irreversible, involuntary, dyskinetic movements, may appear in some patients on long-term therapy or may occur after drug therapy has been discontinued. The risk appears to be greater in elderly patients on high-dose therapy, especially females. The symptoms are persistent and in some patients appear irreversible. The syndrome is characterized by rhythmical involuntary movements of tongue, face, mouth or jaw (*e.g.,* protrusion of tongue, puffing of cheeks, puckering of mouth, chewing movements). Sometimes these may be accompanied by involuntary movements of extremities and the trunk.

There is no known effective treatment for tardive dyskinesia; antiparkinson agents usually do not alleviate the symptoms of this syndrome. It is suggested that all antipsychotic agents be discontinued if these symptoms appear. Should it be necessary to reinstitute treatment, or increase the dosage of the agent, or switch to a different antipsychotic agent, this syndrome may be masked.

It has been reported that fine vermicular movement of the tongue may an early sign of tardive dyskinesia and if the medication is stopped at that time the full syndrome may not develop.

Tardive Dystonia

Tardive dystonia, not associated with the above syndrome, has also been reported. Tardive dystonia is characterized by delayed onset of choreic or dystonic movements, is often persistent, and has the potential of becoming irreversible.

Other CNS Effects: Insomnia, restlessness, anxiety, euphoria, agitation, drowsiness, depression, lethargy, headache, confusion, vertigo, grand mal seizures, exacerbation of psychotic symptoms including hallucinations, and catatonic-like behavioral states which may be responsive to drug withdrawal and/or treatment with anticholinergic drugs.

Body as a Whole: Neuroleptic malignant syndrome (NMS), hyperpyrexia and heat stroke have been reported with haloperidol. (See WARNINGS for further information concerning NMS.)

Cardiovascular Effects: Tachycardia, hypotension, hypertension and ECG changes including prolongation of the Q-T interval and ECG pattern changes compatible with the polymorphous configuration of torsades de pointes.

Hematologic Effects: Reports have appeared citing the occurrence of mild and usually transient leukopenia and leukocytosis, minimal decreases in red blood cell counts, anemia, or a tendency toward lymphomonocytosis. Agranulocytosis has rarely been reported to have occurred with the use of haloperidol, and then only in association with other medication.

Liver Effects: Impaired liver function and/or jaundice have been reported.

Dermatologic Reactions: Maculopapular and acneiform skin reactions and isolated cases of photosensitivity and loss of hair.

Endocrine Disorders: Lactation, breast engorgement, mastalgia, menstrual irregularities, gynecomastia, impotence, increased libido, hyperglycemia, hypoglycemia and hyponatremia.

Gastrointestinal Effects: Anorexia, constipation, diarrhea, hypersalivation, dyspepsia, nausea and vomiting.

Autonomic Reactions: Dry mouth, blurred vision, urinary retention, diaphoresis and priapism.

Respiratory Effects: Laryngospasm, bronchospasm and increased depth of respiration.

Special Senses: Cataracts, retinopathy and visual disturbances.

OTHER

Cases of sudden and unexpected death have been reported in association with the administration of haloperidol. The nature of the evidence makes it impossible to determine definitively what role, if any, haloperidol played in the outcome of the reported cases. The possibility that haloperidol caused death cannot, of course, be excluded, but it is to be kept in mind that sudden and unexpected death may occur in psychotic patients when they go untreated or when they are treated with other antipsychotic drugs.

POSTMARKETING EVENTS

Hyperammonemia has been reported in a 5½ year old child with citrullinemia, an inherited disorder of ammonia excretion, following treatment with haloperidol.

DOSAGE AND ADMINISTRATION

There is considerable variation from patient to patient in the amount of medication required for treatment. As with all antipsychotic drugs, dosage should be individualized according to the needs and response of each patient. Dosage adjustments, either upward or downward, should be carried out as rapidly as practicable to achieve optimum therapeutic control.

To determine the initial dosage, consideration should be given to the patient's age, severity of illness, previous response to other antipsychotic drugs, and any concomitant medication or disease state. Children, debilitated or geriatric patients, as well as those with a history of adverse reactions to antipsychotic drugs, may require less haloperidol. The optimal response in such patients is usually obtained with more gradual dosage adjustments and at lower dosage levels, as recommended below.

ORAL ADMINISTRATION

Clinical experience suggests the following recommendations:

Initial Oral Dosage Range

Adults

Moderate Symptomatology: 0.5-2.0 mg bid or tid.

Severe Symptomatology: 3.0-5.0 mg bid or tid.

To achieve prompt control, higher doses may be required in some cases.

Geriatric or Debilitated Patients: 0.5-2.0 mg bid or tid.
Chronic or Resistant Patients: 3.0-5.0 mg bid or tid.

Patients who remain severely disturbed or inadequately controlled may require dosage adjustment. Daily dosages up to 100 mg may be necessary in some cases to achieve an optimal response. Infrequently, haloperidol has been used in doses above 100 mg for severely resistant patients; however, the limited clinical usage has not demonstrated the safety of prolonged administration of such doses.

Children

The following recommendations apply to children between the ages of 3 and 12 years (weight range 15-40 kg). Haloperidol is not intended for children under 3 years old. Therapy should begin at the lowest dose possible (0.5 mg/day). If required, the dose should be increased by an increment of 0.5 mg at 5-7 day intervals until the desired therapeutic effect is obtained. (See list below.)

The total dose may be divided, to be given bid or tid.
Psychotic Disorders: 0.05-0.15 mg/kg/day
Non-Psychotic Behavior Disorders and Tourette's Disorder: 0.05-0.075 mg/kg/day

Severely disturbed psychotic children may require higher doses. In severely disturbed, non-psychotic children or in hyperactive children with accompanying conduct disorders, who have failed to respond to psychotherapy or medications other than antipsychotics, it should be noted that since these behaviors may be short-lived, short-term administration of haloperidol may suffice. There is no evidence establishing a maximum effective dosage. There is little evidence that behavior improvement is further enhanced in dosages beyond 6 mg/day.

H

Maintenance Dosage

Upon achieving a satisfactory therapeutic response, dosage should then be gradually reduced to the lowest effective maintenance level.

INTRAMUSCULAR ADMINISTRATION

Adults

Parenteral medication, administered intramuscularly in doses of 2-5 mg, is utilized for prompt control of the acutely agitated patient with moderately severe to very severe symptoms. Depending on the response of the patient, subsequent doses may be given, administered as often as every hour, although 4-8 hour intervals may be satisfactory.

Controlled trials to establish the safety and effectiveness of intramuscular administration in children have not been conducted.

Parenteral drug products should be inspected visually for particulate matter and discoloration prior to administration, whenever solution and container permit.

SWITCHOVER PROCEDURE

The oral form should supplant the injectable as soon as practicable. In the absence of bioavailability studies establishing bioequivalence between these two dosage forms the following guidelines for dosage are suggested. For an initial approximation of the total daily dose required, the parenteral dose administered in the preceding 24 hours may be used. Since this dose is only an initial estimate, it is recommended that careful monitoring of clinical signs and symptoms, including clinical efficacy, sedation, and adverse effects, be carried out periodically for the first several days following the initiation of switchover. In this way, dosage adjustments, either upward or downward, can be quickly accomplished. Depending on the patient's clinical status, the first oral dose should be given within 12-24 hours following the last parenteral dose.

HOW SUPPLIED

HALDOL TABLETS

Haldol brand of haloperidol tablets with a cut-out "H" design are scored, imprinted with "McNEIL" and "HALDOL" and are available in the following strengths and colors:

½ mg: White.
1 mg: Yellow.
2 mg: Pink.
5 mg: Green.
10 mg: Aqua.
20 mg: Salmon.

Storage: Store at controlled room temperature (15-30°C, 59-86°F). Protect from light. Dispense in a tight, light-resistant container.

HALDOL CONCENTRATE

2 mg per ml (as the lactate) is a colorless, odorless, and tasteless solution.
Storage: Store at controlled room temperature (15-30°C, 59-86°F). Do not freeze.

HALDOL INJECTION

Haldol for immediate release is 5 mg per ml (as the lactate).
Storage: Store at controlled room temperature (15-30°C, 59-86°F). Do not freeze.

PRODUCT LISTING - RATED THERAPEUTICALLY EQUIVALENT

Size	Price	Manufacturer	NDC
Concentrate - Oral - 1 mg/ml			
5 ml x 50	$45.50	GENERIC, Udl Laboratories Inc	51079-0797-10
Concentrate - Oral - 2 mg/ml			
5 ml x 100	$100.00	GENERIC, Pharmaceutical Assoc Inc Div Beach Products	00121-0581-05
10 ml x 100	$538.00	GENERIC, Pharmaceutical Assoc Inc Div Beach Products	00121-0581-10
15 ml	$6.00	GENERIC, Raway Pharmacal Inc	00686-0604-15
15 ml	$9.48	GENERIC, Silarx Pharmaceuticals Inc	54838-0501-15
15 ml	$9.60	GENERIC, Major Pharmaceuticals Inc	00904-1729-35
15 ml	$9.76	GENERIC, Roxane Laboratories Inc	00054-3350-41
15 ml	$12.22	GENERIC, Warner Chilcott Laboratories	00047-2913-35
15 ml	$12.50	GENERIC, Alpharma Uspd Makers Of Barre and Nmc	00472-0766-99
15 ml	$13.00	GENERIC, Teva Pharmaceuticals Usa	00093-9604-23
120 ml	$15.00	GENERIC, Pharmaceutical Assoc Inc Div Beach Products	00121-0581-04
120 ml	$15.75	GENERIC, Raway Pharmacal Inc	00686-0604-14
120 ml	$18.00	FEDERAL UPPER LIMIT, H.C.F.A. F F P	99999-1418-20
120 ml	$31.84	GENERIC, Roxane Laboratories Inc	00054-3350-50
120 ml	$32.70	GENERIC, Geneva Pharmaceuticals	00781-6205-04
120 ml	$32.75	GENERIC, Qualitest Products Inc	00603-1290-54
120 ml	$32.95	GENERIC, Major Pharmaceuticals Inc	00904-1729-20
120 ml	$36.84	GENERIC, Silarx Pharmaceuticals Inc	54838-0501-40
120 ml	$36.84	GENERIC, Boca Pharmacal Inc	64376-0403-40
120 ml	$45.20	GENERIC, Alpharma Uspd Makers Of Barre and Nmc	00472-0766-94
120 ml	$54.32	GENERIC, Teva Pharmaceuticals Usa	00093-9604-12
120 ml	$54.32	GENERIC, Ivax Corporation	00182-6059-71
Solution - Injectable - Decanoate 50 mg/ml			
1 ml	$27.00	GENERIC, American Pharmaceutical Partners	63323-0469-01
1 ml	$28.10	GENERIC, Superior Pharmaceutical Company	00144-0444-51
1 ml x 10	$270.00	GENERIC, Gensia Sicor Pharmaceuticals Inc	00703-7011-03
1 ml x 10	$281.00	GENERIC, Able Laboratories Inc	53265-0444-51
1 ml x 10	$288.00	GENERIC, Bedford Laboratories	55390-0412-01
1 ml x 10	$288.00	GENERIC, Bedford Laboratories	55390-0422-01
5 ml	$135.00	GENERIC, Gensia Sicor Pharmaceuticals Inc	00703-7013-01
5 ml	$135.00	GENERIC, American Pharmaceutical Partners	63323-0469-05
5 ml	$140.00	GENERIC, Bedford Laboratories	60505-0702-01
5 ml	$140.50	GENERIC, Superior Pharmaceutical Company	00144-0444-56
5 ml	$140.50	GENERIC, Able Laboratories Inc	53265-0444-56
5 ml	$144.00	GENERIC, Bedford Laboratories	55390-0412-05
5 ml	$144.00	GENERIC, Bedford Laboratories	55390-0422-05
Solution - Injectable - Decanoate 100 mg/ml			
1 ml	$49.50	GENERIC, American Pharmaceutical Partners	63323-0471-01
1 ml	$52.50	GENERIC, Superior Pharmaceutical Company	00144-0544-51
1 ml x 10	$495.00	GENERIC, Gensia Sicor Pharmaceuticals Inc	00703-7021-03
1 ml x 10	$525.00	GENERIC, Able Laboratories Inc	53265-0544-51
1 ml x 10	$576.00	HALOPERIDOL DECANOATE, Bedford Laboratories	55390-0413-01
1 ml x 10	$576.00	GENERIC, Bedford Laboratories	55390-0423-01
5 ml	$247.25	GENERIC, Apotex Usa Inc	60505-0703-01
5 ml	$247.50	GENERIC, Gensia Sicor Pharmaceuticals Inc	00703-7023-01
5 ml	$247.50	GENERIC, American Pharmaceutical Partners	63323-0471-05
5 ml	$262.50	GENERIC, Superior Pharmaceutical Company	00144-0544-56
5 ml	$288.00	GENERIC, Bedford Laboratories	55390-0423-05
5 ml x 10	$288.00	HALOPERIDOL DECANOATE, Bedford Laboratories	55390-0413-05
Solution - Injectable - 5 mg/ml			
1 ml x 10	$63.00	GENERIC, Solo Pak Medical Products Inc	39769-0088-02
1 ml x 10	$71.88	GENERIC, Bedford Laboratories	55390-0147-01
1 ml x 10	$74.90	GENERIC, Bedford Laboratories	55390-0147-10
1 ml x 10	$77.00	GENERIC, Bedford Laboratories	55390-0447-10
1 ml x 10	$78.75	GENERIC, Gensia Sicor Pharmaceuticals Inc	00703-7041-03
1 ml x 10	$99.00	HALDOL, Janssen Pharmaceuticals	00045-0255-01
1 ml x 25	$187.25	GENERIC, American Pharmaceutical Partners	63323-0474-01
1 ml x 50	$75.00	GENERIC, Raway Pharmacal Inc	00686-0088-02
10 ml	$71.88	GENERIC, American Pharmaceutical Partners	63323-0474-10
10 ml	$75.00	GENERIC, Bedford Laboratories	55390-0447-01
10 ml	$76.25	GENERIC, Gensia Sicor Pharmaceuticals Inc	00703-7045-01
10 ml	$96.45	HALDOL, Janssen Pharmaceuticals	00045-0255-49
Tablet - Oral - 0.5 mg			
15's	$4.17	GENERIC, Heartland Healthcare Services	61392-0263-15
30 x 25	$192.45	GENERIC, Sky Pharmaceuticals Packaging, Inc	63739-0120-01
30 x 25	$192.45	GENERIC, Sky Pharmaceuticals Packaging, Inc	63739-0120-03
30's	$8.35	GENERIC, Heartland Healthcare Services	61392-0263-30
30's	$8.35	GENERIC, Heartland Healthcare Services	61392-0263-39
31 x 10	$88.80	GENERIC, Vangard Labs	00615-2594-63
31's	$8.62	GENERIC, Heartland Healthcare Services	61392-0263-31
32's	$8.90	GENERIC, Heartland Healthcare Services	61392-0263-32
45's	$12.52	GENERIC, Heartland Healthcare Services	61392-0263-45
60's	$16.69	GENERIC, Heartland Healthcare Services	61392-0263-60
90's	$25.04	GENERIC, Heartland Healthcare Services	61392-0263-90
100's	$6.75	GENERIC, Cmc-Consolidated Midland Corporation	00223-1020-01
100's	$11.50	GENERIC, Major Pharmaceuticals Inc	00904-1730-60
100's	$13.44	GENERIC, Roxane Laboratories Inc	00054-8342-25
100's	$13.49	GENERIC, Purepac Pharmaceutical Company	00228-2289-10
100's	$13.78	GENERIC, Roxane Laboratories Inc	00054-4342-25
100's	$14.95	GENERIC, Major Pharmaceuticals Inc	00904-1830-60

Package	Price	Product / Manufacturer	NDC
100's	$17.65	GENERIC, Mova Pharmaceutical Corporation	55370-0802-07
100's	$17.68	GENERIC, Aligen Independent Laboratories Inc	00405-4459-01
100's	$17.79	GENERIC, Auro Pharmaceutical	55829-0294-10
100's	$18.55	GENERIC, Qualitest Products Inc	00603-3782-21
100's	$19.00	GENERIC, Ivax Corporation	00182-1262-01
100's	$19.00	GENERIC, Watson/Schein Pharmaceuticals Inc	00364-2204-01
100's	$19.51	GENERIC, Moore, H.L. Drug Exchange Inc	00839-7346-06
100's	$23.59	GENERIC, Geneva Pharmaceuticals	00781-1391-01
100's	$24.20	GENERIC, Major Pharmaceuticals Inc	00904-1730-61
100's	$24.35	GENERIC, Vangard Labs	00615-2594-13
100's	$24.80	GENERIC, Mylan Pharmaceuticals Inc	00378-0351-01
100's	$28.47	GENERIC, Major Pharmaceuticals Inc	00904-1830-61
100's	$29.49	GENERIC, Geneva Pharmaceuticals	00781-1391-13
200 x 5	$286.45	GENERIC, Vangard Labs	00615-2594-43

Tablet - Oral - 1 mg

Package	Price	Product / Manufacturer	NDC
10's	$7.77	GENERIC, Pharma Pac	52959-0518-10
10's	$11.75	HALDOL, Pharma Pac	52959-0356-10
15's	$5.37	GENERIC, Heartland Healthcare Services	61392-0266-15
30 x 25	$286.05	GENERIC, Sky Pharmaceuticals Packaging, Inc	63739-0121-03
30 x 25	$313.32	GENERIC, Sky Pharmaceuticals Packaging, Inc	63739-0121-01
30's	$10.75	GENERIC, Heartland Healthcare Services	61392-0266-30
30's	$10.75	GENERIC, Heartland Healthcare Services	61392-0266-39
31 x 10	$140.83	GENERIC, Vangard Labs	00615-2595-53
31 x 10	$140.83	GENERIC, Vangard Labs	00615-2595-63
31's	$11.10	GENERIC, Heartland Healthcare Services	61392-0266-31
32's	$11.46	GENERIC, Heartland Healthcare Services	61392-0266-32
45's	$16.12	GENERIC, Heartland Healthcare Services	61392-0266-45
60's	$16.34	GENERIC, Global Source Management	60429-0087-60
60's	$21.49	GENERIC, Heartland Healthcare Services	61392-0266-60
90's	$32.24	GENERIC, Heartland Healthcare Services	61392-0266-90
100's	$7.95	GENERIC, Cmc-Consolidated Midland Corporation	00223-1021-01
100's	$18.50	GENERIC, Major Pharmaceuticals Inc	00904-1731-60
100's	$18.50	GENERIC, Major Pharmaceuticals Inc	00904-1831-60
100's	$18.55	GENERIC, Mova Pharmaceutical Corporation	55370-0803-07
100's	$19.13	GENERIC, Roxane Laboratories Inc	00054-8343-25
100's	$20.15	GENERIC, Purepac Pharmaceutical Company	00228-2280-10
100's	$20.22	GENERIC, Roxane Laboratories Inc	00054-4343-25
100's	$22.87	GENERIC, Mutual/United Research Laboratories	00677-1116-01
100's	$23.68	GENERIC, Aligen Independent Laboratories Inc	00405-4460-01
100's	$26.76	GENERIC, Auro Pharmaceutical	55829-0295-10
100's	$27.00	GENERIC, Parmed Pharmaceuticals Inc	00349-8945-01
100's	$27.25	GENERIC, Qualitest Products Inc	00603-3783-21
100's	$27.90	GENERIC, Watson/Schein Pharmaceuticals Inc	00364-2205-01
100's	$28.25	GENERIC, Ivax Corporation	00182-1263-01
100's	$29.29	GENERIC, Moore, H.L. Drug Exchange Inc	00839-7347-06
100's	$35.15	GENERIC, Mylan Pharmaceuticals Inc	00378-0257-01
100's	$35.18	GENERIC, Geneva Pharmaceuticals	00781-1392-01
100's	$38.42	GENERIC, Vangard Labs	00615-2595-13
100's	$38.62	GENERIC, Major Pharmaceuticals Inc	00904-1731-61
100's	$45.43	GENERIC, Geneva Pharmaceuticals	00781-1392-13
100's	$45.43	GENERIC, Major Pharmaceuticals Inc	00904-1831-61

Tablet - Oral - 2 mg

Package	Price	Product / Manufacturer	NDC
15's	$7.26	GENERIC, Heartland Healthcare Services	61392-0269-15
25 x 30	$385.05	GENERIC, Sky Pharmaceuticals Packaging, Inc	63739-0122-03
30's	$14.53	GENERIC, Heartland Healthcare Services	61392-0269-30
30's	$15.43	GENERIC, Heartland Healthcare Services	61392-0269-39
31's	$15.01	GENERIC, Heartland Healthcare Services	61392-0269-31
32's	$15.49	GENERIC, Heartland Healthcare Services	61392-0269-32
45's	$21.79	GENERIC, Heartland Healthcare Services	61392-0269-45
60's	$22.28	GENERIC, Global Source Management	60429-0088-60
60's	$29.05	GENERIC, Heartland Healthcare Services	61392-0269-60
90's	$33.42	GENERIC, Global Source Management	60429-0088-90
90's	$43.58	GENERIC, Heartland Healthcare Services	61392-0269-90
100's	$10.95	GENERIC, Cmc-Consolidated Midland Corporation	00223-1022-01
100's	$22.50	GENERIC, Major Pharmaceuticals Inc	00904-1732-60
100's	$25.82	GENERIC, Roxane Laboratories Inc	00054-8344-25
100's	$27.37	GENERIC, Purepac Pharmaceutical Company	00228-2281-10
100's	$28.08	GENERIC, Roxane Laboratories Inc	00054-4344-25
100's	$30.65	GENERIC, Major Pharmaceuticals Inc	00904-1832-60
100's	$35.88	GENERIC, Auro Pharmaceutical	55829-0296-10
100's	$36.10	GENERIC, Mova Pharmaceutical Corporation	55370-0804-07
100's	$36.20	GENERIC, Aligen Independent Laboratories Inc	00405-4461-01
100's	$37.00	GENERIC, Parmed Pharmaceuticals Inc	00349-8946-01
100's	$37.60	GENERIC, Qualitest Products Inc	00603-3784-21
100's	$38.60	GENERIC, Watson/Schein Pharmaceuticals Inc	00364-2206-01
100's	$38.85	GENERIC, Ivax Corporation	00182-1264-01
100's	$39.76	GENERIC, Moore, H.L. Drug Exchange Inc	00839-7348-06
100's	$47.60	GENERIC, Major Pharmaceuticals Inc	00904-1732-61
100's	$47.75	GENERIC, Vangard Labs	00615-2596-13
100's	$48.15	GENERIC, Mylan Pharmaceuticals Inc	00378-0214-01
100's	$48.15	GENERIC, Geneva Pharmaceuticals	00781-1393-01
100's	$56.80	GENERIC, Major Pharmaceuticals Inc	00904-1832-61
100's	$60.19	GENERIC, Geneva Pharmaceuticals	00781-1393-13
200 x 5	$554.42	GENERIC, Vangard Labs	00615-2596-43

Tablet - Oral - 5 mg

Package	Price	Product / Manufacturer	NDC
25 x 30	$644.33	GENERIC, Sky Pharmaceuticals Packaging, Inc	63739-0123-03
30's	$2.40	GENERIC, Heartland Healthcare Services	61392-0272-30
30's	$24.00	GENERIC, Heartland Healthcare Services	61392-0272-39
31 x 10	$275.14	GENERIC, Vangard Labs	00615-2597-53
31 x 10	$275.14	GENERIC, Vangard Labs	00615-2597-63
31's	$24.80	GENERIC, Heartland Healthcare Services	61392-0272-31
32's	$25.60	GENERIC, Heartland Healthcare Services	61392-0272-32
45's	$3.60	GENERIC, Heartland Healthcare Services	61392-0272-45
60's	$4.80	GENERIC, Heartland Healthcare Services	61392-0272-60
60's	$35.92	GENERIC, Global Source Management	60429-0089-60
90's	$7.20	GENERIC, Heartland Healthcare Services	61392-0272-90
90's	$53.89	GENERIC, Global Source Management	60429-0089-90
100's	$36.50	GENERIC, Major Pharmaceuticals Inc	00904-1733-60
100's	$38.95	GENERIC, Major Pharmaceuticals Inc	00904-1833-60
100's	$39.84	GENERIC, Purepac Pharmaceutical Company	00228-2282-10
100's	$41.23	GENERIC, Roxane Laboratories Inc	00054-8345-25
100's	$45.96	GENERIC, Roxane Laboratories Inc	00054-4345-25
100's	$56.28	GENERIC, Auro Pharmaceutical	55829-0297-10
100's	$59.00	GENERIC, Qualitest Products Inc	00603-3785-21
100's	$59.02	GENERIC, Aligen Independent Laboratories Inc	00405-4462-01
100's	$59.80	GENERIC, Watson/Schein Pharmaceuticals Inc	00364-2207-01
100's	$65.05	GENERIC, Ivax Corporation	00182-1265-01
100's	$67.56	GENERIC, Moore, H.L. Drug Exchange Inc	00839-7349-06
100's	$77.99	GENERIC, Geneva Pharmaceuticals	00781-1396-01
100's	$78.00	GENERIC, Mylan Pharmaceuticals Inc	00378-0327-01
100's	$80.41	GENERIC, Vangard Labs	00615-2597-13
100's	$81.00	GENERIC, Major Pharmaceuticals Inc	00904-1733-61
100's	$95.29	GENERIC, Major Pharmaceuticals Inc	00904-1833-61
100's	$97.49	GENERIC, Geneva Pharmaceuticals	00781-1396-13
200 x 5	$887.55	GENERIC, Vangard Labs	00615-2597-43

Tablet - Oral - 10 mg

Package	Price	Product / Manufacturer	NDC
30's	$32.18	GENERIC, Heartland Healthcare Services	61392-0275-30
30's	$32.18	GENERIC, Heartland Healthcare Services	61392-0275-39
31's	$33.25	GENERIC, Heartland Healthcare Services	61392-0275-31
32's	$34.32	GENERIC, Heartland Healthcare Services	61392-0275-32
45's	$48.26	GENERIC, Heartland Healthcare Services	61392-0275-45
60's	$39.62	GENERIC, Global Source Management	60429-0090-60
60's	$64.35	GENERIC, Heartland Healthcare Services	61392-0275-60
90's	$60.80	GENERIC, Global Source Management	60429-0090-90
90's	$96.53	GENERIC, Heartland Healthcare Services	61392-0275-90
100's	$22.50	GENERIC, Cmc-Consolidated Midland Corporation	00223-1024-01
100's	$42.67	GENERIC, Purepac Pharmaceutical Company	00228-2286-10
100's	$46.40	GENERIC, Major Pharmaceuticals Inc	00904-1734-60
100's	$62.55	GENERIC, Roxane Laboratories Inc	00054-8346-25
100's	$64.20	GENERIC, Parmed Pharmaceuticals Inc	00349-8948-01
100's	$65.00	GENERIC, Roxane Laboratories Inc	00054-4346-25
100's	$65.00	GENERIC, Mova Pharmaceutical Corporation	55370-0806-07
100's	$65.63	GENERIC, Aligen Independent Laboratories Inc	00405-4463-01
100's	$65.70	GENERIC, Qualitest Products Inc	00603-3786-21
100's	$69.55	GENERIC, Ivax Corporation	00182-1854-01
100's	$71.62	GENERIC, Moore, H.L. Drug Exchange Inc	00839-7398-06
100's	$75.28	GENERIC, Auro Pharmaceutical	55829-0298-10
100's	$101.25	GENERIC, Major Pharmaceuticals Inc	00904-1834-61
100's	$119.17	GENERIC, Major Pharmaceuticals Inc	00904-1734-61
100's	$131.00	GENERIC, Geneva Pharmaceuticals	00781-1397-01
100's	$163.75	GENERIC, Geneva Pharmaceuticals	00781-1397-13

Tablet - Oral - 20 mg

Package	Price	Product / Manufacturer	NDC
30's	$37.48	GENERIC, Heartland Healthcare Services	61392-0121-30
30's	$37.48	GENERIC, Heartland Healthcare Services	61392-0121-39
31's	$38.73	GENERIC, Heartland Healthcare Services	61392-0121-31
32's	$39.97	GENERIC, Heartland Healthcare Services	61392-0121-32
45's	$56.21	GENERIC, Heartland Healthcare Services	61392-0121-45
60's	$74.95	GENERIC, Heartland Healthcare Services	61392-0121-60
90's	$112.43	GENERIC, Heartland Healthcare Services	61392-0121-90
100's	$35.40	GENERIC, Major Pharmaceuticals Inc	00904-1735-61
100's	$63.52	GENERIC, Purepac Pharmaceutical Company	00228-2287-10
100's	$97.15	GENERIC, Auro Pharmaceutical	55829-0299-10
100's	$112.50	GENERIC, Roxane Laboratories Inc	00054-8347-25
100's	$115.57	GENERIC, Roxane Laboratories Inc	00054-4347-25
100's	$126.56	GENERIC, Major Pharmaceuticals Inc	00904-1835-61
100's	$251.78	GENERIC, Geneva Pharmaceuticals	00781-1398-01

PRODUCT LISTING - EQUIVALENTS NOT AVAILABLE

Concentrate - Oral - 2 mg/ml

Package	Price	Product / Manufacturer	NDC
15 ml	$7.75	GENERIC, Cmc-Consolidated Midland Corporation	00223-6525-15

H

15 ml	$10.32	GENERIC, Southwood Pharmaceuticals Inc	58016-8691-01
120 ml	$32.00	GENERIC, Cmc-Consolidated Midland Corporation	00223-6525-04
Solution - Injectable - Decanoate 50 mg/ml			
1 ml x 3	$125.22	HALDOL DECANOATE, Janssen Pharmaceuticals	00045-0253-03
1 ml x 10	$417.40	HALDOL DECANOATE, Janssen Pharmaceuticals	00045-0253-01
5 ml	$208.75	HALDOL DECANOATE, Janssen Pharmaceuticals	00045-0253-46
Solution - Injectable - Decanoate 100 mg/ml			
1 ml x 5	$382.95	HALDOL DECANOATE, Janssen Pharmaceuticals	00045-0254-14
5 ml	$262.50	GENERIC, Able Laboratories Inc	53265-0544-56
5 ml	$382.93	HALDOL DECANOATE, Janssen Pharmaceuticals	00045-0254-46
Solution - Injectable - 5 mg/ml			
1 ml x 10	$17.83	GENERIC, Physicians Total Care	54868-3459-00
Tablet - Oral - 0.5 mg			
30's	$2.64	GENERIC, Physicians Total Care	54868-2570-01
100's	$4.09	GENERIC, Physicians Total Care	54868-2570-00
Tablet - Oral - 1 mg			
12's	$7.32	GENERIC, Southwood Pharmaceuticals Inc	58016-0716-12
15's	$9.16	GENERIC, Southwood Pharmaceuticals Inc	58016-0716-15
20's	$12.21	GENERIC, Southwood Pharmaceuticals Inc	58016-0716-20
30's	$3.02	GENERIC, Physicians Total Care	54868-0091-01
30's	$18.31	GENERIC, Southwood Pharmaceuticals Inc	58016-0716-30
100's	$6.18	GENERIC, Physicians Total Care	54868-0091-02
100's	$61.04	GENERIC, Southwood Pharmaceuticals Inc	58016-0716-00
Tablet - Oral - 5 mg			
12's	$16.51	GENERIC, Southwood Pharmaceuticals Inc	58016-0312-12
15's	$20.64	GENERIC, Southwood Pharmaceuticals Inc	58016-0312-15
20's	$27.52	GENERIC, Southwood Pharmaceuticals Inc	58016-0312-20
30's	$3.42	GENERIC, Physicians Total Care	54868-2296-02
30's	$41.28	GENERIC, Southwood Pharmaceuticals Inc	58016-0312-30
60's	$42.54	GENERIC, Allscripts Pharmaceutical Company	54569-2883-02
100's	$6.68	GENERIC, Physicians Total Care	54868-2296-00
100's	$16.00	GENERIC, Cmc-Consolidated Midland Corporation	00223-1023-01
100's	$137.60	GENERIC, Southwood Pharmaceuticals Inc	58016-0312-00
Tablet - Oral - 10 mg			
100's	$11.18	GENERIC, Physicians Total Care	54868-2306-00

H

Haloperidol Decanoate *(001419)*

Categories: Psychosis; Schizophrenia; Pregnancy Category C; FDA Approved 1986 Jan
Drug Classes: Antipsychotics
Brand Names: Haldol Decanoas; **Haldol Decanoate**
Foreign Brand Availability: Aloperidin (Greece); Haldol (New-Zealand); Haldol Decanoas (Bahamas; Bahrain; Barbados; Belgium; Belize; Benin; Bermuda; Bulgaria; Burkina-Faso; Costa-Rica; Curacao; Cyprus; Czech-Republic; Dominican-Republic; Egypt; Ethiopia; France; Gambia; Ghana; Guatemala; Guinea; Guyana; Honduras; Hong-Kong; Indonesia; Iran; Iraq; Italy; Ivory-Coast; Jamaica; Jordan; Kenya; Kuwait; Lebanon; Liberia; Libya; Malawi; Mali; Mauritania; Mauritius; Mexico; Morocco; Netherland-Antilles; Nicaragua; Niger; Nigeria; Oman; Panama; Peru; Qatar; Republic-of-Yemen; Saudi-Arabia; Senegal; Seychelles; Sierra-Leone; Sudan; Surinam; Switzerland; Syria; Taiwan; Tanzania; Thailand; Trinidad; Tunia; Uganda; United-Arab-Emirates; Zambia; Zimbabwe); Haldol Decanoat (Austria; Germany); Haldol Decanoaat (Netherlands); Halidol Decanoas (Israel); Halopidol decanoato (Colombia); Haridol Decanoate (Thailand); Pericate (Israel); Senorm L.A. (Thailand); Serenase (Finland); Serenase Dekanoat (Denmark)
Cost of Therapy: $41.74 (Schizophrenia; Haldol Decanoate Injection; 50 mg/ml; 1ml; 1 injection; variable day supply)
$27.00 (Schizophrenia; Generic Injection; 50 mg/ml; 1ml; 1 injection; variable day supply)
HCFA JCODE(S): J1631 per 50 mg IM

DESCRIPTION

Haloperidol decanoate is the decanoate ester of the butyrophenone, Haldol (haloperidol). It has a markedly extended duration of effect. It is available in sesame oil in sterile form for intramuscular (IM) injection. The structural formula of haloperidol decanoate is 4-(4-chlorophenyl)-1-[4-(4-fluorophenyl)-4-oxobutyl]-4 piperidinyl decanoate.

Haloperidol decanoate is almost insoluble in water (0.01 mg/ml), but is soluble in most organic solvents.

Each ml of haloperidol decanoate 50 for IM injection contains 50 mg haloperidol (present as haloperidol decanoate 70.52 mg) in a sesame oil vehicle, with 1.2% (w/v) benzyl alcohol as a preservative.

Each ml of haloperidol decanoate 100 for IM injection contains 100 mg haloperidol (present as haloperidol decanoate 141.04 mg) in a sesame oil vehicle, with 1.2% (w/v) benzyl alcohol as a preservative.

CLINICAL PHARMACOLOGY

Haloperidol decanoate is the long-acting form of haloperidol. The basic effects of haloperidol decanoate are no different from those of haloperidol with the exception of duration of action. Haloperidol blocks the effects of dopamine and increases its turnover rate; however, the precise mechanism of action is unknown.

Administration of haloperidol decanoate in sesame oil results in slow and sustained release of haloperidol. The plasma concentrations of haloperidol gradually rise, reaching a peak at about 6 days after the injection, and falling thereafter, with an apparent half-life of about 3 weeks. Steady state plasma concentrations are achieved after the third or fourth dose. The relationship between dose of haloperidol decanoate and plasma haloperidol concentration is roughly linear for doses below 450 mg. It should be noted, however, that pharmacokinetics of haloperidol decanoate following intramuscular injections can be quite variable between subjects.

INDICATIONS AND USAGE

Haloperidol decanoate 50 and 100 are indicated for the treatment of schizophrenic patients who require prolonged parenteral antipsychotic therapy.

CONTRAINDICATIONS

Since the pharmacologic and clinical actions of haloperidol decanoate are attributed to haloperidol as the active medication, CONTRAINDICATIONS, WARNINGS, and additional information are those of haloperidol, modified only to reflect the prolonged action.

Haloperidol is contraindicated in severe toxic central nervous system depression or comatose states from any cause and in individuals who are hypersensitive to this drug or have Parkinson's disease.

WARNINGS

TARDIVE DYSKINESIA

A syndrome consisting of potentially irreversible, involuntary, dyskinetic movements may develop in patients treated with antipsychotic drugs. Although the prevalence of the syndrome appears to be highest among the elderly, especially elderly women, it is impossible to rely upon prevalence estimates to predict, at the inception of antipsychotic treatment, which patients are likely to develop the syndrome. Whether antipsychotic drug products differ in their potential to cause tardive dyskinesia is unknown.

Both the risk of developing tardive dyskinesia and the likelihood that it will become irreversible are believed to increase as the duration of treatment and the total cumulative dose of antipsychotic drugs administered to the patient increase. However, the syndrome can develop, although much less commonly, after relatively brief treatment periods at low doses.

There is no known treatment for established cases of tardive dyskinesia, although the syndrome may remit, partially or completely, if antipsychotic treatment is withdrawn. Antipsychotic treatment, itself, however, may suppress (or partially suppress) the signs and symptoms of the syndrome and thereby may possibly mask the underlying process. The effect that symptomatic suppression has upon the long-term course of the syndrome is unknown.

Given these considerations, antipsychotic drugs should be prescribed in a manner that is most likely to minimize the occurrence of tardive dyskinesia. Chronic antipsychotic treatment should generally be reserved for patients who suffer from a chronic illness that (1) is known to respond to antipsychotic drugs, and (2) for whom alternative, equally effective, but potentially less harmful treatments are **not** available or appropriate. In patients who do require chronic treatment, the smallest dose and the shortest duration of treatment producing a satisfactory clinical response should be sought. The need for continued treatment should be reassessed periodically.

If signs and symptoms of tardive dyskinesia appear in a patient on antipsychotics, drug discontinuation should be considered. However, some patients may require treatment despite the presence of the syndrome. (For further information about description of tardive dyskinesia and its clinical detection, please refer ADVERSE REACTIONS.)

NEUROLEPTIC MALIGNANT SYNDROME (NMS)

A potentially fatal symptom complex sometimes referred to as Neuroleptic Malignant Syndrome (NMS) has been reported in association with antipsychotic drugs. Clinical manifestations of NMS are hyperpyrexia, muscle rigidity, altered mental status (including catatonic signs), and evidence of autonomic instability (irregular pulse or blood pressure, tachycardia, diaphoresis, and cardiac dysrhythmias). Additional signs may include elevated creatine phosphokinase, myoglobinuria (rhabdomyolysis), and acute renal failure.

The diagnostic evaluation of patients with this syndrome is complicated. In arriving at a diagnosis, it is important to identify cases where the clinical presentation includes both serious medical illness (*e.g.*, pneumonia, systemic infection, etc.) and untreated or inadequately treated extrapyramidal signs and symptoms (EPS). Other important considerations in the differential diagnosis include central anticholinergic toxicity, heat stroke, drug fever, and primary central nervous system (CNS) pathology.

The management of NMS should include (1) immediate discontinuation of antipsychotic drugs and other drugs not essential to concurrent therapy, (2) intensive symptomatic treatment and medical monitoring, and (3) treatment of any concomitant serious medical problems for which specific treatments are available. There is no general agreement about specific pharmacological treatment regimens for uncomplicated NMS.

If a patient requires antipsychotic drug treatment after recovery from NMS, the potential reintroduction of drug therapy should be carefully considered. The patient should be carefully monitored, since recurrences of NMS have been reported.

Hyperpyrexia and heat stroke, not associated with the above symptom complex, have also been reported with haloperidol.

GENERAL

A number of cases of bronchopneumonia, some fatal, have followed the use of antipsychotic drugs, including haloperidol. It has been postulated that lethargy and decreased sensation of thirst due to central inhibition may lead to dehydration, hemoconcentration and reduced pulmonary ventilation. Therefore, if the above signs and symptoms appear, especially in the elderly, the physician should institute remedial therapy promptly.

Although not reported with haloperidol, decreased serum cholesterol and/or cutaneous and ocular changes have been reported in patients receiving chemically-related drugs.

PRECAUTIONS

Haloperidol decanoate should be administered cautiously to patients:

- With severe cardiovascular disorders, because of the possibility of transient hypotension and/or precipitation of anginal pain. Should hypotension occur and a vasopressor be required, epinephrine should not be used since haloperidol may block its vasopressor activity, and paradoxical further lowering of the blood pressure may occur. Instead, metaraminol, phenylephrine or norepinephrine should be used.
- Receiving anticonvulsant medications, with a history of seizures, or with EEG abnormalities, because haloperidol may lower the convulsive threshold. If indicated, adequate anticonvulsant therapy should be concomitantly maintained.
- With known allergies, or with a history of allergic reactions to drugs.

- Receiving anticoagulants, since an isolated instance of interference occurred with the effects of one anticoagulant (phenindione).

If concomitant antiparkinson medication is required, it may have to be continued after haloperidol decanoate is discontinued because of the prolonged action of haloperidol decanoate. If both drugs are discontinued simultaneously, extrapyramidal symptoms may occur. The physician should keep in mind the possible increase in intraocular pressure when anticholinergic drugs, including antiparkinson agents, are administered concomitantly with haloperidol decanoate.

In patients with thyrotoxicosis who are also receiving antipsychotic medication, including haloperidol decanoate, severe neurotoxicity (rigidity, inability to walk or talk) may occur.

When haloperidol is used to control mania in bipolar disorders, there may be a rapid mood swing to depression.

INFORMATION FOR THE PATIENT

Haloperidol decanoate may impair the mental or physical abilities required for the performance of hazardous tasks such as operating machinery or driving a motor vehicle. The ambulatory patient should be warned accordingly.

The use of alcohol with this drug should be avoided due to possible additive effects and hypotension.

CARCINOGENESIS, MUTAGENESIS, AND IMPAIRMENT OF FERTILITY

No mutagenic potential of haloperidol decanoate was found in the Ames *Salmonella* microsomal activation assay. Negative or inconsistent positive findings have been obtained *in vitro* and *in vivo* studies of effects of short-acting haloperidol on chromosome structure and number. The available cytogenic evidence is considered too inconsistent to be conclusive at this time.

Carcinogenicity studies using oral haloperidol were conducted in Wistar rats (dosed at up to 5 mg/kg daily for 24 months) and in Albino Swiss mice (dosed at up to 5 mg/kg daily for 18 months). In the rat study survival was less than optimal in all dose groups, reducing the number of rats at risk for developing tumors. However, although a relatively greater number of rats survived to the end of the study in high-dose male and female groups, these animals did not have a greater incidence of tumors than control animals. Therefore, although not optimal, this study does suggest the absence of a haloperidol related increase in the incidence of neoplasia in rats at doses up to 20 times the usual daily human dose for chronic or resistant patients.

In female mice at 5 and 20 times the highest initial daily dose for chronic or resistant patients, there was a statistically significant increase in mammary gland neoplasia and total tumor incidence; at 20 times the same daily dose there was a statistically significant increase in pituitary gland neoplasia. In male mice, no statistically significant differences in incidences of total tumors or specific tumor types were noted.

Antipsychotic drugs elevate prolactin levels; the elevation persists during chronic administration. Tissue culture experiments indicated that approximately one-third of human breast cancers are prolactin dependent *in vitro*, a factor of potential importance if the prescription of these drugs is contemplated in a patient with a previously detected breast cancer. Although disturbances such as galactorrhea, amenorrhea, gynecomastia, and impotence have been reported, the clinical significance of elevated serum prolactin levels is unknown for most patients.

An increase in mammary neoplasms has been found in rodents after chronic administration of antipsychotic drugs. Neither clinical studies nor epidemiologic studies conducted to date, however, have shown an association between chronic administration of these drugs and mammary tumorigenesis; the available evidence is considered too limited to be conclusive at this time.

PREGNANCY CATEGORY C

Rodents given up to 3 times the usual maximum human dose of haloperidol decanoate showed an increase in incidence of resorption, fetal mortality, and pup mortality. No fetal abnormalities were observed.

Cleft palate has been observed in mice given oral haloperidol at 15 times the usual maximum human dose. Cleft palate in mice appears to be a nonspecific response to stress or nutritional imbalance as well as to a variety of drugs, and there is no evidence to relate this phenomenon to predictable human risk for most of these agents.

There are no adequate and well-controlled studies in pregnant women. There are reports, however, of cases of limb malformations observed following maternal use of haloperidol along with other drugs which have suspected teratogenic potential during the first trimester of pregnancy. Causal relationships were not established with these cases. Since such experience does not exclude the possibility of fetal damage due to haloperidol, haloperidol decanoate should be used during pregnancy or in women likely to become pregnant only if the benefit clearly justifies a potential risk to the fetus.

NURSING MOTHERS

Since haloperidol is excreted in human breast milk, infants should not be nursed during drug treatment with haloperidol decanoate.

PEDIATRIC USE

Safety and effectiveness of haloperidol decanoate in children have not been established.

GERIATRIC USE

Clinical studies of haloperidol did not include sufficient numbers of subjects aged 65 and over to determine whether they respond differently from younger subjects. Other reported clinical experience has not consistently identified differences in responses between the elderly and younger patients. However, the prevalence of tardive dyskinesia appears to be highest among the elderly, especially elderly women (see WARNINGS, Tardive dyskinesia). Also, the pharmacokinetics of haloperidol in geriatric patients generally warrants the use of lower doses (see DOSAGE AND ADMINISTRATION).

DRUG INTERACTIONS

An encephalopathic syndrome (characterized by weakness, lethargy, fever, tremulousness and confusion, extrapyramidal symptoms, leukocytosis, elevated serum enzymes, BUN, and FBS) followed by irreversible brain damage has occurred in a few patients treated with lithium plus haloperidol. A causal relationship between these events and the concomitant administration of lithium and haloperidol has not been established; however, patients receiving such combined therapy should be monitored closely for early evidence of neurological toxicity and treatment discontinued promptly if such signs appear.

As with other antipsychotic agents, it should be noted that haloperidol may be capable of potentiating CNS depressants such as anesthetics, opiates, and alcohol.

In a study of 12 schizophrenic patients coadministered oral haloperidol and rifampin, plasma haloperidol levels were decreased by a mean of 70% and mean scores on the Brief Psychiatric Rating Scale were increased from baseline. In 5 other schizophrenic patients treated with oral haloperidol and rifampin, discontinuation of rifampin produced a mean 3.3-fold increase in haloperidol concentrations. Thus, careful monitoring of clinical status is warranted when rifampin is administered or discontinued in haloperidol-treated patients.

ADVERSE REACTIONS

Adverse reactions following the administration of haloperidol decanoate are those of haloperidol. Since vast experience has accumulated with haloperidol, the adverse reactions are reported for that compound as well as for haloperidol decanoate. As with all injectable medications, local tissue reactions have been reported with haloperidol decanoate.

CNS EFFECTS

Extrapyramidal Symptoms (EPS)

EPS during the administration of haloperidol have been reported frequently, often during the first few days of treatment. EPS can be categorized generally as Parkinson-like symptoms, akathisia, or dystonia (including opisthotonos and oculogyric crisis). While all can occur at relatively low doses, they occur more frequently and with greater severity at higher doses. The symptoms may be controlled with dose reductions or administration of antiparkinson drugs such as benztropine mesylate or trihexyphenidyl HCl. It should be noted that persistent EPS have been reported; the drug may have to be discontinued in such cases.

Withdrawal Emergent Neurological Signs

Generally, patients receiving short-term therapy experience no problems with abrupt discontinuation of antipsychotic drugs. However, some patients on maintenance treatment experience transient dyskinetic signs after abrupt withdrawal. In certain of these cases the dyskinetic movements are indistinguishable from the syndrome described in Tardive Dyskinesia except for duration. Although the long-acting properties of haloperidol decanoate provide gradual withdrawal, it is not known whether gradual withdrawal of antipsychotic drugs will reduce the rate of occurrence of withdrawal emergent neurological signs.

Tardive Dyskinesia

As with all antipsychotic agents haloperidol has been associated with persistent dyskinesias. Tardive dyskinesia, a syndrome consisting of potentially irreversible, involuntary, dyskinetic movements, may appear in some patients on long-term therapy with haloperidol decanoate or may occur after drug therapy has been discontinued. The risk appears to be greater in elderly patients on high-dose therapy, especially females. The symptoms are persistent and in some patients appear irreversible. The syndrome is characterized by rhythmical involuntary movements of tongue, face, mouth, or jaw (*e.g.*, protrusion of tongue, puffing of cheeks, puckering of mouth, chewing movements). Sometimes these may be accompanied by involuntary movements of extremities and the trunk.

There is no known effective treatment for tardive dyskinesia; antiparkinson agents usually do not alleviate the symptoms of this syndrome. It is suggested that all antipsychotic agents be discontinued if these symptoms appear. Should it be necessary to reinstitute treatment, or increase the dosage of the agent, or switch to a different antipsychotic agent, this syndrome may be masked.

It has been reported that fine vermicular movement of the tongue may be an early sign of tardive dyskinesia and if the medication is stopped at that time the full syndrome may not develop.

Tardive Dystonia

Tardive dystonia, not associated with the above syndrome, has also been reported. Tardive dystonia is characterized by delayed onset of choreic or dystonic movements, is often persistent, and has the potential of becoming irreversible.

Other CNS Effects

Insomnia, restlessness, anxiety, euphoria, agitation, drowsiness, depression, lethargy, headache, confusion, vertigo, grand mal seizures, exacerbation of psychotic symptoms including hallucinations, and catatonic-like behavioral states which may be responsive to drug withdrawal and/or treatment with anticholinergic drugs.

Body as a Whole: Neuroleptic malignant syndrome (NMS), hyperpyrexia and heat stroke have been reported with haloperidol. (See WARNINGS for further information concerning NMS.)

Cardiovascular Effects: Tachycardia, hypotension, hypertension, and ECG changes including prolongation of the Q-T interval and ECG pattern changes compatible with the polymorphous configuration of torsades de pointes.

Hematologic Effects: Reports have appeared citing the occurrence of mild and usually transient leukopenia and leukocytosis, minimal decreases in red blood cell counts, anemia, or a tendency toward lymphomonocytosis. Agranulocytosis has rarely been reported to have occurred with the use of haloperidol, and then only in association with other medication.

Liver Effects: Impaired liver function and/or jaundice have been reported.

Dermatologic Reactions: Maculopapular and acneiform skin reactions and isolated cases of photosensitivity and loss of hair.

Endocrine Disorders: Lactation, breast engorgement, mastalgia, menstrual irregularities, gynecomastia, impotence, increased libido, hyperglycemia, hypoglycemia, and hyponatremia.

Gastrointestinal Effects: Anorexia, constipation, diarrhea, hypersalivation, dyspepsia, nausea, and vomiting.

Autonomic Reactions: Dry mouth, blurred vision, urinary retention, diaphoresis, and priapism.

Respiratory Effects: Laryngospasm, bronchospasm, and increased depth of respiration.

Special Senses: Cataracts, retinopathy, and visual disturbances.

Other: Cases of sudden and unexpected death have been reported in association with the administration of haloperidol. The nature of the evidence makes it impossible to determine definitively what role, if any, haloperidol played in the outcome of the reported cases. The possibility that haloperidol caused death cannot, of course, be excluded, but it is to be kept in mind that sudden and unexpected death may occur in psychotic patients when they go untreated or when they are treated with other antipsychotic drugs.

POSTMARKETING EVENTS

Hyperammonemia has been reported in a 5½-year-old child with citrullinemia, an inherited disorder of ammonia excretion, following treatment with haloperidol.

DOSAGE AND ADMINISTRATION

Haloperidol decanoate should be administered by deep intramuscular injection. A 21 gauge needle is recommended. The maximum volume per injection site should not exceed 3 ml. DO NOT ADMINISTER INTRAVENOUSLY.

Parenteral drug products should be inspected visually for particulate matter and discoloration prior to administration, whenever solution and container permit.

Haloperidol decanoate is intended for use in schizophrenic patients who require prolonged parenteral antipsychotic therapy. These patients should be previously stabilized on antipsychotic medication before considering a conversion to haloperidol decanoate. Furthermore, it is recommended that patients being considered for haloperidol decanoate therapy have been treated with, and tolerate well, short-acting haloperidol in order to reduce the possibility of an unexpected adverse sensitivity to haloperidol. Close clinical supervision is required during the initial period of dose adjustment in order to minimize the risk of overdosage or reappearance of psychotic symptoms before the next injection. During dose adjustment or episodes of exacerbation of symptoms of schizophrenia, haloperidol decanoate therapy can be supplemented with short-acting forms of haloperidol.

The dose of haloperidol decanoate should be expressed in terms of its haloperidol content. The starting dose of haloperidol decanoate should be based on the patient's age, clinical history, physical condition, and response to previous antipsychotic therapy. The preferred approach to determining the minimum effective dose is to begin with lower initial doses and to adjust the dose upward as needed. For patients previously maintained on low doses of antipsychotics (*e.g.*, up to the equivalent of 10 mg/day oral haloperidol), it is recommended that the initial dose of haloperidol decanoate be 10-15 times the previous daily dose in oral haloperidol equivalents, limited clinical experience suggests that lower initial doses may be adequate.

INITIAL THERAPY

Conversion from oral haloperidol to haloperidol decanoate can be achieved by using an initial dose of haloperidol decanoate that is 10-20 times the previous daily dose in oral haloperidol equivalents.

In patients who are elderly, debilitated, or stable on low doses of oral haloperidol (*e.g.*, up to the equivalent of 10 mg/day oral haloperidol), a range of 10-15 times the previous daily dose in oral haloperidol equivalents is appropriate for initial conversion.

In patients previously maintained on higher doses of antipsychotics for whom a low dose approach risks recurrence of psychiatric decompensation and in patients whose long-term use of haloperidol has resulted in a tolerance to the drug, 20 times the previous daily dose in oral haloperidol equivalents should be considered for initial conversion, with downward titration on succeeding injections.

The initial dose of haloperidol decanoate should not exceed 100 mg regardless of previous antipsychotic dose requirements. If, therefore, conversion requires more than 100 mg of haloperidol decanoate as an initial dose, that dose should be administered in two injections (*i.e.*, a maximum of 100 mg initially followed by the balance in 3-7 days).

MAINTENANCE THERAPY

The maintenance dosage of haloperidol decanoate must be individualized with titration upward or downward based on therapeutic response. The usual maintenance range is 10-15 times the previous daily dose in oral haloperidol equivalents dependent on the clinical response of the patient (see TABLE 1).

TABLE 1 *Haloperidol Decanoate Dosing Recommendations*

Patients	1st Month	Monthly Maintenance
Stabilized on low daily oral doses (up to 10 mg/day) Elderly or debilitated	10-15× Daily oral dose	10-15× Previous daily oral dose
High dose Risk of relapse Tolerent to oral haloperidol	20× Daily oral dose	10-15× Previous daily oral dose

Close clinical supervision is required during initiation and stabilization of haloperidol decanoate therapy.

Haloperidol decanoate is usually administered monthly or every 4 weeks. However, variation in patient response may dictate a need for adjustment of the dosing interval as well as the dose. (See CLINICAL PHARMACOLOGY.)

Clinical experience with haloperidol decanoate at doses greater than 450 mg/month has been limited.

HOW SUPPLIED

Haldol Deconoate for IM injection is available as:

50 mg injection: Haldol (haloperidol) Decanoate 50 for IM injection, 50 mg haloperidol as 70.5 mg/ml haloperidol decanoate, 10 × 1 ml ampuls, 3 × 1 ml ampuls and 5 ml multiple dose vials.

100 mg injection: Haldol (haloperidol) Decanoate 100 for IM injection, 100 mg haloperidol as 141.04 mg/ml haloperidol decanoate, 5 × 1 ml ampuls and 5 ml multiple dose vials.

STORAGE

Store at controlled room temperature 15-30°C (59-86°F). Do not refrigerate or freeze.

Protect from light.

Heparin Sodium *(001428)*

Categories: Arrhythmias, atrial, with embolism; Disseminated intravascular coagulation; Embolism, arterial; Embolism, arterial, prophylaxis; Embolism, pulmonary; Embolism, pulmonary, prophylaxis; Thrombosis, deep vein, prophylaxis; Thrombosis, venous; Thrombosis, venous, prophylaxis; Pregnancy Category C; FDA Approved 1942 Feb; WHO Formulary

Drug Classes: Anticoagulants

Brand Names: Heparin Flush; Heparin Lok-Pak; Heparin Porcine; Hepflush; Liquaemin Sodium; Sodium Heparin

Foreign Brand Availability: Beparine (India); Helberina (Mexico); Hepaflex (Finland; Norway); Hepalean (Canada); Heparin (Austria; Benin; Bulgaria; Burkina-Faso; Czech-Republic; England; Ethiopia; Finland; Gambia; Germany; Ghana; Greece; Guinea; Hungary; Israel; Ivory-Coast; Kenya; Liberia; Malawi; Mali; Mauritania; Mauritius; Morocco; Niger; Nigeria; Norway; Senegal; Seychelles; Sierra-Leone; Sudan; Sweden; Switzerland; Tanzania; Tunia; Uganda; Zambia; Zimbabwe); Heparin Injection B.P. (Australia); Heparin Leo (Canada; Denmark; Hong-Kong; Indonesia; Malaysia; New-Zealand; Philippines; Taiwan); Heparin Novo (South-Africa; Taiwan; Thailand); Heparin Sodium B Braun (Indonesia; Malaysia); Heparin Subcutaneous (New-Zealand); Heparina Leo (Costa-Rica; Dominican-Republic; El-Salvador; Guatemala; Honduras; Panama); Heparina (Spain); Heparine (Belgium; Netherlands); Heparine Choay (France); Heparine Novo (Belgium; Netherlands); Inhepar (Mexico); Inviclot (Indonesia); Liquemin (Germany; Italy; Switzerland); Liquemine (Belgium; Ecuador); Monoparin (New-Zealand); Multiparin (New-Zealand); Thromboliquine (Israel); Thrombophob (Germany); Thromboreduct (Germany); Uniparin (Australia)

Cost of Therapy: $13.44 (Deep Vein Thrombosis; Generic Injection; 5000 μg/ml; 1 ml; 2 ml/day; 7 day supply)

HCFA JCODE(S): J1644 1,000 units IV, SC

DESCRIPTION

Heparin is a heterogenous group of straight-chain anionic mucopolysaccharides, called glycosaminoglycans, having anticoagulant properties. Although others may be present, the main sugars occurring in heparin are: (1) α-L-iduronic acid 2-sulfate, (2) 2-deoxy-2-sulfamino-α-D-glucose 6-sulfate, (3) β-D-glucuronic acid, (4) 2-acetamido-2-deoxy-α-D-glucose, and (5) α-L-iduronic acid. These sugars are present in decreasing amounts, usually in the order: (2) > (1) > (4) > (3) > (5), and are joined by glycosidic linkages, forming polymers of varying sizes. Heparin is strongly acidic because of its content of covalently linked sulfate and carboxylic acid groups. In heparin sodium, the acidic protons of the sulfate units are partially replaced by sodium ions.

Heparin sodium injection is a sterile solution of heparin sodium derived from bovine lung tissue, standardized for anticoagulant activity. It is to be administered by intravenous or deep subcutaneous routes. The potency is determined by a biological assay using a USP reference standard based on units of heparin activity per milligram. Heparin is pyrogen-free.

Each ml of the 1000 and 5000 USP units per ml preparations contains: Heparin sodium 1000 or 5000 USP units; 9 mg sodium chloride; 9.45 mg benzyl alcohol added as preservative.

Each ml of the 10,000 USP units per ml preparations contains: Heparin sodium 10,000 USP units; 9.45 mg benzyl alcohol added as preservative.

When necessary, the pH of heparin sodium injection was adjusted with hydrochloric acid and/or sodium hydroxide. The pH range is 5.0-7.5.

CLINICAL PHARMACOLOGY

Heparin inhibits reactions that lead to the clotting of blood and the formation of fibrin clots both *in vitro* and *in vivo*. Heparin acts at multiple sites in the normal coagulation system. Small amounts of heparin in combination with antithrombin III (heparin cofactor) can inhibit thrombosis by inactivating activated Factor X and inhibiting the conversion of prothrombin to thrombin. Once active thrombosis has developed, larger amounts of heparin can inhibit further coagulation by inactivating thrombin and preventing the conversion of fibrinogen to fibrin. Heparin also prevents the formation of a stable fibrin clot by inhibiting the activation of the fibrin stabilizing factor.

Bleeding time is usually unaffected by heparin. Clotting time is prolonged by full therapeutic doses of heparin; in most cases, it is not measurably affected by low doses of heparin.

Peak plasma levels of heparin are achieved 2-4 hours following subcutaneous administration, although there are considerable individual variations. Loglinear plots of heparin plasma concentrations with time for a wide range of dose levels are linear which suggests the absence of zero order processes. Liver and the reticulo-endothelial system are the site of biotransformation. The biphasic elimination curve, a rapidly declining alpha phase (t½ = 10 minutes) and after the age of 40 a slower beta phase, indicates uptake in organs. The absence of a relationship between anticoagulant half-life and concentration half-life may reflect factors such as protein binding of heparin.

Heparin does not have fibrinolytic activity; therefore, it will not lyse existing clots.

INDICATIONS AND USAGE

Heparin sodium is indicated for anticoagulant therapy in prophylaxis and treatment of venous thrombosis and its extension; (in a low-dose regimen) for prevention of postoperative deep venous thrombosis and pulmonary embolism in patients undergoing major abdomino-thoracic surgery or who for other reasons, are at risk of developing thromboembolic disease (see DOSAGE AND ADMINISTRATION); for prophylaxis and treatment of pulmonary embolism; for atrial fibrillation with embolization; for diagnosis and treatment of acute and chronic consumption coagulopathies (disseminated intravascular coagulation);

for prevention of clotting in arterial and heart surgery; for prophylaxis and treatment of peripheral arterial embolism; as an anticoagulant in blood transfusions, extracorporeal circulation and dialysis procedures, and in blood samples for laboratory purposes.

NON-FDA APPROVED INDICATIONS

Although not FDA approved, heparin has been used to reduce mortality in unstable angina, following myocardial infarction to prevent mural thrombosis and reinfarction, and for anticoagulation during pregnancy.

CONTRAINDICATIONS

Heparin sodium should not be used in patients:

- With severe thrombocytopenia.
- In whom suitable blood coagulation tests — *e.g.*, the whole-blood clotting time, partial thromboplastic time, etc. — cannot be performed at appropriate intervals (this contraindication refers to full dose heparin; there is usually no need to monitor coagulation parameters in patients receiving low-dose heparin).
- With an uncontrollable active bleeding state (see WARNINGS), except when this is due to disseminated intravascular coagulation.

WARNINGS

Heparin is not intended for intramuscular use.

HYPERSENSITIVITY

Patients with documented hypersensitivity to heparin should be given the drug only in clearly life-threatening situations.

HEMORRHAGE

Hemorrhage can occur at virtually any site in patients receiving heparin. An unexplained fall in hematocrit, fall in blood pressure, or any other unexplained symptom should lead to serious consideration of a hemorrhagic event.

Heparin sodium should be used with extreme caution in disease states in which there is increased danger of hemorrhage. Some of the conditions in which increased danger of hemorrhage exists are:

- ***Cardiovascular:*** Subacute bacterial endocarditis. Severe hypertension.
- ***Surgical:*** During and immediately following (a) spinal tap or spinal anesthesia or (b) major surgery, especially involving the brain, spinal cord, or eye.
- ***Hematologic:*** Conditions associated with increased bleeding tendencies, such as hemophilia, thrombocytopenia, and some vascular purpuras.
- ***Gastrointestinal:*** Ulcerative lesions and continuous tube drainage of the stomach or small intestine.
- ***Other:*** Menstruation, liver disease with impaired hemostasis.

COAGULATION TESTING

When heparin sodium is administered in therapeutic amounts, its dosage should be regulated by frequent blood coagulation tests. If the coagulation test is unduly prolonged or if hemorrhage occurs, heparin sodium should be discontinued promptly.

THROMBOCYTOPENIA

Thrombocytopenia has been reported to occur in patients receiving heparin with a reported incidence of 0% to 30%. Mild thrombocytopenia (count greater than 100,000/mm^3) may remain stable or reverse even if heparin is continued. However, reduction in platelet count of any degree should be monitored closely. If the count falls below 100,000/mm^3 or if recurrent thrombosis develops (see PRECAUTIONS, General, White Clot Syndrome), the heparin product should be discontinued. If continued heparin therapy is essential, administration of heparin from a different organ source can be reinstituted with caution.

MISCELLANEOUS

This product contains benzyl alcohol as preservative. Benzyl alcohol has been reported to be associated with a fatal "Gasping Syndrome" in premature infants.

PRECAUTIONS

GENERAL

White Clot Syndrome

It has been reported that patients on heparin may develop new thrombus formation in association with thrombocytopenia resulting from irreversible aggregation of platelets induced by heparin, the so-called "white clot syndrome". The process may lead to severe thromboembolic complications like skin necrosis, gangrene of the extremities that may lead to amputation, myocardial infarction, pulmonary embolism, stroke, and possibly death. Therefore, heparin administration should be promptly discontinued if a patient develops new thrombosis in association with a reduction in platelet count.

Heparin Resistance

Increased resistance to heparin is frequently encountered in fever, thrombosis, thrombophlebitis, infections with thrombosing tendencies, myocardial infarction, cancer, in postsurgical patients, and patients with antithrombin III deficiency.

Increased Risk in Older Women

A higher incidence of bleeding has been reported in women over 60 years of age.

LABORATORY TESTS

Periodic platelet counts, hematocrits, and tests for occult blood in stool are recommended during the entire course of heparin therapy, regardless of the route of administration (see DOSAGE AND ADMINISTRATION).

DRUG/LABORATORY TEST INTERACTIONS

Hyperaminotransferasemia

Significant elevations of aminotransferase (SGOT [S-AST] and SGPT [S-ALT]) levels have occurred in a high percentage of patients (and healthy subjects) who have received heparin.

Since aminotransferase determinations are important in the differential diagnosis of myocardial infarction, liver disease, and pulmonary emboli, rises that might be caused by drugs (like heparin) should be interpreted with caution.

CARCINOGENESIS, MUTAGENESIS, AND IMPAIRMENT OF FERTILITY

No long-term studies in animals have been performed to evaluate the carcinogenic potential of heparin. Also, no reproduction studies in animals have been performed concerning mutagenesis or impairment of fertility.

PREGNANCY CATEGORY C

Teratogenic Effects: Animal reproduction studies have not been conducted with heparin sodium. It is also not known whether heparin sodium can cause fetal harm when administered to a pregnant woman or can affect reproduction capacity. Heparin sodium should be given to a pregnant woman only if clearly needed.
Nonteratogenic Effects: Heparin does not cross the placental barrier.

NURSING MOTHERS

Heparin is not excreted in human milk.

PEDIATRIC USE

See DOSAGE AND ADMINISTRATION.

DRUG INTERACTIONS

DRUG ENHANCING HEPARIN EFFECT

Oral Anticoagulants

Heparin sodium may prolong the one-stage prothrombin time. Therefore, when heparin sodium is given with dicumarol or warfarin sodium, a period of at least 5 hours after the last intravenous dose or 24 hours after the last subcutaneous dose should elapse before blood is drawn if a valid prothrombin time is to be obtained.

Platelet Inhibitors

Drugs such as acetylsalicylic acid, dextran, phenylbutazone, ibuprofen, indomethacin, dipyridamole, hydroxychloroquine and others that interfere with platelet-aggregation reactions (the main hemostatic defense of heparinized patients) may induce bleeding and should be used with caution in patients receiving heparin sodium.

The anticoagulant effect of heparin is enhanced by concurrent treatment with antithrombin III (human) in patients with hereditary antithrombin III deficiency. Thus in order to avoid bleeding, reduced dosage of heparin is recommended during treatment with antithrombin III (human).

DRUGS DECREASING HEPARIN EFFECT

Digitalis, tetracyclines, nicotine, or antihistamines may partially counteract the anticoagulant action of heparin sodium. Heparin sodium injection should not be mixed with doxorubicin, droperidol, ciprofloxacin, or mitoxantrone, since it has been reported that these drugs are incompatible with heparin and a precipitate may form.

ADVERSE REACTIONS

HEMORRHAGE

Hemorrhage is the chief complication that may result from heparin therapy (see WARNINGS). An overly prolonged clotting time or minor bleeding during therapy can usually be controlled by withdrawing the drug. **It should be appreciated that gastrointestinal or urinary tract bleeding during anticoagulant therapy may indicate the presence of an underlying occult lesion.** Bleeding can occur at any site but certain specific hemorrhagic complications may be difficult to detect:

- Adrenal hemorrhage, with resultant acute adrenal insufficiency, has occurred during anticoagulant therapy. Therefore, such treatment should be discontinued in patients who develop signs and symptoms of acute adrenal hemorrhage and insufficiency. Initiation of corrective therapy should not depend on laboratory confirmation of the diagnosis, since any delay in an acute situation may result in the patient's death.
- Ovarian (corpus luteum) hemorrhage developed in a number of women of reproductive age receiving short- or long-term anticoagulant therapy. This complication if unrecognized may be fatal.
- Retroperitoneal hemorrhage.

LOCAL IRRITATION

Local irritation, erythema, mild pain, hematoma or ulceration may follow deep subcutaneous (intrafat) injection of heparin sodium. These complications are much more common after intramuscular use, and such use is not recommended.

HYPERSENSITIVITY

Generalized hypersensitivity reactions have been reported, with chills, fever, and urticaria as the most usual manifestations, and asthma, rhinitis, lacrimation, headache, nausea and vomiting, and anaphylactoid reactions, including shock, occurring more rarely. Itching and burning, especially on the plantar site of the feet, may occur.

Thrombocytopenia has been reported to occur in patients receiving heparin with a reported incidence of 0-30%. While often mild and of no obvious clinical significance, a reduction in platelet count can be accompanied by severe thromboembolic complications such as skin necrosis, gangrene of the extremities that may lead to amputation, myocardial infarction, pulmonary embolism, stroke, and possibly death. (See WARNINGS and PRECAUTIONS.)

Certain episodes of painful, ischemic, and cyanosed limbs have in the past been attributed to allergic vasospastic reactions. Whether these are in fact identical to the thrombocytopenia associated complications remains to be determined.

MISCELLANEOUS

Osteoporosis following long-term administration of high-doses of heparin, cutaneous necrosis after systemic administration, suppression of aldosterone synthesis, delayed transient alopecia, priapism, and rebound hyperlipemia on discontinuation of heparin sodium have also been reported.

Significant elevations of aminotransferase (SGOT [S-AST] and SGPT [S-ALT]) levels have occurred in a high percentage of patients (and healthy subjects) who have received heparin.

DOSAGE AND ADMINISTRATION

Parenteral drug products should be inspected visually for particulate matter and discoloration prior to administration, whenever solution and container permit. Slight discoloration does not alter potency.

When heparin is added to an infusion solution for continuous intravenous administration, the container should be inverted at least 6 times to insure adequate mixing and prevent pooling of the heparin in the solution.

Heparin sodium is not effective by oral administration and should be given by intermittent intravenous injection, intravenous infusion, or deep subcutaneous (intrafat, *i.e.,* above the iliac crest or abdominal fat layer) injection. **The intramuscular route of administration should be avoided because of the frequent occurrence of hematoma at the injection site.**

The dosage of heparin sodium should be adjusted according to the patient's coagulation test results. When heparin is given by continuous intravenous infusion, the coagulation time should be determined approximately every 4 hours in the early stages of treatment. When the drug is administered intermittently by intravenous injection, coagulation tests should be performed before each injection during the early stages of treatment and at appropriate intervals thereafter. Dosage is considered adequate when the activated partial thromboplastin time (APTT) is 1.5 to 2 times normal or when the whole blood clotting time is elevated approximately 2.5 to 3 times the control value. After deep subcutaneous (intrafat) injections, tests for adequacy of dosage are best performed on samples drawn 4-6 hours after the injections.

Periodic platelet counts, hematocrits, and tests for occult blood in stool are recommended during the entire course of heparin therapy, regardless of the route of administration.

Heparin sodium injection should not be mixed with doxorubicin, droperidol, ciprofloxacin, or mitoxantrone, since it has been reported that these drugs are incompatible with heparin and a precipitate may form.

CONVERTING TO ORAL ANTICOAGULANT

When an oral anticoagulant of the coumarin or similar type is to be begun in patients already receiving heparin sodium, baseline and subsequent tests of prothrombin activity must be determined at a time when heparin activity is too low to affect the prothrombin time. This is about 5 hours after the last IV bolus and 24 hours after the last subcutaneous dose. If continuous IV heparin infusion is used, prothrombin time can usually be measured at any time.

In converting from heparin to an oral anticoagulant, the dose of the oral anticoagulant should be the usual initial amount and thereafter prothrombin time should be determined at the usual intervals. To ensure continuous anticoagulation, it is advisable to continue full heparin therapy for several days after the prothrombin time has reached the therapeutic range. Heparin therapy may then be discontinued without tapering.

THERAPEUTIC ANTICOAGULANT EFFECT WITH FULL-DOSE HEPARIN

Although dosage must be adjusted for the individual patient according to the results of suitable laboratory tests, the dosage schedules found in TABLE 1 may be used as guidelines.

TABLE 1

Method of Administration	Frequency	Recommended Dose*
Deep subcutaneous (intrafat) injection	Initial dose	5000 units by IV injection, followed by 10,000 to 20,000 units of a concentrated solution, subcutaneously
A different site should be used for each injection to prevent the development of massive hematoma.	Every 8 h or	8000-10,000 units of a concentrated solution
	Every 12 h	15,000-20,000 units of a concentrated solution
Intermittent intravenous injection	Initial dose	10,000 units, either undiluted or in 50-100 ml of sodium chloride injection, 0.9%
	Every 4-6 hours	5000-10,000 units, either undiluted or in 50-100 ml of sodium chloride injection 0.9%
Continuous intravenous infusion	Initial dose	5000 units by IV Injection
	Continuous	20,000-40,000 units/24 hours in 1000 ml of sodium chloride injection 0.9% (or in any compatible solution) for infusion

* Based on 150 lb (68 kg) patient.

PEDIATRIC USE

Follow recommendations of appropriate pediatric reference texts. In general, the following dosage schedule may be used as a guideline:

Initial Dose: 50 units/kg (IV, drip).

Maintenance Dose: 100 units/kg (IV, drip) every 4 hours, or 20,000 units/M^2/24 hours continuously.

SURGERY OF THE HEART AND BLOOD VESSELS

Patients undergoing total body perfusion for open-heart surgery should receive an initial dose of not less than 150 units of heparin sodium per kilogram of body weight. Frequently, a dose of 300 units per kilogram is used for procedures estimated to last less than 60 minutes or 400 units per kilogram for those estimated to last longer than 60 minutes.

LOW-DOSE PROPHYLAXIS OF POSTOPERATIVE THROMBOEMBOLISM

A number of well-controlled clinical trials have demonstrated that low-dose heparin prophylaxis, given just prior to and after surgery, will reduce the incidence of postoperative deep vein thrombosis in the legs (as measured by the I-125 fibrinogen technique and venography) and of clinical pulmonary embolism. The most widely used dosage has been 5000 units 2 hours before surgery and 5000 units every 8-12 hours thereafter for 7 days or until the patient is fully ambulatory, whichever is longer. The heparin is given by deep subcutaneous (intrafat, *i.e.,* above the iliac crest or abdominal fat layer, arm, or thigh) injection with a fine (25-26 gauge) needle to minimize tissue trauma. A concentrated solution of heparin sodium is recommended. Such prophylaxis should be reserved for patients over the age of 40 who are undergoing major surgery. Patients with bleeding disorders and those having brain or spinal cord surgery, spinal anesthesia, eye surgery, or potentially sanguineous operations should be excluded, as should patients receiving oral anticoagulants or platelet-active drugs (see WARNINGS). The value of such prophylaxis in hip surgery has not been established. The possibility of increased bleeding during surgery or postoperatively should be borne in mind. If such bleeding occurs, discontinuance of heparin and neutralization with protamine sulfate are advisable. If clinical evidence of thromboembolism develops despite low-dose prophylaxis, full therapeutic doses of anticoagulants should be given unless contraindicated. Prior to initiating heparinization the physician should rule out bleeding disorders by appropriate history and laboratory tests, and appropriate coagulation tests should be repeated just prior to surgery. Coagulation tests values should be normal or only slightly elevated at these times.

EXTRACORPOREAL DIALYSIS

Follow equipment manufacturers' operating directions carefully.

BLOOD TRANSFUSION

Addition of 400-600 USP units per 100 ml of whole blood is usually employed to prevent coagulation. Usually, 7500 USP units of heparin sodium are added to 100 ml of sodium chloride injection 0.9% (or 75,000 USP units per 1000 ml of sodium chloride injection 0.9%) and mixed; from this sterile solution, 6-8 ml are added per 100 ml of whole blood.

LABORATORY SAMPLES

Addition of 70-150 units of heparin sodium per 10-20 ml sample of whole blood is usually employed to prevent coagulation of the sample. Leukocyte counts should be performed on heparinized blood within 2 hours after addition of the heparin. Heparinized blood should not be used for isoagglutinin, complement, or erythrocyte fragility tests or platelet counts.

HOW SUPPLIED

Heparin sodium injection is derived **from beef lung.**

Storage: Store the product at controlled room temperature 20-25°C (68-77°F).

PRODUCT LISTING - RATED THERAPEUTICALLY EQUIVALENT

Size	Price	Manufacturer	NDC
Kit - Injectable - 10 U/ml			
1 ml x 50	$121.72	GENERIC, Abbott Pharmaceutical	00074-1282-02
1 ml x 50	$160.23	GENERIC, Esi Lederle Generics	00008-2528-50
1 ml x 50	$188.10	GENERIC, Esi Lederle Generics	00008-2528-52
2.50 ml x 30	$134.75	GENERIC, Esi Lederle Generics	00008-2528-51
3 ml x 25	$28.50	GENERIC, Abbott Pharmaceutical	00074-1280-03
10 ml x 25	$17.25	GENERIC, American Pharmaceutical Partners	63323-0544-11
30 ml x 25	$42.75	GENERIC, American Pharmaceutical Partners	63323-0544-31
Kit - Injectable - 100 U/ml			
1 ml x 30	$57.00	GENERIC, Abbott Pharmaceutical	00074-1389-32
Solution - Injectable - Beef Lung 1000 U/ml			
10 ml	$3.70	GENERIC, Pharmacia and Upjohn	00009-0268-01
10 ml x 25	$79.75	GENERIC, American Pharmaceutical Partners	63323-0038-10
10 ml x 25	$92.50	GENERIC, Pharmacia and Upjohn	00009-0268-12
30 ml	$10.56	GENERIC, Pharmacia and Upjohn	00009-0268-02
30 ml x 25	$160.00	GENERIC, American Pharmaceutical Partners	63323-0038-30
Solution - Injectable - Beef Lung 5000 U/ml			
10 ml	$17.19	GENERIC, Pharmacia and Upjohn	00009-0291-01
Solution - Injectable - Beef Lung 10000 U/ml			
1 ml x 25	$92.56	GENERIC, Pharmacia and Upjohn	00009-0317-10
4 ml	$13.79	GENERIC, Pharmacia and Upjohn	00009-0317-02
4 ml x 25	$344.75	GENERIC, Pharmacia and Upjohn	00009-0317-11
Solution - Injectable - 10 U/ml			
1 ml x 25	$13.25	GENERIC, Esi Lederle Generics	00641-0392-25
1 ml x 25	$15.50	GENERIC, Esi Lederle Generics	00641-0414-25
1 ml x 25	$20.00	GENERIC, American Pharmaceutical Partners	63323-0544-01
1 ml x 25	$37.50	GENERIC, Cmc-Consolidated Midland Corporation	00223-7861-01
1 ml x 25	$58.44	GENERIC, Abbott Pharmaceutical	00074-4822-01
1 ml x 50	$39.19	GENERIC, Abbott Pharmaceutical	00074-1280-01
1 ml x 50	$62.34	GENERIC, Abbott Pharmaceutical	00074-1280-31
1 ml x 50	$67.69	GENERIC, Abbott Pharmaceutical	00074-1280-11
1 ml x 50	$67.69	GENERIC, Abbott Pharmaceutical	00074-1280-21
1 ml x 50	$121.72	GENERIC, Abbott Pharmaceutical	00074-1389-01
2 ml x 25	$13.75	GENERIC, Esi Lederle Generics	00641-0393-25
2 ml x 25	$25.00	GENERIC, Cmc-Consolidated Midland Corporation	00223-7863-02
2 ml x 50	$54.00	GENERIC, Abbott Pharmaceutical	00074-1280-02
2 ml x 50	$57.28	GENERIC, Sanofi Winthrop Pharmaceuticals	00024-0721-02
2 ml x 50	$67.09	GENERIC, Abbott Pharmaceutical	00074-1280-32
2 ml x 50	$69.47	GENERIC, Abbott Pharmaceutical	00074-1280-12
2 ml x 50	$69.47	GENERIC, Abbott Pharmaceutical	00074-1280-22
3 ml	$2.23	GENERIC, Becton Dickinson	08290-3065-12

3 ml	$2.23	GENERIC, Becton Dickinson	08290-3065-21
3 ml	$2.76	GENERIC, Baxter Healthcare Corporation	00338-8106-69
3 ml	$3.07	GENERIC, Becton Dickinson	08290-0340-03
3 ml	$3.27	GENERIC, Becton Dickinson	08290-0360-03
3 ml x 25	$36.22	GENERIC, Abbott Pharmaceutical	00074-1280-33
3 ml x 25	$40.00	GENERIC, Abbott Pharmaceutical	00074-1280-23
3 ml x 25	$45.72	GENERIC, Abbott Pharmaceutical	00074-1280-13
5 ml	$2.53	GENERIC, Becton Dickinson	08290-3065-10
5 ml	$2.53	GENERIC, Becton Dickinson	08290-3065-11
5 ml	$3.00	GENERIC, Baxter Healthcare Corporation	00338-8110-70
5 ml	$3.28	GENERIC, Becton Dickinson	08290-3065-25
5 ml	$3.36	GENERIC, Becton Dickinson	08290-0350-05
5 ml	$3.36	GENERIC, Becton Dickinson	08290-0360-05
5 ml	$4.11	GENERIC, Becton Dickinson	08290-0361-05
5 ml x 25	$36.22	GENERIC, Abbott Pharmaceutical	00074-1280-35
5 ml x 25	$36.52	GENERIC, Abbott Pharmaceutical	00074-1280-05
5 ml x 25	$55.52	GENERIC, Abbott Pharmaceutical	00074-1280-15
6 ml	$2.55	GENERIC, Becton Dickinson	08290-3065-09
6 ml	$3.48	GENERIC, Becton Dickinson	08290-0360-06
10 ml x 25	$15.44	GENERIC, Abbott Pharmaceutical	00074-1151-70
10 ml x 25	$15.73	GENERIC, Abbott Pharmaceutical	00074-1151-12
10 ml x 25	$17.25	GENERIC, Esi Lederle Generics	00641-2438-45
10 ml x 25	$97.00	GENERIC, American Pharmaceutical Partners	63323-0017-10
30 ml x 25	$32.66	GENERIC, Abbott Pharmaceutical	00074-1151-78
30 ml x 25	$43.25	GENERIC, Esi Lederle Generics	00641-2442-45

Solution - Injectable - 100 U/ml

1 ml x 25	$13.25	GENERIC, Esi Lederle Generics	00641-0389-25
1 ml x 25	$15.50	GENERIC, Esi Lederle Generics	00641-0411-25
1 ml x 25	$20.00	GENERIC, American Pharmaceutical Partners	63323-0545-01
1 ml x 50	$67.09	GENERIC, Abbott Pharmaceutical	00074-1281-31
1 ml x 50	$69.47	GENERIC, Abbott Pharmaceutical	00074-1281-11
1 ml x 50	$69.47	GENERIC, Abbott Pharmaceutical	00074-1281-21
2 ml x 25	$13.50	GENERIC, Esi Lederle Generics	00641-0387-25
2 ml x 30	$93.34	GENERIC, Abbott Pharmaceutical	00074-1389-02
2 ml x 50	$65.00	GENERIC, Abbott Pharmaceutical	00074-1281-22
2 ml x 50	$67.09	GENERIC, Abbott Pharmaceutical	00074-1281-32
2 ml x 50	$69.47	GENERIC, Abbott Pharmaceutical	00074-1281-12
3 ml	$2.23	GENERIC, Becton Dickinson	08290-3065-14
3 ml	$2.23	GENERIC, Becton Dickinson	08290-3065-16
3 ml	$2.23	GENERIC, Becton Dickinson	08290-3065-17
3 ml	$2.76	GENERIC, Baxter Healthcare Corporation	00338-8206-69
3 ml	$3.07	GENERIC, Becton Dickinson	08290-0370-03
3 ml	$3.07	GENERIC, Becton Dickinson	08290-0380-03
3 ml	$3.27	GENERIC, Becton Dickinson	08290-0390-03
3 ml x 25	$28.75	GENERIC, Abbott Pharmaceutical	00074-1281-03
3 ml x 25	$44.53	GENERIC, Abbott Pharmaceutical	00074-1281-23
3 ml x 25	$44.83	GENERIC, Abbott Pharmaceutical	00074-1281-13
5 ml	$2.53	GENERIC, Becton Dickinson	08290-3065-13
5 ml	$2.53	GENERIC, Becton Dickinson	08290-3065-15
5 ml	$3.28	GENERIC, Becton Dickinson	08290-3065-31
5 ml	$3.36	GENERIC, Becton Dickinson	08290-0380-05
5 ml	$3.36	GENERIC, Becton Dickinson	08290-0390-05
5 ml	$4.11	GENERIC, Becton Dickinson	08290-0391-05
5 ml x 25	$36.22	GENERIC, Abbott Pharmaceutical	00074-1281-33
5 ml x 25	$36.22	GENERIC, Abbott Pharmaceutical	00074-1281-35
5 ml x 25	$52.25	GENERIC, Abbott Pharmaceutical	00074-1281-25
5 ml x 25	$57.30	GENERIC, Abbott Pharmaceutical	00074-1281-15
5 ml x 25	$105.00	GENERIC, American Pharmaceutical Partners	63323-0545-05
5 ml x 50	$91.44	GENERIC, Abbott Pharmaceutical	00074-3454-25
5 ml x 180	$138.24	GENERIC, Baxter Healthcare Corporation	00338-8210-70
10 ml x 25	$14.84	GENERIC, Abbott Pharmaceutical	00074-1152-70
10 ml x 25	$16.63	GENERIC, Abbott Pharmaceutical	00074-1152-12
10 ml x 25	$18.75	GENERIC, Esi Lederle Generics	00641-2436-45
30 ml x 25	$32.66	GENERIC, Abbott Pharmaceutical	00074-1152-78
30 ml x 25	$33.84	GENERIC, Abbott Pharmaceutical	00074-1152-14
30 ml x 25	$48.75	GENERIC, Esi Lederle Generics	00641-2443-45

Solution - Injectable - 1000 U/ml

1 ml x 10	$9.50	GENERIC, Esi Lederle Generics	00008-0275-01
1 ml x 25	$15.00	GENERIC, Esi Lederle Generics	00641-0391-25
1 ml x 25	$20.00	GENERIC, Cmc-Consolidated Midland Corporation	00223-7801-01
1 ml x 25	$27.00	GENERIC, American Pharmaceutical Partners	63323-0540-01
2 ml x 25	$92.25	GENERIC, American Pharmaceutical Partners	63323-0276-02
10 ml	$4.50	GENERIC, Cmc-Consolidated Midland Corporation	00223-7843-10
10 ml	$4.75	GENERIC, Cmc-Consolidated Midland Corporation	00223-7810-10
10 ml x 25	$25.00	GENERIC, Esi Lederle Generics	00641-2440-45
10 ml x 25	$37.50	GENERIC, American Pharmaceutical Partners	63323-0540-11
30 ml	$12.50	GENERIC, Cmc-Consolidated Midland Corporation	00223-7844-30
30 ml x 25	$56.75	GENERIC, Esi Lederle Generics	00641-2450-45
30 ml x 25	$87.50	GENERIC, American Pharmaceutical Partners	63323-0540-31

Solution - Injectable - 2500 U/ml

0.25 ml x 10	$12.59	GENERIC, Abbott Pharmaceutical	00074-1316-02

Solution - Injectable - 5000 U/ml

1 ml x 10	$10.60	GENERIC, Abbott Pharmaceutical	00074-1402-01
1 ml x 10	$16.00	GENERIC, Esi Lederle Generics	00008-0278-02
1 ml x 10	$60.00	GENERIC, Abbott Pharmaceutical	00074-1402-31
1 ml x 25	$24.00	GENERIC, Esi Lederle Generics	00641-0400-25
1 ml x 25	$32.25	GENERIC, American Pharmaceutical Partners	63323-0262-01
1 ml x 50	$53.00	GENERIC, Abbott Pharmaceutical	00074-1402-11
10 ml	$5.50	GENERIC, Pegasus Laboratories Inc	10974-0010-10
10 ml	$5.93	GENERIC, Interstate Drug Exchange Inc	00814-3655-40
10 ml	$17.50	GENERIC, Cmc-Consolidated Midland Corporation	00223-7820-10
10 ml x 25	$77.50	GENERIC, Esi Lederle Generics	00641-2460-45
10 ml x 25	$112.25	GENERIC, American Pharmaceutical Partners	63323-0047-10

Solution - Injectable - 7500 U/ml

1 ml x 10	$12.10	GENERIC, Sanofi Winthrop Pharmaceuticals	00024-0733-04

Solution - Injectable - 10000 U/ml

0.50 ml x 10	$10.60	GENERIC, Abbott Pharmaceutical	00074-1316-13
0.50 ml x 50	$49.50	GENERIC, Abbott Pharmaceutical	00074-1316-14
0.75 ml x 10	$18.88	GENERIC, Abbott Pharmaceutical	00074-1316-12
1 ml	$4.75	GENERIC, Cmc-Consolidated Midland Corporation	00223-7846-01
1 ml x 10	$17.90	GENERIC, Abbott Pharmaceutical	00074-1316-01
1 ml x 10	$23.63	GENERIC, Esi Lederle Generics	00008-0277-01
1 ml x 25	$22.75	GENERIC, Esi Lederle Generics	00641-0410-25
1 ml x 25	$42.25	GENERIC, American Pharmaceutical Partners	63323-0542-01
1 ml x 50	$95.59	GENERIC, Abbott Pharmaceutical	00074-1316-11
1 ml x 50	$96.78	GENERIC, Abbott Pharmaceutical	00074-1316-31
4 ml	$8.00	GENERIC, C.O. Truxton Inc	00463-1034-05
4 ml x 25	$72.50	GENERIC, Esi Lederle Generics	00641-2470-45
5 ml	$3.90	GENERIC, Cmc-Consolidated Midland Corporation	00223-7831-05
5 ml	$30.42	GENERIC, Lilly, Eli and Company	00002-7217-01
5 ml x 25	$74.52	GENERIC, Abbott Pharmaceutical	00074-2581-02
5 ml x 25	$140.75	GENERIC, American Pharmaceutical Partners	63323-0542-07
10 ml	$11.50	GENERIC, Cmc-Consolidated Midland Corporation	00223-7832-10
10 ml	$14.53	GENERIC, Pasadena Research Laboratories Inc	00418-4351-41
25 ml	$35.00	GENERIC, Cmc-Consolidated Midland Corporation	00223-7828-01
100 ml	$90.00	GENERIC, Cmc-Consolidated Midland Corporation	00223-7830-04
125 ml	$125.25	GENERIC, Pasadena Research Laboratories Inc	00418-4351-05

Solution - Injectable - 12500 U/ml

5 ml x 25	$67.50	GENERIC, Abbott Pharmaceutical	00074-2582-02

Solution - Injectable - 20000 U/ml

1 ml x 25	$120.25	GENERIC, American Pharmaceutical Partners	63323-0915-01
5 ml	$11.95	GENERIC, Cmc-Consolidated Midland Corporation	00223-7840-05
5 ml	$13.92	GENERIC, Pasadena Research Laboratories Inc	00418-4341-05
10 ml	$22.75	GENERIC, Pasadena Research Laboratories Inc	00418-4341-41
10 ml x 25	$86.88	GENERIC, Abbott Pharmaceutical	00074-2583-02
500 ml	$165.60	GENERIC, Baxter I.V. Systems Division	00338-0549-03

Solution - Injectable - 25000 U/ml

10 ml x 25	$123.80	GENERIC, Abbott Pharmaceutical	00074-2584-02

Solution - Injectable - 40000 U/ml

5 ml	$16.00	GENERIC, Pegasus Laboratories Inc	10974-0002-05
5 ml	$23.38	GENERIC, Pasadena Research Laboratories Inc	00418-4461-05

Solution - Intravenous - 5%;10,000 U/100 ml

100 ml x 12	$127.05	GENERIC, Abbott Pharmaceutical	00074-6286-11
100 ml x 24	$179.55	GENERIC, Abbott Pharmaceutical	00074-7793-23
150 ml x 24	$362.88	GENERIC, Abbott Pharmaceutical	00074-7793-61
250 ml x 24	$145.07	GENERIC, Abbott Pharmaceutical	00074-7793-62
250 ml x 24	$238.56	GENERIC, Baxter I.V. Systems Division	00338-0550-02
250 ml x 48	$625.80	GENERIC, B. Braun/Mcgaw Inc	00264-9587-20

Solution - Intravenous - 5%;4000 U/100 ml

500 ml x 24	$121.13	GENERIC, Abbott Pharmaceutical	00074-7760-03
500 ml x 24	$567.99	GENERIC, B. Braun/Mcgaw Inc	00264-9567-10

Solution - Intravenous - 5%;5000 U/100 ml

100 ml x 24	$302.40	GENERIC, Abbott Pharmaceutical	00074-7794-23
200 ml x 24	$377.60	GENERIC, Abbott Pharmaceutical	00074-7794-12
250 ml x 24	$164.73	GENERIC, Abbott Pharmaceutical	00074-7794-62
500 ml	$24.93	GENERIC, B. Braun/Mcgaw Inc	00264-9577-10
500 ml x 18	$178.92	GENERIC, Baxter I.V. Systems Division	00338-0550-03
500 ml x 24	$135.60	GENERIC, Abbott Pharmaceutical	00074-7761-03

Solution - Intravenous - 200 U/100 ml;0.9%

500 ml	$15.31	GENERIC, B. Braun/Mcgaw Inc	00264-9872-10
500 ml x 18	$70.11	GENERIC, Abbott Pharmaceutical	00074-7620-03
500 ml x 18	$123.66	GENERIC, Baxter I.V. Systems Division	00338-0431-03
1000 ml x 12	$80.80	GENERIC, Abbott Pharmaceutical	00074-7620-59
1000 ml x 12	$87.84	GENERIC, Baxter I.V. Systems Division	00338-0433-04

Solution - Intravenous - 5000 U/100 ml;0.45%

250 ml x 24	$144.21	GENERIC, Abbott Pharmaceutical	00074-7651-62
500 ml x 24	$201.78	GENERIC, Abbott Pharmaceutical	00074-7651-03

Solution - Intravenous - 10000 U/100 ml;0.45%

250 ml x 24	$188.10	GENERIC, Abbott Pharmaceutical	00074-7650-62

PRODUCT LISTING - EQUIVALENTS NOT AVAILABLE

Kit - Injectable - 10 U/ml

3 ml x 25	$27.52	GENERIC, Sanofi Winthrop Pharmaceuticals	00024-0721-14

H

5 ml x 25	$32.87	GENERIC, Sanofi Winthrop Pharmaceuticals	00024-0721-15
Solution - Injectable - 100 U/ml			
1 ml	$2.51	GENERIC, Medefil Inc	64253-0333-11
1 ml	$2.71	GENERIC, Medefil Inc	64253-0333-21
1 ml x 25	$13.75	GENERIC, Cmc-Consolidated Midland Corporation	00223-7865-01
2 ml	$2.80	GENERIC, Medefil Inc	64253-0333-12
2 ml	$2.95	GENERIC, Medefil Inc	64253-0333-22
2 ml x 25	$20.00	GENERIC, Cmc-Consolidated Midland Corporation	00223-7867-02
3 ml	$3.09	GENERIC, Medefil Inc	64253-0333-23
3 ml	$3.39	GENERIC, Medefil Inc	64253-0333-33
3 ml x 180	$138.24	GENERIC, Baxter Healthcare Corporation	00338-8209-69
5 ml	$3.49	GENERIC, Medefil Inc	64253-0333-25
5 ml	$3.71	GENERIC, Medefil Inc	64253-0333-35
10 ml	$3.95	GENERIC, Medefil Inc	64253-0333-30
Solution - Injectable - 1000 U/ml			
10 ml	$4.50	GENERIC, International Technidyne Corporation	11743-0210-02
30 ml	$2.69	GENERIC, Mcguff Company	49072-0291-30
Solution - Injectable - 5000 U/ml			
1 ml x 25	$25.00	GENERIC, Cmc-Consolidated Midland Corporation	00223-7818-01
10 ml	$3.49	GENERIC, Mcguff Company	49072-0297-10
Solution - Injectable - 10000 U/ml			
4 ml	$3.29	GENERIC, Mcguff Company	49072-0299-05
4 ml	$4.80	GENERIC, C.O. Truxton Inc	00463-1034-04
4 ml	$5.00	GENERIC, Cmc-Consolidated Midland Corporation	00223-7847-04
4 ml x 25	$100.00	GENERIC, Cmc-Consolidated Midland Corporation	00223-7847-25
Solution - Injectable - 20000 U/ml			
5 ml	$14.95	GENERIC, Cmc-Consolidated Midland Corporation	00223-7840-01

Hepatitis A Inactivated; Hepatitis B (Recombinant) Vaccine (003521)

For complete prescribing information, refer to the CD-ROM included with the book.

Categories: Immunization, hepatitis A; Immunization, hepatitis B; Pregnancy Category C; FDA Approved 2001 May
Drug Classes: Vaccines
Brand Names: Twinrix

DESCRIPTION

Note: The trade name has been used throughout this monograph for clarity.

Twinrix [hepatitis A inactivated and hepatitis B (recombinant) vaccine] is a sterile bivalent vaccine containing the antigenic components used in producing Havrix (Hepatitis A Vaccine, Inactivated) and Engerix-B [Hepatitis B Vaccine (Recombinant)]. Twinrix is a sterile suspension of inactivated hepatitis A virus (strain HM175) propagated in MRC-5 cells, and combined with purified surface antigen of the hepatitis B virus. The purified hepatitis B surface antigen (HBsAg) is obtained by culturing genetically engineered *Saccharomyces cerevisiae* cells, which carry the surface antigen gene of the hepatitis B virus, in synthetic media containing inorganic salts, amino acids, dextrose, and vitamins. Bulk preparations of each antigen are adsorbed separately onto aluminum salts and then pooled during formulation.

A 1.0 ml dose of vaccine contains not less than 720 ELISA units of inactivated hepatitis A virus and 20 µg of recombinant HBsAg protein. One dose of vaccine also contains 0.45 mg of aluminum in the form of aluminum phosphate and aluminum hydroxide as adjuvants, amino acids, 5.0 mg 2-phenoxyethanol as a preservative, sodium chloride, phosphate buffer, polysorbate 20, water for injection, traces of formalin (not more than 0.1 mg), a trace amount of thimerosal (<1 µg mercury) from the manufacturing process, and residual MRC-5 cellular proteins (not more than 2.5 µg). Neomycin sulfate, an aminoglycoside antibiotic, is included in the cell growth media; only trace amounts (not more than 20 ng/dose) remain following purification. The manufacturing procedures used to manufacture Twinrix result in a product that contains no more than 5% yeast protein.

Twinrix is supplied as a sterile suspension for intramuscular administration. The vaccine is ready for use without reconstitution; it must be shaken before administration since a fine white deposit with a clear colorless supernatant may form on storage. After shaking, the vaccine is a slightly turbid white suspension.

INDICATIONS AND USAGE

Twinrix is indicated for active immunization of persons 18 years of age or older against disease caused by hepatitis A virus and infection by all known subtypes of hepatitis B virus. As with any vaccine, vaccination with Twinrix may not protect 100% of recipients. As hepatitis D (caused by the delta virus) does not occur in the absence of HBV infection, it can be expected that hepatitis D will also be prevented by vaccination with Twinrix.

Twintrix will not prevent hepatitis caused by other agents such as hepatitis C virus, hepatitis E virus or other pathogens known to infect the liver.

Immunization is recommended for all susceptible persons 18 years of age or older who are, or will be, at risk of exposure to both hepatitis A and B viruses, including but not limited to:

Travelers to areas of high/intermediate endemicity for *both* HAV and HBV (see TABLE 4) *who are at increased risk of HBV infection due to behavioral or occupational factors.*

TABLE 4 *Hepatitis A and B Endemicity by Region*

Geographic Region	HAV	HBV
Africa	High	High (most)
Caribbean	High	Intermediate
Central America	High	Intermediate
South America (temperate)	High	Intermediate
South America (tropical)	High	High
South and Southwest Asia*	High	High
Middle East†	High	High
Eastern Europe	Intermediate	Intermediate
Southern Europe	Intermediate	Intermediate
Former Soviet Union	Intermediate	Intermediate

* *Japan:* Low HAV and intermediate HBV endemicity.
† *Israel:* Intermediate HBV endemicity.

Patients with chronic liver disease, including:

- Alcoholic cirrhosis
- Chronic hepatitis C
- Autoimmune hepatitis
- Primary biliary cirrhosis

Persons at risk through their work:

Laboratory workers who handle live hepatitis A and hepatitis B virus.
Police and other personnel who render first-aid or medical assistance.
Workers who come in contact with feces or sewage.
Healthcare personnel who render first-aid or emergency medical assistance.
Personnel employed in day-care centers and correctional facilities. Residents of drug and alcohol treatment centers. Staff of hemodialysis units.
People living in, or relocating to, areas of high/intermediate endemicity of HAV and who have risk factors for HBV.
Men who have sex with men.
Persons at increased risk of disease due to their sexual practices.[20,21]
Patients frequently receiving blood products including persons who have clotting-factor disorders (hemophiliacs and other recipients of therapeutic blood products).
Military recruits and other military personnel at increased risk for HBV.
Users of injectable illicit drugs.
Individuals who are at increased risk for HBV infection and who are close household contacts of patients with acute or relapsing hepatitis A and individuals who are at increased risk for HAV infection and who are close household contacts of individuals with acute or chronic hepatitis B infection.

CONTRAINDICATIONS

Twintrix is contraindicated in people with known hypersensitivity to any component of the vaccine or to subjects having shown signs of hypersensitivity after previous administration of Twinrix or monovalent hepatitis A or hepatitis B vaccines.

WARNINGS

There have been rare reports of anaphylaxis/anaphylactoid reactions following routine clinical use of Havrix. (See CONTRAINDICATIONS.)

Hepatitis A and B have relatively long incubation periods. The vaccine may not prevent hepatitis A or B infection in individuals who have an unrecognized hepatitis A or B infection at the time of vaccination. Additionally, it may not prevent infection in individuals who do not achieve protective antibody titers.

DOSAGE AND ADMINISTRATION

Twintrix should be administered by IM injection. *Do not inject intravenously or intradermally.* In adults, the injection should be given in the deltoid region. Twinrix should not be administered in the gluteal region; such injections may result in a suboptimal response.

For individuals with clotting-factor disorders who are at risk of hemorrhage following IM injection, the ACIP recommends that when any IM vaccine is indicated for such patients, "...it should be administered intramuscularly if, in the opinion of a physician familiar with the patient's bleeding risk, the vaccine can be administered with reasonable safety by this route. If the patient receives antihemophilia or other similar therapy, IM vaccination can be scheduled shortly after such therapy is administered. A fine needle (23 gauge or smaller) can be used for the vaccination and firm pressure applied to the site (without rubbing) for at least 2 minutes. The patient should be instructed concerning the risk of hematoma from the injection."[28]

When concomitant administration of other vaccines or immunoglobulin (IG) is required, they should be given with different syringes and at different injection sites.

PREPARATION FOR ADMINISTRATION

Shake vial or syringe well before withdrawal and use. Parenteral drug products should be inspected visually for particulate matter or discoloration prior to administration. With thorough agitation, Twinrix is a slightly white turbid suspension. Discard if it appears otherwise.

The vaccine should be used as supplied; no dilution or reconstitution is necessary. The full recommended dose of the vaccine should be used. After removal of the appropriate volume from a single-dose vial, any vaccine remaining in the vial should be discarded.

Primary immunization for adults consists of 3 doses, given on a 0, 1 and 6 month schedule. Each 1 ml dose contains 720 EL.U. of inactivated hepatitis A virus and 20 µg of hepatitis B surface antigen.

PRODUCT LISTING - EQUIVALENTS NOT AVAILABLE

Solution - Intramuscular - 720 U;20 mcg/ml			
1 ml	$98.15	TWINRIX, Glaxosmithkline	58160-0850-01
1 ml x 5	$484.50	TWINRIX, Glaxosmithkline	58160-0850-35
1 ml x 5	$484.50	TWINRIX, Glaxosmithkline	58160-0850-46
1 ml x 10	$965.80	TWINRIX, Glaxosmithkline	58160-0850-11

Hepatitis A Vaccine (003158)

For complete prescribing information, refer to the CD-ROM included with the book.

Categories: Immunization, hepatitis A; Pregnancy Category C; FDA Approved 1995 Feb
Drug Classes: Vaccines
Brand Names: Havrix
Foreign Brand Availability: Avaxim (Australia; Canada; Colombia; England; Hong-Kong; Ireland; New-Zealand; South-Africa; Thailand); Epaxal (Canada; New-Zealand; Peru); HAVpur (Germany); Vaqta (Australia; Canada; England; Germany; Ireland; Israel; Mexico)

DESCRIPTION

Note: The trade names have been used throughout this monograph for clarity.

HAVRIX

Havrix (Hepatitis A Vaccine, Inactivated) is a noninfectious hepatitis A vaccine developed and manufactured by SmithKline Beecham Biologicals. The virus (strain HM175) is propagated in MRC_5 human diploid cells. After removal of the cell culture medium, the cells are lysed to form a suspension. This suspension is purified through ultrafiltration and gel permeation chromatography procedures. Treatment of this lysate with formalin ensures viral inactivation. Havrix contains a sterile suspension of inactivated virus; viral antigen activity is referenced to a standard using an enzyme linked immunosorbent assay (ELISA), and is therefore expressed in terms of ELISA Units (EL.U.).

Havrix is supplied as a sterile suspension for intramuscular administration. The vaccine is ready for use without reconstitution; it must be shaken before administration to assure a uniform suspension. After shaking, the vaccine is a homogeneous white turbid suspension.

Each 1 ml adult dose of vaccine consists of not less than 1440 EL.U. of viral antigen, adsorbed on 0.5 mg of aluminum, as aluminum hydroxide.

There are two pediatric dose formulations, each with its own dosing schedule (see DOSAGE AND ADMINISTRATION, Havrix). The formulations are: not less than 360 EL.U. of viral antigen/0.5 ml; not less than 720 EL.U. of viral antigen/0.5 ml. Each dose is adsorbed onto 0.25 mg of aluminum, as aluminum hydroxide.

The vaccine preparations also contain 0.5% (w/v) of 2-phenoxyethanol as a preservative. Other excipients are: amino acid supplement (0.3% w/v) in a phosphate-buffered saline solution and polysorbate 20 (0.05 mg/ml). Residual MRC_5 cellular proteins (not more than 5 μg/adult dose) and traces of formalin (not more than 0.1 mg/ml) are present.

VAQTA

Vaqta [Hepatitis A Vaccine, Inactivated] is an inactivated whole virus vaccine derived from hepatitis A virus (HAV) grown in cell culture in human MRC-5 diploid fibroblasts. It contains inactivated virus of a strain which was originally derived by further serial passage of a proven attenuated strain. The virus is grown, harvested, purified by a combination of physical and high performance liquid chromatographic techniques developed at the Merck Research Laboratories, formalin inactivated, and then adsorbed onto aluminum hydroxide. One milliliter (1 ml) of the vaccine contains approximately 50 units (U) of hepatitis A virus antigen, which is purified and formulated without a preservative. Within the limits of current assay variability, the 50 U dose of Vaqta contains less than 0.1 μg of non-viral protein, less than 4×10^{-6} μg of DNA, less than 10^{-4} μg of bovine albumin, and less than 0.8 μg of formaldehyde. Other process chemical residuals are less than 10 parts per billion (ppb).

Vaqta is a sterile suspension for intramuscular injection.

Vaqta is supplied in two formulations:

Pediatric/Adolescent Formulation: Each 0.5 ml dose contains approximately 25 U of hepatitis A virus antigen adsorbed onto approximately 0.225 mg of aluminum provided as aluminum hydroxide, and 35 μg of sodium borate as a pH stabilizer, in 0.9% sodium chloride.

Adult Formulation: Each 1 ml dose contains approximately 50 U of hepatitis A virus antigen adsorbed onto approximately 0.45 mg of aluminum provided as aluminum hydroxide, and 70 μg of sodium borate as a pH stabilizer, in 0.9% sodium chloride.

INDICATIONS AND USAGE

HAVRIX

Havrix is indicated for active immunization of persons ≥2 years of age against disease caused by hepatitis A virus (HAV).

Havrix will not prevent hepatitis caused by other agents such as hepatitis B virus, hepatitis C virus, hepatitis E virus or other pathogens known to infect the liver.

Immunization with Havrix is indicated for those people desiring protection against hepatitis A. Primary immunization should be completed at least 2 weeks prior to expected exposure to HAV.

Individuals who are, or will be, at increased risk of infection by HAV include:

Travelers: Persons traveling to areas of higher endemicity for hepatitis A. These areas include, but are not limited to, Africa, Asia (except Japan), the Mediterranean basin, eastern Europe, the Middle East, Central and South America, Mexico, and parts of the Caribbean. Current CDC advisories should be consulted with regard to specific locales.

Military personnel.

People living in, or relocating to, areas of high endemicity.

Certain ethnic and geographic populations that experience cyclic hepatitis A epidemics such as: Native peoples of Alaska and the Americas.

People with chronic liver disease, including:

- Alcoholic cirrhosis
- Chronic hepatitis B
- Chronic hepatitis C
- Autoimmune hepatitis
- Primary biliary cirrhosis

Others:

- Persons engaging in high-risk sexual activity (such as men having sex with men)[17]
- Residents of a community experiencing an outbreak of hepatitis A
- Users of illicit injectable drugs
- Persons who have clotting-factor disorders (hemophiliacs and other recipients of therapeutic blood products). Hepatitis A transmission has been documented in persons with clotting disorders. Susceptible persons in this category, especially those who receive solvent-detergent-treated clotting-factor concentrates, should be vaccinated against hepatitis A[18] (see DOSAGE AND ADMINISTRATION, Havrix).

Although the epidemiology of hepatitis A does not permit the identification of other specific populations at high risk of disease, outbreaks of hepatitis A or exposure to hepatitis A virus have been described in a variety of populations in which Havrix may be useful:

- Certain institutional workers (*e.g.,* caretakers for the developmentally challenged).
- Employees of child day-care centers.
- Laboratory workers who handle live hepatitis A virus.
- Handlers of primate animals that may be harboring HAV.

People Exposed to Hepatitis A

For those requiring both immediate and long-term protection, Havrix may be administered concomitantly with IG. The ACIP has issued the following recommendations regarding food handlers: "Persons who work as food handlers can contract hepatitis A and transmit HAV to others. To decrease the frequency of evaluations of food handlers with hepatitis A and the need for postexposure prophylaxis of patrons, vaccination may be considered where state or local health authorities or private employers determine that such vaccination is cost-effective."[18]

VAQTA

Vaqta is indicated for active pre-exposure prophylaxis against disease caused by hepatitis A virus in persons 2 years of age and older. Primary immunization should be given at least 2 weeks prior to expected exposure to HAV.

Individuals who are or will be at increased risk of infection by HAV include:[23-35,37,38]

Travelers: Persons traveling to areas of higher endemicity for hepatitis A. These areas include, but are not limited to, Africa, Asia (except Japan), the Mediterranean basin, Eastern Europe, the Middle East, Central and South America, Mexico, and parts of the Caribbean. Current CDC (Centers for Disease Control and Prevention) advisories should be consulted with regard to specific locales.

Military personnel.

People living in, or relocating to, areas of high endemicity.

Certain ethnic and geographic populations that experience cyclic hepatitis A epidemics such as: Native peoples of Alaska and the Americas.

Others:

Persons engaging in high-risk sexual activity (such as homosexually active males); users of illicit injectable drugs; residents of a community experiencing an outbreak of hepatitis A.

Hemophiliacs and other recipients of therapeutic blood products (see DOSAGE AND ADMINISTRATION, Vaqta).

Persons who test positive for hepatitis C virus and have diagnosed liver disease.[45]

Although the epidemiology of hepatitis A does not permit the identification of other specific populations at high risk of disease, outbreaks of hepatitis A or exposure to hepatitis A virus have been described in a variety of populations in which Vaqta may be useful:

- Certain institutional workers (*e.g.,* caretakers for the developmentally challenged).
- Employees of child day-care centers.
- Laboratory workers who handle live hepatitis A virus.
- Handlers of primate animals that may be harboring HAV.

People Exposed to Hepatitis A

For those requiring both immediate and long-term protection, Vaqta may be administered concomitantly with IG.

Revaccination

See DOSAGE AND ADMINISTRATION, Vaqta, Dosage.

Use With Other Vaccines

Vaqta may be given concomitantly at separate injection sites with typhoid and yellow fever vaccines. The GMTs for hepatitis A when Vaqta, typhoid and yellow fever vaccines were administered concomitantly were reduced when compared to Vaqta alone. Following receipt of the booster dose of Vaqta, the GMTs for hepatitis A in these two groups were observed to be comparable. (See DOSAGE AND ADMINISTRATION, Vaqta, Dosage, Use With Other Vaccines.)

The Advisory Committee on Immunization Practices has stated that limited data from studies conducted among adults indicate that simultaneous administration of hepatitis A vaccine with diphtheria, poliovirus (oral and inactivated), tetanus, oral typhoid, cholera, Japanese encephalitis, rabies, or yellow fever vaccine does not decrease the immune response to either vaccine or increase the frequency of reported adverse events. Studies indicate that hepatitis B vaccine can be administered with Vaqta without affecting immunogenicity or increasing the frequency of adverse events.[46]

Use With Immune Globulin

For individuals requiring either post-exposure prophylaxis or combined immediate and longer-term protection (*e.g.,* travelers departing on short notice to endemic areas), Vaqta may be administered concomitantly with IG using separate sites and syringes (see DOSAGE AND ADMINISTRATION, Vaqta).

VAQTA IS NOT RECOMMENDED FOR USE IN INFANTS YOUNGER THAN 2 YEARS OF AGE SINCE DATA ON USE IN THIS AGE GROUP ARE NOT CURRENTLY AVAILABLE.

CONTRAINDICATIONS

HAVRIX

Havrix is contraindicated in people with known hypersensitivity to any component of the vaccine.

VAQTA

Hypersensitivity to any component of the vaccine.

WARNINGS

HAVRIX

There have been rare reports of anaphylaxis/anaphylactoid reactions following commercial use of the vaccine in other countries. Patients experiencing hypersensitivity reactions after a Havrix injection should not receive further Havrix injections. (See CONTRAINDICATIONS, Havrix.)

Hepatitis A has a relatively long incubation period (15-50 days). Hepatitis A vaccine may not prevent hepatitis A infection in individuals who have an unrecognized hepatitis A infection at the time of vaccination. Additionally, it may not prevent infection in individuals who do not achieve protective antibody titers (although the lowest titer needed to confer protection has not been determined).

VAQTA

Individuals who develop symptoms suggestive of hypersensitivity after an injection of Vaqta should not receive further injections of the vaccine (see CONTRAINDICATIONS, Vaqta).

If Vaqta is used in individuals with malignancies or those receiving immunosuppressive therapy or who are otherwise immunocompromised, the expected immune response may not be obtained.

DOSAGE AND ADMINISTRATION

HAVRIX

Havrix should be administered by intramuscular injection. *Do not inject intravenously, intradermally or subcutaneously.*

In adults, the injection should be given in the deltoid region. Havrix should not be administered in the gluteal region; such injections may result in suboptimal response.

Havrix may be administered concomitantly with IG, although the ultimate antibody titer obtained is likely to be lower than when the vaccine is given alone. Havrix has been administered simultaneously with Engerix-B without interference with their respective immune responses.

For individuals with clotting-factor disorders who are at risk of hemorrhage following intramuscular injection, the ACIP recommends that when any intramuscular vaccine is indicated for such patients, "...it should be administered intramuscularly if, in the opinion of a physician familiar with the patient's bleeding risk, the vaccine can be administered with reasonable safety by this route. If the patient receives antihemophilia or other similar therapy, intramuscular vaccination can be scheduled shortly after such therapy is administered. A fine needle (≤23 gauge) can be used for the vaccination and firm pressure applied to the site (without rubbing) for at least 2 minutes. The patient or family should be instructed concerning the risk of hematoma from the injection."[21] When concomitant administration of other vaccines or IG is required, they should be given with different syringes and at different injection sites.

Preparation for Administration

Shake vial or syringe well before withdrawal and use. Parenteral drug products should be inspected visually for particulate matter or discoloration prior to administration. With thorough agitation, Havrix is a turbid white suspension. Discard if it appears otherwise.

The vaccine should be used as supplied; no dilution or reconstitution is necessary. The full recommended dose of the vaccine should be used. After removal of the appropriate volume from a single-dose vial, any vaccine remaining in the vial should be discarded.

Primary immunization for adults consists of a single dose of 1440 EL.U. in 1 ml. Primary immunization for children and adolescents (2-18 years of age) may follow either of the two schedules outlined in TABLE 6.

TABLE 6 *Children and Adolescents (2-18 years of age)*

Dose	Schedule
Primary Course: 360 EL.U./0.5 ml	*Primary Course:* Two doses given 1 month apart (month 0 and month 1)
Booster: 360 EL.U./0.5 ml	*Booster:* 6-12 months after primary course
OR	
Primary Course: 720 EL.U./0.5 ml	*Primary Course:* One dose (month 0)
Booster: 720 EL.U./0.5 ml	*Booster:* 6-12 months after primary course

Individuals should not be alternated between the 360 EL.U. and 720 EL.U. doses. Those who receive an initial 360 EL.U. dose should continue on the 360 EL.U. dosing schedule. Likewise, those individuals who receive a single 720 EL.U. primary dose should receive a 720 EL.U. booster dose.

For all age groups, a booster dose is recommended anytime between 6 and 12 months after the initiation of the primary dose in order to ensure the highest antibody titers.

In those with an impaired immune system, adequate anti-HAV response may not be obtained after the primary immunization course. Such patients may therefore require administration of additional doses of vaccine.

VAQTA

Do not inject intravenously, intradermally, or subcutaneously.

Vaqta is for intramuscular injection. The deltoid muscle is the preferred site for intramuscular injection.

Dosage

The vaccination regimen consists of 1 primary dose and 1 booster dose for healthy children, adolescents, and adults, as follows:

Pediatric/Adolescent

Individuals 2-18 years of age should receive a single 0.5 ml (~25 U) dose of vaccine at elected date and a booster dose of 0.5 ml (~25 U) 6-18 months later.

A 1.0 ml (~50 U) dose also was evaluated in individuals 18 years of age and was found to be immunogenic and generally well tolerated.

Adult

Adults 19 years of age and older should receive a single 1.0 ml (~50 U) dose of vaccine at elected date and a booster dose of 1.0 ml (~50 U) 6-12 months later.

Interchangeability of the Booster Dose

A booster dose of Vaqta may be given at 6-12 months following the initial dose of other inactivated hepatitis A vaccines (*e.g.,* Havrix).

Use With Other Vaccines

Vaqta may be given concomitantly with typhoid and yellow fever vaccines. The GMTs for hepatitis A when Vaqta, typhoid and yellow fever vaccines were administered concomitantly were reduced when compared to Vaqta alone. Following receipt of the booster dose of Vaqta, the GMTs for hepatitis A in these two groups were observed to be comparable. Data on concomitant use with other vaccines are limited. Separate injection sites and syringes should be used for concomitant administration of injectable vaccines. (See INDICATIONS AND USAGE, Vaqta, Use With Other Vaccines.)

Use With Immune Globulin

Vaqta may be administered concomitantly with IG using separate sites and syringes. The vaccination regimen for Vaqta should be followed as stated above. Consult the manufacturer's product circular for the appropriate dosage of IG. A booster dose of Vaqta should be administered at the appropriate time as outlined above.

Administration

Known or Presumed Exposure to HAV/Travel to Endemic Areas

For individuals requiring either post-exposure prophylaxis or combined immediate and longer term protection (*e.g.,* travelers departing on short notice to endemic areas), Vaqta may be administered concomitantly with IG using separate sites and syringes (see Use With Immune Globulin).

Injection must be accomplished with a needle long enough to ensure intramuscular deposition of the vaccine. The Advisory Committee on Immunization Practices (ACIP) has recommended that "For all intramuscular injections, the needle should be long enough to reach the muscle mass and prevent vaccine from seeping into subcutaneous tissue, but not so long as to endanger underlying neurovascular structures or bone." For toddlers and older children they further state that "...the deltoid may be used if the muscle mass is adequate. The needle size can range from 22-25 gauge and from 5/8 to 1 1/4 inches, based on the size of the muscle...the anterolateral thigh may be used, but the needle should be longer — generally ranging from 7/8 to 1 1/4 inches." For adults they state that "...the deltoid is recommended for routine intramuscular vaccination among adults...The suggested needle size is 1 to 1 1/2 inches and 20-25 gauge."[42]

For individuals with bleeding disorders who are at risk of hemorrhage following intramuscular injection, the ACIP recommends that when any intramuscular vaccine is indicated for such patients, "...it should be administered intramuscularly if, in the opinion of a physician familiar with the patient's bleeding risk, the vaccine can be administered with reasonable safety by this route. If the patient receives antihemophilia or other similar therapy, intramuscular vaccination can be scheduled shortly after such therapy is administered. A fine needle ≤23 gauge) can be used for the vaccination and firm pressure applied to the site (without rubbing) for at least 2 minutes. The patient or family should be instructed concerning the risk of hematoma from the injection."[42]

The vaccine should be used as supplied; no reconstitution is necessary.

Shake well before withdrawal and use. Thorough agitation is necessary to maintain suspension of the vaccine. Discard if the suspension does not appear homogenous.

Parenteral drug products should be inspected visually for extraneous particulate matter and discoloration prior to administration whenever solution and container permit. After thorough agitation, Vaqta is a slightly opaque, white suspension.

It is important to use a separate sterile syringe and needle for each individual to prevent transmission of infectious agents from one person to another.

PRODUCT LISTING - EQUIVALENTS NOT AVAILABLE

Solution - Intramuscular - 25 U/0.5 ml			
0.50 ml	$39.23	VAQTA, Merck & Company Inc	00006-4831-00
0.50 ml	$39.23	VAQTA, Merck & Company Inc	00006-4845-00
0.50 ml x 5	$169.53	VAQTA, Merck & Company Inc	00006-4831-38
0.50 ml x 5	$169.53	VAQTA, Merck & Company Inc	00006-4845-38
0.50 ml x 10	$339.05	VAQTA, Merck & Company Inc	00006-4831-41
Solution - Intramuscular - 50 U/ml			
1 ml	$65.58	VAQTA, Allscripts Pharmaceutical Company	54569-4469-00
1 ml	$78.45	VAQTA, Merck & Company Inc	00006-4841-00
1 ml	$78.45	VAQTA, Merck & Company Inc	00006-4844-00
1 ml x 5	$309.31	VAQTA, Allscripts Pharmaceutical Company	54569-4351-00
1 ml x 5	$370.25	VAQTA, Merck & Company Inc	00006-4841-38
1 ml x 5	$370.25	VAQTA, Merck & Company Inc	00006-4844-38
Solution - Intramuscular - 1440 U/ml			
0.50 ml	$20.40	HAVRIX PEDIATRIC, Allscripts Pharmaceutical Company	54569-4068-00
0.50 ml	$20.40	HAVRIX PEDIATRIC, Glaxosmithkline	58160-0836-01
0.50 ml	$29.75	HAVRIX PEDIATRIC, Glaxosmithkline	58160-0837-02

0.50 ml	$34.16	HAVRIX PEDIATRIC, Glaxosmithkline	58160-0837-01
0.50 ml x 5	$148.60	HAVRIX PEDIATRIC, Glaxosmithkline	58160-0837-05
0.50 ml x 5	$163.35	HAVRIX PEDIATRIC, Glaxosmithkline	58160-0837-35
0.50 ml x 5	$163.35	HAVRIX PEDIATRIC, Glaxosmithkline	58160-0837-46
0.50 ml x 10	$326.70	HAVRIX PEDIATRIC, Glaxosmithkline	58160-0837-11
0.50 ml x 25	$784.16	HAVRIX PEDIATRIC, Glaxosmithkline	58160-0837-50
0.50 ml x 25	$784.16	HAVRIX PEDIATRIC, Glaxosmithkline	58160-0837-56
0.50 ml x 25	$816.84	HAVRIX PEDIATRIC, Glaxosmithkline	58160-0837-26
0.50 ml x 25	$816.84	HAVRIX PEDIATRIC, Glaxosmithkline	58160-0837-58
1 ml	$55.45	HAVRIX, Compumed Pharmaceuticals	00403-4969-18
1 ml	$59.45	HAVRIX, Allscripts Pharmaceutical Company	54569-3987-00
1 ml	$59.45	HAVRIX, Glaxosmithkline	58160-0835-02
1 ml	$65.50	HAVRIX, Glaxosmithkline	58160-0835-32
1 ml	$65.50	HAVRIX, Glaxosmithkline	58160-0835-41
1 ml	$66.94	HAVRIX, Glaxosmithkline	58160-0835-01
1 ml x 5	$327.50	HAVRIX, Glaxosmithkline	58160-0835-35
1 ml x 5	$327.50	HAVRIX, Glaxosmithkline	58160-0835-46
1 ml x 10	$297.30	HAVRIX, Glaxosmithkline	58160-0835-05
10 ml	$594.58	HAVRIX, Glaxosmithkline	58160-0835-07

Hepatitis B Immune Globulin *(001429)*

For complete prescribing information, refer to the CD-ROM included with the book.

Categories: Hepatitis B, Post-Exposure prophylaxis; Pregnancy Category C; FDA Pre 1938 Drugs; WHO Formulary
Drug Classes: Immune globulins
Brand Names: H-Big; **Hep-B-Gammagee**; Hyperhep
Foreign Brand Availability: Bayhep B (Canada); Euvax-B (Thailand); Hepuman Berna (Peru); IVheBex (France)

DESCRIPTION

Hepatitis B immune globulin (human) injection is available in standard as well as solvent/detergent treated and filtered forms. When differentiation between these forms is necessary, the brand names "H-BIG" (standard form) and "Nabi-HB" (solvent/detergent treated and filtered form) will be used for clarity.

H-BIG

H-BIG is a sterile solution of immunoglobulin (16.5 ± 1.5% protein) which is prepared from the pooled plasma of individuals with high titers of antibody to the hepatitis B surface antigen (anti-HBs), by the Cohn-Oncley cold alcohol fractionation process. **Hepatitis B immune globulin (human) is intended only for intramuscular injection.** The product is stabilized with 0.3M glycine and contains 1:10,000 thimerosal (a mercury derivative) as a preservative. The solution has been adjusted to a pH of 6.8 ± 0.4 with sodium hydroxide or hydrochloric acid. Each vial of H-BIG contains anti-HBs equivalent to or exceeding the potency of anti-HBs in a US Reference hepatitis B immune globulin (Center for Biologics Evaluation and Research, FDA). The high titer plasma was fractionated by Centeon. The plasma used to make Fraction II powder for potency adjustment was fractionated by Centeon and/or Michigan Department of Public Health.

NABI-HB

Nabi-HB is a sterile solution of immunoglobulin (5 ± 1% protein) containing antibodies to hepatitis B surface antigen (anti-HBs). It is prepared from plasma donated by individuals with high titers of anti-HBs. The plasma is purified by an anion-exchange column chromatography method[1,2] with two added viral reduction steps described below. The product is formulated in 0.075 M sodium chloride, 0.15 M glycine, and 0.01% polysorbate 80, pH 6.25. It contains no preservative and is intended for single use by the intramuscular route only. The product appears as a clear to opalescent, nonturbid liquid.

The manufacturing steps are designed to reduce the risk of transmission of viral disease. The solvent/detergent treatment step, using tri-n-butyl phosphate and Triton X-100, is effective in inactivating known enveloped viruses such as hepatitis B virus (HBV), hepatitis C virus (HCV), and human immunodeficiency virus (HIV).[3] Virus filtration, using a Planova 35 nm Virus Filter, is effective in reducing some known enveloped and non-enveloped viruses.[4] The inactivation and reduction of known enveloped and non-enveloped model viruses were validated in laboratory studies as summarized in TABLE 1.

***TABLE 1** Log Reduction of Test Viruses[5]*

	Test Virus				
	HIV	BVD	PRV	Polio	BPV
Model Virus:	HIV	HCV	HBV	Hepatitis A	PVB19
Envelope/Genome:	yes/RNA	yes/RNA	yes/DNA	no/RNA	no/DNA
Manufacturing Step					
Dextran Sulfate	NT	NT	NT	3.32	<1
Anion-Exchange	NT	NT	NT	>3.52	>5.34
Solvent/Detergent	>4.67	>7.43	>5.26	2.7	>5.81
Virus Filtration	>6.02	>7.30	>6.77	4.25	>4.97

BVD Bovine Viral Diarrhea.
PRV Pseudorabies Virus.
Polio Poliovirus.
BPV Bovine Parvovirus.
PVB19 Parvovirus B19.
NT Not tested.

The product potency is expressed in international units (IU) by comparison to the World Health Organization (WHO) standard. Each vial contains greater than 312 IU/ml anti-HBs. The potency of each vial of Nabi-HB exceeds the potency of anti-HBs in a US reference hepatitis B immune globulin (FDA). The US reference has been tested by Nabi against the WHO standard and found to be equal to 208 IU/ml.

INDICATIONS AND USAGE

H-BIG

H-BIG is indicated for post-exposure prophylaxis[10,11] following either parenteral exposure (accidental "needlestick"), direct mucous membrane contact (accidental splash), sexual exposure[11], or oral ingestion (pipetting accident) involving HBsAg positive materials such as blood, plasma, and serum. H-BIG is also indicated in post-exposure prophylaxis in infants born to hepatitis B surface antigen positive (HBsAg positive) mothers.[10-12] Such infants are at risk of becoming chronic carriers.[17,22,25] The risk is especially great if the mother is also HBeAg positive.[18,26] The carrier state can be prevented in about 75% of such exposures if newborns are given hepatitis B immune globulin (human), immediately after birth and in the early months of life.[10,11] Concurrent H-BIG and hepatitis B vaccine administration does not appear to interfere with antibody responses to hepatitis B vaccine and increases efficacy to about 94%.[11,12,15]

NABI-HB

Nabi-HB is indicated for treatment of acute exposure to blood containing HBsAg, perinatal exposure of infants born to HBsAg-positive mothers, sexual exposure to HBsAg-positive persons and household exposure to persons with acute HBV infection in the following settings:

- ***Acute exposure to blood containing HBsAg:*** Following either parenteral exposure (needlestick, bite, sharps), direct mucous membrane contact (accidental splash), or oral ingestion (pipetting accident), involving HBsAg-positive materials such as blood, plasma or serum.
- ***Perinatal exposure of infants born to HBsAg-positive mothers:*** Infants born to mothers positive for HBsAg with or without HBeAg.[11]
- ***Sexual exposure to HBsAg-positive persons:*** Sexual partners of HBsAg-positive persons.
- ***Household exposure to persons with acute HBV infection:*** Infants less than 12 months old whose mother or primary caregiver is positive for HBsAg. Other household contacts with an identifiable blood exposure to the index patient.

Nabi-HB is indicated for intramuscular use only.

CONTRAINDICATIONS

H-BIG

There are no specific contraindications for H-BIG. No adverse reactions have been seen in individuals with preexisting hepatitis B surface antigen (HBsAg) although data regarding this occurrence are limited. Some individuals may demonstrate hypersensitivity to the glycine and/or thimerosal components used to stabilize and preserve this product.

NABI-HB

Individuals known to have had an anaphylactic or severe systemic reaction to human globulin should not receive Nabi-HB, or any other human immune globulin. Nabi-HB contains less than 40 micrograms/ml IgA. Individuals who are deficient in IgA may have the potential to develop IgA antibodies and have an anaphylactoid reaction. The physician must weigh the potential benefit of treatment with Nabi-HB against the potential for hypersensitivity reactions.

WARNINGS

H-BIG

H-BIG should be given with caution to patients with a history of prior systemic allergic reactions following the administration of human immunoglobulin preparations. Persons with an isolated deficiency of Immunoglobulin A (IgA) have the potential for developing antibodies to such immunoglobulin, which could result in anaphylactic reactions to subsequent administration of any blood products containing IgA.[27] As with any other immune globulin preparation, H-BIG should be given to such persons only if the expected benefits outweigh the potential risks. In patients who have severe thrombocytopenia or any coagulation disorder that would contraindicate intramuscular injections, H-BIG should be given only if the expected benefits outweigh the potential risks.

NABI-HB

In patients who have severe thrombocytopenia or any coagulation disorder that would contraindicate intramuscular injections, Nabi-HB should be given only if the expected benefits outweigh the potential risks.

Nabi-HB is made from human plasma. Products made from human plasma may contain infectious agents, such as viruses, that can cause disease. The risk that such products can transmit an infectious agent has been reduced by screening plasma donors for prior exposure to certain viruses, by testing for the presence of certain current viral infections, and by inactivating and/or reducing certain viruses. The Nabi-HB manufacturing process includes a solvent/detergent treatment step (using tri-n-butyl phosphate and Triton X-100) that is effective in inactivating known enveloped viruses such as HBV, HCV, and HIV. Nabi-HB is filtered using a Planova 35 nm virus filter that is effective in reducing the levels of some enveloped and non-enveloped viruses. These two processes are designed to increase product safety. Despite these measures, such products can still potentially transmit disease. There is also the possibility that unknown infectious agents may be present in such products. ALL infections thought by a physician possibly to have been transmitted by this product should be reported by the physician or other health care provider to Nabi at 1-800-458-4244. The physician should discuss the risks and benefits of this product with the patient.

DOSAGE AND ADMINISTRATION

H-BIG

Parenteral drug products should be inspected visually for particulate matter and discoloration prior to administration whenever solution and container permit. H-BIG is a clear, very slightly amber, moderately viscous liquid. **H-BIG should be administered intramuscularly, preferably in the gluteal or deltoid region.** H-BIG should never be administered into or near blood vessels or nerves. DO NOT INJECT INTRAVENOUSLY.

If blood or any unusual discoloration is present in the syringe, H-BIG should not be injected. The needle should be withdrawn and syringe discarded. A new dose of hepatitis B immune globulin (human) should be prepared and the procedure for administration repeated at a different site, using a new syringe and needle. It is important to use a separate sterile syringe and needle for each individual patient, in order to prevent transmission of hepatitis B and other infectious agents from one person to another. **Any vial that has been entered into should be used promptly. Partially used vials should be discarded and not saved for future use.**

Adults

The Immunization Practices Advisory Committee (ACIP) recommends that hepatitis B immune globulin (human) and hepatitis B vaccine be given concurrently.[11]

Recommendations for adults who have not been previously vaccinated against hepatitis B are the following: H-BIG (0.06 ml/kg) should be administered intramuscularly as soon as possible after exposure and within 24 hours if possible. Hepatitis B vaccine (see appropriate product information for dosage recommendations), should be given intramuscularly, within 7 days of exposure. Second and third doses should be administered at 1 and 6 months, respectively, after the first dose.

H

Recommendations for adults who have been previously vaccinated against hepatitis B are the following: Persons should have their anti-HBs titers checked promptly. For those with known adequate antibody levels (10 mIU/ml anti-HBs are approximately equal to 10 SRU), no injection is required.[11] Those with inadequate or unknown titers should receive a dose of hepatitis B immune globulin (human) and one of hepatitis B vaccine simultaneously at 2 different sites. The recommended dose of H-BIG is 0.06 ml/kg (usually 3-5 ml), administered as soon as possible after exposure (preferably within 24 hours). Doses over 5 ml should be administered in the multiple sites to minimize discomfort. Immunization with hepatitis B vaccine should begin as soon as possible, but within 7 days. For use of Hepatitis B vaccine, see appropriate product information. If the individual refuses the hepatitis B vaccine, a second dose of H-BIG (0.06 ml/kg) should be given 1 month after the first dose.

Newborns

Infants born to HBsAg positive mothers are at high risk of becoming chronic carriers of hepatitis B virus and of developing the chronic sequelae of hepatitis B virus infection. Controlled studies have shown that administration of three 0.5 ml doses of H-BIG starting at birth is 75% effective in preventing establishment of the chronic carrier state in these infants during the first year of life.[34] Protection can be transient, whereupon the effectiveness of the hepatitis B immune globulin (human) would decline thereafter. Results from clinical studies indicate that the administration of one 0.5 ml dose of H-BIG at birth and the recommended 3 doses of hepatitis B vaccine be given concurrently to infants born to HBsAg positive mothers (especially those mothers who are HBeAg positive).[10-12,15,21] The recommended dose of H-BIG for at risk newborns is 0.5 ml as soon after birth as possible, preferably no later than 12 hours. Immunization with hepatitis B vaccine should begin promptly within 7 days of birth. For information on hepatitis B vaccine, refer to the appropriate product information. If administration of the first dose of hepatitis B vaccine is delayed for as long as 3 months, then a 0.5 ml dose of H-BIG should be repeated at 3 months. If the hepatitis B vaccine is refused, then the 0.5 ml dose of H-BIG should be repeated at 3 and 6 months.

Testing for HBsAg and anti-HBs is recommended at 12-15 months of age. If HBsAg is not detectable and anti-HBs is present, the child has been protected.[11] The recommended dosage for infants born to HBsAg positive mothers is shown in TABLE 2.

TABLE 2

	Birth	Within 7 days	1 month	6 months
Hepatitis B Vaccine*	—	0.5 ml†	0.5 ml	0.5 ml
H-Big	0.5 ml	—	—	—

* See DOSAGE AND ADMINISTRATION in the product information for the hepatitis B vaccine that you are utilizing.
† The first dose of hepatitis B vaccine may be given at birth at the same time as hepatitis B immune globulin (human); but should be administered in the anterolateral aspect of the opposite thigh.

NABI-HB

This product is for intramuscular use only. The use of this product by the intravenous route is not indicated. Parenteral drug products should be inspected visually for particulate matter and discoloration prior to administration.

It is important to use a separate vial, sterile syringe, and needle for each individual patient, in order to prevent transmission of infectious agents from one person to another. **Any vial of Nabi-HB that has been entered should be used promptly. Do not reuse or save for future use. This product contains no preservative; therefore, partially used vials should be discarded immediately.**

Hepatitis B immune globulin (human) may be administered at the same time (but at a different site), or up to 1 month preceding hepatitis B vaccination without impairing the active immune response to hepatitis B vaccine.[14]

Acute Exposure to Blood Containing HBsAg

TABLE 3 summarizes prophylaxis for percutaneous (needlestick, bite, sharps), ocular, or mucous membrane exposure to blood according to the source of exposure and vaccination status of the exposed person. For greatest effectiveness, passive prophylaxis with hepatitis B immune globulin (human) should be given as soon as possible after exposure, as its value after 7 days following exposure is unclear.[11] An injection of 0.06 ml/kg of body weight should be administered intramuscularly as soon as possible after exposure and within 24 hours, if possible. Consult the hepatitis B vaccine product information for dosage information regarding the vaccine.

For persons who refuse hepatitis B vaccine or are known non-responders to vaccine, a second dose of hepatitis B immune globulin (human) should be given 1 month after the first dose.[11]

***TABLE 3** Recommendations for Hepatitis B Prophylaxis Following Percutaneous or Permucosal Exposure[11]*

	Exposed Person	
Source	**Unvaccinated**	**Vaccinated**
HBsAg-positive	1. Hepatitis B immune globulin (human) × 1 immediately* 2. Initiate HB vaccine series†	1. Test exposed person for anti-HBs 2. If inadequate antibody‡, hepatitis B immune globulin (human) × 1 immediately plus HB vaccine booster dose
Known Source — High Risk for HBsAg-positive	1. Initiate HB vaccine series 2. Test source for HBsAg. If positive, hepatitis B immune globulin (human) × 1	1. Test source for HBsAg only if exposed is vaccine nonresponder; if source is HBsAg-positive, give hepatitis B immune globulin (human) × 1 immediately plus HB vaccine booster dose
Known Source — Low Risk for HBsAg-positive	Initiate HB vaccine series	Nothing required.
Unknown Source	Initiate HB vaccine series	Nothing required.

* Hepatitis B immune globulin (human) dose of 0.06 ml/kg IM.
† See manufacturers' recommendation for appropriate dose.
‡ Less than 10 mIU/ml anti-HBs by radioimmunoassay, negative by enzyme immunoassay.

Prophylaxis of Infants Born to Mothers who are Positive for HBsAg with or without HBeAg

TABLE 4 contains the recommended schedule of hepatitis B prophylaxis for infants born to mothers that are either known to be positive for HBsAg or have not been screened. Infants born to mothers known to be HBsAg-positive should receive 0.5 ml hepatitis B immune globulin (human) after physiologic stabilization of the infant and preferably within 12 hours of birth. The hepatitis B vaccine series should be initiated simultaneously, if not contraindicated, with the first dose of the vaccine given concurrently with the hepatitis B immune globulin (human), but at a different site. Subsequent doses of the vaccine should be administered in accordance with the recommendations of the manufacturer.

Women admitted for delivery, who were not screened for HBsAg during the prenatal period, should be tested. While test results are pending, the newborn infant should receive hepatitis B vaccine within 12 hours of birth (see manufacturers' recommendations for dose). If the mother is later found to be HBsAg positive, the infant should receive 0.5 ml hepatitis B immune globulin (human) as soon as possible and within 7 days of birth; however, the efficacy of hepatitis B immune globulin (human) administered after 48 hours of age is not known.[13,23] Testing for HBsAg and anti-HBs is recommended at 12-15 months of age. If HBsAg is not detectable and anti-HBs is present, the child has been protected.[11]

***TABLE 4** Recommended Schedule of Hepatitis B Immunoprophylaxis to Prevent Perinatal Transmission of Hepatitis B Virus Infection[23]*

	Age of Infant	
Administer	**Infant born to mother known to be HBsAg positive**	**Infant born to mother not screened for HBsAg**
First vaccination*	Birth (within 12 hours)	Birth (within 12 hours)
Hepatitis B immune globulin (human)†	Birth (within 12 hours)	If mother is found to be HBsAg positive, administer dose to infant as soon as possible, not later than 1 week after birth
Second vaccination*	1 month	1-2 months
Third vaccination*	6 months‡	6 months ‡

* See manufacturers' recommendations for appropriate dose.
† 0.5 ml administered IM at a site different from that used for the vaccine.
‡ See ACIP recommendation.

Sexual Exposure to HBsAg-positive Persons

All susceptible persons whose sexual partners have acute hepatitis B infection should receive a single dose of hepatitis B immune globulin (human) (0.06 ml/kg) and should begin the hepatitis B vaccine series, if not contraindicated, within 14 days of the last sexual contact or if sexual contact with the infected person will continue. Administering the vaccine with hepatitis B immune globulin (human) may improve the efficacy of post exposure treatment. The vaccine has the added advantage of conferring long-lasting protection.[23]

Household Exposure to Persons With Acute HBV Infection

Prophylaxis of an infant less than 12 months of age with 0.5 ml hepatitis B immune globulin (human) and hepatitis B vaccine is indicated if the mother or primary caregiver has acute HBV infection. Prophylaxis of other household contacts of persons with acute HBV infection is not indicated unless they had an identifiable blood exposure to the index patient, such as by sharing toothbrushes or razors. Such exposures should be treated like sexual exposures. If the index patient becomes an HBV carrier, all household contacts should receive hepatitis B vaccine.[23]

PRODUCT LISTING - EQUIVALENTS NOT AVAILABLE

Solution - Intramuscular - Strength n/a

0.50 ml	$54.00	HYPERHEP, Bayer	00192-0616-00
0.50 ml	$78.75	BAYHEP B, Bayer	00026-0636-03
0.50 ml	$118.80	BAYHEP B, Bayer	00026-0636-00
0.50 ml	$167.50	H-BIG, Nabi	59730-8399-02
1 ml	$102.00	HYPERHEP, Bayer	00026-0616-01
1 ml	$107.25	H-BIG, Nabi	59730-8399-01
1 ml	$142.56	BAYHEP B, Bayer	00026-0636-02
1 ml	$175.00	NABI-HB, Nabi	59730-4402-01
1 ml	$1199.99	BAYHEP B, Bayer	00026-0636-01
5 ml	$162.19	NABI-HB, Nabi	59730-4202-01
5 ml	$182.88	H-BIG, Allscripts Pharmaceutical Company	54569-3829-00
5 ml	$360.00	HYPERHEP, Bayer	00192-0616-05
5 ml	$700.00	NABI-HB, Allscripts Pharmaceutical Company	54569-4739-00
5 ml	$700.00	NABI-HB, Nabi	59730-4403-01
5 ml	$710.00	NABI-HB, Nabi	59730-4203-01
5 ml	$1199.99	BAYHEP B, Bayer	00026-0636-05

Hepatitis B Vaccine, Recombinant *(001431)*

For complete prescribing information, refer to the CD-ROM included with the book.

Categories: Immunization, hepatitis B; Pregnancy Category C; Recombinant DNA Origin; FDA Approved 1986 Jul; WHO Formulary

Drug Classes: Vaccines

Brand Names: Engerix-B; Recombivax Hb; **Recombivax-HB**

Foreign Brand Availability: Bio-Hep-B (Israel); H-B-Vax II (Australia; Austria; Belgium; Bulgaria; Czech-Republic; Denmark; Finland; France; Germany; Greece; Hungary; Italy; Mexico; Netherlands; New-Zealand; Norway; Poland; Portugal; Slovenia; Spain; Sweden; Switzerland; Turkey); HBvaxPRO (England; Ireland); Heberbiovac HB (Mexico); Hepacare (Austria; Belgium; Bulgaria; Czech-Republic; Denmark; England; Finland; France; Germany; Greece; Hungary; Ireland; Italy; Netherlands; Norway; Poland; Portugal; Slovenia; Spain; Sweden; Switzerland; Turkey); Hepavax Gene (Colombia)

DESCRIPTION

Note: The trade names have been used throughout this monograph for clarity.

ENGERIX-B

Engerix-B is a noninfectious recombinant DNA hepatitis B vaccine developed and manufactured by SmithKline Beecham Biologicals. It contains purified surface antigen of the virus obtained by culturing genetically engineered *Saccharomyces cerevisiae* cells, which carry the surface antigen gene of the hepatitis B virus. The surface antigen expressed in *Saccharomyces cerevisiae* cells is purified by several physicochemical steps and formulated as a suspension of the antigen adsorbed on aluminum hydroxide. The procedures used to manufacture Engerix-B result in a product that contains no more than 5% yeast protein. No substances of human origin are used in its manufacture.

Engerix-B is supplied as a sterile suspension for intramuscular administration. The vaccine is ready for use without reconstitution; it must be shaken before administration since a fine white deposit with a clear colorless supernatant may form on storage.

Pediatric/Adolescent

Each 0.5 ml of vaccine consists of 10 µg of hepatitis B surface antigen adsorbed on 0.25 mg aluminum as aluminum hydroxide. The pediatric/adolescent vaccine is formulated without preservatives. The pediatric formulation contains a trace amount of thimerosal (<0.5 µg mercury) from the manufacturing process, sodium chloride (9 mg/ml) and phosphate buffers (disodium phosphate dihydrate, 0.98 mg/ml; sodium dihydrogen phosphate dihydrate, 0.71 mg/ml).

Adult

Each 1 ml adult dose consists of 20 µg of hepatitis B surface antigen adsorbed on 0.5 mg aluminum as aluminum hydroxide. The adult vaccine is formulated without preservatives. The adult formulation contains a trace amount of thimerosal (<1.0 µg mercury) from the manufacturing process, sodium chloride (9 mg/ml) and phosphate buffers (disodium phosphate dihydrate, 0.98 mg/ml; sodium dihydrogen phosphate dihydrate, 0.71 mg/ml).

RECOMBIVAX HB

Recombivax HB is a non-infectious subunit viral vaccine derived from hepatitis B surface antigen (HBsAg) produced in yeast cells. A portion of the hepatitis B virus gene, coding for HBsAg, is cloned into yeast, and the vaccine for hepatitis B is produced from cultures of this recombinant yeast strain according to methods developed in the Merck Research Laboratories.

The antigen is harvested and purified from fermentation cultures of a recombinant strain of the yeast *Saccharomyces cerevisiae* containing the gene for the *adw* subtype of HBsAg. The HBsAg protein is released from the yeast cells by cell disruption and purified by a series of physical and chemical methods. The vaccine contains no detectable yeast DNA but may contain not more than 1% yeast protein. The vaccine produced by the Merck method has been shown to be comparable to the plasma-derived vaccine in terms of animal potency (mouse, monkey, and chimpanzee) and protective efficacy (chimpanzee and human).

The vaccine against hepatitis B, prepared from recombinant yeast cultures, is free of association with human blood or blood products.

Each lot of hepatitis B vaccine is tested for safety, in mice and guinea pigs, and for sterility.

Recombivax HB is a sterile suspension for intramuscular injection. However, for persons at risk of hemorrhage following intramuscular injection, the vaccine may be administered subcutaneously. (See DOSAGE AND ADMINISTRATION, Recombivax HB.)

Recombivax HB is supplied in three formulations.

Pediatric/Adolescent Formulation (with and without preservative), 10 µg/ml: each 0.5 ml dose contains 5 µg of hepatitis B surface antigen.

Adult Formulation, 10 µg/ml: each 1 ml dose contains 10 µg of hepatitis B surface antigen.

Dialysis Formulation, 40 µg/ml: each 1 ml dose contains 40 µg of hepatitis B surface antigen.

Formulations that contain a preservative include thimerosal, a mercury derivative, at 1:20,000 or 50 µg/ml. All formulations have been treated with formaldehyde prior to adsorption onto aluminum hydroxide. In each formulation, hepatitis B surface antigen is adsorbed onto approximately 0.5 mg of aluminum (provided as aluminum hydroxide) per ml of vaccine. The vaccine is of the *adw* subtype. Recombivax HB is indicated for vaccination of persons at risk of infection from hepatitis B virus including all known subtypes. Recombivax HB Dialysis Formulation is indicated for vaccination of adult predialysis and dialysis patients against infection caused by all known subtypes of hepatitis B virus.

INDICATIONS AND USAGE

ENGERIX-B

Engerix-B is indicated for immunization against infection caused by all known subtypes of hepatitis B virus. As hepatitis D (caused by the delta virus) does not occur in the absence of hepatitis B infection, it can be expected that hepatitis D will also be prevented by Engerix-B vaccination.

Engerix-B will not prevent hepatitis caused by other agents, such as hepatitis A, C and E viruses, or other pathogens known to infect the liver.

Immunization is recommended in persons of all ages, especially those who are, or will be, at increased risk of exposure to hepatitis B virus,[1] for example:

Infants, including those born of HBsAg-positive mothers: See DOSAGE AND ADMINISTRATION, Engerix-B.

Adolescents.

Health care personnel: Dentists and oral surgeons. Dental, medical and nursing students. Physicians, surgeons and podiatrists. Nurses. Paramedical and ambulance personnel and custodial staff who may be exposed to the virus via blood or other patient specimens. Dental hygienists and dental nurses. Laboratory and blood-bank personnel handling blood, blood products, and other patient specimens. Hospital cleaning staff who handle waste.

Selected patients and patient contacts: Patients and staff in hemodialysis units and hematology/oncology units. Patients requiring frequent and/or large volume blood transfusions or clotting factor concentrates (*e.g.*, persons with hemophilia, thalassemia, sickle-cell anemia, cirrhosis). Clients (residents) and staff of institutions for the mentally handicapped. Classroom contacts of deinstitutionalized mentally handicapped persons who have persistent hepatitis B surface antigenemia and who show aggressive behavior. Household and other intimate contacts of persons with persistent hepatitis B surface antigenemia.

Subpopulations with a known high incidence of the disease, such as: Alaskan Eskimos. Pacific Islanders. Indochinese immigrants. Haitian immigrants. Refugees from other HBV endemic areas. All infants of women born in areas where the infection is highly endemic.

Individuals with chronic hepatitis C: Risk factors for hepatitis C are similar to those for hepatitis B. Consequently, immunization with hepatitis B vaccine is recommended for individuals with chronic hepatitis C.

Persons who may be exposed to the hepatitis B virus by travel to high-risk areas: See ACIP Guidelines, 1990.

Military personnel identified as being at increased risk.

Morticians and embalmers.

Persons at increased risk of the disease due to their sexual practices,[1,16] such as: Persons with more than 1 sexual partner in a 6 month period. Persons who have contracted a sexually transmitted disease. Homosexually active males. Female prostitutes.

Prisoners.

Users of illicit injectable drugs.

Others: Police and fire department personnel who render first aid or medical assistance, and any others who, through their work or personal life-style, may be exposed to the hepatitis B virus. Adoptees from countries of high HBV endemicity.

Use With Other Vaccines

The Immunization Practices Advisory Committee states that, in general, simultaneous administration of certain live and inactivated pediatric vaccines has not resulted in impaired antibody responses or increased rates of adverse reactions.[17] Separate sites and syringes should be used for simultaneous administration of injectable vaccines.

RECOMBIVAX HB

Recombivax HB is indicated for vaccination against infection caused by all known subtypes of hepatitis B virus. **Recombivax HB Dialysis Formulation** is indicated for vaccination of adult predialysis and dialysis patients against infection caused by all known subtypes of hepatitis B virus.

Vaccination with Recombivax HB is recommended for:

1. Infants including those born to HBsAg positive mothers (high-risk infants).
2. Children born after November 21, 1991.[49]
3. Adolescents.
4. Other persons of all ages in areas of high prevalence or those who are or may be at increased risk of infection with hepatitis B virus, such as:[49]
   - ***Health care personnel:***
     Dentists and oral surgeons.
     Physicians and surgeons.

H

Nurses.
Paramedical personnel and custodial staff who may be exposed to the virus via blood or other patient specimens.
Dental hygienists and dental nurses.
Laboratory personnel handling blood, blood products, and other patient specimens.
Dental, medical and nursing students.

- ***Selected patients and patient contacts:***

Staff in hemodialysis units and hematology/oncology units.
Hemodialysis patients and patients with early renal failure before they require hemodialysis.
Patients requiring frequent and/or large volume blood transfusions or clotting factor concentrates (*e.g.*, persons with hemophilia, thalassemia).
Clients (residents) and staff of institutions for the mentally handicapped.
Classroom contacts of deinstitutionalized mentally handicapped persons who have persistent hepatitis B surface antigenemia and who show aggressive behavior.
Household and other intimate contacts of persons with persistent hepatitis B surface antigenemia.

- ***Sub-populations with a known high incidence of the disease, such as:***

Alaskan Natives.
Pacific Islanders.
Refugees from areas where hepatitis B virus infection is endemic.
Adoptees from countries where hepatitis B virus infection is endemic.

- ***International travelers.***
- ***Military personnel identified as being at increased risk.***
- ***Morticians and embalmers.***
- ***Blood bank and plasma fractionation workers.***
- ***Persons at increased risk of the disease due to their sexual practices, such as:***

Persons who have heterosexual activity with multiple partners.
Persons who repeatedly contract sexually transmitted diseases.
Homosexual and bisexual adolescent and adult men.
Female prostitutes.

- ***Prisoners.***
- ***Injection drug users.***

Neither dosage strength will prevent hepatitis caused by other agents, such as hepatitis A virus, hepatitis C virus, hepatitis E virus or other viruses known to infect the liver.

Use With Other Vaccines

Results from clinical studies indicate that Recombivax HB can be administered concomitantly with DTP (Diphtheria, Tetanus and whole cell Pertussis), OPV (oral Poliomyelitis vaccine), M-M-RII (Measles, Mumps, and Rubella Virus Vaccine Live), Liquid PedvaxHIB [Haemophilus b Conjugate Vaccine (Meningococcal Protein Conjugate)] or a booster dose of DTaP [Diphtheria, Tetanus, acellular Pertussis], using separate sites and syringes for injectable vaccines. No impairment of immune response to individual tested vaccine antigens was demonstrated.

The type, frequency and severity of adverse experiences observed in these studies with Recombivax HB were similar to those seen when the other vaccines were given alone.

In addition, a HBsAg-containing product, Comvax [Haemophilus b Conjugate (Meningococcal Protein Conjugate) and Hepatitis B (Recombinant) Vaccine], was given concomitantly with eIPV (enhanced inactivated Poliovirus vaccine) or Varivax [Varicella Virus Vaccine Live (Oka/Merck)], using separate sites and syringes for injectable vaccines. No impairment of immune response to these individually tested vaccine antigens was demonstrated. No serious vaccine-related adverse events were reported.

Comvax has also been administered concomitantly with the primary series of DTaP to a limited number of infants. No serious vaccine-related adverse events were reported.[29]

Separate sites and syringes should be used for simultaneous administration of injectable vaccines.

CONTRAINDICATIONS

ENGERIX-B

Hypersensitivity to yeast or any other component of the vaccine is a contraindication for use of the vaccine. Patients experiencing hypersensitivity after an Engerix-B injection should not receive further injections of Engerix-B.

RECOMBIVAX HB

Hypersensitivity to yeast or any component of the vaccine.

WARNINGS

ENGERIX-B

Hepatitis B has a long incubation period. Hepatitis B vaccination may not prevent hepatitis B infection in individuals who had an unrecognized hepatitis B infection at the time of vaccine administration. Additionally, it may not prevent infection in individuals who do not achieve protective antibody titers.

RECOMBIVAX HB

Patients who develop symptoms suggestive of hypersensitivity after an injection should not receive further injections of the vaccine (see CONTRAINDICATIONS, Recombivax HB).

Because of the long incubation period for hepatitis B, it is possible for unrecognized infection to be present at the time the vaccine is given. The vaccine may not prevent hepatitis B in such patients.

DOSAGE AND ADMINISTRATION

ENGERIX-B

Injection

Engerix-B should be administered by intramuscular injection. *Do not inject intravenously or intradermally.* In adults, the injection should be given in the deltoid region but it may be preferable to inject in the anterolateral thigh in neonates and infants, who have smaller deltoid muscles. Engerix-B should not be administered in the gluteal region; such injections may result in suboptimal response. The attending physician should determine final selection of the injection site and needle size, depending upon the patient's age and the size of the target muscle. A 1 inch 23 gauge needle is sufficient to penetrate the anterolateral thigh in infants younger than 12 months of age. A 5/8 inch 25 gauge needle may be used to administer the vaccine in the deltoid region of toddlers and children up to, and including, 10 years of age. The 1 inch 23 gauge needle is appropriate for use in older children and adults.[17]

Engerix-B may be administered subcutaneously to persons at risk of hemorrhage (*e.g.*, hemophiliacs). However, hepatitis B vaccines administered subcutaneously are known to result in lower GMTs. Additionally, when other aluminum-adsorbed vaccines have been administered subcutaneously, an increased incidence of local reactions including subcutaneous nodules has been observed. Therefore, subcutaneous administration should be used only in persons who are at risk of hemorrhage with intramuscular injections.

Dosing Schedules

The usual immunization regimen (see TABLE 1) consists of three doses of vaccine given according to the following schedule: *1st Dose:* At elected date; *2nd Dose:* 1 month later; *3rd Dose:* 6 months after first dose.

TABLE 1 *Recommended Dosage and Administration Schedule*

Group	Dose	Schedule
Infants born of:		
HBsAg-negative mothers	10 μg/0.5 ml	0, 1, 6 months
HBsAg-positive mothers	10 μg/0.5 ml	0, 1, 6 months
Children:		
Birth through 10 years of age	10 μg/0.5 ml	0, 1, 6 months
Adolescents:		
11 through 19 years of age	10 μg/0.5 ml	0, 1, 6 months
Adults (>19 years)	20 μg/1.0 ml	0, 1, 6 months
Adult hemodialysis	40 μg/2.0 ml*	0, 1, 2, 6 months

* 2 × 20 μg in 1 or 2 injections.

For hemodialysis patients, in whom vaccine-induced protection is less complete and may persist only as long as antibody levels remain above 10 mIU/ml, the need for booster doses should be assessed by annual antibody testing. 40 μg (2 × 20 μg) booster doses with Engerix-B should be given when antibody levels decline below 10 mIU/ml.[1] Data show individuals given a booster with Engerix-B achieve high antibody titers.

There are alternate dosing and administration schedules which may be used for specific populations (see TABLE 2 and accompanying explanations).

TABLE 2 *Alternate Dosage and Administration Schedules*

Group	Dose	Schedule
Infants born of:		
HBsAg-positive mothers	10 μg/0.5 ml	0, 1, 2, 12 months*
Children:		
Birth through 10 years of age	10 μg/0.5 ml	0, 1, 2, 12 months*
5 through 10 years of age	10 μg/0.5 ml	0, 12, 24 months†
Adolescents:		
11 through 16 years of age	10 μg/0.5 ml	0, 12, 24 months†
11 through 19 years of age	20 μg/1.0 ml	0, 1, 6 months
11 through 19 years of age	20 μg/1.0 ml	0, 1, 2, 12 months*
Adults (>19 years)	20 μg/1.0 ml	0, 1, 2, 12 months*

* This schedule is designed for certain populations (*e.g.*, neonates born of hepatitis B infected mothers, others who have or might have been recently exposed to the virus, certain travelers to high-risk areas. See INDICATIONS AND USAGE, Engerix-B.). On this alternate schedule, an additional dose at 12 months is recommended for prolonged maintenance of protective titers.
† For children and adolescents for whom an extended administration schedule is acceptable based on risk of exposure.

Booster Vaccinations

Whenever administration of a booster dose is appropriate, the dose of Engerix-B is 10 μg for children 10 years of age and under; 20 μg for adolescents 11-19 years of age and 20 μg for adults. Studies have demonstrated a substantial increase in antibody titers after Engerix-B booster vaccination following an initial course with both plasma- and yeast-derived vaccines. See previous section for discussion on booster vaccination for adult hemodialysis patients.

Known or Presumed Exposure to Hepatitis B Virus

Unprotected individuals with known or presumed exposure to the hepatitis B virus (*e.g.*, neonates born of infected mothers, others experiencing percutaneous or permucosal exposure) should be given hepatitis B immune globulin (HBIG) in addition to Engerix-B in accordance with ACIP recommendations[1] and with the package insert for HBIG. Engerix-B can be given on either dosing schedule (see above).

RECOMBIVAX HB

Do not inject intravenously or intradermally.

RECOMBIVAX HB DIALYSIS FORMULATION (40 μg/ml) IS INTENDED ONLY FOR ADULT PREDIALYSIS/DIALYSIS PATIENTS.

RECOMBIVAX HB PEDIATRIC/ADOLESCENT (WITH AND WITHOUT PRESERVATIVE) and ADULT FORMULATIONS ARE NOT INTENDED FOR USE IN PREDIALYSIS/DIALYSIS PATIENTS.

RECOMBIVAX HB PEDIATRIC/ADOLESCENT FORMULATION (WITHOUT PRESERVATIVE) IS AVAILABLE FOR USE IN INDIVIDUALS FOR WHOM A THIMEROSAL-FREE VACCINE IS ADVISABLE (*e.g.*, INFANTS 0-6 MONTHS OF AGE WHO MAY RECEIVE OTHER VACCINES CONTAINING THIMEROSAL).[50]

Three-Dose Regimen

The vaccination regimen for each population consists of 3 doses of vaccine given according to the following schedule:

First Dose: At elected date.

Second Dose: 1 month later.

Third Dose: 6 months after the first dose.

For infants born of mothers who are HBsAg positive or mothers of unknown HBsAg status, treatment recommendations are described in the subsection titled: Guidelines For Treatment of Infants Born of HBsAg Positive Mothers or Mothers of Unknown HBsAg Status.

Two-Dose Regimen — Adolescents (11-15 years of age)

An alternate two-dose regimen is available for routine vaccination of adolescents (11-15 years of age). The regimen consists of two doses of vaccine (10 µg) given according to the following schedule:

First Injection: At elected date.

Second Injection: 4-6 months later.

TABLE 3 summarizes the dose and formulation of Recombivax HB for specific populations, regardless of the risk of infection with hepatitis B virus.

TABLE 3

Group	Dose/Regimen*	Formulation	Color Code
Infants, children & adolescents 0-19 years of age	5 µg (0.5 ml) 3 × 5 µg	Pediatric/Adolescent	Yellow
Adolescents† 11-15 years of age	10 µg (1.0 ml) 2 × 10 µg	Adult	Green
Adults ≥20 years of age	10 µg (1.0 ml) 3 × 10 µg	Adult	Green
Predialysis & dialysis patients‡	40 µg (1.0 ml) 3 × 40 µg	Dialysis	Blue

* If the suggested formulation is not available, the appropriate dosage can be achieved from another formulation provided that the total volume of vaccine administered does not exceed 1 ml (see text above regarding use of the Pediatric/Adolescent Formulation Without Preservative). However, the Dialysis Formulation may be used only for adult predialysis/dialysis patients.

† Adolescents (11-15 years of age) may receive either regimen: the 3 × 5 µg (Pediatric/Adolescent Formulation) or the 2 × 10 µg (Adult Formulation).

‡ See also recommendations for revaccination of predialysis and dialysis patients in Revaccination.

Recombivax HB is for intramuscular injection. The *deltoid muscle* is the preferred site for intramuscular injection in adults. Data suggest that injections given in the buttocks frequently are given into fatty tissue instead of into muscle. Such injections have resulted in a lower seroconversion rate than was expected. The *anterolateral thigh* is the recommended site for intramuscular injection in infants and young children.

For persons at risk of hemorrhage following intramuscular injection, Recombivax HB may be administered subcutaneously. However, when other aluminum-adsorbed vaccines have been administered subcutaneously, an increased incidence of local reactions including subcutaneous nodules has been observed. Therefore, subcutaneous administration should be used only in persons (*e.g.,* hemophiliacs) who are at risk of hemorrhage following intramuscular injections.

The vaccine should be used as supplied; no dilution or reconstitution is necessary. The full recommended dose of the vaccine should be used.

For the Pediatric/Adolescent Formulation (without preservative): Once the single-dose vial has been penetrated, the withdrawn vaccine should be used promptly, and the vial must be discarded.

For Vial and Pre-Filled Single Dose Syringe: Shake well before use. Thorough agitation at the time of administration is necessary to maintain suspension of the vaccine.

Parenteral drug products should be inspected visually for particulate matter and discoloration prior to administration. After thorough agitation, the vaccine is a slightly opaque, white suspension.

For Vial: Withdraw the recommended dose from the vial using a sterile needle and syringe free of preservatives, antiseptics, and detergents.

It is important to use a separate sterile syringe and needle for each individual patient to prevent transmission of hepatitis and other infectious agents from one person to another. Needles should be disposed of properly and should not be recapped.

Injection must be accomplished with a needle long enough to ensure intramuscular deposition of the vaccine.

Guidelines For Treatment of Infants Born of HBsAg Positive Mothers or Mothers of Unknown HBsAg Status

Each infant should receive three 5 µg doses of Recombivax HB irrespective of the mother's HBsAg status (see TABLE 3). The ACIP recommends that if the mother is determined to be HBsAg positive within 7 days of delivery, the infant also should be given a dose of HBIG (0.5 ml) immediately. The first dose of Recombivax HB may be given at the same time as HBIG, but it should be administered in the opposite anterolateral thigh.[26]

Revaccination

The duration of the protective effect of Recombivax HB in healthy vaccinees is unknown at present and the need for booster doses is not yet defined.

A booster dose or revaccination with Recombivax HB Dialysis Formulation (blue color code) may be considered in predialysis/dialysis patients if the anti-HBs level is less than 10 mIU/ml 1-2 months after the third dose.[42] The ACIP recommends that the need for booster doses of vaccine should be assessed by annual antibody testing and a booster dose given when antibody levels decline to <10 mIU/ml.[49]

Known or Presumed Exposure to HBsAg

There are no prospective studies directly testing the efficacy of a combination of HBIG and Recombivax HB in preventing clinical hepatitis B following percutaneous, ocular or mucous membrane exposure to hepatitis B virus. However, since most persons with such exposures (*e.g.,* health-care workers) are candidates for Recombivax HB and since combined HBIG plus vaccine is more efficacious than HBIG alone in perinatal exposures, the following guidelines are recommended for persons who have been exposed to hepatitis B virus such as through (1) percutaneous (needlestick), ocular, mucous membrane exposure to blood known or presumed to contain HBsAg, (2) human bites by known or presumed HBsAg carriers, that penetrate the skin, or (3) following intimate sexual contact with known or presumed HBsAg.

HBIG (0.06 ml/kg) should be given intramuscularly as soon as possible after exposure and within 24 hours if possible. Recombivax HB (see dosage recommendation) should be given intramuscularly at a separate site within 7 days of exposure and second and third doses given 1 and 6 months, respectively, after the first dose.

PRODUCT LISTING - EQUIVALENTS NOT AVAILABLE

Solution - Intramuscular - 10 mcg/ml

0.50 ml	$27.70	RECOMBIVAX HB, Merck & Company Inc	00006-4769-00
0.50 ml	$30.48	RECOMBIVAX HB, Merck & Company Inc	00006-4980-00
0.50 ml x 5	$138.60	RECOMBIVAX HB, Merck & Company Inc	00006-4969-00
0.50 ml x 5	$145.60	RECOMBIVAX HB, Merck & Company Inc	00006-4849-00
0.50 ml x 10	$284.71	RECOMBIVAX HB, Merck & Company Inc	00006-4876-00
0.50 ml x 10	$290.10	RECOMBIVAX HB, Merck & Company Inc	00006-4981-00
1 ml	$70.29	RECOMBIVAX HB, Physicians Total Care	54868-2219-01
1 ml	$74.44	RECOMBIVAX HB, Merck & Company Inc	00006-4995-00
1 ml	$74.63	RECOMBIVAX HB, Merck & Company Inc	00006-4775-00
1 ml x 5	$373.20	RECOMBIVAX HB, Merck & Company Inc	00006-4848-00
1 ml x 10	$736.80	RECOMBIVAX HB, Merck & Company Inc	00006-4995-41
1 ml x 10	$738.70	RECOMBIVAX HB, Merck & Company Inc	00006-4872-00
3 ml	$209.46	RECOMBIVAX HB, Physicians Total Care	54868-2219-00
3 ml	$223.69	RECOMBIVAX HB, Merck & Company Inc	00006-4773-00
3 ml x 10	$2216.70	RECOMBIVAX HB, Merck & Company Inc	00006-4873-00

Solution - Intramuscular - 20 mcg/ml

0.50 ml	$26.52	ENGERIX-B, Glaxosmithkline	58160-0856-01
0.50 ml	$27.55	ENGERIX-B PEDIATRIC, Compumed Pharmaceuticals	00403-4195-18
0.50 ml	$27.84	ENGERIX-B PEDIATRIC, Physicians Total Care	54868-3236-00
0.50 ml x 5	$121.00	ENGERIX-B PEDIATRIC, Glaxosmithkline	58160-0859-35
0.50 ml x 5	$121.00	ENGERIX-B PEDIATRIC, Glaxosmithkline	58160-0859-36
0.50 ml x 5	$132.60	ENGERIX-B PEDIATRIC, Glaxosmithkline	58160-0856-46
0.50 ml x 5	$159.12	ENGERIX-B, Glaxosmithkline	58160-0856-35
0.50 ml x 10	$265.20	ENGERIX-B, Glaxosmithkline	58160-0856-11
0.50 ml x 25	$605.00	ENGERIX-B PEDIATRIC, Glaxosmithkline	58160-0859-26
0.50 ml x 25	$605.00	ENGERIX-B PEDIATRIC, Glaxosmithkline	58160-0859-27
0.50 ml x 25	$641.02	ENGERIX-B PEDIATRIC, Glaxosmithkline	58160-0856-57
0.50 ml x 25	$641.02	ENGERIX-B PEDIATRIC, Glaxosmithkline	58160-0856-58
0.50 ml x 25	$663.00	ENGERIX-B PEDIATRIC, Glaxosmithkline	58160-0856-50
0.50 ml x 25	$663.25	ENGERIX-B PEDIATRIC, Glaxosmithkline	58160-0856-56
0.50 ml x 25	$1515.75	ENGERIX-B, Glaxosmithkline	58160-0857-16
1 ml	$49.40	ENGERIX-B, Compumed Pharmaceuticals	00403-3839-18
1 ml	$55.10	ENGERIX-B, Glaxosmithkline	58160-0860-01
1 ml	$60.86	ENGERIX-B, Prescript Pharmaceuticals	00247-0290-01
1 ml	$62.20	ENGERIX-B, Glaxosmithkline	58160-0857-01
1 ml x 5	$246.50	ENGERIX-B, Compumed Pharmaceuticals	00403-4923-18
1 ml x 5	$275.55	ENGERIX-B, Allscripts Pharmaceutical Company	54569-4729-00
1 ml x 5	$275.55	ENGERIX-B, Glaxosmithkline	58160-0861-35
1 ml x 5	$304.75	ENGERIX-B, Glaxosmithkline	58160-0857-46
1 ml x 25	$1523.75	ENGERIX-B, Glaxosmithkline	58160-0857-50
2.50 ml x 5	$121.00	ENGERIX-B PEDIATRIC, Allscripts Pharmaceutical Company	54569-4213-00

Solution - Intramuscular - 40 mcg/ml

1 ml	$207.36	RECOMBIVAX HB, Merck & Company Inc	00006-4992-00
1 ml	$207.55	RECOMBIVAX HB, Merck & Company Inc	00006-4776-00

Hydralazine Hydrochloride *(001450)*

Categories: Hypertension, essential; Pregnancy Category C; FDA Approved 1952 Aug; WHO Formulary
Drug Classes: Vasodilators
Brand Names: **Apresoline**; Apresrex; Dralzine; Hyperex; Ipolina; Naselin; Nepresol; Solezorin; Sulesorin; Supres; Zinepress
Foreign Brand Availability: Alphapress (Australia; Israel); Apdormin (Japan); Apresolin (Denmark; Norway; Sweden; Turkey); Apresolina (Ecuador; Mexico; Portugal); Aprezin (Taiwan); Deselazin (Japan); Hydrapres (Spain); Hypatol (Japan); Hyperphen (South-Africa); Nonpolin (Japan); Novo-Hylazin (Canada); Resporidin (Japan); Slow-Apresoline (Bahamas; Bahrain; Barbados; Belize; Benin; Bermuda; Burkina-Faso; Curacao; Cyprus; Egypt; Ethiopia; Gambia; Ghana; Guinea; Guyana; Iran; Iraq; Ivory-Coast; Jamaica; Jordan; Kenya; Kuwait; Lebanon; Liberia; Libya; Malawi; Mali; Mauritania; Mauritius; Morocco; Netherland-Antilles; Niger; Nigeria; Oman; Qatar; Republic-of-Yemen; Saudi-Arabia; Senegal; Seychelles; Sierra-Leone; Sudan; Surinam; Syria; Tanzania; Trinidad; Tunia; Uganda; United-Arab-Emirates; Zambia; Zimbabwe); Solesorin (Japan); Tetrasoline (Japan); Travinon (Japan)
Cost of Therapy: $3.16 (Hypertension; Generic Tablets; 10 mg; 4 tablets/day; 30 day supply)
HCFA JCODE(S): J0360 up to 20 mg IV, IM

DESCRIPTION

Hydralazine HCl is an antihypertensive. Its chemical name is 1-hydrazinophthalazine monohydrochloride.

Hydralazine HCl is a white to off-white, odorless crystalline powder. It is soluble in water, slightly soluble in alcohol, and very slightly soluble in ether. It melts at about 275°C, with decomposition, and has a molecular weight of 196.64. The molecular formula is $C_8H_8N_4 \cdot HCl$.

TABLETS

Hydralazine HCl is available as 10, 25, 50 and 100 mg tablets for oral administration.

Inactive Ingredients: Acacia, D&C yellow no. 10 (10 mg tablets), FD&C blue no. 1 (25 and 50 mg tablets), FD&C yellow no. 5 and FD&C yellow no. 6 (100 mg tablets), lactose, magnesium stearate, mannitol, polyethylene glycol, sodium starch glycolate, starch, and stearic acid.

Storage: Store at controlled room temperature 15-30°C (59-86°F). Dispense in tight, light-resistant container.

INJECTION

Hydralazine HCl is available in 1 ml ampuls for intravenous and intramuscular administration. Each milliliter of the sterile, colorless solution contains hydralazine HCl, 20 mg; methylparaben, 0.65 mg; propylparaben, 0.35 mg; propene glycol, 103.6 mg. The pH of the solution is 3.4-4.0.

Storage: Store between 15-30°C (59-86°F).

CLINICAL PHARMACOLOGY

Although the precise mechanism of action of hydralazine is not fully understood, the major effects are on the cardiovascular system. Hydralazine apparently lowers blood pressure by exerting a peripheral vasodilating effect through a direct relaxation of vascular smooth muscle. Hydralazine, by altering cellular calcium metabolism, interferes with calcium movements within the vascular smooth muscle that are responsible for initiating or maintaining the contractile state.

The peripheral vasodilating effect of hydralazine results in decreased arterial blood pressure (diastolic more than systolic); decreased peripheral vascular resistance; and an increased heart rate, stroke volume, and cardiac output. The preferential dilatation of arterioles, as compared to veins, minimizes postural hypotension and promotes the increase in cardiac output. Hydralazine usually increases renin activity in plasma, presumably as a result of increased secretion of renin by the renal juxtaglomerular cells in response to reflex sympathetic discharge. This increase in renin activity leads to the production of angiotensin II, which then causes stimulation of aldosterone and consequent sodium reabsorption. Hydralazine also maintains or increases renal and cerebral blood flow.

ADDITIONAL INFORMATION FOR TABLETS

Hydralazine is rapidly absorbed after oral administration, and peak plasma levels are reached at 1-2 hours. Plasma levels of apparent hydralazine decline with a half-life of 3-7 hours. Binding to human plasma protein is 87%. Plasma levels of hydralazine vary widely among individuals. Hydralazine is subject to polymorphic acetylation; slow acetylators generally have higher plasma levels of hydralazine and require lower doses to maintain control of blood pressure. Hydralazine undergoes extensive hepatic metabolism; it is excreted mainly in the form of metabolites in the urine.

ADDITIONAL INFORMATION FOR INJECTION

The average maximal decrease in blood pressure usually occurs 10-80 minutes after administration of parenteral hydralazine HCl. No other pharmacokinetic data on parenteral hydralazine HCl are available.

INDICATIONS AND USAGE

Essential hypertension, alone or as an adjunct.

NON-FDA APPROVED INDICATIONS

While it is not approved for the treatment of congestive heart failure (CHF), hydralazine is commonly used to increase cardiac output in patients with CHF due to some causes, including severe aortic valvular insufficiency.

CONTRAINDICATIONS

Hypersensitivity to hydralazine; coronary artery disease; mitral valvular rheumatic heart disease.

WARNINGS

In a few patients hydralazine may produce a clinical picture simulating systemic lupus erythematosus including glomerulonephritis. In such patients hydralazine should be discontinued unless the benefit-to-risk determination requires continued antihypertensive therapy with this drug. Symptoms and signs usually regress when the drug is discontinued, but residua have been detected many years later. Long-term treatment with steroids may be necessary. (See PRECAUTIONS, Laboratory Tests.)

PRECAUTIONS

GENERAL

Myocardial stimulation produced by hydralazine HCl can cause anginal attacks and ECG changes of myocardial ischemia. The drug has been implicated in the production of myocardial infarction. It must, therefore, be used with caution in patients with suspected coronary artery disease.

The "hyperdynamic" circulation caused by hydralazine HCl may accentuate specific cardiovascular inadequacies. For example, hydralazine HCl may increase pulmonary artery pressure in patients with mitral valvular disease. The drug may reduce the pressor responses to epinephrine. Postural hypotension may result from hydralazine HCl but is less common than with ganglionic blocking agents. It should be used with caution in patients with cerebral vascular accidents.

In hypertensive patients with normal kidneys who are treated with hydralazine HCl, there is evidence of increased renal blood flow and a maintenance of glomerular filtration rate. In some instances where control values were below normal, improved renal function has been noted after administration of hydralazine HCl. However, as with any antihypertensive agent, hydralazine HCl should be used with caution in patients with advanced renal damage.

Peripheral neuritis, evidenced by paresthesia, numbness, and tingling, has been observed. Published evidence suggests an antipyridoxine effect, and that pyridoxine should be added to the regimen if symptoms develop.

INFORMATION FOR THE PATIENT

Patients should be informed of possible side effects and advised to take the medication regularly and continuously as directed.

LABORATORY TESTS

Complete blood counts and antinuclear antibody titer determinations are indicated before and periodically during prolonged therapy with hydralazine even though the patient is asymptomatic. These studies are also indicated if the patient develops arthralgia, fever, chest pain, continued malaise, or other unexplained signs or symptoms.

A positive antinuclear antibody titer requires that the physician carefully weigh the implications of the test results against the benefits to be derived from antihypertensive therapy with hydralazine.

Blood dyscrasias, consisting of reduction in hemoglobin and red cell count, leukopenia, agranulocytosis, and purpura, have been reported. If such abnormalities develop, therapy should be discontinued.

CARCINOGENESIS, MUTAGENESIS, AND IMPAIRMENT OF FERTILITY

In a lifetime study in Swiss albino mice, there was a statistically significant increase in the incidence of lung tumors (adenomas and adenocarcinomas) of both male and female mice given hydralazine continuously in their drinking water at a dosage of about 250 mg/kg/day (about 80 times the maximum recommended human dose). In a 2 year carcinogenicity study of rats given hydralazine by gavage at dose levels of 15, 30, and 60 mg/kg/day (approximately 5-20 times the recommended human daily dosage), microscopic examination of the liver revealed a small, but statistically significant, increase in benign neoplastic nodules in male and female rats from the high-dose group and in female rats from the intermediate-dose group. Benign interstitial cell tumors of the testes were also significantly increased in male rats from the high-dose group. The tumors observed are common in aged rats and a significantly increased incidence was not observed until 18 months of treatment. Hydralazine was shown to be mutagenic in bacterial systems (Gene Mutation and DNA Repair) and in 1 of 2 rat and 1 rabbit hepatocyte *in vitro* DNA repair studies. Additional *in vivo* and *in vitro* studies using lymphoma cells, germinal cells, and fibroblasts from mice, bone marrow cells from Chinese hamsters, and fibroblasts from human cell lines did not demonstrate any mutagenic potential for hydralazine.

The extent to which these findings indicate a risk to man is uncertain. While long-term clinical observation has not suggested that human cancer is associated with hydralazine use, epidemiologic studies have so far been insufficient to arrive at any conclusions.

PREGNANCY CATEGORY C

Animal studies indicate that hydralazine is teratogenic in mice at 20-30 times the maximum daily human dose of 200-300 mg and possibly in rabbits at 10-15 times the maximum daily human dose, but that it is nonteratogenic in rats. Teratogenic effects observed were cleft palate and malformations of facial and cranial bones.

There are no adequate and well-controlled studies in pregnant women. Although clinical experience does not include any positive evidence of adverse effects on the human fetus, hydralazine should be used during pregnancy only if the expected benefit justifies the potential risk to the fetus.

NURSING MOTHERS

Hydralazine has been shown to be excreted in breast milk.

PEDIATRIC USE

Safety and effectiveness in pediatric patients have not been established in controlled clinical trails, although there is experience with the use of hydralazine HCl in these patients. The usual recommended oral starting dosage is 0.75 mg/kg of body weight daily in 4 divided doses. Dosage may be increased gradually over the next 3-4 weeks to a maximum of 7.5 mg/kg or 200 mg daily.

Tablets

The usual recommended oral starting dosage is 0.75 mg/kg of body weight daily in 4 divided doses. Dosage may be increased gradually over the next 3-4 weeks to a maximum of 7.5 mg/kg or 200 mg daily.

Injection

The usual recommended parenteral dosage, administered intramuscularly or intravenously, is 1.7-3.5 mg/kg of body weight daily, divided into 4-6 doses.

DRUG INTERACTIONS

MAO inhibitors should be used with caution in patients receiving hydralazine.

When other potent parenteral antihypertensive drugs, such as diazoxide, are used in combination with hydralazine, patients should be continuously observed for several hours for any excessive fall in blood pressure. Profound hypotensive episodes may occur when diazoxide injection and hydralazine HCl are used concomitantly.

DRUG/FOOD INTERACTIONS WITH TABLETS

Administration of hydralazine with food results in higher plasma levels.

ADVERSE REACTIONS

Adverse reactions with hydralazine HCl are usually reversible when dosage is reduced. However, in some cases it may be necessary to discontinue the drug.

The following adverse reactions have been observed, but there has not been enough systematic collection of data to support an estimate of their frequency.

Common: Headache, anorexia, vomiting, diarrhea, palpitations, tachycardia, angina pectoris.

Less Frequent:

Digestive: Constipation, paralytic ileus.

Cardiovascular: Hypotension, paradoxical pressor response, edema.

Respiratory: Dyspnea.

Neurologic: Peripheral neuritis, evidenced by paresthesia, numbness, and tingling; dizziness; tremors; muscle cramps; psychotic reactions characterized by depression, disorientation, or anxiety.

Genitourinary: Difficulty in urination.

Hematologic: Blood dyscrasias, consisting of reduction in hemoglobin and red cell count, leukopenia, agranulocytosis, purpura; lymphadenopathy; splenomegaly.

Hypersensitive Reactions: Rash, urticaria, pruritus, fever, chills, arthralgia, eosinophilia, and rarely, hepatitis.

Other: Nasal congestion, flushing, lacrimation, conjunctivitis.

DOSAGE AND ADMINISTRATION

TABLETS

Initiate therapy in gradually increasing dosages; adjust according to individual response. Start with 10 mg four times daily for the first 2-4 days, increase to 25 mg four times daily for the balance of the first week. For the second and subsequent weeks, increase dosage to 50 mg four times daily. For maintenance, adjust dosage to the lowest effective levels.

The incidence of toxic reactions, particularly the L.E. cell syndrome, is high in the group of patients receiving large doses of hydralazine HCl.

In a few resistant patients, up to 300 mg of hydralazine HCl daily may be required for a significant antihypertensive effect. In such cases, a lower dosage of hydralazine HCl combined with a thiazide and/or reserpine or a beta blocker may be considered. However, when combining therapy, individual titration is essential to ensure the lowest possible therapeutic dose of each drug.

INJECTION

When there is urgent need, therapy in the hospitalized patient may be initiated intramuscularly or as a rapid intravenous bolus injection directly into the vein. Parenteral hydralazine HCl should be used only when the drug cannot be given orally. The usual dose is 20-40 mg, repeated as necessary. Certain patients (especially those with marked renal damage) may require a lower dose. Blood pressure should be checked frequently. It may begin to fall within a few minutes after injection, with the average maximal decrease occurring in 10-80 minutes. In cases where there has been increased intracranial pressure, lowering the blood pressure may increase cerebral ischemia. Most patients can be transferred to oral hydralazine HCl within 24-48 hours.

The product should be used immediately after the ampul is opened. It should not be added to infusion solutions. Apresoline hydrochloride parenteral may discolor upon contact with metal; discolored solutions should be discarded.

Parenteral drug products should be inspected visually for particulate matter and discoloration prior to administration, whenever solution and container permit.

PRODUCT LISTING - RATED THERAPEUTICALLY EQUIVALENT

Solution - Injectable - 20 mg/ml

1 ml x 25	$243.75	GENERIC, Solo Pak Medical Products Inc	39769-0021-01
1 ml x 25	$375.00	GENERIC, American Pharmaceutical Partners	63323-0614-01
1 ml x 25	$468.75	GENERIC, American Regent Laboratories Inc	00517-0901-25
1 ml x 25	$468.75	GENERIC, Gensia Sicor Pharmaceuticals Inc	00703-8201-04

Tablet - Oral - 10 mg

100's	$2.63	GENERIC, Moore, H.L. Drug Exchange Inc	00839-6114-06
100's	$2.75	GENERIC, Cmc-Consolidated Midland Corporation	00223-1060-01
100's	$3.00	GENERIC, Major Pharmaceuticals Inc	00904-2338-60
100's	$3.50	GENERIC, Aligen Independent Laboratories Inc	00405-4469-01
100's	$3.54	FEDERAL UPPER LIMIT, H.C.F.A. F F P	99999-1450-01
100's	$4.00	GENERIC, Martec Pharmaceuticals Inc	52555-0029-01
100's	$4.14	GENERIC, Major Pharmaceuticals Inc	00904-5169-60
100's	$4.18	GENERIC, Qualitest Products Inc	00603-3830-21
100's	$4.20	GENERIC, Sidmak Laboratories Inc	50111-0398-01
100's	$4.41	GENERIC, Par Pharmaceutical Inc	49884-0029-01
100's	$4.58	GENERIC, Major Pharmaceuticals Inc	00904-2338-61
100's	$4.88	GENERIC, Pd-Rx Pharmaceuticals	55289-0326-01
100's	$4.95	GENERIC, Raway Pharmacal Inc	00686-0074-20
100's	$5.42	GENERIC, Camall Company	00147-0255-10
100's	$5.83	GENERIC, Ivax Corporation	00182-0905-89
100's	$7.31	GENERIC, Auro Pharmaceutical	55829-0300-10

Tablet - Oral - 25 mg

25's	$5.19	GENERIC, Pd-Rx Pharmaceuticals	55289-0133-97
30's	$4.58	GENERIC, Heartland Healthcare Services	61392-0043-30
30's	$4.58	GENERIC, Heartland Healthcare Services	61392-0043-39
31's	$4.73	GENERIC, Heartland Healthcare Services	61392-0043-31
32's	$4.89	GENERIC, Heartland Healthcare Services	61392-0043-32
60's	$9.16	GENERIC, Heartland Healthcare Services	61392-0043-60
90's	$5.33	GENERIC, Pd-Rx Pharmaceuticals	55289-0133-90
90's	$13.74	GENERIC, Heartland Healthcare Services	61392-0043-90
100's	$1.02	GENERIC, Global Pharmaceutical Corporation	00115-3660-01
100's	$3.25	GENERIC, Cmc-Consolidated Midland Corporation	00223-1061-01
100's	$3.38	GENERIC, Interstate Drug Exchange Inc	00814-3709-14
100's	$3.95	GENERIC, Major Pharmaceuticals Inc	00904-2339-60
100's	$4.26	GENERIC, Allscripts Pharmaceutical Company	54569-0515-00
100's	$4.32	GENERIC, Aligen Independent Laboratories Inc	00405-4470-01
100's	$4.50	FEDERAL UPPER LIMIT, H.C.F.A. F F P	99999-1450-03
100's	$4.94	GENERIC, Major Pharmaceuticals Inc	00904-5170-60
100's	$4.99	GENERIC, Martec Pharmaceuticals Inc	52555-0027-01
100's	$5.00	GENERIC, Raway Pharmacal Inc	00686-0075-20
100's	$5.19	GENERIC, Sidmak Laboratories Inc	50111-0327-01
100's	$5.97	GENERIC, Qualitest Products Inc	00603-3831-21
100's	$6.21	GENERIC, Major Pharmaceuticals Inc	00904-2339-61
100's	$6.79	GENERIC, Camall Company	00147-0256-10
100's	$6.87	GENERIC, Pd-Rx Pharmaceuticals	55289-0133-01
100's	$7.27	GENERIC, Par Pharmaceutical Inc	49884-0027-01
100's	$8.75	GENERIC, Auro Pharmaceutical	55829-0301-10
100's	$17.07	GENERIC, Ivax Corporation	00182-0554-89

Tablet - Oral - 50 mg

90's	$4.64	GENERIC, Pd-Rx Pharmaceuticals	55289-0134-90
100's	$1.48	GENERIC, Global Pharmaceutical Corporation	00115-3662-01
100's	$3.50	GENERIC, Cmc-Consolidated Midland Corporation	00223-1062-01
100's	$4.20	GENERIC, Interstate Drug Exchange Inc	00814-3710-14
100's	$4.66	GENERIC, Moore, H.L. Drug Exchange Inc	00839-1363-06
100's	$4.75	GENERIC, Aligen Independent Laboratories Inc	00405-4471-01
100's	$5.00	GENERIC, Major Pharmaceuticals Inc	00904-2340-60
100's	$5.29	GENERIC, Martec Pharmaceuticals Inc	52555-0028-01
100's	$5.75	GENERIC, Raway Pharmacal Inc	00686-0076-20
100's	$5.75	GENERIC, Sidmak Laboratories Inc	50111-0328-01
100's	$6.04	GENERIC, Par Pharmaceutical Inc	49884-0028-01
100's	$7.45	GENERIC, Major Pharmaceuticals Inc	00904-2340-61
100's	$7.75	GENERIC, Qualitest Products Inc	00603-3832-21
100's	$8.21	GENERIC, Camall Company	00147-0257-10
100's	$8.85	GENERIC, Major Pharmaceuticals Inc	00904-5171-60
100's	$9.73	GENERIC, Auro Pharmaceutical	55829-0302-10
100's	$18.42	GENERIC, Vangard Labs	00615-0532-13
100's	$21.31	GENERIC, Ivax Corporation	00182-0555-89
100's	$63.30	APRESOLINE, Physicians Total Care	54868-3369-00

Tablet - Oral - 100 mg

100's	$6.90	GENERIC, Major Pharmaceuticals Inc	00904-2341-60
100's	$7.20	GENERIC, Udl Laboratories Inc	51079-0183-40
100's	$8.11	GENERIC, Aligen Independent Laboratories Inc	00405-4472-01
100's	$8.29	GENERIC, Ivax Corporation	00182-1553-01
100's	$8.46	GENERIC, Martec Pharmaceuticals Inc	52555-0026-01
100's	$8.51	GENERIC, Moore, H.L. Drug Exchange Inc	00839-6761-06
100's	$8.75	GENERIC, Raway Pharmacal Inc	00686-0183-20
100's	$10.29	GENERIC, Camall Company	00147-0258-10
100's	$10.34	GENERIC, Qualitest Products Inc	00603-3833-21
100's	$10.34	GENERIC, Par Pharmaceutical Inc	49884-0121-01
100's	$10.34	GENERIC, Sidmak Laboratories Inc	50111-0397-01
100's	$11.97	GENERIC, Major Pharmaceuticals Inc	00904-5172-60
100's	$19.12	GENERIC, Auro Pharmaceutical	55829-0303-10

PRODUCT LISTING - EQUIVALENTS NOT AVAILABLE

Tablet - Oral - 10 mg

12's	$2.47	GENERIC, Southwood Pharmaceuticals Inc	58016-0505-12
15's	$3.09	GENERIC, Southwood Pharmaceuticals Inc	58016-0505-15
20's	$4.12	GENERIC, Southwood Pharmaceuticals Inc	58016-0505-20
30's	$6.18	GENERIC, Southwood Pharmaceuticals Inc	58016-0505-30
100's	$20.60	GENERIC, Southwood Pharmaceuticals Inc	58016-0505-00

Tablet - Oral - 25 mg

12's	$3.53	GENERIC, Southwood Pharmaceuticals Inc	58016-0506-12
15's	$4.42	GENERIC, Southwood Pharmaceuticals Inc	58016-0506-15
20's	$5.89	GENERIC, Southwood Pharmaceuticals Inc	58016-0506-20
30's	$1.58	GENERIC, Allscripts Pharmaceutical Company	54569-0515-01
30's	$8.83	GENERIC, Southwood Pharmaceuticals Inc	58016-0506-30
45's	$6.87	GENERIC, Heartland Healthcare Services	61392-0043-45
100's	$29.44	GENERIC, Southwood Pharmaceuticals Inc	58016-0506-00
100's	$43.50	GENERIC, Southwood Pharmaceuticals Inc	58016-0507-00
120's	$18.32	GENERIC, Heartland Healthcare Services	61392-0043-34

Tablet - Oral - 50 mg

12's	$5.22	GENERIC, Southwood Pharmaceuticals Inc	58016-0507-12

15's	$6.53	GENERIC, Southwood Pharmaceuticals Inc	58016-0507-15
20's	$8.70	GENERIC, Southwood Pharmaceuticals Inc	58016-0507-20
30's	$13.05	GENERIC, Southwood Pharmaceuticals Inc	58016-0507-30
60's	$3.79	GENERIC, Allscripts Pharmaceutical Company	54569-0517-01

Hydrochlorothiazide *(001456)*

Categories: Edema; Hypertension, essential; Pregnancy Category B; WHO Formulary; FDA Approved 1963 Aug
Drug Classes: Diuretics, thiazide and derivatives
Brand Names: Aquazide H; Carozide; **Esidrix**; Hydro Par; Hydro-T; Hydrocot; Hydrodiuril; Microzide; Oretic; Zide
Foreign Brand Availability: Apo-Hydro (Canada; Malaysia); Clothia (Japan); Dichlothiazide (Russia); Dichlotride (Australia; Belgium; Denmark; Hong-Kong; Japan; Netherlands; New-Zealand; Norway; Philippines; Sweden; Taiwan; Thailand); Dichlozid (Korea); Didralin (Malaysia; Thailand); Di-Ertride (Singapore); Disothiazide (Israel); Diurace (Peru); Diuret-P (Thailand); Diurex (Argentina); Esidrex (Austria; Bahamas; Bahrain; Barbados; Belize; Benin; Bermuda; Burkina-Faso; Curacao; Cyprus; Egypt; Ethiopia; France; Gambia; Ghana; Guinea; Guyana; India; Iran; Iraq; Italy; Ivory-Coast; Jamaica; Japan; Jordan; Kenya; Kuwait; Lebanon; Liberia; Libya; Malawi; Mali; Mauritania; Mauritius; Morocco; Netherland-Antilles; Netherlands; Niger; Nigeria; Norway; Oman; Puerto-Rico; Qatar; Republic-of-Yemen; Saudi-Arabia; Senegal; Seychelles; Sierra-Leone; South-Africa; Spain; Sudan; Surinam; Sweden; Switzerland; Syria; Tanzania; Trinidad; Tunia; Uganda; United-Arab-Emirates; Zambia; Zimbabwe); H.C.T. (Indonesia); Hidrenox (Argentina); Hidrosaluretil (Spain); Hydrex (Finland); Hydrex-semi (Finland); Hydrochlorzide (Malaysia); Hydrosaluric (England); Hydrozide (Hong-Kong; Thailand); Maschitt (Japan); Newtolide (Japan); Pantemon (Japan); Ridaq (South-Africa); Tandiur (Argentina)
Cost of Therapy: $1.79 (Hypertension; Oretic; 25 mg; 1 tablet/day; 30 day supply)
$0.21 (Hypertension; Generic Tablets; 25 mg; 1 tablet/day; 30 day supply)

H

DESCRIPTION

Hydrochlorothiazide is a diuretic and antihypertensive. It is the 3,4-dihydro derivative of chlorothiazide. Its chemical name is 6-chloro-3,4-dihydro-2*H*-1,2,4-benzothiadiazine-7-sulfonamide 1,1-dioxide. Its molecular formula is $C_7H_8ClN_3O_4S_2$. Its molecular weight is 297.75.

It is a white, or practically white, crystalline powder, which is slightly soluble in water but freely soluble in sodium hydroxide solution.

Hydrochlorothiazide is supplied as 25 or 50 mg tablets for oral use. The inactive ingredients in hydrochlorothiazide 25 and 50 mg tablets are calcium phosphate, FD&C yellow no. 6, gelatin, lactose, magnesium stearate, starch, and talc.

Microzide is supplied as 12.5 mg capsules. Each capsule contains 12.5 mg hydrochlorothiazide. The inactive ingredients in microzide 12.5 mg capsules colloidal silicon dioxide, corn starch, D&C red no. 28, D&C yellow no. 10, FD&C blue no. 1, gelatin, lactose monohydrate, magnesium stearate, titanium dioxide, and other ingredients.

CLINICAL PHARMACOLOGY

MECHANISM OF ACTION

The mechanism of the antihypertensive effect of thiazides is unknown. Hydrochlorothiazide does not usually affect normal blood pressure.

Hydrochlorothiazide affects the distal renal tubular mechanism of electrolyte reabsorption. At maximal therapeutic dosage all thiazides are approximately equal in their diuretic efficacy.

Hydrochlorothiazide increases excretion of sodium and chloride in approximately equivalent amounts. Natriuresis may be accompanied by some loss of potassium and bicarbonate.

After oral use, diuresis begins within 2 hours, peaks in about 4 hours, and lasts about 6-12 hours.

Hydrochlorothiazide blocks the reabsorption of sodium and chloride ions, and it thereby increases the quantity of sodium traversing the distal tubule and the volume of water excreted. A portion of the additional sodium presented to the distal tubule is exchanged there for potassium and hydrogen ions. With continued use of hydrochlorothiazide and depletion of sodium, compensatory mechanisms tend to increase this exchange and may produce excessive loss of potassium, hydrogen, and chloride ions. Hydrochlorothiazide also *decreases* the excretion of calcium and uric acid, may *increase* the excretion of iodide, and may *reduce* glomerular filtration rate. Metabolic toxicities associated with excessive electrolyte changes caused by hydrochlorothiazide have been shown to be dose-related.

PHARMACOKINETICS AND METABOLISM

Tablets

Hydrochlorothiazide is not metabolized but is eliminated rapidly by the kidney. When plasma levels have been followed for at least 24 hours, the plasma half-life has been observed to vary between 5.6 and 14.8 hours. At least 61% of the oral dose is eliminated unchanged within 24 hours. Hydrochlorothiazide crosses the placental barrier (but not the blood-brain barrier) and is excreted in breast milk.

Capsules

Hydrochlorothiazide is well absorbed (65-75%) following oral administration. Absorption of hydrochlorothiazide is reduced in patients with congestive heart failure.

Peak plasma concentrations are observed within 1-5 hours of dosing and range from 70-490 ng/ml following oral doses of 12.5-100 mg. Plasma concentrations are linearly related to the administered dose. Concentrations of hydrochlorothiazide are 1.6-1.8 times higher in whole blood than in plasma. Binding to serum proteins has been reported to be approximately 40-68%. The plasma elimination half-life has been reported to be 6-15 hours. Hydrochlorothiazide is eliminated primarily by renal pathways. Following oral doses of 12.5-100 mg, 55-77% of the administered dose appears in urine and more than 95% of the absorbed dose is excreted in urine as unchanged drug. In patients with renal disease, plasma concentrations of hydrochlorothiazide are increased and the elimination half-life is prolonged.

When hydrochlorothiazide is administered with food, its bioavailability is reduced by 10%, the maximum plasma concentration is reduced by 20%, and the time to maximum concentration increases from 1.6-2.9 hours.

PHARMACODYNAMICS

Acute antihypertensive effects of thiazides are thought to result from a reduction in blood volume and cardiac output, secondary to a natriuretic effect, although a direct vasodilatory mechanism has also been proposed. With chronic administration, plasma volume returns toward normal, but peripheral vascular resistance is decreased. The exact mechanism of the antihypertensive effect of hydrochlorothiazide is not known.

Thiazides do not affect normal blood pressure. Onset of action occurs within 2 hours of dosing, peak effect is observed at about 4 hours, and activity persists for up to 24 hours.

INDICATIONS AND USAGE

TABLETS

Hydrochlorothiazide is indicated as adjunctive therapy in edema associated with congestive heart failure, hepatic cirrhosis, and corticosteroid and estrogen therapy.

Hydrochlorothiazide has also been found useful in edema due to various forms of renal dysfunction such as nephrotic syndrome, acute glomerulonephritis, and chronic renal failure.

CAPSULES

Hydrochlorothiazide is indicated in the management of hypertension, either as the sole therapeutic agent or to enhance the effectiveness of other antihypertensive drugs, in the more severe forms of hypertension.

Unlike potassium-sparing combination diuretic products, hydrochlorothiazide may be used in those patients in whom the development of hyperkalemia cannot be risked, including patients taking ACE inhibitors.

USE IN PREGNANCY

The routine use of diuretics in an otherwise healthy woman is inappropriate and exposes mother and fetus to unnecessary hazard. Diuretics do not prevent development of toxemia of pregnancy, and there is no satisfactory evidence that they are useful in the treatment of developed toxemia.

Edema during pregnancy may arise from pathological causes or from the physiologic and mechanical consequences of pregnancy. Diuretics are indicated in pregnancy when edema is due to pathology causes, just as they are in the absence of pregnancy (see PRECAUTIONS, Pregnancy, Teratogenic Effects, Pregnancy Category B). Dependent edema in pregnancy, resulting from restriction of venous return by the expanded uterus, is properly treated through elevation of the lower extremities and use of support hose. The use of diuretics to lower intravascular volume in this case is illogical and unnecessary. There is hypervolemia during normal pregnancy, which is harmful to neither the fetus nor the mother (in the absence of cardiovascular disease), but which is associated with edema, including generalized edema in the majority of pregnant women. If this edema causes discomfort, increased recumbency will often provide relief. In rare instances, this edema may cause extreme discomfort, that is not relieved by rest. In these cases, a short course of diuretics may provide relief and be appropriate.

NON-FDA APPROVED INDICATIONS

Non FDA-approved uses of hydrochlorothiazide include treatment of hypercalciuric states, osteoporosis, and diabetes insipidus.

CONTRAINDICATIONS

Hydrochlorothiazide is contraindicated in patients with anuria. Hypersensitivity to this product or other sulfonamide-derived drugs is also contraindicated.

WARNINGS

Diabetes and Hyperglycemia: Latent diabetes mellitus may become manifest, and diabetic patients given thiazides may require adjustment of their insulin dose.

Renal Disease: Cumulative effects of the thiazides may develop in patients with impaired renal function. In such patients, thiazides may precipitate azotemia.

Hepatic Function: Use with caution in patients with impaired hepatic function or progressive liver disease, since minor alterations of fluid and electrolyte balance may precipitate hepatic coma (see PRECAUTIONS, Impaired Hepatic Function).

Antihypertensive Drugs: Thiazides may add to or potentiate the action of other antihypertensive drugs.

Allergy/Asthma: Sensitivity reactions may occur in patients with or without a history of allergy or bronchial asthma.

Lupus: The possibility of exacerbation or activation of systemic lupus erythematosus has been reported.

Lithium: Generally, lithium should not be given with diuretics (see DRUG INTERACTIONS).

PRECAUTIONS

ELECTROLYTE AND HYPOKALEMIA

All patients receiving diuretic therapy should be observed for evidence of fluid or electrolyte imbalance: namely, hyponatremia, hypochloremic alkalosis, and hypokalemia. Serum and urine electrolyte determinations are particularly important when the patient is vomiting excessively or receiving parenteral fluids.

Warning signs or symptoms of fluid and electrolyte imbalance include dryness of mouth, thirst, weakness, lethargy, drowsiness, restlessness, confusion, seizures, muscle pains or cramps, muscular fatigue, hypotension, oliguria, tachycardia, and gastrointestinal disturbances such as nausea and vomiting.

Hypokalemia may develop, especially with brisk diuresis, when severe cirrhosis is present during concomitant use of corticosteroid or adrenocorticotropic hormone (ACTH), or after prolonged therapy.

Interference with adequate oral electrolyte intake will also contribute to hypokalemia. Hypokalemia and hypomagnesemia can provoke ventricular arrhythmias or sensitize or exaggerate the response of the heart to the toxic effects of digitalis (*e.g.*, increased ventricular irritability). Hypokalemia may be avoided or treated by potassium supplementation or increased intake of potassium-rich foods.

Although any chloride deficit is generally mild and usually does not require specific treatment, except under extraordinary circumstances (as in liver disease or renal disease), chloride replacement may be required in the treatment of metabolic alkalosis.

Dilutional hyponatremia is life-threatening and may occur in edematous patients in hot weather; appropriate therapy is water restriction rather than salt administration, except in rare instances when the hyponatremia is life-threatening. In actual salt depletion, appropriate replacement is the therapy of choice.

LABORATORY TESTS

Periodic determination of serum electrolytes to detect possible electrolyte imbalance should be done at appropriate intervals.

Capsules (12.5 mg)

In published studies, clinically significant hypokalemia has been consistently less common in patients who received 12.5 mg of hydrochlorothiazide than in patients who received higher doses. Nevertheless, periodic determination of serum electrolytes should be performed in patients who may be at risk for the development of hypokalemia. Patients should be observed for signs of fluid or electrolyte disturbances, (*i.e.,* hyponatremia, hypochloremic alkalosis, hypokalemia, and hypomagnesemia).

HYPERURICEMIA

Hyperuricemia or acute gout may be precipitated in certain patients receiving thiazides diuretics.

HEPATIC EFFECTS

Thiazides should be used with caution in patients with impaired hepatic function. They can precipitate hepatic coma in patients with severe liver disease.

PARATHYROID DISEASE

Calcium excretion is decreased by thiazides, and pathological changes in parathyroid glands, with hypercalcemia and hypophosphatemia, have been observed in a few patients on prolonged thiazide therapy.

Thiazides may cause intermittent and slight elevation of serum calcium in the absence of known disorders of calcium metabolism. Marked hypercalcemia may be evidence of hidden hyperparathyroidism. Thiazides should be discontinued before carrying out tests for parathyroid function (see Drug/Laboratory Test Interactions).

DIABETES

In diabetic patients, dosage adjustments of insulin or oral hypoglycemic agents may be required. Hyperglycemia may occur with thiazide diuretics. Thus latent diabetes mellitus may become manifest during thiazide therapy.

ANTIHYPERTENSIVE DRUGS

The antihypertensive effects of the drug may be enhanced in the postsympathectomy patient.

RENAL EFFECTS

If progressive renal impairment becomes evident, consider withholding or discontinuing diuretic therapy.

HYPOMAGNESEMIA

Thiazides have been shown to increase the urinary excretion of magnesium; this may result in hypomagnesemia.

CHOLESTEROL/TRIGLYCERIDE LEVELS

Increases in cholesterol and triglyceride levels may be associated with thiazide diuretic therapy.

DRUG/LABORATORY TEST INTERACTIONS

Thiazides should be discontinued before carrying out tests for parathyroid function (see Parathyroid Disease).

CARCINOGENESIS, MUTAGENESIS, AND IMPAIRMENT OF FERTILITY

Two year feeding studies in mice and rats conducted under the auspices of the National Toxicology Program (NTP) uncovered no evidence of a carcinogenic potential of hydrochlorothiazide in female mice (at doses of up to approximately 600 mg/kg/day) or in male and female rats (at doses of up to approximately 100 mg/kg/day). The NTP, however, found equivocal evidence for hepatocarcinogenicity in male mice.

Hydrochlorothiazide was not genotoxic *in vitro* in the Ames mutagenicity assay of *Salmonella typhimurium* strains TA 98, TA 100, TA 1535, TA 1537, and TA 1538 and in the Chinese Hamster Ovary (CHO) test for chromosomal aberrations, or *in vivo* in assays using mouse germinal cell chromosomes, Chinese hamster bone marrow chromosomes, and the *Drosophila* sex-linked recessive lethal trait gene. Positive test results were obtained only in the *in vitro* CHO Sister Chromatid Exchange (clastogenicity) and in the Mouse Lymphoma Cell (mutagenicity) assays, using concentrations of hydrochlorothiazide from 43-1300 µg/ml, and in the *Aspergillus nidulans* nondisjunction assay at an unspecified concentration.

Hydrochlorothiazide had no adverse effects on the fertility of mice and rats of either sex in studies wherein these species were exposed, via their diet, to doses of up to 100 and 4 mg/kg, respectively, prior to conception and throughout gestation.

PREGNANCY, TERATOGENIC EFFECTS, PREGNANCY CATEGORY B

Studies in which hydrochlorothiazide was orally administered to pregnant mice and rats during their respective periods of major organogenesis at doses of up to 3000 and 1000 mg hydrochlorothiazide/kg, respectively, provided no evidence of harm to the fetus.

There are, however, no adequate and well-controlled studies in pregnant women. Because animal reproduction studies are not always predictive of human response, this drug should be used during pregnancy only if clearly needed.

Nonteratogenic Effects: Thiazides cross the placental barrier and appear in cord blood. There is a risk of fetal or neonatal jaundice, thrombocytopenia, and possibly other adverse reactions that have occurred in adults.

NURSING MOTHERS

Thiazides are excreted in breast milk. Because of the potential for serious adverse reactions in nursing infants, a decision should be made whether to discontinue nursing or to discontinue hydrochlorothiazide, taking into account the importance of the drug to the mother.

PEDIATRIC USE

Safety and effectiveness in pediatric patients have not been established.

GERIATRIC USE

A greater blood pressure reduction and an increase in side effects may be observed in the elderly (>65 years) with hydrochlorothiazide. Starting treatment with the lowest available dose of hydrochlorothiazide (12.5 mg) is therefore recommended. If further titration is required, 12.5 mg increments should be utilized.

DRUG INTERACTIONS

When given concurrently, the following drugs may interact with thiazide diuretics:

Alcohol, Barbiturates, or Narcotics: Potentiation of orthostatic hypotension may occur.

Antidiabetic Drugs (oral agents and insulin): Dosage adjustment of the antidiabetic drug may be required.

Other Antihypertensive Drugs: Additive effect or potentiation.

Cholestyramine and Colestipol Resins: Cholestyramine and colestipol resins bind the hydrochlorothiazide and reduce its absorption from the gastrointestinal tract by up to 85 and 43%, respectively.

Corticosteroids, ACTH: Intensified electrolyte depletion, particularly hypokalemia.

Pressor Amines (e.g., norepinephrine): Possible decreased response to pressor amines but not sufficient to preclude their use.

Skeletal Muscle Relaxants, Nondepolarizing (e.g., tubocurarine): Possible increased responsiveness to the muscle relaxant.

Lithium: Generally should not be given with diuretics. Diuretic agents reduce the renal clearance of lithium and greatly increase the risk of lithium toxicity. Refer to the product information for lithium preparations before use of such preparations with hydrochlorothiazide.

Nonsteroidal Antiinflammatory Drugs: In some patients, the administration of a nonsteroidal antiinflammatory agent can reduce the diuretic, natriuretic, and antihypertensive effects of loop, potassium-sparing, and thiazide diuretics. When hydrochlorothiazide and nonsteroidal antiinflammatory agents are used concomitantly, the patients should be observed closely to determine if the desired effect of the diuretic is obtained.

ADVERSE REACTIONS

The adverse reactions associated with hydrochlorothiazide have been shown to be dose-related. In controlled clinical trials, the adverse events reported with doses of 12.5 mg hydrochlorothiazide once daily were comparable to placebo.

The following adverse reactions have been reported for doses of hydrochlorothiazide 25 mg and greater and, within each category, are listed in the order of decreasing severity:

Body as a Whole: Weakness.

Cardiovascular: Hypotension, including orthostatic hypotension (may be aggravated by alcohol, barbiturates, narcotics, or antihypertensive drugs).

Digestive: Pancreatitis, jaundice (intrahepatic cholestatic jaundice), diarrhea, vomiting, sialadenitis, cramping, constipation, gastric irritation, nausea, anorexia.

Hematologic: Aplastic anemia, agranulocytosis, leukopenia, hemolytic anemia, thrombocytopenia.

Hypersensitivity: Anaphylactic reactions, necrotizing angiitis (vasculitis and cutaneous vasculitis), respiratory distress including pneumonitis and pulmonary edema, photosensitivity, fever, urticaria, rash, purpura.

Metabolic: Electrolyte imbalance (see PRECAUTIONS), hyperglycemia, glycosuria, hyperuricemia.

Musculoskeletal: Muscle spasm.

Nervous System/Psychiatric: Vertigo, paresthesias, dizziness, headache, restlessness.

Renal: Renal failure, renal dysfunction, interstitial nephritis. (See WARNINGS.)

Skin: Erythema multiform (including Stevens-Johnson syndrome), exfoliative dermatitis (including toxic epidermal necrolysis), alopecia.

Special Senses: Transient blurred vision, xanthopsia.

Urogenital: Impotence.

Whenever adverse reactions are moderate or severe, thiazide dosage should be reduced or therapy withdrawn.

DOSAGE AND ADMINISTRATION

Therapy should be individualized according to patient response. Use the smallest dosage necessary to achieve the required response.

ADULTS

For Control of Hypertension

Capsules: The adult initial dose of hydrochlorothiazide is 1 capsule given once daily, whether given alone or in combination with other antihypertensives. Total daily doses greater than 50 mg are not recommended.

Tablets: The usual initial dose in adults is 25 mg daily given as a single dose. The dose may be increased to 50 mg daily, given as a single dose or 2 divided doses. Doses greater than 50 mg are often associated with marked reductions in serum potassium (see also PRECAUTIONS).

For Edema

The usual adult dosage is 25-100 mg daily as a single or divided dose. Many patients with edema respond to intermittent therapy, (*i.e.*, administration on alternate days or on 3-5 days each week). With an intermittent schedule, excessive response and the resulting undesirable electrolyte imbalance are less likely to occur.

Patients usually do not require doses in excess of 50 mg of hydrochlorothiazide daily when used concomitantly with other antihypertensive agents.

INFANTS AND CHILDREN

For Diuresis and for Control of Hypertension

The usual pediatric dosage is 0.5-1 mg/lb/day (1-2 mg/kg/day) in a single dose or 2 divided doses, not to exceed 37.5 mg/day in infants up to 2 years of age or 100 mg/day in children 2-12 years of age. In infants less than 6 months of age, doses of up to 1.5 mg/lb/day (3 mg/kg/day) in 2 divided doses may be required.

HOW SUPPLIED

MICROZIDE CAPSULES

Microzide, 12.5 mg: Microzide capsules are #4 teal, opaque/teal, 2-piece, hard gelatin capsules imprinted with "Microzide" and "12.5" mg in black ink.

Storage: Store at room temperature 15-30°C (59-86°F). Protect from light, moisture, and freezing. Dispense in a tight, light-resistant container, using a child-resistant closure.

PRODUCT LISTING - RATED THERAPEUTICALLY EQUIVALENT

Capsule - Oral - 12.5 mg

30's	$14.86	GENERIC, Allscripts Pharmaceutical Company	54569-4912-00
100's	$42.45	GENERIC, Caremark Inc	00339-5148-12
100's	$42.45	GENERIC, Mylan Pharmaceuticals Inc	00378-0810-01
100's	$42.45	GENERIC, Watson Laboratories Inc	00591-0347-01
100's	$42.45	GENERIC, Watson Laboratories Inc	52544-0347-01
100's	$59.99	GENERIC, Watson Laboratories Inc	52544-0622-01

Tablet - Oral - 25 mg

6's	$1.92	GENERIC, Pd-Rx Pharmaceuticals	55289-0136-06
12's	$1.12	GENERIC, Heartland Healthcare Services	61392-0011-12
15's	$1.40	GENERIC, Heartland Healthcare Services	61392-0011-15
16's	$2.84	GENERIC, Pd-Rx Pharmaceuticals	55289-0136-16
20's	$2.25	GENERIC, Pd-Rx Pharmaceuticals	55289-0136-20
25's	$2.65	GENERIC, Udl Laboratories Inc	51079-0049-19
30's	$1.32	GENERIC, Circle Pharmaceuticals Inc	00659-1302-30
30's	$2.00	GENERIC, Pharmaceutical Corporation Of America	51655-0126-24
30's	$2.25	GENERIC, Major Pharmaceuticals Inc	00904-2083-46
30's	$2.50	GENERIC, Pd-Rx Pharmaceuticals	58864-0250-30
30's	$2.81	GENERIC, Heartland Healthcare Services	61392-0011-30
30's	$2.81	GENERIC, Heartland Healthcare Services	61392-0011-39
30's	$3.53	GENERIC, Pd-Rx Pharmaceuticals	55289-0136-30
31 x 10	$33.57	GENERIC, Vangard Labs	00615-1561-53
31 x 10	$33.57	GENERIC, Vangard Labs	00615-1561-63
31's	$2.90	GENERIC, Heartland Healthcare Services	61392-0011-31
32's	$3.00	GENERIC, Heartland Healthcare Services	61392-0011-32
45's	$4.21	GENERIC, Heartland Healthcare Services	61392-0011-45
60's	$2.64	GENERIC, Pharmaceutical Corporation Of America	51655-0126-25
60's	$5.62	GENERIC, Heartland Healthcare Services	61392-0011-60
60's	$5.62	GENERIC, Heartland Healthcare Services	61392-0011-65
90's	$4.00	GENERIC, Pharmaceutical Corporation Of America	51655-0126-26
90's	$4.70	GENERIC, Pd-Rx Pharmaceuticals	58864-0250-90
90's	$5.40	GENERIC, Major Pharmaceuticals Inc	00904-2083-89
90's	$5.52	GENERIC, Pd-Rx Pharmaceuticals	55289-0136-90
90's	$8.42	GENERIC, Heartland Healthcare Services	61392-0011-90
100's	$0.69	GENERIC, Global Pharmaceutical Corporation	00115-3670-01
100's	$1.75	GENERIC, Cmc-Consolidated Midland Corporation	00223-1069-01
100's	$2.00	FEDERAL UPPER LIMIT, H.C.F.A. F F P	99999-1456-03
100's	$3.00	GENERIC, Interstate Drug Exchange Inc	00814-3720-14
100's	$3.11	GENERIC, Moore, H.L. Drug Exchange Inc	00839-5135-06
100's	$3.25	GENERIC, Camall Company	00147-0116-10
100's	$3.60	GENERIC, Allscripts Pharmaceutical Company	54569-0547-01
100's	$4.87	GENERIC, Auro Pharmaceutical	55829-0290-10
100's	$5.00	GENERIC, Raway Pharmacal Inc	00686-0049-20
100's	$5.11	GENERIC, Major Pharmaceuticals Inc	00904-2083-61
100's	$5.15	GENERIC, Pharmaceutical Corporation Of America	51655-0126-21
100's	$5.88	GENERIC, Abbott Pharmaceutical	00074-6978-05
100's	$5.95	GENERIC, Abbott Pharmaceutical	00074-6978-01
100's	$7.13	GENERIC, Ivax Corporation	00172-2083-60
100's	$8.48	GENERIC, Qualitest Products Inc	00603-3856-21
100's	$10.20	GENERIC, Udl Laboratories Inc	51079-0049-20
100's	$10.83	GENERIC, Vangard Labs	00615-1561-13
100's	$14.82	GENERIC, Ivax Corporation	00182-0556-89
100's	$15.12	GENERIC, Pd-Rx Pharmaceuticals	55289-0136-01
120's	$4.89	GENERIC, Pharmaceutical Corporation Of America	51655-0126-82

Tablet - Oral - 50 mg

25's	$5.22	GENERIC, Pd-Rx Pharmaceuticals	55289-0135-97
30's	$1.32	GENERIC, Circle Pharmaceuticals Inc	00659-1303-30
30's	$1.50	GENERIC, Golden State Medical	60429-0213-30
30's	$1.70	GENERIC, Major Pharmaceuticals Inc	00904-2089-46
30's	$2.25	GENERIC, Pharmaceutical Corporation Of America	51655-0077-24
30's	$3.99	GENERIC, Heartland Healthcare Services	61392-0799-30
30's	$3.99	GENERIC, Heartland Healthcare Services	61392-0799-39
30's	$4.65	GENERIC, Pd-Rx Pharmaceuticals	55289-0135-30
30's	$97.40	GENERIC, Medirex Inc	57480-0335-06
31's	$4.12	GENERIC, Heartland Healthcare Services	61392-0799-31
32's	$4.25	GENERIC, Heartland Healthcare Services	61392-0799-32
45's	$5.98	GENERIC, Heartland Healthcare Services	61392-0799-45
60's	$2.50	GENERIC, Pharmaceutical Corporation Of America	51655-0077-25
60's	$7.97	GENERIC, Heartland Healthcare Services	61392-0799-60
90's	$3.60	GENERIC, Pharmaceutical Corporation Of America	51655-0077-26
90's	$4.13	GENERIC, Golden State Medical	60429-0213-90
90's	$11.96	GENERIC, Heartland Healthcare Services	61392-0799-90
100's	$0.74	GENERIC, Global Pharmaceutical Corporation	00115-3675-01
100's	$2.54	FEDERAL UPPER LIMIT, H.C.F.A. F F P	99999-1456-07
100's	$2.60	GENERIC, Major Pharmaceuticals Inc	00904-2205-60
100's	$2.75	GENERIC, Cmc-Consolidated Midland Corporation	00223-1070-01
100's	$3.41	GENERIC, Camall Company	00147-0123-10
100's	$3.50	GENERIC, West Point Pharma	59591-0243-68
100's	$3.55	GENERIC, Roberts/Hauck Pharmaceutical Corporation	43797-0038-03
100's	$3.56	GENERIC, Camall Company	00147-0108-10
100's	$3.80	GENERIC, Columbia Drug Company	11735-0008-11
100's	$3.80	GENERIC, Pharmaceutical Corporation Of America	51655-0077-21
100's	$3.90	GENERIC, Moore, H.L. Drug Exchange Inc	00839-5136-06
100's	$3.94	GENERIC, Economed Pharmaceuticals Inc	38130-0020-01
100's	$4.13	GENERIC, Interstate Drug Exchange Inc	00814-3725-14
100's	$4.47	GENERIC, Allscripts Pharmaceutical Company	54569-0549-01
100's	$5.26	GENERIC, Major Pharmaceuticals Inc	00904-2089-61
100's	$5.50	GENERIC, Raway Pharmacal Inc	00686-0111-20
100's	$6.26	GENERIC, Pd-Rx Pharmaceuticals	55289-0135-01
100's	$6.31	GENERIC, Vangard Labs	00615-1562-13
100's	$8.38	GENERIC, Auro Pharmaceutical	55829-0291-10
100's	$9.80	GENERIC, Seneca Pharmaceuticals	47028-0003-01
100's	$12.33	GENERIC, Udl Laboratories Inc	51079-0111-20
100's	$16.45	GENERIC, Ivax Corporation	00172-2089-60
100's	$16.45	GENERIC, Qualitest Products Inc	00603-3857-21
100's	$17.54	GENERIC, Ivax Corporation	00182-0557-89
100's	$25.45	HYDRODIURIL, Merck & Company Inc	00006-0105-68
120's	$3.90	GENERIC, Pharmaceutical Corporation Of America	51655-0077-82

Tablet - Oral - 100 mg

100's	$1.04	GENERIC, Global Pharmaceutical Corporation	00115-3677-01
100's	$2.75	GENERIC, Cmc-Consolidated Midland Corporation	00223-1068-01
100's	$4.00	GENERIC, Major Pharmaceuticals Inc	00904-2478-61
100's	$5.25	GENERIC, Major Pharmaceuticals Inc	00904-2478-60
100's	$5.40	GENERIC, Interstate Drug Exchange Inc	00814-3726-14
100's	$6.50	GENERIC, Martec Pharmaceuticals Inc	52555-0299-01
100's	$6.87	GENERIC, Moore, H.L. Drug Exchange Inc	00839-6013-06
100's	$39.87	GENERIC, Ivax Corporation	00172-2485-60

PRODUCT LISTING - EQUIVALENTS NOT AVAILABLE

Solution - Oral - 50 mg/5 ml

500 ml	$16.91	GENERIC, Roxane Laboratories Inc	00054-3383-63

Tablet - Oral - 25 mg

2's	$3.44	GENERIC, Prescript Pharmaceuticals	00247-0200-02
3's	$0.22	GENERIC, Allscripts Pharmaceutical Company	54569-0547-06
3's	$3.47	GENERIC, Prescript Pharmaceuticals	00247-0200-03
10's	$3.75	GENERIC, Prescript Pharmaceuticals	00247-0200-10
12's	$1.62	GENERIC, Southwood Pharmaceuticals Inc	58016-0523-12
14's	$3.91	GENERIC, Prescript Pharmaceuticals	00247-0200-14
15's	$2.02	GENERIC, Southwood Pharmaceuticals Inc	58016-0523-15
20's	$2.70	GENERIC, Southwood Pharmaceuticals Inc	58016-0523-20
30's	$2.16	GENERIC, Allscripts Pharmaceutical Company	54569-0547-00
30's	$4.04	GENERIC, Southwood Pharmaceuticals Inc	58016-0523-30
30's	$4.54	GENERIC, Prescript Pharmaceuticals	00247-0200-30
60's	$4.75	GENERIC, Pharma Pac	52959-0132-60
60's	$5.74	GENERIC, Prescript Pharmaceuticals	00247-0200-60
90's	$3.11	GENERIC, Allscripts Pharmaceutical Company	54569-8540-00
90's	$6.93	GENERIC, Prescript Pharmaceuticals	00247-0200-90
100's	$6.10	GENERIC, Pharma Pac	52959-0132-00
100's	$7.33	GENERIC, Prescript Pharmaceuticals	00247-0200-00
100's	$13.48	GENERIC, Southwood Pharmaceuticals Inc	58016-0523-00
150's	$19.13	GENERIC, Sky Pharmaceuticals Packaging, Inc	63739-0128-15

Tablet - Oral - 50 mg

12's	$2.56	GENERIC, Southwood Pharmaceuticals Inc	58016-0524-12
15's	$3.20	GENERIC, Southwood Pharmaceuticals Inc	58016-0524-15
20's	$4.27	GENERIC, Southwood Pharmaceuticals Inc	58016-0524-20
30's	$3.63	GENERIC, Allscripts Pharmaceutical Company	54569-0549-00
30's	$6.41	GENERIC, Southwood Pharmaceuticals Inc	58016-0524-30
30's	$7.25	GENERIC, Pharma Pac	52959-0133-30

60's	$7.25	GENERIC, Allscripts Pharmaceutical Company	54569-0549-03
90's	$3.56	GENERIC, Allscripts Pharmaceutical Company	54569-8587-00
100's	$7.95	GENERIC, Pharma Pac	52959-0133-00
100's	$21.35	GENERIC, Southwood Pharmaceuticals Inc	58016-0524-00
150's	$23.12	GENERIC, Sky Pharmaceuticals Packaging, Inc	63739-0129-15
Tablet - Oral - 100 mg			
100's	$5.63	GENERIC, Vangard Labs	00615-2511-13

Hydrochlorothiazide; Irbesartan *(003486)*

For complete prescribing information, refer to the CD-ROM included with the book.

Categories: Hypertension, essential; FDA Approved 1998 Aug; Pregnancy Category C, 1st Trimester; Pregnancy Category D, 2nd & 3rd Trimesters

Drug Classes: Angiotensin II receptor antagonists; Diuretics, thiazide and derivatives

Brand Names: **Avalide**

Foreign Brand Availability: Aprovel HCT (Thailand); Avapro HCT (Australia); Coaprovel (Austria; Belgium; Bulgaria; Colombia; Czech-Republic; Denmark; England; Finland; France; Germany; Greece; Hong-Kong; Hungary; Ireland; Italy; Korea; Netherlands; Norway; Philippines; Poland; Portugal; Singapore; Slovenia; Spain; Sweden; Switzerland; Taiwan; Turkey); CoApprovel (Germany); Irban Plus (Israel); Karvezide (Australia; Austria; Belgium; Bulgaria; Czech-Republic; Denmark; England; Finland; France; Germany; Greece; Hungary; Ireland; Italy; Netherlands; Norway; Poland; Portugal; Slovenia; Spain; Sweden; Switzerland; Turkey)

Cost of Therapy: $57.12 (Hypertension; Avalide; 12.5 mg; 150 mg; 1 tablet/day; 30 day supply)

WARNING

Note: The trade name has been used throughout this monograph for clarity.

USE IN PREGNANCY

When used in pregnancy during the second and third trimesters, drugs that act directly on the renin-angiotensin system can cause injury and even death to the developing fetus. When pregnancy is detected, Avalide tablets should be discontinued as soon as possible. (See WARNINGS, Fetal/Neonatal Morbidity and Mortality.)

DESCRIPTION

Avalide (irbesartan-hydrochlorothiazide) tablets are a combination of an angiotensin II receptor antagonist (AT_1 subtype), irbesartan and a thiazide diuretic, hydrochlorothiazide (HCTZ).

Irbesartan is a nonpeptide compound, chemically described as a 2-butyl-3-[[2′-(1*H*-tetrazol-5-yl) [1,1′-biphenyl]-4-yl]methyl]-1,3-diazaspiro[4,4]non-1-en-4-one. Its empirical formula is $C_{25}H_{28}N_6O$.

Irbesartan is a white to off-white crystalline powder with a molecular weight of 428.5. It is a nonpolar compound with a partition coefficient (octanol/water) of 10.1 at pH of 7.4. Irbesartan is slightly soluble in alcohol and methylene chloride and practically insoluble in water.

Hydrochlorothiazide is 6-chloro-3,4-dihydro-2*H*-1,2,4-benzo-thiadiazine-7-sulfonamide 1,1-dioxide. Its empirical formula is $C_7H_8ClN_3O_4S_2$.

Hydrochlorothiazide is a white, or practically white, crystalline powder with a molecular weight of 297.7. Hydrochlorothiazide is slightly soluble in water and freely soluble in sodium hydroxide solution.

Avalide is available for oral administration in tablets containing 12.5 mg of hydrochlorothiazide combined with 150 or 300 mg of irbesartan. Inactive ingredients include: lactose monohydrate, microcrystalline cellulose, pregelatinized starch, croscarmellose sodium, ferric oxide red, ferric oxide yellow, silicon dioxide, and magnesium stearate.

INDICATIONS AND USAGE

Avalide tablets are indicated for the treatment of hypertension. This fixed dose combination is not indicated for initial therapy (see DOSAGE AND ADMINISTRATION).

CONTRAINDICATIONS

Avalide is contraindicated in patients who are hypersensitive to any component of this product.

Because of the hydrochlorothiazide component, this product is contraindicated in patients with anuria or hypersensitivity to other sulfonamide-derived drugs.

WARNINGS

FETAL/NEONATAL MORBIDITY AND MORTALITY

Drugs that act directly on the renin-angiotensin system can cause fetal and neonatal morbidity and death when administered to pregnant women. Several dozen cases have been reported in the world literature in patients who were taking angiotensin converting enzyme inhibitors. When pregnancy is detected, Avalide tablets should be discontinued as soon as possible.

The use of drugs that act directly on the renin-angiotensin system during the second and third trimesters of pregnancy has been associated with fetal and neonatal injury, including hypotension, neonatal skull hypoplasia, anuria, reversible or irreversible renal failure, and death. Oligohydramnios has also been reported, presumably resulting from decreased fetal renal function; oligohydramnios in this setting has been associated with fetal limb contractures, craniofacial deformation, and hypoplastic lung development. Prematurity, intrauterine growth retardation, and patent ductus arteriosus have also been reported, although it is not clear whether these occurrences were due to exposure to the drug.

These adverse effects do not appear to have resulted from intrauterine drug exposure that has been limited to the first trimester.

Mothers whose embryos and fetuses are exposed to an angiotensin II receptor antagonist only during the first trimester should be so informed. Nonetheless, when patients become pregnant, physicians should have the patient discontinue the use of Avalide as soon as possible.

Rarely (probably less often than once in every thousand pregnancies), no alternative to a drug acting on the renin-angiotensin system will be found. In these rare cases, the mothers should be apprised of the potential hazards to their fetuses, and serial ultrasound examinations should be performed to assess the intraamniotic environment.

If oligohydramnios is observed, Avalide tablets should be discontinued unless it is considered life-saving for the mother. Contraction stress testing (CST), a nonstress test (NST), or biophysical profiling (BPP) may be appropriate depending upon the week of pregnancy. Patients and physicians should be aware, however, that oligohydramnios may not appear until after the fetus has sustained irreversible injury.

Infants with histories of *in utero* exposure to an angiotensin II receptor antagonist should be closely observed for hypotension, oliguria, and hyperkalemia. If oliguria occurs, attention should be directed toward support of blood pressure and renal perfusion. Exchange transfusion or dialysis may be required as a means of reversing hypotension and/or substituting for disordered renal function.

When pregnant rats were treated with irbesartan from day 0 to day 20 of gestation (oral doses of 50, 180, and 650 mg/kg/day), increased incidences of renal pelvic cavitation, hydroureter and/or absence of renal papilla were observed in fetuses at doses ≥50 mg/kg/day (approximately equivalent to the maximum recommended human dose [MRHD], 300 mg/day, on a body surface area basis). Subcutaneous edema was observed in fetuses at doses ≥180 mg/kg/day (about 4 times the MRHD on a body surface area basis). As these anomalies were not observed in rats in which irbesartan exposure (oral doses of 50, 150 and 450 mg/kg/day) was limited to gestation days 6-15, they appear to reflect late gestational effects of the drug. In pregnant rabbits, oral doses of 30 mg irbesartan/kg/day were associated with maternal mortality and abortion. Surviving females receiving this dose (about 1.5 times the MRHD on a body surface area basis) had a slight increase in early resorptions and a corresponding decrease in live fetuses. Irbesartan was found to cross the placental barrier in rats and rabbits.

Radioactivity was present in the rat and rabbit fetus during late gestation and in rat milk following oral doses of radiolabeled irbesartan.

Studies in which hydrochlorothiazide was administered to pregnant mice and rats during their respective periods of major organogenesis at doses up to 3000 and 1000 mg/kg/day, respectively, provided no evidence of harm to the fetus.

A development toxicity study was performed in rats with doses of 50/50 and 150/150 mg/kg/day Avalide. Although the high dose combination appeared to be more toxic to the dams than either drug alone, there did not appear to be an increase in toxicity to the developing embryos.

Thiazides cross the placental barrier and appear in cord blood. There is a risk of fetal or neonatal jaundice, thrombocytopenia, and possibly other adverse reactions that have occurred in adults.

HYPOTENSION IN VOLUME- OR SALT-DEPLETED PATIENTS

Excessive reduction of blood pressure was rarely seen in patients with uncomplicated hypertension treated with irbesartan alone (<0.1%) or with Avalide (approximately 1%). Initiation of antihypertensive therapy may cause symptomatic hypotension in patients with intravascular volume- or sodium-depletion, *e.g.*, in patients treated vigorously with diuretics or in patients on dialysis. Such volume depletion should be corrected prior to administration of antihypertensive therapy.

If hypotension occurs, the patient should be placed in the supine position and, if necessary, given an intravenous infusion of normal saline. A transient hypotensive response is not a contraindication to further treatment, which usually can be continued without difficulty once the blood pressure has stabilized.

HYDROCHLOROTHIAZIDE

Hepatic Impairment: Thiazides should be used with caution in patients with impaired hepatic function or progressive liver disease, since minor alterations of fluid and electrolyte balance may precipitate hepatic coma.

Hypersensitivity Reaction: Hypersensitivity reactions to hydrochlorothiazide may occur in patients with or without a history of allergy or bronchial asthma, but are more likely in patients with such a history.

Systemic Lupus Erythematosus: Thiazide diuretics have been reported to cause exacerbation or activation of systemic lupus erythematosus.

Lithium Interaction: Lithium generally should not be given with thiazides.

DOSAGE AND ADMINISTRATION

Hydrochlorothiazide is effective in doses of 12.5 to 50 mg once daily.

The recommended initial dose of irbesartan is 150 mg once daily. Patients requiring further reduction in blood pressure should be titrated to 300 mg once daily.

A lower initial dose of irbesartan (75 mg) is recommended in patients with depletion of intravascular volume (*e.g.*, patients treated vigorously with diuretics or on hemodialysis) (see WARNINGS, Hypotension in Volume- or Salt-Depleted Patients). Patients not adequately treated by the maximum dose of 300 mg once daily are unlikely to derive additional benefit from a higher dose or twice-daily dosing.

To minimize dose-independent side effects, it is usually appropriate to begin combination therapy only after a patient has failed to achieve the desired effect with monotherapy.

The side effects (see WARNINGS) of irbesartan are generally rare and apparently independent of dose; those of hydrochlorothiazide are a mixture of dose-dependent (primarily hypokalemia) and dose-independent phenomena (*e.g.*, pancreatitis), the former much more common than the latter. Therapy with any combination of hydrochlorothiazide and irbesartan will be associated with both sets of dose-independent side effects.

Avalide may be administered with other antihypertensive agents.

Avalide may be administered with or without food.

REPLACEMENT THERAPY

The combination may be substituted for the titrated components.

DOSE TITRATION BY CLINICAL EFFECT

A patient whose blood pressure is inadequately controlled by hydrochlorothiazide or irbesartan alone may be switched to once daily Avalide. Recommended doses of Avalide, in order of increasing mean effect, are (irbesartan-hydrochlorothiazide) 150/12.5 mg, 300/12.5 mg, and 300/25 mg (two 150/12.5 mg tablets). The largest incremental effect will likely be in the transition from monotherapy to 150/12.5 mg. It takes 2-4 weeks for the blood pressure to stabilize after a change in the dose of Avalide.

The usual dose of Avalide is 1 tablet once daily. More than 2 tablets once daily is not recommended. The maximal antihypertensive effect is attained about 2-4 weeks after initiation of therapy.

USE IN PATIENTS WITH RENAL IMPAIRMENT

The usual regimens of therapy with Avalide may be followed as long as the patient's creatinine clearance is >30 ml/min. In patients with more severe renal impairment, loop diuretics are preferred to thiazides, so Avalide is not recommended.

PATIENTS WITH HEPATIC IMPAIRMENT

No dosage adjustment is necessary in patients with hepatic impairment.

PRODUCT LISTING - EQUIVALENTS NOT AVAILABLE

Tablet - Oral - 12.5 mg;150 mg

30's	$57.13	AVALIDE, Bristol-Myers Squibb	00087-2775-31
90's	$171.35	AVALIDE, Bristol-Myers Squibb	00087-2775-32

Tablet - Oral - 12.5 mg;300 mg

30's	$61.08	AVALIDE, Bristol-Myers Squibb	00087-2776-31
90's	$183.23	AVALIDE, Bristol-Myers Squibb	00087-2776-32

H

Hydrochlorothiazide; Lisinopril *(001458)*

For complete prescribing information, refer to the CD-ROM included with the book.

Categories: Hypertension, essential; Pregnancy Category C, 1st Trimester; Pregnancy Category D, 2nd & 3rd Trimesters; FDA Approved 1989 Feb
Drug Classes: Angiotensin converting enzyme inhibitors; Diuretics, thiazide and derivatives
Brand Names: Prinzide; Zestoretic
Foreign Brand Availability: Acercomp (Germany); Carace Plus (England); Cipril - H (India); Coric Plus (Germany); Novazyd (Netherlands); Vivazid (Denmark)
Cost of Therapy: $37.35 (Hypertension; Prinzide; 12.5 mg; 10 mg; 1 tablet/day; 30 day supply)
$32.22 (Hypertension; Generic Tablets; 12.5 mg; 10 mg; 1 tablet/day; 30 day supply)
$38.40 (Hypertension; Zestoretic; 12.5 mg; 10 mg; 1 tablet/day; 30 day supply)

WARNING

Note: The trade name has been used throughout this monograph for clarity.

USE IN PREGNANCY

When used in pregnancy during the second and third trimesters, ACE inhibitors can cause injury and even death to the developing fetus. When pregnancy is detected, Prinzide should be discontinued as soon as possible. See WARNINGS, Pregnancy, Lisinopril — Fetal/Neonatal Morbidity and Mortality.

DESCRIPTION

Prinzide (lisinopril-hydrochlorothiazide) combines an angiotensin converting enzyme inhibitor, lisinopril, and a diuretic, hydrochlorothiazide.

Lisinopril, a synthetic peptide derivative, is an oral long-acting angiotensin converting enzyme inhibitor. It is chemically described as (*S*)-1-[N^2-(1-carboxy-3-phenylpropyl)-L-lysyl]-L-proline dihydrate. Its empirical formula is $C_{21}H_{31}N_3O_5 \cdot 2H_2O$.

Lisinopril is a white to off-white, crystalline powder, with a molecular weight of 441.52. It is soluble in water, sparingly soluble in methanol, and practically insoluble in ethanol.

Hydrochlorothiazide is 6-chloro-3,4-dihydro-2*H*-1,2,4-benzothiadiazine-7-sulfonamide 1,1-dioxide. Its empirical formula is $C_7H_8ClN_3O_4S_2$.

Hydrochlorothiazide is a white, or practically white, crystalline powder with a molecular weight of 297.73, which is slightly soluble in water, but freely soluble in sodium hydroxide solution.

Prinzide is available for oral use in 3 tablet combinations of lisinopril with hydrochlorothiazide:

Prinzide 10-12.5, containing 10 mg lisinopril and 12.5 mg hydrochlorothiazide.
Prinzide 20-12.5, containing 20 mg lisinopril and 12.5 mg hydrochlorothiazide.
Prinzide 20-25, containing 20 mg lisinopril and 25 mg hydrochlorothiazide.

Inactive ingredients are calcium phosphate, magnesium stearate, mannitol, and starch. Prinzide 10-12.5 also contains FD&C blue no. 2 aluminum lake. Prinzide 20-12.5 and Prinzide 20-25 also contain iron oxide.

INDICATIONS AND USAGE

Prinzide is indicated for the treatment of hypertension.

These fixed-dose combinations are not indicated for initial therapy (see DOSAGE AND ADMINISTRATION).

In using Prinzide, consideration should be given to the fact that an angiotensin converting enzyme inhibitor, captopril, has caused agranulocytosis, particularly in patients with renal impairment or collagen vascular disease, and that available data are insufficient to show that lisinopril does not have a similar risk. (See WARNINGS.)

In considering use of Prinzide, it should be noted that black patients receiving ACE inhibitors have been reported to have a higher incidence of angioedema compared to non-blacks. (See WARNINGS, General, Lisinopril, Angioedema.)

CONTRAINDICATIONS

Prinzide is contraindicated in patients who are hypersensitive to any component of this product and in patients with a history of angioedema related to previous treatment with an angiotensin converting enzyme inhibitor and in patients with hereditary or idiopathic angioedema. Because of the hydrochlorothiazide component, this product is contraindicated in patients with anuria or hypersensitivity to other sulfonamide-derived drugs.

WARNINGS

GENERAL

Lisinopril

Anaphylactoid and Possibly Related Reactions

Presumably because angiotensin-converting enzyme inhibitors affect the metabolism of eicosanoids and polypeptides, including endogenous bradykinin, patients receiving ACE inhibitors (including Prinzide) may be subject to a variety of adverse reactions, some of them serious.

Angioedema

Angioedema of the face, extremities, lips, tongue, glottis and/or larynx has been reported rarely in patients treated with angiotensin converting enzyme inhibitors, including lisinopril. This may occur at any time during treatment. In such cases Prinzide should be promptly discontinued and appropriate therapy and monitoring should be provided until complete and sustained resolution of signs and symptoms has occurred. In instances where swelling has been confined to the face and lips the condition has generally resolved without treatment, although antihistamines have been useful in relieving symptoms. Angioedema associated with laryngeal edema may be fatal. **Where there is involvement of the tongue, glottis or larynx, likely to cause airway obstruction, subcutaneous epinephrine solution 1:1000 (0.3-0.5 ml) and/or measures necessary to ensure a patent airway, should be promptly provided.**

Patients with a history of angioedema unrelated to ACE inhibitor therapy may be at increased risk of angioedema while receiving an ACE inhibitor (see also INDICATIONS AND USAGE and CONTRAINDICATIONS).

Anaphylactoid Reactions During Desensitization

Two patients undergoing desensitizing treatment with hymenoptera venom while receiving ACE inhibitors sustained life-threatening anaphylactoid reactions. In the same patients, these reactions were avoided when ACE inhibitors were temporarily withheld, but they reappeared upon inadvertent rechallenge.

Anaphylactoid Reactions During Membrane Exposure

Anaphylactoid reactions have been reported in patients dialyzed with high-flux membranes and treated concomitantly with an ACE inhibitor. Anaphylactoid reactions have also been reported in patients undergoing low-density lipoprotein apheresis with dextran sulfate absorption.

Hypotension and Related Effects

Excessive hypotension was rarely seen in uncomplicated hypertensive patients but is a possible consequence of lisinopril use in salt/volume-depleted persons, such as those treated vigorously with diuretics or patients on dialysis.

Syncope has been reported in 0.8% of patients receiving Prinzide. In patients with hypertension receiving lisinopril alone, the incidence of syncope was 0.1%. The overall incidence of syncope may be reduced by proper titration of the individual components. (See DOSAGE AND ADMINISTRATION.)

In patients with severe congestive heart failure, with or without associated renal insufficiency, excessive hypotension has been observed and may be associated with oliguria and/or progressive azotemia, and rarely with acute renal failure and/or death. Because of the potential fall in blood pressure in these patients, therapy should be started under very close medical supervision. Such patients should be followed closely for the first 2 weeks of treatment and whenever the dose of lisinopril and/or diuretic is increased. Similar considerations apply to patients with ischemic heart or cerebrovascular disease in whom an excessive fall in blood pressure could result in a myocardial infarction or cerebrovascular accident.

If hypotension occurs, the patient should be placed in supine position and, if necessary, receive an intravenous infusion of normal saline. A transient hypotensive response is not a contraindication to further doses which usually can be given without difficulty once the blood pressure has increased after volume expansion.

Neutropenia/Agranulocytosis

Another angiotensin converting enzyme inhibitor, captopril, has been shown to cause agranulocytosis and bone marrow depression, rarely in uncomplicated patients but more frequently in patients with renal impairment, especially if they also have a collagen vascular disease. Available data from clinical trials of lisinopril are insufficient to show that lisinopril does not cause agranulocytosis at similar rates. Marketing experience has revealed rare cases of neutropenia and bone marrow depression in which a causal relationship to lisinopril cannot be excluded. Periodic monitoring of white blood cell counts in patients with collagen vascular disease and renal disease should be considered.

Hepatic Failure

Rarely, ACE inhibitors have been associated with a syndrome that starts with cholestatic jaundice and progresses to fulminant hepatic necrosis, and (sometimes) death. The mechanism of this syndrome is not understood. Patients receiving ACE inhibitors who develop jaundice or marked elevations of hepatic enzymes should discontinue the ACE inhibitor and receive appropriate medical follow-up.

Hydrochlorothiazide

Thiazides should be used with caution in severe renal disease. In patients with renal disease, thiazides may precipitate azotemia. Cumulative effects of the drug may develop in patients with impaired renal function.

Thiazides should be used with caution in patients with impaired hepatic function or progressive liver disease, since minor alterations of fluid and electrolyte balance may precipitate hepatic coma.

Sensitivity reactions may occur in patients with or without a history of allergy or bronchial asthma.

The possibility of exacerbation or activation of systemic lupus erythematosus has been reported.

Lithium generally should not be given with thiazides.

PREGNANCY

Lisinopril-Hydrochlorothiazide

Teratogenicity studies were conducted in mice and rats with up to 90 mg/kg/day of lisinopril in combination with 10 mg/kg/day of hydrochlorothiazide. This dose of lisinopril is 5 times (in mice) and 10 times (in rats) the maximum recommended human daily dose (MRHDD) when compared on a body surface area basis (mg/m^2); the dose of hydrochlorothiazide is 0.9 times (in mice) and 1.8 times (in rats) the MRHDD. Maternal or fetotoxic effects were not seen in mice with the combination. In rats decreased maternal weight gain and decreased fetal weight occurred down to 3/10 mg/kg/day (the lowest dose tested). Associated with the decreased fetal weight was a delay in fetal ossification. The decreased fetal weight and delay in fetal ossification were not seen in saline-supplemented animals given 90/10 mg/kg/day.

When used in pregnancy during the second and third trimesters, ACE inhibitors can cause injury and even death to the developing fetus. When pregnancy is detected, Prinzide should be discontinued as soon as possible. (See Lisinopril — Fetal/Neonatal Morbidity and Mortality.)

Lisinopril — Fetal/Neonatal Morbidity and Mortality

ACE inhibitors can cause fetal and neonatal morbidity and death when administered to pregnant women. Several dozen cases have been reported in the world literature. When pregnancy is detected, ACE inhibitors should be discontinued as soon as possible.

The use of ACE inhibitors during the second and third trimesters of pregnancy has been associated with fetal and neonatal injury, including hypotension, neonatal skull hypoplasia, anuria, reversible or irreversible renal failure, and death. Oligohydramnios has also been reported, presumably resulting from decreased fetal renal function; oligohydramnios in this setting has been associated with fetal limb contractures, craniofacial deformation, and hypoplastic lung development. Prematurity, intrauterine growth retardation, and patent ductus arteriosus have also been reported, although it is not clear whether these occurrences were due to the ACE-inhibitor exposure.

These adverse effects do not appear to have resulted from intrauterine ACE-inhibitor exposure that has been limited to the first trimester. Mothers whose embryos and fetuses are exposed to ACE inhibitors only during the first trimester should be so informed. Nonetheless, when patients become pregnant, physicians should make every effort to discontinue the use of Prinzide as soon as possible.

Rarely (probably less often than once in every thousand pregnancies), no alternative to ACE inhibitors will be found. In these rare cases, the mothers should be apprised of the potential hazards to their fetuses, and serial ultrasound examinations should be performed to assess the intraamniotic environment.

If oligohydramnios is observed, Prinzide should be discontinued unless it is considered lifesaving for the mother. Contraction stress testing (CST), a non-stress test (NST), or biophysical profiling (BPP) may be appropriate, depending upon the week of pregnancy. Patients and physicians should be aware, however, that oligohydramnios may not appear until after the fetus has sustained irreversible injury.

Infants with histories of *in utero* exposure to ACE inhibitors should be closely observed for hypotension, oliguria, and hyperkalemia. If oliguria occurs, attention should be directed toward support of blood pressure and renal perfusion. Exchange transfusion or dialysis may be required as means of reversing hypotension and/or substituting for disordered renal function. Lisinopril, which crosses the placenta, has been removed from neonatal circulation by peritoneal dialysis with some clinical benefit, and theoretically may be removed by exchange transfusion, although there is no experience with the latter procedure.

No teratogenic effects of lisinopril were seen in studies of pregnant mice, rats, and rabbits. On a body surface area basis, the doses used were up 55 times, 33 times, and 0.15 times, respectively, the MRHDD.

Hydrochlorothiazide

Studies in which hydrochlorothiazide was orally administered to pregnant mice and rats during their respective periods of major organogenesis at doses up to 3000 and 1000 mg/kg/day, respectively, provided no evidence of harm to the fetus. These doses are more than 150 times the MRHDD on a body surface area basis. Thiazides cross the placental barrier and appear in cord blood. There is a risk of fetal or neonatal jaundice, thrombocytopenia and possibly other adverse reactions that have occurred in adults.

DOSAGE AND ADMINISTRATION

Lisinopril is an effective treatment of hypertension in once-daily doses of 10-80 mg, while hydrochlorothiazide is effective in doses of 12.5-50 mg. In clinical trials of lisinopril/hydrochlorothiazide combination therapy using lisinopril doses of 10-80 mg and hydrochlorothiazide doses of 6.25-50 mg, the antihypertensive response rates generally increased with increasing dose of either component.

The side effects (see WARNINGS) of lisinopril are generally rare and apparently independent of dose; those of hydrochlorothiazide are a mixture of dose-dependent phenomena (primarily hypokalemia) and dose-independent phenomena (*e.g.*, pancreatitis), the former much more common than the latter. Therapy with any combination of lisinopril and hydrochlorothiazide will be associated with both sets of dose-independent side effects, but addition of lisinopril in clinical trials blunted the hypokalemia normally seen with diuretics.

To minimize dose-independent side effects, it is usually appropriate to begin combination therapy only after a patient has failed to achieve the desired effect with monotherapy.

DOSE TITRATION GUIDED BY CLINICAL EFFECT

A patient whose blood pressure is not adequately controlled with either lisinopril or hydrochlorothiazide monotherapy may be switched to Prinzide 10/12.5 or Prinzide 20/12.5. Further increases of either or both components could depend on clinical response. The hydrochlorothiazide dose should generally not be increased until 2-3 weeks have elapsed. Patients whose blood pressures are adequately controlled with 25 mg of daily hydrochlorothiazide, but who experience significant potassium loss with this regimen, may achieve similar or greater blood pressure control with less potassium loss if they are switched to Prinzide 10/12.5. Dosage higher than lisinopril 80 mg and hydrochlorothiazide 50 mg should not be used.

REPLACEMENT THERAPY

The combination may be substituted for the titrated individual components.

USE IN RENAL IMPAIRMENT

The usual regimens of therapy with Prinzide need not be adjusted as long as the patient's creatinine clearance is >30 ml/min/1.73 m^2 (serum creatinine approximately ≤3 mg/dl or 265 µmol/L). In patients with more severe renal impairment, loop diuretics are preferred to thiazides, so Prinzide is not recommended (see WARNINGS, General, Lisinopril, Anaphylactoid Reactions During Membrane Exposure).

USE IN ELDERLY

In general, blood pressure response and adverse experiences were similar in younger and older patients given Prinzide. However, in a multiple dose pharmacokinetic study in elderly versus young patients using the lisinopril/hydrochlorothiazide combination, area under the plasma concentration time curve (AUC) increased approximately 120% for lisinopril and approximately 80% for hydrochlorothiazide in older patients. Therefore, dosage adjustments in elderly patients should be made with particular caution.

PRODUCT LISTING - RATED THERAPEUTICALLY EQUIVALENT

Tablet - Oral - 12.5 mg;10 mg

30's	$32.20	GENERIC, Purepac Pharmaceutical Company	00228-2706-03
30's	$32.29	ZESTORETIC, Allscripts Pharmaceutical Company	54569-4829-00
100's	$94.34	ZESTORETIC, Astra-Zeneca Pharmaceuticals	00038-0141-10
100's	$107.40	GENERIC, Purepac Pharmaceutical Company	00228-2706-11
100's	$110.40	GENERIC, Ivax Corporation	00172-5033-60
100's	$110.80	GENERIC, Teva Pharmaceuticals Usa	00093-1035-01
100's	$110.90	GENERIC, Mylan Pharmaceuticals Inc	00378-1012-01
100's	$111.00	GENERIC, Eon Labs Manufacturing Inc	00185-7100-01
100's	$111.50	GENERIC, West Ward Pharmaceutical Corporation	00143-1262-01
100's	$112.04	GENERIC, Geneva Pharmaceuticals	00781-1848-01
100's	$128.00	ZESTORETIC, Pharma Pac	52959-0498-00
100's	$128.14	ZESTORETIC, Astra-Zeneca Pharmaceuticals	00310-0141-10

Tablet - Oral - 12.5 mg;20 mg

30's	$34.85	GENERIC, Purepac Pharmaceutical Company	00228-2707-03
100's	$102.11	ZESTORETIC, Astra-Zeneca Pharmaceuticals	00038-0142-10
100's	$116.30	GENERIC, Purepac Pharmaceutical Company	00228-2707-11
100's	$119.50	GENERIC, Ivax Corporation	00172-5034-60
100's	$119.75	GENERIC, West Ward Pharmaceutical Corporation	00143-1263-01
100's	$119.94	GENERIC, Teva Pharmaceuticals Usa	00093-1036-01
100's	$120.05	GENERIC, Mylan Pharmaceuticals Inc	00378-2012-01
100's	$120.15	GENERIC, Eon Labs Manufacturing Inc	00185-0152-01
100's	$121.28	GENERIC, Geneva Pharmaceuticals	00781-1176-01
100's	$138.71	ZESTORETIC, Astra-Zeneca Pharmaceuticals	00310-0142-10

Tablet - Oral - 25 mg;20 mg

30's	$35.30	GENERIC, Purepac Pharmaceutical Company	00228-2708-03
30's	$37.20	PRINZIDE, Pd-Rx Pharmaceuticals	55289-0573-30
30's	$40.91	PRINZIDE, Merck & Company Inc	00006-0142-31
100's	$103.37	ZESTORETIC, Astra-Zeneca Pharmaceuticals	00038-0145-10
100's	$117.70	GENERIC, Purepac Pharmaceutical Company	00228-2708-11
100's	$120.90	GENERIC, Ivax Corporation	00172-5032-60
100's	$120.95	GENERIC, West Point Pharma	00143-1264-01
100's	$121.39	GENERIC, Teva Pharmaceuticals Usa	00093-1037-01
100's	$121.50	GENERIC, Mylan Pharmaceuticals Inc	00378-2025-01
100's	$121.60	GENERIC, Eon Labs Manufacturing Inc	00185-0173-01
100's	$122.75	GENERIC, Geneva Pharmaceuticals	00781-1178-01
100's	$136.39	PRINZIDE, Merck & Company Inc	00006-0142-58
100's	$140.39	ZESTORETIC, Astra-Zeneca Pharmaceuticals	00310-0145-10

PRODUCT LISTING - EQUIVALENTS NOT AVAILABLE

Tablet - Oral - 12.5 mg;10 mg

30's	$37.34	PRINZIDE, Merck & Company Inc	00006-0145-31
100's	$124.49	PRINZIDE, Merck & Company Inc	00006-0145-58

Tablet - Oral - 12.5 mg;20 mg

30's	$40.43	PRINZIDE, Merck & Company Inc	00006-0140-31
100's	$134.76	PRINZIDE, Merck & Company Inc	00006-0140-58

Hydrochlorothiazide; Losartan Potassium (003260)

For complete prescribing information, refer to the CD-ROM included with the book.

Categories: Hypertension, essential; FDA Approved 1995 Apr; Pregnancy Category D
Drug Classes: Angiotensin II receptor antagonists; Diuretics, thiazide and derivatives
Brand Names: Hyzaar
Foreign Brand Availability: Fortzaar (France; Thailand); Hyzaar DS (Canada; Philippines); Hyzaar forte (Hong-Kong; Singapore; Taiwan); Satoren H (Colombia); Tensarten-HCT (Colombia); Zaart-H (India)
Cost of Therapy: $47.57 (Hypertension; Hyzaar; 50 mg; 12.5 mg; 1 tablet/day; 30 day supply)

WARNING

Note: The trade name has been used throughout this monograph for clarity.

USE IN PREGNANCY

When used in pregnancy during the second and third trimesters, drugs that act directly on the renin-angiotensin system can cause injury and even death to the developing fetus. When pregnancy is detected, Hyzaar should be discontinued as soon as possible. See WARNINGS, Fetal/Neonatal Morbidity and Mortality.

H

DESCRIPTION

Hyzaar 50-12.5 (losartan potassium-hydrochlorothiazide) and Hyzaar 100-25 (losartan potassium-hydrochlorothiazide), combine an angiotensin II receptor (type AT_1) antagonist and a diuretic, hydrochlorothiazide.

Losartan potassium, a non-peptide molecule, is chemically described as 2-butyl-4-chloro-1-[*p*-(*o*-1*H*-tetrazol-5-ylphenyl)benzyl]imidazole-5-methanol monopotassium salt. Its empirical formula is $C_{22}H_{22}ClKN_6O$.

Losartan potassium is a white to off-white free-flowing crystalline powder with a molecular weight of 461.01. It is freely soluble in water, soluble in alcohols, and slightly soluble in common organic solvents, such as acetonitrile and methyl ethyl ketone.

Oxidation of the 5-hydroxymethyl group on the imidazole ring results in the active metabolite of losartan.

Hydrochlorothiazide is 6-chloro-3,4-dihydro-2*H*-1,2,4-benzothiadiazine-7-sulfonamide 1,1-dioxide. Its empirical formula is $C_7H_8ClN_3O_4S_2$.

Hydrochlorothiazide is a white, or practically white, crystalline powder with a molecular weight of 297.74, which is slightly soluble in water, but freely soluble in sodium hydroxide solution.

Hyzaar is available for oral administration in 2 tablet combinations of losartan and hydrochlorothiazide. Hyzaar 50-12.5 contains 50 mg of losartan potassium and 12.5 mg of hydrochlorothiazide. Hyzaar 100-25 contains 100 mg of losartan potassium and 25 mg of hydrochlorothiazide. Inactive ingredients are microcrystalline cellulose, lactose hydrous, pregelatinized starch, magnesium stearate, hydroxypropyl cellulose, hydroxypropyl methylcellulose, titanium dioxide and D&C yellow no. 10 aluminum lake.

Hyzaar 50-12.5 contains 4.24 mg (0.108 mEq) of potassium and Hyzaar 100-25 contains 8.48 mg (0.216 mEq) of potassium.

INDICATIONS AND USAGE

Hyzaar is indicated for the treatment of hypertension. This fixed dose combination is not indicated for initial therapy (see DOSAGE AND ADMINISTRATION).

CONTRAINDICATIONS

Hyzaar is contraindicated in patients who are hypersensitive to any component of this product.

Because of the hydrochlorothiazide component, this product is contraindicated in patients with anuria or hypersensitivity to other sulfonamide-derived drugs.

WARNINGS

FETAL/NEONATAL MORBIDITY AND MORTALITY

Drugs that act directly on the renin-angiotensin system can cause fetal and neonatal morbidity and death when administered to pregnant women. Several dozen cases have been reported in the world literature in patients who were taking angiotensin converting enzyme inhibitors. When pregnancy is detected, Hyzaar should be discontinued as soon as possible.

The use of drugs that act directly on the renin-angiotensin system during the second and third trimesters of pregnancy has been associated with fetal and neonatal injury, including hypotension, neonatal skull hypoplasia, anuria, reversible or irreversible renal failure, and death. Oligohydramnios has also been reported, presumably resulting from decreased fetal renal function; oligohydramnios in this setting has been associated with fetal limb contractures, craniofacial deformation, and hypoplastic lung development. Prematurity, intrauterine growth retardation, and patent ductus arteriosus have also been reported, although it is not clear whether these occurrences were due to exposure to the drug.

These adverse effects do not appear to have resulted from intrauterine drug exposure that has been limited to the first trimester.

Mothers whose embryos and fetuses are exposed to an angiotensin II receptor antagonist only during the first trimester should be so informed. Nonetheless, when patients become pregnant, physicians should have the patient discontinue the use of Hyzaar as soon as possible.

Rarely (probably less often than once in every 1000 pregnancies), no alternative to an angiotensin II receptor antagonist will be found. In these rare cases, the mothers should be apprised of the potential hazards to their fetuses, and serial ultrasound examinations should be performed to assess the intra-amniotic environment.

If oligohydramnios is observed, Hyzaar should be discontinued unless it is considered life-saving for the mother. Contraction stress testing (CST), a non-stress test (NST), or biophysical profiling (BPP) may be appropriate, depending upon the week of pregnancy. Patients and physicians should be aware, however, that oligohydramnios may not appear until after the fetus has sustained irreversible injury.

Infants with histories of *in utero* exposure to an angiotensin II receptor antagonist should be closely observed for hypotension, oliguria, and hyperkalemia. If oliguria occurs, attention should be directed toward support of blood pressure and renal perfusion. Exchange transfusion or dialysis may be required as means of reversing hypotension and/or substituting for disordered renal function.

There was no evidence of teratogenicity in rats or rabbits treated with a maximum losartan potassium dose of 10 mg/kg/day in combination with 2.5 mg/kg/day of hydrochlorothiazide. At these dosages, respective exposures (AUCs) of losartan, its active metabolite, and hydrochlorothiazide in rabbits were approximately 5, 1.5, and 1.0 times those achieved in humans with 100 mg losartan in combination with 25 mg hydrochlorothiazide. AUC values for losartan, its active metabolite and hydrochlorothiazide, extrapolated from data obtained with losartan administered to rats at a dose of 50 mg/kg/day in combination with 12.5 mg/kg/day of hydrochlorothiazide, were approximately 6, 2, and 2 times greater than those achieved in humans with 100 mg of losartan in combination with 25 mg of hydrochlorothiazide. Fetal toxicity in rats, as evidenced by a slight increase in supernumerary ribs, was observed when females were treated prior to and throughout gestation with 10 mg/kg/day losartan in combination with 2.5 mg/kg/day hydrochlorothiazide. As also observed in studies with losartan alone, adverse fetal and neonatal effects, including decreased body weight, renal toxicity, and mortality, occurred when pregnant rats were treated during late gestation and/or lactation with 50 mg/kg/day losartan in combination with 12.5 mg/kg/day hydrochlorothiazide. Respective AUCs for losartan, its active metabolite and hydrochlorothiazide at these dosages in rats were approximately 35, 10 and 10 times greater than those achieved in humans with the administration of 100 mg of losartan in combination with 25 mg hydrochlorothiazide. When hydrochlorothiazide was administered without losartan to pregnant mice and rats during their respective periods of major organogenesis, at doses up to 3000 and 1000 mg/kg/day, respectively, there was no evidence of harm to the fetus.

Thiazides cross the placental barrier and appear in cord blood. There is a risk of fetal or neonatal jaundice, thrombocytopenia, and possibly other adverse reactions that have occurred in adults.

HYPOTENSION — VOLUME-DEPLETED PATIENTS

In patients who are intravascularly volume-depleted (*e.g.,* those treated with diuretics), symptomatic hypotension may occur after initiation of therapy with Hyzaar. This condition should be corrected prior to administration of Hyzaar (see DOSAGE AND ADMINISTRATION).

IMPAIRED HEPATIC FUNCTION

Losartan Potassium-Hydrochlorothiazide

Hyzaar is not recommended for patients with hepatic impairment who require titration with losartan. The lower starting dose of losartan recommended for use in patients with hepatic impairment cannot be given using Hyzaar.

Hydrochlorothiazide

Thiazides should be used with caution in patients with impaired hepatic function or progressive liver disease, since minor alterations of fluid and electrolyte balance may precipitate hepatic coma.

HYPERSENSITIVITY REACTION

Hypersensitivity reactions to hydrochlorothiazide may occur in patients with or without a history of allergy or bronchial asthma, but are more likely in patients with such a history.

SYSTEMIC LUPUS ERYTHEMATOSUS

Thiazide diuretics have been reported to cause exacerbation or activation of systemic lupus erythematosus.

LITHIUM INTERACTION

Lithium generally should not be given with thiazides.

DOSAGE AND ADMINISTRATION

Dosing must be individualized. The usual starting dose of losartan is 50 mg once daily, with 25 mg recommended for patients with intravascular volume depletion (*e.g.,* patients treated with diuretics) (see WARNINGS, Hypotension — Volume-Depleted Patients) and patients with a history of hepatic impairment (see WARNINGS, Impaired Hepatic Function). Losartan can be administered once or twice daily at total daily doses of 25-100 mg. If the antihypertensive effect measured at trough using once-a-day dosing is inadequate, a twice-a-day regimen at the same total daily dose or an increase in dose may give a more satisfactory response.

Hydrochlorothiazide is effective in doses of 12.5 to 50 mg once daily and can be given at doses of 12.5 to 25 mg as Hyzaar.

To minimize dose-independent side effects, it is usually appropriate to begin combination therapy only after a patient has failed to achieve the desired effect with monotherapy.

The side effects (see WARNINGS) of losartan are generally rare and apparently independent of dose; those of hydrochlorothiazide are a mixture of dose-dependent (primarily hypokalemia) and dose-independent phenomena (*e.g.,* pancreatitis), the former much more common than the latter. Therapy with any combination of losartan and hydrochlorothiazide will be associated with both sets of dose-independent side effects.

REPLACEMENT THERAPY

The combination may be substituted for the titrated components.

DOSE TITRATION BY CLINICAL EFFECT

A patient whose blood pressure is not adequately controlled with losartan monotherapy (see preceding) or hydrochlorothiazide alone, may be switched to Hyzaar 50-12.5 (losartan 50 mg/hydrochlorothiazide 12.5 mg) once daily. If blood pressure remains uncontrolled after about 3 weeks of therapy, the dose may be increased to 2 tablets of Hyzaar 50-12.5 once daily or 1 tablet of Hyzaar 100-25 (losartan 100 mg/hydrochlorothiazide 25 mg) once daily.

A patient whose blood pressure is inadequately controlled by 25 mg once daily of hydrochlorothiazide, or is controlled but who experiences hypokalemia with this regimen, may be switched to Hyzaar 50-12.5 (losartan 50 mg/hydrochlorothiazide 12.5 mg) once daily, reducing the dose of hydrochlorothiazide without reducing the overall expected antihypertensive response. The clinical response to Hyzaar 50-12.5 should be subsequently evaluated and if blood pressure remains uncontrolled after about 3 weeks of therapy, the dose may be increased to 2 tablets of Hyzaar 50-12.5 once daily or 1 tablet of Hyzaar 100-25 (losartan 100 mg/hydrochlorothiazide 25 mg) once daily.

The usual dose of Hyzaar is 1 tablet of Hyzaar 50-12.5 once daily. More than 2 tablets of Hyzaar 50-12.5 once daily or more than 1 tablet of Hyzaar 100-25 once daily is not recommended. The maximal antihypertensive effect is attained about 3 weeks after initiation of therapy.

USE IN PATIENTS WITH RENAL IMPAIRMENT

The usual regimens of therapy with Hyzaar may be followed as long as the patient's creatinine clearance is >30 ml/min. In patients with more severe renal impairment, loop diuretics are preferred to thiazides, so Hyzaar is not recommended.

PATIENTS WITH HEPATIC IMPAIRMENT

Hyzaar is not recommended for titration in patients with hepatic impairment (see WARNINGS, Impaired Hepatic Function) because the appropriate 25 mg starting dose of losartan cannot be given.

Hyzaar may be administered with other antihypertensive agents.

Hyzaar may be administered with or without food.

PRODUCT LISTING - EQUIVALENTS NOT AVAILABLE

Tablet - Oral - 12.5 mg;50 mg

30's	$38.99	HYZAAR, Allscripts Pharmaceutical Company	54569-4722-01
30's	$45.20	HYZAAR, Physicians Total Care	54868-3866-00
30's	$47.58	HYZAAR, Merck & Company Inc	00006-0717-31
60's	$77.99	HYZAAR, Allscripts Pharmaceutical Company	54569-4722-00
90's	$142.71	HYZAAR, Merck & Company Inc	00006-0717-54
100's	$151.45	HYZAAR, Merck & Company Inc	00006-0717-28
100's	$158.56	HYZAAR, Merck & Company Inc	00006-0717-58

Tablet - Oral - 25 mg;100 mg

30's	$64.80	HYZAAR, Merck & Company Inc	00006-0747-31
30's	$66.60	HYZAAR, Physicians Total Care	54868-4341-00
100's	$206.30	HYZAAR, Merck & Company Inc	00006-0747-28
100's	$215.99	HYZAAR, Merck & Company Inc	00006-0747-58

Hydrochlorothiazide; Metoprolol Tartrate *(001460)*

Categories: Hypertension, essential; Pregnancy Category C; FDA Approved 1984 Dec
Drug Classes: Antiadrenergics, beta blocking; Diuretics, thiazide and derivatives
Brand Names: **Lopressor HCT**; Selokomb
Foreign Brand Availability: Beloc Comp (Austria; Germany); Betoprolol (Colombia); Co-Betaloc (England; Ireland); Seloken Retard Comp. (Austria); Selokomb 200 (Netherlands); Selokomb Zoc 100 (Netherlands); Selopres Zok (Mexico)
Cost of Therapy: $51.00 (Hypertension; Lopressor HCT ; 25 mg; 100 mg; 1 tablet/day; 30 day supply)

DESCRIPTION

Lopressor HCT has the antihypertensive effect of Lopressor, metoprolol tartrate, a selective $beta_1$-adrenoreceptor blocking agent, and the antihypertensive and diuretic actions of hydrochlorothiazide. It is available as tablets for oral administration. The 50/25 tablets contain 50 mg of metoprolol tartrate and 25 mg of hydrochlorothiazide; the 100/25 tablets contain 100 mg of metoprolol tartrate and 25 mg of hydrochlorothiazide; and the 100/50 tablets contain 100 mg of metoprolol tartrate and 50 mg of hydrochlorothiazide.

Metoprolol tartrate is (±)-1-isopropylamino-3-(*p*-(2-methoxyethyl)phenoxy)-2-propanol 2:1 *dextro*-tartrate salt.

FOR COMPLETE PRESCRIBING INFORMATION REFER TO THE INDIVIDUAL DRUG MONOGRAPHS (HYDROCHLOROTHIAZIDE; METOPROLOL TARTRATE).

INDICATIONS AND USAGE

Lopressor HCT is indicated for the management of hypertension.

This fixed-combination drug is not indicated for initial therapy of hypertension. If the fixed combination represents the dose titrated to the individual patient's needs, therapy with the fixed combination may be more convenient than with the separate components.

DOSAGE AND ADMINISTRATION

Dosage should be determined by individual titration.

Hydrochlorothiazide is usually given at a dosage of 25-100 mg/day. The usual initial dosage of Lopressor is 100 mg daily in single or divided doses. Dosage may be increased gradually until optimum blood pressure control is achieved. The effective dosage range is 100-450 mg/day. While once-daily dosing is effective and can maintain a reduction in blood pressure throughout the day, lower doses (especially 100 mg) may not maintain a full effect at the end of the 24 hour period, and larger or more frequent daily doses may be required. This can be evaluated by measuring blood pressure near the end of the dosing interval to determine whether satisfactory control is being maintained throughout the day. $Beta_1$ selectivity diminishes as dosage of Lopressor is increased.

The following dosage schedule may be used to administer from 100-200 mg of Lopressor per day and from 25-50 mg of hydrochlorothiazide per day (see TABLE 1).

TABLE 1

Lopressor HCT	Dosage
Tablets of 50/25	2 tablets per day in single or divided doses
Tablets of 100/25	1-2 tablets per day in single or divided doses
Tablets of 100/50	1 tablet per day in single or divided doses

Dosing regimens that exceed 50 mg of hydrochlorothiazide per day are not recommended. When necessary, another antihypertensive agent may be added gradually, beginning with 50% of the usual recommended starting dose to avoid an excessive fall in blood pressure.

STORAGE

Store between 15-30°C (59-86°F). Protect from moisture.

Dispense in tight, light-resistant container.

PRODUCT LISTING - EQUIVALENTS NOT AVAILABLE

Tablet - Oral - 25 mg;50 mg

100's	$108.79	LOPRESSOR HCT, Novartis Pharmaceuticals	00028-0035-01

Tablet - Oral - 25 mg;100 mg

100's	$170.00	LOPRESSOR HCT, Novartis Pharmaceuticals	00028-0053-01

Tablet - Oral - 50 mg;100 mg

100's	$180.29	LOPRESSOR HCT, Novartis Pharmaceuticals	00028-0073-01

Hydrochlorothiazide; Moexipril Hydrochloride *(003342)*

For complete prescribing information, refer to the CD-ROM included with the book.

Categories: Hypertension, essential; Pregnancy Category C, 1st Trimester; Pregnancy Category D, 2nd & 3rd Trimesters
Drug Classes: Angiotensin converting enzyme inhibitors; Diuretics, thiazide and derivatives
Brand Names: **Uniretic**
Cost of Therapy: $32.35 (Hypertension; Uniretic; 12.5 mg; 7.5 mg; 1 tablet/day; 30 day supply)

WARNING

Note: The trade name has been used throughout this monograph for clarity.

USE IN PREGNANCY

When used in pregnancy during the second and third trimesters, ACE inhibitors can cause injury and even death to the developing fetus. When pregnancy is detected, Uniretic should be discontinued as soon as possible. See WARNINGS, Fetal/Neonatal Morbidity and Mortality.

DESCRIPTION

Uniretic (moexipril hydrochloride/hydrochlorothiazide) is a combination of an angiotensin-converting enzyme (ACE) inhibitor, moexipril hydrochloride, and a diuretic, hydrochlorothiazide. Moexipril hydrochloride is a fine white to off-white powder. It is soluble (about 10% weight-to-volume) in distilled water at room temperature. It has the empirical formula $C_{27}H_{34}N_2O_7 \cdot HCl$ and a molecular weight of 535.04. It is chemically described as [3S-[2[R*(R*)],3R*]]-2-[2-[[1-(Ethoxycarbonyl)-3-phenyl-propyl]amino]-1-oxopropyl]-1,2,3,4-tetrahydro-6,7-dimethoxy-3-isoquinolinecarboxylic acid, monohydrochloride. Moexipril hydrochloride is a non-sulfhydryl containing precursor of the active ACE inhibitor moexiprilat.

Hydrochlorothiazide is a white, or practically white, crystalline powder. It is slightly soluble in water, freely soluble in sodium hydroxide solution, in n-butylamine and in dimethylformamide. Hydrochlorothiazide has the empirical formula $C_7H_8ClN_3O_4S_2$ and a molecular weight of 297.75. It is chemically described as 2*H*-1,2,4-Benzothiadiazine-7-sulfonamide,6-chloro-3,4-dihydro-,1,1-dioxide. Hydrochlorothiazide is a thiazide diuretic.

Uniretic is available for oral administration in three tablet strengths. The inactive ingredients in all strengths are lactose, magnesium oxide, crospovidone, magnesium stearate and gelatin. The film coating in all strengths contains hydroxypropyl methylcellulose, hydroxypropyl cellulose, polyethylene glycol 6000, magnesium stearate and titanium dioxide. In addition, the film coating for Uniretic 7.5/12.5 and Uniretic 15/25 contains ferric oxide.

INDICATIONS AND USAGE

Uniretic is indicated for treatment of patients with hypertension. **This fixed combination is not indicated for the initial therapy of hypertension (see DOSAGE AND ADMINISTRATION).**

In using Uniretic, consideration should be given to the fact that another ACE inhibitor, captopril, has caused agranulocytosis, particularly in patients with renal impairment or collagen-vascular disease. Available data are insufficient to show that Uniretic does not have a similar risk (see WARNINGS, Neutropenia/Agranulocytosis). In addition, ACE inhibitors, for which adequate data are available, cause a higher rate of angioedema in black than in nonblack patients (see WARNINGS, Anaphylactoid and Possibly Related Reactions, Angioedema).

H

CONTRAINDICATIONS

Uniretic is contraindicated in patients who are hypersensitive to any component of this product and in patients with a history of angioedema related to previous treatment with an ACE inhibitor. Because of the hydrochlorothiazide component, this product is contraindicated in patients with anuria or hypersensitivity to other sulfonamide-derived drugs. Hypersensitivity reactions are more likely to occur in patients with a history of allergy or bronchial asthma.

WARNINGS

ANAPHYLACTOID AND POSSIBLY RELATED REACTIONS

Presumably because angiotensin-converting enzyme inhibitors affect the metabolism of eicosanoids and polypeptides, including endogenous bradykinin, patients receiving ACE inhibitors, including Uniretic, may be subject to a variety of adverse reactions, some of them serious.

Angioedema

Angioedema involving the face, extremities, lips, tongue, glottis, and/or larynx has been reported in patients treated with ACE inhibitors, including moexipril. Symptoms suggestive of angioedema or facial edema occurred in <0.5% of moexipril-treated patients in placebo-controlled trials. None of the cases were considered life-threatening and all resolved either without treatment or with medication (antihistamines or glucocorticoids). One patient treated with hydrochlorothiazide alone experienced laryngeal edema. No instances of angioedema were reported in placebo-treated patients.

In cases of angioedema, treatment with Uniretic should be promptly discontinued and the patient carefully observed until the swelling disappears. In instances where swelling has been confined to the face and lips, the condition has generally resolved without treatment, although antihistamines have been useful in relieving symptoms.

Angioedema associated with involvement of the tongue, glottis, or larynx may be fatal due to airway obstruction. Appropriate therapy, *e.g.*, subcutaneous epinephrine solution 1:1000 (0.3-0.5 ml) and/or measures to ensure a patent airway, should be promptly provided.

Anaphylactoid Reactions During Desensitization

Two patients undergoing desensitizing treatment with hymenoptera venom while receiving ACE inhibitors sustained life-threatening anaphylactoid reactions. In the same patients, these reactions did not occur when ACE inhibitors were temporarily withheld, but they reappeared when the ACE inhibitors were inadvertently readministered.

Anaphylactoid Reactions During Membrane Exposure

Anaphylactoid reactions have been reported in patients dialyzed with high-flux membranes and treated concomitantly with an ACE inhibitor. Anaphylactoid reactions have also been reported in patients undergoing low-density lipoprotein apheresis with dextran sulfate absorption.

HYPOTENSION

Uniretic can cause symptomatic hypotension, although, as with other ACE inhibitors, this is unusual in uncomplicated hypertensive patients treated with Uniretic alone. Symptomatic hypotension is most likely to occur in patients who have been salt- and/or volume-depleted as a result of prolonged diuretic therapy, dietary salt restriction, dialysis, diarrhea, or vomiting. Volume- and/or salt-depletion should be corrected before initiating therapy with Uniretic.

The thiazide component of Uniretic may potentiate the action of other antihypertensive drugs, especially ganglionic or peripheral adrenergic-blocking drugs. The antihypertensive effects of the thiazide component may also be enhanced in the postsympathectomy patient.

In patients with congestive heart failure, with or without associated renal insufficiency, ACE inhibitor therapy may cause excessive hypotension, which may be associated with oliguria or progressive azotemia, and rarely, with acute renal failure and death. In these patients, Uniretic therapy should be started under close medical supervision, and patients should be followed closely for the first 2 weeks of treatment and whenever the dose of Uniretic is increased. Care in avoiding hypotension should also be taken in patients with ischemic heart disease, aortic stenosis, or cerebrovascular disease, in whom an excessive decrease in blood pressure could result in a myocardial infarction or a cerebrovascular accident.

If hypotension occurs, the patient should be placed in a supine position and, if necessary, treated with an intravenous infusion of normal saline. Uniretic treatment usually can be continued following restoration of blood pressure and volume.

IMPAIRED RENAL FUNCTION

Uniretic should be used with caution in patients with severe renal disease. Thiazide diuretics may precipitate azotemia in such patients and the effects of repeated dosing may be cumulative.

As a consequence of inhibition of the renin-angiotensin-aldosterone system, changes in renal function may be anticipated in susceptible individuals. There is no clinical experience of Uniretic in the treatment of hypertension in patients with renal failure.

Some hypertensive patients with no apparent preexisting renal vascular disease have developed increases in blood urea nitrogen and serum creatinine, usually minor and transient, especially when moexipril has been given concomitantly with a thiazide diuretic. This is more likely to occur in patients with preexisting renal impairment. There may be a need for dose adjustment of Uniretic. **Evaluation of hypertensive patients should always include assessment of renal function** (see DOSAGE AND ADMINISTRATION).

In hypertensive patients with severe congestive heart failure, whose renal function may depend on the activity of the renin-angiotensin-aldosterone system, treatment with ACE inhibitors, including moexipril, may be associated with oliguria and/or progressive azotemia and, rarely, acute renal failure and/or death.

In hypertensive patients with unilateral or bilateral renal artery stenosis, increases in blood urea nitrogen and serum creatinine have been observed in some patients following ACE inhibitor therapy. These increases were almost always reversible upon discontinuation of the ACE inhibitor and/or diuretic therapy. In such patients, renal function should be monitored during the first few weeks of therapy.

NEUTROPENIA/AGRANULOCYTOSIS

Another ACE inhibitor, captopril, has been shown to cause agranulocytosis and bone marrow depression, rarely in patients with uncomplicated hypertension, but more frequently in hypertensive patients with renal impairment, especially if they also have a collagen-vascular disease such as systemic lupus erythematosus or scleroderma. Although there were no instances of severe neutropenia (absolute neutrophil count $<500/mm^3$) among patients given moexipril, as with other ACE inhibitors, monitoring of white blood cell counts should be considered for patients who have collagen-vascular disease, especially if the disease is associated with impaired renal function. Available data from clinical trials of moexipril are insufficient to show that moexipril does not cause agranulocytosis at rates similar to captopril.

FETAL/NEONATAL MORBIDITY AND MORTALITY

ACE inhibitors can cause fetal and neonatal morbidity and death when administered to pregnant women. Several dozen cases have been reported in the world literature.When pregnancy is detected, ACE inhibitors should be discontinued as soon as possible.

The use of ACE inhibitors during the second and third trimesters of pregnancy has been associated with fetal and neonatal injury, including hypotension, neonatal skull hypoplasia, anuria, reversible or irreversible renal failure, and death. Oligohydramnios has also been reported, presumably resulting from decreased fetal renal function; oligohydramnios in this setting has been associated with fetal limb contractures, craniofacial deformation, and hypoplastic lung development. Prematurity, intrauterine growth retardation, and patent ductus arteriosus have also been reported, although it is not clear whether these were caused by the ACE inhibitor exposure.

Fetal and neonatal morbidity do not appear to have resulted from intrauterine ACE inhibitor exposure limited to the first trimester. Mothers who have used ACE inhibitors only during the first trimester should be informed of this. Nonetheless, when patients become pregnant, physicians should make every effort to discontinue the use of Uniretic as soon as possible.

Rarely (probably less often than once in every thousand pregnancies), no alternative to ACE inhibitors will be found. In these rare cases, the mothers should be apprised of the potential hazards to their fetuses, and serial ultrasound examinations should be performed to assess the intraamniotic environment.

If oligohydramnios is observed, Uniretic should be discontinued unless it is considered life-saving for the mother. Contraction stress testing (CST), a non-stress test (NST), or biophysical profiling (BPP) may be appropriate, depending upon the week of pregnancy. Patients and physicians should be aware, however, that oligohydramnios may not be detected until after the fetus has sustained irreversible injury.

Infants with histories of *in utero* exposure to ACE inhibitors should be closely observed for hypotension, oliguria, and hyperkalemia. If oliguria occurs, attention should be directed toward support of blood pressure and renal perfusion. Exchange transfusion or peritoneal dialysis may be required as means of reversing hypotension and/or substituting for disordered renal function. Theoretically, the ACE inhibitor could be removed from the neonatal circulation by exchange transfusion, but no experience with this procedure has been reported.

Intrauterine exposure to thiazide diuretics is associated with fetal or neonatal jaundice, thrombocytopenia, and possibly other adverse reactions that have occurred in adults.

Reproduction studies with the combination of moexipril HCl and hydrochlorothiazide (ratio 7.5:12.5) indicated that the combination possessed no teratogenic properties up to the lethal dose of 800 mg/kg/day in rats and up to the maternotoxic dose of 160 mg/kg/day in rabbits.

HEPATIC FAILURE

Rarely, ACE inhibitors have been associated with a syndrome that starts with cholestatic jaundice and progresses to fulminant hepatic necrosis and sometimes death. The mechanism of this syndrome is not understood. Patients receiving ACE inhibitors who develop jaundice or marked elevations of hepatic enzymes should discontinue the ACE Inhibitor and receive appropriate medical follow-up.

IMPAIRED HEPATIC FUNCTION

Uniretic should be used with caution in patients with impaired hepatic function or progressive liver disease, since minor alterations of fluid and electrolyte balance may precipitate hepatic coma. In patients with mild to moderate cirrhosis given single 15 mg doses of moexipril, the C_{max} of moexipril was increased by about 50% and the AUC increased by about 120%, while the C_{max} for moexiprilat was decreased by about 50% and the AUC increased by almost 300%. No formal pharmacokinetic studies have been carried out with Uniretic in hypertensive patients with impaired liver function.

SYSTEMIC LUPUS ERYTHEMATOSUS

Thiazide diuretics have been reported to cause exacerbation or activation of systemic lupus erythematosus.

DOSAGE AND ADMINISTRATION

Moexipril and hydrochlorothiazide are effective treatments for hypertension. The recommended dosage range of moexipril is 7.5 to 30 mg daily, administered in a single or two divided doses 1 hour before meals, while hydrochlorothiazide is effective in a dosage of 12.5 to 50 mg daily.

The side effects (see WARNINGS) of moexipril are generally rare and apparently independent of dose; those of hydrochlorothiazide are a mixture of dose-dependent phenomena (primarily hypokalemia) and dose-independent phenomena (*e.g.*, pancreatitis), the former much more common than the latter. Therapy with any combination of moexipril and hydrochlorothiazide will be associated with both sets of dose-independent side effects, but regimens in which moexipril is combined with low doses of hydrochlorothiazide produce minimal effects on serum potassium. In Uniretic controlled clinical trials, the average change in serum potassium was near zero in subjects who received 3.75/6.25 mg or 7.5/12.5

mg, but subjects who received 15/12.5 mg or 15/25 mg experienced a mild decrease in serum potassium, similar to that experienced by subjects who received the same dose of hydrochlorothiazide monotherapy. To minimize dose-independent side effects, it is usually appropriate to begin combination therapy only after a patient has failed to achieve the desired effect with monotherapy.

DOSE TITRATION GUIDED BY CLINICAL EFFECT

A patient whose blood pressure is not adequately controlled with either moexipril or hydrochlorothiazide monotherapy may be given Uniretic 7.5/12.5, Uniretic 15/12.5 or Uniretic 15/25 one hour before a meal. Further increases of moexipril, hydrochlorothiazide or both depend on clinical response. The hydrochlorothiazide dose should generally not be increased until 2-3 weeks have elapsed.

Total daily doses above 30 mg/50 mg a day have not been studied in hypertensive patients. Patients whose blood pressures are adequately controlled with 25 mg of hydrochlorothiazide daily, but who experience significant potassium loss with this regimen, may achieve blood pressure control without electrolyte disturbance if they are switched to moexipril 3.75 mg/hydrochlorothiazide 6.25 mg (one-half of the Uniretic 7.5/12.5 tablet). For patients who experience an excessive reduction in blood pressure with Uniretic 7.5/12.5, the physician may consider prescribing moexipril 3.75 mg/hydrochlorothiazide 6.25 mg.

REPLACEMENT THERAPY

The combination may be substituted for the titrated individual active ingredients.

USE IN RENAL IMPAIRMENT

The usual dosage regimen of Uniretic does not need to be adjusted as long as the patient's creatinine clearance is >40 ml/min/1.73 ^{2} (serum creatinine approximately ≤3 mg/dl or 265 µmol/L). In patients with more severe renal impairment, loop diuretics are preferred to thiazides, so Uniretic is not recommended.

PRODUCT LISTING - EQUIVALENTS NOT AVAILABLE

Tablet - Oral - 12.5 mg;7.5 mg

100's $107.83 UNIRETIC, Schwarz Pharma 00091-3712-01

Tablet - Oral - 12.5 mg;15 mg

100's $107.83 UNIRETIC, Schwarz Pharma 00091-3720-01

Tablet - Oral - 25 mg;15 mg

100's $107.83 UNIRETIC, Schwarz Pharma 00091-3725-01

Hydrochlorothiazide; Propranolol Hydrochloride *(001461)*

For complete prescribing information, refer to the CD-ROM included with the book.

Categories: Hypertension, essential; Pregnancy Category C; FDA Approval Pre 1982
Drug Classes: Antiadrenergics, beta blocking; Diuretics, thiazide and derivatives
Brand Names: **Inderide**; Inderide LA
Foreign Brand Availability: Artensol H (Colombia); Ciplar-H (India)
Cost of Therapy: $52.17 (Hypertension; Inderide; 25 mg; 80 mg; 1 tablet/day; 30 day supply)
$10.86 (Hypertension; Generic Tablets; 25 mg; 80 mg; 1 tablet/day; 30 day supply)
$42.65 (Hypertension; Inderide LA; 50 mg; 80 mg; 1 tablet/day; 30 day supply)

DESCRIPTION

Note: The trade names have been used throughout this monograph for clarity.

INDERIDE

Inderide tablets for oral administration combine two antihypertensive agents: Propranolol hydrochloride, a beta-adrenergic blocking agent, and hydrochlorothiazide, a thiazide diuretic-antihypertensive. Inderide 40/25 tablets contain 40 mg propranolol hydrochloride and 25 mg hydrochlorothiazide; Inderide 80/25 tablets contain 80 mg propranolol hydrochloride and 25 mg hydrochlorothiazide. Propranolol hydrochloride is a synthetic betaadrenergic receptor-blocking agent chemically described as 1-(isopropylamino)-3-(1-naphthyloxy)-2-propanol hydrochloride.

Propranolol hydrochloride is a stable, white, crystalline solid which is readily soluble in water and ethanol. Its molecular weight is 295.81.

Hydrochlorothiazide is a white, or practically white, practically odorless, crystalline powder. It is slightly soluble in water; freely soluble in sodium hydroxide solution; sparingly soluble in methanol; insoluble in ether, chloroform, benzene, and dilute mineral acids. Its chemical name is: 6-chloro-3,4-dihydro-2H-1,2,4-benzothiadiazine-7-sulfonamide 1,1-dioxide.

The inactive ingredients contained in Inderide tablets are lactose, magnesium stearate, microcrystalline cellulose, stearic acid, and yellow ferric oxide.

INDERIDE LA

Inderide LA is indicated in the once-daily management of hypertension.

Inderide LA combines two antihypertensive agents: Propranolol hydrochloride, a beta-adrenergic receptor-blocking agent, and hydrochlorothiazide, a thiazide diuretic-antihypertensive. Inderide LA is formulated to provide a sustained release of propranolol hydrochloride. Hydrochlorothiazide in Inderide LA exists in a conventional (not sustained-release) formulation.

Propranolol hydrochloride is a synthetic betaadrenergic receptor-blocking agent chemically described as 1-(Isopropylamino)-3-(1-naphthyloxy)-2-propanol hydrochloride. Propranolol hydrochloride is a stable, white, crystalline solid which is readily soluble in water and ethanol. Its molecular weight is 295.81.

Hydrochlorothiazide is a white, or practically white, practically odorless, crystalline powder. It is slightly soluble in water; freely soluble in sodium hydroxide solution; sparingly soluble in methanol; insoluble in ether, chloroform, benzene, and dilute mineral acids. Its chemical name is 6-Chloro-3, 4-dihydro-2H-1,2,4-benzothiadiazine-7-sulfonamide 1,1-dioxide.

Inderide LA contains the following inactive ingredients: calcium carbonate, ethylcellulose, gelatin capsules, hydroxypropyl methylcellulose, lactose, magnesium stearate, microcrystalline cellulose, sodium lauryl sulfate, sodium starch glycolate, titanium dioxide, and D&C yellow no. 10. In addition, Inderide LA 80/50 mg and 120/50 mg capsules contain D&C red no. 33; Inderide LA 120/50 mg and 160/50 mg capsules contain FD&C blue no. 1 and FD&C red no. 40.

INDICATIONS AND USAGE

INDERIDE

Inderide is indicated in the management of hypertension.

This fixed combination is not indicated for initial therapy of hypertension. Hypertension requires therapy titrated to the individual patient. If the fixed combination represents the dosage so determined, its use may be more convenient in patient management.

INDERIDE LA

Inderide LA is indicated in the management of hypertension.

This fixed-combination drug is not indicated for initial therapy of hypertension. Hypertension requires therapy titrated to the individual patient. If the fixed combination represents the dosage so determined, its use may be more convenient in patient management. The treatment of hypertension is not static, but must be reevaluated as conditions in each patient warrant.

CONTRAINDICATIONS

INDERIDE

Propranolol HCl

Propranolol is contraindicated in (1) cardiogenic shock; (2) sinus bradycardia and greater than first-degree block; (3) bronchial asthma; (4) congestive heart failure (see WARNINGS) unless the failure is secondary to a tachyarrhythmia treatable with propranolol.

Hydrochlorothiazide

Hydrochlorothiazide is contraindicated in patients with anuria or hypersensitivity to this or other sulfonamide-derived drugs.

INDERIDE LA

Propranolol HCl

Propranolol is contraindicated in: (1) cardiogenic shock; (2) sinus bradycardia and greater than first-degree block; (3) bronchial asthma; (4) congestive heart failure (see WARNINGS), unless the failure is secondary to a tachyarrhythmia treatable with propranolol.

Hydrochlorothiazide

Hydrochlorothiazide is contraindicated in patients with anuria or hypersensitivity to this or other sulfonamide-derived drugs.

WARNINGS

INDERIDE

Propranolol HCl

Cardiac Failure

Sympathetic stimulation is a vital component supporting circulatory function in congestive heart failure, and inhibition with beta blockade always carries the potential hazard of further depressing myocardial contractility and precipitating cardiac failure. Propranolol acts selectively without abolishing the inotropic action of digitalis on the heart muscle (*i.e.,* that of supporting the strength of myocardial contractions). In patients already receiving digitalis, the positive inotropic action of digitalis may be reduced by propranolol's negative inotropic effect. The effects of propranolol and digitalis are additive in depressing av conduction.

Patients Without a History of Heart Failure

Continued depression of the myocardium over a period of time can, in some cases, lead to cardiac failure. In rare instances, this has been observed during propranolol therapy. Therefore, at the first sign or symptom of impending cardiac failure, patients should be fully digitalized and/or given additional diuretic, and the response observed closely: (a) if cardiac failure continues, despite adequate digitalization and diuretic therapy, propranolol therapy should be withdrawn (gradually, if possible); (b) if tachyarrhythmia is being controlled, patients should be maintained on combined therapy and the patient closely followed until threat of cardiac failure is over.

Angina Pectoris

There have been reports of exacerbation of angina and, in some cases, myocardial infarction following abrupt discontinuation of propranolol therapy. Therefore, when discontinuance of propranolol is planned, the dosage should be gradually reduced and the patient should be carefully monitored. In addition, when propranolol is prescribed for angina pectoris, the patient should be cautioned against interruption or cessation of therapy without the physician's advice. If propranolol therapy is interrupted and exacerbation of angina occurs, it usually is advisable to reinstitute propranolol therapy and take other measures appropriate for the management of unstable angina pectoris. Since coronary artery disease may be unrecognized, it may be prudent to follow the above advice in patients considered at risk of having occult atherosclerotic heart disease, who are given propranolol for other indications.

Nonallergic Bronchospasm (e.g., chronic bronchitis, emphysema)

Patients with bronchospastic diseases should, in general, not receive beta blockers. Propranolol should be administered with caution since it may block bronchodilation produced by endogenous and exogenous catecholamine stimulation of beta receptors.

Major Surgery

The necessity or desirability of withdrawal of beta-blocking therapy prior to major surgery is controversial. It should be noted, however, that the impaired ability of the heart to respond to reflex adrenergic stimuli may augment the risks of general anesthesia and surgical procedures.

Propranolol, like other beta blockers, is a competitive inhibitor of beta-receptor agonists, and its effects can be reversed by administration of such agents, *e.g.*, dobutamine or isoproterenol. However, such patients may be subject to protracted severe hypotension. Difficulty in starting and maintaining the heartbeat has also been reported with beta blockers.

Diabetes and Hypoglycemia

Beta-adrenergic blockade may prevent the appearance of certain premonitory signs and symptoms (pulse rate and pressure changes) of acute hypoglycemia in labile insulin-dependent diabetes. In these patients, it may be more difficult to adjust the dosage of insulin. Hypoglycemic attack may be accompanied by a precipitous elevation of blood pressure in patients on propranolol.

Propranolol therapy, particularly in infants and children, diabetic or not, has been associated with hypoglycemia especially during fasting as in preparation for surgery. Hypoglycemia also has been found after this type of drug therapy and prolonged physical exertion and has occurred in renal insufficiency, both during dialysis and sporadically, in patients on propranolol.

Acute increases in blood pressure have occurred after insulin induced hypoglycemia in patients on propranolol.

Thyrotoxicosis

H

Beta blockade may mask certain clinical signs of hyperthyroidism. Therefore, abrupt withdrawal of propranolol may be followed by an exacerbation of symptoms of hyperthyroidism, including thyroid storm. Propranolol may change thyroid-function tests, increasing T4 and reverse T3, and decreasing T3.

Wolff-Parkinson-White Syndrome

Several cases have been reported in which, after propranolol, the tachycardia was replaced by a severe bradycardia requiring a demand pacemaker. In one case this resulted after an initial dose of 5 mg propranolol.

Hydrochlorothiazide

Thiazides should be used with caution in severe renal disease. In patients with renal disease, thiazides may precipitate azotemia. In patients with impaired renal function, cumulative effects of the drug may develop.

Thiazides should also be used with caution in patients with impaired hepatic function or progressive liver disease, since minor alterations of fluid and electrolyte balance may precipitate hepatic coma.

Thiazides may add to or potentiate the action of other antihypertensive drugs. Potentiation occurs with ganglionic or peripheral adrenergic-blocking drugs.

Sensitivity reactions may occur in patients with a history of allergy or bronchial asthma. The possibility of exacerbation or activation of systemic lupus erythematosus has been reported.

INDERIDE LA

Propranolol HCl

Cardiac Failure: Sympathetic stimulation may be a vital component supporting circulatory function in patients with congestive heart failure, and its inhibition by beta blockade may precipitate more severe failure. Although beta blockers should be avoided in overt congestive heart failure, if necessary, they can be used with close follow-up in patients with a history of failure who are well compensated and are receiving digitalis and diuretics. Beta-adrenergic blocking agents do not abolish the inotropic action of digitalis on heart muscle.

In Patients Without a History of Heart Failure, continued use of beta blockers can, in some cases, lead to cardiac failure. Therefore, at the first sign or symptom of heart failure, the patient should be digitalized and/or treated with diuretics, and the response observed closely, or propranolol should be discontinued (gradually, if possible).

In Patients With Angina Pectoris, there have been reports of exacerbation of angina and, in some cases, myocardial infarction, following abrupt discontinuance of propranolol therapy. Therefore, when discontinuance of propranolol is planned, the dosage should be gradually reduced and the patient carefully monitored. In addition, when propranolol is prescribed for angina pectoris, the patient should be cautioned against interruption or cessation of therapy without the physician's advice. If propranolol therapy is interrupted and exacerbation of angina occurs, it usually is advisable to reinstitute propranolol therapy and take other measures appropriate for the management of unstable angina pectoris. Since coronary artery disease may be unrecognized, it may be prudent to follow the above advice in patients considered at risk of having occult atherosclerotic heart disease who are given propranolol for other indications.

Thyrotoxicosis: Beta blockade may mask certain clinical signs of hyperthyroidism. Therefore, abrupt withdrawal of propranolol may be followed by an exacerbation of symptoms of hyperthyroidism, including thyroid storm. Propranolol does not distort thyroid function tests.

In Patients With Wolff-Parkinson-White Syndrome, several cases have been reported in which, after propranolol, the tachycardia was replaced by a severe bradycardia requiring a demand pacemaker. In one case this resulted after an initial dose of 5 mg propranolol.

Major Surgery: The necessity or desirability of withdrawal of beta-blocking therapy prior to major surgery is controversial. It should be noted, however, that the impaired ability of the heart to respond to reflex adrenergic stimuli may augment the risks of general anesthesia and surgical procedures.

Nonallergic Bronchospasm (e.g., chronic bronchitis, emphysema): PATIENTS WITH BRONCHOSPASTIC DISEASES SHOULD, IN GENERAL, NOT RECEIVE BETA BLOCKERS. Propranolol HCl should be administered with caution since it may block bronchodilation produced by endogenous and exogenous catecholamine stimulation of beta receptors.

Diabetes and Hypoglycemia: Beta-adrenergic blockade may prevent the appearance of certain premonitory signs and symptoms (pulse rate and pressure changes) of acute hypoglycemia in labile insulin-dependent diabetes. In these patients, it may be more difficult to adjust the dosage of insulin. Hypoglycemic attacks may be accompanied by a precipitous elevation of blood pressure in patients on propranolol.

Propranolol therapy, particularly in infants and children, diabetic or not, has been associated with hypoglycemia especially during fasting as in preparation for surgery. Hypoglycemia also has been found after this type of drug therapy and prolonged physical exertion and has occured in renal insufficiency, both during dialysis and sporadically, in patients on propranolol.

Acute increases in blood pressure have occurred after insulin-induced hypoglycemia in patients on propranolol.

Hydrochlorothiazide

Thiazides should be used with caution in severe renal disease. In patients with renal disease, thiazides may precipitate azotemia. In patients with impaired renal function, cumulative effects of the drug may develop. Thiazides should also be used with caution in patients with impaired hepatic function or progressive liver disease, since minor alterations of fluid and electrolyte balance may precipitate hepatic coma.

Thiazides may add to or potentiate the action of other antihypertensive drugs. Potentiation occurs with ganglionic or peripheral adrenergic-blocking drugs.

Sensitivity reactions may occur in patients with a history of allergy or bronchial asthma. The possibility of exacerbation or activation of systemic lupus erythematosus has been reported.

DOSAGE AND ADMINISTRATION

INDERIDE

The dosage must be determined by individual titration. Hydrochlorothiazide can be given at doses of 12.5 to 50 mg/day when used alone. The initial dose of propranolol is 80 mg daily, and it may be increased gradually until optimal blood pressure control is achieved. The usual effective dose when used alone is 160-480 mg/day.

One Inderide tablet twice daily can be used to administer up to 160 mg of propranolol and 50 mg of hydrochlorothiazide. For doses of propranolol greater than 160 mg the combination products are not appropriate, because their use would lead to an excessive dose of the thiazide component.

When necessary, another antihypertensive agent may be added gradually beginning with 50% of the usual recommended starting dose to avoid an excessive fall in blood pressure.

INDERIDE LA

The dosage must be determined by individual titration. Hydrochlorothiazide can be given at doses of 12.5 to 50 mg/day when used alone. The initial dose of propranolol is 80 mg daily, and it may be increased gradually until optimal blood pressure control is achieved. The usual effective dose, when used alone, is 160-480 mg/day.

One Inderide LA capsule once a day can be used to administer up to 160 mg of propranolol and 50 mg of hydrochlorothiazide. For doses of propranolol greater than 160 mg, the combination products are not appropriate because their use would lead to an excessive dose of the thiazide component.

Inderide LA provides propranolol HCl in a sustained-release form and hydrochlorothiazide in conventional formulation, for once-daily administration. If patients are switched from Inderide tablets (or propranolol HCl plus hydrochlorothiazide) to Inderide LA, care should be taken to ensure that the desired therapeutic effect is maintained. Inderide LA should not be considered a mg-for-mg substitute for Inderide or propranolol HCl plus hydrochlorothiazide. Inderide LA has different kinetics and produces lower blood levels. Retitration may be necessary, especially to maintain effectiveness at the end of the 24 hour dosing interval.

When necessary, another antihypertensive agent may be added gradually, beginning with 50% of the usual recommended starting dose, to avoid an excessive fall in blood pressure.

PRODUCT LISTING - RATED THERAPEUTICALLY EQUIVALENT

Tablet - Oral - 25 mg;40 mg

100's	$7.71	FEDERAL UPPER LIMIT, H.C.F.A. F F P	99999-1461-01
100's	$24.90	GENERIC, Ivax Corporation	00182-1833-01
100's	$26.50	GENERIC, Major Pharmaceuticals Inc	00904-0434-60
100's	$29.24	GENERIC, Major Pharmaceuticals Inc	00904-0434-61
100's	$31.12	GENERIC, Geneva Pharmaceuticals	00781-1431-01
100's	$31.12	GENERIC, Moore, H.L. Drug Exchange Inc	00839-7197-06
100's	$33.95	GENERIC, Mylan Pharmaceuticals Inc	00378-0731-01
100's	$33.95	GENERIC, Sidmak Laboratories Inc	50111-0473-01
100's	$35.58	GENERIC, Aligen Independent Laboratories Inc	00405-4894-01
100's	$40.70	GENERIC, Purepac Pharmaceutical Company	00228-2358-10
100's	$96.90	GENERIC, Major Pharmaceuticals Inc	00904-0434-80
100's	$138.44	INDERIDE, Wyeth-Ayerst Laboratories	00046-0484-81

Tablet - Oral - 25 mg;80 mg

100's	$11.70	FEDERAL UPPER LIMIT, H.C.F.A. F F P	99999-1461-04
100's	$36.20	GENERIC, Geneva Pharmaceuticals	00781-1432-01
100's	$36.52	GENERIC, Ivax Corporation	00182-1834-01
100's	$37.90	GENERIC, Major Pharmaceuticals Inc	00904-0438-60
100's	$38.47	GENERIC, Mutual/United Research Laboratories	00677-1107-01
100's	$38.48	GENERIC, Moore, H.L. Drug Exchange Inc	00839-7198-06
100's	$38.95	GENERIC, Aligen Independent Laboratories Inc	00405-4895-01
100's	$41.75	GENERIC, Mylan Pharmaceuticals Inc	00378-0347-01
100's	$41.75	GENERIC, Sidmak Laboratories Inc	50111-0474-01

100's	$45.40	GENERIC, Purepac Pharmaceutical Company	00228-2360-10
100's	$173.90	INDERIDE, Wyeth-Ayerst Laboratories	00046-0488-81

PRODUCT LISTING - EQUIVALENTS NOT AVAILABLE

Capsule, Extended Release - Oral - 50 mg;80 mg

30's	$42.65	INDERIDE LA, Pd-Rx Pharmaceuticals	55289-0485-30

Hydrochlorothiazide; Quinapril Hydrochloride *(003487)*

For complete prescribing information, refer to the CD-ROM included with the book.

Categories: Hypertension, essential; FDA Approved 2000 Jan; Pregnancy Category C, 1st Trimester; Pregnancy Category D, 2nd & 3rd Trimesters

Drug Classes: Angiotensin converting enzyme inhibitors; Diuretics, thiazide and derivatives

Foreign Brand Availability: Accuretic (Canada; Colombia; New-Zealand; Peru; Tanzania; Uganda; Zambia; Zimbabwe); Accuzide (Bahrain; Cyprus; Egypt; Germany; Iran; Iraq; Israel; Jordan; Kuwait; Lebanon; Libya; Oman; Qatar; Republic-of-Yemen; Saudi-Arabia; Syria; United-Arab-Emirates); Aculix (France; Mauritius)

Cost of Therapy: $35.61 (Hypertension; Accuretic; 12.5 mg; 10 mg; 1 tablet/day; 30 day supply)

WARNING

USE IN PREGNANCY

When used in pregnancy during the second and third trimesters, ACE inhibitors can cause injury and even death to the developing fetus. When pregnancy is detected, hydrochlorothiazide; quinapril should be discontinued as soon as possible. (See WARNINGS, Fetal/Neonatal Morbidity and Mortality.)

DESCRIPTION

Accuretic is a fixed-combination tablet that combines an angiotensin-converting enzyme (ACE) inhibitor, quinapril hydrochloride, and a thiazide diuretic, hydrochlorothiazide.

Quinapril hydrochloride is chemically described as [3S-[2[R*(R*)],3R*]]-2-[2-[[1-(ethoxycarbonyl)-3-phenylpropyl]amino]-1-oxopropyl]-1,2,3,4-tetrahydro-3-isoquinolinecarboxylic acid, monohydrochloride. Its empirical formula is $C_{25}H_{30}N_2O_5{\cdot}HCl$.

Quinapril hydrochloride is a white to off-white amorphous powder that is freely soluble in aqueous solvents.

Hydrochlorothiazide is chemically described as: 6-Chloro-3,4-dihydro-2H-1,2,4-benzothiadiazine-7-sulfonamide 1,1-dioxide. Its empirical formula is $C_7H_8ClN_3O_4S_2$.

Hydrochlorothiazide is a white to off-white, crystalline powder which is slightly soluble in water but freely soluble in sodium hydroxide solution.

Accuretic is available for oral use as fixed combination tablets in 3 strengths of quinapril with hydrochlorothiazide: 10 mg with 12.5 mg (Accuretic 10/12.5), 20 mg with 12.5 mg (Accuretic 20/12.5), and 20 mg with 25 mg (Accuretic 20/25). Inactive ingredients: candelilla wax, crospovidone, hydroxypropyl cellulose, hydroxypropylmethyl cellulose, iron oxide red, iron oxide yellow, lactose, magnesium carbonate, magnesium stearate, polyethylene glycol, povidone, and titanium dioxide.

INDICATIONS AND USAGE

Hydrochlorothiazide; quinapril is indicated for the treatment of hypertension. This fixed combination is not indicated for the initial therapy of hypertension (see DOSAGE AND ADMINISTRATION).

In using hydrochlorothiazide; quinapril, consideration should be given to the fact that another angiotensin-converting enzyme inhibitor, captopril, has caused agranulocytosis, particularly in patients with renal impairment or collagen vascular disease. Available data are insufficient to show that quinapril does not have a similar risk (see WARNINGS: Neutropenia/Agranulocytosis).

ANGIOEDEMA IN BLACK PATIENTS

Black patients receiving ACE inhibitor monotherapy have been reported to have a higher incidence of angioedema compared to non-blacks. It should also be noted that in controlled clinical trials, ACE inhibitors have an effect on blood pressure that is less in black patients than in non-blacks.

CONTRAINDICATIONS

Hydrochlorothiazide; quinapril is contraindicated in patients who are hypersensitive to quinapril or hydrochlorothiazide and in patients with a history of angioedema related to previous treatment with an ACE inhibitor.

Because of the hydrochlorothiazide components, this product is contraindicated in patients with anuria or hypersensitivity to other sulfonamide-derived drugs.

WARNINGS

ANAPHYLACTOID AND POSSIBLY RELATED REACTIONS

Presumably because angiotensin converting inhibitors affect the metabolism of eicosanoids and polypeptides, including endogenous bradykinin, patients receiving ACE inhibitors (including quinapril) may be subject to a variety of adverse reactions, some of them serious.

ANGIOEDEMA

Angioedema of the face, extremities, lips, tongue, glottis, and larynx has been reported in patients treated with ACE inhibitors and has been seen in 0.1% of patients receiving quinapril. In two similarly sized US postmarketing quinapril trials that, combined, enrolled over 3,000 black patients and over 19,000 non-blacks, angioedema was reported in 0.30% and 0.55% of blacks (in Study 1 and 2, respectively) and 0.39% and 0.17% of non-blacks.

Angioedema associated with laryngeal edema can be fatal. If laryngeal stridor or angioedema of the face, tongue, or glottis occurs, treatment with hydrochlorothiazide; quinapril should be discontinued immediately, the patient treated in accordance with accepted medical care, and carefully observed until the swelling disappears. In instances where swelling is confined to the face and lips, the condition generally resolves without treatment; antihistamines may be useful in relieving symptoms. **Where there is involvement of the tongue, glottis, or larynx likely to cause airway obstruction, emergency therapy including, but not limited to, subcutaneous epinephrine solution 1:1000 (0.3-0.5 ml) should be promptly administered.**

PATIENTS WITH A HISTORY OF ANGIOEDEMA

Patients with a history of angioedema unrelated to ACE inhibitor therapy may be at increased risk of angioedema while receiving an ACE inhibitor (see also CONTRAINDICATIONS).

ANAPHYLACTOID REACTIONS DURING DESENSITIZATION

Two patients undergoing desensitizing treatment with Hymenoptera venom while receiving ACE inhibitors sustained life-threatening anaphylactoid reactions. In the same patients, these reactions were avoided when ACE inhibitors were temporarily withheld, but they reappeared upon inadvertent challenge.

ANAPHYLACTOID REACTIONS DURING MEMBRANE EXPOSURE

Anaphylactoid reactions have been reported in patients dialyzed with high-flux membranes and treated concomitantly with an ACE inhibitor. Anaphylactoid reactions have also been reported in patients undergoing low-density lipoprotein apheresis with dextran sulfate absorption.

HEPATIC FAILURE

Rarely, ACE inhibitors have been associated with a syndrome that starts with cholestatic jaundice and progresses to fulminant hepatic necrosis and (sometimes) death. The mechanism of this syndrome is not understood. Patients receiving ACE inhibitors who develop jaundice or marked elevations of hepatic enzymes should discontinue the ACE inhibitor and receive appropriate medical follow-up.

HYPOTENSION

Hydrochlorothiazide; quinapril can cause symptomatic hypotension, probably not more frequently than either monotherapy. It was reported in 1.2% of 1571 patients receiving hydrochlorothiazide; quinapril during clinical trials. Like other ACE inhibitors, quinapril has been only rarely associated with hypotension in uncomplicated hypertensive patients.

Symptomatic hypotension sometimes associated with oliguria and/or progressive azotemia, and rarely acute renal failure and/or death, include patients with the following conditions or characteristics: heart failure, hyponatremia, high dose diuretic therapy, recent intensive diuresis or increase in diuretic dose, renal dialysis or severe volume and/or salt depletion of any etiology. Volume and/or salt depletion should be corrected before initiating therapy with hydrochlorothiazide; quinapril.

Hydrochlorothiazide; quinapril should be used cautiously in patients receiving concomitant therapy with other antihypertensives. The thiazide component of hydrochlorothiazide; quinapril may potentiate the action of other antihypertensive drugs, especially ganglionic or peripheral adrenergic-blocking drugs. The antihypertensive effects of the thiazide component may also be enhanced in the postsympathectomy patients.

In patients at risk of excessive hypotension, therapy with hydrochlorothiazide; quinapril should be started under close medical supervision. Such patients should be followed closely for the first 2 weeks of treatment and whenever the dosage of quinapril or diuretic is increased. Similar considerations may apply to patients with ischemic heart or cerebrovascular disease in whom an excessive fall in blood pressure could result in myocardial infarction or cerebrovascular accident.

If excessive hypotension occurs, the patient should be placed in a supine position and, if necessary, treated with intravenous infusion of normal saline. Hydrochlorothiazide; quinapril treatment usually can be continued following restoration of blood pressure and volume. If symptomatic hypotension develops, a dose reduction or discontinuation of hydrochlorothiazide; quinapril may be necessary.

IMPAIRED RENAL FUNCTION

Hydrochlorothiazide; quinapril should be used with caution in patients with severe renal disease. Thiazides may precipitate azotemia in such patients, and the effects of repeated dosing may be cumulative.

When the renin-angiotensin-aldosterone system is inhibited by quinapril, changes in renal function may be anticipated in susceptible individuals. In patients with severe congestive heart failure, whose renal function may depend on the activity of the renin-angiotensin-aldosterone system, treatment with angiotensin-converting enzyme inhibitors (including quinapril) may be associated with oliguria and/or progressive azotemia and (rarely) with acute renal failure and/or death.

In clinical studies in hypertensive patients with unilateral renal artery stenosis, treatment with ACE inhibitors was associated with increases in blood urea nitrogen and serum creatinine; these increases were reversible upon discontinuation of ACE inhibitor, concomitant diuretic, or both. When such patients are treated with hydrochlorothiazide; quinapril, renal function should be monitored during the first few weeks of therapy.

Some quinapril-treated hypertensive patients with no apparent preexisting renal vascular diseases have developed increases in blood urea nitrogen and serum creatinine, usually minor and transient, especially when quinapril has been given concomitantly with a diuretic. This is more likely to occur in patients with pre-existing renal impairment. Dosage reduction of hydrochlorothiazide; quinapril may be required. **Evaluation of the hypertensive patients should also include assessment of the renal function (see DOSAGE AND ADMINISTRATION).**

H

NEUTROPENIA/AGRANULOCYTOSIS

Another ace inhibitor, captopril, has been shown to cause agranulocytosis and bone marrow depression rarely in patients with uncomplicated hypertension, but more frequently in patients with renal impairment, especially if they also have a collagen vascular disease, such as systemic lupus erythematosus or scleroderma. Agranulocytosis did occur during quinapril treatment in 1 patient with a history of neutropenia during previous captopril therapy. Available data from clinical trials of quinapril are insufficient to show that, in patients without prior reactions to other ace inhibitors, quinapril does not cause agranulocytosis at similar rates. As with other ace inhibitors, periodic monitoring of white blood cell counts in patients with collagen vascular disease and/or renal disease should be considered.

FETAL/NEONATAL MORBIDITY AND MORTALITY

ACE inhibitors can cause fetal and neonatal morbidity and death when administered to pregnant women. Several dozen cases have been reported in the world literature. When pregnancy is detected, hydrochlorothiazide; quinapril should be discontinued as soon as possible.

The use of ACE inhibitors during the second and third trimesters of pregnancy has been associated with fetal and neonatal injury, including hypotension, neonatal skull hypoplasia, anuria, reversible or irreversible renal failure, and death. Oligohydramnios has also been reported, presumably resulting from decreased fetal renal function; oligohydramnios in this setting has been associated with fetal limb contractures, craniofacial deformation, and hypoplastic lung development. Prematurity, intrauterine growth retardation, and patent ductus arteriosus have also been reported, although it is not clear whether these occurrences were due to the ACE inhibitor exposure.

H

These adverse effects do not appear to have resulted from intrauterine ACE inhibitor exposure that has been limited to the first trimester. Mothers whose embryos and fetuses are exposed to ACE inhibitors only during the first trimester should be so informed. Nonetheless, when patients become pregnant, physicians should make every effort to discontinue the use of quinapril as soon as possible.

Rarely (probably less often than once in every thousand pregnancies), no alternative to ACE inhibitors will be found. In these rare cases, the mothers should be apprised of the potential hazards to their fetuses, and serial ultrasound examinations should be performed to assess the intra-amniotic environment.

If oligohydramnios is observed, quinapril should be discontinued unless it is considered life-saving for the mother. Contraction stress testing (CST), a nonstress test (NST), or biophysical profiling (BPP) may be appropriate, depending upon the week of pregnancy. Patients and physicians should be aware, however, that oligohydramnios may not appear until after the fetus has sustained irreversible injury.

Infants with histories of *in utero* exposure to ACE inhibitors should be closely observed for hypotension, oliguria, and hyperkalemia. If oliguria occurs, attention should be directed toward support of blood pressure and renal perfusion. Exchange transfusion or peritoneal dialysis may be required as a means of reversing hypotension and/or substituting for disordered renal function. Removal of quinapril, which crosses the placenta, from the neonatal circulation is not significantly accelerated by these means.

Intrauterine exposure to thiazide diuretics is associated with fetal or neonatal jaundice, thrombocytopenia, and possibly other adverse reactions that occurred in adults.

No teratogenic effects of quinapril were seen in studies of pregnant rats and rabbits. On a mg/kg basis, the doses used were up to 180 times (in rats) and one time (in rabbits) the maximum recommended human dose. No teratogenic effects of hydrochlorothiazide; quinapril were seen in studies of pregnant rats and rabbits. On a mg/kg (hydrochlorothiazide; quinapril) basis, the doses used were up to 188/94 times (in rats) and 0.6/0.3 times (in rabbits) the maximum recommended human dose.

IMPAIRED HEPATIC FUNCTION

Hydrochlorothiazide; quinapril should be used with caution in patients with impaired hepatic function or progressive liver disease, since minor alterations of fluid and electrolyte balance may precipitate hepatic coma. Also, since the metabolism of quinapril to quinaprilat is normally dependent upon hepatic esterases, patients with impaired liver function could develop markedly elevated plasma levels of quinapril. No normal pharmacokinetic studies have been carried out in hypertensive patients with impaired liver function.

SYSTEMIC LUPUS ERYTHEMATOSUS

Thiazide diuretics have been reported to cause exacerbation or activation of systemic lupus erythematosus.

DOSAGE AND ADMINISTRATION

As individual monotherapy, quinapril is an effective treatment of hypertension in once-daily doses of 10 to 80 mg and hydrochlorothiazide is effective in doses of 12.5-50 mg. In clinical trials of hydrochlorothiazide; quinapril combination therapy using hydrochlorothiazide doses of 6.25-25 mg andquinapril doses of 2.5-40 mg, the antihypertensive effects increased with increasing dose of either component.

The side effects (see WARNINGS) of quinapril are generally rare and apparently independent of dose; those of hydrochlorothiazide are a mixture of dose-dependent phenomena (primarily hypokalemia) and dose-independent phenomena (*e.g.*, pancreatitis), the former much more common than the latter. Therapy with any combination of hydrochlorothiazide and quinapril will be associated with both sets of dose-independent side effects, but regimens that combine low doses of hydrochlorothiazide with quinapril produce minimal effects on serum potassium. In clinical trials of hydrochlorothiazide; quinapril, the average change in serum potassium was near zero in subjects who received HCTZ 6.25 mg in the combination, and the average subject who received 10-40/12.5-25 mg experienced a milder reduction in serum potassium than that experienced by the average subject receiving the same dose of hydrochlorothiazide monotherapy.

To minimize dose-independent side effects, it is usually appropriate to begin combination therapy only after a patient has failed to achieve the desired effect with monotherapy.

THERAPY GUIDED BY CLINICAL EFFECT

Patients whose blood pressures are not adequately controlled with quinapril monotherapy may instead be given hydrochlorothiazide; quinapril 12.5/10 or 12.5/20. Further increases of either or both components could depend on clinical response. The hydrochlorothiazide dose should generally not be increased until 2-3 weeks have elapsed. Patients whose blood pressures are adequately controlled with 25 mg of daily hydrochlorothiazide, but who experience significant potassium loss with this regimen, may achieve blood pressure control with less electrolyte disturbance if they are switched to hydrochlorothiazide; quinapril 12.5/10 or 12.5/20.

REPLACEMENT THERAPY

For convenience, patients who are adequately treated with 20 mg of quinapril and 25 mg of hydrochlorothiazide and experience no significant electrolyte disturbances may instead wish to receive hydrochlorothiazide; quinapril 25/20.

USE IN RENAL IMPAIRMENT

Regimens of therapy with hydrochlorothiazide; quinapril need not take account of renal function as long as the patient's creatinine clearance is >30 ml/min/1.73 m^2 (serum creatinine roughly ≤3 mg/dl or 265 μmol/L). In patients with more severe renal impairment, loop diuretics are preferred to thiazides. Therefore, hydrochlorothiazide; quinapril is not recommended for use in these patients.

PRODUCT LISTING - EQUIVALENTS NOT AVAILABLE

Tablet - Oral - 10 mg;12.5 mg			
30's	$33.76	ACCURETIC, Parke-Davis	00071-0222-06
90's	$106.84	ACCURETIC, Pfizer U.S. Pharmaceuticals	00071-0222-23
Tablet - Oral - 20 mg;12.5 mg			
30's	$33.76	ACCURETIC, Parke-Davis	00071-0220-06
90's	$106.84	ACCURETIC, Pfizer U.S. Pharmaceuticals	00071-0220-23
Tablet - Oral - 20 mg;25 mg			
90's	$106.84	ACCURETIC, Pfizer U.S. Pharmaceuticals	00071-0223-23

Hydrochlorothiazide; Telmisartan *(002215)*

For complete prescribing information, refer to the CD-ROM included with the book.

Categories: Hypertension, essential; FDA Approved 2000 Nov; Pregnancy Category C, 1st Trimester; Pregnancy Category D, 2nd & 3rd Trimesters
Drug Classes: Angiotensin II receptor antagonists; Diuretics, thiazide and derivatives
Brand Names: **Micardis HCT**
Foreign Brand Availability: Micardis Plus (Philippines); Pritorplus (France)
Cost of Therapy: $49.13 (Hypertension; Micardis HCT; 12.5 mg; 40 mg; 1 tablet/day; 30 day supply)

WARNING

USE IN PREGNANCY

When used in pregnancy during the second and third trimesters, drugs that act directly on the renin-angiotensin system can cause injury and even death to the developing fetus. When pregnancy is detected, hydrochlorothiazide; telmisartan tablets should be discontinued as soon as possible (see WARNINGS, Fetal/Neonatal Morbidity and Mortality).

DESCRIPTION

Micardis HCT is a combination of telmisartan, an orally active angiotensin II antagonist acting on the AT_1 receptor subtype, and hydrochlorothiazide, a diuretic.

Telmisartan, a nonpeptide molecule, is chemically described as 4′-[(1,4′-dimethyl-2′-propyl[2,6′-bi-1H-benzimidazol]-1′-yl]-[1,1′-biphenyl]-2-carboxylic acid. Its empirical formula is $C_{33}H_{30}N_4O_2$, and its molecular weight is 514.63.

Telmisartan is a white to off-white, odorless crystalline powder. It is practically insoluble in water and in the pH range of 3-9, sparingly soluble in strong acid (except insoluble in hydrochloric acid), and soluble in strong base.

Hydrochlorothiazide is a white, or practically white, practically odorless, crystalline powder with a molecular weight of 297.74. It is slightly soluble in water, and freely soluble in sodium hydroxide solution. Hydrochlorothiazide is chemically described as 6-chloro-3,4-dihydro-2*H*-2,4-benzothiadiazine-7-sulfonamide 1,1-dioxide. Its empirical formula is $C_7H_8ClN_3O_4S_2$.

Micardis HCT tablets are formulated for oral administration with a combination of 40 or 80 mg of telmisartan and 12.5 mg hydrochlorothiazide. The tablets contain the following inactive ingredients: sodium hydroxide, meglumine, povidone, sorbitol, magnesium stearate, lactose monohydrate, microcrystalline cellulose, maize starch, iron oxide red, sodium starch glycolate. Micardis HCT tablets are hygroscopic and require protection from moisture.

INDICATIONS AND USAGE

Hydrochlorothiazide; telmisartan is indicated for the treatment of hypertension. This fixed dose combination is not indicated for initial therapy (see DOSAGE AND ADMINISTRATION).

CONTRAINDICATIONS

Hydrochlorothiazide; telmisartan is contraindicated in patients who are hypersensitive to any component of this product.

Because of the hydrochlorothiazide component, this product is contraindicated in patients with anuria or hypersensitivity to other sulfonamide-derived drugs.

WARNINGS

FETAL/NEONATAL MORBIDITY AND MORTALITY

Drugs that act directly on the renin-angiotensin system can cause fetal and neonatal morbidity and death when administered to pregnant women. Several dozen cases have been reported in the world literature in patients who were taking angiotensin converting enzyme inhibitors. When pregnancy is detected, hydrochlorothiazide; telmisartan tablets should be discontinued as soon as possible.

The use of drugs that act directly on the renin-angiotensin system during the second and third trimesters of pregnancy has been associated with fetal and neonatal injury, including hypotension, neonatal skull hypoplasia, anuria, reversible or irreversible renal failure, and death. Oligohydramnios has also been reported, presumably resulting from decreased fetal renal function; oligohydramnios in this setting has been associated with fetal limb contractures, craniofacial deformation, and hypoplastic lung development. Prematurity, intrauterine growth retardation, and patent ductus arteriosus have also been reported, although it is not clear whether these occurrences were due to exposure to the drug.

These adverse effects do not appear to have resulted from intrauterine drug exposure that has been limited to the first trimester. Mothers whose embryos and fetuses are exposed to an angiotensin II receptor antagonist only during the first trimester should be so informed. Nonetheless, when patients become pregnant, physicians should have the patient discontinue the use of hydrochlorothiazide; telmisartan tablets as soon as possible.

Rarely (probably less often than once in every 1000 pregnancies), no alternative to an angiotensin II receptor antagonist will be found. In these rare cases, the mothers should be apprised of the potential hazards to their fetuses, and serial ultrasound examination should be performed to assess the intra-amniotic environment.

If oligohydramnios is observed, hydrochlorothiazide; telmisartan tablets should be discontinued unless they are considered life-saving for the mother. Contraction stress testing (CST), a non-stress test (NTS), or biophysical profiling (BPP) may be appropriate, depending upon the week of pregnancy. Patients and physicians should be aware, however, that oligohydramnios may not appear until after the fetus has sustained irreversible injury.

Infants with histories of *in utero* exposure to an angiotensin II receptor antagonist should be closely observed for hypotension, oliguria, and hyperkalemia. If oliguria occurs, attention should be directed toward support of blood pressure and renal perfusion. Exchange transfusion or dialysis may be required as a means of reversing hypotension and/or substituting for disordered renal function.

TELMISARTAN AND HYDROCHLOROTHIAZIDE IN ANIMALS

A developmental toxicity study was performed in rats with hydrochlorothiazide; telmisartan doses of 1.0/3.2, 4.7/15, 15.6/50, and 15.6/0 mg/kg/day. Although the two higher dose combinations appeared to be more toxic (significant decrease in body weight gain) to the dams than either drug alone, there did not appear to be an increase in toxicity to the developing embryos.

TELMISARTAN IN ANIMALS

No teratogenic effects were observed when telmisartan was administered to pregnant rats at oral doses of up to 50 mg/kg/day and to pregnant rabbits at oral doses up to 45 mg/kg/day. In rabbits, embryolethality associated with maternal toxicity (reduced body weight gain and food consumption) was observed at 45 mg/kg/day [about 12 times the maximum recommended human dose (MRHD) of 80 mg on a mg/m^2 basis]. In rats, maternally toxic (reduction in body weight gain and food consumption) telmisartan doses of 15 mg/kg/day (about 1.9 times the MRHD on a mg/m^2 basis), administered during late gestation and lactation, were observed to produce adverse effects in neonates, including reduced viability, low birth weight, delayed maturation, and decreased weight gain. Telmisartan has been shown to be present in rat fetuses during late gestation and in rat milk. The no observed effect doses for developmental toxicity in rats and rabbits, 5 and 15 mg/kg/day, respectively, are about 0.64 and 3.7 times, on a mg/m^2 basis, the MRHD dose of telmisartan (80 mg/day).

HYDROCHLOROTHIAZIDE IN ANIMALS

Studies in which hydrochlorothiazide was administered to pregnant mice and rats during their respective periods of major organogenesis at doses up to 3000 and 1000 mg/kg/day, respectively, provided no evidence of harm to the fetus.

Thiazides cross the placental barrier and appear in cord blood. There is a risk of fetal or neonatal jaundice, thrombocytopenia, and possibly other adverse reactions that have occurred in adults.

HYPOTENSION IN VOLUME-DEPLETED PATIENTS

Initiation of antihypertensive therapy in patients whose renin-angiotensin system are activated such as patients who are intravascular volume- or sodium-depleted, *e.g.,* in patients treated vigorously with diuretics, should only be approached cautiously. These conditions should be corrected prior to administration of hydrochlorothiazide; telmisartan. Treatment should be started under close medical supervision (see DOSAGE AND ADMINISTRATION). If hypotension occurs, the patients should be placed in the supine position and, if necessary, given an intravenous infusion of normal saline. A transient hypotensive response is not a contraindication to further treatment which usually can be continued without difficulty once the blood pressure has stabilized.

HYDROCHLOROTHIAZIDE

Hepatic Impairment: Thiazide diuretics should be used with caution in patients with impaired hepatic function or progressive liver disease, since minor alterations of fluid and electrolyte balance may precipitate hepatic coma.

Hypersensitivity Reaction: Hypersensitivity reactions to hydrochlorothiazide may occur in patients with or without a history of allergy or bronchial asthma, but are more likely in patients with such a history.

Systemic Lupus Erythematosus: Thiazide diuretics have been reported to cause exacerbation or activation of systemic lupus erythematosus.

Lithium Interaction: Lithium generally should not be given with thiazides.

DOSAGE AND ADMINISTRATION

The usual starting dose of telmisartan is 40 mg once a day; blood pressure response is dose related over the range of 20-80 mg. Patients with depletion of intravascular volume should have the condition corrected or telmisartan tablets should be initiated under close medical supervision (see WARNINGS, Hypotension in Volume Depleted Patients). Patients with biliary obstructive disorders or hepatic insufficiency should have treatment started under close medical supervision.

Hydrochlorothiazide is effective in doses of 12.5 to 50 mg once daily.

To minimize dose-independent side effects, it is usually appropriate to begin combination therapy only after a patient has failed to achieve the desired effect with monotherapy. The side effects (see WARNINGS) of telmisartan are generally rare and apparently independent of dose; those of hydrochlorothiazide are a mixture of dose-dependent phenomena (primarily hypokalemia) and dose-independent phenomena (*e.g.,* pancreatitis), the former much more common than the latter. Therapy with any combination of telmisartan and hydrochlorothiazide will be associated with both sets of dose-independent side effects.

Hydrochlorothiazide; telmisartan tablets may be administered with other antihypertensive agents.

Hydrochlorothiazide; telmisartan tablets may be administered with or without food.

REPLACEMENT THERAPY

The combination may be substituted for the titrated components.

DOSE TITRATION BY CLINICAL EFFECT

Micardis HCT is available as tablets containing either telmisartan 40 or 80 mg and hydrochlorothiazide 12.5 mg. A patient whose blood pressure is not adequately controlled with telmisartan monotherapy 80 mg (see above) may be switched to hydrochlorothiazide 12.5 mg/telmisartan 80 mg once daily, and finally titrated up to 25/160 mg, if necessary.

A patient whose blood pressure is inadequately controlled by 25 mg once daily of hydrochlorothiazide, or is controlled but who experiences hypokalemia with this regimen, may be switched to hydrochlorothiazide 12.5 mg/telmisartan 80 mg once daily, reducing the dose of hydrochlorothiazide without reducing the overall expected antihypertensive response. The clinical response to hydrochlorothiazide; telmisartan should be subsequently evaluated and if blood pressure remains uncontrolled after 2-4 weeks of therapy, the dose may be titrated up to 160/25 mg, if necessary.

PATIENTS WITH RENAL IMPAIRMENT

The usual regimens of therapy with hydrochlorothiazide; telmisartan may be followed as long as the patient's creatinine clearance is >30 ml/min. In patients with more severe renal impairment, loop diuretics are preferred to thiazides, so hydrochlorothiazide; telmisartan it not recommended.

PATIENTS WITH HEPATIC IMPAIRMENT

Hydrochlorothiazide; telmisartan is not recommended for patients with severe hepatic impairment. Patients with biliary obstructive disorders or hepatic insufficiency should have treatment started under close medical supervision using the 12.5/40 mg combination.

PRODUCT LISTING - EQUIVALENTS NOT AVAILABLE

Tablet - Oral - 12.5 mg;40 mg

7 x 4	$45.85	MICARDIS HCT, Abbott Pharmaceutical	00597-0043-28

Tablet - Oral - 12.5 mg;80 mg

7 x 4	$48.08	MICARDIS HCT, Abbott Pharmaceutical	00597-0044-28

Hydrochlorothiazide; Timolol Maleate *(001464)*

For complete prescribing information, refer to the CD-ROM included with the book.

Categories: Hypertension, essential; Pregnancy Category C; FDA Approval Pre 1982
Drug Classes: Antiadrenergics, beta blocking; Diuretics, thiazide and derivatives
Brand Names: Timolide
Cost of Therapy: $48.72 (Hypertension; Timolide; 25 mg; 10 mg; 2 tablets/day; 30 day supply)

DESCRIPTION

Timolide (hydrochlorothiazide; timolol maleate) is for the treatment of hypertension. It combines the antihypertensive activity of two agents: a non-selective beta-adrenergic receptor blocking agent (timolol maleate) and a diuretic (hydrochlorothiazide).

Timolol maleate is (*S*)-1-[(1,1-dimethylethyl)amino]-3-[[4-(4-morpholinyl)-1,2,5-thiadiazol-3-yl]oxy]-2-propanol(*Z*)-2-butenedioate (1:1) salt. Its empirical formula is $C_{13}H_{24}N_4O_3S{\cdot}C_4H_4O_4$.

Timolol maleate has a molecular weight of 432.50. It is a white, odorless, crystalline powder which is soluble in water, methanol, and alcohol.

Hydrochlorothiazide is 6-chloro-3,4-dihydro-2*H*-1,2,4-benzothiadiazine-7-sulfonamide 1,1-dioxide. Its empirical formula is $C_7H_8ClN_3O_4S_2$.

Hydrochlorothiazide has a molecular weight of 297.73. It is a white, or practically white, crystalline powder which is slightly soluble in water, but freely soluble in sodium hydroxide solution.

Timolide is supplied as tablets containing 10 mg of timolol maleate and 25 mg of hydrochlorothiazide for oral administration. Inactive ingredients are cellulose, FD&C blue 2, magnesium stearate, and starch.

INDICATIONS AND USAGE

Hydrochlorothiazide; timolol maleate is indicated for the treatment of hypertension.

This fixed combination drug is not indicated for initial therapy of hypertension. If the fixed combination represents the dose titrated to an individual patient's needs, it may be more convenient than the separate components.

CONTRAINDICATIONS

Hydrochlorothiazide; timolol maleate is contraindicated in patients with bronchial asthma or with a history of bronchial asthma, or severe chronic obstructive pulmonary disease (see

WARNINGS); sinus bradycardia; second and third degree atrioventricular block; overt cardiac failure (see WARNINGS); cardiogenic shock; anuria; hypersensitivity to this product or to sulfonamide-derived drugs.

WARNINGS

CARDIAC FAILURE

Sympathetic stimulation may be essential for support of the circulation in individuals with diminished myocardial contractility, and its inhibition by beta-adrenergic receptor blockade may precipitate more severe failure. Although beta-blockers should be avoided in overt congestive heart failure, they can be used, if necessary, with caution in patients with a history of failure who are well-compensated, usually with digitalis and diuretics. Both digitalis and timolol maleate slow AV conduction. If cardiac failure persists, therapy with hydrochlorothiazide; timolol maleate should be withdrawn.

In Patients Without a History of Cardiac Failure

Continued depression of the myocardium with beta-blocking agents over a period of time can, in some cases, lead to cardiac failure. At the first sign or symptom of cardiac failure, patients receiving hydrochlorothiazide; timolol maleate should be digitalized and/or be given additional diuretic therapy. Observe the patient closely. If cardiac failure continues, despite adequate digitalization and diuretic therapy, hydrochlorothiazide; timolol maleate should be withdrawn.

RENAL AND HEPATIC DISEASE AND ELECTROLYTE DISTURBANCES

Since timolol maleate is partially metabolized in the liver and excreted mainly by the kidneys, dosage reductions may be necessary when hepatic and/or renal insufficiency is present.

Although the pharmacokinetics of timolol maleate are not greatly altered by renal impairment, marked hypotensive responses have been seen in patients with marked renal impairment undergoing dialysis after 20 mg doses. Dosing in such patients should therefore be especially cautious.

In patients with renal disease, thiazides may precipitate azotemia, and cumulative effects may develop in the presence of impaired renal function. If progressive renal impairment becomes evident, hydrochlorothiazide; timolol maleate should be discontinued.

In patients with impaired hepatic function or progressive liver disease, even minor alterations in fluid and electrolyte balance may precipitate hepatic coma. Hepatic encephalopathy, manifested by tremors, confusion, and coma, has been reported in association with diuretic therapy including hydrochlorothiazide.

Exacerbation of Ischemic Heart Disease Following Abrupt Withdrawal:

Hypersensitivity to catecholamines has been observed in patients withdrawn from beta-blocker therapy; exacerbation of angina and, in some cases, myocardial infarction have occurred after *abrupt* discontinuation of such therapy. When discontinuing chronically administered timolol maleate, particularly in patients with ischemic heart disease, the dosage should be gradually reduced over a period of 1-2 weeks and the patient should be carefully monitored. If angina markedly worsens or acute coronary insufficiency develops, timolol maleate administration should be reinstituted promptly, at least temporarily, and other measures appropriate for the management of unstable angina should be taken. Patients should be warned against interruption or discontinuation of therapy without the physician's advice. Because coronary artery disease is common and may be unrecognized, it may be prudent not to discontinue timolol maleate therapy abruptly even in patients treated only for hypertension.

OBSTRUCTIVE PULMONARY DISEASE

PATIENTS WITH CHRONIC OBSTRUCTIVE PULMONARY DISEASE (*e.g.*, CHRONIC BRONCHITIS, EMPHYSEMA) OF MILD OR MODERATE SEVERITY, BRONCHOSPASTIC DISEASE OR A HISTORY OF BRONCHOSPASTIC DISEASE (OTHER THAN BRONCHIAL ASTHMA OR A HISTORY OF BRONCHIAL ASTHMA, IN WHICH HYDROCHLOROTHIAZIDE; TIMOLOL MALEATE IS CONTRAINDICATED, SEE CONTRAINDICATIONS), SHOULD IN GENERAL NOT RECEIVE BETA-BLOCKERS, INCLUDING HYDROCHLOROTHIAZIDE; TIMOLOL MALEATE. However, if hydrochlorothiazide; timolol maleate is necessary in such patients, then the drug should be administered with caution since it may block bronchodilation produced by endogenous and exogenous catecholamine stimulation of beta$_2$ receptors.

MAJOR SURGERY

The necessity or desirability of withdrawal of beta-blocking therapy prior to major surgery is controversial. Beta-adrenergic receptor blockade impairs the ability of the heart to respond to beta-adrenergically mediated reflex stimuli. This may augment the risk of general anesthesia in surgical procedures. Some patients receiving beta-adrenergic receptor blocking agents have been subject to protracted severe hypotension during anesthesia. Difficulty in restarting and maintaining the heartbeat has also been reported. For these reasons, in patients undergoing elective surgery, some authorities recommend gradual withdrawal of beta-adrenergic receptor blocking agents.

If necessary during surgery, the effects of beta-adrenergic blocking agents may be reversed by sufficient doses of such agonists as isoproterenol, dopamine, dobutamine or levarterenol.

METABOLIC AND ENDOCRINE EFFECTS

Beta-adrenergic blockade may mask certain clinical signs (*e.g.*, tachycardia) of hyperthyroidism. Patients suspected of developing thyrotoxicosis should be managed carefully to avoid abrupt withdrawal of beta-blockade which might precipitate a thyroid storm. Thiazides may decrease serum PBI levels without signs of thyroid disturbance.

Beta-adrenergic receptor blocking agents may mask the signs and symptoms of acute hypoglycemia. Therefore, hydrochlorothiazide; timolol maleate should be administered with caution to patients subject to spontaneous hypoglycemia, or to diabetic patients (especially those with labile diabetes) who are receiving insulin or oral hypoglycemic agents. Insulin requirements in diabetic patients may be increased, decreased, or unchanged by thiazides. Diabetes mellitus that has been latent may become manifest during administration of thiazide diuretics.

Because calcium excretion is decreased by thiazides, hydrochlorothiazide; timolol maleate should be discontinued before carrying out tests for parathyroid function. Pathologic changes in the parathyroid glands, with hypercalcemia and hypophosphatemia, have been observed in a few patients on prolonged thiazide therapy; however, the common complications of hyperparathyroidism such as renal lithiasis, bone resorption, and peptic ulceration have not been seen.

Hyperuricemia may occur or acute gout may be precipitated in certain patients receiving thiazide therapy.

DOSAGE AND ADMINISTRATION

The recommended starting and maintenance dosage is 1 tablet twice a day or 2 tablets once a day. Hydrochlorothiazide can be given at doses of 12.5 to 50 mg/day when used alone. If the antihypertensive response is not satisfactory, another nondiuretic antihypertensive agent may be added.

PRODUCT LISTING - EQUIVALENTS NOT AVAILABLE

Tablet - Oral - 25 mg;10 mg

100's $81.20 TIMOLIDE 10-25, Merck & Company Inc 00006-0067-68

Hydrochlorothiazide; Triamterene *(001465)*

Categories: Edema; Hypertension, essential; Pregnancy Category C; FDA Approval Pre 1982
Drug Classes: Diuretics, potassium sparing; Diuretics, thiazide and derivatives
Brand Names: **Dyazide**; Maxzide
Foreign Brand Availability: Anjal (Taiwan); Apo-triazide (Canada); Dazid (Taiwan; Thailand); Dinazide (Thailand); Diuracet-K (Peru); Dyberzide (Greece); Dytenzide (Belgium; Netherlands); Dytide H (Austria; Germany); Esiteren (Germany); Hydrene (Australia; New-Zealand); Renezide (South-Africa); Triamizide (New-Zealand; Taiwan); Triazide (Taiwan); Trizid (New-Zealand); Turfa (Germany)
Cost of Therapy: $17.23 (Hypertension; Maxzide; 25 mg; 37.5 mg; 1 tablet/day; 30 day supply)
$14.36 (Hypertension; Dyazide; 25 mg; 37.5 mg; 1 tablet/day; 30 day supply)
$8.97 (Hypertension; Generic Tablets; 25 mg; 37.5 mg; 1 tablet/day; 30 day supply)

DESCRIPTION

Each Dyazide capsule for oral use, with opaque red cap and opaque white body, contains hydrochlorothiazide 25 mg and triamterene 37.5 mg, and is imprinted with the product name "DYAZIDE" and "SB". Hydrochlorothiazide is a diuretic/antihypertensive agent and triamterene is an antikaliuretic agent.

Hydrochlorothiazide is slightly soluble in water. It is soluble in dilute ammonia, dilute aqueous sodium hydroxide and dimethylformamide. It is sparingly soluble in methanol.

Hydrochlorothiazide is 6-chloro-3,4-dihydro-2H-1, 2, 4-benzothiadiazine-7-sulfonamide 1,1-dioxide.

At 50°C, triamterene is practically insoluble in water (less than 0.1%). It is soluble in formic acid, sparingly soluble in methoxyethanol and very slightly soluble in alcohol.

Triamterene is 2, 4, 7-triamino-6-phenylpteridine.

Inactive ingredients consist of benzyl alcohol, cetylpyridinium chloride, D&C red no. 33, FD&C yellow no. 6, gelatin, glycine, lactose, magnesium stearate, microcrystalline cellulose, povidone, polysorbate 80, sodium starch glycolate, titanium dioxide, and trace amounts of other inactive ingredients.

Storage: Store at controlled room temperature 20-25°C (68-77°F). Protect from light. Dispense in a tight, light-resistant container.

CLINICAL PHARMACOLOGY

Hydrochlorothiazide; triamterene is a diuretic/antihypertensive drug product that combines natriuretic and antikaliuretic effects. Each component complements the action of the other. The hydrochlorothiazide component blocks the reabsorption of sodium and chloride ions, and thereby increases the quantity of sodium traversing the distal tubule and the volume of water excreted. A portion of the additional sodium presented to the distal tubule is exchanged there for potassium and hydrogen ions. With continued use of hydrochlorothiazide and depletion of sodium, compensatory mechanisms tend to increase this exchange and may produce excessive loss of potassium, hydrogen, and chloride ions. Hydrochlorothiazide also decreases the excretion of calcium and uric acid, may increase the excretion of iodide and may reduce glomerular filtration rate. The exact mechanism of the antihypertensive effect of hydrochlorothiazide is not known.

The triamterene component of hydrochlorothiazide; triamterene exerts its diuretic effect on the distal renal tubule to inhibit the reabsorption of sodium in exchange for potassium and hydrogen ions. Its natriuretic activity is limited by the amount of sodium reaching its site of action. Although it blocks the increase in this exchange that is stimulated by mineralocorticoids (chiefly aldosterone) it is not a competitive antagonist of aldosterone and its activity can be demonstrated in adrenalectomized rats and patients with Addison's disease. As a result, the dose of triamterene required is not proportionally related to the level of mineralocorticoid activity, but is dictated by the response of the individual patients, and the kaliuretic effect of concomitantly administered drugs. By inhibiting the distal tubular exchange mechanism, triamterene maintains or increases the sodium excretion and reduces the excess loss of potassium, hydrogen, and chloride ions induced by hydrochlorothiazide. As with hydrochlorothiazide, triamterene may reduce glomerular filtration and renal plasma flow. Via this mechanism it may reduce uric acid excretion although it has no tubular effect on uric acid reabsorption or secretion. Triamterene does not affect calcium excretion. No predictable antihypertensive effect has been demonstrated for triamterene.

Duration of diuretic activity and effective dosage range of the hydrochlorothiazide and triamterene components of hydrochlorothiazide; triamterene are similar. Onset of diuresis with hydrochlorothiazide; triamterene takes place within 1 hour, peaks at 2-3 hours and tapers off during the subsequent 7-9 hours.

Hydrochlorothiazide; triamterene capsule is well absorbed.

Upon administration of a single oral dose to fasted normal male volunteers, the following mean pharmacokinetic parameters were determined (see TABLE 1).

TABLE 1

	AUC(0-48) ng*h/ml (±SD)	C_{max} ng/ml (±SD)	Median T_{max} h	Ae mg (±SD)
Triamterene	148.7 (87.9)	46.4 (29.4)	1.1	2.7 (1.4)
Hydroxytriamterene sulfate	1865 (471)	720 (364)	1.3	19.7 (6.1)
Hydrochlorothiazide	834 (177)	135.1 (35.7)	2.0	14.3 (3.8)

AUC(0-48), C_{max}, T_{max} and Ae represent area under the plasma concentration versus time plot, maximum plasma concentration, time to reach C_{max} and amount excreted in urine over 48 hours.

Hydrochlorothiazide; triamterene capsule is bioequivalent to a single-entity 25 mg hydrochlorothiazide tablet and 37.5 mg triamterene capsule used in the double-blind clinical trial.

In a limited study involving 12 subjects, coadministration of hydrochlorothiazide; triamterene with a high-fat meal resulted in: (1) an increase in the mean bioavailability of triamterene by about 67% (90% confidence interval = 0.99, 1.90), p-hydroxytriamterene sulfate by about 50% (90% confidence interval = 1.06, 1.77), hydrochlorothiazide by about 17% (90% confidence interval = 0.90, 1.34); (2) increases in the peak concentrations of triamterene and p-hydroxytriamterene; and (3) a delay of up to 2 hours in the absorption of the active constituents.

INDICATIONS AND USAGE

This fixed combination drug is not indicated for the initial therapy of edema or hypertension except in individuals in whom the development of hypokalemia cannot be risked.

Hydrochlorothiazide; triamterene is indicated for the treatment of hypertension or edema in patients who develop hypokalemia on hydrochlorothiazide alone.

Hydrochlorothiazide; triamterene is also indicated for those patients who require a thiazide diuretic and in whom the development of hypokalemia cannot be risked.

Hydrochlorothiazide; triamterene may be used alone or as an adjunct to other antihypertensive drugs, such as beta-blockers. Since hydrochlorothiazide; triamterene may enhance the action of these agents, dosage adjustments may be necessary.

USAGE IN PREGNANCY

The routine use of diuretics in an otherwise healthy woman is inappropriate and exposes mother and fetus to unnecessary hazard. Diuretics do not prevent development of toxemia of pregnancy, and there is no satisfactory evidence that they are useful in the treatment of developed toxemia.

Edema during pregnancy may arise from pathological causes or from the physiologic and mechanical consequences of pregnancy. Diuretics are indicated in pregnancy when edema is due to pathologic causes, just as they are in the absence of pregnancy. Dependent edema in pregnancy resulting from restriction of venous return by the expanded uterus is properly treated through elevation of the lower extremities and use of support hose; use of diuretics to lower intravascular volume in this case is illogical and unnecessary. There is hypervolemia during normal pregnancy which is harmful to neither the fetus nor the mother (in the absence of cardiovascular disease), but which is associated with edema, including generalized edema in the majority of pregnant women. If this edema produces discomfort, increased recumbency will often provide relief. In rare instances this edema may cause extreme discomfort which is not relieved by rest. In these cases a short course of diuretics may provide relief and may be appropriate.

CONTRAINDICATIONS

ANTIKALIURETIC THERAPY AND POTASSIUM SUPPLEMENTATION

Hydrochlorothiazide; triamterene should not be given to patients receiving other potassium-sparing agents such as spironolactone, amiloride or other formulations containing triamterene. Concomitant potassium-containing salt substitutes should also not be used.

Potassium supplementation should not be used with hydrochlorothiazide; triamterene except in severe cases of hypokalemia. Such concomitant therapy can be associated with rapid increases in serum potassium levels. If potassium supplementation is used, careful monitoring of the serum potassium level is necessary.

IMPAIRED RENAL FUNCTION

Hydrochlorothiazide; triamterene is contraindicated in patients with anuria, acute and chronic renal insufficiency or significant renal impairment.

HYPERSENSITIVITY

Hypersensitivity to either drug in the preparation or to other sulfonamide-derived drugs is a contraindication.

HYPERKALEMIA

Hydrochlorothiazide; triamterene should not be used in patients with preexisting elevated serum potassium.

WARNINGS

HYPERKALEMIA

Abnormal elevation of serum potassium levels (greater than or equal to 5.5 mEq/L) can occur with all potassium-sparing diuretic combinations, including hydrochlorothiazide; triamterene. Hyperkalemia is more likely to occur in patients with renal impairment and diabetes (even without evidence of renal impairment), and in the elderly or severely ill. Since uncorrected hyperkalemia may be fatal, serum potassium levels must be monitored at frequent intervals especially in patients first receiving hydrochlorothiazide; triamterene, when dosages are changed or with any illness that may influence renal function.

If hyperkalemia is suspected (warning signs include paresthesias, muscular weakness, fatigue, flaccid paralysis of the extremities, bradycardia, and shock), an electrocardiogram (ECG) should be obtained. However, it is important to monitor serum potassium levels because hyperkalemia may not be associated with ECG changes. If hyperkalemia is present, hydrochlorothiazide; triamterene should be discontinued immediately and a thiazide alone should be substituted. If the serum potassium exceeds 6.5 mEq/L more vigorous therapy is required. The clinical situation dictates the procedures to be employed. These include the intravenous administration of calcium chloride solution, sodium bicarbonate solution and/or the oral or parenteral administration of glucose with a rapid-acting insulin preparation. Cationic exchange resins such as sodium polystyrene sulfonate may be orally or rectally administered. Persistent hyperkalemia may require dialysis.

The development of hyperkalemia associated with potassium-sparing diuretics is accentuated in the presence of renal impairment (see CONTRAINDICATIONS). Patients with mild renal functional impairment should not receive this drug without frequent and continuing monitoring of serum electrolytes. Cumulative drug effects may be observed in patients with impaired renal function. The renal clearances of hydrochlorothiazide and the pharmacologically active metabolite of triamterene, the sulfate ester of hydroxytriamterene, have been shown to be reduced and the plasma levels increased following hydrochlorothiazide; triamterene administration to elderly patients and patients with impaired renal function.

Hyperkalemia has been reported in diabetic patients with the use of potassium-sparing agents even in the absence of apparent renal impairment. Accordingly, serum electrolytes must be frequently monitored if hydrochlorothiazide; triamterene is used in diabetic patients.

METABOLIC OR RESPIRATORY ACIDOSIS

Potassium-sparing therapy should also be avoided in severely ill patients in whom respiratory or metabolic acidosis may occur. Acidosis may be associated with rapid elevations in serum potassium levels. If hydrochlorothiazide; triamterene is employed, frequent evaluations of acid/base balance and serum electrolytes are necessary.

H

PRECAUTIONS

DIABETES

Caution should be exercised when administering hydrochlorothiazide; triamterene to patients with diabetes, since thiazides may cause hyperglycemia, glycosuria, and alter insulin requirements in diabetes. Also, diabetes mellitus may become manifest during thiazide administration.

IMPAIRED HEPATIC FUNCTION

Thiazides should be used with caution in patients with impaired hepatic function. They can precipitate hepatic coma in patients with severe liver disease. Potassium depletion induced by the thiazide may be important in this connection. Administer hydrochlorothiazide; triamterene cautiously and be alert for such early signs of impending coma as confusion, drowsiness, and tremor; if mental confusion increases discontinue hydrochlorothiazide; triamterene for a few days. Attention must be given to other factors that may precipitate hepatic coma, such as blood in the gastrointestinal tract or preexisting potassium depletion.

HYPOKALEMIA

Hypokalemia is uncommon with hydrochlorothiazide; triamterene; but, should it develop, corrective measures should be taken such as potassium supplementation or increased intake of potassium-rich foods. Institute such measures cautiously with frequent determinations of serum potassium levels, especially in patients receiving digitalis or with a history of cardiac arrhythmias. If serious hypokalemia (serum potassium less than 3.0 mEq/L) is demonstrated by repeat serum potassium determinations. Hydrochlorothiazide; triamterene should be discontinued and potassium chloride supplementation initiated. Less serious hypokalemia should be evaluated with regard to other coexisting conditions and treated accordingly.

ELECTROLYTE IMBALANCE

Electrolyte imbalance, often encountered in such conditions as heart failure, renal disease or cirrhosis of the liver, may also be aggravated by diuretics and should be considered during hydrochlorothiazide; triamterene therapy when using high doses for prolonged periods or in patients on a salt-restricted diet. Serum determinations of electrolytes should be performed, and are particularly important if the patient is vomiting excessively or receiving fluids parenterally. Possible fluid and electrolyte imbalance may be indicated by such warning signs as: dry mouth, thirst, weakness, lethargy, drowsiness, restlessness, muscle pain or cramps, muscular fatigue, hypotension, oliguria, tachycardia, and gastrointestinal symptoms.

HYPOCHLOREMIA

Although any chloride deficit is generally mild and usually does not require specific treatment except under extraordinary circumstances (as in liver disease or renal disease), chloride replacement may be required in the treatment of metabolic alkalosis. Dilutional hyponatremia may occur in edematous patients in hot weather; appropriate therapy is water restriction, rather than administration of salt, except in rare instances when the hyponatremia is life threatening. In actual salt depletion, appropriate replacement is the therapy of choice.

RENAL STONES

Triamterene has been found in renal stones in association with the other usual calculus components. Hydrochlorothiazide; triamterene should be used with caution in patients with a history of renal stones.

LABORATORY TESTS

Serum Potassium

The normal adult range of serum potassium is 3.5-5.0 mEq/L with 4.5 mEq often being used for a reference point. If hypokalemia should develop, corrective measures should be taken such as potassium supplementation or increased dietary intake of potassium-rich foods.

Institute such measures cautiously with frequent determinations of serum potassium levels. Potassium levels persistently above 6 mEq/L require careful observation and treatment. Serum potassium levels do not necessarily indicate true body potassium concentration. A rise in plasma pH may cause a decrease in plasma potassium concentration and an increase in the intracellular potassium concentration. Discontinue corrective measures for hypokalemia immediately if laboratory determinations reveal an abnormal elevation of serum potassium. Discontinue hydrochlorothiazide; triamterene and substitute a thiazide diuretic alone until potassium levels return to normal.

Serum Creatinine and BUN

Hydrochlorothiazide; triamterene may produce an elevated blood urea nitrogen level, creatinine level or both. This apparently is secondary to a reversible reduction of glomerular filtration rate or a depletion of intravascular fluid volume (prerenal azotemia) rather than renal toxicity; levels usually return to normal when hydrochlorothiazide; triamterene is discontinued. If azotemia increases, discontinue hydrochlorothiazide; triamterene. Periodic BUN or serum creatinine determinations should be made, especially in elderly patients and in patients with suspected or confirmed renal insufficiency.

Serum PBI

Thiazide may decrease serum PBI levels without sign of thyroid disturbance.

Parathyroid Function

Thiazides should be discontinued before carrying out tests for parathyroid function. Calcium excretion is decreased by thiazides. Pathologic changes in the parathyroid glands with hypercalcemia and hypophosphatemia have been observed in a few patients on prolonged thiazide therapy. The common complications of hyperparathyroidism such as bone resorption and peptic ulceration have not been seen.

DRUG/LABORATORY TEST INTERACTIONS

Triamterene and quinidine have similar fluorescence spectra; thus, hydrochlorothiazide; triamterene will interfere with the fluorescent measurement of quinidine.

CARCINOGENESIS, MUTAGENESIS, AND IMPAIRMENT OF FERTILITY

Carcinogenesis

Long-term studies have not been conducted with hydrochlorothiazide; triamterene, or with triamterene alone.

Hydrochlorothiazide

Two year feeding studies in mice and rats, conducted under the auspices of the National Toxicology Program (NTP), treated mice and rats with doses of hydrochlorothiazide up to 600 and 100 mg/kg/day, respectively. On a body-weight basis, these doses are 600 times (in mice) and 100 times (in rats) the Maximum Recommended Human Dose (MRHD) for the hydrochlorothiazide component of hydrochlorothiazide; triamterene at 50 mg/day (or 1.0 mg/kg/day based on 50 kg individuals). On the basis of body-surface area, these doses are 56 times (in mice) and 21 times (in rats) the MRHD. These studies uncovered no evidence of carcinogenic potential of hydrochlorothiazide in rats or female mice, but there was equivocal evidence of hepatocarcinogenicity in male mice.

Mutagenesis

Studies of the mutagenic potential of hydrochlorothiazide; triamterene, or of triamterene alone have not been performed.

Hydrochlorothiazide

Hydrochlorothiazide was not genotoxic in *in vitro* assays using strains TA 98, TA 100, TA 1535, TA 1537, and TA 1538 of *Salmonella typhimurium* (the Ames test); in the Chinese Hamster Ovary (CHO) test for chromosomal aberrations; or in *in vivo* assays using mouse germinal cell chromosomes, Chinese hamster bone marrow chromosomes, and the *Drosophila* sex-linked recessive lethal trait gene. Positive test results were obtained in the *in vitro* CHO Sister Chromatid Exchange (clastogenicity) test, and in the mouse Lymphoma Cell (mutagenicity) assays, using concentrations of hydrochlorothiazide of 43-1300 μg/ml. Positive test results were also obtained in the *Aspergillus nidulans* nondisjunction assay, using an unspecified concentration of hydrochlorothiazide.

Impairment of Fertility

Studies of the effects of hydrochlorothiazide; triamterene, or of triamterene alone on animal reproductive function have not been conducted.

Hydrochlorothiazide

Hydrochlorothiazide had no adverse effects on the fertility of mice and rats of either sex in studies wherein these species were exposed, via their diet, to doses of up to 100 and 4 mg/kg/day, respectively, prior to mating and throughout gestation. Corresponding multiples of the MRHD are 100 (mice) and 4 (rats) on the basis of body-weight and 9.4 (mice) and 0.8 (rats) on the basis of body-surface area.

PREGNANCY CATEGORY C

Teratogenic Effects

Hydrochlorothiazide; Triamterene

Animal reproduction studies to determine the potential for fetal harm by hydrochlorothiazide; triamterene have not been conducted. However, a One Generation Study in the rat approximated hydrochlorothiazide; triamterene composition by using a 1:1 ratio of triamterene to hydrochlorothiazide (30:30 mg/kg/day); there was no evidence of teratogenicity at those doses which were, on a body-weight basis, 15 and 30 times, respectively, the MRHD, and on the basis of body-surface area, 3.1 and 6.2 times, respectively, the MRHD.

The safe use of hydrochlorothiazide; triamterene in pregnancy has not been established since there are no adequate and well-controlled studies with hydrochlorothiazide; triamterene in pregnant women. Hydrochlorothiazide; triamterene should be used during pregnancy only if the potential benefit justifies the risk to the fetus.

Triamterene

Reproduction studies have been performed in rats at doses as high as 20 times the MRHD on the basis of body-weight, and 6 times the human dose on the basis of body-surface area without evidence of harm to the fetus due to triamterene.

Because animal reproduction studies are not always predictive of human response, this drug should be used during pregnancy only if clearly needed.

Hydrochlorothiazide

Hydrochlorothiazide was orally administered to pregnant mice and rats during respective periods of major organogenesis at doses up to 3000 and 1000 mg/kg/day, respectively. At these doses, which are multiples of the MRHD equal to 3000 for mice and 1000 for rats, based on body-weight, and equal to 282 for mice and 206 for rats, based on body-surface area, there was no evidence of harm to the fetus.

There are, however, no adequate and well-controlled studies in pregnant women. Because animal reproduction studies are not always predictive of human response, this drug should be used during pregnancy only if clearly needed.

Nonteratogenic Effects

Thiazides and triamterene have been shown to cross the placental barrier and appear in cord blood. The use of thiazides and triamterene in pregnant women requires that the anticipated benefit be weighed against possible hazards to the fetus. These hazards include fetal or neonatal jaundice, pancreatitis, thrombocytopenia, and possible other adverse reactions which have occurred in the adult.

NURSING MOTHERS

Thiazides and triamterene in combination have not been studied in nursing mothers. Triamterene appears in animal milk; this may occur in humans. Thiazides are excreted in human breast milk. If use of the combination drug product is deemed essential, the patient should stop nursing.

PEDIATRIC USE

Safety and effectiveness in pediatric patients have not been established.

DRUG INTERACTIONS

ANGIOTENSIN-CONVERTING ENZYME INHIBITORS

Potassium-sparing agents should be used with caution in conjunction with angiotensin-converting enzyme (ACE) inhibitors due to an increased risk of hyperkalemia.

ORAL HYPOGLYCEMIC DRUGS

Concurrent use with chlorpropamide may increase the risk of severe hyponatremia.

NONSTEROIDAL ANTI-INFLAMMATORY DRUGS

A possible interaction resulting in acute renal failure has been reported in a few patients on hydrochlorothiazide; triamterene when treated with indomethacin, a nonsteroidal anti-inflammatory agent. Caution is advised in administering nonsteroidal anti-inflammatory agents with hydrochlorothiazide; triamterene.

LITHIUM

Lithium generally should not be given with diuretics because they reduce its renal clearance and increase the risk of lithium toxicity. Read circulars for lithium preparations before use of such concomitant therapy with hydrochlorothiazide; triamterene.

SURGICAL CONSIDERATIONS

Thiazides have been shown to decrease arterial responsiveness to norepinephrine (an effect attributed to loss of sodium). This diminution is not sufficient to preclude effectiveness of the pressor agent for therapeutic use. Thiazides have also been shown to increase the paralyzing effect of nondepolarizing muscle relaxants such as tubocurarine (an effect attributed to potassium loss); consequently caution should be observed in patients undergoing surgery.

OTHER CONSIDERATIONS

Concurrent use of hydrochlorothiazide with amphotericin B or corticosteroids or corticotropin (ACTH) may intensify electrolyte imbalance, particularly hypokalemia, although the presence of triamterene minimizes the hypokalemic effect.

Thiazides may add to or potentiate the action of other antihypertensive drugs. See INDICATIONS AND USAGE for concomitant use with other antihypertensive drugs.

The effect of oral anticoagulants may be decreased when used concurrently with hydrochlorothiazide; dosage adjustments may be necessary.

Hydrochlorothiazide; triamterene may raise the level of blood uric acid; dosage adjustments of antigout medication may be necessary to control hyperuricemia and gout.

The following agents given together with triamterene may promote serum potassium accumulation and possibly result in hyperkalemia because of the potassium-sparing nature of triamterene, especially in patients with renal insufficiency: blood from blood bank (may contain up to 30 mEq of potassium per liter of plasma or up to 65 mEq/L of whole blood when stored for more than 10 days); low-salt milk (may contain up to 60 mEq of potassium per liter); potassium-containing medications (such as parenteral penicillin G potassium); salt substitutes (most contain substantial amounts of potassium).

Exchange resins, such as sodium polystyrene sulfonate, whether administered orally or rectally, reduce serum potassium levels by sodium replacement of the potassium; fluid retention may occur in some patients because of the increased sodium intake.

Chronic or overuse of laxatives may reduce serum potassium levels by promoting excessive potassium loss from the intestinal tract; laxatives may interfere with the potassium-retaining effects of triamterene.

The effectiveness of methenamine may be decreased when used concurrently with hydrochlorothiazide because of alkalinization of the urine.

ADVERSE REACTIONS

Adverse effects are listed in decreasing order of frequency; however, the most serious adverse effects are listed first regardless of frequency. The serious adverse effects associated with hydrochlorothiazide; triamterene have commonly occurred in less than 0.1% of patients treated with this product.

Hypersensitivity: Anaphylaxis, rash, urticaria, photosensitivity.
Cardiovascular: Arrhythmia, postural hypotension.
Metabolic: Diabetes, mellitus, hyperkalemia, hyperglycemia, glycosuria, hyperuricemia, hypokalemia, hyponatremia, acidosis, hypochloremia.
Gastrointestinal: Jaundice and/or liver enzyme abnormalities, pancreatitis, nausea and vomiting, diarrhea, constipation, abdominal pain.
Renal: Acute renal failure (one case of irreversible renal failure has been reported), interstitial nephritis, renal stones composed primarily of triamterene, elevated BUN and serum creatinine, abnormal urinary sediment.
Hematologic: Leukopenia, thrombocytopenia and purpura, megaloblastic anemia.
Musculoskeletal: Muscle cramps.
Central Nervous System: Weakness, fatigue, dizziness, headache, dry mouth.
Miscellaneous: Impotence, sialadenitis.

Thiazides alone have been shown to cause the following additional adverse reactions:
Central Nervous System: Paresthesias, vertigo.
Ophthalmic: Xanthopsia, transient blurred vision.
Respiratory: Allergic pneumonitis, pulmonary edema, respiratory distress.
Other: Necrotizing vasculitis, exacerbation of lupus.
Hematologic: Aplastic anemia, agranulocytosis, hemolytic anemia.
Neonate and Infancy: Thrombocytopenia and pancreatitis—rarely, in newborns whose mothers have received thiazides during pregnancy.

DOSAGE AND ADMINISTRATION

The usual dose of hydrochlorothiazide; triamterene is 1 or 2 capsules given once daily, with appropriate monitoring of serum potassium and of the clinical effect (see WARNINGS, Hyperkalemia).

PRODUCT LISTING - RATED THERAPEUTICALLY EQUIVALENT

Capsule - Oral - 25 mg;37.5 mg

31 x 10	$114.40	GENERIC, Vangard Labs	00615-1333-53
31 x 10	$114.40	GENERIC, Vangard Labs	00615-1333-63
90's	$36.09	DYAZIDE, Allscripts Pharmaceutical Company	54569-8533-00
100's	$31.77	FEDERAL UPPER LIMIT, H.C.F.A. F F P	99999-1465-09
100's	$37.53	GENERIC, Mylan Pharmaceuticals Inc	00378-2537-01
100's	$37.53	GENERIC, Barr Laboratories Inc	00555-0488-02
100's	$37.53	GENERIC, Barr Laboratories Inc	00555-0875-02
100's	$37.53	GENERIC, Geneva Pharmaceuticals	00781-2074-01
100's	$47.85	DYAZIDE, Allscripts Pharmaceutical Company	54569-3824-01
100's	$53.95	DYAZIDE, Glaxosmithkline	00007-3650-22
100's	$55.35	DYAZIDE, Glaxosmithkline	00007-3650-21

Capsule - Oral - 25 mg;50 mg

30's	$9.25	GENERIC, Allscripts Pharmaceutical Company	54569-0543-01
30's	$10.89	GENERIC, Heartland Healthcare Services	61392-0165-30
30's	$10.89	GENERIC, Heartland Healthcare Services	61392-0165-39
30's	$89.10	GENERIC, Golden State Medical	60429-0190-30
31's	$11.26	GENERIC, Heartland Healthcare Services	61392-0165-31
32's	$11.62	GENERIC, Heartland Healthcare Services	61392-0165-32
45's	$16.34	GENERIC, Heartland Healthcare Services	61392-0165-45
60's	$18.50	GENERIC, Allscripts Pharmaceutical Company	54569-0543-02
60's	$21.79	GENERIC, Heartland Healthcare Services	61392-0165-60
90's	$25.90	GENERIC, Allscripts Pharmaceutical Company	54569-8015-00
90's	$25.90	GENERIC, Allscripts Pharmaceutical Company	54569-8502-00
90's	$32.68	GENERIC, Heartland Healthcare Services	61392-0165-90
100's	$9.95	GENERIC, Raway Pharmacal Inc	00686-0433-20
100's	$27.95	GENERIC, Geneva Pharmaceuticals	00781-2540-01
100's	$27.95	GENERIC, Moore, H.L. Drug Exchange Inc	00839-8043-06
100's	$28.10	GENERIC, Ivax Corporation	00172-2950-60
100's	$28.50	GENERIC, Martec Pharmaceuticals Inc	52555-0648-01
100's	$28.78	GENERIC, Allscripts Pharmaceutical Company	54569-8015-01
100's	$29.95	GENERIC, Major Pharmaceuticals Inc	00904-1936-60
100's	$30.83	GENERIC, Allscripts Pharmaceutical Company	54569-0543-00
100's	$32.00	GENERIC, Geneva Pharmaceuticals	00781-2715-13
100's	$34.50	GENERIC, Medirex Inc	57480-0372-01
100's	$48.54	GENERIC, Geneva Pharmaceuticals	00781-2715-01
180's	$51.80	GENERIC, Allscripts Pharmaceutical Company	54569-8502-01

Tablet - Oral - 25 mg;37.5 mg

30's	$11.81	GENERIC, Pd-Rx Pharmaceuticals	55289-0090-30
30's	$16.41	MAXZIDE, Allscripts Pharmaceutical Company	54569-2320-01
30's	$18.82	MAXZIDE, Physicians Total Care	54868-0907-01
30's	$19.86	MAXZIDE, Pd-Rx Pharmaceuticals	55289-0382-30
60's	$36.46	MAXZIDE, Physicians Total Care	54868-0907-02
90's	$30.29	GENERIC, Allscripts Pharmaceutical Company	54569-8596-00
100's	$19.32	FEDERAL UPPER LIMIT, H.C.F.A. F F P	99999-1465-03
100's	$29.90	GENERIC, Qualitest Products Inc	00603-6180-21
100's	$31.50	GENERIC, Sidmak Laboratories Inc	50111-0534-01
100's	$32.48	GENERIC, Aligen Independent Laboratories Inc	00405-5049-01
100's	$32.67	GENERIC, Watson/Rugby Laboratories Inc	00536-5665-01
100's	$32.89	GENERIC, Caremark Inc	00339-5837-12
100's	$33.50	GENERIC, Creighton Products Corporation	50752-0300-05
100's	$33.65	GENERIC, Major Pharmaceuticals Inc	00904-7873-60
100's	$33.95	GENERIC, Barr Laboratories Inc	00555-0643-02
100's	$33.95	GENERIC, Geneva Pharmaceuticals	00781-1123-01
100's	$33.95	GENERIC, Moore, H.L. Drug Exchange Inc	00839-7950-06
100's	$33.96	GENERIC, Watson Laboratories Inc	52544-0424-01
100's	$35.70	GENERIC, Watson Laboratories Inc	00591-0424-01
100's	$45.20	GENERIC, Udl Laboratories Inc	51079-0935-20
100's	$57.42	MAXZIDE, Bertek Pharmaceuticals Inc	62794-0464-01
100's	$63.21	MAXZIDE, Bertek Pharmaceuticals Inc	62794-0464-88

Tablet - Oral - 50 mg;75 mg

15's	$2.40	GENERIC, Major Pharmaceuticals Inc	00904-1965-48
15's	$4.04	GENERIC, Pd-Rx Pharmaceuticals	55289-0488-15
30's	$3.45	GENERIC, Major Pharmaceuticals Inc	00904-1965-46
30's	$8.70	GENERIC, Pd-Rx Pharmaceuticals	55289-0488-30
30's	$10.11	GENERIC, Golden State Medical	60429-0191-30
30's	$32.36	MAXZIDE, Physicians Total Care	54868-0866-02
60's	$67.21	MAXZIDE, Physicians Total Care	54868-0866-03
90's	$29.18	GENERIC, Golden State Medical	60429-0191-90
100's	$4.88	FEDERAL UPPER LIMIT, H.C.F.A. F F P	99999-1465-06
100's	$8.93	GENERIC, Interstate Drug Exchange Inc	00814-8011-14
100's	$14.69	GENERIC, Pd-Rx Pharmaceuticals	55289-0488-01
100's	$28.46	GENERIC, Qualitest Products Inc	00603-6182-21
100's	$28.50	GENERIC, Major Pharmaceuticals Inc	00904-1965-60
100's	$28.78	GENERIC, Barr Laboratories Inc	00555-0444-02
100's	$28.90	GENERIC, Aligen Independent Laboratories Inc	00405-5048-01
100's	$33.10	GENERIC, Creighton Products Corporation	50752-0304-05
100's	$40.24	GENERIC, Caremark Inc	00339-5625-12
100's	$46.77	GENERIC, Major Pharmaceuticals Inc	00904-1965-61
100's	$49.98	GENERIC, Par Pharmaceutical Inc	49884-0279-01
100's	$49.98	GENERIC, Martec Pharmaceuticals Inc	52555-0974-01
100's	$50.02	GENERIC, Moore, H.L. Drug Exchange Inc	00839-7422-06
100's	$55.60	GENERIC, Watson/Rugby Laboratories Inc	00536-4927-01
100's	$55.60	GENERIC, Sidmak Laboratories Inc	50111-0505-01
100's	$69.03	GENERIC, Ivax Corporation	00182-1872-89
100's	$84.75	GENERIC, Par Pharmaceutical Inc	49884-0017-01
100's	$88.70	GENERIC, Geneva Pharmaceuticals	00781-1008-01
100's	$91.36	GENERIC, Udl Laboratories Inc	51079-0433-20
100's	$91.68	GENERIC, Watson Laboratories Inc	00591-0348-01
100's	$91.68	GENERIC, Watson Laboratories Inc	52544-0348-01
100's	$96.68	GENERIC, Watson/Schein Pharmaceuticals Inc	00364-2242-01
100's	$124.06	MAXZIDE, Bertek Pharmaceuticals Inc	62794-0460-01

PRODUCT LISTING - EQUIVALENTS NOT AVAILABLE

Capsule - Oral - 25 mg;37.5 mg

15's	$6.18	GENERIC, Southwood Pharmaceuticals Inc	58016-0368-15
30's	$11.45	GENERIC, Allscripts Pharmaceutical Company	54569-3967-00
30's	$11.48	GENERIC, Heartland Healthcare Services	61392-0162-30
30's	$11.86	GENERIC, Heartland Healthcare Services	61392-0162-39
30's	$12.37	GENERIC, Southwood Pharmaceuticals Inc	58016-0368-30
31's	$11.86	GENERIC, Heartland Healthcare Services	61392-0162-31
32's	$12.25	GENERIC, Heartland Healthcare Services	61392-0162-32
45's	$17.22	GENERIC, Heartland Healthcare Services	61392-0162-45
60's	$22.96	GENERIC, Heartland Healthcare Services	61392-0162-60
60's	$24.75	GENERIC, Southwood Pharmaceuticals Inc	58016-0368-60
90's	$34.44	GENERIC, Heartland Healthcare Services	61392-0162-90
100's	$37.53	GENERIC, Allscripts Pharmaceutical Company	54569-3967-01
100's	$41.26	GENERIC, Southwood Pharmaceuticals Inc	58016-0368-00

Capsule - Oral - 25 mg;50 mg

12's	$9.61	GENERIC, Southwood Pharmaceuticals Inc	58016-0520-12
15's	$6.60	GENERIC, Pharma Pac	52959-0395-15
15's	$12.02	GENERIC, Southwood Pharmaceuticals Inc	58016-0520-15
20's	$16.02	GENERIC, Southwood Pharmaceuticals Inc	58016-0520-20
30's	$9.07	GENERIC, Pharmaceutical Corporation Of America	51655-0510-24
30's	$24.03	GENERIC, Southwood Pharmaceuticals Inc	58016-0520-30
60's	$48.06	GENERIC, Southwood Pharmaceuticals Inc	58016-0520-60
100's	$32.25	GENERIC, Interstate Drug Exchange Inc	00814-8010-14
100's	$80.10	GENERIC, Southwood Pharmaceuticals Inc	58016-0520-00
120's	$96.12	GENERIC, Southwood Pharmaceuticals Inc	58016-0520-02

Tablet - Oral - 25 mg;37.5 mg

100's	$33.96	GENERIC, Mylan Pharmaceuticals Inc	00378-1352-01

Tablet - Oral - 50 mg;75 mg

14's	$12.05	GENERIC, Allscripts Pharmaceutical Company	54569-2545-04
15's	$12.50	GENERIC, Southwood Pharmaceuticals Inc	58016-0545-15
30's	$10.50	GENERIC, Pharma Pac	52959-0172-30
30's	$24.75	GENERIC, Southwood Pharmaceuticals Inc	58016-0545-30
30's	$25.81	GENERIC, Allscripts Pharmaceutical Company	54569-2545-00
60's	$51.62	GENERIC, Allscripts Pharmaceutical Company	54569-2545-03
60's	$58.81	GENERIC, Quality Care Pharmaceuticals Inc	49999-0094-60
90's	$30.70	GENERIC, Allscripts Pharmaceutical Company	54569-8526-00
100's	$82.50	GENERIC, Southwood Pharmaceuticals Inc	58016-0545-00

100's	$84.50	GENERIC, Mylan Pharmaceuticals Inc	00378-1355-01
100's	$86.04	GENERIC, Allscripts Pharmaceutical Company	54569-2545-02

Hydrochlorothiazide; Valsartan *(003520)*

For complete prescribing information, refer to the CD-ROM included with the book.

Categories: Hypertension, essential; FDA Approved 1998 Mar; Pregnancy Category C, 1st Trimester; Pregnancy Category D, 2nd & 3rd Trimesters
Drug Classes: Angiotensin II receptor antagonists; Diuretics, thiazide and derivatives
Brand Names: **Diovan HCT**
Foreign Brand Availability: Co-Diovan (Hong-Kong; Indonesia; Israel; Korea; Philippines; Singapore; Thailand); CoDiovan (Germany; Mexico; South-Africa); Cotareg (France); Nisisco (France)
Cost of Therapy: $53.65 (Hypertension; Diovan HCT; 12.5 mg; 80 mg; 1 tablet/day; 30 day supply)

WARNING

Note: The trade name has been used throughout this monograph for clarity.

USE IN PREGNANCY

When used in pregnancy during the second and third trimesters, drugs that act directly on the renin-angiotensin system can cause injury and even death to the developing fetus. When pregnancy is detected, Diovan HCT should be discontinued as soon as possible. See WARNINGS, Fetal/Neonatal Morbidity and Mortality.

H

DESCRIPTION

Diovan HCT is a combination of valsartan, an orally active, specific angiotensin II antagonist acting on the AT_1 receptor subtype, and hydrochlorothiazide, a diuretic.

Valsartan, a nonpeptide molecule, is chemically described as *N*-(1-oxopentyl)-*N*-[[2'-(1*H*-tetrazol-5-yl)[1,1'-biphenyl]-4-yl]methyl]-L-Valine. Its empirical formula is $C_{24}H_{29}N_5O_3$, its molecular weight is 435.5.

Valsartan is a white to practically white fine powder. It is soluble in ethanol and methanol and slightly soluble in water.

Hydrochlorothiazide is a white, or practically white, practically odorless, crystalline powder. It is slightly soluble in water; freely soluble in sodium hydroxide solution, in *n*-butylamine, and in dimethylformamide; sparingly soluble in methanol; and insoluble in ether, in chloroform, and in dilute mineral acids. Hydrochlorothiazide is chemically described as 6-chloro-3,4-dihydro-2*H*-1,2,4-benzothiadiazine-7-sulfonamide 1,1-dioxide. Hydrochlorothiazide is a thiazide diuretic. Its empirical formula is $C_7H_8ClN_3O_4S_2$, its molecular weight is 297.73.

Diovan HCT tablets are formulated for oral administration to contain valsartan and hydrochlorothiazide 80/12.5 mg, 160/12.5 mg and 160/25 mg. The inactive ingredients of the tablets are colloidal silicon dioxide, crospovidone, hydroxypropyl methylcellulose, iron oxides, magnesium stearate, microcrystalline cellulose, polyethylene glycol, talc, and titanium dioxide.

INDICATIONS AND USAGE

Diovan HCT is indicated for the treatment of hypertension. This fixed dose combination is not indicated for initial therapy (see DOSAGE AND ADMINISTRATION).

CONTRAINDICATIONS

Diovan HCT is contraindicated in patients who are hypersensitive to any component of this product.

Because of the hydrochlorothiazide component, this product is contraindicated in patients with anuria or hypersensitivity to other sulfonamide-derived drugs.

WARNINGS

FETAL/NEONATAL MORBIDITY AND MORTALITY

Drugs that act directly on the renin-angiotensin system can cause fetal and neonatal morbidity and death when administered to pregnant women. Several dozen cases have been reported in the world literature in patients who were taking angiotensin-converting enzyme inhibitors. When pregnancy is detected, Diovan HCT should be discontinued as soon as possible.

The use of drugs that act directly on the renin-angiotensin system during the second and third trimesters of pregnancy has been associated with fetal and neonatal injury, including hypotension, neonatal skull hypoplasia, anuria, reversible or irreversible renal failure, and death. Oligohydramnios has also been reported, presumably resulting from decreased fetal renal function; oligohydramnios in this setting has been associated with fetal limb contractures, craniofacial deformation, and hypoplastic lung development. Prematurity, intrauterine growth retardation, and patent ductus arteriosus have also been reported, although it is not clear whether these occurrences were due to exposure to the drug.

These adverse effects do not appear to have resulted from intrauterine drug exposure that has been limited to the first trimester.

Mothers whose embryos and fetuses are exposed to an angiotensin II receptor antagonist only during the first trimester should be so informed. Nonetheless, when patients become pregnant, physicians should advise the patient to discontinue the use of Diovan HCT as soon as possible.

Rarely (probably less often than once in every thousand pregnancies), no alternative to a drug acting on the renin-angiotensin system will be found. In these rare cases, the mothers should be apprised of the potential hazards to their fetuses, and serial ultrasound examinations should be performed to assess the intraamniotic environment.

If oligohydramnios is observed, Diovan HCT should be discontinued unless it is considered life-saving for the mother. Contraction stress testing (CST), a nonstress test (NST), or biophysical profiling (BPP) may be appropriate, depending upon the week of pregnancy. Patients and physicians should be aware, however, that oligohydramnios may not appear until after the fetus has sustained irreversible injury.

Infants with histories of *in utero* exposure to an angiotensin II receptor antagonist should be closely observed for hypotension, oliguria, and hyperkalemia. If oliguria occurs, attention should be directed toward support of blood pressure and renal perfusion. Exchange transfusion or dialysis may be required as means of reversing hypotension and/or substituting for disordered renal function.

VALSARTAN - HYDROCHLOROTHIAZIDE IN ANIMALS

There was no evidence of teratogenicity in mice, rats, or rabbits treated orally with valsartan at doses up to 600, 100 and 10 mg/kg/day, respectively, in combination with hydrochlorothiazide at doses up to 188, 31 and 3 mg/kg/day. These non-teratogenic doses in mice, rats and rabbits, respectively, represent 18, 7 and 1 times the maximum recommended human dose (MRHD) of valsartan and 38, 13 and 2 times the MRHD of hydrochlorothiazide on a mg/m^2 basis. (Calculations assume an oral dose of 160 mg/day valsartan in combination with 25 mg/day hydrochlorothiazide and a 60 kg patient.)

Fetotoxicity was observed in association with maternal toxicity in rats and rabbits at valsartan doses of ≥200 and 10 mg/kg/day, respectively, in combination with hydrochlorothiazide doses of ≥63 and 3 mg/kg/day. Fetotoxicity in rats was considered to be related to decreased fetal weights and included fetal variations of sternebrae, vertebrae, ribs and/or renal papillae. Fetotoxicity in rabbits included increased numbers of late resorptions with resultant increases in total resorptions, postimplantation losses and decreased number of live fetuses. The no observed adverse effect doses in mice, rats and rabbits for valsartan were 600, 100 and 3 mg/kg/day, respectively, in combination with hydrochlorothiazide doses of 188, 31 and 1 mg/kg/day. These no adverse effect doses in mice, rats and rabbits, respectively, represent 5, 1.5 and 0.06 times the MRHD of valsartan and 38, 13 and 0.5 times the MRHD of hydrochlorothiazide on a mg/m^2 basis. (Calculations assume an oral dose of 160 mg/day valsartan in combination with 25 mg/day hydrochlorothiazide and a 60 kg patient.)

VALSARTAN IN ANIMALS

No teratogenic effects were observed when valsartan was administered to pregnant mice and rats at oral doses up to 600 mg/kg/day and to pregnant rabbits at oral doses up to 10 mg/kg/day. However, significant decreases in fetal weight, pup birth weight, pup survival rate, and slight delays in developmental milestones were observed in studies in which parental rats were treated with valsartan at oral, maternally toxic (reduction in body weight gain and food consumption) doses of 600 mg/kg/day during organogenesis or late gestation and lactation. In rabbits, fetotoxicity (*i.e.*, resorptions, litter loss, abortions, and low body weight) associated with maternal toxicity (mortality) was observed at doses of 5 and 10 mg/kg/day. The no observed adverse effect doses of 600, 200 and 2 mg/kg/day in mice, rats and rabbits represent 18, 12 and 0.2 times, respectively, the maximum recommended human dose on a mg/m^2 basis. (Calculations assume an oral dose of 160 mg/day and a 60 kg patient.)

HYDROCHLOROTHIAZIDE IN ANIMALS

Under the auspices of the National Toxicology Program, pregnant mice and rats that received hydrochlorothiazide via gavage at doses up to 3000 and 1000 mg/kg/day, respectively, on gestation days 6 through 15 showed no evidence of teratogenicity. These doses of hydrochlorothiazide in mice and rats represent 608 and 405 times, respectively, the maximum recommended human dose on a mg/m^2 basis. (Calculations assume an oral dose of 25 mg/day and a 60 kg patient.)

Intrauterine exposure to thiazide diuretics is associated with fetal or neonatal jaundice, thrombocytopenia, and possibly other adverse reactions that have occurred in adults.

HYPOTENSION IN VOLUME- AND/OR SALT-DEPLETED PATIENTS

Excessive reduction of blood pressure was rarely seen (0.5%) in patients with uncomplicated hypertension treated with Diovan HCT. In patients with an activated renin-angiotensin system, such as volume- and/or salt-depleted patients receiving high doses of diuretics, symptomatic hypotension may occur. This condition should be corrected prior to administration of Diovan HCT, or the treatment should start under close medical supervision.

If hypotension occurs, the patient should be placed in the supine position and, if necessary, given an intravenous infusion of normal saline. A transient hypotensive response is not a contraindication to further treatment, which usually can be continued without difficulty once the blood pressure has stabilized.

HYDROCHLOROTHIAZIDE

Impaired Hepatic Function

Thiazide diuretics should be used with caution in patients with impaired hepatic function or progressive liver disease, since minor alterations of fluid and electrolyte balance may precipitate hepatic coma.

Hypersensitivity Reaction

Hypersensitivity reactions to hydrochlorothiazide may occur in patients with or without a history of allergy or bronchial asthma, but are more likely in patients with such a history.

Systemic Lupus Erythematosus

Thiazide diuretics have been reported to cause exacerbation or activation of systemic lupus erythematosus.

Lithium Interaction

Lithium generally should not be given with thiazides.

DOSAGE AND ADMINISTRATION

The recommended starting dose of valsartan is 80 mg once daily when used as monotherapy in patients who are not volume depleted. Valsartan may be used over a dose range of 80-320 mg daily, administered once-a-day. Hydrochlorothiazide is effective in doses of 12.5 to 50 mg once daily, and can be given at doses of 12.5 to 25 mg as Diovan HCT.

To minimize dose-independent side effects, it is usually appropriate to begin combination therapy only after a patient has failed to achieve the desired effect with monotherapy.

The side effects (see WARNINGS) of valsartan are generally rare and apparently independent of dose; those of hydrochlorothiazide are a mixture of dose-dependent phenomena (primarily hypokalemia) and dose-independent phenomena (*e.g.,* pancreatitis), the former much more common than the latter. Therapy with any combination of valsartan and hydrochlorothiazide will be associated with both sets of dose-independent side effects.

REPLACEMENT THERAPY

The combination may be substituted for the titrated components.

DOSE TITRATION BY CLINICAL EFFECT

Diovan HCT is available as tablets containing either valsartan 80 mg or 160 mg and hydrochlorothiazide 12.5 mg. A patient whose blood pressure is not adequately controlled with valsartan monotherapy (see above) may be switched to Diovan HCT, valsartan 80 mg/hydrochlorothiazide 12.5 mg once daily. If blood pressure remains uncontrolled after about 3-4 weeks of therapy, either valsartan or both components may be increased depending on clinical response. There are no studies evaluating doses of valsartan greater than 160 mg in combination with hydrochlorothiazide 25 mg.

A patient whose blood pressure is inadequately controlled by 25 mg once daily of hydrochlorothiazide, or is controlled but who experiences hypokalemia with this regimen, may be switched to Diovan HCT (valsartan 80 mg/hydrochlorothiazide 12.5 mg) once daily, reducing the dose of hydrochlorothiazide without reducing the overall expected antihypertensive response. The clinical response to Diovan HCT should be subsequently evaluated and if blood pressure remains uncontrolled after 3-4 weeks of therapy, the dose may be titrated up to valsartan 160 mg/hydrochlorothiazide 25 mg.

The maximal antihypertensive effect is attained about 4 weeks after initiation of therapy.

PATIENTS WITH RENAL IMPAIRMENT

The usual regimens of therapy with Diovan HCT may be followed as long as the patient's creatinine clearance is >30 ml/min. In patients with more severe renal impairment, loop diuretics are preferred to thiazides, so Diovan HCT is not recommended.

PATIENTS WITH HEPATIC IMPAIRMENT

Care should be exercised with dosing of Diovan HCT in patients with hepatic impairment.

OTHER

No initial dosage adjustment is required for elderly patients.

Diovan HCT may be administered with other antihypertensive agents.

Diovan HCT may be administered with or without food.

PRODUCT LISTING - EQUIVALENTS NOT AVAILABLE

Tablet - Oral - 12.5 mg;80 mg

30's	$42.09	DIOVAN HCT, Allscripts Pharmaceutical Company	54569-4766-00
100's	$147.30	DIOVAN HCT, Novartis Pharmaceuticals	00078-0314-06
100's	$178.83	DIOVAN HCT, Novartis Pharmaceuticals	00078-0314-05

Tablet - Oral - 12.5 mg;160 mg

30's	$44.10	DIOVAN HCT, Allscripts Pharmaceutical Company	54569-4767-00
100's	$152.27	DIOVAN HCT, Novartis Pharmaceuticals	00078-0315-06
100's	$194.58	DIOVAN HCT, Novartis Pharmaceuticals	00078-0315-05

Tablet - Oral - 25 mg;160 mg

10 x 10	$220.65	DIOVAN HCT, Novartis Pharmaceuticals	00078-0383-06
100's	$220.65	DIOVAN HCT, Novartis Pharmaceuticals	00078-0383-05

Hydrocodone Bitartrate; Ibuprofen (000227)

Categories: Pain; DEA Class CIII; FDA Pre 1938 Drugs; Pregnancy Category C
Drug Classes: Analgesics, narcotic; Nonsteroidal anti-inflammatory drugs
Brand Names: Vicoprofen
Cost of Therapy: $32.20 (Pain; Vicoprofen; 7.5 mg; 200 mg; 4 tablets/day; 7 day supply)

DESCRIPTION

Each Vicoprofen tablet contains: Hydrocodone bitartrate, 7.5 mg (WARNING: May be habit forming); ibuprofen, 200 mg.

Hydrocodone bitartrate; ibuprofen is supplied in a fixed combination tablet form for oral administration. Hydrocodone bitartrate; ibuprofen combines the opioid analgesic agent, hydrocodone bitartrate, with the nonsteroidal anti-inflammatory (NSAID) agent, ibuprofen.

Hydrocodone bitartrate is a semisynthetic and centrally acting opioid analgesic. Its chemical name is: 4,5 α-epoxy-3-methoxy-17-methylmorphinan-6-one tartrate (1:1) hydrate (2:5). Its chemical formula is: $C_{18}H_{21}NO_3 \cdot C_4H_6O_6 \cdot 2\frac{1}{2}\ H_2O$, and the molecular weight is 494.50.

Ibuprofen is a nonsteroidal anti-inflammatory drug with analgesic and antipyretic properties. Its chemical name is: (±)-2-(*p*-isobutylphenyl) propionic acid. Its chemical formula is: $C_{13}H_{18}O_2$, and the molecular weight is 206.29.

Inactive ingredients in Vicoprofen tablets include: Colloidal silicon dioxide, corn starch, croscarmellose sodium, hydroxypropyl methylcellulose, magnesium stearate, microcrystalline cellulose, polyethylene glycol, polysorbate 80, and titanium dioxide.

CLINICAL PHARMACOLOGY

HYDROCODONE COMPONENT

Hydrocodone is a semisynthetic opioid analgesic and antitussive with multiple actions qualitatively similar to those of codeine. Most of these involve the central nervous system and smooth muscle. The precise mechanism of action of hydrocodone and other opioids is not known, although it is believed to relate to the existence of opiate receptors in the central nervous system. In addition to analgesia, opioids may produce drowsiness, changes in mood, and mental clouding.

IBUPROFEN COMPONENT

Ibuprofen is a non-steroidal anti-inflammatory agent that possesses analgesic and antipyretic activities. Its mode action, like that of other NSAIDs, is not completely understood, but may be related to inhibition of cyclooxygenase activity and prostaglandin synthesis. Ibuprofen is a peripherally acting analgesic. Ibuprofen does not have any known effects on opiate receptors.

PHARMACOKINETICS

Absorption

After oral dosing with the hydrocodone bitartrate; ibuprofen tablets, a peak hydrocodone plasma level of 27 ng/ml is achieved at 1.7 hours, and a peak ibuprofen plasma level of 30 μg/ml is achieved at 1.8 hours. The effect of food on the absorption of either component from the hydrocodone bitartrate; ibuprofen tablets has not been established.

Distribution

Ibuprofen is highly protein-bound (99%) like most other non- steroidal anti-inflammatory agents. Although the extent of protein binding of hydrocodone in human plasma has not been definitely determined, structural similarities to related opioid analgesics suggest that hydrocodone is not extensively protein bound. As most agents in the 5-ring morphinan group of semisynthetic opioids bind plasma protein to a similar degree (range 19% [hydromorphone] to 45% [oxycodone]), hydrocodone is expected to fall within this range.

Metabolism

Hydrocodone exhibits a complex pattern of metabolism, including *O*-demethylation, *N*-demethylation, and 6-keto reduction to the corresponding 6-α-and 6-β-hydroxy metabolites. Hydromorphone, a potent opioid, is formed from the *O*-demethylation of hydrocodone and contributes to the total analgesic effect of hydrocodone. The *O*- and *N*- demethylation processes are mediated by separate P-450 isoenzymes: CYP2D6 and CYP3A4, respectively.

Ibuprofen is present in this product as a racemate, and following absorption it undergoes interconversion in the plasma from the R-isomer to the S-isomer. Both the R- and S-isomers are metabolized to two primary metabolites: (+)-2-4′-(2hydroxy-2-methyl-propyl) phenyl propionic acid and (+)-2-4′-(2carboxypropyl) phenyl propionic acid, both of which circulate in the plasma at low levels relative to the parent.

Elimination

Hydrocodone and its metabolites are eliminated primarily in the kidneys, with a mean plasma half-life of 4.5 hours. Ibuprofen is excreted in the urine, 50-60% as metabolites and approximately 15% as unchanged drug and conjugate. The plasma half-life is 2.2 hours.

SPECIAL POPULATIONS

No significant pharmacokinetic differences based on age or gender have been demonstrated. The pharmacokinetics of hydrocodone and ibuprofen from hydrocodone bitartrate; ibuprofen has not been evaluated in children.

RENAL IMPAIRMENT

The effect of renal insufficiency on the pharmacokinetics of the hydrocodone bitartrate; ibuprofen dosage form has not been determined.

INDICATIONS AND USAGE

Hydrocodone bitartrate; ibuprofen tablets are indicated for the short-term (generally less than 10 days) management of acute pain. Hydrocodone bitartrate; ibuprofen is not indicated for the treatment of such conditions as osteoarthritis or rheumatoid arthritis.

CONTRAINDICATIONS

Hydrocodone bitartrate; ibuprofen should not be administered to patients who previously have exhibited hypersensitivity to hydrocodone or ibuprofen. Hydrocodone bitartrate; ibuprofen should not be given to patients who have experienced asthma, urticaria, or allergic-type reactions after taking aspirin or other NSAIDs. Severe, rarely fatal, anaphylactic-like reactions to NSAIDs have been reported in such patients (see WARNINGS, Anaphylactoid Reactions and PRECAUTIONS, Pre-Existing Asthma).

Patients known to be hypersensitive to other opioids may exhibit cross-sensitivity to hydrocodone.

WARNINGS

ABUSE AND DEPENDENCE

Hydrocodone can produce drug dependence of the morphine type and therefore has the potential for being abused. Psychic and physical dependence as well as tolerance may develop upon repeated administration of this drug and it should be prescribed and administered with the same degree of caution as other narcotic drugs.

RESPIRATORY DEPRESSION

At high doses or in opioid-sensitive patients, hydrocodone may produce dose-related respiratory depression by acting directly on the brain stem respiratory centers. Hydrocodone also affects the center that controls respiratory rhythm, and may produce irregular and periodic breathing.

HEAD INJURY AND INCREASED INTRACRANIAL PRESSURE

The respiratory depressant effects of opioids and their capacity to elevate cerebrospinal fluid pressure may be markedly exaggerated in the presence of head injury, intracranial lesions or a pre-existing increase in intracranial pressure. Furthermore, opioids produce adverse reactions which may obscure the clinical course of patients with head injuries.

ACUTE ABDOMINAL CONDITIONS
The administration of opioids may obscure the diagnosis or clinical course of patients with acute abdominal conditions.

GASTROINTESTINAL (GI) EFFECTS—RISK OF GI ULCERATION, BLEEDING AND PERFORATION
Serious gastrointestinal toxicity, such as inflammation, bleeding, ulceration, and perforation of the stomach, small intestine or large intestine, can occur at any time, with or without warning symptoms, in patients treated with nonsteroidal anti-inflammatory drugs (NSAIDs). Minor upper GI problems, such as dyspepsia, are common and may also occur at any time during NSAID therapy. Therefore, physicians and patients should remain alert for ulceration and bleeding even in the absence of previous GI tract symptoms. Patients should be informed about the signs and/or symptoms of serious GI toxicity and what steps to take if they occur. The utility of periodic laboratory monitoring has not been demonstrated, nor has it been adequately assessed. Only 1 in 5 patients, who develop a serious upper GI adverse event of NSAID therapy, is symptomatic. Even short term therapy is not without risk.

ANAPHYLACTIC REACTIONS
Anaphylactoid reactions may occur in patients without known prior exposure to hydrocodone bitartrate and ibuprofen. Hydrocodone bitartrate; ibuprofen should not be given to patients with the aspirin triad. The triad typically occurs in asthmatic patients who experience rhinitis with or without nasal polyps, or who exhibit severe, potentially fatal bronchospasm after taking aspirin or other NSAIDs. Fatal reactions to NSAIDs have been reported in such patients (see CONTRAINDICATIONS and PRECAUTIONS, Pre-Existing Asthma). Emergency help should be sought when anaphylactoid reaction occurs.

ADVANCED RENAL DISEASE
In cases with advanced kidney disease, treatment with hydrocodone bitartrate; ibuprofen is not recommended. If NSAID therapy, however, must be initiated, close monitoring of the patient's kidney function is advisable (see PRECAUTIONS, Renal Effects).

USE IN PREGNANCY
As with other NSAID-containing products, hydrocodone bitartrate; ibuprofen should be avoided in late pregnancy because it may cause premature closure of the ductus arteriosus.

NSAIDs should be prescribed with extreme caution in those with a prior history of ulcer disease or gastrointestinal bleeding. Most spontaneous reports of fatal GI events are in elderly or debilitated patients and therefore special care should be taken in treating this population. To minimize the potential risk for an adverse GI event, the lowest effective dose should be used for the shortest possible duration. For high risk patients, alternate therapies that do not involve NSAIDs should be considered.

Studies have shown that patients with a prior history of peptic ulcer disease and/or gastrointestinal bleeding and who use NSAIDs, have a greater than tenfold risk for developing a GI bleed than patients with neither of these risk factors. In addition to a past history of ulcer disease, pharmacoepidemiological studies have identified several other cotherapies or comorbid conditions that may increase the risk for GI bleeding such as: treatment with oral corticosteroids, treatment with anticoagulants, longer duration of NSAID therapy, smoking, alcoholism, older age, and poor general health status.

PRECAUTIONS

GENERAL

Special Risk Patients
As with any opioid analgesic agent, hydrocodone bitartrate; ibuprofen tablets should be used with caution in elderly or debilitated patients, and those with severe impairment of hepatic or renal function, hypothyroidism, Addison's disease, prostatic hypertrophy or urethral stricture. The usual precautions should be observed and the possibility of respiratory depression should be kept in mind.

Cough Reflex
Hydrocodone suppresses the cough reflex; as with opioids, caution should be exercised when hydrocodone bitartrate; ibuprofen is used postoperatively and in patients with pulmonary disease.

Effect on Diagnostic Signs
The antipyretic and anti-inflammatory activity of ibuprofen may reduce fever and inflammation, thus diminishing their utility as diagnostic signs in detecting complications of presumed noninfectious, noninflammatory painful conditions.

Hepatic Effects
as with other nsaids, ibuprofen has been reported to cause borderline elevations of one or more liver enzymes; this may occur in up to 15% of patients. These abnormalities may progress, may remain essentially unchanged, or may be transient with continued therapy. Notable (3 times the upper limit of normal) elevations of sgpt (alt) or sgot (ast) occurred in controlled clinical trials in less than 1% of patients. A patient with symptoms and/or signs suggesting liver dysfunction, or in whom an abnormal liver test has occurred, should be evaluated for evidence of the development of more severe hepatic reactions while on therapy with hydrocodone bitartrate; ibuprofen. Severe hepatic reactions, including jaundice and cases of fatal hepatitis, have been reported with ibuprofen as with other nsaids. Although such reactions are rare, if abnormal liver tests persist or worsen, if clinical signs and symptoms consistent with liver disease develop, or if systemic manifestations occur (*e.g.,* eosinophilia, rash, etc.), hydrocodone bitartrate; ibuprofen should be discontinued.

Fluid Retention and Edema
Fluid retention and edema have been reported in association with ibuprofen; therefore, the drug should be used with caution in patients with a history of cardiac decompensation, hypertension or heart failure.

Pre-Existing Asthma
Patient with asthma may have aspirin-sensitive asthma. The use of aspirin in patients with aspirin-sensitive asthma has been associated with severe bronchospasm, which may be fatal. Since cross-reactivity between aspirin and other NSAIDs has been reported in such aspirin-sensitive patients, hydrocodone bitartrate; ibuprofen should not be administered to patients with this form of aspirin sensitivity and should be used with caution in patients with pre-existing asthma.

Aseptic Meningitis
Aseptic meningitis with fever and coma has been observed on rare occasions in patients on ibuprofen therapy. Although it is probably more likely to occur in patients with systemic lupus erythematous and related connective tissue diseases, it has been reported in patients who do not have an underlying chronic disease. If signs or symptoms of meningitis develop in a patient on hydrocodone bitartrate; ibuprofen, the possibility of its being related to ibuprofen should be considered.

Renal Effects
Caution should be used when initiating treatment with hydrocodone bitartrate; ibuprofen in patients with considerable dehydration. It is advisable to rehydrate patients first and then start therapy with hydrocodone bitartrate; ibuprofen. Caution is also recommended in patients with pre-existing kidney disease (see WARNINGS, Advanced Renal Disease).

As with other NSAIDs, long-term administration of ibuprofen has resulted in renal papillary necrosis and other renal pathologic changes. Renal toxicity has also been seen in patients in which renal prostaglandins have a compensatory role in the maintenance of renal perfusion. In these patients, administration of a nonsteroidal anti-inflammatory drug may cause a dose-dependent reduction in prostaglandin formation and, secondarily, in renal blood flow, which may precipitate overt renal decompensation. Patients at greatest risk of this reaction are those with impaired renal function, heart failure, liver dysfunction, those taking diuretics and ACE inhibitors, and the elderly. Discontinuation of nonsteroidal anti-inflammatory drug therapy is usually followed by recovery to the pretreatment state.

Ibuprofen metabolites are eliminated primarily by the kidneys. The extent to which the metabolites may accumulate in patients with renal failure has not been studied. Patients with significantly impaired renal function should be more closely monitored.

Hematological Effects
Ibuprofen, like other NSAIDs, can inhibit platelet aggregation but the effect is quantitatively less and of shorter duration than that seen with aspirin. Ibuprofen has been shown to prolong bleeding time in normal subjects. Because this prolonged bleeding effect may be exaggerated in patients with underlying hemostatic defects, hydrocodone bitartrate; ibuprofen should be used with caution in persons with intrinsic coagulation defects and those on anticoagulant therapy.

Anemia is sometimes seen in patients receiving NSAIDs, including ibuprofen. This may be due to fluid retention, GI loss, or an incompletely described effect upon erythropoiesis.

LABORATORY TESTS
A decrease in hemoglobin may occur during hydrocodone bitartrate; ibuprofen therapy, and elevations of liver enzymes may be seen in a small percentage of patients during hydrocodone bitartrate; ibuprofen therapy (see Hematological Effects and Hepatic Effects).

In patients with severe hepatic or renal disease, effects of therapy should be monitored with liver and/or renal function tests.

CARCINOGENESIS, MUTAGENESIS, AND IMPAIRMENT OF FERTILITY
The carcinogenic and mutagenic potential of hydrocodone bitartrate; ibuprofen has not been investigated. The ability of hydrocodone bitartrate; ibuprofen to impair fertility has not been assessed.

PREGNANCY CATEGORY C
Pregnancy, Teratogenic Effects: Hydrocodone bitartrate; ibuprofen, administered to rabbits at 95 mg/kg (5.72 and 1.9 times the maximum clinical dose based on body weight and surface area, respectively), a maternally toxic dose, resulted in an increase in the percentage of litters and fetuses with any major abnormality and an increase in the number of litters and fetuses with one or more nonossified metacarpals (a minor abnormality). Hydrocodone bitartrate; ibuprofen, administered to rats at 166 mg/kg (10.0 and 1.66 times the maximum clinical dose based on body weight and surface area, respectively), a maternally toxic dose, did not result in any reproductive toxicity. There are no adequate and well-controlled studies in pregnant women. Hydrocodone bitartrate; ibuprofen should be used during pregnancy only if the potential benefit justifies the potential risk to the fetus.
Pregnancy, Nonteratogenic Effects: Because of the known effects of nonsteroidal anti-inflammatory drugs on the fetal cardiovascular system (closure of the ductus arteriosus), use during pregnancy (particularly late pregnancy) should be avoided. Babies born to mothers who have been taking opioids regularly prior to delivery will be physically dependent. The withdrawal signs include irritability and excessive crying, tremors, hyperactive reflexes, increased respiratory rate, increased stools, sneezing, yawning, vomiting, and fever. The intensity of the syndrome does not always correlate with the duration of maternal opioid use or dose. There is no consensus on the best method of managing withdrawal.

LABOR AND DELIVERY
As with other drugs known to inhibit prostaglandin synthesis, an increased incidence of dystocia and delayed parturition occurred in rats. Administration of hydrocodone bitartrate; ibuprofen is not recommended during labor and delivery.

NURSING MOTHERS
It is not known whether hydrocodone is excreted in human milk. In limited studies, an assay capable of detecting 1 μg/ml did not demonstrate ibuprofen in the milk of lactating mothers. However, because of the limited nature of the studies, and the possible adverse effects of prostaglandin-inhibiting drugs on neonates, hydrocodone bitartrate; ibuprofen is not recommended for use in nursing mothers.

PEDIATRIC USE

The safety and effectiveness of hydrocodone bitartrate; ibuprofen in pediatric patients below the age of 16 have not been established.

GERIATRIC USE

In controlled clinical trials there was no difference in tolerability between patients <65 years of age and those ≥65, apart from an increased tendency of the elderly to develop constipation. However, because the elderly may be more sensitive to the renal and gastrointestinal effects of nonsteroidal anti-inflammatory agents as well as possible increased risk of respiratory depression with opioids, extra caution and reduced dosages should be used when treating the elderly with hydrocodone bitartrate; ibuprofen.

DRUG INTERACTIONS

ACE-Inhibitors: Reports suggest that NSAIDs may diminish the antihypertensive effect of ACE-inhibitors. This interaction should be given consideration in patients taking hydrocodone bitartrate; ibuprofen concomitantly with ACE-inhibitors.

Anticholinergics: The concurrent use of anticholinergics with hydrocodone preparations may produce paralytic ileus.

Antidepressants: The use of MAO inhibitors or tricyclic antidepressants with hydrocodone bitartrate; ibuprofen may increase the effect of either the antidepressant or hydrocodone.

Aspirin: As with other products containing NSAIDs, concomitant administration of hydrocodone bitartrate; ibuprofen and aspirin is not generally recommended because of the potential of increased adverse effects.

CNS Depressants: Patients receiving other opioids, antihistamines, antipsychotics, antianxiety agents, or other CNS depressants (including alcohol) concomitantly with hydrocodone bitartrate; ibuprofen may exhibit an additive CNS depression. When combined therapy is contemplated, the dose of one or both agents should be reduced.

Furosemide: Ibuprofen has been shown to reduce the natriuretic effect of furosemide and thiazides in some patients. This response has been attributed to inhibition of renal prostaglandin synthesis. During concomitant therapy with hydrocodone bitartrate; ibuprofen the patient should be observed closely for signs of renal failure (see PRECAUTIONS, Renal Effects), as well as diuretic efficacy.

Lithium: Ibuprofen has been shown to elevate plasma lithium concentration and reduce renal lithium clearance. This effect has been attributed to inhibition of renal prostaglandin synthesis by ibuprofen. Thus, when hydrocodone bitartrate; ibuprofen and lithium are administered concurrently, patients should be observed for signs of lithium toxicity.

Methotrexate: Ibuprofen, as well as other NSAIDs, has been reported to competitively inhibit methotrexate accumulation in rabbit kidney slices. This may indicate that ibuprofen could enhance the toxicity of methotrexate. Caution should be used when hydrocodone bitartrate; ibuprofen is administered concomitantly with methotrexate.

Warfarin: The effects of warfarin and NSAIDs on GI bleeding are synergistic, such that users of both drugs together have a risk of serious GI bleeding higher than users of either drug alone.

ADVERSE REACTIONS

Hydrocodone bitartrate; ibuprofen was administered to approximately 300 pain patients in a safety study that employed dosages and a duration of treatment sufficient to encompass the recommended usage (see DOSAGE AND ADMINISTRATION). Adverse event rates generally increased with increasing daily dose. The event rates reported below are from approximately 150 patients who were in a group that received 1 tablet of hydrocodone bitartrate; ibuprofen an average of 3-4 times daily. The overall incidence rates of adverse experiences in the trials were fairly similar for this patient group and those who received the comparison treatment, acetaminophen 600 mg with codeine 60 mg.

The following lists adverse events that occurred with an incidence of 1% or greater in clinical trials of hydrocodone bitartrate; ibuprofen, without regard to the causal relationship of the events to the drug. To distinguish different rates of occurrence in clinical studies, the adverse events are listed as follows:

Body as a Whole: Abdominal pain*, asthenia*, fever, flu syndrome, headache (27%), infection*, pain.

Cardiovascular: Palpitations, vasodilation.

Central Nervous System: Anxiety*, confusion, dizziness (14%), hypertonia, insomnia*, nervousness*, paresthesia, somnolence (22%), thinking abnormalities.

Digestive: Anorexia, constipation (22%), diarrhea*, dry mouth*, dyspepsia (12%), flatulence*, gastritis, melena, mouth ulcers, nausea (21%), thirst, vomiting.*

Metabolic and Nutritional Disorders: Edema.*

Respiratory: Dyspnea, hiccups, pharyngitis, rhinitis.

Skin and Appendages: Pruritus*, sweating.*

Special Senses: Tinnitus.

Urogenital: Urinary frequency.

Name of adverse event = less than 3%.

Adverse events marked with an asterisk*=3-9%.

Adverse event rates over 9% are in parentheses.

Incidence Less Than 1%

Body as a Whole: Allergic reaction.

Cardiovascular: Arrhythmia, hypotension, tachycardia.

Central Nervous System: Agitation, abnormal dreams, decreased libido, depression, euphoria, mood changes, neuralgia, slurred speech, tremor, vertigo.

Digestive: Chalky stool, "clenching teeth", dysphagia, esophageal spasm, esophagitis, gastroenteritis, glossitis, liver enzyme elevation.

Metabolic and Nutritional: Weight decrease.

Musculoskeletal: Arthralgia, myalgia.

Respiratory: Asthma, bronchitis, hoarseness, increased cough, pulmonary congestion, pneumonia, shallow breathing, sinusitis.

Skin and Appendages: Rash, urticaria.

Special Senses: Altered vision, bad taste, dry eyes.

Urogenital: Cystitis, glycosuria, impotence, urinary incontinence, urinary retention.

DOSAGE AND ADMINISTRATION

For the short-term (generally less than 10 days) management of acute pain, the recommended dose of hydrocodone bitartrate; ibuprofen is 1 tablet every 4-6 hours, as necessary. Dosage should not exceed 5 tablets in a 24 hour period. It should be kept in mind that tolerance to hydrocodone can develop with continued use and that the incidence of untoward effects is dose related.

The lowest effective dose or the longest dosing interval should be sought for each patient, especially in the elderly. After observing the initial response to therapy with hydrocodone bitartrate; ibuprofen, the dose and frequency of dosing should be adjusted to suit the individual patient's need, without exceeding the total daily dose recommended.

HOW SUPPLIED

Vicoprofen tablets are available as: White film-coated round convex tablets, engraved with "VP" over the Knoll triangle on one side and plain on the other side.

STORAGE

Store at 25°C (77°F); excursions permitted to 15-30°C (59-86°F).

Dispense in a tight, light-resistant container.

PRODUCT LISTING - EQUIVALENTS NOT AVAILABLE

Tablet - Oral - 7.5 mg;200 mg

Qty	Price	Product	NDC
2's	$2.30	VICOPROFEN, Southwood Pharmaceuticals Inc	58016-0422-02
12's	$22.50	VICOPROFEN, Pharma Pac	52959-0522-12
15's	$17.25	VICOPROFEN, Southwood Pharmaceuticals Inc	58016-0422-15
15's	$27.12	VICOPROFEN, Pharma Pac	52959-0522-15
20's	$23.00	VICOPROFEN, Southwood Pharmaceuticals Inc	58016-0422-20
20's	$33.96	VICOPROFEN, Pharma Pac	52959-0522-20
25 x 4	$133.19	VICOPROFEN, Abbott Pharmaceutical	00074-2277-12
30's	$34.50	VICOPROFEN, Southwood Pharmaceuticals Inc	58016-0422-30
30's	$45.31	VICOPROFEN, Pharma Pac	52959-0522-30
40's	$46.00	VICOPROFEN, Southwood Pharmaceuticals Inc	58016-0422-40
40's	$58.63	VICOPROFEN, Pharma Pac	52959-0522-40
60's	$69.00	VICOPROFEN, Southwood Pharmaceuticals Inc	58016-0422-60
100's	$115.00	VICOPROFEN, Southwood Pharmaceuticals Inc	58016-0422-00
100's	$115.80	VICOPROFEN, Abbott Pharmaceutical	00074-2277-14
100's	$133.19	VICOPROFEN, Knoll Pharmaceutical Company	00044-0723-41

H

Hydrocortisone *(001476)*

For related information, see the comparative table section in Appendix A.

Categories: Adrenocortical insufficiency; Anemia, acquired hemolytic; Anemia, congenital hypoplastic; Anemia, erythroblastopenia; Ankylosing spondylitis; Arthritis, gouty; Arthritis, post-traumatic; Arthritis, psoriatic; Arthritis, rheumatoid; Asthma; Berylliosis; Bursitis; Carditis, rheumatic; Chorioretinitis; Choroiditis; Colitis, ulcerative; Conjunctivitis, allergic; Crohn's disease; Dermatitis herpetiformis, bullous; Dermatitis, atopic; Dermatitis, contact; Dermatitis, exfoliative; Dermatitis, seborrheic; Dermatomyositis, systemic; Dermatosis, corticosteroid-responsive; Epicondylitis; Erythema multiforme; Herpes zoster ophthalmicus; Hypercalcemia, secondary to neoplasia; Hypersensitivity reactions; Inflammation, anterior segment, ophthalmic; Inflammation, ophthalmic; Inflammatory bowel disease; Iridocyclitis; Iritis; Keratitis; Leukemia; Loffler's syndrome; Lupus erythematosus, systemic; Lymphoma; Meningitis, tuberculous; Multiple sclerosis; Mycosis fungoides; Nephrotic syndrome; Neuritis, optic; Ophthalmia, sympathetic; Pemphigus; Pneumonitis, aspiration; Polymyositis; Psoriasis; Rhinitis, perennial allergic; Rhinitis, seasonal allergic; Sarcoidosis; Serum sickness; Stevens-Johnson syndrome; Synovitis, secondary to osteoarthritis; Tenosynovitis; Thrombocytopenia, secondary; Thyroiditis, nonsuppurative; Trichinosis; Tuberculosis, disseminated; Tuberculosis, fulminating; Tuberculosis, meningitis; Ulcer, allergic corneal marginal; Uveitis; Pregnancy Category C; FDA Approved 1952 Dec; WHO Formulary

Drug Classes: Corticosteroids; Corticosteroids, topical; Dermatologics

Brand Names: Acticort; Aeroseb-Hc; Ala-Cort; Ala-Scalp; Albacort; Allercort; Alphaderm; Anusol-Hc; Balneol-Hc; Beta-Hc; Cetacort; Coracin; Coreton; Cort-Dome; Cortef; Cortenema; Cortes; Cortril; Cotacort; Dermol Hc; Eldecort; Epicort; Flexicort; Glycort; H-Cort; Hi-Cor; Hidroaltesona; Hidromar; Hidrotisona; Hycort; Hycortole; Hydro-Tex; Hydrocortemel; Hydrocortone; Hymac; Hytone; IVocort; Lacticare; Lemoderm; Lidex; Nogenic Hc; **Nutracort**; Otozonbase; Penecort; Procto-Hc; Proctocort; Rederm; S-T Cort; Stie-Cort; Synacort; Tega-Cort; Texacort; Topisone

Foreign Brand Availability: Algicortis (Italy); Cortate (Canada); Covocort (South-Africa); Cremicort-H (Belgium); Cutaderm (South-Africa); Dermaid (Australia); Dermaid Soft Cream (Australia); Dermocortal (Italy); Derm-Aid Cream (Australia; New-Zealand; Singapore); Dioderm (England); Eczacort (Philippines); Efcortelan (Bahrain; Benin; Burkina-Faso; Cyprus; Egypt; Ethiopia; Gambia; Ghana; Guinea; Iran; Iraq; Ivory-Coast; Jordan; Kenya; Kuwait; Lebanon; Liberia; Libya; Malawi; Mali; Mauritania; Mauritius; Morocco; Niger; Nigeria; Oman; Qatar; Republic-of-Yemen; Saudi-Arabia; Senegal; Seychelles; Sierra-Leone; Sudan; Syria; Tanzania; Tunia; Uganda; United-Arab-Emirates; Zambia; Zimbabwe); Egocort Cream (Australia; Hong-Kong; Malaysia; New-Zealand); Emo-Cort (Canada); Ficortril (Germany; Sweden); Filocot (Greece); Hycor (Australia); Hydrocortison (Finland; Germany; Hungary); Hydrocortisone (Belgium; France); Hydrocortisone Astier (France; Switzerland); Hydrocortisonum (Netherlands); Hydrocortisyl (Bahrain; Cyprus; Egypt; England; Iran; Iraq; Jordan; Kuwait; Lebanon; Libya; Oman; Qatar; Republic-of-Yemen; Saudi-Arabia; Syria; United-Arab-Emirates); Hydroderm (Austria; Germany); Hydrogalen (Germany); Hydrokort (Norway); Hydrokortison (Denmark; Norway; Sweden); Hydrotopic (Philippines); Hytisone (Hong-Kong); Hytone Lotion (Korea); Kyypakkaus (Finland); Lacticare HC (Mexico; Philippines; Taiwan); Lemnis Fatty Cream HC (New-Zealand); Lenirit (Italy); Mildison (Denmark; England; Sweden); Mildison-Fatty (Finland); Mildison fet krem (Norway); Mildison Lipocream (England; Ireland; New-Zealand); Mitocortyl Demangeaisons (France); Prevex HC (Thailand); Procutan (South-Africa); Sanatison (Germany); Schericur (Austria); Schericur 0.25% (Spain); Sistral Hydrocort (Germany); Skincalm (New-Zealand); Unicort (Colombia); Uniderm (Denmark; Finland; Sweden)

Cost of Therapy: $22.48 (Asthma; Cortef; 20 mg; 1 tablet/day; 30 day supply)
$2.78 (Asthma; Generic Tablets; 20 mg; 1 tablet/day; 30 day supply)

DESCRIPTION

TABLETS

Hydrocortisone is a glucocorticoid. Glucocorticoids are adrenocortical steroids, both naturally occurring and synthetic, which are readily absorbed from the gastrointestinal tract. Hydrocortisone is white to practically white, odorless, crystalline powder with a melting point of about 215°C. It is very slightly soluble in water and ether; sparingly soluble in acetone and in alcohol; slightly soluble in chloroform.

The chemical name for hydrocortisone is pregn-4-ene-3, 20-dione,11,17,21-trihydroxy-,(11β). Its molecular weight is 362.46.

Cortef tablets are available for oral administration in three strengths: each tablet contains either 5, 10, or 20 mg of hydrocortisone. *Inactive Ingredients:* Calcium stearate, corn starch, lactose, mineral oil, sorbic acid, sucrose.

CREAM

The topical corticosteroids constitute a class of primarily synthetic steroids used as antiinflammatory and antipruritic agents.

Hydrocortisone Cream, 1%: A topical corticosteroid containing hydrocortisone 1% in a pH-adjusted cream containing stearyl alcohol, cetyl alcohol, isopropyl palmitate, citric acid anhydrous, polyoxyl 40 stearate, dibasic sodium phosphate dried, propylene glycol, water, and benzyl alcohol as a preservative.

Hydrocortisone Cream, 2.5%: A topical corticosteroid with hydrocortisone 2.5% (active ingredient) in a water-washable cream containing the following inactive ingredients: benzyl alcohol, petrolatum, stearyl alcohol, propylene glycol, isopropyl myristate, polyoxyl 40 stearate, carbomer 934, sodium lauryl sulfate, edetate disodium, sodium hydroxide to adjust the pH, and purified water.

Hydrocortisone has the chemical name Pregn-4-ene-3,20-dione, 11, 17, 21-trihydroxy-(11β)-; it has a molecular formula of $C_{21}H_{30}O_5$; a molecular weight of 362.47.

CLINICAL PHARMACOLOGY

TABLETS

Naturally occurring glucocorticoids (hydrocortisone and cortisone), which also have salt-retaining properties, are used as replacement therapy in adrenocortical deficiency states. Their synthetic analogs are primarily used for their potent anti-inflammatory effects in disorders of many organ systems.

Glucocorticoids cause profound and varied metabolic effects. In addition, they modify the body's immune responses to diverse stimuli.

CREAM

Topical corticosteroids share antiinflammatory, antipruritic and vasoconstrictive actions.

The mechanism of antiinflammatory activity of the topical corticosteroids is unclear. Various laboratory methods, including vasoconstrictor assays, are used to compare and predict potencies and/or clinical efficacies of the topical corticosteroids. There is some evidence to suggest that a recognizable correlation exists between vasoconstrictor potency and therapeutic efficacy in man.

Pharmacokinetics

The extent of percutaneous absorption of topical corticosteroids is determined by many factors including the vehicle, the integrity of the epidermal barrier, and the use of occlusive dressings.

Topical corticosteroids can be absorbed from normal intact skin. Inflammation and/or other disease processes in the skin increase percutaneous absorption. Occlusive dressings substantially increase the percutaneous absorption of topical corticosteroids. Thus, occlusive dressings may be a valuable therapeutic adjunct for treatment of resistant dermatoses (see DOSAGE AND ADMINISTRATION).

Once absorbed through the skin, topical corticosteroids are handled through pharmacokinetic pathways similar to systemically administered corticosteroids. Corticosteroids are bound to plasma proteins in varying degrees. Corticosteroids are metabolized primarily in the liver and are then excreted by the kidneys. Some of the topical corticosteroids and their metabolites are also excreted into the bile.

INDICATIONS AND USAGE

TABLETS

Hydrocortisone tablets are indicated in the following conditions:

Endocrine Disorders: Primary or secondary adrenocortical insufficiency (hydrocortisone or cortisone is the first choice; synthetic analogs may used in conjunction with mineralocorticoids where applicable; in infancy mineralocorticoid supplementation is of particular importance), congenital adrenal hyperplasia, nonsuppurative thyroiditis and hypercalcemia associated with cancer.

Rheumatic Disorders: As adjunctive therapy for short-term administration (to tide the patient over an acute episode or exacerbation) in: psoriatic arthritis, rheumatoid arthritis, including juvenile rheumatoid arthritis (selected cases may require low-dose maintenance therapy), ankylosing spondylitis, acute and subacute bursitis, acute nonspecific tenosynovitis, acute gouty arthritis, post-traumatic osteoarthritis, synovitis of osteoarthritis and epicondylitis.

Collagen Diseases: During an exacerbation or as maintenance therapy in selected cases of: Systemic lupus erythematosus, systemic dermatomyositis (polymyositis), acute rheumatic carditis.

Dermatologic Diseases: Pemphigus, bullous dermatitis herpetiformis, severe erythema multiforme (Stevens-Johnson syndrome), exfoliative dermatitis, mycosis fungoides, severe psoriasis, and severe seborrheic dermatitis.

Allergic States: Control of severe or incapacitating allergic conditions intractable to adequate trials of conventional treatment: Seasonal or perennial allergic rhinitis, serum sickness, bronchial asthma, contact dermatitis, atopic dermatitis, and drug hypersensitivity reactions.

Ophthalmic Diseases: Severe acute and chronic allergic and inflammatory processes involving the eye and its adnexa such as: Allergic conjunctivitis, keratitis, allergic corneal marginal ulcers, herpes zoster ophthalmicus, iritis and iridocyclitis, chorioretinitis, anterior segment inflammation, diffuse posterior uveitis and choroiditis, optic neuritis, and sympathetic ophthalmia.

Respiratory Diseases: Symptomatic sarcoidosis, Loeffler's syndrome not manageable by other means, berylliosis, fulminating or disseminated pulmonary tuberculosis when used concurrently with appropriate antituberculous chemotherapy, and aspiration pneumonitis.

Hematologic Disorders: Idiopathic thrombocytopenic purpura in adults, secondary thrombocytopenia in adults, acquired (autoimmune) hemolytic anemia, erythroblastopenia (RBC anemia), and congenital (erythroid) hypoplastic anemia.

Neoplastic Diseases: For palliative management of: Leukemias and lymphomas in adults, and acute leukemia of childhood.

Edematous States: To induce a diuresis or remission of proteinuria in the nephrotic syndrome, without uremia, of the idiopathic type or that due to lupus erythematosus.

Gastrointestinal Diseases: To tide the patient over a critical period of the disease in: Ulcerative colitis, and regional enteritis.

Nervous System: Acute exacerbations of multiple sclerosis.

Miscellaneous: Tuberculous meningitis with subarachnoid block or impending block when used concurrently with appropriate antituberculous chemotherapy, and trichinosis with neurologic or myocardial involvement.

CREAM

Topical corticosteroids are indicated for the relief of the inflammatory and pruritic manifestations of corticosteroid-responsive dermatoses.

CONTRAINDICATIONS

TABLETS

Systemic fungal infections and known hypersensitivity to components.

CREAM

Topical corticosteroids are contraindicated in those patients with a history of hypersensitivity to any of the components of the preparation.

WARNINGS

TABLETS

In patients on corticosteroid therapy subjected to unusual stress, increased dosage of rapidly acting corticosteroids before, during, and after the stressful situation is indicated.

Corticosteroids may mask some signs of infection, and new infections may appear during their use. Infections with any pathogen including viral, bacterial, fungal, protozoan or helminthic infections, in any location of the body, may be associated with the use of corticosteroids alone or in combination with other immunosuppressive agents that affect cellular immunity, humoral immunity, or neutrophil function.[1]

These infections may be mild, but can be severe and at times fatal. With increasing doses of corticosteroids, the rate of occurrence of infectious complications increases.[2] There may be decreased resistance and inability to localize infection when corticosteroids are used.

Prolonged use of corticosteroids may produce posterior subcapsular cataracts, glaucoma with possible damage to the optic nerves, and may enhance the establishment of secondary ocular infections due to fungi or viruses.

Use in Pregnancy: Since adequate human reproduction studies have not been done with corticosteroids, the use of these drugs in pregnancy, nursing mothers or women of child-bearing potential requires that the possible benefits of the drug be weighed against the potential hazards to the mother and embryo or fetus. Infants born of mothers who have received substantial doses of corticosteroids during pregnancy, should be carefully observed for signs of hypoadrenalism.

Average and large doses of hydrocortisone or cortisone can cause elevation of blood pressure, salt and water retention, and increased excretion of potassium. These effects are less likely to occur with the synthetic derivatives except when used in large doses. Dietary salt restriction and potassium supplementation may be necessary. All corticosteroids increase calcium excretion.

Administration of live or live, attenuated vaccines is contraindicated in patients receiving immunosuppressive doses of corticosteroids. Killed or inactivated vaccines may be administered to patients receiving immunosuppressive doses of corticosteroids; however, the response to such vaccines may be diminished. Indicated immunization procedures may be undertaken in patients receiving nonimmunosuppressive doses of corticosteroids.

The use of hydrocortisone in active tuberculosis should be restricted to those cases of fulminating or disseminated tuberculosis in which the corticosteroid is used for the management of the disease in conjunction with an appropriate antituberculous regimen.

If corticosteroids are indicated in patients with latent tuberculosis or tuberculin reactivity, close observation is necessary as reactivation of the disease may occur. During prolonged corticosteroid therapy, these patients should receive chemoprophylaxis.

Persons who are on drugs which suppress the immune system are more susceptible to infections than healthy individuals. Chicken pox and measles, for example, can have a more serious or even fatal course in non-immune children or adults on corticosteroids. In such children or adults who have not had these diseases, particular care should be taken to avoid exposure. How the dose, route and duration of corticosteroid administration affects the risk of developing a disseminated infection is not known. The contribution of the underlying disease and/or prior corticosteroid treatment to the risk is also not known. If exposed to chicken pox, prophylaxis with varicella zoster immune globulin (VZIG) may be indicated. If exposed to measles, prophylaxis with pooled intramuscular immunoglobulin (IG) may be indicated. (See the respective prescribing information for complete VZIG and IG for complete information.) If chicken pox develops, treatment with antiviral agents may be considered. Similarly, corticosteroids should be used with great care in patients with known or suspected Strongyloides (threadworm) infestation. In such patients, corticosteroid-induced immunosuppression may lead to Strongyloides hyperinfection and dissemination with widespread larval migration, often accompanied by severe enterocolitis and potentially fatal gram-negative septicemia.

PRECAUTIONS

TABLETS

General

Drug-induced secondary adrenocortical insufficiency may be minimized by gradual reduction of dosage. This type of relative insufficiency may persist for months after discontinuation of therapy; therefore, in any situation of stress occurring during that period, hormone therapy should be reinstituted. Since mineralocorticoid secretion may be impaired, salt and/or a mineralocorticoid should be administered concurrently.

There is an enhanced effect of corticosteroids on patients with hypothyroidism and in those with cirrhosis.

Corticosteroids should be used cautiously in patients with ocular herpes simplex because of possible corneal perforation.

The lowest possible dose of corticosteroid should be used to control the condition under treatment, and when reduction in dosage is possible, the reduction should be gradual.

Psychic derangements may appear when corticosteroids are used, ranging from euphoria, insomnia, mood swings, personality changes, and severe depression, to frank psychotic manifestations. Also, existing emotional instability or psychotic tendencies may be aggravated by corticosteroids.

Steroids should be used with caution in nonspecific ulcerative colitis, if there is a probability of impending perforation, abscess or other pyogenic infection; diverticulitis; fresh intestinal anastomoses; active or latent peptic ulcer; renal insufficiency; hypertension; osteoporosis; and myasthenia gravis.

Growth and development of infants and children on prolonged corticosteroid therapy should be carefully observed.

Kaposi's sarcoma has been reported to occur in patients receiving corticosteroid therapy. Discontinuation of corticosteroids may result in clinical remission.

Although controlled clinical trials have shown corticosteroids to be effective in speeding the resolution of acute exacerbations of multiple sclerosis, they do not show that corticosteroids affect the ultimate outcome or natural history of the disease. The studies do show that relatively high doses of corticosteroids are necessary to demonstrate a significant effect. (See DOSAGE AND ADMINISTRATION.)

Since complications of treatment with glucocorticosteroids are dependent on the size of the dose and the duration of treatment, a risk/benefit decision must be made in each individual case as to dose and duration of treatment and as to whether daily or intermittent therapy should be used.

Information for the Patient

Persons who are on immunosuppressant doses of corticosteroids should be warned to avoid exposure to chicken pox or measles. Patients should also be advised that if they are exposed, medical advice should be sought without delay.

CREAM

General

Systemic absorption of topical corticosteroids has produced reversible hypothalamic-pituitary-adrenal (HPA) axis suppression, manifestations of Cushing's syndrome, hyperglycemia, and glucosuria in some patients.

Conditions which augment systemic absorption include the application of the more potent steroids, use over large surface areas, prolonged use, and the addition of occlusive dressings.

Therefore, patients receiving a large dose of a potent topical steroid applied to a large surface area or under an occulsive dressing should be evaluated periodically for evidence of HPA axis suppression by using the urinary-free cortisol and ACTH stimulation tests. If HPA axis suppression is noted an attempt should be made to withdraw the drug or to reduce the frequency of application or substitute a less potent steroid.

Recovery of HPA axis function is generally prompt and complete upon discontinuation of the drug. Infrequently, signs and symptoms of steroid withdrawal may occur, requiring supplemental systemic corticosteroids.

Pediatric patients may absorb proportionally larger amounts of topical corticosteroids and thus be more susceptible to systemic toxicity (see Pediatric Use).

If irritation develops, topical corticosteroids should be discontinued and appropriate therapy instituted. In the presence of dermatological infections, the use of an appropriate antifungal or antibacterial agent should be instituted. If a favorable response does not occur promptly, the corticosteroid should be discontinued until the infection had been adequately controlled.

Information for the Patient

Patients using topical corticosteroids should receive the following information and instructions:

1. This medication is to be used as directed by the physician. It is for external use only. Avoid contact with the eyes.
2. Patients should be advised not to use this medication for any disorder other than that for which it has been prescribed.
3. The treated skin area should not be bandaged or otherwise covered or wrapped as to be occlusive unless directed by the physician.
4. Patients should report any signs of local adverse reactions especially under occlusive dressing.
5. Parents of pediatric patients should be advised not to use tight-fitting diapers or plastic pants on a pediatric patient being treated in the diaper area, as these garments may constitute occlusive dressings.

Laboratory Tests

The following tests may be helpful in evaluating the HPA axis suppression: Urinary-free cortisol test, and ACTH stimulation test.

Carcinogenesis, Mutagenesis, and Impairment of Fertility

Long-term animal studies have not been performed to evaluate the carcinogenic potential or the effect on fertility of topical corticosteroids. Studies to determine mutagenicity with prednisolone and hydrocortisone have revealed negative results.

Pregnancy Category C

Corticosteroids are generally teratogenic in laboratory animals when administered systemically at relatively low dosage levels. The more potent corticosteroids have been shown to be teratogenic after dermal application in laboratory animals. There are no adequate and well-controlled studies in pregnant women on teratogenic effects from topically applied corticosteroids.

Therefore, topical corticosteroids should be used during pregnancy only if the potential benefit justifies the potential risk to the fetus. Drugs of this class should not be used extensively on pregnant patients, in large amounts, or for prolonged periods of time.

Nursing Mothers

It is not known whether topical administration of corticosteroids could result in sufficient systemic absorption to produce detectable quantities in breast milk. Systemically administered corticosteroids are secreted into breast milk in quantities not likely to have a deleterious effect on the infant. Nevertheless, caution should be exercised when topical corticosteroids are administered to a nursing woman.

Pediatric Use

Pediatric patients may demonstrate greater susceptibility to topical corticosteroid-induced HPA axis suppression and Cushing's syndrome than mature patients because of a larger skin surface area to body weight ratio.

Hypothalamic-pituitary-adrenal (HPA) axis suppression, Cushing's syndrome, and intracranial hypertension have been reported in pediatric patients receiving topical corticosteroids. Manifestations of adrenal suppression in pediatric patients include linear growth retardation, delayed weight gain, low plasma cortisol levels, and absence of response ACTH stimulation. Manifestations of intracranial hypertension include bulging fontanelles, headaches, and bilateral papilledema.

Administration of topical corticosteroids to pediatric patients should be limited to the least amount compatible with an effective therapeutic regimen. Chronic corticosteroid therapy may interfere with the growth and development of pediatric patients.

DRUG INTERACTIONS

TABLETS

The pharmacokinetic interactions listed below are potentially clinically important. Drugs that induce hepatic enzymes such as phenobarbital, phenytoin and rifampin may increase the clearance of corticosteroids and may require increases in corticosteroid dose to achieve the desired response. Drugs such as troleandomycin and ketoconazole may inhibit the metabolism of corticosteroids and thus decrease their clearance. Therefore, the dose of corticosteroid should be titrated to avoid steroid toxicity. Corticosteroids may increase the clearance of chronic high dose aspirin. This could lead to decreased salicylate serum levels or increase the risk of salicylate toxicity when corticosteroid is withdrawn. Aspirin should be used cautiously in conjunction with corticosteroids in patients suffering from hypoprothrombinemia. The effect of corticosteroids on oral anticoagulants is variable. There are reports of enhanced as well as diminished effects of anticoagulants when given concurrently with corticosteroids. Therefore, coagulation indices should be monitored to maintain the desired anticoagulant effect.

ADVERSE REACTIONS

TABLETS

Fluid and Electrolyte Disturbances: Sodium retention, fluid retention, congestive heart failure in susceptible patients, potassium loss, hypokalemic alkalosis, hypertension.

Musculoskeletal: Muscle weakness, steroid myopathy, loss of muscle mass, osteoporosis, tendon rupture, particularly of the Achilles tendon, vertebral compression fractures, aseptic necrosis of femoral and humeral heads, pathologic fracture of long bones.

Gastrointestinal: Peptic ulcer with possible perforation and hemorrhage, pancreatitis, abdominal distention, ulcerative esophagitis, increases in alanine transaminase (ALT, SGPT), aspartate transaminase (AST, SGOT) and alkaline phosphatase have been observed following corticosteroid treatment. These changes are usually small, not associated with any clinical sydrome and are reversible upon discontinuation.

Dermatologic: Impaired wound healing, thin fragile skin, petechiae and ecchymoses, facial erythema, increased sweating, may suppress reactions to skin tests.

Neurological: Increased intracranial pressure with papilledema (pseudotumor cerebri) usually after treatment, convulsions, vertigo, headache.

Endocrine: Development of cushingoid state, suppression of growth in children, secondary adrenocortical and pituitary unresponsiveness, particularly in times of stress, as in trauma, surgery or illness, menstrual irregularities, decreased carbohydrate tolerance, manifestations of latent diabetes mellitus, increased requirements for insulin or oral hypoglycemic agents in diabetics.

Ophthalmic: Posterior subcapsular cataracts, increased intraocular pressure, glaucoma, exophthalmos.

Metabolic: Negative nitrogen balance due to protein catabolism.

CREAM

The following local adverse reactions are reported infrequently with topical corticosteroids, but may occur more frequently with the use of occlusive dressings. These reactions are listed in an approximate decreasing order of occurrence:

Burning, itching, irritation, dryness, folliculitis, hypertrichosis, acneiform eruptions, hypopigmentation, perioral dermatitis, allergic contact dermatitis, maceration of the skin, secondary infection, skin atrophy, striae and miliaria.

DOSAGE AND ADMINISTRATION

TABLETS

The initial dosage may vary from 20-240 mg of hydrocortisone per day depending on the specific disease entity being treated. In situations of less severity lower doses will generally suffice while in selected patients higher initial doses may be required. The initial dosage should be maintained or adjusted until a satisfactory response is noted. If after a reasonable period of time there is a lack of satisfactory clinical response, hydrocortisone should be discontinued and the patient transferred to other appropriate therapy. IT SHOULD BE EMPHASIZED THAT DOSAGE REQUIREMENTS ARE VARIABLE AND MUST BE INDIVIDUALIZED ON THE BASIS OF THE DISEASE UNDER TREATMENT AND THE

RESPONSE OF THE PATIENT. After a favorable response is noted, the proper maintenance dosage should be determined by decreasing the initial drug dosage in small decrements at appropriate time intervals until the lowest dosage which will maintain an adequate clinical response is reached. It should be kept in mind that constant monitoring is needed in regard to drug dosage. Included in the situations which may make dosage adjustments necessary are changes in clinical status secondary to remissions or exacerbations in the disease process, the patient's individual drug responsiveness, and the effect of patient exposure to stressful situations not directly related to the disease entity under treatment; in this latter situation it may be necessary to increase the dosage of hydrocortisone for a period of time consistent with the patient's condition. If after long-term therapy the drug is to be stopped, it is recommended that it be withdrawn gradually, rather than abruptly.

Multiple Sclerosis

In treatment of acute exacerbations of multiple sclerosis, daily doses of 200 mg of prednisolone for a week followed by 80 mg every other day for 1 month have been shown to be effective (20 mg of hydrocortisone is equivalent to 5 mg of prednisolone).

CREAM

1% Hydrocortisone Cream: Topical corticosteroids are generally applied to the affected area as a thin film from 3 or 4 times daily depending on the severity of the condition.

2.5% Hydrocortisone Cream: Apply to the affected area 2-4 times daily depending on the severity of the condition.

Occlusive dressings may be used for the management of psoriasis or recalcitrant conditions.

H

If an infection develops, the use of occlusive dressings should be discontinued and appropriate antimicrobial therapy instituted.

HOW SUPPLIED

TABLETS

Cortef tablets are available in the following strengths:

5 mg: White, round, scored, imprinted "CORTEF 5".
10 mg: White, round, scored, imprinted "CORTEF 10".
20 mg: White, round, scored, imprinted "CORTEF 20".

Storage: Store at controlled room temperature 20-25°C (68-77°F).

CREAM

Store hydrocortisone cream at controlled room temperature 15-30°C (59-86°F). Store away from heat. Protect from freezing.

PRODUCT LISTING - RATED THERAPEUTICALLY EQUIVALENT

Size	Price	Product	NDC
Cream - Topical - 0.5%			
30 gm	$1.13	FEDERAL UPPER LIMIT, H.C.F.A. F F P	99999-1476-16
Cream - Topical - 1%			
30 gm	$1.76	FEDERAL UPPER LIMIT, H.C.F.A. F F P	99999-1476-24
Cream - Topical - 2.5%			
5 gm	$2.25	GENERIC, Cmc-Consolidated Midland Corporation	00223-4125-05
20 gm	$3.71	GENERIC, Moore, H.L. Drug Exchange Inc	00839-6376-45
20 gm	$3.80	GENERIC, Thames Pharmacal Company Inc	49158-0200-07
20 gm	$4.65	GENERIC, Major Pharmaceuticals Inc	00904-0756-29
20 gm	$4.75	GENERIC, Cmc-Consolidated Midland Corporation	00223-4159-20
20 gm	$4.90	GENERIC, Clay-Park Laboratories Inc	45802-0004-02
20 gm	$4.95	GENERIC, Cmc-Consolidated Midland Corporation	00223-4125-20
20 gm	$5.45	GENERIC, Ivax Corporation	00182-5005-48
20 gm	$5.45	GENERIC, Mutual/United Research Laboratories	00677-0718-38
20 gm	$5.49	GENERIC, Geneva Pharmaceuticals	00781-7011-22
20 gm	$5.55	GENERIC, Interstate Drug Exchange Inc	00814-3779-94
20 gm	$5.85	GENERIC, Interstate Drug Exchange Inc	00814-3762-94
20 gm	$5.88	GENERIC, Watson/Rugby Laboratories Inc	00536-0611-99
20 gm	$5.95	GENERIC, Major Pharmaceuticals Inc	00904-0757-29
20 gm	$6.75	GENERIC, Alpharma Uspd Makers Of Barre and Nmc	00472-0337-20
20 gm	$35.63	GENERIC, Ambix Laboratories	10038-0030-06
20 gm	$35.63	GENERIC, Ambix Laboratories	10038-0112-06
28 gm	$22.53	PROCTOCREAM-HC, Prescript Pharmaceuticals	00247-0235-29
28 gm	$38.95	HYTONE, Aventis Pharmaceuticals	00066-0095-01
30 gm	$5.25	GENERIC, Watson/Schein Pharmaceuticals Inc	00364-2446-56
30 gm	$5.46	FEDERAL UPPER LIMIT, H.C.F.A. F F P	99999-1476-37
30 gm	$6.75	GENERIC, Major Pharmaceuticals Inc	00904-0756-30
30 gm	$6.75	GENERIC, Major Pharmaceuticals Inc	00904-0756-31
30 gm	$7.24	GENERIC, Clay-Park Laboratories Inc	45802-0004-03
30 gm	$8.22	GENERIC, Moore, H.L. Drug Exchange Inc	00839-6376-49
30 gm	$8.34	GENERIC, C and M	00398-0019-01
30 gm	$8.39	GENERIC, Thames Pharmacal Company Inc	49158-0200-08
30 gm	$8.84	GENERIC, Fougera	00168-0080-31
30 gm	$8.95	GENERIC, Alpharma Uspd Makers Of Barre and Nmc	00472-0337-30
30 gm	$23.65	PROCTOCREAM-HC, Prescript Pharmaceuticals	00247-0235-30
30 gm	$33.10	GENERIC, Qualitest Products Inc	00603-7781-78
30 gm	$36.90	PROCTOCREAM-HC, Schwarz Pharma	00091-4640-24
30 gm	$42.53	GENERIC, King Pharmaceuticals Inc	60793-0313-11
30 gm	$44.21	HYTONE, Physicians Total Care	54868-2234-00
56 gm	$62.26	HYTONE, Aventis Pharmaceuticals	00066-0095-02
60 gm	$13.68	GENERIC, C and M	00398-0019-02
454 gm	$56.69	GENERIC, Thames Pharmacal Company Inc	49158-0200-16
454 gm	$57.02	GENERIC, Ambix Laboratories	10038-0030-16
454 gm	$58.32	GENERIC, Clay-Park Laboratories Inc	45802-0004-05
454 gm	$68.24	GENERIC, Alpharma Uspd Makers Of Barre and Nmc	23317-0322-16
454 gm	$72.00	GENERIC, Alpharma Uspd Makers Of Barre and Nmc	00472-0337-16
454 gm	$74.86	GENERIC, C and M	00398-0019-16
454 gm	$90.00	GENERIC, Fougera	00168-0080-16
480 gm	$57.02	GENERIC, Ambix Laboratories	10038-0112-16
Cream with Applicator - Rectal - 1%			
28 gm	$14.97	GENERIC, American Generics Inc	58634-0024-01
28 gm	$29.49	GENERIC, Ranbaxy Laboratories	63304-0405-01
30 gm	$43.09	PROCTOCORT, Monarch Pharmaceuticals Inc	61570-0028-01
30 gm	$46.54	PROCTOCORT, Monarch Pharmaceuticals Inc	61570-0070-01
Cream with Applicator - Rectal - 2.5%			
28 gm	$14.15	GENERIC, American Generics Inc	58634-0025-01
28 gm	$24.94	GENERIC, Ranbaxy Laboratories	63304-0407-01
30 gm	$24.95	GENERIC, Rising Pharmaceuticals	64980-0301-30
30 gm	$26.40	GENERIC, Allscripts Pharmaceutical Company	54569-4329-00
30 gm	$30.13	ANUSOL-HC, Southwood Pharmaceuticals Inc	58016-3004-01
30 gm	$34.38	ANUSOL-HC, Allscripts Pharmaceutical Company	54569-3346-00
30 gm	$36.95	GENERIC, American Generics Inc	58634-0028-01
30 gm	$36.95	GENERIC, Ranbaxy Laboratories	63304-0406-01
30 gm	$37.13	ANUSOL-HC, Monarch Pharmaceuticals Inc	61570-0313-11
Lotion - Topical - 0.5%			
60 ml	$16.25	CETACORT, Galderma Laboratories Inc	00299-3948-02
120 ml	$5.00	GENERIC, C.O. Truxton Inc	00463-8010-04
Lotion - Topical - 1%			
120 ml	$8.10	FEDERAL UPPER LIMIT, H.C.F.A. F F P	99999-1476-45
Lotion - Topical - 2.5%			
59 ml	$40.20	FEDERAL UPPER LIMIT, H.C.F.A. F F P	99999-1476-65
59 ml	$58.13	HYTONE, Aventis Pharmaceuticals	00066-0098-02
59 ml	$67.13	GENERIC, Stiefel Laboratories Inc	00145-2538-02
59.20 ml	$36.22	GENERIC, Thames Pharmacal Company Inc	49158-0348-32
60 ml	$29.67	GENERIC, Qualitest Products Inc	00603-7785-52
60 ml	$35.86	GENERIC, Major Pharmaceuticals Inc	00904-5454-03
60 ml	$52.03	GENERIC, Fougera	00168-0288-02
60 ml	$54.10	NUTRACORT, Healthpoint	00064-2210-02
118 ml	$120.85	GENERIC, Stiefel Laboratories Inc	00145-2538-04
120 ml	$76.49	GENERIC, Glades Pharmaceuticals	59366-2708-04
120 ml	$83.15	NUTRACORT, Healthpoint	00064-2210-04
Ointment - Topical - 1%			
20 gm	$2.36	GENERIC, Moore, H.L. Drug Exchange Inc	00839-5208-45
25 gm x 12	$5.00	HYDROCORTISONE 1% IN ABSORBASE, Carolina Medical Products Company	46287-0003-01
28 gm	$3.54	GENERIC, Fougera	00168-0020-31
30 gm	$1.68	FEDERAL UPPER LIMIT, H.C.F.A. F F P	99999-1476-54
30 gm	$1.78	GENERIC, Home Aid Healthcare	65557-0206-30
30 gm	$2.00	GENERIC, Thames Pharmacal Company Inc	49158-0103-08
30 gm	$2.69	GENERIC, Moore, H.L. Drug Exchange Inc	00839-5208-49
30 gm	$4.10	GENERIC, Alpharma Uspd Makers Of Barre and Nmc	00472-1326-26
30 gm	$10.24	HYTONE, Aventis Pharmaceuticals	00066-0087-01
120 gm	$7.14	GENERIC, Moore, H.L. Drug Exchange Inc	00839-5208-53
120 gm x 12	$9.00	HYDROCORTISONE 1% IN ABSORBASE, Carolina Medical Products Company	46287-0003-04
454 gm	$21.74	GENERIC, Moore, H.L. Drug Exchange Inc	00839-5208-60
454 gm	$23.75	GENERIC, Clay-Park Laboratories Inc	45802-0013-05
454 gm	$31.78	HYDROCORTISONE 1% IN ABSORBASE, Carolina Medical Products Company	46287-0003-16
454 gm	$31.87	GENERIC, Fougera	00168-0020-16
454 gm	$42.75	GENERIC, Thames Pharmacal Company Inc	49158-0103-16
Ointment - Topical - 2.5%			
20 gm	$4.90	GENERIC, Suppositoria Laboratories Inc	00414-0014-02
20 gm	$4.90	GENERIC, Clay-Park Laboratories Inc	45802-0014-02
20 gm	$5.70	GENERIC, Mutual/United Research Laboratories	00677-0724-38
30 gm	$8.84	GENERIC, Fougera	00168-0146-30
30 gm	$20.66	HYTONE, Aventis Pharmaceuticals	00066-0085-01
454 gm	$36.45	GENERIC, Clay-Park Laboratories Inc	45802-0014-05
454 gm	$58.32	GENERIC, Suppositoria Laboratories Inc	00414-0014-05
454 gm	$58.32	GENERIC, Clay-Park Laboratories Inc	00414-0014-06
454 gm	$90.00	GENERIC, Fougera	00168-0146-16
Solution - Topical - 1%			
30 ml	$11.22	TEXACORT, Bioglan Pharmaceutical Inc	62436-0247-01

60 ml	$7.81	GENERIC, Heran Pharmaceutical Inc	50434-0003-02
120 ml	$6.13	GENERIC, Harmony Laboratories	52512-0692-04
120 ml	$8.00	GENERIC, Med Derm Pharmaceuticals Inc	45565-0502-22
120 ml	$8.10	GENERIC, Clay-Park Laboratories Inc	45802-0023-06
120 ml	$8.22	GENERIC, Moore, H.L. Drug Exchange Inc	00839-6233-53
120 ml	$8.75	GENERIC, Qualitest Products Inc	00603-7784-54
120 ml	$9.00	GENERIC, Interstate Drug Exchange Inc	00814-3733-76
Solution - Topical - 2.5%			
30 ml	$21.61	TEXACORT, Bioglan Pharmaceutical Inc	62436-0293-01
Suspension - Rectal - 100 mg/60 ml			
60 ml	$12.40	GENERIC, Paddock Laboratories Inc	00574-2020-01
60 ml x 7	$84.84	GENERIC, Paddock Laboratories Inc	00574-2020-07

PRODUCT LISTING - RATED NOT THERAPEUTICALLY EQUIVALENT

Lotion - Topical - 2.5%			
59 ml	$53.47	GENERIC, Glades Pharmaceuticals	59366-2708-02
Suspension - Rectal - 100 mg/60 ml			
60 ml	$8.24	GENERIC, Copley	38245-0168-12
60 ml x 7	$84.84	GENERIC, Teva Pharmaceuticals Usa	00093-9168-71
Tablet - Oral - 10 mg			
100's	$23.93	HYDROCORTONE, Allscripts Pharmaceutical Company	54569-0328-00
100's	$25.09	HYDROCORTONE, Merck & Company Inc	00006-0619-68
100's	$39.53	CORTEF, Pharmacia and Upjohn	00009-0031-01
Tablet - Oral - 20 mg			
100's	$9.25	GENERIC, Moore, H.L. Drug Exchange Inc	00839-1365-06
100's	$9.75	GENERIC, Interstate Drug Exchange Inc	00814-3735-14
100's	$11.25	GENERIC, Major Pharmaceuticals Inc	00904-2674-60
100's	$12.00	GENERIC, West Ward Pharmaceutical Corporation	00143-1254-01
100's	$38.35	HYDROCORTONE, Merck & Company Inc	00006-0625-68
100's	$42.50	GENERIC, Cmc-Consolidated Midland Corporation	00223-1063-01
100's	$74.94	CORTEF, Pharmacia and Upjohn	00009-0044-01

PRODUCT LISTING - EQUIVALENTS NOT AVAILABLE

Cream - Topical - Buteprate 0.1%			
15 gm	$23.14	PANDEL, Savage Laboratories	00281-0153-15
45 gm	$43.75	PANDEL, Savage Laboratories	00281-0153-46
80 gm	$79.91	PANDEL, Savage Laboratories	00281-0153-80
Cream - Topical - 2.5%			
3.50 gm	$7.13	GENERIC, Pharma Pac	52959-0019-03
5 gm	$2.25	GENERIC, Cmc-Consolidated Midland Corporation	00223-4159-05
20 gm	$5.40	GENERIC, C.O. Truxton Inc	00463-8058-20
20 gm	$5.58	GENERIC, Allscripts Pharmaceutical Company	54569-2299-00
20 gm	$5.80	GENERIC, Prescript Pharmaceuticals	00247-0174-20
20 gm	$10.02	GENERIC, Pharma Pac	52959-0019-01
28 gm	$6.82	GENERIC, Prescript Pharmaceuticals	00247-0174-29
28 gm	$6.84	GENERIC, Prescript Pharmaceuticals	00247-0174-34
30 gm	$5.25	GENERIC, Watson/Schein Pharmaceuticals Inc	00591-2446-30
30 gm	$7.02	GENERIC, Prescript Pharmaceuticals	00247-0174-30
30 gm	$9.54	GENERIC, Southwood Pharmaceuticals Inc	58016-3186-01
30 gm	$10.69	GENERIC, Pharma Pac	52959-0019-02
30 gm	$15.69	GENERIC, Allscripts Pharmaceutical Company	54569-1154-00
120 gm	$16.50	GENERIC, Cmc-Consolidated Midland Corporation	00223-4159-03
454 gm	$77.50	GENERIC, Cmc-Consolidated Midland Corporation	00223-4159-13
Cream with Applicator - Rectal - 2.5%			
30 gm	$14.15	GENERIC, Ferndale Laboratories Inc	00496-0859-04
30 gm	$21.68	GENERIC, Southwood Pharmaceuticals Inc	58016-3005-30
Foam with Applicator - Rectal - 10%			
15 gm	$86.14	CORTIFOAM, Schwarz Pharma	00091-0695-20
Lotion - Topical - 2%			
30 ml	$7.71	GENERIC, Del Ray Laboratories Inc	00316-0140-01
Ointment - Topical - 1%			
28 gm	$4.64	GENERIC, Prescript Pharmaceuticals	00247-0217-29
30 gm	$2.40	GENERIC, Ivax Corporation	00182-5061-34
30 gm	$2.70	GENERIC, Raway Pharmacal Inc	00686-0013-02
30 gm	$4.71	GENERIC, Prescript Pharmaceuticals	00247-0217-30
60 gm	$4.90	GENERIC, Ivax Corporation	00182-5061-43
454 gm	$29.50	GENERIC, Cmc-Consolidated Midland Corporation	00223-4161-13
Ointment - Topical - 2.5%			
20 gm	$5.30	GENERIC, Allscripts Pharmaceutical Company	54569-4030-00
28.40 gm	$38.95	HYTONE, Aventis Pharmaceuticals	00066-9997-01
454 gm	$77.50	GENERIC, Cmc-Consolidated Midland Corporation	00223-4125-13
Solution - Topical - 1%			
30 ml	$9.92	GENERIC, Allergan Inc	00023-0889-30
44 ml	$4.20	GENERIC, Fougera	00168-0296-51
60 ml	$12.46	GENERIC, Baker Cummins Dermatologicals	58174-0114-02
60 ml	$16.06	GENERIC, Allergan Inc	00023-0889-60
74 ml	$7.20	GENERIC, Fougera	00168-0296-52
75 ml	$7.95	GENERIC, Major Pharmaceuticals Inc	00904-7854-99
120 ml	$9.98	GENERIC, Clay-Park Laboratories Inc	45802-0283-06
Solution - Topical - 2.5%			
30 ml	$21.61	TEXACORT, Sirius Laboratories	65880-0293-01
Spray - Topical - 0.5%			
58 gm	$18.61	AEROSEB-HC, Allergan Inc	00023-0804-90
Suppository - Rectal - 30 mg			
12's	$45.63	GENERIC, Upsher-Smith Laboratories Inc	00245-0112-12
12's	$45.64	GENERIC, Qualitest Products Inc	00603-8136-11
12's	$51.75	PROCTOCORT, Monarch Pharmaceuticals Inc	61570-0025-12
24's	$85.60	GENERIC, Qualitest Products Inc	00603-8136-18
24's	$97.08	GENERIC, Upsher-Smith Laboratories Inc	00245-0112-24
24's	$97.10	PROCTOCORT, Monarch Pharmaceuticals Inc	61570-0025-25
Suspension - Rectal - 100 mg/60 ml			
60 ml	$13.38	CORTENEMA, Solvay Pharmaceuticals Inc	00032-1904-73
60 ml x 7	$78.19	CORTENEMA, Solvay Pharmaceuticals Inc	00032-1904-82
Tablet - Oral - 5 mg			
50's	$11.16	CORTEF, Pharmacia and Upjohn	00009-0012-01

Hydrocortisone Acetate *(001477)*

Categories: Alopecia areata; Arthritis, gouty; Arthritis, post-traumatic; Arthritis, rheumatoid; Bursitis; Colitis, ulcerative, adjunct; Cryptitis; Dermatosis, corticosteroid-responsive; Epicondylitis; Granuloma annulare; Hemorrhoids; Lichen planus; Lichen simplex chronicus; Lupus erythematosus, discoid; Necrobiosis lipoidica diabeticorum; Neurodermatitis; Proctitis, post irradiation; Proctitis, ulcerative, adjunct; Pruritus ani; Psoriasis; Synovitis, secondary to osteoarthritis; Tenosynovitis; FDA Approved 1956 Jul; Pregnancy Category C

Drug Classes: Corticosteroids; Corticosteroids, topical; Dermatologics

Brand Names: Anucort-Hc; Anurx Hc; Anusol + H; Anusol Hc; Cort-Dome Suppository; Corta-Plex Hc; Cortef Acetate; Cortifoam; Dricort; Hemorrhoidal Hc; Hemril-Hc; Hemsol-Hc; Hydrocorten-A; **Hydrocortone Acetate**; Orabase Hca; Proctosol-Hc; Rectasol-Hc

Foreign Brand Availability: Apocort (Finland); Biocort (South-Africa); Calacort (Indonesia); Colifoam (Australia; Austria; Belgium; Denmark; England; Finland; Germany; Greece; Ireland; Israel; Italy; New-Zealand; Norway; Portugal; Sweden; Switzerland); Colofoam (France); Cordes H (Germany); Cortaid (New-Zealand); Cortamed (Canada); Cortef (Canada); Cortef Cream (Australia); Cortic Cream (Australia); Cortoderm (Canada); Cortril (Belgium); DHAcort (Malaysia); Dilucort (South-Africa); Ekzemsalbe (Austria); Enkacort (Indonesia); Fenistil hydrocortison (Germany); Ficortril (Germany); Glycortison (Germany); Hycor Eye Ointment (Australia); Hyderm (Canada); Hydrocort (Singapore); Hydrocortison (Germany); Hydrocortison Berco (Germany); Hydrocortison Dispersa (Switzerland); Hydrocortison Streuli (Germany; Switzerland); Hydrocutan (Germany); Hydrokortison (Denmark); Hytisone (Thailand); Lanacort (Israel); Mylocort (South-Africa); Nutracort (Finland); Pannocort (Belgium); Proctocort (France); Siquent Hycor (Australia); Squibb-HC (Australia); Steroderm (Indonesia); Stopitch (South-Africa); Wycort (India)

HCFA JCODE(S): J1700 up to 25 mg IV, IM, SC

DESCRIPTION

The topical corticosteroids constitute a class of primarily synthetic steroids used as anti-inflammatory and anti-pruritic agents. Hydrocortisone acetate has the chemical name pregn-4-ene-3,20-dione,21-(acetyloxy)-11,17-dihydroxy-,(11β)-.

TOPICAL CREAM

Hydrocortisone acetate cream 1% is a topical corticosteroid with micronized hydrocortisone acetate 1% (active ingredient) in a buffered, water-washable cream containing the following inactive ingredients: citric acid; glyceryl stearate; imidurea; methylparaben; mineral oil; PEG-100 stearate; polysorbate 60; propylene glycol; propylparaben; purified water; sodium citrate, hydrous; sorbitan monostearate; and white petrolatum.

SUPPOSITORIES

Each hydrocortisone acetate 25 mg suppository contains 25 mg hydrocortisone acetate in a hydrogenated cocoglyceride base. Each 30 mg suppository contains 30 mg hydrocortisone acetate in a specially blended hydrogenated vegetable oil base. Hydrocortisone acetate is a corticosteroid.

STERILE SUSPENSION

Hydrocortisone acetate sterile suspension is a sterile suspension of hydrocortisone acetate (pH 5.0-7.0) in a suitable aqueous medium. It is supplied in 2 strengths, one containing 25 mg hydrocortisone acetate/ml, the other containing 50 mg/ml. Inactive ingredients per ml: sodium chloride, 9 mg; polysorbate 80, 4 mg; sodium carboxymethylcellulose, 5 mg; and water for injection, qs, 1 ml. Benzyl alcohol, 9 mg, added as a preservative.

ORAL PASTE

Hydrocortisone acetate oral paste is an adrenocorticoid topical dental paste for application to the oral mucosa. Each gram contains hydrocortisone acetate 5 g (0.5%) in a paste vehicle containing pectin, gelatin, sodium carboxymethylcellulose dispersed in a plasticized hydrocarbon gel composed of 5% polyethylene in mineral oil, flavored with imitation vanilla. Hydrocortisone acetate is also known as cortisol acetate.

RECTAL FOAM

Cortifoam (hydrocortisone acetate rectal aerosol) contains hydrocortisone acetate 10% in a base containing propylene glycol, emulsifying wax, polyoxyethylene-10-stearytl ether, cetyl alcohol, methylparaben, propylparaben, trolamine, purified water and inert propellants: isobutane and propane.

Each application delivers approximately 900 mg of foam containing 80 mg of hydrocortisone (90 mg of hydrocortisone acetate).

The molecular weight of hydrocortisone acetate is 404.50. It is designated chemically as pregn-4-ene-3,20-dione,21-(acetyloxy)-11,17-dihydroxy-,(11β)-. The empirical formula is $C_{23}H_{32}O_6$.

Hydrocortisone acetate, a synthetic adrenocortical steroid, is a white to practically white, odorless, crystalline powder. It is insoluble in water (1 mg/100 ml) and slightly soluble in alcohol and chloroform.

CLINICAL PHARMACOLOGY

Topical corticosteroids are primarily effective because of their anti-inflammatory, antipruritic and vasoconstrictive actions.

TOPICAL CREAM

The mechanism of anti-inflammatory activity of the topical corticosteroids is unclear. Various laboratory methods, including vasoconstrictor assays, are used to compare and predict potencies and/or clinical efficacies of the topical corticosteroids. There is some evidence to suggest that a recognizable correlation exists between vasoconstrictor potency and therapeutic efficacy in man.

Pharmacokinetics

The extent of percutaneous absorption of topical corticosteroids is determined by many factors including the vehicle, the integrity of the epidermal barrier, and the use of occlusive dressings.

Topical corticosteroids can be absorbed from normal intact skin. Inflammation and/or other disease processes in the skin increase percutaneous absorption. Occlusive dressings substantially increase the percutaneous absorption of topical corticosteroids. Thus, occlusive dressings may be a valuable therapeutic adjunct for treatment of resistant dermatoses (see DOSAGE AND ADMINISTRATION).

Once absorbed through the skin, topical corticosteroids are handled through pharmacokinetic pathways similar to systemically administered corticosteroids. Corticosteroids are bound to plasma proteins in varying degrees. Corticosteroids are metabolized primarily in the liver and are then excreted by the kidneys. Some of the topical corticosteroids and their metabolites are also excreted into the bile.

H

SUPPOSITORIES

In normal subjects, about 26% of hydrocortisone acetate is absorbed when the hydrocortisone acetate suppository is applied to the rectum. Absorption of hydrocortisone acetate may vary across abraded or inflamed surfaces.

STERILE SUSPENSION

Hydrocortisone Acetate sterile suspension has a slow onset but long duration of action when compared with more soluble preparations. Because of its insolubility, it is suitable for intra-articular, intralesional, and soft tissue injection where its anti-inflammatory effects are confined mainly to the area in which it has been injected, although it is capable of producing systemic hormonal effects.

Naturally occurring glucocorticoids (hydrocortisone and cortisone), which also have salt-retaining properties, are used as replacement therapy in adrenocortical deficiency states. They are also used for their potent anti-inflammatory effect in disorders of many organ systems.

Glucocorticoids cause profound and varied metabolic effects. In addition, they modify the body's immune responses to diverse stimuli.

ORAL PASTE

The paste acts as an adhesive vehicle for applying the active medication to oral tissues. The protective action of the adhesive vehicle may serve to reduce oral irritation.

The mechanism of anti-inflammatory activity of the topical steroids is unclear. Various laboratory methods, including vasoconstrictor assays, are used to compare and predict potencies and/or clinical efficacies of the topical corticosteroids. There is some evidence to suggest that a recognizable correlation exists between vasoconstrictor potency and therapeutic efficacy in man.

Once absorbed, topical corticosteroids are handled through pharmacokinetic pathways similar to systemically administered corticosteroids. Corticosteroids are bound to plasma proteins in varying degrees. Corticosteroids are metabolized primarily in the liver and are then excreted by the kidneys. Some of the topical corticosteroids and their metabolites are also excreted into the bile.

RECTAL FOAM

Hydrocortisone acetate rectal aerosol, 10%, provides effective topical administration of an anti-inflammatory corticosteroid as adjunctive therapy of ulcerative proctitis. Direct observations of methylene blue-containing foam have shown staining about 10 cm into the rectum.

INDICATIONS AND USAGE

TOPICAL CREAM

Topical corticosteroids are indicated for the relief of the inflammatory and pruritic manifestations of corticosteroid-responsive dermatoses.

SUPPOSITORIES

For use in inflamed hemorrhoids, post irradiation (factitial) proctitis, as an adjunct in the treatment of chronic ulcerative colitis, cryptitis, other inflammatory conditions of the anorectum and pruritus ani.

STERILE SUSPENSION

By intra-articular or soft tissue injection: As adjunctive therapy for short-term administration (to tide the patient over an acute episode or exacerbation) in: Synovitis of osteoarthritis, rheumatoid arthritis, acute and sub acute bursitis, acute gouty arthritis, epicondylitis, acute nonspecific tenosynovitis, post-traumatic osteoarthritis.

By intralesional injection: Keloids, localized hypertrophic, infiltrated, inflammatory lesions of: lichen planus, psoriatic plaques, granuloma annulare, and lichen simplex chronicus (neurodermatitis), discoid lupus erythematosus, necrobiosis lipoidica diabeticorum, alopecia areata, may also be useful in cystic tumors of an aponeurosis or tendon (ganglia).

ORAL PASTE

Indicated for adjunctive treatment and for temporary relief of symptoms associated with oral inflammatory lesions and ulcerative lesions resulting from trauma.

RECTAL FOAM

Hydrocortisone acetate rectal aerosol, 10%, is indicated as adjunctive therapy in the topical treatment of ulcerative proctitis of the distal portion of the rectum in patients who cannot retain hydrocortisone or other corticosteroid enemas.

CONTRAINDICATIONS

TOPICAL CREAM AND SUPPOSITORIES

Topical/suppository corticosteroids are contraindicated in those patients having a history of hypersensitivity to hydrocortisone or any of the components.

STERILE SUSPENSION

Systemic fungal infections.
Hypersensitivity to any component of this product.

ORAL PASTE

Topical corticosteroids are contraindicated in those patients with a history of hypersensitivity to any of the components of the preparation. Because it contains a corticosteroid, the preparation is contraindicated in the presence of fungal, viral, or bacterial infections of the mouth or throat.

RECTAL FOAM

Hydrocortisone acetate rectal aerosol, 10%, is contraindicated in patients who are hypersensitive to any components of this product.

Local contraindications to the use of intrarectal steroids include obstruction, abscess, perforation, peritonitis, fresh intestinal anastomoses, extensive fistulas and sinus tracts.

WARNINGS

STERILE SUSPENSION

Because rare instances of anaphylactoid reactions have occurred in patients receiving corticosteroid therapy, appropriate precautionary measures should be taken prior to administration, especially when the patient has a history of allergy to any drug.

In patients on corticosteroid therapy subjected to any unusual stress, increased dosage of rapidly acting corticosteroids before, during, and after the stressful situation is indicated.

Drug-induced secondary adrenocortical insufficiency may result from too rapid withdrawal of corticosteroids and may be minimized by gradual reduction of dosage. This type of relative insufficiency may persist for months after discontinuation of therapy; therefore, in any situation of stress occurring during that period, hormone therapy should be reinstituted. If the patient is receiving steroids already, dosage may have to be increased. Since mineralocorticoid secretion may be impaired, salt and/or a mineralocorticoid should be administered concurrently.

Corticosteroids may mask some signs of infection, and new infections may appear during their use. There may be decreased resistance and inability to localize infection when corticosteroids are used. Moreover, corticosteroids may affect the nitroblue-tetrazolium test for bacterial infection and produce false negative results.

In cerebral malaria, a double-blind trial has shown that the use of corticosteroids is associated with prolongation of coma and a higher incidence of pneumonia and gastrointestinal bleeding.

Corticosteroids may activate latent amebiasis. Therefore, it is recommended that latent or active amebiasis be ruled out before initiating corticosteroid therapy in any patient who has spent time in the tropics or any patient with unexplained diarrhea.

Prolonged use of corticosteroids may produce posterior subcapsular cataracts, glaucoma with possible damage to the optic nerves, and may enhance the establishment of secondary ocular infections due to fungi or viruses.

Use in Pregnancy: Since adequate human reproduction studies have not been done with corticosteroids, use of these drugs in pregnancy or in women of childbearing potential requires that the anticipated benefits be weighed against the possible hazards to the mother and embryo or fetus. Infants born of mothers who have received substantial doses of corticosteroids during pregnancy should be carefully observed for signs of hypoadrenalism. Corticosteroids appear in breast milk and could suppress growth, interfere with endogenous corticosteroid production, or cause other unwanted effects. Mothers taking pharmacologic doses of corticosteroids should be advised not to nurse.

Average and large doses of cortisone or hydrocortisone can cause elevation of blood pressure, salt and water retention, and increased excretion of potassium. These effects are less likely to occur with the synthetic derivatives except when used in large doses. Dietary salt restriction and potassium supplementation may be necessary. All corticosteroids increase calcium excretion.

Administration of live virus vaccines, including smallpox, is contraindicated in individuals receiving immunosuppressive doses of corticosteroids. If inactivated viral or bacterial vaccines are administered to individuals receiving immunosuppressive doses of corticosteroids, the expected serum antibody response may not be obtained.

If corticosteroids are indicated in patients with latent tuberculosis or tuberculin reactivity, close observation is necessary as reactivation of the disease may occur. During prolonged corticosteroid therapy, these patients should receive chemoprophylaxis.

Literature reports suggest an apparent association between use of corticosteroids and left ventricular free wall rupture after a recent myocardial infarction; therefore, therapy with corticosteroids should be used with great caution in these patients.

RECTAL FOAM

General

Do not insert any part of the aerosol container directly into the anus. Contents of the container are under pressure. Do not burn or puncture the aerosol container. Do not store at temperatures above 120°F. Because hydrocortisone acetate rectal aerosol, 10%, is not expelled, systemic hydrocortisone absorption may be greater from hydrocortisone acetate rectal aerosol, 10%, than from corticosteroid enema formulations. If there is not evidence of clinical or proctologic improvement within 2 or 3 weeks after starting hydrocortisone acetate rectal aerosol, 10%, therapy, or if the patient's condition worsens, discontinue the drug.

Rare instances of anaphylactoid reactions have occurred in patients receiving corticosteroid therapy (see ADVERSE REACTIONS).

Cardiorenal

Corticosteroids can cause elevation of blood pressure, salt and water retention, and increased excretion of potassium. These effects are less likely to occur with the synthetic derivatives except when used in large doses. Dietary salt restriction and potassium supplementation may be necessary. All corticosteroids increase calcium excretion.

Literature reports suggest an apparent association between use of corticosteroids and left ventricular free wall rupture after a recent myocardial infarction; therefore, therapy with corticosteroids should be used with great caution in these patients.

Endocrine

Corticosteroids can produce reversible hypothalamic-pituitary adrenal (HPA) axis suppression with the potential for glucocorticosteroid insufficiency after withdrawal of treatment.

Metabolic clearance of corticosteroids is decreased in hypothyroid patients and increased in hyperthyroid patients. Changes in thyroid status of the patient may necessitate adjustment in dosage.

Infections

General

Patients who are on corticosteroids are more susceptible to infections than are healthy individuals. There may be decreased resistance and inability to localize infection when corticosteroids are used. Infection with any pathogen (viral, bacterial, fungal, protozoan or helminthic) in any location of the body may be associated with the use of corticosteroids alone or in combination with other immunosuppressive agents. These infections may be mild to severe. With increasing doses of corticosteroids, the rate of occurrence of infectious complications increases. Corticosteroids may also mask some signs of current infection.

Fungal Infections

Corticosteroids may exacerbate systemic fungal infections and therefore should not be used in the presence of such infections unless they are needed to control drug reactions. There have been cases reported in which concomitant use of amphotericin B and hydrocortisone was followed by cardiac enlargement and congestive heart failure (see DRUG INTERACTIONS, Amphotericin B Injection and Potassium-Depleting Agents).

Special Pathogens

Latent disease may be activated or there may be an exacerbation of intercurrent infections due to pathogens, including those caused by *Amoeba, Candida, Cryptococcus, Mycobacterium, Nocardia, Pneumocystis,* and *Toxoplasma*.

It is recommended that latent amebiasis or active amebiasis be ruled out before initiating corticosteroid therapy in any patient who has spent time in the tropics or in any patient with unexplained diarrhea.

Similarly, corticosteroids should be used with great care in patients with known or suspected *Strongyloides* (threadworm) infestation. In such patients, corticosteroid-induced immunosuppression may lead to *Strongyloides* hyperinfection and dissemination with widespread larval migration, often accompanied by severe enterocolitis and potentially fatal gram-negative septicemia.

Corticosteroids should not be used in cerebral malaria.

Tuberculosis

If corticosteroids are indicated in patients with latent tuberculosis or tuberculin reactivity, close observation is necessary as reactivation of the disease may occur. During prolonged corticosteroid therapy, these patients should receive chemoprophylaxis.

Vaccination

Administration of live or live, attenuated vaccines is contraindicated in patients receiving immunosuppressive doses of corticosteroids. Killed or inactivated vaccines may be administered. However, the response to such vaccines cannot be predicted. Immunization procedures may be undertaken in patients who are receiving corticosteroids as replacement therapy, *e.g.,* for Addison's disease.

Viral Infections

Chicken pox and measles can have a more serious or even fatal course in pediatric and adult patients on corticosteroids in pediatric and adult patients on corticosteroids. In pediatric and adult patients who have not had these diseases, particular care should be taken to avoid exposure. The contribution of the underlying disease and/or prior corticosteroid treatment to the risk is also not known. If exposed to chicken pox, prophylaxis with varicella zoster immune globulin (VZIG) may be indicated. If exposed to measles, prophylaxis with immunoglobulin (IG) may be indicated. (See the respective package inserts for complete VZIG and IG prescribing information.) If chicken pox develops, treatment with antiviral agents should be considered.

Ophthalmic

Use of corticosteroids may produce posterior subcapsular cataracts, glaucoma with possible damage to the optic nerves, and may enhance the establishment of secondary ocular infections due to bacteria, fungi, or viruses. The use of oral corticosteroids is not recommended in the treatment of optic neuritis and may lead to an increase in the risk of new episodes. Corticosteroids should not be used in active ocular herpes simplex.

PRECAUTIONS

GENERAL

Topical Cream and Oral Paste

Systemic absorption of topical corticosteroids has produced reversible hypothalamic-pituitary-adrenal (HPA) axis suppression, manifestations of Cushing's syndrome, hyperglycemia, and glucosuria in some patients.

Conditions which augment systemic absorption include the application of the more potent steroids, use over large surface areas, prolonged use, and the addition of occlusive dressings.

Therefore, patients receiving a large dose of a potent topical steroid applied to a large surface area or under an occlusive dressing should be evaluated periodically for evidence of HPA axis suppression by using the urinary free cortisol and ACTH stimulation tests. If HPA axis suppression is noted, an attempt should be made to withdraw the drug, to reduce the frequency of application, or to substitute a less potent steroid.

Recovery of HPA axis function is generally prompt and complete upon discontinuation of the drug. Infrequently, signs and symptoms of steroid withdrawal may occur, requiring supplemental systemic corticosteroids.

Children may absorb proportionally larger amounts of topical corticosteroids and thus be more susceptible to systemic toxicity (see Pediatric Use).

If irritation develops, topical corticosteroids should be discontinued and appropriate therapy instituted. In the presence of dermatological infections, the use of an appropriate antifungal or antibacterial agent should be instituted. If a favorable response does not occur promptly, the corticosteroid should be discontinued until the infection has been adequately controlled.

Suppositories

Do not use unless adequate proctologic examination is made.

If irritation develops, the product should be discontinued and appropriate therapy instituted.

In the presence of an infection, the use of an appropriate antifungal or antibacterial agent should be instituted. If a favorable response does not occur promptly, the suppositories should be discontinued until the infection has been adequately controlled.

No long-term studies in animals have been performed to evaluate the carcinogenic potential of corticosteroid suppositories.

Sterile Suspension

This product, like many other steroid formulations, is sensitive to heat. Therefore, it should not be autoclaved when it is desirable to sterilize the exterior of the vial.

Following prolonged therapy, withdrawal of corticosteroids may result in symptoms of the corticosteroid withdrawal syndrome including fever, myalgia, arthralgia, and malaise. This may occur in patients even without evidence of adrenal insufficiency.

There is an enhanced effect of corticosteroids in patients with hypothyroidism and in those with cirrhosis.

Corticosteroids should be used cautiously in patients with ocular herpes simplex for fear of corneal perforation.

Psychic derangements may appear when corticosteroids are used, ranging from euphoria, insomnia, mood swings, personality changes, and severe depression to frank psychotic manifestations. Also, existing emotional instability or psychotic tendencies may be aggravated by corticosteroids.

Aspirin should be used cautiously in conjunction with corticosteroids in hypothrombinemia.

Steroids should be used with caution in nonspecific ulcerative colitis, if there is a probability of impending perforation, abscess, or other pyogenic infection, also in diverticulitis, fresh intestinal anastomoses, active or latent peptic ulcer, renal insufficiency, hypertension, osteoporosis, and myasthenia gravis. Signs of peritoneal irritation following gastrointestinal perforation in patients receiving large doses of corticosteroids may be minimal or absent. Fat embolism has been reported as a possible complication of hypercortisonism.

When large doses are given, some authorities advise that antacids be administered between meals to prevent peptic ulcer.

Growth and development of infants and children on prolonged corticosteroid therapy should be carefully followed.

Steroids may increase or decrease motility and number of spermatozoa in some patients.

Phenytoin, phenobarbital, ephedrine, and rifampin may enhance the metabolic clearance of corticosteroids resulting in decreased blood levels and lessened physiologic activity, thus requiring adjustment in corticosteroid dosage.

The prothrombin time should be checked frequently in patients who are receiving corticosteroids and coumarin anticoagulants at the same time because of reports that corticosteroids have altered the response to these anticoagulants. Studies have shown that the usual effect produced by adding corticosteroids is inhibition of response to coumarins, although there have been some conflicting reports of potentiation not substantiated by studies.

When corticosteroids are administered concomitantly with potassium-depleting diuretics, patients should be observed closely for development of hypokalemia.

Intra-articular injection of a corticosteroid may produce systemic as well as local effects.

Appropriate examination of any joint fluid present is necessary to exclude a septic process.

A marked increase in pain accompanied by local swelling, further restriction of joint motion, fever, and malaise is suggestive of septic arthritis. If this complication occurs and the diagnosis of sepsis is confirmed, appropriate antimicrobial therapy should be instituted.

Injection of a steroid into an infected site is to be avoided.

Corticosteroids should not be injected into unstable joints.

Patients should be impressed strongly with the importance of not overusing joints in which symptomatic benefit has been obtained as long as the inflammatory process remains active.

Frequent intra-articular injection may result in damage to joint tissues.

Rectal Foam

The lowest possible dose of corticosteroid should be used to control the condition under treatment. When reduction in dosage is possible, the reduction should be gradual.

Since complications of treatment with glucocorticoids are dependent on the size of the dose and the duration of treatment, a risk/benefit decision must be made in each individual case as to dose and duration of treatment and as to whether daily or intermittent therapy should be used.

Kaposi's sarcoma has been reported to occur in patients receiving corticosteroid therapy, most often for chronic conditions. Discontinuation of corticosteroids may result in clinical improvement.

Cardiorenal

As sodium retention with resultant edema and potassium loss may occur in patients receiving corticosteroids, these agents should be used with caution in patients with congestive heart failure, hypertension, or renal insufficiency.

Endocrine

Drug-induced secondary adrenocortical insufficiency may be minimized by gradual reduction of dosage. This type of relative insufficiency may persist for months after discontinuation of therapy; therefore, in any situation of stress occurring during that period, hormone therapy should be reinstituted. Since mineralocorticoid secretion may be impaired, salt and/or a mineralocorticoid should be administered concurrently.

Gastrointestinal

Steroids should be used with caution in active or latent peptic ulcers, diverticulitis, fresh intestinal anastomoses, and nonspecific ulcerative colitis, since they may increase the risk of a perforation. Where surgery is imminent, it is hazardous to wait more than a few days for a satisfactory response to medical treatment.

H

Do not employ in immediate or early postoperative period following ileorectostomy.

Signs of peritoneal irritation following gastrointestinal perforation in patients receiving corticosteroids may be minimal or absent.

There is an enhanced effect of corticosteroids in patients with cirrhosis.

Musculoskeletal

Corticosteroids decrease bone formation and increase bone resorption both through their effect on calcium regulation (*i.e.*, decreasing absorption and increasing excretion) and inhibition of osteoblast function. This, together with a decrease in the protein matrix of the bone secondary to an increase in protein catabolism, and reduced sex hormone production, may lead to inhibition of bone growth in pediatric patients and the development of osteoporosis at any age. Special consideration should be given to patients at increased risk of osteoporosis (*i.e.*, postmenopausal women) before initiating corticosteroid therapy.

Neuropsychiatric

An acute myopathy has been observed with the use of high doses of corticosteroids, most often occurring in patients with disorders of neuromuscular transmission (*e.g.*, myasthenia gravis), or in patients receiving concomitant therapy with neuromuscular blocking drugs (*e.g.*, pancuronium). This acute myopathy is generalized, may involve ocular and respiratory muscles, and may result in quadriparesis. Elevation of creatinine kinase may occur. Clinical improvement or recovery after stopping corticosteroids may require weeks to years.

Psychic derangements may appear when corticosteroids are used, ranging from euphoria, insomnia, mood swings, personality changes, and severe depression to frank psychotic manifestations. Also, existing emotional instability or psychotic tendencies may be aggravated by corticosteroids.

Ophthalmic

Intraocular pressure may become elevated in some individuals. If steroid therapy is continued for more than 6 weeks, intraocular pressure should be monitored.

INFORMATION FOR THE PATIENT

Patients who are on immunosuppressive doses of corticosteroids should be warned to avoid exposure to chicken pox or measles and, if exposed, to obtain medical advice.

Topical Cream and Oral Paste

Patients using topical corticosteroids should receive the following information and instructions:

- This medication is to be used as directed by the dentist or physician. (The **topical cream** is for external use only.) Avoid contact with the eyes.
- Patients should be advised not to use this medication for any disorder other than for which it has been prescribed.
- The treated skin area should not be bandaged or otherwise covered or wrapped as to be occlusive unless directed by the physician.
- Patients should report any signs of local adverse reactions especially under occlusive dressing.
- Parents of pediatric patients should be advised not to use tight-fitting diapers or plastic pants on a child being treated in the diaper area, as these garments may constitute occlusive dressings.

Suppository

Staining of fabric may occur with use of the suppository. Precautionary measures are recommended.

Rectal Foam

Patients should be warned not to discontinue the use of corticosteroids abruptly or without medical supervision, to advise any medical attendants that they are taking corticosteroids and to seek medical advice at once should they develop fever or other signs of infection.

Persons who are on corticosteroids should be warned to avoid exposure to chicken pox or measles. Patients should also be advised that if they are exposed, medical advice should be sought without delay.

LABORATORY TESTS

Topical Cream and Oral Paste

The following tests may be helpful in evaluating the HPA axis suppression:

Urinary free cortisol test.
ACTH stimulation test.

CARCINOGENESIS, MUTAGENESIS, AND IMPAIRMENT OF FERTILITY

Topical Cream and Oral Paste

Long-term animal studies have not been performed to evaluate the carcinogenic potential or the effect on fertility of topical corticosteroids. Studies to determine mutagenicity with prednisolone and hydrocortisone have revealed negative results.

Suppositories

No long-term studies in animals have been performed to evaluate the carcinogenic potential of corticosteroid suppositories.

Rectal Foam

No adequate studies have been conducted in animals to determine whether corticosteroids have a potential for carcinogenesis or mutagenesis.

Steroids may increase or decrease motility and number of spermatozoa in some patients.

PEDIATRIC USE

Topical Cream and Oral Paste

PEDIATRIC PATIENTS MAY DEMONSTRATE GREATER SUSCEPTIBILITY TO TOPICAL CORTICOSTEROID-INDUCED HPA AXIS SUPPRESSION AND CUSHING'S SYNDROME THAN MATURE PATIENTS BECAUSE OF A LARGER SKIN SURFACE AREA TO BODY WEIGHT RATIO.

Hypothalamic-pituitary-adrenal (HPA) axis suppression, Cushing's syndrome, and intracranial hypertension have been reported in children receiving topical corticosteroids. Manifestations of adrenal suppression in children include linear growth retardation, delayed weight gain, low plasma cortisol levels, and absence of response to ACTH stimulation. Manifestations of intracranial hypertension include bulging fontanelles, headaches, and bilateral papilledema.

Administration of topical corticosteroids to children should be limited to the least amount compatible with an effective therapeutic regimen. Chronic corticosteroid therapy may interfere with the growth and development of children.

Rectal Foam

Safety and effectiveness in pediatric patients have not been established.

PREGNANCY, TERATOGENIC EFFECTS, PREGNANCY CATEGORY C

Topical Cream and Oral Paste

Corticosteroids are generally teratogenic in laboratory animals when administered systemically at relatively low dosage levels. The more potent corticosteroids have been shown to be teratogenic after dermal application in laboratory animals. There are no adequate and well-controlled studies in pregnant women on teratogenic effects from topically applied corticosteroids. Therefore, topical corticosteroids should be used during pregnancy only if the potential benefit justifies the potential risk to the fetus. Drugs of this class should not be used extensively on pregnant patients, in large amounts, or for prolonged periods of time.

Suppositories

In laboratory animals, topical steroids have been associated with an increase in the incidence of fetal abnormalities when gestating females have been exposed to rather low dosage levels. There are no adequate and well-controlled studies in pregnant women. Hydrocortisone acetate suppositories should only be used during pregnancy if the potential benefit justifies the risk to the fetus. Drugs of this class should not be used extensively on pregnant patients, in large amounts, or for prolonged periods of time.

Rectal Foam

Corticosteroids have been shown to be teratogenic in many species when given in doses equivalent to the human dose. Animal studies in which corticosteroids have been given to pregnant mice, rats, and rabbits have yielded an increased incidence of cleft palate in the offspring. There are no adequate and well-controlled studies in pregnant women. Corticosteroids should be used during pregnancy only if the potential benefit justifies the potential risk to the fetus. Infants born to mothers who have received corticosteroids during pregnancy should be carefully observed for signs of hypoadrenalism.

NURSING MOTHERS

Topical Cream and Oral

It is not known whether topical administration of corticosteroids could result in sufficient systemic absorption to produce detectable quantities in breast milk. Systemically administered corticosteroids are secreted into breast milk in quantities not likely to have a deleterious effect on the infant. Nevertheless, caution should be exercised when topical corticosteroids are administered to a nursing woman.

Suppositories

It is not known whether this drug is excreted in human milk, and because many drugs are excreted in human milk and because of the potential for serious adverse reactions in nursing infants from hydrocortisone acetate, a decision should be made whether to discontinue nursing or to discontinue the drug, taking into account the importance of the drug to the mother.

Rectal Foam

Systemically administered corticosteroids appear in human milk and could suppress growth, interfere with endogenous corticosteroid production, or cause other untoward effects. Caution should be exercised when corticosteroids are administered to a nursing woman.

GERIATRIC USE

Rectal Foam

No overall differences in safety or effectiveness were observed between elderly subjects and younger subjects, and other reported clinical experience has not identified differences in responses between the elderly and younger patients, but greater sensitivity of some older individuals cannot be ruled out.

DRUG INTERACTIONS

RECTAL FOAM

Aminoglutethimide: Aminoglutethimide may lead to a loss of corticosteroid-induced adrenal suppression.

Amphotericin B injection and potassium-depleting agents: When corticosteroids are administered concomitantly with potassium-depleting agents (*i.e.,* amphotericin B, diuretics), patients should be observed closely for development of hypokalemia. There have been cases reported in which concomitant use of amphotericin B and hydrocortisone was followed by cardiac enlargement and congestive heart failure.

Antibiotics: Macrolide antibiotics have been reported to cause a significant decrease in corticosteroid clearance.

Anticholinesterases: Concomitant use of anticholinesterase agents and corticosteroids may produce severe weakness in patients with myasthenia gravis. If possible, anticholinesterase agents should be withdrawn at least 24 hours before initiating corticosteroid therapy.

Anticoagulants, oral: Coadministration of corticosteroids and warfarin result in inhibition of response to warfarin. Therefore, coagulation indices should be monitored to maintain the desired anticoagulant effect.

Antidiabetics: Because corticosteroids may increase blood glucose concentrations, dosage adjustments of antidiabetic agents may be required.

Antitubercular drugs: Serum concentration of isoniazid may be decreased.

Cholestyramine: Cholestyramine may increase the clearance of corticosteroids.

Cyclosporine: Increased activity of both cyclosporine and corticosteroids may occur when the 2 are used concurrently. Convulsions have been reported with this concurrent use.

Digitalis glycosides: Patients on digitalis glycosides may be at increased risk of arrhythmias due to hypokalemia.

Estrogens, including oral contraceptives: Estrogens may decrease the hepatic metabolism of certain corticosteroids, thereby increasing their effect.

Hepatic enzyme inducers (e.g., barbiturates, phenytoin, carbamazepine, rifampin): Drugs which induce hepatic microsomal drug metabolizing enzyme activity may enhance the metabolism of corticosteroids and require that the dosage of the corticosteroid be increased.

Ketoconazole: Ketoconazole has been reported to decrease the metabolism of certain corticosteroids by up to 60%, leading to an increased risk of corticosteroid side effects.

Nonsteroidal anti-inflammatory agents (NSAIDS): Concomitant use of aspirin (or other nonsteroidal anti-inflammatory agents) and corticosteroids increases the risk of gastrointestinal side effects. Aspirin should be used cautiously in conjunction with corticosteroids in hypoprothrombinemia. The clearance of salicylates may be increased with concurrent use of corticosteroids.

Skin tests: Corticosteroids may suppress reactions to skin tests.

Vaccines: Patients on prolonged corticosteroid therapy may exhibit a diminished response to toxoids and live or inactivated vaccines due to inhibition of antibody response. Corticosteroids may also potentiate the replication of some organisms contained in live attenuated vaccines. Routine administration of vaccines or toxoids should be deferred until corticosteroid therapy is discontinued if possible (see WARNINGS, Infections, Vaccination).

ADVERSE REACTIONS

TOPICAL CREAM

The following local adverse reactions are reported infrequently with topical corticosteroids, but may occur more frequently with the use of occlusive dressings. These reactions are listed in an approximate decreasing order of occurrence.

Burning, itching, irritation, dryness, folliculitis, hypertrichosis, acneiform eruptions, hypopigmentation, perioral dermatitis, allergic contact dermatitis, maceration of the skin, secondary infection, skin atrophy, striae, and miliaria.

SUPPOSITORIES

The following local adverse reactions have been reported with corticosteroid suppositories:

Burning, itching, irritation, dryness, folliculitis, hypopigmentation, allergic contact dermatitis, and secondary infection.

STERILE SUSPENSION

Fluid and electrolyte disturbances: Sodium retention; fluid retention; congestive heart failure in susceptible patients; potassium loss; hypokalemic alkalosis; hypertension.

Musculoskeletal: Muscle weakness; steroid myopathy; loss of muscle mass; osteoporosis; vertebral compression fractures; aseptic necrosis of femoral and humeral heads; pathologic fracture of long bones; tendon rupture.

Gastrointestinal: Peptic ulcer with possible subsequent perforation and hemorrhage; perforation of the small and large bowel, particularly in patients with inflammatory bowel disease; pancreatitis; abdominal distension; ulcerative esophagitis.

Dermatologic: Impaired wound healing; thin fragile skin; petechiae and ecchymoses; erythema; increased sweating; may suppress reactions to skin tests; other cutaneous reactions, such as allergic dermatitis, urticaria, angioneurotic edema.

Neurologic: Convulsions; increased intracranial pressure with papilledema (pseudotumor cerebri) usually after treatment; vertigo; headache; psychic disturbances.

Endocrine: Menstrual irregularities; development of cushingoid state; suppression of growth in children; secondary adrenocortical and pituitary unresponsiveness, particularly in times of stress, as in trauma, surgery or illness; decreased carbohydrate tolerance; manifestation of latent diabetes mellitus; increased requirements for insulin or oral hypoglycemic agents in diabetics; hirsutism.

Ophthalmic: Posterior subcapsular cataracts; increased intraocular pressure; glaucoma; exophthalmos.

Metabolic: Negative nitrogen balance due to protein catabolism.

Cardiovascular: Myocardial rupture following recent myocardial infarction (see WARNINGS).

Other: Anaphylactoid or hypersensitivity reactions; thromboembolism; weight gain; increased appetite; nausea; malaise.

The following *additional* adverse reactions are related to injection of corticosteroids: Rare instances of blindness associated with intralesional therapy around the face and head; hyperpigmentation or hypopigmentation; subcutaneous (SC) and cutaneous atrophy; sterile abscess; postinjection flare (following intra-articular use); Charcot-like arthropathy.

ORAL PASTE

The following local adverse reactions are reported infrequently with topical corticosteroids. These reactions are listed in an approximate decreasing order of occurrence: Burning, itching, irritation, dryness, hypopigmentation, perioral dermatitis, allergic contact dermatitis, secondary infection, striae, miliaria.

RECTAL FOAM

Adverse reactions listed alphabetically under each subsection:

Allergic Reactions: Anaphylactoid reaction, anaphylaxis, angioedema.

Cardiovascular: Bradycardia, cardiac arrest, cardiac arrhythmias, cardiac enlargement, circulatory collapse, congestive heart failure, fat embolism, hypertension, hypertrophic cardiomyopathy in premature infants, myocardial rupture following recent myocardial infarction (see WARNINGS), pulmonary edema, syncope, tachycardia, thromboembolism, thrombophlebitis, vasculitis.

Dermatologic: Acne, allergic dermatitis, cutaneous and SC atrophy, dry scaly skin, ecchymoses and petechiae, edema, erythema, hyperpigmentation, hypopigmentation, impaired wound healing, increased sweating, rash, sterile abscess, striae, suppressed reactions to skin tests, thin fragile skin, thinning scalp hair, urticaria.

Endocrine: Decreased carbohydrate and glucose tolerance, development of cushingoid state, glycosuria, hirsutism, hypertrichosis, increased requirement for insulin or oral hypoglycemic agents in diabetes, manifestations of latent diabetes mellitus, menstrual irregularities, secondary adrenocortical and pituitary unresponsiveness (particularly in times of stress, as in trauma, surgery, or illness), suppression of growth in pediatric patients.

Fluid and Electrolyte Disturbances: Congestive heart failure in susceptible patients, fluid retention, hypokalemic alkalosis, potassium loss, sodium retention.

Where hypokalemia and other symptoms associated with fluid and electrolyte imbalance call for potassium supplementation and salt poor or salt-free diets, these may be instituted and are compatible with diet requirements for ulcerative proctitis.

Gastrointestinal: Abdominal distention, elevation in serum liver enzyme levels (usually reversible upon discontinuation), hepatomegaly, increased appetite, nausea, pancreatitis, peptic ulcer with possible perforation and hemorrhage, perforation of the small and large intestine (particularly in patients with inflammatory bowel disease), ulcerative esophagitis.

Metabolic: Negative nitrogen balance due to protein catabolism.

Musculoskeletal: Aseptic necrosis of femoral and humeral heads, Charcot-like arthropathy, loss of muscle mass, muscle weakness, osteoporosis, pathologic fracture of long bones, steroid myopathy, tendon rupture, vertebral compression fractures.

Neurologic/Psychiatric: Convulsions, depression, emotional instability, euphoria, headache, increased intracranial pressure with papilledema (pseudotumor cerebri) usually following discontinuation of treatment, insomnia, mood swings, neuritis, neuropathy, paresthesia, personality changes, psychic disorders, vertigo.

Ophthalmic: Exophthalmos, glaucoma, increased intraocular pressure, posterior subcapsular cataracts, rare instances of blindness associated with periocular injections.

Other: Abnormal fat deposits, decreased resistance to infection, hiccups, increased or decreased motility and number of spermatozoa, malaise, moon face, weight gain.

DOSAGE AND ADMINISTRATION

TOPICAL CREAM

Topical corticosteroids are generally applied to the affected area as a thin film from 2-4 times daily depending on the severity of the condition.

Occlusive dressings may be used for the management of psoriasis or recalcitrant conditions. If an infection develops, the use of occlusive dressings should be discontinued and appropriate antimicrobial therapy instituted.

SUPPOSITORIES

For rectal administration. Insert 1 suppository in the rectum twice daily, morning and night for 2 weeks, in nonspecific proctitis. In more severe cases, 1 suppository 3 times a day or 2 suppositories twice daily. In factitial proctitis, the recommended duration of therapy is 6-8 weeks or less, according to the response of the individual case.

STERILE SUSPENSION

For intra-articular, intralesional, and soft tissue injection only. NOT FOR INTRAVENOUS USE.

DOSAGE AND FREQUENCY OF INJECTION ARE VARIABLE AND MUST BE INDIVIDUALIZED ON THE BASIS OF THE DISEASE AND THE RESPONSE OF THE PATIENT.

The initial dose varies from 5-75 mg depending on the disease being treated and the size of the area to be injected. Frequency of injection depends on symptomatic response, and usually is once every 2 or 3 weeks. Severe conditions may require injection once a week. Frequent intra-articular injection may result in damage to joint tissues. If satisfactory clinical response does not occur after a reasonable period of time, discontinue hydrocortisone acetate sterile suspension and transfer the patient to other therapy.

Patients should be observed closely for signs that might require dosage adjustment, including changes in clinical status resulting from remissions or exacerbations of the disease, and individual responsiveness.

Some of the usual single doses are:

Large Joints (e.g., knee): 25 mg, occasionally 37.5 mg. Doses over 50 mg not recommended.

Small Joints (e.g., interphalangeal, temporomandibular): 10 to 25 mg.

Bursae: 25 to 37.5 mg.

Tendon Sheaths: 5 to 12.5 mg.

Soft Tissue Infiltration: 25 to 50 mg, occasionally 75 mg.

Ganglia: 12.5 to 25 mg.

For rapid onset of action, a soluble adrenocortical hormone preparation, such as dexamethasone sodium phosphate injection or prednisolone sodium phosphate injection, may be given with hydrocortisone acetate sterile suspension.

If desired, a local anesthetic may be used, and may be injected before hydrocortisone acetate sterile suspension or mixed in a syringe with hydrocortisone acetate sterile suspension and given simultaneously.

If used prior to intra-articular injection of the steroid, inject most of the anesthetic into the soft tissues of the surrounding area and instill a small amount into the joint.

If given together, mixing should be done in the injection syringe by drawing the steroid in *first,* then the anesthetic. In this way, the anesthetic will not be introduced inadvertently into the vial of steroid. *The mixture must be used immediately and any unused portion discarded.*

ORAL PASTE

Dab, **do not rub,** on the lesion until the paste adheres. (Rubbing this preparation on lesions may result in a granular, gritty sensation.) After application, a smooth, slippery film develops.

Usual Adult Dose: Topical, to the oral mucous membrane, 2 or 3 times a day following meals and at bedtime.

Usual Pediatric Dose: Dosage has not been established.

RECTAL FOAM

The usual dose is 1 applicatorful once or twice daily for 2 or 3 weeks, and every second day thereafter, administered rectally. **Directions for Use,** on the carton describe how to use the aerosol container and applicator. Satisfactory response usually occurs within 5-7 days marked by a decrease in symptoms. Symptomatic improvement in ulcerative proctitis should not be used as the sole criterion for evaluating efficacy. Sigmoidoscopy is also recommended to judge dosage adjustment, duration of therapy, and rate of improvement.

It should be emphasized that dosage requirements are variable and must be individualized on the basis of the disease under treatment and the response of the patient. After a favorable response is noted, the proper maintenance dosage should be determined by decreasing the initial drug dosage in small decrements at appropriate time intervals until the lowest dosage which will maintain an adequate clinical response is reached. Situation which may make dosage adjustments necessary are changes in clinical status secondary to remissions or exacerbations in the disease process, the patient's individual drug responsiveness, and the effect of patient exposure to stressful situations not directly related to the disease entity under treatment. In this latter situation it may be necessary to increase the dosage of the corticosteroid for a period of time consistent with the patient's condition. If after long-term therapy the drug is to be stopped, it is recommended that it be withdrawn gradually rather than abruptly.

HOW SUPPLIED

TOPICAL CREAM

Cortifoam cream 1% is a topical corticosteroid with micronized hydrocortisone acetate 1% (active ingredient) in a buffered, water-washable cream.

Storage: Store at controlled room temperature 15-30°C (59-86°F).

SUPPOSITORIES

Each Cortifoam 25 mg suppository contains 25 mg hydrocortisone acetate in a hydrogenated cocoglyceride base. Each 30 mg suppository contains 30 mg hydrocortisone acetate in a specially blended hydrogenated vegetable oil base.

Storage: Store below 30°C (86°F). Protect from freezing.

STERILE SUSPENSION

Cortifoam sterile suspension is supplied in 2 strengths, one containing 25 mg hydrocortisone acetate/ml, the other containing 50 mg/ml.

Storage: Sensitive to heat. Do not autoclave. Protect from freezing.

ORAL PASTE

Each g of Cortifoam paste contains hydrocortisone acetate 5 g (0.5%) in a paste vehicle containing pectin, gelatin, sodium carboxymethylcellulose dispersed in a plasticized hydrocarbon gel composed of 5% polyethylene in mineral oil, flavored with imitation vanilla.

RECTAL FOAM

Cortifoam rectal foam is supplied in an aerosol container with a special rectal applicator. Each applicator delivers approximately 900 mg of foam containing approximately 80 mg of hydrocortisone as 90 mg of hydrocortisone acetate. When used correctly, the aerosol container will deliver a minimum of 14 applications.

Storage: Store at controlled room temperature, 20-25°C (68-77°F).

DO NOT REFRIGERATE.

PRODUCT LISTING - RATED THERAPEUTICALLY EQUIVALENT

Cream - Topical - 1%

Size	Price	Product	NDC
15 gm	$1.50	GENERIC, Ambix Laboratories	10038-0031-05
15 gm	$1.95	GENERIC, Cmc-Consolidated Midland Corporation	00223-4161-15
20 gm	$1.73	GENERIC, Clay-Park Laboratories Inc	45802-0013-02
20 gm	$1.90	GENERIC, Thames Pharmacal Company Inc	49158-0101-07
20 gm	$2.06	GENERIC, Clay-Park Laboratories Inc	45802-0003-02
20 gm	$2.15	GENERIC, Moore, H.L. Drug Exchange Inc	00839-5207-45
20 gm	$2.25	GENERIC, Cmc-Consolidated Midland Corporation	00223-4161-20
20 gm	$2.40	GENERIC, Interstate Drug Exchange Inc	00814-3756-94
20 gm	$2.40	GENERIC, Interstate Drug Exchange Inc	00814-3776-94
30 gm	$1.90	GENERIC, Ambix Laboratories	10038-0031-07
30 gm	$1.92	GENERIC, Alpharma Uspd Makers Of Barre and Nmc	23317-0343-29
30 gm	$2.16	GENERIC, Clay-Park Laboratories Inc	45802-0013-03
30 gm	$2.31	GENERIC, Qualitest Products Inc	00603-0534-50
30 gm	$2.42	GENERIC, Moore, H.L. Drug Exchange Inc	00839-5207-49
30 gm	$2.50	GENERIC, Cmc-Consolidated Midland Corporation	00223-4161-30
30 gm	$2.63	GENERIC, Interstate Drug Exchange Inc	00814-3776-72
30 gm	$2.95	GENERIC, Major Pharmaceuticals Inc	00904-0749-31
30 gm	$3.06	GENERIC, Clay-Park Laboratories Inc	45802-0003-03
30 gm	$3.42	GENERIC, Fougera	00168-0015-31
30 gm	$3.95	GENERIC, Syosset Laboratories Company	47854-0660-05
30 gm	$4.10	GENERIC, Alpharma Uspd Makers Of Barre and Nmc	00472-0321-26
30 gm	$4.20	GENERIC, Thames Pharmacal Company Inc	49158-0101-08
30 gm	$4.28	GENERIC, Dermol Pharmaceuticals Inc	50744-0104-05
30 gm	$4.28	GENERIC, Dermol Pharmaceuticals Inc	50744-0567-05
30 gm	$5.70	GENERIC, C and M	00398-0050-01
30 gm	$6.71	GENERIC, Del Ray Laboratories Inc	00316-0126-01
30 gm	$8.00	HYTONE, Aventis Pharmaceuticals	00066-0083-01
30 gm	$9.50	GENERIC, Allergan Inc	00023-0510-30
57 gm	$6.50	GENERIC, Syosset Laboratories Company	47854-0660-07
90 gm	$11.18	GENERIC, Del Ray Laboratories Inc	00316-0126-03
100 gm	$2.00	GENERIC, Cmc-Consolidated Midland Corporation	00223-4124-15
100 gm	$2.40	GENERIC, Cmc-Consolidated Midland Corporation	00223-4124-20
100 gm	$2.50	GENERIC, Cmc-Consolidated Midland Corporation	00223-4124-30
120 gm	$7.13	GENERIC, Moore, H.L. Drug Exchange Inc	00839-5207-53
120 gm	$7.45	GENERIC, Clay-Park Laboratories Inc	45802-0003-04
120 gm	$7.50	GENERIC, Major Pharmaceuticals Inc	00904-0749-22
120 gm	$7.50	GENERIC, Ambix Laboratories	10038-0031-12
120 gm	$7.50	GENERIC, Thames Pharmacal Company Inc	49158-0101-12
120 gm	$7.88	GENERIC, Clay-Park Laboratories Inc	45802-0013-04
120 gm	$8.75	GENERIC, Cmc-Consolidated Midland Corporation	00223-4124-11
120 gm	$9.38	GENERIC, Interstate Drug Exchange Inc	00814-3776-76
454 gm	$20.02	GENERIC, Ambix Laboratories	10038-0031-16
454 gm	$21.60	GENERIC, Thames Pharmacal Company Inc	49158-0101-16
454 gm	$22.52	GENERIC, Syosset Laboratories Company	47854-0660-18
454 gm	$24.99	GENERIC, Clay-Park Laboratories Inc	45802-0278-05
454 gm	$27.38	GENERIC, Allscripts Pharmaceutical Company	54569-2607-00
454 gm	$29.10	GENERIC, Interstate Drug Exchange Inc	00814-3776-84
454 gm	$31.45	GENERIC, Fougera	00168-0015-16
454 gm	$53.21	GENERIC, C and M	00398-0050-16
480 gm	$23.76	GENERIC, Clay-Park Laboratories Inc	45802-0003-05
480 gm	$24.34	GENERIC, Major Pharmaceuticals Inc	00904-0749-27

Lotion - Topical - 1%

Size	Price	Product	NDC
60 ml	$18.75	CETACORT, Galderma Laboratories Inc	00299-3949-02
60 ml	$24.33	NUTRACORT, Healthpoint	00064-2200-02
60 ml	$30.03	CETACORT, Healthpoint	00064-2000-02
118 ml	$40.26	GENERIC, Stiefel Laboratories Inc	00145-2537-04
120 ml	$4.65	GENERIC, Mericon Industries Inc	00394-0859-32
120 ml	$8.70	GENERIC, Mutual/United Research Laboratories	00677-1428-41
120 ml	$13.88	GENERIC, Del Ray Laboratories Inc	00316-0131-04
120 ml	$20.20	GENERIC, Glades Pharmaceuticals	59366-2707-04
120 ml	$36.40	NUTRACORT, Healthpoint	00064-2200-04

PRODUCT LISTING - RATED NOT THERAPEUTICALLY EQUIVALENT

Size	Price	Product	NDC
Suspension - Injectable - acetate 25 mg/ml			
5 ml	$4.75	GENERIC, Cmc-Consolidated Midland Corporation	00223-7880-05
Suspension - Injectable - acetate 50 mg/ml			
10 ml	$5.50	GENERIC, C.O. Truxton Inc	00463-1037-10

PRODUCT LISTING - EQUIVALENTS NOT AVAILABLE

Cream - Topical - 1%

Size	Price	Product	NDC
1 gm x 144	$14.80	GENERIC, Ivax Corporation	00182-5060-30
5 gm	$1.40	GENERIC, Cmc-Consolidated Midland Corporation	00223-4124-05
15 gm	$1.58	GENERIC, Alpharma Uspd Makers Of Barre and Nmc	23317-0330-14
15 gm	$1.58	GENERIC, Alpharma Uspd Makers Of Barre and Nmc	23317-0331-14
15 gm	$2.86	GENERIC, Pro Metic Pharma	62174-0157-26

Size	Price	Product	NDC
15 gm	$2.86	GENERIC, Pro Metic Pharma	62174-0158-26
15 gm	$3.94	GENERIC, Prescript Pharmaceuticals	00247-0111-15
20 gm	$2.38	GENERIC, Allscripts Pharmaceutical Company	54569-1771-01
20 gm	$4.14	GENERIC, Prescript Pharmaceuticals	00247-0111-20
20 gm	$9.15	GENERIC, Pharma Pac	52959-0039-01
28 gm	$4.47	GENERIC, Prescript Pharmaceuticals	00247-0111-29
28 gm	$4.48	GENERIC, Prescript Pharmaceuticals	00247-0111-34
30 gm	$1.19	GENERIC, Leader Brand Products	37205-0161-10
30 gm	$1.19	GENERIC, Leader Brand Products	37205-0162-10
30 gm	$1.50	GENERIC, Leader Brand Products	37205-0272-10
30 gm	$1.80	GENERIC, Heritage Consumer Products	63736-0646-03
30 gm	$2.00	GENERIC, Everett Laboratories Inc	00642-0071-01
30 gm	$2.00	GENERIC, Everett Laboratories Inc	00642-0073-01
30 gm	$2.27	GENERIC, G and W Laboratories Inc	00713-0289-31
30 gm	$2.35	GENERIC, G and W Laboratories Inc	00713-0288-31
30 gm	$2.35	GENERIC, G and W Laboratories Inc	00713-0291-31
30 gm	$2.40	GENERIC, Ivax Corporation	00182-5060-34
30 gm	$2.46	GENERIC, G and W Laboratories Inc	00713-0290-31
30 gm	$2.58	GENERIC, G and W Laboratories Inc	00713-0626-31
30 gm	$3.91	GENERIC, Allscripts Pharmaceutical Company	54569-1096-00
30 gm	$4.00	GENERIC, Altaire Pharmaceuticals Inc	59390-0049-17
30 gm	$4.14	GENERIC, Pro Metic Pharma	62174-0157-28
30 gm	$4.14	GENERIC, Pro Metic Pharma	62174-0158-28
30 gm	$4.54	GENERIC, Prescript Pharmaceuticals	00247-0111-30
30 gm	$10.13	GENERIC, Pharma Pac	52959-0039-03
30 gm	$21.41	CARMOL HC, Doak Dermatologics Division	10337-0550-52
45 gm	$2.04	GENERIC, Alpharma Uspd Makers Of Barre and Nmc	23317-0330-43
45 gm	$2.04	GENERIC, Alpharma Uspd Makers Of Barre and Nmc	23317-0331-43
50 gm	$5.33	GENERIC, Prescript Pharmaceuticals	00247-0111-50
60 gm	$2.70	GENERIC, Alpharma Uspd Makers Of Barre and Nmc	23317-0330-57
60 gm	$5.30	GENERIC, Ivax Corporation	00182-5060-43
60 gm	$5.73	GENERIC, Prescript Pharmaceuticals	00247-0111-60
60 gm	$6.95	GENERIC, Rexall Group	60814-0163-02
144.90 gm	$14.30	GENERIC, Allscripts Pharmaceutical Company	54569-4090-00
454 gm	$13.92	GENERIC, Clay-Park Laboratories Inc	45802-0276-05
454 gm	$27.52	GENERIC, Alpharma Uspd Makers Of Barre and Nmc	00472-0321-16
454 gm	$30.00	GENERIC, Cmc-Consolidated Midland Corporation	00223-4124-04
454 gm	$30.70	GENERIC, Ivax Corporation	00182-5060-45

Lotion - Topical - 1%

Size	Price	Product	NDC
120 ml	$12.06	GENERIC, Allscripts Pharmaceutical Company	54569-2830-00
120 ml	$13.00	GENERIC, Fougera	00168-0287-04
120 ml	$14.26	GENERIC, Blansett Pharmacal Company Inc	51674-0110-04
120 ml	$15.46	GENERIC, Southwood Pharmaceuticals Inc	58016-3223-01

Paste - Topical - 0.5%

Size	Price	Product	NDC
5 gm	$6.41	ORABASE HCA, Colgate Oral Pharmaceuticals Inc	00126-0101-45

Suppository - Rectal - 25 mg

Size	Price	Product	NDC
2's	$3.59	GENERIC, Prescript Pharmaceuticals	00247-0223-02
4's	$3.84	GENERIC, Prescript Pharmaceuticals	00247-0223-04
6's	$4.07	GENERIC, Prescript Pharmaceuticals	00247-0223-06
10's	$4.55	GENERIC, Prescript Pharmaceuticals	00247-0223-10
12's	$4.14	GENERIC, Alpharma Uspd Makers Of Barre and Nmc	23317-0511-12
12's	$4.25	GENERIC, Bio Pharm Inc	59741-0301-12
12's	$4.79	GENERIC, Prescript Pharmaceuticals	00247-0223-12
12's	$4.84	GENERIC, Pro Metic Pharma	62174-0091-82
12's	$4.85	GENERIC, Paddock Laboratories Inc	00574-7090-12
12's	$5.93	GENERIC, Upsher-Smith Laboratories Inc	00245-0111-12
12's	$5.95	GENERIC, Raway Pharmacal Inc	00686-0503-12
12's	$6.10	GENERIC, Compumed Pharmaceuticals	00403-0298-18
12's	$6.48	GENERIC, Moore, H.L. Drug Exchange Inc	00839-7603-12
12's	$6.75	GENERIC, Major Pharmaceuticals Inc	00904-0160-12
12's	$7.35	GENERIC, Vintage Pharmaceuticals Inc	00254-8400-06
12's	$7.35	GENERIC, Qualitest Products Inc	00603-8127-11
12's	$8.99	GENERIC, Cypress Pharmaceutical Inc	60258-0501-12
12's	$9.00	GENERIC, Allscripts Pharmaceutical Company	54569-5586-00
12's	$9.15	GENERIC, Pharma Pac	52959-0250-03
12's	$9.20	GENERIC, Southwood Pharmaceuticals Inc	58016-2023-01
12's	$9.49	GENERIC, Allscripts Pharmaceutical Company	54569-2586-00
12's	$9.50	GENERIC, Clay-Park Laboratories Inc	45802-0725-30
12's	$9.55	GENERIC, G and W Laboratories Inc	00713-0503-12
12's	$9.90	GENERIC, Mutual/United Research Laboratories	00677-1377-12
12's	$10.75	GENERIC, Ivax Corporation	00182-7038-11
12's	$10.95	GENERIC, Cmc-Consolidated Midland Corporation	00223-5555-12
12's	$11.25	GENERIC, Alpharma Uspd Makers Of Barre and Nmc	00472-0511-12
12's	$11.70	GENERIC, Able Laboratories Inc	53265-0761-12
12's	$14.90	GENERIC, Elge Inc	58298-0150-12
12's	$18.38	GENERIC, American Generics Inc	58634-0036-01
12's	$18.38	GENERIC, Ranbaxy Laboratories	63304-0408-12
12's	$24.12	GENERIC, Southwood Pharmaceuticals Inc	58016-2023-12
12's	$40.66	CORT-DOME HIGH POTENCY, Bayer	00026-5005-12
12's	$41.31	ANUSOL-HC, Monarch Pharmaceuticals Inc	61570-0303-61
24's	$13.97	GENERIC, Vintage Pharmaceuticals Inc	00254-8400-15
24's	$13.97	GENERIC, Qualitest Products Inc	00603-8127-18
24's	$14.94	GENERIC, Geneva Pharmaceuticals	00781-7700-40
24's	$17.85	GENERIC, Able Laboratories Inc	53265-0761-24
24's	$18.50	GENERIC, Clay-Park Laboratories Inc	45802-0725-31
24's	$18.71	GENERIC, G and W Laboratories Inc	00713-0503-24
24's	$21.50	GENERIC, Ivax Corporation	00182-7038-16
24's	$21.50	GENERIC, Alpharma Uspd Makers Of Barre and Nmc	00472-0511-24
24's	$25.00	GENERIC, Elge Inc	58298-0150-24
24's	$26.95	GENERIC, Bio Pharm Inc	59741-0301-24
24's	$32.19	GENERIC, American Generics Inc	58634-0036-02
24's	$32.19	GENERIC, Ranbaxy Laboratories	63304-0408-24
24's	$72.36	ANUSOL-HC, Monarch Pharmaceuticals Inc	61570-0303-62
50's	$42.50	GENERIC, Elge Inc	58298-0150-50
50's	$49.50	GENERIC, Bio Pharm Inc	59741-0301-50
100's	$39.95	GENERIC, Bio Pharm Inc	59741-0301-49
100's	$43.80	GENERIC, Major Pharmaceuticals Inc	00904-0160-60
100's	$61.24	GENERIC, Able Laboratories Inc	53265-0761-10
100's	$82.33	GENERIC, G and W Laboratories Inc	00713-0503-01
100's	$89.50	GENERIC, Cmc-Consolidated Midland Corporation	00223-5555-01
100's	$125.00	GENERIC, Raway Pharmacal Inc	00686-0503-01

Suspension - Injectable - acetate 25 mg/ml

Size	Price	Product	NDC
10 ml	$3.60	GENERIC, C.O. Truxton Inc	00463-1036-10

H

Hydrocortisone Sodium Succinate *(001485)*

Categories: Adrenocortical insufficiency; Anemia, acquired hemolytic; Anemia, congenital hypoplastic; Anemia, erythroblastopenia; Ankylosing spondylitis; Arthritis, gouty; Arthritis, post-traumatic; Arthritis, psoriatic; Arthritis, rheumatoid; Asthma; Berylliosis; Bursitis; Carditis, rheumatic; Chorioretinitis; Choroiditis; Colitis, ulcerative; Conjunctivitis, allergic; Crohn's disease; Dermatitis herpetiformis, bullous; Dermatitis, atopic; Dermatitis, contact; Dermatitis, exfoliative; Dermatitis, seborrheic; Dermatomyositis, systemic; Epicondylitis; Erythema multiforme; Herpes zoster ophthalmicus; Hypercalcemia, secondary to neoplasia; Hypersensitivity reactions; Inflammation, anterior segment, ophthalmic; Inflammation, ophthalmic; Inflammatory bowel disease; Iridocyclitis; Iritis; Keratitis; Leukemia; Loffler's syndrome; Lupus erythematosus, systemic; Lymphoma; Meningitis, tuberculous; Multiple sclerosis; Mycosis fungoides; Nephrotic syndrome; Neuritis, optic; Ophthalmia, sympathetic; Pemphigus; Pneumonitis, aspiration; Polymyositis; Psoriasis; Rhinitis, perennial allergic; Rhinitis, seasonal allergic; Sarcoidosis; Serum sickness; Stevens-Johnson syndrome; Synovitis, secondary to osteoarthritis; Tenosynovitis; Thrombocytopenia, secondary; Thyroiditis, nonsuppurative; Trichinosis; Tuberculosis, disseminated; Tuberculosis, fulminating; Tuberculosis, meningitis; Ulcer, allergic corneal marginal; Uveitis; FDA Approved 1955 Apr; Pregnancy Category C

Drug Classes: Corticosteroids

Brand Names: A-Hydrocort; **Solu-Cortef**

Foreign Brand Availability: Corticap (Korea); Efcortelan Soluble (Bahrain; Cyprus; Egypt; Iran; Iraq; Jordan; Kuwait; Lebanon; Libya; Oman; Qatar; Republic-of-Yemen; Saudi-Arabia; Syria; United-Arab-Emirates); Flebocortid (Ecuador; Mexico); Hycortil (Philippines); Hydro-Adreson Aquosum (Benin; Burkina-Faso; Ethiopia; Gambia; Ghana; Guinea; Ivory-Coast; Kenya; Liberia; Malawi; Mali; Mauritania; Mauritius; Morocco; Niger; Nigeria; Senegal; Seychelles; Sierra-Leone; Sudan; Tanzania; Tunia; Uganda; Zambia; Zimbabwe); Hydro Adreson Aquosum (Malaysia); Hydrocortison (Germany); Hydrocortisone Roussel (France); Hydrocortisone Upjohn (France); Hydrotopic (Philippines); Nositrol (Mexico); Radicortin (Bahrain; Benin; Burkina-Faso; Cyprus; Egypt; Ethiopia; Gambia; Ghana; Guinea; Iran; Iraq; Ivory-Coast; Jordan; Kenya; Kuwait; Lebanon; Liberia; Libya; Malawi; Mali; Mauritania; Mauritius; Morocco; Niger; Nigeria; Oman; Qatar; Republic-of-Yemen; Saudi-Arabia; Senegal; Seychelles; Sierra-Leone; Sudan; Syria; Tanzania; Tunia; Uganda; United-Arab-Emirates; Zambia; Zimbabwe); Solu Cortef (Bahrain; Belgium; Benin; Burkina-Faso; Canada; Colombia; Costa-Rica; Cyprus; Czech-Republic; Denmark; Egypt; El-Salvador; England; Ethiopia; Finland; Gambia; Ghana; Greece; Guatemala; Guinea; Honduras; Hong-Kong; Hungary; Indonesia; Iran; Iraq; Ireland; Israel; Italy; Ivory-Coast; Jordan; Kenya; Kuwait; Lebanon; Liberia; Libya; Malawi; Malaysia; Mali; Mauritania; Mauritius; Morocco; Netherlands; Nicaragua; Niger; Nigeria; Norway; Oman; Panama; Peru; Philippines; Qatar; Republic-of-Yemen; Russia; Saudi-Arabia; Senegal; Seychelles; Sierra-Leone; South-Africa; Sudan; Sweden; Switzerland; Syria; Taiwan; Tanzania; Thailand; Tunia; Uganda; United-Arab-Emirates; Zambia; Zimbabwe); Solu Cortef M.O.V. (Bahrain; Cyprus; Egypt; Iran; Iraq; Jordan; Kuwait; Lebanon; Libya; Oman; Qatar; Republic-of-Yemen; Saudi-Arabia; Syria; United-Arab-Emirates)

HCFA JCODE(S): J1720 up to 100 mg IV, IM, SC

DESCRIPTION

Solu-Cortef sterile powder contains hydrocortisone sodium succinate as the active ingredient. Hydrocortisone sodium succinate is a white or nearly white, odorless, hygroscopic amorphous solid. It is very soluble in water and in alcohol, very slightly soluble in acetone and insoluble in chloroform. The chemical name is pregn-4-ene-3,20-dione,21-(3-carboxy-1-oxopropoxy)-11,17-dihydroxy-, monosodium salt, (11β)- and its molecular weight is 484.52.

Hydrocortisone sodium succinate is an anti-inflammatory adrenocortical steroid. This highly water-soluble sodium succinate ester of hydrocortisone permits the immediate IV administration of high doses of hydrocortisone in a small volume of diluent and is particularly useful where high blood levels of hydrocortisone are required rapidly.

Solu-Cortef sterile powder is available in several packages for IV or IM administration.

100 mg plain: Vials containing hydrocortisone sodium succinate equivalent to 100 mg hydrocortisone, also 0.8 mg monobasic sodium phosphate anhydrous, 8.73 mg dibasic sodium phosphate dried (see TABLE 1).

When necessary, the pH of each formula was adjusted with sodium hydroxide so that the pH of the reconstituted solution is within the USP specified range of 7-8.

Storage: Store unreconstituted product at controlled room temperature 20-25°C (68-77°F). Store solution at controlled room temperature 20-25°C (68-77°F) and protect from light. Use solution only if it is clear. Unused solution should be discarded after 3 days.

CLINICAL PHARMACOLOGY

Naturally occurring glucocorticoids (hydrocortisone and cortisone), which also have salt-retaining properties, are used as replacement therapy in adrenocortical deficiency states. Their synthetic analogs are primarily used for their potent anti-inflammatory effects in disorders of many organ systems.

TABLE 1 *Solu-Cortef Act-O-Vial System (Single-Dose Vial) in Four Strengths:*

	100 mg	250 mg	500 mg	1000 mg
	Each 2 ml contains: (when mixed)	Each 2 ml contains: (when mixed)	Each 4 ml contains: (when mixed)	Each 8 ml contains: (when mixed)
Hydrocortisone sodium succinate	equiv. to 100 mg hydrocortisone	equiv. to 250 mg hydrocortisone	equiv. to 500 mg hydrocortisone	equiv. to 1000 mg hydrocortisone
Monobasic sodium phosphate anhydrous	0.8 mg	2 mg	4 mg	8 mg
Dibasic sodium phosphate dried	8.76 mg	21.8 mg	44 mg	87.32 mg
Benzyl alcohol added as preservative	18.1 mg	16.4 mg	33.4 mg	66.9 mg

Glucocorticoids cause profound and varied metabolic effects. In addition, they modify the body's immune response to diverse stimuli.

Hydrocortisone sodium succinate has the same metabolic and anti-inflammatory actions as hydrocortisone. When given parenterally and in equimolar quantities, the two compounds are equivalent in biologic activity. Following the IV injection of hydrocortisone sodium succinate, demonstrable effects are evident within 1 hour and persist for a variable period. Excretion of the administered dose is nearly complete within 12 hours. Thus, if constantly high blood levels are required, injections should be made every 4-6 hours. This preparation is also rapidly absorbed when administered intramuscularly and is excreted in a pattern similar to that observed after IV injection.

INDICATIONS AND USAGE

When oral therapy is not feasible, and the strength, dosage form and route of administration of the drug reasonably lend the preparation to the treatment of the condition, hydrocortisone sodium succinate sterile powder is indicated for IV or IM use in the following conditions:

Endocrine disorders:

Primary or secondary adrenocortical insufficiency (hydrocortisone or cortisone is the drug of choice; synthetic analogs may be used in conjunction with mineralocorticoids where applicable; in infancy, mineralocorticoid supplementation is of particular importance).

Acute adrenocortical insufficiency (hydrocortisone or cortisone is the drug of choice; mineralocorticoid supplementation may be necessary, particularly when synthetic analogs are used).

Preoperatively, and in the event of serious trauma or illness, in patients with known adrenal insufficiency or when adrenocortical reserve is doubtful.

Shock unresponsive to conventional therapy if adrenocortical insufficiency exists or is suspected.

Congenital adrenal hyperplasia.

Hypercalcemia associated with cancer.

Nonsuppurative thyroiditis.

Rheumatic disorders: As adjunctive therapy for short-term administration (to tide the patient over an acute or exacerbation) in:

Post-traumatic osteoarthritis.

Synovitis of osteoarthritis.

Rheumatoid arthritis, including juvenile rheumatoid arthritis (selected cases may require low-dose maintenance therapy).

Acute and subacute bursitis.

Epicondylitis.

Acute nonspecific tenosynovitis.

Acute gouty arthritis.

Psoriatic arthritis.

Ankylosing spondylitis.

Collagen diseases: During an exacerbation or as maintenance therapy in selected cases of:

Systemic lupus erythematosus.

Systemic dermatomyositis (polymyositis).

Acute rheumatic carditis.

Dermatologic diseases:

Pemphigus.

Severe erythema multiforme (Stevens-Johnson syndrome).

Exfoliative dermatitis.

Bullous dermatitis herpetiformis.

Severe seborrheic dermatitis.

Severe psoriasis.

Mycosis fungoides.

Allergic states: Control of severe or incapacitating allergic conditions intractable to adequate trials of conventional treatment in:

Bronchial asthma.

Contact dermatitis.

Atopic dermatitis.

Serum sickness.

Seasonal or perennial allergic rhinitis.

Drug hypersensitivity reactions.

Urticarial transfusion reactions.

Acute noninfectious laryngeal edema (epinephrine is the drug of first choice).

Ophthalmic diseases: Severe acute and chronic allergic and inflammatory processes involving the eye, such as:

Herpes zoster ophthalmicus.

Iritis, iridocyclitis.

Chorioretinitis.

Diffuse posterior uveitis and choroiditis.

Optic neuritis.

Sympathetic ophthalmia.

Anterior segment inflammation.

Allergic conjunctivitis.

Allergic corneal marginal ulcers.

Keratitis.

Gastrointestinal diseases: To tide the patient over a critical period of the disease in:

Ulcerative colitis (systemic therapy).

Regional enteritis (systemic therapy).

Respiratory diseases:

Symptomatic sarcoidosis.

Berylliosis.

Fulminating or disseminated pulmonary tuberculosis when used concurrently with appropriate antituberculous chemotherapy.

Loeffler's syndrome not manageable by other means.

Aspiration pneumonitis.

Hematologic disorders:

Acquired (autoimmune) hemolytic anemia.

Idiopathic thrombocytopenic purpura in adults (IV only; IM administration is contraindicated).

Secondary thrombocytopenia in adults.

Erythroblastopenia (RBC anemia).

Congenital (erythroid) hypoplastic anemia.

Neoplastic diseases: For palliative management of:

Leukemias and lymphomas in adults.

Acute leukemia of childhood.

Edematous states: To induce diuresis or remission of proteinuria in the nephrotic syndrome, without uremia, of the idiopathic type, or that due to lupus erythematosus.

Nervous sytem: Acute exacerbations of multiple sclerosis.

Miscellaneous:

Tuberculous meningitis with subarachnoid block or impending block when used concurrently with appropriate antituberculous chemotherapy.

Trichinosis with neurologic or myocardial involvement.

CONTRAINDICATIONS

The use of hydrocortisone sodium succinate sterile powder is contraindicated in premature infants because the 100, 250, 500and 1000 mg ACT-O-VIAL System contain benzyl alcohol. Benzyl alcohol has been reported to be associated with a fatal "Gasping Syndrome" in premature infants. Hydrocortisone sodium succinate sterile powder is also contraindicated in systemic fungal infections and patients with known hypersensitivity to the product and its constituents.

WARNINGS

In patients on corticosteroid therapy subjected to unusual stress, increased dosage of rapidly acting corticosteroids before, during, and after the stressful situation is indicated.

Corticosteroids may mask some signs of infection, and new infections may appear during their use. There may be decreased resistance and inability to localize infection when corticosteroids are used. Infections with any pathogen including viral, bacterial, fungal, protozoan or helminthic infections, in any location of the body, may be associated with the use of corticosteroids alone or in combination with other immunosuppressive agents that affect cellular immunity, or neutrophil function.[1]

These infections may be mild, but can be severe and at times fatal. With increasing doses of corticosteroids, the rate of occurrence of infectious complications increases.[2]

Prolonged use of corticosteroids may produce posterior subcapsular cataracts, glaucoma with possible damage to the optic nerves, and may enhance the establishment of secondary ocular infections due to fungi or viruses.

Usage in Pregnancy: Since adequate human reproduction studies have not been done with corticosteroids, the use of these drugs in pregnancy, nursing mothers, or women of childbearing potential requires that the possible benefits of the drug be weighed against the potential hazards to the mother and embryo or fetus. Infants born of mothers who have received substantial doses of corticosteroids during pregnancy should be carefully observed for signs of hypoadrenalism.

Average and large doses of hydrocortisone can cause elevation of blood pressure, salt and water retention, and increased excretion of potassium. These effects are less likely to occur with the synthetic derivatives except when used in large doses. Dietary salt restriction and potassium supplementation may be necessary. All corticosteroids increase calcium excretion.

Administration of live or live, attenuated vaccines is contraindicated in patients receiving immunosuppressive doses of corticosteroids. Killed or inactivated vaccines may be administered to patients receiving immunosuppressive doses of corticosteroids; however, the response to such vaccines may be diminished. Indicated immunization procedures may be undertaken in patients receiving nonimmunosuppresive doses of corticosteroids.

The use of hydrocortisone sodium succinate sterile powder in active tuberculosis should be restricted to those cases of fulminating or disseminated tuberculosis in which the corticosteroid is used for the management of the disease in conjunction with appropriate antituberculous regimen.

If corticosteroids are indicated in patients with latent tuberculosis or tuberculin reactivity, close observation is necessary as reactivation of the disease may occur. During prolonged corticosteroid therapy, these patients should receive chemoprophylaxis.

Because rare instances of anaphylactoid reactions (*e.g.,* bronchospasm) have occurred in patients receiving parenteral corticosteroid therapy, appropriate precautionary measures should be taken prior to administration, especially when the patient has a history of allergy to any drug.

Persons who are on drugs which suppress the immune system are more susceptible to infections than healthy individuals. Chicken pox and measles, for example, can have a more serious or even fatal course in non-immune children or adults on corticosteroids. In such children or adults who have not had these diseases, particular care should be taken to avoid exposure. How the dose, route and duration of corticosteroid administration affects the risk of developing a disseminated infection is not known. The contribution of the underlying disease and/or prior corticosteroid treatment to the risk is also not known. If exposed to chicken pox, prophylaxis with varicella zoster immune globulin (VZIG) may be indicated. If exposed to measles, prophylaxis with pooled IM immunoglobulin (IG) may be indicated. (See the respective prescribing information for complete VZIG and IG information.) If chicken pox develops, treatment with antiviral agents may be considered. Similarly, corticosteroids should be used with great care in patients with known or suspected Stongyloides (threadworm) infestation. In such patients, corticosteroid-induced immunosuppression may lead to Strongyloides hyperinfection and dissemination with widespread larval migration, often accompanied by severe enterocolitis and potentially fatal gram-negative septicemia.

PRECAUTIONS

GENERAL

Drug-induced secondary adrenocortical insufficiency may be minimized by gradual reduction of dosage. This type of relative insufficiency may persist for months after discontinuation of therapy; therefore, in any situation of stress occurring during that period, hormone therapy should be reinstituted. Since mineralocorticoid secretion may be impaired, salt and/or a mineralocorticoid should be administered concurrently.

There is an enhanced effect of corticosteroids in patients with hypothyroidism and in those with cirrhosis.

Corticosteroids should be used cautiously in patients with ocular herpes simplex for fear of corneal perforation.

The lowest possible dose of corticosteroid should be used to control the condition under treatment, and when reduction in dosage is possible, the reduction must be gradual.

Psychic derangements may appear when corticosteroids are used, ranging from euphoria, insomnia, mood swings, personality changes, and severe depression to frank psychotic manifestations. Also, existing emotional instability or psychotic tendencies may be aggravated by corticosteroids.

Steroids should be used with caution in nonspecific ulcerative colitis, if there is a probability of impending perforation, abscess or other pyogenic infection, also in diverticulitis, fresh intestinal anastomoses, active or latent peptic ulcer, renal insufficiency, hypertension, osteoporosis, and myasthenia gravis.

Growth and development of infants and children on prolonged corticosteroid therapy should be carefully followed.

Kaposi's sarcoma has been reported to occur in patients receiving corticosteroid therapy. Discontinuation of corticosteroids may result in clinical remission.

Although controlled clinical trials have shown corticosteroids to be effective in speeding the resolution of acute exacerbations of multiple sclerosis, they do not show that corticosteroids affect the ultimate outcome or natural history of the disease. The studies do show that relatively high doses of corticosteroids are necessary to demonstrate a significant effect. (See DOSAGE AND ADMINISTRATION.)

An acute myopathy has been observed with the use of high doses of corticosteroids, most often occurring in patients with disorders of neuromuscular transmission (*e.g.,* myasthenia gravis), or in patients receiving concomitant therapy with neuromuscular blocking drugs (*e.g.,* pancuronium). This acute myopathy is generalized, may involve ocular and respiratory muscles, and may result in quadriparesis. Elevations of creatine kinase may occur. Clinical improvement or recovery after stopping corticosteroids may require weeks to years.

Since complications of treatment with glucocorticoids are dependent on the size of the dose and the duration of treatment, a risk/benefit decision must be made in each individual case as to dose and duration of treatment and as to whether daily or intermittent therapy should be used.

INFORMATION FOR THE PATIENT

Persons who are on immunosuppressant doses of corticosteroids should be warned to avoid exposure to chickenpox or measles. Patients should be advised that if they are exposed, medical advice should be sought without delay.

DRUG INTERACTIONS

The pharmacokinetic interactins listed below are potentially clinically important. Drugs that induce hepatic enzymes such as phenobarbital, phenytoin and rifampin may increase the clearance of corticosteroids and may require increases in corticosteroid dose to achieve the desired response. Drugs such as troleandomycin and ketoconazole may inhibit the metabolism of corticosteroids and thus decrease their clearance. Therefore, the dose of corticosteroid should be titrated to avoid steroid toxicity. Corticosteroids may increase the clearance of chronic high dose aspirin. This could lead to decreased salicylate serum levels or increase the risk of salicylate toxicity when corticosteroid is withdrawn. Aspirin should be used cautiously in conjunction with corticosteroids in patients suffering from hypoprothrombinemia. The effect of corticosteroids on oral anticoagulants is variable. There are reports of enhanced as well as diminished effects of anticoagulants when given concurrently with corticosteroids. Therefore, coagulation indices should be monitored to maintain the desired anticoagulant effect.

ADVERSE REACTIONS

Fluid and Electrolyte Disturbances: Sodium retention; fluid retention; congestive heart failure in susceptible patients; potassium loss; hypokalemic alkalosis; hypertension.

Musculoskeletal: Muscle weakness; steroid myopathy, loss of muscle mass; osteoporosis; tendon rupture, particularly of the Achilles tendon; vertebral compression fractures; aseptic necrosis of femoral and humeral heads; pathologic fracture of long bones.

Gastrointestinal: Peptic ulcer with possible perforation and hemorrhage; pancreatitis; abdominal distention; ulcerative esophagitis; increases in alanine transaminase (ALT, SGPT), aspartate transaminase (AST, SGOT) and alkaline phosphatase have been observed following corticosteroid treatment. These changes are usually small, not associated with any clinical syndrome and are reversible upon discontinuation.

Dermatologic: Impaired wound healing; thin fragile skin; petechiae and ecchymoses; facial erythema; increased sweating; may suppress reactions to skin tests.

Neurological: Convulsions; increased intracranial pressure with papilledema (pseudotumor cerebri) usually after treatment; vertigo; headache.

Endocrine: Menstrual irregularities; development of Cushingoid state; suppression of growth in children; secondary adrenocortical and pituitary unresponsiveness, particularly in times of stress, as in trauma, surgery or illness; decreased carbohydrate tolerance; manifestations of latent diabetes mellitus; increased requirements for insulin or oral hypoglycemic agents in diabetics.

Ophthalmic: Posterior subcapsular cataracts; increased intraocular pressure; glaucoma; exophthalmos.

Metabolic: Negative nitrogen balance due to protein catabolism.

The following additional reactions are related to parenteral corticosteroid therapy:

Allergic, anaphylactic or other hypersensitivity reactions.
Hyperpigmentation or hypopigmentation.
Subcutaneous and cutaneous atrophy.
Sterile abscess.

DOSAGE AND ADMINISTRATION

This preparation may be administered by IV injection, by IV infusion, or by IM injection, the preferred method for initial emergency use being IV injection. Following the initial emergency period, consideration should be given to employing a longer acting injectable preparation or an oral preparation.

Therapy is initiated by administering hydrocortisone sodium succinate sterile powder intravenously over a period of 30 seconds (*e.g.,* 100 mg) to 10 minutes (*e.g.,* 500 mg or more). In general, high dose corticosteroid therapy should be continued only until the patient's condition has stabilized — usually not beyond 48-72 hours. Although adverse effects associated with high dose, short-term corticoid therapy are uncommon, peptic ulceration may occur. Prophylactic antacid therapy may be indicated.

When high dose hydrocortisone therapy must be continued beyond 48-72 hours, hypernatremia may occur. Under such circumstances it may be desirable to replace hydrocortisone sodium succinate with a corticoid such as methylprednisolone sodium succinate which causes little or no sodium retention.

The initial dose of hydrocortisone sodium succinate sterile powder is 100 mg to 500 mg, depending on the severity of the condition. This dose may be repeated at intervals of 2, 4 or 6 hours as indicated by the patient's response and clinical condition. While the dose may be reduced for infants and children, it is governed more by the severity of the condition and response of the patient than by age or body weight but should not be less than 25 mg daily.

Patients subjected to severe stress following corticosteroid therapy should be observed closely for signs and symptoms of adrenocortical insufficiency.

Corticoid therapy is an adjunct to, and not a replacement for, conventional therapy.

PREPARATION OF SOLUTIONS

100 mg Plain: For IV or IM injection, prepare solution by aseptically adding **not more than 2 ml** of bacteriostatic water for injection or bacteriostatic sodium chloride injection to the contents of one vial. *For IV infusion,* first prepare solution by adding **not more than 2 ml** of bacteriostatic water for injection to the vial; this solution may then be added to 100 to 1000 ml of the following: 5% dextrose in water (or isotonic saline solution or 5% dextrose in isotonic saline solution if patient is not on sodium restriction).

Further dilution is not necessary for IV or IM injection. For IV infusion, first prepare solution as just described. The **100 mg** solution may then be added to 100 to 1000 ml of 5% dextrose in water (or isotonic saline solution or 5% dextrose in isotonic saline solution if patient is not on sodium restriction). The **250 mg** solution may be added to 250 to 1000 ml, the **500 mg** solution may be added to 500 to 1000 ml and the **1000 mg** solution to 1000 ml of the same diluents. In cases where administration of a small volume of fluid is desirable, 100 mg to 3000 mg of hydrocortisone sodium succinate may be added to 50 ml of the above diluents. The resulting solutions are stable for at least 4 hours and may be administered either directly or by IV piggyback.

When reconstituted as directed, pH's of the solutions range from 7-8 and the tonicities are: 100 mg Act-O-Vial, 0.36 osmolar; 250 mg Act-O-Vial, 500 mg Act-O-Vial, and the 1000 mg Act-O-Vial, 0.57 osmolar. (Isotonic saline = 0.28 osmolar.)

PRODUCT LISTING - RATED THERAPEUTICALLY EQUIVALENT

Powder For Injection - Injectable - 1 Gm

1's	$29.00	SOLU-CORTEF, Pharmacia and Upjohn	00009-0920-03
1's	$30.00	GENERIC, Cmc-Consolidated Midland Corporation	00223-7899-08

Powder For Injection - Injectable - 100 mg

1's	$2.00	SOLU-CORTEF, Allscripts Pharmaceutical Company	54569-1384-00
1's	$2.18	SOLU-CORTEF, Pharmacia and Upjohn	00009-0825-01
1's	$2.29	SOLU-CORTEF, Pharmacia and Upjohn	00009-0900-13
1's	$3.34	SOLU-CORTEF, Pharmacia and Upjohn	00009-0900-15
1's	$3.75	GENERIC, Cmc-Consolidated Midland Corporation	00223-7893-02
2's	$4.08	SOLU-CORTEF, Physicians Total Care	54868-0605-00
10's	$18.18	A-HYDROCORT, Abbott Pharmaceutical	00074-5671-02
25's	$56.00	SOLU-CORTEF, Pharmacia and Upjohn	00009-0900-20

Powder For Injection - Injectable - 250 mg

1's	$3.51	SOLU-CORTEF, Allscripts Pharmaceutical Company	54569-3133-00
1's	$4.03	SOLU-CORTEF, Pharmacia and Upjohn	00009-0909-08
1's	$9.50	GENERIC, Cmc-Consolidated Midland Corporation	00223-7894-02
1's	$189.06	SOLU-CORTEF, Pharmacia and Upjohn	00009-0909-09
10's	$23.28	A-HYDROCORT, Abbott Pharmaceutical	00074-5672-02

H

25's $99.01 SOLU-CORTEF, Pharmacia and Upjohn 00009-0909-16

Powder For Injection - Injectable - 500 mg
1's $8.95 SOLU-CORTEF, Pharmacia and Upjohn 00009-0912-05
25's $174.86 A-HYDROCORT, Abbott Pharmaceutical 00074-5673-04

PRODUCT LISTING - EQUIVALENTS NOT AVAILABLE

Powder For Injection - Injectable - 500 mg
1's $15.00 GENERIC, Cmc-Consolidated Midland Corporation 00223-7898-08

Hydrocortisone Valerate (001486)

Categories: Dermatosis, corticosteroid-responsive; Pregnancy Category C; FDA Approved 1978 Mar
Drug Classes: Corticosteroids, topical; Dermatologics
Brand Names: Westcort
Foreign Brand Availability: Hydcort (Korea)

H

DESCRIPTION

WESTCORT CREAM

Westcort cream contains hydrocortisone valerate, 11,2l-dihydroxy-17-[(loxopentyl)oxy]-(11β)-pregn-4-ene-3,20-dione, a synthetic corticosteroid for topical dermatologic use. The corticosteroids constitute a class of primarily synthetic steroids used topically as anti-inflammatory and antipruritic agents.

Chemically, hydrocortisone valerate is $C_{26}H_{38}O_6$.

Hydrocortisone valerate has a molecular weight of 446.58. It is a white, crystalline solid, soluble in ethanol and methanol, sparingly soluble in propylene glycol and insoluble in water.

Each gram of Wescort cream contains 2 mg hydrocortisone valerate in a hydrophilic base composed of amphoteric-9, carbomer 940, dried sodium phosphate, propylene glycol, sodium lauryl sulfate, sorbic acid, stearyl alcohol, water and white petrolatum.

WESTCORT OINTMENT

For Dermatologic Use Only. Not for Ophthalmic Use.

Westcort ointment contains hydrocortisone valerate, 11,2l-dihydroxy-17-[(loxopentyl)oxy]-(11β)-pregn-4-ene-3,20-dione, a synthetic corticosteroid for topical dermatologic use. The corticosteroids constitute a class of primarily synthetic steroids used topically as anti-inflammatory and antipruritic agents.

Chemically, hydrocortisone valerate is $C_{26}H_{38}O_6$.

Hydrocortisone valerate has a molecular weight of 446.58. It is a white, crystalline solid, soluble in ethanol and methanol, sparingly soluble in propylene glycol and insoluble in water.

Each gram of Westcort ointment contains 2.0 mg hydrocortisone valerate in a hydrophilic base composed of white petrolatum, stearyl alcohol, propylene glycol, sorbic acid, sodium lauryl sulfate, carbomer 934, dried sodium phosphate, mineral oil, steareth-2, steareth-100, and water.

Storage: Store between 15-26°C (59-78°F).

CLINICAL PHARMACOLOGY

HYDROCORTISONE VALERATE CREAM

Like other topical corticosteroids, hydrocortisone valerate has anti-inflammatory, antipruritic and vasoconstrictive properties. The mechanism of the anti-inflammatory activity of the topical steroids, in general, is unclear. However, corticosteroids are thought to act by the induction of phospholipase A^2 inhibitory proteins, collectively called lipocortins. It is postulated that these proteins control the biosynthesis of potent mediators of inflammation such as prostaglandins and leukotrienes by inhibiting the release of their common precursor arachidonic acid. Arachidonic acid is released from membrane phospholipids by phospholipase A^2.

Pharmacokinetics

The extent of percutaneous absorption of topical corticosteroids is determined by many factors including the vehicle and the integrity of the epidermal barrier. Occlusive dressings with hydrocortisone for up to 24 hours have not been demonstrated to increase penetration; however, occlusion of hydrocortisone for 96 hours markedly enhances penetration. Topical corticosteroids can be absorbed from normal intact skin. Inflammation and/or other disease processes in the skin may increase percutaneous absorption.

Studies performed with hydrocortisone valerate cream indicate that it is in the medium range of potency as compared with other topical corticosteroids.

HYDROCORTISONE VALERATE OINTMENT

Like other topical corticosteroids, hydrocortisone valerate has anti-inflammatory, antipruritic and vasoconstrictive properties. The mechanism of the anti-inflammatory activity of the topical steroids, in general, is unclear. However, corticosteroids are thought to act by the induction of phospholipase A_2 inhibitory proteins, collectively called lipocortins. It is postulated that these proteins control the biosynthesis of potent mediators of inflammation such as prostaglandins and leukotrienes by inhibiting the release of their common precursor arachidonic acid. Arachidonic acid is released from membrane phospholipids by phospholipase A_2.

Pharmacokinetics

The extent of percutaneous absorption of topical corticosteroids is determined by many factors including the vehicle and the integrity of the epidermal barrier. Occlusive dressings with hydrocortisone for up to 24 hours have not been demonstrated to increase penetration; however, occlusion of hydrocortisone for 96 hours markedly enhances penetration. Topical corticosteroids can be absorbed from normal intact skin. Inflammation and/or other disease processes in the skin may increase percutaneous absorption.

Studies performed with hydrocortisone valerate ointment indicate that it is in the medium range of potency as compared with other topical corticosteroids.

INDICATIONS AND USAGE

HYDROCORTISONE VALERATE CREAM

Hydrocortisone valerate cream is a medium potency corticosteroid indicated for the relief of the inflammatory and pruritic manifestations of corticosteroid responsive dermatoses in adult patients.

HYDROCORTISONE VALERATE OINTMENT

Hydrocortisone valerate ointment is a medium potency corticosteroid indicated for the relief of the inflammatory and pruritic manifestations of corticosteroid responsive dermatoses in adult patients.

CONTRAINDICATIONS

HYDROCORTISONE VALERATE CREAM AND OINTMENT

Topical corticosteroids are contraindicated in those patients with a history of hypersensitivity to any of the components of the preparation.

PRECAUTIONS

HYDROCORTISONE VALERATE CREAM

General

Systemic absorption of topical corticosteroids can produce reversible hypothalamic-pituitary-adrenal (HPA) axis suppression with the potential for glucocorticosteroid insufficiency after withdrawal of treatment. Manifestations of Cushing's syndrome, hyperglycemia, and glucosuria can also be produced in some patients by systemic absorption of topical corticosteroids while on treatment.

Patients applying a topical steroid to a large surface area or to areas under occlusion should be evaluated periodically for evidence of HPA axis suppression. This may be done by using the ACTH stimulation, AM plasma cortisol, and urinary free cortisol tests.

Hydrocortisone valerate cream has produced mild, reversible adrenal suppression in adult patients when used under occlusion for 5 days, 15 g twice a day over 25-60% body surface area or when used 3 times a day over 20-30% body surface area to treat psoriasis for 3-4 weeks.

If HPA axis suppression is noted, an attempt should be made to withdraw the drug, to reduce the frequency of application, or to substitute a less potent corticosteroid. Recovery of HPA axis function is generally prompt upon discontinuation of topical corticosteroids. Infrequently, signs and symptoms of glucocorticosteroid insufficiency may occur, requiring supplemental systemic corticosteroids. For information on systemic supplementation, see prescribing information for these products.

Pediatric patients may be more susceptible to systemic toxicity from equivalent doses due to their larger skin surface to body mass ratios. (See Hydrocortisone Valerate Cream, Pediatric Use.)

If irritation develops, hydrocortisone valerate cream should be discontinued and appropriate therapy instituted. Allergic contact dermatitis with corticosteroids is usually diagnosed by observing a failure to heal rather than noting a clinical exacerbation, as with most topical products not containing corticosteroids. Such an observation should be corroborated with appropriate diagnostic patch testing.

If concomitant skin infections are present or develop, an appropriate antifungal or antibacterial agent should be used. If a favorable response does not occur promptly, use of hydrocortisone valerate cream should be discontinued until the infection has been adequately controlled.

Information for the Patient

Patients using topical corticosteroids should receive the following information and instructions:

- This medication is to be used as directed by the physician. It is for external use only. Avoid contact with the eyes.
- This medication should not be used for any disorder other than that for which it was prescribed.
- The treated skin area should not be bandaged, otherwise covered or wrapped, so as to be occlusive unless directed by the physician.
- Patients should report to their physician any signs of local adverse reactions.
- Hydrocortisone valerate cream should not be applied in the diaper areas as diapers or plastic pants may constitute occlusive dressings. (See DOSAGE AND ADMINISTRATION, Hydrocortisone Valerate Cream.)
- This medication should not be used on the face, underarms, or groin areas unless directed by the physician.
- As with other corticosteroids, therapy should be discontinued when control is achieved. If no improvement is seen within 2 weeks, contact the physician.

Laboratory Tests

The following tests may be helpful in evaluating the HPA axis suppression:

- ACTH stimulation test
- AM plasma cortisol test
- Urinary free cortisol test

Carcinogenesis, Mutagenesis, and Impairment of Fertility

Long-term animal studies have not been performed to evaluate the carcinogenic potential of hydrocortisone valerate. Hydrocortisone valerate cream was shown to be non-mutagenic in the Ames-*Salmonella*/Microsome Plate Test. There are no studies which assess the effects of hydrocortisone valerate on fertility and general reproductive performance.

Pregnancy, Teratogenic Effects, Pregnancy Category C

Corticosteroids have been shown to be teratogenic in laboratory animals when administered systemically at relatively low dosage levels. Some corticosteroids have been shown to be teratogenic after dermal application in laboratory animals.

Dermal embryofetal developmental studies were conducted in rabbits and rats with hydrocortisone valerate cream, 0.2%. Hydrocortisone valerate cream, 0.2%, was administered topically for 4 h/day, rather than the preferred 24 h/day, during the period of organogenesis in rats (gestational Days 5-16) and rabbits (gestational Days 6-19). Topical doses of hydrocortisone valerate up to 9 mg/kg/day (54 mg/m^2/day) were administered to rats and 5 mg/kg/day (60 mg/m^2/day) were administered to rabbits. In the absence of maternal toxicity, a significant increase in delayed skeletal ossification in fetuses was noted at 9 mg/kg/day [2.5× the Maximum Recommended Human Dose (MRHD) based on body surface area (BSA) comparisons] in the rat study. No malformations in the fetuses were noted at 9 mg/kg/day (2.5× MRHD based on BSA comparisons) in the rat study. Indicators of embryofetal toxicity, significant decrease in fetal weight at 2 mg/kg/day (1× MRHD based on BSA) and a significant increase in post-implantation loss and embryo resorption at 5 mg/kg (3× MRHD based on BSA), were noted in the rabbit study. A significant increase in delayed skeletal ossification in fetuses was noted at 5 mg/kg/day (3× the MRHD based on BSA comparisons) in the rabbit study. Increased numbers of fetal malformations (*e.g.*, cleft palate, omphalocele and clubbed feet) were noted at 5 mg/kg/day (3× MRHD based on BSA comparisons) in the rabbit study.

There are no adequate and well-controlled studies in pregnant women. Hydrocortisone valerate cream should be used during pregnancy only if the potential benefit justifies the potential risk to the fetus.

Nursing Mothers

Systemically administered corticosteroids appear in human milk and could suppress growth, interfere with endogenous corticosteroid production, or cause other untoward effects. It is not known whether topical administration of corticosteroids could result in sufficient systemic absorption to produce detectable quantities in human milk. Because many drugs are excreted in human milk, caution should be exercised when hydrocortisone valerate cream is administered to a nursing woman.

Pediatric Use

Safety of this product in pediatric patients has not been established. There is no data on adrenal suppression and/or growth suppression.

Because of a higher ratio of skin surface area to body mass, pediatric patients are at a greater risk than adults of HPA axis suppression and Cushing's syndrome when they are treated with topical corticosteroids. They are therefore also at a greater risk of adrenal insufficiency during and/or after withdrawal of treatment. Adverse effects including striae have been reported with inappropriate use of topical corticosteroids in infants and children. (See PRECAUTIONS, Hydrocortisone Valerate Cream.)

HPA axis suppression, Cushing's syndrome, linear growth retardation, delayed weight gain, and intracranial hypertension have been reported in children receiving topical corticosteroids. Manifestations of adrenal suppression in children include low plasma cortisol levels, and an absence of response to ACTH stimulation. Manifestations of intracranial hypertension include bulging fontanelles, headaches, and bilateral papilledema.

Geriatric Use

Clinical studies of hydrocortisone valerate cream did not include sufficient numbers of subjects aged 65 and over to determine whether they respond differently from younger subjects. Other reported clinical experience has not identified differences in responses between the elderly and younger patients.

HYDROCORTISONE VALERATE OINTMENT

General

Systemic absorption of topical corticosteroids can produce reversible hypothalamic-pituitary-adrenal (HPA) axis suppression with the potential for glucocorticosteroid insufficiency after withdrawal of treatment. Manifestations of Cushing's syndrome, hyperglycemia, and glucosuria can also be produced in some patients by systemic absorption of topical corticosteroids while on treatment.

Patients applying a topical steroid to a large surface area or to areas under occlusion should be evaluated periodically for evidence of HPA axis suppression. This may be done by using the ACTH stimulation, AM plasma cortisol, and urinary free cortisol tests.

Hydrocortisone valerate ointment has produced mild, reversible adrenal suppression in adult patients when used under occlusion for 5 days, 15 g twice a day over 25-60% body surface area or when used 3 times a day over 20-30% body surface area to treat psoriasis for 3-4 weeks.

If HPA axis suppression is noted, an attempt should be made to withdraw the drug, to reduce the frequency of application, or to substitute a less potent corticosteroid. Recovery of HPA axis function is generally prompt upon discontinuation of topical corticosteroids. Infrequently, signs and symptoms of glucocorticosteroid insufficiency may occur, requiring supplemental systemic corticosteroids. For information on systemic supplementation, see prescribing information for these products.

Pediatric patients may be more susceptible to systemic toxicity from equivalent doses due to their larger skin surface to body mass ratios. (See Hydrocortisone Valerate Ointment, Pediatric Use.)

If irritation develops, hydrocortisone valerate ointment should be discontinued and appropriate therapy instituted. Allergic contact dermatitis with corticosteroids is usually diagnosed by observing a failure to heal rather than noting a clinical exacerbation, as with most topical products not containing corticosteroids. Such an observation should be corroborated with appropriate diagnostic patch testing.

If concomitant skin infections are present or develop, an appropriate antifungal or antibacterial agent should be used. If a favorable response does not occur promptly, use of hydrocortisone valerate ointment should be discontinued until the infection has been adequately controlled.

Information for the Patient

Patients using topical corticosteroids should receive the following information and instructions:

- This medication is to be used as directed by the physician. It is for external use only. Avoid contact with the eyes.
- This medication should not be used for any disorder other than that for which it was prescribed.
- The treated skin area should not be bandaged, otherwise covered or wrapped, so as to be occlusive unless directed by the physician.
- Patients should report to their physician any signs of local adverse reactions.
- Hydrocortisone valerate ointment should not be applied in the diaper areas as diapers or plastic pants may constitute occlusive dressings. (See DOSAGE AND ADMINISTRATION, Hydrocortisone Valerate Ointment.)
- This medication should not be used on the face, underarms, or groin areas unless directed by the physician.
- As with other corticosteroids, therapy should be discontinued when control is achieved. If no improvement is seen within 2 weeks, contact the physician.

Laboratory Tests

The following tests may be helpful in evaluating patients for HPA axis suppression:

- ACTH stimulation test
- AM plasma cortisol test
- Urinary free cortisol test

Carcinogenesis, Mutagenesis, and Impairment of Fertility

Long-term animal studies have not been performed to evaluate the carcinogenic potential of hydrocortisone valerate. Hydrocortisone valerate ointment was shown to be non-mutagenic in the Ames-Salmonella/Microsome Plate Test. There are no studies which assess the effects of hydrocortisone valerate on fertility and general reproductive performance.

H

Pregnancy, Teratogenic Effects, Pregnancy Category C

Corticosteroids have been shown to be teratogenic in laboratory animals when administered systemically at relatively low dosage levels. Some corticosteroids have been shown to be teratogenic after dermal application in laboratory animals.

Dermal embryofetal developmental studies were conducted in rabbits and rats with hydrocortisone valerate cream, 0.2%. Hydrocortisone valerate cream, 0.2%, was administered topically for 4 h/day, rather than the preferred 24 h/day, during the period of organogenesis in rats (gestational Days 5-16) and rabbits (gestational Days 6-19). Topical doses of hydrocortisone valerate up to 9 mg/kg/day (54 mg/m^2/day) were administered to rats and 5 mg/kg/day (60 mg/m^2/day) were administered to rabbits. In the absence of maternal toxicity, a significant increase in delayed skeletal ossification in fetuses was noted at 9 mg/kg/day [2.5× the Maximum Recommended Human Dose (MRHD) based on body surface area (BSA) comparisons] in the rat study. No malformations in the fetuses were noted at 9 mg/kg/day (2.5× MRHD based on BSA comparisons) in the rat study. Indicators of embryofetal toxicity, significant decrease in fetal weight at 2 mg/kg/day (1× MRHD based on BSA) and a significant increase in post-implantation loss and embryo resorption at 5 mg/kg (3× MRHD based on BSA), were noted in the rabbit study. A significant increase in delayed skeletal ossification in fetuses was noted at 5 mg/kg/day (3× the MRHD based on BSA comparisons) in the rabbit study. Increased numbers of fetal malformations (*e.g.*, cleft palate, omphalocele and clubbed feet) were noted at 5 mg/kg/day (3× MRHD based on BSA comparisons) in the rabbit study.

There are no adequate and well-controlled studies in pregnant women. Hydrocortisone valerate ointment should be used during pregnancy only if the potential benefit justifies the potential risk to the fetus.

Nursing Mothers

Systemically administered corticosteroids appear in human milk and could suppress growth, interfere with endogenous corticosteroid production, or cause other untoward effects. It is not known whether topical administration of corticosteroids could result in sufficient systemic absorption to produce detectable quantities in human milk. Because many drugs are excreted in human milk, caution should be exercised when hydrocortisone valerate ointment is administered to a nursing woman.

Pediatric Use

Safety of this product in pediatric patients has not been established. There is no data on adrenal suppression and/or growth suppression.

Because of a higher ratio of skin surface area to body mass, pediatric patients are at a greater risk than adults of HPA axis suppression and Cushing's syndrome when they are treated with topical corticosteroids. They are therefore also at a greater risk of adrenal insufficiency during and/or after withdrawal of treatment. Adverse effects including striae have been reported with inappropriate use of topical corticosteroids in infants and children. (See PRECAUTIONS, Hydrocortisone Valerate Ointment.)

HPA axis suppression, Cushing's syndrome, linear growth retardation, delayed weight gain, and intracranial hypertension have been reported in children receiving topical corticosteroids. Manifestations of adrenal suppression in children include low plasma cortisol levels, and an absence of response to ACTH stimulation. Manifestations of intracranial hypertension include bulging fontanelles, headaches, and bilateral papilledema.

Geriatric Use

Clinical studies of hydrocortisone valerate ointment, 0.2% did not include sufficient numbers of subjects aged 65 and over to determine whether they respond differently from younger subjects. Other reported clinical experience has not identified differences in responses between the elderly and younger patients.

ADVERSE REACTIONS

HYDROCORTISONE VALERATE CREAM

The following local adverse reactions have been reported with topical corticosteroids, and they may occur more frequently with the use of occlusive dressings. These reactions are listed in an approximate decreasing order of occurrence: burning, itching, irritation, dryness, folliculitis, hypertrichosis, acneiform eruptions, hypopigmentation, perioral dermatitis, allergic contact dermatitis, maceration of the skin, secondary infection, skin atrophy, striae, and miliaria.

In controlled clinical studies involving pediatric patients 1 month to 2 years of age (n=29), the incidence of adverse experiences, regardless of relationship to the use of hydrocortisone valerate cream, was approximately 21%. Reported reactions included stinging (10%), eczema (7%), fungal infection (3%), and gastrointestinal disorder (3%).

In controlled clinical studies involving pediatric patients 2-12 years of age (n=153), the sincidence of adverse experiences, regardless of relationship to the use of hydrocortisone valerate cream, was approximately 10%. Reported reactions included stinging (3%), burning skin (2%), infection (body as a whole) (2%). Skin irritation, eczema, pruritus, application site reaction, rash, rash maculopapular, and dry skin were all reported at incidences of approximately 1%.

HYDROCORTISONE VALERATE OINTMENT

In controlled clinical trials, the total incidence of adverse reactions associated with the use of hydrocortisone valerate ointment was approximately 12%. These included worsening of condition (2%), transient itching (2%), irritation (1%) and redness (1%).

In controlled clinical studies involving pediatric atopic dermatitis patients 2-12 years of age (n=64), the incidence of adverse experiences was approximately 28.1%, which is higher than that seen in adult patients. Reported reactions included eczema (12.5%), pruritis (6%), stinging (2%), and dry skin (2%). Patients were not specifically evaluated for signs of atrophy (thinning, telangiectasia, erythema). No studies were performed to assess adrenal suppression and/or growth suppression.

The following additional local adverse reactions have been reported with topical corticosteroids, and they may occur more frequently with the use of occlusive dressings. These reactions are listed in an approximate decreasing order of occurrence: burning, dryness, folliculitis, acneiform eruptions, hypopigmentation, perioral dermatitis, allergic contact dermatitis, secondary infection, skin atrophy, striae, and miliaria.

DOSAGE AND ADMINISTRATION

HYDROCORTISONE VALERATE CREAM

Hydrocortisone valerate cream should be applied to the affected area as a thin film 2 or 3 times daily depending on the severity of the condition.

Occlusive dressings may be used for management of psoriasis or recalcitrant conditions.

As with other corticosteroids, therapy should be discontinued when control is achieved. If no improvement is seen within 2 weeks, reassessment of the diagnosis may be necessary. Hydrocortisone valerate cream should not be used with occlusive dressings unless directed by a physician. Hydrocortisone valerate cream should not be applied in the diaper area if the patient requires diapers or plastic pants as these garments may constitute occlusive dressing.

HYDROCORTISONE VALERATE OINTMENT

Hydrocortisone valerate ointment should be applied to the affected area as a thin film 2 or 3 times daily depending on the severity of the condition. As with other corticosteroids, therapy should be discontinued when control is achieved. If no improvement is seen within 2 weeks, reassessment of the diagnosis may be necessary. Hydrocortisone valerate ointment should not be used with occlusive dressings unless directed by a physician. Hydrocortisone valerate ointment should not be applied in the diaper area if the patient requires diapers or plastic pants as these garments may constitute occlusive dressing.

HOW SUPPLIED

WESTCORT CREAM

Westcort, 0.2%, is supplied in 15, 45 and 60 g tube sizes.

Storage

Store between 20-25°C (68-77°F); excursions permitted between 15 and 30°C.

WESTCORT OINTMENT

Westcort ointment is supplied in 15 and 60 g tubes.

Storage

Store between 15-26°C (59-78°F)

PRODUCT LISTING - RATED THERAPEUTICALLY EQUIVALENT

Cream - Topical - Valerate 0.2%

15 gm	$14.40	GENERIC, Taro Pharmaceuticals U.S.A. Inc	51672-1290-01
15 gm	$15.02	GENERIC, Allscripts Pharmaceutical Company	54569-4814-00
15 gm	$15.25	GENERIC, Bristol-Myers Squibb	59772-8100-07
15 gm	$15.31	WESTCORT, Southwood Pharmaceuticals Inc	58016-3102-01
15 gm	$15.50	GENERIC, Clay-Park Laboratories Inc	45802-0455-35
15 gm	$16.69	WESTCORT, Allscripts Pharmaceutical Company	54569-1098-00
15 gm	$17.53	WESTCORT, Bristol-Myers Squibb	00072-8100-15
15 gm	$20.23	WESTCORT, Physicians Total Care	54868-2229-03
45 gm	$27.25	GENERIC, Teva Pharmaceuticals Usa	38245-0679-72
45 gm	$29.70	GENERIC, Taro Pharmaceuticals U.S.A. Inc	51672-1290-06
45 gm	$31.16	GENERIC, Teva Pharmaceuticals Usa	54569-4815-00
45 gm	$32.15	GENERIC, Clay-Park Laboratories Inc	45802-0455-42
45 gm	$32.15	GENERIC, Bristol-Myers Squibb	59772-8100-04
45 gm	$34.62	WESTCORT, Allscripts Pharmaceutical Company	54569-0791-00
45 gm	$36.35	WESTCORT, Bristol-Myers Squibb	00072-8100-45
45 gm	$41.32	WESTCORT, Physicians Total Care	54868-2229-02
60 gm	$36.00	GENERIC, Taro Pharmaceuticals U.S.A. Inc	51672-1290-03
60 gm	$38.50	GENERIC, Bristol-Myers Squibb	59772-8100-05
60 gm	$38.70	GENERIC, Clay-Park Laboratories Inc	45802-0455-37
60 gm	$43.73	WESTCORT, Bristol-Myers Squibb	00072-8100-60
60 gm	$49.57	WESTCORT, Physicians Total Care	54868-2229-01

Ointment - Topical - Valerate 0.2%

15 gm	$15.25	GENERIC, Bristol-Myers Squibb	59772-7800-02
15 gm	$15.52	GENERIC, Taro Pharmaceuticals U.S.A. Inc	51672-1292-01
15 gm	$17.53	WESTCORT, Westwood Squibb Pharmaceutical Corporation	00072-7800-15
15 gm	$18.96	WESTCORT, Physicians Total Care	54868-2230-00
45 gm	$32.15	GENERIC, Bristol-Myers Squibb	59772-7800-04
45 gm	$32.20	GENERIC, Taro Pharmaceuticals U.S.A. Inc	51672-1292-06
45 gm	$36.35	WESTCORT, Bristol-Myers Squibb	00072-7800-45
60 gm	$38.50	GENERIC, Bristol-Myers Squibb	59772-7800-07
60 gm	$38.73	GENERIC, Taro Pharmaceuticals U.S.A. Inc	51672-1292-03
60 gm	$43.73	WESTCORT, Bristol-Myers Squibb	00072-7800-60

PRODUCT LISTING - EQUIVALENTS NOT AVAILABLE

Ointment - Topical - Valerate 0.2%

15 gm	$15.02	GENERIC, Allscripts Pharmaceutical Company	54569-4906-00

Hydrocortisone; Neomycin Sulfate; Polymyxin B Sulfate *(001490)*

Categories: Burns, ophthalmic; Conjunctivitis, infectious; Dermatitis; Infection, ear, external; Inflammation, ophthalmic; Trauma, ophthalmic; Uveitis; Pregnancy Category C; FDA Approval Pre 1982

Drug Classes: Antibiotics, aminoglycosides; Antibiotics, polymyxins; Anti-infectives, ophthalmic; Anti-infectives, otic; Anti-infectives, topical; Corticosteroids, ophthalmic; Corticosteroids, otic; Corticosteroids, topical; Dermatologics; Ophthalmics; Otics

Brand Names: Aerocortin; Ak-Spore HC; Antibiotic Ear; Aural Acute; Bacticort; Biocot; Biotis; C-Sporin; Cobiron; Cort-Biotic; Cortatrigen; Cortiotic; **Cortisporin**; Cortomycin; Deltabiox; Drotic; Ear-Eze; Equi-C-Sporin; Genasporin H.C.; Hydromycin; I-Neocort; Infa-Otic; Lazersporin-C; Masporin Otic; Mayotic; Medisol-Sp; Neo-Otosol-Hc; Neocin Pb-Hc; Neomycin Polymyxin Hc; Neosporin-H; Octicair; Octigen; Ocusporin Hc; Ocutricin Hc; Ortega-Otic-M; Oti-Sone; Otic-Care; Oticair; Oticin Hc; Oticrex; Otimar; Otisol Hc; Otitricin; Oto K Plus; Otobione; Otocidin; Otocort; Otomycin-Hpn; Otosporin; Pediotic; Phn-Otic; Pocin-H; Poly Otic; Qrp Ear Suspension; Spectro-Sporin; Storz H-P-N; Tex Sporin-Hc; Tri-Otic; Triple-Gen; Uad Otic; Visporin

Foreign Brand Availability: Cortisporin Ear (Philippines); Isonep H (Philippines)

TOPICAL

DESCRIPTION

Cortisporin cream (neomycin and polymyxin B sulfates and hydrocortisone acetate cream) is a topical antibacterial cream. *Each gram contains:* Neomycin sulfate equivalent to 3.5 mg neomycin base, polymyxin B sulfate equivalent to 10,000 polymyxin B units, and hydrocortisone acetate 5 mg (0.5%). The inactive ingredients are liquid petrolatum, white petrolatum, propylene glycol, polyoxyethylene polyoxypropylene compound, emulsifying wax, purified water, and 0.25% methylparaben added as a preservative. Sodium hydroxide or sulfuric acid may be added to adjust pH.

Neomycin sulfate is the sulfate salt of neomycin B and C, which are produced by the growth of *Streptomyces fradiae* Waksman (Fam. Streptomycetaceae). It has a potency equivalent of not less than 600 µg of neomycin standard per mg, calculated on an anhydrous basis.

Polymyxin B sulfate is the sulfate salt of polymyxin B_1 and B_2, which are produced by the growth of *Bacillus polymyxa* (Prazmowski) Migula (Fam. Bacillaceae). It has a potency of not less than 6000 polymyxin B units per mg, calculated on an anhydrous basis.

Hydrocortisone acetate is the acetate ester of hydrocortisone, an anti-inflammatory hormone. Its chemical name is 21-(acetyloxy)-11β,17-dihydroxypregn-4-ene-3,20-dione.

The base is a smooth vanishing cream with a pH of approximately 5.0.

CLINICAL PHARMACOLOGY

Corticoids suppress the inflammatory response to a variety of agents and they may delay healing. Since corticoids may inhibit the body's defense mechanism against infection, a concomitant antimicrobial drug may be used when this inhibition is considered to be clinically significant in a particular case. The anti-infective components in the combination are included to provide action against specific organisms susceptible to them. Polymyxin B sulfate and neomycin sulfate together are considered active against the following microorganisms: *Staphylococcus aureus, Escherichia coli, Haemophilus influenzae, Klebsiella-Enterobacter* species, *Neisseria species,* and *Pseudomonas aeruginosa.* The product does not provide adequate coverage against *Serratia marcescens* and streptococci, including *Streptococcus pneumoniae.*

The relative potency of corticosteroids depends on the molecular structure, concentration, and release from the vehicle.

The acid pH helps restore normal cutaneous acidity. Owing to its excellent spreading and penetrating properties, the cream facilitates treatment of hairy and intertriginous areas. It may also be of value in selective cases where the lesions are moist.

INDICATIONS AND USAGE

For the treatment of corticosteroid-responsive dermatoses with secondary infection. It has not been demonstrated that this steroid-antibiotic combination provides greater benefit than the steroid component alone after 7 days of treatment (see WARNINGS).

CONTRAINDICATIONS

Not for use in the eyes or in the external ear canal if the eardrum is perforated. This product is contraindicated in tuberculous, fungal, or viral lesions of the skin (herpes simplex, vaccinia, and varicella). This product is contraindicated in those individuals who have shown hypersensitivity to any of its components.

WARNINGS

Because of the concern of nephrotoxicity and ototoxicity associated with neomycin, this combination should not be used over a wide area or for extended periods of time.

PRECAUTIONS

GENERAL

As with any antibacterial preparation, prolonged use may result in overgrowth of nonsusceptible organisms, including fungi. Appropriate measures should be taken if this occurs. Use of steroids on infected areas should be supervised with care as anti-inflammatory steroids may encourage spread of infection. If this occurs, steroid therapy should be stopped and appropriate antibacterial drugs used. Generalized dermatological conditions may require systemic corticosteroid therapy.

Signs and symptoms of exogenous hyperadrenocorticism can occur with the use of topical corticosteroids, including adrenal suppression. Systemic absorption of topically applied steroids will be increased if extensive body surface areas are treated or if occlusive dressings are used. Under these circumstances, suitable precautions should be taken when long-term use is anticipated.

Specifically, sufficient percutaneous absorption of hydrocortisone can occur in pediatric patients during prolonged use to cause cessation of growth, as well as other systemic signs and symptoms of hyperadrenocorticism.

INFORMATION FOR THE PATIENT

If redness, irritation, swelling or pain persists or increases, discontinue use and notify physician. Do not use in the eyes.

LABORATORY TESTS

Systemic effects of excessive levels of hydrocortisone may include a reduction in the number of circulating eosinophils and a decrease in urinary excretion of 17-hydroxycorticosteroids.

CARCINOGENESIS, MUTAGENESIS, AND IMPAIRMENT OF FERTILITY

Long-term studies in animals (rats, rabbits, mice) showed no evidence of carcinogenicity attributable to oral administration of corticosteroids.

PREGNANCY, TERATOGENIC EFFECTS, PREGNANCY CATEGORY C

Corticosteroids have been shown to be teratogenic in rabbits when applied topically at concentrations of 0.5% on days 6-18 of gestation and in mice when applied topically at a concentration of 15% on days 10-13 of gestation. There are no adequate and well-controlled studies in pregnant women. Corticosteroids should be used during pregnancy only if the potential benefit justifies the potential risk to the fetus.

NURSING MOTHERS

Hydrocortisone acetate appears in human milk following oral administration of the drug. Since systemic absorption of hydrocortisone may occur when applied topically, caution should be exercised when hydrocortisone; neomycin sulfate; polymyxin B sulfate cream is used by a nursing woman.

PEDIATRIC USE

Safety and effectiveness in pediatric patients have not been established (see General).

ADVERSE REACTIONS

Neomycin occasionally causes skin sensitization. Ototoxicity and nephrotoxicity have also been reported (see WARNINGS). Adverse reactions have occurred with topical use of antibiotic combinations including neomycin and polymyxin B. Exact incidence figures are not available since no denominator of treated patients is available. The reaction occurring most often is allergic sensitization. In one clinical study, using a 20% neomycin patch, neomycin-induced allergic skin reactions occurred in 2 of 2175 (0.09%) individuals in the general population.[1] In another study, the incidence was found to be approximately 1%.[2]

The following local adverse reactions have been reported with topical corticosteroids, especially under occlusive dressings: Burning, itching, irritation, dryness, folliculitis, hypertrichosis, acneiform eruptions, hypopigmentation, perioral dermatitis, allergic contact dermatitis, maceration of the skin, secondary infection, skin atrophy, striae, and miliaria. When steroid preparations are used for long periods of time in intertriginous areas or over extensive body areas, with or without occlusive non-permeable dressings, striae may occur; also there exists the possibility of systemic side effects when steroid preparations are used over large areas or for a long period of time.

DOSAGE AND ADMINISTRATION

A small quantity of the cream should be applied 2-4 times daily, as required. The cream should, if conditions permit, be gently rubbed into the affected areas.

HOW SUPPLIED

Cortisporin cream is supplied in a tube of 7.5 g.
Storage: Store at 15-25°C (59-77°F).

OPHTHALMIC

DESCRIPTION

Cortisporin ophthalmic suspension (neomycin and polymyxin B sulfates and hydrocortisone ophthalmic suspension) is a sterile antimicrobial and anti-inflammatory suspension for ophthalmic use. *Each ml contains:* Neomycin sulfate equivalent to 3.5 mg neomycin base, polymyxin B sulfate equivalent to 10,000 polymyxin B units, and hydrocortisone 10 mg (1%). The vehicle contains thimerosal 0.001% (added as a preservative) and the inactive ingredients cetyl alcohol, glyceryl monostearate, mineral oil, polyoxyl 40 stearate, propylene glycol, and water for injection. Sulfuric acid may be added to adjust pH.

Neomycin sulfate is the sulfate salt of neomycin B and C, which are produced by the growth of *Streptomyces fradiae* Waksman (Fam. Streptomycetaceae). It has a potency equivalent of not less than 600 μg of neomycin standard per mg, calculated on an anhydrous basis.

Polymyxin B sulfate is the sulfate salt of polymyxin B_1 and B_2, which are produced by the growth of *Bacillus polymyxa* (Prazmowski) Migula (Fam. Bacillaceae). It has a potency of not less than 6000 polymyxin B units per mg, calculated on an anhydrous basis.

Hydrocortisone, 11β,17,21-trihydroxypregn-4-ene-3,20-dione, is an anti-inflammatory hormone.

CLINICAL PHARMACOLOGY

Corticosteroids suppress the inflammatory response to a variety of agents, and they probably delay or slow healing. Since corticosteroids may inhibit the body's defense mechanism against infection, concomitant antimicrobial drugs may be used when this inhibition is considered to be clinically significant in a particular case.

When a decision to administer both a corticosteroid and antimicrobials is made, the administration of such drugs in combination has the advantage of greater patient compliance and convenience, with the added assurance that the appropriate dosage of all drugs is administered. When each type of drug is in the same formulation, compatibility of ingredients is assured and the correct volume of drug is delivered and retained.

The relative potency of corticosteroids depends on the molecular structure, concentration, and release from the vehicle.

MICROBIOLOGY

The anti-infective components in hydrocortisone; neomycin sulfate; polymyxin B sulfate ophthalmic suspension are included to provide action against specific organisms susceptible to it. Neomycin sulfate and polymyxin B sulfate are active *in vitro* against susceptible strains of the following microorganisms: *Staphylococcus aureus, Escherichia coli, Haemophilus influenzae, Klebsiella/Enterobacter* species, *Neisseria* species, and *Pseudomonas aeruginosa.* The product does not provide adequate coverage against *Serratia marcescens* and streptococci, including *Streptococcus pneumoniae* (see INDICATIONS AND USAGE).

INDICATIONS AND USAGE

Hydrocortisone; neomycin sulfate; polymyxin B sulfate ophthalmic suspension is indicated for steroid-responsive inflammatory ocular conditions for which a corticosteroid is indicated and where bacterial infection or a risk of bacterial infection exists.

Ocular corticosteroids are indicated in inflammatory conditions of the palpebral and bulbar conjunctiva, cornea, and anterior segment of the globe where the inherent risk of corticosteroid use in certain infective conjunctivitides is accepted to obtain a diminution in edema and inflammation. They are also indicated in chronic anterior uveitis and corneal injury from chemical, radiation, or thermal burns, or penetration of foreign bodies.

The use of a combination drug with an anti-infective component is indicated where the risk of infection is high or where there is an expectation that potentially dangerous numbers of bacteria will be present in the eye (see CLINICAL PHARMACOLOGY, Microbiology).

The particular anti-infective drugs in this product are active against the following common bacterial eye pathogens: *Staphylococcus aureus, Escherichia coli, Haemophilus influenzae, Klebsiella/Enterobacter* species, *Neisseria* species, and *Pseudomonas aeruginosa.*

The product does not provide adequate coverage against *Serratia marcescens* and streptococci, including *Streptococcus pneumoniae.*

CONTRAINDICATIONS

Hydrocortisone; neomycin sulfate; polymyxin B sulfate ophthalmic suspension is contraindicated in most viral diseases of the cornea and conjunctiva including: epithelial herpes simplex keratitis (dendritic keratitis), vaccinia and varicella, and also in mycobacterial infection of the eye and fungal diseases of ocular structures.

Hydrocortisone; neomycin sulfate; polymyxin B sulfate ophthalmic suspension is also contraindicated in individuals who have shown hypersensitivity to any of its components. Hypersensitivity to the antibiotic component occurs at a higher rate than for other components.

WARNINGS

NOT FOR INJECTION INTO THE EYE. Hydrocortisone; neomycin sulfate; polymyxin B sulfate ophthalmic suspension should never be directly introduced into the anterior chamber of the eye.

Prolonged use of corticosteroids may result in ocular hypertension and/or glaucoma, with damage to the optic nerve, defects in visual acuity and fields of vision, and in posterior subcapsular cataract formation. Prolonged use may suppress the host response and thus increase the hazard of secondary ocular infections. In those diseases causing thinning of the cornea or sclera, perforations have been known to occur with the use of topical corticosteroids. In acute purulent conditions of the eye, corticosteroids may mask infection or enhance existing infection.

If these products are used for 10 days or longer, intraocular pressure should be routinely monitored even though it may be difficult in uncooperative patients. Corticosteroids should be used with caution in the presence of glaucoma. The use of corticosteroids after cataract surgery may delay healing and increase the incidence of filtering blebs. Use of ocular corticosteroids may prolong the course and may exacerbate the severity of many viral infections of the eye (including herpes simplex). Employment of corticosteroid medication in the treatment of herpes simplex requires great caution.

Topical antibiotics, particularly, neomycin sulfate, may cause cutaneous sensitization. A precise incidence of hypersensitivity reactions (primarily skin rash) due to topical antibiotics is not known. The manifestations of sensitization to topical antibiotics are usually itching, reddening, and edema of the conjunctiva and eyelid. A sensitization reaction may manifest simply as a failure to heal. During long-term use of topical antibiotic products, periodic examination for such signs is advisable, and the patient should be told to discontinue the product if they are observed. Symptoms usually subside quickly on withdrawing the medication. Application of products containing these ingredients should be avoided for the patient thereafter (see PRECAUTIONS, General).

PRECAUTIONS

GENERAL

The initial prescription and renewal of the medication order beyond 20 ml should be made by a physician only after examination of the patient with the aid of magnification, such as slit lamp biomicroscopy and, where appropriate, fluorescein staining. If signs and symptoms fail to improve after 2 days, the patient should be re-evaluated.

The possibility of fungal infections of the cornea should be considered after prolonged corticosteroid dosing. Fungal cultures should be taken when appropriate.

If this product is used for 10 days or longer, intraocular pressure should be monitored (see WARNINGS). There have been reports of bacterial keratitis associated with the use of topical ophthalmic products in multiple-dose containers which have been inadvertently contaminated by patients, most of whom had a concurrent corneal disease or a disruption of the ocular epithelial surface (see Information for the Patient).

Allergic cross-reactions may occur which could prevent the use of any or all of the following antibiotics for the treatment of future infections: kanamycin, paromomycin, streptomycin, and possibly gentamicin.

INFORMATION FOR THE PATIENT

Patients should be instructed to avoid allowing the tip of the dispensing container to contact the eye, eyelid, fingers, or any other surface. The use of this product by more than one person may spread infection.

Patients should also be instructed that ocular products, if handled improperly, can become contaminated by common bacteria known to cause ocular infections. Serious damage to the eye and subsequent loss of vision may result from using contaminated products (see General).

H

If the condition persists or gets worse, or if a rash or allergic reaction develops, the patient should be advised to stop use and consult a physician. Do not use this product if you are allergic to any of the listed ingredients. Keep tightly closed when not in use. Keep out of reach of children.

CARCINOGENESIS, MUTAGENESIS, AND IMPAIRMENT OF FERTILITY

Long-term studies in animals to evaluate carcinogenic or mutagenic potential have not been conducted with polymyxin B sulfate. Treatment of cultured human lymphocytes *in vitro* with neomycin increased the frequency of chromosome aberrations at the highest concentrations (80 μg/ml) tested; however, the effects of neomycin on carcinogenesis and mutagenesis in humans are unknown.

Long-term studies in animals (rats, rabbits, mice) showed no evidence of carcinogenicity or mutagenicity attributable to oral administration of corticosteroids. Long-term animal studies have not been performed to evaluate the carcinogenic potential of topical corticosteroids. Studies to determine mutagenicity with hydrocortisone have revealed negative results.

Polymyxin B has been reported to impair the motility of equine sperm, but its effects on male or female fertility are unknown. Long-term animal studies have not been performed to evaluate the effect on fertility of topical corticosteroids.

PREGNANCY, TERATOGENIC EFFECTS, PREGNANCY CATEGORY C

Corticosteroids have been found to be teratogenic in rabbits when applied topically at concentrations of 0.5% on days 6-18 of gestation and in mice when applied topically at a concentration of 15% on days 10-13 of gestation. There are no adequate and well-controlled studies in pregnant women. Hydrocortisone; neomycin sulfate; polymyxin B sulfate ophthalmic suspension should be used during pregnancy only if the potential benefit justifies the potential risk to the fetus.

NURSING MOTHERS

It is not known whether topical administration of corticosteroids could result in sufficient systemic absorption to produce detectable quantities in human milk. Systemically administered corticosteroids appear in human milk and could suppress growth, interfere with endogenous corticosteroid production, or cause other untoward effects. Because of the potential for serious adverse reactions in nursing infants from hydrocortisone; neomycin sulfate; polymyxin B sulfate ophthalmic suspension, a decision should be made whether to discontinue nursing or to discontinue the drug, taking into account the importance of the drug to the mother.

PEDIATRIC USE

Safety and effectiveness in pediatric patients have not been established.

ADVERSE REACTIONS

Adverse reactions have occurred with corticosteroid/anti-infective combination drugs which can be attributed to the corticosteroid component, the anti-infective component, or the combination. The exact incidence is not known. Reactions occurring most often from the presence of the anti-infective ingredient are allergic sensitization reactions including itching, swelling, and conjunctival erythema (see WARNINGS). More serious hypersensitivity reactions, including anaphylaxis, have been reported rarely.

The reactions due to the corticosteroid component in decreasing order of frequency are: Elevation of intraocular pressure (IOP) with possible development of glaucoma, and infrequent optic nerve damage; posterior subcapsular cataract formation; and delayed wound healing.

Secondary Infection: The development of secondary infection has occurred after use of combinations containing corticosteroids and antimicrobials. Fungal and viral infections of the cornea are particularly prone to develop coincidentally with long-term applications of a corticosteroid. The possibility of fungal invasion must be considered in any persistent corneal ulceration where corticosteroid treatment has been used.

Local irritation on instillation has also been reported.

DOSAGE AND ADMINISTRATION

One (1) or 2 drops in the affected eye every 3 or 4 hours, depending on the severity of the condition. The suspension may be used more frequently if necessary.

Not more than 20 ml should be prescribed initially and the prescription should not be refilled without further evaluation as outlined in PRECAUTIONS.

SHAKE WELL BEFORE USING.

HOW SUPPLIED

Cortisporin ophthalmic suspension is supplied in plastic Drop Dose dispenser bottle of 7.5 ml.

Storage: Store at 15-25°C (59-77°F).

OTIC

DESCRIPTION

Hydrocortisone; neomycin sulfate; polymyxin B sulfate otic solution and suspensions are sterile antibacterial and anti-inflammatory solutions for otic use.

Neomycin sulfate is the sulfate salt of neomycin B and C, which are produced by the growth of *Streptomyces fradiae* Waksman (Fam. Streptomycetaceae). It has a potency equivalent of not less than 600 μg of neomycin standard per mg, calculated on an anhydrous basis.

Polymyxin B sulfate is the sulfate salt of polymyxin B_1 and B_2, which are produced by the growth of *Bacillus polymyxa* (Prazmowski) Migula (Fam. Bacillaceae). It has a potency of not less than 6000 polymyxin B units per mg, calculated on an anhydrous basis.

Hydrocortisone, 11β,17,21-trihydroxypregn-4-ene-3, 20-dione, is an anti-inflammatory hormone.

CORTISPORIN OTIC SOLUTION

Each ml contains: Neomycin sulfate equivalent to 3.5 mg neomycin base, polymyxin B sulfate equivalent to 10,000 polymyxin B units, and hydrocortisone 10 mg (1%). The vehicle contains potassium metabisulfite 0.1% (added as a preservative) and the inactive ingredients cupric sulfate, glycerin, hydrochloric acid, propylene glycol, and water for injection.

CORTISPORIN OTIC SUSPENSION

Each ml contains: Neomycin sulfate equivalent to 3.5 mg neomycin base, polymyxin B sulfate equivalent to 10,000 polymyxin B units, and hydrocortisone 10 mg (1%). The vehicle contains thimerosal 0.01% (added as a preservative) and the inactive ingredients cetyl alcohol, propylene glycol, polysorbate 80, and water for injection. Sulfuric acid may be added to adjust pH.

PEDIOTIC SUSPENSION

Each ml contains: Neomycin sulfate equivalent to 3.5 mg neomycin base, polymyxin B sulfate equivalent to 10,000 polymyxin B units, and hydrocortisone 10 mg (1%). The vehicle contains thimerosal 0.001% (added as a preservative) and the inactive ingredients cetyl alcohol, glyceryl monostearate, mineral oil, polyoxyl 40 stearate, propylene glycol, and water for injection. Sulfuric acid may be added to adjust pH. Pediotic suspension has a minimum pH of 4.1, which is less acidic than the minimum pH of 3.0 for Cortisporin otic suspension.

CLINICAL PHARMACOLOGY

Corticoids suppress the inflammatory response to a variety of agents and they may delay healing. Since corticoids may inhibit the body's defense mechanism against infection, a concomitant antimicrobial drug may be used when this inhibition is considered to be clinically significant in a particular case.

The anti-infective components in the combination are included to provide action against specific organisms susceptible to them. Neomycin sulfate and polymyxin B sulfate together are considered active against the following microorganisms: *Staphylococcus aureus, Escherichia coli, Haemophilus influenzae, Klebsiella-Enterobacter* species, *Neisseria* species, and *Pseudomonas aeruginosa.* This product does not provide adequate coverage against *Serratia marcescens* and streptococci, including *Streptococcus pneumoniae.*

The relative potency of corticosteroids depends on the molecular structure, concentration, and release from the vehicle.

INDICATIONS AND USAGE

SOLUTION

For the treatment of superficial bacterial infections of the external auditory canal caused by organisms susceptible to the action of the antibiotics.

SUSPENSIONS

For the treatment of superficial bacterial infections of the external auditory canal caused by organisms susceptible to the action of the antibiotics, and for the treatment of infections of mastoidectomy and fenestration cavities caused by organisms susceptible to the antibiotics.

CONTRAINDICATIONS

SOLUTION

This product is contraindicated in those individuals who have shown hypersensitivity to any of its components.

This product should not be used if the external auditory canal disorder is suspected or known to be due to cutaneous viral infection (for example, herpes simplex virus or varicella zoster virus).

SUSPENSIONS

This product is contraindicated in those individuals who have shown hypersensitivity to any of its components, and in herpes simplex, vaccinia, and varicella infections.

WARNINGS

SOLUTION

Neomycin can induce permanent sensorineural hearing loss due to cochlear damage, mainly destruction of hair cells in the organ of Corti. The risk of ototoxicity is greater with pro-

pending on tolerance and dose. Dose should be adjusted so that 3-4 hours of path relief may be achieved.

TABLETS AND ORAL SOLUTION

The dosage of opioid analgesics like hydromorphone should be individualized for any given patient, since adverse events can occur at doses that may not provide complete freedom from pain.

Pharmacokinetics

In a single-dose crossover study in 27 normal subjects the pharmacokinetics of hydromorphone HCl tablets was compared was compared to that of 8 ml of hydromorphone HCl oral liquid (1 mg/ml). Plasma hydromorphone concentration was determined using a sensitive and specific assay. The pharmacokinetic parameters from this study are outlined below.

TABLE 1

Parameter Mean & (CV)	8 mg Tablet	8 ml Oral Liquid (1 mg/ml)
C_{max} (ng/ml)	5.5 (33%)	5.7 (31%)
T_{max} (h)	0.74 (34%)	0.73 (71%)
AUC_O (ng·h/ml)	23.7 (28%)	24.6 (29%)
T½ (h)	2.6 (18%)	2.8 (20%)

Dose proportionally between the 8 mg hydromorphone HCl tablets and other strengths of hydromorphone HCl tablets has not been established.

In normal human volunteers hydromorphone is metabolized primarily in the liver. It is excreted in the urine primarily as the glucuronidated conjugate, with small amounts of parent drug and minor amounts of 6-hydroxy reduction metabolites. The effects of renal disease on the clearance of hydromorphone are unknown, but caution should be taken to guard against unanticipated accumulation if renal and/or hepatic functions are seriously impaired. Hydromorphone has been shown to cross placental membranes.

INDICATIONS AND USAGE

INJECTION

Hydromorphone HCl high potency is indicated for the relief of moderate-to-severe pain in narcotic-tolerant patients who require larger than usual doses of narcotics to provide adequate pain relief. Because hydromorphone HCl high potency contains 10 mg of hydromorphone per ml, a smaller injection volume can be used than with other parenteral narcotic formulations. Discomfort associated with the intramuscular or subcutaneous injection of an unusually large volume of solution can therefore be avoided.

TABLETS AND ORAL SOLUTION

Hydromorphone HCl oral liquid and tablets are indicated for the management of pain in patients where an opioid analgesic is appropriate.

NON-FDA APPROVED INDICATIONS

Hydromorphone has been used as an adjunct in general anesthesia, although this use is not approved by the FDA.

CONTRAINDICATIONS

Hydromorphone HCl is contraindicated in patients with known hypersensitivity to the drug, patients with respiratory depression in the absence of resuscitative equipment, and in patients with status asthmaticus. Hydromorphone HCl is also contraindicated for use in obstetrical analgesia.

INJECTION

Hydromorphone HCl high potency is also contraindicated in patients who are not already receiving large amounts of parenteral narcotics.

WARNINGS

DRUG DEPENDENCE

Hydromorphone HCl high potency, hydromorphone HCl tablets, and hydromorphone HCl oral solution can produce drug dependence of the morphine type and therefore has the potential for being abused. Psychic dependence, physical dependence and tolerance may develop upon repeated administration of hydromorphone HCl high potency, and it should be prescribed and administered with the same degree of caution appropriate for the use of morphine. Since hydromorphone HCl high potency is indicated for use in patients who are already tolerant to and hence physically dependent on narcotics, abrupt discontinuance in the administration of hydromorphone HCl high potency is likely to result in a withdrawal syndrome.

IMPAIRED RESPIRATION

Respiratory depressing is the chief hazard of hydromorphone HCl. Respiratory depression occurs most frequently in the elderly, in the debilitated, and in those suffering from conditions accompanied by hypoxia or hypercapnia when even moderate therapeutic doses may dangerously decrease pulmonary ventilation.

Hydromorphone HCl high potency, hydromorphone HCl tablets, and hydromorphone HCl oral solution should be used with extreme caution in patients with chronic obstructive pulmonary disease or cor pulmonale, patient having a substantially decreased respiratory reserve, hypoxia, hypercapnia, or preexisting respiratory depression. In such patients even usual therapeutic doses of narcotic analgesics may decrease respiratory drive while simultaneously increasing airway resistance to the point of apnea.

ADDITIONAL INFORMATION FOR INJECTION

Infants born to mothers physically dependent on hydromorphone HCl high potency will also be physically dependent and may exhibit respiratory difficulties and withdrawal symptoms.

Head Injury and Increased Intracranial Pressure

The respiratory depressant effect of hydromorphone HCl with carbon dioxide retention and secondary elevation of cerebrospinal fluid pressure may be markedly exaggerated in the presence of head injury, other intracranial lesions, or preexisting increase in intracranial pressure. Narcotic analgesics including hydromorphone HCl may produce effects which can obscure the clinical course and neurologic signs of further increasing pressure in patients with head injuries.

Hypotensive Effect

Narcotic analgesics, including hydromorphone HCl high potency, may cause severe hypotension in an individual whose ability to maintain his blood pressure has already been compromised by a depleted blood volume, or a concurrent administration of drugs such as phenothiazines or general anesthetics (see also DRUG INTERACTIONS). Hydromorphone HCl high potency may produce orthostatic hypotension in ambulatory patients.

Hydromorphone HCl high potency should be administered with caution to patients in circulatory shock, since vasodilation produced by the drug may further reduce cardiac output and blood pressure.

ADDITIONAL INFORMATION FOR TABLETS AND ORAL SOLUTION

Sulfites

Contains sodium bisulfite, a sulfite that may cause allergic-type reactions including anaphylactic symptoms and life-threatening or less severe asthmatic episodes in certain susceptible people. The overall prevalence of sulfite sensitivity in the general population is unknown and probably low. Sulfite sensitivity is seen more frequently in asthmatic than in non-asthmatic people.

H

PRECAUTIONS

In general, narcotics should be given with caution and the initial dose should be reduced in the elderly or debilitated and those with severe impairment of hepatic, pulmonary or renal function; myxedema or hypothyroidism; adrenocortical insufficiency (*e.g.,* Addison's disease); CNS depression or coma; toxic psychoses; prostatic hypertrophy or urethral stricture; gall bladder disease; acute alcoholism; delirium tremens; or kyphoscoliosis.

The administration of narcotic analgesics including hydromorphone HCl may obscure the diagnosis or clinical course in patients with acute abdominal conditions and may aggravate preexisting convulsions in patients with convulsive disorders.

Narcotic analgesics including hydromorphone HCl should also be used with caution in patients about to undergo surgery of the biliary tract since it may cause spasm of the sphincter of Oddi.

LABOR AND DELIVERY

Hydromorphone HCl high potency, hydromorphone HCl tablets, and hydromorphone HCl oral solution are contraindicated in Labor and Delivery (see CONTRAINDICATIONS).

NURSING MOTHERS

Low levels of narcotic analgesics have been detected in human milk. As a general rule, nursing should not be undertaken while a patient is receiving hydromorphone HCl since they, and other drugs in this class, may be excreted in the milk.

PEDIATRIC USE

Safety and effectiveness in children have not been established.

ADDITIONAL INFORMATION FOR INJECTION

General

Because of its high concentration, the delivery of precise doses of hydromorphone HCl high potency may be difficult if low doses of hydromorphone are required. Therefore, hydromorphone HCl high potency should be used only if the amount of hydromorphone required can be delivered accurately with this formulation.

In the case of hydromorphone HCl high potency, however, the patient is presumed to be receiving a narcotic to which he or she exhibits tolerance and that initial dose of hydromorphone HCl high potency selected should be estimated based on the relative potency of hydromorphone and the narcotic previously used by the patient. See DOSAGE AND ADMINISTRATION.

Pregnancy Category C

Human

Adequate animal studies on reproduction have not been performed to determine whether hydromorphone affects fertility in males or females. There are no well-controlled studies in women. Reports based on marketing experience do not identity any specific teratogenic risks following routine (short-term) clinical use. Although there is no clearly defined risk, such reports do not exclude the possibility of infrequent of subtle damage to the human fetus. Hydromorphone HCl high potency should be used in pregnant women only when clearly needed (see Labor and Delivery).

Animal

Literature reports of hydromorphone HCl administration to pregnant Syrian hamsters show that hydromorphone HCl is teratogenic at a dose of 20 mg/kg which is 600 times the human dose. A maximal teratogenic effect (50% of fetuses affected) in the Syrian hamster was observed at a dose of 125 mg/kg.

TABLETS AND ORAL SOLUTION

Head Injury and Increased Intracranial Pressure

The respiratory depressant effects of hydromorphone HCl oral liquid and tablets with carbon dioxide retention and secondary elevation of cerebrospinal fluid pressure may be markedly exaggerated in the presence of head injury, other intracranial lesions, or preexisting increase in intracranial pressure. Opioid analgesics including hydromorphone HCl oral liquid and hydromorphone HCl tablets may produce effects which can obscure the clinical course and neurologic signs of further increase in intracranial pressure in patients with head injuries.

Hypotensive Effect

Opioid analgesics, including hydromorphone HCl oral liquid and tablets, may cause severe hypotension in an individual whose ability to maintain blood pressure has already been compromised by a depleted blood volume, or a concurrent administration of drugs such as phenothiazines or general anesthetics (see DRUG INTERACTIONS). Therefore, hydromorphone HCl oral liquid and tablets should be administered with caution to patients in circulatory shock, since vasodilation produced by the drug may further reduce cardiac output and blood pressure.

Use in Ambulatory Patients

Hydromorphone HCl oral liquid and tablets may impair mental and/or physical ability required for the performance of potentially hazardous tasks (*e.g.*, driving, operating machinery). Patients should be cautioned accordingly. Hydromorphone HCl may produce orthostatic hypotension in ambulatory patients. The addition of other CNS depressants to hydromorphone HCl therapy may produce additive depressant effects, and hydromorphone HCl should not be taken with alcohol.

Use in Drug and Alcohol Dependent Patients

Hydromorphone HCl should be used with caution in patients with alcoholism and other drug dependencies due to the increased frequency of narcotic tolerance, dependence, and risk of addiction observed in these patient populations. Abuse of hydromorphone HCl in combination with other CNS depressant drugs can result in serious risk to the patient.

Carcinogenesis, Mutagenesis, and Impairment of Fertility

Studies in animals to evaluate the drug's carcinogenic and mutagenic potential or the effect on fertility have not been conducted.

Pregnancy Category C

Literature reports of hydromorphone HCl administration to pregnant Syrian hamsters show that hydromorphone HCl is teratogenic at a dose of 20 mg/kg which is 600 times the human dose. A maximal teratogenic effect (50% of fetuses affected) in the Syrian hamster was observed at a dose of 125 mg/kg (738 mg/m2). There are no well-controlled studies in women. Hydromorphone is known to cross placental membranes. Hydromorphone HCl oral liquid and tablets should be used in pregnant women only if the potential benefit justifies the potential risk to the fetus (see Labor and Delivery).

Geriatric Use

Hydromorphone HCl has not been studied in geriatric patients. Elderly subjects have been shown to have at least twice the sensitivity (as measured by EEG changes) of young adults for some opioids. When administering hydromorphone HCl to the elderly, the initial dose should be reduced (see PRECAUTIONS).

DRUG INTERACTIONS

The concomitant use of other central nervous system depressants including sedatives or hypnotics, general anesthetics, phenothiazines, tranquilizers and alcohol may produce additive depressant effects. Respiratory depression, hypotension and profound sedation or coma may occur. When such combined therapy is contemplated, the dose of one or both agents should be reduced. Narcotic analgesics, including hydromorphone HCl high potency, hydromorphone HCl tablets, and hydromorphone HCl oral liquid may enhance the action of neuromuscular blocking agents and produce an increased degree of respiratory depression.

ADVERSE REACTIONS

INJECTION, TABLETS, AND ORAL SOLUTION

The adverse effects of hydromorphone HCl high potency, hydromorphone HCl tablets and hydromorphone HCl oral liquid are similar to those of other narcotic analgesics, and represent established pharmacological effects of the drug class. The major hazards include respiratory depression and apnea. To a lesser degree, circulatory depression, respiratory arrest, shock and cardiac arrest have occurred.

The most frequently observed adverse effects are lightheadedness, dizziness, sedation, nausea, vomiting, and sweating. These effects seem to be more prominent in ambulatory patients and in those not experiencing severe pain. Some adverse reactions in ambulatory patients may be alleviated if the patient lies down.

Less frequently observed with narcotic analgesics:

General and CNS: Dysphonia, euphoria, weakness, headache, agitation, tremor, uncoordinated muscle movements, alterations of mood (nervousness, apprehension, depression, floating feelings, dreams), muscle rigidity, paresthesia, muscle tremor, blurred vision, nystagmus, diplopia and miosis, transient hallucinations and disorientation, visual disturbances, insomnia and increased intracranial pressure may occur.

Cardiovascular: Chills, tachycardia, bradycardia, palpitation, faintness, syncope, hypotension and hypertension have been reported.

Respiratory: Bronchospasm and laryngospasm have been known to occur.

Gastrointestinal: Constipation, biliary tract spasm, anorexia, diarrhea, cramps and taste alterations have been reported.

Genitourinary: Urinary retention or hesitancy, and antidiuretic effects have been reported.

Dermatologic: Pruritus, urticaria, other skin rashes, and diaphoresis.

INJECTION

General and CNS: Hallucinations, although unusual with pure agonist narcotics, have been observed in 1 patient following both a 6 and a 4 mg hydromorphone HCl high potency dose. However, the patient was receiving several concomitant medications during the second episode and a causal relationship cannot be established.

Cardiovascular: Flushing of the face.

Gastrointestinal: Dry mouth.

Dermatologic: Wheal and flare over the vein with intravenous injection have been reported with narcotic analgesics.

Other: In clinical trials, neither local tissue irritation nor induration was observed at the site of subcutaneous injection of hydromorphone HCl high potency; pain at the injection site was rarely observed. However, local irritation and induration have been seen following parenteral injection of other narcotic drug products.

DOSAGE AND ADMINISTRATION

INJECTION

Parenteral: HYDROMORPHONE HCl HIGH POTENCY SHOULD BE GIVEN ONLY TO PATIENTS WHO ARE ALREADY RECEIVING LARGE DOSES OF NARCOTICS. Hydromorphone HCl high potency is indicated for relief of moderate-to-severe pain in narcotic-tolerant patients. Thus, these patients will already have been treated with other narcotic analgesics. If the patient is being changed from regular hydromorphone HCl to hydromorphone HCl high potency, similar doses should be used, depending on the patient's clinical response to the drug. If hydromorphone HCl high potency is substituted for a different narcotic analgesic, TABLE 3, an equivalency table, should be used as a guide to determine the appropriate starting dose of hydromorphone HCl high potency (hydromorphone HCl).

TABLE 3 *Strong Analgesics and Structurally Related Drugs Used in the Treatment of Cancer Pain**

IM or SC Administration

Nonproprietary Names	Dose, mg Equianalgesic to 10 mg of IM Morphine†	Duration Compared with Morphine
Morphine sulfate	10	Same
Papaveretum	20	Same
Hydromorphone HCl	1.3	Slightly Shorter
Oxymorphone HCl	1.1	Slightly Shorter
Nalbuphine HCl	12	Same
Heroin, diamorphine HCl (NA in US)	4-5	Slightly Shorter
Levorphanol tartrate	2.3	Same
Butorphanol tartrate	1.5-2.5	Same
Pentazocine lactate or HCl	60	Shorter
Meperidine, pethidine HCl	80	Shorter
Methadone HCl	10	Same

* From Beaver WT, Management of Cancer Pain with Parenteral Medication J. Am. Med. Assoc. 244:2653-2657 (1980)

† In terms of the area under the analgesic time-effect curve.

In open clinical trials with hydromorphone HCl high potency in patients with terminal cancer, doses ranged from 1-14 mg subcutaneously or intramuscularly; 1 patient received 30 mg subcutaneously on two occasions. In these trials, both subcutaneous and intramuscular injections of hydromorphone HCl high potency were well-tolerated, with minimal pain and/or burning at the injection site. Mild erythema was rarely noted after intramuscular injection. There was no induration after either intramuscular or subcutaneous administration of hydromorphone HCl high potency. Subcutaneous injections of hydromorphone HCl high potency were particularly well accepted when administered with a short, 30 gauge needle.

Experience with administration of hydromorphone HCl high potency by the intravenous route is limited. Should intravenous administration be necessary, the injection should be given slowly, over at least 2-3 minutes. The intravenous route is usually painless. A gradual increase in dose may be required if analgesia is inadequate, tolerance occurs, or if pain severity increases. The first sign of tolerance is usually a reduced duration of effect.

Note: Parenteral drug products should be inspected visually for particulate matter and discoloration prior to administration, whenever solution and container permit. A slight yellowish discoloration may develop in hydromorphone HCl high potency ampules. No loss of potency has been demonstrated. Hydromorphone HCl injection is physically compatible and chemically stable for at least 24 hours at 25°C protected from light in most common large volume parenteral solutions.

TABLETS AND ORAL SOLUTION

A gradual increase in dose may be required if analgesia is inadequate, as tolerance develops, or if pain severity increases. The first sign of tolerance is usually a decreased duration of effect.

Tablets: The usual starting dose for hydromorphone HCl tablets is 2-4 mg, orally, every 4-6 hours. Appropriate use of the 8 mg tablet must be decided by careful evaluation of each clinical situation.

Oral Solution: The usual adult oral dosage of hydromorphone HCl oral liquid is one-half (2.5 ml) to 2 teaspoonfuls (10 ml) (2.5-10 mg) every 3-6 hours as directed by the clinical situation. Oral dosages higher than the usual dosages may be required in some patients.

Safety and Handling Instructions

Hydromorphone HCl oral liquid and tablets pose little risk of direct exposure to health care personnel and should be handled and disposed of prudently in accordance with hospital or institutional policy. Significant absorption from dermal exposure is unlikely; accidental dermal exposure to hydromorphone HCl oral liquid should be treated by removal of any contaminated clothing and rinsing the affected area with water. Patients and their families should be instructed to flush any hydromorphone HCl oral liquid and tablets that are no longer needed.

Access to abusable drugs such as hydromorphone HCl oral liquid and tablets presents an occupational hazard for addiction in the health care industry. Routine procedures for handling controlled substances developed to protect the public may not be adequate to protect health care workers. Implementation of more effective accounting procedures and measures to restrict access to drugs of this class (appropriate to the practice setting) may minimize the risk of self-administration by health care providers.

HOW SUPPLIED

ORAL SOLUTION

Dilaudid oral liquid is a clear, sweet, slightly viscous liquid.

Storage: Dilaudid oral liquid and tablets should be stored at 15-25°C (59-77°F). Protect from light.

TABLETS

Dilaudid tablets are triangular shaped, embossed with the number of milligrams on one side and bisected and embossed with a double "Knoll" triangle on the other side.

1 mg: Contains 1 mg hydromorphone HCl (green tablet).
2 mg: Contains 2 mg hydromorphone HCl (orange tablet).
3 mg: Contains 3 mg hydromorphone HCl (pink tablet).
4 mg: Contains 4 mg hydromorphone HCl (yellow tablet).
8 mg: Contains 8 mg hydromorphone HCl (white tablet).

Storage: Dilaudid oral liquid and tablets should be stored at 15-25°C (59-77°F). Protect from light.

INJECTION

Storage: Parenteral forms of hydromorphone HCl should be stored at 15-30°C (59-86°F). Protect from light.

PRODUCT LISTING - RATED THERAPEUTICALLY EQUIVALENT

Size	Price	Product	NDC
Liquid - Oral - 1 mg/ml			
120 ml	$23.98	GENERIC, Roxane Laboratories Inc	00054-3387-50
500 ml	$95.17	GENERIC, Roxane Laboratories Inc	00054-3387-63
Solution - Injectable - 10 mg/ml			
1 ml x 10	$35.40	DILAUDID-HP, Abbott Pharmaceutical	00074-2453-11
5 ml x 10	$167.90	DILAUDID-HP, Abbott Pharmaceutical	00074-2453-27
50 ml	$172.50	DILAUDID-HP, Abbott Pharmaceutical	00074-2453-51
Tablet - Oral - 8 mg			
100's	$121.98	GENERIC, Roxane Laboratories Inc	00054-4370-25
100's	$146.59	DILAUDID, Abbott Pharmaceutical	00074-2426-14

PRODUCT LISTING - EQUIVALENTS NOT AVAILABLE

Size	Price	Product	NDC
Liquid - Oral - 1 mg/ml			
480 ml	$108.18	DILAUDID-5, Knoll Pharmaceutical Company	00044-1085-01
Powder For Injection - Injectable - 250 mg			
1's	$83.76	DILAUDID-HP, Knoll Pharmaceutical Company	00044-1911-01
1's	$85.24	DILAUDID-HP, Abbott Pharmaceutical	00074-2455-31
Solution - Injectable - 1 mg/ml			
1 ml x 10	$10.09	GENERIC, Abbott Pharmaceutical	00074-1283-01
1 ml x 10	$10.40	GENERIC, Abbott Pharmaceutical	00074-1283-31
1 ml x 10	$12.60	DILAUDID, Abbott Pharmaceutical	00074-2332-11
1 ml x 10	$12.70	DILAUDID, Knoll Pharmaceutical Company	00044-1011-01
10 ml	$14.70	GENERIC, Sanofi Winthrop Pharmaceuticals	00024-0726-01
Solution - Injectable - 2 mg/ml			
1 ml x 10	$10.45	GENERIC, Abbott Pharmaceutical	00074-1312-01
1 ml x 10	$11.50	GENERIC, Abbott Pharmaceutical	00074-1312-02
1 ml x 10	$11.99	GENERIC, Abbott Pharmaceutical	00074-1312-31
1 ml x 10	$12.94	GENERIC, Abbott Pharmaceutical	00074-1312-12
1 ml x 10	$13.30	GENERIC, Abbott Pharmaceutical	00074-1312-30
1 ml x 10	$14.00	DILAUDID, Knoll Pharmaceutical Company	00044-1012-01
1 ml x 10	$14.00	DILAUDID, Abbott Pharmaceutical	00074-2333-11
1 ml x 25	$26.00	GENERIC, Esi Lederle Generics	00641-0121-25
1 ml x 25	$33.25	DILAUDID, Knoll Pharmaceutical Company	00044-1012-09
1 ml x 25	$33.50	DILAUDID, Abbott Pharmaceutical	00074-2333-26
10 ml	$15.32	GENERIC, Sanofi Winthrop Pharmaceuticals	00024-0728-12
20 ml	$10.63	GENERIC, Esi Lederle Generics	00641-2341-41
20 ml	$21.56	DILAUDID, Knoll Pharmaceutical Company	00044-1062-05
20 ml	$21.56	DILAUDID, Abbott Pharmaceutical	00074-2414-21
Solution - Injectable - 4 mg/ml			
1 ml x 10	$10.00	GENERIC, Abbott Pharmaceutical	00074-1304-01
1 ml x 10	$12.83	GENERIC, Abbott Pharmaceutical	00074-1304-31
1 ml x 10	$16.90	DILAUDID, Knoll Pharmaceutical Company	00044-1014-01
1 ml x 10	$17.00	DILAUDID, Abbott Pharmaceutical	00074-2334-11
10 ml	$15.94	GENERIC, Sanofi Winthrop Pharmaceuticals	00024-0727-04
20 ml x 10	$125.00	GENERIC, International Medication Systems, Limited	00548-1940-10
Solution - Injectable - 10 mg/ml			
1 ml x 10	$35.40	DILAUDID-HP, Knoll Pharmaceutical Company	00044-1017-10
5 ml x 10	$167.90	DILAUDID-HP, Knoll Pharmaceutical Company	00044-1017-25
50 ml	$172.50	DILAUDID-HP, Knoll Pharmaceutical Company	00044-1017-06
Suppository - Rectal - 3 mg			
6's	$21.58	GENERIC, Paddock Laboratories Inc	00574-7224-06
6's	$23.97	DILAUDID, Knoll Pharmaceutical Company	00044-1053-01
Tablet - Oral - 2 mg			
100's	$23.33	GENERIC, Rexar Pharmacal	00478-5402-01
100's	$28.12	GENERIC, Vintage Pharmaceuticals Inc	00254-3611-28
100's	$28.12	GENERIC, Qualitest Products Inc	00603-3925-21
100's	$32.20	GENERIC, Shire Richwood Pharmaceutical Company Inc	58521-0002-01
100's	$36.95	GENERIC, Mallinckrodt Medical Inc	00406-3243-01
100's	$37.13	GENERIC, Endo Laboratories Llc	60951-0752-70
100's	$37.18	GENERIC, Roxane Laboratories Inc	00054-4392-25
100's	$42.64	GENERIC, Ethex Corporation	58177-0298-04
100's	$47.17	GENERIC, Roxane Laboratories Inc	00054-8392-24
100's	$47.17	GENERIC, Ethex Corporation	58177-0298-11
100's	$49.34	DILAUDID, Knoll Pharmaceutical Company	00044-1022-02
100's	$49.34	DILAUDID, Abbott Pharmaceutical	00074-2415-14
100's	$62.39	DILAUDID, Knoll Pharmaceutical Company	00044-1022-45
100's	$62.39	DILAUDID, Abbott Pharmaceutical	00074-2415-12
Tablet - Oral - 4 mg			
100's	$39.17	GENERIC, Rexar Pharmacal	00478-5404-01
100's	$45.45	GENERIC, Vintage Pharmaceuticals Inc	00254-3612-28
100's	$45.45	GENERIC, Qualitest Products Inc	00603-3926-21
100's	$52.30	GENERIC, Shire Richwood Pharmaceutical Company Inc	58521-0004-01
100's	$52.75	GENERIC, Ivax Corporation	00182-9178-01
100's	$60.95	GENERIC, Mallinckrodt Medical Inc	00406-3244-01
100's	$61.25	GENERIC, Endo Laboratories Llc	60951-0757-70
100's	$61.31	GENERIC, Roxane Laboratories Inc	00054-4394-25
100's	$69.61	GENERIC, Ethex Corporation	58177-0299-04
100's	$71.71	GENERIC, Roxane Laboratories Inc	00054-8394-24
100's	$71.71	GENERIC, Ethex Corporation	58177-0299-11
100's	$80.54	DILAUDID, Knoll Pharmaceutical Company	00044-1024-02
100's	$80.54	DILAUDID, Abbott Pharmaceutical	00074-2416-14
100's	$94.86	DILAUDID, Knoll Pharmaceutical Company	00044-1024-45
100's	$94.86	DILAUDID, Abbott Pharmaceutical	00074-2416-12
Tablet - Oral - 8 mg			
100's	$146.59	DILAUDID, Knoll Pharmaceutical Company	00044-1028-02

Hydroquinone (001503)

Categories: Freckles; Lentigines, senile; Melasma; Pregnancy Category C; FDA Pre 1938 Drugs
Drug Classes: Dermatologics; Depigmenting agents
Brand Names: Banquin; Eldopaque Forte; **Eldoquin Forte**; Hydroxyquinone; Melanex; Melanol; Melpaque Hp; Melquin; Nuquin Hp; Solaquin Forte
Foreign Brand Availability: Aldoquin 2 (Colombia); Crema Blanca Bustillos (Mexico); Eldopaque (Bahrain; Costa-Rica; Cyprus; Dominican-Republic; Egypt; El-Salvador; Greece; Guatemala; Honduras; Hong-Kong; Iran; Iraq; Jordan; Kuwait; Lebanon; Libya; Nicaragua; Oman; Panama; Philippines; Qatar; Republic-of-Yemen; Saudi-Arabia; Syria; United-Arab-Emirates); Eldoquin (Bahrain; Canada; Costa-Rica; Cyprus; Dominican-Republic; Egypt; El-Salvador; Guatemala; Honduras; Hong-Kong; Iran; Iraq; Jordan; Kuwait; Lebanon; Libya; Mexico; Nicaragua; Oman; Panama; Philippines; Qatar; Republic-of-Yemen; Saudi-Arabia; Syria; United-Arab-Emirates); Eldoquin Cream (New-Zealand); Esomed (Israel); Ginomi (Korea); Melanox (Indonesia); Melquin HP (Korea); Melquine (Taiwan); Polyquin Forte (Singapore); Solaquin (Bahrain; Canada; Cyprus; Egypt; Hong-Kong; Iran; Iraq; Jordan; Kuwait; Lebanon; Libya; Oman; Qatar; Republic-of-Yemen; Saudi-Arabia; Syria; United-Arab-Emirates); Ultraquin (Canada; China); Zumae (Taiwan)

DESCRIPTION

Topical Solution 3%: Each ml of hydroquinone 3% topical solution contains 30 mg of hydroquinone in a vehicle containing SD alcohol 40-B (45%), propylene glycol, laureth-4, isopropyl alcohol (4%), purified water, and ascorbic acid. Chemically, hydroquinone is $C_6H_6O_2$ and has a molecular weight of 110.11. The chemical name is 1, 4 dihydroxybenzene.

Solaquin Forte 4% Cream: Each gram of Solaquin Forte 4% cream contains 40 mg of hydroquinone, 80 mg octyl dimethyl-p-aminobenzoate and 30 mg dioxybenzone USP and 20 mg oxybenzone USP in a vanishing cream base of purified water, glyceryl monostearate, octyldodecyl stearoyl stearate, glyceryl dilaurate, quaternium-26, coceth-6, stearyl alcohol, diethylaminoethyl stearate, dimethicone, polysorbate-80, lactic acid, ascorbic acid, hydroxyethylcellulose, quaternium 14, myristylkonium chloride, disodium EDTA, and sodium metabisulfite.

Eldopaque Forte 4% Cream: Each gram of Eldopaque Forte contains 40 mg of hydroquinone in a tinted sunblocking cream base of water, stearic acid, talc, PEG-40 stearate, PEG-25 propylene glycol stearate, propylene glycol, glyceryl stearate, iron oxides, mineral oil, squalene, disodium EDTA, sodium metabisulfite, and potassium sorbate.

Eldoquin Forte 4% Cream: Each gram of Eldoquin Forte contains 40 mg of hydroquinone in a vanishing cream base of purified water, stearic acid, propylene glycol, polyoxyl 40 stearate, propylene glycol monostearate, glyceryl monostearate, mineral oil, squalene, propylparaben, and sodium metabisulfite.

Solaquin Forte 4% Gel: Each gram of Solaquin Forte gel contains 40 mg of hydroquinone, 50 mg of octyl dimethyl p-aminobenzoate, and 30 mg dioxybenzone, in a hydro-alcoholic base of ethyl alcohol, purified water, propylene glycol, tetrahydroxypropyl ethylenediamine, carbomer 940, disodium EDTA, and sodium metabisulfite.

CLINICAL PHARMACOLOGY

Topical application of hydroquinone produces a reversible depigmentation of the skin by inhibition of the enzymatic oxidation of tyrosine to 3,4-dihydroxyphenylalanine (dopa)[1] and suppression of other melanocyte metabolic processes.[2] Exposure to sunlight or ultraviolet light will cause repigmentation of bleached areas.[3]

INDICATIONS AND USAGE

All forms are indicated for the gradual bleaching of hyperpigmented skin conditions such as chloasma, melasma, freckles, senile lentigines, and other unwanted areas of melanin hyperpigmentation.

Eloquin Forte 4% Cream: This cream is intended for night-time use only since it contains no sunblocking agents. For daytime usage, Solaquin Forte 4% cream, Solaquin Forte 4% gel or Eldopaque Forte 4% cream should be prescribed.

CONTRAINDICATIONS

Prior history of sensitivity or allergic reaction to hydroquinone or any of the ingredients of the products. The safety of topical hydroquinone use during pregnancy or in children (12 years and under) has not been established.

WARNINGS

Cream and Gel

A. *Caution:* Hydroquinone is a skin bleaching agent which may produce unwanted cosmetic effects if not used as directed. The physician should be familiar with the contents of this insert before prescribing or dispensing these medications.

B. Test for skin sensitivity before using these medications by applying a small amount to an unbroken patch of skin and check in 24 hours. Minor redness is not a contraindication, but where there is itching or vesicle formation of excessive inflammatory response further treatment is not advised. Close patient supervision is recommended. Contact with the eyes should be avoided. If no bleaching or lightening effect is noted after 2 months of treatment use, the medication should be discontinued. Hydroquinone 4% cream or gel are formulated for use as a skin bleaching agent and should not be used for the prevention of sunburn.

C. Sunscreen use is an essential aspect of hydroquinone therapy because even minimal sunlight exposure sustains melanocytic activity. The sunscreens in Hydroquinone 4% cream or gel provide the necessary sun protection during skin bleaching therapy. After clearing and during maintenance therapy, sun exposure should be avoided on bleached skin by application of a sunscreen or sunblock agent or protective clothing to prevent repigmentation.

D. Keep this and all medication out of the reach of children. In case of accidental ingestion, call a physician or a poison control center immediately.

E. *Warning:* Contains sodium metabisulfite, a sulfite that may cause serious allergic type reactions (*e.g.*, hives, itching, wheezing, anaphylaxis, severe asthma attack) in certain susceptible persons.

PRECAUTIONS

For cream and gel, see also WARNINGS.

General: For external use only. Avoid contact with eyes and mucous membranes.

Pregnancy Category C: Animal reproduction studies have not been conducted with topical hydroquinone. It is also not known whether hydroquinone can cause fetal harm when administered to a pregnant woman or can affect reproduction capacity. It is not known to what degree, if any, topical hydroquinone is absorbed systemically. Topical hydroquinone should be given to a pregnant women only if clearly needed.

Nursing Mothers: It is not known whether this drug is excreted in human milk. Because many drugs are excreted in human milk, caution should be exercised when topical hydroquinone is administered to a nursing mother.

Pediatric Usage: Safety and effectiveness in pediatric patients below the age of 12 years have not been established.

ADVERSE REACTIONS

The Following Adverse Reactions Have Been Reported: Dryness and fissuring of paranasal and infraorbital areas, erythema, and stinging. Occasional hypersensitivity (localized contact dermatitis) may develop. If this occurs, the medication should be discontinued and the physician notified immediately.

DOSAGE AND ADMINISTRATION

Topical Solution 3%: Hydroquinone topical solution 3% should be applied to affected areas and rubbed in well twice daily, in the morning and before bedtime, or as directed by a physician. Since this product contains no sunscreen, an effective broad spectrum sun blocking agent should be used and unnecessary solar exposure avoided, or protective clothing should be worn to cover bleached skin in order to prevent repigmentation from occurring during the day. If no improvement is seen after 3 months of treatment, use of this product should be discontinued.

Solaquin Forte 4% Cream and Solaquin Forte 4% Gel: These forms should be applied to the affected area and rubbed in well twice daily or as directed by a physician to achieve maximum therapeutic potential.

Eldopaque Forte 4% Cream: This form should be applied with a thin application to the affected area twice daily or as directed by a physician. Do not rub in.

Eldoquin Forte 4% Cream: This form is indicated to be used during night hours as the product contains no sunblocking agent. Apply to affected area and rub in well twice daily or as directed by a physician.

There is no recommended dosage for children under 12 years of age except under the advice and supervision of a physician.

HOW SUPPLIED

Storage: Store at controlled room temperature 15-30°C (59-86°F).

PRODUCT LISTING - EQUIVALENTS NOT AVAILABLE

Size	Price	Product	NDC
Cream - Topical - 4%			
15 gm	$11.25	GENERIC, Stratus Pharmaceuticals Inc	58980-0473-05
15 gm	$11.90	GENERIC, Stratus Pharmaceuticals Inc	58980-0574-05
15 gm	$17.60	GENERIC, Stratus Pharmaceuticals Inc	58980-0472-05
15 gm	$18.56	SOLAQUIN FORTE, Southwood Pharmaceuticals Inc	58016-3189-01
28 gm	$48.95	ELDOQUIN FORTE, Icn Pharmaceuticals Inc	00187-0394-31
28 gm	$48.95	ELDOPAQUE FORTE, Icn Pharmaceuticals Inc	00187-0395-31
28 gm	$48.95	SOLAQUIN FORTE, Icn Pharmaceuticals Inc	00187-0396-31
28 gm	$52.50	GLYQUIN, Icn Pharmaceuticals Inc	00187-0420-46
28.35 gm	$45.03	GENERIC, Glades Pharmaceuticals	59366-2785-03
28.35 gm	$45.03	GENERIC, Glades Pharmaceuticals	59366-2787-03
28.40 gm	$48.25	GENERIC, Glades Pharmaceuticals	59366-2789-03
30 gm	$3.40	GENERIC, Syosset Laboratories Company	47854-0717-05
30 gm	$19.75	GENERIC, Stratus Pharmaceuticals Inc	58980-0473-10
30 gm	$30.75	GENERIC, Qualitest Products Inc	00603-7788-78
30 gm	$30.75	GENERIC, Qualitest Products Inc	00603-7789-78
30 gm	$35.50	GENERIC, Stratus Pharmaceuticals Inc	58980-0472-10
30 gm	$35.50	GENERIC, Stratus Pharmaceuticals Inc	58980-0574-10
30 gm	$38.84	ELDOQUIN, Southwood Pharmaceuticals Inc	58016-3527-30
30 gm	$40.04	GENERIC, Ethex Corporation	58177-0801-02
30 gm	$40.04	GENERIC, Ethex Corporation	58177-0802-02
30 gm	$43.49	LUSTRA, Allscripts Pharmaceutical Company	54569-4633-00
30 gm	$44.00	GENERIC, Stratus Pharmaceuticals Inc	58980-0580-10
30 gm	$47.83	LUSTRA, Allscripts Pharmaceutical Company	54569-4826-00
30 gm	$59.93	LUSTRA, Medicis Dermatologics Inc	99207-0250-10
30 gm	$65.90	LUSTRA-AF, Medicis Dermatologics Inc	99207-0255-10
30 gm	$77.79	ALUSTRA, Medicis Dermatologics Inc	99207-0251-10
45 gm	$118.69	CLARIPEL, Stiefel Laboratories Inc	00145-2516-05
60 gm	$2.75	GENERIC, Cmc-Consolidated Midland Corporation	00223-4330-02
60 gm	$39.00	GENERIC, Stratus Pharmaceuticals Inc	58980-0574-20
60 gm	$70.75	GENERIC, Stratus Pharmaceuticals Inc	58980-0580-20
60 gm	$113.85	LUSTRA, Medicis Dermatologics Inc	99207-0250-20
60 gm	$125.19	LUSTRA-AF, Medicis Dermatologics Inc	99207-0255-20
120 gm	$4.00	GENERIC, Cmc-Consolidated Midland Corporation	00223-4330-04
Gel - Topical - 4%			
15 gm	$11.90	GENERIC, Stratus Pharmaceuticals Inc	58980-0475-05
28.35 gm	$45.03	GENERIC, Glades Pharmaceuticals	59366-2783-03
30 gm	$29.00	GENERIC, Stratus Pharmaceuticals Inc	58980-0475-10
30 gm	$48.95	SOLAQUIN FORTE, Icn Pharmaceuticals Inc	00187-0523-31
60 gm	$32.13	GENERIC, Stratus Pharmaceuticals Inc	58980-0475-20
Solution - Topical - 3%			
30 ml	$8.70	MELQUIN-3, Stratus Pharmaceuticals Inc	58980-0476-10
30 ml	$12.07	GENERIC, Glades Pharmaceuticals	59366-2781-03
30 ml	$12.91	MELANEX, Neutrogena Corporation	10812-0930-00
30 ml	$13.13	MELANEX, Neutrogena Corporation	10812-0930-01
Solution - Topical - 4%			
30 ml	$27.95	GENERIC, Glades Pharmaceuticals	59366-2788-01

Hydroxychloroquine Sulfate *(001506)*

Categories: Arthritis, rheumatoid; Lupus erythematosus, discoid; Lupus erythematosus, systemic; Malaria; Malaria, prophylaxis; FDA Approved 1955 Apr; Pregnancy Category C

Drug Classes: Antiprotozoals; Disease modifying antirheumatic drugs

Brand Names: **Plaquenil**

Foreign Brand Availability: Dimard (Colombia); Ercoquin (Denmark; Japan; Norway); Geniquin (Taiwan); Oxiklorin (Finland; Korea); Plaquenil Sulfate (Canada); Plaquinol (Colombia; Costa-Rica; Dominican-Republic; El-Salvador; Guatemala; Honduras; Nicaragua; Panama; Peru; Portugal); Quensyl (Germany); Toremonil (Japan); Yuma (Korea)

Cost of Therapy: $54.58 (Malaria Treatment; Plaquenil; 200 mg; 10 tablets; 3 day supply)
$31.31 (Malaria Treatment; Generic Tablets; 200 mg; 10 tablets; 3 day supply)
$54.58 (Rheumatoid Arthritis; Plaquenil; 200 mg; 1 tablet/day; 30 day supply)
$31.31 (Rheumatoid Arthritis; Generic Tablets; 200 mg; 1 tablet/day; 30 day supply)

WARNING

PHYSICIANS SHOULD COMPLETELY FAMILIARIZE THEMSELVES WITH THE COMPLETE CONTENTS OF THIS LEAFLET BEFORE PRESCRIBING HYDROXYCHLOROQUINE.

DESCRIPTION

Hydroxychloroquine sulfate is a colorless crystalline solid, soluble in water to at least 20%; chemically the drug is 2-[[4-[(7-Chloro-4-quinolyl)amino]pentyl]ethylamino]ethanol sulfate (1:1). Plaquenil (hydroxychloroquine sulfate) tablets contain 200 mg hydroxychloroquine sulfate, equivalent to 155 mg base, and are for oral administration.

Inactive Ingredients: Dibasic calcium phosphate, hydroxypropyl methylcellulose, magnesium stearate, polyethylene glycol 400, polysorbate 80, starch, titanium dioxide.

CLINICAL PHARMACOLOGY

ACTIONS

The drug possesses antimalarial actions and also exerts a beneficial effect in lupus erythematosus (chronic discoid or systemic) and acute or chronic rheumatoid arthritis. The precise mechanism of action is not known.

Malaria

Like chloroquine phosphate, hydroxychloroquine sulfate is highly active against the erythrocytic forms of *Plasmodium vivax* and *malariae* and most strains of *P. falciparum* (but not the gametocytes of *P. falciparum*). Hydroxychloroquine sulfate does not prevent relapses in patients with *vivax* or *malariae* malaria because it is not effective against exo-erythrocytic forms of the parasite, nor will it prevent *vivax* or *malariae* infection when administered as a prophylactic. It is highly effective as a suppressive agent in patients with *vivax* or *malariae* malaria, in terminating acute attacks, and significantly lengthening the interval between treatment and relapse. In patients with *falcparum* malaria, it abolishes the acute attack and effects complete cure of the infection, unless due to a resistant strain of *P. falciparum.*

INDICATIONS AND USAGE

Hydroxychloroquine sulfate is indicated for the suppressive treatment and treatment of acute attacks of malaria due to *Plasmodium vivax, P. malariae, P. ovale,* and susceptible strains of *P. falciparum.* It is also indicated for the treatment of discoid and systemic lupus erythematosus, and rheumatoid arthritis.

MALARIA

Hydroxychloroquine sulfate is indicated for the treatment of acute attacks and suppression of malaria.

LUPUS ERYTHEMATOSUS AND RHEUMATOID ARTHRITIS

Hydroxychloroquine sulfate is useful in patients with the following disorders who have not responded satisfactorily to drugs with less potential for serious side effects: lupus erythernatosus (chronic discoid and systemic) and acute or chronic rheumatoid arthritis.

NON-FDA APPROVED INDICATIONS

Although not approved by the FDA, hydroxychloroquine is recommended by the CDC for malaria prophylaxis for travel to areas of risk where chloroquine-resistant P. falciparum has not been reported.

CONTRAINDICATIONS

Use of this drug is contraindicated (1) in the presence of retinal or visual field changes attributable to any 4-aminoquinoline compound, (2) in patients with known hypersensitivity to 4-aminoquinoline compounds, and (3) for long-term therapy in children.

WARNINGS

GENERAL

Hydroxychloroquine sulfate is not effective against chloroquine-resistant strains of *P. falciparum.*

Children are especially sensitive to the 4-aminoquinoline compounds. A number of fatalities have been reported following the accidental ingestion of chloroquine, sometimes in relatively small doses (0.75 or 1 g in one 3-year-old child). Patients should be strongly warned to keep these drugs out of the reach of children.

Use of hydroxychloroquine sulfate in patients with psoriasis may precipitate a severe attack of psoriasis. When used in patients with porphyria the condition may be exacerbated. The preparation should not be used in these conditions unless in the judgment of the physician the benefit to the patient outweighs the possible hazard.

Use in Pregnancy

Usage of this drug during pregnancy should be avoided except in the suppression or treatment of malaria when in the judgment of the physician the benefit outweighs the possible hazard. It should be noted that radioactively-tagged chloroquine administered intravenously to pregnant, pigmented CBA mice passed rapidly across the placenta. It accumulated selectively in the melanin structures of the fetal eyes and was retained in the ocular tissues for 5 months after the drug had been eliminated from the rest of the body.

MALARIA

In recent years, it has been found that certain strains of *P. falciparum* have become resistant to 4-aminoquinoline compounds (including hydroxychloroquine) as shown by the fact that normally adequate doses have failed to prevent or cure clinical malaria or parasitemia. Treatment with quinine or other specific forms of therapy is therefore advised for patients infected with a resistant strain of parasites.

LUPUS ERYTHEMATOSUS AND RHEUMATOID ARTHRITIS

PHYSICIANS SHOULD COMPLETELY FAMILIARIZE THEMSELVES WITH THE COMPLETE CONTENTS OF THIS PRESCRIBING INFORMATION BEFORE PRESCRIBING HYDROXYCHLOROQUINE SULFATE.

Irreversible retinal damage has been observed in some patients who had received long-term or high-dosage 4-aminoquinoline therapy for discoid and systemic lupus erythematosus, or rheumatoid arthritis. Retinopathy has been reported to be dose-related.

When prolonged therapy with any antimalarial compound is contemplated, initial (base line) and periodic (every 3 months) ophthalmologic examinations (including visual acuity, expert slit-lamp, funduscopic, and visual field tests) should be performed.

If there is any indication of abnormality in the visual acuity, visual field, or retinal macular areas (such as pigmentary changes, loss of foveal reflex), or any visual symptoms (such as light flashes and streaks) which are not fully explainable by difficulties of accommodation or corneal opacities, the drug should be discontinued immediately and the patient closely observed for possible progression. Retinal changes (and visual disturbances) may progress even after cessation of therapy.

All patients on long-term therapy with this preparation should be questioned and examined periodically, including the testing of knee and ankle reflexes, to detect any evidence of muscular weakness. If weakness occurs, discontinue the drug.

In the treatment of rheumatoid arthritis, if objective improvement (such as reduced joint swelling, increased mobility) does not occur within 6 months, the drug should be discontinued.

Safe use of the drug in the treatment of juvenile arthritis has not been established.

PRECAUTIONS

GENERAL

Antimalarial compounds should be used with caution in patients with hepatic disease or alcoholism or in conjunction with known hepatotoxic drugs.

Periodic blood cell counts should be made if patients are given prolonged therapy. If any severe blood disorder appears which is not attributable to the disease under treatment, discontinuation of the drug should be considered. The drug should be administered with caution in patients having G-6-PD (glucose-6-phosphate dehydrogenase) deficiency.

LUPUS ERYTHEMATOSUS AND RHEUMATOID ARTHRITIS

Dermatologic reactions to hydroxychloroquine sulfate may occur and, therefore, proper care should be exercised when it is administered to any patient receiving a drug with a significant tendency to produce dermatitis.

The methods recommended for early diagnosis of "chloroquine retinopathy" consist of (1) funduscopic examination of the macula for fine pigmentary disturbances or loss of the foveal reflex and (2) examination of the central visual field with a small red test object for pericentral or paracentral scotoma or determination of retinal thresholds to red. Any unexplained visual symptoms, such as light flashes or streaks should also be regarded with suspicion as possible manifestations of retinopathy. If serious toxic symptoms occur from overdosage or sensitivity, it has been suggested that ammonium chloride (8 g daily in divided doses for adults) be administered orally 3 or 4 days a week for several months after therapy has been stopped, as acidification of the urine increases renal excretion of the 4-aminoquinoline compounds by 20-90%. However, caution must be exercised in patients with impaired renal function and/or metabolic acidosis.

ADVERSE REACTIONS

MALARIA

Following the administration in doses adequate for the treatment of an acute malarial attack, mild and transient headache, dizziness, and gastrointestinal complaints (diarrhea, anorexia, nausea, abdominal cramps and, on rare occasions, vomiting) may occur.

Cardiomyopathy has been rarely reported with high daily dosages of hydroxychloroquine.

H

LUPUS ERYTHEMATOSUS AND RHEUMATOID ARTHRITIS

Not all of the following reactions have been observed with every 4-aminoquinoline compound during long-term therapy, but they have been reported with one or more and should be borne in mind when drugs of this class are administered. Adverse effects with different compounds vary in type and frequency.

CNS Reactions: Irritability, nervousness, emotional changes, nightmares, psychosis, headache, dizziness, vertigo, tinnitus, nystagmus, nerve deafness, convulsions, ataxia.

Neuromuscular Reactions: Skeletal muscle palsies or skeletal muscle myopathy or neuromyopathy leading to progressive weakness and atrophy of proximal muscle groups which may be associated with mild sensory changes, depression of tendon reflexes and abnormal nerve conduction.

Ocular Reactions:

Ciliary Body: Disturbance of accommodation with symptoms of blurred vision. This reaction is dose-related and reversible with cessation of therapy.

Cornea: Transient edema, punctate to lineal opacities, decreased corneal sensitivity. The corneal changes, with or without accompanying symptoms (blurred vision, halos around lights, photophobia), are fairly common, but reversible. Corneal deposits may appear as early as 3 weeks following initiation of therapy.

The incidence of corneal changes and visual side effects appears to be considerably lower with hydroxychloroquine than with chloroquine.

Retina: *Macula:* Edema, atrophy, abnormal pigmentation (mild pigment stippling to a "bull's-eye" appearance), loss of foveal reflex, increased macular recovery time following exposure to a bright light (photo-stress test), elevated retinal threshold to red light in macular, paramacular, and peripheral retinal areas.

Other fundus changes include optic disc pallor and atrophy, attenuation of retinal arterioles, fine granular pigmentary disturbances in the peripheral retina and prominent choroidal patterns in advanced stage.

Visual Field Defects: Pericentral or paracentral scotoma, central scotoma with decreased-visual acuity, rarely field constriction.

The most common visual symptoms attributed to the retinopathy are: reading and seeing difficulties (words, letters, or parts of objects missing), photophobia, blurred distance vision, missing or blacked out areas in the central or peripheral visual field, light flashes and streaks.

Retinopathy appears to be dose related and has occurred within several months (rarely) to several years of daily therapy; a small number of cases have been reported several years after antimalarial drug therapy was discontinued. It has not been noted during prolonged use of weekly doses of the 4-aminoquinoline compounds for suppression of malaria.

Patients with retinal changes may have visual symptoms or may be asymptomatic (with or without visual field changes). Rarely scotomatous vision or field defects may occur without obvious retinal change.

Retinopathy may progress even after the drug is discontinued. In a number of patients, early retinopathy (macular pigmentation sometimes with central field defects) diminished or regressed completely after therapy was discontinued. Paracentral scotoma to red targets (sometimes called "premaculopathy") is indicative of early retinal dysfunction which is usually reversible with cessation of therapy.

A small number of cases of retinal changes have been reported as occurring in patients who received only hydroxychloroquine. These usually consisted of alteration in retinal pigmentation which was detected on periodic ophthalmologic examination; visual field defects were also present in some instances. A case of delayed retinopathy has been reported with loss of vision starting 1 year after administration of hydroxychloroquine had been discontinued.

Dermatologic Reactions: Bleaching of hair, alopecia, pruritus, skin and mucosal pigmentation, photosensitivity, and skin eruptions (urticarial, morbilliform, lichenoid, maculopapular, purpuric, erythema annulare centrifugum, Stevens-Johnson syndrome, acute generalized exanthematous pustulosis, and exfoliative dermatitis).

Hematologic Reactions: Various blood dyscrasias such as aplastic anemia, agranulocytosis, leukopenia, thrombocytopenia (hemolysis in individuals with glucose-6-phosphate dehydrogenase (G6-PD) deficiency).

Gastrointestinal Reactions: Anorexia, nausea, vomiting, diarrhea, and abdominal cramps. Isolated cases of abnormal liver function and fulminant hepatic failure.

Miscellaneous Reactions: Weight loss, lassitude, exacerbation or precipitation of porphyria and nonlight-sensitive psoriasis.

Cardiomyopathy has been rarely reported with high daily dosages of hydroxychloroquine.

DOSAGE AND ADMINISTRATION

One (1) tablet of 200 mg of hydroxychloroquine sulfate is equivalent to 155 mg base.

MALARIA

Supression

In adults, 400 mg (= 310 mg base) on exactly the same day of each week. *In infants and children,* the weekly suppressive dosage is 5 mg, calculated as base, per kg of body weight, but should not exceed the adult dose regardless of weight.

If circumstances permit, suppressive therapy should begin 2 weeks prior to exposure.

However, failing this, in adults an initial double (loading) dose of 800 mg (= 620 mg base), or in children 10 mg base/kg may be taken in 2 divided doses, 6 hours apart. The suppressive therapy should be continued for 8 weeks after leaving the endemic area.

Treatment of the Acute Attack

In adults, an initial dose of 800 mg (= 620 mg base) followed by 400 mg (= 310 mg base) in 6-8 hours and 400 mg (= 310 mg base) on each of 2 consecutive days (total 2 g hydroxychloroquine sulfate or 1.55 g base). An alternative method, employing a single dose of 800 mg (= 620 mg base), has also proved effective.

The dosage for adults may also be calculated on the basis of body weight; this method is preferred for infants and children.

A total dose representing 25 mg of base per kg of body weight is administered in 3 days, as follows:

First Dose: 10 mg base per kg (but not exceeding a single dose of 620 mg base).

Second Dose: 5 mg base per kg (but not exceeding a single dose of 310 mg base) 6 hours after first dose.

Third Dose: 5 mg base per kg 18 hours after second dose.

Fourth Dose: 5 mg base per kg 24 hours after third dose.

For radical cure of *vivax* and *malariae* malaria concomitant therapy with an 8-aminoquinoline compound is necessary.

LUPUS ERYTHEMATOSUS AND RHEUMATOID ARTHRITIS

One (1) tablet of hydroxychloroquine sulfate, 200 mg, is equivalent to 155 mg base.

Lupus Erythematosus

Initially, the average *adult* dose is 400 mg (= 310 mg base) once or twice daily. This may be continued for several weeks or months, depending on the response of the patient. For prolonged maintenance therapy, a smaller dose, from 200-400 mg (155-310 mg base) daily will frequently suffice.

The incidence of retinopathy has been reported to be higher when this maintenance dose is exceeded.

Rheumatoid Arthritis

The compound is cumulative in action and will require several weeks to exert its beneficial therapeutic effects, whereas minor side effects may occur relatively early.

Several months of therapy may be required before maximum effects can be obtained. If objective improvement (such as reduced joint swelling, increased mobility) does not occur within 6 months, the drug should be discontinued. Safe use of the drug in the treatment of juvenile rheumatoid arthritis has not been established.

Initial Dosage

In adults, from 400-600 mg (= 310-465 mg base) daily, each dose to be taken with a meal or a glass of milk. In a small percentage of patients, troublesome side effects may require temporary reduction of the initial dosage. Later (usually from 5-10 days), the dose may gradually be increased to the optimum response level, often without return of side effects.

Maintenance Dosage

When a good response is obtained (usually in 4-12 weeks), the dosage is reduced by 50% and continued at a usual maintenance level of 200-400 mg (= 155-310 mg base) daily, each dose to be taken with a meal or a glass of milk. The incidence of retinopathy has been reported to be higher when this maintenance dose is exceeded. Should a relapse occur after medication is withdrawn, therapy may be resumed or continued on an intermittent schedule if there are no ocular contraindications.

Corticosteroids and salicylates may be used in conjunction with this compound, and they can generally be decreased gradually in dosage or eliminated after the drug has been used for several weeks. When gradual reduction of steroid dosage is indicated, it may be done by reducing every 4-5 days the dose of cortisone by no more than from 5-15 mg; of hydrocortisone from 5-10 mg; of prednisolone and prednisone from 1-2.5 mg; of methylprednisolone and triamcinolone from 1-2 mg; and of dexamethasone from 0.25-0.5 mg.

HOW SUPPLIED

Plaquenil tablets are white, to off-white, film coated tablets imprinted "PLAQUENIL" on one face in black ink. Each tablet contains 200 mg hydroxychloroquine sulfate (equivalent to 155 mg base).

Storage: Dispense in a tight, light-resistant container. Store at room temperature up to 30°C (86°F).

PRODUCT LISTING - RATED THERAPEUTICALLY EQUIVALENT

Tablet - Oral - 200 mg

30's	$31.72	GENERIC, Golden State Medical	60429-0700-30
60's	$63.05	GENERIC, Golden State Medical	60429-0700-60
100's	$85.35	FEDERAL UPPER LIMIT, H.C.F.A. F F P	99999-1506-01
100's	$104.36	GENERIC, Moore, H.L. Drug Exchange Inc	00839-7963-06
100's	$104.93	GENERIC, Dixon-Shane Inc	17236-0610-01
100's	$106.95	GENERIC, Major Pharmaceuticals Inc	00904-5107-60
100's	$109.55	GENERIC, Ivax Corporation	00182-2609-01
100's	$109.55	GENERIC, Geneva Pharmaceuticals	00781-1407-01
100's	$110.53	GENERIC, Martec Pharmaceuticals Inc	52555-0642-01
100's	$117.10	GENERIC, Sanofi Winthrop Pharmaceuticals	00955-0790-01
100's	$117.35	GENERIC, Teva Pharmaceuticals Usa	00093-9774-01
100's	$123.20	GENERIC, Mylan Pharmaceuticals Inc	00378-0373-01
100's	$123.20	GENERIC, Watson Laboratories Inc	00591-0698-01
100's	$123.20	GENERIC, Watson Laboratories Inc	52544-0698-01
100's	$181.93	PLAQUENIL SULFATE, Sanofi Winthrop Pharmaceuticals	00024-1562-10

PRODUCT LISTING - EQUIVALENTS NOT AVAILABLE

Tablet - Oral - 200 mg

30's	$36.96	GENERIC, Allscripts Pharmaceutical Company	54569-4981-00
60's	$65.50	GENERIC, Pharma Pac	52959-0176-60
60's	$73.92	GENERIC, Allscripts Pharmaceutical Company	54569-4981-01
100's	$108.35	GENERIC, Apothecon Inc	62269-0250-24
100's	$108.35	GENERIC, Geneva Pharmaceuticals	62269-1407-01

Hydroxyurea *(001512)*

Categories: Anemia, sickle cell; Leukemia, chronic granulocytic; Leukemia, chronic myelogenous; Melanoma, malignant; FDA Approved 1967 Dec; Pregnancy Category D; Orphan Drugs

Drug Classes: Antineoplastics, miscellaneous

Brand Names: Hydrea

Foreign Brand Availability: Litalir (Czech-Republic; Germany; Hungary; Philippines; Switzerland); Neodrea (India); Onco-Carbide (Italy)

Cost of Therapy: $85.16 (Ovarian Carcinoma; Hydrea; 500 mg; 2 capsules/day; 30 day supply)
$24.35 (Ovarian Carcinoma; Generic Capsules; 500 mg; 2 capsules/day; 30 day supply)
$81.00 (Sickle Cell Anemia; Droxia; 400 mg; 3 capsules/day; 30 day supply)

WARNING

Note: The trade names have been used throughout this monograph for clarity.

DROXIA

Treatment of patients with Droxia may be complicated by severe, sometimes life-threatening, adverse effects. Droxia should be administered under the supervision of a physician experienced in the use of this medication for the treatment of sickle cell anemia.

Hydroxyurea is mutagenic and clastogenic, and causes cellular transformation to a tumorigenic phenotype. Hydroxyurea is thus unequivocally genotoxic and a presumed transspecies carcinogen which implies a carcinogenic risk to humans. In patients receiving long-term hydroxyurea for myeloproliferative disorders, such as polycythemia vera and thrombocythemia, secondary leukemias have been reported. It is unknown whether this leukemogenic effect is secondary to hydroxyurea or is associated with the patients' underlying disease. The physician and patient must very carefully consider the potential benefits of Droxia relative to the undefined risk of developing secondary malignancies.

DESCRIPTION

DROXIA

Droxia (hydroxyurea capsules) is available for oral use as capsules providing 200, 300, and 400 mg hydroxyurea. *Inactive Ingredients:* Citric acid, gelatin, lactose, magnesium stearate, sodium phosphate, titanium dioxide and capsule colorants; FD&C blue no. 1 and FD&C green no. 3 (200 mg capsules); D&C red no. 28, D&C red no. 33 and FD&C blue no. 1 (300 mg capsules); D&C red no. 28, D&C red no. 33 and D&C yellow no. 10 (400 mg capsules).

Hydroxyurea is an essentially tasteless, white crystalline powder.

HYDREA

Hydrea (hydroxyurea capsules) is an antineoplastic agent, available for oral use as capsules providing 500 mg hydroxyurea. *Inactive Ingredients:* Citric acid, colorants (D&C yellow no. 10, FD&C blue no. 1, FD&C red 40 and D&C red 28), gelatin, lactose, magnesium stearate, sodium phosphate, and titanium dioxide.

Hydroxyurea occurs as an essentially tasteless, white crystalline powder.

CLINICAL PHARMACOLOGY

DROXIA

Mechanism of Action

The precise mechanism by which hydroxyurea produces its cytotoxic and cytoreductive effects is not known. However, various studies support the hypothesis that hydroxyurea causes an immediate inhibition of DNA synthesis by acting as a ribonucleotide reductase inhibitor, without interfering with the synthesis of ribonucleic acid or of protein.

The mechanisms by which Droxia produces its beneficial effects in patients with sickle cell anemia (SCA) are uncertain. Known pharmacologic effects of Droxia that may contribute to its beneficial effects include increasing hemoglobin F levels in RBCs, decreasing neutrophils, increasing the water content of RBCs, increasing deformability of sickled cells, and altering the adhesion of RBCs to endothelium.

Pharmacokinetics

Absorption

Hydroxyurea is readily absorbed after oral administration. Peak plasma levels are reached in 1-4 hours after an oral dose. With increasing doses, disproportionately greater mean peak plasma concentrations and AUCs are observed.

There are no data on the effect of food on the absorption of hydroxyurea.

Distribution

Hydroxyurea distributes rapidly and widely in the body with an estimated volume of distribution approximating total body water.

Plasma to ascites fluid ratios range from 2:1 to 7.5:1. Hydroxyurea concentrates in leukocytes and erythrocytes.

Metabolism

Up to 50% of an oral dose undergoes conversion through metabolic pathways that are not fully characterized. In one minor pathway, hydroxyurea may be degraded by urease found in intestinal bacteria. Acetohydroxamic acid was found in the serum of 3 leukemic patients receiving hydroxyurea and may be formed from hydroxylamine resulting from action of urease on hydroxyurea.

Excretion

Excretion of hydroxyurea in humans is a nonlinear process occurring through two pathways. One is saturable, probably hepatic metabolism; the other is first-order renal excretion. In adults with SCA, mean cumulative urinary hydroxyurea excretion was 62% of the administered dose at 8 hours.

Special Populations

Geriatric, Gender, Race

No information is available regarding pharmacokinetic differences due to age, gender or race.

Pediatric

No pharmacokinetic data are available in pediatric patients treated with hydroxyurea for SCA.

Renal Insufficiency

There are no data that support specific guidance for dosage adjustment in patients with renal impairment. As renal excretion is a pathway of elimination, consideration should be given to decreasing the dosage of hydroxyurea in patients with renal impairment. Close monitoring of hematologic parameters is advised in these patients.

Hepatic Insufficiency

There are no data that support specific guidance for dosage adjustment in patients with hepatic impairment. Close monitoring of hematologic parameters is advised in these patients.

Drug Interactions

There are no data on concomitant use of hydroxyurea with other drugs in humans.

HYDREA

Mechanism of Action

The precise mechanism by which hydroxyurea produces its antineoplastic effects cannot, at present, be described. However, the reports of various studies in tissue culture in rats and man lend support to the hypothesis that hydroxyurea causes an immediate inhibition of DNA synthesis without interfering with the synthesis of ribonucleic acid or of protein. This hypothesis explains why, under certain conditions, hydroxyurea may induce teratogenic effects.

Three mechanisms of action have been postulated for the increased effectiveness of concomitant use of hydroxyurea therapy with irradiation on squamous cell (epidermoid) carcinomas of the head and neck. *In vitro* studies utilizing Chinese hamster cells suggest that hydroxyurea (1) is lethal to normally radioresistant S-stage cells, and (2) holds other cells of the cell cycle in the G1 or pre-DNA synthesis stage where they are most susceptible to the effects of irradiation. The third mechanism of action has been theorized on the basis of *in vitro* studies of HeLa cells: it appears that hydroxyurea, by inhibition of DNA synthesis, hinders the normal repair process of cells damaged but not killed by irradiation, thereby decreasing their survival rate; RNA and protein syntheses have shown no alteration.

Pharmacokinetics

Absorption

Hydroxyurea is readily absorbed after oral administration. Peak plasma levels are reached in 1-4 hours after an oral dose. With increasing doses, disproportionately greater mean peak plasma concentrations and AUCs are observed.

There are no data on the effect of food on the absorption of hydroxyurea.

Distribution

Hydroxyurea distributes rapidly and widely in the body with an estimated volume of distribution approximating total body water.

Plasma to ascites fluid ratios range from 2:1 to 7.5:1. Hydroxyurea concentrates in leukocytes and erythrocytes.

Metabolism

Up to 50% of an oral dose undergoes conversion through metabolic pathways that are not fully characterized. In one minor pathway, hydroxyurea may be degraded by urease found in intestinal bacteria. Acetohydroxamic acid was found in the serum of 3 leukemic patients receiving hydroxyurea and may be formed from hydroxylamine resulting from action of urease on hydroxyurea.

Excretion

Excretion of hydroxyurea in humans is a nonlinear process occurring through two pathways. One is saturable, probably hepatic metabolism; the other is first-order renal excretion.

Special Populations

Geriatric, Gender, Race

No information is available regarding pharmacokinetic differences due to age, gender or race.

Pediatric

No pharmacokinetic data are available in pediatric patients treated with hydroxyurea.

Renal Insufficiency

There are no data that support specific guidance for dosage adjustment in patients with renal impairment. As renal excretion is a pathway of elimination, consideration should be given to decreasing the dosage of hydroxyurea in patients with renal impairment. Close monitoring of hematologic parameters is advised in these patients.

Hepatic Insufficiency

There are no data that support specific guidance for dosage adjustment in patients with hepatic impairment. Close monitoring of hematologic parameters is advised in these patients.

Drug Interactions

There are no data on concomitant use of hydroxyurea with other drugs in humans.

H

INDICATIONS AND USAGE

DROXIA

Droxia is indicated to reduce the frequency of painful crises and to reduce the need for blood transfusions in adult patients with sickle cell anemia with recurrent moderate to severe painful crises (generally at least 3 during the preceding 12 months).

HYDREA

Significant tumor response to Hydrea has been demonstrated in melanoma, resistant chronic myelocytic leukemia, and recurrent, metastatic, or inoperable carcinoma of the ovary.

Hydroxyurea used concomitantly with irradiation therapy is intended for use in the local control of primary squamous cell (epidermoid) carcinomas of the head and neck, excluding the lip.

NON-FDA APPROVED INDICATIONS

Non-FDA approved uses of hydroxyurea include the treatment of polycythemia vera and essential thrombocytopenia.

CONTRAINDICATIONS

DROXIA

Droxia is contraindicated in patients who have demonstrated a previous hypersensitivity to hydroxyurea or any other component of its formulation.

HYDREA

Hydroxyurea is contraindicated in patients with marked bone marrow depression, *i.e.,* leukopenia (<2500 WBC) or thrombocytopenia (<100,000), or severe anemia.

Hydrea is contraindicated in patients who have demonstrated a previous hypersensitivity to hydroxyurea or any other component of its formulation.

WARNINGS

DROXIA

Droxia is a cytotoxic and myelosuppressive agent. Droxia should not be given if bone marrow function is markedly depressed, as indicated by neutrophils below 2000 $cells/mm^3$; a platelet count below $80,000/mm^3$; a hemoglobin level below 4.5 g/dl; or reticulocytes below $80,000/mm^3$ when the hemoglobin concentration is below 9 g/dl. Neutropenia is generally the first and most common manifestation of hematologic suppression. (See DOSAGE AND ADMINISTRATION.) Thrombocytopenia and anemia occur less often, and are seldom seen without a preceding leukopenia. Recovery from myelosuppression is usually rapid when therapy is interrupted. Droxia causes macrocytosis, which may mask the incidental development of folic acid deficiency. Prophylactic administration of folic acid is recommended.

Hydroxyurea should be used with caution in patients with renal dysfunction. (See DOSAGE AND ADMINISTRATION.)

Fatal and nonfatal pancreatitis have occurred in HIV-infected patients during therapy with hydroxyurea and didanosine, with or without stavudine. Hepatotoxicity and hepatic failure resulting in death have been reported during post-marketing surveillance in HIV-infected patients treated with hydroxyurea and other antiretroviral agents. Fatal hepatic events were reported most often in patients treated with the combination of hydroxyurea, didanosine, and stavudine. Peripheral neuropathy, which was severe in some cases, has been reported in HIV-infected patients receiving hydroxyurea in combination with antiretroviral agents, including didanosine, with or without stavudine.

Carcinogenesis and Mutagenesis

See BOXED WARNING.

Hydroxyurea is genotoxic in a wide range of test systems and is thus presumed to be a human carcinogen. In patients receiving long-term hydroxyurea for myeloproliferative disorders, such as polycythemia vera and thrombocythemia, secondary leukemia has been reported. It is unknown whether this leukemogenic effect is secondary to hydroxyurea or is associated with the patients' underlying disease. Skin cancer has also been reported in patients receiving long-term hydroxyurea.

Conventional long-term studies to evaluate the carcinogenic potential of Droxia have not been performed. However, intraperitoneal administration of 125-250 mg/kg hydroxyurea (about 0.6-1.2 times the maximum recommended human oral daily dose on a mg/m^2 basis) twice weekly for 6 months to female rats increased the incidence of mammary tumors in rats surviving to 18 months compared to control. Hydroxyurea is mutagenic *in vitro* to bacteria, fungi, protozoa, and mammalian cells. Hydroxyurea is clastogenic *in vitro* (hamster cells, human lymphoblasts) and *in vivo* (SCE assay in rodents, mouse micronucleus assay). Hydroxyurea causes the transformation of rodent embryo cells to a tumorigenic phenotype.

Pregnancy

Droxia can cause fetal harm when administered to a pregnant woman. Hydroxyurea has been demonstrated to be a potent teratogen in a wide variety of animal models, including mice, hamsters, cats, miniature swine, dogs and monkeys at doses within 1-fold of the human dose given on a mg/m^2 basis. Hydroxyurea is embryotoxic and causes fetal malformations (partially ossified cranial bones, absence of eye sockets, hydrocephaly, bipartite sternebrae, missing lumbar vertebrae) at 180 mg/kg/day (about 0.8 times the maximum recommended human daily dose on a mg/m^2 basis) in rats and at 30 mg/kg/day (about 0.3 times the maximum recommended human daily dose on a mg/m^2 basis) in rabbits. Embryotoxicity was characterized by decreased fetal viability, reduced live litter sizes, and developmental delays. Hydroxyurea crosses the placenta. Single doses of ≥375 mg/kg (about 1.7 times the maximum recommended human daily dose on a mg/m^2 basis) to rats caused growth retardation and impaired learning ability. There are no adequate and well-controlled studies in pregnant women. If this drug is used during pregnancy or if the patient becomes pregnant while taking this drug, the patient should be apprised of the potential harm to the fetus. Women of childbearing potential should be advised to avoid becoming pregnant.

HYDREA

Treatment with hydroxyurea should not be initiated if bone marrow function is markedly depressed (see CONTRAINDICATIONS). Bone marrow suppression may occur, and leukopenia is generally its first and most common manifestation. Thrombocytopenia and anemia occur less often, and are seldom seen without a preceding leukopenia. However, the recovery from myelosuppression is rapid when therapy is interrupted. It should be borne in mind that bone marrow depression is more likely in patients who have previously received radiotherapy or cytotoxic cancer chemotherapeutic agents; hydroxyurea should be used cautiously in such patients.

Patients who have received irradiation therapy in the past may have an exacerbation of postirradiation erythema.

Fatal and nonfatal pancreatitis have occurred in HIV-infected patients during therapy with hydroxyurea and didanosine, with or without stavudine. Hepatotoxicity and hepatic failure resulting in death have been reported during post-marketing surveillance in HIV-infected patients treated with hydroxyurea and other antiretroviral agents. Fatal hepatic events were reported most often in patients treated with the combination of hydroxyurea, didanosine, and stavudine. Peripheral neuropathy, which was severe in some cases, has been reported in HIV-infected patients receiving hydroxyurea in combination with antiretroviral agents, including didanosine, with or without stavudine.

Severe anemia must be corrected before initiating therapy with hydroxyurea.

Erythrocytic abnormalities: megaloblastic erythropoiesis, which is self-limiting, is often seen early in the course of hydroxyurea therapy. The morphologic change resembles pernicious anemia, but is not related to vitamin B_{12} or folic acid deficiency. Hydroxyurea may also delay plasma iron clearance and reduce the rate of iron utilization by erythrocytes, but it does not appear to alter the red blood cell survival time.

Hydroxyurea should be used with caution in patients with marked renal dysfunction.

Elderly patients may be more sensitive to the effects of hydroxyurea, and may require a lower dose regimen.

In patients receiving long-term hydroxyurea for myeloproliferative disorders, such as polycythemia vera and thrombocythemia, secondary leukemia has been reported. It is unknown whether this leukemogenic effect is secondary to hydroxyurea or associated with the patients' underlying disease.

Carcinogenesis and Mutagenesis

Hydroxyurea is genotoxic in a wide range of test systems and is thus presumed to be a human carcinogen. In patients receiving long-term hydroxyurea for myeloproliferative disorders, such as polycythemia vera and and thrombocythemia, secondary leukemia has been reported. It is unknown whether this leukemogenic effect is secondary to hydroxyurea or is associated with the patients' underlying disease. Skin cancer has also been reported in patients receiving long-term hydroxyurea.

Conventional long-term studies to evaluate the carcinogenic potential of hydroxyurea have not been performed. However, intraperitoneal administration of 125-250 mg/kg hydroxyurea (about 0.6-1.2 times the maximum recommended human oral daily dose on a mg/m^2 basis) twice weekly for 6 months to female rats increased the incidence of mammary tumors in rats surviving to 18 months compared to control. Hydroxyurea is mutagenic *in vitro* to bacteria, fungi, protozoa, and mammalian cells. Hydroxyurea is clastogenic *in vitro* (hamster cells, human lymphoblasts) and *in vivo* (SCE assay in rodents, mouse micronucleus assay). Hydroxyurea causes the transformation of rodent embryo cells to a tumorigenic phenotype.

Pregnancy

Drugs which affect DNA synthesis, such as hydroxyurea, may be potential mutagenic agents. The physician should carefully consider this possibility before administering this drug to male or female patients who may contemplate conception.

Hydrea can cause fetal harm when administered to a pregnant woman. Hydroxyurea has been demonstrated to be a potent teratogen in a wide variety of animal models, including mice, hamsters, cats, miniature swine, dogs and monkeys at doses within 1-fold of the human dose given on a mg/m^2 basis. Hydroxyurea is embryotoxic and causes fetal malformations (partially ossified cranial bones, absence of eye sockets, hydrocephaly, bipartite sternebrae, missing lumbar vertebrae) at 180 mg/kg/day (about 0.8 times the maximum recommended human daily dose on a mg/m^2 basis) in rats and at 30 mg/kg/day (about 0.3 times the maximum recommended human daily dose on a mg/m^2 basis) in rabbits. Embryotoxicity was characterized by decreased fetal viability, reduced live litter sizes, and developmental delays. Hydroxyurea crosses the placenta. Single doses of ≥375 mg/kg (about 1.7 times the maximum recommended human daily dose on a mg/m^2 basis) to rats caused growth retardation and impaired learning ability. There are no adequate and well-controlled studies in pregnant women. If this drug is used during pregnancy or if the patient becomes pregnant while taking this drug, the patient should be apprised of the potential harm to the fetus. Women of childbearing potential should be advised to avoid becoming pregnant.

PRECAUTIONS

DROXIA

Therapy with Droxia requires close supervision. Some patients treated at the recommended initial dose of 15 mg/kg/day have experienced severe or life-threatening myelosuppression, requiring interruption of treatment and dose reduction. The hematologic status of the patient, as well as kidney and liver function should be determined prior to, and repeatedly during treatment. Treatment should be interrupted if neutrophil levels fall to <2000/mm^3; platelets fall to <80,000/mm^3; hemoglobin declines to less than 4.5 g/dl; or if reticulocytes fall below 80,000/mm^3 when the hemoglobin concentration is below 9 g/dl. Following recovery, treatment may be resumed at lower doses (see DOSAGE AND ADMINISTRATION).

Patients must be able to follow directions regarding drug administration and their monitoring and care.

Hydroxyurea is not indicated for the treatment of HIV infection; however, if HIV-infected patients are treated with hydroxyurea, and in particular, in combination with didanosine and/or stavudine, close monitoring for signs and symptoms of pancreatitis and hepatotoxicity is recommended. Patients who develop signs and symptoms of pancreatitis or hepatotoxicity should permanently discontinue therapy with hydroxyurea. (See WARNINGS and ADVERSE REACTIONS.)

Carcinogenesis, Mutagenesis, and Impairment of Fertility

See WARNINGS and BOXED WARNING for Carcinogenesis and Mutagenesis information.

Impairment of Fertility

Hydroxyurea administered to male rats at 60 mg/kg/day (about 0.3 times the maximum recommended human daily dose on a mg/m^2 basis) produced testicular atrophy, decreased spermatogenesis, and significantly reduced their ability to impregnate females.

Pregnancy Category D

See WARNINGS.

Nursing Mothers

Hydroxyurea is excreted in human milk. Because of the potential for serious adverse reactions with hydroxyurea, a decision should be made either to discontinue nursing or to discontinue the drug, taking into account the importance of the drug to the mother.

Pediatric Use

Safety and effectiveness in pediatric patients have not been established.

Information for the Patient

See the Patient Information that is distributed with the prescription for complete instructions.

Patients should be reminded that this medication must be handled with care. People who are not taking hydroxyurea should not be exposed to it. If the powder from the capsule is spilled, it should be wiped up immediately with a damp disposable towel and discarded in a closed container, such as a plastic bag. The medication should be kept away from children and pets.

The necessity of monitoring blood counts every 2 weeks, throughout the duration of therapy, should be emphasized. For additional information, see the Patient Information that is distributed with the prescription.

HYDREA

Therapy with hydroxyurea requires close supervision. The complete status of the blood, including bone marrow examination, if indicated, as well as kidney function and liver function should be determined prior to, and repeatedly during, treatment. The determination of the hemoglobin level, total leukocyte counts, and platelet counts should be performed at least once a week throughout the course of hydroxyurea therapy. If the white blood cell count decreases to less than 2500/mm^3, or the platelet count to less than 100,000/mm^3, therapy should be interrupted until the values rise significantly toward normal levels. Severe anemia, if it occurs, should be managed without interrupting hydroxyurea therapy.

Hydroxyurea is not indicated for the treatment of HIV infection; however, if HIV-infected patients are treated with hydroxyurea, and in particular, in combination with didanosine and/or stavudine, close monitoring for signs and symptoms of pancreatitis and hepatotoxicity is recommended. Patients who develop signs and symptoms of pancreatitis or hepatotoxicity should permanently discontinue therapy with hydroxyurea. (See WARNINGS and ADVERSE REACTIONS.)

Carcinogenesis, Mutagenesis, and Impairment of Fertility

See WARNINGS for Carcinogenesis and Mutagenesis information.

Impairment of Fertility

Hydroxyurea administered to male rats at 60 mg/kg/day (about 0.3 times the maximum recommended human daily dose on a mg/m^2 basis) produced testicular atrophy, decreased spermatogenesis, and significantly reduced their ability to impregnate females.

Pregnancy Category D

See WARNINGS.

Nursing Mothers

Hydroxyurea is excreted in human milk.

Because of the potential for serious adverse reactions with hydroxyurea, a decision should be made whether to discontinue nursing or to discontinue the drug, taking into account the importance of the drug to the mother.

Pediatric Use

Safety and effectiveness in pediatric patients have not been established.

Information for the Patient

Hydrea is a medication that must be handled with care. People who are not taking Hydrea should not be exposed to it. If the powder from the capsule is spilled, it should be wiped up immediately with a damp disposable towel and discarded in a closed container, such as a plastic bag. The medication should be kept away from children and pets.

DRUG INTERACTIONS

DROXIA

Prospective studies on the potential for hydroxyurea to interact with other drugs have not been performed.

HYDREA

Prospective studies on the potential for hydroxyurea to interact with other drugs have not been performed.

Concurrent use of hydroxyurea and other myelosuppressive agents or radiation therapy may increase the likelihood of bone marrow depression or other adverse events. (See WARNINGS and ADVERSE REACTIONS.)

Since hydroxyurea may raise the serum uric acid level, dosage adjustment of uricosuric medication may be necessary.

ADVERSE REACTIONS

DROXIA

Sickle Cell Anemia

In patients treated for sickle cell anemia in the Multicenter Study of Hydroxyurea in Sickle Cell Anemia,[1] the most common adverse reactions were hematologic, with neutropenia, and low reticulocyte and platelet levels necessitating temporary cessation in almost all patients. Hematologic recovery usually occurred in 2 weeks.

Non-hematologic events that possibly were associated with treatment include hair loss, skin rash, fever, gastrointestinal disturbances, weight gain, bleeding and parvovirus B-19 infection; however, these non-hematologic events occurred with similar frequencies in the hydroxyurea and placebo treatment groups. Melanonychia has also been reported in patients receiving Droxia for SCA.

Other

Adverse events associated with the use of hydroxyurea in the treatment of neoplastic diseases, in addition to hematologic effects include: gastrointestinal symptoms (stomatitis, anorexia, nausea, vomiting, diarrhea, and constipation), and dermatological reactions such as maculopapular rash, skin ulceration, dermatomyositis-like skin changes, peripheral erythema and facial erythema. Hyperpigmentation, atrophy of skin and nails, scaling and violet papules have been observed in some patients after several years of long-term daily maintenance therapy with hydroxyurea. Skin cancer has been reported. Dysuria and alopecia occur very rarely. Large doses may produce moderate drowsiness. Neurological disturbances have occurred extremely rarely and were limited to headache, dizziness, disorientation, hallucinations, and convulsions. Hydroxyurea occasionally may cause temporary impairment of renal tubular function accompanied by elevations in serum uric acid, BUN, and creatinine levels. Abnormal BSP retention has been reported. Fever, chills, malaise, edema, asthenia, and elevation of hepatic enzymes have also been reported.

The association of hydroxyurea with the development of acute pulmonary reactions consisting of diffuse pulmonary infiltrates, fever and dyspnea has been rarely reported. Pulmonary fibrosis also has been reported rarely.

Fatal and nonfatal pancreatitis and hepatotoxicity, and severe peripheral neuropathy have been reported in HIV-infected patients who received hydroxyurea in combination with antiretroviral agents, in particular, didanosine plus stavudine. Patients treated with hydroxyurea in combination with didanosine, stavudine, and indinavir in study ACTG 5025 showed a median decline in CD4 cells of approximately 100/mm^3. (See WARNINGS and PRECAUTIONS.)

HYDREA

Adverse reactions have been primarily bone marrow depression (leukopenia, anemia, and occasionally thrombocytopenia), and less frequently gastrointestinal symptoms (stomatitis, anorexia, nausea, vomiting, diarrhea, and constipation), and dermatological reactions such as maculopapular rash, skin ulceration, dermatomyositis-like skin changes, peripheral, and facial erythema. Hyperpigmentation, atrophy of skin and nails, scaling and violet papules have been observed in some patients after several years of long-term daily maintenance therapy with Hydrea. Skin cancer has been reported. Dysuria and alopecia occur very rarely. Large doses may produce moderate drowsiness. Neurological disturbances have occurred extremely rarely and were limited to headache, dizziness, disorientation, hallucinations, and convulsions. Hydrea occasionally may cause temporary impairment of renal tubular function accompanied by elevations in serum uric acid, BUN, and creatinine levels. Abnormal BSP retention has been reported. Fever, chills, malaise, edema, asthenia, and elevation of hepatic enzymes have also been reported.

Adverse reactions observed with combined hydroxyurea and irradiation therapy are similar to those reported with the use of hydroxyurea or radiation treatment alone. These effects primarily include bone marrow depression (anemia and leukopenia), gastric irritation, and mucositis. Almost all patients receiving an adequate course of combined hydroxyurea and irradiation therapy will demonstrate concurrent leukopenia. Platelet depression (<100,000 cells/mm^3) has occurred rarely and only in the presence of marked leukopenia. Hydrea may potentiate some adverse reaction usually seen with irradiation alone, such as gastric distress and mucositis.

The association of hydroxyurea with the development of acute pulmonary reactions consisting of diffuse pulmonary infiltrates, fever and dyspnea has been rarely reported. Pulmonary fibrosis also has been reported rarely.

Fatal and nonfatal pancreatitis and hepatotoxicity, and severe peripheral neuropathy have been reported in HIV-infected patients who received hydroxyurea in combination with antiretroviral agents, in particular, didanosine plus stavudine. Patients treated with hydroxyurea in combination with didanosine, stavudine, and indinavir in study ACTG 5025 showed a median decline in CD4 cells of approximately 100/mm^3. (See WARNINGS and PRECAUTIONS.)

DOSAGE AND ADMINISTRATION

DROXIA

Dosage should be based on the patient's actual or ideal weight, whichever is less. The initial dose of Droxia is 15 mg/kg/day as a single dose. The patient's blood count must be monitored every 2 weeks. (See WARNINGS.)

If blood counts are in an **acceptable range***, the dose may be increased by 5 mg/kg/day every 12 weeks until a maximum tolerated dose (the highest dose that does not produce **toxic†** blood counts over 24 consecutive weeks), or 35 mg/kg/day, is reached.

If blood counts are between the **acceptable range*** and **toxic†**, the dose is not increased.

If blood counts are considered **toxic†**, Droxia should be discontinued until hematologic recovery. Treatment may then be resumed after reducing the dose by 2.5 mg/kg/day from the dose associated with hematologic toxicity. Droxia may then be titrated up or down, every 12 weeks in 2.5 mg/kg/day increments, until the patient is at a stable dose that does not result in hematologic toxicity for 24 weeks. Any dosage on which a patient develops hematologic toxicity twice should not be tried again.

***acceptable range =**
- neutrophils ≥2500 cells/mm^3,
- platelets ≥95,000/mm^3,
- hemoglobin >5.3 g/dl and
- reticulocytes ≥95,000/mm^3 if the hemoglobin concentration <9 g/dl.

†toxic =
- neutrophils <2000 cells/mm^3,
- platelets <80,000/mm^3,
- hemoglobin <4.5 g/dl and
- reticulocytes <80,000/mm^3 if the hemoglobin concentration <9 g/dl.

Renal Insufficiency

There are no data that support specific guidance for dosage adjustment in patients with renal impairment. As renal excretion is a pathway of elimination, consideration should be given to decreasing the dosage of Droxia in patients with renal impairment. Close monitoring of hematologic parameters is advised in these patients.

Hepatic Insufficiency

There are no data that support specific guidance for dosage adjustment in patients with hepatic impairment. Close monitoring of hematologic parameters is advised in these patients.

Procedures for proper handling and disposal of cytotoxic drugs should be considered. Several guidelines on this subject have been published.[2-8] There is no general agreement that all of the procedures recommended in the guidelines are necessary or appropriate.

HYDREA

Procedures for proper handling and disposal of antineoplastic drugs should be considered. Several guidelines on this subject have been published.[9-15] There is no general agreement that all of the procedures recommended in the guidelines are necessary or appropriate.

Because of the rarity of melanoma, resistant chronic myelocytic leukemia, carcinoma of the ovary, and carcinomas of the head and neck in pediatric patients, dosage regimens have not been established.

All dosage should be based on the patient's actual or ideal weight, whichever is less. Concurrent use of hydroxyurea with other myelosuppressive agents may require adjustment of dosages.

Solid Tumors

Intermittent Therapy

80 mg/kg administered orally as a *single dose* every *third* day.

Continuous Therapy

20-30 mg/kg administered orally as a *single dose daily.*

Concomitant Therapy With Irradiation

Carcinoma of the Head and Neck: 80 mg/kg administered orally as a *single dose* every *third* day.

Administration of hydroxyurea should begin at least 7 days before initiation of irradiation and continued during radiotherapy as well as indefinitely afterwards provided that the patient may be kept under adequate observation and evidences no unusual or severe reactions.

Resistant Chronic Myelocytic Leukemia

Until the intermittent therapy regimen has been evaluated, CONTINUOUS therapy (20-30 mg/kg administered orally as a *single dose daily*) is recommended.

An adequate trial period for determining the antineoplastic effectiveness of hydroxyurea is 6 weeks of therapy. When there is regression in tumor size or arrest in tumor growth, therapy should be continued indefinitely. Therapy should be interrupted if the white blood cell count drops below 2500/mm^3, or the platelet count below 100,000/mm^3. In these cases, the counts should be re-evaluated after 3 days, and therapy resumed when the counts rise significantly toward normal values. Since the hematopoietic rebound is prompt, it is usually necessary to omit only a few doses. If prompt rebound has not occurred during combined

Hydrea and irradiation therapy, irradiation may also be interrupted. However, the need for postponement of irradiation has been rare; radiotherapy has usually been continued using the recommended dosage and technique. Severe anemia, if it occurs, should be corrected without interrupting hydroxyurea therapy. Because hematopoiesis may be compromised by extensive irradiation or by other antineoplastic agents, it is recommended that hydroxyurea be administered cautiously to patients who have recently received extensive radiation therapy or chemotherapy with other cytotoxic drugs.

Pain or discomfort from inflammation of the mucous membranes at the irradiated site (mucositis) is usually controlled by measures such as topical anesthetics and orally administered analgesics. If the reaction is severe, hydroxyurea therapy may be temporarily interrupted; if it is extremely severe, irradiation dosage may, in addition, be temporarily postponed. However, it has rarely been necessary to terminate these therapies.

Severe gastric distress, such as nausea, vomiting, and anorexia, resulting from combined therapy may usually be controlled by temporary interruption of hydroxyurea administration.

Renal Insufficiency

There are no data that support specific guidance for dosage adjustments in patients with renal impairment. As renal excretion is a pathway of elimination, consideration should be given to decreasing the dosage of Hydrea in patients with renal impairment. Close monitoring of hematologic parameters is advised in these patients.

Hepatic Insufficiency

There are no data that support specific guidance for dosage adjustment in patients with hepatic impairment. Close monitoring of hematologic parameters is advised in these patients.

H

ANIMAL PHARMACOLOGY

HYDREA

The oral LD_{50} of hydroxyurea is 7330 mg/kg in mice and 5780 mg/kg in rats, given as a single dose.

In subacute and chronic toxicity studies in the rat, the most consistent pathological findings were an apparent dose-related mild to moderate bone marrow hypoplasia as well as pulmonary congestion and mottling of the lungs. At the highest dosage levels (1260 mg/kg/day for 37 days then 2520 mg/kg/day for 40 days), testicular atrophy with absence of spermatogenesis occurred; in several animals, hepatic cell damage with fatty metamorphosis was noted. In the dog, mild to marked bone marrow depression was a consistent finding except at the lower dosage levels. Additionally, at the higher dose levels (140-420 mg or 140-1260 mg/kg/week given 3 or 7 days weekly for 12 weeks), growth retardation, slightly increased blood glucose values, and hemosiderosis of the liver or spleen were found; reversible spermatogenic arrest was noted. In the monkey, bone marrow depression, lymphoid atrophy of the spleen, and degenerative changes in the epithelium of the small and large intestines were found. At the higher, often lethal, doses (400-800 mg/kg/day for 7-15 days), hemorrhage and congestion were found in the lungs, brain, and urinary tract. Cardiovascular effects (changes in heart rate, blood pressure, orthostatic hypotension, EKG changes) and hematological changes (slight hemolysis, slight methemoglobinemia) were observed in some species of laboratory animals at doses exceeding clinical levels.

HOW SUPPLIED

DROXIA

200 mg Capsules: The cap and body are opaque blue-green. The capsule is marked in black ink on both the cap and body with "DROXIA" and "6335".

300 mg Capsules: The cap and body are opaque purple. The capsule is marked in black ink on both the cap and body with "DROXIA" and "6336".

400 mg Capsules: The cap and body are opaque reddish-orange. The capsule is marked in black ink on both the cap and body with "DROXIA"and "6337".

Storage: Store at 25°C (77°F); excursions permitted to 15-30°C (59-86°F). Keep tightly closed.

HYDREA

Hydrea is supplied in 500 mg capsules. The cap is opaque green and the body is opaque pink. They are imprinted on both sections in black ink with "HYDREA" and "830".

Storage: Store at 25°C (77°F); excursions permitted to 15-30°C (59-86°F). Keep tightly closed.

PRODUCT LISTING - RATED THERAPEUTICALLY EQUIVALENT

Capsule - Oral - 200 mg

60's	$54.00	DROXIA, Bristol-Myers Squibb	00003-6335-17

Capsule - Oral - 300 mg

60's	$56.76	DROXIA, Bristol-Myers Squibb	00003-6336-17

Capsule - Oral - 400 mg

60's	$54.00	DROXIA, Bristol-Myers Squibb	00003-6337-17

Capsule - Oral - 500 mg

30's	$42.57	HYDREA, Allscripts Pharmaceutical Company	54569-0378-02
60's	$85.16	HYDREA, Allscripts Pharmaceutical Company	54569-0378-01
100's	$40.59	GENERIC, Richmond Pharmaceuticals	54738-0547-01
100's	$116.65	FEDERAL UPPER LIMIT, H.C.F.A. F F P	99999-1512-01
100's	$127.70	GENERIC, Major Pharmaceuticals Inc	00904-5394-60
100's	$127.73	GENERIC, Roxane Laboratories Inc	00054-2247-25
100's	$127.73	GENERIC, Barr Laboratories Inc	00555-0882-02
100's	$127.73	GENERIC, Qualitest Products Inc	00603-3946-21
100's	$127.73	GENERIC, Par Pharmaceutical Inc	49884-0724-01
100's	$127.73	GENERIC, Duramed Pharmaceuticals Inc	51285-0548-02
100's	$130.58	GENERIC, United Research Laboratories, Inc.	00677-1680-01
100's	$132.27	GENERIC, Roxane Laboratories Inc	00054-8247-25
100's	$141.93	HYDREA, Bristol-Myers Squibb	00003-0830-50
100's	$141.93	HYDREA, Allscripts Pharmaceutical Company	54569-0378-00

Tablet - Oral - 1000 mg

60's	$150.00	MYLOCEL, Mgi Pharma Inc	58063-0979-09

Hydroxyzine (001513)

Categories: Alcohol withdrawal; Anxiety; Delirium tremens; Dermatitis, atopic; Dermatitis, contact; Nausea; Pain, adjunct; Pruritus; Urticaria, chronic; Vomiting; FDA Approved 1956 Apr; Pregnancy Category C

Drug Classes: Antiemetics/antivertigo; Antihistamines, H1; Anxiolytics; Sedatives/hypnotics

Brand Names: **Atarax**; Hyzine; Neucalm 50; Vistacot; Vistaril; Vistazine

Foreign Brand Availability: AH3 N (Germany); Abacus (Thailand); Apo-Hydroxyzine (Canada); Atarax P (Japan); Aterax (South-Africa); Bestalin (Indonesia); Bobsule (Japan); Cedar (Colombia); Centilax (Korea); Cerax (Thailand); Darax (Thailand); Disron P (Japan); Dormirex (Colombia); Drazine (Thailand); Hiderax (Colombia); Histan (Thailand); Hizin (Thailand); Iremofar (Greece); Iterax (Indonesia; Philippines); Novohydroxyzin (Canada); Otarex (Israel); Paxistil (Belgium); Phymorax (Singapore); Postarax (Thailand); R-Rax (Thailand); Trandozine (Thailand); Tranquijust (Japan); Unamine (Thailand)

Cost of Therapy: $91.97 (Pruritis; Atarax; 25 mg; 3 tablets/day; 30 day supply)
$6.26 (Pruritis; Generic Tablets; 25 mg; 3 tablets/day; 30 day supply)
$86.53 (Pruritis; Vistaril; 25 mg; 3 capsules/day; 30 day supply)
$7.16 (Pruritis; Generic Capsules; 25 mg; 3 capsules/day; 30 day supply)

HCFA JCODE(S): J3410 up to 25 mg IM

INTRAMUSCULAR

DESCRIPTION

Note: The trade names have been used throughout this monograph for clarity.

For Intramuscular Use Only.

Hydroxyzine hydrochloride is designated chemically as 1-(p-chlorobenzhydryl) 4-[2-(2-hydroxyethoxy)ethyl] piperazine dihydrochloride.

TABLE 1

	Dosage Strength	
	25 mg/1 ml	50 mg/1 ml & 100 mg/2 ml
Hydroxyzine hydrochloride	25 mg/ml	50 mg/ml
Benzyl alcohol	0.9%	0.9%
	Sodium hydroxide to adjust to optimum pH	

CLINICAL PHARMACOLOGY

MECHANISM OF ACTION

Vistaril is unrelated chemically to phenothiazine, reserpine, and meprobamate. Hydroxyzine has demonstrated its clinical effectiveness in the chemotherapeutic aspect of the total management of neuroses and emotional disturbances manifested by anxiety, tension, agitation, apprehension or confusion.

Hydroxyzine has been shown clinically to be a rapid-acting true ataraxic with a wide margin of safety. It induces a calming effect in anxious, tense, psychoneurotic adults and also in anxious, hyperkinetic children without impairing mental alertness. It is not a cortical depressant, but its action may be due to a suppression of activity in certain key regions of the subcortical area of the central nervous system.

Primary skeletal muscle relaxation has been demonstrated experimentally.

Hydroxyzine has been shown experimentally to have antispasmodic properties, apparently mediated through interference with the mechanism that responds to spasmogenic agents such as serotonin, acetylcholine, and histamine.

Antihistaminic effects have been demonstrated experimentally and confirmed clinically.

An antiemetic effect, both by the apomorphine test and the veriloid test, has been demonstrated. Pharmacological and clinical studies indicate that hydroxyzine in therapeutic dosage does not increase gastric secretion or acidity and in most cases provides mild antisecretory benefits.

INDICATIONS AND USAGE

The total management of anxiety, tension, and psychomotor agitation in conditions of emotional stress requires in most instances a combined approach of psychotherapy and chemotherapy. Hydroxyzine has been found to be particularly useful for this latter phase of therapy in its ability to render the disturbed patient more amenable to psychotherapy in long term treatment of the psychoneurotic and psychotic, although it should not be used as the sole treatment of psychosis or of clearly demonstrated cases of depression.

Hydroxyzine is also useful in alleviating the manifestations of anxiety and tension as in the preparation for dental procedures and in acute emotional problems. It has also been recommended for the management of anxiety associated with organic disturbances and as adjunctive therapy in alcoholism and allergic conditions with strong emotional overlay, such as in asthma, chronic urticaria, and pruritus.

Vistaril intramuscular solution is useful in treating the following types of patients when intramuscular administration is indicated:

1. The acutely disturbed or hysterical patient.
2. The acute or chronic alcoholic with anxiety withdrawal symptoms or delirium tremens.
3. As pre- and postoperative and pre- and postpartum adjunctive medication to permit reduction in narcotic dosage, allay anxiety and control emesis.

Vistaril has also demonstrated effectiveness in controlling nausea and vomiting, excluding nausea and vomiting of pregnancy. (See CONTRAINDICATIONS.)

In prepartum states, the reduction in narcotic requirement effected by hydroxyzine is of particular benefit to both mother and neonate.

Hydroxyzine benefits the cardiac patient by its ability to allay the associated anxiety and apprehension attendant to certain types of heart disease. Hydroxyzine is not known to interfere with the action of digitalis in any way and may be used concurrently with this agent.

The effectiveness of hydroxyzine in long term use, that is, more than 4 months, has not been assessed by systematic clinical studies. The physician should reassess periodically the usefulness of the drug for the individual patient.

CONTRAINDICATIONS

Hydroxyzine hydrochloride intramuscular solution is intended only for intramuscular administration and should not, under any circumstances, be injected subcutaneously, intra-arterially, or intravenously.

This drug is contraindicated for patients who have shown a previous hypersensitivity to it.

Hydroxyzine, when administered to the pregnant mouse, rat, and rabbit, induced fetal abnormalities in the rat at doses substantially above the human therapeutic range. Clinical data in human beings are inadequate to establish safety in early pregnancy. Until such data are available, hydroxyzine is contraindicated in early pregnancy.

PRECAUTIONS

THE POTENTIATING ACTION OF HYDROXYZINE MUST BE CONSIDERED WHEN THE DRUG IS USED IN CONJUNCTION WITH CENTRAL NERVOUS SYSTEM DEPRESSANTS SUCH AS NARCOTICS, BARBITURATES, AND ALCOHOL. Rarely, cardiac arrests and death have been reported in association with the combined use of hydroxyzine hydrochloride IM and other CNS depressants. Therefore when central nervous system depressants are administered concomitantly with hydroxyzine their dosage should be reduced up to 50%. The efficacy of hydroxyzine as adjunctive pre- and postoperative sedative medication has also been well established, especially as regards its ability to allay anxiety, control emesis, and reduce the amount of narcotic required.

HYDROXYZINE MAY POTENTIATE NARCOTICS AND BARBITURATES, so their use in preanesthetic adjunctive therapy should be modified on an individual basis. Atropine and other belladonna alkaloids are not affected by the drug.

When hydroxyzine is used preoperatively or prepartum, narcotic requirements may be reduced as much as 50%. Thus, when 50 mg of Vistaril intramuscular solution is employed, meperidine dosage may be reduced from 100 mg to 50 mg. The administration of meperidine may result in severe hypotension in the postoperative patient or any individual whose ability to maintain blood pressure has been compromised by a depleted blood volume. Meperidine should be used with great caution and in reduced dosage in patients who are receiving other pre- and/or postoperative medications and in whom there is a risk of respiratory depression, hypotension, and profound sedation or coma occurring. Before using any medications concomitant with hydroxyzine, the manufacturer's prescribing information should be read carefully.

Since drowsiness may occur with the use of this drug, patients should be warned of this possibility and cautioned against driving a car or operating dangerous machinery while taking this drug.

As with all intramuscular preparations, Vistaril intramuscular solution should be injected well within the body of a relatively large muscle. Inadvertent subcutaneous injection may result in significant tissue damage.

Adults: The preferred site is the upper outer quadrant of the buttock, (*i.e.,* gluteus maximus), or the mid-lateral thigh.

Children: It is recommended that intramuscular injections be given preferably in the midlateral muscles of the thigh. In infants and small children the periphery of the upper outer quadrant of the gluteal region should be used only when necessary, such as in burn patients, in order to minimize the possibility of damage to the sciatic nerve.

The deltoid area should be used only if well developed such as in certain adults and older children, and then only with caution to avoid radial nerve injury. Intramuscular injections should not be made into the lower and mid-third of the upper arm. As with all intramuscular injections, aspiration is necessary to help avoid inadvertent injection into a blood vessel.

GERIATRIC USE

A determination has not been made whether controlled clinical studies of Vistaril included sufficient numbers of subjects aged 65 and over to define a difference in response from younger subjects. Other reported clinical experience has not identified differences in responses between the elderly and younger patients. In general, dose selection for an elderly patient should be cautious, usually starting at the low end of the dosing range, reflecting the greater frequency of decreased hepatic, renal or cardiac function, and of concomitant disease or other drug therapy.

The extent of renal excretion of Vistaril has not been determined. Because elderly patients are more likely to have decreased renal function, care should be taken in dose selections.

Sedating drugs may cause confusion and over sedation in the elderly; elderly patients generally should be started on low doses of Vistaril and observed closely.

ADVERSE REACTIONS

Therapeutic doses of hydroxyzine seldom produce impairment of mental alertness. However, drowsiness may occur; if so, it is usually transitory and may disappear in a few days of continued therapy or upon reduction of the dose. Dryness of the mouth may be encountered at higher doses. Extensive clinical use has substantiated the absence of toxic effects on the liver or bone marrow when administered in the recommended doses for over 4 years of uninterrupted therapy. The absence of adverse effects has been further demonstrated in experimental studies in which excessively high doses were administered.

Involuntary motor activity, including rare instances of tremor and convulsions, has been reported, usually with doses considerably higher than those recommended. Continuous therapy with over 1 g/day has been employed in some patients without these effects having been encountered.

DOSAGE AND ADMINISTRATION

The recommended dosages for Vistaril intramuscular solution are listed in TABLE 2.

As with all potent medications, the dosage should be adjusted according to the patient's response to therapy.

TABLE 2

For adult psychiatric and emotional emergencies, including acute alcoholism.	IM: 50-100 mg stat, and q4-6h, prn
Nausea and vomiting excluding nausea and vomiting of pregnancy.	Adults: 25-100 mg IM Children: 0.5 mg/lb body weight IM
Pre- and postoperaive adjunctive medication.	Adults: 25-100 mg IM Children: 0.5 mg/lb body weight IM
Pre- and postpartum adjunctive therapy.	25-100 mg IM

FOR ADDITIONAL INFORMATION OF THE ADMINISTRATION AND SITE OF SELECTION SEE PRECAUTIONS. *Note:* Vistaril intramuscular solution may be administered without further dilution.

Patients may be started on intramuscular therapy when indicated. They should be maintained on oral therapy whenever this route is practicable.

HOW SUPPLIED

Vistaril intramuscular solution is available in:

Multi-Dose Vials: 25 and 50 mg/ml containing 10 ml.

Unit Dose Vials: 1 ml vial containing 50 mg/ml and 2 ml vial containing 100 mg/2 ml.

Storage: Store below 30°C (86°F). Protect from freezing.

H

ORAL

DESCRIPTION

Note: The trade names have been used throughout this monograph for clarity.

ATARAX

Hydroxyzine hydrochloride is designated chemically as 1-(p-chlorobenzhydryl) 4-[2-(2-hydroxyethoxy)-ethyl] piperazine dihydrochloride.

Atarax Tablets

Inert ingredients for the tablets are: acacia; carnauba wax; dibasic calcium phosphate; gelatin; lactose; magnesium stearate; precipitated calcium carbonate; shellac; sucrose; talc; white wax. The 10 mg tablets also contain: sodium hydroxide; starch; titanium dioxide; yellow 6 lake. The 25 mg tablets also contain: starch, velo dark green. The 50 mg tablets also contain: starch; velo yellow. The 100 mg tablets also contain: alginic acid; blue 1; polyethylene glycol; red 3.

Atarax Syrup

The inert ingredients for the syrup are: alcohol; menthol; peppermint oil; sodium benzoate; spearmint oil; sucrose; water.

VISTARIL

Hydroxyzine pamoate is designated chemically as 1-(p-chlorobenzhydryl) 4-[2-(2-hydroxyethoxy)ethyl] diethylenediamine salt of 1,1′-methylene bis(2-hydroxy-3-naphthalene carboxylic acid).

Inert ingredients for the capsule formulations are: hard gelatin capsules (which may contain yellow 10, green 3, yellow 6, red 33, and other inert ingredients); magnesium stearate; sodium lauryl sulfate; starch; sucrose.

Inert ingredients for the oral suspension formulation are: carboxymethylcellulose sodium; lemon flavor; propylene glycol; sorbic acid; sorbitol solution; water.

CLINICAL PHARMACOLOGY

ATARAX

Atarax is unrelated chemically to the phenothiazines, reserpine, meprobamate, or the benzodiazepines.

Atarax is not a cortical depressant, but its action may be due to a suppression of activity in certain key regions of the subcortical area of the central nervous system. Primary skeletal muscle relaxation has been demonstrated experimentally. Bronchodilator activity, and antihistaminic and analgesic effects have been demonstrated experimentally and confirmed clinically. An antiemetic effect, both by the apomorphine test and the veriloid test, has been demonstrated. Pharmacological and clinical studies indicate that hydroxyzine in therapeutic dosage does not increase gastric secretion or acidity and in most cases has mild antisecretory activity. Hydroxyzine is rapidly absorbed from the gastrointestinal tract and Atarax's clinical effects are usually noted within 15-30 minutes after oral administration.

VISTARIL

Vistaril is unrelated chemically to the phenothiazines, reserpine, meprobamate, or the benzodiazepines.

Vistaril is not a cortical depressant, but its action may be due to a suppression of activity in certain key regions of the subcortical area of the central nervous system. Primary skeletal muscle relaxation has been demonstrated experimentally. Bronchodilator activity, and antihistaminic and analgesic effects have been demonstrated experimentally and confirmed clinically. An antiemetic effect, both by the apomorphine test and the veriloid test, has been demonstrated. Pharmacological and clinical studies indicate that hydroxyzine in therapeutic dosage does not increase gastric secretion or acidity and in most cases has mild antisecretory activity. Hydroxyzine is rapidly absorbed from the gastrointestinal tract and Vistaril's clinical effects are usually noted within 15-30 minutes after oral administration.

INDICATIONS AND USAGE

ATARAX

For symptomatic relief of anxiety and tension associated with psychoneurosis and as an adjunct in organic disease states in which anxiety is manifested.

Useful in the management of pruritus due to allergic conditions such as chronic urticaria and atopic and contact dermatoses, and in histamine-mediated pruritus.

As a sedative when used as premedication and following general anesthesia, **hydroxyzine may potentiate meperidine and barbiturates,** so their use in pre-anesthetic adjunctive therapy should be modified on an individual basis. Atropine and other belladonna alkaloids are not affected by the drug. Hydroxyzine is not known to interfere with the action of digitalis in any way and it may be used concurrently with this agent.

The effectiveness of hydroxyzine as an antianxiety agent for long term use, that is more than 4 months, has not been assessed by systematic clinical studies. The physician should reassess periodically the usefulness of the drug for the individual patient.

VISTARIL

For symptomatic relief of anxiety and tension associated with psychoneurosis and as an adjunct in organic disease states in which anxiety is manifested.

Useful in the management of pruritus due to allergic conditions such as chronic urticaria and atopic and contact dermatoses, and in histamine-mediated pruritus.

As a sedative when used as premedication and following general anesthesia, **hydroxyzine may potentiate meperidine and barbiturates,** so their use in pre-anesthetic adjunctive therapy should be modified on an individual basis. Atropine and other belladonna alkaloids are not affected by the drug. Hydroxyzine is not known to interfere with the action of digitalis in any way and it may be used concurrently with this agent.

The effectiveness of hydroxyzine as an antianxiety agent for long-term use, that is, more than 4 months, has not been assessed by systematic clinical studies. The physician should reassess periodically the usefulness of the drug for the individual patient.

CONTRAINDICATIONS

ATARAX

Hydroxyzine, when administered to the pregnant mouse, rat, and rabbit, induced fetal abnormalities in the rat and mouse at doses substantially above the human therapeutic range. Clinical data in human beings are inadequate to establish safety in early pregnancy. Until such data are available, hydroxyzine is contraindicated in early pregnancy.

Hydroxyzine is contraindicated for patients who have shown a previous hypersensitivity to it.

VISTARIL

Hydroxyzine, when administered to the pregnant mouse, rat, and rabbit, induced fetal abnormalities in the rat and mouse at doses substantially above the human therapeutic range. Clinical data in human beings are inadequate to establish safety in early pregnancy. Until such data are available, hydroxyzine is contraindicated in early pregnancy.

Hydroxyzine pamoate is contraindicated for patients who have shown a previous hypersensitivity to it.

WARNINGS

ATARAX

Nursing Mothers

It is not known whether this drug is excreted in human milk. Since many drugs are so excreted, hydroxyzine should not be given to nursing mothers.

For Tablets Only

This product is manufactured with 1,1,1-trichloroethane, a substance which harms public health and the environment by destroying ozone in the upper atmosphere.

VISTARIL

Nursing Mothers

It is not known whether this drug is excreted in human milk. Since many drugs are so excreted, hydroxyzine should not be given to nursing mothers.

PRECAUTIONS

ATARAX

THE POTENTIATING ACTION OF HYDROXYZINE MUST BE CONSIDERED WHEN THE DRUG IS USED IN CONJUNCTION WITH CENTRAL NERVOUS SYSTEM DEPRESSANTS SUCH AS NARCOTICS, NON-NARCOTIC ANALGESICS AND BARBITURATES. Therefore when central nervous system depressants are administered concomitantly with hydroxyzine their dosage should be reduced.

Since drowsiness may occur with use of this drug, patients should be warned of this possibility and cautioned against driving a car or operating dangerous machinery while taking Atarax. Patients should be advised against the simultaneous use of other CNS depressant drugs, and cautioned that the effect of alcohol may be increased.

Geriatric Use

A determination has not been made whether controlled clinical studies of Atarax included sufficient numbers of subjects aged 65 and over to define a difference in response from younger subjects. Other reported clinical experience has not identified differences in responses between the elderly and younger patients. In general, dose selection for an elderly patient should be cautious, usually starting at the low end of the dosing range, reflecting the greater frequency of decreased hepatic, renal or cardiac function, and of concomitant disease or other drug therapy.

The extent of renal excretion of Atarax has not been determined. Because elderly patients are more likely to have decreased renal function, care should be taken is dose selections.

Sedating drugs may cause confusion and over sedation in the elderly; elderly patients generally should be started on low doses of Atarax and observed closely.

VISTARIL

THE POTENTIATING ACTION OF HYDROXYZINE MUST BE CONSIDERED WHEN THE DRUG IS USED IN CONJUNCTION WITH CENTRAL NERVOUS SYSTEM DEPRESSANTS SUCH AS NARCOTICS, NON-NARCOTIC ANALGESICS AND BARBITURATES. Therefore, when central nervous system depressants are administered concomitantly with hydroxyzine, their dosage should be reduced. Since drowsiness may occur with use of the drug, patients should be warned of this possibility and cautioned against driving a car or operating dangerous machinery while taking Vistaril. Patients should be advised against the simultaneous use of other CNS depressant drugs, and cautioned that the effect of alcohol may be increased.

Geriatric Use

A determination has not been made whether controlled clinical studies of Vistaril included sufficient numbers of subjects aged 65 and over to define a difference in response from younger subjects. Other reported clinical experience has not identified differences in responses between the elderly and younger patients. In general, dose selection for an elderly patient should be cautious, usually starting at the low end of the dosing range, reflecting the greater frequency of decreased hepatic, renal or cardiac function, and of concomitant disease or other drug therapy.

The extent of renal excretion of Vistaril has not been determined. Because elderly patients are more likely to have decreased renal function, care should be taken in dose selections.

Sedating drugs may cause confusion and over sedation in the elderly; elderly patients generally should be started on low doses of Vistaril and observed closely.

ADVERSE REACTIONS

ATARAX

Side effects reported with the administration of Atarax are usually mild and transitory in nature.

Anticholinergic: Dry mouth.

Central Nervous System: Drowsiness is usually transitory and may disappear in a few days of continued therapy or upon reduction of the dose. Involuntary motor activity including rare instances of tremor and convulsions have been reported, usually with doses considerably higher than those recommended. Clinically significant respiratory depression has not been reported at recommended doses.

VISTARIL

Side effects reported with the administration of Vistaril are usually mild and transitory in nature.

Anticholinergic: Dry mouth.

Central Nervous System: Drowsiness is usually transitory and may disappear in a few days of continued therapy or upon reduction of the dose. Involuntary motor activity, including rare instances of tremor and convulsions, has been reported, usually with doses considerably higher than those recommended. Clinically significant respiratory depression has not been reported at recommended doses.

DOSAGE AND ADMINISTRATION

ATARAX

For symptomatic relief of anxiety and tension associated with psychoneurosis and as an adjunct in organic disease states in which anxiety is manifested:

In adults, 50-100 mg qid.
Children under 6 years, 50 mg daily in divided doses.
Children over 6 years, 50-100 mg daily in divided doses.

For use in the management of pruritus due to allergic conditions such as chronic urticaria and atopic and contact dermatoses, and in histamine-mediated pruritus:

In adults, 25 mg tid or qid.
Children under 6 years, 50 mg daily in divided doses.
Children over 6 years, 50-100 mg daily in divided doses.

As a sedative when used as a premedication and following general anesthesia:

50-100 mg in adults.
0.6 mg/kg in children.

When treatment is initiated by the intramuscular route of administration, subsequent doses may be administered orally.

As with all medications, the dosage should be adjusted according to the patient's response to therapy.

VISTARIL

For symptomatic relief of anxiety and tension associated with psychoneurosis and as an adjunct in organic disease states in which anxiety is manifested:

In adults, 50-100 mg qid.
Children under 6 years, 50 mg daily in divided doses.
Children over 6 years, 50-100 mg daily in divided doses.

For use in the management of pruritus due to allergic conditions such as chronic urticaria and atopic and contact dermatoses, and in histamine-mediated pruritus:

In adults, 25 mg tid or qid.
Children under 6 years, 50 mg daily in divided doses.
Children over 6 years, 50-100 mg daily in divided doses.

As a sedative when used as a premedication and following general anesthesia:

50-100 mg in adults.
0.6 mg/kg in children.

When treatment is initiated by the intramuscular route of administration, subsequent doses may be administered orally.

As with all medications, the dosage should be adjusted according to the patient's response to therapy.

HOW SUPPLIED

ATARAX

Atarax Tablets

10 mg: Orange tablets.
25 mg: Green tablets.
50 mg: Yellow tablets.
100 mg: Red tablets.

Atarax Syrup

10 mg per teaspoon (5 ml): 1 pint bottles. *Alcohol Content:* Ethyl alcohol, 0.5% v/v.

VISTARIL

Vistaril Capsules

25 mg: Two-tone green capsules.
50 mg: Green and white capsules.
100 mg: Green and gray capsules.

Vistaril Oral Suspension

25 mg hydroxyzine hydrochloride per teaspoonful (5 ml). Shake vigorously until product is completely resuspended.

PRODUCT LISTING - RATED THERAPEUTICALLY EQUIVALENT

Capsule - Oral - Pamoate 25 mg

10's	$3.68	GENERIC, Pd-Rx Pharmaceuticals	55289-0226-10
30's	$16.46	GENERIC, Heartland Healthcare Services	61392-0123-30
30's	$16.46	GENERIC, Heartland Healthcare Services	61392-0123-39
31 x 10	$132.58	GENERIC, Vangard Labs	00615-0331-53
31 x 10	$132.58	GENERIC, Vangard Labs	00615-0331-63
31's	$17.01	GENERIC, Heartland Healthcare Services	61392-0123-31
32's	$17.56	GENERIC, Heartland Healthcare Services	61392-0123-32
45's	$24.69	GENERIC, Heartland Healthcare Services	61392-0123-45
60's	$32.92	GENERIC, Heartland Healthcare Services	61392-0123-60
90's	$49.37	GENERIC, Heartland Healthcare Services	61392-0123-90
100's	$7.95	GENERIC, Cmc-Consolidated Midland Corporation	00223-1049-01
100's	$15.15	GENERIC, Major Pharmaceuticals Inc	00904-0362-60
100's	$15.20	GENERIC, Raway Pharmacal Inc	00686-0077-20
100's	$15.40	GENERIC, Qualitest Products Inc	00603-3994-21
100's	$16.50	GENERIC, Interstate Drug Exchange Inc	00814-3775-14
100's	$17.82	GENERIC, Martec Pharmaceuticals Inc	52555-0326-01
100's	$18.75	GENERIC, Geneva Pharmaceuticals	00781-2252-01
100's	$18.75	GENERIC, Mova Pharmaceutical Corporation	55370-0517-07
100's	$20.46	GENERIC, Aligen Independent Laboratories Inc	00405-4518-01
100's	$20.60	GENERIC, Watson/Schein Pharmaceuticals Inc	00591-5726-01
100's	$20.60	GENERIC, Moore, H.L. Drug Exchange Inc	00839-6270-06
100's	$20.80	GENERIC, Martec Pharmaceuticals Inc	52555-0562-01
100's	$21.94	GENERIC, Ivax Corporation	00172-2911-60
100's	$22.89	GENERIC, Eon Labs Manufacturing Inc	00185-0613-01
100's	$23.14	GENERIC, Auro Pharmaceutical	55829-0665-10
100's	$29.94	GENERIC, Barr Laboratories Inc	00555-0323-02
100's	$29.94	GENERIC, Watson Laboratories Inc	52544-0800-01
100's	$32.19	GENERIC, Barr Laboratories Inc	00555-0302-02
100's	$35.56	GENERIC, Major Pharmaceuticals Inc	00904-0362-61
100's	$44.31	GENERIC, Udl Laboratories Inc	51079-0077-20
100's	$46.00	GENERIC, Ivax Corporation	00182-1098-89
100's	$105.86	VISTARIL, Pfizer U.S. Pharmaceuticals	00069-5410-66
100's	$106.32	VISTARIL, Physicians Total Care	54868-0169-01

Capsule - Oral - Pamoate 50 mg

10's	$3.98	GENERIC, Pd-Rx Pharmaceuticals	55289-0195-10
15's	$4.87	GENERIC, Heartland Healthcare Services	61392-0010-15
30's	$16.46	GENERIC, Heartland Healthcare Services	61392-0010-30
30's	$16.46	GENERIC, Heartland Healthcare Services	61392-0010-39
30's	$376.60	GENERIC, Medirex Inc	57480-0396-06
31 x 10	$203.36	GENERIC, Vangard Labs	00615-0332-53
31 x 10	$203.36	GENERIC, Vangard Labs	00615-0332-63
31's	$17.01	GENERIC, Heartland Healthcare Services	61392-0010-31
32's	$17.56	GENERIC, Heartland Healthcare Services	61392-0010-32
45's	$14.62	GENERIC, Heartland Healthcare Services	61392-0010-45
60's	$32.92	GENERIC, Heartland Healthcare Services	61392-0010-60
90's	$49.37	GENERIC, Heartland Healthcare Services	61392-0010-90
100's	$11.25	GENERIC, Cmc-Consolidated Midland Corporation	00223-1050-01
100's	$16.00	GENERIC, Raway Pharmacal Inc	00686-0078-20
100's	$16.50	GENERIC, Major Pharmaceuticals Inc	00904-0363-60
100's	$18.00	GENERIC, Interstate Drug Exchange Inc	00814-3774-14
100's	$18.01	GENERIC, Qualitest Products Inc	00603-3995-21
100's	$18.83	GENERIC, Martec Pharmaceuticals Inc	52555-0327-01
100's	$19.98	GENERIC, Geneva Pharmaceuticals	00781-2254-01
100's	$20.00	GENERIC, Mova Pharmaceutical Corporation	55370-0519-07
100's	$21.93	GENERIC, Mutual/United Research Laboratories	00677-0597-01
100's	$21.95	GENERIC, Moore, H.L. Drug Exchange Inc	00839-6271-06
100's	$22.20	GENERIC, Watson Laboratories Inc	00591-0801-01
100's	$22.20	GENERIC, Martec Pharmaceuticals Inc	52555-0563-01
100's	$22.79	GENERIC, Aligen Independent Laboratories Inc	00405-4519-01
100's	$23.30	GENERIC, Ivax Corporation	00172-2909-60
100's	$24.13	GENERIC, Vangard Labs	00615-0332-13
100's	$24.39	GENERIC, Eon Labs Manufacturing Inc	00185-0615-01
100's	$26.31	GENERIC, Auro Pharmaceutical	55829-0666-10
100's	$32.19	GENERIC, Watson/Schein Pharmaceuticals Inc	00364-0484-01
100's	$32.19	GENERIC, Watson Laboratories Inc	52544-0801-01
100's	$41.66	GENERIC, Major Pharmaceuticals Inc	00904-0363-61
100's	$62.72	GENERIC, Udl Laboratories Inc	51079-0078-20
100's	$63.60	GENERIC, Ivax Corporation	00182-1099-89
100's	$129.06	VISTARIL, Pfizer U.S. Pharmaceuticals	00069-5420-66

Capsule - Oral - Pamoate 100 mg

100's	$18.50	GENERIC, Major Pharmaceuticals Inc	00904-0364-61
100's	$18.95	GENERIC, Cmc-Consolidated Midland Corporation	00223-1051-01
100's	$24.00	GENERIC, Raway Pharmacal Inc	00686-0058-20
100's	$28.85	GENERIC, Geneva Pharmaceuticals	00781-2256-01
100's	$34.00	GENERIC, Ivax Corporation	00182-1991-01
100's	$34.00	GENERIC, Moore, H.L. Drug Exchange Inc	00839-6272-06
100's	$34.13	GENERIC, Interstate Drug Exchange Inc	00814-3772-14
100's	$39.75	GENERIC, Major Pharmaceuticals Inc	00904-0360-60
100's	$39.75	GENERIC, Major Pharmaceuticals Inc	00904-0364-60
100's	$41.71	GENERIC, Aligen Independent Laboratories Inc	00405-4520-01
100's	$56.99	GENERIC, Barr Laboratories Inc	00555-0324-02
100's	$158.59	VISTARIL, Pfizer U.S. Pharmaceuticals	00069-5430-66

Solution - Intramuscular - Hydrochloride 25 mg/ml

1 ml x 10	$7.00	GENERIC, Abbott Pharmaceutical	00074-1277-01
1 ml x 25	$18.50	GENERIC, American Regent Laboratories Inc	00517-4201-25
1 ml x 25	$38.25	GENERIC, American Pharmaceutical Partners	63323-0021-01
10 ml	$2.03	GENERIC, Moore, H.L. Drug Exchange Inc	00839-6337-30
10 ml	$3.00	GENERIC, Cmc-Consolidated Midland Corporation	00223-7877-10
10 ml	$3.45	GENERIC, Major Pharmaceuticals Inc	00904-0361-10
10 ml	$6.38	GENERIC, Watson/Rugby Laboratories Inc	00536-5050-70
25 ml	$25.00	GENERIC, Cmc-Consolidated Midland Corporation	00223-7885-01

Solution - Intramuscular - Hydrochloride 50 mg/ml

1 ml x 10	$8.00	GENERIC, Abbott Pharmaceutical	00074-1278-01
1 ml x 25	$22.25	GENERIC, American Regent Laboratories Inc	00517-5601-25
1 ml x 25	$44.50	GENERIC, American Pharmaceutical Partners	63323-0051-01
2 ml x 10	$9.10	GENERIC, Abbott Pharmaceutical	00074-1279-02
2 ml x 25	$32.25	GENERIC, American Regent Laboratories Inc	00517-5602-25
2 ml x 25	$50.75	GENERIC, American Pharmaceutical Partners	63323-0051-02
10 ml	$2.63	GENERIC, Moore, H.L. Drug Exchange Inc	00839-6338-30
10 ml	$3.50	GENERIC, Cmc-Consolidated Midland Corporation	00223-7878-10
10 ml	$3.53	GENERIC, Interstate Drug Exchange Inc	00814-3805-40
10 ml	$3.55	GENERIC, Vita-Rx Corporation	49727-0734-10
10 ml	$3.60	GENERIC, Keene Pharmaceuticals Inc	00588-5602-70
10 ml	$3.90	GENERIC, Ivax Corporation	00182-1182-63
10 ml	$4.35	GENERIC, Major Pharmaceuticals Inc	00904-0365-10
10 ml	$4.95	GENERIC, Roberts/Hauck Pharmaceutical Corporation	43797-0137-12
10 ml	$5.00	GENERIC, C.O. Truxton Inc	00463-1101-10
10 ml	$6.00	GENERIC, Bolan Pharmaceutical Inc	44437-0171-10
10 ml	$7.26	GENERIC, Hyrex Pharmaceuticals	00314-1400-70
10 ml	$15.10	GENERIC, Merz Pharmaceuticals	00259-0340-10
10 ml	$19.31	VISTARIL IM, Allscripts Pharmaceutical Company	54569-1749-01
10 ml	$21.26	VISTARIL IM, Pfizer U.S. Pharmaceuticals	00049-5460-74
10 ml x 25	$78.50	GENERIC, American Regent Laboratories Inc	00517-5610-25
25 ml	$25.00	GENERIC, Cmc-Consolidated Midland Corporation	00223-7883-01
50 ml	$25.00	GENERIC, Cmc-Consolidated Midland Corporation	00223-7884-02

Syrup - Oral - Hydrochloride 10 mg/5 ml

120 ml	$3.85	GENERIC, Circle Pharmaceuticals Inc	00659-3005-54
120 ml	$12.70	GENERIC, Morton Grove Pharmaceuticals Inc	60432-0150-04
473 ml	$24.15	GENERIC, Hi-Tech Pharmacal Company Inc	50383-0796-16
473 ml	$65.93	ATARAX, Pfizer U.S. Pharmaceuticals	00049-5590-93
480 ml	$11.50	GENERIC, Cmc-Consolidated Midland Corporation	00223-6525-01
480 ml	$12.77	GENERIC, Interstate Drug Exchange Inc	00814-3792-82
480 ml	$12.79	GENERIC, Watson/Rugby Laboratories Inc	00536-1002-85
480 ml	$14.59	GENERIC, Moore, H.L. Drug Exchange Inc	00839-6476-69
480 ml	$18.07	GENERIC, Mutual/United Research Laboratories	00677-1421-33
480 ml	$22.25	GENERIC, Ivax Corporation	00182-1376-40
480 ml	$25.46	GENERIC, Morton Grove Pharmaceuticals Inc	60432-0150-16
480 ml	$25.50	GENERIC, Alpharma Uspd Makers Of Barre and Nmc	00472-0771-16
480 ml	$25.50	GENERIC, Qualitest Products Inc	00603-1310-58
480 ml	$28.95	GENERIC, Major Pharmaceuticals Inc	00904-0379-16
3840 ml	$85.56	GENERIC, Alpharma Uspd Makers Of Barre and Nmc	00472-0771-28

Syrup - Oral - 10 mg/5 ml

480 ml	$14.74	FEDERAL UPPER LIMIT, H.C.F.A. F F P	99999-1513-02

Tablet - Oral - Hydrochloride 10 mg

10's	$1.73	GENERIC, Pd-Rx Pharmaceuticals	55289-0912-10
10's	$8.79	GENERIC, Pharma Pac	52959-0481-10
12's	$10.56	GENERIC, Pharma Pac	52959-0481-12

20's	$3.28	GENERIC, St. Mary'S Mpp	60760-0307-20
20's	$12.49	GENERIC, Pharma Pac	52959-0481-20
30's	$4.05	GENERIC, Pd-Rx Pharmaceuticals	55289-0912-30
30's	$9.71	GENERIC, Heartland Healthcare Services	61392-0012-30
30's	$9.71	GENERIC, Heartland Healthcare Services	61392-0012-39
30's	$18.77	GENERIC, Pharma Pac	52959-0481-30
31's	$10.03	GENERIC, Heartland Healthcare Services	61392-0012-31
32's	$10.36	GENERIC, Heartland Healthcare Services	61392-0012-32
45's	$14.57	GENERIC, Heartland Healthcare Services	61392-0012-45
60's	$5.78	GENERIC, Pd-Rx Pharmaceuticals	55289-0912-60
60's	$19.42	GENERIC, Heartland Healthcare Services	61392-0012-60
90's	$29.14	GENERIC, Heartland Healthcare Services	61392-0012-90
100's	$5.63	GENERIC, Interstate Drug Exchange Inc	00814-3793-14
100's	$6.75	GENERIC, Major Pharmaceuticals Inc	00904-0357-60
100's	$6.98	GENERIC, Pd-Rx Pharmaceuticals	55289-0912-01
100's	$7.55	GENERIC, Royce Laboratories Inc	51875-0345-01
100's	$7.56	GENERIC, Moore, H.L. Drug Exchange Inc	00839-7437-06
100's	$7.58	GENERIC, Aligen Independent Laboratories Inc	00405-4511-01
100's	$7.75	GENERIC, Ivax Corporation	00182-1492-01
100's	$7.75	GENERIC, Qualitest Products Inc	00603-3970-21
100's	$8.90	GENERIC, Allscripts Pharmaceutical Company	54569-0406-01
100's	$9.75	GENERIC, Martec Pharmaceuticals Inc	52555-0557-01
100's	$10.13	GENERIC, Watson/Schein Pharmaceuticals Inc	00364-0494-01
100's	$12.63	GENERIC, Mutual/United Research Laboratories	00677-0604-01
100's	$12.66	GENERIC, Watson Laboratories Inc	52544-0699-01
100's	$15.55	GENERIC, Vangard Labs	00615-1525-13
100's	$15.99	GENERIC, Auro Pharmaceutical	55829-0306-10
100's	$31.15	GENERIC, Major Pharmaceuticals Inc	00904-0357-61
100's	$62.36	GENERIC, Watson Laboratories Inc	00591-5522-01
100's	$62.36	GENERIC, Sidmak Laboratories Inc	50111-0307-01
100's	$69.68	ATARAX, Pfizer U.S. Pharmaceuticals	00049-5600-66
120's	$38.85	GENERIC, Heartland Healthcare Services	61392-0012-34
250's	$15.20	GENERIC, Major Pharmaceuticals Inc	00904-0357-70

Tablet - Oral - Hydrochloride 25 mg

6's	$1.58	GENERIC, Pd-Rx Pharmaceuticals	55289-0139-06
15's	$5.72	GENERIC, Heartland Healthcare Services	61392-0013-15
20's	$3.90	GENERIC, Pd-Rx Pharmaceuticals	55289-0139-20
20's	$4.05	GENERIC, Dhs Inc	55887-0985-20
25's	$6.08	GENERIC, Pd-Rx Pharmaceuticals	55289-0139-97
30's	$4.35	GENERIC, Pd-Rx Pharmaceuticals	55289-0139-30
30's	$5.03	GENERIC, Dhs Inc	55887-0985-30
30's	$11.45	GENERIC, Heartland Healthcare Services	61392-0013-30
30's	$11.45	GENERIC, Heartland Healthcare Services	61392-0013-39
31 x 10	$133.26	GENERIC, Vangard Labs	00615-1526-53
31 x 10	$133.26	GENERIC, Vangard Labs	00615-1526-63
31's	$11.83	GENERIC, Heartland Healthcare Services	61392-0013-31
32's	$12.21	GENERIC, Heartland Healthcare Services	61392-0013-32
40's	$4.80	GENERIC, Pd-Rx Pharmaceuticals	55289-0139-40
45's	$17.17	GENERIC, Heartland Healthcare Services	61392-0013-45
60's	$22.90	GENERIC, Heartland Healthcare Services	61392-0013-60
90's	$34.34	GENERIC, Heartland Healthcare Services	61392-0013-90
100's	$8.25	GENERIC, Interstate Drug Exchange Inc	00814-3794-14
100's	$8.70	GENERIC, Pd-Rx Pharmaceuticals	55289-0139-01
100's	$10.33	GENERIC, Moore, H.L. Drug Exchange Inc	00839-7438-06
100's	$10.37	GENERIC, Aligen Independent Laboratories Inc	00405-4512-01
100's	$10.98	GENERIC, Economed Pharmaceuticals Inc	38130-0044-01
100's	$11.40	GENERIC, Martec Pharmaceuticals Inc	52555-0558-01
100's	$11.54	GENERIC, Major Pharmaceuticals Inc	00904-0358-60
100's	$11.85	GENERIC, Ivax Corporation	00182-1493-01
100's	$11.90	GENERIC, Qualitest Products Inc	00603-3971-21
100's	$14.93	GENERIC, Watson/Schein Pharmaceuticals Inc	00364-0495-01
100's	$18.66	GENERIC, Watson Laboratories Inc	52544-0700-01
100's	$20.95	GENERIC, Auro Pharmaceutical	55829-0307-10
100's	$37.91	GENERIC, Major Pharmaceuticals Inc	00904-0358-61
100's	$91.46	GENERIC, Watson/Schein Pharmaceuticals Inc	00591-5523-01
100's	$91.46	GENERIC, Sidmak Laboratories Inc	50111-0308-01
100's	$91.97	GENERIC, Mutual/United Research Laboratories	00677-0605-01
100's	$91.97	GENERIC, Mutual Pharmaceutical Co Inc	53489-0127-01
100's	$102.19	ATARAX, Pfizer U.S. Pharmaceuticals	00049-5610-66
200 x 5	$429.87	GENERIC, Vangard Labs	00615-1526-43
250's	$21.40	GENERIC, Major Pharmaceuticals Inc	00904-0358-70

Tablet - Oral - Hydrochloride 50 mg

3's	$3.55	GENERIC, Prescript Pharmaceuticals	00247-1074-03
6's	$3.75	GENERIC, Prescript Pharmaceuticals	00247-1074-06
20's	$4.68	GENERIC, Prescript Pharmaceuticals	00247-1074-20
20's	$9.10	GENERIC, Pd-Rx Pharmaceuticals	55289-0138-20
30's	$4.82	GENERIC, Pd-Rx Pharmaceuticals	55289-0138-30
30's	$10.80	GENERIC, Heartland Healthcare Services	61392-0122-30
30's	$10.80	GENERIC, Heartland Healthcare Services	61392-0122-39
31's	$11.16	GENERIC, Heartland Healthcare Services	61392-0122-31
32's	$11.52	GENERIC, Heartland Healthcare Services	61392-0122-32
45's	$16.20	GENERIC, Heartland Healthcare Services	61392-0122-45
60's	$21.60	GENERIC, Heartland Healthcare Services	61392-0122-60
90's	$32.40	GENERIC, Heartland Healthcare Services	61392-0122-90
100's	$9.75	GENERIC, Interstate Drug Exchange Inc	00814-3795-14
100's	$10.70	GENERIC, Major Pharmaceuticals Inc	00904-0359-60
100's	$11.54	GENERIC, Moore, H.L. Drug Exchange Inc	00839-7439-06
100's	$12.11	GENERIC, Aligen Independent Laboratories Inc	00405-4513-01
100's	$12.59	GENERIC, Royce Laboratories Inc	51875-0347-01
100's	$12.60	GENERIC, Martec Pharmaceuticals Inc	52555-0559-01
100's	$13.10	GENERIC, Ivax Corporation	00182-1494-01
100's	$14.85	GENERIC, Qualitest Products Inc	00603-3972-21
100's	$16.87	GENERIC, Major Pharmaceuticals Inc	00904-0359-61
100's	$18.56	GENERIC, Watson/Schein Pharmaceuticals Inc	00364-0496-01
100's	$23.20	GENERIC, Watson/Schein Pharmaceuticals Inc	00591-5565-01
100's	$23.20	GENERIC, Watson Laboratories Inc	52544-0704-01
100's	$25.15	GENERIC, Auro Pharmaceutical	55829-0308-10
100's	$72.00	GENERIC, Richmond Pharmaceuticals	54738-0309-01
100's	$111.50	GENERIC, Sidmak Laboratories Inc	50111-0309-01
100's	$112.12	GENERIC, Mutual/United Research Laboratories	00677-0606-01
100's	$112.12	GENERIC, Mutual Pharmaceutical Co Inc	53489-0128-01
100's	$124.58	ATARAX, Pfizer U.S. Pharmaceuticals	00049-5620-66
250's	$19.90	GENERIC, Major Pharmaceuticals Inc	00904-0359-70

Tablet - Oral - Hydrochloride 100 mg

100's	$153.08	ATARAX, Pfizer U.S. Pharmaceuticals	00049-5630-66

Tablet - Oral - 10 mg

100's	$5.25	FEDERAL UPPER LIMIT, H.C.F.A. F F P	99999-1513-04

Tablet - Oral - 25 mg

100's	$4.81	FEDERAL UPPER LIMIT, H.C.F.A. F F P	99999-1513-08

Tablet - Oral - 50 mg

100's	$5.57	FEDERAL UPPER LIMIT, H.C.F.A. F F P	99999-1513-12

PRODUCT LISTING - EQUIVALENTS NOT AVAILABLE

Capsule - Oral - Pamoate 25 mg

6's	$1.24	GENERIC, Allscripts Pharmaceutical Company	54569-2353-03
10's	$10.50	GENERIC, Southwood Pharmaceuticals Inc	58016-0259-10
20's	$4.12	GENERIC, Allscripts Pharmaceutical Company	54569-2353-02
20's	$21.00	GENERIC, Southwood Pharmaceuticals Inc	58016-0259-20
30's	$6.18	GENERIC, Allscripts Pharmaceutical Company	54569-2353-05
30's	$31.50	GENERIC, Southwood Pharmaceuticals Inc	58016-0259-30
40's	$13.75	GENERIC, Pharma Pac	52959-0433-40
50's	$52.50	GENERIC, Southwood Pharmaceuticals Inc	58016-0259-50
60's	$63.00	GENERIC, Southwood Pharmaceuticals Inc	58016-0259-60
100's	$12.11	GENERIC, Physicians Total Care	54868-2892-00
100's	$105.00	GENERIC, Southwood Pharmaceuticals Inc	58016-0259-00

Capsule - Oral - Pamoate 50 mg

10's	$28.63	GENERIC, Southwood Pharmaceuticals Inc	58016-0464-10
15's	$42.95	GENERIC, Southwood Pharmaceuticals Inc	58016-0464-15
20's	$5.71	GENERIC, Allscripts Pharmaceutical Company	54569-2571-01
20's	$57.27	GENERIC, Southwood Pharmaceuticals Inc	58016-0464-20
30's	$4.95	GENERIC, Physicians Total Care	54868-1854-01
30's	$85.90	GENERIC, Southwood Pharmaceuticals Inc	58016-0464-30
60's	$8.56	GENERIC, Physicians Total Care	54868-1854-03
100's	$13.71	GENERIC, Physicians Total Care	54868-1854-00

Capsule - Oral - Pamoate 100 mg

100's	$26.88	GENERIC, Physicians Total Care	54868-4108-00
100's	$33.60	GENERIC, Physicians Total Care	54868-4109-00

Solution - Intramuscular - Hydrochloride 25 mg/ml

1 ml x 25	$28.30	GENERIC, Physicians Total Care	54868-0858-00

Solution - Intramuscular - Hydrochloride 50 mg/ml

10 ml	$3.56	GENERIC, Allscripts Pharmaceutical Company	54569-1924-00
10 ml	$4.63	GENERIC, Physicians Total Care	54868-0231-00
10 ml	$4.75	GENERIC, Southwood Pharmaceuticals Inc	58016-9299-01
10 ml	$5.50	GENERIC, Cmc-Consolidated Midland Corporation	00223-7882-10
10 ml	$8.50	GENERIC, Clint Pharmaceutical Inc	55553-0171-10

Suspension - Oral - Pamoate 25 mg/5 ml

120 ml	$28.00	GENERIC, Monument Pharmaceutical Inc	62927-0621-04
120 ml x 4	$161.56	VISTARIL, Pfizer U.S. Pharmaceuticals	00069-5440-97
480 ml	$100.00	GENERIC, Monument Pharmaceutical Inc	62927-0621-16

Syrup - Oral - Hydrochloride 10 mg/5 ml

5 ml	$3.47	GENERIC, Prescript Pharmaceuticals	00247-0332-05
10 ml	$3.60	GENERIC, Prescript Pharmaceuticals	00247-0332-10
60 ml	$4.82	GENERIC, Prescript Pharmaceuticals	00247-0332-60
118 ml	$6.25	GENERIC, Prescript Pharmaceuticals	00247-0332-52
120 ml	$7.17	GENERIC, Physicians Total Care	54868-4336-00
120 ml	$7.90	GENERIC, Pharma Pac	52959-0582-03
120 ml	$8.75	GENERIC, Alpharma Uspd Makers Of Barre and Nmc	63874-0718-12
120 ml	$12.70	GENERIC, Allscripts Pharmaceutical Company	54569-1640-01
480 ml	$12.19	GENERIC, Aligen Independent Laboratories Inc	00405-2900-16
480 ml	$14.86	GENERIC, Physicians Total Care	54868-2032-00
3840 ml	$75.00	GENERIC, Cmc-Consolidated Midland Corporation	00223-6525-02

Tablet - Oral - Hydrochloride 10 mg

6's	$3.79	GENERIC, Southwood Pharmaceuticals Inc	58016-0405-06
10's	$3.62	GENERIC, Prescript Pharmaceuticals	00247-0127-10
10's	$6.31	GENERIC, Southwood Pharmaceuticals Inc	58016-0405-10
12's	$3.68	GENERIC, Prescript Pharmaceuticals	00247-0127-12

15's	$1.34	GENERIC, Allscripts Pharmaceutical Company	54569-0406-05
15's	$3.76	GENERIC, Prescript Pharmaceuticals	00247-0127-15
15's	$9.47	GENERIC, Southwood Pharmaceuticals Inc	58016-0405-15
20's	$1.78	GENERIC, Allscripts Pharmaceutical Company	54569-0406-03
20's	$3.89	GENERIC, Prescript Pharmaceuticals	00247-0127-20
20's	$3.93	GENERIC, Physicians Total Care	54868-0229-01
20's	$12.62	GENERIC, Southwood Pharmaceuticals Inc	58016-0405-20
24's	$3.26	GENERIC, Pharmaceutical Corporation Of America	51655-0078-30
30's	$2.67	GENERIC, Allscripts Pharmaceutical Company	54569-0406-00
30's	$3.39	GENERIC, Physicians Total Care	54868-0229-02
30's	$4.05	GENERIC, Pharmaceutical Corporation Of America	51655-0078-24
30's	$4.16	GENERIC, Prescript Pharmaceuticals	00247-0127-30
30's	$18.93	GENERIC, Southwood Pharmaceuticals Inc	58016-0405-30
30's	$31.20	GENERIC, Alpharma Uspd Makers Of Barre and Nmc	63874-0303-30
50's	$4.71	GENERIC, Prescript Pharmaceuticals	00247-0127-50
60's	$5.11	GENERIC, Physicians Total Care	54868-0229-04
100's	$5.25	GENERIC, Cmc-Consolidated Midland Corporation	00223-1006-01
100's	$6.58	GENERIC, Physicians Total Care	54868-0229-03
100's	$63.10	GENERIC, Southwood Pharmaceuticals Inc	58016-0405-00

Tablet - Oral - Hydrochloride 25 mg

2's	$3.44	GENERIC, Prescript Pharmaceuticals	00247-0105-02
3's	$3.47	GENERIC, Prescript Pharmaceuticals	00247-0105-03
4's	$3.52	GENERIC, Prescript Pharmaceuticals	00247-0105-04
5's	$3.55	GENERIC, Prescript Pharmaceuticals	00247-0105-05
6's	$0.74	GENERIC, Allscripts Pharmaceutical Company	54569-0413-08
6's	$3.59	GENERIC, Prescript Pharmaceuticals	00247-0105-06
7's	$3.64	GENERIC, Prescript Pharmaceuticals	00247-0105-07
8's	$0.98	GENERIC, Allscripts Pharmaceutical Company	54569-4825-01
8's	$3.67	GENERIC, Prescript Pharmaceuticals	00247-0105-08
9's	$8.09	GENERIC, Southwood Pharmaceuticals Inc	58016-0406-09
10's	$1.23	GENERIC, Allscripts Pharmaceutical Company	54569-0413-05
10's	$3.75	GENERIC, Prescript Pharmaceuticals	00247-0105-10
12's	$2.90	GENERIC, Pharmaceutical Corporation Of America	51655-0079-27
12's	$3.84	GENERIC, Prescript Pharmaceuticals	00247-0105-12
12's	$10.79	GENERIC, Southwood Pharmaceuticals Inc	58016-0406-12
12's	$18.68	GENERIC, Pharma Pac	52959-0074-12
13's	$20.22	GENERIC, Pharma Pac	52959-0074-13
14's	$1.72	GENERIC, Allscripts Pharmaceutical Company	54569-4825-00
14's	$3.91	GENERIC, Prescript Pharmaceuticals	00247-0105-14
15's	$1.84	GENERIC, Allscripts Pharmaceutical Company	54569-0413-06
15's	$3.95	GENERIC, Prescript Pharmaceuticals	00247-0105-15
15's	$13.49	GENERIC, Southwood Pharmaceuticals Inc	58016-0406-15
15's	$22.49	GENERIC, Pharma Pac	52959-0074-15
16's	$23.96	GENERIC, Pharma Pac	52959-0074-16
20's	$2.45	GENERIC, Allscripts Pharmaceutical Company	54569-0413-00
20's	$3.39	GENERIC, Physicians Total Care	54868-0063-02
20's	$4.15	GENERIC, Prescript Pharmaceuticals	00247-0105-20
20's	$17.98	GENERIC, Southwood Pharmaceuticals Inc	58016-0406-20
20's	$27.08	GENERIC, Pharma Pac	52959-0074-20
20's	$28.08	GENERIC, Alpharma Uspd Makers Of Barre and Nmc	63874-0303-20
21's	$4.19	GENERIC, Prescript Pharmaceuticals	00247-0105-21
21's	$28.35	GENERIC, Pharma Pac	52959-0074-21
24's	$4.31	GENERIC, Prescript Pharmaceuticals	00247-0105-24
24's	$32.15	GENERIC, Pharma Pac	52959-0074-24
30's	$3.68	GENERIC, Allscripts Pharmaceutical Company	54569-0413-01
30's	$4.26	GENERIC, Physicians Total Care	54868-0063-03
30's	$4.54	GENERIC, Prescript Pharmaceuticals	00247-0105-30
30's	$5.50	GENERIC, Pharmaceutical Corporation Of America	51655-0079-24
30's	$9.30	GENERIC, St. Mary'S Mpp	60760-0971-30
30's	$26.97	GENERIC, Southwood Pharmaceuticals Inc	58016-0406-30
30's	$29.12	GENERIC, Alpharma Uspd Makers Of Barre and Nmc	63874-0304-30
30's	$40.14	GENERIC, Pharma Pac	52959-0074-30
35's	$4.74	GENERIC, Prescript Pharmaceuticals	00247-0105-35
40's	$4.92	GENERIC, Allscripts Pharmaceutical Company	54569-0413-09
40's	$5.12	GENERIC, Physicians Total Care	54868-0063-07
40's	$35.96	GENERIC, Southwood Pharmaceuticals Inc	58016-0406-40
40's	$51.90	GENERIC, Pharma Pac	52959-0074-40
60's	$7.37	GENERIC, Allscripts Pharmaceutical Company	54569-0413-04
60's	$54.36	GENERIC, Alpharma Uspd Makers Of Barre and Nmc	63874-0305-60
90's	$9.44	GENERIC, Physicians Total Care	54868-0063-00
100's	$6.95	GENERIC, Cmc-Consolidated Midland Corporation	00223-1007-01
100's	$7.33	GENERIC, Prescript Pharmaceuticals	00247-0105-00
100's	$10.13	GENERIC, Physicians Total Care	54868-0063-05
100's	$89.90	GENERIC, Southwood Pharmaceuticals Inc	58016-0406-00

Tablet - Oral - Hydrochloride 50 mg

20's	$3.27	GENERIC, Physicians Total Care	54868-1804-02
20's	$11.32	GENERIC, Southwood Pharmaceuticals Inc	58016-0452-20
30's	$4.46	GENERIC, Allscripts Pharmaceutical Company	54569-0409-01
30's	$16.98	GENERIC, Southwood Pharmaceuticals Inc	58016-0452-30
30's	$33.80	GENERIC, Alpharma Uspd Makers Of Barre and Nmc	63874-0077-30
100's	$8.75	GENERIC, Cmc-Consolidated Midland Corporation	00223-1008-01
100's	$56.60	GENERIC, Southwood Pharmaceuticals Inc	58016-0452-00

Tablet - Oral - Hydrochloride 100 mg

100's	$22.50	GENERIC, Cmc-Consolidated Midland Corporation	00223-1009-01

Hylan G-F 20 *(003371)*

Categories: Arthritis, osteoarthritis; FDA Approved 1997 Aug
Drug Classes: Hyaluronic acid derivatives
Brand Names: Synvisc
Cost of Therapy: $736.23 (Arthritis; Synvisc Injection; 8 mg/ml; 2 ml; 1 injection/week; 21 day supply)
HCFA JCODE(S): J7320 16 mg OTH

H

DESCRIPTION

Hylan G-F 20 is an elastoviscous fluid containing hylan polymers produced from chicken combs. Hylans are derivatives of hyaluronan (sodium hyaluronate), a natural complex sugar of the glycosaminoglycan family. Hyaluronan is a long-chain polymer containing repeating disaccharide units of Na-glucuronate-N-acetylglucosamine.

Detailed Device Description: Synvisc contains hylan A (average molecular weight 6,000,000) and hylan B hydrated gel in a buffered physiological sodium chloride solution, pH 7.2. Synvisc has an elasticity (storage modulus G') at 2.5 Hz of 111 ± 13 Pascals (Pa) and a viscosity (loss modulus G") of 25 ± 2 Pa (elasticity and viscosity of knee synovial fluid of 18-27 year old humans measured with a comparable method at 2.5 Hz: G' = 117 ± 13 Pa; G" = 45 ± 8 Pa.)

Each syringe of Synvisc contains:

- ***Hylan polymers (hylan A + hylan B):*** 16 mg
- ***Sodium chloride:*** 17 mg
- ***Disodium hydrogen phosphate:*** 0.32 mg
- ***Sodium dihydrogen phosphate monohydrate:*** 0.08 mg
- ***Water for injection:*** qs to 2.0 ml

INDICATIONS AND USAGE

Hylan G-F 20 is indicated for the treatment of pain in osteoarthritis (OA) of the knee in patients who have failed to respond adequately to conservative nonpharmacologic therapy and simple analgesics (*e.g.,* acetaminophen).

CONTRAINDICATIONS

- Do not administer to patients with known hypersensitivity (allergy) to hyaluronan (sodium hyaluronate) preparations.
- Do not inject hylan G-F 20 in the knees of patients having knee joint infections or skin diseases or infections in the area of the injection site.

WARNINGS

- Do not concomitantly use disinfectants containing quaternary ammonium salts for skin preparation because hyaluronan can precipitate in their presence.
- Do not inject hylan G-F 20 extra-articularly or into the synovial tissues and capsule. One such systemic adverse event occurred following extra-articular injections of hylan G-F 20 in clinical use outside the US.
- Intravascular injections of hylan G-F 20 may cause systemic adverse events.

PRECAUTIONS

GENERAL

- The effectiveness of a single treatment cycle of less than three injections of hylan G-F 20 has not been established.
- The safety and effectiveness of hylan G-F 20 in locations other than the knee and for conditions other than osteoarthritis have not been established.
- Do not inject anesthetics or other medications into the knee joint during hylan G-F 20 therapy. Such medications may dilute hylan G-F 20 and affect its safety and effectiveness.
- Use caution when injecting hylan G-F 20 into patients who are allergic to avian proteins, feathers, and egg products.
- The safety and effectiveness of hylan G-F 20 in severely inflamed knee joints have not been established.
- Strict aseptic administration technique must be followed.
- STERILE CONTENTS. The syringe is intended for single use. The contents of the syringe must be used immediately after its packaging is opened. Discard any unused hylan G-F 20.
- Do not use hylan G-F 20 if package is opened or damaged. Store in original packaging (protected from light) at room temperature below 30°C (86°F). DO NOT FREEZE.
- Remove synovial fluid or effusion, if present, before injecting hylan G-F 20.
- Hylan G-F 20 should be used with caution when there is evidence of lymphatic or venous stasis in that leg.

INFORMATION FOR THE PATIENT

- Provide patients with a copy of the patient labeling prior to use.
- Transient pain and/or swelling of the injected joint may occur after intra-articular injection of hylan G-F 20.

- As with any invasive joint procedure, it is recommended that the patient avoid any strenuous activities or prolonged weight-bearing activities such as jogging or tennis following the intra-articular injection.
- The safety and effectiveness of repeat treatment cycles of hylan G-F 20 have not been established.

PREGNANCY

The safety and effectiveness of hylan G-F 20 have not been established in pregnant women.

NURSING MOTHERS

It is not known if hylan G-F 20 is excreted in human milk. The safety and effectiveness of hylan G-F 20 have not been established in lactating women.

PEDIATRIC USE

The safety and effectiveness of hylan G-F 20 have not been established in children.

ADVERSE REACTIONS

H

A total of 511 patients (559 knees) received 1771 injections in seven clinical trials of hylan G-F 20. There were 39 reports in 37 patients (2.2% of injections, 7.2% of patients) of knee pain and/or swelling after these injections.

Ten patients (10 knees) were treated with arthrocentesis and removal of joint effusion. Two additional patients (2 knees) received treatment with intra-articular steroids. Two patients (2 knees) received NSAIDs. One of these patients also received arthrocentesis. One patient was treated with arthroscopy. The remaining patients with adverse events localized to the knee received no treatment or only analgesics.

Systemic adverse events each occurred in 10 (2.0%) of the hylan G-F 20-treated patients. There was one case each of rash (thorax and back) and itching of the skin following hylan G-F 20 injections in these studies. These symptoms did not recur when these patients received additional hylan G-F 20 injections. The remaining generalized adverse events reported were calf cramps, hemorrhoid problems, ankle edema, muscle pain, tonsillitis with nausea, tachyarrhythmia, phlebitis with varicosities and low back sprain.

In three concurrently controlled clinical trials with a total of 112 patients who received hylan G-F 20 and 110 patients who received either saline or arthrocentesis, there were no statistically significant differences in the numbers or types of adverse events between the group of patients that received hylan G-F 20 and the group that received control treatments.

In clinical use in Canada (since 1992) and Sweden (since 1995), the most common adverse events reported have been pain, swelling, and/or effusion in the injected knees. Other adverse events reported were one case each of: generalized urticaria: recurring small hives: pain on one side of the body with nausea, anxiety and listlessness; facial flush with swelling of lips; nausea with dizziness; and shivering with headache, nausea, respiratory difficulties; and prickling in body which did not recur after subsequent hylan G-F 20 injections. No cases of anaphylaxis or anaphylactoid reactions have been reported. No deaths have been associated with the use of hylan G-F 20. Intra-articular infections did not occur in any of the clinical trials, but have occurred in clinical use following hylan G-F 20 injections.

DOSAGE AND ADMINISTRATION

DIRECTIONS FOR USE

Hylan G-F 20 is administered by intra-articular injection once a week (1 week apart) for a total of three injections.

Note these precautions:

- Do not use hylan G-F 20 if the package has been opened or damaged. Store in original packaging (protected from light) at room temperature below 30°C (86°F). DO NOT FREEZE.
- Strict aseptic administration technique must be followed.
- Do not concomitantly use disinfectants containing quaternary ammonium salts for skin preparation because hyaluronan can precipitate in their presence.
- Remove synovial fluid or effusion, if present, before injecting hylan G-F 20.
- Do not use the same syringe for removing synovial fluid and for injecting hylan G-F 20, but the same needle should be used.
- Take particular care to remove the tip cap of the syringe and needle aseptically.
- Inject hylan G-F 20 into the knee joint through an 18 to 22 gauge needle.
- Do not inject anesthetics or any other medications intra-articularly into the knee while administering hylan G-F 20 therapy. This may dilute hylan G-F 20 and affect its safety and effectiveness.
- The syringe containing hylan G-F 20 is intended for single use. The contents of the syringe must be used immediately after the syringe has been removed from its packaging. Inject the full 2 ml in one knee only. If treatment is bilateral, a separate syringe must be used for each knee. Discard any unused hylan G-F 20.

PRODUCT LISTING - EQUIVALENTS NOT AVAILABLE

Solution - Intra-Articular - 8 mg/ml

2 ml	$235.00	SYNVISC, Wyeth-Ayerst Laboratories	00008-9149-01
2 ml x 3	$736.23	SYNVISC, Wyeth-Ayerst Laboratories	00008-9149-02
6 ml	$675.38	SYNVISC, Allscripts Pharmaceutical Company	54569-4771-00

Hyoscyamine Sulfate (001516)

Categories: Anesthesia, adjunct; Bladder, neurogenic, adjunct; Bladder, spastic; Bowel, neurogenic, adjunct; Colic, biliary; Colic, renal; Colitis, spastic; Colon, neurogenic, adjunct; Cramps, abdominal; Diverticulitis; Dysentery; Enterocolitis; Heart block; Imaging, renal, adjunct; Irritable bowel syndrome; Pancreatitis, adjunct; Parkinson's disease; Poisoning, anticholinesterase; Pylorospasm; Rhinitis, acute; Ulcer, peptic, adjunct; Pregnancy Category C; FDA Pre 1938 Drugs

Drug Classes: Anticholinergics; Gastrointestinals

Brand Names: A-Spas S L; Anaspaz; Cystospaz-M; Donnamar; Ed-Spaz; Gastrosed; Hyco; Hyosol Sl; Hyospaz; Levbid; **Levsin**; Levsinex; Liqui-Sooth; Medispaz; NuLev; Pasmex; Setamine; Spasdel

Foreign Brand Availability: Levsin SL (Hong-Kong)

Cost of Therapy: $35.14 (Gastrointestinal Disorders; Levsin; 0.125 mg; 2 tablets/day; 30 day supply)
$5.92 (Gastrointestinal Disorders; Generic Tablets; 0.125 mg; 2 tablets/day; 30 day supply)

HCFA JCODE(S): J1980 up to 0.25 mg SC, IM, IV

DESCRIPTION

Hyoscyamine sulfate is one of the principal anticholinergic/antispasmodic components of belladonna alkaloids. The empirical formula is $(C_{17}H_{23}NO_3)_2 \cdot H_2SO_4 \cdot 32H_2O$ and the molecular weight is 712.85. Chemically, it is benzeneacetic acid, α-(hydroxymethyl)-,8-methyl-8-azabicyclo[3.2.1.]oct-3-yl ester,(3(S)-endo)-,sulfate (2:1),dihydrate.

LEVSIN SUBLINGUAL TABLETS

Contain 0.125 mg hyoscyamine sulfate formulated for sublingual administration. However, the tablets may also be chewed or taken orally.

Inactive ingredients: Colloidal silicon dioxide, dextrates, FD&C green no. 3, flavor, mannitol, and stearic acid.

LEVSIN TABLETS

Contain 0.125 mg hyoscyamine sulfate formulated for oral administration.

Inactive ingredients: Acacia, confectioner's sugar, corn starch, lactose, powdered cellulose, and stearic acid.

LEVSIN ELIXIR

Contains 0.125 mg hyoscyamine sulfate per 5 ml (teaspoonful) with 20% alcohol for oral use.

Inactive ingredients: FD&C red no. 40, FD&C yellow no. 6, flavor, glycerin, purified water, sorbitol solution, and sucrose.

LEVSIN DROPS AND ORAL SOLUTION

Contain 0.125 mg hyoscyamine sulfate per ml with 5% alcohol.

Inactive ingredients: FD&C red no. 40, FD&C yellow no. 6, flavor, glycerin, purified water, sodium citrate, sorbitol solution, and sucrose.

LEVSIN INJECTION

A sterile solution containing 0.5 mg hyoscyamine sulfate per ml.

The 1 ml ampuls contain as inactive ingredients: Water for injection, pH is adjusted with hydrochloric acid when necessary.

LEVSIN EXTENDED-RELEASE TABLETS

Contain 0.375 mg hyoscyamine sulfate in a timed-release formulation designed for oral bid dosage.

Each capsule may also contain as inactive ingredients: Corn starch, D&C red no. 28, FD&C blue no. 1, FD&C blue no. 2, FD&C red no. 40, FD&C yellow no. 6, gelatin, sucrose, titanium dioxide and other ingredients.

NULEV ORALLY DISINTEGRATING TABLETS

NuLev orally disintegrating tablets 0.125 mg is formulated for oral administration using patented DuraSolv technology. NuLev disintegrates within seconds after placement on the tongue, allowing it to be swallowed with or without water.

Each tablet also contains as inactive ingredients: Aspartame, colloidal silicon dioxide, crospovidone, flavor, magnesium stearate, mannitol, microcrystalline cellulose.

CLINICAL PHARMACOLOGY

Hyoscyamine inhibits specifically the actions of acetylcholine on structures innervated by postganglionic cholinergic nerves and on smooth muscles that respond to acetylcholine but lack cholinergic innervation. These peripheral cholinergic receptors are present in the autonomic effector cells of the smooth muscle, cardiac muscle, the sinoatrial node, the atrioventricular node, and the exocrine glands.

At therapeutic doses, it is completely devoid of any action in the autonomic ganglia. Hyoscyamine inhibits gastrointestinal propulsive motility and decreases gastric acid secretion. Hyoscyamine also controls excessive pharyngeal, tracheal, and bronchial secretions.

Hyoscyamine is absorbed totally and completely by sublingual administration as well as oral administration. Once absorbed, hyoscyamine disappears rapidly from the blood and is distributed throughout the entire body. The half-life of hyoscyamine is 3.5 hours. Hyoscyamine is partly hydrolyzed to tropic acid and tropine but the majority of the drug is excreted in the urine unchanged within the first 12 hours. Only traces of this drug are found in breast milk. Hyoscyamine passes the blood-brain barrier and the placental barrier.

Hyoscyamine sublingual tablets can be taken orally with the same pharmacological effects occurring; however, the effects may not occur as rapidly as with sublingual administration.

Hyoscyamine extended-release tablets release 0.375 mg hyoscyamine sulfate at a controlled and predictable rate for 12 hours. Peak blood levels occur in 2.5 hours and the apparent plasma half-life is approximately 7 hours. The urinary excretion from both the immediate-release dosage form and the timed-release dosage form is equal and uniform over a 24 hour period.

INDICATIONS AND USAGE

Hyoscyamine is effective as adjunctive therapy in the treatment of peptic ulcer. It can also be used to control gastric secretion, visceral spasm and hypermotility in spastic colitis, spastic bladder, cystitis, pylorospasm, and associated abdominal cramps. May be used in functional intestinal disorders to reduce symptoms such as those seen in mild dysenteries, diverticulitis, and acute enterocolitis. For use as adjunctive therapy in the treatment of irritable bowel syndrome (irritable colon, spastic colon, mucous colitis) and functional gastrointestinal disorders. Also as adjunctive therapy in the treatment of neurogenic bladder and neurogenic bowel disturbances including the splenic flexure syndrome and neurogenic colon. Also used in the treatment of infant colic (elixir and drops). Hyoscyamine is indicated along with morphine or other narcotics in symptomatic relief of biliary and renal colic; as a "drying agent" in the relief of symptoms of acute rhinitis; in the therapy of parkinsonism to reduce rigidity and tremors and to control associated sialorrhea and hyperhidrosis. May be used in the therapy of poisoning by anticholinesterase agents.

Parenterally administered hyoscyamine is also effective in reducing gastrointestinal motility to facilitate diagnostic procedures such as endoscopy or hypotonic duodenography. Hyoscyamine may be used to reduce pain and hypersecretion in pancreatitis.

Hyoscyamine may also be used in certain cases of partial heart block associated with vagal activity.

In anesthesia: Hyoscyamine injection is indicated as a preoperative antimuscarinic to reduce salivary, tracheobronchial, and pharyngeal secretions; to reduce the volume and acidity of gastric secretions, and to block cardiac vagal inhibitory reflexes during induction of anesthesia and intubation. Hyoscyamine protects against the peripheral muscarinic effects such as bradycardia and excessive secretions produced by halogenated hydrocarbons and cholinergic agents such as physostigmine, neostigmine, and pyridostigmine given to reverse the actions of curariform agents.

In urology: Hyoscyamine injection may also be used intravenously to improve radiologic visibility of the kidneys.

CONTRAINDICATIONS

Glaucoma; obstructive uropathy (for example, bladder neck obstruction due to prostatic hypertrophy); obstructive disease of the gastrointestinal tract (as in achalasia, pyloroduodenal stenosis); paralytic ileus, intestinal atony of elderly or debilitated patients; unstable cardiovascular status in acute hemorrhage; severe ulcerative colitis; toxic megacolon complicating ulcerative colitis; myasthenia gravis.

WARNINGS

In the presence of high environmental temperature, heat prostration can occur with drug use (fever and heat stroke due to decreased sweating). Diarrhea may be an early symptom of incomplete intestinal obstruction, especially in patients with ileostomy or colostomy. In this instance, treatment with this drug would be inappropriate and possibly harmful. Like other anticholinergic agents, hyoscyamine may produce drowsiness or blurred vision. In this event, the patient should be warned not to engage in activities requiring mental alertness such as operating a motor vehicle or other machinery or to perform hazardous work while taking this drug.

Psychosis has been reported in sensitive individuals given anticholinergic drugs. CNS signs and symptoms include confusion, disorientation, short-term memory loss, hallucinations, dysarthria, ataxia, coma, euphoria, decreased anxiety, fatigue, insomnia, agitation and mannerisms, and inappropriate affect. These CNS signs and symptoms usually resolve within 12-48 hours after discontinuation of the drug.

PRECAUTIONS

GENERAL

Use with caution in patients with: Autonomic neuropathy, hyperthyroidism, coronary heart disease, congestive heart failure, cardiac arrhythmias, hypertension, and renal disease. Investigate any tachycardia before giving any anticholinergic drug since they may increase the heart rate. Use with caution in patients with hiatal hernia associated with reflux esophagitis.

INFORMATION FOR THE PATIENT

Like other anticholingeric agents hyoscyamine may produce drowsiness, dizziness, or blurred vision. In this event, the patient should be warned not to engage in activities requiring mental alertness such as operating a motor vehicle or other machinery or to perform hazardous work while taking this drug.

Use of hyoscyamine may decrease sweating resulting in heat prostration, fever, or heat stroke; febrile patients or those who may be exposed to elevated environmental temperatures should use caution.

PHENYLKETONURICS

Phenylketonuric patients should be informed that hyoscyamine sulfate contains phenylalanine 1.7 mg per orally disintegrating tablet.

CARCINOGENESIS, MUTAGENESIS, AND IMPAIRMENT OF FERTILITY

No long-term studies in animals have been performed to determine the carcinogenic, mutagenic, or impairment of fertility potential of hyoscyamine; however, over 30 years of marketing experience with hyoscyamine sulfate shows no demonstrable evidence of a problem.

PREGNANCY CATEGORY C

Animal reproduction studies have not been conducted with hyoscyamine. It is also not known whether hyoscyamine can cause fetal harm when administered to a pregnant woman or can affect reproduction capacity. Hyoscyamine should be given to a pregnant woman only if clearly needed.

NURSING MOTHERS

Hyoscyamine is excreted in human milk. Caution should be exercised when hyoscyamine is administered to a nursing woman.

DRUG INTERACTIONS

Additive adverse effects resulting from cholinergic blockade may occur when hyoscyamine is administered concomitantly with other antimuscarinics, amantadine, haloperidol, phenothiazines, monoamine oxidase (MAO) inhibitors, tricyclic antidepressants, or some antihistamines.

Antacids may interfere with the absorption of hyoscyamine; take hyoscyamine before meals and antacids after meals.

ADVERSE REACTIONS

Not all of the following adverse reactions have been reported with hyoscyamine sulfate. The following adverse reactions have been reported for pharmacologically similar drugs with anticholinergic/antispasmodic action. Adverse reactions may include dryness of the mouth; urinary hesitancy and retention; blurred vision; tachycardia; palpitations; mydriasis; cycloplegia, increased ocular tension; loss of taste; headache; nervousness; drowsiness; weakness; dizziness; insomnia; nausea; vomiting; impotence; suppression of lactation; constipation; bloated feeling; allergic reactions or drug idiosyncrasies; urticaria and other dermal manifestations; ataxia; speech disturbance; some degree of mental confusion and/or excitement (especially in elderly persons); and decreased sweating.

H

DOSAGE AND ADMINISTRATION

Dosage may be adjusted according to the conditions and severity of symptoms.

SUBLINGUAL TABLETS

The tablets may be taken sublingually, orally, or chewed.

Adults and pediatric patients 12 years of age and older: 1-2 tablets every 4 hours or as needed. Do not exceed 12 tablets in 24 hours.

Pediatric patients 2 to under 12 years of age: ½-1 tablet every 4 hours or as needed. Do not exceed 6 tablets in 24 hours.

TABLETS

Adults and pediatric patients 12 years of age and older: 1-2 tablets every 12 hours. Do not exceed 12 tablets in 24 hours.

Pediatric patients 2 to under 12 years of age: ½-1 tablet every 4 hours or as needed. Do not exceed 6 tablets in 24 hours.

ELIXIR

Adults and pediatric patients 12 years of age and older: 1-2 teaspoonfuls every 4 hours or as needed. Do not exceed 12 teaspoonfuls in 24 hours.

Pediatric patients 2 to under 12 years of age: Please see the following dosage guide based on body weight. The doses may be repeated every 4 hours or as needed. Do not exceed 6 teaspoonfuls in 24 hours.

TABLE 1

Body Weight	Usual Dose
10 kg (22 lb)	¼ tsp
20 kg (44 lb)	½ tsp
40 kg (88 lb)	¾ tsp
50 kg (110 lb)	1 tsp

DROPS

Adults and pediatric patients 12 years of age and older: 1-2 ml every 4 hours or as needed. Do not exceed 12 ml in 24 hours.

Pediatric patients 2 to under 12 years of age: ¼-1 ml every 4 hours or as needed. Do not exceed 6 ml in 24 hours.

Pediatric patients under 2 years of age: The following dosage guide is based upon body weight. The doses may be repeated every 4 hours or as needed.

TABLE 2

Body Weight	Usual Dose	Do Not Exceed in 24 Hours
3.4 kg (7.5 lb)	4 drops	24 drops
5 kg (11 lb)	5 drops	30 drops
7 kg (15 lb)	6 drops	36 drops
10 kg (22 lb)	8 drops	48 drops

INJECTION

The dose may be administered subcutaneously, intramuscularly, or intravenously without dilution.

Gastrointestinal Disorders

The usual adult recommended dose is 0.5-1.0 ml (0.25-0.5 mg). Some patients may need only a single dose; others may require administration 2, 3, or 4 times a day at 4 hour intervals.

Diagnostic Procedures
The usual adult recommended dose is 0.5-1.0 ml (0.25-0.5 mg) administered intravenously 5-10 minutes prior to the diagnostic procedure.

Anesthesia
Adults and pediatric patients over 2 years of age: As a preanesthetic medication, the recommended dose is 5 µg (0.005 mg) per kg of body weight. This dose is usually given 30-60 minutes prior to the anticipated time of induction of anesthesia or at the time the preanesthetic narcotic or sedative is administered.
Hyoscyamine injection may be used during surgery to reduce drug-induced bradycardia. It should be administered intravenously in increments of 0.25 ml and repeated as needed. To achieve reversal of neuromuscular blockade, the recommended dose is 0.2 mg (0.4 ml) hyoscyamine injection for every 1 mg neostigmine or the equivalent dose of physostigmine or pyridostigmine.

Parenteral drug products should be inspected visually for particulate matter and discoloration prior to administration, whenever solution and container permit.

EXTENDED-RELEASE TABLETS
Adults and pediatric patients 12 years of age and older: 1-2 capsules every 12 hours. Dosage may be adjusted to 1 capsule every 8 hours if needed. Do not exceed 4 capsules in 24 hours.

ORALLY DISINTEGRATING TABLETS
Dosage may be adjusted according to the conditions and severity of symptoms. Place tablet on tongue, allowing the tablet to rapidly disintegrate and be swallowed. May be taken with or without water.
Adults and pediatric patients 12 years of age and older: 1-2 tablets every 4 hours or as needed. Do not exceed 12 tablets in 24 hours.
Pediatric patients 2 to under 12 years of age: ½ to 1 tablet every 4 hours or as needed. Do not exceed 6 tablets in 24 hours.

HOW SUPPLIED

Storage: Store at controlled room temperature 15-30°C (59-86°F). Dispense in a tight, light-resistant container.

PRODUCT LISTING - EQUIVALENTS NOT AVAILABLE

Capsule, Extended Release - Oral - 0.375 mg

20's	$6.85	GENERIC, Physicians Total Care	54868-3215-01
20's	$20.51	LEVSINEX SR, Allscripts Pharmaceutical Company	54569-3496-00
100's	$39.95	GENERIC, Superior Pharmaceutical Company	00144-0716-01
100's	$48.19	CYSTOSPAZ-M, Polymedica Pharmaceuticals Usa Inc	61451-2260-01
100's	$49.95	GENERIC, Moore, H.L. Drug Exchange Inc	00839-8071-06
100's	$49.95	GENERIC, Major Pharmaceuticals Inc	00904-7833-60
100's	$51.00	GENERIC, Watson/Rugby Laboratories Inc	00536-5592-01
100's	$51.00	GENERIC, Moore, H.L. Drug Exchange Inc	00839-7910-06
100's	$52.95	GENERIC, Amide Pharmaceutical Inc	52152-0163-02
100's	$53.20	GENERIC, Ivax Corporation	00182-1993-01
100's	$54.22	GENERIC, Ethex Corporation	58177-0017-04
100's	$54.28	GENERIC, Qualitest Products Inc	00603-4005-21
100's	$56.75	GENERIC, Kremers Urban	62175-0103-01
100's	$85.92	GENERIC, Duramed Pharmaceuticals Inc	51285-0938-02
100's	$128.36	LEVSINEX SR, Schwarz Pharma	00091-3537-01

Liquid - Oral - 0.125 mg/5 ml

15 ml	$14.60	GENERIC, Vintage Pharmaceuticals Inc	00254-9216-43
473 ml	$26.25	HYOSYNE, Silarx Pharmaceuticals Inc	54838-0511-80
473 ml	$88.58	LEVSIN, Schwarz Pharma	00091-4532-16
480 ml	$11.45	GENERIC, Ivax Corporation	00182-6136-40
480 ml	$15.74	GENERIC, Marlop Pharmaceuticals Inc	12939-0346-16
480 ml	$20.00	GENERIC, Marlop Pharmaceuticals Inc	12939-0775-16
480 ml	$29.70	GENERIC, Liquipharm Inc	54198-0147-16
480 ml	$38.10	GENERIC, Qualitest Products Inc	00603-1315-58

Solution - Injectable - 0.5 mg/ml

1 ml x 5	$90.05	LEVSIN, Schwarz Pharma	00091-1536-05

Solution - Oral - 0.125 mg/ml

15 ml	$8.40	GENERIC, Marlop Pharmaceuticals Inc	12939-0345-15
15 ml	$9.70	GENERIC, Kremers Urban	62175-0105-15
15 ml	$10.25	GENERIC, Econolab	55053-0380-15
15 ml	$10.50	HYOSYNE, Silarx Pharmaceuticals Inc	54838-0506-15
15 ml	$10.70	GENERIC, Liquipharm Inc	54198-0146-15
15 ml	$10.79	GENERIC, Aligen Independent Laboratories Inc	00405-2910-61
15 ml	$14.60	GENERIC, Qualitest Products Inc	00603-1314-73
15 ml	$14.60	GENERIC, Morton Grove Pharmaceuticals Inc	60432-0103-15
15 ml	$14.99	GENERIC, Cypress Pharmaceutical Inc	60258-0802-15
15 ml	$34.21	LEVSIN, Schwarz Pharma	00091-4538-15
480 ml	$25.96	GENERIC, Cypress Pharmaceutical Inc	60258-0801-16
480 ml	$38.30	GENERIC, Kremers Urban	62175-0104-16

Tablet - Oral - 0.125 mg

10's	$3.36	ANASPAZ, Physicians Total Care	54868-3451-00
20's	$3.17	GENERIC, Physicians Total Care	54868-2209-02
20's	$5.71	GENERIC, Allscripts Pharmaceutical Company	54569-3763-02
30's	$16.01	LEVSIN, Allscripts Pharmaceutical Company	54569-0428-00
40's	$5.01	GENERIC, Physicians Total Care	54868-2209-00
100's	$9.86	GENERIC, Physicians Total Care	54868-2209-03
100's	$11.25	GENERIC, Alphagen Laboratories Inc	59743-0026-01
100's	$12.37	GENERIC, Liquipharm Inc	57779-0101-04
100's	$12.95	GENERIC, Major Pharmaceuticals Inc	00904-2496-60
100's	$13.50	GENERIC, Aligen Independent Laboratories Inc	00405-4521-01
100's	$13.50	GENERIC, Marnel Pharmaceuticals Inc	00682-0106-01
100's	$15.50	GENERIC, Marlop Pharmaceuticals Inc	12939-0347-10
100's	$16.50	GENERIC, Trinity Technologies Corporation	61355-0002-10
100's	$18.00	ANASPAZ, Edwards Pharmaceuticals Inc	00485-0056-01
100's	$18.00	GENERIC, Marlop Pharmaceuticals Inc	12939-0773-60
100's	$19.78	GENERIC, Moore, H.L. Drug Exchange Inc	00839-7521-06
100's	$20.00	GENERIC, Liquipharm Inc	10267-1621-01
100's	$20.22	ANASPAZ, Ascher, B.F. and Company Inc	00225-0295-15
100's	$20.89	MEDISPAZ, Med Tek Pharmaceuticals Inc	52349-0240-10
100's	$24.15	GENERIC, Integrity Pharmaceutical Corporation	64731-0300-01
100's	$28.66	GENERIC, Ivax Corporation	00182-1607-01
100's	$29.24	GENERIC, Mutual Pharmaceutical Co Inc	00677-1662-01
100's	$29.25	GENERIC, Ethex Corporation	58177-0274-04
100's	$34.50	GENERIC, Qualitest Products Inc	00603-4003-21
100's	$36.15	GENERIC, Amide Pharmaceutical Inc	52152-0143-02
100's	$36.15	GENERIC, Kremers Urban	62175-0101-01
100's	$58.57	LEVSIN, Physicians Total Care	54868-1555-02
100's	$70.00	LEVSIN, Schwarz Pharma	00091-3531-01

Tablet - Oral - 0.15 mg

100's	$21.25	GENERIC, Expert-Med Inc	51991-0135-01
100's	$21.25	GENERIC, Econolab	55053-0111-01
100's	$24.25	GENERIC, Trinity Technologies Corporation	61355-0004-10
100's	$38.82	GENERIC, Prasco Laboratories	66993-0402-02
100's	$42.55	GENERIC, Integrity Pharmaceutical Corporation	64731-0295-01
100's	$47.81	CYSTOSPAZ, Polymedica Pharmaceuticals Usa Inc	61451-2225-01

Tablet - Sublingual - 0.125 mg

100's	$13.66	GENERIC, Hyrex Pharmaceuticals	00314-0011-01
100's	$17.77	LEVSIN SL, Physicians Total Care	54868-1767-00
100's	$18.25	GENERIC, Iomed Laboratories Inc	61646-0156-01
100's	$18.95	GENERIC, Econolab	55053-0170-01
100's	$18.95	HYOSOL/SL, Econolab	55053-0717-01
100's	$19.95	GENERIC, Aligen Independent Laboratories Inc	00405-4523-01
100's	$20.25	GENERIC, Liquipharm Inc	57779-0140-04
100's	$20.40	GENERIC, Trinity Technologies Corporation	61355-0003-10
100's	$20.99	GENERIC, Amide Pharmaceutical Inc	52152-0155-02
100's	$21.65	GENERIC, Watson/Rugby Laboratories Inc	00536-5575-01
100's	$22.94	GENERIC, Moore, H.L. Drug Exchange Inc	00839-7806-06
100's	$24.50	GENERIC, Major Pharmaceuticals Inc	00904-5120-60
100's	$25.35	GENERIC, Integrity Pharmaceutical Corporation	64731-0305-01
100's	$27.45	GENERIC, Mutual/United Research Laboratories	00677-1665-01
100's	$28.99	GENERIC, Ethex Corporation	58177-0255-04
100's	$30.00	SYMAX SL, Ion Laboratories Inc	11808-0111-01
100's	$33.37	SYMAX SL, Capellon Pharmaceuticals	64543-0111-01
100's	$34.50	GENERIC, Qualitest Products Inc	00603-4002-21
100's	$36.15	GENERIC, Kremers Urban	62175-0102-01
100's	$63.69	GENERIC, Ethex Corporation	58177-0423-04
100's	$67.48	LEVSIN SL, Schwarz Pharma	00091-3532-01

Tablet, Disintegrating - Oral - 0.125 mg

100's	$60.55	GENERIC, Breckenridge Inc	51991-0171-01
100's	$70.78	NULEV, Schwarz Pharma	00091-3111-01

Tablet, Extended Release - Oral - 0.375 mg

100's	$30.00	GENERIC, Dayton Laboratories Inc	52041-0017-15
100's	$39.95	GENERIC, Superior Pharmaceutical Company	00144-0717-01
100's	$39.95	GENERIC, Amide Pharmaceutical Inc	52152-0156-02
100's	$50.00	SYMAX SR, Ion Laboratories Inc	11808-0112-01
100's	$51.25	GENERIC, Iomed Laboratories Inc	61646-0155-01
100's	$53.39	GENERIC, Major Pharmaceuticals Inc	00904-5387-60
100's	$53.67	GENERIC, Watson/Rugby Laboratories Inc	00536-5900-01
100's	$53.95	GENERIC, Econolab	55053-0310-01
100's	$54.28	GENERIC, Qualitest Products Inc	00603-4004-21
100's	$54.28	GENERIC, Duramed Pharmaceuticals Inc	51285-0937-02
100's	$66.13	GENERIC, Mutual/United Research Laboratories	00677-1717-01
100's	$66.14	GENERIC, Ethex Corporation	58177-0237-04
100's	$66.74	SYMAX SR, Capellon Pharmaceuticals	64543-0112-01
100's	$69.15	GENERIC, Kremers Urban	62175-0108-01
100's	$114.13	LEVBID, Schwarz Pharma	00091-3538-01

Ibritumomab Tiuxetan (003550)

Categories: Lymphoma, non-Hodgkin's; FDA Approved 2002 Feb; Pregnancy Category D; Orphan Drugs
Drug Classes: Antineoplastics, monoclonal antibodies; Antineoplastics, radiopharmaceuticals; Monoclonal antibodies
Brand Names: Zevalin

WARNING

Note: The trade name has been used throughout this monograph for clarity.

Fatal Infusion Reactions

Deaths have occurred within 24 hours of rituximab infusion, an essential component of the Zevalin therapeutic regimen. These fatalities were associated with an infusion reaction symptom complex that included hypoxia, pulmonary infiltrates, acute respiratory distress syndrome, myocardial infarction, ventricular fibrillation, or cardiogenic shock. Approximately 80% of fatal infusion reactions occurred in association with the first rituximab infusion (see WARNINGS and ADVERSE REACTIONS). Patients who develop severe infusion reactions should have rituximab, In-111 Zevalin, and Y-90 Zevalin infusions discontinued and receive medical treatment.

Prolonged and Severe Cytopenias

Y-90 Zevalin administration results in severe and prolonged cytopenias in most patients. The Zevalin therapeutic regimen should not be administered to patients with ≥25% lymphoma marrow involvement and/or impaired bone marrow reserve (see ADVERSE REACTIONS).

Dosing:

- **The prescribed, measured, and administered dose of Y-90 Zevalin should not exceed the absolute maximum allowable dose of 32.0 mCi (1184 MBq).**
- **Y-90 Zevalin should not be administered to patients with altered biodistribution as determined by imaging with In-111 Zevalin.**

In-111 Zevalin and Y-90 Zevalin are radiopharmaceuticals and should be used only by physicians and other professionals qualified by training and experienced in the safe use and handling of radionuclides.

DESCRIPTION

ZEVALIN

Zevalin (ibritumomab tiuxetan) is the immunoconjugate resulting from a stable thiourea covalent bond between the monoclonal antibody ibritumomab and the linker-chelator tiuxetan [N-[2-bis(carboxymethyl)amino]-3-(p-isothiocyanatophenyl)-propyl]-[N-[2-bis(carboxymethyl)amino]-2-(methyl)-ethyl]glycine. This linker-chelator provides a high affinity, conformationally restricted chelation site for indium-111 or yttrium-90. The approximate molecular weight of ibritumomab tiuxetan is 148 kD.

The antibody moiety of Zevalin is ibritumomab, a murine IgG_1 kappa monoclonal antibody directed against the CD20 antigen, which is found on the surface of normal and malignant B lymphocytes. Ibritumomab is produced in Chinese hamster ovary cells and is composed of two murine gamma 1 heavy chains of 445 amino acids each and two kappa light chains of 213 amino acids each.

ZEVALIN THERAPEUTIC REGIMEN

The Zevalin therapeutic regimen is administered in two steps: Step 1 includes one infusion of rituximab preceding In-111 Zevalin. Step 2 follows Step 1 by 7-9 days and consists of a second infusion of rituximab followed by Y-90 Zevalin.

Zevalin is supplied as two separate and distinctly labeled kits that contain all of the non-radioactive ingredients necessary to produce a single dose of In-111 Zevalin and a single dose of Y-90 Zevalin, both essential components of the Zevalin therapeutic regimen. Indium-111 chloride and rituximab must be ordered separately from the Zevalin kit. Yttrium-90 chloride sterile solution is supplied by MDS Nordion when the Y-90 Zevalin kit is ordered.

ZEVALIN KITS

Each of the two Zevalin kits contains four vials that are used to produce a single dose of either In-111 Zevalin or Y-90 Zevalin, as indicated on the outer container label:

1. One (1) Zevalin vial containing 3.2 mg of ibritumomab tiuxetan in 2 ml of 0.9% sodium chloride solution; a sterile, pyrogen-free, clear, colorless solution that may contain translucent particles; no preservative present.
2. One (1) 50 mM Sodium Acetate Vial containing 13.6 mg of sodium acetate trihydrate in 2 ml of water for injection; a sterile, pyrogen-free, clear, colorless solution; no preservative present.
3. One (1) Formulation Buffer Vial containing 750 mg of albumin (human), 76 mg of sodium chloride, 21 mg of sodium phosphate dibasic heptahydrate, 4 mg of pentetic acid, 2 mg of potassium phosphate monobasic and 2 mg of potassium chloride in 10 ml of water for injection adjusted to pH 7.1 with either sodium hydroxide or hydrochloric acid; a sterile, pyrogen-free, clear yellow to amber colored solution; no preservative present.
4. One (1) empty Reaction Vial, sterile, pyrogen-free.

Physical/Radiochemical Characteristics of In-111

Indium-111 decays by electron capture, with a physical half-life of 67.3 hours (2.81 days).[1] The product of radioactive decay is nonradioactive cadmium-111. Radiation emission data for In-111 are summarized in TABLE 1.

TABLE 1 *Principal In-111 Radiation Emission Data*

Radiation	Mean % per Disintegration	Mean Energy (keV)
Gamma-2	90.2	171.3
Gamma-3	94.0	245.4

External Radiation

The exposure rate constant for 37 MBq (1 mCi) of In-111 is 8.3×10^{-4} C/kg/h (3.2 R/h) at 1 cm. Adequate shielding should be used with this gamma-emitter, in accordance with institutional good radiation safety practices.

To allow correction for physical decay of In-111, the fractions that remain at selected intervals before and after the time of calibration are shown in TABLE 2.

TABLE 2 *Physical Decay Chart: In-111 Half-Life 2.81 Days (67.3 Hours)*

Calibration Time	Fraction Remaining
-48 hours	1.64
-42 hours	1.54
-36 hours	1.45
-24 hours	1.28
-12 hours	1.13
-6 hours	1.06
0 hours	1.00
6 hours	0.94
12 hours	0.88
24 hours	0.78
36 hours	0.69
42 hours	0.65
48 hours	0.61

Physical/Radiochemical Characteristics of Y-90

Yttrium-90 decays by emission of beta particles, with a physical half-life of 64.1 hours (2.67 days).[1] The product of radioactive decay is non-radioactive zirconium-90. The range of beta particles in soft tissue (χ_{90}) is 5 mm. Radiation emission data for Y-90 are summarized in TABLE 3.

TABLE 3 *Principal Y-90 Radiation Emission Data*

Radiation	Mean % per Disintegration	Mean Energy (keV)
Beta minus	100	750-935

External Radiation

The exposure rate for 37 MBq (1 mCi) of Y-90 is 8.3×10^{-3} C/kg/h (32 R/h) at the mouth of an open Y-90 vial. Adequate shielding should be used with this beta-emitter, in accordance with institutional good radiation safety practices.

To allow correction for physical decay of Y-90, the fractions that remain at selected intervals before and after the time of calibration are shown in TABLE 4.

TABLE 4 *Physical Decay Chart: Y-90 Half-Life 2.67 Days (64.1 Hours)*

Calibration Time	Fraction Remaining	Calibration Time	Fraction Remaining
-36 hours	1.48	0 hours	1.00
-24 hours	1.30	1 hours	0.99
-12 hours	1.14	2 hours	0.98
-8 hours	1.09	3 hours	0.97
-7 hours	1.08	4 hours	0.96
-6 hours	1.07	5 hours	0.95
-5 hours	1.06	6 hours	0.94
-4 hours	1.04	7 hours	0.93
-3 hours	1.03	8 hours	0.92
-2 hours	1.02	12 hours	0.88
-1 hours	1.01	24 hours	0.77
0 hours	1.00	36 hours	0.68

CLINICAL PHARMACOLOGY

GENERAL PHARMACOLOGY

Ibritumomab tiuxetan binds specifically to the CD20 antigen (human B-lymphocyte-restricted differentiation antigen, Bp35).[2,3] The apparent affinity (K_D) of ibritumomab tiuxetan for the CD20 antigen ranges between approximately 14-18 nM.

The CD20 antigen is expressed on pre-B and mature B lymphocytes and on >90% of B-cell non-Hodgkin's lymphomas (NHL).[4,5] The CD20 antigen is not shed from the cell surface and does not internalize upon antibody binding.[6]

Mechanism of Action

The complementarity-determining regions of ibritumomab bind to the CD20 antigen on B lymphocytes. Ibritumomab, like rituximab, induces apoptosis in CD20+ B-cell lines *in vitro*.[6] The chelate tiuxetan, which tightly binds In-111 or Y-90, is covalently linked to the amino groups of exposed lysines and arginines contained within the antibody. The beta emission from Y-90 induces cellular damage by the formation of free radicals in the target and neighboring cells.[7]

Normal Human Tissue Cross-Reactivity

Ibritumomab tiuxetan binding was observed *in vitro* on lymphoid cells of the bone marrow, lymph node, thymus, red and white pulp of the spleen, and lymphoid follicles of the tonsil, as well as lymphoid nodules of other organs such as the large and small intestines. Binding was not observed on the nonlymphoid tissues or gonadal tissues (see Radiation Dosimetry).

PHARMACOKINETICS/PHARMACODYNAMICS

Pharmacokinetic and biodistribution studies were performed using In-111 Zevalin (5 mCi [185 MBq] In-111, 1.6 mg ibritumomab tiuxetan). In a study designed to assess the need for pre-administration of unlabeled antibody, only 18% of known sites of disease were imaged when In-111 Zevalin was administered without unlabeled ibritumomab. When preceded by unlabeled ibritumomab (1.0 or 2.5 mg/kg), In-111 Zevalin detected 56% and 92% of known disease sites, respectively.

In pharmacokinetic studies of patients receiving the Zevalin therapeutic regimen, the mean effective half-life for Y-90 activity in blood was 30 hours, and the mean area under the fraction of injected activity (FIA) vs time curve in blood was 39 hours. Over 7 days, a median of 7.2% of the injected activity was excreted in urine.

In clinical studies, administration of the Zevalin therapeutic regimen resulted in sustained depletion of circulating B cells. At 4 weeks, the median number of circulating B cells was zero (range, 0-1084 cell/mm^3). B-cell recovery began at approximately 12 weeks following treatment, and the median level of B cells was within the normal range (32-341 cells/mm^3) by 9 months after treatment. Median serum levels of IgG and IgA remained within the normal range throughout the period of B-cell depletion. Median IgM serum levels dropped below normal (median 49 mg/dl, range 13-3990 mg/dl) after treatment and recovered to normal values by 6 month post therapy.

RADIATION DOSIMETRY

Estimations of radiation-absorbed doses for In-111 Zevalin and Y-90 Zevalin were performed using sequential whole body images and the MIRDOSE 3 software program.[8,9] The estimated radiation absorbed doses to organs and marrow from a course of the Zevalin therapeutic regimen are summarized in TABLE 5. Absorbed dose estimates for the lower large intestine, upper large intestine, and small intestine have been modified from the standard MIRDOSE 3 output to account for the assumption that activity is within the intestine wall rather than the intestine contents.

TABLE 5 *Estimated Radiation Absorbed Doses From Y-90 Zevalin and In-111 Zevalin*

	Y-90 Zevalin (mGy/MBq)		In-111 Zevalin (mGy/MBq)	
Organ	**Median**	**Range**	**Median**	**Range**
Spleen*	9.4	1.8-14.4	0.9	0.2-1.2
Testes*	9.1	5.4-11.4	0.6	0.4-0.8
Liver*	4.8	2.3-8.1	0.7	0.3-1.1
Lower large intestinal wall*	4.8	3.1-8.2	0.4	0.2-0.6
Upper large intestinal wall*	3.6	2.0-6.7	0.3	0.2-0.6
Heart wall*	2.8	1.5-3.2	0.4	0.2-0.5
Lungs*	2.0	1.2-3.4	0.2	0.1-0.4
Small intestine*	1.4	0.8-2.1	0.2	0.1-0.3
Red marrow†	1.3	0.7-1.8	0.2	0.1-0.2
Urinary bladder wall‡	0.9	0.7-2.1	0.2	0.1-0.2
Bone surfaces†	0.9	0.5-1.2	0.2	0.1-0.2
Ovaries‡	0.4	0.3-0.5	0.2	0.2-0.2
Uterus‡	0.4	0.3-0.5	0.2	0.1-0.2
Adrenals‡	0.3	0.0-0.5	0.2	0.1-0.3
Brain‡	0.3	0.0-0.5	0.1	0.0-0.1
Breasts‡	0.3	0.0-0.5	0.1	0.0-0.1
Gallbladder wall‡	0.3	0.0-0.5	0.3	0.1-0.4
Muscle‡	0.3	0.0-0.5	0.1	0.0-0.1
Pancreas‡	0.3	0.0-0.5	0.2	0.1-0.3
Skin‡	0.3	0.0-0.5	0.1	0.0-0.1
Stomach‡	0.3	0.0-0.5	0.1	0.1-0.2
Thymus‡	0.3	0.0-0.5	0.1	0.1-0.2
Thyroid‡	0.3	0.0-0.5	0.1	0.0-0.1
Kidneys*	0.1	0.0-0.2	0.2	0.1-0.2
Total body‡	0.5	0.2-0.7	0.1	0.1-0.2

* Organ region of interest.
† Sacrum region of interest.[10]
‡ Whole body region of interest.

INDICATIONS AND USAGE

Zevalin, as part of the Zevalin therapeutic regimen (see DOSAGE AND ADMINISTRATION), is indicated for the treatment of patients with relapsed or refractory low-grade, follicular, or transformed B-cell non-Hodgkin's lymphoma, including patients with rituximab refractory follicular non-Hodgkin's lymphoma. Determination of the effectiveness of the Zevalin therapeutic regimen in a relapsed or refractory patient population is based on overall response rates. The effects of the Zevalin therapeutic regimen on survival are not known.

CONTRAINDICATIONS

The Zevalin therapeutic regimen is contraindicated in patients with known Type I hypersensitivity or anaphylactic reactions to murine proteins or to any component of this product, including rituximab, yttrium chloride, and indium chloride.

WARNINGS

SEE BOXED WARNING.

ALTERED BIODISTRIBUTION

Y-90 Zevalin should not be administered to patients with altered biodistribution of In-111 Zevalin. The expected biodistribution of In-111 Zevalin includes easily detectable uptake in the blood pool areas on the first day image, with less activity in the blood pool areas on the second or third day image; moderately high to high uptake in normal liver and spleen during the first day and the second or third day image; and moderately low or very low uptake in normal kidneys, urinary bladder, and normal bowel on the first day image and the second or third day image. Altered biodistribution of In-111 Zevalin can be characterized by diffuse uptake in normal lung more intense than the cardiac blood pool on the first day image or more intense than the liver on the second or third day image; kidneys with greater intensity than the liver on the posterior view of the second or third day image; or intense areas of uptake throughout the normal bowel comparable to uptake by the liver on the second or third day images.

SEVERE INFUSION REACTIONS

See PRECAUTIONS, Hypersensitivity.

The Zevalin therapeutic regimen may cause severe, and potentially fatal, infusion reactions. These severe reactions typically occur during the first rituximab infusion with time to onset of 30-120 minutes. Signs and symptoms of severe infusion reaction may include hypotension, angioedema, hypoxia, or bronchospasm, and may require interruption of rituximab, In-111 Zevalin, or Y-90 Zevalin administration. The most severe manifestations and sequelae may include pulmonary infiltrates, acute respiratory distress syndrome, myocardial infarction, ventricular fibrillation, and cardiogenic shock. **Because the Zevalin therapeutic regimen includes the use of rituximab, see also prescribing information for Rituxan (rituximab).**

CYTOPENIAS

See ADVERSE REACTIONS, Hematologic Events.

The most common severe adverse events reported with the Zevalin therapeutic regimen were thrombocytopenia (61% of patients with platelet counts <50,000 cells/mm^3) and neutropenia (57% of patients with absolute neutrophil count (ANC) <1,000 cells/mm^3) in patients with ≥150,000 platelets/mm^3 prior to treatment. Both incidences of severe thrombocytopenia and neutropenia increased to 78% and 74% for patients with mild thrombocytopenia at baseline (platelet count of 100,000-149,000 cells/mm^3). For all patients, the median time to nadir was 7-9 weeks and the median duration of cytopenias was 22-35 days. In <5% of cases, patients experienced severe cytopenia that extended beyond the prospectively defined protocol treatment period of 12 weeks following administration of the Zevalin therapeutic regimen. Some of these patients eventually recovered from cytopenia, while others experienced progressive disease, received further anti-cancer therapy, or died of their lymphoma without having recovered from cytopenia. The cytopenias may have influenced subsequent treatment decisions.

Hemorrhage, including fatal cerebral hemorrhage, and severe infections have occurred in a minority of patients in clinical studies. Careful monitoring for and management of cytopenias and their complications (*e.g.,* febrile neutropenia, hemorrhage) for up to 3 months after use of the Zevalin therapeutic regimen are necessary. Caution should be exercised in treating patients with drugs that interfere with platelet function or coagulation following the Zevalin therapeutic regimen and patients receiving such agents should be closely monitored.

The Zevalin therapeutic regimen should not be administered to patients with ≥25% lymphoma marrow involvement and/or impaired bone marrow reserve, *e.g.,* prior myeloablative therapies; platelet count <100,000 cells/mm^3; neutrophil count <1,500 cells/mm^3; hypocellular bone marrow (≤15% cellularity or marked reduction in bone marrow precursors); or to patients with a history of failed stem cell collection.

SECONDARY MALIGNANCIES

Out of 349 patients treated with the Zevalin therapeutic regimen, 3 cases of acute myelogenous leukemia and 2 cases of myelodysplastic syndrome have been reported following the Zevalin therapeutic regimen (see ADVERSE REACTIONS).

PREGNANCY CATEGORY D

Y-90 Zevalin can cause fetal harm when administered to a pregnant woman. There are no adequate and well-controlled studies in pregnant women. If this drug is used during pregnancy, or if the patient becomes pregnant while receiving this drug, the patient should be apprised of the potential hazard to the fetus. Women of childbearing potential should be advised to avoid becoming pregnant.

CREUTZFELDT-JAKOB DISEASE (CJD)

This product contains albumin, a derivative of human blood. Based on effective donor screening and product manufacturing processes, it carries an extremely remote risk for transmission of viral diseases. A theoretical risk for transmission of Creutzfeldt-Jakob Disease (CJD) also is considered extremely remote. No cases of transmission of viral diseases or CJD have ever been identified for albumin.

PRECAUTIONS

The Zevalin therapeutic regimen is intended as a single course treatment. The safety and toxicity profile from multiple courses of the Zevalin therapeutic regimen or of other forms of therapeutic irradiation preceding, following, or in combination with the Zevalin therapeutic regimen have not been established.

RADIONUCLIDE PRECAUTIONS

The contents of the Zevalin kit are not radioactive. However, during and after radiolabeling Zevalin with In-111 or Y-90, care should be taken to minimize radiation exposure to patients and to medical personnel, consistent with institutional good radiation safety practices and patient management procedures.

HYPERSENSITIVITY

Anaphylactic and other hypersensitivity reactions have been reported following the intravenous administration of proteins to patients. Medications for the treatment of hypersensitivity reactions, *e.g.,* epinephrine, antihistamines and corticosteroids, should be available for immediate use in the event of an allergic reaction during administration of Zevalin. Patients who have received murine proteins should be screened for human anti-mouse antibodies (HAMA). Patients with evidence of HAMA have not been studied and may be at increased risk of allergic or serious hypersensitivity reactions during Zevalin therapeutic regimen administrations.

IMMUNIZATION

The safety of immunization with live viral vaccines following the Zevalin therapeutic regimen has not been studied. Also, the ability of patients who received the Zevalin therapeutic regimen to generate a primary or anamnestic humoral response to any vaccine has not been studied.

LABORATORY MONITORING

Complete blood counts (CBC) and platelet counts should be obtained weekly following the Zevalin therapeutic regimen and should continue until levels recover. CBC and platelet counts should be monitored more frequently in patients who develop severe cytopenia, or as clinically indicated.

CARCINOGENESIS, MUTAGENESIS, AND IMPAIRMENT OF FERTILITY

No long-term animal studies have been performed to establish the carcinogenic or mutagenic potential of the Zevalin therapeutic regimen, or to determine its effects on fertility in males or females. However, radiation is a potential carcinogen and mutagen. The Zevalin therapeutic regimen results in a significant radiation dose to the testes. The radiation dose to the ovaries has not been established. There have been no studies to evaluate whether the Zevalin therapeutic regimen causes hypogonadism, premature menopause, azoospermia and/or mutagenic alterations to germ cells. There is a potential risk that the Zevalin therapeutic regimen could cause toxic effects on the male and female gonads. Effective contraceptive methods should be used during treatment and for up to 12 months following the Zevalin therapeutic regimen.

PREGNANCY CATEGORY D

SEE WARNINGS.

NURSING MOTHERS

It is not known whether Zevalin is excreted in human milk. Because human IgG is excreted in human milk and the potential for Zevalin exposure in the infant is unknown, women should be advised to discontinue nursing and formula feeding should be substituted for breast feedings (see CLINICAL PHARMACOLOGY).

GERIATRIC USE

Of 349 patients treated with the Zevalin therapeutic regimen in clinical studies, 38% (132 patients) were age 65 years and over, while 12% (41 patients) were age 75 years and over. No overall differences in safety or effectiveness were observed between these subjects and younger subjects, but greater sensitivity of some older individuals cannot be ruled out.

PEDIATRIC USE

The safety and effectiveness of the Zevalin therapeutic regimen in children have not been established.

DRUG INTERACTIONS

No formal drug interaction studies have been performed with Zevalin. Due to the frequent occurrence of severe and prolonged thrombocytopenia, the potential benefits of medications which interfere with platelet function and/or anticoagulation should be weighed against the potential increased risks of bleeding and hemorrhage. Patients receiving medications that interfere with platelet function or coagulation should have more frequent laboratory monitoring for thrombocytopenia. In addition, the transfusion practices for such patients may need to be modified given the increased risk of bleeding.

ADVERSE REACTIONS

Safety data, except where indicated, are based upon 349 patients treated in 5 clinical studies with the Zevalin therapeutic regimen (see DOSAGE AND ADMINISTRATION). Because the Zevalin therapeutic regimen includes the use of rituximab, also see prescribing information for Rituxan (rituximab).

The most serious adverse reactions caused by the Zevalin therapeutic regimen include infections (predominantly bacterial in origin), allergic reactions (bronchospasm and angioedema), and hemorrhage while thrombocytopenic (resulting in deaths). In addition, patients who have received the Zevalin therapeutic regimen have developed myeloid malignancies and dysplasias. Fatal infusion reactions have occurred following the infusion of rituximab. Please refer to the BOXED WARNING and WARNINGS sections for detailed descriptions of these reactions.

The most common toxicities reported were neutropenia, thrombocytopenia, anemia, gastrointestinal symptoms (nausea, vomiting, abdominal pain, and diarrhea), increased cough, dyspnea, dizziness, arthralgia, anorexia, anxiety, and ecchymosis. Hematologic toxicity was often severe and prolonged, whereas most non-hematologic toxicity was mild in severity. TABLE 7 lists adverse events that occurred in ≥5% of patients. A more detailed description of the incidence and duration of hematologic toxicities, according to baseline platelet count (as an indicator of bone marrow reserve) is provided in TABLE 8.

The following adverse events (except for those noted in TABLE 7) occurred in between 1 and 4% of patients during the treatment period: urticaria (4%), anxiety (4%), dyspepsia (4%), sweats (4%), petechia (3%), epistaxis (3%), allergic reaction (2%), and melena (2%).

Severe or life-threatening adverse events occurred in 1-5% of patients (except for those noted in TABLE 7) consisted of pancytopenia (2%), allergic reaction (1%), gastrointestinal hemorrhage (1%), melena (1%), tumor pain (1%), and apnea (1%). The following severe or life threatening events occurred in <1% of patients: angioedema, tachycardia, urticaria, arthritis, lung edema, pulmonary embolus, encephalopathy, hematemesis, subdural hematoma, and vaginal hemorrhage.

HEMATOLOGIC EVENTS

Hematologic toxicity was the most frequently observed adverse event in clinical trials. TABLE 8 presents the incidence and duration of severe hematologic toxicity for patients with normal baseline platelet count (≥150,000 cells/mm^3) treated with the Zevalin therapeutic regimen and patients with mild thrombocytopenia (platelet count 100,000-149,000 cells/mm^3) at baseline who were treated with a modified Zevalin therapeutic regimen that included a lower specific activity Y-90 Zevalin dose at 0.3 mCi/kg (11.1 MBq/kg).

Median time to ANC nadir was 62 days, to platelet nadir was 53 days, and to hemoglobin nadir was 68 days. Information on growth factor use and platelet transfusions is based on 211 patients for whom data were collected. Filgrastim was given to 13% of patients and erythropoietin to 8%. Platelet transfusions were given to 22% of patients and red blood cell transfusions to 20%.

INFECTIOUS EVENTS

During the first 3 months after initiating the Zevalin therapeutic regimen, 29% of patients developed infections. Three percent (3%) of patients developed serious infections comprising urinary tract infection, febrile neutropenia, sepsis, pneumonia, cellulitis, colitis, diarrhea, osteomyelitis, and upper respiratory tract infection. Life threatening infections were reported for 2% of patients that included sepsis, empyema, pneumonia, febrile neutropenia, fever, and biliary stent-associated cholangitis. During follow-up from 3 months to 4 years after the start of treatment with Zevalin, 6% of patients developed infections. Two percent (2%) of patients had serious infections comprising urinary tract infection, bacterial or viral pneumonia, febrile neutropenia, perihilar infiltrate, pericarditis, and intravenous drug-associated viral hepatitis. One percent (1%) of patients had life threatening infections that included bacterial pneumonia, respiratory disease, and sepsis.

TABLE 7 *Incidence of Adverse Events in ≥5% of Patients Receiving the Zevalin Therapeutic Regimen* (n=349)*

	All Grades	Grade 3/4
Any Adverse Event	**99%**	**89%**
Body as a Whole	**80%**	**12%**
Asthenia	43%	3%
Infection	29%	5%
Chills	24%	<1%
Fever	17%	1%
Abdominal pain	16%	3%
Pain	13%	1%
Headache	12%	1%
Throat irritation	10%	0%
Back pain	8%	1%
Flushing	6%	0%
Cardiovascular System	**17%**	**3%**
Hypotension	6%	1%
Digestive System	**48%**	**3%**
Nausea	31%	1%
Vomiting	12%	0%
Diarrhea	9%	<1%
Anorexia	8%	0%
Abdominal enlargement	5%	0%
Constipation	5%	0%
Hemic and Lymphatic System	**98%**	**86%**
Thrombocytopenia	95%	63%
Neutropenia	77%	60%
Anemia	61%	17%
Ecchymosis	7%	<1%
Metabolic and Nutritional Disorders	**23%**	**3%**
Peripheral edema	8%	1%
Angioedema	5%	<1%
Musculoskeletal System	**18%**	**1%**
Arthralgia	7%	1%
Myalgia	7%	<1%
Nervous System	**27%**	**2%**
Dizziness	10%	<1%
Insomnia	5%	0%
Respiratory System	**36%**	**3%**
Dyspnea	14%	2%
Increased cough	10%	0%
Rhinitis	6%	0%
Bronchospasm	5%	0%
Skin and Appendages	**28**	**1**
Pruritus	9%	<1%
Rash	8%	<1%
Special Senses	**7%**	**<1%**
Urogenital System	**6%**	**<1%**

* Adverse events were followed for a period of 12 weeks following the first rituximab infusion of the Zevalin therapeutic regimen.

Note: All adverse events are included, regardless of relationship.

TABLE 8 *Severe Hematologic Toxicity*

	Zevalin Therapeutic Regimen Using 0.4 mCi/kg Y-90 Dose (14.8 MBq/kg)	Modified Zevalin Therapeutic Regimen Using 0.3 mCi/kg Y-90 Dose (11.1 MBq/kg)
ANC		
Median nadir (cells/mm^3)	800	600
Per patient incidence ANC <1000 cells/mm^3	57%	74%
Per patient incidence ANC <500 cells/mm^3	30%	35%
Median duration (days)* ANC <1000 cells/mm^3	22	29
Platelets		
Median nadir (cells/mm^3)	41,000	24,000
Per patient incidence Platelets <50,000 cells/mm^3	61%	78%
Per patient incidence Platelets <10,000 cells/mm^3	10%	14%
Median duration (days)† Platelets <50,000 cells/mm^3	24	35

* Median duration of neutropenia for patients with ANC <1000 cells/mm^3 (Date from last laboratory value showing ANC ≥1000 cells/mm^3 to date of first laboratory value following nadir showing ANC ≥1000 cells/mm^3, censored at initiation of next treatment or death).

† Median duration of thrombocytopenia for patients with platelets <50,000 cells/mm^3 (Date from last laboratory value showing platelet count ≥50,000 cells/mm^3 to date of first laboratory value following nadir showing platelet count ≥50,000 cells/mm^3, censored at initiation of next treatment or death).

SECONDARY MALIGNANCIES

A total of 2% of patients developed secondary malignancies following the Zevalin therapeutic regimen. One patient developed a Grade 1 meningioma, three developed acute myelogenous leukemia, and two developed a myelodysplastic syndrome. The onset of a second cancer was 8-34 months following the Zevalin therapeutic regimen and 4-14 years following the patients' diagnosis of NHL.

IMMUNOGENICITY

Of 211 patients who received the Zevalin therapeutic regimen in clinical trials and who were followed for 90 days, there were eight (3.8%) patients with evidence of human anti-mouse antibody (HAMA) (n=5) or human anti-chimeric antibody (HACA) (n=4) at any time during the course of the study. Two patients had low titers of HAMA prior to initiation of the Zevalin therapeutic regimen; one remained positive without an increase in titer while the other had a negative titer post-treatment. Three patients had evidence of HACA responses prior to initiation of the Zevalin therapeutic regimen; one had a marked increase in HACA titer while the other two had negative titers post-treatment. Of the three patients who had negative HAMA or HACA titers prior to the Zevalin therapeutic regimen, two developed HAMA in absence of HACA titers, and one had both HAMA and HACA positive titers post-treatment. Evidence of immunogenicity may be masked in patients who are lymphopenic. There has not been adequate evaluation of HAMA and HACA at delayed timepoints, concurrent with the recovery from lymphopenia at 6-12 months, to establish whether masking of the immunogenicity at early timepoints occurs. The data reflect the percentage of patients whose test results were considered positive for antibodies to ibritumomab or rituximab using kinetic enzyme immunoassays to ibritumomab and rituximab. The observed incidence of antibody positivity in an assay is highly dependent on the sensitivity and specificity of the assay and may be influenced by several factors including sample handling and concomitant medications. Comparisons of the incidence of HAMA/HACA to the Zevalin therapeutic regimen with the incidence of antibodies to other products may be misleading.

DOSAGE AND ADMINISTRATION

The Zevalin therapeutic regimen is administered in two steps: Step 1 includes a single infusion of 250 mg/mm^2 rituximab (not included in the Zevalin kits) preceding a fixed dose of 5.0 mCi (1.6 mg total antibody dose) of In-111 Zevalin administered as a 10 minute IV push. Step 2 follows step 1 by 7-9 days and consists of a second infusion of 250 mg/mm^2 of rituximab prior to 0.4 mCi/kg of Y-90 Zevalin administered as a 10 minute IV push.

RITUXIMAB ADMINISTRATION

NOTE THAT THE DOSE OF RITUXIMAB IS LOWER WHEN USED AS PART OF THE ZEVALIN THERAPEUTIC REGIMEN, AS COMPARED TO THE DOSE OF RITUXIMAB WHEN USED AS A SINGLE AGENT. DO NOT ADMINISTER RITUXIMAB AS AN INTRAVENOUS PUSH OR BOLUS. Hypersensitivity reactions may occur (see WARNINGS). Premedication, consisting of acetaminophen and diphenhydramine, should be considered before each infusion of rituximab.

ZEVALIN THERAPEUTIC REGIMEN DOSE MODIFICATION IN PATIENTS WITH MILD THROMBOCYTOPENIA

The Y-90 Zevalin dose should be reduced to 0.3 mCi/kg (11.1 MBq/kg) for patients with a baseline platelet count between 100,000 and 149,000 cells/mm^3.

Two separate and distinctly-labeled kits are ordered for the preparation of a single dose each of In-111 Zevalin and Y-90 Zevalin. In-111 Zevalin and Y-90 Zevalin are radiopharmaceuticals and should be used only by physicians and other professionals qualified by training and experienced in the safe use and handling of radionuclides. **Changing the ratio of any of the reactants in the radiolabeling process may adversely impact therapeutic results. In-111 Zevalin and Y-90 Zevalin should not be used in the absence of the rituximab pre-dose.**

ZEVALIN THERAPEUTIC REGIMEN ADMINISTRATION

Step 1:

First Rituximab Infusion: Rituximab at a dose of 250 mg/mm^2 should be administered intravenously at an initial rate of 50 mg/h. Rituximab should not be mixed or diluted with other drugs. If hypersensitivity or infusion-related events do not occur, escalate the infusion rate in 50 mg/h increments every 30 minutes, to a maximum of 400 mg/h. If hypersensitivity or an infusion-related event develops, the infusion should be temporarily slowed or interrupted (see WARNINGS). The infusion can continue at one-half the previous rate upon improvement of patient symptoms.

In-111 Zevalin Injection: Within 4 hours following completion of the rituximab dose, 5.0 mCi (1.6 mg total antibody dose) of In-111 Zevalin is injected intravenously (IV) over a period of 10 minutes.

Assess Biodistribution: 1st image 2-24 hours after In-111 Zevalin, 2nd image 48-72 hours after In-111 Zevalin, optional: 3rd image 90-120 hours after In-111 Zevalin. If biodistribution is acceptable continue with Step 2. If biodistribution is not acceptable, DO NOT PROCEED with Step 2 (see Image Acquisition and Interpretation).

Step 2:

Step 2 of the Zevalin therapeutic regimen is initiated 7-9 days following Step 1 administrations.

Second Rituximab Infusion: Rituximab at a dose of 250 mg/mm^2 is administered IV at an initial rate of 100 mg/h (50 mg/h if infusion related events were documented during the first rituximab administration) and increased by 100 mg/h increments at 30 minute intervals, to a maximum of 400 mg/h, as tolerated.

Y-90 ZEVALIN INJECTION

Within 4 hours following completion of the rituximab dose, Y-90 Zevalin at a dose of 0.4 mCi/kg (14.8 MBq/kg) actual body weight for patients with a platelet count >150,000 cells/mm^3, and 0.3 mCi/kg (11.1 MBq/kg) actual body weight for patients with a platelet count of 100,000-149,000 cells/mm^3 is injected intravenously (IV) over a period of 10 minutes. Precautions should be taken to avoid extravasation. A free flowing IV line should be established prior to Y-90 Zevalin injection. Close monitoring for evidence of extravasation during the injection of Y-90 Zevalin is required. If any signs or symptoms of extravasation have occurred, the infusion should be immediately terminated and restarted in another vein. **The prescribed, measured, and administered dose of Y-90 Zevalin must not exceed the absolute maximum allowable dose of 32.0 mCi (1184 MBq), regardless of the patient's body weight. Do not give Y-90 Zevalin to patients with a platelet count <100,000/mm^3 (see WARNINGS).**

IMAGE ACQUISITION AND INTERPRETATION

The biodistribution of In-111 Zevalin should be assessed by a visual evaluation of whole body planar view anterior and posterior gamma images at 2-24 hours and 48-72 hours after injection. To resolve ambiguities, a third image at 90-120 hours may be necessary. Images should be acquired using a large field of view gamma camera equipped with a medium energy collimator. The gamma camera should be calibrated using the 171 and 245 keV photopeaks for In-111 with a 15-20% symmetric window. Using a 256 × 1024 computer acquisition matrix, the scan speed should be 10 cm/min for the first scan, 7 cm/min for the second scan, and 5 cm/min for the optional third scan.

The radiopharmaceutical is expected to be easily detectable in the blood pool areas at the first time point, with less activity in the blood pool on later images. Moderately high to high uptake is seen in the normal liver and spleen, with low uptake in the lungs, kidneys, and urinary bladder. Localization to lymphoid aggregates in the bowel wall has been reported. Tumor uptake may be visualized in soft tissue as areas of increased intensity, and tumor-bearing areas in normal organs may be seen as areas of increased or decreased intensity.

If a visual inspection of the gamma images reveals an altered biodistribution, the patient should not proceed to the Y-90 Zevalin dose. The patient may be considered to have an altered biodistribution if the blood pool is not visualized on the first image indicating rapid clearance of the radiopharmaceutical by the reticuloendothelial system to the liver, spleen, and/or marrow. Other potential examples of altered biodistribution may include diffuse uptake in the normal lungs or kidneys more intense than the liver on the second or third image.

During Zevalin clinical development, individual tumor radiation absorbed dose estimates as high as 778 cGy/mCi have been reported. Although solid organ toxicity has not been directly attributed to radiation from adjacent tumors, careful consideration should be applied before proceeding with treatment in patients with very high tumor uptake next to critical organs or structures.

HOW SUPPLIED

The In-111 Zevalin kit provides for the radiolabeling of ibritumomab tiuxetan with In-111. The Y-90 Zevalin kit provides for the radiolabeling of ibritumomab tiuxetan with Y-90.

The kit for the preparation of a single dose of In-111 Zevalin includes four vials: one Zevalin vial containing 3.2 mg of ibritumomab tiuxetan in 2 ml of 0.9% sodium chloride solution; one 50 mM Sodium Acetate vial; one Formulation Buffer vial; one empty Reaction vial and four identification labels.

The kit for the preparation of a single dose of Y-90 Zevalin includes four vials: one Zevalin vial containing 3.2 mg of ibritumomab tiuxetan in 2 ml of 0.9% sodium chloride solution; one 50 mM Sodium Acetate vial; one Formulation Buffer vial; one empty Reaction vial and four identification labels.

The contents of all vials are sterile, pyrogen-free and contain no preservatives.

The indium-111 chloride sterile solution (In-111 chloride) must be ordered separately from either Amersham Health, Inc. or Mallinckrodt, Inc. at the time the In-111 Zevalin kit is ordered. The yttrium-90 chloride sterile solution will be shipped directly from MDS Nordion upon placement of an order for the Y-90 Zevalin kit.

Storage: Store at 2-8°C (36-46°F). Do not freeze.

PRODUCT LISTING - EQUIVALENTS NOT AVAILABLE

Kit - Intravenous - 3.2 mg/2 ml

1's	$2915.40	IN-111 ZEVALIN, Idec Pharmaceuticals Corporation	64406-0104-04
1's	$25238.85	Y-90 ZEVALIN, Idec Pharmaceuticals Corporation	64406-0103-03

Ibuprofen

(001520)

For related information, see the comparative table section in Appendix A.

Categories: Arthritis, osteoarthritis; Arthritis, rheumatoid; Dysmenorrhea; Fever; Pain, mild to moderate; FDA Approved 1985 May; Pregnancy Category B; Pregnancy Category D, 3rd Trimester; WHO Formulary

Drug Classes: Analgesics, non-narcotic; Antipyretics; Nonsteroidal anti-inflammatory drugs

Brand Names: Advil; Ibren; Ibu-Tab; Ibuprohm; Ifen; **Motrin**; Profen

Foreign Brand Availability: Act-3 (Australia; New-Zealand); Adex 200 (Israel); Advil Infantil (Mexico); Advil Liqui-Gels (Israel); Afebril (Peru); Algofen (Italy); Allipen (Korea); Am-Fam 400 (India); Ampifen (Singapore); Anadvil (France); Anbifen (Thailand); Anco (Germany); Andran (Japan); Anflagen (Japan); Antarene (France); Antiflam (South-Africa); Apo-Ibuprofen (Canada); Atril 300 (Brazil); Balkaprofen (Benin; Burkina-Faso; Ethiopia; Gambia; Ghana; Guinea; Ivory-Coast; Kenya; Liberia; Malawi; Mali; Mauritania; Mauritius; Morocco; Niger; Nigeria; Senegal; Seychelles; Sierra-Leone; Sudan; Tanzania; Tunia; Uganda; Zambia; Zimbabwe); Bestafen (Mexico); Betaprofen (South-Africa); Bifen (Hong-Kong; Singapore); Bluton (Japan); Brufanic (Japan); Brufen (Australia; Austria; Bahrain; Belgium; Bulgaria; Cyprus; Czech-Republic; Denmark; Egypt; England; Finland; France; Germany; Greece; Hong-Kong; Iran; Iraq; Ireland; Italy; Japan; Jordan; Korea; Kuwait; Lebanon; Libya; Malaysia; Netherlands; New-Zealand; Norway; Oman; Philippines; Portugal; Qatar; Republic-of-Yemen; Saudi-Arabia; South-Africa; Sweden; Switzerland; Syria; Taiwan; Thailand; Turkey; United-Arab-Emirates); Brufen Retard (New-Zealand); Brufen 400 (Israel); Brufort (Italy); Brugesic (South-Africa); Brumed (Thailand); Buburone (Japan); Bufect (Indonesia); Bufect Forte (Indonesia); Bupogesic (Hong-Kong); Burana (Finland); Butacortelone (Mexico); Carol (Korea); Children's Motrin (Indonesia); Codral Period Pain (Australia; New-Zealand); Combiflam (India); Cuprofen (Thailand); Dibufen (Mexico); Diffutab SR 600 (Korea); Dolan FP (Philippines); Dolgit (Bahrain; Cyprus; Egypt; Germany; Iran; Iraq; Israel; Jordan; Kuwait; Lebanon; Libya; Oman; Qatar; Republic-of-Yemen; Saudi-Arabia; Syria; Taiwan; United-Arab-Emirates); Dolocyl (Switzerland); Dolofen-F (Indonesia); Dolomax (Peru); Dolval (Mexico); Donjust B (Japan); Dorival (Spain); Drin (Greece); Easifon (Taiwan); Emflam-200 (India); Emodin (Argentina); Epobron (Japan); Expanfen (France); Febratic (Mexico); Febryn (Indonesia); Fenbid (Bahrain; Benin; Burkina-Faso; Cyprus; Egypt; England; Ethiopia; Gambia; Ghana; Guinea; Iran; Iraq; Israel; Ivory-Coast; Jordan; Kenya; Kuwait; Lebanon; Liberia; Libya; Malawi; Mali; Mauritania; Mauritius; Morocco; Niger; Nigeria; Oman; Qatar; Republic-of-Yemen; Saudi-Arabia; Senegal; Seychelles; Sierra-Leone; South-Africa; Sudan; Syria; Tanzania; Tunia; Uganda; United-Arab-Emirates; Zambia; Zimbabwe); Focus (Italy); Gyno-neuralgin (Germany); H-Loniten (Colombia); IB-100 (Japan); Ibosure (Netherlands); Ibufen (Israel; Malaysia); Ibuflam (Mexico); Ibufug (Germany); Ibugesic (India); Ibulgan (Bahamas; Bahrain; Barbados; Belize; Benin; Bermuda; Burkina-Faso; Curacao; Cyprus; Egypt; Ethiopia; Gambia; Ghana; Guinea; Guyana; Iran; Iraq; Israel; Ivory-Coast; Jamaica; Jordan; Kenya; Kuwait; Lebanon; Liberia; Libya; Malawi; Mali; Mauritania; Mauritius; Morocco; Netherland-Antilles; Niger; Nigeria; Oman; Puerto-Rico; Qatar; Republic-of-Yemen; Saudi-Arabia; Senegal; Seychelles; Sierra-Leone; South-Africa; Sudan; Surinam; Syria; Tanzania; Trinidad; Tunia; Uganda; United-Arab-Emirates; Zambia; Zimbabwe); Ibuloid (Singapore); Ibumetin (Denmark; Finland; Netherlands; Norway; Sweden); Ibupen (Hong-Kong); Ibupirac (Argentina); Ibuprocin (Japan); Ibuprofen (Hong-Kong); Iburon (Korea); Ibusal (Finland); Ibu-slow (Belgium); Idyl SR (Philippines); Infibu (Colombia); Ipren (Denmark; Korea; Russia; Sweden); Irfen (Bahrain; Cyprus; Egypt; Iran; Iraq; Israel; Jordan; Kuwait; Lebanon; Libya; Oman; Qatar; Republic-of-Yemen; Saudi-Arabia; Switzerland; Syria; United-Arab-Emirates); Isodol (Spain); Lamidon (Japan); Librofem (Spain); Liptan (Bahrain; Cyprus; Egypt; Iran; Iraq; Israel; Japan; Jordan; Kuwait; Lebanon; Libya; Oman; Qatar; Republic-of-Yemen; Saudi-Arabia; Syria; United-Arab-Emirates); Lopane (Thailand); Mensoton (Germany); Mobilat (China); Mynosedin (Japan); Nagifen-D (Japan); Napacetin (Japan); Nobfelon (Japan); Nobgen (Japan); Norflam-T (South-Africa); Noritis (Benin; Burkina-Faso; Ethiopia; Gambia; Ghana; Guinea; Ivory-Coast; Kenya; Liberia; Malawi; Mali; Mauritania; Mauritius; Morocco; Niger; Nigeria; Senegal; Seychelles; Sierra-Leone; South-Africa; Sudan; Tanzania; Tunia; Uganda; Zambia; Zimbabwe); Norton (South-Africa); Novogent (Germany); Novoprofen (Canada); Nureflex (France); Nurofen (Australia; Austria; Belgium; Benin; Burkina-Faso; Czech-Republic; Denmark; England; Ethiopia; Gambia; Ghana; Guinea; Ivory-Coast; Kenya; Liberia; Malawi; Mali; Mauritania; Mauritius; Morocco; Netherlands; New-Zealand; Niger; Nigeria; Philippines; Senegal; Seychelles; Sierra-Leone; Singapore; South-Africa; Sudan; Sweden; Tanzania; Tunia; Turkey; Uganda; Zambia; Zimbabwe); Optifen (Switzerland); Opturem (Germany); Oren (Colombia); Ostarin (Indonesia); Ostofen (Thailand); Panafen (New-Zealand); Pantrop (Japan); Perofen (Bahamas; Barbados; Belize; Bermuda; Curacao; Guyana; Jamaica; Malaysia; Netherland-Antilles; Puerto-Rico; Surinam; Trinidad); Proartinal (Mexico); Profeno (Thailand); Proris (Indonesia); Provon (Peru); Quadrax (Mexico); Rafen (Australia; New-Zealand); Ranofen (South-Africa); Roidenin (Japan); Rupan (Bahrain; Cyprus; Egypt; Iran; Iraq; Jordan; Kuwait; Lebanon; Libya; Oman; Qatar; Republic-of-Yemen; Saudi-Arabia; Syria; Thailand; United-Arab-Emirates); Schufen (Hong-Kong); Solufen Lidose (Singapore); Syntofene (France); Tabalon (Ecuador); Tabalon 400 (Mexico); Tatanal (Korea); Tofen (Thailand); Upfen (France); Uprofen (Taiwan); Urem (Germany); Zofen (Malaysia)

Cost of Therapy: $24.11 (Osteoarthritis; Motrin; 400 mg; 3 tablets/day; 30 day supply)
$3.56 (Osteoarthritis; Generic Tablets; 400 mg; 3 tablets/day; 30 day supply)

DESCRIPTION

Motrin tablets and ibuprofen children's suspension contain the active ingredient ibuprofen, which is (±)-2-(*p*-isobutylphenyl) propionic acid. Ibuprofen is a white powder with a melting point of 74-77°C and is very slightly soluble in water (<1 mg/ml) and readily soluble in organic solvents such as ethanol and acetone.

SUSPENSION

Ibuprofen children's suspension is a nonsteroidal anti-inflammatory agent. It is available for oral administration as a sucrose-sweetened, fruit-flavored liquid suspension containing 100 mg of ibuprofen per 5 ml.

Inactive Ingredients: Cellulose gum, citric acid, disodium EDTA, FD&C red no. 40, flavors, glycerin, microcrystalline cellulose, polysorbate 80, sodium benzoate, sorbitol, sucrose, water, xanthan gum.

TABLETS

Ibuprofen, a nonsteroidal anti-inflammatory agent, is available in 400, 600, and 800 mg tablets for oral administration.

Inactive Ingredients: Carnauba wax, colloidal silicon dioxide, croscarmellose sodium, hydroxypropyl methylcellulose, lactose, magnesium stearate, microcrystalline cellulose, propylene glycol, titanium dioxide.

CLINICAL PHARMACOLOGY

Ibuprofen tablets and ibuprofen children's suspension contain ibuprofen which possesses analgesic and antipyretic activities. Its mode of action, like that of other nonsteroidal anti-inflammatory agents, is not completely understood, but may be related to prostaglandin synthetase inhibition.

PHARMACOKINETICS

Ibuprofen is rapidly metabolized and eliminated in the urine. The excretion of ibuprofen is virtually complete 24 hours after the last dose. The serum half-life is 1.8-2 hours.

Suspension

Ibuprofen is rapidly absorbed when administered orally. As is true with most tablet and suspension formulations, ibuprofen children's suspension is absorbed somewhat faster than the tablet with a time to peak serum level generally within 1 hour. Peak serum ibuprofen levels are generally attained 1-2 hours after administration of ibuprofen tablets and within about 1 hour after the suspension. With single, oral, solid doses up to 800 mg, in adults, a linear relationship exists between the amount of drug administered and the integrated area under the serum drug concentration versus time curve. Above 800 mg, however, the area under the curve increase is less than proportional to the increase in dose. There is no evidence of age-dependent kinetics in patients 2-11 years old. With single doses of ibuprofen children's suspension ranging up to 10 mg/kg, a dose/response relationship exists between the amount of drug administered to febrile children and the serum concentration versus time curve. There is also a correlation between reduction of fever and drug concentration over time, although the peak reduction in fever occurs 2-4 hours after dosing.

No absorption differences are noticeable when ibuprofen tablets or suspension are given under fasting conditions or immediately before meals. When either product is taken with food, however, the peak levels are somewhat lower (up to 30%) and the time to reach peak levels is slightly prolonged (up to 30 min) although the extent of absorption is unchanged. A bioavailability study has shown that there was no interference with the absorption of ibuprofen when given in conjunction with an antacid containing both aluminum hydroxide and magnesium hydroxide.

Studies have shown that following ingestion of the drug, 45-79% of the dose was recovered in the urine within 24 hours as metabolite A (25%), (+)-2-4′-(2-hydroxy-2-methylpropyl)-phenylpropionic acid and metabolite B (37%), (+)-2-4′-(2-carboxypropyl)-phenylpropionic acid; the percentages of free and conjugated ibuprofen were approximately 1% and 14%, respectively.

Tablets

Ibuprofen is rapidly absorbed. Peak serum ibuprofen levels are generally attained 1-2 hours after administration. With single doses up to 800 mg, a linear relationship exists between amount of drug administered and the integrated area under the serum drug concentration versus time curve. Above 800 mg, however, the area under the curve increases less than proportional to increases in dose. There is no evidence of drug accumulation or enzyme induction.

The administration of ibuprofen tablets either under fasting conditions or immediately before meals yields quite similar serum ibuprofen concentration-time profiles. When ibuprofen is administered immediately after a meal, there is a reduction in the rate of absorption but no appreciable decrease in the extent of absorption. The bioavailability of the drug is minimally altered by the presence of food.

A bioavailability study has shown that there was no interference with the absorption of ibuprofen when ibuprofen was given in conjunction with an antacid containing both aluminum hydroxide and magnesium hydroxide.

Studies have shown that following ingestion of the drug, 49-79% of the dose was recovered in the urine within 24 hours as metabolite A (25%), (+)-2-[*p*-(2 hydroxymethyl-propyl) phenyl] propionic acid and metabolite B (37%), (+)-2-[*p*-(2 carboxypropyl)phenyl] propionic acid; the percentages of free and conjugated ibuprofen were approximately 1% and 14%, respectively.

INDICATIONS AND USAGE

SUSPENSION

Ibuprofen children's suspension is indicated for relief of the signs and symptoms of juvenile arthritis, rheumatoid arthritis and osteoarthritis.

Ibuprofen children's suspension is indicated for the relief of mild to moderate pain in adults and of primary dysmenorrhea.

Ibuprofen children's suspension is also indicated for the reduction of fever in patients ages 6 months and older.

Since there have been no controlled trials to demonstrate whether there is any beneficial effect or harmful interaction with the use of ibuprofen in conjunction with aspirin, the combination cannot be recommended (see DRUG INTERACTIONS).

TABLETS

Ibuprofen tablets are indicated for relief of the signs and symptoms of rheumatoid arthritis and osteoarthritis.

Ibuprofen is indicated for relief of mild to moderate pain.

Ibuprofen is also indicated for the treatment of primary dysmenorrhea.

Since there have been no controlled clinical trials to demonstrate whether or not there is any beneficial effect or harmful interaction with the use of ibuprofen in conjunction with aspirin, the combination cannot be recommended (see DRUG INTERACTIONS).

Controlled clinical trials to establish the safety and effectiveness of ibuprofen in children have not been conducted.

CONTRAINDICATIONS

Ibuprofen tablets or ibuprofen children's suspension should not be used in patients who have previously exhibited hypersensitivity to the drug, or in individuals with the syndrome of nasal polyps, angioedema, and bronchospastic reactivity to aspirin or other nonsteroidal anti-inflammatory agents. Anaphylactoid reactions have occurred in such patients.

WARNINGS

RISK OF GI ULCERATION, BLEEDING AND PERFORATION WITH NONSTEROIDAL ANTI-INFLAMMATORY THERAPY

Serious gastrointestinal toxicity such as bleeding, ulceration, and perforation, can occur at any time, with or without warning symptoms, in patients treated chronically with nonsteroidal anti-inflammatory drugs. Although minor upper gastrointestinal problems, such as dyspepsia, are common, usually developing early in therapy, physicians should remain alert for ulceration and bleeding in patients treated chronically with nonsteroidal anti-inflammatory drugs even in the absence of previous GI tract symptoms. In patients observed in clinical trials of several months to 2 years duration, symptomatic upper GI ulcers, gross bleeding or perforation appear to occur in approximately 1% of patients treated for 3-6 months, and in about 2-4% of patients treated for 1 year. Physicians should inform patients about the signs and/or symptoms of serious GI toxicity and what steps to take if they occur.

Studies to date have not identified any subset of patients not at risk of developing peptic ulceration and bleeding. Except for a prior history of serious GI events and other risk factors known to be associated with peptic ulcer disease, such as alcoholism, smoking, etc., no risk factors (*e.g.*, age, sex) have been associated with increased risk. Elderly or debilitated patients seem to tolerate ulceration or bleeding less well than other individuals and most spontaneous reports of fatal GI events are in this population. Studies to date are inconclusive concerning the relative risk of various nonsteroidal anti-inflammatory agents in causing such reactions. High doses of any such agents probably carry a greater risk of these reactions, although controlled clinical trials showing this do not exist in most cases. In considering the use of relatively large doses (within the recommended dosage range), sufficient benefit should be anticipated to offset the potential increased risk of GI toxicity.

PRECAUTIONS

GENERAL

Blurred and/or diminished vision, scotomata, and/or changes in color vision have been reported. If a patient develops such complaints while receiving ibuprofen, the drug should be discontinued, and the patient should have an ophthalmologic examination which includes central visual fields and color vision testing.

Fluid retention and edema have been reported in association with ibuprofen; therefore, the drug should be used with caution in patients with a history of cardiac decompensation or hypertension.

Ibuprofen, like other nonsteroidal anti-inflammatory agents, can inhibit platelet aggregation but the effect is quantitatively less and of shorter duration than that seen with aspirin. Ibuprofen has been shown to prolong bleeding time (but within the normal range) in normal subjects. Because this prolonged bleeding effect may be exaggerated in patients with underlying hemostatic defects, ibuprofen should be used with caution in persons with intrinsic coagulation defects and those on anticoagulant therapy.

Patients on ibuprofen should report to their physicians signs or symptoms of gastrointestinal ulceration or bleeding, blurred vision or other eye symptoms, skin rash, weight gain, or edema.

In order to avoid exacerbation of disease or adrenal insufficiency, patients who have been on prolonged corticosteroid therapy should have their therapy tapered slowly rather than discontinued abruptly when ibuprofen is added to the treatment program.

The antipyretic and anti-inflammatory activity of ibuprofen may reduce fever and inflammation, thus diminishing their utility as diagnostic signs in detecting complications of presumed noninfectious, noninflammatory painful conditions.

Liver Effects

As with other nonsteroidal anti-inflammatory drugs, borderline elevations of one or more liver function tests may occur in up to 15% of patients. These abnormalities may progress, may remain essentially unchanged, or may be transient with continued therapy. The SGPT (ALT) test is probably the most sensitive indicator of liver dysfunction. Meaningful (3 times the upper limit of normal) elevations of SGPT or SGOT (AST) occurred in controlled clinical trials in less than 1% of patients. A patient with symptoms and/or signs suggesting liver dysfunction, or in whom an abnormal liver test has occurred, should be evaluated for evidence of the development of more severe hepatic reactions while on therapy with ibuprofen. Severe hepatic reactions, including jaundice and cases of fatal hepatitis, have been reported with ibuprofen as with other nonsteroidal anti-inflammatory drugs. Although such reactions are rare, if abnormal liver tests persist or worsen, if clinical signs and symptoms consistent with liver disease develop, or if systemic manifestations occur (*e.g.*, eosinophilia, rash, etc.), ibuprofen should be discontinued.

Hemoglobin Levels

In cross-study comparisons with doses ranging from 1200-3200 mg daily for several weeks, a slight dose-response decrease in hemoglobin/hematocrit was noted. This has been observed with other nonsteroidal anti-inflammatory drugs; the mechanism is unknown. With daily doses of 3200 mg, the total decrease in hemoglobin may exceed 1 g; if there are no signs of bleeding, it is probably not clinically important.

In two postmarketing clinical studies the incidence of a decreased hemoglobin level was greater than previously reported. Decrease in hemoglobin of 1 g or more was observed in 17.1% of 193 patients on 1600 mg ibuprofen daily (osteoarthritis), and in 22.8% of 189 patients taking 2400 mg of ibuprofen daily (rheumatoid arthritis). Positive stool occult blood tests and elevated serum creatinine levels were also observed in these studies.

Aseptic Meningitis

Aseptic meningitis with fever and coma has been observed on rare occasions in patients on ibuprofen therapy. Although it is probably more likely to occur in patients with systemic lupus erythematosus and related connective tissue diseases, it has been reported in patients who do not have an underlying chronic disease. If signs or symptoms of meningitis develop in a patient on ibuprofen, the possibility of its being related to ibuprofen should be considered.

Renal Effects

As with other nonsteroidal anti-inflammatory drugs, long-term administration of ibuprofen to animals has resulted in renal papillary necrosis and other abnormal renal pathology. In humans, there have been reports of acute interstitial nephritis with hematuria, proteinuria, and occasionally nephrotic syndrome.

A second form of renal toxicity has been seen in patients with prerenal conditions leading to a reduction in renal blood flow or blood volume, where the renal prostaglandins have a supportive role in the maintenance of renal perfusion. In these patients administration of a nonsteroidal anti-inflammatory drug may cause a dose dependent reduction in prostaglandin formation and may precipitate overt renal decompensation. Patients at greatest risk of this reaction are those with impaired renal function, heart failure, liver dysfunction, those taking diuretics and the elderly. Discontinuation of nonsteroidal anti-inflammatory drug therapy is typically followed by recovery to the pretreatment state. Those patients at high risk who chronically take ibuprofen should have renal function monitored if they have signs or symptoms which may be consistent with mild azotemia, such as malaise, fatigue, loss of appetite, etc. Occasional patients may develop some elevation of serum creatinine and BUN levels without signs or symptoms.

Since ibuprofen is eliminated primarily by the kidneys, patients with significantly impaired renal function should be closely monitored; and a reduction in dosage should be anticipated to avoid drug accumulation. Prospective studies on the safety of ibuprofen in patients with chronic renal failure have not been conducted.

INFORMATION FOR THE PATIENT

Ibuprofen, like other drugs of its class, is not free of side effects. The side effects of these drugs can cause discomfort and, rarely, there are more serious side effects, such as gastrointestinal bleeding, which may result in hospitalization and even fatal outcomes.

Nonsteroidal anti-inflammatory drugs are often essential agents in the management of arthritis and have a major role in the treatment of pain, but they also may be commonly employed for conditions which are less serious.

Physicians may wish to discuss with their patients the potential risks (see WARNINGS, Renal Effects, and ADVERSE REACTIONS) and likely benefits of nonsteroidal anti-inflammatory drug treatment, particularly when the drugs are used for less serious conditions where treatment without such agents may represent an acceptable alternative to both the patient and physician.

LABORATORY TESTS

Because serious GI tract ulcerations and bleeding can occur without warning symptoms, physicians should follow chronically treated patients for the signs and symptoms of ulcerations and bleeding and should inform them of the importance of this follow-up (see WARNINGS, Risk of GI Ulceration, Bleeding and Perforation With Nonsteroidal Anti-inflammatory Therapy).

PREGNANCY

Reproductive studies conducted in rats and rabbits at doses somewhat less than the maximal clinical dose did not demonstrate evidence of developmental abnormalities. However, animal reproduction studies are not always predictive of human response. As there are no adequate and well-controlled studies in pregnant women, this drug should be used during pregnancy only if clearly needed. Because of the known effects of nonsteroidal anti-inflammatory drugs on the fetal cardiovascular system (closure of ductus arteriosus), use during late pregnancy should be avoided. As with other drugs known to inhibit prostaglandin synthesis, an increased incidence of dystocia and delayed parturition occurred in rats. Administration of ibuprofen is not recommended during pregnancy.

NURSING MOTHERS

In limited studies, an assay capable of detecting 1 μg/ml did not demonstrate ibuprofen in the milk of lactating mothers. However, because of the limited nature of the studies, and the possible adverse effects of prostaglandin-inhibiting drugs on neonates, ibuprofen is not recommended for use in nursing mothers.

PEDIATRIC USE

Suspension

Infants: Safety and efficacy of ibuprofen children's suspension in children below the age of 6 months has not been established.

DRUG INTERACTIONS

Coumarin-Type Anticoagulants: Several short-term controlled studies failed to show that ibuprofen significantly affected prothrombin times or a variety of other clotting factors when administered to individuals on coumarin-type anticoagulants. However, because bleeding has been reported when ibuprofen and other nonsteroidal anti-inflammatory agents have been administered to patients on coumarin-type anticoagulants, the physician should be cautious when administering ibuprofen to patients on anticoagulants.

Aspirin: Animal studies show that aspirin given with nonsteroidal anti-inflammatory agents, including ibuprofen, yields a net decrease in anti-inflammatory activity with lowered blood levels of the non-aspirin drug. Single dose bioavailability studies in normal volunteers have failed to show an effect of aspirin on ibuprofen blood levels. Correlative clinical studies have not been performed.

Methotrexate: Ibuprofen, as well as other nonsteroidal anti-inflammatory drugs, probably reduces the tubular secretion of methotrexate based on *in vitro* studies in rabbit kidney slices. This may indicate that ibuprofen could enhance the toxicity of methotrexate. Caution should be used if ibuprofen is administered concomitantly with methotrexate.

H-2 Antagonists: In studies with human volunteers, co-administration of cimetidine or ranitidine with ibuprofen had no substantive effect on ibuprofen serum concentrations.

Furosemide: Clinical studies, as well as random observations, have shown that ibuprofen can reduce the natriuretic effect of furosemide and thiazides in some patients. This response has been attributed to inhibition of renal prostaglandin synthesis. During concomitant therapy with ibuprofen, the patient should be observed closely for signs of renal failure (see PRECAUTIONS, General, Renal Effects), as well as to assure diuretic efficacy.

Lithium: Ibuprofen produced an elevation of plasma lithium levels and a reduction in renal lithium clearance in a study of eleven normal volunteers. The mean minimum lithium concentration increased 15% and the renal clearance of lithium was decreased by 19% during this period of concomitant drug administration.

This effect has been attributed to inhibition of renal prostaglandin synthesis by ibuprofen. Thus, when ibuprofen and lithium are administered concurrently, subjects should be observed carefully for signs of lithium toxicity. (Read circular for lithium preparation before use of such concurrent therapy).

ADVERSE REACTIONS

TABLETS AND SUSPENSION

The most frequent type of adverse reaction occurring with ibuprofen is gastrointestinal. In controlled clinical trials, the percentage of patients reporting one or more gastrointestinal complaints ranged from 4% to 16%.

In controlled studies when ibuprofen was compared to aspirin and indomethacin in equally effective doses, the overall incidence of gastrointestinal complaints was about half that seen in either the aspirin- or indomethacin-treated patients.

Adverse reactions observed during controlled clinical trials at an incidence greater than 1% are listed in TABLE 1A and TABLE 1B. Those reactions listed in column one encompass observations in approximately 3000 patients. More than 500 of these patients were treated for periods of at least 54 weeks.

Still other reactions occurring less frequently than 1 in 100 were reported in controlled clinical trials and from marketing experience. These reactions have been divided into two categories: column two of TABLE 1A and TABLE 1B lists reactions with therapy with ibuprofen where the probability of a causal relationship exists; for the reactions in column three, a causal relationship with ibuprofen has not been established.

Reported side effects were higher at doses of 3200 mg/day than at doses of 2400 mg or less per day in clinical trials of patients with rheumatoid arthritis. The increases in incidence were slight and still within the ranges reported in TABLE 1A and TABLE 1B.

TABLE 1A

Incidence Greater than 1% (but less than 3%) Probable Causal Relationship	Precise Incidence Unknown (but less than 1%) Probable Causal Relationship*	Precise Incidence Unknown (but less than 1%) Causal Relationship Unknown*
Gastrointestinal		
Nausea†, epigastric pain†, heartburn†, diarrhea, abdominal distress, nausea and vomiting, indigestion, constipation, abdominal cramps or pain, fullness of GI tract (bloating and flatulence)	Gastric or duodenal ulcer with bleeding and/or perforation, gastrointestinal hemorrhage, melena, gastritis, hepatitis, jaundice, abnormal liver function tests; pancreatitis	
Central Nervous System		
Dizziness†, headache, nervousness	Depression, insomnia, confusion, emotional lability, somnolence, aseptic meningitis with fever and coma (See PRECAUTIONS)	Paresthesias, hallucinations, dream abnormalities, pseudotumor cerebri
Dermatologic		
Rash† (including maculopapular type), pruritus	Vesiculobullous eruptions, urticaria, erythema multiform, Stevens-Johnson syndrome, alopecia	Toxic epidermal necrolysis, photoallergic skin reactions
Special Senses		
Tinnitus	Hearing loss, amblyopia (blurred and/or diminished vision, scotomata and/or changes in color vision) (see PRECAUTIONS)	Conjunctivitis, diplopia, optic neuritis, cataracts

* Reactions are classified under *"Probable Causal Relationship (PCR)"* if there has been 1 positive rechallenge or if 3 or more cases occur which might be causally related. Reactions are classified under *"Causal Relationship Unknown"* if 7 or more events have been reported but the criteria for PCR have not been met.

† Reactions occurring in 3-9% of patients treated with ibuprofen. (Those reactions occurring in less than 3% of the patients are unmarked.)

SUSPENSION

In a 12 week comparison of ibuprofen children's suspension (n=45) and aspirin (n=47) in children with juvenile arthritis, the most common adverse experiences were also gastrointestinal in nature, usually of mild severity. Abdominal pain of possible drug relationship was reported in about 25% of patients on ibuprofen and/or aspirin; other possibly drug-related effects associated with the digestive system were reported in 42% of the children taking ibuprofen and in 70% of those taking aspirin.

DOSAGE AND ADMINISTRATION

TABLETS

Do not exceed 3200 mg total daily dose. If gastrointestinal complaints occur, administer ibuprofen tablets with meals or milk.

Rheumatoid Arthritis and Osteoarthritis, Including Flare-Ups of Chronic Disease

Suggested Dosage

1200-3200 mg daily (300 mg qid; 400 , 600 or 800 mg tid or qid). Individual patients may show a better response to 3200 mg daily, as compared with 2400 mg, although in well-controlled clinical trials patients on 3200 mg did not show a better mean response in terms of efficacy. Therefore, when treating patients with 3200 mg/day, the physician should observe sufficient increased clinical benefits to offset potential increased risk.

The dose should be tailored to each patient, and may be lowered or raised depending on the severity of symptoms either at time of initiating drug therapy or as the patient responds or fails to respond.

In general, patients with rheumatoid arthritis seem to require higher doses of ibuprofen than do patients with osteoarthritis.

The smallest dose of ibuprofen that yields acceptable control should be employed. A linear blood level dose-response relationship exists with single doses up to 800 mg (see CLINICAL PHARMACOLOGY) for effects of food on rate of absorption.

The availability of four tablet strengths facilitates dosage adjustment.

In Chronic Conditions

A therapeutic response to therapy with ibuprofen is sometimes seen in a few days to a week but most often is observed by 2 weeks. After a satisfactory response has been achieved, the patient's dose should be reviewed and adjusted as required.

TABLE 1B

Incidence Greater than 1% (but less than 3%) Probable Causal Relationship	Precise Incidence Unknown (but less than 1%) Probable Causal Relationship*	Precise Incidence Unknown (but less than 1%) Causal Relationship Unknown*
Hematologic		
	Neutropenia, agranulocytosis, aplastic anemia, hemolytic anemia (sometimes Coombs positive), thrombocytopenia with or without purpura, eosinophilia, decreases in hemoglobin and hematocrit (see PRECAUTIONS)	Bleeding episodes (*e.g.*, epistaxis, menorrhagia)
Metabolic/Endocrine		
Decreased appetite		Gynecomastia, hypoglycemic reaction, acidosis
Cardiovascular		
Edema, fluid retention (generally responds promptly to drug discontinuation) (see PRECAUTIONS)	Congestive heart failure in patients with marginal cardiac function, elevated blood pressure, palpitations	Arrhythmias (sinus tachycardia, sinus bradycardia)
Allergic		
	Syndrome of abdominal pain, fever, chills, nausea and vomiting; anaphylaxis; bronchospasm (see CONTRAINDICATIONS)	Serum sickness, lupus erythematosus syndrome, Henoch-Schonlein vasculitis, angioedema
Renal		
	Acute renal failure (see PRECAUTIONS), decreased creatinine clearance, polyuria, azotemia, cystitis, hematuria	Renal papillary necrosis
Miscellaneous		
	Dry eyes and mouth, gingival ulcer, rhinitis	

* Reactions are classified under *"Probable Causal Relationship (PCR)"* if there has been 1 positive rechallenge or if 3 or more cases occur which might be causally related. Reactions are classified under *"Causal Relationship Unknown"* if 7 or more events have been reported but the criteria for PCR have not been met.

SUSPENSION

Shake well prior to administration.

Do not exceed 3200 mg total daily dose. If gastrointestinal complaints occur, administer ibuprofen with meals or milk.

Juvenile Arthritis

The usual dose is 30-40 mg/kg/day divided into 3 or 4 doses. Patients with milder disease may be adequately treated with 20 mg/kg/day.

Doses above 50 mg/kg/day are not recommended because they have not been studied and because side effects appear to be dose related.

Therapeutic response may require from a few days to several weeks to be achieved. Once a clinical response is obtained, dosage should be lowered to the smallest dose of ibuprofen children's suspension needed to maintain adequate control of disease.

Rheumatoid Arthritis and Osteoarthritis, Including Flare-Ups of Chronic Disease

Suggested Adult Dosage: 1200-3200 mg daily (300 mg qid, or 400, 600 or 800 mg tid or qid). Individual patients may show a better response to 3200 mg daily, as compared with 2400 mg, although in well-controlled clinical trials patients on 3200 mg did not show a better mean response in terms of efficacy. Therefore, when treating patients with 3200 mg/day, the physician should observe sufficient increased clinical benefits to offset potential increased risk.

The dose of ibuprofen children's suspension should be tailored to each patient, and may be lowered or raised from the suggested doses depending on the severity of symptoms either at the time of initiating drug therapy or as the patient responds to fails to respond.

In general, patients with rheumatoid arthritis seem to require higher doses of ibuprofen than do patients with osteoarthritis.

The smallest dose of ibuprofen children's suspension that yields acceptable control should be employed. A linear blood level dose-response relationship exists with single doses up to 800 mg (see CLINICAL PHARMACOLOGY, Pharmacokinetics for effects of food on rate of absorption).

In chronic conditions, a therapeutic response to ibuprofen therapy is sometimes seen in a few days to a week but most often is observed by 2 weeks. After a satisfactory response has been achieved, the patient's dose should be reviewed and adjusted as required.

Fever Reduction in Children 6 Months to 12 Years of Age

Dosage should be adjusted on the basis of the initial temperature level. The recommended dose is 5 mg/kg if the baseline temperature is 102.5°F or below or 10 mg/kg if the baseline temperature is greater than 102.5°F. The duration of fever reduction is generally 6-8 hours and is longer with the higher dose. The recommended maximum daily dose is 40 mg/kg (see TABLE 2).

Fever Reduction in Adults

400 mg every 4-6 hours as necessary.

Information for Patients

Ibuprofen, like other drugs of its class, is not free of side effects. The side effects of these drugs can cause discomfort and, rarely, there are more serious side effects, such as gastrointestinal bleeding, which may result in hospitalization and even fatal outcomes.

TABLE 2

Age	Weight (lb)	5 mg/kg (Fever ≤102.5° F) (mg)	(tsp)	10 mg/kg (Fever >102.5° F) (mg)	(tsp)
6-11 months	13-17	25	¼	50	½
12-23 months	18-23	50	½	100	1
2-3 years	24-35	75	¾	150	1½
4-5 years	36-47	100	1	200	2
6-8 years	48-59	125	1¼	250	2½
9-10 years	60-71	150	1½	300	3
11-12 years	72-95	200	2	400	4

Nonsteroidal anti-inflammatory drugs are often essential agents in the management of arthritis and have a major role in the treatment of pain, but they also may be commonly employed for conditions which are less serious.

Physicians may wish to discuss with their patients the potential risks (see WARNINGS, PRECAUTIONS, and ADVERSE REACTIONS) and likely benefits of nonsteroidal anti-inflammatory drug treatment, particularly when the drugs are used for less serious conditions where treatment without such agents may represent an acceptable alternative to both the patient and physician.

TABLETS AND SUSPENSION

Mild to Moderate Pain: 400 mg every 4-6 hours as necessary for the relief of pain in adults.

In controlled analgesic clinical trials, doses of ibuprofen greater than 400 mg were no more effective than the 400 mg dose.

Dysmenorrhea: For the treatment of dysmenorrhea, beginning with the earliest onset of such pain, ibuprofen children's suspension should be given in a dose of 400 mg every 4 hours as necessary for the relief of pain.

HOW SUPPLIED

MOTRIN TABLETS

400 mg: White, round, and imprinted with "Motrin 400".
600 mg: White, elliptical, and imprinted with "Motrin 600".
800 mg: White, elliptical, and imprinted with "Motrin 800".

Storage

Store at controlled room temperature 20-25°C (68-77°F).

MOTRIN CHILDREN'S SUSPENSION

Motrin Children's Suspension is available for oral administration as a sucrose-sweetened, fruit-flavored liquid suspension containing 100 mg of ibuprofen per 5 ml.

Storage

Ibuprofen children's suspension should be stored at controlled room temperature; 20-25°C (68-77°F).

Shake well before use. Keep container tightly closed.

PRODUCT LISTING - RATED THERAPEUTICALLY EQUIVALENT

Tablet - Oral - 300 mg

50's	$5.20	GENERIC, Major Pharmaceuticals Inc	00904-1638-51
100's	$6.00	GENERIC, Major Pharmaceuticals Inc	00904-1638-60

Tablet - Oral - 400 mg

8's	$6.72	GENERIC, Pd-Rx Pharmaceuticals	55289-0590-08
12's	$7.70	GENERIC, Pd-Rx Pharmaceuticals	55289-0590-12
15's	$8.02	GENERIC, Pd-Rx Pharmaceuticals	55289-0590-15
20's	$3.12	GENERIC, Alpharma Uspd Makers Of Barre and Nmc	63874-0322-20
20's	$3.40	MOTRIN, Allscripts Pharmaceutical Company	54569-4321-02
20's	$5.47	MOTRIN, Prescript Pharmaceuticals	00247-0162-20
20's	$8.30	GENERIC, Pd-Rx Pharmaceuticals	55289-0590-20
21's	$4.16	GENERIC, Alpharma Uspd Makers Of Barre and Nmc	63874-0322-21
21's	$8.82	GENERIC, Pd-Rx Pharmaceuticals	55289-0590-21
25 x 30	$165.38	GENERIC, Sky Pharmaceuticals Packaging, Inc	63739-0135-03
25's	$3.22	GENERIC, Udl Laboratories Inc	51079-0291-19
25's	$5.52	GENERIC, Udl Laboratories Inc	51079-0281-19
25's	$7.53	GENERIC, Pd-Rx Pharmaceuticals	55289-0590-97
30's	$4.53	GENERIC, Golden State Medical	60429-0092-30
30's	$5.66	MOTRIN, Physicians Total Care	54868-0438-00
30's	$6.24	GENERIC, Alpharma Uspd Makers Of Barre and Nmc	63874-0322-30
30's	$6.53	MOTRIN, Prescript Pharmaceuticals	00247-0162-30
30's	$6.67	GENERIC, Heartland Healthcare Services	61392-0527-30
30's	$6.67	GENERIC, Heartland Healthcare Services	61392-0527-39
30's	$7.94	MOTRIN, Allscripts Pharmaceutical Company	54569-4321-00
30's	$9.91	GENERIC, Pd-Rx Pharmaceuticals	55289-0590-30
31 x 10	$62.00	GENERIC, Vangard Labs	00615-2525-53
31 x 10	$62.00	GENERIC, Vangard Labs	00615-2525-63
31's	$6.89	GENERIC, Heartland Healthcare Services	61392-0527-31
32's	$7.11	GENERIC, Heartland Healthcare Services	61392-0527-32
36's	$10.64	GENERIC, Pd-Rx Pharmaceuticals	55289-0590-36
40's	$6.81	MOTRIN, Allscripts Pharmaceutical Company	54569-4321-03
40's	$7.59	MOTRIN, Prescript Pharmaceuticals	00247-0162-40
40's	$8.32	GENERIC, Alpharma Uspd Makers Of Barre and Nmc	63874-0322-40
40's	$11.20	GENERIC, Pd-Rx Pharmaceuticals	55289-0590-40
45's	$10.00	GENERIC, Heartland Healthcare Services	61392-0527-45
50's	$8.51	MOTRIN, Allscripts Pharmaceutical Company	54569-4321-01
60's	$13.33	GENERIC, Heartland Healthcare Services	61392-0527-60
60's	$15.42	GENERIC, Alpharma Uspd Makers Of Barre and Nmc	63874-0322-60
60's	$15.75	GENERIC, Pd-Rx Pharmaceuticals	55289-0590-60
60's	$58.13	GENERIC, Udl Laboratories Inc	51079-0281-98
90's	$17.15	GENERIC, Interpharm Inc	53746-0131-90
90's	$18.47	GENERIC, Allscripts Pharmaceutical Company	54569-3820-00
90's	$20.00	GENERIC, Heartland Healthcare Services	61392-0527-90
90's	$20.83	GENERIC, Pd-Rx Pharmaceuticals	55289-0590-90
100's	$3.95	GENERIC, Raway Pharmacal Inc	00686-1809-01
100's	$3.95	GENERIC, Major Pharmaceuticals Inc	00904-5185-60
100's	$4.25	GENERIC, Knoll Pharmaceutical Company	00044-0165-01
100's	$4.93	FEDERAL UPPER LIMIT, H.C.F.A. F F P	99999-1520-02
100's	$5.68	GENERIC, Richmond Pharmaceuticals	54738-0119-13
100's	$6.00	GENERIC, Interstate Drug Exchange Inc	00814-3813-14
100's	$6.50	GENERIC, Raway Pharmacal Inc	00686-0281-20
100's	$11.00	GENERIC, Baker Norton Pharmaceuticals	50732-0744-01
100's	$11.60	GENERIC, Major Pharmaceuticals Inc	00904-1648-60
100's	$11.60	GENERIC, Major Pharmaceuticals Inc	00904-1748-60
100's	$11.69	GENERIC, Purepac Pharmaceutical Company	00228-2124-10
100's	$11.95	GENERIC, Marlop Pharmaceuticals Inc	12939-0814-01
100's	$12.12	GENERIC, Invamed Inc	52189-0223-24
100's	$12.38	GENERIC, Aligen Independent Laboratories Inc	00405-4527-01
100's	$12.39	GENERIC, Par Pharmaceutical Inc	49884-0162-01
100's	$13.00	GENERIC, Alra	51641-0214-01
100's	$16.70	GENERIC, Pd-Rx Pharmaceuticals	55289-0590-01
100's	$17.43	GENERIC, Auro Pharmaceutical	55829-0312-10
100's	$19.48	GENERIC, Interpharm Inc	53746-0131-01
100's	$19.50	GENERIC, Dixon-Shane Inc	17236-0568-01
100's	$19.76	GENERIC, Alpharma Uspd Makers Of Barre and Nmc	63874-0322-01
100's	$20.50	GENERIC, Qualitest Products Inc	00603-4018-21
100's	$20.50	GENERIC, Par Pharmaceutical Inc	49884-0467-01
100's	$20.50	GENERIC, Par Pharmaceutical Inc	49884-0777-01
100's	$21.55	GENERIC, Major Pharmaceuticals Inc	00904-1748-61
100's	$22.10	GENERIC, Udl Laboratories Inc	51079-0281-20
100's	$22.95	GENERIC, Watson/Schein Pharmaceuticals Inc	00364-0765-90
100's	$26.79	MOTRIN, Pharmacia and Upjohn	00009-7385-01
100's	$29.10	MOTRIN, Pharmacia and Upjohn	00009-7385-04
100's	$30.16	GENERIC, Ivax Corporation	00182-1809-89
100's	$32.19	GENERIC, Alra	51641-0214-11
120's	$23.81	MOTRIN, Pharmacia and Upjohn	00009-0750-26

Tablet - Oral - 600 mg

4's	$0.96	MOTRIN, Allscripts Pharmaceutical Company	54569-4319-06
6's	$7.00	GENERIC, Pd-Rx Pharmaceuticals	55289-0142-06
10's	$7.56	GENERIC, Pd-Rx Pharmaceuticals	55289-0142-10
12's	$4.26	GENERIC, Alpharma Uspd Makers Of Barre and Nmc	63874-0324-12
12's	$8.12	GENERIC, Pd-Rx Pharmaceuticals	55289-0142-12
14's	$9.03	GENERIC, Pd-Rx Pharmaceuticals	55289-0142-14
15's	$5.03	GENERIC, Alpharma Uspd Makers Of Barre and Nmc	63874-0324-15
15's	$9.21	GENERIC, Pd-Rx Pharmaceuticals	55289-0142-15
18's	$9.42	GENERIC, Pd-Rx Pharmaceuticals	55289-0142-18
20's	$5.30	GENERIC, Alpharma Uspd Makers Of Barre and Nmc	63874-0324-20
20's	$6.53	MOTRIN, Prescript Pharmaceuticals	00247-0161-20
20's	$7.74	MOTRIN, Allscripts Pharmaceutical Company	54569-4319-00
20's	$10.47	GENERIC, Pd-Rx Pharmaceuticals	55289-0142-20
21's	$6.14	GENERIC, Alpharma Uspd Makers Of Barre and Nmc	63874-0324-21
21's	$10.68	GENERIC, Pd-Rx Pharmaceuticals	55289-0142-21
24's	$6.24	GENERIC, Alpharma Uspd Makers Of Barre and Nmc	63874-0324-24
24's	$11.73	GENERIC, Pd-Rx Pharmaceuticals	55289-0142-24
25 x 30	$229.58	GENERIC, Sky Pharmaceuticals Packaging, Inc	63739-0136-03
25's	$7.40	GENERIC, Udl Laboratories Inc	51079-0282-19
25's	$14.35	GENERIC, Pd-Rx Pharmaceuticals	55289-0142-97
30's	$2.95	GENERIC, Major Pharmaceuticals Inc	00904-1758-46
30's	$3.24	GENERIC, Pd-Rx Pharmaceuticals	58864-0286-30
30's	$5.00	GENERIC, Golden State Medical	60429-0093-30
30's	$7.37	MOTRIN, Physicians Total Care	54868-0439-03
30's	$8.12	MOTRIN, Prescript Pharmaceuticals	00247-0161-30
30's	$8.84	GENERIC, Alpharma Uspd Makers Of Barre and Nmc	63874-0324-30
30's	$11.56	GENERIC, Heartland Healthcare Services	61392-0529-30
30's	$11.56	GENERIC, Heartland Healthcare Services	61392-0529-39
30's	$11.61	MOTRIN, Allscripts Pharmaceutical Company	54569-4319-04
30's	$12.81	GENERIC, Pd-Rx Pharmaceuticals	55289-0142-30
31 x 10	$86.03	GENERIC, Vangard Labs	00615-2526-53
31 x 10	$86.03	GENERIC, Vangard Labs	00615-2526-63
31's	$11.94	GENERIC, Heartland Healthcare Services	61392-0529-31

Qty	Price	Product	NDC
32's	$12.33	GENERIC, Heartland Healthcare Services	61392-0529-32
40's	$8.65	GENERIC, St. Mary'S Mpp	60760-0076-40
40's	$11.44	GENERIC, Alpharma Uspd Makers Of Barre and Nmc	63874-0324-40
40's	$16.63	GENERIC, Pd-Rx Pharmaceuticals	55289-0142-40
60's	$4.60	GENERIC, Major Pharmaceuticals Inc	00904-1758-52
60's	$4.90	GENERIC, Pd-Rx Pharmaceuticals	58864-0286-60
60's	$13.53	MOTRIN, Physicians Total Care	54868-0439-04
60's	$16.64	GENERIC, Alpharma Uspd Makers Of Barre and Nmc	63874-0324-60
60's	$20.55	GENERIC, Pd-Rx Pharmaceuticals	55289-0142-60
60's	$23.11	GENERIC, Heartland Healthcare Services	61392-0529-60
60's	$58.13	GENERIC, Udl Laboratories Inc	51079-0282-98
90's	$15.38	GENERIC, Golden State Medical	60429-0093-90
90's	$25.10	GENERIC, Interpharm Inc	53746-0132-90
90's	$26.21	MOTRIN, Pharmacia and Upjohn	00009-0742-08
90's	$31.12	MOTRIN, Pharmacia and Upjohn	00009-7386-05
90's	$34.67	GENERIC, Heartland Healthcare Services	61392-0529-90
100's	$4.45	GENERIC, Raway Pharmacal Inc	00686-1810-01
100's	$5.56	GENERIC, Knoll Pharmaceutical Company	00044-0162-01
100's	$5.73	FEDERAL UPPER LIMIT, H.C.F.A. F F P	99999-1520-10
100's	$6.95	GENERIC, Raway Pharmacal Inc	00686-0282-20
100's	$7.20	GENERIC, Interstate Drug Exchange Inc	00814-3814-14
100's	$7.75	GENERIC, Cmc-Consolidated Midland Corporation	00223-1092-01
100's	$14.75	GENERIC, Baker Norton Pharmaceuticals	50732-0747-01
100's	$16.75	GENERIC, Major Pharmaceuticals Inc	00904-1658-60
100's	$16.75	GENERIC, Major Pharmaceuticals Inc	00904-1758-60
100's	$16.75	GENERIC, Par Pharmaceutical Inc	49884-0163-01
100's	$16.83	GENERIC, Aligen Independent Laboratories Inc	00405-4528-01
100's	$16.85	GENERIC, Warner Chilcott Laboratories	00047-0922-24
100's	$17.19	GENERIC, Invamed Inc	52189-0224-24
100's	$17.43	GENERIC, Auro Pharmaceutical	55829-0313-10
100's	$17.55	GENERIC, Moore, H.L. Drug Exchange Inc	00839-7113-06
100's	$18.50	GENERIC, Alra	51641-0213-01
100's	$22.89	GENERIC, Pd-Rx Pharmaceuticals	55289-0142-01
100's	$26.80	GENERIC, St. Mary'S Mpp	60760-0076-00
100's	$27.39	GENERIC, Major Pharmaceuticals Inc	00904-5186-60
100's	$27.64	GENERIC, Watson/Schein Pharmaceuticals Inc	00364-0766-01
100's	$27.64	GENERIC, Watson Laboratories Inc	00591-4011-01
100's	$27.64	GENERIC, Dixon-Shane Inc	17236-0569-01
100's	$27.65	GENERIC, Interpharm Inc	53746-0132-01
100's	$28.45	GENERIC, Major Pharmaceuticals Inc	00904-1758-61
100's	$29.04	GENERIC, Qualitest Products Inc	00603-4019-21
100's	$29.04	GENERIC, Par Pharmaceutical Inc	49884-0468-01
100's	$29.04	GENERIC, Par Pharmaceutical Inc	49884-0778-01
100's	$29.60	GENERIC, Udl Laboratories Inc	51079-0282-20
100's	$29.75	GENERIC, Pd-Rx Pharmaceuticals	55289-0142-17
100's	$30.45	GENERIC, Major Pharmaceuticals Inc	00904-5186-61
100's	$31.33	GENERIC, Vangard Labs	00615-2526-13
100's	$31.45	GENERIC, Watson/Schein Pharmaceuticals Inc	00364-0766-90
100's	$34.55	MOTRIN, Pharmacia and Upjohn	00009-7386-01
100's	$38.69	MOTRIN, Pharmacia and Upjohn	00009-7386-04
100's	$40.00	GENERIC, Alra	51641-0213-11
100's	$40.64	GENERIC, Ivax Corporation	00182-1810-89
100's	$41.45	GENERIC, American Health Packaging	62584-0747-01
100's	$45.90	GENERIC, Alpharma Uspd Makers Of Barre and Nmc	63874-0324-01
120's	$7.28	GENERIC, Pd-Rx Pharmaceuticals	58864-0286-98
120's	$7.70	GENERIC, Major Pharmaceuticals Inc	00904-1758-18
180's	$12.55	GENERIC, Major Pharmaceuticals Inc	00904-1758-93
270's	$62.85	MOTRIN, Allscripts Pharmaceutical Company	54569-8588-00

Tablet - Oral - 800 mg

Qty	Price	Product	NDC
15's	$3.30	GENERIC, Pd-Rx Pharmaceuticals	58864-0287-15
15's	$5.13	GENERIC, Dhs Inc	55887-0976-15
15's	$6.61	GENERIC, Alpharma Uspd Makers Of Barre and Nmc	63874-0323-15
15's	$9.91	GENERIC, Pd-Rx Pharmaceuticals	55289-0140-15
20's	$8.84	GENERIC, Alpharma Uspd Makers Of Barre and Nmc	63874-0323-20
20's	$9.80	MOTRIN, Allscripts Pharmaceutical Company	54569-4320-00
20's	$11.90	GENERIC, Pd-Rx Pharmaceuticals	55289-0140-20
21's	$7.42	GENERIC, Dhs Inc	55887-0976-21
21's	$8.91	MOTRIN, Pd-Rx Pharmaceuticals	55289-0041-21
21's	$12.64	GENERIC, Pd-Rx Pharmaceuticals	55289-0140-21
25 x 30	$241.58	GENERIC, Sky Pharmaceuticals Packaging, Inc	63739-0137-03
25's	$4.76	GENERIC, Udl Laboratories Inc	51079-0596-19
25's	$14.84	GENERIC, Pd-Rx Pharmaceuticals	55289-0140-97
30's	$4.20	GENERIC, Pd-Rx Pharmaceuticals	58864-0287-30
30's	$7.56	GENERIC, Golden State Medical	60429-0094-30
30's	$9.35	MOTRIN, Physicians Total Care	54868-0437-03
30's	$9.40	GENERIC, Heartland Healthcare Services	61392-0528-30
30's	$9.40	GENERIC, Heartland Healthcare Services	61392-0528-39
30's	$9.56	GENERIC, Dhs Inc	55887-0976-30
30's	$10.77	MOTRIN, Pd-Rx Pharmaceuticals	55289-0041-30
30's	$13.58	GENERIC, Alpharma Uspd Makers Of Barre and Nmc	63874-0323-30
30's	$13.70	GENERIC, St. Mary'S Mpp	60760-0135-30
30's	$14.07	GENERIC, Pd-Rx Pharmaceuticals	55289-0140-30
30's	$14.70	MOTRIN, Allscripts Pharmaceutical Company	54569-4320-01
30's	$33.95	GENERIC, Major Pharmaceuticals Inc	00904-1760-46
30's	$189.80	GENERIC, Medirex Inc	57480-0338-06
31 x 10	$112.53	GENERIC, Vangard Labs	00615-2528-53
31 x 10	$112.53	GENERIC, Vangard Labs	00615-2528-63
31's	$9.72	GENERIC, Heartland Healthcare Services	61392-0528-31
32's	$10.03	GENERIC, Heartland Healthcare Services	61392-0528-32
40's	$18.63	GENERIC, Alpharma Uspd Makers Of Barre and Nmc	63874-0323-40
40's	$19.60	MOTRIN, Allscripts Pharmaceutical Company	54569-4320-06
40's	$20.13	GENERIC, Pd-Rx Pharmaceuticals	55289-0140-40
42's	$12.66	GENERIC, Dhs Inc	55887-0976-42
42's	$20.86	GENERIC, Pd-Rx Pharmaceuticals	55289-0140-42
50's	$23.46	GENERIC, Pd-Rx Pharmaceuticals	55289-0140-50
60's	$6.90	GENERIC, Pd-Rx Pharmaceuticals	58864-0287-60
60's	$17.49	MOTRIN, Physicians Total Care	54868-0437-04
60's	$18.81	GENERIC, Heartland Healthcare Services	61392-0528-60
60's	$22.40	GENERIC, St. Mary'S Mpp	60760-0135-60
60's	$28.18	GENERIC, Pd-Rx Pharmaceuticals	55289-0140-60
60's	$28.51	GENERIC, Alpharma Uspd Makers Of Barre and Nmc	63874-0323-60
60's	$60.00	GENERIC, Udl Laboratories Inc	51079-0596-98
90's	$9.20	GENERIC, Major Pharmaceuticals Inc	00904-1760-89
90's	$9.70	GENERIC, Pd-Rx Pharmaceuticals	58864-0287-90
90's	$22.32	GENERIC, Golden State Medical	60429-0094-90
90's	$28.21	GENERIC, Heartland Healthcare Services	61392-0528-90
90's	$31.22	GENERIC, Interpharm Inc	53746-0137-90
90's	$40.82	MOTRIN, Pharmacia and Upjohn	00009-7387-05
100's	$6.65	GENERIC, Richmond Pharmaceuticals	57438-0121-13
100's	$8.50	GENERIC, Knoll Pharmaceutical Company	00044-0173-01
100's	$10.50	GENERIC, Interstate Drug Exchange Inc	00814-3816-14
100's	$10.65	FEDERAL UPPER LIMIT, H.C.F.A. F F P	99999-1520-19
100's	$13.25	GENERIC, Cmc-Consolidated Midland Corporation	00223-1093-01
100's	$21.50	GENERIC, Alra	51641-0212-01
100's	$21.95	GENERIC, Major Pharmaceuticals Inc	00904-1760-60
100's	$22.07	GENERIC, Purepac Pharmaceutical Company	00228-2111-10
100's	$22.57	GENERIC, Invamed Inc	52189-0225-24
100's	$23.00	GENERIC, Baker Norton Pharmaceuticals	50732-0781-01
100's	$23.18	GENERIC, Aligen Independent Laboratories Inc	00405-4529-01
100's	$23.89	GENERIC, Par Pharmaceutical Inc	49884-0216-01
100's	$24.95	GENERIC, Parmed Pharmaceuticals Inc	00349-8609-01
100's	$25.04	GENERIC, Moore, H.L. Drug Exchange Inc	00839-7236-06
100's	$27.77	GENERIC, Auro Pharmaceutical	55829-0314-10
100's	$28.35	MOTRIN, Physicians Total Care	54868-0437-00
100's	$29.52	GENERIC, Vangard Labs	00615-2528-13
100's	$31.60	GENERIC, Udl Laboratories Inc	51079-0596-20
100's	$34.02	GENERIC, St. Mary'S Mpp	60760-0135-00
100's	$35.93	GENERIC, Major Pharmaceuticals Inc	00904-1760-61
100's	$35.95	GENERIC, Major Pharmaceuticals Inc	00904-5187-60
100's	$36.27	GENERIC, Watson/Schein Pharmaceuticals Inc	00364-2137-01
100's	$36.27	GENERIC, Dixon-Shane Inc	17236-0570-01
100's	$36.28	GENERIC, Interpharm Inc	53746-0137-01
100's	$36.37	GENERIC, Watson Laboratories Inc	00591-2137-01
100's	$37.05	GENERIC, Watson/Schein Pharmaceuticals Inc	00364-2137-90
100's	$38.10	GENERIC, Par Pharmaceutical Inc	49884-0469-01
100's	$38.10	GENERIC, Par Pharmaceutical Inc	49884-0779-01
100's	$38.54	GENERIC, Qualitest Products Inc	00603-4020-21
100's	$39.95	GENERIC, Major Pharmaceuticals Inc	00904-5187-61
100's	$41.29	MOTRIN, Pharmacia and Upjohn	00009-0725-02
100's	$41.67	GENERIC, Alpharma Uspd Makers Of Barre and Nmc	63874-0323-01
100's	$42.39	GENERIC, Pd-Rx Pharmaceuticals	55289-0140-01
100's	$42.83	GENERIC, Ivax Corporation	00182-1297-89
100's	$43.69	GENERIC, American Health Packaging	62584-0748-01
100's	$45.34	MOTRIN, Pharmacia and Upjohn	00009-7387-01
100's	$46.15	GENERIC, Alra	51641-0212-11
100's	$49.01	MOTRIN, Pharmacia and Upjohn	00009-7387-04
270's	$67.32	GENERIC, Golden State Medical	60429-0094-27
270's	$79.71	MOTRIN, Allscripts Pharmaceutical Company	54569-8560-00

PRODUCT LISTING - EQUIVALENTS NOT AVAILABLE

Qty	Price	Product	NDC
Suspension - Oral - 40 mg/ml			
15 ml	$4.44	ADVIL PEDIATRIC, Whitehall-Robins	00573-0172-20
15 ml	$4.44	ADVIL PEDIATRIC, Whitehall-Robins	00573-0173-20
15 ml	$4.50	PEDIACARE FEVER, Pharmacia and Upjohn	00009-4513-01
15 ml	$4.89	GENERIC, Major Pharmaceuticals Inc	00904-5463-35
15 ml	$4.97	MOTRIN CHILDRENS, Johnson and Johnson/Merck	50580-0100-15
Suspension - Oral - 100 mg/5 ml			
5 ml x 50	$96.00	GENERIC, Alpharma Uspd Makers Of Barre and Nmc	50962-0475-60
119 ml	$6.00	ADVIL, Wyeth-Ayerst Laboratories	00008-0900-01
120 ml	$4.79	GENERIC, Bergen Brunswig Drug Company	24385-0905-26
120 ml	$7.26	GENERIC, Alpharma Uspd Makers Of Barre and Nmc	00472-1270-94

I

120 ml	$8.16	MOTRIN CHILDRENS, Johnson and Johnson/Merck	00045-0448-04
120 ml x 24	$151.34	MOTRIN CHILDRENS, Johnson and Johnson/Merck	00045-0448-03
473 ml	$21.53	ADVIL, Wyeth-Ayerst Laboratories	00008-0900-03
480 ml	$22.73	MOTRIN CHILDRENS, Johnson and Johnson/Merck	00045-0448-17
480 ml	$24.28	GENERIC, Alpharma Uspd Makers Of Barre and Nmc	00472-1270-16
480 ml	$27.28	MOTRIN CHILDRENS, Johnson and Johnson/Merck	00045-0448-16

Tablet - Oral - 200 mg

100's	$6.68	GENERIC, Auro Pharmaceutical	55829-0311-10

Tablet - Oral - 400 mg

2's	$0.41	GENERIC, Allscripts Pharmaceutical Company	54569-3820-04
2's	$3.40	GENERIC, Prescript Pharmaceuticals	00247-0080-02
3's	$3.42	GENERIC, Prescript Pharmaceuticals	00247-0080-03
4's	$0.82	GENERIC, Allscripts Pharmaceutical Company	54569-3820-01
4's	$3.45	GENERIC, Prescript Pharmaceuticals	00247-0080-04
6's	$1.23	GENERIC, Allscripts Pharmaceutical Company	54569-3820-03
6's	$3.49	GENERIC, Prescript Pharmaceuticals	00247-0080-06
8's	$3.28	GENERIC, Southwood Pharmaceuticals Inc	58016-0241-08
8's	$3.54	GENERIC, Prescript Pharmaceuticals	00247-0080-08
10's	$3.59	GENERIC, Prescript Pharmaceuticals	00247-0080-10
12's	$2.46	GENERIC, Allscripts Pharmaceutical Company	54569-0285-07
12's	$3.64	GENERIC, Prescript Pharmaceuticals	00247-0080-12
12's	$4.92	GENERIC, Southwood Pharmaceuticals Inc	58016-0241-12
14's	$5.74	GENERIC, Southwood Pharmaceuticals Inc	58016-0241-14
15's	$2.67	GENERIC, Physicians Total Care	54868-0079-00
15's	$3.08	GENERIC, Allscripts Pharmaceutical Company	54569-0285-09
15's	$3.71	GENERIC, Prescript Pharmaceuticals	00247-0080-15
15's	$6.15	GENERIC, Southwood Pharmaceuticals Inc	58016-0241-15
16's	$3.28	GENERIC, Allscripts Pharmaceutical Company	54569-0285-00
16's	$3.73	GENERIC, Prescript Pharmaceuticals	00247-0080-16
16's	$6.56	GENERIC, Southwood Pharmaceuticals Inc	58016-0241-16
20's	$3.01	GENERIC, Physicians Total Care	54868-0079-05
20's	$3.82	GENERIC, Prescript Pharmaceuticals	00247-0080-20
20's	$4.10	GENERIC, Allscripts Pharmaceutical Company	54569-0285-04
20's	$4.23	GENERIC, Pharmaceutical Corporation Of America	51688-0049-52
20's	$8.20	GENERIC, Southwood Pharmaceuticals Inc	58016-0241-20
20's	$8.72	GENERIC, Pharma Pac	52959-0075-20
21's	$3.85	GENERIC, Prescript Pharmaceuticals	00247-0080-21
21's	$4.31	GENERIC, Allscripts Pharmaceutical Company	54569-0285-06
21's	$8.61	GENERIC, Southwood Pharmaceuticals Inc	58016-0241-21
21's	$9.19	GENERIC, Pharma Pac	52959-0075-21
28's	$4.01	GENERIC, Prescript Pharmaceuticals	00247-0080-28
28's	$5.75	GENERIC, Allscripts Pharmaceutical Company	54569-3820-02
30's	$3.67	GENERIC, Physicians Total Care	54868-0079-07
30's	$4.06	GENERIC, Prescript Pharmaceuticals	00247-0080-30
30's	$5.85	GENERIC, Pharmaceutical Corporation Of America	51688-0049-24
30's	$6.16	GENERIC, Allscripts Pharmaceutical Company	54569-0285-01
30's	$12.30	GENERIC, Southwood Pharmaceuticals Inc	58016-0241-30
30's	$13.07	GENERIC, Pharma Pac	52959-0075-30
35's	$4.18	GENERIC, Prescript Pharmaceuticals	00247-0080-35
40's	$4.29	GENERIC, Prescript Pharmaceuticals	00247-0080-40
40's	$7.48	GENERIC, Pharmaceutical Corporation Of America	51688-0049-51
40's	$8.21	GENERIC, Allscripts Pharmaceutical Company	54569-0285-05
40's	$16.40	GENERIC, Southwood Pharmaceuticals Inc	58016-0241-40
40's	$17.38	GENERIC, Pharma Pac	52959-0075-40
50's	$4.53	GENERIC, Prescript Pharmaceuticals	00247-0080-50
50's	$10.26	GENERIC, Allscripts Pharmaceutical Company	54569-0285-02
50's	$20.50	GENERIC, Southwood Pharmaceuticals Inc	58016-0241-50
56's	$4.67	GENERIC, Prescript Pharmaceuticals	00247-0080-56
56's	$22.96	GENERIC, Southwood Pharmaceuticals Inc	58016-0241-56
60's	$4.76	GENERIC, Prescript Pharmaceuticals	00247-0080-60
60's	$5.68	GENERIC, Physicians Total Care	54868-0079-02
60's	$10.70	GENERIC, Pharmaceutical Corporation Of America	51688-0049-25
60's	$12.31	GENERIC, Allscripts Pharmaceutical Company	54569-0285-08
60's	$24.60	GENERIC, Southwood Pharmaceuticals Inc	58016-0241-60
60's	$25.99	GENERIC, Pharma Pac	52959-0075-60
90's	$15.54	GENERIC, Pharmaceutical Corporation Of America	51688-0049-26
90's	$30.90	GENERIC, Pharma Pac	52959-0075-90
90's	$36.90	GENERIC, Southwood Pharmaceuticals Inc	58016-0241-90
100's	$4.50	GENERIC, Richmond Pharmaceuticals	54738-0119-01
100's	$5.71	GENERIC, Prescript Pharmaceuticals	00247-0080-00
100's	$6.92	GENERIC, Physicians Total Care	54868-0079-04
100's	$12.00	GENERIC, Greenstone Limited	59762-3886-01
100's	$20.52	GENERIC, Allscripts Pharmaceutical Company	54569-0285-03
100's	$20.52	GENERIC, Greenstone Limited	59762-7378-01
100's	$31.50	GENERIC, Pharma Pac	52959-0075-00
100's	$41.00	GENERIC, Southwood Pharmaceuticals Inc	58016-0241-00
120's	$20.39	GENERIC, Pharmaceutical Corporation Of America	51688-0049-82

Tablet - Oral - 600 mg

2's	$3.44	GENERIC, Prescript Pharmaceuticals	00247-0058-02
3's	$3.47	GENERIC, Prescript Pharmaceuticals	00247-0058-03
4's	$1.16	GENERIC, Allscripts Pharmaceutical Company	54569-4002-02
4's	$3.52	GENERIC, Prescript Pharmaceuticals	00247-0058-04
5's	$3.55	GENERIC, Prescript Pharmaceuticals	00247-0058-05
6's	$2.69	GENERIC, Southwood Pharmaceuticals Inc	58016-0242-06
6's	$3.59	GENERIC, Prescript Pharmaceuticals	00247-0058-06
8's	$3.20	GENERIC, Southwood Pharmaceuticals Inc	58016-0242-08
8's	$3.67	GENERIC, Prescript Pharmaceuticals	00247-0058-08
10's	$2.91	GENERIC, Allscripts Pharmaceutical Company	54569-0287-00
10's	$3.69	GENERIC, Southwood Pharmaceuticals Inc	58016-0242-10
10's	$3.75	GENERIC, Prescript Pharmaceuticals	00247-0058-10
10's	$4.10	GENERIC, Pharma Pac	52959-0076-10
12's	$3.49	GENERIC, Allscripts Pharmaceutical Company	54569-0287-01
12's	$3.84	GENERIC, Prescript Pharmaceuticals	00247-0058-12
12's	$4.08	GENERIC, Southwood Pharmaceuticals Inc	58016-0242-12
12's	$6.25	GENERIC, Pharma Pac	52959-0076-12
15's	$2.92	GENERIC, Physicians Total Care	54868-0080-04
15's	$3.95	GENERIC, Prescript Pharmaceuticals	00247-0058-15
15's	$4.36	GENERIC, Allscripts Pharmaceutical Company	54569-4002-00
15's	$4.84	GENERIC, Southwood Pharmaceuticals Inc	58016-0242-15
15's	$6.83	GENERIC, Pharma Pac	52959-0076-15
16's	$3.99	GENERIC, Prescript Pharmaceuticals	00247-0058-16
16's	$4.65	GENERIC, Allscripts Pharmaceutical Company	54569-0287-02
16's	$7.35	GENERIC, Pharma Pac	52959-0076-16
20's	$3.34	GENERIC, Physicians Total Care	54868-0080-02
20's	$4.15	GENERIC, Prescript Pharmaceuticals	00247-0058-20
20's	$5.62	GENERIC, Southwood Pharmaceuticals Inc	58016-0242-20
20's	$5.82	GENERIC, Allscripts Pharmaceutical Company	54569-0287-08
20's	$8.82	GENERIC, Pharma Pac	52959-0076-20
21's	$4.19	GENERIC, Prescript Pharmaceuticals	00247-0058-21
21's	$5.90	GENERIC, Southwood Pharmaceuticals Inc	58016-0242-21
21's	$6.11	GENERIC, Allscripts Pharmaceutical Company	54569-4002-01
21's	$9.45	GENERIC, Pharma Pac	52959-0076-21
24's	$4.31	GENERIC, Prescript Pharmaceuticals	00247-0058-24
24's	$6.98	GENERIC, Allscripts Pharmaceutical Company	54569-0287-09
24's	$10.92	GENERIC, Pharma Pac	52959-0076-24
25's	$4.34	GENERIC, Prescript Pharmaceuticals	00247-0058-25
25's	$11.29	GENERIC, Pharma Pac	52959-0076-25
28's	$4.47	GENERIC, Prescript Pharmaceuticals	00247-0058-28
28's	$8.14	GENERIC, Allscripts Pharmaceutical Company	54569-4002-04
30's	$3.10	GENERIC, Circle Pharmaceuticals Inc	00659-0422-30
30's	$4.17	GENERIC, Physicians Total Care	54868-0080-08
30's	$4.54	GENERIC, Prescript Pharmaceuticals	00247-0058-30
30's	$7.87	GENERIC, Pharmaceutical Corporation Of America	51655-0050-24
30's	$8.43	GENERIC, Southwood Pharmaceuticals Inc	58016-0242-30
30's	$8.72	GENERIC, Allscripts Pharmaceutical Company	54569-0287-03
30's	$13.49	GENERIC, Pharma Pac	52959-0076-30
40's	$4.94	GENERIC, Prescript Pharmaceuticals	00247-0058-40
40's	$5.01	GENERIC, Physicians Total Care	54868-0080-03
40's	$11.24	GENERIC, Southwood Pharmaceuticals Inc	58016-0242-40
40's	$11.63	GENERIC, Allscripts Pharmaceutical Company	54569-0287-07
40's	$18.17	GENERIC, Pharma Pac	52959-0076-40
42's	$5.02	GENERIC, Prescript Pharmaceuticals	00247-0058-42
45's	$5.14	GENERIC, Prescript Pharmaceuticals	00247-0058-45
45's	$19.75	GENERIC, Pharma Pac	52959-0076-45
50's	$5.34	GENERIC, Prescript Pharmaceuticals	00247-0058-50
50's	$14.05	GENERIC, Southwood Pharmaceuticals Inc	58016-0242-50
50's	$22.68	GENERIC, Pharma Pac	52959-0076-50
60's	$5.74	GENERIC, Prescript Pharmaceuticals	00247-0058-60
60's	$6.68	GENERIC, Physicians Total Care	54868-0080-05
60's	$14.73	GENERIC, Pharmaceutical Corporation Of America	51655-0050-25
60's	$16.87	GENERIC, Southwood Pharmaceuticals Inc	58016-0242-60
60's	$17.45	GENERIC, Allscripts Pharmaceutical Company	54569-0287-04
60's	$26.93	GENERIC, Pharma Pac	52959-0076-60
80's	$22.49	GENERIC, Southwood Pharmaceuticals Inc	58016-0242-80
90's	$6.93	GENERIC, Prescript Pharmaceuticals	00247-0058-90
90's	$9.19	GENERIC, Physicians Total Care	54868-0080-00
90's	$21.59	GENERIC, Pharmaceutical Corporation Of America	51655-0050-26
90's	$25.30	GENERIC, Southwood Pharmaceuticals Inc	58016-0242-90
90's	$26.17	GENERIC, Allscripts Pharmaceutical Company	54569-4002-05
90's	$40.32	GENERIC, Pharma Pac	52959-0076-90

100's	$5.69	GENERIC, Richmond Pharmaceuticals	54738-0120-13
100's	$7.05	GENERIC, Richmond Pharmaceuticals	54738-0120-01
100's	$7.33	GENERIC, Prescript Pharmaceuticals	00247-0058-00
100's	$10.03	GENERIC, Physicians Total Care	54868-0080-06
100's	$12.90	GENERIC, Ampharco Inc	59015-0522-01
100's	$13.96	IBREN, Economed Pharmaceuticals Inc	38130-0053-01
100's	$16.50	GENERIC, Greenstone Limited	59762-3887-01
100's	$28.11	GENERIC, Southwood Pharmaceuticals Inc	58016-0242-00
100's	$29.08	GENERIC, Allscripts Pharmaceutical Company	54569-0287-05
100's	$29.08	GENERIC, Greenstone Limited	59762-7379-01
100's	$44.10	GENERIC, Pharma Pac	52959-0076-00
118's	$8.04	GENERIC, Prescript Pharmaceuticals	00247-0058-52
120's	$28.71	GENERIC, Pharmaceutical Corporation Of America	51655-0050-82
120's	$33.73	GENERIC, Southwood Pharmaceuticals Inc	58016-0242-02
180's	$35.83	GENERIC, Pharmaceutical Corporation Of America	51655-0050-83
270's	$63.03	GENERIC, Pharmaceutical Corporation Of America	51655-0050-92

Tablet - Oral - 800 mg

1's	$3.41	GENERIC, Prescript Pharmaceuticals	00247-0062-01
2's	$3.46	GENERIC, Prescript Pharmaceuticals	00247-0062-02
3's	$3.52	GENERIC, Prescript Pharmaceuticals	00247-0062-03
4's	$1.43	GENERIC, Allscripts Pharmaceutical Company	54569-3332-00
4's	$3.56	GENERIC, Prescript Pharmaceuticals	00247-0062-04
6's	$2.29	GENERIC, Allscripts Pharmaceutical Company	54569-3332-06
6's	$3.67	GENERIC, Prescript Pharmaceuticals	00247-0062-06
8's	$3.05	GENERIC, Allscripts Pharmaceutical Company	54569-3332-03
8's	$3.78	GENERIC, Prescript Pharmaceuticals	00247-0062-08
9's	$3.84	GENERIC, Prescript Pharmaceuticals	00247-0062-09
10's	$3.82	GENERIC, Allscripts Pharmaceutical Company	54569-0289-00
10's	$3.88	GENERIC, Prescript Pharmaceuticals	00247-0062-10
10's	$5.82	GENERIC, Pharma Pac	52959-0077-10
12's	$3.99	GENERIC, Prescript Pharmaceuticals	00247-0062-12
12's	$4.58	GENERIC, Allscripts Pharmaceutical Company	54569-0289-08
12's	$5.44	GENERIC, Southwood Pharmaceuticals Inc	58016-0243-12
12's	$7.81	GENERIC, Pharma Pac	52959-0077-12
14's	$6.35	GENERIC, Southwood Pharmaceuticals Inc	58016-0243-14
14's	$8.53	GENERIC, Pharma Pac	52959-0077-14
15's	$3.52	GENERIC, Physicians Total Care	54868-0133-01
15's	$4.15	GENERIC, Prescript Pharmaceuticals	00247-0062-15
15's	$5.35	GENERIC, Pharmaceutical Corporation Of America	51655-0051-54
15's	$5.72	GENERIC, Allscripts Pharmaceutical Company	54569-0289-01
15's	$6.80	GENERIC, Southwood Pharmaceuticals Inc	58016-0243-15
15's	$9.92	GENERIC, Pharma Pac	52959-0077-15
16's	$4.20	GENERIC, Prescript Pharmaceuticals	00247-0062-16
16's	$6.10	GENERIC, Allscripts Pharmaceutical Company	54569-3332-01
16's	$7.25	GENERIC, Southwood Pharmaceuticals Inc	58016-0243-16
16's	$9.71	GENERIC, Pharma Pac	52959-0077-16
18's	$10.67	GENERIC, Pharma Pac	52959-0077-18
20's	$4.14	GENERIC, Physicians Total Care	54868-0133-05
20's	$4.41	GENERIC, Prescript Pharmaceuticals	00247-0062-20
20's	$7.63	GENERIC, Allscripts Pharmaceutical Company	54569-3332-07
20's	$9.07	GENERIC, Southwood Pharmaceuticals Inc	58016-0243-20
20's	$11.62	GENERIC, Pharma Pac	52959-0077-20
21's	$4.47	GENERIC, Prescript Pharmaceuticals	00247-0062-21
21's	$8.01	GENERIC, Allscripts Pharmaceutical Company	54569-0289-07
21's	$9.52	GENERIC, Southwood Pharmaceuticals Inc	58016-0243-21
21's	$12.10	GENERIC, Pharma Pac	52959-0077-21
24's	$4.62	GENERIC, Prescript Pharmaceuticals	00247-0062-24
24's	$10.88	GENERIC, Southwood Pharmaceuticals Inc	58016-0243-24
24's	$13.53	GENERIC, Pharma Pac	52959-0077-24
28's	$4.84	GENERIC, Prescript Pharmaceuticals	00247-0062-28
28's	$10.68	GENERIC, Allscripts Pharmaceutical Company	54569-3332-04
28's	$12.70	GENERIC, Southwood Pharmaceuticals Inc	58016-0243-28
28's	$15.44	GENERIC, Pharma Pac	52959-0077-28
30's	$4.94	GENERIC, Prescript Pharmaceuticals	00247-0062-30
30's	$5.37	GENERIC, Physicians Total Care	54868-0133-06
30's	$9.71	GENERIC, Pharmaceutical Corporation Of America	51655-0051-24
30's	$11.45	GENERIC, Allscripts Pharmaceutical Company	54569-0289-02
30's	$13.60	GENERIC, Southwood Pharmaceuticals Inc	58016-0243-30
30's	$16.38	GENERIC, Pharma Pac	52959-0077-30
40's	$5.47	GENERIC, Prescript Pharmaceuticals	00247-0062-40
40's	$6.61	GENERIC, Physicians Total Care	54868-0133-02
40's	$15.26	GENERIC, Allscripts Pharmaceutical Company	54569-0289-09
40's	$18.14	GENERIC, Southwood Pharmaceuticals Inc	58016-0243-40
40's	$21.15	GENERIC, Pharma Pac	52959-0077-40
42's	$5.58	GENERIC, Prescript Pharmaceuticals	00247-0062-42
42's	$16.02	GENERIC, Allscripts Pharmaceutical Company	54569-3332-02
42's	$19.04	GENERIC, Southwood Pharmaceuticals Inc	58016-0243-42
42's	$22.05	GENERIC, Pharma Pac	52959-0077-42
45's	$5.74	GENERIC, Prescript Pharmaceuticals	00247-0062-45
45's	$17.17	GENERIC, Allscripts Pharmaceutical Company	54569-0289-03
45's	$20.40	GENERIC, Southwood Pharmaceuticals Inc	58016-0243-45
45's	$23.39	GENERIC, Pharma Pac	52959-0077-45
50's	$6.00	GENERIC, Prescript Pharmaceuticals	00247-0062-50
50's	$22.67	GENERIC, Southwood Pharmaceuticals Inc	58016-0243-50
50's	$25.90	GENERIC, Pharma Pac	52959-0077-50
56's	$25.39	GENERIC, Southwood Pharmaceuticals Inc	58016-0243-56
60's	$6.53	GENERIC, Prescript Pharmaceuticals	00247-0062-60
60's	$9.08	GENERIC, Physicians Total Care	54868-0133-04
60's	$18.41	GENERIC, Pharmaceutical Corporation Of America	51655-0051-25
60's	$22.89	GENERIC, Allscripts Pharmaceutical Company	54569-0289-04
60's	$27.20	GENERIC, Southwood Pharmaceuticals Inc	58016-0243-60
60's	$30.66	GENERIC, Pharma Pac	52959-0077-60
80's	$36.27	GENERIC, Southwood Pharmaceuticals Inc	58016-0243-80
84's	$38.09	GENERIC, Southwood Pharmaceuticals Inc	58016-0243-84
90's	$8.12	GENERIC, Prescript Pharmaceuticals	00247-0062-90
90's	$12.79	GENERIC, Physicians Total Care	54868-0133-03
90's	$27.12	GENERIC, Pharmaceutical Corporation Of America	51655-0051-26
90's	$34.34	GENERIC, Allscripts Pharmaceutical Company	54569-3332-05
90's	$40.81	GENERIC, Southwood Pharmaceuticals Inc	58016-0243-90
90's	$45.45	GENERIC, Pharma Pac	52959-0077-90
100's	$8.31	GENERIC, Richmond Pharmaceuticals	54738-0121-13
100's	$8.65	GENERIC, Prescript Pharmaceuticals	00247-0062-00
100's	$10.35	GENERIC, Richmond Pharmaceuticals	54738-0121-01
100's	$14.03	GENERIC, Physicians Total Care	54868-0133-00
100's	$38.15	GENERIC, Allscripts Pharmaceutical Company	54569-0289-05
100's	$38.15	GENERIC, Greenstone Limited	59762-7380-01
100's	$45.34	GENERIC, Southwood Pharmaceuticals Inc	58016-0243-00
100's	$49.71	GENERIC, Pharma Pac	52959-0077-00
120's	$54.41	GENERIC, Southwood Pharmaceuticals Inc	58016-0243-02
180's	$53.24	GENERIC, Pharmaceutical Corporation Of America	51655-0051-83
270's	$79.85	GENERIC, Pharmaceutical Corporation Of America	51655-0051-92

Tablet, Chewable - Oral - 100 mg

100's	$25.95	MOTRIN CHILDRENS, Johnson and Johnson/Merck	00045-0431-10

Idarubicin Hydrochloride *(003013)*

Categories: Leukemia, acute myelogenous; Pregnancy Category D; FDA Approved 1990 Sep; Orphan Drugs
Drug Classes: Antineoplastics, antibiotics
Brand Names: Idamycin
Foreign Brand Availability: Damycin (Mexico); Idaralem (Mexico); Zavedos (Australia; Austria; Bahrain; Bulgaria; China; Colombia; Costa-Rica; Cyprus; Czech-Republic; Denmark; Dominican-Republic; Egypt; El-Salvador; England; Finland; France; Germany; Greece; Guatemala; Honduras; Hong-Kong; Hungary; Iran; Iraq; Ireland; Israel; Italy; Jordan; Korea; Kuwait; Lebanon; Libya; Malaysia; Netherlands; New-Zealand; Nicaragua; Norway; Oman; Panama; Philippines; Portugal; Qatar; Republic-of-Yemen; Saudi-Arabia; South-Africa; Spain; Sweden; Switzerland; Syria; Taiwan; Thailand; Turkey; United-Arab-Emirates)
HCFA JCODE(S): J9211 5 mg IV

WARNING

Note: Trade names have been use in this monograph for clarity.

FOR INTRAVENOUS USE ONLY.

Idarubicin should be given slowly into a freely flowing intravenous infusion. It must *never* be given intramuscularly or subcutaneously. Severe local tissue necrosis can occur if there is extravasation during administration.

As is the case with other anthracyclines the use of Idarubicin can cause myocardial toxicity leading to congestive heart failure. Cardiac toxicity is more common in patients who have received prior anthracyclines or who have pre-existing cardiac disease.

As is usual with antileukemic agents, severe myelosuppression occurs when Idamycin or Idamycin PFS is used at effective therapeutic doses.

It is recommended that Idarubicin be administered only under the supervision of a physician who is experienced in leukemia chemotherapy and in facilities with laboratory and supportive resources adequate to monitor drug tolerance and protect and maintain a patient compromised by drug toxicity. The physician and institution must be capable of responding rapidly and completely to severe hemorrhagic conditions and/or overwhelming infection.

Dosage should be reduced in patients with impaired hepatic or renal function. (See DOSAGE AND ADMINISTRATION.)

DESCRIPTION

IDAMYCIN

Idamycin (idarubicin hydrochloride for injection) is a sterile, semi-synthetic antineoplastic anthracycline for intravenous (IV) use. Chemically, idarubicin hydrochloride is 5,12-Naphthacenedione, 9-acetyl-7-[(3-amino-2,3,6-trideoxy-α-L-*lyxo*-hexopyranosyl)oxy]-7,8,9,10-tetrahydro-6,9,11-trihydroxyhydrochloride, (7S-*cis*).

The empirical formula is $C_{26}H_{27}NO_9 \cdot HCl$. The molecular weight is 533.96.

Idamycin, a sterile lyophilized powder for reconstitution and IV administration, is available in a 20 mg single use only vial.

Each 20 mg vial contains 20 mg idarubicin hydrochloride, and 200 mg of lactose (hydrous) as an orange-red, lyophilized powder.

IDAMYCIN PFS

Idamycin PFS injection contains idarubicin hydrochloride and is a sterile, semi-synthetic, preservative-free solution (PFS) antineoplastic anthracycline for intravenous use. Chemically, idarubicin hydrochloride is 5,12-Naphthacenedione, 9-acetyl-7-[(3-amino-2,3,6-trideoxy-α-L-*lyxo*-hexopyranosyl)oxy]-7,8,9,10-tetrahydro-6,9,11-trihydroxyhydrochloride, (7S-*cis*).

The empirical formula is $C_{26}H_{27}NO_9 \cdot HCl$. The molecular weight is 533.96.

Idamycin PFS is a sterile, red-orange, isotonic parenteral preservative-free solution, available in 5 ml (5 mg), 10 ml (10 mg) and 20 ml (20 mg) single-use-only vials.

Each ml contains idarubicine hydrochloride 1 mg and the following inactive ingredients: glycerin, 25 mg and water for injection. Hydrochloric acid is used to adjust the pH to a target of 3.5.

CLINICAL PHARMACOLOGY

MECHANISM OF ACTION

Idarubicin HCl is a DNA-intercalating analog of daunorubicin which has an inhibitory effect on nucleic acid synthesis and interacts with the enzyme topoisomerase II. The absence of a methoxy group at position 4 of the anthracycline structure gives the compound a high lipophilicity which results in an increased rate of cellular uptake compared with other anthracyclines.

PHARMACOKINETICS

General

Pharmacokinetic studies have been performed in adult leukemia patients with normal renal and hepatic function following IV administration of 10-12 mg/m^2 of idarubicin daily for 3-4 days as a single agent or combined with cytarabine. The plasma concentrations of idarubicin are best described by a two or three compartment open model. The elimination rate of idarubicin from plasma is slow with an estimated mean terminal half-life of 22 hours (range, 4-48 hours) when used as a single agent and 20 hours (range, 7-38 hours) when used in combination with cytarabine. The elimination of the primary active metabolite, idarubicinol, is considerably slower than that of the parent drug with an estimated mean terminal half-life that exceeds 45 hours; hence, its plasma levels are sustained for a period greater than 8 days.

Distribution

The disposition profile shows a rapid distributive phase with a very high volume of distribution presumably reflecting extensive tissue binding. Studies of cellular (nucleated blood and bone marrow cells) drug concentrations in leukemia patients have shown that peak cellular idarubicin concentrations are reached a few minutes after injection. Concentrations of idarubicin and idarubicinol in nucleated blood and bone marrow cells are more than 100 times the plasma concentrations. Idarubicin disappearance rates in plasma and cells were comparable with a terminal half-life of about 15 hours. The terminal half-life of idarubicinol in cells was about 72 hours. The extent of drug and metabolite accumulation predicted in leukemia patients for Days 2 and 3 of dosing, based on the mean plasma levels and half-life obtained after the first dose, is 1.7- and 2.3-fold, respectively, and suggests no change in kinetics following a daily × 3 regimen. The percentages of idarubicin and idarubicinol bound to human plasma proteins averaged 97% and 94%, respectively, at concentrations similar to maximum plasma levels obtained in the pharmacokinetic studies. The binding is concentration independent. The plasma clearance is twice the expected hepatic plasma flow indicating extensive extrahepatic metabolism.

Metabolism

The primary active metabolite formed is idarubicinol. As idarubicinol has cytotoxic activity, it presumably contributes to the effects of idarubicin.

Elimination

The drug is eliminated predominately by biliary and to a lesser extent by renal excretion, mostly in the form of idarubicinol.

PHARMACOKINETICS IN SPECIAL POPULATIONS

Pediatric Patients

Idarubicin studies in pediatric leukemia patients, at doses of 4.2-13.3 mg/m^2/day × 3, suggest dose independent kinetics. There is no difference between the half-lives of the drug following daily × 3 or weekly × 3 administration. Cerebrospinal fluid (CSF) levels of idarubicin and idarubicinol were measured in pediatric leukemia patients treated intravenously. Idarubicin was detected in 2 of 21 CSF samples (0.14 and 1.57 ng/ml), while idarubicinol was detected in 20 of these 21 CSF samples obtained 18-30 hours after dosing (mean = 0.51 ng/ml; range, 0.22-1.05 ng/ml). The clinical relevance of these findings is unknown.

Hepatic and Renal Impairment

The pharmacokinetics of idarubicin have not been evaluated in leukemia patients with hepatic impairment. It is expected that in patients with moderate or severe hepatic dysfunction, the metabolism of idarubicin may be impaired and lead to higher systemic drug levels. The disposition of idarubicin may be also affected by renal impairment. Therefore, a dose reduction should be considered in patients with hepatic and/or renal impairment (see DOSAGE AND ADMINISTRATION).

DRUG-DRUG INTERACTIONS

No formal drug interactions studies have been performed.

INDICATIONS AND USAGE

Idamycin or Idamycin PFS in combination with other approved antileukemic drugs is indicated for the treatment of acute myeloid leukemia (AML) in adults. This includes French-American-British (FAB) classifications M1 through M7.

NON-FDA APPROVED INDICATIONS

Although not approved by the FDA, clinical trials have reported that idarubicin may have a role in the treatment of advanced breast cancer.

WARNINGS

Idarubicin is intended for administration under the supervision of a physician who is experienced in leukemia chemotherapy.

Idarubicin is a potent bone marrow suppressant. Idarubicin should not be given to patients with pre-existing bone marrow suppression induced by previous drug therapy or radiotherapy unless the benefit warrants the risk.

Severe myelosuppression will occur in all patients given a therapeutic dose of this agent for induction, consolidation or maintenance. Careful hematologic monitoring is required. Deaths due to infection and/or bleeding have been reported during the period of severe myelosuppression. Facilities with laboratory and supportive resources adequate to monitor drug tolerability and protect and maintain a patient compromised by drug toxicity should be available. It must be possible to treat rapidly and completely a severe hemorrhagic condition and/or a severe infection.

Pre-existing heart disease and previous therapy with anthracyclines at high cumulative doses or other potentially cardiotoxic agents are co-factors for increased risk of idarubicin-induced cardiac toxicity and the benefit to risk ratio of idarubicin therapy in such patients should be weighed before starting treatment with idarubicin.

Myocardial toxicity as manifested by potentially fatal congestive heart failure, acute life-threatening arrhythmias or other cardiomyopathies may occur following therapy with idarubicin. Appropriate therapeutic measures for the management of congestive heart failure and/or arrhythmias are indicated.

Cardiac function should be carefully monitored during treatment in order to minimize the risk of cardiac toxicity of the type described for other anthracycline compounds. The risk of such myocardial toxicity may be higher following concomitant or previous radiation to the mediastinal-pericardial area or in patients with anemia, bone marrow depression, infections, leukemic pericarditis and/or myocarditis. While there are no reliable means for predicting congestive heart failure, cardiomyopathy induced by anthracyclines is usually associated with a decrease of the left ventricular ejection fraction (LVEF) from pretreatment baseline values.

Since hepatic and/or renal function impairment can affect the disposition of idarubicin, liver and kidney function should be evaluated with conventional clinical laboratory tests (using serum bilirubin and serum creatinine as indicators) prior to and during treatment. In a number of Phase III clinical trials, treatment was not given if bilirubin and/or creatinine serum levels exceeded 2 mg%. However, in one Phase III trial, patients with bilirubin levels between 2.6 and 5 mg% received the anthracycline with a 50% reduction in dose. Dose reduction of idarubicin should be considered if the bilirubin and/or creatinine levels are above the normal range. (See DOSAGE AND ADMINISTRATION.)

PREGNANCY CATEGORY D

Idarubicin was embryotoxic and teratogenic in the rat at a dose of 1.2 mg/m^2/day or one-tenth the human dose, which was nontoxic to dams. Idarubicin was embryotoxic but not teratogenic in the rabbit even at a dose of 2.4 mg/m^2/day or two-tenths the human dose, which was toxic to dams. There is no conclusive information about idarubicin adversely affecting human fertility or causing teratogenesis. There has been 1 report of a fetal fatality after maternal exposure to idarubicin during the second trimester.

There are no adequate and well-controlled studies in pregnant women. If idarubicin is to be used during pregnancy, or if the patient becomes pregnant during therapy, the patient should be apprised of the potential hazard to the fetus. Women of childbearing potential should be advised to avoid pregnancy.

PRECAUTIONS

GENERAL

Therapy with idarubicin requires close observation of the patient and careful laboratory monitoring. Hyperuricemia secondary to rapid lysis of leukemic cells may be induced. Appropriate measures must be taken to prevent hyperuricemia and to control any systemic infection before beginning therapy.

Extravasation of idarubicin can cause severe local tissue necrosis. Extravasation may occur with or without an accompanying stinging or burning sensation even if blood returns well on aspiration of the infusion needle. If signs or symptoms of extravasation occur the injection or infusion should be terminated immediately and restarted in another vein. (See DOSAGE AND ADMINISTRATION.)

LABORATORY TESTS

Frequent complete blood counts and monitoring of hepatic and renal function tests are recommended.

CARCINOGENESIS, MUTAGENESIS, AND IMPAIRMENT OF FERTILITY

Formal long-term carcinogenicity studies have not been conducted with idarubicin. Idarubicin and related compounds have been shown to have mutagenic and carcinogenic properties when tested in experimental models (including bacterial systems, mammalian cells in culture and female Sprague-Dawley rats).

In male dogs given 1.8 mg/m^2/day 3 times/week (about one-seventh the weekly human dose on a mg/m^2 basis) for 13 weeks, or 3 times the human dose, testicular atrophy was observed with inhibition of spermatogenesis and sperm maturation, with few or no mature sperm. These effects were not readily reversed after recovery of 8 weeks.

PREGNANCY CATEGORY D

(See WARNINGS.)

NURSING MOTHERS

It is not known whether this drug is excreted in human milk. Because many drugs are excreted in human milk and because of the potential for serious adverse reactions in nursing infants from idarubicin, mothers should discontinue nursing prior to taking this drug.

PEDIATRIC USE

Safety and effectiveness in children have not been established.

ADVERSE REACTIONS

Approximately 550 patients with AML have received idarubicin in combination with cytarabine in controlled clinical trials worldwide. In addition, over 550 patients with acute leukemia have been treated in uncontrolled trials utilizing idarubicin as a single agent or in combination. TABLE 2 lists the adverse experiences reported in US Study 2 and is representative of the experiences in other studies. These adverse experiences constitute all reported or observed experiences, including those not considered to be drug related. Patients undergoing induction therapy for AML are seriously ill due to their disease, are receiving multiple transfusions, and concomitant medications including potentially toxic antibiotics and antifungal agents. The contribution of the study drug to the adverse experience profile is difficult to establish.

TABLE 2

Induction Phase Adverse Experiences	IDR (n=110)	DNR (n=118)
Infection	95%	97%
Nausea and vomiting	82%	80%
Hair loss	77%	72%
Abdominal cramps/diarrhea	73%	68%
Hemorrhage	63%	65%
Mucositis	50%	55%
Dermatologic	46%	40%
Mental status	41%	34%
Pulmonary-clinical	39%	39%
Fever (not elsewhere classified)	26%	28%
Headache	20%	24%
Cardiac-clinical	16%	24%
Neurologic-peripheral nerves	7%	9%
Pulmonary allergy	2%	4%
Seizure	4%	5%
Cerebellar	4%	4%

The duration of aplasia and incidence of mucositis were greater on the IDR arm than the DNR arm, especially during consolidation in some US controlled trials.

The following information reflects experience based on US controlled clinical trials.

Myelosuppression: Severe myelosuppression is the major toxicity associated with idarubicin therapy, but this effect of the drug is required in order to eradicate the leukemic clone. During the period of myelosuppression, patients are at risk of developing infection and bleeding which may be life-threatening or fatal.

Gastrointestinal: Nausea and/or vomiting, mucositis, abdominal pain and diarrhea were reported frequently, but were severe (equivalent to WHO Grade 4) in less than 5% of patients. Severe enterocolitis with perforation has been reported rarely. The risk of perforation may be increased by instrumental intervention. The possibility of perforation should be considered in patients who develop severe abdominal pain and appropriate steps for diagnosis and management should be taken.

Dermatologic: Alopecia was reported frequently and dermatologic reactions including generalized rash, urticaria, and a bullous erythrodermatous rash of the palms and soles have occurred. The dermatologic reactions were usually attributed to concomitant antibiotic therapy. Local reactions including hives at the injection site have been reported. Recall of skin reaction due to prior radiotherapy has occurred with idarubicin administration.

Hepatic and Renal: Changes in hepatic and renal function tests have been observed. These changes were usually transient and occurred in the setting of sepsis and while patients were receiving potentially hepatotoxic and nephrotoxic antibiotics and antifungal agents. Severe changes in renal function (equivalent to WHO Grade 4) occurred in no more than 1% of patients, while severe changes in hepatic function (equivalent to WHO Grade 4) occurred in less than 5% of patients.

Cardiac: Congestive heart failure (frequently attributed to fluid overload), serious arrhythmias including atrial fibrillation, chest pain, myocardial infarction, and asymptomatic declines in LVEF have been reported in patients undergoing induction therapy for AML. Myocardial insufficiency and arrhythmias were usually reversible and occurred in the setting of sepsis, anemia and aggressive IV fluid administration. The events were reported more frequently in patients over age 60 years and in those with pre-existing cardiac disease.

DOSAGE AND ADMINISTRATION

IDAMYCIN

See WARNINGS.

For induction therapy in adult patients with AML the following dose schedule is recommended:

Idamycin 12 mg/m^2 daily for 3 days by slow (10-15 min) IV injection in combination with cytarabine. The cytarabine may be given as 100 mg/m^2 daily by continuous infusion for 7 days or as cytarabine 25 mg/^{2} IV bolus followed by cytarabine 200 mg/m^2 daily for 5 days continuous infusion. In patients with unequivocal evidence of leukemia after the first induction course, a second course may be administered. Administration of the second course should be delayed in patients who experience severe mucositis, until recovery from this toxicity has occurred, and a dose reduction of 25% is recommended. In patients with hepatic and/or renal impairment, a dose reduction of Idamycin should be considered. Idamycin should not be administered if the bilirubin level exceeds 5 mg%. (See WARNINGS.)

The benefit of consolidation in prolonging the duration of remissions and survival is not proven. There is no consensus regarding optional regimens to be used for consolidation.

Preparation of Solution

Caution in handling of the powder and preparation of the solution must be exercised as skin reactions associated with Idamycin may occur. Skin accidentally exposed to Idamycin should be washed thoroughly with soap and water and if the eyes are involved, standard irrigation techniques should be used immediately. The use of goggles, gloves, and protective gowns is recommended during preparation and administration of the drug.

Idamycin 20 mg vials should be reconstituted with 20 ml of water for injection to give a final concentration of 1 mg/ml of idarubicin hydrochloride. Bacteriostatic diluents are not recommended. The reconstituted solution is hypotonic, and the recommended administration procedure via a freely flowing IV infusion must be followed.

The vial contents are under a negative pressure to minimize aerosol formation during reconstitution; therefore, particular care should be taken when the needle is inserted. Inhalation of any aerosol produced during reconstitution must be avoided.

Reconstituted solutions are physically and chemically stable for 72 hours (3 days) under refrigeration (2-8°C, 36-46°F) and at controlled room temperature, (15-30°C, 59-86°F). Discard unused solutions in an appropriate manner. (See Handling and Disposal.)

Care in the administration of Idamycin will reduce the chance of perivenous infiltration. It may also decrease the chance of local reactions such as urticaria and erythematous streaking. During IV administration of Idamycin extravasation may occur with or without an accompanying stinging or burning sensation even if blood returns well on aspiration of the infusion needle. If any signs or symptoms of extravasation have occurred, the injection or infusion should be immediately terminated and restarted in another vein. If it is known or suspected that subcutaneous extravasation has occurred, it is recommended that intermittent ice packs (½ hour immediately, then ½ hour 4 times/day for 3 days) be placed over the area of extravasation and that the affected extremity be elevated. Because of the progressive nature of extravasation reactions, the area of injection should be frequently examined and plastic surgery consultation obtained early if there is any sign of a local reaction such as pain, erythema, edema or vesication. If ulceration begins or there is severe persistent pain at the site of extravasation, early wide excision of the involved area should be considered.[1]

Idamycin should be administered slowly (over 10-15 minutes) into the tubing of a freely running IV infusion of sodium chloride injection (0.9%) or 5% dextrose injection. The tubing should be attached to a Butterfly needle or other suitable device and inserted preferably into a large vein.

Incompatibility

Unless specific compatibility data are available, Idamycin should not be mixed with other drugs. Precipitation occurs with heparin. Prolonged contact with any solution of an alkaline pH will result in degradation of the drug.

Parenteral drug products should be inspected visually for particulate matter and discoloration prior to administration whenever solution and containers permit.

Handling and Disposal

Procedures for handling and disposal of anticancer drugs should be considered. Several guidelines on this subject have been published.[2-8] There is no general agreement that all of the procedures recommended in the guidelines are necessary or appropriate.

IDAMYCIN PFS

See WARNINGS.

For induction therapy in adult patients with AML the following dose schedule is recommended:

Idamycin PFS injection 12 mg/m^2 daily for 3 days by slow (10-15 min) IV injection in combination with cytarabine. The cytarabine may be given as 100 mg/m^2 daily by continuous infusion for 7 days or as cytarabine 25 mg/m^2 IV bolus followed by cytarabine 200 mg/m^2 daily for 5 days continuous infusion. In patients with unequivocal evidence of leukemia after the first induction course, a second course may be administered. Administration of the second course should be delayed in patients who experience severe mucositis, until recovery from this toxicity has occurred, and a dose reduction of 25% is recommended. In patients with hepatic and/or renal impairment, a dose reduction of Idamycin PFS should be considered. Idamycin PFS should not be administered if the bilirubin level exceeds 5 mg%. (See WARNINGS.)

The benefit of consolidation in prolonging the duration of remissions and survival is not proven. There is no consensus regarding optional regimens to be used for consolidation.

Preparation and Administration Precautions

Caution in handling of the solution must be exercised as skin reactions associated with Idamycin PFS may occur. Skin accidentally exposed to Idamycin PFS should be washed thoroughly with soap and water and if the eyes are involved, standard irrigation techniques should be used immediately. The use of goggles, gloves, and protective gowns is recommended during preparation and administration of the drug.

Care in the administration of Idamycin PFS will reduce the chance of perivenous infiltration. It may also decrease the chance of local reactions such as urticaria and erythematous streaking. During IV administration of Idamycin PFS extravasation may occur with or without an accompanying stinging or burning sensation even if blood returns well on aspiration of the infusion needle. If any signs or symptoms of extravasation have occurred, the injection or infusion should be immediately terminated and restarted in another vein. If it is known or suspected that subcutaneous extravasation has occurred, it is recommended that intermittent ice packs (½ hour immediately, then ½ hour 4 times/day for 3 days) be placed over the area of extravasation and that the affected extremity be elevated. Because of the progressive nature of extravasation reactions, the area of injection should be frequently examined and plastic surgery consultation obtained early if there is any sign of a local reaction such as pain, erythema, edema or vesication. If ulceration begins or if there is severe persistent pain at the site of extravasation, early wide excision of the involved area should be considered.

Idamycin PFS should be administered slowly (over 10-15 minutes) into the tubing of a freely running IV infusion of sodium chloride injection (0.9%) or 5% dextrose injection. The tubing should be attached to a Butterfly needle or other suitable device and inserted preferably into a large vein.

Incompatibility

Unless specific compatibility data are available, Idamycin PFS should not be mixed with other drugs. Precipitation occurs with heparin. Prolonged contact with any solution of an alkaline pH will result in degradation of the drug.

Parenteral drug products should be inspected visually for particulate matter and discoloration prior to administration whenever solution and containers permit.

Handling and Disposal

Procedures for handling and disposal of anticancer drugs should considered. Several guidelines on this subject have been published.[2-9] There is no general agreement that all of the procedures recommended in the guidelines are necessary or appropriate.

HOW SUPPLIED

IDAMYCIN

Idamycin for injection is available in 20 mg single dose vials.

Storage: Store at controlled room temperature, 15-30°C (59-86°F), and protect from light.

IDAMYCIN PFS

Idamycin PFS injection is available in single dose glass vials (sterile single use only, contains no preservative) as follows:

5 mg/5 ml vial (1 mg/ml), single vials.
10 mg/10 ml vial (1 mg/ml), single vials.
20 mg/20 ml vial (1 mg/ml), single vials.

Single dose Cytosafe vials (sterile single use only, contains no preservative) as follows:

5 mg/5 ml vial (1 mg/ml), single vials.
10 mg/10 ml vial (1 mg/ml), single vials.
20 mg/20 ml vial (1 mg/ml), single vials.

Storage: Store under refrigeration 2-8°C (36-46°F), and protect from light. Retain in carton until time of use.

PRODUCT LISTING - RATED THERAPEUTICALLY EQUIVALENT

Solution - Intravenous - 1 mg/ml

5 ml	$442.04	GENERIC, Gensia Sicor Pharmaceuticals Inc	00703-4154-11
10 ml	$884.06	GENERIC, Gensia Sicor Pharmaceuticals Inc	00703-4155-11
20 ml	$1767.81	GENERIC, Gensia Sicor Pharmaceuticals Inc	00703-4156-11

PRODUCT LISTING - EQUIVALENTS NOT AVAILABLE

Solution - Intravenous - 1 mg/ml

5 ml	$455.61	IDAMYCIN PFS, Pharmacia and Upjohn	00013-2536-78
5 ml	$491.15	IDAMYCIN PFS, Pharmacia and Upjohn	00013-2200-01
5 ml	$491.15	IDAMYCIN PFS, Pharmacia Corporation	00013-2576-91
10 ml	$982.29	IDAMYCIN PFS, Pharmacia and Upjohn	00013-2546-86
10 ml	$982.29	IDAMYCIN PFS, Pharmacia Corporation	00013-2586-91
20 ml	$1964.61	IDAMYCIN PFS, Pharmacia and Upjohn	00013-2202-01
20 ml	$1964.61	IDAMYCIN PFS, Pharmacia Corporation	00013-2596-91

Ifosfamide (001524)

For complete prescribing information, refer to the CD-ROM included with the book.

Categories: Carcinoma, testicular; Pregnancy Category D; FDA Approved 1988 Dec; Orphan Drugs
Drug Classes: Antineoplastics, alkylating agents
Brand Names: Ifex; Ifex Mesnex
Foreign Brand Availability: Formamide (Germany); Holoxan (Australia; Austria; Bahrain; Belgium; Costa-Rica; Cyprus; Czech-Republic; Denmark; Dominican-Republic; Egypt; El-Salvador; Finland; France; Germany; Greece; Guatemala; Honduras; Hong-Kong; Hungary; Indonesia; Iran; Iraq; Italy; Jordan; Kuwait; Lebanon; Libya; Malaysia; Netherlands; New-Zealand; Nicaragua; Norway; Oman; Panama; Philippines; Portugal; Qatar; Republic-of-Yemen; Russia; Saudi-Arabia; South-Africa; Sweden; Switzerland; Syria; Taiwan; Thailand; Turkey; United-Arab-Emirates); Ifo-cell (Germany); Ifolem (Mexico); Ifomide (Japan); Ifoxan (Israel; Mexico); Mitoxana (England); Tronoxal (Spain)
HCFA JCODE(S): J9208 per 1 g IV

WARNING

Ifosfamide should be administered under the supervision of a qualified physician experienced in the use of cancer chemotherapeutic agents. Urotoxic side effects, especially hemorrhagic cystitis, as well as CNS toxicities such as confusion and coma have been associated with the use of ifosfamide. When they occur, they may require cessation of ifosfamide therapy. Severe myelosuppression has been reported.

DESCRIPTION

Ifosfamide is a white crystalline powder that is soluble in water. Ifosfamide is a chemotherapeutic agent chemically related to the nitrogen mustards and a synthetic analog of cyclophosphamide. Ifosfamide is 3-(2-chloroethyl)-2-[(2-chloroethyl)amino]tetrahydro-2H-1,3,2-oxazaphosphorine 2-oxide. The molecular formula is $C_7H_{15}Cl_2N_2O_2P$ and its molecular weight is 261.1.

Ifex single-dose vials for constitution and administration by intravenous infusion each contain 1 or 3 g of sterile ifosfamide.

INDICATIONS AND USAGE

Ifosfamide, used in combination with certain other approved antineoplastic agents, is indicated for third line chemotherapy of germ cell testicular cancer. It should ordinarily be used in combination with a prophylactic agent for hemorrhagic cystitis, such as mesna.

NON-FDA APPROVED INDICATIONS

This drug is also used in combination with other antineoplastic agents without FDA approval for the treatment of a wide variety of neoplasms, especially lymphomas and sarcomas. Ifosfamide has been used to treat both small cell and non-small cell lung cancer, ovarian cancer, and cervical cancer. It should ordinarily be used in combination with a prophylactic agent for hemorrhagic cystitis, such as mesna.

CONTRAINDICATIONS

Continued use of ifosfamide is contraindicated in patients with severely depressed bone marrow function (see WARNINGS). Ifosfamide is also contraindicated in patients who have demonstrated a previous hypersensitivity to it.

WARNINGS

URINARY SYSTEM

Urotoxic side effects, especially hemorrhagic cystitis, have been frequently associated with the use of ifosfamide. It is recommended that a urinalysis should be obtained prior to each dose of ifosfamide. If microscopic hematuria, (greater than 10 RBCs per high power field), is present, then subsequent administration should be withheld until complete resolution.

Further administration of ifosfamide should be given with vigorous oral or parenteral hydration.

HEMATOPOIETIC SYSTEM

When ifosfamide is given in combination with other chemotherapeutic agents, severe myelosuppression is frequently observed. Close hematologic monitoring is recommended. White blood cell (WBC) count, platelet count and hemoglobin should be obtained prior to each administration had at appropriate intervals. Unless clinically essential, ifosfamide should not be given to patients with a WBC count below 2,000/µl and/or a platelet count below 50,000/µl.

CENTRAL NERVOUS SYSTEM

Neurologic manifestations consisting of somnolence, confusion, hallucinations and in some instances, coma, have been reported following ifosfamide therapy. The occurrence of these symptoms requires discontinuing ifosfamide therapy. The symptoms have usually been reversible and supportive therapy should be maintained until their complete resolution.

PREGNANCY

Animal studies indicate that the drug is capable of causing gene mutations and chromosomal damage *in vivo*. Embryotoxic and teratogenic effects have been observed in mice, rats and rabbits at doses 0.05 to 0.075 times the human dose. Ifosfamide can cause fetal damage when administered to a pregnant woman. If ifosfamide is used during pregnancy, or if the patient becomes pregnant while taking this drug, the patient should be apprised of the potential hazard to the fetus.

DOSAGE AND ADMINISTRATION

Ifosfamide should be administered intravenously at a dose of 1.2 g/m²/day for 5 consecutive days. Treatment is repeated every 3 weeks or after recovery from hematologic toxicity (Platelets ≥100,000/µl, WBC ≥4000/µl). In order to prevent bladder toxicity, ifosfamide should be given with extensive hydration consisting of at least 2 liters of oral or intravenous fluid per day. A protector, such as mesna, should also be used to prevent hemorrhagia cystitis. Ifosfamide should be administered as a slow intravenous infusion lasting a minimum of 30 minutes. Although ifosfamide has been administered to a small number of patients with compromised hepatic and/or renal function, studies to establish optimal dose schedules of ifosfamide in such patients have not been conducted.

PREPARATION FOR INTRAVENOUS ADMINISTRATION/STABILITY

Injections are prepared for parenteral use by adding *Sterile water for injection* or *Bacteriostatic water for injection* (benzyl alcohol or parabens preserved) to the vial and shaking to dissolve. Use the quantity of diluent shown in TABLE 2 to constitute the product.

TABLE 2

Dosage Strength	Quantity of Diluent	Final Concentration
1 gram	20 ml	50 mg/ml
3 gram	60 ml	50 mg/ml

Solutions of ifosfamide may be diluted further to achieve concentrations of 0.6 to 20 mg/ml in the following fluids:

- 5% Dextrose injection
- 0.9% Sodium chloride injection
- Lactated ringer's injection
- Sterile water for injection

Such admixtures, when stored in large volume parenteral glass bottles, Viaflex bags, or PAB bags, are physically and chemically stable for at least 1 week at 30°C or 6 weeks at 5°C.

Because essentially identical stability results were obtained for sterile water admixtures as for the other admixtures (5% dextrose injection, 0.9% sodium chloride injection, and lactated Ringer's injection), the use of large volume parenteral glass bottles, Viaflex bags or PAB bags that contain intermediate concentrations or mixtures of excipients (*e.g.*, 2.5% dextrose injection, 0.45% sodium chloride injection, or 5% dextrose and 0.9% sodium chloride injection) is also acceptable.

Constituted or constituted and further diluted solution of ifosfamide should be refrigerated and used within 24 hours.

Parenteral drug products should be inspected visually for particulate matter and discoloration prior to administration.

PRODUCT LISTING - EQUIVALENTS NOT AVAILABLE

Powder For Injection - Intravenous - 1 Gm

1's	$97.86	IFEX, Bristol-Myers Squibb	00015-0556-41
1's	$164.89	GENERIC, American Pharmaceutical Partners	63323-0142-10
1's	$169.84	IFEX, Bristol-Myers Squibb	00015-0556-05

Powder For Injection - Intravenous - 3 Gm

1's	$509.51	IFEX, Bristol-Myers Squibb	00015-0557-41

Imatinib Mesylate (003519)

Categories: FDA Approved 2000 May; Pregnancy Category D; Leukemia, chronic myelogenous; Gastrointestinal stromal tumors; Orphan Drugs
Drug Classes: Antineoplastics, signal transduction inhibitors
Brand Names: Gleevec
Foreign Brand Availability: Glivec (Australia; Colombia; England; France; Hong-Kong; Indonesia; Ireland; Israel; Korea; Philippines); Glivic (New-Zealand)
Cost of Therapy: $365.13 (CML; Gleevec; 100 mg; 4 capsules/day; 30 day supply)

DESCRIPTION

Gleevec capsules contain imatinib mesylate equivalent to 100 mg of imatinib free base. Imatinib mesylate is designated chemically as 4-[(4-methyl-1-piperazinyl)methyl]-N-[4-methyl-3-[[4-(3-pyridinyl)-2-pyrimidinyl]amino]-phenyl]benzamide methanesulfonate.

Imatinib mesylate is a white to off-white to brownish or yellowish tinged crystalline powder. Its molecular formula is $C_{29}H_{31}N_7O \cdot CH_4SO_3$ and its relative molecular mass is 589.7. Imatinib mesylate is very soluble in water and soluble in aqueous buffers $\leq$ pH 5.5 but is very slightly soluble to insoluble in neutral/alkaline aqueous buffers. In non-aqueous solvents, the drug substance is freely soluble to very slightly soluble in dimethyl sulfoxide, methanol and ethanol, but is insoluble in n-octanol, acetone and acetonitrile.

Inactive Ingredients: Colloidal silicon dioxide, crospovidone, magnesium stearate and microcrystalline cellulose. *Capsule Shell:* Gelatin, iron oxide, red (E172); iron oxide, yellow (E172); titanium dioxide (E171).

CLINICAL PHARMACOLOGY

MECHANISM OF ACTION

Imatinib mesylate is a protein-tyrosine kinase inhibitor that inhibits the Bcr-Abl tyrosine kinase, the constitutive abnormal tyrosine kinase created by the Philadelphia chromosome abnormality in chronic myeloid leukemia (CML). It inhibits proliferation and induces apoptosis in Bcr-Abl positive cell lines as well as fresh leukemic cells from Philadelphia chromosome positive chronic myeloid leukemia. In colony formation assays using *ex vivo* peripheral blood and bone marrow samples, imatinib shows inhibition of Bcr-Abl positive colonies from CML patients.

In vivo, it inhibits tumor growth of Bcr-Abl transfected murine myeloid cells as well as Bcr-Abl positive leukemia lines derived from CML patients in blast crisis.

Imatinib is also an inhibitor of the receptor tyrosine kinases for platelet-derived growth factor (PDGF) and stem cell factor (SCF), c-kit, and inhibits PDGF- and SCF-mediated cellular events. *In vitro,* imatinib inhibits proliferation and induces apoptosis in gastrointestinal stromal tumor (GIST) cells, which express an activating c-kit mutation.

PHARMACOKINETICS

The pharmacokinetics of imatinib mesylate have been evaluated in studies in healthy subjects and in population pharmacokinetic studies in over 500 patients. Imatinib is well absorbed after oral administration with C_{max} achieved within 2-4 hours post-dose. Mean absolute bioavailability for the capsule formulation is 98%. Following oral administration in healthy volunteers, the elimination half-lives of imatinib and its major active metabolite, the N-desmethyl derivative, were approximately 18 and 40 hours, respectively. Mean imatinib AUC increased proportionally with increasing dose in the range 25-1000 mg. There was no significant change in the pharmacokinetics of imatinib on repeated dosing, and accumulation is 1.5- to 2.5-fold at steady state when imatinib mesylate is dosed once daily. At clinically relevant concentrations of imatinib, binding to plasma proteins in *in vitro* experiments is approximately 95%, mostly to albumin and α_1-acid glycoprotein.

The pharmacokinetics of imatinib were similar in CML and GIST patients.

METABOLISM AND ELIMINATION

CYP3A4 is the major enzyme responsible for metabolism of imatinib. Other cytochrome P450 enzymes, such as CYP1A2, CYP2D6, CYP2C9, and CYP2C19, play a minor role in its metabolism. The main circulating active metabolite in humans is the N-demethylated piperazine derivative, formed predominantly by CYP3A4. It shows *in vitro* potency similar to the parent imatinib. The plasma AUC for this metabolite is about 15% of the AUC for imatinib.

Elimination is predominately in the feces, mostly as metabolites. Based on the recovery of compound(s) after an oral ^{14}C-labelled dose of imatinib, approximately 81% of the dose was eliminated within 7 days, in feces (68% of dose) and urine (13% of dose). Unchanged imatinib accounted for 25% of the dose (5% urine, 20% feces), the remainder being metabolites.

Typically, clearance of imatinib in a 50-year-old patient weighing 50 kg is expected to be 8 L/h, while for a 50-year-old patient weighing 100 kg the clearance will increase to 14 L/h. However, the inter-patient variability of 40% in clearance does not warrant initial dose adjustment based on body weight and/or age but indicates the need for close monitoring for treatment related toxicity.

SPECIAL POPULATIONS

Pediatric

There are no pharmacokinetic data in pediatric patients.

Hepatic Insufficiency

No clinical studies were conducted with imatinib mesylate in patients with impaired hepatic function.

Renal Insufficiency

No clinical studies were conducted with imatinib mesylate in patients with decreased renal function (studies excluded patients with serum creatinine concentration more than 2 times the upper limit of the normal range). Imatinib and its metabolites are not significantly excreted via the kidney.

DRUG-DRUG INTERACTIONS

CYP3A4 Inhibitors: There was a significant increase in exposure to imatinib (mean C_{max} and AUC increased by 26% and 40%, respectively) in healthy subjects when imatinib mesylate was coadministered with a single dose of ketoconazole (a CYP3A4 inhibitor). (See DRUG INTERACTIONS.)

CYP3A4 Substrates: Imatinib increased the mean C_{max} and AUC of simvastatin (CYP3A4 substrate) by 2- and 3.5-fold, respectively, indicating an inhibition of CYP3A4 by imatinib. (See DRUG INTERACTIONS.)

CYP3A4 Inducers: No formal study of CYP3A4 inducers has been conducted, but a patient on chronic therapy with phenytoin (a CYP3A4 inducer) given 350 mg daily dose of imatinib mesylate had an AUC(0-24) about one-fifth of the typical AUC(0-24) of 20 μg·h/ml. This probably reflects the induction of CYP3A4 by phenytoin. (See DRUG INTERACTIONS.)

In Vitro Studies of CYP Enzyme Inhibition: Human liver microsome studies demonstrated that imatinib is a potent competitive inhibitor of CYP2C9, CYP2D6, and CYP3A4/5 with Ki values of 27, 7.5, and 8 μM, respectively. Imatinib is likely to increase the blood level of drugs that are substrates of CYP2C9, CYP2D6 and CYP3A4/5. (See DRUG INTERACTIONS.)

I

INDICATIONS AND USAGE

Imatinib mesylate is indicated for the treatment of patients with Philadelphia chromosome positive chronic myeloid leukemia (CML) in blast crisis, accelerated phase, or in chronic phase after failure of interferon-alpha therapy. Imatinib mesylate is also indicated for the treatment of patients with Kit (CD117) positive unresectable and/or metastatic malignant gastrointestinal stromal tumors (GIST).

The effectiveness of imatinib mesylate is based on overall hematologic and cytogenetic response rates in CML and objective response rate in GIST. There are no controlled trials demonstrating a clinical benefit, such as improvement in disease-related symptoms or increased survival.

NON-FDA APPROVED INDICATIONS

Due to its ability to inhibit other tyrosine kinases, imatinib is also under investigation for the treatment of acute lymphocytic leukemia, gliomas, small cell lung cancer, refractory prostate cancer, and soft tissue sarcomas. However, none of these uses is approved by the FDA.

CONTRAINDICATIONS

Use of imatinib mesylate is contraindicated in patients with hypersensitivity to imatinib or to any other component of imatinib mesylate.

WARNINGS

PREGNANCY

Women of childbearing potential should be advised to avoid becoming pregnant.

Imatinib mesylate was teratogenic in rats when administered during organogenesis at doses $\geq$100 mg/kg, approximately equal to the maximum clinical dose of 800 mg/day, based on body surface area. Teratogenic effects included exencephaly or encephalocele, absent/reduced frontal and absent parietal bones. Female rats administered this dose also experienced significant post-implantation loss in the form of early fetal resorption. At doses higher than 100 mg/kg, total fetal loss was noted in all animals. These effects were not seen at doses $\leq$30 mg/kg (one-third the maximum human dose of 800 mg).

There are no adequate and well-controlled studies in pregnant women. If imatinib mesylate is used during pregnancy, or if the patient becomes pregnant while taking (receiving) imatinib mesylate, the patient should be apprised of the potential hazard to the fetus.

PRECAUTIONS

GENERAL

Fluid Retention and Edema

Imatinib mesylate is often associated with edema and occasionally serious fluid retention (see ADVERSE REACTIONS). Patients should be weighed and monitored regularly for signs and symptoms of fluid retention. An unexpected rapid weight gain should be carefully investigated and appropriate treatment provided. The probability of edema was increased with higher imatinib dose and age >65 years in the CML studies. Severe fluid retention (*e.g.,* pleural effusion, pericardial effusion, pulmonary edema, and ascites) was reported in 2-8% of patients taking imatinib mesylate for CML. In addition, severe superficial edema was reported in 2-5% of the patients with CML.

Severe superficial edema and severe fluid retention (pleural effusion, pulmonary edema and ascites) were reported in 1-6% of patients taking imatinib mesylate for GIST.

GI Irritation

Imatinib mesylate is sometimes associated with GI irritation. Imatinib mesylate should be taken with food and a large glass of water to minimize this problem.

Hemorrhage

In the GIST clinical trial seven patients (5%), four in the 600 mg dose group and three in the 400 mg dose group, had a total of eight events of CTC grade 3/4 — gastrointestinal (GI) bleeds (3 patients), intra-tumoral bleeds (3 patients) or both (1 patient). Gastrointestinal tumor sites may have been the source of GI bleeds.

Hematologic Toxicity

Treatment with imatinib mesylate is often associated with neutropenia or thrombocytopenia. Complete blood counts should be performed weekly for the first month, biweekly for the second month, and periodically thereafter as clinically indicated (for example every 2-3 months). The occurrence of these cytopenias is dependent on the stage of disease and is more frequent in patients with accelerated phase CML or blast crisis than in patients with chronic phase CML. (See DOSAGE AND ADMINISTRATION.)

Hepatotoxicity

Hepatotoxocity, occasionally severe, may occur with imatinib mesylate (see ADVERSE REACTIONS). Liver function (transaminases, bilirubin, and alkaline phosphatase) should be monitored before initiation of treatment and monthly or as clinically indicated. Laboratory abnormalities should be managed with interruption and/or dose reduction of the treatment with imatinib mesylate. (See DOSAGE AND ADMINISTRATION.) Patients with hepatic impairment should be closely monitored because exposure to imatinib mesylate may be increased. As there are no clinical studies of imatinib mesylate in patients with impaired liver function, no specific advice concerning initial dosing adjustment can be given.

Toxicities From Long-Term Use

Because follow-up of most patients treated with imatinib is relatively short, there are no long-term safety data on imatinib mesylate treatment. It is important to consider potential toxicities suggested by animal studies, specifically, *liver and kidney toxicity and immunosupression.* Severe liver toxicity was observed in dogs treated for 2 weeks, with elevated liver enzymes, hepatocellular necrosis, bile duct necrosis, and bile duct hyperplasia. Renal toxicity was observed in monkeys treated for 2 weeks, with focal mineralization and dilation of the renal tubules and tubular nephrosis. Increased BUN and creatinine were observed in several of these animals. An increased rate of opportunistic infections was observed with chronic imatinib treatment. In a 39 week monkey study, treatment with imatinib resulted in worsening of normally suppressed malarial infections in these animals. Lymphopenia was observed in animals (as in humans).

CARCINOGENESIS, MUTAGENESIS, AND IMPAIRMENT OF FERTILITY

Carcinogenicity studies have not been performed with imatinib mesylate.

Positive genotoxic effects were obtained for imatinib in an *in vitro* mammalian cell assay (Chinese hamster ovary) for clastogenicity (chromosome aberrations) in the presence of metabolic activation. Two intermediates of the manufacturing process, which are also present in the final product, are positive for mutagenesis in the Ames assay. One of these intermediates was also positive in the mouse lymphoma assay. Imatinib was not genotoxic when tested in an *in vitro* bacterial cell assay (Ames test), an *in vitro* mammalian cell assay (mouse lymphoma) and an *in vivo* rat micronucleus assay.

In a study of fertility, in male rats dosed for 70 days prior to mating, testicular and epididymal weights and percent motile sperm were decreased at 60 mg/kg, approximately equal to the maximum clinical dose of 800 mg/day, based on body surface area. This was not seen at doses ≤20 mg/kg (one-fourth the maximum human dose of 800 mg). When female rats were dosed 14 days prior to mating and through to gestational day 6, there was no effect on mating or on number of pregnant females. At a dose of 60 mg/kg (approximately equal to the human dose of 800 mg), female rats had significant post-implantation fetal loss and a reduced number of live fetuses. This was not seen at doses ≤20 mg/kg (one-fourth the maximum human dose of 800 mg).

PREGNANCY CATEGORY D

See WARNINGS.

NURSING MOTHERS

It is not known whether imatinib mesylate or its metabolites are excreted in human milk. However, in lactating female rats administered 100 mg/kg, a dose approximately equal to the maximum clinical dose of 800 mg/day based on body surface area, imatinib and/or its metabolites were extensively excreted in milk. It is estimated that approximately 1.5% of a maternal dose is excreted into milk, which is equivalent to a dose to the infant of 30% the maternal dose per unit body weight. Because many drugs are excreted in human milk and because of the potential for serious adverse reactions in nursing infants, women should be advised against breastfeeding while taking imatinib mesylate.

PEDIATRIC USE

The safety and effectiveness of imatinib mesylate in pediatric patients have not been established.

GERIATRIC USE

In the CML clinical studies, approximately 40% of patients were older than 60 years and 10% were older than 70 years. No difference was observed in the safety profile in patients older than 65 years as compared to younger patients, with the exception of a higher frequency of edema. (See PRECAUTIONS.) The efficacy of imatinib mesylate was similar in older and younger patients.

In the GIST study, 29% of patients were older than 60 years and 10% of patients were older than 70 years. No obvious differences in the safety or efficacy profile were noted in patients older than 65 years as compared to younger patients, but the small number of patients does not allow a formal analysis.

DRUG INTERACTIONS

DRUGS THAT MAY ALTER IMATINIB PLASMA CONCENTRATIONS

Drugs That May Increase Imatinib Plasma Concentrations

Caution is recommended when administering imatinib mesylate with inhibitors of the CYP3A4 family (*e.g.,* ketoconazole, itraconazole, erythromycin, clarithromycin). Substances that inhibit the cytochrome P450 isoenzyme (CYP3A4) activity may decrease metabolism and increase imatinib concentrations. There is a significant increase in exposure to imatinib when imatinib mesylate is co-administered with ketoconazole (CYP3A4 inhibitor).

Drugs That May Decrease Imatinib Plasma Concentrations

Substances that are inducers of CYP3A4 activity may increase metabolism and decrease imatinib plasma concentrations. Co-medications that induce CYP3A4 (*e.g.,* dexamethasone, phenytoin, carbamazepine, rifampicin, phenobarbital or St. John's Wort) may reduce exposure to imatinib mesylate. No formal study of CYP3A4 inducers has been conducted, but a patient on chronic therapy with phenytoin (a CYP3A4 inducer) given 350 mg daily dose of imatinib mesylate had an AUC(0-24) about one-fifth of the typical AUC(0-24) of 20 μg·h/ml. This probably reflects the induction of CYP3A4 by phenytoin. (See PRECAUTIONS.)

DRUGS THAT MAY HAVE THEIR PLASMA CONCENTRATION ALTERED BY IMATINIB MESYLATE

Imatinib increases the mean C_{max} and AUC of simvastatin (CYP3A4 substrate) 2- and 3.5-fold, respectively, suggesting an inhibition of the CYP3A4 by imatinib. Particular caution is recommended when administering imatinib mesylate with CYP3A4 substrates that have a narrow therapeutic window (*e.g.,* cyclosporine or pimozide). Imatinib mesylate will increase plasma concentration of other CYP3A4 metabolized drugs (*e.g.,* triazolo-benzodiazepines, dihydropyridine calcium channel blockers, certain HMG-CoA reductase inhibitors, etc.)

Because *warfarin* is metabolized by CYP2C9 and CYP3A4, patients who require anticoagulation should receive low-molecular weight or standard heparin.

In vitro, imatinib mesylate inhibits the cytochrome P450 isoenzyme CYP2D6 activity at similar concentrations that affect CYP3A4 activity. Systemic exposure to substrates of CYP2D6 is expected to be increased when co-administered with imatinib mesylate. No specific studies have been performed and caution is recommended.

ADVERSE REACTIONS

CHRONIC MYELOID LEUKEMIA

The majority of imatinib mesylate-treated patients experienced adverse events at some time. Most events were of mild to moderate grade, but drug was discontinued for adverse events in 2% of patients in chronic phase, 3% in accelerated phase and 5% in blast crisis.

The most frequently reported drug-related adverse events were nausea, vomiting, diarrhea, edema, and muscle cramps (TABLE 3). Edema was most frequently periorbital or in lower limbs and was managed with diuretics, other supportive measures, or by reducing the dose of imatinib mesylate. (See DOSAGE AND ADMINISTRATION.) The frequency of severe edema was 2-5%.

A variety of adverse events represent local or general fluid retention including pleural effusion, ascites, pulmonary edema and rapid weight gain with or without superficial edema. These events appear to be dose related, were more common in the blast crisis and accelerated phase studies (where the dose was 600 mg/day), and are more common in the elderly. These events were usually managed by interrupting imatinib mesylate treatment and with diuretics or other appropriate supportive care measures. However, a few of these events may be serious or life threatening, and one patient with blast crisis died with pleural effusion, congestive heart failure, and renal failure.

Adverse events, regardless of relationship to study drug, that were reported in at least 10% of the patients treated in the imatinib mesylate studies are shown in TABLE 3.

HEMATOLOGIC TOXICITY

Cytopenias, and particularly neutropenia and thrombocytopenia, were a consistent finding in all studies, with a higher frequency at doses ≥750 mg (Phase 1 study). The occurrence of cytopenias in CML patients was also dependent on the stage of the disease, with a frequency of Grade 3 or 4 neutropenia and thrombocytopenia between 2- and 3-fold higher in blast crisis and accelerated phase compared to chronic phase (see TABLE 4). The median duration of the neutropenic and thrombocytopenic episodes ranged usually from 2-3 weeks, and from 3-4 weeks, respectively. These events can usually be managed with either a reduction of the dose or an interruption of treatment with imatinib mesylate, but in rare cases require permanent discontinuation of treatment.

HEPATOTOXICITY

Severe elevation of transaminases or bilirubin occurred in 1-4% (see TABLE 4) and were usually managed with dose reduction or interruption (the median duration of these episodes was approximately 1 week). Treatment was discontinued permanently because of liver laboratory abnormalities in less than 0.5% of patients. However, one patient, who was taking acetaminophen regularly for fever, died of acute liver failure.

ADVERSE EFFECTS IN SUBPOPULATIONS

With the exception of edema, where it was more frequent, there was no evidence of an increase in the incidence or severity of adverse events in older patients (≥65 years old). With the exception of a slight increase in the frequency of Grade 1/2 periorbital edema, headache and fatigue in women, there was no evidence of a difference in the incidence or severity of adverse events between the sexes. No differences were seen related to race but the subsets were too small for proper evaluation.

GASTROINTESTINAL STROMAL TUMORS

The majority of imatinib mesylate-treated patients experienced adverse events at some time. The most frequently reported adverse events were edema, nausea, diarrhea, abdominal pain, muscle cramps, fatigue and rash. Most events were of mild to moderate severity. Drug was discontinued for adverse events in 6 patients (8%) in both dose levels studied. Superficial

TABLE 3 *Adverse Experiences Reported in CML Clinical Trials (≥10% of all patients in any trial)**

Preffered Term	Myeloid Blast Crisis (n=260) All Grades	Myeloid Blast Crisis (n=260) Grades 3/4	Accelerated Phase (n=235) All Grades	Accelerated Phase (n=235) Grades 3/4	Chronic Phase, IFN Failure (n=532) All Grades	Chronic Phase, IFN Failure (n=532) Grades 3/4
Nausea	70%	4%	71%	5%	60%	2%
Fluid retention	71%	12%	73%	6%	66%	3%
Superficial edema	67%	5%	71%	4%	64%	2%
Other fluid retention events†	22%	8%	10%	3%	7%	2%
Muscle cramps	27%	0.8%	42%	0.4%	55%	1%
Diarrhea	42%	4%	55%	4%	43%	2%
Vomiting	54%	4%	56%	3%	32%	1%
Hemorrhage	52%	19%	44%	9%	22%	2%
CNS hemorrhage	7%	5%	2%	0.9%	1%	1%
Gastorintestinal hemorrhage	8%	3%	5%	3%	2%	0.4%
Musculoskeletal pain	43%	9%	46%	9%	35%	2%
Skin rash	35%	5%	44%	4%	42%	3%
Headache	27%	5%	30%	2%	34%	0.2%
Fatigue	29%	3%	41%	4%	40%	1%
Arthralgia	25%	4%	31%	6%	36%	1%
Dyspepsia	11%	0%	21%	0%	24%	0%
Myalgia	8%	0%	22%	2%	25%	0.2%
Weight increase	5%	0.8%	14%	3%	30%	5%
Pyrexia	41%	7%	39%	8%	17%	1%
Abdominal pain	31%	6%	33%	3%	29%	0.6%
Cough	14%	0.8%	26%	0.9%	17%	0%
Dyspnea	14%	4%	20%	7%	9%	0.6%
Anorexia	14%	2%	17%	2%	6%	0%
Constipation	15%	2%	15%	0.9%	6%	0.2%
Nasopharingitis	8%	0%	16%	0%	18%	0.2%
Night sweats	12%	0.8%	14%	1%	10%	0.2%
Pruritus	8%	1%	13%	0.9%	12%	0.8%
Epistaxis	13%	3%	13%	0%	5%	0.2%
Hypokalemia	13%	4%	8%	2%	5%	0.2%
Petechiae	10%	2%	5%	0.9%	1%	0%
Pneumonia	12%	6%	8%	6%	3%	0.8%
Weakness	12%	3%	9%	3%	7%	0.2%
Upper respiratory tract infection	3%	0%	9%	0.4%	15%	0%
Dizziness	11%	0.4%	12%	0%	13%	0.2%
Insomnia	10%	0%	13%	0%	13%	0.2%
Sore throat	8%	0%	11%	0%	11%	0%
Ecchymosis	11%	0.4%	6%	0.9%	2%	0%
Rigors	10%	0%	11%	0.4%	8%	0%
Asthenia	5%	2%	11%	2%	6%	0%
Influenza	0.8%	0.4%	6%	0%	10%	0.2%

* All adverse events occurring in ≥10% of patients are listed regardless of suspected relationship to treatment.

† Other fluid retention events include pleural effusion, ascites, pulmonary edema, pericardial effusion, anasarca, edema aggravated, and fluid retention not otherwise specified.

TABLE 4 *Lab Abnormalities in CML Clinical Trials*

	Myeloid Blast Crisis (n=260)		Accelerated Phase (n=235)		Chronic Phase, IFN Failure (n=532)	
	600 mg	n=223	600 mg	n=158		
	400 mg	n=37	400 mg	n=77	400 mg	400 mg
CTC Grade	**Grade 3**	**Grade 4**	**Grade 3**	**Grade 4**	**Grade 3**	**Grade 4**
Hematology Parameters						
Neutropenia	16%	48%	23%	36%	27%	8%
Thrombocytopenia	29%	33%	31%	13%	19%	<1%
Anemia	41%	11%	34%	6%	6%	1%
Biochemistry Parameters						
Elevated creatinine	1.5%	0%	1.3%	0%	0.2%	0%
Elevated bilirubin	3.8%	0%	2.1%	0%	0.8%	0%
Elevated alkaline phosphatase	4.6%	0%	5.1%	0.4%	0.2%	0%
Elevated SGOT (AST)	1.9%	0%	3.0%	0%	2.3%	0%
Elevated SGPT (ALT)	2.3%	0.4%	3.8%	0%	1.9%	0%

CTC grades: Neutropenia (Grade 3 ≥0.5-1.0 × 10^9/L), Grade 4 <0.5 × 10^9/L), thrombocytopenia (Grade 3 ≥10-50 × 10^9/L, Grade 4 <10 × 10^9/L), anemia (hemoglobin ≥65-80 g/L, Grade 4 <65 g/L), elevated creatinine (Grade 3 >3-6 × upper limit normal range (ULN), Grade 4 >6 × ULN), elevated bilirubin (Grade 3 >3-10 × ULN, Grade 4 >10 × ULN), elevated alkaline phosphatase (Grade 3 >5-20 × ULN, Grade 4 >20 × ULN), elevated SGOT or SGPT (Grade 3 >5-20 × ULN, Grade 4 >20 × ULN).

edema, most frequently periorbital or lower limb edema, was managed with diuretics, other supportive measures, or by reducing the dose of imatinib mesylate. (See DOSAGE AND ADMINISTRATION.) Severe (CTC grade 3/4) superficial edema was observed in 3 patients (2%), including face edema in 1 patient. Grade 3/4 pleural effusion or ascites was observed in 3 patients (2%).

Adverse events, regardless of relationship to study drug, that were reported in at least 10% of the patients treated with imatinib mesylate are shown in TABLE 5. No major differences were seen in the severity of adverse events between the 400 or 600 mg treatment groups, although overall incidence of diarrhea, muscle cramps, headache, dermatitis and edema was somewhat higher in the 600 mg treatment group.

TABLE 5 *Adverse Experiences Reported in GIST Trial (≥10% of all patients at either dose)**

Preferred Term	All CTC Grades 400 mg (n=73)	All CTC Grades 600 mg (n=74)	CTC Grade 3/4 400 mg (n=73)	CTC Grade 3/4 600 mg (n=74)
Fluid retention	71%	76%	6%	3%
Superficial edema	71%	76%	4%	0%
Pleural effusion or ascites	6%	4%	1%	3%
Diarrhea	56%	60%	1%	4%
Nausea	53%	56%	3%	3%
Fatigue	33%	38%	1%	0%
Muscle cramps	30%	41%	0%	0%
Abdominal pain	37%	37%	7%	3%
Skin rash	26%	38%	3%	3%
Headache	25%	35%	0%	0%
Vomiting	22%	23%	1%	3%
Musculoskeletal pain	19%	11%	3%	0%
Flatulence	16%	23%	0%	0%
Any hemorrhage	18%	19%	5%	8%
Tumor hemorrhage	1%	4%	1%	4%
Cerebral hemorrhage	1%	0%	1%	0%
GI tract hemorrhage	6%	4%	4%	1%
Nasopharyngitis	12%	14%	0%	0%
Pyrexia	12%	5%	0%	0%
Insomnia	11%	11%	0%	0%
Back pain	11%	10%	1%	0%
Lacrimation increased	6%	11%	0%	0%
Upper respiratory tract infection	6%	11%	0%	0%
Taste disturbance	1%	14%	0%	0%

* All adverse events occurring in ≥10% of patients are listed regardless of suspected relationship to treatment.

Clinically relevant or severe abnormalities of routine hematologic or biochemistry laboratory values are presented in TABLE 6.

TABLE 6 *Laboratory Abnormalities in GIST Trial*

Parameter	400 mg (n=73)		600 mg (n=74)	
CTC Grade	**Grade 3**	**Grade 4**	**Grade 3**	**Grade 4**
Hematology Parameters				
Anemia	3%	0%	4%	1%
Thrombocytopenia	0%	0%	1%	0%
Neutropenia	3%	3%	5%	4%
Biochemistry Parameters				
Elevated creatinine	0%	1%	3%	0%
Reduced albumin	3%	0%	4%	0%
Elevated bilirubin	1%	0%	1%	3%
Elevated alkaline phosphatase	0%	0%	1%	0%
Elevated SGOT (AST)	3%	0%	1%	1%
Elevated SGPT (ALT)	3%	0%	4%	0%

CTC Grades: Neutropenia (Grade 3 ≥0.5 - 1.0 × 10^9/L, Grade 4 <0.5 × 10^9/L), thrombocytopenia (Grade 3 ≥10-50 × 10^9/L, Grade 4 <10 × 10^9/L), anemia (Grade 3 ≥65-80 g/L, Grade 4 <65 g/L), elevated creatinine (Grade 3 >3-6 × upper limit normal range (ULN), Grade 4 >6 × ULN), elevated bilirubin (Grade 3 >3-10 × ULN, Grade 4 >10 × ULN), elevated alkaline phosphatase, SGOT or SGPT (Grade 3 >5-20 × ULN, Grade 4 >20 × ULN), albumin (Grade 3 <20 g/L)

DOSAGE AND ADMINISTRATION

Therapy should be initiated by a physician experienced in the treatment of patients with chronic myeloid leukemia or gastrointestinal stromal tumors.

The prescribed dose should be administered orally, with a meal and a large glass of water. Doses of 400 or 600 mg should be administered once daily, whereas a dose of 800 mg should be administered as 400 mg twice a day.

Treatment may be continued as long as there is no evidence of progressive disease or unacceptable toxicity.

The recommended dosage of imatinib mesylate is 400 mg/day for patients in chronic phase CML and 600 mg/day for patients in accelerated phase or blast crisis. The recommended dosage of imatinib mesylate is 400 or 600 mg/day for patients with unresectable and/or metastatic, malignant GIST.

In CML, dose increase from 400 to 600 mg in patients with chronic phase disease, or from 600 to 800 mg (given as 400 mg twice daily) in patients in accelerated phase or blast crisis may be considered in the absence of severe adverse drug reaction and severe non-leukemia related neutropenia or thrombocytopenia in the following circumstances: disease progression (at any time); failure to achieve a satisfactory hematologic response after at least 3 months of treatment; loss of a previously achieved hematologic response.

DOSE ADJUSTMENT FOR HEPATOTOXICITY AND OTHER NON-HEMATOLOGIC ADVERSE REACTIONS

If a severe non-hematologic adverse reaction develops (such as severe hepatotoxicity or severe fluid retention), imatinib mesylate should be withheld until the event has resolved. Thereafter, treatment can be resumed as appropriate depending on the initial severity of the event.

If elevations in bilirubin >3 × institutional upper limit of normal (IULN) or in liver transaminases >5 × IULN occur, imatinib mesylate should be withheld until bilirubin levels have returned to a <1.5 × IULN and transaminase levels to <2.5 × IULN. Treatment with imatinib mesylate may then be continued at a reduced daily dose (*i.e.*, 400 to 300 mg or 600 to 400 mg).

HEMATOLOGIC ADVERSE REACTIONS

Dose reduction or treatment interruptions for severe neutropenia and thrombocytopenia are recommended as indicated in TABLE 7.

TABLE 7 *Dose Adjustments for Neutropenia and Thrombocytopenia*

Chronic Phase CML or GIST (starting dose 400 mg)	
ANC <1.0 × 10^9/L and/or Platelets <50 × 10^9/L	1. Stop imatinib mesylate until ANC ≥1.5 × 10^9/L and platelets ≥75 × 10^9/L 2. Resume treatment with imatinib mesylate at dose of 400 mg 3. If recurrence of ANC <1.0 × 10^9/L and/or platelets <50 × 10^9/L, repeat step 1 and resume imatinib mesylate at reduced dose of 300 mg
Accelerated Phase CML and Blast Crisis or GIST (starting dose 600 mg)	
*ANC <0.5 × 10^9/L and/or Platelets <10 × 10^9/L	1. Check if cytopenia is related to leukemia (marrow aspirate or biopsy) 2. If cytopenia is unrelated to leukemia, reduce dose of imatinib mesylate to 400 mg 3. If cytopenia persist 2 weeks, reduce further to 300 mg 4. If cytopenia persist 4 weeks and is still unrelated to leukemia, stop imatinib mesylate until ANC ≥1 × 10^9/L and platelets ≥20 × 10^9/L and then resume treatment at 300 mg

* Occurring after at least 1 month of treatment.

PEDIATRIC

The safety and efficacy of imatinib mesylate in patients under the age of 18 years have not been established.

HOW SUPPLIED

Each Gleevec hard gelatin capsule contains 100 mg of imatinib free base.

100 mg Capsules: Orange to grayish orange opaque capsule with "NVR SI" printed in red ink.

STORAGE

Store at 25°C (77°F); excursions permitted to 15-30°C (59-86°F).

Dispense in a tight container.

PRODUCT LISTING - EQUIVALENTS NOT AVAILABLE

Capsule - Oral - 100 mg

120's $2555.94 GLEEVEC, Novartis Pharmaceuticals 00078-0373-66

Imipenem; Cilastatin Sodium *(000819)*

Categories: Endocarditis; Infection, bone; Infection, gynecologic; Infection, intra-abdominal; Infection, joint; Infection, lower respiratory tract; Infection, polymicrobic; Infection, skin and skin structures; Infection, urinary tract; Septicemia; Abscess, cutaneous; Pneumonia; Cellulitis; Infection, endomyometrial, postpartum; Pregnancy Category C; FDA Approved 1985 Nov; WHO Formulary

Drug Classes: Antibiotics, carbapenems

Brand Names: **Primaxin**

Foreign Brand Availability: Prepenem (Korea); Tenacid (Italy); Tienam (Bangladesh; Belgium; Bulgaria; Colombia; Czech-Republic; Denmark; Ecuador; Finland; France; Hong-Kong; Hungary; Indonesia; Israel; Italy; Korea; Malaysia; Mexico; Netherlands; Norway; Pakistan; Peru; Philippines; Portugal; Spain; Sweden; Switzerland; Taiwan; Thailand); Tienam 500 (South-Africa); Zienam (Austria; Germany)

Cost of Therapy: $1257.34 (Infection; Primaxin Injection; 500 mg;500 mg; 2 g/day; 10 day supply)

HCFA JCODE(S): J0743 per 250 mg IV, IM

DESCRIPTION

IV

Primaxin IV is a sterile formulation of imipenem (a thienamycin antibiotic) and cilastatin sodium (the inhibitor of the renal dipeptidase, dehydropeptidase I), with sodium bicarbonate added as a buffer. Cilastatin sodium; imipenem IV is a potent broad spectrum antibacterial agent for intravenous administration.

Cilastatin sodium; imipenem IV is buffered to provide solutions in the pH range of 6.5-7.5. There is no significant change in pH when solutions are prepared and used as directed. (See DOSAGE AND ADMINISTRATION, Compatibility and Stability.) Primaxin IV 250 contains 18.8 mg of sodium (0.8 mEq) and Primaxin IV 500 contains 37.5 mg of sodium (1.6 mEq). Solutions of Primaxin IV range from colorless to yellow. Variations of color within this range do not affect the potency of the product.

IM

Sterile Primaxin IM is a formulation of imipenem (a thienamycin antibiotic) and cilastatin sodium (the inhibitor of the renal dipeptidase, dehydropeptidase I). Cilastatin sodium; imipenem IM is a potent broad spectrum antibacterial agent for intramuscular administration.

Primaxin IM 500 contains 32 mg of sodium (1.4 mEq) and Primaxin 750 contains 48 mg of sodium (2.1 mEq). Prepared Primaxin IM suspensions are white to light tan in color. Variations of color within this range do not effect the potency of the product.

IV AND IM INJECTION

Imipenem (N-formimidoylthienamycin monohydrate) is a crystalline derivative of thienamycin, which is produced by *Streptomyces cattleya.* Its chemical name is (5*R*,6*S*)-3-[[2-(formimidoylamino)ethyl]thio]-6-[(*R*)-1-hydroxyethyl]-7-oxo-1-azabicyclo[3.2.0]hept-2-ene-2-carboxylic acid monohydrate. It is an off-white, nonhygroscopic crystalline compound with a molecular weight of 317.37. It is sparingly soluble in water, and slightly soluble in methanol. Its empirical formula is $C_{12}H_{17}N_3O_4S{\cdot}H_2O$.

Cilastatin sodium is the sodium salt of a derivatized heptenoic acid. Its chemical name is sodium (*Z*)-7-[[(*R*)-2-amino-2-carboxyethyl]thio]-2-[(*S*)-2,2-dimethylcyclopropanecarboxamido]-2-heptenoate. It is an off-white to yellowish-white, hygroscopic, amorphous compound with a molecular weight of 380.43. It is very soluble in water and in methanol. Its empirical formula is $C_{16}H_{25}N_2O_5S$ Na.

CLINICAL PHARMACOLOGY

GENERAL

IV

Intravenous infusion of cilastatin sodium; imipenem IV over 20 minutes results in peak plasma levels of imipenem antimicrobial activity that range from 14-24 μg/ml for the 250 mg dose, from 21-58 μg/ml for the 500 mg dose, and from 41-83 μg/ml for the 1000 mg dose. At these doses, plasma levels of imipenem antimicrobial activity decline to below 1 μg/ml or less in 4-6 hours. Peak plasma levels of cilastatin IV following a 20 minute intravenous infusion of cilastatin sodium; imipenem IV, range from 15-25 μg/ml for the 250 mg dose, from 31-49 μg/ml for the 500 mg dose and from 56-88 μg/ml for the 1000 mg dose.

The plasma half-life of each component is approximately 1 hour. The binding of imipenem to human serum proteins is approximately 20% and that of cilastatin is approximately 40%. Approximately, 70% of the administered imipenem is recovered in the urine within 10 hours after which no further urinary excretion is detectable. Urine concentrations of imipenem in excess of 10 μg/ml can be maintained for up to 8 hours with cilastatin sodium; imipenem IV at the 500 mg dose. Approximately, 70% of the cilastatin sodium dose is recovered in the urine within 10 hours of administration of cilastatin sodium; imipenem.

No accumulation of cilastatin sodium; imipenem IV in plasma or urine is observed with regimens administered as frequently as every 6 hours in patients with normal renal function.

Imipenem, when administered alone, is metabolized in the kidneys by dehydropeptidase I resulting in relatively low levels in urine. Cilastatin sodium, an inhibitor of this enzyme, effectively prevents renal metabolism of imipenem so that when imipenem and cilastatin sodium are given concomitantly, fully adequate antibacterial levels of imipenem are achieved in the urine.

After a 1 g dose of cilastatin sodium; imipenem IV, the following average levels of imipenem were measured (usually at 1 hour post dose except where indicated) in the tissues and fluids listed in TABLE 1.

TABLE 1

Tissue or Fluid		Imipenem level μg/ml or μg/g	Range
Vitreous humor	n=3	3.4 (3.5 hours post dose)	2.88-3.6
Aqueous humor	n=5	2.99 (2 hours post dose)	2.4-3.9
Lung tissue	n=8	5.6 (median)	3.5-15.5
Sputum	n=1	2.1	—
Pleural	n=1	22.0	—
Peritoneal	n=12	23.9 SD± 5.3 (2 hours post dose)	—
Bile	n=2	5.3 (2.25 hours post dose)	4.6-6.0
CSF (uninflamed)	n=5	1.0 (4 hours post dose)	0.26-2.0
CSF (inflamed)	n=7	2.6 (2 hours post dose)	0.5-5.5
Fallopian tubes	n=1	13.6	—
Endometrium	n=1	11.1	—
Myometrium	n=1	5.0	—
Bone	n=10	2.6	0.4-5.4
Interstitial fluid	n=12	16.4	10.0-22.6
Skin	n=12	4.4	NA
Fascia	n=12	4.4	NA

Cilastatin sodium; imipenem is hemodialyzable. However, usefulness of this procedure in the overdosage setting is questionable.

IM

Following intramuscular administrations of 500 or 750 mg doses of imipenem-cilastatin sodium in a 1:1 ratio with 1% lidocaine, peak plasma levels of imipenem antimicrobial activity occur within 2 hours and average 10 and 12 μg/ml, respectively. For cilastatin, peak plasma levels average 24 and 33 μg/ml respectively, and occur within 1 hour. When compared to intravenous administration of imipenem-cilastatin sodium is approximately 75% bioavailable following intramuscular administration while cilastatin is approximately 95% bioavailable. The absorption of imipenem-cilastatin sodium from the IM injection site continues for 6-8 hours while that for cilastatin is essentially complete within 4 hours. This prolonged absorption of cilastatin sodium; imipenem following the administration of the intramuscular formulation of cilastatin sodium; imipenem results in an effective plasma half-life of imipenem of approximately 2-3 hours and plasma levels of the antibiotic which remain above 2 μg/ml for at least 6-8 hours, following a 500 or 750 mg dose, respectively. This plasma profile for imipenem permits IM administration of the intramuscular formulation of cilastatin sodium; imipenem every 12 hours with no accumulation of cilastatin and only slight accumulation of imipenem.

A comparison of plasma levels of imipenem after a single dose of 500 or 750 mg of cilastatin sodium; imipenem (intravenous formulation) administered intravenously or of cilastatin sodium; imipenem (intramuscular formulation) diluted with 1% lidocaine and administered intramuscularly as seen in TABLE 2.

Imipenem urine levels remain above 10 μg/ml for the 12 hour dosing interval following the administration of 500 or 750 mg doses of the intramuscular formulation of cilastatin sodium; imipenem. Total urinary excretion of imipenem averages 50% while that for cilastatin averages 75% following either dose of the intramuscular formulation of imipenem-cilastatin sodium.

TABLE 2 *Plasma Concentrations of Imipenem (μg/ml)*

	500 mg		750 mg	
Time	IV	IM	IV	IM
25 min	45.1	6.0	57.0	6.7
1 h	21.6	9.4	28.1	10.0
2 h	10.0	9.9	12.0	11.4
4 h	0.6	2.5	1.1	3.8
12 h	ND*	0.5	ND*	0.8

* ND: Not Detectable (<0.3 μg/ml).

Imipenem, when administered alone, is metabolized in the kidneys by dehydropeptidase I resulting in relatively low levels in urine. Cilastatin sodium, an inhibitor of this enzyme, effective prevents renal metabolism of imipenem so that when imipenem and cilastatin sodium are given concomitantly increased levels of imipenem are achieved in the urine. The binding of imipenem to human serum proteins is approximately 20% and that of cilastatin is approximately 40%.

In a clinical study in which a 500 mg dose of the intramuscular formulation of cilastatin sodium; imipenem was administered to healthy subjects, the average peak level of imipenem in interstitial fluid (skin blister fluid) was approximately 5.0 μg/ml within 3.5 hours after administration

Cilastatin sodium; imipenem is hemodialyzable. However, usefulness of this procedure in the overdosage setting is questionable.

MICROBIOLOGY

The bactericidal activity of imipenem results from the inhibition of cell wall synthesis. Its greatest affinity is for penicillin binding proteins (PBPs) 1A, 1B, 2, 4, 5, and 6 of *Escherichia coli*, and 1A, 1B, 2, 4, and 5 of *Pseudomonas aeruginosa*. The lethal effect is related to binding to PBP 2 and PBP 1B.

Imipenem has a high degree of stability in the presence of beta-lactamases, both penicillinases and cephalosporinases produced by gram-negative and gram-positive bacteria. It is a potent inhibitor of beta-lactamases from certain gram-negative bacteria which are inherently resistant to most beta-lactam antibiotics (*e.g., Pseudomonas aeruginosa, Serratia* spp., and *Enterobacter* spp.

Imipenem has *in vitro* activity against a wide range of gram-positive and gram-negative organisms. Imipenem is active against most strains of the following microorganisms *in vitro* and in clinical infections treated with cilistatin sodium; imipenem (see INDICATIONS AND USAGE).

Gram-Positive Aerobes:

Enterococcus faecalis (formerly *S. faecalis*). *NOTE:* Imipenem is inactive *in vitro* against *Enterococcus faecium* [formerly *S. faecium*]
Staphylococcus aureus including penicillinase-producing strains
Staphylococcus epidermidis including penicillinase-producing strains. *NOTE:* Methicillin-resistant staphylococci should be reported as resistant to imipenem
Streptococcus agalactiae (Group B Streptococcus)
Streptococcus pneumoniae
Streptococcus pyogenes

Gram-Negative Aerobes:

Acinetobacter spp
Citrobacter spp
Enterobacter spp
Escherichia coli
Gardnerella vaginalis
Haemophilus influenzae
Haemophilus parainfluenzae
Klebsiella spp
Morganella morganii
Proteus vulgaris
Providencia rettgeri
Pseudomonas aeruginosa NOTE: Imipenem is inactive *in vitro* against *Xanthomonas (Pseudomonas) maltophilia* and some strains of *P. cepacia*
Serratia spp., including *S. marcescens*

Gram-Positive Anaerobes:

Bifidobacterium spp
Clostridium spp
Eubacterium spp
Peptococcus spp
Peptostreptococcus spp
Propionibacterium spp

Gram-Negative Anaerobes:

Bacteroides spp., including *B. fragilis*
Fusobacterium spp

The following *in vitro* data are available, **but their clinical significance is unknown.** Imipenem exhibits *in vitro* minimum inhibitory concentrations (MICs) of 4 μg/ml or less against most (≥90%) strains of the following microorganisms; however, the safety and effectiveness of imipenem in treating clinical infections due to these microorganisms have not been established in adequate and well-controlled clinical trials.

Gram-Positive Aerobes:

Listeria monocytogenes
Nocardia spp
Group C *streptococcus*
Group G *streptococcus*
Viridans group *streptococci*

Gram-Negative Aerobes:

Achromobacter spp
Aeromonas hydrophila
Alcaligenes spp
Bordetella bronchiseptica
Campylobacter spp
Hafnia lave
Klebsiella oxytoca
Klebsiella pneumoniae
Moraxella spp
Neisseria gonorrhoeae including penicillinase-producing strains
Pasteurella multocida
Plesiomonas shigelloides
Proteus mirabilis
Providencia stuartii
Salmonella spp
Serratia proteamaculans (formerly *S. liquefaciens*)
Shigella spp
Yersinia spp., including *Y. enterocolitica* and *Y. pseudotuberculosis*

Gram-Positive Anaerobes:

Actinomyces spp
Clostridium perfringens
Propionibacterium acnes

Gram-Negative Anaerobes:

Bacteroides spp., including *B. bivius, B. disiens, B. distasonis, B. intermedius* (formerly *B. melaninogenicus intermedius*) *B. ovatus, B. thetaiotaomicron,* and *B. vulgatus*
Porphyromonas asaccharolytica (formerly *B. asaccharolyticus*)
Veillonella spp

In vitro tests show imipenem to act synergistically with aminoglycoside antibiotics against some isolates of *Pseudomonas aeruginosa.*

SUSCEPTIBILITY TESTING

Measurement of MIC or minimum bactericidal concentration (MBC) and achieved antimicrobial compound concentrations may be appropriate to guide therapy in some infections. (See CLINICAL PHARMACOLOGY for further information on drug concentrations achieved in infected body sites and other pharmacokinetic properties of this antimicrobial drug product.)

DIFFUSION TECHNIQUES

Quantitative methods that require measurement of zone diameters provide reproducible estimates of the susceptibility of bacteria to antimicrobial compounds. One such standardized procedure,[1] that has been recommended for use with disks to test the susceptibility of microorganisms to imipenem, uses the 10 mg imipenem disk. Interpretation involves the correlation of the diameter obtained in the disk test with the MIC for imipenem.

Reports from the laboratory providing results of the standard single-disk susceptibility test with a 10 μg imipenem disk should be interpreted according to the criteria found in TABLE 3.

TABLE 3

Zone Diameter (mm)	Interpretation
≥16	Susceptible (S)
14-15	Intermediate (I)
≤13	Resistant (R)

A report of "Susceptible" indicates that the pathogen is likely to be inhibited by usually achievable concentrations of the antimicrobial compound in blood. A report of "Intermediate" indicates that the result should be considered equivocal, and, if the microorganism is not fully susceptible to alternative, clinically feasible drugs, the test should be repeated. This category implies possible clinical applicability in body sites where the drug is physiologically concentrated or in situations where high dosage of drug can be used. This category also provides a buffer zone that prevents small uncontrolled technical factors from causing major discrepancies in interpretation. A report of "Resistant" indicates that usually achievable concentrations of the antimicrobial compound in the blood are unlikely to be inhibitory and that other therapy should be selected.

Standardized susceptibility test procedures require the use of laboratory control microorganisms. The 10 μg imipenem disk should provide the diameters shown in TABLE 4 in these laboratory test quality control strains.

TABLE 4

Microorganism	Zone Diameter (mm)
E. coli ATCC 25922	26-32
P. aeruginosa ATCC 27853	20-28

DILUTION TECHNIQUES

Quantitative methods that are used to determine MICs provide reproducible estimates of the susceptibility of bacteria to antimicrobial compounds. One such procedure uses a standardized dilution method[2] (broth, agar, or microdilution) or equivalent with imipenem powder.

The MIC values obtained should be interpreted according to the criteria found in TABLE 5.

TABLE 5

MIC (μg/ml)	Interpretation
≤4	Susceptible (S)
8	Intermediate (I)
≥16	Resistant (R)

Interpretation should be as stated above for results using diffusion techniques.

As with standard diffusion techniques, dilution methods require the use of laboratory control microorganisms. Standard imipenem powder should provide the MIC values shown in TABLE 6.

TABLE 6

Microorganism	MIC (μg/ml)
E. coli ATCC 25922	0.06-0.25
S. aureus ATCC 29213	0.015-0.06
E. faecalis ATCC 29212	0.5-2.0
P. aeruginosa ATCC 27853	1.0-4.0

ANAEROBIC TECHNIQUES

For anaerobic bacteria, the susceptibility to imipenem can be determined by the reference agar dilution method or by alternate standardized test methods.[3]

As with other susceptibility techniques, the use of laboratory control microorganisms is required. Standard imipenem powder should provide the MIC values as shown in TABLE 7 and TABLE 8.

TABLE 7 Reference Agar Dilution Testing

Microorganism	MIC (μg/ml)
B. fragilis ATCC 25285	0.03-0.12
B. thetaiotaomicron ATCC 29741	0.06-0.25
E. lentum ATCC 43055	0.25-1.0

TABLE 8 Broth Microdilution Testing

Microorganism	MIC (μg/ml)
B. thetaiotaomicron ATCC 29741	0.06-0.25
E. lentum ATCC 43055	0.12-0.5

INDICATIONS AND USAGE

IV

Cilastatin sodium; imipenem IV is indicated for the treatment of serious infections caused by susceptible strains of the designated microorganisms in the diseases listed below:

1. ***Lower Respiratory Tract Infections:*** *Staphylococcus aureus* (penicillinase-producing strains), *Acinetobacter* species, *Enterobacter* species, *Escherichia coli, Haemophilus influenzae, Haemophilus parainfluenzae**, *Klebsiella* species, *Serratia marcescens.*
2. ***Urinary Tract Infections (Complicated and Uncomplicated):*** *Enterococcus faecalis, Staphylococcus aureus* (penicillinase-producing strains)*, *Enterobacter* species, *Escherichia coli, Klebsiella* species, *Morganella morganii**, *Proteus vulgaris**, *Providencia rettgeri**, *Pseudomonas aeruginosa.*
3. ***Intra-Abdominal Infections:*** *Enterococcus faecalis, Staphylococcus aureus* (penicillinase-producing strains)*, *Staphylococcus epidermidis, Citrobacter* species,*Enterobacter* species, *Escherichia coli, Klebsiella* species, *Morganella morganii**, *Proteus* species, *Pseudomonas aeruginosa, Bifidobacterium* species, *Clostridium* species, *Eubacterium* species, *Peptococcus* species, *Peptostreptococcus* species, *Propionibacterium* species*, *Bacteroides* species including *B. fragilis, Fusobacterium* species.
4. ***Gynecologic Infections:*** *Enterococcus faecalis, Staphylococcus aureus* (penicillinase-producing strains)*, *Staphylococcus epidermidis, Streptococcus agalactiae* (Group B streptococcus), *Enterobacter* species*, *Escherichia coli, Gardnerella vaginalis, Klebsiella* species*, *Proteus* species, *Bifidobacterium* species*, *Peptococcus* species*, *Peptostreptococcus* species, *Propionibacterium* species*, *Bacteroides* species including *B. fragilis**.
5. ***Bacterial Septicemia:*** *Enterococcus faecalis, Staphylococcus aureus* (penicillinase-producing strains), *Enterobacter* species, *Escherichia coli, Klebsiella* species, *Pseudomonas aeruginosa, Serratia* species*, *Bacteroides* species including *B. fragilis**.
6. ***Bone and Joint Infections:*** *Enterococcus faecalis, Staphylococcus aureus* (penicillinase-producing strains), *Staphylococcus epidermidis, Enterobacter* species, *Pseudomonas aeruginosa.*
7. ***Skin and Skin Structure Infections:*** *Enterococcus faecalis, Staphylococcus aureus* (penicillinase-producing strains), *Staphylococcus epidermidis, Acinetobacter* species, *Citrobacter* species, *Enterobacter* species, *Escherichia coli, Klebsiella* species, *Morganella morganii, Proteus vulgaris, Providencia rettgeri**, *Pseudomonas aeruginosa, Serratia* species, *Peptococcus* species, *Peptostreptococcus* species, *Bacteroides* species including *B. fragilis, Fusobacterium* species*.
8. ***Endocarditis:*** *Staphylococcus aureus* (penicillinase-producing strains).
9. ***Polymicrobic Infections:*** Cilastatin sodium; imipenem IV is indicated for polymicrobic infections including those in which *S. pneumoniae* (pneumonia, septicemia), *S. pyogenes* (skin and skin structure), or nonpenicillinase-producing *S. aureus* is one of the causative organisms. However monobacterial infections due to these organisms are usually treated with narrower spectrum antibiotics, such as penicillin G.

*Efficacy for this organism in this organ system was studied in fewer than 10 infections.

Cilastatin sodium; imipenem IV is not indicated in patients with meningitis because safety and efficacy have not been established.

For pediatric use information, see PRECAUTIONS, Pediatric Use and DOSAGE AND ADMINISTRATION.

Because of its broad spectrum of bactericidal activity against gram-positive and gram-negative aerobic and anaerobic bacteria, cilastatin sodium; imipenem is useful for the treatment of mixed infections and as presumptive therapy prior to the identification of the causative organisms.

Although clinical improvement has been observed in patients with cystic fibrosis, chronic pulmonary disease, and lower respiratory tract infections caused by *Pseudomonas aeruginosa,* bacterial eradication may not necessarily be achieved.

As with other beta-lactam antibiotics, some strains of *Pseudomonas aeruginosa* may develop resistance fairly rapidly on treatment with cilastatin sodium; imipenem IV. During therapy of *Pseudomonas aeruginosa* infections, periodic susceptibility testing should be done when clinically appropriate.

Infections resistant to other antibiotics, for example, cephalosporins, penicillin, and aminoglycosides, have been shown to respond to treatment with cilastatin sodium; imipenem IV.

IM

Cilastatin sodium; imipenem IM is indicated for the treatment of serious infections (listed below) of mild to moderate severity for which intramuscular therapy is appropriate. **Cilastatin sodium; imipenem IM is not intended for the therapy of severe or life-threatening infections, including bacterial sepsis or endocarditis, or in instances of major physiological impairments such as shock.**

Cilastatin sodium; imipenem IM is indicated for the treatment of infections caused by susceptible strains of the designated microorganisms in the conditions listed below:

1. ***Lower Respiratory Tract Infections:*** Including pneumonia and bronchitis as an exacerbation of COPD, caused by *Streptococcus pneumoniae* and *Haemophilus influenzae.*
2. ***Intra-Abdominal Infections:*** Including acute gangrenous or perforated appendicitis and appendicitis with peritonitis, caused by Group D streptococcus including *Enterococcus faecalis**; *Streptococcus viridans* group*; *Escherichia coli; Klebsiella pneumoniae**; *Pseudomonas aeruginosa**; *Bacteroides* species including *B fragilis, B. distasonis**, *B. intermedius** and *B. thetaiotaomicron**; *Fusobacterium* species and *Peptostreptococcus** species.
3. ***Skin and Skin Structure Infections:*** Including abscesses, cellulitis, infected skin ulcers and wound infections caused by *Staphylococcus aureus* including penicillinase-producing strains; *Streptococcus pyogenes**; Group D *streptococcus* including *Enterococcus faecalis; Acinetobacter* species* including *A. calcoaceticus**; *Citrobacter* species*; *Escherichia coli; Enterobacter cloacae; Klebsiella pneumoniae**; *Pseudomonas aeruginosa** and *Bacteroides* species* including *B. fragilis**.
4. ***Gynecologic Infections:*** Including postpartum endomyometritis, caused by Group D streptococcus including *Enterococcus faecalis**; *Escherichia coli; Klebsiella pneumoniae**; *Bacteroides intermedius**; and *Peptostreptococcus* species*.

As with other beta-lactam antibiotics, some strains of *Pseudomonas aeruginosa* may develop resistance fairly rapidly during treatment with cilastatin sodium; imipenem IM. During therapy of *Pseudomonas aeruginosa* infections, periodic susceptibility testing should be done when clinically appropriate. Efficacy for this organism in this organ system was studied in fewer than 10 infections.

*Efficacy for this organism in this organ system was studied in fewer than 10 infections.

NON-FDA APPROVED INDICATIONS

Although not approved by the FDA, imipenem-cilastatin has been used in the treatment of febrile neutropenia and bacterial meningitis.

CONTRAINDICATIONS

IV and IM Injection: Cilastatin sodium; imipenem IV and IM are contraindicated in patients who have shown hypersensitivity to any component of this product.

Additional Information for IM: Due to the use of lidocaine HCl diluent, cilastatin sodium; imipenem IM is contraindicated in patients with a known hypersensitivity to local anesthetics of the amide type and in patients with severe shock or heart block. (Refer to the package circular for lidocaine HCl.)

WARNINGS

SERIOUS AND OCCASIONALLY FATAL HYPERSENSITIVITY (ANAPHYLACTIC) REACTIONS HAVE BEEN REPORTED IN PATIENTS RECEIVING THERAPY WITH BETA-LACTAMS. THESE REACTIONS ARE MORE APT TO OCCUR IN PERSONS WITH A HISTORY OF SENSITIVITY TO MULTIPLE ALLERGENS.

THERE HAVE BEEN REPORTS OF PATIENTS WITH A HISTORY OF PENICILLIN HYPERSENSITIVITY WHO HAVE EXPERIENCED SEVERE HYPERSENSITIVITY REACTIONS WHEN TREATED WITH ANOTHER BETA-LACTAM. BEFORE INITIATING THERAPY WITH CILASTATIN-IMIPENEM IV OR IM, CAREFUL INQUIRY SHOULD BE MADE CONCERNING PREVIOUS HYPERSENSITIVITY REACTIONS TO PENICILLINS, CEPHALOSPORINS, OTHER BETA-LACTAMS, AND OTHER ALLERGENS. IF AN ALLERGIC REACTION OCCURS, CILASTATIN SODIUM; IMIPENEM SHOULD BE DISCONTINUED.

SERIOUS ANAPHYLACTIC REACTIONS REQUIRE IMMEDIATE EMERGENCY TREATMENT WITH EPINEPHRINE. OXYGEN, INTRAVENOUS STEROIDS, AND AIRWAY MANAGEMENT, INCLUDING INTUBATION, MAY ALSO BE ADMINISTERED AS INDICATED.

Seizures and other CNS adverse experiences, such as confusional states and myoclonic activity, have been reported during treatment with cilastatin sodium; imipenem IV. (See PRECAUTIONS.)

Pseudomembranous colitis has been reported with nearly all antibacterial agents, including cilastatin sodium; imipenem, and may range in severity from mild to life threatening. Therefore, it is important to consider this diagnosis in patients who present with diarrhea subsequent to the administration of antibacterial agents.

Treatment with antibacterial agents alters the normal flora of the colon and may permit overgrowth of clostridia. Studies indicate that a toxin produced by *Clostridium difficile* is one primary cause of "antibiotic-associated colitis."

After the diagnosis of pseudomembranous colitis has been established, therapeutic measures should be initiated. Mild cases of pseudomembranous colitis usually respond to drug discontinuation alone. In moderate to severe cases, consideration should be given to management with fluids and electrolytes, protein supplementation, and treatment with an antibacterial drug clinically effective against *C. difficile colitis.*

Additional Information for IM: *Lidocaine HCl:* Refer to the prescribing information for lidocaine HCl.

PRECAUTIONS

GENERAL

IV

CNS adverse experiences such as confusional states, myoclonic activity, and seizures have been reported during treatment with cilastatin sodium; imipenem IV especially when recommended dosages were exceeded. These experiences occurred most commonly in patients with CNS disorders (*e.g.,* brain lesions or history of seizures) and/or compromised renal function. However, there have been reports of CNS adverse experiences in patients who had no recognized or documented underlying CNS disorder or compromised renal function.

When recommended doses were exceeded, adult patients with creatinine clearances of $\leq$20 ml/min/1.73 m^2, whether or not undergoing hemodialysis, had a higher risk of seizure activity than those without impairment of renal function. Therefore, close adherence to the dosing guidelines for these patients is recommended (see DOSAGE AND ADMINISTRATION).

Patients with creatinine clearances of $\leq$5 ml/min/1.73 m^2 should not receive cilastatin sodium; imipenem IV unless hemodialysis is instituted within 48 hours.

For patients on hemodialysis, cilastatin sodium; imipenem IV is recommended only when the benefit outweighs the potential risk of seizures.

Close adherence to the recommended dosage and dosage schedules is urged, especially in patients with known factors that predispose to convulsive activity. Anticonvulsant therapy should be continued in patients with known seizure disorders. If focal tremors, myoclonus, or seizures occur, patients should be evaluated neurologically, placed on anticonvulsant therapy if not already instituted, and the dosage of cilastatin sodium; imipenem IV reexamined to determine whether it should be decreased or the antibiotic discontinued.

As with other antibiotics, prolonged use of cilastatin sodium; imipenem IV may result in overgrowth of nonsusceptible organisms. Repeated evaluation of the patient's condition is essential. If superinfection occurs during therapy, appropriate measures should be taken.

IM

CNS adverse experiences such as confusional states, myoclonic activity, or seizures have been reported with cilastatin sodium; imipenem IV. These experiences have occurred most commonly in patients with CNS disorders (*e.g.,* brain lesions or history of seizures) who also have comprised renal function. However, there were reports in which there was no recognized or documented underlying CNS disorder. These adverse CNS effects have not been seen with cilastatin sodium; imipenem IM; however, should they occur during treatment, cilastatin sodium; imipenem IM should be discontinued. Anticonvulsant therapy should be discontinued in patients with a known seizure disorder.

As with other antibiotics, prolonged use of cilastatin sodium; imipenem IM may result in overgrowth of nonsusceptible organisms. Repeated evaluation of the patient's condition is essential. If superinfection occurs during therapy, approximate measures should be taken.

Caution should be taken to avoid inadvertent injection into a blood vessel (see DOSAGE AND ADMINISTRATION). For additional precautions, refer to the prescribing information for lidocaine HCl.

LABORATORY TESTS

While cilastatin sodium; imipenem IV possesses the characteristic low toxicity of the beta-lactam group of antibiotics, periodic assessment of organ system functions, including renal, hepatic, and hematopoietic, is advisable during prolonged therapy.

CARCINOGENESIS, MUTAGENESIS, AND IMPAIRMENT OF FERTILITY

Long term studies in animals have not been performed to evaluate carcinogenic potential of cilastatin sodium; imipenem. Genetic toxicity studies were performed in a variety of bacterial and mammalian tests *in vivo* and *in vitro.* The tests used were: V79 mammalian cell mutagenesis assay (cilastatin sodium; imipenem alone and imipenem alone), Ames test (cilastatin sodium alone and imipenem alone), unscheduled DNA synthesis assay (cilastatin sodium; imipenem) and *in vivo* mouse cytogenetics test (cilastatin sodium; imipenem). None of these tests showed any evidence of genetic alterations.

Reproductive tests in male and female rats were performed with cilastatin sodium; imipenem at dosage levels up to 11 times the usual human dose of the intravenous formulation (on a mg/kg basis), IM at doses up to 11 times† the maximum daily recommended human dose (on a mg/kg basis). Slight decreases in live fetal body weight were restricted to the highest dosage level. No other adverse effects were observed on fertility, reproductive performance, fetal viability, growth or postnatal development of pups. Similarly, no adverse effects on the fetus or on lactation were observed when cilastatin sodium; imipenem was administered to rats late in gestation.

PREGNANCY, TERATOGENIC EFFECTS, PREGNANCY CATEGORY C

IV

Teratology studies with cilastatin sodium in rabbits and rats at 6-20 times* the maximum recommended human dose of the intravenous formulation of cilastatin sodium; imipenem (50 mg/kg/day*), respectively, showed no evidence of adverse effect on the fetus. No evidence of teratogenicity was observed in rabbits and rats given imipenem at doses up to 1 and 18 times the maximum recommended daily human dose of the intravenous formulation of cilastatin sodium; imipenem, respectively.

Teratology studies with cilastatin sodium; imipenem at doses up to 11 times the usual recommended human dose of the intravenous formulation (30 mg/kg/day*) in pregnant mice and rats during the period of major organogenesis revealed no evidence of teratogenicity.

Cilastatin sodium; imipenem, when administered to pregnant rabbits at dosages equivalent to the usual human dose of the intravenous formulation and higher, caused body weight loss, diarrhea, and maternal deaths. When comparable doses of cilastatin sodium; imipenem were given to non-pregnant rabbits, body weight loss, diarrhea, and deaths were also observed. This intolerance is not unlike that seen with other beta-lactam antibiotics in this species and is probably due to alteration of gut flora.

A teratology study in pregnant cynomolgus monkeys given cilastatin sodium; imipenem at doses of 40 mg/kg/day (bolus intravenous injection) or 160 mg/kg/day (subcutaneous injection) resulted in maternal toxicity including emesis, inappetence, body weight loss, diarrhea, abortion, and death in some cases. In contrast, no significant toxicity was observed when non-pregnant cynomolgus monkeys were given doses of cilastatin sodium; imipenem up to 180 mg/kg/day (subcutaneous injection). When doses of cilastatin sodium; imipenem (approximately 100 mg/kg/day or approximately 2 times the maximum recommended daily human dose of the intravenous formulation) were administered to pregnant cynomolgus monkeys at an intravenous infusion rate which mimics human clinical use, there was minimal maternal intolerance (occasional emesis), no maternal deaths, no evidence of teratogenicity, but an increase in embryonic loss relative to control groups.

There are, however, no adequate and well-controlled studies in pregnant women. Cilastatin sodium; imipenem should be used during pregnancy only if the potential benefit justifies the potential risk to the mother and fetus.

*Based on a patient weight of 70 kg.

IM

Teratology studies with cilastatin sodium in rabbits and rats at 10 and 33 times† the maximum recommended daily human dose of the intramuscular formulation (30 mg/kg/day) of cilastatin sodium; imipenem, respectively, showed no evidence of adverse effects on the fetus. No evidence of teratogenicity was observed in rabbits and rats given imipenem at doses up to 2 and 30 times† the maximum recommended daily human dose of the intramuscular formulation of cilastatin sodium; imipenem, respectively.

Teratology studies with cilastatin sodium; imipenem at doses up to 11 times† the maximum recommended human dose in pregnant mice and rats during the period of major organogenesis revealed no evidence of teratogenicity.

Cilastatin sodium; imipenem, when administered to pregnant rabbits at dosages above the usual human dose of the intramuscular formulation (1000-1500 mg/day) caused body weight loss, diarrhea, and maternal deaths. When comparable doses of cilastatin sodium; imipenem were given to non-pregnant rabbits, body weight loss, diarrhea, and deaths were also observed. This intolerance is not unlike that seen with other beta-lactam antibiotics in this species and is probably due to alteration of gut flora.

A teratology study in pregnant cynomolgus monkeys given cilastatin sodium; imipenem at doses of 40 mg/kg/day (bolus intravenous injection) or 160 mg/kg/day (subcutaneous injection) resulted in maternal toxicity including emesis, inappetence, body weight loss, diarrhea, abortion and death in some cases. In contrast, no significant toxicity was observed when non-pregnant cynomolgus monkeys were given doses of cilastatin sodium; imipenem up to 180 mg/kg/day (subcutaneous injection). When doses of cilastatin sodium; imipenem (approximately 100 mg/kg/day or approximately 3 times† the maximum daily recommended human dose of the intramuscular formulation) were administered to pregnant cynomolgus monkeys at an intravenous infusion rate which mimics human clinical use, there was minimal maternal intolerance (occasional emesis), no maternal deaths, no evidence of teratogenicity, but an increase in embryonic loss relative to the control groups.

There are, however, no adequate and well-controlled studies in pregnant women. Cilastatin sodium; imipenem IM should be used during pregnancy only if the potential benefit justifies the potential risk to the mother and fetus.

†Based on patient weight of 50 kg.

NURSING MOTHERS

It is not known whether cilastatin sodium; imipenem is excreted in human milk. Because many drugs are excreted in human milk, caution should be exercised when cilastatin sodium; imipenem IV or IM is administered to a nursing woman.

PEDIATRIC USE

IV

Use of cilastatin sodium; imipenem in pediatric patients neonates to 16 years of age is supported by evidence from adequate and well-controlled studies of cilastatin sodium; imipenem IV in adults and by the following clinical studies and published literature in pediatric patients: Based on published studies of 178* pediatric patients $\geq$3 months of age (with non-CNS infections), the recommended dose of cilastatin sodium; imipenem IV is 15-25 mg/kg/dose administered every 6 hours. Doses of 25 mg/kg/dose in patients 3 months to <3 years of age, and 15 mg/kg/dose in patients 3-12 years of age were associated with mean trough plasma concentrations of imipenem of 1.1 $\pm$ 0.4 μg/ml and 0.6 $\pm$ 0.2 μg/ml following multiple 60 minute infusions, respectively; trough urinary concentrations of imipenem were in excess of 10 μg/ml for both doses. These doses have provided adequate plasma and urine concentrations for the treatment of non-CNS infections. Based on studies in adults, the maximum daily dose for treatment of infections with fully susceptible organisms is 2.0 g/day, and of infections with moderately susceptible organisms (primarily some strains of *P. aeruginosa* is 4.0 g/day (see TABLE 13). Higher doses (up to 90 mg/kg/day in older children) have been used in patients with cystic fibrosis (see DOSAGE AND ADMINISTRATION).

Based on studies of 135† pediatric patients $\leq$3 months of age (weighing $\geq$1500 g), the following dosage schedule is recommended for non-CNS infections:

<1 Week of Age: 25 mg/kg every 12 hours.

1-4 Weeks of Age: 25 mg/kg every 8 hours.

4 Weeks to 3 Months of Age: 25 mg/kg every 6 hours.

In a published dose-ranging study of smaller premature infants (670-1890 g) in the first week of life, a dose of 20 mg/kg q12h by 15-30 minutes infusion was associated with mean peak and trough plasma imipenem concentrations of 43 μg/ml and 1.7 μg/ml after multiple doses, respectively. However, moderate accumulation of cilastatin in neonates may occur following multiple doses of cilastatin sodium; imipenem IV. The safety of this accumulation is unknown.

Cilastatin sodium; imipenem IV is not recommended in pediatric patients with CNS infections because of the risk of seizures.

Cilastatin sodium; imipenem IV is not recommended in pediatric patients <30 kg with impaired renal function, as no data are available.

*Two patients were less than 3 months of age.

†One patient was greater than 3 months of age.

DRUG INTERACTIONS

Since concomitant administration of cilastatin sodium; imipenem and probenecid results in only minimal increases in plasma levels of imipenem and plasma half-life, it is not recommended that probenecid be given with cilastatin sodium; imipenem.

Cilastatin sodium; imipenem should not be mixed with or physically added to other antibiotics. However, cilastatin sodium; imipenem may be administered concomitantly with other antibiotics, such as aminoglycosides.

Additional Information for IV: Generalized seizures have been reported in patients who received ganciclovir and cilastatin sodium; imipenem. These drugs should not be used concomitantly unless the potential benefits outweigh the risks.

ADVERSE REACTIONS

SYSTEMIC ADVERSE REACTIONS

Additional adverse systemic clinical reactions reported as possibly, probably, or definitely drug related occurring in less than 0.2% of the patients or reported since the drug was marketed are listed within each body system in order of decreasing severity.

Gastrointestinal: Pseudomembranous colitis (the onset of pseudomembranous colitis symptoms may occur during or after antibacterial treatment, see WARNINGS), hemorrhagic colitis, hepatitis, jaundice, gastroenteritis, abdominal pain, glossitis, tongue papillar hypertrophy, staining of the teeth and/or tongue, heartburn, pharyngeal pain, increased salivation.

Hematologic: Pancytopenia, bone marrow depression, thrombocytopenia, neutropenia, leukopenia, hemolytic anemia.

CNS: Encephalopathy, tremor, confusion, myoclonus, paresthesia, vertigo, headache, psychic disturbances including hallucinations.

Special Senses: Hearing loss, tinnitus, taste perversion.

Respiratory: Chest discomfort, dyspnea, hyperventilation, thoracic spine pain.

Cardiovascular: Palpitations, tachycardia.

Skin: Stevens-Johnson syndrome, toxic epidermal necrolysis, erythema multiforme, angioneurotic edema, flushing, cyanosis, hyperhidrosis, skin texture changes, candidiasis, pruritus vulvae.

Body as a Whole: Polyarthralgia, asthenia/weakness, drug fever.

Renal: Acute renal failure, oliguria/anuria, polyuria, urine discoloration. The role of cilastatin sodium; imipenem IV in changes in renal function is difficult to assess, since factors predisposing to pre-renal azotemia or to impaired renal function usually have been present.

IV ONLY

Cilastatin sodium; imipenem IV is generally well tolerated. Many of the 1723 patients treated in clinical trials were severely ill and had multiple background diseases and physiological impairments, making it difficult to determine causal relationship of adverse experiences to therapy with cilastatin sodium; imipenem IV.

Local Adverse Reactions

Adverse local clinical reactions that were reported as possibly, probably or definitely related to therapy with cilastatin sodium; imipenem IV were:

Phlebitis/Thrombophlebitis: 3.1%
Pain at the Injection Site: 0.7%
Erythema at the Injection Site: 0.4%
Vein Induration: 0.2%
Infused Vein Infection: 0.1%

Systemic Adverse Reactions

The most frequently reported systemic adverse clinical reactions that were reported as possibly, probably, or definitely related to cilastatin sodium; imipenem IV were nausea (2.0%), diarrhea (1.8%), vomiting (1.5%), rash (0.9%), fever (0.5%), hypotension (0.4%), seizures (0.4%) (see PRECAUTIONS), dizziness (0.3%), pruritus (0.3%), urticaria (0.2%), somnolence (0.2%).

Adverse Laboratory Changes

Adverse laboratory changes without regard to drug relationship that were reported during clinical trials or reported since the drug was marketed were:

Hepatic: Increased ALT (SGPT), AST (SGOT), alkaline phosphatase, bilirubin, and LDH.

Hemic: Increased eosinophils, positive Coombs test, increased WBC, increased platelets, decreased hemoglobin and hematocrit, agranulocytosis, increased monocytes, abnormal prothrombin time, increased lymphocytes, increased basophils.

Electrolytes: Decreased serum sodium, increased potassium, increased chloride.

Renal: Increased BUN, creatinine.

Urinalysis: Presence of urine protein, urine red blood cells, urine white blood cells, urine casts, urine bilirubin, and urine urobilinogen.

PEDIATRIC PATIENTS

In studies of 178 pediatric patients, ≥3 months of age the adverse events shown in TABLE 9 were noted.

In studies of 135 patients (newborn to 3 months of age), the adverse events shown in TABLE 10 were noted.

Examination of published literature and spontaneous adverse event reports suggested a similar spectrum of adverse events in adult and pediatric patients.

IM ONLY

In 686 patients in multiple dose clinical trials of cilastatin sodium; imipenem IM, the following adverse reactions were reported:

Local Adverse Reactions: The most frequent adverse local clinical reaction that was reported as possibly, probably or definitely related to therapy with cilastatin sodium; imipenem IM was pain at the injection site (1.2%)

***TABLE 9** The Most Common Clinical Adverse Experiences Without Regard to Drug Relationship (patient incidence >1%)*

Adverse Experience	Number of Patients
Digestive System	
Diarrhea	7* (3.9%)
Gastroenteritis	2 (1.1%)
Vomiting	2* (1.1%)
Skin	
Rash	4 (2.2%)
Irritation, IV site	2 (1.1%)
Urogenital System	
Urine discoloration	2 (1.1%)
Cardiovascular System	
Phlebitis	4 (2.2%)

* One patient had both vomiting and diarrhea and is counted in each category.

***TABLE 10** The Most Common Clinical Adverse Experiences Without Regard to Drug Relationship (Patient Incidence >1%)*

Adverse Experience	Number of Patients
Digestive System	
Diarrhea	4 (3.0%)
Oral candidiasis	2 (1.5%)
Skin	
Rash	2 (1.5%)
Urogenital System	
Oliguria/anuria	3 (2.2%)
Cardiovascular System	
Tachycardia	2 (1.5%)
Nervous System	
Convulsions	8 (5.9%)

***TABLE 11** Patients ≥3 Months of Age With Normal Pretherapy But Abnormal During Therapy Laboratory Values*

Laboratory Parameter	Abnormality	No. of Patients with Abnormalities/No. of Patients with Lab Done	
Hemoglobin	<4-5 mos. of age: <10 g %; 6 mos.-12 yrs of age: <11.5 g %	19/129	(14.7%)
Hematocrit	<1-5 mos. of age: <30 vol %; 6 mos.-12 yrs of age: <34.5 vol %	23/129	(17.8%)
Neutrophils	≤1000/mm³ (absolute)	4/123	(3.3%)
Eosinophils	≥7%	15/117	(12.8%)
Platelet count	≥500 ths/mm³	16/119	(13.4%)
Urine protein	≥1	8/97	(8.2%)
Serum creatinine	>1.2 mg/dl	0/105	(0%)
BUN	>22 mg/dl	0/108	(0%)
AST (SGOT)	>36 IU/L	14/78	(17.9%)
ALT (SGPT)	>30 IU/L	10/93	(10.8%)

***TABLE 12** Patients (<3 months of age) With Normal Pretherapy But Abnormal During Therapy Laboratory Values*

Laboratory Parameter	No. of Patients with Abnormalities*
Eosinophil count increase	11 (9.0%)
Hematocrit decrease	3 (2.0%)
Hematocrit increase	1 (1.0%)
Platelet count increase	5 (4.0%)
Platelet count decrease	2 (2.0%)
Serum creatinine increase	5 (5.0%)
Bilirubin increase	3 (3.0%)
Bilirubin decrease	1 (1.0%)
AST (SGOT) increase	5 (6.0%)
ALT (SGPT) increase	3 (3.0%)
Serum alkaline phosphate increase	2 (3.0%)

* The denominator used for percentages was the number of patients for whom the test was performed during or post treatment and, therefore, varies by test.

Systemic Adverse Reactions: The most frequently reported systemic adverse clinical reactions that were reported as possibly, probably, or definitely related to therapy with the IM formula were nausea (0.6%), diarrhea (0.6%), vomiting (0.3%) and rash (0.4%).

Adverse Laboratory Changes: Adverse laboratory changes without regard to drug relationship that were reported during clinical trials were:

Hemic: Decreased hemoglobin and hematocrit, eosinophil, increased and decreased WBC, increased and decreased platelets, decreased erythrocytes, and increased prothrombin time.

Hepatic: Increased AST, ALT, alkaline phosphatase, and bilirubin.

Renal: Increased BUN and creatine.

Urinalysis: Presence of red blood cells, white blood cells, casts, and bacteria in the urine.

Potential Adverse Effects: In addition, a variety of adverse effects, not observed in clinical trials with cilastatin sodium; imipenem IM, have been reported with intravenous administration of cilastatin sodium; imipenem IV. Those listed above are to serve as alerting information to physicians.

Adverse Laboratory Changes: Adverse laboratory changes without regard to drug relationship that were reported during clinical trials or reported since the drug was marketed were:

Hepatic: Increased LDH.

Hemic: Positive Coombs test, decreased neutrophils, agranulocytosis, increased monocytes, abnormal prothrombin time, increased lymphocytes, increased basophils.

Electrolytes: Decreased serum sodium, increased potassium, increased chloride.

Urinalysis: Presence of urine protein, urine bilirubin, and urine urobilinogen.

Lidocaine HCl: Refer to the prescribing information for lidocaine HCl.

DOSAGE AND ADMINISTRATION

IV FOR ADULTS

The dosage recommendations for cilastatin sodium; imipenem IV represent the quantity of imipenem to be administered. An equivalent amount of cilastatin is also present in the solution. Each 125, 250 or 500 mg dose should be given by intravenous administration over 20-30 minutes. Each 750 or 1000 mg dose should be infused over 40-60 minutes. In patients who develop nausea during the infusion, the rate of infusion may be slowed.

The total daily dosage for cilastatin sodium; imipenem IV should be based on the type or severity of infection and given in equally divided doses based on consideration of degree of susceptibility of the pathogen(s), renal function, and body weight. Adult patients with impaired renal function, as judged by creatinine clearance ≤70 ml/min/1.73 m², require adjustment of dosage as described in the succeeding section of these guidelines.

Intravenous Dosage Schedule for Adults With Normal Renal Function and Body Weight ≥70 kg

Doses cited in TABLE 13 are based on a patient with normal renal function and a body weight of 70 kg. These doses should be used for a patient with a creatinine clearance of ≥71 ml/min/1.73 m² and a body weight of ≥70 kg. A reduction in dose must be made for a patient with a creatinine clearance ≤70 ml/min/1.73 m² and/or a body weight less than 70 kg (see TABLE 14A, TABLE 14B, TABLE 14C, TABLE 15A, and TABLE 15B).

Dosage regimens in column A in TABLE 13 are recommended for infections caused by fully susceptible organisms which represent the majority of pathogenic species. Dosage regimens in column B of TABLE 13 are recommended for infections caused by organisms with moderate susceptibility to imipenem, primarily some strains of *P. aeruginosa*.

TABLE 13 *Intravenous Dosage Schedule for Adults With Normal Renal Function and Body Weight ≥70 kg*

Type or Severity of Infection	A Fully susceptible organisms including gram-positive and gram-negative aerobes and anaerobes	B Moderately susceptible organisms, primarily some strains of *P. aeruginosa*
Mild	250 mg q6h (TOTAL DAILY DOSE = 1.0 g)	500 mg q6h (TOTAL DAILY DOSE = 2.0 g)
Moderate	500 mg q8h (TOTAL DAILY DOSE = 1.5 g) or 500 mg q6h (TOTAL DAILY DOSE = 2.0g)	500 mg q6h (TOTAL DAILY DOSE = 2.0 g) or 1 g q8h (TOTAL DAILY DOSE = 3.0 g)
Severe, life threatening only	500 mg q6h (TOTAL DAILY DOSE = 2.0 g)	1 g q8h (TOTAL DAILY DOSE = 3.0 g) or 1 g q6h (TOTAL DAILY DOSE = 4.0 g)
Uncomplicated urinary tract infection	250 mg q6h (TOTAL DAILY DOSE = 1.0 g)	250 mg q6h (TOTAL DAILY DOSE = 1.0 g)
Complicated urinary tract infection	500 mg q6h (TOTAL DAILY DOSE = 2.0 g)	500 mg q6h (TOTAL DAILY DOSE = 2.0 g)

Due to the high antimicrobial activity of cilastatin sodium; imipenem IV, it is recommended that the maximum total daily dosage not exceed 50 mg/kg/day or 4.0 g/day, whichever is lower. There is no evidence that higher doses provide greater efficacy. However, patients over 12 years of age with cystic fibrosis and normal renal function have been treated with cilastatin sodium; imipenem IV at doses up to 90 mg/kg/day in divided doses, not exceeding 4.0 g/day.

Reduced Intravenous Dosage Schedule for Adults With Impaired Renal Function and/or Body Weight <70 kg

Patients with creatinine clearance of ≤70 ml/min/1.73 m² and/or body weight less than 70 kg require dosage reduction of cilastatin sodium; imipenem IV as indicated in TABLE 14A, TABLE 14B, and TABLE 14C. Creatinine clearance may be calculated from serum creatinine concentration by the equation found in the following formula:

Tcc (Males) = [(wt. in kg) (140 - age)] ÷ [(72) (creatinine in mg/dl)]

Tcc (Females) = 0.85 × above value

To determine the dose for adults with impaired renal function and/or reduced body weight:

1. Choose a total daily dose from TABLE 13 based on infection characteristics.
   a) If the total daily dose is 1.0, 1.5 or 2.0 g, use the appropriate subsection of TABLE 14A, TABLE 14B, or TABLE 14C and continue with step 3.
   b) If the total daily dose is 3.0 g or 4.0 g, use the appropriate subsection of TABLE 15A and TABLE 15B and continue with step 3.
3. From TABLE 14A, TABLE 14B, and TABLE 14C or TABLE 15A and TABLE 15B:
   a) Select the body weight on the far left which is closest to the patient's body weight (kg).
   b) Select the patient's creatinine clearance category.
   c) Where the row and column intersect is the reduced dosage regimen.

Patients with creatinine clearances of 6-20 ml/min/1.73 m² should be treated with cilastatin sodium; imipenem IV 125 or 250 mg every 12 hours for most pathogens. There may be an increased risk of seizures when doses of 500 mg every 12 hours are administered to these patients.

TABLE 14A *Reduced Intravenous Dosage of Cilastatin Sodium; Imibenem IV in Adult Patients With Impaired Renal Function and/or Body Weight <70 kg*

If total daily dose from TABLE 13 is 1.0 g/day:

And Body Weight is:	And Creatinine Clearance (ml/min/1.73m²) is: ≥71	41-70	21-40	6-20
	Then the reduced dosage regimen (mg) is:			
≥70 kg	250 q6h	250 q8h	250 q12h	250 q12h
60 kg	250 q8h	125 q6h	250 q12h	125 q12h
50 kg	125 q6h	125 q6h	125 q8h	125 q12h
40 kg	125 q6h	125 q8h	125 q12h	125 q12h
30 kg	125 q8h	125 q8h	125 q12h	125 q12h

TABLE 14B *Reduced Intravenous Dosage of Cilastatin Sodium; Imibenem IV in Adult Patients With Impaired Renal Function and/or Body Weight <70 kg*

If total daily dose from TABLE 13 is 1.5 g/day:

And Body Weight is:	And Creatinine Clearance (ml/min/1.73m²) is: ≥71	41-70	21-40	6-20
	Then the reduced dosage regimen (mg) is:			
≥70 kg	500 q8h	250 q6h	250 q8h	250 q12h
60 kg	250 q6h	250 q8h	250 q8h	250 q12h
50 kg	250 q6h	250 q8h	250 q12h	250 q12h
40 kg	250 q8h	125 q6h	125 q8h	125 q12h
30 kg	125 q6h	125 q8h	125 q8h	125 q12h

TABLE 14C *Reduced Intravenous Dosage of Cilastatin Sodium; Imibenem IV in Adult Patients With Impaired Renal Function and/or Body Weight <70 kg*

If total daily dose from TABLE 13 is 2.0 g/day:

And Body Weight is:	And Creatinine Clearance (ml/min/1.73m²) is: ≥71	41-70	21-40	6-20
	Then the reduced dosage regimen (mg) is:			
≥70 kg	500 q6h	500 q8h	250 q6h	250 q12h
60 kg	500 q8h	250 q6h	250 q8h	250 q12h
50 kg	250 q6h	250 q6h	250 q8h	250 q12h
40 kg	250 q6h	250 q8h	250 q12h	250 q12h
30 kg	250 q8h	125 q6h	125 q8h	125 q12h

TABLE 15A *Reduced Intravenous Dosage of Cilastatin Sodium; Imibenem IV in Adult Patients With Impaired Renal Function and/or Body Weight <70 kg*

If total daily dose from TABLE 13 is 3.0 g/day:

And Body Weight is:	And Creatinine Clearance (ml/min/1.73m²) is: ≥71	41-70	21-40	6-20
	Then the reduced dosage regimen (mg) is:			
≥70 kg	1000 q8h	500 q6h	500 q8h	500 q12h
60 kg	750 q8h	500 q8h	500 q8h	500 q12h
50 kg	500 q6h	500 q8h	250 q6h	250 q12h
40 kg	500 q8h	250 q6h	250 q8h	250 q12h
30 kg	250 q6h	250 q8h	250 q8h	250 q12h

TABLE 15B *Reduced Intravenous Dosage of Cilastatin Sodium; Imibenem IV in Adult Patients With Impaired Renal Function and/or Body Weight <70 kg*

If total daily dose from TABLE 13 is 4.0 g/day:

And Body Weight is:	And Creatinine Clearance (ml/min/1.73m²) is: ≥71	41-70	21-40	6-20
	Then the reduced dosage regimen (mg) is:			
≥70 kg	1000 q6h	750 q8h	500 q6h	500 q12h
60 kg	1000 q8h	750 q8h	500 q8h	500 q12h
50 kg	750 q8h	500 q6h	500 q8h	500 q12h
40 kg	500 q6h	500 q8h	250 q6h	250 q12h
30 kg	500 q8h	250 q6h	250 q8h	250 q12h

Patients with creatinine clearance ≤5 ml/min/1.73 m² should not receive cilastatin sodium; imipenem IV unless hemodialysis is instituted within 48 hours. There is inadequate information to recommend usage of cilastatin sodium; imipenem IV for patients undergoing peritoneal dialysis.

Hemodialysis

When treating patients with creatinine clearances of ≤5 ml/min/1.73 m² who are undergoing hemodialysis, use the dosage recommendations for patients with creatinine clearances of 6-20 ml/min/1.73 m². (See Reduced Intravenous Dosage Schedule for Adults With Impaired Renal Function and/or Body Weight <70 kg.) Both imipenem and cilastatin are cleared from the circulation during hemodialysis. The patient should receive cilastatin sodium; imipenem IV after hemodialysis and at 12 hour intervals timed from the end of that hemodialysis session. Dialysis patients, especially those with background CNS disease, should be carefully monitored; for patients on hemodialysis, cilastatin sodium; imipenem IV is recommended only when the benefit outweighs the potential risk of seizures. (See PRECAUTIONS.)

Pediatric Use

See PRECAUTIONS, Pediatric Use.

For pediatric patients, ≥3 months of age, the recommended dose for non-CNS infections is 15-25 mg/kg/dose administered every 6 hours. Based on studies in adults, the maximum daily dose for treatment of infections with fully susceptible organisms is 2.0 g/day, and of infections with moderately susceptible organisms (primarily some strains of *P. aeruginosa*) is 4.0 g/day. Higher doses (up to 90 mg/kg/day in older children) have been used in patients with cystic fibrosis (see DOSAGE AND ADMINISTRATION).

For pediatric patients ≤3 months of age (weighing ≤1500 g), the following dosage schedule is recommended for non-CNS infections:

<1 Week of Age: 25 mg/kg every 12 hours.
1-4 Weeks of Age: 25 mg/kg every 8 hours.
4 Weeks-3 Months of Age: 25 mg/kg every 6 hours.

Doses less than or equal to 500 mg should be given by intravenous infusion over 15-30 minutes. Doses greater than 500 mg should be given by intravenous infusion over 40-60 minutes.

Cilastatin-imibenem is not recommended in pediatric patients with CNS infections because of the risk of seizures.

Cilastatin-imibenem is not recommended in pediatric patients <30 kg with impaired renal function, as no data are available.

I

Preparation of Solution

Infusion Bottles: Contents of the infusion bottles of cilastatin; sodium imibenem IV powder should be restored with 100 ml of diluent (see list of diluents under Compatibility and Stability) and shaken until a clear solution is obtained.

Vials: Contents of the vials must be suspended and transferred to 100 ml of an appropriate infusion solution.

A suggested procedure is to add approximately 10 ml from the appropriate infusion solution (see list of diluents under Compatibility and Stability) to the vial. Shake well and transfer the resulting suspension to the infusion solution container.

Benzyl alcohol as a preservative has been associated with toxicity in neonates. While toxicity has not been demonstrated in pediatric patients greater than 3 months of age, small pediatric patients in this age range may also be at risk for benzyl alcohol toxicity. Therefore, diluents containing benzyl alcohol should not be used when cilastatin; sodium imibenem IV is constituted for administration to pediatric patients in this age range.

CAUTION: THE SUSPENSION IS NOT FOR DIRECT INFUSION.

Repeat with an additional 10 ml of infusion solution to ensure complete transfer of vial contents to the infusion solution. **The resulting mixture should be agitated until clear.**

ADD-Vantage Vials: See INSTRUCTIONS FOR USE OF PRIMAXIN IV IN ADD-Vantage VIALS included with packaging.

Primaxin IV in ADD-Vantage vials should be reconstituted with ADD-Vantage diluent containers containing 100 ml of either 0.9% sodium chloride injection or 100 ml 5% dextrose injection.

Compatibility and Stability

Before Reconstitution: The dry powder should be stored at a temperature below 25°C (77°F).

Reconstituted Solutions: Solutions of Primaxin IV range from colorless to yellow. Variations of color within this range do not affect the potency of the product.

Primaxin IV, as supplied in infusion bottles and vials and reconstituted as above with the following diluents, maintains satisfactory potency for 4 hours at room temperature or for 24 hours under refrigeration (5°C). Solutions of Primaxin IV should not be frozen.

0.9% sodium chloride injection
5% or 10% dextrose injection
5% dextrose and 0.9% sodium chloride injection
5% dextrose injection with 0.225% or 0.45% saline solution
5% dextrose injection with 0.15% potassium chloride solution
Mannitol 5% and 10%

Primaxin IV is supplied in single dose ADD-Vantage vials and should be prepared as directed in the INSTRUCTIONS FOR USE OF PRIMAXIN IV IN ADD-Vantage VIALS accompanying the product, using ADD-Vantage diluent containers containing 100 ml of either 0.9% sodium chloride injection or 5% dextrose injection. When prepared with either of these diluents, Primaxin IV maintains satisfactory potency for 4 hours at room temperature.

Cilastatin; sodium imibenem IV should not be mixed with or physically added to other antibiotics. However, cilastatin; sodium imibenem IV may be administered concomitantly with other antibiotics, such as aminoglycosides.

IM

Cilastatin sodium; imipenem IM is for intramuscular use only.

The dosage recommendations for cilastatin sodium; imipenem IM represents the quantity of imipenem to be administered. An equivalent amount of cilastatin is also present.

Patients with lower respiratory tract infections, skin and skin structure infections, and gynecologic infections of mild to moderate severity may be treated with 500 or 750 mg administered every 12 hours depending on the severity of the infection.

Intra-abdominal infection may be treated with 750 mg every 12 hours (see TABLE 16.)

Total daily IM dosages greater than 1500 mg/day are not recommended.

The dosage for any particular patient should be based on the location of and severity of the infection, the susceptibility of the infecting pathogen(s), and renal function.

TABLE 16 *Dosage Guidelines*

Type*/Location of Infection	Severity	Dosage Regimen
Lower respiratory tract	Mild/Moderate	500 or 750 mg q12h depending on the severity of infection
Skin and skin structure	Mild/Moderate	500 or 750 mg q12h depending on the severity of infection
Gynecologic	Mild/Moderate	500 or 750 mg q12h depending on the severity of infection
Intra-abdominal	Mild/Moderate	750 mg q12h

* See INDICATIONS AND USAGE.

The duration of therapy depends upon the type and severity of the infection. Generally, cilastatin sodium; imipenem IM should be continued for at least two days after the signs and symptoms of infection have resolved. Safety and efficacy of treatment beyond 14 days have not been established.

Cilastatin sodium; imipenem IM should be administered by deep intramuscular injection into a large muscle mass (such as the gluteal muscles or lateral part of the thigh) with a 21 gauge 2″ needle. Aspiration is necessary to avoid inadvertent injection into a blood vessel.

Preparation for Administration

Primaxin IM should be prepared for use with 1.0% lidocaine HCl solution† (without epinephrine). Primaxin IM 500 should be prepared with 2 ml and Primaxin IM 750 with 3 ml of lidocaine HCl. Agitate to form a suspension then withdraw the entire contents of vial intramuscularly. The suspension of Primaxin IM in lidocaine HCl should be used within one hour of preparation. **Note: The IM formulation is not for IV use.**

Compatibility and Stability

Before Reconstitution: The dry powder should be stored at a temperature below 30°C (86°F).

Suspensions for IM Administration: Suspensions of Primaxin IM are white to light tan in color. Variations of color within this range do not affect the potency of the product.

The suspension of Primaxin IM in lidocaine HCl should be used within one hour after preparation.

Primaxin IM should not be mixed with or physically added to other antibiotics. However, Primaxin IM may be administered concomitantly but at separate sites with other antibiotics, such as aminoglycosides.

†Refer to the monograph for lidocaine HCl for detailed information concerning CONTRAINDICATIONS, WARNINGS, PRECAUTIONS, and ADVERSE REACTIONS.

HOW SUPPLIED

IV

Primaxin IV is supplied as a sterile powder mixture in vials and infusion bottles containing imipenem (anhydrous equivalent) and cilastatin sodium as follows:

250 mg imipenem equivalent and 250 mg cilastatin equivalent and 10 mg sodium bicarbonate as a buffer.

500 mg imipenem equivalent and 500 mg cilastatin equivalent and 20 mg sodium bicarbonate as a buffer.

IM

Primaxin IM is supplied as a sterile powder mixture in vials for IM administration as follows:

500 mg imipenem equivalent and 500 mg cilastatin equivalent.
750 mg imipenem equivalent and 750 mg cilastatin equivalent.

PRODUCT LISTING - EQUIVALENTS NOT AVAILABLE

Powder For Injection - Injectable - 250 mg;250 mg

10's	$1576.60	PRIMAXIN IV, Merck & Company Inc	00006-3514-74
25's	$417.50	PRIMAXIN IV, Merck & Company Inc	00006-3514-58
25's	$433.53	PRIMAXIN IV, Merck & Company Inc	00006-3551-58

Powder For Injection - Injectable - 500 mg;500 mg

10's	$314.34	PRIMAXIN IM, Merck & Company Inc	00006-3582-75
10's	$331.01	PRIMAXIN IV, Merck & Company Inc	00006-3517-75
25's	$785.84	PRIMAXIN IV, Merck & Company Inc	00006-3516-59
25's	$801.31	PRIMAXIN IV, Merck & Company Inc	00006-3552-59
25's	$845.69	PRIMAXIN IV, Merck & Company Inc	00006-3666-59

Powder For Injection - Intramuscular - 750 mg;750 mg

10's	$431.99	PRIMAXIN IM, Merck & Company Inc	00006-3583-76

Imipramine Hydrochloride (001525)

For related information, see the comparative table section in Appendix A.

Categories: Depression; Enuresis; FDA Approved 1959 Oct; Pregnancy Category D
Drug Classes: Antidepressants, tricyclic
Brand Names: Imipramine Hcl; Imiprin; Janimine; **Tofranil**
Foreign Brand Availability: Antidep (India); Apo-Imipramine (Canada); Chrytemin (Japan); Daypress (Japan); Depsol (India); Depsonil (India); Ethipramine (South-Africa); Fronil (Taiwan); Imidol (Japan); Imiprex (Bahrain; Cyprus; Egypt; Iran; Iraq; Jordan; Kuwait; Lebanon; Libya; Oman; Qatar; Republic-of-Yemen; Saudi-Arabia; Syria; United-Arab-Emirates); Melipramine (Australia); Primonil (Israel); Pryleugan (Germany); Sermonil (Thailand); Talpramin (Mexico); Tofranil-PM (Colombia; Mexico); Venefon (Greece)
Cost of Therapy: $163.23 (Depression; Tofranil; 50 mg; 2 tablets/day; 30 day supply)
$3.45 (Depression; Generic Tablets; 50 mg; 2 tablets/day; 30 day supply)
$48.06 (Childhood Enuresis; Tofranil; 25 mg; 1 tablet/day; 30 day supply)
$1.35 (Childhood Enuresis; Generic Tablets; 25 mg; 1 tablet/day; 30 day supply)
HCFA JCODE(S): J3270 up to 25 mg IM

DESCRIPTION

Imipramine HCl, the original tricyclic antidepressant, is a member of the dibenzazepine group of compounds. It is designated 5-[3-(dimethylamino) propyl]-10,11-dihydro-5H-dibenz(b,f)-azepine monohydrochloride.

Imipramine HCl is a white to off-white, odorless, or practically odorless crystalline powder. It is freely soluble in water and in alcohol, soluble in acetone, and insoluble in ether and in benzene. Its molecular weight is 316.87. The molecular formula is $C_{19}H_{24}N \cdot HCl$.

Tofranil tablets inactive ingredients: Calcium phosphate, cellulose compounds, docusate sodium, iron oxides, magnesium stearate, polyethylene glycol, povidone, sodium starch glycolate, sucrose, talc and titanium dioxide.

Each 2 cc ampul (for IM injection) contains imipramine HCl, 25 mg; ascorbic acid, 2 mg; sodium bisulfite, 1 mg; sodium sulfite, anhydrous, 1 mg.

STORAGE

Store tablets and ampules (for injection) between 59-86°F (15-30°C).

Dispense tablets in tight container.

CLINICAL PHARMACOLOGY

The mechanism of action of imipramine HCl is not definitely known. However, it does not act primarily by stimulation of the central nervous system. The clinical effect is hypothesized as being due to potentiation of adrenergic synapses by blocking uptake of norepinephrine at nerve endings. The mode of action of the drug in controlling childhood enuresis is thought to be apart from its antidepressant effect.

INDICATIONS AND USAGE

DEPRESSION

For the relief of symptoms of depression. Endogenous depression is more likely to be alleviated than other depressive states. One (1) to 3 weeks of treatment may be needed before optimal therapeutic effects are evident.

CHILDHOOD ENURESIS

May be useful as temporary adjunctive therapy in reducing enuresis in children aged 6 years and older, after possible organic causes have been excluded by appropriate tests. In patients having daytime symptoms of frequency and urgency, examination should include voiding cystourethrography and cystoscopy, as necessary. The effectiveness of treatment may decrease with continued drug administration.

NON-FDA APPROVED INDICATIONS

Imipramine has also been used in the treatment of dysthymia, neuropathic and chronic pain, and bulimia One study has suggested that imipramine may be useful in decreasing the frequency of chest pain in patients with the syndrome of chest pain and normal coronary angiograms. Another small study has reported that imipramine can modify small intestinal motor function and may have therapeutic actions in irritable bowel syndrome (which is unrelated to mood improvement). None of these uses have been approved by the FDA.

CONTRAINDICATIONS

The concomitant use of monoamine oxidase inhibiting compounds is contraindicated. Hyperpyretic crises or severe convulsive seizures may occur in patients receiving such combinations. The potentiation of adverse effects can be serious, or even fatal. When it is desired to substitute imipramine HCl in patients receiving a monoamine oxidase inhibitor, as long an interval should elapse as the clinical situation will allow, with a minimum of 14 days. Initial dosage should be low and increases should be gradual and cautiously prescribed.

The drug is contraindicated during the acute recovery period after a myocardial infarction. Patients with a known hypersensitivity to this compound should not be given the drug. The possibility of cross-sensitivity to other dibenzazepine compounds should be kept in mind.

WARNINGS

Children: A dose of 2.5 mg/kg/day of imipramine HCl should not be exceeded in childhood. ECG changes of unknown significance have been reported in pediatric patients with doses twice this amount.

Extreme caution should be used when this drug is given to:

1. Patients with cardiovascular disease because of the possibility of conduction defects, arrhythmias, congestive heart failure, myocardial infarction, strokes, and tachycardia. These patients require cardiac surveillance at all dosage levels of the drug.
2. Patients with increased intraocular pressure, history of urinary retention, or history of narrow-angle glaucoma because of the drug's anticholinergic properties.
3. Hyperthyroid patients or those on thyroid medication because of the possibility of cardiovascular toxicity.
4. Patients with a history of seizure disorder because this drug has been shown to lower the seizure threshold.
5. Patients receiving guanethidine, clonidine, or similar agents, since imipramine HCl may block the pharmacologic effects of these drugs.
6. Patients receiving methylphenidate HCl. Since methylphenidate HCl may inhibit the metabolism of imipramine HCl, downward dosage adjustment of imipramine HCl may be required when given concomitantly with methylphenidate HCl.

Imipramine HCl may enhance the CNS depressant effects of alcohol. Therefore, it should be borne in mind that the dangers inherent in a suicide attempt or accidental overdosage with the drug may be increased for the patient who uses excessive amounts of alcohol (see PRECAUTIONS).

Since imipramine HCl may impair the mental and/or physical abilities required for the performance of potentially hazardous tasks, such as operating an automobile or machinery, the patient should be cautioned accordingly.

Additional Information for Injection: Contains sodium sulfite and sodium bisulfite, that may cause allergic-type reactions including anaphylactic symptoms and life-threatening or less severe asthmatic episodes in certain susceptible people. The overall prevalence of sulfite sensitivity in the general population is unknown and probably low. Sulfite sensitivity is seen more frequently in asthmatic than in nonasthmatic people.

PRECAUTIONS

TABLETS

An ECG recording should be taken prior to the initiation of larger-than-usual doses of imipramine HCl and at appropriate intervals thereafter until steady state is achieved. Patients with any evidence of cardiovascular disease require cardiac surveillance at all dosage levels of the drug (see WARNINGS). Elderly patients and patients with cardiac disease or a prior history of cardiac disease are at special risk of developing the cardiac abnormalities associated with the use of imipramine HCl.

It should be kept in mind that the possibility of suicide in seriously depressed patients is inherent in the illness and may persist until significant remission occurs. Such patients should be carefully supervised during the early phase of treatment with imipramine HCl, and may require hospitalization. Prescriptions should be written for the smallest amount feasible. Hypomanic or manic episodes may occur, particularly in patients with cyclic disorders. Such reactions may necessitate discontinuation of the drug. If needed, imipramine HCl may be resumed in lower dosage when these episodes are relieved.

Administration of a tranquilizer may be useful in controlling such episodes.

An activation of the psychosis may occasionally be observed in schizophrenic patients and may require reduction of dosage and the addition of a phenothiazine.

Concurrent administration of imipramine HCl with electroshock therapy may increase the hazards; such treatment should be limited to those patients for whom it is essential, since there is limited clinical experience.

Pregnancy

Animal reproduction studies have yielded inconclusive results (see also ANIMAL PHARMACOLOGY).

There have been no well-controlled studies conducted with pregnant women to determine the effect of imipramine HCl on the fetus. However, there have been clinical reports of congenital malformations associated with the use of the drug. Although a causal relationship between these effects and the drug could not be established, the possibility of fetal risk from the maternal ingestion of imipramine HCl cannot be excluded. Therefore, imipramine HCl should be used in women who are or might become pregnant only if the clinical condition clearly justifies potential risk to the fetus.

Nursing Mothers

Limited data suggest that imipramine HCl is likely to be excreted in human breast milk. As a general rule, a woman taking a drug should not nurse since the possibility exists that the drug may be excreted in breast milk and be harmful to the child.

Pediatric Use

The effectiveness of the drug in children for conditions other than nocturnal enuresis has not been established.

The safety and effectiveness of the drug as temporary adjunctive therapy for nocturnal enuresis in children less than 6 years of age has not been established.

The safety of the drug for long-term, chronic use as adjunctive therapy for nocturnal enuresis in children 6 years of age or older has not been established; consideration should be given to instituting a drug-free period following an adequate therapeutic trial with a favorable response.

A dose of 2.5 mg/kg/day should not be exceeded in childhood. ECG changes of unknown significance have been reported in pediatric patients with doses twice this amount.

Patients should be warned that imipramine HCl may enhance the CNS depressant effects of alcohol (see WARNINGS).

Imipramine HCl should be used with caution in patients with significantly impaired renal or hepatic function.

Patients who develop a fever and sore throat during therapy with imipramine HCl should have leukocyte and differential blood counts performed. Imipramine HCl should be discontinued if there is evidence of pathological neutrophil depression.

Prior to elective surgery, imipramine HCl should be discontinued for as long as the clinical situation will allow.

In occasional susceptible patients or in those receiving anticholinergic drugs (including antiparkinsonism agents) in addition, the atropine-like effects may become more pronounced (*e.g.*, paralytic ileus).

Close supervision and careful adjustment of dosage is required when imipramine HCl is administered concomitantly with anticholinergic drugs.

Avoid the use of preparations, such as decongestants and local anesthetics, which contain any sympathomimetic amine (*e.g.*, epinephrine, norepinephrine), since it has been reported that tricyclic antidepressants can potentiate the effects of catecholamines.

Caution should be exercised when imipramine HCl is used with agents that lower blood pressure.

Imipramine HCl may potentiate the effects of CNS depressant drugs.

The plasma concentration of imipramine HCl may increase when the drug is given concomitantly with hepatic enzyme inhibitors (*e.g.*, cimetidine, fluoxetine) and decrease by concomitant administration of hepatic enzyme inducers (*e.g.*, barbiturates, phenytoin), and adjustment of the dosage of imipramine HCl may therefore be necessary.

Patients taking imipramine HCl should avoid excessive exposure to sunlight since there have been reports of photosensitization.

Both elevation and lowering of blood sugar levels have been reported with imipramine HCl use.

DRUG INTERACTIONS

DRUGS METABOLIZED BY P450 2D6

The biochemical activity of the drug metabolizing isozyme cytochrome P450 2D6 (debrisoquin hydroxylase) is reduced in a subset of the Caucasian population (about 7-10% of Caucasians are so-called "poor metabolizers"). Reliable estimates of the prevalence of reduced P450 2D6 isozyme activity among Asian, African, and other populations are not yet available. Poor metabolizers have higher than expected plasma concentrations of tricyclic antidepressants (TCAs) when given usual doses. Depending on the fraction of drug metabolized by P450 2D6, the increase in plasma concentration may be small or quite large (8-fold increase in plasma AUC of the TCA).

In addition, certain drugs inhibit the activity of this isozyme and make normal metabolizers resemble poor metabolizers. An individual who is stable on a given dose of TCA may become abruptly toxic when given one of these inhibiting drugs as concomitant therapy. The drugs that inhibit cytochrome P450 2D6 include some that are not metabolized by the enzyme (quinidine; cimetidine) and many that are substrates for P450 2D6 (many other antidepressants, phenothiazines, and the Type 1C antiarrhythmics propafeonone and flecainide). While all the selective serotonin reuptake inhibitors (SSRIs), (*e.g.*, fluoxetine, sertraline, and paroxetine) inhibit P450 2D6, they may vary in the extent of inhibition. The extent to which SSRI-TCA interactions may pose clinical problems will depend on the degree of inhibition and the pharmacokinetics of the SSRI involved. Nevertheless, caution is indicated in the coadministration of TCAs with any of the SSRIs and also in switching from one class to the other. Of particular importance, sufficient time must elapse before initiating TCA treatment in a patient being withdrawn from fluoxetine, given the long half-life of the parent and active metabolite (at least 5 weeks may be necessary).

Concomitant use of tricyclic antidepressants with drugs that can inhibit cytochrome P450 2D6 may require lower doses than usually prescribed for either the tricyclic antidepressant or the other drug. Furthermore, whenever one of these other drugs is withdrawn from co-therapy, an increased dose of tricyclic antidepressant may be required. It is desirable to monitor TCA plasma levels whenever a TCA is going to be coadministered with another drug known to be an inhibitor of P450 2D6.

ADVERSE REACTIONS

Note: Although the listing which follows includes a few adverse reactions which have not been reported with this specific drug, the pharmacological similarities among the tricyclic antidepressant drugs require that each of the reactions be considered when imipramine HCl is administered.

Cardiovascular: Orthostatic hypotension, hypertension, tachycardia, palpitation, myocardial infarction, arrhythmias, heart block, ECG changes, precipitation of congestive heart failure, stroke.

Psychiatric: Confusional states (especially in the elderly) with hallucinations, disorientation, delusions; anxiety, restlessness, agitation; insomnia and nightmares; hypomania; exacerbation of psychosis.

Neurological: Numbness, tingling, paresthesia of extremities; incoordination, ataxia, tremors; peripheral neuropathy; extrapyramidal symptoms; seizures, alterations in EEG patterns; tinnitus.

Anticholinergic: Dry mouth, and rarely, associated sublingual adenitis; blurred vision, disturbances of accommodation, mydriasis; constipation, paralytic ileus; urinary retention, delayed micturition, dilation of the urinary tract.

Allergic: Skin rash, petechiae, urticaria, itching, photosensitization, edema (general or of face and tongue); drug fever; cross-sensitivity with desipramine.

Hematologic: Bone marrow depression including agranulocytosis; eosinophilia; purpura; thrombocytopenia.

Gastrointestinal: Nausea and vomiting, anorexia, epigastric distress, diarrhea; peculiar taste, stomatitis, abdominal cramps, black tongue.

Endocrine: Gynecomastia in the male; breast enlargement and galactorrhea in the female; increased or decreased libido, impotence; testicular swelling; elevation or depression of blood sugar levels; inappropriate antidiuretic hormone (ADH) secretion syndrome.

Other: Jaundice (simulating obstructive); altered liver function; weight gain or loss; perspiration; flushing; urinary frequency; drowsiness; dizziness; weakness and fatigue; headache; parotid swelling; alopecia; proneness to falling.

Withdrawal Symptoms: Though not indicative of addiction, abrupt cessation of treatment after prolonged therapy may produce nausea, headache, and malaise.

Note: In enuretic children treated with imipramine HCl the most common adverse reactions have been nervousness, sleep disorders, tiredness, and mild gastrointestinal disturbances. These usually disappear during continued drug administration or when dosage is decreased. Other reactions which have been reported include constipation, convulsions, anxiety, emotional instability, syncope, and collapse. All of the adverse effects reported with adult use should be considered.

DOSAGE AND ADMINISTRATION

TABLETS

Depression

Lower dosages are recommended for elderly patients and adolescents. Lower dosages are also recommended for outpatients as compared to hospitalized patients who will be under close supervision. Dosage should be initiated at a low level and increased gradually, noting carefully the clinical response and any evidence of intolerance. Following remission, maintenance, medication may be required for a longer period of time, at the lowest dose that will maintain remission.

Usual Adult Dose

Hospitalized Patients: Initially, 100 mg/day in divided doses gradually increased to 200 mg/day as required. If no response after 2 weeks, increase to 250-300 mg/day.

Outpatients: Initially, 75 mg/day increased to 150 mg/day. Dosages over 200 mg/day are not recommended. Maintenance, 50-150 mg/day.

Adolescent and Geriatric Patients: Initially, 30-40 mg/day; it is generally not necessary to exceed 100 mg/day.

Childhood Enuresis

Initially, an oral dose of 25 mg/day should be tried in children aged 6 and older. Medication should be given 1 hour before bedtime. If a satisfactory response does not occur within 1 week, increase the dose to 50 mg nightly in children under 12 years; children over 12 may receive up to 75 mg nightly. A daily dose greater than 75 mg does not enhance efficacy and tends to increase side effects. Evidence suggests that in early night bed-wetters, the drug is more effective given earlier and in divided amounts (*i.e.*, 25 mg in midafternoon repeated at bedtime). Consideration should be given to instituting a drug-free period following an adequate therapeutic trial with a favorable response. Dosage should be tapered off gradually rather than abruptly discontinued; this may reduce the tendency to relapse. Children who relapse when the drug is discontinued do not always respond to a subsequent course of treatment.

A dose of 2.5 mg/kg/day should not be exceeded. ECG changes of unknown significance have been reported in pediatric patients with doses twice this amount.

The safety and effectiveness of imipramine HCl as temporary adjunctive therapy for nocturnal enuresis in children less than 6 years of age has not been established.

INJECTION

Initially, up to 100 mg/day intramuscularly in divided doses.

Parenteral administration should be used for starting therapy in patients unable or unwilling to use oral medication. The oral form should supplant the injectable as soon as possible.

Lower dosages are recommended for elderly patients and adolescents. Lower dosages are also recommended for outpatients as compared to hospitalized patients who will be under close supervision. Dosage should be initiated at a low level and gradually increased, noting carefully the clinical response and any evidence of intolerance. Following remission, oral maintenance medication may be required for a longer period of time, at the lowest dose that will maintain remission.

Note: Upon storage of ampules, minute crystals may form. This has no influence on the therapeutic efficacy of the preparation, and the crystals redissolve when the affected ampules are immersed in hot tap water for 1 minute.

ANIMAL PHARMACOLOGY

ACUTE

Oral LD_{50} ranges are as follows: *Rat:* 355-682 mg/kg, *Dog:* 100-215 mg/kg. Depending on the dosage in both species, toxic signs proceeded progressively from depression, irregular respiration, and ataxia to convulsions and death.

REPRODUCTION/TERATOGENIC

The overall evaluation may be summed up in the following manner:

Oral: Independent studies in three species (rat, mouse, and rabbit) revealed that when imipramine HCl is administered orally in doses up to approximately 2½ times the maximum human dose in the first 2 species and up to 25 times the maximum human dose in the third species, the drug is essentially free from teratogenic potential. In the three species studied, only one instance of fetal abnormality occurred (in the rabbit) and in that study there was likewise an abnormality in the control group. However, evidence does exist from the rat studies that some systemic and embryotoxic potential is demonstrable. This is manifested by reduced litter size, a slight increase in the stillborn rate, and a reduction in the mean birth weight.

Parenteral: In contradistinction to the oral data, imipramine HCl does exhibit a slight but definite teratogenic potential when administered by the subcutaneous route. Drug effects on both the mother and fetus in the rabbit are manifested in higher resorption rates and decreases in mean fetal birth weights, while teratogenic findings occurred at a level of 5 times the maximum human dose. In the mouse, teratogenicity occurred at 1½ and 6½ the maximum human dose, but no teratogenic effects were seen at levels 3 times the maximum human dose. Thus, in the mouse, the findings are equivocal.

PRODUCT LISTING - RATED THERAPEUTICALLY EQUIVALENT

Tablet - Oral - 10 mg

Qty	Price	Product	NDC
30's	$2.57	GENERIC, Heartland Healthcare Services	61392-0025-30
30's	$2.57	GENERIC, Heartland Healthcare Services	61392-0025-39
30's	$3.00	GENERIC, Pd-Rx Pharmaceuticals	55289-0149-30
30's	$13.15	GENERIC, Mutual/United Research Laboratories	00677-0421-07
31's	$2.65	GENERIC, Heartland Healthcare Services	61392-0025-31
32's	$2.74	GENERIC, Heartland Healthcare Services	61392-0025-32
45's	$3.85	GENERIC, Heartland Healthcare Services	61392-0025-45
60's	$4.50	GENERIC, Pd-Rx Pharmaceuticals	55289-0149-60
60's	$5.13	GENERIC, Heartland Healthcare Services	61392-0025-60
60's	$26.04	GENERIC, Mutual/United Research Laboratories	00677-0421-06
90's	$7.70	GENERIC, Heartland Healthcare Services	61392-0025-90
100's	$3.25	GENERIC, Cmc-Consolidated Midland Corporation	00223-1103-01

100's	$4.46	GENERIC, Moore, H.L. Drug Exchange Inc	00839-1370-06
100's	$5.30	GENERIC, Martec Pharmaceuticals Inc	52555-0254-01
100's	$5.95	GENERIC, Raway Pharmacal Inc	00686-0079-20
100's	$14.85	FEDERAL UPPER LIMIT, H.C.F.A. F F P	99999-1525-02
100's	$28.36	GENERIC, Qualitest Products Inc	00603-4043-21
100's	$28.37	GENERIC, Mutual Pharmaceutical Co Inc	53489-0330-01
100's	$42.95	GENERIC, Geneva Pharmaceuticals	00781-1762-01
100's	$42.95	GENERIC, Par Pharmaceutical Inc	49884-0054-01
100's	$95.89	TOFRANIL, Novartis Pharmaceuticals	00028-0032-01
250's	$6.70	GENERIC, Major Pharmaceuticals Inc	00904-0925-70
Tablet - Oral - 25 mg			
14's	$4.59	GENERIC, Pd-Rx Pharmaceuticals	55289-0144-14
30's	$3.16	GENERIC, Heartland Healthcare Services	61392-0026-30
30's	$3.16	GENERIC, Heartland Healthcare Services	61392-0026-39
30's	$6.36	GENERIC, Pd-Rx Pharmaceuticals	55289-0144-30
30's	$14.51	GENERIC, Mutual/United Research Laboratories	00677-0422-07
31's	$3.27	GENERIC, Heartland Healthcare Services	61392-0026-31
32's	$3.37	GENERIC, Heartland Healthcare Services	61392-0026-32
45's	$4.74	GENERIC, Heartland Healthcare Services	61392-0026-45
60's	$6.32	GENERIC, Heartland Healthcare Services	61392-0026-60
60's	$43.48	GENERIC, Mutual/United Research Laboratories	00677-0422-06
90's	$9.49	GENERIC, Heartland Healthcare Services	61392-0026-90
90's	$13.26	GENERIC, Pd-Rx Pharmaceuticals	55289-0144-90
100's	$4.50	GENERIC, Cmc-Consolidated Midland Corporation	00223-1102-01
100's	$4.93	GENERIC, Moore, H.L. Drug Exchange Inc	00839-1371-06
100's	$6.55	GENERIC, Raway Pharmacal Inc	00686-0080-20
100's	$11.20	GENERIC, Martec Pharmaceuticals Inc	52555-0255-01
100's	$16.77	FEDERAL UPPER LIMIT, H.C.F.A. F F P	99999-1525-06
100's	$47.39	GENERIC, Qualitest Products Inc	00603-4044-21
100's	$71.75	GENERIC, Par Pharmaceutical Inc	49884-0055-01
100's	$71.76	GENERIC, Geneva Pharmaceuticals	00781-1764-01
100's	$87.30	GENERIC, Geneva Pharmaceuticals	00781-1764-13
100's	$88.03	GENERIC, American Health Packaging	62584-0750-01
100's	$160.19	TOFRANIL, Novartis Pharmaceuticals	00028-0140-01
100's	$160.19	TOFRANIL, Mallinckrodt Medical Inc	00406-9921-01
250's	$7.65	GENERIC, Major Pharmaceuticals Inc	00904-0927-70
Tablet - Oral - 50 mg			
30's	$6.05	GENERIC, Heartland Healthcare Services	61392-0027-30
30's	$6.05	GENERIC, Heartland Healthcare Services	61392-0027-39
30's	$8.45	GENERIC, Pd-Rx Pharmaceuticals	55289-0839-30
30's	$21.12	GENERIC, Mutual/United Research Laboratories	00677-0423-07
31's	$6.25	GENERIC, Heartland Healthcare Services	61392-0027-31
32's	$6.46	GENERIC, Heartland Healthcare Services	61392-0027-32
45's	$9.08	GENERIC, Heartland Healthcare Services	61392-0027-45
60's	$12.10	GENERIC, Heartland Healthcare Services	61392-0027-60
60's	$42.68	GENERIC, Mutual/United Research Laboratories	00677-0423-06
90's	$18.16	GENERIC, Heartland Healthcare Services	61392-0027-90
100's	$5.75	GENERIC, Cmc-Consolidated Midland Corporation	00223-1104-01
100's	$5.93	GENERIC, Moore, H.L. Drug Exchange Inc	00839-1372-06
100's	$7.00	GENERIC, Raway Pharmacal Inc	00686-0081-20
100's	$12.90	GENERIC, Martec Pharmaceuticals Inc	52555-0256-01
100's	$20.48	FEDERAL UPPER LIMIT, H.C.F.A. F F P	99999-1525-10
100's	$69.00	GENERIC, Qualitest Products Inc	00603-4045-21
100's	$69.00	GENERIC, Mutual Pharmaceutical Co Inc	53489-0332-01
100's	$121.85	GENERIC, Par Pharmaceutical Inc	49884-0056-01
100's	$121.88	GENERIC, Geneva Pharmaceuticals	00781-1766-01
100's	$130.12	GENERIC, American Health Packaging	62584-0751-01
100's	$146.26	GENERIC, Geneva Pharmaceuticals	00781-1766-13
100's	$272.05	TOFRANIL, Novartis Pharmaceuticals	00028-0136-01
250's	$11.10	GENERIC, Major Pharmaceuticals Inc	00904-0929-70

PRODUCT LISTING - EQUIVALENTS NOT AVAILABLE

Tablet - Oral - 10 mg			
12's	$3.13	GENERIC, Southwood Pharmaceuticals Inc	58016-0839-12
15's	$3.91	GENERIC, Southwood Pharmaceuticals Inc	58016-0839-15
20's	$5.22	GENERIC, Southwood Pharmaceuticals Inc	58016-0839-20
30's	$7.83	GENERIC, Southwood Pharmaceuticals Inc	58016-0839-30
50's	$14.19	GENERIC, Allscripts Pharmaceutical Company	54569-2726-00
100's	$26.09	GENERIC, Southwood Pharmaceuticals Inc	58016-0839-00
Tablet - Oral - 25 mg			
12's	$5.24	GENERIC, Southwood Pharmaceuticals Inc	58016-0841-12
15's	$6.54	GENERIC, Southwood Pharmaceuticals Inc	58016-0841-15
20's	$8.73	GENERIC, Southwood Pharmaceuticals Inc	58016-0841-20
30's	$5.22	GENERIC, Physicians Total Care	54868-1344-00
30's	$13.09	GENERIC, Southwood Pharmaceuticals Inc	58016-0841-30
30's	$14.22	GENERIC, Allscripts Pharmaceutical Company	54569-0194-00
40's	$9.30	GENERIC, Pharmaceutical Corporation Of America	51655-0148-51
50's	$7.81	GENERIC, Physicians Total Care	54868-1344-02
50's	$11.05	GENERIC, Pharmaceutical Corporation Of America	51655-0148-77
100's	$10.61	GENERIC, Physicians Total Care	54868-1344-03
100's	$43.63	GENERIC, Southwood Pharmaceuticals Inc	58016-0841-00
100's	$47.40	GENERIC, Allscripts Pharmaceutical Company	54569-0194-02
Tablet - Oral - 50 mg			
12's	$8.89	GENERIC, Southwood Pharmaceuticals Inc	58016-0866-12
15's	$11.12	GENERIC, Southwood Pharmaceuticals Inc	58016-0866-15
20's	$14.82	GENERIC, Southwood Pharmaceuticals Inc	58016-0866-20
30's	$6.07	GENERIC, Physicians Total Care	54868-2221-03
30's	$20.70	GENERIC, Allscripts Pharmaceutical Company	54569-0196-03
30's	$22.24	GENERIC, Southwood Pharmaceuticals Inc	58016-0866-30
40's	$10.80	GENERIC, Pharmaceutical Corporation Of America	51655-0223-51
60's	$10.80	GENERIC, Physicians Total Care	54868-2221-01
100's	$16.44	GENERIC, Physicians Total Care	54868-2221-00
100's	$69.00	GENERIC, Allscripts Pharmaceutical Company	54569-0196-04
100's	$74.12	GENERIC, Southwood Pharmaceuticals Inc	58016-0866-00

Imiquimod *(003328)*

For complete prescribing information, refer to the CD-ROM included with the book.

Categories: Condyloma acuminata; Pregnancy Category B; FDA Approved 1997 Mar
Drug Classes: Dermatologics; Immunomodulators
Brand Names: **Aldara**
Foreign Brand Availability: Zartra (Austria; Belgium; Bulgaria; Czech-Republic; Denmark; England; Finland; France; Germany; Greece; Hungary; Ireland; Italy; Netherlands; Norway; Poland; Portugal; Slovenia; Spain; Sweden; Switzerland; Turkey)
Cost of Therapy: $10.40 (Genital Warts; Aldara; 5%; 0.25 g; 3 applications/week; variable day supply)

DESCRIPTION

For Dermatologic Use Only - Not for Ophthalmic Use.

Aldara is the brand name for imiquimod which is an immune response modifier. Each gram of the 5% cream contains 50 mg of imiquimod in an off-white oil-in-water vanishing cream base consisting of isostearic acid, cetyl alcohol, stearyl alcohol, white petrolatum, polysorbate 60, sorbitan monostearate, glycerin, xanthan gum, purified water, benzyl alcohol, methylparaben, and propylparaben.

Chemically, imiquimod is 1-(2-methylpropyl)-1*H*-imidazo[4,5-*c*]quinolin-4-amine. Imiquimod has a molecular formula of $C_{14}H_{16}N_4$ and a molecular weight of 240.3.

INDICATIONS AND USAGE

Imiquimod 5% cream is indicated for the treatment of external genital and perianal warts/condyloma acuminata in individuals 12 years old and above.

CONTRAINDICATIONS

None known.

WARNINGS

Imiquimod cream has not been evaluated for the treatment of urethral, intra-vaginal, cervical, rectal, or intra-anal human papilloma viral disease and is not recommended for these conditions.

DOSAGE AND ADMINISTRATION

Imiquimod cream is to be applied 3 times/week, prior to normal sleeping hours, and left on the skin for 6-10 hours. Following the treatment period cream should be removed by washing the treated area with mild soap and water. Examples of 3 times/week application schedules are: Monday, Wednesday, Friday; or Tuesday, Thursday, Saturday application prior to sleeping hours. Imiquimod treatment should continue until there is total clearance of the genital/perianal warts or for a maximum of 16 weeks. Local skin reactions (erythema) at the treatment site are common. A rest period of several days may be taken if required by the patient's discomfort or severity of the local skin reaction. Treatment may resume once the reaction subsides. Non-occlusive dressings such as cotton gauze or cotton underwear may be used in the management of skin reactions. The technique for proper dose administration should be demonstrated by the prescriber to maximize the benefit of imiquimod therapy. Handwashing before and after cream application is recommended. Imiquimod 5% cream is packaged in single-use packets which contain sufficient cream to cover a wart area of up to 20 cm^2; use of excessive amounts of cream should be avoided. Patients should be instructed to apply imiquimod cream to external genital/perianal warts. A thin layer is applied to the wart area and rubbed in until the cream is no longer visible. The application site is not to be occluded.

PRODUCT LISTING - EQUIVALENTS NOT AVAILABLE

Cream - Topical - 5%			
0.25 gm x 12	$124.80	ALDARA, Allscripts Pharmaceutical Company	54569-4894-00
0.25 gm x 12	$165.38	ALDARA, 3M Pharmaceuticals	00089-0610-12

Immune Globulin (Human) *(001527)*

For complete prescribing information, refer to the CD-ROM included with the book.

Categories: Agammaglobulinemia; Hepatitis A, prophylaxis; Hypogammaglobulinemia; Immunization, rubeola; Immunoglobulin deficiency; Varicella, passive immunity; Pregnancy Category C; FDA Pre 1938 Drugs; Orphan Drugs; WHO Formulary

Drug Classes: Immune globulins

Brand Names: Gamastan; Gamimune-N; Gamma Globulin; Gammagard; **Gammar**; IG; Immune Globulin; IGIM; IGIV; Iveegam; Sandoglobulin; Venoglobulin; WinRho SD

Foreign Brand Availability: Allerglobuline (Benin; Burkina-Faso; Ethiopia; Gambia; Ghana; Guinea; Ivory-Coast; Kenya; Liberia; Malawi; Mali; Mauritania; Mauritius; Morocco; Niger; Nigeria; Senegal; Seychelles; Sierra-Leone; Sudan; Tanzania; Tunia; Uganda; Zambia; Zimbabwe); Aunativ (Bahrain; Cyprus; Egypt; Iran; Iraq; Jordan; Kuwait; Lebanon; Libya; Oman; Qatar; Republic-of-Yemen; Saudi-Arabia; Syria; United-Arab-Emirates); Baygam (Canada); Beriglobin (Austria; Bahrain; Cyprus; Egypt; Germany; Iran; Iraq; Jordan; Kuwait; Lebanon; Libya; Oman; Qatar; Republic-of-Yemen; Saudi-Arabia; Sweden; Syria; United-Arab-Emirates); Beriglobin P (Taiwan); Beriglobin-P (South-Africa); Beriglobina (Ecuador; Spain); Citax F (Mexico); Endobulin (Czech-Republic; England; Finland; South-Africa); Endobuline (France); Gamafine (India); Gamastan Immune Globulin (Israel); Gamma 16 (Israel); Gammabulin (Hong-Kong); Gammagard S D (Canada; Hong-Kong; Israel); Gammonativ (Bahrain; Cyprus; Denmark; Egypt; Germany; Iran; Iraq; Jordan; Kuwait; Lebanon; Libya; Norway; Oman; Qatar; Republic-of-Yemen; Saudi-Arabia; Sweden; Syria; United-Arab-Emirates); Globuman Berna (Hong-Kong; Malaysia; Peru; Philippines; South-Africa; Taiwan; Thailand); IG Gamma (Israel; Philippines); Intraglobin (Germany; Italy; Switzerland; Taiwan); Intraglobin F (Israel; Thailand); IV Globulin-S (Korea); Octagam (France); Pentaglobin (Austria; Germany; Thailand); Sandoglobulina (Italy; Mexico); Sandoglobuline (Belgium; France); Venoglobulin-I (Malaysia); Venoglobulin S (Taiwan)

HCFA JCODE(S): J1460 1 cc IM; J1470 2 cc IM; J1480 3 cc IM; J1490 4 cc IM; J1500 5 cc IM; J1510 6 cc IM; J1520 7 cc IM; J1530 8 cc IM; J1540 9 cc IM; J1550 10 cc IM; J1560 over 10 cc IM; J1561 per 500 mg IV; J1562 per 500 mg IV

DESCRIPTION

SOLVENT DETERGENT TREATED

Immune Globulin Intravenous (Human) [IGIV] Gammagard S/D is a solvent/detergent treated, sterile, freeze-dried preparation of highly purified immunoglobulin G (IgG) derived from large pools of human plasma. The product is manufactured by the Cohn-Oncley cold ethanol fractionation process followed by ultrafiltration and ion exchange chromatography. Source material for fractionation may be obtained from another US licensed manufacturer. The manufacturing process includes treatment with an organic solvent/detergent mixture,[1,2] composed of tri-n-butyl phosphate, octoxynol 9 and polysorbate 80.[3] The Gammagard S/D manufacturing process provides a significant viral reduction in *in vitro* studies.[3] These studies, summarized in TABLE 1, demonstrate virus clearance during Gammagard S/D manufacturing using infectious human immunodeficiency virus, Types 1 and 2 (HIV-1, HIV-2); bovine viral diarrhea virus (BVD), a model virus for hepatitis C virus; sindbis virus (SIN), a model virus for lipid-enveloped viruses; pseudorabies virus (PRV), a model virus for lipid-enveloped DNA viruses such as herpes; vesicular stomatitis virus (VSV), a model virus for lipid-enveloped RNA viruses; hepatitis A virus (HAV) and encephalomyocarditis virus (EMC), a model virus for non-lipid enveloped RNA viruses; and porcine parvovirus (PPV), a model virus for non-lipid enveloped DNA viruses.[3] These reductions are achieved through a combination of process chemistry, partitioning and/or inactivation during cold ethanol fractionation and the solvent/detergent treatment.[3]

TABLE 1 *In Vitro Virus Clearance During Gammagard S/D Manufacturing*

	Process Step Evaluated				
	Step 1	**Step 2**	**Step 3**	**Step 4**	**Cumulative**
			Virus Clearance (log_{10})		
Lipid Enveloped Viruses					
BVD	0.6*	1.3	0.7*	>4.9	**6.2**
HIV-1	5.7	4.9	4.0	>3.7	**18.3**
HIV-2	NT	NT	NT	5.7	**5.7**
PRV	1.0*	3.7	4.5	>4.1	**12.3**
SIN	NT	NT	NT	5.1	**5.1**
VSV	NT	NT	NT	6.0	**6.0**
Non-Lipid Enveloped Viruses					
EMC	NT	3.7	3.0	NA	**6.7**
HAV	0.5*	4.1	3.9	NA	**8.0**
PPV	0.2*	3.5	3.9	NA	**7.4**

Step 1: Processing of Cryo-Poor Plasma to Fraction I+II+III Precipitate
Step 2: Processing of Resuspended Suspension A Precipitate to Suspension B Filter Press Filtrate
Step 3: Processing of Suspension B Filter Press to Suspension B Cuno 70 Filtrate
Step 4: Solvent/Detergent Treatment
Cumulative: Cumulative Reduction of Virus (log_{10})
* These values are not included in the computation of the cumulative reduction of virus since the virus clearance is within the variability limit of the assay (#1.0).
NA Not Applicable. Solvent/detergent treatment does not effect non-lipid enveloped viruses.
NT Not Tested.

When reconstituted with the total volume of diluent (sterile water for injection) supplied, this preparation contains approximately 50 mg of protein per ml (5%), of which at least 90% is gamma globulin. The product, reconstituted to 5%, contains a physiological concentration of sodium chloride (approximately 8.5 mg/ml) and has a pH of 6.8 ± 0.4. Stabilizing agents and additional components are present in the following maximum amounts for a 5% solution: 3 mg/ml Albumin (Human), 22.5 mg/ml glycine, 20 mg/ml glucose, 2 mg/ml polyethylene glycol (PEG), 1 μg/ml tri-n-butyl phosphate, 1 μg/ml octoxynol 9, and 100 μg/ml polysorbate 80. If it is necessary to prepare a 10% (100 mg/ml) solution for infusion, half the volume of diluent should be added. In this case, the stabilizing agents and other components will be present at double the concentrations given for the 5% solution. The manufacturing process for Gammagard S/D, isolates IgG without additional chemical or enzymatic modification, and the Fc portion is maintained intact. Gammagard S/D contains all of the IgG antibody activities which are present in the donor population. On the average, the distribution of IgG subclasses present in this product is similar to that in normal plasma.[3] Gammagard S/D contains only trace amounts of IgA (<3.7 μg/ml in a 5% solution). IgM is also present in trace amounts.

Immune Globulin Intravenous (Human), Gammagard S/D contains no preservative.

INDICATIONS AND USAGE

Gammagard S/D is not indicated in patients with selective IgA deficiency where the IgA deficiency is the only abnormality of concern (see WARNINGS).

PRIMARY IMMUNODEFICIENCY DISEASES

Gammagard S/D is indicated for the treatment of primary immunodeficient states, such as: congenital agammaglobulinemia, common variable immunodeficiency, Wiskott-Aldrich syndrome, and severe combined immunodeficiencies.[6,7] This indication was supported by a clinical trial of 17 patients with primary immunodeficiency who received a total of 341 infusions. Gammagard S/D is especially useful when high levels or rapid elevation of circulating IgG are desired or when intramuscular injections are contraindicated (*e.g.*, small muscle mass).

B-CELL CHRONIC LYMPHOCYTIC LEUKEMIA (CLL)

Gammagard S/D is indicated for prevention of bacterial infections in patients with hypogammaglobulinemia and/or recurrent bacterial infections associated with B-cell Chronic Lymphocytic Leukemia (CLL). In a study of 81 patients, 41 of whom were treated with Immune Globulin Intravenous (Human), Gammagard, bacterial infections were significantly reduced in the treatment group.[8,9] In this study, the placebo group had approximately twice as many bacterial infections as the IGIV group. The median time to first bacterial infection for the IGIV group was greater than 365 days. By contrast, the time to first bacterial infection in the placebo group was 192 days. The number of viral and fungal infections, which were for the most part minor, was not statistically different between the two groups.

IDIOPATHIC THROMBOCYTOPENIC PURPURA (ITP)

When a rapid rise in platelet count is needed to prevent and/or to control bleeding in a patient with Idiopathic Thrombocytopenic Purpura, the administration of Gammagard S/D, should be considered.

The efficacy of Gammagard has been demonstrated in a clinical study involving 16 patients. Of these 16 patients, 13 had chronic ITP (11 adults, 2 children), and 3 patients had acute ITP (1 adult, 2 children). All 16 patients (100%) demonstrated a clinically significant rise in platelet count to a level greater than 40,000/mm^3 following the administration of Gammagard. Ten of the 16 patients (62.5%) exhibited a significant rise to greater than 80,000 platelets/mm^3. Of these 10 patients, 7 had chronic ITP (5 adults, 2 children), and 3 patients had acute ITP (1 adult, 2 children).

The rise in platelet count to greater than 40,000/mm^3 occurred after a single 1 g/kg infusion of Gammagard in 8 patients with chronic ITP (6 adults, 2 children), and in 2 patients with acute ITP (1 adult, 1 child). A similar response was observed after two 1 g/kg infusions in 3 adult patients with chronic ITP, and 1 child with acute ITP. The remaining 2 adult patients with chronic ITP received more than two 1 g/kg infusions before achieving a platelet count greater than 40,000/mm^3. The rise in platelet count was generally rapid, occurring within 5 days. However, this rise was transient and not considered curative. Platelet count rises lasted 2-3 weeks, with a range of 12 days to 6 months. It should be noted that childhood ITP may resolve spontaneously without treatment.

KAWASAKI SYNDROME

Gammagard S/D, is indicated for the prevention of coronary artery aneurysms associated with Kawasaki syndrome. The percentage incidence of coronary artery aneurysm in patients with Kawasaki syndrome receiving Gammagard either at a single dose of 1 g/kg (n=22) or at a dose of 400 mg/kg for four consecutive days (n=22), beginning within 7 days of onset of fever, was 3/44 (6.8%). This was significantly different (p=0.008) from a comparable group of patients that received aspirin only in previous trials and of whom 42/185 (22.7%) experienced coronary artery aneurysms.[10,11,12] All patients in the Gammagard trial received concomitant aspirin therapy and none experienced hypersensitivity-type reactions (urticaria, bronchospasm or generalized anaphylaxis).[13]

Several studies have documented the efficacy of intravenous gammaglobulin in reducing the incidence of coronary artery abnormalities resulting from Kawasaki syndrome.[10-12,14-17]

NON-FDA APPROVED INDICATIONS

Although not FDA approved, immune globulin intravenous (human) has also been used with varying degrees of success in myasthenia gravis, glomerulonephritis due to Henoch-Scholein purpura, Guillain-Barre syndrome, amyotrophic lateral sclerosis, cytomegalovirus infections, other autoimmune cytopenias, hypogammaglobulinemia associated with multiple myeloma, severe dermatomyositis, suppression of recurrent genital herpes simplex virus, intractable seizures, antiphospholipid syndrome in pregnancy, chronic fatigue syndrome, and prophylaxis against hepatitis A and measles. Well-controlled data are lacking for many of these uses.

Although not FDA approved, immune globulin intramuscular (human) has also been used with varying success to prevent bacterial infections in burn patients and in the treatment of asthma or allergic disorders. Well controlled data are lacking and the efficacy for such uses has not been established.

CONTRAINDICATIONS

Patients may experience severe hypersensitivity reactions or anaphylaxis in the setting of detectable IgA levels following infusion of Gammagard S/D. The occurrence of severe hypersensitivity reactions or anaphylaxis under such conditions should prompt consideration of an alternative therapy. Gammagard S/D is contraindicated in patients with selective IgA deficiency where the IgA deficiency is the only abnormality of concern (see INDICATIONS AND USAGE and WARNINGS).

WARNINGS

Warning

Immune Globulin Intravenous (Human) products have been reported to be associated with renal dysfunction, acute renal failure, osmotic nephrosis, and death.[16,18] Patients predisposed to acute renal failure include patients with any degree of pre-existing renal insufficiency, diabetes mellitus, age greater than 65, volume depletion,

> **Cont'd**
>
> **sepsis, paraproteinemia, or patients receiving known nephrotoxic drugs. Especially in such patients, IGIV products should be administered at the minimum concentration available and the minimum rate of infusion practicable. While these reports of renal dysfunction and acute renal failure have been associated with the use of many of the licensed IGIV products, those containing sucrose as a stabilizer accounted for a disproportionate share of the total number.***
>
> **See DOSAGE AND ADMINISTRATION for important information intended to reduce the risk of acute renal failure.**
>
> ***Gammagard S/D does not contain sucrose.**

Immune Globulin Intravenous (Human), Gammagard S/D is made from human plasma. Products made from human plasma may contain infectious agents, such as viruses, that can cause disease. The risk that such products will transmit an infectious agent has been reduced by screening plasma donors for prior exposure to certain viruses, by testing for the presence of certain current virus infections, and by inactivating and/or removing certain viruses. (See DESCRIPTION.) Despite these measures, such products can still potentially transmit disease. Because this product is made from human blood, it may carry a risk of transmitting infectious agents, *e.g.,* viruses and theoretically, the Creutzfeldt-Jakob disease (CJD) agent. ALL infections thought by a physician possibly to have been transmitted by this product should be reported by the physician or other healthcare provider to Baxter Healthcare Corporation, Hyland Immuno at 1-800-423-2862 (in the US). The physician should discuss the risks and benefits of this product with the patient.

Immune Globulin Intravenous (Human), Gammagard S/D, should only be administered intravenously. Other routes of administration have not been evaluated.

Immediate anaphylactic and hypersensitivity reactions are a remote possibility. Epinephrine should be available for treatment of any acute anaphylactoid reactions.

Gammagard S/D contains only trace amounts of IgA (<3.7 μg/ml in a 5% solution). Gammagard S/D is not indicated in patients with selective IgA deficiency where the IgA deficiency is the only abnormality of concern. It should be given with caution to patients with antibodies to IgA or IgA deficiencies, that are a component of an underlying primary immunodeficiency disease for which IGIV therapy is indicated.[7,19] In such instances, a risk of anaphylaxis may exist despite the fact that Gammagard S/D contains only trace amounts of IgA.

DOSAGE AND ADMINISTRATION

PRIMARY IMMUNODEFICIENCY DISEASES

For patients with primary immunodeficiencies, monthly doses of at least 100 mg/kg are recommended. Initially, patients may receive 200-400 mg/kg. As there are significant differences in the half-life of IgG among patients with primary immunodeficiencies, the frequency and amount of immunoglobulin therapy may vary from patient to patient. The proper amount can be determined by monitoring clinical response. The minimum serum concentration of IgG necessary for protection has not been established.

B-CELL CHRONIC LYMPHOCYTIC LEUKEMIA (CLL)

For patients with hypogammaglobulinemia and/or recurrent bacterial infections due to B-cell Chronic Lymphocytic Leukemia, a dose of 400 mg/kg every 3-4 weeks is recommended.

KAWASAKI SYNDROME

For patients with Kawasaki syndrome, either a single 1 g/kg dose or a dose of 400 mg/kg for 4 consecutive days beginning within 7 days of the onset of fever, administered concomitantly with appropriate aspirin therapy (80-100 mg/kg/day in four divided doses) is recommended.

IDIOPATHIC THROMBOCYTOPENIC PURPURA (ITP)

For patients with acute or chronic Idiopathic Thrombocytopenic Purpura, a dose of 1 g/kg is recommended. The need for additional doses can be determined by clinical response and platelet count. Up to three separate doses may be given on alternate days if required. No prospective data are presently available to identify a maximum safe dose, concentration, and rate of infusion in patients determined to be at increased risk of acute renal failure. In the absence of prospective data, the recommended doses should not be exceeded and the concentration and infusion rate selected should be the minimum level practicable. Reduction in dose, concentration, and/or rate of administration in patients at risk of acute renal failure has been proposed in the literature in order to reduce the risk of acute renal failure.[32]

RECONSTITUTION

Use Aseptic Technique

When reconstitution is performed aseptically outside of a sterile laminar air flow hood, administration should begin as soon as possible, but not more than 2 hours after reconstitution.

When reconstitution is performed aseptically in a sterile laminar air flow hood, the reconstituted product may be either maintained in the original glasscontainer or pooled into Viaflex bags and stored under constant refrigeration (2-8°C), for up to 24 hours. (The date and time of reconstitution/pooling should be recorded.) If these conditions are not met, sterility of the reconstituted product cannot be maintained. Partially used vials should be discarded.

RATE OF ADMINISTRATION

It is recommended that initially a 5% solution be infused at a rate of 0.5 ml/kg/h. If infusion at this rate and concentration causes the patient no distress, the administration rate may be gradually increased to a maximum rate of 4 ml/kg/h. Patients who tolerate the 5% concentration at 4 ml/kg/h can be infused with the 10% concentration starting at 0.5 ml/kg/h. If no adverse effects occur, the rate can be increased gradually up to a maximum of 8 ml/kg/h. For patients judged to be at risk for developing renal dysfunction, it may be prudent to reduce the amount of product infused per unit time by infusing Gammagard S/D, at a rate less than 13.3 mg IG/kg/min (<0.27 ml/kg/min of 5% or <0.13 ml/kg/min of 10%).

It is recommended that antecubital veins be used especially for 10% solutions, if possible. This may reduce the likelihood of the patient experiencing discomfort at the infusion site.

A rate of administration which is too rapid may cause flushing and changes in pulse rate and blood pressure. Slowing or stopping the infusion usually allows the symptoms to disappear promptly.

DRUG INTERACTIONS

Admixtures of Immune Globulin Intravenous (Human), Gammagard S/D, with other drugs and intravenous solutions have not been evaluated. It is recommended that Gammagard S/D be administered separately from other drugs or medications which the patient may be receiving. The product should not be mixed with Immune Globulin Intravenous (Human) from other manufacturers.

Antibodies in immune globulin preparations may interfere with patient responses to live vaccines, such as those for measles, mumps, and rubella. The immunizing physician should be informed of recent therapy with Immune Globulin Intravenous (Human) so that appropriate precautions can be taken.

ADMINISTRATION

Gammagard S/D should be administered as soon after reconstitution as possible, or as described in DOSAGE AND ADMINISTRATION.

The reconstituted material should be at room temperature during administration.

Parenteral drug products should be inspected visually for particulate matter and discoloration prior to administration, whenever solution and container permit.

Reconstituted material should be a clear to slightly opalescent and colorless to pale yellow solution. Do not use if particulate matter and/or discoloration is observed.

Follow directions for use which accompany the administration set provided. If another administration set is used, ensure that the set contains a similar filter.

PRODUCT LISTING - EQUIVALENTS NOT AVAILABLE

Quantity	Price	Product	NDC
Powder For Injection - Intravenous - 0.5 Gm			
1's	$118.80	GAMMAGARD S/D, Baxter Healthcare Corporation	00944-2620-01
Powder For Injection - Intravenous - 1 Gm			
1's	$95.19	SANDOGLOBULIN, Novartis Pharmaceuticals	00078-0120-94
1's	$118.80	GAMMAR-P I.V., Centeon	00053-7486-01
Powder For Injection - Intravenous - 2.5 Gm			
1's	$118.80	GAMMAR-P I.V., Centeon	00053-7486-02
1's	$118.80	GAMMAGARD S/D, Baxter Healthcare Corporation	00944-2620-02
1's	$118.80	GENERIC, American Red Cross	52769-0471-72
Powder For Injection - Intravenous - 3 Gm			
1's	$247.50	CARIMUNE, Zlb Bioplasma Inc	44206-0506-53
Powder For Injection - Intravenous - 5 Gm			
1's	$118.80	GAMMAR-P I.V., Centeon	00053-7486-05
1's	$118.80	IVEEGAM EN, Baxter Healthcare Corporation	64193-0250-50
1's	$303.13	GAMMAR-P I.V., Centeon	00053-7486-06
1's	$1198.80	GENERIC, American Red Cross	52769-0471-75
1's	$1249.99	GAMMAGARD S/D, Baxter Healthcare Corporation	00944-2620-03
Powder For Injection - Intravenous - 6 Gm			
1's	$51.76	CARIMUNE, Zlb Bioplasma Inc	44206-0507-56
1's	$118.80	PANGLOBULIN, American Red Cross Blood Services	52769-0268-66
1's	$118.80	PANGLOBULIN, American Red Cross	52769-0270-76
1's	$363.15	SANDOGLOBULIN, Novartis Pharmaceuticals	00078-0124-96
10's	$1249.99	SANDOGLOBULIN, Novartis Pharmaceuticals	00078-0124-19
Powder For Injection - Intravenous - 10 Gm			
1's	$1249.99	GAMMAGARD S/D, Baxter Healthcare Corporation	00944-2620-04
1's	$1249.99	GENERIC, American Red Cross	05276-9471-80
1's	$1674.00	GAMMAR-P I.V., Centeon	00053-7486-10
1's	$1674.00	GENERIC, American Red Cross	52769-0471-80
Powder For Injection - Intravenous - 12 Gm			
1's	$118.80	PANGLOBULIN, American Red Cross	52769-0269-72
1's	$118.80	PANGLOBULIN, American Red Cross	52769-0270-82
1's	$990.00	CARIMUNE, Zlb Bioplasma Inc	44206-0508-62
1's	$1249.99	SANDOGLOBULIN, Novartis Pharmaceuticals	00078-0244-93
10's	$1249.99	SANDOGLOBULIN, Novartis Pharmaceuticals	00078-0244-19
Solution - Intramuscular - Strength n/a			
2 ml	$31.88	BAYGAM, Bayer	00026-0635-04
2 ml	$34.47	BAYGAM, Physicians Total Care	54868-4193-00
2 ml	$42.50	BIOGAM, Bioport Corporation	64678-0113-02
2 ml	$118.80	IMMUNE GLOBULIN, American Red Cross Blood Services	52769-0576-22
2 ml	$118.80	GENERIC, Bioport Corporation	64678-0101-02
2 ml	$119.99	GENERIC, American Red Cross Blood Services	14362-0011-52
10 ml	$128.13	BAYGAM, Bayer	00026-0635-12
Solution - Intravenous - 50 mg/ml			
10 ml	$36.00	GAMIMUNE N 5%, Bayer	00026-0640-12
10 ml	$45.00	GAMIMUNE N 5%, Bayer	00026-0646-12
10 ml	$45.60	GAMIMUNE N 5%, Bayer	00192-0640-12
50 ml	$86.40	GAMIMUNE N 5%, Bayer	00026-0640-20
50 ml	$126.00	GAMIMUNE N 5%, Bayer	00026-0646-20
50 ml	$225.00	GAMIMUNE N 5%, Bayer	00192-0640-20
50 ml	$287.50	GENERIC, Alpha Therapeutic Corporation	49669-1612-01
100 ml	$172.80	GAMIMUNE N 5%, Bayer	00026-0640-71

100 ml	$450.00	GAMIMUNE N 5%, Bayer	00026-0646-71
100 ml	$450.00	GAMIMUNE N 5%, Bayer	00192-0640-71
100 ml	$575.00	GENERIC, Alpha Therapeutic Corporation	49669-1613-01
200 ml	$900.00	GAMIMUNE N 5%, Bayer	00026-0646-24
200 ml	$1150.00	GENERIC, Alpha Therapeutic Corporation	49669-1614-01
250 ml	$714.00	GAMIMUNE N 5%, Bayer	00192-0640-25
250 ml	$1125.00	GAMIMUNE N 5%, Bayer	00026-0646-25
Solution - Intravenous - 100 mg/ml			
10 ml	$54.00	GAMIMUNE N 10%, Bayer	00026-0649-12
10 ml	$90.00	GAMIMUNE N 10%, Bayer	00192-0649-12
10 ml	$118.80	GAMIMUNE N 10%, Bayer	00026-0648-12
25 ml	$1249.99	GAMIMUNE N 10%, Bayer	00026-0648-15
50 ml	$270.00	GAMIMUNE N 10%, Bayer	00026-0649-20
50 ml	$450.00	GAMIMUNE N 10%, Bayer	00192-0649-20
50 ml	$506.25	GAMIMUNE N 10%, Bayer	00026-0648-20
50 ml	$594.00	GENERIC, Alpha Therapeutic Corporation	49669-1622-01
100 ml	$900.00	GAMIMUNE N 10%, Bayer	00192-0649-71
100 ml	$1012.50	GAMIMUNE N 10%, Bayer	00026-0648-71
100 ml	$1188.00	GENERIC, Alpha Therapeutic Corporation	49669-1623-01
100 ml	$1249.99	GAMIMUNE N 10%, Bayer	00026-0649-71
200 ml	$1800.00	GAMIMUNE N 10%, Bayer	00192-0649-24
200 ml	$2025.00	GAMIMUNE N 10%, Bayer	00026-0648-24
200 ml	$2376.00	GENERIC, Alpha Therapeutic Corporation	49669-1624-01

Indapamide *(001529)*

Categories: Edema; Hypertension, essential; Pregnancy Category B; FDA Approved 1983 Jul

Drug Classes: Diuretics, thiazide and derivatives

Brand Names: Depermide; **Lozol**; Natralix

Foreign Brand Availability: Agelan (Hong-Kong; Ireland); Damide (Italy); Dapa (Malaysia); Dapa-tabs (Australia; New-Zealand); Dapamax (South-Africa; Tanzania; Uganda; Zambia; Zimbabwe); Diflerix (Hong-Kong; Taiwan); Dixamid (Greece); Extur (Spain); Fludex (Austria; Belgium; Denmark; France; Greece; Netherlands; Portugal; Switzerland; Turkey); Fludex SR (Korea); Frumeron (Thailand); Hydro-Less (South-Africa); Indahexal (Australia); Indalix (Hong-Kong; South-Africa); Indicontin Continus (Hong-Kong); Insig (Australia); Ipamix (Italy); Lorvas (India); Lozide (Canada); Magniton-R (Greece); Millibar (China; Singapore; Taiwan); Napamide (Singapore; Thailand); Naplin (New-Zealand); Natrilix (Australia; Bahamas; Bahrain; Barbados; Belize; Benin; Bermuda; Burkina-Faso; China; Colombia; Costa-Rica; Curacao; Cyprus; Egypt; El-Salvador; England; Ethiopia; Finland; Gambia; Germany; Ghana; Guatemala; Guinea; Guyana; Honduras; Hong-Kong; India; Indonesia; Iran; Iraq; Ireland; Israel; Italy; Ivory-Coast; Jamaica; Jordan; Kenya; Kuwait; Lebanon; Liberia; Libya; Malawi; Malaysia; Mali; Mauritania; Mauritius; Morocco; Netherland-Antilles; New-Zealand; Nicaragua; Niger; Nigeria; Oman; Panama; Peru; Puerto-Rico; Qatar; Republic-of-Yemen; Saudi-Arabia; Senegal; Seychelles; Sierra-Leone; South-Africa; Sudan; Surinam; Syria; Taiwan; Tanzania; Trinidad; Tunia; Uganda; United-Arab-Emirates; Zambia; Zimbabwe); Natrilix SR (Australia; Germany; India; Philippines; Singapore); Natrix (Japan); Natrix SR (Korea); Pamid (Israel); Rinalix (Singapore); Sicco (Germany); Tandix (Portugal); Tertensif (Czech-Republic; Finland; Spain)

Cost of Therapy: $29.75 (Hypertension; Lozol; 1.25 mg; 1 tablet/day; 30 day supply)
$18.42 (Hypertension; Generic Tablets; 1.25 mg; 1 tablet/day; 30 day supply)

DESCRIPTION

Lozol (indapamide) is an oral antihypertensive/diuretic. Its molecule contains both a polar sulfamoyl chlorobenzamide moiety and a liquid-soluble methylindoline moiety. It differs chemically from the thiazides in that it does not possess the thiazide ring system and contains only one sulfonamide group. The chemical name of indapamide is 4-chloro-N-(2-methyl-1-indolinyl)-3-sulfamoylbenzamide, and its molecular weight is 365.84. The compound is a weak acid, pKa=8.8, and is soluble in aqueous solutions of strong bases. It is a white to yellow-white crystalline (tetragonal) powder.

CLINICAL PHARMACOLOGY

Indapamide is the first of a new class of antihypertensive/diuretics, the indolines. It has been reported that the oral administration of 2.5 mg (two 1.25 mg tablets) of indapamide to male subjects produced peak concentrations of approximately 115 ng/ml of the drug in blood within 2 hours. It has been reported that the oral administration of 5 mg (two 2.5 mg tablets) of indapamide to healthy male subjects produced peak concentrations of approximately 260 ng/ml of the drug in the blood within 2 hours. A minimum of 70% of a single oral dose is eliminated by the kidneys and an additional 23% by the gastrointestinal tract, probably including the biliary route. The half-life of indapamide in whole blood is approximately 14 hours.

Indapamide is preferentially and reversibly taken up by the erythrocytes in the peripheral blood. The whole blood/plasma ratio is approximately 6:1 at the time of peak concentration and decreases to 3.5:1 at 8 hours. From 71-79% of the indapamide in plasma is reversibly bound to plasma proteins.

Indapamide is an extensively metabolized drug with only about 7% of the total dose administered, recovered in the urine as unchanged drug during the first 48 hours after administration. The urinary elimination of ^{14}C-labeled indapamide and metabolites is biphasic with a terminal half-life of excretion of total radioactivity of 26 hours.

In a parallel design double-blind, placebo controlled trial in hypertension, daily doses of indapamide between 1.25 and 10 mg produced dose-related antihypertensive effects. Doses of 5 and 10 mg were not distinguishable from each other although each was differentiated from placebo and 1.25 mg indapamide. At daily doses of 1.25, 5 and 10 mg, a mean decrease of serum potassium of 0.28, 0.61 and 0.76 mEq/L, respectively, was observed and uric acid increased by about 0.69 mg/100 ml.

In other parallel design, dose-ranging clinical trials in hypertension and edema, daily doses of indapamide between 0.5 and 5 mg produced dose-related effects. Generally, doses of 2.5 and 5 mg were not distinguishable from each other although each was differentiated from placebo and from 0.5 or 1 mg indapamide. At daily doses of 2.5 and 5 mg a mean decrease of serum potassium of 0.5 and 0.6 mEq/L, respectively, was observed and uric acid increased by about 1 mg/100 ml.

At these doses, the effects of indapamide on blood pressure and edema are approximately equal to those obtained with conventional doses of other antihypertensive/diuretics.

In hypertensive patients daily doses of 1.25, 2.5 and 5 mg of indapamide have no appreciable cardiac inotropic or chronotropic effect. The drug decreases peripheral resistance, with little or no effect on cardiac output, rate or rhythm. Chronic administration of indapamide to hypertensive patients has little or no effect on glomerular filtration rate or renal plasma flow.

Indapamide had an antihypertensive effect in patients with varying degrees of renal impairment, although in general, diuretic effects declined as renal function decreased.

In a small number of controlled studies, indapamide taken with other antihypertensive drugs such as hydralazine, propranolol, guanethidine and methyldopa, appeared to have the additive effect typical of thiazide type diuretics.

INDICATIONS AND USAGE

Indapamide is indicated for the treatment of hypertension, alone or in combination with other antihypertensive drugs.

Indapamide is also indicated for the treatment of salt and fluid retention associated with congestive heart failure.

USAGE IN PREGNANCY

The routine use of diuretics in an otherwise healthy woman is inappropriate and exposes mother and fetus to unnecessary hazard (see PRECAUTIONS). Diuretics do not prevent development of toxemia of pregnancy, and there is no satisfactory evidence that they are useful in the treatment of developed toxemia.

Edema during pregnancy may arise from pathological causes or from the physiologic and mechanical consequences of pregnancy. Indapamide is indicated in pregnancy when edema is due to pathologic causes, just as it is in the absence of pregnancy (see PRECAUTIONS). Dependent edema in pregnancy, resulting from restriction of venous return by the expanded uterus, is properly treated through elevation of the lower extremities and use of support hose; use of diuretics to lower intravascular volume in this case is illogical and unnecessary. There is hypervolemia during normal pregnancy which is not harmful to either the fetus or the mother (in the absence of cardiovascular disease), but which is associated with edema, including generalized edema in the majority of pregnant women. If this edema produces discomfort, increased recumbency will often provide relief. In rare instances, this edema may cause extreme discomfort which is not relieved by rest. In these cases, a short course of diuretics may provide relief and may be appropriate.

CONTRAINDICATIONS

Anuria.

Known hypersensitivity to indapamide or to other sulfonamide-derived drugs.

WARNINGS

Severe cases of hyponatremia, accompanied by hypokalemia, have been reported with recommended doses of indapamide. This occurred primarily in elderly females. This appears to be dose-related. Also a large case-controlled pharmacoepidemiology study indicates that there is an increased risk of hyponatremia with indapamide 2.5 and 5 mg doses. Hyponatremia considered possibly clinically significant (less than 125 mEq/L) has not been observed in clinical trials with the 1.25 mg dosage (see PRECAUTIONS). Thus patients should be started at the 1.25 mg dose and maintained at the lowest possible dose. (See DOSAGE AND ADMINISTRATION.)

Hypokalemia occurs commonly with diuretics (see ADVERSE REACTIONS), and electrolyte monitoring is essential, particularly in patients who would be at increased risk from hypokalemia, such as those with cardiac arrhythmias or who are receiving concomitant cardiac glycosides.

In general, diuretics should not be given concomitantly with lithium because they reduce its renal clearance and add a high risk of lithium toxicity. Read prescribing information for lithium preparations before use of such concomitant therapy.

PRECAUTIONS

GENERAL

Hypokalemia, Hyponatremia, and Other Fluid and Electrolyte Imbalances

Periodic determinations of serum electrolytes should be performed at appropriate intervals. In addition, patients should be observed for clinical signs of fluid or electrolyte imbalance, such as hyponatremia, hypochloremic alkalosis, or hypokalemia. Warning signs include dry mouth, thirst, weakness, fatigue, lethargy, drowsiness, restlessness, muscle pains or cramps, hypotension, oliguria, tachycardia and gastrointestinal disturbance. Electrolyte determinations are particularly important in patients who are vomiting excessively or receiving parenteral fluids, in patients subject to electrolyte imbalance (including those with heart failure, kidney disease, and cirrhosis), and in patients on a salt-restricted diet.

The risk of hypokalemia secondary to diuresis and natriuresis is increased when larger doses are used, when the diuresis is brisk, when severe cirrhosis is present and during concomitant use of corticosteroids or ACTH. Interference with adequate oral intake of electrolytes will also contribute to hypokalemia. Hypokalemia can sensitize or exaggerate the response of the heart to the toxic effects of digitalis, such as increased ventricular irritability.

Dilutional hyponatremia may occur in edematous patients; the appropriate treatment is restriction of water rather than administration of salt, except in rare instances when the hyponatremia is life threatening. However, in actual salt depletion, appropriate replacement is the treatment of choice. Any chloride deficit that may occur during treatment is generally mild and usually does not require specific treatment except in extraordinary circumstances as in liver or renal disease. Thiazide-like diuretics have been shown to increase the urinary excretion of magnesium; this may result in hypomagnesemia.

Hyperuricemia and Gout

Serum concentrations of uric acid increased by an average of 0.69 mg/100 ml in patients treated with indapamide 1.25 mg, and by an average of 1 mg/100 ml in patients treated with indapamide 2.5 and 5 mg, and frank gout may be precipitated in certain patients receiving indapamide (see ADVERSE REACTIONS). Serum concentrations of uric acid should, therefore, be monitored periodically during treatment.

Renal Impairment

Indapamide, like the thiazides, should be used with caution in patients with severe renal disease, as reduced plasma volume may exacerbate or precipitate azotemia. If progressive renal impairment is observed in a patient receiving indapamide, withholding or discontinuing diuretic therapy should be considered. Renal function tests should be performed periodically during treatment with indapamide.

Impaired Hepatic Function

Indapamide, like the thiazides, should be used with caution in patients with impaired hepatic function or progressive liver disease, since minor alterations of fluid and electrolyte balance may precipitate hepatic coma.

Glucose Tolerance

Latent diabetes may become manifest and insulin requirements in diabetic patients may be altered during thiazide administration. A mean increase in glucose of 6.47 mg/dl was observed in patients treated with indapamide 1.25 mg, which was not considered clinically significant in these trials. Serum concentrations of glucose should be monitored routinely during treatment with indapamide.

Calcium Excretion

Calcium excretion is decreased by diuretics pharmacologically related to indapamide. After 6-8 weeks of indapamide 1.25 mg treatment and in long-term studies of hypertensive patients, with higher doses of indapamide, however, serum concentrations of calcium increased only slightly with indapamide. Prolonged treatment with drugs pharmacologically related to indapamide may in rare instances be associated with hypercalcemia and hypophosphatemia secondary to physiologic changes in the parathyroid gland; however, the common complications of hyperparathyroidism, such as renal lithiasis, bone resorption, and peptic ulcer, have not been seen. Treatment should be discontinued before tests for parathyroid function are performed. Like the thiazides, indapamide may decrease serum PBI levels without signs of thyroid disturbance.

Interaction With Systemic Lupus Erythematosus

Thiazides have exacerbated or activated systemic lupus erythematosus and this possibility should be considered with indapamide as well.

CARCINOGENESIS, MUTAGENESIS, AND IMPAIRMENT OF FERTILITY

Both mouse and rat lifetime carcinogenicity studies were conducted. There was no significant difference in the incidence of tumors between the indapamide-treated animals and the control groups.

PREGNANCY, TERATOGENIC EFFECTS, PREGNANCY CATEGORY B

Reproduction studies have been performed in rats, mice and rabbits at doses up to 6250 times the therapeutic human dose and have revealed no evidence of impaired fertility or harm to the fetus due to indapamide. Postnatal development in rats and mice was unaffected by pre-treatment of parent animals during gestation. There are, however, no adequate and well-controlled studies in pregnant women. Moreover, diuretics are known to cross the placental barrier and appear in cord blood. Because animal reproduction studies are not always predictive of human response, this drug should be used during pregnancy only if clearly needed. There may be hazards associated with this use such as fetal or neonatal jaundice, thrombocytopenia, and possibly other adverse reactions that have occurred in the adult.

NURSING MOTHERS

It is not known whether this drug is excreted in human milk. Because most drugs are excreted in human milk, if use of this drug is deemed essential, the patient should stop nursing.

PEDIATRIC USE

Safety and effectiveness of indapamide in pediatric patients have not been established.

DRUG INTERACTIONS

Other Antihypertensives: Indapamide may add to or potentiate the action of other antihypertensive drugs. In limited controlled trials that compared the effect of indapamide combined with other antihypertensive drugs with the effect of the other drugs administered alone, there was no notable change in the nature or frequency of adverse reactions associated with the combined therapy.

Lithium: See WARNINGS.

Post-Sympathectomy Patient: The antihypertensive effect of the drug may be enhanced in the post-sympathectomized patient.

Norepinephrine: Indapamide, like the thiazides, may decrease arterial responsiveness to norepinephrine, but this diminution is not sufficient to preclude effectiveness of the pressor agent for therapeutic use.

ADVERSE REACTIONS

Most adverse effects have been mild and transient.

The clinical adverse reactions in the first list represent data from Phase 2/3 placebo-controlled studies (306 patients given indapamide 1.25 mg). The clinical adverse reactions in the second list represent data from Phase 2 placebo-controlled studies and long-term controlled clinical trials (426 patients given indapamide 2.5 or 5 mg). The reactions are arranged into two groups: (1) a cumulative incidence equal to or greater than 5%; (2) a cumulative incidence less than 5%. Reactions are counted regardless of relation to drug.

Adverse reactions from studies of 1.25 mg (incidence ≥5%):

Body as a Whole: Headache, infection, pain, back pain.

Central Nervous System: Dizziness.

Respiratory System: Rhinitis.

Adverse reactions from studies of 1.25 mg (incidence <5%):

Body as a Whole: Asthenia, flu syndrome, abdominal pain, chest pain.

Gastrointestinal: Constipation, diarrhea, dyspepsia, nausea.

Metabolic System: Peripheral edema.

Central Nervous System: Nervousness, hypertonia.

Respiratory System: Cough, pharyngitis, sinusitis.

Special Senses: Conjunctivitis.

Other: *All other clinical adverse reactions occurred at an incidence of <1%.

Approximately 4% of patients given indapamide 1.25 mg compared to 5% of the patients given placebo discontinued treatment in the trials of up to 8 weeks because of adverse reactions.

In controlled clinical trials of 6-8 weeks in duration, 20% of patients receiving indapamide 1.25 mg, 61% of patients receiving indapamide 5 mg, and 80% of patients receiving indapamide 10 mg had at least one potassium value below 3.4 mEq/L. In the indapamide 1.25 mg group, about 40% of those patients who reported hypokalemia as a laboratory adverse event returned to normal serum potassium values without intervention. Hypokalemia with concomitant clinical signs or symptoms occurred in 2% of patients receiving indapamide 1.25 mg.

Adverse reactions from studies of 2.5 and 5 mg (incidence ≥5%):

Central Nervous System/Neuromuscular: Headache, dizziness, fatigue, weakness, loss of energy, lethargy, tiredness or malaise, muscle cramps or spasm, numbness of the extremities, nervousness, tension, anxiety, irritability, or agitation.

Adverse reactions from studies of 2.5 and 5 mg (incidence <5%):

Central Nervous System/Neuromuscular: Lightheadedness, drowsiness, vertigo, insomnia, depression, blurred vision.

Gastrointestinal System: Constipation, nausea, vomiting, diarrhea, gastric irritation, abdominal pain or cramps, anorexia.

Cardiovascular System: Orthostatic hypotension, premature ventricular contractions, irregular heart beat, palpitations.

Genitourinary System: Frequency of urination, nocturia, polyuria.

Dermatologic/Hypersensitivity: Rash, hives, pruritus, vasculitis.

Other: Impotence or reduced libido, rhinorrhea, flushing, hyperuricemia, hyperglycemia, hyponatremia, hypochloremia, increase in serum urea nitrogen (BUN) or creatinine, glycosuria, weight loss, dry mouth, tingling of extremities.

Because most of these data are from long-term studies (up to 40 weeks of treatment), it is probable that many of the adverse experiences reported are due to causes other than the drug. Approximately 10% of patients given indapamide discontinued treatment in long-term trials because of reactions either related or unrelated to the drug.

Hypokalemia with concomitant clinical signs or symptoms occurred in 3% of patients receiving indapamide 2.5 mg qd and 7% of patients receiving indapamide 5 mg qd. In long-term controlled clinical trials comparing the hypokalemic effects of daily doses of indapamide and hydrochlorothiazide, however, 47% of patients receiving indapamide 2.5 mg, 72% of patients receiving indapamide 5 mg, and 44% of patients receiving hydrochlorothiazide 50 mg had at least one potassium value (out of a total of 11 taken during the study) below 3.5 mEq/L. In the indapamide 2.5 mg group, over 50% of those patients returned to normal serum potassium values without intervention.

In clinical trials of 6-8 weeks, the mean changes in selected values are shown in TABLE 1 and TABLE 2.

TABLE 1 *Mean Changes From Baseline After 8 Weeks of Treatment*

	Indapamide 1.25 mg (n=255-257)	Placebo (n=263-266)
Serum electrolytes		
Potassium (mEq/L)	-0.28	0.00
Sodium (mEq/L)	-0.63	-0.11
Chloride (mEq/L)	-2.60	-0.21
Serum uric acid (mg/dl)	0.69	0.06
BUN (mg/dl)	1.46	0.06

No patients receiving indapamide 1.25 mg experienced hyponatremia considered possibly clinically significant (<125 mEq/L).

Indapamide had no adverse effects on lipids.

TABLE 2 *Mean Changes From Baseline After 40 Weeks of Treatment*

	Indapamide	
	2.5 mg (n=76)	5 mg (n=81)
Serum electrolytes		
Potassium (mEq/L)	-0.4	-0.6
Sodium (mEq/L)	-0.6	-0.7
Chloride (mEq/L)	-3.6	-5.1
Serum uric acid (mg/dl)	0.7	1.1
BUN (mg/dl)	-0.1	1.4

The following reactions have been reported with clinical usage of indapamide: Jaundice (intrahepatic cholestatic jaundice), hepatitis, pancreatitis, and abnormal liver function tests. These reactions were reversible with discontinuance of the drug.

Also reported are erythema multiforme, Stevens-Johnson syndrome, bullous eruptions, purpura, photosensitivity, fever, pneumonitis, anaphylactic reactions, agranulocytosis, leukopenia, thrombocytopenia and aplastic anemia. Other adverse reactions reported with antihypertensive/diuretics are necrotizing angitis, respiratory distress, sialadenitis, xanthopsia.

DOSAGE AND ADMINISTRATION

HYPERTENSION

The adult starting indapamide dose for hypertension is 1.25 mg as a single daily dose taken in the morning. If the response to 1.25 mg is not satisfactory after 4 weeks, the daily dose may be increased to 2.5 mg taken once daily. If the response to 2.5 mg is not satisfactory after 4 weeks, the daily dose may be increased to 5 mg taken once daily, but adding another antihypertensive should be considered.

EDEMA OF CONGESTIVE HEART FAILURE

The adult starting indapamide dose for edema of congestive heart failure is 2.5 as a single daily dose taken in the morning. If the response to 2.5 mg is not satisfactory after 1 week, the daily dose may be increased to 5 mg once daily.

If the antihypertensive response to indapamide is insufficient, indapamide may be combined with other antihypertensive drugs, with careful monitoring of blood pressure. It is recommended that the usual dose of other agents be reduced by 50% during initial combination therapy. As the blood pressure response becomes evident, further dosage adjustments may be necessary.

In general, doses of 5 mg and larger have not appeared to provide additional effects on blood pressure or heart failure, but are associated with a greater degree of hypokalemia. There is minimal clinical trial experience in patients with doses greater than 5 mg once a day.

HOW SUPPLIED

Lozol 1.25 mg: Orange, film-coated, octagon shaped, marked with an "R" and a "7".
Lozol 2.5 mg: White, film-coated, octagon shaped, marked with an "R" and an "8".

Storage: Keep tightly closed. Store at controlled room temperature 20-25°C (68-77°F). Avoid excessive heat. This product should be dispensed in a container with a child resistant cap.

PRODUCT LISTING - RATED THERAPEUTICALLY EQUIVALENT

Tablet - Oral - 1.25 mg

Qty	Price	Product	NDC
30's	$18.40	GENERIC, Ivax Corporation	00172-4262-46
100's	$10.35	FEDERAL UPPER LIMIT, H.C.F.A. F F P	99999-1529-01
100's	$61.40	GENERIC, Major Pharmaceuticals Inc	00904-5333-60
100's	$61.65	GENERIC, Apothecon Inc	62269-0246-24
100's	$63.90	GENERIC, Teva Pharmaceuticals Usa	00536-3971-01
100's	$67.70	GENERIC, Mylan Pharmaceuticals Inc	00378-0069-01
100's	$67.70	GENERIC, Lannett Company Inc	00527-1299-01
100's	$67.90	GENERIC, Ivax Corporation	00172-4262-60
100's	$67.90	GENERIC, Ivax Corporation	00182-8201-89
100's	$67.95	GENERIC, Purepac Pharmaceutical Company	00228-2597-11
100's	$83.25	GENERIC, Par Pharmaceutical Inc	49884-0589-01
100's	$83.27	GENERIC, Watson Laboratories Inc	52544-0527-01

Tablet - Oral - 2.5 mg

Qty	Price	Product	NDC
30's	$22.72	GENERIC, Heartland Healthcare Services	61392-0124-30
30's	$22.72	GENERIC, Heartland Healthcare Services	61392-0124-39
30's	$34.71	LOZOL, Allscripts Pharmaceutical Company	54569-0579-00
30's	$36.74	LOZOL, Physicians Total Care	54868-1295-01
30's	$43.29	LOZOL, Pd-Rx Pharmaceuticals	55289-0276-30
31's	$23.47	GENERIC, Heartland Healthcare Services	61392-0124-31
32's	$24.23	GENERIC, Heartland Healthcare Services	61392-0124-32
45's	$34.07	GENERIC, Heartland Healthcare Services	61392-0124-45
60's	$45.43	GENERIC, Heartland Healthcare Services	61392-0124-60
90's	$68.15	GENERIC, Heartland Healthcare Services	61392-0124-90
90's	$73.21	LOZOL, Allscripts Pharmaceutical Company	54569-8536-00
100's	$11.25	FEDERAL UPPER LIMIT, H.C.F.A. F F P	99999-1529-02
100's	$65.98	GENERIC, Aligen Independent Laboratories Inc	00405-4538-01
100's	$73.12	GENERIC, Geneva Pharmaceuticals	00781-1051-01
100's	$74.45	GENERIC, Moore, H.L. Drug Exchange Inc	00839-8030-06
100's	$76.20	GENERIC, Apothecon Inc	62269-0247-24
100's	$77.50	GENERIC, Major Pharmaceuticals Inc	00904-5074-60
100's	$77.50	GENERIC, Major Pharmaceuticals Inc	00904-5334-60
100's	$82.80	GENERIC, Mylan Pharmaceuticals Inc	00378-0080-01
100's	$83.00	GENERIC, Ivax Corporation	00172-4259-60
100's	$83.00	GENERIC, Ivax Corporation	00182-2610-89
100's	$83.00	GENERIC, Lannett Company Inc	00527-1300-01
100's	$83.05	GENERIC, Purepac Pharmaceutical Company	00228-2571-11
100's	$101.80	GENERIC, Par Pharmaceutical Inc	49884-0590-01
100's	$101.84	GENERIC, Watson Laboratories Inc	52544-0504-01
100's	$122.65	LOZOL, Aventis Pharmaceuticals	00075-0082-00

PRODUCT LISTING - EQUIVALENTS NOT AVAILABLE

Tablet - Oral - 1.25 mg

Qty	Price	Product	NDC
30's	$8.40	GENERIC, Physicians Total Care	54868-3885-00
100's	$99.16	LOZOL, Aventis Pharmaceuticals	00075-0700-00

Tablet - Oral - 2.5 mg

Qty	Price	Product	NDC
30's	$9.61	GENERIC, Physicians Total Care	54868-3106-00
90's	$66.35	GENERIC, Allscripts Pharmaceutical Company	54569-8604-00
100's	$77.96	GENERIC, Arcola Laboratories	00070-3000-00
100's	$79.42	GENERIC, Udl Laboratories Inc	51079-0868-20

Indinavir Sulfate *(003252)*

For related information, see the comparative table section in Appendix A.

Categories: Infection, human immunodeficiency virus; FDA Approved 1996 Feb; Pregnancy Category C; WHO Formulary
Drug Classes: Antivirals; Protease inhibitors
Brand Names: Crixivan
Cost of Therapy: $546.37 (HIV; Crixivan; 400 mg; 6 capsules/day; 30 day supply)

DESCRIPTION

Crixivan (indinavir sulfate) is an inhibitor of the human immunodeficiency virus (HIV) protease. Crixivan capsules are formulated as a sulfate salt and are available for oral administration in strengths of 100, 200, 333, and 400 mg of indinavir (corresponding to 125, 250, 416.3, and 500 mg indinavir sulfate, respectively). Each capsule also contains the inactive ingredients anhydrous lactose and magnesium stearate. The capsule shell has the following inactive ingredients and dyes: gelatin, titanium dioxide, silicon dioxide and sodium lauryl sulfate.

The chemical name for indinavir sulfate is [1(1*S*,2*R*),5(*S*)]-2,3,5-trideoxy-*N*-(2,3-dihydro-2-hydroxy-1*H*-inden-1-yl)-5-[2-[[(1,1-dimethylethyl)amino]carbonyl]-4-(3-pyridinylmethyl)-1-piperazinyl]-2-(phenylmethyl)-D-*erythro*-pentonamide sulfate (1:1) salt.

Indinavir sulfate is a white to off-white, hygroscopic, crystalline powder with the molecular formula $C_{36}H_{47}N_5O_4 \cdot H_2SO_4$ and a molecular weight of 711.88. It is very soluble in water and in methanol.

CLINICAL PHARMACOLOGY

MICROBIOLOGY

Mechanism of Action

HIV-1 protease is an enzyme required for the proteolytic cleavage of the viral polyprotein precursors into the individual functional proteins found in infectious HIV-1. Indinavir binds to the protease active site and inhibits the activity of the enzyme. This inhibition prevents cleavage of the viral polyproteins resulting in the formation of immature non-infectious viral particles.

Antiretroviral Activity In Vitro

The *in vitro* activity of indinavir was assessed in cell lines of lymphoblastic and monocytic origin and in peripheral blood lymphocytes. HIV-1 variants used to infect the different cell types include laboratory-adapted variants, primary clinical isolates and clinical isolates resistant to nucleoside analogue and nonnucleoside inhibitors of the HIV-1 reverse transcriptase. The IC_{95} (95% inhibitory concentration) of indinavir in these test systems was in the range of 25-100 nM. In drug combination studies with the nucleoside analogues zidovudine and didanosine, indinavir showed synergistic activity in cell culture. The relationship between *in vitro* susceptibility of HIV-1 to indinavir and inhibition of HIV-1 replication in humans has not been established.

Drug Resistance

Isolates of HIV-1 with reduced susceptibility to the drug have been recovered from some patients treated with indinavir. Viral resistance was correlated with the accumulation of mutations that resulted in the expression of amino acid substitutions in the viral protease. Eleven (11) amino acid residue positions, (L10I/V/R, K20I/M/R, L24I, M46I/L, I54A/V, L63P, I64V, A71T/V, V82A/F/T, I84V, and L90M), at which substitutions are associated with resistance, have been identified. Resistance was mediated by the co-expression of multiple and variable substitutions at these positions. No single substitution was either necessary or sufficient for measurable resistance (≥4-fold increase in IC_{95}). In general, higher levels of resistance were associated with the co-expression of greater numbers of substitutions, although their individual effects varied and were not additive. At least 3 amino acid substitutions must be present for phenotypic resistance to indinavir to reach measurable levels. In addition, mutations in the p7/p1 and p1/p6 gag cleavage sites were observed in some indinavir resistant HIV-1 isolates.

In vitro phenotypic susceptibilities to indinavir were determined for 38 viral isolates from 13 patients who experienced virologic rebounds during indinavir monotherapy. Pretreatment isolates from 5 patients exhibited indinavir IC_{95} values of 50-100 nM. At or following viral RNA rebound (after 12-76 weeks of therapy), IC_{95} values ranged from 25 to >3000 nM, and the viruses carried 2-10 mutations in the protease gene relative to baseline.

Cross-Resistance to Other Antiviral Agents

Varying degrees of HIV-1 cross-resistance have been observed between indinavir and other HIV-1 protease inhibitors. In studies with ritonavir, saquinavir, and amprenavir, the extent and spectrum of cross-resistance varied with the specific mutational patterns observed. In general, the degree of cross-resistance increased with the accumulation of resistance-associated amino acid substitutions. Within a panel of 29 viral isolates from indinavir-treated patients that exhibited measurable (≥4-fold) phenotypic resistance to indinavir, all were resistant to ritonavir. Of the indinavir resistant HIV-1 isolates, 63% showed resistance to saquinavir and 81% to amprenavir.

PHARMACOKINETICS

Absorption

Indinavir was rapidly absorbed in the fasted state with a time to peak plasma concentration (T_{max}) of 0.8 ± 0.3 hours (mean ± SD) (n=11). A greater than dose-proportional increase in indinavir plasma concentrations was observed over the 200-1000 mg dose range. At a dosing regimen of 800 mg every 8 hours, steady-state area under the plasma concentration time curve (AUC) was 30,691 ± 11,407 nM·h (n=16), peak plasma concentration (C_{max}) was 12,617 ± 4,037 nM (n=16), and plasma concentration 8 hours post dose (trough) was 251 ± 178 nM (n=16).

Effect of Food on Oral Absorption

Administration of indinavir with a meal high in calories, fat, and protein (784 kcal, 48.6 g fat, 31.3 g protein) resulted in a 77 ± 8% reduction in AUC and an 84 ± 7% reduction in C_{max} (n=10). Administration with lighter meals (*e.g.,* a meal of dry toast with jelly, apple juice, and coffee with skim milk and sugar or a meal of corn flakes, skim milk and sugar) resulted in little or no change in AUC, C_{max} or trough concentration.

Distribution

Indinavir was approximately 60% bound to human plasma proteins over a concentration range of 81 to 16,300 nM.

Metabolism

Following a 400 mg dose of ^{14}C-indinavir, 83 ± 1% (n=4) and 19 ± 3% (n=6) of the total radioactivity was recovered in feces and urine, respectively; radioactivity due to parent drug in feces and urine was 19.1% and 9.4%, respectively. Seven metabolites have been identified, one glucuronide conjugate and six oxidative metabolites. *In vitro* studies indicate that cytochrome P450 3A4 (CYP3A4) is the major enzyme responsible for formation of the oxidative metabolites.

Elimination

Less than 20% of indinavir is excreted unchanged in the urine. Mean urinary excretion of unchanged drug was 10.4 ± 4.9% (n=10) and 12.0 ± 4.9% (n=10) following a single 700 mg and 1000 mg dose, respectively. Indinavir was rapidly eliminated with a half-life of 1.8 ± 0.4 hours (n=10). Significant accumulation was not observed after multiple dosing at 800 mg every 8 hours.

SPECIAL POPULATIONS

Hepatic Insufficiency

Patients with mild to moderate hepatic insufficiency and clinical evidence of cirrhosis had evidence of decreased metabolism of indinavir resulting in approximately 60% higher mean AUC following a single 400 mg dose (n=12). The half-life of indinavir increased to 2.8 ± 0.5 hours. Indinavir pharmacokinetics have not been studied in patients with severe hepatic insufficiency (see DOSAGE AND ADMINISTRATION, Hepatic Insufficiency).

Renal Insufficiency

The pharmacokinetics of indinavir have not been studied in patients with renal insufficiency.

Gender

The effect of gender on the pharmacokinetics of indinavir was evaluated in 10 HIV seropositive women who received indinavir sulfate 800 mg every 8 hours with zidovudine 200 mg every 8 hours and lamivudine 150 mg twice a day for 1 week. Indinavir pharmacokinetic parameters in these women were compared to those in HIV seropositive men (pooled historical control data). Differences in indinavir exposure, peak concentrations, and trough concentrations between males and females are shown in TABLE 1.

TABLE 1

PK Parameter	% Change in PK Parameter*	90% Confidence Interval
AUC(0-8h) (nM·h)	dec 13%	(dec 32%, inc 12%)
C_{max} (nM)	dec 13%	(dec 32%, inc 10%)
C_{8h} (nM)	dec 22%	(dec 47%, inc 15%)

* For females relative to males.
dec: Indicates a decrease in the PK parameter; inc: indicates an increase in the PK parameter.

The clinical significance of these gender differences in the pharmacokinetics of indinavir is not known.

Race

Pharmacokinetics of indinavir appear to be comparable in Caucasians and Blacks based on pharmacokinetic studies including 42 Caucasians (26 HIV-positive) and 16 Blacks (4 HIV-positive).

Pediatric

The optimal dosing regimen for use of indinavir in pediatric patients has not been established. In HIV-infected pediatric patients (age 4-15 years), a dosage regimen of indinavir capsules, 500 mg/m^2 every 8 hours, produced AUC(0-8h) of 38,742 ± 24,098 nM·h (n=34), C_{max} of 17,181 ± 9,809 nM (n=34), and trough concentrations of 134 ± 91 nM (n=28). The pharmacokinetic profiles of indinavir in pediatric patients were not comparable to profiles previously observed in HIV-infected adults receiving the recommended dose of 800 mg every 8 hours. The AUC and C_{max} values were slightly higher and the trough concentrations were considerably lower in pediatric patients. Approximately 50% of the pediatric patients had trough values below 100 nM; whereas, approximately 10% of adult patients had trough levels below 100 nM. The relationship between specific trough values and inhibition of HIV replication has not been established.

DRUG INTERACTIONS

Also see DRUG INTERACTIONS.

Specific drug interaction studies were performed with indinavir and a number of drugs.

Drugs That Should Not Be Coadministered With Indinavir Sulfate

Administration of indinavir (800 mg every 8 hours) with rifampin (600 mg once daily) for 1 week resulted in an 89 ± 9% decrease in indinavir AUC.

In a published study, 8 HIV-negative volunteers received indinavir 800 mg every 8 hours for 4 doses prior to and at the end of a 14 day course of St. John's wort (*Hypericum perforatum,* standardized to 0.3% hypericin) 300 mg three times daily. Indinavir plasma pharmacokinetics were determined following the fourth dose of indinavir prior to and following St. John's wort. Following the course of St. John's wort, the AUC(0-8h) of indinavir was decreased 57% ± 19% and the C(8h) of indinavir was decreased 81% ± 16% compared to when indinavir was taken alone. All subjects demonstrated a decrease in AUC(0-8h) (range 36-79%) and a decrease in C(8h) (range 49-99%). (See WARNINGS.)

Drugs Requiring Dose Modification

Delavirdine

Preliminary data (n=14) indicate that delavirdine inhibits the metabolism of indinavir such that coadministration of a 400 mg single dose of indinavir with delavirdine (400 mg three times a day) resulted in indinavir AUC values slightly less than those observed following administration of an 800 mg dose of indinavir alone. Also, coadministration of a 600 mg dose of indinavir with delavirdine (400 mg three times a day) resulted in indinavir AUC values approximately 40% greater than those observed following administration of an 800 mg dose of indinavir alone. Indinavir had no effect on delavirdine pharmacokinetics (see DOSAGE AND ADMINISTRATION, Concomitant Therapy, Delavirdine).

Efavirenz

When indinavir (800 mg every 8 hours) was given with efavirenz (200 mg once daily) for 2 weeks, the indinavir AUC and C_{max} were decreased by approximately 31% and 16%, respectively, as a result of enzyme induction. (See DOSAGE AND ADMINISTRATION, Concomitant Therapy, Efavirenz.)

Sildenafil

The results of one published study in HIV-infected men (n=6) indicated that coadministration of indinavir (800 mg every 8 hours chronically) with a single 25 mg dose of sildenafil resulted in an 11% increase in average AUC(0-8h) of indinavir and a 48% increase in average indinavir peak concentration (C_{max}) compared to 800 mg every 8 hours alone. Average sildenafil AUC was increased by 340% following coadministration of sildenafil and indinavir compared to historical data following administration of sildenafil alone (see DRUG INTERACTIONS).

Itraconazole

In a multiple-dose study, administration in the fasted state of itraconazole capsules 200 mg twice daily with indinavir 600 mg every 8 hours resulted in an indinavir AUC similar to that observed during administration of indinavir 800 mg every 8 hours alone for 1 week (see DOSAGE AND ADMINISTRATION, Concomitant Therapy, Itraconazole).

Ketoconazole

In a single-dose study, administration of a 400 mg dose of ketoconazole with a 400 mg dose of indinavir resulted in a 68% ± 48% increase in indinavir AUC compared to a 400 mg dose of indinavir alone. In a multiple-dose study, administration of ketoconazole 400 mg once daily with indinavir 600 mg every 8 hours resulted in an 18% ± 17% decrease in indinavir AUC compared to an 800 mg dose of indinavir alone every 8 hours (see DOSAGE AND ADMINISTRATION, Concomitant Therapy, Ketoconazole).

Rifabutin

The coadministration of indinavir 800 mg every 8 hours with rifabutin either 300 mg once daily or 150 mg once daily was evaluated in 2 separate clinical studies. The results of these studies showed a decrease in indinavir AUC (32% ± 19% and 31% ± 15%, respectively) versus indinavir 800 mg every 8 hours alone and an increase in rifabutin AUC (204% ± 142% and 60% ± 47%, respectively) versus rifabutin 300 mg once daily alone. (See DOSAGE AND ADMINISTRATION, Concomitant Therapy, Rifabutin.)

Drugs Not Requiring Dose Modification

Cimetidine, Quinidine, Grapefruit Juice

Administration of a single 400 mg dose of indinavir following 6 days of cimetidine (600 mg every 12 hours) did not affect indinavir AUC. Administration of a single 400 mg dose of indinavir with 8 oz of grapefruit juice resulted in a decrease in indinavir AUC (26% ± 18%). Administration of a single 400 mg dose of indinavir with 200 mg of quinidine sulfate resulted in a 10% ± 26% increase in indinavir AUC.

Methadone

Administration of indinavir (800 mg every 8 hours) with methadone (20-60 mg daily) for 1 week resulted in no change in methadone AUC and little or no change in indinavir AUC.

Nucleoside Analogue Antiretroviral Agents

Administration of indinavir (1000 mg every 8 hours) with zidovudine (200 mg every 8 hours) for 1 week resulted in a 13% ± 48% increase in indinavir AUC and a 17% ± 23% increase in zidovudine AUC. In another study, administration of indinavir (800 mg every 8 hours) with zidovudine (200 mg every 8 hours) in combination with lamivudine (150 mg twice daily) for 1 week resulted in no change in indinavir AUC, a 36% increase in zidovudine AUC, and a 6% decrease in lamivudine AUC. Administration of indinavir (800 mg every 8 hours) in combination with stavudine (40 mg every 12 hours) for 1 week resulted in no change in indinavir AUC and a 25% ± 26% increase in stavudine AUC.

Ethinyl Estradiol; Norethindrone (0.035 mg/1 mg)

Administration of indinavir (800 mg every 8 hours) with ethinyl estradiol; norethindrone (0.035 mg/1 mg) for 1 week resulted in a 24% ± 17% increase in ethinyl estradiol AUC and a 26% ± 14% increase in norethindrone AUC.

Trimethoprim/Sulfamethoxazole, Fluconazole, Isoniazid, Clarithromycin

Administration of indinavir (400 mg every 6 hours) with trimethoprim/sulfamethoxazole (1 double strength tablet every 12 hours) for 1 week resulted in no change in indinavir AUC, a 19% ± 31% increase in trimethoprim AUC, and no change in sulfamethoxazole AUC. Administration of indinavir (1000 mg every 8 hours) with fluconazole (400 mg once daily) for 1 week resulted in a 19% ± 33% decrease in indinavir AUC and no change in fluconazole AUC. Administration of indinavir (800 mg every 8 hours) with isoniazid (300 mg once daily) for 1 week resulted in no change in indinavir AUC and a 13% ± 15% increase in isoniazid AUC. Administration of indinavir (800 mg every 8 hours) with clarithromycin

(500 mg every 12 hours) for 1 week resulted in a 29% ± 42% increase in indinavir AUC and a 53% ± 36% increase in clarithromycin AUC.

INDICATIONS AND USAGE

Indinavir sulfate in combination with antiretroviral agents is indicated for the treatment of HIV infection.

This indication is based on two clinical trials of approximately 1 year duration that demonstrated: (1) a reduction in the risk of AIDS-defining illnesses or death; (2) a prolonged suppression of HIV RNA.

NON-FDA APPROVED INDICATIONS

Indinavir sulfate in combination with other antiretroviral agents is recommended by the Public Health Service interagency working group for use in postexposure prophylaxis of HIV although, this is not FDA approved.

CONTRAINDICATIONS

Indinavir sulfate is contraindicated in patients with clinically significant hypersensitivity to any of its components.

Indinavir sulfate should not be administered concurrently with terfenadine, cisapride, astemizole, triazolam, midazolam, pimozide, or ergot derivatives. Inhibition of CYP3A4 by indinavir sulfate could result in elevated plasma concentrations of these drugs, potentially causing serious or life-threatening reactions.

WARNINGS

ALERT: Find out about medicines that should not be taken with indinavir sulfate. This statement is included on the product's bottle label.

NEPHROLITHIASIS/UROLITHIASIS

Nephrolithiasis/urolithiasis has occurred with indinavir sulfate therapy. The cumulative frequency of nephrolithiasis is substantially higher in pediatric patients (29%) than in adult patients (12.4%; range across individual trials: 4.7-34.4%). The cumulative frequency of nephrolithiasis events increases with increasing exposure to indinavir sulfate; however, the risk over time remains relatively constant. In some cases, nephrolithiasis/urolithiasis has been associated with renal insufficiency or acute renal failure, pyelonephritis with or without bacteremia. If signs or symptoms of nephrolithiasis/urolithiasis occur, (including flank pain, with or without hematuria or microscopic hematuria), temporary interruption (*e.g.,* 1-3 days) or discontinuation of therapy may be considered. **Adequate hydration is recommended in all patients treated with indinavir. (See ADVERSE REACTIONS and DOSAGE AND ADMINISTRATION, Nephrolithiasis/Urolithiasis.)**

HEMOLYTIC ANEMIA

Acute hemolytic anemia, including cases resulting in death, has been reported in patients treated with indinavir sulfate. Once a diagnosis is apparent, appropriate measures for the treatment of hemolytic anemia should be instituted, including discontinuation of indinavir sulfate.

HEPATITIS

Hepatitis including cases resulting in hepatic failure and death has been reported in patients treated with indinavir sulfate. Because the majority of these patients had confounding medical conditions and/or were receiving concomitant therapy(ies), a causal relationship between indinavir sulfate and these events has not been established.

HYPERGLYCEMIA

New onset diabetes mellitus, exacerbation of pre-existing diabetes mellitus and hyperglycemia have been reported during post-marketing surveillance in HIV-infected patients receiving protease inhibitor therapy. Some patients required either initiation or dose adjustments of insulin or oral hypoglycemic agents for treatment of these events. In some cases, diabetic ketoacidosis has occurred. In those patients who discontinued protease inhibitor therapy, hyperglycemia persisted in some cases. Because these events have been reported voluntarily during clinical practice, estimates of frequency cannot be made and a causal relationship between protease inhibitor therapy and these events has not been established.

DRUG INTERACTIONS

Concomitant use of indinavir sulfate with lovastatin or simvastatin is not recommended. Caution should be exercised if HIV protease inhibitors, including indinavir sulfate, are used concurrently with other HMG-CoA reductase inhibitors that are also metabolized by the CYP3A4 pathway (*e.g.,* atorvastatin or cerivastatin). The risk of myopathy including rhabdomyolysis may be increased when HIV protease inhibitors, including indinavir sulfate, are used in combination with these drugs.

Particular caution should be used when prescribing sildenafil in patients receiving indinavir. Coadministration of indinavir sulfate with sildenafil is expected to substantially increase sildenafil plasma concentrations and may result in an increase in sildenafil-associated adverse events, including hypotension, visual changes, and priapism (see DRUG INTERACTIONS and PRECAUTIONS, Information for the Patient, and the manufacturer's complete prescribing information for sildenafil).

Concomitant use of indinavir sulfate and St. John's wort (*Hypericum perforatum*) or products containing St. John's wort is not recommended. Coadministration of indinavir and St. John's wort has been shown to substantially decrease indinavir sulfate concentrations (see CLINICAL PHARMACOLOGY, Drug Interactions, Drugs That Should Not Be Coadministered With Indinavir Sulfate) and may lead to loss of virologic response and possible resistance to indinavir sulfate or to the class of protease inhibitors.

PRECAUTIONS

GENERAL

Indirect hyperbilirubinemia has occurred frequently during treatment with indinavir sulfate and has infrequently been associated with increases in serum transaminases (see also ADVERSE REACTIONS: Clinical Trials in Adults and Post-Marketing Experience). It is not known whether indinavir sulfate will exacerbate the physiologic hyperbilirubinemia seen in neonates. (See Pregnancy Category C.)

COEXISTING CONDITIONS

Patients with hemophilia: There have been reports of spontaneous bleeding in patients with hemophilia A and B treated with protease inhibitors. In some patients, additional factor VIII was required. In many of the reported cases, treatment with protease inhibitors was continued or restarted. A causal relationship between protease inhibitor therapy and these episodes has not been established. (See ADVERSE REACTIONS, Post-Marketing Experience.)

Patients with hepatic insufficiency due to cirrhosis: In these patients, the dosage of indinavir sulfate should be lowered because of decreased metabolism of indinavir sulfate (see DOSAGE AND ADMINISTRATION).

Patients with renal insufficiency: Patients with renal insufficiency have not been studied.

FAT REDISTRIBUTION

Redistribution/accumulation of body fat including central obesity, dorsocervical fat enlargement (buffalo hump), peripheral wasting, facial wasting, breast enlargement, and "cushingoid appearance" have been observed in patients receiving antiretroviral therapy. The mechanism and long-term consequences of these events are currently unknown. A causal relationship has not been established.

INFORMATION FOR THE PATIENT

A statement to patients and health care providers is included on the product's bottle label. **ALERT: Find out about medicines that should NOT be taken with indinavir sulfate.** A Patient Package Insert (PPI) for indinavir sulfate is available for patient information.

Indinavir sulfate is not a cure for HIV infection and patients may continue to develop opportunistic infections and other complications associated with HIV disease. The long-term effects of indinavir sulfate are unknown at this time. Indinavir has not been shown to reduce the risk of transmission of HIV to others through sexual contact or blood contamination.

Patients should be advised to remain under the care of a physician when using indinavir and should not modify or discontinue treatment without first consulting the physician. Therefore, if a dose is missed, patients should take the next dose at the regularly scheduled time and should not double this dose. Therapy with indinavir should be initiated and maintained at the recommended dosage.

Indinavir sulfate may interact with some drugs; therefore, patients should be advised to report to their doctor the use of any other prescription, non-prescription medication or herbal products, particularly St. John's wort.

For optimal absorption, indinavir sulfate should be administered without food but with water 1 hour before or 2 hours after a meal. Alternatively, indinavir sulfate may be administered with other liquids such as skim milk, juice, coffee, or tea, or with a light meal, *e.g.,* dry toast with jelly, juice, and coffee with skim milk and sugar; or corn flakes, skim milk and sugar (see CLINICAL PHARMACOLOGY, Pharmacokinetics, Effect of Food on Oral Absorption and DOSAGE AND ADMINISTRATION). Ingestion of indinavir sulfate with a meal high in calories, fat, and protein reduces the absorption of indinavir.

Patients receiving sildenafil should be advised that they may be at an increased risk of sildenafil-associated adverse events including hypotension, visual changes, and priapism, and should promptly report any symptoms to their doctors.

Patients should be informed that redistribution or accumulation of body fat may occur in patients receiving antiretroviral therapy and that the cause and long-term health effects of these conditions are not known at this time.

Indinavir sulfate capsules are sensitive to moisture. Patients should be informed that indinavir sulfate should be stored and used in the original container and the desiccant should remain in the bottle.

CARCINOGENESIS, MUTAGENESIS, AND IMPAIRMENT OF FERTILITY

Carcinogenicity studies were conducted in mice and rats. In mice, no increased incidence of any tumor type was observed. The highest dose tested in rats was 640 mg/kg/day; at this dose a statistically significant increased incidence of thyroid adenomas was seen only in male rats. At that dose, daily systemic exposure in rats was approximately 1.3 times higher than daily systemic exposure in humans. No evidence of mutagenicity or genotoxicity was observed in *in vitro* microbial mutagenesis (Ames) tests, *in vitro* alkaline elution assays for DNA breakage, *in vitro* and *in vivo* chromosomal aberration studies, and *in vitro* mammalian cell mutagenesis assays. No treatment-related effects on mating, fertility, or embryo survival were seen in female rats and no treatment-related effects on mating performance were seen in male rats at doses providing systemic exposure comparable to or slightly higher than that with the clinical dose. In addition, no treatment-related effects were observed in fecundity or fertility of untreated females mated to treated males.

PREGNANCY CATEGORY C

Developmental toxicity studies were performed in rabbits (at doses up to 240 mg/kg/day), dogs (at doses up to 80 mg/kg/day), and rats (at doses up to 640 mg/kg/day). The highest doses in these studies produced systemic exposures in these species comparable to or slightly greater than human exposure. No treatment-related external, visceral, or skeletal changes were observed in rabbits or dogs. No treatment-related external or visceral changes were observed in rats. Treatment-related increases over controls in the incidence of supernumerary ribs (at exposures at or below those in humans) and of cervical ribs (at exposures comparable to or slightly greater than those in humans) were seen in rats. In all 3 species, no treatment-related effects on embryonic/fetal survival or fetal weights were observed.

In rabbits, at a maternal dose of 240 mg/kg/day, no drug was detected in fetal plasma 1 hour after dosing. Fetal plasma drug levels 2 hours after dosing were approximately 3% of maternal plasma drug levels. In dogs, at a maternal dose of 80 mg/kg/day, fetal plasma drug levels were approximately 50% of maternal plasma drug levels both 1 and 2 hours after dosing. In rats, at maternal doses of 40 and 640 mg/kg/day, fetal plasma drug levels were approximately 10-15% and 10-20% of maternal plasma drug levels 1 and 2 hours after dosing, respectively.

Indinavir was administered to Rhesus monkeys during the third trimester of pregnancy (at doses up to 160 mg/kg twice daily) and to neonatal Rhesus monkeys (at doses up to 160 mg/kg twice daily). When administered to neonates, indinavir caused an exacerbation of the transient physiologic hyperbilirubinemia seen in this species after birth; serum bilirubin values were approximately 4-fold above controls at 160 mg/kg twice daily. A similar exacerbation did not occur in neonates after *in utero* exposure to indinavir during the third trimester of pregnancy. In Rhesus monkeys, fetal plasma drug levels were approximately 1-2% of maternal plasma drug levels approximately 1 hour after maternal dosing at 40, 80, or 160 mg/kg twice daily.

Hyperbilirubinemia has occurred during treatment with indinavir sulfate (see PRECAUTIONS and ADVERSE REACTIONS). It is unknown whether indinavir sulfate administered to the mother in the perinatal period will exacerbate physiologic hyperbilirubinemia in neonates.

There are no adequate and well-controlled studies in pregnant women. Indinavir sulfate should be used during pregnancy only if the potential benefit justifies the potential risk to the fetus.

Antiviral Pregnancy Registry: To monitor maternal-fetal outcomes of pregnant women exposed to indinavir sulfate, an Antiretroviral Pregnancy Registry has been established. Physicians are encouraged to register patients by calling 1-800-258-4263.

NURSING MOTHERS

Studies in lactating rats have demonstrated that indinavir is excreted in milk. Although it is not known whether indinavir sulfate is excreted in human milk, there exists the potential for adverse effects from indinavir in nursing infants. Mothers should be instructed to discontinue nursing if they are receiving indinavir sulfate. This is consistent with the recommendation by the US Public Health Service Centers for Disease Control and Prevention that HIV-infected mothers not breast-feed their infants to avoid risking postnatal transmission of HIV.

PEDIATRIC USE

The optimal dosing regimen for use of indinavir in pediatric patients has not been established. A dose of 500 mg/m^2 every 8 hours has been studied in uncontrolled studies of 70 children, 3-18 years of age. The pharmacokinetic profiles of indinavir at this dose were not comparable to profiles previously observed in adults receiving the recommended dose (see CLINICAL PHARMACOLOGY, Special Populations, Pediatric). Although viral suppression was observed in some of the 32 children who were followed on this regimen through 24 weeks, a substantially higher rate of nephrolithiasis was reported when compared to adult historical data (see WARNINGS, Nephrolithiasis/Urolithiasis). Physicians considering the use of indinavir in pediatric patients without other protease inhibitor options should be aware of the limited data available in this population and the increased risk of nephrolithiasis.

GERIATRIC USE

Clinical studies of indinavir sulfate did not include sufficient numbers of subjects aged 65 and over to determine whether they respond differently from younger subjects. In general, dose selection for an elderly patient should be cautious, reflecting the greater frequency of decreased hepatic, renal or cardiac function and of concomitant disease or other drug therapy.

DRUG INTERACTIONS

DELAVIRDINE

Due to an increase in indinavir plasma concentrations (preliminary results), a dosage reduction of indinavir should be considered when indinavir sulfate and delavirdine are coadministered. (See DOSAGE AND ADMINISTRATION, Concomitant Therapy, Delavirdine and CLINICAL PHARMACOLOGY, Drug Interactions, Drugs Requiring Dose Modification, Delavirdine.)

EFAVIRENZ

Due to a decrease in the plasma concentrations of indinavir, a dosage increase of indinavir is recommended when indinavir sulfate and efavirenz are coadministered. No adjustment of the dose of efavirenz is necessary when given with indinavir. (See DOSAGE AND ADMINISTRATION, Concomitant Therapy, Efavirenz and CLINICAL PHARMACOLOGY, Drug Interactions, Drugs Requiring Dose Modification, Efavirenz.)

ERECTILE DYSFUNCTION AGENTS

Particular caution should be used when prescribing sildenafil for patients receiving indinavir. The results of one published study in 6 HIV-infected subjects indicated that coadministration of indinavir (800 mg every 8 hours chronically) and sildenafil (25 mg as a single dose) resulted in increased indinavir and sildenafil concentrations. In 2 of the 6 subjects, prolonged clinical effects of sildenafil were noted for 72 hours after a single dose of sildenafil in combination with indinavir. Based on the results of this study, the dose of sildenafil should not exceed 25 mg in a 48 hour period. Patients receiving sildenafil should be advised that they are at an increased risk of sildenafil-associated adverse events including hypotension, visual changes, and priapism, and should promptly report any symptoms to their health care providers (see CLINICAL PHARMACOLOGY, Drug Interactions and WARNINGS).

ITRACONAZOLE

Itraconazole is an inhibitor of P450 3A4 that increases plasma concentrations of indinavir. Therefore, a dosage reduction of indinavir is recommended when indinavir sulfate and itraconazole are coadministered (see DOSAGE AND ADMINISTRATION, Concomitant Therapy, Itraconazole and CLINICAL PHARMACOLOGY, Drug Interactions, Drugs Requiring Dose Modification, Itraconazole).

KETOCONAZOLE

Ketoconazole is an inhibitor of P450 3A4 that increases plasma concentrations of indinavir. Therefore, a dosage reduction of indinavir is recommended when indinavir sulfate and ketoconazole are coadministered (see DOSAGE AND ADMINISTRATION, Concomitant Therapy, Ketoconazole and CLINICAL PHARMACOLOGY, Drug Interactions, Drugs Requiring Dose Modification, Ketoconazole).

RIFABUTIN

When rifabutin and indinavir sulfate are coadministered, there is an increase in the plasma concentrations of rifabutin and a decrease in the plasma concentrations of indinavir. A dosage reduction of rifabutin and a dosage increase of indinavir sulfate are necessary when rifabutin is coadministered with indinavir sulfate. The suggested dose adjustments are expected to result in rifabutin concentrations at least 50% higher than typically observed when rifabutin is administered alone at its usual dose (300 mg/day) and indinavir concentrations which may be slightly less than typically observed when indinavir is administered alone at its usual dose (800 mg every 8 hours). (See DOSAGE AND ADMINISTRATION, Concomitant Therapy, Rifabutin and CLINICAL PHARMACOLOGY, Drug Interactions, Drugs Requiring Dose Modification, Rifabutin.)

RIFAMPIN

Rifampin is a potent inducer of P450 3A4 that markedly diminishes plasma concentrations of indinavir. Therefore, indinavir sulfate and rifampin should not be coadministered (see CLINICAL PHARMACOLOGY, Drug Interactions, Drugs That Should Not Be Coadministered With Indinavir).

CALCIUM CHANNEL BLOCKERS

Calcium channel blockers are metabolized by CYP3A4 which is inhibited by indinavir. Coadministration of indinavir sulfate with calcium channel blockers may result in increased plasma concentrations of the calcium channel blockers which could increase or prolong their therapeutic and adverse effects.

OTHER

If indinavir sulfate and didanosine are administered concomitantly, they should be administered at least 1 hour apart on an empty stomach; a normal (acidic) gastric pH may be necessary for optimum absorption of indinavir, whereas acid rapidly degrades didanosine which is formulated with buffering agents to increase pH (consult the manufacturer's prescribing information for didanosine).

Interactions between indinavir and less potent CYP3A4 inducers than rifampin, such as phenobarbital, phenytoin, carbamazepine, and dexamethasone have not been studied. These agents should be used with caution if administered concomitantly with indinavir because decreased indinavir plasma concentrations may result.

ADVERSE REACTIONS

CLINICAL TRIALS IN ADULTS

Nephrolithiasis/urolithiasis, including flank pain with or without hematuria (including microscopic hematuria), has been reported in approximately 12.4% (301/2429; range across individual trials: 4.7-34.4%) of patients receiving indinavir sulfate at the recommended dose in clinical trials with a median follow-up of 47 weeks (range: 1 day to 242 weeks; 2238 patient-years follow-up). The cumulative frequency of nephrolithiasis events increases with duration of exposure to indinavir sulfate; however, the risk over time remains relatively constant. Of the patients treated with indinavir sulfate who developed nephrolithiasis/urolithiasis in clinical trials during the double-blind phase, 2.8% (7/246) were reported to develop hydronephrosis and 4.5% (11/246) underwent stent placement. Following the acute episode, 4.9% (12/246) of patients discontinued therapy. (See WARNINGS and DOSAGE AND ADMINISTRATION, Nephrolithiasis/Urolithiasis.)

Asymptomatic hyperbilirubinemia (total bilirubin ≥2.5 mg/dl), reported predominantly as elevated indirect bilirubin, has occurred in approximately 14% of patients treated with indinavir sulfate. In <1% this was associated with elevations in ALT or AST.

Hyperbilirubinemia and nephrolithiasis/urolithiasis occurred more frequently at doses exceeding 2.4 g/day compared to doses ≤2.4 g/day.

Clinical adverse experiences reported in ≥2% of patients treated with indinavir sulfate alone, indinavir sulfate in combination with zidovudine or zidovudine plus lamivudine, zidovudine alone, or zidovudine plus lamivudine are presented in TABLE 5A and TABLE 5B.

In Phase 1 and 2 controlled trials, the following adverse events were reported significantly more frequently by those randomized to nucleoside analogues: Rash, upper respiratory infection, dry skin, pharyngitis, taste perversion.

Selected laboratory abnormalities of severe or life-threatening intensity reported in patients treated with indinavir sulfate alone, indinavir sulfate in combination with zidovudine or zidovudine plus lamivudine, zidovudine alone, or zidovudine plus lamivudine are presented in TABLE 6A and TABLE 6B.

POST-MARKETING EXPERIENCE

Body as a Whole: Redistribution/accumulation of body fat (see PRECAUTIONS, Fat Redistribution).

Cardiovascular System: Cardiovascular disorders including myocardial infarction and angina pectoris; cerebrovascular disorder.

Digestive System: Liver function abnormalities; hepatitis including reports of hepatic failure (see WARNINGS); pancreatitis; jaundice; abdominal distention; dyspepsia.

Hematologic: Increased spontaneous bleeding in patients with hemophilia (see PRECAUTIONS); acute hemolytic anemia (see WARNINGS).

Endocrine/Metabolic: New onset diabetes mellitus, exacerbation of pre-existing diabetes mellitus, hyperglycemia (see WARNINGS).

Hypersensitivity: Anaphylactoid reactions; urticaria; vasculitis.

Musculoskeletal System: Arthralgia.

Nervous System/Psychiatric: Oral paresthesia; depression.

Skin and Skin Appendage: Rash including erythema multiforme and Stevens-Johnson Syndrome; hyperpigmentation; alopecia; ingrown toenails and/or paronychia; pruritus.

Urogenital System: Nephrolithiasis/urolithiasis; in some cases resulting in renal insufficiency or acute renal failure; pyelonephritis with or without bacteremia (see WARNINGS); interstitial nephritis sometimes with indinavir crystal deposits; in

TABLE 5A *Clinical Adverse Experiences Reported in ≥2% of Patients — Study 028: Considered Drug-Related and of Moderate or Severe Intensity*

Adverse Experience	Indinavir Sulfate (n=332)	Indinavir Sulfate + Zidovudine (n=332)	Zidovudine (n=332)
Body as a Whole			
Abdominal pain	16.6%	16.0%	12.0%
Asthenia/fatigue	2.1%	4.2%	3.6%
Fever	1.5%	1.5%	2.1%
Malaise	2.1%	2.7%	1.8%
Digestive System			
Nausea	11.7%	31.9%	19.6%
Diarrhea	3.3%	3.0%	2.4%
Vomiting	8.4%	17.8%	9.0%
Acid regurgitation	2.7%	5.4%	1.8%
Anorexia	2.7%	5.4%	3.0%
Appetite increase	2.1%	1.5%	1.2%
Dyspepsia	1.5%	2.7%	0.9%
Jaundice	1.5%	2.1%	0.3%
Hemic and Lymphatic System			
Anemia	0.6%	1.2%	2.1%
Musculoskeletal System			
Back pain	8.4%	4.5%	1.5%
Nervous System/Psychiatric			
Headache	5.4%	9.6%	6.0%
Dizziness	3.0%	3.9%	0.9%
Somnolence	2.4%	3.3%	3.3%
Skin and Skin Appendage			
Pruritus	4.2%	2.4%	1.8%
Rash	1.2%	0.6%	2.4%
Respiratory System			
Cough	1.5%	0.3%	0.6%
Difficulty breathing/dyspnea/ shortness of breath	0%	0.6%	0.3%
Urogenital System			
Nephrolithiasis/urolithiasis*	8.7%	7.8%	2.1%
Dysuria	1.5%	2.4%	0.3%
Special Senses			
Taste perversion	2.7%	8.4%	1.2%

* Including renal colic, and flank pain with and without hematuria.

TABLE 5B *Clinical Adverse Experiences Reported in ≥2% of Patients — Study ACTG 320 of Unknown Drug Relationship and of Severe or Life-Threatening Intensity*

Adverse Experience	Indinavir Sulfate + Zidovudine + Lamivudine (n=571)	Zidovudine + Lamivudine (n=575)
Body as a Whole		
Abdominal pain	1.9%	0.7%
Asthenia/fatigue	2.4%	4.5%
Fever	3.8%	3.0%
Malaise	0%	0%
Digestive System		
Nausea	2.8%	1.4%
Diarrhea	0.9%	1.2%
Vomiting	1.4%	1.4%
Acid regurgitation	0.4%	0%
Anorexia	0.5%	0.2%
Appetite increase	0%	0%
Dyspepsia	0%	0%
Jaundice	0%	0%
Hemic and Lymphatic System		
Anemia	2.4%	3.5%
Musculoskeletal System		
Back pain	0.9%	0.7%
Nervous System/Psychiatric		
Headache	2.4%	2.8%
Dizziness	0.5%	0.7%
Somnolence	0%	0%
Skin and Skin Appendage		
Pruritus	0.5%	0%
Rash	1.1%	0.5%
Respiratory System		
Cough	1.6%	1.0%
Difficulty breathing/dyspnea/ shortness of breath	1.8%	1.0%
Urogenital System		
Nephrolithiasis/urolithiasis*	2.6%	0.3%
Dysuria	0.4%	0.2%
Special Senses		
Taste perversion	0.2%	0%

* Including renal colic, and flank pain with and without hematuria.

some patients, the interstitial nephritis did not resolve following discontinuation of indinavir sulfate; crystalluria; dysuria.

LABORATORY ABNORMALITIES

Increased serum triglycerides; increased serum cholesterol.

TABLE 6A *Selected Laboratory Abnormalities of Severe or Life-Threatening Intensity — Reported in Study 028*

	Indinavir Sulfate (n=329)	Indinavir Sulfate + Zidovudine (n=320)	Zidovudine (n=330)
Hematology			
Decreased hemoglobin <7.0 g/dl	0.6%	0.9%	3.3%
Decreased platelet count <50 THS/mm^3	0.9%	0.9%	1.8%
Decreased neutrophils <0.75 THS/mm^3	2.4%	2.2%	6.7%
Blood Chemistry			
Increased ALT >500% ULN	4.9%	4.1%	3.0%
Increased AST >500% ULN	3.7%	2.8%	2.7%
Total serum bilirubin >250% ULN	11.9%	9.7%	0.6%
Increased serum amylase >200% ULN	2.1%	1.9%	1.8%
Increased glucose >250 mg/dl	0.9%	0.9%	0.6%
Increased creatinine >300% ULN	0%	0%	0.6%

ULN = Upper limit of the normal range.

TABLE 6B *Selected Laboratory Abnormalities of Severe or Life-Threatening Intensity — Reported in Study ACTG 320*

	Indinavir Sulfate + Zidovudine + Lamivudine (n=571)	Zidovudine + Lamivudine (n=575)
Hematology		
Decreased hemoglobin <7.0 g/dl	2.4%	3.5%
Decreased platelet count <50 THS/mm^3	0.2%	0.9%
Decreased neutrophils <0.75 THS/mm^3	5.1%	14.6%
Blood Chemistry		
Increased ALT >500% ULN	2.6%	2.6%
Increased AST >500% ULN	3.3%	2.8%
Total serum bilirubin >250% ULN	6.1%	1.4%
Increased serum amylase >200% ULN	0.9%	0.3%
Increased glucose >250 mg/dl	1.6%	1.9%
Increased creatinine >300% ULN	0.2%	0%

ULN = Upper limit of the normal range.

DOSAGE AND ADMINISTRATION

The recommended dosage of indinavir sulfate is 800 mg (usually **two** 400 mg capsules) orally every 8 hours.

Indinavir sulfate must be taken at intervals of 8 hours. For optimal absorption, indinavir sulfate should be administered without food but with water 1 hour before or 2 hours after a meal. Alternatively, indinavir sulfate may be administered with other liquids such as skim milk, juice, coffee, or tea, or with a light meal, *e.g.*, dry toast with jelly, juice, and coffee with skim milk and sugar; or corn flakes, skim milk and sugar. (See CLINICAL PHARMACOLOGY, Pharmacokinetics, Effect of Food on Oral Absorption.)

To ensure adequate hydration, it is recommended that adults drink at least 1.5 liters (approximately 48 ounces) of liquids during the course of 24 hours.

CONCOMITANT THERAPY

See CLINICAL PHARMACOLOGY, Drug Interactions and/or DRUG INTERACTIONS.

Delavirdine: Dose reduction of indinavir sulfate to 600 mg every 8 hours should be considered when administering delavirdine 400 mg 3 times a day.

Didanosine: If indinavir and didanosine are administered concomitantly, they should be administered at least 1 hour apart on an empty stomach (consult the manufacturer's product circular for didanosine).

Efavirenz: Dose increase of indinavir sulfate to 1000 mg every 8 hours is recommended when administering efavirenz concurrently (consult the manufacturer's product circular for efavirenz).

Itraconazole: Dose reduction of indinavir sulfate to 600 mg every 8 hours is recommended when administering itraconazole 200 mg twice daily concurrently.

Ketoconazole: Dose reduction of indinavir sulfate to 600 mg every 8 hours is recommended when administering ketoconazole concurrently.

Rifabutin: Dose reduction of rifabutin to half the standard dose (consult the manufacturer's product circular for rifabutin) and a dose increase of indinavir sulfate to 1000 mg (**three** 333 mg capsules) every 8 hours are recommended when rifabutin and indinavir sulfate are coadministered.

HEPATIC INSUFFICIENCY

The dosage of indinavir sulfate should be reduced to 600 mg every 8 hours in patients with mild-to-moderate hepatic insufficiency due to cirrhosis.

NEPHROLITHIASIS/UROLITHIASIS

In addition to adequate hydration, medical management in patients who experience nephrolithiasis/urolithiasis may include temporary interruption (*e.g.*, 1-3 days) or discontinuation of therapy.

HOW SUPPLIED

Crixivan capsules are supplied as follows:

100 mg: Semi-translucent white capsules coded "CRIXIVAN 100 mg" in green.

200 mg: Semi-translucent white capsules coded "CRIXIVAN 200 mg" in blue.

333 mg: Semi-translucent white capsules coded "CRIXIVAN 333 mg" in red and a radial red band on the body.

400 mg: Semi-translucent white capsules coded "CRIXIVAN 400 mg" in green.

STORAGE

Bottles

Store in a tightly-closed container at room temperature, 15-30°C (59-86°F). Protect from moisture.

Crixivan capsules are sensitive to moisture. Crixivan should be dispensed and stored in the original container. The desiccant should remain in the original bottle.

Unit-Dose Packages

Store at room temperature, 15-30°C (59-86°F). Protect from moisture.

PRODUCT LISTING - EQUIVALENTS NOT AVAILABLE

Package	Price	Product, Manufacturer	NDC
Capsule - Oral - 200 mg			
270's	$375.98	CRIXIVAN, Merck & Company Inc	00006-0571-42
Capsule - Oral - 333 mg			
135's	$341.14	CRIXIVAN, Merck & Company Inc	00006-0574-65
Capsule - Oral - 400 mg			
12's	$41.45	CRIXIVAN, Pharma Pac	52959-0507-12
18's	$48.01	CRIXIVAN, Merck & Company Inc	00006-0573-18
18's	$61.84	CRIXIVAN, Pharma Pac	52959-0507-18
24's	$77.28	CRIXIVAN, Pharma Pac	52959-0507-24
42's	$127.49	CRIXIVAN, Merck & Company Inc	00006-0573-42
90's	$273.19	CRIXIVAN, Merck & Company Inc	00006-0573-54
120's	$348.90	CRIXIVAN, Merck & Company Inc	00006-0573-40
180's	$546.37	CRIXIVAN, Merck & Company Inc	00006-0573-62

Indomethacin *(001532)*

For related information, see the comparative table section in Appendix A.

Categories: Ankylosing spondylitis; Arthritis, gouty; Arthritis, osteoarthritis; Arthritis, rheumatoid; Bursitis; Patent ductus arteriosus; Tendonitis, shoulder; FDA Approved 1965 Jun; Pregnancy Category B; Pregnancy Category D, 3rd Trimester

Drug Classes: Analgesics, non-narcotic; Nonsteroidal anti-inflammatory drugs

Brand Names: Indameth; **Indocin**; Indomethegan

Foreign Brand Availability: Amuno (Germany); Amuno Retard (Germany); Antalgin Dialicels (Mexico); Apo-Indomethacin (Canada); Areumatin (Indonesia); Argilex (Argentina); Arthrexin (Australia; South-Africa); Articulen (South-Africa); Artrinovo (Spain); Asimet (Malaysia); Benocid (Indonesia); Betacin (South-Africa); Bonidon (Costa-Rica; Dominican-Republic; Ecuador; El-Salvador; Guatemala; Nicaragua; Panama); Catlep (Japan); Chrono-Indocid (France); Confortid (Bahrain; Cyprus; Denmark; Egypt; Finland; Iran; Iraq; Jordan; Kuwait; Lebanon; Libya; Norway; Oman; Qatar; Republic-of-Yemen; Saudi-Arabia; Sweden; Switzerland; Syria; United-Arab-Emirates); Confortid Retard (Denmark); Confortid Retardkapseln (Switzerland); Dolazal (Netherlands); Dometin (Netherlands); Durametacin (Germany); Elmego Spray (Thailand); Elmetacin (Germany; New-Zealand); Flamaret (South-Africa); Grindocin (Mexico); IDC (Thailand); Idicin (India); IM-75 (Argentina); Imbrilon (England; Ireland); Imet (Benin; Burkina-Faso; Ethiopia; Gambia; Ghana; Guinea; Italy; Ivory-Coast; Kenya; Liberia; Malawi; Mali; Mauritania; Mauritius; Morocco; Niger; Nigeria; Senegal; Seychelles; Sierra-Leone; Sudan; Tanzania; Tunia; Uganda; Zambia; Zimbabwe); Inacid (Spain); Indacin (Japan); Indo (Malaysia); Indocap (India); Indocap S.R. (India); Indocid (Argentina; Australia; Austria; Bahrain; Belgium; Benin; Burkina-Faso; Canada; Cyprus; Denmark; Egypt; England; Ethiopia; France; Gambia; Ghana; Greece; Guinea; Hong-Kong; Iran; Iraq; Ivory-Coast; Jordan; Kenya; Kuwait; Lebanon; Liberia; Libya; Malawi; Malaysia; Mali; Mauritania; Mauritius; Mexico; Morocco; Netherlands; New-Zealand; Niger; Nigeria; Norway; Oman; Philippines; Portugal; Qatar; Republic-of-Yemen; Saudi-Arabia; Senegal; Seychelles; Sierra-Leone; South-Africa; Sudan; Switzerland; Syria; Taiwan; Tanzania; Thailand; Tunia; Uganda; United-Arab-Emirates; Zambia; Zimbabwe); Indocid R (Hong-Kong); Indocid-R (New-Zealand); Indocolir (Germany); Indocollyre (France; Israel; Korea); Indogesic (Bahrain; Cyprus; Egypt; Hong-Kong; Iran; Iraq; Jordan; Kuwait; Lebanon; Libya; Oman; Qatar; Republic-of-Yemen; Saudi-Arabia; Syria; United-Arab-Emirates); Indolag (Bahamas; Bahrain; Barbados; Belize; Benin; Bermuda; Burkina-Faso; Curacao; Cyprus; Egypt; Ethiopia; Gambia; Ghana; Guinea; Guyana; Iran; Iraq; Ivory-Coast; Jamaica; Jordan; Kenya; Kuwait; Lebanon; Liberia; Libya; Malawi; Mali; Mauritania; Mauritius; Morocco; Netherland-Antilles; Niger; Nigeria; Oman; Qatar; Republic-of-Yemen; Saudi-Arabia; Senegal; Seychelles; Sierra-Leone; Sudan; Surinam; Syria; Tanzania; Trinidad; Tunia; Uganda; United-Arab-Emirates; Zambia; Zimbabwe); Indolar SR (England); Indomecin (Colombia); Indomed (Israel); Indomed F (Thailand); Indomee (Sweden); Indomelan (Austria); Indometicina McKesson (Costa-Rica; Dominican-Republic; El-Salvador; Guatemala; Honduras; Nicaragua; Panama); Indometin (Finland); Indomin (Bahrain; Cyprus; Egypt; Iran; Iraq; Jordan; Kuwait; Lebanon; Libya; Oman; Qatar; Republic-of-Yemen; Saudi-Arabia; Syria; United-Arab-Emirates); Indono (Thailand); Indo-Phlogont (Germany); Indorem (Bahamas; Barbados; Belize; Bermuda; Curacao; Guyana; Jamaica; Netherland-Antilles; Surinam; Trinidad); Indo-Tablinen (Germany); Indotard (Israel); Indovis (Israel); Indoy (Taiwan); Indrenin (Czech-Republic); Indylon (Benin; Burkina-Faso; Ethiopia; Gambia; Ghana; Guinea; Ivory-Coast; Kenya; Liberia; Malawi; Mali; Mauritania; Mauritius; Morocco; Niger; Nigeria; Senegal; Seychelles; Sierra-Leone; Sudan; Tanzania; Tunia; Uganda; Zambia; Zimbabwe); Inflazon (Japan); Lauzit (Japan); Malival (Mexico); Malival AP (Mexico); Metacen (Italy); Methacin (Malaysia); Methocaps (South-Africa); Metindol (Thailand); Novomethacin (Canada); Reumacid (Bahrain; Cyprus; Egypt; Iran; Iraq; Jordan; Kuwait; Lebanon; Libya; Oman; Qatar; Republic-of-Yemen; Saudi-Arabia; Syria; United-Arab-Emirates); Reusin (Spain); Rheumacid (Benin; Burkina-Faso; Ethiopia; Gambia; Ghana; Guinea; Ivory-Coast; Kenya; Liberia; Malawi; Mali; Mauritania; Mauritius; Morocco; Niger; Nigeria; Senegal; Seychelles; Sierra-Leone; Sudan; Tanzania; Tunia; Uganda; Zambia; Zimbabwe); Rheumacin (New-Zealand); Rheumacin SR (New-Zealand); Salinac (Japan); Sidocin (Taiwan); Vonum (Germany)

Cost of Therapy: $60.71 (Osteoarthritis; Indocin; 25 mg; 3 capsules/day; 30 day supply)
$3.72 (Osteoarthritis; Generic Capsules; 25 mg; 3 capsules/day; 30 day supply)
$71.23 (Osteoarthritis; Indocin SR; 75 mg; 1 capsule/day; 30 day supply)
$21.40 (Osteoarthritit; Generic Extended Release Capsules; 75 mg; 1 capsule/day; 30 day supply)

DESCRIPTION

CAPSULES, ORAL SUSPENSION AND SUPPOSITORIES

Indomethacin cannot be considered a simple analgesic and should not be used in conditions other than those recommended under INDICATIONS AND USAGE.

Indomethacin is supplied in four dosage forms. Indomethacin capsules for oral administration contain either 25 or 50 mg of indomethacin and the following inactive ingredients: colloidal silicon dioxide, FD&C blue 1, FD&C red 3, gelatin, lactose, lecithin, magnesium stearate, and titanium dioxide. Indomethacin extended-release capsules for sustained release oral administration contain 75 mg of indomethacin and the following inactive ingredients: cellulose, confectioner's sugar, FD& C blue 1, FD&C blue 2, FD&C red 3, gelatin, hydroxypropyl methylcellulose, magnesium stearate, polyvinyl acetate-crotonic acid copolymer, starch, and titanium dioxide. Suspension indomethacin for oral use contains 25 mg of indomethacin per 5 ml, alcohol 1%, and sorbic acid 0.1% added as a preservative and the following inactive ingredients: antifoam AF emulsion, flavors, purified water, sodium hydroxide or hydrochloric acid to adjust pH, sorbitol solution, tragacanth. Suppositories indomethacin for rectal use contain 50 mg of indomethacin and the following inactive ingredients: butylated hydroxyanisole, butylated hydroxytoluene, edetic acid, glycerin, polyethylene glycol 3350, polyethylene glycol 8000 and sodium chloride.

Indomethacin is a non-steroidal anti-inflammatory indole derivative designated chemically as 1-(4-chlorobenzoyl)-5-methoxy-2-methyl-1*H*-indole-3-acetic acid. Indomethacin is practically insoluble in water and sparingly soluble in alcohol. It has a pKa of 4.5 and is stable in neutral or slightly acidic media and decomposes in strong alkali. The suspension has a pH of 4.0-5.0.

Storage

Store capsules and extended-release capsules below 30°C (86°F). *Protect from light.* Store container in carton until contents have been used.

Store oral suspension indomethacin below 30°C (86°F). Avoid temperatures above 50°C (122°F). Protect from freezing.

Store suppositories indomethacin below 30°C (86°F). Avoid transient temperatures above 40°C (104°F).

INTRAVENOUS

Sterile indomethacin IV (indomethacin sodium trihydrate) for intravenous administration is lyophilized indomethacin sodium trihydrate. Each vial contains indomethacin sodium trihydrate equivalent to 1 mg indomethacin as a white to yellow lyophilized powder or plug. Variations in the size of the lyophilized plug and the intensity of color have no relationship to the quality or amount of indomethacin present in the vial.

Indomethacin sodium trihydrate is designated chemically as 1-(4-chlorobenzoyl)-5-methoxy-2-methyl-1*H*-indole-3-acetic acid, sodium salt, trihydrate. Its molecular weight is 433.82. Its empirical formula is $C_{19}H_{15}ClNNaO_4 \cdot 3H_2O$.

CLINICAL PHARMACOLOGY

CAPSULES, ORAL SUSPENSION AND SUPPOSITORIES

Indomethacin is a non-steroidal drug with anti-inflammatory, antipyretic and analgesic properties. Its mode of action, like that of other anti-inflammatory drugs, is not known. However, its therapeutic action is not due to pituitary-adrenal stimulation.

Indomethacin is a potent inhibitor of prostaglandin synthesis *in vitro.* Concentrations are reached during therapy which have been demonstrated to have an effect *in vivo* as well. Prostaglandins sensitize afferent nerves and potentiate the action of bradykinin in inducing pain in animal models. Moreover, prostaglandins are known to be among the mediators of inflammation. Since indomethacin is an inhibitor of prostaglandin synthesis, its mode of action may be due to a decrease of prostaglandins in peripheral tissues.

Indomethacin has been shown to be an effective anti-inflammatory agent, appropriate for long-term use in rheumatoid arthritis, ankylosing spondylitis, and osteoarthritis.

Indomethacin affords relief of symptoms; it does not alter the progressive course of the underlying disease.

Indomethacin suppresses inflammation in rheumatoid arthritis as demonstrated by relief of pain, and reduction of fever, swelling and tenderness. Improvement in patients treated with indomethacin for rheumatoid arthritis has been demonstrated by a reduction in joint swelling, average number of joints involved, and morning stiffness; by increased motility as demonstrated by a decrease in walking time; and by improved functional capability as demonstrated by an increase in grip strength.

Indomethacin has been reported to diminish basal and CO_2 stimulated cerebral blood flow in healthy volunteers following acute oral and intravenous administration. In one study after 1 week of treatment with orally administered indomethacin, this effect on basal cerebral blood flow had disappeared. The clinical significance of this effect has not been established.

Indomethacin capsules have been found effective in relieving the pain, reducing the fever, swelling, redness, and tenderness of acute gouty arthritis. Indomethacin capsules rather than indomethacin extended-release capsules are recommended for treatment of acute gouty arthritis (see INDICATIONS AND USAGE).

Following single oral doses of indomethacin capsules 25 or 50 mg, indomethacin is readily absorbed, attaining peak plasma concentrations of about 1 and 2 μg/ml, respectively, at about 2 hours. Orally administered indomethacin capsules are virtually 100% bioavailable, with 90% of the dose absorbed within 4 hours.

Indomethacin extended-release capsules 75 mg are designed to release 25 mg of the drug initially and the remaining 50 mg over approximately 12 hours (90% of dose absorbed by 12 hours). When measured over a 24 hour period, the cumulative amount and time-course of indomethacin absorption from a single indomethacin extended-release capsule are comparable to those of 3 doses of 25 mg indomethacin capsules given at 4-6 hour intervals.

Plasma concentrations of indomethacin fluctuate less and are more sustained following administration of indomethacin extended-release capsules than following administration of 25 mg indomethacin capsules given at 4-6 hour intervals. In multiple-dose comparisons, the mean daily steady-state plasma level of indomethacin attained with daily administration of indomethacin extended-release capsules 75 mg was indistinguishable from that following indomethacin capsules 25 mg given at 0, 6 and 12 hours daily. However, there was a significant difference in indomethacin plasma levels between the two dosage regimens especially after 12 hours.

Controlled clinical studies of safety and efficacy in patients with osteoarthritis have shown that 1 capsule indomethacin extended-release was clinically comparable to one 25 mg capsule indomethacin tid; and in controlled clinical studies in patients with rheumatoid arthritis, 1 indomethacin extended-release capsule taken in the morning and 1 in the evening were clinically indistinguishable from one 50 mg indomethacin capsule tid.

Indomethacin is eliminated via renal excretion, metabolism, and biliary excretion. Indomethacin undergoes appreciable enterohepatic circulation. The mean half-life of indomethacin is estimated to be about 4.5 hours. With a typical therapeutic regimen of 25 mg or 50 mg tid, the steady-state plasma concentrations of indomethacin are an average 1.4 times those following the first dose.

The rate of absorption is more rapid from the rectal suppository than from indomethacin capsules. Ordinarily, therefore, the total amount absorbed from the suppository would be expected to be at least equivalent to the capsule. In controlled clinical trials, however, the amount of indomethacin absorbed was found to be somewhat less (80-90%) than that absorbed from indomethacin capsules. This is probably because some subjects did not retain the material from the suppository for the 1 hour necessary to assure complete absorption. Since the suppository dissolves rather quickly rather than melting slowly, it is seldom recovered in recognizable form if the patient retains the suppository for more than a few minutes.

Indomethacin exists in the plasma as the parent drug and its desmethyl, desbenzoyl, and desmethyl-desbenzoyl metabolites, all in the unconjugated form. About 60% of an oral dosage is recovered in urine as drug and metabolites (26% as indomethacin and its glucuronide), and 33% is recovered in feces (1.5% as indomethacin).

About 99% of indomethacin is bound to protein in plasma over the expected range of therapeutic plasma concentrations. Indomethacin has been found to cross the blood-brain barrier and the placenta.

In a gastroscopic study in 45 healthy subjects, the number of gastric mucosal abnormalities was significantly higher in the group receiving indomethacin capsules than in the group taking indomethacin suppositories or placebo.

In a double-blind comparative clinical study involving 175 patients with rheumatoid arthritis, however, the incidence of upper gastrointestinal adverse effects with indomethacin suppositories or capsules was comparable. The incidence of lower gastrointestinal adverse effects was greater in the suppository group.

INTRAVENOUS

Although the exact mechanism of action through which indomethacin causes closure of a patent ductus arteriosus is not known, it is believed to be through inhibition of prostaglandin synthesis. Indomethacin has been shown to be a potent inhibitor of prostaglandin synthesis, both *in vitro* and *in vivo*. In human newborns with certain congenital heart malformations, PGE 1 dilates the ductus arteriosus. In fetal and newborn lambs, E type prostaglandins have also been shown to maintain the patency of the ductus, and as in human newborns, indomethacin causes its constriction.

Studies in healthy young animals and in premature infants with patent ductus arteriosus indicated that, after the first dose of intravenous indomethacin, there was a transient reduction in cerebral blood flow velocity and cerebral blood flow. The clinical significance of this effect has not been established.

In double-blind placebo-controlled studies of indomethacin IV in 460 small pre-term infants, weighing 1750 g or less, the infants treated with placebo had a ductus closure rate after 48 hours of 25-30%, whereas those treated with indomethacin IV had a 75-80% closure rate. In one of these studies, a multicenter study, involving 405 pre-term infants, later reopening of the ductus arteriosus occurred in 26% of infants treated with indomethacin IV, however, 70% of these closed subsequently without the need for surgery or additional indomethacin.

Pharmacokinetics and Metabolism

The disposition of indomethacin following intravenous administration (0.2 mg/kg) in preterm neonates with patent ductus arteriosus has not been extensively evaluated. Even though the plasma half-life of indomethacin was variable among premature infants, it was shown to vary inversely with postnatal age and weight. In one study, of 28 infants who could be evaluated, the plasma half-life in those infants less than 7 days old averaged 20 hours (range: 3-60 hours, n=18). In infants older than 7 days, the mean plasma half-life of indomethacin was 12 hours (range: 4-38 hours, n=10). Grouping the infants by weight, mean plasma half-life in those weighing less than 1000 g was 21 hours (range: 9-60 hours, n=10); in those infants weighing more than 1000 g, the mean plasma half-life was 15 hours (range: 3-52 hours, n=18).

Following IV administration in adults, indomethacin is eliminated via renal excretion, metabolism, and biliary excretion. Indomethacin undergoes appreciable enterohepatic circulation. The mean plasma half-life of indomethacin is 4.5 hours. In the absence of enterohepatic circulation, it is 90 minutes.

In adults, about 99% of indomethacin is bound to protein in plasma over the expected range of therapeutic plasma concentrations. The percent bound in neonates has not been studied. In controlled trials in premature infants, however, no evidence of bilirubin displacement has been observed as evidenced by increased incidence of bilirubin encephalopathy (kernicterus).

INDICATIONS AND USAGE

CAPSULES, ORAL SUSPENSION AND SUPPOSITORIES

Indomethacin has been found effective in active stages of the following:

1. Moderate to severe rheumatoid arthritis including acute flares of chronic disease.
2. Moderate to severe ankylosing spondylitis.
3. Moderate to severe osteoarthritis.
4. Acute painful shoulder (bursitis and/or tendinitis).
5. Acute gouty arthritis.

Indomethacin extended-release capsules are recommended for all of the indications for indomethacin capsules except acute gouty arthritis.

Indomethacin may enable the reduction of steroid dosage in patients receiving steroids for the more severe forms of rheumatoid arthritis. In such instances the steroid dosage should be reduced slowly and the patients followed very closely for any possible adverse effects.

The use of indomethacin in conjunction with aspirin or other salicylates is not recommended. Controlled clinical studies have shown that the combined use of indomethacin and aspirin does not produce any greater therapeutic effect than the use of indomethacin alone. Furthermore, in one of these clinical studies, the incidence of gastrointestinal side effects was significantly increased with combined therapy (see DRUG INTERACTIONS).

INTRAVENOUS

Indomethacin IV is indicated to close a hemodynamically significant patent ductus arteriosus in premature infants weighing between 500 and 1750 g when after 48 hours usual medical management (*e.g.,* fluid restriction, diuretics, digitalis, respiratory support, etc.) is ineffective. Clear-cut clinical evidence of a hemodynamically significant patent ductus arteriosus should be present, such as respiratory distress, a continuous murmur, a hyperactive precordium, cardiomegaly and pulmonary plethora on chest x-ray.

NON-FDA APPROVED INDICATIONS

While not an FDA approved indication, indomethacin is also used in the management of cluster headaches. Indomethacin may also be opiate and steroid sparing. Indomethacin has also been used to treat Sweet's syndrome (acute febrile neutrophilic dermatosis).

CONTRAINDICATIONS

CAPSULES, ORAL SUSPENSION AND SUPPOSITORIES

Indomethacin should not be used in:

Patients who are hypersensitive to this product.

Patients in whom acute asthmatic attacks, urticaria, or rhinitis are precipitated by aspirin or other non-steroidal anti-inflammatory agents.

Indomethacin suppositories are contraindicated in patients with a history of proctitis or recent rectal bleeding.

INTRAVENOUS

Indomethacin IV Is Contraindicated in:

Infants with proven or suspected infection that is untreated.

Infants who are bleeding, especially those with active intracranial hemorrhage or gastrointestinal bleeding.

Infants with thrombocytopenia.

Infants with coagulation defects.

Infants with or who are suspected of having necrotizing enterocolitis.

Infants with significant impairment of renal function.

Infants with congenital heart disease in whom patency of the ductus arteriosus is necessary for satisfactory pulmonary or systemic blood flow (*e.g.,* pulmonary atresia, severe tetralogy of Fallot, severe coarctation of the aorta).

WARNINGS

CAPSULES, ORAL SUSPENSION AND SUPPOSITORIES

General

Because of the variability of the potential of indomethacin to cause adverse reactions in the individual patient, the following are strongly recommended:

1. The lowest possible effective dose for the individual patient should be prescribed. Increased dosage tends to increase adverse effects, particularly in doses over 150-200 mg/day, without corresponding increase in clinical benefits.
2. Careful instructions to, and observations of, the individual patient are essential to the prevention of serious adverse reactions. As advancing years appear to increase the possibility of adverse reactions, indomethacin should be used with greater care in the aged.
3. Effectiveness of indomethacin in pediatric patients has not been established. Indomethacin should not be prescribed for pediatric patients 14 years of age and younger unless toxicity or lack of efficacy associated with other drugs warrants the risk. In experience with more than 900 pediatric patients reported in the literature or to Merck who were treated with indomethacin capsules, side effects in pediatric patients were comparable to those reported in adults. Experience in pediatric patients has been confined to the use of indomethacin capsules. If a decision is made to use indomethacin for pediatric patients 2 years of age or older, such patients should be monitored closely and periodic assessment of liver function is recommended. There have been cases of hepatotoxicity reported in pediatric patients with juvenile rheumatoid arthritis, including fatalities. If indomethacin treatment is instituted, a suggested starting dose is 2 mg/kg/day given in divided doses. Maximum daily dosage should not exceed 4 mg/kg/day or 150-200 mg/day, whichever is less. As symptoms subside, the total daily dosage should be reduced to the lowest level required to control symptoms, or the drug should be discontinued.
4. If indomethacin extended-release capsules are used for initial therapy or during dosage adjustment, observe the patient closely (see DOSAGE AND ADMINISTRATION).

Gastrointestinal Effects

Single or multiple ulcerations, including perforation and hemorrhage of the esophagus, stomach, duodenum or small and large intestine, have been reported to occur with indomethacin. Fatalities have been reported in some instances. Rarely, intestinal ulceration has been associated with stenosis and obstruction.

Gastrointestinal bleeding without obvious ulcer formation and perforation of pre-existing sigmoid lesions (diverticulum, carcinoma, etc.) have occurred. Increased abdominal pain in ulcerative colitis patients or the development of ulcerative colitis and regional ileitis have been reported to occur rarely.

Because of the occurrence, and at times severity, of gastrointestinal reactions to indomethacin, the prescribing physician must be continuously alert for any sign or symptom signaling a possible gastrointestinal reaction. The risks of continuing therapy with indomethacin in the face of such symptoms must be weighed against the possible benefits to the individual patient.

Indomethacin should not be given to patients with active gastrointestinal lesions or with a history of recurrent gastrointestinal lesions except under circumstances which warrant the very high risk and where patients can be monitored very closely.

The gastrointestinal effects may be reduced by giving indomethacin capsules or indomethacin extended-release capsules immediately after meals, with food, or with antacids.

Risk of GI Ulcerations, Bleeding and Perforation With NSAID Therapy

Serious gastrointestinal toxicity such as bleeding, ulceration, and perforation, can occur at any time, with or without warning symptoms, in patients treated chronically with NSAID therapy. Although minor upper gastrointestinal problems, such as dyspepsia, are common, usually developing early in therapy, physicians should remain alert for ulceration and bleeding in patients treated chronically with NSAIDs even in the absence of previous GI tract symptoms. In patients observed in clinical trials of several months to 2 years duration, symptomatic upper GI ulcers, gross bleeding or perforation appear to occur in approximately 1% of patients treated for 3-6 months, and in about 2-4% of patients treated for 1 year. Physicians should inform patients about the signs and/or symptoms of serious GI toxicity and what steps to take if they occur.

Studies to date have not identified any subset of patients not at risk of developing peptic ulceration and bleeding. Except for a prior history of serious GI events and other risk factors known to be associated with peptic ulcer disease, such as alcoholism, smoking, etc., no risk factors (*e.g.*, age, sex) have been associated with increased risk. Elderly or debilitated patients seem to tolerate ulceration or bleeding less well than other individuals and most spontaneous reports of fatal GI events are in this population. Studies to date are inconclusive concerning the relative risk of various NSAIDs in causing such reactions. High doses of any NSAID probably carry a greater risk of these reactions, although controlled clinical trials showing this do not exist in most cases. In considering the use of relatively large doses (within the recommended dosage range), sufficient benefit should be anticipated to offset the potential increased risk of GI toxicity.

Renal Effects

As with other non-steroidal anti-inflammatory drugs, long term administration of indomethacin to animals has resulted in renal papillary necrosis and other abnormal renal pathology. In humans, there have been reports of acute interstitial nephritis with hematuria, proteinuria, and occasionally nephrotic syndrome.

A second form of renal toxicity has been seen in patients with prerenal and renal conditions leading to a reduction in renal blood flow or blood volume, where the renal prostaglandins have a supportive role in the maintenance of renal perfusion. In these patients administration of an NSAID may cause a dose dependent reduction in prostaglandin formation and may precipitate overt renal decompensation. Patients at greatest risk of this reaction are those with conditions such as renal or hepatic dysfunction, diabetes mellitus, advanced age, extracellular volume depletion from any cause, congestive heart failure, septicemia, pyelonephritis, or concomitant use of any nephrotoxic drug. Indomethacin or other NSAIDs should be given with caution and renal function should be monitored in any patient who may have reduced renal reserve. Discontinuation of NSAID therapy is typically followed by recovery to the pretreatment state.

Increases in serum potassium concentration, including hyperkalemia, have been reported, even in some patients without renal impairment. In patients with normal renal function, these effects have been attributed to a hyporeninemic-hypoaldosteronism state (see PRECAUTIONS and DRUG INTERACTIONS).

Since indomethacin is eliminated primarily by the kidneys, patients with significantly impaired renal function should be closely monitored; a lower daily dosage should be anticipated to avoid excessive drug accumulation.

Ocular Effects

Corneal deposits and retinal disturbances, including those of the macula, have been observed in some patients who had received prolonged therapy with indomethacin. The prescribing physician should be alert to the possible association between the changes noted and indomethacin. It is advisable to discontinue therapy if such changes are observed. Blurred vision may be a significant symptom and warrants a thorough ophthalmological examination. Since these changes may be asymptomatic, ophthalmologic examination at periodic intervals is desirable in patients where therapy is prolonged.

Central Nervous System Effects

Indomethacin may aggravate depression or other psychiatric disturbances, epilepsy, and parkinsonism, and should be used with considerable caution in patients with these conditions. If severe CNS adverse reactions develop, indomethacin should be discontinued.

Indomethacin may cause drowsiness; therefore, patients should be cautioned about engaging in activities requiring mental alertness and motor coordination, such as driving a car. Indomethacin may also cause headache. Headache which persists despite dosage reduction requires cessation of therapy with indomethacin.

Use in Pregnancy and the Neonatal Period

Indomethacin is not recommended for use in pregnant women, since safety for use has not been established. The known effects of indomethacin and other drugs of this class on the human fetus during the third trimester of pregnancy include: constriction of the ductus arteriosus prenatally, tricuspid incompetence, and pulmonary hypertension; non-closure of the ductus arteriosus postnatally which may be resistant to medical management; myocardial degenerative changes, platelet dysfunction with resultant bleeding, intracranial bleeding, renal dysfunction or failure, renal injury/dysgenesis which may result in prolonged or permanent renal failure, oligohydramnios, gastrointestinal bleeding or perforation, and increased risk of necrotizing enterocolitis.

Teratogenic studies were conducted in mice and rats at dosages of 0.5, 1.0, 2.0, and 4.0 mg/kg/day. Except for retarded fetal ossification at 4 mg/kg/day considered secondary to the decreased average fetal weights, no increase in fetal malformations was observed as compared with control groups. Other studies in mice reported in the literature using higher doses (5-15 mg/kg/day) have described maternal toxicity and death, increased fetal resorptions, and fetal malformations. Comparable studies in rodents using high doses of aspirin have shown similar maternal and fetal effects.

As with other non-steroidal anti-inflammatory agents which inhibit prostaglandin synthesis, indomethacin has been found to delay parturition in rats.

In rats and mice, 4.0 mg/kg/day given during the last three days of gestation caused a decrease in maternal weight gain and some maternal and fetal deaths. An increased incidence of neuronal necrosis in the diencephalon in the live-born fetuses was observed. At 2.0 mg/kg/day, no increase in neuronal necrosis was observed as compared to the control groups. Administration of 0.5 or 4.0 mg/kg/day during the first three days of life did not cause an increase in neuronal necrosis at either dose level.

Use in Nursing Mothers

Indomethacin is excreted in the milk of lactating mothers. Indomethacin is not recommended for use in nursing mothers.

INTRAVENOUS

Gastrointestinal Effects

In the collaborative study, major gastrointestinal bleeding was no more common in those infants receiving indomethacin than in those infants on placebo. However, minor gastrointestinal bleeding (*i.e.*, chemical detection of blood in the stool) was more commonly noted in those infants treated with indomethacin. Severe gastrointestinal effects have been reported in adults with various arthritic disorders treated chronically with oral indomethacin. (For further information, see package circular for indomethacin capsules).

Central Nervous System Effects

Prematurity per se, is associated with an increased incidence of spontaneous intraventricular hemorrhage. Because indomethacin may inhibit platelet aggregation, the potential for intraventricular bleeding may be increased. However, in the large multi-center study of indomethacin IV (see CLINICAL PHARMACOLOGY), the incidence of intraventricular hemorrhage in babies treated with indomethacin IV was not significantly higher than in the control infants.

Renal Effects

Indomethacin IV may cause significant reduction in urine output (50% or more) with concomitant elevations of blood urea nitrogen and creatinine, and reductions in glomerular filtration rate and creatinine clearance. These effects in most infants are transient, disappearing with cessation of therapy with indomethacin IV. However, because adequate renal function can depend upon renal prostaglandin synthesis, indomethacin IV may precipitate renal insufficiency, including acute renal failure, especially in infants with other conditions that may adversely affect renal function (*e.g.*, extracellular volume depletion from any cause, congestive heart failure, sepsis, concomitant use of any nephrotoxic drug, hepatic dysfunction). When significant suppression of urine volume occurs after a dose of indomethacin IV, no additional dose should be given until the urine output returns to normal levels.

Indomethacin IV in pre-term infants may suppress water excretion to a greater extent than sodium excretion. When this occurs, a significant reduction in serum sodium values (*i.e.*, hyponatremia) may result. Infants should have serum electrolyte determinations done during therapy with indomethacin IV. Renal function and serum electrolytes should be monitored (see PRECAUTIONS, DRUG INTERACTIONS, and DOSAGE AND ADMINISTRATION).

PRECAUTIONS

CAPSULES, ORAL SUSPENSION AND SUPPOSITORIES

General

Non-steroidal anti-inflammatory drugs, including indomethacin, may mask the usual signs and symptoms of infection. Therefore, the physician must be continually on the alert for this and should use the drug with extra care in the presence of existing infection.

Fluid retention and peripheral edema have been observed in some patients taking indomethacin. Therefore, as with other non-steroidal anti-inflammatory drugs, indomethacin should be used with caution in patients with cardiac dysfunction, hypertension, or other conditions predisposing to fluid retention.

In a study of patients with severe heart failure and hyponatremia, indomethacin was associated with significant deterioration of circulatory hemodynamics, presumably due to inhibition of prostaglandin dependent compensatory mechanisms.

Indomethacin, like other non-steroidal anti-inflammatory agents, can inhibit platelet aggregation. This effect is of shorter duration than that seen with aspirin and usually disappears within 24 hours after discontinuation of indomethacin. Indomethacin has been shown to prolong bleeding time (but within the normal range) in normal subjects. Because this effect may be exaggerated in patients with underlying hemostatic defects, indomethacin should be used with caution in persons with coagulation defects.

As with other non-steroidal anti-inflammatory drugs, borderline elevation of one or more liver tests may occur in up to 15% of patients. These abnormalities may progress, may remain essentially unchanged, or may be transient with continued therapy. The SGPT (ALT) test is probably the most sensitive indicator of liver dysfunction. Meaningful (3 times the upper limit of normal) elevations of SGPT or SGOT (AST) occurred in controlled clinical trials in less than 1% of patients. A patient with symptoms and/or signs suggesting liver dysfunction, or in whom an abnormal liver test has occurred, should be evaluated for evidence of the development of more severe hepatic reaction while on therapy with indomethacin. Severe hepatic reactions, including jaundice and cases of fatal hepatitis, have been reported with indomethacin as with other non-steroidal anti-inflammatory drugs. Although such reactions are rare, if abnormal liver tests persist or worsen, if clinical signs and symptoms consistent with liver disease develop, or if systemic manifestations occur (*e.g.*, eosinophilia, rash, etc.), indomethacin should be discontinued.

Information for the Patient

Indomethacin, like other drugs of its class, is not free of side effects. The side effects of these drugs can cause discomfort and, rarely, there are more serious side effects such as gastrointestinal bleeding, which may result in hospitalization and even fatal outcomes.

NSAIDs are often essential agents in the management of arthritis; but they also may be commonly employed for conditions which are less serious.

Physicians may wish to discuss with their patients the potential risks (see WARNINGS, PRECAUTIONS and ADVERSE REACTIONS) and likely benefits of NSAID treatment, particularly when the drugs are used for less serious conditions where treatment without NSAIDs may represent an acceptable alternative to both the patient and physician.

Laboratory Tests

Because serious GI tract ulceration and bleeding can occur without warning symptoms, physicians should follow chronically treated patients for the signs and symptoms of ulceration and bleeding and should inform them of the importance of this follow-up (see WARNINGS, Risk of GI Ulcerations, Bleeding and Perforation With NSAID Therapy).

Carcinogenesis, Mutagenesis, and Impairment of Fertility

In an 81 week chronic oral toxicity study in the rat at doses up to 1 mg/kg/day, indomethacin had no tumorigenic effect.

Indomethacin produced no neoplastic or hyperplastic changes related to treatment in carcinogenic studies in the rat (dosing period 73-110 weeks) and the mouse (dosing period 62-88 weeks) at doses up to 1.5 mg/kg/day.

Indomethacin did not have any mutagenic effect in *in vitro* bacterial tests (Ames test and *E. coli* with or without metabolic activation) and a series of *in vivo* tests including the host-mediated assay, sex-linked recessive lethals in *Drosophila,* and the micronucleus test in mice.

Indomethacin at dosage levels up to 0.5 mg/kg/day had no effect on fertility in mice in a two generation reproduction study or a two litter reproduction study in rats.

Pediatric Use

Effectiveness in pediatric patients 14 years of age and younger has not been established (see WARNINGS).

INTRAVENOUS

General

Indomethacin may mask the usual signs and symptoms of infection. Therefore, the physician must be continually on the alert for this and should use the drug with extra care in the presence of existing controlled infection.

Severe hepatic reactions have been reported in adults treated chronically with oral indomethacin for arthritic disorders. (For further information, see package circular for capsules, indomethacin). If clinical signs and symptoms consistent with liver disease develop in the neonate, or if systemic manifestations occur, indomethacin IV should be discontinued.

Indomethacin IV may inhibit platelet aggregation. In one small study, platelet aggregation was grossly abnormal after indomethacin therapy (given orally to premature infants to close the ductus arteriosus). Platelet aggregation returned to normal by the tenth day. Premature infants should be observed for signs of bleeding.

The drug should be administered carefully to avoid extravascular injection or leakage as the solution may be irritating to tissue.

Neonatal Effects

In rats and mice, oral indomethacin 4.0 mg/kg/day given during the last three days of gestation caused a decrease in maternal weight gain and some maternal and fetal deaths. An increased incidence of neuronal necrosis in the diencephalon in the live-born fetuses was observed. At 2.0 mg/kg/day, no increase in neuronal necrosis was observed as compared to the control groups. Administration of 0.5 or 4.0 mg/kg/day during the first three days of life did not cause an increase in neuronal necrosis at either dose level.

Pregnant rats, given 2.0 mg/kg/day and 4.0 mg/kg/day during the last trimester of gestation, delivered offspring whose pulmonary blood vessels were both reduced in number and excessively muscularized. These findings are similar to those observed in the syndrome of persistent pulmonary hypertension of the newborn.

DRUG INTERACTIONS

CAPSULES, ORAL SUSPENSION AND SUPPOSITORIES

In normal volunteers receiving indomethacin, the administration of diflunisal decreased the renal clearance and significantly increased the plasma levels of indomethacin. In some patients, combined use of indomethacin and diflunisal has been associated with fatal gastrointestinal hemorrhage. Therefore, diflunisal and indomethacin should not be used concomitantly.

In a study in normal volunteers, it was found that chronic concurrent administration of 3.6 g of aspirin per day decreases indomethacin blood levels approximately 20%.

The concomitant use of indomethacin with other NSAIDs is not recommended due to the increased possibility of gastrointestinal toxicity, with little or no increase in efficacy.

Clinical studies have shown that indomethacin does not influence the hypoprothrombinemia produced by anticoagulants. However, when any additional drug, including indomethacin, is added to the treatment of patients on anticoagulant therapy, the patients should be observed for alterations of the prothrombin time.

When indomethacin is given to patients receiving probenecid, the plasma levels of indomethacin are likely to be increased. Therefore, a lower total daily dosage of indomethacin may produce a satisfactory therapeutic effect. When increases in the dose of indomethacin are made, they should be made carefully and in small increments.

Caution should be used if indomethacin is administered simultaneously with methotrexate. Indomethacin has been reported to decrease the tubular secretion of methotrexate and to potentiate its toxicity.

Administration of non-steroidal anti-inflammatory drugs concomitantly with cyclosporine has been associated with an increase in cyclosporine-induced toxicity, possibly due to decreased synthesis of renal prostacyclin. NSAIDs should be used with caution in patients taking cyclosporine, and renal function should be carefully monitored.

Indomethacin capsules 50 mg tid produced a clinically relevant elevation of plasma lithium and reduction in renal lithium clearance in psychiatric patients and normal subjects with steady state plasma lithium concentrations. This effect has been attributed to inhibition of prostaglandin synthesis. As a consequence, when indomethacin and lithium are given concomitantly, the patient should be carefully observed for signs of lithium toxicity. (Read circulars for lithium preparations before use of such concomitant therapy.) In addition, the frequency of monitoring serum lithium concentration should be increased at the outset of such combination drug treatment.

Indomethacin given concomitantly with digoxin has been reported to increase the serum concentration and prolong the half-life of digoxin. Therefore, when indomethacin and digoxin are used concomitantly, serum digoxin levels should be closely monitored.

In some patients, the administration of indomethacin can reduce the diuretic, natriuretic, and, antihypertensive effects of loop, potassium-sparing, and thiazide diuretics. Therefore, when indomethacin and diuretics are used concomitantly, the patient should be observed closely to determine if the desired effect of the diuretic is obtained.

Indomethacin reduces basal plasma renin activity (PRA), as well as those elevations of PRA induced by furosemide administration, or salt or volume depletion. These facts should be considered when evaluating plasma renin activity in hypertensive patients.

It has been reported that the addition of triamterene to a maintenance schedule of indomethacin resulted in reversible acute renal failure in 2 of 4 healthy volunteers. Indomethacin and triamterene should not be administered together.

Indomethacin and potassium-sparing diuretics each may be associated with increased serum potassium levels. The potential effects of indomethacin and potassium-sparing diuretics on potassium kinetics and renal function should be considered when these agents are administered concurrently.

Most of the above effects concerning diuretics have been attributed, at least in part, to mechanisms involving inhibition of prostaglandin synthesis by indomethacin.

Blunting of the antihypertensive effect of beta-adrenoceptor blocking agents by non-steroidal anti-inflammatory drugs including indomethacin has been reported. Therefore, when using these blocking agents to treat hypertension, patients should be observed carefully in order to confirm that the desired therapeutic effect has been obtained. There are reports that indomethacin can reduce the antihypertensive effect of captopril in some patients.

False-negative results in the dexamethasone suppression test (DST) in patients being treated with indomethacin have been reported. Thus, results of the DST should be interpreted with caution in these patients.

INTRAVENOUS

Since renal function may be reduced by indomethacin IV, consideration should be given to reduction in dosage of those medications that rely on adequate renal function for their elimination. Because the half-life of digitalis (given frequently to pre-term infants with patent ductus arteriosus and associated cardiac failure) may be prolonged when given concomitantly with indomethacin, the infant should be observed closely; frequent ECGs and serum digitalis levels may be required to prevent or detect digitalis toxicity early. Furthermore, in one study of premature infants treated with indomethacin IV and also receiving either gentamicin or amikacin, both peak and trough levels of these aminoglycosides were significantly elevated.

Therapy with indomethacin may blunt the natriuretic effect of furosemide. This response has been attributed to inhibition of prostaglandin synthesis by non-steroidal anti-inflammatory drugs. In a study of 19 premature infants with patent ductus arteriosus treated with either indomethacin IV alone or a combination of indomethacin IV and furosemide, results showed that infants receiving both indomethacin IV and furosemide had significantly higher urinary output, higher levels of sodium and chloride excretion, and higher glomerular filtration rates than did those infants receiving indomethacin IV alone. In this study, the data suggested that therapy with furosemide helped to maintain renal function in the premature infant when indomethacin IV was added to the treatment of patent ductus arteriosus.

ADVERSE REACTIONS

CAPSULES, ORAL SUSPENSION AND SUPPOSITORIES

The adverse reactions for indomethacin capsules listed below have been arranged into two groups: (1) incidence greater than 1%; and (2) incidence less than 1%. The incidence for group (1) was obtained from 33 double-blind controlled clinical trials reported in the literature (1092 patients). The incidence for group (2) was based on reports in clinical trials, in the literature, and on voluntary reports since marketing. The probability of a causal relationship exists between indomethacin and these adverse reactions, some of which have been reported only rarely.

In controlled clinical trials, the incidence of adverse reactions to indomethacin extended-release capsules and equal 24 hour doses of indomethacin capsules were similar.

The adverse reactions reported with indomethacin capsules may occur with use of the suppositories. In addition, rectal irritation and tenesmus have been reported in patients who have received the suppositories.

The adverse reactions reported with indomethacin capsules may also occur with use of the suspension.

Gastrointestinal: *Incidence greater than 1%:* Nausea* with or without vomiting, dyspepsia* (including indigestion, hearburn and epigastric pain etc.), diarrhea, abdominal distress or pain, constipation. *Incidence less than 1%:* Anorexia; bloating (includes distension); flatulence; peptic ulcer; gastroenteritis; rectal bleeding; proctitis; single or multiple ulcerations, including perforation and hemorrhage of the esophagus, stomach, duodenum, or small and large intestines; intestinal ulceration associated with stenosis and obstruction; gastrointestinal bleeding without obvious ulcer formation and perforation of preexisting sigmoid lesions (diverticulum, carcinoma, development of ulcerative colitis and regional ileitis); ulcerative stomatitis; toxic hepatitis and jaundice (some fatal cases have been reported); intestinal strictures (diaphragms).

Central Nervous System: *Incidence greater than 1%:* Headache (11.7%), dizziness*, vertigo, somnolence, depression and fatigue (including malaise and listlessness). *Incidence less than 1%:* Anxiety (includes nervousness); muscle weakness; involuntary muscle movements; insomnia; muzziness; psychic disturbances including psychotic episodes; mental confusion; drowsiness; light-headedness; syncope; paresthesia of epilepsy and parkinsonism; depersonalization; coma; peripheral neuropathy, convulsion; dysarthria.

Special Senses: *Incidence greater than 1%:* Tinnitus. *Incidence less than 1%:* Ocular — corneal deposits and retinal disturbances, including those of the macula, have been reported in some patients on prolonged therapy with indomethacin; blurred vision,; diplopia; hearing distrubances; deafness.

Cardiovascular: *Incidence greater than 1%:* None. *Incidence less than 1%:* Hypertension, hypotensioin, tachycardia, chest pain, congestive heart failure, arrhythmia, palpitations.

Metabolic: *Incidence greater than 1%:* None. *Incidence less than 1%:* Edema, weight gain, fluid retention, flushing or sweating, hyperglycemia, glycosuria, hyperkalemia.

Integumentary: *Incidence greater than 1%:* None. *Incidence less than 1%:* Pruritus rash, urticaria, petechiae or ecchymosis, exfoliative dermatitis, erythema nodosum, loss of hair, Stevens-Johnson syndrome, erythema multiforme, toxic epidermal necrolysis.

Hematologic: *Incidence greater than 1%:* None. *Incidence less than 1%:* Leukopenia, bone marrow depression, anemia secondary to obvious or occult gastrointestinal bleeding, aplastic anemia, hemolytic anemia, agranulocytosis, thrombocytopenic purpura, disseminated intravascular coagulation.

Hypersensitivity: *Incidence Greater Than 1%:* None. *Incidence less than 1%:* Acute anaphylaxis, acute respiratory distress, rapid fall in blood pressure resembling a shocklike state fever, angioedema, dyspnea, astham, purpura, angitis, pulmonary edema.

Genitourinary: *Incidence greater than 1%:* None. *Incidence less than 1%:* Hematuria, vaginal bleeding, proteinuria, nephrotic syndrome, interstitial nephritis, BUN elevation, renal insufficiency (including renal failure).

Miscellaneous: *Incidence greater than 1%:* None. *Incidence less than 1%:* Epistaxis; breast changes, including enlargement and tenderness, or gynecomastia.

*Reactions occurring in 3-9% of patients treated with indomethacin. (Those reactions occurring in less than 3% of the patients are unmarked.)

Causal Relationship Unknown

Other reactions have been reported but occurred under circumstances where a causal relationship could not be established. However, in these rarely reported events, the possibility cannot be excluded. Therefore, these observations are being listed to serve as alerting information to physicians:

Cardiovascular: Thrombophlebitis.

Hematologic: Although there have been several reports of leukemia, the supporting information is weak.

Genitourinary: Urinary frequency.

A rare occurrence of fulminant necrotizing fasciitis, particularly in association with Group A β-hemolytic streptococcus, has been described in persons treated with non-steroidal anti-inflammatory agents, including indomethacin, sometimes with fatal outcomes (see PRECAUTIONS, General).

INTRAVENOUS

In a double-blind placebo-controlled trial of 405 premature infants weighing less than or equal to 1750 g with evidence of large ductal shunting, in those infants treated with indomethacin (n=206), there was a statistically significantly greater incidence of bleeding problems, including gross or microscopic bleeding into the gastrointestinal tract, oozing from the skin after needle stick, pulmonary hemorrhage, and disseminated intravascular coagulopathy. There was no statistically significant difference between treatment groups with reference to intracranial hemorrhage.

The infants treated with indomethacin sodium trihydrate also had a significantly higher incidence of transient oliguria and elevations of serum creatinine (greater than or equal to 1.8 mg/dl) than did the infants treated with placebo.

The incidences of retrolental fibroplasia (grades III and IV) and pneumothorax in infants treated with indomethacin IV were no greater than in placebo controls and were statistically significantly lower than in surgically-treated infants.

The following additional adverse reactions in infants have been reported from the collaborative study, anecdotal case reports, and from other studies using rectal, oral, or intravenous indomethacin for treatment of patent ductus arteriosus. The rates are based on the experience of 849 indomethacin-treated infants reported in the medical literature, regardless of the route of administration. One (1) year follow-up is available on 175 infants and shows no long-term sequelae which could be attributed to indomethacin. In controlled clinical studies, only electrolyte imbalance and renal dysfunction (of the reactions listed below) occurred statistically significantly more frequently after indomethacin IV than after placebo.

Renal: Renal dysfunction in 41% of infants, including one or more of the following: reduced urinary output; reduced urine sodium, chloride, or potassium, urine osmolality, free water clearance, or glomerular filtration rate; elevated serum creatinine or BUN; uremia.

Cardiovascular: Intracranial bleeding†, pulmonary hypertension.

Gastrointestinal: Gastrointestinal bleeding*, vomiting, abdominal distention, transient ileus, localized perforation(s) of the small and/or large intestine.

Metabolic: Hyponatremia*, elevated serum potassium*, reduction in blood sugar, including hypoglycemia, increased weight gain (fluid retention).

Coagulation: Decreased platelet aggregation (see PRECAUTIONS).

The following adverse reactions have also been reported in infants treated with indomethacin, however, a causal relationship to therapy with indomethacin IV has not been established:

Cardiovascular: Bradycardia.

Respiratory: Apnea, exacerbation of pre-existing pulmonary infection.

Metabolic: Acidosis/alkalosis.

Hematologic: Disseminated intravascular coagulation.

Gastrointestinal: Necrotizing enterocolitis.

Ophthalmic: Retrolental fibroplasia.†

A variety of additional adverse experiences have been reported in adults treated with oral indomethacin for moderate to severe rheumatoid arthritis, osteoarthritis, ankylosing spondylitis, acute painful shoulder and acute gouty arthritis. Their relevance to the pre-term neonate receiving indomethacin for patent ductus arteriosus is unknown, however, the possibility exists that these experiences may be associated with the use of indomethacin IV in pre-term neonates.

*Incidence 3-9%. Those reactions which are unmarked occurred in 1-3% of patients.

†Incidence in both indomethacin and placebo-treated infants 3-9%. Those reactions which are unmarked occurred in less than 3%.

DOSAGE AND ADMINISTRATION

CAPSULES, ORAL SUSPENSION AND SUPPOSITORIES

Indomethacin is available as 25 and 50 mg indomethacin capsules, 75 mg indomethacin extended-release capsules for oral use, oral suspension indomethacin, containing 25 mg of indomethacin per 5 ml, and 50 mg suppositories indomethacin for rectal use. Indomethacin extended-release capsules 75 mg once a day can be substituted for indomethacin capsules 25 mg tid However, there will be significant differences between the two dosage regimens in indomethacin blood levels, especially after 12 hours (see CLINICAL PHARMACOLOGY). In addition, indomethacin extended-release capsules 75 mg bid can be substituted for indomethacin capsules 50 mg tid Indomethacin extended-release capsules may be substituted for all the indications for indomethacin capsules except acute gouty arthritis.

Adverse reactions appear to correlate with the size of the dose of indomethacin in most patients but not all. Therefore, every effort should be made to determine the smallest effective dosage for the individual patient.

Always give indomethacin capsules, indomethacin extended-release capsules, or oral suspension indomethacin with food, immediately after meals, or with antacids to reduce gastric irritation.

Pediatric Use

Indomethacin ordinarily should not be prescribed for pediatric patients 14 years of age and under (see WARNINGS).

Adult Use

Dosage recommendations for active stages of the following: Moderate to severe rheumatoid arthritis including acute flares of chronic disease; moderate to severe ankylosing spondylitis; and moderate to severe osteoarthritis.

Suggested dosage: Indomethacin capsules 25 mg bid or tid If this is well tolerated, increase the daily dosage by 25 or by 50 mg, if required by continuing symptoms, at weekly intervals until a satisfactory response is obtained or until a total daily dose of 150-200 mg is reached. DOSES ABOVE THIS AMOUNT GENERALLY DO NOT INCREASE THE EFFECTIVENESS OF THE DRUG.

In patients who have persistent night pain and/or morning stiffness, the giving of a large portion, up to a maximum of 100 mg, of the total daily dose at bedtime, either orally or by rectal suppositories, may be helpful in affording relief. The total daily dose should not exceed 200 mg. In acute flares of chronic rheumatoid arthritis, it may be necessary to increase the dosage by 25 mg or, if required, by 50 mg daily.

If indomethacin extended-release capsules 75 mg are used for initiating indomethacin treatment, 1 capsule daily should be the usual starting dose in order to observe patient tolerance since 75 mg/day is the maximum recommended starting dose for indomethacin. If indomethacin extended-release capsules are used to increase the daily dose, patients should be observed for possible signs and symptoms of intolerance since the daily increment will exceed the daily increment recommended for the other dosage forms. For patients who require 150 mg of indomethacin per day and have demonstrated acceptable tolerance, indomethacin extended-release may be prescribed as 1 capsule twice daily.

If minor adverse effects develop as the dosage is increased, reduce the dosage rapidly to a tolerated dose and OBSERVE THE PATIENT CLOSELY.

If severe adverse reactions occur, STOP THE DRUG. After the acute phase of the disease is under control, an attempt to reduce the daily dose should be made repeatedly until the patient is receiving the smallest effective dose or the drug is discontinued.

Careful instructions to, and observations of, the individual patient are essential to the prevention of serious, irreversible, including fatal, adverse reactions.

As advancing years appear to increase the possibility of adverse reactions, indomethacin should be used with greater care in the aged.

Acute Painful Shoulder (Bursitis and/or Tendinitis)

Initial Dose: 75-150 mg daily in 3 or 4 divided doses.

The drug should be discontinued after the signs and symptoms of inflammation have been controlled for several days. The usual course of therapy is 7-14 days.

Acute Gouty Arthritis

Suggested Dosage: Indomethacin capsules 50 mg tid until pain is tolerable. The dose should then be rapidly reduced to complete cessation of the drug. Definite relief of pain has been reported within 2-4 hours. Tenderness and heat usually subside in 24-36 hours, and swelling gradually disappears in 3-5 days.

INTRAVENOUS

FOR INTRAVENOUS ADMINISTRATION ONLY.

Dosage recommendations for closure of the ductus arteriosus depends on the age of the infant at the time of therapy. A course of therapy is defined as three intravenous doses of indomethacin IV given at 12-24 hour intervals, with careful attention to urinary output. If anuria or marked oliguria (urinary output <0.6 ml/kg/h) is evident at the scheduled time of the second or third dose of indomethacin IV, no additional doses should be given until laboratory studies indicate that renal function has returned to normal (see WARNINGS, Renal Effects).

Dosage according to age is shown in TABLE 1.

TABLE 1

Age at 1st Dose	Dosage (mg/kg) 1st	2nd	3rd
Less than 48 hours	0.2	0.1	0.1
2-7 days	0.2	0.2	0.2
Over 7 days	0.2	0.25	0.25

If the ductus arteriosus closes or is significantly reduced in size after an interval of 48 hours or more from completion of the first course of indomethacin IV, no further doses are necessary. If the ductus arteriosus re-opens, a second course of 1-3 doses may be given, each dose separated by a 12-24 hour interval as described above.

If the infant remains unresponsive to therapy with indomethacin IV after 2 courses, surgery may be necessary for closure of the ductus arteriosus. If severe adverse reactions occur, STOP THE DRUG.

PRODUCT LISTING - RATED THERAPEUTICALLY EQUIVALENT

Capsule - Oral - 25 mg

Qty	Price	Product	NDC
20's	$5.60	GENERIC, Pd-Rx Pharmaceuticals	55289-0147-20
20's	$12.21	GENERIC, Dhs Inc	55887-0917-20
20's	$15.15	INDOCIN, Physicians Total Care	54868-0738-02
21's	$5.70	GENERIC, Pd-Rx Pharmaceuticals	55289-0147-21
21's	$12.82	GENERIC, Dhs Inc	55887-0917-21
25's	$3.90	GENERIC, Udl Laboratories Inc	51079-0190-19
25's	$5.20	GENERIC, Pd-Rx Pharmaceuticals	55289-0147-97
30's	$3.42	GENERIC, Circle Pharmaceuticals Inc	00659-0406-30
30's	$6.20	GENERIC, Pd-Rx Pharmaceuticals	55289-0147-30
30's	$18.28	GENERIC, Dhs Inc	55887-0917-30
90's	$4.15	GENERIC, Major Pharmaceuticals Inc	00904-1175-89
100's	$4.13	GENERIC, Interstate Drug Exchange Inc	00814-3837-14
100's	$6.50	GENERIC, Cmc-Consolidated Midland Corporation	00223-1195-01
100's	$6.95	GENERIC, Raway Pharmacal Inc	00686-0190-20
100's	$8.45	GENERIC, Watson Laboratories Inc	52544-0303-01
100's	$10.85	GENERIC, West Point Pharma	59591-0172-68
100's	$14.90	GENERIC, Par Pharmaceutical Inc	49884-0067-01
100's	$16.46	GENERIC, Aligen Independent Laboratories Inc	00405-4541-01
100's	$19.96	GENERIC, Moore, H.L. Drug Exchange Inc	00839-6762-06
100's	$20.90	GENERIC, Qualitest Products Inc	00603-4067-21
100's	$20.90	GENERIC, Sidmak Laboratories Inc	50111-0406-01
100's	$20.90	GENERIC, Novopharm Usa Inc	55953-0420-40
100's	$29.93	GENERIC, Major Pharmaceuticals Inc	00904-1175-61
100's	$31.81	GENERIC, Udl Laboratories Inc	51079-0190-20
100's	$33.18	GENERIC, Auro Pharmaceutical	55829-0681-10
100's	$33.22	GENERIC, Geneva Pharmaceuticals	00781-2325-13
100's	$36.75	GENERIC, Major Pharmaceuticals Inc	00904-1175-60
100's	$37.11	GENERIC, Ivax Corporation	00172-4029-60
100's	$39.00	GENERIC, Mylan Pharmaceuticals Inc	00378-0143-01
100's	$53.80	GENERIC, Ivax Corporation	00182-1681-89
100's	$67.46	INDOCIN, Merck & Company Inc	00006-0025-68

Capsule - Oral - 50 mg

Qty	Price	Product	NDC
20's	$5.90	GENERIC, Pd-Rx Pharmaceuticals	55289-0663-20
21's	$5.00	GENERIC, Circle Pharmaceuticals Inc	00659-0407-21
30's	$6.80	GENERIC, Pd-Rx Pharmaceuticals	55289-0663-30
100's	$5.85	GENERIC, Interstate Drug Exchange Inc	00814-3838-14
100's	$7.50	GENERIC, Cmc-Consolidated Midland Corporation	00223-1196-01
100's	$9.20	GENERIC, Raway Pharmacal Inc	00686-0191-20
100's	$14.07	GENERIC, Watson Laboratories Inc	52544-0304-01
100's	$15.04	GENERIC, Pd-Rx Pharmaceuticals	55289-0663-01
100's	$17.70	GENERIC, West Point Pharma	59591-0159-68
100's	$22.40	GENERIC, Par Pharmaceutical Inc	49884-0068-01
100's	$31.82	GENERIC, Aligen Independent Laboratories Inc	00405-4542-01
100's	$31.98	GENERIC, Moore, H.L. Drug Exchange Inc	00839-6763-06
100's	$37.65	GENERIC, Mutual/United Research Laboratories	00677-0873-01
100's	$37.65	GENERIC, Geneva Pharmaceuticals	00781-2350-01
100's	$37.65	GENERIC, Sidmak Laboratories Inc	50111-0407-01
100's	$37.66	GENERIC, Qualitest Products Inc	00603-4068-21
100's	$44.88	GENERIC, Major Pharmaceuticals Inc	00904-1176-61
100's	$52.37	GENERIC, Auro Pharmaceutical	55829-0682-10
100's	$53.71	GENERIC, Geneva Pharmaceuticals	00781-2350-13
100's	$62.15	GENERIC, Major Pharmaceuticals Inc	00904-1176-60
100's	$62.75	GENERIC, Ivax Corporation	00172-4030-60
100's	$65.90	GENERIC, Mylan Pharmaceuticals Inc	00378-0147-01
100's	$67.88	GENERIC, Udl Laboratories Inc	51079-0191-20
100's	$74.64	GENERIC, Ivax Corporation	00182-1682-89
100's	$110.14	INDOCIN, Merck & Company Inc	00006-0050-68

Capsule, Extended Release - Oral - 75 mg

Qty	Price	Product	NDC
10's	$12.80	GENERIC, Pd-Rx Pharmaceuticals	55289-0469-10
14's	$13.44	GENERIC, Pd-Rx Pharmaceuticals	55289-0469-14
14's	$26.22	INDOCIN SR, Allscripts Pharmaceutical Company	54569-0279-02
15's	$14.44	GENERIC, Pd-Rx Pharmaceuticals	55289-0469-15
20's	$19.20	GENERIC, Pd-Rx Pharmaceuticals	55289-0469-20
30's	$30.00	GENERIC, Pd-Rx Pharmaceuticals	55289-0469-30
30's	$63.04	INDOCIN SR, Physicians Total Care	54868-0878-00
60's	$57.00	GENERIC, Qualitest Products Inc	00603-4070-20
60's	$59.15	GENERIC, Major Pharmaceuticals Inc	00904-1178-52
60's	$67.13	GENERIC, Interstate Drug Exchange Inc	00814-3839-10
60's	$69.50	GENERIC, Brightstone Pharma	62939-7012-07
60's	$71.48	GENERIC, Moore, H.L. Drug Exchange Inc	00839-7374-05
60's	$85.67	GENERIC, Inwood Laboratories Inc	00258-3607-06
60's	$116.08	GENERIC, Eon Labs Manufacturing Inc	00185-0720-60
60's	$116.80	GENERIC, Able Laboratories Inc	53265-0269-60
60's	$142.46	INDOCIN SR, Eon Labs Manufacturing Inc	64814-0695-60
100's	$88.03	GENERIC, Qualitest Products Inc	00603-4070-21
100's	$88.61	GENERIC, Aligen Independent Laboratories Inc	00405-4547-01
100's	$92.60	GENERIC, Moore, H.L. Drug Exchange Inc	00839-7374-06
100's	$98.50	GENERIC, Brightstone Pharma	62939-7012-01
100's	$99.80	GENERIC, Major Pharmaceuticals Inc	00904-1178-60
100's	$150.48	GENERIC, Inwood Laboratories Inc	00258-3607-01
100's	$193.00	GENERIC, Able Laboratories Inc	53265-0269-10
100's	$193.47	GENERIC, Eon Labs Manufacturing Inc	00185-0720-01

Suppository - Rectal - 50 mg

Qty	Price	Product	NDC
15's	$35.42	GENERIC, Pd-Rx Pharmaceuticals	55289-0114-15
30's	$46.20	GENERIC, Ivax Corporation	00182-7031-17
30's	$49.90	GENERIC, G and W Laboratories Inc	00713-0176-30

Suspension - Oral - 25 mg/5 ml

Qty	Price	Product	NDC
237 ml	$50.65	INDOCIN, Merck & Company Inc	00006-3376-66
500 ml	$61.89	GENERIC, Roxane Laboratories Inc	00054-3423-63

PRODUCT LISTING - EQUIVALENTS NOT AVAILABLE

Capsule - Oral - 25 mg

Qty	Price	Product	NDC
3's	$3.52	GENERIC, Prescript Pharmaceuticals	00247-0202-03
4's	$3.56	GENERIC, Prescript Pharmaceuticals	00247-0202-04
5's	$3.62	GENERIC, Prescript Pharmaceuticals	00247-0202-05
8's	$4.94	GENERIC, Southwood Pharmaceuticals Inc	58016-0235-08
10's	$2.09	GENERIC, Allscripts Pharmaceutical Company	54569-0277-09
10's	$3.88	GENERIC, Prescript Pharmaceuticals	00247-0202-10
12's	$2.51	GENERIC, Allscripts Pharmaceutical Company	54569-0277-06
12's	$3.99	GENERIC, Prescript Pharmaceuticals	00247-0202-12
15's	$3.14	GENERIC, Allscripts Pharmaceutical Company	54569-0277-04
15's	$4.15	GENERIC, Prescript Pharmaceuticals	00247-0202-15
15's	$4.15	GENERIC, Pharmaceutical Corporation Of America	51655-0128-54
20's	$4.18	GENERIC, Allscripts Pharmaceutical Company	54569-0277-00
20's	$4.41	GENERIC, Prescript Pharmaceuticals	00247-0202-20
20's	$12.36	GENERIC, Southwood Pharmaceuticals Inc	58016-0235-20
20's	$18.11	GENERIC, Pharma Pac	52959-0080-20
21's	$4.39	GENERIC, Allscripts Pharmaceutical Company	54569-4123-01
21's	$4.47	GENERIC, Prescript Pharmaceuticals	00247-0202-21
21's	$19.00	GENERIC, Pharma Pac	52959-0080-21
25's	$11.96	GENERIC, Alpharma Uspd Makers Of Barre and Nmc	63874-0318-25
28's	$4.84	GENERIC, Prescript Pharmaceuticals	00247-0202-28
28's	$5.85	GENERIC, Allscripts Pharmaceutical Company	54569-4123-02
30's	$3.84	GENERIC, Physicians Total Care	54868-0074-03
30's	$4.94	GENERIC, Prescript Pharmaceuticals	00247-0202-30
30's	$6.27	GENERIC, Allscripts Pharmaceutical Company	54569-0277-01
30's	$16.82	GENERIC, Alpharma Uspd Makers Of Barre and Nmc	63874-0318-30
30's	$18.54	GENERIC, Southwood Pharmaceuticals Inc	58016-0235-30
30's	$25.86	GENERIC, Pharma Pac	52959-0080-30
40's	$4.56	GENERIC, Physicians Total Care	54868-0074-04
40's	$5.47	GENERIC, Prescript Pharmaceuticals	00247-0202-40
40's	$31.94	GENERIC, Pharma Pac	52959-0080-40
60's	$6.01	GENERIC, Physicians Total Care	54868-0074-05
60's	$6.53	GENERIC, Prescript Pharmaceuticals	00247-0202-60
60's	$37.08	GENERIC, Southwood Pharmaceuticals Inc	58016-0235-60
75's	$46.35	GENERIC, Southwood Pharmaceuticals Inc	58016-0235-75
90's	$19.90	GENERIC, Pharmaceutical Corporation Of America	51655-0128-26
100's	$8.90	GENERIC, Physicians Total Care	54868-0074-02
100's	$20.90	GENERIC, Allscripts Pharmaceutical Company	54569-0277-03
100's	$61.80	GENERIC, Southwood Pharmaceuticals Inc	58016-0235-00

Capsule - Oral - 50 mg

Qty	Price	Product	NDC
3's	$3.55	GENERIC, Prescript Pharmaceuticals	00247-0203-03
4's	$3.62	GENERIC, Prescript Pharmaceuticals	00247-0203-04
14's	$13.35	GENERIC, Southwood Pharmaceuticals Inc	58016-0236-14
15's	$4.34	GENERIC, Prescript Pharmaceuticals	00247-0203-15
15's	$5.65	GENERIC, Allscripts Pharmaceutical Company	54569-0275-05
15's	$16.54	GENERIC, Alpharma Uspd Makers Of Barre and Nmc	63874-0394-15
20's	$4.68	GENERIC, Prescript Pharmaceuticals	00247-0203-20
20's	$19.07	GENERIC, Southwood Pharmaceuticals Inc	58016-0236-20
20's	$20.36	GENERIC, Pharma Pac	52959-0081-20
21's	$4.74	GENERIC, Prescript Pharmaceuticals	00247-0203-21
21's	$7.91	GENERIC, Allscripts Pharmaceutical Company	54569-0275-00
21's	$20.02	GENERIC, Southwood Pharmaceuticals Inc	58016-0236-21
21's	$21.35	GENERIC, Pharma Pac	52959-0081-21
24's	$4.94	GENERIC, Prescript Pharmaceuticals	00247-0203-24
30's	$3.67	GENERIC, Physicians Total Care	54868-0875-02
30's	$5.34	GENERIC, Prescript Pharmaceuticals	00247-0203-30
30's	$11.30	GENERIC, Allscripts Pharmaceutical Company	54569-0275-01
30's	$27.46	GENERIC, Alpharma Uspd Makers Of Barre and Nmc	63874-0394-30
30's	$28.60	GENERIC, Southwood Pharmaceuticals Inc	58016-0236-30
30's	$29.57	GENERIC, Pharma Pac	52959-0081-30
40's	$4.78	GENERIC, Physicians Total Care	54868-0875-04
40's	$37.70	GENERIC, Pharma Pac	52959-0081-40
40's	$38.13	GENERIC, Southwood Pharmaceuticals Inc	58016-0236-40
60's	$7.33	GENERIC, Prescript Pharmaceuticals	00247-0203-60
60's	$7.52	GENERIC, Physicians Total Care	54868-0875-00
60's	$57.20	GENERIC, Southwood Pharmaceuticals Inc	58016-0236-60
100's	$9.95	GENERIC, Physicians Total Care	54868-0875-01
100's	$69.09	GENERIC, Pharma Pac	52959-0081-00

100's	$95.33	GENERIC, Southwood Pharmaceuticals Inc	58016-0236-00
Capsule, Extended Release - Oral - 75 mg			
7's	$11.43	GENERIC, Southwood Pharmaceuticals Inc	58016-0237-07
7's	$11.80	GENERIC, Allscripts Pharmaceutical Company	54569-1518-01
7's	$14.43	GENERIC, Pharma Pac	52959-0082-07
10's	$8.92	GENERIC, Prescript Pharmaceuticals	00247-0321-10
10's	$16.33	GENERIC, Southwood Pharmaceuticals Inc	58016-0237-10
10's	$16.86	GENERIC, Allscripts Pharmaceutical Company	54569-1518-06
12's	$19.60	GENERIC, Southwood Pharmaceuticals Inc	58016-0237-12
14's	$11.14	GENERIC, Prescript Pharmaceuticals	00247-0321-14
14's	$22.86	GENERIC, Southwood Pharmaceuticals Inc	58016-0237-14
14's	$23.60	GENERIC, Allscripts Pharmaceutical Company	54569-1518-02
14's	$25.32	GENERIC, Pharma Pac	52959-0082-14
14's	$28.60	GENERIC, St. Mary'S Mpp	60760-0607-14
15's	$24.50	GENERIC, Southwood Pharmaceuticals Inc	58016-0237-15
15's	$25.91	GENERIC, Pharma Pac	52959-0082-15
20's	$12.82	GENERIC, Physicians Total Care	54868-0922-03
20's	$32.67	GENERIC, Southwood Pharmaceuticals Inc	58016-0237-20
20's	$33.18	GENERIC, Pharma Pac	52959-0082-20
20's	$33.71	GENERIC, Allscripts Pharmaceutical Company	54569-1518-03
21's	$34.30	GENERIC, Southwood Pharmaceuticals Inc	58016-0237-21
21's	$34.82	GENERIC, Pharma Pac	52959-0082-21
24's	$39.20	GENERIC, Southwood Pharmaceuticals Inc	58016-0237-24
28's	$45.73	GENERIC, Southwood Pharmaceuticals Inc	58016-0237-28
30's	$29.11	GENERIC, Physicians Total Care	54868-0922-01
30's	$48.88	GENERIC, Pharma Pac	52959-0082-30
30's	$49.00	GENERIC, Southwood Pharmaceuticals Inc	58016-0237-30
30's	$50.57	GENERIC, Allscripts Pharmaceutical Company	54569-1518-00
40's	$38.25	GENERIC, Physicians Total Care	54868-0922-06
40's	$65.33	GENERIC, Southwood Pharmaceuticals Inc	58016-0237-40
60's	$42.80	GENERIC, Physicians Total Care	54868-0922-02
60's	$74.53	GENERIC, Pharma Pac	52959-0082-60
60's	$98.00	GENERIC, Southwood Pharmaceuticals Inc	58016-0237-60
100's	$71.17	GENERIC, Physicians Total Care	54868-0922-00
Powder For Injection - Intravenous - 1 mg			
3's	$97.21	INDOCIN, Merck & Company Inc	00006-3406-17

Infliximab *(003410)*

Categories: Arthritis, rheumatoid; Crohn's disease; FDA Approved 1998 Aug; Pregnancy Category C; Orphan Drugs
Drug Classes: Disease modifying antirheumatic drugs; Gastrointestinals; Immunomodulators; Monoclonal antibodies; Tumor necrosis factor modulators
Brand Names: Remicade
Foreign Brand Availability: Revellex (South-Africa)
Cost of Therapy: $1,452.38 (Rheumatoid Arthritis; Remicade; 100 mg; 210 mg; 1 day supply)
$2,420.64 (Crohn's Disease; Remicade; 100 mg; 350 mg; 1 day supply)

WARNING

RISK OF INFECTIONS

Tuberculosis (frequently disseminated or extrapulmonary at clinical presentation), invasive fungal infections, and other opportunistic infections, have been observed in patients receiving infliximab. Some of these infections have been fatal (see WARNINGS).

Patients should be evaluated for latent tuberculosis infection with a tuberculin skin test.[1] Treatment of latent tuberculosis infection should be initiated prior to therapy with infliximab.

DESCRIPTION

Infliximab is a chimeric IgG1k monoclonal antibody with an approximate molecular weight of 149,100 daltons. It is composed of human constant and murine variable regions. Infliximab binds specifically to human tumor necrosis factor alpha (TNFα) with an association constant of 10^{10} M^{-1}. Infliximab is produced by a recombinant cell line cultured by continuous perfusion and is purified by a series of steps that includes measures to inactivate and remove viruses.

Remicade is supplied as a sterile, white, lyophilized powder for intravenous infusion. Following reconstitution with 10 ml of sterile water for injection, the resulting pH is approximately 7.2. Each single-use vial contains 100 mg infliximab, 500 mg sucrose, 0.5 mg polysorbate 80, 2.2 mg monobasic sodium phosphate, monohydrate, and 6.1 mg dibasic sodium phosphate, dihydrate. No preservatives are present.

CLINICAL PHARMACOLOGY

GENERAL

Infliximab neutralizes the biological activity of TNFα by binding with high affinity to the soluble and transmembrane forms of TNFα and inhibits binding of TNFα with its receptors.[2-5] Infliximab does not neutralize TNFβ (lymphotoxin α), a related cytokine that utilizes the same receptors as TNFα. Biological activities attributed to TNFα include: induction of pro-inflammatory cytokines such as interleukins (IL) 1 and 6, enhancement of leukocyte migration by increasing endothelial layer permeability and expression of adhesion molecules by endothelial cells and leukocytes, activation of neutrophil and eosinophil functional activity, induction of acute phase reactants and other liver proteins, as well as tissue degrading enzymes produced by synoviocytes and/or chondrocytes. Cells expressing transmembrane TNFα bound by infliximab can be lysed *in vitro* by complement or effector cells.[3] Infliximab inhibits the functional activity of TNFα in a wide variety of *in vitro* bioassays utilizing human fibroblasts, endothelial cells, neutrophils,[4] B and T lymphocytes and epithelial cells. Anti-TNFα antibodies reduce disease activity in the cotton-top tamarin colitis model, and decrease synovitis and joint erosions in a murine model of collagen-induced arthritis. Infliximab prevents disease in transgenic mice that develop polyarthritis as a result of constitutive expression of human TNFα, and, when administered after disease onset, allows eroded joints to heal.

PHARMACODYNAMICS

Elevated concentrations of TNFα have been found in the joints of rheumatoid arthritis patients[6] and the stools of Crohn's disease patients[7] and correlate with elevated disease activity. In rheumatoid arthritis, treatment with infliximab reduced infiltration of inflammatory cells into inflamed areas of the joint as well as expression of molecules mediating cellular adhesion [E-selectin, intercellular adhesion molecule-1 (ICAM-1) and vascular cell adhesion molecule-1 (VCAM-1)], chemoattraction [IL-8 and monocyte chemotactic protein (MCP-1)] and tissue degradation [matrix metalloproteinase (MMP) 1 and 3].[5] In Crohn's disease, treatment with infliximab reduced infiltration of inflammatory cells and TNFα production in inflamed areas of the intestine, and reduced the proportion of mononuclear cells from the lamina propria able to express TNFα and interferon.[5] After treatment with infliximab, patients with rheumatoid arthritis or Crohn's disease exhibited decreased levels of serum IL-6 and C-reactive protein (CRP) compared to baseline. Peripheral blood lymphocytes from infliximab-treated patients showed no significant decrease in number or in proliferative responses to *in vitro* mitogenic stimulation when compared to cells from untreated patients.

PHARMACOKINETICS

Single intravenous (IV) infusions of 3-20 mg/kg showed a predictable and linear relationship between the dose administered and the maximum serum concentration and area under the concentration-time curve. The volume of distribution at steady state was independent of dose and indicated that infliximab was distributed primarily within the vascular compartment. Median pharmacokinetic results for doses of 3-10 mg/kg in rheumatoid arthritis and 5 mg/kg in Crohn's disease indicate that the terminal half-life of infliximab is 8.0-9.5 days.

Following an initial dose of infliximab, repeated infusions at 2 and 6 weeks in fistulizing Crohn's disease and rheumatoid arthritis patients resulted in predictable concentration-time profiles following each treatment. No systemic accumulation of infliximab occurred upon continued repeated treatment with 3 or 10 mg/kg at 4 or 8 week intervals in rheumatoid arthritis patients or patients with moderate or severe Crohn's disease retreated with 4 infusions of 10 mg/kg infliximab at 8 week intervals. The proportion of patients with rheumatoid arthritis who had undetectable infliximab concentrations at 8 weeks following an infusion was approximately 25% for those receiving 3 mg/kg every 8 weeks, 15% for patients administered 3 mg/kg every 4 weeks, and 0% for patients receiving 10 mg/kg every 4 or 8 weeks. No major differences in clearance or volume of distribution were observed in patient subgroups defined by age or weight. It is not known if there are differences in clearance or volume of distribution between gender subgroups or in patients with marked impairment of hepatic or renal function.

INDICATIONS AND USAGE

RHEUMATOID ARTHRITIS

Infliximab, in combination with methotrexate, is indicated for reducing signs and symptoms and inhibiting the progression of structural damage in patients with moderately to severely active rheumatoid arthritis who have had an inadequate response to methotrexate.

CROHN'S DISEASE

Infliximab is indicated for the reduction in signs and symptoms of Crohn's disease in patients with moderately to severely active Crohn's disease who have had an inadequate response to conventional therapy.

The safety and efficacy of therapy continued beyond a single dose have not been established (see DOSAGE AND ADMINISTRATION).

Infliximab is indicated for the reduction in the number of draining enterocutaneous fistulas in patients with fistulizing Crohn's disease.

The safety and efficacy of therapy continued beyond 3 doses have not been established (see DOSAGE AND ADMINISTRATION).

CONTRAINDICATIONS

Infliximab should not be administered to patients with known hypersensitivity to any murine proteins or other component of the product.

WARNINGS

RISK OF INFECTIONS

See BOXED WARNING.

SERIOUS INFECTIONS, INCLUDING SEPSIS, HAVE BEEN REPORTED IN PATIENTS RECEIVING TNF-BLOCKING AGENTS. SOME OF THESE INFECTIONS HAVE BEEN FATAL. MANY OF THE SERIOUS INFECTIONS IN PATIENTS TREATED WITH INFLIXIMAB HAVE OCCURRED IN PATIENTS ON CONCOMITANT IMMUNOSUPPRESSIVE THERAPY THAT, IN ADDITION TO THEIR CROHN'S DISEASE OR RHEUMATOID ARTHRITIS, COULD PREDISPOSE THEM TO INFECTIONS.

INFLIXIMAB SHOULD NOT BE GIVEN TO PATIENTS WITH A CLINICALLY IMPORTANT, ACTIVE INFECTION. CAUTION SHOULD BE EXERCISED WHEN CONSIDERING THE USE OF INFLIXIMAB IN PATIENTS WITH A CHRONIC INFECTION OR A HISTORY OF RECURRENT INFECTION. PATIENTS SHOULD BE MONITORED FOR SIGNS AND SYMPTOMS OF INFECTION WHILE ON OR AFTER TREATMENT WITH INFLIXIMAB. NEW INFECTIONS SHOULD BE CLOSELY MONITORED. IF A PATIENT DEVELOPS A SERIOUS INFECTION, INFLIXIMAB THERAPY SHOULD BE DISCONTINUED (see ADVERSE REACTIONS, Infections).

CASES OF HISTOPLASMOSIS, LISTERIOSIS, PNEUMOCYSTOSIS AND TUBERCULOSIS, HAVE BEEN OBSERVED IN PATIENTS RECEIVING INFLIX-

I

IMAB. FOR PATIENTS WHO HAVE RESIDED IN REGIONS WHERE HISTOPLASMOSIS IS ENDEMIC, THE BENEFITS AND RISKS OF INFLIXIMAB TREATMENT SHOULD BE CAREFULLY CONSIDERED BEFORE INITIATION OF INFLIXIMAB THERAPY.

HYPERSENSITIVITY

Infliximab has been associated with hypersensitivity reactions that vary in their time of onset. Most hypersensitivity reactions, which include urticaria, dyspnea, and/or hypotension, have occurred during or within 2 hours of infliximab infusion. However, in some cases, serum sickness-like reactions have been observed in Crohn's disease patients 3-12 days after infliximab therapy was reinstituted following an extended period without infliximab treatment. Symptoms associated with these reactions include fever, rash, headache, sore throat, myalgias, polyarthralgias, hand and facial edema and/or dysphagia. These reactions were associated with marked increase in antibodies to infliximab, loss of detectable serum concentrations of infliximab, and possible loss of drug efficacy. Infliximab should be discontinued for severe reactions. Medications for the treatment of hypersensitivity reactions (*e.g.,* acetaminophen, antihistamines, corticosteroids and/or epinephrine) should be available for immediate use in the event of a reaction (see ADVERSE REACTIONS, Infusion-Related Reactions).

NEUROLOGIC EVENTS

Infliximab and other agents that inhibit TNF have been associated in rare cases with exacerbation of clinical symptoms and/or radiographic evidence of de-myelinating disease. Prescribers should exercise caution in considering the use of infliximab in patients with pre-existing or recent onset of central nervous system de-myelinating disorders.

PRECAUTIONS

AUTOIMMUNITY

Treatment with infliximab may result in the formation of autoantibodies and, rarely, in the development of a lupus-like syndrome. If a patient develops symptoms suggestive of a lupus-like syndrome following treatment with infliximab, treatment should be discontinued (see ADVERSE REACTIONS, Autoantibodies/Lupus-Like Syndrome).

MALIGNANCY

Patients with long duration of Crohn's disease or rheumatoid arthritis and chronic exposure to immunosuppressant therapies are more prone to develop lymphomas (see ADVERSE REACTIONS, Malignancies/Lymphoproliferative Disease). The impact of treatment with infliximab on these phenomena is unknown.

IMMUNOGENICITY

Treatment with infliximab can be associated with the development of antibodies to infliximab. One hundred thirty-four (134) of the 199 Crohn's disease patients treated with infliximab were evaluated for the development of infliximab-specific antibodies; 18 (13%) were antibody-positive (the majority at low titer, <1:20). Patients who were antibody-positive were more likely to experience an infusion reaction (see ADVERSE REACTIONS, Infusion-Related Reactions). Antibody development was lower among rheumatoid arthritis and Crohn's disease patients receiving immunosuppressant therapies such as 6-MP, AZA or MTX. With repeated dosing of infliximab, serum concentrations of infliximab were higher in rheumatoid arthritis patients who received concomitant MTX. There are limited data available on the development of antibodies to infliximab in patients receiving long-term treatment with infliximab. Because immunogenicity analyses are product-specific, comparison of antibody rates to those from other products is not appropriate.

VACCINATIONS

No data are available on the response to vaccination or on the secondary transmission of infection by live vaccines in patients receiving anti-TNF therapy. It is recommended that live vaccines not be given concurrently.

CARCINOGENESIS, MUTAGENESIS, AND IMPAIRMENT OF FERTILITY

Long-term studies in animals have not been performed to evaluate the carcinogenic potential. No clastogenic or mutagenic effects of infliximab were observed in the *in vivo* mouse micronucleus test or the *Salmonella-Escherichia coli* (Ames) assay, respectively. Chromosomal aberrations were not observed in an assay performed using human lymphocytes. Tumorigenicity studies in mice deficient in TNFα demonstrated no increase in tumors when challenged with known tumor initiators and/or promoters. It is not known whether infliximab can impair fertility in humans. No impairment of fertility was observed in a fertility and general reproduction toxicity study conducted in mice using an analogous antibody that selectively inhibits the functional activity of mouse TNFα.

PREGNANCY CATEGORY B

Since infliximab does not cross-react with TNFα in species other than humans and chimpanzees, animal reproduction studies have not been conducted with infliximab. No evidence of maternal toxicity, embryotoxicity or teratogenicity was observed in a developmental toxicity study conducted in mice using an analogous antibody that selectively inhibits the functional activity of mouse TNFα. Doses of 10-15 mg/kg in pharmacodynamic animal models with the anti-TNF analogous antibody produced maximal pharmacologic effectiveness. Doses up to 40 mg/kg were shown to produce no adverse effects in animal reproduction studies. It is not known whether infliximab can cause fetal harm when administered to a pregnant woman or can affect reproduction capacity. Infliximab should be given to a pregnant woman only if clearly needed.

NURSING MOTHERS

It is not known whether infliximab is excreted in human milk or absorbed systemically after ingestion. Because many drugs and immunoglobulins are excreted in human milk, and because of the potential for adverse reactions in nursing infants from infliximab, a decision should be made whether to discontinue nursing or to discontinue the drug, taking into account the importance of the drug to the mother.

PEDIATRIC USE

Safety and effectiveness of infliximab in patients with juvenile rheumatoid arthritis and in pediatric patients with Crohn's disease have not been established.

GERIATRIC USE

In the ATTRACT study, no overall differences were observed in effectiveness or safety in 72 patients aged 65 or older compared to younger patients. In Crohn's disease studies, there were insufficient numbers of patients aged 65 and over to determine whether they respond differently from patients aged 18-65. Because there is a higher incidence of infections in the elderly population in general, caution should be used in treating the elderly (see ADVERSE REACTIONS, Infections).

DRUG INTERACTIONS

Specific drug interaction studies, including interactions with MTX, have not been conducted. The majority of patients in rheumatoid arthritis or Crohn's disease clinical studies received one or more concomitant medications. In rheumatoid arthritis, concomitant medications besides MTX were nonsteroidal anti-inflammatory agents, folic acid, corticosteroids and/or narcotics. Concomitant Crohn's disease medications were antibiotics, antivirals, corticosteroids, 6-MP/AZA and aminosalicylates. Patients with Crohn's disease who received immunosuppressants tended to experience fewer infusion reactions compared to patients on no immunosuppressants (see PRECAUTIONS, Immunogenicity and ADVERSE REACTIONS, Infusion-Related Reactions).

ADVERSE REACTIONS

A total of 771 patients were treated with infliximab in clinical studies. In both rheumatoid arthritis and Crohn's disease studies, approximately 6% of patients discontinued infliximab because of adverse experiences. The most common reasons for discontinuation of treatment were dyspnea, urticaria and headache. Adverse events have been reported in a higher proportion of patients receiving the 10 mg/kg dose than the 3 mg/kg dose.

INFUSION-RELATED REACTIONS

Acute Infusion Reactions

An infusion reaction was defined as any adverse event occurring during the infusion or within 1-2 hours after the infusion. Nineteen percent (19%) of infliximab-treated patients in all clinical studies experienced an infusion reaction compared to 8% of placebo-treated patients. Among the 4797 infliximab infusions, 3% were accompanied by nonspecific symptoms such as fever or chills, 1% were accompanied by cardiopulmonary reactions (primarily chest pain, hypotension, hypertension or dyspnea), <1% were accompanied by pruritus, urticaria, or the combined symptoms of pruritus/urticaria and cardiopulmonary reactions. Serious infusion reactions including anaphylaxis were infrequent. Less than 2% of patients discontinued infliximab because of infusion reactions, and all patients recovered with treatment and/or discontinuation of infusion. Infliximab infusions beyond the initial infusion in rheumatoid arthritis patients were not associated with a higher incidence of reactions.

Patients with Crohn's disease who became positive for antibodies to infliximab were more likely to develop infusion reactions than were those who were negative (36% vs 11% respectively). Use of concomitant immunosuppressant agents appeared to reduce the frequency of antibodies to infliximab and infusion reactions (see PRECAUTIONS, Immunogenicity and DRUG INTERACTIONS).

Reactions Following Readministration

In a clinical study of 40 patients with Crohn's disease retreated with infliximab following a 2-4 year period without infliximab treatment, 10 patients experienced adverse events manifesting 3-12 days following infusion of which 6 were considered serious. Signs and symptoms included myalgia and/or arthralgia with fever and/or rash, with some patients also experiencing pruritus, facial, hand or lip edema, dysphagia, urticaria, sore throat, and headache. Patients experiencing these adverse events had not experienced infusion-related adverse events associated with their initial infliximab therapy. Of the 40 patients enrolled, these adverse events occurred in 9 of 23 (39%) who had received liquid formulation which is no longer in use and 1 of 17 (6%) who received lyophilized formulation. The clinical data are not adequate to determine if occurrence of these reactions is due to differences in formulation. Patients' signs and symptoms improved substantially or resolved with treatment in all cases. There are insufficient data on the incidence of these events after drug-free intervals of less than 2 years. However, these events have been observed infrequently in clinical studies and post-marketing surveillance at intervals of less than 1 year.

INFECTIONS

In infliximab clinical studies, treated infections were reported in 32% of infliximab-treated patients (average of 37 weeks of follow-up) and in 22% of placebo-treated patients (average of 29 weeks of follow-up). The infections most frequently reported were upper respiratory tract infections (including sinusitis, pharyngitis, and bronchitis) and urinary tract infections. No increased risk of serious infections or sepsis were observed with infliximab compared to placebo in the ATTRACT study. Among infliximab-treated patients, these serious infections included pneumonia, cellulitis and sepsis. In the ATTRACT study, 1 patient died with miliary tuberculosis and 1 died with disseminated coccidioidomycosis. Other cases of tuberculosis, including disseminated tuberculosis, also have been reported post-marketing. Most of the cases of tuberculosis occurred within the first 2 months after initiation of therapy with infliximab and may reflect recrudescence of latent disease (see WARNINGS, Risk of Infections). Twelve percent (12%) of patients with fistulizing Crohn's disease developed a new abscess 8-16 weeks after the last infusion of infliximab.

In post-marketing experience, infections have been observed with various pathogens including viral, bacterial, fungal, and protozoal organisms. Infections have been noted in all organ systems and have been reported in patients receiving infliximab alone or in combination with immunosuppressive agents.

AUTOANTIBODIES/LUPUS-LIKE SYNDROME

In the ATTRACT rheumatoid arthritis study through week 54, 49% of infliximab-treated patients developed antinuclear antibodies (ANA) between screening and last evaluation, compared to 21% of placebo-treated patients. Anti-dsDNA antibodies developed in approximately 10% of infliximab-treated patients, compared to none of the placebo-treated patients. No association was seen between infliximab dose/schedule and development of ANA or anti-dsDNA.

Of Crohn's disease patients treated with infliximab who were evaluated for antinuclear antibodies (ANA), 34% developed ANA between screening and last evaluation. Anti-dsDNA antibodies developed in approximately 9% of Crohn's disease patients treated with infliximab. The development of anti-dsDNA antibodies was not related to either the dose or duration of infliximab treatment. However, baseline therapy with an immunosuppressant in Crohn's disease patients was associated with reduced development of anti-dsDNA antibodies (3% compared to 21% in patients not receiving any immunosuppressant). Crohn's disease patients were approximately 2 times more likely to develop anti-dsDNA antibodies if they were ANA-positive at study entry.

In clinical studies, 3 patients developed clinical symptoms consistent with a lupus-like syndrome, 2 with rheumatoid arthritis and 1 with Crohn's disease. All 3 patients improved following discontinuation of therapy and appropriate medical treatment. No cases of lupus-like reactions have been observed in up to 3 years of long-term follow-up (see PRECAUTIONS, Autoimmunity).

MALIGNANCIES/LYMPHOPROLIFERATIVE DISEASE

In completed clinical studies of infliximab for up to 54 weeks, 7 of 771 patients developed 8 new or recurrent malignancies. These were non-Hodgkin's B-cell lymphoma, breast cancer, melanoma, squamous, rectal adenocarcinoma and basal cell carcinoma. There are insufficient data to determine whether infliximab contributed to the development of these malignancies. The observed rates and incidences were similar to those expected for the populations studied[16,17] (see PRECAUTIONS, Malignancy).

OTHER ADVERSE REACTIONS

Adverse events occurring at a frequency of at least 5% in all patients treated with infliximab are shown in TABLE 4. Patients with Crohn's disease who were treated with infliximab were more likely than patients with rheumatoid arthritis to experience adverse events associated with gastrointestinal symptoms.

TABLE 4 *Adverse Events in Rheumatoid Arthritis and Crohn's Disease Studies*

	Rheumatoid Arthritis		Crohn's Disease	
	Placebo (n=133)	Infliximab (n=555)	Placebo (n=56)	Infliximab (n=199)
Avg. weeks of follow-up	35.9	41.2	14.7	27.0
Respiratory				
Upper respiratory infection	17%	26%	9%	16%
Coughing	7%	13%	0%	5%
Sinusitis	4%	13%	2%	5%
Pharyngitis	6%	11%	5%	9%
Rhinitis	7%	9%	4%	6%
Bronchitis	5%	6%	2%	7%
Gastrointestinal				
Nausea	18%	17%	4%	17%
Diarrhea	14%	13%	2%	3%
Abdominal pain	8%	10%	4%	12%
Vomiting	10%	7%	0%	9%
Dyspepsia	5%	6%	0%	5%
Other				
Headache	14%	22%	21%	23%
Rash	5%	12%	5%	6%
Dizziness	10%	10%	9%	8%
Urinary tract infection	7%	8%	4%	3%
Fatigue	5%	8%	5%	11%
Fever	6%	8%	7%	10%
Pain	8%	8%	5%	9%
Back pain	3%	6%	4%	5%
Pruritus	0%	6%	2%	5%
Arthralgia	2%	6%	2%	5%
Chest pain	5%	5%	5%	6%

Serious adverse events (all occurred at frequencies <2%) by body system in all patients treated with infliximab are as follows:

Body as a Whole: Abdominal hernia, asthenia, chest pain, diaphragmatic hernia, edema, fall, pain.

Blood: Splenic infarction, splenomegaly.

Cardiovascular: Hypertension, hypotension, syncope.

Central & Peripheral Nervous: Encephalopathy, dizziness, headache, spinal stenosis, upper motor neuron lesion.

Autoimmunity: Lupus erythematosus syndrome, worsening rheumatoid arthritis, rheumatoid nodules.

Ear and Hearing: Ceruminosis.

Eye and Vision: Endophthalmitis.

Gastrointestinal: Abdominal pain, appendicitis, Crohn's disease, diarrhea, gastric ulcer, gastrointestinal hemorrhage, intestinal obstruction, intestinal perforation, intestinal stenosis, nausea, pancreatitis, peritonitis, proctalgia, vomiting.

Heart Rate and Rhythm: Arrhythmia, atrioventricular block, bradycardia, cardiac arrest, palpitation, tachycardia.

Liver and Biliary: Biliary pain, cholecystitis, cholelithiasis, hepatitis cholestatic.

Metabolic and Nutritional: Dehydration, pancreatic insufficiency, weight decrease.

Musculoskeletal: Arthralgia, arthritis, back pain, bone fracture, hemarthrosis, intervertebral disk herniation, joint cyst, joint degeneration, myalgia, osteoarthritis, osteoporosis, spondylolisthesis, symphyseolysis, tendon disorder, tendon injury.

Myo-, Endo-, Pericardial and Coronary Valve: Angina pectoris, cardiac failure, myocardial ischemia.

Neoplasms: Basal cell, breast, lymphoma, melanoma, rectal adenocarcinoma, skin.

Platelet, Bleeding and Clotting: Thrombocytopenia.

Psychiatric: Anxiety, confusion, delirium, depression, somnolence, suicide attempt.

Red Blood Cell: Anemia.

Reproductive: Endometriosis.

Resistance Mechanism: Abscess, bacterial infection, cellulitis, fever, fungal infection, herpes zoster, infection, inflammation, sepsis.

Respiratory: Adult respiratory distress syndrome, bronchitis, coughing, dyspnea, pleural effusion, pleurisy, pneumonia, pneumothorax, pulmonary edema, pulmonary infiltration, respiratory insufficiency, upper respiratory tract infection.

Skin and Appendages: Furunculosis, increased sweating, injection site inflammation, rash, ulceration.

Urinary: Azotemia, dysuria, hydronephrosis, kidney infarction, pyelonephritis, renal calculus, renal failure, ureteral obstruction.

Vascular (Extracardiac): Brain infarction, peripheral ischemia, pulmonary embolism, thrombophlebitis deep.

White Cell and Reticuloendothelial: Leukopenia, lymphadenopathy, lymphangitis.

A greater proportion of patients enrolled into the ATTRACT study who received infliximab plus MTX experienced mild, transient elevations (<2 times the upper limit of normal) in AST or ALT (35% and 32% respectively) compared to patients treated with placebo with MTX (24% each). Six (1.8%) patients treated with infliximab and MTX experienced more prolonged elevations in their ALT.

Additional adverse events reported from worldwide post-marketing experience with infliximab include Guillain-Barre syndrome, optic neuritis, and polyneuropathy (see ADVERSE REACTIONS, Infections).

DOSAGE AND ADMINISTRATION

RHEUMATOID ARTHRITIS

The recommended dose of infliximab is 3 mg/kg given as an IV infusion followed with additional similar doses at 2 and 6 weeks after the first infusion then every 8 weeks thereafter. Infliximab should be given in combination with methotrexate. For patients who have an incomplete response, consideration may be given to adjusting the dose up to 10 mg/kg or treating as often as every 4 weeks.

CROHN'S DISEASE

The recommended dose of infliximab is 5 mg/kg given as a single IV infusion for treatment of moderately to severely active Crohn's disease. In patients with fistulizing disease, an initial 5 mg/kg dose should be followed with additional 5 mg/kg doses at 2 and 6 weeks after the first infusion.

There are insufficient safety and efficacy data for the use of infliximab in Crohn's disease beyond the recommended duration (see WARNINGS, Hypersensitivity; ADVERSE REACTIONS, Infusion-Related Reactions; and INDICATIONS AND USAGE).

HOW SUPPLIED

Remicade lyophilized concentrate for IV injection is supplied in single-use vials containing 100 mg infliximab in a 20 ml vial.

Storage: Store the lyophilized product under refrigeration at 2-8°C (36-46°F). Do not freeze. Do not use beyond the expiration date. This product contains no preservative.

PRODUCT LISTING - EQUIVALENTS NOT AVAILABLE

Powder For Injection - Intravenous - 100 mg

1's $691.61 REMICADE, Centocor Inc 57894-0030-01

Influenza Virus Vaccine *(001533)*

For complete prescribing information, refer to the CD-ROM included with the book.

Categories: Immunization, influenza; Pregnancy Category C; FDA Pre 1938 Drugs; WHO Formulary

Drug Classes: Vaccines

Brand Names: Flu Shield; **Fluimmune**; Fluogen; Flushield; Fluvirin; Fluzone

Foreign Brand Availability: Agrippal (England; Ireland; Italy; Philippines; South-Africa); Alorbat (Germany); Begrivac (Austria; Germany); Begrivac F (Israel); Fluarix (Australia; Bahamas; Barbados; Belize; Bermuda; Curacao; Guyana; Hong-Kong; Jamaica; Mexico; Netherland-Antilles; New-Zealand; Puerto-Rico; Surinam; Trinidad); Fluvax (Australia; New-Zealand); Fluviral S/F (Canada); Fluvirine (France); Hiberix (Australia; Bahamas; Barbados; Belize; Bermuda; Curacao; Guyana; India; Jamaica; Netherland-Antilles; Peru; Puerto-Rico; Surinam; Taiwan; Thailand; Trinidad); Inflexal (Austria; Italy; Spain); Inflexal Berna (Philippines; South-Africa); Inflexal Berna Polyvalent Vaccine (Malaysia); Inflexal V (England; Ireland); Influvac (Bahrain; Benin; Burkina-Faso; Cyprus; Egypt; Ethiopia; Gambia; Ghana; Guinea; Iran; Iraq; Israel; Ivory-Coast; Jordan; Kenya; Kuwait; Lebanon; Liberia; Libya; Malawi; Mali; Mauritania; Mauritius; Morocco; Niger; Nigeria; Oman; Qatar; Republic-of-Yemen; Saudi-Arabia; Senegal; Seychelles; Sierra-Leone; Sudan; Syria; Tanzania; Tunia; Uganda; United-Arab-Emirates; Zambia; Zimbabwe); Mutagrip (Belgium; France; Germany; Netherlands; Spain); Sandovac (Austria); Vaxigrip (Austria; Belgium; Bulgaria; Denmark; France; Greece; Hong-Kong; Israel; Netherlands; New-Zealand; Norway; Philippines; South-Africa); X-Flu (South-Africa)

DESCRIPTION

Influenza Virus Vaccine, Trivalent, Types A and B (chromatograph- and filter-purified subvirion antigen)

1993-94 FORMULA

DO NOT INJECT INTRAVENOUSLY Influenza virus vaccine, trivalent, types A and B (purified subvirion) is a sterile injectable for administration intramuscularly.

Influenza virus vaccine, trivalent, types A and B (purified subvirion) is prepared from the allantoic fluids of chick embryos inoculated with a specific type of influenza virus. During processing, not more than 5 mcg of gentamicin sulfate per ml is added. The harvested virus is inactivated with formaldehyde and is concentrated and purified.

Influenza virus vaccine, trivalent, types A and B (purified subvirion) is concentrated and refined by a column-chromatographic procedure. At the same time, addition of tri(n-)butylphosphate and polysorbate 80, to the column-eluting fluids effects disruption and inactivation of a significant proportion of the virus to smaller subunit particles. The recovered subvirion (split-virus) suspension is freed of substantial portions of the disrupting agents by dialysis and of other undesirable materials by selective filtration through membranes of controlled pore size.

The viral antigen content has been standardized by immunodiffusion tests, according to current U.S. Public Health Service requirements. Each dose (0.5 ml) contains the proportions and not less than the microgram amounts of hemagglutinin antigens (mcg HA) representative of the specific components recommended for the current influenza season.

The vaccine contains 1:10,000 thimerosal (mercury derivative) as a preservative. Gentamicin sulfate is used during manufacturing but is not detectable in the final product by current assay procedures.

INDICATIONS AND USAGE

Influenza virus vaccine is recommended for 1) high-risk persons 6 months of age or older and for their medical-care providers or household contacts; 2) for children and teenagers receiving long-term aspirin therapy who, therefore, may be at increased risk of developing Reye's syndrome after an influenza virus infection; and 3) for other persons who wish to reduce their chances of acquiring influenza.

Guidelines for the use of vaccine among different groups are given below.

TARGET GROUPS FOR VACCINATION

Groups at Increased Risk for Influenza-Related Complications:

1. Otherwise healthy persons 65 years of age or older.
2. Residents of nursing homes and other chronic-care facilities housing patients of any age with chronic medical conditions.
3. Adults and children with chronic disorders of the pulmonary or cardiovascular systems requiring regular medical follow-up or hospitalization during the preceding year, including children with asthma.
4. Adults and children who have required regular medical follow-up or hospitalization during the preceding year because of chronic metabolic diseases (including diabetes mellitus), renal dysfunction, hemoglobinopathies, or immunosuppression (including immunosuppression caused by medications).
5. Children and teenagers (aged 6 months to 18 years) who are receiving long-term aspirin therapy and, therefore, may be at risk of developing Reye's syndrome after influenza infection.

Elderly persons and persons with certain chronic diseases may develop lower post-vaccination antibody titers than healthy young adults and thus may remain susceptible to influenza upper-respiratory-tract infections. Nevertheless, even if such persons develop influenza illness, the vaccine has been shown to be effective in preventing lower-respiratory-tract involvement or other complications, thereby reducing the risk of hospitalization and death.

GROUPS POTENTIALLY CAPABLE OF NOSOCOMIAL TRANSMISSION OF INFLUENZA TO HIGH-RISK PERSONS

Individuals attending high-risk persons can transmit influenza infections to them while they are themselves incubating infection, undergoing subclinical infection, or working despite the existence of symptoms. Some high-risk persons, (*e.g.,* the elderly, transplant recipients, persons with acquired immunodeficiency syndrome (AIDS)), can have relatively low antibody responses to influenza vaccine. Efforts to protect them against influenza may be improved by reducing the chances that their care providers may expose them to influenza. Therefore, the following groups should be vaccinated:

1. Physicians, nurses, and other personnel in both hospital and outpatient settings.
2. Providers of home care to high-risk persons (*e.g.,* visiting nurses, volunteer workers) as well as all household members of high-risk persons, including children, whether or not they provide care.

VACCINATION OF OTHER GROUPS

General Population: Physicians should administer influenza vaccine to any person who wishes to reduce his/her chances of acquiring influenza infection. Persons who provide essential community services and students or other healthy individuals in institutional settings (*i.e.,* schools and colleges) should be encouraged to receive vaccine to minimize the disruption of routine activity during outbreaks.

Pregnant Women: Influenza-associated excess mortality among pregnant women has not been documented, except in the largest pandemics of 1918-19 and 1957-58. However, pregnant women who have medical conditions increasing their risks of complications from influenza should be vaccinated, as the vaccine is considered safe for pregnant women. Administering the vaccine after the first trimester is a reasonable precaution to minimize any concern over the theoretical possibility of teratogenicity. However, it is undesirable to delay vaccination of pregnant women with high-risk conditions who will still be in the first trimester of pregnancy when the influenza season begins.

Persons Infected With Human Immunodeficiency Virus (HIV): Little information exists regarding the frequency and severity of influenza illness in human immunodeficiency virus (HIV)-infected persons, but recent reports suggest that symptoms may be prolonged and the risk of complications increased for this high-risk group. Because influenza may result in serious illness and complications, vaccination is a prudent precaution and will result in protective antibody levels in many recipients. However, the antibody response to vaccine may be low in persons with advanced HIV-related illnesses; a booster dose of vaccine has not improved the immune response for these individuals.

Foreign Travelers: The risk of exposure to influenza during foreign travel varies, depending on, among other factors, season of travel and destination. Influenza can occur throughout the year in the tropics; the season of greatest influenza activity in the Southern Hemisphere is April-September. Because of the short incubation period for influenza, exposure to the virus during travel will often result in clinical illness that begins during travel, an inconvenience or potential danger, especially for persons at increased risk for complications. Persons preparing to travel to the tropics at any time of year or to the Southern Hemisphere during April-September should review their vaccination histories. If not vaccinated the previous fall/winter, they should be considered for influenza vaccination prior to travel. Persons in the high-risk categories especially should be encouraged to receive the vaccine. The most current available vaccine should be used. High-risk persons given the previous season's vaccine prior to travel should be revaccinated in the fall/winter with current vaccine.[1]

IMMUNIZATION PROGRAMS

If this product is to be used in an immunization program sponsored by an organization WHERE A TRADITIONAL PHYSICIAN/PATIENT RELATIONSHIP DOES NOT EXIST, each participant (or legal guardian) should be made aware of the possible risks that have been associated with the use of influenza virus vaccines, including the possible risk of a form of paralysis sometimes known as Guillain-Barre syndrome. Information about possible side effects and adverse reactions is presented below, and consent, preferably written, should be obtained from the intended recipient (or legal guardian) before vaccine administration.

Simultaneous Administration of Pneumoccal or Pediatric Vaccines: Pneumococcal vaccine and influenza vaccine can be given at the same time at different sites without increased side effects. However, it should be emphasized that whereas influenza vaccine is given annually, it is currently recommended that, with few exceptions, pneumococcal vaccine be given only once.[1]

It may be desirable to simultaneously administer influenza vaccine, if indicated, with routine pediatric vaccine but at different sites. Although studies have not been done, no diminution of immunogenicity or enhancement of adverse reactions should be expected.[1] Influenza vaccine should not be given within 3 days of vaccination with pertussis vaccine.

CONTRAINDICATIONS

INFLUENZA VIRUS VACCINE SHOULD NOT BE ADMINISTERED TO INDIVIDUALS WITH A HISTORY OF HYPERSENSITIVITY (ALLERGY) TO CHICKEN EGG OR OTHER COMPONENTS OF INFLUENZA VIRUS VACCINES WITHOUT FIRST CONSULTING A PHYSICIAN. Before being vaccinated, persons known to be hypersensitive to egg protein should be given a skin test or other allergy-evaluating test, using the Influenza Virus Vaccine as the antigen. Persons with adverse reactions to such testing should not be vaccinated. Chemoprophylaxis may be indicated for prevention of influenza A in such persons. However, persons with a history of anaphylactic hypersensitivity to vaccine components but who are also at highest risk for complications of influenza infections may benefit from vaccine after appropriate evaluation and desensitization.[1]

Although gentamicin sulfate is not detectable in the final product by current assay procedures, the vaccine should not be administered to persons with known sensitivity to gentamicin or other aminoglycosides.

Persons with a past history of Guillain-Barre syndrome (GBS) should not be given influenza virus vaccine.

Persons with acute febrile illnesses usually should not be vaccinated until their symptoms have abated. However, minor illness with or without fever should not contraindicate the use of influenza vaccine, particularly in children with a mild upper-respiratory-tract infection or allergic rhinitis.[3]

WARNINGS

Patients with impaired immune responsiveness, whether due to the use of immunosuppressive therapy (including irradiation, large amounts of corticosteroids, antimetabolites, alkylating agents, and cytotoxic agents), a genetic defect, human immunodeficiency virus (HIV) infection, leukemia, lymphoma, generalized malignancy, or other causes, may have a reduced antibody response to active immunization procedures.[1] Short-term (less than 2 weeks) corticosteroid therapy or intra-articular, bursal, or tendon injections with corticosteroids should not be immunosuppressive. Inactivated vaccines are not a risk to immunocompromised individuals, although their efficacy may be substantially reduced. Because patients with immunodeficiencies may not have an adequate response to immunizing agents, they may remain susceptible despite having received an appropriate vaccine. If feasible, specific serum antibody titers or other immunologic responses may be determined after immunization to assess immunity.[3] Chemoprophylaxis may be indicated for high-risk persons who are expected to have a poor antibody response to influenza vaccine.[1]

DOSAGE AND ADMINISTRATION

Although influenza virus vaccine often contains one or more antigens used in previous years, immunity declines during the year following vaccination. Therefore, a history of vaccination in any previous year with a vaccine containing one or more antigens included in the current vaccine does NOT preclude the need for revaccination for the 1993-1994 influenza season to provide optimal protection. REMAINING VACCINE FROM THE PREVIOUS YEAR SHOULD NOT BE USED.

Influenza vaccine may be offered to high-risk persons presenting for routine care or hospitalization beginning in September, but not until new vaccine is available (see INDICATIONS AND USAGE, Vaccination of Other Groups for foreign travel, related exceptions). Opportunities to vaccinate persons at high risk for complications of influenza should not be missed. In the United States, influenza activity generally peaks between late December and early March, and high levels of influenza activity infrequently occur in the contiguous 48 states before December. Therefore, the optimal time for organized vaccination campaigns for high-risk persons usually is the period between mid-October and mid-November. In facilities such as nursing homes it is particularly important to avoid administering vaccine too far in advance of the influenza season because antibody may begin to decline within a few months. Such vaccination programs may be undertaken as soon as current vaccine is available in September or October if regional influenza activity is expected to begin earlier than normal.

Children less than 9 years of age who have not been vaccinated previously should receive two doses with at least 1 month between doses to maximize the chance of a satisfactory antibody response to all three vaccine antigens. The second dose should be given before December if possible. Vaccine should continue to be offered to both children and adults up to and even after influenza virus activity is documented in a community which may be as late as April in some years.

Parenteral drug products should be inspected visually for particulate matter and discoloration, whenever solution and container permit.

DO NOT INJECT INTRAVENOUSLY. Injections of FluShield are recommended to be given intramuscularly. The recommended site is the deltoid muscle for adults and older children. The preferred site for infants and young children is the anterolateral aspect of the thigh musculature. Because of lack of adequate evaluation of other route in high-risk persons, the preferred route of vaccination is intramuscularly whenever possible. Before injection, the skin over the site to be injected should be cleansed with a suitable germicide. After insertion of the needle, aspirate to help avoid inadvertent injection into a blood vessel. SeeTABLE 1 for pediatric dosages.

TABLE 1

AGE GROUP	DOSAGE SCHEDULE
9 years and older	0.5 ml (one dose)
3 to 8 years	0.5 ml (1 or 2 doses)*
6 to 35 months	0.25 ml (1 or 2 doses)*
For those under 13 years, only split-virus (subvirion) vaccine is recommended.	

* A single dose is considered sufficient for those under 9 years who have received at least 1 dose of influenza virus vaccine. With the 2-dose regimen, allow 4 weeks or more between doses. Both doses are recommended for maximum protection.

Immunogenicity and reactogenicity of split- and whole-virus vaccines are similar in adults when used according to the recommended dosage.[1]

Storage: Store between 2°-8°C (35°-46° F). Potency is destroyed by freezing; do not use Influenza Virus Vaccine that has been frozen.

PRODUCT LISTING - EQUIVALENTS NOT AVAILABLE

Suspension - Intramuscular - Strength n/a

0.50 ml x 10	$55.95	GENERIC, Medeva Pharmaceuticals Inc	19650-0103-01
0.50 ml x 10	$55.95	FLUVIRIN, Allscripts Pharmaceutical Company	54569-5137-00
0.50 ml x 10	$80.73	GENERIC, Wyeth-Ayerst Laboratories	00008-0985-02
0.50 ml x 10	$89.64	FLUVIRIN, Evans Vaccines	66521-0105-01
0.50 ml x 10	$111.56	FLUZONE PFS, Aventis Pharmaceuticals	49281-0368-11
0.50 ml x 10	$123.38	FLUZONE, Aventis Pharmaceuticals	49281-0370-11
5 ml	$44.95	FLUVIRIN, Allscripts Pharmaceutical Company	54569-5136-00
5 ml	$53.21	GENERIC, Wyeth-Ayerst Laboratories	00008-0985-01
5 ml	$66.19	GENERIC, Wyeth-Ayerst Laboratories	00008-0986-01
5 ml	$67.50	GENERIC, Wyeth-Ayerst Laboratories	00008-0987-01
5 ml	$69.12	FLUVIRIN, Evans Vaccines	66521-0105-10
5 ml	$75.00	FLUZONE SV, Aventis Pharmaceuticals	49281-0368-15
5 ml	$87.50	FLUZONE, Aventis Pharmaceuticals	49281-0370-15

Influenza Virus Vaccine Live (003601)

For complete prescribing information, refer to the CD-ROM included with the book.

Categories: Immunization, influenza; Pregnancy Category C; FDA Approved 2003 Jun
Drug Classes: Vaccines
Brand Names: FluMist

DESCRIPTION

FOR NASAL ADMINISTRATION ONLY.

Influenza virus vaccine live, intranasal (FluMist) is a live trivalent nasally administered vaccine intended for active immunization for the prevention of influenza.

Each 0.5 ml dose is formulated to contain $10^{6.5-7.5}$ $TCID_{50}$ (median tissue culture infectious dose) of live attenuated influenza virus reassortants of the strains recommended by the US Public Health Service (USPHS) for the 2003-2004 season: A/New Caledonia/20/99 (H1N1), A/Panama/2007/99 (H3N2) (A/Moscow/10/99-like), and B/Hong Kong/330/2001.[1] These strains are (a) *antigenically representative* of influenza viruses that may circulate in humans during the 2003-2004 influenza season; (b) *cold-adapted (ca)* (*i.e.,* they replicate efficiently at 25°C, a temperature that is restrictive for replication of many wild-type viruses); (c) *temperature-sensitive (ts)* (*i.e.,* they are restricted in replication at 37°C (Type B strains) or 39°C (Type A strains), temperatures at which many wild-type influenza viruses grow efficiently); and (d) *attenuated (att)* so as not to produce classic influenza-like illness in the ferret model of human influenza infection. The cumulative effect of the antigenic properties and the *ca, ts,* and *att* phenotype is that the vaccine viruses replicate in the nasopharynx to produce protective immunity.

Each of the three influenza virus strains contained in influenza virus vaccine live, intranasal is a genetic reassortant of a Master Donor Virus (MDV) and a wild-type influenza virus. The MDVs (A/Ann Arbor/6/60 and B/Ann Arbor/1/66) were developed by serial passage at sequentially lower temperatures in specific pathogen-free (SPF) primary chick kidney cells.[2] During this process, the MDVs acquired the *ca, ts,* and *att* phenotype and multiple mutations in the gene segments that encode viral proteins other than the surface glycoproteins. The individual contribution of the genetic sequences of the six non-glycoprotein MDV genes ("internal gene segments") to the *ca, ts,* and *att* phenotype is not completely understood. However, at least five genetic loci in three different internal gene segments of the Type A MDV and at least three genetic loci in two different internal gene segments of the Type B MDV contribute to the *ts* property.[3,4] For each of the three strains in influenza virus vaccine live, intranasal, the six internal gene segments responsible for *ca, ts,* and *att* phenotypes are derived from the MDV, and the two segments that encode the two surface glycoproteins, hemagglutinin (HA) and neuraminidase (NA), are derived from the corresponding antigenically relevant wild-type influenza viruses that have been recommended by the USPHS for inclusion in the annual vaccine formulation. Thus, the three viruses contained in influenza virus vaccine live, intranasal maintain the replication characteristics and phenotypic properties of the MDV and express the HA and NA of wild-type viruses that are related to strains expected to circulate during the 2003-2004 influenza season.

Viral harvests used in the production of influenza virus vaccine live, intranasal are produced by inoculating each of the three reassortant viruses into specific pathogen-free (SPF) eggs that are incubated to allow for vaccine virus replication. The allantoic fluid of these eggs is harvested, clarified by centrifugation, and stabilized with buffer containing sucrose, potassium phosphate, and monosodium glutamate (0.47 mg/dose). Viral harvests from the three strains (H1N1, H3N2, and B) are subsequently blended and diluted to desired potency with allantoic fluid derived from uninfected SPF eggs to produce trivalent bulk vaccine. Each lot of viral harvest is tested for *ca, ts,* and *att* and is also tested extensively by *in vitro* and *in vivo* methods to detect adventitious agents. The bulk vaccine is then filled directly into individual sprayers for nasal administration. These sprayers are labeled and stored at ≤-15°C.

Gentamicin sulfate is added early in the manufacturing process during preparation of reassortant viruses at a calculated concentration of approximately 1 μg/ml. Later steps of the manufacturing process do not use gentamicin, resulting in a diluted residual concentration in the final product of <0.015 μg/ml (limit of detection of the assay). FluMist does not contain any preservatives.

Each pre-filled FluMist sprayer contains a single 0.5 ml dose. The teflon tip attached to the sprayer is equipped with a one-way valve that produces a fine mist that is primarily deposited in the nose and nasopharynx. When thawed for administration, FluMist is a colorless to pale yellow liquid and is clear to slightly cloudy (see DOSAGE AND ADMINISTRATION).

INDICATIONS AND USAGE

FOR NASAL ADMINISTRATION ONLY.

Influenza virus vaccine live, intranasal is indicated for active immunization for the prevention of disease caused by influenza A and B viruses in healthy children and adolescents, 5-17 years of age, and healthy adults, 18-49 years of age.

Influenza virus vaccine live, intranasal is not indicated for immunization of individuals less than 5 years of age, or 50 years of age and older, or for therapy of influenza, nor will it protect against infections and illness caused by infectious agents other than influenza A or B viruses.

I

CONTRAINDICATIONS

Under no circumstances should influenza virus vaccine live, intranasal be administered parenterally.

Individuals with a history of hypersensitivity, especially anaphylactic reactions, to any component of influenza virus vaccine live, intranasal, including eggs or egg products, should not receive influenza virus vaccine live, intranasal (see DESCRIPTION).

Influenza virus vaccine live, intranasal is contraindicated in children and adolescents (5-17 years of age) receiving aspirin therapy or aspirin-containing therapy, because of the association of Reye syndrome with aspirin and wild-type influenza infection.

Influenza virus vaccine live, intranasal should not be administered to individuals who have a history of Guillain-Barré syndrome.

As with other live virus vaccines, influenza virus vaccine live, intranasal should not be administered to individuals with known or suspected immune deficiency diseases such as combined immunodeficiency, agammaglobulinemia, and thymic abnormalities and conditions such as human immunodeficiency virus infection, malignancy, leukemia, or lymphoma. Influenza virus vaccine live, intranasal is also contraindicated in patients who may be immunosuppressed or have altered or compromised immune status as a consequence of treatment with systemic corticosteroids, alkylating drugs, antimetabolites, radiation, or other immunosuppressive therapies.

WARNINGS

The safety of influenza virus vaccine live, intranasal in individuals with asthma or reactive airways disease has not been established. In a large safety study in children 1-17 years of age, children <5 years of age who received influenza virus vaccine live, intranasal were found to have an increased rate of asthma within 42 days of vaccination when compared to placebo recipients. Influenza virus vaccine live, intranasal should not be administered to individuals with a history of asthma or reactive airways disease.

The safety of influenza virus vaccine live, intranasal in individuals with underlying medical conditions that may predispose them to severe disease following wild-type influenza infection has not been established. Influenza virus vaccine live, intranasal is not indicated for these individuals. According to the Advisory Committee on Immunization Practices (ACIP), such individuals include, but are not limited to, adults and children with chronic disorders of the cardiovascular and pulmonary systems, including asthma; pregnant women who will be in their second or third trimesters during influenza season; adults and children who required regular medical follow-up or hospitalization during the preceding year because of chronic metabolic diseases (including diabetes), renal dysfunction, or hemoglobinopathies; and adults and children with congenital or acquired immunosuppression caused by underlying disease or immunosuppressive therapy (see CONTRAINDICATIONS). Intramuscularly administered inactivated influenza vaccines are available to immunize high-risk individuals.[1]

As with any vaccine, influenza virus vaccine live, intranasal may not protect 100% of individuals receiving the vaccine.

DOSAGE AND ADMINISTRATION

FOR NASAL USE ONLY. DO NOT ADMINISTER PARENTERALLY.

Influenza virus vaccine live, intranasal should be administered according to the schedule in TABLE 5.

For healthy children age 5 years through 8 years who have not previously received influenza virus vaccine live, intranasal, the recommended dosage schedule for nasal administration is one 0.5 ml dose followed by a second 0.5 ml dose given at least 6 weeks later. Only limited data are available on the degree of protection in children who receive 1 dose.

For all other healthy individuals, including children age 5-8 years who have previously received at least 1 dose of influenza virus vaccine live, intranasal, the recommended schedule is 1 dose.

TABLE 5

Age Group	Vaccination Status	Dosage Schedule
Children age 5 years through 8 years	Not previously vaccinated with influenza virus vaccine live, intranasal	2 doses (0.5 ml each, 60 days apart ±14 days) for initial season
Children age 5 years through 8 years	Previously vaccinated with influenza virus vaccine live, intranasal	1 dose (0.5 ml) per season
Children and Adults age 9 through 49 years	Not applicable	1 dose (0.5 ml) per season

Influenza virus vaccine live, intranasal should be administered prior to exposure to influenza. The peak of influenza activity is variable from year to year, but generally occurs in the US between late December and early March. Because the duration of protection induced by influenza virus vaccine live, intranasal is not known and yearly antigenic variation in the influenza strains is possible, annual revaccination may increase the likelihood of protection.

Influenza virus vaccine live, intranasal must be thawed prior to administration. Influenza virus vaccine live, intranasal may be thawed by holding the sprayer in the palm of the hand and supporting the plunger rod with the thumb (see Administration Instructions that are distributed with the prescription); the vaccine should be administered immediately thereafter. Alternatively, influenza virus vaccine live, intranasal may be thawed in a refrigerator and stored at 2-8°C (36-46°F) for no more than 24 hours prior to use. When thawed for administration, influenza virus vaccine live, intranasal is a colorless to pale yellow liquid and is clear to slightly cloudy; some proteinaceous particulates may be present but do not affect the use of the product.

Approximately 0.25 ml (*i.e.*, half of the dose from a single influenza virus vaccine live, intranasal sprayer) is administered into each nostril while the recipient is in an upright position. Insert the tip of the sprayer just inside the nose and depress the plunger to spray. The dose-divider clip is removed from the sprayer to administer the second half of the dose (approximately 0.25 ml) into the other nostril. Once influenza virus vaccine live, intranasal has been administered, the used sprayer should be disposed of according to the standard procedures for biohazardous waste products.

Insulin (Human Recombinant) *(001544)*

For related information, see the comparative table section in Appendix A.

Categories: Diabetes mellitus; Recombinant DNA Origin; FDA Approved 1982 Oct; Pregnancy Category B; WHO Formulary

Drug Classes: Antidiabetic agents; Insulins

Brand Names: **Humulin**; Humulin Br; Humulin R; Insulin Human; Mixtard Human 70 30; Novolin 70 30 Penfill; Novolin N Penfill; Novolin R; Velosulin Human; Velosulin Human R

Foreign Brand Availability: Actrapid (Australia; Finland; New-Zealand); Actrapid HM (Bahamas; Bahrain; Barbados; Belize; Benin; Bermuda; Burkina-Faso; Curacao; Cyprus; Egypt; Ethiopia; France; Gambia; Germany; Ghana; Guinea; Guyana; Hong-Kong; Iran; Iraq; Israel; Italy; Ivory-Coast; Jamaica; Jordan; Kenya; Kuwait; Lebanon; Liberia; Libya; Malawi; Malaysia; Mali; Mauritania; Mauritius; Morocco; Netherland-Antilles; Niger; Nigeria; Oman; Philippines; Puerto-Rico; Qatar; Republic-of-Yemen; Saudi-Arabia; Senegal; Seychelles; Sierra-Leone; South-Africa; Sudan; Surinam; Syria; Taiwan; Tanzania; Thailand; Trinidad; Tunia; Uganda; United-Arab-Emirates; Zambia; Zimbabwe); Actrapid Human (Indonesia; Japan; Korea); Berlinsulin Actrapid Normal U-40 (Germany); Berlinsulin H Basal U-40 (Germany); Biohulin (Korea); Human Actrapid (India; Ireland); Human Nordisulin (India); Huminsulin "Lilly" Normal (Austria); Huminsulin Normal (Germany; Switzerland); Humulina Regular (Spain); Humulin C (Ecuador; Peru); Humulin-R (Canada; Colombia; Dominican-Republic; El-Salvador; Guatemala; Honduras; Nicaragua; Panama); Humulin Regular (Denmark; Finland; Norway; Portugal; Sweden; Taiwan); Humulin (Regular) (Greece); Humuline Regular (Sweden); Insulina (Spain); Insulina Actrapid HM (Spain); Insulina Velosulin HM (Spain); Insulin Hoechst-Rapid U-100 (Switzerland); Insulin Human Actrapid (England); Insulin Actrapid HM (Bulgaria); Insulin "Novo Nordisk" Actrapid HM (Austria); Insulin "Novo Nordisk" Velosulin HM (Austria); Insulin Velosulin HM (Israel); Insuline (Netherlands); Insuline Actrapid (Belgium; Netherlands); Insuline Humuline Regular (Netherlands); Insuline Velosulin Humaan (Netherlands); Insuman (Austria; Belgium; Bulgaria; Czech-Republic; Denmark; England; Finland; France; Germany; Greece; Hungary; Ireland; Italy; Netherlands; Norway; Poland; Portugal; Slovenia; Spain; Sweden; Switzerland; Turkey); Insuman Basal (France); Insuman Infusat (Germany); Insuman Rapid (France); Orgasulin Rapid (France); Umuline Profil 10 (France); Umuline Profil 20 (France); Umuline Profil 30 (France); Umuline Profil 40 (France); Umuline Profil 50 (France); Velosulin (Denmark; Finland); Velosuline Humaine (France)

HCFA JCODE(S): J1820 up to 100 units SC

WARNING

THIS LILLY HUMAN INSULIN PRODUCT DIFFERS FROM ANIMAL-SOURCE INSULINS BECAUSE IT IS STRUCTURALLY IDENTICAL TO THE INSULIN PRODUCED BY YOUR BODY'S PANCREAS AND BECAUSE OF ITS UNIQUE MANUFACTURING PROCESS.

ANY CHANGE OF INSULIN SHOULD BE MADE CAUTIOUSLY AND ONLY UNDER MEDICAL SUPERVISION. CHANGES IN STRENGTH, MANUFACTURER, TYPE (*e.g.*, REGULAR, NPH, LENTE), SPECIES (BEEF, PORK, BEEF-PORK, HUMAN), OR METHOD OF MANUFACTURE (rDNA VERSUS ANIMAL-SOURCE INSULIN) MAY RESULT IN THE NEED FOR A CHANGE IN DOSAGE.

SOME PATIENTS TAKING HUMULIN (HUMAN INSULIN, rDNA ORIGIN, LILLY) MAY REQUIRE A CHANGE IN DOSAGE FROM THAT USED WITH ANIMAL-SOURCE INSULINS. IF AN ADJUSTMENT IS NEEDED, IT MAY OCCUR WITH THE FIRST DOSE OR DURING THE FIRST SEVERAL WEEKS OR MONTHS.

PATIENT PACKAGE INSERT

DIABETES

Insulin is a hormone produced by the pancreas, a large gland that lies near the stomach. This hormone is necessary for the body's correct use of food, especially sugar. Diabetes occurs when the pancreas does not make enough insulin to meet your body's needs.

To control your diabetes, your doctor has prescribed injections of insulin to keep your blood glucose at a nearly normal level. Proper control of your diabetes requires dose and constant cooperation with your doctor. In spite of diabetes, you can lead an active, healthy, and useful life if you eat a balanced diet daily, exercise regularly, and take your insulin injections as prescribed.

You have been instructed to test your blood and/or your urine regularly for glucose. If your blood tests consistently show above- or below-normal glucose levels or your urine tests consistently show the presence of glucose, your diabetes is not properly controlled and you must let your doctor know.

Always keep an extra supply of insulin as well as a spare syringe and needle on hand. Always wear diabetic identification so that appropriate treatment can be given if complications occur away from home.

DESCRIPTION

Humulin is synthesized in a special non-disease-producing laboratory strain of *Escherichia coli* bacteria that has been genetically altered by the addition of the gene for human insulin production.

The time course of action of any insulin may vary considerably in different individuals or at different times in the same individual. As with all insulin preparation, the duration of action of all forms of Humulin is dependent on dose, site of injection, blood supply, temperature, and physical activity. Humulin is a sterile solution and is for subcutaneous injection. The concentration of all forms of Humulin is 100 units/ml (U-100).

Humulin R consists of zinc-insulin crystals dissolved in a clear fluid. Humulin R has nothing added to change the speed or length of its action. It takes effect rapidly and has a relatively short duration of activity (4-12 hours) as compared with other insulins. It should not be used intramuscularly.

Humulin N is a crystalline suspension of human insulin with protamine and zinc providing an intermediate-acting insulin with a slower onset of action and a longer duration of activity (up to 24 hours) than that of regular insulin. It should not be used intravenously or intramuscularly.

Humulin L is an amorphous and crystalline suspension of human insulin with zinc providing an intermediate -acting insulin with a slower onset and a longer duration of activity (up to 24 hours) than regular insulin. It should not be used intravenously or intramuscularly.

Humulin U is a crystalline suspension of human insulin with zinc providing a slower onset and a longer and less intense duration of activity (up to 28 hours) than regular insulin or the intermediate-acting insulins (NPH and Lente). It should not be used intravenously or intramuscularly.

Humulin 50/50 is a mixture of 50% Human Insulin Isophane Suspension and 50% Human Insulin Injection. It is an intermediate-acting insulin combined with the more rapid onset of action than regular insulin. The duration of activity may last up to 24 hours following injection. It should not be used intravenously or intramuscularly.

Humulin 70/30 is a mixture of 70% human insulin isophane suspension and 30% human insulin injection. It is an intermediate-acting insulin combined with the more rapid onset of action of regular insulin. The duration of activity may last up to 24 hours following injection. It should not be used intravenously or intramuscularly.

IDENTIFICATION

Human insulin manufactured by Eli Lilly and Company has the trademark Humulin and is available in 6 formulations — Regular (R), NPH (N), Lente (L), Ultralente (U), 50% Human Insulin Isophane Suspension [NPH]/50% Human Insulin Injection [buffered regular] (50/50), and 70% Human Insulin Isophane Suspension [NPH]/30% Human Insulin Injection [buffered regular] (70/30). Your doctor has prescribed the type of insulin that he/she believes is best for you. **DO NOT USE ANY OTHER INSULIN EXCEPT ON HIS/HER ADVICE AND DIRECTION.**

Always check the carton and the bottle label for the name and letter designation of the insulin you receive from your pharmacy to make sure it is the same as that your doctor has prescribed. Always examine the appearance of your bottle of insulin before withdrawing each dose.

Humulin R can be identified as follows: Humulin R is a clear and colorless liquid with a water-like appearance and consistency. Do not use if it appears cloudy, thickened, or slightly colored or if solid particles are visible.

Humulin N can be identified as follows: A bottle of Humulin N must be carefully shaken or rotated before each injection so that the contents are uniformly mixed. Humulin N should look uniformly cloudy or milky after mixing. Do not use it if the insulin substance (the white material) remains at the bottom of the bottle after mixing. Do not use a bottle of Humulin N if there are clumps in the insulin after mixing. Do not use a bottle of Humulin N if solid white particles stick to the bottom or wall of the bottle, giving it a frosted appearance.

Humulin L can be identified as follows: A bottle of Humulin L must be carefully shaken or rotated before each injection so that the contents are uniformly mixed. Humulin L should look uniformly cloudy or milky after mixing. Do not use it if the insulin substance (the white material) remains at the bottom of the bottle after mixing. Do not use a bottle of Humulin L if there are clumps in the insulin after mixing.

Humulin U can be identified as follows: A bottle of Humulin U must be carefully shaken or rotated before each injection so that the contents are uniformly mixed. Humulin U should look uniformly cloudy or milky after mixing. Do not use it if the insulin substance (the white material) remains at the bottom of the bottle after mixing. Do not use a bottle of Humulin U if there are clumps in the insulin after mixing.

Humulin 50/50 can be identified as follows: A bottle of Humulin 50/50 must be carefully shaken or rotated before each injection so that the contents are uniformly mixed. Humulin 50/50 should look uniformly cloudy or milky after mixing. Do not use it if the insulin substance (the white material) remains at the bottom of the bottle after mixing. Do not use a bottle of Humulin 50/50 if there are clumps in the insulin after mixing. Do not use a bottle of Humulin 50/50 if solid white particles stick to the bottom or wall of the bottle, giving it a frosted appearance.

Humulin 70/30 can be identified as follows: A bottle of Humulin 70/30 must be carefully shaken or rotated before each injection so that the contents are uniformly mixed. Humulin 70/30 should look uniformly cloudy or milky after mixing. Do not use it if the insulin substance (the white material) remains at the bottom of the bottle after mixing. Do not use a bottle of Humulin 70/30 if there are clumps in the insulin after mixing. Do not use a bottle of Humulin 70/30 if solid white particles stick to the bottom or wall of the bottle, giving it a frosted appearance.

Always check the appearance of your bottle of insulin before using, and if you note anything unusual in the appearance of your insulin or notice your insulin requirements changing markedly, consult your doctor.

STORAGE

Insulin should be stored in a refrigerator but not in the freezer. If refrigeration is not possible, the bottle of insulin that you are currently using can be kept unrefrigerated as long as it is kept as cool as possible (below 86°F [30°C]) and away from heat and light. Do not use insulin if it has been frozen. Do not use a bottle of insulin after the expiration date on the label.

DOSAGE

Your doctor has told you which insulin to use, how much, and when and how often to inject it. Because each patient's case of diabetes is different, this schedule has been individualized for you.

Your usual insulin dose may be affected by changes in your food, activity, or work schedule. Carefully follow your doctor's instructions to allow for these changes. Other things that may affect your insulin dose are:

Illness: Illness, especially with nausea and vomiting, may cause your insulin requirements to change. Even if you are not eating, you will still require insulin. You and your doctor should establish a sick day plan for you to use in case of illness. When you are sick, test your blood/urine frequently and call your doctor as instructed.

Pregnancy: Good control of diabetes is especially important for you and your unborn baby. Pregnancy may make managing your diabetes more difficult. If you are planning to have a baby, are pregnant, or are nursing a baby, consult your doctor.

Medication: Insulin requirements may be increased if you are taking other drugs with hyperglycemic activity, such as oral contraceptives, corticosteroids, or thyroid replacement therapy. Insulin requirements may be reduced in the presence of drugs with hypoglycemic activity, such as oral hypoglycemics, salicylates (for example, aspirin), sulfa antibiotics, and certain antidepressants. Always discuss any medications you are taking with your doctor.

Exercise: Exercise may lower your body's need for insulin during and for some time after the activity. Exercise may also help speed up the effect of an insulin dose, especially if the exercise involves the area of injection site (for example, the leg should not be used for injection just prior to running). Discuss with your doctor how you should adjust your regimen to accommodate exercise.

Travel: Persons traveling across more than 2 time zones should consult their doctor concerning adjustments in their insulin schedule.

COMMON PROBLEMS OF DIABETES

Hypoglycemia (Insulin Reaction)

Hypoglycemia (too little glucose in the blood) is one of the most frequent adverse events experienced by insulin users. It can be brought about by:

1. Taking too much insulin.
2. Missing or delaying meals.
3. Exercising or working more than usual.
4. An infection or illness (especially with diarrhea or vomiting).
5. A change in the body's need for insulin.
6. Diseases of the adrenal, pituitary, or thyroid gland, or progression of kidney or liver disease.
7. Interactions with other drugs that lower blood glucose such as oral hypoglycemics, salicylates (for example, aspirin), sulfa antibiotics, and certain antidepressants.
8. Consumption of alcoholic beverages.

Symptoms of mild to moderate hypoglycemia may occur suddenly and can include: Sweating; dizziness; palpitation; tremor; hunger; restlessness; tingling in the hands, feet, lips, or tongue; lightheadedness; inability to concentrate; headache; drowsiness; sleep disturbances; anxiety; blurred vision; slurred speech; depressive mood; irritability; abnormal behavior; unsteady movement; personality changes.

Signs of severe hypoglycemia can include: Disorientation, unconsciousness, seizures, death.

Therefore, it is important that assistance be obtained immediately.

Early warning symptoms of hypoglycemia may be different or less pronounced under certain conditions, such as long duration of diabetes, diabetic nerve disease, medications such as beta-blockers, change in insulin preparations, or intensified control (3 or more insulin injections per day) of diabetes.

A few patients who have experienced hypoglycemic reactions after transfer from animal-source insulin to human insulin have reported that the early warning symptoms of hypoglycemia were less pronounced or different from those experienced with their previous insulin.

Without recognition of early warning symptoms, you may not be able to take steps to avoid more serious hypoglycemia. Be alert for all of the various types of symptoms that may indicate hypoglycemia. Patients who experience hypoglycemia without early warning symptoms should monitor their blood glucose frequently, especially prior to activities such as driving. If the blood glucose is below your normal fasting glucose, you should consider eating or drinking sugar-containing foods to treat your hypoglycemia.

Mild to moderate hypoglycemia may be treated by eating foods or drinks that contain sugar. Patients should always carry a quick source of sugar, such as candy mints or glucose tablets. More severe hypoglycemia may require the assistance of another person. Patients who are unable to take sugar orally or who are unconscious require an injection of glucagon or should be treated with intravenous administration of glucose at a medical facility.

You should learn to recognize your own symptoms of hypoglycemia. If you are uncertain about these symptoms, you should monitor your blood glucose frequently to help you learn to recognize the symptoms that you experience with hypoglycemia.

If you have frequent episodes of hypoglycemia or experience difficultly in recognizing the symptoms, you should consult your doctor to discuss possible changes in therapy, meal plans, and/or exercise programs to help you avoid hypoglycemia.

Hyperglycemia and Diabetic Acidosis

Hyperglycemia (too much glucose in the blood) may develop if your body has too little insulin. Hyperglycemia can be brought about by:

1. Omitting your insulin or taking less than the doctor has prescribed.
2. Eating significantly more than your meal plan suggests.
3. Developing a fever, infection, or other significant stressful situation.

In patients with insulin-dependent diabetes, prolonged hyperglycemia can result in diabetic acidosis. The first symptoms of diabetic acidosis usually come on gradually, over a period of hours or days, and include a drowsy feeling, flushed face, thirst, loss of appetite, and fruity odor on the breath. With acidosis, urine tests show large amounts of glucose and acetone. Heavy breathing and a rapid pulse are more severe symptoms. If uncorrected, prolonged hyperglycemia or diabetic acidosis can lead to nausea, vomiting, dehydration, loss of consciousness or death. Therefore, it is important that you obtain medical assistance immediately.

Lipodystrophy

Rarely, administration of insulin subcutaneously can result in lipoatrophy (depression in the skin) or lipohypertrophy (enlargement or thickening of tissue). If you notice either of these conditions, consult your doctor. A change in your injection technique may help alleviate the problem.

Allergy to Insulin

Local Allergy

Patients occasionally experience redness, swelling, and itching at the site of injection of insulin. This condition, called local allergy, usually clears up in a few days to a few weeks. In some instances, this condition may be related to factors other than insulin, such as irritants in the skin cleansing agent or poor injection technique. If you have local reactions, contact your doctor.

Systemic Allergy

Less common, but potentially more serious, is generalized allergy to insulin, which may cause rash over the whole body, shortness of breath, wheezing, reduction in blood pressure, fast pulse, or sweating. Severe cases of generalized allergy may be life threatening. If you think you are having a generalized allergic reaction to insulin, notify a doctor immediately.

ADDITIONAL INFORMATION

Additional information about diabetes may be obtained from your diabetes educator.

Diabetes Forecast is a national magazine designed especially for patients with diabetes and their families and is available by subscription from the American Diabetes Association, National Service Center, 1660 Duke Street, Alexandria, Virginia 22314, 1-800-DIABETES (1-800-342-2383).

Another publication, *Diabetes Countdown,* is available from the Juvenile Diabetes Foundation, 432 Park Avenue South, New York, New York 10016-8013, 1-800-JDF-CURE (1-800-533-2873).

PRODUCT LISTING - EQUIVALENTS NOT AVAILABLE

Solution - Injectable - Human Recombinant 500 U/ml

20 ml	$200.65	HUMULIN R, Lilly, Eli and Company	00002-8501-01

Insulin (Human, Isophane) *(001541)*

Categories: Diabetes mellitus; Recombinant DNA Origin; FDA Pre 1938 Drugs; Pregnancy Category B; WHO Formulary
Drug Classes: Antidiabetic agents; Insulins
Brand Names: **Humulin N**; Insulatard NPH Human; Insulin Human; Insuline; Novolin N
Foreign Brand Availability: Basal-H-Insulin (Germany); Human Insulatard (India); Human Protaphane (England; Ireland); Huminsulin Basal (NPH) (Germany; Switzerland); Huminsulin "Lilly" Basal (NPH) (Austria); Humulin I (Italy); Humulin NPH (Australia; Denmark; Greece; New-Zealand; Philippines; Sweden; Taiwan); Humulina NPH (Spain); Humuline NPH (Belgium); Insulatard (Denmark; Switzerland); Insulatard HM (Bahamas; Bahrain; Barbados; Belgium; Belize; Benin; Bermuda; Burkina-Faso; Curacao; Cyprus; Egypt; Ethiopia; Gambia; Ghana; Guinea; Guyana; Iran; Iraq; Israel; Ivory-Coast; Jamaica; Jordan; Kenya; Kuwait; Lebanon; Liberia; Libya; Malawi; Mali; Mauritania; Mauritius; Morocco; Netherland-Antilles; Niger; Nigeria; Oman; Puerto-Rico; Qatar; Republic-of-Yemen; Saudi-Arabia; Senegal; Seychelles; Sierra-Leone; Spain; Sudan; Surinam; Syria; Taiwan; Tanzania; Trinidad; Tunia; Uganda; United-Arab-Emirates; Zambia; Zimbabwe); Insulin Insulatard HM (Switzerland); Insulin Insulatard Human (Germany; Thailand); Insulin "Novo Nordisk" Insulatard HM (Austria); Insulin Protaphane HM (Germany; Switzerland); Insuline Humuline NPH (Netherlands); Insuline Isuhuman Basal (Netherlands); Insuline Insulatard (Netherlands); Insuman Basal (Germany); Novolin ge NPH (Canada); Orgasuline NPH (France); Protaphane (New-Zealand); Protaphane HM (Bahrain; Benin; Burkina-Faso; Cyprus; Egypt; Ethiopia; Gambia; Ghana; Guinea; Hong-Kong; Iran; Iraq; Israel; Ivory-Coast; Jordan; Kenya; Kuwait; Lebanon; Liberia; Libya; Malawi; Malaysia; Mali; Mauritania; Mauritius; Morocco; Niger; Nigeria; Oman; Philippines; Qatar; Republic-of-Yemen; Saudi-Arabia; Senegal; Seychelles; Sierra-Leone; South-Africa; Sudan; Syria; Tanzania; Thailand; Tunia; Uganda; United-Arab-Emirates; Zambia; Zimbabwe); Umuline Protamine Isophane (France)
HCFA JCODE(S): J1820 up to 100 units SC

DESCRIPTION

For complete prescribing information, please refer to Insulin (Human Recombinant).

Insulin (Human, Isophane/Regular) *(001542)*

For related information, see the comparative table section in Appendix A.

Categories: Diabetes mellitus; Recombinant DNA Origin; FDA Pre 1938 Drugs; Pregnancy Category B; WHO Formulary

Drug Classes: Antidiabetic agents; Insulins

Brand Names: Humulin 50 50; **Humulin 70 30**; Insuman; Novolin 70 30

Foreign Brand Availability: Actraphane HM (Benin; Burkina-Faso; Ethiopia; Gambia; Ghana; Guinea; Ivory-Coast; Kenya; Liberia; Malawi; Malaysia; Mali; Mauritania; Mauritius; Morocco; Niger; Nigeria; Philippines; Senegal; Seychelles; Sierra-Leone; South-Africa; Sudan; Taiwan; Tanzania; Thailand; Tunia; Uganda; Zambia; Zimbabwe); Berlinsulin H 10 90 (Germany); Berlinsulin H 20 80 (Germany); Berlinsulin H 30 70 (Germany); Berlinsulin H 40 60 (Germany); Huminsulin "Lilly" Long (Austria); Huminsulin Profil I (Germany; Switzerland); Huminsulin Profil II (Germany; Switzerland); Huminsulin Profil III (Germany; Switzerland); Huminsulin Profil IV (Germany; Switzerland); Humulin 10 90 (Canada; Italy; Malaysia); Humulin 20 80 (Australia; Canada; Italy; Malaysia; South-Africa); Humulin 30 70 (Australia; Canada; Italy; Malaysia; Mexico; South-Africa); Humulin 40 60 (Canada; Italy; Malaysia; South-Africa); Humulin 60 40 (Korea; New-Zealand; Thailand); Humulin 80 20 (New-Zealand; Thailand); Humulin 90 10 (Korea; New-Zealand); Humulin M3 (England); Humulin M2 (England); Humulin M1 (England); Humulin M4 (England); Humulina 10 90 (Spain); Humulina 20 80 (Spain); Humulina 30 70 (Spain); Humulina 40 60 (Spain); Humulina 50 50 (Spain); Humulina 70 30 (Spain); Humuline 20 80 (Belgium); Humuline 30 70 (Belgium); Humuline 40 60 (Belgium); Insulin Actraphan HM (Switzerland); Insulin Actraphane HM (Hungary); Insulin Actraphane HM 30 70 (Germany); Insulin Actraphane HM 10 90 (Germany); Insulin Actraphane HM 20 80 (Germany); Insulin Actraphane HM 40 60 (Germany); Insulin Actraphane HM 50 50 (Germany); Insulin Hoechst-Komb 15 U-100 (Switzerland); Insulin Hoechst-Komb 25 U-100 (Switzerland); Insulin Hoechst-Komb 50 U-100 (Switzerland); Insulin Mixtard 10 HM (Switzerland); Insulin Mixtard 20 HM (Switzerland); Insulin Mixtard 30 HM (Israel; Switzerland); Insulin Mixtard 40 HM (Switzerland); Insulin Mixtard 50 HM (Switzerland); Insulin Mixtard 50 50 HM (Israel); Insulin Mixtard 30 70 Human (Germany); Insulin Mixtard 50 50 Human (Germany); Insulin Mixtard 15 85 Human (Israel); Insulin "Novo Nordisk" Mixtard HM 15 85 (Austria); Insulin "Novo Nordisk" Mixtard HM 30 70 (Austria); Insulin "Novo Nordisk" Mixtard HM 50 50 (Austria); Insulina Combi HM 85 15 (Spain); Insulina Mixt HM 30 70 (Spain); Insuline Humaan (Netherlands); Insuline Humuline 10 90 (Netherlands); Insuline Humuline 20 80 (Netherlands); Insuline Humuline 30 70 (Netherlands); Insuline Humuline 40 60 (Netherlands); Mixtard 15 85 (Australia; New-Zealand); Mixtard 20 80 (South-Africa); Mixtard 30 70 (Australia; New-Zealand); Mixtard 30 HM (Bahrain; Benin; Burkina-Faso; Cyprus; Egypt; Ethiopia; Gambia; Ghana; Guinea; Hong-Kong; Iran; Iraq; Ivory-Coast; Jordan; Kenya; Kuwait; Lebanon; Liberia; Libya; Malawi; Mali; Mauritania; Mauritius; Morocco; Niger; Nigeria; Oman; Qatar; Republic-of-Yemen; Saudi-Arabia; Senegal; Seychelles; Sierra-Leone; Sudan; Syria; Taiwan; Tanzania; Tunia; Uganda; United-Arab-Emirates; Zambia; Zimbabwe); Mixtard 50 50 (Australia; New-Zealand); Mixtard Human (Korea); Mixtard 30 Human (Indonesia); Mixtard 10 Penfill (France); Mixtard 20 Penfill (France); Mixtard 30 Penfill (France); Mixtard 40 Penfill (France); Mixtard 50 Penfill (France); Orgasuline 30/70 (France); Novolet 30 70 (Korea); Novolin ge 30/70 (Canada); Umuline Profil 10 (France); Umuline Profil 20 (France); Umuline Profil 30 (France); Umuline Profil 40 (France)

HCFA JCODE(S): J1820 up to 100 units SC

DESCRIPTION

For complete prescribing information, please refer to Insulin (Human Recombinant).

Insulin (Human, Lente) *(001543)*

For related information, see the comparative table section in Appendix A.

Categories: Diabetes mellitus; Recombinant DNA Origin; FDA Pre 1938 Drugs; Pregnancy Category B; WHO Formulary

Drug Classes: Antidiabetic agents; Insulins

Brand Names: **Humulin L**; Humulin U; Humulin U Hi-610 Ultralente; Novolin L

Foreign Brand Availability: Human Monosulin (India); Human Monotard (India); Huminsulin Long 100 (Germany); Insuline Humuline Zink (Netherlands); Insulin Lente MC (Bulgaria); Insulin Monotard HM (Germany); Insulin "Novo Nordisk" Monotard HM (Austria); Insulina Monotard HM (Spain); Monotard (Australia); Monotard HM (Bahamas; Bahrain; Barbados; Belize; Benin; Bermuda; Burkina-Faso; Curacao; Cyprus; Egypt; Ethiopia; Gambia; Ghana; Guinea; Guyana; Hong-Kong; Iran; Iraq; Ivory-Coast; Jamaica; Jordan; Kenya; Kuwait; Lebanon; Liberia; Libya; Malawi; Malaysia; Mali; Mauritania; Mauritius; Morocco; Netherland-Antilles; New-Zealand; Niger; Nigeria; Oman; Philippines; Qatar; Republic-of-Yemen; Saudi-Arabia; Senegal; Seychelles; Sierra-Leone; Sudan; Surinam; Syria; Taiwan; Tanzania; Thailand; Trinidad; Tunia; Uganda; United-Arab-Emirates; Zambia; Zimbabwe); Monotard Human (Indonesia); Novolin ge Lente (Canada); Umuline Zinc (France)

HCFA JCODE(S): J1820 up to 100 units SC

DESCRIPTION

For complete prescribing information, please refer to Insulin (Human Recombinant).

Insulin Aspart *(003494)*

For related information, see the comparative table section in Appendix A.

Categories: Diabetes mellitus; FDA Approved 2000 Jun; Pregnancy Category C

Drug Classes: Antidiabetic agents; Insulins

Brand Names: **NovoLog**

Foreign Brand Availability: NovoMix 30 (Austria; Belgium; Bulgaria; Czech-Republic; Denmark; England; Finland; France; Germany; Greece; Hungary; Ireland; Italy; Netherlands; Norway; Poland; Portugal; Slovenia; Spain; Sweden; Switzerland; Turkey); Novorapid (Australia; Austria; Belgium; Bulgaria; Czech-Republic; Denmark; England; Finland; France; Germany; Greece; Hungary; Ireland; Israel; Italy; Netherlands; New-Zealand; Norway; Poland; Portugal; Slovenia; Spain; Sweden; Switzerland; Turkey)

DESCRIPTION

Note: The trade names have been used throughout this monograph for clarity.

NovoLog (insulin aspart [rDNA origin] injection) is a human insulin analog that is a rapid-acting, parenteral blood glucose-lowering agent. NovoLog is homologous with regular human insulin with the exception of a single substitution of the amino acid proline by aspartic acid in position B28, and is produced by recombinant DNA technology utilizing *Saccharomyces cerevisiae* (baker's yeast) as the production organism. Insulin aspart has the empirical formula $C_{256}H_{381}N_{65}O_{79}S_6$ and a molecular weight of 5825.8.

NovoLog is a sterile, aqueous, clear, and colorless solution, that contains insulin aspart (B28 asp regular human insulin analog) 100 Units/ml, glycerin 16 mg/ml, phenol 1.50 mg/ml, metacresol 1.72 mg/ml, zinc 19.6 μg/ml, disodium hydrogen phosphate dihydrate 1.25 mg/ml, and sodium chloride 0.58 mg/ml. NovoLog has a pH of 7.2-7.6. Hydrochloric acid 10% and/or sodium hydroxide 10% may be added to adjust pH.

CLINICAL PHARMACOLOGY

MECHANISM OF ACTION

The primary activity of NovoLog is the regulation of glucose metabolism. Insulins, including NovoLog, bind to the insulin receptors on muscle and fat cells and lower blood glucose by facilitating the cellular uptake of glucose and simultaneously inhibiting the output of glucose from the liver.

In standard biological assays in mice and rabbits, 1 unit of NovoLog has the same glucose-lowering effect as 1 unit of regular human insulin. In humans, the effect of NovoLog is more rapid in onset and of shorter duration, compared to regular human insulin, due to its faster absorption after subcutaneous (SC) injection.

PHARMACOKINETICS

The single substitution of the amino acid proline with aspartic acid at position B28 in NovoLog reduces the molecule's tendency to form hexamers as observed with regular human insulin. NovoLog is therefore more rapidly absorbed after SC injection compared to regular human insulin.

Bioavailability and Absorption

NovoLog has a faster absorption, a faster onset of action, and a shorter duration of action than regular human insulin after SC injection. The relative bioavailability of NovoLog compared to regular human insulin indicates that the two insulins are absorbed to a similar extent.

In studies in healthy volunteers (total n=l07) and patients with Type 1 diabetes (total n=40), NovoLog consistently reached peak serum concentrations approximately twice as fast as regular human insulin. The median time to maximum concentration in these trials was 40-50 minutes for NovoLog versus 80-120 minutes for regular human insulin. In a clinical trial in patients with Type 1 diabetes, NovoLog and regular human insulin, both administered subcutaneously at a dose of 0.15 U/kg body weight, reached mean maximum concentrations of 82.1 and 35.9 mU/L, respectively. Pharmacokinetic/pharmacodynamic characteristics of insulin aspart have not been established in patients with Type 2 diabetes.

The intra-individual variability in time to maximum serum insulin concentration for healthy male volunteers was significantly less for NovoLog than for regular human insulin. The clinical significance of this observation has not been established.

In a clinical study in healthy non-obese subjects, the pharmacokinetic differences between NovoLog and regular human insulin described above, were observed independent of the injection site (abdomen, thigh, or upper arm). Differences in pharmacokinetics between NovoLog and regular human insulin are not associated with differences in overall glycemic control.

Distribution and Elimination

NovoLog has a low binding to plasma proteins, 0-9%, similar to regular human insulin. After SC administration in normal male volunteers (n=24), NovoLog was more rapidly eliminated than regular human insulin with an average apparent half-life of 81 minutes compared to 141 minutes for regular human insulin.

PHARMACODYNAMICS

Studies in normal volunteers and patients with diabetes demonstrated that NovoLog has a more rapid onset of action than regular human insulin.

In a 6 hour study in patients with Type 1 diabetes (n= 22), the maximum glucose-lowering effect of NovoLog occurred between 1 and 3 hours after SC injection. The duration of action for NovoLog is 3-5 hours compared to 5-8 hours for regular human insulin. The time course of action of insulin and insulin analogs such as NovoLog may vary considerably in different individuals or within the same individual. The rate of insulin absorption and consequently the onset of activity is known to be affected by the site of injection, exercise, and other variables (see PRECAUTIONS, General). Differences in pharmacodynamics between NovoLog and regular human insulin are not associated with differences in overall glycemic control.

SPECIAL POPULATIONS

Children and Adolescents

The pharmacokinetic and pharmacodynamic properties of NovoLog and regular human insulin were evaluated in a single dose study in 18 children (6-12 years, n=9) and adolescents (13-17 years [Tanner grade ≥2], n=9) with Type 1 diabetes. The relative differences in pharmacokinetics and pharmacodynamics in children and adolescents with Type 1 diabetes between NovoLog and regular human insulin were similar to those in healthy adult subjects and adults with Type 1 diabetes.

Geriatrics

The effect of age on the pharmacokinetics and pharmacodynamics of NovoLog has not been studied.

Gender

In healthy volunteers, no difference in insulin aspart levels was seen between men and women when body weight differences were taken into account. There was no significant difference in efficacy noted (as assessed by HbA1c) between genders in a trial in patients with Type 1 diabetes.

Obesity

In a study of 23 patients with Type 1 diabetes and a wide range of body mass index (BMI, 22-39 kg/m^2), the pharmacokinetic parameters, AUC and C_{max}, of NovoLog were generally unaffected by BMI. Clearance of NovoLog was reduced by 28% in patients with BMI >32 compared to patients with BMI <23 when single dose of 0.1 u/kg NovoLog was administered. However, only 3 patients with BMI <23 were studied.

Ethnic Origin

The effect of ethnic origin on the pharmacokinetics of NovoLog has not been studied.

Renal Impairment

Some studies with human insulin have shown increased circulating levels of insulin in patients with renal failure. A single SC dose of NovoLog was administered in a study of 18 patients with creatinine clearance values ranging from normal to <30 ml/min and not requiring hemodialysis. No apparent effect of creatinine clearance values on AUC and C_{max} of NovoLog was found. However, only 2 patients with severe renal impairment were studied (<30 ml/min). Careful glucose monitoring and dose adjustments of insulin, including NovoLog, may be necessary in patients with renal dysfunction (see PRECAUTIONS, General, Renal Impairment).

Hepatic Impairment

Some studies with human insulin have shown increased circulating levels of insulin in patients with liver failure. In an open-label, single dose study of 24 patients with Child-Pugh Scores ranging from 0 (healthy volunteers) to 12 (severe hepatic impairment), no correlation was found between the degree of hepatic failure and any NovoLog pharmacokinetic parameter. Careful glucose monitoring and dose adjustments of insulin, including NovoLog, may be necessary in patients with hepatic dysfunction (see PRECAUTIONS, General, Hepatic Impairment).

Pregnancy

The effect of pregnancy on the pharmacokinetics and glucodynamics of NovoLog has not been studied (see PRECAUTIONS, Pregnancy, Teratogenic Effects, Pregnancy Category C).

Smoking

The effect of smoking on the pharmacokinetics/pharmacodynamics of NovoLog has not been studied.

INDICATIONS AND USAGE

NovoLog is indicated for the treatment of adult patients with diabetes mellitus, for the control of hyperglycemia. Because NovoLog has a more rapid onset and a shorter duration of activity than human regular insulin, NovoLog given by injection should normally be used in regimens with an intermediate or long-acting insulin. NovoLog may also be infused subcutaneously by external insulin pumps. (See WARNINGS; PRECAUTIONS: [especially General, Usage in Pumps], Information for the Patient [especially For Patients Using Pumps]; DRUG INTERACTIONS, Mixing of Insulins; DOSAGE AND ADMINISTRATION; and HOW SUPPLIED, Recommended Storage.)

CONTRAINDICATIONS

NovoLog is contraindicated during episodes of hypoglycemia and in patients hypersensitive to NovoLog or one of its excipients.

WARNINGS

NovoLog differs from regular human insulin by a more rapid onset and a shorter duration of activity. Because of the fast onset of action, the injection of NovoLog should immediately be followed by a meal. Because of the short duration of action of NovoLog, patients with diabetes also require a longer-acting insulin to maintain adequate glucose control. Glucose monitoring is recommended for all patients with diabetes and is particularly important for patients using external pump infusion therapy.

Hypoglycemia is the most common adverse effect of insulin therapy, including NovoLog. As with all insulins, the timing of hypoglycemia may differ among various insulin formulations.

Any change of insulin dose should be made cautiously and only under medical supervision. Changes in insulin strength, manufacturer, type (*e.g.,* regular, NPH, analog), species (animal, human), or method of manufacture (rDNA versus animal-source insulin) may result in the need for a change in dosage.

INSULIN PUMPS

When used in an external insulin pump for SC infusion, NovoLog should not be diluted or mixed with any other insulin. Physicians and patients should carefully evaluate information on pump use in the NovoLog physician and patient package inserts and in the pump manufacturer's manual (*e.g.,* NovoLog-specific information should be followed for in-use time, frequency of changing infusion sets, or other details specific to NovoLog usage, because NovoLog-specific information may differ from general pump manual instructions). Pump or infusion set malfunctions or insulin degradation can lead to hyperglycemia and ketosis in a short time because of the small SC depot of insulin. This is especially pertinent for rapid-acting insulin analogs that are more rapidly absorbed through skin and have shorter duration of action. These differences may be particularly relevant when patients are switched from multiple injection therapy or infusion with buffered regular insulin. Prompt identification and correction of the cause of hyperglycemia or ketosis is necessary. Interim therapy with SC injection may be required. (See PRECAUTIONS, Information for the Patient; DRUG INTERACTIONS, Mixing of Insulins; DOSAGE AND ADMINISTRATION; and HOW SUPPLIED, Recommended Storage.)

PRECAUTIONS

GENERAL

Hypoglycemia and hypokalemia are among the potential clinical adverse effects associated with the use of all insulins. Because of differences in the action of NovoLog and other insulins, care should be taken in patients in whom such potential side effects might be clinically relevant (*e.g.,* patients who are fasting, have autonomic neuropathy, or are using potassium-lowering drugs or patients taking drugs sensitive to serum potassium level). Lipodystrophy and hypersensitivity are among other potential clinical adverse effects associated with the use of all insulins.

As with all insulin preparations, the time course of NovoLog action may vary in different individuals or at different times in the same individual and is dependent on site of injection, blood supply, temperature, and physical activity.

Adjustment of dosage of any insulin may be necessary if patients change their physical activity or their usual meal plan. Insulin requirements may be altered during illness, emotional disturbances, or other stresses.

Hypoglycemia

As with all insulin preparations, hypoglycemic reactions may be associated with the administration of NovoLog. Rapid changes in serum glucose levels may induce symptoms of hypoglycemia in persons with diabetes, regardless of the glucose value. Early warning symptoms of hypoglycemia may be different or less pronounced under certain conditions, such as long duration of diabetes, diabetic nerve disease, use of medications such as beta-blockers, or intensified diabetes control (see DRUG INTERACTIONS). Such situations may result in severe hypoglycemia (and, possibly, loss of consciousness) prior to patients' awareness of hypoglycemia.

Renal Impairment

As with other insulins, the dose requirements for NovoLog may be reduced in patients with renal impairment (see CLINICAL PHARMACOLOGY, Pharmacokinetics).

Hepatic Impairment

As with other insulins, the dose requirements for NovoLog may be reduced in patients with hepatic impairment (see CLINICAL PHARMACOLOGY, Pharmacokinetics).

Allergy

Local Allergy

As with other insulin therapy, patients may experience redness, swelling, or itching at the site of injection. These minor reactions usually resolve in a few days to a few weeks, but in some occasions, may require discontinuation of NovoLog. In some instances, these reactions may be related to factors other than insulin, such as irritants in a skin cleansing agent or poor injection technique.

Systemic Allergy

Less common, but potentially more serious, is generalized allergy to insulin, which may cause rash (including pruritus) over the whole body, shortness of breath, wheezing, reduction in blood pressure, rapid pulse, or sweating. Severe cases of generalized allergy, including anaphylactic reaction, may be life threatening.

Localized reactions and generalized myalgias have been reported with the use of cresol as an injectable excipient.

In controlled clinical trials using injection therapy, allergic reactions were reported in 3 of 735 patients (0.4%) who received regular human insulin and 10 of 1394 patients (0.7%) who received NovoLog. During these and other trials, 3 of 2341 patients treated with NovoLog were discontinued due to allergic reactions.

Antibody Production

Increases in levels of anti-insulin antibodies that react with both human insulin and insulin aspart have been observed in patients treated with NovoLog. The number of patients treated with insulin aspart experiencing these increases is greater than the number among those treated with human regular insulin. Data from a 12 month controlled trial in patients with Type 1 diabetes suggest that the increase in these antibodies is transient. The differences in antibody levels between the human regular insulin and insulin aspart treatment groups observed at 3 and 6 months were no longer evident at 12 months. The clinical significance of these antibodies is not known. The do not appear to cause deterioration in HbA1c or to necessitate increases in insulin dose.

Pregnancy and Lactation

Female patients should be advised to tell their physician if they intend to become, or if they become pregnant. Information is not available on the use of NovoLog during pregnancy or lactation.

Usage in Pumps

NovoLog is recommended for use in Disetronic H-TRON plus V100 with Disetronic 3.15 plastic cartridges and Classic or Tender infusion sets; MiniMed Models 505, 506, or 507 with MiniMed 3 ml syringes and Polyfin or Sof-set infusion sets.

In vitro studies have shown that pump malfunction, loss of cresol, and insulin degradation, may occur with the use of NovoLog for more than 2 days at 37°C (98.6°F) in infusion sets and reservoirs. NovoLog in clinical use should not be exposed to temperatures greater than 37°C (98.6°F). **NovoLog should not be mixed with other insulins or with a diluent when it is used in the pump.** (See WARNINGS; PRECAUTIONS, Information for the Patient; DRUG INTERACTIONS, Mixing of Insulins; DOSAGE AND ADMINISTRATION; and HOW SUPPLIED, Recommended Storage.)

INFORMATION FOR THE PATIENT

For All Patients

Patients should be informed about potential risks and advantages of NovoLog therapy including the possible side effects. Patients should also be offered continued education and advice on insulin therapies, injection technique, life-style management, regular glucose monitoring, periodic glycosylated hemoglobin testing, recognition and management of hypo- and hyperglycemia, adherence to meal planning, complications of insulin therapy, timing of dose, instruction in the use of injection or SC infusion devices, and proper storage of insulin. Patients should be informed that frequent, patient-performed blood glucose measurements are needed to achieve optimal glycemic control and avoid both hyper- and hypoglycemia.

Female patients should be advised to tell their physician if they intend to become, or if they become pregnant. Information is not available on the use of NovoLog during pregnancy or lactation (see Pregnancy, Teratogenic Effects, Pregnancy Category C).

For Patients Using Pumps

Patients using external pump infusion therapy should be trained in intensive insulin therapy with multiple injections and in the function of their pump and pump accessories. NovoLog is recommended for use with Disetronic H-TRON plus V100 with Disetronic 3.15 plastic cartridges and Classic or Tender infusion sets; MiniMed Models 505, 506, and 507 with MiniMed 3 ml syringes and Polyfin or Sof-set infusion sets. The use of NovoLog in quick-release infusion sets and cartridge adapters has not been assessed.

To avoid insulin degradation, infusion set occlusion, and loss of the preservative (cresol), the infusion sets (reservoir syringe, tubing, and catheter) and the NovoLog in the reservoir should be replaced, and a new infusion site selected every 48 hours or less. Insulin exposed to temperatures higher than 37°C (98.6°F) should be discarded. The temperature of the insulin may exceed ambient temperature when the pump housing, cover, tubing, or sport case is exposed to sunlight or radiant heat. Infusion sites that are erythematous, pruritic, or thickened should be reported to medical personnel, and a new site selected because continued infusion may increase the skin reaction and/or alter the absorption of NovoLog.

Pump or infusion set malfunctions or insulin degradation can lead to hyperglycemia and ketosis in a short time because of the small SC depot of insulin. This is especially pertinent for rapid-acting insulin analogs that are more rapidly absorbed through skin and have shorter duration of action. These differences are particularly relevant when patients are switched from infused buffered regular insulin or multiple injection therapy. Prompt identification and correction of the cause of hyperglycemia or ketosis is necessary. Problems include pump malfunction, infusion set occlusion, leakage, disconnection or kinking, and degraded insulin. Less commonly, hypoglycemia from pump malfunction may occur. If these problems cannot be promptly corrected, patients should resume therapy with SC insulin injection and contact their physician. (See WARNINGS; DRUG INTERACTIONS, Mixing of Insulins; DOSAGE AND ADMINISTRATION; and HOW SUPPLIED, Recommended Storage.)

I

LABORATORY TESTS

As with all insulin therapy, the therapeutic response to NovoLog should be monitored by periodic blood glucose tests. Periodic measurement of glycosylated hemoglobin is recommended for the monitoring of long-term glycemic control.

CARCINOGENESIS, MUTAGENESIS, AND IMPAIRMENT OF FERTILITY

Standard 2 year carcinogenicity studies in animals have not been performed to evaluate the carcinogenic potential of NovoLog. In 52 week studies, Sprague-Dawley rats were dosed subcutaneously with NovoLog at 10, 50, and 200 U/kg/day (approximately 2, 8, and 32 times the human SC dose of 1.0 U/kg/day, based on U/body surface area, respectively). At a dose of 200 U/kg/day, NovoLog increased the incidence of mammary gland tumors in females when compared to untreated controls. The incidence of mammary tumors for NovoLog was not significantly different than for regular human insulin. The relevance of these findings to humans is not known. NovoLog was not genotoxic in the following tests: Ames test, mouse lymphoma cell forward gene mutation test, human peripheral blood lymphocyte chromosome aberration test, *in vivo* micronucleus test in mice, and in *ex vivo* UDS test in rat liver hepatocytes. In fertility studies in male and female rats, at SC doses up to 200 U/kg/day (approximately 32 times the human SC dose, based on U/body surface area), no direct adverse effects on male and female fertility, or general reproductive performance of animals was observed.

PREGNANCY, TERATOGENIC EFFECTS, PREGNANCY CATEGORY C

There are no adequate well-controlled clinical studies of the use of NovoLog in pregnant women. NovoLog should be used during pregnancy only if the potential benefit justifies the potential risk to the fetus.

It is essential for patients with diabetes or history of gestational diabetes to maintain good metabolic control before conception and throughout pregnancy. Insulin requirements may decrease during the first trimester, generally increase during the second and third trimesters, and rapidly decline after delivery. Careful monitoring of glucose control is essential in such patients.

Subcutaneous reproduction and teratology studies have been performed with NovoLog and regular human insulin in rats and rabbits. In these studies, NovoLog was given to female rats before mating, during mating, and throughout pregnancy, and to rabbits during organogenesis. The effects of NovoLog did not differ from those observed with SC regular human insulin. NovoLog, like human insulin, caused pre- and post-implantation losses and visceral/skeletal abnormalities in rats at a dose of 200 U/kg/day (approximately 32 times the human SC dose of 1.0 U/kg/day, based on U/body surface area) and in rabbits at a dose of 10 U/kg/day (approximately 3 times the human SC dose of 1.0 U/kg/day, based on U/body surface area). The effects are probably secondary to maternal hypoglycemia at high doses. No significant effects were observed in rats at a dose of 50 U/kg/day and rabbits at a dose of 3 U/kg/day. These doses are approximately 8 times the human SC dose of 1.0 U/kg/day for rats and equal to the human SC dose of 1.0 U/kg/day for rabbits, based on U/body surface area.

NURSING MOTHERS

It is unknown whether insulin aspart is excreted in human milk. Many drugs, including human insulin, are excreted in human milk. For this reason, caution should be exercised when NovoLog is administered to a nursing mother.

PEDIATRIC USE

Safety and effectiveness of NovoLog in children have not been studied.

GERIATRIC USE

In the large controlled clinical trials, 36 patients ≥65 years of age were treated with NovoLog. No conclusions regarding the safety and efficacy of NovoLog in the elderly patients compared to younger adults can be reached from this limited data set.

DRUG INTERACTIONS

A number of substances affect glucose metabolism and may require insulin dose adjustment and particularly close monitoring.

The following are examples of substances that may increase the blood-glucose-lowering effect and susceptibility to hypoglycemia: Oral antidiabetic products, ACE inhibitors, disopyramide, fibrates, fluoxetine, monoamine oxidase (MAO) inhibitors, propoxyphene, salicylates, somatostatin analog (*e.g.,* octreotide), sulfonamide antibiotics.

The following are examples of substances that may reduce the blood-glucose-lowering effect: Corticosteroids, niacin, danazol, diuretics, sympathomimetic agents (*e.g.,* epinephrine, salbutamol, terbutaline), isoniazid, phenothiazine derivatives, somatropin, thyroid hormones, estrogens, progestogens (*e.g.,* in oral contraceptives).

Beta-blockers, clonidine, lithium salts, and alcohol may either potentiate or weaken the blood-glucose-lowering effect of insulin. Pentamidine may cause hypoglycemia, which may sometimes be followed by hyperglycemia.

In addition, under the influence of sympatholytic medicinal products such as beta-blockers, clonidine, guanethidine, and reserpine, the signs of hypoglycemia may be reduced or absent (see CLINICAL PHARMACOLOGY).

MIXING OF INSULINS

- A clinical study in healthy male volunteers (n=24) demonstrated that mixing NovoLog with NPH human insulin immediately before injection produced some attenuation in the peak concentration of NovoLog, but that the time to peak and the total bioavailability of NovoLog were not significantly affected. If NovoLog is mixed with NPH human insulin, NovoLog should be drawn into the syringe first. The injection should be made immediately after mixing. Because there are no data on the compatibility of NovoLog and crystalline zinc insulin preparations, NovoLog should not be mixed with these preparations.
- The effects of mixing NovoLog with insulins of animal source or insulin preparations produced by other manufacturers have not been studied (see WARNINGS).
- Mixtures should not be administered intravenously.
- When used in external SC infusion pumps for insulin, NovoLog should not be mixed with any other insulins or diluent.

ADVERSE REACTIONS

Clinical trials comparing NovoLog with regular human insulin did not demonstrate a difference in frequency of adverse events between the two treatments.

Adverse events commonly associated with human insulin therapy include the following:

Body as a Whole: Allergic reactions (see PRECAUTIONS, General, Allergy).

Skin and Appendages: Injection site reaction, lipodystrophy, pruritus, rash (see PRECAUTIONS: General, Allergy, Information for the Patient, and General, Usage in Pumps).

Other: Hypoglycemia, hyperglycemia and ketosis (see WARNINGS and PRECAUTIONS).

In controlled clinical trials, small, but persistent elevations in alkaline phosphatase result were observed in some patients treated with NovoLog. The clinical significance of this finding is unknown.

DOSAGE AND ADMINISTRATION

NovoLog should generally be given immediately before a meal (start of meal within 5-10 minutes after injection) because of its fast onset of action. The dosage of NovoLog should be individualized and determined, based on the physician's advice, in accordance with the needs of the patient. The total daily individual insulin requirement is usually between 0.5-1.0 units/kg/day. When used in a meal-related SC injection treatment regimen, 50-70% of total insulin requirements may be provided by NovoLog and the remainder provided by an intermediate-acting or long-acting insulin. When used in external insulin infusion pumps, the initial programming of the pump is based on the total daily insulin dose of the previous regimen. Although there is significant interpatient variability, approximately 50% of the total dose is given as meal-related boluses of NovoLog and the remainder as basal infusion.

Because of NovoLog's comparatively rapid onset and short duration of glucose lowering activity, some patients may require more basal insulin and more total insulin to prevent pre-meal hyperglycemia when using NovoLog than when using human regular insulin. Additional basal insulin injections, or higher basal rates in external SC infusion pumps may be necessary. **Infusion sets and the insulin in the infusion sets must be changed every 48 hours or sooner to assure the activity of NovoLog and proper pump function.** (See WARNINGS and PRECAUTIONS, Information for the Patient.)

NovoLog should be administered by SC injection in the abdominal wall, the thigh, or the upper arm, or by continuous SC infusion in the abdominal wall. Injection sites and infusion sites should be rotated within the same region. As with all insulins, the duration of action will vary according to the dose, injection site, blood flow, temperature, and level of physical activity.

Parenteral drug products should be inspected visually for particulate matter and discoloration prior to administration, whenever solution and container permit. Never use any NovoLog if it has become viscous (thickened) or cloudy; use it only if it is clear and colorless. NovoLog should not be used after the printed expiration date.

HOW SUPPLIED

NovoLog is available in 10 ml vials and 3 ml PenFill cartridges, each presentation contains 100 Units of insulin aspart per ml (U-100).

RECOMMENDED STORAGE

NovoLog in unopened vials and cartridges should be stored between 2 and 8°C (36-46°F). *Do not freeze.* **Do not use NovoLog if it has been frozen or exposed to temperatures that exceed 37°C (98.6°F).** After a vial or cartridge has been punctured, it may be kept at temperatures below 30°C (86°F) for up to 28 days, but should not be exposed to excessive heat or sunlight. Opened vials may be refrigerated. Cartridges should not be refrigerated after insertion into the NovoPen 3. Infusion sets (reservoirs, tubing, and catheters) and the NovoLog in the reservoir should be discarded after no more than 48 hours of use or after exposure to temperatures that exceed 37°C (98.6°F).

PRODUCT LISTING - EQUIVALENTS NOT AVAILABLE

Solution - Subcutaneous - 100 U/ml

3 ml x 5	$114.20	NOVOLOG PENFILL, Novo Nordisk Pharmaceuticals Inc	00169-3303-12
3 ml x 5	$114.20	NOVOLOG PENFILL, Novo Nordisk Pharmaceuticals Inc	00169-3682-13
3 ml x 5	$118.70	NOVOLOG, Novo Nordisk Pharmaceuticals Inc	00169-3696-19
10 ml	$61.43	NOVOLOG, Novo Nordisk Pharmaceuticals Inc	00169-7501-11

Insulin Aspart Protamine; Insulin Aspart (003554)

Categories: Diabetes mellitus; FDA Approved 2001 Nov; Pregnancy Category C
Drug Classes: Antidiabetic agents; Insulins
Brand Names: **NovoLog Mix 70/30**

DESCRIPTION

Note: The trade name has been used throughout this monograph for clarity.

NovoLog Mix 70/30 (70% insulin aspart protamine suspension and 30% insulin aspart [rDNA origin]) is a human insulin analogue suspension containing 70% insulin aspart protamine crystals and 30% soluble insulin aspart. NovoLog Mix 70/30 is a blood glucose-lowering agent with a rapid onset and an intermediate duration of action. Insulin aspart is homologous with regular human insulin with the exception of a single substitution of the amino acid proline by aspartic acid in position B28, and is produced by recombinant DNA technology utilizing *Saccharomyces cerevisiae* (baker's yeast) as the production organism. Insulin aspart (NovoLog) has the empirical formula $C_{256}H_{381}N_{65}O_{79}S_6$ and a molecular weight of 5825.8 Da.

NovoLog Mix 70/30 is a uniform, white, sterile suspension that contains insulin aspart (B28 asp regular human insulin analogue) 100 Units/ml, mannitol 36.4 mg/ml, phenol 1.50 mg/ml, metacresol 1.72 mg/ml, zinc 19.6 µg/ml, disodium hydrogen phosphate dihydrate 1.25 mg/ml, sodium chloride 0.58 mg/ml, and protamine sulfate 0.33 mg/ml. NovoLog Mix 70/30 has a pH of 7.20-7.44. Hydrochloric acid or sodium hydroxide may be added to adjust pH.

CLINICAL PHARMACOLOGY

MECHANISM OF ACTION

The primary activity of NovoLog Mix 70/30 is the regulation of glucose metabolism. Insulins, including NovoLog Mix 70/30, exert their specific action through binding to insulin receptors. Insulin binding activates mechanisms to lower blood glucose by facilitating cellular uptake of glucose into skeletal muscle and fat, simultaneously inhibiting the output of glucose from the liver.

In standard biological assays in mice and rabbits, one unit of NovoLog has the same glucose-lowering effect as one unit of regular human insulin. However, the effect of NovoLog Mix 70/30 is more rapid in onset compared to Novolin (human insulin) 70/30 due to its faster absorption after subcutaneous injection.

PHARMACOKINETICS

Bioavailability and Absorption

The single substitution of the amino acid proline with aspartic acid at position B28 in insulin aspart (NovoLog) reduces the molecule's tendency to form hexamers as observed with regular human insulin. The rapid absorption characteristics of NovoLog are maintained by NovoLog Mix 70/30. The insulin aspart in the soluble component of NovoLog Mix 70/30 is absorbed more rapidly from the subcutaneous layer than regular human insulin. The remaining 70% is in crystalline form as insulin aspart protamine which has a prolonged absorption profile after subcutaneous injection.

The relative bioavailability of NovoLog Mix 70/30 compared to NovoLog and Novolin 70/30 indicates that they are absorbed to similar degrees. In euglycemic clamp studies in healthy volunteers (n=23) after dosing with 0.2 U/kg of NovoLog Mix 70/30, a mean maximum serum concentration (C_{max}) of 23.4 ± 5.3 mU/L was reached after 60 minutes. The mean half-life ($T_{½}$) of NovoLog Mix 70/30 was about 8-9 hours. Serum insulin levels returned to baseline 15-18 hours after a subcutaneous dose. Similar data were seen in a separate euglycemic clamp study in healthy volunteers (n=24) after dosing with 0.3 U/kg of NovoLog Mix 70/30. A C_{max} of 61.3 ± 20.1 mU/L was reached after 85 minutes. Serum insulin levels returned to baseline 12 hours after a subcutaneous dose.

The C_{max} and the area under the insulin concentration-time curve (AUC) after administration of NovoLog Mix 70/30 differed by approximately 20% from those after administration of NovoLog Mix 50/50 (investigational drug, not marketed) and Novolin 70/30.

Pharmacokinetic measurements were generated in clamp studies employing insulin doses of 0.3 U/kg. Insulin kinetics exhibit significant inter- and intra-patient variability. The rate of insulin absorption and consequently the onset of activity is known to be affected by the site of injection, exercise, and other variables (see PRECAUTIONS, General). Differences in pharmacokinetics between NovoLog Mix 70/30 and products to which it has been compared are not associated with differences in overall glycemic control.

Distribution and Elimination

NovoLog has a low binding to plasma proteins, 0-9%, similar to regular human insulin. After subcutaneous administration in normal male volunteers (n=24), NovoLog was more rapidly eliminated than regular human insulin with an average apparent half-life of 81 minutes compared to 141 minutes for regular human insulin.

PHARMACODYNAMICS

The two euglycemic clamp studies described above assessed glucose utilization after dosing of healthy volunteers. NovoLog Mix 70/30 has a more rapid onset of action than regular human insulin in studies of normal volunteers and patients with diabetes. The peak pharmacodynamic effect of NovoLog Mix 70/30 occurs between 1 and 4 hours after injection. The duration of action may be as long as 24 hours.

Pharmacodynamic measurements were generated in clamp studies employing insulin doses of 0.3 U/kg. Insulin pharmacodynamics exhibit significant inter- and intra-patient variability. The rate of insulin absorption and consequently the onset of activity is known to be affected by the site of injection, exercise, and other variables (see PRECAUTIONS, General). Differences in pharmacodynamics between NovoLog Mix 70/30 and products to which it has been compared are not associated with differences in overall glycemic control.

SPECIAL POPULATIONS

Children and Adolescents

The pharmacokinetic and pharmacodynamic properties of NovoLog Mix 70/30 have not been assessed in children and adolescents less than 18 years of age.

Geriatrics

The effect of age on the pharmacokinetics and pharmacodynamics of NovoLog Mix 70/30 has not been studied.

Gender

The effect of gender on the pharmacokinetics and pharmacodynamics of NovoLog Mix 70/30 has not been studied.

Obesity

The effect of obesity and/or subcutaneous fat thickness on the pharmacokinetics and pharmacodynamics of NovoLog Mix 70/30 has not been studied but data on the rapid acting component (NovoLog) show no significant effect.

Ethnic Origin

The effect of ethnic origin on the pharmacokinetics and pharmacodynamics of NovoLog Mix 70/30 has not been studied.

Renal Impairment

The effect of renal function on the pharmacokinetics and pharmacodynamics of NovoLog Mix 70/30 has not been studied but data on the rapid acting component (NovoLog) show no significant effect. Some studies with human insulin have shown increased circulating levels of insulin in patients with renal failure. Careful glucose monitoring and dose adjustments of insulin, including NovoLog Mix 70/30, may be necessary in patients with renal dysfunction (see PRECAUTIONS, Renal Impairment).

Hepatic Impairment

The effect of hepatic impairment on the pharmacokinetics and pharmacodynamics of NovoLog Mix 70/30 has not been studied but data on the rapid-acting component (NovoLog) show no significant effect. Some studies with human insulin have shown increased circulating levels of insulin in patients with liver failure. Careful glucose monitoring and dose adjustments of insulin, including NovoLog Mix 70/30, may be necessary in patients with hepatic dysfunction (see PRECAUTIONS, Hepatic Impairment).

Pregnancy

The effect of pregnancy on the pharmacokinetics and pharmacodynamics of NovoLog Mix 70/30 has not been studied (see PRECAUTIONS, Pregnancy, Teratogenic Effects, Pregnancy Category C).

Smoking

The effect of smoking on the pharmacokinetics and pharmacodynamics of NovoLog Mix 70/30 has not been studied.

INDICATIONS AND USAGE

NovoLog Mix 70/30 is indicated for the treatment of patients with diabetes mellitus for the control of hyperglycemia.

CONTRAINDICATIONS

NovoLog Mix 70/30 is contraindicated during episodes of hypoglycemia and in patients hypersensitive to NovoLog Mix 70/30 or one of its excipients.

WARNINGS

Because NovoLog Mix 70/30 has peak pharmacodynamic activity 1 hour after injection, it should be administered with meals.

NovoLog Mix 70/30 should not be administered intravenously.

NovoLog Mix 70/30 is not to be used in insulin infusion pumps.

NovoLog Mix 70/30 should not be mixed with any other insulin product.

Hypoglycemia is the most common adverse effect of insulin therapy, including NovoLog Mix 70/30. As with all insulins, the timing of hypoglycemia may differ among various insulin formulations.

Glucose monitoring is recommended for all patients with diabetes.

Any change of insulin dose should be made cautiously and only under medical supervision. Changes in insulin strength, manufacturer, type (*e.g.*, regular, NPH, analog), species (animal, human), or method of manufacture (rDNA versus animal-source insulin) may result in the need for a change in dosage.

PRECAUTIONS

GENERAL

Hypoglycemia and hypokalemia are among the potential clinical adverse effects associated with the use of all insulins. Because of differences in the action of NovoLog Mix 70/30 and other insulins, care should be taken in patients in whom such potential side effects might be clinically relevant (*e.g.*, patients who are fasting, have autonomic neuropathy, or are using potassium-lowering drugs or patients taking drugs sensitive to serum potassium level).

Fixed ratio insulins are typically dosed on a twice daily basis, *i.e.*, before breakfast and supper, with each dose intended to cover two meals or a meal and snack (see DOSAGE AND ADMINISTRATION). Because there is diurnal variation in insulin resistance and endogenous insulin secretion, variability in the time and content of meals, and variability in the time and extent of exercise, fixed ratio insulin mixtures may not provide optimal glycemic control for all patients. The dose of insulin required to provide adequate glycemic control for one of the meals may result in hyper- or hypoglycemia for the other meal. The pharmacodynamic profile may also be inadequate for patients (*e.g.*, pregnant women) who require more frequent meals.

Adjustments in insulin dose or insulin type may be needed during illness, emotional stress, and other physiologic stress in addition to changes in meals and exercise.

The pharmacokinetic and pharmacodynamic profiles of all insulins may be altered by the site used for injection and the degree of vascularization of the site. Smoking, temperature, and exercise contribute to variations in blood flow and insulin absorption. These and other factors contribute to inter- and intra-patient variability.

Lipodystrophy and hypersensitivity are among other potential clinical adverse effects associated with the use of all insulins.

HYPOGLYCEMIA

As with all insulin preparations, hypoglycemic reactions may be associated with the administration of NovoLog Mix 70/30. Rapid changes in serum glucose concentrations may induce symptoms of hypoglycemia in persons with diabetes, regardless of the glucose value. Early warning symptoms of hypoglycemia may be different or less pronounced under certain conditions, such as long duration of diabetes, diabetic nerve disease, use of medications such as beta-blockers, or intensified diabetes control.

I

RENAL IMPAIRMENT

Clinical or pharmacology studies with NovoLog Mix 70/30 in diabetic patients with various degrees of renal impairment have not been conducted. As with other insulins, the requirements for NovoLog Mix 70/30 may be reduced in patients with renal impairment.

HEPATIC IMPAIRMENT

Clinical or pharmacology studies with NovoLog Mix 70/30 in diabetic patients with various degrees of hepatic impairment have not been conducted. As with other insulins, the requirements for NovoLog Mix 70/30 may be reduced in patients with hepatic impairment.

ALLERGY

Local Reactions

Erythema, swelling, and pruritus at the injection site have been observed with NovoLog Mix 70/30 as with other insulin therapy. Reactions may be related to the insulin molecule, other components in the insulin preparation including protamine and cresol, components in skin cleansing agents, or injection techniques.

Systemic Reactions

Less common, but potentially more serious, is generalized allergy to insulin, which may cause rash (including pruritus) over the whole body, shortness of breath, wheezing, reduction in blood pressure, rapid pulse, or sweating. Severe cases of generalized allergy, including anaphylactic reaction, may be life threatening. Localized reactions and generalized myalgias have been reported with the use of cresol as an injectable excipient.

ANTIBODY PRODUCTION

Specific anti-insulin antibodies as well as cross-reacting anti-insulin antibodies were monitored in the 3 month open-label comparator trial as well as in a long-term extension trial. Changes in cross-reactive antibodies were more common after NovoLog Mix 70/30 than with Novolin 70/30 but these changes did not correlate with change in HbA1c or increase in insulin dose. The clinical significance of these antibodies has not been established. Antibodies did not increase further after long-term exposure (>6 months) to NovoLog Mix 70/30.

INFORMATION FOR THE PATIENT

Patients should be informed about potential risks and advantages of NovoLog Mix 70/30 therapy including the possible side effects. Patients should also be offered continued education and advice on insulin therapies, injection technique, life-style management, regular glucose monitoring, periodic glycosylated hemoglobin testing, recognition and management of hypo- and hyperglycemia, adherence to meal planning, complications of insulin therapy, timing of dose, instruction for use of injection devices, and proper storage of insulin.

Female patients should be advised to discuss with their physician if they intend to, or if they become, pregnant because information is not available on the use of NovoLog Mix 70/30 during pregnancy or lactation (see Pregnancy, Teratogenic Effects, Pregnancy Category C).

LABORATORY TESTS

The therapeutic response to NovoLog Mix 70/30 should be assessed by measurement of serum or blood glucose and glycosylated hemoglobin.

CARCINOGENESIS, MUTAGENESIS, AND IMPAIRMENT OF FERTILITY

Standard 2 year carcinogenicity studies in animals have not been performed to evaluate the carcinogenic potential of NovoLog Mix 70/30. In 52 week studies, Sprague-Dawley rats were dosed subcutaneously with NovoLog, the rapid-acting component of NovoLog Mix 70/30, at 10, 50, and 200 U/kg/day (approximately 2, 8, and 32 times the human subcutaneous dose of 1.0 U/kg/day, based on U/body surface area, respectively). At a dose of 200 U/kg/day, NovoLog increased the incidence of mammary gland tumors in females when compared to untreated controls. The incidence of mammary tumors for NovoLog was not significantly different than for regular human insulin. The relevance of these findings to humans is not known. NovoLog was not genotoxic in the following tests: Ames test, mouse lymphoma cell forward gene mutation test, human peripheral blood lymphocyte chromosome aberration test, *in vivo* micronucleus test in mice, and in *ex vivo* UDS test in rat liver hepatocytes. In fertility studies in male and female rats, NovoLog at subcutaneous doses up to 200 U/kg/day (approximately 32 times the human subcutaneous dose, based on U/body surface area) had no direct adverse effects on male and female fertility, or on general reproductive performance of animals.

PREGNANCY, TERATOGENIC EFFECTS, PREGNANCY CATEGORY C

Animal reproduction studies have not been conducted with NovoLog Mix 70/30. However, reproductive toxicology and teratology studies have been performed with NovoLog (the rapid-acting component of NovoLog Mix 70/30) and regular human insulin in rats and rabbits. In these studies, NovoLog was given to female rats before mating, during mating, and throughout pregnancy, and to rabbits during organogenesis. The effects of NovoLog did not differ from those observed with subcutaneous regular human insulin. NovoLog, like human insulin, caused pre- and post-implantation losses and visceral/skeletal abnormalities in rats at a dose of 200 U/kg/day (approximately 32 times the human subcutaneous dose of 1.0 U/kg/day, based on U/body surface area), and in rabbits at a dose of 10 U/kg/day (approximately 3 times the human subcutaneous dose of 1.0 U/kg/day, based on U/body surface area). The effects are probably secondary to maternal hypoglycemia at high doses. No significant effects were observed in rats at a dose of 50 U/kg/day and rabbits at a dose of 3 U/kg/day.

These doses are approximately 8 times the human subcutaneous dose of 1.0 U/kg/day for rats and equal to the human subcutaneous dose of 1.0 U/kg/day for rabbits based on U/body surface area.

It is not known whether NovoLog Mix 70/30 can cause fetal harm when administered to a pregnant woman or can affect reproductive capacity. There are no adequate and well-controlled studies of the use of NovoLog Mix 70/30 or NovoLog in pregnant women. NovoLog Mix 70/30 should be used during pregnancy only if the potential benefit justifies the potential risk to the fetus.

NURSING MOTHERS

It is unknown whether NovoLog Mix 70/30 is excreted in human milk as is human insulin. There are no adequate and well-controlled studies of the use of NovoLog Mix 70/30 or NovoLog in lactating women.

PEDIATRIC USE

Safety and effectiveness of NovoLog Mix 70/30 in children have not been established.

GERIATRIC USE

Clinical studies of NovoLog Mix 70/30 did not include sufficient numbers of patients aged 65 and over to determine whether they respond differently than younger patients. In general, dose selection for an elderly patient should be cautious, usually starting at the low end of the dosing range reflecting the greater frequency of decreased hepatic, renal, or cardiac function, and of concomitant disease or other drug therapy in this population.

DRUG INTERACTIONS

A number of substances affect glucose metabolism and may require insulin dose adjustment and particularly close monitoring. The following are examples of substances that may increase the blood-glucose-lowering effect and susceptibility to hypoglycemia: oral antidiabetic products, ACE inhibitors, disopyramide, fibrates, fluoxetine, monoamine oxidase (MAO) inhibitors, propoxyphene, salicylates, somatostatin analog (*e.g.*, octreotide), sulfonamide antibiotics.

The following are examples of substances that may reduce the blood-glucose-lowering effect: corticosteroids, niacin, danazol, diuretics, sympathomimetic agents (*e.g.*, epinephrine, salbutamol, terbutaline), isoniazid, phenothiazine derivatives, somatropin, thyroid hormones, estrogens, progestogens (*e.g.*, in oral contraceptives).

Beta-blockers, clonidine, lithium salts, and alcohol may either potentiate or weaken the blood-glucose-lowering effect of insulin.

Pentamidine may cause hypoglycemia, which may sometimes be followed by hyperglycemia.

In addition, under the influence of sympatholytic medical products such as beta-blockers, clonidine, guanethidine, and reserpine, the signs of hypoglycemia may be reduced or absent (see CLINICAL PHARMACOLOGY).

MIXING OF INSULINS

NovoLog Mix 70/30 should not be mixed with any other insulin product.

ADVERSE REACTIONS

Clinical trials comparing NovoLog Mix 70/30 with Novolin 70/30 did not demonstrate a difference in frequency of adverse events between the two treatments.

Adverse events commonly associated with human insulin therapy include the following:

Body as Whole: *Allergic reactions* (see PRECAUTIONS, Allergy).

Skin and Appendages: *Local injection site reactions or rash or pruritus, as with other insulin therapies, occurred in 7% of all patients on NovoLog Mix 70/30 and 5% on Novolin 70/30. Rash led to withdrawal of therapy in <1% of patients on either drug* (see PRECAUTIONS, Allergy).

Hypoglycemia: See WARNINGS and PRECAUTIONS.

Other: Small elevations in alkaline phosphatase were observed in patients treated in NovoLog controlled clinical trials. There have been no clinical consequences of these laboratory findings.

DOSAGE AND ADMINISTRATION

GENERAL

Fixed ratio insulins are typically dosed on a twice daily basis, *i.e.*, before breakfast and supper, with each dose intended to cover two meals or a meal and snack. NovoLog Mix 70/30 is intended only for subcutaneous injection (into the abdominal wall, thigh, or upper arm). NovoLog Mix 70/30 should not be administered intravenously. The absorption rate of NovoLog Mix 70/30 from the subcutaneous tissue allows dosing within 15 minutes of meal initiation.

Dose regimens of NovoLog Mix 70/30 will vary among patients and should be determined by the health care professional familiar with the patient's metabolic needs, eating habits, and other lifestyle variables. As with all insulins, the duration of action may vary according to the dose, injection site, blood flow, temperature, and level of physical activity and conditioning.

TABLE 2 *Summary of Pharmacodynamic Properties of Insulin Products (Pooled Cross-Study Comparison) and Recommended Interval Between Dosing and Meal Initiation*

Insulin Products	Dose* (U/kg)	Interval† (minutes)	Time of Peak Activity‡ (h) (mean ± SD)	Total Activity§ (mean, range)
NovoLog	0.3	10-20	2.2 ± 0.98	65% ± 11%
Novolin R	0.2	30	3.3	60% ± 16%
Novolin 50/50	0.5	30	4.0 ± 0.6	54% ± 12%
NovoLog Mix 70/30	0.3	10-20	2.4 ± 0.80	45% ± 22%
Novolin 70/30	0.3	30	4.2 ± 0.39	25% ± 5%
Novolin N	0.3	n/a	8.0 ± 5.3	21% ± 11%

* Dose used in study.
† Recommended interval between dosing and meal initiation; applicable only to Novolin R and NovoLog alone or as components of insulin mixes.
‡ Hours after dosing.
§ Percent of total activity occurring in the first 4 hours.

ADMINISTRATION USING PENFILL CARTRIDGES FOR 3 ML PENFILL CARTRIDGE COMPATIBLE DELIVERY DEVICES, NOVOLOG MIX 70/30 FLEXPEN PREFILLED SYRINGES, OR VIALS

*PenFill Cartridges for 3 ml PenFill Cartridge Compatible Delivery Devices**

NovoLog Mix 70/30 PenFill suspension should be visually inspected and resuspended immediately before use. The resuspended NovoLog Mix 70/30 must appear uniformly white and cloudy. Before inserting the cartridge into the insulin delivery system, roll the cartridge between your palms 10 times. Thereafter, turn the cartridge upside down so that the glass ball moves from one end of the cartridge to the other. Do this at least 10 times. The rolling and turning procedure must be repeated until the suspension appears uniformly white and cloudy. Inject immediately. Before each subsequent injection, turn the 3 ml PenFill cartridge compatible delivery devices* upside down so that the glass ball moves from one end of the cartridge to the other. Repeat this 10 times until the suspension appears uniformly white and cloudy. Inject immediately. **After use, needles on the insulin pen delivery devices should not be recapped. Used syringes, needles, or lancets should be placed in sharps containers (such as red biohazard containers), hard plastic containers (such as detergent bottles), or metal containers (such as empty coffee can). Such containers should be sealed and disposed of properly.**

*NovoLog Mix 70/30 PenFill cartridges are for use with the following 3 ml PenFill cartridge compatible delivery devices: NovoPen 3, Innovo, and InDuo.

Disposable NovoLog Mix 70/30 FlexPen Prefilled Syringes

NovoLog Mix 70/30 suspension should be visually inspected and resuspended immediately before use. The resuspended NovoLog Mix 70/30 must appear uniformly white and cloudy. Before use, roll the disposable NovoLog Mix 70/30 FlexPen prefilled syringe between your palms 10 times. Thereafter, turn the disposable NovoLog Mix 70/30 FlexPen prefilled syringe upside down so that the glass ball moves from one end of the reservoir to the other. Do this at least 10 times. The rolling and turning procedure must be repeated until the suspension appears uniformly white and cloudy. Inject immediately. Before each subsequent injection, turn the disposable NovoLog Mix 70/30 FlexPen Prefilled syringe upside down so that the glass ball moves from one end of the reservoir to the other at least 10 times and until the suspension appears uniformly white and cloudy. Inject immediately. **After use, needles on the disposable NovoLog Mix 70/30 FlexPen prefilled syringes should not be recapped. Used syringes, needles, or lancets should be placed in sharps containers (such as red biohazard containers), hard plastic containers (such as detergent bottles), or metal containers (such as empty coffee can). Such containers should be sealed and disposed of properly.**

Vial

NovoLog Mix 70/30 vial must be resuspended immediately before use. Roll the vial gently 10 times in your hand to mix it. The resuspended NovoLog Mix 70/30 must appear uniformly white and cloudy.

HOW SUPPLIED

NovoLog Mix 70/30 is available as follows: each presentation containing 100 Units of insulin aspart per ml (U-100).

10 ml vials
3 ml PenFill cartridges*
3 ml NovoLog Mix 70/30 FlexPen Prefilled syringe

*NovoLog Mix 70/30 PenFill cartridges are for use with the following 3 ml PenFill cartridge compatible delivery devices: NovoPen 3, Innovo, and InDuo.

RECOMMENDED STORAGE

NovoLog Mix 70/30 should be stored between 2 and 8°C (36-46°F). *Do not freeze.* **Do not use NovoLog Mix 70/30 if it has been frozen.**

Vials

The vials should be stored in a refrigerator, not in a freezer. If refrigeration is not possible, the bottle in use can be kept unrefrigerated at room temperature below 30°C (86°F) for up to 28 days, as long as it is kept as cool as possible and away from direct heat and light.

Unpunctured vials can be used until the expiration date printed on the label if they are stored in a refrigerator. Keep unused vials in the carton so they will stay clean and protected from light.

PenFill Cartridges or NovoLog Mix 70/30 FlexPen Prefilled Syringes

Once a cartridge or a NovoLog Mix 70/30 FlexPen prefilled syringe is punctured, it may be used for up to 14 days if it is kept at room temperature below 30°C (86°F). Cartridges or NovoLog Mix 70/30 FlexPen prefilled syringes in use must NOT be stored in the refrigerator. Keep all PenFill cartridges and disposable NovoLog Mix 70/30 FlexPen Prefilled syringes away from direct heat and sunlight. Unpunctured PenFill cartridges and NovoLog Mix 70/30 FlexPen Prefilled syringes can be used until the expiration date printed on the label if they are stored in a refrigerator. Keep unused PenFill cartridges and NovoLog Mix 70/30 FlexPen Prefilled syringes in the carton so they will stay clean and protected from light.

PRODUCT LISTING - EQUIVALENTS NOT AVAILABLE

Suspension - Subcutaneous - 30 U;70 U/ml

3 ml x 5	$118.70	NOVOLOG MIX 70/30 FLEXPEN, Novo Nordisk Pharmaceuticals Inc	00169-6339-10
10 ml	$61.43	NOVOLOG MIX 70/30, Novo Nordisk Pharmaceuticals Inc	00169-3685-12

Insulin Glargine *(003483)*

I

For related information, see the comparative table section in Appendix A.

Categories: Diabetes mellitus; FDA Approved 2000 Apr; Pregnancy Category C
Drug Classes: Antidiabetic agents; Insulins
Foreign Brand Availability: Lantus (Austria; Belgium; Bulgaria; Czech-Republic; Denmark; England; Finland; France; Germany; Greece; Hungary; Ireland; Italy; Netherlands; Norway; Poland; Portugal; Slovenia; Spain; Sweden; Switzerland; Turkey); Optisulin (Austria; Belgium; Bulgaria; Czech-Republic; Denmark; England; Finland; France; Germany; Greece; Hungary; Ireland; Italy; Netherlands; Norway; Poland; Portugal; Slovenia; Spain; Sweden; Switzerland; Turkey)

DESCRIPTION

Lantus must not be diluted or mixed with any other insulin or solution.

Lantus (insulin glargine [rDNA origin] injection) is a sterile solution of insulin glargine for use as an injection. Insulin glargine is a recombinant human insulin analog that is a long-acting (up to 24 hour duration of action), parenteral blood-glucose-lowering agent. (See CLINICAL PHARMACOLOGY.) Insulin glargine is produced by recombinant DNA technology utilizing a non-pathogenic laboratory strain of *Escherichia coli* (K12) as the production organism. Insulin glargine differs from human insulin in that the amino acid asparagine at position A21 is replaced by glycine and two arginines are added to the C-terminus of the B-chain. Chemically, it is 21^{A}-Gly-30^{B}a-L-Arg-30^{B}b-L-Arg-human insulin and has the empirical formula $C_{267}H_{404}N_{72}O_{78}S_6$ and a molecular weight of 6063.

Lantus consists of insulin glargine dissolved in a clear aqueous fluid. Each milliliter of Lantus (insulin glargine injection) contains 100 IU (3.6378 mg) insulin glargine, 30 μg zinc, 2.7 mg m-cresol, 20 mg glycerol 85%, and water for injection. The pH is adjusted by addition of aqueous solutions of hydrochloric acid and sodium hydroxide. Lantus has a pH of approximately 4.

STORAGE

Unopened Insulin glargine vials and cartridges should be stored in a refrigerator, 36-46°F (2-8°C). Insulin glargine should not be stored in the freezer and it should not be allowed to freeze.

If refrigeration is not possible, the 10 ml vial or cartridge of Lantus in use can be kept unrefrigerated for up to 28 days away from direct heat and light, as long as the temperature is not greater than 86°F (30°C). Unrefrigerated 10 ml vials and cartridges must be used within the 28-day period or they must be discarded.

If refrigeration is not possible, 5 ml vials of Lantus in use can be kept unrefrigerated for up to 14 days away from direct heat and light, as long as the temperature is not greater than 86°F (30°C). Unrefrigerated 5 ml vials must be used within the 14-day period or they must be discarded. If refrigerated, the 5 ml vial of Lantus in use can be kept for up to 28 days.

Once the cartridge is placed in an OptiPen One, it should not be put in the refrigerator.

CLINICAL PHARMACOLOGY

MECHANISM OF ACTION

The primary activity of insulin, including insulin glargine, is regulation of glucose metabolism. Insulin and its analogs lower blood glucose levels by stimulating peripheral glucose uptake, especially by skeletal muscle and fat, and by inhibiting hepatic glucose production. Insulin inhibits lipolysis in the adipocyte, inhibits proteolysis, and enhances protein synthesis.

PHARMACODYNAMICS

Insulin glargine is a human insulin analog that has been designed to have low aqueous solubility at neutral pH. At pH 4, as in the insulin glargine injection solution, it is completely soluble. After injection into the subcutaneous tissue, the acidic solution is neutralized, leading to formation of micro-precipitates from which small amounts of insulin glargine are slowly released, resulting in a relatively constant concentration/time profile over 24 hours with no pronounced peak. This profile allows once-daily dosing as a patient's basal insulin.

In clinical studies, the glucose-lowering effect on a molar basis (*i.e.*, when given at the same doses) of intravenous insulin glargine is approximately the same as human insulin. In euglycemic clamp studies in healthy subjects or in patients with Type 1 diabetes, the onset of action of subcutaneous insulin glargine was slower than NPH human insulin. The effect profile of insulin glargine was relatively constant with no pronounced peak and the duration of its effect was prolonged compared to NPH human insulin. Figure 1 shows results from a study in patients with Type 1 diabetes conducted for a maximum of 24 hours after the injection. The median time between injection and the end of pharmacological effect was 14.5 hours (range: 9.5-19.3 hours) for NPH human insulin, and 24 hours (range: 10.8 to >24.0 hours) (24 hours was the end of the observation period) for insulin glargine.

The longer duration of action (up to 24 hours) of insulin glargine is directly related to its slower rate of absorption and supports once-daily subcutaneous administration. The time course of action of insulins, including insulin glargine, may vary between individuals and/or within the same individual.

PHARMACOKINETICS

Absorption and Bioavailability

After subcutaneous injection of insulin glargine in healthy subjects and in patients with diabetes, the insulin serum concentrations indicated a slower, more prolonged absorption and a relatively constant concentration/time profile over 24 hours with no pronounced peak in comparison to NPH human insulin. Serum insulin concentrations were thus consistent with the time profile of the pharmacodynamic activity of insulin glargine.

After subcutaneous injection of 0.3 IU/kg insulin glargine in patients with Type 1 diabetes, a relatively constant concentration/time profile has been demonstrated. The duration of action after abdominal, deltoid, or thigh subcutaneous administration was similar.

Metabolism

A metabolism study in humans indicates that insulin glargine is partly metabolized at the carboxyl terminus of the B chain in the subcutaneous depot to form 2 active metabolites with *in vitro* activity similar to that of insulin, M1 (21^A-Gly-insulin) and M2 (21^A-Gly-des-30^B-Thr- insulin). Unchanged drug and these degradation products are also present in the circulation.

I

SPECIAL POPULATIONS

Age, Race, and Gender

Information on the effect of age, race, and gender on the pharmacokinetics of insulin glargine is not available. However, in controlled clinical trials in adults (n=3890) and a controlled clinical trial in pediatric patients (n=349), subgroup analyses based on age, race, and gender did not show differences in safety and efficacy between insulin glargine and NPH human insulin.

Smoking

The effect of smoking on the pharmacokinetics/pharmacodynamics of insulin glargine has not been studied.

Pregnancy

The effect of pregnancy on the pharmacokinetics and pharmacodynamics of insulin glargine has not been studied. (See PRECAUTIONS, Pregnancy, Teratogenic Effects, Pregnancy Category C.)

Obesity

In controlled clinical trials, which included patients with Body Mass Index (BMI) up to and including 49.6 kg/m^2, subgroup analyses based on bmi did not show any differences in safety and efficacy between insulin glargine and NPH human insulin.

Renal Impairment

The effect of renal impairment on the pharmacokinetics of insulin glargine has not been studied. However, some studies with human insulin have shown increased circulating levels of insulin in patients with renal failure. Careful glucose monitoring and dose adjustments of insulin, including insulin glargine, may be necessary in patients with renal dysfunction. (See PRECAUTIONS, Renal Impairment.)

Hepatic Impairment

The effect of hepatic impairment on the pharmacokinetics of insulin glargine has not been studied. However, some studies with human insulin have shown increased circulating levels of insulin in patients with liver failure. Careful glucose monitoring and dose adjustments of insulin, including insulin glargine, may be necessary in patients with hepatic dysfunction. (See PRECAUTIONS, Hepatic Impairment.)

INDICATIONS AND USAGE

Insulin glargine is indicated for once-daily subcutaneous administration at bedtime in the treatment of adult and pediatric patients with Type 1 diabetes mellitus or adult patients with Type 2 diabetes mellitus who require basal (long-acting) insulin for the control of hyperglycemia.

CONTRAINDICATIONS

Insulin glargine is contraindicated in patients hypersensitive to insulin glargine or the excipients.

WARNINGS

Hypoglycemia is the most common adverse effect of insulin, including insulin glargine. As with all insulins, the timing of hypoglycemia may differ among various insulin formulations. Glucose monitoring is recommended for all patients with diabetes.

Any change of insulin should be made cautiously and only under medical supervision. Changes in insulin strength, manufacturer, type (*e.g.,* regular, NPH, or insulin analogs), species (animal, human), or method of manufacture (recombinant DNA versus animal-source insulin) may result in the need for a change in dosage. Concomitant oral antidiabetic treatment may need to be adjusted.

PRECAUTIONS

GENERAL

Insulin glargine is not intended for intravenous administration. The prolonged duration of activity of insulin glargine is dependent on injection into subcutaneous tissue. Intravenous administration of the usual subcutaneous dose could result in severe hypoglycemia.

Insulin glargine must not be diluted or mixed with any other insulin or solution. If insulin glargine is diluted or mixed, the solution may become cloudy, and the pharmacokinetic/pharmacodynamic profile (*e.g.,* onset of action, time to peak effect) of insulin glargine and/or the mixed insulin may be altered in an unpredictable manner. When insulin glargine and regular human insulin were mixed immediately before injection in dogs, a delayed onset of action and time to maximum effect for regular human insulin was observed. The total bioavailability of the mixture was also slightly decreased compared to separate injections of insulin glargine and regular human insulin. The relevance of these observations in dogs to humans is not known.

As with all insulin preparations, the time course of insulin glargine action may vary in different individuals or at different times in the same individual and the rate of absorption is dependent on blood supply, temperature, and physical activity.

Insulin may cause sodium retention and edema, particularly if previously poor metabolic control is improved by intensified insulin therapy.

HYPOGLYCEMIA

As with all insulin preparations, hypoglycemic reactions may be associated with the administration of insulin glargine. Hypoglycemia is the most common adverse effect of insulins. Early warning symptoms of hypoglycemia may be different or less pronounced under certain conditions, such as long duration of diabetes, diabetic nerve disease, use of medications such as beta-blockers, or intensified diabetes control. (See DRUG INTERACTIONS.) Such situations may result in severe hypoglycemia (and, possibly, loss of consciousness) prior to patients' awareness of hypoglycemia.

The time of occurrence of hypoglycemia depends on the action profile of the insulins used and may, therefore, change when the treatment regimen is changed. Patients being switched from twice daily NPH insulin to once-daily insulin glargine should have their insulin glargine dose reduced by 20% from the previous total daily NPH dose to reduce the risk of hypoglycemia. (See DOSAGE AND ADMINISTRATION, Changeover to Insulin Glargine.)

The prolonged effect of subcutaneous insulin glargine may delay recovery from hypoglycemia.

In a clinical study, symptoms of hypoglycemia or counter-regulatory hormone responses were similar after intravenous insulin glargine and regular human insulin both in healthy subjects and patients with Type 1 diabetes.

RENAL IMPAIRMENT

Although studies have not been performed in patients with diabetes and renal impairment, insulin glargine requirements may be diminished because of reduced insulin metabolism, similar to observations found with other insulins. (See CLINICAL PHARMACOLOGY, Special Populations.)

HEPATIC IMPAIRMENT

Although studies have not been performed in patients with diabetes and hepatic impairment, insulin glargine requirements may be diminished due to reduced capacity for gluconeogenesis and reduced insulin metabolism, similar to observations found with other insulins. (See CLINICAL PHARMACOLOGY, Special Populations.)

INJECTION SITE AND ALLERGIC REACTIONS

As with any insulin therapy, lipodystrophy may occur at the injection site and delay insulin absorption. Other injection site reactions with insulin therapy include redness, pain, itching, hives, swelling, and inflammation. Continuous rotation of the injection site within a given area may help to reduce or prevent these reactions. Most minor reactions to insulins usually resolve in a few days to a few weeks.

Reports of injection site pain were more frequent with insulin glargine than NPH human insulin (2.7% insulin glargine versus 0.7% NPH). The reports of pain at the injection site were usually mild and did not result in discontinuation of therapy.

Immediate-type allergic reactions are rare. Such reactions to insulin (including insulin glargine) or the excipients may, for example, be associated with generalized skin reactions, angioedema, bronchospasm, hypotension, or shock and may be life threatening.

INTERCURRENT CONDITIONS

Insulin requirements may be altered during intercurrent conditions such as illness, emotional disturbances, or stress.

INFORMATION FOR THE PATIENT

Insulin glargine must only be used if the solution is clear and colorless with no particles visible. (See DOSAGE AND ADMINISTRATION, Preparation and Handling.)

Patients must be advised that insulin glargine must not be diluted or mixed with any other insulin or solution. (See PRECAUTIONS, General.) Patients should be instructed on self-management procedures including glucose monitoring, proper injection technique, and hypoglycemia and hyperglycemia management. Patients must be instructed on handling of special situations such as intercurrent conditions (illness, stress, or emotional disturbances), an inadequate or skipped insulin dose, inadvertent administration of an increased insulin dose, inadequate food intake, or skipped meals. Refer patients to the insulin glargine information for the patient circular for additional information.

As with all patients who have diabetes, the ability to concentrate and/or react may be impaired as a result of hypoglycemia or hyperglycemia.

Patients with diabetes should be advised to inform their doctor if they are pregnant or are contemplating pregnancy.

CARCINOGENESIS, MUTAGENESIS, AND IMPAIRMENT OF FERTILITY

In mice and rats, standard 2 year carcinogenicity studies with insulin glargine were performed at doses up to 0.455 mg/kg, which is for the rat approximately 10 times and for the mouse approximately 5 times the recommended human subcutaneous starting dose of 10 IU (0.008 mg/kg/day), based on mg/m^2. The findings in female mice were not conclusive due to excessive mortality in all dose groups during the study. Histiocytomas were found at injection sites in male rats (statistically significant) and male mice (not statistically significant) in acid vehicle containing groups. These tumors were not found in female animals, in saline control, or insulin comparator groups using a different vehicle. The relevance of these findings to humans is unknown.

Insulin glargine was not mutagenic in tests for detection of gene mutations in bacteria and mammalian cells (Ames- and HGPRT-test) and in tests for detection of chromosomal aberrations (cytogenetics *in vitro* in V79 cells and *in vivo* in Chinese hamsters).

In a combined fertility and prenatal and postnatal study in male and female rats at subcutaneous doses up to 0.36 mg/kg/day, which is approximately 7 times the recommended human subcutaneous starting dose of 10 IU (0.008 mg/kg/day), based on mg/m^2, maternal toxicity due to dose-dependent hypoglycemia, including some deaths, was observed. Consequently, a reduction of the rearing rate occurred in the high-dose group only. Similar effects were observed with NPH human insulin.

PREGNANCY, TERATOGENIC EFFECTS, PREGNANCY CATEGORY C

Subcutaneous reproduction and teratology studies have been performed with insulin glargine and regular human insulin in rats and Himalayan rabbits. The drug was given to female rats before mating, during mating, and throughout pregnancy at doses up to 0.36 mg/kg/day, which is approximately 7 times the recommended human subcutaneous starting dose of 10 IU (0.008 mg/kg/day), based on mg/m^2. In rabbits, doses of 0.072 mg/kg/day, which is approximately 2 times the recommended human subcutaneous starting dose of 10 IU (0.008 mg/kg/day), based on mg/m^2, were administered during organogenesis. The effects of insulin glargine did not generally differ from those observed with regular human insulin in rats or rabbits. However, in rabbits, 5 fetuses from 2 litters of the high-dose group exhibited dilation of the cerebral ventricles. Fertility and early embryonic development appeared normal.

There are no well-controlled clinical studies of the use of insulin glargine in pregnant women. It is essential for patients with diabetes or a history of gestational diabetes to maintain good metabolic control before conception and throughout pregnancy. Insulin requirements may decrease during the first trimester, generally increase during the second and third trimesters, and rapidly decline after delivery. Careful monitoring of glucose control is essential in such patients. Because animal reproduction studies are not always predictive of human response, this drug should be used during pregnancy only if clearly needed.

NURSING MOTHERS

It is unknown whether insulin glargine is excreted in significant amounts in human milk. Many drugs, including human insulin, are excreted in human milk. For this reason, caution should be exercised when insulin glargine is administered to a nursing woman. Lactating women may require adjustments in insulin dose and diet.

PEDIATRIC USE

Safety and effectiveness of insulin glargine have been established in the age group 6-15 years with Type 1 diabetes.

GERIATRIC USE

In controlled clinical studies comparing insulin glargine to NPH human insulin, 593 of 3890 patients with Type 1 and Type 2 diabetes were 65 years and older. The only difference in safety or effectiveness in this subpopulation compared to the entire study population was an expected higher incidence of cardiovascular events in both insulin glargine and NPH human insulin-treated patients.

In elderly patients with diabetes, the initial dosing, dose increments, and maintenance dosage should be conservative to avoid hypoglycemic reactions. Hypoglycemia may be difficult to recognize in the elderly. (See Hypoglycemia.)

DRUG INTERACTIONS

A number of substances affect glucose metabolism and may require insulin dose adjustment and particularly close monitoring.

The following are examples of substances that may increase the blood-glucose-lowering effect and susceptibility to hypoglycemia: oral antidiabetic products, ACE inhibitors, disopyramide, fibrates, fluoxetine, MAO inhibitors, propoxyphene, salicylates, somatostatin analog (*e.g.*, octreotide), sulfonamide antibiotics.

The following are examples of substances that may reduce the blood-glucose-lowering effect of insulin: corticosteroids, danazol, diuretics, sympathomimetic agents (*e.g.*, epinephrine, albuterol, terbutaline), isoniazid, phenothiazine derivatives, somatropin, thyroid hormones, estrogens, progestogens (*e.g.*, in oral contraceptives).

Beta-blockers, clonidine, lithium salts, and alcohol may either potentiate or weaken the blood-glucose-lowering effect of insulin. Pentamidine may cause hypoglycemia, which may sometimes be followed by hyperglycemia.

In addition, under the influence of sympatholytic medicinal products such as beta-blockers, clonidine, guanethidine, and reserpine, the signs of hypoglycemia may be reduced or absent.

ADVERSE REACTIONS

The adverse events commonly associated with insulin glargine include the following:

Body as a Whole: Allergic reactions (see PRECAUTIONS).

Skin and Appendages: Injection site reaction, lipodystrophy, pruritus, rash (see PRECAUTIONS).

Other: Hypoglycemia (see WARNINGS and PRECAUTIONS).

In clinical studies in adult patients, there was a higher incidence of treatment-emergent injection site pain in insulin glargine-treated patients (2.7%) compared to NPH insulin-treated patients (0.7%). The reports of pain at the injection site were usually mild and did not result in discontinuation of therapy. Other treatment-emergent injection site reactions occurred at similar incidences with both insulin glargine and NPH human insulin.

Retinopathy was evaluated in the clinical studies by means of retinal adverse events reported and fundus photography. The numbers of retinal adverse events reported for insulin glargine and NPH treatment groups were similar for patients with Type 1 and Type 2 diabetes. Progression of retinopathy was investigated by fundus photography using a grading protocol derived from the Early Treatment Diabetic Retinopathy Study (ETDRS). In one clinical study involving patients with Type 2 diabetes, a difference in the number of subjects with ≥3-step progression in ETDRS scale over a 6 month period was noted by fundus photography (7.5% in insulin glargine group versus 2.7% in NPH treated group). The overall relevance of this isolated finding cannot be determined due to the small number of patients involved, the short follow-up period, and the fact that this finding was not observed in other clinical studies.

DOSAGE AND ADMINISTRATION

Insulin glargine is a recombinant human insulin analog. Its potency is approximately the same as human insulin. It exhibits a relatively constant glucose-lowering profile over 24 hours that permits once-daily dosing. Insulin glargine should be administered subcutaneously once a day at bedtime.

Insulin glargine is not intended for intravenous administration. (See PRECAUTIONS.) Intravenous administration of the usual subcutaneous dose could result in severe hypoglycemia. The desired blood glucose levels as well as the doses and timing of antidiabetic medications must be determined individually. Blood glucose monitoring is recommended for all patients with diabetes. The prolonged duration of activity of insulin glargine is dependent on injection into subcutaneous space.

As with all insulins, injection sites within an injection area (abdomen, thigh or deltoid) must be rotated from one injection to the next.

In clinical studies, there was no relevant difference in insulin glargine absorption after abdominal, deltoid, or thigh subcutaneous administration. As for all insulins, the rate of absorption, and consequently the onset and duration of action, may be affected by exercise and other variables.

Insulin glargine is not the insulin of choice for the treatment of diabetic ketoacidosis. Intravenous short-acting insulin is the preferred treatment.

PEDIATRIC USE

Insulin glargine can be safely administrated to pediatric patients ≥6 years of age. Administration to pediatric patients <6 years has not been studied. Based on the results of a study in pediatric patients, the dose recommendation for changeover to insulin glargine is the same as described for adults in Changeover to Insulin Glargine.

INITIATION OF INSULIN GLARGINE THERAPY

In a clinical study with insulin naïve patients with Type 2 diabetes already treated with oral antidiabetic drugs, insulin glargine was started at an average dose of 10 IU once daily, and subsequently adjusted according to the patient's need to a total daily dose ranging from 2-100 IU.

CHANGEOVER TO INSULIN GLARGINE

If changing from a treatment regimen with an intermediate- or long-acting insulin to a regimen with insulin glargine, the amount and timing of short- or fast-acting insulin analog or the dose of any oral antidiabetic drug may need to be adjusted. In clinical studies, when patients were transferred from once-daily NPH human insulin or ultralente human insulin to once-daily insulin glargine, the initial dose was usually not changed. However, when patients were transferred from twice-daily NPH human insulin to insulin glargine once daily at bedtime, to reduce the risk of hypoglycemia, the initial dose (IU) was usually reduced by approximately 20% (compared to total daily IU of NPH human insulin) within the first week of treatment and then adjusted based on patient response. (See PRECAUTIONS, Hypoglycemia.)

A program of close metabolic monitoring under medical supervision is recommended during transfer and in the initial weeks thereafter. The amount and timing of short- or fast-acting insulin analog may need to be adjusted. This is particularly true for patients with acquired antibodies to human insulin needing high insulin doses and occurs with all insulin analogs. Dose adjustment of insulin glargine and other insulins or oral antidiabetic drugs may be required; for example, if the patient's weight or lifestyle changes or other circumstances arise that increase susceptibility to hypoglycemia or hyperglycemia. (See PRECAUTIONS, Hypoglycemia.)

The dose may also have to be adjusted during intercurrent illness. (See PRECAUTIONS, Intercurrent Conditions)

PREPARATION AND HANDLING

Parenteral drug products should be inspected visually prior to administration whenever the solution and the container permit. Insulin glargine must only be used if the solution is clear and colorless with no particles visible.

The syringes must not contain any other medicinal product or residue.

Mixing and Diluting: **Insulin glargine must not be diluted or mixed with any other insulin or solution. (See PRECAUTIONS, General.)**

Cartridge Version Only: If the OptiPen One Insulin Delivery Device malfunctions, Insulin glargine may be drawn from the cartridge into a U 100 syringe and injected.

PRODUCT LISTING - EQUIVALENTS NOT AVAILABLE

Solution - Subcutaneous - 100 U/ml

10 ml $51.21 LANTUS, Aventis Pharmaceuticals 00088-2220-33

Insulin Lispro (Human Analog) *(003293)*

For related information, see the comparative table section in Appendix A.

Categories: Diabetes mellitus; FDA Approved 1996 Jun; Pregnancy Category B
Drug Classes: Antidiabetic agents; Insulins
Brand Names: **Humalog**
Foreign Brand Availability: Humalog Lispro (Costa-Rica; El-Salvador; France; Guatemala; Honduras; Israel; Korea; Mexico; Nicaragua; Panama; Peru); Humalog Mix NPL (Austria; Belgium; Bulgaria; Czech-Republic; Denmark; England; Finland; France; Germany; Greece; Hungary; Ireland; Italy; Netherlands; Norway; Poland; Portugal; Slovenia; Spain; Sweden; Switzerland; Turkey); Insuline Lispro Humalog (France)

DESCRIPTION

Insulin lispro, rDNA origin is a human insulin analog that is a rapid-acting, parenteral blood glucose-lowering agent. Chemically, it is Lys(B28), Pro(B29) human insulin analog, created when the amino acids at positions 28 and 29 on the insulin B-chain are reversed. Humalog is synthesized in a special non-pathogenic laboratory strain of *Escherichia coli* bacteria that has been genetically altered by the addition of the gene for insulin lispro.

Humalog has the empirical formula $C_{257}H_{383}N_{65}O_{77}S_6$ and a molecular weight of 5808, both identical to that of human insulin.

The vials and cartridges contain a sterile solution of Humalog for use as an injection. Humalog injection consists of zinc-insulin lispro crystals dissolved in a clear aqueous fluid.

Each milliliter of Humalog injection contains insulin lispro 100 units, 16 mg glycerin, 1.88 mg dibasic sodium phosphate, 3.15 mg *m*-cresol, zinc oxide content adjusted to provide 0.0197 mg zinc ion, trace amounts of phenol, and water for injection. Insulin lispro has a pH of 7.0-7.8. Hydrochloric acid 10% and/or sodium hydroxide 10% may be added to adjust pH.

CLINICAL PHARMACOLOGY

ANTIDIABETIC ACTIVITY

The primary activity of insulin, including insulin lispro, is the regulation of glucose metabolism. In addition, all insulins have several anabolic and anti-catabolic actions on many tissues in the body. In muscle and other tissues (except the brain), insulin causes rapid transport of glucose and amino acids intracellularly, promotes anabolism, and inhibits protein catabolism. In the liver, insulin promotes the uptake and storage of glucose in the form of glycogen, inhibits gluconeogenesis, and promotes the conversion of excess glucose into fat.

Insulin lispro has been shown to be equipotent to human insulin on a molar basis. One (1) unit of insulin lispro has the same glucose-lowering effect as 1 unit of human regular insulin, but its effect is more rapid and of shorter duration. The glucose-lowering activity of insulin lispro and human regular insulin is comparable when administered to normal volunteers by the intravenous (IV) route.

PHARMACOKINETICS

Absorption and Bioavailability

Insulin lispro is as bioavailable as human regular insulin, with absolute bioavailability ranging between 55% and 77% with doses between 0.1 and 0.2 U/kg, inclusive. Studies in normal volunteers and patients with Type 1 (insulin-dependent) diabetes demonstrated that insulin lispro is absorbed faster than human regular insulin (U100). In normal volunteers given subcutaneous doses of insulin lispro ranging from 0.1-0.4 U/kg, peak serum levels were seen 30- 90 minutes after dosing. When normal volunteers received equivalent doses of human regular insulin, peak insulin doses occurred between 50 and 120 minutes after dosing. Similar results were seen in patients with Type 1 diabetes. The pharmacokinetic profiles of insulin lispro and human regular insulin are comparable to one another when administered to normal volunteers by the IV route. Insulin lispro was absorbed at a consistently faster rate than human regular insulin in healthy male volunteers given 0.2 U/kg human regular insulin or insulin lispro at abdominal, deltoid, or femoral sites, the three sites often used by patients with diabetes. After abdominal administration of insulin lispro, serum drug levels are higher and the duration of action is slightly shorter than after deltoid or thigh administration (see DOSAGE AND ADMINISTRATION). Insulin lispro has less intra- and inter-patient variability compared to human regular insulin.

Distribution

The volume of distribution for insulin lispro is identical to that of human regular insulin, with a range of 0.26-0.36 L/kg.

Metabolism

Human metabolism studies have not been conducted. However, animal studies indicate that the metabolism of insulin lispro is identical to that of human regular insulin.

Elimination

When insulin lispro is given subcutaneously, its T½ is shorter than that of human regular insulin (1 vs 1.5 hours, respectively). When given intravenously, humalog and human regular insulin show identical dose-dependent elimination, with a T½ of 26 and 52 minutes at 0.1 and 0.2 U/kg, respectively.

PHARMACODYNAMICS

Studies in normal volunteers and patients with diabetes demonstrated that insulin lispro has a more rapid onset of glucose lowering activity, an earlier peak for glucose-lowering, and a shorter duration of glucose-lowering activity than human regular insulin. The earlier onset of activity of insulin lispro is directly related to its more rapid rate of absorption. The time course of action of insulin and insulin analogs such as insulin lispro may vary considerably in different individuals or within the same individual. The rate of insulin absorption and consequently the onset of activity is known to be affected by the site of injection, exercise, and other variables (see Absorption and Bioavailability).

In open-label, crossover studies of 1008 patients with Type 1 diabetes and 722 patients with Type 2 (non-insulin-dependent) diabetes, insulin lispro reduced postprandial glucose compared with human regular insulin (see TABLE 1). The clinical significance of improvement in postprandial hyperglycemia has not been established.

TABLE 1 *Comparison of Means of Glycemic Parameters at the End of Combined Treatment Periods. All Randomized Patients in Cross-Over Studies (3 months for each treatment)*

Type 1, n=1008*†	Insulin Lispro‡	Regular Insulin Human Injection§	*p*-value
Premeal blood glucose	11.64 ± 5.09	11.34 ± 4.96	.274
1 hour postprandial	12.91 ± 5.43	13.89 ± 5.37	<.001
2 hour postprandial	11.16 ± 5.30	12.87 ± 5.77	<.001
HbA1c (%)	8.24 ± 1.49	8.17 ± 1.46	.089
Type 2*†, n=722	**Insulin Lispro‡**	**Regular Insulin Human Injection§**	***p*-value**
Premeal blood glucose	10.67 ± 3.77	10.17 ± 3.67	.002
1 hour postprandial	13.23 ± 4.43	13.89 ± 4.18	<.001
2 hour postprandial	12.08 ± 4.62	13.14 ± 4.48	<.001
HbA1c (%)	8.18 ± 1.30	8.18 ± 1.38	.924

* mg/dl=mmol/L × 18.0.
† Glycemic parameter, (mmol/l).
‡ Mean ±standard deviation.
§ Humulin (regular insulin human injection, [recombinant DNA origin]).

In 12 month parallel studies of Type 1 and Type 2 patients, hemoglobin A_{1c} did not differ between patients treated with human regular insulin and those treated with insulin lispro.

While the overall rate of hypoglycemia did not differ between patients with Type 1 and Type 2 diabetes treated with insulin lispro compared with human regular insulin, patients with Type 1 diabetes treated with insulin lispro had fewer hypoglycemic episodes between midnight and 6 AM. The lower rate of hypoglycemia in the humalog-treated group may have been related to higher nocturnal blood glucose levels, as reflected by a small increase in mean fasting blood glucose levels.

SPECIAL POPULATIONS

Age and Gender: Information on the effect of age and gender on the pharmacokinetics of insulin lispro is unavailable. However, in large clinical trials, subgroup analysis based on age and gender did not indicate any difference in postprandial glucose parameters between insulin lispro and human regular insulin.

Smoking: The effect of smoking on the pharmacokinetics and glucodynamics of insulin lispro has not been studied.

Pregnancy: The effect of pregnancy on the pharmacokinetics and glucodynamics of insulin lispro has not been studied.

Obesity: The effect of obesity and/or subcutaneous fat thickness on the pharmacokinetics and glucodynamics of insulin lispro has not been studied. In large clinical trials, which included patients with Body-Mass-Index up to and including 35 kg/m^2, no consistent differences were seen between insulin lispro and regular insulin human injection with respect to postprandial glucose parameters.

Renal Impairment: Some studies with human insulin have shown increased circulating levels of insulin in patients with renal failure. Information on the effect of renal impairment on the pharmacokinetics of insulin lispro is limited. Careful glucose monitoring and dose adjustments of insulin, including insulin lispro, may be necessary in patients with renal dysfunction.

Hepatic Impairment: Some studies with human insulin have shown increased circulating levels of insulin in patients with hepatic failure. Careful glucose monitoring and dose adjustments of insulin, including insulin lispro, may be necessary in patients with hepatic dysfunction.

INDICATIONS AND USAGE

Insulin lispro is an insulin analog that is indicated in the treatment of patients with diabetes mellitus for the control of hyperglycemia. Insulin lispro has a more rapid onset and a shorter duration of action than human regular insulin. Therefore, insulin lispro should be used in regimens including a longer-acting insulin.

CONTRAINDICATIONS

Insulin lispro is contraindicated during episodes of hypoglycemia and in patients sensitive to insulin lispro or one of its excipients.

WARNINGS

This human insulin analog differs from human regular insulin by its rapid onset of action as well as a shorter duration of activity. When used as a mealtime insulin, the dose of insulin lispro should be given within 15 minutes before the meal. Because of the short duration of action of insulin lispro, patients with Type 1 diabetes also require a longer-acting insulin to maintain glucose control.

Hypoglycemia is the most common adverse effect associated with insulins, including insulin lispro. As with all insulins, the timing of hypoglycemia may differ among various insulin formulations. Glucose monitoring is recommended for all patients with diabetes[1].

Any change of insulin should be made cautiously and only under medical supervision. Changes in insulin strength, manufacturer, type (*e.g.*, regular, NPH, analog), species (animal, human), or method of manufacture (rDNA versus animal-source insulin) may result in the need for a change in dosage.

PRECAUTIONS

GENERAL

Hypoglycemia and hypokalemia are among the potential clinical adverse effects associated with the use of all insulins. Because of differences in the action of insulin lispro and other insulins, care should be taken in patients in whom such potential side effects might be clinically relevant (*e.g.*, patients who are fasting, have autonomic neuropathy, or are using potassium-lowering drugs). Lipodystrophy and hypersensitivity are among other potential clinical adverse effects associated with the use of all insulins.

As with all insulin preparations, the time course of insulin lispro action may vary in different individuals or at different times in the same individual and is dependent on site of injection, blood supply, temperature, and physical activity.

Adjustment of dosage of any insulin may be necessary if patients change their physical activity or their usual meal plan. Insulin requirements may be altered during illness, emotional disturbances, or other stress.

HYPOGLYCEMIA

As with all insulin preparations, hypoglycemic reactions may be associated with the administration of insulin lispro. Rapid changes in serum glucose levels may induce symptoms of hypoglycemia in persons with diabetes, regardless of the glucose value. Early warning symptoms of hypoglycemia may be different or less pronounced under certain conditions, such as long duration of diabetes, diabetic nerve disease, use of medications such as beta-blockers, or intensified diabetes control.

RENAL IMPAIRMENT

Although there are no specific data in patients with diabetes, insulin lispro requirements may be reduced in the presence of renal impairment, similar to observations found with other insulins.

HEPATIC IMPAIRMENT

Although studies have not been performed in diabetes patients with hepatic disease, insulin lispro requirements may be reduced in the presence of impaired hepatic function, similar to observations found with other insulins.

ALLERGY

Local Allergy: As with any insulin therapy, patients may experience redness, swelling, or itching at the site of injection. These minor reactions usually resolve in a few days to a few weeks. In some instances, these reactions may be related to factors other than insulin, such as irritants in a skin cleansing agent or poor injection technique.

Systemic Allergy: Less common, but potentially more serious, is generalized allergy to insulin, which may cause rash (including pruritus) over the whole body, shortness of breath, wheezing, reduction in blood pressure, rapid pulse, or sweating. Severe cases of generalized allergy, including anaphylactic reaction, may be life-threatening. In controlled clinical trials, pruritus (with or without rash) was seen in 17 patients receiving regular insulin human injection (n=2969) and 30 patients receiving insulin lispro (n=2944) (p=.053). Localized reactions and generalized myalgias have been reported with the use of cresol as an injectable excipient.

Antibody Production: In large clinical trials, antibodies that cross react with human insulin and insulin lispro were observed in both regular insulin human injection- and insulin lispro-treatment groups. As expected, the largest increase in the antibody levels during the 12 month clinical trials was observed with patients new to insulin therapy.

INFORMATION FOR THE PATIENT

Patients should be informed of the potential risks and advantages of insulin lispro and alternative therapies. Patients should also be informed about the importance of proper insulin storage, injection technique, timing of dosage, adherence to meal planning, regular physical activity, regular blood glucose monitoring, periodic glycosylated hemoglobin testing, recognition and management of hypo- and hyperglycemia, and periodic assessment for diabetes complications.

Patients should be advised to inform their physician if they are pregnant or intend to become pregnant.

Refer patients to the Information for the Patient circular distributed with the prescription for information on proper injection technique, timing of insulin lispro dosing (≤15 minutes before a meal), storing and mixing insulin, and common adverse effects.

LABORATORY TESTS

As with all insulins, the therapeutic response to insulin lispro should be monitored by periodic blood glucose tests. Periodic measurement of glycosylated hemoglobin is recommended for the monitoring of long-term glycemic control.

MIXING OF INSULINS

Care should be taken when mixing all insulins as a change in peak action may occur. The American Diabetes Association warns in its Position Statement on Insulin Administration, "On mixing, physiochemical changes in the mixture may occur (either immediately or over time). As a result, the physiological response to the insulin mixture may differ from that of the injection of the insulins separately[1]." A decrease in the absorption rate, but not total bioavailability, was seen when insulin lispro was mixed with insulin human isophene. This decrease in absorption rate was not seen when insulin lispro was mixed with insulin ultralente. When insulin lispro is mixed with either insulin ultralente or insulin human isophene, the mixture should be given within 15 minutes before a meal.

The effects of mixing insulin lispro with insulins of animal source or insulin preparations produced by other manufacturers have not been studied (see WARNINGS).

If insulin lispro is mixed with a longer-acting insulin, insulin lispro should be drawn into the syringe first to prevent clouding of the insulin lispro by the longer-acting insulin. Injection should be made immediately after mixing. Mixtures should not be administered intravenously.

CARCINOGENESIS, MUTAGENESIS, AND IMPAIRMENT OF FERTILITY

Long-term studies in animals have not been performed to evaluate the carcinogenic potential of insulin lispro. Insulin lispro was not mutagenic in a battery of *in vitro* and *in vivo* genetic toxicity assays (bacterial mutation tests, unscheduled DNA synthesis, mouse lymphoma assay, chromosomal aberration tests, and a micronucleus test). There is no evidence from animal studies of insulin lispro-induced impairment of fertility.

PREGNANCY, TERATOGENIC EFFECTS, PREGNANCY CATEGORY B

Reproduction studies have been performed in pregnant rats and rabbits at parenteral doses up to 4 and 0.3 times, respectively, the average human dose (40 U/day) based on body surface area. The results have revealed no evidence of impaired fertility or harm to the fetus due to insulin lispro. There are, however, no adequate and well-controlled studies in pregnant women. Because animal reproduction studies are not always predictive of human response, this drug should be used during pregnancy only if clearly needed.

Although there are no clinical studies of the use of insulin lispro in pregnancy, published studies with human insulins suggest that optimizing overall glycemic control, including postprandial control, before conception and during pregnancy improves fetal outcome. Although the fetal complications of maternal hyperglycemia have been well documented, fetal toxicity also has been reported with maternal hypoglycemia. Insulin requirements usually fall during the first trimester and increase during the second and third trimesters. Careful monitoring of the patient is required throughout pregnancy. During the perinatal period, careful monitoring of infants born to mothers with diabetes is warranted.

NURSING MOTHERS

It is unknown whether insulin lispro is excreted in significant amounts in human milk. Many drugs, including human insulin, are excreted in human milk. For this reason, caution should be exercised when insulin lispro is administered to a nursing woman. Patients with diabetes who are lactating may require adjustments in insulin lispro dose, meal plan, or both.

PEDIATRIC USE

Safety and effectiveness in patients less than 12 years of age have not been established.

DRUG INTERACTIONS

See CLINICAL PHARMACOLOGY. Insulin requirements may be increased by medications with hyperglycemic activity such as corticosteroids, isoniazid, certain lipid-lowering drugs (*e.g.*, niacin), estrogens, oral contraceptives, phenothiazines, and thyroid replacement therapy.

Insulin requirements may be decreased in the presence of drugs with hypoglycemic activity, such as oral hypoglycemic agents, salicylates, sulfa antibiotics, and certain antidepressants (monoamine oxidase inhibitors), certain angiotensin-converting-enzyme inhibitors, beta-adrenergic blockers, inhibitors of pancreatic function (*e.g.*, octreotide), and alcohol. Beta-adrenergic blockers may mask the symptoms of hypoglycemia in some patients.

ADVERSE REACTIONS

Clinical studies comparing insulin lispro with human regular insulin did not demonstrate a difference in frequency of adverse events between the two treatments.

Adverse events commonly associated with human insulin therapy include the following:

Body as a Whole: Allergic reactions (see PRECAUTIONS).

Skin and Appendages: Injection site reaction, lipodystrophy, pruritus, rash.

Other: Hypoglycemia (see WARNINGS and PRECAUTIONS).

DOSAGE AND ADMINISTRATION

Insulin lispro is intended for subcutaneous administration. Dosage regimens of insulin lispro will vary among patients and should be determined by the health care professional familiar with the patient's metabolic needs, eating habits, and other lifestyle variables. Pharmacokinetic and pharmacodynamic studies showed insulin lispro to be equipotent to human regular insulin (*i.e.*, one unit of insulin lispro has the same glucose-lowering capability as one unit of human regular insulin), but with more rapid activity. The quicker glucose-lowering effect of insulin lispro is related to the more rapid absorption rate from subcutaneous tissue. An adjustment of dose or schedule of basal insulin may be needed when a patient changes from other insulins to insulin lispro, particularly to prevent pre-meal hyperglycemia.

When used as a meal-time insulin, insulin lispro should be given within 15 minutes before a meal. Human regular insulin is best given 30-60 minutes before a meal. To achieve optimal glucose control, the amount of longer acting insulin being given may need to be adjusted when using insulin lispro.

The rate of insulin absorption and consequently the onset of activity is known to be affected by the site of injection, exercise, and other variables. Insulin lispro was absorbed at a consistently faster rate than human regular insulin in healthy male volunteers given 0.2 U/kg human regular insulin or insulin lispro at abdominal, deltoid, or femoral sites, the three sites often used by patients with diabetes. When not mixed in the same syringe with other insulins, insulin lispro maintains its rapid onset of action and has less variability in its onset of action among injection sites compared with human regular insulin (see PRECAUTIONS). After abdominal administration, insulin lispro concentrations are higher than those following deltoid or thigh injections. Also, the duration of action of insulin lispro is slightly shorter following abdominal injection, compared with deltoid and femoral injections. As with all insulin preparations, the time course of action of insulin lispro may vary considerably in different individuals or within the same individual. Patients must be educated to use proper injection techniques.

Parenteral drug products should be inspected visually prior to administration whenever the solution and the container permit. If the solution is cloudy, contains particulate matter, is thickened, or is discolored, the contents must not be injected. Insulin lispro should not be used after its expiration date.

HOW SUPPLIED

Storage: Humalog should be stored in a refrigerator (2-8°C [36-46°F]), but not in the freezer. If refrigeration is impossible, the vial or cartridge of Humalog in use can be unrefrigerated for up to 28 days, as long as it is kept as cool as possible (not greater than 30°C [86°F]) and away from direct heat and light. Unrefrigerated vials and cartridges must be used within this time period or be discarded. Do not use Humalog if it has been frozen.

PRODUCT LISTING - EQUIVALENTS NOT AVAILABLE

Injection - Subcutaneous - 100 U/ml

1.50 ml x 5	$61.80	HUMALOG, Lilly, Eli and Company	00002-7515-59
3 ml x 5	$118.70	HUMALOG PEN, Lilly, Eli and Company	00002-8725-59
3 ml x 5	$123.65	HUMALOG, Lilly, Eli and Company	00002-7516-59
10 ml	$61.43	HUMALOG, Lilly, Eli and Company	00002-7510-01

Insulin Lispro; Insulin Lispro Protamine (003489)

Categories: Diabetes mellitus; FDA Approved 2000 Apr; Pregnancy Category B
Drug Classes: Antidiabetic agents; Insulins
Foreign Brand Availability: Humalog Mix (France; Germany; Israel); Humalog Mix 25 (New-Zealand)

DESCRIPTION

Humalog Mix 50/50 [50% insulin lispro protamine suspension and 50% insulin lispro injection, (rDNA origin)] and Humalog Mix 75/25 [75% insulin lispro protamine suspension and 25% insulin lispro injection, (rDNA origin)] are mixtures of insulin lispro solution, a rapid-acting blood glucose-lowering agent and insulin lispro protamine suspension, an intermediate-acting blood glucose-lowering agent. Chemically, insulin lispro is Lys(B28), Pro(B29) human insulin analog, created when the amino acids at positions 28 and 29 on the insulin B-chain are reversed. Insulin lispro is synthesized in a special non-pathogenic laboratory strain of *Escherichia coli* bacteria that has been genetically altered by the addition of the gene for insulin lispro. Insulin lispro protamine suspension (NPL component) is a suspension of crystals produced from combining insulin lispro and protamine sulfate under appropriate conditions for crystal formation.

Insulin lispro has the empirical formula $C_{257}H_{383}N_{65}O_{77}S_6$ and a molecular weight of 5808, both identical to that of human insulin.

Humalog Mix 50/50 and Humalog Mix 75/25 vials, cartridges, and disposable insulin delivery devices contain a sterile suspension of insulin lispro protamine suspension mixed with soluble insulin lispro for use as an injection.

50/50 Mix: Each milliliter of Humalog Mix 50/50 injection contains insulin lispro 100 Units, 0.19 mg protamine sulfate, 16 mg glycerin, 3.78 mg dibasic sodium phosphate, 2.20 mg *m*-cresol, zinc oxide content adjusted to provide 0.0305 mg zinc ion, 0.89 mg phenol, and water for injection. Humalog Mix 50/50 has a pH of 7.0-7.8. Hydrochloric acid 10% and/or sodium hydroxide 10% may have been added to adjust pH.

75/25 Mix: Each milliliter of Humalog Mix 75/25 injection contains insulin lispro 100 Units, 0.28 mg protamine sulfate, 16 mg glycerin, 3.78 mg dibasic sodium phosphate, 1.76 mg *m*-cresol, zinc oxide content adjusted to provide 0.025 mg zinc ion, 0.715 mg phenol, and water for injection. Humalog Mix 75/25 has a pH of 7.0-7.8. Hydrochloric acid 10% and/or sodium hydroxide 10% may have been added to adjust pH.

CLINICAL PHARMACOLOGY

ANTIDIABETIC ACTIVITY

The primary activity of insulin, including insulin lispro injection and insulin lispro protamine suspension, is the regulation of glucose metabolism. In addition, all insulins have several anabolic and anticatabolic actions on many tissues in the body. In muscle and other tissues (except the brain), insulin causes rapid transport of glucose and amino acids intracellularly, promotes anabolism, and inhibits protein catabolism. In the liver, insulin promotes the uptake and storage of glucose in the form of glycogen, inhibits gluconeogenesis, and promotes the conversion of excess glucose into fat.

Insulin lispro, the rapid-acting component of insulin lispro injection and insulin lispro protamine suspension, has been shown to be equipotent to regular human insulin on a molar basis. One unit of Humalog has the same glucose-lowering effect as one unit of regular human insulin, but its effect is more rapid and of shorter duration.

75/25 Mix: Humalog Mix 75/25 has a similar glucose-lowering effect as compared to Humulin 70/30 on a unit for unit basis.

PHARMACOKINETICS

Absorption

Studies in nondiabetic subjects and patients with type 1 (insulin-dependent) diabetes demonstrated that Humalog, the rapid-acting component of insulin lispro injection and insulin lispro protamine suspension, is absorbed faster than regular human insulin (U100). In nondiabetic subjects given subcutaneous doses of Humalog ranging from 0.1-0.4 U/kg, peak serum concentrations were observed 30-90 minutes after dosing. When nondiabetic subjects received equivalent doses of regular human insulin, peak insulin concentrations occurred 50-120 minutes after dosing. Similar results were found in patients with type 1 diabetes.

Humalog Mix 50/50 has 2 phases of absorption. The early phase represents insulin lispro and its distinct characteristics of rapid onset. The late phase represents the prolonged action of insulin lispro protamine suspension.The rapid absorption characteristics of Humalog are maintained with insulin lispro injection and insulin lispro protamine suspension.

50/50 Mix

In 30 nondiabetic subjects given subcutaneous doses (0.3U/kg) of insulin lispro injection and insulin lispro protamine suspension, peak serum concentrations were observed 45 minutes to 13.5 hours (median, 60 minutes) after dosing. In patients with type 1 diabetes, peak serum concentrations were observed 45 minutes to 120 minutes (median, 60 minutes) after dosing. Direct comparison of insulin lispro injection and insulin lispro protamine suspension and Humulin 50/50 was not performed. However, a cross-study comparison suggests that insulin lispro injection and insulin lispro protamine suspension has a more rapid absorption than Humulin 50/50.

75/25 Mix

In 30 nondiabetic subjects given subcutaneous doses (0.3 U/kg) of Humalog Mix 75/25, peak serum concentrations were observed 30-240 minutes (median, 60 minutes) after dosing. Identical results were found in patients with type 1 diabetes. Humalog Mix 75/25 has a more rapid absorption than Humulin 70/30, which has been confirmed in patients with type 1 diabetes.

Distribution

Radiolabeled distribution studies of insulin lispro injection and insulin lispro protamine suspension have not been conducted. However, the volume of distribution following injection of Humalog is identical to that of regular human insulin, with a range of 0.26-0.36 L/kg.

Metabolism

Human metabolism studies of insulin lispro injection and insulin lispro protamine suspension have not been conducted. Studies in animals indicate that the metabolism of Humalog, the rapid-acting component of insulin lispro injection and insulin lispro protamine suspension, is identical to that of regular human insulin.

Elimination

Insulin lispro injection and insulin lispro protamine suspension has two absorption phases, a rapid and a prolonged phase, representative of the insulin lispro and insulin lispro protamine suspension components of the mixture. As with other intermediate-acting insulins, a meaningful terminal phase half-life cannot be calculated after administration of insulin lispro injection and insulin lispro protamine suspension because of the prolonged insulin lispro protamine suspension absorption.

PHARMACODYNAMICS

Studies in nondiabetic subjects and patients with diabetes demonstrated that Humalog has a more rapid onset of glucose-lowering activity, an earlier peak for glucose lowering, and a shorter duration of glucose-lowering activity than regular human insulin. The early onset of activity of insulin lispro injection and insulin lispro protamine suspension is directly related to the rapid absorption of Humalog. The time course of action of insulin and insulin analogs such as Humalog (and hence insulin lispro injection and insulin lispro protamine suspension) may vary considerably in different individuals or within the same individual. The parameters of insulin lispro injection and insulin lispro protamine suspension activity (time of onset, peak time, and duration) should be considered only as general guidelines. The rate of insulin absorption and consequently the onset of activity is known to be affected by the site of injection, exercise, and other variables (see PRECAUTIONS, General).

In a glucose clamp study performed in 30 nondiabetic subjects, the onset of action and glucose-lowering activity of Humalog, Humalog Mix 50/50, Humalog Mix 75/25 and insulin lispro protamine suspension were compared. Graphs of mean glucose infusion rate versus time showed a distinct insulin activity profile for each formulation. The rapid onset of glucose-lowering activity characteristic of Humalog was maintained in insulin lispro injection and insulin lispro protamine suspension.

50/50 Mix: Direct comparison between Humalog Mix 50/50 and Humulin 50/50 was not performed. However, a cross-study comparison suggests that Humalog Mix 50/50 has a duration of activity that is similar to Humulin 50/50.

75/25 Mix: In separate glucose clamp studies performed in nondiabetic subjects, glucodynamics of Humalog Mix 75/25 and Humulin 70/30 were assessed. Humalog Mix 75/25 has a duration of activity similar to that of Humulin 70/30.

SPECIAL POPULATIONS

Age and Gender

Information on the effect of age on the pharmacokinetics of insulin lispro injection and insulin lispro protamine suspension is unavailable. Pharmacokinetic and pharmacodynamic comparisons between men and women administered insulin lispro injection and insulin lispro protamine suspension showed no gender differences. In large Humalog clinical trials, subgroup analyses based upon age and gender demonstrated that differences between Humalog and regular human insulin in postprandial glucose parameters are maintained across subgroups.

Smoking

The effect of smoking on the pharmacokinetics and glucodynamics of insulin lispro injection and insulin lispro protamine suspension has not been studied.

Pregnancy

The effect of pregnancy on the pharmacokinetics and glucodynamics of insulin lispro injection and insulin lispro protamine suspension has not been studied.

Obesity

The effect of obesity and/or subcutaneous fat thickness on the pharmacokinetics and glucodynamics of insulin lispro injection and insulin lispro protamine suspension has not been studied. In large clinical trials, which included patients with Body-Mass-Index up to and including 35 kg/m^2, no consistent differences were observed between Humalog and Humulin R with respect to postprandial glucose parameters.

Renal Impairment

The effect of renal impairment on the pharmacokinetics and glucodynamics of insulin lispro injection and insulin lispro protamine suspension has not been studied. In a study of 25 patients with type 2 diabetes and a wide range of renal function, the pharmacokinetic differences between Humalog and human regular insulin were generally maintained. However, the sensitivity of the patients to insulin did change, with an increased response to insulin as the renal function declined. Careful glucose monitoring and dose reductions of insulin, including insulin lispro injection and insulin lispro protamine suspension, may be necessary in patients with renal dysfunction.

Hepatic Impairment

Some studies with human insulin have shown increased circulating levels of insulin in patients with hepatic failure. The effect of hepatic impairment on the pharmacokinetics and glucodynamics of insulin lispro injection and insulin lispro protamine suspension has not been studied. However, in a study of 22 patients with type 2 diabetes, impaired hepatic function did not affect the subcutaneous absorption or general disposition of Humalog when compared to patients with no history of hepatic dysfunction. In that study, Humalog maintained its more rapid absorption and elimination when compared to regular human insulin. Careful glucose monitoring and dose adjustments of insulin, including insulin lispro injection and insulin lispro protamine suspension, may be necessary in patients with hepatic dysfunction.

INDICATIONS AND USAGE

Insulin lispro injection and insulin lispro protamine suspension, a mixture of 50% insulin lispro protamine suspension and 50% insulin lispro, is indicated in the treatment of patients with diabetes mellitus for the control of hyperglycemia.

50/50 MIX

Based on cross-study comparisons of the pharmacodynamics of Humalog Mix 50/50 and Humulin 50/50, it is likely that Humalog Mix 50/50 has a more rapid onset of glucose-lowering activity compared to Humulin 50/50 while having a similar duration of action. This profile is achieved by combining the rapid onset of Humalog with the intermediate action of insulin lispro protamine suspension.

75/25 MIX

Humalog Mix 75/25 has a more rapid onset of glucose-lowering activity compared to Humulin 70/30 while having a similar duration of action. This profile is achieved by combining the rapid onset of Humalog with the intermediate action of insulin lispro protamine suspension.

CONTRAINDICATIONS

Insulin lispro injection and insulin lispro protamine suspension is contraindicated during episodes of hypoglycemia and in patients sensitive to insulin lispro or any of the excipients contained in the formulation.

WARNINGS

Humalog differs from regular human insulin by its rapid onset of action as well as a shorter duration of activity. Therefore, the dose of insulin lispro injection and insulin lispro protamine suspension should be given within 15 minutes before a meal.

Hypoglycemia is the most common adverse effect associated with the use of insulins, including insulin lispro injection and insulin lispro protamine suspension. As with all insulins, the timing of hypoglycemia may differ among various insulin formulations. Glucose monitoring is recommended for all patients with diabetes.

Any change of insulin should be made cautiously and only under medical supervision. Changes in insulin strength, manufacturer, type (*e.g.,* regular, NPH, analog), species (animal, human), or method of manufacture (rDNA versus animal-source insulin) may result in the need for a change in dosage.

PRECAUTIONS

GENERAL

Hypoglycemia and hypokalemia are among the potential clinical adverse effects associated with the use of all insulins. Because of differences in the action of insulin lispro injection and insulin lispro protamine suspension and other insulins, care should be taken in patients in whom such potential side effects might be clinically relevant (*e.g.,* patients who are fasting, have autonomic neuropathy, or are using potassium-lowering drugs or patients taking drugs sensitive to serum potassium level). Lipodystrophy and hypersensitivity are among other potential clinical adverse effects associated with the use of all insulins.

As with all insulin preparations, the time course of action of insulin lispro injection and insulin lispro protamine suspension may vary in different individuals or at different times in the same individual and is dependent on site of injection, blood supply, temperature, and physical activity.

Adjustment of dosage of any insulin may be necessary if patients change their physical activity or their usual meal plan. Insulin requirements may be altered during illness, emotional disturbances, or other stress.

Hypoglycemia

As with all insulin preparations, hypoglycemic reactions may be associated with the administration of insulin lispro injection and insulin lispro protamine suspension. Rapid changes in serum glucose concentrations may induce symptoms of hypoglycemia in persons with diabetes, regardless of the glucose value. Early warning symptoms of hypoglycemia may be different or less pronounced under certain conditions, such as long duration of diabetes, diabetic nerve disease, use of medications such as beta-blockers, or intensified diabetes control.

Renal Impairment

As with other insulins, the requirements for insulin lispro injection and insulin lispro protamine suspension may be reduced in patients with renal impairment.

Hepatic Impairment

Although impaired hepatic function does not affect the absorption or disposition of Humalog, careful glucose monitoring and dose adjustments of insulin, including insulin lispro injection and insulin lispro protamine suspension, may be necessary.

Allergy

Local Allergy: As with any insulin therapy, patients may experience redness, swelling, or itching at the site of injection. These minor reactions usually resolve in a few days to a few weeks. In some instances, these reactions may be related to factors other than insulin, such as irritants in a skin cleansing agent or poor injection technique.

Systemic Allergy: Less common, but potentially more serious, is generalized allergy to insulin, which may cause rash (including pruritus) over the whole body, shortness of breath, wheezing, reduction in blood pressure, rapid pulse, or sweating. Severe cases of generalized allergy, including anaphylactic reaction, may be life threatening. Localized reactions and generalized myalgias have been reported with the use of cresol as an injectable excipient.

Antibody Production: In clinical trials, antibodies that cross-react with human insulin and insulin lispro were observed in both human insulin mixtures and insulin lispro mixtures treatment groups.

INFORMATION FOR THE PATIENT

Patients should be informed of the potential risks and advantages of insulin lispro injection and insulin lispro protamine suspension and alternative therapies. Patients should not mix insulin lispro injection and insulin lispro protamine suspension with any other insulin. They should also be informed about the importance of proper insulin storage, injection technique, timing of dosage, adherence to meal planning, regular physical activity, regular blood glucose monitoring, periodic glycosylated hemoglobin testing, recognition and management of hypo- and hyperglycemia, and periodic assessment for diabetes complications.

Patients should be advised to inform their physician if they are pregnant or intend to become pregnant.

Refer patients to the Information for the Patient insert for information on normal appearance, proper resuspension and injection techniques, timing of dosing (within 15 minutes before a meal), storing, and common adverse effects.

LABORATORY TESTS

As with all insulins, the therapeutic response to insulin lispro injection and insulin lispro protamine suspension should be monitored by periodic blood glucose tests. Periodic measurement of glycosylated hemoglobin is recommended for the monitoring of long-term glycemic control.

CARCINOGENESIS, MUTAGENESIS, AND IMPAIRMENT OF FERTILITY

Long-term studies in animals have not been performed to evaluate the carcinogenic potential of Humalog or insulin lispro injection and insulin lispro protamine suspension. Insulin lispro was not mutagenic in a battery of *in vitro* and *in vivo* genetic toxicity assays (bacterial mutation tests, unscheduled DNA synthesis, mouse lymphoma assay, chromosomal aberration tests, and a micronucleus test). There is no evidence from animal studies of impairment of fertility induced by insulin lispro.

PREGNANCY, TERATOGENIC EFFECTS, PREGNANCY CATEGORY B

Reproduction studies with insulin lispro have been performed in pregnant rats and rabbits at parenteral doses up to 4 and 0.3 times, respectively, the average human dose (40 units/day) based on body surface area. The results have revealed no evidence of impaired fertility or harm to the fetus due to insulin lispro. There are, however, no adequate and well-controlled studies with Humalog or insulin lispro injection and insulin lispro protamine suspension in pregnant women. Because animal reproduction studies are not always predictive of human response, this drug should be used during pregnancy only if clearly needed.

NURSING MOTHERS

It is unknown whether insulin lispro is excreted in significant amounts in human milk. Many drugs, including human insulin, are excreted in human milk. For this reason, caution should be exercised when insulin lispro injection and insulin lispro protamine suspension is administered to a nursing woman. Patients with diabetes who are lactating may require adjustments in insulin lispro injection and insulin lispro protamine suspension dose, meal plan, or both.

PEDIATRIC USE

Safety and effectiveness of insulin lispro injection and insulin lispro protamine suspension in patients less than 18 years of age have not been established.

GERIATRIC USE

Clinical studies of insulin lispro injection and insulin lispro protamine suspension did not include sufficient numbers of patients aged 65 and over to determine whether they respond differently than younger patients. In general, dose selection for an elderly patient should take into consideration the greater frequency of decreased hepatic, renal, or cardiac function, and of concomitant disease or other drug therapy in this population.

DRUG INTERACTIONS

Insulin requirements may be increased by medications with hyperglycemic activity such as corticosteroids, isoniazid, certain lipid-lowering drugs (*e.g.,* niacin), estrogens, oral contraceptives, phenothiazines, and thyroid replacement therapy.

Insulin requirements may be decreased in the presence of drugs with hypoglycemic activity, such as oral antidiabetic agents, salicylates, sulfa antibiotics, certain antidepressants (monoamine oxidase inhibitors), certain angiotensin-converting-enzyme inhibitors, beta-adrenergic blockers, inhibitors of pancreatic function (*e.g.,* octreotide), and alcohol. Beta-adrenergic blockers may mask the symptoms of hypoglycemia in some patients.

ADVERSE REACTIONS

Clinical studies comparing insulin lispro injection and insulin lispro protamine suspension with human insulin mixtures did not demonstrate a difference in frequency of adverse events between the 2 treatments.

Adverse events commonly associated with human insulin therapy include the following:

Body as a Whole: Allergic reactions (see PRECAUTIONS).

Skin and Appendages: Injection site reaction, lipodystrophy, pruritus, rash.

Other: Hypoglycemia (see WARNINGS and PRECAUTIONS).

DOSAGE AND ADMINISTRATION

Insulin lispro injection and insulin lispro protamine suspension is intended only for subcutaneous administration. Insulin lispro injection and insulin lispro protamine suspension

TABLE 1* *Summary of Glucodynamic Properties of Insulin Products (Pooled Cross-Study Comparison)*

Insulin Products	Dose, U/kg	Time of Peak Activity, Hours After Dosing	Percent of Total Activity Occurring in the First 4 Hours
Humalog	0.3	2.4 (0.8-4.3)	70% (49-89%)
Humulin R	0.32 (0.26-0.37)	4.4 (4.0-5.5)	54% (38-65%)
Humalog Mix 75/25	0.3	2.6 (1.0-6.5)	35% (21-56%)
Humulin 70/30	0.3	4.4 (1.5-1.6)	32% (14-60%)
Humalog Mix 50/50	0.3	2.3 (0.8-4.8)	45% (27-69%)
Humulin 50/50	0.3	3.3 (2.0-5.5)	44% (21-60%)
NPH	0.32 (0.27-0.40)	5.5 (3.5-9.5)	14% (3.0-48%)
NPL component	0.3	5.8 (1.3-18.3)	22% (6.3-40%)

* The information supplied in this table indicates when peak insulin activity can be expected and the percent of the total insulin activity occurring during the first 4 hours. The information was derived from 3 separate glucose clamp studies in nondiabetic subjects. Values represent means, with ranges provided in parentheses.

should not be administered intravenously. Dosage regimens of insulin lispro injection and insulin lispro protamine suspension will vary among patients and should be determined by the health care professional familiar with the patient's metabolic needs, eating habits, and other lifestyle variables. Humalog has been shown to be equipotent to regular human insulin on a molar basis. One unit of Humalog has the same glucose-lowering effect as one unit of regular human insulin, but its effect is more rapid and of shorter duration. The quicker glucose-lowering effect of Humalog is related to the more rapid absorption rate of insulin lispro from subcutaneous tissue.

75/25 MIX

Humalog Mix 75/25 has a similar glucose-lowering effect as compared to Humulin 70/30 on a unit for unit basis.

Humalog Mix 75/25 starts lowering blood glucose more quickly than regular human insulin, allowing for convenient dosing immediately before a meal (within 15 minutes). In contrast, mixtures containing regular human insulin should be given 30-60 minutes before a meal.

The rate of insulin absorption and consequently the onset of activity are known to be affected by the site of injection, exercise, and other variables. As with all insulin preparations, the time course of action of insulin lispro injection and insulin lispro protamine suspension may vary considerably in different individuals or within the same individual. Patients must be educated to use proper injection techniques.

Insulin lispro injection and insulin lispro protamine suspension should be inspected visually before use. Insulin lispro injection and insulin lispro protamine suspension should be used only if it appears uniformly cloudy after mixing. Insulin lispro injection and insulin lispro protamine suspension should not be used after its expiration date.

50/50 MIX

Direct comparison between Humalog Mix 50/50 and Humulin 50/50 was not performed. However, a cross-study comparison suggests that Humalog Mix 50/50 has a duration of activity that is similar to Humulin 50/50.

HOW SUPPLIED

50/50 Mix: Humalog Mix 50/50 is available as vials, cartridges, and a disposable insulin delivery device.

75/25 Mix: Humalog Mix 75/25 is available as vials, cartridges, and a disposable insulin delivery device.

STORAGE

Humalog Mix should be stored in a refrigerator (2-8°C [36-46°F]) before use, but not in the freezer. However, vials of Humalog Mix in use can be kept unrefrigerated at room temperature for up to 28 days, as long as they are kept as cool as possible and away from direct heat and light. Cartridges of Humalog Mix or Humalog Mix Pens in use can be kept unrefrigerated at room temperature for up to 10 days, as long as they are kept as cool as possible and away from direct heat and light. Unrefrigerated vials, cartridges, and pens must be used within the specified time periods or be discarded.

Do not use Humalog Mix if it has been frozen.

PRODUCT LISTING - EQUIVALENTS NOT AVAILABLE

Suspension - Subcutaneous - 25 U;75 U/ml

3 ml x 5	$118.70	HUMALOG MIX 75/25 PEN, Lilly, Eli and Company	00002-8794-59
10 ml	$61.43	HUMALOG MIX 75/25, Lilly, Eli and Company	00002-7511-01

Suspension - Subcutaneous - 50 U;50 U/ml

3 ml x 5	$87.64	HUMALOG MIX 50/50 PEN, Lilly, Eli and Company	00002-8793-59

Insulin, (Human, Semi-Synthetic, Buffered) *(003429)*

Categories: Diabetes mellitus; FDA Approved 1997 April; Pregnancy Category B
Drug Classes: Antidiabetic agents; Insulins
Brand Names: Velosulin BR

PATIENT PACKAGE INSERT

INSULIN USE IN DIABETES

Your physician has explained that you have diabetes and that your treatment involves injections of insulin. Insulin is normally produced by the pancreas, a gland that lies behind the stomach. Without insulin, glucose (a simple sugar made from digested food) is trapped in the bloodstream and cannot enter the cells of the body. Some patients who don't make enough of their own insulin, or who cannot use the insulin they do make properly, must take insulin by injection in order to control their blood glucose levels.

Each case of diabetes is different and requires direct and continued medical supervision. Your physician has told you the type, strength, and amount of insulin you should use and the time(s) at which you should inject it, and has also discussed with you a diet and exercise schedule. You should contact your physician if you experience any difficulties or if you have questions.

TYPES OF INSULINS

Standard and purified animal insulins as well as human insulins are available. Standard and purified insulins differ in their degree of purification and content of noninsulin material. Standard and purified insulins also vary in species source: they may be of beef, pork, or mixed beef and pork origin. Human insulin is identical in structure to the insulin produced by the human pancreas, and thus differs from animal insulins. Insulins vary in time of action and in strength, see Product Description and Syringes for additional information. Your physician has prescribed the insulin that is right for you; be sure you have purchased the correct insulin and check it carefully before you use it.

PRODUCT DESCRIPTION

Velosulin BR is a clear solution of insulin in a phosphate buffer. This human insulin is structurally identical to the insulin produced by the pancreas in the human body. This structural identity is obtained by enzymatic conversion of purified pork insulin. When a U-100 insulin syringe is used to deliver the insulin. Velosulin BR has a rapid onset of action, approximately ½ hour after the injection. The effect lasts up to approximately 8 hours with a maximal effect between the 1st and 3rd hour.

The time course of action of any insulin may vary considerably in different individuals, or at different times in the same individual, or if using an external insulin infusion pump to deliver the insulin.

Because of this variation, the time periods listed here should be considered as general guidelines only when using U-100 insulin syringes to deliver the insulin.

FOR USE IN EXTERNAL INSULIN INFUSION PUMPS OR WITH U-100 INSULIN SYRINGES.

WARNINGS

Any change of insulin should be made cautiously and only under medical supervision. Changes in purity, strength (U-40, U-100), brand (manufacturer), type (Lente-, NPH, regular etc.) and/or species source (beef, pork, beef/pork, human) may result in the need for a change in dosage. Adjustment may be needed with the first dose or over a period of several weeks. Be aware that symptoms of hypoglycemia (low blood glucose) or hyperglycemia (high blood glucose) may indicate the need for dosage adjustment. Please see Insulin Reaction and Diabetic Ketoacidosis and Coma.

Insulin, (human, semi-synthetic, buffered) should not be mixed with Lente-type insulin products because the buffering agent in insulin, (human, semi-synthetic, buffered) may interact with the other insulin and result in a change of activity. This change could lead to an unpredictable effect on blood glucose. When used with an external insulin infusion pump insulin, (human, semi-synthetic, buffered) should not be mixed with any other insulin.

Velosulin BR has been tested only in MiniMed Model 504-S pumps, using the accompanying Model MMT-103 syringe as well as both MiniMed Model MMT-106 Polyfin and MiniMed Model 111 Sofset infusion sets. MiniMed Model 504-S and Model 506 pumps are equivalent.

Change the catheter tubing and the insulin in the reservoir every 48 hours.

PREGNANCY

It is particularly important to maintain good control of your diabetes during pregnancy and special attention must be paid to your diet, exercise, and insulin regimens. If you are pregnant or nursing a baby, consult your physician or nurse educator.

INSULIN REACTION

Insulin reaction (too little sugar in the blood, also called hypoglycemia) can occur if you take too much insulin, miss a meal or exercise or work harder than normal. The symptoms, which usually come on suddenly, are hunger, dizziness, and sweating. Personality change or confusion may also occur. Eating sugar or a sugar-sweetened product will normally correct the condition.

If symptoms persist, call a physician: an insulin reaction can lead to unconsciousness. If a reaction results in loss of consciousness, emergency medical care should be obtained immediately. If you have had repeated reactions or if an insulin reaction has led to a loss of consciousness, contact your physician. Severe hypoglycemia can result in temporary or permanent impairment of brain function and death.

In certain cases, the nature and intensity of the warning symptoms of hypoglycemia may change. A few patients have reported that after being transferred to human in-

sulin, the early warning symptoms of hypoglycemia were less pronounced than they had been with animal-source insulin.

DIABETIC KETOACIDOSIS AND COMA

Diabetic ketoacidosis may develop if your body has too little insulin. The most common causes are acute illness, infection or failure to take enough insulin by injection or catheter clogging when used with an external insulin infusion pump. If you are ill, you should check your urine for ketones. The symptoms of diabetic ketoacidosis usually come on gradually, over a period of hours or days, and include a drowsy feeling, flusched face, thirst and loss of appetite. Notify a physician immediately if the urine test is positive for ketones (acetone) or if you have any of these symptoms. More severe symptoms are fast, heavy breathing and rapid pulse: if these symptoms occur, you should have medical attention right away. Severe, sustained hyperglycemia may result in diabetic coma and death.

Insulin allergy occurs very rarely, but when it does, it may cause a serious reaction including a general skin rash over the body, shortness of breath, fast pulse, sweating and a drop in blood pressure. If any of these symptoms develop you should seek emergency medical care. In a very few diabetics, the skin where insulin has been injected may become red, swollen, and itchy. This is called a local reaction. It may occur if the injection is not properly made, if the skin is sensitive to the cleansing solution or if the patient is allergic to insulin. If you have a local reaction, notify your physician.

Patients with severe systemic allergic reactions to insulin (*i.e.,* generalized urticaria, angioedema, anaphylaxis) should be skin tested with each new preparation to be used prior to initiation of therapy with that preparation.

EXTERNAL INSULIN INFUSION PUMPS

Read and follow the instructions that accompany your insulin infusion pump. It is important to follow the instructions from the manufacturer of the pump that you use.

Use the correct reservoir and catheter for the pump that you are using. Catheter clogging with insulin crystals has been known to occur.

You should change the catheter tubing and the insulin in the reservoir every 48 hours. Failure to do so may affect the amount of insulin you receive. This can cause serious problems for you, such as too little or too much glucose in the blood.

When used with an external insulin infusion pump, insulin, (human, semi-synthetic, buffered) should not be mixed with any other insulin.

SYRINGES

Use the Correct Syringe

The volume of the dose depends on the number of units of insulin per ml. veolsulin BR is only available in the U-100 strength (100 units per ml). Make sure that you understand the markings on your syringe and use only syringe marked for U-100.

Novo Nordisk insulin vials are intended for use with standard insulin syringes. Novo Nordisk has not evaluated the use of these vials with other devices for insulin delivery or with devices intended to aid in giving injections. Consult your doctor and the manufacturer of these devices before use with this product.

Disposable Syringes

Disposable syringes and needles require no sterilization provided the package is intact. They should be used only once and discarded.

Reusable Syringes

Reusable syringes and needles must be sterile when used. The best method of sterilization is to boil the syringe, plunger and needle in water for 5 minutes. If this is not possible, as when traveling, the parts may be sterilized by immersion for at least 5 minutes in a sterilizing liquid like ethyl alcohol 70%. Do not use bathing, rubbing or medicated alcohol for sterilization. Remove all liquid from the syringe by pushing the plunger in and out several times and leave it to dry if alcohol has been used for sterilization.

IMPORTANT

Failure to comply with the above and the following antiseptic measures may lead to infections at the injection site.

1. Wipe the rubber stopper with an alcohol swab. (*Note:* Remove the tamper-resistant cap at first use. If the cap has already been removed, do not use this product, return it to your pharmarcy.)
2. Pull back the plunger until the black tip reaches the marking for the number of units you will inject.
3. Push the needle through the rubber stopper into the vial
4. Push the plunger all the way in. This inserts air into the bottle.
5. Turn the vial and syringe upside down and slowly pull the plunger back to a few units beyond the correct dose.
6. If there are air bubbles, flick the syringe firmly with your finger to raise the air bubbles to the needle, then slowly push the plunger to the correct unit marking.
7. Lift the vial off the syringe.

GIVING THE INJECTION

1. ***The following areas are suitable for subcutaneous insulin injection:*** Thighs, upper arms, buttocks, abdomen. Do not change areas without consulting your physician. The actual point of injection should be changed each time; injection sites should be about an inch apart.
2. The injection site should be clean and dry. Pinch up skin area to be injected and hold it firmly.
3. Hold the syringe like a pencil and push the needle quickly and firmly into the pinched-up area.
4. Release the skin and push plunger all the way in to inject insulin beneath the skin. Do not inject into a muscle unless your physician has advised it. You should never inject insulin into a vein.
5. Remove the needle. If slight bleeding occurs, press lightly with a dry cotton swab for a few seconds—do not rub.

MIXING TWO TYPES OF INSULIN

In Syringes Only: When using U-100 insulin syringes, different insulins should be mixed only under instruction from a physician. Hypodermic syringes may vary in the amount of space between the bottom line and the needle ("dead space"), so if you are mixing 2 types of insulin be sure to discuss any change in the model and brand of syringe you are using with your physician or pharmacist. When you are mixing 2 types of insulin, always draw the Regular (clear) insulin into the syringe first.

Insulin, (human, semi-synthetic, buffered) should not be mixed with Lente-type insulin products because the buffering agent in insulin, (human, semi-synthetic, buffered) may interact with the other insulin and result in a change of activity. This change could lead to an unpredictable effect on blood glucose. When used with an external insulin infusion pump insulin, (human, semi-synthetic, buffered) should not be mixed with any other insulin.

IMPORTANT NOTES

1. A change in the type, strength, species or purity of insulin could require a dosage adjustment. Any change in insulin should be made under medical supervision.
2. You may have learned how to test your urine or your blood for glucose. It is important to do these tests regularly and to record the results for review with your physician or nurse educator.
3. If you have an illness, especially with vomiting or fever, continue taking your insulin. If possible, stay on your regular diet. If you have trouble eating, drink fruit juices, regular soft drinks, or clear soups; if you can, eat small amounts of bland foods. Test your urine for glucose and ketones and, if possible, test your blood glucose. Note the results and contact your physician for possible insulin dose adjustment. If you have severe and prolonged vomiting, seek emergency medical care.
4. You should always carry identification which states that you have diabetes.

Always consult your physician if you have any questions about your condition or the use of insulin.

Helpful information for people with diabetes is published by American Diabetes Association, 1660 Duke St., Alexandria, VA 22314.

STORAGE

Insulin should be stored in a cold place, preferably in a refrigerator, but not in the freezing compartment. Do not let it freeze. Keep the insulin vial in its carton so that it will stay clean and protected from light. If refrigeration is not possible, the bottle of insulin which you are currently using can be kept unrefrigerated as long as it is kept as cool as possible and away from heat and sunlight.

Do not use the preparation if the color has become other than water clear or if the liquid has become viscous (thickened).

Never use insulin after expiration date which is printed on the vial label and carton.

Interferon Alfa-2a, Recombinant *(001545)*

For complete prescribing information, refer to the CD-ROM included with the book.

Categories: Leukemia, chronic myelogenous; Leukemia, hairy cell; Sarcoma, Kaposi's; Pregnancy Category C; Recombinant DNA Origin; FDA Approved 1986 Jun; Orphan Drugs

Drug Classes: Antineoplastics, biological response modifiers; Antivirals; Immunomodulators

Brand Names: **Roferon-A**

Foreign Brand Availability: Roceron (Norway); Roceron-A (Sweden); Roferon A (Austria; Bahamas; Barbados; Belgium; Belize; Bermuda; Bulgaria; Canada; Curacao; Guyana; Hungary; Jamaica; Netherland-Antilles; Portugal; Surinam; Trinidad); Roferon-A HSA Free (Singapore); Green-Alpha (Korea)

HCFA JCODE(S): J9213 3 million units SC, IM

DESCRIPTION

Interferon alfa-2a, recombinant is a sterile protein product for use by injection. Roferon-A is manufactured by recombinant DNA technology that employs a genetically engineered *Escherichia coli* bacterium containing DNA that codes for the human protein. Interferon alfa-2a, recombinant is a highly purified protein containing 165 amino acids, and it has an approximate molecular weight of 19,000 daltons. Fermentation is carried out in a defined nutrient medium containing the antibiotic tetracycline HCl, 5 mg/L. However, the presence of the antibiotic is not detectable in the final product. Roferon-A is supplied as an injectable solution in a vial or a prefilled syringe. Each glass syringe barrel contains 0.5 ml of product. In addition, there is a needle which is ½ inch in length.

Single Use Injectable Solution:

3 million IU (11.1 μg/ml) Roferon-A per vial: The solution is colorless and each ml contains 3 MIU of interferon alfa-2a, recombinant, 7.21 mg sodium chloride, 0.2 mg polysorbate 80, 10 mg benzyl alcohol as a preservative and 0.77 mg ammonium acetate.

6 million IU (22.2 μg/ml) Roferon-A per vial: The solution is colorless and each ml contains 6 MIU of interferon alfa-2a, recombinant, 7.21 mg sodium chloride, 0.2 mg polysorbate 80, 10 mg benzyl alcohol as a preservative and 0.77 mg ammonium acetate.

9 million IU (33.3 μg/0.9 ml) Roferon-A per vial: The solution is colorless and each 0.9 ml contains 9 MIU of interferon alfa-2a, recombinant, 6.49 mg sodium chloride, 0.18 mg polysorbate 80, 9 mg benzyl alcohol as a preservative and 0.69 mg ammonium acetate. For single dose administration, withdraw 0.9 ml using a 1 ml syringe. Also can be used as a multidose vial.

36 million IU (133.3 μg/ml) Roferon-A per vial: The solution is colorless and each ml contains 36 MIU of interferon alfa-2a, recombinant, 7.21 mg sodium chloride, 0.2 mg polysorbate 80, 10 mg benzyl alcohol as a preservative and 0.77 mg ammonium acetate.

Single Use Prefilled Syringes:

3 million IU (11.1 μg/0.5 ml) Roferon-A per syringe: The solution is colorless and each 0.5 ml contains 3 MIU of interferon alfa-2a, recombinant, 3.605 mg sodium chloride, 0.1 mg polysorbate 80, 5 mg benzyl alcohol as a preservative and 0.385 mg ammonium acetate.

6 million IU (22.2 μg/0.5 ml) Roferon-A per syringe: The solution is colorless and each 0.5 ml contains 6 MIU of interferon alfa-2a, recombinant, 3.605 mg sodium chloride, 0.1 mg polysorbate 80, 5 mg benzyl alcohol as a preservative and 0.385 mg ammonium acetate.

9 million IU (33.3 μg/0.5 ml) Roferon-A per syringe: The solution is colorless and each 0.5 ml contains 9 MIU of interferon alfa-2a, recombinant, 3.605 mg sodium chloride, 0.1 mg polysorbate 80, 5 mg benzyl alcohol as a preservative and 0.385 mg ammonium acetate.

Multidose Injectable Solution:

9 million IU (33.3 μg/0.9 ml) Roferon-A per vial: The solution is colorless and each 0.9 ml contains 9 MIU of interferon alfa-2a, recombinant, 6.49 mg sodium chloride, 0.18 mg polysorbate 80, 9 mg benzyl alcohol as a preservative and 0.69 mg ammonium acetate. Also can be used as a single use vial.

18 million IU (66.7 μg/3 ml) Roferon-A per vial: The solution is colorless and each ml contains 6 MIU of interferon alfa-2a, recombinant, 7.21 mg sodium chloride, 0.2 mg polysorbate 80, 10 mg benzyl alcohol as a preservative and 0.77 mg ammonium acetate. Each 0.5 ml contains 3 MIU of interferon alfa-2a, recombinant.

Based on the specific activity of 2.7×10^8IU/mg protein, the corresponding quantities of interferon alfa-2a, recombinant in the vials described above are approximately 3 MIU (11.1 μg/ml), 6 MIU (22.2 μg/ml), 9 MIU (33.3 μg/0.9 ml), 18 MIU (66.7 μg/3 ml) and 36 MIU (133.3 μg/ml).

The route of administration for the vial is subcutaneous or intramuscular; the route of administration for the prefilled syringe is subcutaneous only.

I

INDICATIONS AND USAGE

Interferon alfa-2a, recombinant is indicated for the treatment of chronic hepatitis C, hairy cell leukemia and AIDS-related Kaposi's sarcoma in patients 18 years of age or older. In addition, it is indicated for chronic phase, Philadelphia chromosome (Ph) positive chronic myelogenous leukemia (CML) patients who are minimally pretreated (within 1 year of diagnosis).

For patients with Chronic Hepatitis C: Interferon alfa-2a, recombinant is indicated for use in patients with chronic hepatitis C diagnosed by HCV antibody and/or a history of exposure to hepatitis C who have compensated liver disease and are 18 years of age or older. A liver biopsy and a serum test for the presence of antibody to HCV should be performed to establish the diagnosis of chronic hepatitis C. Other causes of hepatitis, including hepatitis B, should be excluded prior to therapy with interferon alfa-2a, recombinant.

For patients with AIDS-Related Kaposi's Sarcoma: Interferon alfa-2a, recombinant is indicated for the treatment of AIDS-related Kaposi's sarcoma in a select group of patients. In determining whether a patient should be treated, the physician should assess the likelihood of response based on the clinical manifestations of HIV infection, including prior opportunistic infections, presence of B symptoms, and CD4 count, and the manifestations of Kaposi's sarcoma requiring treatment.

CONTRAINDICATIONS

Interferon alfa-2a, recombinant is contraindicated in patients with known hypersensitivity to alfa interferon or any component of the product. The injectable solutions contain benzyl alcohol and are contraindicated in any individual with a known allergy to that preservative.

WARNINGS

Interferon alfa-2a, recombinant should be administered under the guidance of a qualified physician (see DOSAGE AND ADMINISTRATION). Appropriate management of the therapy and its complications is possible only when adequate facilities are readily available.

DEPRESSION AND SUICIDAL BEHAVIOR INCLUDING SUICIDAL IDEATION, SUICIDAL ATTEMPTS AND SUICIDES HAVE BEEN REPORTED IN ASSOCIATION WITH TREATMENT WITH ALFA INTERFERONS, INCLUDING INTERFERON ALFA-2A, RECOMBINANT. Patients to be treated with interferon alfa-2a, recombinant should be informed that depression and suicidal ideation may be side effects of treatment and should be advised to report these side effects immediately to the prescribing physician. Patients receiving interferon alfa-2a, recombinant therapy should receive close monitoring for the occurrence of depressive symptomatology. Cessation of treatment should be considered for patients experiencing depression. Although dose reduction or treatment cessation may lead to resolution of the depressive symptomatology, depression may persist and suicides have occurred after withdrawing therapy.

Central nervous system adverse reactions have been reported in a number of patients. These reactions included decreased mental status, dizziness, impaired memory, agitation, manic behavior and psychotic reactions. More severe obtundation and coma have been rarely observed. Most of these abnormalities were mild and reversible within a few days to 3 weeks upon dose reduction or discontinuation of interferon alfa-2a, recombinant therapy. Careful periodic neuropsychiatric monitoring of all patients is recommended.

Interferon alfa-2a, recombinant should be used with caution in patients with severe preexisting cardiac disease, severe renal or hepatic disease, seizure disorders and/or compromised central nervous system function.

Interferon alfa-2a, recombinant should be administered with caution to patients with cardiac disease or with any history of cardiac illness. Acute, self-limited toxicities (*i.e.*, fever, chills) frequently associated with interferon alfa-2a, recombinant administration may exacerbate preexisting cardiac conditions. Rarely, myocardial infarction has occurred in patients receiving interferon alfa-2a, recombinant. Cases of cardiomyopathy have been observed on rare occasions in patients treated with alfa interferons.

Patients with a history of autoimmune hepatitis or a history of autoimmune disease and patients who are immunosuppressed transplant recipients should not be treated with interferon alfa-2a, recombinant. Controlled studies of interferon alfa-2a, recombinant therapy in patients with advanced cirrhosis and/or decompensated liver disease have not been performed. In chronic hepatitis C, initiation of alfa-interferon therapy, including interferon alfa-2a, recombinant, has been reported to cause transient liver abnormalities, which in patients with poorly compensated liver disease can result in increased ascites, hepatic failure or death.

Leukopenia and elevation of hepatic enzymes occurred frequently but were rarely dose-limiting. Thrombocytopenia occurred less frequently. Proteinuria and increased cells in urinary sediment were also seen infrequently. Dose-limiting hepatic or renal toxicities were unusual. Infrequently, severe renal toxicities, sometimes requiring renal dialysis, have been reported with alfa-interferon therapy alone or in combination with IL-2.

Infrequently, severe or fatal gastrointestinal hemorrhage has been reported in association with alfa-interferon therapy.

Caution should be exercised when administering interferon alfa-2a, recombinant to patients with myelosuppression or when interferon alfa-2a, recombinant is used in combination with other agents that are known to cause myelosuppression. Synergistic toxicity has been observed when interferon alfa-2a, recombinant is administered in combination with zidovudine (AZT).[10] The effects of interferon alfa-2a, recombinant when combined with other drugs used in the treatment of AIDS-related disease are not known.

Hyperglycemia has been observed rarely in patients treated with interferon alfa-2a, recombinant. Symptomatic patients should have their blood glucose measured and followed-up accordingly. Patients with diabetes mellitus may require adjustment of their anti-diabetic regimen.

Interferon alfa-2a, recombinant should not be used for the treatment of visceral AIDS-related Kaposi's sarcoma associated with rapidly progressive or life-threatening disease.

The injectable solutions contain benzyl alcohol and should not be used by patients with a known allergy to benzyl alcohol. This product is not indicated for use in neonates or infants and should not be used by patients in that age group. There have been rare reports of death in neonates and infants associated with excessive exposure to benzyl alcohol. The amount of benzyl alcohol at which toxicity or adverse effects may occur in neonates or infants is not known (see CONTRAINDICATIONS).

DOSAGE AND ADMINISTRATION

The recommended dosages of interferon alfa-2a, recombinant differ for chronic hepatitis C, hairy cell leukemia, AIDS-related Kaposi's sarcoma and chronic myelogenous leukemia. See indication-specific dosages below.

Note: Parenteral drug products should be inspected visually for particulate matter and discoloration before administration, whenever solution and container permit.

Roferon-A vials are administered either subcutaneously or intramuscularly. The Roferon-A prefilled syringe is administered subcutaneously only, due to the length of the syringe needle (½ inch) provided in the packaging.

CHRONIC HEPATITIS C

The recommended dosage of interferon alfa-2a, recombinant for the treatment of chronic hepatitis C is 3 MIU three times a week (tiw) administered subcutaneously or intramuscularly for 12 months (48-52 weeks). Normalization of serum ALT generally occurs within a few weeks after initiation of treatment in responders. Approximately 90% of patients who respond to interferon alfa-2a, recombinant do so within the first 3 months of treatment; however, patients responding to interferon alfa-2a, recombinant with a reduction in ALT should complete 12 months of treatment. Patients who have no response to interferon alfa-2a, recombinant within the first 3 months of therapy are not likely to respond with continued treatment; treatment discontinuation should be considered in these patients.

Patients who tolerate and partially or completely respond to therapy with interferon alfa-2a, recombinant but relapse following its discontinuation may be re-treated. Re-treatment with either 3 MIU tiw or with 6 MIU tiw for 6-12 months may be considered.

Temporary dose reduction by 50% is recommended in patients who do not tolerate the prescribed dose. If adverse events resolve, treatment with the original prescribed dose can be re-initiated. In patients who cannot tolerate the reduced dose, cessation of therapy, at least temporarily, is recommended.

HAIRY CELL LEUKEMIA

Prior to initiation of therapy, tests should be performed to quantitate peripheral blood hemoglobin, platelets, granulocytes, and hairy cells and bone marrow hairy cells. These parameters should be monitored periodically (*e.g.*, monthly) during treatment to determine whether response to treatment has occurred. If a patient does not respond within 6 months, treatment should be discontinued. If a response to treatment does occur, treatment should be continued until no further improvement is observed and these laboratory parameters have been stable for about 3 months. Patients with hairy cell leukemia have been treated for up to 24 consecutive months. The optimal duration of treatment for this disease has not been determined.

The induction dose of interferon alfa-2a, recombinant is 3 MIU daily for 16-24 weeks, administered as a subcutaneous or intramuscular injection. Subcutaneous administration is particularly suggested for, but not limited to, thrombocytopenic patients (platelet count <50,000) or for patients at risk for bleeding. The recommended maintenance dose is 3 MIU, three times a week (tiw). Dose reduction by one-half or withholding of individual doses may be needed when severe adverse reactions occur. The use of doses higher than 3 MIU is not recommended in hairy cell leukemia.

AIDS-RELATED KAPOSI'S SARCOMA

Interferon alfa-2a, recombinant is useful for the treatment of AIDS-related Kaposi's sarcoma in a select group of patients. In determining whether a patient should be treated, the physician should assess the likelihood of response based on the clinical manifestations of HIV infection and the manifestations of Kaposi's sarcoma requiring treatment.

Indicator lesion measurements and total lesion count should be performed before initiation of therapy. These parameters should be monitored periodically (*e.g.*, monthly) during treatment to determine whether response to treatment or disease stabilization has occurred. When disease stabilization or a response to treatment occurs, treatment should continue until there is no further evidence of tumor or until discontinuation is required because of a severe opportunistic infection or adverse effects. The optimal duration of treatment for this disease has not been determined.

The recommended induction dose of interferon alfa-2a, recombinant is 36 MIU daily for 10-12 weeks, administered as an intramuscular or subcutaneous injection. Subcutaneous administration is particularly suggested for, but not limited to, patients who are thrombocytopenic (platelet count <50,000) or who are at risk for bleeding. The recommended maintenance dose is 36 MIU, three times a week (tiw). If severe reactions occur, the dose should be modified (50% reduction) or therapy should be temporarily discontinued until the adverse reactions abate. An escalating schedule of 3 MIU, 9 MIU, and 18 MIU each daily for 3 days followed by 36 MIU daily for the remainder of the 10-12 week induction period has also produced equivalent therapeutic benefit with some amelioration of the acute toxicity in some patients.

CHRONIC MYELOGENOUS LEUKEMIA

For Patients With Ph-Positive CML in Chronic Phase

Prior to initiation of therapy, a diagnosis of Philadelphia chromosome positive CML in chronic phase by the appropriate peripheral blood, bone marrow and other diagnostic testing should be made. Monitoring of hematologic parameters should be done regularly (*e.g.*, monthly). Since significant cytogenetic changes are not readily apparent until after hematologic response has occurred, and usually not until several months of therapy have elapsed, cytogenetic monitoring may be performed at less frequent intervals. Achievement of complete cytogenetic response has been observed up to 2 years following the start of interferon alfa-2a, recombinant treatment.

The recommended initial dose of interferon alfa-2a, recombinant is 9 MIU daily administered as a subcutaneous or intramuscular injection. Based on clinical experience,[3] short-term tolerance may be improved by gradually increasing the dose of interferon alfa-2a, recombinant over the first week of administration from 3 MIU daily for 3 days to 6 MIU daily for 3 days to the target dose of 9 MIU daily for the duration of the treatment period.

The optimal dose and duration of therapy have not yet been determined. Even though the median time to achieve a complete hematologic response was 5 months in study MI400, hematologic responses have been observed up to 18 months after treatment start. Treatment should be continued until disease progression. If severe side effects occur, a treatment interruption or a reduction in either the dose or the frequency of injections may be necessary to achieve the individual maximally tolerated dose.

Limited data are available on the use of interferon alfa-2a, recombinant in children with CML. In one report of 15 children with Ph-positive, adult-type CML doses between 2.5 to 5 MIU/m^2/day given intramuscularly were tolerated.[9] In another study, severe adverse effects including deaths were noted in children with previously untreated, Ph-negative, juvenile CML, who received interferon doses of 30 MIU/m^2/day.[14]

PRODUCT LISTING - EQUIVALENTS NOT AVAILABLE

Solution - Injectable - 3000000 U/0.5 ml

0.50 ml	$38.25	ROFERON-A, Roche Laboratories	00004-2015-09
0.50 ml x 6	$229.49	ROFERON-A, Roche Laboratories	00004-2015-07

Solution - Injectable - 6000000 U/ml

3 ml	$229.26	ROFERON-A, Roche Laboratories	00004-2011-09

Solution - Injectable - 6000000 U/0.5 ml

0.50 ml	$76.48	ROFERON-A, Roche Laboratories	00004-2016-09
0.50 ml x 6	$419.47	ROFERON-A, Roche Laboratories	00004-2016-07

Solution - Injectable - 9000000 U/0.5 ml

0.50 ml x 6	$107.68	ROFERON-A, Roche Laboratories	00004-2017-09

Solution - Injectable - 9000000 U/0.9 ml

0.90 ml x 6	$645.99	ROFERON-A, Roche Laboratories	00004-2017-07

Solution - Injectable - 36000000 U/ml

1 ml	$419.26	ROFERON-A, Roche Laboratories	00004-2012-09

Interferon Alfa-2b, Recombinant *(001546)*

For complete prescribing information, refer to the CD-ROM included with the book.

Categories: Condyloma acuminata; Hepatitis B; Hepatitis C; Leukemia, hairy cell; Lymphoma, follicular; Melanoma, malignant; Sarcoma, Kaposi's; Pregnancy Category C; Recombinant DNA Origin; FDA Approved 1986 Jun; Orphan Drugs
Drug Classes: Antineoplastics, biological response modifiers; Antivirals; Immunomodulators
Brand Names: Intron A
Foreign Brand Availability: Bioferon (Thailand); Intron-A (Canada; Ecuador; Greece; Indonesia; Mexico; Peru; Singapore; Thailand); Introna (Austria; Denmark; Finland; France; Norway; Sweden); Peg-Intron (Hong-Kong; Israel); Reaferon (Korea); Rebetron (Peru); Viraferon (Austria; Belgium; Bulgaria; Czech-Republic; Denmark; England; Finland; France; Germany; Greece; Hungary; Ireland; Italy; Netherlands; Norway; Poland; Portugal; Slovenia; Spain; Sweden; Switzerland; Turkey)
HCFA JCODE(S): J9214 1 million units SC, IM

WARNING

Alpha interferons, including interferon alfa-2b, recombinant, cause or aggravate fatal or life-threatening neuropsychiatric, autoimmune, ischemic, and infectious disorders. Patients should be monitored closely with periodic clinical and laboratory evaluations. Patients with persistently severe or worsening signs or symptoms of these conditions should be withdrawn from therapy. In many but not all cases these disorders resolve after stopping interferon alfa-2b, recombinant therapy. See WARNINGS.

DESCRIPTION

Interferon alfa-2b, recombinant for intramuscular, subcutaneous, intralesional, or intravenous injection is a purified sterile recombinant interferon product.

Interferon alfa-2b, recombinant for injection has been classified as an alfa interferon and is a water-soluble protein with a molecular weight of 19,271 daltons produced by recombinant DNA techniques. It is obtained from the bacterial fermentation of a strain of *Escherichia coli* bearing a genetically engineered plasmid containing an interferon alfa-2b gene from human leukocytes. The fermentation is carried out in a defined nutrient medium containing the antibiotic tetracycline HCl at a concentration of 5-10 mg/L; the presence of this antibiotic is not detectable in the final product. The specific activity of interferon alfa-2b, recombinant is approximately 2.6 × 10^8 IU/mg protein as measured by the HPLC assay.

TABLE 1 *Powder for Injection*

Vial Strength	Diluent	Final Concentration After Reconstitution million IU/ml*	Intron A†	Route of Administration
3 MIU	1 ml	3	0.012 mg	IM, SC, IV
5 MIU	1 ml	5	0.019 mg	IM, SC, IV
10 MIU	2 ml	5	0.038 mg	IM, SC, IV, IL‡
18 MIU	1 ml	18	0.069 mg	IM, SC, IV
25 MIU	5 ml	5	0.096 mg	IM, SC, IV
50 MIU	1 ml	50	0.192 mg	IM, SC, IV

* Each ml also contains 20 mg glycine, 2.3 mg sodium phosphate dibasic, 0.55 mg sodium phosphate monobasic, and 1.0 mg human albumin.
† Based on the specific activity of approximately 2.6 × 10^8 IU/mg protein, as measured by HPLC assay.
‡ The 10 MIU vial for intralesional use should be reconstituted with 1 ml of the provided diluent.

Prior to administration, the Intron A powder for injection is to be reconstituted with the provided diluent for interferon alfa-2b, recombinant for injection (bacteriostatic water for injection) containing 0.9% benzyl alcohol as a preservative. (See DOSAGE AND ADMINISTRATION.) Intron A powder for injection is a white to cream-colored powder.

TABLE 2 *Solution Vials for Injection*

Vial Strength	Final Concentration*	Intron A†	Route of Administration
3 MIU	3 million IU/0.5 ml	0.012 mg	IM, SC
5 MIU	5 million IU/0.5 ml	0.019 mg	IM, SC, IL
10 MIU	10 million IU/1.0 ml	0.038 mg	IM, SC, IL
18‡ MIU multidose	3 million IU/0.5 ml	0.088 mg	IM, SC
25§ MIU multidose	5 million IU/0.5 ml	0.123 mg	IM, SC, IL

* Each ml contains 7.5 mg sodium chloride, 1.8 mg sodium phosphate dibasic, 1.3 mg sodium phosphate monobasic, 0.1 mg edetate disodium, 0.1 mg polysorbate 80, and 1.5 mg m-cresol as a preservative.
† Based on the specific activity of approximately 2.6 × 10^8 IU/mg protein as measured by HPLC assay.
‡ This is a multidose vial which contains a total of 22.8 million IU of interferon alfa-2b, recombinant/3.8 ml in order to provide the delivery of six 0.5 ml doses, each containing 3 million IU of interferon alfa-2b, recombinant for injection (for a label strength of 18 million IU).
§ This is a multidose vial which contains a total of 32.0 million IU of interferon alfa-2b, recombinant/3.2 ml in order to provide the delivery of five 0.5 ml doses, each containing 5 million IU of interferon alfa-2b, recombinant for injection (for a label strength of 25 million IU).

TABLE 3 *Solution in Multidose Pens for Injection*

Pen Strength	Final Concentration*	Intron A Dose Delivered†	Intron A‡	Route of Administration
18 MIU	22.5 MIU/1.5 ml	3 MIU/dose	0.087 mg	SC
30 MIU	37.5 MIU/1.5 ml	5 MIU/dose	0.144 mg	SC
60 MIU	75 MIU/1.5 ml	10 MIU/dose	0.288 mg	SC

* Each ml also contains 7.5 mg sodium chloride, 1.8 mg sodium phosphate dibasic, 1.3 mg sodium phosphate monobasic, 0.1 mg edetate disodium, 0.1 mg polysorbate 80, and 1.5 mg m-cresol as a preservative.
† 6 doses, 0.2 ml each.
‡ Based on the specific activity of approximately 2.6 × 10^8 IU/mg protein as measured by HPLC assay.

These packages do not require reconstitution prior to administration (see DOSAGE AND ADMINISTRATION). Intron A solution for injection is a clear, colorless solution.

INDICATIONS AND USAGE

HAIRY CELL LEUKEMIA

Interferon alfa-2b, recombinant for injection is indicated for the treatment of patients 18 years of age or older with hairy cell leukemia.

MALIGNANT MELANOMA

Interferon alfa-2b, recombinant for injection is indicated as adjuvant to surgical treatment in patients 18 years of age or older with malignant melanoma who are free of disease but at high risk for systemic recurrence, within 56 days of surgery.

FOLLICULAR LYMPHOMA

Interferon alfa-2b, recombinant for injection is indicated for the initial treatment of clinically aggressive follicular non-Hodgkin's lymphoma in conjunction with anthracycline-containing combination chemotherapy in patients 18 years of age or older. Efficacy of interferon alfa-2b, recombinant in patients with low-grade, low-tumor burden follicular Non-Hodgkin's Lymphoma has not been demonstrated.

CONDYLOMATA ACUMINATA

Interferon alfa-2b, recombinant for injection is indicated for intralesional treatment of selected patients 18 years of age or older with condylomata acuminata involving external surfaces of the genital and perianal areas. (See DOSAGE AND ADMINISTRATION.)

The use of this product in adolescents has not been studied.

AIDS-RELATED KAPOSI'S SARCOMA

Interferon alfa-2b, recombinant for injection is indicated for the treatment of selected patients 18 years of age or older with AIDS-Related Kaposi's Sarcoma. The likelihood of response to interferon alfa-2b, recombinant therapy is greater in patients who are without systemic symptoms, who have limited lymphadenopathy and who have a relatively intact immune system as indicated by total CD4 count.

CHRONIC HEPATITIS C

Interferon alfa-2b, recombinant for injection is indicated for the treatment of chronic hepatitis C in patients 18 years of age or older with compensated liver disease who have a history of blood or blood-product exposure and/or are HCV antibody positive. Studies in these patients demonstrated that interferon alfa-2b, recombinant therapy can produce clinically meaningful effects on this disease, manifested by normalization of serum alanine aminotransferase (ALT) and reduction in liver necrosis and degeneration.

A liver biopsy should be performed to establish the diagnosis of chronic hepatitis. Patients should be tested for the presence of antibody to HCV. Patients with other causes of chronic hepatitis, including autoimmune hepatitis, should be excluded. Prior to initiation of interferon alfa-2b, recombinant therapy, the physician should establish that the patient has compensated liver disease. The following patient entrance criteria for compensated liver disease were used in the clinical studies and should be considered before interferon alfa-2b, recombinant treatment of patients with chronic hepatitis C:

- No history of hepatic encephalopathy, variceal bleeding, ascites, or other clinical signs of decompensation.
- ***Bilirubin:*** ≤2 mg/dl.
- ***Albumin:*** Stable and within normal limits.
- ***Prothrombin Time:*** <3 seconds prolonged.
- ***WBC:*** ≥3000/mm^3.
- ***Platelets:*** ≥70,000/mm^3.
- Serum creatinine should be normal or near normal.

Prior to initiation of interferon alfa-2b, recombinant therapy, CBC and platelet counts should be evaluated in order to establish baselines for monitoring potential toxicity. These tests should be repeated at Weeks 1 and 2 following initiation of interferon alfa-2b, recombinant therapy, and monthly thereafter. Serum ALT should be evaluated at approximately 3 month intervals to assess response to treatment. (See DOSAGE AND ADMINISTRATION.)

Patients with preexisting thyroid abnormalities may be treated if thyroid-stimulating hormone (TSH) levels can be maintained in the normal range by medication. TSH levels must be within normal limits upon initiation of interferon alfa-2b, recombinant treatment and TSH testing should be repeated at 3 and 6 months.

Interferon alfa-2b, recombinant in combination with ribavirin capsules is indicated for the treatment of chronic hepatitis C in patients with compensated liver disease previously untreated with alfa interferon therapy or who have relapsed following alfa interferon therapy. See Rebetron Combination Therapy package insert for additional information.

CHRONIC HEPATITIS B

Interferon alfa-2b, recombinant for injection is indicated for the treatment of chronic hepatitis B in patients 1 year of age or older with compensated liver disease. Patients who have been serum HBsAg positive for at least 6 months and have evidence of HBV replication (serum HBeAg positive) with elevated serum ALT are candidates for treatment. Studies in these patients demonstrated that interferon alfa-2b, recombinant therapy can produce virologic remission of this disease (loss of serum HBeAg), and normalization of serum aminotransferases. Interferon alfa-2b, recombinant therapy resulted in the loss of serum HBsAg in some responding patients. Prior to initiation of interferon alfa-2b, recombinant therapy, it is recommended that a liver biopsy be performed to establish the presence of chronic hepatitis and the extent of liver damage. The physician should establish that the patient has compensated liver disease. The following patient entrance criteria for compensated liver disease were used in the clinical studies and should be considered before interferon alfa-2b, recombinant treatment of patients with chronic hepatitis B:

- No history of hepatic encephalopathy, variceal bleeding, ascites, or other signs of clinical decompensation.
- ***Bilirubin:*** Normal.
- ***Albumin:*** Stable and within normal limits.
- ***Prothrombin Time:*** *Adults:* <3 seconds prolonged; *Pediatrics:* <2 seconds prolonged.
- ***WBC:*** ≥4000/mm^3.
- ***Platelets:*** *Adults:* ≥100,000/mm^3; *Pediatrics:* >150,000/mm^3.

Patients with causes of chronic hepatitis other than chronic hepatitis B or chronic hepatitis C should not be treated with interferon alfa-2b, recombinant injection. CBC and platelet counts should be evaluated prior to initiation of interferon alfa-2b, recombinant therapy in order to establish baselines for monitoring potential toxicity. These tests should be repeated at treatment Weeks 1, 2, 4, 8, 12, and 16. Liver function tests, including serum ALT, albumin, and bilirubin, should be evaluated at treatment Weeks 1, 2, 4, 8, 12, and 16. HBeAg, HBsAg, and ALT should be evaluated at the end of therapy, as well as 3 and 6 months posttherapy, since patients may become virologic responders during the 6 month period following the end of treatment. In clinical studies in adults, 39% (15/38) of responding patients lost HBeAg 1-6 months following the end of interferon alfa-2b, recombinant therapy. Of responding patients who lost HBsAg, 58% (7/12) did so 1-6 months posttreatment.

A transient increase in ALT >2 × baseline value (flare) can occur during interferon alfa-2b, recombinant therapy for chronic hepatitis B. In clinical trials in adults and pediatrics, this flare generally occurred 8-12 weeks after initiation of therapy and was more frequent in interferon alfa-2b, recombinant responders (*Adults:* 63%, 24/38; *Pediatrics:* 59%, 10/17) than in nonresponders (*Adults:* 27%, 13/48; *Pediatrics:* 35%, 19/55). However, in adults and pediatrics, elevations in bilirubin >3 mg/dl (>2 times ULN) occurred infrequently (*Adults:* 2%, 2/86; *Pediatrics:* 3%, 2/72) during therapy. When ALT flare occurs, in general, interferon alfa-2b, recombinant therapy should be continued unless signs and symptoms of liver failure are observed. During ALT flare, clinical symptomatology and liver function tests including ALT, prothrombin time, alkaline phosphatase, albumin, and bilirubin, should be monitored at approximately 2 week intervals. (See WARNINGS.)

CONTRAINDICATIONS

Interferon alfa-2b, recombinant for injection is contraindicated in patients with a history of hypersensitivity to interferon alfa or any component of the injection. Rebetron combination therapy containing interferon alfa-2b, recombinant and ribavirin capsules must not be used by women who are pregnant or by men whose female partners are pregnant. Extreme care must be taken to avoid pregnancy in female patients and in female partners of patients taking combination interferon alfa-2b, recombinant/ribavirin therapy. Patients with autoimmune hepatitis must not be treated with combination interferon alfa-2b, recombinant/ribavirin therapy. See Rebetron Combination Therapy package insert for additional information.

WARNINGS

GENERAL

Moderate to severe adverse experiences may require modification of the patient's dosage regimen, or in some cases termination of interferon alfa-2b, recombinant therapy. Because of the fever and other "flu-like" symptoms associated with interferon alfa-2b, recombinant administration, it should be used cautiously in patients with debilitating medical conditions, such as those with a history of pulmonary disease (*e.g.,* chronic obstructive pulmonary disease), or diabetes mellitus prone to ketoacidosis. Caution should also be observed in patients with coagulation disorders (*e.g.,* thrombophlebitis, pulmonary embolism) or severe myelosuppression.

Patients with platelet counts of less than 50,000/mm^3 should not be administered interferon alfa-2b, recombinant for injection intramuscularly, but instead by subcutaneous administration.

Interferon alfa-2b, recombinant therapy should be used cautiously in patients with a history of cardiovascular disease. Those patients with a history of myocardial infarction and/or previous or current arrhythmic disorder who require interferon alfa-2b, recombinant therapy should be closely monitored. Cardiovascular adverse experiences, which include hypotension, arrhythmia, or tachycardia of 150 beats/min or greater, and rarely, cardiomyopathy and myocardial infarction have been observed in some interferon alfa-2b, recombinant treated patients. Some patients with these adverse events had no history of cardiovascular disease. Transient cardiomyopathy was reported in approximately 2% of the AIDS-Related Kaposi's Sarcoma patients treated with interferon alfa-2b, recombinant for injection. Hypotension may occur during interferon alfa-2b, recombinant administration, or up to 2 days post-therapy, and may require supportive therapy including fluid replacement to maintain intravascular volume.

Supraventricular arrhythmias occurred rarely and appeared to be correlated with preexisting conditions and prior therapy with cardiotoxic agents. These adverse experiences were controlled by modifying the dose or discontinuing treatment, but may require specific additional therapy.

DEPRESSION AND SUICIDAL BEHAVIOR INCLUDING SUICIDAL IDEATION, SUICIDAL ATTEMPTS, AND COMPLETED SUICIDES HAVE BEEN REPORTED IN ASSOCIATION WITH TREATMENT WITH ALFA INTERFERONS, INCLUDING INTERFERON ALFA-2B, RECOMBINANT THERAPY. Patients with a preexisting psychiatric condition, especially depression, or a history of severe psychiatric disorder should not be treated with interferon alfa-2b, recombinant for injection.[11] Interferon alfa-2b, recombinant therapy should be discontinued for any patient developing severe depression or other psychiatric disorder during treatment. Obtundation and coma have also been observed in some patients, usually elderly, treated at higher doses. While these effects are usually rapidly reversible upon discontinuation of therapy, full resolution of symptoms has taken up to 3 weeks in a few severe episodes. Narcotics, hypnotics, or sedatives may be used concurrently with caution and patients should be closely monitored until the adverse effects have resolved.

Bone marrow toxicity interferon alfa-2b, recombinant therapy suppresses bone marrow function and may result in severe cytopenias including very rare events of aplastic anemia. It is advised that complete blood counts (CBC) be obtained pretreatment and monitored routinely during therapy. Interferon alfa-2b, recombinant therapy should be discontinued in patients who develop severe decreases in neutrophil (<0.5 × 109/L) or platelet counts (<25 × 109/L) (see TABLE 9.

Infrequently, patients receiving interferon alfa-2b, recombinant therapy developed thyroid abnormalities, either hypothyroid or hyperthyroid. The mechanism by which interferon alfa-2b, recombinant for injection may alter thyroid status is unknown. Patients with preexisting thyroid abnormalities whose thyroid function cannot be maintained in the normal range by medication should not be treated with interferon alfa-2b, recombinant for injection. Prior to initiation of interferon alfa-2b, recombinant therapy, serum TSH should be evaluated. Patients developing symptoms consistent with possible thyroid dysfunction during the course of interferon alfa-2b, recombinant therapy should have their thyroid function evaluated and appropriate treatment instituted. Therapy should be discontinued for patients developing thyroid abnormalities during treatment whose thyroid function cannot be normalized by medication. Discontinuation of interferon alfa-2b, recombinant therapy has not always reversed thyroid dysfunction occurring during treatment.

Hepatotoxicity, including fatality, has been observed in interferon alfa treated patients, including those treated with interferon alfa-2b, recombinant for injection. Any patient developing liver function abnormalities during treatment should be monitored closely and if appropriate, treatment should be discontinued.

Pulmonary infiltrates, pneumonitis and pneumonia, including fatality, have been observed in interferon alfa treated patients, including those treated with interferon alfa-2b, recombinant for injection. The etiologic explanation for these pulmonary findings has yet to be established. Any patient developing fever, cough, dyspnea, or other respiratory symptoms should have a chest X-ray taken. If the chest X-ray shows pulmonary infiltrates or there is evidence of pulmonary function impairment, the patient should be closely monitored, and, if appropriate, interferon alfa treatment should be discontinued. While this has been reported more often in patients with chronic hepatitis C treated with interferon alfa, it has also been reported in patients with oncologic diseases treated with interferon alfa.

Retinal hemorrhages, cotton-wool spots, and retinal artery or vein obstruction have been observed rarely in patients treated with interferon alfa, including those treated with interferon alfa-2b, recombinant for injection. The etiologic explanation for these findings has not yet been established. These events appear to occur after use of the drug for several months, but also have been reported after shorter treatment periods. Diabetes mellitus or hypertension have been present in some patients. Any patient complaining of changes in visual acuity or visual fields, or reporting other ophthalmologic symptoms during treatment with interferon alfa-2b, recombinant for injection, should have an eye examination. Because the retinal events may have to be differentiated from those seen with diabetic or hypertensive retinopathy, a baseline ocular examination is recommended prior to treatment with interferon in patients with diabetes mellitus or hypertension.

Rare cases of autoimmune diseases including thrombocytopenia, vasculitis, Raynaud's phenomenon, rheumatoid arthritis, lupus erythematosus, and rhabdomyolysis have been observed in patients treated with alfa interferons, including patients treated with interferon alfa-2b, recombinant for injection. In very rare cases the event resulted in fatality. The mechanism by which these events develop and their relationship to interferon alfa therapy is not clear. Any patient developing an autoimmune disorder during treatment should be closely monitored and, if appropriate, treatment should be discontinued.

Diabetes mellitus and hyperglycemia have been observed rarely in patients treated with interferon alfa-2b, recombinant for injection. Symptomatic patients should have their blood glucose measured and followed up accordingly. Patients with diabetes mellitus may require adjustment of their antidiabetic regimen.

The 50 million IU strength of the interferon alfa-2b, recombinant powder for injection is not to be used for the treatment of hairy cell leukemia, condylomata acuminata, follicular lymphoma, chronic hepatitis C, or chronic hepatitis B. The 3, 5, 18, and 25 million IU strengths of the interferon alfa-2b, recombinant powder for injection are not to be used for the intralesional treatment of condylomata acuminata since the dilution required for the intralesional use would result in a hypertonic solution.

The interferon alfa-2b, recombinant multidose pens, the 3 million IU vial, and the 18 million IU multidose vial of interferon alfa-2b, recombinant solution for injection are not to be used for the treatment of condylomata acuminata. The interferon alfa-2b, recombinant multidose pens and the 18 million and 25 million IU multidose vials of interferon alfa-2b, recombinant solution for injection are not to be used for the treatment of AIDS-Related Kaposi's Sarcoma. Interferon alfa-2b, recombinant solution for injection is not recommended for the IV treatment of malignant melanoma.

The powder formulations of this product contain albumin, a derivative of human blood. Based on effective donor screening and product manufacturing processes, it carries an extremely remote risk for transmission of viral diseases. A theoretical risk for transmission of Creutzfeldt-Jakob disease (CJD) also is considered extremely remote. No cases of transmission of viral diseases or CJD have ever been identified for albumin.

AIDS-RELATED KAPOSI'S SARCOMA

Interferon alfa-2b, recombinant therapy should not be used for patients with rapidly progressive visceral disease. Also of note, there may be synergistic adverse effects between interferon alfa-2b, recombinant for injection and zidovudine. Patients receiving concomitant zidovudine have had a higher incidence of neutropenia than that expected with zidovudine alone. Careful monitoring of the WBC count is indicated in all patients who are myelosuppressed and in all patients receiving other myelosuppressive medications. The effects of interferon alfa-2b, recombinant for injection when combined with other drugs used in the treatment of AIDS-Related disease are unknown.

CHRONIC HEPATITIS C AND CHRONIC HEPATITIS B

Patients with decompensated liver disease, autoimmune hepatitis or a history of autoimmune disease, and patients who are immunosuppressed transplant recipients should not be treated with interferon alfa-2b, recombinant for injection. There are reports of worsening liver disease, including jaundice, hepatic encephalopathy, hepatic failure, and death following interferon alfa-2b, recombinant therapy in such patients. Therapy should be discontinued for any patient developing signs and symptoms of liver failure.

Chronic hepatitis B patients with evidence of decreasing hepatic synthetic functions, such as decreasing albumin levels or prolongation of prothrombin time, who nevertheless meet the entry criteria to start therapy, may be at increased risk of clinical decompensation if a flare of aminotransferases occurs during interferon alfa-2b, recombinant treatment. In such patients, if increases in ALT occur during interferon alfa-2b, recombinant therapy for chronic hepatitis B, they should be followed carefully including close monitoring of clinical symptomatology and liver function tests, including ALT, prothrombin time, alkaline phosphatase, albumin, and bilirubin. In considering these patients for interferon alfa-2b, recombinant therapy, the potential risks must be evaluated against the potential benefits of treatment.

Interferon alfa-2b, recombinant powder for injection when reconstituted with the provided diluent for interferon alfa-2b, recombinant for injection (bacteriostatic water for injection) contains benzyl alcohol. There have been rare reports of death in infants associated with excessive exposure to benzyl alcohol. The amount of benzyl alcohol at which toxicity or adverse effects may occur in infants is not known. Interferon alfa-2b, recombinant **powder for injection** is not indicated for use in infants and should not be used in pediatric patients in this age group.

Rebetron combination therapy containing interferon alfa-2b, recombinant and ribavirin capsules was associated with hemolytic anemia. Hemoglobin <10 g/dl was observed in approximately 10% of patients in clinical trials. Anemia occurred within 1-2 weeks of initiation of ribavirin therapy. Rebetron combination therapy containing interferon alfa-2b, recombinant and ribavirin is not recommended in patients with severe renal impairment and should be used with caution in patients with moderate renal impairment. See Rebetron Combination Therapy package insert for additional information.

DOSAGE AND ADMINISTRATION

IMPORTANT

Interferon alfa-2b, recombinant is packaged as (1) powder for reconstitution/injection; (2) solution for injection; and (3) solution in prefilled, multidose cartridges in a multidose pen device for subcutaneous injection. Not all dosage forms and strengths are appropriate for some indications. It is important that you carefully read the instructions below for the indication you are treating to ensure you are using an appropriate dosage form and strength.

INTERFERON ALFA-2B, RECOMBINANT SOLUTION FOR INJECTION IS NOT RECOMMENDED FOR IV ADMINISTRATION.

HAIRY CELL LEUKEMIA

The recommended dosage of interferon alfa-2b, recombinant for injection for the treatment of hairy cell leukemia is 2 million IU/m^2 administered intramuscularly (see WARNINGS) or subcutaneously 3 times/week for up to 6 months. Responding patients may benefit from continued treatment. **NOTE: The 50 million IU strength of the interferon alfa-2b, recombinant powder for injection is NOT to be used for the treatment of hairy cell leukemia.** Higher doses are not recommended.

If severe adverse reactions develop, the dosage should be modified (50% reduction) or therapy should be temporarily discontinued until the adverse reactions abate. If persistent or recurrent intolerance develops following adequate dosage adjustment, or disease progresses, interferon alfa-2b, recombinant treatment should be discontinued. The minimum effective interferon alfa-2b, recombinant dose has not been established.

MALIGNANT MELANOMA

The recommended interferon alfa-2b, recombinant treatment regimen includes induction treatment 5 consecutive days/week for 4 weeks as an IV infusion at a dose of 20 million IU/m^2, followed by maintenance treatment 3 times/week for 48 weeks as a subcutaneous (SC) injection, at a dose of 10 million IU/m^2.

In the clinical trial, the median daily interferon alfa-2b, recombinant doses administered to patients were 19.1 million IU/m^2 during the induction phase and 9.1 million IU/m^2 during the maintenance phase. **NOTE: Interferon alfa-2b, recombinant solution for injection is NOT recommended for IV administration and should not be used for the induction phase of malignant melanoma.**

Regular laboratory testing should be performed to monitor laboratory abnormalities for the purposes of dose modification. If adverse reactions develop during interferon alfa-2b, recombinant treatment, particularly if granulocytes decrease to <500/mm^3 or SGPT/SGOT rises to >5 × upper limit of normal, treatment should be temporarily discontinued until the adverse reactions abate. Interferon alfa-2b, recombinant treatment should be restarted at 50% of the previous dose. If intolerance persists after dose adjustments or if granulocytes decrease to <250/mm^3 or SGPT/SGOT rises to >10 × upper limit of normal, interferon alfa-2b, recombinant therapy should be discontinued.

FOLLICULAR LYMPHOMA

The recommended dosage of interferon alfa-2b, recombinant for injection is 5 million IU subcutaneously 3 times/week for up to 18 months in conjunction with an anthracycline-containing chemotherapy regimen.

In published reports, the doses of myelosuppressive drugs were reduced by 25% from those utilized in a full-dose CHOP regimen, and cycle length increased by 33% (*e.g.*, from 21-28 days) when an alfa interferon was added to the regimen.[1,4] The dosing regimen should be modified for evidence of serious toxicity. The following dose modification guidelines for hematologic toxicity were used in the clinical trial: the chemotherapy regimen was delayed if either the neutrophil count was <1500/mm^3 or the platelet count was <75,000/mm^3. Administration of interferon alfa-2b, recombinant was temporarily interrupted for a neutrophil count <1000/mm^3, or a platelet count <50,000/mm^3, or reduced by 50% to 2.5 MIU tiw for a neutrophil count >1000/mm^3 but <1500/mm^3.

Reinstitution of the initial interferon alfa-2b, recombinant dose (5 million IU tiw) was tolerated after resolution of hematologic toxicity (≥1500/mm^3).

Interferon alfa-2b, recombinant therapy should be discontinued if SGOT exceeds >5 × the upper limit of normal or serum creatinine >2.0 mg/dl. (See WARNINGS.)

CONDYLOMATA ACUMINATA

The 10 million IU vial of interferon alfa-2b, recombinant powder for injection must be reconstituted with 1 ml of diluent for interferon alfa-2b, recombinant for injection (bacteriostatic water for injection). Do not reconstitute the 10 million IU vial of interferon alfa-2b, recombinant powder for injection with more than 1 ml of diluent since the injection would be subpotent. Do not use the 3, 5, 18, 25, or 50 million IU vials of interferon alfa-2b, recombinant powder for injection for the treatment of condylomata acuminata since the resulting reconstituted solution would be either hypertonic or an inappropriate concentration. Do not use the 3 million IU vial or the 18 million IU multidose vial of interferon alfa-2b, recombinant solution for injection for the intralesional treatment of condylomata acuminata since the concentrations are inappropriate for such use.

Inject 1.0 million IU of interferon alfa-2b, recombinant for injection (either 0.1 ml of reconstituted 10 million IU interferon alfa-2b, recombinant powder for injection or 0.1 ml of the 5 million IU, 10 million IU, or 25 million IU strengths of interferon alfa-2b, recombinant solution for injection, each having a final concentration of 10 million IU/ml) into each lesion 3 times/week on alternate days, for 3 weeks. The injection should be administered intralesionally using a Tuberculin or similar syringe and a 25- to 30-gauge needle. The needle should be directed at the center of the base of the wart and at an angle almost parallel to the plane of the skin (approximating that in the commonly used PPD test). This will deliver the interferon to the dermal core of the lesion, infiltrating the lesion and causing a small wheal. Care should be taken not to go beneath the lesion too deeply; subcutaneous injection should be avoided, since this area is below the base of the lesion. Do not inject too superficially since this will result in possible leakage, infiltrating only the keratinized layer, and not the dermal core. As many as 5 lesions can be treated at 1 time. To reduce side effects, interferon alfa-2b, recombinant injections may be administered in the evening, when possible. Additionally, acetaminophen may be administered at the time of injection to alleviate some of the potential side effects.

The maximum response usually occurs 4-8 weeks after initiation of the first treatment course. If results at 12-16 weeks after the initial treatment course has concluded are not satisfactory, a second course of treatment using the above dosage schedule may be instituted providing that clinical symptoms and signs, or changes in laboratory parameters (liver function tests, WBC, and platelets) do not preclude such a course of action.

Patients with 6-10 condylomata may receive a second (sequential) course of treatment at the above dosage schedule, to treat up to 5 additional condylomata per course of treatment. Patients with greater than 10 condylomata may receive additional sequences depending on how large a number of condylomata are present.

AIDS-RELATED KAPOSI'S SARCOMA

The recommended interferon alfa-2b, recombinant dosage is 30 million IU/m^2 3 times/week administered subcutaneously or intramuscularly. **NOTE: Interferon alfa-2b, recombinant solution for injection should NOT be used for AIDS-Related Kaposi's Sarcoma since the concentrations are inappropriate.** The 18 and 25 million IU multidose strengths of the interferon alfa-2b, recombinant solution for injection should not be used for the treatment of AIDS-Related Kaposi's Sarcoma since the concentrations are inappropriate.

The selected dosage regimen should be maintained unless the disease progresses rapidly or severe intolerance is manifested. If severe adverse reactions develop, the dosage should be modified (50% reduction) or therapy should be temporarily discontinued until the adverse reactions abate. When patients initiate therapy at 30 million IU/m^2 tiw, the average dose tolerated at the end of 12 weeks of therapy is 110 million IU/week and 75 million IU/week at the end of 24 weeks of therapy.

When disease stabilization or a response to treatment occurs, treatment should continue until there is no further evidence of tumor or until discontinuation is required by evidence of a severe opportunistic infection or adverse effect.

CHRONIC HEPATITIS C

The recommended dosage of interferon alfa-2b, recombinant for injection for the treatment of chronic hepatitis C is 3 million IU 3 times/week (tiw) administered subcutaneously or intramuscularly. **NOTE: The 10 million IU vial of interferon alfa-2b, recombinant solution for injection should NOT be used for chronic hepatitis C.** In patients tolerating therapy with normalization of ALT at 16 weeks of treatment, interferon alfa-2b, recombinant therapy should be extended to 18-24 months (72-96 weeks) at 3 million IU tiw to improve the sustained response rate. Patients who do not normalize their ALTs after 16 weeks of therapy rarely achieve a sustained response with extension of treatment. Consideration should be given to discontinuing these patients from therapy.

If severe adverse reactions develop during interferon alfa-2b, recombinant treatment, the dose should be modified (50% reduction) or therapy should be temporarily discontinued as indicated below. If intolerance persists after dose adjustment, interferon alfa-2b, recombinant therapy should be discontinued.

See Rebetron Combination Therapy package insert for dosing when used in combination with ribavirin capsules.

CHRONIC HEPATITIS B

Adults

The recommended dosage of interferon alfa-2b, recombinant for injection for the treatment of chronic hepatitis B is 30-35 million IU/week, administered subcutaneously or intramuscularly, either as 5 million IU daily (qd) or as 10 million IU 3 times/week (tiw) for 16 weeks.

Pediatrics

The recommended dosage of interferon alfa-2b, recombinant for injection for the treatment of chronic hepatitis B is 3 million IU/m^2 3 times/week (tiw) for the first week of therapy followed by dose escalation to 6 million IU/m^2 tiw (maximum of 10 million IU tiw) administered subcutaneously for a total therapy duration of 16-24 weeks. **NOTE: The 3 million IU single-use vial and the 18 million IU multidose vial of interferon alfa-2b, recombinant solution for injection should NOT be used for chronic hepatitis B.**

If severe adverse reactions or laboratory abnormalities develop during interferon alfa-2b, recombinant therapy the dose should be modified (50% reduction), or discontinued if appropriate, until the adverse reactions abate. If intolerance persists after dose adjustment, interferon alfa-2b, recombinant therapy should be discontinued.

For patients with decreases in white blood cell, granulocyte, or platelet counts, the following guidelines for dose modification should be followed. (See TABLE 9.)

TABLE 9 *Guidelines for Dose Modification*

Interferon alfa-2b, recombinant Dose	White Blood Cell Count	Granulocyte Count	Platelet Count
Reduce 50%	$<1.5 \times 10^9$/L	$<0.75 \times 10^9$/L	$<50 \times 10^9$/L
Permanently discontinue	$<1.0 \times 10^9$/L	$<0.5 \times 10^9$/L	$<25 \times 10^9$/L

Interferon alfa-2b, recombinant therapy was resumed at up to 100% of the initial dose when white blood cell, granulocyte, and/or platelet counts returned to normal or baseline values.

At the discretion of the physician, the patient may self-administer the medication.

PRODUCT LISTING - EQUIVALENTS NOT AVAILABLE

Powder For Injection - Injectable - 3000000 IU

1's	$35.63	INTRON A, Caremark Inc	00339-6511-99
6's	$245.93	INTRON A, Caremark Inc	00339-6512-99
6's	$255.77	INTRON A, Schering Corporation	00085-0647-05

Powder For Injection - Injectable - 5000000 IU

1's	$68.30	INTRON A, Caremark Inc	00339-6513-99
1's	$71.04	INTRON A, Schering Corporation	00085-0120-02

Powder For Injection - Injectable - 10000000 IU

1's	$136.62	INTRON A, Caremark Inc	00339-6514-99
1's	$155.49	INTRON A, Schering Corporation	00085-0571-02
1's	$388.78	INTRON A, Schering Corporation	00085-1133-01
6's	$933.05	INTRON A, Schering Corporation	00085-1179-02

Powder For Injection - Injectable - 18000000 IU

1's	$245.93	INTRON A, Caremark Inc	00339-6515-99
1's	$279.90	INTRON A, Schering Corporation	00085-1110-01

Powder For Injection - Injectable - 25000000 IU

1's	$341.59	INTRON A, Caremark Inc	00339-6516-99
1's	$355.25	INTRON A, Schering Corporation	00085-0285-02

Powder For Injection - Injectable - 50000000 IU

1's	$683.16	INTRON A, Caremark Inc	00339-6517-99
1's	$777.54	INTRON A, Schering Corporation	00085-0539-01

Solution - Injectable - 3000000 U/0.2 ml

1.50 ml	$245.93	INTRON A, Caremark Inc	00339-6501-99
1.50 ml	$279.90	INTRON A, Schering Corporation	00085-1242-01

Solution - Injectable - 5000000 U/0.2 ml

1.50 ml	$409.90	INTRON A, Caremark Inc	00339-6502-99
1.50 ml	$466.51	INTRON A, Schering Corporation	00085-1235-01

Solution - Injectable - 5000000 U/0.5 ml

0.50 ml	$59.38	INTRON A, Caremark Inc	00339-6505-99
0.50 ml x 6	$409.90	INTRON A, Caremark Inc	00339-6509-99
0.50 ml x 6	$426.29	INTRON A, Schering Corporation	00085-1191-02

Solution - Injectable - 6000000 IU/ml

0.50 ml	$35.63	INTRON A, Caremark Inc	00339-6504-99
0.50 ml x 6	$245.93	INTRON A, Caremark Inc	00339-6508-99
0.50 ml x 6	$255.77	INTRON A, Schering Corporation	00085-1184-02
3 ml	$245.93	INTRON A, Caremark Inc	00339-6503-99
3 ml	$279.89	INTRON A, Schering Corporation	00085-1168-01

Solution - Injectable - 10000000 U/0.2 ml

1.50 ml	$819.80	INTRON A, Caremark Inc	00339-6500-99
1.50 ml	$933.05	INTRON A, Schering Corporation	00085-1254-01

Interferon Alfa-2b; Ribavirin *(003409)*

For complete prescribing information, refer to the CD-ROM included with the book.

Categories: Hepatitis C; FDA Approved 1998 May; Pregnancy Category X
Drug Classes: Antivirals; Immunomodulators
Brand Names: Rebetron
Foreign Brand Availability: Rebetron Combination Therapy (Australia)

WARNING

Note: The trade names have been used throughout this monograph for clarity.

Combination Rebetol/Intron A therapy is contraindicated in females who are pregnant and in the male partners of females who are pregnant. Extreme care must be taken to avoid pregnancy during therapy and for 6 months after completion of treatment in female patients, and in female partners of male patients who are taking combination Rebetol/Intron A therapy. Females of childbearing potential and males must use two reliable forms of effective contraception during treatment and during the 6 month posttreatment follow-up period. Significant teratogenic and/or embryocidal effects have been demonstrated for ribavirin in all animal species studied. See CONTRAINDICATIONS and WARNINGS. Rebetol monotherapy is not effective for the treatment of chronic hepatitis C and should not be used for this indication. See WARNINGS.

Alpha interferons, including Intron A, cause or aggravate fatal or life-threatening neuropsychiatric, autoimmune, ischemic, and infectious disorders. Patients should be monitored closely with periodic clinical and laboratory evaluations. Patients with persistently severe or worsening signs or symptoms of these conditions should be withdrawn from therapy. In many but not all cases these disorders resolve after stopping Intron A therapy. See WARNINGS.

DESCRIPTION

REBETOL

Rebetol is Schering Corporation's brand name for ribavirin, a nucleoside analog with antiviral activity. The chemical name of ribavirin is 1-β-D-ribofuranosyl-1*H*-1,2,4-triazole-3-carboxamide.

Ribavirin is a white, crystalline powder. It is freely soluble in water and slightly soluble in anhydrous alcohol. The empirical formula is $C_8H_{12}N_4O_5$ and the molecular weight is 244.21.

Rebetol capsules consist of a white powder in a white, opaque, gelatin capsule. Each capsule contains 200 mg ribavirin and the inactive ingredients microcrystalline cellulose, lactose monohydrate, croscarmellose sodium, and magnesium stearate. The capsule shell consists of gelatin, sodium lauryl sulfate, silicon dioxide, and titanium dioxide. The capsule is printed with edible blue pharmaceutical ink which is made of shellac, anhydrous ethyl alcohol, isopropyl alcohol, n-butyl alcohol, propylene glycol, ammonium hydroxide, and FD&C blue no. 2 aluminum lake.

INTRON A

Intron A is Schering Corporation's brand name for interferon alfa-2b, recombinant, a purified, sterile, recombinant interferon product.

Interferon alfa-2b, recombinant has been classified as an alpha interferon and is a water-soluble protein composed of 165 amino acids with a molecular weight of 19,271 daltons produced by recombinant DNA techniques. It is obtained from the bacterial fermentation of a strain of *Escherichia coli* bearing a genetically engineered plasmid containing an interferon alfa-2b gene from human leukocytes. The fermentation is carried out in a defined nutrient medium containing the antibiotic tetracycline hydrochloride at a concentration of 5-10 mg/L; the presence of this antibiotic is not detectable in the final product.

Intron A injection is a clear, colorless solution. The 3 million IU vial of Intron A injection contains 3 million IU of interferon alfa-2b, recombinant per 0.5 ml. The 18 million IU multidose vial of Intron A injection contains a total of 22.8 million IU of interferon alfa-2b, recombinant per 3.8 ml (3 million IU/0.5 ml) in order to provide the delivery of six 0.5 ml doses, each containing 3 million IU of Intron A (for a label strength of 18 million IU). The 18 million IU Intron A injection multidose pen contains a total of 22.5 million IU of interferon alfa-2b, recombinant per 1.5 ml (3 million IU/0.2 ml) in order to provide the delivery of six 0.2 ml doses, each containing 3 million IU of Intron A (for a label strength of 18 million IU). Each ml also contains 7.5 mg sodium chloride, 1.8 mg sodium phosphate dibasic, 1.3 mg sodium phosphate monobasic, 0.1 mg edetate disodium, 0.1 mg polysorbate 80, and 1.5 mg m-cresol as a preservative.

Based on the specific activity of approximately 2.6×10^8 IU/mg protein as measured by HPLC assay, the corresponding quantities of interferon alfa-2b, recombinant in the vials and pen described above are approximately 0.012 mg, 0.088 mg, and 0.087 mg protein, respectively.

INDICATIONS AND USAGE

Rebetol capsules are indicated in combination with Intron A (interferonn alfa-2b, recombinant) injection for the treatment of chronic hepatitis C in patients with compensated liver disease previously untreated with alpha interferon or who have relapsed following alpha interferon therapy.

CONTRAINDICATIONS

Combination Rebetol/Intron A therapy must not be used by females who are pregnant or by males whose female partners are pregnant. Extreme care must be taken to avoid pregnancy in female patients and in female partners of male patients taking combination Rebetol/Intron A therapy. Combination Rebetol/Intron A therapy should not be initiated until a report of a negative pregnancy test has been obtained immediately prior to initiation of therapy. Females of childbearing potential and males must use two forms of effective contraception during treatment and during the 6 months after treatment has been concluded. Significant teratogenic and/or embryocidal effects have been demonstrated for ribavirin in all animal species in which adequate studies have been conducted. These effects occurred at doses as low as one-twentieth of the recommended human dose of Rebetol capsules. If pregnancy occurs in a patient or partner of a patient during treatment or during the 6 months after treatment stops, physicians are encouraged to report such cases by calling 800-727-7064. **See BOXED WARNING and WARNINGS.**

Rebetol capsules in combination with Intron A injection is contraindicated in patients with a history of hypersensitivity to ribavirin and/or alpha interferon or any component of the capsule and/or injection.

Patients with autoimmune hepatitis must not be treated with combination Rebetol/Intron A therapy.

WARNINGS

PREGNANCY

Category X, may cause birth defects. See BOXED WARNING and CONTRAINDICATIONS.

ANEMIA

HEMOLYTIC ANEMIA (HEMOGLOBIN <10 g/dl) WAS OBSERVED IN APPROXIMATELY 10% OF REBETOL/INTRON A-TREATED PATIENTS IN CLINICAL TRIALS. ANEMIA OCCURRED WITHIN 1-2 WEEKS OF INITIATION OF RIBAVIRIN THERAPY. BECAUSE OF THIS INITIAL ACUTE DROP IN HEMOGLOBIN, IT IS ADVISED THAT COMPLETE BLOOD COUNTS (CBC) SHOULD BE OBTAINED PRETREATMENT AND AT WEEK 2 AND WEEK 4 OF THERAPY OR MORE FREQUENTLY IF CLINICALLY INDICATED. PATIENTS SHOULD THEN BE FOLLOWED AS CLINICALLY APPROPRIATE.

The anemia associated with Rebetol/Intron A therapy may result in deterioration of cardiac function and/or exacerbation of the symptoms of coronary disease. Patients should be assessed before initiation of therapy and should be appropriately monitored during therapy. If there is any deterioration of cardiovascular status, therapy should be suspended or discontinued. (See DOSAGE AND ADMINISTRATION.) Because cardiac disease may be worsened by drug induced anemia, patients with a history of significant or unstable cardiac disease should not use combination Rebetol/Intron A therapy.

Similarly, patients with hemoglobinopathies (*e.g.*, thalassemia, sickle-cell anemia) should not be treated with combination Rebetol/Intron A therapy.

PSYCHIATRIC

Severe psychiatric adverse events, including depression, psychoses, aggressive behavior, hallucinations, violent behavior (suicidal ideation, suicidal attempts, suicides) and rare instances of homicidal ideation have occurred during combination Rebetol/Intron A therapy, both in patients with and without a previous psychiatric disorder. Rebetol/Intron A therapy should be used with extreme caution in patients with a history of pre-existing psychiatric disorders, and all patients should be carefully monitored for evidence of depression and other psychiatric symptoms. Suspension of Rebetol/Intron A therapy should be considered if psychiatric intervention and/or dose reduction is unsuccessful in controlling psychiatric symptoms. In severe cases, therapy should be stopped immediately and psychiatric intervention sought.

PULMONARY

Pulmonary symptoms, including dyspnea, pulmonary infiltrates, pneumonitis and pneumonia, including fatality, have been reported during therapy with Rebetol/Intron A. If there is evidence of pulmonary infiltrates or pulmonary function impairment, the patient should be closely monitored, and, if appropriate, combination Rebetol/Intron A treatment should be discontinued.

OTHER

Rebetol capsule monotherapy is not effective for the treatment of chronic hepatitis C and should not be used for this indication.

Fatal and nonfatal pancreatitis has been observed in patients treated with Rebetol/Intron A therapy. Rebetol/Intron A therapy should be suspended in patients with signs and symptoms of pancreatitis and discontinued in patients with confirmed pancreatitis.

Combination Rebetol/Intron A therapy should be used with caution in patients with creatinine clearance <50 ml/min.

Diabetes mellitus and hyperglycemia have been observed in patients treated with Intron A.

Ophthalmologic disorders have been reported with treatment with alpha interferons (including Intron A therapy). Investigators using alpha interferons have reported the occurrence of retinal hemorrhages, cotton wool spots, and retinal artery or vein obstruction in rare instances. Any patient complaining of loss of visual acuity or visual field should have an eye examination. Because these ocular events may occur in conjunction with other disease states, a visual exam prior to initiation of combination Rebetol/Intron A therapy is recommended in patients with diabetes mellitus or hypertension.

Acute serious hypersensitivity reactions (*e.g.*, urticaria, angioedema, bronchoconstriction, anaphylaxis) have been observed in Intron A-treated patients; if such an acute reaction develops, combination Rebetol/Intron A therapy should be discontinued immediately and appropriate medical therapy instituted.

Combination Rebetol/Intron A therapy should be discontinued for patients developing thyroid abnormalities during treatment whose thyroid function cannot be controlled by medication.

DOSAGE AND ADMINISTRATION

Intron A injection should be administered subcutaneously and Rebetol capsules should be administered orally. Rebetol may be administered without regard to food, but should be administered in a consistent manner.

ADULTS

The recommended dose of Rebetol capsules depends on the patient's body weight. The recommended doses of Rebetol and Intron A for adults are given in TABLE 7.

The recommended duration of treatment for patients previously untreated with interferon is 24-48 weeks. The duration of treatment should be individualized to the patient depending on baseline disease characteristics, response to therapy, and tolerability of the regimen. After 24 weeks of treatment virologic response should be assessed. Treatment discontinuation should be considered in any patient who has not achieved an HCV-RNA below the limit of detection of the assay by 24 weeks. There are no safety and efficacy data on treatment for longer than 48 weeks in the previously untreated patient population.

In patients who relapse following interferon therapy, the recommended duration of treatment is 24 weeks. There are no safety and efficacy data on treatment for longer than 24 weeks in the relapse patient population.

TABLE 7 *Recommended Adult Dosing*

Body Weight	Rebetol Capsules	Intron A Injection
≤75 kg	2 × 200 mg capsules AM 3 × 200 mg capsules PM daily PO	3 million IU 3 times weekly SC
>75 kg	3 × 200 mg capsules AM 3 × 200 mg capsules PM daily PO	3 million IU 3 times weekly SC

PEDIATRICS

Efficacy of Rebetol and Intron A for pediatric patients has not been established. Based on pharmacokinetic data, the following doses of Rebetol and Intron A provide similar exposures in pediatric patients as observed in adult patients treated with the approved doses of Rebetol and Intron A (see TABLE 8).

TABLE 8 *Pediatric Dosing*

Body Weight	Rebetol Capsules	Intron A Injection
25-36 kg	1 × 200 mg capsule AM 1 × 200 mg capsule PM Daily PO	3 million IU/m² 3 times weekly SC
37-49 kg	1 × 200 mg capsule AM 2 × 200 mg capsules PM Daily PO	3 million IU/m² 3 times weekly SC
50-61 kg	2 × 200 mg capsules AM 2 × 200 mg capsules PM Daily PO	3 million IU/m² 3 times weekly SC
>61 kg	Refer to adult dosing table	Refer to adult dosing table

Under no circumstances should Rebetol capsules be opened, crushed or broken (see CONTRAINDICATIONS and WARNINGS).

DOSE MODIFICATION

See TABLE 9.

In clinical trials, approximately 26% of patients required modification of their dose of Rebetol capsules, Intron A injection, or both agents. If severe adverse reactions or laboratory abnormalities develop during combination Rebetol/Intron A therapy the dose should be modified, or discontinued if appropriate, until the adverse reactions abate. If intolerance persists after dose adjustment, Rebetol/Intron A therapy should be discontinued.

Rebetol/Intron A therapy should be administered with caution to patients with pre-existing cardiac disease. Patients should be assessed before commencement of therapy and should be appropriately monitored during therapy. If there is any deterioration of cardiovascular status, therapy should be stopped. (See WARNINGS.)

For patients with a history of stable cardiovascular disease, a permanent dose reduction is required if the hemoglobin decreases by ≥2 g/dl during any 4 week period. In addition, for these cardiac history patients, if the hemoglobin remains <12 g/dl after 4 weeks on a reduced dose, the patient should discontinue combination Rebetol/Intron A therapy.

It is recommended that a patient whose hemoglobin level falls below 10 g/dl have his/her Rebetol dose reduced to 600 mg daily (1 × 200 mg capsule AM, 2 × 200 mg capsules PM). A patient whose hemoglobin level falls below 8.5 g/dl should be permanently discontinued from Rebetol/Intron A therapy. (See WARNINGS.)

It is recommended that a patient who experiences moderate depression (persistent low mood, loss of interest, poor self image, and/or hopelessness) have his/her Intron A dose temporarily reduced and/or be considered for medical therapy. A patient experiencing severe depression or suicidal ideation/attempt should be discontinued from Rebetol/Intron A therapy and followed closely with appropriate medical management. (See WARNINGS.)

TABLE 9 *Guidelines for Dose Modifications*

	Dose Reduction* **Rebetol - Adults 600 mg daily** **Rebetol - Pediatrics: half the dose** **Intron A - Adults 1.5 million IU tiw** **Intron A - Pediatrics: 1.5 million IU/m^2 tiw**	**Permanent Discontinuation of Treatment Rebetol and Intron A**
Hemoglobin	<10 g/dl (Rebetol) **Cardiac History Patients Only. ≥2 g/dl decrease during any 4 week period during treatment (Rebetol/Intron A)**	<8.5 g/dl **Cardiac History Patients Only. <12 g/dl after 4 weeks of dose reduction**
White blood count	<1.5 × 10^9/L (Intron A)	<1.0 × 10^9/L
Neutrophil count	<0.75 × 10^9/L (Intron A)	<0.5 × 10^9/L
Platelet count	Adults: <50 × 10^9/L (Intron A)	Adults: <25 × 10^9/L
Platelet count	Pediatrics: <80 × 10^9/L (Intron A)	Pediatrics: <50 × 10^9/L

* Study medication to be dose reduced is shown in parenthesis.

Parenteral drug products should be inspected visually for particulate matter and discoloration prior to administration, whenever solution and container permit. Intron A injection may be administered using either sterilized glass or plastic disposable syringes.

STABILITY

Intron A injection provided in vials is stable at 35°C (95°F) for up to 7 days and at 30°C (86°F) for up to 14 days. Intron A injection provided in a multidose pen is stable at 30°C (86°F) for up to 2 days. The solution is clear and colorless.

PRODUCT LISTING - EQUIVALENTS NOT AVAILABLE

Kit - Oral and Injectable - Multiple Dose 600 mg/Day

1's	$658.70	REBETRON, Schering Corporation	00085-1236-03
1's	$658.70	REBETRON, Schering Corporation	00085-1258-03

Kit - Oral and Injectable - Multiple Dose 1000 mg/Day

1's	$804.32	REBETRON, Schering Corporation	00085-1236-02
1's	$804.32	REBETRON, Schering Corporation	00085-1258-02

Kit - Oral and Injectable - Multiple Dose 1200 mg/Day

1's	$888.76	REBETRON, Schering Corporation	00085-1236-01
1's	$888.76	REBETRON, Schering Corporation	00085-1258-01

Kit - Oral and Injectable - Single Dose 600 mg/Day

1's	$658.70	REBETRON, Schering Corporation	00085-1241-03

Kit - Oral and Injectable - Single Dose 1000 mg/Day

1's	$804.32	REBETRON, Schering Corporation	00085-1241-02

Kit - Oral and Injectable - Single Dose 1200 mg/Day

1's	$888.76	REBETRON, Schering Corporation	00085-1241-01

Interferon Alfa-N3 *(003048)*

For complete prescribing information, refer to the CD-ROM included with the book.

Categories: Condyloma acuminata; Pregnancy Category C; FDA Approved 1990 Jun
Drug Classes: Antivirals; Immunomodulators
Brand Names: Alferon N
HCFA JCODE(S): J9215 250,000 IU IM

DESCRIPTION

Interferon alfa-n3 (human leukocyte derived) is a sterile aqueous formulation of purified, natural, human interferon alpha proteins for use by injection. Alferon N injection consists of interferon alpha proteins comprising approximately 166 amino acids ranging in molecular weights from 16,000-27,000 daltons. The specific activity of interferon alfa-n3 is approximately equal to, or greater than 2 × 10^4 IU/mg of protein.

Alferon N injection is manufactured from pooled units of human leukocytes which have been induced by incomplete infection with an avian virus (Sendai virus) to produce interferon alfa-n3. The manufacturing process includes immunoaffinity chromatography with a murine monoclonal antibody, acidification (pH 2) for 5 days at 4°C, and gel filtration chromatography.

Since Alferon N injection is manufactured using source leukocytes, human, donor screening is performed to minimize the risk that the leukocytes could contain infectious agents. In addition, the manufacturing process contains steps which have been shown to inactivate viruses, and there has been no evidence of infection transmission to recipients in clinical trials. The laboratory and clinical data obtained support the conclusion that Alferon N injection is equivalent to other products derived from human blood or plasma which are free of risk of transmission of infectious agents, such as immunoglobulin and albumin.

Each unit of leukocytes used in the production of Alferon N injection is from a donor whose serum is tested and found negative for hepatitis B surface antigen (HBsAg) and antibodies to human immunodeficiency virus (HIV-1) and human T lymphotropic virus-1 (HTLV-1) by FDA approved tests: the donor's serum has also been screened for ALT (alanine aminotransferase) levels. All donors are screened to eliminate those in high risk groups for transmission of diseases caused by retroviruses and hepatitis viruses.

The Alferon N injection manufacturing process was evaluated for quantitative removal or inactivation of model pathogenic viruses. The viruses were deliberately added to the leukocytes in amounts far exceeding those present in contaminated blood, (*i.e.*, ≥10^9 infectious units per milliliter. The manufacturing process yielded a cumulative reduction of ≥10^{14} of infectious HIV-1, *i.e.*, ≥$10^{6.5}$ removal by acid inactivation and ≥$10^{7.9}$ removal by the purification process. In the validation studies, there was 10^8 reduction in the titer of hepatitis B virus as determined by HBsAg assay, and a 10^9 reduction in the infectious titer of herpes simplex virus-1 (HSV-1). Cultivation of Alferon N Injection Purified Drug Concentrate with human indicator cells, (*i.e.*, MRC-5 cells, peripheral blood leukocytes in the presence of Cyclosporin A, and fetal cord blood cells), did not defect the presence of infectious viruses.

As part of a validation study, Alferon N injection was examined for the presence of the following viruses: Sendai virus (SV), HIV-1, HTLV-I, HBV, HSV-1, CMV, and EBV. Alferon N injection contained no detectable quantities of these viruses. In addition other studies. *i.e.*, Polymerase Chain Reaction (PCR) and Dot Blot Hybridization (DBH), have shown no detectable genetic material from these viruses in interferon alfa-n3 injection. The sensitivity of the PCR was 10 copies for HIV-1 (envgene probe) and 10 copies for HBV (S/P gene probe). The sensitivity of the DBH was 1 pg for EBV, <10 pg for CMV, <10 pg for HSV-1, and <2 pg for SV. Furthermore, sera from 105 patients treated with interferon alfa-n3 injection (95 with condylomata acuminata and 10 with cancer) were tested for antibody to HIV-1 and HIV p24 antigen. there was no evidence to suggest transmission of HIV-1 by interferon alfa-n3 injection. Sera from 135 patients with condylomata acuminata treated with interferon alfa-n3 injection were tested to determine abnormal SGOT laboratory values. There was no evidence to suggest transmission of hepatitis by interferon alfa-n3 injection based on both SGOT results and patient data collected during clinical trials.

Alferon N injection has been extensively purified using immunoaffinity chromatography with a murine monoclonal antibody, acidification (pH 2) for 5 days at 4°C, and gel filtration chromatography. Alferon N injection has been subjected to the acid treatment for five days during its manufacture in order to reduce the risk of viral transmission. Subsequent analyses of the Alferon N injection Purified Drug Concentrate confirm the absence of detectable infectious or non-infectious viral particles.

The leukocyte nutrient medium contains the antibiotic neomycin sulfate at a concentration of 35 mg/l: however, neomycin sulfate is not detectable in the final product, (*i.e.* <0.64 μg/ml).

Murine immunoglobulin (IgG) is detected in the Alferon N Injection Purified Drug Concentrate at levels below 0.15% of the interferon alfa-n3 protein. This equates to levels less than 8 ng of murine IgG per million IU interferon alfa-n3 (range of 0.9-5.6 ng typically found).

Interferon alfa-n3 (human leukocyte derived) is available in an injectable solution containing 5 million IU Alferon N injection per vial for intralesional injection. The solution is clear and colorless. Each milliliter (ml) contains five million IU of interferon alfa-n3 in phosphate buffered saline (8.0 mg sodium chloride, 1.74 mg sodium phosphate dibasic, 0.20 mg potassium phosphate monobasic, and 0.20 mg potassium chloride) containing 3.3 mg phenol as a preservative and 1 mg Albumin (Human) as a stabilizer.

Storage: Alferon N injection should be stored at 2-8°C (36-46°F). Do not freeze. Do not shake.

INDICATIONS AND USAGE

Interferon alfa-n3 injection is indicated for the intralesional treatment of refractory or recurring external condylomata acuminata in patients 18 years of age or older (see DOSAGE AND ADMINISTRATION).

The physician should select patients for treatment with interferon alfa-n3 injection after consideration of a number of factors: The locations and sizes of the lesions, past treatment and response thereto, and the patient's ability to comply with the treatment regimen. Interferon alfa-n3 injection is particularly useful for patients who have not responded satisfactorily to other treatment modalities, (*e.g.*, podophyllin resin, surgery, laser or cryotherapy).

There have been no studies with this product in adolescents. This product is not recommended for use in patients less than 18 years of age.

CONTRAINDICATIONS

Interferon alfa-n3 injection is contraindicated in patients with known hypersensitivity to human interferon alpha or any component of the product. The product also is contraindicated in patients who have anaphylactic sensitivity to mouse immunoglobulin (IgG), egg protein or neomycin.

WARNINGS

Because of the fever and other "flu-like" symptoms associated with interferon alfa-n3 injection, it should be used cautiously in patients with debilitating medical conditions such as cardiovascular disease (*e.g.*, unstable angina and uncontrolled congestive heart failure), severe pulmonary disease (*e.g.*, chronic obstructive pulmonary disease), or diabetes mellitus with ketoacidosis. Interferon alfa-n3 injection should be used cautiously in patients with coagulation disorders (*e.g.*, thrombophlebitis, pulmonary embolism and hemophilia), severe myelosuppression, or seizure disorders. Acute, serious hypersensitivity reactions (*e.g.*, urticaria, angioedema, bronchoconstriction, and anaphylaxis) have not been observed in patients receiving interferon alfa-n3 injection. However, if such reactions develop, drug administration should be discontinued immediately and appropriate medical therapy should be instituted.

DOSAGE AND ADMINISTRATION

The recommended dose of interferon alfa-n3 injection (human leukocyte derived) for the treatment of condylomata acuminata is 0.05 ml (250,000 IU) per wart. Interferon alfa-n3 injection should be administered twice weekly for up to 8 weeks. The maximum recommended dose per treatment session is 0.5 ml (2.5 million IU). Interferon alfa-n3 injection should be injected into the base of each wart, preferably using a 30 gauge needle. For large warts, interferon alfa-n3 injection may be injected at several points around the periphery of the wart, using a total dose of 0.05 ml per wart.

The minimum effective dose of interferon alfa-n3 injection for the treatment of condylomata acuminata has not been established. Moderate to severe adverse experiences may require modification of the dosage regimen or, in some cases, termination of therapy with interferon alfa-n3 injection.

Genital warts usually begin to disappear after several weeks of treatment with interferon alfa-n3 injection. Treatment should continue for a maximum of 8 weeks. In clinical trials with interferon alfa-n3 injection, many patients who had partial resolution of warts during treatment experienced further resolution of their warts after cessation of treatment. Of the patients who had complete resolution of warts due to treatment, half the patients had complete resolution of warts by the end of the treatment and half had complete resolution of warts during the 3 months after cessation of treatment. Thus, it is recommended that no further therapy (interferon alfa-n3 injection or conventional therapy) be administered for 3 months after the initial 8 week course of treatment unless the warts enlarge or new warts appear. Studies to determine the safety and efficacy of a second course of treatment with interferon alfa-n3 injection (human leukocyte derived) have not been conducted.

Parenteral drug products should be inspected visually for particulate matter and discoloration prior to administration, whenever solution and container permit.

PRODUCT LISTING - EQUIVALENTS NOT AVAILABLE

Solution - Injectable - 5000000 IU/ml

1 ml	$159.00	ALFERON N, Interferon Sciences Inc	54746-0001-01

Interferon Alfacon-1 *(003357)*

For complete prescribing information, refer to the CD-ROM included with the book.

Categories: Hepatitis C; Pregnancy Category C; FDA Approved 1997 Oct
Drug Classes: Antivirals; Immunomodulators
Brand Names: Infergen

DESCRIPTION

Interferon alfacon-1 is a recombinant non-naturally occurring type-I interferon. The 166-amino acid sequence of interferon alfacon-1 was derived by scanning the sequences of several natural interferon alpha subtypes and assigning the most frequently observed amino acid in each corresponding position.[1] Four additional amino acid changes were made to facilitate the molecular construction, and a corresponding synthetic DNA sequence was constructed using chemical synthesis methodology. Interferon alfacon-1 differs from interferon alpha-2 at 20/166 amino acids (88% homology), and comparison with interferon-beta shows identity at over 30% of the amino acid positions. Interferon alfacon- 1 is produced in *Escherichia coli (E coli)* cells that have been genetically altered by insertion of a synthetically constructed sequence that codes for interferon alfacon-1. Prior to final purification, interferon alfacon-1 is allowed to oxidize to its native state, and its final purity is achieved by sequential passage over a series of chromatography columns. This protein has a molecular weight of 19,434 daltons.

Infergen is a sterile, clear, colorless, preservative-free liquid formulated with 100 mM sodium chloride and 25 mM sodium phosphate at pH 7.0 ± 0.2. The product is available in single-use vials and prefilled syringes containing 9 µg and 15 µg interferon alfacon-1 at a fill volume of 0.3 ml and 0.5 ml, respectively. Infergen vials and prefilled syringes contain 0.03 mg/ml of interferon alfacon-1, 5.9 mg/ml sodium chloride, and 3.8 mg/ml sodium phosphate in water for injection. The Infergen SingleJect prefilled syringe has a glass barrel and a 26 gauge, 5/8-inch needle. Infergen is to be administered undiluted by subcutaneous (SC) injection.

INDICATIONS AND USAGE

Interferon alfacon-1 is indicated for the treatment of chronic HCV infection in patients 18 years of age or older with compensated liver disease who have anti-HCV serum antibodies and/or the presence of HCV RNA. Other causes of hepatitis, such as viral hepatitis B or autoimmune hepatitis should be ruled out prior to initiation of therapy with interferon alfacon-1. In some patients with chronic HCV infection, interferon alfacon-1 normalizes serum ALT concentrations, reduces serum HCV RNA concentrations to undetectable quantities (<100 copies/ml), and improves liver histology.

CONTRAINDICATIONS

Interferon alfacon-1 is contraindicated in patients with known hypersensitivity to alpha interferons, to *E coli*-derived products, or to any component of the product.

WARNINGS

Treatment with interferon alfacon-1 should be administered under the guidance of a qualified physician, and may lead to moderate-to-severe adverse experiences requiring dose reduction, temporary dose cessation, or discontinuation of further therapy.

Withdrawal from study for adverse events occurred in 7% of patients treated with 9 µg interferon alfacon-1 (including 4% due to psychiatric events).

SEVERE PSYCHIATRIC ADVERSE EVENTS MAY MANIFEST IN PATIENTS RECEIVING THERAPY WITH INTERFERON, INCLUDING INTERFERON ALFACON-1. DEPRESSION, SUICIDAL IDEATION, AND SUICIDE ATTEMPT MAY OCCUR. The incidence of psychiatric events of suicidal ideation was small (1%) for patients treated with 9 µg interferon alfacon-1 compared to the overall incidence (55%) of psychiatric events. Interferon alfacon-1 be used with caution in patients who report a history of depression and physicians should monitor all patients for evidence of depression. Physicians should inform patients of the possible development of depression prior to initiation of interferon alfacon-1 therapy, and patients should report any sign or symptom of depression immediately. Other prominent psychiatric adverse events may also occur, including nervousness, anxiety, emotional lability, abnormal thinking, agitation, or apathy.

INTERFERON ALFACON-1 SHOULD BE ADMINISTERED WITH CAUTION TO PATIENTS WITH PRE-EXISTING CARDIAC DISEASE. Hypertension and supraventricular arrhythmias, chest pain, and myocardial infarction have been associated with interferon therapies.[6]

No studies with interferon alfacon-1 have been conducted in patients with decompensated hepatic disease. Patients with decompensated hepatic disease should not be treated with interferon alfacon-1, and patients who develop symptoms of hepatic decompensation, such as jaundice, ascites, coagulopathy, or decreased serum albumin, should halt further interferon therapy.

DOSAGE AND ADMINISTRATION

The recommended dose of interferon alfacon-1 for treatment of chronic HCV infection is 9 µg TIW administered SC as a single injection for 24 weeks. At least 48 hours should elapse between doses of interferon alfacon-1. Should a patient miss a scheduled dose, the missed dose should be taken as soon as possible, and the administration schedule revised at the physician's discretion.

Patients who tolerated previous interferon therapy and did not respond or relapsed following its discontinuation may be subsequently treated with 15 µg of interferon alfacon-1 TIW for 6 months. Patients should not be treated with 15 µg of interferon alfacon-1 TIW if they have not received, or have not tolerated, an initial course of interferon therapy.

There are significant differences in specific activities among interferons. Health care providers should be aware that changes in interferon brand may require adjustments of dosage and/or change in route of administration. Patients should be warned not to change brands of interferon without medical consultation. Patients should also be instructed by their physician not to reduce the dosage of interferon alfacon-1 prior to medical consultation.

DOSE REDUCTION

For patients who experience a severe adverse reaction on interferon alfacon-1, dosage should be withheld temporarily. If the adverse reaction does not become tolerable, therapy should be discontinued. Dose reduction to 7.5 µg may be necessary following an intolerable adverse event. In the pivotal study, 11% of patients (26/231) who initially received interferon alfacon-1 at a dose of 9 µg (0.3 ml) were dose-reduced to 7.5 µg (0.25 ml).

If adverse reactions continue to occur at the reduced dosage, the physician may discontinue treatment or reduce dosage further. However, decreased efficacy may result from continued treatment at dosages below 7.5 µg.

During subsequent treatment with 15 µg of interferon alfacon-1, 33% of patients required dose reductions in 3 µg increments.

ADMINISTRATION OF INTERFERON ALFACON-1

If home use is determined to be desirable by the physician, instructions on appropriate use should be given by a health care professional. After administration of interferon alfacon-1, it is essential to follow the procedure for proper disposal of syringes and needles. See "Information For Patients" leaflet for detailed instructions provided separately.

PRODUCT LISTING - EQUIVALENTS NOT AVAILABLE

Solution - Injectable - 9 mcg/0.3 ml			
0.30 ml	$38.80	GENERIC, Amgen	55513-0554-01
0.30 ml	$252.00	GENERIC, Intermune Pharmaceuticals	64116-0039-06
0.30 ml x 6	$252.00	GENERIC, Amgen	55513-0554-06
Solution - Injectable - 15 mcg/0.5 ml			
0.50 ml	$64.70	GENERIC, Amgen	55513-0562-01
0.50 ml x 6	$369.96	GENERIC, Amgen	55513-0562-06
0.50 ml x 6	$420.24	GENERIC, Intermune Pharmaceuticals	64116-0031-06

Interferon Beta-1a *(003287)*

For complete prescribing information, refer to the CD-ROM included with the book.

Categories: Multiple sclerosis; Pregnancy Category C; Orphan Drugs; FDA Approved 1996 May
Drug Classes: Immunomodulators
Brand Names: Avonex
Foreign Brand Availability: Rebif (Australia; Canada; France; Hong-Kong; Israel; Mexico; Peru; Taiwan)
HCFA JCODE(S): J1825 33 µg IM

DESCRIPTION

Note: The trade names have been used throughout this monograph for clarity.

AVONEX

Avonex (interferon beta-1a) is produced by recombinant DNA technology. Interferon beta-1a is a 166 amino acid glycoprotein with a predicted molecular weight of approximately 22,500 daltons. It is produced by mammalian cells (Chinese Hamster Ovary cells) into which the human interferon beta gene has been introduced. The amino acid sequence of Avonex is identical to that of natural human interferon beta.

Using the World Health Organization (WHO) natural interferon beta standard, Second International Standard for Interferon, Human Fibroblast (Gb-23-902-531), Avonex has a specific activity of approximately 200 million international units (IU) of antiviral activity per mg; 30 µg of Avonex contains 6 million IU of antiviral activity. The activity against other standards is not known.

I

Avonex is formulated as a sterile, white to off-white lyophilized powder for intramuscular injection after reconstitution with supplied diluent or sterile water for injection, preservative-free.

Each 1.0 ml (1.0 cc) of reconstituted Avonex contains 30 µg of interferon beta-1a, 15 mg albumin human, 5.8 mg sodium chloride, 5.7 mg dibasic sodium phosphate, and 1.2 mg monobasic sodium phosphate, at a pH of approximately 7.3.

REBIF

Rebif (interferon beta-1a) is a purified 166 amino acid glycoprotein with a molecular weight of approximately 22,500 daltons. It is produced by recombinant DNA technology using genetically engineered Chinese Hamster Ovary cells into which the human interferon beta gene has been introduced. The amino acid sequence of Rebif is identical to that of natural fibroblast derived human interferon beta. Natural interferon beta and interferon beta-1a (Rebif) are glycosylated with each containing a single N-linked complex carbohydrate moiety.

Using a reference standard calibrated against the World Health Organization natural interferon beta standard (Second International Standard for Interferon, Human Fibroblast GB 23 902 531), Rebif has a specific activity of approximately 270 million international units (MIU) of antiviral activity per mg of interferon beta-1a determined specifically by an *in vitro* cytopathic effect bioassay using WISH cells and Vesicular Stomatitis virus. Rebif 44 µg contains approximately 12 MIU of antiviral activity using this method.

Rebif is formulated as a sterile solution in a pre-filled syringe intended for subcutaneous (SC) injection. Each 0.5 ml (0.5 cc) of Rebif contains either 44 µg or 22 µg of interferon beta-1a, 4 or 2 mg albumin (human), 27.3 mg mannitol, 0.4 mg sodium acetate, water for injection.

INDICATIONS AND USAGE

AVONEX

Avonex is indicated for the treatment of relapsing forms of multiple sclerosis to slow the accumulation of physical disability and decrease the frequency of clinical exacerbations. Safety and efficacy in patients with chronic progressive multiple sclerosis have not been evaluated.

REBIF

Rebif is indicated for the treatment of patients with relapsing forms of multiple sclerosis to decrease the frequency of clinical exacerbations and delay the accumulation of physical disability. Efficacy of Rebif in chronic progressive multiple sclerosis has not been established.

CONTRAINDICATIONS

AVONEX

Avonex is contraindicated in patients with a history of hypersensitivity to natural or recombinant interferon beta, human albumin, or any other component of the formulation.

REBIF

Rebif is contraindicated in patients with a history of hypersensitivity to natural or recombinant interferon, human albumin, or any other component of the formulation.

WARNINGS

AVONEX

Avonex should be used with caution in patients with depression. Depression and suicide have been reported to occur in patients receiving other interferon compounds. Depression and suicidal ideation are known to occur at an increased frequency in the multiple sclerosis population. A relationship between occurrence of depression and/or suicidal ideation and the use of Avonex has not been established. An equal incidence of depression was seen in the placebo-treated and Avonex-treated patients in the placebo-controlled multiple sclerosis study. Patients treated with Avonex should be advised to report immediately any symptoms of depression and/or suicidal ideation to their prescribing physicians. If a patient develops depression, cessation of Avonex therapy should be considered.

REBIF

Depression

Rebif should be used with caution in patients with depression, a condition that is common in people with multiple sclerosis. Depression, suicidal ideation, and suicide attempts have been reported to occur with increased frequency in patients receiving interferon compounds, including Rebif. Patients should be advised to report immediately any symptoms of depression and/or suicidal ideation to the prescribing physician. If a patient develops depression, cessation of treatment with Rebif should be considered.

Hepatic Injury

A case of fulminant hepatic failure requiring liver transplantation in a patient who initiated Rebif therapy while taking another potentially hepato-toxic medication has been reported from a non-US postmarketing source. Symptomatic hepatic dysfunction, primarily presenting as jaundice, has been reported as a rare complication of Rebif use. Asymptomatic elevation of hepatic transaminases (particularly SGPT) is common with interferon therapy. Rebif should be initiated with caution in patients with active liver disease, alcohol abuse, increased serum SGPT (<2.5 times ULN), or a history of significant liver disease. Dose reduction should be considered if SGPT rises above 5 times the upper limit of normal. The dose may be gradually re-escalated when enzyme levels have normalized. Treatment with Rebif should be stopped if jaundice or other clinical symptoms of liver dysfunction appear.

Anaphylaxis

Anaphylaxis has been reported as a rare complication of Rebif use. Other allergic reactions have included skin rash and urticaria, and have ranged from mild to severe without a clear relationship to dose or duration of exposure. Several allergic reactions, some severe, have occurred after prolonged use.

Albumin (Human)

This product contains albumin, a derivative of human blood. Based on effective donor screening and product manufacturing processes, it carries an extremely remote risk for transmission of viral diseases. A theoretical risk for transmission of Creutzfeldt-Jakob disease (CJD) also is considered extremely remote. No cases of transmission of viral diseases or CJD have ever been identified for albumin.

DOSAGE AND ADMINISTRATION

AVONEX

The recommended dosage of Avonex for the treatment of relapsing forms of multiple sclerosis is 30 µg injected intramuscularly once a week.

Avonex is intended for use under the guidance and supervision of a physician. Patients may self-inject only if their physician determines that it is appropriate and with medical follow-up, as necessary, after proper training in intramuscular injection technique.

REBIF

The recommended dosage of Rebif is 44 µg injected subcutaneously 3 times per week. Rebif should be administered, if possible, at the same time (preferably in the late afternoon or evening) on the same 3 days (*e.g.*, Monday, Wednesday, and Friday) at least 48 hours apart each week. Generally, patients should be started at 8.8 µg SC tiw and increased over a 4 week period to 44 µg tiw (see TABLE 6). A Rebif "Starter Kit" containing 22 µg syringes, is available for use in titrating the dose during the first 4 weeks of treatment. Following the administration of each dose, any residual product remaining in the syringe should be discarded in a safe and proper manner.

TABLE 6 *Schedule for Patient Titration*

	Recommended Titration	Rebif Dose	Volume	Syringe Strength (per 0.5 ml)
Weeks 1-2	20%	8.8 µg	0.2 ml	22 µg
Weeks 3-4	50%	22 µg	0.5 ml	22 µg
Weeks 5+	100%	44 µg	0.5 ml	44 µg

Leukopenia or elevated liver function tests may necessitate dose reductions of 20-50% until toxicity is resolved (see WARNINGS, Rebif, Hepatic Injury).

Rebif is intended for use under the guidance and supervision of a physician. It is recommended that physicians or qualified medical personnel train patients in the proper technique for self-administering subcutaneous injections using the pre-filled syringe. Patients should be advised to rotate sites for SC injections. Concurrent use of analgesics and/or antipyretics may help ameliorate flu-like symptoms on treatment days. Rebif should be inspected visually for particulate matter and discoloration prior to administration.

Stability and Storage

Rebif should be stored refrigerated between 2-8°C (36-46°F). DO NOT FREEZE. If a refrigerator is temporarily not available, such as while you are traveling, Rebif should be kept cool (*i.e.*, below 25°C/77°F) and away from heat and light.

Do not use beyond the expiration date printed on packages. Rebif contains no preservatives. Each syringe is intended for single use. Unused portions should be discarded.

PRODUCT LISTING - EQUIVALENTS NOT AVAILABLE

Solution - Injectable - 22 mcg
1 x 12 $1334.16 REBIF, Serono Laboratories Inc 44087-0022-03
Solution - Injectable - 30 mcg
1's $1076.25 AVONEX, Biogen 59627-0001-03
Solution - Injectable - 44 mcg
1 x 12 $1334.16 REBIF, Serono Laboratories Inc 44087-0044-03

Interferon Beta-1b, Recombinant *(003154)*

For complete prescribing information, refer to the CD-ROM included with the book.

Categories: Multiple sclerosis; Recombinant DNA Origin; FDA Approved 1993 Jul; Pregnancy Category C; Orphan Drugs
Drug Classes: Immunomodulators
Brand Names: **Betaseron**
Foreign Brand Availability: Beneseron (Korea); Betaferon (Australia; Austria; Belgium; Bulgaria; Canada; Czech-Republic; Denmark; England; Finland; France; Germany; Greece; Hungary; Ireland; Israel; Italy; Mexico; Netherlands; New-Zealand; Norway; Peru; Poland; Portugal; Slovenia; South-Africa; Spain; Sweden; Switzerland; Turkey)
HCFA JCODE(S): J1830 0.25 mg SC

DESCRIPTION

Interferon beta-1b is a purified, sterile, lyophilized protein product produced by recombinant DNA techniques and formulated for use by injection. Interferon beta-1b is manufactured by bacterial fermentation of a strain of *Escherichia coli* that bears a genetically engineered plasmid containing the gene for human interferon beta $_{ser17}$. The native gene was obtained from human fibroblasts and altered in a way that substitutes serine for the cysteine residue found at position 17. Interferon beta-1b is a highly purified protein that has 165 amino acids and an approximate molecular weight of 18,500 daltons. It does not include the carbohydrate side chains found in the natural material.

The specific activity of interferon beta-1b, recombinant is approximately 32 million international units (IU)/mg Interferon beta-1b. Each vial contains 0.3 mg (9.6 million IU) of Interferon beta-1b. The unit measurement is derived by comparing the antiviral activity of the product to the World Health Organization (WHO) reference standard of recombinant human interferon beta. Dextrose and albumin human (15 mg each/vial) are added as stabilizers. Prior to 1993, a different analytical standard was used to determine potency. It assigned 54 million IU to 0.3 mg Interferon beta- 1b.

Lyophilized interferon beta-1b, recombinant is a sterile, white to off-white powder intended for subcutaneous injection after reconstitution with the diluent supplied (sodium chloride, 0.54% solution).

INDICATIONS AND USAGE

Interferon beta-1b, recombinant is indicated for use in ambulatory patients with relapsing-remitting multiple sclerosis to reduce the frequency of clinical exacerbations. Relapsing-remitting MS is characterized by recurrent attacks of neurologic dysfunction followed by complete or incomplete recovery. The safety and efficacy of interferon beta-1b, recombinant in chronic-progressive MS has not been evaluated.

CONTRAINDICATIONS

Interferon beta-1b, recombinant is contraindicated in patients with a history of hypersensitivity to natural or recombinant interferon beta, albumin human, or any other component of the formulation.

WARNINGS

One suicide and 4 attempted suicides were observed among 372 study patients during a 3 year period. All five patients received interferon beta-1b, recombinant (three in the 0.05 mg [1.6 million IU] group and two in the 0.25 mg [8 million IU] group). There were no attempted suicides in patients on study who did not receive interferon beta-1b, recombinant. Depression and suicide have been reported to occur in patients receiving interferon alfa, a related compound. Patients to be treated with interferon beta-1b, recombinant should be informed that depression and suicidal ideation may be a side effect of the treatment and should report these symptoms immediately to the prescribing physician. Patients exhibiting depression should be monitored closely and cessation of therapy should be considered.

DOSAGE AND ADMINISTRATION

The recommended dose of interferon beta-1b, recombinant for the treatment of ambulatory relapsing-remitting MS is 0.25 mg (8 million IU) injected subcutaneously every other day. Limited data regarding the activity of a lower dose are presented above.

Evidence of efficacy beyond 2 years is not known since the primary evidence of efficacy derives from a 2 year, double-blind, placebo-controlled clinical trial. Safety data are not available beyond the third year. Patients were discontinued from this trial due to unremitting disease progression of 6 months or greater.

To reconstitute lyophilized interferon beta-1b, recombinant for injection, use a sterile syringe and needle to inject 1.2 ml of the diluent supplied, sodium chloride, 0.54% solution, into the interferon beta-1b, recombinant vial. Gently swirl the vial of interferon beta-1b, recombinant to dissolve the drug completely; do not shake. Inspect the reconstituted product visually and discard the product before use if it contains particulate matter or is discolored. After reconstitution with accompanying diluent, interferon beta-1b, recombinant vials contain 0.25 mg (8 million IU) Interferon beta-1b/ml of solution.

Withdraw 1 ml of reconstituted solution from the vial into a sterile syringe fitted with a 27-gauge needle and inject the solution subcutaneously. Sites for self-injection include arms, abdomen, hips, and thighs. A vial is suitable for single use only; unused portions should be discarded.

Stability: The reconstituted product contains no preservative. Before and after reconstitution with diluent, store at 2-8°C (36-46°F). Product should be used within 3 hours of reconstitution.

PRODUCT LISTING - EQUIVALENTS NOT AVAILABLE

Powder For Injection - Injectable - 0.3 mg

1's	$72.00	BETASERON, Berlex Laboratories	50419-0521-03
15's	$1125.00	BETASERON, Berlex Laboratories	50419-0521-15
15's	$1273.63	BETASERON, Berlex Laboratories	50419-0523-15

Interferon Gamma-1b, Recombinant (003049)

For complete prescribing information, refer to the CD-ROM included with the book.

Categories: Granulomatous disease, chronic; Osteopetrosis, malignant; Pregnancy Category C; Recombinant DNA Origin; FDA Approved 1990 Dec; Orphan Drugs
Drug Classes: Immunomodulators
Brand Names: Actimmune
Foreign Brand Availability: Immukin (Hong-Kong); Imufor (Austria; Germany); Imukin (Australia; Austria; Czech-Republic; Denmark; Finland; France; Germany; Greece; Italy; Norway; Spain; Sweden; Switzerland); Imukin Inj. (New-Zealand)
HCFA JCODE(S): J9216 3 million units SC

DESCRIPTION

Interferon gamma-1b, a biologic response modifier, is a single-chain polypeptide containing 140 amino acids. Production of Actimmune is achieved by fermentation of a genetically engineered *Escherichia coli* bacterium containing the DNA which encodes for the human protein. Purification of the product is achieved by conventional column chromatography. Actimmune is a highly purified sterile solution consisting of non-covalent dimers of two identical 16,465 dalton monomers; with a specific activity of 20 million International Units (IU)/mg (2×10^6 IU per 0.5 ml) which is equivalent to 30 million units/mg.

Actimmune is a sterile, clear, colorless solution filled in a single-dose vial for subcutaneous injection. *Each 0.5 ml of Actimmune Contains:* 100 μg (2 million IU) of interferon gamma-1b, formulated in 20 mg mannitol, 0.36 mg sodium succinate, 0.05 mg polysorbate 20 and sterile water for injection. *Note that the above activity is expressed in International Units (1 million IU/50 μg). This is equivalent to what was previously expressed as units (1.5 million U/50 μg).*

INDICATIONS AND USAGE

Interferon gamma-1b, recombinant is indicated for reducing the frequency and severity of serious infections associated with Chronic Granulomatous Disease.

Interferon gamma-1b, recombinant is indicated for delaying time to disease progression in patients with severe, malignant osteopetrosis.

NON-FDA APPROVED INDICATIONS

Although not an approved indication by the FDA, several studies have reported the efficacy of interferon gamma-1b in the treatment of rheumatoid arthritis.

CONTRAINDICATIONS

Interferon gamma-1b, recombinant is contraindicated in patients who develop or have known hypersensitivity to interferon-gamma, *E. coli* derived products, or any component of the product.

WARNINGS

Interferon gamma-1b, recombinant should be used with caution in patients with pre-existing cardiac disease, including symptoms of ischemia, congestive heart failure or arrhythmia. No direct cardiotoxic effect has been demonstrated but it is possible that acute and transient "flu-like" or constitutional symptoms such as fever, and chills frequently associated with interferon gamma-1b, recombinant administration at doses of 250 μg/m²/day or higher may exacerbate pre-existing cardiac conditions.

Caution should be exercised when treating patients with known seizure disorders and/or compromised central nervous system function. Central nervous system adverse reactions including decreased mental status, gait disturbance and dizziness have been observed, particularly in patients receiving doses greater than 250 μg/m²/day. Most of these abnormalities were mild and reversible within a few days upon dose reduction or discontinuation of therapy.

Caution should be exercised when administering interferon gamma-1b, recombinant to patients with myelosuppression. Reversible neutropenia and elevation of hepatic enzymes can be dose limiting above 250 μg/m²/day. Thrombocytopenia and proteinuria have also been seen rarely.

I

DOSAGE AND ADMINISTRATION

The recommended dosage of interferon gamma-1b, recombinant for the treatment of patients with Chronic Granulomatous Disease and severe, malignant osteopetrosis is 50 μg/m²(1 million IU/m²) for patients whose body surface area is greater than 0.5 m² and 1.5 μg/kg/dose for patients whose body surface area is equal to or less than 0.5 m². Note that the above activity is expressed in International Units (1 million IU/50 μg). *This is equivalent to what was previously expressed as units (1.5 million U/50 μg).* Injections should be administered subcutaneously 3 times weekly (for example, Monday, Wednesday, Friday). The optimum sites of injection are the right and left deltoid and anterior thigh. Interferon gamma-1b, recombinant can be administered by a physician, nurse, family member or patient when trained in the administration of subcutaneous injections. Parenteral drug products should be inspected visually for particulate matter and discoloration prior to administration, whenever solution and container permit.

The formulation does not contain a preservative. A vial of interferon gamma-1b, recombinant is suitable for a single dose only. The unused portion of any vial should be discarded.

Higher doses are not recommended. Safety and efficacy has not been established for interferon gamma-1b, recombinant given in doses greater or less than the recommended dose of 50 μg/m². The minimum effective dose of interferon gamma-1b, recombinant has not been established.

If severe reactions occur, the dosage should be modified (50% reduction) or therapy should be discontinued until the adverse reaction abates.

Interferon gamma-1b, recombinant may be administered using either sterilized glass or plastic disposable syringes.

PRODUCT LISTING - EQUIVALENTS NOT AVAILABLE

Solution - Injectable - 2000000 IU/0.5 ml

0.50 ml	$223.49	ACTIMMUNE, Connetics Inc	64116-0011-01
0.50 ml x 12	$2438.10	ACTIMMUNE, Connetics Inc	64116-0011-12

Ipecac Syrup (001575)

Categories: Overdose, drug; Poisoning; FDA Pre 1938 Drugs; WHO Formulary
Drug Classes: Vitamins/minerals
Brand Names: Ipecac

DESCRIPTION

Ipecac syrup contains 7 g of ipecac per 100 ml.

INDICATIONS AND USAGE

It is useful as an emetic to induce vomiting in poisoning.

CONTRAINDICATIONS

It should not be given to unconscious patients.

WARNINGS

Ipecac syrup may not be effective in those cases in which the ingested substance is an antiemetic.

The drug can exert a cardiotoxic effect if it is not vomited but is absorbed.

PRECAUTIONS

Emesis is not the proper treatment in all cases of potential poisoning; it should not be induced when such substances as petroleum distillates, strong alkali, acids, or strychnine are ingested.

DOSAGE AND ADMINISTRATION

Children less than 1 year of age: 1-2 teaspoonfuls.
Children over 1 year of age and adults: 3 teaspoonfuls.

The dosage may be repeated in 20 minutes if vomiting does not occur. Then, if the patient does not vomit, the dosage should be recovered (lavage).

HOW SUPPLIED

Ipecac syrup is supplied in 16 fl oz bottles.

Ipratropium Bromide *(001578)*

For related information, see the comparative table section in Appendix A.

Categories: Bronchitis, chronic; Emphysema; FDA Approved 1986 Dec; Pregnancy Category B; WHO Formulary
Drug Classes: Anticholinergics; Bronchodilators
Brand Names: Atrovent
Foreign Brand Availability: Aerovent (Bahrain; Cyprus; Egypt; Iran; Iraq; Israel; Jordan; Kuwait; Lebanon; Libya; Oman; Qatar; Republic-of-Yemen; Saudi-Arabia; Syria; United-Arab-Emirates); Apovent (Israel); Aproven (Australia); Atem (Bahrain; Cyprus; Egypt; Iran; Iraq; Italy; Jordan; Kuwait; Lebanon; Libya; Oman; Qatar; Republic-of-Yemen; Saudi-Arabia; Syria; United-Arab-Emirates); Atronase (Belgium); Atrovent Aerosol (Australia; New-Zealand); Atrovent Nasal (Australia; Hong-Kong; New-Zealand); Ipra Uni-dose (New-Zealand); Ipravent (Hong-Kong; India); Ipvent (South-Africa); Narilet (Spain); Tropium (Costa-Rica; Dominican-Republic; El-Salvador; Guatemala; Honduras; Nicaragua; Panama)
Cost of Therapy: \$38.87 (Emphysema; Atrovent Inhaler; 18 µg/inh; 14 g; 8 inhalations/day; 25 day supply)
\$42.46 (Allergic Rhinitis; Atrovent Nasal; 21 µg/spray; 12 sprays/day; 28 day supply)
HCFA JCODE(S): J7645 per ml INH

I

INHALATION

DESCRIPTION

The active ingredient in Atrovent is ipratropium bromide monohydrate. It is an anticholinergic bronchodilator chemically described as 8-azoniabicyclo(3.2.1)-octane,3-(3-hydroxy-1-oxo-2-phenylpropoxy)-8-methyl-8-(1-methylethyl)-, bromide, monohydrate *(endo, syn)*-, (±)-; a synthetic quaternary ammonium compound, chemically related to atropine.

Ipratropium bromide is a white to off-white crystalline substance, freely soluble in water and lower alcohols. It is a quaternary ammonium compound and thus exists in an ionized state in aqueous solutions. It is relatively insoluble in non-polar media.

Atrovent Inhalation Aerosol is an inhalation aerosol for oral administration. The net weight is 14 g; it yields 200 inhalations. Each actuation of the valve delivers 18 µg of ipratropium bromide from the mouthpiece. The inert ingredients are dichlorodifluoromethane, dichlorotetrafluoroethane, and trichlorofluoromethane as propellants and soya lecithin.

Atrovent Inhalation Solution is administered by oral inhalation with the aid of a nebulizer. It contains ipratropium bromide 0.02% (anhydrous basis) in a sterile, preservative-free, isotonic saline solution, pH-adjusted to 3.4 (3-4) with hydrochloric acid.

CLINICAL PHARMACOLOGY

Ipratropium bromide is an anticholinergic (parasympatholytic) agent that, based on animal studies, appears to inhibit vagally-mediated reflexes by antagonizing the action of acetylcholine, the transmitter agent released from the vagus nerve.

Anticholinergics prevent the increases in intracellular concentration of cyclic guanosine monophosphate (cyclic GMP) that are caused by interaction of acetylcholine with the muscarinic receptor on bronchial smooth muscle.

The bronchodilation following inhalation of ipratropium bromide is primarily a local, site-specific effect, not a systemic one. Much of an administered dose is swallowed but not absorbed, as shown by fecal excretion studies.

Following nebulization of a 2 mg dose, a mean 7% of the dose was absorbed into the systemic circulation either from the surface of the lung or from the gastrointestinal tract. The half-life of elimination is about 1.6 hours after intravenous administration. Ipratropium bromide is minimally (0-9% *in vitro*) bound to plasma albumin and α_1-acid glycoproteins. It is partially metabolized. Autoradiographic studies in rats have shown that ipratropium bromide does not penetrate the blood-brain barrier. Ipratropium bromide has not been studied in patients with hepatic or renal insufficiency. It should be used with caution in those patient populations.

In controlled 12 week studies in patients with bronchospasm associated with chronic obstructive pulmonary disease (chronic bronchitis and emphysema) significant improvements in pulmonary function (FEV_1 increases of 15% or more) occurred within 15-30 minutes, reached a peak in 1-2 hours, and persisted for periods of 4-5 hours in the majority of patients, with about 25-38% of the patients demonstrating increases of 15% or more for at least 7-8 hours. Continued effectiveness of ipratropium bromide inhalation solution was demonstrated throughout the 12 week period. In addition, significant increases in forced vital capacity (FVC) have been demonstrated. However, ipratropium bromide did not consistently produce significant improvement in subjective symptom scores nor in quality of life scores over the 12 week duration of study.

Additional controlled 12 week studies were conducted to evaluate the safety and effectiveness of ipratropium bromide inhalation solution administered concomitantly with the beta adrenergic bronchodilator solutions metaproterenol and albuterol compared with the administration of each of the beta agonists alone. Combined therapy produced significant additional improvement in FEV_1 and FVC. On combined therapy, the median duration of 15% improvement in FEV_1 was 5-7 hours, compared with 3-4 hours in patients receiving a beta agonist alone.

INDICATIONS AND USAGE

Ipratropium bromide inhalation solution administered either alone or with other bronchodilators, especially beta adrenergics, is indicated as a bronchodilator for maintenance treatment of bronchospasm associated with chronic obstructive pulmonary disease, including chronic bronchitis and emphysema.

CONTRAINDICATIONS

Ipratropium bromide inhalation aerosol is contraindicated in patients with a history of hypersensitivity to soya lecithin or related food products such as soybean and peanut.

Ipratropium bromide is contraindicated in known or suspected cases of hypersensitivity to ipratropium bromide, or to atropine and its derivatives.

WARNINGS

The use of ipratropium bromide inhalation solution as a single agent for the relief of bronchospasm in acute COPD exacerbation has not been adequately studied. Drugs with faster onset of action may be preferable as initial therapy in this situation. Combination of ipratropium bromide and beta agonists has not been shown to be more effective than either drug alone in reversing the bronchospasm associated with acute COPD exacerbation.

PRECAUTIONS

GENERAL

Ipratropium bromide should be used with caution in patients with narrow-angle glaucoma, prostatic hypertrophy or bladder-neck obstruction.

INFORMATION FOR THE PATIENT

Patients should be advised that temporary blurring of vision, precipitation or worsening of narrow-angle glaucoma or eye pain may result if the solution comes into direct contact with the eyes. Use of a nebulizer with mouthpiece rather than face mask may be preferable, to reduce the likelihood of the nebulizer solution reaching the eyes. Patients should be advised that ipratropium bromide inhalation solution can be mixed in the nebulizer with albuterol if used within 1 hour. Compatibility data are not currently available with other drugs. Patients should be reminded that ipratropium bromide Inhalation Solution should be used consistently as prescribed throughout the course of therapy.

CARCINOGENESIS, MUTAGENESIS, AND IMPAIRMENT OF FERTILITY

Two (2) year oral carcinogenicity studies in rats and mice have revealed no carcinogenic potential at dietary doses up to 6 mg/kg/day of ipratropium bromide.

Results of various mutagenicity studies (Ames test, mouse dominant lethal test, mouse micronucleus test and chromosome aberration of bone marrow in Chinese hamsters) were negative.

Fertility of male or female rats at oral doses up to 50 mg/kg/day was unaffected by ipratropium bromide administration. At doses above 90 mg/kg, increased resorption and decreased conception rates were observed.

PREGNANCY, TERATOGENIC EFFECTS, PREGNANCY CATEGORY B

Oral reproduction studies performed in mice, rats and rabbits at doses 10, 100, and 125 mg/kg respectively, and inhalation reproduction studies in rats and rabbits at doses of 1.5 and 1.8 mg/kg (or approximately 38 and 45 times the recommended human daily dose) respectively, have demonstrated no evidence of teratogenic effects as a result of ipratropium bromide. However, no adequate or well-controlled studies have been conducted in pregnant women. Because animal reproduction studies are not always predictive of human response, ipratropium bromide should be used during pregnancy only if clearly needed.

NURSING MOTHERS

It is not known whether ipratropium bromide is excreted in human milk. Although lipid-insoluble quaternary bases pass into breast milk, it is unlikely that ipratropium bromide would reach the infant to a significant extent, especially when taken by inhalation since ipratropium bromide is not well absorbed systematically after inhalation or oral administration. However, because many drugs are excreted in human milk, caution should be exercised when ipratropium bromide is administered to a nursing woman.

PEDIATRIC USE

Safety and effectiveness in children below the age of 12 have not been established.

DRUG INTERACTIONS

Ipratropium bromide has been shown to be a safe and effective bronchodilator when used in conjunction with beta adrenergic bronchodilators. Ipratropium bromide has also been used with other pulmonary medications, including methylxanthines and corticosteroids, without adverse drug interactions.

ADVERSE REACTIONS

Adverse reaction information concerning ipratropium bromide inhalation solution is derived from 12 week active-controlled clinical trials. Additional information is derived from foreign post-marketing experience and the published literature.

All adverse events, regardless of drug relationship, reported by 3% or more patients in the 12 week controlled clinical trials appear in TABLE 1A, TABLE 1B and TABLE 1C.

Additional adverse reactions reported in less than 3% of the patients treated with ipratropium bromide include tachycardia, palpitations, eye pain, urinary retention, urinary tract infection and urticaria. A single case of anaphylaxis thought to be possibly related to ipratropium bromide has been reported. Cases of precipitation or worsening of narrow-angle glaucoma and acute eye pain have been reported.

Lower respiratory adverse reactions (bronchitis, dyspnea and bronchospasm) were the most common events leading to discontinuation of ipratropium bromide therapy in the 12 week trials. Headache, mouth dryness and aggravation of COPD symptoms are more common when the total daily dose of ipratropium bromide equals or exceeds 2000 µg.

*TABLE 1A All Adverse Events, From a Double-Blind, Parallel, 12 Week Study of Patients With COPD**

	Ipratropium Bromide (500 μg tid) n=219	Metaproterenol (15 mg tid) n=212
Body as a Whole — General Disorders		
Headache	6.4%	5.2%
Pain	4.1%	3.3%
Influenza-like symptoms	3.7%	4.7%
Back pain	3.2%	1.9%
Chest pain	3.2%	4.2%
Cardiovascular Disorders		
Hypertension/hypertension aggravated	0.9%	1.9%
Central & Peripheral Nervous System		
Dizziness	2.3%	3.3%
Insomnia	0.9%	0.5%
Tremor	0.9%	7.1%
Nervousness	0.5%	4.7%
Gastrointestinal System Disorders		
Mouth dryness	3.2%	0.0%
Nausea	4.1%	3.8%
Constipation	0.9%	0.0%
Musculo-Skeletal System Disorders		
Arthritis	0.9%	1.4%
Respiratory System Disorders (Lower)		
Coughing	4.6%	8.0%
Dyspnea	9.6%	13.2%
Bronchitis	14.6%	24.5%
Bronchospasm	2.3%	2.8%
Sputum increased	1.4%	1.4%
Respiratory disorder	0.0%	6.1%
Respiratory System Disorders (Upper)		
Upper respiratory tract infection	13.2%	11.3%
Pharyngitis	3.7%	4.2%
Rhinitis	2.3%	4.2%
Sinusitis	2.3%	2.8%

* All adverse events, regardless of drug relationship, reported by 3% or more patients in the 12 week controlled clinical trials.

*TABLE 1B All Adverse Events, From a Double-Blind, Parallel, 12 Week Study of Patients With COPD**

	Ipratropium Bromide / Metaprotrenol (500 μg tid/15 mg tid) n=108	Albuterol (2.5 mg tid) n=205
Body as a Whole — General Disorders		
Headache	6.5%	6.3%
Pain	0.9%	2.9%
Influenza-like symptoms	6.5%	0.5%
Back pain	1.9%	2.4%
Chest pain	5.6%	2.0%
Cardiovascular Disorders		
Hypertension/hypertension aggravated	0.9%	1.5%
Central & Peripheral Nervous System		
Dizziness	1.9%	3.9%
Insomnia	4.6%	1.0%
Tremor	8.3%	1.0%
Nervousness	6.5%	1.0%
Gastrointestinal System Disorders		
Mouth dryness	1.9%	2.0%
Nausea	1.9	2.9%
Constipation	3.7%	1.0%
Musculo-Skeletal System Disorders		
Arthritis	0.9%	0.5%
Respiratory System Disorders (Lower)		
Coughing	6.5%	5.4%
Dyspnea	16.7%	12.7%
Bronchitis	15.7%	16.6%
Bronchospasm	4.6%	5.4%
Sputum increased	4.6%	3.4%
Respiratory disorder	6.5%	2.0%
Respiratory System Disorders (Upper)		
Upper respiratory tract infection	9.3%	12.2%
Pharyngitis	5.6%	2.9%
Rhinitis	1.9%	2.4%
Sinusitis	0.9%	5.4%

* All adverse events, regardless of drug relationship, reported by 3% or more patients in the 12 week controlled clinical trials.

DOSAGE AND ADMINISTRATION

The usual dosage of ipratropium bromide inhalation solution is 500 μg (1 Unit-Dose Vial) administered 3-4 times a day by oral nebulization, with doses 6-8 hours apart. Ipratropium bromide inhalation solution unit-dose vials contain 500 μg ipratropium bromide anhydrous in 2.5 ml normal saline. Ipratropium bromide inhalation solution can be mixed in the nebulizer with albuterol if used within 1 hour. Compatibility data are not currently available with other drugs.

HOW SUPPLIED

Ipratropium bromide inhalation solution unit dose vial is supplied as a 0.02% clear, colorless solution containing 2.5 ml with 25 vials per foil pouch.

Each vial is made from a low density polyethylene (LDPE) resin.

*TABLE 1C All Adverse Events, From a Double-Blind, Parallel, 12 WEEK Study of Patients With COPD**

	Ipratropium Bromide/Albuterol (500 μg tid/2.5 mg tid) n=100
Body as a Whole — General Disorders	
Headache	9.0%
Pain	5.0%
Influenza-like symptoms	1.0%
Back pain	0.0%
Chest pain	1.0%
Cardiovascular Disorders	
Hypertension/hypertension aggravated	4.0%
Central & Peripheral Nervous System	
Dizziness	4.0%
Insomnia	1.0%
Tremor	0.0%
Nervousness	1.0%
Gastrointestinal System Disorders	
Mouth dryness	3.0%
Nausea	2.0%
Constipation	1.0%
Musculo-Skeletal System Disorders	
Arthritis	3.0%
Respiratory System Disorders (Lower)	
Coughing	6.0%
Dyspnea	9.0%
Bronchitis	20.0%
Bronchospasm	5.0%
Sputum increased	0.0%
Respiratory disorder	4.0%
Respiratory System Disorders (Upper)	
Upper respiratory tract infection	16.0%
Pharyngitis	4.0%
Rhinitis	0.0%
Sinusitis	4.0%

* All adverse events, regardless of drug relationship, reported by 3% or more patients in the 12 week controlled clinical trials.

Ipratropium bromide inhalation aerosol is supplied as a metered dose inhaler with a white mouthpiece which has a clear, colorless sleeve and a green protective cap. Ipratropium bromide inhalation aerosol with mouthpiece, net contents 14 g. Ipratropium bromide inhalation aerosol refill, net contents 14 g. Each 14 g vial provides sufficient medication for 200 inhalations. Each actuation delivers 18 μg of ipratropium bromide from the mouthpiece.

Storage: Store between 15-30°C (59-86°F). Protect from light. Avoid excessive humidity. Store unused vials in the foil pouch.

Note: The statement below is required by the federal Clean Air Act for all products containing chlorofluorocarbons (CFCs), including products such as this one:

Warning: Contains trichloromonofluoromethane (CFC-11), dichlorodifluoromethane (CFC-12) and dichlorotetrafluoroethane (CFC-114), substances which harm public health and the environment by destroying ozone in the upper atmosphere.

INTRANASAL

DESCRIPTION

The active ingredient in Atrovent nasal spray is ipratropium bromide monohydrate. It is an anticholinergic agent chemically described as 8-azoniabicyclo (3.2.1) octane,3-(3-hydroxy-1-oxo-2-phenylpropoxy)-8-methyl-8-(1-methylethyl)-, bromide, monohydrate *(endo,syn)*-, (±)- :a synthetic quaternary ammonium compound, chemically related to atropine.

Ipratropium bromide has the chemical formula $C_{20}H_{30}BrNO_3 \cdot H_2O$ and a molecular weight of 430.4.

Ipratropium bromide is a white to off-white, crystalline substance. It is freely soluble in lower alcohols and water, existing in an ionized state in aqueous solutions, and relatively insoluble in non-polar media.

Atrovent nasal spray 0.03% is a metered-dose, manual pump spray unit which delivers 21 μg (70 μl) ipratropium bromide per spray on an anhydrous basis in an isotonic, aqueous solution with pH adjusted to 4.7. It also contains benzalkonium chloride, edetate disodium, sodium chloride, sodium hydroxide, hydrochloric acid, and purified water. Each bottle contains 345 sprays.

Atrovent nasal spray 0.06% is intended for local administration to the nasal mucosa to control rhinorrhea in patients with the common cold. It contains 0.06% ipratropium bromide on an anhydrous basis (42 μg/spray) in an isotonic, aqueous solution with pH-adjusted to 4.7, which also contains benzalkonium cholride, edetate disodium, sodium chloride, sodium hyrdroxide, hydrochloric acid, and purified water.

CLINICAL PHARMACOLOGY

MECHANISM OF ACTION

Ipratropium bromide is an anticholinergic agent that inhibits vagally-mediated reflexes by antagonizing the action of acetylcholine at the cholinergic receptor. In humans, ipratropium bromide has anti-secretory properties and, when applied locally, inhibits secretions from the serous and seromucous glands lining the nasal mucosa. Ipratropium bromide is a quaternary amine that minimally crosses the nasal and gastrointestinal membrane and the blood-brain barrier, resulting in a reduction of the systemic anticholinergic effects (*e.g.*, neurologic, ophthalmic, cardiovascular, and gastrointestinal effects) that are seen with tertiary anticholinergic amines.

PHARMACOKINETICS

Ipratropium Bromide Nasal Spray 0.03%

Absorption

Ipratropium bromide is poorly absorbed into the systemic circulation following oral administration (2-3%). Less than 20% of an 84 μg per nostril dose was absorbed from the nasal mucosa of normal volunteers, induced-cold patients, or perennial rhinitis patients.

Distribution

Ipratropium bromide is minimally bound (0-9% *in vitro*) to plasma albumin and α_1-acid glycoprotein. Its blood/plasma concentration ratio was estimated to be about 0.89. Studies in rats have shown that ipratropium bromide does not penetrate the blood-brain barrier.

Metabolism

Ipratropium bromide is partially metabolized to ester hydrolysis products, tropic acid and tropane. These metabolites appear to be inactive based on *in vitro* receptor affinity studies using rat brain tissue homogenates.

Elimination

After intravenous administration of 2 mg ipratropium bromide to 10 healthy volunteers, the terminal half-life of ipratropium was approximately 1.6 hours. The total body clearance and renal clearance were estimated to be 2505 and 1019 ml/min, respectively. The amount of the total dose excreted unchanged in the urine (Ae) within 24 hours was approximately one-half of the administered dose.

Pediatrics

Following administration of 42 μg of ipratropium bromide per nostril 2 or 3 times a day in perennial rhinitis patients 6-18 years old, the mean amounts of the total dose excreted in the urine (8.6-11.1%) were higher than those reported in adult volunteers or adult perennial rhinitis patients (3.7-5.6%). Plasma ipratropium were relatively low (ranging from undetectable up to 0.49 ng/ml). No correlation of the amount of the total dose excreted unchanged in the urine (Ae) with age or gender was observed in the pediatric population.

I

Special Populations

Gender does not appear to influence the absorption or excretion of nasally administered ipratropium bromide. The pharmacokinetics of ipratropium bromide have not been studied in patients with hepatic or renal insufficiency or in the elderly.

Drug-Drug Interactions

No specific pharmacokinetic studies were conducted to evaluate potential drug-drug interactions.

Pharmacodynamics

In two single-dose trials (n=17), doses up to 336 μg of ipratropium bromide did not significantly affect pupillary diameter, hear rate, or systolic/diastolic blood pressure. Similarly, in patients with induced-colds, ipratropium bromide nasal spray 0.06% (84 μg/nostril 4 times a day), had no significant effects on pupillary diameter, heart rate or systolic/diastolic blood pressure.

Two nasal provocation trials in perennial rhinitis patients (n=44) using ipratropium bromide nasal spray showed a dose-dependent increase in inhibition of methacholine induced nasal secretion with an onset of action within 15 minutes (time of first observation).

Controlled clinical trials demonstrated that intranasal fluorocarbon-propelled ipratropium bromide does not alter physiologic nasal functions (*e.g.,* sense of smell, ciliary beat frequency, mucociliary clearance, or the air conditioning capacity of the nose).

Ipratropium Bromide Nasal Spray 0.06%

Ipratropium bromide is a quaternary amine that is poorly absorbed into the systemic circulation from the nasal mucosa. Less than 20% of an 84 μg per nostril dose is absorbed from the nasal mucosa of normal volunteers, induced-cold patients or perennial rhinitis patients, but the amount of ipratropium bromide which is systemically absorbed from nasal administration exceeds the amount of ipratropium bromide absorbed from either ipratropium bromide inhalation solution (2% of a 500 μg dose) or ipratropium bromide inhalation aerosol (20% of a 36 μg mouthpiece dose).

The half-life of elimination of ipratropium is about 1.6 hours after intravenous administration. Ipratropium bromide is minimally bound (0-9% *in vitro*) to plasma albumin and a_1-acid glycoprotein. It is partially metabolized to inactive ester hydrolysis products. Following intravenous administration, approximately one-half of the dose is excreted unchanged in the urine. Studies in rats have shown that ipratropium bromide does not penetrate the blood-brain barrier. The pharmacokinetics of ipratropium bromide have not been studied in patients with hepatic or renal insufficiency or in the elderly. Gender does not seem to influence the absorption or excretion of nasally administered ipratropium bromide.

Pharmacodynamic data also indicate little systemic absorption. In two single dose, pharmacokinetic trials (n=17), solutions of up to 0.12% ipratropium bromide (336 μg total nasal dose) did not significantly affect pupillary diameter, heart rate or systolic/diastolic blood pressure. Similarly, in an induced-cold, pharmacokinetic trial with ipratropium bromide nasal spray 0.06% (84 μg/nostril 4 times a day) no significant effects on pupillary diameter, heart rate, or systolic/diastolic blood pressures were observed.

Controlled clinical trials demonstrated that intranasal fluorocarbon-propelled ipratropium bromide does not alter physiologic nasal functions (*e.g.,* sense of smell, ciliary beat frequency, mucocilliary clearance, or the air conditioning capacity of the nose).

INDICATIONS AND USAGE

IPRATROPIUM BROMIDE NASAL SPRAY 0.03%

Indicated for the symptomatic relief of rhinorrhea associated with allergic and nonallergic perennial rhinitis in adults and children age 6 years and older. Ipratropium bromide nasal spray 0.03% does not relieve nasal congestion, sneezing or postnasal drip associated with allergic or nonallergic perennial rhinitis.

IPRATROPIUM BROMIDE NASAL SPRAY 0.06%

Indicated for the symptomatic relief of rhinorrhea associated with the common cold for adults and children age 12 years and older. Ipratropium bromide nasal spray 0.03% does not relieve nasal congestion or sneezing associated with the common cold.

The safety and effectiveness of the use of ipratropium bromide nasal spray 0.06% beyond 4 days in patients with the common cold has not been established.

CONTRAINDICATIONS

Ipratropium bromide nasal spray is contraindicated in patients with a history of hypersensitivity to atropine or its derivatives, or to any of the other ingredients.

WARNINGS

Immediate hypersensitivity reactions may occur after administration of ipratropium bromide, as demonstrated by rare cases of urticaria, angioedema, rash, bronchospasm and oropharyngeal edema.

PRECAUTIONS

GENERAL

Ipratropium bromide nasal spray should be used with caution in patients with narrow-angle glaucoma, prostatic hypertrophy or bladder neck obstruction, particularly if they are receiving an anticholinergic by another route. Cases of precipitation or worsening of narrow-angle glaucoma and acute eye pain have been reported with direct eye contact of ipratropium bromide administered by oral inhalation.

INFORMATION FOR THE PATIENT

Patients should be advised that temporary blurring of vision, precipitation or worsening of narrow-angle glaucoma or eye pain may result if ipratropium bromide nasal spray comes into direct contact with the eyes. Patients should be instructed to avoid spraying ipratropium bromide nasal spray in or around their eyes. Patients who experience eye pain, blurred vision, excessive nasal dryness or episodes of nasal bleeding should be instructed to contact their doctor.

CARCINOGENESIS, MUTAGENESIS, AND IMPAIRMENT OF FERTILITY

Ipratropium Bromide Nasal Spray 0.03%

In 2 year carcinogenicity studies in rats and mice, ipratropium bromide at oral doses up to 6 mg/kg (approximately 190 and 95 times the maximum recommended daily intranasal dose in adults, respectively, and approximately 110 and 60 times the maximum recommended daily intranasal dose in children, respectively, on a mg/m^2 basis) showed no carcinogenic activity.

Results of various mutagenicity studies (Ames test, mouse dominant lethal test, mouse micronucleus test, and chromosome aberration of bone marrow in Chinese hamsters) were negative.

Fertility of male or female rats was unaffected by ipratropium bromide at oral doses up to 50 mg/kg/day (about 1600 times the maximum recommended daily intranasal dose in adults on a mg/m^2 basis). At an oral dose of 500 mg/kg (approximately 16,000 times the maximum recommended daily intranasal doses in adults on a mg/m^2 basis), ipratropium bromide produced a decrease in the conception rate.

Ipratropium Bromide Nasal Spray 0.06%

Two (2) year oral carcinogenicity studies in rats and mice have revealed no carcinogenic activity at doses up to 6 mg/kg/day. This dose corresponds, in rats and mice respectively, to about 70 and 40 times the maximum recommended human daily dose (MRHD) on a mg/m^2 basis of ipratropium bromide nasal spray 0.06%. Results of various mutagenicity studies (Ames test, mouse dominant lethal test, mouse micronucleus test and chromosome aberration of bone marrow in Chinese hamsters) were negative.

Fertility of male or female rats at oral doses up to 50 mg/kg/day (about 600 times the MRHD on a mg/m^2 basis) was unaffected by ipratropium bromide administration. At doses above 90 mg/kg/day (about 1000 times the MRHD on a mg/m^2 basis), a decreased conception rate was observed.

PREGNANCY, TERATOGENIC EFFECTS, PREGNANCY CATEGORY B

Oral reproduction studies were performed at doses of 10 mg/kg/day in mice, 100 mg/kg/day in rats and 125 mg/kg/day in rabbits. These doses correspond, in each species respectively, to about 160, 3000 and 8000 times the maximum recommended daily intranasal dose of ipratropium bromide nasal spray 0.03% and to about 60, 1200, and 3000 times the MRHD of ipratropium bromide nasal spray 0.06% in the common cold (672 μg/day) on a mg/m^2 basis. Inhalation reproduction studies in rats and rabbits at doses of 1.5 and 1.8 mg/kg/day (about 50 and 120 times the MRHD for 0.03% nasal spray and 20 and 40 the MRHD for 0.06% nasal spray, on a mg/m^2 basis for each species, respectively) have demonstrated no evidence of teratogenic effects as a result of ipratropium bromide. At oral doses above 90 mg/kg/day in rats (about 3000 times the MRHD for 0.03% nasal spray and 1000 times the MRHD for 0.06% nasal spray, on a mg/m^2 basis) embryotoxicity was observed as increased resorption. This effect is not considered relevant to human use due to the large doses at which it was observed and the difference in route of administration. However, no adequate or well controlled studies have been conducted in pregnant women. Because animal reproduction studies are not always predictive of human response, ipratropium bromide nasal spray should be used during pregnancy only if clearly needed.

NURSING MOTHERS

It is known that some ipratropium bromide is systemically absorbed following nasal administration; however the portion which may be excreted in human milk is unknown. Although lipid-insoluble quatemary bases pass into breast milk, the minimal systemic absorption makes it unlikely that ipratropium bromide would reach the infant in an amount sufficient to cause a clinical effect. However, because many drugs are excreted in human milk, caution should be exercised when ipratropium bromide nasal spray is administered to a nursing woman.

PEDIATRIC USE

Ipratropium Bromide Nasal Spray 0.03%

The safety of ipratropium bromide nasal spray 0.03% at a dose of two sprays (42 μg) per nostril 2 or 3 times daily (total dose 168 to 252 μg/day) has been demonstrated in 77 pediatric patients 6-12 years of age in placebo-controlled, 4 week trials and in 55 pediatric patients in active-controlled, 6 month trials. The effectiveness of ipratropium bromide nasal spray 0.03% for the treatment of rhinorrhea associated with allergic and nonallergic perennial rhinitis in this pediatric age group is based on an extrapolation of the demonstrated efficacy of ipratropium bromide nasal spray 0.03% in adults with these conditions and the likelihood that the disease course, pathophysiology, and the drug's effects are substantially similar to that of the adults. The recommended dose for the pediatric population is based on within and cross-study comparisons of the efficacy of ipratropium bromide nasal spray 0.03% in adults and pediatric patients and on its safety profile in both adults and pediatric patients. The safety and effectiveness of ipratropium bromide nasal spray 0.03% in patients under 6 years of age have not been established.

Ipratropium Bromide Nasal Spray 0.06%

Safety and effectiveness of ipratropium bromide nasal spray 0.06% in patients below the age of 12 years have not been established.

DRUG INTERACTIONS

No controlled clinical trials were conducted to investigate drug-drug interactions. Ipratropium bromide nasal spray, 0.03%and 0.06%, is minimally absorbed into the systemic circulation; nonetheless, there is some potential for an additive interaction with other concomitantly administered anticholinergic medications, including ipratropium bromide for oral inhalation.

ADVERSE REACTIONS

IPRATROPIUM BROMIDE NASAL SPRAY 0.03%

Adverse reaction information on ipratropium bromide nasal spray 0.03% in patients with perennial rhinitis was derived from four multicenter, vehicle-controlled clinical trials involving 703 patients (356 patients on ipratropium bromide nasal spray 0.03% and 347 patients on vehicle), and a 1 year, open-label, follow-up trial. In three of the trials, patients received ipratropium bromide nasal spray 0.03% three times daily, for 8 weeks. In the other trial, ipratropium bromide nasal spray 0.03% was given to patients 2 times daily for 4 weeks. Of the 285 patients who entered the open-label, follow-up trial, 232 were treated for 3 months, 200 for 6 months, and 159 up to 1 year. The majority (>86%) of patients treated for 1 year were maintained on 42 μg per nostril, 2 or 3 times daily, of ipratropium bromide nasal spray 0.03%.

TABLE 1 shows adverse events, and the frequency that these adverse events led to the discontinuation of treatment, reported for patients who received ipratropium bromide nasal spray 0.03% at the recommended dose of 42 μg per nostril, or vehicle 2 or 3 times daily for 4 or 8 weeks. Only adverse events reported with an incidence of at least 2.0% in the ipratropium bromide nasal spray 0.03% group and higher in the ipratropium bromide nasal spray 0.03% group than in the vehicle group are shown.

TABLE 1 *Percent of Patients Reporting Events**

	Nasal Spray 0.03% (n=356)		Vehicle Control (n=347)	
	Incidence	Discontinued	Incidence	Discontinued
Headache	9.8%	0.6%	9.2%	0%
Upper respiratory tract infection	9.8%	1.4%	7.2%	1.4%
Epistaxis†	9.0%	0.3%	4.6%	0.3%
Rhinitis‡				
Nasal dryness	5.1%	0%	0.9%	0.3%
Nasal irritation§	2.0%	0%	1.7%	0.6%
Other nasal symptoms¤	3.1%	1.1%	1.7%	0.3%
Pharyngitis	8.1%	0.3%	4.6%	0%
Nausea	2.2%	0.3%	0.9%	0%

* This table includes adverse events which occurred at an incidence rate of at least 2.0% in the ipratropium bromide nasal spray 0.03% group and more frequently in the ipratropium bromide nasal spray 0.03% group than in the vehicle group.

† Epistaxis reported by 7.0% of ipratropium bromide patients and 2.3% of vehicle patients, blood-tinged mucus by 2.0% of ipratropium bromide patients and 2.3% of vehicle patients.

‡ All events are listed by their WHO term; rhinitis has been presented by descriptive terms for clarification.

§ Nasal irritation includes reports of nasal itching, nasal burning, nasal irritation and ulcerative rhinitis.

¤ Other nasal symptoms include reports of nasal congestion, increased rhinorrhea, increased rhinitis, posterior nasal drip, sneezing, nasal polyps and nasal edema.

Ipratropium bromide nasal spray 0.03% was well tolerated by most patients. The most frequently reported nasal adverse events were transient episodes of nasal dryness or epistaxis. These adverse events were mild or moderate in nature, none was considered serious, none resulted in hospitalization and most resolved spontaneously or following a dose reduction. Treatment for nasal dryness and epistaxis was required infrequently (2% or less) and consisted of local application of pressure or a moisturizing agent (*e.g.,* petroleum jelly or saline nasal spray). Patient discontinuation for epistaxis or nasal dryness was infrequent in both the controlled (0.3% or less) and 1 year, open-label (2% or less) trials. There was no evidence of nasal rebound (*i.e.,* a clinically significant increase in rhinorrhea, posterior nasal drip, sneezing or nasal congestion severity compared to baseline) upon discontinuation of double-blind therapy in these trials.

Adverse events reported by less than 2% of the patients receiving ipratropium bromide nasal spray 0.03% during the controlled clinical trials or during the open-label follow-up trial, which are potentially related to ipratropium bromide's local effects or systemic anticholinergic effects include: dry mouth/throat, dizziness, ocular irritation, blurred vision, conjunctivitis, hoarseness, cough and taste perversion. Additional anticholinergic effects noted with other ipratropium bromide dosage forms (ipratropium bromide inhalation solution, ipratropium bromide inhalation aerosol, and ipratropium bromide nasal spray 0.06%) include: precipitation or worsening of narrow angle glaucoma, urinary retention, prostatic disorders, tachycardia, constipation, and bowel obstruction.

There were infrequent reports of skin rash in both the controlled and uncontrolled clinical studies. Other allergic-type reactions such as angioedema of the throat, tongue, lips and face, urticaria, laryngospasm and anaphylactic reactions have been reported with other ipratropium bromide products.

No controlled trial was conducted to address the relative incidence of adverse events of bid versus tid therapy.

IPRATROPIUM BROMIDE NASAL SPRAY 0.06%

Adverse reaction information on ipratropium bromide nasal spray 0.06% in patients with the common cold was derived from two multi-center, vehicle-controlled clinical trials involving 1276 patients (195 patients on ipratropium bromide nasal spray 0.03%, 352 patients on ipratropium bromide nasal spray 0.06%, 189 patients on ipratropium bromide nasal spray 0.12%, 351 patients on vehicle and 189 patients receiving no treatment).

TABLE 2 shows adverse events reported for patients who received ipratropium bromide nasal spray 0.06% at the recommended dose of 84 μg per nostril, or vehicle, administered 3 or 4 times daily, where the incidence is 1% or greater in the ipratropium bromide group and higher in the ipratropium bromide group than in the vehicle group.

TABLE 2 *Percent of Patients Reporting Events**

	Nasal Spray 0.06% (n=352)	Vehicle Control (n=351)
Epistaxis†	8.2%	2.3%
Dry mouth/throat	1.4%	0.3%
Nasal congestion	1.1%	0.0%
Nasal dryness	4.8%	2.8%

* This table includes adverse events for which the incidence was 1% or greater in the ipratropium bromide group and higher in the ipratropium bromide than in the vehicle group.

† Epistaxis reported by 5.4% of ipratropium bromide patients and 1.4% of vehicle patients, blood tinged mucus by 2.8% of ipratropium bromide patients and 0.9% of vehicle patients.

Ipratropium bromide nasal spray 0.06% was well tolerated by most patients. The most frequently reported adverse events were transient episodes of nasal dryness or epistaxis. The majority of these adverse events (96%) were mild or moderate in nature, none was considered serious, and none resulted in hospitalization. No patient required treatment for nasal dryness, and only 3 patients (<1%) required treatment for epistaxis, which consisted of local application of pressure or a moisturizing agent (*e.g.,* petroleum jelly). No patient receiving ipratropium bromide nasal spray 0.06% was discontinued from the trial due to either nasal dryness or bleeding.

Adverse events reported by less than 1% of the patients receiving ipratropium bromide nasal spray 0.06% during the controlled clinical trials which are potentially related to the local or systemic anticholinergic effects of ipratropium bromide nasal spray 0.06% include: taste perversion, nasal burning, conjunctivitis, coughing, dizziness, hoarseness, palpitation, pharyngitis, tachycardia, thirst, tinnitus and blurred vision. Additional anticholinergic effects noted with other ipratropium bromide dosage forms (ipratropium bromide inhalation solution, ipratropium bromide inhalation aerosol and ipratropium bromide nasal spray 0.03%) include: precipitation or worsening of narrow-angle glaucoma, urinary retention, prostate disorders, constipation and bowel obstruction.

There were no reports of allergic-type reactions in the controlled clinical trials. Allergic-type reactions such as skin rash, angioedema of the tongue, lips and face, urticaria, laryngospasm and anaphylactic reactions have been reported with other ipratropium bromide products.

No controlled trial was conducted to address the relative incidence of adverse events for tid versus qid therapy.

DOSAGE AND ADMINISTRATION

The recommended dose of ipratropium bromide nasal spray 0.03% is two sprays (42 μg) per nostril 2 or 3 times daily (total dose 168-252 μg/day) for the symptomatic relief of rhinorrhea associated with allergic and nonallergic perennial rhinitis in adults and children age 6 years and older. Optimum dosage varies with the response of the individual patient.

The recommended dose of ipratropium bromide nasal spray 0.06% is two sprays (84 μg) per nostril 3 or 4 times daily (total dose 504-672 μg/day) for the symptomatic relief of rhinorrhea associated with the common cold in adults and children age 12 years and older. Optimum dosage varies with the response of the individual patient.

The safety and effectiveness of the use of ipratropium bromide nasal spray 0.06% beyond 4 days in patients with the common cold have not been established.

Initial pump priming requires 7 actuations of the pump. If used regularly as recommended, no further priming is required. If not used for more than 24 hours, the pump will require 2 actuations, or if not used for more than 7 days, the pump will require 7 actuations to reprime.

HOW SUPPLIED

Atrovent nasal spray 0.03% is supplied in a white high density polyethylene (HDPE) bottle fitted with a white and clear metered nasal spray pump, a green safety clip to prevent accidental discharge of the spray, and a clear plastic dust cap. It contains as 31.1 g of product formulation, 345 sprays, each delivering 21 μg (70 μl) of ipratropium per spray, or 28 days of therapy at the maximum recommended dose (2 sprays per nostril 3 times a day).

Atrovent nasal spray 0.06% is supplied as 15 ml of solution in a high density polyethylene (HDPE) bottle fitted with a metered nasal spray pump, a safety clip to prevent accidental discharge of the spray, and a clear plastic dust cap. The 15 ml bottle of Atrovent nasal spray is designed to deliver 165 sprays of 0.07 ml each (42 μg ipratropium bromide).

Storage: Store tightly closed between 15-30°C (59-86°F). Avoid freezing. Keep out of reach of children. Avoid spraying in or around the eyes.

PRODUCT LISTING - RATED THERAPEUTICALLY EQUIVALENT

Solution - Inhalation - 0.02%

2.50 ml x 25	$44.00	GENERIC, Ivax Corporation	00172-6407-44
2.50 ml x 25	$44.00	GENERIC, Dey Laboratories	49502-0685-03
2.50 ml x 25	$44.06	GENERIC, Roxane Laboratories Inc	00054-8404-11
2.50 ml x 25	$56.00	GENERIC, Apotex Usa Inc	60505-0806-01
2.50 ml x 25	$56.50	GENERIC, Alpharma Uspd Makers Of Barre and Nmc	00472-0751-23
2.50 ml x 25	$87.50	ATROVENT, Boehringer-Ingelheim	00597-0080-62
2.50 ml x 30	$39.60	GENERIC, Nephron	00487-9801-01
2.50 ml x 30	$39.60	GENERIC, Nephron	00487-9801-30
2.50 ml x 30	$52.80	GENERIC, Dey Laboratories	49502-0685-33
2.50 ml x 30	$52.87	GENERIC, Roxane Laboratories Inc	00054-8404-13
2.50 ml x 60	$79.20	GENERIC, Nephron	00487-9801-60
2.50 ml x 60	$105.60	GENERIC, Ivax Corporation	00172-6407-49
2.50 ml x 60	$105.60	GENERIC, Dey Laboratories	49502-0685-60
2.50 ml x 60	$105.74	GENERIC, Roxane Laboratories Inc	00054-8404-21
2.50 ml x 60	$118.80	GENERIC, Alpharma Uspd Makers Of Barre and Nmc	00472-0751-60

PRODUCT LISTING - EQUIVALENTS NOT AVAILABLE

Aerosol - Inhalation - 18 mcg/Inh			
14 gm	$38.87	ATROVENT, Allscripts Pharmaceutical Company	54569-1006-00
14 gm	$46.32	ATROVENT, Physicians Total Care	54868-1439-01
14 gm	$52.24	ATROVENT, Boehringer-Ingelheim	00597-0082-14
Solution - Inhalation - 0.02%			
2.50 ml x 25	$18.62	GENERIC, Allscripts Pharmaceutical Company	54569-4910-00
2.50 ml x 25	$26.31	GENERIC, Physicians Total Care	54868-4082-01
2.50 ml x 25	$44.00	GENERIC, Roxane Laboratories Inc	00054-8402-11
2.50 ml x 25	$52.75	GENERIC, Rxelite	66794-0002-25
2.50 ml x 30	$52.80	GENERIC, Roxane Laboratories Inc	00054-8402-13
2.50 ml x 30	$63.30	GENERIC, Rxelite	66794-0002-30
2.50 ml x 30	$67.80	GENERIC, Alpharma Uspd Makers Of Barre and Nmc	00472-0751-30
2.50 ml x 60	$53.95	GENERIC, Physicians Total Care	54868-4082-00
2.50 ml x 60	$105.60	GENERIC, Roxane Laboratories Inc	00054-8402-21
2.50 ml x 60	$126.60	GENERIC, Rxelite	66794-0002-60
Spray - Nasal - 21 mcg/Inh			
30 ml	$42.46	ATROVENT NASAL, Allscripts Pharmaceutical Company	54569-4420-00
30 ml	$57.56	ATROVENT NASAL, Boehringer Mannheim	00597-0081-30
Spray - Nasal - 42 mcg/Inh			
15 ml	$36.38	ATROVENT NASAL, Allscripts Pharmaceutical Company	54569-4421-00
15 ml	$49.35	ATROVENT NASAL, Boehringer Mannheim	00597-0086-76

Irbesartan (003356)

For related information, see the comparative table section in Appendix A.

Categories: Nephropathy, diabetic; Hypertension, essential; Pregnancy Category C, 1st Trimester; Pregnancy Category D, 2nd & 3rd Trimesters; FDA Approved 1997 Oct
Drug Classes: Angiotensin II receptor antagonists
Brand Names: Avapro
Foreign Brand Availability: Approvel (Germany); Aprovel (Austria; Belgium; Bulgaria; Colombia; Czech-Republic; Denmark; England; Finland; France; Germany; Greece; Hong-Kong; Hungary; Indonesia; Ireland; Italy; Mexico; Netherlands; Norway; Peru; Philippines; Poland; Portugal; Singapore; Slovenia; South-Africa; Spain; Sweden; Switzerland; Taiwan; Thailand; Turkey); Irban (Israel); Irovel (India); Irvell (Indonesia); Karvea (Australia; Austria; Belgium; Bulgaria; Czech-Republic; Denmark; England; Finland; France; Germany; Greece; Hungary; Ireland; Italy; Netherlands; Norway; Poland; Portugal; Slovenia; Spain; Sweden; Switzerland; Turkey)
Cost of Therapy: $47.52 (Hypertension; Avapro; 150 mg; 1 tablet/day; 30 day supply)

WARNING

USE IN PREGNANCY

When used in pregnancy during the second and third trimesters, drugs that act directly on the renin-angiotensin system can cause injury and even death to the developing fetus. When pregnancy is detected, irbesartan should be discontinued as soon as possible. See WARNINGS, Fetal/Neonatal Morbidity and Mortality.

DESCRIPTION

Irbesartan is an angiotensin II receptor (AT_1 subtype) antagonist.

Irbesartan is a non-peptide compound, chemically described as a 2-butyl-3-[*p*-(*o*-1*H*-tetrazol-5-ylphenyl)benzyl]-1,3-diazaspiro[4.4]non-1-en-4-one.

Its empirical formula is $C_{25}H_{28}N_6O$.

Irbesartan is a white to off-white crystalline powder with a molecular weight of 428.5. It is a nonpolar compound with a partition coefficient (octanol/water) of 10.1 at pH of 7.4. Irbesartan is slightly soluble in alcohol and methylene chloride and practically insoluble in water.

Avapro is available for oral administration in unscored tablets containing 75, 150, or 300 mg of irbesartan. *Inactive Ingredients Include:* Lactose, microcrystalline cellulose, pregelatinized starch, croscarmellose sodium, poloxamer 188, silicon dioxide, and magnesium stearate.

CLINICAL PHARMACOLOGY

MECHANISM OF ACTION

Angiotensin II is a potent vasoconstrictor formed from angiotensin I in a reaction catalyzed by angiotensin-converting enzyme (ACE, kininase II). Angiotensin II is the principal pressor agent of the renin-angiotensin system (RAS) and also stimulates aldosterone synthesis and secretion by adrenal cortex, cardiac contraction, renal resorption of sodium, activity of the sympathetic nervous system, and smooth muscle cell growth. Irbesartan blocks the vasoconstrictor and aldosterone-secreting effects of angiotensin II by selectively binding to the AT_1 angiotensin II receptor. There is also an AT_2 receptor in many tissues, but it is not involved in cardiovascular homeostasis.

Irbesartan is a specific competitive antagonist of AT_1 receptors with a much greater affinity (more than 8500-fold) for the AT_1 receptor than for the AT_2 receptor and no agonist activity.

Blockade of the AT_1 receptor removes the negative feedback of angiotensin II on renin secretion, but the resulting increased plasma renin activity and circulating angiotensin II do not overcome the effects of irbesartan on blood pressure.

Irbesartan does not inhibit ACE or renin or affect other hormone receptors or ion channels known to be involved in the cardiovascular regulation of blood pressure and sodium homeostasis. Because irbesartan does not inhibit ACE, it does not affect the response to bradykinin; whether this has clinical relevance is not known.

PHARMACOKINETICS

Irbesartan is an orally active agent that does not require biotransformation into an active form. The oral absorption of irbesartan is rapid and complete with an average absolute bioavailability of 60-80%. Following oral administration of irbesartan, peak plasma concentrations of irbesartan are attained at 1.5-2 hours after dosing. Food does not affect the bioavailability of irbesartan.

Irbesartan exhibits linear pharmacokinetics over the therapeutic dose range.

The terminal elimination half-life of irbesartan averaged 11-15 hours. Steady-state concentrations are achieved within 3 days. Limited accumulation of irbesartan (<20%) is observed in plasma upon repeated once-daily dosing.

METABOLISM AND ELIMINATION

Irbesartan is metabolized via glucuronide conjugation and oxidation. Following oral or IV administration of ^{14}C-labeled irbesartan, more than 80% of the circulating plasma radioactivity is attributable to unchanged irbesartan. The primary circulating metabolite is the inactive irbesartan glucuronide conjugate (approximately 6%). The remaining oxidative metabolites do not add appreciably to irbesartan's pharmacologic activity.

Irbesartan and its metabolites are excreted by both biliary and renal routes. Following either oral or IV administration of ^{14}C-labeled irbesartan, about 20% of radioactivity is recovered in the urine and the remainder in the feces, as irbesartan or irbesartan glucuronide.

In vitro studies of irbesartan oxidation by cytochrome P450 isoenzymes indicated irbesartan was oxidized primarily by 2C9; metabolism by 3A4 was negligible. Irbesartan was neither metabolized by, nor did it substantially induce or inhibit, isoenzymes commonly associated with drug metabolism (1A1, 1A2, 2A6, 2B6, 2D6, 2E1). There was no induction or inhibition of 3A4.

DISTRIBUTION

Irbesartan is 90% bound to serum proteins (primarily albumin and α_1-acid glycoprotein) with negligible binding to cellular components of blood. The average volume of distribution is 53-93 L. Total plasma and renal clearances are in the range of 157-176 ml/min and 3.0-3.5 ml/min, respectively. With repetitive dosing, irbesartan accumulates to no clinically relevant extent.

Studies in animals indicate that radiolabeled irbesartan weakly crosses the blood brain barrier and placenta. Irbesartan is excreted in the milk of lactating rats.

SPECIAL POPULATIONS

Pediatric

The pharmacokinetics of irbesartan were studied in hypertensive children (age 6-12, n=9) and adolescents (age 13-16, n=12) following single and multiple daily doses of 2 mg/kg (maximum dose of 150 mg/day) for 4 weeks. Accumulation with repeated doses was limited (18%) in both age groups. Clearance rates, AUC values, and C_{max} values were comparable to adults receiving 150 mg daily. Irbesartan pharmacokinetics have not been investigated in patients <6 years of age.

Gender

No gender related differences in pharmacokinetics were observed in healthy elderly (age 65-80 years) or in healthy young (age 18-40 years) subjects. In studies of hypertensive patients, there was no gender difference in half-life or accumulation, but somewhat higher plasma concentrations of irbesartan were observed in females (11-44%). No gender-related dosage adjustment is necessary.

Geriatric

In elderly subjects (age 65-80 years), irbesartan elimination half-life was not significantly altered, but AUC and C_{max} values were about 20-50% greater than those of young subjects (age 18-40 years). No dosage adjustment is necessary in the elderly.

Race

In healthy black subjects, irbesartan AUC values were approximately 25% greater than whites; there were no differences in C_{max} values.

Renal Insufficiency

The pharmacokinetics of irbesartan were not altered in patients with renal impairment or in patients on hemodialysis. Irbesartan is not removed by hemodialysis. No dosage adjustment is necessary in patients with mild to severe renal impairment unless a patient with renal impairment is also volume depleted (see WARNINGS, Hypotension in Volume- or Salt-Depleted Patients and DOSAGE AND ADMINISTRATION).

Hepatic Insufficiency

The pharmacokinetics of irbesartan following repeated oral administration were not significantly affected in patients with mild to moderate cirrhosis of the liver. No dosage adjustment is necessary in patients with hepatic insufficiency.

Drug Interactions

See DRUG INTERACTIONS.

PHARMACODYNAMICS

In healthy subjects, single oral irbesartan doses of up to 300 mg produced dose-dependent inhibition of the pressor effect of angiotensin II infusions. Inhibition was complete (100%) 4 hours following oral doses of 150 or 300 mg and partial inhibition was sustained for 24 hours (60% and 40% at 300 mg and 150 mg, respectively).

In hypertensive patients, angiotensin II receptor inhibition following chronic administration of irbesartan causes a 1.5- to 2-fold rise in angiotensin II plasma concentration and a 2- to 3-fold increase in plasma renin levels. Aldosterone plasma concentrations generally decline following irbesartan administration, but serum potassium levels are not significantly affected at recommended doses.

In hypertensive patients, chronic oral doses of irbesartan (up to 300 mg) had no effect on glomerular filtration rate, renal plasma flow or filtration fraction. In multiple dose studies in hypertensive patients, there were no clinically important effects on fasting triglycerides, total cholesterol, HDL-cholesterol, or fasting glucose concentrations. There was no effect on serum uric acid during chronic oral administration, and no uricosuric effect.

INDICATIONS AND USAGE

HYPERTENSION

Irbesartan is indicated for the treatment of hypertension. It may be used alone or in combination with other antihypertensive agents.

Nephropathy in Type 2 Diabetic Patients

Irbesartan is indicated for the treatment of diabetic nephropathy with an elevated serum creatinine and proteinuria (>300 mg/day) in patients with Type 2 diabetes and hypertension. In this population, irbesartan reduces the rate of progression of nephropathy as measured by the occurrence of doubling of serum creatinine or end-stage renal disease (need for dialysis or renal transplantation).

NON-FDA APPROVED INDICATIONS

Irbesartan has been investigated in the management of hyperaldosteronism, and for its ability to significantly reduce levels of inflammatory markers (superoxide, tumor necrosis factor aRII, and vascular cell adhesion molecule-1) without affecting blood pressure in normotensive patients with premature atherosclerosis; however, these uses are not approved by the FDA.

CONTRAINDICATIONS

Irbesartan is contraindicated in patients who are hypersensitive to any component of this product.

WARNINGS

FETAL/NEONATAL MORBIDITY AND MORTALITY

Drugs that act directly on the renin-angiotensin system can cause fetal and neonatal morbidity and death when administered to pregnant women. Several dozen cases have been reported in the world literature in patients who were taking angiotensin-converting-enzyme inhibitors. When pregnancy is detected, irbesartan should be discontinued as soon as possible.

The use of drugs that act directly on the renin-angiotensin system during the second and third trimesters of pregnancy has been associated with fetal and neonatal injury, including hypotension, neonatal skull hypoplasia, anuria, reversible or irreversible renal failure, and death. Oligohydramnios has also been reported, presumably resulting from decreased fetal renal function; oligohydramnios in this setting has been associated with fetal limb contractures, craniofacial deformation, and hypoplastic lung development. Prematurity, intrauterine growth retardation, and patent ductus arteriosus have also been reported, although it is not clear whether these occurrences were due to exposure to the drug.

These adverse effects do not appear to have resulted from intrauterine drug exposure that has been limited to the first trimester.

Mothers whose embryos and fetuses are exposed to an angiotensin II receptor antagonist only during the first trimester should be so informed. Nonetheless, when patients become pregnant, physicians should have the patient discontinue the use of irbesartan as soon as possible.

Rarely (probably less often than once in every thousand pregnancies), no alternative to a drug acting on the renin-angiotensin system will be found. In these rare cases, the mothers should be apprised of the potential hazards to their fetuses, and serial ultrasound examinations should be performed to assess the intraamniotic environment.

If oligohydramnios is observed, irbesartan should be discontinued unless it is considered life-saving for the mother. Contraction stress testing (CST), a non-stress test (NST), or biophysical profiling (BPP) may be appropriate depending upon the week of pregnancy. Patients and physicians should be aware, however, that oligohydramnios may not appear until after the fetus has sustained irreversible injury.

Infants with histories of *in utero* exposure to an angiotensin II receptor antagonist should be closely observed for hypotension, oliguria, and hyperkalemia. If oliguria occurs, attention should be directed toward support of blood pressure and renal perfusion. Exchange transfusion or dialysis may be required as means of reversing hypotension and/or substituting for disordered renal function.

When pregnant rats were treated with irbesartan from day 0 to day 20 of gestation (oral doses of 50, 180, and 650 mg/kg/day), increased incidences of renal pelvic cavitation, hydroureter and/or absence of renal papilla were observed in fetuses at doses ≥50 mg/kg/day (approximately equivalent to the maximum recommended human dose [MRHD], 300 mg/day, on a body surface area basis). Subcutaneous edema was observed in fetuses at doses ≥180 mg/kg/day (about 4 times the MRHD on a body surface area basis). As these anomalies were not observed in rats in which irbesartan exposure (oral doses of 50, 150, and 450 mg/kg/day) was limited to gestation days 6-15, they appear to reflect late gestational effects of the drug. In pregnant rabbits, oral doses of 30 mg irbesartan/kg/day were associated with maternal mortality and abortion. Surviving females receiving this dose (about 1.5 times the MRHD on a body surface area basis) had a slight increase in early resorptions and a corresponding decrease in live fetuses. Irbesartan was found to cross the placental barrier in rats and rabbits.

Radioactivity was present in the rat and rabbit fetus during late gestation and in rat milk following oral doses of radiolabeled irbesartan.

HYPOTENSION IN VOLUME- OR SALT-DEPLETED PATIENTS

Excessive reduction of blood pressure was rarely seen (<0.1%) in patients with uncomplicated hypertension. Initiation of antihypertensive therapy may cause symptomatic hypotension in patients with intravascular volume- or sodium-depletion, *e.g.*, in patients treated vigorously with diuretics or in patients on dialysis). Such volume depletion should be corrected prior to administration of irbesartan, or a low starting dose should be used (see DOSAGE AND ADMINISTRATION).

If hypotension occurs, the patient should be placed in the supine position and, if necessary, given an IV infusion of normal saline. A transient hypotensive response is not a contraindication to further treatment, which usually can be continued without difficulty once the blood pressure has stabilized.

PRECAUTIONS

IMPAIRED RENAL FUNCTION

As a consequence of inhibiting the renin-angiotensin-aldosterone system, changes in renal function may be anticipated in susceptible individuals. In patients whose renal function may depend on the activity of the renin-angiotensin-aldosterone system (*e.g.*, patients with severe congestive heart failure), treatment with angiotensin-converting-enzyme inhibitors has been associated with oliguria and/or progressive azotemia and (rarely) with acute renal failure and/or death. Irbesartan would be expected to behave similarly.

In studies of ACE inhibitors in patients with unilateral or bilateral renal artery stenosis, increases in serum creatinine or BUN have been reported. There has been no known use of irbesartan in patients with unilateral or bilateral renal artery stenosis, but a similar effect should be anticipated.

INFORMATION FOR THE PATIENT

Pregnancy

Female patients of childbearing age should be told about the consequences of second- and third-trimester exposure to drugs that act on the renin-angiotensin system, and they should also be told that these consequences do not appear to have resulted from intrauterine drug exposure that has been limited to the first trimester. These patients should be asked to report pregnancies to their physicians as soon as possible.

CARCINOGENESIS, MUTAGENESIS, AND IMPAIRMENT OF FERTILITY

No evidence of carcinogenicity was observed when irbesartan was administered at doses of up to 500/1000 mg/kg/day (males/females, respectively) in rats and 1000 mg/kg/day in mice for up to 2 years. For male and female rats, 500 mg/kg/day provided an average systemic exposure to irbesartan [AUC(0-24h) bound plus unbound] about 3 and 11 times, respectively, the average systemic exposure in humans receiving the maximum recommended dose (MRD) or 300 mg irbesartan/day, whereas 1000 mg/kg/day (administered to females only) provided an average systemic exposure about 21 times that reported for humans at the MRD. For male and female mice, 1000 mg/kg/day provided an exposure to irbesartan about 3 and 5 times, respectively, the human exposure at 300 mg/day.

Irbesartan was not mutagenic in a battery of *in vitro* tests (Ames microbial test, rat hepatocyte DNA repair test, V79 mammalian-cell forward gene-mutation assay). Irbesartan was negative in several tests for induction of chromosomal aberrations (*in vitro*-human lymphocyte assay; *in vivo*-mouse micronucleus study).

Irbesartan had no adverse effects on fertility or mating of male or female rats at oral doses ≤650 mg/kg/day, the highest dose providing a systemic exposure to irbesartan [AUC(0-24h) bound plus unbound] about 5 times that found in humans receiving the maximum recommended dose of 300 mg/day.

PREGNANCY CATEGORY C (FIRST TRIMESTER) AND PREGNANCY CATEGORY D (SECOND AND THIRD TRIMESTERS)

See WARNINGS, Fetal/Neonatal Morbidity and Mortality.

NURSING MOTHERS

It is not known whether irbesartan is excreted in human milk, but irbesartan or some metabolite of irbesartan is secreted at low concentration in the milk of lactating rats. Because of the potential for adverse effects on the nursing infant, a decision should be made whether to discontinue nursing or discontinue the drug, taking into account the importance of the drug to the mother.

PEDIATRIC USE

Safety and effectiveness in pediatric patients have not been established.

Pharmacokinetic parameters in pediatric subjects (age 6-16, n=21) were comparable to adults. At doses up to 150 mg daily for 4 weeks, irbesartan was well tolerated in hypertensive children and adolescents (see CLINICAL PHARMACOLOGY, Special Populations). Blood pressure reductions were comparable to adults receiving 150 mg daily; however, greater sensitivity in some patients cannot be ruled out (see DOSAGE AND ADMINISTRATION, Pediatric Patients). Irbesartan has not been studied in pediatric patients less than 6 years old.

GERIATRIC USE

Of 4925 subjects receiving irbesartan in controlled clinical studies of hypertension, 911 (18.5%) were 65 years and over, while 150 (3.0%) were 75 years and over. No overall differences in effectiveness or safety were observed between these subjects and younger subjects, but greater sensitivity of some older individuals cannot be ruled out. (See CLINICAL PHARMACOLOGY: Pharmacokinetics and Special Populations.)

DRUG INTERACTIONS

No significant drug-drug pharmacokinetic (or pharmacodynamic) interactions have been found in interaction studies with hydrochlorothiazide, digoxin, warfarin, and nifedipine.

In vitro studies show significant inhibition of the formation of oxidized irbesartan metabolites with the known cytochrome CYP 2C9 substrates/inhibitors sulphenazole, tolbutamide, and nifedipine. However, in clinical studies the consequences of concomitant irbesartan on the pharmacodynamics of warfarin were negligible. Based on *in vitro* data, no interaction would be expected with drugs whose metabolism is dependent upon cytochrome P450 isozymes 1A1, 1A2, 2A6, 2B6, 2D6, 2E1, or 3A4.

In separate studies of patients receiving maintenance doses of warfarin, hydrochlorothiazide, or digoxin, irbesartan administration for 7 days had no effect on the pharmacodynamics of warfarin (prothrombin time) or pharmacokinetics of digoxin. The pharmacokinetics of irbesartan were not affected by coadministration of nifedipine or hydrochlorothiazide.

ADVERSE REACTIONS

HYPERTENSION

Irbesartan has been evaluated for safety in more than 4300 patients with hypertension and about 5000 subjects overall. This experience includes 1303 patients treated for over 6 months and 407 patients for 1 year or more. Treatment with irbesartan was well-tolerated, with an incidence of adverse events similar to placebo. These events generally were mild and transient with no relationship to the dose of irbesartan.

I

In placebo-controlled clinical trials, discontinuation of therapy due to a clinical adverse event was required in 3.3% of patients treated with irbesartan, versus 4.5% of patients given placebo.

In placebo-controlled clinical trials, the adverse event experiences reported in at least 1% of patients treated with irbesartan (n=1965) and at a higher incidence versus placebo (n=641), excluding those too general to be informative and those not reasonably associated with the use of drug because they were associated with the condition being treated or are very common in the treated population include: diarrhea (3% vs 2%), dyspepsia/heartburn (2% vs 1%), and fatigue (4% vs 3%).

The following adverse events occurred at an incidence of 1% or greater in patients treated with irbesartan, but were at least as frequent or more frequent in patients receiving placebo: Abdominal pain, anxiety/nervousness, chest pain, dizziness, edema, headache, influenza, musculoskeletal pain, pharyngitis, nausea/vomiting, rash, rhinitis, sinus abnormality, tachycardia, and urinary tract infection.

Irbesartan use was not associated with an increased incidence of dry cough, as is typically associated with ACE inhibitor use. In placebo controlled studies, the incidence of cough in irbesartan treated patients was 2.8% vs 2.7% in patients receiving placebo.

The incidence of hypotension or orthostatic hypotension was low in irbesartan treated patients (0.4%), unrelated to dosage, and similar to the incidence among placebo treated patients (0.2%). Dizziness, syncope, and vertigo were reported with equal or less frequency in patients receiving irbesartan compared with placebo.

In addition, the following potentially important events occurred in less than 1% of the 1965 patients and at least 5 patients (0.3%) receiving irbesartan in clinical studies, and those less frequent, clinically significant events (listed by body system). It cannot be determined whether these events were causally related to irbesartan:

Body as a Whole: Fever, chills, facial edema, upper extremity edema.

Cardiovascular: Flushing, hypertension, cardiac murmur, myocardial infarction, angina pectoris, arrhythmic/conduction disorder, cardio-respiratory arrest, heart failure, hypertensive crisis.

Dermatologic: Pruritus, dermatitis, ecchymosis, erythema face, urticaria.

Endocrine/Metabolic/Electrolyte Imbalances: Sexual dysfunction, libido change, gout.

Gastrointestinal: Constipation, oral lesion, gastroenteritis, flatulence, abdominal distention.

Musculoskeletal/Connective Tissue: Extremity swelling, muscle cramp, arthritis, muscle ache, musculoskeletal chest pain, joint stiffness, bursitis, muscle weakness.

Nervous System: Sleep disturbance, numbness, somnolence, emotional disturbance, depression, paresthesia, tremor, transient ischemic attack, cerebrovascular accident.

Renal/Genitourinary: Abnormal urination, prostate disorder.

Respiratory: Epistaxis, tracheobronchitis, congestion, pulmonary congestion, dyspnea, wheezing.

Special Senses: Vision disturbance, hearing abnormality, ear infection, ear pain, conjunctivitis, other eye disturbance, eyelid abnormality, ear abnormality.

NEPHROPATHY IN TYPE 2 DIABETIC PATIENTS

In clinical studies in patients with hypertension and Type 2 diabetic renal disease, the adverse drug experiences were similar to those seen in patients with hypertension with the exception of an increased incidence of orthostatic symptoms (dizziness, orthostatic dizziness, and orthostatic hypotension) observed in IDNT (proteinuria ≥900 mg/day, and serum creatinine ranging from 1.0-3.0 mg/dl). In this trial, orthostatic symptoms occurred more frequently in the irbesartan group (dizziness 10.2%, orthostatic dizziness 5.4%, orthostatic hypotension 5.4%) than in the placebo group (dizziness 6.0%, orthostatic dizziness 2.7%, orthostatic hypotension 3.2%).

POST-MARKETING EXPERIENCE

The following have been very rarely reported in post-marketing experience: Urticaria; angiodema (involving swelling of the face, lips, pharynx, and/or tongue); increased liver function tests; jaundice. Hyperkalemia has been rarely reported.

LABORATORY TEST FINDINGS

Hypertension

In controlled clinical trials, clinically important differences in laboratory tests were rarely associated with administration of irbesartan.

Creatinine, Blood Urea Nitrogen

Minor increases in blood urea nitrogen (BUN) or serum creatinine were observed in less than 0.7% of patients with essential hypertension treated with irbesartan alone vs 0.9% on placebo. (See PRECAUTIONS, Impaired Renal Function.)

Hematologic

Mean decreases in hemoglobin of 0.2 g/dl were observed in 0.2% of patients receiving irbesartan compared to 0.3% of placebo treated patients. Neutropenia (<1000 cells/mm^3) occurred at similar frequencies among patients receiving irbesartan (0.3%) and placebo treated patients (0.5%).

NEPHROPATHY IN TYPE 2 DIABETIC PATIENTS

Hyperkalemia

In IDNT (proteinuria ≥900 mg/day, and serum creatinine ranging from 1.0-3.0 mg/dl), the percent of patients with hyperkalemia (>6 mEq/L) was 18.6% in the irbesartan group vs 6.0% in the placebo group. Discontinuations due to hyperkalemia in the irbesartan group were 2.1% vs 0.4% in the placebo group.

DOSAGE AND ADMINISTRATION

Irbesartan may be administered with other antihypertensive agents and with or without food.

HYPERTENSION

The recommended initial dose of irbesartan is 150 mg once daily. Patients requiring further reduction in blood pressure should be titrated to 300 mg once daily.

A low dose of a diuretic may be added, if blood pressure is not controlled by irbesartan alone. Hydrochlorothiazide has been shown to have an additive effect. Patients not adequately treated by the maximum dose of 300 mg once daily are unlikely to derive additional benefit from a higher dose or twice-daily dosing.

No dosage adjustment is necessary in elderly patients, or in patients with hepatic impairment or mild to severe renal impairment.

NEPHROPATHY IN TYPE 2 DIABETIC PATIENTS

The recommended target maintenance dose is 300 mg once daily. There are no data on the clinical effects of lower doses of irbesartan on diabetic nephropathy.

PEDIATRIC PATIENTS

Children (<6 years): Safety and effectiveness have not been established.

Children (6-12 years): An initial dose of 75 mg once daily is reasonable. Patients requiring further reduction in blood pressure should be titrated to 150 mg once daily (see PRECAUTIONS, Pediatric Use).

Adolescent patients (13-16 years): An initial dose of 150 mg once daily is reasonable. Patients requiring further reduction in blood pressure should be titrated to 300 mg once daily. Higher doses are not recommended (see PRECAUTIONS, Pediatric Use).

VOLUME- AND SALT-DEPLETED PATIENTS

A lower initial dose of irbesartan (75 mg) is recommended in patients with depletion of intravascular volume or salt (*e.g.*, patients treated vigorously with diuretics or on hemodialysis) (see WARNINGS, Hypotension in Volume- or Salt-Depleted Patients).

HOW SUPPLIED

Avapro is available in:

75 mg tablets: White to off-white biconvex oval tablets, debossed with a heart shape on one side and "2771" on the other.

150 mg tablets: White to off-white biconvex oval tablets, debossed with a heart shape on one side and "2772" on the other.

300 mg tablets: White to off-white biconvex oval tablets, debossed with a heart shape on one side and "2773" on the other.

Storage: Store at a temperature between 15 and 30°C (59 and 86°F).

PRODUCT LISTING - EQUIVALENTS NOT AVAILABLE

Size	Price	Product	NDC
Tablet - Oral - 75 mg			
30's	$45.14	AVAPRO, Bristol-Myers Squibb	00087-2771-31
90's	$135.43	AVAPRO, Bristol-Myers Squibb	00087-2771-32
Tablet - Oral - 150 mg			
30's	$39.10	AVAPRO, Allscripts Pharmaceutical Company	54569-4572-00
30's	$47.51	AVAPRO, Bristol-Myers Squibb	00087-2772-31
90's	$142.56	AVAPRO, Bristol-Myers Squibb	00087-2772-32
100's	$158.40	AVAPRO, Bristol-Myers Squibb	00087-2772-35
Tablet - Oral - 300 mg			
30's	$47.00	AVAPRO, Allscripts Pharmaceutical Company	54569-4895-00
30's	$57.13	AVAPRO, Bristol-Myers Squibb	00087-2773-31
90's	$171.35	AVAPRO, Bristol-Myers Squibb	00087-2773-32
100's	$210.88	AVAPRO, Bristol-Myers Squibb	00087-2773-35

Irinotecan Hydrochloride *(003296)*

Categories: Carcinoma, colorectal; Pregnancy Category D; FDA Approved 1996 Jun
Drug Classes: Antineoplastics, topoisomerase inhibitors
Brand Names: Camptosar
Foreign Brand Availability: Campto (Benin; Burkina-Faso; Ethiopia; France; Gambia; Germany; Ghana; Guinea; Hong-Kong; Indonesia; Israel; Ivory-Coast; Japan; Kenya; Korea; Liberia; Malawi; Mali; Mauritania; Mauritius; Morocco; Niger; Nigeria; Philippines; Senegal; Seychelles; Sierra-Leone; South-Africa; Sudan; Tanzania; Thailand; Tunia; Uganda; Zambia; Zimbabwe); Irinotel (India); Topotecin (Japan)
HCFA JCODE(S): J9206 20 mg IV

WARNING

Irinotecan HCl injection should be administered only under the supervision of a physician who is experienced in the use of cancer chemotherapeutic agents. Appropriate management of complications is possible only when adequate diagnostic and treatment facilities are readily available.

Irinotecan HCl can induce both early and late forms of diarrhea that appear to be mediated by different mechanisms. Both forms of diarrhea may be severe.

Early diarrhea (occurring during or shortly after infusion of irinotecan HCl) may be accompanied by cholinergic symptoms of rhinitis, increased salivation, miosis, lacrimation, diaphoresis, flushing, and intestinal hyperperistalsis that can cause abdominal cramping. Early diarrhea and other cholinergic symptoms may be prevented or ameliorated by atropine (see PRECAUTIONS, General). Late diarrhea (generally occurring more than 24 hours after administration of irinotecan HCl) can be life threatening since it may be prolonged and may lead to dehydration, electrolyte imbalance, or sepsis. Late diarrhea should be treated promptly with loperamide. Patients with diarrhea should be carefully monitored and given fluid and electrolyte replacement if they become dehydrated or antibiotic therapy if they develop ileus, fever, or severe neutropenia (see WARNINGS). Administration of irinotecan HCl should be interrupted and subsequent doses reduced if severe diarrhea occurs (see DOSAGE AND ADMINISTRATION).

Severe myelosuppression may occur (see WARNINGS).

DESCRIPTION

Irinotecan hydrochloride injection is an antineoplastic agent of the topoisomerase I inhibitor class. Irinotecan hydrochloride was clinically investigated as CPT-11.

Camptosar is supplied as a sterile, pale yellow, clear, aqueous solution. It is available in two single-dose sizes: 2 ml fill vials contain 40 mg irinotecan hydrochloride and 5 ml fill vials contain 100 mg irinotecan hydrochloride. Each ml of solution contains 20 mg of irinotecan hydrochloride (on the basis of the trihydrate salt), 45 mg of sorbitol powder, and 0.9 mg of lactic acid. The pH of the solution has been adjusted to 3.5 (range, 3.0-3.8) with sodium hydroxide or hydrochloric acid. Irinotecan HCl is intended for dilution with 5% dextrose injection (D5W), or 0.9% sodium chloride injection, prior to intravenous infusion. The preferred diluent is 5% dextrose injection.

Irinotecan hydrochloride is a semisynthetic derivative of camptothecin, an alkaloid extract from plants such as *Camptotheca acuminata.* The chemical name is *(S)*-4,11-diethyl-3,4,12,14-tetrahydro-4-hydroxy-3,14-dioxo-1*H*-pyrano[3′,4′:6,7]-indolizino[1,2-b]quinolin-9-yl-[1,4′-bipiperidine]-1′-carboxylate, monohydrochloride, trihydrate.

Irinotecan hydrochloride is a pale yellow to yellow crystalline powder, with the empirical formula $C_{33}H_{38}N_4O_6 \cdot HCl \cdot 3H_2O$ and a molecular weight of 677.19. It is slightly soluble in water and organic solvents.

CLINICAL PHARMACOLOGY

Irinotecan is a derivative of camptothecin. Camptothecins interact specifically with the enzyme topoisomerase I which relieves torsional strain in DNA by inducing reversible single-strand breaks. Irinotecan and its active metabolite SN-38 bind to the topoisomerase I-DNA complex and prevent religation of these single-strand breaks. Current research suggests that the cytotoxicity of irinotecan is due to double-strand DNA damage produced during DNA synthesis when replication enzymes interact with the ternary complex formed by topoisomerase I, DNA, and either irinotecan or SN-38. Mammalian cells cannot efficiently repair these double-strand breaks.

Irinotecan serves as a water-soluble precursor of the lipophilic metabolite SN-38. SN-38 is formed from irinotecan by carboxylesterase-mediated cleavage of the carbamate bond between the camptothecin moiety and the dipiperidino side chain. SN-38 is approximately 1000 times as potent as irinotecan as an inhibitor of topoisomerase I purified from human and rodent tumor cell lines. *In vitro* cytotoxicity assays show that the potency of SN-38 relative to irinotecan varies from 2- to 2000-fold. However, the plasma area under the concentration versus time curve (AUC) values for SN-38 are 2-8% of irinotecan and SN-38 is 95% bound to plasma proteins compared to approximately 50% bound to plasma proteins for irinotecan (see Pharmacokinetics). The precise contribution of SN-38 to the activity of irinotecan HCl is thus unknown. Both irinotecan and SN-38 exist in an active lactone form and an inactive hydroxy acid anion form. A pH-dependent equilibrium exists between the two forms such that an acid pH promotes the formation of the lactone, while a more basic pH favors the hydroxy acid anion form.

Administration of irinotecan has resulted in antitumor activity in mice bearing cancers of rodent origin and in human carcinoma xenografts of various histological types.

PHARMACOKINETICS

After intravenous infusion of irinotecan in humans, irinotecan plasma concentrations decline in a multiexponential manner, with a mean terminal elimination half-life of about 6-12 hours. The mean terminal elimination half-life of the active metabolite SN-38 is about 10-20 hours. The half-lives of the lactone (active) forms of irinotecan and SN-38 are similar to those of total irinotecan and SN-38, as the lactone and hydroxy acid forms are in equilibrium.

Over the recommended dose range of 50-350 mg/m^2, the AUC of irinotecan increases linearly with dose; the AUC of SN-38 increases less than proportionally with dose. Maximum concentrations of the active metabolite SN-38 are generally seen within 1 hour following the end of a 90 minute infusion of irinotecan. Pharmacokinetic parameters for irinotecan and SN-38 following a 90 minute infusion of irinotecan at dose levels of 125 and 340 mg/m^2 determined in two clinical studies in patients with solid tumors are summarized in TABLE 1.

TABLE 1 *Summary of Mean (±SD) Irinotecan and SN-38 Pharmacokinetic Parameters in Patients With Solid Tumors*

	Dose	
	125 mg/m^2 n=64	340 mg/m^2 n=6
Irinotecan		
C_{max} (ng/ml)	1,660 ± 797	3,392 ± 874
AUC(0-24) (ng·h/ml)	10,200 ± 3,270	20,604 ± 6,027
T½ (h)	5.8* ± 0.7	11.7† ± 1.0
Vz (L/m^2)	110 ± 48.5	234 ± 69.6
CL (L/h/m^2)	13.3 ± 6.01	13.9 ± 4.0
SN-38		
C_{max} (ng/ml)	26.3 ± 11.9	56.0 ± 28.2
AUC(0-24) (ng·h/ml)	229 ± 108	474 ± 245
T½ (h)	10.4* ± 3.1	21.0† ± 4.3

* Plasma specimens collected for 24 hours following the end of the 90 minute infusion.
† Plasma specimens collected for 48 hours following the end of the 90 minute infusion. Because of the longer collection period, these values provide a more accurate reflection of the terminal elimination half-life of irinotecan and SN-38.
C_{max} = Maximum plasma concentration.
AUC(0-24) = Area under the plasma concentration-time curve from time 0 to 24 hours after the end of the 90 minute infusion.
T½ = Terminal elimination half-life.
Vz = Volume of distribution of terminal elimination phase.
CL = Total systemic clearance.

Irinotecan exhibits moderate plasma protein binding (30-68% bound). SN-38 is highly bound to human plasma proteins (approximately 95% bound). The plasma protein to which irinotecan and SN-38 predominantly binds is albumin.

Metabolism and Excretion

The metabolic conversion of irinotecan to the active metabolite SN-38 is mediated by carboxylesterase enzymes and primarily occurs in the liver. SN-38 subsequently undergoes conjugation to form a glucuronide metabolite. SN-38 glucuronide had 1/50 to 1/100 the activity of SN-38 in cytotoxicity assays using two cell lines *in vitro.* The disposition of irinotecan has not been fully elucidated in humans. The urinary excretion of irinotecan is 11-20%; SN-38, <1%; and SN-38 glucuronide, 3%. The cumulative biliary and urinary excretion of irinotecan and its metabolites (SN-38 and SN-38 glucuronide) over a period of 48 hours following administration of irinotecan in 2 patients ranged from approximately 25% (100 mg/m^2) to 50% (300 mg/m^2).

PHARMACOKINETICS IN SPECIAL POPULATIONS

Geriatric

In studies using the weekly schedule, the terminal half-life of irinotecan was 6.0 hours in patients who were 65 years or older and 5.5 hours in patients younger than 65 years. Dose-normalized AUC(0-24) for SN-38 in patients who were at least 65 years of age was 11% higher than in patients younger than 65 years. No change in the starting dose is recommended for geriatric patients receiving the weekly dosage schedule of irinotecan. The pharmacokinetics of irinotecan given once every 3 weeks has not been studied in the geriatric population; a lower starting dose is recommended in patients 70 years or older based on clinical toxicity experience with this schedule (see DOSAGE AND ADMINISTRATION).

Pediatric

Information regarding the pharmacokinetics of irinotecan is not available.

Gender

The pharmacokinetics of irinotecan do not appear to be influenced by gender.

Race

The influence of race on the pharmacokinetics of irinotecan has not been evaluated.

Hepatic Insufficiency

The influence of hepatic insufficiency on the pharmacokinetic characteristics of irinotecan and its metabolites has not been formally studied. Among patients with known hepatic tumor involvement (a majority of patients), irinotecan and SN-38 AUC values were somewhat higher than values for patients without liver metastases (see PRECAUTIONS).

Renal Insufficiency

The influence of renal insufficiency on the pharmacokinetics of irinotecan has not been evaluated.

DRUG-DRUG INTERACTIONS

In a Phase 1 clinical study involving irinotecan, 5-fluorouracil (5-FU), and leucovorin (LV) in 26 patients with solid tumors, the disposition of irinotecan was not substantially altered when the drugs were co-administered. Although the C_{max} and AUC(0-24) of SN-38, the active metabolite, were reduced (by 14% and 8%, respectively) when irinotecan was followed by 5-FU and LV administration compared with when irinotecan was given alone, this sequence of administration was used in the combination trials and is recommended (see DOSAGE AND ADMINISTRATION). Formal *in vivo* or *in vitro* drug interaction studies to

I

evaluate the influence of irinotecan on the disposition of 5-FU and LV have not been conducted.

Possible pharmacokinetic interactions of irinotecan HCl with other concomitantly administered medications have not been formally investigated.

INDICATIONS AND USAGE

Irinotecan HCl injection is indicated as a component of first-line therapy in combination with 5-fluorouracil and leucovorin for patients with metastatic carcinoma of the colon or rectum. Irinotecan HCl is also indicated for patients with metastatic carcinoma of the colon or rectum whose disease has recurred or progressed following initial fluorouracil-based therapy.

NON-FDA APPROVED INDICATIONS

Irinotecan has been tested in studies for the treatment of patients with squamous cell carcinoma of the cervix, brain tumors, leukemia, pancreatic cancer, gastric cancer, ovarian cancer and both non-small cell lung cancer and small cell lung cancer. While preliminary results are promising, additional confirmatory trials are needed.

CONTRAINDICATIONS

Irinotecan HCl injection is contraindicated in patients with a known hypersensitivity to the drug.

WARNINGS

GENERAL

Outside of a well-designed clinical study, irinotecan HCl injection should not be used in combination with the "Mayo Clinic" regimen of 5-FU/LV (administration for 4-5 consecutive days every 4 weeks) because of reports of increased toxicity, including toxic deaths. Irinotecan HCl should be used as recommended (see TABLE 10).

In patients receiving either irinotecan/5-FU/LV or 5-FU/LV in the clinical trials, higher rates of hospitalization, neutropenic fever, thromboembolism, first-cycle treatment discontinuation, and early deaths were observed in patients with a baseline performance status of 2 than in patients with a baseline performance status of 0 or 1.

DIARRHEA

Irinotecan HCl can induce both early and late forms of diarrhea that appear to be mediated by different mechanisms. Early diarrhea (occurring during or shortly after infusion of irinotecan HCl) is cholinergic in nature. It is usually transient and only infrequently is severe. It may be accompanied by symptoms of rhinitis, increased salivation, miosis, lacrimation, diaphoresis, flushing, and intestinal hyperperistalsis that can cause abdominal cramping. Early diarrhea and other cholinergic symptoms may be prevented or ameliorated by administration of atropine (see PRECAUTIONS, General, for dosing recommendations for atropine).

Late diarrhea (generally occurring more than 24 hours after administration of irinotecan HCl) can be life threatening since it may be prolonged and may lead to dehydration, electrolyte imbalance, or sepsis. Late diarrhea should be treated promptly with loperamide (see PRECAUTIONS, Information for the Patient, for dosing recommendations for loperamide). Patients with diarrhea should be carefully monitored, should be given fluid and electrolyte replacement if they become dehydrated, and should be given antibiotic support if they develop ileus, fever, or severe neutropenia. After the first treatment, subsequent weekly chemotherapy treatments should be delayed in patients until return of pretreatment bowel function for at least 24 hours without need for anti-diarrhea medication. If Grade 2, 3, or 4 late diarrhea occurs subsequent doses of irinotecan HCl should be decreased within the current cycle (see DOSAGE AND ADMINISTRATION).

NEUTROPENIA

Deaths due to sepsis following severe neutropenia have been reported in patients treated with irinotecan HCl. Neutropenic complications should be managed promptly with antibiotic support (see PRECAUTIONS). Therapy with irinotecan HCl should be temporarily omitted during a cycle of therapy if neutropenic fever occurs or if the absolute neutrophil count drops $<1500/mm^3$. After the patient recovers to an absolute neutrophil count $\geq 1500/mm^3$, subsequent doses of irinotecan HCl should be reduced depending upon the level of neutropenia observed (see DOSAGE AND ADMINISTRATION).

Routine administration of a colony-stimulating factor (CSF) is not necessary, but physicians may wish to consider CSF use in individual patients experiencing significant neutropenia.

HYPERSENSITIVITY

Hypersensitivity reactions including severe anaphylactic or anaphylactoid reactions have been observed.

COLITIS/ILEUS

Cases of colitis complicated by ulceration, bleeding, ileus, and infection have been observed. Patients experiencing ileus should receive prompt antibiotic support (see PRECAUTIONS).

RENAL IMPAIRMENT/RENAL FAILURE

Rare cases of renal impairment and acute renal failure have been identified, usually in patients who became volume depleted from severe vomiting and/or diarrhea.

THROMBOEMBOLISM

Thromboembolic events have been observed in patients receiving irinotecan-containing regimens; the specific cause of these events has not been determined.

PREGNANCY

Irinotecan HCl may cause fetal harm when administered to a pregnant woman. Radioactivity related to ^{14}C-irinotecan crosses the placenta of rats following intravenous administration of 10 mg/kg (which in separate studies produced an irinotecan C_{max} and AUC about 3 and 0.5 times, respectively, the corresponding values in patients administered 125 mg/m^2). Administration of 6 mg/kg/day intravenous irinotecan to rats (which in separate studies produced an irinotecan C_{max} and AUC about 2 and 0.2 times, respectively, the corresponding values in patients administered 125 mg/m^2) and rabbits (about one-half the recommended human weekly starting dose on a mg/m^2 basis) during the period of organogenesis, is embryotoxic as characterized by increased post-implantation loss and decreased numbers of live fetuses. Irinotecan was teratogenic in rats at doses greater than 1.2 mg/kg/day (which in separate studies produced an irinotecan C_{max} and AUC about 2/3 and 1/40th, respectively, of the corresponding values in patients administered 125 mg/m^2) and in rabbits at 6.0 mg/kg/day (about one-half the recommended human weekly starting dose on a mg/m^2 basis). Teratogenic effects included a variety of external, visceral, and skeletal abnormalities. Irinotecan administered to rat dams for the period following organogenesis through weaning at doses of 6 mg/kg/day caused decreased learning ability and decreased female body weights in the offspring. There are no adequate and well-controlled studies of irinotecan in pregnant women. If the drug is used during pregnancy, or if the patient becomes pregnant while receiving this drug, the patient should be apprised of the potential hazard to the fetus. Women of childbearing potential should be advised to avoid becoming pregnant while receiving treatment with irinotecan HCl.

PRECAUTIONS

GENERAL

Care of Intravenous Site

Irinotecan HCL injection is administered by intravenous infusion. Care should be taken to avoid extravasation, and the infusion site should be monitored for signs of inflammation. Should extravasation occur, flushing the site with sterile water and applications of ice are recommended.

Premedication With Antiemetics

Irinotecan is emetigenic. It is recommended that patients receive premedication with antiemetic agents. In clinical studies of the weekly dosage schedule, the majority of patients received 10 mg of dexamethasone given in conjunction with another type of antiemetic agent, such as a 5-HT^3 blocker (*e.g.,* ondansetron or granisetron). Antiemetic agents should be given on the day of treatment, starting at least 30 minutes before administration of irinotecan HCl. Physicians should also consider providing patients with an antiemetic regimen (*e.g.,* prochlorperazine) for subsequent use as needed.

Treatment of Cholinergic Symptoms

Prophylactic or therapeutic administration of 0.25 to 1 mg of intravenous or subcutaneous atropine should be considered (unless clinically contraindicated) in patients experiencing rhinitis, increased salivation, miosis, lacrimation, diaphoresis, flushing, abdominal cramping, or diarrhea (occurring during or shortly after infusion of irinotecan HCl). These symptoms are expected to occur more frequently with higher irinotecan doses.

Patients at Particular Risk

In patients receiving either irinotecan/5-FU/LV or 5-FU/LV in the clinical trials, higher rates of hospitalization, neutropenic fever, thromboembolism, first-cycle treatment discontinuation, and early deaths were observed in patients with a baseline performance status of 2 than in patients with a baseline performance status of 0 or 1. Patients who had previously received pelvic/abdominal radiation and elderly patients with comorbid conditions should be closely monitored.

The use of irinotecan HCl in patients with significant hepatic dysfunction has not been established. In clinical trials of either dosing schedule, irinotecan was not administered to patients with serum bilirubin >2.0 mg/dl, or transaminase >3 times the upper limit of normal if no liver metastasis, or transaminase >5 times the upper limit of normal with liver metastasis. However in clinical trials of the weekly dosage schedule, it has been noted that patients with modestly elevated baseline serum total bilirubin levels (1.0-2.0 mg/dl) have had a significantly greater likelihood of experiencing first-cycle Grade 3 or 4 neutropenia than those with bilirubin levels that were less than 1.0 mg/dl (50.0% [19/38] vs 17.7% [47/226]; $p < 0.001$). Patients with abnormal glucuronidation of bilirubin, such as those with Gilbert's syndrome, may also be at greater risk of myelosuppression when receiving therapy with irinotecan HCl. An association between baseline bilirubin elevations and an increased risk of late diarrhea has not been observed in studies of the weekly dosage schedule.

INFORMATION FOR THE PATIENT

Patients and patients' caregivers should be informed of the expected toxic effects of irinotecan HCl, particularly of its gastrointestinal complications, such as nausea, vomiting, abdominal cramping, diarrhea, and infection. Each patient should be instructed to have loperamide readily available and to begin treatment for late diarrhea (generally occurring more than 24 hours after administration of irinotecan HCl) at the first episode of poorly formed or loose stools or the earliest onset of bowel movements more frequent than normally expected for the patient. One dosage regimen for loperamide used in clinical trials consisted of the following (Note: This dosage regimen exceeds the usual dosage recommendations for loperamide.): 4 mg at the first onset of late diarrhea and then 2 mg every 2 hours until the patient is diarrhea-free for at least 12 hours. During the night, the patient may take 4 mg of loperamide every 4 hours. Premedication with loperamide is not recommended. The use of drugs with laxative properties should be avoided because of the potential for exacerbation of diarrhea. Patients should be advised to contact their physician to discuss any laxative use.

Patients should be instructed to contact their physician or nurse if any of the following occur: Diarrhea for the first time during treatment; black or bloody stools; symptoms of dehydration such as lightheadedness, dizziness, or faintness; inability to take fluids by mouth due to nausea or vomiting; inability to get diarrhea under control within 24 hours; or fever or evidence of infection.

Patients should be alerted to the possibility of alopecia.

LABORATORY TESTS

Careful monitoring of the white blood cell count with differential, hemoglobin, and platelet count is recommended before each dose of irinotecan HCl.

DRUG/LABORATORY TEST INTERACTIONS

There are no known interactions between irinotecan HCl and laboratory tests.

CARCINOGENESIS, MUTAGENESIS, AND IMPAIRMENT OF FERTILITY

Long-term carcinogenicity studies with irinotecan were not conducted. Rats were, however, administered intravenous doses of 2 mg/kg or 25 mg/kg irinotecan once per week for 13 weeks (in separate studies, the 25 mg/kg dose produced an irinotecan C_{max} and AUC that were about 7.0 times and 1.3 times the respective values in patients administered 125 mg/m^2 weekly) and were then allowed to recover for 91 weeks. Under these conditions, there was a significant linear trend with dose for the incidence of combined uterine horn endometrial stromal polyps and endometrial stromal sarcomas. Neither irinotecan nor SN-38 was mutagenic in the *in vitro* Ames assay. Irinotecan was clastogenic both *in vitro* (chromosome aberrations in Chinese hamster ovary cells) and *in vivo* (micronucleus test in mice). No significant adverse effects on fertility and general reproductive performance were observed after intravenous administration of irinotecan in doses of up to 6 mg/kg/day to rats and rabbits. However, atrophy of male reproductive organs was observed after multiple daily irinotecan doses both in rodents at 20 mg/kg (which in separate studies produced an irinotecan C_{max} and AUC about 5 and 1 times, respectively, the corresponding values in patients administered 125 mg/m^2 weekly) and dogs at 0.4 mg/kg (which in separate studies produced an irinotecan C_{max} and AUC about one-half and 1/15th, respectively, the corresponding values in patients administered 125 mg/m^2 weekly).

PREGNANCY CATEGORY D

See WARNINGS.

NURSING MOTHERS

Radioactivity appeared in rat milk within 5 minutes of intravenous administration of radiolabeled irinotecan and was concentrated up to 65-fold at 4 hours after administration relative to plasma concentrations. Because many drugs are excreted in human milk and because of the potential for serious adverse reactions in nursing infants, it is recommended that nursing be discontinued when receiving therapy with irinotecan HCl.

PEDIATRIC USE

The safety and effectiveness of irinotecan HCl in pediatric patients have not been established.

GERIATRIC USE

Patients greater than 65 years of age should be closely monitored because of a greater risk of late diarrhea in this population (see CLINICAL PHARMACOLOGY, Pharmacokinetics in Special Populations and ADVERSE REACTIONS, Overview of Adverse Events). The starting dose of irinotecan HCl in patients 70 years and older for the once-every-3-week dosage schedule should be 300 mg/m^2 (see DOSAGE AND ADMINISTRATION).

DRUG INTERACTIONS

The adverse effects of irinotecan HCl, such as myelosuppression and diarrhea, would be expected to be exacerbated by other antineoplastic agents having similar adverse effects.

Patients who have previously received pelvic/abdominal irradiation are at increased risk of severe myelosuppression following the administration of irinotecan HCl. The concurrent administration of irinotecan HCl with irradiation has not been adequately studied and is not recommended.

Lymphocytopenia has been reported in patients receiving irinotecan HCl, and it is possible that the administration of dexamethasone as antiemetic prophylaxis may have enhanced the likelihood of this effect. However, serious opportunistic infections have not been observed, and no complications have specifically been attributed to lymphocytopenia.

Hyperglycemia has also been reported in patients receiving irinotecan HCl. Usually, this has been observed in patients with a history of diabetes mellitus or evidence of glucose intolerance prior to administration of irinotecan HCl. It is probable that dexamethasone, given as antiemetic prophylaxis, contributed to hyperglycemia in some patients.

The incidence of akathisia in clinical trials of the weekly dosage schedule was greater (8.5%, 4/47 patients) when prochlorperazine was administered on the same day as irinotecan HCl than when these drugs were given on separate days (1.3%, 1/80 patients). The 8.5% incidence of akathisia, however, is within the range reported for use of prochlorperazine when given as a premedication for other chemotherapies.

It would be expected that laxative use during therapy with irinotecan HCl would worsen the incidence or severity of diarrhea, but this has not been studied.

In view of the potential risk of dehydration secondary to vomiting and/or diarrhea induced by irinotecan HCl, the physician may wish to withhold diuretics during dosing with irinotecan HCl and, certainly, during periods of active vomiting or diarrhea.

ADVERSE REACTIONS

FIRST-LINE COMBINATION THERAPY

A total of 955 patients with metastatic colorectal cancer received the recommended regimens of irinotecan in combination with 5-FU/LV, 5-FU/LV alone, or irinotecan alone. In the two Phase 3 studies, 370 patients received irinotecan in combination with 5-FU/LV, 362 patients received 5-FU/LV alone, and 223 patients received irinotecan alone. (See TABLE 10 for recommended combination-agent regimens.)

In Study 1, 49 (7.3%) patients died within 30 days of last study treatment: 21 (9.3%) received irinotecan in combination with 5-FU/LV, 15 (6.8%) received 5-FU/LV alone, and 13 (5.8%) received irinotecan alone. Deaths potentially related to treatment occurred in 2 (0.9%) patients who received irinotecan in combination with 5-FU/LV (2 neutropenic fever/sepsis), 3 (1.4%) patients who received 5-FU/LV alone (1 neutropenic fever/sepsis, 1 CNS bleeding during thrombocytopenia, 1 unknown) and 2 (0.9%) patients who received irinotecan alone (2 neutropenic fever). Deaths from any cause within 60 days of first study treatment were reported for 15 (6.7%) patients who received irinotecan in combination with 5-FU/LV, 16 (7.3%) patients who received 5-FU/LV alone, and 15 (6.7%) patients who received irinotecan alone. Discontinuations due to adverse events were reported for 17 (7.6%) patients who received irinotecan in combination with 5-FU/LV, 14 (6.4%) patients who received 5-FU/LV alone, and 26 (11.7%) patients who received irinotecan alone.

In Study 2, 10 (3.5%) patients died within 30 days of last study treatment: 6 (4.1%) received irinotecan in combination with 5-FU/LV and 4 (2.8%) received 5-FU/LV alone. There was one potentially treatment-death, which occurred in a patient who received irinotecan in combination with 5-FU/LV (0.7%, neutropenic sepsis). Deaths from any cause within 60 days of first study treatment were reported for 3 (2.1%) patients who received irinotecan in combination with 5-FU/LV and 2 (1.4%) patients who received 5-FU/LV alone. Discontinuations due to adverse events were reported for 9 (6.2%) patients who received irinotecan in combination with 5-FU/LV and 1 (0.7%) patient who received 5-FU/LV alone.

The most clinically significant adverse events for patients receiving irinotecan-based therapy were diarrhea, nausea, vomiting, neutropenia, and alopecia. The most clinically significant adverse events for patients receiving 5-FU/LV therapy were diarrhea, neutropenia, neutropenic fever, and mucositis. In Study 1, Grade 4 neutropenia, neutropenic fever (defined as Grade 2 fever and Grade 4 neutropenia), and mucositis were observed less often with weekly irinotecan/5-FU/LV than with monthly administration of 5-FU/LV.

TABLE 6 and TABLE 7 list the clinically relevant adverse events reported in Studies 1 and 2, respectively.

TABLE 6 *Study 1: Percent of Patients Experiencing Clinically Relevant Adverse Events in Combination Therapies**

	Irinotecan + Bolus 5-FU/LV		Bolus 5-FU/LV		Irinotecan	
	Weekly × 4 q 6 Weeks		Daily × 5 q 4 Weeks		Weekly × 4 q 6 Weeks	
	n=225		n=219		n=223	
Adverse Event	**Grade 1-4**	**Grade 3 & 4**	**Grade 1-4**	**Grade 3 & 4**	**Grade 1-4**	**Grade 3 & 4**
Total Adverse Events	100	53.3	100	45.7	99.6	45.7
Gastrointestinal						
Diarrhea						
Late	84.9%	22.7%	69.4%	13.2%	83.0%	31.0%
Grade 3	—	15.1%	—	5.9%	—	18.4%
Grade 4	—	7.6%	—	7.3%	—	12.6%
Early	45.8%	4.9%	31.5%	1.4%	43.0%	6.7%
Nausea	79.1%	15.6%	67.6%	8.2%	81.6%	16.1%
Abdominal pain	63.1%	14.6%	50.2%	11.5%	67.7%	13.0%
Vomiting	60.4%	9.7%	46.1%	4.1%	62.8%	12.1%
Anorexia	34.2%	5.8%	42.0%	3.7%	43.9%	7.2%
Constipation	41.3%	3.1%	31.5%	1.8%	32.3%	0.4%
Mucositis	32.4%	2.2%	76.3%	16.9%	29.6%	2.2%
Hematologic						
Neutropenia	96.9%	53.8%	98.6%	66.7%	96.4%	31.4%
Grade 3	—	29.8%	—	23.7%	—	19.3%
Grade 4	—	24.0%	—	42.5%	—	12.1%
Leukopenia	96.9%	37.8%	98.6%	23.3%	96.4%	21.5%
Anemia	96.9%	8.4%	98.6%	5.5%	96.9%	4.5%
Neutropenic fever	—	7.1%	—	14.6%	—	5.8%
Thrombocytopenia	96.0%	2.6%	98.6%	2.7%	96.0%	1.7%
Neutropenic infection	—	1.8%	—	0%	—	2.2%
Body as a Whole						
Asthenia	70.2%	19.5%	64.4%	11.9%	69.1%	13.9%
Pain	30.7%	3.5%	26.9%	3.6%	22.9%	2.2%
Fever	42.2%	1.7%	32.4%	3.6%	43.5%	0.4%
Infection	22.2%	0%	16.0%	1.4%	13.9%	0.4%
Metabolic & Nutritional						
inc Bilirubin	87.6%	7.1%	92.2%	8.2%	83.9%	7.2%
Dermatologic						
Exfoliative dermatitis	0.9%	0%	3.2%	0.5%	0%	0%
Rash	19.1%	0%	26.5%	0.9%	14.3%	0.4%
Alopecia†	43.1%	—	26.5%	—	46.1%	—
Respiratory						
Dyspnea	27.6%	6.3%	16.0%	0.5%	22.0%	2.2%
Cough	26.7%	1.3%	18.3%	0%	20.2%	0.4%
Pneumonia	6.2%	2.7%	1.4%	1.0%	3.6%	1.3%
Neurologic						
Dizziness	23.1%	1.3%	16.4%	0%	21.1%	1.8%
Somnolence	12.4%	1.8%	4.6%	1.0%	9.4%	1.3%
Confusion	7.1%	1.8%	4.1%	0%	2.7%	0%
Cardiovascular						
Vasodilation	9.3%	0.9%	5.0%	0%	9.0%	0%
Hypotension	5.8%	1.3%	2.3%	0.5%	5.8%	1.7%
Thromboembolic events‡	9.3%	—	11.4%	—	5.4%	—

* Severity of adverse events based on NCI CTC (version 1.0).
† Complete hair loss = Grade 2.
‡ Includes angina pectoris, arterial thrombosis, cerebral infarct, cerebrovascular accident, deep thrombophlebitis, embolus lower extremity, heart arrest, myocardial infarct, myocardial ischemia, peripheral vascular disorder, pulmonary embolus, sudden death, thrombophlebitis, thrombosis, vascular disorder.

SECOND-LINE SINGLE-AGENT THERAPY

Weekly Dosage Schedule

In three clinical studies evaluating the weekly dosage schedule, 304 patients with metastatic carcinoma of the colon or rectum that had recurred or progressed following 5-FU-based therapy were treated with irinotecan HCl. Seventeen (17) of the patients died within 30 days of the administration of irinotecan HCl; in five cases (1.6%, 5/304), the deaths were potentially drug-related. These 5 patients experienced a constellation of medical events that included known effects of irinotecan HCl. One of these patients died of neutropenic sepsis

TABLE 7 *Study 2: Percent of Patients Experiencing Clinically Relevant Adverse Events in Combination Therapies**

	Irinotecan + 5-FU/LV Infusional Days 1 & 2 q 2 Weeks		5-FU/LV Infusional Days 1 & 2 q 2 Weeks	
	Grade 1-4	Grade 3 & 4	Grade 1-4	Grade 3 & 4
Adverse Event	**n=145**	**n=145**	**n=143**	**n=143**
Total Adverse Events	100	72.4	100	39.2
Gastrointestinal				
Diarrhea				
Late	72.4%	14.4%	44.8%	6.3%
Grade 3	—	10.3%	—	4.2%
Grade 4	—	4.1%	—	2.1%
Cholinergic syndrome†	28.3%	1.4%	0.7%	0%
Nausea	66.9%	2.1%	55.2%	3.5%
Abdominal pain	17.2%	2.1%	16.8%	0.7%
Vomiting	44.8%	3.5%	32.2%	2.8%
Anorexia	35.2%	2.1%	18.9%	0.7%
Constipation	30.3%	0.7%	25.2%	1.4%
Mucositis	40.0%	4.1%	28.7%	2.8%
Hematologic				
Neutropenia	82.5%	46.2%	47.9%	13.4%
Grade 3	—	36.4%	—	12.7%
Grade 4	—	9.8%	—	0.7%
Leukopenia	81.3%	17.4%	42.0%	3.5%
Anemia	97.2%	2.1%	90.9%	2.1%
Neutropenic fever	—	3.4%	—	0.7%
Thrombocytopenia	32.6%	0%	32.2%	0%
Neutropenic infection	—	2.1%	—	0%
Body as a Whole				
Asthenia	57.9%	9.0%	48.3%	4.2%
Pain	64.1%	9.7%	61.5%	8.4%
Fever	22.1%	0.7%	25.9%	0.7%
Infection	35.9%	7.6%	33.6%	3.5%
Metabolic & Nutritional				
inc Bilirubin	19.1%	3.5%	35.9%	10.6%
Dermatologic				
Hand & foot syndrome	10.3%	0.7%	12.6%	0.7%
Cutaneous signs	17.2%	0.7%	20.3%	0%
Alopecia‡	56.6%	—	16.8%	—
Respiratory				
Dyspnea	9.7%	1.4%	4.9%	0%
Cardiovascular				
Hypotension	3.4%	1.4%	0.7%	0%
Thromboembolic events§	11.7%	—	5.6%	—

* Severity of adverse events based on NCI CTC (version 1.0).
† Includes rhinitis, increased salivation, miosis, lacrimation, diaphoresis, flushing, abdominal cramping or diarrhea (occurring during or shortly after infusion of irinotecan).
‡ Complete hair loss = Grade 2.
§ Includes angina pectoris, arterial thrombosis, cerebral infarct, cerebrovascular accident, deep thrombophlebitis, embolus lower extremity, heart arrest, myocardial infarct, myocardial ischemia, peripheral vascular disorder, pulmonary embolus, sudden death, thrombophlebitis, thrombosis, vascular disorder.
inc = Increase.

without fever. Neutropenic fever occurred in nine (3.0%) other patients; these patients recovered with supportive care.

One hundred nineteen (39.1%) of the 304 patients were hospitalized a total of 156 times because of adverse events; 81 (26.6%) patients were hospitalized for events judged to be related to administration of irinotecan HCl. The primary reasons for drug-related hospitalization were diarrhea, with or without nausea and/or vomiting (18.4%); neutropenia/leukopenia, with or without diarrhea and/or fever (8.2%); and nausea and/or vomiting (4.9%).

Adjustments in the dose of irinotecan HCl were made during the cycle of treatment and for subsequent cycles based on individual patient tolerance. The first dose of at least one cycle of irinotecan HCl was reduced for 67% of patients who began the studies at the 125 mg/m^2 starting dose. Within-cycle dose reductions were required for 32% of the cycles initiated at the 125 mg/m^2 dose level. The most common reasons for dose reduction were late diarrhea, neutropenia, and leukopenia. Thirteen (4.3%) patients discontinued treatment with irinotecan HCl because of adverse events. The adverse events in TABLE 8 are based on the experience of the 304 patients enrolled in the CLINICAL STUDIES section, Second-Line Treatment for Recurrent or Progressive Metastatic Colorectal Cancer After 5-FU Based Treatment, Weekly Dosage Schedule studies (available on enclosed CD-ROM).

Once-Every-3-Week Dosage Schedule

A total of 535 patients with metastatic colorectal cancer whose disease had recurred or progressed following prior 5-FU therapy participated in the two Phase 3 studies: 316 received irinotecan, 129 received 5-FU, and 90 received best supportive care. Eleven (3.5%) patients treated with irinotecan died within 30 days of treatment. In three cases (1%, 3/316), the deaths were potentially related to irinotecan treatment and were attributed to neutropenic infection, Grade 4 diarrhea, and asthenia, respectively. One (0.8%, 1/129) patient treated with 5-FU died within 30 days of treatment; this death was attributed to Grade 4 diarrhea.

Hospitalizations due to serious adverse events (whether or not related to study treatment) occurred at least once in 60% (188/316) of patients who received irinotecan, 63% (57/90) who received best supportive care, and 39% (50/129) who received 5-FU-based therapy. Eight percent (8%) of patients treated with irinotecan and 7% treated with 5-FU-based therapy discontinued treatment due to adverse events.

Of the 316 patients treated with irinotecan, the most clinically significant adverse events (all grades, 1-4) were diarrhea (84%), alopecia (72%), nausea (70%), vomiting (62%), cholinergic symptoms (47%), and neutropenia (30%). TABLE 9 lists the Grade 3 and 4 adverse events reported in the patients enrolled to all treatment arms of the two studies.

TABLE 8 *Adverse Events Occurring in >10% of 304 Previously Treated Patients With Metastatic Carcinoma of the Colon or Rectuma**

Body System/Event	NCI Grades 1-4	NCI Grades 3 & 4
Gastrointestinal		
Diarrhea (late)†	88%	31%
7-9 Stools/day (Grade 3)	—	(16%)
≥10 Stools/day (Grade 4)	—	(14%)
Nausea	86%	17%
Vomiting	67%	12%
Anorexia	55%	6%
Diarrhea (early)‡	51%	8%
Constipation	30%	2%
Flatulence	12%	0%
Stomatitis	12%	1%
Dyspepsia	10%	0%
Hematologic		
Leukopenia	63%	28%
Anemia	60%	7%
Neutropenia	54%	26%
500 to <1000/mm^3 (Grade 3)	—	(15)
<500/mm^3 (Grade 4)	—	(12)
Body as a Whole		
Asthenia	76%	12%
Abdominal cramping/pain	57%	16%
Fever	45%	1%
Pain	24%	2%
Headache	17%	1%
Back pain	14%	2%
Chills	14%	0%
Minor infection§	14%	0%
Edema	10%	1%
Abdominal enlargement	10%	0%
Metabolic & Nutritional		
dec Body weight	30%	1%
Dehydration	15%	4%
inc Alkaline phosphatase	13%	4%
inc SGOT	10%	1%
Dermatologic		
Alopecia	60%	NA
Sweating	16%	0%
Rash	13%	1%
Respiratory		
Dyspnea	22%	4%
inc Coughing	17%	0%
Rhinitis	16%	0%
Neurologic		
Insomnia	19%	0%
Dizziness	15%	0%
Cardiovascular		
Vasodilation (flushing)	11%	0%

* Severity of adverse events based on NCI CTC (version 1.0).
† Occurring >24 hours after administration of irinotecan HCl.
‡ Occurring ≤24 hours after administration of irinotecan HCl.
§ Primarily upper respiratory infections.
NA Not applicable; complete hair loss = NCI Grade 2.
inc = Increase.
dec = Decrease.

OVERVIEW OF ADVERSE EVENTS

Gastrointestinal

Nausea, vomiting, and diarrhea are common adverse events following treatment with irinotecan HCl and can be severe. When observed, nausea and vomiting usually occur during or shortly after infusion of irinotecan HCl. In the clinical studies testing the every 3-week-dosage schedule, the median time to the onset of late diarrhea was 5 days after irinotecan infusion. In the clinical studies evaluating the weekly dosage schedule, the median time to onset of late diarrhea was 11 days following administration of irinotecan HCl. For patients starting treatment at the 125 mg/m^2 weekly dose, the median duration of any grade of late diarrhea was 3 days. Among those patients treated at the 125 mg/m^2 weekly dose who experienced Grade 3 or 4 late diarrhea, the median duration of the entire episode of diarrhea was 7 days. The frequency of Grade 3 or 4 late diarrhea was somewhat greater in patients starting treatment at 125 mg/m^2 than in patients given a 100 mg/m^2 weekly starting dose (34% [65/193] vs 23% [24/102]; p=0.08). The frequency of Grade 3 and 4 late diarrhea by age was significantly greater in patients ≥65 years than in patients <65 years (40% [53/133] vs 23% [40/171]; p=0.002). In one study of the weekly dosage treatment, the frequency of Grade 3 and 4 late diarrhea was significantly greater in male than in female patients (43% [25/58] vs 16% [5/32]; p=0.01), but there were no gender differences in the frequency of Grade 3 and 4 late diarrhea in the other two studies of the weekly dosage treatment schedule. Colonic ulceration, sometimes with gastrointestinal bleeding, has been observed in association with administration of irinotecan HCl.

Hematology

Irinotecan HCl commonly causes neutropenia, leukopenia (including lymphocytopenia), and anemia. Serious thrombocytopenia is uncommon. When evaluated in the trials of weekly administration, the frequency of Grade 3 and 4 neutropenia was significantly higher in patients who received previous pelvic/abdominal irradiation than in those who had not received such irradiation (48% [13/27] vs 24% [67/277]; p=0.04). In these same studies, patients with baseline serum total bilirubin levels of 1.0 mg/dl or more also had a significantly greater likelihood of experiencing first-cycle Grade 3 or 4 neutropenia than those with bilirubin levels that were less than 1.0 mg/dl (50% [19/38] vs 18% [47/266]; p <0.001). There were no significant differences in the frequency of Grade 3 and 4 neutropenia by age or gender. In the clinical studies evaluating the weekly dosage schedule, neutropenic fever (concurrent NCI Grade 4 neutropenia and fever of Grade 2 or greater) occurred in 3% of the patients; 6% of patients received G-CSF for the treatment of neutropenia. NCI Grade 3 or 4 anemia was noted in 7% of the patients receiving weekly treatment; blood transfusions were given to 10% of the patients in these trials.

TABLE 9 *Percent of Patients Experiencing Grade 3 & 4 Adverse Events in Comparative Studies of Once-Every-3 Week Irinotecan Therapy**

	Study 1		Study 2	
	Irinotecan	BSC†	Irinotecan	5-FU
Adverse Event	**n=189**	**n=90**	**n=127**	**n=129**
Total Grade 3/4 Adverse Events	79	67	69	54
Gastrointestinal				
Diarrhea	22%	6%	22%	11%
Vomiting	14%	8%	14%	5%
Nausea	14%	3%	11%	4%
Abdominal pain	14%	16%	9%	8%
Constipation	10%	8%	8%	6%
Anorexia	5%	7%	6%	4%
Mucositis	2%	1%	2%	5%
Hematologic				
Leukopenia/neutropenia	22%	0%	14%	2%
Anemia	7%	6%	6%	3%
Hemorrhage	5%	3%	1%	3%
Thrombocytopenia	1%	0%	4%	2%
Infection				
Without Grade 3/4 neutropenia	8%	3%	1%	4%
With Grade 3/4 neutropenia	1%	0%	2%	0%
Fever				
Without Grade 3/4 neutropenia	2%	1%	2%	0%
With Grade 3/4 neutropenia	2%	0%	4%	2%
Body as a Whole				
Pain	19%	22%	17%	13%
Asthenia	15%	19%	13%	12%
Metabolic & Nutritional				
Hepatic‡	9%	7%	9%	6%
Dermatologic				
Hand & foot syndrome	0%	0%	0%	5%
Cutaneous signs§	2%	0%	1%	3%
Respiratory¤	10%	8%	5%	7%
Neurologic¶	12%	13%	9%	4%
Cardiovascular**	9%	3%	4%	2%
Other††	32%	28%	12%	14%

* Severity of adverse events based on NCI CTC (version 1.0).
† BSC = best supportive care.
‡ Hepatic includes events such as ascites and jaundice.
§ Cutaneous signs include events such as rash.
¤ Respiratory includes events such as dyspnea and cough.
¶ Neurologic includes events such as somnolence.
** Cardiovascular includes events such as dysrhythmias, ischemia, and mechanical cardiac dysfunction.
†† Other includes events such as accidental injury, hepatomegaly, syncope, vertigo, and weight loss.

Body as a Whole

Asthenia, fever, and abdominal pain are generally the most common events of this type.

Cholinergic Symptoms

Patients may have cholinergic symptoms of rhinitis, increased salivation, miosis, lacrimation, diaphoresis, flushing, and intestinal hyperperistalsis that can cause abdominal cramping and early diarrhea. If these symptoms occur, they manifest during or shortly after drug infusion. They are thought to be related to the anticholinesterase activity of the irinotecan parent compound and are expected to occur more frequently with higher irinotecan doses.

Hepatic

In the clinical studies evaluating the weekly dosage schedule, NCI Grade 3 or 4 liver enzyme abnormalities were observed in fewer than 10% of patients. These events typically occur in patients with known hepatic metastases.

Dermatologic

Alopecia has been reported during treatment with irinotecan HCl. Rashes have also been reported but did not result in discontinuation of treatment.

Respiratory

Severe pulmonary events are infrequent. In the clinical studies evaluating the weekly dosage schedule, NCI Grade 3 or 4 dyspnea was reported in 4% of patients. Over half the patients with dyspnea had lung metastases; the extent to which malignant pulmonary involvement or other preexisting lung disease may have contributed to dyspnea in these patients is unknown.

Neurologic

Insomnia and dizziness can occur, but are not usually considered to be directly related to the administration of irinotecan HCl. Dizziness may sometimes represent symptomatic evidence of orthostatic hypotension in patients with dehydration.

Cardiovascular

Vasodilation (flushing) may occur during administration of C. Bradycardia may also occur, but has not required intervention. These effects have been attributed to the cholinergic syndrome sometimes observed during or shortly after infusion of irinotecan HCl. Thromboembolic events have been observed in patients receiving irinotecan HCl; the specific cause of these events has not been determined.

OTHER NON-US CLINICAL TRIALS

Irinotecan has been studied in over 1100 patients in Japan. Patients in these studies had a variety of tumor types, including cancer of the colon or rectum, and were treated with several different doses and schedules. In general, the types of toxicities observed were similar to those seen in US trials with irinotecan HCl. There is some information from Japanese trials that patients with considerable ascites or pleural effusions were at increased risk for neutropenia or diarrhea. A potentially life-threatening pulmonary syndrome, consisting of dyspnea, fever, and a reticulonodular pattern on chest x-ray, was observed in a small percentage of patients in early Japanese studies. The contribution of irinotecan to these preliminary events was difficult to assess because these patients also had lung tumors and some had preexisting nonmalignant pulmonary disease. As a result of these observations, however, clinical studies in the US have enrolled few patients with compromised pulmonary function, significant ascites, or pleural effusions.

POST-MARKETING EXPERIENCE

The following events have been identified during postmarketing use of irinotecan HCl in clinical practice. Cases of colitis complicated by ulceration, bleeding, ileus, or infection have been observed. There have been rare cases of renal impairment and acute renal failure, generally in patients who became infected and/or volume depleted from severe gastrointestinal toxicities (see WARNINGS).

Hypersensitivity reactions including severe anaphylactic or anaphylactoid reactions have also been observed (see WARNINGS).

DOSAGE AND ADMINISTRATION

COMBINATION-AGENT DOSAGE

Dosage Regimens

Irinotecan HCl Injection in Combination With 5-Fluorouracil (5-FU) and Leucovorin (LV)

Irinotecan HCl should be administered as an intravenous infusion over 90 minutes (see Preparation of Infusion Solution). For all regimens, the dose of LV should be administered immediately after irinotecan HCl, with the administration of 5-FU to occur immediately after receipt of LV. Irinotecan HCl should be used as recommended; the currently recommended regimens are shown in TABLE 10.

TABLE 10 *Combination-Agent Dosage Regimens & Dose Modifications**

	Starting Dose	Dose Level -1	Dose Level -2
Regimen 1: 6 Wk Cycle With Bolus 5-FU/LV (next cycle begins on day 43)			
Irinotecan HCl‡ (125 mg/m² IV over 90 min)	125 mg/m²	100 mg/m²	75 mg/m²
LV‡ (20 mg/m² IV bolus)	20 mg/m²	20 mg/m²	20 mg/m²
5-FU‡ (500 mg/m² IV bolus)	500 mg/m²	400 mg/m²	300 mg/m²
Regimen 2: 6 Wk Cycle With Infusional 5-FU/LV (next cycle begins on day 43)			
Irinotecan HCl§ (180 mg/m² IV over 90 min)	180 mg/m²	150 mg/m²	120 mg/m²
LV§ (200 mg/m² IV over 2 h)	200 mg/m²	200 mg/m²	200 mg/m²
5-FU¤ bolus (400 mg/m² IV bolus)	400 mg/m²	320 mg/m²	240 mg/m²
5-FU¤ Infusion† (600 mg/m² IV over 22 h)	600 mg/m²	480 mg/m²	360 mg/m²

* Dose reductions beyond dose level -2 by decrements of ~20% may be warranted for patients continuing to experience toxicity. Provided intolerable toxicity does not develop, treatment with additional cycles may be continued indefinitely as long as patients continue to experience clinical benefit.
† Infusion follows bolus administration.
‡ Dosing on days 1, 8, 15, 22.
§ Dosing on days 1, 15, 29.
¤ Dosing on days 1, 2, 15, 16, 29, 30.

Dosing for patients with bilirubin >2 mg/dl cannot be recommended since such patients were not included in clinical studies. It is recommended that patients receive premedication with antiemetic agents. Prophylactic or therapeutic administration of atropine should be considered in patients experiencing cholinergic symptoms. See PRECAUTIONS, General.

Dose Modification

Patients should be carefully monitored for toxicity and assessed prior to each treatment. Doses of irinotecan HCl and 5-FU should be modified as necessary to accommodate individual patient tolerance to treatment. Based on the recommended dose-levels described in TABLE 10, subsequent doses should be adjusted as suggested in TABLE 11. All dose modifications should be based on the worst preceding toxicity. After the first treatment, patients with active diarrhea should return to pre-treatment bowel function without requiring antidiarrhea medications for at least 24 hours before the next chemotherapy administration.

A new cycle of therapy should not begin until the toxicity has recovered to NCI Grade 1 or less. Treatment may be delayed 1-2 weeks to allow for recovery from treatment- related toxicity. If the patient has not recovered, consideration should be given to discontinuing therapy. Provided intolerable toxicity does not develop, treatment with additional cycles of irinotecan HCl/5-FU/LV may be continued indefinitely as long as patients continue to experience clinical benefit.

SINGLE-AGENT DOSAGE SCHEDULES

Dosage Regimens

Irinotecan HCl should be administered as an intravenous infusion over 90 minutes for both the weekly and once-every-3-week dosage schedules (see Preparation of Infusion Solution). Single-agent dosage regimens are shown in TABLE 12.

TABLE 11 *Recommended Dose Modifications for Irinotecan HCl/5-Fluorouracil (5-FU)/Leucovorin (LV) Combination Schedules**

Toxicity NCI CTC Grade† (value)	During a Cycle of Therapy	At the Start of Subsequent Cycles of Therapy‡
No toxicity	Maintain dose level	Maintain dose level
Neutropenia		
1 (1500-1999/mm^3)	Maintain dose level	Maintain dose level
2 (1000-1499/mm^3)	dec 1 dose level	Maintain dose level
3 (500-999/mm^3)	Omit dose until resolved to ≤Grade 2, then dec 1 dose level	dec 1 dose level
4 (<500/mm^3)	Omit dose until resolved to ≤Grade 2, then dec 2 dose levels	dec 2 dose levels
Neutropenic Fever	Omit dose until resolved, then dec 2 dose levels	
Other Hematologic Toxicities	Dose modifications for leukopenia or thrombocytopenia during a cycle of therapy and at the start of subsequent cycles of therapy are also based on NCI toxicity criteria and are the same as recommended for neutropenia above.	
Diarrhea		
1 (2-3 stools/day >pretx§)	Delay dose until resolved to baseline, then give same dose	Maintain dose level
2 (4-6 stools/day >pretx)	Omit dose until resolved to baseline, then dec 1 dose level	Maintain dose level
3 (7-9 stools/day >pretx)	Omit dose until resolved to baseline, then dec 1 dose level	dec 1 dose level
4 (≥10 stools/day >pretx)	Omit dose until resolved to baseline, then dec 2 dose levels	dec 2 dose levels
Other Nonhematologic Toxicities¤		
1	Maintain dose level	Maintain dose level
2	Omit dose until resolved to ≤Grade 1, then dec 1 dose level	Maintain dose level
3	Omit dose until resolved to ≤Grade 2, then dec 1 dose level	dec 1 dose level
4	Omit dose until resolved to ≤Grade 2, then dec 2 dose levels	dec 2 dose levels
	For mucositis/stomatitis decrease only 5-FU, not irinotecan HCl	*For mucositis/stomatitis decrease only 5-FU, not irinotecan HCl*

* **Patients should return to pre-treatment bowel function without requiring antidiarrhea medications for at least 24 hours before the next chemotherapy administration. A new cycle of therapy should not begin until the granulocyte count has recovered to ≥1500/mm^3, and the platelet count has recovered to ≥100,000/mm^3, and treatment-related diarrhea is fully resolved. Treatment should be delayed 1-2 weeks to allow for recovery from treatment-related toxicities. If the patient has not recovered after a 2 week delay, consideration should be given to discontinuing therapy.**
† National Cancer Institute Common Toxicity Criteria (version 1.0).
‡ Relative to the starting dose used in the previous cycle.
§ Pretreatment.
¤ Excludes alopecia, anorexia, asthenia.

A reduction in the starting dose by one dose level of irinotecan HCl may be considered for patients with any of the following conditions: age ≥65 years, prior pelvic/abdominal radiotherapy, performance status of 2, or increased bilirubin levels. Dosing for patients with bilirubin >2 mg/dl cannot be recommended since such patients were not included in clinical studies.

It is recommended that patients receive premedication with antiemetic agents. Prophylactic or therapeutic administration of atropine should be considered in patients experiencing cholinergic symptoms. See PRECAUTIONS, General.

Dose Modification

Patients should be carefully monitored for toxicity and doses of irinotecan HCl should be modified as necessary to accommodate individual patient tolerance to treatment. Based on recommended dose-levels described in TABLE 12, subsequent doses should be adjusted as suggested in TABLE 13. All dose modifications should be based on the worst preceding toxicity.

A new cycle of therapy should not begin until the toxicity has recovered to NCI Grade 1 or less. Treatment may be delayed 1-2 weeks to allow for recovery from treatment-related toxicity. If the patient has not recovered, consideration should be given to discontinuing this combination therapy. Provided intolerable toxicity does not develop, treatment with additional cycles of irinotecan HCl may be continued indefinitely as long as patients continue to experience clinical benefit.

TABLE 12 *Single-Agent Regimens of Irinotecan HCl & Dose Modifications*

	Starting Dose	Dose Level -1	Dose Level -2
Weekly Regimen*			
Irinotecan HCl† (125 mg/m^2 IV over 90 min)	125 mg/m^2	100 mg/m^2	75 mg/m^2
Once-Every-3-Week Regimen‡			
Irinotecan HCl§ (350 mg/m^2 IV over 90 min)¤	350 mg/m^2	300 mg/m^2	250 mg/m^2

* Subsequent doses may be adjusted as high as 150 mg/m^2 or to as low as 50 mg/m^2 in 25-50 mg/m^2 decrements depending upon individual patient tolerance.
† Dosing on days 1, 8, 15, 22, then 2 week rest.
‡ Subsequent doses may be adjusted as low as 200 mg/m^2 in 50 mg/m^2 decrements depending upon individual patient tolerance.
§ Once every 3 weeks.‡
¤ Provided intolerable toxicity does not develop, treatment with additional cycles may be continued indefinitely as long as patients continue to experience clinical benefit.

TABLE 13 *Recommended Dose Modifications for Single-Agent Schedules**

Worst Toxicity NCI Grade‡(value)	During a Cycle of Therapy: Weekly	At the Start of the Next Cycles of Therapy (after adequate recovery), Compared With the Starting Dose in the Previous Cycle*: Weekly	Once Every 3 Weeks
No toxicity	Maintain dose level	inc 25 mg/m^2 up to a maximum dose of 150 mg/m^2	Maintain dose level
Neutropenia			
1 (1500-1999/mm^3)	Maintain dose level	Maintain dose level	Maintain dose level
2 (1000-1499/mm^3)	dec 25 mg/m^2	Maintain dose level	Maintain dose level
3 (500-999/mm^3)	Omit dose until resolved to ≤ Grade 2, then dec 25 mg/m^2	dec 25 mg/m^2	dec 50 mg/m^2
4 (<500/mm^3)	Omit dose until resolved to ≤ Grade 2, then dec 50 mg/m^2	dec 50 mg/m^2	dec 50 mg/m^2
Neutropenic Fever	Omit dose until resolved, then dec 50 mg/m^2 when resolved	dec 50 mg/m^2	dec 50 mg/m^2
Other Hematologic Toxicities	Dose modifications for leukopenia, thrombocytopenia, and anemia during a cycle of therapy and at the start of subsequent cycles of therapy are also based on NCI toxicity criteria and are the same as recommended for neutropenia above.		
Diarrhea			
1 (2-3 stools/day >pretx§)	Maintain dose level	Maintain dose level	Maintain dose level
2 (4-6 stools/day >pretx)	dec 25 mg/m^2	Maintain dose level	Maintain dose level
3 (7-9 stools/day >pretx)	Omit dose until resolved to ≤ Grade 2, then dec 25 mg/m^2	dec 25 mg/m^2	dec 50 mg/m^2
4 (≥10 stools/day >pretx)	Omit dose until resolved to ≤ Grade 2, then dec 50 mg/m^2	dec 50 mg/m^2	dec 50 mg/m^2
Other Nonhematologic Toxicities¤			
1	Maintain dose level	Maintain dose level	Maintain dose level
2	dec 25 mg/m^2	dec 25 mg/m^2	dec 50 mg/m^2
3	Omit dose until resolved to ≤ Grade 2, then dec 25 mg/m^2	dec 25 mg/m^2	dec 50 mg/m^2
4	Omit dose until resolved to ≤ Grade 2, then dec 50 mg/m^2	dec 50 mg/m^2	dec 50 mg/m^2

* All dose modifications should be based on the worst preceding toxicity.
† **A new cycle of therapy should not begin until the granulocyte count has recovered to ≥1500/mm^3, and the platelet count has recovered to ≥100,000/mm^3, and treatment-related diarrhea is fully resolved. Treatment should be delayed 1-2 weeks to allow for recovery from treatment-related toxicities. If the patient has not recovered after a 2 week delay, consideration should be given to discontinuing irinotecan HCl.**
‡ National Cancer Institute Common Toxicity Criteria (version 1.0).
§ Pretreatment.
¤ Excludes alopecia, anorexia, asthenia.
inc = Increase.
dec = Decrease.

PREPARATION & ADMINISTRATION PRECAUTIONS

As with other potentially toxic anticancer agents, care should be exercised in the handling and preparation of infusion solutions prepared from irinotecan HCl injection. The use of gloves is recommended. If a solution of irinotecan HCl contacts the skin, wash the skin immediately and thoroughly with soap and water. If irinotecan HCl contacts the mucous membranes, flush thoroughly with water. Several published guidelines for handling and disposal of anticancer agents are available.[1-7]

PREPARATION OF INFUSION SOLUTION

Inspect vial contents for particulate matter and repeat inspection when drug product is withdrawn from vial into syringe.

Irinotecan HCl injection must be diluted prior to infusion. Irinotecan HCl should be diluted in 5% dextrose injection (preferred) or 0.9% sodium chloride injection, to a final concentration range of 0.12-2.8 mg/ml. In most clinical trials, irinotecan HCl was administered in 250-500 ml of 5% dextrose injection.

The solution is physically and chemically stable for up to 24 hours at room temperature (approximately 25°C) and in ambient fluorescent lighting. Solutions diluted in 5% dextrose injection, and stored at refrigerated temperatures (approximately 2 to 8°C), and protected from light are physically and chemically stable for 48 hours. Refrigeration of admixtures using 0.9% sodium chloride injection, is not recommended due to a low and sporadic incidence of visible particulates. Freezing irinotecan HCl and admixtures of irinotecan HCl may result in precipitation of the drug and should be avoided. Because of possible microbial contamination during dilution, it is advisable to use the admixture prepared with 5% dextrose injection, within 24 hours if refrigerated (2-8°C, 36-46°F). In the case of admixtures prepared with 5% dextrose injection, or sodium chloride injection, the solutions should be used within 6 hours if kept at room temperature (15-30°C, 59-86°F).

Other drugs should not be added to the infusion solution. Parenteral drug products should be inspected visually for particulate matter and discoloration prior to administration whenever solution and container permit.

HOW SUPPLIED

Each ml of Camptosar Injection contains 20 mg irinotecan (on the basis of the trihydrate salt); 45 mg sorbitol; and 0.9 mg lactic acid. When necessary, pH has been adjusted to 3.5 (range, 3.0-3.8) with sodium hydroxide or hydrochloric acid.

Camptosar Injection is available in 2 or 5 ml single-dose amber glass vials.

This is packaged in a backing/plastic blister to protect against inadvertent breakage and leakage. The vial should be inspected for damage and visible signs of leaks before removing the backing/plastic blister. If damaged, incinerate the unopened package.

Storage: Store at controlled room temperature 15-30°C (59-86°F). Protect from light. It is recommended that the vial (and backing/plastic blister) should remain in the carton until the time of use.

PRODUCT LISTING - EQUIVALENTS NOT AVAILABLE

Solution - Intravenous - 20 mg/ml

2 ml	$319.60	CAMPTOSAR, Pharmacia and Upjohn	00009-7529-02
5 ml	$799.03	CAMPTOSAR, Pharmacia and Upjohn	00009-7529-01

Isocarboxazid *(001581)*

For related information, see the comparative table section in Appendix A.

Categories: Depression; FDA Pre 1938 Drugs; Pregnancy Category C
Drug Classes: Antidepressants, monoamine oxidase inhibitors
Brand Names: Marplan
Foreign Brand Availability: Enerzer (Japan)
Cost of Therapy: $42.40 (Depression; Marplan; 10 mg; 2 tablets/day; 30 day supply)

DESCRIPTION

Marplan, a monoamine oxidase inhibitor, is available for oral administration in 10-mg tablets. Each tablet also contains gelatin, lactose, magnesium stearate, corn starch, talc, FD&C red no. 3 and FD&C yellow no. 6. Chemically, isocarboxazid is 5-methyl-3-isoxazolecarboxylic acid 2-benzylhydrazide.

Isocarboxazid is a colorless, crystalline substance with very little taste.

CLINICAL PHARMACOLOGY

PHARMACODYNAMICS

Isocarboxazid is a non-selective hydrazine monoamine oxidase (MAO) inhibitor. *In vivo* and *in vitro* studies demonstrated inhibition of MAO in the brain, heart, and liver. The mechanism by which MAO inhibitors act as antidepressants is not fully understood, but is thought to involve the elevation of brain levels of biogenic amines. However, MAO is a complex enzyme system, widely distributed throughout the body, and drugs that inhibit MAO in the laboratory are associated with a number of clinical effects. Thus, it is unknown whether MAO inhibition per se, other pharmacologic actions, or an interaction of both is responsible for the antidepressant effects observed.

PHARMACOKINETICS

Isocarboxazid pharmacokinetic information is not available.

INDICATIONS AND USAGE

Isocarboxazid is indicated for the treatment of depression. Because of its potentially serious side effects, isocarboxazid is not an antidepressant of first choice in the treatment of newly diagnosed depressed patients.

The efficacy of isocarboxazid in the treatment of depression was established in 6 week controlled trials of depressed outpatients. These patients had symptoms that corresponded to the DSM-IV category of major depressive disorder; however, they often also had signs and symptoms of anxiety (anxious mood, panic, and/or phobic symptoms). (See CLINICAL PHARMACOLOGY.)

A major depressive episode (DSM-IV) implies a prominent and relatively persistent (nearly every day for at least 2 weeks) depressed or dysphoric mood that usually interferes with daily functioning, and includes at least five of the following nine symptoms: depressed mood, loss of interest in usual activities, significant change in weight and/or appetite, insomnia or hypersomnia, psychomotor agitation or retardation, increased fatigue, feelings of guilt or worthlessness, slowed thinking or impaired concentration, and a suicide attempt or suicidal ideation.

The antidepressant effectiveness of isocarboxazid in hospitalized depressed patients, or in endogenomorphically retarded and delusionally depressed patients, has not been adequately studied.

The effectiveness of isocarboxazid in long-term use, that is, for more than 6 weeks, has not been systematically evaluated in controlled trials. Therefore, the physician who elects to use isocarboxazid for extended periods should periodically evaluate the long-term usefulness of the drug for the individual patient.

CONTRAINDICATIONS

Isocarboxazid should not be administered in combination with any of the following: MAO inhibitors or dibenzazepine derivatives; sympathomimetics (including amphetamines); some central nervous system depressants (including narcotics and alcohol); antihypertensive, diuretic, antihistaminic, sedative or anesthetic drugs, buproprion HCl, buspirone HCl, dextromethorphan, cheese or other foods with a high tyramine content; or excessive quantities of caffeine.

Isocarboxazid should not be administered to any patient with a confirmed or suspected cerebrovascular defect or to any patient with cardiovascular disease, hypertension, or history of headache.

Contraindicated Patient Populations:

Hypersensitivity: Isocarboxazid should not be used in patients with known hypersensitivity to isocarboxazid.

Cerebrovascular Disorders: Isocarboxazid should not be administered to any patient with a confirmed or suspected cerebrovascular defect or to any patient with cardiovascular disease or hypertension.

Pheochromocytoma: Isocarboxazid should not be used in the presence of pheochromocytoma, as such tumors secrete pressor substances whose metabolism may be inhibited by isocarboxazid.

Liver Disease: Isocarboxazid should not be used in patients with a history of liver disease, or in those with abnormal liver function tests.

Renal Impairment: Isocarboxazid should not be used in patients with severe impairment of renal function.

Patients with Severe/Frequent Headaches: Patients with severe or frequent headaches should not be considered candidates for therapy with isocarboxazid, because headaches during therapy may be the first symptom of a hypertensive reaction to the drug.

Contraindicated MAOI-Other Drug Combinations:

Other MAO Inhibitors or with Dibenzazepine-Related Entities: Isocarboxazid should not be administered together with, or in close proximity to, other MAO inhibitors or dibenzazepine-related entities. Hypertensive crises, severe convulsive seizures, coma, or circulatory collapse may occur in patients receiving such combinations.

In patients being transferred to isocarboxazid from another MAO inhibitor or from a dibenzazepine-related entity, a medication-free interval of at least 1 week should be allowed, after which isocarboxazid therapy should be started using half the normal starting dosage for at least the first week of therapy. Similarly, at least 1 week should elapse between the discontinuation of isocarboxazid and initiation of another MAO inhibitor or dibenzazepine-related entity, or the readministration of isocarboxazid. The following list includes some other MAO inhibitors, dibenzazepine-related entities, and tricyclic antidepressants.

Other MAO Inhibitors: Furazolidone, pargyline HCl, methyclothiazide; pargyline HCl, phenelzine sulfate; procarbazine; tranylcypromine sulfate.

Dibenzazepine-Related and Other Tricyclics: Amitriptyline HCl, amitriptyline HCl; perphenazine, clomipramine HCl, desipramine HCl, imipramine HCl, nortriptyline HCl, protripyline HCl, doxepin HCl, carbamazepine, cyclobenzaprine HCl, amoxapine, maprotiline HCl, trimipramine maleate.

Bupropion: The concurrent administration of an MAO inhibitor and bupropion HCl is contraindicated. At least 14 days should elapse between discontinuation of an MAO inhibitor and initiation of treatment with bupropion HCl.

Selective Serotonin Reuptake Inhibitors (SSRIs): Isocarboxazid should not be administered in combination with any SSRI. There have been reports of serious, sometimes fatal, reactions (including hyperthermia, rigidity, myoclonus, autonomic instability with possible rapid fluctuations of vital signs, and mental status changes that include extreme agitation and confusion progressing to delirium and coma) in patients receiving fluoxetine in combination with a monoamine oxidase inhibitor (MAOI), and in patients who have recently discontinued fluoxetine and are then started on an MAOI. Some cases presented with features resembling neuroleptic malignant syndrome. Fluoxetine and other SSRIs should therefore not be used in combination with isocarboxazid, or within 14 days of discontinuing therapy with isocarboxazid. As fluoxetine and its major metabolite have very long elimination half-lives, at least 5 weeks should be allowed after stopping fluoxetine before starting isocarboxazid. At least 2 weeks should be allowed after stopping sertraline or paroxetine before starting isocarboxazid. In addition, there should be an interval of at least 10 days between discontinuation of isocarboxazid and initiation of fluoxetine or other SSRIs.

Buspirone: Isocarboxazid should not be used in combination with buspirone HCl; several cases of elevated blood pressure have been reported in patients taking MAO inhibitors who were then given buspirone HCl. At least 10 days should elapse between the discontinuation of isocarboxazid and the institution of buspirone HCl.

Sympathomimetics: Isocarboxazid should not be administered in combination with sympathomimetics, including amphetamines, or with over-the-counter drugs such as cold, hay fever, or weight-reducing preparations that contain vasoconstrictors.

During isocarboxazid therapy, it appears that some patients are particularly vulnerable to the effects of sympathomimetics when the activity of metabolizing enzymes is inhibited. Use of sympathomimetics and compounds such as guanethidine, methyldopa, methylphenidate, reserpine, epinephrine, norepinephrine, phenylalanine, dopamine, levodopa, tyrosine, and tryptophan with isocarboxazid may precipitate hypertension, headache, and related symptoms. The combination of MAO inhibitors and tryptophan has been reported to cause behavioral and neurologic symptoms, including disorientation, confusion, amnesia, delirium, agitation, hypomanic signs, ataxia, myoclonus, hyperreflexia, shivering, ocular oscillations, and Babinski signs.

Meperidine: Meperidine should not be used concomitantly with MAO inhibitors or within 2 or 3 weeks following MAO therapy. Serious reactions have been precipitated with concomitant use, including coma, severe hypertension or hypotension, severe respiratory depression, convulsions, malignant hyperpyrexia, excitation, peripheral vascular collapse, and death. It is thought that these reactions may be mediated by accumulation of 5-HT (serotonin) consequent to MAO inhibition.

Dextromethorphan: Isocarboxazid should not be used in combination with dextromethorphan. The combination of MAO inhibitors and dextromethorphan has been reported to cause brief episodes of psychosis or bizarre behavior.

Cheese or Other Foods with a High Tyramine Content: Hypertensive crises have sometimes occurred during isocarboxazid therapy after ingestion of foods with a high tyramine content. In general, patients should avoid protein foods in which aging or protein breakdown is used to increase flavor. In particular, patients should be instructed not to take foods such as cheese (particularly strong or aged varieties), sour cream, Chianti wine, sherry, beer (including non-alcoholic beer), liqueurs, pickled herring, anchovies, caviar, liver, canned figs, raisins, bananas or avocados (particularly if overripe), chocolate, soy sauce, sauerkraut, the pods of broad beans (fava beans), yeast extracts, yogurt, meat extracts, meat prepared with tenderizers, or dry sausage.

Anesthetic Agents: Patients taking isocarboxazid should not undergo elective surgery requiring general anesthesia. Also, they should not be given cocaine or local anesthesia containing sympathomimetic vasoconstrictors. The possible combined hypotensive effects of isocarboxazid and spinal anesthesia should be kept in mind. Isocarboxazid should be discontinued at least 10 days before elective surgery.

CNS Depressants: Isocarboxazid should not be used in combination with some central nervous system depressants, such as narcotics, barbiturates, or alcohol.

Antihypertensives: Isocarboxazid should not be used in combination with antihypertensive agents, including thiazide diuretics. A marked potentiating effect on these drugs has been reported, resulting in hypotension.

Caffeine: Excessive use of caffeine in any form should be avoided in patients receiving isocarboxazid.

WARNINGS

SECOND LINE STATUS

Isocarboxazid can cause serious side effects. It is not recommended as initial therapy but should be reserved for patients who have not responded satisfactorily to other antidepressants.

HYPERTENSIVE CRISES

The most important reaction associated with MAO inhibitors is the occurrence of hypertensive crises, which have sometimes been fatal, resulting from the co-administration of MAOIs and certain drugs and foods (see CONTRAINDICATIONS). These crises are characterized by some or all of the following symptoms: Occipital headache which may radiate frontally, palpitation, neck stiffness or soreness, nausea or vomiting, sweating (sometimes with fever and sometimes with cold, clammy skin), and photophobia. Either tachycardia or bradycardia may be present, and associated constricting chest pain and dilated pupils may occur. Intracranial bleeding, sometimes fatal, has been reported in association with the increase in blood pressure.

Blood pressure should be followed closely in patients taking isocarboxazid to detect any pressor response.

Therapy should be discontinued immediately if palpitations or frequent headaches occur during isocarboxazid therapy as these symptoms may be prodromal of a hypertensive crisis.

If a hypertensive crisis occurs, isocarboxazid should be discontinued, and therapy to lower blood pressure should be instituted immediately. Although there has been no systematic study of treatment of hypertensive crises, phentolamine has been used and is recommended at a dosage of 5 mg IV. Care should be taken to administer the drug slowly in order to avoid producing an excessive hypotensive effect. Fever should be managed by means of external cooling. Other symptomatic and supportive measures may be desirable in particular cases. Parenteral reserpine should not be used.

WARNINGS TO THE PATIENT

Patients should be instructed to report promptly the occurrence of headache or other unusual symptoms, *i.e.*, palpitation and/or tachycardia, a sense of constriction in the throat or chest, sweating, dizziness, neck stiffness, nausea, or vomiting. Patients should be warned against eating the foods listed in CONTRAINDICATIONS while on isocarboxazid therapy and should also be told not to drink alcoholic beverages. The patient should also be warned about the possibility of hypotension and faintness, as well as drowsiness sufficient to impair performance of potentially hazardous tasks, such as driving a car or operating machinery.

Patients should also be cautioned not to take concomitant medications, whether prescription or over-the-counter drugs such as cold, hay fever, or weight-reducing preparations, without the advice of a physician. They should be advised not to consume excessive amounts of caffeine in any form. Likewise, they should inform their physicians and their dentist about the use of isocarboxazid.

LIMITED EXPERIENCE WITH ISOCARBOXAZID AT HIGHER DOSES

Because of the limited experience with systematically monitored patients receiving isocarboxazid at the higher end of the currently recommended dose range of up to 60 mg/day, caution is indicated in patients for whom a dose of 40 mg/day is exceeded (see ADVERSE REACTIONS).

PRECAUTIONS

GENERAL

Hypotension

Hypotension has been observed during isocarboxazid therapy. Symptoms of postural hypotension are seen most commonly, but not exclusively, in patients with preexistent hypertension; blood pressure usually returns rapidly to pretreatment levels upon discontinuation of the drug. Dosage increases should be made more gradually in patients showing a tendency toward hypotension at the beginning of therapy. Postural hypotension may be relieved by having the patient lie down until blood pressure returns to normal. When isocarboxazid is combined with phenothiazine derivatives or other compounds known to cause hypotension, the possibility of additive hypotensive effects should be considered.

Lowered Seizure Threshold

Because isocarboxazid lowers the convulsive threshold in some animal experiments, suitable precautions should be taken if epileptic patients are treated. Isocarboxazid appears to have varying effects in epileptic patients; while some have a decrease in frequency of seizures, others have more seizures.

Drugs that lower the seizure threshold, including MAO inhibitors, should not be used with metrizamide. As with other MAO inhibitors, isocarboxazid should be discontinued at least 48 hours before myelography and should not be resumed for at least 24 hours postprocedure.

Hepatotoxicity

There is a low incidence of altered liver function or jaundice in patients treated with isocarboxazid. In the past, it was difficult to differentiate most cases of drug-induced hepatocellular jaundice from viral hepatitis although this is no longer true. Periodic liver chemistry tests should be performed during isocarboxazid therapy; use of the drug should be discontinued at the first sign of hepatic dysfunction or jaundice.

Suicide

In depressed patients, the possibility of suicide should always be considered and adequate precautions taken. Exclusive reliance on drug therapy to prevent suicidal attempts is unwarranted, as there may be a delay in the onset of therapeutic effect or an increase in anxiety or agitation. Also, some patients fail to respond to drug therapy or may respond only temporarily. The strictest supervision, and preferably hospitalization, are required.

Use in Patients With Concomitant Illness

MAO inhibitors can suppress anginal pain that would otherwise serve as a warning of myocardial ischemia.

In patients with impaired renal function, isocarboxazid should be used cautiously to prevent accumulation.

Some MAO inhibitors have contributed to hypoglycemic episodes in diabetic patients receiving insulin or glycemic agents. Isocarboxazid should therefore be used with caution in diabetics using these drugs.

Isocarboxazid may aggravate coexisting symptoms in depression, such as anxiety and agitation.

Use isocarboxazid with caution in hyperthyroid patients because of their increased sensitivity to pressor amines.

Isocarboxazid should be used cautiously in hyperactive or agitated patients, as well as in schizophrenic patients, because it may cause excessive stimulation. Activation of mania/hypomania has been reported in a small proportion of patients with major affective disorder who were treated with marketed antidepressants.

CARCINOGENESIS, MUTAGENESIS, AND IMPAIRMENT OF FERTILITY

Long term studies to evaluate carcinogenic potential have not been conducted with this drug, and there is no information concerning mutagenesis or impairment of fertility.

PREGNANCY CATEGORY C

The potential reproductive toxicity of isocarboxazid has not been adequately evaluated in animals. It is also not known whether isocarboxazid can cause embryo/fetal harm when administered to a pregnant woman or can affect reproductive capacity. Isocarboxazid should be given to a pregnant woman only if clearly needed.

NURSING MOTHERS

Levels of excretion of isocarboxazid and/or its metabolites in human milk have not been determined, and effects on the nursing infant are unknown. Isocarboxazid should be used in women who are nursing only if clearly needed.

PEDIATRIC USE

Isocarboxazid is not recommended for use in patients under 16 years of age, as safety and effectiveness in pediatric populations have not been demonstrated.

DRUG INTERACTIONS

See CONTRAINDICATIONS, WARNINGS, and PRECAUTIONS for information on drug interactions.

Isocarboxazid should be administered with caution to patients receiving disulfiram. In a single study, rats given high intraperitoneal doses of an MAO inhibitor plus disulfiram experienced severe toxicity, including convulsions and death.

Concomitant use of isocarboxazid and other psychotropic agents is generally not recommended because of possible potentiating effects. This is especially true in patients who may subject themselves to an overdosage of drugs. If combination therapy is needed, careful consideration should be given to the pharmacology of all agents to be used. The monoamine oxidase inhibitory effects of isocarboxazid may persist for a substantial period after discontinuation of the drug, and this should be borne in mind when another drug is prescribed following isocarboxazid. To avoid potentiation, the physician wishing to terminate treatment with isocarboxazid and begin therapy with another agent should allow for an interval of 10 days.

ADVERSE REACTIONS

ADVERSE FINDINGS OBSERVED IN SHORT-TERM, PLACEBO-CONTROLLED TRIALS

Systematically collected data are available from only 86 patients exposed to isocarboxazid, of whom only 52 received doses of ≥50 mg/day, including only 11 who were dosed at ≥60 mg/day. Because of the limited experience with systematically monitored patients receiving isocarboxazid at the higher end of the currently recommended dose range of up to 60 mg/day, caution is indicated in patients for whom a dose of 40 mg/day is exceeded (see WARNINGS).

TABLE 2 enumerates the incidence, rounded to the nearest percent, of treatment emergent adverse events that occurred among 86 depressed patients who received isocarboxazid at doses ranging from 20-80 mg/day in placebo-controlled trials of 6 weeks in duration. Events included are those occurring in 1% or more of patients treated with isocarboxazid and for which the incidence in patients treated with isocarboxazid was greater than the incidence in placebo-treated patients.

The prescriber should be aware that these figures cannot be used to predict the incidence of adverse events in the course of usual medical practice where patient characteristics and other factors differ from those which prevailed in the clinical trials. Similarly, the cited frequencies cannot be compared with figures obtained from other clinical investigations involving different treatments, uses, and investigators. The cited figures, however, do provide the prescribing physician with some basis for estimating the relative contribution of drug and non-drug factors to the adverse event incidence rate in the population studied.

The commonly observed adverse event that occurred in isocarboxazid patients with an incidence of 5% or greater and at least twice the incidence in placebo patients were nausea, dry mouth, and dizziness (see TABLE 2).

In three clinical trials for which the data were pooled, 4 of 85 (5%) patients who received placebo, 10 of 86 (12%) who received <50 mg of isocarboxazid per day, and 1 of 52 (2%) who received ≥50 mg of isocarboxazid per day prematurely discontinued treatment. The most common reasons for discontinuation were dizziness, orthostatic hypotension, syncope, and dry mouth.

TABLE 2 *Treatment-Emergent Adverse Events*

*Incidence in placebo-controlled clinical trials with isocarboxazid doses of 40-80 mg/day**

Body System/Adverse Event	Placebo (n=85)	Isocarboxazid <50 mg (n=86)	Isocarboxazid ≥50 mg (n=52)†
Miscellaneous			
Drowsy	0%	4%	0%
Anxiety	1%	2%	0%
Chills	0%	2%	0%
Forgetful	1%	2%	2%
Hyperactive	0%	2%	0%
Lethargy	0%	2%	2%
Sedation	1%	2%	0%
Syncope	0%	2%	0%
Integumentary			
Sweating	0%	2%	2%
Musculoskeletal			
Heavy feeling	0%	2%	0%
Cardiovascular			
Orthostatic hypotension	1%	4%	4%
Palpitations	1%	2%	0%
Gastrointestinal			
Dry mouth	4%	9%	6%
Constipation	6%	7%	4%
Nausea	2%	6%	4%
Diarrhea	1%	2%	0%
Urogenital			
Impotence	0%	2%	0%
Urinary frequency	1%	2%	0%
Urinary hesitancy	0%	1%	4%
Central Nervous			
Headache	13%	15%	6%
Insomnia	4%	4%	6%
Sleep disturbance	0%	5%	2%
Tremor	0%	4%	4%
Myoclonic jerks	0%	2%	0%
Paresthesia	1%	2%	0%
Special Senses			
Dizziness	14%	29%	15%

* Events reported by at least 1% of patients treated with isocarboxazid are presented, except for those which had an incidence on placebo greater than or equal to that on isocarboxazid.
† All patients also received isocarboxazid at doses 50 mg.

OTHER EVENTS OBSERVED DURING THE POSTMARKETING EVALUATION OF ISOCARBOXAZID

Isolated cases of akathisia, ataxia, black tongue, coma, dysuria, euphoria, hematologic changes, incontinence, neuritis, photosensitivity, sexual disturbances, spider telangiectases, and urinary retention have been reported. These side effects sometimes necessitate discontinuation of therapy. In rare instances, hallucinations have been reported with high dosages, but they have disappeared upon reduction of dosage or discontinuation of therapy. Toxic amblyopia was reported in 1 psychiatric patient who had received isocarboxazid for about a year; no causal relationship to isocarboxazid was established. Impaired water excretion compatible with the syndrome of inappropriate secretion of antidiuretic hormone (SIADH) has been reported.

DOSAGE AND ADMINISTRATION

For maximum therapeutic effect, the dosage of isocarboxazid must be individually adjusted on the basis of careful observation of the patient. Dosage should be started with 1 tablet (10 mg) of isocarboxazid twice daily. If tolerated, dosage may be increased by increments of 1 tablet (10 mg) every 2-4 days to achieve a dosage of 4 tablets daily (40 mg) by the end of the first week of treatment. Dosage can then be increased by increments of up to 20 mg/week, if needed and tolerated, to a maximum recommended dosage of 60 mg/day. Daily dosage should be divided into 2-4 doses. After maximum clinical response is achieved, an attempt should be made to reduce the dosage slowly over a period of several weeks without jeopardizing the therapeutic response. Beneficial effect may not be seen in some patients for 3-6 weeks. If no response is obtained by then, continued administration is unlikely to help.

Because of the limited experience with systematically monitored patients receiving isocarboxazid at the higher end of the currently recommended dose range of up to 60 mg/day, caution is indicated in patients for whom a dose of 40 mg/day is exceeded (see ADVERSE REACTIONS).

HOW SUPPLIED

Marplan is available in tablets of 10 mg isocarboxazid each, that are peach-colored and scored.

PRODUCT LISTING - EQUIVALENTS NOT AVAILABLE

Tablet - Oral - 10 mg

100's	$70.66	MARPLAN, Oxford Pharmaceutical Services	64803-0032-01

Isoetharine Hydrochloride *(001582)*

For related information, see the comparative table section in Appendix A.

Categories: Asthma; Bronchitis, chronic; Emphysema; Pregnancy Category C; FDA Approved 1961 Dec
Drug Classes: Adrenergic agonists; Bronchodilators
Brand Names: Arm-A-Med; Beta-2; Bisorine; **Bronkosol**; Dey-Lute
Foreign Brand Availability: Numotac (Benin; Burkina-Faso; Ethiopia; Gambia; Ghana; Guinea; Ivory-Coast; Kenya; Liberia; Malawi; Mali; Mauritania; Mauritius; Morocco; Niger; Nigeria; Senegal; Seychelles; Sierra-Leone; Sudan; Tanzania; Tunia; Uganda; Zambia; Zimbabwe)
HCFA JCODE(S): J7651 0.125% per ml INH; J7650 0.1% per ml INH; J7652 0.167% per ml INH; J7653 0.2% per ml INH; J7654 0.25% per ml INH; J7655 1.0% per ml INH

DESCRIPTION

BRONCHODILATOR SOLUTION FOR ORAL INHALATION.

Isoetharine hydrochloride, 1% also contains: acetone sodium bisulfite, glycerin, parabens, purified water, sodium chloride, and sodium citrate.

STORAGE

Store at controlled room temperature, 15-30°C (59-86°F).

PROTECT FROM LIGHT. Store vial in pouch until time of use. Do not use solution if its color is pinkish or darker than slightly yellow or if it contains a precipitate.

CLINICAL PHARMACOLOGY

Isoetharine is a sympathomimetic amine with preferential affinity for $beta_2$ adrenergic receptor sites of bronchial and certain arteriolar musculature and a lower order of affinity for $beta_1$ adrenergic receptors. Its activity in symptomatic relief of bronchospasm is rapid and of relatively long duration. By relieving bronchospasm, isoetharine helps give prompt relief and significantly increases vital capacity.

I

INDICATIONS AND USAGE

Isoetharine hydrochloride is indicated for use as a bronchodilator for bronchial asthma and for reversible bronchospasm that may occur in association with bronchitis and emphysema.

CONTRAINDICATIONS

Isoetharine inhalation solution should not be administered to patients who are hypersensitive to any of its ingredients.

WARNINGS

Contains acetone sodium bisulfite, a sulfite that may cause allergic-type reactions including anaphylactic symptoms and life-threatening or less severe asthmatic episodes in certain susceptible people. The overall prevalence of sulfite sensitivity in the general population is unknown and probably low. Sulfite sensitivity is seen more frequently in asthmatic than in nonasthmatic people.

Excessive use of an adrenergic aerosol should be discouraged as it may lose its effectiveness. Occasional patients have been reported to develop severe paradoxical airway resistance with repeated excessive use of an aerosol adrenergic inhalation preparation. The cause of this refractory state is unknown. It is advisable that in such instances the use of the aerosol adrenergic be discontinued immediately and alternative therapy instituted, since in the reported cases the patients did not respond to other forms of therapy until the drug was withdrawn. Cardiac arrest has been noted in several instances.

Isoetharine hydrochloride should not be administered along with epinephrine or other sympathomimetic amines, since these drugs are direct cardiac stimulants and may cause excessive tachycardia. They may, however, be alternated if desired.

Usage in Pregnancy: Although there has been no evidence of teratogenic effects with this drug, use of any drug in pregnancy, lactation, or in women of childbearing potential requires that the potential benefit of the drug be weighed against its possible hazard to the mother or child.

PRECAUTIONS

GENERAL

Dosage must be carefully adjusted in patients with hyperthyroidism, hypertension, acute coronary disease, cardiac asthma, limited cardiac reserve and in individuals sensitive to sympathomimetic amines since overdosage may result in tachycardia, palpitations, nausea, headache or epinephrine like side effects.

ADVERSE REACTIONS

Although isoetharine hydrochloride is relatively free of toxic side effects, too frequent use may cause tachycardia, palpitation, nausea, headache, changes in blood pressure, anxiety, tension, restlessness, insomnia, tremor, weakness, dizziness, and excitement, as is the case with other sympathomimetic amines.

DOSAGE AND ADMINISTRATION

Isoetharine hydrochloride can be administered by hand nebulizer, oxygen aerosolization, or intermittent positive pressure breathing (IPPB). Usually treatment need not be repeated more often than every 4 hours, although in severe cases more frequent administration may be necessary. (See TABLE 1 and TABLE 2.)

TABLE 1

Method of Administration	Usual Dose (1% Solution)*	Range
Oxygen aerosolization†	0.50 ml	0.25-0.50 ml
IPPB‡	0.50 ml	0.25-1 ml

* The doses given are for the 1% solution which must be suitably diluted prior to administration. See TABLE 2 for dose equivalents for the entire prediluted and ready-to-use line.
† Administered with oxygen flow adjusted to 4-6 L/min over a period of 15-20 minutes
‡ Usually an inspiratory flow rate of 15 L/min at a cycling pressure of 15 cm H_2O is recommended. It may be necessary, according to patient and type of IPPB apparatus to adjust flow rate to 6-30 L/min, cycling pressure to 10-15 cm H_2O and further dilution according to needs of patient.

TABLE 2

Product Strength	Volume (ml)	Equivalent to - ml of Isoetharine HCl 1%
0.062%	4 ml	0.25 ml
0.125%	4 ml	0.5 ml
0.167%	3 ml	0.5 ml
0.2%	2.5 ml	0.5 ml
0.25%	2 ml	0.5 ml

PRODUCT LISTING - RATED THERAPEUTICALLY EQUIVALENT

Solution - Inhalation - 1%
30 ml $96.11 GENERIC, Physicians Total Care 54868-3682-00

Isoniazid *(001585)*

Categories: Tuberculosis; FDA Approved 1952 Nov; Pregnancy Category C; WHO Formulary
Drug Classes: Antimycobacterials
Brand Names: INH; Laniazid; Niazid; Nydrazid; Rimifon
Foreign Brand Availability: Curazid Forte (Philippines); Dianicotyl (Greece); Diazid (Japan); Europlex (Philippines); Hidrazida (Portugal); Hydra (Japan); Hydrazide (Japan); Hydrazin (Taiwan); Iscotin (Japan; Taiwan); Isokin (India); Isonex (India; Indonesia); Isoniazid (Australia; New-Zealand); Isoniazid Atlantic (Hong-Kong); Isoniazida N.T. (Ecuador); Isotamine (Canada); Isozid (Germany); Medic Aid Isoniazid (Philippines); Nicetal (Ecuador); Nicotibine (Belgium); Nicozid (Italy); PMS Isoniazid (Canada); Rimicid (Bulgaria); Tibinide (Sweden); Tubilysin (Finland); Valifol (Mexico); Yuhan-Zid (Korea)
Cost of Therapy: $2.09 (Tuberculosis; Generic Tablets; 300 mg; 1 tablet/day; 30 day supply)

WARNING

Severe and sometimes fatal hepatitis associated with isoniazid therapy may occur and may develop even after many months of treatment. The risk of developing hepatitis is age related. Approximate case rates by age are: 0 per 1000 for persons under 20 years of age, 3 per 1000 for persons in the 20-34 year age group, 12 per 1000 for persons in the 35-49 year age group, 23 per 1000 for persons in the 50-64 year age group, and 8 per 1000 for persons over 65 years of age.

The risk of hepatitis is increased with daily consumption of alcohol. Precise data to provide a fatality rate for isoniazid-related hepatitis is not available; however, in a US Public Health Service Surveillance Study of 13,838 persons taking isoniazid, there were 8 deaths among 174 cases of hepatitis.

Therefore, patients given isoniazid should be carefully monitored and interviewed at monthly intervals. Serum transaminase concentration becomes elevated in about 10-20% of patients, usually during the first few months of therapy but it can occur at any time. Usually enzyme levels return to normal despite continuance of drug but in some cases progressive liver dysfunction occurs.

Patients should be instructed to report immediately any of the prodromal symptoms of hepatitis, such as fatigue, weakness, malaise, anorexia, nausea, or vomiting. If these symptoms appear or if signs suggestive of hepatic damage are detected, isoniazid should be discontinued promptly, since continued use of the drug in these cases has been reported to cause a more severe form of liver damage.

Patients with tuberculosis should be given appropriate treatment with alternative drugs. If isoniazid must be reinstituted, it should be reinstituted only after symptoms and laboratory abnormalities have cleared. The drug should be restarted in very small and gradually increasing doses and should be withdrawn immediately if there is any indication of recurrent liver involvement.

Preventive treatment should be deferred in persons with acute hepatic diseases.

DESCRIPTION

INJECTION

Isoniazid Injection provides 100 mg isoniazid per ml with 0.25% chlorobutanol (chloral derivative) as a preservative; the pH has been adjusted to 6.0-7.0 with sodium hydroxide or hydrochloric acid. At the time of manufacture, the air in the container is replaced by nitrogen.

Storage

Store at room temperature.

Isoniazid for injection may crystallize at low temperatures. If this occurs, warm the vial to room temperature before use to redissolve the crystals.

ORAL TABLETS

Isoniazid is an antibiotic available as 100 and 300 mg tablets for oral administration. Isoniazid is isonicotinic acid hydrazide.

Isoniazid is colorless or white crystals or white crystalline powder. It is odorless and slowly affected by exposure to air and light. It is freely soluble in water, sparingly soluble in alcohol, and slightly soluble in chloroform and in ether. Its molecular weight is 137.14.

ORAL SYRUP

This product produced by Carolina is an orange flavored syrup containing 50 mg of isoniazid per 5 ml of syrup. Sorbitol solution (containing 70% sorbitol) is used as the vehicle.

CLINICAL PHARMACOLOGY

Isoniazid acts against actively growing tubercle bacilli.

Within 1-2 hours after oral administration isoniazid produces peak blood levels which decline to 50% or less within 6 hours. It diffuses readily into all body fluids (cerebrospinal, pleural, and ascitic), tissues, organs, and excreta (saliva, sputum, and feces). The drug also passes through the placental barrier and into milk in concentrations comparable to those in the plasma. From 50-70% of a dose of isoniazid is excreted in the urine in 24 hours.

Isoniazid is metabolized primarily by acetylation and dehydrazination. The rate of acetylation is genetically determined. Approximately 50% of Blacks and Caucasians are "slow acetylators" and the rest are rapid acetylators; the majority of Eskimos and Orientals are "rapid acetylators".

The rate of acetylation does not significantly alter the effectiveness of isoniazid. However, slow acetylation may lead to higher blood levels of the drug, and thus an increase in toxic reactions.

Pyridoxine (B_6) deficiency is sometimes observed in adults with high doses of isoniazid and is considered probably due to its competition with pyridoxal phosphate for the enzyme apotryptophanase.

INDICATIONS AND USAGE

For all forms of tuberculosis in which organisms are susceptible.

For preventive therapy for the following groups, in order of priority:

1. Household members and other close associates of persons with recently diagnosed tuberculous disease.
2. Positive tuberculin skin test reactors with findings on the chest roentgenogram consistent with nonprogressive tuberculous disease, in whom there are neither positive bacteriologic findings nor a history of adequate chemotherapy.
3. Newly infected persons.
4. Positive tuberculin skin test reactors in the following special clinical situations: prolonged therapy with adrenocorticosteroids; immunosuppressive therapy; some hematologic and reticuloendothelial diseases, such as leukemia or Hodgkin's disease; diabetes mellitus; silicosis; after gastrectomy.
5. Other positive tuberculin reactors under 35 years of age. The risk of hepatitis must be weighed against the risk of tuberculosis in positive tuberculin reactors over the age of 35. However, the use of isoniazid is recommended for those with the additional risk factors listed above (1-4) and on an individual basis in situations where there is likelihood of serious consequences to contacts who may become infected.

CONTRAINDICATIONS

Isoniazid is contraindicated in patients who develop severe hypersensitivity reactions, including drug-induced hepatitis. Previous isoniazid-associated hepatic injury: severe adverse reactions to isoniazid, such as drug fever, chills, and arthritis; acute liver disease of any etiology.

WARNINGS

See BOXED WARNING.

PRECAUTIONS

All drugs should be stopped and an evaluation made at the first sign of a hypersensitivity reaction. If isoniazid therapy must be reinstituted, the drug should be given only after symptoms have cleared. The drug should be restarted in very small and gradually increasing doses and should be withdrawn immediately if there is any indication of recurrent hypersensitivity reaction.

Use of isoniazid should be carefully monitored in the following:

1. Patients who are receiving phenytoin concurrently. Isoniazid may decrease the excretion of phenytoin or may enhance its effects. To avoid phenytoin intoxication, appropriate adjustment of the anticonvulsant should be made.
2. Daily users of alcohol. Daily ingestion of alcohol may be associated with a higher incidence of isoniazid hepatitis.
3. Patients with current chronic liver disease or severe renal dysfunction.

Ophthalmologic examinations (including ophthalmoscopy) should be done *before* isoniazid is started and periodically thereafter, even without occurrence of visual symptoms.

USAGE IN PREGNANCY AND LACTATION

It has been reported that in both rats and rabbits, isoniazid may exert an embryocidal effect when administered orally during pregnancy, although no isoniazid-related congenital anomalies have been found in reproduction studies in mammalian species (mice, rats, and rabbits). Isoniazid should be prescribed during pregnancy only when therapeutically necessary. The benefit of preventive therapy should be weighed against a possible risk to the fetus. Preventive treatment generally should be started after delivery because of the increased risk of tuberculosis for new mothers.

Since isoniazid is known to cross the placental barrier and to pass into maternal breast milk, neonates and breast-fed infants of isoniazid-treated mothers should be carefully observed for any evidence of adverse effects.

CARCINOGENESIS

Isoniazid has been reported to induce pulmonary tumors in a number of strains of mice.

ADVERSE REACTIONS

The most frequent reactions are those affecting the nervous system and the liver.

Nervous System Reactions: Peripheral neuropathy is the most common toxic effect. It is dose-related, occurs most often in the malnourished and in those predisposed to neuritis (*e.g.,* alcoholics and diabetics), and is usually preceded by paresthesias of the feet and hands. The incidence is higher in "slow inactivators".

Other neurotoxic effects, which are uncommon with conventional doses, are convulsions, toxic encephalopathy, optic neuritis and atrophy, memory impairment, and toxic psychosis.

Gastrointestinal Reactions: Nausea, vomiting, epigastric distress.

Hepatic Reactions: Elevated serum transaminases (SGOT; SGPT), bilirubinemia, bilirubinuria, jaundice and occasionally severe and sometimes fatal hepatitis. The common prodromal symptoms are anorexia, nausea, vomiting, fatigue, malaise, and weakness. Mild and transient elevation of serum transaminase levels, occurs in 10-20% of persons taking isoniazid. The abnormality usually occurs in the first 4-6 months of treatment but can occur at any time during therapy. In most instances, enzyme levels return to normal with no necessity to discontinue medication. In occasional instances, progressive liver damage occurs, with accompanying symptoms. In these cases, the drug should be discontinued immediately. The frequency of progressive liver damage increases with age. It is rare in persons under 20, but occurs in up to 2.3% of those over 50 years of age.

Hematologic Reactions: Agranulocytosis; hemolytic, sideroblastic, or aplastic anemia; thrombocytopenia; and eosinophilia.

Hypersensitivity Reactions: Fever, skin eruptions (morbilliform, maculopapular, purpuric, or exfoliative), lymphadenopathy and vasculitis.

Metabolic and Endocrine Reactions: Pyridoxine deficiency, pellagra, hyperglycemia, metabolic acidosis, and gynecomastia.

Miscellaneous Reactions: Rheumatic syndrome and systemic lupus erythematosus-like syndrome. Local irritation has been observed at the site of intramuscular injection.

DOSAGE AND ADMINISTRATION

INJECTION

Isoniazid injection is used in conjunction with other effective antituberculosis agents. If the bacilli become resistant, therapy must be changed to agents to which the bacilli are susceptible.

Usual Parenteral Dosage

For Treatment of Tuberculosis:

Adults: 5 mg/kg up to 300 mg daily in a single dose.

Infants and Children: 10 to 20 mg/kg depending on severity of infection (up to 300 to 500 mg daily) in a single dose.

For Preventive Therapy:

Adults: 300 mg per day in a single.

Infants and Children: 10 mg/kg (up to 300 mg daily) in a single dose.

Continuous administration of isoniazid for a sufficient period of time is an essential part of the regimen because relapse rate are higher if chemotherapy is stopped prematurely. In the treatment of tuberculosis, resistant organisms may multiply and their emergence during the treatment may necessitate a change in the regimen.

Concomitant administration of pyridoxine (B_6) is recommended in the malnourished and in those predisposed to neuropathy (*e.g.,* alcoholics and diabetics).

ORAL TABLETS AND SYRUP

For Treatment of Active Tuberculosis: Isoniazid is used in conjunction with other effective antituberculous agents.

If the bacilli become resistant, therapy must be changed to agents to which the bacilli are susceptible.

Usual Oral Dosage

Adults: 5 mg/kg up to 300 mg daily in a single dose.

Infants and children: 10-20 mg/kg depending on severity of infection, (up to 300-500 mg daily) in a single dose.

For Preventive Therapy

Adults: 300 mg per day in a single dose.

Infants and Children: 10 mg/kg (up to 300 mg daily) in a single dose.

Continuous administration of isoniazid for a sufficient period is an essential part of the regimen because relapse rates are higher if chemotherapy is stopped prematurely. In the treatment of tuberculosis, resistant organisms may multiply and the emergence of resistant organisms during the treatment may necessitate a change in the regimen.

Concomitant administration of pyridoxine (B_6) is recommended in the malnourished and in those predisposed to neuropathy (*e.g.,* alcoholics and diabetics).

PRODUCT LISTING - RATED THERAPEUTICALLY EQUIVALENT

Package	Price	Product, Manufacturer	NDC
Solution - Intramuscular - 100 mg/ml			
10 ml	$20.26	NYDRAZID, Bristol-Myers Squibb	00003-0643-50
Syrup - Oral - 50 mg/5 ml			
473 ml	$20.00	GENERIC, Carolina Medical Products Company	46287-0009-01
480 ml	$20.00	GENERIC, Allscripts Pharmaceutical Company	54569-2900-00
480 ml	$22.50	GENERIC, Versapharm Inc	61748-0017-16
Tablet - Oral - 100 mg			
30's	$2.48	GENERIC, Eon Labs Manufacturing Inc	00185-4351-30
30's	$2.90	GENERIC, Pd-Rx Pharmaceuticals	58864-0298-30
30's	$2.95	GENERIC, Allscripts Pharmaceutical Company	54569-2942-01
30's	$6.89	GENERIC, Pd-Rx Pharmaceuticals	55289-0055-30
45's	$7.28	GENERIC, Pd-Rx Pharmaceuticals	55289-0055-45
60's	$3.90	GENERIC, Pd-Rx Pharmaceuticals	58864-0298-60
60's	$8.25	GENERIC, Pd-Rx Pharmaceuticals	55289-0055-60
75's	$11.37	GENERIC, Pd-Rx Pharmaceuticals	55289-0055-75
90's	$4.50	GENERIC, Pd-Rx Pharmaceuticals	58864-0298-90
100's	$0.68	GENERIC, Global Pharmaceutical Corporation	00115-3706-01
100's	$4.20	GENERIC, Paddock Laboratories Inc	00574-0100-01
100's	$4.95	GENERIC, Cmc-Consolidated Midland Corporation	00223-1150-01
100's	$5.16	GENERIC, Dixon-Shane Inc	17236-0180-01
100's	$5.40	GENERIC, Versapharm Inc	61748-0016-01
100's	$5.70	GENERIC, Major Pharmaceuticals Inc	00904-2095-60
100's	$5.80	GENERIC, Ivax Corporation	00182-0559-01
100's	$5.92	GENERIC, Aligen Independent Laboratories Inc	00405-4552-01
100's	$6.55	GENERIC, Eon Labs Manufacturing Inc	00185-4351-01
100's	$6.60	GENERIC, Halsey Drug Company Inc	00879-0113-01
100's	$7.90	GENERIC, West Ward Pharmaceutical Corporation	00143-1260-25
100's	$8.20	GENERIC, West Ward Pharmaceutical Corporation	00143-1260-01
100's	$9.83	GENERIC, Barr Laboratories Inc	00555-0066-02
100's	$9.95	GENERIC, Raway Pharmacal Inc	00686-0082-20
100's	$12.60	GENERIC, Udl Laboratories Inc	51079-0082-20
100's	$15.45	GENERIC, Pd-Rx Pharmaceuticals	55289-0055-01
Tablet - Oral - 300 mg			
10 x 10	$12.00	GENERIC, Versapharm Inc	61748-0013-11
30's	$1.95	GENERIC, Major Pharmaceuticals Inc	00904-2096-46
30's	$3.65	GENERIC, Dixon-Shane Inc	17236-0182-30
30's	$4.06	GENERIC, Versapharm Inc	61748-0013-30
30's	$6.43	GENERIC, West Ward Pharmaceutical Corporation	00143-1261-30
30's	$7.20	GENERIC, Pd-Rx Pharmaceuticals	55289-0742-30
30's	$9.06	GENERIC, Eon Labs Manufacturing Inc	00185-4350-30
30's	$10.15	GENERIC, Barr Laboratories Inc	00555-0071-01
30's	$11.44	GENERIC, Pharma Pac	52959-0145-30
35's	$4.25	GENERIC, Dixon-Shane Inc	17236-0182-35
35's	$4.49	GENERIC, Pd-Rx Pharmaceuticals	55289-0742-35
50's	$9.42	GENERIC, Pd-Rx Pharmaceuticals	55289-0742-50
50's	$18.00	GENERIC, Pharma Pac	52959-0145-50
60's	$18.40	GENERIC, Pd-Rx Pharmaceuticals	55289-0742-60
100's	$4.66	GENERIC, Major Pharmaceuticals Inc	00904-2096-61
100's	$6.95	GENERIC, Cmc-Consolidated Midland Corporation	00223-1151-01
100's	$8.43	GENERIC, Aligen Independent Laboratories Inc	00405-4553-01
100's	$8.90	FEDERAL UPPER LIMIT, H.C.F.A. F F P	99999-1585-06
100's	$9.75	GENERIC, West Ward Pharmaceutical Corporation	00143-1261-25
100's	$10.96	GENERIC, Versapharm Inc	61748-0013-01
100's	$11.50	GENERIC, Raway Pharmacal Inc	00686-0083-20
100's	$13.06	GENERIC, Eon Labs Manufacturing Inc	00185-4350-01
100's	$13.06	GENERIC, Lannett Company Inc	00527-1109-01
100's	$13.11	GENERIC, Major Pharmaceuticals Inc	00904-2096-60
100's	$14.15	GENERIC, West Ward Pharmaceutical Corporation	00143-1261-01
100's	$14.51	GENERIC, Pd-Rx Pharmaceuticals	55289-0742-01
100's	$15.51	GENERIC, Dixon-Shane Inc	17236-0182-01
100's	$17.66	GENERIC, Udl Laboratories Inc	51079-0083-20
100's	$20.63	GENERIC, Barr Laboratories Inc	00555-0071-02
180's	$39.68	GENERIC, Pharma Pac	52959-0145-81

PRODUCT LISTING - EQUIVALENTS NOT AVAILABLE

Package	Price	Product, Manufacturer	NDC
Tablet - Oral - 100 mg			
60's	$1.89	GENERIC, Pharmaceutical Corporation Of America	51655-0394-25
60's	$5.90	GENERIC, Allscripts Pharmaceutical Company	54569-2942-02
100's	$9.83	GENERIC, Allscripts Pharmaceutical Company	54569-2942-00
100's	$9.93	GENERIC, Southwood Pharmaceuticals Inc	58016-0912-00
Tablet - Oral - 300 mg			
10's	$1.27	GENERIC, Southwood Pharmaceuticals Inc	58016-0913-10
12's	$1.53	GENERIC, Southwood Pharmaceuticals Inc	58016-0913-12
14's	$1.78	GENERIC, Southwood Pharmaceuticals Inc	58016-0913-14
15's	$1.91	GENERIC, Southwood Pharmaceuticals Inc	58016-0913-15
15's	$4.54	GENERIC, Prescript Pharmaceuticals	00247-0150-15
20's	$2.55	GENERIC, Southwood Pharmaceuticals Inc	58016-0913-20
21's	$2.68	GENERIC, Southwood Pharmaceuticals Inc	58016-0913-21
24's	$3.06	GENERIC, Southwood Pharmaceuticals Inc	58016-0913-24
24's	$5.26	GENERIC, Prescript Pharmaceuticals	00247-0150-24
28's	$3.57	GENERIC, Southwood Pharmaceuticals Inc	58016-0913-28
30's	$3.17	GENERIC, Allscripts Pharmaceutical Company	54569-2509-03
30's	$3.22	GENERIC, Physicians Total Care	54868-2416-02
30's	$3.36	GENERIC, Heartland Healthcare Services	61392-0126-30
30's	$3.36	GENERIC, Heartland Healthcare Services	61392-0126-39
30's	$3.64	GENERIC, Cardinal Pharmaceuticals	63874-0366-30
30's	$3.82	GENERIC, Southwood Pharmaceuticals Inc	58016-0913-30
30's	$4.75	GENERIC, Cmc-Consolidated Midland Corporation	00223-1151-30
30's	$5.25	GENERIC, Pharmaceutical Corporation Of America	51655-0391-24
30's	$5.39	GENERIC, Huffman Laboratories Division Pharmed Group	54252-0109-30
30's	$5.74	GENERIC, Prescript Pharmaceuticals	00247-0150-30
31's	$3.47	GENERIC, Heartland Healthcare Services	61392-0126-31

32's	$3.58	GENERIC, Heartland Healthcare Services	61392-0126-32
35's	$3.70	GENERIC, Allscripts Pharmaceutical Company	54569-2509-02
35's	$6.13	GENERIC, Prescript Pharmaceuticals	00247-0150-35
36's	$6.21	GENERIC, Prescript Pharmaceuticals	00247-0150-36
40's	$5.10	GENERIC, Southwood Pharmaceuticals Inc	58016-0913-40
45's	$5.04	GENERIC, Heartland Healthcare Services	61392-0126-45
48's	$7.16	GENERIC, Prescript Pharmaceuticals	00247-0150-48
50's	$5.65	GENERIC, Allscripts Pharmaceutical Company	54569-2509-00
60's	$6.71	GENERIC, Heartland Healthcare Services	61392-0126-60
60's	$7.64	GENERIC, Southwood Pharmaceuticals Inc	58016-0913-60
60's	$8.12	GENERIC, Prescript Pharmaceuticals	00247-0150-60
90's	$10.07	GENERIC, Heartland Healthcare Services	61392-0126-90
100's	$7.61	GENERIC, Physicians Total Care	54868-2416-00
100's	$9.62	GENERIC, Allscripts Pharmaceutical Company	54569-2509-01
100's	$11.29	GENERIC, Prescript Pharmaceuticals	00247-0150-00
100's	$12.74	GENERIC, Southwood Pharmaceuticals Inc	58016-0913-00
100's	$13.25	GENERIC, Cardinal Pharmaceuticals	63874-0366-01
100's	$20.75	GENERIC, Pharma Pac	52959-0145-00

Isoniazid; Pyrazinamide; Rifampin (003210)

Categories: Tuberculosis; Pregnancy Category C; FDA Approved 1994 May; Orphan Drugs; WHO Formulary
Drug Classes: Antimycobacterials
Brand Names: Rifater
Foreign Brand Availability: Rimactazide + Z (Switzerland)
Cost of Therapy: $343.44 (Tuberculosis; Rifater; 50 mg; 300 mg; 120 mg; 6 tablets/day; 30 day supply)

DESCRIPTION

FOR COMPLETE PRESCRIBING INFORMATION, REFER TO THE INDIVIDUAL DRUG MONOGRAPHS (ISONIAZID; PYRAZINAMIDE; RIFAMPIN).

INDICATIONS AND USAGE

This combination drug is indicated in the initial phase of the short-course treatment of pulmonary tuberculosis. During this phase, which should last 2 months, Rifater should be administered on a daily, continuous basis.

Following and initial phase and treatment with this combination drug, treatment should be continued with rifampin and isoniazid (*e.g.,* Rifamate) for at least 4 months. Treatment should be continued for a longer period of time if the patient is still sputum or culture positive, if resistant organisms are present, or if the patient is HIV positive.

In the treatment of tuberculosis, the small number of cells present within large populations of susceptible cells can rapidly become the predominant type. Since resistance can emerge rapidly, susceptibility tests should be performed in the event of persistent positive cultures during the course of treatment. Bacteriologic smears or cultures should be obtained before the start of therapy to confirm the susceptibility of the organism to rifampin, isoniazid, and pyrazinamide and they should be repeated throughout therapy to monitor response to the treatment. If test results show resistance to any of the components of this combination drug and the patient is not responding to therapy, the drug regimen should be modified.

DOSAGE AND ADMINISTRATION

Adults: Patients should be given the following single daily dose of Rifater either 1 hour before or 2 hours after a meal with a full glass of water.

Patients weighing ≤44 kg - 4 tablets
Patients weighing between 45-54 kg - 5 tablets
Patients weighing ≥55 kg - 6 tablets

Children: The ratio of the drugs in this combination may not be appropriate in children or adolescents under the age of 15 (*e.g.,* higher mg/kg doses of isoniazid are usually given in children than adults).

This combination drug is recommended in the initial phase of short-course therapy which is usually continued for 2 months. The Advisory Council for the Elimination of Tuberculosis, the American Thoracic Society, and the Centers for Disease Control and Prevention recommend that either streptomycin or ethambutol be added as a fourth drug in a regimen containing isoniazid (INH), rifampin and pyrazinamide for initial treatment of tuberculosis unless the likelihood of INH or rifampin resistance is very low. The need for fourth drug should be reassessed when the results of susceptibility testing are known. If community rates of INH resistance are currently less than 4%, an initial treatment regimen with less than four drugs maybe considered.

Following the initial phase, treatment should be continued with rifampin and isoniazid (*e.g.,* Rifamate) for at least 4 months. Treatment should be continued for longer if the patient is still sputum or culture positive, if resistant organisms are present, or if the patient is HIV positive. Concomitant administration of pyridoxine (B_6) is recommended in the malnourished, in those predisposed to neuropathy (*e.g.,* alcoholics and diabetics), and in adolescents.

HOW SUPPLIED

Rifater tablets are light beige, smooth, round, and shiny sugar-coated tablets imprinted with "RIFATER" in black ink and contain 120 mg rifampin, 50 mg isoniazid, and 300 mg pyrazinamide, and are supplied as:

Bottles of 60 tablets.

Unit dose blister packages of 100 tablets.

Storage Conditions: Store at controlled room temperature 59°-86°F (15°-30°C). Protect from excessive humidity.

PRODUCT LISTING - EQUIVALENTS NOT AVAILABLE

Tablet - Oral - 50 mg;300 mg;120 mg

60's	$114.48	RIFATER, Glaxosmithkline	00088-0576-41

Isoniazid; Rifampin (001587)

Categories: Tuberculosis; FDA Approval Pre 1982; Pregnancy Category C; WHO Formulary
Drug Classes: Antimycobacterials
Brand Names: Refinah; Rifamate; **Rimactane INH**; Rimactizid
Foreign Brand Availability: Dipicin-INH (Philippines); Ramicin-ISO (Indonesia; Philippines); R-Cinex 600 (India); Refinah 300 (Malaysia; Philippines; Thailand); Ricinis (Hong-Kong; Thailand); Rif Plus (Indonesia); Rifaina (Taiwan); Rifamiso (Thailand); Rifazida (Spain); Rifinah (Bahrain; Benin; Burkina-Faso; Cyprus; Egypt; England; Ethiopia; France; Gambia; Germany; Ghana; Greece; Guinea; Hong-Kong; Iran; Iraq; Ivory-Coast; Jordan; Kenya; Kuwait; Lebanon; Liberia; Libya; Malawi; Mali; Mauritania; Mauritius; Mexico; Morocco; Niger; Nigeria; Oman; Qatar; Republic-of-Yemen; Saudi-Arabia; Senegal; Seychelles; Sierra-Leone; South-Africa; Spain; Sudan; Syria; Tanzania; Tunia; Uganda; United-Arab-Emirates; Zambia; Zimbabwe); Rifinah 300 (New-Zealand; Taiwan); Rifoldin 300MG + INH (Austria); Rimactazid (Bahamas; Bahrain; Barbados; Belize; Benin; Bermuda; Burkina-Faso; Colombia; Curacao; Cyprus; Ecuador; Egypt; England; Ethiopia; Gambia; Ghana; Greece; Guinea; Guyana; Iran; Iraq; Ireland; Ivory-Coast; Jamaica; Jordan; Kenya; Kuwait; Lebanon; Liberia; Libya; Malawi; Malaysia; Mali; Mauritania; Mauritius; Morocco; Netherland-Antilles; Niger; Nigeria; Oman; Qatar; Republic-of-Yemen; Saudi-Arabia; Senegal; Seychelles; Sierra-Leone; Spain; Sudan; Surinam; Syria; Taiwan; Tanzania; Thailand; Trinidad; Tunia; Uganda; United-Arab-Emirates; Zambia; Zimbabwe); Rimactazid 300 (Philippines); Rimpazid 450 (Benin; Burkina-Faso; Ethiopia; Gambia; Ghana; Guinea; Ivory-Coast; Kenya; Liberia; Malawi; Mali; Mauritania; Mauritius; Morocco; Niger; Nigeria; Senegal; Seychelles; Sierra-Leone; Sudan; Tanzania; Tunia; Uganda; Zambia; Zimbabwe)
Cost of Therapy: $154.68 (Tuberculosis; Rifamate; 150 mg; 300 mg; 2 capsules/day; 30 day supply)

DESCRIPTION

FOR COMPLETE PRESCRIBING INFORMATION, REFER TO THE INDIVIDUAL DRUG MONOGRAPHS (ISONIAZID; RIFAMPIN).

INDICATIONS AND USAGE

For pulmonary tuberculosis in which organisms are susceptible, and when the patient has been titrated on the individual components and it has therefore been established that this fixed dosage is therapeutically effective.

This fixed-dosage combination drug is not recommended for initial therapy of tuberculosis or for preventive therapy.

In the treatment of tuberculosis, small numbers of resistant cells, present within large populations of susceptible cells, can rapidly become the predominating type. Since rapid emergence of resistance can occur, culture and susceptibility tests should be performed in the event of persistent positive cultures.

This drug is not indicated for the treatment of meningococcal infections or asymptomatic carriers of *N. meningitidis* to eliminate meningococci from the nasopharynx.

DOSAGE AND ADMINISTRATION

In general, therapy should be continued until bacterial conversion and maximal improvement have occurred.

Adults: Two rifampin-isoniazid capsules (600 mg rifampin, 300 mg isoniazid) once daily, administered 1 hour before or 2 hours after a meal.

Concomitant administration of pyridoxine (B_6) is recommended in the malnourished, in those predisposed to neuropathy (*e.g.,* diabetics) and in adolescents.

SUSCEPTIBILITY TESTING-RIFAMPIN

Rifampin susceptibility powders are available for both direct and indirect methods of determining the susceptibility of strains of mycobacteria. The MICs of susceptible clinical isolates when determined in 7H10 or other non-egg-containing media have ranged from 0.1 to 2 μg/ml.

Quantitative methods that require measurement of zone diameters give the most precise estimates of antibiotic susceptibility. One such procedure has been recommended for use with discs for testing susceptibility to rifampin. Interpretations correlate zone diameters from the disc test with MIC (minimal inhibitory concentration) values for rifampin.

PRODUCT LISTING - EQUIVALENTS NOT AVAILABLE

Capsule - Oral - 150 mg;300 mg

60's	$154.68	RIFAMATE, Aventis Pharmaceuticals	00068-0509-60

Isoproterenol Hydrochloride (001590)

Categories: Adams-Stokes; Asthma; Bronchitis, chronic; Bronchospasm, secondary to anesthesia; Cardiac arrest; Emphysema; Heart block; Heart failure, congestive; Shock, cardiogenic; Shock, hypovolemic; Shock, septic; Pregnancy Category C; FDA Approved 1947 Nov; WHO Formulary
Drug Classes: Adrenergic agonists; Bronchodilators
Brand Names: Aerolone; Dispos-A-Med Isoproterenol HCC; Isopro Aerometer ; **Isuprel**; Medihaler-Iso; Norisodrine; Vapo-Iso
Foreign Brand Availability: Isolin (India); Isuprel Mistometer (Bahrain; Cyprus; Egypt; Iran; Iraq; Jordan; Kuwait; Lebanon; Libya; Oman; Qatar; Republic-of-Yemen; Saudi-Arabia; Syria; United-Arab-Emirates); Isuprel Nebulimetro (Peru); Isoprenalin (Sweden); Saventrine (Finland; Greece; Singapore)
Cost of Therapy: $30.52 (Asthma; Isuprel Mistometer; 0.131 mg; 16.8 g; 6 inhalations/day; day supply)
HCFA JCODE(S): J7660 0.5% per ml INH; J7665 1.0% per ml INH

DESCRIPTION

Chemically, isoproterenol hydrochloride is 3,4-dihydroxy-α-[(isopropylamino) methyl]-benzyl alcohol hydrochloride, a synthetic sympathomimetic amine that is structurally related to epinephrine but acts almost exclusively on beta receptors.

Isoproterenol hydrochloride is a racemic compound with a molecular weight of 247.72 and the molecular formula $C_{11}H_{17}NO_3 \cdot HCl$.

INJECTION

Each milliliter of the sterile 1:5000 Isuprel solution contains:
Isoproterenol hydrochloride injection 0.2 mg
Lactic acid 0.12 mg
Sodium chloride 7.0 mg
Sodium lactate 1.8 mg
Sodium metabisulfite (as preservative) 1.0 mg
Water for injection qs ad 1.0 ml

The pH is adjusted between 3.5 and 4.5 with hydrochloric acid. The air in the ampuls has been displaced by nitrogen gas.

The sterile 1:5000 solution can be administered by intravenous, intramuscular, subcutaneous, or intracardiac routes.

Storage

Store in a cool place between 8-15°C (46-50°F).

Do not use if the injection is pinkish to brownish in color or contains a precipitate.

INHALATION AEROSOL

Isuprel Mistometer is a beta agonist sympathomimetic bronchodilator. It is a complete nebulizing unit consisting of a plastic-coated vial of aerosol solution, detachable plastic mouthpiece with built-in nebulizer, and protective cap. The vial contains isoproterenol hydrochloride 0.25% (w/w) with inert ingredients of alcohol 33% (w/w) and ascorbic acid 0.1% (w/w) and, as propellants, dichlorodifluoromethane and dichlorotetrafluoroethane.

The contents permit the delivery of not less than 200 actuations from the 11.2 g (10 ml) vial and not less than 300 actuations from the 16.8 (15 ml) vial. The Mistometer delivers a measured dose of 131 μg of the bronchodilator in a fine, even mist for inhalation.

Storage

Store at controlled room temperature 15°C to -30°C (59-86°F).

INHALATION SOLUTION

Isuprel hydrochloride, brand of isoproterenol inhalation solution, is a beta agonist sympathomimetic bronchodilator.

Solution 1:200: Contains isoproterenol hydrochloride 5 mg/ml. *Inactive Ingredients:* Chlorobutanol 0.5% and sodium metabisulfite 0.3% as preservatives, citric acid, glycerin, purified water, and sodium chloride.

Solution 1:100: Contains isoproterenol hydrochloride 10 mg/ml. *Inactive Ingredients:* Chlorobutanol 0.5% and sodium metabisulfite 0.3% as preservatives, citric acid, purified water, saccharin sodium, sodium chloride, and sodium citrate.

Isoproterenol hydrochloride is soluble in water (1 g isoproterenol hydrochloride dissolves in 3 ml H_2O). The solutions have a pH range of 3-4.5.

The air in the bottles has been displaced by nitrogen gas.

Storage

Protect from light. Do not use the inhalation solution of their color are pinkish to brownish or if they contain a precipitate. Although solutions of isoproterenol HCl left in nebulizers will remain clear and potent for many days, for sanitary reasons it is recommended that they be changed daily.

Store at controlled room temperature 15-30°C (59-86°F).

CLINICAL PHARMACOLOGY

INJECTION

Isoproterenol HCl injection acts primarily on the heart and on smooth muscle of bronchi, skeletal muscle vasculature, and alimentary tract. The positive inotropic and chronotropic actions of the drug result in an increase in minute blood flow. There is an increase in heart rate, an approximately unchanged stroke volume, and an increase in ejection velocity. The rate of discharge of cardiac pacemakers is increased with isoproterenol HCl injection. Venous return to the heart is increased through a decreased compliance of the venous bed. Systemic resistance and pulmonary vascular resistance are decreased, and there is an increase in coronary and renal blood flow. Systolic blood pressure may increase and diastolic blood pressure may decrease. Mean arterial blood pressure is usually unchanged or reduced. The peripheral and coronary vasodilating effects of the drug may aid tissue perfusion.

Isoproterenol HCl injection relaxes most smooth muscle, the most pronounced effect being on bronchial and gastrointestinal smooth muscle. It produces marked relaxation in the smaller bronchi and may even dilate the trachea and main bronchi past the resting diameter.

Isoproterenol HCl injection is metabolized primarily in the liver by COMT. The duration of action of isoproterenol HCl injection may be longer than epinephrine, but it is still brief.

INHALATION AEROSOL AND INHALATION SOLUTION

Isoproterenol HCl relaxes bronchial spasm and facilitates expectoration of pulmonary secretions by acting almost exclusively on beta receptors. It is frequently effective when epinephrine and other drugs fail, and it has a wide margin of safety.

Isoproterenol HCl is readily absorbed when given as an aerosol. It is metabolized primarily in the liver and other tissues by catechol-0-methyltransferase (COMT).

Recent studies in laboratory animals (minipigs, rodents, and dogs) recorded the occurrence of cardiac arrhythmias and sudden death (with histologic evidence of myocardial necrosis) when beta agonists and methylxanthines were concomitantly administered. The significance of these findings when applied to human usage is currently unknown.

INDICATIONS AND USAGE

INJECTION:

Isoproterenol HCl injection is indicated:

- For mild or transient episodes of heart block that do not require electric shock or pacemaker therapy.
- For serious episodes of heart block and Adams-Stokes attacks (except when caused by ventricular tachycardia or fibrillation). (See CONTRAINDICATIONS.)
- For use in cardiac arrest until electric shock or pacemaker therapy, the treatments of choice, is available. (See CONTRAINDICATIONS.)
- For bronchospasm occurring during anesthesia.
- As an adjunct to fluid and electrolyte replacement therapy and the use of other drugs and procedures in the treatment of hypovolemic and septic shock, low cardiac output (hypoperfusion) states, congestive heart failure, and cardiogenic shock. (See WARNINGS.)

INHALATION AEROSOL AND INHALATION SOLUTION

Isoproterenol HCl is indicated for the relief of bronchospasm associated with acute and chronic asthma and reversible bronchospasm which may be associated with chronic bronchitis or emphysema.

NON-FDA APPROVED INDICATIONS

Isoproterenol is used without FDA approval to support the transplanted heart postoperatively since both chronotropic and inotropic effects are desirous.

CONTRAINDICATIONS

INJECTION

Use of isoproterenol HCl injection is contraindicated in patients with tachyarrhythmias; tachycardia or heart block caused by digitalis intoxication; ventricular arrhythmias which require inotropic therapy; and angina pectoris.

INHALATION AEROSOL AND INHALATION SOLUTION

Use of isoproterenol in patients with preexisting cardiac arrhythmias associated with tachycardia is generally considered contraindicated because the cardiac stimulant effect of the drug may aggravate such disorders. The use of this medication is contraindicated in those patients who have a known hypersensitivity to isoproterenol or to any of the other components of this drug.

WARNINGS

INJECTION

Isoproterenol HCl injection, by increasing myocardial oxygen requirements while decreasing effective coronary perfusion, may have a deleterious effect on the injured or failing heart. Most experts discourage its use as the initial agent in treating cardiogenic shock following myocardial infarction. However, when a low arterial pressure has been elevated by other means, isoproterenol HCl injection may produce beneficial hemodynamic and metabolic effects.

In a few patients, presumably with organic disease of the AV node and its branches, isoproterenol HCl injection has paradoxically been reported to worsen heart block or to precipitate Adams-Stokes attacks during normal sinus rhythm or transient heart block.

Contains sodium metabisulfite, a sulfite that may cause allergic-type reactions including anaphylactic symptoms and life-threatening or less severe asthmatic episodes in certain susceptible people. The overall prevalence of sulfite sensitivity in the general population is unknown and probably low. Sulfite sensitivity is seen more frequently in asthmatic than in nonasthmatic people.

INHALATION SOLUTION

Contains sodium metabisulfite, a sulfite that may cause allergic-type reactions including anaphylactic symptoms and life-threatening or less severe asthmatic episodes in certain susceptible people. The overall prevalence of sulfite sensitivity in the general population is unknown and probably low. Sulfite sensitivity is seen more frequently in asthmatic than in nonasthmatic people.

Excessive use of an adrenergic aerosol should be discouraged as it may lose its effectiveness.

Isoproterenol administration as a solution for nebulization has been associated with a decrease in arterial pO_2 in asthmatic patients as a result of ventilation-perfusion abnormalities despite improvement in airway obstruction. The clinical significance of this relative hypoxemia is unclear.

As with other inhaled beta adrenergic agonists, isoproterenol HCl can produce paradoxical bronchospasm, that can be life threatening. If this occurs, the product should be discontinued immediately and alternative therapy instituted.

Deaths have been reported following excessive use of isoproterenol inhalation preparations and the exact cause is unknown. Cardiac arrest was noted in several instances. It is therefore essential that the physician instruct the patient in the need for further evaluation if his/her asthma worsens.

INHALATION AEROSOL

Excessive use of an adrenergic aerosol should be discouraged as it may lose its effectiveness.

In patients with status asthmaticus and abnormal blood gas tensions, improvement in vital capacity and in blood gas tensions may not accompany apparent relief of bronchospasm. Facilities for administering oxygen mixtures and ventilatory assistance are necessary for such patients.

Occasional patients have been reported to develop severe paradoxical airway resistance with repeated, excessive use of isoproterenol inhalation preparations. The cause of this refractory state is unknown. It is advisable that in such instances the use of this preparation be discontinued immediately and alternative therapy instituted, since in the reported cases the patients did not respond to other forms of therapy until the drug was withdrawn.

Deaths have been reported following excessive use of isoproterenol inhalation preparations and the exact cause is unknown. Cardiac arrest was noted in several instances. It is therefore essential that the physician instruct the patient in the need for further evaluation if his/her asthma worsens.

PRECAUTIONS

GENERAL

Injection

Isoproterenol HCl injection should generally be started at the lowest recommended dose. This may be gradually increased if necessary while carefully monitoring the patient. Doses sufficient to increase the heart rate to more than 130 beats per minute may increase the likelihood of inducing ventricular arrhythmias. Such increases in heart rate will also tend to increase cardiac work and oxygen requirements which may adversely affect the failing heart or the heart with a significant degree of arteriosclerosis.

Particular caution is necessary in administering isoproterenol HCl injection to patients with coronary artery disease, coronary insufficiency, diabetes, hyperthyroidism, and sensitivity to sympathomimetic amines.

Adequate filling of the intravascular compartment by suitable volume expanders is of primary importance in most cases of shock and should precede the administration of vasoactive drugs. In patients with normal cardiac function, determination of central venous pressure is a reliable guide during volume replacement. If evidence of hypoperfusion persists after adequate volume replacement, isoproterenol HCl injection may be given.

In addition to the routine monitoring of systemic blood pressure, heart rate, urine flow, and the electrocardiograph, the response to therapy should also be monitored by frequent determination of the central venous pressure and blood gases. Patients in shock should be closely observed during isoproterenol HCl injection administration. If the heart rate exceeds 110 beats per minute, it may be advisable to decrease the infusion rate or temporarily discontinue the infusion. Determinations of cardiac output and circulation time may also be helpful. Appropriate measures should be taken to ensure adequate ventilation. Careful attention should be paid to acid-base balance and to the correction of electrolyte disturbances. In cases of shock associated with bacteremia, suitable antimicrobial therapy is, of course, imperative.

I

Inhalation Aerosol

Isoproterenol should be used with caution in patients with cardiovascular disorders including coronary insufficiency, diabetes, or hyperthyroidism, and in persons sensitive to sympathomimetic amines.

A single treatment with the isoproterenol HCl aerosol is usually sufficient for controlling isolated attacks of asthma.

Any patient who requires more than 3 aerosol treatments within a 24 hour period should be under the close supervision of a physician. Further therapy with the bronchodilator aerosol alone is inadvisable when 3-5 treatments within 6-12 hours produce minimal or no relief.

Inhalation Solution

Isoproterenol HCl, as with all sympathomimetic amines, should be used with caution in patients with cardiovascular disorders, especially coronary insufficiency, cardiac arrhythmias, and hypertension; in patients with convulsive disorders, hyperthyroidism, or diabetes mellitus; and in patients who are unusually responsive to sympathomimetic amines. Clinically significant changes in systolic and diastolic blood pressure have been seen in some patients after use of any beta adrenergic bronchodilator.

When compressed oxygen is employed as the aerosol propellant, the percentage of oxygen used should be determined by the patient's individual requirements to avoid depression of respiratory drive.

Any patient who requires more than 3 aerosol treatments within a 24 hour period should be under the close supervision of a physician. Further therapy with the bronchodilator aerosol alone is inadvisable when 3-5 treatments within 6-12 hours produce minimal or no relief.

CARCINOGENESIS, MUTAGENESIS, AND IMPAIRMENT OF FERTILITY

Long-term studies in animals to evaluate the carcinogenic potential of isoproterenol HCl have not been done. Mutagenic potential and effect on fertility have not been determined. There is no evidence from human experience that isoproterenol HCl injection may be carcinogenic or mutagenic or that it impairs fertility.

PREGNANCY CATEGORY C

Animal reproduction studies have not been conducted with isoproterenol HCl. It is also not known whether isoproterenol HCl can cause fetal harm when administered to a pregnant woman or can affect reproduction capacity. Isoproterenol HCl should be given to a pregnant woman only if clearly needed.

NURSING MOTHERS

It is not known whether this drug is excreted in human milk. Because many drugs are excreted in human milk, caution should be exercised when isoproterenol HCl is administered to a nursing woman.

INFORMATION FOR THE PATIENT

Inhalation Aerosol

Do not inhale more often than directed by your physician. Read instructions enclosed with the prescription before using. Do not exceed the dose prescribed by your physician. If difficulty in breathing persists, contact your physician immediately. Avoid spraying in eyes. Contents under pressure. Do not break or incinerate. Do not store at temperatures above 120°F. Keep out of reach of children.

PEDIATRIC USE

Inhalation Aerosol and Inhalation Solution

In general, the technique of isoproterenol HCl aerosol and isoproterenol HCl solution in administration to children is similar to that of adults, since children's smaller ventilatory exchange capacity automatically provides proportionally smaller aerosol intake. However, it is generally recommended that the 1:200 solution (rather than the 1:100) be used for an acute attack of bronchospasm, and no more than 0.25 ml of the 1:200 solution should be used for each 10-15 minute programmed treatment in chronic bronchospastic disease.

DRUG INTERACTIONS

INJECTION

Isoproterenol HCl injection and epinephrine should not be administered simultaneously because both drugs are direct cardiac stimulants and their combined effects may induce serious arrhythmias. The drugs may, however, be administered alternately provided a proper interval has elapsed between doses.

Isoproterenol HCl should be used with caution, if at all, when potent inhalational anesthetics such as halothane are employed because of potential to sensitize the myocardium to effects of sympathomimetic amines.

INHALATION AEROSOL

Epinephrine should not be administered concomitantly with isoproterenol HCl, as both drugs are direct cardiac stimulants and their combined effects may induce serious arrhythmia. If desired they may, however, be alternated, provided an interval of at least 4 hours has elapse.

INHALATION SOLUTION

Other sympathomimetic aerosol bronchodilators or epinephrine should not be used concomitantly with isoproterenol HCl. If additional adrenergic drugs are to be administered by any route to the patient using isoproterenol HCl, they should be used with caution to avoid deleterious cardiovascular effects.

Beta adrenergic agonists should be administered with caution to patients being treated with MAO inhibitors or tricyclic antidepressants since the action of the beta adrenergic agonists on the vascular system may be potentiated.

Beta receptor blocking agents and isoproterenol HCl inhibit the effects of each other.

ADVERSE REACTIONS

INJECTION

The following reactions to isoproterenol HCl have been reported:

CNS: Nervousness, headache, dizziness.

Cardiovascular: Tachycardia, palpitations, angina, Adams-Stokes attacks, pulmonary edema, hypertension, hypotension, ventricular arrhythmias, tachyarrhythmias.

In a few patients, presumably with organic disease of the AV node and its branches, isoproterenol HCl injection has been reported to precipitate Adams-Stokes seizures during normal sinus rhythm or transient heart block.

Other: Flushing of the skin, sweating, mild tremors, weakness.

INHALATION AEROSOL AND INHALATION SOLUTION

The mist from the isoproterenol HCl aerosol contains alcohol but is generally very well tolerated. An occasional patient may experience some transient throat irritation which has been attributed to the alcohol content.

Serious reactions to isoproterenol HCl are infrequent. The following reactions, however, have been reported:

CNS: Nervousness, headache, dizziness, weakness.

Gastrointestinal: Nausea, vomiting.

Cardiovascular: Tachycardia, palpitations, precordial distress, angina-type pain.

Other: Flushing of the skin, tremor, and sweating.

The inhalation route is usually accompanied by a minimum of side effects. These untoward reactions disappear quickly and do not as a rule, inconvenience the patient to the extent that the drug must be discontinued. No cumulative effects have been reported.

DOSAGE AND ADMINISTRATION

INJECTION

Isoproterenol HCl injection 1:5000 should generally be started at the lowest recommended dose and the rate of administration gradually increased if necessary while carefully monitoring the patient. The usual route of administration is by intravenous infusion or bolus intravenous injection. In dire emergencies, the drug may be administered by intracardiac injection. If time is not of the utmost importance, initial therapy by intramuscular or subcutaneous injection is preferred (see TABLE 1).

TABLE 1 *Recommended Dosage for Adults With Heart Block, Adams-Stokes Attacks, and Cardiac Arrest*

Route of Administration	Preparation of Dilution	Initial Dose	Subsequent Dose Range*
Bolus intravenous injection	Dilute 1 ml (0.2 mg) to 10 ml with sodium chloride injection, or 5% dextrose injection	0.02-0.06 mg (1-3 ml of diluted solution)	0.01-0.2 mg (0.5-10 ml of diluted solution)
Intravenous infusion	Dilute 10 ml (2 mg) in 500 ml of 5% dextrose injection	5 μg/min. (1.25 ml of diluted solution per minute)	
Intramuscular	Use Solution 1:5000 undiluted	0.2 mg (1 ml)	0.02-1 mg (0.1-5 ml)
Subcutaneous	Use Solution 1:5000 undiluted	0.2 mg (1 ml)	0.15-0.2 mg (0.75-1 ml)
Intracardiac	Use Solution 1:5000 undiluted	0.02 mg (0.1 ml)	

* Subsequent dosage and method of administration depend on the ventricular rate and the rapidity with which the cardiac pacemaker can take over when the drug is gradually withdrawn.

There are no well-controlled studies in children to establish appropriate dosing; however, the American Heart Association recommends an initial infusion rate of 0.1 μg/kg/min, with the usual range being 0.1-1.0 μg/kg/min (see TABLE 2).

Parenteral drug products should be inspected visually for particulate matter and discoloration prior to administration, whenever solution and container permit. Such solution should not be used.

TABLE 2 *Recommended Dosage for Adults With Shock and Hypoperfusion States*

Route of Administration	Preparation of Dilution*	Infusion Rate†
Intravenous infusion	Dilute 5 ml (1 mg) in 500 ml of 5% dextrose injection	0.5-5 µg/min (0.25-2.5 ml of diluted solution)

* Concentrations up to 10 times greater have been used when limitation of volume is essential.
† Rates over 30 µg/min have been used in advanced stages of shock. The rate of infusion should be adjusted on the basis of heart rate, central venous pressure, systemic blood pressure, and urine flow. If the heart rate exceeds 110 beats per minute, it may be advisable to decrease or temporarily discontinue the infusion (see TABLE 3).

TABLE 3 *Recommended Dosage for Adults With Bronchospasm Occurring During Anesthesia*

Route of Administration	Preparation of Dilution	Initial Dose	Subsequent Dose
Bolus intravenous injection	Dilute 1 ml (0.2 mg) to 10 ml with sodium chloride injection, or 5% dextrose injection	0.01-0.02 mg (0.5-1 ml of diluted solution)	The initial dose may be repeated when necessary

INHALATION AEROSOL

Acute Bronchial Asthma

Hold the aerosol in an inverted position. Close lips and teeth around open end of mouthpiece. Breathe out, expelling as much air from the lungs as possible; then inhale deeply while pressing down on the bottle to activate spray mechanism. Try to hold breath for a few seconds before exhaling. Wait one full minute in order to determine the effect before considering a second inhalation. A treatment may be repeated up to 5 times daily if necessary. (See PRECAUTIONS.) If carefully instructed, children quickly learn to keep the stream of mist clear of the teeth and tongue, thereby assuring inhalation into the lungs. Occlusion of the nares of very young children may be advisable to make inhalation certain.

Warm water should be run through the mouthpiece once daily to wash it and prevent clogging.

The mouthpiece may also be sanitized by immersion in alcohol.

Bronchospasm in Chronic Obstructive Lung Disease

The aerosol provides a convenient aerosol method for delivering isoproterenol HCl. The treatment described above for Acute Bronchial Asthma may be repeated at not less than 3-4 hour intervals as part of a programmed regimen of treatment of obstructive lung disease complicated by a reversible bronchospastic component. One application from the aerosol may be regarded as equivalent in effectiveness to 5-7 operations of a hand-bulb nebulizer using a 1:100 solution.

Children's Dosage

In general, the technique of isoproterenol HCl aerosol in administration to children is similar to that of adults, since children's smaller ventilatory exchange capacity automatically provides proportionally smaller aerosol intake.

INHALATION SOLUTION

Isoproterenol HCl HCl solutions can be administered as an aerosol mist by hand-bulb nebulizer, compressed air or oxygen operated nebulizer, or by intermittent positive pressure breathing (IPPB) devices. The method of delivery, and the treatment regimen employed in the management of the reversible bronchospastic element accompanying bronchial asthma, chronic bronchitis, and chronic obstructive lung diseases, will depend on such factors as the severity of the bronchospasm, patient age, tolerance to the medication, complicating cardiopulmonary conditions, and whether therapy is for an intermittent acute attack of bronchospasm or is part of a programmed treatment regimen for constant bronchospasm.

Acute Bronchial Asthma Hand-Bulb Nebulizer

Depending on the frequency of treatment and the type of nebulizer used, a volume of solution of isoproterenol HCl, sufficient for not more than one day's treatment, should be placed in the nebulizer using the dropper provided. In time, the patient can learn to adjust the volume required. For adults and children, the 1:200 solution is administered by hand-bulb nebulization in a dosage of 5-15 deep inhalations (using an all glass or plastic nebulizer). In adults, the 1:100 solution may be used if a stronger solution seems to be indicated. The dose is 3-7 deep inhalations. If after about 5-10 minutes inadequate relief is observed, these doses may be repeated one more time. If the acute attack recurs, treatments may be repeated up to 5 times daily if necessary. (See PRECAUTIONS.)

Bronchospasm in Chronic Obstructive Lung Disease Hand-Bulb Nebulizer

A solution of 1:200 or 1:100 of isoproterenol HCl may be administered daily at not less than 3-4 hour intervals for subacute bronchospastic attacks or as part of a programmed treatment regimen in patients with chronic obstructive lung disease with a reversible bronchospastic component. An adequate dose is usually 5-15 deep inhalations, using the 1:200 solution. Some patients with severe attacks of bronchospasm may require 3-7 deep inhalations using the 1:100 solution of isoproterenol HCl.

Nebulization by Compressed Air or Oxygen

A method often used in patients with severe chronic obstructive lung disease is to deliver the isoproterenol mist *in more dilute form over a longer period of time.* The purpose is, not so much to increase the dose supplied, as to achieve progressively deeper bronchodilation and thus insure that the mist achieves maximum penetration of the finer bronchioles. In this method, 0.5 ml of a 1:200 solution of isoproterenol HCl is diluted to 2 ml to 2.5 ml with water or isotonic saline to achieve a use concentration of 1:800 to 1:1000. If desired, 0.25 ml of the 1:100 solution may be similarly diluted to achieve the same use concentration. The diluted solution is placed in a nebulizer (*e.g.*, DeVilbiss #640 unit) connected to either a source of compressed air or oxygen. The flow rate is regulated to suit the particular nebulizer so that the diluted solution of isoproterenol HCl will be delivered over approximately 10-20 minutes. A treatment may be repeated up to 5 times daily if necessary. Although the total delivered dose of isoproterenol HCl is somewhat higher than with the treatment regimen employing the hand-bulb nebulizer, patients usually tolerate it well because of the greater dilution and longer application-time factors.

Intermittent Positive Pressure Breathing (IPPB)

Diluted solutions of 1:200 or 1:100 of isoproterenol HCl are used in a programmed regimen for the treatment of reversible bronchospasm in patients with chronic obstructive lung disease who require intermittent positive pressure breathing therapy. These devices generally have a small nebulizer, usually of 3 ml to 5 ml capacity, on a patient-operated side arm. The effectiveness of IPPB therapy is greatly enhanced by the simultaneous use of aerosolized bronchodilators. As with compressed air or oxygen operated nebulizers, the usual regimen is to place 0.5 ml of 1:200 solution of isoproterenol HCl diluted to 2 ml to 2.5 ml with water or isotonic saline in the nebulizer cup and follow the IPPB manufacturer's operating instructions. IPPB-bronchodilator treatments are usually administered over 15-20 minutes, up to 5 times if necessary.

Children's Dosage

In general, the technique of isoproterenol HCl solution in administration to children is similar to that of adults, since children's smaller ventilatory exchange capacity automatically provides proportionally smaller aerosol intake. However, it is generally recommended that the 1:200 solution (rather than the 1:100) be used for an acute attack of bronchospasm, and no more than 0.25 ml of the 1:200 solution should be used for each 10-15 minute programmed treatment in chronic bronchospastic disease.

PRODUCT LISTING - RATED THERAPEUTICALLY EQUIVALENT

Solution - Inhalation - 0.5%

Size	Price	Product	NDC
10 ml	$24.80	ISUPREL HCL, Sanofi Winthrop Pharmaceuticals	00024-0871-01

Solution - Intravenous - 0.2 mg/ml

Size	Price	Product	NDC
5 ml x 10	$131.28	GENERIC, Abbott Pharmaceutical	00074-4978-01
5 ml x 10	$157.80	GENERIC, Abbott Pharmaceutical	00074-4978-15
5 ml x 25	$95.75	GENERIC, Esi Lederle Generics	00641-1438-35
10 ml x 10	$133.80	GENERIC, Abbott Pharmaceutical	00074-4905-01
10 ml x 10	$177.36	GENERIC, Abbott Pharmaceutical	00074-4977-01
10 ml x 10	$213.50	GENERIC, Abbott Pharmaceutical	00074-4977-18
125 ml	$125.00	GENERIC, Cmc-Consolidated Midland Corporation	00223-7910-05

PRODUCT LISTING - EQUIVALENTS NOT AVAILABLE

Aerosol - Inhalation - 0.131 mg/Inh

Size	Price	Product	NDC
15 ml	$30.52	ISUPREL MISTOMETER, Sanofi Winthrop Pharmaceuticals	00024-0879-01
15 ml	$34.44	ISUPREL MISTOMETER, Sanofi Winthrop Pharmaceuticals	00024-0878-01

Solution - Intravenous - 0.2 mg/ml

Size	Price	Product	NDC
1 ml x 25	$141.00	ISUPREL HCL, Abbott Pharmaceutical	00074-1410-01
5 ml x 10	$203.90	ISUPREL HCL, Abbott Pharmaceutical	00074-1410-05

Isosorbide Dinitrate *(001593)*

Categories: Angina pectoris; Pregnancy Category C; FDA Approved 1986 Sep; WHO Formulary
Drug Classes: Nitrates; Vasodilators
Brand Names: Dilatrate-Sr; Dinisor; Isd; Iso-Bid; Isonate; Iso-Par; Isorbid; **Isorem**; Isotrate; Sorbitrate
Foreign Brand Availability: Acordin (Switzerland); Angiolong (China); Angitrit (Thailand); APO-ISDN (Canada; Malaysia); Bideren (Philippines); Caranil (Japan); Cardopax (Denmark); Cardopax Retard (Denmark); Carsodil (Korea); Carvasin (Italy); Cedocard (Austria; Belgium; England; Netherlands; Philippines; Switzerland); Cedocard Retard (Austria; England; Indonesia; Netherlands; Russia); Cedocard SR (Canada); Conducil (Argentina); Cordil (Israel); Cordil 40 SR (Israel); Cornilat (Slovenia); Coronex (New-Zealand); Corosorbide (Argentina); Corovliss (Germany); Corovliss Retard (Germany); Difutrat (Slovenia); Dilanid (South-Africa); Duranitrat (Germany); Hartsorb (Thailand); ISDN (Germany); Ismo 20 (Ecuador); Isobar (Philippines); Isobide (Taiwan); Isobinate (Thailand); Isocard Retard (Bahrain; Cyprus; Egypt; Iran; Iraq; Jordan; Kuwait; Lebanon; Libya; Oman; Qatar; Republic-of-Yemen; Saudi-Arabia; Syria; United-Arab-Emirates); Isocardide (Israel); Isocord (Colombia); Isoday 40 (Bahrain; Cyprus; Egypt; Iran; Iraq; Jordan; Kuwait; Lebanon; Libya; Oman; Qatar; Republic-of-Yemen; Saudi-Arabia; Syria; United-Arab-Emirates); Isogen (Australia); Isoket (Bulgaria; China; Czech-Republic; Germany; Hong-Kong; Indonesia; Israel; Philippines; Portugal; Russia; Switzerland); Isoket Retard (Bulgaria; Czech-Republic; England; Germany; Hong-Kong; India; Korea; Malaysia; Portugal; Switzerland); Isoket Spray (Korea); Isomack (Austria; Korea); Iso-Mack (Denmark); Iso Mack (Germany; Switzerland); Isomack Retard (China; Hong-Kong); Isomack Spray (Korea); Iso-Mack Retard (Malaysia); Iso Mack Retard (Bahrain; Cyprus; Ecuador; Egypt; Indonesia; Iran; Iraq; Jordan; Kuwait; Lebanon; Libya; Oman; Qatar; Republic-of-Yemen; Saudi-Arabia; Syria; Thailand; United-Arab-Emirates); Isonit (Finland); Iso-Puren (Germany); Isorbide (Peru); Isordil (Argentina; Bahrain; Belgium; Benin; Burkina-Faso; Canada; Colombia; Costa-Rica; Cyprus; Dominican-Republic; Ecuador; Egypt; El-Salvador; Ethiopia; Gambia; Ghana; Guatemala; Guinea; Honduras; Hong-Kong; Hungary; India; Indonesia; Iran; Iraq; Ireland; Israel; Ivory-Coast; Jordan; Kenya; Kuwait; Lebanon; Liberia; Libya; Malawi; Malaysia; Mali; Mauritania; Mauritius; Morocco; Netherlands; Nicaragua; Niger; Nigeria; Oman; Panama; Philippines; Portugal; Qatar; Republic-of-Yemen; Saudi-Arabia; Senegal; Seychelles; Sierra-Leone; South-Africa; Sudan; Syria; Taiwan; Tanzania; Thailand; Tunia; Turkey; Uganda; United-Arab-Emirates; Zambia; Zimbabwe); Isostenase (Germany); Isotard 20 (Israel); Isotard 40 (Israel); Izo (Thailand); Langoran (France); Langoran LP (France); Lomilan (Slovenia); Maycor (Argentina; Czech-Republic; Germany); Maycor Retard (Czech-Republic; Spain); Mono Mack (Costa-Rica; Dominican-Republic; El-Salvador; Guatemala; Honduras; Panama); Nitorol (Malaysia; Philippines; Taiwan); Nitrol (Japan); Nitrol R (Japan); Nitrosid (Finland); Nitrosid Retard (Finland); Nitrosorbide (Benin; Burkina-Faso; Ethiopia; Gambia; Ghana; Guinea; Italy; Ivory-Coast; Kenya; Liberia; Malawi; Mali; Mauritania; Mauritius; Morocco; Niger; Nigeria; Senegal; Seychelles; Sierra-Leone; Sudan; Tanzania; Tunia; Uganda; Zambia; Zimbabwe); Nitrosorbon (Germany); Nosim (Argentina); Pensordil (Greece); Risordan (France; Greece); Sigillum (Argentina); Soni-Slo (Bahrain; Benin; Burkina-Faso; Cyprus; Egypt; England; Ethiopia; Gambia; Ghana; Guinea; Iran; Iraq; Ivory-Coast; Jordan; Kenya; Kuwait; Lebanon; Liberia; Libya; Malawi; Mali; Mauritania; Mauritius; Morocco; Niger; Nigeria; Oman; Qatar; Republic-of-Yemen; Saudi-Arabia; Senegal; Seychelles; Sierra-Leone; Sudan; Syria; Tanzania; Tunia; Uganda; United-Arab-Emirates; Zambia; Zimbabwe); Sorbangil (Norway; Sweden); Sorbichew (England); Sorbid (Turkey); Sorbidilat (Austria; Switzerland); Sorbidilat Retard (Austria); Sorbidilat SR (Switzerland); Sorbidin (Australia); Sorbonit (Hungary); Storo (Japan); Surantol (Argentina); Tinidil (Slovenia); U-Sorbide (Taiwan); Vascardin (Bahamas; Bahrain; Barbados; Belize; Benin; Bermuda; Burkina-Faso; Curacao; Cyprus; Egypt; Ethiopia; Gambia; Ghana; Guinea; Guyana; Indonesia; Iran; Iraq; Ivory-Coast; Jamaica; Jordan; Kenya; Kuwait; Lebanon; Liberia; Libya; Malawi; Mali; Mauritania; Mauritius; Morocco; Netherland-Antilles; Niger; Nigeria; Oman; Puerto-Rico; Qatar; Republic-of-Yemen; Saudi-Arabia; Senegal; Seychelles; Sierra-Leone; Sudan; Surinam; Syria; Tanzania; Trinidad; Tunia; Uganda; United-Arab-Emirates; Zambia; Zimbabwe); Vasodilat (Argentina)
Cost of Therapy: $34.59 (Angina; Isordil; 10 mg; 3 tablets/day; 30 day supply)
$1.69 (Angina; Generic Tablets; 10 mg; 3 tablets/day; 30 day supply)

DESCRIPTION

Note: The trade names have been used throughout this monograph for clarity.

Isosorbide dinitrate (ISDN) is 1,4:3,6-dianhydro-D-glucitol 2,5-dinitrate, an organic nitrate whose molecular weight is 236.14. The organic nitrates are vasodilators, active on both arteries and veins.

Isosorbide dinitrate is a white, crystalline, odorless compound which is stable in air and in solution, has a melting point of 70°C and has an optical rotation of +134° (c=1.0, alcohol, 20°C). Isosorbide dinitrate is freely soluble in organic solvents such as acetone, alcohol, and ether, but is only sparingly soluble in water.

DILATRATE-SR SUSTAINED RELEASE CAPSULES

Each Dilatrate-SR sustained-release capsule contains 40 mg of isosorbide dinitrate, in a microdialysis delivery system that causes the active drug to be released over an extended period. Each capsule also contains ethylcellulose, lactose, pharmaceutical glaze, starch, sucrose and talc. The capsule shells contain D&C red 33, D&C yellow 10, gelatin and titanium dioxide.

ISORDIL SUBLINGUAL TABLETS

Each Isordil Sublingual tablet contains 2.5, 5, or 10 mg of isosorbide dinitrate. The inactive ingredients in each tablet are cellulose, lactose, magnesium stearate, and starch. The 2.5 mg dosage strength also contains D&C yellow 10 and FD&C yellow 6, and the 5 mg dosage strength also contains FD&C red 40.

ISORDIL TITRADOSE TABLETS

Each Isordil Titradose tablet contains 5, 10, 20, 30, or 40 mg of isosorbide dinitrate. The inactive ingredients in each tablet are lactose, cellulose, and magnesium stearate. The 5, 20, 30, and 40 mg dosage strengths also contain the following: *5 mg:* FD&C red 40; *20 and 40 mg:* D&C yellow 10, FD&C blue 1, and FD&C yellow 6; *30 mg:* FD&C blue 1.

CLINICAL PHARMACOLOGY

DILATRATE-SR SUSTAINED RELEASE CAPSULES

The principal pharmacological action of isosorbide dinitrate is relaxation of vascular smooth muscle and consequent dilatation of peripheral arteries and veins, especially the latter. Dilatation of the veins promotes peripheral pooling of blood and decreases venous return to the heart, thereby reducing left ventricular end-diastolic pressure and pulmonary capillary wedge pressure (preload). Arteriolar relaxation reduces systemic vascular resistance, systolic arterial pressure, and mean arterial pressure (afterload). Dilatation of the coronary arteries also occurs. The relative importance of preload reduction, afterload reduction, and coronary dilatation remains undefined.

Dosing regimens for most chronically used drugs are designed to provide plasma concentrations that are continuously greater than a minimally effective concentration. This strategy is inappropriate for organic nitrates. Several well-controlled clinical trials have used exercise testing to assess the antianginal efficacy of continuously-delivered nitrates. In the large majority of these trials, active agents were no more effective than placebo after 24 hours (or less) of continuous therapy. Attempts to overcome nitrate tolerance by dose escalation, even to doses far in excess of those used acutely, have consistently failed. Only after nitrates have been absent from the body for several hours has their antianginal efficacy been restored.

Pharmacokinetics

The kinetics of absorption of isosorbide dinitrate from Dilatrate-SR sustained-release capsules have not been well studied. Studies of immediate-release formulations of ISDN have found highly variable bioavailability (10-90%), with extensive first-pass metabolism in the liver. Most such studies have observed progressive increases in bioavailability during chronic therapy; it is not known whether similar increases in bioavailability appear during the course of chronic therapy with Dilatrate-SR sustained-release capsules.

Once absorbed, the distribution volume of isosorbide dinitrate is 2-4 L/kg and this volume is cleared at the rate of 2-4 L/min, so ISDN's half-life in serum is about an hour. Since the clearance exceeds hepatic blood flow, considerable extrahepatic metabolism must also occur. Clearance is affected primarily by denitration to the 2-mononitrate (15-25%) and the 5-mononitrate (75-85%).

Both metabolites have biological activity, especially the 5-mononitrate. With an overall half-life of about 5 hours, the 5-mononitrate is cleared from the serum by denitration to isosorbide; glucuronidation to the 5-mononitrate glucuronide; and denitration/hydration to sorbitol. The 2-mononitrate has been less well studied, but it appears to participate in the same metabolic pathways, with a half-life of about 2 hours.

The interdosing interval sufficient to avoid tolerance to ISDN has not been well defined. Studies of nitroglycerin (an organic nitrate with a very short half-life) have shown that dosing intervals of 10-12 hours are usually sufficient to prevent or attenuate tolerance. Dosing intervals that have succeeded in avoiding tolerance during trials of moderate doses (*e.g.*, 30 mg) of immediate-release ISDN have generally been somewhat longer (at least 14 hours), but this is consistent with the longer half-lives of ISDN and its active metabolites.

An interdosing interval sufficient to avoid tolerance with Dilatrate-SR has not been demonstrated. In an eccentric dosing study, 40 mg capsules of Dilatrate-SR were administered daily at 0800 and 1400 hours. After 2 weeks of this regimen, Dilatrate-SR was statistically indistinguishable from placebo. Thus, the necessary interdosing interval sufficient to avoid tolerance remains unknown, but it must be greater than 18 hours.

Few well-controlled clinical trials of organic nitrates have been designed to detect rebound or withdrawal effects. In one such trial, however, subjects receiving nitroglycerin had less exercise tolerance at the end of the daily interdosing interval than the parallel group receiving placebo. The incidence, magnitude, and clinical significance of similar phenomena in patients receiving ISDN have not been studied.

ISORDIL SUBLINGUAL TABLETS

The principal pharmacological action of isosorbide dinitrate is relaxation of vascular smooth muscle and consequent dilatation of peripheral arteries and veins, especially the latter. Dilatation of the veins promotes peripheral pooling of blood and decreases venous return to the heart, thereby reducing left ventricular end-diastolic pressure and pulmonary capillary wedge pressure (preload). Arteriolar relaxation reduces systemic vascular resistance, systolic arterial pressure, and mean arterial pressure (afterload). Dilatation of the coronary arteries also occurs. The relative importance of preload reduction, afterload reduction, and coronary dilatation remains undefined.

Dosing regimens for most chronically used drugs are designed to provide plasma concentrations that are continuously greater than a minimally effective concentration. This strategy is inappropriate for organic nitrates. Several well-controlled clinical trials have used exercise testing to assess the anti-anginal efficacy of continuously-delivered nitrates. In the large majority of these trials, active agents were no more effective than placebo after 24 hours (or less) of continuous therapy. Attempts to overcome nitrate tolerance by dose escalation, even to doses far in excess of those used acutely, have consistently failed. Only after nitrates have been absent from the body for several hours has their anti-anginal efficacy been restored.

Pharmacokinetics

Bioavailability of ISDN after single sublingual doses is 40-50%.

Multiple-dose studies of sublingual ISDN pharmacokinetics have not been reported; multiple-dose studies of ingested ISDN have observed progressive increases in bioavailability during chronic therapy. Serum levels of ISDN reach their maxima 10-15 minutes after sublingual dosing.

Once absorbed, the volume of distribution of isosorbide dinitrate is 2-4 L/kg, and this volume is cleared at the rate of 2-4 L/min, so ISDN's half-life in serum is about an hour. Since the clearance exceeds hepatic blood flow, considerable extrahepatic metabolism must also occur. Clearance is affected primarily by denitration to the 2-mononitrate (15-25%) and the 5-mononitrate (75-85%).

Both metabolites have biological activity, especially the 5-mononitrate. With an overall half-life of about 5 hours, the 5-mononitrate is cleared from the serum by denitration to isosorbide, glucuronidation to the 5-mononitrate glucuronide, and denitration/hydration to sorbitol. The 2-mononitrate has been less well studied, but it appears to participate in the same metabolic pathways, with a half-life of about 2 hours.

The daily dose-free interval sufficient to avoid tolerance to organic nitrates has not been well defined. Studies of nitroglycerin (an organic nitrate with a very short half-life) have shown that daily dose-free intervals of 10-12 hours are usually sufficient to minimize tolerance. Daily dose-free intervals that have succeeded in avoiding tolerance during trials of moderate doses (*e.g.*, 30 mg) of immediate-release ISDN have generally been somewhat longer (at least 14 hours), but this is consistent with the longer half-lives of ISDN and its active metabolites.

Few well-controlled clinical trials of organic nitrates have been designed to detect rebound or withdrawal effects. In one such trial, however, subjects receiving nitroglycerin had less exercise tolerance at the end of the daily dose-free interval than the parallel group receiving placebo. The incidence, magnitude, and clinical significance of similar phenomena in patients receiving ISDN have not been studied.

ISORDIL TITRADOSE TABLETS

The principal pharmacological action of isosorbide dinitrate is relaxation of vascular smooth muscle and consequent dilatation of peripheral arteries and veins, especially the latter. Dilatation of the veins promotes peripheral pooling of blood and decreases venous return to the heart, thereby reducing left ventricular end-diastolic pressure and pulmonary capillary wedge pressure (preload). Arteriolar relaxation reduces systemic vascular resistance, systolic arterial pressure, and mean arterial pressure (afterload). Dilatation of the coronary arteries also occurs. The relative importance of preload reduction, afterload reduction, and coronary dilatation remains undefined.

Dosing regimens for most chronically used drugs are designed to provide plasma concentrations that are continuously greater than a minimally effective concentration. This strategy is inappropriate for organic nitrates. Several well-controlled clinical trials have used exercise testing to assess the anti-anginal efficacy of continuously-delivered nitrates. In the large majority of these trials, active agents were no more effective than placebo after 24 hours (or less) of continuous therapy. Attempts to overcome nitrate tolerance by dose escalation, even to doses far in excess of those used acutely, have consistently failed. Only after nitrates have been absent from the body for several hours has their anti-anginal efficacy been restored.

Pharmacokinetics

Absorption of isosorbide dinitrate after oral dosing is nearly complete, but bioavailability is highly variable (10-90%), with extensive first-pass metabolism in the liver. Serum levels reach their maxima about an hour after ingestion. The average bioavailability of ISDN is about 25%; most studies have observed progressive increases in bioavailability during chronic therapy.

Once absorbed, the volume of distribution of isosorbide dinitrate is 2-4 L/kg, and this volume is cleared at the rate of 2-4 L/min, so ISDN's half-life in serum is about an hour. Since the clearance exceeds hepatic blood flow, considerable extrahepatic metabolism must also occur. Clearance is affected primarily by denitration to the 2-mononitrate (15-25%) and the 5-mononitrate (75-85%).

Both metabolites have biological activity, especially the 5-mononitrate. With an overall half-life of about 5 hours, the 5-mononitrate is cleared from the serum by denitration to isosorbide, glucuronidation to the 5-mononitrate glucuronide, and denitration/hydration to sorbitol. The 2-mononitrate has been less well studied, but it appears to participate in the same metabolic pathways, with a half-life of about 2 hours.

The daily dose-free interval sufficient to avoid tolerance to organic nitrates has not been well defined. Studies of nitroglycerin (an organic nitrate with a very short half-life) have shown that daily dose-free intervals of 10-12 hours are usually sufficient to minimize tolerance. Daily dose-free intervals that have succeeded in avoiding tolerance during trials of moderate doses (*e.g.*, 30 mg) of immediate-release ISDN have generally been somewhat longer (at least 14 hours), but this is consistent with the longer half-lives of ISDN and its active metabolites.

Few well-controlled clinical trials of organic nitrates have been designed to detect rebound or withdrawal effects. In one such trial, however, subjects receiving nitroglycerin had less exercise tolerance at the end of the daily dose-free interval than the parallel group receiving placebo. The incidence, magnitude, and clinical significance of similar phenomena in patients receiving ISDN have not been studied.

INDICATIONS AND USAGE

DILATRATE-SR SUSTAINED RELEASE CAPSULES

Dilatrate-SR sustained-release capsules are indicated for the prevention of angina pectoris due to coronary artery disease. The onset of action of controlled-release oral isosorbide dinitrate is not sufficiently rapid for this product to be useful in aborting an acute anginal episode.

ISORDIL SUBLINGUAL TABLETS

Isordil Sublingual tablets are indicated for the prevention and treatment of angina pectoris due to coronary artery disease. However, because the onset of action of sublingual ISDN is significantly slower than that of sublingual nitroglycerin, sublingual ISDN is not the drug of first choice for abortion of an acute anginal episode.

ISORDIL TITRADOSE TABLETS

Isordil Titradose tablets are indicated for the prevention of angina pectoris due to coronary artery disease. The onset of action of immediate-release oral isosorbide dinitrate is not sufficiently rapid for this product to be useful in aborting an acute anginal episode.

NON-FDA APPROVED INDICATIONS

Non-FDA approved uses of isosorbide dinitrate include treatment of pulmonary hypertension, congestive heart failure, and diffuse esophageal spasm without gastroesophageal reflux. Isosorbide dinitrate is used to reduce portal hypertension to prevent bleeding in some patients with liver cirrhosis.

CONTRAINDICATIONS

DILATRATE-SR SUSTAINED RELEASE CAPSULES

Allergic reactions to organic nitrates are extremely rare, but they do occur. Isosorbide dinitrate is contraindicated in patients who are allergic to it.

ISORDIL SUBLINGUAL TABLETS

Allergic reactions to organic nitrates are extremely rare, but they do occur. Isordil is contraindicated in patients who are allergic to isosorbide dinitrate or any of its other ingredients.

ISORDIL TITRADOSE TABLETS

Allergic reactions to organic nitrates are extremely rare, but they do occur. Isordil is contraindicated in patients who are allergic to isosorbide dinitrate or any of its other ingredients.

WARNINGS

DILATRATE-SR SUSTAINED RELEASE CAPSULES

Amplification of the vasodilatory effects of Dilatrate-SR by sildenafil can result in severe hypotension. The time course and dose dependence of this interaction have not been studied. Appropriate supportive care has not been studied, but it seems reasonable to treat this as a nitrate overdose, with elevation of the extremities and with central volume expansion.

The benefits of extended-release oral isosorbide dinitrate in patients with acute myocardial infarction or congestive heart failure have not been established. If one elects to use isosorbide dinitrate in these conditions, careful clinical or hemodynamic monitoring must be used to avoid the hazards of hypotension and tachycardia. Because the effects of extended-release oral isosorbide dinitrate are so difficult to terminate rapidly, this formulation is not recommended in these settings.

ISORDIL SUBLINGUAL TABLETS

Amplification of the vasodilatory effects of Isordil by sildenafil can result in severe hypotension. The time course and dose dependence of this interaction have not been studied. Appropriate supportive care has not been studied, but it seems reasonable to treat this as a nitrate overdose, with elevation of the extremities and with central volume expansion.

The benefits of sublingual isosorbide dinitrate in patients with acute myocardial infarction or congestive heart failure have not been established. If one elects to use isosorbide dinitrate in these conditions, careful clinical or hemodynamic monitoring must be used to avoid the hazards of hypotension and tachycardia.

ISORDIL TITRADOSE TABLETS

Amplification of the vasodilatory effects of Isordil by sildenafil can result in severe hypotension. The time course and dose dependence of this interaction have not been studied. Appropriate supportive care has not been studied, but it seems reasonable to treat this as a nitrate overdose, with elevation of the the extremities and with central volume expansion.

The benefits of immediate-release oral isosorbide dinitrate in patients with acute myocardial infarction or congestive heart failure have not been established. If one elects to use isosorbide dinitrate in these conditions, careful clinical or hemodynamic monitoring must be used to avoid the hazards of hypotension and tachycardia. Because the effects of oral isosorbide dinitrate are so difficult to terminate rapidly, this formulation is not recommended in these settings.

PRECAUTIONS

DILATRATE-SR SUSTAINED RELEASE CAPSULES

General

Severe hypotension, particularly with upright posture, may occur with even small doses of isosorbide dinitrate. This drug should therefore be used with caution in patients who may be volume depleted or who, for whatever reason, are already hypotensive. Hypotension induced by isosorbide dinitrate may be accompanied by paradoxical bradycardia and increased angina pectoris.

Nitrate therapy may aggravate the angina caused by hypertrophic cardiomyopathy.

As tolerance to isosorbide dinitrate develops, the effect of sublingual nitroglycerin on exercise tolerance, although still observable, is somewhat blunted.

Some clinical trials in angina patients have provided nitroglycerin for about 12 continuous hours of every 24 hour day. During the interdosing intervals in some of these trials, anginal attacks have been more easily provoked than before treatment and patients have demonstrated hemodynamic rebound and decreased exercise tolerance. The importance of these observations to the routine, clinical use of controlled-release oral isosorbide dinitrate is not known.

In industrial workers who have had long-term exposure to unknown (presumably high) doses of organic nitrates, tolerance clearly occurs. Chest pain, acute myocardial infarction, and even sudden death have occurred during temporary withdrawal of nitrates from these workers demonstrating the existence of true physical dependence.

Information for the Patient

Patients should be told that the antianginal efficacy of isosorbide dinitrate is strongly related to its dosing regimen, so the prescribed schedule of dosing should be followed carefully. In particular, daily headaches sometimes accompany treatment with isosorbide dinitrate. In patients who get these headaches, the headaches are a marker of the activity of the drug. Patients should resist the temptation to avoid headaches by altering the schedule of their treatment with isosorbide dinitrate, since loss of headache may be associated with simultaneous loss of antianginal efficacy. Aspirin and/or acetaminophen, on the other hand, often successfully relieve isosorbide dinitrate-induced headaches with no deleterious effect on isosorbide dinitrate's antianginal efficacy.

Treatment with isosorbide dinitrate may be associated with lightheadedness on standing, especially just after rising from a recumbent or seated position. This effect may be more frequent in patients who have also consumed alcohol.

Carcinogenesis, Mutagenesis, and Impairment of Fertility

No long-term studies in animals have been performed to evaluate the carcinogenic potential of isosorbide dinitrate. In a modified 2 L reproduction study, there was no remarkable gross pathology and no altered fertility or gestation among rats fed isosorbide dinitrate at 25 or 100 mg/kg/day.

Pregnancy Category C

At oral doses 35 and 150 times the daily Maximum Recommended Human Dose (MRHD), isosorbide dinitrate has been shown to cause a dose related increase in embryotoxicity (increase in mummified pups) in rabbits. There are no adequate, well-controlled studies in pregnant women. Isosorbide dinitrate should be used during pregnancy only if the potential benefit justifies the potential risk to the fetus.

Nursing Mothers

It is not known whether isosorbide dinitrate is excreted in human milk. Because many drugs are excreted in human milk, caution should be exercised when isosorbide dinitrate is administered to a nursing woman.

Pediatric Use

Safety and effectiveness in pediatric patients have not been established.

ISORDIL SUBLINGUAL TABLETS

General

Severe hypotension, particularly with upright posture, may occur with even small doses of isosorbide dinitrate. This drug should therefore be used with caution in patients who may be volume depleted or who, for whatever reason, are already hypotensive. Hypotension induced by isosorbide dinitrate may be accompanied by paradoxical bradycardia and increased angina pectoris.

Nitrate therapy may aggravate the angina caused by hypertrophic cardiomyopathy.

As tolerance to isosorbide dinitrate develops, the effect of sublingual nitroglycerin on exercise tolerance, although still observable, is somewhat blunted.

Some clinical trials in angina patients have provided nitroglycerin for about 12 continuous hours of every 24 hour day. During the daily dose-free interval in some of these trials, anginal attacks have been more easily provoked than before treatment, and patients have demonstrated hemodynamic rebound and *decreased* exercise tolerance. The importance of these observations to the routine, clinical use of sublingual isosorbide dinitrate is not known.

In industrial workers who have had long-term exposure to unknown (presumably high) doses of organic nitrates, tolerance clearly occurs. Chest pain, acute myocardial infarction, and even sudden death have occurred during temporary withdrawal of nitrates from these workers, demonstrating the existence of true physical dependence.

Information for the Patient

Patients should be told that the anti-anginal efficacy of isosorbide dinitrate is strongly related to its dosing regimen, so the prescribed schedule of dosing should be followed carefully. In particular, daily headaches sometimes accompany treatment with isosorbide dinitrate. In patients who get these headaches, the headaches are a marker of the activity of the drug. Patients should resist the temptation to avoid headaches by altering the schedule of their treatment with isosorbide dinitrate, since loss of headache may be associated with simultaneous loss of anti-anginal efficacy. Aspirin and/or acetaminophen, on the other hand, often successfully relieve isosorbide dinitrate-induced headaches with no deleterious effect on isosorbide dinitrate's antianginal efficacy.

Treatment with isosorbide dinitrate may be associated with lightheadedness on standing, especially just after rising from a recumbent or seated position. This effect may be more frequent in patients who have also consumed alcohol.

Carcinogenesis, Mutagenesis, and Impairment of Fertility

No long-term studies in animals have been performed to evaluate the carcinogenic potential of isosorbide dinitrate. In a modified two-litter reproduction study, there was no remarkable gross pathology and no altered fertility or gestation among rats fed isosorbide dinitrate at 25 or 100 mg/kg/day.

Pregnancy Category C

At oral doses 35 and 150 times the maximum recommended human daily dose, isosorbide dinitrate has been shown to cause a dose-related increase in embryotoxicity (increase in mummified pups) in rabbits. There are no adequate, well-controlled studies in pregnant women. Isosorbide dinitrate should be used during pregnancy only if the potential benefit justifies the potential risk to the fetus.

Nursing Mothers

It is not known whether isosorbide dinitrate is excreted in human milk. Because many drugs are excreted in human milk, caution should be exercised when isosorbide dinitrate is administered to a nursing woman.

Pediatric Use

Safety and effectiveness in pediatric patients have not been established.

Geriatric Use

Clinical studies of Isordil Sublingual did not include sufficient numbers of subjects aged 65 and over to determine whether they respond differently from younger subjects. Other reported clinical experience has not identified differences in responses between the elderly and younger patients. In general, dose selection for an elderly patient should be cautious, usually starting at the low end of the dosing range, reflecting the greater frequency of decreased hepatic, renal, or cardiac function, and of concomitant disease or other drug therapy.

ISORDIL TITRADOSE TABLETS

General

Severe hypotension, particularly with upright posture, may occur with even small doses of isosorbide dinitrate. This drug should therefore be used with caution in patients who may be volume depleted or who, for whatever reason, are already hypotensive. Hypotension induced by isosorbide dinitrate may be accompanied by paradoxical bradycardia and increased angina pectoris.

Nitrate therapy may aggravate the angina caused by hypertrophic cardiomyopathy.

As tolerance to isosorbide dinitrate develops, the effect of sublingual nitroglycerin on exercise tolerance, although still observable, is somewhat blunted.

Some clinical trials in angina patients have provided nitroglycerin for about 12 continuous hours of every 24 hour day. During the daily dose-free interval in some of these trials, anginal attacks have been more easily provoked than before treatment, and patients have demonstrated hemodynamic rebound and *decreased* exercise tolerance. The importance of these observations to the routine, clinical use of immediate-release oral isosorbide dinitrate is not known.

In industrial workers who have had long-term exposure to unknown (presumably high) doses of organic nitrates, tolerance clearly occurs. Chest pain, acute myocardial infarction, and even sudden death have occurred during temporary withdrawal of nitrates from these workers, demonstrating the existence of true physical dependence.

Information for the Patient

Patients should be told that the anti-anginal efficacy of isosorbide dinitrate is strongly related to its dosing regimen, so the prescribed schedule of dosing should be followed carefully. In particular, daily headaches sometimes accompany treatment with isosorbide dinitrate. In patients who get these headaches, the headaches are a marker of the activity of the drug. Patients should resist the temptation to avoid headaches by altering the schedule of their treatment with isosorbide dinitrate, since loss of headache may be associated with simultaneous loss of anti-anginal efficacy. Aspirin and/or acetaminophen, on the other hand, often successfully relieve isosorbide dinitrate-induced headaches with no deleterious effect on isosorbide dinitrate's anti-anginal efficacy.

Treatment with isosorbide dinitrate may be associated with lightheadedness on standing, especially just after rising from a recumbent or seated position. This effect may be more frequent in patients who have also consumed alcohol.

Carcinogenesis, Mutagenesis, and Impairment of Fertility

No long-term studies in animals have been performed to evaluate the carcinogenic potential of isosorbide dinitrate. In a modified two-litter reproduction study, there was no remarkable gross pathology and no altered fertility or gestation among rats fed isosorbide dinitrate at 25 or 100 mg/kg/day.

Pregnancy Category C

At oral doses 35 and 150 times the maximum recommended human daily dose, isosorbide dinitrate has been shown to cause a dose-related increase in embryotoxicity (increase in mummified pups) in rabbits. There are no adequate, well-controlled studies in pregnant women. Isosorbide dinitrate should be used during pregnancy only if the potential benefit justifies the potential risk to the fetus.

Nursing Mothers

It is not known whether isosorbide dinitrate is excreted in human milk. Because many drugs are excreted in human milk, caution should be exercised when isosorbide dinitrate is administered to a nursing woman.

Pediatric Use

Safety and effectiveness in pediatric patients have not been established.

Geriatric Use

Clinical studies of Isordil Titradose did not include sufficient numbers of subjects aged 65 and over to determine whether they respond differently from younger subjects. Other reported clinical experience has not identified differences in responses between the elderly and younger patients. In general, dose selection for an elderly patient should be cautious, usually starting at the low end of the dosing range, reflecting the greater frequency of decreased hepatic, renal, or cardiac function, and of concomitant disease or other drug therapy.

DRUG INTERACTIONS

DILATRATE-SR SUSTAINED RELEASE CAPSULES

The vasodilating effects of isosorbide dinitrate may be additive with those of other vasodilators. Alcohol, in particular, has been found to exhibit additive effects of this variety.

ISORDIL SUBLINGUAL TABLETS

The vasodilating effects of isosorbide dinitrate may be additive with those of other vasodilators. Alcohol, in particular, has been found to exhibit additive effects of this variety.

ISORDIL TITRADOSE TABLETS

The vasodilating effects of isosorbide dinitrate may be additive with those of other vasodilators. Alcohol, in particular, has been found to exhibit additive effects of this variety.

ADVERSE REACTIONS

DILATRATE-SR SUSTAINED RELEASE CAPSULES

Adverse reactions to isosorbide dinitrate are generally dose related, and almost all of these reactions are the result of isosorbide dinitrate's activity as a vasodilator. Headache, which may be severe, is the most commonly reported side effect. Headache may be recurrent with each daily dose, especially at higher doses. Transient episodes of lightheadedness, occasionally related to blood pressure changes, may also occur. Hypotension occurs infrequently, but in some patients it may be severe enough to warrant discontinuation of therapy. Syncope, crescendo angina, and rebound hypertension have been reported but are uncommon.

Extremely rarely, ordinary doses of organic nitrates have caused methemoglobinemia in normal-seeming patients.

Data are not available to allow estimation of the frequency of adverse reactions during treatment with Dilatrate-SR sustained-release capsules.

ISORDIL SUBLINGUAL TABLETS

Adverse reactions to isosorbide dinitrate are generally dose-related, and almost all of these reactions are the result of isosorbide dinitrate's activity as a vasodilator. Headache, which may be severe, is the most commonly reported side effect. Headache may be recurrent with each daily dose, especially at higher doses. Transient episodes of lightheadedness, occasionally related to blood pressure changes, may also occur. Hypotension occurs infrequently, but in some patients it may be severe enough to warrant discontinuation of therapy. Syncope, crescendo angina, and rebound hypertension have been reported but are uncommon.

Extremely rarely, ordinary doses of organic nitrates have caused methemoglobinemia in normal-seeming patients.

Data are not available to allow estimation of the frequency of adverse reactions during treatment with Isordil Sublingual tablets.

ISORDIL TITRADOSE TABLETS

Adverse reactions to isosorbide dinitrate are generally dose-related, and almost all of these reactions are the result of isosorbide dinitrate's activity as a vasodilator. Headache, which may be severe, is the most commonly reported side effect. Headache may be recurrent with each daily dose, especially at higher doses. Transient episodes of lightheadedness, occasionally related to blood pressure changes, may also occur. Hypotension occurs infrequently, but in some patients it may be severe enough to warrant discontinuation of therapy. Syncope, crescendo angina, and rebound hypertension have been reported but are uncommon.

Extremely rarely, ordinary doses of organic nitrates have caused methemoglobinemia in normal-seeming patients.

Data are not available to allow estimation of the frequency of adverse reactions during treatment with Isordil Titradose tablets.

DOSAGE AND ADMINISTRATION

DILATRATE-SR SUSTAINED RELEASE CAPSULES

As noted in CLINICAL PHARMACOLOGY, Dilatrate-SR Sustained Release Capsules, multiple studies with ISDN and other nitrates have shown that maintenance of continuous 24 hour plasma levels results in refractory tolerance. Every dosing regimen for organic nitrates including Dilatrate-SR must provide a daily nitrate-free interval to avoid the development of tolerance. To achieve the necessary nitrate-free interval with immediate-release oral ISDN, it appears that at least one of the daily interdose intervals must be at least 14 hours long. The necessary interdose interval for Dilatrate-SR has not been clearly identified, but it must be greater than 18 hours.

As noted under CLINICAL PHARMACOLOGY, Dilatrate-SR Sustained Release Capsules, only one trial has ever studied the use of extended-release isosorbide dinitrate for more than one dose. In that trial, 40 mg of Dilatrate-SR was administered twice daily in doses given 6 hours apart. After 4 weeks, Dilatrate-SR could not be distinguished from placebo.

Large controlled studies with other nitrates suggest that no dosing regimen with Dilatrate-SR should be expected to provide more than about 12 hours of continuous anti-anginal efficacy per day.

In clinical trials, immediate-release oral isosorbide dinitrate has been administered in a variety of regimens, with total daily doses ranging from 30-480 mg.

Do not exceed 160 mg (4 capsules) per day.

ISORDIL SUBLINGUAL TABLETS

As noted under CLINICAL PHARMACOLOGY, Isordil Sublingual Tablets, multiple-dose studies with ISDN and other nitrates have shown that maintenance of continuous 24 hour plasma levels results in refractory tolerance. Every dosing regimen for ISDN must provide a daily dose-free interval to minimize the development of this tolerance. In the case of sublingual tablets, it is probably true that one of the daily dose-free intervals must be somewhat longer than 14 hours.

As also noted under CLINICAL PHARMACOLOGY, Isordil Sublingual Tablets, the efficacy of daily doses after the first has never been demonstrated.

Large controlled studies with other nitrates suggest that no dosing regimen with Isordil Sublingual tablets should be expected to provide more than about 12 hours of continuous anti-anginal efficacy per day.

A patient anticipating activity likely to cause angina should take one Isordil Sublingual tablet (2.5 to 5 mg) about 15 minutes before the activity is expected to begin. Isordil Sublingual tablets may be used to abort an acute anginal episode, but its use is recommended only in patients who fail to respond to sublingual nitroglycerin.

ISORDIL TITRADOSE TABLETS

As noted under CLINICAL PHARMACOLOGY, Isordil Titradose Tablets, multiple-dose studies with ISDN and other nitrates have shown that maintenance of continuous 24 hour plasma levels results in refractory tolerance. Every dosing regimen for Isordil Titradose tablets must provide a daily dose-free interval to minimize the development of this tolerance. With immediate-release ISDN, it appears that one daily dose-free interval must be at least 14 hours long.

As also noted under CLINICAL PHARMACOLOGY, Isordil Titradose Tablets, the effects of the second and later doses have been smaller and shorter-lasting than the effects of the first.

Large controlled studies with other nitrates suggest that no dosing regimen with Isordil Titradose tablets should be expected to provide more than about 12 hours of continuous anti-anginal efficacy per day.

As with all titratable drugs, it is important to administer the minimum dose which produces the desired clinical effect. The usual starting dose of Isordil Titradose is 5-20 mg, two or three times daily. For maintenance therapy, 10-40 mg, two or three times daily is recommended. Some patients may require higher doses. A daily dose-free interval of at least 14 hours is advisable to minimize tolerance. The optimal interval will vary with the individual patient, dose and regimen.

HOW SUPPLIED

DILATRATE-SR SUSTAINED RELEASE CAPSULES

Dilatrate-SR 40 mg sustained-release capsules are opaque pink and colorless capsules with white beadlets and are imprinted "Schwarz" and "0920".

Storage: Store at controlled room temperature at 15-30°C (59-86°F) in a dry place.

ISORDIL SUBLINGUAL TABLETS

Isordil Sublingual tablets are available as follows:

2.5 mg: Round, yellow tablets imprinted "2.5" on one side and "W" on reverse side.

5 mg: Round, pink tablets imprinted "5" on one side and "W" on reverse side.

10 mg: Round, white tablets imprinted "10" on one side and "Wyeth" on reverse side.

Storage

Store at room temperature, approximately 25°C (77°F).

Protect from light.

Keep bottles tightly closed.

Dispense in a light-resistant, tight container.

Use carton to protect blisters from light.

ISORDIL TITRADOSE TABLETS

Isordil Oral Titradose tablets are available as follows:

5 mg: Round, pink tablets imprinted "WYETH 4152" on one side and deeply scored on reverse side.

10 mg: Round, white tablets imprinted "WYETH 4153" on one side and deeply scored on reverse side.

20 mg: Round, green tablets imprinted "WYETH 4154" on one side and deeply scored on reverse side.

30 mg: Round, blue tablets imprinted "WYETH 4159" on one side and deeply scored on reverse side.

40 mg: Round, light green tablets imprinted "WYETH 4192" on one side and deeply scored on reverse side.

Storage

Store at room temperature, approximately 25°C (77°F).

Protect from light.

Keep bottles tightly closed.

Dispense in a light-resistant, tight container.

Use carton to protect blisters from light.

PRODUCT LISTING - RATED THERAPEUTICALLY EQUIVALENT

Package	Price	Description	NDC
Tablet - Oral - 5 mg			
25 x 30	$111.68	GENERIC, Sky Pharmaceuticals Packaging, Inc	63739-0147-03
30's	$4.04	GENERIC, Heartland Healthcare Services	61392-0311-30
30's	$4.04	GENERIC, Heartland Healthcare Services	61392-0311-39
30's	$89.80	GENERIC, Medirex Inc	57480-0339-06
31 x 10	$48.41	GENERIC, Vangard Labs	00615-1564-53
31 x 10	$48.41	GENERIC, Vangard Labs	00615-1564-63
31's	$4.18	GENERIC, Heartland Healthcare Services	61392-0311-31
32's	$4.31	GENERIC, Heartland Healthcare Services	61392-0311-32
45's	$6.06	GENERIC, Heartland Healthcare Services	61392-0311-45
60's	$8.08	GENERIC, Heartland Healthcare Services	61392-0311-60
90's	$12.12	GENERIC, Heartland Healthcare Services	61392-0311-90
100's	$2.42	FEDERAL UPPER LIMIT, H.C.F.A. F F P	99999-1593-09
100's	$2.96	GENERIC, Moore, H.L. Drug Exchange Inc	00839-1378-06
100's	$4.35	GENERIC, Aligen Independent Laboratories Inc	00405-4558-01
100's	$4.70	GENERIC, Major Pharmaceuticals Inc	00904-2150-60
100's	$4.75	GENERIC, West Ward Pharmaceutical Corporation	00143-1769-01
100's	$5.35	GENERIC, Caremark Inc	00339-5572-12
100's	$5.50	GENERIC, Raway Pharmacal Inc	00686-0084-20
100's	$5.60	GENERIC, West Ward Pharmaceutical Corporation	00143-1767-01
100's	$7.25	GENERIC, Qualitest Products Inc	00603-4116-21
100's	$13.74	GENERIC, Geneva Pharmaceuticals	00781-1635-01
100's	$14.40	GENERIC, West Ward Pharmaceutical Corporation	00143-1769-25
100's	$14.95	GENERIC, Ivax Corporation	00182-0550-89
100's	$15.20	GENERIC, Medirex Inc	57480-0339-01
100's	$15.69	GENERIC, Major Pharmaceuticals Inc	00904-2150-61
100's	$16.24	GENERIC, Par Pharmaceutical Inc	49884-0020-01
100's	$16.49	GENERIC, Geneva Pharmaceuticals	00781-1635-13
100's	$34.35	ISORDIL TITRADOSE, Wyeth-Ayerst Laboratories	00008-4152-01
200 x 5	$156.16	GENERIC, Vangard Labs	00615-1564-43
Tablet - Oral - 10 mg			
8's	$2.93	GENERIC, Pd-Rx Pharmaceuticals	55289-0667-08
15's	$2.46	GENERIC, Heartland Healthcare Services	61392-0305-15
25 x 30	$142.73	GENERIC, Sky Pharmaceuticals Packaging, Inc	63739-0148-03
25's	$5.05	GENERIC, Pd-Rx Pharmaceuticals	55289-0667-97
30 x 20	$109.20	GENERIC, Medirex Inc	57480-0340-06
30's	$4.91	GENERIC, Heartland Healthcare Services	61392-0305-30
30's	$4.91	GENERIC, Heartland Healthcare Services	61392-0305-39
31 x 10	$55.38	GENERIC, Vangard Labs	00615-1560-53
31 x 10	$55.38	GENERIC, Vangard Labs	00615-1560-63
31's	$5.08	GENERIC, Heartland Healthcare Services	61392-0305-31
32's	$5.24	GENERIC, Heartland Healthcare Services	61392-0305-32
45's	$7.37	GENERIC, Heartland Healthcare Services	61392-0305-45
60's	$9.83	GENERIC, Heartland Healthcare Services	61392-0305-60
90's	$5.60	GENERIC, Golden State Medical	60429-0101-90
90's	$14.74	GENERIC, Heartland Healthcare Services	61392-0305-90
100's	$2.78	GENERIC, Interstate Drug Exchange Inc	00814-3985-14
100's	$2.81	FEDERAL UPPER LIMIT, H.C.F.A. F F P	99999-1593-12
100's	$2.95	GENERIC, Cmc-Consolidated Midland Corporation	00223-1096-01
100's	$4.17	GENERIC, Moore, H.L. Drug Exchange Inc	00839-1381-06
100's	$4.79	GENERIC, Pd-Rx Pharmaceuticals	55289-0667-01
100's	$4.85	GENERIC, Aligen Independent Laboratories Inc	00405-4559-01
100's	$4.85	GENERIC, Mova Pharmaceutical Corporation	55370-0807-07
100's	$5.64	GENERIC, Caremark Inc	00339-5573-12
100's	$5.75	GENERIC, Major Pharmaceuticals Inc	00904-2151-60

Qty	Price	Product	NDC
100's	$5.80	GENERIC, West Ward Pharmaceutical Corporation	00143-1771-01
100's	$5.95	GENERIC, Raway Pharmacal Inc	00686-0029-20
100's	$7.69	GENERIC, Qualitest Products Inc	00603-4117-21
100's	$15.37	GENERIC, Geneva Pharmaceuticals	00781-1556-01
100's	$17.02	GENERIC, Par Pharmaceutical Inc	49884-0021-01
100's	$17.15	GENERIC, West Ward Pharmaceutical Corporation	00143-1771-25
100's	$18.20	GENERIC, Ivax Corporation	00182-0514-89
100's	$18.50	GENERIC, Medirex Inc	57480-0340-01
100's	$19.56	GENERIC, Geneva Pharmaceuticals	00781-1556-13
100's	$19.56	GENERIC, Major Pharmaceuticals Inc	00904-2151-61
100's	$26.41	SORBITRATE, Astra-Zeneca Pharmaceuticals	00310-0780-39
100's	$26.86	SORBITRATE, Astra-Zeneca Pharmaceuticals	00310-0780-10
100's	$38.43	ISORDIL TITRADOSE, Wyeth-Ayerst Laboratories	00008-4153-01
100's	$40.43	ISORDIL TITRADOSE, Physicians Total Care	54868-0682-01
120's	$62.00	GENERIC, Golden State Medical	60429-0101-12
270's	$17.95	GENERIC, Golden State Medical	60429-0101-27

Tablet - Oral - 20 mg

Qty	Price	Product	NDC
25's	$6.23	GENERIC, Pd-Rx Pharmaceuticals	55289-0174-97
30 x 25	$147.53	GENERIC, Sky Pharmaceuticals Packaging, Inc	63739-0149-01
30 x 25	$147.53	GENERIC, Sky Pharmaceuticals Packaging, Inc	63739-0149-03
30's	$5.97	GENERIC, Heartland Healthcare Services	61392-0321-30
30's	$5.97	GENERIC, Heartland Healthcare Services	61392-0321-39
31 x 10	$71.71	GENERIC, Vangard Labs	00615-1575-53
31 x 10	$71.71	GENERIC, Vangard Labs	00615-1575-63
31's	$6.17	GENERIC, Heartland Healthcare Services	61392-0321-31
32's	$6.36	GENERIC, Heartland Healthcare Services	61392-0321-32
45's	$8.95	GENERIC, Heartland Healthcare Services	61392-0321-45
60's	$11.93	GENERIC, Heartland Healthcare Services	61392-0321-60
90's	$3.05	GENERIC, Major Pharmaceuticals Inc	00904-2154-89
90's	$5.25	GENERIC, Golden State Medical	60429-0102-90
90's	$17.90	GENERIC, Heartland Healthcare Services	61392-0321-90
100's	$2.91	FEDERAL UPPER LIMIT, H.C.F.A. F F P	99999-1593-16
100's	$3.23	GENERIC, Interstate Drug Exchange Inc	00814-3988-14
100's	$4.25	GENERIC, Cmc-Consolidated Midland Corporation	00223-1099-01
100's	$4.31	GENERIC, Moore, H.L. Drug Exchange Inc	00839-6017-06
100's	$5.50	GENERIC, Aligen Independent Laboratories Inc	00405-4560-01
100's	$5.50	GENERIC, Mova Pharmaceutical Corporation	55370-0808-07
100's	$6.59	GENERIC, Major Pharmaceuticals Inc	00904-2154-60
100's	$6.65	GENERIC, West Ward Pharmaceutical Corporation	00143-1772-01
100's	$6.85	GENERIC, Caremark Inc	00339-5574-12
100's	$8.99	GENERIC, Qualitest Products Inc	00603-4118-21
100's	$20.05	GENERIC, Par Pharmaceutical Inc	49884-0022-01
100's	$21.15	GENERIC, West Ward Pharmaceutical Corporation	00143-1772-25
100's	$21.92	GENERIC, Major Pharmaceuticals Inc	00904-2154-61
100's	$22.45	GENERIC, Ivax Corporation	00182-0868-89
100's	$24.80	GENERIC, Geneva Pharmaceuticals	00781-1695-01
100's	$29.76	GENERIC, Geneva Pharmaceuticals	00781-1695-13
100's	$40.97	SORBITRATE, Astra-Zeneca Pharmaceuticals	00310-0820-10
100's	$42.04	SORBITRATE, Astra-Zeneca Pharmaceuticals	00310-0820-39
100's	$62.00	ISORDIL TITRADOSE, Wyeth-Ayerst Laboratories	00008-4154-01
120's	$3.60	GENERIC, Major Pharmaceuticals Inc	00904-2154-18
180's	$4.64	GENERIC, Major Pharmaceuticals Inc	00904-2154-93
240's	$5.76	GENERIC, Major Pharmaceuticals Inc	00904-2154-34
270's	$20.30	GENERIC, Golden State Medical	60429-0102-27

Tablet - Oral - 30 mg

Qty	Price	Product	NDC
30's	$1.50	GENERIC, Heartland Healthcare Services	61392-0318-30
30's	$1.50	GENERIC, Heartland Healthcare Services	61392-0318-39
31's	$1.55	GENERIC, Heartland Healthcare Services	61392-0318-31
32's	$1.60	GENERIC, Heartland Healthcare Services	61392-0318-32
45's	$2.25	GENERIC, Heartland Healthcare Services	61392-0318-45
60's	$3.00	GENERIC, Heartland Healthcare Services	61392-0318-60
90's	$4.50	GENERIC, Heartland Healthcare Services	61392-0318-90
100's	$6.48	GENERIC, Aligen Independent Laboratories Inc	00405-4561-01
100's	$7.09	GENERIC, Moore, H.L. Drug Exchange Inc	00839-6618-06
100's	$17.97	GENERIC, Major Pharmaceuticals Inc	00904-2682-61
100's	$52.65	GENERIC, Major Pharmaceuticals Inc	00904-2682-60
100's	$52.97	GENERIC, Caremark Inc	00339-5653-12
100's	$53.15	GENERIC, Par Pharmaceutical Inc	49884-0009-01
100's	$69.70	ISORDIL TITRADOSE, Wyeth-Ayerst Laboratories	00008-4159-01
100's	$132.15	GENERIC, Kremers Urban	62175-0128-86

Tablet - Oral - 40 mg

Qty	Price	Product	NDC
90's	$14.13	GENERIC, Pharmaceutical Corporation Of America	51655-0601-26
100's	$4.95	GENERIC, Cmc-Consolidated Midland Corporation	00223-1097-01
100's	$6.47	GENERIC, Mova Pharmaceutical Corporation	55370-0809-07
100's	$9.68	GENERIC, Interstate Drug Exchange Inc	00814-3977-14
100's	$12.69	GENERIC, Major Pharmaceuticals Inc	00904-2153-61
100's	$47.96	SORBITRATE, Astra-Zeneca Pharmaceuticals	00310-0774-10
100's	$53.02	SORBITRATE, Astra-Zeneca Pharmaceuticals	00310-0774-39
100's	$75.61	ISORDIL TITRADOSE, Wyeth-Ayerst Laboratories	00008-4192-01

Tablet - Sublingual - 2.5 mg

Qty	Price	Product	NDC
100's	$4.35	GENERIC, Geneva Pharmaceuticals	00781-1515-01
100's	$4.44	GENERIC, Moore, H.L. Drug Exchange Inc	00839-5044-06
100's	$5.20	GENERIC, Major Pharmaceuticals Inc	00904-2342-60
100's	$5.25	GENERIC, West Ward Pharmaceutical Corporation	00143-1765-01
100's	$6.91	GENERIC, Caremark Inc	00339-5655-12
100's	$8.00	GENERIC, Geneva Pharmaceuticals	00781-1515-13
100's	$10.28	GENERIC, Qualitest Products Inc	00603-4122-21
100's	$31.98	ISORDIL, Wyeth-Ayerst Laboratories	00008-4139-01

Tablet - Sublingual - 5 mg

Qty	Price	Product	NDC
100's	$2.50	GENERIC, Cmc-Consolidated Midland Corporation	00223-1094-01
100's	$4.60	GENERIC, Mutual/United Research Laboratories	00677-0409-01
100's	$4.66	GENERIC, Geneva Pharmaceuticals	00781-1565-01
100's	$4.85	GENERIC, Major Pharmaceuticals Inc	00904-2343-61
100's	$5.06	GENERIC, Moore, H.L. Drug Exchange Inc	00839-5043-06
100's	$5.55	GENERIC, Major Pharmaceuticals Inc	00904-2343-60
100's	$5.92	GENERIC, Aligen Independent Laboratories Inc	00405-4570-01
100's	$6.65	GENERIC, Geneva Pharmaceuticals	00781-1565-13
100's	$7.93	GENERIC, Caremark Inc	00339-5657-12
100's	$10.28	GENERIC, Qualitest Products Inc	00603-4123-21

Tablet, Chewable - Oral - 5 mg

Qty	Price	Product	NDC
100's	$22.45	SORBITRATE, Astra-Zeneca Pharmaceuticals	00310-0810-10

Tablet, Extended Release - Oral - 40 mg

Qty	Price	Product	NDC
100's	$11.18	GENERIC, Pd-Rx Pharmaceuticals	55289-0970-01
100's	$56.60	GENERIC, Inwood Laboratories Inc	00258-3613-01

Tablet, Sublingual - Sublingual - 2.5 mg

Qty	Price	Product	NDC
100's	$4.88	FEDERAL UPPER LIMIT, H.C.F.A. F F P	99999-1593-01

PRODUCT LISTING - RATED NOT THERAPEUTICALLY EQUIVALENT

Capsule, Extended Release - Oral - 40 mg

Qty	Price	Product	NDC
60's	$37.34	DILATRATE-SR, Schwarz Pharma	00021-0920-02
60's	$37.34	DILATRATE-SR, Schwarz Pharma	00091-0920-02
100's	$59.48	ISORDIL TEMBIDS, Wyeth-Ayerst Laboratories	00008-4140-01
100's	$60.38	DILATRATE-SR, Schwarz Pharma	00021-0920-01
100's	$83.31	DILATRATE-SR, Schwarz Pharma	00091-0920-01

PRODUCT LISTING - EQUIVALENTS NOT AVAILABLE

Tablet - Oral - 5 mg

Qty	Price	Product	NDC
100's	$2.60	GENERIC, Caremark Inc	00223-1095-01
100's	$3.73	GENERIC, Physicians Total Care	54868-2297-00
200's	$5.97	GENERIC, Physicians Total Care	54868-2297-02

Tablet - Oral - 10 mg

Qty	Price	Product	NDC
90's	$6.07	GENERIC, Pharmaceutical Corporation Of America	51655-0406-26
100's	$1.88	GENERIC, Allscripts Pharmaceutical Company	54569-0455-00
100's	$3.67	GENERIC, Physicians Total Care	54868-0681-01
100's	$6.75	GENERIC, Pharmaceutical Corporation Of America	51655-0406-21

Tablet - Oral - 20 mg

Qty	Price	Product	NDC
8's	$7.80	GENERIC, Pharmaceutical Corporation Of America	51655-0547-80
30's	$17.99	GENERIC, Southwood Pharmaceuticals Inc	58016-0707-30
60's	$35.98	GENERIC, Southwood Pharmaceuticals Inc	58016-0707-60
90's	$6.40	GENERIC, Pharmaceutical Corporation Of America	51655-0547-26
90's	$53.96	GENERIC, Southwood Pharmaceuticals Inc	58016-0707-90
100's	$3.88	GENERIC, Physicians Total Care	54868-2127-01
100's	$5.72	GENERIC, Allscripts Pharmaceutical Company	54569-0450-00
100's	$7.03	GENERIC, Allscripts Pharmaceutical Company	54569-0452-00
100's	$9.00	GENERIC, Pharmaceutical Corporation Of America	51655-0547-21
100's	$59.96	GENERIC, Southwood Pharmaceuticals Inc	58016-0707-00
270's	$17.82	GENERIC, Pharmaceutical Corporation Of America	51655-0547-92

Tablet - Oral - 30 mg

Qty	Price	Product	NDC
100's	$7.24	GENERIC, Physicians Total Care	54868-2590-02

Tablet - Sublingual - 10 mg

Qty	Price	Product	NDC
100's	$39.95	ISORDIL, Wyeth-Ayerst Laboratories	00008-4161-01

Tablet, Extended Release - Oral - 40 mg

Qty	Price	Product	NDC
30's	$3.16	GENERIC, Allscripts Pharmaceutical Company	54569-0454-00

60's	$6.31	GENERIC, Allscripts Pharmaceutical Company	54569-0454-03
90's	$8.70	GENERIC, Major Pharmaceuticals Inc	00904-2149-89
90's	$9.47	GENERIC, Allscripts Pharmaceutical Company	54569-0454-04
100's	$6.00	GENERIC, Cmc-Consolidated Midland Corporation	00223-1116-01
100's	$6.21	GENERIC, Aligen Independent Laboratories Inc	00405-4564-01
100's	$6.75	GENERIC, Moore, H.L. Drug Exchange Inc	00839-6188-06
100's	$7.45	GENERIC, Major Pharmaceuticals Inc	00904-2149-60
100's	$9.03	GENERIC, Physicians Total Care	54868-2711-00
100's	$10.05	GENERIC, Ivax Corporation	00182-0879-01
100's	$10.52	GENERIC, Allscripts Pharmaceutical Company	54569-0454-01
100's	$11.10	GENERIC, Caremark Inc	00339-5833-12
100's	$15.08	GENERIC, Inwood Laboratories Inc	00258-3549-01
100's	$24.35	GENERIC, Major Pharmaceuticals Inc	00904-2149-61
100's	$52.51	GENERIC, Southwood Pharmaceuticals Inc	58016-0584-00
100's	$76.18	GENERIC, Forest Pharmaceuticals	00456-0637-01

Isosorbide Mononitrate *(003106)*

Categories: Angina pectoris; Pregnancy Category C; FDA Approved 1991 Dec
Drug Classes: Nitrates; Vasodilators
Brand Names: Imdur; **Ismo**; Monoket
Foreign Brand Availability: Angistad (Philippines); Cincordil (Colombia); Conpin (Germany); Conpin Retardkaps (Germany); Corangin (China; New-Zealand); Corangin SR (Taiwan); Coxime (Taiwan); Coxine SR (Taiwan); Duride (Australia; New-Zealand); Elan (Italy); Elantan (Austria; Czech-Republic; Dominican-Republic; El-Salvador; England; Germany; Guatemala; Honduras; Hong-Kong; Indonesia; Ireland; Korea; Malaysia; Mexico; Panama; Peru; Philippines; Switzerland; Taiwan; Thailand); Elantan Long (China; Czech-Republic; Germany; Hong-Kong; Malaysia; Peru; Philippines); Elantan Retard (Switzerland); Elonton SR (Korea); Etimonis (China); Imdex CR (Singapore); Imdur 60 (Mexico; Taiwan); Imdur Durules (Australia); Imtrate (Australia; New-Zealand); ISMN (Austria; Germany); Ismexin (Finland); Ismo-20 (Benin; Burkina-Faso; Ethiopia; Gambia; Ghana; Guinea; Ivory-Coast; Kenya; Liberia; Malawi; Mali; Mauritania; Mauritius; Morocco; Niger; Nigeria; Senegal; Seychelles; Sierra-Leone; South-Africa; Sudan; Tanzania; Tunia; Uganda; Zambia; Zimbabwe); Ismo 20 (Bahamas; Barbados; Belize; Bermuda; Curacao; Guyana; Hong-Kong; India; Indonesia; Jamaica; Malaysia; Netherland-Antilles; New-Zealand; South-Africa; Surinam; Taiwan; Thailand; Trinidad); Ismox (Finland); Isobid (Korea); Isomon (Greece); Isomonat (Austria; Czech-Republic); Isomonit (Germany); Isonite (Korea); Isopen-20 (Thailand); Isotril ER (Korea); Iturol (Japan); Medocor (Ecuador); Monicor (France); Monis (Colombia); Monit 20 (India); Mono Corax (Germany); Mono Corax Retard (Germany); Monoclair (Germany); Monocord 20 (Israel); Monocord 40 (Israel); Monocord 50 SR (Israel); Monodur Durules (Australia); Monoket OD (Norway; Sweden); Monoket Retard (Austria; Italy); Monolong (Germany); Monolong 40 (Israel); Monolong 60 (Israel); Mono-Mack (Czech-Republic); Mono Mack (China; Ecuador; Mexico; Peru; South-Africa); Mononit (Bulgaria; Poland); Monopront (Finland); Mono-Sanorania (Germany); Monosorbitrate (India); Monosordil (Greece); Monotrate (India); Mononit 20 (Israel); Mononit 40 (Israel); Mononit Retard 50 (Israel); Nitramin (Greece); Pentacard (Belgium; China; Indonesia); Vasotrate (India)
Cost of Therapy: $54.84 (Angina; Ismo; 20 mg; 2 tablets/day; 30 day supply)
$32.02 (Angina; Generic Tablets; 20 mg; 2 tablets/day; 30 day supply)
$57.78 (Angina; Imdur Extended Release; 30 mg; 1 tablet/day; 30 day supply)
$33.47 (Angina; Generic Extended Release tablets; 30 mg; 1 tablet/day; 30 day supply)

DESCRIPTION

Isosorbide mononitrate, an organic nitrate and the major biologically active metabolite of isosorbide dinitrate, is a vasodilator with effects on both arteries and veins.

The chemical name for isosorbide mononitrate is 1,4:3,6-dianhydro-,D-glucitol 5-nitrate. Isosorbide mononitrate is a white, crystalline, odorless compound which is stable in air and in solution, has a melting point of about 90°C, and an optical rotation of +144° (2% in water, 20°C).

Isosorbide mononitrate is freely soluble in water, ethanol, methanol, chloroform, ethyl acetate, and dichloromethane.

Each Ismo tablet contains 20 mg of isosorbide mononitrate. The inactive ingredients in each tablet are D&C yellow 10 aluminum lake, FD&C yellow 6 aluminum lake, hydroxypropyl methylcellulose, lactose, magnesium stearate, microcrystalline cellulose, polyethylene glycol, polysorbate 20, povidone, silicon dioxide, sodium starch glycolate, titanium dioxide and hydroxypropyl cellulose.

Imdur tablets contain 30, 60, or 120 mg of isosorbide mononitrate in an extended-release formulation. The inactive ingredients are aluminum silicate, colloidal silicon dioxide, hydroxypropyl cellulose, hydroxypropyl methylcellulose, iron oxide, magnesium stearate, paraffin wax, polyethylene glycol, titanium dioxide, and trace amounts of ethanol.

CLINICAL PHARMACOLOGY

MECHANISM OF ACTION

The isosorbide mononitrate extended release tablets product is an oral extended-release formulation of isosorbide mononitrate, the major active metabolite of isosorbide dinitrate; most of the clinical activity of the dinitrate is attributable to the mononitrate.

The principal pharmacological action of isosorbide mononitrate and all organic nitrates in general is relaxation of vascular smooth muscle, producing dilatation of peripheral arteries and veins, especially the latter. Dilatation of the veins promotes peripheral pooling of blood, decreases venous return to the heart, thereby reducing left ventricular end-diastolic pressure and pulmonary capillary wedge pressure (preload). Arteriolar relaxation reduces systemic vascular resistance, and systolic arterial pressure and mean arterial pressure (afterload). Dilatation of the coronary arteries also occurs. The relative importance of preload reduction, afterload reduction, and coronary dilatation remains undefined.

Isosorbide mononitrate is the major active metabolite of isosorbide dinitrate, and most of the clinical activity of the dinitrate is attributable to the mononitrate.

PHARMACODYNAMICS

Dosing regimens for most chronically used drugs are designed to provide plasma concentrations that are continuously greater than a minimally effective concentration. This strategy is inappropriate for organic nitrates. Several well-controlled clinical trials have used exercise testing to assess the antianginal efficacy of continuously-delivered nitrates. In the large majority of these trials, active agents were indistinguishable from placebo after 24 hours (or less) of continuous therapy. Attempts to overcome tolerance by dose escalation, even to doses far in excess of those used acutely, have consistently failed. Only after nitrates have been absent from the body for several hours has their antianginal efficacy been restored.

Immediate Release Tablets

The drug-free interval sufficient to avoid tolerance to isosorbide mononitrate has not been completely defined. In the only regimen of twice-daily isosorbide mononitrate that has been shown to avoid development of tolerance, the 2 doses of isosorbide mononitrate tablets are given 7 hours apart, so there is a gap of 17 hours between the second dose of each day and the first dose of the next day. Taking account of the relatively long half-life of isosorbide mononitrate this result is consistent with those obtained for other organic nitrates.

The same twice-daily regimen of isosorbide mononitrate tablets successfully avoided significant rebound/withdrawal effects. The incidence and magnitude of such phenomena have appeared, in studies of other nitrates, to be highly dependent upon the schedule of nitrate administration.

Extended Release Tablets

The isosorbide mononitrate extended release tablets during long-term use over 42 days dosed at 120 mg once daily continued to improve exercise performance at 4 hours and at 12 hours after dosing but its effects (although better than placebo) are less than or at best equal to the effects of the first dose of 60 mg.

PHARMACOKINETICS

Immediate Release Tablets

In humans, isosorbide mononitrate is not subject to first pass metabolism in the liver. The absolute bioavailability of isosorbide mononitrate from isosorbide mononitrate tablets is nearly 100%. Maximum serum concentrations of isosorbide mononitrate are achieved 30 to 60 minutes after ingestion of isosorbide mononitrate.

The volume of distribution of isosorbide mononitrate is approximately 0.6 L/kg, and less than 4% is bound to plasma proteins. It is cleared from the serum by denitration to isosorbide; glucuronidation to the mononitrate glucuronide; and denitration/hydration to sorbitol. None of these metabolites is vasoactive. Less than 1% of administered isosorbide mononitrate is eliminated in the urine.

The overall elimination half-life of isosorbide mononitrate is about 5 hours; the rate of clearance is the same in healthy young adults, in patients with various degrees of renal, hepatic, or cardiac dysfunction, and in the elderly. In a single-dose study, the pharmacokinetics of isosorbide mononitrate were dose-proportional up to at least 60 mg.

PHARMACOKINETICS AND METABOLISM

Extended Release Tablets

After intravenous administration, isosorbide mononitrate is distributed into total body water in about 9 minutes with a volume of distribution of approximately 0.6-0.7 L/kg. Isosorbide mononitrate is approximately 5% bound to human plasma proteins and is distributed into blood cells and saliva. Isosorbide mononitrate is primarily metabolized by the liver, but unlike oral isosorbide dinitrate, it is not subject to first-pass metabolism. Isosorbide mononitrate is cleared by denitration to isosorbide and glucuronidation as the mononitrate, with 96% of the administered dose excreted in the urine within 5 days and only about 1% eliminated in the feces. At least 6 different compounds have been detected in urine, with about 2% of the dose excreted as the unchanged drug and at least five metabolites. The metabolites are not pharmacologically active. Renal clearance accounts for only about 4% of total body clearance. The mean plasma elimination half-life of isosorbide mononitrate is approximately 5 hours.

The disposition of isosorbide mononitrate in patients with various degrees of renal insufficiency, liver cirrhosis, or cardiac dysfunction was evaluated and found to be similar to that observed in healthy subjects. The elimination half-life of isosorbide mononitrate was not prolonged, and there was no drug accumulation in patients with chronic renal failure after multiple oral dosing.

The pharmacokinetics and/or bioavailability of isosorbide mononitrate extended release tablets have been studied in both normal volunteers and patients following single- and multiple-dose administration. Data from these studies suggest that the pharmacokinetics of isosorbide mononitrate administered as isosorbide mononitrate extended release tablets are similar between normal healthy volunteers and patients with angina pectoris. In single- and multiple-dose studies, the pharmacokinetics of isosorbide mononitrate were dose proportional between 30 mg and 240 mg.

In a multiple-dose study, the effect of age on the pharmacokinetic profile of isosorbide mononitrate extended release tablets 60 mg and 120 mg (2 × 60 mg) tablets was evaluated in subjects ≥45 years. The results of that study indicate that there are no significant differences in any of the pharmacokinetic variables of isosorbide mononitrate between elderly (≥65 years) and younger individuals (45-64 years) for the isosorbide mononitrate extended release tablets 60 mg dose. The administration of extended release tablet 120 mg (2 × 60 mg tablets every 24 hours for 7 days) produced a dose-proportional increase in C_{max} and AUC, without changes in T_{max} or the terminal half-life. The older group (65-74 years) showed 30% lower apparent oral clearance (Cl/F) following the higher dose, ie, 120 mg, compared to the younger group (45-64 years); Cl/F was not different between the 2 groups following the 60 mg regimen. While Cl/F was independent of dose in the younger group, the older group showed slightly lower Cl/F following the 120 mg regimen compared to the 60 mg regimen. Differences between the 2 age groups, however, were not statistically significant. In the same study, females showed a slight (15%) reduction in clearance when the dose was increased. Females showed higher AUCs and C_{max} compared to males, but these differences were accounted for by differences in body weight between the 2 groups. When the data were analyzed using age as a variable, the results indicated that there were no significant differences in any of the pharmacokinetic variables of isosorbide mononitrate between older (≥65 years) and younger individuals (45-64 years). The results of this study, however, should be viewed with caution due to the small numbers of subjects in each age subgroup and consequently the lack of sufficient statistical power.

I

TABLE 1 summarizes key pharmacokinetic parameters of isosorbide mononitrate after single- and multiple-dose administration of isosorbide mononitrate as an oral solution or isosorbide mononitrate extended release tablets.

TABLE 1

Parameter	Single-Dose Studies: Isosorbide Mononitrate 60 mg	Single-Dose Studies: Isosorbide Mononitrate Extended Release Tablets 60 mg	Multiple-Dose Studies: Isosorbide Mononitrate Extended Release Tablets 60 mg	Multiple-Dose Studies: Isosorbide Mononitrate Extended Release Tablets 120 mg
C_{max} (ng/ml)	1242-1534	424-541	557-572	1151-1180
T_{max} (h)	0.6-0.7	3.1-4.5	2.9-4.2	3.1-3.2
AUC (ng·h/ml)	8189-8313	5990-7452	6625-7555	14241-16800
T½ (h)	4.8-5.1	6.3-6.6	6.2-6.3	6.2-6.4
Cl/F (ml/min)	120-122	151-187	132-151	119-140

Food Effects

The influence of food on the bioavailability of isosorbide mononitrate after single-dose administration of isosorbide mononitrate extended release tablets 60 mg was evaluated in three different studies involving either a "light" breakfast or a high-calorie, high-fat breakfast. Results of these studies indicate that concomitant food intake may decrease the rate (increase in T_{max}) but not the extent (AUC) of absorption of isosorbide mononitrate.

INDICATIONS AND USAGE

isosorbide mononitrate tablets are indicated for the prevention of angina pectoris due to coronary artery disease. The onset of action of oral isosorbide mononitrate is not sufficiently rapid for this product to be useful in aborting an acute anginal episode.

NON-FDA APPROVED INDICATIONS

Nitrates are used without FDA approval to treat portal hypertension, which, in some cases, reduces the frequency of esophageal hemorrhage.

CONTRAINDICATIONS

Immediate Release Tablets: Allergic reactions to organic nitrates are extremely rare, but they do occur. Isosorbide mononitrate is contraindicated in patients who are allergic to it.
Extended Release Tablets: Isosorbide mononitrate extended release tablets are contraindicated in patients who have shown hypersensitivity or idiosyncratic reactions to other nitrates or nitrites.

WARNINGS

The benefits of isosorbide mononitrate in patients with acute myocardial infarction or congestive heart failure have not been established; because the effects of isosorbide mononitrate are difficult to terminate rapidly, this drug is not recommended in these settings.

If isosorbide mononitrate is used in these conditions, careful clinical or hemodynamic monitoring must be used to avoid the hazards of hypotension and tachycardia.

PRECAUTIONS

GENERAL

Severe hypotension, particularly with upright posture, may occur with even small doses of isosorbide mononitrate. This drug should therefore be used with caution in patients who may be volume depleted or who, for whatever reason, are already hypotensive. Hypotension induced by isosorbide mononitrate may be accompanied by paradoxical bradycardia and increased angina pectoris.

Nitrate therapy may aggravate the angina caused by hypertrophic cardiomyopathy.

In industrial workers who have had long-term exposure to unknown (presumably high) doses of organic nitrates, tolerance clearly occurs. Chest pain, acute myocardial infarction, and even sudden death have occurred during temporary withdrawal of nitrates from these workers, demonstrating the existence of true physical dependence. The importance of these observations to the routine, clinical use of oral isosorbide mononitrate is not known.

INFORMATION FOR THE PATIENT

Patients should be told that the antianginal efficacy of isosorbide mononitrate tablets can be maintained by carefully following the prescribed schedule of dosing (2 doses taken 7 hours apart). For most patients, this can be accomplished by taking the first dose on awakening and the second dose 7 hours later. For patients taking the isosorbide mononitrate extended release tablets, this can be accomplished by taking the dose on arising.

As with other nitrates, daily headaches sometimes accompany treatment with isosorbide mononitrate. In patients who get these headaches, the headaches are a marker of the activity of the drug. Patients should resist the temptation to avoid headaches by altering the schedule of their treatment with isosorbide mononitrate, since loss of headache may be associated with simultaneous loss of antianginal efficacy. Aspirin and/or acetaminophen, on the other hand, often successfully relieve isosorbide mononitrate-induced headaches with no deleterious effect on isosorbide mononitrate's antianginal efficacy.

Treatment with isosorbide mononitrate may be associated with light-headedness on standing, especially just after rising from a recumbent or seated position. This effect may be more frequent in patients who have also consumed alcohol.

DRUG/LABORATORY TEST INTERACTIONS

Nitrates and nitrites may interfere with the Zlatkis-Zak color reaction, causing falsely low readings in serum cholesterol determinations.

CARCINOGENESIS, MUTAGENESIS, AND IMPAIRMENT OF FERTILITY

Immediate Release Tablets

No carcinogenic effects were observed in mice exposed to oral isosorbide mononitrate for 104 weeks at doses of up to 900 mg/kg/day (102 X the human exposure comparing body surface area). Rats treated with 900 mg/kg/day for 26 weeks (225 X the human exposure comparing body surface area) and 500 mg/kg/day for the remaining 95-111 weeks (males and females, respectively) showed no evidence of tumors.

No mutagenic activity was seen in a variety of *in vitro* and *in vivo* assays.

No adverse effects on fertility were observed when isosorbide mononitrate was administered to male and female rats at doses of up to 500 mg/kg/day (125 X the human exposure comparing body surface area).

Extended Release Tablets

No evidence of carcinogenicity was observed in rats exposed to isosorbide mononitrate in their diets at doses of up to 900 mg/kg/day for the first 6 months and 500 mg/kg/day for the remaining duration of a study in which males were dosed for up to 121 weeks and females were dosed for up to 137 weeks.

Isosorbide mononitrate did not produce gene mutations (Ames test, mouse lymphoma test) or chromosome aberrations (human lymphocyte and mouse micronucleus tests) at biologically relevant concentrations.

No effects on fertility were observed in a study in which male and female rats were administered doses of up to 750 mg/kg/day beginning, in males, 9 weeks prior to mating, and in females, 2 weeks prior to mating.

PREGNANCY CATEGORY C

Immediate Release Tablets

Isosorbide mononitrate has been shown to be associated with stillbirths and neonatal death in rats receiving 500 mg/kg/day of isosorbide mononitrate (125 × the human exposure comparing body surface area). At 250 mg/kg/day, no adverse effects on reproduction and development were reported.

In rats and rabbits receiving isosorbide mononitrate at up to 250 mg/kg/day, no developmental abnormalities, fetal abnormalities, or other effects upon reproductive performance were detected; these doses are larger than the maximum recommended human dose by factors between 70 (body-surface-area basis in rabbits) and 310 (body-weight basis, either species). In rats receiving 500 mg/kg/day, there were small but statistically significant increases in the rates of prolonged gestation, prolonged parturition, stillbirth, and neonatal death; and there were small but statistically significant decreases in birth weight, live litter size, and pup survival.

There are no adequate and well-controlled studies in pregnant women. Isosorbide mononitrate should be used during pregnancy only if the potential benefit justifies the potential risk to the fetus.

PREGNANCY CATEGORY B

Extended Release Tablets

Teratogenic Effects

In studies designed to detect effects of isosorbide mononitrate on embryo-fetal development, doses of up to 240 or 248 mg/kg/day, administered to pregnant rats and rabbits, were unassociated with evidence of such effects. These animal doses are about 100 times the maximum recommended human dose (120 mg in a 50 kg woman) when comparison is based on body weight; when comparison is based on body surface area, the rat dose is about 17 times the human dose and the rabbit dose is about 38 times the human dose. There are, however, no adequate and well-controlled studies in pregnant women. Because animal reproduction studies are not always predictive of human response, isosorbide mononitrate extended release tablets should be used during pregnancy only if clearly needed.

Nonteratogenic Effects

Neonatal survival and development and incidence of stillbirths were adversely affected when pregnant rats were administered oral doses of 750 (but not 300) mg isosorbide mononitrate/kg/day during late gestation and lactation. This dose (about 312 times the human dose when comparison is based on body weight and 54 times the human dose when comparison is based on body surface area) was associated with decreases in maternal weight gain and motor activity and evidence of impaired lactation.

NURSING MOTHERS

It is not known whether isosorbide mononitrate is excreted in human milk. Because many drugs are excreted in human milk, caution should be exercised when isosorbide mononitrate is administered to a nursing woman.

PEDIATRIC USE

The safety and effectiveness of isosorbide mononitrate in children have not been established.

DRUG INTERACTIONS

The vasodilating effects of isosorbide mononitrate may be additive with those of other vasodilators. Alcohol, in particular, has been found to exhibit additive effects of this variety.

Marked symptomatic orthostatic hypotension has been reported when calcium channel blockers and organic nitrates were used in combination. Dose adjustments of either class of agents may be necessary.

ADVERSE REACTIONS

IMMEDIATE RELEASE TABLETS

TABLE 2 shows the frequencies of the adverse reactions observed in more than 1% of the subjects (a) in 6 placebo-controlled domestic studies in which patients in the active-treatment arm received 20 mg of isosorbide mononitrate twice daily, and (b) in all studies in which patients received isosorbide mononitrate in a variety of regimens. In parentheses, the same table shows the frequencies with which these adverse reactions led to discontinuation of treatment. Overall, eleven percent of the patients who received isosorbide mononitrate in the six controlled US studies discontinued treatment because of adverse reactions. Most of these discontinued because of headache. "Dizziness" and nausea were also frequently associated with withdrawal from these studies (see TABLE 2).

Other adverse reactions, each reported by fewer than 1% of exposed patients, and in many cases of uncertain relation to drug treatment, were:

TABLE 2 *Frequency of Adverse Reactions (discontinuations)**

Dose	6 Controlled Studies Placebo	20 mg	92 Clinical Studies (Varied)
Patients	204	219	3344
Headache	9% (0%)	38% (9%)	19% (4.3%)
Dizziness	1% (0%)	5% (1%)	3% (0.2%)
Nausea, vomiting	<1% (0%)	4% (3%)	2% (0.2%)

* Some individuals discontinued for multiple reasons.

Cardiovascular: Angina pectoris, arrhythmias, atrial fibrillation, hypotension, palpitations, postural hypotension, premature ventricular contractions, supraventricular tachycardia, syncope.
Dermatologic: Pruritus, rash.
Gastrointestinal: Abdominal pain, diarrhea, dyspepsia, tenesmus, tooth disorder, vomiting.
Genitourinary: Dysuria, impotence, urinary frequency.
Miscellaneous: Asthenia, blurred vision, cold sweat, diplopia, edema, malaise, neck stiffness, rigors.
Musculoskeletal: Arthralgia.
Neurologic: Agitation, anxiety, confusion, dyscoordination, hypoesthesia, hypokinesia, increased appetite, insomnia, nervousness, nightmares.
Respiratory: Bronchitis, pneumonia, upper respiratory tract infection.
Extremely rarely, ordinary doses of organic nitrates have caused methemoglobinemia in normal-seeming patients.

EXTENDED RELEASE TABLETS

TABLE 3 shows the frequencies of the adverse events that occurred in >5% of the subjects in three placebo-controlled North American studies, in which patients in the active treatment arm received 30 mg, 60 mg, 120 mg, or 240 mg of isosorbide mononitrate as isosorbide mononitrate extended release tablets once daily. In parentheses, TABLE 3 shows the frequencies with which these adverse events were associated with the discontinuation of treatment. Overall, 8% of the patients who received 30 mg, 60 mg, 120 mg, or 240 mg of isosorbide mononitrate in the three placebo-controlled North American studies discontinued treatment because of adverse events. Most of these discontinued because of headache. Dizziness was rarely associated with withdrawal from these studies. Since headache appears to be a dose-related adverse effect and tends to disappear with continued treatment, it is recommended that isosorbide mononitrate extended release tablets treatment be initiated at low doses for several days before being increased to desired levels.

TABLE 3 *Frequency and Adverse Events (discontinued)**
Three Controlled North American Studies

Dose	Placebo	30 mg	60 mg	120 mg†	240 mg†
Patients	96	60	102	65	65
Headache	15% (0%)	38% (5%)	51% (8%)	42% (5%)	57% (8%)
Dizziness	4% (0%)	8% (0%)	11% (1%)	9% (2%)	9% (2%)

* Some individuals discontinued for multiple reasons.
† Patients were started on 60 mg and titrated to their final dose.

In addition, the three North American trials were pooled with 11 controlled trials conducted in Europe. Among the 14 controlled trials, a total of 711 patients were randomized to isosorbide mononitrate extended release tablets. When the pooled data were reviewed, headache and dizziness were the only adverse events that were reported by >5% of patients. Other adverse events, each reported by ≤5% of exposed patients, and in many cases of uncertain relation to drug treatment, were:
Autonomic Nervous System Disorders: Dry mouth, hot flushes.
Body as a Whole: Asthenia, back pain, chest pain, edema, fatigue, fever, flu-like symptoms, malaise, rigors.
Cardiovascular Disorders, General: Cardiac failure, hypertension, hypotension.
Central and Peripheral Nervous System Disorders: Dizziness, headache, hypoesthesia, migraine, neuritis, paresis, paresthesia, ptosis, tremor, vertigo.
Gastrointestinal System Disorders: Abdominal pain, constipation, diarrhea, dyspepsia, flatulence, gastric ulcer, gastritis, glossitis, hemorrhagic gastric ulcer, hemorrhoids, loose stools, melena, nausea, vomiting.
Hearing and Vestibular Disorders: Earache, tinnitus, tympanic membrane perforation.
Heart Rate and Rhythm Disorders: Arrhythmia, arrhythmia atrial, atrial fibrillation, bradycardia, bundle branch block, extrasystole, palpitation, tachycardia, ventricular tachycardia.
Liver and Biliary System Disorders: SGOT increase, SGPT increase.
Metabolic and Nutritional Disorders: Hyperuricemia, hypokalemia.
Musculoskeletal Disorders: Arthralgia, frozen shoulder, muscle weakness, musculoskeletal pain, myalgia, myositis, tendon disorder, torticollis.
Myo-, Endo-, Pericardial and Valve Disorders: Angina pectoris aggravated, heart murmur, heart sound abnormal, myocardial infarction, Q-Wave abnormality.
Platelet, Bleeding, and Clotting Disorders: Purpura, thrombocytopenia.
Psychiatric Disorders: Anxiety, concentration impaired, confusion, decreased libido, depression, impotence, insomnia, nervousness, paroniria, somnolence.
Red Blood Cell Disorder: Hypochromic anemia.
Reproductive Disorders, Female: Atrophic vaginitis, breast pain.
Resistance Mechanism Disorders: Bacterial infection, moniliasis, viral infection.
Respiratory System Disorders: Bronchitis, bronchospasm, coughing, dyspnea, increased sputum, nasal congestion, pharyngitis, pneumonia, pulmonary infiltration, rales, rhinitis, sinusitis.
Skin and Appendages Disorders: Acne, hair texture abnormal, increased sweating, pruritus, rash, skin nodule.
Urinary System Disorders: Polyuria, renal calculus, urinary tract infection.
Vascular (Extracardiac) Disorders: Flushing, intermittent claudication, leg ulcer, varicose vein.
Vision Disorders: Conjunctivitis, photophobia, vision abnormal.
In addition, the following spontaneous adverse event has been reported during the marketing of isosorbide mononitrate: Syncope.

DOSAGE AND ADMINISTRATION

IMMEDIATE RELEASE TABLETS

The recommended regimen of isosorbide mononitrate tablets is 20 mg (1 tablet) twice daily, with the 2 doses given 7 hours apart. For most patients, this can be accomplished by taking the first dose on awakening and the second dose 7 hours later. Dosage adjustments are not necessary for elderly patients or patients with altered renal or hepatic function.

As noted in CLINICAL PHARMACOLOGY, multiple studies of organic nitrates have shown that maintenance of continuous 24 hour plasma levels results in refractory tolerance. The dosing regimen for isosorbide mononitrate tablets provides a daily nitrate-free interval to avoid the development of this tolerance.

As also noted in CLINICAL PHARMACOLOGY, well-controlled studies have shown that tolerance to isosorbide mononitrate tablets is avoided when using the twice-daily regimen in which the 2 doses are given 7 hours apart. This regimen has been shown to have antianginal efficacy beginning 1 hour after the first dose and lasting at least 5 hours after the second dose. The duration (if any) of antianginal activity beyond twelve hours has not been studied; large controlled studies with other nitrates suggest that no dosing regimen should be expected to provide more than about twelve hours of continuous antianginal efficacy per day.

In clinical trials, isosorbide mononitrate tablets have been administered in a variety of regimens. Single doses less than 20 mg have not been adequately studied, while single doses greater than 20 mg have demonstrated no greater efficacy than doses of 20 mg.

EXTENDED RELEASE TABLETS

The recommended starting dose of isosorbide mononitrate extended release tablets is 30 mg (given as a single 30 mg tablet or as ½ of a 60 mg tablet) or 60 mg (given as a single tablet) once daily. After several days the dosage may be increased to 120 mg (given as a single 120 mg tablet or as two 60 mg tablets) once daily. Rarely, 240 mg may be required. The daily dose of isosorbide mononitrate extended release tablets should be taken in the morning on arising. Isosorbide mononitrate extended release tablets should not be chewed or crushed and should be swallowed together with a half-glassful of fluid.

HOW SUPPLIED

ISMO TABLETS

Each 20 mg Ismo tablet is orange, round, film-coated and engraved with "ISMO 20" on one side and "W" on the reverse side.
Storage: Store at controlled room temperature between 15-30°C (59-86°F).
Dispense in tight container.

IMDUR EXTENDED RELEASE TABLETS

30 mg: Rose-colored tablets, scored on both sides and branded with the tradename ("IMDUR") on one side and the strength on the other.
60 mg: Yellow-colored tablets, scored on both sides and branded with the tradename ("IMDUR") on one side and the strength on the other, repeated on both sides of the score.
120 mg: White-colored tablets, branded with the tradename ("IMDUR") on one side and the strength on the other.
Storage: Store between 2-30°C (36-86°F).
Protect unit dose from excessive moisture.

PRODUCT LISTING - RATED THERAPEUTICALLY EQUIVALENT

Package	Price	Product	NDC
Tablet - Oral - 10 mg			
100's	$61.10	FEDERAL UPPER LIMIT, H.C.F.A. F F P	99999-3106-01
100's	$81.02	GENERIC, Kremers Urban	62175-0106-01
100's	$98.46	MONOKET, Schwarz Pharma	00091-3610-01
Tablet - Oral - 20 mg			
30's	$28.42	ISMO, Physicians Total Care	54868-3001-03
30's	$39.60	ISMO, Pd-Rx Pharmaceuticals	55289-0580-30
60's	$48.21	MONOKET, Schwarz Pharma	00091-3620-60
60's	$55.66	ISMO, Physicians Total Care	54868-3001-01
100's	$49.50	FEDERAL UPPER LIMIT, H.C.F.A. F F P	99999-3106-02
100's	$72.40	GENERIC, Teva Pharmaceuticals Usa	00093-0076-01
100's	$73.50	GENERIC, West Ward Pharmaceutical Corporation	00143-1333-01
100's	$74.52	GENERIC, Purepac Pharmaceutical Company	00228-2620-11
100's	$81.25	GENERIC, Kremers Urban	62175-0107-01
100's	$91.40	ISMO, Physicians Total Care	54868-3001-04
100's	$108.61	MONOKET, Schwarz Pharma	00091-3620-01
100's	$114.33	ISMO, Wyeth-Ayerst Laboratories	00008-0771-02
100's	$119.43	MONOKET, Schwarz Pharma	00091-3620-11
100's	$142.91	ISMO, Wyeth-Ayerst Laboratories	00008-0771-01
120's	$110.15	ISMO, Physicians Total Care	54868-3001-02
180's	$195.46	MONOKET, Schwarz Pharma	00091-3620-18
Tablet, Extended Release - Oral - 30 mg			
25 x 30	$782.76	GENERIC, Sky Pharmaceuticals Packaging, Inc	63739-0277-03
31 x 10	$409.67	GENERIC, Vangard Labs	00615-4546-53
31 x 10	$409.67	GENERIC, Vangard Labs	00615-4546-63
100's	$111.56	GENERIC, Warrick Pharmaceuticals Corporation	59930-1502-01
100's	$120.16	GENERIC, Kremers Urban	62475-0128-37
100's	$126.06	GENERIC, Caremark Inc	00339-6531-12

100's	$132.15	GENERIC, Kremers Urban	62475-0128-86
100's	$144.81	GENERIC, Purepac Pharmaceutical Company	00228-2713-11
100's	$144.82	GENERIC, Kremers Urban	62175-0128-37
100's	$192.60	IMDUR, Schering Corporation	00085-3306-03
100's	$211.83	IMDUR, Schering Corporation	00085-3306-01
Tablet, Extended Release - Oral - 60 mg			
25 x 30	$824.04	GENERIC, Sky Pharmaceuticals Packaging, Inc	63739-0278-03
30's	$54.43	IMDUR, Physicians Total Care	54868-3245-00
31 x 10	$396.71	GENERIC, Vangard Labs	00615-4544-53
31 x 10	$396.71	GENERIC, Vangard Labs	00615-4544-63
100's	$74.92	FEDERAL UPPER LIMIT, H.C.F.A. F F P	99999-3106-03
100's	$117.40	GENERIC, Warrick Pharmaceuticals Corporation	59930-1549-01
100's	$132.67	GENERIC, Caremark Inc	00339-6532-12
100's	$135.75	GENERIC, Ivax Corporation	00182-2687-89
100's	$152.41	GENERIC, Bristol-Myers Squibb	00228-2711-11
100's	$152.42	GENERIC, Kremers Urban	62175-0119-37
100's	$202.14	IMDUR, Schering Corporation	00085-4110-01
100's	$202.70	IMDUR, Schering Corporation	00085-4110-03
200 x 5	$1279.70	GENERIC, Vangard Labs	00615-4544-43
Tablet, Extended Release - Oral - 120 mg			
100's	$210.74	IMDUR, Schering Corporation	00085-1153-04
100's	$213.38	GENERIC, Kremers Urban	62175-0129-37
100's	$283.75	IMDUR, Schering Corporation	00085-1153-03

PRODUCT LISTING - EQUIVALENTS NOT AVAILABLE

Tablet - Oral - 10 mg			
60's	$30.00	MONOKET, Schwarz Pharma	00091-3610-60
100's	$55.00	MONOKET, Schwarz Pharma	00091-3610-11
180's	$90.00	MONOKET, Schwarz Pharma	00091-3610-18
Tablet - Oral - 20 mg			
30's	$18.86	GENERIC, Allscripts Pharmaceutical Company	54569-4444-00
100's	$53.36	GENERIC, Physicians Total Care	54868-3822-01
Tablet, Extended Release - Oral - 30 mg			
100's	$129.13	GENERIC, Ethex Corporation	58177-0222-04
100's	$132.85	GENERIC, Ethex Corporation	58177-0222-11
Tablet, Extended Release - Oral - 60 mg			
100's	$135.90	GENERIC, Ethex Corporation	58177-0238-04
100's	$136.25	GENERIC, Ethex Corporation	58177-0238-11
Tablet, Extended Release - Oral - 120 mg			
100's	$195.70	GENERIC, Ethex Corporation	58177-0201-04

I

Isotretinoin *(001595)*

Categories: Acne, nodular; Pregnancy Category X; FDA Approved 1982 May
Drug Classes: Retinoids
Brand Names: Accutane
Foreign Brand Availability: Accure (Australia); Accutane Roche (Canada); Akinol (Korea); Curacne Ge (France); Curatane (Israel); Isotren (Korea); Isotrex (Australia; Benin; Burkina-Faso; England; Ethiopia; Gambia; Ghana; Guinea; Ivory-Coast; Kenya; Korea; Liberia; Malawi; Mali; Mauritania; Mauritius; Morocco; Niger; Nigeria; Senegal; Seychelles; Sierra-Leone; South-Africa; Sudan; Taiwan; Tanzania; Tunia; Uganda; Zambia; Zimbabwe); Isotrex Gel (Colombia; France; Germany; Hong-Kong; Israel; Malaysia; Mexico; New-Zealand; Philippines; Spain; Thailand); Nimegen (Singapore); Oratane (Australia; Hong-Kong; New-Zealand; Singapore); Pinple (Korea); Procuta Ge (France); Roaccutan (Mexico); Roaccutane (Australia; Bahamas; Bahrain; Barbados; Belgium; Belize; Bermuda; Bulgaria; China; Costa-Rica; Curacao; Cyprus; Czech-Republic; Dominican-Republic; Egypt; El-Salvador; England; France; Ghana; Greece; Guatemala; Guyana; Honduras; Hong-Kong; Iran; Iraq; Ireland; Israel; Jamaica; Jordan; Kenya; Korea; Kuwait; Lebanon; Libya; Malaysia; Netherland-Antilles; Netherlands; New-Zealand; Nicaragua; Oman; Panama; Philippines; Qatar; Republic-of-Yemen; Saudi-Arabia; South-Africa; Surinam; Switzerland; Syria; Taiwan; Tanzania; Thailand; Trinidad; Uganda; United-Arab-Emirates; Zambia); Roaccutan (Austria; Colombia; Denmark; Finland; Germany; Italy; Portugal); Roaccuttan (Colombia); Roacutan (Spain); Roacuttan (Hungary)
Cost of Therapy: $1948.19 (Acne vulgaris; Accutane; 20 mg; 2 capsules/day; 105 day supply)
$1488.04 (Acne vulgaris; Generic Capsules; 20 mg; 2 capsules/day; 105 day supply)

WARNING

Note: The trade name has been used throughout this monograph for clarity.

CAUSES BIRTH DEFECTS.

DO NOT GET PREGNANT.

Accutane must not be used by females who are pregnant. Although not every fetus exposed to Accutane has resulted in a deformed child, there is an extremely high risk that a deformed infant can result if pregnancy occurs while taking Accutane in any amount even for short periods of time. Potentially any fetus exposed during pregnancy can be affected. Presently, there are no accurate means of determining, after Accutane exposure, which fetus has been affected and which fetus has not been affected.

Major human fetal abnormalities related to Accutane administration in females have been documented. There is an increased risk of spontaneous abortion. In addition, premature births have been reported.

Documented external abnormalities include: skull abnormality; ear abnormalities (including anotia, micropinna, small or absent external auditory canals); eye abnormalities (including microphthalmia), facial dysmorphia; cleft palate. Documented internal abnormalities include: CNS abnormalities (including cerebral abnormalities, cerebellar malformation, hydrocephalus, microcephaly, cranial nerve deficit); cardiovascular abnormalities; thymus gland abnormality; parathyroid hormone deficiency. In some cases death has occurred with certain of the abnormalities previously noted.

Cases of IQ scores less than 85 with or without obvious CNS abnormalities have also been reported.

WARNING — *Cont'd*

Accutane is contraindicated in females of childbearing potential unless the patient meets all of the following conditions:

- **Must NOT be pregnant or breast feeding.**
- **Must be capable of complying with the mandatory contraceptive measures required for Accutane therapy and understand behaviors associated with an increased risk of pregnancy.**
- **Must be reliable in understanding and carrying out instructions.**

Accutane must be prescribed under the *System to Manage Accutane Related Teratogenicity* (S.M.A.R.T.).

To prescribe Accutane, the prescriber must obtain a supply of yellow self-adhesive Accutane Qualification Stickers. To obtain these stickers:

1. **Read the booklet entitled *System to Manage Accutane Related Teratogenicity* (S.M.A.R.T.) *Guide to Best Practices.***
2. **Sign and return the completed S.M.A.R.T. *Letter of Understanding* containing the following Prescriber Checklist:**
   - **I know the risk and severity of fetal injury/birth defects from Accutane.**
   - **I know how to diagnose and treat the various presentations of acne.**
   - **I know the risk factors for unplanned pregnancy and the effective measures for avoidance of unplanned pregnancy.**
   - **It is the informed patient's responsibility to avoid pregnancy during Accutane therapy and for 1 month after stopping Accutane. To help patients have the knowledge and tools to do so: Before beginning treatment of female patients with Accutane I will refer for expert, detailed pregnancy prevention counseling and prescribing, reimbursed by the manufacturer, OR I have the expertise to perform this function and elect to do so.**
   - **I understand, and will properly use throughout the Accutane treatment course, the S.M.A.R.T. procedures for Accutane, including monthly pregnancy avoidance counseling, pregnancy testing and use of the yellow self-adhesive Accutane Qualification Stickers.**
3. **To use the yellow self-adhesive Accutane Qualification Sticker Accutane should not be prescribed or dispensed to any patient (male or female) without a yellow self-adhesive Accutane Qualification Sticker.**

For female patients, the yellow self-adhesive Accutane Qualification Sticker signifies that she:

- **Must have had 2 negative urine or serum pregnancy tests with a sensitivity of at least 25 mIU/ml before receiving the initial Accutane prescription. The first test (a screening test) is obtained by the prescriber when the decision is made to pursue qualification of the patient for Accutane. The second pregnancy test, (a confirmation test) should be done during the first 5 days of the menstrual period immediately preceding the beginning of Accutane therapy. For patients with amenorrhea, the second test should be done at least 11 days after the last act of unprotected sexual intercourse (without using 2 effective forms of contraception). Each month of therapy, the patient must have a negative result from a urine or serum pregnancy test. A pregnancy test must be repeated every month prior to the female patient receiving each prescription. The manufacturer will make available urine pregnancy test kits for female Accutane patients for the initial, second and monthly testing during therapy.**
- **Must have selected and have committed to use 2 forms of effective contraception simultaneously, at least 1 of which must be a primary form, unless absolute abstinence is the chosen method, or the patient has undergone a hysterectomy. Patients must use 2 forms of effective contraception for at least 1 month prior to initiation of Accutane therapy, during Accutane therapy, and for 1 month after discontinuing Accutane therapy. Counseling about contraception and behaviors associated with an increased risk of pregnancy must be repeated on a monthly basis.**

Effective forms of contraception include both primary and secondary forms of contraception. Primary forms of contraception include: tubal ligation, partner's vasectomy, intrauterine devices, birth control pills, and injectable/implantable/insertable hormonal birth control products. Secondary forms of contraception include diaphragms, latex condoms, and cervical caps; each must be used with a spermicide.

Any birth control method can fail. Therefore, it is critically important that women of childbearing potential use 2 effective forms of contraception simultaneously. A drug interaction that decreases effectiveness of hormonal contraceptives has not been entirely ruled out for Accutane. Although hormonal contraceptives are highly effective, there have been reports of pregnancy from women who have used oral contraceptives, as well as injectable/implantable contraceptive products. These reports occurred while these patients were taking Accutane. These reports are more frequent for women who use only a single method of contraception. Patients must receive written warnings about the rates of possible contraception failure (included in patient education kits).

Prescribers are advised to consult the package insert of any medication administered concomitantly with hormonal contraceptives, since some medications may decrease the effectiveness of these birth control products. Patients should be prospectively cautioned not to self-medicate with the herbal supplement St. John's Wort because a possible interaction has been suggested with hormonal contraceptives based on reports of breakthrough bleeding on oral contraceptives shortly after starting St. John's Wort. Pregnancies have been reported by users of combined hormonal contraceptives who also used some form of St. John's Wort (see PRECAUTIONS).

- **Must have signed a Patient Information/Consent form that contains warnings about the risk of potential birth defects if the fetus is exposed to isotretinoin.**
- **Must have been informed of the purpose and importance of participating in the Accutane Survey and has been given the opportunity to enroll (see PRECAUTIONS).**

The yellow self-adhesive Accutane Qualification Sticker documents that the female patient is qualified, and includes the date of qualification, patient gender, cut-off date for filling the prescription, and up to a 30 day supply limit with no refills.

These yellow self-adhesive Accutane Qualification Stickers should also be used for male patients. See TABLE 1.

If a pregnancy does occur during treatment of a woman with Accutane, the prescriber and patient should discuss the desirability of continuing the pregnancy. Prescribers are strongly encouraged to report all cases of pregnancy to Roche 1-800-526-6367 where a Roche Pregnancy Prevention Program

WARNING — Cont'd

Specialist will be available to discuss Roche pregnancy information, or prescribers may contact the Food and Drug Administration MedWatch Program 1-800-FDA-1088.

Accutane should be prescribed only by prescribers who have demonstrated special competence in the diagnosis and treatment of severe recalcitrant nodular acne, are experienced in the use of systemic retinoids, have read the S.M.A.R.T. *Guide to Best Practices,* signed and returned the *completed* S.M.A.R.T. *Letter of Understanding,* and obtained yelow self-adhesive Accutane Qualification Stickers. Accutane should not be prescribed or dispensed without a yellow self-adhesive Accutane Qualification Sticker.

INFORMATION FOR PHARMACISTS:

ACCUTANE MUST ONLY BE DISPENSED:

- **IN NO MORE THAN A 30 DAY SUPPLY.**
- **ONLY ON PRESENTATION OF AN ACCUTANE PRESCRIPTION WITH A YELLOW SELF-ADHESIVE ACCUTANE QUALIFICATION STICKER.**
- **WRITTEN WITHIN THE PREVIOUS 7 DAYS.**
- **REFILLS REQUIRE A NEW PRESCRIPTION WITH A YELLOW SELF-ADHESIVE ACCUTANE QUALIFICATION STICKER.**
- **NO TELEPHONE OR COMPUTERIZED PRESCRIPTIONS ARE PERMITTED.**

AN ACCUTANE MEDICATION GUIDE MUST BE GIVEN TO THE PATIENT EACH TIME ACCUTANE IS DISPENSED, AS REQUIRED BY LAW. THIS ACCUTANE MEDICATION GUIDE IS AN IMPORTANT PART OF THE RISK MANAGEMENT PROGRAM FOR THE PATIENT.

TABLE 1 *Use of Pregnancy Tests and Accutane Qualification Stickers for Patients*

Pregnancy Test Required	Qualification Date	Accutane Qualification Sticker Necessary	Dispense Within 7 Days of Qualification Date
All Males:			
No	Date prescription written	Yes	Yes
Females of Childbearing Potential:			
Yes	Date of confirmatory negative pregnancy test	Yes	Yes
Females* Not of Childbearing Potential:			
No	Date prescription written	Yes	Yes

* Females who have had a hysterectomy or who are postmenopausal are not considered to be of childbearing potential.

DESCRIPTION

Isotretinoin, a retinoid, is available as Accutane in 10, 20, and 40 mg soft gelatin capsules for oral administration. Each capsule contains beeswax, butylated hydroxyanisole, edetate disodium, hydrogenated soybean oil flakes, hydrogenated vegetable oil, and soybean oil. Gelatin capsules contain glycerin and parabens (methyl and propyl), with the following dye systems: *10 mg:* Iron oxide (red) and titanium dioxide; *20 mg:* FD&C red no. 3, FD&C blue no. 1, and titanium dioxide; *40 mg:* FD&C yellow no. 6, D&C yellow no. 10, and titanium dioxide.

Chemically, isotretinoin is 13-*cis*-retinoic acid and is related to both retinoic acid and retinol (vitamin A). It is a yellow to orange crystalline powder with a molecular weight of 300.44.

CLINICAL PHARMACOLOGY

Isotretinoin is a retinoid, which when administered in pharmacologic dosages of 0.5-1.0 mg/kg/day (see DOSAGE AND ADMINISTRATION), inhibits sebaceous gland function and keratinization. The exact mechanism of action of isotretinoin is unknown.

NODULAR ACNE

Clinical improvement in nodular acne patients occurs in association with a reduction in sebum secretion. The decrease in sebum secretion is temporary and is related to the dose and duration of treatment with Accutane, and reflects a reduction in sebaceous gland size and an inhibition of sebaceous gland differentiation.[1]

PHARMACOKINETICS

Absorption

Due to its high lipophilicity, oral absorption of isotretinoin is enhanced when given with a high-fat meal. In a crossover study, 74 healthy adult subjects received a single 80 mg oral dose (2 × 40 mg capsules) of Accutane under fasted and fed conditions. Both peak plasma concentration (C_{max}) and the total exposure (AUC) of isotretinoin were more than doubled following a standardized high-fat meal when compared with Accutane given under fasted conditions (see TABLE 2). The observed elimination half-life was unchanged. This lack of change in half-life suggests that food increases the bioavailability of isotretinoin without altering its disposition. The time to peak concentration (T_{max}) was also increased with food and may be related to a longer absorption phase. Therefore, Accutane capsules should always be taken with food (see DOSAGE AND ADMINISTRATION). Clinical studies have shown that there is no difference in the pharmacokinetics of isotretinoin between patients with nodular acne and healthy subjects with normal skin.

Distribution

Isotretinoin is more than 99.9% bound to plasma proteins, primarily albumin.

Metabolism

Following oral administration of isotretinoin, at least three metabolites have been identified in human plasma: 4-*oxo*-isotretinoin, retinoic acid (tretinoin), and 4-*oxo*-retinoic acid (4-*oxo*-tretinoin). Retinoic acid and 13-*cis*-retinoic acid are geometric isomers and show reversible interconversion. The administration of one isomer will give rise to the other. Isotretinoin is also irreversibly oxidized to 4-*oxo*-isotretinoin, which forms its geometric isomer 4-*oxo*-tretinoin.

TABLE 2 *Pharmacokinetic Parameters of Isotretinoin — Mean (%CV)*

	Accutane 2 × 40 mg Capsules (n=74)	
	Fed*	Fasted
AUC(0-∞) (ng·h/ml)	10,004 (22%)	3,703 (46%)
C_{max} (ng/ml)	862 (22%)	301 (63%)
T_{max} (h)	5.3 (77%)	3.2 (56%)
$T_{½}$ (h)	21 (39%)	21 (30%)

* Eating a standardized high-fat meal.

After a single 80 mg oral dose of Accutane to 74 healthy adult subjects, concurrent administration of food increased the extent of formation of all metabolites in plasma when compared to the extent of formation under fasted conditions.

All of these metabolites possess retinoid activity that is in some *in vitro* models more than that of the parent isotretinoin. However, the clinical significance of these models is unknown. After multiple oral dose administration of isotretinoin to adult cystic acne patients (≥18 years), the exposure of patients to 4-*oxo*-isotretinoin at steady-state under fasted and fed conditions was approximately 3.4 times higher than that of isotretinoin.

In vitro studies indicate that the primary P450 isoforms involved in isotretinoin metabolism are 2C8, 2C9, 3A4, and 2B6. Isotretinoin and its metabolites are further metabolized into conjugates, which are then excreted in urine and feces.

Elimination

Following oral administration of an 80 mg dose of ^{14}C-isotretinoin as a liquid suspension, ^{14}C-activity in blood declined with a half-life of 90 hours. The metabolites of isotretinoin and any conjugates are ultimately excreted in the feces and urine in relatively equal amounts (total of 65% to 83%). After a single 80 mg oral dose of Accutane to 74 healthy adult subjects under fed conditions, the mean ±SD elimination half-lives ($T_{½}$) of isotretinoin and 4-*oxo*-isotretinoin were 21.0 ± 8.2 hours and 24.0 ± 5.3 hours, respectively. After both single and multiple doses, the observed accumulation ratios of isotretinoin ranged from 0.90-5.43 in patients with cystic acne.

SPECIAL PATIENT POPULATIONS

Pediatric Patients

The pharmacokinetics of isotretinoin were evaluated after single and multiple doses in 38 pediatric patients (12-15 years) and 19 adult patients (≥18 years) who received Accutane for the treatment of severe recalcitrant nodular acne. In both age groups, 4-*oxo*-isotretinoin was the major metabolite; tretinoin and 4-*oxo*-tretinoin were also observed. The dose-normalized pharmacokinetic parameters for isotretinoin following single and multiple doses are summarized in TABLE 3 for pediatric patients. There were no statistically significant differences in the pharmacokinetics of isotretinoin between pediatric and adult patients.

TABLE 3 *Pharmacokinetic Parameters of Isotretinoin Following Single and Multiple Dose Administration in Pediatric Patients, 12-15 Years of Age — Mean (±SD), n=38**

Parameter	Isotretinoin (Single Dose)	Isotretinoin (Steady-State)
C_{max} (ng/ml)	573.25 (278.79)	731.98 (361.86)
AUC(0-12) (ng·h/ml)	3033.37 (1394.17)	5082.00 (2184.23)
AUC(0-24) (ng·h/ml)	6003.81 (2885.67)	—
T_{max} (h)†	6.00 (1.00-24.60)	4.00 (0-12.00)
Css_{min} (ng/ml)	—	352.32 (184.44)
$T_{½}$ (h)	—	15.69 (5.12)
CL/F (L/h)	—	17.96 (6.27)

* The single and multiple dose data in this table were obtained following a non-standardized meal that is not comparable to the high-fat meal that was used in the study in TABLE 2.
† Median (range).

In pediatric patients (12-15 years), the mean ±SD elimination half-lives ($T_{½}$) of isotretinoin and 4-*oxo*-isotretinoin were 15.7 ± 5.1 hours and 23.1 ± 5.7 hours, respectively. The accumulation ratios of isotretinoin ranged from 0.46-3.65 for pediatric patients.

INDICATIONS AND USAGE

SEVERE RECALCITRANT NODULAR ACNE

Accutane is indicated for the treatment of severe recalcitrant nodular acne. Nodules are inflammatory lesions with a diameter of 5 mm or greater. The nodules may become suppurative or hemorrhagic. "Severe," by definition,[2] means "many" as opposed to "few or several" nodules. Because of significant adverse effects associated with its use, Accutane should be reserved for patients with severe nodular acne who are unresponsive to conventional therapy, including systemic antibiotics. In addition, Accutane is indicated only for those females who are not pregnant, because Accutane can cause severe birth defects (see BOXED WARNING).

A single course of therapy for 15-20 weeks has been shown to result in complete and prolonged remission of disease in many patients.[1,3,4] If a second course of therapy is needed, it should not be initiated until at least 8 weeks after completion of the first course, because experience has shown that patients may continue to improve while off Accutane. The optimal interval before retreatment has not been defined for patients who have not completed skeletal growth (see WARNINGS, Skeletal: Bone Mineral Density, Hyperostosis, and Premature Epiphyseal Closure).

CONTRAINDICATIONS

PREGNANCY CATEGORY X

See BOXED WARNING.

ALLERGIC REACTIONS

Accutane is contraindicated in patients who are hypersensitive to this medication or to any of its components. Accutane should not be given to patients who are sensitive to parabens, which are used as preservatives in the gelatin capsule (see PRECAUTIONS, Hypersensitivity).

WARNINGS

PSYCHIATRIC DISORDERS

Accutane may cause depression, psychosis and, rarely, suicidal ideation, suicide attempts, suicide, and aggressive and/or violent behaviors. Discontinuation of Accutane therapy may be insufficient; further evaluation may be necessary. No mechanism of action has been established for these events (see ADVERSE REACTIONS, Dose Relationship, Psychiatric). Prescribers should read the brochure, *Recognizing Psychiatric Disorders in Adolescents and Young Adults: A Guide for Prescribers of Accutane (isotretinoin).*

PSEUDOTUMOR CEREBRI

Accutane use has been associated with a number of cases of pseudotumor cerebri (benign intracranial hypertension), some of which involved concomitant use of tetracyclines. Concomitant treatment with tetracyclines should therefore be avoided. Early signs and symptoms of pseudotumor cerebri include papilledema, headache, nausea and vomiting, and visual disturbances. Patients with these symptoms should be screened for papilledema and, if present, they should be told to discontinue Accutane immediately and be referred to a neurologist for further diagnosis and care (see ADVERSE REACTIONS, Dose Relationship, Neurological).

I

PANCREATITIS

Acute pancreatitis has been reported in patients with either elevated or normal serum triglyceride levels. **In rare instances, fatal hemorrhagic pancreatitis has been reported.** Accutane should be stopped if hypertriglyceridemia cannot be controlled at an acceptable level or if symptoms of pancreatitis occur.

LIPIDS

Elevations of serum triglycerides have been reported in patients treated with Accutane. Marked elevations of serum triglycerides in excess of 800 mg/dl were reported in approximately 25% of patients receiving Accutane in clinical trials. In addition, approximately 15% developed a decrease in high-density lipoproteins and about 7% showed an increase in cholesterol levels. In clinical trials, the effects on triglycerides, HDL, and cholesterol were reversible upon cessation of Accutane therapy. Some patients have been able to reverse triglyceride elevation by reduction in weight, restriction of dietary fat and alcohol, and reduction in dose while continuing Accutane.[5]

Blood lipid determinations should be performed before Accutane is given and then at intervals until the lipid response to Accutane is established, which usually occurs within 4 weeks. Especially careful consideration must be given to risk/benefit for patients who may be at high risk during Accutane therapy (patients with diabetes, obesity, increased alcohol intake, lipid metabolism disorder or familial history of lipid metabolism disorder). If Accutane therapy is instituted, more frequent checks of serum values for lipids and/or blood sugar are recommended (see PRECAUTIONS, Laboratory Tests).

The cardiovascular consequences of hypertriglyceridemia associated with Accutane are unknown.

ANIMAL STUDIES

In rats given 8 or 32 mg/kg/day of isotretinoin (1.3-5.3 times the recommended clinical dose of 1.0 mg/kg/day after normalization for total body surface area) for 18 months or longer, the incidences of focal calcification, fibrosis and inflammation of the myocardium, calcification of coronary, pulmonary and mesenteric arteries, and metastatic calcification of the gastric mucosa were greater than in control rats of similar age. Focal endocardial and myocardial calcifications associated with calcification of the coronary arteries were observed in 2 dogs after approximately 6-7 months of treatment with isotretinoin at a dosage of 60-120 mg/kg/day (30-60 times the recommended clinical dose of 1.0 mg/kg/day, respectively, after normalization for total body surface area).

HEARING IMPAIRMENT

Impaired hearing has been reported in patients taking Accutane; in some cases, the hearing impairment has been reported to persist after therapy has been discontinued. Mechanism(s) and causality for this event have not been established. Patients who experience tinnitus or hearing impairment should discontinue Accutane treatment and be referred for specialized care for further evaluation (see ADVERSE REACTIONS, Dose Relationship, Special Senses).

HEPATOTOXICITY

Clinical hepatitis considered to be possibly or probably related to Accutane therapy has been reported. Additionally, mild to moderate elevations of liver enzymes have been observed in approximately 15% of individuals treated during clinical trials, some of which normalized with dosage reduction or continued administration of the drug. If normalization does not readily occur or if hepatitis is suspected during treatment with Accutane, the drug should be discontinued and the etiology further investigated.

INFLAMMATORY BOWEL DISEASE

Accutane has been associated with inflammatory bowel disease (including regional ileitis) in patients without a prior history of intestinal disorders. In some instances, symptoms have been reported to persist after Accutane treatment has been stopped. Patients experiencing abdominal pain, rectal bleeding or severe diarrhea should discontinue Accutane immediately (see ADVERSE REACTIONS, Dose Relationship, Gastrointestinal).

SKELETAL

Bone Mineral Density

Effects of multiple courses of Accutane on the developing musculoskeletal system are unknown. There is some evidence that long-term, high-dose, or multiple courses of therapy with isotretinoin have more of an effect than a single course of therapy on the musculoskeletal system. In an open-label clinical trial (n=217) of a single course of therapy with Accutane for severe recalcitrant nodular acne, bone density measurements at several skeletal sites were not significantly decreased (lumbar spine change >-4% and total hip change >-5%) or were increased in the majority of patients. One patient had a decrease in lumbar spine bone mineral density >4% based on unadjusted data. Sixteen (7.9%) patients had decreases in lumbar spine bone mineral density >4%, and all the other patients (92%) did not have significant decreases or had increases (adjusted for body mass index). Nine patients (4.5%) had a decrease in total hip bone mineral density >5% based on unadjusted data. Twenty-one (10.6%) patients had decreases in total hip bone mineral density >5%, and all the other patients (89%) did not have significant decreases or had increases (adjusted for body mass index). Follow-up studies performed in 8 of the patients with decreased bone mineral density for up to 11 months thereafter demonstrated increasing bone density in 5 patients at the lumbar spine, while the other 3 patients had lumbar spine bone density measurements below baseline values. Total hip bone mineral densities remained below baseline (range -1.6% to -7.6%) in 5 of 8 patients (62.5%).

In a separate open-label extension study of 10 patients, ages 13-18 years, who started a second course of Accutane 4 months after the first course, 2 patients showed a decrease in mean lumbar spine bone mineral density up to 3.25% (adjusted for body mass index).

Spontaneous reports of osteoporosis, osteopenia, bone fractures, and delayed healing of bone fractures have been seen in the Accutane population. While causality to Accutane has not been established, an effect cannot be ruled out. Longer term effects have not been studied. It is important that Accutane be given at the recommended doses for no longer than the recommended duration.

Hyperostosis

A high prevalence of skeletal hyperostosis was noted in clinical trials for disorders of keratinization with a mean dose of 2.24 mg/kg/day. Additionally, skeletal hyperostosis was noted in 6 of 8 patients in a prospective study of disorders of keratinization.[6] Minimal skeletal hyperostosis and calcification of ligaments and tendons have also been observed by x-ray in prospective studies of nodular acne patients treated with a single course of therapy at recommended doses. The skeletal effects of multiple Accutane treatment courses for acne are unknown.

In a clinical study of 217 pediatric patients (12-17 years) with severe recalcitrant nodular acne, hyperostosis was not observed after 16-20 weeks of treatment with approximately 1 mg/kg/day of Accutane given in 2 divided doses. Hyperostosis may require a longer time frame to appear. The clinical course and significance remain unknown.

Premature Epiphyseal Closure

There are spontaneous reports of premature epiphyseal closure in acne patients receiving recommended doses of Accutane. The effect of multiple courses of Accutane on epiphyseal closure is unknown.

VISION IMPAIRMENT

Visual problems should be carefully monitored. All Accutane patients experiencing visual difficulties should discontinue Accutane treatment and have an ophthalmological examination (see ADVERSE REACTIONS, Dose Relationship, Special Senses).

Corneal Opacities

Corneal opacities have occurred in patients receiving Accutane for acne and more frequently when higher drug dosages were used in patients with disorders of keratinization. The corneal opacities that have been observed in clinical trial patients treated with Accutane have either completely resolved or were resolving at follow-up 6-7 weeks after discontinuation of the drug (see ADVERSE REACTIONS, Dose Relationship, Special Senses).

Decreased Night Vision

Decreased night vision has been reported during Accutane therapy and in some instances the event has persisted after therapy was discontinued. Because the onset in some patients was sudden, patients should be advised of this potential problem and warned to be cautious when driving or operating any vehicle at night.

PRECAUTIONS

The Accutane Pregnancy Prevention and Risk Management Programs consist of the *System to Manage Accutane Related Teratogenicity* (S.M.A.R.T.) and the Accutane Pregnancy Prevention Program (PPP). S.M.A.R.T. should be followed for prescribing Accutane with the goal of preventing fetal exposure to isotretinoin. It consists of (1) reading the booklet entitled *System to Manage Accutane Related Teratogenicity* (S.M.A.R.T.) *Guide to Best Practices,* (2) signing and returning the completed S.M.A.R.T. *Letter of Understanding* containing the Prescriber Checklist, (3) a yellow self-adhesive Accutane Qualification Sticker to be affixed to the prescription page. In addition, the patient educational material, *Be Smart, Be Safe, Be Sure,* should be used with each patient.

The following further describes each component:

The S.M.A.R.T. *Guide to Best Practices* includes: Accutane teratogenic potential, information on pregnancy testing, specific information about effective contraception, the limitations of contraceptive methods and behaviors associated with an increased risk of contraceptive failure and pregnancy, the methods to evaluate pregnancy risk, and the method to complete a qualified Accutane prescription.

The S.M.A.R.T. *Letter of Understanding* attests that Accutane prescribers understand that Accutane is a teratogen, have read the S.M.A.R.T. *Guide to Best Practices,* understand their responsibilities in preventing exposure of pregnant females to Accutane and the procedures for qualifying female patients as defined in the BOXED WARNING.

The Prescriber Checklist attests that Accutane prescribers know the risk and severity of injury/birth defects from Accutane; know how to diagnose and treat the various presentations of acne; know the risk factors for unplanned pregnancy and the effective measures for avoidance; will refer the patient for, or provide, detailed pregnancy prevention counseling to help the patient have knowledge and tools needed to fulfill their ultimate responsibility to avoid becoming pregnant; understand and properly use throughout the Accutane treatment course, the revised risk management procedures, including monthly pregnancy avoidance counseling, pregnancy testing, and use of qualified prescriptions with the yellow self-adhesive Accutane Qualification Sticker.

The yellow self-adhesive Accutane Qualification Sticker is used as documentation that the prescriber has qualified the female patient according to the qualification criteria (see BOXED WARNING).

Accutane Pregnancy Prevention Program (PPP) is a systematic approach to comprehensive patient education about their responsibilities and includes education for contraception compliance and reinforcement of educational messages. The PPP includes information on the risks and benefits of Accutane which is linked to the Accutane Medication Guide dispensed by pharmacists with each prescription.

Male and female patients are provided with separate booklets. Each booklet contains information on Accutane therapy, including precautions and warnings, an Informed Consent/Patient Agreement form, and a toll-free line which provides Accutane information in 13 languages.

The booklet for male patients, *Be Smart, Be Safe, Be Sure, Accutane Risk Management Program for Men,* also includes information about male reproduction, a warning not to share Accutane with others or to donate blood during Accutane therapy and for 1 month following discontinuation of Accutane.

The booklet for female patients, *Be Smart, Be Safe, Be Sure, Accutane Pregnancy Prevention and Risk Management Program for Women,* also includes a referral program that offers females free contraception counseling, reimbursed by the manufacturer, by a reproductive specialist; a second Patient Information/Consent form concerning birth defects, obtaining her consent to be treated within this agreement; an enrollment form for the Accutane Survey; and a qualification checklist affirming the conditions under which female patients may receive Accutane. In addition, there is information on the types of contraceptive methods, the selection and use of appropriate, effective contraception, and the rates of possible contraceptive failure; a toll-free contraception counseling line; and a video about the most common reasons for unplanned pregnancies.

GENERAL

Although an effect of Accutane on bone loss is not established, physicians should use caution when prescribing Accutane to patients with a genetic predisposition for age-related osteoporosis, a history of childhood osteoporosis conditions, osteomalacia, or other disorders of bone metabolism. This would include patients diagnosed with anorexia nervosa and those who are on chronic drug therapy that causes drug-induced osteoporosis/osteomalacia and/or affects vitamin D metabolism, such as systemic corticosteroids and any anticonvulsant.

Patients may be at increased risk when participating in sports with repetitive impact where the risks of spondylolisthesis with and without pars fractures and hip growth plate injuries in early and late adolescence are known. There are spontaneous reports of fractures and/or delayed healing in patients while on treatment with Accutane or following cessation of treatment with Accutane while involved in these activities. While causality to Accutane has not been established, an effect cannot be ruled out.

INFORMATION FOR PATIENTS AND PRESCRIBERS

Patients should be instructed to read the Medication Guide supplied as required by law when Accutane is dispensed. For additional information, patients should also read the *Patient Product Information, Important Information Concerning Your Treatment with Accutane (isotretinoin).* All patients should sign the Informed Consent/Patient Agreement.

Females of childbearing potential should be instructed that they must not be pregnant when Accutane therapy is initiated, and that they should use 2 forms of effective contraception 1 month before starting Accutane, while taking Accutane, and for 1 month after Accutane has been stopped. They should also sign a consent form prior to beginning Accutane therapy. They should be given an opportunity to enroll in the Accutane Survey and to review the patient videotape provided by the manufacturer to the prescriber. It includes information about contraception, the most common reasons that contraception fails, and the importance of using 2 forms of effective contraception when taking teratogenic drugs. Female patients should be seen by their prescribers monthly and have a urine or serum pregnancy test performed each month during treatment to confirm negative pregnancy status before another Accutane prescription is written (see BOXED WARNING).

Accutane is found in the semen of male patients taking Accutane, but the amount delivered to a female partner would be about 1 million times lower than an oral dose of 40 mg. While the no-effect limit for isotretinoin-induced embryopathy is unknown, 20 years of postmarketing reports include 4 with isolated defects compatible with features of retinoid exposed fetuses. None of these cases had the combination of malformations characteristic of retinoid exposure, and all had other possible explanations for the defects observed.

Patients may report mental health problems or family history of psychiatric disorders. These reports should be discussed with the patient and/or the patient's family. A referral to a mental health professional may be necessary. The physician should consider whether or not Accutane therapy is appropriate in this setting (see WARNINGS, Psychiatric Disorders).

Patients should be informed that they must not share Accutane with anyone else because of the risk of birth defects and other serious adverse events.

Patients should not donate blood during therapy and for 1 month following discontinuance of the drug because the blood might be given to a pregnant woman whose fetus must not be exposed to Accutane.

Patients should be reminded to take Accutane with a meal (see DOSAGE AND ADMINISTRATION). To decrease the risk of esophageal irritation, patients should swallow the capsules with a full glass of liquid.

Patients should be informed that transient exacerbation (flare) of acne has been seen, generally during the initial period of therapy.

Wax epilation and skin resurfacing procedures (such as dermabrasion, laser) should be avoided during Accutane therapy and for at least 6 months thereafter due to the possibility of scarring (see ADVERSE REACTIONS, Dose Relationship, Skin and Appendages).

Patients should be advised to avoid prolonged exposure to UV rays or sunlight.

Patients should be informed that they may experience decreased tolerance to contact lenses during and after therapy.

Patients should be informed that approximately 16% of patients treated with Accutane in a clinical trial developed musculoskeletal symptoms (including arthralgia) during treatment. In general, these symptoms were mild to moderate, but occasionally required discontinuation of the drug. Transient pain in the chest has been reported less frequently. In the clinical trial, these symptoms generally cleared rapidly after discontinuation of Accutane, but in some cases persisted (see ADVERSE REACTIONS, Dose Relationship, Musculoskeletal). There have been rare postmarketing reports of rhabdomyolysis, some associated with strenuous physical activity (see Laboratory Tests, Pregnancy Test, CPK).

Pediatric patients and their caregivers should be informed that approximately 29% (104/358) of pediatric patients treated with Accutane developed back pain. Back pain was severe in 13.5% (14/104) of the cases and occurred at a higher frequency in female than male patients. Arthralgias were experienced in 22% (79/358) of pediatric patients. Arthralgias were severe in 7.6% (6/79) of patients. Appropriate evaluation of the musculoskeletal system should be done in patients who present with these symptoms during or after a course of Accutane. Consideration should be given to discontinuation of Accutane if any significant abnormality is found.

Neutropenia and rare cases of agranulocytosis have been reported. Accutane should be discontinued if clinically significant decreases in white cell counts occur.

HYPERSENSITIVITY

Anaphylactic reactions and other allergic reactions have been reported. Cutaneous allergic reactions and serious cases of allergic vasculitis, often with purpura (bruises and red patches) of the extremities and extracutaneous involvement (including renal) have been reported. Severe allergic reaction necessitates discontinuation of therapy and appropriate medical management.

LABORATORY TESTS

Pregnancy Test

Female patients of childbearing potential must have negative results from 2 urine or serum pregnancy tests with a sensitivity of at least 25 mIU/ml before receiving the initial Accutane prescription. The first test is obtained by the prescriber when the decision is made to pursue qualification of the patient for Accutane (a screening test). The second pregnancy test (a confirmation test) should be done during the first 5 days of the menstrual period immediately preceding the beginning of Accutane therapy. For patients with amenorrhea, the second test should be done at least 11 days after the last act of unprotected sexual intercourse (without using 2 effective forms of contraception).

Each month of therapy, the patient must have a negative result from a urine or serum pregnancy test. A pregnancy test must be repeated each month prior to the female patient receiving each prescription.

Lipids: Pretreatment and follow-up blood lipids should be obtained under fasting conditions. After consumption of alcohol, at least 36 hours should elapse before these determinations are made. It is recommended that these tests be performed at weekly or biweekly intervals until the lipid response to Accutane is established. The incidence of hypertriglyceridemia is 1 patient in 4 on Accutane therapy (see WARNINGS, Lipids).

Liver Function Tests: Since elevations of liver enzymes have been observed during clinical trials, and hepatitis has been reported, pretreatment and follow-up liver function tests should be performed at weekly or biweekly intervals until the response to Accutane has been established (see WARNINGS, Hepatotoxicity).

Glucose: Some patients receiving Accutane have experienced problems in the control of their blood sugar. In addition, new cases of diabetes have been diagnosed during Accutane therapy, although no causal relationship has been established.

CPK: Some patients undergoing vigorous physical activity while on Accutane therapy have experienced elevated CPK levels; however, the clinical significance is unknown. There have been rare postmarketing reports of rhabdomyolysis, some associated with strenuous physical activity. In a clinical trial of 217 pediatric patients (12-17 years) with severe recalcitrant nodular acne, transient elevations in CPK were observed in 12% of patients, including those undergoing strenuous physical activity in association with reported musculoskeletal adverse events such as back pain, arthralgia, limb injury, or muscle sprain. In these patients, approximately half of the CPK elevations returned to normal within 2 weeks and half returned to normal within 4 weeks. No cases of rhabdomyolysis were reported in this trial.

CARCINOGENESIS, MUTAGENESIS, AND IMPAIRMENT OF FERTILITY

In male and female Fischer 344 rats given oral isotretinoin at dosages of 8 or 32 mg/kg/day (1.3 to 5.3 times the recommended clinical dose of 1.0 mg/kg/day, respectively, after normalization for total body surface area) for greater than 18 months, there was a dose-related increased incidence of pheochromocytoma relative to controls. The incidence of adrenal medullary hyperplasia was also increased at the higher dosage in both sexes. The relatively high level of spontaneous pheochromocytomas occurring in the male Fischer 344 rat makes it an equivocal model for study of this tumor; therefore, the relevance of this tumor to the human population is uncertain.

The Ames test was conducted with isotretinoin in two laboratories. The results of the tests in one laboratory were negative while in the second laboratory a weakly positive response (less than 1.6× background) was noted in *S. typhimurium* TA100 when the assay was conducted with metabolic activation. No dose-response effect was seen and all other strains were negative. Additionally, other tests designed to assess genotoxicity (Chinese hamster cell assay, mouse micronucleus test, *S. cerevisiae* D7 assay, *in vitro* clastogenesis assay with human-derived lymphocytes, and unscheduled DNA synthesis assay) were all negative.

In rats, no adverse effects on gonadal function, fertility, conception rate, gestation or parturition were observed at oral dosages of isotretinoin of 2, 8, or 32 mg/kg/day (0.3, 1.3, or 5.3 times the recommended clinical dose of 1.0 mg/kg/day, respectively, after normalization for total body surface area).

In dogs, testicular atrophy was noted after treatment with oral isotretinoin for approximately 30 weeks at dosages of 20 or 60 mg/kg/day (10 or 30 times the recommended clinical dose of 1.0 mg/kg/day, respectively, after normalization for total body surface area). In general, there was microscopic evidence for appreciable depression of spermatogenesis but some sperm were observed in all testes examined and in no instance were completely atrophic tubules seen. In studies of 66 men, 30 of whom were patients with nodular acne under treatment with oral isotretinoin, no significant changes were noted in the count or motility of spermatozoa in the ejaculate. In a study of 50 men (ages 17-32 years) receiving Accutane therapy for nodular acne, no significant effects were seen on ejaculate volume, sperm count, total sperm motility, morphology or seminal plasma fructose.

PREGNANCY CATEGORY X

See BOXED WARNING.

NURSING MOTHERS

It is not known whether this drug is excreted in human milk. Because of the potential for adverse effects, nursing mothers should not receive Accutane.

I

PEDIATRIC USE

The use of Accutane in pediatric patients less than 12 years of age has not been studied. The use of Accutane for the treatment of severe recalcitrant nodular acne in pediatric patients ages 12-17 years should be given careful consideration, especially for those patients where a known metabolic or structural bone disease exists (see General). Use of Accutane in this age group for severe recalcitrant nodular acne is supported by evidence from a clinical study comparing 103 pediatric patients (13-17 years) to 197 adult patients (≥18 years). Results from this study demonstrated that Accutane, at a dose of 1 mg/kg/day given in 2 divided doses, was equally effective in treating severe recalcitrant nodular acne in both pediatric and adult patients.

In studies with Accutane, adverse reactions reported in pediatric patients were similar to those described in adults except for the increased incidence of back pain and arthralgia (both of which were sometimes severe) and myalgia in pediatric patients (see ADVERSE REACTIONS).

In an open-label clinical trial (n=217) of a single course of therapy with Accutane for severe recalcitrant nodular acne, bone density measurements at several skeletal sites were not significantly decreased (lumbar spine change >-4% and total hip change >-5%) or were increased in the majority of patients. One patient had a decrease in lumbar spine bone mineral density >4% based on unadjusted data. Sixteen (7.9%) patients had decreases in lumbar spine bone mineral density >4%, and all the other patients (92%) did not have significant decreases or had increases (adjusted for body mass index). Nine patients (4.5%) had a decrease in total hip bone mineral density >5% based on unadjusted data. Twenty-one (10.6%) patients had decreases in total hip bone mineral density >5%, and all the other patients (89%) did not have significant decreases or had increases (adjusted for body mass index). Follow-up studies performed in 8 of the patients with decreased bone mineral density for up to 11 months thereafter demonstrated increasing bone density in 5 patients at the lumbar spine, while the other 3 patients had lumbar spine bone density measurements below baseline values. Total hip bone mineral densities remained below baseline (range -1.6% to -7.6%) in 5 of 8 patients (62.5%).

GERIATRIC USE

Clinical studies of isotretinoin did not include sufficient numbers of subjects aged 65 years and over to determine whether they respond differently from younger subjects. Although reported clinical experience has not identified differences in responses between elderly and younger patients, effects of aging might be expected to increase some risks associated with isotretinoin therapy (see WARNINGS and PRECAUTIONS).

DRUG INTERACTIONS

- ***Vitamin A:*** Because of the relationship of Accutane to vitamin A, patients should be advised against taking vitamin supplements containing vitamin A to avoid additive toxic effects.
- ***Tetracyclines:*** Concomitant treatment with Accutane and tetracyclines should be avoided because Accutane use has been associated with a number of cases of pseudotumor cerebri (benign intracranial hypertension), some of which involved concomitant use of tetracyclines.
- ***Micro-Dosed Progesterone Preparations:*** Micro-dosed progesterone preparations ("minipills" that do not contain an estrogen) may be an inadequate method of contraception during Accutane therapy. Although other hormonal contraceptives are highly effective, there have been reports of pregnancy from women who have used combined oral contraceptives, as well as injectable/implantable contraceptive products. These reports are more frequent for women who use only a single method of contraception. It is not known if hormonal contraceptives differ in their effectiveness when used with Accutane. Therefore, it is critically important for women of childbearing potential to select and commit to use 2 forms of effective contraception simultaneously, at least 1 of which must be a primary form, unless absolute abstinence is the chosen method, or the patient has undergone a hysterectomy (see BOXED WARNING).
- ***Phenytoin:*** Accutane has not been shown to alter the pharmacokinetics of phenytoin in a study in 7 healthy volunteers. These results are consistent with the *in vitro* finding that neither isotretinoin nor its metabolites induce or inhibit the activity of the CYP 2C9 human hepatic P450 enzyme. Phenytoin is known to cause osteomalacia. No formal clinical studies have been conducted to assess if there is an interactive effect on bone loss between phenytoin and Accutane. Therefore, caution should be exercised when using these drugs together.
- ***Systemic Corticosteroids:*** Systemic corticosteroids are known to cause osteoporosis. No formal clinical studies have been conducted to assess if there is an interactive effect on bone loss between systemic corticosteroids and Accutane. Therefore, caution should be exercised when using these drugs together.

Prescribers are advised to consult the package insert of medication administered concomitantly with hormonal contraceptives, since some medications may decrease the effectiveness of these birth control products. **Accutane use is associated with depression in some patients. (See WARNINGS, Psychiatric Disorders and ADVERSE REACTIONS, Dose Relationship, Psychiatric.)** Patients should be prospectively cautioned not to self-medicate with the herbal supplement St. John's Wort because a possible interaction has been suggested with hormonal contraceptives based on reports of breakthrough bleeding on oral contraceptives shortly after starting St. John's Wort. Pregnancies have been reported by users of combined hormonal contraceptives who also used some form of St. John's Wort.

ADVERSE REACTIONS

CLINICAL TRIALS AND POSTMARKETING SURVEILLANCE

The adverse reactions listed below reflect the experience from investigational studies of Accutane, and the postmarketing experience. The relationship of some of these events to Accutane therapy is unknown. Many of the side effects and adverse reactions seen in patients receiving Accutane are similar to those described in patients taking very high doses of vitamin A (dryness of the skin and mucous membranes, *e.g.*, of the lips, nasal passage, and eyes).

DOSE RELATIONSHIP

Cheilitis and hypertriglyceridemia are usually dose related. Most adverse reactions reported in clinical trials were reversible when therapy was discontinued; however, some persisted after cessation of therapy (see WARNINGS and ADVERSE REACTIONS).

Body as a Whole: Allergic reactions, including vasculitis, systemic hypersensitivity (see PRECAUTIONS, Hypersensitivity), edema, fatigue, lymphadenopathy, weight loss.

Cardiovascular: Palpitation, tachycardia, vascular thrombotic disease, stroke.

Endocrine/Metabolic: Hypertriglyceridemia (see WARNINGS, Lipids), alterations in blood sugar levels (see PRECAUTIONS, Laboratory Tests).

Gastrointestinal: Inflammatory bowel disease (see WARNINGS, Inflammatory Bowel Disease), hepatitis (see WARNINGS, Hepatotoxicity), pancreatitis (see WARNINGS, Lipids), bleeding and inflammation of the gums, colitis, esophagitis/esophageal ulceration, ileitis, nausea, other nonspecific gastrointestinal symptoms.

Hematologic: Allergic reactions (see PRECAUTIONS, Hypersensitivity), anemia, thrombocytopenia, neutropenia, rare reports of agranulocytosis (see PRECAUTIONS, Information for Patients and Prescribers). See PRECAUTIONS, Laboratory Tests for other hematological parameters.

Musculoskeletal: Skeletal hyperostosis, calcification of tendons and ligaments, premature epiphyseal closure, decreases in bone mineral density (see WARNINGS, Skeletal), musculoskeletal symptoms (sometimes severe) including back pain and arthralgia (see PRECAUTIONS, Information for Patients and Prescribers), transient pain in the chest (see PRECAUTIONS, Information for Patients and Prescribers), arthritis, tendonitis, other types of bone abnormalities, elevations of CPK/rare reports of rhabdomyolysis (see PRECAUTIONS, Laboratory Tests).

Neurological: Pseudotumor cerebri (see WARNINGS, Pseudotumor Cerebri), dizziness, drowsiness, headache, insomnia, lethargy, malaise, nervousness, paresthesias, seizures, stroke, syncope, weakness.

Psychiatric: Suicidal ideation, suicide attempts, suicide, depression, psychosis, aggression, violent behaviors (see WARNINGS, Psychiatric Disorders), emotional instability.

Note: Of the patients reporting depression, some reported that the depression subsided with discontinuation of therapy and recurred with reinstitution of therapy.

Reproductive System: Abnormal menses.

Respiratory: Bronchospasms (with or without a history of asthma), respiratory infection, voice alteration.

Skin and Appendages: Acne fulminans, alopecia (which in some cases persists), bruising, cheilitis (dry lips), dry mouth, dry nose, dry skin, epistaxis, eruptive xanthomas,[7] flushing, fragility of skin, hair abnormalities, hirsutism, hyperpigmentation and hypopigmentation, infections (including disseminated herpes simplex), nail dystrophy, paronychia, peeling of palms and soles, photoallergic/photosensitizing reactions, pruritus, pyogenic granuloma, rash (including facial erythema, seborrhea, and eczema), sunburn susceptibility increased, sweating, urticaria, vasculitis (including Wegener's granulomastosis; see PRECAUTIONS, Hypersensitivity), abnormal wound healing (delayed healing or exuberant granulation tissue with crusting; see PRECAUTIONS, Information for Patients and Prescribers).

Special Senses: *Hearing:* Hearing impairment (see WARNINGS, Hearing Impairment), tinnitus. *Vision:* Corneal opacities (see WARNINGS, Vision Impairment, Corneal Opacities), decreased night vision which may persist (see WARNINGS, Vision Impairment, Decreased Night Vision), cataracts, color vision disorder, conjunctivitis, dry eyes, eyelid inflammation, keratitis, optic neuritis, photophobia, visual disturbances.

Urinary System: Glomerulonephritis (see PRECAUTIONS, Hypersensitivity), nonspecific urogenital findings (see PRECAUTIONS, Laboratory Tests for other urological parameters).

LABORATORY

Elevation of plasma triglycerides (see WARNINGS, Lipids), decrease in serum high-density lipoprotein (HDL) levels, elevations of serum cholesterol during treatment.

Increased alkaline phosphatase, SGOT (AST), SGPT (ALT), GGTP or LDH (see WARNINGS, Hepatotoxicity).

Elevation of fasting blood sugar, elevations of CPK (see PRECAUTIONS, Laboratory Tests), hyperuricemia.

Decreases in red blood cell parameters, decreases in white blood cell counts (including severe neutropenia and rare reports of agranulocytosis; see PRECAUTIONS, Information for Patients and Prescribers), elevated sedimentation rates, elevated platelet counts, thrombocytopenia.

White cells in the urine, proteinuria, microscopic or gross hematuria.

DOSAGE AND ADMINISTRATION

Accutane should be administered with a meal (see PRECAUTIONS, Information for Patients and Prescribers).

The recommended dosage range for Accutane is 0.5-1.0 mg/kg/day given in 2 divided doses with food for 15-20 weeks. In studies comparing 0.1, 0.5, and 1.0 mg/kg/day,[8] it was found that all dosages provided initial clearing of disease, but there was a greater need for retreatment with the lower dosages. During treatment, the dose may be adjusted according to response of the disease and/or the appearance of clinical side effects — some of which may be dose related. Adult patients whose disease is very severe with scarring or is primarily manifested on the trunk may require dose adjustments up to 2.0 mg/kg/day, as tolerated. Failure to take Accutane with food will significantly decrease absorption. Before upward dose adjustments are made, the patients should be questioned about their compliance with food instructions.

The safety of once daily dosing with Accutane has not been established. Once daily dosing is **not** recommended.

If the total nodule count has been reduced by more than 70% prior to completing 15-20 weeks of treatment, the drug may be discontinued. After a period of 2 months or more off therapy, and if warranted by persistent or recurring severe nodular acne, a second course of therapy may be initiated. The optimal interval before retreatment has not been defined for patients who have not completed skeletal growth Long-term use of Accutane, even in low doses, has not been studied, and is not recommended. It is important that Accutane be given at the recommended doses for no longer than the recommended duration. The effect of long-term use of Accutane on bone loss is unknown (see WARNINGS, Skeletal: Bone Mineral Density, Hyperostosis, and Premature Epiphyseal Closure).

Contraceptive measures must be followed for any subsequent course of therapy (see BOXED WARNING).

TABLE 4 *Accutane Dosing by Body Weight (Based on Administration With Food)*

Body Weight		Total mg/day		
kilograms	pounds	0.5 mg/kg	1 mg/kg	2 mg/kg*
40	88	20	40	80
50	110	25	50	100
60	132	30	60	120
70	154	35	70	140
80	176	40	80	160
90	198	45	90	180
100	220	50	100	200

* See DOSAGE AND ADMINISTRATION: the recommended dosage range is 0.5-1.0 mg/kg/day.

Information for Pharmacists: Accutane must only be dispensed in no more than a 30 day supply and only on presentation of an Accutane prescription with a yellow self-adhesive Accutane Qualification Sticker written within the previous 7 days. REFILLS REQUIRE A NEW WRITTEN PRESCRIPTION WITH A YELLOW SELF-ADHESIVE ACCUTANE QUALIFICATION STICKER WITHIN THE PREVIOUS 7 DAYS. No telephone or computerized prescriptions are permitted.

An Accutane Medication Guide must be given to the patient each time Accutane is dispensed, as required by law. This Accutane Medication Guide is an important part of the risk management program for the patient.

HOW SUPPLIED

Accutane is available in:

10 mg: Light pink soft gelatin capsules, imprinted "ACCUTANE 10 ROCHE".
20 mg: Maroon soft gelatin capsules, imprinted "ACCUTANE 20 ROCHE".
40 mg: Yellow soft gelatin capsules, imprinted "ACCUTANE 40 ROCHE".

Storage: Store at controlled room temperature (15-30°C, 59-86°F). Protect from light.

PRODUCT LISTING - EQUIVALENTS NOT AVAILABLE

Capsule - Oral - 10 mg

100's	$703.31	GENERIC, Bertek Pharmaceuticals Inc	62794-0611-88
100's	$782.33	ACCUTANE, Roche Laboratories	00004-0155-49

Capsule - Oral - 20 mg

30's	$260.21	GENERIC, Bertek Pharmaceuticals Inc	62794-0612-93
100's	$834.01	GENERIC, Bertek Pharmaceuticals Inc	62794-0612-88
100's	$927.71	ACCUTANE, Roche Laboratories	00004-0169-49

Capsule - Oral - 40 mg

30's	$295.63	ACCUTANE, Allscripts Pharmaceutical Company	54569-0482-00
30's	$302.31	GENERIC, Bertek Pharmaceuticals Inc	62794-0614-93
100's	$968.95	GENERIC, Bertek Pharmaceuticals Inc	62794-0614-88
100's	$1077.81	ACCUTANE, Roche Laboratories	00004-0156-49
100's	$1121.90	ACCUTANE, Physicians Total Care	54868-0955-00

Isradipine *(003014)*

For related information, see the comparative table section in Appendix A.

Categories: Hypertension, essential; Pregnancy Category C; FDA Approved 1990 Dec
Drug Classes: Calcium channel blockers
Brand Names: **Dynacirc**
Foreign Brand Availability: Dynacirc SRO (Colombia; Ecuador; Hong-Kong; Malaysia; Mexico; New-Zealand; Peru; Philippines; Thailand); Icaz SRO (Philippines); Lomir (Austria; Bahrain; Belgium; Benin; Bulgaria; Burkina-Faso; Cyprus; Czech-Republic; Denmark; Egypt; Ethiopia; Finland; Gambia; Germany; Ghana; Greece; Guinea; Hungary; Iran; Iraq; Ireland; Ivory-Coast; Jordan; Kenya; Kuwait; Lebanon; Liberia; Libya; Malawi; Mali; Mauritania; Mauritius; Morocco; Netherlands; Niger; Nigeria; Norway; Oman; Portugal; Qatar; Republic-of-Yemen; Saudi-Arabia; Senegal; Seychelles; Sierra-Leone; Spain; Sudan; Sweden; Switzerland; Syria; Tanzania; Tunia; Uganda; United-Arab-Emirates; Zambia; Zimbabwe); Lomir Retard (Denmark); Lomir SRO (Austria; Czech-Republic; Finland; Hungary; Italy; Netherlands; Norway; Portugal; Spain; Sweden; Switzerland); Prescal (England; Ireland); Vascal (Netherlands)
Cost of Therapy: $80.61 (Hypertension; Dynacirc; 2.5 mg; 2 capsules/day; 30 day supply)
$43.00 (Hypertension; Dynacirc CR; 5 mg; 1 tablet/day; 30 day supply)

DESCRIPTION

Isradipine is a calcium antagonist available for oral administration in capsules containing 2.5 or 5 mg.

Chemically, isradipine is 3,5-Pyridinedicarboxylic acid, 4-(4-benzofurazanyl) -1,4-dihydro-2,6-dimethyl-,methyl 1-methylethyl ester. Isradipine is a yellow, fine crystalline powder which is odorless or has a faint characteristic odor. Isradipine is practically insoluble in water (<10 mg/L at 37°C), but is soluble in ethanol and freely soluble in acetone, chloroform and methylene chloride.

Active Ingredient: Isradipine

Dynacirc Inactive Ingredients: colloidal silicon dioxide, D&C red no. 7 calcium lake, FD&C red no. 40 (5 mg capsule only), FD&C yellow no. 6 aluminum Lake, gelatin, lactose, starch, titanium dioxide and other ingredients.

The 2.5 and 5 mg capsules may also contain: benzyl alcohol, butylparaben, edetate calcium disodium, methylparaben, propylparaben, sodium propionate.

CLINICAL PHARMACOLOGY

MECHANISM OF ACTION

Isradipine is a dihydropyridine calcium channel blocker. It binds to calcium channels with high affinity and specificity and inhibits calcium flux into cardiac and smooth muscle. The effects observed in mechanistic experiments *in vitro* and studied in intact animals and man are compatible with this mechanism of action and are typical of the class.

Except for diuretic activity, the mechanism of which is not clearly understood, the pharmacodynamic effects of isradipine observed in whole animals can also be explained by calcium channel blocking activity, especially dilating effects in arterioles which reduce systemic resistance and lower blood pressure, with a small increase in resting heart rate. Although like other dihydropyridine calcium channel blockers, isradipine has negative inotropic effects *in vitro*, studies conducted in intact anesthetized animals have shown that the vasodilating effect occurs at doses lower than those which affect contractility. In patients with normal ventricular function, isradipine's afterload reducing properties lead to some increase in cardiac output.

Effects in patients with impaired ventricular function have not been fully studied.

Clinical Effects

Dose-related reductions in supine and standing blood pressure are achieved within 2-3 hours following single oral doses of 2.5, 5, 10, and 20 mg isradipine, with a duration of action (at least 50% of peak response) of more than 12 hours following administration of the highest dose.

Isradipine has been shown in controlled, double blind clinical trials to be an effective antihypertensive agent when used as monotherapy, or when added to therapy with thiazide-type diuretics. During chronic administration, divided doses (bid) in the range of 5-20 mg daily have shown to be effective, with response at trough(prior to next dose) over 50% of the peak blood pressure effect. The response is dose-related between 5-10 mg daily. Isradipine is equally effective in reducing supine, sitting and standing blood pressure.

On chronic administration, increases in resting pulse rate averaged about 3-5 beats/min. These increases were not dose-related.

HEMODYNAMICS

In man, peripheral vasodilation produced by isradipine is reflected by decreased systemic vascular resistance and increased cardiac output. Hemodynamic studies conducted in patients with normal left ventricular function produced, following intravenous isradipine administration, increases in cardiac index, stroke volume index, coronary sinus blood flow, heart rate, and peak positive left ventricular dP/dt. Systemic, coronary, and pulmonary vascular resistance were decreased. These studies were conducted with doses of isradipine which produced clinically significant decreases in blood pressure. The clinical consequences of these hemodynamic effects, if any, have not been evaluated.

Effects on heart rate are variable, dependent upon rate of administration and presence of underlying cardiac condition. While increases in both peak positive dP/dt and LV ejection fraction are seen when intravenous isradipine is given, it is impossible to conclude that these represent a positive inotropic effect due to simultaneous changes in preload and afterload. In patients with coronary artery disease, undergoing atrial pacing during cardiac catheterization, intravenous isradipine diminished abnormalities of systolic performance. In patients with moderate left ventricular dysfunction, oral and intravenous isradipine in doses which reduce blood pressure by 12-30% percent, resulted in improvement in cardiac index without increase in heart rate, and with no change or reduction in pulmonary capillary wedge pressure, Combination of isradipine and propranolol did not significantly effect left ventricular dP/dt max. The clinical consequences of these effects have not been evaluated.

ELECTROPHYSIOLOGIC EFFECTS

In general, no detrimental effects on the cardiac conduction system were seen with the use of isradipine. Electrophysiologic studies were conducted on patients with normal sinus and atrioventricular node function. Intravenous isradipine in doses which reduce systolic blood pressure did not effect PR, QRS, AH* or HV* intervals.

No changes were seen in Wenckebach cycle length, atrial, and ventricular refractory periods. Slight prolongation of QT_c interval of 3% was seen in one study. Effects on sinus node recovery time (CSNRT) were mild or not seen.

In patients with sick sinus syndrome, at doses which significantly reduced blood pressure, intravenous isradipine resulted in no depressant effect on sinus and atrioventricular node function.

*AH= conduction time from low right atrium to His bundle deflection, or AV nodal conduction time;

HV= conduction time through the His bundle and the bundle branch-Purkinje system.

PHARMACOKINETICS AND METABOLISM

Isradipine is 90-95% absorbed and is subject to extensive first-pass metabolism, resulting in a bioavailability of about 15-24%. Isradipine is detectable in plasma within 20 minutes after administration of single oral doses of 2.5-20 mg, and peak concentrations of approximately 1 ng/ml/mg dosed occur about 1.5 hours after drug administration. Administration of isradipine with food significantly increases the time to peak by about an hour, but has no effect on the total bioavailability (area under the curve)of the drug. Isradipine is 95% bound to plasma proteins. Both peak plasma concentration and AUC exhibit a linear relationship to dose over the 0-20 mg dose range. The elimination of isradipine is biphasic with an early half-life of 1.5-2 hours, and a terminal half-life of about 8 hours. The total body clearance of isradipine is 1.4 L/min and the apparent volume of distribution is 3 L/kg.

Isradipine is completely metabolized prior to excretion and no unchanged drug is detected in the urine. Six metabolites have been characterized in blood and urine, with the mono acids of the pyridine derivative and a cyclic lactone product accounting for >75% of the material identified. Approximately 60-65% of an administered dose is excreted in the urine and 25-30% in the feces. Mild renal impairment (creatinine clearance 30-80 mL/min) increases the bioavailability (AUC) of isradipine by 45%. Progressive deterioration reverses this trend, and patients with severe renal failure (creatinine clearance <10mL/min) who have been on hemodialysis show a 20-50% lower AUC than healthy volunteers. No pharmacokinetic information is available on drug therapy during hemodialysis. In elderly patients, $C_{max}$and AUC are increased by 13% and 40%, respectively; in patients with hepatic impairment, C_{max} and AUC are increased by 32% and 52%, respectively (see DOSAGE AND ADMINISTRATION).

INDICATIONS AND USAGE

Hypertension: Isradipine is indicated in the management of hypertension. It may be used alone or concurrently with thiazide-type diuretics.

NON-FDA APPROVED INDICATIONS

Non-FDA-approved uses include angina pectoris prophylaxis.

CONTRAINDICATIONS

Isradipine is contraindicated in individuals who have shown hypersensitivity to any of the ingredients in the formulation.

WARNINGS

None.

PRECAUTIONS

GENERAL

Blood Pressure

Because isradipine decreases peripheral resistance, like other calcium blockers isradipine may occasionally produce symptomatic hypotension. However, symptoms like syncope and severe dizziness have rarely been reported in hypertensive patients administered isradipine, particularly at the initial recommended doses (see DOSAGE AND ADMINISTRATION).

Use in Patients With Congestive Heart Failure

Although acute hemodynamic studies in patients with congestive heart failure have shown that isradipine reduced afterload without impairing myocardial contractility, it has a negative inotropic effect at high doses *in vitro*, and possibly in some patients. Caution should be exercised when using the drug in congestive heart failure patients, particularly in combination with a beta-blocker.

CARCINOGENESIS, MUTAGENESIS, AND IMPAIRMENT OF FERTILITY

Treatment of male rats for 2 years with 2.5, 12.5, or 62.5 mg/kg/day isradipine admixed with the diet (approximately 6, 31, and 156 times the maximum recommended daily dose based on a 50 kg man) resulted in dose dependent increases in the incidence of benign Leydig cell tumors and testicular hyperplasia relative to untreated control animals. These findings, which were replicated in a subsequent experiment, may have been indirectly related to an effect of isradipine on circulating gonadotropin levels in the rats; a comparable endocrine effect was not evident in male patients receiving therapeutic doses of the drug on a chronic basis. Treatment of mice for 2 years with 2.5, 15, or 80 mg/kg/day isradipine in the diet (approximately 6, 38, and 200 times the maximum recommended daily dose based on a 50 kg man) showed no evidence of oncogenicity. There was no evidence of mutagenic potential based on the results of a battery of mutagenicity tests. No effect on fertility was observed in male and female rats treated with up to 60 mg/kg/day isradipine.

PREGNANCY CATEGORY C

Isradipine was administered orally to rats and rabbits during organogenesis. Treatment of pregnant rats with doses of 6, 20, or 60 mg/kg/day produced a significant reduction in maternal weight gain during treatment with the highest dose (150 times the maximum recommended human daily dose) but with no lasting effects on the mother or the offspring. Treatment of pregnant rabbits with doses of 1, 3, or 10 mg/kg/day (2.5, 7.5, and 25 times the maximum recommended human daily dose) produced decrements in maternal body weight gain and increased fetal resorptions at the 2 higher doses. There was no evidence of embryotoxicity at doses which were not maternotoxic and no evidence of teratogenicity at any dose tested. In a peri/postnatal administration study in rats, reduced maternal body weight gain during late pregnancy at oral doses of 20 and 60 mg/kg/day isradipine was associated with reduced birth weights and decreased peri and postnatal pup survival.

There are no adequate and well controlled studies in pregnant women. The use of isradipine during pregnancy should only be considered if the potential benefit outweighs potential risks.

NURSING MOTHERS

It is not known whether isradipine is excreted in human milk. Because many drugs are excreted in human milk, and because of the potential for adverse effects of isradipine on nursing infants, a decision should be made as to whether to discontinue nursing or discontinue the drug, taking into account the importance of the drug to the mother.

PEDIATRIC USE

Safety and effectiveness have not been established in children.

DRUG INTERACTIONS

Nitroglycerin: Isradipine has been safely coadministered with nitroglycerin.

Hydrochlorothiazide: A study in normal healthy volunteers has shown that concomitant administration of isradipine and hydrochlorothiazide does not result in altered pharmacokinetics of either drug. In a study in hypertensive patients, addition of isradipine to existing hydrochlorothiazide therapy did not result in any unexpected adverse effects, and isradipine had an additional antihypertensive effect.

Propranolol: In a single dose study in normal volunteers, coadministration of propranolol had a small effect on the rate but no effect on the extent of isradipine bioavailability. Significant increases in AUC (27%) and C_{max} (58%) and decreases in t_{max} (23%) of propranolol were noted in this study. However, concomitant administration of 5 mg bid isradipine and 40 mg bid propranolol, to healthy volunteers under steady-state conditions had no relevant effect on either drug's bioavailability. AUC and C_{max} differences were <20% between isradipine given singly and in combination with propanolol, and between propranolol given singly and in combination with isradipine.

Cimetidine: In a study in healthy volunteers, a 1 week course of cimetidine at 400 mg bid with a single 5 mg dose of isradipine on the sixth day showed an increase in isradipine mean peak plasma concentrations (36%) and significant increase in area under the curve (50%). If isradipine therapy is initiated in a patient currently receiving cimetidine, careful monitoring for adverse reactions is advised and downward dose adjustment may be required.

Rifampicin: In a study in healthy volunteers, a six-day course of rifampicin at 600 mg/day followed by a single 5 mg dose of isradipine resulted in a reduction in isradipine levels to below detectable limits. If rifampicin therapy is required, isradipine concentrations and therapeutic effects are likely to be markedly reduced or abolished as a consequence of increased metabolism and higher clearance of isradipine.

Warfarin: In a study in healthy volunteers, no clinically relevant pharmacokinetic or pharmacodynamic interaction between isradipine and racemic warfarin was seen when 2 single oral doses of warfarin (0.7 mg/kg body weight) were administered during 11 days of multiple-dose treatment with 5 mg bid isradipine. Neither racemic warfarin nor isradipine binding to plasma proteins *in vitro* was altered by the addition of the other drug.

Digoxin: The concomitant administration of DynaCirc (isradipine) and digoxin in a single-dose pharmacokinetic study did not affect renal, non-renal and total body clearance of digoxin.

Fentanyl Anesthesia: Severe hypotension has been reported during fentanyl anesthesia with concomitant use of a beta blocker and a calcium channel blocker. Even though such interactions have not been seen in clinical studies with DynaCirc (isradipine), an increased volume of circulating fluids might be required if such an interaction were to occur.

ADVERSE REACTIONS

In multiple dose US studies in hypertension, 1228 patients received Isradipine alone or in combination with other agents, principally a thiazide diuretic, 934 of them in controlled comparisons with placebo or active agents. An additional 652 patients (which includes 374 normal volunteers) received isradipine in US studies of conditions other than hypertension, and 1321 patients received isradipine in non-US studies. About 500 patients received isradipine in long-term hypertension studies, 410 of them for at least 6 months. The adverse reaction rates given below are principally based on controlled hypertension studies, but rarer serious events are derived from all exposures to isradipine, including foreign marketing experience.

Most adverse reactions were mild and related to the vasodilatory effects of isradipine (dizziness, edema, palpitations, flushing, tachycardia) and many were transient. About 5% of isradipine patients left studies prematurely because of adverse reactions (versus 3% of placebo patients and 6% of active control patients), principally due to headache, edema, dizziness, palpitations and gastrointestinal disturbances.

TABLE 1 below shows the most common adverse reactions, volunteered or elicited, considered by the investigator to be at least possibly drug related. The results for the isradipine treated patients are presented for all doses pooled together (reported by 1% or greater of patients receiving any dose of isradipine, and also for the two treatment regimens most applicable to the treatment of hypertension with Isradipine: (1) initial and maintenance dose of 2.5 mg bid, and (2) initial dose of 2.5 mg bid followed by maintenance dose of 5.0 mg bid.

Except for headache, which is not clearly drug-related (see TABLE 1), the more frequent adverse reactions listed above show little change, or increase slightly, in frequency over time, as shown in TABLE 2

TABLE 1

Adverse Experience	All Doses	2.5 mg bid	5 mg bid*	10 mg bid†	Placebo	Active Controls‡
	n=934	n=199	n=150	n=59	n=297	n=414
Headache	13.7%	12.6%	10.7%	22.0%	14.1%	9.4%
Dizziness	7.3%	8.0%	5.3%	3.4%	4.4%	8.2%
Edema	7.2%	3.5%	8.7%	8.5%	3.0%	2.9%
Palpitations	4.0%	1.0%	4.7%	5.1%	1.4%	1.5%
Fatigue	3.9%	2.5%	2.0%	8.5%	0.3%	6.3%
Flushing	2.6%	3.0%	2.0%	5.1%	0.0%	1.2%
Chest pain	2.4%	2.5%	2.7%	1.7%	2.4%	2.9%
Nausea	1.8%	1.0%	2.7%	5.1%	1.7%	3.1%
Dyspnea	1.8%	0.5%	2.7%	3.4%	1.0%	2.2%
Abdominal discomfort	1.7%	0.0%	3.3%	1.7%	1.7%	3.9%
Tachycardia	1.5%	1.0%	1.3%	3.4%	0.3%	0.5%
Rash	1.5%	1.5%	2.0%	1.7%	0.3%	0.7%
Pollakiuria	1.5%	2.0%	1.3%	3.4%	0.0%	<1.0%
Weakness	1.2%	0.0%	0.7%	0.0%	0.0%	1.2%
Vomiting	1.1%	1.0%	1.3%	0.0%	0.3%	0.2%
Diarrhea	1.1%	0.0%	2.7%	3.4%	2.0%	1.9%

* Initial dose of 2.5 mg bid followed by maintenance dose of 5.0 mg bid.
† Initial dose of 2.5 mg bid followed by sequential titration to 5.0 mg bid, 7.5 mg bid, and maintenance dose of 10.0 mg bid.
‡ Propranolol, prazosin, hydrochlorothiazide, enalapril, captopril.

***TABLE 2** Incidence Rates for Isradipine (All Doses) by Week*

Week	1	2	3	4	5	6
N	694	906	649	847	432	494
Adverse Reaction						
Headache	6.5%	6.1%	5.2%	5.2%	5.8%	4.5%
Dizziness	1.6%	1.9%	1.7%	2.2%	2.3%	2.0%
Edema	1.2%	2.5%	3.2%	3.2%	5.3%	5.5%
Palpitations	1.2%	1.3%	1.4%	1.9%	2.1%	1.4%
Fatigue	0.4%	1.0%	1.4%	1.2%	1.2%	1.6%
Flushing	1.2%	1.3%	2.0%	1.4%	2.1%	1.4%
Week	**7**	**8**	**9**	**10**	**11**	**12**
N	**153**	**377**	**261**	**362**	**107**	**105**
Headache	20.0%	2.7%	1.9%	2.8%	2.8%	3.8%
Dizziness	2.0%	1.9%	2.3%	3.9%	4.7%	3.8%
Edema	5.9%	5.0%	4.6%	4.7%	3.8%	3.8%
Palpitations	1.3%	0.8%	0.8%	1.7%	1.9%	2.9%
Fatigue	2.0%	2.7%	1.5%	1.4%	0.9%	1.9%
Flushing	3.3%	1.3%	1.1%	0.8%	0.0%	0.0%

Edema, palpitations, fatigue, and flushing appear to be dose-related, especially at the higher doses of 15-20 mg/day.

In open-label, long-term studies of up to 2 years in duration, the adverse events reported were generally the same as those reported in the short-term controlled trials. The overall frequencies of these adverse events were slightly higher in the long-term than in the controlled studies, but as in the controlled trials most adverse reactions were mild and transient.

The following adverse events were reported in 0.5-1.0% of the isradipine treated patients in hypertension studies, or are rare. More serious events from this and other data sources, including postmarketing exposure, are shown in italics. The relationship of these adverse events to isradipine administration is uncertain.

Skin: Pruritus, *urticaria*

Musculoskeletal: Cramps of legs/feet

Respiratory: Cough

Cardiovascular: Shortness of breath, hypotension, *atrial fibrillation, ventricular fibrillation, myocardial infarction, heart failure*

Gastrointestinal: Abdominal discomfort, constipation, diarrhea

Urogenital: Nocturia

Nervous System: Drowsiness, insomnia, lethargy, nervousness, impotence, decreased libido, depression, *syncope, paresthesia* (which includes numbness and tingling), *transient ischemic attack, stroke*

Autonomic: Hyperhidrosis, visual disturbance, dry mouth, numbness

Miscellaneous: Throat discomfort, *leukopenia, elevated liver function tests*

DOSAGE AND ADMINISTRATION

The dosage of isradipine should be individualized. The recommended initial dose of isradipine is 2.5 mg bid alone or in combination with a thiazide diuretic. An antihypertensive response usually occurs within 2-3 hours. Maximal response may require 2-4 weeks. If a satisfactory reduction in blood pressure does not occur after this period, the dose may be adjusted in increments of 5 mg/day at 2-4 week intervals up to a maximum of 20 mg per day. Most patients, however, show no additional response to doses above 10 mg/day, and adverse effects are increased in frequency above 10 mg/day.

The bioavailability of increased AUC is increased in elderly patients (above 65 years of age), patients with hepatic functional impairment, and patients with mild renal impairment. Ordinarily, the starting dose should still be 2.5 mg bid in these patients.

HOW SUPPLIED

DynaCirc Capsules 2.5 mg: White, imprinted twice with the DynaCirc (isradipine) logo and "DynaCirc" on one end, and "2.5" and "S" (within a triangle) on the other.

DynaCirc Capsules 5 mg: Light pink, imprinted twice with the DynaCirc (isradipine) logo and "DynaCirc" on one end, and "5" and "S" (within a triangle) on the other.

Store and Dispense: Below 30°C (86°F) in a tight container. Protect from light.

PRODUCT LISTING - EQUIVALENTS NOT AVAILABLE

Capsule - Oral - 2.5 mg

60's	$56.86	DYNACIRC, Novartis Pharmaceuticals	00078-0226-44
60's	$80.61	DYNACIRC, Reliant Pharmaceuticals, Llc.	65726-0226-15
100's	$93.18	DYNACIRC, Novartis Pharmaceuticals	00078-0226-05
100's	$132.11	DYNACIRC, Reliant Pharmaceuticals, Llc.	65726-0226-25

Capsule - Oral - 5 mg

60's	$82.82	DYNACIRC, Novartis Pharmaceuticals	00078-0227-44
60's	$117.43	DYNACIRC, Reliant Pharmaceuticals, Llc.	65726-0227-15
100's	$135.64	DYNACIRC, Novartis Pharmaceuticals	00078-0227-05
100's	$192.28	DYNACIRC, Reliant Pharmaceuticals, Llc.	65726-0227-25

Tablet, Extended Release - Oral - 5 mg

30's	$39.12	DYNACIRC CR, Novartis Pharmaceuticals	00078-0235-15
30's	$43.00	DYNACIRC CR, Reliant Pharmaceuticals, Llc.	65726-0235-10
100's	$127.60	DYNACIRC CR, Novartis Pharmaceuticals	00078-0235-05
100's	$140.23	DYNACIRC CR, Reliant Pharmaceuticals, Llc.	65726-0235-25

Tablet, Extended Release - Oral - 10 mg

30's	$62.19	DYNACIRC CR, Novartis Pharmaceuticals	00078-0236-15
30's	$68.34	DYNACIRC CR, Reliant Pharmaceuticals, Llc.	65726-0236-10
30's	$68.34	DYNACIRC CR, Reliant Pharmaceuticals, Llc.	65726-0236-15
100's	$203.32	DYNACIRC CR, Novartis Pharmaceuticals	00078-0236-05
100's	$223.44	DYNACIRC CR, Reliant Pharmaceuticals, Llc.	65726-0236-05
100's	$223.44	DYNACIRC CR, Reliant Pharmaceuticals, Llc.	65726-0236-25

Itraconazole *(003133)*

For related information, see the comparative table section in Appendix A.

Categories: Aspergillosis; Blastomycosis; Candidiasis; Histoplasmosis; Tinea unguium; Pregnancy Category C; FDA Approved 1992 Sep

Drug Classes: Antifungals

Brand Names: Sporanox

Foreign Brand Availability: Candistat (India); Canditral (Singapore); Carexa (Mexico); Forcanox (Indonesia); Fungitrazol (Indonesia); Furolnok (Indonesia); Irta (Korea); Isox (Mexico); Itodal (Peru); Itra (Thailand); Itracon (Thailand); Itranax (Mexico); Itrizole (Japan); Itzol (Indonesia); Micoral (Peru); Norspor (Thailand); Nufatrac (Indonesia); Sempera (Germany); Sinozol (Mexico); Spazol (Thailand); Sporacid (Indonesia); Sporal (Thailand); Sporanox 15 D (Costa-Rica; Dominican-Republic; El-Salvador; Guatemala; Honduras; Mexico; Nicaragua; Panama; Peru); Sporlab (Thailand); Spornar (Thailand); Spyrocon (Indonesia); Trachon (Indonesia)

Cost of Therapy: $1212.74 (Onychomycosis; Sporanox; 100 mg; 2 capsules/day; 84 day supply)

INTRAVENOUS

WARNING

Congestive Heart Failure

When itraconazole was administered intravenously to dogs and healthy human volunteers, negative inotropic effects were seen. If signs or symptoms of congestive heart failure occur during administration of itraconazole injection, continued itraconazole use should be reassessed. (See CLINICAL PHARMACOLOGY, Special Populations; CONTRAINDICATIONS; WARNINGS; DRUG INTERACTIONS; and ADVERSE REACTIONS, Post-Marketing Experience for more information.)

Drug Interactions

Coadministration of cisapride, pimozide, quinidine, or dofetilide with itraconazole capsules, injection or oral solution is contraindicated. Itraconazole, a potent cytochrome P450 3A4 isoenzyme system (CYP3A4) inhibitor, may increase plasma concentrations of drugs metabolized by this pathway. Serious cardiovascular events, including QT prolongation, torsades de pointes, ventricular tachycardia, cardiac arrest, and/or sudden death have occurred in patients using cisapride, pimozide, or quinidine, concomitantly with itraconazole and/or other CYP3A4 inhibitors. (See CONTRAINDICATIONS, WARNINGS, and DRUG INTERACTIONS for more information.)

DESCRIPTION

For intravenous (IV) infusion (NOT FOR IV BOLUS INJECTION).

Itraconazole is a synthetic triazole antifungal agent. Itraconazole is a 1:1:1:1 racemic mixture of four diastereomers (two enantiomeric pairs), each possessing three chiral centers. It may be represented by the following nomenclature: (±)-1-[(R*)-sec-butyl]-4-[p-[4-[p-[[(2R*,4S*)-2-(2,4-dichlorophenyl)-2-(1H-1,2,4-triazol-1-ylmethyl)-1,3-dioxolan-4-yl]methoxy]phenyl]-1-piperazinyl]phenyl]-Δ^2-1,2,4-triazolin-5-one mixture with (±)-1-[(R*)-sec-butyl]-4-[p-[4-[p-[[(2S*4,R*)-2-(2,4,-dichlorophenyl)-2-(1H-1,2,4-triazol-1-ylmethyl)-1,3-dioxolan-4-yl]methoxy]phenyl]-1-piperazinyl]phenyl]-Δ^2-1,2,4-triazolin-5-one **or** (±)-1-[(RS)-sec-butyl]-4-[p-[4-[p-[[(2R,4S)-2-(2,4-dichlorophenyl)-2-(1H-1,2,4-triazol-1-ylmethyl)-1,3,-dioxolan-4-yl]methoxy]phenyl]-1-piperazinyl]phenyl]-Δ^2-1,2,4-triazolin-5-one.

Itraconazole has a molecular formula of $C_{35}H_{38}Cl_2N_8O_4$ and a molecular weight of 705.64. It is a white to slightly yellowish powder. It is insoluble in water, very slightly soluble in alcohols, and freely soluble in dichloromethane. It has a pKa of 3.70 (based on extrapolation of values obtained from methanolic solutions) and a log (n-octanol/water) partition coefficient of 5.66 at pH 8.1.

Sporanox (itraconazole) injection is a sterile pyrogen-free clear, colorless to slightly yellow solution for IV infusion. Each ml contains 10 mg of itraconazole, solubilized by hydroxypropyl-β-cyclodextrin (400 mg) as a molecular inclusion complex, with 3.8 μl hydrochloric acid, 25 μl propylene glycol, and sodium hydroxide for pH adjustment to 4.5, in water for injection. Sporanox injection is packaged in 25 ml colorless glass ampules, containing 250 mg of itraconazole, contents of which are diluted in 50 ml 0.9% sodium chloride injection (normal saline) prior to infusion. When properly administered, contents of 1 ampule will supply 200 mg of itraconazole.

CLINICAL PHARMACOLOGY

MICROBIOLOGY

Mechanism of Action

In vitro studies have demonstrated that itraconazole inhibits the cytochrome P450-dependent synthesis of ergosterol, which is a vital component of fungal cell membranes.

Activity In Vitro and In Vivo

Itraconazole exhibits *in vitro* activity against *Blastomyces dermatitidis, Histoplasma capsulatum, Histoplasma duboisii, Aspergillus flavus, Aspergillus fumigatus, Candida albicans,* and *Cryptococcus neoformans.* Itraconazole also exhibits varying *in vitro* activity against *Sporothrix schenckii, Trichophyton* species, *Candida krusei,* and other *Candida* species. The bioactive metabolite, hydroxyitraconazole, has not been evaluated against *Histoplasma capsulatum* and *Blastomyces dermatitidis.* Correlation between minimum inhibitory concentration (MIC) results *in vitro* and clinical outcome has yet to be established for azole antifungal agents.

Itraconazole administered orally was active in a variety of animal models of fungal infection using standard laboratory strains of fungi. Fungistatic activity has been demonstrated against disseminated fungal infections caused by *Blastomyces dermatitidis, Histoplasma duboisii, Aspergillus fumigatus, Coccidioides immitis, Cryptococcus neoformans, Paracoccidioides brasiliensis, Sporothrix schenckii, Trichophyton rubrum,* and *Trichophyton mentagrophytes.*

Itraconazole administered at 2.5 and 5 mg/kg via the oral and parenteral routes increased survival rates and sterilized organ systems in normal and immunosuppressed guinea pigs with disseminated *Aspergillus fumigatus* infections. Oral itraconazole administered daily at 40 mg/kg and 80 mg/kg increased survival rates in normal rabbits with disseminated disease and in immunosuppressed rats with pulmonary *Aspergillus fumigatus* infection, respectively. Itraconazole has demonstrated antifungal activity in a variety of animal models infected with *Candida albicans* and other *Candida* species.

Resistance

Isolates from several fungal species with decreased susceptibility to itraconazole have been isolated *in vitro* and from patients receiving prolonged therapy.

Several *in vitro* studies have reported that some fungal clinical isolates, including *Candida* species, with reduced susceptibility to one azole antifungal agent may also be less susceptible to other azole derivatives. The finding of cross-resistance is dependent on a number of factors, including the species evaluated, its clinical history, the particular azole compounds compared, and the type of susceptibility test that is performed. The relevance of these *in vitro* susceptibility data to clinical outcome remains to be elucidated.

Studies (both *in vitro* and *in vivo*) suggest that the activity of amphotericin B may be suppressed by prior azole antifungal therapy. As with other azoles, itraconazole inhibits the ^{14}C-demethylation step in the synthesis of ergosterol, a cell wall component of fungi. Ergosterol is the active site for amphotericin B. In one study the antifungal activity of amphotericin B against *Aspergillus fumigatus* infections in mice was inhibited by ketoconazole therapy. The clinical significance of test results obtained in this study is unknown.

PHARMACOKINETICS AND METABOLISM

Note: The plasma concentrations reported below were measured by high-performance liquid chromatography (HPLC) specific for itraconazole. When itraconazole in plasma is measured by a bioassay, values reported may be higher than those obtained by HPLC due to the presence of the bioactive metabolite, hydroxyitraconazole. (See Microbiology.)

The pharmacokinetics of itraconazole injection (200 mg bid for 2 days, then 200 mg qd for 5 days) followed by oral dosing of itraconazole capsules were studied in patients with advanced HIV infection. Steady-state plasma concentrations were reached after the fourth dose for itraconazole and by the seventh dose for hydroxyitraconazole. Steady-state plasma concentrations were maintained by administration of itraconazole capsules, 200 mg bid. Pharmacokinetic parameters for itraconazole and hydroxyitraconazole are presented in TABLE 1.

TABLE 1

	Injection Day 7 n=29		Capsules, 200 mg bid Day 36 n=12	
Parameter	Itraconazole	Hydroxyitraconazole	Itraconazole	Hydroxyitraconazole
C_{max} (ng/ml)	2856 ± 866*	1906 ± 612	2010 ± 1420	2614 ± 1703
T_{max} (h)	1.08 ± 0.14	8.53 ± 6.36	3.92 ± 1.83	5.92 ± 6.14
AUC(0-12h) (ng·h/ml)	—	—	18,768 ± 13,933	28,516 ± 19,149
AUC(0-24h) (ng·h/ml)	30,605 ± 8,961	42,445 ± 13,282	—	—

* Mean ± standard deviation.

The estimated mean ±SD half-life at steady-state of itraconazole after IV infusion was 35.4 ± 29.4 hours. In previous studies, the mean elimination half-life for itraconazole at steady-state after daily oral administration of 100-400 mg was 30-40 hours. Approximately 93-101% of hydroxypropyl-β-cyclodextrin was excreted unchanged in the urine within 12 hours after dosing.

The plasma protein binding of itraconazole is 99.8% and that of hydroxyitraconazole is 99.5%. Following IV administration, the volume of distribution of itraconazole averaged 796 ± 185 L.

Itraconazole is metabolized predominately by the cytochrome P450 3A4 isoenzyme system (CYP3A4), resulting in the formation of several metabolites, including hydroxyitraconazole, the major metabolite. Results of a pharmacokinetics study suggest that itraconazole may undergo saturable metabolism with multiple dosing. Fecal excretion of the parent drug varies between 3-18% of the dose. Renal excretion of the parent drug is less than 0.03% of the dose. About 40% of the dose is excreted as inactive metabolites in the urine. No single excreted metabolite represents more than 5% of a dose. Itraconazole total plasma clearance averaged 381 ± 95 ml/min following IV administration. Approximately 80-90% of hydroxypropyl-β-cyclodextrin is eliminated through the kidneys. (See CONTRAINDICATIONS and DRUG INTERACTIONS for more information.)

SPECIAL POPULATIONS

Renal Insufficiency

Plasma concentrations of itraconazole in patients with mild to moderate renal insufficiency were comparable to those obtained in healthy subjects. The majority of the 8 g dose of hydroxypropyl-β-cyclodextrin was eliminated in the urine during the 120 hour collection period in normal subjects and in patients with mild to severe renal insufficiency. Following a single IV dose of 200 mg to subjects with severe renal impairment (creatinine clearance ≤19 ml/min), clearance of hydroxypropyl-β-cyclodextrin was reduced 6-fold compared with subjects with normal renal function. Itraconazole injection should not be used in patients with creatinine clearance <30 ml/min.

Hepatic Insufficiency

Patients with impaired hepatic function should be carefully monitored when taking itraconazole. The prolonged elimination half-life of itraconazole observed in a clinical trial with itraconazole capsules in cirrhotic patients should be considered when deciding to initiate therapy with other medications metabolized by CYP3A4. (See BOXED WARNING, CONTRAINDICATIONS, and DRUG INTERACTIONS.)

Decreased Cardiac Contractility

When itraconazole was administered intravenously to anesthetized dogs, a dose-related negative inotropic effect was documented. In a healthy volunteer study of itraconazole injection (IV infusion), transient, asymptomatic decreases in left ventricular ejection fraction were observed using gated SPECT imaging; these resolved before the next infusion, 12 hours later. If signs or symptoms of congestive heart failure appear during administration of itraconazole injection, monitor carefully and consider other treatment alternatives which may include discontinuation of itraconazole injection administration. (See WARNINGS; DRUG INTERACTIONS; and ADVERSE REACTIONS, Post-Marketing Experience for more information.)

INDICATIONS AND USAGE

Itraconazole injection/oral solution is indicated for empiric therapy of febrile neutropenic patients with suspected fungal infections. (*Note:* In a comparative trial, the overall response rate for itraconazole-treated subjects was higher than for amphotericin B-treated subjects. However, compared to amphotericin B-treated subjects, a larger number of itraconazole-treated subjects discontinued treatment due to persistent fever and a change in antifungal medication due to fever. Whereas, a larger number of amphotericin B-treated subjects discontinued due to drug intolerance.

Itraconazole injection is also indicated for the treatment of the following fungal infections in immunocompromised and non-immunocompromised patients:

- Blastomycosis, pulmonary and extrapulmonary;
- Histoplasmosis, including chronic cavitary pulmonary disease and disseminated, non-meningeal histoplasmosis; and
- Aspergillosis, pulmonary and extrapulmonary, in patients who are intolerant of or who are refractory to amphotericin B therapy.

Specimens for fungal cultures and other relevant laboratory studies (wet mount, histopathology, serology) should be obtained prior to therapy to isolate and identify causative organisms. Therapy may be instituted before the results of the cultures and other laboratory studies are known; however, once these results become available, anti-infective therapy should be adjusted accordingly.

(See CLINICAL PHARMACOLOGY, Special Populations; WARNINGS; and ADVERSE REACTIONS, Post-Marketing Experience for more information.)

NON-FDA APPROVED INDICATIONS

Itraconazole has demonstrated clinical utility for the treatment of a number of other fungal infections including coccidioidomycosis, paracoccidioidomycosis, vaginal candidiasis, tinea versicolor, cryptococcosis, and sporotrichosis, although none of these indications are approved by the FDA.

CONTRAINDICATIONS

Drug Interactions: Concomitant administration of itraconazole capsules, injection, or oral solution and certain drugs metabolized by the cytochrome P450 3A4 isoenzyme system (CYP3A4) may result in increased plasma concentrations of those drugs, leading to potentially serious and/or life-threatening adverse events. Cisapride, oral midazolam, pimozide, quinidine, dofetilide and triazolam are contraindicated with itraconazole. HMG CoA-reductase inhibitors metabolized by CYP3A4, such as lovastatin and simvastatin, are also contraindicated with itraconazole. (See BOXED WARNING and DRUG INTERACTIONS.)

Itraconazole is contraindicated for patients who have shown hypersensitivity to itraconazole or its excipients. There is no information regarding cross-hypersensitivity between itraconazole and other azole antifungal agents. Caution should be used when prescribing itraconazole to patients with hypersensitivity to other azoles.

WARNINGS

Itraconazole injection contains the excipient hydroxypropyl-β-cyclodextrin which produced pancreatic adenocarcinomas in a rat carcinogenicity study. These findings were not observed in a similar mouse carcinogenicity study. The clinical relevance of these findings is unknown. (See PRECAUTIONS, Carcinogenesis, Mutagenesis, and Impairment of Fertility.)

HEPATIC EFFECTS

Itraconazole has been associated with rare cases of serious hepatotoxicity, including liver failure and death. Some of these cases had neither pre-existing liver disease nor a serious underlying medical condition and some of these cases developed within the first week of treatment. If clinical signs or symptoms develop that are consistent with liver disease, treatment should be discontinued and liver function testing performed. Continued itraconazole use or reinstitution of treatment with itraconazole is strongly discouraged unless there is a serious or life threatening situation where the expected benefit exceeds the risk. (See PRECAUTIONS, Information for the Patient; and ADVERSE REACTIONS.)

CARDIAC DYSRHYTHMIAS

Life-threatening cardiac dysrhythmias and/or sudden death have occurred in patients using cisapride, pimozide or quinidine concomitantly with itraconazole and/or other CYP3A4 inhibitors. Concomitant administration of these drugs with itraconazole is contraindicated. (See BOXED WARNING, CONTRAINDICATIONS, and DRUG INTERACTIONS.)

CARDIAC DISEASE

Itraconazole injection should not be used in patients with evidence of ventricular dysfunction unless the benefit clearly outweighs the risk. For patients with risk factors for congestive heart failure, physicians should carefully review the risks and benefits of itraconazole therapy. These risk factors include cardiac disease such as ischemic and valvular disease; significant pulmonary disease such as chronic obstructive pulmonary disease; and renal failure and other edematous disorders. Such patients should be informed of the signs and symptoms of CHF, should be treated with caution, and should be monitored for signs and symptoms of CHF during treatment. If signs or symptoms of CHF appear during administration of itraconazole injection, monitor carefully and consider other treatment alternatives which may include discontinuation of itraconazole injection administration.

When itraconazole was administered intravenously to anesthetized dogs, a dose-related negative inotropic effect was documented. In a healthy volunteer study of itraconazole injection (IV infusion), transient, asymptomatic decreases in left ventricular ejection fraction were observed using gated SPECT imaging; these resolved before the next infusion, 12 hours later.

Cases of CHF, peripheral edema, and pulmonary edema have been reported in the post-marketing period among patients being treated for onychomycosis and/or systemic fungal infections. (See CLINICAL PHARMACOLOGY, Special Populations; DRUG INTERACTIONS; and ADVERSE REACTIONS, Post-Marketing Experience for more information.)

PRECAUTIONS

GENERAL

Rare cases of serious hepatotoxicity have been observed with itraconazole treatment, including some cases within the first week. In patients with elevated or abnormal liver enzymes or active liver disease, or who have experienced liver toxicity with other drugs, treatment with itraconazole is strongly discouraged unless there is a serious or life threatening situation where the expected benefit exceeds the risk. Liver function monitoring should be done in patients with pre-existing hepatic function abnormalities or those who have experienced liver toxicity with other medications and should be considered in all patients receiving itraconazole. Treatment should be stopped immediately and liver function testing should be conducted in patients who develop signs and symptoms suggestive of liver dysfunction.

If neuropathy occurs that may be attributable to itraconazole injection, the treatment should be discontinued.

As severe renal impairment prolongs the elimination rate of hydroxypropyl-β-cyclodextrin, itraconazole injection should not be used in patients with severe renal dysfunction (creatinine clearance <30 ml/min). (See CLINICAL PHARMACOLOGY, Special Populations.)

INFORMATION FOR THE PATIENT

Itraconazole injection contains the excipient hydroxypropyl-β-cyclodextrin which produced pancreatic adenocarcinomas in a rat carcinogenicity study. These findings were not observed in a similar mouse carcinogenicity study. The clinical relevance of these findings is unknown. (See Carcinogenesis, Mutagenesis, and Impairment of Fertility.)

CARCINOGENESIS, MUTAGENESIS, AND IMPAIRMENT OF FERTILITY

Itraconazole showed no evidence of carcinogenicity potential in mice treated orally for 23 months at dosage levels up to 80 mg/kg/day (approximately 10× the maximum recommended human dose [MRHD]). Male rats treated with 25 mg/kg/day (3.1× MRHD) had a slightly increased incidence of soft tissue sarcoma. These sarcomas may have been a consequence of hypercholesterolemia, which is a response of rats, but not dogs or humans, to chronic itraconazole administration. Female rats treated with 50 mg/kg/day (6.25× MRHD) had an increased incidence of squamous cell carcinoma of the lung (2/50) as compared to the untreated group. Although the occurrence of squamous cell carcinoma in the lung is extremely uncommon in untreated rats, the increase in this study was not statistically significant.

Hydroxypropyl-β-cyclodextrin (HP-β-CD), the solubilizing excipient used in itraconazole injection and oral solution, was found to produce pancreatic exocrine hyperplasia and neoplasia when administered orally to rats at doses of 500, 2000 or 5000 mg/kg/day for 25 months. Adenocarcinomas of the exocrine pancreas produced in the treated animals were not seen in the untreated group and are not reported in the historical controls. Development of these tumors may be related to a mitogenic action of cholecystokinin. This finding was not observed in the mouse carcinogenicity study at doses of 500, 2000 or 5000 mg/kg/day for 22-23 months; however, the clinical relevance of these findings is unknown. Based on body surface area comparisons, the exposure to humans of HP-β-CD at the recommended clinical dose of itraconazole oral solution, is approximately equivalent to 1.7 times the exposure at the lowest dose in the rat study. The relevance of the findings with orally administered HP-β-CD to potential carcinogenic effects for itraconazole injection is uncertain.

Itraconazole produced no mutagenic effects when assayed in a DNA repair test (unscheduled DNA synthesis) in primary rat hepatocytes, in Ames tests with *Salmonella typhimurium* (6 strains) and *Escherichia coli*, in the mouse lymphoma gene mutation tests, in a sex-linked recessive lethal mutation (*Drosophila melanogaster*) test, in chromosome aberration tests in human lymphocytes, in a cell transformation test with C3H/10T½C18 mouse embryo fibroblasts cells, in a dominant lethal mutation test in male and female mice, and in micronucleus tests in mice and rats.

Itraconazole did not affect the fertility of male or female rats treated orally with dosage levels of up to 40 mg/kg/day (5× MRHD), even though parental toxicity was present at this dosage level. More severe signs of parental toxicity, including death, were present in the next higher dosage level, 160 mg/kg/day (20× MRHD).

PREGNANCY, TERATOGENIC EFFECTS, PREGNANCY CATEGORY C

Itraconazole was found to cause a dose-related increase in maternal toxicity, embryotoxicity, and teratogenicity in rats at dosage levels of approximately 40-160 mg/kg/day (5-20× MRHD), and in mice at dosage levels of approximately 80 mg/kg/day (10× MRHD). In rats, the teratogenicity consisted of major skeletal defects; in mice, it consisted of encephaloceles and/or macroglossia.

There are no studies in pregnant women. Itraconazole should be used for the treatment of systemic fungal infections in pregnancy only if the benefit outweighs the potential risk.

NURSING MOTHERS

Itraconazole is excreted in human milk; therefore, the expected benefits of itraconazole therapy for the mother should be weighed against the potential risk from exposure of itraconazole to the infant. The US Public Health Service Centers for Disease Control and Prevention advises HIV-infected women not to breast-feed to avoid potential transmission of HIV to uninfected infants.

PEDIATRIC USE

The efficacy and safety of itraconazole have not been established in pediatric patients. No pharmacokinetic data on itraconazole capsules or injection are available in children. A small number of patients ages 3-16 years have been treated with 100 mg/day of itraconazole capsules for systemic fungal infections, and no serious unexpected adverse effects have been reported. Itraconazole oral solution (5 mg/kg/day) has been administered to pediatric patients (n=26, ages 6 months to 12 years) for 2 weeks and no serious unexpected adverse events were reported.

The long-term effects of itraconazole on bone growth in children are unknown. In three toxicology studies using rats, itraconazole induced bone defects at dosage levels as low as 20 mg/kg/day (2.5× MRHD). The induced defects included reduced bone plate activity, thinning of the zona compacta of the large bones, and increased bone fragility. At a dosage level of 80 mg/kg/day (10× MRHD) over 1 year or 160 mg/kg/day (20× MRHD) for 6 months, itraconazole induced small tooth pulp with hypocellular appearance in some rats. No such bone toxicity has been reported in adult patients.

GERIATRIC USE

Clinical studies of itraconazole injection did not include sufficient numbers of subjects aged 65 and over to determine whether they respond differently from younger subjects. Other reported clinical experience has not identified differences in responses between the elderly and younger patients. In general, dose selection for an elderly patient should be cautious, reflecting the greater frequency of decreased hepatic, renal, or cardiac function, and of concomitant disease or other drug therapy.

DRUG INTERACTIONS

Itraconazole and its major metabolite, hydroxyitraconazole, are inhibitors of CYP3A4. Therefore, the following drug interactions may occur (see TABLE 3 and the following drug class subheadings that follow):

Itraconazole may decrease the elimination of drugs metabolized by CYP3A4, resulting in increased plasma concentrations of these drugs when they are administered with itraconazole. These elevated plasma concentrations may increase or prolong both therapeutic and adverse effects of these drugs. Whenever possible, plasma concentrations of these drugs should be monitored, and dosage adjustments made after concomitant itraconazole therapy is initiated. When appropriate, clinical monitoring for signs or symptoms of increased or prolonged pharmacologic effects is advised. Upon discontinuation, depending on the dose and duration of treatment, itraconazole plasma concentrations decline gradually (especially in patients with hepatic cirrhosis or in those receiving CYP3A4 inhibitors). This is particularly important when initiating therapy with drugs whose metabolism is affected by itraconazole.

Inducers of CYP3A4 may decrease the plasma concentrations of itraconazole. Itraconazole may not be effective in patients concomitantly taking itraconazole and one of these drugs. Therefore, administration of these drugs with itraconazole is not recommended.

Other inhibitors of CYP3A4 may increase the plasma concentrations of itraconazole. Patients who must take itraconazole concomitantly with one of these drugs should be monitored closely for signs or symptoms of increased or prolonged pharmacologic effects of itraconazole.

ANTIARRHYTHMICS

The Class IA antiarrhythmic quinidine and Class III antiarrhythmic dofetilide are known to prolong the QT interval. Coadministration of quinidine or dofetilide with itraconazole may increase plasma concentrations of quinidine or dofetilide which could result in serious cardiovascular events. Therefore, concomitant administration of itraconazole and quinidine or

I

TABLE 3 *Selected Drugs That Are Predicted to Alter the Plasma Concentration of Itraconazole or Have Their Plasma Concentration Altered by Itraconazole**

Drug Plasma Concentration Increased by Itraconazole	
Antiarrhythmics	Digoxin, dofetilide†, quinidine†
Anticonvulsants	Carbamazepine
Antimycobacterials	Rifabutin
Antineoplastics	Busulfan, docetaxel, vinca alkaloids
Antipsychotics	Pimozide†
Benzodiazepines	Alprazolam, diazepam, midazolam†‡, triazolam†
Calcium channel blockers	Dihydropyridines, verapamil
Gastrointestinal motility agents	Cisapride†
HMG CoA-reductase inhibitors	Atorvastatin, cerivastatin, lovastatin†, simvastatin†
Immunosuppressants	Cyclosporine, tacrolimus, sirolimus
Oral hypoglycemics	Oral hypoglycemics
Protease inhibitors	Indinavir, ritonavir, saquinavir
Other	Alfentanil, buspirone, methylprednisolone, trimetrexate, warfarin
Decrease Plasma Concentration of Itraconazole	
Anticonvulsants	Carbamazepine, phenobarbital, phenytoin
Antimycobacterials	Isoniazid, rifabutin, rifampin
Reverse transcriptase inhibitors	Nevirapine
Increase Plasma Concentration of Itraconazole	
Macrolide antibiotics	Clarithromycin, erythromycin
Protease inhibitors	Indinavir, ritonavir

* This list is not all-inclusive.
† Contraindicated with itraconazole based on clinical and/or pharmacokinetics studies. (See WARNINGS and below.)
‡ For information on parenterally administered midazolam, see Benzodiazepines.

dofetilide is contraindicated. (See BOXED WARNING, CONTRAINDICATIONS, and WARNINGS.)

Concomitant administration of digoxin and itraconazole has led to increased plasma concentrations of digoxin.

ANTICONVULSANTS

Reduced plasma concentrations of itraconazole were reported when itraconazole was administered concomitantly with phenytoin. Carbamazepine, phenobarbital, and phenytoin are all inducers of CYP3A4. Although interactions with carbamazepine and phenobarbital have not been studied, concomitant administration of itraconazole and these drugs would be expected to result in decreased plasma concentrations of itraconazole. In addition, *in vivo* studies have demonstrated an increase in plasma carbamazepine concentrations in subjects concomitantly receiving ketoconazole. Although there are no data regarding the effect of itraconazole on carbamazepine metabolism, because of the similarities between ketoconazole and itraconazole, concomitant administration of itraconazole and carbamazepine may inhibit the metabolism of carbamazepine.

ANTIMYCOBACTERIALS

Drug interaction studies have demonstrated that plasma concentrations of azole antifungal agents and their metabolites, including itraconazole and hydroxyitraconazole, were significantly decreased when these agents were given concomitantly with rifabutin or rifampin. *In vivo* data suggest that rifabutin is metabolized in part by CYP3A4. Itraconazole may inhibit the metabolism of rifabutin. Although no formal study data are available for isoniazid, similar effects should be anticipated. Therefore, the efficacy of itraconazole could be substantially reduced if given concomitantly with one of these agents. Coadministration is not recommended.

ANTINEOPLASTICS

Itraconazole may inhibit the metabolism of busulfan, docetaxel, and vinca alkaloids.

ANTIPSYCHOTICS

Pimozide is known to prolong the QT interval and is partially metabolized by CYP3A4. Coadministration of pimozide with itraconazole could result in serious cardiovascular events. Therefore, concomitant administration of itraconazole and pimozide is contraindicated. (See BOXED WARNING, CONTRAINDICATIONS, and WARNINGS.)

BENZODIAZEPINES

Concomitant administration of itraconazole and alprazolam, diazepam, oral midazolam, or triazolam could lead to increased plasma concentrations of these benzodiazepines. Increased plasma concentrations could potentiate and prolong hypnotic and sedative effects. Concomitant administration of itraconazole and oral midazolam or triazolam is contraindicated. (See CONTRAINDICATIONS and WARNINGS.) If midazolam is administered parenterally, special precaution and patient monitoring is required since the sedative effect may be prolonged.

CALCIUM CHANNEL BLOCKERS

Edema has been reported in patients concomitantly receiving itraconazole and dihydropyridine calcium channel blockers. Appropriate dosage adjustment may be necessary.

Calcium channel blockers can have a negative inotropic effect which may be additive to those of itraconazole; itraconazole can inhibit the metabolism of calcium channel blockers such as dihydropyridines (*e.g.*, nifedipine and felodipine) and verapamil. Therefore, caution should be used when coadministering itraconazole and calcium channel blockers. (See CLINICAL PHARMACOLOGY, Special Populations; WARNINGS; and ADVERSE REACTIONS, Post-Marketing Experience for more information.)

GASTROINTESTINAL MOTILITY AGENTS

Coadministration of itraconazole with cisapride can elevate plasma cisapride concentrations which could result in serious cardiovascular events. Therefore, concomitant administration of itraconazole with cisapride is contraindicated. (See BOXED WARNING, CONTRAINDICATIONS, and WARNINGS.)

HMG COA-REDUCTASE INHIBITORS

Human pharmacokinetic data suggest that itraconazole inhibits the metabolism of atorvastatin, cerivastatin, lovastatin, and simvastatin, which may increase the risk of skeletal muscle toxicity, including rhabdomyolysis. Concomitant administration of itraconazole with HMG CoA-reductase inhibitors, such as lovastatin and simvastatin, is contraindicated. (See CONTRAINDICATIONS and WARNINGS.)

IMMUNOSUPPRESSANTS

Concomitant administration of itraconazole and cyclosporine or tacrolimus has led to increased plasma concentrations of these immunosuppressants. Concomitant administration of itraconazole and sirolimus could increase plasma concentrations of sirolimus.

MACROLIDE ANTIBIOTICS

Erythromycin and clarithromycin are known inhibitors of CYP3A4 (see TABLE 3) and may increase plasma concentrations of itraconazole. In a small pharmacokinetic study involving HIV infected patients, clarithromycin was shown to increase plasma concentrations of itraconazole. Similarly, following administration of 1 g of erythromycin ethyl succinate and 200 mg itraconazole as single doses, the mean C_{max} and AUC(0-∞) of itraconazole increased by 44% (90% CI: 119-175%) and 36% (90% CI: 108-171%), respectively.

ORAL HYPOGLYCEMIC AGENTS

Severe hypoglycemia has been reported in patients concomitantly receiving azole antifungal agents and oral hypoglycemic agents. Blood glucose concentrations should be carefully monitored when itraconazole and oral hypoglycemic agents are coadministered.

POLYENES

Prior treatment with itraconazole, like other azoles, may reduce or inhibit the activity of polyenes such as amphotericin B. However, the clinical significance of this drug effect has not been clearly defined.

PROTEASE INHIBITORS

Concomitant administration of itraconazole and protease inhibitors metabolized by CYP3A4, such as indinavir, ritonavir, and saquinavir, may increase plasma concentrations of these protease inhibitors. In addition, concomitant administration of itraconazole and indinavir and ritonavir (but not saquinavir) may increase plasma concentrations of itraconazole. Caution is advised when itraconazole and protease inhibitors must be given concomitantly.

REVERSE TRANSCRIPTASE INHIBITORS

Nevirapine is an inducer of CYP3A4. *In vivo* studies have shown that nevirapine induces the metabolism of ketoconazole, significantly reducing the bioavailability of ketoconazole. Studies involving nevirapine and itraconazole have not been conducted. However, because of the similarities between ketoconazole and itraconazole, concomitant administration of itraconazole and nevirapine is not recommended. In a clinical study, when 8 HIV-infected subjects were treated concomitantly with itraconazole capsules 100 mg twice daily and the nucleoside reverse transcriptase inhibitor zidovudine 8 ± 0.4 mg/kg/day, the pharmacokinetics of zidovudine were not affected. Other nucleoside reverse transcriptase inhibitors have not been studied.

OTHER

- *In vitro* data suggest that alfentanil is metabolized by CYP3A4. Administration with itraconazole may increase plasma concentrations of alfentanil.
- Human pharmacokinetic data suggest that concomitant administration of itraconazole and buspirone results in significant increases in plasma concentrations of buspirone.
- Itraconazole may inhibit the metabolism of methylprednisolone.
- *In vitro* data suggest that trimetrexate is extensively metabolized by CYP3A4. *In vitro* animal models have demonstrated that ketoconazole potently inhibits the metabolism of trimetrexate. Although there are no data regarding the effect of itraconazole on trimetrexate metabolism, because of the similarities between ketoconazole and itraconazole, concomitant administration of itraconazole and trimetrexate may inhibit the metabolism of trimetrexate.
- Itraconazole enhances the anticoagulant effect of coumarin-like drugs, such as warfarin.

ADVERSE REACTIONS

Itraconazole has been associated with rare cases of serious hepatotoxicity, including liver failure and death. Some of these cases had neither pre-existing liver disease nor a serious underlying medical condition. If clinical signs or symptoms develop that are consistent with liver disease, treatment should be discontinued and liver function testing performed. The risks and benefits of itraconazole use should be reassessed. (See WARNINGS, Hepatic Effects; and PRECAUTIONS: General and Information for the Patient.)

ADVERSE EVENTS REPORTED IN TRIALS IN PATIENTS WITH ITRACONAZOLE INJECTION

Adverse events considered at least possibly drug related are shown in TABLE 4 and are based on the experience of 360 patients treated with itraconazole injection in four pharmacokinetic, one uncontrolled and four active controlled studies where the control was amphotericin B or fluconazole. Nearly all patients were neutropenic or were otherwise immunocompromised and were treated empirically for febrile episodes, for documented systemic fungal infections, or in trials to determine pharmacokinetics. The dose of itraconazole injection was 200 mg twice daily for the first 2 days followed by a single daily dose of 200 mg for the remainder of the IV treatment period. The majority of patients received between 7 and 14 days of itraconazole injection.

TABLE 4 *Summary of Possibly or Definitely Drug-Related Adverse Events Reported by ≥2% of Subjects*

Adverse Event	Total Itraconazole Injection (n=360)	Comparative Studies: Itraconazole Injection (n=234)	IV Fluconazole (n=32)	IV Amphotericin B (n=202)
Gastrointestinal System Disorders				
Nausea	8%	9%	0%	15%
Diarrhea	6%	6%	3%	9%
Vomiting	4%	6%	0%	10%
Abdominal pain	2%	2%	0%	3%
Constipation	0%	1%	3%	0%
Metabolic and Nutritional Disorders				
Hypokalemia	5%	8%	0%	29%
Alkaline phosphatase increased	1%	2%	3%	2%
Serum creatinine increased	2%	2%	3%	26%
Hypomagnesemia	1%	1%	0%	5%
Blood urea nitrogen increased	0%	1%	0%	7%
Fluid overload	0%	0%	0%	3%
Hypocalcemia	0%	0%	0%	3%
Liver and Biliary System Disorders				
Bilirubinemia	4%	6%	9%	3%
SGPT/ALT increased	2%	3%	3%	1%
Hepatic function abnormal	1%	2%	0%	2%
Jaundice	1%	2%	0%	0%
SGOT/AST increased	1%	2%	0%	0%
Body as a Whole — General Disorders				
Pain	1%	2%	0%	0%
Rigors	0%	0%	0%	34%
Fever	0%	0%	0%	6%
Skin and Appendages Disorders				
Rash	3%	3%	3%	3%
Sweating increased	1%	2%	0%	0%
Respiratory System Disorder				
Dyspnea	0%	0%	0%	3%
Central and Peripheral Nervous System Disorders				
Dizziness	1%	2%	0%	1%
Headache	2%	2%	0%	3%
Urinary System Disorders				
Renal function abnormal	1%	1%	0%	11%
Application Site Disorder				
Application site reaction	4%	0%	0%	0%
Cardiovascular Disorders, General				
Hypotension	0%	0%	0%	3%
Hypertension	0%	0%	0%	2%
Heart Rate and Rythym Disorders				
Tachycardia	0%	1%	0%	3%
Vascular (Extracardiac) Disorders				
Vein disorder	3%	0%	0%	0%

The following adverse events occurred in less than 2% of patients in clinical trials of itraconazole injection: LDH increased, edema, albuminuria, hyperglycemia, and hepatitis.

POST-MARKETING EXPERIENCE

Worldwide post-marketing experiences with the use of itraconazole include adverse events of gastrointestinal origin, such as dyspepsia, nausea, vomiting, diarrhea, abdominal pain and constipation. Other reported adverse events include peripheral edema, congestive heart failure and pulmonary edema, headache, dizziness, peripheral neuropathy, menstrual disorders, reversible increases in hepatic enzymes, hepatitis, liver failure, hypokalemia, hypertriglyceridemia, alopecia, allergic reactions (such as pruritus, rash, urticaria, angioedema, anaphylaxis), Stevens-Johnson syndrome, and neutropenia. (See CLINICAL PHARMACOLOGY, Special Populations; CONTRAINDICATIONS; WARNINGS; and DRUG INTERACTIONS for more information.)

DOSAGE AND ADMINISTRATION

Use only the components [itraconazole injection ampule, 0.9% sodium chloride injection (normal saline) bag and filtered infusion set] provided in the kit: **DO NOT SUBSTITUTE.**

Itraconazole injection should not be diluted with 5% dextrose injection or with lactated Ringer's injection alone or in combination with any other diluent. The compatibility of itraconazole injection with diluents other than 0.9% sodium chloride injection (normal saline) is not known. **NOT FOR IV BOLUS INJECTION.**

Note: After reconstitution, the diluted itraconazole injection may be stored refrigerated (2-8°C) or at room temperature (15-25°C) for up to 48 hours, when protected from direct light. During administration, exposure to normal room light is acceptable.

Note: Use only a dedicated infusion line for administration of itraconazole injection. Do not introduce concomitant medication in the same bag nor through the same line as itraconazole injection. Other medications may be administered after flushing the line/catheter with 0.9% sodium chloride injection as described below, and removing and replacing the entire infusion line. Alternatively, utilize another lumen, in the case of a multi-lumen catheter.

Correct preparation and administration of itraconazole injection are necessary to ensure maximal efficacy and safety. A precise mixing ratio is required in order to obtain a stable admixture. It is critical to maintain a 3.33 mg/ml itraconazole:diluent ratio. Failure to maintain this concentration will lead to the formation of a precipitate.

Add the full contents (25 ml) of the itraconazole injection ampule into the infusion bag provided, which contains 50 ml of 0.9% sodium chloride injection (normal saline). Mix gently after the solution is completely transferred. Withdraw and discard 15 ml of the solution before administering to the patient. Using a flow control device, infuse 60 ml of the dilute solution (3.33 mg/ml = 200 mg itraconazole, pH apx. 4.8) intravenously over 60 minutes, using an extension line and the infusion set provided. After administration, flush the infusion set with 15-20 ml of 0.9% sodium chloride injection over 30 seconds to 15 minutes, via the two-way stopcock. Do not use bacteriostatic sodium chloride injection. The compatibility of itraconazole injection with flush solutions other than 0.9% sodium chloride injection (normal saline) is not known. Discard the entire infusion line.

Parenteral drug products should be inspected visually for particulate matter and discoloration prior to administration, whenever solution and container permit.

EMPIRIC THERAPY IN FEBRILE, NEUTROPENIC PATIENTS WITH SUSPECTED FUNGAL INFECTIONS (ETFN)

The recommended dose of itraconazole injection is 200 mg bid for 4 doses, followed by 200 mg once daily for up to 14 days. Each IV dose should be infused over 1 hour. Treatment should be continued with itraconazole oral solution 200 mg (20 ml) bid until resolution of clinically significant neutropenia. The safety and efficacy of itraconazole use exceeding 28 days in ETFN is not known.

TREATMENT OF BLASTOMYCOSIS, HISTOPLASMOSIS AND ASPERGILLOSIS

The recommended IV dose is 200 mg bid for 4 doses, followed by 200 mg qd. Each IV dose should be infused over 1 hour.

For the treatment of blastomycosis, histoplasmosis and aspergillosis, itraconazole can be given as oral capsules or intravenously. The safety and efficacy of itraconazole injection administered for greater than 14 days is not known.

Total itraconazole therapy (itraconazole injection followed by itraconazole capsules) should be continued for a minimum of 3 months and until clinical parameters and laboratory tests indicate that the active fungal infection has subsided. An inadequate period of treatment may lead to recurrence of active infection.

Itraconazole injection should not be used in patients with creatinine clearance <30 ml/min.

HOW SUPPLIED

Sporanox (itraconazole) injection for IV infusion is supplied as a kit, containing one 25 ml colorless glass ampule of itraconazole 10 mg/ml sterile, pyrogen-free solution, one 50 ml bag (100 ml capacity) of 0.9% sodium chloride injection (normal saline) and 1 filtered infusion set.

Storage: Store at or below 25°C (77°F). Protect from light and freezing.

ORAL

WARNING

Congestive Heart Failure

Itraconazole capsules should not be administered for the treatment of onychomycosis in patients with evidence of ventricular dysfunction such as congestive heart failure (CHF) or a history of CHF. If signs or symptoms of congestive heart failure occur during administration of itraconazole oral solution, continued itraconazole use should be reassessed. If signs or symptoms of congestive heart failure occur during administration of itraconazole capsules, discontinue administration. When itraconazole was administered intravenously to dogs and healthy human volunteers, negative inotropic effects were seen. (See CLINICAL PHARMACOLOGY, Special Populations; CONTRAINDICATIONS; WARNINGS; DRUG INTERACTIONS; and ADVERSE REACTIONS, Post-Marketing Experience: Capsules and Oral Solution for more information.)

Drug Interactions

Coadministration of cisapride, pimozide, quinidine, or dofetilide with itraconazole capsules, injection or oral solution is contraindicated. Itraconazole, a potent cytochrome P450 3A4 isoenzyme system (CYP3A4) inhibitor, may increase plasma concentrations of drugs metabolized by this pathway. Serious cardiovascular events, including QT prolongation, torsades de pointes, ventricular tachycardia, cardiac arrest, and/or sudden death have occurred in patients using cisapride, pimozide, or quinidine, concomitantly with itraconazole and/or other CYP3A4 inhibitors. (See CONTRAINDICATIONS, WARNINGS, and DRUG INTERACTIONS for more information.)

DESCRIPTION

Itraconazole is a synthetic triazole antifungal agent. Itraconazole is a 1:1:1:1 racemic mixture of four diastereomers (two enantiomeric pairs), each possessing three chiral centers. It may be represented by the following nomenclature:

(±)-1-[(R*)-sec-butyl]-4-[p-[4-[p-[[(2R*,4S*)-2-(2,4-dichlorophenyl)-2-(1H-1,2,4-triazol-1-ylmethyl)-1,3-dioxolan-4-yl]methoxy]phenyl]-1-piperazinyl]phenyl]-Δ^2-1,2,4-triazolin-5-one mixture with (±)-1-[(R*)-sec-butyl]-4-[p-[4-[p-[[(2S*,4R*)-2-(2,4-dichlorophenyl)-2-(1H-1,2,4-triazol-1-ylmethyl)-1,3-dioxolan-4-yl]methoxy]phenyl]-1-piperazinyl]phenyl]-Δ^2-1,2,4-triazolin-5-one **or** (±)-1-[(RS)-sec-butyl]-4-[p-[4-[p-[[(2R,4S)-2-(2,4-dichlorophenyl)-2-(1H-1,2,4-triazol-1-ylmethyl)-1,3-dioxolan-4-yl]methoxy]phenyl]-1-piperazinyl]phenyl]-Δ^2-1,2,4-triazolin-5-one.

Itraconazole has a molecular formula of $C_{35}H_{38}Cl_2N_8O_4$ and a molecular weight of 705.64. It is a white to slightly yellowish powder. It is insoluble in water, very slightly soluble in alcohols, and freely soluble in dichloromethane. It has a pKa of 3.70 (based on extrapolation of values obtained from methanolic solutions) and a log (n-octanol/water) partition coefficient of 5.66 at pH 8.1.

CAPSULES

Sporanox capsules contain 100 mg of itraconazole coated on sugar spheres. Inactive ingredients are gelatin, hydroxypropyl methylcellulose, polyethylene glycol (PEG) 20,000, starch, sucrose, titanium dioxide, FD&C blue no. 1, FD&C blue no. 2, D&C red no. 22 and D&C red no. 28.

ORAL SOLUTION

Sporanox (itraconazole) oral solution contains 10 mg of itraconazole per ml, solubilized by hydroxypropyl-β-cyclodextrin (400 mg/ml) as a molecular inclusion complex. Sporanox oral solution is clear and yellowish in color with a target pH of 2. Other ingredients are hydrochloric acid, propylene glycol, purified water, sodium hydroxide, sodium saccharin, sorbitol, cherry flavor 1, cherry flavor 2 and caramel flavor.

CLINICAL PHARMACOLOGY

MICROBIOLOGY

Mechanism of Action

In vitro studies have demonstrated that itraconazole inhibits the cytochrome P450-dependent synthesis of ergosterol, which is a vital component of fungal cell membranes.

Activity In Vitro and In Vivo

Itraconazole exhibits *in vitro* activity against *Blastomyces dermatitidis, Histoplasma capsulatum, Histoplasma duboisii, Aspergillus flavus, Aspergillus fumigatus, Candida albicans,* and *Cryptococcus neoformans.* Itraconazole also exhibits varying *in vitro* activity against *Sporothrix schenckii, Trichophyton* species, *Candida krusei,* and other *Candida* species. The bioactive metabolite, hydroxyitraconazole, has not been evaluated against *Histoplasma capsulatum* and *Blastomyces dermatitidis.* Correlation between minimum inhibitory concentration (MIC) results *in vitro* and clinical outcome has yet to be established for azole antifungal agents.

Itraconazole administered orally was active in a variety of animal models of fungal infection using standard laboratory strains of fungi. Fungistatic activity has been demonstrated against disseminated fungal infections caused by *Blastomyces dermatitidis, Histoplasma duboisii, Aspergillus fumigatus, Coccidioides immitis, Cryptococcus neoformans, Paracoccidioides brasiliensis, Sporothrix schenckii, Trichophyton rubrum,* and *Trichophyton mentagrophytes.*

I

Itraconazole administered at 2.5 and 5 mg/kg via the oral and parenteral routes increased survival rates and sterilized organ systems in normal and immunosuppressed guinea pigs with disseminated *Aspergillus fumigatus* infections. Oral itraconazole administered daily at 40 mg/kg and 80 mg/kg increased survival rates in normal rabbits with disseminated disease and in immunosuppressed rats with pulmonary *Aspergillus fumigatus* infection, respectively. Itraconazole has demonstrated antifungal activity in a variety of animal models infected with *Candida albicans* and other *Candida* species.

Resistance

Isolates from several fungal species with decreased susceptibility to itraconazole have been isolated *in vitro* and from patients receiving prolonged therapy.

Several *in vitro* studies have reported that some fungal clinical isolates, including *Candida* species, with reduced susceptibility to one azole antifungal agent may also be less susceptible to other azole derivatives. The finding of cross-resistance is dependent on a number of factors, including the species evaluated, its clinical history, the particular azole compounds compared, and the type of susceptibility test that is performed. The relevance of these *in vitro* susceptibility data to clinical outcome remains to be elucidated.

Studies (both *in vitro* and *in vivo*) suggest that the activity of amphotericin B may be suppressed by prior azole antifungal therapy. As with other azoles, itraconazole inhibits the ^{14}C-demethylation step in the synthesis of ergosterol, a cell wall component of fungi. Ergosterol is the active site for amphotericin B. In one study the antifungal activity of amphotericin B against *Aspergillus fumigatus* infections in mice was inhibited by ketoconazole therapy. The clinical significance of test results obtained in this study is unknown.

PHARMACOKINETICS AND METABOLISM

Capsules

NOTE: The plasma concentrations reported below were measured by high-performance liquid chromatography (HPLC) specific for itraconazole. When itraconazole in plasma is measured by a bioassay, values reported are approximately 3.3 times higher than those obtained by HPLC due to the presence of the bioactive metabolite, hydroxyitraconazole. (See Microbiology.)

The pharmacokinetics of itraconazole after IV administration and its absolute oral bioavailability from an oral solution were studied in a randomized crossover study in 6 healthy male volunteers. The observed absolute oral bioavailability of itraconazole was 55%.

The oral bioavailability of itraconazole is maximal when itraconazole capsules are taken with a full meal. The pharmacokinetics of itraconazole were studied in 6 healthy male volunteers who received, in a crossover design, single 100 mg doses of itraconazole as a polyethylene glycol capsule, with or without a full meal. The same 6 volunteers also received 50 or 200 mg with a full meal in a crossover design. In this study, only itraconazole plasma concentrations were measured. The respective pharmacokinetic parameters for itraconazole are presented in TABLE 5.

TABLE 5

	50 mg (fed)	100 mg (fed)	100 mg (fasted)	200 mg (fed)
C_{max} (ng/ml)	45 ± 16*	132 ± 67	38 ± 20	289 ± 100
T_{max} (hours)	3.2 ± 1.3	4.0 ± 1.1	3.3 ± 1.0	4.7 ± 1.4
AUC(0-∞) (ng·h/ml)	567 ± 264	1899 ± 838	722 ± 289	5211 ± 2116

* Mean ± standard deviation.

Doubling the itraconazole dose results in approximately a 3-fold increase in the itraconazole plasma concentrations.

Values given in TABLE 6 represent data from a crossover pharmacokinetics study in which 27 healthy male volunteers each took a single 200 mg dose of itraconazole capsules with or without a full meal.

Absorption of itraconazole under fasted conditions in individuals with relative or absolute achlorhydria, such as patients with AIDS or volunteers taking gastric acid secretion suppressors (*e.g.,* H_2 receptor antagonists), was increased when itraconazole capsules were administered with a cola beverage. Eighteen (18) men with AIDS received single 200 mg doses of itraconazole capsules under fasted conditions with 8 oz of water or 8 oz of a cola beverage in a crossover design. The absorption of itraconazole was increased when itraconazole capsules were coadministered with a cola beverage, with AUC(0-24) and C_{max} increasing 75% ± 121% and 95% ± 128%, respectively.

TABLE 6

	Itraconazole		Hydroxyitraconazole	
	Fed	Fasted	Fed	Fasted
C_{max} (ng/ml)	239 ± 85*	140 ± 65	397 ± 103	286 ± 101
T_{max} (hours)	4.5 ± 1.1	3.9 ± 1.0	5.1 ± 1.6	4.5 ± 1.1
AUC(0-∞) (ng·h/ml)	3423 ± 1154	2094 ± 905	7978 ± 2648	5191 ± 2489
T½ (hours)	21 ± 5	21 ± 7	12 ± 3	12 ± 3

* Mean ± standard deviation.

Thirty (30) healthy men received single 200 mg doses of itraconazole capsules under fasted conditions either (1) with water; (2) with water, after ranitidine 150 mg bid for 3 days; or (3) with cola, after ranitidine 150 mg bid for 3 days. When itraconazole capsules were administered after ranitidine pretreatment, itraconazole was absorbed to a lesser extent than when itraconazole capsules were administered alone, with decreases in AUC(0-24) and C_{max} of 39% ± 37% and 42% ± 39%, respectively. When itraconazole capsules were administered with cola after ranitidine pretreatment, itraconazole absorption was comparable to that observed when itraconazole capsules were administered alone. (See DRUG INTERACTIONS.)

Steady-state concentrations were reached within 15 days following oral doses of 50-400 mg daily. Values given in TABLE 7 are data at steady-state from a pharmacokinetics study in which 27 healthy male volunteers took 200 mg itraconazole capsules bid (with a full meal) for 15 days.

TABLE 7

	Itraconazole	Hydroxyitraconazole
C_{max} (ng/ml)	2282 ± 514*	3488 ± 742
C_{min} (ng/ml)	1855 ± 535	3349 ± 761
T_{max} (hours)	4.6 ± 1.8	3.4 ± 3.4
AUC(0-12h) (ng·h/ml)	22,569 ± 5,375	38,572 ± 8,450
T½ (hours)	64 ± 32	56 ± 24

* Mean ± standard deviation.

The plasma protein binding of itraconazole is 99.8% and that of hydroxyitraconazole is 99.5%. Following IV administration, the volume of distribution of itraconazole averaged 796 ± 185 L.

Itraconazole is metabolized predominately by the cytochrome P450 3A4 isoenzyme system (CYP3A4), resulting in the formation of several metabolites, including hydroxyitraconazole, the major metabolite. Results of a pharmacokinetics study suggest that itraconazole may undergo saturable metabolism with multiple dosing. Fecal excretion of the parent drug varies between 3-18% of the dose. Renal excretion of the parent drug is less than 0.03% of the dose. About 40% of the dose is excreted as inactive metabolites in the urine. No single excreted metabolite represents more than 5% of a dose. Itraconazole total plasma clearance averaged 381 ± 95 ml/min following IV administration. (See CONTRAINDICATIONS and DRUG INTERACTIONS for more information.)

Oral Solution

Note: The plasma concentrations reported below were measured by high-performance liquid chromatography (HPLC) specific for itraconazole. When itraconazole in plasma is measured by a bioassay, values reported may be higher than those obtained by HPLC due to the presence of the bioactive metabolite, hydroxyitraconazole. (See Microbiology.)

The absolute bioavailability of itraconazole administered as a non-marketed solution formulation under fed conditions was 55% in 6 healthy male volunteers. However, the bioavailability of itraconazole oral solution is increased under fasted conditions reaching higher maximum plasma concentrations (C_{max}) in a shorter period of time. In 27 healthy male volunteers, the steady-state area under the plasma concentration versus time curve [AUC(0-24h)] of itraconazole (itraconazole oral solution, 200 mg daily for 15 days) under fasted conditions was 131 ± 30% of that obtained under fed conditions. Therefore, unlike itraconazole capsules, it is recommended that itraconazole oral solution be administered without food. Presented in TABLE 8 are the steady-state (Day 15) pharmacokinetic parameters for itraconazole and hydroxyitraconazole (itraconazole oral solution) under fasted and fed conditions.

TABLE 8

	Itraconazole		Hydroxyitraconazole	
	Fasted	Fed	Fasted	Fed
C_{max} (ng/ml)	1963 ± 601*	1435 ± 477	2055 ± 487	1781 ± 397
T_{max} (hours)	2.5 ± 0.8	4.4 ± 0.7	5.3 ± 4.3	4.3 ± 1.2
AUC(0-24h) (ng·h/ml)	29,271 ± 10,285	22,815 ± 7,098	45,184 ± 10,981	38,823 ± 8,907
T½ (hours)	39.7 ± 13	37.4 ± 13	27.3 ± 13	26.1 ± 10

* Mean ± standard deviation.

The bioavailability of itraconazole oral solution relative to itraconazole capsules was studied in 30 healthy male volunteers who received 200 mg of itraconazole as the oral solution and capsules under fed conditions. The AUC(0-∞) from itraconazole oral solution was 149 ± 68% of that obtained from itraconazole capsules; a similar increase was observed for hydroxyitraconazole. In addition, a cross study comparison of itraconazole and hydroxyitraconazole pharmacokinetics following the administration of single 200 mg doses of itraconazole oral solution (under fasted conditions) or itraconazole capsules (under fed conditions) indicates that when these two formulations are administered under conditions which optimize their systemic absorption, the bioavailability of the solution relative to capsules is expected to be increased further. Therefore, it is recommended that itraconazole oral solution and itraconazole capsules not be used interchangeably. TABLE 9 contains pharmacokinetic parameters for itraconazole and hydroxyitraconazole following single 200 mg doses of itraconazole oral solution (n=27) or itraconazole capsules (n=30) administered to healthy male volunteers under fasted and fed conditions, respectively.

TABLE 9

	Itraconazole		Hydroxyitraconazole	
	Oral Solution	Capsules	Oral Solution	Capsules
	Fasted	Fed	Fasted	Fed
C_{max} (ng/ml)	544 ± 213*	302 ± 119	622 ± 116	504 ± 132
T_{max} (hours)	2.2 ± 0.8	5 ± 0.8	3.5 ± 1.2	5 ± 1
AUC(0-24h) (ng·h/ml)	4505 ± 1670	2682 ± 1084	9552 ± 1835	7293 ± 2144

* Mean ± standard deviation.

The plasma protein binding of itraconazole is 99.8% and that of hydroxyitraconazole is 99.5% Following IV administration, the volume of distribution of itraconazole averaged 796 ± 185 L.

Itraconazole is metabolized predominately by the cytochrome P450 3A4 isoenzyme system (CYP3A4), resulting in the formation of several metabolites, including hydroxyitraconazole, the major metabolite. Results of a pharmacokinetics study suggest that itraconazole may undergo saturable metabolism with multiple dosing. Fecal excretion of the parent drug varies between 3-18% of the dose. Renal excretion of the parent drug is less than 0.03% of the dose. About 40% of the dose is excreted as inactive metabolites in the urine. No single excreted metabolite represents more than 5% of a dose. Itraconazole total plasma clearance averaged 381 ± 95 ml/min following IV administration. (See CONTRAINDICATIONS and DRUG INTERACTIONS for more information.)

SPECIAL POPULATIONS

Pediatrics — Oral Solution

The pharmacokinetics of itraconazole oral solution were studied in 26 pediatric patients requiring systemic antifungal therapy. Patients were stratified by age: 6 months to 2 years (n=8), 2-5 years (n=7) and 5-12 years (n=11), and received itraconazole oral solution 5 mg/kg once daily for 14 days. Pharmacokinetic parameters at steady-state (Day 14) were not significantly different among the age strata and are summarized in TABLE 10 for all 26 patients.

TABLE 10

	Itraconazole	Hydroxyitraconazole
C_{max} (ng/ml)	582.5 ± 382.4*	692.4 ± 355.0
C_{min} (ng/ml)	187.5 ± 161.4	403.8 ± 336.1
AUC(0-24h) (ng·h/ml)	7,706.7 ± 5,245.2	13,356.4 ± 8,942.4
$T_{½}$ (hours)	35.8 ± 35.6	17.7 ± 13.0

* Mean ± standard deviation.

Renal Insufficiency

A pharmacokinetic study using a single 200 mg dose of itraconazole (four 50 mg capsules) was conducted in 3 groups of patients with renal impairment (uremia: n=7; hemodialysis: n=7; and continuous ambulatory peritoneal dialysis: n=5). In uremic subjects with a mean creatinine clearance of 13 ml/min × 1.73 m^2, the bioavailability was slightly reduced compared with normal population parameters. This study did not demonstrate any significant effect of hemodialysis or continuous ambulatory peritoneal dialysis on the pharmacokinetics of itraconazole [T_{max}, C_{max}, and AUC(0-8)]. Plasma concentration-versus-time profiles showed wide intersubject variation in all 3 groups.

Hepatic Insufficiency

Capsules

A pharmacokinetic study using a single 100 mg dose of itraconazole (one 100 mg capsule) was conducted in 6 healthy and 12 cirrhotic subjects. No statistically significant differences in AUC were seen between these 2 groups. A statistically significant reduction in mean C_{max} (47%) and a 2-fold increase in the elimination half-life (37 ± 17 hours) of itraconazole were noted in cirrhotic subjects compared with healthy subjects. Patients with impaired hepatic function should be carefully monitored when taking itraconazole. The prolonged elimination half-life of itraconazole observed in cirrhotic patients should be considered when deciding to initiate therapy with other medications metabolized by CYP3A4. (See BOXED WARNING, CONTRAINDICATIONS, and DRUG INTERACTIONS.)

Oral Solution

Patients with impaired hepatic function should be carefully monitored when taking itraconazole. The prolonged elimination half-life of itraconazole observed in cirrhotic patients should be considered when deciding to initiate therapy with other medications metabolized by CYP3A4. (See BOXED WARNING, CONTRAINDICATIONS, and DRUG INTERACTIONS.)

Decreased Cardiac Contractility

When itraconazole was administered intravenously to anesthetized dogs, a dose-related negative inotropic effect was documented. In a healthy volunteer study of itraconazole injection (IV infusion), transient, asymptomatic decreases in left ventricular ejection fraction were observed using gated SPECT imaging; these resolved before the next infusion, 12 hours later. If signs or symptoms of congestive heart failure appear during administration of itraconazole capsules, itraconazole capsules should be discontinued. If signs or symptoms of congestive heart failure appear during administration of itraconazole oral solution, monitor carefully and consider other treatment alternatives which may include discontinuation of itraconazole oral solution administration. (See CONTRAINDICATIONS; WARNINGS; DRUG INTERACTIONS; and ADVERSE REACTIONS, Post-Marketing Experience: Capsules and Oral Solution for more information.)

Cystic Fibrosis — Oral Solution

Seventeen (17) cystic fibrosis patients, ages 7-28 years old, were administered itraconazole oral solution 2.5 mg/kg bid for 14 days in a pharmacokinetic study. Steady-state trough concentrations >250 ng/ml were achieved in 7 out of 12 patients greater than 16 years of age but in none of the 5 patients less than 16 years of age. Large variability was observed in the pharmacokinetic data (%CV = 88% and 65% for >16 and <16 years, respectively for trough concentrations). If a patient does not respond to itraconazole oral solution, consideration should be given to switching to alternative therapy.

INDICATIONS AND USAGE

CAPSULES

Itraconazole capsules are indicated for the treatment of the following fungal infections in immunocompromised and non-immunocompromised patients:

- Blastomycosis, pulmonary and extrapulmonary;
- Histoplasmosis, including chronic cavitary pulmonary disease and disseminated, non-meningeal histoplasmosis; and
- Aspergillosis, pulmonary and extrapulmonary, in patients who are intolerant of or who are refractory to amphotericin B therapy.

Specimens for fungal cultures and other relevant laboratory studies (wet mount, histopathology, serology) should be obtained before therapy to isolate and identify causative organisms. Therapy may be instituted before the results of the cultures and other laboratory studies are known; however, once these results become available, anti-infective therapy should be adjusted accordingly.

Itraconazole capsules are also indicated for the treatment of the following fungal infections in non-immunocompromised patients:

- Onychomycosis of the toenail, with or without fingernail involvement, due to dermatophytes (tinea unguium), and
- Onychomycosis of the fingernail due to dermatophytes (tinea unguium).

Prior to initiating treatment, appropriate nail specimens for laboratory testing (KOH preparation, fungal culture, or nail biopsy) should be obtained to confirm the diagnosis of onychomycosis.

(See CLINICAL PHARMACOLOGY, Special Populations; CONTRAINDICATIONS; WARNINGS; and ADVERSE REACTIONS, Post-Marketing Experience: Capsules and Oral Solution for more information.)

ORAL SOLUTION

Itraconazole injection/oral solution is indicated for empiric therapy of febrile neutropenic patients with suspected fungal infections. (*NOTE:* In a comparative trial, the overall response rate for itraconazole-treated subjects was higher than for amphotericin B-treated subjects. However, compared to amphotericin B-treated subjects, a larger number of itraconazole-treated subjects discontinued treatment due to persistent fever and a change in antifungal medication due to fever. Whereas, a larger number of amphotericin B-treated subjects discontinued due to drug intolerance.

Itraconazole oral solution is also indicated for the treatment of oropharyngeal and esophageal candidiasis.

(See CLINICAL PHARMACOLOGY, Special Populations; WARNINGS; and ADVERSE REACTIONS, Post-Marketing Experience: Capsules and Oral Solution for more information.)

NON-FDA APPROVED INDICATIONS

Itraconazole has demonstrated clinical utility for the treatment of a number of other fungal infections including coccidioidomycosis, paracoccidioidomycosis, vaginal candidiasis, tinea versicolor, cryptococcosis, and sporotrichosis, although none of these indications are approved by the FDA.

CONTRAINDICATIONS

CONGESTIVE HEART FAILURE — CAPSULES

Itraconazole capsules should not be administered for the treatment of onychomycosis in patients with evidence of ventricular dysfunction such as congestive heart failure (CHF) or a history of CHF. (See CLINICAL PHARMACOLOGY, Special Populations; WARNINGS; DRUG INTERACTIONS, Calcium Channel Blockers; and ADVERSE REACTIONS, Post-Marketing Experience: Capsules and Oral Solution.)

DRUG INTERACTIONS

Concomitant administration of itraconazole capsules, injection, or oral solution and certain drugs metabolized by the cytochrome P450 3A4 isoenzyme system (CYP3A4) may result in increased plasma concentrations of those drugs, leading to potentially serious and/or life-threatening adverse events. Cisapride, oral midazolam, pimozide, quinidine, dofetilide, and triazolam are contraindicated with itraconazole. HMG CoA-reductase inhibitors metabolized by CYP3A4, such as lovastatin and simvastatin, are also contraindicated with itraconazole. (See BOXED WARNING and DRUG INTERACTIONS.)

Itraconazole should not be administered for the treatment of onychomycosis to pregnant patients or to women contemplating pregnancy.

I

Itraconazole is contraindicated for patients who have shown hypersensitivity to itraconazole or its excipients. There is no information regarding cross-hypersensitivity between itraconazole and other azole antifungal agents. Caution should be used when prescribing itraconazole to patients with hypersensitivity to other azoles.

WARNINGS

Itraconazole capsules and oral solution should not be used interchangeably. This is because drug exposure is greater with the oral solution than with the capsules when the same dose of drug is given. In addition, the topical effects of mucosal exposure may be different between the two formulations. Only the oral solution has been demonstrated effective for oral and/or esophageal candidiasis. Itraconazole oral solution contains the excipient hydroxypropyl-β-cyclodextrin which produced pancreatic adenocarcinomas in a rat carcinogenicity study. These findings were not observed in a similar mouse carcinogenicity study. The clinical relevance of these findings is unknown. (See PRECAUTIONS, Carcinogenesis, Mutagenesis, and Impairment of Fertility.)

HEPATIC EFFECTS

Itraconazole has been associated with rare cases of serious hepatotoxicity, including liver failure and death. Some of these cases had neither pre-existing liver disease nor a serious underlying medical condition and some of these cases developed within the first week of treatment. If clinical signs or symptoms develop that are consistent with liver disease, treatment should be discontinued and liver function testing performed. Continued itraconazole use or reinstitution of treatment with itraconazole is strongly discouraged unless there is a serious or life threatening situation where the expected benefit exceeds the risk. (See PRECAUTIONS, Information for the Patient; and ADVERSE REACTIONS.)

CARDIAC DYSRHYTHMIAS

Life-threatening cardiac dysrhythmias and/or sudden death have occurred in patients using cisapride, pimozide, or quinidine concomitantly with itraconazole and/or other CYP3A4 inhibitors. Concomitant administration of these drugs with itraconazole is contraindicated. (See BOXED WARNING, CONTRAINDICATIONS, and DRUG INTERACTIONS.)

CARDIAC DISEASE

Itraconazole capsules should not be administered for the treatment of onychomycosis in patients with evidence of ventricular dysfunction such as congestive heart failure (CHF) or a history of CHF. Itraconazole capsules and oral solution should not be used for other indications in patients with evidence of ventricular dysfunction unless the benefit clearly outweighs the risk.

For patients with risk factors for congestive heart failure, physicians should carefully review the risks and benefits of itraconazole therapy. These risk factors include cardiac disease such as ischemic and valvular disease; significant pulmonary disease such as chronic obstructive pulmonary disease; and renal failure and other edematous disorders. Such patients should be informed of the signs and symptoms of CHF, should be treated with caution, and should be monitored for signs and symptoms of CHF during treatment. If signs or symptoms of CHF appear during administration of itraconazole capsules, discontinue administration of itraconazole capsules. If signs or symptoms of CHF appear during administration of itraconazole oral solution, monitor carefully and consider other treatment alternatives which may include discontinuation of itraconazole oral solution administration.

When itraconazole was administered intravenously to anesthetized dogs, a dose-related negative inotropic effect was documented. In a healthy volunteer study of itraconazole injection (IV infusion), transient, asymptomatic decreases in left ventricular ejection fraction were observed using gated SPECT imaging; these resolved before the next infusion, 12 hours later.

Cases of CHF, peripheral edema, and pulmonary edema have been reported in the post-marketing period among patients being treated for onychomycosis and/or systemic fungal infections. (See CLINICAL PHARMACOLOGY, Special Populations; CONTRAINDICATIONS; DRUG INTERACTIONS; and ADVERSE REACTIONS, Post-Marketing Experience: Capsules and Oral Solution for more information.)

PRECAUTIONS

GENERAL

Rare cases of serious hepatotoxicity have been observed with itraconazole treatment, including some cases within the first week. In patients with elevated or abnormal liver enzymes or active liver disease, or who have experienced liver toxicity with other drugs, treatment with itraconazole is strongly discouraged unless there is a serious or life threatening situation where the expected benefit exceeds the risk. Liver function monitoring should be done in patients with pre-existing hepatic function abnormalities or those who have experienced liver toxicity with other medications and should be considered in all patients receiving itraconazole. Treatment should be stopped immediately and liver function testing should be conducted in patients who develop signs and symptoms suggestive of liver dysfunction.

If neuropathy occurs that may be attributable to itraconazole capsules, the treatment should be discontinued.

Capsules

Itraconazole capsules should be administered after a full meal. (See CLINICAL PHARMACOLOGY, Pharmacokinetics and Metabolism, Capsules.)

Under fasted conditions, itraconazole absorption was decreased in the presence of decreased gastric acidity. The absorption of itraconazole may be decreased with the concomitant administration of antacids or gastric acid secretion suppressors. Studies conducted under fasted conditions demonstrated that administration with 8 oz of a cola beverage resulted in increased absorption of itraconazole in AIDS patients with relative or absolute achlorhydria. This increase relative to the effects of a full meal is unknown. (See CLINICAL PHARMACOLOGY, Pharmacokinetics and Metabolism, Capsules.)

INFORMATION FOR THE PATIENT

- The topical effects of mucosal exposure may be different between the itraconazole capsules and oral solution. Only the oral solution has been demonstrated effective for oral and/or esophageal candidiasis. Itraconazole capsules should not be used interchangeably with itraconazole oral solution. Itraconazole oral solution contains the excipient hydroxypropyl-β-cyclodextrin which produced pancreatic adenocarcinomas in a rat carcinogenicity study. These findings were not observed in a similar mouse carcinogenicity study. The clinical relevance of these findings is unknown. (See Carcinogenesis, Mutagenesis, and Impairment of Fertility.)
- Instruct patients about the signs and symptoms of congestive heart failure, and if these signs or symptoms occur during itraconazole administration, they should discontinue itraconazole and contact their healthcare provider immediately.
- Instruct patients to report any signs and symptoms that may suggest liver dysfunction so that the appropriate laboratory testing can be done. Such signs and symptoms may include unusual fatigue, anorexia, nausea and/or vomiting, jaundice, dark urine, or pale stools.
- Instruct patients to stop itraconazole treatment immediately and contact their healthcare provider if any signs and symptoms suggestive of liver dysfunction develop. Such signs and symptoms may include unusual fatigue, anorexia, nausea and/or vomiting, jaundice, dark urine, or pale stools.
- Instruct patients to contact their physician before taking any concomitant medications with itraconazole to ensure there are no potential drug interactions.
- ***Capsules:*** Instruct patients to take itraconazole capsules with a full meal.
- ***Oral Solution:*** Taking itraconazole oral solution under fasted conditions improves the systemic availability of itraconazole. Instruct patients to take itraconazole oral solution without food, if possible.
- ***Oral Solution:*** Itraconazole oral solution should not be used interchangeably with itraconazole capsules.

CARCINOGENESIS, MUTAGENESIS, AND IMPAIRMENT OF FERTILITY

Itraconazole showed no evidence of carcinogenicity potential in mice treated orally for 23 months at dosage levels up to 80 mg/kg/day (approximately 10× the maximum recommended human dose [MRHD]). Male rats treated with 25 mg/kg/day (3.1× MRHD) had a slightly increased incidence of soft tissue sarcoma. These sarcomas may have been a consequence of hypercholesterolemia, which is a response of rats, but not dogs or humans, to chronic itraconazole administration. Female rats treated with 50 mg/kg/day (6.25× MRHD) had an increased incidence of squamous cell carcinoma of the lung (2/50) as compared to the untreated group. Although the occurrence of squamous cell carcinoma in the lung is extremely uncommon in untreated rats, the increase in this study was not statistically significant.

Hydroxypropyl-β-cyclodextrin (HP-β-CD), the solubilizing excipient used in itraconazole oral solution, was found to produce pancreatic exocrine hyperplasia and neoplasia when administered orally to rats at doses of 500, 2000 or 5000 mg/kg/day for 25 months. Adenocarcinomas of the exocrine pancreas produced in the treated animals were not seen in the untreated group and are not reported in the historical controls. Development of these tumors may be related to a mitogenic action of cholecystokinin. This finding was not observed in the mouse carcinogenicity study at doses of 500, 2000 or 5000 mg/kg/day for 22-23 months; however, the clinical relevance of these findings is unknown. Based on body surface area comparisons, the exposure to humans of HP-β-CD at the recommended clinical dose of itraconazole oral solution, is approximately equivalent to 1.7 times the exposure at the lowest dose in the rat study.

Itraconazole produced no mutagenic effects when assayed in DNA repair test (unscheduled DNA synthesis) in primary rat hepatocytes, in Ames tests with *Salmonella typhimurium* (6 strains) and *Escherichia coli*, in the mouse lymphoma gene mutation tests, in a sex-linked recessive lethal mutation *(Drosophila melanogaster)* test, in chromosome aberration tests in human lymphocytes, in a cell transformation test with C3H/10T½ C18 mouse embryo fibroblasts cells, in a dominant lethal mutation test in male and female mice, and in micronucleus tests in mice and rats.

Itraconazole did not affect the fertility of male or female rats treated orally with dosage levels of up to 40 mg/kg/day (5× MRHD), even though parental toxicity was present at this dosage level. More severe signs of parental toxicity, including death, were present in the next higher dosage level, 160 mg/kg/day (20× MRHD).

PREGNANCY, TERATOGENIC EFFECTS, PREGNANCY CATEGORY C

Itraconazole was found to cause a dose-related increase in maternal toxicity, embryotoxicity, and teratogenicity in rats at dosage levels of approximately 40-160 mg/kg/day (5-20× MRHD), and in mice at dosage levels of approximately 80 mg/kg/day (10× MRHD). In rats, the teratogenicity consisted of major skeletal defects; in mice, it consisted of encephaloceles and/or macroglossia.

There are no studies in pregnant women. Itraconazole should be used for the treatment of systemic fungal infections in pregnancy only if the benefit outweighs the potential risk. Itraconazole capsules should not be administered for the treatment of onychomycosis to pregnant patients or to women contemplating pregnancy. Itraconazole capsules should not be administered to women of childbearing potential for the treatment of onychomycosis unless they are using effective measures to prevent pregnancy and they begin therapy on the second or third day following the onset of menses. Effective contraception should be continued throughout itraconazole therapy and for 2 months following the end of treatment.

NURSING MOTHERS

Itraconazole is excreted in human milk; therefore, the expected benefits of itraconazole therapy for the mother should be weighed against the potential risk from exposure of itraconazole to the infant. The US Public Health Service Centers for Disease Control and Prevention advises HIV-infected women not to breastfeed to avoid potential transmission of HIV to uninfected infants.

PEDIATRIC USE

The efficacy and safety of itraconazole have not been established in pediatric patients. No pharmacokinetic data on itraconazole capsules are available in children. A small number of patients ages 3-16 years have been treated with 100 mg/day of itraconazole capsules for systemic fungal infections, and no serious unexpected adverse effects have been reported. Itraconazole oral solution (5 mg/kg/day) has been administered to pediatric patients (n=26; ages 6 months to 12 years) for 2 weeks and no serious unexpected adverse events were reported. (See CLINICAL PHARMACOLOGY.)

The long-term effects of itraconazole on bone growth in children are unknown. In three toxicology studies using rats, itraconazole induced bone defects at dosage levels as low as 20 mg/kg/day (2.5× MRHD). The induced defects included reduced bone plate activity, thinning of the zona compacta of the large bones, and increased bone fragility. At a dosage level of 80 mg/kg/day (10× MRHD) over 1 year or 160 mg/kg/day (20× MRHD) for 6 months, itraconazole induced small tooth pulp with hypocellular appearance in some rats. No such bone toxicity has been reported in adult patients.

HIV-INFECTED PATIENTS — CAPSULES

Because hypochlorhydria has been reported in HIV-infected individuals, the absorption of itraconazole in these patients may be decreased.

DRUG INTERACTIONS

Itraconazole and its major metabolite, hydroxyitraconazole, are inhibitors of CYP3A4. Therefore, the following drug interactions may occur (see TABLE 12 below and the following drug class subheadings that follow):

Itraconazole may decrease the elimination of drugs metabolized by CYP3A4, resulting in increased plasma concentrations of these drugs when they are administered with itraconazole. These elevated plasma concentrations may increase or prolong both therapeutic and adverse effects of these drugs. Whenever possible, plasma concentrations of these drugs should be monitored, and dosage adjustments made after concomitant itraconazole therapy is initiated. When appropriate, clinical monitoring for signs or symptoms of increased or prolonged pharmacologic effects is advised. Upon discontinuation, depending on the dose and duration of treatment, itraconazole plasma concentrations decline gradually (especially in patients with hepatic cirrhosis or in those receiving CYP3A4 inhibitors). This is particularly important when initiating therapy with drugs whose metabolism is affected by itraconazole.

Inducers of CYP3A4 may decrease the plasma concentrations of itraconazole. Itraconazole may not be effective in patients concomitantly taking itraconazole and one of these drugs. Therefore, administration of these drugs with itraconazole is not recommended.

Other inhibitors of CYP3A4 may increase the plasma concentrations of itraconazole. Patients who must take itraconazole concomitantly with one of these drugs should be monitored closely for signs or symptoms of increased or prolonged pharmacologic effects of itraconazole.

TABLE 12 *Selected Drugs That Are Predicted to Alter the Plasma Concentration of Itraconazole or Have Their Plasma Concentration Altered by Itraconazole**

Drug Plasma Concentration Increased by Itraconazole	
Antiarrhythmics	Digoxin, dofetilide†, quinidine†
Anticoagulants	Warfarin
Anticonvulsants	Carbamazepine
Antimycobacterials	Rifabutin
Antineoplastics	Busulfan, docetaxel, vinca alkaloids
Antipsychotics	Pimozide†
Benzodiazepines	Alprazolam, diazepam, midazolam†‡, triazolam†
Calcium channel blockers	Dihydropyridines, verapamil
Gastrointestinal motility agents	Cisapride†
HMG CoA-reductase inhibitors	Atorvastatin, cerivastatin, lovastatin†, simvastatin†
Immunosuppressants	Cyclosporine, tacrolimus, sirolimus
Oral hypoglycemics	Oral hypoglycemics
Protease inhibitors	Indinavir, ritonavir, saquinavir
Other	Alfentanil, buspirone, methylprednisolone, trimetrexate
Decrease Plasma Concentration of Itraconazole	
Anticonvulsants	Carbamazepine, phenobarbital, phenytoin
Antimycobacterials	Isoniazid, rifabutin, rifampin
Gastric acid suppressors/neutralizers	Antacids, H_2-receptor antagonists, proton pump inhibitors
Non-nucleoside reverse transcriptase inhibitors	Nevirapine
Increase Plasma Concentration of Itraconazole	
Macrolide antibiotics	Clarithromycin, erythromycin
Protease inhibitors	Indinavir, ritonavir

* This list is not all-inclusive.
† Contraindicated with itraconazole based on clinical and/or pharmacokinetics studies. (See WARNINGS and below.)
‡ For information on parenterally administered midazolam, see Benzodiazepines.

ANTIARRHYTHMICS

The Class IA antiarrhythmic quinidine and Class III antiarrhythmic dofetilide are known to prolong the QT interval. Coadministration of quinidine or dofetilide with itraconazole may increase plasma concentrations of quinidine or dofetilide which could result in serious cardiovascular events. Therefore, concomitant administration of itraconazole and quinidine or dofetilide is contraindicated. (See BOXED WARNING, CONTRAINDICATIONS, and WARNINGS.)

Concomitant administration of digoxin and itraconazole has led to increased plasma concentrations of digoxin.

ANTICOAGULANTS

Itraconazole enhances the anticoagulant effect of coumarin-like drugs, such as warfarin.

ANTICONVULSANTS

Reduced plasma concentrations of itraconazole were reported when itraconazole was administered concomitantly with phenytoin. Carbamazepine, phenobarbital, and phenytoin are all inducers of CYP3A4. Although interactions with carbamazepine and phenobarbital have not been studied, concomitant administration of itraconazole and these drugs would be expected to result in decreased plasma concentrations of itraconazole. In addition, *in vivo* studies have demonstrated an increase in plasma carbamazepine concentrations in subjects concomitantly receiving ketoconazole. Although there are no data regarding the effect of itraconazole on carbamazepine metabolism, because of the similarities between ketoconazole and itraconazole, concomitant administration of itraconazole and carbamazepine may inhibit the metabolism of carbamazepine.

ANTIMYCOBACTERIALS

Drug interaction studies have demonstrated that plasma concentrations of azole antifungal agents and their metabolites, including itraconazole and hydroxyitraconazole, were significantly decreased when these agents were given concomitantly with rifabutin or rifampin. *In vivo* data suggest that rifabutin is metabolized in part by CYP3A4. Itraconazole may inhibit the metabolism of rifabutin. Although no formal study data are available for isoniazid, similar effects should be anticipated. Therefore, the efficacy of itraconazole could be substantially reduced if given concomitantly with one of these agents. Coadministration is not recommended.

ANTINEOPLASTICS

Itraconazole may inhibit the metabolism of busulfan, docetaxel, and vinca alkaloids.

ANTIPSYCHOTICS

Pimozide is known to prolong the QT interval and is partially metabolized by CYP3A4. Coadministration of pimozide with itraconazole could result in serious cardiovascular events. Therefore, concomitant administration of itraconazole and pimozide is contraindicated. (See BOXED WARNING, CONTRAINDICATIONS, and WARNINGS.)

BENZODIAZEPINES

Concomitant administration of itraconazole and alprazolam, diazepam, oral midazolam, or triazolam could lead to increased plasma concentrations of these benzodiazepines. Increased plasma concentrations could potentiate and prolong hypnotic and sedative effects. Concomitant administration of itraconazole and oral midazolam or triazolam is contraindicated. (See CONTRAINDICATIONS and WARNINGS.) If midazolam is administered parenterally, special precaution and patient monitoring is required since the sedative effect may be prolonged.

CALCIUM CHANNEL BLOCKERS

Edema has been reported in patients concomitantly receiving itraconazole and dihydropyridine calcium channel blockers. Appropriate dosage adjustment may be necessary.

Calcium channel blockers can have a negative inotropic effect which may be additive to those of itraconazole; itraconazole can inhibit the metabolism of calcium channel blockers such as dihydropyridines (*e.g.*, nifedipine and felodipine) and verapamil. Therefore, caution should be used when coadministering itraconazole and calcium channel blockers. (See CLINICAL PHARMACOLOGY, Special Populations; CONTRAINDICATIONS; WARNINGS; and ADVERSE REACTIONS, Post-Marketing Experience: Capsules and Oral Solution for more information.)

GASTRIC ACID SUPPRESSORS/NEUTRALIZERS

Reduced plasma concentrations of itraconazole were reported when itraconazole capsules were administered concomitantly with H_2-receptor antagonists. Studies have shown that absorption of itraconazole is impaired when gastric acid production is decreased. Therefore, itraconazole should be administered with a cola beverage if the patient has achlorhydria or is taking H_2-receptor antagonists or other gastric acid suppressors. Antacids should be administered at least 1 hour before or 2 hours after administration of itraconazole capsules. In a clinical study, when itraconazole capsules were administered with omeprazole (a proton pump inhibitor), the bioavailability of itraconazole was significantly reduced. However, as itraconazole is already dissolved in itraconazole oral solution, the effect of H_2 antagonists is expected to be substantially less than with the capsules. Nevertheless, caution is advised when the two drugs are coadministered.

GASTROINTESTINAL MOTILITY AGENTS

Coadministration of itraconazole with cisapride can elevate plasma cisapride concentrations which could result in serious cardiovascular events. Therefore, concomitant administration of itraconazole with cisapride is contraindicated. (See BOXED WARNING, CONTRAINDICATIONS, and WARNINGS.)

HMG COA-REDUCTASE INHIBITORS

Human pharmacokinetic data suggest that itraconazole inhibits the metabolism of atorvastatin, cerivastatin, lovastatin, and simvastatin, which may increase the risk of skeletal muscle toxicity, including rhabdomyolysis. Concomitant administration of itraconazole with HMG CoA-reductase inhibitors, such as lovastatin and simvastatin, is contraindicated. (See CONTRAINDICATIONS and WARNINGS.)

IMMUNOSUPPRESSANTS

Concomitant administration of itraconazole and cyclosporine or tacrolimus has led to increased plasma concentrations of these immunosuppressants. Concomitant administration of itraconazole and sirolimus could increase plasma concentrations of sirolimus.

MACROLIDE ANTIBIOTICS

Erythromycin and clarithromycin are known inhibitors of CYP3A4 (see TABLE 12) and may increase plasma concentrations of itraconazole. In a small pharmacokinetic study involving HIV infected patients, clarithromycin was shown to increase plasma concentrations of itraconazole. Similarly, following administration of 1 g of erythromycin ethyl succinate and 200 mg itraconazole as single doses, the mean C_{max} and AUC(0-∞) of itraconazole increased by 44% (90% CI: 119-175%) and 36% (90% CI: 108-171%), respectively.

NON-NUCLEOSIDE REVERSE TRANSCRIPTASE INHIBITORS

Nevirapine is an inducer of CYP3A4. *In vivo* studies have shown that nevirapine induces the metabolism of ketoconazole, significantly reducing the bioavailability of ketoconazole. Studies involving nevirapine and itraconazole have not been conducted. However, because of the similarities between ketoconazole and itraconazole, concomitant administration of itraconazole and nevirapine is not recommended.

In a clinical study, when 8 HIV-infected subjects were treated concomitantly with itraconazole capsules 100 mg twice daily and the nucleoside reverse transcriptase inhibitor zidovudine 8 ± 0.4 mg/kg/day, the pharmacokinetics of zidovudine were not affected. Other nucleoside reverse transcriptase inhibitors have not been studied.

ORAL HYPOGLYCEMIC AGENTS

Severe hypoglycemia has been reported in patients concomitantly receiving azole antifungal agents and oral hypoglycemic agents. Blood glucose concentrations should be carefully monitored when itraconazole and oral hypoglycemic agents are coadministered.

POLYENES

Prior treatment with itraconazole, like other azoles, may reduce or inhibit the activity of polyenes such as amphotericin B. However, the clinical significance of this drug effect has not been clearly defined.

PROTEASE INHIBITORS

Concomitant administration of itraconazole and protease inhibitors metabolized by CYP3A4, such as indinavir, ritonavir, and saquinavir, may increase plasma concentrations of these protease inhibitors. In addition, concomitant administration of itraconazole and indinavir and ritonavir (but not saquinavir) may increase plasma concentrations of itraconazole. Caution is advised when itraconazole and protease inhibitors must be given concomitantly.

OTHER

- *In vitro* data suggest that alfentanil is metabolized by CYP3A4. Administration with itraconazole may increase plasma concentrations of alfentanil.
- Human pharmacokinetic data suggest that concomitant administration of itraconazole and buspirone results in significant increases in plasma concentrations of buspirone.
- Itraconazole may inhibit the metabolism of methylprednisolone.
- *In vitro* data suggest that trimetrexate is extensively metabolized by CYP3A4. *In vitro* animal models have demonstrated that ketoconazole potently inhibits the metabolism of trimetrexate. Although there are no data regarding the effect of itraconazole on trimetrexate metabolism, because of the similarities between ketoconazole and itraconazole, concomitant administration of itraconazole and trimetrexate may inhibit the metabolism of trimetrexate.
- Itraconazole enhances the anticoagulant effect of coumarin-like drugs, such as warfarin.

ADVERSE REACTIONS

CAPSULES

Itraconazole has been associated with rare cases of serious hepatotoxicity, including liver failure and death. Some of these cases had neither pre-existing liver disease nor a serious underlying medical condition. If clinical signs or symptoms develop that are consistent with liver disease, treatment should be discontinued and liver function testing performed. The risks and benefits of itraconazole use should be reassessed. (See WARNINGS, Hepatic Effects; and PRECAUTIONS: General and Information for the Patient.)

Adverse Events in the Treatment of Systemic Fungal Infections

Adverse event data were derived from 602 patients treated for systemic fungal disease in US clinical trials who were immunocompromised or receiving multiple concomitant medications. Treatment was discontinued in 10.5% of patients due to adverse events. The median duration before discontinuation of therapy was 81 days (range: 2-776 days). TABLE 13 lists adverse events reported by at least 1% of patients.

Adverse events infrequently reported in all studies included constipation, gastritis, depression, insomnia, tinnitus, menstrual disorder, adrenal insufficiency, gynecomastia, and male breast pain.

Adverse Events Reported in Toenail Onychomycosis Clinical Trials

Patients in these trials were on a continuous dosing regimen of 200 mg once daily for 12 consecutive weeks.

The following adverse events led to temporary or permanent discontinuation of therapy (see TABLE 14).

The following adverse events occurred with an incidence of greater than or equal to 1% (n=112): Headache: 10%; rhinitis: 9%; upper respiratory tract infection: 8%; sinusitis, injury: 7%; diarrhea, dyspepsia, flatulence, abdominal pain, dizziness, rash: 4%; cystitis, urinary tract infection, liver function abnormality, myalgia, nausea: 3%; appetite increased, constipation, gastritis, gastroenteritis, pharyngitis, asthenia, fever, pain, tremor, herpes zoster, abnormal dreaming: 2%.

Adverse Events Reported in Fingernail Onychomycosis Clinical Trials

Patients in these trials were on a pulse regimen consisting of two 1 week treatment periods of 200 mg twice daily, separated by a 3 week period without drug.

The following adverse events led to temporary or permanent discontinuation of therapy (see TABLE 15).

The following adverse events occurred with an incidence of greater than or equal to 1% (n=37): Headache: 8%; pruritus, nausea, rhinitis: 5%; rash, bursitis, anxiety, depression, constipation, abdominal pain, dyspepsia, ulcerative stomatitis, gingivitis, hypertriglyceridemia, sinusitis, fatigue, malaise, pain, injury: 3%.

TABLE 13 *Clinical Trials of Systemic Fungal Infections: Adverse Events Occurring With an Incidence of Greater Than or Equal to 1%*

Body System / Adverse Event	Incidence (n=602)
Gastrointestinal	
Nausea	11%
Vomiting	5%
Diarrhea	3%
Abdominal pain	2%
Anorexia	1%
Body as a Whole	
Edema	4%
Fatigue	3%
Fever	3%
Malaise	1%
Skin and Appendages	
Rash*	9%
Pruritus	3%
Central/Peripheral Nervous System	
Headache	4%
Dizziness	2%
Psychiatric	
Libido decreased	1%
Somnolence	1%
Cardiovascular	
Hypertension	3%
Metabolic/Nutritional	
Hypokalemia	2%
Urinary System	
Albuminuria	1%
Liver and Biliary System	
Hepatic function abnormal	3%
Reproductive System, Male	
Impotence	1%

* Rash tends to occur more frequently in immunocompromised patients receiving immunosuppressive medications.

TABLE 14 *Clinical Trials of Onychomycosis of the Toenail: Adverse Events Leading to Temporary or Permanent Discontinuation of Therapy*

Adverse Event	Incidence Itraconazole (n=112)
Elevated liver enzymes (greater than twice the upper limit of normal)	4%
Gastrointestinal disorders	4%
Rash	3%
Hypertension	2%
Orthostatic hypotension	1%
Headache	1%
Malaise	1%
Myalgia	1%
Vasculitis	1%
Vertigo	1%

TABLE 15 *Clinical Trials of Onychomycosis of the Fingernail: Adverse Events Leading to Temporary or Permanent Discontinuation of Therapy*

Adverse Event	Incidence Itraconazole (n=37)
Rash/pruritus	3%
Hypertriglyceridemia	3%

Post-Marketing Experience

Worldwide post-marketing experiences with the use of itraconazole include adverse events of gastrointestinal origin, such as dyspepsia, nausea, vomiting, diarrhea, abdominal pain and constipation. Other reported adverse events include peripheral edema, congestive heart failure and pulmonary edema, headache, dizziness, peripheral neuropathy, menstrual disorders, reversible increases in hepatic enzymes, hepatitis, liver failure, hypokalemia, hypertriglyceridemia, alopecia, allergic reactions (such as pruritus, rash, urticaria, angioedema, anaphylaxis), Stevens-Johnson syndrome, and neutropenia. (See CLINICAL PHARMACOLOGY, Special Populations; CONTRAINDICATIONS; WARNINGS; and DRUG INTERACTIONS for more information.)

ORAL SOLUTION

Itraconazole has been associated with rare cases of serious hepatotoxicity, including liver failure and death. Some of these cases had neither pre-existing liver disease nor a serious underlying medical condition. If clinical signs or symptoms develop that are consistent with liver disease, treatment should be discontinued and liver function testing performed. The risks and benefits of itraconazole use should be reassessed. (See WARNINGS, Hepatic Effects; and PRECAUTIONS: General and Information for the Patient.)

Adverse Events Reported in Empiric Therapy in Febrile Neutropenic (ETFN) Patients

Adverse events considered at least possibly drug related in a clinical trial of empiric therapy in 384 febrile, neutropenic patients (192 treated with itraconazole and 192 with amphotericin B) with suspected fungal infections are listed in TABLE 16. Patients received a regimen of itraconazole injection followed by itraconazole oral solution. The dose of itraconazole injection was 200 mg twice daily for the first 2 days followed by a single daily dose of 200 mg for the remainder of the IV treatment period. The majority of patients received between

7 and 14 days of itraconazole injection. The dose of itraconazole oral solution was 200 mg (20 ml) bid for the remainder of therapy.

TABLE 16 *Summary of Possibly or Definitely Drug-Related Adverse Events Reported in ≥2% of Subjects (Empiric Therapy Trial in Febrile Neutropenic Patients)*

Adverse Event	Itraconazole (n=192)	Amphotericin B (n=192)
Gastrointestinal System Disorders		
Nausea	11%	15%
Diarrhea	10%	9%
Vomiting	7%	10%
Abdominal pain	3%	3%
Metabolic and Nutritional Disorders		
Hypokalemia	9%	28%
Serum creatinine increased	3%	25%
LDH increased	2%	0%
Alkaline phosphatase increased	2%	2%
Hypomagnesemia	2%	4%
Blood urea nitrogen increased	1%	6%
Fluid overload	1%	3%
Hypocalcemia	1%	2%
Liver and Biliary System Disorders		
Bilirubinemia	6%	3%
Hepatic function abnormal	3%	2%
SGPT/ALT increased	3%	1%
Jaundice	2%	1%
SGOT/AST increased	2%	1%
Skin and Appendage Disorders		
Rash	5%	3%
Sweating increased	2%	1%
CNS and Peripheral Nervous System		
Headache	2%	2%
Body as a Whole		
Edema	2%	2%
Rigors	1%	34%
Fever	0%	7%
Respiratory System Disorder		
Dyspnea	1%	3%
Urinary System Disorder		
Renal function abnormal	1%	12%
Cardiovascular Disorders, General		
Hypotension	1%	3%
Hypertension	0%	2%
Heart Rate and Rhythm Disorders		
Tachycardia	1%	3%

The following additional adverse events considered at least possibly related occurred in between 1 and 2% of patients who received itraconazole injection and oral solution: Constipation, hypophosphatemia, gamma-GT increased, erythematous rash, pruritus, dizziness, tremor, and pulmonary infiltration.

Adverse Events Reported in Oropharyngeal or Esophageal Candidiasis Trials

US adverse experience data are derived from 350 immunocompromised patients (332 HIV seropositive/AIDS) treated for oropharyngeal or esophageal candidiasis. TABLE 17 lists adverse events reported by at least 2% of patients treated with itraconazole oral solution in US clinical trials. Data on patients receiving comparator agents in these trials are included for comparison.

Adverse events reported by less than 2% of patients in US clinical trials with itraconazole included: Adrenal insufficiency, asthenia, back pain, dehydration, dyspepsia, dysphagia, flatulence, gynecomastia, hematuria, hemorrhoids, hot flushes, implantation complication, infection unspecified, injury, insomnia, male breast pain, myalgia, pharyngitis, pruritus, rhinitis, rigors, stomatitis ulcerative, taste perversion, tinnitus, upper respiratory tract infection, vision abnormal, and weight decrease. Edema, hypokalemia and menstrual disorders have been reported in clinical trials with itraconazole capsules.

Post-Marketing Experience

Worldwide post-marketing experiences with the use of itraconazole include adverse events of gastrointestinal origin, such as dyspepsia, nausea, vomiting, diarrhea, abdominal pain and constipation. Other reported adverse events include peripheral edema, congestive heart failure and pulmonary edema, headache, dizziness, peripheral neuropathy, menstrual disorders, reversible increases in hepatic enzymes, hepatitis, liver failure, hypokalemia, hypertriglyceridemia, alopecia, allergic reactions (such as pruritus, rash, urticaria, angioedema, anaphylaxis), Stevens-Johnson syndrome, and neutropenia. (See CLINICAL PHARMACOLOGY, Special Populations; CONTRAINDICATIONS; WARNINGS; and DRUG INTERACTIONS for more information.)

DOSAGE AND ADMINISTRATION

CAPSULES

Itraconazole capsules should be taken with a full meal to ensure maximal absorption.

Itraconazole capsules are a different preparation than itraconazole oral solution and should not be used interchangeably.

Treatment of Blastomycosis and Histoplasmosis

The recommended dose is 200 mg once daily (2 capsules). If there is no obvious improvement, or there is evidence of progressive fungal disease, the dose should be increased in 100 mg increments to a maximum of 400 mg daily. Doses above 200 mg/day should be given in 2 divided doses.

Treatment of Aspergillosis

A daily dose of 200-400 mg is recommended.

TABLE 17 *Summary of Adverse Events Reported by ≥2% of Itraconazole Treated Patients in US Clinical Trials (Total)*

Body System / Adverse Event	Itraconazole Total (n=350*)	Itraconazole All Controlled Studies (n=272)	Fluconazole (n=125†)	Clotrimazol (n=81‡)
Gastrointestinal Disorders				
Nausea	11%	10%	11%	5%
Diarrhea	11%	10%	10%	4%
Vomiting	7%	6%	8%	1%
Abdominal pain	6%	4%	7%	7%
Constipation	2%	2%	1%	0%
Body as a Whole				
Fever	7%	6%	8%	5%
Chest pain	3%	3%	2%	0%
Pain	2%	2%	4%	0%
Fatigue	2%	1%	2%	0%
Respiratory Disorders				
Coughing	4%	4%	10%	0%
Dyspnea	2%	3%	5%	1%
Pneumonia	2%	2%	0%	0%
Sinusitis	2%	2%	4%	0%
Sputum increased	2%	3%	3%	1%
Skin and Appendages Disorders				
Rash	4%	5%	4%	6%
Increased sweating	3%	4%	6%	1%
Skin disorder, unspecified	2%	2%	2%	1%
Central/Peripheral Nervous System				
Headache	4%	4%	6%	6%
Dizziness	2%	2%	4%	1%
Resistance Mechanism Disorders				
Pneumocystis carinii infection	2%	2%	2%	0%
Psychiatric Disorders				
Depression	2%	1%	0%	1%

* Of the 350 patients, 209 were treated for oropharyngeal candidiasis in controlled studies, 63 were treated for esophageal candidiasis in controlled studies and 78 were treated for oropharyngeal candidiasis in an open study.
† Of the 125 patients, 62 were treated for oropharyngeal candidiasis and 63 were treated for esophageal candidiasis.
‡ All 81 patients were treated for oropharyngeal candidiasis.

Treatment in Life-Threatening Situations

In life-threatening situations, a loading dose should be used whether given as oral capsules or intravenously.

IV Injection: The recommended IV dose is 200 mg bid for 4 consecutive doses, followed by 200 mg once daily thereafter. Each IV dose should be infused over 1 hour. The safety and efficacy of itraconazole injection administered for greater than 14 days is not known. See complete prescribing information for itraconazole injection.

Capsules: Although clinical studies did not provide for a loading dose, it is recommended, based on pharmacokinetic data, that a loading dose of 200 mg (2 capsules) three times daily (600 mg/day) be given for the first 3 days of treatment.

Treatment should be continued for a minimum of 3 months and until clinical parameters and laboratory tests indicate that the active fungal infection has subsided. An inadequate period of treatment may lead to recurrence of active infection.

Itraconazole capsules and oral solution should not be used interchangeably. Only the oral solution has been demonstrated effective for oral and/or esophageal candidiasis.

Treatment of Onychomycosis

Toenails with or without fingernail involvement: The recommended dose is 200 mg (2 capsules) once daily for 12 consecutive weeks.

Treatment of Onychomycosis

Fingernails only: The recommended dosing regimen is 2 treatment pulses, each consisting of 200 mg (2 capsules) bid (400 mg/day) for 1 week. The pulses are separated by a 3 week period without itraconazole.

ORAL SOLUTION

Empiric Therapy in Febrile, Neutropenic Patients With Suspected Fungal Infections (ETFN)

The recommended dose of itraconazole injection is 200 mg bid for 4 doses, followed by 200 mg once daily for up to 14 days. Each IV dose should be infused over 1 hour. Treatment should be continued with itraconazole oral solution 200 mg (20 ml) bid until resolution of clinically significant neutropenia. The safety and efficacy of itraconazole use exceeding 28 days in ETFN is not known.

Itraconazole oral solution is a different preparation than itraconazole capsules and should not be used interchangeably.

Treatment of Oropharyngeal and Esophageal Candidiasis

The solution should be vigorously swished in the mouth (10 ml at a time) for several seconds and swallowed.

The recommended dosage of itraconazole oral solution for oropharyngeal candidiasis is 200 mg (20 ml) daily for 1-2 weeks. Clinical signs and symptoms of oropharyngeal candidiasis generally resolve within several days.

For patients with oropharyngeal candidiasis unresponsive/refractory to treatment with fluconazole tablets, the recommended dose is 100 mg (10 ml) bid. For patients responding to therapy, clinical response will be seen in 2-4 weeks. Patients may be expected to relapse shortly after discontinuing therapy. Limited data on the safety of long-term use (>6 months) of itraconazole oral solution are available at this time.

The recommended dosage of itraconazole oral solution for esophageal candidiasis is 100 mg (10 ml) daily for a minimum treatment of 3 weeks. Treatment should continue for 2 weeks following resolution of symptoms. Doses up to 200 mg (20 ml) per day may be used based on medical judgement of the patient's response to therapy.

Itraconazole oral solution and capsules should not be used interchangeably. Patients should be instructed to take itraconazole oral solution without food, if possible. Only itraconazole oral solution has been demonstrated effective for oral and/or esophageal candidiasis.

HOW SUPPLIED

SPORANOX CAPSULES

Sporanox (itraconazole) capsules are available containing 100 mg of itraconazole, with a blue opaque cap and pink transparent body, imprinted with "JANSSEN" and "SPORANOX 100".

Storage: Store at controlled room temperature 15-25°C (59-77°F). Protect from light and moisture.

SPROANOX ORAL SOLUTION

Sporanox (itraconazole) oral solution is available in 150 ml amber glass bottles containing 10 mg of itraconazole per ml.

Storage: Store at or below 25°C (77°F). Do not freeze.

PRODUCT LISTING - EQUIVALENTS NOT AVAILABLE

Capsule - Oral - 100 mg

7 x 4	$256.90	SPORANOX, Janssen Pharmaceuticals	50458-0290-28
14's	$103.81	SPORANOX, Allscripts Pharmaceutical Company	54569-4869-00
30's	$216.56	SPORANOX, Physicians Total Care	54868-3706-00
30's	$268.25	SPORANOX, Janssen Pharmaceuticals	50458-0290-01
30's	$268.25	SPORANOX, Janssen Pharmaceuticals	50458-0290-04

Kit - Intravenous - 250 mg

10's	$202.01	SPORANOX, Ortho Biotech Inc	50458-0298-01

Suspension - Oral - 10 mg/ml

150 ml	$133.63	SPORANOX, Janssen Pharmaceuticals	50458-0295-15

K

Ivermectin *(003134)*

For complete prescribing information, refer to the CD-ROM included with the book.

Categories: Onchocerciasis; Strongyloidiasis; FDA Approved 1996 Nov; Pregnancy Category C; WHO Formulary
Drug Classes: Antihelmintics
Brand Names: **Mectizan**; Stromectol
Cost of Therapy: $21.76 (Helminth Infection; Stromectol; 3 mg; 4 tablets/day; 1 day supply)

DESCRIPTION

Stromectol (ivermectin) is a semisynthetic, anthelmintic agent for oral administration. Ivermectin is derived from the avermectins, a class of highly active broad-spectrum antiparasitic agents isolated from the fermentation products of *Streptomyces avermitilis*. Ivermectin is a mixture containing at least 90% 5-*O*-demethyl-22,23-dihydroavermectin A_{1a} and less than 10% 5-*O*-demethyl-25-de(1-methylpropyl)-22,23-dihydro-25-(1-methylethyl)avermectin A_{1a}, generally referred to as 22,23-dihydroavermectin B_{1a} and B_{1b}, or H_2B_{1a} and H_2B_{1b}, respectively. The respective empirical formulas are $C_{48}H_{74}O_{14}$ and $C_{47}H_{72}O_{14}$, with molecular weights of 875.10 and 861.07, respectively.

Ivermectin is a white to yellowish-white, nonhygroscopic, crystalline powder with a melting point of about 155°C. It is insoluble in water but is freely soluble in methanol and soluble in 95% ethanol.

Stromectol is available in 3 mg tablets and 6 mg scored tablets. Each tablet contains the following inactive ingredients: microcrystalline cellulose, pregelatinized starch, magnesium stearate, butylated hydroxyanisole, and citric acid powder (anhydrous).

INDICATIONS AND USAGE

Ivermectin is indicated for the treatment of the following infections:

Strongyloidiasis of the intestinal tract. Ivermectin is indicated for the treatment of intestinal (*i.e.*, nondisseminated) strongyloidiasis due to the nematode parasite *Strongyloides stercoralis*.

This indication is based on clinical studies of both comparative and open-label designs, in which from 64-100% of infected patients were cured following a single 200 μg/kg dose of ivermectin.

Onchocerciasis. Ivermectin is indicated for the treatment of onchocerciasis due to the nematode parasite *Onchocerca volvulus*.

This indication is based on randomized, double-blind, placebo-controlled and comparative studies conducted in 1427 patients in onchocerciasis-endemic areas of West Africa. The comparative studies used diethylcarbamazine citrate (DEC-C).

Note: Ivermectin has no activity against adult *Onchocerca volvulus* parasites. The adult parasites reside in subcutaneous nodules which are infrequently palpable. Surgical excision of these nodules (nodulectomy) may be considered in the management of patients with onchocerciasis, since this procedure will eliminate the microfilariae-producing adult parasites.

NON-FDA APPROVED INDICATIONS

Although not FDA-approved, ivermectin has also been used for treatment of many other helminth infections including Pediculus capitus, Sarcoptes scabiei (scabies), Loa loa, and Ascariasis lumbricoides (roundworm).

CONTRAINDICATIONS

Ivermectin is contraindicated in patients who are hypersensitive to any component of this product.

WARNINGS

Historical data have shown that microfilaricidal drugs, such as diethylcarbamazine citrate (DEC-C), might cause cutaneous and/or systemic reactions of varying severity (the Mazzotti reaction) and ophthalmological reactions in patients with onchocerciasis. These reactions are probably due to allergic and inflammatory responses to the death of microfilariae. Patients treated with ivermectin for onchocerciasis may experience these reactions in addition to clinical adverse reactions possibly, probably, or definitely related to the drug itself.

The treatment of severe Mazzotti reactions has not been subjected to controlled clinical trials. Oral hydration, recumbency, intravenous normal saline, and/or parenteral corticosteroids have been used to treat postural hypotension. Antihistamines and/or aspirin have been used for most mild to moderate cases.

DOSAGE AND ADMINISTRATION

STRONGYLOIDIASIS

The recommended dosage of ivermectin for the treatment of strongyloidiasis is a single oral dose designed to provide approximately 200 μg of ivermectin per kg of body weight. See TABLE 2 for dosage guidelines. Patients should take tablets with water. In general, additional doses are not necessary. However, follow-up stool examinations should be performed to verify eradication of infection.

TABLE 2 *Dosage Guidelines for Ivermectin for Strongyloidiasis*

	Single Oral Dose	
Body Weight (kg)	**Number of 3 mg Tablet**	**Number of 6 mg Tablets**
15-24	1 tablet	½ tablet
25-35	2 tablets	1 tablet
36-50	3 tablets	1½ tablets
51-65	4 tablets	2 tablets
66-79	5 tablets	2½ tablets
≥80	200 μg/kg	200 μg/kg

ONCHOCERCIASIS

The recommended dosage of ivermectin for the treatment of onchocerciasis is a single oral dose designed to provide approximately 150 μg of ivermectin per kg of body weight. See TABLE 3 for dosage guidelines. Patients should take tablets with water. In mass distribution campaigns in international treatment programs, the most commonly used dose interval is 12 months. For the treatment of individual patients, retreatment may be considered at intervals as short as 3 months.

TABLE 3 *Dosage Guidelines for Ivermectin for Onchocerciasis*

	Single Oral Dose	
Body Weight (kg)	**Number of 3 mg Tablet**	**Number of 6 mg Tablets**
15-25	1 tablet	½ tablet
26-44	2 tablets	1 tablet
45-64	3 tablets	1½ tablets
65-84	4 tablets	2 tablets
≥85	150 μg/kg	150 μg/kg

PRODUCT LISTING - EQUIVALENTS NOT AVAILABLE

Tablet - Oral - 3 mg

20's	$108.80	STROMECTOL, Merck & Company Inc	00006-0032-20

Tablet - Oral - 6 mg

10's	$99.74	STROMECTOL, Merck & Company Inc	00006-0139-10

Ketamine Hydrochloride *(001604)*

For complete prescribing information, refer to the CD-ROM included with the book.

Categories: Anesthesia, adjunct; Anesthesia, general; FDA Approved 1970 Feb; Pregnancy Category C; WHO Formulary
Drug Classes: Anesthetics, general
Brand Names: **Ketalar**
Foreign Brand Availability: Anesject (Indonesia); Calypsol (Bahamas; Bahrain; Barbados; Belize; Bermuda; Curacao; Cyprus; Egypt; Guyana; Iran; Iraq; Jamaica; Jordan; Kuwait; Lebanon; Libya; Netherland-Antilles; Oman; Qatar; Republic-of-Yemen; Saudi-Arabia; Surinam; Syria; Thailand; Trinidad; United-Arab-Emirates); Keta-Hameln (Thailand); Ketalin (Mexico); Ketamax (Philippines); Ketanest (Bulgaria; Czech-Republic; Germany); Ketmin (India); Ketolar (Spain); Soon-Soon (Taiwan); Tekam (Bahrain; Cyprus; Egypt; Iran; Iraq; Jordan; Kuwait; Lebanon; Libya; Oman; Qatar; Republic-of-Yemen; Saudi-Arabia; Syria; United-Arab-Emirates)

WARNING

SPECIAL NOTE

EMERGENCE REACTIONS HAVE OCCURRED IN APPROXIMATELY 12% OF PATIENTS.

THE PSYCHOLOGICAL MANIFESTATIONS VARY IN SEVERITY BETWEEN PLEASANT DREAM-LIKE STATES, VIVID IMAGERY, HALLUCINATIONS, AND EMERGENCE DELIRIUM. IN SOME CASES THESE STATES HAVE BEEN ACCOMPANIED BY CONFUSION, EXCITEMENT, AND IRRATIONAL BEHAVIOR WHICH A FEW PATIENTS RECALL AS AN UNPLEASANT EXPERIENCE. THE DURATION ORDINARILY IS NO MORE THAN A FEW HOURS; IN A FEW CASES, HOWEVER, RECURRENCES HAVE TAKEN PLACE UP TO 24

WARNING — Cont'd

HOURS POSTOPERATIVELY. NO RESIDUAL PSYCHOLOGICAL EFFECTS ARE KNOWN TO HAVE RESULTED FROM USE OF KETAMINE HCl.

THE INCIDENCE OF THESE EMERGENCE PHENOMENA IS LEAST IN THE YOUNG (15 YEARS OF AGE OR LESS) AND ELDERLY (OVER 65 YEARS OF AGE) PATIENT. ALSO, THEY ARE LESS FREQUENT WHEN THE DRUG IS GIVEN INTRAMUSCULARLY AND THE INCIDENCE IS REDUCED AS EXPERIENCE WITH THE DRUG IS GAINED.

THE INCIDENCE OF PSYCHOLOGICAL MANIFESTATIONS DURING EMERGENCE, PARTICULARLY DREAM-LIKE OBSERVATIONS AND EMERGENCE DELIRIUM, MAY BE REDUCED BY USING LOWER RECOMMENDED DOSAGES OF KETAMINE HCl IN CONJUNCTION WITH INTRAVENOUS DIAZEPAM DURING INDUCTION AND MAINTENANCE OF ANESTHESIA. (see DOSAGE AND ADMINISTRATION.) ALSO, THESE REACTIONS MAY BE REDUCED IF VERBAL, TACTILE AND VISUAL STIMULATION OF THE PATIENT IS MINIMIZED DURING THE RECOVERY PERIOD. THIS DOES NOT PRECLUDE THE MONITORING OF VITAL SIGNS.

IN ORDER TO TERMINATE A SEVERE EMERGENCE REACTION THE USE OF A SMALL HYPNOTIC DOSE OF A SHORT-ACTING OR ULTRA SHORT-ACTING BARBITURATE MAY BE REQUIRED.

WHEN KETAMINE HCl IS USED ON AN OUTPATIENT BASIS, THE PATIENT SHOULD NOT BE RELEASED UNTIL RECOVERY FROM ANESTHESIA IS COMPLETE AND THEN SHOULD BE ACCOMPANIED BY A RESPONSIBLE ADULT.

DESCRIPTION

Ketamine HCl is a nonbarbiturate anesthetic chemically designated *dl*2-(o-chlorophenyl)-2-(methylamino) cyclohexanone hydrochloride. It is formulated as a slightly acid (pH 3.5-5.5) sterile solution for intravenous or intramuscular injection in concentrations containing the equivalent of either 10, 50, or 100 mg ketamine base per milliliter and contains not more than 0.1 mg/ml benzethonium chloride added as a preservative. The 10 mg/ml solution has been made isotonic with sodium chloride.

INDICATIONS AND USAGE

Ketamine HCl is indicated as the sole anesthetic agent for diagnostic and surgical procedures that do not require skeletal muscle relaxation. Ketamine HCl is best suited for short procedures but it can be used, with additional doses, for longer procedures.

Ketamine HCl is indicated for the induction of anesthesia prior to the administration of other general anesthetic agents.

Ketamine HCl is indicated to supplement low-potency agents, such as nitrous oxide.

CONTRAINDICATIONS

Ketamine HCl is contraindicated in those in whom a significant elevation of blood pressure would constitute a serious hazard and in those who have shown hypersensitivity to the drug.

WARNINGS

Cardiac function should be continually monitored during the procedure in patients found to have hypertension or cardiac decompensation.

Postoperative confusional states may occur during the recovery period. (See BOXED WARNING.)

Respiratory depression may occur with overdosage or too rapid a rate of administration of ketamine HCl, in which case supportive ventilation should be employed. Mechanical support of respiration is preferred to administration of analeptics.

DOSAGE AND ADMINISTRATION

Note: Barbiturates and ketamine HCl, being chemically incompatible because of precipitate formation, *should not* be injected from the same syringe.

If the ketamine HCl dose is augmented with diazepam, the two drugs must be given separately. Do not mix ketamine HCl and diazepam in syringe or infusion flask. For additional information on the use of diazepam, refer to the WARNINGS and DOSAGE AND ADMINISTRATION sections of the diazepam insert.

PREOPERATIVE PREPARATIONS

1. While vomiting has been reported following ketamine HCl administration, some airway protection may be afforded because of active laryngeal-pharyngeal reflexes. However, since aspiration may occur with ketamine HCl and since protective reflexes may also be diminished by supplementary anesthetics and muscle relaxants, the possibility of aspiration must be considered. ketamine HCl is recommended for use in the patient whose stomach is not empty when, in the judgment of the practitioner, the benefits of the drug outweigh the possible risks.
2. Atropine, scopolamine, or another drying agent should be given at an appropriate interval prior to induction.

ONSET AND DURATION

Because of rapid induction following the initial intravenous injection, the patient should be in a supported position during administration.

The onset of action of ketamine HCl is rapid; an intravenous dose of 2 mg/kg (1 mg/lb) of body weight usually produces surgical anesthesia within 30 seconds after injection, with the anesthetic effect usually lasting 5-10 minutes. If a longer effect is desired, additional increments can be administered intravenously or intramuscularly to maintain anesthesia without producing significant cumulative effects.

Intramuscular doses, from experience primarily in pediatric patients, in a range of 9-13 mg/kg (4-6 mg/lb) usually produce surgical anesthesia within 3-4 minutes following injection, with the anesthetic effect usually lasting 12-25 minutes.

DOSAGE

As with other general anesthetic agents, the individual response to ketamine HCl is somewhat varied depending on the dose, route of administration, and age of patient, so that dosage recommendation cannot be absolutely fixed. The drug should be titrated against the patient's requirements.

INDUCTION

Intravenous Route

The initial dose of ketamine HCl administered intravenously may range from 1 to 4.5 mg/kg (0.5 to 2 mg/lb). The average amount required to produce 5-10 minutes of surgical anesthesia has been 2 mg/kg (1 mg/lb).

Alternatively, in adult patients an induction dose of 1-2 mg/kg intravenous ketamine at a rate of 0.5 mg/kg/min may be used for induction of anesthesia. In addition, diazepam in 2-5 mg doses, administered in a separate syringe over 60 seconds, may be used. In most cases, 15 mg of intravenous diazepam *or less* will suffice. The incidence of psychological manifestations during emergence, particularly dream-like observations and emergence delirium, may be reduced by this induction dosage program.

Note: The 100 mg/ml concentration of ketamine HCl *should not* be injected intravenously without proper dilution. It is recommended the drug be diluted with an equal volume of either sterile water for injection, normal saline, or 5% dextrose in water.

Rate of Administration: It is recommended that ketamine HCl be administered slowly (over a period of 60 seconds). More rapid administration may result in respiratory depression and enhanced pressor response.

Intramuscular Route

The initial dose of ketamine HCl administered intramuscularly may range from 6.5 to 13 mg/kg (3-6 mg/lb). A dose of 10 mg/kg (5 mg/lb) will usually produce 12-25 minutes of surgical anesthesia.

MAINTENANCE OF ANESTHESIA

The maintenance dose should be adjusted according to the patient's anesthetic needs and whether an additional anesthetic agent is employed.

Increments of one-half to the full induction dose may be repeated as needed for maintenance of anesthesia. However, it should be noted that purposeless and tonic-clonic movements of extremities may occur during the course of anesthesia. These movements do not imply a light plane and are not indicative of the need for additional doses of the anesthetic.

It should be recognized that the larger the total dose of ketamine HCl administered, the longer will be the time to complete recovery.

Adult patients induced with ketamine HCl augmented with intravenous diazepam may be maintained on ketamine HCl given by slow microdrip infusion technique at a dose of 0.1-0.5 mg/min, augmented with diazepam 2-5 mg administered intravenously as needed. In many cases 20 mg *or less* of intravenous diazepam total for combined induction and maintenance will suffice. However, slightly more diazepam may be required depending on the nature and duration of the operation, physical status of the patient, and other factors. The incidence of psychological manifestations during emergence, particularly dream-like observations and emergence delirium, may be reduced by this maintenance dosage program.

Dilution

To prepare a dilute solution containing 1 mg of ketamine per ml, aseptically transfer 10 ml (50 mg/ml Steri-Vial) or 5 ml (100 mg/ml Steri-Vial) to 500 ml of 5% dextrose injection or sodium chloride (0.9%) injection (normal saline) and mix well. The resultant solution will contain 1 mg of ketamine per ml.

The fluid requirements of the patient and duration of anesthesia must be considered when selecting the appropriate dilution of ketamine HCl. If fluid restriction is required, ketamine HCl can be added to a 250 ml infusion as described above to provide a ketamine HCl concentration of 2 mg/ml.

Ketalar Steri-Vials, 10 mg/ml are not recommended for dilution.

SUPPLEMENTARY AGENTS

Ketamine HCl is clinically compatible with the commonly used general and local anesthetic agents when an adequate respiratory exchange is maintained.

The regimen of a reduced dose of ketamine HCl supplemented with diazepam can be used to produce balanced anesthesia by combination with other agents such as nitrous oxide and oxygen.

PRODUCT LISTING - RATED THERAPEUTICALLY EQUIVALENT

Package	Price	Product	NDC
Solution - Injectable - 10 mg/ml			
20 ml x 10	$149.90	KETALAR, Monarch Pharmaceuticals Inc	61570-0581-10
20 ml x 10	$177.85	GENERIC, King Pharmaceuticals Inc	60793-0581-10
Solution - Injectable - 50 mg/ml			
10 ml x 10	$77.07	GENERIC, Abbott Pharmaceutical	00074-2053-10
10 ml x 10	$162.50	GENERIC, Bedford Laboratories	55390-0475-10
10 ml x 10	$278.50	KETALAR, Monarch Pharmaceuticals Inc	61570-0582-10
Solution - Injectable - 100 mg/ml			
5 ml x 10	$97.97	GENERIC, Abbott Pharmaceutical	00074-2051-05
5 ml x 10	$273.10	KETALAR, Monarch Pharmaceuticals Inc	61570-0585-10

Ketoconazole *(001605)*

For related information, see the comparative table section in Appendix A.

Categories: Blastomycosis; Candidiasis; Chromomycosis; Coccidioidomycosis; Dandruff; Dermatitis, seborrheic; Histoplasmosis; Paracoccidioidomycosis; Tinea corporis; Tinea cruris; Tinea pedis; Tinea versicolor; Pregnancy Category C; FDA Approved 1981 Jun

Drug Classes: Antifungals; Antifungals, topical; Dermatologics

Brand Names: **Nizoral**

Foreign Brand Availability: Akorazol (Mexico); Anfuhex (Indonesia); Antanazol (Singapore); Aquarius (Greece); Beatoconazole (Singapore); Bigazol (Korea); Comozol (Korea); Conazol (Mexico); Cremosan (Mexico); Diazon (Hong-Kong; Thailand); Daktagold (New-Zealand); Dezoral (Singapore); Diazon (Singapore); Fazol (Colombia); Formyco (Indonesia); Funazole Tabs (India); Funet (Indonesia); Fungarest (Spain); Fungazol Tabs (Hong-Kong; Thailand); Fungaway (Taiwan); Fugen (Costa-Rica; El-Salvador; Guatemala; Honduras; Nicaragua; Panama); Fungicide (Thailand); Fungicide Tabs (Bahrain; India; Republic-Of-Yemen); Fungiderm-K (Thailand); Funginoc (Bahrain); Funginox Tabs (Thailand); Fungoral (Greece; Norway; Sweden); Kenazol (Thailand); Kenazole (Bahrain; Cyprus; Egypt; Iran; Iraq; Jordan; Kuwait; Lebanon; Libya; Oman; Qatar; Republic-of-Yemen; Saudi-Arabia; Syria; United-Arab-Emirates); Kesnazol (Korea); Ketazol (Bahrain; Cyprus; Egypt; Iran; Iraq; Jordan; Kuwait; Lebanon; Libya; Oman; Qatar; Republic-of-Yemen; Saudi-Arabia; South-Africa; Syria; United-Arab-Emirates); Keto-Comp (Peru); Ketoconazol (Costa-Rica; Dominican-Republic; El-Salvador; Guatemala; Honduras; Nicaragua; Panama); Keto-Crema (Peru); Ketoderm (France); Ketoisdin (Spain); Ketomed (Colombia); Ketomicin (Peru); Ketomicol (Peru); Ketona (China; Taiwan); Keto-Shampoo (Peru); Ketozal (Thailand); Ketozol (India); Kezon (Thailand); Konaturil (Mexico); Lama (Thailand); Larry (Thailand); Lusanoc (Indonesia); Mizole (Korea); Mizoron (Thailand); Mycofebrin (Greece); Nastil (Mexico); Nazole (Korea); Neutrogena T/Sal (Peru); Niz Creme (South-Africa); Niz Shampoo (South-Africa); Nizoral 2% Cream (Australia; New-Zealand; Philippines); Nizoral Cream and Tablets (England; Mexico; Netherlands); Nizoral Shampoo (Australia; Germany; New-Zealand; Philippines); Nizoral Tablets (Australia; Colombia; Costa-Rica; Dominican-Republic; Ecuador; El-Salvador; France; Guatemala; Honduras; Mexico; New-Zealand; Nicaragua; Panama; Peru); Nizoral Tabs and Cream (Taiwan); Oxonazol (Peru); Panfungol (Spain); Pasalen (Thailand); Picamic (Indonesia); Prenalon (Mexico); Pristine (Hong-Kong); Pristinex (Hong-Kong); Profungal (Singapore); Sebizole (Australia; Hong-Kong); Spike (Korea); Sporium (Colombia); Sporoxyl (Thailand); Sporozol (India); Termizol (Mexico); Triatop Lotion (China); Zoralin Tabs (Indonesia)

Cost of Therapy: \$27.39 (Candidiasis; Nizoral; 200 mg; 1 tablets/day; 7 day supply)
\$21.27 (Candidiasis; Generic Tablets; 200 mg; 1 tablets/day; 7 day supply)

WARNING

When used orally, ketoconazole has been associated with hepatic toxicity, including some fatalities. Patients receiving this drug should be informed by the physician of the risk and should be closely monitored. See WARNINGS and PRECAUTIONS.

Coadministration of terfenadine with ketoconazole tablets is contraindicated. Rare cases of serious cardiovascular adverse events including death, ventricular tachycardia, and torsades de pointes have been observed in patients taking ketoconazole concomitantly with terfenadine, due to increased terfenadine concentrations induced by ketoconazole tablets. See CONTRAINDICATIONS, WARNINGS, and PRECAUTIONS.

Pharmacokinetic data indicate that oral ketoconazole inhibits the metabolism of astemizole, resulting in elevated plasma levels of astemizole and its active metabolite desmethylastemizole, which may prolong QT intervals. Coadministration of astemizole with ketoconazole tablets is therefore contraindicated. See CONTRAINDICATIONS, WARNINGS, and PRECAUTIONS.

Coadministration of cisapride with ketoconazole is contraindicated. Serious cardiovascular adverse events including ventricular tachycardia, ventricular fibrillation and torsades de pointes have occurred in patients taking ketoconazole concomitantly with cisapride. See CONTRAINDICATIONS, WARNINGS, and PRECAUTIONS.

DESCRIPTION

Ketoconazole is cis-1-acetyl-4-[4-[[2-(2,4-dichlorophenyl)-2-(1H-imidazol-1-ylmethyl)-1,3-dioxolan-4-yl]methoxyl]phenyl] piperazine.

Ketoconazole is a white to slightly beige, odorless powder soluble in acids. It has a molecular weight of 531.44. It molecular formula is $C_{26}H_{28}Cl_2N_4O_4$.

CREAM

Ketoconazole 2% cream contains the broad-spectrum synthetic antifungal agent ketoconazole 2% formulated in an aqueous cream vehicle consisting of propylene glycol, stearyl and cetyl alcohols, sorbitan monostearate, polysorbate 60, isopropyl myristate, sodium sulfite anhydrous, polysorbate 80, and purified water.

SHAMPOO

Ketoconazole 2% shampoo is a red-orange liquid for topical application, which contains the broad-spectrum synthetic antifungal agent ketoconazole in a concentration of 2% in an aqueous suspension. It also contains: coconut fatty acid diethanolamide, disodium monolauryl ether sulfosuccinate, FD&C red no. 40, hydrochloric acid, imidurea, laurdimonium hydrolyzed animal collagen, macrogol 120 methyl glucose dioleate, perfume bouquet, sodium chloride, sodium hydroxide, sodium lauryl ether sulphate, and purified water.

TABLETS

Ketoconazole is a synthetic broad-spectrum antifungal agent available in scored white tablets, each containing 200 mg ketoconazole base for oral administration. *Inactive Ingredients:* Colloidal silicon dioxide, corn starch, lactose, magnesium stearate, microcrystalline cellulose, and povidone.

CLINICAL PHARMACOLOGY

CREAM

When ketoconazole 2% cream was applied dermally to intact or abraded skin of Beagle dogs for 28 consecutive days at a dose of 80 mg, there were no detectable plasma levels using an assay method having a lower detection limit of 2 ng/ml.

After a single topical application to the chest, back, and arms of normal volunteers, systemic absorption of ketoconazole was not detected at the 5 ng/ml level in blood over a 72 hour period.

Two dermal irritancy studies, a human sensitization test, a phototoxicity study, and a photoallergy study conducted in 38 male and 62 female volunteers showed no contact sensitization of the delayed hypersensitivity type, no irritation, no phototoxicity, and no photoallergic potential due to ketoconazole 2% cream.

SHAMPOO

When ketoconazole 2% shampoo was applied dermally to intact or abraded skin of rabbits for 28 days at doses up to 50 mg/kg and allowed to remain 1 hour before being washed away, there were no detectable plasma ketoconazole levels using an assay method having a lower detection limit of 5 ng/ml. Ketoconazole was not detected in plasma in 39 patients who shampooed 4-10 times per week for 6 months or in 33 patients who shampooed 2-3 times per week for 3-26 months (mean: 16 months).

Twelve (12) hours after a single shampoo, hair samples taken from 6 patients showed that high amounts of ketoconazole were present on the hair but only about 5% penetrated into the hair keratin. Chronic shampooing (twice weekly for 2 months) increased the ketoconazole levels in the hair keratin to 20% but did not increase levels on the hair. There were no detectable plasma levels.

An exaggerated-use washing test on the sensitive antecubital skin of 10 subjects twice daily for 5 consecutive days showed that the irritancy potential of ketoconazole 2% shampoo was significantly less than that of 2.5% selenium sulfide shampoo.

A human sensitization test, a phototoxicity study, and a photoallergy study conducted in 38 male and 22 female volunteers showed no contact sensitization of the delayed hypersensitivity type, no phototoxicity and no photoallergic potential due to ketoconazole 2% shampoo.

TABLETS

Mean peak plasma levels of approximately 3.5 μg/ml are reached within 1-2 hours, following oral administration of a single 200 mg dose taken with a meal. Subsequent plasma elimination is biphasic with half-life of 2 hours during the first 10 hours and 8 hours thereafter. Following absorption from the gastrointestinal tract, ketoconazole is converted into several inactive metabolites. The major identified metabolic pathways are oxidation and degradation of the imidazole and piperazine rings, oxidative O-dealkylation and aromatic hydroxylation. About 13% of the dose is excreted in the urine, of which 2-4% is unchanged drug. The major route of excretion is through the bile into the intestinal tract. *In vitro*, the plasma protein-binding is about 99%, mainly to the albumin fraction. Only a negligible proportion of ketoconazole reaches the cerebrospinal fluid. Ketoconazole is a weak dibasic agent and thus requires acidity for dissolution and absorption.

Ketoconazole tablets are active against clinical infections with *Blastomyces dermatitidis, Candida spp., Coccidioides immitis, Histoplasma capsulatum, Paracoccidioides brasiliensis,* and *Phialophora spp.* Ketoconazole tablets are also active against *Trichophyton spp., Epidermophyton spp.,* and *Microsporum spp.* Ketoconazole is also active *in vitro* against a variety of fungi and yeast. In animal models, activity has been demonstrated against *Candida spp., Blastomyces dermatitidis, Histoplasma capsulatum, Malassezia furfur, Coccidioides immitis,* and *Cryptococcus neoformans.*

MODE OF ACTION

Tablets, Shampoo, and Cream

In vitro studies suggest that ketoconazole impairs the synthesis of ergosterol, which is a vital component of fungal cell membranes.

Shampoo

It is postulated that the therapeutic effect of ketoconazole in dandruff is due to the reduction of *Pityrosporum ovale (Malassezia ovale),* but this has not been proven. Support for this hypothesis comes from a 4-week, double-blind, placebo controlled clinical trial in which the decrease in *P. ovale* on the scalp was significantly greater with ketoconazole (36 patients) than with placebo (20 patients) and was comparable to that with selenium sulfide (42 patients). In the same study, ketoconazole and selenium sulfide reduced the severity of adherent dandruff significantly more than placebo did. Ketoconazole produced significantly higher proportions of patients with at least 50% reductions in adherent dandruff (50% vs 15%) and in loose dandruff (67% vs 15%) than did the placebo.

Cream

It is postulated that the therapeutic effect of ketoconazole in seborrheic dermatitis is due to the reduction of *M. ovale,* but this has not been proven.

MICROBIOLOGY

Shampoo and Cream

Ketoconazole is a broad spectrum synthetic antifungal agent which inhibits the *in vitro* growth of the following common dermatophytes and yeast by altering the permeability of the cell membrane: dermatophytes: *Trichophyton rubrum, T. mentagrophytes, T. tonsurans, Microsporum canis, M. audouini, M. gypseum* and *Epidermophyton floccosum;* yeasts: *Candida albicans, Malassezia ovale (pityrosporum ovale),* and *C. tropicalis.* Development of resistance by these microorganisms to ketoconazole has not been reported.

Cream Only

In the cream form ketoconazole also inhibits the *in vitro* growth of the following additional yeast by altering the permeability of the cell: the organism responsible for tinea versicolor, *Malassezia furfur (Pityrosporum orbiculare).* Only those organisms listed in INDICATIONS AND USAGE have been proven to be clinically affected. Development of resistance to ketoconazole has not been reported.

INDICATIONS AND USAGE

CREAM

Ketoconazole 2% cream is indicated for the topical treatment of tinea corporis, tinea cruris, and tinea pedis caused by *Trichophyton rubrum, T. mentagrophytes,* (efficacy for this organism in this organ system was studied in fewer than 10 infections), and *Epidermophyton floccosum;* in the treatment of tinea (pityriasis) versicolor caused by *Malassezia furfur (Pityrosporum orbiculare);* in the treatment of cutaneous candidiasis caused by *Candida spp.,* and in the treatment of seborrheic dermatitis.

SHAMPOO

Ketoconazole 2% shampoo is indicated for the reduction of scaling due to dandruff.

TABLETS

Ketoconazole tablets are indicated for the treatment of the following systemic fungal infections: Candidiasis, chronic mucocutaneous candidiasis, oral thrush, candiduria, blastomycosis, coccidioidomycosis, histoplasmosis, chromomycosis, and paracoccidioidomycosis. Ketoconazole should not be used for fungal meningitis because it penetrates poorly into the cerebrospinal fluid.

Ketoconazole tablets are also indicated for the treatment of patients with severe recalcitrant cutaneous dermatophyte infections who have not responded to topical therapy or oral griseofulvin, or who are unable to take griseofulvin.

CONTRAINDICATIONS

CREAM AND SHAMPOO

Ketoconazole is contraindicated in patients who have shown hypersensitivity to the drug or excipients of the formulation(s).

TABLETS

Ketoconazole is contraindicated in patients who have shown hypersensitivity to the drug or excipients of the formulation(s).

Coadministration of terfenadine or astemizole with ketoconazole tablets is contraindicated. (See BOXED WARNING, WARNINGS, and PRECAUTIONS.)

Concomitant administration of ketoconazole tablets with cisapride is contraindicated. (See BOXED WARNING, WARNINGS, and PRECAUTIONS.)

WARNINGS

CREAM

Ketoconazole 2% cream is not for ophthalmic use.

Ketoconazole 2% cream contains sodium sulfite anhydrous, a sulfite that may cause allergic-type reactions including anaphylactic symptoms and life-threatening or less severe asthmatic episodes in certain susceptible people. The overall prevalence of sulfite sensitivity in the general population is unknown and probably low. Sulfite sensitivity is seen more frequently in asthmatic than in nonasthmatic people.

TABLETS

Hepatotoxicity, primarily of the hepatocellular type, has been associated with the use of ketoconazole tablets, including rare fatalities. The reported incidence of hepatotoxicity has been about 1:10,000 exposed patients, but this probably represents some degree of under-reporting, as is the case for most reported adverse reactions to drugs. The median duration of ketoconazole therapy in patients who developed symptomatic hepatotoxicity was about 28 days, although the range extended to as low as 3 days. The hepatic injury has usually, but not always, been reversible upon discontinuation of ketoconazole treatment. Several cases of hepatitis have been reported in children.

Prompt recognition of liver injury is essential. Liver function tests (such as SGGT, alkaline phosphatase, SGPT, SGOT and bilirubin) should be measured before starting treatment and at frequent intervals during treatment. Patients receiving ketoconazole concurrently with other potentially hepatotoxic drugs should be carefully monitored, particularly those patients requiring prolonged therapy or those who have had a history of liver disease.

Most of the reported cases of hepatotoxicity have to date been in patients treated for onychomycosis. Of 180 patients worldwide developing idiosyncratic liver dysfunction during ketoconazole tablet therapy, 61.3% had onychomycosis and 16.8% had chronic recalcitrant dermatophytoses.

Transient minor elevations in liver enzymes have occurred during ketoconazole treatment. The drug should be discontinued if these persist, if the abnormalities worsen, or if the abnormalities become accompanied by symptoms of possible liver injury.

In rare cases anaphylaxis has been reported after the first dose. Several cases of hypersensitivity reactions including urticaria have also been reported.

Coadministration of ketoconazole tablets and terfenadine has led to elevated plasma concentrations of terfenadine, which may prolong QT intervals, sometimes resulting in life-threatening cardiac dysrhythmias. Cases of torsades de pointes and other serious ventricular dysrhythmias, in rare cases leading to fatality, have been reported among patients taking terfenadine concurrently with ketoconazole tablets. Coadministration of ketoconazole tablets and terfenadine is contraindicated.

Coadministration of astemizole with ketoconazole tablets is contraindicated. (See BOXED WARNING, CONTRAINDICATIONS, and PRECAUTIONS.)

Concomitant administration of ketoconazole tablets with cisapride is contraindicated in markedly elevated cisapride plasma concentrations and prolonged QT interval, and has rarely been associated with ventricular arrhythmias and torsades de pointes. (See BOXED WARNING, CONTRAINDICATIONS, and PRECAUTIONS.)

In European clinical trials involving 350 patients with metastatic prostatic cancer, 11 deaths were reported within 2 weeks of starting treatment with a high dose of ketoconazole (1200 mg/day). It is not possible to ascertain from the information available whether death was related to ketoconazole therapy in these patients with serious underlying disease. However, high doses of ketoconazole tablets are known to suppress adrenal corticosteroid secretion.

In female rats treated 3-6 months with ketoconazole at dose levels of 80 mg/kg and higher, increased fragility of long bones, in some cases leading to fracture, was seen. The maximum "no effect" dose level in these studies was 20 mg/kg (2.5 times the maximum recommended human dose). The mechanisms responsible for this phenomenon is obscure. Limited studies in dogs failed to demonstrate such an effect on the metacarpals and ribs.

PRECAUTIONS

GENERAL

Shampoo

If a reaction suggesting sensitivity or chemical irritation should occur, use of the medication should be discontinued.

Tablets

Ketoconazole tablets have been demonstrated to lower serum testosterone. Once therapy with ketoconazole has been discontinued, serum testosterone levels return to baseline values. Testosterone levels are impaired with doses of 800 mg/day and abolished by 1600 mg/day. Ketoconazole tablets also decrease ACTH-induced corticosteroid serum levels at similar high doses. The recommended dose of 200-400 mg daily should be followed closely.

In 4 subjects with drug-induced achlorhydria, a marked reduction in ketoconazole absorption was observed. Ketoconazole tablets require acidity for dissolution. If concomitant antacids, anticholinergics, and H_2-blockers are needed, they should be given at least 2 hours after administration of ketoconazole tablets. In cases of achlorhydria, the patients should be instructed to dissolve each tablet in 4 ml aqueous solution of 0.2 N HCl. For ingesting the resulting mixture, they should use a drinking straw so as to avoid contact with the teeth. This administration should be followed with a cup of tap water.

INFORMATION FOR THE PATIENT

Shampoo

May be irritating to mucous membranes of the eyes, and contact with this area should be avoided.

There have been reports that use of the shampoo resulted in removal of the curl from permanently waved hair.

Tablets

Patients should be instructed to report any signs and symptoms which may suggest liver dysfunction so that appropriate biochemical testing can be done. Such signs and symptoms may include unusual fatigue, anorexia, nausea and/or vomiting, jaundice, dark urine or pale stools (see WARNINGS).

CARCINOGENESIS, MUTAGENESIS, AND IMPAIRMENT OF FERTILITY

The dominant lethal mutation test in male and female mice revealed that single oral doses of ketoconazole as high as 80 mg/kg produced no mutation in any stage of germ cell development. The Ames *Salmonella* microsomal activator assay was also negative. A long-term feeding study in Swiss Albino mice and in Wistar rats showed no evidence of oncogenic activity.

PREGNANCY CATEGORY C

Teratogenic Effects

Shampoo

Ketoconazole is not detected in plasma after chronic shampooing.

Tablets

Ketoconazole has been shown to be teratogenic (syndactylia and oligodactylia) in the rat when given in the diet at 80 mg/kg/day (10 times the maximum recommended human dose). However, these effects may be related to maternal toxicity, evidence of which also was seen at this and higher dose levels. There are no adequate and well-controlled studies in pregnant women.

Ketoconazole should be used during pregnancy only if the potential benefit justifies the potential risk to the fetus.

Nonteratogenic Effects

Tablets

Ketoconazole has also been found to be embryotoxic in the rat when given in the diet at doses higher than 80 mg/kg during the first trimester of gestation.

In addition, dystocia (difficult labor) was noted in rats administered oral ketoconazole during the third trimester of gestation. This occurred when ketoconazole was administered at doses higher than 10 mg/kg (higher than 1.25 times the maximum human dose).

It is likely that both the malformations and the embryotoxicity resulting from the administration of oral ketoconazole during gestation are a reflection of the particular sensitivity of the female rat to this drug. For example, the oral LD_{50} of ketoconazole given by gavage to the female rat is 166 mg/kg, whereas in the male rat the oral LD_{50} is 287 mg/kg.

NURSING MOTHERS

Cream

It is not known whether ketoconazole 2% cream administered topically could result in sufficient systemic absorption to produce detectable quantities in breast milk. Nevertheless, a decision should be made whether to discontinue nursing or discontinue the drug, taking into account the importance of the drug to the mother.

Shampoo

Ketoconazole is not detected in plasma after chronic shampooing. Nevertheless, caution should be exercised when ketoconazole 2% shampoo is administered to a nursing woman.

Tablets

Since ketoconazole is probably excreted in the milk, mothers who are under treatment should not breastfeed.

PEDIATRIC USE

Cream and Shampoo

Safety and effectiveness in children have not been established.

Tablets

Ketoconazole tablets have not been systematically studied in children of any age, and essentially no information is available on children under 2 years. Ketoconazole tablets should not be used in pediatric patients unless the potential benefit outweighs the risks.

DRUG INTERACTIONS

TABLETS

Ketoconazole is a potent inhibitor of the cytochrome P450 3A4 enzyme system. Coadministration of ketoconazole tablets and drugs primarily metabolized by the cytochrome P450 3A4 enzyme system may result in increased plasma concentrations of the drugs that could increase or prolong both therapeutic and adverse effects. Therefore, unless otherwise specified, appropriate dosage adjustments may be necessary. The following drug interactions have been identified involving ketoconazole tablets and other drugs metabolized by the cytochrome P450 3A4 enzyme system:

Ketoconazole tablets inhibit the metabolism of terfenadine, resulting in an increased plasma concentration of terfenadine and a delay in the elimination of its acid metabolite. The increased plasma concentration of terfenadine or its acid metabolite may result in prolonged QT intervals. (See BOXED WARNING, CONTRAINDICATIONS, and WARNINGS.)

Pharmacokinetic data indicate that oral ketoconazole inhibits the metabolism of astemizole, resulting in elevated plasma levels of astemizole and its active metabolite desmethylastemizole which may prolong QT intervals. Coadministration of astemizole with ketoconazole tablets is therefore contraindicated. (See BOXED WARNING, CONTRAINDICATIONS, and WARNINGS.)

Human pharmacokinetics data indicate that oral ketoconazole potently inhibits the metabolism of cisapride resulting in a mean 8-fold increase in AUC of cisapride. Data suggest that coadministration of oral ketoconazole and cisapride can result in prolongation of the QT interval on the ECG. Therefore, concomitant administration of ketoconazole tablets with cisapride is contraindicated (see BOXED WARNING, CONTRAINDICATIONS, and WARNINGS).

Ketoconazole tablets may alter the metabolism of cyclosporine, tacrolimus, and methylprednisolone, resulting in elevated plasma concentrations of the latter drugs. Dosage adjustment may be required if cyclosporine, tacrolimus, or methylprednisolone are given concomitantly with ketoconazole tablets.

Coadministration of ketoconazole tablets with midazolam or triazolam has resulted in elevated plasma concentrations of the latter two drugs. This may potentiate and prolong hypnotic and sedative effects, especially with repeated dosing or chronic administration of these agents. These agents should not be used in patients treated with ketoconazole tablets. If midazolam is administered parenterally, special precaution is required since the sedative effect may be prolonged.

K

Rare cases of elevated plasma concentrations of digoxin have been reported. It is not clear whether this was due to the combination of therapy. It is, therefore, advisable to monitor digoxin concentrations in patients receiving ketoconazole.

When taken orally, imidazole compounds like ketoconazole may enhance the anticoagulant effect of coumarin-like drugs. In simultaneous treatment with imidazole drugs and coumarin drugs, the anticoagulant effect should be carefully titrated and monitored.

Because severe hypoglycemia has been reported in patients concomitantly receiving oral miconazole (an imidazole) and oral hypoglycemic agents, such a potential interaction involving the latter agents when used concomitantly with ketoconazole (an imidazole) cannot be ruled out.

Concomitant administration of ketoconazole with phenytoin may alter the metabolism of one or both of the drugs. It is suggested to monitor both ketoconazole and phenytoin.

Concomitant administration of rifampin with ketoconazole tablets reduces the blood levels of the latter. INH (isoniazid) is also reported to affect ketoconazole concentrations adversely. These drugs should not be given concomitantly.

After the coadministration of 200 mg oral ketoconazole twice daily and one 20 mg dose of loratadine to 11 subjects, the AUC and C_{max} of loratadine averaged 302% (± 142 SD) and 251% (± 68 SD), respectively, of those obtained after cotreatment with placebo. The AUC and C_{max} of descarboethoxyloratadine, an active metabolite, averaged 155% (± 27 SD) and 141% (± 35 SD), respectively. However, no related changes were noted in the QTc on ECG taken at 2, 6, and 24 hours after coadministration. Also, there were no clinically significant differences in adverse events when loratadine was administered with or without ketoconazole.

Rare cases of a disulfiram-like reaction to alcohol have been reported. These experiences have been characterized by flushing, rash, peripheral edema, nausea, and headache. Symptoms resolved within a few hours.

ADVERSE REACTIONS

CREAM

During clinical trials 45 (5%) of 905 patients treated with ketoconazole 2% cream and 5 (2.4%) of 208 patients treated with placebo reported side effects consisting mainly of severe irritation, pruritus, and stinging. One (1) of the patients treated with ketoconazole cream developed a painful allergic reaction.

SHAMPOO

In eleven double-blind trials in 264 patients using ketoconazole 2% shampoo, an increase in normal hair loss and irritation occurred in less than 1% of patients. In three open-label safety trials in which 41 patients shampooed 4-10 times weekly for 6 months, the following adverse experiences each occurred once: abnormal hair texture, scalp pustules, mild dryness of the skin, and itching. As with other shampoos, oiliness and dryness of hair and scalp have been reported.

TABLETS

In rare cases anaphylaxis has been reported after the first dose. Several cases of hypersensitivity reactions including urticaria have also been reported. However, the most frequent adverse reactions were nausea and/or vomiting in approximately 3%, abdominal pain in 1.2%, pruritus in 1.5%, and the following in less than 1% of the patients: headache, dizziness, somnolence, fever and chills, photophobia, diarrhea, gynecomastia, impotence, thrombocytopenia, leukopenia, hemolytic anemia, and bulging fontanelles. Oligospermia has been reported in investigational studies with the drug at dosages above those currently approved. Oligospermia has not been reported at dosages up to 400 mg daily; however, sperm counts have been obtained infrequently in patients treated with these dosages. Most of these reactions were mild and transient and rarely required discontinuation of ketoconazole tablets. In contrast, the rare occurrences of hepatic dysfunction require special attention (see WARNINGS).

In worldwide postmarketing experience with ketoconazole tablets there have been rare reports of alopecia, paresthesia, and signs of increased intracranial pressure including bulging fontanelles and papilledema. Hypertriglyceridemia has also been reported but a causal association with ketoconazole tablets is uncertain.

Neuropsychiatric disturbances, including suicidal tendencies and severe depression, have occurred rarely in patients using ketoconazole tablets.

Ventricular dysrhythmias (prolonged QT intervals) have occurred with the concomitant use of terfenadine with ketoconazole tablets. (See BOXED WARNING, CONTRAINDICATIONS, and WARNINGS.) Data suggest that coadministration of ketoconazole tablets and cisapride can result in prolongation of the QT interval and has rarely been associated with ventricular arrhythmias. (See CONTRAINDICATIONS, WARNINGS, and PRECAUTIONS.)

DOSAGE AND ADMINISTRATION

CREAM

Cutaneous Candidiasis, Tinea Corporis, Tinea Cruris, and Tinea (Pityriasis) Versicolor

It is recommended that ketoconazole 2% cream be applied once daily to cover the affected and immediate surrounding area. Clinical improvement may be seen fairly soon after treatment is begun; however, candidal infections and tinea cruris and corporis should be treated for 2 weeks in order to reduce the possibility of recurrence. Patients with tinea versicolor usually require 2 weeks of treatment. Patients with tinea pedis require 6 weeks of treatment.

Seborrheic Dermatitis

Ketoconazole 2% cream should be applied to the affected area twice daily for 4 weeks or until clinical clearing.

If a patient shows no clinical improvement after the treatment period, the diagnosis should be redetermined.

SHAMPOO

Shampoo twice a week for 4 weeks with at least 3 days between each shampooing and then intermittently as needed to maintain control.

TABLETS

Adults: The recommended starting dose of ketoconazole tablets is a single daily administration of 200 mg (1 tablet). In very serious infections or if clinical responsiveness is insufficient within the expected time, the dose of ketoconazole may be increased to 400 mg (2 tablets) once daily.

Children: In small numbers of children over 2 years of age, a single daily dose of 3.3-6.6 mg/kg has been used. Ketoconazole tablets have not been studied in children under 2 years of age.

There should be laboratory as well as clinical documentation of infection prior to starting ketoconazole therapy. Treatment should be continued until tests indicate that active fungal infection has subsided. Inadequate periods of treatment may yield poor response and lead to early recurrence of clinical symptoms. Minimum treatment for candidiasis is 1 or 2 weeks. Patients with chronic mucocutaneous candidiasis usually require maintenance therapy. Minimum treatment for the other indicated systemic mycoses is 6 months.

Minimum treatment for recalcitrant dermatophyte infections is 4 weeks in cases involving glabrous skin. Palmar and plantar infections may respond more slowly. Apparent cures may subsequently recur after discontinuation of therapy in some cases.

HOW SUPPLIED

CREAM

Nizoral 2% cream is supplied in 15, 30, and 60 g tubes.

SHAMPOO

Nizoral 2% shampoo is a red-orange liquid.

Storage: Store at a temperature not above 25°C (77°F). Protect from light.

TABLETS

Nizoral is available as white, scored tablets containing 200 mg of ketoconazole debossed "JANSSEN" and on the reverse side debossed "NIZORAL".

Storage: Store at room temperature 15-25°C (59-77°F). Protect from moisture.

PRODUCT LISTING - RATED THERAPEUTICALLY EQUIVALENT

Cream - Topical - 2%

Size	Price	Product	NDC
15 gm	$16.46	GENERIC, Teva Pharmaceuticals Usa	00093-0840-15
15 gm	$18.29	NIZORAL TOPICAL, Allscripts Pharmaceutical Company	54569-2440-00
15 gm	$20.45	NIZORAL TOPICAL, Southwood Pharmaceuticals Inc	58016-1051-01
15 gm	$20.96	NIZORAL TOPICAL, Janssen Pharmaceuticals	50458-0221-15
15 gm	$21.85	NIZORAL TOPICAL, Prescript Pharmaceuticals	00247-0340-15
15 gm	$23.84	NIZORAL TOPICAL, Physicians Total Care	54868-1879-01
15 gm	$26.46	NIZORAL TOPICAL, Pharma Pac	52959-0556-00
15 gm	$26.75	GENERIC, Pharma Pac	52959-0497-15
30 gm	$27.70	GENERIC, Teva Pharmaceuticals Usa	00093-0840-30
30 gm	$28.25	NIZORAL TOPICAL, Southwood Pharmaceuticals Inc	58016-3181-01
30 gm	$30.78	NIZORAL TOPICAL, Allscripts Pharmaceutical Company	54569-1103-00
30 gm	$35.11	NIZORAL TOPICAL, Physicians Total Care	54868-1879-02

30 gm	$35.29	NIZORAL TOPICAL, Janssen Pharmaceuticals	50458-0221-30
60 gm	$42.08	GENERIC, Teva Pharmaceuticals Usa	00093-0840-92
60 gm	$53.03	NIZORAL TOPICAL, Physicians Total Care	54868-1879-03
60 gm	$53.60	NIZORAL TOPICAL, Janssen Pharmaceuticals	50458-0221-60
Tablet - Oral - 200 mg			
6's	$25.96	NIZORAL, Physicians Total Care	54868-0940-03
10's	$42.48	NIZORAL, Physicians Total Care	54868-0940-02
14's	$59.99	NIZORAL, Pharma Pac	52959-0197-14
20's	$61.88	NIZORAL, Southwood Pharmaceuticals Inc	58016-0168-20
20's	$83.79	NIZORAL, Physicians Total Care	54868-0940-06
20's	$85.36	NIZORAL, Pharma Pac	52959-0197-20
30's	$90.04	NIZORAL, Southwood Pharmaceuticals Inc	58016-0168-30
30's	$91.19	GENERIC, Mutual Pharmaceutical Co Inc	53489-0554-07
30's	$94.80	GENERIC, Mutual/United Research Laboratories	00677-1700-07
30's	$94.80	GENERIC, Taro Pharmaceuticals U.S.A. Inc	51672-4026-06
30's	$125.10	NIZORAL, Physicians Total Care	54868-0940-01
30's	$127.39	NIZORAL, Pharma Pac	52959-0197-30
30's	$316.00	GENERIC, Taro Pharmaceuticals U.S.A. Inc	51672-4026-01
100's	$277.50	FEDERAL UPPER LIMIT, H.C.F.A. F F P	99999-1605-01
100's	$303.85	GENERIC, Mutual Pharmaceutical Co Inc	53489-0554-01
100's	$308.98	GENERIC, Mova Pharmaceutical Corporation	55370-0558-07
100's	$313.98	GENERIC, Teva Pharmaceuticals Usa	00093-0900-01
100's	$315.80	GENERIC, Mylan Pharmaceuticals Inc	00378-0261-01
100's	$316.00	GENERIC, Mutual/United Research Laboratories	00677-1700-01
100's	$391.29	NIZORAL, Physicians Total Care	54868-0940-04
100's	$447.53	NIZORAL, Janssen Pharmaceuticals	50458-0220-10

PRODUCT LISTING - EQUIVALENTS NOT AVAILABLE

Cream - Topical - 2%			
15 gm	$16.83	GENERIC, Taro Pharmaceuticals U.S.A. Inc	51672-1298-01
30 gm	$28.32	GENERIC, Taro Pharmaceuticals U.S.A. Inc	51672-1298-02
60 gm	$43.02	GENERIC, Taro Pharmaceuticals U.S.A. Inc	51672-1298-03
Shampoo - Topical - 2%			
120 ml	$22.62	NIZORAL TOPICAL, Pharma Pac	54569-3394-00
120 ml	$23.84	NIZORAL TOPICAL, Physicians Total Care	54868-2239-00
120 ml	$27.48	NIZORAL TOPICAL, Janssen Pharmaceuticals	50458-0223-04
120 ml	$33.22	NIZORAL TOPICAL, Pharma Pac	52959-0554-03
Tablet - Oral - 200 mg			
100's	$303.83	GENERIC, Sidmak Laboratories Inc	50111-0621-01

Ketoprofen (001606)

For related information, see the comparative table section in Appendix A.

Categories: Arthritis, osteoarthritis; Arthritis, rheumatoid; Dysmenorrhea; Pain; Pregnancy Category B; FDA Approved 1986 Jan
Drug Classes: Analgesics, non-narcotic; Nonsteroidal anti-inflammatory drugs
Brand Names: Alrhumat; Kefenid; **Orudis**; Oruvail
Foreign Brand Availability: Alrheumat (Denmark; England; Ireland); Alrheumun (Germany); Aneol (Japan); Anzema (Indonesia); Apo-Keto (Canada); Arcental (Spain); Bi-Profenid (France); Bi-Rofenid (Belgium); Dolomax (Colombia); Efiken (Mexico); Epatec (Japan); Fastum (Italy; Spain); Fetik (Indonesia); Gabrilen Retard (Germany); Kaltrofen (Indonesia); Kebanon (Korea); Keduril (Costa-Rica; Dominican-Republic; El-Salvador; Guatemala; Honduras; Mexico; Nicaragua; Panama); Kefen (New-Zealand); Kehancer (Singapore); Kenofen Gel (Korea); Keprofen (Japan); Ketadom (Hong-Kong); Ketin (Taiwan); Ketofen (Thailand); Keto Film (Korea); Ketoflam (South-Africa); Ketolgin (Bahrain; Cyprus; Egypt; Iran; Iraq; Jordan; Kuwait; Lebanon; Libya; Oman; Qatar; Republic-of-Yemen; Saudi-Arabia; Syria; United-Arab-Emirates); Ketolgin SR (Bahrain; Cyprus; Egypt; Iran; Iraq; Jordan; Kuwait; Lebanon; Libya; Oman; Qatar; Republic-of-Yemen; Saudi-Arabia; Syria; United-Arab-Emirates); Ketolgin Gel (Bahrain; Cyprus; Egypt; Iran; Iraq; Jordan; Kuwait; Lebanon; Libya; Oman; Qatar; Republic-of-Yemen; Saudi-Arabia; Syria; United-Arab-Emirates); Ketomex (Finland); Ketonal (Israel); Ketorin (Finland); Keotsan (Peru); Ketosolan (Spain); Ketum (Colombia); Kevadon (Argentina); Knavon (Greece); Mohrus (Japan); Naxal (Japan); Novo-Keto-EC (Canada); Orucote (South-Africa); Orudis E-100 (Malaysia); Orudis EC (Philippines); Orudis R-PR (Bahamas; Barbados; Belize; Bermuda; Curacao; Guyana; Jamaica; Netherland-Antilles; Puerto-Rico; Surinam; Trinidad); Orudis SR (Australia; New-Zealand; Switzerland); Oruvail EC (New-Zealand); Oruvail SR (Australia; New-Zealand); Ostofen (India); Ovurila (Indonesia); Ovurila E (Indonesia); Profenid (Austria; Bulgaria; China; Colombia; Czech-Republic; Ecuador; Indonesia; Israel; Mexico; Peru; Poland; Portugal; Russia; Switzerland; Taiwan; Turkey); Profenid 50 (India); Profenil (Italy); Provail CR (Singapore); Rhetoflam (Indonesia); Rheuna PAP (Korea); Rofenid (Belgium); Toprec (France); Treosin (Japan)
Cost of Therapy: $147.30 (Osteoarthritis; Orudis; 50 mg; 4 capsules/day; 30 day supply)
$96.74 (Osteoarthritis; Generic Capsules; 50 mg; 4 capsules/day; 30 day supply)
$100.94 (Osteoarthritis; Oruvail Extended-Release; 200 mg; 1 capsule/day; 30 day supply)
$74.70 (Osteoarthritis; Generic Extended-Release Capsules; 200 mg; 1 capsule/day; 30 day supply)

DESCRIPTION

Ketoprofen is a nonsteroidal anti-inflammatory drug. The chemical name for ketoprofen is 2-(3-benzoylphenyl)-propionic acid.

Its empirical formula is $C_{16}H_{14}O_3$, with a molecular weight of 254.29. It has a pKa of 5.94 in methanol:water (3:1) and an n-octanol:water partition coefficient of 0.97 (buffer pH 7.4).

Ketoprofen is a white or off-white, odorless, non-hygroscopic, fine to granular powder, melting at about 95°C. It is freely soluble in ethanol, chloroform, acetone, ether and soluble in benzene and strong alkali, but practically insoluble in water at 20°C.

ORUDIS CAPSULES

Orudis capsules contain 25, 50, or 75 mg of ketoprofen for oral administration. The inactive ingredients present are D&C yellow no. 10, FD&C blue no. 1, FD&C yellow no. 6, gelatin, lactose, magnesium stearate, and titanium dioxide. The 25 mg dosage strength also contains D&C red no. 28 and FD&C red no.40.

ORUVAIL EXTENDED-RELEASE CAPSULES

Oruvail extended-release capsules 100, 150, or 200 mg capsule contains ketoprofen in the form of hundreds of coated pellets. The dissolution of the pellets is pH dependent with optimum dissolution occurring at pH 6.5-7.5. There is no dissolution at pH 1.

In addition to the active ingredient, each 100, 150, or 200 mg capsule of Oruvail contains the following inactive ingredients: D&C red no. 22, D&C red no. 28, FD&C blue no. 1, ethyl cellulose, gelatin, shellac, silicon dioxide, sodium lauryl sulfate, starch, sucrose, talc, titanium dioxide, and other proprietary ingredients. The 100 and 150 mg capsules also contain D&C yellow no. 10 and FD&C green no. 3.

CLINICAL PHARMACOLOGY

Ketoprofen is a nonsteroidal anti-inflammatory drug with analgesic and antipyretic properties.

The anti-inflammatory, analgesic, and antipyretic properties of ketoprofen have been demonstrated in classical animal and *in vitro* test systems. In anti-inflammatory models ketoprofen has been shown to have inhibitory effects on prostaglandin and leukotriene synthesis, to have antibradykinin activity, as well as to have lysosomal membrane-stabilizing action. However, its mode of action, like that of other nonsteroidal anti-inflammatory drugs, is not fully understood.

PHARMACODYNAMICS

Ketoprofen is a racemate with only the S enantiomer possessing pharmacological activity. The enantiomers have similar concentration time curves and do not appear to interact with one another.

An analgesic effect-concentration relationship for ketoprofen was established in an oral surgery pain study with ketoprofen capsules. The effect-site rate constant (k_{eo}) was estimated to be 0.9 $hour^{-1}$ (95% confidence limits: 0 to 2.1), and the concentration (Ce_{50}) of ketoprofen that produced one-half the maximum PID (pain intensity difference) was 0.3 μg/ml (95% confidence limits: 0.1 to 0.5). Thirty-three (33) to 68% of patients had an onset of action (as measured by reporting some pain relief) within 30 minutes following a single oral dose in post-operative pain and dysmenorrhea studies. Pain relief (as measured by remedication) persisted for up to 6 hours in 26-72% of patients in these studies.

K

PHARMACOKINETICS

General

Ketoprofen capsules and ketoprofen extended-release capsules differ only in their release characteristics. Ketoprofen capsules release drug in the stomach whereas the pellets in ketoprofen extended-release capsules are designed to resist dissolution in the low pH of gastric fluid but release drug at a controlled rate in the higher pH environment of the small intestine (see DESCRIPTION).

Irrespective of the pattern of release, the systemic availability (Fs) when either oral formulation is compared with IV administration is approximately 90% in humans. For 75-200 mg single doses, the area under the curve has been shown to be dose proportional.

Ketoprofen is >99% bound to plasma proteins, mainly to albumin.

Separate sections follow which delineate differences between ketoprofen capsules and ketoprofen extended-release capsules.

Absorption

Capsules

Ketoprofen is rapidly and well-absorbed, with peak plasma levels occurring within 0.5 to 2 hours.

Food intake reduces C_{max} by approximately one-half and increases the mean time to peak concentration (T_{max}) from 1.2 hours for fasting subjects (range, 0.5 to 3 hours) to 2.0 hours for fed subjects (range, 0.75 to 3 hours). The fluctuation of plasma peaks may also be influenced by circadian changes in the absorption process.

Concomitant administration of magnesium hydroxide and aluminum hydroxide does not interfere with absorption of ketoprofen from ketoprofen capsules.

Extended-Release Capsules

Ketoprofen is also well-absorbed from this dosage form, although an observable increase in plasma levels does not occur until approximately 2-3 hours after taking the formulation. Peak plasma levels are usually reached 6-7 hours after dosing. (See TABLE 1.)

When ketoprofen is administered with food, its total bioavailability (AUC) is not altered; however, the rate of absorption from either dosage form is slowed.

Administration of ketoprofen extended-release capsules with a high-fat meal causes a delay of about 2 hours in reaching the C_{max}; neither the total bioavailability (AUC) nor the C_{max} is affected. Circadian changes in the absorption process have not been studied.

The administration of antacids or other drugs which may raise stomach pH would not be expected to change the rate or extent of absorption of ketoprofen from ketoprofen extended-release capsules.

Multiple Dosing

Steady-state concentrations of ketoprofen are attained within 24 hours after commencing treatment with either formulation. In studies with healthy male volunteers, trough levels at 24 hours following administration of ketoprofen extended-release capsules were 0.4 mg/L compared with 0.07 mg/ml at 24 hours following administration of ketoprofen 50 mg capsules qid (12 hours) or 0.13 mg/L following administration of ketoprofen 75 mg capsules tid for 12 hours. Thus, relative to the peak plasma concentration, the accumulation of ketoprofen after multiple doses of either formulation is minimal.

***TABLE 1** Comparison of Pharmacokinetic Parameters* for Ketoprofen Capsules and Ketoprofen Extended-Release Capsules*

Kinetic Parameters	Capsules (4 × 50 mg)	Extended-Release Capsules (1 × 200 mg)
Extent of oral absorption (bioavailability Fs (%)	~90	~90
Peak plasma levels C_{max} (mg/L)		
Fasted	3.9 ± 1.3	3.1 ± 1.2
Fed	2.4 ± 1.0	3.4 ± 1.3
Time to peak concentration T_{max} (h)		
Fasted	1.2 ± 0.6	6.8 ± 2.1
Fed	2.0 ± 0.8	9.2 ± 2.6
Fasted	32.1 ± 7.2	30.1 ± 7.9
Fed	36.6 ± 8.1	31.3 ± 8.1
Oral-dose clearance		
Cl/F (L/h)	6.9 ± 0.8	6.8 ± 1.8
Half-life T½ (h)†	2.1 ± 1.2	5.4 ± 2.2

* Values expressed are mean ± standard deviation
† In the case of ketoprofen extended-release capsules, absorption is slowed, intrinsic clearance is unchanged, but because the rate of elimination is dependent on absorption, the half-life is prolonged.

Metabolism

The metabolism fate of ketoprofen is glucuronide conjugation to form an unstable acyl-glucuronide. The glucuronic acid moiety can be converted back to the parent compound. Thus, the metabolite serves as a potential reservoir for parent drug, and this may be important in persons with renal insufficiency, whereby the conjugate may accumulate in the serum and undergo deconjugation back to the parent drug (see Special Populations, Renally Impaired). The conjugates are reported to appear only in trace amounts in plasma in healthy adults, but are higher in elderly subjects—presumably because of reduced renal clearance. It has been demonstrated that in elderly subjects following multiple doses (50 mg every 6 hours), the ratio of conjugated to parent ketoprofen AUC was 30% and 3%, respectively for the S & R enantiomers.

There are no known active metabolites of ketoprofen. Ketoprofen has been shown not to induce drug-metabolizing enzymes.

K

Elimination

The plasma clearance of ketoprofen is approximately 0.08 L/kg/h with a Vd of 0.1 L/kg after IV administration. The elimination half-life of ketoprofen has been reported to be 2.05 ± 0.58 hours (Mean ± SD) following IV administration, from 2-4 hours following administration of ketoprofen capsules, and 5.4 ± 2.2 hours after administration of ketoprofen extended-release capsules. In cases of slow drug absorption, the elimination rate is dependent on the absorption rate and thus T½ relative to an IV dose appears prolonged.

After a single 200 mg dose of ketoprofen extended-release capsules, the plasma levels decline slowly, the average 0.4 mg/L after 24 hours.

In a 24 hour period, approximately 80% of an administered dose of ketoprofen is excreted in the urine, primarily as the glucuronide metabolite.

Enterohepatic recirculation of the drug has been postulated, although biliary levels have never measured to confirm this.

Special Populations

Elderly — Clearance and Unbound Fraction

The plasma and renal clearance of ketoprofen is reduced in the elderly (mean age, 73 years) compared to a younger normal population (mean age, 27 years). Hence, ketoprofen peak concentration and AUC increase with increasing age. In addition, there is a corresponding increase in unbound fraction with increasing age. Data from one trial suggest that the increase is greater in women than in men. It has not been determined whether age-related changes in absorption among the elderly contribute to the changes in bioavailability of ketoprofen.

Capsules

In a study conducted with young and elderly men and women, results for subjects older than 75 years of age showed that free drug AUC increased by 40% and C_{max} increased by 60% as compared with estimates of the same parameters in young subjects (those younger than 35 years of age; see DOSAGE AND ADMINISTRATION, Individualization Of Dosage).

Also in the elderly, the rate of intrinsic clearance/availability decreased by 35% and plasma half-life was prolonged by 26%. This reduction is thought to be due to a decrease in hepatic extraction associated with aging.

Extended-Release Capsules

The effects of age and gender on ketoprofen disposition were investigated in 2 small studies in which elderly male and female subjects received ketoprofen extended-release capsules. The results were compared with those from another study conducted in healthy young men.

Compared to the younger subject group, the elimination half-life in the elderly was prolonged by 54% and total drug C_{max} and AUC were 40% and 70% higher, respectively. Plasma concentrations in the elderly after single doses and at steady state were essentially the same. Thus, no drug accumulation occurs.

In comparison to younger subjects taking the immediate-release formulation, there was a decrease of 16% and 25% in the total drug C_{max} and AUC, respectively, among the elderly. Free drug data are not available for ketoprofen extended-release capsules.

Renally Impaired

Studies of the effects of renal-function impairment have been small. They indicate a decrease in clearance in patients with impaired renal function. In 23 patients with renal impairment, free ketoprofen peak concentration was not significantly elevated, but free ketoprofen clearance was reduced from 15 L/kg/h for normal subjects to 7 L/kg/h in patients with mildly impaired renal function, and to 4 L/kg/h in patients with moderately to severely impaired renal function. The elimination T½ was prolonged from 1.6 hours in normal subjects to approximately 3 hours in patients with mild renal impairment, and to approximately 5-9 hours in patients with moderately to severely impaired renal function.

No studies have been conducted in patients with renal impairment taking ketoprofen extended-release capsules. It is recommended that only the immediate-release formulation of ketoprofen be used to treat patients with significant renal impairment (see DOSAGE AND ADMINISTRATION, Individualization Of Dosage).

Hepatically Impaired

For patients with alcoholic cirrhosis, no significant changes in the kinetic disposition of ketoprofen capsules were observed relative to age-matched normal subjects: the plasma clearance of drug was 0.07 L/kg/h in 26 hepatically impaired patients. The elimination half-life was comparable to that observed for normal subjects. However, the unbound (biologically active) fraction was approximately doubled, probably due to hypoalbuminemia and high variability which was observed in the pharmacokinetics for cirrhotic patients. Therefore, these patients should be carefully monitored and daily doses of ketoprofen kept at the minimum providing the desired therapeutic effect.

No studies have been conducted in patients with hepatic impairment taking ketoprofen extended-release capsules. It is recommended that only the immediate-release formulation of ketoprofen be used to treat patients who have hepatic impairment and serum albumin levels below 3.5 g/dl (see DOSAGE AND ADMINISTRATION, Individualization Of Dosage).

INDICATIONS AND USAGE

Ketoprofen capsules or extended-release capsules are indicated for the management of the signs and symptoms of rheumatoid arthritis and osteoarthritis. Ketoprofen extended-release capsules are not recommended for treatment of acute pain because of their controlled-release characteristics (see CLINICAL PHARMACOLOGY, Pharmacokinetics).

Ketoprofen capsules are indicated for the management of pain. Ketoprofen capsules are also indicated for treatment of primary dysmenorrhea.

CONTRAINDICATIONS

Ketoprofen is contraindicated in patients who have shown hypersensitivity to it. Ketoprofen should not be given to patients in whom aspirin or other nonsteroidal anti-inflammatory drugs induce asthma, urticaria, or other allergic-type reactions, because severe, rarely fatal, anaphylactic reactions to ketoprofen have been reported in such patients.

WARNINGS

RISK OF GI ULCERATION, BLEEDING AND PERFORATION WITH NSAID THERAPY

Serious gastrointestinal toxicity, such as bleeding, ulceration, and perforation, can occur at any time with or without warning symptoms, in patients treated chronically with NSAID therapy. Although minor upper-gastrointestinal problems, such as dyspepsia, are common, usually developing early in therapy, physicians should remain alert for ulceration and bleeding in patients treated chronically with NSAIDs even in the absence of previous GI-tract symptoms. In patients observed in clinical trials of several months to 2 years' duration, symptomatic upper-GI ulcers, gross bleeding, or perforation appear to occur in approximately 1% of patients treated for 3 to 6 months, and in about 2-4% of patients treated for 1 year. Physicians should inform patients about the signs and/or symptoms of serious GI toxicity and what steps to take if they occur.

Studies to date have not identified any subset of patients not at risk of developing peptic ulceration and bleeding. Except for a prior history of serious GI events and other risk factors known to be associated with peptic ulcer disease, such as alcoholism, smoking, etc., no other risk factors (*e.g.,* age, sex) have been associated with increased risk. Elderly or debilitated patients seem to tolerate ulceration or bleeding less well than other individuals, and most spontaneous reports of fatal GI events are in this population. Studies to date are inconclusive concerning the relative risk of various NSAIDs in causing such reactions. High doses of any NSAID probably carry a greater risk of these reactions, although controlled clinical trials showing this do not exist in most cases. In considering the use of relatively large doses (within the recommended dosage range), sufficient benefit should be anticipated to offset the potential increased risk of GI toxicity.

PRECAUTIONS

GENERAL

Ketoprofen and other nonsteroidal anti-inflammatory drugs cause nephritis in mice and rats associated with chronic administration. Rare cases of interstitial nephritis or nephrotic syndrome have been reported in humans with ketoprofen since it has been marketed.

A second form of renal toxicity has been seen in patients with conditions leading to a reduction in renal blood flow or blood volume, where renal prostaglandins have a supportive role in the maintenance of renal blood flow. In these patients, administration of a nonsteroidal anti-inflammatory drug results in a dose-dependent decrease in prostaglandin synthesis and, secondarily, in renal blood flow which may precipitate overt renal failure. Patients at greatest risk of this reaction are those with impaired renal function, heart failure, liver dysfunction, those taking diuretics, and the elderly. Discontinuation of nonsteroidal anti-inflammatory drug therapy is typically followed by recovery to the pretreatment state.

Since ketoprofen is primarily eliminated by the kidneys and its pharmacokinetics are altered by renal failure (see CLINICAL PHARMACOLOGY), patients with significantly impaired renal function should be closely monitored, and a reduction of dosage should be anticipated to avoid accumulation of ketoprofen and/or its metabolites (see DOSAGE AND ADMINISTRATION, Individualization Of Dosage).

As with other nonsteroidal anti-inflammatory drugs, borderline elevations of one or more liver function tests may occur in up to 15% of patients. These abnormalities may progress, may remain essentially unchanged, or may disappear with continued therapy. The ALT (SGPT) test is probably the most sensitive indicator of liver dysfunction. Meaningful (3 times the upper limit of normal) elevations of ALT or AST (SGOT) occurred in controlled clinical trials in less than 1% of patients. A patient with symptoms and/or signs suggesting liver dysfunction, or in whom an abnormal liver test has occurred, should be evaluated for evidence of the development of a more severe hepatic reaction while on therapy with ketoprofen. Serious hepatic reactions, including jaundice, have been reported from post-marketing experience with ketoprofen as well as with other nonsteroidal anti-inflammatory drugs.

In patients with chronic liver disease with reduced serum albumin levels, ketoprofen's pharmacokinetics are altered (see CLINICAL PHARMACOLOGY). Such patients should be closely monitored, and a reduction of dosage should be anticipated to avoid high blood levels of ketoprofen and/or its metabolites (see DOSAGE AND ADMINISTRATION, Individualization Of Dosage).

If steroid dosage is reduced or eliminated during therapy, it should be reduced slowly and the patients observed closely for any evidence of adverse effects, including adrenal insufficiency and exacerbation of symptoms of arthritis.

Anemia is commonly observed in rheumatoid arthritis and is sometimes aggravated by nonsteroidal anti-inflammatory drugs, which may produce fluid retention or significant gastrointestinal blood loss in some patients. Patients on long-term treatment with NSAIDs, including ketoprofen capsules or ketoprofen extended-release capsules, should have their hemoglobin or hematocrit checked if they develop signs or symptoms of anemia.

Peripheral edema has been observed in approximately 2% of patients taking ketoprofen. Therefore, as with other nonsteroidal anti-inflammatory drugs, ketoprofen should be used with caution in patients with fluid retention, hypertension, or heart failure.

INFORMATION FOR THE PATIENT

The capsules and extended-release capsules contain ketoprofen. Like other drugs of its class, ketoprofen, is not free of side effects. The side effects of these drugs can cause discomfort and, rarely, there are more serious side effects, such as gastrointestinal bleeding, which may result in hospitalization and even fatal outcomes.

NSAIDs are often essential agents in the management of arthritis and have a major role in the treatment of pain, but they also may be commonly employed for conditions which are less serious. Physicians may wish to discuss with their patients the potential risks (see WARNINGS, PRECAUTIONS, and ADVERSE REACTIONS) and likely benefits of NSAID treatment, particularly when the drugs are used for less serious conditions where treatment without NSAIDs might represent an acceptable alternative to both the patient and physician.

Because aspirin causes an increase in the level of unbound ketoprofen, patients should be advised not to take aspirin while taking ketoprofen (see DRUG INTERACTIONS). It is possible that minor adverse symptoms of gastric intolerance may be prevented by administering ketoprofen capsules with antacids, food, or milk. Ketoprofen extended-release capsules have not been studied with antacids. Because food and milk do affect the rate but not the extent of absorption (see CLINICAL PHARMACOLOGY), physicians may want to make specific recommendations to patients about when they should take ketoprofen in relation to food and/or what patients should do if they experience minor GI symptoms associated with ketoprofen therapy.

LABORATORY TESTS

Because serious GI-tract ulceration and bleeding can occur without warning symptoms, physicians should follow chronically treated patients for the signs and symptoms of ulceration and bleeding and should inform them of the importance of this follow-up (see WARNINGS).

DRUG/LABORATORY TEST INTERACTIONS

Effect on Blood Coagulation

Ketoprofen decreases platelet adhesion and aggregation. Therefore, it can prolong bleeding time by approximately 3 to 4 minutes from baseline values. There is no significant change in platelet count, prothrombin time, partial thromboplastin time, or thrombin time.

CARCINOGENESIS, MUTAGENESIS, AND IMPAIRMENT OF FERTILITY

Chronic oral toxicity studies in mice (up to 32 mg/kg/day; 96 mg/m^2/day) did not indicate a carcinogenic potential for ketoprofen. The maximum recommended human therapeutic dose is 300 mg/day for a 60 kg patient with a body surface area of 1.6 m^2, which is 5 mg/kg/day or 185 mg/m^2/day. Thus the mice were treated at 0.5 times the maximum human daily dose based on surface area.

A 2 year carcinogenicity study in rats, using doses up to 6.0 mg/kg/day (36 mg/m^2/day), showed no evidence of tumorigenic potential. All groups were treated for 104 weeks except the females receiving 6.0 mg/kg/day (36 mg/m^2/day) where the drug treatment was terminated in week 81 because of low survival; the remaining rats were sacrificed after week 87. Their survival in the groups treated for 104 weeks was within 6% of the control group. An earlier 2 year study with doses up to 12.5 mg/kg/day (75 mg/m^2/day) also showed no evidence of tumorigenicity, but the survival rate was low and the study was therefore judged inconclusive. Ketoprofen did not show mutagenic potential in the Ames Test. Ketoprofen administered to male rats (up to 9 mg/kg/day; or 54 mg/m^2/day) had no significant effect on reproductive performance or fertility. In female rats administered 6 or 9 mg/kg/day (36 or 54 mg/m^2/day), a decrease in the number of implantation sites has been noted. The dosages of 36 mg/m^2/day in rats represent 0.2 times the maximum recommended human dose of 185 mg/m^2/day.

Abnormal spermatogenesis or inhibition of spermatogenesis developed in rats and dogs at high doses, and a decrease in the weight of the testes occurred in dogs and baboons at high doses.

PREGNANCY, TERATOGENIC EFFECTS, PREGNANCY CATEGORY B

In teratology studies ketoprofen administered to mice at doses up to 12 mg/kg/day (36 mg/m^2/day) and rats at doses up to 9 mg/kg/day (54 mg/m^2/day), the approximate equivalent of 0.2 times the maximum recommended therapeutic dose of 185 mg/m^2/day, showed no teratogenic or embryotoxic effects. In separate studies in rabbits, maternally toxic doses were associated with embryotoxicity but not teratogenicity.

There are no adequate and well-controlled studies in pregnant women. Because animal teratology studies are not always predictive of the human response, ketoprofen should be used during pregnancy only if the potential benefit justifies the risk.

LABOR AND DELIVERY

The effects of ketoprofen on labor and delivery in pregnant women are unknown. Studies in rats have shown ketoprofen at doses of 6 mg/kg (36 mg/m^2/day, approximately equal to 0.2 times the maximum recommended human dose) prolong pregnancy when given before the onset of labor. Because of the known effects of prostaglandin-inhibiting drugs on the fetal cardiovascular system (closure of ductus arteriosus), use of ketoprofen during late pregnancy should be avoided.

NURSING MOTHERS

Data on secretion in human milk after ingestion of ketoprofen do not exist. In rats, ketoprofen at doses of 9 mg/kg (54 mg/m^2/day; approximately 0.3 times the maximum human therapeutic dose) did not affect perinatal development. Upon administration to lactating dogs, the milk concentration of ketoprofen was found to be 4-5% of the plasma drug level. As with other drugs that are excreted in milk, ketoprofen is not recommended for use in nursing mothers.

PEDIATRIC USE

Ketoprofen is not recommended for use in children, because its safety and effectiveness have not been studied in children.

DRUG INTERACTIONS

The following drug interactions were studied with ketoprofen doses of 200 mg/day. The possibility of increased interaction should be kept in mind when doses of ketoprofen capsules greater than 50 mg as a single dose or 200 mg of ketoprofen per day are used concomitantly with highly bound drugs.

Antacids: Concomitant administration of magnesium hydroxide and aluminum hydroxide does not interfere with the rate or extent of the absorption of ketoprofen administered as ketoprofen capsules.

Aspirin: Ketoprofen does not alter aspirin absorption; however, in a study of 12 normal subjects, concurrent administration of aspirin decreased ketoprofen protein binding and increased ketoprofen plasma clearance from 0.07 L/kg/h without aspirin to 0.11 L/kg/h with aspirin. The clinical significance of these changes has not been adequately studied. Therefore, concurrent use of aspirin and ketoprofen is not recommended.

Diuretic: Hydrochlorothiazide, given concomitantly with ketoprofen, produces a reduction in urinary potassium and chloride excretion compared to hydrochlorothiazide alone. Patients taking diuretics are at greater risk of developing renal failure secondary to a decrease in renal blood flow caused by prostaglandin inhibition (see PRECAUTIONS, General).

Digoxin: In a study in 12 patients with congestive heart failure where ketoprofen and digoxin were concomitantly administered, ketoprofen did not alter the serum levels of digoxin.

Warfarin: In a short-term controlled study in 14 normal volunteers, ketoprofen did not significantly interfere with the effect of warfarin on prothrombin time. Bleeding from a number of sites may be a complication of warfarin treatment and GI bleeding a complication of ketoprofen treatment. Because prostaglandins play an important role in hemostasis and ketoprofen has an effect on platelet function as well (see PRECAUTIONS, Drug/Laboratory Test Interactions, Effect on Blood Coagulation), concurrent therapy with ketoprofen and warfarin requires close monitoring of patients on both drugs.

Probenecid: Probenecid increases both free and bound ketoprofen by reducing the plasma clearance of ketoprofen to about one-third, as well as decreasing its protein binding. Therefore, the combination of ketoprofen and probenecid is not recommended.

Methotrexate: Ketoprofen, like other NSAIDs, may cause changes in the elimination of methotrexate leading to elevated serum levels of the drug and increased toxicity.

Lithium: Nonsteroidal anti-inflammatory agents have been reported to increase steady-state plasma lithium levels. It is recommended that plasma lithium levels be monitored when ketoprofen is co-administered with lithium.

ADVERSE REACTIONS

The incidence of common adverse reactions (above 1%) was obtained from a population of 835 patients treated with ketoprofen capsules in double-blind trials lasting from 4-54 weeks and in 622 ketoprofen extended-release capsules (200 mg/day) patients in trials lasting from 4-16 weeks.

Minor gastrointestinal side effects predominated; upper gastrointestinal symptoms were more common than lower gastrointestinal symptoms. In crossover trials in 321 patients with rheumatoid arthritis or osteoarthritis, there was no difference in either upper or lower gastrointestinal symptoms between patients treated with 200 mg of ketoprofen extended-release capsules once a day or 75 mg of ketoprofen capsules tid (225 mg/day). Peptic ulcer or GI bleeding occurred in controlled clinical trials in less than 1% of 1076 patients; however, in open label continuation studies in 1292 patients the rate was greater than 2%.

The incidence of peptic ulceration in patients on NSAIDs is dependent on many risk factors including age, sex, smoking, alcohol use, diet, stress, concomitant drugs such as aspirin and corticosteroids, as well as the dose and duration of treatment with NSAIDs (see WARNINGS).

Gastrointestinal reactions were followed in frequency by central nervous system side effects, such as headache, dizziness, or drowsiness. The incidence of some adverse reactions appears to be dose-related (see DOSAGE AND ADMINISTRATION). Rare adverse reactions (incidence less than 1%) were collected from foreign reports to manufacturers and regulatory agencies, publications, and US clinical trials.

Reactions are listed below under body system, then by incidence or number of cases in decreasing incidence.

Incidence Greater Than 1% (probable causal relationship):

Digestive: Dyspepsia (11%), nausea*, abdominal pain*, diarrhea*, constipation*, flatulence*, anorexia, vomiting, stomatitis.

K

Nervous System: Headache*, dizziness, CNS inhibition (*i.e.*, pooled reports of somnolence, malaise, depression, etc.) or excitation (*i.e.*, insomnia, nervousness, dreams, etc.).*

Special Senses: Tinnitus, visual disturbance.

Skin and Appendages: Rash.

Urogenital: Impairment of renal function (edema, increased BUN)*, signs or symptoms of urinary-tract irritation.

*Adverse events occurring in 3-9% of patients.

Incidence Less Than 1% (probable causal relationship):

Body as a Whole: Chills, facial edema, infection, pain, allergic reaction, anaphylaxis.

Cardiovascular: Hypertension, palpitation, tachycardia, congestive heart failure, peripheral vascular disease, vasodilation.

Digestive: Appetite increased, dry mouth, eructation, gastritis, rectal hemorrhage, melena, fecal occult blood, salivation, peptic ulcer, gastrointestinal perforation, hematemesis, intestinal ulceration.

Hemic: Hypocoagulability, agranulocytosis, anemia, hemolysis, purpura, thrombocytopenia.

Metabolic and Nutritional: Thirst, weight gain, weight loss, hepatic dysfunction, hyponatremia.

Musculoskeletal: Myalgia.

Nervous System: Amnesia, confusion, impotence, migraine, paresthesia, vertigo.

Respiratory: Dyspnea, hemoptysis, epistaxis, pharyngitis, rhinitis, bronchospasm, laryngeal edema.

Skin and Appendages: Alopecia, eczema, pruritus, purpuric rash, sweating, urticaria, bullous rash, exfoliative dermatitis, photosensitivity, skin discoloration, onycholysis.

Special Senses: Conjunctivitis, conjunctivitis sicca, eye pain, hearing impairment, retinal hemorrhage and pigmentation change, taste perversion.

Urogenital: Menometrorrhagia, hematuria, renal failure, interstitial nephritis, nephrotic syndrome.

Incidence Less Than 1% (causal relationship unknown): The following rare adverse reactions, whose causal relationship to ketoprofen is uncertain, are being listed to serve as alerting information to the physician.

Body as a Whole: Septicemia, shock.

Cardiovascular: Arrhythmias, myocardial infarction.

Digestive: Buccal necrosis, ulcerative colitis, microvesicular steatosis, jaundice, pancreatitis.

Endocrine: Diabetes mellitus (aggravated).

Nervous System: Dysphoria, hallucination, libido disturbance, nightmares, personality disorder, aseptic meningitis.

Urogenital: Acute tubulopathy, gynecomastia.

DOSAGE AND ADMINISTRATION

RHEUMATOID ARTHRITIS AND OSTEOARTHRITIS

The recommended starting dose of ketoprofen in otherwise healthy patients is for ketoprofen capsules 75 mg three times or 50 mg four times a day or for ketoprofen extended-release capsules 200 mg administered once a day. Smaller doses of ketoprofen capsules and ketoprofen extended-release capsules should be utilized initially in small individuals or in debilitated or elderly patients. The recommended maximum daily dose of ketoprofen is 300 mg/day for ketoprofen or 200 mg/day for ketoprofen extended-release capsules (see Individualization Of Dosage).

Dosage higher than 300 mg/day of ketoprofen capsules or 200 mg/day of ketoprofen extended-release capsules are not recommended because the have not been studied.

Concomitant use of ketoprofen capsules and ketoprofen extended-release capsules is not recommended. Relatively smaller people may need smaller doses (see Individualization Of Dosage).

MANAGEMENT OF PAIN AND DYSMENORRHEA

The usual dose of ketoprofen capsules recommended for mild-to-moderate pain and dysmenorrhea is 25-50 mg every 6-8 hours as necessary. A smaller dose should be utilized initially in small individuals, in debilitated or elderly patients, or in patients with renal or liver disease (see PRECAUTIONS, General). A larger dose may be tried if the patient's response to a previous dose was less than satisfactory, but doses above 75 mg have not been shown to give added analgesia. Daily doses above 300 mg are not recommended because they have not been adequately studied. Because of its typical nonsteroidal anti-inflammatory drug-side-effect profile, including as its principal adverse effect GI side effects (see WARNINGS and ADVERSE REACTIONS), higher doses of ketoprofen capsules should be used with caution and patients receiving them observed carefully (see Individualization Of Dosage).

Ketoprofen extended-release capsules are not recommended for use in treating acute pain because of their controlled-release characteristics.

INDIVIDUALIZATION OF DOSAGE

The recommended starting dose of ketoprofen in otherwise healthy patients is ketoprofen capsules, 75 mg three times or 50 mg four times a day, or ketoprofen extended-release capsules, 200 mg administered once a day. Smaller doses of ketoprofen capsules or ketoprofen extended-release capsules should be utilized initially in small individuals or in debilitated or elderly patients. The recommended maximum daily dose of ketoprofen is 300 mg/day for ketoprofen capsules or 200 mg/day for ketoprofen extended-release capsules is not recommended.

If minor side effects appear, they may disappear at a lower dose which may still have an adequate therapeutic effect. If well tolerated but not optimally effective, the dosage may be increased. Individual patients may show a better response to 300 mg of ketoprofen daily as compared to 200 mg, although in well-controlled clinical trials patients on 300 mg did not show greater mean effectiveness. They did, however, show an increased frequency of upper- and lower-GI distress and headaches. It is of interest that women also had an increased frequency of these adverse effects compared to men. When treating patients with 300 mg/day, the physician should observe sufficient increased clinical benefit to offset potential increased risk.

In patients with mildly impaired renal function, the maximum recommended total daily dose of ketoprofen capsules or ketoprofen extended-release capsules is 150 mg. In patients with a more severe renal impairment (GFR less than 25 ml/min/1.73 m^2 or end-stage renal impairment), the maximum daily dose of ketoprofen capsules or ketoprofen extended-release-capsules should not exceed 100 mg.

In elderly patients, renal function may be reduced with apparently normal serum creatinine and/or BUN levels. Therefore, it is recommended that the initial dosage of ketoprofen capsules or ketoprofen extended-release capsules should be reduced for patients over 75 years of age.

It is recommended that for patients with impaired liver function and serum albumin concentration less than 3.5 g/dl, the maximum initial total daily dose of ketoprofen capsules and ketoprofen extended-release capsules should be 100 mg. All patients with metabolic impairment, particularly those with both hypoalbuminemia and reduced renal function, may have increased levels of free (biologically active) ketoprofen and should be closely monitored. The dosage may be increased to the range recommended for the general population, if necessary, only after good individual tolerance has been ascertained.

Because hypoalbuminemia and reduced renal function both increase the fraction of free drug (biologically active form), patients who have both conditions may be at greater risk of adverse effects. Therefore, it is recommended that such patients also be started on lower doses of ketoprofen capsules and ketoprofen extended-release capsules and closely monitored.

As with other nonsteroidal anti-inflammatory drugs, the predominant adverse effects of ketoprofen are gastrointestinal. To attempt to minimize these effects, physicians may wish to prescribe that ketoprofen capsules or ketoprofen extended-release capsules be taken with antacids, food, or milk. Although food delays the absorption of both formulations (see CLINICAL PHARMACOLOGY), in most of the clinical trials ketoprofen was taken with food or milk.

Physicians may want to make specific recommendations to patients about when they should take ketoprofen capsules or ketoprofen extended-release capsules in relation to food and/or what patients should do if they experience minor GI symptoms associated with either formulation.

HOW SUPPLIED

ORUDIS CAPSULES

Orudis capsules are available as follows:

25 mg: Dark-green and red capsule marked "WYETH 4186" on one side and "ORUDIS 25" on the reverse side.

50 mg: Dark-green and light-green capsule marked "WYETH 4181" on one side and "ORUDIS 50" on the reverse side.

75 mg: Dark-green and white capsule marked "WYETH 4187" on one side and "ORUDIS 75" on the reverse side.

Storage: Keep tightly closed. Store at room temperature, approximately 25°C (77°F). Dispense in a tight container. Protect from direct light and excessive heat and humidity.

ORUVAIL EXTENDED-RELEASE CAPSULES

Orudis extended-release capsules are available as follows:

100 mg: Opaque pink and dark-green capsule marked with two radial bands and "ORUVAIL 100".

150 mg: Opaque pink and light-green capsule marked with two radial bands and "ORUVAIL 150".

200 mg: Opaque pink and off-white capsule marked with two radial bands and "ORUVAIL 200".

Storage: Keep tightly closed. Store at room temperature, approximately 25°C (77°F). Dispense in a tight container.

PRODUCT LISTING - RATED THERAPEUTICALLY EQUIVALENT

Capsule - Oral - 25 mg			
100's	$65.68	GENERIC, Ivax Corporation	00182-1958-01
100's	$70.98	GENERIC, Geneva Pharmaceuticals	00781-2409-01
100's	$72.15	GENERIC, West Point Pharma	59591-0001-68
100's	$74.35	GENERIC, Esi Lederle Generics	00005-3284-43
100's	$78.50	GENERIC, Aligen Independent Laboratories Inc	00405-4578-01
100's	$99.99	ORUDIS, Wyeth-Ayerst Laboratories	00008-4186-01
Capsule - Oral - 50 mg			
30's	$12.38	GENERIC, Pd-Rx Pharmaceuticals	55289-0287-30
30's	$36.83	ORUDIS, Pharma Pac	54569-2178-00
100's	$47.49	FEDERAL UPPER LIMIT, H.C.F.A. F F P	99999-1606-01
100's	$80.62	GENERIC, Qualitest Products Inc	00603-4177-21
100's	$89.11	GENERIC, Mutual/United Research Laboratories	00677-1463-01
100's	$89.15	GENERIC, West Point Pharma	59591-0002-68
100's	$89.25	GENERIC, Major Pharmaceuticals Inc	00904-7711-60
100's	$90.44	GENERIC, Ivax Corporation	00182-1959-01
100's	$91.00	GENERIC, Geneva Pharmaceuticals	00781-2410-01
100's	$91.91	GENERIC, Esi Lederle Generics	00005-3285-43
100's	$92.20	GENERIC, Aligen Independent Laboratories Inc	00405-4579-01
100's	$96.50	GENERIC, Teva Pharmaceuticals Usa	00093-3193-01
100's	$96.50	GENERIC, Mylan Pharmaceuticals Inc	00378-4070-01
100's	$122.75	ORUDIS, Wyeth-Ayerst Laboratories	00008-4181-01
Capsule - Oral - 75 mg			
12's	$17.93	GENERIC, Dhs Inc	55887-0912-12
15's	$13.96	GENERIC, Pd-Rx Pharmaceuticals	55289-0181-15
18's	$27.76	ORUDIS, Physicians Total Care	54868-1052-04
20's	$11.96	GENERIC, Pd-Rx Pharmaceuticals	55289-0181-20
21's	$12.23	GENERIC, Pd-Rx Pharmaceuticals	55289-0181-21
21's	$31.66	GENERIC, Dhs Inc	55887-0912-21

30's $14.94 GENERIC, Pd-Rx Pharmaceuticals 55289-0181-30
30's $42.11 GENERIC, Dhs Inc 55887-0912-30
100's $23.11 GENERIC, Esi Lederle Generics 00005-3286-43
100's $40.58 FEDERAL UPPER LIMIT, H.C.F.A. F F P 99999-1606-02
100's $98.90 GENERIC, Qualitest Products Inc 00603-4178-21
100's $99.15 GENERIC, West Point Pharma 59591-0003-68
100's $99.29 GENERIC, Aligen Independent Laboratories Inc 00405-4580-01
100's $99.30 GENERIC, Major Pharmaceuticals Inc 00904-7712-60
100's $100.30 GENERIC, Ivax Corporation 00182-1960-01
100's $102.19 GENERIC, Geneva Pharmaceuticals 00781-2411-01
100's $107.30 GENERIC, Teva Pharmaceuticals Usa 00093-3195-01
100's $107.30 GENERIC, Mylan Pharmaceuticals Inc 00378-5750-01
100's $136.53 ORUDIS, Wyeth-Ayerst Laboratories 00008-4187-01

Capsule, Extended Release - Oral - 200 mg

7's $21.11 ORUVAIL, Allscripts Pharmaceutical Company 54569-3792-01
10's $36.74 ORUVAIL, Physicians Total Care 54868-3380-03
10's $41.18 ORUVAIL, Pd-Rx Pharmaceuticals 55289-0369-10
10's $42.34 GENERIC, Pharma Pac 52959-0520-10
15's $45.24 ORUVAIL, Allscripts Pharmaceutical Company 54569-3792-02
15's $54.52 ORUVAIL, Physicians Total Care 54868-3380-02
15's $54.91 ORUVAIL, Pharma Pac 52959-0347-15
15's $63.06 GENERIC, Pharma Pac 52959-0520-15
20's $70.58 ORUVAIL, Pharma Pac 52959-0347-20
20's $83.62 GENERIC, Pharma Pac 52959-0520-20
30's $94.47 ORUVAIL, Allscripts Pharmaceutical Company 54569-3792-00
30's $98.05 ORUVAIL, Pharma Pac 52959-0347-30
30's $107.87 ORUVAIL, Physicians Total Care 54868-3380-01
30's $124.67 GENERIC, Pharma Pac 52959-0520-30
100's $219.85 GENERIC, Esi Lederle Generics 59911-5889-01
100's $249.08 GENERIC, Andrx Pharmaceuticals 62037-0520-01
100's $336.47 ORUVAIL, Physicians Total Care 54868-3380-00
100's $339.91 ORUVAIL, Wyeth-Ayerst Laboratories 00008-0690-01

PRODUCT LISTING - EQUIVALENTS NOT AVAILABLE

Capsule - Oral - 25 mg

100's $67.49 GENERIC, Moore, H.L. Drug Exchange Inc 00839-7768-06

Capsule - Oral - 50 mg

10's $11.13 GENERIC, Southwood Pharmaceuticals Inc 58016-0262-10
15's $16.69 GENERIC, Southwood Pharmaceuticals Inc 58016-0262-15
20's $22.25 GENERIC, Southwood Pharmaceuticals Inc 58016-0262-20
21's $23.44 GENERIC, Pharma Pac 52959-0503-21
28's $31.15 GENERIC, Southwood Pharmaceuticals Inc 58016-0262-28
30's $8.86 GENERIC, Physicians Total Care 54868-2414-00
30's $33.38 GENERIC, Southwood Pharmaceuticals Inc 58016-0262-30
40's $38.58 GENERIC, Pharma Pac 52959-0503-40
60's $66.75 GENERIC, Southwood Pharmaceuticals Inc 58016-0262-60
100's $90.44 GENERIC, Moore, H.L. Drug Exchange Inc 00839-7769-06
100's $111.25 GENERIC, Southwood Pharmaceuticals Inc 58016-0262-00

Capsule - Oral - 75 mg

3's $4.39 GENERIC, Prescript Pharmaceuticals 00247-0366-03
4's $4.73 GENERIC, Prescript Pharmaceuticals 00247-0366-04
10's $6.80 GENERIC, Prescript Pharmaceuticals 00247-0366-10
10's $12.40 GENERIC, Southwood Pharmaceuticals Inc 58016-0380-10
12's $11.34 GENERIC, Allscripts Pharmaceutical Company 54569-3688-02
12's $14.88 GENERIC, Southwood Pharmaceuticals Inc 58016-0380-12
14's $17.36 GENERIC, Southwood Pharmaceuticals Inc 58016-0380-14
15's $8.52 GENERIC, Prescript Pharmaceuticals 00247-0366-15
15's $14.17 GENERIC, Allscripts Pharmaceutical Company 54569-3688-03
15's $18.60 GENERIC, Southwood Pharmaceuticals Inc 58016-0380-15
20's $6.63 GENERIC, Physicians Total Care 54868-2415-00
20's $10.24 GENERIC, Prescript Pharmaceuticals 00247-0366-20
20's $18.90 GENERIC, Allscripts Pharmaceutical Company 54569-3688-01
20's $24.80 GENERIC, Southwood Pharmaceuticals Inc 58016-0380-20
20's $25.79 GENERIC, Cardinal Pharmaceuticals 63874-0418-20
20's $27.44 GENERIC, Pharma Pac 52959-0245-20
21's $10.58 GENERIC, Prescript Pharmaceuticals 00247-0366-21
21's $19.84 GENERIC, Allscripts Pharmaceutical Company 54569-3688-04
21's $26.04 GENERIC, Southwood Pharmaceuticals Inc 58016-0380-21
21's $28.85 GENERIC, Pharma Pac 52959-0245-21
24's $29.76 GENERIC, Southwood Pharmaceuticals Inc 58016-0380-24
28's $34.72 GENERIC, Southwood Pharmaceuticals Inc 58016-0380-28
30's $9.28 GENERIC, Physicians Total Care 54868-2415-02
30's $13.68 GENERIC, Prescript Pharmaceuticals 00247-0366-30
30's $28.34 GENERIC, Allscripts Pharmaceutical Company 54569-3688-00
30's $37.20 GENERIC, Southwood Pharmaceuticals Inc 58016-0380-30
30's $38.69 GENERIC, Cardinal Pharmaceuticals 63874-0418-30
30's $39.22 GENERIC, Pharma Pac 52959-0245-30
40's $49.60 GENERIC, Southwood Pharmaceuticals Inc 58016-0380-40
50's $62.00 GENERIC, Southwood Pharmaceuticals Inc 58016-0380-50
60's $17.23 GENERIC, Physicians Total Care 54868-2415-01
60's $24.00 GENERIC, Prescript Pharmaceuticals 00247-0366-60
60's $74.40 GENERIC, Southwood Pharmaceuticals Inc 58016-0380-60
90's $111.60 GENERIC, Southwood Pharmaceuticals Inc 58016-0380-90
100's $98.40 GENERIC, Moore, H.L. Drug Exchange Inc 00839-7770-06
100's $124.00 GENERIC, Southwood Pharmaceuticals Inc 58016-0380-00

Capsule, Extended Release - Oral - 100 mg

15's $33.83 GENERIC, Southwood Pharmaceuticals Inc 58016-0496-15
20's $45.10 GENERIC, Southwood Pharmaceuticals Inc 58016-0496-20
30's $67.65 GENERIC, Southwood Pharmaceuticals Inc 58016-0496-30
40's $90.20 GENERIC, Southwood Pharmaceuticals Inc 58016-0496-40
50's $112.75 GENERIC, Southwood Pharmaceuticals Inc 58016-0496-50
60's $135.30 GENERIC, Southwood Pharmaceuticals Inc 58016-0496-60
100's $189.46 GENERIC, Esi Lederle Generics 59911-5887-01
100's $225.50 GENERIC, Southwood Pharmaceuticals Inc 58016-0496-00
100's $247.69 ORUVAIL, Wyeth-Ayerst Laboratories 00008-0821-01

Capsule, Extended Release - Oral - 150 mg

100's $230.27 GENERIC, Esi Lederle Generics 59911-5888-01
100's $301.05 ORUVAIL, Wyeth-Ayerst Laboratories 00008-0822-01

Capsule, Extended Release - Oral - 200 mg

15's $37.36 GENERIC, Allscripts Pharmaceutical Company 54569-4581-00
30's $74.71 GENERIC, Allscripts Pharmaceutical Company 54569-4581-01
30's $84.07 GENERIC, Southwood Pharmaceuticals Inc 58016-0754-30
100's $249.00 GENERIC, Watson/Schein Pharmaceuticals Inc 00364-2667-01

Ketorolac Tromethamine *(001607)*

For related information, see the comparative table section in Appendix A.

Categories: Conjunctivitis, allergic; Inflammation, ophthalmic; Pain, moderate to severe; Pain, ophthalmic; Photophobia, post-operative; Pruritus, ocular; Pregnancy Category C; FDA Approved 1989 Nov

Drug Classes: Analgesics, non-narcotic; Nonsteroidal anti-inflammatory drugs; Ophthalmics

Brand Names: Acular; **Toradol**

Foreign Brand Availability: Acdol (Colombia); Acular PF (China); Alidol (Mexico); Burten (Peru); Dolac (Benin; Burkina-Faso; Ethiopia; Gambia; Ghana; Guinea; Ivory-Coast; Kenya; Liberia; Malawi; Mali; Mauritania; Mauritius; Mexico; Morocco; Niger; Nigeria; Senegal; Seychelles; Sierra-Leone; South-Africa; Sudan; Tanzania; Tunia; Uganda; Zambia; Zimbabwe); Dolorex (Peru); Estopein (Mexico); Kelac (India); Kerola (Korea); Ketanov (India); Ketodrol (Colombia); Ketonic (India); Ketorac (Korea); Ketron (Colombia); Onemer (Mexico); Rolesen (Ecuador; Peru); Tabel (Korea); Tarasyn (Korea); Toloran (Mexico); Toral (Mexico); Supradol (Mexico); Tora-Dol (South-Africa); Torolac (India); Tradak (Japan); Tromedal (Mexico)

Cost of Therapy: $132.00 (Pain; Toradol Injection; 30 mg/ml; 1 ml; 4 injections/day; 5 day supply)
$21.98 (Pain; Toradol Tablet; 10 mg; 4 tablets/day; 5 day supply)
$18.59 (Pain; Generic Tablets; 10 mg; 4 tablets/day; 5 day supply)
$100.00 (Pain; Generic Injection; 30 mg/ml; 1 ml; 4 injections/day; 5 day supply)
$31.46 (Allergic Conjunctivitis; Acular Ophth. Solution; 0.5%; 5ml; 4 drops/day; variable day supply)

HCFA JCODE(S): J1885 per 15 mg IM, IV

IM-IV

WARNING

Note: The trade names have been used throughout this monograph for clarity.

Note: The IM/IV section also includes the oral prescribing information.

Toradol, a nonsteroidal anti-inflammatory drug (NSAID), is indicated for the short-term (up to 5 days in adults) management of moderately severe acute pain that requires analgesia at the opioid level. It is NOT indicated for minor or chronic painful conditions. Toradol is a potent NSAID analgesic, and its administration carries many risks. The resulting NSAID-related adverse events can be serious in certain patients for whom Toradol is indicated, especially when the drug is used inappropriately. Increasing the dose of Toradol beyond the label recommendations will not provide better efficacy but will result in increasing the risk of developing serious adverse events.

Gastrointestinal Effects:

Toradol can cause peptic ulcers, gastrointestinal bleeding and/or perforation. Therefore, Toradol is CONTRAINDICATED in patients with active peptic ulcer disease, in patients with recent gastrointestinal bleeding or perforation, and in patients with a history of peptic ulcer disease or gastrointestinal bleeding.

Renal Effects:

Toradol is CONTRAINDICATED in patients with advanced renal impairment and in patients at risk for renal failure due to volume depletion (see WARNINGS).

Risk of Bleeding:

Toradol inhibits platelet function and is, therefore, CONTRAINDICATED in patients with suspected or confirmed cerebrovascular bleeding, patients with hemorrhagic diathesis, incomplete hemostasis and those at high risk of bleeding (see WARNINGS and PRECAUTIONS).

Toradol is CONTRAINDICATED as prophylactic analgesic before any major surgery and is CONTRAINDICATED intraoperatively when hemostasis is critical because of the increased risk of bleeding.

Hypersensitivity:

Hypersensitivity reactions, ranging from bronchospasm to anaphylactic shock, have occurred and appropriate counteractive measures must be available when administering the first dose of Toradol IV/IM (see CONTRAINDICATIONS and WARNINGS). Toradol is CONTRAINDICATED in patients with previously demonstrated hypersensitivity to ketorolac tromethamine or allergic manifestations to aspirin or other nonsteroidal anti-inflammatory drugs (NSAIDs).

Intrathecal or Epidural Administration:

Toradol is CONTRAINDICATED for intrathecal or epidural administration due to its alcohol content.

Labor, Delivery and Nursing:

The use of Toradol in labor and delivery is CONTRAINDICATED because it may adversely affect fetal circulation and inhibit uterine contractions.

The use of Toradol is CONTRAINDICATED in nursing mothers because of the potential adverse effects of prostaglandin-inhibiting drugs on neonates.

K

WARNING — Cont'd

Concomitant Use With NSAIDs:

Toradol is CONTRAINDICATED in patients currently receiving ASA or NSAIDs because of the cumulative risk of inducing serious NSAID-related side effects.

Dosage and Administration:

Toradol Oral:

Toradol oral is indicated only as continuation therapy to Toradol IV/IM, and the combined duration of use of Toradol IV/IM and Toradol oral is not to exceed 5 days because of the increased risk of serious adverse events.

The recommended total daily dose of Toradol oral (maximum 40 mg) is significantly lower than for Toradol IV/IM (maximum 120 mg) (see DOSAGE AND ADMINISTRATION, Toradol IV/IM, Transition From Toradol IV/IM to Toradol Oral).

Special Populations:

Dosage should be adjusted for patients 65 years or older, for patients under 50 kg (110 lb) of body weight (see DOSAGE AND ADMINISTRATION) and for patients with moderately elevated serum creatinine (see WARNINGS). Doses of Toradol IV/IM are not to exceed 60 mg (total dose per day) in these patients. Toradol IV/IM is indicated as a single dose therapy in pediatric patients (see DOSAGE AND ADMINISTRATION); not to exceed 30 mg for IM administration and 15 mg for IV administration.

DESCRIPTION

Toradol (ketorolac tromethamine) is a member of the pyrrolo-pyrrole group of nonsteroidal anti-inflammatory drugs (NSAIDs). The chemical name for ketorolac tromethamine is (±)-5-benzoyl-2,3-dihydro-1H-pyrrolizine-1-carboxylic acid, compound with 2-amino-2-(hydroxymethyl)-1,3-propanediol.

Toradol is a racemic mixture of [-]S and [+]R ketorolac tromethamine. Ketorolac tromethamine may exist in three crystal forms. All forms are equally soluble in water. Ketorolac tromethamine has a pKa of 3.5 and an n-octanol/water partition coefficient of 0.26. The molecular weight of ketorolac tromethamine is 376.41. Its molecular formula is $C_{19}H_{24}N_2O_6$.

Toradol is available for intravenous (IV) or intramuscular (IM) administration as: 15 mg in 1 ml (1.5%) and 30 mg in 1 ml (3%) in sterile solution; 60 mg in 2 ml (3%) of ketorolac tromethamine in sterile solution is available for IM administration only. The solutions contain 0.1% citric acid, 10% (w/v) alcohol, and 6.68 mg, 4.35 mg and 8.70 mg, respectively, of sodium chloride in sterile water. The pH is adjusted with sodium hydroxide or hydrochloric acid, and the solutions are packaged with nitrogen. The sterile solutions are clear and slightly yellow in color.

Toradol oral is available as round, white, film-coated, red-printed tablets. Each tablet contains 10 mg ketorolac tromethamine, the active ingredient, with added lactose, magnesium stearate and microcrystalline cellulose. The white film-coating contains hydroxypropyl methylcellulose, polyethylene glycol and titanium dioxide.

The tablets are printed with red ink that includes FD&C red no. 40 aluminum lake as the colorant. There is a large "T" printed on both sides of the tablet, as well as the word "TORADOL" on one side, and the word "ROCHE" on the other.

CLINICAL PHARMACOLOGY

PHARMACODYNAMICS

Ketorolac tromethamine is a nonsteroidal anti-inflammatory drug (NSAID) that exhibits analgesic activity in animal models. Ketorolac tromethamine inhibits synthesis of prostaglandins and may be considered a peripherally acting analgesic. The biological activity of ketorolac tromethamine is associated with the S-form. Ketorolac tromethamine possesses no sedative or anxiolytic properties.

The peak analgesic effect of Toradol occures within 2-3 hours and is not statistically significantly different over the recommended dosage range of Toradol. The greatest difference between large and small doses of Toradol by either route was in the duration of analgesia.

PHARMACOKINETICS

Ketorolac tromethamine is a racemic mixture of [-]S- and [+]R-enantiomeric forms, with the S-form having analgesic activity.

Comparison of IV, IM and Oral Pharmacokinetics

The pharmacokinetics of ketorolac tromethamine, following IV, IM and oral doses of Toradol, are compared in TABLE 1. In adults, the extent of bioavailability following administration of the oral and IM forms of Toradol was equal to that following an IV bolus.

Linear Kinetics

In adults, following administration of single oral, IM or IV doses of Toradol in the recommended dosage ranges, the clearance of the racemate does not change. This implies that the pharmacokinetics of ketorolac tromethamine in adults, following single or multiple IM, IV or recommended oral doses of Toradol, are linear. At the higher recommended doses, there is a proportional increase in the concentrations of free and bound racemate.

Absorption

Toradol is 100% absorbed after oral administration (see TABLE 1). Oral administration of Toradol after a high-fat meal resulted in decreased peak and delayed time-to-peak concentrations of ketorolac tromethatmine by about 1 hour. Antacids did not affect the extent of absorption.

Distribution

The mean apparent volume (Vβ) of ketorolac tromethamine following complete distribution was approximately 13 L. This parameter was determined from single-dose data. The ketorolac tromethamine racemate has been shown to be highly protein bound (99%). Nevertheless, even plasma concentrations as high as 10 µg/ml will only occupy approximately 5% of the albumin binding sites. Thus, the unbound fraction for each enantiomer will be constant over the therapeutic range. A decrease in serum albumin, however, will result in increased free drug concentrations.

Ketorolac tromethamine is excreted in human milk (see PRECAUTIONS, Lactation and Nursing).

Metabolism

Ketorolac tromethamine is largely metabolized in the liver. The metabolic products are hydroxylated and conjugated forms of the parent drug. The products of metabolism, and some unchanged drug, are excreted in the urine.

Excretion

The principal route of elimination of ketorolac and its metabolites is renal. About 92% of a given dose is found in the urine, approximately 40% as metabolites and 60% as unchanged ketorolac. Approximately 6% of a dose is excreted in the feces. A single-dose study with 10 mg Toradol (n=9) demonstrated that the S-enantiomer is cleared approximately 2 times faster than the R-enantiomer and that the clearance was independent of the route of administration. This means that the ratio of S/R plasma concentrations decreases with time after each dose. There is little or no inversion of the R- to S-form in humans. The clearance of the racemate in normal subjects, elderly individuals and in hepatically and renally impaired patients is outlined in TABLE 2 (see Kinetics in Special Populations).

The half-life of the ketorolac tromethamine S-enantiomer was approximately 2.5 hours (SD ±0.4) compared with 5 hours (SD ±1.7) for the R-enantiomer. In other studies, the half-life for the racemate has been reported to lie within the range of 5-6 hours.

Accumulation

Toradol administered as an IV bolus every 6 hours for 5 days to healthy subjects (n=13), showed no significant difference in C_{max} on Day 1 and Day 5. Trough levels averaged 0.29 µg/ml (SD ±0.13) on Day 1 and 0.55 µg/ml (SD ±0.23) on Day 6. Steady state was approached after the fourth dose.

Accumulation of ketorolac tromethamine has not been studied in special populations (geriatric, pediatric, renal failure or hepatic disease patients).

Kinetics in Special Populations

Geriatric Patients

Based on single-dose data only, the half-life of the ketorolac tromethamine racemate increased from 5-7 hours in the elderly (65-78 years) compared with young healthy volunteers (24-35 years) (see TABLE 2). There was little difference in the C_{max} for the 2 groups (elderly, 2.52 µg/ml ± 0.77; young, 2.99 µg/ml ± 1.03) (see PRECAUTIONS, Geriatric Use).

Pediatric Patients

Following a single intravenous bolus dose of 0.5 mg/kg in 10 children 4-8 years old, the half-life was 6 hours (range: 3.5-10 h), the average clearance was 0.042 L/h/kg and the Vd was 0.26 L/kg (range: 0.19-0.44 L/kg). In a second study, following a single IV dose of 0.6 mg/kg in 24 children 3-18 years old, C_{max} was 4.3 ± 1.7 µg/ml, T_{max} was 10.25 ± 1.15 minutes, half-life was 3.8 ± 2.6 hours, CL was 0.06778 L/h/kg and Vd was 0.25 L/kg. The volume of distribution and clearance of ketorolac in pediatric patients was twice that observec in adult subjects (see TABLE 1 and TABLE 2). There are no pharmacokinetic data available for Toradol administration by the IM route in pediatric patients.

Renal Insufficiency

Based on single-dose data only, the mean half-life of ketorolac tromethamine in renally impaired patients is between 6 and 19 hours and is dependent on the extent of the impairment. There is poor correlation between creatinine clearance and total ketorolac tromethamine clearance in the elderly and populations with renal impairment (r=0.5).

In patients with renal disease, the AUC(∞) of each enantiomer increased by approximately 100% compared with healthy volunteers. The volume of distribution doubles for the S-enantiomer and increases by 1/5th for the R-enantiomer. The increase in volume of distribution of ketorolac tromethamine implies an increase in unbound fraction.

The AUC(∞)-ratio of the ketorolac tromethamine enantiomers in healthy subjects and patients remained similar, indicating there was no selective excretion of either enantiomer in patients compared to healthy subjects (see WARNINGS, Renal Effects and TABLE 2).

Hepatic Insufficiency

There was no significant difference in estimates of half-life, AUC(∞) and C_{max} in 7 patients with liver disease compared to healthy volunteers (see PRECAUTIONS, General, Hepatic Effects and TABLE 2).

Race

Pharmacokinetic differences due to race have not been identified.

IV ADMINISTRATION

In normal subjects (n=37), the total clearance of 30 mg IV-administered Toradol was 0.030 (0.017-0.051) L/h/kg. The terminal half-life was 5.6 (4.0-7.9) hours. (See Kinetics in Special Populations for use of Toradol IV in pediatric patients.)

INDICATIONS AND USAGE

ADULT PATIENTS

Toradol is indicated for the short-term (≤5 days) management of moderately severe acute pain that requires analgesia at the opioid level, usually in a postoperative setting. Therapy should always be initiated with Toradol IV/IM, and Toradol oral is to be used only as continuation treatment, if necessary. Combined use of Toradol IV/IM and Toradol oral is not to exceed 5 days of use because of the potential of increasing the frequency and severity of adverse reactions associated with the recommended doses (see WARNINGS, PRECAUTIONS, DOSAGE AND ADMINISTRATION and ADVERSE REACTIONS). Patients should be switched to alternative analgesics as soon as possible, but Toradol therapy is not to exceed 5 days.

***TABLE 1** Table of Approximate Average Pharmacokinetic Parameters (Mean ±SD) Following Oral, IM and IV Doses of Toradol*

Pharmacokinetic Parameters (units)	Oral* 10 mg	IM† 15 mg	IM† 30 mg	IM† 60 mg	IV Bolus‡ 15 mg	IV Bolus‡ 30 mg
Bioavailability (extent)	100%					
T_{max}¶ (min)	44 ± 34	33 ± 21§	44 ± 29	33 ± 21	1.1 ± 0.7§	2.9 ± 1.8
C_{max}** (μg/ml) [single-dose]	0.87 ± 0.22	1.14 ± 0.32§	2.42 ± 0.68	4.55 ± 1.27§	2.47 ± 0.51§	4.65 ± 0.96
C_{max} (μg/ml) [steady state qid]	1.05 ± 0.26§	1.56 ± 0.44§	3.11 ± 0.87§	N/A¤	3.09 ± 1.17§	6.85 ± 2.61
C_{min}†† (μg/ml) [steady state qid]	0.29 ± 0.07§	0.47 ± 0.13§	0.93 ± 0.26§	N/A	0.61 ± 0.21§	1.04 ± 0.35
C_{avg}‡‡ (μg/ml) [steady state qid]	0.59 ± 0.20§	0.94 ± 0.29§	1.88 ± 0.59§	N/A	1.09 ± 0.30§	2.17 ± 0.59
Vβ§§ (L/kg)	0.175 ± 0.039				0.210 ± 0.044	

% Dose metabolized = <50.
% Dose excreted in urine = 91.
% Dose excreted in feces = 6.
% Plasma protein binding = 99.
* Derived from PO pharmacokinetic studies in 77 normal fasted volunteers.
† Derived from IM pharmacokinetic studies in 54 normal volunteers.
‡ Derived from IV pharmacokinetic studies in 24 normal volunteers.
§ Mean value was simulated from observed plasma concentration data and standard deviation was simulated from percent coefficient of variation for observed C_{max} and T_{max} data.
¤ Not applicable because 60 mg is only recommended as a single dose.
¶ Time-to-peak plasma concentration.
** Peak plasma concentration.
†† Trough plasma concentration.
‡‡ Average plasma concentration.
§§ Volume of distribution.

***TABLE 2** The Influence of Age, Liver and Kidney Function on the Clearance and Terminal Half-Life of Toradol (IM* and Oral†) in Adult Populations*

Type of Subjects	Total Clearance [in L/h/kg]‡ IM Mean (range)	Total Clearance [in L/h/kg]‡ Oral Mean (range)	Terminal Half-Life [in hours] IM Mean (range)	Terminal Half-Life [in hours] Oral Mean (range)
Normal subjects§	0.023 (0.010-0.046)	0.025 (0.013-0.050)	5.3 (3.5-9.2)	5.3 (2.4-9.0)
Healthy elderly subjects¤	0.019 (0.013-0.034)	0.024 (0.018-0.034)	7.0 (4.7-8.6)	6.1 (4.3-7.6)
Patients with hepatic dysfunction¶	0.029 (0.013-0.066)	0.033 (0.019-0.051)	5.4 (2.2-6.9)	4.5 (1.6-7.6)
Patients with renal impairment**	0.015 (0.005-0.043)	0.016 (0.007-0.052)	10.3 (5.9-19.2)	10.8 (3.4-18.9)
Renal dialysis patients††	0.016 (0.003-0.036)	—	13.6 (8.0-39.1)	—

* Estimated from 30 mg single IM doses of ketorolac tromethamine.
† Estimated from 10 mg single oral doses of ketorolac tromethamine.
‡ L/h/kg.
§ IM (n=54) mean age = 32, range 18-60; Oral (n=77) mean age = 32, range 20-60.
¤ IM (n=13), oral (n=12) mean age = 72, range 65-78.
¶ IM and oral (n=7) mean age = 51, range 43-64.
** IM (n=25), oral (n=9) serum creatinine = 1.9-5.0 mg/dl, mean age (IM) = 54, range 35-71, mean age (oral) = 57, range 39-70.
†† IM and oral (n=9) mean age = 40, range 27-63.

PEDIATRIC PATIENTS

The safety and effectiveness of single doses of Toradol IV/IM have been established in pediatric patients between the ages of 2 and 16 years. Toradol, as a single injectable dose, has been shown to be effective in the management of moderately severe acute pain that requires analgesia at the opioid level, usually in the postoperative setting. There is limited data available to support the use of multiple doses of Toradol in pediatric patients. Safety and effectiveness have not been established in pediatric patients below the age of 2 years. Use of Toradol in pediatric patients is supported by evidence from adequate and well-controlled studies of Toradol in adults with additional pharmacokinetic, efficacy and safety data on its use in pediatric patients available in the published literature (see WARNINGS and PRECAUTIONS).

Toradol IV/IM has been used concomitantly with morphine and meperidine and has shown an opioid-sparing effect. For breakthrough pain, it is recommended to supplement the lower end of the Toradol IV/IM dosage range with low doses of narcotics prn, unless otherwise contraindicated. Toradol IV/IM and narcotics should not be administered in the same syringe (see DOSAGE AND ADMINISTRATION, Toradol IV/IM, Pharmaceutical Information for Toradol IV/IM).

CONTRAINDICATIONS

See also BOXED WARNING.

Toradol is CONTRAINDICATED in patients with active peptic ulcer disease, in patients with recent gastrointestinal bleeding or perforation and in patients with a history of peptic ulcer disease or gastrointestinal bleeding.

Toradol is CONTRAINDICATED in patients with advanced renal impairment or in patients at risk for renal failure due to volume depletion (see WARNINGS for correction of volume depletion).

Toradol is CONTRAINDICATED in labor and delivery because, through its prostaglandin synthesis inhibitory effect, it may adversely affect fetal circulation and inhibit uterine contractions, thus increasing the risk of uterine hemorrhage.

The use of Toradol is CONTRAINDICATED in nursing mothers because of the potential adverse effects of prostaglandin-inhibiting drugs on neonates.

Toradol is CONTRAINDICATED in patients with previously demonstrated hypersensitivity to ketorolac tromethamine, allergic manifestations to aspirin or other nonsteroidal anti-inflammatory drugs (NSAIDs).

Toradol is CONTRAINDICATED as prophylactic analgesic before any major surgery and is CONTRAINDICATED intraoperatively when hemostasis is critical because of the increased risk of bleeding.

Toradol inhibits platelet function and is, therefore, CONTRAINDICATED in patients with suspected or confirmed cerebrovascular bleeding, hemorrhagic diathesis, incomplete hemostasis and those at high risk of bleeding (see WARNINGS and PRECAUTIONS).

Toradol is CONTRAINDICATED in patients currently receiving ASA or NSAIDs because of the cumulative risks of inducing serious NSAID-related adverse events.

Toradol IV/IM is CONTRAINDICATED for neuraxial (epidural or intrathecal) administration due to its alcohol content.

The concomitant use of Toradol and probenecid is CONTRAINDICATED.

WARNINGS

See also BOXED WARNING.

The combined use of Toradol IV/IM and Toradol oral is not to exceed 5 days in adults. Only single doses of Toradol IV/IM are recommended for use in pediatric patients.

The most serious risks associated with Toradol are as follows.

GASTROINTESTINAL (GI) EFFECTS — RISK OF GI ULCERATIONS, BLEEDING AND PERFORATION

Toradol is CONTRAINDICATED in patients with previously documented peptic ulcers and/or GI bleeding. Serious gastrointestinal toxicity, such as bleeding, ulceration and perforation, can occur at any time, with or without warning symptoms, in patients treated with Toradol. Studies to date with NSAIDs have not identified any subset of patients not at risk of developing peptic ulceration and bleeding. Elderly or debilitated patients seem to tolerate ulceration or bleeding less well than other individuals, and most spontaneous reports of fatal GI events are in this population. Postmarketing experience with parenterally administered Toradol suggests that there may be a greater risk of gastrointestinal ulcerations, bleeding and perforation in the elderly.

The incidence and severity of gastrointestinal complications increases with increasing dose of, and duration of treatment with, Toradol. In a nonrandomized, in-hospital postmarketing surveillance study comparing parenteral Toradol to parenteral opioids, higher rates of clinically serious GI bleeding were seen in adult patients <65 years of age who received an average total daily dose of more than 90 mg of Toradol IV/IM per day.

The same study showed that elderly (≥65 years of age) and debilitated patients are more susceptible to gastrointestinal complications. A history of peptic ulcer disease was revealed as another risk factor that increases the possibility of developing serious gastrointestinal complications during Toradol therapy.

HEMORRHAGE

Because prostaglandins play an important role in hemostasis and NSAIDs affect platelet aggregation as well, use of Toradol in patients who have coagulation disorders should be undertaken very cautiously, and those patients should be carefully monitored. Patients on therapeutic doses of anticoagulants (*e.g.,* heparin or dicumarol derivatives) have an increased risk of bleeding complications if given Toradol concurrently; therefore, physicians should administer such concomitant therapy only extremely cautiously. The concurrent use of Toradol and prophylactic low-dose heparin (2500-5000 units q12h), warfarin and dextrans have not been studied extensively, but may also be associated with an increased risk of bleeding. Until data from such studies are available, physicians should carefully weigh the benefits against the risks and use such concomitant therapy in these patients only extremely cautiously. In patients who receive anticoagulants for any reason, there is an increased risk of intramuscular hematoma formation from administered Toradol IM (see DRUG INTERACTIONS). Patients receiving therapy that affects hemostasis should be monitored closely.

In postmarketing experience, postoperative hematomas and other signs of wound bleeding have been reported in association with the perioperative use of Toradol IV/IM. Therefore, perioperative use of Toradol should be avoided and postoperative use be undertaken with caution when hemostasis is critical (see WARNINGS and PRECAUTIONS).

PEDIATRICS AND TONSILLECTOMY

Physicians should consider the increased risk of bleeding before deciding to administer Toradol in patients following tonsillectomy. Toradol IV/IM is not recommended for use in pediatric patients below the age of 2 years. In a retrospective analysis of patients having undergone tonsillectomy with or without adenoidectomy, the risk of bleeding was 10.1% in patients administered Toradol IV/IM compared to 2.2% in hose receiving opioids. The postoperative hemorrhage rate in patients 12 years and younget was 6.5% and 3.3% with and without Toradol, respectively. In a prospective study of Toradol in pediatric patients (ages 3-9 years) undergoing tonsillectomy with or without adenoidectomy, the overall incidence of bleeding was similar between the patients receiving Toradol and morphine (16.3% vs 17%, respectively). However, during the first 24 hours after surgery, a higher incidence o fbleeding was observed in the Toradol IV/IM group (14.3%) versus the morphine group (4.2%).

ANAPHYLACTOID REACTIONS

Anaphylactoid reactions may occur in patients without a known previous exposure or hypersensitivity to aspirin, Toradol or other NSAIDs, or in individuals with a history of angioedema, bronchospastic reactivity (*e.g.,* asthma) and nasal polyps. Anaphylactoid reactions, like anaphylaxis, may have a fatal outcome.

K

IMPAIRED RENAL FUNCTION

Toradol should be used with caution in patients with impaired renal function or a history of kidney disease because it is a potent inhibitor of prostaglandin synthesis. Renal toxicity with Toradol has been seen in patients with conditions leading to a reduction in blood volume and/or renal blood flow where renal prostaglandins have a supportive role in the maintenance of renal perfusion. In these patients administration of Toradol may cause a dose-dependent reduction in renal prostaglandin formation and may precipitate acute renal failure. Patients at greatest risk of this reaction are those with impaired renal function, dehydration, heart failure, liver dysfunction, those taking diuretics and the elderly. Discontinuation of Toradol therapy is usually followed by recovery to the pretreatment state.

RENAL EFFECTS

Toradol and its metabolites are eliminated primarily by the kidneys, which, in patients with reduced creatinine clearance, will result in diminished clearance of the drug (see CLINICAL PHARMACOLOGY). Therefore, Toradol should be used with caution in patients with impaired renal function (see DOSAGE AND ADMINISTRATION) and such patients should be followed closely. With the use of Toradol, there have been reports of acute renal failure, nephritis and nephrotic syndrome.

Because patients with underlying renal insufficiency are at increased risk of developing acute renal failure, the risks and benefits should be assessed prior to giving Toradol to these patients. Hence, in patients with moderately elevated serum creatinine, it is recommended that the daily dose of Toradol IV/IM be reduced by half, not to exceed 60 mg/day. **TORADOL IS CONTRAINDICATED IN PATIENTS WITH SERUM CREATININE CONCENTRATIONS INDICATING ADVANCED RENAL IMPAIRMENT (see CONTRAINDICATIONS).**

Hypovolemia should be corrected before treatment with Toradol is initiated.

FLUID RETENTION AND EDEMA

Fluid retention, edema, retention of NaCl, oliguria, elevations of serum urea nitrogen and creatinine have been reported in clinical trials with Toradol. Therefore, Toradol should be used only very cautiously in patients with cardiac decompensation, hypertension or similar conditions.

PREGNANCY

In late pregnancy, as with other NSAIDs, Toradol should be avoided because it may cause premature closure of the ductus arteriosus.

K

PRECAUTIONS

GENERAL

Hepatic Effects

Toradol should be used with caution in patients with impaired hepatic function or a history of liver disease. Treatment with Toradol may cause elevations of liver enzymes, and, in patients with pre-existing liver dysfunction, it may lead to the development of a more severe hepatic reaction. The administration of Toradol should be discontinued in patients in whom an abnormal liver test has occurred as a result of Toradol therapy.

Hematologic Effects

Toradol inhibits platelet aggregation and may prolong bleeding time; therefore, it is contraindicated as a preoperative medication, and caution should be used when hemostasis is critical. Unlike aspirin, the inhibition of platelet function by Toradol disappears within 24-48 hours after the drug is discontinued. Toradol does not appear to affect platelet count, prothrombin time (PT) or partial thromboplastin time (PTT). In controlled clinical studies, where Toradol was administered intramuscularly or intravenously postoperatively, the incidence of clinically significant postoperative bleeding was 0.4% for Toradol compared to 0.2% in the control groups receiving narcotic analgesics.

INFORMATION FOR THE PATIENT

Toradol is a potent NSAID and may cause serious side effects such as gastrointestinal bleeding or kidney failure, which may result in hospitalization and even fatal outcome.

Physicians, when prescribing Toradol, should inform their patients or their guardians of the potential risks of Toradol treatment (see BOXED WARNING; WARNINGS; PRECAUTIONS; and ADVERSE REACTIONS). *Advise patients not to give Toradol oral to other family members and to discard any unused drug.*

Remember that the total duration of Toradol therapy is not to exceed 5 days in adults or a single dose in pediatric patients ages 2-16 years.

CARCINOGENESIS, MUTAGENESIS, AND IMPAIRMENT OF FERTILITY

An 18 month study in mice with oral doses of ketorolac tromethamine at 2 mg/kg/day (0.9 times the human systemic exposure at the recommended IM or IV dose of 30 mg qid, based on area-under-the-plasma-concentration curve [AUC]), and a 24 month study in rats at 5 mg/kg/day (0.5 times the human AUC) showed no evidence of tumorigenicity.

Ketorolac tromethamine was not mutagenic in the Ames test, unscheduled DNA synthesis and repair, and in forward mutation assays. Ketorolac tromethamine did not cause chromosome breakage in the *in vivo* mouse micronucleus assay. At 1590 µg/ml and at higher concentrations, ketorolac tromethamine increased the incidence of chromosomal aberrations in Chinese hamster ovarian cells.

Impairment of fertility did not occur in male or female rats at oral doses of 9 mg/kg (0.9 times the human AUC) and 16 mg/kg (1.6 times the human AUC) of ketorolac tromethamine, respectively.

PREGNANCY CATEGORY C

Reproduction studies have been performed during organogenesis using daily oral doses of ketorolac tromethamine at 3.6 mg/kg (0.37 times the human AUC) in rabbits and at 10 mg/kg (1.0 times the human AUC) in rats. Results of these studies did not reveal evidence of teratogenicity to the fetus. Oral doses of ketorolac tromethamine at 1.5 mg/kg (0.14 times the human AUC), administered after gestation Day 17, caused dystocia and higher pup mortality in rats. There are no adequate and well-controlled studies of Toradol in pregnant women. Toradol should be used during pregnancy only if the potential benefit justifies the potential risk to the fetus.

LABOR AND DELIVERY

The use of Toradol is contraindicated in labor and delivery because, through its prostaglandin synthesis inhibitory effect, it may adversely affect fetal circulation and inhibit uterine contractions, thus increasing the risk of uterine hemorrhage (see CONTRAINDICATIONS).

LACTATION AND NURSING

After a single administration of 10 mg of Toradol oral to humans, the maximum milk concentration observed was 7.3 ng/ml, and the maximum milk-to-plasma ratio was 0.037. After 1 day of dosing (qid), the maximum milk concentration was 7.9 ng/ml, and the maximum milk-to-plasma ratio was 0.025. Because of the possible adverse effects of prostaglandin-inhibiting drugs on neonates, use in nursing mothers is contraindicated.

PEDIATRIC USE

The safety and effectiveness of single doses of Toradol IV/IM have been established in pediatric patients between the ages of 2 and 16 years. Toradol IV/IM has been shown to be effective in the management of moderately severe acute pain that requires analgesia at the opioid level, usually in a postoperative setting. Safety and efficacy in pediatric patients below the age of 2 have nto been established. Therefore, Toradol IV/IM is not recommended in pediatric patients below the age of 2. The risk of bleeding was greater in those patients administered Toradol IV/IM following tonsillectomy. Physicians should consider the increased risk of bleeding before deciding to administer Toradol IV/IM in patients following tonsillectomy (see WARNINGS: Hemorrhage and Pediatrics and Tonsillectomy).

The risks identified in the adult population with Toradol IV/IM use also apply to pediatric patients. Therefore, consult CONTRAINDICATIONS, WARNINGS, PRECAUTIONS, and ADVERSE REACTIONS when prescribing Toradol IV/IM to pediatric patients.

GERIATRIC USE (≥65 YEARS OF AGE)

Because ketorolac tromethamine may be cleared more slowly by the elderly (see CLINICAL PHARMACOLOGY) who are also more sensitive to the adverse effects of NSAIDs (see WARNINGS, Renal Effects), extra caution and reduced dosages (see DOSAGE AND ADMINISTRATION) must be used when treating the elderly with Toradol IV/IM. The lower end of the Toradol IV/IM dosage range is recommended for patients over 65 years of age, and total daily dose is not to exceed 60 mg. The incidence and severity of gastrointestinal complications increases with increasing dose of, and duration of treatment with, Toradol.

DRUG INTERACTIONS

Ketorolac is highly bound to human plasma protein (mean 99.2%).

WARFARIN, DIGOXIN, SALICYLATE, AND HEPARIN

The *in vitro* binding of ***warfarin*** to plasma proteins is only slightly reduced by ketorolac tromethamine (99.5% control vs 99.3%) when ketorolac plasma concentrations reach 5-10 µg/ml. Ketorolac does not alter ***digoxin*** protein binding. *In vitro* studies indicate that, at therapeutic concentrations of ***salicylate*** (300 µg/ml), the binding of ketorolac was reduced from approximately 99.2% to 97.5%, representing a potential 2-fold increase in unbound ketorolac plasma levels. Therapeutic concentrations of ***digoxin, warfarin, ibuprofen, naproxen, piroxicam, acetaminophen, phenytoin*** and ***tolbutamide*** did not alter ketorolac tromethamine protein binding.

In a study involving 12 adult volunteers, Toradol oral was coadministered with a single dose of 25 mg ***warfarin,*** causing no significant changes in pharmacokinetics or pharmacodynamics of warfarin. In another study, Toradol IV/IM was given with 2 doses of 5000 U of ***heparin*** to 11 healthy volunteers, resulting in a mean template bleeding time of 6.4 minutes (3.2-11.4 min) compared to a mean of 6.0 minutes (3.4-7.5 min) for heparin alone and 5.1 minutes (3.5-8.5 min) for placebo. Although these results do not indicate a significant interaction between Toradol and warfarin or heparin, the administration of Toradol to patients taking anticoagulants should be done extremely cautiously, and patients should be closely monitored (see WARNINGS and PRECAUTIONS).

FUROSEMIDE

Toradol IV/IM reduced the diuretic response to ***furosemide*** in normovolemic healthy subjects by approximately 20% (mean sodium and urinary output decreased 17%).

PROBENECID

Concomitant administration of Toradol oral and ***probenecid*** resulted in decreased clearance of ketorolac and significant increases in ketorolac plasma levels (total AUC increased approximately 3-fold from 5.4 to 17.8 µg/h/ml) and terminal half-life increased approximately 2-fold from 6.6 to 15.1 hours. Therefore, concomitant use of Toradol and probenecid is contraindicated.

LITHIUM

Inhibition of renal ***lithium*** clearance, leading to an increase in plasma lithium concentration, has been reported with some prostaglandin synthesis-inhibiting drugs. The effect of Toradol on plasma lithium has not been studied, but cases of increased lithium plasma levels during Toradol therapy have been reported.

METHOTREXATE

Concomitant administration of ***methotrexate*** and some NSAIDs has been reported to reduce the clearance of methotrexate, enhancing the toxicity of methotrexate. The effect of Toradol on methotrexate clearance has not been studied.

NONDEPOLARIZING MUSCLE RELAXANTS

In postmarketing experience there have been reports of a possible interaction between Toradol IV/IM and ***nondepolarizing muscle relaxants*** that resulted in apnea. The concurrent use of Toradol with muscle relaxants has not been formally studied.

ACE INHIBITORS
Concomitant use of ***ACE inhibitors*** may increase the risk of renal impairment, particularly in volume-depleted patients.

ANTIEPILEPTIC DRUGS
Sporadic cases of seizures have been reported during concomitant use of Toradol and ***antiepileptic drugs*** (phenytoin, carbamazepine).

PSYCHOACTIVE DRUGS
Hallucinations have been reported when Toradol was used in patients taking ***psychoactive drugs*** (fluoxetine, thiothixene, alprazolam).

MORPHINE
Toradol IV/IM has been administered concurrently with ***morphine*** in several clinical trials of postoperative pain without evidence of adverse interactions. Do not mix Toradol and morphine in the same syringe.

There is no evidence in animal or human studies that Toradol induces or inhibits hepatic enzymes capable of metabolizing itself or other drugs.

ADVERSE REACTIONS

Adverse reaction rates increase with higher doses of Toradol. Practitioners should be alert for the severe complications of treatment with Toradol, such as GI ulceration, bleeding and perforation, postoperative bleeding, acute renal failure, anaphylactic and anaphylactoid reactions and liver failure (see BOXED WARNING, WARNINGS, PRECAUTIONS, and DOSAGE AND ADMINISTRATION). These NSAID-related complications can be serious in certain patients for whom Toradol is indicated, especially when the drug is used inappropriately.

THE ADVERSE REACTIONS LISTED BELOW WERE REPORTED IN CLINICAL TRIALS AS PROBABLY RELATED TO TORADOL

Incidence Greater Than 1%

Percentage of incidence in parentheses for those events reported in 3% or more patients:

Body as a Whole: Edema (4%).
Cardiovascular: Hypertension.
Dermatologic: Pruritus, rash.
Gastrointestinal: Nausea (12%), dyspepsia (12%), gastrointestinal pain (13%), diarrhea (7%), constipation, flatulence, gastrointestinal fullness, vomiting, stomatitis.
Hemic and Lymphatic: Purpura.
Nervous System: Headache (17%), drowsiness (6%), dizziness (7%), sweating.
Injection-Site Pain was reported by 2% of patients in multidose studies.

Incidence 1% or Less

Body as a Whole: Weight gain, fever, infections, asthenia.
Cardiovascular: Palpitation, pallor, syncope.
Dermatologic: Urticaria.
Gastrointestinal: Gastritis, rectal bleeding, eructation, anorexia, increased appetite.
Hemic and Lymphatic: Epistaxis, anemia, eosinophilia.
Nervous System: Tremors, abnormal dreams, hallucinations, euphoria, extrapyramidal symptoms, vertigo, paresthesia, depression, insomnia, nervousness, excessive thirst, dry mouth, abnormal thinking, inability to concentrate, hyperkinesis, stupor.
Respiratory: Dyspnea, pulmonary edema, rhinitis, cough.
Special Senses: Abnormal taste, abnormal vision, blurred vision, tinnitus, hearing loss.
Urogenital: Hematuria, proteinuria, oliguria, urinary retention, polyuria, increased urinary frequency.

THE FOLLOWING ADVERSE EVENTS WERE REPORTED FROM POSTMARKETING EXPERIENCE

Body as a Whole: Hypersensitivity reactions such as anaphylaxis, anaphylactoid reaction, laryngeal edema, tongue edema (see BOXED WARNING and WARNINGS), angioedema, myalgia.
Cardiovascular: Hypotension, flushing.
Dermatologic: Lyell's syndrome, Stevens-Johnson syndrome, exfoliative dermatitis, maculopapular rash, urticaria.
Gastrointestinal: Peptic ulceration, GI hemorrhage, GI perforation (see BOXED WARNING and WARNINGS), melena, acute pancreatitis, hematemesis, esophagitis.
Hemic and Lymphatic: Postoperative wound hemorrhage (rarely requiring blood transfusion - see BOXED WARNING, WARNINGS, and PRECAUTIONS), thrombocytopenia, leukopenia.
Hepatic: Hepatitis, liver failure, cholestatic jaundice.
Nervous System: Convulsions, psychosis, aseptic meningitis.
Respiratory: Asthma, bronchospasm.
Urogenital: Acute renal failure (see BOXED WARNING and WARNINGS), flank pain with or without hematuria and/or azotemia, interstitial nephritis, hyponatremia, hyperkalemia, hemolytic uremic syndrome.

DOSAGE AND ADMINISTRATION

IN ADULTS, THE COMBINED DURATION OF USE OF TORADOL IV/IM AND TORADOL ORAL IS NOT TO EXCEED 5 DAYS. IN ADULTS, THE USE OF TORADOL ORAL IS ONLY INDICATED AS CONTINUATION THERAPY TO TORADOL IV/IM.

TORADOL IV/IM

Adult Patients

Toradol IV/IM may be used as a single or multiple dose on a regular or prn schedule for the management of moderately severe acute pain that requires analgesia at the opioid level, usually in a postoperative setting. Hypovolemia should be corrected prior to the administration of Toradol (see WARNINGS, Renal Effects). Patients should be switched to alternative analgesics as soon as possible, but Toradol therapy is not to exceed 5 days.

When administering Toradol IV/IM, the IV bolus must be given over no less than 15 seconds. The IM administration should be given slowly and deeply into the muscle. The analgesic effect begins in ~30 minutes with maximum effect in 1-2 hours after dosing IV or IM. Duration of analgesic effect is usually 4-6 hours.

Single-Dose Treatment

The following regimen should be limited to single administration use only.

Adult Patients

IM Dosing:
Patients <65 years of age: One dose of 60 mg.
Patients ≥65 years of age, renally impaired and/or less than 50 kg (110 lb) of body weight: One dose of 30 mg.

IV Dosing:
Patients <65 years of age: One dose of 30 mg.
Patients ≥65 years of age, renally impaired and/or less than 50 kg (110 lb) of body weight: One dose of 15 mg.

Pediatric Patients (2-16 years of age)

The pediatric population should receive only a single dose of Toradol injection, as follows:
IM Dosing: One dose of 1 mg/kg up to a maximym of 30 mg.
IV Dosing: One dose of 0.5 mg/kg up to a maximum of 15 mg.

Multiple-Dose Treatment (IV or IM) in Adults

Patients <65 years of age: The recommended dose is 30 mg Toradol IV/IM every 6 hours. The maximum daily dose should not exceed 120 mg.
For patients ≥65 years of age, renally impaired patients (see WARNINGS) and patients less than 50 kg (110 lb): The recommended dose is 15 mg Toradol IV/IM every 6 hours. The maximum daily dose for these populations should not exceed 60 mg.

For breakthrough pain do not increase the dose or the frequency of Toradol. Consideration should be given to supplementing these regimens with low doses of opioids prn unless otherwise contraindicated.

Pharmaceutical Information for Toradol IV/IM

Parenteral drug products should be inspected visually for particulate matter and discoloration prior to administration whenever solution and container permit.

Toradol IV/IM should not be mixed in a small volume (*e.g.*, in a syringe) with morphine sulfate, meperidine hydrochloride, promethazine hydrochloride or hydroxyzine hydrochloride; this will result in precipitation of ketorolac from solution.

Toradol oral is indicated ONLY as continuation therapy to Toradol IV/IM for the management of moderately severe acute pain that requires analgesia at the opioid level (see also PRECAUTIONS, Information for the Patient).

Transition From Toradol IV/IM to Toradol Oral in Adults

The recommended Toradol oral dose is as follows:

Patients <65 years of age: 2 tablets as a first oral dose for patients who received **60 mg IM single dose, 30 mg IV single dose or 30 mg multiple dose.** Toradol IV/IM followed by 1 tablet Toradol oral every 4-6 hours, not to exceed 40 mg/24 h of Toradol oral.
Patients ≥65 years of age, renally impaired and/or less than 50 kg (110 lb) of body weight: 1 tablet as a first oral dose for patients who received **30 mg IM single dose, 15 IV single dose or 15 mg multiple dose.** Toradol IV/IM followed by 1 tablet Toradol oral every 4-6 hours, not to exceed 40 mg/24 h of Toradol oral.

Shortening the recommended dosing intervals may result in increased frequency and severity of adverse reactions.

In adults, the maximum combined duration of use (parenteral and oral Toradol) is limited to 5 days.

HOW SUPPLIED

TORADOL IV/IM

Toradol IV/IM for intramuscular or intravenous use is available in a sterile vial:
15 mg: 15 mg/ml, 1 ml fill per 2 ml single use vial.
30 mg: 30 mg/ml, 1 ml fill per 2 ml single use vial.

For IM single-dose use only; not intended for IV use:
60 mg: 30 mg/ml, 2 ml fill per 2 ml single use vial.

Storage

Store vials at 15-30°C (59-86°F) with protection from light.

TORADOL ORAL

Toradol oral is available as 10 mg round, white, film-coated, red-printed tablets. There is a large "T" printed on both sides of the tablet, with "TORADOL" on one side, and "ROCHE" on the other.

Storage

Store bottles at 15-30°C (59-86°F).

OPHTHALMIC

DESCRIPTION

Note: The trade names have been used throughout this monograph for clarity.

ACULAR

Acular (ketorolac tromethamine ophthalmic solution) is a member of the pyrrolo-pyrrole group of nonsteroidal anti-inflammatory drugs (NSAIDs) for ophthalmic use. Its chemical name is (±)-5-benzoyl-2,3-dihydro-1H-pyrrolizine-1-carboxylic acid, compound with 2-amino-2-(hydroxymethyl)-1,3-propanediol(1:1).

K

Acular ophthalmic solution is supplied as a sterile isotonic aqueous 0.5% solution, with a pH of 7.4. Acular ophthalmic solution is a racemic mixture of R-(+) and S-(-)-ketorolac tromethamine. Ketorolac tromethamine may exist in three crystal forms. All forms are equally soluble in water. The pKa of ketorolac is 3.5. This white to off-white crystalline substance discolors on prolonged exposure to light. The molecular weight of ketorolac tromethamine is 376.41. The osmolality of Acular ophthalmic solution is 290 mOsmol/kg. **Each ml of Acular ophthalmic solution contains:** *Active:* Ketorolac tromethamine 0.5%. *Preservative:* Benzalkonium chloride 0.01%. *Inactives:* Edetate disodium 0.1%; octoxynol 40; sodium chloride; hydrochloric acid and/or sodium hydroxide to adjust the pH.

ACULAR PF

Acular PF (ketorolac tromethamine ophthalmic solution) preservative-free is a member of the pyrrolo-pyrrole group of nonsteroidal anti-inflammatory drugs (NSAIDs) for ophthalmic use. Its chemical name is (±)-5-benzoyl-2, 3-dihydro-1H pyrrolizine-1-carboxylic acid compound with 2-amino-2-(hydroxymethyl)-1,3-propanediol (1:1).

Acular PF is a racemic mixture of R-(+) and S-(-)-ketorolac tromethamine. Ketorolac tromethamine may exist in three crystal forms. All forms are equally soluble in water. The pKa of ketorolac is 3.5. This white to off-white crystalline substance discolors on prolonged exposure to light. The molecular weight of ketorolac tromethamine is 376.41. The osmolality of Acular PF is 290 mOsmol/kg.

Each ml of Acular PF contains: *Active Ingredient:* Ketorolac tromethamine 0.5%. *Inactives:* Sodium chloride; hydrochloric acid and/or sodium hydroxide to adjust the pH to 7.4; and purified water.

ACULAR LS

Acular LS (ketorolac tromethamine ophthalmic solution) 0.4% is a member of the pyrrolo-pyrrole group of nonsteroidal anti-inflammatory drugs (NSAIDs) for ophthalmic use.

The molecular formula is C19H24N2O6. The molecular weight is 376.41.

The chemical name is (±)-5-Benzoyl-2,3-dihydro-1H-pyrrolizine-1-carboxylic acid, compound with 2-amino-2-(hydroxymethyl)-1,3-propanediol (1:1).

Acular LS contains: *Active:* Ketorolac tromethamine 0.4%. Preservative: benzalkonium chloride 0.006%. *Inactives:* Sodium chloride; edetate disodium 0.015%; octoxynol 40; purified water; and hydrochloric acid and/or sodium hydroxide to adjust the pH.

Acular LS ophthalmic solution is supplied as a sterile isotonic aqueous 0.4% solution, with a pH of approximately 7.4. Acular LS ophthalmic solution is a racemic mixture of R-(+) and S-(-)-ketorolac tromethamine. Ketorolac tromethamine may exist in three crystal forms. All forms are equally soluble in water. The pKa of ketorolac is 3.5. This white to off-white crystalline substance discolors on prolonged exposure to light. The osmolality of Acular LS ophthalmic solution is approximately 290 mOsml/kg.

CLINICAL PHARMACOLOGY

ACULAR

Ketorolac tromethamine is a nonsteroidal anti-inflammatory drug which, when administered systemically, has demonstrated analgesic, anti-inflammatory, and anti-pyretic activity. The mechanism of its action is thought to be due to its ability to inhibit prostaglandin biosynthesis. Ketorolac tromethamine given systemically does not cause pupil constriction.

Prostaglandins have been shown in many animal models to be mediators of certain kinds of intraocular inflammation. In studies performed in animal eyes, prostaglandins have been shown to produce disruption of the blood-aqueous humor barrier, vasodilation, increased vascular permeability, leukocytosis, and increased intraocular pressure. Prostaglandins also appear to play a role in the miotic response produced during ocular surgery by constricting the iris sphincter independently of cholinergic mechanisms.

Two drops (0.1 ml) of 0.5% Acular ophthalmic solution instilled into the eyes of patients 12 hours and 1 hour prior to cataract extraction achieved measurable levels in 8 of 9 patients' eyes (mean ketorolac concentration 95 ng/ml aqueous humor, range 40-170 ng/ml). Ocular administration of ketorolac tromethamine reduces prostaglandin E2 (PGE2) levels in aqueous humor. The mean concentration of PGE2 was 80 pg/ml in the aqueous humor of eyes receiving vehicle and 28 pg/ml in the eyes receiving Acular 0.5% ophthalmic solution.

One drop (0.05 ml) of 0.5% Acular ophthalmic solution was instilled into 1 eye and 1 drop of vehicle into the other eye tid in 26 normal subjects. Only 5 of 26 subjects had a detectable amount of ketorolac in their plasma (range 10.7-22.5 ng/ml) at day 10 during topical ocular treatment. When ketorolac tromethamine 10 mg is administered systemically every 6 hours, peak plasma levels at steady state are around 960 ng/ml.

Two controlled clinical studies showed that Acular ophthalmic solution was significantly more effective than its vehicle in relieving ocular itching caused by seasonal allergic conjunctivitis.

Two controlled clinical studies showed that patients treated for 2 weeks with Acular ophthalmic solution were less likely to have measurable signs of inflammation (cell and flare) than patients treated with its vehicle.

Results from clinical studies indicate that ketorolac tromethamine has no significant effect upon intraocular pressure; however, changes in intraocular pressure may occur following cataract surgery.

ACULAR PF

Ketorolac tromethamine is a nonsteroidal anti-inflammatory drug which, when administered systemically, has demonstrated analgesic, anti-inflammatory, and anti-pyretic activity. The mechanism of its action is thought to be due to its ability to inhibit prostaglandin biosynthesis. Ketorolac tromethamine given systemically does not cause pupil constriction.

One drop (0.05 ml) of ketorolac tromethamine (preserved) was instilled into 1 eye and 1 drop of vehicle into the other eye tid in 26 normal subjects. Only 5 of 26 subjects had a detectable amount of ketorolac in their plasma (range 10.7-22.5 ng/ml) at Day 10 during topical ocular treatment. When ketorolac tromethamine 10 mg is administered systemically every 6 hours, peak plasma levels at steady state are around 960 ng/ml.

In two double-masked, multi-centered, parallel-group studies, 340 patients who had undergone incisional refractive surgery received Acular PF or its vehicle qid for up to 3 days. Significant differences favored Acular PF for the treatment of ocular pain and photophobia. Results from clinical studies indicate that ketorolac tromethamine has no significant effect upon intraocular pressure.

ACULAR LS

Mechanism of Action

Ketorolac tromethamine is a nonsteroidal anti-inflammatory drug which, when administered systemically, has demonstrated analgesic, anti-inflammatory, and anti-pyretic activity. The mechanism of its action is thought to be due to its ability to inhibit prostaglandin biosynthesis. Ketorolac tromethamine given systemically does not cause pupil constriction.

Pharmacokinetics

One drop (0.05 ml) of 0.5% ketorolac tromethamine ophthalmic solution was instilled into 1 eye and 1 drop of vehicle into the other eye tid in 26 normal subjects. Only 5 of 26 subjects had a detectable amount of ketorolac in their plasma (range 10.7-22.5 ng/ml) at Day 10 during topical ocular treatment. When ketorolac tromethamine 10 mg is administered systemically every 6 hours, peak plasma levels at steady state are around 960 ng/ml.

INDICATIONS AND USAGE

ACULAR

Acular ophthalmic solution is indicated for the temporary relief of ocular itching due to seasonal allergic conjunctivitis. Acular ophthalmic solution is also indicated for the treatment of postoperative inflammation in patients who have undergone cataract extraction.

ACULAR PF

Acular PF ophthalmic solution is indicated for the reduction of ocular pain and photophobia following incisional refractive surgery.

ACULAR LS

Acular LS ophthalmic solution is indicated for the reduction of ocular pain and burning/stinging following corneal refractive surgery.

NON-FDA APPROVED INDICATIONS

Ketorolac ophthalmic solution has been investigated as an adjunct in the treatment of non-infective, non-contact lens related traumatic corneal abrasions; however, this use is not approved by the FDA.

CONTRAINDICATIONS

ACULAR

Acular ophthalmic solution is contraindicated in patients with previously demonstrated hypersensitivity to any of the ingredients in the formulation.

ACULAR PF

Acular PF ophthalmic solution is contraindicated in patients with previously demonstrated hypersensitivity to any of the ingredients in the formulation.

ACULAR LS

Acular LS ophthalmic solution is contraindicated in patients with previously demonstrated hypersensitivity to any of the ingredients in the formulation.

WARNINGS

ACULAR

There is the potential for cross-sensitivity to acetylsalicylic acid, phenylacetic acid derivatives, and other nonsteroidal anti-inflammatory agents. Therefore, caution should be used when treating individuals who have previously exhibited sensitivities to these drugs.

With some nonsteroidal anti-inflammatory drugs, there exists the potential for increased bleeding time due to interference with thrombocyte aggregation. There have been reports that ocularly applied nonsteroidal anti-inflammatory drugs may cause increased bleeding of ocular tissues (including hyphemas) in conjunction with ocular surgery.

ACULAR PF

There is the potential for cross-sensitivity to acetylsalicylic acid, phenylacetic acid derivatives, and other nonsteroidal anti-inflammatory agents. Therefore, caution should be used when treating individuals who have previously exhibited sensitivities to these drugs.

With some nonsteroidal anti-inflammatory drugs, there exists the potential for increased bleeding time due to interference with thrombocyte aggregation. There have been reports that ocularly applied nonsteroidal anti-inflammatory drugs may cause increased bleeding of ocular tissues (including hyphemas) in conjunction with ocular surgery.

ACULAR LS

There is the potential for cross-sensitivity to acetylsalicylic acid, phenylacetic acid derivatives, and other nonsteroidal anti-inflammatory agents. Therefore, caution should be used when treating individuals who have previously exhibited sensitivities to these drugs.

With some nonsteroidal anti-inflammatory drugs there exists the potential for increased bleeding time due to interference with thrombocyte aggregation. There have been reports that ocularly applied nonsteroidal anti-inflammatory drugs may cause increased bleeding of ocular tissues (including hyphemas) in conjunction with ocular surgery.

PRECAUTIONS

ACULAR

General

All topical nonsteroidal anti-inflammatory drugs (NSAIDs) may slow or delay healing. Topical corticosteroids are also known to slow or delay healing. Concomitant use of topical NSAIDs and topical steroids may increase the potential for healing problems.

Use of topical NSAIDs may result in keratitis. In some susceptible patients, continued use of topical NSAIDs may result in epithelial breakdown, corneal thinning, corneal erosion, corneal ulceration or corneal perforation . These events may be sight threatening. Patients with evidence of corneal epithelial breakdown should immediately discontinue use of topical NSAIDs and should be closely monitored for corneal health.

Postmarketing experience with topical NSAIDs suggests that patients with complicated ocular surgeries, corneal denervation, corneal epithelial defects, diabetes mellitus, ocular surface diseases (*e.g.*, dry eye syndrome), rheumatoid arthritis, or repeat ocular surgeries within a short period of time may be at increased risk for corneal adverse events which may become sight threatening. Topical NSAIDs should be used with caution in these patients.

Postmarketing experience with topical NSAIDs also suggests that use more than 24 hours prior to surgery or use beyond 14 days post-surgery may increase patient risk for the occurrence and severity of corneal adverse events.

It is recommended that Acular ophthalmic solution be used with caution in patients with known bleeding tendencies or who are receiving other medications which may prolong bleeding time.

Information for the Patient

Acular ophthalmic solution should not be administered while wearing contact lenses.

Carcinogenesis, Mutagenesis, and Impairment of Fertility

Ketorolac tromethamine was not carcinogenic in rats given up to 5 mg/kg/day orally for 24 months (151 times the maximum recommended human topical ophthalmic dose, on a mg/kg basis, assuming 100% absorption in humans and animals) nor in mice given 2 mg/kg/day orally for 18 months (60 times the maximum recommended human topical ophthalmic dose, on a mg/kg basis, assuming 100% absorption in humans and animals).

Ketorolac tromethamine was not mutagenic *in vitro* in the Ames assay or in forward mutation assays. Similarly, it did not result in an *in vitro* increase in unscheduled DNA synthesis or an *in vivo* increase in chromosome breakage in mice. However, ketorolac tromethamine did result in an increased incidence in chromosomal aberrations in Chinese hamster ovary cells.

Ketorolac tromethamine did not impair fertility when administered orally to male and female rats at doses up to 272 and 484 times the maximum recommended human topical ophthalmic dose, respectively, on a mg/kg basis, assuming 100% absorption in humans and animals.

Pregnancy Category C

Teratogenic Effects

Ketorolac tromethamine, administered during organogenesis, was not teratogenic in rabbits or rats at oral doses up to 109 times and 303 times the maximum recommended human topical ophthalmic dose, respectively, on a mg/kg basis assuming 100% absorption in humans and animals. When administered to rats after Day 17 of gestation at oral doses up to 45 times the maximum recommended human topical ophthalmic dose, respectively, on a mg/kg basis, assuming 100% absorption in humans and animals, ketorolac tromethamine resulted in dystocia and increased pup mortality. There are no adequate and well-controlled studies in pregnant women. Acular ophthalmic solution should be used during pregnancy only if the potential benefit justifies the potential risk to the fetus.

Nonteratogenic Effects

Because of the known effects of prostaglandin-inhibiting drugs on the fetal cardiovascular system (closure of the ductus arteriosus), the use of Acular ophthalmic solution during late pregnancy should be avoided.

Nursing Mothers

Caution should be exercised when Acular ophthalmic solution is administered to a nursing woman.

Pediatric Use

Safety and efficacy in pediatric patients below the age of 3 have not been established.

Geriatric Use

No overall differences in safety or effectiveness have been observed between elderly and younger patients.

ACULAR PF

General

All topical nonsteroidal anti-inflammatory drugs (NSAIDs) may slow or delay healing. Topical corticosteroids are also known to slow or delay healing. Concomitant use of topical NSAIDs and topical steroids may increase the potential for healing problems.

Use of topical NSAIDs may result in keratitis. In some susceptible patients, continued use of topical NSAIDs may result in epithelial breakdown, corneal thinning, corneal erosion, corneal ulceration or corneal perforation . These events may be sight threatening. Patients with evidence of corneal epithelial breakdown should immediately discontinue use of topical NSAIDs and should be closely monitored for corneal health.

Postmarketing experience with topical NSAIDs suggests that patients with complicated ocular surgeries, corneal denervation, corneal epithelial defects, diabetes mellitus, ocular surface diseases (*e.g.*, dry eye syndrome), rheumatoid arthritis, or repeat ocular surgeries within a short period of time may be at increased risk for corneal adverse events which may become sight threatening. Topical NSAIDs should be used with caution in these patients.

Post marketing experience with topical NSAIDs also suggests that use more than 24 hours prior to surgery or use beyond 14 days post surgery may increase patient risk for the occurrence and severity of corneal adverse events.

It is recommended that Acular PF ophthalmic solution be used with caution in patients with known bleeding tendencies or who are receiving other medications which may prolong bleeding time.

Information for the Patient

Acular PF should not be administered while wearing contact lenses.

The solution from 1 individual single-use vial is to be used immediately after opening for administration to 1 or both eyes, and the remaining contents should be discarded immediately after administration. To avoid contamination, do not touch tip of unit-dose vial to eye or any other surface.

Carcinogenesis, Mutagenesis, and Impairment of Fertility

Ketorolac tromethamine was not carcinogenic in rats given up to 5 mg/kg/day orally for 24 months (151 times the maximum recommended human topical ophthalmic dose, on a mg/kg basis, assuming 100% absorption in humans and animals) nor in mice given 2 mg/kg/day orally for 18 months (60 times the maximum recommended human topical ophthalmic dose, on a mg/kg basis, assuming 100% absorption in humans and animals).

Ketorolac tromethamine was not mutagenic *in vitro* in the Ames assay or in forward mutation assays. Similarly, it did not result in an *in vitro* increase in unscheduled DNA synthesis or an *in vivo* increase in chromosome breakage in mice. However, ketorolac tromethamine did result in an increased incidence in chromosomal aberrations in Chinese hamster ovary cells.

Ketorolac tromethamine did not impair fertility when administered orally to male and female rats at doses up to 272 and 484 times the maximum recommended human topical ophthalmic dose, respectively, on a mg/kg basis, assuming 100% absorption in humans and animals.

Pregnancy Category C

Teratogenic Effects

Ketorolac tromethamine, administered during organogenesis, was not teratogenic in rabbits or rats at oral doses up to 109 times and 303 times the maximum recommended human topical ophthalmic dose, respectively, on a mg/kg basis assuming 100% absorption in humans and animals. When administered to rats after Day 17 of gestation at oral doses up to 45 times the maximum recommended human topical ophthalmic dose, respectively, on a mg/kg basis, assuming 100% absorption in humans and animals, ketorolac tromethamine resulted in dystocia and increased pup mortality. There are no adequate and well-controlled studies in pregnant women. Acular PF ophthalmic solution should be used during pregnancy only if the potential benefit justifies the potential risk to the fetus.

Nonteratogenic Effects

Because of the known effects of prostaglandin-inhibiting drugs on the fetal cardiovascular system (closure of the ductus arteriosus), the use of Acular PF ophthalmic solution during late pregnancy should be avoided.

Nursing Mothers

Caution should be exercised when Acular PF is administered to a nursing woman.

Pediatric Use

Safety and efficacy in pediatric patients below the age of 3 have not been established.

Geriatric Use

No overall differences in safety or effectiveness have been observed between elderly and younger patients.

ACULAR LS

General

All topical nonsteroidal anti-inflammatory drugs (NSAIDs), including ketorolac tromethamine ophthalmic solution, may slow or delay healing. Topical corticosteroids are also known to slow or delay healing. Concomitant use of topical NSAIDs and topical steroids may increase the potential for healing problems.

Use of topical NSAIDs may result in keratitis. In some susceptible patients, continued use of topical NSAIDs may result in epithelial breakdown, corneal thinning, corneal erosion, corneal ulceration or corneal perforation. These events may be sight threatening. Patients with evidence of corneal epithelial breakdown should immediately discontinue use of topical NSAIDs and should be closely monitored for corneal health.

Postmarketing experience with topical NSAIDs suggests that patients with complicated ocular surgeries, corneal denervation, corneal epithelial defects, diabetes mellitus, ocular surface diseases (*e.g.*, dry eye syndrome), rheumatoid arthritis, or repeat ocular surgeries within a short period of time may be at increased risk for corneal adverse events which may become sight threatening. Topical NSAIDs should be used with caution in these patients.

Postmarketing experience with topical NSAIDs also suggests that use more than 24 hours prior to surgery or use beyond 14 days post-surgery may increase patient risk for the occurrence and severity of corneal adverse events.

It is recommended that Acular LS ophthalmic solution be used with caution in patients with known bleeding tendencies or who are receiving other medications, which may prolong bleeding time.

Information for the Patient

Acular LS ophthalmic solution should not be administered while wearing contact lenses.

Carcinogenesis, Mutagenesis, and Impairment of Fertility

Ketorolac tromethamine was neither carcinogenic in rats given up to 5 mg/kg/day orally for 24 months (156 times the maximum recommended human topical ophthalmic dose, on a mg/kg basis, assuming 100% absorption in humans and animals) nor in mice given 2 mg/kg/day orally for 18 months (62.5 times the maximum recommended human topical ophthalmic dose, on a mg/kg basis, assuming 100% absorption in humans and animals).

Ketorolac tromethamine was not mutagenic *in vitro* in the Ames assay or in forward mutation assays. Similarly, it did not result in an *in vitro* increase in unscheduled DNA synthesis or an *in vivo* increase in chromosome breakage in mice. However, ketorolac tromethamine did result in an increased incidence in chromosomal aberrations in Chinese hamster ovary cells.

Ketorolac tromethamine did not impair fertility when administered orally to male and female rats at doses up to 280 and 499 times the maximum recommended human topical ophthalmic dose, respectively, on a mg/kg basis, assuming 100% absorption in humans and animals.

K

Pregnancy Category C

Teratogenic Effects

Ketorolac tromethamine, administered during organogenesis, was not teratogenic in rabbits or rats at oral doses up to 112 times and 312 times the maximum recommended human topical ophthalmic dose, respectively, on a mg/kg basis assuming 100% absorption in humans and animals. When administered to rats after Day 17 of gestation at oral doses up to 46 times the maximum recommended human topical ophthalmic dose on a mg/kg basis, assuming 100% absorption in humans and animals, ketorolac tromethamine resulted in dystocia and increased pup mortality. There are no adequate and well-controlled studies in pregnant women. Acular LS ophthalmic solution should be used during pregnancy only if the potential benefit justifies the potential risk to the fetus.

Nonteratogenic Effects

Because of the known effects of prostaglandin-inhibiting drugs on the fetal cardiovascular system (closure of the ductus arteriosus), the use of Acular LS ophthalmic solution during late pregnancy should be avoided.

Nursing Mothers

Caution should be exercised when Acular LS ophthalmic solution is administered to a nursing woman.

Pediatric Use

Safety and effectiveness of ketorolac tromethamine in pediatric patients below the age of 3 have not been established.

Geriatric Use

No overall differences in safety or effectiveness have been observed between elderly and younger patients.

ADVERSE REACTIONS

ACULAR

The most frequent adverse events reported with the use of ketorolac tromethamine ophthalmic solutions have been transient stinging and burning on instillation. These events were reported by up to 40% of patients participating in clinical trials.

Other adverse events occurring approximately 1-10% of the time during treatment with ketorolac tromethamine ophthalmic solutions included allergic reactions, corneal edema, iritis, ocular inflammation, ocular irritation, superficial keratitis and superficial ocular infections.

Other adverse events reported rarely with the use of ketorolac tromethamine ophthalmic solutions included: corneal infiltrates, corneal ulcer, eye dryness, headaches, and visual disturbance (blurry vision).

Clinical Practice

The following events have been identified during postmarketing use of ketorolac tromethamine ophthalmic solution 0.5% in clinical practice. Because they are reported voluntarily from a population of unknown size, estimates of frequency cannot be made. The events, which have been chosen for inclusion due to either their seriousness, frequency of reporting, possible causal connection to topical ketorolac tromethamine ophthalmic solution 0.5%, or a combination of these factors, include corneal erosion, corneal perforation, corneal thinning, and epithelial breakdown (see PRECAUTIONS, Acular, General).

ACULAR PF

The most frequent adverse events reported with the use of ketorolac tromethamine ophthalmic solutions have been transient stinging and burning on instillation. These events were reported by approximately 20% of patients participating in clinical trials.

Other adverse events occurring approximately 1-10% of the time during treatment with ketorolac tromethamine ophthalmic solutions included allergic reactions, corneal edema, iritis, ocular inflammation, ocular irritation, superficial keratitis, and superficial ocular infections.

Other adverse events reported rarely with the use of ketorolac tromethamine ophthalmic solutions include: corneal infiltrates, corneal ulcer, eye dryness, headaches, and visual disturbance (blurry vision).

Clinical Practice

The following events have been identified during postmarketing use of topical ketorolac tromethamine ophthalmic solution 0.5% in clinical practice. Because they are reported voluntarily from a population of unknown size, estimates of frequency cannot be made. The events, which have been chosen for inclusion due to either their seriousness, frequency of reporting, possible causal connection to topical ketorolac tromethamine ophthalmic solution 0.5%, or a combination of these factors, include corneal erosion, corneal perforation, corneal thinning, and epithelial breakdown (see PRECAUTIONS, Acular PF,General).

ACULAR LS

The most frequently reported adverse reactions for Acular LS ophthalmic solution occurring in approximately 1-5% of the overall study population were conjunctival hyperemia, corneal infiltrates, headache, ocular edema and ocular pain.

The most frequent adverse events reported with the use of ketorolac tromethamine ophthalmic solutions have been transient stinging and burning on instillation. These events were reported by 20-40% of patients participating in these other clinical trials.

Other adverse events occurring approximately 1-10% of the time during treatment with ketorolac tromethamine ophthalmic solutions included allergic reactions, corneal edema, iritis, ocular inflammation, ocular irritation, ocular pain, superficial keratitis, and superficial ocular infections.

Clinical Practice

The following events have been identified during postmarketing use of ketorolac tromethamine ophthalmic solutions in clinical practice. Because they are reported voluntarily from a population of unknown size, estimates of frequency cannot be made. The events, which have been chosen for inclusion due to either their seriousness, frequency of reporting, possible causal connection to topical ketorolac tromethamine ophthalmic solutions, or a combination of these factors, include corneal erosion, corneal perforation, corneal thinning and epithelial breakdown (see PRECAUTIONS, Acular LS, General).

DOSAGE AND ADMINISTRATION

ACULAR

The recommended dose of Acular ophthalmic solution is 1 drop (0.25 mg) 4 times a day for relief of ocular itching due to seasonal allergic conjunctivitis.

For the treatment of postoperative inflammation in patients who have undergone cataract extraction, 1 drop of Acular ophthalmic solution should be applied to the affected eye(s) 4 times daily beginning 24 hours after cataract surgery and continuing through the first 2 weeks of the postoperative period.

Acular ophthalmic solution has been safely administered in conjunction with other ophthalmic medications such as antibiotics, beta blockers, carbonic anhydrase inhibitors, cycloplegics, and mydriatics.

ACULAR PF

The recommended dose of Acular PF is 1 drop (0.25 mg) 4 times a day in the operated eye as needed for pain and photophobia for up to 3 days after incisional refractive surgery.

ACULAR LS

The recommended dose of Acular LS ophthalmic solution is 1 drop 4 times a day in the operated eye as needed for pain and burning/stinging for up to 4 days following corneal refractive surgery.

Ketorolac tromethamine ophthalmic solution has been safely administered in conjunction with other ophthalmic medications such as antibiotics, beta blockers, carbonic anhydrase inhibitors, cycloplegics, and mydriatics.

HOW SUPPLIED

ACULAR

Acular (ketorolac tromethamine ophthalmic solution) is supplied sterile in opaque white LDPE plastic bottles with droppers with gray high impact polystyrene (HIPS) caps as follows:

3 ml in 6 ml bottle.
5 ml in 10 ml bottle.
10 ml in 10 ml bottle.

Storage: Store at room temperature 15-30°C (59-86°F) with protection from light.

ACULAR PF

Acular PF (ketorolac tromethamine ophthalmic solution) 0.5% preservative-free is available as a sterile solution supplied in single-use vials of 0.4 ml each.

Storage: Store Acular PF between 15-30°C (59-86°F) with protection from light.

ACULAR LS

Acular LS (ketorolac tromethamine ophthalmic solution) 0.4% is supplied sterile in an opaque white LDPE plastic bottle with a white dropper with a gray high impact polystyrene (HIPS) cap as follows:

5 ml in 10 ml bottle.

Storage: Store at 15-25°C (59-77°F).

PRODUCT LISTING - RATED THERAPEUTICALLY EQUIVALENT

Size	Price	Product, Manufacturer	NDC
Solution - Injectable - 15 mg/ml			
1 ml	$3.62	GENERIC, Baxter Pharmaceutical Products, Inc	10019-0021-09
1 ml x 10	$80.00	GENERIC, Bedford Laboratories	55390-0480-01
1 ml x 10	$87.16	GENERIC, Abbott Pharmaceutical	00074-2288-01
1 ml x 10	$87.38	GENERIC, Abbott Pharmaceutical	00074-2023-02
1 ml x 10	$89.06	GENERIC, Abbott Pharmaceutical	00074-2288-31
1 ml x 10	$90.25	GENERIC, Abbott Pharmaceutical	00074-2288-11
1 ml x 25	$93.75	GENERIC, Abbott Pharmaceutical	00074-3793-01
1 ml x 25	$93.75	GENERIC, American Pharmaceutical Partners	63323-0161-01
1 ml x 25	$191.88	GENERIC, Abbott Pharmaceutical	00074-3793-49
2 ml x 10	$97.00	GENERIC, Vha Supply	00074-2023-49
Solution - Injectable - 30 mg/ml			
1 ml	$3.89	GENERIC, Baxter Pharmaceutical Products, Inc	10019-0022-09
1 ml	$9.95	GENERIC, Prescript Pharmaceuticals	00247-0236-01
1 ml	$11.01	TORADOL IV/IM, Physicians Total Care	54868-3843-00
1 ml x 10	$65.08	GENERIC, Abbott Pharmaceutical	00074-2287-01
1 ml x 10	$66.10	TORADOL, Roche Laboratories	00004-6926-06
1 ml x 10	$70.85	TORADOL IV/IM, Allscripts Pharmaceutical Company	54569-3822-00
1 ml x 10	$73.60	TORADOL, Roche Laboratories	00004-6922-06
1 ml x 10	$73.98	GENERIC, Abbott Pharmaceutical	00074-2287-31
1 ml x 10	$84.00	GENERIC, Bedford Laboratories	55390-0481-01
1 ml x 10	$91.20	GENERIC, Abbott Pharmaceutical	00074-2287-11
1 ml x 10	$91.38	GENERIC, Abbott Pharmaceutical	00074-2036-02
1 ml x 10	$91.38	GENERIC, Vha Supply	00074-2036-49
1 ml x 10	$108.81	TORADOL IV/IM, Physicians Total Care	54868-1763-00
1 ml x 25	$91.00	GENERIC, Abbott Pharmaceutical	00074-3795-01
1 ml x 25	$125.00	GENERIC, American Pharmaceutical Partners	63323-0162-01
1 ml x 25	$201.56	GENERIC, Vha Supply	00074-3795-49
2 ml	$4.15	GENERIC, Baxter Pharmaceutical Products, Inc	10019-0022-32
2 ml	$6.67	TORADOL, Roche Laboratories	00004-6927-09

2 ml	$7.44	TORADOL IM, Allscripts Pharmaceutical Company	54569-3736-01
2 ml	$8.44	TORADOL IM, Physicians Total Care	54868-4133-00
2 ml	$9.00	GENERIC, Prescript Pharmaceuticals	00247-0124-02
2 ml x 10	$83.71	TORADOL IM, Syntex Laboratories Inc	00033-2444-50
2 ml x 10	$88.00	GENERIC, Bedford Laboratories	55390-0481-02
2 ml x 10	$96.78	GENERIC, Abbott Pharmaceutical	00074-2287-02
2 ml x 10	$96.78	GENERIC, Abbott Pharmaceutical	00074-2287-61
2 ml x 10	$97.00	GENERIC, Abbott Pharmaceutical	00074-2039-02
2 ml x 10	$97.00	GENERIC, Vha Supply	00074-2039-49
2 ml x 25	$112.50	GENERIC, Abbott Pharmaceutical	00074-3796-01
2 ml x 25	$156.25	GENERIC, American Pharmaceutical Partners	63323-0162-02
2 ml x 25	$211.56	GENERIC, Vha Supply	00074-3796-49
10 ml	$69.40	GENERIC, Prescript Pharmaceuticals	00247-0236-10
10 ml x 10	$440.00	GENERIC, Bedford Laboratories	55390-0481-10
20 ml	$59.80	GENERIC, Prescript Pharmaceuticals	00247-0124-20
50 ml	$144.48	GENERIC, Prescript Pharmaceuticals	00247-0124-50
Tablet - Oral - 10 mg			
1's	$4.82	TORADOL, Prescript Pharmaceuticals	00247-0121-01
2's	$1.96	GENERIC, Allscripts Pharmaceutical Company	54569-4494-04
2's	$6.29	TORADOL, Prescript Pharmaceuticals	00247-0121-02
3's	$7.76	TORADOL, Prescript Pharmaceuticals	00247-0121-03
4's	$9.24	TORADOL, Prescript Pharmaceuticals	00247-0121-04
6's	$12.16	TORADOL, Prescript Pharmaceuticals	00247-0121-06
8's	$7.84	GENERIC, Allscripts Pharmaceutical Company	54569-4494-01
8's	$8.44	TORADOL, Allscripts Pharmaceutical Company	54569-3539-02
8's	$11.50	TORADOL, Southwood Pharmaceuticals Inc	58016-0371-08
8's	$14.08	GENERIC, Pharma Pac	52959-0512-08
8's	$15.11	TORADOL, Prescript Pharmaceuticals	00247-0121-08
8's	$16.10	TORADOL, Pharma Pac	52959-0224-08
8's	$17.97	TORADOL, Pd-Rx Pharmaceuticals	55289-0985-08
10's	$9.80	GENERIC, Allscripts Pharmaceutical Company	54569-4494-03
10's	$10.55	TORADOL, Allscripts Pharmaceutical Company	54569-3539-07
10's	$13.34	GENERIC, Dhs Inc	55887-0880-10
10's	$17.10	TORADOL, Southwood Pharmaceuticals Inc	58016-0371-10
10's	$17.22	GENERIC, Pharma Pac	52959-0512-10
10's	$18.05	TORADOL, Prescript Pharmaceuticals	00247-0121-10
10's	$20.01	TORADOL, Pharma Pac	52959-0224-10
12's	$19.35	TORADOL, Southwood Pharmaceuticals Inc	58016-0371-12
12's	$20.64	GENERIC, Pharma Pac	52959-0512-12
12's	$20.99	TORADOL, Prescript Pharmaceuticals	00247-0121-12
12's	$23.81	TORADOL, Pharma Pac	52959-0224-12
14's	$22.46	TORADOL, Southwood Pharmaceuticals Inc	58016-0371-14
14's	$23.98	GENERIC, Pharma Pac	52959-0512-14
14's	$27.69	TORADOL, Pharma Pac	52959-0224-14
15's	$14.69	GENERIC, Allscripts Pharmaceutical Company	54569-4494-02
15's	$15.83	TORADOL, Allscripts Pharmaceutical Company	54569-3539-03
15's	$20.82	GENERIC, Pd-Rx Pharmaceuticals	55289-0328-15
15's	$24.06	TORADOL, Southwood Pharmaceuticals Inc	58016-0371-15
15's	$24.45	TORADOL, Physicians Total Care	54868-2285-02
15's	$25.39	TORADOL, Prescript Pharmaceuticals	00247-0121-15
15's	$25.65	GENERIC, Pharma Pac	52959-0512-15
15's	$26.25	TORADOL, Pd-Rx Pharmaceuticals	55289-0985-15
15's	$29.62	TORADOL, Pharma Pac	52959-0224-15
16's	$26.86	TORADOL, Prescript Pharmaceuticals	00247-0121-16
20's	$19.59	GENERIC, Allscripts Pharmaceutical Company	54569-4494-00
20's	$20.59	GENERIC, St. Mary'S Mpp	60760-0314-20
20's	$21.10	TORADOL, Allscripts Pharmaceutical Company	54569-3539-01
20's	$26.98	GENERIC, Dhs Inc	55887-0880-20
20's	$27.39	GENERIC, Pd-Rx Pharmaceuticals	55289-0328-20
20's	$27.91	TORADOL, Southwood Pharmaceuticals Inc	58016-0371-20
20's	$30.98	TORADOL, Pd-Rx Pharmaceuticals	55289-0985-20
20's	$32.21	TORADOL, Physicians Total Care	54868-2285-01
20's	$32.74	TORADOL, Prescript Pharmaceuticals	00247-0121-20
20's	$34.15	GENERIC, Pharma Pac	52959-0512-20
20's	$38.68	TORADOL, Pharma Pac	52959-0224-20
20's	$39.86	TORADOL, Dhs Inc	55887-0915-20
21's	$29.31	TORADOL, Southwood Pharmaceuticals Inc	58016-0371-21
21's	$34.20	TORADOL, Prescript Pharmaceuticals	00247-0121-21
28's	$44.49	TORADOL, Prescript Pharmaceuticals	00247-0121-28
30's	$39.31	TORADOL, Southwood Pharmaceuticals Inc	58016-0371-30
30's	$41.64	GENERIC, Pd-Rx Pharmaceuticals	55289-0328-30
30's	$45.14	TORADOL, Physicians Total Care	54868-2285-04
30's	$46.80	TORADOL, Pd-Rx Pharmaceuticals	55289-0985-30
30's	$47.42	TORADOL, Prescript Pharmaceuticals	00247-0121-30
30's	$50.99	GENERIC, Pharma Pac	52959-0512-30
30's	$57.13	TORADOL, Pharma Pac	52959-0224-30
40's	$42.04	TORADOL, Southwood Pharmaceuticals Inc	58016-0371-40
40's	$62.12	TORADOL, Prescript Pharmaceuticals	00247-0121-40
40's	$63.25	TORADOL, Physicians Total Care	54868-2285-03
40's	$65.16	GENERIC, Pharma Pac	52959-0512-40
40's	$69.42	TORADOL, Pd-Rx Pharmaceuticals	55289-0985-40
40's	$73.88	TORADOL, Pharma Pac	52959-0224-40
60's	$94.80	GENERIC, Pharma Pac	52959-0512-60
60's	$109.26	TORADOL, Pharma Pac	52959-0224-60
100's	$67.73	FEDERAL UPPER LIMIT, H.C.F.A. F F P	99999-1607-01
100's	$92.97	GENERIC, Teva Pharmaceuticals Usa	00093-0314-01
100's	$92.98	GENERIC, Ethex Corporation	58177-0301-04
100's	$102.00	GENERIC, Mylan Pharmaceuticals Inc	00378-1134-01
100's	$102.50	GENERIC, Sidmak Laboratories Inc	50111-0608-01
100's	$109.91	TORADOL, Roche Laboratories	00004-0273-01
100's	$118.87	TORADOL, Southwood Pharmaceuticals Inc	58016-0371-00
100's	$150.27	TORADOL, Prescript Pharmaceuticals	00247-0121-00

PRODUCT LISTING - EQUIVALENTS NOT AVAILABLE

Solution - Injectable - 15 mg/ml			
1 ml x 10	$60.50	TORADOL, Roche Laboratories	00004-6925-06
1 ml x 10	$67.60	TORADOL IV/IM, Roche Laboratories	00004-6921-06
1 ml x 10	$70.30	TORADOL, Roche Laboratories	00004-6920-06
Solution - Injectable - 30 mg/ml			
1 ml x 10	$50.00	GENERIC, Allscripts Pharmaceutical Company	54569-4954-00
2 ml	$116.64	GENERIC, Southwood Pharmaceuticals Inc	58016-9413-01
2 ml x 10	$56.25	GENERIC, Allscripts Pharmaceutical Company	54569-4955-00
Solution - Ophthalmic - 0.5%			
0.40 ml x 12	$44.26	ACULAR, Allergan Inc	00023-9055-04
3 ml	$27.36	ACULAR, Allscripts Pharmaceutical Company	54569-4573-00
3 ml	$29.74	ACULAR, Physicians Total Care	54868-3950-00
3 ml	$33.74	ACULAR, Allergan Inc	00023-2181-03
5 ml	$31.46	ACULAR, Allscripts Pharmaceutical Company	54569-4083-00
5 ml	$49.90	ACULAR, Southwood Pharmaceuticals Inc	58016-6461-01
5 ml	$56.26	ACULAR, Allergan Inc	00023-2181-05
5 ml	$67.08	ACULAR, Pharma Pac	52959-0114-05
10 ml	$99.80	ACULAR, Southwood Pharmaceuticals Inc	58016-6461-02
10 ml	$112.45	ACULAR, Allergan Inc	00023-2181-10
Tablet - Oral - 10 mg			
4's	$5.11	GENERIC, Prescript Pharmaceuticals	00247-1571-04
6's	$5.99	GENERIC, Prescript Pharmaceuticals	00247-1571-06
10's	$7.74	GENERIC, Prescript Pharmaceuticals	00247-1571-10
10's	$10.51	GENERIC, Southwood Pharmaceuticals Inc	58016-0247-10
12's	$12.61	GENERIC, Southwood Pharmaceuticals Inc	58016-0247-12
15's	$9.93	GENERIC, Prescript Pharmaceuticals	00247-1571-15
15's	$15.77	GENERIC, Southwood Pharmaceuticals Inc	58016-0247-15
15's	$19.76	GENERIC, Cardinal Pharmaceuticals	63874-0472-15
20's	$12.13	GENERIC, Prescript Pharmaceuticals	00247-1571-20
20's	$14.75	GENERIC, Physicians Total Care	54868-4171-00
20's	$21.02	GENERIC, Southwood Pharmaceuticals Inc	58016-0247-20
20's	$26.00	GENERIC, Cardinal Pharmaceuticals	63874-0472-20
21's	$22.07	GENERIC, Southwood Pharmaceuticals Inc	58016-0247-21
30's	$16.51	GENERIC, Prescript Pharmaceuticals	00247-1571-30
30's	$31.53	GENERIC, Southwood Pharmaceuticals Inc	58016-0247-30
30's	$39.52	GENERIC, Cardinal Pharmaceuticals	63874-0472-30
40's	$42.04	GENERIC, Southwood Pharmaceuticals Inc	58016-0247-40
100's	$105.10	GENERIC, Southwood Pharmaceuticals Inc	58016-0247-00
100's	$116.00	GENERIC, Cardinal Pharmaceuticals	63874-0472-01

Labetalol Hydrochloride *(001613)*

For related information, see the comparative table section in Appendix A.

Categories: Hypertension, essential; Pregnancy Category C; FDA Approved 1984 Aug
Drug Classes: Antiadrenergics, beta blocking
Brand Names: Coreton; Normodate; **Normodyne**; Trandate
Foreign Brand Availability: Abetol (Italy); Albetol (Finland); Amipress (Italy); Hybloc (New-Zealand); Ipolab (Italy); Labelol (Argentina); Labesine (Korea); Lamitol (Slovenia); Liondox (Argentina); Presolol (Australia; Taiwan); Pressalolo (Italy); Salmagne (Greece)
Cost of Therapy: $39.04 (Hypertension; Normodyne; 100 mg; 2 tablets/day; 30 day supply)
$28.81 (Hypertension; Generic Tablets; 100 mg; 2 tablets/day; 30 day supply)

DESCRIPTION

Labetalol hydrochloride is an adrenergic receptor blocking agent that has both selective alpha$_1$-adrenergic and nonselective beta-adrenergic receptor blocking actions in a single substance.

Labetalol hydrochloride is a racemate, chemically designated as 2-hydroxy-5-[1-hydroxy-2-[(1-methyl-3-phenylpropyl)amino]ethyl]benzamide monohydrochloride.

Labetalol hydrochloride has the empirical formula $C_{19}H_{24}N_2O_3{\cdot}HCl$ and a molecular weight of 364.9. It has two asymmetric centers and therefore exists as a molecular complex of two diastereoisomeric pairs. Dilevalol, the R,R′ stereoisomer, makes up 25% of racemic labetalol.

Labetalol hydrochloride is a white or off-white crystalline powder, soluble in water.

INJECTION

Labetalol hydrochloride injection is a clear, colorless to light yellow, aqueous, sterile, isotonic solution for intravenous (IV) injection. It has a pH range of 3-4. Each ml contains 5 mg labetalol hydrochloride, 45 mg anhydrous dextrose, 0.1 mg edetate disodium; 0.8 mg methylparaben and 0.1 mg propylparaben as preservatives, citric acid monohydrate and sodium hydroxide, as necessary, to bring the solution into the pH range.

TABLETS

Labetalol hydrochloride tablets contain 100, 200 or 300 mg labetalol hydrochloride and are taken orally.

The tablets also contain the inactive ingredients corn starch, FD&C yellow no. 6 (100 and 300 mg tablets only), hydroxypropyl methylcellulose, lactose, magnesium stearate, methylparaben, pregelatinized corn starch, propylparaben, sodium benzoate (200 mg tablet only), talc (100 mg tablet only), and titanium dioxide.

CLINICAL PHARMACOLOGY

Labetalol HCl combines both selective, competitive, $alpha_1$- adrenergic blocking and nonselective, competitive, beta-adrenergic blocking activity in a single substance. In man, the ratios of alpha- to beta-blockade have been estimated to be approximately 1:3 and 1:7 following oral and IV administration, respectively. $Beta_2$-agonist activity has been demonstrated in animals with minimal $beta_1$-agonist (ISA) activity detected. In animals, at doses greater than those required for alpha- or beta-adrenergic blockade, a membrane stabilizing effect has been demonstrated.

PHARMACODYNAMICS

The capacity of labetalol HCl to block alpha receptors in man has been demonstrated by attenuation of the pressor effect of phenylephrine and by a significant reduction of the pressor response caused by immersing the hand in ice-cold water ("cold-pressor test"). Labetalol HCl's $beta_1$-receptor blockade in man was demonstrated by a small decrease in the resting heart rate, attenuation of tachycardia produced by isoproterenol or exercise, and by attenuation of the reflex tachycardia to the hypotension produced by amyl nitrite. $Beta_2$-receptor blockade was demonstrated by inhibition of the isoproterenol-induced fall in diastolic blood pressure. Both the alpha- and beta-blocking actions of orally administered labetalol HCl contribute to a decrease in blood pressure in hypertensive patients. Labetalol HCl consistently, in dose-related fashion, blunted increases in exercise-induced blood pressure and heart rate, and in their double product. The pulmonary circulation during exercise was not affected by labetalol HCl dosing.

Single oral doses of labetalol HCl administered to patients with coronary artery disease had no significant effect on sinus rate, intraventricular conduction, or QRS duration. The atrioventricular (AV) conduction time was modestly prolonged in 2 of 7 patients. In another study, IV labetalol HCl slightly prolonged AV nodal conduction time and atrial effective refractory period with only small changes in heart rate. The effects on AV nodal refractoriness were inconsistent.

Labetalol HCl produces dose-related falls in blood pressure without reflex tachycardia and without significant reduction in heart rate, presumably through a mixture of its alpha- and beta-blocking effects. Hemodynamic effects are variable, with small, nonsignificant changes in cardiac output seen in some studies but not others, and small decreases in total peripheral resistance. Elevated plasma renins are reduced.

Doses of labetalol HCl that controlled hypertension did not affect renal function in mildly to severely hypertensive patients with normal renal function.

Exacerbation of angina and, in some cases, myocardial infarction and ventricular dysrhythmias have been reported after abrupt discontinuation of therapy with beta-adrenergic blocking agents in patients with coronary artery disease. Abrupt withdrawal of these agents in patients without coronary artery disease has resulted in transient symptoms, including tremulousness, sweating, palpitation, headache, and malaise. Several mechanisms have been proposed to explain these phenomena, among them increased sensitivity to catecholamines because of increased numbers of beta receptors.

Although beta-adrenergic receptor blockade is useful in the treatment of angina and hypertension, there are also situations in which sympathetic stimulation is vital. For example, in patients with severely damaged hearts, adequate ventricular function may depend on sympathetic drive. Beta-adrenergic blockade may worsen AV block by preventing the necessary facilitating effects of sympathetic activity on conduction. $Beta_2$-adrenergic blockade results in passive bronchial constriction by interfering with endogenous adrenergic bronchodilator activity in patients subject to bronchospasm, and may also interfere with exogenous bronchodilators in such patients.

Injection

Due to the $alpha_1$-receptor blocking activity of labetalol HCl, blood pressure is lowered more in the standing than in the supine position, and symptoms of postural hypotension can occur. During dosing with IV labetalol HCl, the contribution of the postural component should be considered when positioning patients for treatment, and patients should not be allowed to move to an erect position unmonitored until their ability to do so is established.

In a clinical pharmacologic study in severe hypertensives, an initial 0.25 mg/kg injection of labetalol HCl, administered to patients in the supine position, decreased blood pressure by an average of 11/7 mm Hg. Additional injections of 0.5 mg/kg at 15 minute intervals up to a total cumulative dose of 1.75 mg/kg of labetalol HCl caused further dose-related decreases in blood pressure. Some patients required cumulative doses of up to 3.25 mg/kg. The maximal effect of each dose level occurred within 5 minutes. Following discontinuation of IV treatment with labetalol HCl, the blood pressure rose gradually and progressively, approaching pretreatment baseline values within an average of 16-18 hours in the majority of patients.

Similar results were obtained in the treatment of patients with severe hypertension requiring urgent blood pressure reduction with an initial dose of 20 mg (which corresponds to 0.25 mg/kg for an 80 kg patient) followed by additional doses of either 40 or 80 mg at 10 minute intervals to achieve the desired effect, or up to a cumulative dose of 300 mg.

Labetalol HCl administered as a continuous IV infusion, with a mean dose of 136 mg (27-300 mg) over a period of 2-3 hours (mean of 2 hours and 39 minutes) lowered the blood pressure by an average of 60/35 mmHg.

Tablets

Due to the $alpha_1$-receptor blocking activity of labetalol HCl, blood pressure is lowered more in the standing than in the supine position, and symptoms of postural hypotension (2%), including rare instances of syncope, can occur. Following oral administration, when postural hypotension has occurred, it has been transient and is uncommon when the recommended starting dose and titration increments are closely followed (see DOSAGE AND ADMINISTRATION). Symptomatic postural hypotension is more likely to occur 2-4 hours after a dose, especially following the use of large initial doses or upon large changes in dose.

The peak effects of single oral doses of labetalol HCl occur within 2-4 hours. The duration of effect depends upon dose, lasting at least 8 hours following single oral doses of 100 mg and more than 12 hours following single oral doses of 300 mg. The maximum, steady-state blood pressure response upon oral, twice-a-day dosing occurs within 24-72 hours.

The antihypertensive effect of labetalol has a linear correlation with the logarithm of labetalol plasma concentration, and there is also a linear correlation between the reduction in exercise-induced tachycardia occurring at 2 hours after oral administration of labetalol HCl and the logarithm of the plasma concentration.

About 70% of the maximum beta-blocking effect is present for 5 hours after the administration of a single oral dose of 400 mg, with suggestion that about 40% remains at 8 hours.

The antianginal efficacy of labetalol HCl has not been studied. In 37 patients with hypertension and coronary artery disease, labetalol HCl did not increase the incidence or severity of angina attacks.

PHARMACOKINETICS AND METABOLISM

The metabolism of labetalol is mainly through conjugation to glucuronide metabolites. These metabolites are present in plasma and are excreted in the urine and, via the bile, into the feces. Approximately 55-60% of a dose appears in the urine as conjugates or unchanged labetalol within the first 24 hours of dosing.

Labetalol has been shown to cross the placental barrier in humans. Only negligible amounts of the drug crossed the blood-brain barrier in animal studies. Labetalol is approximately 50% protein bound. Neither hemodialysis nor peritoneal dialysis removes a significant amount of labetalol HCl from the general circulation (<1%).

Injection

Following IV infusion of labetalol, the elimination half-life is about 5.5 hours and the total body clearance is approximately 33 ml/min/kg. The plasma half-life of labetalol following oral administration is about 6-8 hours. In patients with decreased hepatic or renal function, the elimination half-life of labetalol is not altered; however, the relative bioavailability in hepatically impaired patients is increased due to decreased "first-pass" metabolism.

Tablets

Labetalol HCl is completely absorbed from the gastrointestinal tract with peak plasma levels occurring 1-2 hours after oral administration. The relative bioavailability of labetalol HCl tablets compared to an oral solution is 100%. The absolute bioavailability (fraction of drug reaching systemic circulation) of labetalol when compared to an IV infusion is 25%; this is due to extensive "first-pass" metabolism. Despite "first-pass" metabolism there is a linear relationship between oral doses of 100-3000 mg and peak plasma levels. The absolute bioavailability of labetalol is increased when administered with food.

The plasma half-life of labetalol following oral administration is about 6-8 hours. Steady-state plasma levels of labetalol during repetitive dosing are reached by about the third day of dosing. In patients with decreased hepatic or renal function, the elimination half-life of labetalol is not altered; however, the relative bioavailability in hepatically impaired patients is increased due to decreased "first-pass" metabolism.

Elderly Patients

Some pharmacokinetic studies indicate that the elimination of labetalol is reduced in elderly patients. Therefore, although elderly patients may initiate therapy at the currently recommended dosage of 100 mg bid, elderly patients will generally require lower maintenance dosages than nonelderly patients.

INDICATIONS AND USAGE

INJECTION

Labetalol HCl injection is indicated for control of blood pressure in severe hypertension.

TABLETS

Labetalol HCl tablets are indicated in the management of hypertension. Labetalol tablets may be used alone or in combination with other antihypertensive agents, especially thiazide and loop diuretics.

NON-FDA APPROVED INDICATIONS

Labetalol is also used without FDA approval for the treatment of hypertensive emergencies and for hypertension and tachycardia associated with pheochromocytoma.

CONTRAINDICATIONS

Labetalol HCl injection and tablets are contraindicated in bronchial asthma, overt cardiac failure, greater-than-first-degree heart block, cardiogenic shock, severe bradycardia, other conditions associated with severe and prolonged hypotension, and in patients with a history of hypersensitivity to any component of the product (see WARNINGS).

Beta-blockers, even those with apparent cardioselectivity, should not be used in patients with a hisory of obstructive airway diesease, including asthma.

WARNINGS

HEPATIC INJURY

Severe hepatocellular injury, confirmed by rechallenge in at least one case, occurs rarely with labetalol therapy. The hepatic injury is usually reversible, but hepatic necrosis and death have been reported. Injury has occurred after both short- and long-term treatment and may be slowly progressive despite minimal symptomatology. Similar hepatic events have been reported with a related compound, dilevalol HCl, including 2 deaths. Dilevalol HCl is

1 of the 4 isomers of labetalol HCl. Thus, for patients taking labetalol, periodic determination of suitable hepatic laboratory tests would be appropriate. Appropriate laboratory testing should also be done at the very first symptom or sign of liver dysfunction (*e.g.*, pruritus, dark urine, persistent anorexia, jaundice, right upper quadrant tenderness, or unexplained "flu-like" symptoms). If the patient has laboratory evidence of liver injury or jaundice, labetalol HCl should be stopped and not restarted.

CARDIAC FAILURE

Sympathetic stimulation is a vital component supporting circulatory function in congestive heart failure. Beta-blockade carries a potential hazard of further depressing myocardial contractility and precipitating more severe failure. Although beta-blockers should be avoided in overt congestive heart failure, if necessary, labetalol HCl can be used with caution in patients with a history of heart failure who are well compensated. Congestive heart failure has been observed in patients receiving labetalol HCl. Labetalol HCl does not abolish the inotropic action of digitalis on heart muscle.

IN PATIENTS WITHOUT A HISTORY OF CARDIAC FAILURE

In patients with latent cardiac insufficiency, continued depression of the myocardium with beta-blocking agents over a period of time can, in some cases, lead to cardiac failure. At the first sign or symptom of impending cardiac failure, patients should be fully digitalized and/or be given a diuretic, and the response observed closely. If cardiac failure continues, despite adequate digitalization and diuretic, labetalol HCl therapy should be withdrawn (gradually, if possible).

PHEOCHROMOCYTOMA

Labetalol HCl has been shown to be effective in lowering the blood pressure and relieving symptoms in patients with pheochromocytoma; higher than usual doses may be required-(Injection). However, paradoxical hypertensive responses have been reported in a few patients with this tumor; therefore, use caution when administering labetalol HCl to patients with pheochromocytoma.

DIABETES MELLITUS AND HYPOGLYCEMIA

Beta-adrenergic blockade may prevent the appearance of premonitory signs and symptoms (*e.g.*, tachycardia) of acute hypoglycemia. This is especially important with labile diabetics. Beta-blockade also reduces the release of insulin in response to hyperglycemia; it may therefore be necessary to adjust the dose of antidiabetic drugs.

MAJOR SURGERY

The necessity of desirability of withdrawing beta-blocking therapy before a major surgery is controversial. Protracted severe hypotension and difficulty in restarting or maintaining a heartbeat have been reported with beta-blockers. The effect of labetalol HCl's alpha-adrenergic activity has not been evaluated in this setting.

A synergism between labetalol HCl and halothane anesthesia has been shown (see DRUG INTERACTIONS).

INJECTION

Ischemic Heart Disease

Angina pectoris has not been reported upon labetalol HCl discontinuation. However, following abrupt cessation of therapy with some beta-blocking agents in patients with coronary artery disease, exacerbations of angina pectoris and, in some cases, myocardial infarction have been reported. Therefore, such patients should be cautioned against interruption of therapy without the physician's advice. Even in the absence of overt angina pectoris, when discontinuation of labetalol HCl is planned, the patient should be carefully observed and should be advised to limit physical activity. If angina markedly worsens or acute coronary insufficiency develops, labetalol HCl administration should be reinstituted promptly, at least temporarily, and other measures appropriate for the management of unstable angina should be taken.

Nonallergic Bronchospasm (e.g., chronic bronchitis and emphysema)

Since labetalol HCl injection at the usual IV therapeutic doses has not been studied in patients with nonallergic bronchospastic disease, it should not be used in such patients.

Major Surgery

Several deaths have occurred when labetalol HCl was used during surgery (including when used in cases to control bleeding).

Rapid Decreases of Blood Pressure

Caution must be observed when reducing severely elevated blood pressure. A number of adverse reactions, including cerebral infarction, optic nerve infarction, angina, and ischemic changes in the electrocardiogram have been reported with other agents when severely elevated blood pressure was reduced over time courses of several hours to as long as 1 or 2 days. The desired blood pressure lowering should therefore be achieved over as long a period of time as is compatible with the patient's status.

TABLETS

Exacerbation of Ischemic Heart Disease Following Abrupt Withdrawal

Angina pectoris has not been reported upon labetalol HCl discontinuation. However, hypersensitivity to catecholamines has been observed in patients withdrawn from beta-blocker therapy; exacerbation of angina and, in some cases, myocardial infarction have occurred after *abrupt* discontinuation of such therapy. When discontinuing chronically administered labetalol HCl tablets, particularly in patients with ischemic heart disease, the dosage should be gradually reduced over a period of 1-2 weeks and the patient should be carefully monitored. If angina markedly worsens or acute coronary insufficiency develops, labetalol HCl administration should be reinstituted promptly, at least temporarily, and other measures appropriate for the management of unstable angina should be taken. Patients should be warned against interruption or discontinuation of therapy without the physician's advice. Because coronary artery disease is common and may be unrecognized, it may be prudent not to discontinue labetalol HCl therapy abruptly even in patients treated only for hypertension.

Nonallergic Bronchospasm (e.g., chronic bronchitis and emphysema):

Patients with bronchospastic disease should, in general, not receive beta-blockers. Labetalol HCl tablets may be used with caution, however, in patients who do not respond to, or cannot tolerate, other antihypertensive agents. It is prudent, if labetalol HCl is used, to use the smallest effective dose, so that inhibition of endogenous or exogenous beta-agonists is minimized.

PRECAUTIONS

GENERAL

Impaired Hepatic Function: Labetalol HCl should be used with caution in patients with impaired hepatic function since metabolism of the drug may be diminished.

Jaundice or Hepatic Dysfunction: See WARNINGS.

Injection

Following Coronary Artery Bypass Surgery

In one uncontrolled study, patients with low cardiac indices and elevated systemic vascular resistance following IV labetalol HCl experienced significant declines in cardiac output with little change in systemic vascular resistance. One of these patients developed hypotension following labetalol treatment. Therefore, use of labetalol HCl should be avoided in such patients.

High-Dose Labetalol HCl

Administration of up to 3 g/day as an infusion for up to 2-3 days has been anecdotally reported; several patients experienced hypotension or bradycardia.

Hypotension

Symptomatic postural hypotension (incidence 58%) is likely to occur if patients are tilted or allowed to assume the upright position within 3 hours of receiving labetalol HCl injection. Therefore, the patient's ability to tolerate an upright position should be established before permitting any ambulation.

INFORMATION FOR THE PATIENT

As with all drugs with beta-blocking activity, certain advice to patients being treated with labetalol HCl is warranted. This information is intended to aid in the safe and effective use of this medication. It is not a disclosure of all possible adverse or intended effects. While no incident of the abrupt withdrawal phenomenon (exacerbation of angina pectoris) has been reported with labetalol HCl, dosing with labetalol HCl tablets should not be interrupted or discontinued without a physician's advice. Patients being treated with labetalol HCl tablets should consult a physician at any signs or symptoms of impending cardiac failure or hepatic dysfunction (see WARNINGS). Also, transient scalp tingling may occur, usually when treatment with labetalol HCl tablets is initiated (see ADVERSE REACTIONS).

Injection

The following information is intended to aid in the safe and effective use of this medication. It is not a disclosure of all possible adverse or intended effects. During and immediately following (for up to 3 hours) labetalol HCl injection, the patient should remain supine. Subsequently, the patient should be advised on how to proceed gradually to become ambulatory, and should be observed at the time of first ambulation.

When the patient is started on labetalol HCl tablets, following adequate control of blood pressure with labetalol HCl injection, appropriate directions for titration of dosage should be provided (see DOSAGE AND ADMINISTRATION).

LABORATORY TESTS

Injection

Routine laboratory tests are ordinarily not required before or after IV labetalol HCl. In patients with concomitant illnesses, such as impaired renal function, appropriate tests should be done to monitor these conditions.

Tablets

As with any new drug given over prolonged periods, laboratory parameters should be observed over regular intervals. In patients with concomitant illnesses, such as impaired renal function, appropriate tests should be done to monitor these conditions.

DRUG/LABORATORY TEST INTERACTIONS

The presence of labetalol metabolites in the urine may result in falsely elevated levels of urinary catecholamines, metanephrine, normetanephrine, and vanillylmandelic acid when measured by fluorimetric or photometric methods. In screening patients suspected of having a pheochromocytoma and being treated with labetalol HCl, a specific method, such as a high performance liquid chromatographic assay with solid phase extraction (*e.g., J Chromatogr* 385:241, 1987) should be employed in determining levels of catecholamines.

Labetalol HCl has also been reported to produce a false-positive test for amphetamine when screening urine for the presence of drugs using the commercially available assay methods Toxi-Lab A (thin-layer chromatographic assay) and Emit-d.a.u. (radioenzymatic assay). When patients being treated with labetalol HCl have a positive urine test for amphetamine using these techniques, confirmation should be made by using more specific methods, such as a gas chromatographic-mass spectrometer technique.

CARCINOGENESIS, MUTAGENESIS, AND IMPAIRMENT OF FERTILITY

Long-term oral dosing studies with labetalol HCl for 18 months in mice and for 2 years in rats showed no evidence of carcinogenesis. Studies with labetalol HCl using dominant lethal assays in rats and mice, and exposing microorganisms according to modified Ames tests, showed no evidence of mutagenesis.

PREGNANCY CATEGORY C

Teratogenic Effects

Teratogenic studies have been performed with labetalol HCl in rats and rabbits at oral doses up to approximately 6 and 4 times the maximum recommended human dose (MRHD), re-

L

spectively. No reproducible evidence of fetal malformations was observed. Increased fetal resorptions were seen in both species at doses approximating the MRHD. A teratology study performed with labetalol HCl in rabbits at IV doses up to 1.7 times the MRHD revealed no evidence of drug- related harm to the fetus. There are no adequate and well-controlled studies in pregnant women. Labetalol HCl should be used during pregnancy only if the potential benefit justifies the potential risk to the fetus.

Nonteratogenic Effects

Hypotension, bradycardia, hypoglycemia, and respiratory depression have been reported in infants of mothers who were treated with labetalol HCl for hypertension during pregnancy. Oral administration of labetalol to rats during late gestation through weaning at doses of 2-4 times the MRHD caused a decrease in neonatal survival.

LABOR AND DELIVERY

Labetalol HCl given to pregnant women with hypertension did not appear to affect the usual course of labor and delivery.

NURSING MOTHERS

Small amounts of labetalol (approximately 0.004% of the maternal dose) are excreted in human milk. Caution should be exercised when labetalol HCl injection or tablets are administered to a nursing woman.

PEDIATRIC USE

Safety and effectiveness in children have not been established.

GERIATRIC USE

Tablets

As in the general population, some elderly patients (60 years of age and older) have experienced orthostatic hypotension, dizziness, or lightheadedness during treatment with labetalol. Because elderly patients are generally more likely than younger patients to experience orthostatic symptoms, they should be cautioned about the possibility of such side effects during treatement with labetalol.

DRUG INTERACTIONS

In one survey, 2.3% of patients taking labetalol HCl orally in combination with tricyclic antidepressants experienced tremor, as compared to 0.7% reported to occur with labetalol HCl alone. The contribution of each of the treatments to this adverse reaction is unknown but the possibility of a drug interaction cannot be excluded.

Drugs possessing beta-blocking properties can blunt the bronchodilator effect of beta-receptor agonist drugs in patients with bronchospasm; therefore, doses greater than the normal anti-asthmatic dose of beta-agonist bronchodilator drugs may be required.

Cimetidine has been shown to increase the bioavailability of labetalol HCl administered orally. Since this could be explained either by enhanced absorption or by an alteration of hepatic metabolism of labetalol HCl, special care should be used in establishing the dose required for blood pressure control in such patients.

Synergism has been shown between halothane anesthesia and intravenously administered labetalol HCl. During controlled hypotensive anesthesia using labetalol HCl in association with halothane, high concentrations (3% or above) of halothane should not be used because the degree of hypotension will be increased and because of the possibility of a large reduction in cardiac output and an increase in central venous pressure. The anesthesiologist should be informed when a patient is receiving labetalol HCl.

Labetalol HCl blunts the reflex tachycardia produced by nitroglycerin without preventing its hypotensive effect. If labetalol HCl is used with nitroglycerin in patients with angina pectoris, additional antihypertensive effects may occur.

Care should be taken if labetalol HCl is used concomitantly with calcium antagonists of the verapamil type.

Risk of Anaphylactic Reaction: While taking beta-blockers, patients with a history of severe anaphylactic reactions to a variety of allergens may be more reactive to repeated challenge, either accidental, diagnostic, or therapeutic. Such patients may be unresponsive to the usual doses of epinephrine used to treat allergic reaction.

INJECTION

Since labetalol HCl injection may be administered to patients already being treated with other medications, including other antihypertensive agents, careful monitoring of these patients is necessary to detect and treat promptly any undesired effect from concomitant administration.

ADVERSE REACTIONS

INJECTION

Labetalol HCl injection is usually well tolerated. Most adverse effects have been mild and transient and, in controlled trials involving 92 patients, did not require labetalol HCl withdrawal. Symptomatic postural hypotension (incidence, 58%) is likely to occur if patients are tilted or allowed to assume the upright position within 3 hours of receiving labetalol HCl injection. Moderate hypotension occurred in 1 of 100 patients while supine. Increased sweating was noted in 4 of 100 patients, and flushing occurred in 1 of 100 patients.

The following also were reported with labetalol HCl injection with the incidence per 100 patients as noted:

Cardiovascular System: Ventricular arrhythmia in 1.

Central and Peripheral Nervous Systems: Dizziness in 9; tingling of the scalp/skin in 7; hypoesthesia (numbness) and vertigo in 1 each.

Gastrointestinal System: Nausea in 13; vomiting in 4; dyspepsia and taste distortion in 1 each.

Metabolic Disorders: Transient increases in blood urea nitrogen and serum creatinine levels occurred in 8 of 100 patients; these were associated with drops in blood pressure, generally in patients with prior renal insufficiency.

Psychiatric Disorders: Somnolence/yawning in 3.

Respiratory System: Wheezing in 1.

Skin: Pruritus in 1.

The incidence of adverse reactions depends upon the dose of labetalol HCl. The largest experience is with oral labetalol HCl (see labetalol HCl tablet information for details).

TABLETS

Most adverse effects are mild and transient and occur early in the course of treatment. In controlled clinical trials of 3-4 months duration, discontinuation of labetalol HCl tablets due to one or more adverse effects was required in 7% of all patients. In these same trials, other agents with solely beta-blocking activity used in the control groups led to discontinutation in 8-10% of patients, and a centrally acting alpha-agonist in 30% of patients.

The incidence rates of adverse reactions listed in TABLE 1 were derived from multicenter, controlled clinical trials comparing labetalol HCl, placebo, metoprolol, and propranolol over treatment periods of 3 and 4 months. Where the frequency of adverse effects for labetalol HCl and placebo is similar, causal relationship is uncertain. The rates are based on adverse reactions considered probably drug related by the investigator. If all reports are considered, the rates are somewhat higher (*e.g.,* dizziness 20%, nausea 14%, fatigue 11%), but the overall conclusions are unchanged.

TABLE 1

	Labetalol HCl (n=227)	Placebo (n=98)	Propranolol (n=84)	Metoprolol (n=49)
Body as a Whole				
Fatigue	5%	0%	12%	12%
Asthenia	1%	1%	1%	0%
Headache	2%	1%	1%	2%
Gastrointestinal				
Nausea	6%	1%	1%	2%
Vomiting	<1%	0%	0%	0%
Dyspepsia	3%	1%	1%	0%
Abdominal pain	0%	0%	1%	2%
Diarrhea	<1%	0%	2%	0%
Taste distortion	1%	0%	0%	0%
Central and Peripheral Nervous Systems				
Dizziness	11%	3%	4%	4%
Paresthesia	<1%	0%	0%	0%
Drowsiness	<1%	2%	2%	2%
Autonomic Nervous System				
Nasal stuffiness	3%	0%	0%	0%
Ejaculation failure	2%	0%	0%	0%
Impotence	1%	0%	1%	3%
Increased sweating	<1%	0%	0%	0%
Cardiovascular				
Edema	1%	0%	0%	0%
Postural hypotension	1%	0%	0%	0%
Bradycardia	0%	0%	5%	12%
Respiratory				
Dyspnea	2%	0%	1%	2%
Skin				
Rash	1%	0%	0%	0%
Special Senses				
Vision abnormality	1%	0%	0%	0%
Vertigo	2%	1%	0%	0%

The adverse effects were reported spontaneously and are representative of the incidence of adverse effects that may be observed in a properly selected hypertensive patient population, *i.e.,* a group excluding patients with bronchospastic disease, overt congestive heart failure, or other contraindications to beta-blocker therapy.

Clinical trials also included studies utilizing daily doses up to 2400 mg in more severely hypertensive patients. Certain of the side effects increased with increasing dose, as shown in TABLE 2 which depicts the entire US therapeutic trials data base for adverse reactions that are clearly or possibly drug related.

TABLE 2

	Labetolol HCl Daily Dose (mg)								
	200	300	400	600	800	900	1200	1600	2400
n=	522	181	606	608	503	117	411	242	175
Dizziness	2%	3%	3%	3%	5%	1%	9%	13%	16%
Fatigue	2%	1%	4%	4%	5%	3%	7%	6%	10%
Nausea	<1%	0%	1%	2%	4%	0%	7%	11%	19%
Vomiting	0%	0%	<1%	<1%	<1%	0%	1%	2%	3%
Dyspepsia	1%	0%	2%	1%	1%	0%	2%	2%	4%
Paresthesia	2%	0%	2%	2%	1%	1%	2%	5%	5%
Nasal stuffiness	1%	1%	2%	2%	2%	2%	4%	5%	6%
Ejaculation failure	0%	2%	1%	2%	3%	0%	4%	3%	5%
Impotence	1%	1%	1%	1%	2%	4%	3%	4%	3%
Edema	1%	0%	1%	1%	1%	0%	1%	2%	2%

In addition, a number of the less common adverse events have been reported:

Body as a Whole: Fever.

Cardiovascular: Hypotension, and rarely, syncope, bradycardia, heart block.

Central and Peripheral Nervous Systems: Paresthesia, most frequently described as scalp tingling. In most cases, it was mild and transient and usually occurred at the beginning of treatment.

Collagen Disorders: Systemic lupus erythematosus, positive antinuclear factor.

Eyes: Dry eyes.

Immunological System: Antimitochondrial antibodies.

Liver and Biliary System: Hepatic necrosis, hepatitis, cholestatic jaundice, elevated liver function tests.

Musculoskeletal System: Muscle cramps, toxic myopathy.

Respiratory System: Bronchospasm.

Skin and Appendages: Rashes of various types, such as generalized maculopapular, lichenoid, urticarial, bullous lichen planus, psoriaform, facial erythema, Peyronie's disease, reversible alopecia.

Urinary System: Difficulty in micturition, including acute urinary bladder retention.

Hypersensitivity: Rare reports of hypersensitivity (*e.g.,* rash, urticaria, pruritus, angioedema, dyspnea) and anaphylactoid reactions.

Following approval for marketing in the United Kingdom, a monitored release survey involving approximately 6800 patients was conducted for further safety and efficacy evaluation of this product. Results of this survey indicate that the type, severity, and incidence of adverse effects were comparable to those cited above.

Potential Adverse Effects

In addition, other adverse effects not listed above have been reported with other beta-adrenergic blocking agents.

Central Nervous System: Reversible mental depression progressing to catatonia, an acute reversible syndrome characterized by disorientation for time and place, short-term memory loss, emotional lability, slightly cloudy sensorium, and decreased performance on psychometrics.

Cardiovascular: Intensification of AV block (see CONTRAINDICATIONS).

Allergic: Fever combined with aching and sore throat, laryngospasm, respiratory distress.

Hematologic: Agranulocytosis, thrombocytopenic or nonthrombocytopenic purpura.

Gastrointestinal: Mesenteric artery thrombosis, ischemic colitis.

The oculomucocutaneous syndrome associated with the beta-blocker practolol has not been reported with labetalol HCl.

Clinical Laboratory Tests

There have been reversible increases of serum transaminases in 4% of patients treated with labetalol HCl and tested, and more rarely, reversible increases in blood urea.

DOSAGE AND ADMINISTRATION

INJECTION

Labetalol HCl injection is intended for IV use in hospitalized patients. DOSAGE MUST BE INDIVIDUALIZED depending upon the severity of hypertension and the response of the patient during dosing.

Patients should always be kept in a supine position during the period of IV drug administration. A substantial fall in blood pressure on standing should be expected in these patients. The patient's ability to tolerate an upright position should be established before permitting any ambulation, such as using toilet facilities.

Either of two methods of administration of labetalol HCl injection may be used: a) repeated IV injection, b) slow continuous infusion.

Repeated Intravenous Injection

Initially, labetalol HCl injection should be given in a 20 mg dose (which corresponds to 0.25 mg/kg for an 80 kg patient) by slow IV injection over a 2 minute period.

Immediately before the injection and at 5 and 10 minutes after injection, supine blood pressure should be measured to evaluate response. Additional injections of 40 or 80 mg can be given at 10 minute intervals until a desired supine blood pressure is achieved or a total of 300 mg labetalol HCl has been injected. The maximum effect usually occurs within 5 minutes of each injection.

Slow Continuous Infusion

Labetalol HCl injection is prepared for continuous IV infusion by diluting the vial contents with commonly used IV fluids (see Compatibility With Commonly Used Intravenous Fluids). Examples of methods of preparing the infusion solution are:

Add 40 ml labetalol HCl injection to 160 ml of a commonly used IV fluid such that the resultant 200 ml of solution contains 200 mg of labetalol HCl, 1 mg/ml. The diluted solution should be administered at a rate of 2 ml/min to deliver 2 mg/min.

Alternatively, add 40 ml of labetalol HCl injection to 250 ml of a commonly used IV fluid. The resultant solution will contain 200 mg of labetalol HCl, approximately 2 mg/3 ml. The diluted solution should be administered at a rate of 3 ml/min to deliver approximately 2 mg/min.

The rate of infusion of the diluted solution may be adjusted according to the blood pressure response, at the discretion of the physician. To facilitate a desired rate of infusion, the diluted solution can be infused using a controlled administration mechanism, *e.g.,* graduated burette or mechanically driven infusion pump.

Since the half-life of labetalol is 5-8 hours, steady-state blood levels (in the face of a constant rate of infusion) would not be reached during the usual infusion time period. The infusion should be continued until a satisfactory response is obtained and should then be stopped and oral labetalol HCl started (see Initiation of Dosing With Labetalol HCl Tablets). The effective IV dose is usually in the range of 50-200 mg. A total dose of up to 300 mg may be required in some patients.

Blood Pressure Monitoring

The blood pressure should be monitored during and after completion of the infusion or IV injections. Rapid or excessive falls in either systolic or diastolic blood pressure during IV treatment should be avoided. In patients with excessive systolic hypertension, the decrease in systolic pressure should be used as an indicator of effectiveness in addition to the response of the diastolic pressure.

Initiation of Dosing With Labetalol HCl Tablets

Subsequent oral dosing with labetalol HCl tablets should begin when it has been established that the supine diastolic blood pressure has begun to rise. The recommended initial dose is 200 mg, followed in 6-12 hours by an additional dose of 200 or 400 mg, depending on the blood pressure response. Thereafter, **inpatient titration with labetalol HCl tablets** may proceed as shown in TABLE 3.

TABLE 3 *Inpatient Titration Instructions*

Regimen	Daily Dose*
200 mg bid	400 mg
400 mg bid	800 mg
800 mg bid	1600 mg
1200 mg bid	2400 mg

* If needed, the total daily dose may be given in 3 divided doses.

The dosage of labetalol HCl tablets used in the hospital may be increased at 1 day intervals to achieve the desired blood pressure reduction.

For subsequent outpatient titration or maintenance dosing see the labetalol HCl tablets section for additional recommendations.

Compatibility With Commonly Used Intravenous Fluids

Parenteral drug products should be inspected visually for particulate matter and discoloration prior to administration, whenever solution and container permit.

Labetalol HCl injection was tested for compatibility with commonly used IV fluids at final concentrations of 1.25-3.75 mg labetalol HCl per ml of the mixture. Labetalol HCl injection was found to be compatible with and stable (for 24 hours refrigerated or at room temperature) in mixtures with the following solutions: Ringers injection, lactated Ringers injection, 5% dextrose and Ringers injection, 5% lactated Ringers and 5% dextrose injection, 5% dextrose injection, 0.9% sodium chloride injection, 5% dextrose and 0.2% sodium chloride injection, 2.5% dextrose and 0.45% sodium chloride injection, 5% dextrose and 0.9% sodium chloride injection, 5% dextrose and 0.33% sodium chloride injection.

Labetalol HCl injection was NOT compatible with 5% sodium bicarbonate injection. Care should be taken when administering alkaline drugs, including furosemide, in combination with labetalol. Compatibility should be assured prior to administering these drugs together.

TABLETS

DOSAGE MUST BE INDIVIDUALIZED. The recommended *initial* dose is 100 mg *twice* daily whether used alone or added to a diuretic regimen. After 2 or 3 days, using standing blood pressure as an indicator, dosage may be titrated in increments of 100 mg bid every 2 or 3 days. The usual *maintenance* dosage of labetalol HCl is between 200 and 400 mg *twice* daily.

Since the full antihypertensive effect of labetalol HCl is usually seen within the first 1-3 hours of the initial dose or dose increment, the assurance of a lack of an exaggerated hypotensive response can be clinically established in the office setting. The antihypertensive effects of continued dosing can be measured at subsequent visits, approximately 12 hours after a dose, to determine whether future titration is necessary.

Patients with severe hypertension may require from 1200-2400 mg per day, with or without thiazide diuretics. Should side effects (principally nausea or dizziness) occur with these doses administered twice daily, the same total daily dose administered 3 times daily may improve tolerability and facilitate further titration. Titration increments should not exceed 200 mg twice daily.

When a diuretic is added, an additive antihypertensive effect can be expected. In some cases this may necessitate a labetalol HCl dosage adjustment. As with most antihypertensive drugs, optimal dosages of labetalol HCl tablets are usually lower in patients also receiving a diuretic.

When transferring patients from other antihypertensive drugs, labetalol HCl tablets should be introduced as recommended and the dosage of the existing therapy progressively decreased.

Elderly Patients

As in the general patient population, labetalol therapy may be initiated at 100 mg twice daily and titrated upwards in increments of 100 mg bid as required for control of blood pressure. Since some elderly patients eliminate labetalol more slowly, however, adequate control of blood pressure may be achieved at a lower maintenace dosage compared to the general population. The majority of elderly patients will require between 100 and 200 mg bid.

HOW SUPPLIED

INJECTION

Trandate injection, 5 mg/ml, is supplied in 20 ml (100 mg) and 40 ml (200 mg) vials.

Storage: Store between 2-30°C (36-86°F). Do not freeze. Protect from light.

TABLETS

Trandate tablets are available in:

100 mg: Light orange, round, scored, film-coated tablets engraved on one side with "TRANDATE 100".

200 mg: White, round, scored, film-coated tablets engraved on one side with "TRANDATE 200".

300 mg: Peach, round, scored, film-coated tablets engraved on one side with "TRANDATE 300".

Storage: Store between 2-30°C (36-86°F). Labetalol HCl tablets in the unit-dose boxes should be protected from excessive moisture.

PRODUCT LISTING - RATED THERAPEUTICALLY EQUIVALENT

Solution - Intravenous - 5 mg/ml

4 ml	$19.57	NORMODYNE, Schering Corporation	00085-0362-08
4 ml x 10	$47.62	GENERIC, Abbott Pharmaceutical	00074-2339-05
4 ml x 10	$48.21	GENERIC, Abbott Pharmaceutical	00074-2339-34
4 ml x 10	$48.81	GENERIC, Abbott Pharmaceutical	00074-2339-11
4 ml x 10	$58.78	GENERIC, Abbott Pharmaceutical	00074-2267-05
4 ml x 10	$58.78	GENERIC, Abbott Pharmaceutical	00074-2267-11
4 ml x 10	$58.78	GENERIC, Abbott Pharmaceutical	00074-2267-34
8 ml	$29.40	NORMODYNE, Schering Corporation	00085-0362-09

Size	Price	Description	NDC
20 ml	$5.28	GENERIC, Baxter Pharmaceutical Products, Inc	10019-0210-02
20 ml	$6.12	GENERIC, Abbott Pharmaceutical	00074-2267-20
20 ml	$18.75	TRANDATE, Faro Pharmaceuticals Inc	60976-0350-58
20 ml	$34.46	TRANDATE, Prometheus Inc	65483-0355-02
20 ml	$45.35	NORMODYNE, Schering Corporation	00085-0362-07
20 ml x 10	$12.50	GENERIC, Bedford Laboratories	55390-0130-20
20 ml x 10	$350.00	GENERIC, Faulding Pharmaceutical Company	61703-0233-22
40 ml	$10.56	GENERIC, Baxter Pharmaceutical Products, Inc	10019-0210-04
40 ml	$12.25	GENERIC, Abbott Pharmaceutical	00074-2267-54
40 ml	$37.50	TRANDATE, Faro Pharmaceuticals Inc	60976-0350-57
40 ml	$66.76	TRANDATE, Prometheus Inc	65483-0355-04
40 ml	$87.85	NORMODYNE, Schering Corporation	00085-0362-06
40 ml x 10	$24.00	GENERIC, Bedford Laboratories	55390-0130-40
40 ml x 10	$650.00	GENERIC, Faulding Pharmaceutical Company	61703-0233-41
Tablet - Oral - 100 mg			
60's	$38.82	TRANDATE, Physicians Total Care	54868-2864-01
100's	$31.41	FEDERAL UPPER LIMIT, H.C.F.A. F F P	99999-1613-01
100's	$48.01	GENERIC, United Research Laboratories, Inc.	00677-1701-01
100's	$48.01	GENERIC, Mutual Pharmaceutical Co Inc	53489-0354-01
100's	$48.20	GENERIC, Udl Laboratories Inc	51079-0928-20
100's	$50.28	GENERIC, Eon Labs Manufacturing Inc	00185-0010-01
100's	$50.28	GENERIC, Watson Laboratories Inc	52544-0605-01
100's	$63.34	TRANDATE, Physicians Total Care	54868-2864-00
100's	$63.42	TRANDATE, Prometheus Inc	65483-0391-11
100's	$65.06	NORMODYNE, Schering Corporation	00085-0244-04
100's	$66.32	NORMODYNE, Schering Corporation	00085-0244-08
100's	$66.59	TRANDATE, Faro Pharmaceuticals Inc	60976-0346-47
100's	$70.88	TRANDATE, Faro Pharmaceuticals Inc	60976-0346-43
100's	$70.88	TRANDATE, Prometheus Inc	65483-0391-10
Tablet - Oral - 200 mg			
30's	$25.38	NORMODYNE, Allscripts Pharmaceutical Company	54569-0590-00
60's	$56.47	NORMODYNE, Physicians Total Care	54868-1004-01
100's	$44.37	FEDERAL UPPER LIMIT, H.C.F.A. F F P	99999-1613-03
100's	$68.10	GENERIC, United Research Laboratories, Inc.	00677-1702-01
100's	$68.10	GENERIC, Mutual Pharmaceutical Co Inc	53489-0355-01
100's	$68.10	GENERIC, Warrick Pharmaceuticals Corporation	59930-1636-01
100's	$68.20	GENERIC, Udl Laboratories Inc	51079-0929-20
100's	$71.07	GENERIC, Warrick Pharmaceuticals Corporation	59930-1636-04
100's	$71.33	GENERIC, Eon Labs Manufacturing Inc	00185-0117-01
100's	$71.33	GENERIC, Watson Laboratories Inc	00591-0606-01
100's	$71.33	GENERIC, Watson Laboratories Inc	52544-0606-01
100's	$75.67	TRANDATE, Glaxo Wellcome	00173-0347-43
100's	$88.39	TRANDATE, Prometheus Inc	65483-0392-22
100's	$88.60	NORMODYNE, Schering Corporation	00085-0752-04
100's	$89.77	NORMODYNE, Schering Corporation	00085-0752-08
100's	$100.06	TRANDATE, Faro Pharmaceuticals Inc	60976-0347-43
100's	$100.06	TRANDATE, Prometheus Inc	65483-0392-10
100's	$104.41	TRANDATE, Faro Pharmaceuticals Inc	60976-0347-47
Tablet - Oral - 300 mg			
100's	$59.19	FEDERAL UPPER LIMIT, H.C.F.A. F F P	99999-1613-05
100's	$90.61	GENERIC, Mutual/United Research Laboratories	00677-1703-01
100's	$90.61	GENERIC, Mutual Pharmaceutical Co Inc	53489-0356-01
100's	$90.61	GENERIC, Warrick Pharmaceuticals Corporation	59930-1653-01
100's	$92.89	GENERIC, Ivax Corporation	00172-4366-60
100's	$93.59	GENERIC, Warrick Pharmaceuticals Corporation	59930-1653-03
100's	$94.89	GENERIC, Eon Labs Manufacturing Inc	00185-0118-01
100's	$94.89	GENERIC, Watson Laboratories Inc	00591-0607-01
100's	$94.89	GENERIC, Watson Laboratories Inc	52544-0607-01
100's	$107.63	NORMODYNE, Schering Corporation	00085-0438-06
100's	$116.40	TRANDATE, Prometheus Inc	65483-0393-33
100's	$122.78	NORMODYNE, Schering Corporation	00085-0438-03
100's	$123.23	TRANDATE, Prometheus Inc	65483-0393-10
100's	$127.31	TRANDATE, Prometheus Inc	60676-0348-47
100's	$127.31	TRANDATE, Faro Pharmaceuticals Inc	60976-0348-47
100's	$133.10	TRANDATE, Faro Pharmaceuticals Inc	60976-0348-43

Lactulose *(001621)*

Categories: Constipation; Encephalopathy, hepatic; Pregnancy Category B; FDA Approved 1976 Mar

Drug Classes: Gastrointestinals; Laxatives

Brand Names: C-Cephulose; **Cephulac**; Cholac; Constilac; Constulose; Duphalac; Enulose; Evalose; Generlac; Heptalac; Laxilose

Foreign Brand Availability: Actilax (Australia); Alpha-Lactulose (New-Zealand); Avilac (Israel); Bifinorma (Germany); Bifinorma Granulat (Germany); Bifiteral (Belgium; Germany); Danilax (Hong-Kong); Dhactulose (Singapore); Dia-Colon (Italy); Genlac (Australia); Hepalac (Thailand); Lacson (South-Africa); Lactocur (Germany); Lactulax (Indonesia; Israel; Mexico; Peru); Lactulen (Colombia); Lactuverlan (Germany); Laevolac (Austria; Czech-Republic; Hungary; Israel; Italy; Portugal; Switzerland); Laxette (South-Africa); Laximed (Germany); Levolac (Finland; Norway); Lipebin (Bahrain; Cyprus; Egypt; Iran; Iraq; Israel; Jordan; Kuwait; Lebanon; Libya; Oman; Peru; Qatar; Republic-of-Yemen; Saudi-Arabia; Syria; United-Arab-Emirates); Livo Luk (India); Monilac (Japan; Korea); Normolax (Bahrain; Cyprus; Egypt; Iran; Iraq; Jordan; Kuwait; Lebanon; Libya; Oman; Qatar; Republic-of-Yemen; Saudi-Arabia; Syria; United-Arab-Emirates); Pralax (Indonesia); Regulact (Mexico); Sirolax (Israel)

DESCRIPTION

Note: The trade name has been used throughout this monograph for clarity.

CEPHULAC

Cephulac (lactulose) is a synthetic disaccharide in solution form for oral or rectal administration. Cephulac is a colonic acidifier for treatment and prevention of portal-systemic encephalopathy.

Each 15 ml of Cephulac contains: 10 g lactulose (and less than 2.2 g galactose, less than 1.2 g lactose, and 1.2 g or less of other sugars). Also contains FD&C blue no. 1, FD&C yellow no. 6, water, and flavoring. A minimal quantity of sodium hydroxide is used to adjust pH when necessary.

The chemical name for lactulose is 4-*O*-β-D-galactopyranosyl-D-fructofuranose.

The molecular weight is 342.30. It is freely soluble in water.

CHRONULAC

Chronulac (lactulose) is a synthetic disaccharide in solution form for oral administration. Chronulac is a colonic acidifier that promotes laxation. The pH range is 3.0 to 7.0.

Each 15 ml of Chronulac contains: 10 g lactulose (and less than 2.2 g galactose, less than 1.2 g lactose, and 1.2 g or less of other sugars). Also contains FD&C blue no. 1, FD&C yellow no. 6, water, and flavoring. A minimal quantity of sodium hydroxide is used to adjust pH when necessary.

The chemical name for lactulose is 4-*O*-β-D-galactopyranosyl-D-fructofuranose.

The molecular weight is 342.30. It is freely soluble in water.

STORAGE

Store at room temperature, 15-30°C (59-86°F).

Under recommended storage conditions, a normal darkening of color may occur. Such darkening is characteristic of sugar solutions and does not affect therapeutic action. Prolonged exposure to temperatures above 30°C (86°F) or to direct light may cause extreme darkening and turbidity which may be pharmaceutically objectionable. If this condition develops, do not use.

Prolonged exposure to freezing temperatures may cause change to a semisolid, too viscous to pour. Viscosity will return to normal upon warming to room temperature.

CLINICAL PHARMACOLOGY

CEPHULAC

Lactulose causes a decrease in blood ammonia concentration and reduces the degree of portalsystemic encephalopathy. These actions are considered to be results of the following:

- Bacterial degradation of lactulose in the colon acidifies the colonic contents.
- This acidification of colonic contents results in the retention of ammonia in the colon as the ammonium ion. Since the colonic contents are then more acid than the blood, ammonia can be expected to migrate from the blood into the colon to form the ammonium ion.
- The acid colonic contents convert NH_3 to the ammonium ion $(NH_4)^+$, trapping it and preventing its absorption.
- The laxative action of the metabolites of lactulose then expels the trapped ammonium ion from the colon.

Experimental data indicate that lactulose is poorly absorbed. Lactulose given orally to man and experimental animals resulted in only small amounts reaching the blood. Urinary excretion has been determined to be 3% or less and is essentially complete within 24 hours.

When incubated with extracts of human small intestinal mucosa, lactulose was not hydrolyzed during a 24 hour period and did not inhibit the activity of these extracts on lactose. Lactulose reaches the colon essentially unchanged. There it is metabolized by bacteria with the formation of low molecular weight acids that acidify the colon contents.

CHRONULAC

Chronulac is poorly absorbed from the gastrointestinal tract and no enzyme capable of hydrolysis of this disaccharide is present in human gastrointestinal tissue. As a result, oral doses of Chronulac reach the colon virtually unchanged. In the colon, Chronulac is broken down primarily to lactic acid, and also to small amounts of formic and acetic acids, by the action of colonic bacteria, which results in an increase in osmotic pressure and slight acidification of the colonic contents. This in turn causes an increase in stool water content and softens the stool.

Since Chronulac does not exert its effect until it reaches the colon, and since transit time through the colon may be slow, 24 to 48 hours may be required to produce the desired bowel movement.

Chronulac given orally to man and experimental animals resulted in only small amounts reaching the blood. Urinary excretion has been determined to be 3% or less and is essentially complete within 24 hours.

INDICATIONS AND USAGE

CEPHULAC

For the prevention and treatment of portal-systemic encephalopathy, including the stages of hepatic pre-coma and coma.

Controlled studies have shown that lactulose solution therapy reduces the blood ammonia levels by 25-50%; this is generally paralleled by an improvement in the patients' mental state and by an improvement in EEG patterns. The clinical response has been observed in about 75% of patients, which is at least as satisfactory as that resulting from neomycin therapy. An increase in patients' protein tolerance is also frequently observed with lactulose therapy. In the treatment of chronic portal-systemic encephalopathy, Cephulac has been given for over 2 years in controlled studies.

CHRONULAC

For the treatment of constipation. In patients with a history of chronic constipation, Chronulac therapy increases the number of bowel movements per day and the number of days on which bowel movements can occur.

NON-FDA APPROVED INDICATIONS

While not FDA approved indications, lactulose is also used to promote normal bowel movements following hemorrhoidectomy or barium studies.

CONTRAINDICATIONS

Since Cephulac and Chronulac contain galactose (less than 2.2 g/15 ml), it is contraindicated in patients who require a low galactose diet.

WARNINGS

A theoretical hazard may exist for patients being treated with lactulose solution who may be required to undergo electrocautery procedures during proctoscopy or colonoscopy. Accumulation of H_2 gas in significant concentration in the presence of an electrical spark may result in an explosive reaction. Although this complication has not been reported with lactulose, patients on lactulose therapy undergoing such procedures should have a thorough bowel cleansing with a nonfermentable solution. Insufflation of CO_2 as an additional safeguard may be pursued but is considered to be a redundant measure.

PRECAUTIONS

GENERAL

Since Cephulac and Chronulac contains galactose (less than 2.2 g/15 ml) and lactose (less than 1.2 g/15 ml), it should be used with caution in diabetics.

Cephulac

In the overall management of portal-systemic encephalopathy, it should be recognized that there is serious underlying liver disease with complications such as electrolyte disturbance (*e.g.*, hypokalemia) for which other specific therapy may be required.

INFORMATION FOR THE PATIENT

Chronulac

In the event that an unusual diarrheal condition occurs, contact your physician.

LABORATORY TESTS

Infants receiving lactulose may develop hyponatremia and dehydration.

Chronulac

Elderly, debilitated patients who receive Chronulac for more than 6 months should have serum electrolytes (potassium, chloride, carbon dioxide) measured periodically.

CARCINOGENESIS, MUTAGENESIS, AND IMPAIRMENT OF FERTILITY

There are no known human data on long-term potential for carcinogenicity, mutagenicity, or impairment of fertility.

There are no known animal data on long-term potential for mutagenicity.

Administration of lactulose solution in the diet of mice for 18 months in concentrations of 3 and 10% (V/W) did not produce any evidence of carcinogenicity.

In studies in mice, rats, and rabbits, doses of lactulose solution up to 6 or 12 ml/kg/day produced no deleterious effects on breeding, conception, or parturition.

PREGNANCY, TERATOGENIC EFFECTS, PREGNANCY CATEGORY B

Reproduction studies have been performed in mice, rats, and rabbits at doses up to 2 or 4 times the usual human oral dose (Cephulac) and 3 or 6 times the usual human oral dose (Chronulac) and have revealed no evidence of impaired fertility or harm to the fetus due to Cephulac. There are, however, no adequate and well-controlled studies in pregnant women. Because animal reproduction studies are not always predictive of human response, this drug should be used during pregnancy only if clearly needed.

NURSING MOTHERS

It is not known whether this drug is excreted in human milk. Because many drugs are excreted in human milk, caution should be exercised when Cephulac is administered to a nursing woman.

PEDIATRIC USE

Cephulac

Very little information on the use of lactulose in young children and adolescents has been recorded. (See DOSAGE AND ADMINISTRATION.)

Chronulac

Safety and effectiveness in pediatric patients have not been established.

DRUG INTERACTIONS

CEPHULAC

There have been conflicting reports about the concomitant use of neomycin and lactulose solution. Theoretically, the elimination of certain colonic bacteria by neomycin and possibly other anti-infective agents may interfere with the desired degradation of lactulose and thus prevent the acidification of colonic contents. Thus the status of the lactulose-treated patient should be closely monitored in the event of concomitant oral anti-infective therapy.

Results of preliminary studies in humans and rats suggest that nonabsorbable antacids given concurrently with lactulose may inhibit the desired lactulose-induced drop in colonic pH. Therefore, a possible lack of desired effect of treatment should be taken into consideration before such drugs are given concomitantly with Cephulac.

Other laxatives should not be used, especially during the initial phase of therapy for portal-systemic encephalopathy, because the loose stools resulting from their use may falsely suggest that adequate Cephulac dosage has been achieved.

CHRONULAC

Results of preliminary studies in humans and rats suggest that nonabsorbable antacids given concurrently with lactulose may inhibit the desired lactulose-induced drop in colonic pH. therefore, a possible lack of desired effect of treatment should be taken into consideration before such drugs are given concomitantly with Chronulac.

ADVERSE REACTIONS

Precise frequency data are not available.

Excessive dosage can lead to diarrhea with potential complications such as loss of fluids, hypokalemia, and hypernatremia. Nausea and vomiting have been reported.

CEPHULAC

Cephulac may produce gaseous distention with flatulence or belching and abdominal discomfort such as cramping in about 20% of patients.

CHRONULAC

Initial dosing of Chronulac may produce flatulence and intestinal cramps, which are usually transient.

DOSAGE AND ADMINISTRATION

ORAL CEPHULAC

Adult

The usual adult, oral dosage is 2-3 tablespoonfuls (30-45 ml, containing 2-30 g of lactulose) 3 or 4 times daily. The dosage may be adjusted every day or two to produce 2 or 3 soft stools daily.

Hourly doses of 30-45 ml of Cephulac may be used to induce the rapid laxation indicated in the initial phase of the therapy of portal-systemic encephalopathy. When the laxative effect has been achieved, the dose of Cephulac may then be reduced to the recommended daily dose. Improvement in the patient's condition may occur within 24 hours but may not begin before 48 hours or even later.

Continuous long-term therapy is indicated to lessen the severity and prevent the recurrence of portal-systemic encephalopathy. The dose of Cephulac for this purpose is the same as the recommended daily dose.

Pediatric

Very little information on the use of lactulose in pediatric patients has been recorded. As with adults, the subjective goal in proper treatment is to produce 2-3 soft stools daily. On the basis of information available, the recommended initial daily oral dose in infants is 2.5 to 10 ml in divided doses. For older children and adolescents, the total daily dose is 40-90 ml. If the initial dose causes diarrhea, the dose should be reduced immediately. If diarrhea persists, lactulose should be discontinued.

RECTAL CEPHULAC

When the adult patient is in the impending coma or coma stage of portal-systemic encephalopathy and the danger of aspiration exists, or when the necessary endoscopic or intubation procedures physically interfere with the administration of the recommended oral doses, Cephulac may be given as a retention enema via a rectal balloon catheter. Cleansing enemas containing soapsuds or other alkaline agents should not be used.

Three hundred (300) ml of Cephulac should be mixed with 700 ml of water or physiologic saline and retained for 30-60 minutes. Cephulac enema may be repeated every 4-6 hours. If the enema is inadvertently evacuated too promptly, it may be repeated immediately.

The goal of treatment is reversal of the coma stage in order that the patient may be able to take oral medication. Reversal of coma may take place within 2 hours of the first enema in some patients. Cephulac, given orally in the recommended doses, should be started before Cephulac by enema is stopped entirely.

CHRONULAC

The usual dose is 1-2 tablespoonfuls (15-30 ml, containing 10-20 g of lactulose) daily. The dose may be increased to 60 ml daily if necessary. Twenty-four (24) to 48 hours may be required to produce a normal bowel movement.

Note: Some patients have found that Chronulac may be more acceptable when mixed with fruit juice, water, or milk.

PRODUCT LISTING - RATED THERAPEUTICALLY EQUIVALENT

Syrup - Oral - 10 Gm/15 ml

Size	Price	Manufacturer	NDC
15 ml x 50	$53.94	GENERIC, Xactdose Inc	50962-0032-15
15 ml x 50	$55.11	GENERIC, Mylan Pharmaceuticals Inc	50962-0033-60
15 ml x 100	$150.00	GENERIC, Xactdose Inc	50962-0031-61
30 ml	$2.09	GENERIC, Alra	51641-0224-61
30 ml	$2.09	GENERIC, Alra	51641-0225-61
30 ml x 40	$115.60	GENERIC, Roxane Laboratories Inc	00054-8486-16
30 ml x 50	$75.00	GENERIC, Mylan Pharmaceuticals Inc	50962-0031-60
30 ml x 50	$147.00	GENERIC, Mylan Pharmaceuticals Inc	50962-0034-60
30 ml x 50	$150.00	GENERIC, Alpharma Uspd Makers Of Barre and Nmc	50962-0032-60
30 ml x 100	$119.16	GENERIC, Pharmaceutical Assoc Inc Div Beach Products	00121-0577-30
30 ml x 100	$300.00	GENERIC, Alpharma Uspd Makers Of Barre and Nmc	50962-0032-61
45 ml x 25	$115.16	GENERIC, Roxane Laboratories Inc	00054-8483-11
237 ml	$14.00	GENERIC, Hi-Tech Pharmacal Company Inc	50383-0779-08
240 ml	$13.50	GENERIC, Watson/Schein Pharmaceuticals Inc	00364-2519-76
240 ml	$13.51	GENERIC, Ivax Corporation	00182-6075-44
240 ml	$13.70	GENERIC, Alra	51641-0224-68
240 ml	$13.91	GENERIC, Morton Grove Pharmaceuticals Inc	60432-0037-08
240 ml	$13.95	GENERIC, Major Pharmaceuticals Inc	00904-2117-09
240 ml	$13.97	GENERIC, Geneva Pharmaceuticals	00781-6406-08
240 ml	$14.40	GENERIC, Roxane Laboratories Inc	00054-3486-58
240 ml	$15.48	GENERIC, Pharmaceutical Assoc Inc Div Beach Products	00121-0577-08
240 ml	$16.97	GENERIC, Alra	51641-0225-68
240 ml	$17.23	GENERIC, Copley	38245-0661-19

240 ml	$17.90	GENERIC, Mylan Pharmaceuticals Inc	00378-3331-70
240 ml	$17.90	GENERIC, Mylan Pharmaceuticals Inc	00472-0208-08
240 ml	$18.28	GENERIC, Qualitest Products Inc	00603-1378-56
240 ml	$20.20	GENERIC, Alpharma Uspd Makers Of Barre and Nmc	00472-1358-08
250 ml	$14.40	GENERIC, Apotex Usa Inc	60505-0360-00
473 ml	$34.40	HEPTALAC, Copley	38245-0670-07
473 ml	$36.50	GENERIC, Hi-Tech Pharmacal Company Inc	50383-0795-16
480 ml	$23.95	GENERIC, Alra	51641-0224-76
480 ml	$25.75	GENERIC, Watson/Schein Pharmaceuticals Inc	00364-2347-16
480 ml	$25.85	GENERIC, Morton Grove Pharmaceuticals Inc	60432-0038-16
480 ml	$26.05	GENERIC, Qualitest Products Inc	00603-1648-58
480 ml	$26.35	GENERIC, Mutual/United Research Laboratories	00677-1098-33
480 ml	$30.38	GENERIC, Moore, H.L. Drug Exchange Inc	00839-7196-69
480 ml	$32.45	GENERIC, Major Pharmaceuticals Inc	00904-2115-16
480 ml	$32.95	GENERIC, Alra	51641-0225-76
480 ml	$34.70	GENERIC, Ivax Corporation	00182-6072-40
480 ml	$34.70	GENERIC, Mylan Pharmaceuticals Inc	00378-3331-72
480 ml	$34.70	GENERIC, Alpharma Uspd Makers Of Barre and Nmc	00472-0208-16
480 ml	$36.35	GENERIC, Alpharma Uspd Makers Of Barre and Nmc	00472-1360-16
500 ml	$25.95	GENERIC, Roxane Laboratories Inc	00054-3486-63
500 ml	$32.40	GENERIC, Apotex Usa Inc	60505-0360-01
946 ml	$65.64	GENERIC, Hi-Tech Pharmacal Company Inc	50383-0779-32
960 ml	$48.75	GENERIC, Alra	51641-0224-82
960 ml	$49.95	GENERIC, Morton Grove Pharmaceuticals Inc	60432-0037-32
960 ml	$50.30	GENERIC, Moore, H.L. Drug Exchange Inc	00839-7199-62
960 ml	$51.46	GENERIC, Major Pharmaceuticals Inc	00904-2117-69
960 ml	$54.69	GENERIC, Mylan Pharmaceuticals Inc	00378-3331-74
960 ml	$54.70	GENERIC, Mylan Pharmaceuticals Inc	00472-0208-32
960 ml	$56.99	GENERIC, Ivax Corporation	00182-6075-58
960 ml	$59.78	GENERIC, Copley	38245-0661-13
960 ml	$65.44	GENERIC, Alpharma Uspd Makers Of Barre and Nmc	00472-1358-32
960 ml	$65.89	GENERIC, Alra	51641-0225-82
960 ml	$67.40	GENERIC, Qualitest Products Inc	00603-1378-59
1000 ml	$47.00	GENERIC, Roxane Laboratories Inc	00054-3486-68
1000 ml	$58.00	GENERIC, Apotex Usa Inc	60505-0360-02
1890 ml	$49.27	HEPTALAC, Copley	38245-0670-83
1893 ml	$96.92	GENERIC, Hi-Tech Pharmacal Company Inc	50383-0795-64
1920 ml	$86.59	GENERIC, Alra	51641-0224-94
1920 ml	$96.96	GENERIC, Alra	51641-0225-94
1920 ml	$97.75	GENERIC, Ivax Corporation	00182-6072-97
1920 ml	$97.75	GENERIC, Watson/Schein Pharmaceuticals Inc	00364-2347-64
1920 ml	$98.76	GENERIC, Morton Grove Pharmaceuticals Inc	60432-0038-64
1920 ml	$109.50	GENERIC, Major Pharmaceuticals Inc	00904-2115-74
1920 ml	$117.79	GENERIC, Alpharma Uspd Makers Of Barre and Nmc	00472-1360-64
3840 ml	$170.88	GENERIC, Alra	51641-0224-97
3840 ml	$170.88	GENERIC, Alra	51641-0225-97
Syrup - Oral - 10 gm/15 ml			
480 ml	$10.51	FEDERAL UPPER LIMIT, H.C.F.A. F F P	99999-1621-01

PRODUCT LISTING - EQUIVALENTS NOT AVAILABLE

Powder For Reconstitution - Oral - 10 Gm			
1's	$1.01	KRISTALOSE, Bertek Pharmaceuticals Inc	62794-0501-17
30's	$31.50	KRISTALOSE, Bertek Pharmaceuticals Inc	62794-0501-93
Powder For Reconstitution - Oral - 20 Gm			
1's	$1.56	KRISTALOSE, Bertek Pharmaceuticals Inc	62794-0502-17
30's	$48.90	KRISTALOSE, Bertek Pharmaceuticals Inc	62794-0502-93
Syrup - Oral - 10 Gm/15 ml			
15 ml x 50	$75.00	GENERIC, Raway Pharmacal Inc	00686-0636-10
30 ml x 20	$95.00	GENERIC, Raway Pharmacal Inc	00686-0637-10
240 ml	$8.75	GENERIC, Physicians Total Care	54868-3101-00
437 ml	$14.41	GENERIC, Allscripts Pharmaceutical Company	54569-4952-00
960 ml	$48.89	GENERIC, Watson/Schein Pharmaceuticals Inc	00364-2519-32

Lamivudine *(003253)*

For related information, see the comparative table section in Appendix A.

Categories: Hepatitis B; Infection, human immunodeficiency virus; Pregnancy Category C; FDA Approved 1995 Nov; WHO Formulary

Drug Classes: Antivirals; Nucleoside reverse transcriptase inhibitors

Brand Names: 3TC; Epivir

Foreign Brand Availability: 3TC-HBV (Indonesia); Heptodin (China); Heptovir (Canada); Inhavir (Colombia); Ladiwin (Benin; Burkina-Faso; Ethiopia; Gambia; Ghana; Guinea; Ivory-Coast; Kenya; Liberia; Malawi; Mali; Mauritania; Mauritius; Morocco; Niger; Nigeria; Senegal; Seychelles; Sierra-Leone; Sudan; Tanzania; Tunia; Uganda; Zambia; Zimbabwe); Lamidac (India); Zeffix (Australia; Austria; Belgium; Bulgaria; Czech-Republic; Denmark; England; Finland; France; Germany; Greece; Hungary; Ireland; Israel; Italy; Netherlands; Norway; Philippines; Poland; Portugal; Singapore; Slovenia; Spain; Sweden; Switzerland; Taiwan; Thailand; Turkey)

Cost of Therapy: $208.35 (HIV; Epivir; 150 mg; 2 tablets/day; 30 day supply)

WARNING

Note: The trade names have been used throughout this monograph for clarity.

EPIVIR

LACTIC ACIDOSIS AND SEVERE HEPATOMEGALY WITH STEATOSIS, INCLUDING FATAL CASES, HAVE BEEN REPORTED WITH THE USE OF NUCLEOSIDE ANALOGUES ALONE OR IN COMBINATION, INCLUDING LAMIVUDINE AND OTHER ANTIRETROVIRALS (SEE WARNINGS, Epivir).

EPIVIR TABLETS AND ORAL SOLUTION (USED TO TREAT HIV INFECTION) CONTAIN A HIGHER DOSE OF THE ACTIVE INGREDIENT (LAMIVUDINE) THAN EPIVIR-HBV TABLETS AND ORAL SOLUTION (USED TO TREAT CHRONIC HEPATITIS B). PATIENTS WITH HIV INFECTION SHOULD RECEIVE ONLY DOSING FORMS APPROPRIATE FOR TREATMENT OF HIV (SEE WARNINGS, Epivir AND PRECAUTIONS, Epivir).

EPIVIR-HBV

LACTIC ACIDOSIS AND SEVERE HEPATOMEGALY WITH STEATOSIS, INCLUDING FATAL CASES, HAVE BEEN REPORTED WITH THE USE OF NUCLEOSIDE ANALOGUES ALONE OR IN COMBINATION, INCLUDING LAMIVUDINE AND OTHER ANTIRETROVIRALS (SEE WARNINGS, Epivir-HBV).

HUMAN IMMUNODEFICIENCY VIRUS (HIV) COUNSELING AND TESTING SHOULD BE OFFERED TO ALL PATIENTS BEFORE BEGINNING EPIVIR-HBV AND PERIODICALLY DURING TREATMENT (SEE WARNINGS, Epivir-HBV), BECAUSE EPIVIR-HBV TABLETS AND ORAL SOLUTION CONTAIN A LOWER DOSE OF THE SAME ACTIVE INGREDIENT (LAMIVUDINE) AS EPIVIR TABLETS AND ORAL SOLUTION USED TO TREAT HIV INFECTION. IF TREATMENT WITH EPIVIR-HBV IS PRESCRIBED FOR CHRONIC HEPATITIS B FOR A PATIENT WITH UNRECOGNIZED OR UNTREATED HIV INFECTION, RAPID EMERGENCE OF HIV RESISTANCE IS LIKELY BECAUSE OF SUBTHERAPEUTIC DOSE AND INAPPROPRIATE MONOTHERAPY.

DESCRIPTION

Epivir (also known as 3TC) is a brand name for lamivudine, a synthetic nucleoside analogue with activity against human immunodeficiency virus-1 (HIV-1) and hepatitis B virus (HBV). The chemical name of lamivudine is (2R,cis)-4-amino-1-(2-hydroxymethyl-1,3-oxathiolan-5-yl)-(1H)-pyrimidin-2-one. Lamivudine is the (-)enantiomer of a dideoxy analogue of cytidine. Lamivudine has also been referred to as (-)2′,3′-dideoxy,3′-thiacytidine. It has a molecular formula of $C_8H_{11}N_3O_3S$ and a molecular weight of 229.3.

Lamivudine is a white to off-white crystalline solid with a solubility of approximately 70 mg/ml in water at 20°C.

EPIVIR

Epivir tablets are for oral administration. Each 150 mg film-coated tablet contains 150 mg of lamivudine and the inactive ingredients hypromellose, magnesium stearate, microcrystalline cellulose, polyethylene glycol, polysorbate 80, sodium starch glycolate, and titanium dioxide.

Each 300 mg film-coated tablet contains 300 mg of lamivudine and the inactive ingredients black iron oxide, hypromellose, magnesium stearate, microcrystalline cellulose, polyethylene glycol, polysorbate 80, sodium starch glycolate, and titanium dioxide.

Epivir oral solution is for oral administration. One milliliter (1 ml) of Epivir oral solution contains 10 mg of lamivudine (10 mg/ml) in an aqueous solution and the inactive ingredients artificial strawberry and banana flavors, citric acid (anhydrous), methylparaben, propylene glycol, propylparaben, sodium citrate (dihydrate), and sucrose.

EPIVIR-HBV

Epivir-HBV tablets are for oral administration. Each tablet contains 100 mg of lamivudine and the inactive ingredients magnesium stearate, microcrystalline cellulose, and sodium starch glycolate. Opadry YS-1-17307-A butterscotch is the coloring agent in the tablet coating.

Epivir-HBV oral solution is for oral administration. One milliliter (1 ml) of Epivir-HBV oral solution contains 5 mg of lamivudine (5 mg/ml) in an aqueous solution and the inactive ingredients artificial strawberry and banana flavors, citric acid (anhydrous), methylparaben, propylene glycol, propylparaben, sodium citrate (dihydrate), and sucrose.

CLINICAL PHARMACOLOGY

EPIVIR

Microbiology

Mechanism of Action

Lamivudine is a synthetic nucleoside analogue. Intracellularly, lamivudine is phosphorylated to its active 5′-triphosphate metabolite, lamivudine triphosphate (L-TP). The principal mode of action of L-TP is the inhibition of HIV-1 reverse transcriptase (RT) via DNA chain termination after incorporation of the nucleoside analogue into viral DNA. L-TP is a weak inhibitor of mammalian DNA polymerases α and β, and mitochondrial DNA polymerase γ.

Antiviral Activity In Vitro

The *in vitro* activity of lamivudine against HIV-1 was assessed in a number of cell lines (including monocytes and fresh human peripheral blood lymphocytes) using standard susceptibility assays. IC_{50} values (50% inhibitory concentrations) were in the range of 2 nM-15 µM. Lamivudine had anti-HIV-1 activity in all acute virus-cell infections tested. In HIV-1-infected MT-4 cells, lamivudine in combination with zidovudine at various ratios exhibited synergistic antiretroviral activity. The relationship between *in vitro* susceptibility of HIV-1 to lamivudine and the inhibition of HIV-1 replication in humans has not been established. Please see the Epivir-HBV package insert for information regarding the inhibitory activity of lamivudine against HBV.

Drug Resistance

Lamivudine-resistant variants of HIV-1 have been selected *in vitro.* Genotypic analysis showed that the resistance was due to a specific amino acid substitution in the HIV-1 reverse transcriptase at codon 184 changing the methionine residue to either isoleucine or valine.

HIV-1 strains resistant to both lamivudine and zidovudine have been isolated from patients. Susceptibility of clinical isolates to lamivudine and zidovudine was monitored in controlled clinical trials. In patients receiving lamivudine monotherapy or combination therapy with lamivudine plus zidovudine, HIV-1 isolates from most patients became phenotypically and genotypically resistant to lamivudine within 12 weeks. In some patients harboring zidovudine-resistant virus at baseline, phenotypic sensitivity to zidovudine was restored by 12 weeks of treatment with lamivudine and zidovudine. Combination therapy with lamivudine plus zidovudine delayed the emergence of mutations conferring resistance to zidovudine.

Mutations in the HBV polymerase YMDD motif have been associated with reduced susceptibility of HBV to lamivudine *in vitro.* In studies of non-HIV-infected patients with chronic hepatitis B, HBV isolates with YMDD mutations were detected in some patients who received lamivudine daily for 6 months or more, and were associated with evidence of diminished treatment response; similar HBV mutants have been reported in HIV-infected patients who received lamivudine-containing antiretroviral regimens in the presence of concurrent infection with hepatitis B virus (see PRECAUTIONS, Epivir and Epivir-HBV package insert).

Cross-Resistance

Lamivudine resistant HIV-1 mutants were cross-resistant to didanosine (ddI) and zalcitabine (ddC). In some patients treated with zidovudine plus didanosine or zalcitabine, isolates resistant to multiple reverse transcriptase inhibitors, including lamivudine, have emerged.

Genotypic and Phenotypic Analysis of On-Therapy HIV-1 Isolates From Patients With Virologic Failure

The clinical relevance of genotypic and phenotypic changes associated with lamivudine therapy has not been fully established.

Study EPV20001

Fifty-three (53) of 554 (10%) patients enrolled in EPV20001 were identified as virological failures (plasma HIV-1 RNA level ≥400 copies/ml) by Week 48. Twenty-eight (28) patients were randomized to the lamivudine once daily treatment group and 25 to the lamivudine twice daily treatment group. The median baseline plasma HIV-1 RNA levels of patients in the lamivudine once daily group and lamivudine twice daily groups were 4.9 $\log_{10}$ copies/ml and 4.6 $\log_{10}$ copies/ml, respectively.

Genotypic analysis of on-therapy isolates from 22 patients identified as virologic failures in the lamivudine once daily group showed that isolates from 0/22 patients contained treatment-emergent mutations associated with zidovudine resistance (M41L, D67N, K70R, L210W, T215Y/F, or K219Q/E), isolates from 10/22 patients contained treatment-emergent mutations associated with efavirenz resistance (L100I, K101E, K103N, V108I, or Y181C), and isolates from 8/22 patients contained a treatment-emergent lamivudine resistance-associated mutation (M184I or M184V).

Genotypic analysis of on-therapy isolates from patients (n=22) in the lamivudine twice daily treatment group showed that isolates from 1/22 patients contained treatment-emergent zidovudine resistance mutations, isolates from 7/22 contained treatment-emergent efavirenz resistance mutations, and isolates from 5/22 contained treatment-emergent lamivudine resistance mutations.

Phenotypic analysis of baseline-matched on-therapy HIV-1 isolates from patients (n=13) receiving lamivudine once daily showed that isolates from 12/13 patients were susceptible to zidovudine; isolates from 8/13 patients exhibited a 25- to 295-fold decrease in susceptibility to efavirenz, and isolates from 7/13 patients showed an 85- to 299-fold decrease in susceptibility to lamivudine.

Phenotypic analysis of baseline-matched on-therapy HIV-1 isolates from patients (n=13) receiving lamivudine twice daily showed that isolates from all 13 patients were susceptible to zidovudine; isolates from 3/13 patients exhibited a 21- to 342-fold decrease in susceptibility to efavirenz, and isolates from 4/13 patients exhibited a 29- to 159-fold decrease in susceptibility to lamivudine.

Study EPV40001

Fifty (50) patients received zidovudine 300 mg twice daily plus abacavir 300 mg twice daily plus lamivudine 300 mg once daily and 50 patients received zidovudine 300 mg plus abacavir 300 mg plus lamivudine 150 mg all twice daily. The median baseline plasma HIV-1 RNA levels for patients in the 2 groups were 4.79 $\log_{10}$ copies/ml and 4.83 $\log_{10}$ copies/ml, respectively. Fourteen (14) of 50 patients in the lamivudine once daily treatment group and 9 of 50 patients in the lamivudine twice daily group were identified as virologic failures.

Genotypic analysis of on-therapy HIV-1 isolates from patients (n=9) in the lamivudine once daily treatment group showed that isolates from 6 patients had abacavir and/or lamivudine resistance-associated mutation M184V alone. On-therapy isolates from patients (n=6) receiving lamivudine twice daily showed that isolates from 2 patients had M184V alone, and isolates from 2 patients harbored the M184V mutation in combination with zidovudine resistance-associated mutations.

Phenotypic analysis of on-therapy isolates from patients (n=6) receiving lamivudine once daily showed that HIV-1 isolates from 4 patients exhibited a 32- to 53-fold decrease in susceptibility to lamivudine. HIV-1 isolates from these 6 patients were susceptible to zidovudine.

Phenotypic analysis of on-therapy isolates from patients (n=4) receiving lamivudine twice daily showed that HIV-1 isolates from 1 patient exhibited a 45-fold decrease in susceptibility to lamivudine and a 4.5-fold decrease in susceptibility to zidovudine.

Pharmacokinetics in Adults

The steady-state pharmacokinetic properties of the Epivir 300 mg tablet once daily for 7 days compared to the Epivir 150 mg tablet twice daily for 7 days were assessed in a cross-over study in 60 healthy volunteers. Epivir 300 mg once daily resulted in lamivudine exposures that were similar to Epivir 150 mg twice daily with respect to plasma $AUC_{24,ss}$; however, $C_{max,ss}$ was 66% higher and the trough value was 53% lower compared to the 150 mg twice daily regimen. Intracellular lamivudine triphosphate exposures in peripheral blood mononuclear cells were also similar with respect to $AUC_{24,ss}$ and $C_{max24,ss}$; however, trough values were lower compared to the 150 mg twice daily regimen. Inter-subject variability was greater for intracellular lamivudine triphosphate concentrations versus lamivudine plasma trough concentrations. The clinical significance of observed differences for both plasma lamivudine concentrations and intracellular lamivudine triphosphate concentrations is not known.

The pharmacokinetic properties of lamivudine have been studied in asymptomatic, HIV-infected adult patients after administration of single intravenous (IV) doses ranging from 0.25 to 8 mg/kg, as well as single and multiple (twice daily regimen) oral doses ranging from 0.25 to 10 mg/kg.

The pharmacokinetic properties of lamivudine have also been studied as single and multiple oral doses ranging from 5-600 mg/day administered to HBV-infected patients.

Absorption and Bioavailability

Lamivudine was rapidly absorbed after oral administration in HIV-infected patients. Absolute bioavailability in 12 adult patients was 86% ± 16% (mean ±SD) for the 150 mg tablet and 87% ± 13% for the oral solution. After oral administration of 2 mg/kg twice a day to 9 adults with HIV, the peak serum lamivudine concentration (C_{max}) was 1.5 ± 0.5 µg/ml (mean ±SD). The area under the plasma concentration versus time curve (AUC) and C_{max} increased in proportion to oral dose over the range from 0.25 to 10 mg/kg.

An investigational 25 mg dosage form of lamivudine was administered orally to 12 asymptomatic, HIV-infected patients on 2 occasions, once in the fasted state and once with food (1099 kcal; 75 g fat, 34 g protein, 72 g carbohydrate). Absorption of lamivudine was slower in the fed state (T_{max}: 3.2 ± 1.3 hours) compared with the fasted state (T_{max}: 0.9 ± 0.3 hours); C_{max} in the fed state was 40% ± 23% (mean ±SD) lower than in the fasted state. There was no significant difference in systemic exposure (AUC∞) in the fed and fasted states; therefore, Epivir tablets and oral solution may be administered with or without food.

The accumulation ratio of lamivudine in HIV-positive asymptomatic adults with normal renal function was 1.50 following 15 days of oral administration of 2 mg/kg twice daily.

Distribution

The apparent volume of distribution after IV administration of lamivudine to 20 patients was 1.3 ± 0.4 L/kg, suggesting that lamivudine distributes into extravascular spaces. Volume of distribution was independent of dose and did not correlate with body weight.

Binding of lamivudine to human plasma proteins is low (<36%). *In vitro* studies showed that, over the concentration range of 0.1 to 100 µg/ml, the amount of lamivudine associated with erythrocytes ranged from 53-57% and was independent of concentration.

Metabolism

Metabolism of lamivudine is a minor route of elimination. In man, the only known metabolite of lamivudine is the trans-sulfoxide metabolite. Within 12 hours after a single oral dose of lamivudine in 6 HIV-infected adults, 5.2% ± 1.4% (mean ±SD) of the dose was excreted as the trans-sulfoxide metabolite in the urine. Serum concentrations of this metabolite have not been determined.

Elimination

The majority of lamivudine is eliminated unchanged in urine. In 9 healthy subjects given a single 300 mg oral dose of lamivudine, renal clearance was 199.7 ± 56.9 ml/min (mean ±SD). In 20 HIV-infected patients given a single IV dose, renal clearance was 280.4 ± 75.2 ml/min (mean ±SD), representing 71% ± 16% (mean ±SD) of total clearance of lamivudine.

In most single dose studies in HIV-infected patients, HBV-infected patients, or healthy subjects with serum sampling for 24 hours after dosing, the observed mean elimination half-life ($T_{1/2}$) ranged from 5-7 hours. In HIV-infected patients, total clearance was 398.5 ± 69.1 ml/min (mean ±SD). Oral clearance and elimination half-life were independent of dose and body weight over an oral dosing range from 0.25 to 10 mg/kg.

Special Populations

Adults With Impaired Renal Function

The pharmacokinetic properties of lamivudine have been determined in a small group of HIV-infected adults with impaired renal function (TABLE 1).

Exposure (AUC∞), C_{max}, and half-life increased with diminishing renal function (as expressed by creatinine clearance). Apparent total oral clearance (Cl/F) of lamivudine decreased as creatinine clearance decreased. T_{max} was not significantly affected by renal function. Based on these observations, it is recommended that the dosage of lamivudine be modified in patients with renal impairment (see DOSAGE AND ADMINISTRATION, Epivir).

Based on a study in otherwise healthy subjects with impaired renal function, hemodialysis increased lamivudine clearance from a mean of 64-88 ml/min; however, the length of time of hemodialysis (4 hours) was insufficient to significantly alter mean lamivudine exposure after a single dose administration. Therefore, it is recommended, following correction of dose for creatinine clearance, that no additional dose modification be made after routine hemodialysis.

L

TABLE 1 *Pharmacokinetic Parameters (Mean ±SD) After a Single 300 mg Oral Dose of Lamivudine in 3 Groups of Adults With Varying Degrees of Renal Function*

	Creatinine Clearance Criterion		
	>60 ml/min	10-30 ml/min	<10 ml/min
Parameter	(n=6)	(n=4)	(n=6)
Creatinine clearance (ml/min)	111 ± 14	28 ± 8	6 ± 2
C_{max} (µg/ml)	2.6 ± 0.5	3.6 ± 0.8	5.8 ± 1.2
AUC∞ (µg·h/ml)	11.0 ± 1.7	48.0 ± 19	157 ± 74
Cl/F (ml/min)	464 ± 76	114 ± 34	36 ± 11

It is not known whether lamivudine can be removed by peritoneal dialysis or continuous (24 hour) hemodialysis.

The effects of renal impairment on lamivudine pharmacokinetics in pediatric patients are not known.

Adults With Impaired Hepatic Function

The pharmacokinetic properties of lamivudine have been determined in adults with impaired hepatic function. Pharmacokinetic parameters were not altered by diminishing hepatic function; therefore, no dose adjustment for lamivudine is required for patients with impaired hepatic function. Safety and efficacy of lamivudine have not been established in the presence of decompensated liver disease.

Pediatric Patients

For pharmacokinetic properties of lamivudine in pediatric patients, see PRECAUTIONS, Epivir, Pediatric Use.

Gender

There are no significant gender differences in lamivudine pharmacokinetics.

Race

There are no significant racial differences in lamivudine pharmacokinetics.

Drug Interactions

No clinically significant alterations in lamivudine or zidovudine pharmacokinetics were observed in 12 asymptomatic HIV-infected adult patients given a single dose of zidovudine (200 mg) in combination with multiple doses of lamivudine (300 mg q12h).

Lamivudine and trimethoprim/sulfamethoxazole (TMP/SMX) were coadministered to 14 HIV-positive patients in a single-center, open-label, randomized, crossover study. Each patient received treatment with a single 300 mg dose of lamivudine and TMP 160 mg/SMX 800 mg once a day for 5 days with concomitant administration of lamivudine 300 mg with the fifth dose in a crossover design. Coadministration of TMP/SMX with lamivudine resulted in an increase of 44% ± 23% (mean ±SD) in lamivudine AUC∞, a decrease of 29% ± 13% in lamivudine oral clearance, and a decrease of 30% ± 36% in lamivudine renal clearance. The pharmacokinetic properties of TMP and SMX were not altered by coadministration with lamivudine.

Lamivudine and zalcitabine may inhibit the intracellular phosphorylation of one another. Therefore, use of lamivudine in combination with zalcitabine is not recommended.

There was no significant pharmacokinetic interaction between lamivudine and interferon alfa in a study of 19 healthy male subjects.

EPIVIR-HBV

Microbiology

Mechanism of Action

Lamivudine is a synthetic nucleoside analogue. Lamivudine is phosphorylated intracellularly to lamivudine triphosphate, L-TP. Incorporation of the monophosphate form into viral DNA by hepatitis B virus (HBV) polymerase results in DNA chain termination. L-TP also inhibits the RNA- and DNA-dependent DNA polymerase activities of HIV-1 reverse transcriptase (RT). L-TP is a weak inhibitor of mammalian alpha-, beta-, and gamma-DNA polymerases.

Antiviral Activity In Vitro

In vitro activity of lamivudine against HBV was assessed in HBV DNA-transfected 2.2.15 cells, HB611 cells, and infected human primary hepatocytes. IC_{50} values (the concentration of drug needed to reduce the level of extracellular HBV DNA by 50%) varied from 0.01 µM (2.3 ng/ml) to 5.6 µM (1.3 µg/ml) depending upon the duration of exposure of cells to lamivudine, the cell model system, and the protocol used. See the Epivir prescribing information for information regarding activity of lamivudine against HIV.

Drug Resistance — HBV

Genotypic analysis of viral isolates obtained from patients who show renewed evidence of replication of HBV while receiving lamivudine suggests that a reduction in sensitivity of HBV to lamivudine is associated with mutations resulting in a methionine to valine or isoleucine substitution in the YMDD motif of the catalytic domain of HBV polymerase (position 552) and a leucine to methionine substitution at position 528. It is not known whether other HBV mutations may be associated with reduced lamivudine susceptibility *in vitro.*

In 4 controlled clinical trials in adults, YMDD-mutant HBV were detected in 81 of 335 patients receiving lamivudine 100 mg once daily for 52 weeks. The prevalence of YMDD mutations was less than 10% in each of these trials for patients studied at 24 weeks and increased to an average of 24% (range in 4 studies: 16-32%) at 52 weeks. In limited data from a long-term follow-up trial in patients who continued 100 mg/day lamivudine after of these studies, YMDD mutations further increased from 16% at 1 year to 42% at 2 years. In small numbers of patients receiving lamivudine for longer periods, further increases in the appearance of YMDD mutations were observed.

In a controlled trial in pediatric patients, YMDD-mutant HBV were detected in 31 of 166 (19%) patients receiving lamivudine for 52 weeks. For a subgroup who remained on lamivudine therapy in a follow-up study, YMDD mutations increased from 24% at 12 months to 45% (53 of 118) at 18 months of lamivudine treatment.

Mutant viruses were associated with evidence of diminished treatment response at 52 weeks relative to lamivudine-treated patients without evidence of YMDD mutations in both adult and pediatric studies (see PRECAUTIONS, Epivir-HBV). The long-term clinical significance of YMDD-mutant HBV is not known.

Drug Resistance — HIV

In studies of HIV-1-infected patients who received lamivudine monotherapy or combination therapy with lamivudine plus zidovudine for at least 12 weeks, HIV-1 isolates with reduced *in vitro* susceptibility to lamivudine were detected in most patients (see WARNINGS, Epivir-HBV).

Pharmacokinetics in Adults

The pharmacokinetic properties of lamivudine have been studied as single and multiple oral doses ranging from 5-600 mg/day administered to HBV-infected patients.

The pharmacokinetic properties of lamivudine have also been studied in asymptomatic, HIV-infected adult patients after administration of single intravenous (IV) doses ranging from 0.25 to 8 mg/kg, as well as single and multiple (twice daily regimen) oral doses ranging from 0.25 to 10 mg/kg.

Absorption and Bioavailability

Lamivudine was rapidly absorbed after oral administration in HBV-infected patients and in healthy subjects. Following single oral doses of 100 mg, the peak serum lamivudine concentration (C_{max}) in HBV-infected patients (steady- state) and healthy subjects (single dose) was 1.28 ± 0.56 µg/ml and 1.05 ± 0.32 µg/ml (mean ±SD), respectively, which occurred between 0.5 and 2 hours after administration. The area under the plasma concentration versus time curve [AUC(0-24h)] following 100 mg lamivudine oral single and repeated daily doses to steady-state was 4.3 ± 1.4 (mean ±SD) and 4.7 ± 1.7 µg·h/ml, respectively. The relative bioavailability of the tablet and solution were then demonstrated in healthy subjects. Although the solution demonstrated a slightly higher peak serum concentration (C_{max}), there was no significant difference in systemic exposure AUC∞ between the solution and the tablet. Therefore, the solution and the tablet may be used interchangeably.

After oral administration of lamivudine once daily to HBV-infected adults, the AUC and peak serum levels (C_{max}) increased in proportion to dose over the range from 5-600 mg once daily.

The 100 mg tablet was administered orally to 24 healthy subjects on 2 occasions, once in the fasted state and once with food (standard meal: 967 kcal; 67 g fat, 33 g protein, 58 g carbohydrate). There was no significant difference in systemic exposure AUC∞ in the fed and fasted states; therefore, Epivir-HBV tablets and oral solution may be administered with or without food.

Lamivudine was rapidly absorbed after oral administration in HIV-infected patients. Absolute bioavailability in 12 adult patients was 86% ± 16% (mean ±SD) for the 150 mg tablet and 87% ± 13% for the 10 mg/ml oral solution.

Distribution

The apparent volume of distribution after IV administration of lamivudine to 20 asymptomatic HIV-infected patients was 1.3 ± 0.4 L/kg, suggesting that lamivudine distributes into extravascular spaces. Volume of distribution was independent of dose and did not correlate with body weight.

Binding of lamivudine to human plasma proteins is low (<36%) and independent of dose. *In vitro* studies showed that, over the concentration range of 0.1 to 100 µg/ml, the amount of lamivudine associated with erythrocytes ranged from 53-57% and was independent of concentration.

Metabolism

Metabolism of lamivudine is a minor route of elimination. In man, the only known metabolite of lamivudine is the trans-sulfoxide metabolite. In 9 healthy subjects receiving 300 mg of lamivudine as single oral doses, a total of 4.2% (range 1.5-7.5%) of the dose was excreted as the trans-sulfoxide metabolite in the urine, the majority of which was excreted in the first 12 hours.

Serum concentrations of the trans-sulfoxide metabolite have not been determined.

Elimination

The majority of lamivudine is eliminated unchanged in urine. In 9 healthy subjects given a single 300 mg oral dose of lamivudine, renal clearance was 199.7 ± 56.9 ml/min (mean ±SD). In 20 HIV-infected patients given a single IV dose, renal clearance was 280.4 ± 75.2 ml/min (mean ±SD), representing 71% ± 16% (mean ±SD) of total clearance of lamivudine.

In most single dose studies in HIV- or HBV-infected patients or healthy subjects with serum sampling for 24 hours after dosing, the observed mean elimination half-life ($T_{1/2}$) ranged from 5-7 hours. In HIV-infected patients, total clearance was 398.5 ± 69.1 ml/min (mean ±SD). Oral clearance and elimination half-life were independent of dose and body weight over an oral dosing range from 0.25 to 10 mg/kg.

Special Populations

Adults With Impaired Renal Function

The pharmacokinetic properties of lamivudine have been determined in healthy subjects and in subjects with impaired renal function, with and without hemodialysis (TABLE 2).

Exposure AUC∞, C_{max}, and half-life increased with diminishing renal function (as expressed by creatinine clearance). Apparent total oral clearance (Cl/F) of lamivudine decreased as creatinine clearance decreased. T_{max} was not significantly affected by renal function. Based on these observations, it is recommended that the dosage of lamivudine be modified in patients with renal impairment (see DOSAGE AND ADMINISTRATION, Epivir-HBV).

TABLE 2 *Pharmacokinetic Parameters (Mean ±SD) Dose-Normalized to a Single 100 mg Oral Dose of Lamivudine in Patients With Varying Degrees of Renal Function*

	Creatinine Clearance Criterion		
	≥80 ml/min	20-59 ml/min	<20 ml/min
Parameter	(n=9)	(n=8)	(n=6)
Creatinine clearance (ml/min)	97 (range 82-117)	39 (range 25-49)	15 (range 13-19)
C_{max} (μg/ml)	1.31 ± 0.35	1.85 ± 0.40	1.55 ± 0.31
AUC∞ (μg·h/ml)	5.28 ± 1.01	14.67 ± 3.74	27.33 ± 6.56
Cl/F (ml/min)	326.4 ± 63.8	120.1 ± 29.5	64.5 ± 18.3

Hemodialysis increases lamivudine clearance from a mean of 64-88 ml/min; however, the length of time of hemodialysis (4 hours) was insufficient to significantly alter mean lamivudine exposure after a single dose administration. Therefore, it is recommended, following correction of dose for creatinine clearance, that no additional dose modification is made after routine hemodialysis.

It is not known whether lamivudine can be removed by peritoneal dialysis or continuous (24 hour) hemodialysis.

The effect of renal impairment on lamivudine pharmacokinetics in pediatric patients with chronic hepatitis B is not known.

Adults With Impaired Hepatic Function

The pharmacokinetic properties of lamivudine have been determined in adults with impaired hepatic function (TABLE 3). Patients were stratified by severity of hepatic functional impairment.

TABLE 3 *Pharmacokinetic Parameters (Mean ±SD) Dose-Normalized to a Single 100 mg Dose of Lamivudine in 3 Groups of Subjects With Normal or Impaired Hepatic Function*

		Impairment*	
	Normal	Moderate	Severe
Parameter	(n=8)	(n=8)	(n=8)
C_{max} (μg/ml)	0.92 ± 0.31	1.06 ± 0.58	1.08 ± 0.27
AUC∞ (μg·h/ml)	3.96 ± 0.58	3.97 ± 1.36	4.30 ± 0.63
T_{max} (h)	1.3 ± 0.8	1.4 ± 0.8	1.4 ± 1.2
Cl/F (ml/min)	424.7 ± 61.9	456.9 ± 129.8	395.2 ± 51.8
CLR (ml/min)	279.2 ± 79.2	323.5 ± 100.9	216.1 ± 58.0

* Hepatic impairment assessed by aminopyrine breath test.

Pharmacokinetic parameters were not altered by diminishing hepatic function. Therefore, no dose adjustment for lamivudine is required for patients with impaired hepatic function. Safety and efficacy of Epivir-HBV have not been established in the presence of decompensated liver disease (see PRECAUTIONS, Epivir-HBV).

Post-Hepatic Transplant

Fourteen (14) HBV-infected patients received liver transplant following lamivudine therapy and completed pharmacokinetic assessments at enrollment, 2 weeks after 100 mg once daily dosing (pre-transplant), and 3 months following transplant; there were no significant differences in pharmacokinetic parameters. The overall exposure of lamivudine is primarily affected by renal dysfunction; consequently, transplant patients with reduced renal function had generally higher exposure than patients with normal renal function. Safety and efficacy of Epivir-HBV have not been established in this population (see PRECAUTIONS, Epivir-HBV).

Pediatric Patients

Lamivudine pharmacokinetics were evaluated in a 28 day dose-ranging study in 53 pediatric patients with chronic hepatitis B. Patients aged 2-12 years were randomized to receive lamivudine 0.35 mg/kg twice daily, 3 mg/kg once daily, 1.5 mg/kg twice daily, or 4 mg/kg twice daily. Patients aged 13-17 years received lamivudine 100 mg once daily. Lamivudine was rapidly absorbed (T_{max} 0.5 to 1 hour). In general, both C_{max} and exposure (AUC) showed dose proportionality in the dosing range studied. Weight-corrected oral clearance was highest at age 2 and declined from 2-12 years, where values were then similar to those seen in adults. A dose of 3 mg/kg given once daily produced a steady-state lamivudine AUC (mean 5953 ng·h/ml ± 1562 SD) similar to that associated with a dose of 100 mg/day in adults.

Gender

There are no significant gender differences in lamivudine pharmacokinetics.

Race

There are no significant racial differences in lamivudine pharmacokinetics.

Drug Interactions

Multiple doses of lamivudine and a single dose of interferon were coadministered to 19 healthy male subjects in a pharmacokinetics study. Results indicated a small (10%) reduction in lamivudine AUC, but no change in interferon pharmacokinetic parameters when the 2 drugs were given in combination. All other pharmacokinetic parameters (C_{max}, T_{max}, and $T_{1/2}$) were unchanged. There was no significant pharmacokinetic interaction between lamivudine and interferon alfa in this study.

Lamivudine and zidovudine were coadministered to 12 asymptomatic HIV-positive adult patients in a single-center, open-label, randomized, crossover study. No significant differences were observed in AUC∞ or total clearance for lamivudine or zidovudine when the 2 drugs were administered together. Coadministration of lamivudine with zidovudine resulted in an increase of 39% ± 62% (mean ±SD) in C_{max} of zidovudine.

Lamivudine and trimethoprim/sulfamethoxazole (TMP/SMX) were coadministered to 14 HIV-positive patients in a single-center, open-label, randomized, crossover study. Each patient received treatment with a single 300 mg dose of lamivudine and TMP 160 mg/SMX 800 mg once a day for 5 days with concomitant administration of lamivudine 300 mg with the fifth dose in a crossover design. Coadministration of TMP/SMX with lamivudine resulted in an increase of 44% ± 23% (mean ±SD) in lamivudine AUC∞, a decrease of 29% ± 13% in lamivudine oral clearance, and a decrease of 30% ± 36% in lamivudine renal clearance. The pharmacokinetic properties of TMP and SMX were not altered by coadministration with lamivudine (see DRUG INTERACTIONS, Epivir-HBV).

Lamivudine and zalcitabine may inhibit the intracellular phosphorylation of one another. Therefore, use of lamivudine in combination with zalcitabine is not recommended.

INDICATIONS AND USAGE

EPIVIR

Epivir in combination with other antiretroviral agents is indicated for the treatment of HIV infection.

EPIVIR-HBV

Epivir-HBV is indicated for the treatment of chronic hepatitis B associated with evidence of hepatitis B viral replication and active liver inflammation. This indication is based on 1 year histologic and serologic responses in adult patients with compensated chronic hepatitis B, and more limited information from a study in pediatric patients ages 2-17 years.

CONTRAINDICATIONS

EPIVIR

Epivir tablets and oral solution are contraindicated in patients with previously demonstrated clinically significant hypersensitivity to any of the components of the products.

EPIVIR-HBV

Epivir-HBV tablets and oral solution are contraindicated in patients with previously demonstrated clinically significant hypersensitivity to any of the components of the products.

WARNINGS

EPIVIR

In pediatric patients with a history of prior antiretroviral nucleoside exposure, a history of pancreatitis, or other significant risk factors for the development of pancreatitis, Epivir should be used with caution. Treatment with Epivir should be stopped immediately if clinical signs, symptoms, or laboratory abnormalities suggestive of pancreatitis occur (see ADVERSE REACTIONS, Epivir).

Lactic Acidosis/Severe Hepatomegaly With Steatosis

Lactic acidosis and severe hepatomegaly with steatosis, including fatal cases, have been reported with the use of nucleoside analogues alone or in combination, including lamivudine and other antiretrovirals. A majority of these cases have been in women. Obesity and prolonged nucleoside exposure may be risk factors. Particular caution should be exercised when administering Epivir to any patient with known risk factors for liver disease; however, cases have also been reported in patients with no known risk factors. Treatment with Epivir should be suspended in any patient who develops clinical or laboratory findings suggestive of lactic acidosis or pronounced hepatotoxicity (which may include hepatomegaly and steatosis even in the absence of marked transaminase elevations).

Important Differences Among Lamivudine-Containing Products

Epivir tablets and oral solution contain a higher dose of the same active ingredient (lamivudine) than in Epivir-HBV tablets and oral solution. Epivir-HBV was developed for patients with chronic hepatitis B. The formulation and dosage of lamivudine in Epivir-HBV are not appropriate for patients dually infected with HIV and HBV. Lamivudine has not been adequately studied for treatment of chronic hepatitis B in patients dually infected with HIV and HBV. If treatment with Epivir-HBV is prescribed for chronic hepatitis B for a patient with unrecognized or untreated HIV infection, rapid emergence of HIV resistance is likely to result because of the subtherapeutic dose and the inappropriateness of monotherapy HIV treatment. If a decision is made to administer lamivudine to patients dually infected with HIV and HBV, Epivir tablets, Epivir oral solution, or Combivir (lamivudine/zidovudine) tablets should be used as part of an appropriate combination regimen. Combivir (a fixed-dose combination tablet of lamivudine and zidovudine) should not be administered concomitantly with Epivir, Epivir-HBV, Retrovir, or Trizivir.

Posttreatment Exacerbations of Hepatitis

In clinical trials in non-HIV-infected patients treated with lamivudine for chronic hepatitis B, clinical and laboratory evidence of exacerbations of hepatitis have occurred after discontinuation of lamivudine. These exacerbations have been detected primarily by serum ALT elevations in addition to re-emergence of HBV DNA. Although most events appear to have been self-limited, fatalities have been reported in some cases. Similar events have been reported from postmarketing experience after changes from lamivudine-containing HIV treatment regimens to non-lamivudine-containing regimens in patients infected with both HIV and HBV. The causal relationship to discontinuation of lamivudine treatment is unknown. Patients should be closely monitored with both clinical and laboratory follow-up for at least several months after stopping treatment. There is insufficient evidence to determine whether re-initiation of lamivudine alters the course of posttreatment exacerbations of hepatitis.

EPIVIR-HBV

Lactic Acidosis/Severe Hepatomegaly With Steatosis

Lactic acidosis and severe hepatomegaly with steatosis, including fatal cases, have been reported with the use of nucleoside analogues alone or in combination, including lamivudine and other antiretrovirals. A majority of these cases have been in women. Obesity and prolonged nucleoside exposure may be risk factors. Most of these reports have described patients receiving nucleoside analogues for treatment of HIV infection, but there have been reports of lactic acidosis in patients receiving lamivudine for hepatitis B. Particular caution should be exercised when administering Epivir or Epivir-HBV to any patient with known risk factors for liver disease; however, cases have also been reported in patients with no known risk factors. Treatment with Epivir or Epivir-HBV should be suspended in any patient who develops clinical or laboratory findings suggestive of lactic acidosis or pronounced hepatotoxicity (which may include hepatomegaly and steatosis even in the absence of marked transaminase elevations).

Important Differences Between Lamivudine-Containing Products, HIV Testing, and Risk of Emergence of Resistant HIV

Epivir-HBV tablets and oral solution contain a lower dose of the same active ingredient (lamivudine) as Epivir tablets and oral solution, Combivir (lamivudine/zidovudine) tablets, and Trizivir (abacavir, lamivudine, and zidovudine) tablets used to treat HIV infection. The formulation and dosage of lamivudine in Epivir-HBV are not appropriate for patients dually infected with HBV and HIV. If a decision is made to administer lamivudine to such patients, the higher dosage indicated for HIV therapy should be used as part of an appropriate combination regimen, and the prescribing information for Epivir , Combivir, or Trizivir as well as for Epivir-HBV should be consulted. HIV counseling and testing should be offered to all patients before beginning Epivir-HBV and periodically during treatment because of the risk of rapid emergence of resistant HIV and limitation of treatment options if Epivir-HBV is prescribed to treat chronic hepatitis B in a patient who has unrecognized or untreated HIV infection or acquires HIV infection during treatment.

Posttreatment Exacerbations of Hepatitis

Clinical and laboratory evidence of exacerbations of hepatitis have occurred after discontinuation of Epivir-HBV (these have been primarily detected by serum ALT elevations, in addition to the re-emergence of HBV DNA commonly observed after stopping treatment; see TABLE 15 for more information regarding frequency of posttreatment ALT elevations). Although most events appear to have been self-limited, fatalities have been reported in some cases. The causal relationship to discontinuation of lamivudine treatment is unknown. Patients should be closely monitored with both clinical and laboratory follow-up for at least several months after stopping treatment. There is insufficient evidence to determine whether re-initiation of therapy alters the course of posttreatment exacerbations of hepatitis.

Pancreatitis

Pancreatitis has been reported in patients receiving lamivudine, particularly in HIV-infected pediatric patients with prior nucleoside exposure.

L

PRECAUTIONS

EPIVIR

Patients With Impaired Renal Function

Reduction of the dosage of Epivir is recommended for patients with impaired renal function (see CLINICAL PHARMACOLOGY, Epivir and DOSAGE AND ADMINISTRATION, Epivir).

Patients With HIV and Hepatitis B Virus Coinfection

Safety and efficacy of lamivudine have not been established for treatment of chronic hepatitis B in patients dually infected with HIV and HBV. In non-HIV-infected patients treated with lamivudine for chronic hepatitis B, emergence of lamivudine-resistant HBV has been detected and has been associated with diminished treatment response (see Epivir-HBV prescribing information for additional information). Emergence of hepatitis B virus variants associated with resistance to lamivudine has also been reported in HIV-infected patients who have received lamivudine-containing antiretroviral regimens in the presence of concurrent infection with hepatitis B virus. Posttreatment exacerbations of hepatitis have also been reported (see WARNINGS, Epivir).

Differences Between Dosing Regimens

Trough levels of lamivudine in plasma and of intracellular lamivudine triphosphate were lower with once daily dosing than with twice daily dosing (see CLINICAL PHARMACOLOGY, Epivir). The clinical significance of this observation is not known.

Fat Redistribution

Redistribution/accumulation of body fat including central obesity, dorsocervical fat enlargement (buffalo hump), peripheral wasting, facial wasting, breast enlargement, and "cushingoid appearance" have been observed in patients receiving antiretroviral therapy. The mechanism and long-term consequences of these events are currently unknown. A causal relationship has not been established.

Information for the Patient

Epivir is not a cure for HIV infection and patients may continue to experience illnesses associated with HIV infection, including opportunistic infections. Patients should remain under the care of a physician when using Epivir. Patients should be advised that the use of Epivir has not been shown to reduce the risk of transmission of HIV to others through sexual contact or blood contamination.

Patients should be advised that Epivir tablets and oral solution contain a higher dose of the same active ingredient (lamivudine) as Epivir-HBV tablets and oral solution. If a decision is made to include lamivudine in the HIV treatment regimen of a patient dually infected with HIV and HBV, the formulation and dosage of lamivudine in Epivir (not Epivir-HBV) should be used.

Patients should be advised that the long-term effects of Epivir are unknown at this time. Epivir tablets and oral solution are for oral ingestion only.

Patients should be advised of the importance of taking Epivir with combination therapy on a regular dosing schedule and to avoid missing doses.

Parents or guardians should be advised to monitor pediatric patients for signs and symptoms of pancreatitis.

Patients should be informed that redistribution or accumulation of body fat may occur in patients receiving antiretroviral therapy and that the cause and long-term health effects of these conditions are not known at this time.

Carcinogenesis, Mutagenesis, and Impairment of Fertility

Long-term carcinogenicity studies with lamivudine in mice and rats showed no evidence of carcinogenic potential at exposures up to 10 times (mice) and 58 times (rats) those observed in humans at the recommended therapeutic dose for HIV infection. Lamivudine was not active in a microbial mutagenicity screen or an *in vitro* cell transformation assay, but showed weak *in vitro* mutagenic activity in a cytogenetic assay using cultured human lymphocytes and in the mouse lymphoma assay. However, lamivudine showed no evidence of *in vivo* genotoxic activity in the rat at oral doses of up to 2000 mg/kg, producing plasma levels of 35-45 times those in humans at the recommended dose for HIV infection. In a study of reproductive performance, lamivudine administered to rats at doses up to 4000 mg/kg/day, producing plasma levels 47-70 times those in humans, revealed no evidence of impaired fertility and no effect on the survival, growth, and development to weaning of the offspring.

Pregnancy Category C

Reproduction studies have been performed in rats and rabbits at orally administered doses up to 4000 mg/kg/day and 1000 mg/kg/day respectively, producing plasma levels up to approximately 35 times that for the adult HIV dose. No evidence of teratogenicity due to lamivudine was observed. Evidence of early embryolethality was seen in the rabbit at exposure levels similar to those observed in humans, but there was no indication of this effect in the rat at exposure levels up to 35 times that in humans. Studies in pregnant rats and rabbits showed that lamivudine is transferred to the fetus through the placenta.

In 2 clinical studies conducted in South Africa, pharmacokinetic measurements were performed on samples from pregnant women who received lamivudine beginning at Week 38 of gestation (10 women who received 150 mg twice daily in combination with zidovudine and 10 who received lamivudine 300 mg twice daily without other antiretrovirals) or beginning at Week 36 of gestation (16 women who received lamivudine 150 mg twice daily in combination with zidovudine). These studies were not designed or powered to provide efficacy information. Lamivudine pharmacokinetics in the pregnant women were similar to those obtained following birth and in non-pregnant adults. Lamivudine concentrations were generally similar in maternal, neonatal, and cord serum samples. In a subset of subjects from whom amniotic fluid specimens were obtained following natural rupture of membranes, amniotic fluid concentrations of lamivudine ranged from 1.2-2.5 μg/ml (150 mg twice daily) and 2.1-5.2 μg/ml (300 mg twice daily) and were typically greater than 2 times the maternal serum levels. See ADVERSE REACTIONS, Epivir for the limited late-pregnancy safety information available from these studies. Lamivudine should be used during pregnancy only if the potential benefits outweigh the risks.

Antiretroviral Pregnancy Registry: To monitor maternal-fetal outcomes of pregnant women exposed to lamivudine, a Pregnancy Registry has been established. Physicians are encouraged to register patients by calling 1-800-258-4263.

Nursing Mothers

The Centers for Disease Control and Prevention recommend that HIV-infected mothers not breastfeed their infants to avoid risking postnatal transmission of HIV infection.

A study in lactating rats administered 45 mg/kg of lamivudine showed that lamivudine concentrations in milk were slightly greater than those in plasma. Lamivudine is also excreted in human milk. Samples of breast milk obtained from 20 mothers receiving lamivudine monotherapy (300 mg twice daily) or combination therapy (150 mg lamivudine twice daily and 300 mg zidovudine twice daily) had measurable concentrations of lamivudine.

Because of both the potential for HIV transmission and the potential for serious adverse reactions in nursing infants, **mothers should be instructed not to breastfeed if they are receiving lamivudine.**

Pediatric Use

HIV

Limited, uncontrolled pharmacokinetic and safety data are available from administration of lamivudine (and zidovudine) to 36 infants up to 1 week of age in 2 studies in South Africa. In these studies, lamivudine clearance was substantially reduced in 1-week-old neonates relative to pediatric patients (>3 months of age) studied previously. There is insufficient information to establish the time course of changes in clearance between the immediate neonatal period and the age ranges >3 months old. See ADVERSE REACTIONS, Epivir for the limited safety information available from these studies.

The safety and effectiveness of twice daily Epivir in combination with other antiretroviral agents have been established in pediatric patients 3 months of age and older.

In Study A2002, pharmacokinetic properties of lamivudine were assessed in a subset of 57 HIV-infected pediatric patients (age range: 4.8 months to 16 years, weight range: 5-66 kg) after oral and IV administration of 1, 2, 4, 8, 12, and 20 mg/kg/day. In the 9 infants and children (range: 5 months to 12 years of age) receiving oral solution 4 mg/kg twice daily (the usual recommended pediatric dose), absolute bioavailability was 66% ± 26% (mean ±SD), which was less than the 86% ± 16% (mean ±SD) observed in adults. The mechanism for the diminished absolute bioavailability of lamivudine in infants and children is unknown.

After oral administration of lamivudine 4 mg/kg twice daily to 11 pediatric patients ranging from 4 months to 14 years of age, C_{max} was 1.1 ± 0.6 μg/ml and half-life was 2.0 ± 0.6 hours. (In adults with similar blood sampling, the half-life was 3.7 ± 1 hours.) Total exposure to lamivudine, as reflected by mean AUC values, was comparable between pediatric patients receiving an 8 mg/kg/day dose and adults receiving a 4 mg/kg/day dose.

Distribution of lamivudine into cerebrospinal fluid (CSF) was assessed in 38 pediatric patients after multiple oral dosing with lamivudine. CSF samples were collected between 2 and 4 hours postdose. At the dose of 8 mg/kg/day, CSF lamivudine concentrations in 8 patients ranged from 5.6-30.9% (mean ±SD of 14.2% ± 7.9%) of the concentration in a simultaneous serum sample, with CSF lamivudine concentrations ranging from 0.04-0.3 µg/ml.

The effect of renal impairment on lamivudine pharmacokinetics in pediatric patients is not known.

The safety and pharmacokinetic properties of Epivir in combination with antiretroviral agents other than zidovudine have not been established in pediatric patients.

See CLINICAL PHARMACOLOGY, Epivir; WARNINGS, Epivir; ADVERSE REACTIONS, Epivir; and DOSAGE AND ADMINISTRATION, Epivir.

HBV

See the complete prescribing information for Epivir-HBV tablets and oral solution for additional information on the pharmacokinetics of lamivudine in HBV-infected children.

Geriatric Use

Clinical studies of Epivir did not include sufficient numbers of subjects aged 65 and over to determine whether they respond differently from younger subjects. In general, dose selection for an elderly patient should be cautious, reflecting the greater frequency of decreased hepatic, renal, or cardiac function, and of concomitant disease or other drug therapy. In particular, because lamivudine is substantially excreted by the kidney and elderly patients are more likely to have decreased renal function, renal function should be monitored and dosage adjustments should be made accordingly (see Patients With Impaired Renal Function and DOSAGE AND ADMINISTRATION, Epivir).

EPIVIR-HBV

General

Patients should be assessed before beginning treatment with Epivir-HBV by a physician experienced in the management of chronic hepatitis B.

Emergence of Resistance-Associated HBV Mutations

In controlled clinical trials, YMDD-mutant HBV were detected in patients with on-lamivudine re-appearance of HBV DNA after an initial decline below the solution hybridization assay limit (see CLINICAL PHARMACOLOGY, Epivir-HBV, Microbiology, Drug Resistance). These mutations can be detected by a research assay and have been associated with reduced susceptibility to lamivudine *in vitro.* Lamivudine-treated patients (adult and pediatric) with YMDD-mutant HBV at 52 weeks showed diminished treatment responses in comparison to lamivudine-treated patients without evidence of YMDD mutations, including lower rates of HBeAg seroconversion and HBeAg loss (no greater than placebo recipients), more frequent return of positive HBV DNA by solution hybridization or branched-chain DNA assay, and more frequent ALT elevations. In the controlled trials, when patients developed YMDD-mutant HBV, they had a rise in HBV DNA and ALT from their own previous on-treatment levels. Progression of hepatitis B, including death, has been reported in some patients with YMDD-mutant HBV, including patients from the liver transplant setting and from other clinical trials. The long-term clinical significance of YMDD-mutant HBV is not known. Increased clinical and laboratory monitoring may aid in treatment decisions if emergence of viral mutants is suspected.

Limitations of Populations Studied

Safety and efficacy of Epivir-HBV have not been established in patients with decompensated liver disease or organ transplants; pediatric patients <2 years of age; patients dually infected with HBV and HCV, hepatitis delta, or HIV; or other populations not included in the principal Phase 3 controlled studies. There are no studies in pregnant women and no data regarding effect on vertical transmission, and appropriate infant immunizations should be used to prevent neonatal acquisition of HBV.

Assessing Patients During Treatment

Patients should be monitored regularly during treatment by a physician experienced in the management of chronic hepatitis B. The safety and effectiveness of treatment with Epivir-HBV beyond 1 year have not been established. During treatment, combinations of such events such as return of persistently elevated ALT, increasing levels of HBV DNA over time after an initial decline below assay limit, progression of clinical signs or symptoms of hepatic disease, and/or worsening of hepatic necroinflammatory findings may be considered as potentially reflecting loss of therapeutic response. Such observations should be taken into consideration when determining the advisability of continuing therapy with Epivir-HBV.

The optimal duration of treatment, the durability of HBeAg seroconversions occurring during treatment, and the relationship between treatment response and long-term outcomes such as hepatocellular carcinoma or decompensated cirrhosis are not known.

Patients With Impaired Renal Function

Reduction of the dosage of Epivir-HBV is recommended for patients with impaired renal function (see CLINICAL PHARMACOLOGY, Epivir-HBV and DOSAGE AND ADMINISTRATION, Epivir-HBV).

Information for the Patient

A Patient Package Insert (PPI) for Epivir-HBV is available for patient information.

Patients should remain under the care of a physician while taking Epivir-HBV. They should discuss any new symptoms or concurrent medications with their physician.

Patients should be advised that Epivir-HBV is not a cure for hepatitis B, that the long-term treatment benefits of Epivir-HBV are unknown at this time, and, in particular, that the relationship of initial treatment response to outcomes such as hepatocellular carcinoma and decompensated cirrhosis is unknown. Patients should be informed that deterioration of liver disease has occurred in some cases if treatment was discontinued, and that they should discuss any change in regimen with their physician. Patients should be informed that emergence of resistant hepatitis B virus and worsening of disease can occur during treatment, and they should promptly report any new symptoms to their physician.

Patients should be counseled on the importance of testing for HIV to avoid inappropriate therapy and development of resistant HIV, and HIV counseling and testing should be offered before starting Epivir-HBV and periodically during therapy. Patients should be advised that Epivir-HBV tablets and oral solution contain a lower dose of the same active ingredient (lamivudine) as Epivir tablets, Epivir oral solution, Combivir tablets, and Trizivir tablets. Epivir-HBV should not be taken concurrently with Epivir, Combivir, or Trizivir (see WARNINGS, Epivir-HBV). Patients infected with both HBV and HIV who are planning to change their HIV treatment regimen to a regimen that does not include Epivir, Combivir, or Trizivir should discuss continued therapy for hepatitis B with their physician.

Patients should be advised that treatment with Epivir-HBV has not been shown to reduce the risk of transmission of HBV to others through sexual contact or blood contamination (see Pregnancy Category C).

Carcinogenesis, Mutagenesis, and Impairment of Fertility

Lamivudine long-term carcinogenicity studies in mice and rats showed no evidence of carcinogenic potential at exposures up to 34 times (mice) and 200 times (rats) those observed in humans at the recommended therapeutic dose for chronic hepatitis B. Lamivudine was not active in a microbial mutagenicity screen or an *in vitro* cell transformation assay, but showed weak *in vitro* mutagenic activity in a cytogenetic assay using cultured human lymphocytes and in the mouse lymphoma assay. However, lamivudine showed no evidence of *in vivo* genotoxic activity in the rat at oral doses of up to 2000 mg/kg producing plasma levels of 60-70 times those in humans at the recommended dose for chronic hepatitis B. In a study of reproductive performance, lamivudine administered to rats at doses up to 4000 mg/kg/day, producing plasma levels 80-120 times those in humans, revealed no evidence of impaired fertility and no effect on the survival, growth, and development to weaning of the offspring.

Pregnancy Category C

Reproduction studies have been performed in rats and rabbits at orally administered doses up to 4000 mg/kg/day and 1000 mg/kg/day, respectively, producing plasma levels up to approximately 60 times that for the adult HBV dose. No evidence of teratogenicity due to lamivudine was observed. Evidence of early embryolethality was seen in the rabbit at exposure levels similar to those observed in humans, but there was no indication of this effect in the rat at exposures up to 60 times that in humans. Studies in pregnant rats and rabbits showed that lamivudine is transferred to the fetus through the placenta. There are no adequate and well-controlled studies in pregnant women. Because animal reproductive toxicity studies are not always predictive of human response, lamivudine should be used during pregnancy only if the potential benefits outweigh the risks.

Lamivudine has not been shown to affect the transmission of HBV from mother to infant, and appropriate infant immunizations should be used to prevent neonatal acquisition of HBV.

Pregnancy Registry: To monitor maternal-fetal outcomes of pregnant women exposed to lamivudine, a Pregnancy Registry has been established. Physicians are encouraged to register patients by calling 1-800-258-4263.

Nursing Mothers

A study in lactating rats showed that lamivudine concentrations in milk were similar to those in plasma. Although it is not known if lamivudine is excreted in human milk, there is the potential for adverse effects from lamivudine in nursing infants. Mothers should be instructed not to breastfeed if they are receiving lamivudine.

Pediatric Use

HBV

Safety and efficacy of lamivudine for treatment of chronic hepatitis B in children have been studied in pediatric patients from 2-17 years of age in a controlled clinical trial (see CLINICAL PHARMACOLOGY, Epivir-HBV; INDICATIONS AND USAGE, Epivir-HBV; and DOSAGE AND ADMINISTRATION, Epivir-HBV).

Safety and efficacy in pediatric patients <2 years of age have not been established.

HIV

See the complete prescribing information for Epivir tablets and oral solution for additional information on pharmacokinetics of lamivudine in HIV-infected children.

Geriatric Use

Clinical studies of Epivir-HBV did not include sufficient numbers of subjects aged 65 and over to determine whether they respond differently from younger subjects. In general, dose selection for an elderly patient should be cautious, reflecting the greater frequency of decreased hepatic, renal, or cardiac function, and of concomitant disease or other drug therapy. In particular, because lamivudine is substantially excreted by the kidney and elderly patients are more likely to have decreased renal function, renal function should be monitored and dosage adjustments should be made accordingly (see Patients With Impaired Renal Function and DOSAGE AND ADMINISTRATION, Epivir-HBV).

DRUG INTERACTIONS

EPIVIR

TMP 160 mg/SMX 800 mg once daily has been shown to increase lamivudine exposure (AUC) by 44% (see CLINICAL PHARMACOLOGY, Epivir). No change in dose of either drug is recommended. There is no information regarding the effect on lamivudine pharmacokinetics of higher doses of TMP/SMX such as those used to treat *Pneumocystis carinii* pneumonia. No data are available regarding the potential for interaction with other drugs that have renal clearance mechanisms similar to that of lamivudine.

Lamivudine and zalcitabine may inhibit the intracellular phosphorylation of one another. Therefore, use of lamivudine in combination with zalcitabine is not recommended.

EPIVIR-HBV

TMP 160 mg/SMX 800 mg once daily has been shown to increase lamivudine exposure (AUC) by 44% (see CLINICAL PHARMACOLOGY, Epivir-HBV). No change in dose of either drug is recommended. There is no information regarding the effect on lamivudine pharmacokinetics of higher doses of TMP/SMX such as those used to treat *Pneumocystis carinii* pneumonia. No data are available regarding the potential for interaction with other drugs that have renal clearance mechanisms similar to that of lamivudine.

L

Lamivudine and zalcitabine may inhibit the intracellular phosphorylation of one another. Therefore, use of lamivudine in combination with zalcitabine is not recommended.

ADVERSE REACTIONS

EPIVIR

Clinical Trials in HIV

Adults

Selected clinical adverse events with a ≥5% frequency during therapy with Epivir 150 mg twice daily plus Retrovir 200 mg 3 times daily compared with zidovudine are listed in TABLE 9.

TABLE 9 *Selected Clinical Adverse Events (≥5% Frequency) in Four Controlled Clinical Trials (A3001, A3002, B3001, B3002)*

Adverse Event	Epivir 150 mg Twice Daily + Retrovir (n=251)	Retrovir* (n=230)
Body as a Whole		
Headache	35%	27%
Malaise & fatigue	27%	23%
Fever or chills	10%	12%
Digestive		
Nausea	33%	29%
Diarrhea	18%	22%
Nausea & vomiting	13%	12%
Anorexia and/or decreased appetite	10%	7%
Abdominal pain	9%	11%
Abdominal cramps	6%	3%
Dyspepsia	5%	5%
Nervous System		
Neuropathy	12%	10%
Insomnia & other sleep disorders	11%	7%
Dizziness	10%	4%
Depressive disorders	9%	4%
Respiratory		
Nasal signs & symptoms	20%	11%
Cough	18%	13%
Skin		
Skin rashes	9%	6%
Musculoskeletal		
Musculoskeletal pain	12%	10%
Myalgia	8%	6%
Arthralgia	5%	5%

* Either zidovudine monotherapy or zidovudine in combination with zalcitabine.

The types and frequencies of clinical adverse events reported in patients receiving Epivir 300 mg once daily or Epivir 150 mg twice daily (in 3-drug combination regimens in EPV20001 and EPV40001) were similar. The most common adverse events in both treatment groups were nausea, dizziness, fatigue and/or malaise, headache, dreams, insomnia and other sleep disorders, and skin rash.

Pancreatitis was observed in 9 of the 2613 adult patients (0.3%) who received Epivir in the controlled clinical trials EPV20001, NUCA3001, NUCB3001, NUCA3002, NUCB3002, and B3007.

Selected laboratory abnormalities observed during therapy are summarized in TABLE 10.

In small, uncontrolled studies in which pregnant women were given lamivudine alone or in combination with zidovudine beginning in the last few weeks of pregnancy (see PRECAUTIONS, Pregnancy Category C), reported adverse events included anemia, urinary tract infections, and complications of labor and delivery. In postmarketing experience, liver function abnormalities and pancreatitis have been reported in women who received lamivudine in combination with other antiretroviral drugs during pregnancy. It is not known whether risks of adverse events associated with lamivudine are altered in pregnant women compared to other HIV-infected patients.

TABLE 10 *Frequencies of Selected Laboratory Abnormalities in Adults in Four 24 Week Surrogate Endpoint Studies (A3001, A3002, B3001, B3002) and a Clinical Endpoint Study (B3007)*

	24 Week Surrogate Endpoint Studies*		Clinical Endpoint Study*	
Test (Threshold Level)	Epivir + Retrovir	Retrovir†	Epivir + Current Therapy	Placebo + Current Therapy‡
Absolute neutrophil count (<750/mm^3)	7.2%	5.4%	15%	13%
Hemoglobin (<8.0 g/dl)	2.9%	1.8%	2.2%	3.4%
Platelets (<50,000/mm^3)	0.4%	1.3%	2.8%	3.8%
ALT (>5.0 × ULN)	3.7%	3.6%	3.8%	1.9%
AST (>5.0 × ULN)	1.7%	1.8%	4.0%	2.1%
Bilirubin (>2.5 × ULN)	0.8%	0.4%	ND	ND
Amylase (>2.0 × ULN)	4.2%	1.5%	2.2%	1.1%

* The median duration on study was 12 months.
† Either zidovudine monotherapy or zidovudine in combination with zalcitabine.
‡ Current therapy was either zidovudine, zidovudine + didanosine, or zidovudine + zalcitabine.
ULN = Upper limit of normal.
ND = Not done.

The frequencies of selected laboratory abnormalities reported in patients receiving Epivir 300 mg once daily or Epivir 150 mg twice daily (in 3-drug combination regimens in EPV20001 and EPV40001) were similar.

Pediatric Patients

Selected clinical adverse events and physical findings with a ≥5% frequency during therapy with Epivir 4 mg/kg twice daily plus Retrovir 160 mg/m^2 three times daily compared with didanosine in therapy-naive (≤56 days of antiretroviral therapy) pediatric patients are listed in TABLE 11.

TABLE 11 *Selected Clinical Adverse Events and Physical Findings (≥5% Frequency) in Pediatric Patients in Study ACTG300*

Adverse Event	Epivir + Retrovir (n=236)	Didanosine (n=235)
Body as a Whole		
Fever	25%	32%
Digestive		
Hepatomegaly	11%	11%
Nausea & vomiting	8%	7%
Diarrhea	8%	6%
Stomatitis	6%	12%
Splenomegaly	5%	8%
Respiratory		
Cough	15%	18%
Abnormal breath sounds/wheezing	7%	9%
Ear, Nose, and Throat		
Signs or symptoms of ears*	7%	6%
Nasal discharge or congestion	8%	11%
Other		
Skin rashes	12%	14%
Lymphadenopathy	9%	11%

* Includes pain, discharge, erythema, or swelling of an ear.

Selected laboratory abnormalities experienced by therapy-naive (≤56 days of antiretroviral therapy) pediatric patients are listed in TABLE 12.

TABLE 12 *Frequencies of Selected Laboratory Abnormalities in Pediatric Patients in Study ACTG300*

Test (Threshold Level)	Epivir + Retrovir	Didanosine
Absolute neutrophil count (<400/mm^3)	8%	3%
Hemoglobin (<7.0 g/dl)	4%	2%
Platelets (<50,000/mm^3)	1%	3%
ALT (>10 × ULN)	1%	3%
AST (>10 × ULN)	2%	4%
Lipase (>2.5 × ULN)	3%	3%
Total amylase (>2.5 × ULN)	3%	3%

ULN = Upper limit of normal.

Pancreatitis, which has been fatal in some cases, has been observed in antiretroviral nucleoside-experienced pediatric patients receiving Epivir alone or in combination with other antiretroviral agents. In an open-label dose-escalation study (A2002), 14 patients (14%) developed pancreatitis while receiving monotherapy with Epivir. Three of these patients died of complications of pancreatitis. In a second open-label study (A2005), 12 patients (18%) developed pancreatitis. In Study ACTG300, pancreatitis was not observed in 236 patients randomized to Epivir plus Retrovir. Pancreatitis was observed in 1 patient in this study who received open-label Epivir in combination with Retrovir and ritonavir following discontinuation of didanosine monotherapy.

Paresthesias and peripheral neuropathies were reported in 15 patients (15%) in Study A2002, 6 patients (9%) in Study A2005, and 2 patients (<1%) in Study ACTG300.

Limited short-term safety information is available from 2 small, uncontrolled studies in South Africa in neonates receiving lamivudine with or without zidovudine for the first week of life following maternal treatment starting at Week 38 or 36 of gestation (see PRECAUTIONS, Epivir, Pediatric Use). Adverse events reported in these neonates included increased liver function tests, anemia, diarrhea, electrolyte disturbances, hypoglycemia, jaundice and hepatomegaly, rash, respiratory infections, sepsis, and syphilis; 3 neonates died (1 from gastroenteritis with acidosis and convulsions, 1 from traumatic injury, and 1 from unknown causes). Two other nonfatal gastroenteritis or diarrhea cases were reported, including 1 with convulsions; 1 infant had transient renal insufficiency associated with dehydration. The absence of control groups further limits assessments of causality, but it should be assumed that perinatally-exposed infants may be at risk for adverse events comparable to those reported in pediatric and adult HIV-infected patients treated with lamivudine-containing combination regimens. Long-term effects of *in utero* and infant lamivudine exposure are not known.

Lamivudine in Patients With Chronic Hepatitis B

Clinical trials in chronic hepatitis B used a lower dose of lamivudine (100 mg daily) than the dose used to treat HIV. The most frequent adverse events with lamivudine versus placebo were ear, nose, and throat infections (25% vs 21%); malaise and fatigue (24% vs 28%); and headache (21% vs 21%), respectively. The most frequent laboratory abnormalities reported with lamivudine were elevated ALT, elevated serum lipase, elevated CPK, and posttreatment elevations of liver function tests. Emergence of HBV viral mutants during lamivudine treatment, associated with reduced drug susceptibility and diminished treatment response, was also reported (also see WARNINGS, Epivir and PRECAUTIONS, Epivir). Please see the complete prescribing information for Epivir-HBV tablets and oral solution for more information.

Observed During Clinical Practice

In addition to adverse events reported from clinical trials, the following events have been identified during post-approval use of lamivudine. Because they are reported voluntarily from a population of unknown size, estimates of frequency cannot be made. These events have been chosen for inclusion due to a combination of their seriousness, frequency of reporting, or potential causal connection to lamivudine.

Body as a Whole: Redistribution/accumulation of body fat (see PRECAUTIONS, Epivir, Fat Redistribution).

Digestive: Stomatitis.

Endocrine and Metabolic: Hyperglycemia.

General: Weakness.

Hemic and Lymphatic: Anemia (including pure red cell aplasia and severe anemias progressing on therapy), lymphadenopathy, splenomegaly.

Hepatic and Pancreatic: Lactic acidosis and hepatic steatosis, pancreatitis, posttreatment exacerbation of hepatitis B (see WARNINGS, Epivir and PRECAUTIONS, Epivir).

Hypersensitivity: Anaphylaxis, urticaria.

Musculoskeletal: Muscle weakness, CPK elevation, rhabdomyolysis.

Nervous: Paresthesia, peripheral neuropathy.

Respiratory: Abnormal breath sounds/wheezing.

Skin: Alopecia, rash, pruritus.

EPIVIR-HBV

Several serious adverse events reported with lamivudine (lactic acidosis and severe hepatomegaly with steatosis, posttreatment exacerbations of hepatitis B, pancreatitis, and emergence of viral mutants associated with reduced drug susceptibility and diminished treatment response) are also described in WARNINGS, Epivir-HBV and PRECAUTIONS, Epivir-HBV.

Clinical Trials in Chronic Hepatitis B

Adults

Selected clinical adverse events observed with a ≥5% frequency during therapy with Epivir-HBV compared with placebo are listed in TABLE 13. Frequencies of specified laboratory abnormalities during therapy with Epivir-HBV compared with placebo are listed in TABLE 14.

TABLE 13 *Selected Clinical Adverse Events (≥5% Frequency) in 3 Placebo-Controlled Clinical Trials During Treatment* — Studies 1-3*

Adverse Event	Epivir-HBV (n=332)	Placebo (n=200)
Non-Site Specific		
Malaise and fatigue	24%	28%
Fever or chills	7%	9%
Ear, Nose, and Throat		
Ear, nose, and throat infections	25%	21%
Sore throat	13%	8%
Gastrointestinal		
Nausea and vomiting	15%	17%
Abdominal discomfort and pain	16%	17%
Diarrhea	14%	12%
Musculoskeletal		
Myalgia	14%	17%
Arthralgia	7%	5%
Neurological		
Headache	21%	21%
Skin		
Skin rashes	5%	5%

* Includes patients treated for 52-68 weeks.

TABLE 14 *Frequencies of Specified Laboratory Abnormalities in 3 Placebo-Controlled Trials in Adults During Treatment*: Studies 1-3*

Test (Abnormal Level)	Patients With Abnormality/Patients With Observations: Epivir-HBV	Placebo
ALT >3 × baseline†	37/331 (11%)	26/199 (13%)
Albumin <2.5 g/dl	0/331 (0%)	2/199 (1%)
Amylase >3 × baseline	2/259 (<1%)	4/167 (2%)
Serum lipase ≥2.5 × ULN‡	19/189 (10%)	9/127 (7%)
CPK ≥7 × baseline	31/329 (9%)	9/198 (5%)
Neutrophils <750/mm^3	0/331 (0%)	1/199 (<1%)
Platelets <50,000/mm^3	10/272 (4%)	5/168 (3%)

* Includes patients treated for 52-68 weeks.
† See TABLE 15 for posttreatment ALT values.
‡ Includes observations during and after treatment in the 2 placebo-controlled trials that collected this information.
ULN = Upper limit of normal.

In patients followed for up to 16 weeks after discontinuation of treatment, posttreatment ALT elevations were observed more frequently in patients who had received Epivir-HBV than in patients who had received placebo. A comparison of ALT elevations between Weeks 52 and 68 in patients who discontinued Epivir-HBV at week 52 and patients in the same studies who received placebo throughout the treatment course is shown in TABLE 15.

TABLE 15 *Posttreatment ALT Elevations in 2 Placebo-Controlled Studies With No-Active-Treatment Follow-Up: Studies 1 and 3*

Abnormal Value	Patients With ALT Elevation/Patients With Observations*: Epivir-HBV	Placebo
ALT ≥2 × baseline value	37/137 (27%)	22/116 (19%)
ALT ≥3 × baseline value†	29/137 (21%)	9/116 (8%)
ALT ≥2 × baseline value and absolute ALT >500 IU/L	21/137 (15%)	8/116 (7%)
ALT ≥2 × baseline value; and bilirubin >2 × ULN and ≥2 × baseline value	1/137 (0.7%)	1/116 (0.9%)

* Each patient may be represented in 1 or more category.
† Comparable to a Grade 3 toxicity in accordance with modified WHO criteria.
ULN = Upper limit of normal.

Lamivudine in Patients With HIV

In HIV-infected patients, safety information reflects a higher dose of lamivudine (150 mg bid) than the dose used to treat chronic hepatitis B in HIV-negative patients. In clinical trials using lamivudine as part of a combination regimen for treatment of HIV infection, several clinical adverse events occurred more often in lamivudine-containing treatment arms than in comparator arms. These included nasal signs and symptoms (20% vs 11%), dizziness (10% vs 4%), and depressive disorders (9% vs 4%). Pancreatitis was observed in 3 of the 656 adult patients (<0.5%) who received Epivir in controlled clinical trials. Laboratory abnormalities reported more often in lamivudine-containing arms included neutropenia and elevations of liver function tests (also more frequent in lamivudine-containing arms for a retrospective analysis of HIV/HBV dually infected patients in 1 study), and amylase elevations. Please see the complete prescribing information for Epivir tablets and oral solution for more information.

Pediatric Patients With Hepatitis B

Most commonly observed adverse events in the pediatric trials were similar to those in adult trials; in addition, respiratory symptoms (cough, bronchitis, and viral respiratory infections) were reported in both lamivudine and placebo recipients. Posttreatment transaminase elevations were observed in some patients followed after cessation of lamivudine.

Pediatric Patients With HIV Infection

In early open-label studies of lamivudine in children with HIV, peripheral neuropathy and neutropenia were reported, and pancreatitis was observed in 14-15% of patients.

Observed During Clinical Practice

The following events have been identified during post-approval use of lamivudine in clinical practice. Because they are reported voluntarily from a population of unknown size, estimates of frequency cannot be made. These events have been chosen for inclusion due to either their seriousness, frequency of reporting, potential causal connection to lamivudine, or a combination of these factors. Postmarketing experience with lamivudine at this time is largely limited to use in HIV-infected patients.

Digestive: Stomatitis.

Endocrine and Metabolic: Hyperglycemia.

General: Weakness.

Hemic and Lymphatic: Anemia, pure red cell aplasia, lymphadenopathy, splenomegaly.

Hepatic and Pancreatic: Lactic acidosis and steatosis, pancreatitis, posttreatment exacerbation of hepatitis (see WARNINGS, Epivir-HBV and PRECAUTIONS, Epivir-HBV).

Hypersensitivity: Anaphylaxis, urticaria.

Musculoskeletal: Rhabdomyolysis.

Nervous: Paresthesia, peripheral neuropathy.

Respiratory: Abnormal breath sounds/wheezing.

Skin: Alopecia, pruritus, rash.

DOSAGE AND ADMINISTRATION

EPIVIR

Adults

The recommended oral dose of Epivir for adults is 300 mg daily, administered as either 150 mg twice daily or 300 mg once daily, in combination with other antiretroviral agents (see PRECAUTIONS, Epivir and CLINICAL PHARMACOLOGY, Epivir). If lamivudine is administered to a patient dually infected with HIV and HBV, the dosage indicated for HIV therapy should be used as part of an appropriate combination regimen (see WARNINGS, Epivir).

Pediatric Patients

The recommended oral dose of Epivir for HIV-infected pediatric patients 3 months up to 16 years of age is 4 mg/kg twice daily (up to a maximum of 150 mg twice a day), administered in combination with other antiretroviral agents.

Dose Adjustment

It is recommended that doses of Epivir be adjusted in accordance with renal function (see TABLE 16). (See CLINICAL PHARMACOLOGY, Epivir.)

Insufficient data are available to recommend a dosage of Epivir in patients undergoing dialysis. Although there are insufficient data to recommend a specific dose adjustment of Epivir in pediatric patients with renal impairment, a reduction in the dose and/or an increase in the dosing interval should be considered.

EPIVIR-HBV

Adults

The recommended oral dose of Epivir-HBV for treatment of chronic hepatitis B in adults is 100 mg once daily (see paragraph below and WARNINGS, Epivir-HBV). Safety and ef-

TABLE 16 *Adjustment of Dosage of Epivir in Adults and Adolescents in Accordance With Creatinine Clearance*

Creatinine Clearance	Recommended Dosage of Epivir
≥50 ml/min	150 mg twice daily or 300 mg once daily
30-49 ml/min	150 mg once daily
15-29 ml/min	150 mg first dose, then 100 mg once daily
5-14 ml/min	150 mg first dose, then 50 mg once daily
<5 ml/min	50 mg first dose, then 25 mg once daily

fectiveness of treatment beyond 1 year have not been established and the optimum duration of treatment is not known (see PRECAUTIONS, Epivir-HBV).

The formulation and dosage of lamivudine in Epivir-HBV are not appropriate for patients dually infected with HBV and HIV. If lamivudine is administered to such patients, the higher dosage indicated for HIV therapy should be used as part of an appropriate combination regimen, and the prescribing information for Epivir as well as Epivir-HBV should be consulted.

Pediatric Patients

The recommended oral dose of Epivir-HBV for pediatric patients 2-17 years of age with chronic hepatitis B is 3 mg/kg once daily up to a maximum daily dose of 100 mg. Safety and effectiveness of treatment beyond 1 year have not been established and the optimum duration of treatment is not known (see PRECAUTIONS, Epivir-HBV).

Epivir-HBV is available in a 5 mg/ml oral solution when a liquid formulation is needed. (Please see information above regarding distinctions between different lamivudine-containing products.)

Dose Adjustment

It is recommended that doses of Epivir-HBV be adjusted in accordance with renal function (TABLE 17) (see CLINICAL PHARMACOLOGY, Epivir-HBV, Special Populations).

TABLE 17 *Adjustment of Adult Dosage of Epivir-HBV in Accordance With Creatinine Clearance*

Creatinine Clearance	Recommended Dosage of Epivir-HBV
≥50 ml/min	100 mg once daily
30-49 ml/min	100 mg first dose, then 50 mg once daily
15-29 ml/min	100 mg first dose, then 25 mg once daily
5-14 ml/min	35 mg first dose, then 15 mg once daily
<5 ml/min	35 mg first dose, then 10 mg once daily

Although there are insufficient data to recommend a specific dose adjustment of Epivir-HBV in pediatric patients with renal impairment, a dose reduction should be considered.

No additional dosing of Epivir-HBV is required after routine (4 hour) hemodialysis. Insufficient data are available to recommend a dosage of Epivir-HBV in patients undergoing peritoneal dialysis (see CLINICAL PHARMACOLOGY, Epivir-HBV, Special Populations).

HOW SUPPLIED

EPIVIR

Epivir Tablets

Epivir tablets are available in:

150 mg: White, modified diamond-shaped, film-coated tablets engraved with "150" on one side and "GX CJ7" on the reverse side.

300 mg: Gray, modified diamond-shaped, film-coated tablets engraved with "GX EJ7" on one side and plain on the reverse side.

Storage: Store at 25°C (77°F), excursions permitted to 15-30°C (59-86°F).

Epivir Oral Solution

Epivir oral solution, a clear, colorless to pale yellow, strawberry-banana flavored liquid, contains 10 mg of lamivudine in each 1 ml in plastic bottles of 240 ml with child-resistant closures. This product does not require reconstitution.

Storage: Store in tightly closed bottles at 25°C (77°F).

EPIVIR-HBV

Epivir-HBV Tablets

Epivir-HBV tablets, 100 mg, are butterscotch-colored, film-coated, biconvex, capsule-shaped tablets imprinted with "GX CG5" on one side.

Storage: Store at controlled room temperature of 20-25°C (68-77°F) in tightly closed bottles.

Epivir-HBV Oral Solution

Epivir-HBV oral solution, a clear, colorless to pale yellow, strawberry-banana flavored liquid, contains 5 mg of lamivudine in each 1 ml.

This product does not require reconstitution.

Storage: Store at controlled room temperature of 20-25°C (68-77°F) in tightly closed bottles.

PRODUCT LISTING - EQUIVALENTS NOT AVAILABLE

Solution - Oral - 5 mg/ml
240 ml $60.67 EPIVIR HBV, Glaxosmithkline 00173-0663-00
Solution - Oral - 10 mg/ml
240 ml $84.28 EPIVIR, Glaxosmithkline 00173-0471-00
Tablet - Oral - 100 mg
60's $345.88 EPIVIR HBV, Glaxosmithkline 00173-0662-00
Tablet - Oral - 150 mg
2's $13.16 EPIVIR, Pharma Pac 52959-0508-02
4's $23.65 EPIVIR, Pharma Pac 52959-0508-04
6's $21.00 EPIVIR, Compumed Pharmaceuticals 00403-4977-06
6's $23.04 EPIVIR, Allscripts Pharmaceutical Company 54569-4221-01
6's $29.76 EPIVIR, Quality Care Pharmaceuticals Inc 60346-1016-06
6's $31.55 EPIVIR, Pharma Pac 52959-0508-06
8's $34.71 EPIVIR, Pharma Pac 52959-0508-08
14's $63.60 EPIVIR, Allscripts Pharmaceutical Company 54569-4221-02
14's $64.37 EPIVIR, Pharma Pac 52959-0508-14
15's $68.96 EPIVIR, Pharma Pac 52959-0508-15
60's $208.35 EPIVIR, Compumed Pharmaceuticals 00403-4977-60
60's $256.60 EPIVIR, Physicians Total Care 54868-3693-00
60's $272.59 EPIVIR, Allscripts Pharmaceutical Company 54569-4221-00
60's $275.45 EPIVIR, Pharma Pac 52959-0508-60
60's $316.04 EPIVIR, Glaxosmithkline 00173-0470-01
Tablet - Oral - 300 mg
30's $316.04 EPIVIR, Glaxosmithkline 00173-0714-00

Lamivudine; Zidovudine (003352)

For complete prescribing information, refer to the CD-ROM included with the book.

For related information, see the comparative table section in Appendix A.

Categories: Infection, human immunodeficiency virus; FDA Approved 1997 Sep; Pregnancy Category C
Drug Classes: Antivirals; Nucleoside reverse transcriptase inhibitors
Brand Names: **Combivir**
Foreign Brand Availability: Combid (Thailand); Lamuzid (Benin; Burkina-Faso; Ethiopia; Gambia; Ghana; Guinea; Ivory-Coast; Kenya; Liberia; Malawi; Mali; Mauritania; Mauritius; Morocco; Niger; Nigeria; Senegal; Seychelles; Sierra-Leone; Sudan; Tanzania; Tunia; Uganda; Zambia; Zimbabwe); Duovir (India); Retrovir/3TC Post-HIV Exposure Prophylaxis (South-Africa); Virdual (Colombia)
Cost of Therapy: $685.28 (HIV; Combivir; 150 mg; 300 mg; 2 tablets/day; 30 day supply)

WARNING

Note: The trade names have been used throughout this monograph for clarity.

ZIDOVUDINE, ONE OF THE TWO ACTIVE INGREDIENTS IN COMBIVIR, HAS BEEN ASSOCIATED WITH HEMATOLOGIC TOXICITY INCLUDING NEUTROPENIA AND SEVERE ANEMIA, PARTICULARLY IN PATIENTS WITH ADVANCED HIV DISEASE (SEE WARNINGS). PROLONGED USE OF ZIDOVUDINE HAS BEEN ASSOCIATED WITH SYMPTOMATIC MYOPATHY.

LACTIC ACIDOSIS AND SEVERE HEPATOMEGALY WITH STEATOSIS, INCLUDING FATAL CASES, HAVE BEEN REPORTED WITH THE USE OF NUCLEOSIDE ANALOGUES ALONE OR IN COMBINATION, INCLUDING LAMIVUDINE, ZIDOVUDINE, AND OTHER ANTIRETROVIRALS (SEE WARNINGS).

DESCRIPTION

COMBIVIR

Combivir tablets are combination tablets containing lamivudine and zidovudine. Lamivudine (Epivir, 3TC) and zidovudine (Retrovir, azidothymidine, AZT, or ZDV) are synthetic nucleoside analogues with activity against human immunodeficiency virus (HIV).

Combivir tablets are for oral administration. Each film-coated tablet contains 150 mg of lamivudine, 300 mg of zidovudine, and the inactive ingredients colloidal silicon dioxide, hydroxypropyl methylcellulose, magnesium stearate, microcrystalline cellulose, polyethylene glycol, polysorbate 80, sodium starch glycolate, and titanium dioxide.

LAMIVUDINE

The chemical name of lamivudine is (2R,cis)-4-amino-1-(2-hydroxymethyl-1,3-oxathiolan-5-yl)-(1H)-pyrimidin-2-one. Lamivudine is the (-)enantiomer of a dideoxy analogue of cytidine. Lamivudine has also been referred to as (-)2′,3′-dideoxy, 3′-thiacytidine. It has a molecular formula of $C_8H_{11}N_3O_3S$ and a molecular weight of 229.3.

Lamivudine is a white to off-white crystalline solid with a solubility of approximately 70 mg/ml in water at 20°C.

ZIDOVUDINE

The chemical name of zidovudine is 3′-azido-3′-deoxythymidine. It has a molecular formula of $C_{10}H_{13}N_5O_4$ and a molecular weight of 267.24.

Zidovudine is a white to beige, odorless, crystalline solid with a solubility of 20.1 mg/ml in water at 25°C.

INDICATIONS AND USAGE

Combivir in combination with other antiretroviral agents is indicated for the treatment of HIV infection.

NON-FDA APPROVED INDICATIONS

Lamivudine-zidovudine is also recommended by the Public Health Service interagency working group for use in postexposure prophylaxis of HIV although this is not approved by the FDA.

CONTRAINDICATIONS

Combivir tablets are contraindicated in patients with previously demonstrated clinically significant hypersensitivity to any of the components of the product.

WARNINGS

Combivir is a fixed-dose combination of lamivudine and zidovudine. Ordinarily, Combivir should not be administered concomitantly with lamivudine, zidovudine, or Trizivir, a fixed-dose combination of abacavir, lamivudine, and zidovudine.

The complete prescribing information for all agents being considered for use with Combivir should be consulted before combination therapy with Combivir is initiated.

BONE MARROW SUPPRESSION

Combivir should be used with caution in patients who have bone marrow compromise evidenced by granulocyte count <1000 cells/mm^3 or hemoglobin <9.5 g/dl.

Frequent blood counts are strongly recommended in patients with advanced HIV disease who are treated with Combivir. For HIV-infected individuals and patients with asymptomatic or early HIV disease, periodic blood counts are recommended.

LACTIC ACIDOSIS/SEVERE HEPATOMEGALY WITH STEATOSIS

Lactic acidosis and severe hepatomegaly with steatosis, including fatal cases, have been reported with the use of nucleoside analogues alone or in combination, including lamivudine, zidovudine, and other antiretrovirals. A majority of these cases have been in women. Obesity and prolonged nucleoside exposure may be risk factors. Particular caution should be exercised when administering Combivir to any patient with known risk factors for liver disease; however, cases have also been reported in patients with no known risk factors. Treatment with Combivir should be suspended in any patient who develops clinical or laboratory findings suggestive of lactic acidosis or pronounced hepatotoxicity (which may include hepatomegaly and steatosis even in the absence of marked transaminase elevations).

MYOPATHY

Myopathy and myositis, with pathological changes similar to that produced by HIV disease, have been associated with prolonged use of zidovudine, and therefore may occur with therapy with Combivir.

POSTTREATMENT EXACERBATIONS OF HEPATITIS

In clinical trials in non-HIV-infected patients treated with lamivudine for chronic hepatitis B, clinical and laboratory evidence of exacerbations of hepatitis have occurred after discontinuation of lamivudine. These exacerbations have been detected primarily by serum ALT elevations in addition to re-emergence of hepatitis B viral DNA (HBV DNA). Although most events appear to have been self-limited, fatalities have been reported in some cases. Similar events have been reported from post-marketing experience after changes from lamivudine-containing HIV treatment regimens to non-lamivudine-containing regimens in patients infected with both HIV and HBV. The causal relationship to discontinuation of lamivudine treatment is unknown. Patients should be closely monitored with both clinical and laboratory follow-up for at least several months after stopping treatment. There is insufficient evidence to determine whether re-initiation of lamivudine alters the course of posttreatment exacerbations of hepatitis.

DOSAGE AND ADMINISTRATION

The recommended oral dose of Combivir for adults and adolescents (at least 12 years of age) is 1 tablet (containing 150 mg of lamivudine and 300 mg of zidovudine) twice daily.

DOSE ADJUSTMENT

Because it is a fixed-dose combination, Combivir should not be prescribed for patients requiring dosage adjustment such as those with reduced renal function (creatinine clearance <50 ml/min) or those experiencing dose-limiting adverse events.

A reduction in the daily dose of zidovudine may be necessary in patients with mild to moderate impaired hepatic function or liver cirrhosis. Because Combivir is a fixed-dose combination that cannot be adjusted for this patient population, Combivir is not recommended for patients with impaired hepatic function.

PRODUCT LISTING - EQUIVALENTS NOT AVAILABLE

Tablet - Oral - 150 mg;300 mg

2's	$29.10	COMBIVIR, Pharma Pac	52959-0546-02
3's	$43.65	COMBIVIR, Pharma Pac	52959-0546-03
4's	$47.50	COMBIVIR, St. Mary'S Mpp	60760-0595-04
4's	$57.80	COMBIVIR, Pharma Pac	52959-0546-04
6's	$59.11	COMBIVIR, Allscripts Pharmaceutical Company	54569-4524-01
6's	$84.23	COMBIVIR, Pharma Pac	52959-0546-06
8's	$112.00	COMBIVIR, Pharma Pac	52959-0546-08
14's	$144.37	COMBIVIR, St. Mary'S Mpp	60760-0595-14
28's	$364.00	COMBIVIR, Pharma Pac	52959-0546-28
60's	$591.07	COMBIVIR, Allscripts Pharmaceutical Company	54569-4524-00
60's	$685.28	COMBIVIR, Glaxosmithkline	00173-0595-00
120's	$1370.55	COMBIVIR, Glaxosmithkline	00173-0595-02

Lamotrigine *(003155)*

Categories: Lennox-Gastaut syndrome; Seizures, partial; FDA Approved 1994 Dec; Pregnancy Category C; Orphan Drugs
Drug Classes: Anticonvulsants
Brand Names: Lamictal
Foreign Brand Availability: Lamictin (South-Africa); Lamogine (Israel)
Cost of Therapy: $191.41 (Epilepsy; Lamictal; 150 mg; 2 tablets/day; 30 day supply)

WARNING

SERIOUS RASHES REQUIRING HOSPITALIZATION AND DISCONTINUATION OF TREATMENT HAVE BEEN REPORTED IN ASSOCIATION WITH THE USE OF LAMOTRIGINE. THE INCIDENCE OF THESE RASHES,

WARNING — Cont'd

WHICH HAVE INCLUDED STEVENS-JOHNSON SYNDROME, IS APPROXIMATELY 0.8 (8/1000) IN PEDIATRIC PATIENTS (AGE <16 YEARS) RECEIVING LAMOTRIGINE AS ADJUNCTIVE THERAPY AND 0.3% (3/1000) IN ADULTS. IN A PROSPECTIVELY FOLLOWED COHORT OF 1983 PEDIATRIC PATIENTS TAKING ADJUNCTIVE LAMOTRIGINE, THERE WAS 1 RASH-RELATED DEATH. IN WORLDWIDE POSTMARKETING EXPERIENCE, RARE CASES OF TOXIC EPIDERMAL NECROLYSIS AND/OR RASH-RELATED DEATH HAVE BEEN REPORTED IN ADULT AND PEDIATRIC PATIENTS, BUT THEIR NUMBERS ARE TOO FEW TO PERMIT A PRECISE ESTIMATE OF THE RATE.

BECAUSE THE RATE OF SERIOUS RASH IS GREATER IN PEDIATRIC PATIENTS THAN IN ADULTS, IT BEARS EMPHASIS THAT LAMOTRIGINE IS APPROVED ONLY FOR USE IN PEDIATRIC PATIENTS BELOW THE AGE OF 16 YEARS WHO HAVE SEIZURES ASSOCIATED WITH THE LENNOX-GASTAUT SYNDROME OR IN PATIENTS WITH PARTIAL SEIZURES (SEE INDICATIONS AND USAGE).

OTHER THAN AGE, THERE ARE AS YET NO FACTORS IDENTIFIED THAT ARE KNOWN TO PREDICT THE RISK OF OCCURRENCE OR THE SEVERITY OF RASH ASSOCIATED WITH LAMOTRIGINE. THERE ARE SUGGESTIONS, YET TO BE PROVEN, THAT THE RISK OF RASH MAY ALSO BE INCREASED BY (1) COADMINISTRATION OF LAMOTRIGINE WITH VALPROIC ACID (VPA), (2) EXCEEDING THE RECOMMENDED INITIAL DOSE OF LAMOTRIGINE, OR (3) EXCEEDING THE RECOMMENDED DOSE ESCALATION FOR LAMOTRIGINE. HOWEVER, CASES HAVE BEEN REPORTED IN THE ABSENCE OF THESE FACTORS.

NEARLY ALL CASES OF LIFE-THREATENING RASHES ASSOCIATED WITH LAMOTRIGINE HAVE OCCURRED WITHIN 2-8 WEEKS OF TREATMENT INITIATION. HOWEVER, ISOLATED CASES HAVE BEEN REPORTED AFTER PROLONGED TREATMENT (*e.g.,* 6 MONTHS). ACCORDINGLY, DURATION OF THERAPY CANNOT BE RELIED UPON AS A MEANS TO PREDICT THE POTENTIAL RISK HERALDED BY THE FIRST APPEARANCE OF A RASH.

ALTHOUGH BENIGN RASHES ALSO OCCUR WITH LAMOTRIGINE, IT IS NOT POSSIBLE TO PREDICT RELIABLY WHICH RASHES WILL PROVE TO BE SERIOUS OR LIFE-THREATENING. ACCORDINGLY, LAMOTRIGINE SHOULD ORDINARILY BE DISCONTINUED AT THE FIRST SIGN OF RASH, UNLESS THE RASH IS CLEARLY NOT DRUG RELATED. DISCONTINUATION OF TREATMENT MAY NOT PREVENT A RASH FROM BECOMING LIFE THREATENING OR PERMANENTLY DISABLING OR DISFIGURING.

DESCRIPTION

Lamotrigine, an antiepileptic drug (AED) of the phenyltriazine class, is chemically unrelated to existing antiepileptic drugs. Its chemical name is 3,5-diamino-6-(2,3-dichlorophenyl)-*as*-triazine, its molecular formula is $C_9H_7N_5Cl_2$, and its molecular weight is 256.09. Lamotrigine is a white to pale cream-colored powder and has a pK_a of 5.7. Lamotrigine is very slightly soluble in water (0.17 mg/ml at 25°C) and slightly soluble in 0.1 M HCl (4.1 mg/ml at 25°C).

Lamictal tablets are supplied for oral administration as 25 mg (white), 100 mg (peach), 150 mg (cream), and 200 mg (blue) tablets. Each tablet contains the labeled amount of lamotrigine and the following inactive ingredients: lactose; magnesium stearate; microcrystalline cellulose; povidone; sodium starch glycolate; FD&C yellow no. 6 lake (100 mg tablet only); ferric oxide, yellow (150 mg tablet only); and FD&C blue no. 2 lake (200 mg tablet only).

Lamictal chewable dispersible tablets are supplied for oral administration. The tablets contain 2 mg (white), 5 mg (white) or 25 mg (white) of lamotrigine and the following inactive ingredients: blackcurrant flavor, calcium carbonate, low-substituted hydroxypropylcellulose, magnesium aluminum silicate, magnesium stearate, povidone, saccharin sodium, and sodium starch glycolate.

CLINICAL PHARMACOLOGY

MECHANISM OF ACTION

The precise mechanism(s) by which lamotrigine exerts its anticonvulsant action are unknown. In animal models designed to detect anticonvulsant activity, lamotrigine was effective in preventing seizure spread in the maximum electroshock (MES) and pentylenetetrazol (scMet) tests, and prevented seizures in the visually and electrically evoked after-discharge (EEAD) tests for antiepileptic activity. The relevance of these models to human epilepsy, however, is not known.

One proposed mechanism of action of lamotrigine, the relevance of which remains to be established in humans, involves an effect on sodium channels. *In vitro* pharmacological studies suggest that lamotrigine inhibits voltage-sensitive sodium channels, thereby stabilizing neuronal membranes and consequently modulating presynaptic transmitter release of excitatory amino acids (*e.g.,* glutamate and aspartate).

Lamotrigine also displayed inhibitory properties in the kindling model in rats both during kindling development and in the fully kindled state. The relevance of this animal model to specific types of human epilepsy is unclear.

PHARMACOLOGICAL PROPERTIES

Although the relevance for human use is unknown, the following data characterize the performance of lamotrigine in receptor binding assays. Lamotrigine had a weak inhibitory effect on the serotonin 5-HT_3 receptor (IC_{50} = 18 μM). It does not exhibit high affinity binding (IC_{50} >100 μM) to the following neurotransmitter receptors: adenosine A_1 and A_2; adrenergic α_1, α_2, and β; dopamine D_1 and D_2; γ-aminobutyric acid (GABA) A and B; histamine H_1; kappa opioid; muscarinic acetylcholine; and serotonin 5-HT_2. Studies have failed to detect an effect of lamotrigine on dihydropyridine-sensitive calcium channels. It had weak effects at sigma opioid receptors (IC_{50} = 145 μM). Lamotrigine did not inhibit the uptake of norepinephrine, dopamine, serotonin, or aspartic acid (IC_{50} >100 μM).

Effect of Lamotrigine on N-Methyl d-Aspartate (NMDA)-Mediated Activity

Lamotrigine did not inhibit NMDA-induced depolarizations in rat cortical slices or NMDA-induced cyclic GMP formation in immature rat cerebellum, nor did lamotrigine displace compounds that are either competitive or noncompetitive ligands at this glutamate receptor complex (CNQX, CGS, TCHP). The IC_{50} for lamotrigine effects on NMDA-induced currents (in the presence of 3 μM of glycine) in cultured hippocampal neurons exceeded 100 μM.

L

Folate Metabolism

In vitro, lamotrigine was shown to be an inhibitor of dihydrofolate reductase, the enzyme that catalyzes the reduction of dihydrofolate to tetrahydrofolate. Inhibition of this enzyme may interfere with the biosynthesis of nucleic acids and proteins. When oral daily doses of lamotrigine were given to pregnant rats during organogenesis, fetal, placental, and maternal folate concentrations were reduced. Significantly reduced concentrations of folate are associated with teratogenesis (see PRECAUTIONS, Pregnancy Category C). Folate concentrations were also reduced in male rats given repeated oral doses of lamotrigine. Reduced concentrations were partially returned to normal when supplemented with folinic acid.

Accumulation in Kidneys

Lamotrigine was found to accumulate in the kidney of the male rat, causing chronic progressive nephrosis, necrosis, and mineralization. These findings are attributed to α-2 microglobulin, a species- and sex-specific protein that has not been detected in humans or other animal species.

Melanin Binding

Lamotrigine binds to melanin-containing tissues, *e.g.*, in the eye and pigmented skin. It has been found in the uveal tract up to 52 weeks after a single dose in rodents.

Cardiovascular

In dogs, lamotrigine is extensively metabolized to a 2-N-methyl metabolite. This metabolite causes dose-dependent prolongations of the PR interval, widening of the QRS complex, and, at higher doses, complete AV conduction block. Similar cardiovascular effects are not anticipated in humans because only trace amounts of the 2-N-methyl metabolite (<0.6% of lamotrigine dose) have been found in human urine (see Drug Disposition). However, it is conceivable that plasma concentrations of this metabolite could be increased in patients with a reduced capacity to glucuronidate lamotrigine (*e.g.*, in patients with liver disease).

PHARMACOKINETICS AND DRUG METABOLISM

The pharmacokinetics of lamotrigine have been studied in patients with epilepsy, healthy young and elderly volunteers, and volunteers with chronic renal failure. Lamotrigine pharmacokinetic parameters for adult and pediatric patients and healthy normal volunteers are summarized in TABLE 1 and TABLE 2.

TABLE 1 *Mean* Pharmacokinetic Parameters in Adult Patients With Epilepsy or Healthy Volunteers*

Adult Study Population		T_{max}† (h)	T½‡ (h)	Cl/F§ (ml/min/kg)
Patients Taking Enzyme-Inducing Antiepileptic Drugs (EIAEDs)¤:				
Single-dose lamotrigine	n=24	2.3 (0.5-5.0)	14.4 (6.4-30.4)	1.10 (0.51-2.22)
Multiple-dose lamotrigine	n=17	2.0 (0.75-5.93)	12.6 (7.5-23.1)	1.21 (0.66-1.82)
Patients Taking EIAEDs + VPA:				
Single-dose lamotrigine	n=25	3.8 (1.0-10.0)	27.2 (11.2-51.6)	0.53 (0.27-1.04)
Patients Taking VPA Only:				
Single-dose lamotrigine	n=4	4.8 (1.8-8.4)	58.8 (30.5-88.8)	0.28 (0.16-0.40)
Healthy Volunteers Taking VPA:				
Single-dose lamotrigine	n=6	1.8 (1.0-4.0)	48.3 (31.5-88.6)	0.30 (0.14-0.42)
Multiple-dose lamotrigine	n=18	1.9 (0.5-3.5)	70.3 (41.9-113.5)	0.18 (0.12-0.33)
Healthy Volunteers Taking No Other Medications:				
Single-dose lamotrigine	n=179	2.2 (0.25-12.0)	32.8 (14.0-103.0)	0.44 (0.12-1.10)
Multiple-dose lamotrigine	n=36	1.7 (0.5-4.0)	25.4 (11.6-61.6)	0.58 (0.24-1.15)

* The majority of parameter means determined in each study had coefficients of variation between 20% and 40% for half-life and Cl/F and between 30% and 70% for T_{max}. The overall mean values were calculated from individual study means that were weighted based on the number of volunteers/patients in each study. The numbers in parentheses below each parameter mean represent the range of individual volunteer/patient values across studies.

† Time of maximum plasma concentration.

‡ Elimination half-life.

§ Apparent plasma clearance.

¤ Examples of EIAEDs are carbamazepine, phenobarbital, phenytoin, and primidone.

The apparent clearance of lamotrigine is affected by the coadministration of AEDs. Lamotrigine is eliminated more rapidly in patients who have been taking hepatic EIAEDs, including carbamazepine, phenytoin, phenobarbital, and primidone. Most clinical experience is derived from this population.

VPA, however, actually decreases the apparent clearance of lamotrigine (*i.e.,* more than doubles the elimination half-life of lamotrigine). Accordingly, if lamotrigine is to be administered to a patient receiving VPA, lamotrigine must be given at a reduced dosage, less than half the dose used in patients not receiving VPA (see DOSAGE AND ADMINISTRATION and DRUG INTERACTIONS).

Absorption

Lamotrigine is rapidly and completely absorbed after oral administration with negligible first-pass metabolism (absolute bioavailability is 98%). The bioavailability is not affected by food. Peak plasma concentrations occur anywhere from 1.4-4.8 hours following drug administration. The lamotrigine chewable/dispersible tablets were found to be equivalent, whether they were administered as dispersed in water, chewed and swallowed, or swallowed as whole, to the lamotrigine compressed tablets in terms of rate and extent of absorption.

Distribution

Estimates of the mean apparent volume of distribution (Vd/F) of lamotrigine following oral administration ranged from 0.9-1.3 L/kg. Vd/F is independent of dose and is similar following single and multiple doses in both patients with epilepsy and in healthy volunteers.

Protein Binding

Data from *in vitro studies* indicate that lamotrigine is approximately 55% bound to human plasma proteins at plasma lamotrigine concentrations from 1-10 μg/ml (10 μg/ml is 4-6 times the trough plasma concentration observed in the controlled efficacy trials). Because lamotrigine is not highly bound to plasma proteins, clinically significant interactions with other drugs through competition for protein binding sites are unlikely. The binding of lamotrigine to plasma proteins did not change in the presence of therapeutic concentrations of phenytoin, phenobarbital, or VPA. Lamotrigine did not displace other AEDs (carbamazepine, phenytoin, phenobarbital) from protein binding sites.

Drug Disposition

Lamotrigine is metabolized predominantly by glucuronic acid conjugation; the major metabolite is an inactive 2-N-glucuronide conjugate. After oral administration of 240 mg of ^{14}C-lamotrigine (15 μCi) to 6 healthy volunteers, 94% was recovered in the urine and 2% was recovered in the feces. The radioactivity in the urine consisted of unchanged lamotrigine (10%), the 2-N-glucuronide (76%), a 5-N-glucuronide (10%), a 2-N-methyl metabolite (0.14%), and other unidentified minor metabolites (4%).

Enzyme Induction

The effects of lamotrigine on specific families of mixed-function oxidase isozymes have not been systematically evaluated.

Following multiple administrations (150 mg twice daily) to normal volunteers taking no other medications, lamotrigine induced its own metabolism, resulting in a 25% decrease in T½ and a 37% increase in Cl/F at steady state compared to values obtained in the same volunteers following a single dose. Evidence gathered from other sources suggests that self-induction by lamotrigine may not occur when lamotrigine is given as adjunctive therapy in patients receiving EIAEDs.

Dose Proportionality

In healthy volunteers not receiving any other medications and given single doses, the plasma concentrations of lamotrigine increased in direct proportion to the dose administered over the range of 50-400 mg. In two small studies (n=7 and 8) of patients with epilepsy who were maintained on other AEDs, there also was a linear relationship between dose and lamotrigine plasma concentrations at steady state following doses of 50-350 mg twice daily.

Elimination

See TABLE 1.

SPECIAL POPULATIONS

Patients With Renal Insufficiency

Twelve (12) volunteers with chronic renal failure (mean creatinine clearance = 13 ml/min; range = 6-23) and another 6 individuals undergoing hemodialysis were each given a single 100 mg dose of lamotrigine. The mean plasma half-lives determined in the study were 42.9 hours (chronic renal failure), 13.0 hours (during hemodialysis), and 57.4 hours (between hemodialysis) compared to 26.2 hours in healthy volunteers. On average, approximately 20% (range = 5.6-35.1) of the amount of lamotrigine present in the body was eliminated by hemodialysis during a 4 hour session.

Hepatic Disease

The pharmacokinetics of lamotrigine following a single 100 mg dose of lamotrigine were evaluated in 24 subjects with moderate to severe hepatic dysfunction and compared with 12 subjects without hepatic impairment. The median apparent clearance of lamotrigine was 0.31, 0.24, or 0.10 ml/kg/min in patients with Grade A, B, or C (Child-Pugh Classification) hepatic impairment, respectively, compared to 0.34 ml/kg/min in the healthy controls. Median half-life of lamotrigine was 36, 60, or 110 hours in patients with Grade A, B, or C hepatic impairment, respectively, versus 32 hours in healthy controls.

Age

Pediatric Patients

The pharmacokinetics of lamotrigine following a single 2 mg/kg dose were evaluated in 2 studies of pediatric patients (n=29 for patients aged 10 months to 5.9 years and n=26 for patients aged 5-11 years). Forty-three (43) patients received concomitant therapy with other AEDS and 12 patients received lamotrigine as monotherapy. Lamotrigine pharmacokinetic parameters for pediatric patients are summarized in TABLE 2.

Population pharmacokinetic analyses involving patients aged 2-18 years demonstrated that lamotrigine clearance was influenced predominantly by total body weight and concurrent AED therapy. The oral clearance of lamotrigine was higher, on a body weight basis, in pediatric patients than in adults. Weight-normalized lamotrigine clearance was higher in those subjects weighing less than 30 kg, compared with those weighing greater than 30 kg. Accordingly, patients weighing less than 30 kg may need an increase of as much as 50% in maintenance doses, based on clinical response, as compared with subjects weighing more than 30 kg being administered the same AEDs (see DOSAGE AND ADMINISTRATION). These analyses also revealed that, after accounting for body weight, lamotrigine clearance was not significantly influenced by age. Thus, the same weight-adjusted doses should be administered to children irrespective of differences in age. Concomitant AEDs which influence lamotrigine clearance in adults were found to have similar effects in children.

Elderly

The pharmacokinetics of lamotrigine following a single 150 mg dose of lamotrigine were evaluated in 12 elderly volunteers between the ages of 65 and 76 years (mean creatinine clearance = 61 ml/min, range = 33-108 ml/min). The mean half-life of lamotrigine in these subjects was 31.2 hours (range 24.5-43.4 hours) and the mean clearance was 0.40 ml/min/kg (range 0.26-0.48 ml/min/kg).

TABLE 2 *Mean Pharmacokinetic Parameters in Pediatric Patients With Epilepsy*

Pediatric Study Population		T_{max} (h)	T½ (h)	Cl/F (ml/min/kg)
Ages 10 months to 5.3 years				
Patients taking EIAEDs	n=10	3.0 (1.0-5.9)	7.7 (5.7-11.4)	3.62 (2.44-5.28)
Patients taking AEDs with no known effect on drug-metabolizing enzymes	n=7	5.2 (2.9-6.1)	19.0 (12.9-27.1)	1.2 (0.75-2.42)
Patients taking VPA only	n=8	2.9 (1.0-6.0)	44.9 (29.5-52.5)	0.47 (0.23-0.77)
Ages 5-11 years				
Patients taking EIAEDs	n=7	1.6 (1.0-3.0)	7.0 (3.8-9.8)	2.54 (1.35-5.58)
Patients taking EIAEDs plus VPA	n=8	3.3 (1.0-6.4)	19.1 (7.0-31.2)	0.89 (0.39-1.93)
Patients taking VPA only*	n=3	4.5 (3.0-6.0)	65.8 (50.7-73.7)	0.24 (0.21-0.26)
Ages 13-18 years				
Patients taking EIAEDs	n=11	†	†	1.3
Patients taking EIAEDs plus VPA	n=8	†	†	0.5
Patients taking VPA only	n=4	†	†	0.3

* Two subjects were included in the calculation for mean T_{max}.
† Parameter not estimated.

Gender

The clearance of lamotrigine is not affected by gender.

Race

The apparent oral clearance of lamotrigine was 25% lower in non-Caucasians than Caucasians.

INDICATIONS AND USAGE

ADJUNCTIVE USE

Lamotrigine is indicated as adjunctive therapy for partial seizures in adults and pediatric patients (≥2 years of age).

Lamotrigine is also indicated as adjunctive therapy for the generalized seizures of Lennox-Gastaut syndrome in adult and pediatric patients (≥2 years of age).

MONOTHERAPY USE

Lamotrigine is indicated for conversion to monotherapy in adults with partial seizures who are receiving treatment with a single EIAED.

Safety and effectiveness of lamotrigine have not been established (1) as initial monotherapy, (2) for conversion to monotherapy from non-enzyme-inducing AEDs (*e.g.,* valproate), or (3) for simultaneous conversion to monotherapy from 2 or more concomitant AEDs (see DOSAGE AND ADMINISTRATION).

Safety and effectiveness in patients below the age of 16 other than those with partial seizures and the generalized seizures of Lennox-Gastaut syndrome have not been established (see BOXED WARNING).

NON-FDA APPROVED INDICATIONS

Lamotrigine has also shown efficacy in the treatment of bipolar disorder, the prophylaxis of migraine with aura, the relief of central post-stroke pain, and the reduction of diabetic neuropathy pain. However, these uses are not approved by the FDA and large controlled studies have not yet been performed.

CONTRAINDICATIONS

Lamotrigine is contraindicated in patients who have demonstrated hypersensitivity to the drug or its ingredients.

WARNINGS

SEE BOXED WARNING REGARDING THE RISK OF SERIOUS RASHES REQUIRING HOSPITALIZATION AND DISCONTINUATION OF LAMOTRIGINE.

ALTHOUGH BENIGN RASHES ALSO OCCUR WITH LAMOTRIGINE, IT IS NOT POSSIBLE TO PREDICT RELIABLY WHICH RASHES WILL PROVE TO BE SERIOUS OR LIFE THREATENING. ACCORDINGLY, LAMOTRIGINE SHOULD ORDINARILY BE DISCONTINUED AT THE FIRST SIGN OF RASH, UNLESS THE RASH IS CLEARLY NOT DRUG RELATED. DISCONTINUATION OF TREATMENT MAY NOT PREVENT A RASH FROM BECOMING LIFE THREATENING OR PERMANENTLY DISABLING OR DISFIGURING.

SERIOUS RASH

Pediatric Population

The incidence of serious rash associated with hospitalization and discontinuation of lamotrigine in a prospectively followed cohort of pediatric patients receiving adjunctive therapy was approximately 0.8% (16 of 1983). When 14 of these cases were reviewed by 3 expert dermatologists, there was considerable disagreement as to their proper classification. To illustrate, one dermatologist considered none of the cases to be Stevens-Johnson syndrome; another assigned 7 of the 14 to this diagnosis. There was 1 rash related death in this 1983 patient cohort. Additionally, there have been rare cases of toxic epidermal necrolysis with and without permanent sequelae and/or death in US and foreign postmarketing experience. It bears emphasis, accordingly, that lamotrigine is only approved for use in those patients below the age of 16 who have partial seizures or generalized seizures associated with the Lennox-Gastaut syndrome (see INDICATIONS AND USAGE).

There is evidence that the inclusion of VPA in a multidrug regimen increases the risk of serious, potentially life-threatening rash in pediatric patients. In pediatric patients who used VPA concomitantly, 1.2% (6 of 482) experienced a serious rash compared to 0.6% (6 of 952) patients not taking VPA.

Adult Population

Serious rash associated with hospitalization and discontinuation of lamotrigine occurred in 0.3% (11/3348) of patients who received lamotrigine in premarketing clinical trials. No fatalities occurred among these individuals. However, in worldwide postmarketing experience, rare cases of rash-related death have been reported, but their numbers are too few to permit a precise estimate of the rate.

Among the rashes leading to hospitalization were Stevens-Johnson syndrome, toxic epidermal necrolysis, angioedema, and a rash associated with a variable number of the following systemic manifestations: fever, lymphadenopathy, facial swelling, hematologic, and hepatologic abnormalities.

There is evidence that the inclusion of VPA in a multidrug regimen increases the risk of serious, potentially life-threatening rash in adults. Specifically, of 584 patients administered lamotrigine with VPA in clinical trials, 6 (1%) were hospitalized in association with rash; in contrast, 4 (0.16%) of 2398 clinical trial patients and volunteers administered lamotrigine in the absence of VPA were hospitalized.

Other examples of serious and potentially life-threatening rash that did not lead to hospitalization also occurred in premarketing development. Among these, 1 case was reported to be Stevens-Johnson-like.

HYPERSENSITIVITY REACTIONS

Hypersensitivity reactions, some fatal or life threatening, have also occurred. Some of these reactions have included clinical features of multiorgan failure/dysfunction, including hepatic abnormalities and evidence of disseminated intravascular coagulation. It is important to note that early manifestations of hypersensitivity (*e.g.,* fever, lymphadenopathy) may be present even though a rash is not evident. If such signs or symptoms are present, the patient should be evaluated immediately. Lamotrigine should be discontinued if an alternative etiology for the signs or symptoms cannot be established.

Prior to initiation of treatment with lamotrigine, the patient should be instructed that a rash or other signs or symptoms of hypersensitivity (*e.g.,* fever, lymphadenopathy) may herald a serious medical event and that the patient should report any such occurrence to a physician immediately.

ACUTE MULTIORGAN FAILURE

Multiorgan failure, which in some cases has been fatal or irreversible, has been observed in patients receiving lamotrigine. Fatalities associated with multiorgan failure and various degrees of hepatic failure have been reported in 2 of 3796 adult patients and 4 of 2435 pediatric patients who received lamotrigine in clinical trials. Rare fatalities from multiorgan failure have also been reported in compassionate plea and postmarketing use. The majority of these deaths occurred in association with other serious medical events, including status epilepticus and overwhelming sepsis, and hantavirus making it difficult to identify the initial cause.

Additionally, 3 patients (a 45-year-old woman, a 3.5-year-old boy, and an 11-year-old girl) developed multiorgan dysfunction and disseminated intravascular coagulation 9-14 days after lamotrigine was added to their AED regimens. Rash and elevated transaminases were also present in all patients and rhabdomyolysis was noted in 2 patients. Both pediatric patients were receiving concomitant therapy with VPA, while the adult patient was being treated with carbamazepine and clonazepam. All patients subsequently recovered with supportive care after treatment with lamotrigine was discontinued.

BLOOD DYSCRASIAS

There have been reports of blood dyscrasias that may or may not be associated with the hypersensitivity syndrome. These have included neutropenia, leukopenia, anemia, thrombocytopenia, pancytopenia, and, rarely, aplastic anemia and pure red cell aplasia.

WITHDRAWAL SEIZURES

As a rule, AEDs should not be abruptly discontinued because of the possibility of increasing seizure frequency. Unless safety concerns require a more rapid withdrawal, the dose of lamotrigine should be tapered over a period of at least 2 weeks (see DOSAGE AND ADMINISTRATION).

PRECAUTIONS

DERMATOLOGICAL EVENTS

See BOXED WARNING and WARNINGS.

Serious rashes associated with hospitalization and discontinuation of lamotrigine have been reported. Rare deaths have been reported, but their numbers are too few to permit a precise estimate of the rate. There are suggestions, yet to be proven, that the risk of rash may also be increased by (1) coadministration of lamotrigine with VPA, (2) exceeding the recommended initial dose of lamotrigine, or (3) exceeding the recommended dose escalation for lamotrigine. However, cases have been reported in the absence of these factors.

In clinical trials, approximately 10% of all patients exposed to lamotrigine developed a rash. Rashes associated with lamotrigine do not appear to have unique identifying features. Typically, rash occurs in the first 2-8 weeks following treatment initiation. However, isolated cases have been reported after prolonged treatment (*e.g.,* 6 months). Accordingly, duration of therapy cannot be relied upon as a means to predict the potential risk heralded by the first appearance of a rash.

Although most rashes resolved even with continuation of treatment with lamotrigine, it is not possible to predict reliably which rashes will prove to be serious or life threatening. **ACCORDINGLY, LAMOTRIGINE SHOULD ORDINARILY BE DISCONTINUED AT THE FIRST SIGN OF RASH, UNLESS THE RASH IS CLEARLY NOT DRUG RELATED. DISCONTINUATION OF TREATMENT MAY NOT PREVENT A RASH FROM BECOMING LIFE THREATENING OR PERMANENTLY DISABLING OR DISFIGURING.**

It is recommended that lamotrigine not be restarted in patients who discontinued due to rash associated with prior treatment with lamotrigine unless the potential benefits clearly outweigh the risks. If the decision is made to restart a patient who has discontinued lam-

L

otrigine, the need to restart with the initial dosing recommendations should be assessed. The greater the interval of time since the previous dose, the greater consideration should be given to restarting with the initial dosing recommendations. If a patient has discontinued lamotrigine for a period of more than 5 half-lives, it is recommended that initial dosing recommendations and guidelines be followed. The half-life of lamotrigine is affected by other concomitant medications (see CLINICAL PHARMACOLOGY, Pharmacokinetics and Drug Metabolism and DOSAGE AND ADMINISTRATION).

SUDDEN UNEXPLAINED DEATH IN EPILEPSY (SUDEP)

During the premarketing development of lamotrigine, 20 sudden and unexplained deaths were recorded among a cohort of 4700 patients with epilepsy (5747 patient-years of exposure).

Some of these could represent seizure-related deaths in which the seizure was not observed, *e.g.,* at night. This represents an incidence of 0.0035 deaths per patient-year. Although this rate exceeds that expected in a healthy population matched for age and sex, it is within the range of estimates for the incidence of sudden unexplained deaths in patients with epilepsy not receiving lamotrigine (ranging from 0.0005 for the general population of patients with epilepsy, to 0.004 for a recently studied clinical trial population similar to that in the clinical development program for lamotrigine, to 0.005 for patients with refractory epilepsy). Consequently, whether these figures are reassuring or suggest concern depends on the comparability of the populations reported upon to the cohort receiving lamotrigine and the accuracy of the estimates provided. Probably most reassuring is the similarity of estimated SUDEP rates in patients receiving lamotrigine and those receiving another antiepileptic drug that underwent clinical testing in a similar population at about the same time. Importantly, that drug is chemically unrelated to lamotrigine. This evidence suggests, although it certainly does not prove, that the high SUDEP rates reflect population rates, not a drug effect.

STATUS EPILEPTICUS

Valid estimates of the incidence of treatment emergent status epilepticus among patients treated with lamotrigine are difficult to obtain because reporters participating in clinical trials did not all employ identical rules for identifying cases. At a minimum, 7 of 2343 adult patients had episodes that could unequivocally be described as status. In addition, a number of reports of variably defined episodes of seizure exacerbation (*e.g.,* seizure clusters, seizure flurries, etc.) were made.

ADDITION OF LAMOTRIGINE TO A MULTIDRUG REGIMEN THAT INCLUDES VPA (DOSAGE REDUCTION)

L

Because VPA reduces the clearance of lamotrigine, the dosage of lamotrigine in the presence of VPA is less than half of that required in its absence (see DOSAGE AND ADMINISTRATION).

USE IN PATIENTS WITH CONCOMITANT ILLNESS

Clinical experience with lamotrigine in patients with concomitant illness is limited. Caution is advised when using lamotrigine in patients with diseases or conditions that could affect metabolism or elimination of the drug, such as renal, hepatic, or cardiac functional impairment.

Hepatic metabolism to the glucuronide followed by renal excretion is the principal route of elimination of lamotrigine (see CLINICAL PHARMACOLOGY).

A study in individuals with severe chronic renal failure (mean creatinine clearance = 13 ml/min) not receiving other AEDs indicated that the elimination half-life of unchanged lamotrigine is prolonged relative to individuals with normal renal function. Until adequate numbers of patients with severe renal impairment have been evaluated during chronic treatment with lamotrigine, it should be used with caution in these patients, generally using a reduced maintenance dose for patients with significant impairment.

Because there is limited experience with the use of lamotrigine in patients with impaired liver function, the use in such patients may be associated with as yet unrecognized risks (see CLINICAL PHARMACOLOGY and DOSAGE AND ADMINISTRATION).

BINDING IN THE EYE AND OTHER MELANIN-CONTAINING TISSUES

Because lamotrigine binds to melanin, it could accumulate in melanin-rich tissues over time. This raises the possibility that lamotrigine may cause toxicity in these tissues after extended use. Although ophthalmological testing was performed in one controlled clinical trial, the testing was inadequate to exclude subtle effects or injury occurring after long-term exposure. Moreover, the capacity of available tests to detect potentially adverse consequences, if any, of lamotrigine's binding to melanin is unknown.

Accordingly, although there are no specific recommendations for periodic ophthalmological monitoring, prescribers should be aware of the possibility of long-term ophthalmologic effects.

INFORMATION FOR THE PATIENT

Prior to initiation of treatment with lamotrigine, the patient should be instructed that a rash or other signs or symptoms of hypersensitivity (*e.g.,* fever, lymphadenopathy) may herald a serious medical event and that the patient should report any such occurrence to a physician immediately. In addition, the patient should notify his or her physician if worsening of seizure control occurs.

Patients should be advised that lamotrigine may cause dizziness, somnolence, and other symptoms and signs of central nervous system (CNS) depression. Accordingly, they should be advised neither to drive a car nor to operate other complex machinery until they have gained sufficient experience on lamotrigine to gauge whether or not it adversely affects their mental and/or motor performance.

Patients should be advised to notify their physicians if they become pregnant or intend to become pregnant during therapy. Patients should be advised to notify their physicians if they intend to breast-feed or are breast-feeding an infant.

Patients should be advised to notify their physician if they stop taking lamotrigine for any reason and not to resume lamotrigine without consulting their physician.

Patients should be informed of the availability of a patient information leaflet, and they should be instructed to read the leaflet prior to taking lamotrigine. See Patient Information at the end of this labeling for the text of the leaflet provided for patients.

LABORATORY TESTS

The value of monitoring plasma concentrations of lamotrigine has not been established. Because of the possible pharmacokinetic interactions between lamotrigine and other AEDs being taken concomitantly (see TABLE 3), monitoring of the plasma levels of lamotrigine and concomitant AEDs may be indicated, particularly during dosage adjustments. In general, clinical judgment should be exercised regarding monitoring of plasma levels of lamotrigine and other anti-seizure drugs and whether or not dosage adjustments are necessary.

DRUG/LABORATORY TEST INTERACTIONS

None known.

CARCINOGENESIS, MUTAGENESIS, AND IMPAIRMENT OF FERTILITY

No evidence of carcinogenicity was seen in one mouse study or two rat studies following oral administration of lamotrigine for up to 2 years at maximum tolerated doses (30 mg/kg/day for mice and 10-15 mg/kg/day for rats, doses that are equivalent to 90 mg/m^2 and 60-90 mg/m^2, respectively). Steady-state plasma concentrations ranged from 1-4 μg/ml in the mouse study and 1-10 μg/ml in the rat study. Plasma concentrations associated with the recommended human doses of 300-500 mg/day are generally in the range of 2-5 μg/ml, but concentrations as high as 19 μg/ml have been recorded.

Lamotrigine was not mutagenic in the presence or absence of metabolic activation when tested in two gene mutation assays (the Ames test and the *in vitro* mammalian mouse lymphoma assay). In two cytogenetic assays (the *in vitro* human lymphocyte assay and the *in vivo* rat bone marrow assay), lamotrigine did not increase the incidence of structural or numerical chromosomal abnormalities.

No evidence of impairment of fertility was detected in rats given oral doses of lamotrigine up to 2.4 times the highest usual human maintenance dose of 8.33 mg/kg/day or 0.4 times the human dose on a mg/m^2 basis. The effect of lamotrigine on human fertility is unknown.

PREGNANCY CATEGORY C

No evidence of teratogenicity was found in mice, rats, or rabbits when lamotrigine was orally administered to pregnant animals during the period of organogenesis at doses up to 1.2, 0.5, and 1.1 times, respectively, on a mg/m^2 basis, the highest usual human maintenance dose (*i.e.,* 500 mg/day). However, maternal toxicity and secondary fetal toxicity producing reduced fetal weight and/or delayed ossification were seen in mice and rats, but not in rabbits at these doses. Teratology studies were also conducted using bolus IV administration of the isethionate salt of lamotrigine in rats and rabbits. In rat dams administered an IV dose at 0.6 times the highest usual human maintenance dose, the incidence of intrauterine death without signs of teratogenicity was increased.

A behavioral teratology study was conducted in rats dosed during the period of organogenesis. At Day 21 postpartum, offspring of dams receiving 5 mg/kg/day or higher displayed a significantly longer latent period for open field exploration and a lower frequency of rearing. In a swimming maze test performed on Days 39-44 postpartum, time to completion was increased in offspring of dams receiving 25 mg/kg/day. These doses represent 0.1 and 0.5 times the clinical dose on a mg/m^2 basis, respectively.

Lamotrigine did not affect fertility, teratogenesis, or postnatal development when rats were dosed prior to and during mating, and throughout gestation and lactation at doses equivalent to 0.4 times the highest usual human maintenance dose on a mg/m^2 basis.

When pregnant rats were orally dosed at 0.1, 0.14, or 0.3 times the highest human maintenance dose (on a mg/m^2 basis) during the latter part of gestation (Days 15-20), maternal toxicity and fetal death were seen. In dams, food consumption and weight gain were reduced, and the gestation period was slightly prolonged (22.6 vs 22.0 days in the control group). Stillborn pups were found in all 3 drug-treated groups with the highest number in the high-dose group. Postnatal death was also seen, but only in the 2 highest doses, and occurred between Day 1 and 20. Some of these deaths appear to be drug-related and not secondary to the maternal toxicity. A no-observed-effect level (NOEL) could not be determined for this study.

Although lamotrigine was not found to be teratogenic in the above studies, lamotrigine decreases fetal folate concentrations in rats, an effect known to be associated with teratogenesis in animals and humans. There are no adequate and well-controlled studies in pregnant women. Because animal reproduction studies are not always predictive of human response, this drug should be used during pregnancy only if the potential benefit justifies the potential risk to the fetus.

Nonteratogenic Effects

As with other antiepileptic drugs, physiological changes during pregnancy may affect lamotrigine concentrations and/or therapeutic effect. There have been reports of decreased lamotrigine concentrations during pregnancy and restoration of pre-partum concentrations after delivery. Dosage adjustments may be necessary to maintain clinical response.

PREGNANCY EXPOSURE REGISTRY

To facilitate monitoring fetal outcomes of pregnant women exposed to lamotrigine, physicians are encouraged to register patients, **before fetal outcome (*e.g.,* ultrasound, results of amniocentesis, birth, etc.) is known,** and can obtain information by calling the Lamotrigine Pregnancy Registry at 800-336-2176 (toll-free). Patients can enroll themselves in the North American Antiepileptic Drug Pregnancy Registry by calling 888-233-2334 (toll free).

Labor and Delivery

The effect of lamotrigine on labor and delivery in humans is unknown.

USE IN NURSING MOTHERS

Preliminary data indicate that lamotrigine passes into human milk. Because the effects on the infant exposed to lamotrigine by this route are unknown, breast-feeding while taking lamotrigine is not recommended.

PEDIATRIC USE

Lamotrigine is indicated as adjunctive therapy for partial seizures in patients above 2 years of age and for the generalized seizures of Lennox-Gastaut syndrome. Safety and effectiveness for other uses in patients below the age of 16 years have not been established (see BOXED WARNING).

GERIATRIC USE

Clinical studies of lamotrigine did not include sufficient numbers of subjects aged 65 and over to determine whether they respond differently from younger subjects. In general, dose selection for an elderly patient should be cautious, usually starting at the low end of the dosing range, reflecting the greater frequency of decreased hepatic, renal, or cardiac function, and of concomitant disease or other drug therapy.

DRUG INTERACTIONS

ANTIEPILEPTIC DRUGS

The use of AEDs in combination is complicated by the potential for pharmacokinetic interactions.

The interaction of lamotrigine with phenytoin, carbamazepine, and VPA has been studied. The net effects of these various AED combinations on individual AED plasma concentrations are summarized in TABLE 3.

TABLE 3 *Summary of AED Interactions With Lamotrigine*

AED	AED Plasma Concentration With Adjunctive Lamotrigine*	Lamotrigine Plasma Concentration With Adjunctive AEDs†
Phenytoin (PHT)	NC	Decreases
Carbamazepine (CBZ)	NC	Decreases
CBZ epoxide‡	?	
Valproic acid (VPA)	Decreases	Increases
VPA + PHT and/or CBZ	NE	NC

* From adjunctive clinical trials and volunteer studies.
† Net effects were estimated by comparing the mean clearance values obtained in adjunctive clinical trials and volunteers studies.
‡ Not administered, but an active metabolite of carbamazepine.
NC = No significant effect.
? = Conflicting data.
NE = Not evaluated.

SPECIFIC EFFECTS OF LAMOTRIGINE ON THE PHARMACOKINETICS OF OTHER AED PRODUCTS

Lamotrigine Added to Phenytoin

Lamotrigine has no appreciable effect on steady-state phenytoin plasma concentration.

Lamotrigine Added to Carbamazepine

Lamotrigine has no appreciable effect on steady-state carbamazepine plasma concentration. Limited clinical data suggest there is a higher incidence of dizziness, diplopia, ataxia, and blurred vision in patients receiving carbamazepine with lamotrigine than in patients receiving other EIAEDs with lamotrigine (see ADVERSE REACTIONS). The mechanism of this interaction is unclear. The effect of lamotrigine on plasma concentrations of carbamazepine-epoxide is unclear. In a small subset of patients (n=7) studied in a placebo-controlled trial, lamotrigine had no effect on carbamazepine-epoxide plasma concentrations, but in a small, uncontrolled study (n=9), carbamazepine-epoxide levels were seen to increase.

Lamotrigine Added to VPA

When lamotrigine was administered to 18 healthy volunteers receiving VPA in a pharmacokinetic study, the trough steady-state VPA concentrations in plasma decreased by an average of 25% over a 3 week period, and then stabilized. However, adding lamotrigine to the existing therapy did not cause a change in plasma VPA concentrations in either adult or pediatric patients in controlled clinical trials.

SPECIFIC EFFECTS OF OTHER AED PRODUCTS ON THE PHARMACOKINETICS OF LAMOTRIGINE

Phenytoin Added to Lamotrigine

The addition of phenytoin decreases lamotrigine steady-state concentrations by approximately 45-54% depending upon the total daily dose of phenytoin (*i.e.*, from 100-400 mg).

Carbamazepine Added to Lamotrigine

The addition of carbamazepine decreases lamotrigine steady-state concentrations by approximately 40%.

Phenobarbital or Primidone Added to Lamotrigine

The addition of phenobarbital or primidone decreases lamotrigine steady-state concentrations by approximately 40%.

VPA Added to Lamotrigine

The addition of VPA increases lamotrigine steady-state concentrations in normal volunteers by slightly more than 2-fold.

INTERACTIONS WITH DRUG PRODUCTS OTHER THAN AEDS

Folate Inhibitors

Lamotrigine is an inhibitor of dihydrofolate reductase. Prescribers should be aware of this action when prescribing other medications that inhibit folate metabolism.

Oral Contraceptives

In women taking lamotrigine, there have been reports of decreased lamotrigine concentrations following introduction of oral contraceptives and reports of increased lamotrigine concentrations following withdrawal of oral contraceptives. Dosage adjustments may be necessary to maintain clinical response when starting or stopping oral contraceptives during lamotrigine therapy.

ADVERSE REACTIONS

SERIOUS RASH REQUIRING HOSPITALIZATION AND DISCONTINUATION OF LAMOTRIGINE, INCLUDING STEVENS-JOHNSON SYNDROME AND TOXIC EPIDERMAL NECROLYSIS, HAVE OCCURRED IN ASSOCIATION WITH THERAPY WITH LAMOTRIGINE. RARE DEATHS HAVE BEEN REPORTED, BUT THEIR NUMBERS ARE TOO FEW TO PERMIT A PRECISE ESTIMATE OF THE RATE (SEE BOXED WARNING).

MOST COMMON ADVERSE EVENTS IN ALL CLINICAL STUDIES

Adjunctive Therapy in Adults

The most commonly observed (≥5%) adverse experiences seen in association with lamotrigine during adjunctive therapy in adults and not seen at an equivalent frequency among placebo-treated patients were: dizziness, ataxia, somnolence, headache, diplopia, blurred vision, nausea, vomiting, and rash. Dizziness, diplopia, ataxia, blurred vision, nausea, and vomiting were dose related. Dizziness, diplopia, ataxia, and blurred vision occurred more commonly in patients receiving carbamazepine with lamotrigine than in patients receiving other EIAEDs with lamotrigine. Clinical data suggest a higher incidence of rash, including serious rash, in patients receiving concomitant VPA than in patients not receiving VPA (see WARNINGS).

Approximately 11% of the 3378 adult patients who received lamotrigine as adjunctive therapy in premarketing clinical trials discontinued treatment because of an adverse experience. The adverse events most commonly associated with discontinuation were rash (3.0%), dizziness (2.8%), and headache (2.5%).

In a dose response study in adults, the rate of discontinuation of lamotrigine for dizziness, ataxia, diplopia, blurred vision, nausea, and vomiting was dose related.

Monotherapy in Adults

The most commonly observed (≥5%) adverse experiences seen in association with the use of lamotrigine during the monotherapy phase of the controlled trial in adults not seen at an equivalent rate in the control group were vomiting, coordination abnormality, dyspepsia, nausea, dizziness, rhinitis, anxiety, insomnia, infection, pain, weight decrease, chest pain, and dysmenorrhea. The most commonly observed (≥5%) adverse experiences associated with the use of lamotrigine during the conversion to monotherapy (add-on) period, not seen at an equivalent frequency among low-dose valproate-treated patients, were dizziness, headache, nausea, asthenia, coordination abnormality, vomiting, rash, somnolence, diplopia, ataxia, accidental injury, tremor, blurred vision, insomnia, nystagmus, diarrhea, lymphadenopathy, pruritus, and sinusitis.

Approximately 10% of the 420 adult patients who received lamotrigine as monotherapy in premarketing clinical trials discontinued treatment because of an adverse experience. The adverse events most commonly associated with discontinuation were rash (4.5%), headache (3.1%), and asthenia (2.4%).

Adjunctive Therapy in Pediatric Patients

The most commonly observed (≥5%) adverse experiences seen in association with the use of lamotrigine as adjunctive treatment in pediatric patients and not seen at an equivalent rate in the control group were infection, vomiting, rash, fever, somnolence, accidental injury, dizziness, diarrhea, abdominal pain, nausea, ataxia, tremor, asthenia, bronchitis, flu syndrome, and diplopia.

In 339 patients age 2-16 years, 4.2% of patients on lamotrigine and 2.9% of patients on placebo discontinued due to adverse experiences. The most commonly reported adverse experiences that led to discontinuation were rash for patients treated with lamotrigine and deterioration of seizure control for patients treated with placebo.

Approximately 11.5% of the 1081 pediatric patients who received lamotrigine as adjunctive therapy in premarketing clinical trials discontinued treatment because of an adverse experience. The adverse events most commonly associated with discontinuation were rash (4.4%), reaction aggravated (1.7%), and ataxia (0.6%).

INCIDENCE IN CONTROLLED CLINICAL STUDIES

The prescriber should be aware that the figures in TABLE 4, TABLE 5, TABLE 6, and TABLE 7 cannot be used to predict the frequency of adverse experiences in the course of usual medical practice where patient characteristics and other factors may differ from those prevailing during clinical studies. Similarly, the cited frequencies cannot be directly compared with figures obtained from other clinical investigations involving different treatments, uses, or investigators. An inspection of these frequencies, however, does provide the prescriber with one basis to estimate the relative contribution of drug and nondrug factors to the adverse event incidences in the population studied.

Incidence in Controlled Adjunctive Clinical Studies in Adults

TABLE 4 lists treatment-emergent signs and symptoms that occurred in at least 2% of adult patients with epilepsy treated with lamotrigine in placebo-controlled trials and were numerically more common in the patients treated with lamotrigine. In these studies, either lamotrigine or placebo was added to the patient's current AED therapy. Adverse events were usually mild to moderate in intensity.

In a randomized, parallel study comparing placebo and 300 and 500 mg/day of lamotrigine, some of the more common drug-related adverse events were dose related (see TABLE 5).

Other events that occurred in more than 1% of patients but equally or more frequently in the placebo group included: Asthenia, back pain, chest pain, flatulence, menstrual disorder, myalgia, paresthesia, respiratory disorder, and urinary tract infection.

The overall adverse experience profile for lamotrigine was similar between females and males, and was independent of age. Because the largest non-Caucasian racial subgroup was only 6% of patients exposed to lamotrigine in placebo-controlled trials, there are insufficient data to support a statement regarding the distribution of adverse experience reports by race. Generally, females receiving either adjunctive lamotrigine or placebo were more likely to report adverse experiences than males. The only adverse experience for which the reports on

TABLE 4 *Treatment-Emergent Adverse Event Incidence in Placebo-Controlled Adjunctive Trials* — Events in at Least 2% of Patients Treated With Lamotrigine and Numerically More Frequent Than in the Placebo Group*

Body System / Adverse Experience†	% Patients Receiving Adjunctive: Lamotrigine (n=711)	Placebo (n=419)
Body as a Whole		
Headache	29%	19%
Flu syndrome	7%	6%
Fever	6%	4%
Abdominal pain	5%	4%
Neck pain	2%	1%
Reaction aggravated (seizure exacerbation)	2%	1%
Digestive		
Nausea	19%	10%
Vomiting	9%	4%
Diarrhea	6%	4%
Dyspepsia	5%	2%
Constipation	4%	3%
Tooth disorder	3%	2%
Anorexia	2%	1%
Musculoskeletal		
Arthralgia	2%	0%
Nervous		
Dizziness	38%	13%
Ataxia	22%	6%
Somnolence	14%	7%
Incoordination	6%	2%
Insomnia	6%	2%
Tremor	4%	1%
Depression	4%	3%
Anxiety	4%	3%
Convulsion	3%	1%
Irritability	3%	2%
Speech disorder	3%	0%
Concentration disturbance	2%	1%
Respiratory		
Rhinitis	14%	9%
Pharyngitis	10%	9%
Cough increased	8%	6%
Skin and Appendages		
Rash	10%	5%
Pruritus	3%	2%
Special Senses		
Diplopia	28%	7%
Blurred vision	16%	5%
Vision abnormality	3%	1%
Urogenital		
Female patients only	(n=365)	(n=207)
Dysmenorrhea	7%	6%
Vaginitis	4%	1%
Amenorrhea	2%	1%

* Patients in these adjunctive studies were receiving 1-3 concomitant EIAEDs in addition to lamotrigine or placebo. Patients may have reported multiple adverse experiences during the study or at discontinuation; thus, patients may be included in more than one category.
† Adverse experiences reported by at least 2% of patients treated with lamotrigine are included.

TABLE 5 *Dose-Related Adverse Events From a Randomized, Placebo-Controlled Trial in Adults*

Adverse Experience	Placebo (n=73)	Lamotrigine 300 mg (n=71)	Lamotrigine 500 mg (n=72)
Ataxia	10%	10%	28%*†
Blurred vision	10%	11%	25%*†
Diplopia	8%	24%*	49%*†
Dizziness	27%	31%	54%*†
Nausea	11%	18%	25%*
Vomiting	4%	11%	18%*

* Significantly greater than placebo group ($P < 0.05$).
† Significantly greater than group receiving lamotrigine 300 mg ($P < 0.05$).

lamotrigine were greater than 10% more frequent in females than males (without a corresponding difference by gender on placebo) was dizziness (difference = 16.5%). There was little difference between females and males in the rates of discontinuation of lamotrigine for individual adverse experiences.

Incidence in a Controlled Monotherapy Trial in Adults With Partial Seizures

TABLE 6 lists treatment-emergent signs and symptoms that occurred in at least 2% of patients with epilepsy treated with monotherapy with lamotrigine in a double-blind trial following discontinuation of either concomitant carbamazepine or phenytoin not seen at an equivalent frequency in the control group.

Incidence in Controlled Adjunctive Trials in Pediatric Patients

TABLE 7 lists adverse events that occurred in at least 2% of 339 pediatric patients who received lamotrigine up to 15 mg/kg/day or a maximum of 750 mg/day. Reported adverse events were classified using COSTART terminology.

TABLE 6 *Treatment-Emergent Adverse Event Incidence in Adults in a Controlled Monotherapy Trial* — Events in at Least 2% of Patients Treated With Lamotrigine and Numerically More Frequent Than in the Valproate (VPA) Group*

Body System / Adverse Experience†	% of Patients Receiving: Lamotrigine Monotherapy‡ (n=43)	Low-Dose VPA§ Monotherapy (n=44)
Body as a Whole		
Pain	5%	0%
Infection	5%	2%
Chest pain	5%	2%
Asthenia	2%	0%
Fever	2%	0%
Digestive		
Vomiting	9%	0%
Dyspepsia	7%	2%
Nausea	7%	2%
Anorexia	2%	0%
Dry mouth	2%	0%
Rectal hemorrhage	2%	0%
Peptic ulcer	2%	0%
Metabolic and Nutritional		
Weight decrease	5%	2%
Peripheral edema	2%	0%
Nervous		
Coordination abnormality	7%	0%
Dizziness	7%	0%
Anxiety	5%	0%
Insomnia	5%	2%
Amnesia	2%	0%
Ataxia	2%	0%
Depression	2%	0%
Hypesthesia	2%	0%
Libido increase	2%	0%
Decreased reflexes	2%	0%
Increased reflexes	2%	0%
Nystagmus	2%	0%
Irritability	2%	0%
Suicidal ideation	2%	0%
Respiratory		
Rhinitis	7%	2%
Epistaxis	2%	0%
Bronchitis	2%	0%
Dyspnea	2%	0%
Skin and Appendages		
Contact dermatitis	2%	0%
Dry skin	2%	0%
Sweating	2%	0%
Special Senses		
Vision abnormality	2%	0%
Urogenital (female patients only)	(n=21)	(n=28)
Dysmenorrhea	5%	0%

* Patients in these studies were converted to lamotrigine or VPA monotherapy from adjunctive therapy with carbamazepine or phenytoin. Patients may have reported multiple adverse experiences during the study; thus, patients may be included in more than one category.
† Adverse experiences reported by at least 2% of patients are included.
‡ Up to 500 mg/day.
§ 1000 mg/day.

OTHER ADVERSE EVENTS OBSERVED DURING ALL CLINICAL TRIALS FOR ADULT AND PEDIATRIC PATIENTS

Lamotrigine has been administered to 3923 individuals for whom complete adverse event data was captured during all clinical trials, only some of which were placebo controlled. During these trials, all adverse events were recorded by the clinical investigators using terminology of their own choosing. To provide a meaningful estimate of the proportion of individuals having adverse events, similar types of events were grouped into a smaller number of standardized categories using modified COSTART dictionary terminology. The frequencies presented represent the proportion of the 3923 individuals exposed to lamotrigine who experienced an event of the type cited on at least 1 occasion while receiving lamotrigine. All reported events are included except those already listed in the previous table, those too general to be informative, and those not reasonably associated with the use of the drug.

Events are further classified within body system categories and enumerated in order of decreasing frequency using the following definitions: *frequent* adverse events are defined as those occurring in at least 1/100 patients; *infrequent* adverse events are those occurring in 1/100 to 1/1000 patients; *rare* adverse events are those occurring in fewer than 1/1000 patients.

Body as a Whole: *Frequent:* Pain. *Infrequent:* Accidental injury, allergic reaction, back pain, chills, face edema, halitosis, infection, and malaise. *Rare:* Abdomen enlarged, abscess, photosensitivity, and suicide attempt.

Cardiovascular System: *Infrequent:* Flushing, hot flashes, migraine, palpitations, postural hypotension, syncope, tachycardia, and vasodilation. *Rare:* Angina pectoris, atrial fibrillation, deep thrombophlebitis, hemorrhage, hypertension, and myocardial infarction.

Dermatologic: *Infrequent:* Acne, alopecia, dry skin, erythema, hirsutism, maculopapular rash, skin discoloration, Stevens-Johnson syndrome, sweating, urticaria, and vesiculobullous rash. *Rare:* Angioedema, erythema multiforme, fungal dermatitis, herpes zoster, leukoderma, petechial rash, pustular rash, and seborrhea.

Digestive System: *Infrequent:* Dry mouth, dysphagia, gingivitis, glossitis, gum hyperplasia, increased appetite, increased salivation, liver function tests abnormal, mouth ulceration, stomatitis, thirst, and tooth disorder. *Rare:* Eructation, gastritis, gastrointestinal hemorrhage, gum hemorrhage, hematemesis, hemorrhagic colitis, hepatitis, melena, stomach ulcer, and tongue edema.

TABLE 7 *Treatment-Emergent Adverse Event Incidence in Placebo-Controlled Adjunctive Trials in Pediatric Patients — Events in at Least 2% of Patients Treated With Lamotrigine and Numerically More Frequent Than in the Placebo Group*

Body System	% of Patients Receiving:	
	Lamotrigine	Placebo
Adverse Experience	(n=168)	(n=171)
Body as a Whole		
Infection	20%	17%
Fever	15%	14%
Accidental injury	14%	12%
Abdominal pain	10%	5%
Asthenia	8%	4%
Flu syndrome	7%	6%
Pain	5%	4%
Facial edema	2%	1%
Photosensitivity	2%	0%
Cardiovascular		
Hemorrhage	2%	1%
Digestive		
Vomiting	20%	16%
Diarrhea	11%	9%
Nausea	10%	2%
Constipation	4%	2%
Dyspepsia	2%	1%
Tooth Disorder	2%	1%
Hemic and Lymphatic		
Lymphadenopathy	2%	1%
Metabolic and Nutritional		
Edema	2%	0%
Nervous System		
Somnolence	17%	15%
Dizziness	14%	4%
Ataxia	11%	3%
Tremor	10%	1%
Emotional lability	4%	2%
Gait abnormality	4%	2%
Thinking abnormality	3%	2%
Convulsions	2%	1%
Nervousness	2%	1%
Vertigo	2%	1%
Respiratory		
Pharyngitis	14%	11%
Bronchitis	7%	5%
Increased cough	7%	6%
Sinusitis	2%	1%
Bronchospasm	2%	1%
Skin		
Rash	14%	12%
Eczema	2%	1%
Pruritus	2%	1%
Special Senses		
Diplopia	5%	1%
Blurred vision	4%	1%
Ear disorder	2%	1%
Visual abnormality	2%	0%
Urogenital		
Male and Female Patients		
Urinary tract infection	3%	0%
Male Patients Only	n=93	n=92
Penis disorder	2%	0%

Endocrine System: *Rare:* Goiter and hypothyroidism.

Hematologic and Lymphatic System: *Infrequent:* Anemia, ecchymosis, leukocytosis, leukopenia, lymphadenopathy, and petechia. *Rare:* Eosinophilia, fibrin decrease, fibrinogen decrease, iron deficiency anemia, lymphocytosis, macrocytic anemia, and thrombocytopenia.

Metabolic and Nutritional Disorders: *Infrequent:* Peripheral edema, weight gain, and weight loss. *Rare:* Alcohol intolerance, alkaline phosphatase increase, bilirubinemia, general edema, and hyperglycemia.

Musculoskeletal System: *Infrequent:* Joint disorder, myasthenia, and twitching. *Rare:* Arthritis, bursitis, leg cramps, pathological fracture, and tendinous contracture.

Nervous System: *Frequent:* Amnesia, confusion, hostility, memory decrease, nervousness, nystagmus, thinking abnormality, and vertigo. *Infrequent:* Abnormal dreams, abnormal gait, agitation, akathisia, apathy, aphasia, CNS depression, depersonalization, dysarthria, dyskinesia, dysphoria, emotional lability, euphoria, faintness, grand mal convulsions, hallucinations, hyperkinesia, hypertonia, hypesthesia, libido increased, mind racing, muscle spasm, myoclonus, panic attack, paranoid reaction, personality disorder, psychosis, sleep disorder, and stupor. *Rare:* Cerebrovascular accident, cerebellar syndrome, cerebral sinus thrombosis, choreoathetosis, CNS stimulation, delirium, delusions, dystonia, hemiplegia, hyperalgesia, hyperesthesia, hypoesthesia, hypokinesia, hypomania, hypotonia, libido decreased, manic depression reaction, movement disorder, neuralgia, neurosis, paralysis, and suicidal ideation.

Respiratory System: *Infrequent:* Dyspnea, epistaxis, and hyperventilation. *Rare:* Bronchospasm, hiccup, and sinusitis.

Special Senses: *Infrequent:* Abnormality of accommodation, conjunctivitis, ear pain, oscillopsia, photophobia, taste perversion, and tinnitus. *Rare:* Deafness, dry eyes, lacrimation disorder, parosmia, ptosis, strabismus, taste loss, and uveitis.

Urogenital System: *Infrequent:* Female lactation, hematuria, polyuria, urinary frequency, urinary incontinence, urinary retention, and vaginal moniliasis. *Rare:* Abnormal ejaculation, acute kidney failure, breast abscess, breast neoplasm, breast pain, creatinine increase, cystitis, dysuria, epididymitis, impotence, kidney failure, kidney pain, menorrhagia, and urine abnormality.

Postmarketing and Other Experience

In addition to the adverse experiences reported during clinical testing of lamotrigine, the following adverse experiences have been reported in patients receiving marketed lamotrigine and from worldwide noncontrolled investigational use. These adverse experiences have not been listed above, and data are insufficient to support an estimate of their incidence or to establish causation.

Blood and Lymphatic: Agranulocytosis, aplastic anemia, disseminated intravascular coagulation, hemolytic anemia, neutropenia, pancytopenia, red cell aplasia.

Gastrointestinal: Esophagitis.

Hepatobiliary Tract and Pancreas: Pancreatitis.

Immunologic: Lupus-like reaction, vasculitis.

Lower Respiratory: Apnea.

Musculoskeletal: Rhabdomyolysis has been observed in patients experiencing hypersensitivity reactions.

Neurology: Exacerbation of parkinsonian symptoms in patients with pre-existing Parkinson's disease, tics.

Non-Site Specific: Hypersensitivity reaction, multiorgan failure, progressive immunosuppression.

DOSAGE AND ADMINISTRATION

ADJUNCTIVE USE

Lamotrigine is indicated as adjunctive therapy for partial seizures in adults and pediatric patients (≥2 years of age). Lamotrigine is also indicated as adjunctive therapy for the generalized seizures of Lennox-Gastaut syndrome in adult and pediatric patients (≥2 years of age).

MONOTHERAPY USE

Lamotrigine is indicated for conversion to monotherapy in adults with partial seizures who are receiving treatment with a single EIAED (*e.g.*, carbamazepine, phenytoin, phenobarbital, etc.).

Safety and effectiveness of lamotrigine have not been established (1) as initial monotherapy, (2) for conversion to monotherapy from non-enzyme-inducing AEDs (*e.g.*, valproate), or (3) for simultaneous conversion to monotherapy from 2 or more concomitant AEDs.

Safety and effectiveness in pediatric patients below the age of 16 years other than those with partial seizures and the generalized seizures of Lennox-Gastaut syndrome have not been established (see BOXED WARNING).

GENERAL DOSING CONSIDERATIONS

The risk of nonserious rash is increased when the recommended initial dose and/or the rate of dose escalation of lamotrigine is exceeded. There are suggestions, yet to be proven, that the risk of severe, potentially life-threatening rash may be increased by (1) coadministration of lamotrigine with valproic acid (VPA), (2) exceeding the recommended initial dose of lamotrigine, or (3) exceeding the recommended dose escalation for lamotrigine. However, cases have been reported in the absence of these factors (see BOXED WARNING). Therefore, it is important that the dosing recommendations be followed closely.

It is recommended that lamotrigine not be restarted in patients who discontinued due to rash associated with prior treatment with lamotrigine, unless the potential benefits clearly outweigh the risks. If the decision is made to restart a patient who has discontinued lamotrigine, the need to restart with the initial dosing recommendations should be assessed. The greater the interval of time since the previous dose, the greater consideration should be given to restarting with the initial dosing recommendations. If a patient has discontinued lamotrigine for a period of more than 5 half-lives, it is recommended that initial dosing recommendations and guidelines be followed. The half-life of lamotrigine is affected by other concomitant medications (see CLINICAL PHARMACOLOGY, Pharmacokinetics and Drug Metabolism).

ADJUNCTIVE THERAPY WITH LAMOTRIGINE

This section provides specific dosing recommendations for patients 2-12 years of age and patients greater than 12 years of age. Within each of these age-groups, specific dosing recommendations are provided depending upon whether or not the patient is receiving VPA (TABLE 8A, TABLE 8B, and TABLE 9 for patients 2-12 years of age, TABLE 10 and TABLE 11 for patients greater than 12 years of age). In addition, the section provides a discussion of dosing for those patients receiving concomitant AEDs that have not been systematically evaluated in combination with lamotrigine.

For dosing guidelines for lamotrigine below, enzyme-inducing antiepileptic drugs (EIAEDs) include phenytoin, carbamazepine, phenobarbital, and primidone.

Patients 2-12 Years of Age

Recommended dosing guidelines for lamotrigine added to an antiepileptic drug (AED) regimen containing VPA are summarized in TABLE 8A and TABLE 8B. Recommended dosing guidelines for lamotrigine added to EIAEDs are summarized in TABLE 9.

Lamotrigine Added to AEDs Other Than EIAEDs and VPA

The effect of AEDs other than EIAEDs and VPA on the metabolism of lamotrigine is not currently known. Therefore, no specific dosing guidelines can be provided in that situation. Conservative starting doses and dose escalations (as with concomitant VPA) would be prudent; maintenance dosing would be expected to fall between the maintenance dose with VPA and the maintenance dose without VPA, but with an EIAED.

Note that the starting doses and dose escalations listed in TABLE 8A, TABLE 8B, and TABLE 9 are different than those used in clinical trials; however, the maintenance doses are the same as in clinical trials. Smaller starting doses and slower dose escalations than those used in clinical trials are recommended because of the suggestions that the risk of rash may be decreased by smaller starting doses and slower dose escalations. Therefore, maintenance doses will take longer to reach in clinical practice than in clinical trials. It may take several weeks to months to achieve an individualized maintenance dose. Maintenance doses in patients weighing less than 30 kg, regardless of age or concomitant AED, may need to be increased as much as 50%, based on clinical response.

The smallest available strength of lamotrigine chewable dispersible tablets is 2 mg, and only whole tablets should be administered. If the calculated dose cannot be achieved using whole tablets, the dose should be rounded down to the nearest whole tablet (see HOW SUPPLIED and the patient package information for a description of the lamotrigine chewable dispersible tablet available sizes).

TABLE 8A *Lamotrigine Added to an AED Regimen Containing VPA in Patients 2-12 Years of Age*

Weeks 1 and 2	0.15 mg/kg/day in 1 or 2 divided doses, rounded down to the nearest whole tablet. Only whole tablets should be used for dosing.
Weeks 3 and 4	0.3 mg/kg/day in 1 or 2 divided doses, rounded down to the nearest whole tablet.

Usual Maintenance Dose: 1-5 mg/kg/day (maximum 200 mg/day in 1 or 2 divided doses). To achieve the usual maintenance dose, subsequent doses should be increased every 1-2 weeks as follows: calculate 0.3 mg/kg/day, round this amount down to the nearest whole tablet, and add this amount to the previously administered daily dose. The usual maintenance dose in patients adding lamotrigine to VPA alone ranges from 1-3 mg/kg/day. The usual maintenance dose in patients adding lamotrigine to VPA alone ranges from 1-3 mg/kg/day. Maintenance doses in patients weighing less than 30 kg may need to be increased by as much as 50%, based on clinical response.

TABLE 8B *Lamotrigine Added to an AED Regimen Containing VPA in Patients 2-12 Years of Age — Weight Based Dosing Can Be Achieved by Using the Following Guide*

If The Patient's Weight Is:		Give This Daily Dose*:	
Greater Than	And Less Than	Weeks 1 and 2	Weeks 3 and 4
6.7 kg	14 kg	2 mg every *other* day	2 mg every day
14.1 kg	27 kg	2 mg every day	4 mg every day
27.1 kg	34 kg	4 mg every day	8 mg every day
34.1 kg	40 kg	5 mg every day	10 mg every day

* Using the most appropriate combination of lamotrigine 2 mg and 5 mg tablets.

Usual Maintenance Dose: 1-5 mg/kg/day (maximum 200 mg/day in 1 or 2 divided doses). To achieve the usual maintenance dose, subsequent doses should be increased every 1-2 weeks as follows: calculate 0.3 mg/kg/day, round this amount down to the nearest whole tablet, and add this amount to the previously administered daily dose. The usual maintenance dose in patients adding lamotrigine to VPA alone ranges from 1-3 mg/kg/day. Maintenance doses in patients weighing less than 30 kg may need to be increased by as much as 50%, based on clinical response.

TABLE 9 *Lamotrigine Added to EIAEDs (Without VPA) in Patients 2-12 Years of Age*

Weeks 1 and 2	0.6 mg/kg/day in 2 divided doses, rounded down to the nearest whole tablet.
Weeks 3 and 4	1.2 mg/kg/day in 2 divided doses, rounded down to the nearest whole tablet.

Usual Maintenance Dose: 5-15 mg/kg/day (maximum 400 mg/day in 2 divided doses). To achieve the usual maintenance dose, subsequent doses should be increased every 1-2 weeks as follows: calculate 1.2 mg/kg/day, round this amount down to the nearest whole tablet, and add this amount to the previously administered daily dose. Maintenance doses in patients weighing less than 30 kg may need to be increased by as much as 50%, based on clinical response.

Patients Over 12 Years of Age

Recommended dosing guidelines for lamotrigine added to VPA are summarized in TABLE 10. Recommended dosing guidelines for lamotrigine added to EIAEDs are summarized in TABLE 11.

Lamotrigine Added to AEDs Other Than EIAEDs and VPA

The effect of AEDs other than EIAEDs and VPA on the metabolism of lamotrigine is not currently known. Therefore, no specific dosing guidelines can be provided in that situation. Conservative starting doses and dose escalations (as with concomitant VPA) would be prudent; maintenance dosing would be expected to fall between the maintenance dose with VPA and the maintenance dose without VPA, but with an EIAED.

TABLE 10 *Lamotrigine Added to an AED Regimen Containing VPA in Patients Over 12 Years of Age*

Weeks 1 and 2	25 mg every *other* day
Weeks 3 and 4	25 mg every day

Usual Maintenance Dose: 100-400 mg/day (1 or 2 divided doses). To achieve maintenance, doses may be increased by 25-50 mg/day every 1-2 weeks. The usual maintenance dose in patients adding lamotrigine to VPA alone ranges from 100-200 mg/day.

TABLE 11 *Lamotrigine Added to EIAEDs (Without VPA) in Patients Over 12 Years of Age*

Weeks 1 and 2	50 mg/day
Weeks 3 and 4	100 mg/day in 2 divided doses

Usual Maintenance Dose: 300-500 mg/day (in 2 divided doses). To achieve maintenance, doses may be increased by 100 mg/day every 1-2 weeks.

CONVERSION FROM A SINGLE EIAED TO MONOTHERAPY WITH LAMOTRIGINE IN PATIENTS ≥16 YEARS OF AGE

The goal of the transition regimen is to effect the conversion to monotherapy with lamotrigine under conditions that ensure adequate seizure control while mitigating the risk of serious rash associated with the rapid titration of lamotrigine.

The conversion regimen involves 2 steps. In the first, lamotrigine is titrated to the targeted dose while maintaining the dose of the EIAED at a fixed level; in the second step, the EIAED is gradually withdrawn over a period of 4 weeks.

The recommended maintenance dose of lamotrigine as monotherapy is 500 mg/day given in 2 divided doses.

Lamotrigine should be added to an EIAED to achieve a dose of 500 mg/day according to the guidelines in TABLE 11. The regimen for the withdrawal of the concomitant EIAED is based on experience gained in the controlled monotherapy clinical trial. In that trial, the concomitant EIAED was withdrawn by 20% decrements each week over a 4 week period.

Because of an increased risk of rash, the recommended initial dose and subsequent dose escalations of lamotrigine should not be exceeded (see BOXED WARNING).

USUAL MAINTENANCE DOSE

The usual maintenance doses identified in TABLE 8A, TABLE 8B, TABLE 9, TABLE 10, and TABLE 11 are derived from dosing regimens employed in the placebo-controlled adjunctive studies in which the efficacy of lamotrigine was established. In patients receiving multidrug regimens employing EIAEDs **without VPA,** maintenance doses of adjunctive lamotrigine as high as 700 mg/day have been used. In patients receiving **VPA alone,** maintenance doses of adjunctive lamotrigine as high as 200 mg/day have been used. The advantage of using doses above those recommended in TABLE 8A, TABLE 8B, TABLE 9, TABLE 10, and TABLE 11 has not been established in controlled trials.

PATIENTS WITH HEPATIC IMPAIRMENT

Experience in patients with hepatic impairment is limited. Based on a clinical pharmacology study in 24 patients with moderate to severe liver dysfunction (see CLINICAL PHARMACOLOGY), the following general recommendations can be made. Initial, escalation, and maintenance doses should generally be reduced by approximately 50% in patients with moderate (Child-Pugh Grade B) and 75% in patients with severe (Child-Pugh Grade C) hepatic impairment. Escalation and maintenance doses should be adjusted according to clinical response.

PATIENTS WITH RENAL FUNCTIONAL IMPAIRMENT

Initial doses of lamotrigine should be based on patients' AED regimen (see above); reduced maintenance doses may be effective for patients with significant renal functional impairment (see CLINICAL PHARMACOLOGY). Few patients with severe renal impairment have been evaluated during chronic treatment with lamotrigine. Because there is inadequate experience in this population, lamotrigine should be used with caution in these patients.

DISCONTINUATION STRATEGY

For patients receiving lamotrigine in combination with other AEDs, a reevaluation of all AEDs in the regimen should be considered if a change in seizure control or an appearance or worsening of adverse experiences is observed.

If a decision is made to discontinue therapy with lamotrigine, a step-wise reduction of dose over at least 2 weeks (approximately 50% per week) is recommended unless safety concerns require a more rapid withdrawal (see PRECAUTIONS).

Discontinuing an EIAED should prolong the half-life of lamotrigine; discontinuing VPA should shorten the half-life of lamotrigine.

TARGET PLASMA LEVELS

A therapeutic plasma concentration range has not been established for lamotrigine. Dosing of lamotrigine should be based on therapeutic response.

ADMINISTRATION OF LAMOTRIGINE CHEWABLE DISPERSIBLE TABLETS

Lamotrigine chewable dispersible tablets may be swallowed whole, chewed, or dispersed in water or diluted fruit juice. If the tablets are chewed, consume a small amount of water or diluted fruit juice to aid in swallowing.

To disperse lamotrigine chewable dispersible tablets, add the tablets to a small amount of liquid (1 teaspoon, or enough to cover the medication). Approximately 1 minute later, when the tablets are completely dispersed, swirl the solution and consume the entire quantity immediately. *No attempt should be made to administer partial quantities of the dispersed tablets.*

HOW SUPPLIED

LAMICTAL TABLETS

25 mg: White, scored, shield-shaped tablets debossed with "LAMICTAL" and "25".

100 mg: Peach, scored, shield-shaped tablets debossed with "LAMICTAL" and "100".

150 mg: Cream, scored, shield-shaped tablets debossed with "LAMICTAL" and "150".

200 mg: Blue, scored, shield-shaped tablets debossed with "LAMICTAL" and "200".

Storage: Store at 25°C (77°F); excursions permitted to 15-30°C (59-86°F) in a dry place and protect from light.

LAMICTAL CHEWABLE DISPERSIBLE TABLETS

2 mg: White to off-white, round tablets debossed with "LTG" over "2".

5 mg: White to off-white, caplet-shaped tablets debossed with "GX CL2".

25 mg: White, super elliptical-shaped tablets debossed with "GX CL5".

Storage: Store at 25°C (77°F); excursions permitted to 15-30°C (59-86°F) in a dry place.

PRODUCT LISTING - EQUIVALENTS NOT AVAILABLE

Tablet - Oral - 25 mg

100's $285.99 LAMICTAL, Glaxosmithkline 00173-0633-02

Tablet - Oral - 100 mg
100's $303.58 LAMICTAL, Glaxosmithkline 00173-0642-55
Tablet - Oral - 150 mg
60's $191.41 LAMICTAL, Glaxosmithkline 00173-0643-60
Tablet - Oral - 200 mg
60's $200.64 LAMICTAL, Glaxosmithkline 00173-0644-60
Tablet, Chewable - Oral - 5 mg
100's $270.25 LAMICTAL, Glaxosmithkline 00173-0526-00
Tablet, Chewable - Oral - 25 mg
100's $283.04 LAMICTAL, Glaxosmithkline 00173-0527-00

Lansoprazole *(003230)*

For related information, see the comparative table section in Appendix A.

Categories: Esophagitis, erosive; Gastroesophageal Reflux Disease; Ulcer, duodenal; Ulcer, gastric; Ulcer, NSAID-associated, prophylaxis; Zollinger-Ellison syndrome; FDA Approved 1995 May; Pregnancy Category B
Drug Classes: Gastrointestinals; Proton pump inhibitors
Brand Names: **Prevacid**
Foreign Brand Availability: Agopton (Austria; Germany; Switzerland); Betalans (Indonesia); Compraz (Indonesia); Digest (Indonesia); Ilsatec (Mexico); Keval (Mexico); Lancid (Korea); Lancopen (Colombia); Lanpraz (Colombia); Lanprol (Bahrain; Cyprus; Egypt; Iran; Iraq; Jordan; Kuwait; Lebanon; Libya; Oman; Qatar; Republic-of-Yemen; Saudi-Arabia; Syria; United-Arab-Emirates); Lanproton (Colombia); Lansazol (Bahrain; Cyprus; Egypt; Iran; Iraq; Jordan; Kuwait; Lebanon; Libya; Oman; Qatar; Republic-of-Yemen; Saudi-Arabia; Syria; United-Arab-Emirates); Lansopep (Colombia); Lanston (Korea); Lanvell (Indonesia); Lanximed (Colombia); Lanz (Philippines); Lanzol-30 (India); Lanzopral (Costa-Rica; Dominican-Republic; El-Salvador; Guatemala; Honduras; Nicaragua; Panama; Peru); Lanzor (France; Germany; South-Africa); Lapraz (Indonesia); Laproton (Indonesia); Laz (Indonesia); Lopral (Colombia; Peru); Neutron (Colombia); Ogast (France); Ogastro (Bahamas; Barbados; Belize; Bermuda; Colombia; Costa-Rica; Curacao; Dominican-Republic; El-Salvador; Guatemala; Guyana; Honduras; Jamaica; Mexico; Netherland-Antilles; Nicaragua; Panama; Peru; Puerto-Rico; Surinam; Trinidad); Prolanz (Indonesia); Prosogan (Indonesia); Suprecid (Philippines); Takepron (Benin; Burkina-Faso; China; Ethiopia; Gambia; Ghana; Guinea; Hong-Kong; Ivory-Coast; Japan; Kenya; Liberia; Malawi; Mali; Mauritania; Mauritius; Morocco; Niger; Nigeria; Senegal; Seychelles; Sierra-Leone; Sudan; Taiwan; Tanzania; Tunia; Uganda; Zambia; Zimbabwe); Ulpax (Mexico); Zoton (Australia; England; Ireland; Israel; New-Zealand)
Cost of Therapy: $136.28 (GERD; Prevacid; 15 mg; 1 tablet/day; 30 day supply)
$138.87 (Gastric Ulcer; Prevacid; 30 mg; 1 tablet/day; 30 day supply)

DESCRIPTION

Note: The trade name has been used throughout this monograph for clarity.

The active ingredient in Prevacid delayed-release capsules, Prevacid for delayed-release oral suspension, and Pravacid SoluTab delayed-release orally disintegrating tablets is a substituted benzimidazole, 2-[[[3-methyl-4-(2,2,2-trifluoroethoxy)-2-pyridyl]methyl]sulfinyl] benzimidazole, a compound that inhibits gastric acid secretion. Its empirical formula is $C_{16}H_{14}F_3N_3O_2S$ with a molecular weight of 369.37.

Lansoprazole is a white to brownish-white odorless crystalline powder which melts with decomposition at approximately 166°C. Lansoprazole is freely soluble in dimethylformamide; soluble in methanol; sparingly soluble in ethanol; slightly soluble in ethyl acetate, dichloromethane and acetonitrile; very slightly soluble in ether; and practically insoluble in hexane and water.

Lansoprazole is stable when exposed to light for up to 2 months. The rate of degradation of the compound in aqueous solution increases with decreasing pH. The degradation half-life of the drug substance in aqueous solution at 25°C is approximately 0.5 hour at pH 5.0 and approximately 18 hours at pH 7.0.

Prevacid is supplied in delayed-release capsules, in delayed-release orally disintegrating tablets for oral administration and in a packet for delayed-release oral suspension.

PREVACID DELAYED-RELEASE CAPSULES

The delayed-release capsules contain the active ingredient, lansoprazole, in the form of enteric-coated granules and are available in two dosage strengths: 15 and 30 mg of lansoprazole per capsule. Each delayed-release capsule contains enteric-coated granules consisting of lansoprazole, hydroxypropyl cellulose, low substituted hydroxypropyl cellulose, colloidal silicon dioxide, magnesium carbonate, methacrylic acid copolymer, starch, talc, sugar sphere, sucrose, polyethylene glycol, polysorbate 80, and titanium dioxide. Components of the gelatin capsule include gelatin, titanium dioxide, D&C red no. 28, FD&C blue no. 1, FD&C green no. 3 (Prevacid 15 mg capsules only), and FD&C red no. 40.

PRAVACID SOLUTAB DELAYED-RELEASE ORALLY DISINTEGRATING TABLETS

Prevacid SoluTab delayed-release orally disintegrating tablets contain the active ingredient, lansoprazole in the form of enteric-coated microgranules. The tablets are available in 15 and 30 mg dosage strengths. Each tablet contains lansoprazole and the following inactive ingredients: lactose monohydrate, microcrystalline cellulose, magnesium carbonate, hydroxypropyl cellulose, hydroxypropyl methylcellulose, titanium dioxide, talc, mannitol, methacrylic acid, polyacrylate, polyethylene glycol, glyceryl monostearate, polysorbate 80, triethyl citrate, ferric oxide, citric acid, crospovidone, aspartame*, strawberry flavor and magnesium stearate.

***Phenylketonurics: Contains phenylalanine 2.5 mg/15 mg tablet and 5.1 mg/30 mg tablet.**

PREVACID FOR DELAYED-RELEASE ORAL SUSPENSION

Prevacid for delayed-release oral suspension is composed of the active ingredient, lansoprazole, in the form of enteric-coated granules and also contains inactive granules. The packets contain lansoprazole granules which are identical to those contained in Prevacid delayed-release capsules and are available in 15 and 30 mg strengths. Inactive granules are composed of the following ingredients: confectioner's sugar, mannitol, docusate sodium, ferric oxide, colloidal silicon dioxide, xanthan gum, crospovidone, citric acid, sodium citrate, magnesium stearate, and artificial strawberry flavor. The lansoprazole granules and inactive granules, present in unit dose packets, are constituted with water to form a suspension and consumed orally.

CLINICAL PHARMACOLOGY

PHARMACOKINETICS AND METABOLISM

Prevacid delayed-release capsules, Prevacid SoluTab delayed-release orally disintegrating tablets and Prevacid for delayed-release oral suspension contain an enteric-coated granule formulation of lansoprazole. Absorption of lansoprazole begins only after the granules leave the stomach. Absorption is rapid, with mean peak plasma levels of lansoprazole occurring after approximately 1.7 hours. Peak plasma concentrations of lansoprazole (C_{max}) and the area under the plasma concentration curve (AUC) of lansoprazole are approximately proportional in doses from 15-60 mg after single-oral administration. Lansoprazole does not accumulate and its pharmacokinetics are unaltered by multiple dosing.

Absorption

The absorption of lansoprazole is rapid, with mean C_{max} occurring approximately 1.7 hours after oral dosing, and relatively complete with absolute bioavailability over 80%. In healthy subjects, the mean (±SD) plasma half-life was 1.5 (±1.0) hours. Both C_{max} and AUC are diminished by about 50-70% if the drug is given 30 minutes after food as opposed to the fasting condition. There is no significant food effect if the drug is given before meals.

Distribution

Lansoprazole is 97% bound to plasma proteins. Plasma protein binding is constant over the concentration range of 0.05 to 5.0 μg/ml.

Metabolism

Lansoprazole is extensively metabolized in the liver. Two metabolites have been identified in measurable quantities in plasma (the hydroxylated sulfinyl and sulfone derivatives of lansoprazole). These metabolites have very little or no antisecretory activity. Lansoprazole is thought to be transformed into 2 active species which inhibit acid secretion by (H^+,K^+)-ATPase within the parietal cell canaliculus, but are not present in the systemic circulation. The plasma elimination half-life of lansoprazole does not reflect its duration of suppression of gastric acid secretion. Thus, the plasma elimination half-life is less than 2 hours, while the acid inhibitory effect lasts more than 24 hours.

Elimination

Following single-dose oral administration of lansoprazole, virtually no unchanged lansoprazole was excreted in the urine. In one study, after a single oral dose of ^{14}C-lansoprazole, approximately one-third of the administered radiation was excreted in the urine and two-thirds was recovered in the feces. This implies a significant biliary excretion of the metabolites of lansoprazole.

Special Populations

Geriatric

The clearance of lansoprazole is decreased in the elderly, with elimination half-life increased approximately 50-100%. Because the mean half-life in the elderly remains between 1.9-2.9 hours, repeated once daily dosing does not result in accumulation of lansoprazole. Peak plasma levels were not increased in the elderly. No dosage adjustment is necessary in the elderly.

Pediatric

The pharmacokinetics of lansoprazole were studied in pediatric patients with GERD aged 1-11 years, with lansoprazole doses of 15 mg qd for subjects weighing ≤30 kg and 30 mg qd for subjects weighing >30 kg. Lansoprazole pharmacokinetics in these pediatric patients were similar to that observed in healthy adult subjects. The mean C_{max} and AUC values were similar between the 2 dose groups and were not affected by weight or age within each weight-adjusted dose group used in this study.

Gender

In a study comparing 12 male and 6 female human subjects, no gender differences were found in pharmacokinetics and intragastric pH results. (Also see PRECAUTIONS, Use in Women.)

Renal Insufficiency

In patients with severe renal insufficiency, plasma protein binding decreased by 1.0-1.5% after administration of 60 mg of lansoprazole. Patients with renal insufficiency had a shortened elimination half-life and decreased total AUC (free and bound). AUC for free lansoprazole in plasma, however, was not related to the degree of renal impairment, and C_{max} and T_{max} were not different from subjects with healthy kidneys. No dosage adjustment is necessary in patients with renal insufficiency.

Hepatic Insufficiency

In patients with various degrees of chronic hepatic disease, the mean plasma half-life of the drug was prolonged from 1.5 hours to 3.2-7.2 hours. An increase in mean AUC of up to 500% was observed at steady state in hepatically-impaired patients compared to healthy subjects. Dose reduction in patients with severe hepatic disease should be considered.

Race

The pooled mean pharmacokinetic parameters of lansoprazole from twelve US Phase 1 studies (n=513) were compared to the mean pharmacokinetic parameters from two Asian studies (n=20). The mean AUCs of lansoprazole in Asian subjects were approximately twice those seen in pooled US data; however, the inter-individual variability was high. The C_{max} values were comparable.

PHARMACODYNAMICS

Mechanism of Action

Lansoprazole belongs to a class of antisecretory compounds, the substituted benzimidazoles, that do not exhibit anticholinergic or histamine H_2-receptor antagonist properties, but that suppress gastric acid secretion by specific inhibition of the (H^+,K^+)-ATPase enzyme system at the secretory surface of the gastric parietal cell. Because this enzyme system is regarded as the acid (proton) pump within the parietal cell, lansoprazole has been characterized as a gastric acid-pump inhibitor, in that it blocks the final step of acid production. This effect is dose-related and leads to inhibition of both basal and stimulated gastric acid secretion irrespective of the stimulus.

Antisecretory Activity

After oral administration, lansoprazole was shown to significantly decrease the basal acid output and significantly increase the mean gastric pH and percent of time the gastric pH was >3 and >4. Lansoprazole also significantly reduced meal-stimulated gastric acid output and secretion volume, as well as pentagastrin-stimulated acid output. In patients with hypersecretion of acid, lansoprazole significantly reduced basal and pentagastrin-stimulated gastric acid secretion. Lansoprazole inhibited the normal increases in secretion volume, acidity and acid output induced by insulin.

In a crossover study that included lansoprazole 15 and 30 mg for 5 days, the following effects on intragastric pH were noted (see TABLE 1).

TABLE 1 *Mean Antisecretory Effects After Single and Multiple Daily Dosing*

Parameter	Baseline Value	Prevacid 15 mg Day 1	Prevacid 15 mg Day 5	Prevacid 30 mg Day 1	Prevacid 30 mg Day 5
Mean 24 hour pH	2.1	2.7*	4.0*	3.6†	4.9†
Mean nighttime pH	1.9	2.4	3.0*	2.6	3.8†
% Time gastric pH >3	18%	33%*	59%*	51%†	72%†
% Time gastric pH >4	12%	22%*	49%*	41%†	66%†

Note: An intragastric pH of >4 reflects a reduction in gastric acid by 99%.
* (p <0.05) versus baseline only.
† (p <0.05) versus baseline and lansoprazole 15 mg.

After the initial dose in this study, increased gastric pH was seen within 1-2 hours with lansoprazole 30 mg and 2-3 hours with lansoprazole 15 mg. After multiple daily dosing, increased gastric pH was seen within the first hour postdosing with lansoprazole 30 mg and within 1-2 hours postdosing with lansoprazole 15 mg.

Acid suppression may enhance the effect of antimicrobials in eradicating *Helicobacter pylori (H. pylori)*. The percentage of time gastric pH was elevated above 5 and 6 was evaluated in a crossover study of Prevacid given qd, bid and tid.

TABLE 2 *Mean Antisecretory Effects After 5 Days of bid and tid Dosing*

Prevacid	Parameter: % Time Gastric pH >5	Parameter: % Time Gastric pH >6
30 mg qd	43%	20%
15 mg bid	47%	23%
30 mg bid	59%*	28%
30 mg tid	77%†	45%†

* (p <0.05) versus Prevacid 30 mg qd.
† (p <0.05) versus Prevacid 30 mg qd, 15 mg bid, and 30 mg bid.

The inhibition of gastric acid secretion as measured by intragastric pH returns gradually to normal over 2-4 days after multiple doses. There is no indication of rebound gastric acidity.

Enterochromaffin-Like (ECL) Cell Effects

During lifetime exposure of rats with up to 150 mg/kg/day of lansoprazole dosed 7 days/week, marked hypergastrinemia was observed followed by ECL cell proliferation and formation of carcinoid tumors, especially in female rats. (See PRECAUTIONS, Carcinogenesis, Mutagenesis, and Impairment of Fertility.)

Gastric biopsy specimens from the body of the stomach from approximately 150 patients treated continuously with lansoprazole for at least 1 year did not show evidence of ECL cell effects similar to those seen in rat studies. Longer term data are needed to rule out the possibility of an increased risk of the development of gastric tumors in patients receiving long-term therapy with lansoprazole.

Other Gastric Effects in Humans

Lansoprazole did not significantly affect mucosal blood flow in the fundus of the stomach. Due to the normal physiologic effect caused by the inhibition of gastric acid secretion, a decrease of about 17% in blood flow in the antrum, pylorus, and duodenal bulb was seen. Lansoprazole significantly slowed the gastric emptying of digestible solids. Lansoprazole increased serum pepsinogen levels and decreased pepsin activity under basal conditions and in response to meal stimulation or insulin injection. As with other agents that elevate intragastric pH, increases in gastric pH were associated with increases in nitrate-reducing bacteria and elevation of nitrite concentration in gastric juice in patients with gastric ulcer. No significant increase in nitrosamine concentrations was observed.

Serum Gastrin Effects

In over 2100 patients, median fasting serum gastrin levels increased 50-100% from baseline but remained within normal range after treatment with lansoprazole given orally in doses of 15-60 mg. These elevations reached a plateau within 2 months of therapy and returned to pretreatment levels within 4 weeks after discontinuation of therapy.

Endocrine Effects

Human studies for up to 1 year have not detected any clinically significant effects on the endocrine system. Hormones studied include testosterone, luteinizing hormone (LH), follicle stimulating hormone (FSH), sex hormone binding globulin (SHBG), dehydroepiandrosterone sulfate (DHEA-S), prolactin, cortisol, estradiol, insulin, aldosterone, parathormone, glucagon, thyroid stimulating hormone (TSH), triiodothyronine (T_3), thyroxine (T_4), and somatotropic hormone (STH). Lansoprazole in oral doses of 15-60 mg for up to 1 year had no clinically significant effect on sexual function. In addition, lansoprazole in oral doses of 15-60 mg for 2-8 weeks had no clinically significant effect on thyroid function.

In 24 month carcinogenicity studies in Sprague-Dawley rats with daily dosages up to 150 mg/kg, proliferative changes in the Leydig cells of the testes, including benign neoplasm, were increased compared to control rates.

Other Effects

No systemic effects of lansoprazole on the central nervous system, lymphoid, hematopoietic, renal, hepatic, cardiovascular or respiratory systems have been found in humans. No visual toxicity was observed among 56 patients who had extensive baseline eye evaluations, were treated with up to 180 mg/day of lansoprazole and were observed for up to 58 months. Other rat-specific findings after lifetime exposure included focal pancreatic atrophy, diffuse lymphoid hyperplasia in the thymus, and spontaneous retinal atrophy.

MICROBIOLOGY

Lansoprazole, clarithromycin and/or amoxicillin have been shown to be active against most strains of *Helicobacter pylori in vitro* and in clinical infections as described in INDICATIONS AND USAGE.

Helicobacter — Helicobacter pylori

Pretreatment Resistance

Clarithromycin pretreatment resistance (≥2.0 μg/ml) was 9.5% (91/960) by E-test and 11.3% (12/106) by agar dilution in the dual and triple therapy clinical trials (M93-125, M93-130, M93-131, M95-392, and M95-399).

Amoxicillin pretreatment susceptible isolates (≤0.25 μg/ml) occurred in 97.8% (936/957) and 98.0% (98/100) of the patients in the dual and triple therapy clinical trials by E-test and agar dilution, respectively. Twenty-one (21) of 957 patients (2.2%) by E-test and 2 of 100 patients (2.0%) by agar dilution had amoxicillin pretreatment MICs of >0.25 μg/ml. One patient on the 14 day triple therapy regimen had an unconfirmed pretreatment amoxicillin minimum inhibitory concentration (MIC) of >256 μg/ml by E-test and the patient was eradicated of *H. pylori*.

TABLE 3 *Clarithromycin Susceptibility Test Results and Clinical/Bacteriological Outcomes**

Clarithromycin Pretreatment Results		Clarithromycin Post-Treatment Results: *H. pylori* Negative — Eradicated	*H. pylori* Positive — Not Eradicated, Post-Treatment Susceptibility Results: S†	I†	R†	No MIC
Triple Therapy 14 Day (lansoprazole 30 mg bid/amoxicillin 1 g bid/clarithromycin 500 mg bid)						
Susceptible†	112	105				7
Intermediate†	3	3				
Resistant†	17	6			7	4
Triple Therapy 10 Day (lansoprazole 30 mg bid/amoxicillin 1 g bid/clarithromycin 500 mg bid (M95-399)						
Susceptible†	42	40	1		1	
Intermediate†						
Resistant†	4	1			3	

* Includes only patients with pretreatment clarithromycin susceptibility test results.
† Susceptible (S) MIC ≤0.25 μg/ml, Intermediate (I) MIC 0.5-1.0 μg/ml, Resistant (R) MIC ≥2 μg/ml.

Patients not eradicated of *H. pylori* following lansoprazole/amoxicillin/clarithromycin triple therapy will likely have clarithromycin resistant *H. pylori*. Therefore, for those patients who fail therapy, clarithromycin susceptibility testing should be done when possible. Patients with clarithromycin resistant *H. pylori* should not be treated with lansoprazole/amoxicillin/clarithromycin triple therapy or with regimens which include clarithromycin as the sole antimicrobial agent.

Amoxicillin Susceptibility Test Results and Clinical/Bacteriological Outcomes

In the dual and triple therapy clinical trials, 82.6% (195/236) of the patients that had pretreatment amoxicillin susceptible MICs (≤0.25 μg/ml) were eradicated of *H. pylori*. Of those with pretreatment amoxicillin MICs of >0.25 μg/ml, 3 of 6 had the *H. pylori* eradicated. A total of 30% (21/70) of the patients failed lansoprazole 30 mg tid/amoxicillin 1 g tid dual therapy and a total of 12.8% (22/172) of the patients failed the 10 and 14 day triple therapy regimens. Post-treatment susceptibility results were not obtained on 11 of the patients who failed therapy. Nine (9) of the 11 patients with amoxicillin post-treatment MICs that failed the triple therapy regimen also had clarithromycin resistant *H. pylori* isolates.

Susceptibility Test for Helicobacter pylori

The reference methodology for susceptibility testing of *H. pylori* is agar dilution MICs.[1] One to three microliters (1-3 μl) of an inoculum equivalent to a No. 2 McFarland standard (1×10^7 to 1×10^8 CFU/ml for *H. pylori*) are inoculated directly onto freshly prepared antimicrobial-containing Mueller-Hinton agar plates with 5% aged defibrinated sheep blood (≥2 weeks old). The agar dilution plates are incubated at 35°C in a microaerobic environment produced by a gas generating system suitable for campylobacters. After 3 days of incubation, the MICs are recorded as the lowest concentration of antimicrobial agent required to inhibit growth of the organism. The clarithromycin and amoxicillin MIC values should be interpreted according to the criteria in TABLE 4.

Standardized susceptibility test procedures require the use of laboratory control microorganisms to control the technical aspects of the laboratory procedures. Standard clarithromycin and amoxicillin powders should provide the MIC values in TABLE 5.

TABLE 4

MIC	Interpretation
Clarithromycin*	
≤0.25 μg/ml	Susceptible (S)
0.5-1.0 μg/ml	Intermediate (I)
≥2.0 μg/ml	Resistant (R)
Amoxicillin†	
≤0.25 μg/ml	Susceptible (S)

* These are tentative breakpoints for the agar dilution methodology and they should not be used to interpret results obtained using alternative methods.
† There were not enough organisms with MICs >0.25 μg/ml to determine a resistance breakpoint.

TABLE 5

Microorganism	Antimicrobial Agent	MIC*
H. pylori ATCC 43504	Clarithromycin	0.015-0.12 μg/ml
H. pylori ATCC 43504	Amoxicillin	0.015-0.12 μg/ml

* These are quality control ranges for the agar dilution methodology and they should not be used to control test results obtained using alternative methods.

INDICATIONS AND USAGE

PREVACID DELAYED-RELEASE CAPSULES, PREVACID SOLUTAB DELAYED-RELEASE ORALLY DISINTEGRATING TABLETS AND PREVACID FOR DELAYED-RELEASE ORAL SUSPENSION ARE INDICATED FOR:

SHORT-TERM TREATMENT OF ACTIVE DUODENAL ULCER

Prevacid is indicated for short-term treatment (up to 4 weeks) for healing and symptom relief of active duodenal ulcer.

H. PYLORI ERADICATION TO REDUCE THE RISK OF DUODENAL ULCER RECURRENCE

Triple Therapy: Prevacid/Amoxicillin/Clarithromycin

Prevacid in combination with amoxicillin plus clarithromycin as triple therapy, is indicated for the treatment of patients with *H. pylori* infection and duodenal ulcer disease (active or 1 year history of a duodenal ulcer) to eradicate *H. pylori*. Eradication of *H. pylori* has been shown to reduce the risk of duodenal ulcer recurrence. (See DOSAGE AND ADMINISTRATION.)

Dual Therapy: Prevacid/Amoxicillin

Prevacid in combination with amoxicillin as dual therapy, is indicated for the treatment of patients with *H. pylori* infection and duodenal ulcer disease (active or 1 year history of a duodenal ulcer) **who are either allergic or intolerant to clarithromycin or in whom resistance to clarithromycin is known or suspected.** (See the clarithromycin package insert, Microbiology.) Eradication of *H. pylori* has been shown to reduce the risk of duodenal ulcer recurrence. (See DOSAGE AND ADMINISTRATION.)

MAINTENANCE OF HEALED DUODENAL ULCERS

Prevacid is indicated to maintain healing of duodenal ulcers. Controlled studies do not extend beyond 12 months.

SHORT-TERM TREATMENT OF ACTIVE BENIGN GASTRIC ULCER

Prevacid is indicated for short-term treatment (up to 8 weeks) for healing and symptom relief of active benign gastric ulcer.

HEALING OF NSAID-ASSOCIATED GASTRIC ULCER

PREVACID IS INDICATED FOR THE TREATMENT OF NSAID-ASSOCIATED GASTRIC ULCER IN PATIENTS WHO CONTINUE NSAID USE. CONTROLLED STUDIES DID NOT EXTEND BEYOND 8 WEEKS.

RISK REDUCTION OF NSAID-ASSOCIATED GASTRIC ULCER

Prevacid is indicated for reducing the risk of NSAID-associated gastric ulcers in patients with a history of a documented gastric ulcer who require the use of an NSAID. Controlled studies did not extend beyond 12 weeks.

GASTROESOPHAGEAL REFLUX DISEASE (GERD)

Short-Term Treatment of Symptomatic GERD

Prevacid is indicated for the treatment of heartburn and other symptoms associated with GERD.

Short-Term Treatment of Erosive Esophagitis

Prevacid is indicated for short-term treatment (up to 8 weeks) for healing and symptom relief of all grades of erosive esophagitis.

For patients who do not heal with Prevacid for 8 weeks (5-10%), it may be helpful to give an additional 8 weeks of treatment.

If there is a recurrence of erosive esophagitis an additional 8 week course of Prevacid may be considered.

MAINTENANCE OF HEALING OF EROSIVE ESOPHAGITIS

Prevacid is indicated to maintain healing of erosive esophagitis. Controlled studies did not extend beyond 12 months.

PATHOLOGICAL HYPERSECRETORY CONDITIONS INCLUDING ZOLLINGER-ELLISON SYNDROME

Prevacid is indicated for the long-term treatment of pathological hypersecretory conditions, including Zollinger-Ellison syndrome.

CONTRAINDICATIONS

Prevacid is contraindicated in patients with known hypersensitivity to any component of the formulations.

Amoxicillin is contraindicated in patients with a known hypersensitivity to any penicillin. (Please refer to full prescribing information for amoxicillin before prescribing.)

Clarithromycin is contraindicated in patients with a known hypersensitivity to any macrolide antibiotic, and in patients receiving terfenadine therapy who have preexisting cardiac abnormalities or electrolyte disturbances. (Please refer to full prescribing information for clarithromycin before prescribing.)

WARNINGS

CLARITHROMYCIN SHOULD NOT BE USED IN PREGNANT WOMEN EXCEPT IN CLINICAL CIRCUMSTANCES WHERE NO ALTERNATIVE THERAPY IS APPROPRIATE. IF PREGNANCY OCCURS WHILE TAKING CLARITHROMYCIN, THE PATIENT SHOULD BE APPRISED OF THE POTENTIAL HAZARD TO THE FETUS. (SEE WARNINGS IN PRESCRIBING INFORMATION FOR CLARITHROMYCIN.)

Pseudomembranous colitis has been reported with nearly all antibacterial agents, including clarithromycin and amoxicillin, and may range in severity from mild to life threatening. Therefore, it is important to consider this diagnosis in patients who present with diarrhea subsequent to the administration of antibacterial agents.

Treatment with antibacterial agents alters the normal flora of the colon and may permit overgrowth of clostridia. Studies indicate that a toxin produced by *Clostridium difficile* is a primary cause of "antibiotic-associated colitis".

After the diagnosis of pseudomembranous colitis has been established, therapeutic measures should be initiated. Mild cases of pseudomembranous colitis usually respond to discontinuation of the drug alone. In moderate to severe cases, consideration should be given to management with fluids and electrolytes, protein supplementation, and treatment with an antibacterial drug clinically effective against *Clostridium difficile* colitis.

Serious and occasionally fatal hypersensitivity (anaphylactic) reactions have been reported in patients on penicillin therapy. These reactions are more apt to occur in individuals with a history of penicillin hypersensitivity and/or a history of sensitivity to multiple allergens.

There have been well-documented reports of individuals with a history of penicillin hypersensitivity reactions who have experienced severe hypersensitivity reactions when treated with a cephalosporin. Before initiating therapy with any penicillin, careful inquiry should be made concerning previous hypersensitivity reactions to penicillins, cephalosporins, and other allergens. If an allergic reaction occurs, amoxicillin should be discontinued and the appropriate therapy instituted.

SERIOUS ANAPHYLACTIC REACTIONS REQUIRE IMMEDIATE EMERGENCY TREATMENT WITH EPINEPHRINE. OXYGEN, INTRAVENOUS STEROIDS, AND AIRWAY MANAGEMENT, INCLUDING INTUBATION, SHOULD ALSO BE ADMINISTERED AS INDICATED.

L

PRECAUTIONS

GENERAL

Symptomatic response to therapy with lansoprazole does not preclude the presence of gastric malignancy.

INFORMATION FOR THE PATIENT

Prevacid delayed-release capsules, Prevacid SoluTab delayed-release orally disintegrating tablets and Prevacid for delayed-release oral suspension should be taken before eating. Prevacid products SHOULD NOT BE CRUSHED OR CHEWED.

Phenylketonurics: Contains phenylalanine 2.5 mg/15 mg tablet and 5.1 mg/30 mg tablet.

ALTERNATIVE ADMINISTRATION OPTIONS

For patients who have difficulty swallowing capsules, there are three options.

Prevacid Delayed-Release Capsules

Prevacid delayed-release capsules can be opened, and the intact granules contained within can be sprinkled on 1 tablespoon of either applesauce, Ensure pudding, cottage cheese, yogurt, or strained pears and swallowed immediately. Alternatively, Prevacid delayed-release capsules may be emptied into a small volume of either apple juice, orange juice or tomato juice (60 ml — approximately 2 oz), mixed briefly and swallowed immediately. To insure complete delivery of the dose, the glass should be rinsed with 2 or more volumes of juice and the contents swallowed immediately. USE IN OTHER FOODS AND LIQUIDS HAS NOT BEEN STUDIED CLINICALLY AND IS THEREFORE NOT RECOMMENDED.

Prevacid SoluTab Delayed-Release Orally Disintegrating Tablets

Prevacid SoluTab delayed-release orally disintegrating tablets are available in 15 and 30 mg strengths. Prevacid SoluTabs are not designed to be swallowed intact or chewed. The tablet typically disintegrates in less than 1 minute.

Place the tablet on the tongue and allow it to disintegrate with or without water until the particles can be swallowed.

Prevacid for Delayed-Release Oral Suspension

Prevacid for delayed-release oral suspension is available in strengths of 15 and 30 mg. *Directions for use:* Empty packet contents into a container containing 2 tablespoons of **WATER.** DO NOT USE OTHER LIQUIDS OR FOODS. Stir well, and drink immediately. If any material remains after drinking, add more water, stir, and drink immediately.

CARCINOGENESIS, MUTAGENESIS, AND IMPAIRMENT OF FERTILITY

In two 24 month carcinogenicity studies, Sprague-Dawley rats were treated orally with doses of 5-150 mg/kg/day, about 1-40 times the exposure on a body surface (mg/m^2) basis, of a 50 kg person of average height (1.46 m^2 body surface area) given the recommended human dose of 30 mg/day (22.2 mg/m^2). Lansoprazole produced dose-related gastric enterochromaffin-like (ECL) cell hyperplasia and ECL cell carcinoids in both male and female rats. It also increased the incidence of intestinal metaplasia of the gastric epithelium in both sexes. In male rats, lansoprazole produced a dose-related increase of testicular interstitial cell adenomas. The incidence of these adenomas in rats receiving doses of 15-150 mg/kg/day (4-40 times the recommended human dose based on body surface area) exceeded the low background incidence (range = 1.4-10%) for this strain of rat. Testicular interstitial cell adenoma also occurred in 1 of 30 rats treated with 50 mg/kg/day (13 times the recommended human dose based on body surface area) in a 1 year toxicity study.

In a 24 month carcinogenicity study, CD-1 mice were treated orally with doses of 15-600 mg/kg/day, 2-80 times the recommended human dose based on body surface area. Lansoprazole produced a dose-related increased incidence of gastric ECL cell hyperplasia. It also produced an increased incidence of liver tumors (hepatocellular adenoma plus carcinoma). The tumor incidences in male mice treated with 300 and 600 mg/kg/day (40-80 times the recommended human dose based on body surface area) and female mice treated with 150-600 mg/kg/day (20-80 times the recommended human dose based on body surface area) exceeded the ranges of background incidences in historical controls for this strain of mice. Lansoprazole treatment produced adenoma of rete testis in male mice receiving 75-600 mg/kg/day (10-80 times the recommended human dose based on body surface area).

Lansoprazole was not genotoxic in the Ames test, the *ex vivo* rat hepatocyte unscheduled DNA synthesis (UDS) test, the *in vivo* mouse micronucleus test or the rat bone marrow cell chromosomal aberration test. It was positive in *in vitro* human lymphocyte chromosomal aberration assays.

Lansoprazole at oral doses up to 150 mg/kg/day (40 times the recommended human dose based on body surface area) was found to have no effect on fertility and reproductive performance of male and female rats.

PREGNANCY, TERATOGENIC EFFECTS

Pregnancy Category B — Lansoprazole

Teratology studies have been performed in pregnant rats at oral doses up to 150 mg/kg/day (40 times the recommended human dose based on body surface area) and pregnant rabbits at oral doses up to 30 mg/kg/day (16 times the recommended human dose based on body surface area) and have revealed no evidence of impaired fertility or harm to the fetus due to lansoprazole.

There are, however, no adequate or well-controlled studies in pregnant women. Because animal reproduction studies are not always predictive of human response, this drug should be used during pregnancy only if clearly needed.

Pregnancy Category C — Clarithromycin

See WARNINGS and full prescribing information for clarithromycin before using in pregnant women.

NURSING MOTHERS

Lansoprazole or its metabolites are excreted in the milk of rats. It is not known whether lansoprazole is excreted in human milk. Because many drugs are excreted in human milk, because of the potential for serious adverse reactions in nursing infants from lansoprazole, and because of the potential for tumorigenicity shown for lansoprazole in rat carcinogenicity studies, a decision should be made whether to discontinue nursing or to discontinue the drug, taking into account the importance of the drug to the mother.

PEDIATRIC USE

The safety and effectiveness of Prevacid have been established in the age group 1-11 years for short-term treatment of symptomatic GERD and erosive esophagitis. Safety and effectiveness have not been established in patients <1 year or 12-17 years of age.

Use of Prevacid in the age group 1-11 years is supported by evidence from adequate and well controlled studies of Prevacid in adults with additional clinical, pharmacokinetic, pharmacodynamic, and safety studies performed in pediatric patients.

In an uncontrolled, open-label, US multicenter study, 66 pediatric patients (1-11 years of age) with GERD were assigned, based on body weight, to receive an initial dose of either Prevacid 15 mg qd if ≤30 kg or Prevacid 30 mg qd if >30 kg administered for 8-12 weeks. The Prevacid dose was increased (up to 30 mg bid) in 24 of 66 pediatric patients after 2 or more weeks of treatment if they remained symptomatic. At baseline 85% of patients had mild to moderate overall GERD symptoms (assessed by investigator interview), 58% had nonerosive GERD and 42% had erosive esophagitis (assessed by endoscopy).

After 8-12 weeks of Prevacid treatment, the intent-to-treat analysis demonstrated an approximate 50% reduction in frequency and severity of GERD symptoms.

Twenty-one (21) of 27 erosive esophagitis patients were healed at 8 weeks and 100% of patients were healed at 12 weeks by endoscopy.

TABLE 19

GERD	Final Visit* (n/N)
Symptomatic GERD	
Improvement in overall GERD symptoms†	76% (47/62‡)
Erosive Esophagitis	
Improvement in overall GERD symptoms†	81% (22/27)
Healing rate	100% (27/27)

* At Week 8 or Week 12.
† Symptoms assessed by patients diary kept by caregiver.
‡ No data were available for 4 pediatric patients.

In a study of 66 pediatric patients in the age group 1-11 years old after treatment with Prevacid given orally in doses of 15 mg qd to 30 mg bid, increases in serum gastrin levels were similar to those observed in adult studies. Median fasting serum gastrin levels increased 89% from 51 pg/ml at baseline to 97 pg/ml [interquartile range (25th-75th percentile) of 71-130 pg/ml] at the final visit.

The pediatric safety of Prevacid delayed-release capsules has been assessed in 66 pediatric patients aged 1-11 years of age. Of the 66 patients with GERD 85% (56/66) took lansoprazole for 8 weeks and 15% (10/66) took it for 12 weeks.

The adverse event profile in these pediatric patients resembled that of adults taking lansoprazole. The most frequently reported (2 or more patients) treatment-related adverse events in patients 1-11 years of age (n=66) were constipation (5%) and headache (3%). There were no adverse events reported in this US clinical study that were not previously observed in adults.

USE IN WOMEN

Over 4000 women were treated with lansoprazole. Ulcer healing rates in females were similar to those in males. The incidence rates of adverse events were also similar to those seen in males.

USE IN GERIATRIC PATIENTS

Ulcer healing rates in elderly patients are similar to those in a younger age group. The incidence rates of adverse events and laboratory test abnormalities are also similar to those seen in younger patients. For elderly patients, dosage and administration of lansoprazole need not be altered for a particular indication.

DRUG INTERACTIONS

Lansoprazole is metabolized through the cytochrome P_{450} system, specifically through the CYP3A and CYP2C19 isozymes. Studies have shown that lansoprazole does not have clinically significant interactions with other drugs metabolized by the cytochrome P_{450} system, such as warfarin, antipyrine, indomethacin, ibuprofen, phenytoin, propranolol, prednisone, diazepam, or clarithromycin in healthy subjects. These compounds are metabolized through various cytochrome P_{450} isozymes including CYP1A2, CYP2C9, CYP2C19, CYP2D6, and CYP3A. When lansoprazole was administered concomitantly with theophylline (CYP1A2, CYP3A), a minor increase (10%) in the clearance of theophylline was seen. Because of the small magnitude and the direction of the effect on theophylline clearance, this interaction is unlikely to be of clinical concern. Nonetheless, individual patients may require additional titration of their theophylline dosage when lansoprazole is started or stopped to ensure clinically effective blood levels.

In a study of healthy subjects neither the pharmacokinetics of warfarin enantiomers nor prothrombin time were affected following single or multiple 60 mg doses of lansoprazole. However, there have been reports of increased International Normalized Ratio (INR) and prothrombin time in patients receiving proton pump inhibitors, including lansoprazole, and warfarin concomitantly. Increases in INR and prothrombin time may lead to abnormal bleeding and even death. Patients treated with proton pump inhibitors and warfarin concomitantly may need to be monitored for increases in INR and prothrombin time.

Lansoprazole has also been shown to have no clinically significant interaction with amoxicillin.

In a single-dose crossover study examining lansoprazole 30 mg and omeprazole 20 mg each administered alone and concomitantly with sucralfate 1 g, absorption of the proton pump inhibitors was delayed and their bioavailability was reduced by 17% and 16%, respectively, when administered concomitantly with sucralfate. Therefore, proton pump inhibitors should be taken at least 30 minutes prior to sucralfate. In clinical trials, antacids were administered concomitantly with Prevacid delayed-release capsules; this did not interfere with its effect.

Lansoprazole causes a profound and long-lasting inhibition of gastric acid secretion; therefore, it is theoretically possible that lansoprazole may interfere with the absorption of drugs where gastric pH is an important determinant of bioavailability (*e.g.*, ketoconazole, ampicillin esters, iron salts, digoxin).

ADVERSE REACTIONS

CLINICAL

Worldwide, over 10,000 patients have been treated with lansoprazole in Phase 2-3 clinical trials involving various dosages and durations of treatment. The adverse reaction profiles for Prevacid delayed-release capsules and Prevacid for delayed-release oral suspension are similar. In general, lansoprazole treatment has been well-tolerated in both short-term and long-term trials.

The following adverse events were reported by the treating physician to have a possible or probable relationship to drug in 1% or more of Prevacid-treated patients and occurred at a greater rate in Prevacid-treated patients than placebo-treated patients (see TABLE 20).

TABLE 20 *Incidence of Possibly or Probably Treatment-Related Adverse Events in Short-Term, Placebo-Controlled Studies*

Body System Adverse Event	Prevacid (n=2768)	Placebo (n=1023)
Body as a Whole		
Abdominal pain	2.1%	1.2%
Digestive System		
Constipation	1.0%	0.4%
Diarrhea	3.8%	2.3%
Nausea	1.3%	1.2%

Headache was also seen at greater than 1% incidence but was more common on placebo. The incidence of diarrhea was similar between patients who received placebo and patients who received lansoprazole 15 and 30 mg, but higher in the patients who received lansoprazole 60 mg (2.9%, 1.4%, 4.2%, and 7.4%, respectively).

The most commonly reported possibly or probably treatment-related adverse event during maintenance therapy was diarrhea.

In the risk reduction study of Prevacid for NSAID-associated gastric ulcers, the incidence of diarrhea for patients treated with Prevacid was 5%, misoprostol 22%, and placebo 3%.

Additional adverse experiences occurring in <1% of patients or subjects in domestic trials are shown below. Refer to Postmarketing for adverse reactions occurring since the drug was marketed.

Body as a Whole: Abdomen enlarged, allergic reaction, asthenia, back pain, candidiasis, carcinoma, chest pain (not otherwise specified), chills, edema, fever, flu syndrome, halitosis, infection (not otherwise specified), malaise, neck pain, neck rigidity, pain, pelvic pain.

Cardiovascular System: Angina, arrhythmia, bradycardia, cerebrovascular accident/cerebral infarction, hypertension/hypotension, migraine, myocardial infarction, palpitations, shock (circulatory failure), syncope, tachycardia, vasodilation.

Digestive System: Abnormal stools, anorexia, bezoar, cardiospasm, cholelithiasis, colitis, dry mouth, dyspepsia, dysphagia, enteritis, eructation, esophageal stenosis, esophageal ulcer, esophagitis, fecal discoloration, flatulence, gastric nodules/fundic gland polyps, gastritis, gastroenteritis, gastrointestinal anomaly, gastrointestinal disorder, gastrointestinal hemorrhage, glossitis, gum hemorrhage, hematemesis, increased appetite, increased salivation, melena, mouth ulceration, nausea and vomiting, nausea and vomiting and diarrhea, oral moniliasis, rectal disorder, rectal hemorrhage, stomatitis, tenesmus, thirst, tongue disorder, ulcerative colitis, ulcerative stomatitis.

Endocrine System: Diabetes mellitus, goiter, hypothyroidism.

Hemic and Lymphatic System: Anemia, hemolysis, lymphadenopathy.

Metabolic and Nutritional Disorders: Gout, dehydration, hyperglycemia/hypoglycemia, peripheral edema, weight gain/loss.

Musculoskeletal System: Arthralgia, arthritis, bone disorder, joint disorder, leg cramps, musculoskeletal pain, myalgia, myasthenia, synovitis.

Nervous System: Abnormal dreams, agitation, amnesia, anxiety, apathy, confusion, convulsion, depersonalization, depression, diplopia, dizziness, emotional lability, hallucinations, hemiplegia, hostility aggravated, hyperkinesia, hypertonia, hypesthesia, insomnia, libido decreased/increased, nervousness, neurosis, paresthesia, sleep disorder, somnolence, thinking abnormality, tremor, vertigo.

Respiratory System: Asthma, bronchitis, cough increased, dyspnea, epistaxis, hemoptysis, hiccup, laryngeal neoplasia, pharyngitis, pleural disorder, pneumonia, respiratory disorder, upper respiratory inflammation/infection, rhinitis, sinusitis, stridor.

Skin and Appendages: Acne, alopecia, contact dermatitis, dry skin, fixed eruption, hair disorder, maculopapular rash, nail disorder, pruritus, rash, skin carcinoma, skin disorder, sweating, urticaria.

Special Senses: Abnormal vision, blurred vision, conjunctivitis, deafness, dry eyes, ear disorder, eye pain, otitis media, parosmia, photophobia, retinal degeneration, taste loss, taste perversion, tinnitus, visual field defect.

Urogenital System: Abnormal menses, breast enlargement, breast pain, breast tenderness, dysmenorrhea, dysuria, gynecomastia, impotence, kidney calculus, kidney pain, leukorrhea, menorrhagia, menstrual disorder, penis disorder, polyuria, testis disorder, urethral pain, urinary frequency, urinary tract infection, urinary urgency, urination impaired, vaginitis.

POSTMARKETING

On-Going Safety Surveillance

ADDITIONAL ADVERSE EXPERIENCES HAVE BEEN REPORTED SINCE LANSOPRAZOLE HAS BEEN MARKETED. THE MAJORITY OF THESE CASES ARE FOREIGN-SOURCED AND A RELATIONSHIP TO LANSOPRAZOLE HAS NOT BEEN ESTABLISHED. BECAUSE THESE EVENTS WERE REPORTED VOLUNTARILY FROM A POPULATION OF UNKNOWN SIZE, ESTIMATES OF FREQUENCY CANNOT BE MADE. THESE EVENTS ARE LISTED BELOW BY COSTART BODY SYSTEM.

Body as a Whole: Anaphylactoid-like reaction.

Digestive System: Hepatotoxicity, vomiting.

Hemic and Lymphatic System: Agranulocytosis, aplastic anemia, hemolytic anemia, leukopenia, neutropenia, pancytopenia, thrombocytopenia, and thrombotic thrombocytopenic purpura.

Special Senses: Speech disorder.

Urogenital System: Urinary retention.

COMBINATION THERAPY WITH AMOXICILLIN AND CLARITHROMYCIN

In clinical trials using combination therapy with Prevacid plus amoxicillin and clarithromycin, and Prevacid plus amoxicillin, no adverse reactions peculiar to these drug combinations were observed. Adverse reactions that have occurred have been limited to those that had been previously reported with Prevacid, amoxicillin, or clarithromycin.

Triple Therapy: Prevacid/Amoxicillin/Clarithromycin

The most frequently reported adverse events for patients who received triple therapy for 14 days were diarrhea (7%), headache (6%), and taste perversion (5%). There were no statistically significant differences in the frequency of reported adverse events between the 10 and 14 day triple therapy regimens. No treatment-emergent adverse events were observed at significantly higher rates with triple therapy than with any dual therapy regimen.

Dual Therapy: Prevacid/Amoxicillin

The most frequently reported adverse events for patients who received Prevacid tid plus amoxicillin tid dual therapy were diarrhea (8%) and headache (7%). No treatment-emergent adverse events were observed at significantly higher rates with Prevacid tid plus amoxicillin tid dual therapy than with Prevacid alone.

For more information on adverse reactions with amoxicillin or clarithromycin, refer to their package inserts, **ADVERSE REACTIONS** sections.

LABORATORY VALUES

The following changes in laboratory parameters for lansoprazole were reported as adverse events:

Abnormal liver function tests, increased SGOT (AST), increased SGPT (ALT), increased creatinine, increased alkaline phosphatase, increased globulins, increased GGTP, increased/decreased/abnormal WBC, abnormal AG ratio, abnormal RBC, bilirubinemia, eosinophilia, hyperlipemia, increased/decreased electrolytes, increased/decreased cholesterol, increased glucocorticoids, increased LDH, increased/decreased/abnormal platelets, and increased gastrin levels. Urine abnormalities such as albuminuria, glycosuria, and hematuria were also reported. Additional isolated laboratory abnormalities were reported.

In the placebo controlled studies, when SGOT (AST) and SGPT (ALT) were evaluated, 0.4% (4/978) placebo patients and 0.4% (11/2677) lansoprazole patients had enzyme elevations greater than 3 times the upper limit of normal range at the final treatment visit. None of these lansoprazole patients reported jaundice at any time during the study.

In clinical trials using combination therapy with Prevacid plus amoxicillin and clarithromycin, and Prevacid plus amoxicillin, no increased laboratory abnormalities particular to these drug combinations were observed.

For more information on laboratory value changes with amoxicillin or clarithromycin, refer to their package inserts, **ADVERSE REACTIONS** section.

DOSAGE AND ADMINISTRATION

Prevacid delayed-release capsules, Prevacid SoluTab delayed-release orally disintegrating tablets and Prevacid for delayed-release oral suspension should be taken before eating. Prevacid products SHOULD NOT BE CRUSHED OR CHEWED. In the clinical trials, antacids were used concomitantly with Prevacid.

No dosage adjustment is necessary in patients with renal insufficiency or the elderly. For patients with severe liver disease, dosage adjustment should be considered.

DUODENAL ULCERS

Short-Term Treatment:

Recommended Adult Dose: 15 mg Prevacid once daily for 4 weeks. (See INDICATIONS AND USAGE.)

Maintenance of Healed:

Recommended Adult Dose: 15 mg Prevacid once daily.

H. PYLORI ERADICATION TO REDUCE THE RISK OF DUODENAL ULCER RECURRENCE*

Triple Therapy:

Recommended Adult Dose: 30 mg Prevacid, 1 g amoxicillin, 500 mg clarithromycin, each twice daily (q12h) for 10 or 14 days. (See INDICATIONS AND USAGE.)

Dual Therapy:

Recommended Adult Dose: 30 mg Prevacid, 1 g amoxicillin, each 3 times daily (q8h) for 14 days. (See INDICATIONS AND USAGE.)

*Please refer to amoxicillin and clarithromycin full prescribing information for CONTRAINDICATIONS and WARNINGS, and for information regarding dosing in elderly and renally-impaired patients.

BENIGN GASTRIC ULCER

Short-Term Treatment:

Recommended Adult Dose: 30 mg Prevacid once daily for up to 8 weeks.

NSAID-ASSOCIATED GASTRIC ULCER

Healing:

Recommended Adult Dose: 30 mg Prevacid once daily for 8 weeks. (Controlled studies did not extend beyond indicated duration.)

Risk Reduction:

Recommended Adult Dose: 15 mg Prevacid once daily for up to 12 weeks. (Controlled studies did not extend beyond indicated duration.)

GASTROESOPHAGEAL REFLUX DISEASE (GERD)

Short-Term Treatment of Symptomatic GERD:

Recommended Adult Dose: 15 mg Prevacid once daily for up to 8 weeks.

Short-Term Treatment of Erosive Esophagitis:

Recommended Adult Dose: 30 mg Prevacid once daily for up to 8 weeks. (For patients who do not heal with Prevacid for 8 weeks [5-10%], it may be helpful to give an additional 8 weeks of treatment. If there is a recurrence of erosive esophagitis, an additional 8 week course of Prevacid may be considered. See INDICATIONS AND USAGE.)

PEDIATRIC (SHORT-TERM TREATMENT OF SYMPTOMATIC GERD, SHORT-TERM TREATMENT OF EROSIVE ESOPHAGITIS) (1-11 YEARS OF AGE)

≤30 kg

Recommended Dose: 15 mg Prevacid once daily for up to 12 weeks. (The Prevacid dose was increased [up to 30 mg bid] in some pediatric patients after 2 or more weeks of treatment if they remained symptomatic. For pediatric patients unable to swallow an intact capsule please see Alternative Administration Options. See PRECAUTIONS, Pediatric Use.

>30 kg

Recommended Dose: 30 mg Prevacid once daily for up to 12 weeks. (The Prevacid dose was increased [up to 30 mg bid] in some pediatric patients after 2 or more weeks of treatment if they remained symptomatic. For pediatric patients unable to swallow an intact capsule please see Alternative Administration Options. See PRECAUTIONS, Pediatric Use.

MAINTENANCE OF HEALING OF EROSIVE ESOPHAGITIS

Recommended Adult Dose: 15 mg Prevacid once daily.

PATHOLOGICAL HYPERSECRETORY CONDITIONS INCLUDING ZOLLINGER-ELLISION SYNDROME

Recommended Adult Dose: 60 mg Prevacid once daily. (Varies with individual patient. Recommended adult starting dose is 60 mg once daily. Doses should be adjusted to individual patient needs and should continue for as long as clinically indicated. Dosages up to 90 mg bid have been administered. Daily dose of greater than 120 mg should be administered in divided doses. Some patients with Zollinger-Ellison syndrome have been treated continuously with Prevacid for more than 4 years.

ALTERNATIVE ADMINISTRATION OPTIONS
For patients who have difficulty swallowing capsules, there are three options.

Prevacid Delayed-Release Capsules
Prevacid delayed-release capsules can be opened, and the intact granules contained within can be sprinkled on 1 tablespoon of either applesauce, Ensure pudding, cottage cheese, yogurt, or strained pears and swallowed immediately. Alternatively, Prevacid delayed-release capsules may be emptied into a small volume of either apple juice, orange juice or tomato juice (60 ml — approximately 2 oz), mixed briefly and swallowed immediately. To insure complete delivery of the dose, the glass should be rinsed with 2 or more volumes of juice and the contents swallowed immediately. USE IN OTHER FOODS AND LIQUIDS HAS NOT BEEN STUDIED CLINICALLY AND IS THEREFORE NOT RECOMMENDED.

For patients who have a nasogastric tube in place, Prevacid delayed-release capsules can be opened and the intact granules mixed in 40 ml of apple juice and injected through the nasogastric tube into the stomach. After administering the granules, the nasogastric tube should be flushed with additional apple juice to clear the tube.

Prevacid SoluTab Delayed-Release Orally Disintegrating Tablets
Prevacid SoluTab delayed-release orally disintegrating tablets are available in 15 and 30 mg strengths. Prevacid SoluTabs are not designed to be swallowed intact or chewed. The tablet typically disintegrates in less than 1 minute.

Place the tablet on the tongue and allow it to disintegrate with or without water until the particles can be swallowed.

Prevacid for Delayed-Release Oral Suspension
Prevacid for delayed-release oral suspension is available in strengths of 15 and 30 mg. *Directions for use:* Empty packet contents into a container containing 2 tablespoons of **WATER.** DO NOT USE OTHER LIQUIDS OR FOODS. Stir well, and drink immediately. If any material remains after drinking, add more water, stir, and drink immediately.

L

HOW SUPPLIED

PREVACID DELAYED-RELEASE CAPSULES

15 mg: Opaque, hard gelatin, colored pink and green with the TAP logo and "PREVACID 15" imprinted on the capsules.

30 mg: Opaque, hard gelatin, colored pink and black with the TAP logo and "PREVACID 30" imprinted on the capsules.

Storage: Store at 25°C (77°F); excursions permitted to 15-30°C (59-86°F).

PREVACID DELAYED-RELEASE ORAL SUSPENSION
Prevacid for delayed-release oral suspension contains white to pale brownish lansoprazole granules and inactive pink granules in a unit dose packet containing 15 or 30 mg of lansoprazole.
Storage: Store at 25°C (77°F); excursions permitted to 15-30°C (59-86°F).

PREVACID SOLUTAB DELAYED-RELEASE ORALLY DISINTEGRATING TABLETS

15 mg: White to yellowish white with orange to dark brown speckles, round, flat-faced, bevel-edged, uncoated, orally disintegrating tablets with no markings on either side and measuring approximately 9 mm (side to side) with a strawberry flavor.

30 mg: White to yellowish white, with orange to dark brown speckles, round, flat-faced, bevel-edged, uncoated, orally disintegrating tablets with no markings on either side and measuring approximately 12 mm (side to side) with a strawberry flavor.

Storage: Store at 25°C (77°F); excursions permitted to 15-30°C (59-86°F).

PRODUCT LISTING - EQUIVALENTS NOT AVAILABLE

Capsule, Enteric Coated - Oral - 15 mg

30's	$102.24	PREVACID, Allscripts Pharmaceutical Company	54569-4450-00
30's	$136.28	PREVACID, Tap Pharmaceuticals Inc	00300-1541-30
100's	$454.26	PREVACID, Tap Pharmaceuticals Inc	00300-1541-11

Capsule, Enteric Coated - Oral - 30 mg

7's	$27.16	PREVACID, Allscripts Pharmaceutical Company	54569-4451-02
14's	$54.32	PREVACID, Allscripts Pharmaceutical Company	54569-4451-01
30's	$104.18	PREVACID, Allscripts Pharmaceutical Company	54569-4451-00
30's	$129.92	PREVACID, Quality Care Pharmaceuticals Inc	60346-0869-30
30's	$130.52	PREVACID, Physicians Total Care	54868-4079-00
30's	$155.11	PREVACID, Pd-Rx Pharmaceuticals	55289-0279-30
100's	$462.90	PREVACID, Tap Pharmaceuticals Inc	00300-3046-11
100's	$462.90	PREVACID, Tap Pharmaceuticals Inc	00300-3046-13

Granule For Reconstitution - Oral - 15 mg/30 ml

30's	$136.28	PREVACID, Tap Pharmaceuticals Inc	00300-7309-30

Granule For Reconstitution - Oral - 30 mg/30 ml

30's	$138.88	PREVACID, Tap Pharmaceuticals Inc	00300-7311-30

Latanoprost *(003299)*

Categories: Glaucoma, open-angle; Hypertension, ocular; Pregnancy Category C; FDA Approved 1996 Aug
Drug Classes: Ophthalmics; Prostaglandins
Brand Names: **Xalatan**
Foreign Brand Availability: Louten (Colombia)
Cost of Therapy: $55.60 (Glaucoma; Xalatan Ophth. Solution; 0.005%; 2.5 ml; 1 drops/day; variable day supply)

DESCRIPTION

Latanoprost is a prostaglandin $F_{2\alpha}$ analogue. Its chemical name is isopropyl-(Z)-7[(1R,2R,3R,5S)3,5-dihydroxy-2-[(3R)-3-hydroxy-5-phenylpentyl]cyclopentyl]-5-heptenoate. Its molecular formula is $C_{26}H_{40}O_5$ and its molecular weight is 432.58.

Latanoprost is a colorless to slightly yellow oil that is very soluble in acetonitrile and freely soluble in acetone, ethanol, ethyl acetate, isopropanol, methanol, and octanol. It is practically insoluble in water.

Xalatan sterile ophthalmic solution is supplied as a sterile, isotonic, buffered aqueous solution of latanoprost with a pH of approximately 6.7 and an osmolality of approximately 267 mOsmol/kg. Each ml of Xalatan contains 50 μg of latanoprost. Benzalkonium chloride, 0.02% is added as a preservative. *The inactive ingredients are:* Sodium chloride, sodium dihydrogen phosphate monohydrate, disodium hydrogen phosphate anhydrous and water for injection. One drop contains approximately 1.5 μg of latanoprost.

CLINICAL PHARMACOLOGY

MECHANISM OF ACTION
Latanoprost is a prostanoid selective FP receptor agonist that is believed to reduce the intraocular pressure (IOP) by increasing the outflow of aqueous humor. Studies in animals and man suggest that the main mechanism of action is increased uveoscleral outflow. Elevated IOP represents a major risk factor for glaucomatous field loss. The higher the level of IOP, the greater the likelihood of optic nerve damage and visual field loss.

PHARMACOKINETICS/PHARMACODYNAMICS

Absorption
Latanoprost is absorbed through the cornea where the isopropyl ester prodrug is hydrolyzed to the acid form to become biologically active. Studies in man indicate that the peak concentration in the aqueous humor is reached about 2 hours after topical administration.

Distribution
The distribution volume in humans is 0.16 ± 0.02 L/kg. The acid of latanoprost can be measured in aqueous humor during the first 4 hours, and in plasma only during the first hour after local administration.

Metabolism
Latanoprost, an isopropyl ester prodrug, is hydrolyzed by esterases in the cornea to the biologically active acid. The active acid of latanoprost reaching the systemic circulation is primarily metabolized by the liver to the 1,2-dinor and 1,2,3,4-tetranor metabolites via fatty acid β-oxidation.

Excretion
The elimination of the acid of latanoprost from human plasma is rapid ($T_{½}$ = 17 min) after both intravenous (IV) and topical administration. Systemic clearance is approximately 7 ml/min/kg. Following hepatic β-oxidation, the metabolites are mainly eliminated via the kidneys. Approximately 88% and 98% of the administered dose is recovered in the urine after topical and IV dosing, respectively.

INDICATIONS AND USAGE

Latanoprost sterile ophthalmic solution is indicated for the reduction of elevated intraocular pressure in patients with open-angle glaucoma or ocular hypertension.

NON-FDA APPROVED INDICATIONS
Latanoprost has been used in the treatment of normal-tension glaucoma, although this use is not approved by the FDA.

CONTRAINDICATIONS

Known hypersensitivity to latanoprost, benzalkonium chloride or any other ingredients in this product.

WARNINGS

Latanoprost sterile ophthalmic solution has been reported to cause changes to pigmented tissues. The most frequently reported changes have been increased pigmentation of the iris, periorbital tissue (eyelid) and eyelashes, and growth of eyelashes. Pigmentation is expected to increase as long as latanoprost is administered. After discontinuation of latanoprost, pigmentation of the iris is likely to be permanent while pigmentation of the periorbital tissue and eyelash changes have been reported to be reversible in some patients. Patients who receive treatment should be informed of the possibility of increased pigmentation. The effects of increased pigmentation beyond 5 years are not known.

PRECAUTIONS

GENERAL
Latanoprost sterile ophthalmic solution may gradually increase the pigmentation of the iris. The eye color change is due to increased melanin content in the stromal melanocytes of the iris rather than to an increase in the number of melanocytes. This change may not be noticeable for several months to years (see WARNINGS). Typically, the brown pigmentation around the pupil spreads concentrically towards the periphery of the iris and the entire iris or parts of the iris become more brownish. Neither nevi nor freckles of the iris appear to be affected by treatment. While treatment with latanoprost can be continued in patients who develop noticeably increased iris pigmentation, these patients should be examined regularly.

During clinical trials, the increase in brown iris pigment has not been shown to progress further upon discontinuation of treatment, but the resultant color change may be permanent.

Eyelid skin darkening, which may be reversible, has been reported in association with the use of latanoprost (see WARNINGS).

Latanoprost may gradually change eyelashes and vellus hair in the treated eye; these changes include increased length, thickness, pigmentation, the number of lashes or hairs, and misdirected growth of eyelashes. Eyelash changes are usually reversible upon discontinuation of treatment.

Latanoprost should be used with caution in patients with a history of intraocular inflammation (iritis/uveitis) and should generally not be used in patients with active intraocular inflammation.

Macular edema, including cystoid macular edema, has been reported during treatment with latanoprost. These reports have mainly occurred in aphakic patients, in pseudophakic patients with a torn posterior lens capsule, or in patients with known risk factors for macular edema. Latanoprost should be used with caution in patients who do not have an intact posterior capsule or who have known risk factors for macular edema.

There is limited experience with latanoprost in the treatment of angle closure, inflammatory or neovascular glaucoma.

There have been reports of bacterial keratitis associated with the use of multiple-dose containers of topical ophthalmic products. These containers had been inadvertently contaminated by patients who, in most cases, had a concurrent corneal disease or a disruption of the ocular epithelial surface (see Information for the Patient).

Contact lenses should be removed prior to the administration of latanoprost, and may be reinserted 15 minutes after administration (see Information for the Patient).

INFORMATION FOR THE PATIENT

See WARNINGS and PRECAUTIONS.

Patients should be advised about the potential for increased brown pigmentation of the iris, which may be permanent. Patients should also be informed about the possibility of eyelid skin darkening, which may be reversible after discontinuation of latanoprost.

Patients should also be informed of the possibility of eyelash and vellus hair changes in the treated eye during treatment with latanoprost. These changes may result in a disparity between eyes in length, thickness, pigmentation, number of eyelashes or vellus hairs, and/or direction of eyelash growth. Eyelash changes are usually reversible upon discontinuation of treatment.

Patients should be instructed to avoid allowing the tip of the dispensing container to contact the eye or surrounding structures because this could cause the tip to become contaminated by common bacteria known to cause ocular infections. Serious damage to the eye and subsequent loss of vision may result from using contaminated solutions.

Patients also should be advised that if they develop an intercurrent ocular condition (*e.g.*, trauma, or infection) or have ocular surgery, they should immediately seek their physician's advice concerning the continued use of the multiple-dose container.

Patients should be advised that if they develop any ocular reactions, particularly conjunctivitis and lid reactions, they should immediately seek their physician's advice.

Patients should also be advised that latanoprost contains benzalkonium chloride, which may be absorbed by contact lenses. Contact lenses should be removed prior to administration of the solution. Lenses may be reinserted 15 minutes following administration of latanoprost.

If more than 1 topical ophthalmic drug is being used, the drugs should be administered at least 5 minutes apart.

CARCINOGENESIS, MUTAGENESIS, AND IMPAIRMENT OF FERTILITY

Latanoprost was not mutagenic in bacteria, in mouse lymphoma or in mouse micronucleus tests.

Chromosome aberrations were observed *in vitro* with human lymphocytes.

Latanoprost was not carcinogenic in either mice or rats when administered by oral gavage at doses of up to 170 μg/kg/day (approximately 2800 times the recommended maximum human dose) for up to 20 and 24 months, respectively.

Additional *in vitro* and *in vivo* studies on unscheduled DNA synthesis in rats were negative. Latanoprost has not been found to have any effect on male or female fertility in animal studies.

PREGNANCY, TERATOGENIC EFFECTS, PREGNANCY CATEGORY C

Reproduction studies have been performed in rats and rabbits. In rabbits an incidence of 4 of 16 dams had no viable fetuses at a dose that was approximately 80 times the maximum human dose, and the highest nonembryocidal dose in rabbits was approximately 15 times the maximum human dose. There are no adequate and well-controlled studies in pregnant women. Latanoprost should be used during pregnancy only if the potential benefit justifies the potential risk to the fetus.

NURSING MOTHERS

It is not known whether this drug or its metabolites are excreted in human milk. Because many drugs are excreted in human milk, caution should be exercised when latanoprost is administered to a nursing woman.

PEDIATRIC USE

Safety and effectiveness in pediatric patients have not been established.

GERIATRIC USE

No overall differences in safety or effectiveness have been observed between elderly and younger patients.

DRUG INTERACTIONS

In vitro studies have shown that precipitation occurs when eye drops containing thimerosal are mixed with latanoprost. If such drugs are used they should be administered at least 5 minutes apart.

ADVERSE REACTIONS

ADVERSE EVENTS REFERRED TO IN OTHER SECTIONS OF THIS INSERT

Eyelash changes (increased length, thickness, pigmentation, and number of lashes); eyelid skin darkening; intraocular inflammation (iritis/uveitis); iris pigmentation changes; and macular edema, including cystoid macular edema (see WARNINGS and PRECAUTIONS).

CONTROLLED CLINICAL TRIALS

The ocular adverse events and ocular signs and symptoms reported in 5-15% of the patients on latanoprost sterile ophthalmic solution in the three 6 month, multi-center, double-masked, active-controlled trials were blurred vision, burning and stinging, conjunctival hyperemia, foreign body sensation, itching, increased pigmentation of the iris, and punctate epithelial keratopathy.

Local conjunctival hyperemia was observed; however, less than 1% of the patients treated with latanoprost required discontinuation of therapy because of intolerance to conjunctival hyperemia.

In addition to the above listed ocular events/signs and symptoms, the following were reported in 1-4% of the patients: Dry eye, excessive tearing, eye pain, lid crusting, lid discomfort/pain, lid edema, lid erythema, and photophobia.

The following events were reported in less than 1% of the patients: Conjunctivitis, diplopia, and discharge from the eye.

During clinical studies, there were extremely rare reports of the following: Retinal artery embolus, retinal detachment, and vitreous hemorrhage from diabetic retinopathy.

The most common systemic adverse events seen with latanoprost were upper respiratory tract infection/cold/flu, which occurred at a rate of approximately 4%. Chest pain/angina pectoris, muscle/joint/back pain, and rash/allergic skin reaction each occurred at a rate of 1-2%.

CLINICAL PRACTICE

The following events have been identified during postmarketing use of latanoprost in clinical practice. Because they are reported voluntarily from a population of unknown size, estimates of frequency cannot be made. The events, which have been chosen for inclusion due to either their seriousness, frequency of reporting, possible causal connection to latanoprost, or a combination of these factors, include: asthma and exacerbation of asthma; corneal edema and erosions; dyspnea; eyelash and vellus hair changes (increased length, thickness, pigmentation, and number); eyelid skin darkening; herpes keratitis; intraocular inflammation (iritis/uveitis); keratitis; macular edema, including cystoid macular edema; misdirected eyelashes sometimes resulting in eye irritation; and toxic epidermal necrolysis.

DOSAGE AND ADMINISTRATION

The recommended dosage is 1 drop (1.5 μg) in the affected eye(s) once daily in the evening.

The dosage of latanoprost sterile ophthalmic solution should not exceed once daily since it has been shown that more frequent administration may decrease the intraocular pressure lowering effect.

Reduction of the intraocular pressure starts approximately 3-4 hours after administration and the maximum effect is reached after 8-12 hours.

Latanoprost may be used concomitantly with other topical ophthalmic drug products to lower intraocular pressure. If more than one topical ophthalmic drug is being used, the drugs should be administered at least 5 minutes apart.

ANIMAL PHARMACOLOGY

In monkeys, latanoprost has been shown to induce increased pigmentation of the iris. The mechanism of increased pigmentation seems to be stimulation of melanin production in melanocytes of the iris, with no proliferative changes observed. The change in iris color may be permanent.

Ocular administration of latanoprost at a dose of 6 μg/eye/day (4 times the daily human dose) to cynomolgus monkeys has also been shown to induce increased palpebral fissure. This effect was reversible upon discontinuation of the drug.

HOW SUPPLIED

Xalatan sterile ophthalmic solution is a clear, isotonic, buffered, preserved, colorless solution of latanoprost 0.005% (50 μg/ml). It is supplied as a 2.5 ml solution.

STORAGE

Protect from light. Store unopened bottle under refrigeration at 2-8°C (36-46°F). Once opened the 2.5 ml container may be stored at room temperature up to 25°C (77°F) for 6 weeks.

PRODUCT LISTING - EQUIVALENTS NOT AVAILABLE

Solution - Ophthalmic - 0.005%

2.50 ml	$55.60	XALATAN, Pharmacia and Upjohn	00013-8303-04
3 ml	$54.48	XALATAN, Physicians Total Care	54868-3881-00
25 ml	$47.73	XALATAN, Pharmacia and Upjohn	54569-4408-00

Leflunomide

(003406)

Categories: Arthritis, rheumatoid; FDA Approved 1998 Sep; Pregnancy Category X
Drug Classes: Disease modifying antirheumatic drugs; Immunomodulators
Brand Names: Arava
Cost of Therapy: $303.68 (Rheumatoid Arthritis; Arava; 20 mg; 1 tablet/day; 30 day supply)

WARNING

PREGNANCY MUST BE EXCLUDED BEFORE THE START OF TREATMENT WITH LEFLUNOMIDE. LEFLUNOMIDE IS CONTRAINDICATED IN PREGNANT WOMEN, OR WOMEN OF CHILDBEARING POTENTIAL WHO

> **WARNING — Cont'd**
> ARE NOT USING RELIABLE CONTRACEPTION. (SEE CONTRAINDICATIONS AND WARNINGS.) PREGNANCY MUST BE AVOIDED DURING LEFLUNOMIDE TREATMENT OR PRIOR TO THE COMPLETION OF THE DRUG ELIMINATION PROCEDURE AFTER LEFLUNOMIDE TREATMENT.

DESCRIPTION

Leflunomide is a pyrimidine synthesis inhibitor. The chemical name for leflunomide is N-(4′-trifluoromethylphenyl)-5-methylisoxazole-4-carboxamide. It has an empirical formula $C_{12}H_9F_3N_2O_2$, and a molecular weight of 270.2.

Arava is available for oral administration as tablets containing 10, 20, or 100 mg of active drug. Combined with leflunomide are the following inactive ingredients: colloidal silicon dioxide, crospovidone, hydroxypropyl methylcellulose, lactose monohydrate, magnesium stearate, polyethylene glycol, povidone, starch, talc, titanium dioxide, and yellow ferric oxide (20 mg tablet only).

CLINICAL PHARMACOLOGY

MECHANISM OF ACTION

Leflunomide is an isoxazole immunomodulatory agent which inhibits dihydroorotate dehydrogenase (an enzyme involved in de novo pyrimidine synthesis) and has antiproliferative activity. Several *in vivo* and *in vitro* experimental models have demonstrated an anti-inflammatory effect.

PHARMACOKINETICS

Following oral administration, leflunomide is metabolized to an active metabolite A77 1726 (hereafter referred to as M1) which is responsible for essentially all of its activity *in vivo.* Plasma levels of leflunomide are occasionally seen, at very low levels. Studies of the pharmacokinetics of leflunomide have primarily examined the plasma concentrations of this active metabolite.

ABSORPTION

Following oral administration, peak levels of the active metabolite, M1, occurred between 6-12 hours after dosing. Due to the very long half-life of M1 (~2 weeks), a loading dose of 100 mg for 3 days was used in clinical studies to facilitate the rapid attainment of steady-state levels of M1. Without a loading dose, it is estimated that attainment of steady-state plasma concentrations would require nearly 2 months of dosing. The resulting plasma concentrations following both loading doses and continued clinical dosing indicate that M1 plasma levels are dose proportional.

TABLE 1 *Pharmacokinetic Parameters for M1 After Administration of Leflunomide at Doses of 5, 10, and 25 mg/day for 24 Days to Patients (n=54) With Rheumatoid Arthritis (Mean ±SD) (Study YU204)*

	Maintenance (Loading) Dose		
Parameter	**5 mg (50 mg)**	**10 mg (100 mg)**	**25 mg (100 mg)**
C_{24} (Day 1) (μg/ml)*	4.0 ± 0.6	8.4 ± 2.1	8.5 ± 2.2
C_{24} (ss) (μg/ml)†	8.8 ± 2.9	18 ± 9.6	63 ± 36
T½ (days)	15 ± 3	14 ± 5	18 ± 9

* Concentration at 24 hours after loading dose.
† Concentration at 24 hours after maintenance doses at steady state.

Relative to an oral solution, leflunomide tablets are 80% bioavailable. Co-administration of leflunomide tablets with a high fat meal did not have a significant impact on M1 plasma levels.

DISTRIBUTION

M1 has a low volume of distribution (Vss = 0.13 L/kg) and is extensively bound (>99.3%) to albumin in healthy subjects. Protein binding has been shown to be linear at therapeutic concentrations. The free fraction of M1 is slightly higher in patients with rheumatoid arthritis and approximately doubled in patients with chronic renal failure; the mechanism and significance of these increases are unknown.

METABOLISM

Leflunomide is metabolized to one primary (M1) and many minor metabolites. Of these minor metabolites, only 4-trifluoromethylaniline (TFMA) is quantifiable, occurring at low levels in the plasma of some patients. The parent compound is rarely detectable in plasma. At the present time the specific site of leflunomide metabolism is unknown. *In vivo* and *in vitro* studies suggest a role for both the GI wall and the liver in drug metabolism. No specific enzyme has been identified as the primary route of metabolism for leflunomide; however, hepatic cytosolic and microsomal cellular fractions have been identified as sites of drug metabolism.

ELIMINATION

The active metabolite M1 is eliminated by further metabolism and subsequent renal excretion as well as by direct biliary excretion. In a 28 day study of drug elimination (n=3) using a single dose of radiolabeled compound, approximately 43% of the total radioactivity was eliminated in the urine and 48% was eliminated in the feces. Subsequent analysis of the samples revealed the primary urinary metabolites to be leflunomide glucuronides and an oxanilic acid derivative of M1. The primary fecal metabolite was M1. Of these 2 routes of elimination, renal elimination is more significant over the first 96 hours after which fecal elimination begins to predominate. In a study involving the intravenous administration of M1, the clearance was estimated to be 31 ml/h.

In small studies using activated charcoal (n=1) or cholestyramine (n=3) to facilitate drug elimination, the *in vivo* plasma half-life of M1 was reduced from >1 week to approximately 1 day (see PRECAUTIONS, General, Need for Drug Elimination). Similar reductions in plasma half-life were observed for a series of volunteers (n=96) enrolled in pharmacokinetic trials who were given cholestyramine. This suggests that biliary recycling is a major contributor to the long elimination half-life of M1. Studies with both hemodialysis and CAPD (chronic ambulatory peritoneal dialysis) indicate that M1 is not dialyzable.

SPECIAL POPULATIONS

Age and Gender

Neither age nor gender have been shown to cause a consistent change in the *in vivo* pharmacokinetics of M1.

Smoking

A population based pharmacokinetic analysis of the phase III data indicates that smokers have a 38% increase in clearance over non-smokers; however, no difference in clinical efficacy was seen between smokers and nonsmokers.

Chronic Renal Insufficiency

In single dose studies in patients (n=6) with chronic renal insufficiency requiring either chronic ambulatory peritoneal dialysis (CAPD) or hemodialysis, neither had a significant impact on circulating levels of M1. The free fraction of M1 was almost doubled, but the mechanism of this increase is not known. In light of the fact that the kidney plays a role in drug elimination, and without adequate studies of leflunomide use in subjects with renal insufficiency, caution should be used when leflunomide is administered to these patients.

Hepatic Insufficiency

Studies of the effect of hepatic insufficiency on M1 pharmacokinetics have not been done. Given the need to metabolize leflunomide into the active species, the role of the liver in drug elimination/recycling, and the possible risk of increased hepatic toxicity, the use of leflunomide in patients with hepatic insufficiency is not recommended.

DRUG INTERACTIONS

In vivo drug interaction studies have demonstrated a lack of a significant drug interaction between leflunomide and tri-phasic oral contraceptives, and cimetidine.

In vitro studies of protein binding indicated that warfarin did not affect M1 protein binding. At the same time M1 was shown to cause increases ranging from 13-50% in the free fraction of diclofenac, ibuprofen and tolbutamide at concentrations in the clinical range. *In vitro* studies of drug metabolism indicate that M1 inhibits CYP 450 2C9, which is responsible for the metabolism of many NSAIDs. M1 has been shown to inhibit the formation of 4′-hydroxydiclofenac from diclofenac *in vitro.* The clinical significance of these findings is unknown, however, there was extensive concomitant use of NSAIDs in clinical studies and no differential effect was observed.

Methotrexate

Coadministration, in 30 patients, of leflunomide (100 mg/day × 2 days followed by 10-20 mg/day) with methotrexate (10-25 mg/week, with folate) demonstrated no pharmacokinetic interaction between the two drugs. However, co-administration increased risk of hepatotoxicity (see DRUG INTERACTIONS, Hepatotoxic Drugs).

Rifampin

Following concomitant administration of a single dose of leflunomide to subjects receiving multiple doses of rifampin, M1 peak levels were increased (~40%) over those seen when leflunomide was given alone. Because of the potential for leflunomide levels to continue to increase with multiple dosing, caution should be used if patients are to receive both leflunomide and rifampin.

INDICATIONS AND USAGE

Leflunomide is indicated in adults for the treatment of active rheumatoid arthritis (RA) to reduce signs and symptoms and to retard structural damage as evidenced by x-ray erosions and joint space narrowing.

Aspirin, nonsteroidal anti-inflammatory agents and/or low dose corticosteroids may be continued during treatment with leflunomide (see DRUG INTERACTIONS, NSAIDs). The combined use of leflunomide with antimalarials, intramuscular or oral gold, D penicillamine, azathioprine, or methotrexate has not been adequately studied (see WARNINGS, Immunosuppression Potential).

CONTRAINDICATIONS

Leflunomide is contraindicated in patients with known hypersensitivity to leflunomide or any of the other components of leflunomide tablets.

Leflunomide can cause fetal harm when administered to a pregnant woman. Leflunomide, when administered orally to rats during organogenesis at a dose of 15 mg/kg, was teratogenic (most notably anophthalmia or microophthalmia and internal hydrocephalus). The systemic exposure of rats at this dose was approximately 1/10 the human exposure level based on AUC. Under these exposure conditions, leflunomide also caused a decrease in the maternal body weight and an increase in embryolethality with a decrease in fetal body weight for surviving fetuses. In rabbits, oral treatment with 10 mg/kg of leflunomide during organogenesis resulted in fused, dysplastic sternebrae. The exposure level at this dose was essentially equivalent to the maximum human exposure level based on AUC. At a 1 mg/kg dose, leflunomide was not teratogenic in rats and rabbits.

When female rats were treated with 1.25 mg/kg of leflunomide beginning 14 days before mating and continuing until the end of lactation, the offspring exhibited marked (greater than 90%) decreases in postnatal survival. The systemic exposure level at 1.25 mg/kg was approximately 1/100 the human exposure level based on AUC.

Leflunomide is contraindicated in women who are or may become pregnant. If this drug is used during pregnancy, or if the patient becomes pregnant while taking this drug, the patient should be apprised of the potential hazard to the fetus.

L

WARNINGS

IMMUNOSUPPRESSION POTENTIAL

Leflunomide is not recommended for patients with severe immunodeficiency, bone marrow dysplasia, or severe, uncontrolled infections.

There have been rare reports of pancytopenia in patients receiving leflunomide. In most of these cases, patients received concomitant treatment with methotrexate or other immunosuppressive agents, or they had recently discontinued these therapies; in some cases, patients had a prior history of a significant hematologic abnormality. If leflunomide is used in such patients, it should be administered with caution and with frequent clinical and hematologic monitoring. The use of leflunomide in combination therapy with methotrexate has not been adequately studied in a controlled setting.

If evidence of bone marrow suppression occurs in a patient taking leflunomide, treatment with leflunomide should be stopped, and cholestyramine or charcoal should be used to reduce the plasma concentration of leflunomide active metabolite (see PRECAUTIONS, General, Need for Drug Elimination).

In any situation in which the decision is made to switch from leflunomide to another anti-rheumatic agent with a known potential for hematologic suppression, it would be prudent to monitor for hematologic toxicity, because there will be overlap of systemic exposure to both compounds. Leflunomide washout with cholestyramine or charcoal may decrease this risk, but also may induce disease worsening if the patient had been responding to leflunomide treatment.

SKIN REACTIONS

Rare cases of Stevens-Johnson syndrome and toxic epidermal necrolysis have been reported in patients receiving leflunomide. If a patient taking leflunomide develops any of these conditions, leflunomide therapy should be stopped, and a drug elimination procedure is recommended (see PRECAUTIONS, General, Need for Drug Elimination).

HEPATOTOXICITY

In clinical trials, leflunomide treatment was associated with elevations of liver enzymes, primarily ALT and AST, in a significant number of patients; these effects were generally reversible. Most transaminase elevations were mild (≤2-fold ULN) and usually resolved while continuing treatment. Marked elevations (>3-fold ULN) occurred infrequently and reversed with dose reduction or discontinuation of treatment. TABLE 6A and TABLE 6B show liver enzyme elevations seen with monthly monitoring in clinical trials US301 and MN301. It was notable that the absence of folate use in MN302 was associated with a considerably greater incidence of liver enzyme elevation on methotrexate.

TABLE 6A *Liver Enzyme Elevations >3-fold Upper Limits of Normal (ULN)*

	US301			MN301		
	LEF	**PL**	**MTX**	**LEF**	**PL**	**SSZ**
ALT (SGPT)						
>3-fold UNL	8	3	5	2	1	2
(n %)	(4.4)	(2.5)	(2.7)	(1.5)	(1.1)	(1.5)
Reversed to ≤2-fold ULN	8	3	5	2	1	2
Timing of Elevation						
0-3 Months	6	1	1	2	1	2
4-6 Months	1	1	3	—	—	—
7-9 Months	1	1	1	—	—	—
10-12 Months	—	—	—	—	—	—
AST (SGOT)						
>3 fold UNL	4	2	1	2	0	5
(n %)	(2.2)	(1.7)	(0.6)	(1.5)	—	(3.8)
Reversed to ≤2-fold ULN	4	2	1	2	—	4
Timing of Elevation						
0-3 Months	2	1	—	2	—	4
4-6 Months	1	1	1	—	—	1
7-9 Months	1	—	—	—	—	—
10-12 Months	—	—	—	—	—	—

* Only 10% of patients in MN302 received folate. All patients in US301 received folate.

TABLE 6B *Liver Enzyme Elevations >3-fold Upper Limits of Normal (ULN)*

	MN302*	
	LEP	**MTX**
ALT (SGPT)		
>3-fold UNL	13	83
(n %)	(2.6)	(16.7)
Reversed to ≤2-fold ULN	12	82
Timing of Elevation		
0-3 Months	7	27
4-6 Months	1	34
7-9 Months	—	16
10-12 Months	5	6
AST (SGOT)		
>3-fold UNL	7	29
(n %)	(1.4)	(5.8)
Reversed to ≤2-fold ULN	5	29
Timing of Elevation		
0-3 Months	3	10
4-6 Months	1	11
7-9 Months	—	8
10-12 Months	3	—

* Only 10% of patients in MN302 received folate. All patients in US301 received folate.

At minimum, ALT (SGPT) should be performed at baseline and monitored initially at monthly intervals then, if stable, at intervals determined by the individual clinical situation.

Guidelines for dose adjustment or discontinuation based on the severity and persistence of ALT elevations are recommended as follows: For confirmed ALT elevations >2-fold ULN, dose reduction to 10 mg/day may allow continued administration of leflunomide. If elevations >2 but ≤3-fold ULN persist despite dose reduction, liver biopsy is recommended if continued treatment is desired. If elevations >3-fold ULN persist despite dose reduction, leflunomide should be discontinued and cholestyramine should be administered (see PRECAUTIONS, General, Need for Drug Elimination) with close monitoring, including retreatment with cholestyramine as indicated.

Rare elevations or alkaline phosphatase and bilirubin have been observed. Trial US301 used ACR Methotrexate Liver Biopsy Guidelines for monitoring therapy. One of 182 patients receiving leflunomide and 1 of 182 patients receiving methotrexate underwent liver biopsy at 106 and 50 weeks respectively. The biopsy for the leflunomide subject was Roegnik Grade IIIA and for the methotrexate subject, Roegnik Grade I.

PRE-EXISTING HEPATIC DISEASE

Given the possible risk of increased hepatotoxicity, and the role of the liver in drug activation, elimination and recycling, the use of leflunomide is not recommended in patients with significant hepatic impairment or positive Hepatitis B or C viruses.

MALIGNANCY

The risk of malignancy, particularly lymphoproliferative disorders, is increased with the use of some immunosuppression medications. There is a potential for immunosuppression with leflunomide. No apparent increase in the incidence of malignancies and lymphoproliferative disorders was reported in the clinical trials of leflunomide, but larger and longer-term studies would be needed to determine whether there is an increased risk of malignancy or lymphoproliferative disorders with leflunomide.

USE IN WOMEN OF CHILDBEARING POTENTIAL

There are no adequate and well-controlled studies evaluating leflunomide in pregnant women. However, based on animal studies, leflunomide may increase the risk of fetal death or teratogenic effects when administered to a pregnant woman (see CONTRAINDICATIONS). Women of childbearing potential must not be started on leflunomide until pregnancy is excluded and it has been confirmed that they are using reliable contraception. Before starting treatment with leflunomide, patients must be fully counseled on the potential for serious risk to the fetus.

The patient must be advised that if there is any delay in onset of menses or any other reason to suspect pregnancy, they must notify the physician immediately for pregnancy testing and, if positive, the physician and patient must discuss the risk to the pregnancy. It is possible that rapidly lowering the blood level of the active metabolite by instituting the drug elimination procedure described below at the first delay of menses may decrease the risk to the fetus from leflunomide.

Upon discontinuing leflunomide, it is recommended that all women of childbearing potential undergo the drug elimination procedure described below. Women receiving leflunomide treatment who wish to become pregnant must discontinue leflunomide and undergo the drug elimination procedure described below which includes verification of M1 metabolite plasma levels less than 0.02 mg/L (0.02 μg/ml). Human plasma levels of the active metabolite (M1) less than 0.02 mg/L (0.02 μg/ml) are expected to have minimal risk based on available animal data.

Drug Elimination Procedure

The following drug elimination procedure is recommended to achieve non-detectable plasma levels (less than 0.02 mg/L or 0.02 μg/ml) after stopping treatment with leflunomide:

Administer cholestyramine 8 g three times daily for 11 days. (The 11 days do not need to be consecutive unless there is a need to lower the plasma level rapidly.)

Verify plasma levels less than 0.02 mg/L (0.02 μg/ml) by 2 separate tests at least 14 days apart. If plasma levels are higher than 0.02 mg/L, additional cholestyramine treatment should be considered.

Without the drug elimination procedure, it may take up to 2 years to reach plasma M1 metabolite levels less than 0.02 mg/L due to individual variation in drug clearance.

PRECAUTIONS

GENERAL

Need for Drug Elimination

The active metabolite of leflunomide is eliminated slowly from the plasma. In instances of any serious toxicity from leflunomide, including hypersensitivity, use of a drug elimination procedure as described in this section is highly recommended to reduce the drug concentration more rapidly after stopping leflunomide therapy. If hypersensitivity is the suspected clinical mechanism, more prolonged cholestyramine or charcoal administration may be necessary to achieve rapid and sufficient clearance. The duration may be modified based on the clinical status of the patient.

Cholestyramine given orally at a dose of 8 g three times a day for 24 hours to 3 healthy volunteers decreased plasma levels of M1 by approximately 40% in 24 hours and by 49 to 65% in 48 hours.

Administration of activated charcoal (powder made into a suspension) orally or via nasogastric tube (50 g every 6 hours for 24 hours) has been shown to reduce plasma concentrations of the active metabolite, M1, by 37% in 24 hours and by 48% in 48 hours.

These drug elimination procedures may be repeated if clinically necessary.

Renal Insufficiency

Single dose studies in dialysis patients show a doubling of the free fraction of M1 in plasma. There is no clinical experience in the use of leflunomide in patients with renal impairment. Caution should be used when administering this drug in this population.

Vaccinations

No clinical data are available on the efficacy and safety of vaccinations during leflunomide treatment. Vaccination with live vaccines is, however, not recommended. The long half-life

L

of leflunomide should be considered when contemplating administration of a live vaccine after stopping leflunomide.

INFORMATION FOR THE PATIENT

The potential for increased risk of birth defects should be discussed with female patients of childbearing potential. It is recommended that physicians advise women that they may be at increased risk of having a child with birth defects if they are pregnant when taking leflunomide, become pregnant while taking leflunomide, or do not wait to become pregnant until they have stopped taking leflunomide and followed the drug elimination procedure (as described in WARNINGS, Use In Women of Childbearing Potential, Drug Elimination Procedure).

Patients should be advised of the possibility of rare, serious skin reactions. Patients should be instructed to inform their physicians promptly if they develop a skin rash or mucous membrane lesions.

Patients should be advised of the potential hepatotoxic effects of leflunomide and of the need for monitoring liver enzymes.

Patients who are receiving other immunosuppressive therapy concurrently with leflunomide, who have recently discontinued such therapy before starting treatment with leflunomide, or who have had a history of a significant hematologic abnormality, should be advised of the potential for pancytopenia and of the need for frequent hematologic monitoring. They should be instructed to notify their physicians promptly if they notice symptoms of pancytopenia (such as easy bruising, proneness to infections, paleness or unusual tiredness).

LABORATORY TESTS

At minimum, ALT (SGPT) should be performed at baseline and monitored initially at monthly intervals then, if stable, at intervals determined by the individual clinical situation. In patients who are at an increased risk of hematologic toxicity (see WARNINGS, Immunosuppression Potential), more vigilant monitoring, including hematologic monitoring, is warranted.

Due to a specific effect on the brush border of the renal proximal tubule, leflunomide has a uricosuric effect. A separate effect of hypophosphaturia is seen in some patients. These effects have not been seen together, nor have there been alterations in renal function.

CARCINOGENESIS, MUTAGENESIS, AND IMPAIRMENT OF FERTILITY

No evidence of carcinogenicity was observed in a 2 year bioassay in rats at oral doses of leflunomide up to the maximally tolerated dose of 6 mg/kg (approximately 1/40 the maximum human M1 systemic exposure based on AUC). However, male mice in a 2 year bioassay exhibited an increased incidence in lymphoma at an oral dose of 15 mg/kg, the highest dose studied (1.7 times the human M1 exposure based on AUC). Female mice, in the same study, exhibited a dose-related increased incidence of bronchoalveolar adenomas and carcinomas combined beginning at 1.5 mg/kg (approximately 1/10 the human M1 exposure based on AUC). The significance of the findings in mice relative to the clinical use of leflunomide is not known.

Leflunomide was not mutagenic in the Ames Assay, the Unscheduled DNA Synthesis Assay, or in the HGPRT Gene Mutation Assay. In addition, leflunomide was not clastogenic in the *in vivo* Mouse Micronucleus Assay nor in the *in vivo* Cytogenetic Test in Chinese Hamster Bone Marrow Cells. However, 4-trifluoromethylaniline (TMFA), a minor metabolite of leflunomide, was mutagenic in the Ames Assay and in the HGPRT Gene Mutation Assay, and was clastogenic in the *in vitro* Assay for Chromosome Aberrations in the Chinese Hamster Cells. TFMA was not clastogenic in the *in vivo* Mouse Micronucleus Assay nor in the *in vivo* Cytogenetic Test in Chinese Hamster Bone Marrow Cells.

Leflunomide had no effect on fertility in either male or female rats at oral doses up to 4.0 mg/kg (approximately 1/30 the human M1 exposure based on AUC).

PREGNANCY CATEGORY X

See CONTRAINDICATIONS.

Pregnancy Registry: To monitor fetal outcomes of pregnant women exposed to leflunomide, health care providers are encouraged to register such patients by calling 1-877-311-8972.

NURSING MOTHERS

Leflunomide should not be used by nursing mothers. It is not known whether leflunomide is excreted in human milk. Many drugs are excreted in human milk, and there is a potential for serious adverse reactions in nursing infants from leflunomide. Therefore, a decision should be made whether to proceed with nursing or to initiate treatment with leflunomide, taking into account the importance of the drug to the mother.

USE IN MALES

Available information does not suggest that leflunomide would be associated with an increased risk of male-mediated fetal toxicity. However, animal studies to evaluate this specific risk have not been conducted. To minimize any possible risk, men wishing to father a child should consider discontinuing use of leflunomide and taking cholestyramine 8 g three times daily for 11 days.

PEDIATRIC USE

The safety and efficacy of leflunomide in the pediatric population has not been studied. Use of leflunomide in patients less than 18 years of age is not recommended.

GERIATRIC USE

No dosage adjustment is needed in patients over 65.

DRUG INTERACTIONS

CHOLESTYRAMINE AND CHARCOAL

Administration of cholestyramine or activated charcoal in patients (n=13) and volunteers (n=96) resulted in a rapid and significant decrease in plasma M1 (the active metabolite of leflunomide) concentration (see PRECAUTIONS, General, Need for Drug Elimination).

TABLE 7A *Percentage of Patients With Adverse Events ≥3% in any Leflunomide Treated Group*

	All RA Studies	Placebo-Controlled Trials MN 301 and US 301			
	LEF (n=1339)†	LEF (n=315)	PBO (n=210)	SSZ (n=133)	MTX (n=182)
Body as a Whole					
Allergic reaction	2%	5%	2%	0%	6%
Asthenia	3%	6%	4%	5%	6%
Flu syndrome	2%	4%	2%	0%	7%
Infection	4%	0%	0%	0%	0%
Injury accident	5%	7%	5%	3%	11%
Pain	2%	4%	2%	2%	5%
Abdominal pain	6%	5%	4%	4%	8%
Back pain	5%	6%	3%	4%	9%
Cardiovascular					
Hypertension‡	10%	9%	4%	4%	3%
Chest Pain	2%	4%	2%	2%	4%
Gastrointestinal					
Anorexia	3%	3%	2%	5%	2%
Diarrhea	17%	27%	12%	10%	20%
Dyspepsia	5%	10%	10%	9%	13%
Gastroenteritis	3%	1%	1%	0%	6%
Abnormal liver enzymes	5%	10%	2%	4%	10%
Nausea	9%	13%	11%	19%	18%
GI/abdominal pain	5%	6%	4%	7%	8%
Mouth ulcer	3%	5%	4%	3%	10%
Vomiting	3%	5%	4%	4%	3%
Metabolic and Nutritional					
Hypokalemia	1%	3%	1%	1%	1%
Weight loss	4%	2%	1%	2%	0%
Musculoskeletal System					
Arthralgia	1%	4%	3%	0%	9%
Leg cramps	1%	4%	2%	2%	6%
Joint disorder	4%	2%	2%	2%	2%
Synovitis	2%	<1%	1%	0%	2%
Tenosynovitis	3%	2%	0%	1%	2%
Nervous System					
Dizziness	4%	5%	3%	6%	5%
Headache	7%	13%	11%	12%	21%
Paresthesia	2%	3%	1%	1%	2%
Respiratory System					
Bronchitis	7%	5%	2%	4%	7%
Increased cough	3%	4%	5%	3%	6%
Respiratory infection	15%	21%	21%	20%	32%
Pharyngitis	3%	2%	1%	2%	1%
Pneumonia	2%	3%	0%	0%	1%
Rhinitis	2%	5%	2%	4%	3%
Sinusitis	2%	5%	5%	0%	10%
Skin and Appendages					
Alopecia	10%	9%	1%	6%	6%
Eczema	2%	1%	1%	1%	1%
Pruritus	4%	5%	2%	3%	2%
Rash	10%	12%	7%	11%	9%
Dry skin	2%	3%	2%	2%	0%
Urogenital System					
Urinary tract infection	5%	5%	7%	4%	2%

* Only 10% of patients in MN302 received folate. All patients in US301 received folate; none in MN301 received folate.
† Includes all controlled and uncontrolled trials with leflunomide.
‡ Hypertension as a preexisting condition was overrepresented in all leflunomide treatment groups in phase III trials. Analysis of new onset hypertension revealed no difference among the treatment groups.

HEPATOTOXIC DRUGS

Increased side effects may occur when leflunomide is given concomitantly with hepatotoxic substances. This is also to be considered when leflunomide treatment is followed by such drugs without a drug elimination procedure. In a small (n=30) combination study of leflunomide with methotrexate, a 2- to 3-fold elevation in liver enzymes was seen in 5 of 30 patients. All elevations resolved, 2 with continuation of both drugs and 3 after discontinuation of leflunomide. A >3-fold increase was seen in another 5 patients. All of these also resolved, 2 with continuation of both drugs and 3 after discontinuation of leflunomide. Three patients met "ACR criteria" for liver biopsy (1: Roegnik Grade I, 2: Roegnik Grade IIIa). No pharmacokinetic interaction was identified (see CLINICAL PHARMACOLOGY).

NSAIDS

In *in vitro* studies, M1 was shown to cause increases ranging from 13-50% in the free fraction of diclofenac and ibuprofen at concentrations in the clinical range. The clinical significance of this finding is unknown, however, there was extensive concomitant use of NSAIDs in clinical studies and no differential effect was observed.

TOLBUTAMIDE

In *in vitro* studies, M1 was shown to cause increases ranging from 13-50% in the free fraction of tolbutamide at concentrations in the clinical range. The clinical significance of this finding is unknown.

RIFAMPIN

Following concomitant administration of a single dose of leflunomide to subjects receiving multiple doses of rifampin, M1 peak levels were increased (~40%) over those seen when leflunomide was given alone. Because of the potential for leflunomide levels to continue to increase with multiple dosing, caution should be used if patients are to be receiving both leflunomide and rifampin.

ADVERSE REACTIONS

Adverse reactions associated with the use of leflunomide in RA include diarrhea, elevated liver enzymes (ALT and AST), alopecia and rash. In the controlled studies, the following adverse events were reported, regardless of causality. (See TABLE 7A and TABLE 7B.)

TABLE 7B *Percentage of Patients With Adverse Events ≥3% in Any Leflunomide Treated Group*

	Active-Controlled Trials MN 302*	
	LEF (n=501)	MTX (n=498)
Body as a Whole		
Allergic reaction	1%	2%
Asthenia	3%	3%
Flu syndrome	0%	0%
Infection	0%	0%
Injury accident	6%	7%
Pain	1%	<1%
Abdominal pain	6%	4%
Back pain	8%	7%
Cardiovascular		
Hypertension‡	10%	4%
Chest pain	1%	2%
Gastrointestinal		
Anorexia	3%	3%
Diarrhea	22%	10%
Dyspepsia	6%	7%
Gastroenteritis	3%	3%
Abnormal liver enzymes	6%	17%
Nausea	13%	18%
GI/abdominal pain	8%	8%
Mouth ulcer	3%	6%
Vomiting	3%	3%
Metabolic and Nutritional		
Hypokalemia	1%	<1%
Weight loss	2%	2%
Musculoskeletal System		
Arthralgia	<1%	1%
Leg cramps	0%	0%
Joint disorder	8%	6%
Synovitis	4%	2%
Tenosynovitis	5%	1%
Nervous System		
Dizziness	7%	6%
Headache	10%	8%
Paresthesia	4%	3%
Respiratory System		
Bronchitis	8%	7%
Increased cough	5%	7%
Respiratory infection	27%	25%
Pharyngitis	3%	3%
Pneumonia	2%	2%
Rhinitis	2%	2%
Sinusitis	1%	1%
Skin and Appendages		
Alopecia	17%	10%
Eczema	3%	2%
Pruritus	6%	2%
Rash	11%	10%
Dry skin	3%	1%
Urogenital System		
Urinary tract infection	5%	6%

* Only 10% of patients in MN302 received folate. All patients in US301 received folate; none in MN301 received folate.
† Includes all controlled and uncontrolled trials with leflunomide.
‡ Hypertension as a preexisting condition was overrepresented in all leflunomide treatment groups in phase III trials. Analysis of new onset hypertension revealed no difference among the treatment groups.

In addition, the following adverse events have been reported in 1% to <3% of the RA patients in the leflunomide treatment group in controlled clinical trials.

Body as a Whole: Abscess, cyst, fever, hernia, malaise, pain, neck pain, pelvic pain.

Cardiovascular: Angina pectoris, migraine, palpitation, tachycardia, vasculitis, vasodilatation, varicose vein.

Gastrointestinal: Cholelithiasis, colitis, constipation, esophagitis, flatulence, gastritis, gingivitis, melena, oral moniliasis, pharyngitis, salivary gland enlarged, stomatitis (or aphthous stomatitis), tooth disorder.

Endocrine: Diabetes mellitus, hyperthyroidism.

Hemic and Lymphatic System: Anemia; (including iron deficiency anemia), ecchymosis.

Metabolic and Nutritional: Creatine phosphokinase increased, peripheral edema, hyperglycemia, hyperlipidemia.

Musculo-Skeletal System: Arthrosis, bursitis, muscle cramps, myalgia, bone necrosis, bone pain, tendon rupture.

Nervous System: Anxiety, depression, dry mouth, insomnia, neuralgia, neuritis, sleep disorder, sweating increased, vertigo.

Respiratory System: Asthma, dyspnea, epistaxis, lung disorder.

Skin and Appendages: Acne, contact dermatitis, fungal dermatitis, hair discoloration, hematoma, herpes simplex, herpes zoster, nail disorder, skin nodule, subcutaneous nodule, maculopapular rash, skin disorder, skin discoloration, ulcer skin.

Special Senses: Blurred vision, cataract, conjunctivitis, eye disorder, taste perversion.

Urogenital System: Albuminuria, cystitis, dysuria, hematuria, menstrual disorder, vaginal moniliasis, prostate disorder, urinary frequency.

Other less common adverse events seen in clinical trials include: 1 case of anaphylactic reaction occurred in Phase 2 following rechallenge of drug after withdrawal due to rash (rare); urticaria; eosinophilia; transient thrombocytopenia (rare); and leukopenia <2000 WBC/mm^3 (rare). In post-marketing experience, rare cases of pancytopenia, Stevens-Johnson syndrome, toxic epidermal necrolysis, and erythema multiforme have been reported.

DOSAGE AND ADMINISTRATION

LOADING DOSE

Due to the long half-life in patients with RA and recommended dosing interval (24 hours), a loading dose is needed to provide steady-state concentrations more rapidly. It is recommended that leflunomide therapy be initiated with a loading dose of one 100 mg tablet per day for 3 days.

MAINTENANCE THERAPY

Daily dosing of 20 mg is recommended for treatment of patients with RA. A small cohort of patients (n=104), treated with 25 mg/day, experienced a greater incidence of side effects: alopecia, weight loss, liver enzyme elevations. Doses higher than 20 mg/day are not recommended. If dosing at 20 mg/day is not well tolerated clinically, the dose may be decreased to 10 mg daily. Liver enzymes should be monitored and dose adjustments may be necessary (see WARNINGS, Hepatotoxicity). Due to the prolonged half-life of the active metabolite of leflunomide, patients should be carefully observed after dose reduction, since it may take several weeks for metabolite levels to decline.

HOW SUPPLIED

Arava tablets are available in:

10 mg: White, round film-coated tablet embossed with "ZBN" on one side.

20 mg: Light yellow, triangular film-coated tablet embossed with "ZBO" on one side.

100 mg: White, round film-coated tablet embossed with "ZBP" on one side.

Storage: Store at 25°C (77°F); excursions permitted to 15-30°C (59-86°F). Protect from light.

PRODUCT LISTING - EQUIVALENTS NOT AVAILABLE

Tablet - Oral - 10 mg
30's $303.68 ARAVA, Aventis Pharmaceuticals 00088-2160-30
Tablet - Oral - 20 mg
30's $303.68 ARAVA, Aventis Pharmaceuticals 00088-2161-30

L

Lepirudin (rDNA) *(003331)*

Categories: Thrombocytopenia, heparin-induced; FDA Approved 1998 Mar; Pregnancy Category B; Orphan Drugs
Drug Classes: Anticoagulants; Thrombin inhibitors
Brand Names: **Refludan**
Foreign Brand Availability: Refludin (South-Africa)

DESCRIPTION

Lepirudin (rDNA) for injection is a highly specific direct inhibitor of thrombin. Lepirudin (chemical designation: [Leu^1, Thr^2]-63-desulfohirudin) is a recombinant hirudin derived from yeast cells. The polypeptide composed of 65 amino acids has a molecular weight of 6979.5 daltons. Natural hirudin is produced in trace amounts as a family of highly homologous isopolypeptides by the leech *Hirudo medicinalis.* The biosynthetic molecule (lepirudin) is identical to natural hirudin except for substitution of leucine for isoleucine at the N-terminal end of the molecule and the absence of a sulfate group on the tyrosine at position 63.

The activity of lepirudin is measured in a chromogenic assay. One antithrombin unit (ATU) is the amount of lepirudin that neutralizes one unit of World Health Organization preparation 89/588 of thrombin. The specific activity of lepirudin is approximately 16000 ATU/mg. Its mode of action is independent of antithrombin III. Platelet factor 4 does not inhibit lepirudin. One molecule of lepirudin binds to one molecule of thrombin and thereby blocks the thrombogenic activity of thrombin. As a result, all thrombin-dependent coagulation assays are affected, *e.g.,* activated partial thromboplastin time (aPTT) values increase in a dose-dependent fashion (*Roethig 1991*).

Refludan is supplied as a sterile, white, freeze-dried powder for injection or infusion and is freely soluble in water for injection or 0.9% sodium chloride injection.

Each vial of Refludan contains 50 mg lepirudin. Other ingredients are 40 mg mannitol and sodium hydroxide for adjustment of pH to approximately 7.

CLINICAL PHARMACOLOGY

PHARMACOKINETICS

The pharmacokinetic properties of lepirudin following intravenous administration are well described by a two-compartment model. Distribution is essentially confined to extracellular fluids and is characterized by an initial half-life of approximately 10 minutes. Elimination follows a first-order process and is characterized by a terminal half-life of about 1.3 hours in young healthy volunteers. As the intravenous dose is increased over the range of 0.1-0.4 mg/kg, the maximum plasma concentration and the area-under-the-curve increase proportionally.

Lepirudin is thought to be metabolized by release of amino acids via catabolic hydrolysis of the parent drug. However, conclusive data are not available. About 48% of the administered dose is excreted in the urine which consists of unchanged drug (35%) and other fragments of the parent drug.

The systemic clearance of lepirudin is proportional to the glomerular filtration rate or creatinine clearance. Dose adjustment based on creatinine clearance is recommended (see DOSAGE AND ADMINISTRATION, Monitoring and Adjusting Therapy — Standard Recommendations and DOSAGE AND ADMINISTRATION, Use in Renal Impairment). In patients with marked renal insufficiency (creatinine clearance below 15 ml/min) and on hemodialysis, elimination half-lives are prolonged up to 2 days.

The systemic clearance of lepirudin in women is about 25% lower than in men. In elderly patients, the systemic clearance of lepirudin is 20% lower than in younger patients. This may be explained by the lower creatinine clearance in elderly patients compared to younger patients.

TABLE 1 summarizes systemic clearance (Cl) and volume of distribution at steady state (Vss) of lepirudin for various study populations.

TABLE 1 *Systemic Clearance (Cl) and Volume of Distribution at Steady State (Vss) of Lepirudin*

	Cl (ml/min) Mean (% CV*)	Vss (L) Mean (% CV*)
Healthy young subjects (n=18, age 18-60 years)	164 (19.3%)	12.2 (16.4%)
Healthy elderly subjects (n=10, age 65-80 years)	139 (22.5%)	18.7 (20.6%)
Renally impaired patients (n=16, creatinine clearance below 80 ml/min)	61 (89.4%)	18.0 (41.1%)
HIT† patients (n=73)	114 (46.8%)	32.1 (98.9%)

* CV: Coefficient of variation.
† HIT: Heparin-induced thrombocytopenia.

PHARMACODYNAMICS

The pharmacodynamic effect of lepirudin on the proteolytic activity of thrombin was routinely assessed as an increase in aPTT. This was observed with increasing plasma concentrations of lepirudin, with no saturable effect up to the highest tested dose (0.5 mg/kg body weight intravenous bolus). Thrombin time (TT) frequently exceeded 200 seconds even at low plasma concentrations of lepirudin, which renders this test unsuitable for routine monitoring of lepirudin therapy.

The pharmacodynamic response defined by the aPTT ratio (aPTT at a time after lepirudin administration over an aPTT reference value, usually median of the laboratory normal range for aPTT) depends on plasma drug levels which in turn depend on the individual patient's renal function (see Pharmacokinetics). For patients undergoing additional thrombolysis, elevated aPTT ratios were already observed at low lepirudin plasma concentrations, and further response to increasing plasma concentrations was relatively flat. In other populations, the response was steeper. At plasma concentrations of 1500 ng/ml, aPTT ratios were nearly 3.0 for healthy volunteers, 2.3 for patients with heparin-induced thrombocytopenia, and 2.1 for patients with deep venous thrombosis.

L

INDICATIONS AND USAGE

Lepirudin is indicated for anticoagulation in patients with heparin-induced thrombocytopenia (HIT) and associated thromboembolic disease in order to prevent further thromboembolic complications.

CONTRAINDICATIONS

Lepirudin is contraindicated in patients with known hypersensitivity to hirudins.

WARNINGS

HEMORRHAGIC EVENTS

Intracranial bleeding following concomitant thrombolytic therapy with rt-PA or streptokinase may be life-threatening (see also ADVERSE REACTIONS, Adverse Events Reported in HIT Patients, Adverse Events Reported in Other Populations and ADVERSE REACTIONS, Intracranial Bleeding).

For patients with increased risk of bleeding, a careful assessment weighing the risk of lepirudin administration vs its anticipated benefit has to be made by the treating physician.

In particular, this includes the following conditions:

- Recent puncture of large vessels or organ biopsy.
- Anomaly of vessels or organs.
- Recent cerebrovascular accident, stroke, intracerebral surgery, or other neuraxial procedures.
- Severe uncontrolled hypertension.
- Bacterial endocarditis.
- Advanced renal impairment (see also Renal Impairment).
- Hemorrhagic diathesis.
- Recent major surgery.
- Recent major bleeding (*e.g.*, intracranial, gastrointestinal, intraocular, or pulmonary bleeding).

RENAL IMPAIRMENT

With renal impairment, relative overdose might occur even with standard dosage regimen. Therefore, the bolus dose and the rate of infusion must be reduced in patients with known or suspected renal insufficiency (see CLINICAL PHARMACOLOGY, Pharmacokinetics and DOSAGE AND ADMINISTRATION, Monitoring and Adjusting Therapy — Standard Recommendations and DOSAGE AND ADMINISTRATION, Use in Renal Impairment).

PRECAUTIONS

GENERAL

Antibodies

Formation of antihirudin antibodies was observed in about 40% of HIT patients treated with lepirudin. This may increase the anticoagulant effect of lepirudin possibly due to delayed renal elimination of active lepirudin-antihirudin complexes (see also ANIMAL PHARMACOLOGY). Therefore, strict monitoring of aPTT is necessary also during prolonged therapy (see also Laboratory Tests and DOSAGE AND ADMINISTRATION, Monitoring and Adjusting Therapy — Standard Recommendations). No evidence of neutralization of lepirudin or of allergic reactions associated with positive antibody test results was found.

Liver Injury

Serious liver injury (*e.g.*, liver cirrhosis) may enhance the anticoagulant effect of lepirudin due to coagulation defects secondary to reduced generation of vitamin K-dependent coagulation factors.

Reexposure

Clinical trials have provided limited information to support any recommendations for reexposure to lepirudin. A total of 13 patients were reexposed in the HAT-1 and HAT-2 studies. One of these patients experienced a mild allergic skin reaction during the second treatment cycle. No further adverse experience was observed in relation to reexposure.

LABORATORY TESTS

In general, the dosage (infusion rate) should be adjusted according to the aPTT ratio (patient aPTT at a given time over an aPTT reference value, usually median of the laboratory normal range for aPTT); for full information, see DOSAGE AND ADMINISTRATION, Monitoring and Adjusting Therapy — Standard Recommendations. Other thrombin-dependent coagulation assays are changed by lepirudin (see also DESCRIPTION).

CARCINOGENESIS, MUTAGENESIS, AND IMPAIRMENT OF FERTILITY

Long-term animal studies to evaluate the potential for carcinogenesis have not been performed with lepirudin. Lepirudin was not genotoxic in the Ames test, the Chinese hamster cell (V79/HGPRT) forward mutation test, the A549 human cell line unscheduled DNA synthesis (UDS) test, the Chinese hamster V79 cell chromosome aberration test, or the mouse micronucleus test. An effect on fertility and reproductive performance of male and female rats was not seen with lepirudin at intravenous doses up to 30 mg/kg/day (180 mg/m^2/day, 1.2 times the recommended maximum human total daily dose based on body surface area of 1.45m^2 for a 50 kg subject).

PREGNANCY, TERATOGENIC EFFECTS, PREGNANCY CATEGORY B

Teratology studies with lepirudin performed in pregnant rats at intravenous doses up to 30 mg/kg/day (180 mg/m^2/day, 1.2 times the recommended maximum human total daily dose based on body surface area) and in pregnant rabbits at intravenous doses up to 30 mg/kg/day (360 mg/m^2/day, 2.4 times the recommended maximum human total daily dose based on body surface area) have revealed no evidence of harm to the fetus due to lepirudin. There are, however, no adequate and well-controlled studies in pregnant women. Because animal reproduction studies are not always predictive of human response, this drug should be used during pregnancy only if clearly needed.

Lepirudin (1 mg/kg) by intravenous administration crosses the placental barrier in pregnant rats. It is not known whether the drug crosses the placental barrier in humans.

Following intravenous administration of lepirudin at 30 mg/kg/day (180 mg/m^2/day, 1.2 times the recommended maximum human total daily dose based on body surface area) during organogenesis and perinatal-postnatal periods, pregnant rats showed an increased maternal mortality due to undetermined causes.

NURSING MOTHERS

It is not known whether lepirudin is excreted in human milk. Because many drugs are excreted in human milk and because of the potential for serious adverse reactions in nursing infants from lepirudin, a decision should be made whether to discontinue nursing or to discontinue the drug, taking into account the importance of the drug to the mother.

PEDIATRIC USE

Safety and effectiveness in pediatric patients have not been established. In the HAT-2 study, two children, an 11-year-old girl and a 12-year-old boy, were treated with lepirudin. Both children presented with TECs at baseline. Lepirudin doses given ranged from 0.15-0.22 mg/kg/h for the girl, and from 0.1 mg/kg/h (in conjunction with urokinase) to 0.7 mg/kg/h for the boy. Treatment with lepirudin was completed after 8 and 58 days, respectively, without serious adverse events (*Schiffmann 1997*).

DRUG INTERACTIONS

Concomitant treatment with thrombolytics (*e.g.*, rt-PA or streptokinase) may:

- Increase the risk of bleeding complications.
- Considerably enhance the effect of lepirudin on aPTT prolongation.

(See also WARNINGS, Hemorrhagic Events; ADVERSE REACTIONS, Adverse Events Reported in HIT Patients, Adverse Events Reported in Other Populations, and ADVERSE REACTIONS, Intracranial Bleeding; and DOSAGE AND ADMINISTRATION, Concomitant Use With Thrombolytic Therapy and DOSAGE AND ADMINISTRATION, Monitoring and Adjusting Therapy — Standard Recommendations).

Concomitant treatment with coumarin derivatives (vitamin K antagonists) and drugs that affect platelet function may also increase the risk of bleeding (see also DOSAGE AND ADMINISTRATION, Use in Patients Scheduled for a Switch to Oral Anticoagulation and DOSAGE AND ADMINISTRATION, Monitoring and Adjusting Therapy — Standard Recommendations).

ADVERSE REACTIONS

ADVERSE EVENTS REPORTED IN HIT PATIENTS

The following safety information is based on all 198 patients treated with lepirudin in the HAT-1 and HAT-2 studies. The safety profile of 113 lepirudin patients from these studies who presented with TECs at baseline is compared to 91 such patients in the historical control.

Hemorrhagic Events

Bleeding was the most frequent adverse event observed in patients treated with lepirudin. TABLE 4 gives an overview of all hemorrhagic events which occurred in at least 2 patients.

TABLE 4 *Hemorrhagic Events**

	HAT-1 HAT-2 (All patients) (n= 198)	Patients with TECs Lepirudine (n=113)	Historical Control (n= 91)
Bleeding from puncture sites and wounds	14.1%	10.6%	4.4%
Anemia or isolated drop in hemoglobin	13.1%	12.4%	1.1%
Other hematoma and unclassified bleeding	11.1%	10.6%	4.4%
Hematuria	6.6%	4.4%	0
Gastrointestinal and rectal bleeding	5.1%	5.3%	6.6%
Epistaxis	3.0%	4.4%	1.1%
Hemothorax	3.0%	0	1.1%
Vaginal bleeding	1.5%	1.8%	0
Intracranial bleeding	0	0	2.2%

* Patients may have suffered more than one event.

Other hemorrhagic events (hemoperitoneum, hemoptysis, liver bleeding, lung bleeding, mouth bleeding, retroperitoneal bleeding) each occurred in 1 individual among all 198 patients treated with lepirudin.

Nonhemorrhagic Events

TABLE 5 gives an overview of the most frequently observed nonhemorrhagic events.

TABLE 5 *Nonhemorrhagic Adverse Events**

	HAT-1 HAT-2 (All patients) (n= 198)	Patients with TECs Lepirudine (n=113)	Historical Control (n= 91)
Fever	6.1%	4.4%	8.8%
Abnormal liver function	6.1%	5.3%	0
Pneumonia	4.0%	4.4%	5.5%
Sepsis	4.0%	3.5%	5.5%
Allergic skin reactions	3.0%	3.5%	1.1%
Heart failure	3.0%	1.8%	2.2%
Abnormal kidney function	2.5%	1.8%	4.4%
Unspecified infections	2.5%	1.8%	1.1%
Multiorgan failure	2.0%	3.5%	0
Pericardial effusion	1.0%	0	1.1%
Ventricular fibrillation	1.0%	0	0

* Patients may have suffered more than one event.

Adverse Events Reported in Other Populations

The following safety information is based on a total of 2302 individuals who were treated with lepirudin in clinical pharmacology studies (n=323) or for clinical indications other than HIT (n=1979).

Intracranial Bleeding

Intracranial bleeding was the most serious adverse reaction found in populations other than HIT patients. However, it only occurred in patients with acute myocardial infarction who were started on both lepirudin and thrombolytic therapy with rt-PA or streptokinase. The overall frequency of this potentially life-threatening complication among patients receiving both lepirudin and thrombolytic therapy was 0.6% (7 out of 1134 patients). No intracranial bleeding was observed in 1168 subjects or patients who did not receive concomitant thrombolysis.

Allergic Reactions

Allergic reactions or suspected allergic reactions in populations other than HIT patients include (in descending order of frequency*):

- ***Airway Reactions (cough, bronchospasm, stridor, dyspnea):*** Common.
- ***Unspecified Allergic Reactions:*** Uncommon.
- ***Skin Reactions (pruritus, urticaria, rash, flushes, chills):*** Uncommon.
- ***General Reactions (anaphylactoid or anaphylactic reactions):*** Uncommon.
- ***Edema (facial edema, tongue edema, larynx edema, angioedema):*** Rare.

The CIOMS (Council for International Organization of Medical Sciences) III standard categories are used for classification of frequencies:

Very Common: 10% or more.
Common (Frequent): 1 to <10%.
Uncommon (Infrequent): 0.1 to <1%.
Rare: 0.01 to <0.1%.
Very Rare: 0.01% or less.

About 53% (n=46) of all allergic reactions or suspected allergic reactions occurred in patients who concomitantly received thrombolytic therapy (*e.g.*, streptokinase) for acute myocardial infarction and/or contrast media for coronary angiography.

DOSAGE AND ADMINISTRATION

INITIAL DOSAGE

Anticoagulation in adult patients with HIT and associated thromboembolic disease:

- 0.4 mg/kg body weight (up to 110 kg) slowly intravenously (*e.g.*, over 15-20 seconds) as a bolus dose,
- Followed by 0.15 mg/kg body weight (up to 110 kg)/hour as a continuous intravenous infusion for 2-10 days or longer if clinically needed.

Normally the initial dosage depends on the patient's body weight. This is valid up to a body weight of 110 kg. In patients with a body weight exceeding 110 kg, the initial dosage should not be increased beyond the 110 kg body weight dose (maximal initial bolus dose of 44 mg, maximal initial infusion dose of 16.5 mg/h; see also Initial Intravenous Bolus, TABLE 7, Intravenous Infusion, and TABLE 8).

In general, therapy with lepirudin is monitored using the aPTT ratio (patient aPTT at a given time over an aPTT reference value, usually median of the laboratory normal range for aPTT, see Monitoring and Adjusting Therapy — Standard Recommendations). A patient baseline aPTT should be determined prior to initiation of therapy with lepirudin, since lepirudin should not be started in patients presenting with a baseline aPTT ratio of 2.5 or more, in order to avoid initial overdosing.

MONITORING AND ADJUSTING THERAPY — STANDARD RECOMMENDATIONS

Monitoring

- **In general, the dosage (infusion rate) should be adjusted according to the aPTT ratio (patient aPTT at a given time over an aPTT reference value, usually median of the laboratory normal range for aPTT).**
- **The target range for the aPTT ratio during treatment (therapeutic window) should be 1.5 to 2.5. Data from clinical trials in HIT patients suggest that with aPTT ratios higher than this target range, the risk of bleeding increases, while there is no incremental increase in clinical efficacy.**
- **As stated in Initial Dosage, lepirudin should not be started in patients presenting with a baseline aPTT ratio of 2.5 or more, in order to avoid initial overdosing.**
- **The first aPTT determination for monitoring treatment should be done 4 hours after start of the lepirudin infusion.**
- **Follow-up aPTT determinations are recommended at least once daily, as long as treatment with lepirudin is ongoing.**
- **More frequent aPTT monitoring is highly recommended in patients with renal impairment or serious liver injury (see Use in Renal Impairment) or with an increased risk of bleeding.**

Dose Modifications

- **Any aPTT ratio out of the target range is to be confirmed at once before drawing conclusions with respect to dose modifications, unless there is a clinical need to react immediately.**
- **If the confirmed aPTT ratio is above the target range, the infusion should be stopped for 2 hours. At restart, the infusion rate should be decreased by 50% (no additional intravenous bolus should be administered). The aPTT ratio should be determined again 4 hours later.**
- **If the confirmed aPTT ratio is below the target range, the infusion rate should be increased in steps of 20%. The aPTT ratio should be determined again 4 hours later.**
- **In general, an infusion rate of 0.21 mg/kg/h should not be exceeded without checking for coagulation abnormalities which might be preventive of an appropriate aPTT response.**

Use in Renal Impairment

As lepirudin is almost exclusively excreted in the kidneys (see also CLINICAL PHARMACOLOGY, Pharmacokinetics), individual renal function should be considered prior to administration. In case of renal impairment, relative overdose might occur even with the standard dosage regimen. Therefore, the bolus dose and the infusion rate must be reduced in case of known or suspected renal insufficiency (creatinine clearance below 60 ml/min or serum creatinine above 1.5 mg/dl).

There is only limited information on the therapeutic use of lepirudin in HIT patients with significant renal impairment. The following dosage recommendations are mainly based on single-dose studies in a small number of patients with renal impairment. Therefore, these recommendations are only tentative.

Dose adjustments should be based on creatinine clearance values, whenever available, as obtained from a reliable method (24 h urine sampling). If creatinine clearance is not available, the dose adjustments should be based on the serum creatinine.

In all patients with renal insufficiency, the bolus dose is to be reduced to 0.2 mg/kg body weight.

The standard initial infusion rate given in Initial Dosage and Administration, Intravenous Infusion, TABLE 8 must be reduced according to the recommendations given in TABLE 6. Additional aPTT monitoring is highly recommended.

TABLE 6 *Reduction of Infusion Rate in Patients With Renal Impairment*

Creatinine Clearance	Serum Creatinine	Adjusted infusion rate (% of standard initial infusion rate)	(mg/kg/h)
45-60 ml/min	1.6-2.0 mg/dl	50%	0.075 mg/kg/h
30-44 ml/min	2.1-3.0 mg/dl	30%	0.045 mg/kg/h
15-29 ml/min	3.1-6.0 mg/dl	15%	0.0225 mg/kg/h
below 15 ml/min*	above 6.0 mg/dl*	avoid or STOP infusion!*	

* In hemodialysis patients or in case of acute renal failure (creatinine clearance below 15 ml/min or serum creatinine above 6.0 mg/dl), infusion of lepirudin is to be avoided or stopped. Additional intravenous bolus doses of 0.1 mg/kg body weight should be considered every other day only if the aPTT ratio falls below the lower therapeutic limit of 1.5 (see also Monitoring and Adjusting Therapy — Standard Recommendations).

Concomitant Use With Thrombolytic Therapy

Clinical trials in HIT patients have provided only limited information on the combined use of lepirudin and thrombolytic agents. The following dosage regimen of lepirudin was used in a total of 9 HIT patients in the HAT-1 and HAT-2 studies who presented with TECs at baseline and were started on both lepirudin and thrombolytic therapy (rt-PA, urokinase or streptokinase):

- ***Initial Intravenous Bolus:*** 0.2 mg/kg body weight.

• *Continuous Intravenous Infusion:* 0.1 mg/kg body weight/h.

The number of patients receiving combined therapy was too small to identify differences in clinical outcome of patients who were started on both lepirudin and thrombolytic therapy as compared to those who were started on lepirudin alone. The combined incidences of death, limb amputation, or new TEC were 22.2% and 20.7%, respectively. While there was a 47% relative increase in the overall bleeding rate in patients who were started on both lepirudin and thrombolytic therapy (55.6% vs 37.9%), there were no differences in the rates of serious bleeding events (fatal or life-threatening bleeds, bleeds that were permanently or significantly disabling, overt bleeds requiring transfusion of 2 or more units of packed red blood cells, bleeds necessitating surgical intervention, intracranial bleeds) between the groups (11.1% vs 11.2%). Although no intracranial bleeding has been observed in any of these patients, the risk of this potentially life-threatening complication may be increased in conjunction with thrombolytic agents (see ADVERSE REACTIONS, Adverse Events Reported in HIT Patients, Adverse Events Reported in Other Populations and ADVERSE REACTIONS, Intracranial Bleeding).

Special attention should be paid to the fact that thrombolytic agents per se may increase the aPTT ratio. Therefore, aPTT ratios with a given plasma level of lepirudin are usually higher in patients who receive concomitant thrombolysis than in those who do not (see also CLINICAL PHARMACOLOGY, Pharmacodynamics).

Use in Patients Scheduled for a Switch to Oral Anticoagulation

If a patient is scheduled to receive coumarin derivatives (vitamin K antagonists) for oral anticoagulation after lepirudin therapy, the dose of lepirudin should first be gradually reduced in order to reach an aPTT ratio just above 1.5 before initiating oral anticoagulation. As soon as an international normalized ratio (INR) of 2.0 is reached, lepirudin therapy should be stopped.

ADMINISTRATION

Directions on Preparation and Dilution: Lepirudin should not be mixed with other drugs except for water for injection, 0.9% sodium chloride injection or 5% dextrose injection. Use lepirudin before the expiration date given on the carton and container.

Reconstitution and further dilution are to be carried out under sterile conditions:

- For reconstitution, water for injection or 0.9% sodium chloride injection are to be used.
- For further dilution, 0.9% sodium chloride injection or 5% dextrose injection are suitable.
- For rapid, complete reconstitution, inject 1 ml of diluent into the vial and shake it gently. After reconstitution a clear, colorless solution is usually obtained in a few seconds, but definitely in less than 3 minutes.
- Parenteral drug products should be inspected visually for particulate matter and discoloration prior to administration whenever solution and container permit. Do not use solutions that are cloudy or contain particles.
- The reconstituted solution is to be used immediately. It remains stable for up to 24 hours at room temperature (*e.g.*, during infusion).
- The preparation should be warmed to room temperature before administration.
- Discard any unused solution appropriately.

Initial Intravenous Bolus

For intravenous bolus injection, use a solution with a concentration of 5 mg/ml.

Preparation of a lepirudin solution with a concentration of 5 mg/ml:

- Reconstitute one vial (50 mg of lepirudin) with 1 ml of water for injection or 0.9% sodium chloride injection.
- The final concentration of 5 mg/ml is obtained by transferring the contents of the vial into a sterile, single-use syringe (of at least 10 ml capacity) and diluting the solution to a total volume of 10 ml, using water for injection, 0.9% sodium chloride injection or 5% dextrose injection.
- The final solution is to be administered according to body weight (see TABLE 7 and Initial Dosage).

Intravenous injection of the bolus is to be carried out slowly (*e.g.*, over 15-20 seconds).

Intravenous Infusion

TABLE 7 *Standard Bolus Injection Volumes According to Body Weight for a 5 mg/ml Concentration*

	Injection Volume	
Body Weight	Dosage 0.4 mg/kg	Dosage 0.2 mg/kg*
50 kg	4.0 ml	2.0 ml
60 kg	4.8 ml	2.4 ml
70 kg	5.6 ml	2.8 ml
80 kg	6.4 ml	3.2 ml
90 kg	7.2 ml	3.6 ml
100 kg	8.0 ml	4.0 ml
≥110 kg	8.8 ml	4.4 ml

* Dosage recommended for all patients with renal insufficiency (see Monitoring and Adjusting Therapy — Standard Recommendations; and Use in Renal Impairment)

For continuous intravenous infusion, solutions with concentration of 0.2 mg/ml or 0.4 mg/ml may be used.

Preparation of a lepirudin solution with a concentration of 0.2 or 0.4 mg/ml:

- Reconstitute two vials (each containing 50 mg of lepirudin) with 1 ml each using either water for injection or 0.9% sodium chloride injection.
- The final concentrations of 0.2 mg/ml or 0.4 mg/ml are obtained by transferring the contents of both vials into an infusion bag containing 500 ml or 250 ml of 0.9% sodium chloride injection or 5% dextrose injection.

The infusion rate (ml/h) is to be set according to body weight (see TABLE 8 and Initial Dosage).

TABLE 8 *Standard Infusion Rates According to Body Weight*

	Infusion Rate at 0.15 mg/kg/h	
Body Weight	500 ml infusion bag 0.2 mg/ml	250 ml infusion bag 0.4 mg/ml
50 kg	38 ml/h	19 ml/h
60 kg	45 ml/h	23 ml/h
70 kg	53 ml/h	26 ml/h
80 kg	60 ml/h	30 ml/h
90 kg	68 ml/h	34 ml/h
100 kg	75 ml/h	38 ml/h
≥110 kg	83 ml/h	41 ml/h

ANIMAL PHARMACOLOGY

GENERAL TOXICITY

Lepirudin caused bleeding in animal toxicity studies. Antibodies against hirudin which appeared in several monkeys treated with lepirudin resulted in a prolongation of the terminal half-life and an increase of AUC plasma values of lepirudin.

HOW SUPPLIED

Refludan is supplied in vials containing 50 mg lepirudin.

Storage: Store unopened vials at 2-25°C (36-77°F). Use Refludan before the expiration date given on the carton and container. Once reconstituted, use Refludan immediately.

PRODUCT LISTING - EQUIVALENTS NOT AVAILABLE

Powder For Injection - Intravenous - 50 mg

10's $1446.90 REFLUDAN, Berlex Laboratories 50419-0150-57

Letrozole (003330)

Categories: Carcinoma, breast; Pregnancy Category D; FDA Approved 1997 Jul
Drug Classes: Antineoplastics, aromatase inhibitors; Hormones/hormone modifiers
Brand Names: Femara
Cost of Therapy: $232.96 (Breast Cancer; Femara; 2.5 mg; 1 tablet/day; 30 day supply)

DESCRIPTION

Letrozole tablets for oral administration contain 2.5 mg of letrozole, a nonsteroidal aromatase inhibitor (inhibitor of estrogen synthesis). It is chemically described as 4,4'-(1H-1,2,4-Triazol-1-ylmethylene)dibenzonitrile.

Letrozole is a white to yellowish crystalline powder, practically odorless, freely soluble in dichloromethane, slightly soluble in ethanol, and practically insoluble in water. It has a molecular weight of 285.31, empirical formula $C_{17}H_{11}N_5$, and a melting range of 184-185°C.

Femara is available as 2.5 mg tablets for oral administration. *Inactive Ingredients:* Colloidal silicon dioxide, ferric oxide, hydroxypropyl methylcellulose, lactose monohydrate, magnesium stearate, maize starch, microcrystalline cellulose, polyethylene glycol, sodium starch glycolate, talc, and titanium dioxide.

CLINICAL PHARMACOLOGY

MECHANISM OF ACTION

The growth of some cancers of the breast is stimulated or maintained by estrogens. Treatment of breast cancer thought to be hormonally responsive (*i.e.,* estrogen and/or progesterone receptor positive or receptor unknown) has included a variety of efforts to decrease estrogen levels (ovariectomy, adrenalectomy, hypophysectomy) or inhibit estrogen effects (antiestrogens and progestational agents). These interventions lead to decreased tumor mass or delayed progression of tumor growth in some women.

In postmenopausal women, estrogens are mainly derived from the action of the aromatase enzyme, which converts adrenal androgens (primarily androstrenedione and testosterone) to estrone and estradiol. The suppression of estrogen biosynthesis in peripheral tissues and in the cancer tissue itself can therefore be achieved by specifically inhibiting the aromatase enzyme.

Letrozole is a nonsteroidal competitive inhibitor of the aromatase enzyme system; it inhibits the conversion of androgens to estrogens. In adult nontumor- and tumor-bearing female animals, letrozole is as effective as ovariectomy in reducing uterine weight, elevating serum LH, and causing the regression of estrogen-dependent tumors. In contrast to ovariectomy, treatment with letrozole does not lead to an increase in serum FSH. Letrozole selectively inhibits gonadal steroidogenesis but has no significant effect on adrenal mineralocorticoid or glucocorticoid synthesis.

Letrozole inhibits the aromatase enzyme by competitively binding to the heme of the cytochrome P450 subunit of the enzyme, resulting in a reduction of estrogen biosynthesis in all tissues. Treatment of women with letrozole significantly lowers serum estrone, estradiol and estrone sulfate and has not been shown to significantly affect adrenal corticosteroid synthesis, aldosterone synthesis, or synthesis of thyroid hormones.

PHARMACOKINETICS

Letrozole is rapidly and completely absorbed from the gastrointestinal tract and absorption is not affected by food. It is metabolized slowly to an inactive metabolite whose glucuronide conjugate is excreted renally, representing the major clearance pathway. About 90% of radiolabeled letrozole is recovered in urine. Letrozole's terminal elimination half-life is about 2 days and steady-state plasma concentration after daily 2.5 mg dosing is reached in 2-6 weeks. Plasma concentrations at steady-state are 1.5 to 2 times higher than predicted from the concentrations measured after a single dose, indicating a slight non-linearity in the pharmacokinetics of letrozole upon daily administration of 2.5 mg. These steady-state levels are maintained over extended periods, however, and continuous accumulation of letrozole does not occur. Letrozole is weakly protein bound and has a large volume of distribution (approximately 1.9 L/kg).

METABOLISM AND EXCRETION

Metabolism to a pharmacologically-inactive carbinol metabolite (4,4′-methanol-bisbenzonitrile) and renal excretion of the glucuronide conjugate of this metabolite is the major pathway of letrozole clearance. Of the radiolabel recovered in urine, at least 75% was the glucuronide of the carbinol metabolite, about 9% was two unidentified metabolites, and 6% was unchanged letrozole.

In human microsomes with specific CYP isozyme activity, CYP3A4 metabolized letrozole to the carbinol metabolite while CYP2A6 formed both this metabolite and its ketone analog. In human liver microsomes, letrozole strongly inhibited CYP2A6 and moderately inhibited CYP2C19.

SPECIAL POPULATIONS

Pediatric, Geriatric, and Race

In the study populations (adults ranging in age from 35 to >80 years), no change in pharmacokinetic parameters was observed with increasing age. Differences in letrozole pharmacokinetics between adult and pediatric populations have not been studied. Differences in letrozole pharmacokinetics due to race have not been studied.

Renal Insufficiency

In a study of volunteers with varying renal function (24 hour creatinine clearance: 9-116 ml/min), no effect of renal function on the pharmacokinetics of single doses of 2.5 mg of letrozole tablets was found. In addition, in a study of 347 patients with advanced breast cancer, about half of whom received 2.5 mg of letrozole and half 0.5 mg letrozole, renal impairment (calculated creatinine clearance: 20-50 ml/min) did not affect steady-state plasma letrozole concentration.

Hepatic Insufficiency

In a study of subjects with varying degrees of non-metastatic hepatic dysfunction (*e.g.*, cirrhosis, Child-Pugh classification A and B), the mean AUC values of the volunteers with moderate hepatic impairment were 37% higher than in normal subjects, but still within the range seen in subjects without impaired function. In a pharmacokinetics study, subjects with liver cirrhosis and severe hepatic impairment (Child-Pugh classification C, which included bilirubins about 2-11 times ULN with minimal to severe ascites) had 2-fold increase in exposure (AUC) and 47% reduction in systemic clearance. Breast cancer patients with severe hepatic impairment are thus expected to be exposed to higher levels of letrozole than patients with normal liver function receiving similar doses of this drug. (See DOSAGE AND ADMINISTRATION, Hepatic Impairment.)

Drug/Drug Interactions

A pharmacokinetic interaction study with cimetidine showed no clinically significant effect on letrozole pharmacokinetics. An interaction study with warfarin showed no clinically significant effect of letrozole on warfarin pharmacokinetics. In *in vitro* experiments, letrozole showed no significant inhibition in the metabolism of diazepam. Similarly, no significant inhibition of letrozole metabolism by diazepam was observed.

Coadministration of letrozole and tamoxifen 20 mg daily resulted in a reduction of letrozole plasma levels of 38% on average. Clinical experience in the second-line breast cancer pivotal trials indicates that the therapeutic effect of letrozole therapy is not impaired if letrozole is administered immediately after tamoxifen.

There is no clinical experience to date on the use of letrozole in combination with other anticancer agents.

PHARMACODYNAMICS

In postmenopausal patients with advanced breast cancer, daily doses of 0.1 to 5 mg letrozole suppress plasma concentrations of estradiol, estrone, and estrone sulfate by 75-95% from baseline with maximal suppression achieved within 2-3 days. Suppression is dose-related, with doses of 0.5 mg and higher giving many values of estrone and estrone sulfate that were below the limit of detection in the assays. Estrogen suppression was maintained throughout treatment in all patients treated at 0.5 mg or higher.

Letrozole is highly specific in inhibiting aromatase activity. There is no impairment of adrenal steroidogenesis. No clinically-relevant changes were found in the plasma concentrations of cortisol, aldosterone, 11-deoxycoritsol, 17-hydroxy-progesterone, ACTH or in plasma renin activity among postmenopausal patients treated with a daily dose of letrozole 0.1 to 5 mg. The ACTH stimulation test performed after 6 and 12 weeks of treatment with daily doses of 0.1, 0.25, 0.5, 1, 2.5, and 5 mg did not indicate any attenuation of aldosterone or cortisol production. Glucocorticoid or mineralocorticoid supplementation is, therefore, not necessary.

No changes were noted in plasma concentrations of androgens (androstenedione and testosterone) among healthy postmenopausal women after 0.1, 0.5, and 2.5 mg single doses of letrozole or in plasma concentrations of androstenedione among postmenopausal patients treated with daily doses of 0.1 to 5 mg. This indicates that the blockade of estrogen biosynthesis does not lead to accumulation of androgenic precursors. Plasma levels of LH and FSH were not affected by letrozole in patients, nor was thyroid function as evaluated by TSH levels, T3 uptake and T4 levels.

INDICATIONS AND USAGE

Letrozole is indicated for first-line treatment of postmenopausal women with hormone receptor positive or hormone receptor unknown locally advanced or metastatic breast cancer. Letrozole is also indicated for the treatment of advanced breast cancer in postmenopausal women with disease progression following antiestrogen therapy.

NON-FDA APPROVED INDICATIONS

Oncologists are now using letrozole to prevent recurrence of early stage breast cancer and prevent new breast cancer based on studies using anastrozole.

CONTRAINDICATIONS

Letrozole is contraindicated in patients with known hypersensitivity to letrozole or any of its excipients.

WARNINGS

PREGNANCY

Letrozole may cause fetal harm when administered to pregnant women. Studies in rats at doses equal to or greater than 0.003 mg/kg (about 1/100 the daily maximum recommended human dose on a mg/m^2 basis) administered during the period of organogenesis, have shown that letrozole is embryotoxic and fetotoxic, as indicated by intrauterine mortality, increased resorption, increased postimplantation loss, decreased numbers of live fetuses and fetal anomalies including absence and shortening of renal papilla, dilation of ureter, edema and incomplete ossification of frontal skull and metatarsals. Letrozole was teratogenic in rats. A 0.03 mg/kg dose (about 1/10 the daily maximum recommended dose in humans on a mg/m^2 basis) caused fetal domed head and cervical/centrum vertebral fusion.

Letrozole is embryotoxic at doses equal to or greater than 0.002 mg/kg and fetotoxic when administered to rabbits at 0.02 mg/kg (about 1/100,000 and 1/10,000 the daily maximum recommended human dose on a mg/m^2 basis, respectively). Fetal anomalies included incomplete ossification of the skull, sternebrae, and fore- and hindlegs.

There are no studies in pregnant women. Letrozole tablets are indicated for postmenopausal women. If there is exposure to letrozole during pregnancy, the patient should be apprised of the potential hazard to the fetus and potential risk for loss of the pregnancy.

PRECAUTIONS

LABORATORY TESTS

No dose-related effect of letrozole on any hematologic or clinical chemistry parameter was evident. Moderate decreases in lymphocyte counts, of uncertain clinical significance, were observed in some patients receiving letrozole 2.5 mg. This depression was transient in about half of those affected. Two patients on letrozole developed thrombocytopenia; relationship to the study drug was unclear. Patient withdrawal due to laboratory abnormalities, whether related to study treatment or not, was infrequent.

Increases in SGOT, SGPT, and gamma GT ≥5 times the upper limit of normal (ULN) and of bilirubin ≥1.5 times the ULN were most often associated with metastatic disease in the liver. About 3% of study participants receiving letrozole had abnormalities in liver chemistries not associated with documented metastases; these abnormalities may have been related to study drug therapy. In the megestrol acetate comparative study about 8% of patients treated with megestrol acetate had abnormalities in liver chemistries that were not associated with documented liver metastases; in the aminoglutethimide study about 10% of aminoglutethimide-treated patients had abnormalities in liver chemistries not associated with hepatic metastases.

HEPATIC INSUFFICIENCY

Subjects with cirrhosis and severe hepatic dysfunction (see CLINICAL PHARMACOLOGY, Special Populations) who were dosed with 2.5 mg of letrozole experienced approximately twice the exposure to letrozole as healthy volunteers with normal liver function. Therefore, a dose reduction is recommended for this patient population. The effect of hepatic impairment on letrozole exposure in cancer patients with elevated bilirubin levels has not been determined. (See DOSAGE AND ADMINISTRATION.)

DRUG/LABORATORY TEST INTERACTIONS

None observed.

CARCINOGENESIS, MUTAGENESIS, AND IMPAIRMENT OF FERTILITY

A conventional carcinogenesis study in mice at doses of 0.6 to 60 mg/kg/day (about 1/100 times the daily maximum recommended human dose on a mg/m^2 basis) administered by oral gavage for up to 2 years revealed a dose-related increase in the incidence of benign ovarian stromal tumors. The incidence of combined hepatocellular adenoma and carcinoma showed a significant trend in females when the high dose group was excluded due to low survival. In a separate study, plasma AUC(0-12h) levels in mice at 60 mg/kg/day were 55 times higher than the AUC(0-24h) level in breast cancer patients at the recommended dose. The carcinogenicity study in rats at oral doses of 0.1 to 10 mg/kg/day (about 0.4 to 40 times the daily maximum recommended human dose on a mg/m^2 basis) for up to 2 years also produced an increase in the incidence of benign ovarian stromal tumors at 10 mg/kg/day. Ovarian hyperplasia was observed in females at doses equal to or greater than 0.1 mg/kg/day. At 10 mg/kg/day, plasma AUC(0-24h) levels in rats were 80 times higher than the level in breast cancer patients at the recommended dose.

Letrozole was not mutagenic in *in vitro* tests (Ames and *E. coli* bacterial tests) but was observed to be a potential clastogen in *in vitro* assays (CHO K1 and CCL 61 Chinese hamster ovary cells). Letrozole was not clastogenic *in vivo* (micronucleus test in rats).

Studies to investigate the effect of letrozole on fertility have not been conducted; however, repeated dosing caused sexual inactivity in females and atrophy of the reproductive tract in males and females at doses of 0.6, 0.1 and 0.03 mg/kg in mice, rats and dogs, respectively (about 1, 0.4 and 0.4 the daily recommended human dose on a mg/m^2 basis, respectively).

PREGNANCY CATEGORY D

See WARNINGS.

NURSING MOTHERS

It is not known if letrozole is excreted in human milk. Because many drugs are excreted in human milk, caution should be exercised when letrozole is administered to a nursing woman (see WARNINGS and PRECAUTIONS).

PEDIATRIC USE

The safety and effectiveness in pediatric patients have not been established.

GERIATRIC USE

The median age of patients in all studies of first-line and second-line treatment for breast cancer was 64-65 years. About 1/3 of the patients were ≥70 years old. In the first-line study patients ≥70 years of age experienced longer time to tumor progression and higher response rates than patients <70.

DRUG INTERACTIONS

Clinical interaction studies with cimetidine and warfarin indicated that the coadministration of letrozole with these drugs does not result in clinically-significant drug interactions. (See CLINICAL PHARMACOLOGY.)

Co-administration of letrozole and tamoxifen 20 mg daily resulted in a reduction of letrozole plasma levels by 38% on average. There is no clinical experience to date on the use of letrozole in combination with other anticancer agents.

ADVERSE REACTIONS

Letrozole was generally well tolerated across all studies as first-line and second-line treatment for breast cancer and adverse reaction rates were similar in both settings.

FIRST-LINE BREAST CANCER

A total of 455 patients was treated for a median time of exposure of 11 months. The incidence of adverse experiences was similar for letrozole and tamoxifen. The most frequently reported adverse experiences were bone pain, hot flushes, back pain, nausea, arthralgia and dyspnea. Discontinuations for adverse experiences other than progression of tumor occurred in 10/455 (2%) of patients on letrozole and in 15/455 (3%) of patients on tamoxifen.

Adverse events, regardless of relationship to study drug, that were reported in at least 5% of the patients treated with letrozole 2.5 mg or tamoxifen 20 mg in the first-line treatment study are shown in TABLE 8.

TABLE 8 *Percentage of Patients With Adverse Events*

Adverse Experience	Letrozole 2.5 mg (n=455)	Tamoxifen 20 mg (n=455)
Body as a Whole		
Fatigue	11%	11%
Chest pain	8%	8%
Weight decreased	6%	4%
Pain-not otherwise specified	5%	6%
Weakness	5%	3%
Cardiovascular		
Hot flushes	18%	15%
Edema-lower limb	5%	5%
Hypertension	5%	4%
Digestive System		
Nausea	15%	16%
Constipation	9%	9%
Diarrhea	7%	4%
Vomiting	7%	7%
Appetite decreased	4%	6%
Pain-abdominal	4%	5%
Infections/Infestations		
Influenza	5%	4%
Musculoskeletal System		
Pain-bone	20%	18%
Pain-back	17%	17%
Arthralgia	14%	13%
Pain-limb	8%	7%
Nervous System		
Headache	8%	7%
Insomnia	6%	4%
Reproductive		
Breast pain	5%	6%
Respiratory System		
Dyspnea	14%	15%
Coughing	11%	10%
Skin and Appendages		
Alopecia/hair thinning	5%	4%
Surgical/Medical Procedures		
Post-mastectomy lymphoedema	7%	6%

Other less frequent (≤2%) adverse experiences considered consequential for both treatment groups, included peripheral thromboembolic events, cardiovascular events, and cerebrovascular events. Peripheral thromboembolic events included venous thrombosis, thrombophlebitis, portal vein thrombosis and pulmonary embolism. Cardiovascular events included angina, myocardial infarction, myocardial ischemia, and coronary heart disease. Cerebrovascular events included transient ischemic attacks, thrombotic or hemorrhagic strokes and development of hemiparesis.

SECOND-LINE BREAST CANCER

Letrozole was generally well tolerated in two controlled clinical trials.

Study discontinuations in the megestrol acetate comparison study for adverse events other than progression of tumor occurred in 5/188 (2.7%) of patients on letrozole 0.5 mg, in 4/174 (2.3%) of the patients on letrozole 2.5 mg, and in 15/190 (7.9%) of patients on megestrol acetate. There were fewer thromboembolic events at both letrozole doses than on the megestrol acetate arm (2 of 362 patients or 0.6% vs 9 of 190 patients or 4.7%). There was also less vaginal bleeding (1 of 362 patients or 0.3% vs 6 of 190 patients or 3.2%) on letrozole than on megestrol acetate. In the aminoglutethimide comparison study, discontinuations for reasons other than progression occurred in 6/193 (3.1%) of patients on 0.5 mg letrozole, 7/185 (3.8%) of patients on 2.5 mg letrozole, and 7/178 (3.9%) of patients on aminoglutethimide.

Comparisons of the incidence of adverse events revealed no significant differences between the high and low dose letrozole groups in either study. Most of the adverse events observed in all treatment groups were mild to moderate in severity and it was generally not possible to distinguish adverse reactions due to treatment from the consequences of the patient's metastatic breast cancer, the effects of estrogen deprivation, or intercurrent illness.

Adverse events, regardless of relationship to study drug, that were reported in at least 5% of the patients treated with letrozole 0.5 mg, letrozole 2.5 mg, megestrol acetate, or aminoglutethimide in the two controlled trials are shown in TABLE 9.

TABLE 9 *Percentage of Patients With Adverse Events*

Adverse Experience	Pooled Letrozole 2.5 mg (n=359)	Pooled Letrozole 0.5 mg (n=380)	Megestrol Acetate 160 mg (n=189)	Aminoglutethimide 500 mg (n=178)
Body as a Whole				
Fatigue	8%	6%	11%	3%
Chest pain	6%	3%	7%	3%
Peripheral edema*	5%	5%	8%	3%
Asthenia	4%	5%	4%	5%
Weight increase	2%	2%	9%	3%
Cardiovascular				
Hypertension	5%	7%	5%	6%
Digestive System				
Nausea	13%	15%	9%	14%
Vomiting	7%	7%	5%	9%
Constipation	6%	7%	9%	7%
Diarrhea	6%	5%	3%	4%
Pain-abdominal	6%	5%	9%	8%
Anorexia	5%	3%	5%	5%
Dyspepsia	3%	4%	6%	5%
Infections/Infestations				
Viral infection	6%	5%	6%	3%
Lab Abnormality				
Hypercholesterolemia	3%	3%	0%	6%
Musculoskeletal System				
Musculoskeletal†	21%	22%	30%	14%
Arthralgia	8%	8%	8%	3%
Nervous System				
Headache	9%	12%	9%	7%
Somnolence	3%	2%	2%	9%
Dizziness	3%	5%	7%	3%
Respiratory System				
Dyspnea	7%	9%	16%	5%
Coughing	6%	5%	7%	5%
Skin and Appendages				
Hot flushes	6%	5%	4%	3%
Rash‡	5%	4%	3%	12%
Pruritus	1%	2%	5%	3%

* Includes peripheral edema, leg edema, dependent edema, edema.
† Includes musculoskeletal pain, skeletal pain, back pain, arm pain, leg pain.
‡ Includes rash, erythematous rash, masculopapular rash, psoriaform rash, vesicular rash.

Other less frequent (<5%) adverse experiences considered consequential and reported in at least 3 patients treated with letrozole, included hypercalcemia, fracture, depression, anxiety, pleural effusion, alopecia, increased sweating and vertigo.

DOSAGE AND ADMINISTRATION

ADULT AND ELDERLY PATIENTS

The recommended dose of letrozole is one 2.5 mg tablet administered once a day, without regard to meals. Treatment with letrozole should continue until tumor progression is evident. No dose adjustment is required for elderly patients. Patients treated with letrozole do not require glucocorticoid or mineralocorticoid replacement therapy.

RENAL IMPAIRMENT

See CLINICAL PHARMACOLOGY. No dosage adjustment is required for patients with renal impairment if creatinine clearance is ≥10 ml/min.

HEPATIC IMPAIRMENT

No dosage adjustment is recommended for patients with mild-to-moderate hepatic impairment, although letrozole blood concentrations were modestly increased in subjects with moderate hepatic impairment due to cirrhosis. The dose of letrozole in patients with cirrhosis and severe hepatic dysfunction should be reduced by 50% (see CLINICAL PHARMACOLOGY). The recommended dose of letrozole for such patients is 2.5 mg administered every other day. The effect of hepatic impairment on letrozole exposure in noncirrhotic cancer patients with elevated bilirubin levels has not been determined. (See CLINICAL PHARMACOLOGY.)

HOW SUPPLIED

Femara Tablets

2.5 mg: Dark yellow, film-coated, round, slightly biconvex, with beveled edges (imprinted with the letters "FV" on one side and "CG" on the other side).

Storage: Store at 25°C (77°F); excursions permitted to 15-30°C (59-86°F).

PRODUCT LISTING - EQUIVALENTS NOT AVAILABLE

Tablet - Oral - 2.5 mg

30's $232.96 FEMARA, Novartis Pharmaceuticals 00078-0249-15

Leucovorin Calcium (001630)

Categories: Anemia, megaloblastic; Carcinoma, colorectal, adjunct; Osteosarcoma; Toxicity, methotrexate; Pregnancy Category C; FDA Approved 1974 Jul; WHO Formulary; Orphan Drugs
Drug Classes: Antidotes; Vitamins/minerals
Brand Names: Calcium Folinate; Ledervorin-Calcium; Lerderfoline; Wellcovorin
Foreign Brand Availability: Antrex (Finland); Calciumfolinat-Ebewe (Taiwan); Calcium Leucovorin (Australia); Citrec (Sweden); Lederfolin (England; Italy; Spain); Lederfoline (France); Lederle Leucovorin (Canada); Ledervorin Calcium (Belgium; Netherlands); Leucovorin (Austria; Czech-Republic; Denmark; England; Finland; Germany; Greece; Hungary; New-Zealand; Norway; Sweden; Switzerland; Thailand); Leucovorin Calcium (Australia; Bahamas; Barbados; Belize; Bermuda; Curacao; Guyana; Hong-Kong; India; Indonesia; Jamaica; Malaysia; Netherland-Antilles; New-Zealand; Surinam; Thailand; Trinidad); Leucovorina Calcica (Peru); Leucovorine Abic (Netherlands); Medsavorin (Mexico); Refolinon (England); Rescufolin (Norway); Rescuvolin (Belgium; Denmark; Germany; Greece; Indonesia; Israel; Korea; Philippines; Sweden; Switzerland; Thailand); Robin (Korea)
HCFA JCODE(S): J0640 per 50 mg IM, IV

DESCRIPTION

Leucovorin is one of several active, chemically reduced derivatives of folic acid. It is useful as an antidote to drugs which act as folic acid antagonists.

Also known as folinic acid, Citrovorum factor, or 5-formyl-5,6,7,8-tetrahydrofolic acid, this compound has the chemical designation of *L*-Glutamic acid, *N*-[4-[[(2-amino-5-formyl-1,4,5,6,7,8-hexahydro-4-oxo-6-pteridinyl)methyl]amino]benzoyl]-, calcium salt (1:1). The formula weight is 511.51.

INJECTION

Leucovorin calcium for injection is indicated for intravenous (IV) or intramuscular (IM) administration and is supplied in 100 mg vials. Each vial of Wellcovorin (leucovorin calcium for injection) sterile powder, when reconstituted with 10 ml of sterile diluent, contains leucovorin (as the calcium salt) 10 mg/ml, and the inactive ingredients sodium chloride 80 mg per vial, and sodium hydroxide and/or hydrochloric acid added to adjust the pH to approximately 8.1. The dry product contains no preservative. Reconstitute with bacteriostatic water for injection, which contains benzyl alcohol (see WARNINGS), or with sterile water for injection.

There is 0.004 mEq of calcium per mg of leucovorin.

TABLETS

Wellcovorin tablets contain either 5 or 25 mg of leucovorin (equivalent to 5.40 or 27.01 mg of anhydrous leucovorin calcium) and the following inactive ingredients: Corn starch, FD&C yellow no. 6 lake (25 mg tablets only), dibasic calcium phosphate, magnesium stearate, and pregelatinized starch.

Leucovorin is a water soluble form of reduced folate in the folate group; it is useful as an antidote to drugs which act as folic acid antagonists. Leucovorin calcium tablets are indicated for oral administration only.

CLINICAL PHARMACOLOGY

Leucovorin is a racemic mixture of the diastereoisomers of the 5-formyl derivative of tetrahydrofolic acid (THF). The biologically active component of the mixture is the (-)-*l*-isomer, known as Citrovorum factor, or (-)-folinic acid. Leucovorin does not require reduction by the enzyme dihydrofolate reductase in order to participate in reactions utilizing folates as a source of "one-carbon" moieties.

INJECTION

l-Leucovorin (*l*-5-formyltetrahydrofolate) is rapidly metabolized (via 5,10-methenyltetrahydrofolate then 5,10-methylenetetrahydrofolate) to *l*,5-methyltetrahydrofolate. *l*,5-Methyltetrahydrofolate can in turn be metabolized via other pathways back to 5,10 methylenetetrahydrofolate, which is converted to 5-methyltetrahydrofolate by an irreversible, enzyme catalyzed reduction using the cofactors $FADH_2$ and NADPH.

Administration of leucovorin can counteract the therapeutic and toxic effects of folic acid antagonists such as methotrexate, which act by inhibiting dihydrofolate reductase.

In contrast, leucovorin can enhance the therapeutic and toxic effects of fluoropyrimidines used in cancer therapy, such as 5-fluorouracil. Concurrent administration of leucovorin does not appear to alter the plasma pharmacokinetics of 5-fluorouracil. 5-Fluorouracil is metabolized to fluorodeoxyuridylic acid, which binds to and inhibits the enzyme thymidylate synthase (an enzyme important in DNA repair and replication).

Leucovorin is readily converted to another reduced folate, 5,10-methylenetetrahydrofolate, which acts to stabilize the binding of fluorodeoxyuridylic acid to thymidylate synthase and thereby enhances the inhibition of this enzyme.

The pharmacokinetics after IV and IM of a 25 mg dose of leucovorin were studied in male volunteers. After IV administration, serum total reduced folates (as measured by *Lactobacillus casei* assay) reached a mean peak of 1259 ng/ml (range 897-1625). The mean time to peak was 10 minutes. This initial rise in total reduced folates was primarily due to the parent compound 5-formyl-THF (measured by *Streptococcus faecalis* assay) which rose to 1206 ng/ml at 10 minutes. A sharp drop in parent compound followed and coincided with the appearance of the active metabolite 5-methyl-THF which became the predominant circulating form of the drug.

The mean peak of 5-methyl-THF was 258 ng/ml and occurred at 1.3 hours. The terminal half-life for total reduced folates was 6.2 hours. The area under the concentration-versus-time curves (AUCs) for *l*-leucovorin,*d*-leucovorin and 5-methyltetrahydrofolate were 28.4 ± 3.5, 956 ± 97 and 129 ± 12 (mg·min/L ± SE). When a higher dose of *d, l*-leucovorin (200 mg/m^2) was used, similar results were obtained. The *d*-isomer persisted in plasma at concentrations greatly exceeding those of the *l*-isomer.

After IM injection, the mean peak of serum total reduced folates was 436 ng/ml (range 240-725) and occurred at 52 minutes. Similar to IV administration, the initial sharp rise due to the parent compound. The mean peak of 5-formyl-THF was 360 ng/ml and occurred at 28 minutes. The level of the metabolite 5-methyl-THF increased subsequently over time until at 1.5 hours it represented 50% of the circulating total folates. The mean peak of 5-methyl-THF was 226 ng/ml at 2.8 hours. The terminal half-life of total reduced folates was 6.2 hours. There was no difference of statistical significance between IM and IV administration in the AUC for total reduced folates, 5-formyl-THF or 5-methyl-THF.

TABLETS

Following oral administration, leucovorin is rapidly absorbed and enters the general body pool of reduced folates. The increase in plasma and serum folate activity (determined microbiologically with *Lactobacillus casei*) seen after oral administration of leucovorin is predominantly due to 5-methyltetrahydrofolate.

Twenty (20) normal men were given a single oral 15 mg dose (7.5 mg/m^2) of leucovorin calcium and serum folate concentrations were assayed with *L. casei*. Mean values observed (± one standard error) were:

a) ***Time to peak serum folate concentration:*** 1.72 ± 0.08 hours.
b) ***Peak serum folate concentration achieved:*** 268 ± 18 mg/ml.
c) ***Serum folate half-disappearance time:*** 3.5 hours.

Oral tablets yielded areas under the serum folate concentration-time curves (AUCs) that were 12% greater than equal amounts of leucovorin given intramuscularly and equal to the same amounts given intravenously.

Oral absorption of leucovorin is saturable at doses above 25 mg. The apparent bioavailability of leucovorin was 97% for 25 mg, 75% for 50 mg and 37% for 100 mg.

INDICATIONS AND USAGE

INJECTION

Leucovorin calcium rescue is indicated after high-dose methotrexate therapy in osteosarcoma. Leucovorin is also indicated for use in combination with 5-fluorouracil to prolong survival in the palliative treatment of patients with advanced colorectal cancer. Leucovorin should not be mixed in the same infusion as 5-fluorouracil because a precipitate may form.

Leucovorin calcium is indicated in the treatment of megaloblastic anemias due to folic acid deficiency when oral therapy is not feasible.

TABLETS

Leucovorin calcium is indicated to diminish the toxicity and counteract the effects of impaired methotrexate elimination and of inadvertent overdosages of folic acid antagonists.

CONTRAINDICATIONS

Leucovorin is improper therapy for pernicious anemia and other megaloblastic anemias secondary to the lack of vitamin B_{12}. A hematologic remission may occur while neurologic manifestations continue to progress.

WARNINGS

In the treatment of accidental overdosage of folic acid antagonists, leucovorin should be administered as promptly as possible. As the time interval between antifolate administration [*e.g.,* methotrexate (MTX)] and leucovorin rescue increases, leucovorin's effectiveness in counteracting hematologic toxicity decreases. In the treatment of accidental overdosages of intrathecally administered folic acid antagonists, do not administer leucovorin intrathecally. LEUCOVORIN MAY BE HARMFUL OR FATAL IF GIVEN INTRATHECALLY.

Monitoring of serum MTX concentration is essential in determining the optimal dose and duration of treatment with leucovorin.

Delayed MTX excretion may be caused by a third space fluid accumulation (*i.e.,* ascites, pleural effusion), renal insufficiency, or inadequate hydration. Under such circumstances, higher doses of leucovorin or prolonged administration may be indicated. Doses higher than those recommended for oral use must be given intravenously.

There have been rare reports of seizures and/or syncope associated with the use of leucovorin, particularly high doses, in combination with fluorouracil for treatment of malignancies in patients with a history of prior seizures or in patients with central nervous system abnormalities.

Leucovorin may enhance the toxicity of fluorouracil. Deaths from severe enterocolitis, diarrhea, and dehydration have been reported in elderly patients receiving leucovorin and fluorouracil.[1] Concomitant granulocytopenia and fever were present in some but not all of the patients.

The concomitant use of leucovorin with trimethoprim-sulfamethoxazole for the acute treatment of *pneumocystis carinii* pneumonia in patients with HIV infection was associated with increased rates of treatment failure and morbidity in a placebo-controlled study.

ADDITIONAL INFORMATION FOR INJECTION

Because of the benzyl alcohol contained in certain diluents used for leucovorin calcium for injection, when doses greater than 10 mg/m^2 are administered, leucovorin calcium for injection should be reconstituted with sterile water for injection, and used immediately (see DOSAGE AND ADMINISTRATION).

Because of the calcium content of the leucovorin solution, no more than 160 mg of leucovorin should be injected intravenously per minute (16 ml of a 10 mg/ml, or 8 ml of a 20 mg/ml solution per minute).

Leucovorin enhances the toxicity of 5-fluorouracil. When these drugs are administered concurrently, the dosage of the 5-fluorouracil must be lower than usually administered. Although the toxicities observed in patients treated with the combination of leucovorin plus 5-fluorouracil are qualitatively similar to those observed in patients treated with 5-fluorouracil alone, gastrointestinal toxicities (particularly stomatitis and diarrhea) are observed more commonly and may be more severe and of prolonged duration in patients treated with the combination.

Therapy with leucovorin and 5-fluorouracil must not be initiated or continued in patients who have symptoms of gastrointestinal toxicity of any severity, until those symptoms have completely resolved. Patients with diarrhea must be monitored with particular care until the diarrhea has resolved, as rapid clinical deterioration leading to death can occur. In a study utilizing higher weekly doses of 5-fluorouracil and leucovorin, elderly and/or debilitated patients were found to be at greater risk for severe gastrointestinal toxicity.[1]

PRECAUTIONS

GENERAL

Parenteral administration is preferable to oral dosing if there is a possibility that the patient may vomit or not absorb the leucovorin. Leucovorin has no effect on non-hematologic toxicities of MTX such as the nephrotoxicity resulting from drug and/or metabolite precipitation in the kidney.

Injection

Since leucovorin enhances the toxicity of fluorouracil, leucovorin/5-fluorouracil combination therapy for advanced colorectal cancer should be administered under the supervision of a physician experienced in the use of antimetabolite cancer chemotherapy. Particular care should be taken in the treatment of elderly or debilitated colorectal cancer patients, as these patients may be at increased risk of severe toxicity.

PREGNANCY, TERATOGENIC EFFECTS, PREGNANCY CATEGORY C

Adequate animal reproduction studies have not been conducted with leucovorin. It is also not known whether leucovorin can cause fetal harm when administered to a pregnant woman or can affect reproduction capacity. Leucovorin should be given to a pregnant woman only if clearly needed.

NURSING MOTHERS

It is not known whether this drug is excreted in human milk. Because many drugs are excreted in human milk, caution should be exercised when leucovorin is administered to a nursing mother.

PEDIATRIC USE

See DRUG INTERACTIONS.

LABORATORY TESTS

Injection

Patients being treated with the leucovorin/5-fluorouracil combination should have a CBC with differential and platelets prior to each treatment. During the first two courses a CBC with differential and platelets has to be repeated weekly and thereafter once each cycle at the time of anticipated WBC nadir. Electrolytes and liver function tests should be performed prior to each treatment for the first three cycles then prior to every other cycle. Dosage modifications of fluorouracil should be instituted as follows, based on the most severe toxicities (see TABLE 1).

TABLE 1

Diarrhea and/or Stomatitis	WBC/mm^3 Nadir	Platelets/mm^3 Nadir	5-FU Dose
Moderate	1000-1900	25-75,000	decrease 20%
Severe	<1000	<25,000	decrease 30%

If no toxicity occurs, the 5-fluorouracil dose may increase 10%.

Treatment should be deferred until WBC's are 4,000/mm^3 and platelets 130,000/mm^3. If blood counts do not reach these levels within 2 weeks, treatment should be discontinued. Patients should be followed up with physical examination prior to each treatment course and appropriate radiological examination as needed. Treatment should be discontinued when there is clear evidence of tumor progression.

DRUG INTERACTIONS

Folic acid in large amounts may counteract the antiepileptic effect of phenobarbital, phenytoin and primidone, and increase the frequency of seizures in susceptible pediatric patients.

Preliminary animal and human studies have shown that small quantities of systemically administered leucovorin enter the CSF primarily as 5-methyltetrahydrofolate and, in humans, remain 1-3 orders of magnitude lower than the usual methotrexate concentrations following intrathecal administration. However, high doses of leucovorin may reduce the efficacy of intrathecally administered methotrexate.

Leucovorin may enhance the toxicity of 5-fluorouracil (see WARNINGS).

ADVERSE REACTIONS

INJECTION

Allergic sensitization, including anaphylactoid reactions and urticaria, has been reported following administration of both oral and parenteral leucovorin. No other adverse reactions have been attributed to the use of leucovorin *per se*.

TABLETS

Allergic sensitization has been reported following both oral and parenteral administration of folic acid.

DOSAGE AND ADMINISTRATION

INJECTION

Leucovorin Rescue After High-Dose Methotrexate Therapy

The recommendations for leucovorin rescue are based on a methotrexate dose of 12-15 g/m^2 administered by IV infusion over 4 hours (see methotrexate package insert for full prescribing information).

Leucovorin rescue at a dose of 15 mg (approximately 10 mg/m^2) every 6 hours for 10 doses starts 24 hours after the beginning of the methotrexate infusion. In the presence of gastrointestinal toxicity, nausea or vomiting, leucovorin should be administered parenterally. Do not administer leucovorin intrathecally.

Serum creatinine and methotrexate levels should be determined at least once daily. Leucovorin administration, hydration, and urinary alkalinization (pH of 7.0 or greater) should be continued until the methotrexate level is below 5×10^{-8} M (0.05 μmol). The leucovorin dose should be adjusted or leucovorin rescue extended based on the guidelines established in TABLE 2.

TABLE 2 *Guidelines For Leucovorin Dosage and Administration*

DO NOT ADMINISTER LEUCOVORIN INTRATHECALLY

Clinical Situation	Laboratory Findings	Leucovorin Dosage and Duration
Normal methotrexate elimination	Serum methotrexate level approximately 10 μmol at 24 hours after administration, 1 μmol at 48 hours, and less than 0.2 μmol at 72 hours.	15 mg PO, IM, or IV q6h for 60 hours (10 doses starting at 24 hours after start of methotrexate infusion).
Delayed late methotrexate elimination	Serum methotrexate level remaining above 0.2 μmol at 72 hours, and more than 0.05 μmol at 96 hours after administration.	Continue 15 mg PO, IM, or IV q6h, until methotrexate level is less than 0.05 μmol.
Delayed early methotrexate elimination and/or evidence of acute renal injury	Serum methotrexate level of 50 μmol or more at 24 hours, or 5 μmol or more at 48 hours after administration, OR; a 100% or greater increase in serum creatinine level at 24 hours after methotrexate administration (*e.g.*, an increase from 0.5 mg/dl to a level of 1 mg/dl or more).	150 mg IV q3h, until methotrexate level is less than 1 μmol; then 15 mg IV q3h until methotrexate level is less than 0.05 μmol.

Patients who experience delayed early methotrexate elimination are likely to develop reversible renal failure. In addition to appropriate leucovorin therapy, these patients require continuing hydration and urinary alkalinization, and close monitoring of fluid and electrolyte status, until the serum methotrexate level has fallen to below 0.05 μmol and the renal failure has resolved.

Some patients will have abnormalities in methotrexate elimination or renal function following methotrexate administration, which are significant but less severe than the abnormalities described in TABLE 2. These abnormalities may or may not be associated with significant clinical toxicity. If significant clinical toxicity is observed, leucovorin rescue should be extended for an additional 24 hours (total of 14 doses over 84 hours) in subsequent courses of therapy. The possibility that the patient is taking other medications which interact with methotrexate (*e.g.*, medications which may interfere with methotrexate elimination or binding to serum albumin) should always be reconsidered when laboratory abnormalities or clinical toxicities are observed.

Impaired Methotrexate Elimination or Inadvertent Overdosage

Leucovorin rescue should begin as soon as possible after an inadvertent overdosage and within 24 hours of methotrexate administration when there is a delayed excretion (see WARNINGS). Leucovorin 15 mg/m^2 should be administered IV, IM, or PO every 6 hours until the serum methotrexate level is less than 10^{-8} M. In the presence of gastrointestinal toxicity, nausea, or vomiting, leucovorin should be administered parenterally. Do not administer leucovorin intrathecally.

Serum creatinine and methotrexate levels should be determined at 24 hour intervals. If the 24 hour serum creatinine has increased 50% over baseline, or if the 24 hour methotrexate level is greater than 5×10^{-6} M or the 48 hour level is greater than 9×10^{-7} M, the doses of leucovorin should be increased to 100 mg/m^2 IV every 3 hours until the methotrexate level is less than 10^{-8} M.[2]

Megaloblastic Anemia Due to Folic Acid Deficiency

Up to 1 mg daily. There is no evidence that doses greater than 1 mg/day have greater efficacy than those of 1 mg; additionally, loss of folate in urine becomes roughly logarithmic as the amount administered exceeds 1 mg.

TABLETS

Leucovorin calcium tablets are intended for oral administration. Because absorption is saturable, oral administration of doses greater than 25 mg is not recommended.

Impaired Methotrexate Elimination or Inadvertent Overdosage

Leucovorin rescue should begin as soon as possible after an inadvertent overdosage and within 24 hours of methotrexate administration when there is a delayed excretion (see WARNINGS). Leucovorin 15 mg/m^2 should be administered IV, IM, or PO every 6 hours until the serum methotrexate level is less than 10^{-8} M. In the presence of gastrointestinal toxicity, nausea, or vomiting, leucovorin should be administered parenterally. Do not administer leucovorin intrathecally.

Serum creatinine and methotrexate levels should be determined at 24 hour intervals. If the 24 hour serum creatinine has increased 50% over baseline, or if the 24 hour methotrexate level is greater than 5×10^{-6} M or the 48 hour level is greater than 9×10^{-7} M, the doses of leucovorin should be increased to 100 mg/m^2 IV every 3 hours until the methotrexate level is less than 10^{-8} M.[2]

Hydration (3 L/day) and urinary alkalinization with sodium bicarbonate solution should be employed concomitantly. The bicarbonate dose should be adjusted to maintain the urine pH at 7.0 or greater.

The recommended dose of leucovorin to counteract hematologic toxicity from folic acid antagonists with less affinity for mammalian dihydrofolate reductase than methotrexate (*i.e.*, trimethoprim, pyrimethamine) is substantially less, and 5-15 mg of leucovorin per day has been recommended by some investigators.

Patients who experience delayed early methotrexate elimination are likely to develop reversible non-oliguric renal failure. In addition to appropriate leucovorin therapy, these patients require continuing hydration and urinary alkalinization, and close monitoring of fluid and electrolyte status, until the serum methotrexate level has fallen to below 0.05 μmol and the renal failure has resolved.

Some patients will have abnormalities in methotrexate elimination or renal function following methotrexate administration, which are significant but less severe. The abnormalities may or may not be associated with significant clinical toxicity. If significant clinical toxicity is observed, leucovorin rescue should be extended for an additional 24 hours (total of 14 doses over 84 hours) is subsequent courses of therapy. The possibility that the patient is taking other medications which interact with methotrexate (*e.g.,* medications which may interfere with methotrexate elimination or binding to serum albumin) should always be reconsidered when laboratory abnormalities or clinical toxicities are observed.

HOW SUPPLIED

WELLCOVORIN TABLETS

Wellcovorin tablets are available in:

5 mg: Off-white, scored tablets containing 5 mg leucovorin as the calcium salt imprinted with "WELLCOVORIN" and "5".

25 mg: Peach. scored tablets containing 25 mg leucovorin as the calcium salt imprinted with 'WELLCOVORIN" and "25".

Storage: Store at 15-25°C (59-77°F). Protect from light and moisture.

WELLCOVORIN INJECTION

Leucovorin calcium is supplied in vials each containing 100 mg/vial.

Storage: Store dry powder and reconstituted solution at controlled room temperature 15-30°C (59-86°F). Protect from light.

PRODUCT LISTING - RATED THERAPEUTICALLY EQUIVALENT

Powder For Injection - Intravenous - 50 mg

10's	$37.50	GENERIC, Bedford Laboratories	55390-0051-10

Powder For Injection - Intravenous - 100 mg

1's	$36.69	GENERIC, Abbott Pharmaceutical	00074-5140-01
1's	$36.69	GENERIC, Gensia Sicor Pharmaceuticals Inc	00703-5140-01
1's	$41.57	GENERIC, Bedford Laboratories	55390-0818-10
10's	$50.00	GENERIC, Bedford Laboratories	55390-0052-10
10's	$350.00	GENERIC, Vha Supply	53905-0818-10

Powder For Injection - Intravenous - 200 mg

1's	$15.00	GENERIC, Bedford Laboratories	55390-0053-01
1's	$77.90	GENERIC, Faulding Pharmaceutical Company	61703-0410-50
1's	$350.00	GENERIC, Bedford Laboratories	55390-0824-01

Powder For Injection - Intravenous - 350 mg

1's	$18.75	GENERIC, Gensia Sicor Pharmaceuticals Inc	00703-5145-01
1's	$137.94	GENERIC, Immunex Corporation	58406-0623-07
1's	$137.94	GENERIC, Xanodyne Pharmacal Inc	66479-0247-25
1's	$137.95	GENERIC, Bedford Laboratories	55390-0054-01
1's	$137.95	GENERIC, Bedford Laboratories	55390-0825-01

Powder For Injection - Intravenous - 500 mg

1's	$195.00	GENERIC, Bedford Laboratories	55390-0009-01

Tablet - Oral - 5 mg

30's	$61.48	GENERIC, Roxane Laboratories Inc	00054-4496-13
30's	$70.81	GENERIC, Barr Laboratories Inc	00555-0484-01
30's	$76.99	GENERIC, Ivax Corporation	00182-1869-17
30's	$149.00	GENERIC, Geneva Pharmaceuticals	00781-1220-31
50's	$140.00	GENERIC, Roxane Laboratories Inc	00054-8496-19
50's	$162.50	GENERIC, Udl Laboratories Inc	51079-0581-06
50's	$190.00	GENERIC, Raway Pharmacal Inc	00686-0581-06
100's	$202.68	GENERIC, Roxane Laboratories Inc	00054-4496-25
100's	$235.20	GENERIC, Barr Laboratories Inc	00555-0484-02
100's	$489.00	GENERIC, Geneva Pharmaceuticals	00781-1220-01
100's	$493.45	GENERIC, Major Pharmaceuticals Inc	00904-2315-60
100's	$551.87	GENERIC, Qualitest Products Inc	00603-4183-21

Tablet - Oral - 10 mg

10's	$66.00	GENERIC, Roxane Laboratories Inc	00054-8497-06
12's	$69.86	GENERIC, Roxane Laboratories Inc	00054-4497-05
24's	$138.33	GENERIC, Roxane Laboratories Inc	00054-4497-10

Tablet - Oral - 15 mg

10's	$82.00	GENERIC, Roxane Laboratories Inc	00054-8498-06
10's	$82.00	GENERIC, Roxane Laboratories Inc	00054-8498-08
12's	$104.00	GENERIC, Roxane Laboratories Inc	00054-4498-05
24's	$195.62	GENERIC, Roxane Laboratories Inc	00054-4498-10

Tablet - Oral - 25 mg

10's	$170.00	GENERIC, Roxane Laboratories Inc	00054-8499-06
20's	$273.75	GENERIC, Udl Laboratories Inc	51079-0582-05
20's	$325.00	GENERIC, Raway Pharmacal Inc	00686-0582-05
25's	$475.07	GENERIC, Roxane Laboratories Inc	00054-4499-11
25's	$600.00	GENERIC, Barr Laboratories Inc	00555-0485-27
25's	$603.00	GENERIC, Geneva Pharmaceuticals	00781-1222-63
25's	$680.34	GENERIC, Qualitest Products Inc	00603-4184-35

PRODUCT LISTING - RATED NOT THERAPEUTICALLY EQUIVALENT

Tablet - Oral - 5 mg

30's	$85.54	GENERIC, Immunex Corporation	58406-0624-62

PRODUCT LISTING - EQUIVALENTS NOT AVAILABLE

Powder For Injection - Intravenous - 100 mg

10's	$80.00	GENERIC, Raway Pharmacal Inc	00686-5140-01

Powder For Injection - Intravenous - 200 mg

1's	$77.95	GENERIC, American Pharmaceutical Partners	63323-0710-50

Powder For Injection - Intravenous - 350 mg

10's	$1379.38	GENERIC, Immunex Corporation	58406-0623-33

Powder For Injection - Intravenous - 500 mg

1's	$195.00	GENERIC, American Pharmaceutical Partners	63323-0711-00

Tablet - Oral - 5 mg

50's	$80.70	GENERIC, Physicians Total Care	54868-3310-01
60's	$96.57	GENERIC, Physicians Total Care	54868-3310-00

Tablet - Oral - 15 mg

12's	$100.56	GENERIC, Immunex Corporation	58406-0626-68

Leuprolide Acetate *(001631)*

Categories: Carcinoma, prostate; Endometriosis; Leiomyoma; Puberty, precocious; Pregnancy Category X; FDA Approved 1985 Apr; Orphan Drugs
Drug Classes: Antineoplastics, hormones/hormone modifiers; Hormones/hormone modifiers
Brand Names: **Lupron**; Lupron Depot; Procren
Foreign Brand Availability: Carcinil (Germany); Enanton Depot (Denmark; Finland; Norway; Sweden); Enantone (France; Germany); Enantone Depot (Italy); Enantone LP (Thailand); Enantone SR (China; Hong-Kong); Leuplin (Korea); Leuplin Depot (Taiwan); Lorelin Depot (Korea); Lucrin (Australia; France; Hong-Kong; Korea; Mexico; New-Zealand; Portugal; Singapore); Lucrin Depot (Belgium; Costa-Rica; Dominican-Republic; El-Salvador; Guatemala; Honduras; Hungary; Israel; Mexico; Netherlands; Nicaragua; Panama; Singapore; Switzerland; Turkey); Lucrin Depot Inj (Australia; New-Zealand); Luprolex (Philippines); Procren Depot (Denmark; Finland; Norway; Sweden); Procrin (Spain); Prostap (England; Ireland); Reliser (Mexico); Tapros (Indonesia)
Cost of Therapy: $540.63 (Prostate Cancer; Lupron Depot; 7.5 mg; 1 injection/month; 30 day supply)
$518.64 (Prostate Cancer; Lupron Depot; 3.75 mg; 1 injection/month; 30 day supply)
HCFA JCODE(S): J1950 3.75 mg IM; J9217 7.5 mg IM; J9218 per 1 mg IM

DESCRIPTION

Lupron, Lupron Depot, Lupron Depot-Ped, and Viadur are each a synthetic nonapeptide analog of naturally occurring gonadotropin releasing hormone (GnRH or LH-RH). The analog possesses greater potency than the natural hormone. The chemical name is 5-Oxo-L-prolyl-L-histidyl-L-tryptophyl-L-seryl-L-tyrosyl-D-leucyl-L-leucyl-L-arginyl-N-ethyl-L-prolinamide acetate (salt).

The molecular weight is 1269.48. The molecular formula is $C_{59}H_{84}N_{16}O_{12} \cdot C_2H_4O_2$.

LUPRON INJECTION

Lupron is a sterile, aqueous solution intended for subcutaneous injection. It is available in a 2.8 ml multiple-dose vial containing 5 mg/ml of leuprolide acetate, sodium chloride for tonicity adjustment, 9 mg/ml of benzyl alcohol as a preservative and water for injection. The pH may have been adjusted with sodium hydroxide and/or acetic acid. The pH range is 4.0-6.0.

LUPRON INJECTION (FOR PEDIATRIC USE)

Lupron injection is a sterile, aqueous solution intended for daily subcutaneous injection.

A 2.8 ml multiple dose vial contains leuprolide acetate (5 mg/ml), sodium chloride (6.3 mg/ml) for tonicity adjustment, benzyl alcohol as a preservative (9 mg/ml), and water for injection. The pH may have been adjusted with sodium hydroxide and/or acetic acid.

LUPRON DEPOT 3.75 MG AND LUPRON DEPOT 7.5 MG

Lupron Depot is supplied in a vial containing sterile lyophilized microspheres, which when mixed with diluent, become a suspension, which is intended as a monthly intramuscular injection.

LUPRON DEPOT 3.75 MG

The single-dose vial of Lupron Depot contains leuprolide acetate (3.75 mg), purified gelatin (0.65 mg), DL-lactic and glycolic acids copolymer (33.1 mg), and D-mannitol (6.6 mg). The accompanying ampule of diluent contains carboxymethylcellulose sodium (7.5 mg), D-mannitol (75 mg), polysorbate 80 (1.5 mg), water for injection, and glacial acetic acid to control pH.

During the manufacturing process of Lupron Depot, acetic acid is lost, leaving the peptide.

LUPRON DEPOT 7.5 MG

The single-dose vial of Lupron Depot contains leuprolide acetate (7.5 mg), purified gelatin (1.3 mg), DL-lactic and glycolic acids copolymer (66.2 mg), and D-mannitol (13.2 mg). The accompanying ampule of diluent contains carboxymethylcellulose sodium (7.5 mg), D-mannitol (75 mg), polysorbate 80 (1.5 mg), water for injection, and acetic acid to control pH.

During the manufacture of Lupron Depot, acetic acid is lost leaving the peptide.

LUPRON DEPOT-PED

Lupron Depot-Ped is supplied in a vial containing sterile lyophilized microspheres, which when mixed with diluent, become a suspension, intended as a single intramuscular injection.

The single-dose vial of Lupron Depot-Ped contains, respectively for each dosage strength, leuprolide acetate (7.5/11.25/15 mg), purified gelatin (1.3/1.95/2.6 mg), DL-lactic and glycolic acids copolymer (66.2/99.3/132.4 mg), and D-mannitol (13.2/19.8/26.4 mg). The accompanying ampule of diluent contains carboxymethylcellulose sodium (7.5 mg), D-mannitol (75 mg), polysorbate 80 (1.5 mg), water for injection, and acetic acid to control pH.

During the manufacture of Lupron Depot-Ped, acetic acid is lost leaving the peptide.

VIADUR

Viadur (leuprolide acetate implant) is a sterile nonbiodegradable, osmotically driven miniaturized implant designed to deliver leuprolide acetate for 12 months at a controlled rate. The system contains 65 mg of leuprolide (free base). The implant is inserted subcutaneously in the inner aspect of the upper arm. After 12 months, the implant must be removed. At the time an implant is removed, another implant may be inserted to continue therapy.

L

Viadur contains 72 mg of leuprolide acetate (equivalent to 65 mg leuprolide free base) dissolved in 104 mg dimethyl sulfoxide. The 4 mm by 45 mm titanium alloy reservoir houses a polyurethane rate-controlling membrane, an elastomeric piston, and a polyethylene diffusion moderator. The reservoir also contains the osmotic tablets, which are not released with the drug formulation. The osmotic tablets are composed of sodium chloride, sodium carboxymethyl cellulose, povidone, magnesium stearate, and sterile water for injection. Polyethylene glycol fills the space between the osmotic tablets and the reservoir. A minute amount of silicone medical fluid is used during manufacture as a lubricant. The weight of the implant is approximately 1.1 g.

CLINICAL PHARMACOLOGY

LEUPROLIDE ACETATE INJECTION AND LEUPROLIDE ACETATE FOR DEPOT SUSPENSION 7.5 MG

Leuprolide acetate, an LH-RH agonist, acts as a potent inhibitor of gonadotropin secretion when given continuously and in therapeutic doses. Animal and human studies indicate that following an initial stimulation, chronic administration of leuprolide acetate results in suppression of ovarian and testicular steroidogenesis. This effect is reversible upon discontinuation of drug therapy. Administration of leuprolide acetate has resulted in inhibition of the growth of certain hormone dependent tumors (prostatic tumors in Noble and Dunning male rats and DMBA-induced mammary tumors in female rats) as well as atrophy of the reproductive organs.

Leuprolide Acetate Injection

In humans, subcutaneous administration of single daily doses of leuprolide acetate results in an initial increase in circulation levels of luteinizing hormone (LH) and follicle stimulating hormone (FSH), leading to a transient increase in levels of the gonadal steroids (testosterone and dihydrotestosterone in males, and estrone and estradiol in pre-menopausal females). However, continuous daily administration of leuprolide acetate results in decreased levels of LH and FSH in all patients. In males, testosterone is reduced to castrate levels. In premenopausal females, estrogens are reduced to post-menopausal levels. These decreases occur within 2-4 weeks after initiation of treatment, and castrate levels of testosterone in prostatic cancer patients have been demonstrated for periods of up to 5 years.

Leuprolide acetate is not active when given orally. Bioavailability by subcutaneous administration is comparable to that by intravenous administration. Leuprolide acetate has a plasma half-life of approximately 3 hours. The metabolism, distribution, and excretion of leuprolide acetate in man have not been determined.

Leuprolide Acetate for Depot Suspension 7.5 mg

In humans, administration of leuprolide acetate results in an initial increase in circulating levels of luteinizing hormone (LH) and follicle stimulating hormone (FSH), leading to a transient increase in levels of the gonadal steroids (testosterone and dihydrotestosterone in males, and estrone and estradiol in pre-menopausal females). However, continuous administration of leuprolide acetate results in decreased levels of LH and FSH. In males, testosterone is reduced to castrate levels. In pre-menopausal females, estrogens are reduced to post-menopausal levels. These decreases occur within 2-4 weeks after initiation of treatment, and castrate levels of testosterone in prostatic cancer patients have been demonstrated for periods of up to 5 years.

Leuprolide acetate is not active when given orally. Following a single leuprolide acetate for depot suspension injection to patients, mean peak leuprolide plasma concentration was almost 20 ng/ml at 4 hours and 0.36 ng/ml at 4 weeks. Nondetectable leuprolide plasma concentrations have been observed during chronic leuprolide acetate administration, but testosterone levels appear to be maintained at castrate levels. The metabolism, distribution, and excretion of leuprolide in humans have not been determined.

LEUPROLIDE ACETATE INJECTION (FOR PEDIATRIC USE) AND LEUPROLIDE ACETATE FOR DEPOT SUSPENSION (FOR PEDIATRIC USE)

Leuprolide acetate, a GnRH agonist, acts as a potent inhibitor of gonadotropin secretion when given continuously and in therapeutic doses. Human studies indicate that following an initial stimulation of gonadotropins, chronic stimulation with leuprolide acetate results in suppression or "downregulation" of these hormones and consequent suppression of ovarian and testicular steroidogenesis. These effects are reversible on discontinuation of drug therapy.

In children with central precocious puberty (CPP), stimulated and basal gonadotropins are reduced to prepubertal levels. Testosterone and estradiol are reduced to prepubertal levels in males and females respectively. Reduction of gonadotropins will allow for normal physical and psychological growth and development. Natural maturation occurs when gonadotropins return to pubertal levels following discontinuation of leuprolide acetate.

The following physiologic effects have been noted with the chronic administration of leuprolide acetate in this patient population.

1. ***Skeletal Growth:*** A measurable increase in body length can be noted since the epiphyseal plates will not close prematurely.
2. ***Organ growth:*** Reproductive organs will return to a prepubertal state.
3. ***Menses:*** Menses, if present, will cease.

Leuprolide Acetate Injection (for Pediatric Use)

Leuprolide acetate is not active when given orally. In adults, bioavailability by subcutaneous administration is comparable to that by intravenous administration; and leuprolide acetate has a plasma half-life of approximately 3 hours. The metabolism, distribution and excretion of leuprolide acetate in humans have not been determined. A pharmacokinetic study of leuprolide acetate in children has not been performed.

Leuprolide Acetate for Depot Suspension (for Pediatric Use)

Leuprolide acetate is not active when given orally. In adults, intramuscular injection of the depot formulation provides plasma concentrations of leuprolide over a period of 1 month. The metabolism, distribution and excretion of leuprolide in humans have not been determined.

In a study of 22 children with central precocious puberty, doses of leuprolide acetate for depot suspension were given every 4 weeks and plasma levels were determined according to weight categories as summarized in TABLE 1.

TABLE 1

Patient Weight Range (kg)	Group Weight Average (kg)	Dose (mg)	Trough Plasma Leuprolide Level Mean ±SD* (ng/ml)
20.2-27.0	22.7	7.5	0.77 ± 0.033
28.4-36.8	32.5	11.25	1.25 ± 1.06
39.3-57.5	44.2	15.0	1.59 ± 0.65

* Group average values determined at Week 4 immediately prior to leuprolide injection. Drug levels at 12 and 24 weeks were similar to respective 4 week levels.

LEUPROLIDE ACETATE FOR DEPOT SUSPENSION 3.75 MG

Leuprolide acetate is a long-acting GnRH analog. A single monthly injection of leuprolide acetate for depot suspension results in an initial stimulation followed by a prolonged suppression of pituitary gonadotropins. Repeated dosing at monthly intervals results in decreased secretion of gonadal steroids; consequently, tissues and functions that depend on gonadal steroids for their maintenance become quiescent. This effect is reversible on discontinuation of drug therapy.

Leuprolide acetate is not active when given orally. Intramuscular injection of the depot formulation provides plasma concentrations of leuprolide over a period of 1 month.

LEUPROLIDE ACETATE IMPLANT

Leuprolide acetate, an LH-RH agonist, acts as a potent inhibitor of gonadotropin secretion when given continuously and in therapeutic doses. Animal and human studies indicate that after an initial stimulation, chronic administration of leuprolide acetate results in suppression of ovarian and testicular steroidogenesis.

In humans, administration of leuprolide acetate results in an initial increase in circulating levels of luteinizing hormone (LH) and follicle-stimulating hormone (FSH), leading to a transient increase in concentrations of gonadal steroids (testosterone and dihydrotestosterone in males, and estrone and estradiol in premenopausal females). However, continuous administration of leuprolide acetate results in decreased levels of LH and FSH. In males, testosterone is reduced to castrate levels. These decreases occur within 2-4 weeks after initiation of treatment.

One (1) leuprolide acetate implant nominally delivers 120 µg of leuprolide acetate per day over 12 months. Leuprolide acetate is not active when given orally.

PHARMACOKINETICS

Absorption

Leuprolide Acetate for Depot Suspension 3.75 mg

A single dose of leuprolide acetate for depot suspension 3.75 mg was administered by intramuscular injection to healthy female volunteers. The absorption of leuprolide was characterized by an initial increase in plasma concentration, with peak concentration ranging from 4.6-10.2 ng/ml at 4 hours postdosing. However, intact leuprolide and an inactive metabolite could not be distinguished by the assay used in the study. Following the initial rise, leuprolide concentrations started to plateau within 2 days after dosing and remained relatively stable for about 4-5 weeks with plasma concentrations of about 0.30 ng/ml.

Leuprolide Acetate Implant

After insertion of leuprolide acetate implant, mean serum leuprolide concentrations were 16.9 ng/ml at 4 hours and 2.4 ng/ml at 24 hours. Thereafter, leuprolide was released at a constant rate. Mean serum leuprolide concentrations were maintained at 0.9 ng/ml (0.3 to 3.1 ng/ml; SD = ± 0.4) for 12 months. Upon removal and insertion of a new leuprolide acetate implant at 12 months, steady-state serum leuprolide concentrations were maintained.

Distribution

The mean steady-state volume of distribution of leuprolide following intravenous bolus administration to healthy male volunteers was 27 l. *In vitro* binding to human plasma proteins ranged from 43-49%.

Metabolism

In healthy male volunteers, a 1 mg bolus of leuprolide administered intravenously revealed that the mean systemic clearance was 7.6 L/h, with a terminal elimination half-life of approximately 3 hours based on two compartment model.

In rats and dogs, administration of ^{14}C-labeled leuprolide was shown to be metabolized to smaller inactive peptides, pentapeptide (Metabolite I), tripeptide (Metabolite II and III) and dipeptide (Metabolite IV). These fragments may be further catabolized.

The major metabolite (M-I) plasma concentrations measured in 5 prostate cancer patients reached mean maximum concentration 2-6 hours after dosing and were approximately 6% of the peak parent drug concentration. One (1) week after dosing, mean plasma M-I concentrations were approximately 20% of leuprolide concentrations.

Excretion

Following administration of leuprolide acetate for depot suspension 3.75 mg to 3 patients, less than 5% of the dose was recovered as parent and M-I metabolite in the urine.

Dose Proportionality

Leuprolide Acetate Implant: In a study comparing 1 leuprolide acetate implant to 2 leuprolide acetate implants, mean serum leuprolide concentrations were proportional to dose.

Special Populations

Geriatrics: The majority (88%) of the 131 patients studied in leuprolide acetate implant clinical trials were age 65 and over.

Pediatrics: The safety and effectiveness of leuprolide acetate implants in pediatric patients have not been established (see CONTRAINDICATIONS).

Race: In the patients studied in leuprolide acetate implant clinical trials (80 Caucasian, 23 Black, 3 Hispanic), mean serum leuprolide concentrations were similar.

Renal and Hepatic Insufficiency: The pharmacokinetics of the drug in hepatically and renally impaired patients have not been determined.

Drug-Drug Interactions: No pharmacokinetic drug-drug interaction studies were conducted with leuprolide acetate implants.

INDICATIONS AND USAGE

LEUPROLIDE ACETATE INJECTION AND LEUPROLIDE ACETATE FOR DEPOT SUSPENSION 7.5 MG

Leuprolide acetate is indicated in the palliative treatment of advanced prostatic cancer. It offers an alternative treatment of prostatic cancer when orchiectomy or estrogen administration are either not indicated or unacceptable to the patient.

Leuprolide Acetate Injection

In a controlled study comparing leuprolide acetate 1 mg/day given subcutaneously to diethylstilbestrol, 3 mg/day, the survival rate for the two groups was comparable after 2 years treatment. The objective response to treatment was also similar for the two groups.

Leuprolide Acetate for Depot Suspension 7.5 mg

In clinical trials, the safety and efficacy of leuprolide acetate for depot suspension does not differ from that of the original daily subcutaneous injection.

LEUPROLIDE ACETATE INJECTION (FOR PEDIATRIC USE) AND LEUPROLIDE ACETATE FOR DEPOT SUSPENSION (FOR PEDIATRIC USE)

Leuprolide acetate is indicated in the treatment of children with central precocious puberty. Children should be selected using the following criteria:

1. Clinical diagnosis of CPP (idiopathic or neurogenic) with onset of secondary sexual characteristics earlier than 8 years in females and 9 years in males.
2. Clinical diagnosis should be confirmed prior to initiation of therapy:
   - Confirmation of diagnosis by a pubertal response to a GnRH stimulation test. The sensitivity and methodology of this assay must be understood.
   - Bone age advanced 1 year beyond the chronological age.
3. Baseline evaluation should also include:
   - Height and weight measurements.
   - Sex steroid levels.
   - Adrenal steroid level to exclude congenital adrenal hyperplasia.
   - Beta human chorionic gonadotropin level to rule out a chorionic gonadotropic secreting tumor.
   - Pelvic/adrenal/testicular ultrasound to rule out a steroid secreting tumor.
   - Computerized tomography of the head to rule out intracranial tumor.

LEUPROLIDE ACETATE FOR DEPOT SUSPENSION 3.75 MG

Endometriosis

Experience with leuprolide acetate for depot suspension in females has been limited to women 18 years of age and older treated for 6 months.

Leuprolide acetate for depot suspension 3.75 mg is indicated for management of endometriosis, including pain relief and reduction of endometriotic lesions.

Uterine Leiomyomata (Fibroids)

Experience with leuprolide acetate for depot suspension in females has been limited to women 18 years of age and older.

Leuprolide acetate for depot suspension 3.75 mg and iron therapy are indicated for the preoperative hematologic improvement of patients with anemia caused by uterine leiomyomata. The clinician may wish to consider a 1 month trial period on iron alone in as much as some of the patients will respond to iron alone. Leuprolide acetate may be added if the response to iron alone is considered inadequate. Recommended duration of therapy with leuprolide acetate for depot suspension is **up to** 3 months (see TABLE 2).

TABLE 2 *Percentage of Patients Achieving Hemoglobin ≥12 g/dl*

Treatment Group	Week 4	Week 8	Week 12
Leuprolide acetate for depot suspension 3.75 mg with iron	41*	71†	79*
Iron alone	17	40	56

* P-Value <0.01
† P-Value <0.001

LEUPROLIDE ACETATE IMPLANT

Leuprolide acetate implant is indicated in the palliative treatment of advanced prostate cancer.

NON-FDA APPROVED INDICATIONS

Experimentally, leuprolide has also been used in the treatment of breast cancer, ovarian cancer, endometrial cancer, leiomyomata uteri, hirsutism, infertility, and benign prostatic hyperplasia.

CONTRAINDICATIONS

LEUPROLIDE ACETATE INJECTION AND LEUPROLIDE ACETATE FOR DEPOT SUSPENSION 7.5 MG

A report of an anaphylactic reaction to synthetic GnRH (Factrel) has been reported in the medical literature.[1]

Leuprolide acetate is contraindicated in women who are or may become pregnant while receiving the drug. When administered on day 6 of pregnancy at test dosages of 0.00024, 0.0024, and 0.024 mg/kg (1/600 to 1/6 the human dose) to rabbits, leuprolide acetate produced a dose-related increase in major fetal abnormalities. Similar studies in rats failed to demonstrate an increase in fetal malformations. There was increased fetal mortality and decreased fetal weights with the 2 higher doses of leuprolide acetate in rabbits and with the highest dose in rats. The effects on fetal mortality are logical consequences of the alterations in hormonal levels brought about by this drug. Therefore, the possibility exists that spontaneous abortion may occur if the drug is administered during pregnancy.

LEUPROLIDE ACETATE INJECTION (FOR PEDIATRIC USE) AND LEUPROLIDE ACETATE FOR DEPOT SUSPENSION (FOR PEDIATRIC USE)

Leuprolide acetate is contraindicated in women who are or may become pregnant while receiving the drug. When administered on day 6 of pregnancy at test dosages of 0.00024, 0.0024, and 0.024 mg/kg (1/1200 to 1/12 the human pediatric dose) to rabbits, leuprolide acetate produced a dose-related increase in major fetal abnormalities. Similar studies in rats failed to demonstrate an increase in fetal malformations. There was increased fetal mortality and decreased fetal weights with the 2 higher doses of leuprolide acetate in rabbits and with the highest dose in rats. The effects on fetal mortality are logical consequences of the alterations in hormonal levels brought about by this drug. Therefore, the possibility exists that spontaneous abortion may occur if the drug is administered during pregnancy.

Leuprolide acetate is contraindicated in children demonstrating hypersensitivity to GnRH, GnRH agonist analogs, or any of the excipients.

A report of an anaphylactic reaction to synthetic GnRH (Factrel) has been reported in the medical literature.[1]

LEUPROLIDE ACETATE FOR DEPOT SUSPENSION 3.75 MG

1. Hypersensitivity to GnRH, GnRH agonist analogs or any of the excipients in leuprolide acetate for depot suspension.
2. Undiagnosed abnormal vaginal bleeding.
3. Leuprolide acetate for depot suspension is contraindicated in women who are or may become pregnant while receiving the drug. Leuprolide acetate for depot suspension may cause fetal harm when administered to a pregnant woman. Major fetal abnormalities were observed in rabbits but not in rats after administration of leuprolide acetate for depot suspension throughout gestation. There was increased fetal mortality and decreased fetal weights in rats and rabbits (see PRECAUTIONS, Pregnancy, Teratogenic Effects, Pregnancy Category X). The effects on fetal mortality are expected consequences of the alterations in hormonal levels brought about by the drug. If this drug is used during pregnancy or if the patient becomes pregnant while taking this drug, she should be apprised of the potential hazard to the fetus.
4. Use in women who are breastfeeding (see PRECAUTIONS, Nursing Mothers).
5. A report of an anaphylactic reaction to synthetic GnRH (Factrel) has been reported in the medical literature.[1]

LEUPROLIDE ACETATE IMPLANT

1. Leuprolide acetate implant is contraindicated in patients with hypersensitivity to GnRH, GnRH agonist analogs, or any of the components in leuprolide acetate implant. Anaphylactic reactions to synthetic GnRH or GnRH agonist analogs have been reported inthe literature.[1]
2. Leuprolide acetate implant is contraindicated in women and in pediatric patients and was not studied in women or children. Moreover, leuprolide acetate can cause fetal harm when administered to a pregnant woman. Major fetal abnormalities were observed in rabbits but not in rats after administration of leuprolide acetate throughout gestation. There were increased fetal mortality and decreased fetal weights in rats and rabbits. The effects on fetal mortality are expected consequences of the alterations in hormonal levels brought about by this drug. The possibility exists that spontaneous abortion may occur.

WARNINGS

LEUPROLIDE ACETATE INJECTION

Isolated cases of worsening of signs and symptoms during the first weeks of treatment have been reported. Worsening of symptoms may contribute to paralysis with or without fatal complications.

LEUPROLIDE ACETATE INJECTION (FOR PEDIATRIC USE) AND LEUPROLIDE ACETATE FOR DEPOT SUSPENSION (FOR PEDIATRIC USE)

During the early phase of therapy, gonadotropins and sex steroids rise above baseline because of the natural stimulatory effect of the drug. Therefore, an increase in clinical signs and symptoms may be observed (see CLINICAL PHARMACOLOGY).

Noncompliance with drug regimen or inadequate dosing may result in inadequate control of the pubertal process. The consequences of poor control include the return of pubertal signs such as menses, breast development, and testicular growth. The long-term consequences of inadequate control of gonadal steroid secretion are unknown, but may include a further compromise of adult stature.

LEUPROLIDE ACETATE FOR DEPOT SUSPENSION 3.75 MG

Safe use of leuprolide acetate in pregnancy has not been established clinically. Before starting treatment with leuprolide acetate for depot suspension, pregnancy must be excluded.

When used monthly at the recommended dose, leuprolide acetate for depot suspension usually inhibits ovulation and stops menstruation. Contraception is not insured, however, by taking leuprolide acetate for depot suspension. Therefore, patients should use nonhormonal methods of contraception. Patients should be advised to see their physician if they believe they may be pregnant. If a patient becomes pregnant during treatment, the drug must be discontinued and the patient must be apprised of the potential risk to the fetus.

During the early phase of therapy, sex steroids temporarily rise above baseline because of the physiologic effect of the drug. Therefore, an increase in clinical signs and symptoms may be observed during the initial days of therapy, but these will dissipate with continued therapy.

LEUPROLIDE ACETATE FOR DEPOT SUSPENSION 7.5 MG

Isolated cases of worsening of signs and symptoms during the first weeks of treatment have been reported with LH-RH analogs. Worsening of symptoms may contribute to paralysis with or without fatal complications. for patients at risk, the physician may consider initiating therapy with daily leuprolide acetate injection for the first 2 weeks to facilitate withdrawal of treatment if that is considered necessary.

LEUPROLIDE ACETATE IMPLANT

Leuprolide acetate implant, like other LH-RH agonists, causes a transient increase in serum concentrations of testosterone during the first week of treatment. Patients may experience worsening of symptoms or onset of new symptoms, including bone pain, neuropathy, hematuria, or ureteral or bladder outlet obstruction (see PRECAUTIONS).

Cases of ureteral obstruction and spinal cord compression, which may contribute to paralysis with or without fatal complications, have been reported with LH-RH agonists.

If spinal cord compression or renal impairment develops, standard treatment of these complications should be instituted.

PRECAUTIONS

GENERAL

Leuprolide Acetate Injection and Leuprolide Acetate for Depot Suspension 7.5 mg

Patients with metastatic vertebral lesions and/or with urinary tract obstruction should be closely observed during the first few weeks of therapy (see WARNINGS and ADVERSE REACTIONS).

Leuprolide Acetate Injection

Patients with known allergies to benzyl alcohol, an ingredient of the drug's vehicle, may present symptoms of hypersensitivity, usually local, in the form of erythema and induration at the injection site.

Leuprolide Acetate Implant

Patients with metastatic vertebral lesions and/or with urinary tract obstruction should be closely observed during the first few weeks of therapy (see WARNINGS).

X-rays do not affect Leuprolide acetate implant functionality. Leuprolide acetate implant is radio-opaque and is well visualized on x-rays.

The titanium alloy reservoir of leuprolide acetate implant is nonferromagnetic and is not affected by magnetic resonance imaging (MRI). Slight image distortion around leuprolide acetate implant may occur during MRI procedures.

LABORATORY TESTS

Leuprolide Acetate Injection and Leuprolide Acetate for Depot Suspension 7.5 mg

Response to leuprolide acetate should be monitored by measuring serum levels of testosterone and acid phosphatase. In the majority of patients, testosterone levels increased above baseline during the first week, declining thereafter to baseline levels or below by the end of the second week of treatment. Castrate levels were reached within 2-4 weeks and once achieved were maintained for as long as drug administration continued (or for as long as the patients received their monthly injection on time for the leuprolide acetate for depot suspension 7.5 mg). Transient increases in acid phosphatase levels occured sometime early in treatment. However, by the fourth week, the elevated levels usually decreased to values at or near baseline.

Leuprolide Acetate Injection (for Pediatric Use) and Leuprolide Acetate for Depot Suspension (for Pediatric Use)

Response to leuprolide acetate should be monitored 1-2 months after the start of therapy with a GnRH stimulation test and sex steroid levels. Measurement of bone age for advancement should be done every 6-12 months.

Sex steroids may increase or rise above prepubertal levels if the dose is inadequate (see WARNINGS). Once a therapeutic dose has been established, gonadotropin and sex steroid levels will decline to prepubertal levels.

Leuprolide Acetate Implant

Response to leuprolide acetate implant should be monitored by measuring serum concentrations of testosterone and prostate-specific antigen periodically.

Results of testosterone determinations are dependent on assay methodology. It is advisable to be aware of the type and precision of the assay methodology to make appropriate clinical and therapeutic decisions.

DRUG/LABORATORY TEST INTERACTIONS

Leuprolide Acetate Injection (for Pediatric Use) and Leuprolide Acetate for Depot Suspension (for Pediatric Use)

Administration of leuprolide acetate in therapeutic doses results in suppression of the pituitary-gonadal system. Normal function is usually restored within 4-12 weeks after treatment is discontinued.

Leuprolide Acetate for Depot Suspension 3.75 mg

Administration of leuprolide acetate for depot suspension in therapeutic doses results in suppression of the pituitary-gonadal system. Normal function is usually restored within 1-3 months after treatment is discontinued. Therefore, diagnostic tests of pituitary gonadotropic and gonadal functions conducted during treatment and up to 1-2 months after discontinuation of leuprolide acetate for depot suspension therapy may be misleading.

Leuprolide Acetate Implant

Therapy with leuprolide results in suppression of the pituitary-gonadal system. Results of diagnostic tests of pituitary gonadotropic and gonadal functions conducted during and after leuprolide therapy may be affected.

INFORMATION FOR THE PATIENT

Leuprolide Acetate Injection

Refer to the Patient Instructions that are distributed with the prescription for complete instructions.

Leuprolide Acetate Injection (for Pediatric Use)

Prior to starting therapy with leuprolide acetate injection, the parent or guardian must be aware of the importance of continuous therapy. Adherence to daily drug administration schedules must be accepted if therapy is to be successful.

Leuprolide Acetate for Depot Suspension (for Pediatric Use)

Prior to starting therapy with leuprolide acetate, the parent or guardian must be aware of the importance of continuous therapy. Adherence to 4 week drug administration schedules must be accepted if therapy is to be successful.

Leuprolide Acetate Injection and Leuprolide Acetate Injection (for Pediatric Use)

Patients with known allergies to benzyl alcohol, an ingredient of the drug's vehicle, may present symptoms of hypersensitivity, usually local, in the form of erythema and induration at the injection site.

Leuprolide Acetate Injection (for Pediatric Use) and Leuprolide Acetate for Depot Suspension (for Pediatric Use)

During the first 2 months of therapy, a female may experience menses or spotting. If bleeding continues beyond the second month, notify the physician.

Any irritation at the injection site should be reported to the physician immediately.

Report any unusual signs or symptoms to the physician.

Leuprolide Acetate for Depot Suspension 3.75 mg

An information pamphlet for patients is included with the product. Patients should be aware of the following information:

1. Since menstruation should stop with effective doses of leuprolide acetate for depot suspension, the patient should notify her physician if regular menstruation persists. Patients missing successive doses of leuprolide acetate for depot suspension may experience breakthrough bleeding.
2. Patients should not use leuprolide acetate for depot suspension if they are pregnant, breastfeeding, have undiagnosed abnormal vaginal bleeding, or are allergic to any of the ingredients in leuprolide acetate for depot suspension.
3. Safe use of the drug in pregnancy has not been established clinically. Therefore, a non-hormonal method of contraception should be used during treatment. Patients should be advised that if they miss successive doses of leuprolide acetate for depot suspension, breakthrough bleeding or ovulation may occur with the potential for contraception. If a patient becomes pregnant during treatment, she should discontinue treatment and consult her physician.
4. Adverse events occurring in clinical studies with leuprolide acetate for depot suspension that are associated with hypoestrogenism include hot flashes, headaches, emotional lability, decreased libido, acne, myalgia, reduction in breast size, and vaginal dryness. Estrogen levels returned to normal after treatment was discontinued.
5. The induced hypoestrogenic state **also** results in a small loss in bone density over the course of treatment, some of which may not be reversible. for a period up to 6 months, this bone loss should not be important. In patients with major risk factors for decreased bone mineral content such as chronic alcohol and/or tobacco use, strong family history of osteoporosis, or chronic use of drugs that can reduce bone mass such as anticonvulsants or corticosteroids, leuprolide acetate for depot suspension therapy may pose an additional risk. In these patients, the risks and benefits must be weighed carefully before therapy with leuprolide acetate for depot suspension is instituted. Repeated courses of therapy with gonadotropin-releasing hormone analogs beyond 6 months are not advisable in patients with major risk factors for loss of bone mineral content.
6. Retreatment cannot be recommended since safety data beyond 6 months are not available.

CARCINOGENESIS, MUTAGENESIS, AND IMPAIRMENT OF FERTILITY

Leuprolide Acetate Injection (for Pediatric Use) and Leuprolide Acetate for Depot Suspension (for Pediatric Use)

Although no clinical studies have been completed in children to assess the full reversibility of fertility suppression, animal studies (prepubertal and adult rats and monkeys) with leuprolide acetate and other GnRH analogs have shown functional recovery. However, following a study with leuprolide acetate, immature male rats demonstrated tubular degeneration in the testes even after a recovery period. In spite of the failure to recover histologically, the treated males proved to be as fertile as the controls. Also, no histologic changes were observed in the female rats following the same protocol. In both sexes, the offspring of the treated animals appeared normal. The effect of the treatment of the parents on the reproductive performance of the F1 generation was not tested. The clinical significance of these findings is unknown.

Leuprolide Acetate Injection, Leuprolide Acetate Injection (for Pediatric Use), Leuprolide Acetate for Depot Suspension 3.75 mg, and Leuprolide Acetate for Depot Suspension (for Pediatric Use)

A 2 year carcinogenicity study was conducted in rats and mice. In rats, a dose-related increase of benign pituitary hyperplasia and benign pituitary adenomas was noted at 24 months when the drug was administered subcutaneously at high daily doses (0.6-4 mg/kg). There was a significant but not dose-related increase of pancreatic islet-cell adenomas in females and of testicular interstitial cell adenomas in males (highest incidence in the low dose group). In mice, no leuprolide acetate-induced tumors or pituitary abnormalities were observed at a dose as high as 60 mg/kg for 2 years. Adult patients have been treated with leuprolide acetate for up to 3 years with doses as high as 10 mg/day and for 2 years with doses as high as 20 mg/day without demonstrable pituitary abnormalities.

Leuprolide Acetate for Depot Suspension 3.75 mg

Mutagenicity studies have been performed with leuprolide acetate using bacterial and mammalian systems. These studies provided no evidence of a mutagenic potential.

Clinical and pharmacologic studies in adults with leuprolide acetate and similar analogs have shown full reversibility of fertility suppression when the drug is discontinued after continuous administration for periods of up to 6 months. Although no clinical studies have been completed in children to assess the full reversibility of fertility suppression, animal studies (prepubertal and adult rats and monkeys) with leuprolide acetate and other GnRH analogs have shown functional recovery.

Two year carcinogenicity studies were conducted in rats and mice. In rats, a dose-related increase of benign pituitary hyperplasia and benign pituitary adenomas was noted at 24 months when the drug was administered subcutaneously at high daily doses (0.6-4 mg/kg). In mice no pituitary abnormalities were observed at a dose as high as 60 mg/kg for 2 years. Patients have been treated with leuprolide acetate for up to 3 years with doses as high as 10 mg/day and for 2 years with doses as high as 20 mg/day without demonstrable pituitary abnormalities.

Leuprolide Acetate Injection and Leuprolide Acetate for Depot Suspension 3.75 mg

Mutagenicity studies have been performed with leuprolide acetate using bacterial and mammalian systems. These studies provided no evidence of a mutagenic potential.

Clinical and pharmacologic studies with leuprolide acetate and similar analogs have shown full reversibility of fertility suppression when the drug is discontinued after continuous administration for periods of up to 24 weeks.

Leuprolide Acetate Injection

No clinical studies have been conducted with leuprolide acetate to assess the reversibility of fertility suppression.

Leuprolide Acetate Implant

Two year carcinogenicity studies were conducted in rats and mice. In rats, dose-related increases of benign pituitary hyperplasia and benign pituitary adenomas were noted at 24 months when the drug was administered subcutaneously at high daily doses (4-24 mg/m^2, 50-300 times the daily human exposure based on body surface area). There were significant but not dose-related increases of pancreatic islet-cell adenomas in females and of testicular interstitial cell adenomas in males (highest incidence in the low dose group). In mice no pituitary abnormalities were observed at up to 180 mg/m^2 (over 2000 times the daily human exposure based on body surface area) for 2 years.

Mutagenicity studies were performed with leuprolide acetate using bacterial and mammalian systems. These studies provided no evidence of a mutagenic potential.

PREGNANCY, TERATOGENIC EFFECTS, PREGNANCY CATEGORY X

Leuprolide Acetate Injection, Leuprolide Acetate Injection (for Pediatric Use), Leuprolide Acetate for Depot Suspension 7.5 mg, Leuprolide Acetate for Depot Suspension (for Pediatric Use), and Leuprolide Acetate Implant

See CONTRAINDICATIONS.

Leuprolide Acetate for Depot Suspension 3.75 mg

See CONTRAINDICATIONS. When administered on day 6 of pregnancy at test dosages of 0.00024, 0.0024, and 0.024 mg/kg (1/300 to 1/3 the human dose) to rabbits, leuprolide acetate for depot suspension produced a dose-related increase in major fetal abnormalities. Similar studies in rats failed to demonstrate an increase in fetal malformations. There was increased fetal mortality and decreased fetal weights with the 2 higher doses of leuprolide acetate for depot suspension in rabbits and with the highest dose (0.024 mg/kg) in rats.

NURSING MOTHERS

Leuprolide Acetate for Depot Suspension 3.75 mg

It is not known whether leuprolide acetate for depot suspension is excreted in human milk. Because many drugs are excreted in human milk, and because the effects of leuprolide acetate for depot suspension on lactation and/or the breastfed child have not been determined, leuprolide acetate for depot suspension should not be used by nursing mothers.

Leuprolide Acetate Injection (for Pediatric Use) and Leuprolide Acetate for Depot Suspension (for Pediatriac Use)

It is not known whether leuprolide acetate is excreted in human milk. Leuprolide acetate should not be used by nursing mothers.

PEDIATRIC USE

Leuprolide Acetate for Depot Suspension 3.75 mg

See leuprolide acetate for depot suspension for the safety and effectiveness in children with central precocious puberty.

Leuprolide Acetate Implan

Leuprolide acetate implant is contraindicated in pediatric patients and was not studied in children (see CONTRAINDICATIONS).

DRUG INTERACTIONS

LEUPROLIDE ACETATE INJECTION AND LEUPROLIDE ACETATE FOR DEPOT SUSPENSION 7.5 MG

None have been reported.

LEUPROLIDE ACETATE INJECTION (FOR PEDIATRIC USE), LEUPROLIDE ACETATE FOR DEPOT SUSPENSION 3.75 MG, AND LEUPROLIDE ACETATE FOR DEPOT SUSPENSION (FOR PEDIATRIC USE)

No pharmacokinetic-based drug-drug interaction studies have been conducted. However, because leuprolide acetate is a peptide that is primarily degraded by peptidase and not by cytochrome P-450 enzymes as noted in specific studies, and the drug is only about 46% bound to plasma proteins, drug interactions would not be expected to occur.

ADVERSE REACTIONS

LEUPROLIDE ACETATE INJECTION

In the majority of patients testosterone levels increased above baseline during the first week, declining thereafter to baseline levels or below by the end of the second week of treatment. This transient increase was occasionally associated with a temporary worsening of signs and symptoms, usually manifested by an increase in bone pain (see WARNINGS). In a few cases a temporary worsening of existing hematuria and urinary tract obstruction occurred during the first week. Temporary weakness and paresthesia of the lower limbs have been reported in a few cases.

Potential exacerbations of signs and symptoms during the first few weeks of treatment is a concern in patients with vertebral metastases and/or urinary obstruction which, if aggravated, may lead to neurological problems or increase the obstruction.

In a comparative trial of leuprolide acetate injection versus diethylstibesterol, in 5% or more of the patients receiving either drug, the following adverse reactions were reported to have a possible or probable relationship to drug as ascribed by the treating physician. Often, causality is difficult to assess in patients with metastatic prostate cancer. Reactions considered not drug related are excluded (see TABLE 3).

TABLE 3

	Number of Reports	
	Leuprolide Acetate (n=98)	DES (n=101)
Cardiovascular System		
Congestive heart failure	1	5
ECG changes/Ischemia	19	22
High blood pressure	8	5
Murmur	3	8
Peripheral edema	12	30
Phlebitis/thrombosis	2	10
Gastrointestinal System		
Anorexia	6	5
Constipation	7	9
Nausea/vomiting	5	17
Endocrine System		
*Decreased testicular size	7	11
*Gynecomastia/breast tenderness or pain	7	63
*Hot flashes	55	12
*Impotence	4	12
Hemic and Lymphatic System		
Anemia	5	5
Musculoskeletal System		
Bone pain	5	2
Myalgia	3	9
Central/Peripheral Nervous System		
Dizziness/lightheadedness	5	7
General pain	13	13
Headache	7	4
Insomnia/sleep disorders	7	5
Respiratory System		
Dyspnea	2	8
Sinus congestion	5	6
Integumentary System		
Dermatitis	5	8
Urogenital System		
Frequency/urgency	6	8
Hematuria	6	4
Urinary tract infection	3	7
Miscellaneous		
Asthenia	10	10

* Physiologic effect of decreased testosterone.

In this same study, the following adverse reactions were reported in less than 5% of the patients on leuprolide acetate.

Cardiovascular System: Angina, cardiac arrhythmias, myocardial infarction, pulmonary emboli.

Gastrointestinal System: Diarrhea, dysphagia, gastrointestinal bleeding, gastrointestinal disturbance, peptic ulcer, rectal polyps.

Endocrine System: Libido decrease, thyroid enlargement.

Musculoskeletal System: Joint pain.

Central/Peripheral Nervous System: Anxiety, blurred vision, lethargy, memory disorder, mood swings, nervousness, numbness, paresthesia, peripheral neuropathy, syncope/blackouts, taste disorders.

Respiratory System: Cough, pleural rub, pneumonia, pulmonary fibrosis.

Integumentary System: Carcinoma of skin/ear, dry skin, ecchymosis, hair loss, itching, local skin reactions, pigmentation, skin lesions.

Urogenital System: Bladder spasms, dysuria, incontinence, testicular pain, urinary obstruction.

Miscellaneous: Depression, diabetes, fatigue, fever/chills, hypoglycemia, increased BUN, increased calcium, increased creatinine, infection/inflammation, ophthalmologic disorders, swelling (temporal bone).

The following additional adverse reactions have been reported with leuprolide acetate or leuprolide acetate for depot suspension during other clinical trials and/or during postmarketing surveillance. Reactions considered as nondrug related by the treating physician are excluded.

Cardiovascular System: Hypotension, transient ischemic attack/stroke.
Gastrointestinal System: Hepatic dysfunction.
Endocrine System: Libido increase.
Hemic and Lymphatic System: Decreased WBC, hemoptysis.
Musculoskeletal System: Ankylosing spondylosis, pelvic fibrosis.
Central/Peripheral Nervous System: Hearing disorder, peripheral neuropathy, spinal fracture/paralysis.
Respiratory System: Pulmonary infiltrate, respiratory disorders.
Integumentary System: Hair growth.
Urogenital System: Penile swelling, prostate pain.
Miscellaneous: Hypoproteinemia, hard nodule in throat, weight gain, increased uric acid.

LEUPROLIDE ACETATE FOR DEPOT SUSPENSION 7.5 MG

In the majority of patients testosterone levels increased above baseline during the first week, declining thereafter to baseline levels or below by the end of the second week of treatment.

Potential exacerbations of signs and symptoms during the first few weeks of treatment is a concern in patients with vertebral metastases and/or urinary obstruction or hematuria which, if aggravated, may lead to neurological problems such as temporary weakness and/or paresthesia of the lower limbs or worsening of urinary symptoms (see WARNINGS).

In a clinical trial of leuprolide acetate for depot suspension, the following adverse reactions were reported to have a possible or probable relationship to drug as ascribed by the treating physician in 5% or more of the patients receiving the drug. Often, causality is difficult to assess in patients with metastatic prostate cancer. Reactions considered not drug related are excluded (see TABLE 4).

TABLE 4

	Leuprolide Acetate for Depot Suspension	
	(n=56)	(Percent)
Cardiovascular System		
Edema	7	(12.5%)
Gastrointestinal System		
Nausea/vomiting	3	(5.4%)
Endocrine System		
*Decreased testicular size	3	(5.4%)
*Hot flashes/sweats	33	(58.9%)
*Impotence	3	(5.4%)
Central/Peripheral Nervous System		
General pain	4	(7.1%)
Respiratory System		
Dyspnea	3	(5.4%)
Miscellaneous		
Asthenia	3	(5.4%)

* Physiologic effect of decreased testosterone.

Laboratory: Elevations of certain parameters were observed, but it is difficult to assess these abnormalities in this population (see TABLE 5).

TABLE 5

SGOT (>2N)	4	(5.4%)
LDH (>2N)	11	(19.6%)
Alkaline phosphatase (>1.5 N)	4	(5.4%)

In this same study, the following adverse reactions were reported in less than 5% of the patients on Leuprolide Acetate for Depot Suspension.

Cardiovascular System: Angina, cardiac arrhythmia.
Gastrointestinal System: Anorexia, diarrhea.
Endocrine System: Gynecomastia, libido decrease.
Musculoskeletal System: Bone pain, myalgia.
Central/Peripheral Nervous System: Paresthesia, insomnia.
Respiratory System: Hemoptysis.
Integumentary System: Dermatitis, local skin reactions, hair growth.
Urogenital System: Dysuria, frequency/urgency, hematuria, testicular pain.
Miscellaneous: Diabetes, fever/chills, hard nodule in throat, increased calcium, weight gain, increased uric acid.

The following additional adverse reactions have been reported with leuprolide acetate injection. Reactions considered by the treating physician as nondrug related are not included.

Cardiovascular System: Congestive heart failure, ECG changes/ischemia, high blood pressure, hypotension, myocardial infarction, murmur, phlebitis/thrombosis, pulmonary emboli, transient ischemic attack/stroke.
Gastrointestinal System: Constipation, dysphagia, gastrointestinal bleeding, gastrointestinal disturbance, hepatic dysfunction, peptic ulcer, rectal polyps.
Endocrine System: Breast tenderness or pain, libido increase, thyroid enlargement.
Hemic and Lymphatic System: Anemia, decreased WBC.
Musculoskeletal System: Ankylosing spondylosis, joint pain, pelvic fibrosis.
Central/Peripheral Nervous System: Anxiety, blurred vision, dizziness/lightheadedness, headache, hearing disorder, sleep disorders, lethargy, memory disorder, mood swings, nervousness, numbness, peripheral neuropathy, spinal fracture/paralysis, syncope/blackouts, taste disorders.
Respiratory System: Cough, pleural rub, pneumonia, pulmonary fibrosis, pulmonary infiltrate, respiratory disorders, sinus congestion.
Integumentary System: Carcinoma of the skin/ear, dry skin, ecchymosis, hair loss, itching, pigmentation, skin lesions.
Urogenital System: Bladder spasms, incontinence, penile swelling, prostrate pain, urinary obstruction, urinary tract infection.
Miscellaneous: Depression, hypoglycemia, hypoproteinemia, increased BUN, increased creatinine, infection/inflammation, ophthalmologic disorders, swelling (temporal bone).

LEUPROLIDE ACETATE INJECTION (FOR PEDIATRIC USE) AND LEUPROLIDE ACETATE FOR DEPOT SUSPENSION (FOR PEDIATRIC USE)

Potential exacerbation of signs and symptoms during the first few weeks of treatment (see PRECAUTIONS) is a concern in patients with rapidly advancing central precocious puberty.

In two studies of children with central precocious puberty, in 2% or more of the patients receiving the drug, the following adverse reactions were reported to have a possible or probable relationship to drug as ascribed by the treating physician. Reactions considered not drug related are excluded (see TABLE 6).

TABLE 6

	Number of Patients	
	n=395	%
Body as a Whole		
General pain	7	2%
Integumentary system acne/seborrhea	7	2%
Injection site reactions including abscess	21	5%
Rash including erythema multiforme	8	2%
Urogenital System		
Vaginitis/bleeding/discharge	7	2%

In those same studies, the following adverse reactions were reported in less than 2% of the patients.

Body as a Whole: Body odor, fever, headache, infection.
Cardiovascular System: Syncope, vasodilation.
Digestive System: Dysphagia, gingivitis, nausea/vomiting.
Endocrine System: Accelerated sexual maturity.
Metabolic and Nutritional Disorders: Peripheral edema, weight gain.
Nervous System: Nervousness, personality disorder, somnolence, emotional lability.
Respiratory System: Epistaxis.
Integumentary System: Alopecia, skin striae.
Urogenital System: Cervix disorder, gynecomastia/breast disorders, urinary incontinence.

LEUPROLIDE ACETATE FOR DEPOT SUSPENSION 3.75 MG

Estradiol levels may increase during the first weeks following the initial injection, but then decline to menopausal levels. This transient increase in estradiol can be associated with a temporary worsening of signs and symptoms (see WARNINGS).

As would be expected with a drug that lowers serum estradiol levels, the most frequently reported adverse reactions were those related to hypoestrogenism.

Endometriosis: In controlled studies comparing leuprolide acetate for depot suspension, 3.75 mg monthly and danazol (800 mg/day), or placebo, adverse reactions most frequently reported and thought to be possibly or probably drug-related.

Cardiovascular System: Palpitations, syncope, tachycardia.
Gastrointestinal System: Dry mouth, thirst, appetite changes.
Central/Peripheral Nervous System: Anxiety,* personality disorder, memory disorder, delusions.
Integumentary System: Ecchymosis, alopecia, hair disorder.
Urogenital System: Dysuria,* lactation.
Miscellaneous: Ophthalmologic disorders,* lymphadenopathy.

Uterine Leiomyomata (Fibroids): In controlled clinical trials comparing leuprolide acetate for depot suspension 3.75 mg and placebo, adverse events reported in >5% of patients and thought to be potentially related to drug are noted in TABLE 7.

TABLE 7

	Leuprolide Acetate for Depot Suspension	Placebo
	n=166	n=163
Body as a Whole		
Asthenia	14 (8.4%)	8 (4.9%)
General pain	14 (8.4%)	10 (6.1%)
Headache*	43 (25.9%)	29 (17.8%)
Cardiovascular System		
Hot flashes/sweats*	121 (72.9%)	29 (17.8%)
Metabolic and Nutritional Disorders		
Edema	9 (5.4%)	2 (1.2%)
Musculoskeletal System		
Joint disorder*	13 (7.8%)	5 (3.1%)
Nervous System		
Depression/emotional lability*	18 (10.8%)	7 (4.3%)
Urogenital System		
Vaginitis*	19 (11.4%)	3 (1.8%)

* Physiologic effect of the drug.

Symptoms reported in <5% of patients included:

Body as Whole : Body odor, flu syndrome, injection site reactions.
Cardiovascular System: Tachycardia.
Digestive System: Appetite changes, dry mouth, GI disturbances, nausea/vomiting.
Metabolic and Nutritional Disorders: Weight changes.
Musculoskeletal System: Myalgia.

Nervous System: Anxiety, decreased libido,* dizziness, insomnia, nervousness,* neuromuscular disorders,* paresthesias.
Respiratory System: Rhinitis.
Integumentary System: Androgen-like effects, nail disorder, skin reactions.
Special Senses: Conjunctivitis, taste perversion.
Urogenital System: Breast changes,* menstrual disorders.
*Physiologic effect of the drug.

In one controlled clinical trial, patients received a higher dose (7.5 mg) of leuprolide acetate for depot suspension. Events seen with this dose that were thought to be potentially related to drug and were not seen at the lower dose included palpitations, syncope, glossitis, ecchymosis, hypesthesia, confusion, lactation, pyelonephritis, and urinary disorders. Generally, a higher incidence of hypoestrogenic effects was observed at the higher dose.

In other clinical trials involving patients with prostate cancer and during postmarketing surveillance, the following adverse reactions were reported to have a possible, probable, or unknown relationship to leuprolide acetate as ascribed by the treating physician. Often, it is difficult to assess causality in patients with prostate cancer. Reactions considered not drug related have been excluded.

Cardiovascular System: Congestive heart failure, ECG changes/ischemia, high blood pressure, murmur, phlebitis/thrombosis, angina, cardiac arrhythmias, myocardial infarction, pulmonary emboli, hypotension, transient ischemic attack/stroke.
Gastrointestinal System: Dysphagia, gastrointestinal bleeding, peptic ulcer, rectal polyps, hepatic dysfunction.
Endocrine System: Decreased testicular size, gynecomastia, impotence, libido increase, thyroid enlargement.
Hemic and Lymphatic System: Anemia, decreased WBC, hemoptysis.
Musculoskeletal System: Bone pain.
Central/Peripheral Nervous System: Peripheral neuropathy, syncope/blackouts, hearing disorder, spinal fracture/paralysis.
Respiratory System: Dyspnea, sinus congestion, cough, pleural rub, pneumonia, pulmonary fibrosis, respiratory disorders.
Urogenital System: Frequency/urgency, hematuria, urinary tract infection, bladder spasm, incontinence, testicular pain, urinary obstruction, penile swelling, prostrate pain.
Miscellaneous: Diabetes, fever, hypoglycemia, increased BUN, increased calcium, increased creatinine, inflammation.

Changes in Bone Density

Endometriosis

A controlled study in endometriosis patients showed that vertebral bone density as measured by dual energy x-ray absorptiometry (DEXA) decreased by an average of 3.9% at 6 months compared with the pretreatment value. Earlier studies in endometriosis patients, utilizing quantitative computed tomography (QCT), demonstrated that in the few patients who were retested at 6 and 12 months, partial to complete recovery of bone density was recorded in the post-treatment period. Use of leuprolide acetate for depot suspension for longer than 6 months or in the presence of other known risk factors for decreased bone mineral content may cause additional bone loss.

Uterine Leiomyomata (Fibroids)

In one study, vertebral trabecular bone mineral density as assessed by quantitative digital radiography (QDR) revealed a mean decrease of 2.7% at 3 months compared with the pretreatment value. It would be anticipated that this loss of bone mineral density would be complete to partially reversible following discontinuation of therapy. Use of leuprolide acetate for depot suspension 3.75 mg for uterine leiomyomata for longer than 3 months or in the presence of other known risk factors for decreased bone mineral content may cause additional bone loss **and is not recommended.**

Changes in Laboratory Values During Treatment

Plasma Enzymes

Endometriosis

During clinical trials with leuprolide acetate for depot suspension, regular laboratory monitoring revealed that SGOT levels were more than twice the upper limit of normal in only 1 patient. There was no other clinical or laboratory evidence of abnormal liver function.

Uterine Leiomyomata (Fibroids)

In clinical trials with leuprolide acetate for depot suspension 3.75 mg, 5 (3%) patients had a post-treatment transaminase value that was at least twice the baseline value and above the upper limit of the normal range. None of the laboratory increases were associated with clinical symptoms.

Lipids

Endometriosis

At enrollment, 4% of the leuprolide acetate for depot suspension patients and 1% of the danazol patients had total cholesterol values above the normal range. These patients also had cholesterol values above the normal range at the end of treatment.

Of those patients whose pretreatment cholesterol values were in the normal range, 7% of the leuprolide acetate for depot suspension patients and 9% of the danazol patients had post-treatment values above the normal range.

The mean (±SEM) pretreatment values for total cholesterol from all patients were 178.8 (2.9) mg/dl in the leuprolide acetate for depot suspension groups and 175.3 (3.0) mg/dl in the danazol group. At the end of treatment, the mean values for total cholesterol from all patients were 193.3 mg/dl in the leuprolide acetate for depot suspension group and 194.4 mg/dl in the danazol group. These increases from the pretreatment values were statistically significant ($p < 0.03$) in both groups.

Triglycerides were increased above the upper limit of normal in 12% of the patients who received leuprolide acetate for depot suspension and in 6% of the patients who received danazol.

At the end of treatment, HDL cholesterol fractions decreased below the lower limit of the normal range in 2% of the leuprolide acetate for depot suspension patients compared with 54% of those receiving danazol. LDL cholesterol fractions increased above the upper limit of the normal range in 6% of the patients receiving leuprolide acetate for depot suspension compared with 23% of those receiving danazol. There was no increase in the LDL/HDL ratio in patients receiving leuprolide acetate for depot suspension but there was approximately a 2-fold increase in the LDL/HDL ratio in patients receiving danazol.

Uterine Leiomyomata (Fibroids)

In patients receiving leuprolide acetate for depot suspension 3.75 mg, mean changes in cholesterol (+11 mg/dl to +29 mg/dl), LDL cholesterol (+8 mg/dl to +22 mg/dl), HDL cholesterol (0 to 6 g/dl), and the LDL/HDL ratio (-0.1 to +0.5) were observed across studies. In the one study in which triglyceride levels were determined, the mean increase from baseline was 32 mg/dl.

Other Changes

Endometriosis

In comparative studies, the following changes were seen in approximately 5-8% of patients. Leuprolide acetate for depot suspension was associated with elevations of LDH and phosphorus, and deceases in WBC counts. Danazol therapy was associated with increases in hematocrit, platelet count, and LDH.

Uterine Leiomyomata (Fibroids): Hematology

In leuprolide acetate for depot suspension treated patients, although there were statistically significant mean decreases in platelet counts from baseline to final visit, the last mean platelet counts were within the normal range. Decreases in total WBC count and neutrophils were observed but were not clinically significant.

Chemistry

Slight to moderate mean increases were noted for glucose, uric acid, BUN, creatinine, total protein, albumin, bilirubin, alkaline phosphatase, LDH, calcium, and phosphorus. None of these increases were clinically significant.

LEUPROLIDE ACETATE IMPLANT

The safety of leuprolide acetate implant was evaluated in 131 patients with prostate cancer treated for up to 24 months in two clinical trials. Leuprolide acetate implant, like other LHRH analogs, caused a transient increase in serum testosterone concentrations during the first 2 weeks of treatment. Therefore, potential exacerbations of signs and symptoms of the disease during the first few weeks of treatment are of concern in patients with vertebral metastases and/or urinary obstruction or hematuria. If these conditions are aggravated, it may lead to neurological problems such as weakness and/or paresthesia of the lower limbs or worsening of urinary symptoms (see WARNINGS and PRECAUTIONS).

In the above-described clinical trials, the transient increase in serum testosterone concentrations was associated with an exacerbation of disease symptoms, manifested by pain or bladder outlet obstructive symptoms (urinary retention or frequency) in 6 (4.6%) patients.

The majority of local reactions associated with initial insertion or removal and insertion of a new implant began and resolved within the first 2 weeks. Reactions persisted in 9.3% of patients. 10.3% of patients developed application-site reactions after the first 2 weeks following insertion.

In these 2 clinical trials, 4 patients had local infection/inflammations that resolved after treatment with oral antibiotics.

Local reactions following insertion of a subsequent implant were comparable to those seen after initial insertion.

In the first 12 months after initial insertion of the implant(s), an implant extruded through the incision site in 3 of 131 patients.

The following possibly or probably related systemic adverse events occurred during clinical trials within 24 months of treatment with leuprolide acetate implant, and were reported in ≥2% of patients (TABLE 8).

In addition, the following possibly or probably related systemic adverse events were reported by <2% of patients using leuprolide acetate implant in clinical studies.

General: General pain, chills, abdominal pain, malaise, dry mucous membranes.
Gastrointestinal: Constipation, nausea.
Hematologic: Iron deficiency anemia.
Metabolic: Edema, weight loss.
Musculoskeletal: Bone pain, arthritis.
Nervous: Dizziness, insomnia, paresthesia, amnesia, anxiety.
Skin: Pruritus, rash, hirsutism.
Urogenital: Urinary urgency, prostatic disorder, urinary tract infection, dysuria, urinary incontinence, urinary retention.

Changes in Bone Density

Decreased bone density has been reported in the medical literature in men who have had orchiectomy or who have been treated with an LH-RH agonist analog. In a clinical trial, 25 men with prostate cancer, 12 of whom had been treated previously with leuprolide acetate for at least 6 months, underwent bone density studies as a result of pain. The leuprolide-treated group had lower bone density scores than the nontreated control group. It can be anticipated that long periods of medical castration in men will have effects on bone density.

DOSAGE AND ADMINISTRATION

LEUPROLIDE ACETATE INJECTION

The recommended dose is 1 mg (0.2 ml) administered as a single daily subcutaneous injection. As with other drugs administered chronically by subcutaneous injection, the injection site should be varied periodically.

Parenteral drug products should be inspected visually for particulate matter, and discoloration prior to administration, whenever solution and container permit.

TABLE 8 *Incidence (%) of Possibley or Probably Related Systemic Adverse Events Reported by ≥2% of Patients Treated With Leuprolide Acetate Implant for up to 24 Months*

Body System / Adverse Event	Number (%)	
Body as a Whole		
Asthenia	10	(7.6%)
Headache	6	(4.6%)
Extremity pain	4	(3.1%)
Cardiovascular		
Vasodilation (hot flashes)*	89	(67.9%)
Digestive		
Diarrhea	3	(2.3%)
Hematology and Lymphatic		
Ecchymosis	6	(4.6%)
Anemia	3	(2.3%)
Metabolic and Nutritional		
Peripheral edema	4	(3.1%)
Weight Gain	3	(2.3%)
Nervous		
Depression	7	(5.3%)
Respiratory		
Dyspnea	3	(2.3%)
Skin		
Sweating*	7	(5.3%)
Alopecia	3	(2.3%)
Urogenital		
Gynecomastia/breast enlargement*	9	(6.9%)
Nocturia	5	(3.8%)
Urinary frequency	5	(3.8%)
Testis atrophy or pain*	5	(3.8%)
Breast pain*	4	(3.1%)
Impotence*	3	(2.3%)

* Expected pharmacologic consequences of testosterone suppression.

LEUPROLIDE ACETATE INJECTION (FOR PEDIATRIC USE)

Leuprolide acetate injection can be administered by a patient/parent or health care professional.

LEUPROLIDE ACETATE FOR DEPOT SUSPENSION (FOR PEDIATRIC USE)

Leuprolide acetate for depot suspension for pediatric use must be administered under the supervision of a physician.

LEUPROLIDE ACETATE INJECTION (FOR PEDIATRIC USE) AND LEUPROLIDE ACETATE FOR DEPOT SUSPENSION (FOR PEDIATRIC USE)

The dose of leuprolide acetate must be individualized for each child. The dose is based on a mg/kg ratio of drug to body weight. Younger children require higher doses on a mg/kg ratio.

for either dosage form, after 1-2 months of initiating therapy or changing doses, the child must be monitored with a GnRH stimulation test, sex steroids, and Tanner staging to confirm downregulation. Measurements of bone age for advancement should be monitored every 6-12 months. The dose should be titrated upward until no progression of the condition is noted either clinically and/or by laboratory parameters.

The first dose found to result in adequate downregulation can probably be maintained for the duration of therapy in most children. However, there are insufficient data to guide dosage adjustment as patients move into higher weight categories after beginning therapy at very young ages and low dosages. It is recommended that adequate downregulation be verified in such patients whose weight has increased significantly while on therapy.

As with other drugs administered by injection, the injection site should be varied periodically.

Discontinuation of leuprolide acetate should be considered before age 11 for females and age 12 for males.

LEUPROLIDE ACETATE INJECTION (FOR PEDIATRIC USE)

The recommended starting dose is 50 μg/kg/day administered as a single subcutaneous injection. If total downregulation is not achieved, the dose should be titrated upward by 10 μg/kg/day. This dose will be considered the maintenance dose.

Note: As with all parenteral products, inspect container's solution for discoloration and particulate matter before each use.

LEUPROLIDE ACETATE FOR DEPOT SUSPENSION (FOR PEDIATRIC USE)

The recommended starting dose is 0.3 mg/kg/4 weeks (minimum 7.5 mg) administered as a single intramuscular injection. The starting dose will be dictated by the child's weight (see TABLE 9).

TABLE 9

Weight	Dose
≤25 kg	7.5 mg
>25-37.5 kg	11.25 mg
> 37.5 kg	15 mg

If total downregulation is not achieved, the dose should be titrated upward in increments of 3.75 mg every 4 weeks. This dose will be considered the maintenance dose.

LEUPROLIDE ACETATE FOR DEPOT SUSPENSION 3.75 MG

Leuprolide acetate for depot suspension must be administered under the supervision of a physician.

The recommended dose of leuprolide acetate for depot suspension is 3.75 mg, incorporated in a depot formulation. The lyophilized microspheres are to be reconstituted and administered monthly as a single intramuscular injection.

Endometriosis

The recommended duration of administration is 6 months. Retreatment cannot be recommended since safety data for retreatment are not available. If the symptoms of endometriosis recur after a course of therapy, and further treatment with leuprolide acetate for depot suspension is contemplated, it is recommended that bone density be assessed before retreatment begins to ensure that values are within normal limits.

Uterine Leiomyomata (Fibroids)

Recommended duration of therapy with leuprolide acetate for depot suspension is **up to** 3 months. The symptoms associated with uterine leiomyomata will recur following discontinuation of therapy. If additional treatment with leuprolide acetate for depot suspension 3.75 mg is contemplated, bone density should be assessed prior to initiation of therapy to ensure that values are within normal limits.

As with other drugs administered by injection, the injection site should be varied periodically.

The vial of leuprolide acetate for depot suspension and the ampule of diluent may be stored at room temperature.

LEUPROLIDE ACETATE FOR DEPOT SUSPENSION 7.5 MG

Leuprolide acetate for depot suspension must be administered under the supervision of a physician.

The recommended dose of leuprolide acetate for depot suspension is 7.5 mg, incorporated in a depot formulation.

As with other drugs administered by injection, the injection site should be varied periodically.

The vial of leuprolide acetate for depot suspension and the ampule of diluent may be stored at room temperature.

LEUPROLIDE ACETATE IMPLANT

The recommended dose of leuprolide acetate implant is 1 implant for 12 months. Each implant contains 65 mg leuprolide. The implant is inserted subcutaneously in the inner aspect of the upper arm and provides continuous release of leuprolide for 12 months of hormonal therapy.

Leuprolide acetate implant must be removed after 12 months of therapy. At the time an implant is removed, another implant may be inserted to continue therapy.

HOW SUPPLIED

LUPRON INJECTION

Each 0.2 ml contains 1 mg of leuprolide acetate, sodium chloride for tonicity adjustment, 1.8 mg of benzyl alcohol as preservative and water for injection. The pH may have been adjusted with sodium hydroxide and/or acetic acid.

Storage

Store below 25°C (77°F). Avoid freezing. Protect from light.

Store vial in carton until use.

LUPRON INJECTION (FOR PEDIATRIC USE)

Lupron injection is a sterile solution.

A 2.8 ml multiple dose vial contains leuprolide acetate (5 mg/ml), sodium chloride (6.3 mg/ml) for tonicity adjustment, benzyl alcohol as a preservative (9 mg/ml), and water for injection. The pH may have been adjusted with sodium hydroxide and/or acetic acid.

Storage

Store below 25°C (77°F). Avoid freezing. Protect from light—store vial in carton until use.

Use the syringes supplied with Lupron injection. Insulin syringes may be substituted for use with Lupron injection. The volume of drug for the dose will vary depending on the syringe used and the concentration of drug.

LUPRON DEPOT 3.75 MG

Lupron Depot 3.75 mg is available in a vial containing sterile lyophilized microspheres which is leuprolide acetate incorporated in a biodegradable copolymer of lactic and glycolic acids.

The single-dose vial of Lupron Depot contains leuprolide acetate (3.75 mg), purified gelatin (0.65 mg), DL-lactic and glycolic acids copolymer (33.1 mg), and D-mannitol (6.6 mg). The accompanying ampule of diluent contains carboxymethylcellulose sodium (7.5 mg), D-mannitol (75 mg), polysorbate 80 (1.5 mg), and water for injection, and glacial acetic acid to control pH. When mixed with 1 ml of diluent, Lupron Depot is administered as a single monthly IM injection.

LUPRON DEPOT 7.5 MG

Lupron Depot 7.5 mg is available in a vial containing sterile lyophilized microspheres which is leuprolide acetate incorporated in a biodegradable copolymer of lactic and glycolic acids.

The single-dose vial of Lupron Depot contains leuprolide acetate (7.5 mg), purified gelatin (1.3 mg), DL-lactic and glycolic acids copolymer (66.2 mg), and D-mannitol (13.2 mg). The accompanying ampule of dilutent contains carboxymethylcellulose sodium (7.5 mg), D-mannitol (75 mg), polysorbate 80 (1.5 mg), water for injection, and acetic acid to control pH. When mixed with 1 ml of diluent, Lupron Depot is administered as a single monthly IM injection.

Storage

No refrigeration necessary. Protect from freezing.

LUPRON DEPOT-PED

Lupron Depot-Ped is available in 3 packages providing a dose of 7.5, 11.25 or 15 mg. Each vial contains sterile lyophilized microspheres which is leuprolide acetate incorporated in a biodegradable copolymer of lactic and glycolic acids.

The single-dose vial of Lupron Depot-Ped contains, respectively for each dosage strength, leuprolide acetate (7.5/11.25,15 mg), purified gelatin (1.3/1.95/2.6 mg), DL-lactic and glycolic acids copolymer (66.2/99.3/132.4 mg), and D-mannitol (13.2/19.8/26.4 mg). The accompanying ampule of diluent contains carboxymethylcellulose sodium (7.5 mg), D-mannitol (75 mg), polysorbate 80 (1.5 mg), water for injection, and acetic acid to control pH.

Storage

The vial of Lupron Depot-Ped and the ampule of diluent may be stored at room temperature. Keep from freezing.

Use the syringes supplied in the Lupron Depot-Ped kits. Any 22 gauge needle may be used with Lupron Depot-Ped.

VIADUR

Viadur is supplied in a box containing 2 inner package trays. One tray contains a sterile Viadur implant in a sealed vial and a sterile Viadur implanter. The other tray constitutes a sterile Viadur Kit, which includes: 1 scalpel, 1 forceps, 1 syringe, povidone swabs, 1 package wound closure strips, 1 22 gauge x 1.5″ needle, 1 25 gauge x 1.5″ needle, 1 ampule lidocaine HCl 2% (10 ml), 6 gauze sponges, 2 alcohol prep pads, 1 package skin protectant, 1 bandage, 1 fenestrated drape, 1 marking pen, 1 ruler, and 1 mosquito clamp. A physician insert, patient information, and insertion and removal instructions are also provided in the box.

Storage

Store at 25°C (77°F); excursions permitted to 15-30°C (59-86°F).

PRODUCT LISTING - RATED THERAPEUTICALLY EQUIVALENT

Package	Price	Product, Manufacturer	NDC
Kit - Subcutaneous - 5 mg/ml			
1's	$383.15	GENERIC, Ivax Corporation	00182-3154-99
2.80 ml	$385.33	GENERIC, Eon Labs Manufacturing Inc	00185-7400-85
2.80 ml	$385.33	GENERIC, Gensia Sicor Pharmaceuticals Inc	00703-4014-18
2.80 ml	$428.15	LUPRON, Allscripts Pharmaceutical Company	54569-4982-00
2.80 ml	$459.09	LUPRON, Tap Pharmaceuticals Inc	00300-3612-28
Solution - Subcutaneous - 5 mg/ml			
2.80 ml x 6	$2219.46	GENERIC, Gensia Sicor Pharmaceuticals Inc	00703-4024-19
2.80 ml x 6	$2219.47	GENERIC, Gensia Sicor Pharmaceuticals Inc	00703-4014-19
2.80 ml x 6	$2311.98	GENERIC, Eon Labs Manufacturing Inc	00185-7400-14

PRODUCT LISTING - EQUIVALENTS NOT AVAILABLE

Package	Price	Product, Manufacturer	NDC
Implant - Subcutaneous - 65 mg			
1's	$5683.75	VIADUR, Bayer	00026-9711-01
1's	$5684.00	VIADUR, Alza	17314-4500-01
Kit - Injectable - 7.5 mg			
1's	$540.63	LUPRON DEPOT-PED, Tap Pharmaceuticals Inc	00300-2106-01
1's	$594.65	LUPRON DEPOT-PED, Allscripts Pharmaceutical Company	54569-2713-00
1's	$643.75	ELIGARD, Sanofi Winthrop Pharmaceuticals	00024-0597-07
1's	$643.75	LUPRON DEPOT-PED, Tap Pharmaceuticals Inc	00300-2108-01
3's	$1931.25	ELIGARD, Sanofi Winthrop Pharmaceuticals	00024-0597-22
Kit - Intramuscular - 3.75 mg			
1's	$556.11	LUPRON DEPOT, Tap Pharmaceuticals Inc	00300-3641-01
Kit - Intramuscular - 11.25 mg			
1's	$931.88	LUPRON DEPOT-PED, Tap Pharmaceuticals Inc	00300-2270-01
1's	$1214.56	LUPRON, Tap Pharmaceuticals Inc	00300-2282-01
1's	$1668.34	LUPRON DEPOT-GYN, Tap Pharmaceuticals Inc	00300-3663-01
Kit - Intramuscular - 15 mg			
1's	$1081.25	LUPRON DEPOT-PED, Tap Pharmaceuticals Inc	00300-2437-01
1's	$1337.71	LUPRON DEPOT-PED, Tap Pharmaceuticals Inc	00300-2440-01
Kit - Intramuscular - 30 mg			
1's	$2575.00	LUPRON DEPOT, Tap Pharmaceuticals Inc	00300-3683-01
Kit - Subcutaneous - 5 mg/ml			
1's	$367.33	OAKLIDE, Oakwood Laboratories Inc	64523-0100-02
Powder For Injection - Injectable - 7.5 mg			
1's	$623.79	LUPRON DEPOT, Allscripts Pharmaceutical Company	54569-4785-00
1's	$643.75	LUPRON DEPOT, Tap Pharmaceuticals Inc	00300-3642-01
Powder For Injection - Intramuscular - 3.75 mg			
1's	$518.64	LUPRON DEPOT, Allscripts Pharmaceutical Company	54569-4547-00
Solution - Intramuscular - 22.5 mg			
1's	$1931.25	LUPRON DEPOT, Tap Pharmaceuticals Inc	00300-3346-01
Solution - Subcutaneous - 5 mg/ml			
2.80 ml	$371.39	LUPRON, Tap Pharmaceuticals Inc	00300-3626-24
2.80 ml x 6	$2204.01	OAKLIDE, Oakwood Laboratories Inc	64523-0100-01
2.80 ml x 6	$2754.54	LUPRON, Tap Pharmaceuticals Inc	00300-3612-24

Levalbuterol Hydrochloride *(003430)*

For related information, see the comparative table section in Appendix A.

Categories: Asthma; FDA Approved 1999 Mar; Pregnancy Category C
Drug Classes: Adrenergic agonists; Bronchodilators
Brand Names: Xopenex
Cost of Therapy: $225.90 (Asthma; Xopenex Solution; 0.63 mg; 3 ml; 3 doses/day; 30 day supply)

DESCRIPTION

Xopenex inhalation solution is a sterile, clear, colorless, preservative-free solution of the hydrochloride salt of levalbuterol, the (R)-enantiomer of the drug substance racemic albuterol. Levalbuterol hydrochloride is a relatively selective beta$_2$-adrenergic receptor agonist (see CLINICAL PHARMACOLOGY). The chemical name for levalbuterol hydrochloride is (R)-α^1-[[(1,1-dimethylethyl)amino]methyl]-4-hydroxy-1,3-benzenedimethanol hydrochloride.

The molecular weight of levalbuterol hydrochloride is 275.8, and its empirical formula is $C_{13}H_{21}NO_3 \cdot HCl$. It is a white to off-white, crystalline solid, with a melting point of approximately 187°C and solubility of approximately 180 mg/ml in water.

Levalbuterol hydrochloride is the USAN modified name for (R)-albuterol hydrochloride in the US.

Xopenex inhalation solution is supplied in unit-dose vials and requires no dilution before administration by nebulization. Each 3 ml unit-dose vial contains either 0.31 mg of levalbuterol (as 0.36 mg of levalbuterol HCl) or 0.63 mg of levalbuterol (as 0.73 mg of levalbuterol HCl) or 1.25 mg of levalbuterol (as 1.44 mg of levalbuterol HCl), sodium chloride to adjust tonicity, and sulfuric acid to adjust the pH to 4.0 (3.3-4.5).

CLINICAL PHARMACOLOGY

Activation of beta$_2$-adrenergic receptors on airway smooth muscle leads to the activation of adenylcyclase and to an increase in the intracellular concentration of cyclic-3′,5′-adenosine monophosphate (cyclic AMP). This increase in cyclic AMP leads to the activation of protein kinase A, which inhibits the phosphorylation of myosin and lowers intracellular ionic calcium concentrations, resulting in relaxation. Levalbuterol relaxes the smooth muscles of all airways, from the trachea to the terminal bronchioles. Levalbuterol acts as a functional antagonist to relax the airway irrespective of the spasmogen involved, thus protecting against all bronchoconstrictor challenges. Increased cyclic AMP concentrations are also associated with the inhibition of release of mediators from mast cells in the airway.

While it is recognized that beta$_2$-adrenergic receptors are the predominant receptors on bronchial smooth muscle, data indicate that there is a population of beta$_2$-receptors in the human heart that comprise between 10 and 50% of cardiac beta-adrenergic receptors. The precise function of these receptors has not been established (see WARNINGS). However, all beta-adrenergic agonist drugs can produce a significant cardiovascular effect in some patients, as measured by pulse rate, blood pressure, symptoms, and/or electrocardiographic changes.

PRECLINICAL STUDIES

Results from an *in vitro* study of binding to human beta-adrenergic receptors demonstrated that levalbuterol has approximately 2-fold greater binding affinity than racemic albuterol and approximately 100-fold greater binding affinity than (S)-albuterol. In guinea pig airways, levalbuterol HCl and racemic albuterol decreased the response to spasmogens (*e.g.*, acetylcholine and histamine), whereas (S)-albuterol was ineffective. These results suggest that most of the bronchodilatory effect of racemic albuterol is due to the (R)-enantiomer.

Intravenous studies in rats with racemic albuterol sulfate have demonstrated that albuterol crosses the blood-brain barrier and reaches brain concentrations amounting to approximately 5.0% of the plasma concentrations. In structures outside the blood-brain barrier (pineal and pituitary glands), albuterol concentrations were found to be 100 times those in the whole brain.

Studies in laboratory animals (minipigs, rodents, and dogs) have demonstrated the occurrence of cardiac arrhythmias and sudden death (with histologic evidence of myocardial necrosis) when beta-agonists and methylxanthines are administered concurrently. The clinical significance of these findings is unknown.

PHARMACOKINETICS — ADULTS AND ADOLESCENTS ≥12 YEARS OLD

The inhalation pharmacokinetics of levalbuterol HCl inhalation solution were investigated in a randomized cross-over study in 30 healthy adults following administration of a single dose of 1.25 mg and a cumulative dose of 5 mg of levalbuterol HCl inhalation solution and a single dose of 2.5 mg and a cumulative dose of 10 mg of racemic albuterol sulfate inhalation solution by nebulization using a PARI LC Jet nebulizer with a Dura-Neb 2000 compressor.

Following administration of a single 1.25 mg dose of levalbuterol HCl inhalation solution, exposure, as measured by C_{max} and area under the curve (AUC) of (R)-albuterol, was 1.5 and 2 times greater, respectively, than that following administration of a single 2.5 mg dose of racemic albuterol sulfate inhalation solution (see TABLE 1). Following administration of a cumulative 5 mg dose of levalbuterol HCl inhalation solution (1.25 mg given every 30 minutes for a total of 4 doses) or a cumulative 10 mg dose of racemic albuterol sulfate inhalation solution (2.5 mg given every 30 minutes for a total of 4 doses) C_{max} and AUC of (R)-albuterol were comparable (see TABLE 1).

PHARMACOKINETICS — CHILDREN 6-11 YEARS OLD

The pharmacokinetic parameters of (R)- and (S)-albuterol in children with asthma were obtained using population pharmacokinetic analysis. These data are presented in TABLE 2. For comparison, adult data obtained by conventional pharmacokinetic analysis from a different study are also presented in TABLE 2.

In children, AUC and C_{max} of (R)-albuterol following administration of 0.63 mg levalbuterol HCl inhalation solution were comparable to that following administration of 1.25 mg racemic albuterol sulfate inhalation solution.

TABLE 1 *Mean (SD) Values for Pharmacokinetic Parameters in Healthy Adults*

	Single Dose		Cumulative Dose	
	Levalbuterol HCl	Racemic albuterol sulfate	Levalbuterol HCl	Racemic albuterol sulfate
	1.25 mg	2.5 mg	5 mg	10 mg
C_{max} (ng/ml)				
(R)-albuterol	1.1 (0.45)	0.8 (0.41)*	4.5 (2.20)	4.2 (1.51)*
T_{max} (h)‡				
(R)-albuterol	0.2 (0.17, 0.37)	0.2 (0.17, 1.50)	0.2 (-0.18†, 1.25)	0.2 (-0.28†, 1.00)
AUC (ng·h/ml)				
(R)-albuterol	3.3 (1.58)	1.7 (0.99)*	17.4 (8.56)	16.0 (7.12)*
T½ (h)				
(R)-albuterol	3.3 (2.48)	1.5 (0.61)	4.0 (1.05)	4.1 (0.97)

* Values reflect only (R)-albuterol and do not include (S)-albuterol.
† A negative T_{max} indicates C_{max} occurred between first and last nebulizations.
‡ Median (Min, Max) reported for T_{max}.

Given the same dose of 0.63 mg of levalbuterol HCl to children and adults, the predicted C_{max} of (R)-albuterol in children was similar to that in adults (0.52 vs 0.56 ng/ml), while predicted AUC in children (2.55 ng·h/ml) was about 1.5-fold higher than that in adults (1.65 ng·h/ml). These data support lower doses for children 6-11 years old compared to the adult doses (see DOSAGE AND ADMINISTRATION).

TABLE 2 *(R)-Albuterol Exposure in Adults and Pediatric Subjects (6-11 years)*

	AUC(0-∞)* (ng·h/ml)	C_{max}† (ng/ml)
Children 6-11 Years		
Levalbuterol HCl 0.31 mg	1.36	0.303
Levalbuterol HCl 0.63 mg	2.55	0.521
Racemic albuterol 1.25 mg	2.65	0.553
Racemic albuterol 2.5 mg	5.02	1.08
Adults ≥12 Years		
Levalbuterol HCl 0.63 mg	1.65‡	0.56‡
Levalbuterol HCl 1.25 mg	3.3§	1.1§

* Area under the plasma concentration curve from time 0 to infinity.
† Maximum plasma concentration.
‡ The values are predicted by assuming linear pharmacokinetics.
§ The data obtained from TABLE 1.

L

PHARMACODYNAMICS — ADULTS AND ADOLESCENTS ≥12 YEARS OLD

In a randomized, double-blind, placebo-controlled, crossover study, 20 adults with mild-to-moderate asthma received single doses of levalbuterol HCl inhalation solution (0.31, 0.63 and 1.25 mg) and racemic albuterol sulfate inhalation solution (2.5 mg). All doses of active treatment produced a significantly greater degree of bronchodilation (as measured by percent change from pre-dose in mean FEV_1) than placebo and there were no significant differences between any of the active treatment arms. The bronchodilator response to 1.25 mg of levalbuterol HCl inhalation solution and 2.5 mg of racemic albuterol sulfate inhalation solution were clinically comparable over the 6 hour evaluation period, except for a slightly longer duration of action (>15% increase in FEV_1 from baseline) after administration of 1.25 mg of levalbuterol HCl inhalation solution. Systemic beta-adrenergic adverse effects were observed with all active doses and were generally dose-related for (R)-albuterol. Lebalbuterol HCl inhalation solution at a dose of 1.25 mg produced a slightly higher rate of systemic beta-adrenergic adverse effects than the 2.5 mg dose of racemic albuterol sulfate inhalation solution.

In a randomized, double-blind, placebo-controlled, cross-over study, 12 adults with mild-to-moderate asthma were challenged with inhaled methacholine chloride 20 and 180 minutes following administration of a single dose of either 2.5 mg of racemic albuterol sulfate, 1.25 mg of levalbuterol HCl, 1.25 mg of (S)-albuterol, or placebo using a PARI LC Jet+ nebulizer. Racemic albuterol sulfate, levalbuterol HCl, and (S)-albuterol had a protective effect against methacholine-induced bronchoconstriction 20 minutes after administration, although the effect of (S)-albuterol was minimal. At 180 minutes after administration, the bronchoprotective effect of 1.25 mg of levalbuterol HCl was comparable to that of 2.5 mg of racemic albuterol sulfate. At 180 minutes after administration, 1.25 mg of (S)-albuterol had no bronchoprotective effect.

In a clinical study in adults with mild-to-moderate asthma, comparable efficacy (as measured by change from baseline in FEV_1) and safety (as measured by heart rate, blood pressure, ECG, serum potassium, and tremor) were demonstrated after a cumulative dose of 5 mg of levalbuterol HCl inhalation solution (4 consecutive doses of 1.25 mg administered every 30 minutes) and 10 mg of racemic albuterol sulfate inhalation solution (4 consecutive doses of 2.5 mg administered every 30 minutes).

INDICATIONS AND USAGE

Levalbuterol HCl inhalation solution is indicated for the treatment or prevention of bronchospasm in adults, adolescents and children 6 years of age and older with reversible obstructive airway disease.

CONTRAINDICATIONS

Levalbuterol HCl inhalation solution is contraindicated in patients with a history of hypersensitivity to levalbuterol HCl or racemic albuterol.

WARNINGS

PARADOXICAL BRONCHOSPASM

Like other inhaled beta-adrenergic agonists, levalbuterol HCl inhalation solution can produce paradoxical bronchospasm, which may be life threatening. If paradoxical bronchospasm occurs, levalbuterol HCl inhalation solution should be discontinued immediately and alternative therapy instituted. It should be recognized that paradoxical bronchospasm, when associated with inhaled formulations, frequently occurs with the first use of a new canister or vial.

DETERIORATION OF ASTHMA

Asthma may deteriorate acutely over a period of hours or chronically over several days or longer. If the patient needs more doses of levalbuterol HCl inhalation solution than usual, this may be a marker of destabilization of asthma and requires reevaluation of the patient and treatment regimen, giving special consideration to the possible need for anti-inflammatory treatment (*e.g.*, corticosteroids).

USE OF ANTI-INFLAMMATORY AGENTS

The use of beta-adrenergic agonist bronchodilators alone may not be adequate to control asthma in many patients. Early consideration should be given to adding anti-inflammatory agents (*e.g.*, corticosteroids, to the therapeutic regimen).

CARDIOVASCULAR EFFECTS

Lebalbuterol HCl inhalation solution, like all other beta-adrenergic agonists, can produce a clinically significant cardiovascular effect in some patients, as measured by pulse rate, blood pressure, and/or symptoms. Although such effects are uncommon after administration of levalbuterol HCl inhalation solution at recommended doses, if they occur, the drug may need to be discontinued. In addition, beta-agonists have been reported to produce ECG changes, such as flattening of the T wave, prolongation of the QTc interval, and ST segment depression. The clinical significance of these findings is unknown. Therefore, levalbuterol HCl inhalation solution, like all sympathomimetic amines, should be used with caution in patients with cardiovascular disorders, especially coronary insufficiency, cardiac arrhythmias, and hypertension.

DO NOT EXCEED RECOMMENDED DOSE

Fatalities have been reported in association with excessive use of inhaled sympathomimetic drugs in patients with asthma. The exact cause of death is unknown, but cardiac arrest following an unexpected development of a severe acute asthmatic crisis and subsequent hypoxia is suspected.

IMMEDIATE HYPERSENSITIVITY REACTIONS

Immediate hypersensitivity reactions may occur after administration of racemic albuterol, as demonstrated by rare cases of urticaria, angioedema, rash, bronchospasm, anaphylaxis, and oropharyngeal edema. The potential for hypersensitivity must be considered in the clinical evaluation of patients who experience immediate hypersensitivity reactions while receiving levalbuterol HCl inhalation solution.

PRECAUTIONS

GENERAL

Levalbuterol HCl, like all sympathomimetic amines, should be used with caution in patients with cardiovascular disorders, especially coronary insufficiency, hypertension, and cardiac arrhythmias; in patients with convulsive disorders, hyperthyroidism, or diabetes mellitus; and in patients who are unusually responsive to sympathomimetic amines. Clinically significant changes in systolic and diastolic blood pressure have been seen in individual patients and could be expected to occur in some patients after the use of any beta-adrenergic bronchodilator.

Large doses of intravenous racemic albuterol have been reported to aggravate preexisting diabetes mellitus and ketoacidosis. As with other beta-adrenergic agonist medications, levalbuterol may produce significant hypokalemia in some patients, possibly through intracellular shunting, which has the potential to produce adverse cardiovascular effects. The decrease is usually transient, not requiring supplementation.

INFORMATION FOR THE PATIENT

See the Patient Instructions that are distributed with the prescription.

The action of levalbuterol HCl inhalation solution may last up to 8 hours. Lebalbuterol HCl inhalation solution should not be used more frequently than recommended. Do not increase the dose or frequency of dosing of levalbuterol HCl inhalation solution without consulting your physician. If you find that treatment with levalbuterol HCl inhalation solution becomes less effective for symptomatic relief, your symptoms become worse, and/or you need to use the product more frequently than usual, you should seek medical attention immediately. While you are taking levalbuterol HCl inhalation solution, other inhaled drugs and asthma medications should be taken only as directed by your physician. Common adverse effects include palpitations, chest pain, rapid heart rate, headache, dizziness, and tremor or nervousness. If you are pregnant or nursing, contact your physician about the use of levalbuterol HCl inhalation solution.

Effective and safe use of levalbuterol HCl inhalation solution requires consideration of the following information in addition to that provided in the Patient Instructions that are distributed with the prescription.

Lebalbuterol HCl inhalation solution single-use low-density polyethylene (LDPE) vials should be protected from light and excessive heat. Store in the protective foil pouch between 20 and 25°C (68 and 77°F). Do not use after the expiration date stamped on the container. Unused vials should be stored in the protective foil pouch. Once the foil pouch is opened, the vials should be used within 2 weeks. Vials removed from the pouch, if not used immediately, should be protected from light and used within 1 week. Discard if the solution is not colorless.

The drug compatibility (physical and chemical), efficacy, and safety of levalbuterol HCl inhalation solution when mixed with other drugs in a nebulizer have not been established.

CARCINOGENESIS, MUTAGENESIS, AND IMPAIRMENT OF FERTILITY

No carcinogenesis or impairment of fertility studies have been carried out with levalbuterol HCl alone. However, racemic albuterol sulfate has been evaluated for its carcinogenic potential and ability to impair fertility.

In a 2 year study in Sprague-Dawley rats, racemic albuterol sulfate caused a significant dose-related increase in the incidence of benign leiomyomas of the mesovarium at and above dietary doses of 2 mg/kg (approximately 2 times the maximum recommended daily inhalation dose of levalbuterol HCl for adults on a mg/m^2 basis). In another study, this effect was blocked by the coadministration of propranolol, a nonselective beta-adrenergic antagonist. In an 18 month study in CD-1 mice, racemic albuterol sulfate showed no evidence of tumorigenicity at dietary doses up to 500 mg/kg (approximately 270 times the maximum recommended daily inhalation dose of levalbuterol HCl for adults on a mg/m^2 basis). In a 22 month study in the Golden hamster, racemic albuterol sulfate showed no evidence of tumorigenicity at dietary doses up to 50 mg/kg (approximately 35 times the maximum recommended daily inhalation dose of levalbuterol HCl for adults on a mg/m^2 basis).

Levalbuterol HCl was not mutagenic in the Ames test or the CHO/HPRT Mammalian Forward Gene Mutation Assay. Although levalbuterol HCl has not been tested for clastogenicity, racemic albuterol sulfate was not clastogenic in a human peripheral lymphocyte assay or in an AH1 strain mouse micronucleus assay. Reproduction studies in rats using racemic albuterol sulfate demonstrated no evidence of impaired fertility at oral doses up to 50 mg/kg (approximately 55 times the maximum recommended daily inhalation dose of levalbuterol HCl for adults on a mg/m^2 basis).

PREGNANCY, TERATOGENIC EFFECTS, PREGNANCY CATEGORY C

A reproduction study in New Zealand White rabbits demonstrated that levalbuterol HCl was not teratogenic when administered orally at doses up to 25 mg/kg (approximately 110 times the maximum recommended daily inhalation dose of levalbuterol HCl for adults on a mg/m^2 basis). However, racemic albuterol sulfate has been shown to be teratogenic in mice and rabbits. A study in CD-1 mice given racemic albuterol sulfate subcutaneously showed cleft palate formation in 5 of 111 (4.5%) fetuses at 0.25 mg/kg (less than the maximum recommended daily inhalation dose of levalbuterol HCl for adults on a mg/m^2 basis) and in 10 of 108 (9.3%) fetuses at 2.5 mg/kg (approximately equal to the maximum recommended daily inhalation dose of levalbuterol HCl for adults on a mg/m^2 basis). The drug did not induce cleft palate formation when administered subcutaneously at a dose of 0.025 mg/kg (less than the maximum recommended daily inhalation dose of levalbuterol HCl for adults on a mg/m^2 basis). Cleft palate also occurred in 22 of 72 (30.5%) fetuses from females treated subcutaneously with 2.5 mg/kg of isoproterenol (positive control).

A reproduction study in Stride Dutch rabbits revealed cranioschisis in 7 of 19 (37%) fetuses when racemic albuterol sulfate was administered orally at a dose of 50 mg/kg (approximately 110 times the maximum recommended daily inhalation dose of levalbuterol HCl for adults on a mg/m^2 basis).

A study in which pregnant rats were dosed with radiolabeled racemic albuterol sulfate demonstrated that drug-related material is transferred from the maternal circulation to the fetus.

There are no adequate and well-controlled studies of levalbuterol HCl inhalation solution in pregnant women. Because animal reproduction studies are not always predictive of human response, levalbuterol HCl inhalation solution should be used during pregnancy only if the potential benefit justifies the potential risk to the fetus.

During marketing experience of racemic albuterol, various congenital anomalies, including cleft palate and limb defects, have been rarely reported in the offspring of patients being treated with racemic albuterol. Some of the mothers were taking multiple medications during their pregnancies. No consistent pattern of defects can be discerned, and a relationship between racemic albuterol use and congenital anomalies has not been established.

USE IN LABOR AND DELIVERY

Because of the potential for beta-adrenergic agonists to interfere with uterine contractility, the use of levalbuterol HCl inhalation solution for the treatment of bronchospasm during labor should be restricted to those patients in whom the benefits clearly outweigh the risk.

TOCOLYSIS

Levalbuterol HCl has not been approved for the management of preterm labor. The benefit:risk ratio when levalbuterol HCl is administered for tocolysis has not been established. Serious adverse reactions, including maternal pulmonary edema, have been reported during or following treatment of premature labor with beta$_2$-agonists, including racemic albuterol.

NURSING MOTHERS

Plasma levels of levalbuterol after inhalation of therapeutic doses are very low in humans, but it is not known whether levalbuterol is excreted in human milk.

Because of the potential for tumorigenicity shown for racemic albuterol in animal studies and the lack of experience with the use of levalbuterol HCl inhalation solution by nursing mothers, a decision should be made whether to discontinue nursing or to discontinue the drug, taking into account the importance of the drug to the mother. Caution should be exercised when levalbuterol HCl inhalation solution is administered to a nursing woman.

PEDIATRICS

The safety and efficacy of levalbuterol HCl inhalation solution have been established in pediatric patients 6 years of age and older in one adequate and well-controlled clinical trial (see CLINICAL PHARMACOLOGY, Pharmacodynamics). Use of levalbuterol HCl in children is also supported by evidence from adequate and well-controlled studies of levalbuterol HCl in adults, considering that the pathophysiology and the drug's exposure level and effects in pediatric and adult patients are substantially similar. Safety and effectiveness of levalbuterol HCl in pediatric patients below the age of 6 years have not been established.

GERIATRICS

Data on the use of levalbuterol HCl in patients 65 years of age and older are very limited. A very small number of patients 65 years of age and older were treated with levalbuterol HCl inhalation solution in a 4 week clinical study (n=2 for 0.63 mg and n=3 for 1.25 mg). In these patients, bronchodilation was observed after the first dose on day 1 and after 4 weeks of treatment. There are insufficient data to determine if the safety and efficacy of levalbuterol HCl inhalation solution are different in patients <65 years of age and patients 65 years of age and older. In general, patients 65 years of age and older should be started at a dose of 0.63 mg of levalbuterol HCl inhalation solution. If clinically warranted due to insufficient bronchodilatoar response, the dose of levalbuterol HCl inhalation solution may be increased in elderly patients as tolerated, in conjunction with frequent clinical and laboratory monitoring, to the maximum recommended daily dose (see DOSAGE AND ADMINISTRATION).

DRUG INTERACTIONS

Other short-acting sympathomimetic aerosol bronchodilators or epinephrine should be used with caution with levalbuterol. If additional adrenergic drugs are to be administered by any route, they should be used with caution to avoid deleterious cardiovascular effects.

Beta-blockers: Beta-adrenergic receptor blocking agents not only block the pulmonary effect of beta agonists such as levalbuterol HCl inhalation solution, but may also produce severe bronchospasm in asthmatic patients. Therefore, patients with asthma should not normally be treated with beta-blockers. However, under certain circumstances, *e.g.*, as prophylaxis after myocardial infarction, there may be no acceptable alternatives to the use of beta-adrenergic blocking agents in patients with asthma. In this setting, cardioselective beta-blockers could be considered, although they should be administered with caution.

Diuretics: The ECG changes and/or hypokalemia that may result from the administration of non-potassium sparing diuretics (such as loop or thiazide diuretics) can be acutely worsened by beta-agonists, especially when the recommended dose of the beta-agonist is exceeded. Although the clinical significance of these effects is not known, caution is advised in the coadministration of beta agonists with non-potassium sparing diuretics.

Digoxin: Mean decreases of 16% and 22% in serum digoxin levels were demonstrated after single-dose intravenous and oral administration of racemic albuterol, respectively, to normal volunteers who had received digoxin for 10 days. The clinical significance of these findings for patients with obstructive airway disease who are receiving levalbuterol HCl and digoxin on a chronic basis is unclear. Nevertheless, it would be prudent to carefully evaluate the serum digoxin levels in patients who are currently receiving digoxin and levalbuterol HCl inhalation solution.

Monoamine oxidase inhibitors or tricyclic antidepressants: Lebalbuterol HCl inhalation solution should be administered with extreme caution to patients being treated with monoamine oxidase inhibitors or tricyclic antidepressants, or within 2 weeks of discontinuation of such agents, because the action of levalbuterol HCl on the vascular system may be potentiated.

L

ADVERSE REACTIONS

ADULTS AND ADOLESCENTS ≥12 YEARS OLD

Adverse events reported in ≥2% of patients receiving levalbuterol HCl inhalation solution or racemic albuterol and more frequently than in patients receiving placebo in a 4 week, controlled clinical trial are listed in TABLE 3.

TABLE 3 *Adverse Events Reported in a 4 Week, Controlled Clinical Trial*

		Lebalbuterol HCl		Racemic albuterol
Body System	**Placebo**	**1.25 mg**	**0.63 mg**	**2.5 mg**
Preferred Term	**(n=75)**	**(n=73)**	**(n=72)**	**(n=74)**
Body as a Whole				
Allergic reaction	1.3%	0%	0%	2.7%
Flu syndrome	0%	1.4%	4.2%	2.7%
Accidental injury	0%	2.7%	0%	0%
Pain	1.3%	1.4%	2.8%	2.7%
Back pain	0%	0%	0%	2.7%
Cardiovascular System				
Tachycardia	0%	2.7%	2.8%	2.7%
Migraine	0%	2.7%	0%	0%
Digestive System				
Dyspepsia	1.3%	2.7%	1.4%	1.4%
Musculoskeletal System				
Leg cramps	1.3%	2.7%	0%	1.4%
Central Nervous System				
Dizziness	1.3%	2.7%	1.4%	0%
Hypertonia	0%	0%	0%	2.7%
Nervousness	0%	9.6%	2.8%	8.1%
Tremor	0%	6.8%	0%	2.7%
Anxiety	0%	2.7%	0%	0%
Respiratory System				
Cough increased	2.7%	4.1%	1.4%	2.7%
Infection viral	9.3%	12.3%	6.9%	12.2%
Rhinitis	2.7%	2.7%	11.1%	6.8%
Sinusitis	2.7%	1.4%	4.2%	2.7%
Turbinate edema	0%	1.4%	2.8%	0%

The incidence of certain systemic beta-adrenergic adverse effects (*e.g.*, tremor, nervousness) was slightly less in the levalbuterol HCl 0.63 mg group as compared to the other active treatment groups. The clinical significance of these small differences is unknown.

Changes in heart rate 15 minutes after drug administration and in plasma glucose and potassium 1 hour after drug administration on Day 1 and Day 29 were clinically comparable in the levalbuterol HCl 1.25 mg and the racemic albuterol 2.5 mg groups (see TABLE 4). Changes in heart rate and plasma glucose were slightly less in the levalbuterol HCl 0.63 mg group compared to the other active treatment groups (see TABLE 4). The clinical significance of these small differences is unknown. After 4 weeks, effects on heart rate, plasma glucose, and plasma potassium were generally diminished compared with Day 1 in all active treatment groups.

TABLE 4 *Mean Changes From Baseline in Heart Rate at 15 Minutes and in Glucose and Potassium at 1 Hour After First Dose (Day 1)*

Treatment	Mean Changes (Day 1) Heart Rate	Glucose	Potassium
Lebalbuterol HCl 0.63 mg, n=72	2.4 bpm	4.6 mg/dl	-0.2 mEq/L
Lebalbuterol HCl 1.25 mg, n=73	6.9 bpm	10.3 mg/dl	-0.3 mEq/L
Racemic albuterol 2.5 mg, n=74	5.7 bpm	8.2 mg/dl	-0.3 mEq/L
Placebo, n=75	-2.8 bpm	-0.2 mg/dl	-0.2 mEq/L

No other clinically relevant laboratory abnormalities related to administration of levalbuterol HCl inhalation solution were observed in this study.

In the clinical trials, a slightly greater number of serious adverse events, discontinuations due to adverse events, and clinically significant ECG changes were reported in patients who received levalbuterol HCl 1.25 mg compared to the other active treatment groups.

The following adverse events, considered potentially related to levalbuterol HCl, occurred in less than 2% of the 292 subjects who received levalbuterol HCl and more frequently than in patients who received placebo in any clinical trial.

Body as a Whole: Chills, pain, chest pain.

Cardiovascular System: ECG abnormal, ECG change, hypertension, hypotension, syncope.

Digestive System: Diarrhea, dry mouth, dry throat, dyspepsia, gastroenteritis, nausea.

Hemic and Lymphatic System: Lymphadenopathy.

Musculoskeletal System: Leg cramps, myalgia.

Nervous System: Anxiety, hypesthesia of the hand, insomnia, paresthesia, tremor.

Special Senses: Eye itch.

The following events, considered potentially related to levalbuterol HCl, occurred in less than 2% of the treated subjects but at a frequency less than in patients who received placebo: Asthma exacerbation, cough increased, wheezing, sweating, and vomiting.

CHILDREN 6-11 YEARS OLD

Adverse events reported in ≥2% of patients in any treatment group and more frequently than in patients receiving placebo in a 3 week, controlled clinical trial are listed in TABLE 5.

TABLE 5 *Most Frequently Reported Adverse Events (≥2% in Any Treatment Group) and More Frequently Than Placebo During the Double-Blind Period (ITT Population, 6-11 Years Old)*

Body System	Placebo	Levalbuterol HCl 0.31 mg	Levalbuterol HCl 0.63 mg	Racemic Albuterol 1.25 mg	Racemic Albuterol 2.5 mg
Preferred Term	(n=59)	(n=66)	(n=67)	(n=64)	(n=60)
Body as a Whole					
Abdominal pain	3.4%	0%	1.5%	3.1%	6.7%
Abdominal injury	3.4%	6.1%	4.5%	3.1%	5.0%
Asthenia	0%	3.0%	3.0%	1.6%	1.7%
Fever	5.1%	9.1%	3.0%	1.6%	6.7%
Headache	8.5%	7.6%	11.9%	9.4%	3.3%
Pain	3.4%	3.0%	1.5%	4.7%	6.7%
Viral infection	5.1%	7.6%	9.0%	4.7%	8.3%
Digestive System					
Diarrhea	0%	1.5%	6.0%	1.6%	0%
Hemic and Lymphatic					
Lymphadenopathy	0%	3.0%	0%	1.6%	0%
Musculoskeletal System					
Myalgia	0%	0%	1.5%	1.6%	3.3%
Respiratory System					
Asthma	5.1%	9.1%	9.0%	6.3%	10.0%
Pharyngitis	6.8%	3.0%	10.4%	0%	6.7%
Rhinitis	1.7%	6.1%	10.4%	3.1%	5.0%
Skin and Appendages					
Eczema	0%	0%	0%	0%	3.3%
Rash	0%	0%	7.5%	1.6%	0%
Urticaria	0%	0%	3.0%	0%	0%
Special Senses					
Otitis media	1.7%	0%	0%	0%	3.3%

Note: Subjects may have more than one adverse event per body system and preferred term.

Changes in heart rate, plasma glucose, and serum potassium are shown in TABLE 6. The clinical significance of these small differences is unknown.

TABLE 6 *Mean Changes From Baseline in Heart Rate at 30 Minutes and in Glucose and Potassium at 1 Hour After First Dose (Day 1) and Last Dose (Day 21) in Children 6-11 Years Old*

Treatment	Heart Rate (bpm)	Glucose (mg/dl)	Potassium (mEq/L)
Mean Changes (Day 1)			
Levalbuterol HCl 0.31 mg, n=66	0.8	4.9	-0.31
Levalbuterol HCl 0.63 mg, n=67	6.7	5.2	-0.36
Racemic albuterol 1.25 mg, n=64	6.4	8.0	-0.27
Racemic albuterol 2.5 mg, n=60	10.9	10.8	-0.56
Placebo, n=59	-1.8	0.6	-0.05
Mean Changes (Day 21)			
Levalbuterol HCl 0.31 mg, n=60	0	2.6	-0.32
Levalbuterol HCl 0.63 mg, n=66	3.8	5.8	-0.34
Racemic albuterol 1.25 mg, n=62	5.8	1.7	-0.18
Racemic albuterol 2.5 mg, n=54	5.7	11.8	-0.26
Placebo, n=55	-1.7	1.1	-0.04

DOSAGE AND ADMINISTRATION

CHILDREN 6-11 YEARS OLD

The recommended dosage of levalbuterol HCl inhalation solution for patients 6-11 years old is 0.31 mg administered 3 times a day, by nebulization. Routine dosing should not exceed 0.63 mg three times a day.

ADULTS AND ADOLESCENTS ≥12 YEARS OLD

The recommended starting dosage of levalbuterol HCl inhalation solution for patients 12 years of age and older is 0.63 mg administered 3 times a day, every 6-8 hours, by nebulization.

Patients 12 years of age and older with more severe asthma or patients who do not respond adequately to a dose of 0.63 mg of levalbuterol HCl inhalation solution may benefit from a dosage of 1.25 mg three times a day.

Patients receiving the highest dose of levalbuterol HCl inhalation solution should be monitored closely for adverse systemic effects, and the risks of such effects should be balanced against the potential for improved efficacy.

The use of levalbuterol HCl inhalation solution can be continued as medically indicated to control recurring bouts of bronchospasm. During this time, most patients gain optimal benefit from regular use of the inhalation solution.

If a previously effective dosage regimen fails to provide the expected relief, medical advice should be sought immediately, since this is often a sign of seriously worsening asthma that would require reassessment of therapy.

The drug compatibility (physical and chemical), efficacy, and safety of levalbuterol HCl inhalation solution when mixed with other drugs in a nebulizer have not been established.

The safety and efficacy of levalbuterol HCl inhalation solution have been established in clinical trials when administered using the PARI LC Jet and the PARI LC Plus nebulizers, and the PARI Master and Dura-Neb 2000 and Dura-Neb 3000 compressors. The safety and efficacy of levalbuterol HCl inhalation solution when administered using other nebulizer systems have not been established.

HOW SUPPLIED

Xopenex inhalation solution is supplied in 3 ml unit-dose, low-density polyethylene (LDPE) vials as a clear, colorless, sterile, preservative-free, aqueous solution in three different strengths of levalbuterol (0.31, 0.63, 1.25 mg).

Storage: Store the Xopenex inhalation solution in the protective foil pouch at 20-25°C (68-77°F). Protect from light and excessive heat. Keep unopened vials in the foil pouch. Once the foil pouch is opened, the vials should be used within 2 weeks. Vials removed from the pouch, if not used immediately, should be protected from light and used within 1 week. Discard any vial if the solution is not colorless.

PRODUCT LISTING - EQUIVALENTS NOT AVAILABLE

Solution - Inhalation - 0.31 mg/3 ml
3 ml x 24 $60.24 XOPENEX, Sepracor Inc 63402-0511-24

Solution - Inhalation - 0.63 mg/3 ml
3 ml x 24 $60.24 XOPENEX, Sepracor Inc 63402-0512-24

Solution - Inhalation - 1.25 mg/3 ml
3 ml x 24 $60.24 XOPENEX, Sepracor Inc 63402-0513-24

Levamisole Hydrochloride *(001632)*

Categories: Carcinoma, colorectal; Pregnancy Category C; FDA Approved 1990 Jun; WHO Formulary

Drug Classes: Antineoplastics, biological response modifiers; Immunomodulators

Brand Names: Ascaryl; Decas; Dewormis; **Ergamisol**; Immunol

Foreign Brand Availability: Ascaridil (Indonesia); Decaris (Bahrain; Benin; Bulgaria; Burkina-Faso; Cyprus; Czech-Republic; Egypt; Ethiopia; Gambia; Ghana; Guinea; Hong-Kong; Hungary; Iran; Iraq; Ivory-Coast; Jordan; Kenya; Kuwait; Lebanon; Liberia; Libya; Malawi; Mali; Mauritania; Mauritius; Mexico; Morocco; Niger; Nigeria; Oman; Qatar; Republic-of-Yemen; Russia; Saudi-Arabia; Senegal; Seychelles; Sierra-Leone; Sudan; Syria; Taiwan; Tanzania; Tunia; Uganda; United-Arab-Emirates; Zambia; Zimbabwe); Detrax 40 (Benin; Burkina-Faso; Ethiopia; Gambia; Ghana; Guinea; Ivory-Coast; Kenya; Liberia; Malawi; Mali; Mauritania; Mauritius; Morocco; Niger; Nigeria; Senegal; Seychelles; Sierra-Leone; Sudan; Tanzania; Tunia; Uganda; Zambia; Zimbabwe); Dewormis 50 (India); Ketrax (India; Ireland); Newkentax (Benin; Burkina-Faso; Ethiopia; Gambia; Ghana; Guinea; Ivory-Coast; Kenya; Liberia; Malawi; Mali; Mauritania; Mauritius; Morocco; Niger; Nigeria; Senegal; Seychelles; Sierra-Leone; Sudan; Tanzania; Tunia; Uganda; Zambia; Zimbabwe); Solaskil (France); Vermisol (India)

Cost of Therapy: $57.24 (Colon Cancer; Ergamisol; 50 mg; 3 tablets/day; 3 day supply)

DESCRIPTION

Levamisole hydrochloride is an immunomodulator available in tablets for oral administration containing the equivalent of 50 mg as levamisole base. Fifty-nine (59) mg of levamisole HCl is equivalent to 50 mg of levamisole base. Inactive ingredients are colloidal silicon dioxide, hydrogenated vegetable oil, hydroxypropyl methylcellulose, lactose, microcrystalline cellulose, polyethylene glycol 6000, polysorbate 80, and talc.

Levamisole hydrochloride is (-)-(S)-2,3,5,6-tetrahydro-6-phenylimidazo [2,1-b] thiazole monohydrochloride.

Levamisole hydrochloride is a white to pale cream colored crystalline powder which is almost odorless and is freely soluble in water. It is quite stable in acid aqueous media but hydrolyzes in alkaline or neutral solutions. It has a molecular weight of 240.75.

CLINICAL PHARMACOLOGY

Two clinical trials having essentially the same design have demonstrated an increase in survival and a reduction in recurrence rate in the subset of patients with resected Dukes' C colon cancer treated with a regimen of Levamisole hydrochloride plus fluorouracil[1,2]. After surgery, patients were randomized to no further therapy, levamisole HCl alone, or levamisole HCl plus fluorouracil.

In one clinical trial in which 408 Dukes' B and C colorectal cancer patients were studied, 262 Dukes' C patients were evaluated for a minimum follow-up of five years[1]. A subset analysis of these Dukes' C patients showed the estimated reduction in death rate was 27% for levamisole HCl plus fluorouracil ($p = 0.11$) and 28% for levamisole HCl alone ($p = 0.11$)[3]. The estimated reduction in recurrence rate was 36% for levamisole HCl plus fluorouracil ($p = 0.025$) and 28% for levamisole HCl alone ($p = 0.11$)[3]. In another clinical trial designed to confirm the above results, 929 Dukes' C colon cancer patients were evaluated for a minimum follow-up of 2 years[2]. The estimated reduction in recurrence rate was 41% for levamisole HCl plus fluorouracil ($p<0.0001$). The levamisole HCl alone group did not show advantage over no treatment on improving recurrence or survival rates. There are presently insufficient data to evaluate the effect of the combination of levamisole HCl plus fluorouracil in Dukes'B patients. There are also insufficient data to evaluate the effect of levamisole HCl plus fluorouracil in patients with rectal cancer because only 12 patients with rectal cancer were treated with the combination in the first study and none in the second study.

The mechanism of action of levamisole HCl in combination with fluorouracil is unknown. The effects of levamisole on the immune system are complex. The drug appears to restore depressed immune function rather than to stimulate response to above-normal levels. Levamisole can stimulate formation of antibodies to various antigens, enhance T-cell responses by stimulating T-cell activation and proliferation, potentiate monocyte and macrophage functions including phagocytosis and chemotaxis, and increase neutrophil mobility, adherence, and chemotaxis. Other drugs have similar short-term effects and the clinical relevance is unclear.

Besides its immunomodulatory function, levamisole has other mammalian pharmacologic activities, including inhibition of alkaline phosphatase, and cholinergic activity.

The pharmacokinetics of levamisole HCl have not been studied in the dosage regimen recommended with fluorouracil not in patients with hepatic insufficiency. After administration of a single oral dose of 50 mg of a research formulation of levamisole HCl, it appears that levamisole is rapidly absorbed from the gastrointestinal tract. Mean peak plasma concentrations of 0.13 mcg/ml are attained within 1.5 to 2 hours. The plasma elimination half-life of levamisole is between 3-4 hours. Following a 150-mg radio-labelled dose, levamisole is extensively metabolized by the liver in humans and the metabolites excreted mainly by the kidneys (70% over 3 days). The elimination half-life of metabolite excretion is 16 hours. Approximately 5% is excreted in the feces. Less than 5% is excreted unchanged in the urine and less than 0.2% in the feces. Approximately 12% is recovered in the urine as the glucuronide of p-hydroxy-levamisole. The clinical significance of these data are unknown since a 150-mg dose may not be proportional to a 50-mg dose.

INDICATIONS AND USAGE

Levamisole hydrochloride is only indicated as adjuvant treatment in combination with fluorouracil after surgical resection in patients with Dukes' stage C colon cancer.

NON-FDA APPROVED INDICATIONS

Levamisole has been used without FDA approval for the treatment of Hodgkin's disease and rheumatoid arthritis. It has also been used as adjuvant treatment in other types of colorectal cancers, advanced breast cancer, and resected melanoma. Because the drug does not directly affect cancer cells, its use as monotherapy for the treatment of cancer is not recommended.

CONTRAINDICATIONS

Levamisole hydrochloride is contraindicated in patients with a known hypersensitivity to the drug or its components.

WARNINGS

Levamisole hydrochloride has been associated with agranulocytosis, sometimes fatal. The onset of agranulocytosis is frequently accompanied by a flu-like syndrome (fever, chills, etc.); however, in a small number of patients it is asymptomatic. A flu-like syndrome may also occur in the absence of agranulocytosis. It is essential that appropriate hematological monitoring be done routinely during therapy with levamisole HCl and fluorouracil. Neutropenia is usually reversible following discontinuation of therapy. Patients should be instructed to report immediately any flu-like symptoms.

Higher than recommended doses of levamisole HCl may be associated with an increased incidence of agranulocytosis, so the recommended dose should not be exceeded.

The combination of levamisole HCl and fluorouracil has been associated with frequent neutropenia, anemia and thrombocytopenia.

PRECAUTIONS

Before beginning this combination adjuvant treatment, the physician should become familiar with the labeling for fluorouracil.

INFORMATION FOR THE PATIENT

The patient should be informed that if flu-like symptoms or malaise occurs, the physician should be notified immediately.

LABORATORY TESTS

On the first day of therapy with levamisole HCl fluorouracil, patients should have a CBC with differential and platelets, electrolytes and liver function tests performed. Thereafter, a CBC with differential and platelets should be performed weekly prior to each treatment with fluorouracil with electrolytes and liver function tests performed every 3 months for a total of one year. Dosage modifications should be instituted as follows: If WBC is 2500-3500/mm^3 defer the fluorouracil dose until WBC is $>3500/mm^3$. If WBC is $<2500/mm^3$, defer the fluorouracil dose until WBC is $>3500/mm^3$; then resume the fluorouracil dose reduced by 20%. If WBC remains $<2500/mm^3$ for over 10 days despite deferring fluorouracil, discontinue administration of levamisole HCl. Both drugs should be deferred unless enough platelets are present ($\geq 100{,}000/mm^3$).

CARCINOGENESIS, MUTAGENESIS, AND IMPAIRMENT OF FERTILITY

Adequate animal carcinogenicity studies have not been conducted with levamisole. Studies of levamisole administered in drinking water at 5, 20, and 80 mg/kg/day to mice for up to 18 months or administered to rats in the diet at 5, 20, and 80 mg/kg/day for 24 months showed no evidence of neoplastic effects. These studies were not conducted at the maximum tolerated dose, therefore the animals may not have been exposed to a reasonable drug challenge. No mutagenic effects were demonstrated in dominant lethal studies in male and female mice, in an Ames test, and in a study to detect chromosomal aberrations in cultured peripheral human lymphocytes.

Adverse effects were not observed on male or female fertility when levamisole was administered to rats in the diet at doses of 2.5, 10, 40 and 160 mg/kg. In a rat gavage study at doses of 20, 60, and 180 mg/kg, the copulation period was increased, the duration of pregnancy was slightly increased, and fertility, pup viability and weight, lactation index, and number of fetuses were decreased at 60 mg/kg. No negative reproductive effects were present when the offspring were allowed to mate and litter.

PREGNANCY CATEGORY C

Teratogenicity studies have been performed in rats and rabbits at oral doses up to 180 mg/kg. Fetal malformations were not observed. In rats, embryotoxicity was present at 160 mg/kg and in rabbits, significant embryotoxicity was observed at 180 mg/kg. There are no adequate and well-controlled studies in pregnant women and levamisole HCl should not be administered unless the potential benefits outweigh the risks. Women taking the combination of levamisole HCl and fluorouracil should be advised not to become pregnant.

NURSING MOTHERS

It is not known whether levamisole HCl is excreted in human milk; it is excreted in cows' milk. Because of the potential for serious adverse reactions in nursing infants from levamisole HCl, a decision should be made whether to discontinue nursing or to discontinue the drug, taking into account the importance of the drug to the mother.

PEDIATRIC USE

Safety and effectiveness of levamisole HCl in children have not been established.

DRUG INTERACTIONS

Levamisole hydrochloride has been reported to produce "Antabuse" -like side effects when given concomitantly with alcohol. Concomitant administration of phenytoin and levamisole HCl plus fluorouracil has led to increased plasma levels of phenytoin. The physician is advised to monitor plasma levels of phenytoin and to decrease the dose if necessary.

Because of reports of prolongation of the prothrombin time beyond the therapeutic range in patients taking concurrent levamisole and warfarin sodium, it is suggested that the prothrombin time be monitored carefully, and the dose of warfarin sodium and other coumarin-like drugs should be adjusted accordingly, in patients taking both drugs.

ADVERSE REACTIONS

Almost all patients receiving Levamisole hydrochloride and fluorouracil reported adverse experiences. Tabulated in TABLE 1 is the incidence of adverse experiences that occurred in at least 1% of patients enrolled in two clinical trials who were adjuvantly treated with either levamisole HCl or levamisole HCl plus fluorouracil following colon surgery. In the larger clinical trial, 66 of 463 patients (14%) discontinued the combination of levamisole HCl plus fluorouracil because of adverse reactions. Forty-three of these patients (9%) developed isolated or a combination of gastrointestinal toxicities (*e.g.*, nausea, vomiting, diarrhea, stomatitis and anorexia). Ten patients developed rash and/or pruritus. Five patients discontinued therapy because of flu-like symptoms or fever with chills; ten patients developed central nervous system symptoms such as dizziness, ataxia, depression, confusion, memory loss, weakness, inability to concentrate, and headache; two patients developed reversible neutropenia and sepsis; one patient because of thrombocytopenia; one patient because of hyperbilirubinemia. One patient in the levamisole HCl plus fluorouracil group developed agranulocytosis and sepsis and died.

In the levamisole HCl alone arm of the trial, 15 of 310 patients (4.8%) discontinued therapy because of adverse experiences. Six of these (2%) discontinued because of rash, six because of arthralgia/myalgia, and one each for fever and neutropenia, urinary infection, and cough (TABLE 1):

In worldwide experience with levamisole HCl, less frequent adverse experiences included exfoliative dermatitis, periorbital edema, vaginal bleeding, anaphylaxis, confusion, convulsions, hallucinations, impaired concentration, renal failure, pancreatitis, elevated serum creatinine, and increased alkaline, phosphatase.

Reports of hyperlipidemia have been observed in patients receiving combination therapy of levamisole HCl and fluorouracil; elevations of triglyceride levels have been greater than increases in cholesterol levels.

Cases of an encephalopathy-like syndrome associated with demyelination have been reported in patients treated with levamisole HCl. Worldwide postmarketing experience with the combination therapy of levamisole HCl and fluorouracil has also included several reports of neurological changes associated with demyelination and several reports of peripheral neuropathy. The onset of symptoms and the clinical presentation in these cases are quite varied. Symptoms may include confusion, speech disturbances, muscle weakness, lethargy, and paresthesia. If an acute neurological syndrome occurs, immediate discontinuation of levamisole HCl and fluorouracil therapy should be considered.

The following additional adverse experiences have been reported for fluorouracil alone: esophagopharyngitis, pancytopenia, myocardial ischemia, angina, gastrointestinal ulceration and bleeding, anaphylaxis and generalized allergic reactions, acute cerebellar syndrome, nystagmus, dry skin, fissuring, photosensitivity, lacrimal duct stenosis, photophobia, euphoria, thrombophlebitis, and nail changes.

DOSAGE AND ADMINISTRATION

The adjuvant use of Levamisole hydrochloride and fluorouracil is limited to the following dosage schedule:

TABLE 1

Adverse Experience	Levamisole HCl N = 440 %	Levamisole HCl plus fluorouracil N = 599 %
Gastrointestinal		
Nausea	22	65
Diarrhea	13	52
Stomatitis	3	39
Vomiting	6	20
Anorexia	2	6
Abdominal pain	2	5
Constipation	2	3
Flatulence	<1	2
Dyspepsia	<1	1
Hematological		
Leukopenia		
<2000/mm^3	<1	1
≥2000 to <4000/mm^3	4	19
≥4000/mm^3	2	33
unscored category	0	<1
Thrombocytopenia		
<50,000/mm^3	0	0
≥50,000 to <130,000/mm^3	1	8
≥130,000/mm^3	1	10
Anemia	0	6
Granulocytopenia	<1	2
Epistaxis	0	1
Skin and Appendages		
Dermatitis	8	23
Alopecia	3	22
Pruritus	1	2
Skin discoloration	0	2
Urticaria	<1	0
Body as a Whole		
Fatigue	6	11
Fever	3	5
Rigors	3	5
Chest pain	<1	1
Edema	1	1
Resistance Mechanisms		
Infection	5	12
Special Sense		
Taste Perversion	8	8
Altered sense of smell	1	1
Musculoskeletal System		
Arthralgia	5	4
Myalgia	3	2
Central and peripheral nervous system		
Dizziness	3	4
Headache	3	4
Paresthesia	2	3
Ataxia	0	2
Psychiatric		
Somnolence	3	2
Depression	1	2
Nervousness	1	2
Insomnia	1	1
Anxiety	1	1
Forgetfulness	0	1
Vision		
Abnormal tearing	0	4
Blurred vision	1	2
Conjunctivitis	<1	2
Liver and biliary system		
Hyperbilirubinemia	<1	1

INITIAL THERAPY:

Levamisole HCl: 50 mg p.o. q8h for 3 days (starting 7-30 days post-surgery)

Fluorouracil: 450 mg/m^2/day IV for 5 days concomitant with a 3-day course of levamisole HCl (starting 21-34 days post-surgery)

MAINTENANCE:

Levamisole HCl: 50 mg p.o. q8h for 3 days every 2 weeks.

Fluorouracil: 450 mg/m^2/day IV once a week beginning 28 days after the initiation of the 5-day course.

Treatment: levamisole HCl, administered orally, should be initiated no earlier than 7 and no later than 30 days post surgery at a dose of 50 mg q8h X 3 days repeated every 14 days for 1 year. Fluorouracil therapy should be initiated no earlier than 21 days and no later than 35 days after surgery providing the patient is out of the hospital, ambulatory, maintaining normal oral nutrition, has well-healed wounds, and is fully recovered from any postoperative complications. If levamisole HCl has been initiated from 7 to 20 days after surgery, initiation of fluorouracil therapy should be coincident with the second course of levamisole HCl, i.e., at 21 to 34 days. If levamisole HCl is initiated from 21 to 30 days after surgery, fluorouracil should be initiated simultaneously with the first course of levamisole HCl.

Fluorouracil should be administered by rapid IV push at a dosage of 450 mg/m^2/day for 5 consecutive days. Dosage calculation is based on actual weight (estimated dry weight if there is evidence of fluid retention). *This course should be discontinued before the full 5 doses are administered if the patient develops any stomatitis or diarrhea* (5 or more loose stools). Twenty-eight days after initiation of this course, weekly fluorouracil should be instituted at a dosage of 450 mg/m^2/week and continued for a total treatment time of 1 year. If stomatitis or diarrhea develop during weekly therapy, the next dose of fluorouracil should be deferred until these side effects have subsided. If these side effects are moderate to severe, the fluorouracil dose should be reduced 20% when it is resumed.

Dosage modifications should be instituted as follows: If WBC is 2500-3500/mm^3 defer the fluorouracil dose until WBC is >3500mm^3. If WBC is <2500/mm^3, defer the fluorouracil dose until WBC is >3500/mm^3; then resume the fluorouracil dose reduced by 20%. If WBC remains <2500/mm^3 for over 10 days despite deferring fluorouracil, discontinue administration of levamisole HCl. Both drugs should be deferred unless platelets are adequate (≥100,000/mm^3).

Levamisole HCl should not be used at doses exceeding the recommended dose or frequency. Clinical studies suggest a relationship between levamisole HCl adverse experiences and increasing dose, and since some of these (e.g., agranulocytosis, may be life-threatening, the recommended dosage regimen should not be exceeded (see WARNINGS.)

Before beginning this combination adjuvant treatment, the physician should become familiar with the labeling for fluorouracil.

HOW SUPPLIED

Ergamisol (levamisole hydrochloride) is available in white, coated tablets containing the equivalent of 50 mg of levamisole base, debossed "JANSSEN" and "L" "50."

Store at room temperature, 15°-30°C (59°-86°F). Protect from moisture.

PRODUCT LISTING - EQUIVALENTS NOT AVAILABLE

Tablet - Oral - 50 mg

36's $228.95 ERGAMISOL, Janssen Pharmaceuticals 50458-0270-36

Levetiracetam (003458)

Categories: Seizures, partial; FDA Approved 1999 Nov; Pregnancy Category C
Drug Classes: Anticonvulsants
Brand Names: Keppra
Cost of Therapy: $121.11 (Epilepsy; Keppra; 500 mg; 2 tablets/day; 30 day supply)

DESCRIPTION

Keppra (levetiracetam) is an antiepileptic drug available as 250 (blue), 500 (yellow), and 750 mg (orange) tablets for oral administration.

The chemical name of levetiracetam, a single enantiomer, is (-)-(S)-α-ethyl-2-oxo-1-pyrrolidine acetamide, its molecular formula is $C_8H_{14}N_2O_2$ and its molecular weight is 170.21. Levetiracetam is chemically unrelated to existing antiepileptic drugs (AEDs).

Levetiracetam is a white to off-white crystalline powder with a faint odor and a bitter taste. It is very soluble in water (104.0 g/100 ml). It is freely soluble in chloroform (65.3 g/100 ml) and in methanol (53.6 g/100 ml), soluble in ethanol (16.5 g/100 ml), sparingly soluble in acetonitrile (5.7 g/100 ml) and practically insoluble in n-hexane.

Keppra tablets contain the labeled amount of levetiracetam. *Inactive Ingredients:* Colloidal silicon dioxide, corn starch, hydroxypropyl methylcellulose, magnesium stearate, polyethylene glycol 4000, povidone, talc, titanium dioxide and coloring agents.

The individual tablets contain the following coloring agents:

250 mg: FD&C blue no. 2.

500 mg: FD&C blue no. 2 and yellow iron oxide.

750 mg: FD&C blue no. 2, FD&C yellow no. 6 and red iron oxide.

CLINICAL PHARMACOLOGY

MECHANISM OF ACTION

The precise mechanism(s) by which levetiracetam exerts its antiepileptic effect is unknown and does not appear to derive from any interaction with known mechanisms involved in inhibitory and excitatory neurotransmission. The antiepileptic activity of levetiracetam was assessed in a number of animal models of epileptic seizures. Levetiracetam did not inhibit single seizures induced by maximal stimulation with electrical current or different chemoconvulsants and showed only minimal activity in submaximal stimulation and in threshold tests. Protection was observed, however, against secondarily generalized activity from focal seizures induced by pilocarpine and kainic acid, two chemoconvulsants that induce seizures that mimic some features of human complex partial seizures with secondary generalization. Levetiracetam also displayed inhibitory properties in the kindling model in rats, another model of human complex partial seizures, both during kindling development and in the fully kindled state. The predictive value of these animal models for specific types of human epilepsy is uncertain.

In vitro studies show that levetiracetam, up to 1700 µg/ml, did not result in significant ligand displacement at known receptor binding sites. Second messenger systems, ion channel proteins, glutamate receptor-mediated neurotransmission, muscimol-induced chloride flux and gamma-aminobutyric acid-transaminase and glutamate decarboxylase activities were unaffected by levetiracetam. Benzodiazepine receptor antagonists had no effect on levetiracetam's protection against seizures. In contrast, a stereoselective binding site for the drug has been demonstrated to exist exclusively in synaptic plasma membranes in the CNS, and not in peripheral tissue.

In vitro and *in vivo* recordings of epileptiform activity from the hippocampus have shown that levetiracetam inhibits burst firing without affecting normal neuronal excitability, suggesting that levetiracetam may selectively prevent hypersynchronization of epileptiform burst firing and propagation of seizure activity.

PHARMACOKINETICS

The pharmacokinetics of levetiracetam have been studied in healthy adult subjects, adults and pediatric patients with epilepsy, elderly subjects and subjects with renal and hepatic impairment.

OVERVIEW

Levetiracetam is rapidly and almost completely absorbed after oral administration. The pharmacokinetics are linear and time-invariant, with low intra- and inter-subject variability. The extent of bioavailability of levetiracetam is not affected by food. Levetiracetam is not protein-bound (<10% bound) and its volume of distribution is close to the volume of intracellular and extracellular water. Sixty-six percent (66%) of the dose is renally excreted unchanged. The major metabolic pathway of levetiracetam (24% of dose) is an enzymatic hydrolysis of the acetamide group. It is not liver cytochrome P450 dependent. The metabolites have no known pharmacological activity and are renally excreted. Plasma half-life of levetiracetam across studies is approximately 6-8 hours. It is increased in the elderly (primarily due to impaired renal clearance) and in subjects with renal impairment.

ABSORPTION AND DISTRIBUTION

Absorption of levetiracetam is rapid, with peak plasma concentrations occurring in about an hour following oral administration in fasted subjects. The oral bioavailability of levetiracetam tablets is 100%. Food does not affect the extent of absorption of levetiracetam but it decreases C_{max} by 20% and delays T_{max} by 1.5 hours. The pharmacokinetics of levetiracetam are linear over the dose range of 500-5000 mg. Steady state is achieved after 2 days of multiple twice daily dosing. Levetiracetam and its major metabolite are less than 10% bound to plasma proteins; clinically significant interactions with other drugs through competition for protein binding sites are therefore unlikely.

METABOLISM

Levetiracetam is not extensively metabolized in humans. The major metabolic pathway is the enzymatic hydrolysis of the acetamide group, which produces the carboxylic acid metabolite, ucb L057 (24% of dose) and is not dependent on any liver cytochrome P450 isoenzymes. The major metabolite is inactive in animal seizure models. Two minor metabolites were identified as the product of hydroxylation of the 2-oxo-pyrrolidine ring (2% of dose) and opening of the 2-oxo-pyrrolidine ring in position 5 (1% of dose). There is no enantiomeric interconversion of levetiracetam or its major metabolite.

ELIMINATION

Levetiracetam plasma half-life in adults is 7 ± 1 hours and is unaffected by either dose or repeated administration. Levetiracetam is eliminated from the systemic circulation by renal excretion as unchanged drug which represents 66% of administered dose. The total body clearance is 0.96 ml/min/kg and the renal clearance is 0.6 ml/min/kg. The mechanism of excretion is glomerular filtration with subsequent partial tubular reabsorption. The metabolite ucb L057 is excreted by glomerular filtration and active tubular secretion with a renal clearance of 4 ml/min/kg. Levetiracetam elimination is correlated to creatinine clearance. Levetiracetam clearance is reduced in patients with impaired renal function (see Special Populations, Renal Impairment and DOSAGE AND ADMINISTRATION, Patients With Impaired Renal Function).

PHARMACOKINETIC INTERACTIONS

In vitro data on metabolic interactions indicate that levetiracetam is unlikely to produce, or be subject to, pharmacokinetic interactions. Levetiracetam and its major metabolite, at concentrations well above C_{max} levels achieved within the therapeutic dose range, are neither inhibitors of, nor high affinity substrates for, human liver cytochrome P450 isoforms, epoxide hydrolase or UDP-glucuronidation enzymes. In addition, levetiracetam does not affect the *in vitro* glucuronidation of valproic acid.

Potential pharmacokinetic interactions were assessed in clinical pharmacokinetic studies (phenytoin, warfarin, digoxin, oral contraceptives) and through pharmacokinetic screening in the placebo-controlled clinical studies in epilepsy patients (see and DRUG INTERACTIONS).

SPECIAL POPULATIONS

Elderly

Pharmacokinetics of levetiracetam were evaluated in 16 elderly subjects (age 61-88 years) with creatinine clearance ranging from 30-74 ml/min. Following oral administration of twice daily dosing for 10 days, total body clearance decreased by 38% and the half-life was 2.5 hours longer in the elderly compared to healthy adults. This is most likely due to the decrease in renal function in these subjects.

Pediatric Patients

Pharmacokinetics of levetiracetam were evaluated in 24 pediatric patients (age 6-12 years) after single dose (20 mg/kg). The apparent clearance of levetiracetam was approximately 40% higher than in adults.

Gender

Levetiracetam C_{max} and AUC were 20% higher in women (n=11) compared to men (n=12). However, clearances adjusted for body weight were comparable.

Race

Formal pharmacokinetic studies of the effects of race have not been conducted. Cross study comparisons involving Caucasians (n=12) and Asians (n=12), however, show that pharmacokinetics of levetiracetam were comparable between the two races. Because levetiracetam is primarily renally excreted and there are no important racial differences in creatinine clearance, pharmacokinetic differences due to race are not expected.

Renal Impairment

The disposition of levetiracetam was studied in subjects with varying degrees of renal function. Total body clearance of levetiracetam is reduced in patients with impaired renal function by 40% in the mild group (CLCR = 50-80 ml/min), 50% in the moderate group (CLCR = 30-50 ml/min) and 60% in the severe renal impairment group (CLCR <30 ml/min). Clearance of levetiracetam is correlated with creatinine clearance.

In anuric (end stage renal disease) patients, the total body clearance decreased 70% compared to normal subjects (CLCR >80ml/min). Approximately 50% of the pool of levetiracetam in the body is removed during a standard 4 hour hemodialysis procedure.

Dosage should be reduced in patients with impaired renal function receiving levetiracetam, and supplemental doses should be given to patients after dialysis (see PRECAUTIONS and DOSAGE AND ADMINISTRATION, Patients With Impaired Renal Function).

Hepatic Impairment

In subjects with mild (Child-Pugh A) to moderate (Child-Pugh B) hepatic impairment, the pharmacokinetics of levetiracetam were unchanged. In patients with severe hepatic impairment (Child-Pugh C), total body clearance was 50% that of normal subjects, but decreased renal clearance accounted for most of the decrease. No dose adjustment is needed for patients with hepatic impairment.

INDICATIONS AND USAGE

Levetiracetam is indicated as adjunctive therapy in the treatment of partial onset seizures in adults with epilepsy.

CONTRAINDICATIONS

This product should not be administered to patients who have previously exhibited hypersensitivity to levetiracetam or any of the inactive ingredients in levetiracetam tablets.

WARNINGS

NEUROPSYCHIATRIC ADVERSE EVENTS

Levetiracetam use is associated with the occurrence of central nervous system adverse events that can be classified into the following categories: (1) somnolence and fatigue, (2) coordination difficulties, and (3) behavioral abnormalities.

In controlled trials of patients with epilepsy, 14.8% of levetiracetam treated patients reported somnolence, compared to 8.4% of placebo patients. There was no clear dose response up to 3000 mg/day. In a study where there was no titration, about 45% of patients receiving 4000 mg/day reported somnolence. The somnolence was considered serious in 0.3% of the treated patients, compared to 0% in the placebo group. About 3% of levetiracetam treated patients discontinued treatment due to somnolence, compared to 0.7% of placebo patients. In 1.4% of treated patients and in 0.9% of placebo patients the dose was reduced, while 0.3% of the treated patients were hospitalized due to somnolence.

In controlled trials of patients with epilepsy, 14.7% of treated patients reported asthenia, compared to 9.1% of placebo patients. Treatment was discontinued in 0.8% of treated patients as compared to 0.5% of placebo patients. In 0.5% of treated patients and in 0.2% of placebo patients the dose was reduced.

A total of 3.4% of levetiracetam treated patients experienced coordination difficulties, (reported as either ataxia, abnormal gait, or incoordination) compared to 1.6% of placebo patients. A total of 0.4% of patients in controlled trials discontinued levetiracetam treatment due to ataxia, compared to 0% of placebo patients. In 0.7% of treated patients and in 0.2% of placebo patients the dose was reduced due to coordination difficulties, while one of the treated patients was hospitalized due to worsening of pre-existing ataxia.

Somnolence, asthenia and coordination difficulties occurred most frequently within the first 4 weeks of treatment.

In controlled trials of patients with epilepsy, 5 (0.7%) of levetiracetam treated patients experienced psychotic symptoms compared to 1 (0.2%) placebo patient. Two (0.3%) levetiracetam treated patients were hospitalized and their treatment was discontinued. Both events, reported as psychosis, developed within the first week of treatment and resolved within 1-2 weeks following treatment discontinuation. Two other events, reported as hallucinations, occurred after 1-5 months and resolved within 2-7 days while the patients remained on treatment. In 1 patient experiencing psychotic depression occurring within a month, symptoms resolved within 45 days while the patient continued treatment. A total of 13.3% of levetiracetam patients experienced other behavioral symptoms (reported as agitation, hostility, anxiety, apathy, emotional lability, depersonalization, depression, etc.) compared to 6.2% of placebo patients. Approximately half of these patients reported these events within the first 4 weeks. A total of 1.7% of treated patients discontinued treatment due to these events, compared to 0.2% of placebo patients. The treatment dose was reduced in 0.8% of treated patients and in 0.5% of placebo patients. A total of 0.8% of treated patients had a serious behavioral event (compared to 0.2% of placebo patients) and were hospitalized.

In addition, 4 (0.5%) of treated patients attempted suicide compared to 0% of placebo patients. One of these patients successfully committed suicide. In the other 3 patients, the events did not lead to discontinuation or dose reduction. The events occurred after patients had been treated for between 4 weeks and 6 months.

WITHDRAWAL SEIZURES

Antiepileptic drugs, including levetiracetam, should be withdrawn gradually to minimize the potential of increased seizure frequency.

PRECAUTIONS

HEMATOLOGIC ABNORMALITIES

Minor, but statistically significant, decreases compared to placebo in total mean RBC count ($0.03 \times 10^6/mm^2$), mean hemoglobin (0.09 g/dl), and mean hematocrit (0.38%), were seen in levetiracetam treated patients in controlled trials.

A total of 3.2% of treated and 1.8% of placebo patients had at least one possibly significant ($\leq 2.8 \times 10^9$/L) decreased WBC, and 2.4% of treated and 1.4% of placebo patients had at least one possibly significant ($\leq 1.0 \times 10^9$/L) decreased neutrophil count. Of the treated patients with a low neutrophil count, all but one rose towards or to baseline with continued treatment. No patient was discontinued secondary to low neutrophil counts.

HEPATIC ABNORMALITIES

There were no meaningful changes in mean liver function tests (LFT) in controlled trials; lesser LFT abnormalities were similar in drug and placebo treated patients in controlled trials (1.4%). No patients were discontinued from controlled trials for LFT abnormalities except for 1 (0.07%) epilepsy patient receiving open treatment.

INFORMATION FOR THE PATIENT

Patients should be instructed to take levetiracetam only as prescribed.

Patients should be advised to notify their physician if they become pregnant or intend to become pregnant during therapy.

Patients should be advised that levetiracetam may cause dizziness and somnolence. Accordingly, patients should be advised not to drive or operate machinery or engage in other hazardous activities until they have gained sufficient experience on levetiracetam to gauge whether it adversely affects their performance of these activities.

LABORATORY TESTS

Although most laboratory tests are not systematically altered with levetiracetam treatment, there have been relatively infrequent abnormalities seen in hematologic parameters and liver function tests.

CARCINOGENESIS, MUTAGENESIS, AND IMPAIRMENT OF FERTILITY

Carcinogenesis

Rats were dosed with levetiracetam in the diet for 104 weeks at doses of 50, 300 and 1800 mg/kg/day. The highest dose corresponds to 6 times the maximum recommended daily human dose (MRHD) of 3000 mg on a mg/m^2 basis and it also provided systemic exposure (AUC) approximately 6 times that achieved in humans receiving the MRHD. There was no evidence of carcinogenicity. A study was conducted in which mice received levetiracetam in the diet for 80 weeks at doses of 60, 240 and 960 mg/kg/day (high dose is equivalent to 2 times the MRHD on a mg/m^2 or exposure basis). Although no evidence for carcinogenicity was seen, the potential for a carcinogenic response has not been fully evaluated in that species because adequate doses have not been studied.

Mutagenesis

Levetiracetam was not mutagenic in the Ames test or in mammalian cells *in vitro* in the Chinese hamster ovary/HGPRT locus assay. It was not clastogenic in an *in vitro* analysis of metaphase chromosomes obtained from Chinese hamster ovary cells or in an *in vivo* mouse micronucleus assay. The hydrolysis product and major human metabolite of levetiracetam (L057) was not mutagenic in the Ames test or the *in vitro* mouse lymphoma assay.

Impairment of Fertility

No adverse effects on male or female fertility or reproductive performance were observed in rats at doses up to 1800 mg/kg/day (approximately 6 times the maximum recommended human dose on a mg/m^2 or exposure basis).

PREGNANCY CATEGORY C

In animal studies, levetiracetam produced evidence of developmental toxicity at doses similar to or greater than human therapeutic doses.

L

Administration to female rats throughout pregnancy and lactation was associated with increased incidences of minor fetal skeletal abnormalities and retarded offspring growth pre- and/or postnatally at doses ≥350 mg/kg/day (approximately equivalent to the maximum recommended human dose of 3000 mg [MRHD] on a mg/m^2 basis) and with increased pup mortality and offspring behavioral alterations at a dose of 1800 mg/kg/day (6 times the MRHD on a mg/m^2 basis). The developmental no effect dose was 70 mg/kg/day (0.2 times the MRHD on a mg/m^2 basis). There was no overt maternal toxicity at the doses used in this study.

Treatment of pregnant rabbits during the period of organogenesis resulted in increased embryofetal mortality and increased incidences of minor fetal skeletal abnormalities at doses ≥600 mg/kg/day (approximately 4 times MRHD on a mg/m^2 basis) and in decreased fetal weights and increased incidences of fetal malformations at a dose of 1800 mg/kg/day (12 times the MRHD on a mg/m^2 basis). The developmental no effect dose was 200 mg/kg/day (1.3 times the MRHD on a mg/m^2 basis). Maternal toxicity was also observed at 1800 mg/kg/day.

When pregnant rats were treated during the period of organogenesis, fetal weights were decreased and the incidence of fetal skeletal variations was increased at a dose of 3600 mg/kg/day (12 times the MRHD). 1200 mg/kg/day (4 times the MRHD) was a developmental no effect dose. There was no evidence of maternal toxicity in this study.

Treatment of rats during the last third of gestation and throughout lactation produced no adverse developmental or maternal effects at doses of up to 1800 mg/kg/day (6 times the MRHD on a mg/m^2 basis).

There are no adequate and well-controlled studies in pregnant women. Levetiracetam should be used during pregnancy only if the potential benefit justifies the potential risk to the fetus.

Pregnancy Exposure Registry

To facilitate monitoring fetal outcomes of pregnant women exposed to levetiracetam physicians are encouraged to register patients, before fetal outcome is known (*e.g.*, ultrasound, results of amniocentesis, etc.), in the Antiepileptic Drug Pregnancy Registry by calling 888-233-2334 (toll free).

LABOR AND DELIVERY

The effect of levetiracetam on labor and delivery in humans is unknown.

NURSING MOTHERS

Levetiracetam is excreted in breast milk. Because of the potential for serious adverse reactions in nursing infants from levetiracetam, a decision should be made whether to discontinue nursing or discontinue the drug, taking into account the importance of the drug to the mother.

PEDIATRIC USE

Safety and effectiveness in patients below the age of 16 have not been established.

GERIATRIC USE

Of the total number of subjects in clinical studies of levetiracetam, 347 were 65 and over. No overall differences in safety were observed between these subjects and younger subjects. There were insufficient numbers of elderly subjects in controlled trials of epilepsy to adequately assess the effectiveness of levetiracetam in these patients.

A study in 16 elderly subjects (age 61-88 years) with oral administration of single dose and multiple twice-daily doses for 10 days showed no pharmacokinetic differences related to age alone.

Levetiracetam is known to be substantially excreted by the kidney, and the risk of adverse reactions to this drug may be greater in patients with impaired renal function. Because elderly patients are more likely to have decreased renal function, care should be taken in dose selection, and it may be useful to monitor renal function.

USE IN PATIENTS WITH IMPAIRED RENAL FUNCTION

Clearance of levetiracetam is decreased in patients with renal impairment and is correlated with creatinine clearance. Caution should be taken in dosing patients with moderate and severe renal impairment and in patients undergoing hemodialysis. The dosage should be reduced in patients with impaired renal function receiving levetiracetam and supplemental doses should be given to patients after dialysis (see CLINICAL PHARMACOLOGY and DOSAGE AND ADMINISTRATION, Patients With Impaired Renal Function).

DRUG INTERACTIONS

In vitro data on metabolic interactions indicate that levetiracetam is unlikely to produce, or be subject to, pharmacokinetic interactions. Levetiracetam and its major metabolite, at concentrations well above C_{max} levels achieved within the therapeutic dose range, are neither inhibitors of nor high affinity substrates for human liver cytochrome P450 isoforms, epoxide hydrolase or UDP-glucuronidation enzymes. In addition, levetiracetam does not affect the *in vitro* glucuronidation of valproic acid.

Levetiracetam circulates largely unbound (<10% bound) to plasma proteins; clinically significant interactions with other drugs through competition for protein binding sites are therefore unlikely.

Potential pharmacokinetic interactions were assessed in clinical pharmacokinetic studies (phenytoin, warfarin, digoxin, oral contraceptive) and through pharmacokinetic screening in the placebo-controlled clinical studies in epilepsy patients.

DRUG-DRUG INTERACTIONS BETWEEN LEVETIRACETAM AND OTHER ANTIEPILEPTIC DRUGS (AEDS)

Potential drug interactions between levetiracetam and other AEDs (phenytoin, carbamazepine, valproic acid, phenobarbital, lamotrigine, gabapentin and primidone) were assessed by evaluating the serum concentrations of levetiracetam and these AEDs during placebo-controlled clinical studies. These data indicate that levetiracetam does not influence the plasma concentration of existing AEDs and that these AEDs do not influence the pharmacokinetics of levetiracetam.

OTHER DRUG INTERACTIONS

Oral Contraceptives: Levetiracetam (500 mg twice daily) did not influence the pharmacokinetics of an oral contraceptive containing 0.03 mg ethinyl estradiol and 0.15 mg levonorgestrel, or of the luteinizing hormone and progesterone levels, indicating that impairment of contraceptive efficacy is unlikely. Coadministration of this oral contraceptive did not influence the pharmacokinetics of levetiracetam.

Digoxin: Levetiracetam (1000 mg twice daily) did not influence the pharmacokinetics and pharmacodynamics (ECG) of digoxin given as a 0.25 mg dose every day. Coadministration of digoxin did not influence the pharmacokinetics of levetiracetam.

Warfarin: Levetiracetam (1000 mg twice daily) did not influence the pharmacokinetics of R and S warfarin. Prothrombin time was not affected by levetiracetam. Coadministration of warfarin did not affect the pharmacokinetics of levetiracetam.

Probenecid: Probenecid, a renal tubular secretion blocking agent, administered at a dose of 500 mg four times a day, did not change the pharmacokinetics of levetiracetam 1000 mg twice daily. Css_{max} of the metabolite, ucb L057, was approximately doubled in the presence of probenecid while the fraction of drug excreted unchanged in the urine remained the same. Renal clearance of ucb L057 in the presence of probenecid decreased 60%, probably related to competitive inhibition of tubular secretion of ucb L057. The effect of levetiracetam on probenecid was not studied.

ADVERSE REACTIONS

In well-controlled clinical studies, the most frequently reported adverse events associated with the use of levetiracetam in combination with other AEDs, not seen at an equivalent frequency among placebo-treated patients, were somnolence, asthenia, infection and dizziness.

TABLE 4 lists treatment-emergent adverse events that occurred in at least 1% of patients with epilepsy treated with levetiracetam participating in placebo-controlled studies and were numerically more common in patients treated with levetiracetam than placebo. In these studies, either levetiracetam or placebo was added to concurrent AED therapy. Adverse events were usually mild to moderate in intensity.

The prescriber should be aware that these figures, obtained when levetiracetam was added to concurrent AED therapy, cannot be used to predict the frequency of adverse experiences in the course of usual medical practice where patient characteristics and other factors may differ from those prevailing during clinical studies. Similarly, the cited frequencies cannot be directly compared with figures obtained from other clinical investigations involving different treatments, uses, or investigators. An inspection of these frequencies, however, does provide the prescriber with one basis to estimate the relative contribution of drug and non-drug factors to the adverse event incidences in the population studied.

Other events reported by 1% or more of patients treated with levetiracetam but as or more frequent in the placebo group were: abdominal pain, accidental injury, amblyopia, arthralgia, back pain, bronchitis, chest pain, confusion, constipation, convulsion, diarrhea, drug level increased, dyspepsia, ecchymosis, fever, flu syndrome, fungal infection, gastroenteritis, gingivitis, grand mal convulsion, insomnia, nausea, otitis media, rash, thinking abnormal, tremor, urinary tract infection, vomiting and weight gain.

TIME COURSE OF ONSET OF ADVERSE EVENTS

Of the most frequently reported adverse events, asthenia, somnolence and dizziness appeared to occur predominantly during the first 4 weeks of treatment with levetiracetam.

TABLE 4 *Incidence (%) of Treatment-Emergent Adverse Events in Placebo-Controlled, Add-On Studies by Body System**

Body System / Adverse Event	Levetiracetam (n=769)	Placebo (n=439)
Body as a Whole		
Asthenia	15%	9%
Headache	14%	13%
Infection	13%	8%
Pain	7%	6%
Digestive System		
Anorexia	3%	2%
Nervous System		
Amnesia	2%	1%
Anxiety	2%	1%
Ataxia	3%	1%
Depression	4%	2%
Dizziness	9%	4%
Emotional lability	2%	0%
Hostility	2%	1%
Nervousness	4%	2%
Paresthesia	2%	1%
Somnolence	15%	8%
Vertigo	3%	1%
Respiratory System		
Cough increased	2%	1%
Pharyngitis	6%	4%
Rhinitis	4%	3%
Sinusitis	2%	1%
Special Senses		
Diplopia	2%	1%

* Adverse events occurred in at least 1% of levetiracetam-treated patients and occurred more frequently than placebo-treated patients.

DISCONTINUATION OR DOSE REDUCTION IN WELL-CONTROLLED CLINICAL STUDIES

In well-controlled clinical studies, 15.0% of patients receiving levetiracetam and 11.6% receiving placebo either discontinued or had a dose reduction as a result of an adverse event. The adverse events most commonly associated (>1%) with discontinuation or dose reduction in either treatment group are presented in TABLE 5.

TABLE 5 *Adverse Events Most Commonly Associated With Discontinuation or Dose Reduction in Placebo-Controlled Studies in Patients With Epilepsy*

	Levetiracetam (n=769)	Placebo (n=439)
Asthenia	10 (1.3%)	3 (0.7%)
Convulsion	23 (3.0%)	15 (3.4%)
Dizziness	11 (1.4%)	0
Somnolence	34 (4.4%)	7 (1.6%)
Rash	0	5 (1.1%)

COMPARISON OF GENDER, AGE AND RACE

The overall adverse experience profile of levetiracetam was similar between females and males. There are insufficient data to support a statement regarding the distribution of adverse experience reports by age and race.

POSTMARKETING EXPERIENCE

In addition to the adverse experiences listed above, the following have been reported in patients receiving marketed levetiracetam worldwide. The listing is alphabetized: aggression, anger, irritability, neutropenia, pancytopenia and thrombocytopenia. These adverse experiences have not been listed above, and data are insufficient to support an estimate of their incidence or to establish causation.

DOSAGE AND ADMINISTRATION

Levetiracetam is indicated as adjunctive treatment of partial onset seizures in adults with epilepsy.

In clinical trials, daily doses of 1000, 2000, and 3000 mg, given as twice a day dosing, were shown to be effective. Although in some studies there was a tendency toward greater response with higher dose, a consistent increase in response with increased dose has not been shown.

Treatment should be initiated with a daily dose of 1000 mg/day, given as twice daily dosing (500 mg bid). Additional dosing increments may be given (1000 mg/day additional every 2 weeks) to a maximum recommended daily dose of 3000 mg. Long term experience at doses greater than 3000 mg/day is relatively minimal, and there is no evidence that doses greater than 3000 mg/day confer additional benefit.

Levetiracetam is given orally with or without food.

PATIENTS WITH IMPAIRED RENAL FUNCTION

Levetiracetam dosing must be individualized according to the patient's renal function status. Recommended doses and adjustment for dose are shown in TABLE 6. To use this dosing table, an estimate of the patient's creatinine clearance (CLCR) in ml/min is needed. CLCR in ml/min may be estimated from serum creatinine (mg/dl) determination using the following formula:

CLCR = {[140-age (years)] × weight (kg)} / {72 × serum creatinine (mg/dl)}
(× 0.85 for female patients)

TABLE 6 *Dosing Adjustment Regimen for Patients With Impaired Renal Function*

Group	Creatinine Clearance	Dosage	Frequency
Normal	>80 ml/min	500-1500 mg	Every 12 h
Mild	50-80 ml/min	500-1000 mg	Every 12 h
Moderate	30-50 ml/min	250-750 mg	Every 12 h
Severe	<30 ml/min	250-500 mg	Every 12 h
ESRD patients using dialysis	—	500-1000 mg	*Every 24 h

* Following dialysis, a 250-500 mg supplemental dose is recommended.

HOW SUPPLIED

Keppra tablets are available in:

250 mg: Blue, oblong-shaped, scored, film-coated tablets debossed with "ucb" and "250" on one side.

500 mg: Yellow, oblong-shaped, scored, film-coated tablets debossed with "ucb" and "500" on one side.

750 mg: Orange, oblong-shaped, scored, film-coated tablets debossed with "ucb" and "750" on one side.

Storage: Store at 25°C (77°F); excursions permitted to 15-30°C (59-86°F).

PRODUCT LISTING - EQUIVALENTS NOT AVAILABLE

Tablet - Oral - 250 mg
120's $198.18 KEPPRA, Ucb Pharma Inc 50474-0591-40
Tablet - Oral - 500 mg
120's $242.22 KEPPRA, Ucb Pharma Inc 50474-0592-40
Tablet - Oral - 750 mg
120's $345.63 KEPPRA, Ucb Pharma Inc 50474-0593-40

Levobunolol Hydrochloride *(001633)*

Categories: Glaucoma, open-angle; Hypertension, ocular; Pregnancy Category C; FDA Approved 1985 Dec
Drug Classes: Antiadrenergics, beta blocking; Ophthalmics
Brand Names: Akbeta; **Betagan**; Levobunolol HCl
Foreign Brand Availability: Bunolgan (Taiwan); Gotensin (Japan); Vistagan (Austria; Bulgaria; Colombia; Czech-Republic; Germany; Greece; Hungary; Italy; Peru; Russia; Switzerland); Vistagen (Japan)
Cost of Therapy: $25.92 (Glaucoma; Betagan Ophthalmic Solution; 0.5%; 5 ml; 1 drops/day; variable day supply)
$7.44 (Glaucoma; Generic Ophthalmic Solution; 0.5%; 5 ml; 1 drops/day; variable day supply)

L

DESCRIPTION

Levobunolol HCl sterile ophthalmic solution is a noncardioselective beta-adrenoceptor blocking agent for ophthalmic use.

The chemical name is (-)-5-(3-(*tert*-Butylamino)-2-hydroxypropoxy)-3, 4-dihydro-)*(2H)*-naphthalenone hydrochloride.

Betagan 0.25% and 0.5% contain: levobunolol HCl 0.25% or 0.5% with liquifilm (polyvinyl alcohol) 1.4%, benzalkonium chloride 0.004%, edetate disodium, sodium metabisulfite, sodium phosphate dibasic, potassium phosphate monobasic, sodium chloride, hydrochloric acid or sodium hydroxide to adjust pH, and purified water.

Storage: Protect from light. Store at controlled room temperature 15-30°C (59-86°F).

CLINICAL PHARMACOLOGY

Levobunolol HCl is a noncardioselective beta-adrenoceptor blocking agent, equipotent at both $beta_1$, and $beta_2$ receptors. Levobunolol HCl is greater than 60 times more potent than its dextro isomer in its beta-blocking activity, yet equipotent in its potential for direct myocardial depression. Accordingly, the levo isomer, levobunolol HCl, is used. Levobunolol HCl does not have significant local anesthetic (membrane-stabilizing) or intrinsic sympathomimetic activity.

Beta-adrenergic receptor blockage reduces cardiac output in both healthy subjects and patients with heart disease in patients with severe impairment of myocardial function, beta-adrenergic receptor blockade may inhibit the stimulatory effect of the sympathetic nervous system necessary to maintain adequate cardiac function.

Beta-adrenergic receptor blockade in the bronchi and bronchioles results in increased airway resistance from unopposed para-sympathetic activity. Such an effect in patients with asthma or other bronchospastic conditions is potentially dangerous.

Levobunolol HCl has been shown to be an active agent in lowering elevated as well as normal intraocular pressure (IOP) whether or not accompanied by glaucoma. Elevated IOP presents a major risk factor in glaucomatous field loss. The higher the level of IOP, the greater the likelihood of optic nerve damage and visual field loss.

The onset of action with 1 drop of levobunolol HCl can be detected within 1 hour after treatment, with maximum effect seen between 2 and 6 hours.

A significant decrease in IOP can be maintained for up to 24 hours following a single dose.

In two, separate, controlled studies (one 3 month and one up to 12 months duration) levobunolol HCl 0.25% bid controlled the IOP of approximately 64% and 70% of the subjects. The overall mean decrease from baseline was 5.4 mm Hg and 5.1 mm Hg respectively. In an open-label study, levobunolol HCl 0.25% qd controlled the IOP of 72% of the subjects while achieving an overall mean decrease of 5.9 mm Hg.

In controlled clinical studies of approximately 2 years duration, intraocular pressure was well-controlled in approximately 80% of subjects treated with levobunolol HCl 0.5% bid. The mean IOP decrease from baseline was between 6.87 and 7.81 mm Hg. No significant effects on pupil size, tear production or corneal sensitivity were observed. Levobunolol HCl at the concentrations tested, when applied topically, decreased heart rate and blood pressure in some patients. The IOP-lowering effect of levobunolol HCl was well maintained over the course of these studies.

In a 3 month clinical study, a single daily application of levobunolol HCl 0.5% controlled the IOP of 72% of subjects achieving an overall mean decrease in IOP of 7.0 mm Hg.

The primary mechanism of the ocular hypotensive action of levobunolol HCl in reducing IOP is most likely a decrease in aqueous humor production. Levobunolol HCl reduces IOP with little or no effect on pupil size or accommodation in contrast to the miosis which cholinergic agents are known to produce. The blurred vision and night blindness often associated with miotics would not be expected and have not been reported with the use of levobunolol HCl. This is particularly important in cataract patients with central lens opacities who would experience decreased visual acuity with pupillary constriction.

INDICATIONS AND USAGE

Levobunolol HCl has been shown to be effective in lowering intraocular pressure and may be used in patients with chronic open-angle glaucoma or ocular hypertension.

CONTRAINDICATIONS

Levobunolol HCl is contraindicated in those individuals with bronchial asthma or with a history of bronchial asthma, or severe chronic obstructive pulmonary disease (see WARNINGS); sinus bradycardia; second and third degree atrioventricular block; overt cardiac failure (see WARNINGS); cardiogenic shock; or hypersensitivity to any component of these products.

WARNINGS

As with other topically applied ophthalmic drugs, levobunolol HCl may be absorbed systemically. The same adverse reactions found with systemic administration of beta-adrenergic blocking agents may occur with topical administration. For example, severe respiratory reactions and cardiac reactions, including death due to bronchospasm in patients with asthma, and rarely death in association with cardiac failure, have been reported with topical application of beta-adrenergic blocking agents (see CONTRAINDICATIONS.)

CARDIAC FAILURE

Sympathetic stimulation may be essential for support of the circulation in individuals with diminished myocardial contractility, and its inhibition by beta-adrenergic receptor blockade may precipitate more severe failure.

In Patients Without a History of Cardiac Failure

Continued depression of the myocardium with beta-blocking agents over a period of time can, in some cases, lead to cardiac failure. At the first sign or symptom of cardiac failure, levobunolol HCl should be discontinued.

OBSTRUCTIVE PULMONARY DISEASE

PATIENTS WITH CHRONIC OBSTRUCTIVE PULMONARY DISEASE (*e.g.*, CHRONIC BRONCHITIS, EMPHYSEMA) OF MILD OR MODERATE SEVERITY, BRONCHOSPASTIC DISEASE OR A HISTORY OF BRONCHOSPASTIC DISEASE (OTHER THAN BRONCHIAL ASTHMA OR A HISTORY OF BRONCHIAL ASTHMA, IN WHICH LEVOBUNOLOL HCl IS CONTRAINDICATED, SEE CONTRAINDICATIONS), SHOULD IN GENERAL NOT RECEIVE BETA BLOCKERS, INCLUDING LEVOBUNOLOL HCl. However, if LEVOBUNOLOL HCl is deemed necessary in such patients, then it should be administered cautiously since it may block bronchodilation produced by endogenous and exogenous catecholamine stimulation of $beta_2$ receptors.

MAJOR SURGERY

The necessity or desirability of withdrawal of beta-adrenergic blocking agents prior to major surgery is controversial. Beta-adrenergic receptor blockade impairs the ability of the heart to respond to beta-adrenergically mediated reflex stimuli. This may augment the risk of general anesthesia in surgical procedures. Some patients receiving beta-adrenergic receptor blocking agents have been subject to protracted severe hypotension during anesthesia. Difficulty in restarting and maintaining the heartbeat has also been reported. For these reasons, in patients undergoing elective surgery, gradual withdrawal of beta-adrenergic receptor blocking agents may be appropriate.

If necessary during surgery, the effects of beta-adrenergic blocking agents may be reversed by sufficient doses of such agonists as isoproterenol, dopamine, dobutamine or levarterenol

DIABETES MELLITUS

Beta-adrenergic blocking agents should be administered with caution in patients subject to spontaneous hypoglycemia or to diabetic patients (especially those with labile diabetes) who are receiving insulin or oral hypoglycemic agents. Beta-adrenergic receptor blocking agents may mask the signs and symptoms of acute hypoglycemia.

THYROTOXICOSIS

Beta-adrenergic blocking agents may mask certain clinical signs (*e.g.*, tachycardia) of hyperthyroidism. Patients suspected of developing thyrotoxicosis should be managed carefully to avoid abrupt withdrawal of beta-adrenergic blocking agents which might precipitate a thyroid storm.

These products contain sodium metabisulfite, a sulfite that may cause allergic-type reactions including anaphylactic symptoms and life-threatening or less severe asthmatic episodes in certain susceptible people. The overall prevalence of sulfite sensitivity in the general population is unknown and probably low. Sulfite sensitivity is seen more frequently in asthmatic than in nonasthmatic people.

PRECAUTIONS

GENERAL

Levobunolol HCl should be used with caution in patients with known hypersensitivity to other beta-adrenoceptor blocking agents.

Use with caution in patients with known diminished pulmonary function.

Levobunolol HCl should be used with caution in patients who are receiving a beta-adrenergic blocking agent orally, because of the potential for additive effects on systemic beta-blockade or on intraocular pressure. Patients should not typically use two or more topical ophthalmic beta-adrenergic blocking agents simultaneously.

Because of the potential effects of beta-adrenergic blocking agents on blood pressure and pulse rates, these medications must be used cautiously in patients with cerebrovascular insufficiency. Should signs or symptoms develop that suggest reduced cerebral blood flow while using levobunolol HCl, alternative therapy should be considered.

In patients with angle-closure glaucoma, the immediate objective of treatment is to reopen the angle. This requires, in most cases, constricting the pupil with a miotic. Levobunolol HCl Liquifilm sterile ophthalmic solution has little or no effect on the pupil. When levobunolol HCl is used to reduce elevated intraocular pressure in angle-closure glaucoma, it should be followed with a miotic and not alone.

Muscle Weakness

Beta-adrenergic blockade has been reported to potentiate muscle weakness consistent with certain myasthenic symptoms (*e.g.*, diplopia, ptosis and generalized weakness).

Animal Studies

No adverse ocular effects were observed in rabbits administered levobunolol HCl topically in studies lasting 1 year in concentrations up to 10 times the human dose concentration.

CARCINOGENESIS, MUTAGENESIS, AND IMPAIRMENT OF FERTILITY

In a lifetime oral study in mice, there were statistically significant ($p \leq 0.05$) increases in the incidence of benign leiomyomas in female mice at 200 mg/kg/day (14,000 times the recommended human dose for glaucoma), but not at 12 or 50 mg/kg/day (850 and 3500 times the human dose). In a 2 year oral study of levobunolol HCl in rats, there was a statistically significant ($p \leq 0.05$) increase in the incidence of benign hepatomas in male rats administered 12,800 times the recommended human dose for glaucoma. Similar differences were not observed in rats administered oral doses equivalent to 350 times to 2000 times the recommended human dose for glaucoma.

Levobunolol did not show evidence of mutagenic activity in a battery of microbiological and mammalian *in vitro* and *in vivo* assays.

Reproduction and fertility studies in rats showed no adverse effect on male or female fertility at doses up to 1800 times the recommended human dose for glaucoma.

PREGNANCY CATEGORY C

Fetotoxicity (as evidenced by a greater number of resorption sites) has been observed in rabbits when doses of levobunolol HCl equivalent to 200 and 700 times the recommended dose for the treatment of glaucoma were given. No fetotoxic effects have been observed in similar studies with rats at up to 1800 times the human dose for glaucoma. Teratogenic studies with levobunolol in rats at doses up to 25 mg/kg/day (1800 times the recommended human dose for glaucoma) showed no evidence of fetal malformations. There were no adverse effects on postnatal development of offspring. It appears when results from studies using rats and studies with other beta-adrenergic blockers are examined, that the rabbit may be a particularly sensitive species. There are no adequate and well-controlled studies in pregnant women. Levobunolol HCl should be used during pregnancy only if the potential benefit justifies the potential risk to the fetus.

NURSING MOTHERS

It is not known whether this drug is excreted in human milk. Systemic beta-blockers and topical timolol maleate are known to be excreted in human milk. Caution should be exercised when levobunolol HCl is administered to a nursing woman.

PEDIATRIC USE

Safety and effectiveness in children have not been established.

DRUG INTERACTIONS

Although levobunolol HCl used alone has little or no effect on pupil size, mydriasis resulting from concomitant therapy with levobunolol HCl and epinephrine may occur.

Close observation of the patient is recommended when a beta-blocker is administered to patients receiving catecholamine-depleting drugs such as reserpine, because of possible additive effects and the production of hypotension and/or marked bradycardia, which may produce vertigo, syncope, or postural hypotension.

Patients receiving beta-adrenergic blocking agents along with either oral or intravenous calcium antagonists should be monitored for possible atrioventricular conduction disturbances, left ventricular failure and hypotension. In patients with impaired cardiac function, simultaneous use should be avoided altogether.

The concomitant use of beta-adrenergic blocking agents with digitalis and calcium antagonists may have additive effects on prolonging atrioventricular conduction time.

Phenothiazine-related compounds and beta-adrenergic blocking agents may have additive hypotensive effects due to the inhibition of each other's metabolism.

RISK OF ANAPHYLACTIC REACTION

While taking beta-blockers, patients with a history of severe anaphylactic reaction to a variety of allergens may be more reactive to repeated challenge, either accidental, diagnostic, or therapeutic. Such patients may be unresponsive to the usual doses of epinephrine used to treat allergic reaction.

ADVERSE REACTIONS

In clinical trials the use of levobunolol HCl has been associated with transient ocular burning and stinging in up to 1 in 3 patients, and with blepharoconjunctivitis in up to 1 in 20 patients. Decreases in heart rate and blood pressure have been reported (see CONTRAINDICATIONS and WARNINGS).

The following adverse effects have been reported rarely with the use of levobunolol HCl: Iridocyclitis, headache, transient ataxia, dizziness, lethargy, urticaria and pruritus.

Decreased corneal sensitivity has been noted in a small number of patients. Although levobunolol has minimal membrane-stabilizing activity, there remains a possibility of decreased corneal sensitivity after prolonged use.

The following additional adverse reactions have been reported either with levobunolol HCl or ophthalmic use of other beta-adrenergic receptor blocking agents:

Body as a Whole: Headache, asthenia, chest pain.
Cardiovascular: Bradycardia, arrhythmia, hypotension, syncope, heart block, cerebral vascular accident, cerebral ischemia, congestive heart failure, palpitation, cardiac arrest.
Digestive: Nausea, diarrhea.
Psychiatric: Depression, increase in signs and symptoms of myasthenia gravis, paresthesia.
Skin: Hypersensitivity, including localized and generalized rash.
Respiratory: Bronchospasm (predominantly in patients with pre-existing bronchospastic disease), respiratory failure, dyspnea, nasal congestion.
Endocrine: Masked symptoms of hypoglycemia in insulin-dependent diabetics (see WARNINGS).
Special Senses: Signs and symptoms of keratitis, blepharoptosis, visual disturbances including refractive changes (due to withdrawal of miotic therapy in some cases), diplopia, ptosis.

Other reactions associated with the oral use of non-selective adrenergic receptor blocking agents should be considered potential effects with ophthalmic use of these agents.

DOSAGE AND ADMINISTRATION

The recommended starting dose is 1-2 drops of levobunolol HCl 0.5% in the affected eye(s) once a day. Typical dosing with levobunolol HCl 0.25% is 1-2 drops twice daily. In patients with more severe or uncontrolled glaucoma, levobunolol HCl 0.5% can be administered bid. As with any new medication, careful monitoring of patients is advised.

Dosages above 1 drop of levobunolol HCl 0.5% b.i.d. are not generally more effective. If the patient's IOP is not at a satisfactory level on this regimen, concomitant therapy with dipivefrin and/or epinephrine, and/or pilocarpine and other miotics, and/or systemically administered carbonic anhydrase inhibitors, such as acetazolamide, can be instituted. Patients should not typically use two or more topical ophthalmic beta-adrenergic blocking agents simultaneously.

PRODUCT LISTING - RATED THERAPEUTICALLY EQUIVALENT

Solution - Ophthalmic - 0.25%

Size	Price	Product	NDC
5 ml	$12.84	GENERIC, Caremark Inc	00339-5931-50
5 ml	$12.85	GENERIC, Ivax Corporation	00182-7003-62
5 ml	$13.37	GENERIC, Akorn Inc	17478-0286-10
5 ml	$14.06	GENERIC, Pacific Pharma	60758-0063-05
5 ml	$15.82	GENERIC, Bausch and Lomb	24208-0545-05
5 ml	$16.63	GENERIC, Apotex Usa Inc	60505-0553-01
10 ml	$12.75	FEDERAL UPPER LIMIT, H.C.F.A. F F P	99999-1633-02
10 ml	$25.51	GENERIC, Caremark Inc	00339-5931-51
10 ml	$25.53	GENERIC, Ivax Corporation	00182-7003-63
10 ml	$26.60	GENERIC, Akorn Inc	17478-0286-11
10 ml	$27.18	GENERIC, Pacific Pharma	60758-0063-10
10 ml	$31.34	GENERIC, Bausch and Lomb	24208-0545-10
10 ml	$32.25	GENERIC, Apotex Usa Inc	60505-0553-02
15 ml	$48.20	GENERIC, Apotex Usa Inc	60505-0553-03

Solution - Ophthalmic - 0.5%

Size	Price	Product	NDC
2 ml	$12.65	BETAGAN, Allergan Inc	11980-0252-02
5 ml	$15.54	GENERIC, Caremark Inc	00339-5933-50
5 ml	$15.54	GENERIC, Caremark Inc	00339-5935-50
5 ml	$16.05	GENERIC, Ivax Corporation	00182-7002-62
5 ml	$16.11	GENERIC, Aligen Independent Laboratories Inc	00405-6065-05
5 ml	$16.50	GENERIC, Major Pharmaceuticals Inc	00904-7887-05
5 ml	$16.64	GENERIC, Bausch and Lomb	24208-0505-05
5 ml	$16.64	GENERIC, Pacific Pharma	60758-0060-05
5 ml	$16.80	GENERIC, Akorn Inc	17478-0287-10
5 ml	$16.86	GENERIC, Moore, H.L. Drug Exchange Inc	00839-7929-85
5 ml	$25.92	BETAGAN, Physicians Total Care	54868-0629-01
5 ml	$27.95	BETAGAN, Physicians Total Care	54868-2624-01
5 ml	$27.96	BETAGAN, Allergan Inc	11980-0252-25
5 ml	$27.96	BETAGAN, Allergan Inc	11980-0252-65
5 ml	$29.36	BETAGAN, Allergan Inc	00023-4385-05
10 ml	$14.93	FEDERAL UPPER LIMIT, H.C.F.A. F F P	99999-1633-04
10 ml	$30.10	GENERIC, Caremark Inc	00339-5933-51
10 ml	$30.10	GENERIC, Caremark Inc	00339-5935-51
10 ml	$30.69	GENERIC, Ivax Corporation	00182-7002-63
10 ml	$31.50	GENERIC, Major Pharmaceuticals Inc	00904-7887-10
10 ml	$31.50	GENERIC, Akorn Inc	17478-0287-11
10 ml	$31.51	GENERIC, Aligen Independent Laboratories Inc	00405-6065-10
10 ml	$32.29	GENERIC, Bausch and Lomb	24208-0505-10
10 ml	$32.29	GENERIC, Pacific Pharma	60758-0060-10
10 ml	$51.36	BETAGAN, Allscripts Pharmaceutical Company	54569-2662-00
10 ml	$55.99	BETAGAN, Allergan Inc	11980-0252-60
10 ml	$58.14	BETAGAN, Allergan Inc	11980-0252-20
10 ml	$61.05	BETAGAN, Allergan Inc	00023-4385-10
15 ml	$43.90	GENERIC, Caremark Inc	00339-5933-52
15 ml	$43.90	GENERIC, Caremark Inc	00339-5935-52
15 ml	$44.50	GENERIC, Major Pharmaceuticals Inc	00904-7887-35
15 ml	$44.63	GENERIC, Ivax Corporation	00182-7002-64
15 ml	$45.92	GENERIC, Aligen Independent Laboratories Inc	00405-6065-15
15 ml	$46.20	GENERIC, Akorn Inc	17478-0287-12
15 ml	$47.99	GENERIC, Moore, H.L. Drug Exchange Inc	00839-7929-61
15 ml	$48.32	GENERIC, Bausch and Lomb	24208-0505-15
15 ml	$48.32	GENERIC, Pacific Pharma	60758-0060-15
15 ml	$84.74	BETAGAN, Allergan Inc	11980-0252-21
15 ml	$88.97	BETAGAN, Allergan Inc	00023-4385-15

PRODUCT LISTING - EQUIVALENTS NOT AVAILABLE

Solution - Ophthalmic - 0.25%

Size	Price	Product	NDC
10 ml	$48.65	BETAGAN, Allergan Inc	00023-4526-10

Solution - Ophthalmic - 0.5%

Size	Price	Product	NDC
5 ml	$7.44	GENERIC, Physicians Total Care	54868-3363-01
5 ml	$16.60	GENERIC, Falcon Pharmaceuticals, Ltd.	61314-0229-05
10 ml	$9.77	GENERIC, Physicians Total Care	54868-3363-00
10 ml	$31.54	GENERIC, Allscripts Pharmaceutical Company	54569-4292-00
10 ml	$32.25	GENERIC, Falcon Pharmaceuticals, Ltd.	61314-0229-10
15 ml	$48.25	GENERIC, Falcon Pharmaceuticals, Ltd.	61314-0229-15

Levobupivacaine *(003445)*

For complete prescribing information, refer to the CD-ROM included with the book.

Categories: Anesthesia, local; Anesthesia, regional; FDA Approved 1999 Aug; Pregnancy Category B
Drug Classes: Anesthetics, local
Brand Names: Chirocaine

DESCRIPTION

Levobupivacaine injection contains a single enantiomer of bupivacaine HCl which is chemically described as (S)-1-butyl-2-piperidylformo-2′,6′-xylidide hydrochloride and it is related chemically and pharmacologically to the amino amide class of local anesthetics.

Levobupivacaine HCl, the S-enantiomer of bupivacaine, is a white crystalline powder with a molecular formula of $C_{18}H_{28}N_2O{\cdot}HCl$, a molecular weight of 324.9.

The solubility of levobupivacaine HCl in water is about 100 mg/ml at 20°C, the partition coefficient (oleyl alcohol/water) is 1624 and the pKa is 8.09. The pKa of levobupivacaine HCl is the same as that of bupivacaine HCl and the partition coefficient is very similar to that of bupivacaine HCl (1565).

Chirocaine is a sterile, non-pyrogenic, colorless solution (pH 4.0-6.5) containing levobupivacaine HCl equivalent to 2.5, 5.0, and 7.5 mg/ml of levobupivacaine, sodium chloride for isotonicity, and water for injection. Sodium hydroxide and/or hydrochloric acid may have been added to adjust pH. Chirocaine is preservative free and is available in 10 ml and 30 ml single dose vials.

Storage: Store Chirocaine at controlled room temperature, 20-25°C (68-77°F), excursions permitted to 15-30°C (59-86°F).

INDICATIONS AND USAGE

Levobupivacaine is indicated for the production of local or regional anesthesia for surgery and obstetrics, and for post-operative pain management.

Surgical Anesthesia: Epidural, peripheral neural blockade; and local infiltration.
Pain Management: Continuous epidural infusion or intermittent epidural neural blockade; continuous or intermittent peripheral neural blockade or local infiltration.

For continuous epidural analgesia, levobupivacaine may be administered in combination with epidural fentanyl or clonidine.

CONTRAINDICATIONS

Levobupivacaine is contraindicated in patients with a known hypersensitivity to levobupivacaine or to any local anesthetic agent of the amide type.

WARNINGS

IN PERFORMING LEVOBUPIVACAINE BLOCKS, UNINTENDED INTRAVENOUS INJECTION IS POSSIBLE AND MAY RESULT IN CARDIAC ARREST. DESPITE RAPID DETECTION AND APPROPRIATE TREATMENT, PROLONGED RESUSCITATION MAY BE REQUIRED. THE RESUSCITABILITY RELATIVE TO BUPIVACAINE IS UNKNOWN AT THIS POINT IN TIME AS IT HAS NOT BEEN STUDIED. AS WITH ALL LOCAL ANESTHETICS OF THE AMIDE TYPE, LEVOBUPIVACAINE SHOULD BE ADMINISTERED IN INCREMENTAL DOSES. SINCE LEVOBUPIVACAINE SHOULD NOT BE INJECTED RAPIDLY IN LARGE DOSES, IT IS NOT RECOMMENDED FOR EMERGENCY SITUATIONS, WHERE A FAST ONSET OF SURGICAL ANESTHESIA IS NECESSARY.

HISTORICALLY, PREGNANT PATIENTS WERE REPORTED TO HAVE A HIGH RISK FOR CARDIAC ARRHYTHMIAS, CARDIAC/CIRCULATORY ARREST AND DEATH WHEN BUPIVACAINE WAS INADVERTENTLY RAPIDLY INJECTED INTRAVENOUSLY. AVOID 0.75% LEVOBUPIVACAINE IN OBSTETRICAL PATIENTS. THIS CONCENTRATION IS INDICATED ONLY FOR NON-OBSTETRICAL SURGERY REQUIRING PROFOUND MUSCLE RELAXATION AND LONG DURATION.

FOR CESARIAN SECTION, THE 5 mg/ml (0.5%) LEVOBUPIVACAINE SOLUTION IN DOSES UP TO 150 mg IS RECOMMENDED.

LOCAL ANESTHETICS SHOULD ONLY BE ADMINISTERED BY CLINICIANS WHO ARE WELL VERSED IN THE DIAGNOSIS AND MANAGEMENT OF DRUG-RELATED TOXICITY AND OTHER ACUTE EMERGENCIES WHICH MIGHT ARISE FROM THE BLOCK BEING ADMINISTERED. THE IMMEDIATE AVAILABILITY OF OXYGEN, OTHER RESUSCITATIVE DRUGS, CARDIOPULMONARY RESUSCITATIVE EQUIPMENT, AND THE PERSONNEL RESOURCES NEEDED FOR PROPER MANAGEMENT OF TOXIC REACTIONS AND RELATED EMERGENCIES MUST BE ENSURED. DELAY IN PROPER MANAGEMENT OF DRUG-RELATED TOXICITY, UNDERVENTILATION FROM ANY CAUSE, AND/OR ALTERED SENSITIVITY MAY LEAD TO THE DEVELOPMENT OF ACIDOSIS, CARDIAC ARREST, AND POSSIBLY DEATH.

SOLUTIONS OF LEVOBUPIVACAINE SHOULD NOT BE USED FOR THE PRODUCTION OF OBSTETRICAL PARACERVICAL BLOCK ANESTHESIA. THERE ARE NO DATA TO SUPPORT SUCH USE AND THERE IS THE ADDITIONAL RISK OF FETAL BRADYCARDIA AND DEATH.

INTRAVENOUS REGIONAL ANESTHESIA (BIER BLOCK) SHOULD NOT BE PERFORMED USING LEVOBUPIVACAINE BECAUSE OF THE LACK OF CLINICAL EXPERIENCE AND THE RISK OF ATTAINING TOXIC BLOOD LEVELS OF LEVOBUPIVACAINE.

It is essential that aspiration for blood or cerebrospinal fluid (where applicable), be done prior to injecting any local anesthetic, both before the original dose and all subsequent doses, to avoid intravascular or intrathecal injection. However, a negative aspiration does *not* ensure against intravascular or intrathecal injection. Levobupivacaine should be used with caution in patients receiving other local anesthetics or agents structurally related to amide-type local anesthetics, since the toxic effects of these drugs are additive.

When contemplating a peripheral nerve block, where large volumes of local anesthetic are needed, caution should be exercised when using the higher mg/ml concentrations of levobupivacaine. Animal studies demonstrate CNS and cardiac toxicity that is dose related, thus equal volumes of higher concentration will be more likely to produce cardiac toxicity.

DOSAGE AND ADMINISTRATION

The rapid injection of a large volume of local anesthetic solution should be avoided and fractional (incremental) doses should always be used. The smallest dose and concentration required to produce the desired result should be administered. The dose of any local anesthetic differs with the anesthetic procedure, the area to be anesthetized, the vascularity of the tissues, the number of neuronal segments to be blocked, the intensity of the block, the degree of muscle relaxation required, the duration of the anesthesia desired, individual tolerance, and the physical condition of the patient. Patients in poor general condition due to aging or other compromising factors such as impaired cardiovascular function, advanced liver disease, or severe renal dysfunction, require special attention.

To reduce the risk of potentially serious adverse reactions, attempts should be made to optimize the patient's condition before major blocks are performed, and the dosage should be adjusted accordingly. Use an adequate test dose (3-5 ml) of a short-acting local anesthetic solution containing epinephrine prior to induction of complete nerve block. This test dose should be repeated if the patient is moved in such a fashion as to have displaced the epidural catheter. It is recommended that adequate time be allowed for the onset of anesthesia following administration of each test dose.

Disinfecting agents containing heavy metals, which cause release of ions (mercury, zinc, copper, etc.), should not be used for skin or mucous membrane disinfection since they have been related to incidents of swelling and edema.

When chemical disinfection of the container surface is desired, either isopropyl alcohol (91%) or ethyl alcohol (70%) is recommended. It is recommended that chemical disinfection be accomplished by wiping the vial stopper thoroughly with cotton or gauze that has been moistened with the recommended alcohol just prior to use.

When a container is required to have a sterile outside, glass containers may be autoclaved once. Stability has been demonstrated following an autoclave cycle at 121°C for 15 minutes.

These products are intended for single use and do not contain preservatives; any solution remaining from an open container should be discarded.

For specific techniques and procedures, refer to standard contemporary textbooks.

LEVOBUPIVACAINE COMPATIBILITY AND ADMIXTURES

Levobupivacaine may not be compatible with alkaline solutions having a pH greater than 8.5. Studies have shown that levobupivacaine is compatible with 0.9% sodium chloride injection and with saline solutions containing morphine, fentanyl, and clonidine. Compatibility studies with other parenteral products have not been studied.

DILUTION STABILITY

Levobupivacaine diluted to 0.625-2.5 mg levobupivacaine per ml in 0.9% sodium chloride injection is physically and chemically stable when stored in PVC (polyvinyl chloride) bags at ambient room temperature for up to 24 hours. Aseptic techniques should be used to prepare the diluted product. Admixtures of levobupivacaine should be prepared for single patient use only and used within 24 hours of preparation. The unused portion of diluted levobupivacaine should be discarded after each use.

Note: Parenteral products should be inspected visually for particulate matter and discoloration prior to administration whenever solution and container permit. Solutions that are not clear and colorless should not be used.

TABLE 4 *Dosage Recommendations*

	Conc.	Dose		Motor Block
Surgical Anesthesia				
Epidural for surgery	0.5-0.75%	10-20 ml	50-150 mg	Moderate to complete
Epidural for cesarean Section	0.5	20-30 ml	100-150 mg	Moderate to complete
Peripheral nerve	0.25-0.5	30 ml	75-150 mg	Moderate to complete
		0.4 ml/kg	1-2 mg/kg	
Ophthalmic	0.75	5-15 ml	37.5-112.5 mg	Moderate to complete
Local infiltration	0.25	60 ml	150 mg	Not Applicable
Pain Management*				
Labor analgesia (epidural bolus)	0.25	10-20 ml	25-50 mg	Minimal to moderate
Post-operative pain (epidural infusion)	0.125-0.25†	4-10 ml/h	5-25 mg/h	Minimal to moderate

* In pain management levobupivacaine can be used epidurally with fentanyl or clonidine.
† Dilutions of levobupivacaine standard solutions should be made with preservative free 0.9% saline according to standard hospital procedures for sterility.

The doses in TABLE 4 are those considered to be necessary to produce a successful block and should be regarded as guidelines for use in adults. Individual variations in onset and duration occur.

Epidural doses of up to 375 mg have been administered incrementally to patients during a surgical procedure.

The maximum dose in 24 hours for intraoperative block and postoperative pain management was 695 mg.

The maximum dose administered as a post-operative epidural infusion over 24 hours was 570 mg.

The maximum dose administered to patients as a single fractionated injection was 300 mg for brachial plexus block.

PRODUCT LISTING - EQUIVALENTS NOT AVAILABLE

Solution - Injectable - 0.25%

10 ml	$83.30	CHIROCAINE, Purdue Frederick Company	59011-0997-10
30 ml	$96.80	CHIROCAINE, Purdue Frederick Company	59011-0997-30

Solution - Injectable - 0.5%

10 ml	$93.30	CHIROCAINE, Purdue Frederick Company	59011-0998-10
30 ml	$107.40	CHIROCAINE, Purdue Frederick Company	59011-0998-30

Solution - Injectable - 0.75%

10 ml	$109.50	CHIROCAINE, Purdue Frederick Company	59011-0999-10
30 ml	$157.80	CHIROCAINE, Purdue Frederick Company	59011-0999-30

Levocabastine Hydrochloride (003187)

Categories: Conjunctivitis, allergic; FDA Approved 1993 Nov; Pregnancy Category C
Drug Classes: Antihistamines, H1; Antihistamines, ophthalmic; Ophthalmics
Brand Names: Livostin
Foreign Brand Availability: Livostin ED (South-Africa); Levophta (Germany)
Cost of Therapy: $39.53 (Allergic Conjunctivitis; Livostin Ophth. Suspension; 0.05%;5 ml; 4 drops/day; variable day supply)

DESCRIPTION

Levocabastine hydrochloride is a selective histamine H_1-receptor antagonist for topical ophthalmic use. Each ml contains 0.54 mg levocabastine hydrochloride equivalent to 0.5 mg levocabastine; 0.15 mg benzalkonium chloride; propylene glycol; polysorbate 80; dibasic sodium phosphate, monohydrate; disodium edetate; hydroxypropyl methylcellulose; and purified water. It has a pH of 6.0-8.0.

The chemical name for levocabastine hydrochloride is (-)-*trans*-1-(*cis*-4-cyano-4-(p-fluorophenyl)cyclohexyl)-3-methyl-4- phenylisonipecotic acid monohydrochloride.

CLINICAL PHARMACOLOGY

Levocabastine is a potent, selective histamine H_1-antagonist.

Antigen challenge studies performed 2-4 hours after initial drug instillation indicated activity was maintained for at least 2 and 4 hours.

In an environmental study, levocabastine HCl instilled 4 times daily was shown to be significantly more effective than its vehicle in reducing ocular itching associated with seasonal allergic conjunctivitis.

After instillation in the eye, levocabastine is systemically absorbed. However, the amount of systemically absorbed levocabastine after therapeutic ocular doses is low (mean plasma concentrations in the range of 1-2 ng/ml).

INDICATIONS AND USAGE

Levocabastine HCl is indicated for the temporary relief of the signs and symptoms of seasonal allergic conjunctivitis.

CONTRAINDICATIONS

This product is contraindicated in persons with known or suspected hypersensitivity to any of its components. It should not be used while soft contact lenses are being worn.

WARNINGS

For topical use only. Not for injection.

PRECAUTIONS

INFORMATION FOR THE PATIENT

SHAKE WELL BEFORE USING. To prevent contaminating the dropper tip and suspension, care should be taken not to touch the eyelids or surrounding areas with the dropper tip of the bottle. Keep bottle tightly closed when not in use. Do not use if the suspension has discolored. Store at controlled room temperature. Protect from freezing.

CARCINOGENESIS, MUTAGENESIS, AND IMPAIRMENT OF FERTILITY

Levocabastine was not carcinogenic in male or female rats or in male mice when administered in the diet for up to 24 months. In female mice, levocabastine doses of 5000 and 21,500 times the maximum recommended ocular human use level resulted in an increased incidence of pituitary gland adenoma and mammary gland adenocarcinoma possibly produced by increased prolactin levels. The clinical relevance of this finding is unknown with regard to the interspecies differences in prolactin physiology and the very low plasma concentrations of levocabastine following ocular administration.

Mutagenic potential was not demonstrated for levocabastine when tested in Ames' *Salmonella* Reversion test or in *Escherichia coli, Drosophila melanogaster,* a mouse Dominant Lethal Assay or in rat Micronucleus test.

In reproduction studies in rats, levocabastine showed no effects on fertility at oral doses of 20 mg/kg/day (8300 times the maximum recommended human ocular dose).

TERATOGENIC EFFECTS

Pregnancy Category C

Levocabastine has been shown to be teratogenic (polydactyly) in rats when given in doses 16,500 times the maximum recommended human ocular dose. Teratogenicity (polydactyly, hydrocephaly, brachygnathia), embryotoxicity, and maternal toxicity were observed in rats at 66,000 times the maximum recommended ocular human dose. There are no adequate and well-controlled studies in pregnant women. Levocabastine should be used during pregnancy only if the potential benefit justifies the potential risk to the fetus.

NURSING MOTHERS

Based on determinations of levocabastine in breast milk after ophthalmic administration of the drug to one nursing woman, it was calculated that the daily dose of levocabastine in the infant was about 0.5 µg.

PEDIATRIC USE

Safety and effectiveness in children below the age of 12 have not been established.

ADVERSE REACTIONS

The most frequent complaint with the use of levocabastine HCl is that of mild, transient stinging and burning (15%) and headache (5%).

Other adverse experiences which have been reported in approximately 1-3% of patients treated with Livostin include visual disturbances, dry mouth, fatigue, pharyngitis, eye pain/dryness, somnolence, red eyes, lacrimation/discharge, cough, nausea, rash/erythema, eyelid edema, and dyspnea.

DOSAGE AND ADMINISTRATION

Shake well before using. The usual dose is 1 drop instilled in affected eyes 4 times per day. Treatment may be continued for up to 2 weeks.

HOW SUPPLIED

Livostin 0.05% 2.5, 5, and 10 ml, is provided in white, polyethylene dropper tip squeeze bottles.

Storage: Keep tightly closed when not in use. Do not use if the suspension has discolored. Store at controlled room temperature 15-30°C (59-86°F). Protect from freezing.

PRODUCT LISTING - EQUIVALENTS NOT AVAILABLE

Suspension - Ophthalmic - 0.05%

5 ml	$39.53	LIVOSTIN, Allscripts Pharmaceutical Company	54569-3948-00
5 ml	$39.98	LIVOSTIN, Pharma Pac	52959-0328-03
5 ml	$53.23	LIVOSTIN, Ciba Vision Ophthalmics	58768-0610-05
10 ml	$81.29	LIVOSTIN, Ciba Vision Ophthalmics	58768-0610-10

Levofloxacin *(003313)*

For related information, see the comparative table section in Appendix A.

Categories: Bronchitis, chronic, acute exacerbation; Conjunctivitis, infectious; Impetigo; Infection, lower respiratory tract; Infection, ophthalmic; Infection, sinus; Infection, skin and skin structures; Infection, upper respiratory tract; Infection, urinary tract; Pneumonia; Pyelonephritis; Pyoderma; Pregnancy Category C; FDA Approved 1996 Dec

Drug Classes: Antibiotics, quinolones; Anti-infectives, ophthalmic; Ophthalmics

Brand Names: **Levaquin**

Foreign Brand Availability: Cravit (China; Indonesia; Japan; Korea; Singapore; Thailand); Cravit Ophthalmic (Hong-Kong); Elequine (Mexico); Floxel (Philippines); Leroxacin (Korea); Lesacin (Korea); Levokacin (Korea); Levox (Philippines); Levoxacin (Korea); Mosardal (Indonesia); Nofaxin (Korea); Reskuin (Indonesia); Tavanic (Bahamas; Barbados; Belize; Bermuda; Colombia; Curacao; England; France; Germany; Guyana; India; Ireland; Israel; Jamaica; Netherland-Antilles; Peru; Puerto-Rico; South-Africa; Surinam; Trinidad); Volequin (Indonesia)

Cost of Therapy: $88.76 (Infection; Levaquin; 500 mg; 1 tablet/day; 10 day supply)

HCFA JCODE(S): J1956 250 mg IV

INTRAVENOUS

DESCRIPTION

See oral route for the prescribing information for Levaquin injection.

OPHTHALMIC

DESCRIPTION

Note: The trade names have been used throughout this monograph for clarity.

Quixin (levofloxacin ophthalmic solution) 0.5% is a sterile topical ophthalmic solution. Levofloxacin is a fluoroquinolone antibacterial active against a broad spectrum of gram-positive and gram-negative ocular pathogens. Levofloxacin is the pure (-)-(S)-enantiomer of the racemic drug substance, ofloxacin. It is more soluble in water at neutral pH than ofloxacin.

The empirical formula is $C_{18}H_{20}FN_3O_4 \cdot ½H_2O$ and the molecular weight is 370.38.

Chemical Name: (-)-(S)-9-fluoro-2,3-dihydro-3-methyl-10-(4-methyl-1-piperazinyl)-7-oxo-*7H*-pyrido[1,2,3-*de*]-1,4 benzoxazine-6-carboxylic acid hemihydrate.

Levofloxacin (hemihydrate) is a yellowish-white crystalline powder.

Each ml of Quixin contains 5.12 mg of levofloxacin hemihydrate equivalent to 5 mg levofloxacin.

Contains: *Active:* Levofloxacin 0.5% (5 mg/ml); *Preservative:* Benzalkonium chloride 0.005%; *Inactives:* Sodium chloride and water. May also contain hydrochloric acid and/or sodium hydroxide to adjust pH.

Quixin solution is isotonic and formulated at pH 6.5 with an osmolality of approximately 300 mOsm/kg. Levofloxacin is a fluorinated 4-quinolone containing a six-member (pyridobenzoxazine) ring from positions 1-8 of the basic ring structure.

CLINICAL PHARMACOLOGY

PHARMACOKINETICS

Levofloxacin concentration in plasma was measured in 15 healthy adult volunteers at various time points during a 15 day course of treatment with Quixin solution. The mean levofloxacin concentration in plasma 1 hour postdose, ranged from 0.86 ng/ml on Day 1 to 2.05 ng/ml on Day 15. The highest maximum mean levofloxacin concentration of 2.5 ng/ml was measured on Day 4 following 2 days of dosing every 2 hours for a total of 8 doses per day. Maximum mean levofloxacin concentrations increased from 0.94 ng/ml on Day 1 to 2.15 ng/ml on Day 15, which is more than 1000 times lower than those reported after standard oral doses of levofloxacin.

Levofloxacin concentration in tears was measured in 30 healthy adult volunteers at various time points following instillation of a single drop of Quixin solution. Mean levofloxacin concentrations in tears ranged from 34.9-221.1 µg/ml during the 60 minute period following the single dose. The mean tear concentrations measured 4 and 6 hours postdose were 17.0 and 6.6 µg/ml. The clinical significance of these concentrations is unknown.

MICROBIOLOGY

Levofloxacin is the L-isomer of the racemate, ofloxacin, a quinolone antimicrobial agent. The antibacterial activity of ofloxacin resides primarily in the L-isomer. The mechanism of action of levofloxacin and other fluoroquinolone antimicrobials involves the inhibition of bacterial topoisomerase IV and DNA gyrase (both of which are Type II topoisomerases), enzymes required for DNA replication, transcription, repair, and recombination.

Levofloxacin has *in vitro* activity against a wide range of gram-negative and gram-positive microorganisms and is often bactericidal at concentrations equal to or slightly greater than inhibitory concentrations.

Fluoroquinolones, including levofloxacin, differ in chemical structure and mode of action from β-lactam antibiotics and aminoglycosides, and therefore may be active against bacteria resistant to β-lactam antibiotics and aminoglycosides. Additionally, β-lactam antibiotics and aminoglycosides may be active against bacteria resistant to levofloxacin.

Resistance to levofloxacin due to spontaneous mutation *in vitro* is a rare occurrence (range: 10^{-9} to 10^{-10}).

Levofloxacin has been shown to be active against most strains of the following microorganisms, both *in vitro* and in clinical infections as described in INDICATIONS AND USAGE.

Aerobic Gram-Positive Microorganisms

Corynebacterium species,* *Staphylococcus aureus, Staphylococcus epidermidis, Streptococcus pneumoniae, Streptococcus* (Groups C/F), *Streptococcus* (Group G), Viridans group streptococci.

*Efficacy for this organism was studied in fewer than 10 infections.

Aerobic Gram-Negative Microorganisms

Acinetobacter lwoffii, Haemophilus influenzae, Serratia marcescens.**

*Efficacy for this organism was studied in fewer than 10 infections.

The following *in vitro* data are also available, but their clinical significance in ophthalmic infections is unknown. The safety and effectiveness of levofloxacin in treating ophthalmological infections due to these microorganisms have not been established in adequate and well-controlled trials.

These organisms are considered susceptible when evaluated using systemic breakpoints. However, a correlation between the *in vitro* systemic breakpoint and ophthalmological efficacy has not been established. The list of organisms is provided as guidance only in assessing the potential treatment of conjunctival infections. Levofloxacin exhibits *in vitro* minimal inhibitory concentrations (MICs) of 2 µg/ml or less (systemic susceptible breakpoint) against most (≥90%) strains of the following ocular pathogens.

Aerobic Gram-Positive Microorganisms

Enterococcus faecalis, Staphylococcus saprophyticus, Streptococcus agalactiae, Streptococcus pyogenes.

Aerobic Gram-Negative Microorganisms

Acinetobacter anitratus, Acinetobacter baumannii, Citrobacter diversus, Citrobacter freundii, Enterobacter aerogenes, Enterobacter agglomerans, Enterobacter cloacae, Escherichia coli, Haemophilus parainfluenzae, Klebsiella oxytoca, Klebsiella pneumoniae, Legionella pneumophila, Moraxella catarrhalis, Morganella morganii, Neisseria gonorrhoeae, Proteus mirabilis, Proteus vulgaris, Providencia rettgeri, Providencia stuartii, Pseudomonas aeruginosa, Pseudomonas fluorescens.

INDICATIONS AND USAGE

Quixin solution is indicated for the treatment of bacterial conjunctivitis caused by susceptible strains of the following organisms:

Aerobic Gram-Positive Microorganisms

Corynebacterium species,* *Staphylococcus aureus, Staphylococcus epidermidis, Streptococcus pneumoniae, Streptococcus* (Groups C/F), *Streptococcus* (Group G), Viridans group streptococci.

*Efficacy for this organism was studied in fewer than 10 infections.

Aerobic Gram-Negative Microorganisms

Acinetobacter lwoffii, Haemophilus influenzae, Serratia marcescens.**

*Efficacy for this organism was studied in fewer than 10 infections.

CONTRAINDICATIONS

Quixin solution is contraindicated in patients with a history of hypersensitivity to levofloxacin, to other quinolones, or to any of the components of this medication.

WARNINGS

NOT FOR INJECTION.

Quixin solution should not be injected subconjunctivally, nor should it be introduced directly into the anterior chamber of the eye.

L

In patients receiving systemic quinolones, serious and occasionally fatal hypersensitivity (anaphylactic) reactions have been reported, some following the first dose. Some reactions were accompanied by cardiovascular collapse, loss of consciousness, angioedema (including laryngeal, pharyngeal or facial edema), airway obstruction, dyspnea, urticaria, and itching. If an allergic reaction to levofloxacin occurs, discontinue the drug. Serious acute hypersensitivity reactions may require immediate emergency treatment. Oxygen and airway management should be administered as clinically indicated.

PRECAUTIONS

GENERAL

As with other anti-infectives, prolonged use may result in overgrowth of non-susceptible organisms, including fungi. If superinfection occurs, discontinue use and institute alternative therapy. Whenever clinical judgment dictates, the patient should be examined with the aid of magnification, such as slit-lamp biomicroscopy and where appropriate, fluorescein staining.

Patients should be advised not to wear contact lenses if they have signs and symptoms of bacterial conjunctivitis.

INFORMATION FOR THE PATIENT

Avoid contaminating the applicator tip with material from the eye, fingers or other source.

Systemic quinolones have been associated with hypersensitivity reactions, even following a single dose. Discontinue use immediately and contact your physician at the first sign of a rash or allergic reaction.

CARCINOGENESIS, MUTAGENESIS, AND IMPAIRMENT OF FERTILITY

In a long term carcinogenicity study in rats, levofloxacin exhibited no carcinogenic or tumorigenic potential following daily dietary administration; the highest dose (100 mg/kg/day) was 875 times the highest recommended human ophthalmic dose.

Levofloxacin was not mutagenic in the following assays: Ames bacterial mutation assay (*S. typhimurium* and *E. coli*), CHO/HGPRT forward mutation assay, mouse micronucleus test, mouse dominant lethal test, rat unscheduled DNA synthesis assay, and the *in vivo* mouse sister chromatid exchange assay. It was positive in the *in vitro* chromosomal aberration (CHL cell line) and *in vitro* sister chromatid exchange (CHL/IU cell line) assays. Levofloxacin caused no impairment of fertility or reproduction in rats at oral doses as high as 360 mg/kg/day, corresponding to 3150 times the highest recommended human ophthalmic dose.

L

PREGNANCY, TERATOGENIC EFFECTS, PREGNANCY CATEGORY C

Levofloxacin at oral doses of 810 mg/kg/day in rats, which corresponds to approximately 7000 times the highest recommended human ophthalmic dose caused decreased fetal body weight and increased fetal mortality.

No teratogenic effect was observed when rabbits were dosed orally as high as 50 mg/kg/day, which corresponds to approximately 400 times the highest recommended maximum human ophthalmic dose, or when dosed intravenously as high as 25 mg/kg/day, corresponding to approximately 200 times the highest recommended human ophthalmic dose.

There are, however, no adequate and well-controlled studies in pregnant women. Levofloxacin should be used during pregnancy only if the potential benefit justifies the potential risk to the fetus.

NURSING MOTHERS

Levofloxacin has not been measured in human milk. Based upon data from ofloxacin, it can be presumed that levofloxacin is excreted in human milk. Caution should be exercised when Quixin is administered to a nursing mother.

PEDIATRIC USE

Safety and effectiveness in infants below the age of 1 year have not been established. Oral administration of quinolones has been shown to cause arthropathy in immature animals. There is no evidence that the ophthalmic administration of levofloxacin has any effect on weight bearing joints.

GERIATRIC USE

No overall differences in safety or effectiveness have been observed between elderly and other adult patients.

DRUG INTERACTIONS

Specific drug interaction studies have not been conducted with Quixin. However, the systemic administration of some quinolones has been shown to elevate plasma concentrations of theophylline, interfere with the metabolism of caffeine, and enhance the effects of the oral anticoagulant warfarin and its derivatives, and has been associated with transient elevations in serum creatinine in patients receiving systemic cyclosporine concomitantly.

ADVERSE REACTIONS

The most frequently reported adverse events in the overall study population were transient decreased vision, fever, foreign body sensation, headache, transient ocular burning, ocular pain or discomfort, pharyngitis and photophobia. These events occurred in approximately 1-3% of patients. Other reported reactions occurring in less than 1% of patients included allergic reactions, lid edema, ocular dryness, and ocular itching.

DOSAGE AND ADMINISTRATION

Days 1 and 2: Instill 1-2 drops in the affected eye(s) every 2 hours while awake up to 8 times per day.

Days 3 through 7: Instill 1-2 drops in the affected eye(s) every 4 hours while awake up to 4 times per day.

HOW SUPPLIED

Quixin (levofloxacin ophthalmic solution) 0.5% is supplied in a white, low density polyethylene bottle with a controlled dropper tip and a tan, high density polyethylene cap.

Storage: Store at 15-25°C (59-77°F).

ORAL

DESCRIPTION

Note: The trade names have been used throughout this monograph for clarity.

Levaquin is a synthetic broad spectrum antibacterial agent for oral and intravenous administration. Chemically, levofloxacin, a chiral fluorinated carboxyquinolone, is the pure (-)-(S)-enantiomer of the racemic drug substance ofloxacin. The chemical name is (-)-(S)-9-fluoro-2,3-dihydro-3-methyl-10-(4-methyl-1-piperazinyl)-7-oxo-7H-pyrido[1,2,3-de]-1,4-benzoxazine-6-carboxylic acid hemihydrate.

Its empirical formula is $C_{18}H_{20}FN_3O_4 \cdot \frac{1}{2}H_2O$ and its molecular weight is 370.38. Levofloxacin is a light yellowish-white to yellow-white crystal or crystalline powder. The molecule exists as a zwitterion at the pH conditions in the small intestine.

The data demonstrate that from pH 0.6-5.8, the solubility of levofloxacin is essentially constant (approximately 100 mg/ml). Levofloxacin is considered *soluble to freely soluble* in this pH range, as defined by USP nomenclature. Above pH 5.8, the solubility increases rapidly to its maximum at pH 6.7 (272 mg/ml) and is considered *freely soluble* in this range. Above pH 6.7, the solubility decreases and reaches a minimum value (about 50 mg/ml) at a pH of approximately 6.9.

Levofloxacin has the potential to form stable coordination compounds with many metal ions. This *in vitro* chelation potential has the following formation order: $Al^{+3}>Cu^{+2}>Zn^{+2}>Mg^{+2}>Ca^{+2}$.

LEVAQUIN TABLETS

Levaquin tablets are available as film-coated tablets and contain the following inactive ingredients:

250 mg (as expressed in the anhydrous form): Hydroxypropyl methylcellulose, crospovidone, microcrystalline cellulose, magnesium stearate, polyethylene glycol, titanium dioxide, polysorbate 80 and synthetic red iron oxide.

500 mg (as expressed in the anhydrous form): Hydroxypropyl methylcellulose, crospovidone, microcrystalline cellulose, magnesium stearate, polyethylene glycol, titanium dioxide, polysorbate 80 and synthetic red and yellow iron oxides.

750 mg (as expressed in the anhydrous form): Hydroxypropyl methylcellulose, crospovidone, microcrystalline cellulose, magnesium stearate, polyethylene glycol, titanium dioxide, polysorbate 80.

LEVAQUIN INJECTION

Levaquin injection in single-use vials is a sterile, preservative-free aqueous solution of levofloxacin with pH ranging from 3.8-5.8. Levaquin injection in premix flexible containers is a sterile, preservative-free aqueous solution of levofloxacin with pH ranging from 3.8-5.8. The appearance of Levaquin injection may range from a clear yellow to a greenish-yellow solution. This does not adversely affect product potency.

Levaquin injection in single-use vials contains levofloxacin in water for injection. Levaquin injection in premix flexible containers is a dilute, non-pyrogenic, nearly isotonic premixed solution that contains levofloxacin in 5% dextrose (D_5W). Solutions of hydrochloric acid and sodium hydroxide may have been added to adjust the pH.

The flexible container is fabricated from a specially formulated non-plasticized, thermoplastic copolyester (CR3). The amount of water that can permeate from the container into the overwrap is insufficient to affect the solution significantly. Solutions in contact with the flexible container can leach out certain of the container's chemical components in very small amounts within the expiration period. The suitability of the container material has been confirmed by tests in animals according to USP biological tests for plastic containers.

CLINICAL PHARMACOLOGY

The mean ±SD pharmacokinetic parameters of levofloxacin determined under single and steady state conditions following oral (po) or intravenous (IV) doses of levofloxacin are summarized in TABLE 1A and TABLE 1B.

ABSORPTION

Levofloxacin is rapidly and essentially completely absorbed after oral administration. Peak plasma concentrations are usually attained 1-2 hours after oral dosing. The absolute bioavailability of a 500 and a 750 mg tablet of levofloxacin are both approximately 99%, demonstrating complete oral absorption of levofloxacin. Following a single intravenous dose of levofloxacin to healthy volunteers, the mean ±SD peak plasma concentration attained was 6.2 ± 1.0 μg/ml after a 500 mg dose infused over 60 minutes and 11.5 ± 4.0 μg/ml after a 750 mg dose infused over 90 minutes.

Levofloxacin pharmacokinetics are linear and predictable after single and multiple oral/or IV dosing regimens. Steady-state conditions are reached within 48 hours following a 500 or 750 mg once-daily dosage regimen. The mean ±SD peak and trough plasma concentrations attained following multiple once-daily oral dosage regimens were approximately 5.7 ± 1.4 and 0.5 ± 0.2 μg/ml after the 500 mg doses, and 8.6 ± 1.9 and 1.1 ± 0.4 μg/ml after the 750 mg doses, respectively. The mean ±SD peak and trough plasma concentrations attained following multiple once-daily IV regimens were approximately 6.4 ± 0.8 and 0.6 ± 0.2 μg/ml after the 500 mg doses, and 12.1 ± 4.1 and 1.3 ± 0.71 μg/ml after the 750 mg doses, respectively.

Oral administration of a 500 mg Levaquin tablet with food slightly prolongs the time to peak concentration by approximately 1 hour and slightly decreases the peak concentration by approximately 14%. Therefore, levofloxacin tablets can be administered without regard to food.

The plasma concentration profile of levofloxacin after IV administration is similar and comparable in extent of exposure (AUC) to that observed for levofloxacin tablets when equal doses (mg/mg) are administered. Therefore, the oral and IV routes of administration can be considered interchangeable.

DISTRIBUTION

The mean volume of distribution of levofloxacin generally ranges from 74-112 L after single and multiple 500 or 750 mg doses, indicating widespread distribution into body tissues. Levofloxacin reaches its peak levels in skin tissues and in blister fluid of healthy subjects at approximately 3 hours after dosing. The skin tissue biopsy to plasma AUC ratio is approximately 2 and the blister fluid to plasma AUC ratio is approximately 1 following multiple once-daily oral administration of 750 mg and 500 mg levofloxacin, respectively, to healthy subjects. Levofloxacin also penetrates well into lung tissues. Lung tissue concentrations were generally 2- to 5-fold higher than plasma concentrations and ranged from approximately 2.4-11.3 μg/g over a 24 hour period after a single 500 mg oral dose.

In vitro, over a clinically relevant range (1-10 μg/ml) of serum/plasma levofloxacin concentrations, levofloxacin is approximately 24-38% bound to serum proteins across all species studied, as determined by the equilibrium dialysis method. Levofloxacin is mainly bound to serum albumin in humans. Levofloxacin binding to serum proteins is independent of the drug concentration.

METABOLISM

Levofloxacin is stereochemically stable in plasma and urine and does not invert metabolically to its enantiomer, D-ofloxacin. Levofloxacin undergoes limited metabolism in humans and is primarily excreted as unchanged drug in the urine. Following oral administration, approximately 87% of an administered dose was recovered as unchanged drug in urine within 48 hours, whereas less than 4% of the dose was recovered in feces in 72 hours. Less than 5% of an administered dose was recovered in the urine as the desmethyl and N-oxide metabolites, the only metabolites identified in humans. These metabolites have little relevant pharmacological activity.

EXCRETION

Levofloxacin is excreted largely as unchanged drug in the urine. The mean terminal plasma elimination half-life of levofloxacin ranges from approximately 6-8 hours following single or multiple doses of levofloxacin given orally or intravenously. The mean apparent total body clearance and renal clearance range from approximately 144-226 ml/min and 96-142 ml/min, respectively. Renal clearance in excess of the glomerular filtration rate suggests that tubular secretion of levofloxacin occurs in addition to its glomerular filtration. Concomitant administration of either cimetidine or probenecid results in approximately 24% and 35% reduction in the levofloxacin renal clearance, respectively, indicating that secretion of levofloxacin occurs in the renal proximal tubule. No levofloxacin crystals were found in any of the urine samples freshly collected from subjects receiving levofloxacin.

SPECIAL POPULATIONS

Geriatric

There are no significant differences in levofloxacin pharmacokinetics between young and elderly subjects when the subjects' differences in creatinine clearance are taken into consideration. Following a 500 mg oral dose of levofloxacin to healthy elderly subjects (66-80 years of age), the mean terminal plasma elimination half-life of levofloxacin was about 7.6 hours, as compared to approximately 6 hours in younger adults. The difference was attributable to the variation in renal function status of the subjects and was not believed to be clinically significant. Drug absorption appears to be unaffected by age. Levofloxacin dose adjustment based on age alone is not necessary.

Pediatric

The pharmacokinetics of levofloxacin in pediatric subjects have not been studied.

Gender

There are no significant differences in levofloxacin pharmacokinetics between male and female subjects when subjects' differences in creatinine clearance are taken into consideration. Following a 500 mg oral dose of levofloxacin to healthy male subjects, the mean terminal plasma elimination half-life of levofloxacin was about 7.5 hours, as compared to approximately 6.1 hours in female subjects. This difference was attributable to the variation in renal function status of the male and female subjects and was not believed to be clinically significant. Drug absorption appears to be unaffected by the gender of the subjects. Dose adjustment based on gender alone is not necessary.

Race

The effect of race on levofloxacin pharmacokinetics was examined through a covariate analysis performed on data from 72 subjects: 48 white and 24 nonwhite. The apparent total body clearance and apparent volume of distribution were not affected by the race of the subjects.

Renal Insufficiency

Clearance of levofloxacin is substantially reduced and plasma elimination half-life is substantially prolonged in patients with impaired renal function (creatinine clearance <50 ml/min), requiring dosage adjustment in such patients to avoid accumulation. Neither hemodialysis nor continuous ambulatory peritoneal dialysis (CAPD) is effective in removal of levofloxacin from the body, indicating that supplemental doses of levofloxacin are not required following hemodialysis or CAPD. (See PRECAUTIONS, General and DOSAGE AND ADMINISTRATION.)

Hepatic Insufficiency

Pharmacokinetic studies in hepatically impaired patients have not been conducted. Due to the limited extent of levofloxacin metabolism, the pharmacokinetics of levofloxacin are not expected to be affected by hepatic impairment.

Bacterial Infection

The pharmacokinetics of levofloxacin in patients with serious community-acquired bacterial infections are comparable to those observed in healthy subjects.

Drug-Drug Interactions

The potential for pharmacokinetic drug interactions between levofloxacin and theophylline, warfarin, cyclosporine, digoxin, probenecid, cimetidine, sucralfate, and antacids has been evaluated. (See DRUG INTERACTIONS.)

TABLE 1A *Mean ± SD Levofloxacin PK Parameters*

Regimen	C_{max} (μg/ml)	T_{max} (h)	AUC (μg·h/ml)
Single Dose			
250 mg po*	2.8 ± 0.4	1.6 ± 1.0	27.2 ± 3.9
500 mg po*§§	5.1 ± 0.8	1.3 ± 0.6	47.9 ± 6.8
500 mg IV*	6.2 ± 1.0	1.0 ± 0.1	48.3 ± 5.4
750 mg po‡§§	9.3 ± 1.6	1.6 ± 0.8	101 ± 20
750 mg IV‡	11.5 ± 4.0	ND	110 ± 40
Multiple Dose			
500 mg q24h po*	5.7 ± 1.4	1.1 ± 0.4	47.5 ± 6.7
500 mg q24h IV*	6.4 ± 0.8	ND	54.6 ± 11.1
500 or 250 mg q24h IV, patients with bacterial infection§	8.7 ± 4.0¤	ND	72.5 ± 51.2¤
750 mg q24h po‡	8.6 ± 1.9	1.4 ± 0.5	90.7 ± 17.6
750 mg q24h IV‡	12.1 ± 4.1†	ND	108 ± 34
500 mg po Single Dose, Effects of Gender and Age			
Male¶	5.5 ± 1.1	1.2 ± 0.4	54.4 ± 18.9
Female**	7.0 ± 1.6	1.7 ± 0.5	67.7 ± 24.2
Young††	5.5 ± 1.0	1.5 ± 0.6	47.5 ± 9.8
Elderly‡‡	7.0 ± 1.6	1.4 ± 0.5	74.7 ± 23.3
500 mg po Single Dose, Patients With Renal Insufficiency			
CLCR 50-80 ml/min	7.5 ± 1.8	1.5 ± 0.5	95.6 ± 11.8
CLCR 20-49 ml/min	7.1 ± 3.1	2.1 ± 1.3	182.1 ± 62.6
CLCR <20 ml/min	8.2 ± 2.6	1.1 ± 1.0	263.5 ± 72.5
Hemodialysis	5.7 ± 1.0	2.8 ± 2.2	ND
CAPD	6.9 ± 2.3	1.4 ± 1.1	ND

* Healthy males 18-53 years of age.
† 60 minute infusion for 250 and 500 mg doses, 90 minute infusion for 750 mg dose.
‡ Healthy male and female subjects 18-54 years of age.
§ 500 mg q48h for patients with moderate renal impairment (CLCR 20-50 ml/min) and infections of the respiratory tract or skin.
¤ Dose-normalized values (to 500 mg dose), estimated by population pharmacokinetic modeling.
¶ Healthy males 22-75 years of age.
** Healthy females 18-80 years of age.
†† Young healthy male and female subjects 18-36 years of age.
‡‡ Healthy elderly male and female subjects 66-80 years of age.
§§ Absolute bioavailability, F = 0.99 ± 0.08 from a 500 mg tablet and F = 0.99 ± 0.06 from a 750 mg tablet; ND = Not Determined.

TABLE 1B *Mean ± SD Levofloxacin PK Parameters*

Regimen	CL/F* (ml/min)	Vd/F† (L)	T½ (h)	CLR (ml/min)
Single Dose				
250 mg po‡	156 ± 20	ND	7.3 ± 0.9	142 ± 21
500 mg po‡§§	178 ± 28	ND	6.3 ± 0.6	103 ± 30
500 mg IV‡	175 ± 20	90 ± 11	6.4 ± 0.7	112 ± 25
750 mg po§,§§	129 ± 24	83 ± 17	7.5 ± 0.9	ND
750 mg IV§¤	126 ± 39	75 ± 13	7.5 ± 1.6	ND
Multiple Dose				
500 mg q24h po‡	175 ± 25	102 ± 22	7.6 ± 1.6	116 ± 31
500 mg q24h IV‡	158 ± 29	91 ± 12	7.0 ± 0.8	99 ± 28
500 or 250 mg q24h IV, patients with bacterial infection¤	154 ± 72	111 ± 58	ND	ND
750 mg q24h po§	143 ± 29	100 ± 16	8.8 ± 1.5	116 ± 28
750 mg q24h IV§	126 ± 37	80 ± 27	7.9 ± 1.9	ND
500 mg po Single Dose, Effects of Gender and Age				
Male¶	166 ± 44	89 ± 13	7.5 ± 2.1	126 ± 38
Female**	136 ± 44	62 ± 16	6.1 ± 0.8	106 ± 40
Young††	182 ± 35	83 ± 18	6.0 ± 0.9	140 ± 33
Elderly‡‡	121 ± 33	67 ± 19	7.6 ± 2.0	91 ± 29
500 mg po Single Dose, Patients With Renal Insufficiency				
CLCR 50-80 ml/min	88 ± 10	ND	9.1 ± 0.9	57 ± 8
CLCR 20-49 ml/min	51 ± 19	ND	27 ± 10	26 ± 13
CLCR <20 ml/min	33 ± 8	ND	35 ± 5	13 ± 3
Hemodialysis	ND	ND	76 ± 42	ND
CAPD	ND	ND	51 ± 24	ND

* Clearance/bioavailability.
† Volume of distribution/bioavailability.
‡ Healthy males 18-53 years of age.
§ Healthy male and female subjects 18-54 years of age.
¤ 500 mg q48h for patients with moderate renal impairment (CLCR 20-50 ml/min) and infections of the respiratory tract or skin.
¶ Healthy males 22-75 years of age.
** Healthy females 18-80 years of age.
†† Young healthy male and female subjects 18-36 years of age.
‡‡ Healthy elderly male and female subjects 66-80 years of age.
§§ Absolute bioavailability, F = 0.99 ± 0.08 from a 500 mg tablet and F = 0.99 ± 0.06 from a 750 mg tablet; ND = Not Determined.

MICROBIOLOGY

Levofloxacin is the L-isomer of the racemate, ofloxacin, a quinolone antimicrobial agent. The antibacterial activity of ofloxacin resides primarily in the L-isomer. The mechanism of action of levofloxacin and other fluoroquinolone antimicrobials involves inhibition of bacterial topoisomerase IV and DNA gyrase (both of which are Type II topoisomerases), enzymes required for DNA replication, transcription, repair and recombination.

Levofloxacin has *in vitro* activity against a wide range of gram-negative and gram-positive microorganisms. Levofloxacin is often bactericidal at concentrations equal to or slightly greater than inhibitory concentrations.

Fluoroquinolones, including levofloxacin, differ in chemical structure and mode of action from aminoglycosides, macrolides and β-lactam antibiotics, including penicillins. Fluoroquinolones may, therefore, be active against bacteria resistant to these antimicrobials.

Resistance to levofloxacin due to spontaneous mutation *in vitro* is a rare occurrence (range: 10^{-9} to 10^{-10}). Although cross-resistance has been observed between levofloxacin and some other fluoroquinolones, some microorganisms resistant to other fluoroquinolones may be susceptible to levofloxacin.

Levofloxacin has been shown to be active against most strains of the following microorganisms both *in vitro* and in clinical infections as described in INDICATIONS AND USAGE.

Aerobic Gram-Positive Microorganisms

Enterococcus faecalis (many strains are only moderately susceptible), *Staphylococcus aureus* (methicillin-susceptible strains), *Staphylococcus saprophyticus, Streptococcus pneumoniae* (including penicillin-resistant strains*), *Streptococcus pyogenes.*

***Note:** Penicillin-resistant *S. pneumoniae* are those strains with a penicillin MIC value of ≥2 µg/ml.

Aerobic Gram-Negative Microorganisms

Enterobacter cloacae, Escherichia coli, Haemophilus influenzae, Haemophilus parainfluenzae, Klebsiella pneumoniae, Legionella pneumophila, Moraxella catarrhalism, Proteus mirabilis, Pseudomonas aeruginosa, Serratia marcescens.

As with other drugs in this class, some strains of *Pseudomonas aeruginosa* may develop resistance fairly rapidly during treatment with levofloxacin.

Other Microorganisms

Chlamydia pneumoniae, Mycoplasma pneumoniae.

The following *in vitro* data are available, **but their clinical significance is unknown.**

Levofloxacin exhibits *in vitro* minimum inhibitory concentrations (MIC values) of 2 µg/ml or less against most (≥90%) strains of the following microorganisms; however, the safety and effectiveness of levofloxacin in treating clinical infections due to these microorganisms have not been established in adequate and well-controlled trials.

Aerobic Gram-Positive Microorganisms

Staphylococcus epidermidis (methicillin-susceptible strains), *Streptococcus* (Group C/F), *Streptococcus* (Group G), *Streptococcus agalactiae, Streptococcus milleri,* Viridans group streptococci.

Aerobic Gram-Negative Microorganisms

Acinetobacter baumannii, Acinetobacter lwoffii, Bordetella pertussis, Citrobacter (diversus) koseri, Citrobacter freundii, Enterobacter aerogenes, Enterobacter sakazakii, Klebsiella oxytoca, Morganella morganii, Pantoea (Enterobacter) agglomerans, Proteus vulgaris, Providencia rettgeri, Providencia stuartii, Pseudomonas fluorescens.

Anaerobic Gram-Positive Microorganisms

Clostridium perfringens.

L

Susceptibility Testing

Susceptibility testing for levofloxacin should be performed, as it is the optimal predictor of activity.

Dilution Techniques

Quantitative methods are used to determine antimicrobial minimal inhibitory concentrations (MIC values). These MIC values provide estimates of the susceptibility of bacteria to antimicrobial compounds. The MIC values should be determined using a standardized procedure. Standardized procedures are based on a dilution method[1] (broth or agar) or equivalent with standardized inoculum concentrations and standardized concentrations of levofloxacin powder. The MIC values should be interpreted according to the criteria in TABLE 2, TABLE 3, TABLE 4, and TABLE 5.

TABLE 2

MIC (µg/ml)	Interpretation
≤2	Susceptible (S)
4	Intermediate (I)
≥8	Resistant (R)

For testing *Haemophilus influenzae* and *Haemophilus parainfluenzae* see TABLE 3.*

TABLE 3

MIC (µg/ml)	Interpretation
≤2	Susceptible (S)

* These interpretative standards are applicable only to broth microdilution susceptibility testing with *Haemophilus influenzae* and *Haemophilus parainfluenzae* using Haemophilus Test Medium.[1]

The current absence of data on resistant strains precludes defining any categories other than "Susceptible". Strains yielding MIC results suggestive of a "nonsusceptible" category should be submitted to a reference laboratory for further testing.

For testing *Streptococcus* spp. including *S. pneumoniae* see TABLE 4.*

A report of "Susceptible" indicates that the pathogen is likely to be inhibited if the antimicrobial compound in the blood reaches the concentrations usually achievable. A report of "Intermediate" indicates that the result should be considered equivocal, and, if the microorganism is not fully susceptible to alternative, clinically feasible drugs, the test should be repeated. This category implies possible clinical applicability in body sites where the drug is physiologically concentrated or in situations where a high dosage of drug can be used. This category also provides a buffer zone which prevents small uncontrolled technical factors from causing major discrepancies in interpretation. A report of "Resistant" indicates that the pathogen is not likely to be inhibited if the antimicrobial compound in the blood reaches the concentrations usually achievable; other therapy should be selected.

TABLE 4

MIC (µg/ml)	Interpretation
≤2	Susceptible (S)
4	Intermediate (I)
≥8	Resistant (R)

* These interpretative standards are applicable only to broth microdilution susceptibility tests using cation-adjusted Mueller-Hinton broth with 2-5% lysed horse blood.

Standardized susceptibility test procedures require the use of laboratory control microorganisms to control the technical aspects of the laboratory procedures. Standard levofloxacin powder should give the MIC values in TABLE 5.

TABLE 5

Microorganism		MIC (µg/ml)
Enterococcus faecalis	ATCC 29212	0.25-2
Escherichia coli	ATCC 25922	0.008-0.06
Escherichia coli	ATCC 35218	0.015-0.06
Haemophilus influenzae	ATCC 49247*	0.008-0.03
Pseudomonas aeruginosa	ATCC 27853	0.5-4
Staphylococcus aureus	ATCC 29213	0.06-0.5
Streptococcus pneumoniae	ATCC 49619†	0.5-2

* This quality control range is applicable to only *H. influenzae* ATCC 49247 tested by a broth microdilution procedure using Haemophilus Test Medium (HTM).[1]

† This quality control range is applicable to only *S. pneumoniae* ATCC 49619 tested by a broth microdulition procedure using cation-adjusted Mueller-Hinton broth with 2-5% lysed horse blood.

Diffusion Techniques

Quantitative methods that require measurement of zone diameters also provide reproducible estimates of the susceptibility of bacteria to antimicrobial compounds. One such standardized procedure[2] requires the use of standardized inoculum concentrations. This procedure uses paper disks impregnated with 5 µg levofloxacin to test the susceptibility of microorganisms to levofloxacin.

Reports from the laboratory providing results of the standard single-disk susceptibility test with a 5 µg levofloxacin disk should be interpreted according to the criteria in TABLE 6, TABLE 7, TABLE 8, and TABLE 9.

For testing *Enterobacteriaceae, Enterococci, Staphylococcus* species, and *Pseudomonas aeruginosa* see TABLE 6.

TABLE 6

Zone Diameter (mm)	Interpretation
≥17	Susceptible (S)
14-16	Intermediate (I)
≤13	Resistant (R)

For *Haemophilus influenzae* and *Haemophilus parainfluenzae* see TABLE 7.*

TABLE 7

Zone Diameter (mm)	Interpretation
≥17	Susceptible (S)

* These interpretative standards are applicable only to disk diffusion susceptibility testing with *Haemophilus influenzae* and *Haemophilus parainfluenzae* using Haemophilus Test Medium.[2]

The current absence of data on resistant strains precludes defining any categories other than "Susceptible". Strains yielding zone diameter results suggestive of a "nonsusceptible" category should be submitted to a reference laboratory for further testing.

For *Streptococcus* spp. including *S. pneumoniae* see TABLE 8.*

TABLE 8

Zone Diameter (mm)	Interpretation
≥17	Susceptible (S)
14-16	Intermediate (I)
≤13	Resistant (R)

* These zone diameter standards for *Streptococcus* spp., including *S. pneumoniae* apply only to tests performed using Mueller-Hinton agar supplemented with 5% sheep blood and incubated in 5% CO_2.

Interpretation should be as stated above for results using dilution techniques. Interpretation involves correlation of the diameter obtained in the disk test with the MIC for levofloxacin.

As with standardized dilution techniques, diffusion methods require the use of laboratory control microorganisms to control the technical aspects of the laboratory procedures. For the diffusion technique, the 5 µg levofloxacin disk should provide the following zone diameters in these laboratory test quality control strains (see TABLE 9).

TABLE 9

Microorganism		Zone Diameter (mm)
Escherichia coli	ATCC 25922	29-37
Haemophilus influenzae	ATCC 49247*	32-40
Pseudomonas aeruginosa	ATCC 27853	19-26
Staphylococcus aureus	ATCC 25923	25-30
Streptococcus pneumoniae	ATCC 49619†	20-25

* This quality control range is applicable only to *H. Influenzae* ATCC 49247 tested by a disk diffusion procedure using Haemophilus Test Medium (HTM).[2]

† This quality control range is applicable to only *S. pneumoniae* ATCC 49619 tested by a disk diffusion procedure using Mueller-Hinton agar supplemented with 5% sheep blood and incubated in 5% CO_2.

INDICATIONS AND USAGE

Levaquin tablets/injection are indicated for the treatment of adults (≥18 years of age) with mild, moderate, and severe infections caused by susceptible strains of the designated microorganisms in the conditions listed below. Levaquin injection is indicated when intravenous administration offers a route of administration advantageous to the patient (*e.g.*, patient cannot tolerate an oral dosage form). Please see DOSAGE AND ADMINISTRATION for specific recommendations.

Acute maxillary sinusitis due to *Streptococcus pneumoniae, Haemophilus influenzae,* or *Moraxella catarrhalis.*

Acute bacterial exacerbation of chronic bronchitis due to *Staphylococcus aureus, Streptococcus pneumoniae, Haemophilus influenzae, Haemophilus parainfluenzae,* or *Moraxella catarrhalis.*

Nosocomial pneumonia due to methicillin-susceptible *Staphylococcus aureus, Pseudomonas aeruginosa, Serratia marcescens, Escherichia coli, Klebsiella pneumoniae, Haemophilus influenzae,* or *Streptococcus pneumoniae.* Adjunctive therapy should be used as clinically indicated. Where *Pseudomonas aeruginosa* is a documented or presumptive pathogen, combination therapy with an anti-pseudomonal β-lactam is recommended.

Community-acquired pneumonia due to *Staphylococcus aureus, Streptococcus pneumoniae* (including penicillin-resistant strains, MIC value for penicillin ≥2 μg/ml), *Haemophilus influenzae, Haemophilus parainfluenzae, Klebsiella pneumoniae, Moraxella catarrhalis, Chlamydia pneumoniae, Legionella pneumophila,* or *Mycoplasma pneumoniae.*

Complicated skin and skin structure infections due to methicillin-susceptible *Staphylococcus aureus, Enterococcus faecalis, Streptococcus pyogenes,* or *Proteus mirabilis.*

Uncomplicated skin and skin structure infections (mild to moderate) including abscesses, cellulitis, furuncles, impetigo, pyoderma, wound infections due to *Staphylococcus aureus,* or *Streptococcus pyogenes.*

Complicated urinary tract infections (mild to moderate) due to *Enterococcus faecalis, Enterobacter cloacae, Escherichia coli, Klebsiella pneumoniae, Proteus mirabilis,* or *Pseudomonas aeruginosa.*

Acute pyelonephritis (mild to moderate) caused by *Escherichia coli.*

Uncomplicated urinary tract infections (mild to moderate) due to *Escherichia coli, Klebsiella pneumoniae,* or *Staphylococcus saprophyticus.*

Appropriate culture and susceptibility tests should be performed before treatment in order to isolate and identify organisms causing the infection and to determine their susceptibility to levofloxacin. Therapy with levofloxacin may be initiated before results of these tests are known; once results become available, appropriate therapy should be selected.

As with other drugs in this class, some strains of *Pseudomonas aeruginosa* may develop resistance fairly rapidly during treatment with levofloxacin. Culture and susceptibility testing performed periodically during therapy will provide information about the continued susceptibility of the pathogens to the antimicrobial agent and also the possible emergence of bacterial resistance.

CONTRAINDICATIONS

Levofloxacin is contraindicated in persons with a history of hypersensitivity to levofloxacin, quinolone antimicrobial agents, or any other components of this product.

WARNINGS

THE SAFETY AND EFFICACY OF LEVOFLOXACIN IN PEDIATRIC PATIENTS, ADOLESCENTS (UNDER THE AGE OF 18 YEARS), PREGNANT WOMEN, AND NURSING WOMEN HAVE NOT BEEN ESTABLISHED. (See PRECAUTIONS: Pediatric Use, Pregnancy, Teratogenic Effects, Pregnancy Category C, and Nursing Mothers.)

In immature rats and dogs, the oral and intravenous administration of levofloxacin increased the incidence and severity of osteochondrosis. Other fluoroquinolones also produce similar erosions in the weight bearing joints and other signs of arthropathy in immature animals of various species. (See ANIMAL PHARMACOLOGY.)

Convulsions and toxic psychoses have been reported in patients receiving quinolones, including levofloxacin. Quinolones may also cause increased intracranial pressure and central nervous system stimulation which may lead to tremors, restlessness, anxiety, lightheadedness, confusion, hallucinations, paranoia, depression, nightmares, insomnia, and, rarely, suicidal thoughts or acts. These reactions may occur following the first dose. If these reactions occur in patients receiving levofloxacin, the drug should be discontinued and appropriate measures instituted. As with other quinolones, levofloxacin should be used with caution in patients with a known or suspected CNS disorder that may predispose to seizures or lower the seizure threshold (*e.g.*, severe cerebral arteriosclerosis, epilepsy) or in the presence of other risk factors that may predispose to seizures or lower the seizure threshold (*e.g.*, certain drug therapy, renal dysfunction.) (See PRECAUTIONS: General and Information for the Patient; DRUG INTERACTIONS; and ADVERSE REACTIONS.)

Serious and occasionally fatal hypersensitivity and/or anaphylactic reactions have been reported in patients receiving therapy with quinolones, including levofloxacin. These reactions often occur following the first dose. Some reactions have been accompanied by cardiovascular collapse, hypotension/shock, seizure, loss of consciousness, tingling, angioedema (including tongue, laryngeal, throat, or facial edema/swelling), airway obstruction (including bronchospasm, shortness of breath, and acute respiratory distress), dyspnea, urticaria, itching, and other serious skin reactions. Levofloxacin should be discontinued immediately at the first appearance of a skin rash or any other sign of hypersensitivity. Serious acute hypersensitivity reactions may require treatment with epinephrine and other resuscitative measures, including oxygen, intravenous fluids, antihistamines, corticosteroids, pressor amines, and airway management, as clinically indicated. (See PRECAUTIONS and ADVERSE REACTIONS.)

Serious and sometimes fatal events, some due to hypersensitivity, and some due to uncertain etiology, have been reported rarely in patients receiving therapy with quinolones, including levofloxacin. These events may be severe and generally occur following the administration of multiple doses. Clinical manifestations may include one or more of the following: fever, rash or severe dermatologic reactions (*e.g.*, toxic epidermal necrolysis, Stevens-Johnson Syndrome); vasculitis; arthralgia; myalgia; serum sickness; allergic pneumonitis; interstitial nephritis; acute renal insufficiency or failure; hepatitis; jaundice; acute hepatic necrosis or failure; anemia, including hemolytic and aplastic; thrombocytopenia, including thrombotic thrombocytopenic purpura; leukopenia; agranulocytosis; pancytopenia; and/or other hematologic abnormalities. The drug should be discontinued immediately at the first appearance of a skin rash or any other sign of hypersensitivity and supportive measures instituted. (See PRECAUTIONS, Information for the Patient and ADVERSE REACTIONS.)

Pseudomembranous colitis has been reported with nearly all antibacterial agents, including levofloxacin, and may range in severity from mild to life-threatening. Therefore, it is important to consider this diagnosis in patients who present with diarrhea subsequent to the administration of any antibacterial agent.

Treatment with antibacterial agents alters the normal flora of the colon and may permit overgrowth of clostridia. Studies indicate that a toxin produced by *Clostridium difficile* is one primary cause of "antibiotic-associated colitis".

After the diagnosis of pseudomembranous colitis has been established, therapeutic measures should be initiated. Mild cases of pseudomembranous colitis usually respond to drug discontinuation alone. In moderate to severe cases, consideration should be given to management with fluids and electrolytes, protein supplementation, and treatment with an antibacterial drug clinically effective against *C. difficile* colitis. (See ADVERSE REACTIONS.)

Ruptures of the shoulder, hand, or Achilles tendons that required surgical repair or resulted in prolonged disability have been reported in patients receiving quinolones, including levofloxacin. Post-marketing surveillance reports indicate that this risk may be increased in patients receiving concomitant corticosteroids, especially in the elderly. Levofloxacin should be discontinued if the patient experiences pain, inflammation, or rupture of a tendon. Patients should rest and refrain from exercise until the diagnosis of tendinitis or tendon rupture has been confidently excluded. Tendon rupture can occur during or after therapy with quinolones, including levofloxacin.

PRECAUTIONS

GENERAL

Because a rapid or bolus intravenous injection may result in hypotension, LEVOFLOXACIN INJECTION SHOULD ONLY BE ADMINISTERED BY SLOW INTRAVENOUS INFUSION OVER A PERIOD OF 60 OR 90 MINUTES DEPENDING ON THE DOSAGE. (See DOSAGE AND ADMINISTRATION.)

Although levofloxacin is more soluble than other quinolones, adequate hydration of patients receiving levofloxacin should be maintained to prevent the formation of a highly concentrated urine.

Administer levofloxacin with caution in the presence of renal insufficiency. Careful clinical observation and appropriate laboratory studies should be performed prior to and during therapy since elimination of levofloxacin may be reduced. In patients with impaired renal function (creatinine clearance <50 ml/min), adjustment of the dosage regimen is necessary to avoid the accumulation of levofloxacin due to decreased clearance. (See CLINICAL PHARMACOLOGY and DOSAGE AND ADMINISTRATION.)

Moderate to severe phototoxicity reactions have been observed in patients exposed to direct sunlight while receiving drugs in this class. Excessive exposure to sunlight should be avoided. However, in clinical trials with levofloxacin, phototoxicity has been observed in less than 0.1% of patients. Therapy should be discontinued if phototoxicity (*e.g.*, a skin eruption) occurs.

As with other quinolones, levofloxacin should be used with caution in any patient with a known or suspected CNS disorder that may predispose to seizures or lower the seizure threshold (*e.g.*, severe cerebral arteriosclerosis, epilepsy) or in the presence of other risk factors that may predispose to seizures or lower the seizure threshold (*e.g.*, certain drug therapy, renal dysfunction). (See WARNINGS and DRUG INTERACTIONS.)

As with other quinolones, disturbances of blood glucose, including symptomatic hyper- and hypoglycemia, have been reported, usually in diabetic patients receiving concomitant treatment with an oral hypoglycemic agent (*e.g.*, glyburide/glibenclamide) or with insulin. In these patients, careful monitoring of blood glucose is recommended. If a hypoglycemic reaction occurs in a patient being treated with levofloxacin, levofloxacin should be discontinued immediately and appropriate therapy should be initiated immediately. (See DRUG INTERACTIONS and ADVERSE REACTIONS.)

Some quinolones, including levofloxacin, have been associated with prolongation of the QT interval on the electrocardiogram and infrequent cases of arrhythmia. During post-marketing surveillance, rare cases of torsades de pointes have been reported in patients taking levofloxacin. These reports generally involved patients with concurrent medical conditions or concomitant medications that may have been contributory. The risk of arrhythmias may be reduced by avoiding concurrent use with other drugs that prolong the QT interval including Class Ia or Class III antiarrhythmic agents; in addition, use of levofloxacin in the presence of risk factors for torsades de pointes such as hypokalemia, significant bradycardia, and cardiomyopathy should be avoided.

As with any potent antimicrobial drug, periodic assessment of organ system functions, including renal, hepatic, and hematopoietic, is advisable during therapy. (See WARNINGS and ADVERSE REACTIONS.)

INFORMATION FOR THE PATIENT

Patients Should Be Advised:

- To drink fluids liberally.
- That antacids containing magnesium, or aluminum, as well as sucralfate, metal cations such as iron, and multivitamin preparations with zinc or didanosine, chewable/buffered tablets or the pediatric powder for oral solution should be taken at least 2 hours before or 2 hours after oral levofloxacin administration. (See DRUG INTERACTIONS.)
- That oral levofloxacin can be taken without regard to meals.
- That levofloxacin may cause neurologic adverse effects (*e.g.*, dizziness, lightheadedness) and that patients should know how they react to levofloxacin before they operate an automobile or machinery or engage in other activities requiring mental alertness and coordination. (See WARNINGS and ADVERSE REACTIONS.)
- To discontinue treatment and inform their physician if they experience pain, inflammation, or rupture of a tendon, and to rest and refrain from exercise until the diagnosis of tendinitis or tendon rupture has been confidently excluded.
- That levofloxacin may be associated with hypersensitivity reactions, even following the first dose, and to discontinue the drug at the first sign of a skin rash, hives or other skin reactions, a rapid heartbeat, difficulty in swallowing or breathing, any swelling suggesting angioedema (*e.g.*, swelling of the lips, tongue, face, tightness of the throat, hoarseness), or other symptoms of an allergic reaction. (See WARNINGS and ADVERSE REACTIONS.)
- To avoid excessive sunlight or artificial ultraviolet light while receiving levofloxacin and to discontinue therapy if phototoxicity (*i.e.*, skin eruption) occurs.
- That if they are diabetic and are being treated with insulin or an oral hypoglycemic agent and a hypoglycemic reaction occurs, they should discontinue levofloxacin and consult a physician. (See PRECAUTIONS, General and DRUG INTERACTIONS.)
- That concurrent administration of warfarin and levofloxacin has been associated with increases of the International Normalized Ratio (INR) or prothrombin time and clinical episodes of bleeding. Patients should notify their physician if they are taking warfarin.
- That convulsions have been reported in patients taking quinolones, including levofloxacin, and to notify their physician before taking this drug if there is a history of this condition.

CARCINOGENESIS, MUTAGENESIS, AND IMPAIRMENT OF FERTILITY

In a lifetime bioassay in rats, levofloxacin exhibited no carcinogenic potential following daily dietary administration for 2 years; the highest dose (100 mg/kg/day) was 1.4 times the highest recommended human dose (750 mg) based upon relative body surface area. Levofloxacin did not shorten the time to tumor development of UV-induced skin tumors in hairless albino (Skh-1) mice at any levofloxacin dose level and was therefore not photo-carcinogenic under conditions of this study. Dermal levofloxacin concentrations in the hairless mice ranged from 25-42 μg/g at the highest levofloxacin dose level (300 mg/kg/day) used in the photo-carcinogenicity study. By comparison, dermal levofloxacin concentrations in human subjects receiving 750 mg of levofloxacin averaged approximately 11.8 μg/g at C_{max}.

Levofloxacin was not mutagenic in the following assays; Ames bacterial mutation assay (*S. typhimurium* and *E. coli*), CHO/HGPRT forward mutation assay, mouse micronucleus test, mouse dominant lethal test, rat unscheduled DNA synthesis assay, and the mouse sister chromatid exchange assay. It was positive in the *in vitro* chromosomal aberration (CHL cell line) and sister chromatid exchange (CHL/IU cell line) assays.

Levofloxacin caused no impairment of fertility or reproductive performance in rats at oral doses as high as 360 mg/kg/day, corresponding to 4.2 times the highest recommended human dose based upon relative body surface area and intravenous doses as high as 100 mg/kg/day, corresponding to 1.2 times the highest recommended human dose based upon relative body surface area.

PREGNANCY, TERATOGENIC EFFECTS, PREGNANCY CATEGORY C

Levofloxacin was not teratogenic in rats at oral doses as high as 810 mg/kg/day which corresponds to 9.4 times the highest recommended human dose based upon relative body surface area, or at intravenous doses as high as 160 mg/kg/day corresponding to 1.9 times the highest recommended human dose based upon relative body surface area. The oral dose of 810 mg/kg/day to rats caused decreased fetal body weight and increased fetal mortality. No teratogenicity was observed when rabbits were dosed orally as high as 50 mg/kg/day which corresponds to 1.1 times the highest recommended human dose based upon relative body surface area, or when dosed intravenously as high as 25 mg/kg/day, corresponding to 0.5 times the highest recommended human dose based upon relative body surface area.

There are, however, no adequate and well-controlled studies in pregnant women. Levofloxacin should be used during pregnancy only if the potential benefit justifies the potential risk to the fetus. (See WARNINGS.)

NURSING MOTHERS

Levofloxacin has not been measured in human milk. Based upon data from ofloxacin, it can be presumed that levofloxacin will be excreted in human milk. Because of the potential for serious adverse reactions from levofloxacin in nursing infants, a decision should be made whether to discontinue nursing or to discontinue the drug, taking into account the importance of the drug to the mother.

PEDIATRIC USE

Safety and effectiveness in pediatric patients and adolescents below the age of 18 years have not been established. Quinolones, including levofloxacin, cause arthropathy and osteochondrosis in juvenile animals of several species. (See WARNINGS.)

GERIATRIC USE

In Phase 3 clinical trials, 1190 levofloxacin-treated patients (25%) were ≥65 years of age. Of these, 675 patients (14%) were between the ages of 65 and 74 and 515 patients (11%) were 75 years or older. No overall differences in safety or effectiveness were observed between these subjects and younger subjects, and other reported clinical experience has not identified differences in responses between the elderly and younger patients, but greater sensitivity of some older individuals cannot be ruled out.

The pharmacokinetic properties of levofloxacin in younger adults and elderly adults do not differ significantly when creatinine clearance is taken into consideration. However since the drug is known to be substantially excreted by the kidney, the risk of toxic reactions to this drug may be greater in patients with impaired renal function. Because elderly patients are more likely to have decreased renal function, care should be taken in dose selection, and it may be useful to monitor renal function.

DRUG INTERACTIONS

ANTACIDS, SUCRALFATE, METAL CATIONS, MULTIVITAMINS

Levaquin Tablets

While the chelation by divalent cations is less marked than with other quinolones, concurrent administration of Levaquin tablets with antacids containing magnesium, or aluminum, as well as sucralfate, metal cations such as iron, and multivitamin preparations with zinc may interfere with the gastrointestinal absorption of levofloxacin, resulting in systemic levels considerably lower than desired. Tablets with antacids containing magnesium, aluminum, as well as sucralfate, metal cations such as iron, and multivitamins preparations with zinc or didanosine, chewable/buffered tablets or the pediatric powder for oral solution may substantially interfere with the gastrointestinal absorption of levofloxacin, resulting in systemic levels considerably lower than desired. These agents should be taken at least 2 hours before or 2 hours after levofloxacin administration.

Levaquin Injection

There are no data concerning an interaction of **intravenous** quinolones with **oral** antacids, sucralfate, multivitamins, didanosine, or metal cations. However, no quinolone should be co-administered with any solution containing multivalent cations, *e.g.*, magnesium, through the same intravenous line. (See DOSAGE AND ADMINISTRATION.)

THEOPHYLLINE

No significant effect of levofloxacin on the plasma concentrations, AUC, and other disposition parameters for theophylline was detected in a clinical study involving 14 healthy volunteers. Similarly, no apparent effect of theophylline on levofloxacin absorption and disposition was observed. However, concomitant administration of other quinolones with theophylline has resulted in prolonged elimination half-life, elevated serum theophylline levels, and a subsequent increase in the risk of theophylline-related adverse reactions in the patient population. Therefore, theophylline levels should be closely monitored and appropriate dosage adjustments made when levofloxacin is co-administered. Adverse reactions, including seizures, may occur with or without an elevation in serum theophylline levels. (See WARNINGS and PRECAUTIONS, General.)

WARFARIN

No significant effect of levofloxacin on the peak plasma concentrations, AUC, and other disposition parameters for R- and S-warfarin was detected in a clinical study involving healthy volunteers. Similarly, no apparent effect of warfarin on levofloxacin absorption and disposition was observed. There have been reports during the post-marketing experience in patients that levofloxacin enhances the effects of warfarin. Elevations of the prothrombin time in the setting of concurrent warfarin and levofloxacin use have been associated with episodes of bleeding. Prothrombin time, International Normalized Ratio (INR), or other suitable anticoagulation tests should be closely monitored if levofloxacin is administered concomitantly with warfarin. Patients should also be monitored for evidence of bleeding.

CYCLOSPORINE

No significant effect of levofloxacin on the peak plasma concentrations, AUC, and other disposition parameters for cyclosporine was detected in a clinical study involving healthy volunteers. However, elevated serum levels of cyclosporine have been reported in the patient population when co-administered with some other quinolones. Levofloxacin C_{max} and ke were slightly lower while T_{max} and $T_{1/2}$ were slightly longer in the presence of cyclosporine than those observed in other studies without concomitant medication. The differences, however, are not considered to be clinically significant. Therefore, no dosage adjustment is required for levofloxacin or cyclosporine when administered concomitantly.

DIGOXIN

No significant effect of levofloxacin on the peak plasma concentrations, AUC, and other disposition parameters for digoxin was detected in a clinical study involving healthy volunteers. Levofloxacin absorption and disposition kinetics were similar in the presence or absence of digoxin. Therefore, no dosage adjustment for levofloxacin or digoxin is required when administered concomitantly.

PROBENECID AND CIMETIDINE

No significant effect of probenecid or cimetidine on the rate and extent of levofloxacin absorption was observed in a clinical study involving healthy volunteers. The AUC and $T_{1/2}$ of levofloxacin were 27-38% and 30% higher, respectively, while CL/F and CLR were 21-35% lower during concomitant treatment with probenecid or cimetidine compared to levofloxacin alone. Although these differences were statistically significant, the changes were not high enough to warrant dosage adjustment for levofloxacin when probenecid or cimetidine is co-administered.

NON-STEROIDAL ANTI-INFLAMMATORY DRUGS

The concomitant administration of a non-steroidal anti-inflammatory drug with a quinolone, including levofloxacin, may increase the risk of CNS stimulation and convulsive seizures. (See WARNINGS and PRECAUTIONS, General.)

ANTIDIABETIC AGENTS

Disturbances of blood glucose, including hyperglycemia and hypoglycemia, have been reported in patients treated concomitantly with quinolones and an antidiabetic agent. Therefore, careful monitoring of blood glucose is recommended when these agents are co-administered.

ADVERSE REACTIONS

The incidence of drug-related adverse reactions in patients during Phase 3 clinical trials conducted in North America was 6.2%. Among patients receiving levofloxacin therapy, 4.1% discontinued levofloxacin therapy due to adverse experiences. The overall incidence, type and distribution of adverse events was similar in patients receiving levofloxacin doses of 750 mg once daily compared to patients receiving doses from 250 mg once daily to 500 mg twice daily.

In clinical trials, the following events were considered likely to be drug-related in patients receiving levofloxacin: Nausea 1.3%, diarrhea 1.0%, vaginitis 0.7%, insomnia 0.4%, abdominal pain 0.4%, flatulence 0.3%, pruritus 0.3%, dizziness 0.3%, dyspepsia 0.3%, rash 0.3%, genital moniliasis 0.2%, taste perversion 0.2%, vomiting 0.2%, constipation 0.1%, fungal infection 0.1%, genital pruritus 0.1%, headache 0.1%, moniliasis 0.1%, nervousness 0.1%, rash erythematous 0.1%, urticaria 0.1%.

In clinical trials, the following events occurred in >3% of patients, regardless of drug relationship: Nausea 7.0%, headache 6.1%, diarrhea 5.7%, insomnia 4.5%, injection site reaction 3.5%, constipation 3.3%.

In clinical trials, the following events occurred in 1-3% of patients, regardless of drug relationship: Dizziness 2.6%, abdominal pain 2.5%, dyspepsia 2.3%, vomiting 2.4%, vaginitis 1.8%, injection site pain 1.7%, flatulence 1.4%, pain 1.4%, pruritus 1.3%, sinusitis 1.3%, chest pain 1.2%, fatigue 1.3%, rash 1.4%, back pain 1.1%, injection site inflammation 1.1%, rhinitis 1.0%, taste perversion 1.0%.

In clinical trials, the following events, of potential medical importance, occurred at a rate of 0.1 to 1.0%, regardless of drug relationship:

Autonomic nervous system disorders: Postural hypotension.

Body as a whole — general disorders: Asthenia, edema, fever, malaise, rigors, substernal chest pain, syncope, enlarged abdomen, allergic reaction, headache, hot flashes, edema, influenza-like symptoms, leg pain, multiple organ failure.

Cardiovascular disorders, general: Cardiac failure, circulatory failure, hypertension, hypotension, postural hypotension.

Central and peripheral nervous system disorders: Abnormal coordination, coma, convulsions (seizures), hyperkinesia, hypertonia, hypoaesthesia, involuntary muscle contractions, paresthesia, paralysis, speech disorder, stupor, tremor, vertigo, encephalopathy, abnormal gait, leg cramps, intracranial hypertension.

Gastrointestinal system disorders: Dry mouth, dysphagia, gastroenteritis, GI hemorrhage, pancreatitis, pseudomembranous colitis, tongue edema, gastritis, gastroesophageal reflux, melena, esophagitis, stomatitis.

Hearing and vestibular disorders: Earache, tinnitus.

Heart rate and rhythm disorders: Arrhythmia, atrial fibrillation, bradycardia, cardiac arrest, palpitation, supraventricular tachycardia, ventricular tacyhcardia, tachycardia.

Liver and biliary system disorders: Elevated bilirubin, abnormal hepatic function, cholelithiasis, jaundice, hepatic failure.

Metabolic and nutritional disorders: Hypomagnesemia, thirst, aggravated diabetes mellitus, dehydration, hyperglycemia, hyperkalemia, hypoglycemia, hypokalemia.

Musculoskeletal system disorders: Arthralgia, arthritis, arthrosis, pathological fracture, myalgia, osteomyelitis, synovitis, tendinitis.

Myo-, endo-, pericardial and valve disorders: Angina pectoris, myocardial infarction.

Neoplasms: Carcinoma.

Other special senses disorders: Parosmia, taste perversion.

Platelet, bleeding and clotting disorders: Pulmonary embolism, hematoma, epistaxis, purpura, thrombocytopenia.

Psychiatric disorders: Abnormal dreaming, agitation, anorexia, anxiety, confusion, depression, hallucination, nervousness, paranoia, sleep disorder, somnolence.

Red blood cell disorders: Anemia.

Reproductive disorders: Dysmenorrhea, leukorrhea.

Resistance mechanism disorders: Abscess, herpes simplex, bacterial infection, viral infection, moniliasis, otitis media, sepsis, fungal infection.

Respiratory system disorders: Bronchitis, epistaxis, pharyngitis, rhinitis, upper respiratory tract infection, asthma, coughing, dyspnea, haemoptysis, hypoxia, pleural effusion, respiratory insufficiency.

Skin and appendages disorders: Rash, dry skin, genital pruritus, increased sweating, skin disorder, skin exfoliation, skin ulceration, urticaria.

Urinary system disorders: Urinary tract infection, abnormal renal function, acute renal failure, hematuria.

Vascular (extracardiac) disorders: Cerebrovascular disorder, phlebitis, purpura, thrombophlebitis (deep).

Vision disorders: Abnormal vision, conjunctivitis.

White cell and RES disorders: Granulocytopenia, leukocytosis, lymphadenopathy, WBC abnormal (not otherwise specified).

In clinical trials using multiple-dose therapy, ophthalmologic abnormalities, including cataracts and multiple punctate lenticular opacities, have been noted in patients undergoing treatment with other quinolones. The relationship of the drugs to these events is not presently established.

Crystalluria and cylindruria have been reported with other quinolones.

The following markedly abnormal laboratory values appeared in >2% of patients receiving levofloxacin. It is not known whether these abnormalities were caused by the drug or the underlying condition being treated.

Blood chemistry: Decreased glucose (2.2%).

Hematology: Decreased lymphocytes (2.4%).

POST-MARKETING ADVERSE REACTIONS

Additional adverse events reported from worldwide post-marketing experience with levofloxacin include: Allergic pneumonitis, anaphylactic shock, anaphylactoid reaction, dysphonia, abnormal EEG, encephalopathy, eosinophilia, erythema multiforme, hemolytic anemia, multi-system organ failure, increased International Normalized Ratio (INR)/prothrombin time, Stevens-Johnson Syndrome, tendon rupture, torsades de pointes, vasodilation.

DOSAGE AND ADMINISTRATION

Levaquin injection should only be administered by intravenous infusion. It is not for intramuscular, intrathecal, intraperitoneal, or subcutaneous administration.

CAUTION: RAPID OR BOLUS INTRAVENOUS INFUSION MUST BE AVOIDED. Levofloxacin injection should be infused intravenously slowly over a period of not less than 60 or 90 minutes, depending on the dosage. (See PRECAUTIONS.)

Single-use vials require dilution prior to administration. (See Preparation of Levofloxacin Injection for Administration.)

The usual dose of Levaquin tablets/injection is 250 or 500 mg administered orally or by slow infusion over 60 minutes every 24 hours or 750 mg administered by slow infusion over 90 minutes every 24 hours, as indicated by infection and described in the following dosing chart. These recommendations apply to patients with normal renal function (*i.e.*, creatinine clearance >80 ml/min). For patients with altered renal function see Patients With Impaired Renal Function. Oral doses should be administered at least 2 hours before or 2 hours after antacids containing magnesium, aluminum, as well as sucralfate, metal cations such as iron, and multivitamin preparations with zinc or didanosine, chewable/buffered tablets or the pediatric powder for oral solution.

PATIENTS WITH NORMAL RENAL FUNCTION

TABLE 12

Infection*	Unit Dose	Freq.	Duration†	Daily Dose
Acute bacterial exacerbation of chronic bronchitis	500 mg	q24h	7 days	500 mg
Nosocomial pneumonia	750 mg	q24h	7-14 days	750 mg
Community acquired pneumonia	500 mg	q24h	7-14 days	500 mg
Acute maxillary sinusitis	500 mg	q24h	10-14 days	500 mg
Complicated SSSI	750 mg	q24h	7-14 days	750 mg
Uncomplicated SSSI	500 mg	q24h	7-10 days	500 mg
Complicated UTI	250 mg	q24h	10 days	250 mg
Acute pyelonephritis	250 mg	q24h	10 days	250 mg
Uncomplicated UTI	250 mg	q24h	3 days	250 mg

* DUE TO THE DESIGNATED PATHOGENS. (See INDICATIONS AND USAGE.)
† Sequential therapy (IV to oral) may be instituted at the discretion of the physician.

PATIENTS WITH IMPAIRED RENAL FUNCTION

TABLE 13

Renal Status	Initial Dose	Subsequent Dose
Acute Bacterial Exacerbation of Chronic Bronchitis/Community-Acquired Pneumonia/Acute Maxillary Sinusitis/Uncomplicated SSSI		
CLCR from 50-80 ml/min	No dosage adjustment required	
CLCR from 20-49 ml/min	500 mg	250 mg q24h
CLCR from 10-19 ml/min	500 mg	250 mg q48h
Hemodialysis	500 mg	250 mg q48h
CAPD	500 mg	250 mg q48h
Complicated SSSI/Nosocomial Pneumonia		
CLCR from 50-80 ml/min	No dosage adjustment required	
CLCR from 20-49 ml/min	750 mg	750 mg q48h
CLCR from 10-19 ml/min	750 mg	500 mg q48h
Hemodialysis	750 mg	500 mg q48h
CAPD	750 mg	500 mg q48h
Complicated UTI/Acute Pyelonephritis		
CLCR ≥20 ml/min	No dosage adjustment required	
CLCR from 10-19 ml/min	250 mg	250 mg q48h
Uncomplicated UTI	No dosage adjustment required	

CLCR = Creatinine clearances.
CAPD = Chronic ambulatory peritoneal dialysis.

When only the serum creatinine is known, the following formula may be used to estimate creatinine clearance:

Men: Creatinine Clearance (ml/min) = [Weight (kg) × (140 - age)] ÷ [72 × serum creatinine (mg/dl)]

Women: 0.85 × the value calculated for men.

The serum creatinine should represent a steady state of renal function.

PREPARATION OF LEVOFLOXACIN INJECTION FOR ADMINISTRATION

Levaquin Injection in Single-Use Vials

Levaquin injection is supplied in single-use vials containing a concentrated levofloxacin solution with the equivalent of 500 mg (20 ml vial) and 750 mg (30 ml vial) of levofloxacin in water for injection. The 20 and 30 ml vials each contain 25 mg of levofloxacin/ml. **THESE LEVAQUIN INJECTION SINGLE-USE VIALS MUST BE FURTHER DILUTED WITH AN APPROPRIATE SOLUTION PRIOR TO INTRAVENOUS ADMINISTRATION.** (See Compatible Intravenous Solutions.) The concentration of the resulting diluted solution should be 5 mg/ml prior to administration.

This intravenous drug product should be inspected visually for particulate matter prior to administration. Samples containing visible particles should be discarded.

Since no preservative or bacteriostatic agent is present in this product, aseptic technique must be used in preparation of the final intravenous solution. **Since the vials are for single-use only, any unused portion remaining in the vial should be discarded. When used to prepare two 250 mg doses from the 20 ml vial containing 500 mg of levofloxacin, the full content of the vial should be withdrawn at once using a single-entry procedure, and a second dose should be prepared and stored for subsequent use.** (See Stability of Levaquin Injection Following Dilution.)

Since only limited data are available on the compatibility of levofloxacin intravenous injection with other intravenous substances, **additives or other medications should not be**

added to Levaquin injection in single-use vials or infused simultaneously through the same intravenous line. If the same intravenous line is used for sequential infusion of several different drugs, the line should be flushed before and after infusion of Levaquin injection with an infusion solution compatible with Levaquin injection and with any other drug(s) administered via this common line.

Compatible Intravenous Solutions

Any of the following intravenous solutions may be used to prepare a 5 mg/ml levofloxacin solution with the approximate pH values (see TABLE 14).

TABLE 14

Intravenous Fluids	Final pH of Levaquin Solution
0.9% Sodium chloride injection	4.71
5% Dextrose injection	4.58
5% Dextrose/0.9% NaCl injection	4.62
5% Dextrose in lactated Ringers	4.92
Plasma-Lyte 56/5% dextrose injection	5.03
5% Dextrose, 0.45% sodium chloride, and 0.15% potassium chloride injection	4.61
Sodium lactate injection (M/6)	5.54

Levaquin Injection Premix in Single-Use Flexible Containers

Levaquin injection is also supplied in flexible containers containing a premixed, ready-to-use levofloxacin solution in D_5W for single-use. The fill volume is either 50 or 100 ml for the 100 ml flexible container or 150 ml for the 150 ml container. **NO FURTHER DILUTION OF THESE PREPARATIONS ARE NECESSARY. Consequently each 50 ml, 100 ml, and 150 ml premix flexible container already contains a dilute solution with the equivalent of 250 mg, 500 mg, and 750 mg of levofloxacin, respectively (5 mg/ml) in 5% dextrose (D_5W).**

This parenteral drug product should be inspected visually for particulate matter prior to administration. Samples containing visible particles should be discarded.

Since the premix flexible containers are for single-use only, any unused portion should be discarded.

Since only limited data are available on the compatibility of levofloxacin intravenous injection with other intravenous substances, **additives or other medications should not be added to Levaquin injection in flexible containers or infused simultaneously through the same intravenous line.** If the same intravenous line is used for sequential infusion of several different drugs, the line should be flushed before and after infusion of Levaquin injection with an infusion solution compatible with Levaquin injection and with any other drug(s) administered via this common line.

Stability of Levaquin Injection as Supplied

When stored under recommended conditions, Levaquin injection, as supplied in 20 and 30 ml vials, or 100 and 150 ml flexible containers, is stable through the expiration date printed on the label.

Stability of Levaquin Injection Following Dilution

Levaquin injection, when diluted in a compatible intravenous fluid to a concentration of 5 mg/ml, is stable for 72 hours when stored at or below 25°C (77°F) and for 14 days when stored under refrigeration at 5°C (41°F) in plastic intravenous containers. Solutions that are diluted in a compatible intravenous solution and frozen in glass bottles or plastic intravenous containers are stable for 6 months when stored at -20°C (-4°F). **THAW FROZEN SOLUTIONS AT ROOM TEMPERATURE 25°C (77°F) OR IN A REFRIGERATOR 8°C (46°F). DO NOT FORCE THAW BY MICROWAVE IRRADIATION OR WATER BATH IMMERSION. DO NOT REFREEZE AFTER INITIAL THAWING.**

ANIMAL PHARMACOLOGY

Levofloxacin and other quinolones have been shown to cause arthropathy in immature animals of most species tested. (See WARNINGS.) In immature dogs (4-5 months old), oral doses of 10 mg/kg/day for 7 days and intravenous doses of 4 mg/kg/day for 14 days of levofloxacin resulted in arthropathic lesions. Administration at oral doses of 300 mg/kg/day for 7 days and intravenous doses of 60 mg/kg/day for 4 weeks produced arthropathy in juvenile rats.

When tested in a mouse ear swelling bioassay, levofloxacin exhibited phototoxicity similar in magnitude to ofloxacin, but less phototoxicity than other quinolones.

While crystalluria has been observed in some intravenous rat studies, urinary crystals are not formed in the bladder, being present only after micturition and are not associated with nephrotoxicity.

In mice, the CNS stimulatory effect of quinolones is enhanced by concomitant administration of non-steroidal anti-inflammatory drugs.

In dogs, levofloxacin administered at 6 mg/kg or higher by rapid intravenous injection produced hypotensive effects. These effects were considered to be related to histamine release.

In vitro and *in vivo* studies in animals indicate that levofloxacin is neither an enzyme inducer or inhibitor in the human therapeutic plasma concentration range; therefore, no drug metabolizing enzyme-related interactions with other drugs or agents are anticipated.

HOW SUPPLIED

LEVAQUIN TABLETS

Levaquin (levofloxacin) tablets are supplied in:

250 mg: Terra cotta pink, modified rectangular, film-coated tablets, debossed "LEVAQUIN" on side 1 and "250" on side 2.

500 mg: Peach, modified rectangular, film-coated tablets, debossed "LEVAQUIN" on side 1 and "500" on side 2.

750 mg: White, modified rectangular, film-coated tablets, debossed "LEVAQUIN" on side 1 and "750" on side 2.

Storage: Levaquin tablets should be stored at 15-30°C (59-86°F) in well-closed containers.

LEVAQUIN INJECTION

Single-Use Vials

Levaquin (levofloxacin) injection is supplied in single-use vials. Each vial contains a concentrated solution of 25 mg/ml with the equivalent of 500 mg of levofloxacin in 20 ml vials and 750 mg of levofloxacin in 30 ml vials.

Storage: Levaquin injection in single-use vials should be stored at controlled room temperature and protected from light.

Premix in Flexible Containers

Levaquin (levofloxacin in 5% dextrose) injection is supplied as a single-use, premixed solution in flexible containers.

Each bag contains a dilute solution of 5 mg/ml with the equivalent of 250 (50 ml flexible container), 500 (100 ml flexible container), or 750 (150 ml flexible container) mg of levofloxacin, respectively, in 5% dextrose (D_5W).

Storage: Levaquin injection premix in flexible containers should be stored at or below 25°C (77°F); however, brief exposure up to 40°C (104°F) does not adversely affect the product. Avoid excessive heat and protect from freezing and light.

PRODUCT LISTING - EQUIVALENTS NOT AVAILABLE

Solution - Intravenous - 25 mg/ml

20 ml	$45.65	LEVAQUIN, Janssen Pharmaceuticals	00045-0069-51
30 ml	$60.59	LEVAQUIN, Janssen Pharmaceuticals	00045-0065-55

Solution - Intravenous - 250 mg/50 ml

50 ml x 24	$547.92	LEVAQUIN, Janssen Pharmaceuticals	00045-0067-01

Solution - Intravenous - 500 mg/100 ml

100 ml x 24	$1095.60	LEVAQUIN, Janssen Pharmaceuticals	00045-0068-01

Solution - Intravenous - 750 mg/150 ml

150 ml x 24	$1373.04	LEVAQUIN, Janssen Pharmaceuticals	00045-0066-01

Solution - Ophthalmic - 0.5%

5 ml	$40.10	QUIXIN, Santen Inc	65086-0135-05

Tablet - Oral - 250 mg

3's	$21.92	LEVAQUIN, Allscripts Pharmaceutical Company	54569-4915-01
10's	$73.07	LEVAQUIN, Allscripts Pharmaceutical Company	54569-4915-00
10's	$87.14	LEVAQUIN, Physicians Total Care	54868-4175-00
50's	$431.36	LEVAQUIN, Janssen Pharmaceuticals	00045-1520-50
100's	$868.76	LEVAQUIN, Janssen Pharmaceuticals	00045-1520-10

Tablet - Oral - 500 mg

1's	$12.61	LEVAQUIN, Pharma Pac	52959-0492-01
2's	$17.17	LEVAQUIN, Allscripts Pharmaceutical Company	54569-4489-01
3's	$25.76	LEVAQUIN, Allscripts Pharmaceutical Company	54569-4489-02
6's	$69.37	LEVAQUIN, Pharma Pac	52959-0492-06
7's	$60.10	LEVAQUIN, Allscripts Pharmaceutical Company	54569-4489-03
7's	$62.13	LEVAQUIN, Southwood Pharmaceuticals Inc	58016-0573-07
7's	$71.46	LEVAQUIN, Physicians Total Care	54868-3923-01
7's	$73.57	LEVAQUIN, Pharma Pac	52959-0492-07
10's	$85.85	LEVAQUIN, Allscripts Pharmaceutical Company	54569-4489-00
10's	$88.76	LEVAQUIN, Southwood Pharmaceuticals Inc	58016-0573-10
10's	$101.58	LEVAQUIN, Physicians Total Care	54868-3923-00
10's	$104.18	LEVAQUIN, Pharma Pac	52959-0492-10
12's	$122.52	LEVAQUIN, Pharma Pac	52959-0492-12
20's	$177.51	LEVAQUIN, Southwood Pharmaceuticals Inc	58016-0573-20
30's	$304.13	LEVAQUIN, Pharma Pac	52959-0492-30
50's	$503.81	LEVAQUIN, Janssen Pharmaceuticals	00045-1525-50
100's	$887.57	LEVAQUIN, Southwood Pharmaceuticals Inc	58016-0573-00
100's	$1013.70	LEVAQUIN, Janssen Pharmaceuticals	00045-1525-10

Tablet - Oral - 750 mg

50's	$614.21	LEVAQUIN, Janssen Pharmaceuticals	00045-1530-50
100's	$1228.45	LEVAQUIN, Janssen Pharmaceuticals	00045-1530-10

Levonorgestrel *(003015)*

Categories: Contraception; Pregnancy Category X; FDA Approved 1990 Dec; WHO Formulary
Drug Classes: Contraceptives; Hormones/hormone modifiers; Progestins
Brand Names: **Norplant**
Foreign Brand Availability: Ange 28 (Japan); duofem (Germany); ECEEZ (India); Levonelle (New-Zealand); Microlut (Colombia); Microval (Colombia); Mirena (Australia; China; Colombia; Germany; Hong-Kong; Israel; Korea; New-Zealand; Philippines; South-Africa; Thailand); Norlevo (France; South-Africa); Norplant 36 (Israel); Plan B (Canada); Postinor-2 (Israel; New-Zealand; Singapore); Vikela (France)

DESCRIPTION

Patients should be counseled that this product does not protect against HIV infection (AIDS) and other sexually transmitted diseases.

The Norplant System kit contains levonorgestrel implants, a set of 6 flexible closed capsules made of silicone rubber tubing (Silastic, dimethylsiloxane/methylvinylsiloxane copolymer), each containing 36 mg of the progestin levonorgestrel contained in an insertion kit to facilitate implantation. The capsules are sealed with Silastic (polydimethylsiloxane) adhesive and sterilized. Each capsule is 2.4 mm in diameter and 34 mm in length. The capsules are inserted in a superficial plane beneath the skin of the upper arm.

Information contained herewith regarding safety and efficacy was derived from studies which used two slightly different Silastic tubing formulations. The formulation being used

L

in the Norplant System has slightly higher release rates of levonorgestrel and at least comparable efficacy.

Evidence indicates that the dose of levonorgestrel provided by the Norplant System is initially about 85 μg/day followed by a decline to about 50 μg/day by 9 months and to about 35 μg/day by 18 months with a further decline thereafter to about 30 μg/day. The Norplant System is a progestin-only product and does not contain estrogen.

Levonorgestrel, (d)(-)-13-beta-ethyl-17-alpha-ethinyl-17-beta-hydroxygon-4-en-3-one), the active ingredient in the Norplant System, has a molecular weight of 312.45.

CLINICAL PHARMACOLOGY

Levonorgestrel is a totally synthetic and biologically active progestin which exhibits no significant estrogenic activity and is highly progestational. The absolute configuration conforms to that of D-natural steroids. Levonorgestrel is not subjected to a "first-pass" effect and is virtually 100% bioavailable. Plasma concentrations average approximately 0.30 ng/ml over 5 years but are highly variable as a function of individual metabolism and body weight.

Diffusion of levonorgestrel through the wall of each capsule provides a continuous low dose of the progestin. Resulting blood levels are substantially below those generally observed among users of combination oral contraceptives containing the progestins norgestrel or levonorgestrel. Because of the range of variability in blood levels and variation in individual response, blood levels alone are not predictive of the risk of pregnancy in an individual woman.

At least two mechanisms are active in preventing pregnancy: ovulation inhibition and thickening of the cervical mucus. Other mechanisms may add to these contraceptive effects.

Levonorgestrel concentrations among women show considerable variation depending on individual clearance rates, body weight, and possibly other factors. Levonorgestrel concentrations reach a maximum, or near maximum, within 24 hours after placement with mean values of 1600 ± 1100 pg/ml. They decline rapidly over the first month partially due to a circulating protein, SHBG, that binds levonorgestrel and which is depressed by the presence of levonorgestrel. At 3 months, mean levels decline to values of around 400 pg/ml while concentrations normalized to a 60 kg body weight were 327 ± 119 (SD) pg/ml at 12 months with further decline by 1.4 pg/ml/month to reach 258 ± 95 (SD) pg/ml at 60 months. Concentrations decreased with an increasing body weight by a mean of 3.3 pg/ml/kg. After capsule removal, mean concentrations drop to below 100 pg/ml by 96 hours and to below assay sensitivity (50 pg/ml) by 5-14 days. Fertility rates return to levels comparable to those seen in the general population of women using no method of contraception. Circulating concentrations can be used to forecast the risk of pregnancy only in a general statistical sense. Mean concentrations associated with pregnancy have been 210 ± 60 (SD) pg/ml. However, in clinical studies, 20% of women had one or more values below 200 pg/ml but an average annual gross pregnancy rate of less than 1.0 per 100 women through 5 years.

Although lipoprotein levels were altered in several clinical studies with the levonorgestrel implant, the long-term clinical effects of these changes have not been determined. A decrease in total cholesterol levels has been reported in all lipoprotein studies and reached statistical significance in several. Both increases and decreases in high-density lipoprotein (HDL) levels have been reported in clinical trials. No statistically significant increases have been reported in the ratio of total cholesterol to HDL-cholesterol. Low-density lipoprotein (LDL) levels decreased during levonorgestrel implant use. Triglyceride levels also decreased from pretreatment values.

INDICATIONS AND USAGE

The levonorgestrel implant is indicated for the prevention of pregnancy and is a long-term (up to 5 years) reversible contraceptive system. The capsules should be removed by the end of the 5th year. New capsules may be inserted at that time if continuing contraceptive protection is desired.

In multicenter trials with the levonorgestrel implant, involving 2470 women, the relationship between body weight and efficacy was investigated. Tabulated in TABLE 1 is the pregnancy experience as a function of body weight. Because levonorgestrel implant is a long-term method of contraception, this is reported over 5 years of use.

***TABLE 1** Annual and 5 Year Cumulative Pregnancy Rates per 100 Users by Weight Class*

Weight Class	Year 1	Year 2	Year 3	Year 4	Year 5	Cumulative
<50 kg (<110 lb)	0.2	0	0	0	0	0.2
50-59 kg (110-130 lb)	0.2	0.5	0.4	2.0	0.4	3.4
60-69 kg (131-153 lb)	0.4	0.5	1.6	1.7	0.8	5.0
≥70 kg (≥154 lb)	0	1.1	5.1	2.5	0	8.5
All	0.2	0.5	1.2	1.6	0.4	3.9

Typically, pregnancy rates with contraceptive methods are reported for only the first year of use as shown in TABLE 2. The efficacy of these contraceptive methods, except the IUD and sterilization, depends in part on the reliability of use. The efficacy of the levonorgestrel implants does not depend on patient compliance. However no contraceptive method is 100% effective.

Levonorgestrel implants gross annual discontinuation and continuation rates are summarized in TABLE 3.

CONTRAINDICATIONS

Active thrombophlebitis or thromboembolic disorders. There is insufficient information regarding women who have had previous thromboembolic disease.

Undiagnosed abnormal genital bleeding.

Known or suspected pregnancy.

Acute liver disease; benign or malignant liver tumors.

Known or suspected carcinoma of the breast.

History of idiopathic intracranial hypertension.

Hypersensitivity to levonorgestrel or any of the other components of the levonorgestrel implants.

***TABLE 2** Percentage of Women Experiencing an Unintended Pregnancy During the First Year of Use of a Contraceptive Method*

Method	Perfect Use	Typical Use
Levonorgestrel implants (6 capsules)	0.05	0.05
Male sterilization	0.1	0.15
Female sterilization	0.5	0.5
DMPA (injectable progestogen)	0.3	0.3
Oral contraceptives		5
Combined	0.1	N/A
Progestin only	0.5	N/A
IUD		
Progesterone	1.5	2.0
Copper T 380A	0.6	0.8
Condom		
(male) without spermicide	3	14
(female) without spermicide	5	21
Cervical cap		
Nulliparous women	9	20
Parous women	26	40
Diaphragm with spermicide cream or jelly	6	20
Spermicides alone (foam, creams, jellies, and vaginal suppositories)	6	26
Periodic abstinence (all methods)	1-9*	25
Withdrawal	4	19
No contraception (planned pregnancy)	85	85

N/A Not available.
* Depending on method (calendar, ovulation, symptothermal, post-ovulation) Adapted from Hatcher, RA *et al. Contraceptive Technology, 17th Revised Edition.* New York, NY: Ardent Media, 1998.

***TABLE 3** Annual and 5 Year Cumulative Rates per 100 Users*

	Year 1	Year 2	Year 3	Year 4	Year 5	Cumulative
Pregnancy	0.2	0.5	1.2	1.6	0.4	3.9
Bleeding irregularities	9.1	7.9	4.9	3.3	2.9	25.1
Medical (excl. bleeding irreg.)	6.0	5.6	4.1	4.0	5.1	22.4
Personal	4.6	7.7	11.7	10.7	11.7	38.7
Continuation	81.0	77.4	79.2	76.7	77.6	29.5

WARNINGS

WARNINGS BASED ON EXPERIENCE WITH THE LEVONORGESTREL IMPLANTS

Insertion and Removal Complications

A surgical incision is required to insert levonorgestrel implant capsules. Complications related to insertion such as pain, edema, and bruising may occur. There also have been reports of infection (including cellulitis and abscess formation), blistering, ulcerations, sloughing, excessive scarring, phlebitis, and hyperpigmentation at the insertion site. There have been reports of arm pain, numbness, and tingling following the insertion and removal procedures. There also have been reports of nerve injury, most commonly associated with deep placement and removal. Expulsion of capsules has been reported more frequently when placement of the capsules was shallow or too close to the incision or when infection was present. There have been reports of capsule displacement (*i.e.,* movement), most of which involved minor changes in the positioning of the capsules. However, infrequent reports (<1%) of significant displacement (a few to several inches) have been received. Some of these reports have been associated with pain and difficult removal. Removal is also a surgical procedure and may take longer, be more difficult, and/or cause more pain than insertion and may be associated with difficulty locating capsules. These complications may lead to the need for additional incisions and/or office visits. See also PRECAUTIONS and ADVERSE REACTIONS.

Bleeding Irregularities

Most women can expect some variation in menstrual bleeding patterns. Irregular menstrual bleeding, intermenstrual spotting, prolonged episodes of bleeding and spotting, and amenorrhea occur in some women. Irregular bleeding patterns associated with the levonorgestrel implants could mask symptoms of cervical or endometrial cancer. Overall, these irregularities diminish with continuing use. Since some levonorgestrel implant users experience periods of amenorrhea, missed menstrual periods cannot serve as the only means of identifying early pregnancy. Pregnancy tests should be performed whenever a pregnancy is suspected. Six weeks or more of amenorrhea after a pattern of regular menses may signal pregnancy. If pregnancy occurs, the capsules must be removed.

Although bleeding irregularities have occurred in clinical trials, proportionately more women had increases rather than decreases in hemoglobin concentrations, a difference that was highly statistically significant. This finding generally indicates that reduced menstrual blood loss is associated with the use of the levonorgestrel implants. In rare instances, patients experienced heavy bleeding that resulted in hemoglobin values consistent with anemia.

Ovarian Cysts (delayed follicular atresia)

If follicular development occurs with the levonorgestrel implants, atresia of the follicle is sometimes delayed, and the follicle may continue to grow beyond the size it would attain in a normal cycle. These enlarged follicles cannot be distinguished clinically from ovarian cysts. In the majority of women, enlarged follicles will spontaneously disappear and should not require surgery. Rarely, they may twist or rupture, sometimes causing abdominal pain, and surgical intervention may be required.

Ectopic Pregnancies

Ectopic pregnancies have occurred among levonorgestrel implant users, although clinical studies have shown no increase in the rate of ectopic pregnancies per year among levonorgestrel implant users as compared with users of no method or of IUDs. The incidence among levonorgestrel implant users was 1.3 per 1000 women-years, a rate significantly below the rate that has been estimated for noncontraceptive users in the US (2.7-3.0 per 1000 woman-years). The risk of ectopic pregnancy may increase with the duration of levonorgestrel implant use and possibly with increased weight of the user. Physicians should be alert to the possibility of an ectopic pregnancy among women using the levonorgestrel implant who become pregnant or complain of lower-abdominal pain. Any patient who presents with lower-abdominal pain must be evaluated to rule out ectopic pregnancy.

Foreign-Body Carcinogenesis

Rarely, cancers have occurred at the site of foreign-body intrusions or old scars. None has been reported in levonorgestrel implant clinical trials. In rodents, which are highly susceptible to such cancers, the incidence decreases with decreasing size of the foreign body. Because of the resistance of human beings to these cancers and because of the small size of the capsules, the risk to users of the levonorgestrel implants is judged to be minimal.

Thromboembolic Disorders and Other Vascular Problems

An increased risk of thromboembolic and thrombotic disease (pulmonary embolism, superficial venous thrombosis, and deep-vein thrombosis) has been found to be associated with the use of combination oral contraceptives. The relative risk has been estimated to be 4- to 11-fold higher for users than for nonusers. There have also been post-marketing reports of these events coincident with levonorgestrel implant use. The reports of thrombophlebitis and superficial phlebitis have more commonly occurred in the arm of insertion. Some of these cases have been associated with trauma to that arm.

Cerebrovascular Disorders

Combination oral contraceptives have been shown to increase both the relative and attributable risks of cerebrovascular events (thrombotic and hemorrhagic strokes), although, in general, the risk is greatest among older (>35 years) hypertensive women who also smoke. Hypertension was found to be a risk factor for both users and nonusers for both types of strokes, while smoking interacted to increase the risk for hemorrhagic strokes. There have been post-marketing reports of stroke coincident with levonorgestrel implant use.

Myocardial Infarction

An increased risk of myocardial infarction has been attributed to combination oral-contraceptive use. This is thought to be primarily thrombotic in origin and is related to the estrogen component of combination oral contraceptives. This increased risk occurs primarily in smokers or in women with other underlying risk factors for coronary-artery disease, such as family history of coronary-artery disease, hypertension, hypercholesterolemia, morbid obesity, and diabetes. The current relative risk of heart attack for combination oral-contraceptive users has been estimated as 2-6 times the risk for nonusers. The absolute risk is very low for women under 30 years of age.

Studies indicate a significant trend toward higher rates of myocardial infarctions and strokes with increasing doses of progestin in combination oral contraceptives. However, a recent study showed no increased risk of myocardial infarction associated with the past use of levonorgestrel-containing combination oral contraceptives. There have been post-marketing reports of myocardial infarction coincident with levonorgestrel implant use.

Patients who develop active thrombophlebitis or thromboembolic disease should have levonorgestrel implant capsules removed. Removal should also be considered in women who will be subjected to prolonged immobilization due to surgery or other illnesses.

Use Before or During Early Pregnancy

Extensive epidemiological studies have revealed no increased risk of birth defects in women who have used oral contraceptives prior to pregnancy. Studies also do not suggest a teratogenic effect, particularly insofar as cardiac anomalies and limb-reduction defects are concerned, when taken inadvertently during early pregnancy. There is no evidence suggesting that the risk associated with levonorgestrel implant use is different.

There have been rare reports of congenital anomalies in offspring of women who were using the levonorgestrel implants inadvertently during early pregnancy. A cause and effect relationship is not believed to exist.

Idiopathic Intracranial Hypertension

Idiopathic intracranial hypertension (pseudotumor cerebri, benign intracranial hypertension) is a disorder of unknown etiology which is seen most commonly in obese females of reproductive age. There have been reports of idiopathic intracranial hypertension in levonorgestrel implant users. A cardinal sign of idiopathic intracranial hypertension is papilledema; early symptoms may include headache (associated with a change in frequency, pattern, severity, or persistence; of particular importance are those headaches that are unremitting in nature) and visual disturbances. Patients with these symptoms, particularly obese patients or those with recent weight gain, should be screened for papilledema and, if present, the patient should be referred to a neurologist for further diagnosis and care. Levonorgestrel implants should be removed from patients experiencing this disorder.

WARNINGS BASED ON EXPERIENCE WITH COMBINATION (PROGESTIN PLUS ESTROGEN) ORAL CONTRACEPTIVES

Cigarette Smoking

Cigarette smoking increases the risk of serious cardiovascular side effects from the use of combination oral contraceptives. This risk increases with age and with the extent of smoking (in epidemiologic studies, 15 or more cigarettes per day was associated with a significantly increased risk) and is quite marked in women over 35 years old. While this is believed to be an estrogen-related effect, it is not known whether a similar risk exists with progestin-only methods such as levonorgestrel; however, women who use the levonorgestrel implants should be advised not to smoke.

Elevated Blood Pressure

Increased blood pressure has been reported in users of combination oral contraceptives. The prevalence of elevated blood pressure increases with long exposure. Although there were no statistically significant trends among levonorgestrel implant users in clinical trials, physicians should be aware of the possibility of elevated blood pressure with the levonorgestrel implants.

Carcinoma

A meta-analysis from 54 epidemiological studies reported that there is a slightly increased relative risk (RR = 1.24) of having breast cancer diagnosed in women who are currently using combination oral contraceptives compared to never-users. The increased risk gradually disappears during the course of the 10 years after cessation of combination oral contraceptive use. These studies do not provide evidence for causation. The observed pattern of increased risk of breast cancer diagnosis may be due to earlier detection of breast cancer in combination oral contraceptive users, the biological effects of combination oral contraceptives, or a combination of both. Because breast cancer is rare in women under 40 years of age, the excess number of breast cancer diagnoses in current and recent combination oral contraceptive users is small in relation to the lifetime risk of breast cancer. Breast cancers diagnosed in ever-users tend to be less advanced clinically than the cancers diagnosed in never-users. Although the results were broadly similar for progestin-only oral contraceptives, the data are based on much smaller numbers of progestin-only oral contraceptive users and therefore are less conclusive than for combination oral contraceptives. This information should be considered when prescribing the levonorgestrel implants.

Some studies suggest that combination oral-contraceptive use has been associated with an increase in the risk of cervical intraepithelial neoplasia or invasive cervical cancer in some populations of women. However, there continues to be controversy about the extent to which such findings may be due to differences in sexual behavior and other factors. In spite of many studies of the relationship between combination oral-contraceptive use and breast and cervical cancers, a cause-and-effect relationship has not been established.

Evidence indicates that combination oral contraceptives may decrease the risk of ovarian and endometrial cancer. Irregular bleeding patterns associated with the levonorgestrel implants could mask symptoms of cervical or endometrial cancer.

Hepatic Tumors

Hepatic adenomas have been found to be associated with the use of combination oral contraceptives with an estimated incidence of about 3 occurrences per 100,000 users per year, a risk that increases after 4 or more years of use. Although benign, hepatic adenomas may rupture and cause death through intra-abdominal hemorrhage. The contribution of the progestin component of oral contraceptives to the development of hepatic adenomas is not known.

Ocular Lesions

There have been clinical case reports of retinal thrombosis associated with the use of oral contraceptives that may lead to partial or complete loss of vision. Although it is believed that this adverse reaction is related to the estrogen component of oral contraceptives, the levonorgestrel implant capsules should be removed if there is unexplained partial or complete loss of vision; onset of proptosis or diplopia; papilledema; or retinal vascular lesions. Appropriate diagnostic and therapeutic measures should be undertaken immediately.

Gallbladder Disease

Earlier studies have reported an increased lifetime relative risk of gallbladder surgery in users of oral contraceptives and estrogens. More recent studies, however, have shown that the relative risk of developing gallbladder disease among oral-contraceptive users may be minimal. The recent findings of minimal risk may be related to the use of oral-contraceptive formulations containing lower hormonal doses of estrogens and progestins. The association of this risk with the use of the levonorgestrel implant progestin-only method is not known.

PRECAUTIONS

GENERAL

Patients should be counseled that this product does not protect against HIV infection (AIDS) and other sexually transmitted diseases.

Physical Examination and Follow-Up

A complete medical history and physical examination should be taken prior to the implantation or reimplantation of levonorgestrel implant capsules and at least annually during its use. These physical examinations should include special reference to the implant site, blood pressure, breasts, abdomen and pelvic organs, including cervical cytology and relevant laboratory tests. In case of undiagnosed, persistent or recurrent abnormal vaginal bleeding, appropriate diagnostic measures should be conducted to rule out malignancy. Women with a strong family history of breast cancer or who have breast nodules should be monitored with particular care.

Insertion and Removal

To be sure that the woman is not pregnant at the time of capsule placement and to assure contraceptive effectiveness during the first cycle of use, it is advisable that insertion be done during the first 7 days of the menstrual cycle or immediately following an abortion. However, levonorgestrel implant capsules may be inserted at any time during the cycle provided pregnancy has been excluded and a nonhormonal contraceptive method is used for at least 7 days following insertion. Insertion is not recommended before 6 weeks postpartum in breast-feeding women.

Insertion and removal instructions must be followed closely. It is strongly advised that all health-care professionals who insert and remove levonorgestrel implant capsules be instructed in the procedures before they attempt them. Proper insertion just under the skin will facilitate removal.

If infection develops after insertion, suitable treatment should be instituted. If infection persists, capsules should be removed.

In the case of capsule expulsion, the expelled capsule must be replaced using a new sterile capsule, as contraceptive efficacy may be inadequate with fewer than 6 capsules. If infection is present, it should be treated and cured before capsule replacement.

Removal should be done upon patient request, for medical indications, or at the end of 5 years of use, by personnel instructed in the removal technique. If the capsules were placed deeply, they may be harder to remove. The use of general anesthesia during removal should generally be avoided.

Before initiating the removal procedure, all levonorgestrel implant capsules should be located via palpation. If all 6 capsules cannot be located by palpation, they may be localized by ultrasound (7 MHz), x-ray, or compression mammography. If all capsules cannot be removed at the first attempt, removal should be attempted later when the site has healed.

Upon removal, levonorgestrel implant capsules should be disposed of in accordance with the Center for Disease Control and Prevention guidelines for the handling of biohazardous waste.

See also WARNINGS, ADVERSE REACTIONS, and "Instructions for Insertion and Removal — Removal Procedure" which is included with the prescription.

Carbohydrate and Lipid Metabolism

An altered glucose tolerance characterized by decreased insulin sensitivity following glucose loading has been found in some users of combination and progestin-only oral contraceptives. The effects of the levonorgestrel implants on carbohydrate metabolism appear to be minimal. In a study in which pretreatment serum-glucose levels were compared with levels after 1 and 2 years of levonorgestrel implant use, no statistically significant differences in mean serum-glucose levels were evident 2 hours after glucose loading. The clinical significance of these findings is unknown, but diabetic patients should be carefully observed while using the levonorgestrel implants.

Women who are being treated for hyperlipidemias should be followed closely if they elect to use the levonorgestrel implants. Some progestins may elevate LDL levels and may render the control of hyperlipidemias more difficult. (See WARNINGS, Warnings Based on Experience With the Levonorgestrel Implants, Thromboembolic Disorders and Other Vascular Problems.)

Liver Function

If jaundice develops in any women while using the levonorgestrel implants, consideration should be given to removing the capsules. Steroid hormones may be poorly metabolized in patients with impaired liver function.

Fluid Retention

Steroid contraceptives may cause some degree of fluid retention. They should be prescribed with caution, and only with careful monitoring, in patients with conditions which might be aggravated by fluid retention.

Emotional Disorders

Consideration should be given to removing levonorgestrel implant capsules in women who become significantly depressed since the symptom may be drug-related. Women with a history of depression should be carefully observed and removal considered if depression recurs to a serious degree.

Contact Lenses

Contact-lens wearers who develop visual changes or changes in lens tolerance should be assessed by an ophthalmologist.

Autoimmune Disease

Autoimmune diseases such as scleroderma, systemic lupus erythematosus and rheumatoid arthritis occur in the general population and more frequently among women of childbearing age. There have been rare reports of various autoimmune diseases, including the above, in levonorgestrel implant users; however, the rate of reporting is significantly less than the expected incidence for these diseases. Studies have raised the possibility of developing antibodies against silicone-containing devices; however, the specificity and clinical relevance of these antibodies are unknown. While it is believed that the occurrence of autoimmune disease among levonorgestrel users is coincidental, health-care providers should be alert to the earliest manifestations.

DRUG/LABORATORY TEST INTERACTIONS

Certain endocrine tests may be affected by levonorgestrel implant use:

Sex-hormone-binding globulin concentrations are decreased.

Thyroxine concentrations may be slightly decreased and triiodothyronine uptake increased.

CARCINOGENESIS

See WARNINGS.

PREGNANCY CATEGORY X

See WARNINGS.

NURSING MOTHERS

Steroids are not considered the contraceptives of first choice for breast-feeding women. Levonorgestrel has been identified in the breast milk. The health of breast-fed infants whose mothers began using the levonorgestrel implants during the 5th to 7th week postpartum was evaluated; no significant effects were observed on the growth or development of infants who were followed to 12 months of age. No data are available on use in breast-feeding mothers earlier than this after parturition.

PEDIATRIC USE

Safety and efficacy of the levonorgestrel implants have been established in women of reproductive age. Safety and efficacy are expected to be similar for postpubertal adolescents under 16 and users 16 and older. Use of this product before menarche is not indicated.

INFORMATION FOR THE PATIENT

See Patient Labeling which is included with the prescription.

Two copies of the Patient Labeling are included to help describe the characteristics of the levonorgestrel implants to the patient. One copy should be provided to the patient. Patients should also be advised that the Prescribing Information is available to them at their request.

It is recommended that prospective users be fully informed about the risks and benefits associated with the use of the levonorgestrel implants, with other forms of contraception, and with no contraception at all. It is also recommended that prospective users be fully informed about the insertion and removal procedures. Health-care providers may wish to obtain informed consent from all patients in light of the techniques involved with insertion and removal.

DRUG INTERACTIONS

Reduced efficacy (pregnancy) has been reported for levonorgestrel implant users taking phenytoin and carbamazepine. These drugs may increase the metabolism of levonorgestrel through induction of microsomal liver enzymes. Levonorgestrel implant users should be warned of the possibility of decreased efficacy with the use of drugs exhibiting enzyme-inducing activity such as those noted above and rifampin. For women receiving long-term therapy with hepatic enzyme inducers, another method of contraception should be considered.

ADVERSE REACTIONS

The following adverse reactions have been associated with the levonorgestrel implants during the first year of use. They include:

Many bleeding days or prolonged bleeding (27.6%); spotting (17.1%); amenorrhea (9.4%); irregular (onsets of) bleeding (7.6%); frequent bleeding onsets (7.0%); scanty bleeding (5.2%); pain or itching near implant site (usually transient) (3.7%); infection at implant site (0.7%).

In addition, removal difficulties affecting subjects (including multiple incisions, capsule fragments remaining, pain, multiple visits, deep placement, lengthy removal procedure, or other) have been reported with a frequency of 6.2%, which is based on 849 removals occurring through 5 years of use. See WARNINGS and PRECAUTIONS.

Clinical studies comparing levonorgestrel implant users with other contraceptive method users suggest that the following adverse reactions occurring during the first year are probably associated with levonorgestrel implant use. These adverse reactions have also been reported post-marketing:

Headache; nervousness/anxiety; nausea/vomiting; dizziness; adnexal enlargement; dermatitis/rash; acne; change of appetite; mastalgia; weight gain; hirsutism, hypertrichosis; and scalp-hair loss.

In addition, the following adverse reactions have been reported with a frequency of 5% or greater during the first year and are possibly related to levonorgestrel implant use:

Breast discharge; cervicitis; musculoskeletal pain; abdominal discomfort; leukorrhea; vaginitis.

The following adverse reactions have been reported post-marketing with an incidence of less than 1% and are possibly related to levonorgestrel implant use:

Emotional lability; idiopathic intracranial hypertension (IIH, pseudotumor cerebri, benign intracranial hypertension); induration; bruising; abscess, cellulitis; dysmenorrhea; migraine; arm pain; numbness; tingling; depression; excessive scarring; hyperpigmentation; nerve injury.

The following adverse reactions have been reported post-marketing with an incidence of less than 1%. These events occurred under circumstances where a causal relationship to the levonorgestrel implants is unknown. These reactions are listed as information for physicians:

Breast cancer; congenital anomalies; pulmonary embolism; superficial venous thrombosis; deep-vein thrombosis; myocardial infarction; blistering, ulcerations, and sloughing; thrombotic thrombocytopenic purpura (TTP); stroke; pruritus; urticaria; asthenia (fatigue/weakness); phlebitis.

DOSAGE AND ADMINISTRATION

The Norplant System consists of 6 Silastic capsules, each containing 36 mg of the progestin, levonorgestrel. The total administered (implanted) dose is 216 mg. Implantation of all 6 capsules should be performed during the first 7 days of the onset of menses by a health-care professional instructed in the Norplant System insertion technique. Insertion is subdermal in the midportion of the upper arm about 8-10 cm above the elbow crease. Distribution should be in a fanlike pattern, about 15° apart, for a total of 75°. Proper insertion will facilitate later removal. See "Instructions for Insertion and Removal" which is included with the prescription.

HOW SUPPLIED

The Norplant System Kit includes the following items: 1 Norplant System (levonorgestrel implants), a set of 6 implants (capsules); 1 Norplant System trocar; 1 scalpel; 1 forceps; 1 syringe; 2 syringe needles; 1 package of skin closures; 3 packages of gauze sponges; 1 stretch bandage; 1 surgical drape (fenestrated); 2 surgical drapes.

Storage: Store at room temperature away from excess heat and moisture.

PRODUCT LISTING - EQUIVALENTS NOT AVAILABLE

Device - Intrauteral - 52 mg

1's	$395.00	MIRENA, Berlex Laboratories	50419-0421-01

Tablet - Oral - 0.75 mg

2's	$21.95	PLAN B, Women'S Capital Corporation	64836-0000-01

Levorphanol Tartrate *(001636)*

For related information, see the comparative table section in Appendix A.

Categories: Pain, moderate to severe; DEA Class CII; Pregnancy Category C; FDA Approved 1991 Dec
Drug Classes: Analgesics, narcotic
Brand Names: Levo-Dromoran
Foreign Brand Availability: Dromoran (Japan)
HCFA JCODE(S): J1960 up to 2 mg SC, IV

DESCRIPTION

Levorphanol tartrate is available as 1 ml ampuls containing 2 mg levorphanol tartrate compounded with 0.2% parabens (methyl and propyl) as preservatives and sodium hydroxide to adjust pH to approximately 4.3; as 10 ml vials containing 2 mg levorphanol tartrate per ml, compounded with 0.45% phenol as preservative and sodium hydroxide to adjust pH to approximately 4.3; and as scored tablets, each containing 2 mg levorphanol tartrate plus lactose, corn starch, stearic acid and talc.

Levorphanol tartrate is a highly potent synthetic analgesic with properties and actions similar to those of morphine. It produces a degree of analgesia at least equal to that of morphine and greater than that of meperidine at far smaller doses than either. It is longer acting than either; from 6-8 hours of pain relief can be expected with levorphanol tartrate whether given orally or by injection. It is almost as effective orally as it is parenterally. Its safety margin is about equal to that of morphine, but it is less likely to produce nausea, vomiting and constipation.

INDICATIONS AND USAGE

Levorphanol tartrate is recommended whenever a narcotic-analgesic is required. It is recommended for the relief of pain whether moderate or severe. For example, it may be used in alleviating pain due to biliary and renal colic, myocardial infarction, and severe trauma; intractable pain due to cancer and other tumors; and for postoperative pain relief. Used preoperatively, it allays apprehension, provides prolonged analgesia, reduces thiopental requirements and shortens recovery-room time. Levorphanol tartrate is compatible with a wide range of anesthetic agents. It is a useful supplement to nitrous oxide-oxygen anesthesia. It has been given by slow intravenous injection for special indications.

L

CONTRAINDICATIONS

As with the use of morphine, levorphanol tartrate is contraindicated in acute alcoholism, bronchial asthma, increased intracranial pressure, respiratory depression and anoxia.

WARNINGS

May be habit forming. Levorphanol tartrate is a narcotic with an addiction liability similar to that of morphine, and for this reason the same precautions should be taken in administering the drug as with morphine. As with all narcotics, levorphanol tartrate should be used in early pregnancy only when expected benefits outweigh risks.

PRECAUTIONS

To counteract narcotic-induced respiratory depression, a narcotic antagonist, such as naloxone HCl, is recommended and should be readily available whenever levorphanol tartrate is used by parenteral administration.

ADVERSE REACTIONS

As is true with the use of any narcotic-analgesic, nausea, emesis and dizziness are not uncommon in the ambulatory patient. Respiratory depression, hypotension, urinary retention and various cardiac arrhythmias have been infrequently reported following the use of levorphanol tartrate, primarily in surgical patients. Occasional allergic reactions in the form of skin rash or urticaria have been reported. Pruritus or sweating are rarely observed.

DOSAGE AND ADMINISTRATION

Good medical practice dictates that the dose of any narcotic-analgesic be appropriate to the degree of pain to be relieved. This is especially important during the postoperative period because (a) residual CNS-depressant effects of anesthetic agents may still be present, and (b) later, gradual lessening of pain may not warrant full narcotizing doses. The average adult dose is 2 mg orally or subcutaneously. The dosage may be increased to 3 mg, if necessary.

PRODUCT LISTING - RATED THERAPEUTICALLY EQUIVALENT

Solution - Injectable - 2 mg/ml

2 ml x 10	$39.60	LEVO-DROMORAN, Roche Laboratories	00187-3072-10

PRODUCT LISTING - EQUIVALENTS NOT AVAILABLE

Solution - Injectable - 2 mg/ml

10 ml	$45.38	LEVO-DROMORAN, Roche Laboratories	00004-1911-06

Tablet - Oral - 2 mg

100's	$56.32	GENERIC, Roxane Laboratories Inc	00054-4494-25

Levothyroxine Sodium *(001612)*

Categories: Carcinoma, thyroid; Goiter; Hypothyroidism; Myxedema coma; Pregnancy Category A; FDA Pre 1938 Drugs; WHO Formulary
Drug Classes: Hormones/hormone modifiers; Thyroid agents
Brand Names: L-Thyroxine; Levo-T; Levothroid; Levoxyl; **Synthroid**; Synthrox; Throxinique; Thyradin; Thyroxine
Foreign Brand Availability: Berlthyrox (Germany); Droxine (Australia; New-Zealand); Eferox (Germany); Elthyrone (Belgium); Eltroxin (Bahamas; Bahrain; Barbados; Belize; Benin; Bermuda; Burkina-Faso; Canada; Curacao; Cyprus; Czech-Republic; Denmark; Egypt; England; Ethiopia; Gambia; Ghana; Guinea; Guyana; Hong-Kong; Hungary; India; Iran; Iraq; Ireland; Israel; Ivory-Coast; Jamaica; Japan; Jordan; Kenya; Kuwait; Lebanon; Liberia; Libya; Malawi; Mali; Mauritania; Mauritius; Morocco; Netherland-Antilles; Netherlands; Niger; Nigeria; Oman; Philippines; Puerto-Rico; Qatar; Republic-of-Yemen; Saudi-Arabia; Senegal; Seychelles; Sierra-Leone; South-Africa; Sudan; Surinam; Switzerland; Syria; Taiwan; Tanzania; Thailand; Trinidad; Tunia; Uganda; United-Arab-Emirates; Zambia; Zimbabwe); Euthyrox (Austria; Belgium; Bulgaria; China; Czech-Republic; Germany; Hungary; Netherlands; Philippines; Singapore); Eutirox (Ireland; Italy; Mexico; Peru); Levaxin (Sweden); Levotirox (Italy); Levothyrox (France); Levotiroxina (Ecuador); Oroxine (Australia; Malaysia; New-Zealand; Singapore); Pondtroxin (Thailand); T4KP (Thailand); Thevier (Germany); Thyradin S (Japan); Thyrax (Belgium; Czech-Republic; Hungary; Indonesia; Netherlands; Philippines; Portugal; Spain); Thyrax Duotab (Benin; Burkina-Faso; Ethiopia; Gambia; Ghana; Guinea; Ivory-Coast; Kenya; Liberia; Malawi; Mali; Mauritania; Mauritius; Morocco; Niger; Nigeria; Senegal; Seychelles; Sierra-Leone; South-Africa; Sudan; Tanzania; Tunia; Uganda; Zambia; Zimbabwe); Thyrex (Austria); Thyro-4 (Bulgaria; Greece); Thyrosit (Thailand); Thyroxin (Finland); Thyroxin-Natrium (Norway); Tiroidine (Mexico); Tiroxin (Colombia)
Cost of Therapy: $11.25 (Hypothyroidism; Synthroid; 0.1 mg; 1 tablet/day; 30 day supply)
$8.28 (Hypothyroidism; Levothroid; 0.1 mg; 1 tablet/day; 30 day supply)
$0.92 (Hypothyroidism; Generic Tablets; 0.1 mg; 1 tablet/day; 30 day supply)

IM-IV

DESCRIPTION

Note: The trade name has been used throughout this monograph for clarity.

Synthroid tablets and injection contain synthetic crystalline L-3,3′,5,5′-tetraiodothyronine sodium salt [levothyroxine (T_4) sodium]. Synthetic T_4 is identical to that produced in the human thyroid gland.

Levothyroxine (T_4) sodium has an empirical formula of $C_{15}H_{10}I_4NNaO_4 \cdot H_2O$, and molecular weight of 798.86 (anhydrous).

Inactive Ingredients: 10 mg mannitol, sodium hydroxide, 0.7 mg tribasic sodium phosphate, anhydrous dodecahydrate. Levothyroxine sodium powder for reconstitution for injection is a sterile preparation.

CLINICAL PHARMACOLOGY

The synthesis and secretion of the major thyroid hormones, L-thyroxine (T_4) and L-triiodothyronine (T_3), from the normally functioning thyroid gland are regulated by complex feedback mechanisms of the hypothalamic-pituitary-thyroid axis. The thyroid gland is stimulated to secrete thyroid hormones by the action of thyrotropin (thyroid stimulating hormone, TSH) which is produced in the anterior pituitary gland. TSH secretion is in turn controlled by thyrotropin-releasing hormone (TRH) produced in the hypothalamus, circulating thyroid hormones, and possibly other mechanisms. Thyroid hormones circulating in the blood act as feedback inhibitors of both TSH and TRH secretion. Thus, when serum concentrations of T_3 and T_4 are increased, secretion of TSH and TRH is increased. Administration of exogenous thyroid hormones to euthyroid individuals results in suppression of endogenous thyroid hormone secretion.

The mechanisms by which thyroid hormones exert their physiologic actions have not been completely elucidated. T_4 and T_3 are transported into cells by passive and active mechanisms. T_3 in cell cytoplasm and T_3 generated from T_4 within the cell diffuse into the nucleus and bind to thyroid receptor proteins, which appear to be primarily attached to DNA. Receptor binding leads to activation or repression of DNA transcription, thereby altering the amounts of mRNA and resultant proteins. Changes in protein concentrations are responsible for the metabolic changes observed in organs and tissues.

Thyroid hormones enhance oxygen consumption of most body tissues and increase the basal metabolic rate and metabolism of carbohydrates, lipids, and proteins. Thus, they exert a profound influence on every organ system and are of particular importance in the development of the central nervous system. Thyroid hormones also appear to have direct effects on tissues, such as increased myocardial contractility and decreased systemic vascular resistance.

The physiologic effects of thyroid hormones are produced primarily by T_3, a large portion of which is derived from the deiodination of T_4 in peripheral tissues. About 70-90% of peripheral T_3 is produced by monodeoidination of T_4 at the 5′ position (outer ring). Peripheral monodeiodination of T_4 at the 5 position (inner ring) results in the formation of reverse triiodothyronine (rT_3), which is calorigenically inactive.

PHARMACOKINETICS

Few clinical studies have evaluated the kinetics of orally administered thyroid hormone. In animals, the most active sites of absorption appear to be the proximal and mid-jejunum. T_4 is not absorbed from the stomach and little, if any, drug is absorbed from the duodenum. There seems to be no absorption of T_4 from the distal colon in animals. A number of human studies have confirmed the importance of an intact jejunum and ileum for T_4 absorption and have shown some absorption from the duodenum. Studies involving radioiodinated T_4 fecal tracer excretion methods, equilibration, and AUC methods have shown that absorption varies from 48-80% of the administered dose. The extent of absorption is increased in the fasting state and decreased in malabsorption syndromes, such as sprue. Absorption may also decrease with age. The degree of T_4 absorption is dependent on the product formulation as well as on the character of the intestinal contents, including plasma protein and soluble dietary factors, which bind thyroid hormone making it unavailable for diffusion. Decreased absorption may result from administration of infant soybean formula, ferrous sulfate, sodium polystyrene sulfonate, aluminum hydroxide sucralfate, or bile acid sequestrants. T_4 absorption following intramuscular administration is variable.

Distribution of thyroid hormones in human body tissues and fluids has not been fully elucidated. More than 99% of circulating hormones is bound to serum proteins, including thyroxine-binding globulin (TBG), thyroxine-binding prealbumin (TBPA), and albumin (TBA). T_4 is more extensively and firmly bound to serum proteins than is T_3. Only unbound thyroid hormone is metabolically active. The higher affinity of TBG and TBPA for T_4 partly explains the higher serum levels, slower metabolic clearance, and longer serum elimination half-life of this hormone.

Certain drugs and physiologic conditions can alter the binding of thyroid hormones to serum proteins and/or the concentrations of the serum proteins available for thyroid hormone binding. These effects must be considered when interpreting the results of thyroid function tests. (See DRUG INTERACTIONS and PRECAUTIONS, Laboratory Test Interactions.)

T_4 is eliminated slowly from the body, with a half-life of 6-7 days. T_3 has a half-life of 1-2 days. The liver is the major site of degradation for both hormones. T_4 and T_3 are conjugated with glucuronic and sulfuric acids and excreted in the bile. There is an enterohepatic circulation of thyroid hormones, as they are liberated by hydrolysis in the intestine and reabsorbed. A portion of the conjugated material reaches the colon unchanged, is hydrolyzed there, and is eliminated as free compounds in the feces. In man, approximately 20-40% of T_4 is eliminated in the stool. About 70% of the T_4 secreted daily is deiodonated to yield equal amounts of T_3 and rT_3. Subsequent deiodination of T_3 and rT_3 yields multiple forms of diiodothyronine. A number of other minor T_4 metabolites have also been identified. Although some of these metabolites have biological activity, their overall contribution to the therapeutic effect of T_4 is minimal.

INDICATIONS AND USAGE

Levothyroxine sodium is indicated:

As replacement or supplemental therapy in patients of any age or state (including pregnancy) with hypothyroidism of any etiology except transient hypothyroidism during the recovery phase of subacute thyroiditis: primary hypothyroidism resulting from thyroid dysfunction, primary atrophy, or partial or total absence of the thyroid gland, or from the effects of surgery, radiation or drugs, with or without the presence of goiter, including subclinical hypothyroidism; secondary (pituitary) hypothyroidism; and tertiary (hypothalamic) hypothyroidism (see CONTRAINDICATIONS and PRECAUTIONS). Synthroid injection can be used intravenously when rapid repletion is required, and either intravenously or intramuscularly when the oral route is precluded.

As a pituitary TSH supressant in the treatment or prevention of various types of euthyroid goiters, including thyroid nodules, subacute or chronic lymphocytic thydroiditis (Hashimoto's), multinodular goiter, and in conjunction with surgery and radioactive iodine therapy in the management of thyrotropin-dependent well-differentiated papillary or follicular carcinoma of the thyroid.

CONTRAINDICATIONS

Synthroid is contraindicated in patients with untreated thyrotoxicosis of any etiology or an apparent hypersensitivity to thyroid hormones or any of the inactive product constituents. (The 50 μg tablet is formulated without color additives for patients who are sensitive to dyes.) There is no well-documented evidence of true allergic or idiosyncratic reactions to thyroid hormone. Synthroid is also contraindicated in the patients with uncorrected adrenal insufficiency, as thyroid hormones increase tissue demands, for adrenocortical hormones and may thereby precipitate acute adrenal crisis (see PRECAUTIONS).

WARNINGS

Thyroid hormones, either alone or together with other therapeutic agents, should not be used for the treatment of obesity. In euthyroid patients, doses within the range of daily hormonal requirements are ineffective for weight reduction. Larger doses may produce serious or even life threatening manifestations of toxicity, particularly when given in association with sympathomimetic amines such as those used for their anorectic effects.

The use of Synthroid in the treatment of obesity, either alone or in combination with other drugs, is unjustified. The use of Synthroid is also unjustified in the treatment of male or female infertility unless this condition is associated with hypothyroidism.

PRECAUTIONS

GENERAL

Synthroid should be used with caution in patients with cardiovascular disorders, including angina, coronary artery disease, and hypertension, and in the elderly who have a greater likelihood of occult cardiac disease. Concomitant administration of thyroid hormone and sympathomimetic agents to patients with coronary artery disease may increase the risk of coronary insufficiency.

Use of Synthroid in patients with concomitant diabetes mellitus, diabetes insipidus or adrenal cortical insufficiency may aggravate the intensity of their symptoms. Appropriate adjustments of the various therapeutic measures directed at these concomitant endocrine diseases may therefore be required. Treatment of myxedema coma may require simultaneous administration of glucocorticoids (see DOSAGE AND ADMINISTRATION).

T_4 enhances the response to anticoagulant therapy. Prothrombin time should be closely monitored in patients taking both Synthroid and oral anticoagulants, and the dosage of anticoagulant adjusted accordingly.

Seizures have been reported rarely in association with the initiation of levothyroxine sodium therapy, and may be related to the effect of thyroid hormone on seizure threshold.

Lithium blocks the TSH-mediated release of T_4 and T_3. Thyroid function should therefore be carefully monitored during lithium initiation, stabilization, and maintenance. If hypothyroidism occurs during lithium treatment, a higher than usual Synthroid dose may be required.

INFORMATION FOR THE PATIENT

Synthroid is intended to replace a hormone that is normally produced by your thyroid gland. It is generally taken for life, except in cases of temporary hypothyroidism associated with an inflammation of the thyroid gland.

Before or at any time while using Synthroid, you should tell your doctor if you are allergic to any foods or medicines, are pregnant or intend to become pregnant, are breast-feeding, are taking or start taking any other prescription or non-prescription (OTC) medications, or have any other medical problems (especially hardening of the arteries, heart disease, high blood pressure, or history of thyroid, adrenal or pituitary gland problems).

Use Synthroid only as prescribed by your doctor. Do not discontinue Synthroid or change the amount you take or how often you take it, except as directed by your doctor.

Synthroid, like all medicines obtained from your doctor, must be used only by you and for the condition determined appropriate by your doctor.

It may take a few weeks for Synthroid to begin working. Until it begins working, you may not notice any change in your symptoms.

You should notify your doctor if you experience any of the following symptoms, or if you experience any other unusual medical event: chest pain, shortness of breath, hives or skin rash, rapid or irregular heartbeat, headache, irritability, nervousness, sleeplessness, diarrhea, excessive sweating, heat intolerance, changes in appetite, vomiting, weight gain or loss, changes in menstrual periods, fever, hand tremors, leg cramps.

You should inform your doctor or dentist that you are taking Synthroid before having any kind of surgery.

You should notify your doctor if you become pregnant while taking Synthroid. Your dose of this medicine will likely have to be increased while you are pregnant.

If you have diabetes, your dose of insulin or oral antidiabetic agent may need to be changed after starting Synthroid. You should monitor your blood or urinary glucose levels as directed by your doctor and report any changes to your doctor immediately.

If you are taking an oral anticoagulant drug such as warfarin, your dose may need to be changed after starting Synthroid. Your coagulation status should be checked often to determine if a change in dose is required.

Partial hair loss may occur rarely during the first few months of levothyroxine sodium therapy, but it is usually temporary.

Synthroid is the trade name for tablets containing the thyroid hormone levothyroxine, manufactured by Knoll Pharmaceutical Company. Other manufactures also make tablets containing levothyroxine. You should not change to another manufacture's product without discussing that change with your doctor first. Repeat blood tests and a change in the amount of levothyroxine sodium you take may be required.

Keep Synthroid out of the reach of children. Store Synthroid away from heat and moisture.

LABORATORY TESTS

Treatment of patients with Synthroid requires periodic assessment of adequacy of titration by appropriate laboratory tests and clinical evaluation. Selection of appropriate tests for the diagnosis and management of thyroid disorders depends on patient variables such as presenting signs and symptoms, pregnancy, and concomitant medications. A combination of sensitive TSH assay and free T_4 estimate (free T_4, free T_4 index) are recommended to confirm a diagnosis of thyroid disease. Normal ranges for these parameters are age-specific in newborns and younger children.

TSH alone or initially may be useful for thyroid disease screening and for monitoring therapy for primary hypothyroidism as a linear inverse correlation exists between serum TSH and free T_4. Measurement of total serum T_4 and T_3, resin T_3 uptake, and free T_3 concentrations may also be useful. Antithyroid microsomal antibodies are an indicator of autoimmune thyroid disease. An elevated serum TSH in the presence of normal T_4 may indicate subclinical hypothyroidism. Intracellular resistance to thyroid hormone is quite rare, and is suggested by clinical signs and symptoms of hypothyroidism in the presence of high serum T_4 levels. Adequacy of Synthroid therapy for hypothyroidism of pituitary or hypothalamic origin should be assessed by measuring free T_4, which should be maintained in the upper half of the normal range. Measurement of TSH is not a reliable indicator of response to therapy for this condition. Adequacy of Synthroid therapy for hypothyroidism of pituitary or hypothalamic origin should be assessed by measuring free T_4, which should be maintained in the upper half of the normal range. Measurement of TSH is not a reliable indicator of response to therapy for this condition. Adequacy of levothyroxine sodium therapy for congenital and acquired pediatric hypothyroidism should be assessed by measuring serum total T_4 or free T_4, which should be maintained in the upper half of the normal range. In congenital hypothyroidism, normalization of serum TSH levels may lag behind normalization of serum T_4 levels by 2-3 months or longer. In rare patients serum TSH remains relatively elevated despite clinical euthyroidism and age-specific normal levels of T_4 or free T_4.

LABORATORY TEST INTERACTIONS

A number of drugs or moieties are known to alter serum levels of TSH, T_4 and T_3 and may thereby influence the interpretation of laboratory tests of thyroid function (see DRUG INTERACTIONS).

Changes in TBG concentration should be taken into consideration when interpreting T_4 and T_3 values. Drugs such as estrogens and estrogen-containing oral contraceptives increase TBG concentrations. TBG may also be increased during pregnancy and in infectious hepatitis. Decreases in TBG concentrations are observed in nephrosis, acromegaly, and after androgen or corticosteroid therapy. Familial hyper- or hypothyroxine-binding-globulinemias have been described. The incidence of TBG deficiency is approximately 1 in 9000. Certain drugs such as salicylates inhibit the protein-binding of T_4. In such cases, the unbound (free) hormone should be measured. Alternatively, an indirect measure of free thyroxine, such as the FT_4I may be used.

Medicinal or dietary iodine interferes with all *in vivo* tests of radioiodine uptake, producing low uptakes which may not indicate a true decrease in hormone synthesis.

Persistent clinical and laboratory evidence of hypothyroidism despite an adequate replacement dose suggests either poor patient compliance, impared absorption, drug interactions, or decreased potency of the preparation due to improper storage.

CARCINOGENESIS, MUTAGENESIS, AND IMPAIRMENT OF FERTILITY

Although animal studies to determine the mutagenic or carcinogenic potential of thyroid hormones have not been performed, synthetic T_4 is identical to that produced by the human thyroid gland. A reported association between prolonged thyroid therapy and breast cancer has not been confirmed and patients receiving levothyroxine sodium for established indications should not discontinue therapy.

PREGNANCY CATEGORY A

Studies in pregnant women have not shown that levothyroxine sodium increases the risk of fetal abnormalities if administered during pregnancy. If levothyroxine sodium is used during pregnancy, the possibility of fetal harm appears remote. Because the studies cannot rule out the possibility of harm, levothyroxine sodium should be used during pregnancy only if clearly needed.

Thyroid hormones cross the placental barrier to some extent. T_4 levels in the cord blood of athyroid fetuses have been shown to be about one-third of maternal levels. Nevertheless, maternal-fetal transfer of T_4 may not prevent *in utero* hypothyroidism.

Hypothyroidism during pregnancy is associated with a higher rate of complications, including spontaneous abortion and preeclampsia, and has been reported to have an adverse effect on fetal and childhood development. On the basis of current knowledge, Synthroid should therefore not be discontinued during pregnancy, and hypothyroidism diagnosed during pregnancy should be treated. Studies have shown that during pregnancy T_4 concentrations may decrease and TSH concentrations may increase to values outside normal ranges. Postpartum values are similar to preconception values. Elevations in TSH may occur as early as at 4 weeks gestation.

Pregnant women who are maintained on Synthroid should have their TSH measured periodically. An elevated TSH should be corrected by an increase in Synthroid dose. After pregnancy, the dose can be decreased to the optimal preconception dose.

NURSING MOTHERS

Minimal amounts of thyroid hormones are excreted in human milk. Thyroid hormones are not associated with serious adverse reactions and do not have known tumorigenic potential. While caution should be exercised when levothyroxine sodium is administered to a nursing woman, adequate replacement doses of Synthroid are generally needed to maintain normal lactation.

PEDIATRIC USE

Congenital Hypothyroidism

Rapid restoration of normal serum T_4 concentrations is essential for preventing the deleterious effects of neonatal thyroid hormone deficiency on intelligence, as well as on overall growth and development. Synthroid should be initiated immediately upon diagnosis, and is generally continued for life. The goal of therapy is to maintain the serum total T_4 or FT_4 in the upper half of the normal range and serum TSH in the normal range.

An initial starting dose of 10-15 μg/kg/day (ages 0-3 months) will generally increase serum T_4 concentrations to the upper half of the normal range in less than 3 weeks. Clinical assessment of growth and development and thyroid status should be monitored frequently. In most cases, the dose of Synthroid per body weight will decrease gradually as the patient grows through infancy and childhood (see TABLE 1). Prolonged use of large doses in infants may be associated with later behavior problems.

Thyroid function tests (serum total T_4 or FT_4 and TSH) should be monitored closely and used to determine the adequacy of Synthroid therapy. Normalization of serum T_4 levels is usually followed by a rapid decline of TSH levels. Nevertheless, normalization of TSH may lag behind normalization of T_4 levels by 2-3 months or longer. The relative elevation of serum TSH is more marked during the early months of therapy, but can persist to some degree throughout life. In rare patients TSH remains relatively elevated despite clinical euthyroidism and age-specific normal levels of total T_4 or FT_4. Increasing the Synthroid dosage to suppress TSH into the normal range may result in overtreatment, with an elevated serum T_4 level and clinical features of hyperthyroidism, including irritability, increased appetite with diarrhea, and sleeplessness. Another risk of prolonged overtreatment in infants is premature cranial synostosis.

Assessment of permanence of hypothyroidism may be done when transient hypothyroidism is suspected. Levothyroxine therapy may be interrupted for 30 days after 3 years of age and serum measurement of T_4 and TSH levels obtained. If T_4 is low and the TSH level is elevated, permanent hypothyroidism is confirmed and therapy should be re-instituted. If T_4 and TSH remain in the normal range, a presumptive diagnosis of transient hypothyroidism can be made. In this instance, continued clinical monitoring and periodic reevaluation of thyroid function may be warranted.

Acquired Hypothyroidism

The initial dose of Synthroid varies with age and body weight, and should be adjusted to maintain serum total T_4 or free T_4 levels in the upper half of the normal range. In general, in the absence of overriding clinical concerns, children should be started on a full replacement dose. Children with underlying heart disease should be started at lower doses, with careful upward titration. Children with severe, long-standing hypothyroidism may also be started on a lower initial dose with upward titration in an attempt to avoid premature closure of epiphyses. The recommended dose per body weight decreases with age (see TABLE 1).

Treated children may resume growth at a rate greater than normal (period of transient catch-up growth). In some cases catch-up growth may be adequate to normalize growth; however, in children with severe and prolonged hypothyroidism, adult height may be reduced. Excessive thyroxine replacement may initiate accelerated bone maturation resulting in disproportionate advancement in skeletal age and shortened adult stature.

Assessment of permanence of hypothyroidism may be done when transient hypothyroidism is suspected. Levothyroxine therapy may be interrupted for 30 days and serum measurement of T_4 and TSH levels obtained. If T_4 is low and the TSH level is elevated, permanent hypothyroidism is confirmed and therapy should be re-instituted. If T_4 and TSH remain in the normal range, a presumptive diagnosis of transient hypothyroidism can be made. In this instance, continued clinical monitoring and periodic reevaluation of thyroid function may be warranted.

DRUG INTERACTIONS

The magnitude and relative importance of the effects noted below are likely to be patient specific and may vary by such factors as age, gender, race, intercurrent illnesses, dose of either agent, additional concomitant medications, and timing of drug administration. Any agent that alters thyroid hormone synthesis, secretion, distribution, effect on target tissues, metabolism, or elimination may alter the optimal therapeutic dose of Synthroid.

Levothyroxine sodium absorption: *The following agents may bind and decrease absorption of levothyroxine sodium from the gastrointestinal tract:* Aluminum hydroxide, cholestyramine resin, colestipol hydrochloride, ferrous sulfate, sodium polystyrene sulfonate, soybean flour (*e.g.*, infant formula), sucralfate.

Binding to serum proteins: *The following agents may either inhibit levothyroxine sodium binding to serum proteins or alter the concentrations of serum binding proteins:* Androgens and related anabolic hormones, asparaginase, clofibrate, estrogens and estrogen-containing compounds, 5-fluorouracil, furosemide, glucocorticoids, meclofenamic acid, mefenamic acid, methadone, perphenazine, phenylbutazone, phenytoin, salicylates, tamoxifen.

Thyroid physiology: *The following agents may alter thyroid hormone or TSH levels, generally by effects on thyroid hormone synthesis, secretion, distribution, metabolism, hormone action, or elimination, or altered TSH secretion:* Aminoglutethimide, p-aminosalicylic acid, amiodarone, androgens and related anabolic hormones, complex anions (thiocyanate, perchlorate, pertechnetate), antithyroid drugs, β-adrenergic blocking agents, carbamazepine, chloral hydrate, diazepam, dopamine and dopamine agonists, ethionamide, glucocorticoids, heparin, hepatic enzyme inducers, insulin, iodinated cholestographic agents, iodine-containing compounds, levodopa, lovastatin, lithium, 6-mercaptopurine, metoclopramide, mitotane, nitroprusside, phenobarbital, phenytoin, resorcinol, rifampin, somatostatin analogs, sulfonamides, sulfonylureas, thiazide diuretics.

Adrenocorticoids: Metabolic clearance of adrenocorticoids is decreased in hypothyroid patients and increased in hyperthyroid patients, and may therefore change with changing thyroid status.

Amiodarone: Amiodarone therapy alone can cause hypothyroidism or hyperthyroidism.

Anticoagulants (oral): The hypoprothrombinemic effect of anticoagulants may be potentiated, apparently by increased catabolism of vitamin K-dependent clotting factors.

Antidiabetic agents (insulin, sulfonylureas): Requirements for insulin or oral antidiabetic agents may be reduced in hypothyroid patients with diabetes mellitus and may subsequently increase with the initiation of thyroid hormone replacement therapy.

β-adrenergic blocking agents: Actions of some of β-blocking agents may be impaired when hypothyroid patients become euthyroid.

Cytokines (interferon, interleukin): Cytokines have been reported to induce both hyperthyroidism and hypothyroidism.

Digitalis glycosides: Therapeutic effects of digitalis glycosides may be reduced. Serum digitalis levels may be decreased in hyperthyroidism or when a hypothyroid patient becomes euthyroid.

Ketamine: Marked hypertension and tachycardia have been reported in association with concomitant administration of levothyroxine sodium and ketamine.

Maprotiline: Risk of cardiac arrhythmias may increase.

Sodium iodide (^{123}I and ^{131}I), sodium pertechnetate Tc99m: Uptake of radiolabeled ions may be decreased.

Somatrem/somatropin: Excessive concurrent use of thyroid hormone may accelerate epiphyseal closure. Untreated hypothyroidism may interfere with the growth response to somatrem or somatropin.

Theophylline: Theophylline clearance may decrease in hypothyroid patients and return toward normal when a euthyroid state is achieved.

Tricyclic antidepressants: Concurrent use may increase the therapeutic and toxic effects of both drugs, possibly due to increased catecholamine sensitivity. Onset of action of tricyclics may be accelerated.

Sympathomimetic agents: Possible increased risk of coronary insufficiency in patients with coronary artery disease.

ADVERSE REACTIONS

Adverse reactions other than those indicative of thyrotoxicosis as a result of therapeutic overdosage, either initially or during the maintenance periods, are rare. Craniosynostosis has been associated with iatrogenic hyperthyroidism in infants receiving thyroid hormone replacement therapy. Inadequate doses of Synthroid may produce or fail to resolve symptoms of hypothyroidism. Hypersensitivity reactions to the product excipients, such as rash and urticaria, may occur. Partial hair loss may occur during the initial months of therapy, but is generally transient. The incidence of continued hair loss is unknown. Pseudotumor cerebri has been reported in pediatric patients receiving thyroid hormone replacement therapy.

DOSAGE AND ADMINISTRATION

The dosage and rate of administration of Synthroid is determined by the indication, and must in every case be individualized according to patient response and laboratory findings.

HYPOTHYROIDISM

The goal of therapy for primary hypothyroidism is to achieve and maintain a clinical and biochemical euthyroid state with consequent resolution of hypothyroid signs and symptoms. The starting dose of Synthroid, the frequency of dose titration, and the optimal full replacement dose must be individualized for every patient, and will be influenced by such factors as age, weight, cardiovascular status, presence of other illness, and the severity and duration of hypothyroid symptoms.

The usual full replacement dose of Synthroid for younger, healthy adults is approximately 1.6 μg/kg/day administered once daily. In the elderly, the full replacement dose may be altered by decreases in T_4 metabolism and levothyroxine sodium absorption. Older patients may require less than 1 μg/kg/day. Children generally require higher doses (see Pediatric Dosage). Women who are maintained on Synthroid during pregnancy may require increased doses (see Pregnancy Category A).

Therapy is usually initiated in younger, healthy adults at the anticipated full replacement dose. Clinical and laboratory evaluations should be performed at 6-8 week intervals (2-3 weeks in severely hypothyroid patients), and the dosage adjusted by 12.5 to 25 μg increments until the serum TSH concentration is normalized and signs and symptoms resolve. In older patients or in younger patients with a history of cardiovascular disease, the starting dose should be 12.5 to 50 μg once daily with adjustments of 12.5 to 25 μg every 3-6 weeks until TSH is normalized. If cardiac symptoms develop or worsen the cardiac disease should be evaluated and the dose of Synthroid reduced. Rarely, worsening angina or other signs of cardiac ischema may prevent achieving a TSH in the normal range.

Treatment of subclinical hypothyroidism, when indicated, may require lower than usual replacement doses, (*e.g.,* 1.0 μg/kg/day). Patients for whom treatment is not initiated should be monitored yearly for changes in clinical status, TSH, and thyroid antibodies.

In patients with hypothyroidism resulting from pituitary or hypothalamic disease, the possibility of secondary adrenal insufficiency should be considered, and if present, treated with glucocorticoids prior to initiation of Synthroid. The adequacy of Synthroid therapy should be assessed in these patients by measuring FT_4I, which should be maintained in the upper half of the normal range, in addition to clinical assessment. Measurement of TSH is not a reliable indicator of response to therapy for this condition.

Few patients require doses greater than 200 μg/day. An inadequate response to daily doses of 300-400 μg/day is rare, and may suggest malabsorption, poor patient compliance, and/or drug interactions.

Once optimal replacement is achieved, clinical and laboratory evaluations should be conducted at least annually or whenever warranted by a change in patient status. Levothyroxine sodium products from different manufacturers should not be used interchangeably unless retesting of the patient and retitration of the dosage, as necessary, accompanies the product switch.

Synthroid injection by the intravenous or intramuscular route can be substituted for the oral dosage form when the oral administration is precluded. The initial parenteral dosage should be approximately one-half the previously established oral dosage of Synthroid tablets. Close observation of the patient is recommended, with adjustment of the dosage as needed. Administration of Synthroid injection by the subcutaneous route is not recommended as studies have shown that the influx of T_4 from the subcutaneous site is very slow, and depends on many factors such as volume of injectate, the anatomic site of injection, ambient temperature, and presence of venospasm.

MYXEDEMA COMA

Myxedema coma represents the extreme expression of severe hypothyroidism and is considered a medical emergency. It is characterized by hypothermia, hypotension, hypoventilation, hyponatremia, and bradycardia. In addition to restoration of normal thyroid hormone levels, therapy should be directed at the correction of electrolyte disturbances and possible infection. Because the mortality rate of patients with untreated myxedema coma is high, treatment must be started immediately, and should include appropriate supportive therapy and corticosteroids to prevent adrenal insufficiency. Possible precipitating factors should also be identified and treated. Synthroid may be given via nasogastric tube, but the preferred route of administration is intravenous. A bolus dose of Synthroid is given immediately to replete the peripheral pool of T_4, usually 300-500 μg. Although such a dose is usually well-tolerated even in the elderly, the rapid IV administration of large doses of levothyroxine sodium to patients with cardiovascular disease is clearly not without risks. Under such circumstances, IV therapy should not be undertaken without weighing the alternate risks of myxedema coma and the cardiovascular disease. Clinical judgement in this situation may dictate smaller IV doses of Synthroid. The initial dose is followed by daily IV doses of 75-100 μg until the patient is stable and oral administration is feasible. Normal T_4 levels are usually achieved in 24 hours, followed by progressive increases in T_3. Improvement in cardiac output, blood pressure, temperature, and mental status generally occur within 24 hours, with improvement in many manifestations of hypothyroidism in 4-7 days.

TSH SUPPRESSION IN THYROID CANCER AND THYROID NODULES

The rationale for TSH suppression therapy is that a reduction in TSH secretion may decrease the growth and function of abnormal thyroid tissue. Exogenous thyroid hormone may inhibit recurrence of tumor growth and may produce regression of metastases from well-differentiated (follicular and papillary) carcinoma of the thyroid. It is used as ancillary therapy of these conditions following surgery or radioactive iodine therapy. Medullary and anaplastic carcinoma of the thyroid is unresponsive to TSH suppression therapy. TSH suppression is also used in treating nontoxic solitary nodules and multinodular goiters.

No controlled studies have compared the various degrees of TSH suppression in the treatment of either benign or malignant thyroid nodular disease. Further, the effectiveness of TSH suppression for benign nodular disease is controversial. The dose of Synthroid used for TSH suppression should therefore be individualized by the nature of the disease, the patient being treated, and the desired clinical response, weighing the potential benefits of therapy against the risks of iatrogenic thyrotoxicosis. In general, Synthroid should be given in the smallest dose that will achieve the desired clinical response.

For well differentiated thyroid cancer, TSH is generally suppressed to less than 0.1 mU/L. Doses of Synthroid greater than 2 μg/kg/day are usually required. The efficacy of TSH suppression in reducing the size of benign thyroid nodules and in preventing nodule regrowth after surgery are controversial. Nevertheless, when treatment with levothyroxine sodium is considered warranted, TSH is generally suppressed to a higher target range (*e.g.,* 0.1-0.3 mU/L) than that employed for the treatment of thyroid cancer. Synthroid therapy may also be considered for patients with nontoxic multinodular goiter who have a TSH in the normal range, to moderately suppress TSH (*e.g.,* 0.1-0.3 mU/L).

Synthroid should be administered with caution to patients in whom there is a suspicion of thyroid gland autonomy, in view of the fact that the effects of exogenous hormone administration will be additive to endogenous thyroid hormone production.

PEDIATRIC DOSAGE

Congenital or Acquired Hypothyroidism

The dosage of Synthroid for pediatric hypothyroidism varies with age and body weight. Synthroid should be given at a dose that maintains the serum total T_4 or free T_4 concentrations in the upper half of the normal range and serum TSH in the normal range (see PRECAUTIONS, Pediatric Use).

Synthroid therapy is usually initiated at the full replacement dose (see TABLE 1). Infants and neonates with very low or undetectable serum T_4 levels (<5 μg/dl) should start at the higher end of the dosage range (*e.g.,* 50 μg daily). A lower starting dosage (*e.g.,* 25 μg daily) should be considered for neonates at risk of cardiac failure, increasing every few days until a full maintenance dose is reached. In children with severe, long-standing hypothyroidism, Synthroid should be initiated gradually, with an initial dose of 25 μg for 2 weeks, and then increasing the dose by 25 μg every 2-4 weeks until the desired dose based on serum T_4 and TSH levels is achieved (see PRECAUTIONS, Pediatric Use).

Serum T_4 and TSH measurements should be evaluated at the following intervals, with subsequent dosage adjustments to normalize serum total T_4 or FT_4 and TSH:

2 and 4 weeks after the initiation of Synthroid treatment.
Every 1-2 months during the first year of life.
Every 2-3 months between 1 and 3 years of age.
Every 3-12 months thereafter until growth is completed.

Evaluation at more frequent intervals is indicated when compliance is questioned or abnormal values are obtained. Patient evaluation is also advisable approximately 6-8 weeks after any change in Synthroid dose.

Synthroid tablets may be given to infants and children who cannot swallow intact tablets by crushing the tablet and suspending the freshly crushed tablet in a small amount of water (5-10 ml), breast milk, or non-soybean formula. The suspension can be given by spoon or dropper. DO NOT STORE THE SUSPENSION FOR ANY PERIOD OF TIME. The crushed tablet may also be sprinkled over a small amount of food, such as apple sauce. Foods or formula containing large amounts of soybean fiber or iron should not be used for administering Synthroid.

TABLE 1 *Dosing Guidelines for Pediatric Hypothyroidism*

Age	Daily Dose*
0-3 months	10-15 μg/kg body weight
3-6 months	8-10 μg/kg body weight
6-12 months	6-8 μg/kg body weight
1-5 years	5-6 μg/kg body weight
6-12 years	4-5 μg/kg body weight
>12 years	2-3 μg/kg body weight
Growth & puberty complete	1.6 μg/kg body weight

* To be adjusted on the basis of clinical response and laboratory tests (see PRECAUTIONS, Laboratory Tests).

HOW SUPPLIED

Synthroid injection is a lyophilized powder. It is supplied in color coded vials as follows:
200 μg: Gray
500 μg: Yellow

Storage: Store at controlled room temperature 15-30°C (59-86°F).

ORAL

DESCRIPTION

Note: The trade name has been used throughout this monograph for clarity.

Synthroid (levothyroxine sodium) tablets contain synthetic crystalline L-3,3′,5,5′-tetraiodothyronine sodium salt [levothyroxine (T_4) sodium]. Synthetic T_4 is identical to that produced in the human thyroid gland. Levothyroxine (T_4) sodium has an empirical formula of $C_{15}H_{10}I_4NNaO_4 \cdot H_2O$, and molecular weight of 798.86 g/mol (anhydrous).

INACTIVE INGREDIENTS

Acacia, confectioner's sugar (contains corn starch), lactose monohydrate, magnesium stearate, povidone, and talc.

The following are the color additives by tablet strength:

25 μg: FD&C yellow no. 6 aluminum lake.
50 μg: None.
75 μg: FD&C red no. 40 aluminum lake, FD&C blue no. 2 aluminum lake.
88 μg: FD&C blue no. 1 aluminum lake, FD&C yellow no. 6 aluminum lake, D&C yellow no. 10 aluminum lake.
100 μg: D&C yellow no. 10 aluminum lake, FD&C yellow no. 6 aluminum lake.
112 μg: D&C red no. 27 & 30 aluminum lake.
125 μg: FD&C yellow no. 6 aluminum lake, FD&C red no. 40 aluminum lake, FD&C blue no. 1 aluminum lake.
150 μg: FD&C blue no. 2 aluminum lake.
175 μg: FD&C blue no. 1 aluminum lake, D&C red no. 27 & 30 aluminum lake.
200 μg: FD&C red no. 40 aluminum lake.
300 μg: D&C yellow no. 10 aluminum lake, FD&C yellow no. 6 aluminum lake, FD&C blue no. 1 aluminum lake.

CLINICAL PHARMACOLOGY

Thyroid hormone synthesis and secretion is regulated by the hypothalamic-pituitary-thyroid axis. Thyrotropin-releasing hormone (TRH) released from the hypothalamus stimulates secretion of thyrotropin-stimulating hormone, TSH, from the anterior pituitary. TSH, in turn, is the physiologic stimulus for the synthesis and secretion of thyroid hormones, L-thyroxine (T_4) and L-triiodothyronine (T_3), by the thyroid gland. Circulating serum T_3 and T_4 levels exert a feedback effect on both TRH and TSH secretion. When serum T_3 and T_4 levels increase, TRH and TSH secretion decrease. When thyroid hormone levels decrease, TRH and TSH secretion increase.

The mechanisms by which thyroid hormones exert their physiologic actions are not completely understood, but it is thought that their principal effects are exerted through control of DNA transcription and protein synthesis. T_3 and T_4 diffuse into the cell nucleus and bind to thyroid receptor proteins attached to DNA. This hormone nuclear receptor complex activates gene transcription and synthesis of messenger RNA and cytoplasmic proteins.

Thyroid hormones regulate multiple metabolic processes and play an essential role in normal growth and development, and normal maturation of the central nervous system and bone. The metabolic actions of thyroid hormones include augmentation of cellular respiration and thermogenesis, as well as metabolism of proteins, carbohydrates and lipids. The protein anabolic effects of thyroid hormones are essential to normal growth and development.

The physiologic actions of thyroid hormones are produced predominately by T_3, the majority of which (approximately 80%) is derived from T_4 by deiodination in peripheral tissues.

Levothyroxine, at doses individualized according to patient response, is effective as replacement or supplemental therapy in hypothyroidism of any etiology, except transient hypothyroidism during the recovery phase of subacute thyroiditis.

Levothyroxine is also effective in the suppression of pituitary TSH secretion in the treatment or prevention of various types of euthyroid goiters, including thyroid nodules, Hashimoto's thyroiditis, multinodular goiter, and adjunctive therapy in the management of thyrotropin-dependent well-differentiated thyroid cancer (see INDICATIONS AND USAGE, PRECAUTIONS, and DOSAGE AND ADMINISTRATION).

PHARMACOKINETICS

Absorption

Absorption of orally administered T_4 from the gastrointestinal (GI) tract ranges from 40-80%. The majority of the levothyroxine dose is absorbed from the jejunum and upper ileum. T_4 absorption is increased by fasting, and decreased in malabsorption syndromes and by certain foods such as soybean infant formula. Dietary fiber decreases bioavailability of T_4. Absorption may also decrease with age. In addition, many drugs and foods affect T_4 absorption (see DRUG INTERACTIONS and PRECAUTIONS, Drug-Food Interactions).

Distribution

Circulating thyroid hormones are greater than 99% bound to plasma proteins, including thyroxine-binding globulin (TBG), thyroxine-binding prealbumin (TBPA), and albumin (TBA), whose capacities and affinities vary for each hormone. The higher affinity of both TBG and TBPA for T_4 partially explains the higher serum levels, slower metabolic clearance, and longer half-life of T_4 compared to T_3. Protein-bound thyroid hormones exist in reverse equilibrium with small amounts of free hormone. Only unbound hormone is metabolically active. Many drugs and physiologic conditions affect the binding of thyroid hormones to serum proteins (see DRUG INTERACTIONS and PRECAUTIONS, Drug/Laboratory Test Interactions). Thyroid hormones do not readily cross the placental barrier (see PRECAUTIONS, Pregnancy Category A).

Metabolism

T_4 is slowly eliminated (see TABLE 2). The major pathway of thyroid hormone metabolism is through sequential deiodination. Approximately 80% of circulating T_3 is derived from peripheral T_4 by monodeiodination. The liver is the major site of degradation for both T_4 and T_3, with T_4 deiodination also occurring at a number of additional sites, including the kidney and other tissues. Approximately 80% of the daily dose of T_4 is deiodinated to yield equal amounts of T_3 and reverse T_3 (rT_3). T_3 and rT_3 are further deiodinated to diiodothyronine. Thyroid hormones are also metabolized via conjugation with glucuronides and sulfates and excreted directly into the bile and gut where they undergo enterohepatic recirculation.

Elimination

Thyroid hormones are primarily eliminated by the kidneys. A portion of the conjugated hormone reaches the colon unchanged and is eliminated in the feces. Approximately 20% of T_4 is eliminated in the stool. Urinary excretion of T_4 decreases with age.

TABLE 2 *Pharmacokinetic Parameters of Thyroid Hormones in Euthyroid Patients*

	Levothyroxine (T_4)	Liothyronine (T_3)
Ratio in thyroglobulin	10-20	1
Biologic potency	1	4
T½ (days)	6-7*	≤2
Protein binding (%)†	99.96	99.5

* 3-4 days in hyperthyroidism, 9-10 days in hypothyroidism.
† Includes TBG, TBPA, and TBA.

INDICATIONS AND USAGE

Levothyroxin sodium is used for the following indications:

Hypothyroidism: As replacement or supplemental therapy in congenital or acquired hypothyroidism of any etiology, except transient hypothyroidism during the recovery phase of subacute thyroiditis. Specific indications include: primary (thyroidal), secondary (pituitary), and tertiary (hypothalamic) hypothyroidism and subclinical hypothyroidism. Primary hypothyroidism may result from functional deficiency, primary atrophy, partial or total congenital absence of the thyroid gland, or from the effects of surgery, radiation, or drugs, with or without the presence of goiter.

Pituitary TSH Suppression: In the treatment or prevention of various types of euthyroid goiters (see WARNINGS and PRECAUTIONS), including thyroid nodules (see WARNINGS and PRECAUTIONS), subacute or chronic lymphocytic thyroiditis (Hashimoto's thyroiditis), multinodular goiter (see WARNINGS and PRECAUTIONS) and, as an adjunct to surgery and radioiodine therapy in the management of thyrotropin-dependent well-differentiated thyroid cancer.

CONTRAINDICATIONS

Levothyroxine is contraindicated in patients with untreated subclinical (suppressed serum TSH level with normal T_3 and T_4 levels) or overt thyrotoxicosis of any etiology and in patients with acute myocardial infarction. Levothyroxine is contraindicated in patients with uncorrected adrenal insufficiency since thyroid hormones may precipitate an acute adrenal crisis by increasing the metabolic clearance of glucocorticoids (see PRECAUTIONS). Synthroid is contraindicated in patients with hypersensitivity to any of the inactive ingredients in Synthroid tablets (see DESCRIPTION, Inactive Ingredients).

WARNINGS

WARNING: Thyroid hormones, including Synthroid, either alone or with other therapeutic agents, should not be used for the treatment of obesity. In euthyroid patients, doses within the range of daily hormonal requirements are ineffective for weight reduction. Larger doses may produce serious or even life threatening manifestations of toxicity, particularly when given in association with sympathomimetic amines such as those used for their anorectic effects.

Levothyroxine sodium should not be used in the treatment of male or female infertility unless this condition is associated with hypothyroidism.

In patients with nontoxic diffuse goiter or nodular thyroid disease, particularly the elderly or those with underlying cardiovascular disease, levothyroxine sodium therapy is contraindicated if the serum TSH level is already suppressed due to the risk of precipitating overt thyrotoxicosis (see CONTRAINDICATIONS). If the serum TSH level is not suppressed, Synthroid should be used with caution in conjunction with careful monitoring of thyroid function for evidence of hyperthyroidism and clinical monitoring for potential associated adverse cardiovascular signs and symptoms of hyperthyroidism.

PRECAUTIONS

GENERAL

Levothyroxine has a narrow therapeutic index. Regardless of the indication for use, careful dosage titration is necessary to avoid the consequences of over- or under-treatment. These consequences include, among others, effects on growth and development, cardiovascular function, bone metabolism, reproductive function, cognitive function, emotional state, gastrointestinal function, and on glucose and lipid metabolism. Many drugs interact with levothyroxine sodium necessitating adjustments in dosing to maintain therapeutic response (see DRUG INTERACTIONS).

Effects on bone mineral density: In women, long-term levothyroxine sodium therapy has been associated with decreased bone mineral density, especially in postmenopausal women on greater than replacement doses or in women who are receiving suppressive doses of levothyroxine sodium. Therefore, it is recommended that patients receiving levothyroxine sodium be given the minimum dose necessary to achieve the desired clinical and biochemical response.

Patients with underlying cardiovascular disease: Exercise caution when administering levothyroxine to patients with cardiovascular disorders and to the elderly in whom there is an increased risk of occult cardiac disease. In these patients, levothyroxine therapy should be initiated at lower doses than those recommended in younger individuals or in patients without cardiac disease (see WARNINGS; PRECAUTIONS, Geriatric Use; and DOSAGE AND ADMINISTRATION). If cardiac symptoms develop or worsen, the levothyroxine dose should be reduced or withheld for 1 week and then cautiously restarted at a lower dose. Overtreatment with levothyroxine sodium may have adverse cardiovascular effects such as an increase in heart rate, cardiac wall thickness, and cardiac contractility and may precipitate angina or arrhythmias. Patients with coronary artery disease who are receiving levothyroxine therapy should be monitored closely during surgical procedures, since the possibility of precipitating cardiac arrhythmias may be greater in those treated with levothyroxine. Concomitant administration of levothyroxine and sympathomimetic agents to patients with coronary artery disease may precipitate coronary insufficiency.

Patients with nontoxic diffuse goiter or nodular thyroid disease: Exercise caution when administering levothyroxine with nontoxic diffuse goiter or nodular thyroid disease in order to prevent precipitation of thyrotoxicosis (see WARNINGS). If the serum TSH is already suppressed, levothyroxine sodium should not be administered (see CONTRAINDICATIONS).

Associated Endocrine Disorders

Hypothalamic/pituitary Hormone Deficiencies

In patients with secondary or tertiary hypothyroidism, additional hypothalamic/pituitary hormone deficiencies should be considered, and if diagnosed, treated (see Autoimmune Polyglandular Syndrome for adrenal insufficiency).

Autoimmune Polyglandular Syndrome

Occasionally, chronic autoimmune thyroiditis may occur in association with other autoimmune disorders such as adrenal insufficiency, pernicious anemia, and insulin-dependent diabetes mellitus. Patients with concomitant adrenal insufficiency should be treated with replacement glucocorticoids prior to initiation of treatment with levothyroxine sodium. Failure to do so may precipitate an acute adrenal crisis when thyroid hormone therapy is initiated, due to increased metabolic clearance of glucocorticoids by thyroid hormone. Patients with diabetes mellitus may require upward adjustments of their antidiabetic therapeutic regimens when treated with levothyroxine (see DRUG INTERACTIONS).

Other Associated Medical Conditions

Infants with congenital hypothyroidism appear to be at increased risk for other congenital anomalies, with cardiovascular anomalies (pulmonary stenosis, atrial septal defect, and ventricular septal defect) being the most common association.

INFORMATION FOR THE PATIENT

Patients should be informed of the following information to aid in the safe and effective use of Synthroid:

Notify your physician if you are allergic to any foods or medicines, are pregnant or intend to become pregnant, are breastfeeding or are taking any other medications, including prescription and over-the-counter preparations.

Notify your physician of any other medical conditions you may have, particularly heart disease, diabetes, clotting disorders, and adrenal or pituitary gland problems. Your dose of medications used to control these other conditions may need to be adjusted while you are taking Synthroid. If you have diabetes, monitor your blood and/or urinary glucose levels as directed by your physician and immediately report any changes to your physician. If you are taking anticoagulants (blood thinners), your clotting status should be checked frequently.

Use Synthroid only as prescribed by your physician. Do not discontinue or change the amount you take or how often you take it, unless directed to do so by your physician.

The levothyroxine in Synthroid is intended to replace a hormone that is normally produced by your thyroid gland. Generally, replacement therapy is to be taken for life, except in cases of transient hypothyroidism, which is usually associated with an inflammation of the thyroid gland (thyroiditis).

Take Synthroid in the morning on an empty stomach, at least one-half hour before eating any food.

It may take several weeks before you notice an improvement in your symptoms.

Notify your physician if you experience any of the following symptoms: rapid or irregular heartbeat, chest pain, shortness of breath, leg cramps, headache, nervousness, irritability, sleeplessness, tremors, change in appetite, weight gain or loss, vomiting, diarrhea, excessive sweating, heat intolerance, fever, changes in menstrual periods, hives or skin rash, or any other unusual medical event.

Notify your physician if you become pregnant while taking Synthroid. It is likely that your dose of Synthroid will need to be increased while you are pregnant.

Notify your physician or dentist that you are taking Synthroid prior to any surgery.

Partial hair loss may occur rarely during the first few months of Synthroid therapy, but this is usually temporary.

Synthroid should not be used as a primary or adjunctive therapy in a weight control program.

Keep Synthroid out of the reach of children. Store Synthroid away from heat, moisture, and light.

LABORATORY TESTS

General

The diagnosis of hypothyroidism is confirmed by measuring TSH levels using a sensitive assay (second generation assay sensitivity $\leq$0.1 mIU/L or third generation assay sensitivity $\leq$0.01 mIU/L) and measurement of free-T_4.

The adequacy of therapy is determined by periodic assessment of appropriate laboratory tests and clinical evaluation. The choice of laboratory tests depends on various factors including the etiology of the underlying thyroid disease, the presence of concomitant medical conditions, including pregnancy, and the use of concomitant medications (see DRUG INTERACTIONS and PRECAUTIONS, Drug/Laboratory Test Interactions). Persistent clinical and laboratory evidence of hypothyroidism despite an apparent adequate replacement dose of Synthroid may be evidence of inadequate absorption, poor compliance, drug interactions, or decreased T_4 potency of the drug product.

Adults

In adult patients with primary (thyroidal) hypothyroidism, serum TSH levels (using a sensitive assay) alone may be used to monitor therapy. The frequency of TSH monitoring during levothyroxine dose titration depends on the clinical situation but it is generally recommended at 6-8 week intervals until normalization. For patients who have recently initiated levothyroxine therapy and whose serum TSH has normalized or in patients who have had their dosage or brand of levothyroxine changed, the serum TSH concentration should be measured after 8-12 weeks. When the optimum replacement dose has been attained, clinical (physical examination) and biochemical monitoring may be performed every 6-12 months, depending on the clinical situation, and whenever there is a change in the patient's status. It is recommended that a physical examination and a serum TSH measurement be performed at least annually in patients receiving levothyroxine sodium (see WARNINGS, PRECAUTIONS, and DOSAGE AND ADMINISTRATION).

Pediatrics

In patients with congenital hypothyroidism, that adequacy of replacement therapy should be assessed by measuring both serum TSH (using a sensitive assay) and total- or free-T_4. During the first 3 years of life, the serum total- or free-T_4 should be maintained at all times in the upper half of the normal range. While the aim of therapy is to also normalize the serum TSH level, this is not always possible in a small percentage of patients, particularly in the first few months of therapy. TSH may not normalize due to a resetting of the pituitary-thyroid feedback threshold as a result of *in utero* hypothyroidism. Failure of the serum T_4 to increase into the upper half of the normal range within 2 weeks of initiation of Synthroid therapy and/or of the serum TSH to decrease below 20 mU/L within 4 weeks should alert the physician to the possibility that the child is not receiving adequate therapy. Careful inquiry should then be made regarding compliance, dose of medication administered, and method of administration prior to raising the dose of Synthroid.

The recommended frequency of monitoring of TSH and total or free T_4 in children is as follows: at 2 and 4 weeks after the initiation of treatment; every 1-2 months during the first year of life; every 2-3 months between 1 and 3 years of age; and every 3-12 months thereafter until growth is completed. More frequent intervals of monitoring may be necessary if poor compliance is suspected or abnormal values are obtained. It is recommended that TSH and T_4 levels, and a physical examination, if indicated, be performed 2 weeks after any change in levothyroxine sodium dosage. Routine clinical examination, including assessment of mental and physical growth and development, and bone maturation, should be performed at regular intervals (see PRECAUTIONS, Pediatric Use and DOSAGE AND ADMINISTRATION).

Secondary (pituitary) and Tertiary (hypothalamic) Hypothyroidism

Adequacy of therapy should be assessed by measuring serum free-T_4 levels, which should be maintained in the upper half of the normal range in these patients.

DRUG-FOOD INTERACTIONS

Consumption of certain foods may affect levothyroxine absorption thereby necessitating adjustments in dosing. Soybean flour (infant formula), cotton seed meal, walnuts, and dietary fiber may bind and decrease the absorption of levothyroxine sodium from the GI tract.

DRUG/LABORATORY TEST INTERACTIONS

Changes in TBG concentration must be considered when interpreting T_4 and T_3 values, which necessitates measurement and evaluation of unbound (free) hormone and/or determination of the free T_4 index (FT_4I). Pregnancy, infectious hepatitis, estrogens, estrogen-containing oral contraceptives, and acute intermittent porphyria increase TBG concentrations. Decreases in TBG concentrations are observed in nephrosis, severe hypoproteinemia, severe liver disease, acromegaly, and after androgen or corticosteroid therapy (see also DRUG INTERACTIONS, Drug-Thyroidal Axis Interactions). Familial hyper- or hypo-thyroxine binding globulinemias have been described, with the incidence of TBG deficiency approximating 1 in 9000.

CARCINOGENESIS, MUTAGENESIS, AND IMPAIRMENT OF FERTILITY

Animal studies have not been performed to evaluate the carcinogenic potential, mutagenic potential or effects on fertility of levothyroxine. The synthetic T_4 in Synthroid is identical to that produced naturally by the human thyroid gland. Although there has been a reported association between prolonged thyroid hormone therapy and breast cancer, this has not been confirmed. Patients receiving Synthroid for appropriate clinical indications should be titrated to the lowest effective replacement dose.

PREGNANCY CATEGORY A

Studies in women taking levothyroxine sodium during pregnancy have not shown an increased risk of congenital abnormalities. Therefore, the possibility of fetal harm appears remote. Synthroid should not be discontinued during pregnancy and hypothyroidism diagnosed during pregnancy should be promptly treated.

Hypothyroidism during pregnancy is associated with a higher rate of complications, including spontaneous abortion, preeclampsia, stillbirth and premature delivery. Maternal hypothyroidism may have an adverse effect on fetal and childhood growth and development. During pregnancy, serum T_4 levels may decrease and serum TSH levels increase to values outside the normal range. Since elevations in serum TSH may occur as early as 4 weeks gestation, pregnant women taking Synthroid should have their TSH measured during each trimester. An elevated serum TSH level should be corrected by an increase in the dose of Synthroid. Since postpartum TSH levels are similar to preconception values, the Synthroid dosage should return to the pre-pregnancy dose immediately after delivery. A serum TSH level should be obtained 6-8 weeks postpartum.

Thyroid hormones do not readily cross the placental barrier; however, some transfer does occur as evidenced by levels in cord blood of athyreotic fetuses being approximately one-third maternal levels. Transfer of thyroid hormone from the mother to the fetus, however, may not be adequate to prevent *in utero* hypothyroidism.

NURSING MOTHERS

Although thyroid hormones are excreted only minimally in human milk, caution should be exercised when Synthroid is administered to a nursing woman. However, adequate replacement doses of levothyroxine are generally needed to maintain normal lactation.

PEDIATRIC USE

General

The goal of treatment in pediatric patients with hypothyroidism is to achieve and maintain normal intellectual and physical growth and development.

The initial dose of levothyroxine varies with age and body weight (see TABLE 3). Dosing adjustments are based on an assessment of the individual patient's clinical and laboratory parameters (see PRECAUTIONS, Laboratory Tests).

In children in whom a diagnosis of permanent hypothyroidism has not been established, it is recommended that levothyroxine administration be discontinued for a 30 day trial period, but only after the child is at least 3 years of age. Serum T_4 and TSH levels should then be obtained. If the T_4 is low and TSH levels are high, the diagnosis of permanent hypothyroidism is established, and levothyroxine therapy should be reinstituted. If the T_4 and TSH levels are normal, euthyroidism may be assumed and, therefore, the hypothyroidism can be considered to have been transient. In this instance, however, the physician should carefully monitor the child and repeat the thyroid function tests if any signs or symptoms of hypothyroidism develop. In this setting, the clinician should have a high index of suspicion of relapse. If the results of the levothyroxine withdrawal test are inconclusive, careful follow-up and subsequent testing will be necessary.

Since some more severely affected children may become clinically hypothyroid when treatment is discontinued for 30 days, an alternate approach is to reduce the replacement dose of levothyroxine by half during the 30 day trial period. If, after 30 days, the serum TSH is elevated above 20 mU/L, the diagnosis of permanent hypothyroidism is confirmed, and full replacement therapy should be resumed. However, if the serum TSH has not risen to greater than 20 mU/L, levothyroxine treatment should be discontinued for another 30 day trial period followed by repeat serum T_4 and TSH.

The presence of concomitant medical conditions should be considered in certain clinical circumstances and, if present, appropriately treated (see PRECAUTIONS).

Congenital Hypothyroidism

See PRECAUTIONS, Laboratory Tests and DOSAGE AND ADMINISTRATION.

Rapid restoration of normal serum T_4 concentrations is essential for preventing the adverse effects of congenital hypothyroidism on intellectual development as well as on overall physical growth and maturation. Therefore, levothyroxine therapy should be initiated immediately upon diagnosis and is generally continued for life.

During the first 2 weeks of Synthroid therapy, infants should be closely monitored for cardiac overload, arrhythmias, and aspiration from avid suckling.

The patient should be monitored closely to avoid undertreatment or overtreatment. Undertreatment may have deleterious effects on intellectual development and linear growth. Overtreatment has been associated with craniosynostosis in infants, and may adversely affect the tempo of brain maturation and accelerate the bone age with resultant premature closure of the epiphyses and compromised adult stature.

Acquired Hypothyroidism in Pediatric Patients

The patient should be monitored closely to avoid undertreatment and overtreatment. Undertreatment may result in poor school performance due to impaired concentration and slowed mentation and in reduced adult height. Overtreatment may accelerate the bone age and result in premature epiphyseal closure and compromised adult stature.

Treated children may manifest a period of catch-up growth, which may be adequate in some cases to normalize adult height. In children with severe or prolonged hypothyroidism, catch-up growth may not be adequate to normalize adult height.

GERIATRIC USE

Because of the increased prevalence of cardiovascular disease among the elderly, levothyroxine therapy should not be initiated at the full replacement dose (see WARNINGS, PRECAUTIONS, and DOSAGE AND ADMINISTRATION).

DRUG INTERACTIONS

Many drugs affect thyroid hormone pharmacokinetics and metabolism (*e.g.*, absorption, synthesis, secretion, catabolism, protein binding, and target tissue response) and may alter the therapeutic response to Synthroid. In addition, thyroid hormones and thyroid status have varied effects on the pharmacokinetics and action of other drugs. A listing of drug-thyroidal axis interactions is contained in Drug-Thyroidal Axis Interactions.

The list of drug-thyroidal axis interactions in Drug-Thyroidal Axis Interactions may not be comprehensive due to the introduction of new drugs that interact with the thyroidal axis or the discovery of previously unknown interactions. The prescriber should be aware of this fact and should consult appropriate reference sources (*e.g.*, package inserts of newly approved drugs, medical literature) for additional information if a drug-drug interaction with levothyroxine is suspected.

DRUG-THYROIDAL AXIS INTERACTIONS

Drugs That May Reduce TSH Secretion — The Reduction Is Not Sustained; Therefore Hypothyroidism Does Not Occur

Dopamine/dopamine agonists, glucocorticoids, octreotide: Use of these agents may result in a transient reduction in TSH secretion when administered at the following doses: dopamine (≥1 μg/kg/min); glucocorticoids (hydrocortisone ≥100 mg/day or equivalent); octreotide (>100 μg/day).

Drugs That Alter Thyroid Hormone Secretion

Drugs that may decrease thyroid hormone secretion, which may result in hypothyroidism:

Aminoglutethimide, amiodarone, iodide (including iodine-containing radiographic contrast agents), lithium, methimazole, propylthiouracil (PTU), sulfonamides, tolbutamide: Long-term lithium therapy can result in goiter in up to 50% of patients, and either subclinical or overt hypothyroidism, each in up to 20% of patients. The fetus, neonate, elderly and euthyroid patients with underlying thyroid disease (*e.g.*, Hashimoto's thyroiditis or with Grave's disease previously treated with radioiodine or surgery) are among those individuals who are particularly susceptible to iodine-induced hypothyroidism. Oral cholecystographic agents and amiodarone are slowly excreted, producing more prolonged hypothyroidism than parenterally administered iodinated contrast agents. Long-term aminoglutethimide therapy may minimally decrease T_4 and T_3 levels and increase TSH, although all values remain within normal limits in most patients.

Drugs that may increase thyroid hormone secretion, which may result in hyperthyroidism:

Amiodarone, iodide (including iodine-containing radiographic contrast agents): Iodide and drugs that contain pharmacologic amounts of iodide may cause hyperthyroidism in euthyroid patients with Grave's disease previously treated with antithyroid drugs or in euthyroid patients with thyroid autonomy (*e.g.*, multinodular goiter or hyperfunctioning thyroid adenoma). Hyperthyroidism may develop over several weeks and may persist for several months after therapy discontinuation. Amiodarone may induce hyperthyroidism by causing thyroiditis.

Drugs that may decrease T_4 absorption, which may result in hypothyroidism:

Antacids (aluminum and magnesium); hydroxides (simethicone); bile acid sequestrants (cholestyramine, colestipol); calcium carbonate; cation exchange resins (kayexalate); ferrous sulfate; sucralfate: Concurrent use may reduce the efficacy of levothyroxine by binding and delaying or preventing absorption, potentially resulting in hypothyroidism. Calcium carbonate may form an insoluble chelate with levothyroxine, and ferrous sulfate likely forms a ferric-thyroxine complex. Administer levothyroxine at least 4 hours apart from these agents.

Drugs That May Alter T_4 and T_3 Serum Transport — But FT_4 Concentration Remains Normal; and Therefore, the Patient Remains Euthyroid

Drugs that may increase serum TBG concentration:

Clofibrate, estrogen-containing oral contraceptives, estrogens (oral), heroin/methadone, 5-fluorouracil, mitotane, tamoxifen.

Drugs that may decrease serum TBG concentration:

Androgens/anabolic steroids, asparaginase, glucocorticoids, slow-release nicotinic acid.

Drugs that may cause protein-binding site displacement:

Furosemide (>80 mg IV); heparin; hydantoins; non-steroidal anti-inflammatory drugs (fenamates, phenylbutazone); salicylates (>2 g/day): Administration of these agents with levothyroxine results in an initial transient increase in FT_4. Continued administration results in a decrease in serum T_4 and normal FT_4 and TSH concentrations and, therefore, patients are clinically euthyroid. Salicylates inhibit binding of T_4 and T_3 to TBG and transthyretin. An initial increase in serum FT_4 is followed by return of FT_4 to normal levels with sustained therapeutic serum salicylate concentrations, although total-T_4 levels may decrease by as much as 30%.

Drugs That May Alter T_4 and T_3 Metabolism

Drugs that may increase hepatic metabolism, which may result in hypothyroidism:

Carbamazepine, hydantoins, phenobarbital, rifampin: Stimulation of hepatic microsomal drug-metabolizing enzyme activity may cause increased hepatic degradation of levothyroxine, resulting in increased levothyroxine requirements. Phenytoin and carbamazepine reduce serum protein binding of levothyroxine, and total- and free-T_4 may be reduced by 20-40%, but most patients have normal serum TSH levels and are clinically euthyroid.

Drugs That May Decrease T_4 5′-Deiodinase Activity

Amiodarone; beta-adrenergic antagonists (e.g., propranolol >160 mg/day); glucocorticoids (e.g., dexamethasone ≥4 mg/day); propylthiouracil (PTU): Administration of these enzyme inhibitors decreases the peripheral conversion of T_4 to T_3, leading to decreased T_3 levels. However, serum T_4 levels are usually normal but may occasionally be slightly increased. In patients treated with large doses of propranolol (>160 mg/day), T_3 and T_4 levels change slightly, TSH levels remain normal, and patients are clinically euthyroid. It should be noted that actions of particular beta-adrenergic antagonists may be impaired when the hypothyroid patient is converted to the euthyroid state. Short-term administration of large doses of glucocorticoids may decrease serum T_3 concentrations by 30% with minimal change in serum T_4 levels. However, long-term glucocorticoid therapy may result in slightly decreased T_3 and T_4 levels due to decreased TBG production (see above).

Miscellaneous

Anticoagulants (oral) — coumarin derivatives, indandione derivatives: Thyroid hormones appear to increase the catabolism of vitamin K-dependent clotting factors, thereby increasing the anticoagulant activity of oral anticoagulants. Concomitant use of these agents impairs the compensatory increases in clotting factor synthesis. Prothrombin time should be carefully monitored in patients taking levothyroxine and oral anticoagulant and the dose of anticoagulant therapy adjusted accordingly.

Antidepressants — tricyclics (e.g., amitriptyline); tetracyclics (e.g., maprotiline); selective serotonin reuptake inhibitors (SSRIs; e.g., sertraline): Concurrent use of tri/tetracyclic antidepressants and levothyroxine may increase the therapeutic and toxic effects of both drugs, possibly due to increased receptor sensitivity to catecholamines. Toxic effects may include increased risk of cardiac arrhythmias and CNS stimulation; onset of action of tricyclics may be accelerated. Administration of sertraline in patients stabilized on levothyroxine may result in increased levothyroxine requirements.

Antidiabetic agents — biguanides, meglitinides, sulfonylureas, thiazolidediones, insulin: Addition of levothyroxine to antidiabetic or insulin therapy may result in increased antidiabetic agent or insulin requirements. Careful monitoring of diabetic control is recommended, especially when thyroid therapy is started, changed, or discontinued.

Cardiac glycosides: Serum digitalis glycoside levels may be reduced in hyperthyroidism or when the hypothyroid patient is converted to the euthyroid state. Therapeutic effect of digitalis glycosides may be reduced.

Cytokines — interferon-α, interleukin-2: Therapy with interferon-α has been associated with the development of antithyroid microsomal antibodies in 20% of patients and some have transient hypothyroidism, hyperthyroidism, or both. Patients who have antithyroid antibodies before treatment are at higher risk for thyroid dysfunction during treatment. Interleukin-2 has been associated with transient painless thyroiditis in 20% of patients. Interferon-β and -γ have not been reported to cause thyroid dysfunction.

Growth hormones — somatrem, somatropin: Excessive use of thyroid hormones with growth hormones may accelerate epiphyseal closure. However, untreated hypothyroidism may interfere with growth response to growth hormone.

Ketamine: Concurrent use may produce marked hypertension and tachycardia; cautious administration to patients receiving thyroid hormone therapy is recommended.

Methylxanthine bronchodilators (e.g., theophylline): Decreased theophylline clearance may occur in hypothyroid patients; clearance returns to normal when the euthyroid state is achieved.

Radiographic agents: Thyroid hormones may reduce the uptake of ^{123}I, ^{131}I, and ^{99m}Tc.

Sympathomimetics: Concurrent use may increase the effects of sympathomimetics or thyroid hormone. Thyroid hormones may increase the risk of coronary insufficiency when sympathomimetic agents are administered to patients with coronary artery disease.

Chloral hydrate, diazepam, ethionamide, lovastatin, metoclopramide, 6-mercaptopurine, nitroprusside, para-aminosalicylate sodium, perphenazine, resorcinol (excessive topical use), thiazide diuretics: These agents have been associated with thyroid hormone and/or TSH level alterations by various mechanisms.

ORAL ANTICOAGULANTS

Levothyroxine increases the response to oral anticoagulant therapy. Therefore, a decrease in the dose of anticoagulant may be warranted with correction of the hypothyroid state or when the Synthroid dose is increased. Prothrombin time should be closely monitored to permit appropriate and timely dosage adjustments (see Drug-Thyroidal Axis Interactions).

DIGITALIS GLYCOSIDES

The therapeutic effects of digitalis glycosides may be reduced by levothyroxine. Serum digitalis glycoside levels may be decreased when a hypothyroid patient becomes euthyroid, necessitating an increase in the dose of digitalis glycosides (see Drug-Thyroidal Axis Interactions).

ADVERSE REACTIONS

Adverse reactions associated with levothyroxine therapy are primarily those of hyperthyroidism due to therapeutic overdosage. They include the following:

General: Fatigue, increased appetite, weight loss, heat intolerance, fever, excessive sweating.

Central Nervous System: Headache, hyperactivity, nervousness, anxiety, irritability, emotional lability, insomnia.

Musculoskeletal: Tremors, muscle weakness.

Cardiac: Palpitations, tachycardia, arrhythmias, increased pulse and blood pressure, heart failure, angina, myocardial infarction, cardiac arrest.

Pulmonary: Dyspnea.
GI: Diarrhea, vomiting, abdominal cramps.
Dermatologic: Hair loss, flushing.
Reproductive: Menstrual irregularities, impaired fertility.

Pseudotumor cerebri has been reported in children receiving levothyroxine therapy.

Seizures have been reported rarely with the institution of levothyroxine therapy.

Inadequate levothyroxine dosage will produce or fail to ameliorate the signs and symptoms of hypothyroidism.

Hypersensitivity reactions to inactive ingredients have occurred in patients treated with thyroid hormone products. These include urticaria, pruritus, skin rash, flushing, angioedema, various GI symptoms (abdominal pain, nausea, vomiting and diarrhea), fever, arthralgia, serum sickness and wheezing. Hypersensitivity to levothyroxine itself is not known to occur.

DOSAGE AND ADMINISTRATION

GENERAL PRINCIPLES

The goal of replacement therapy is to achieve and maintain a clinical and biochemical euthyroid state. The goal of suppressive therapy is to inhibit growth and/or function of abnormal thyroid tissue. The dose of Synthroid that is adequate to achieve these goals depends on a variety of factors including the patient's age, body weight, cardiovascular status, concomitant medical conditions, including pregnancy, concomitant medications, and the specific nature of the condition being treated (see WARNINGS and PRECAUTIONS). Hence, the following recommendations serve only as dosing guidelines. Dosing must be individualized and adjustments made based on periodic assessment of the patients' clinical response and laboratory parameters (see PRECAUTIONS, Laboratory Tests).

Synthroid should be taken in the morning on an empty stomach, at least one-half hour before any food is eaten. Synthroid should be taken at least 4 hours apart from drugs that are known to interfere with its absorption (see DRUG INTERACTIONS).

Due to the long half-life of levothyroxine, the peak therapeutic effect at a given dose of levothyroxine sodium may not be attained for 4-6 weeks.

Caution should be exercised when administering Synthroid to patients with underlying cardiovascular disease, to the elderly, and to those with concomitant adrenal insufficiency (see PRECAUTIONS).

SPECIFIC PATIENT POPULATIONS

Hypothyroidism in Adults and in Children in Whom Growth and Puberty Are Complete

See WARNINGS and PRECAUTIONS, Laboratory Tests.

Therapy may begin at full replacement doses in otherwise healthy individuals less than 50 years old and in those older than 50 years who have been recently treated for hyperthyroidism or who have been hypothyroid for only a short time (such as a few months). The average full replacement dose of levothyroxine sodium is approximately 1.7 µg/kg/day (*e.g.,* **100-125 µg/day** for a 70 kg adult). Older patients may require less than 1 µg/kg/day. Levothyroxine sodium doses greater than 200 µg/day are seldom required. An inadequate response to daily doses ≥3 µg/day is rare and may indicate poor compliance, malabsorption, and/or drug interactions.

For most patients older than 50 years or for patients under 50 years of age with underlying cardiac disease, an initial starting dose of **25-50 µg/day** of levothyroxine sodium is recommended, with gradual increments in dose at 6-8 week intervals, as needed. The recommended starting dose of levothyroxine sodium in elderly patients with cardiac disease is **12.5-25 µg/day,** with gradual dose increments at 4-6 week intervals. The levothyroxine sodium dose is generally adjusted in 12.5-25 µg increments until the patients with primary hypothyroidism is clinically euthyroid and the serum TSH has normalized.

In patients with severe hypothyroidism, the recommended initial levothyroxine sodium dose is **12.5-25 µg/day** with increases of 25 µg/day every 2-4 weeks, accompanied by clinical and laboratory assessment, until the TSH level is normalized.

In patients with secondary (pituitary) or tertiary (hypothalamic) hypothyroidism, the levothyroxine sodium dose should be titrated until the patient is clinically euthyroid and the serum free-T_4 level is restored to the upper half of the normal range.

Pediatric Dosage — Congenital or Acquired Hypothyroidism

See PRECAUTIONS, Laboratory Tests.

General Principles

In general, levothyroxine therapy should be instituted at full replacement doses as soon as possible. Delays in diagnosis and institution of therapy may have deleterious effects on the child's intellectual and physical growth and development.

Undertreatment and overtreatment should be avoided (see PRECAUTIONS, Pediatric Use).

Synthroid may be administered to infants and children who cannot swallow intact tablets by crushing the tablet and suspending the freshly crushed tablet in a small amount (5-10 ml or 1-2 teaspoons) of water. This suspension can be administered by spoon or by dropper. **DO NOT STORE THE SUSPENSION.** Foods that decrease absorption of levothyroxine, such as soybean infant formula, should not be used for administering levothyroxine sodium tablets (see PRECAUTIONS, Drug-Food Interactions).

Newborns

The recommended starting dose of levothyroxine sodium in newborn infants is **10-15 µg/kg/day.** A lower starting dose (*e.g.,* 25 µg/day) should be considered in infants at risk for cardiac failure, and the dose should be increased in 4-6 weeks as needed based on clinical and laboratory response to treatment. In infants with very low (<5 µg/dl) or undetectable serum T_4 concentrations, the recommended initial starting dose is **50 µg/day** of levothyroxine sodium.

Infants and Children

Levothyroxine therapy is usually initiated at full replacement doses, with the recommended dose per body weight decreasing with age (see TABLE 3). However, in children with chronic or severe hypothyroidism, an initial dose of **25 µg/day** of levothyroxine sodium is recommended with increments of 25 µg every 2-4 weeks until the desired effect is achieved.

Hyperactivity in an older child can be minimized if the starting dose is one-fourth of the recommended full replacement dose, and the dose is then increased on a weekly basis by an amount equal to one-fourth the full-recommended replacement dose until the full recommended replacement dose is reached.

TABLE 3 *Levothyroxine Sodium Dosing Guidelines for Pediatric Hypothyroidism*

Age	Daily Dose Per Kg Body Weight*
0-3 months	10-15 µg/kg/day
3-6 months	8-10 µg/kg/day
6-12 months	6-8 µg/kg/day
1-5 years	5-6 µg/kg/day
6-12 years	4-5 µg/kg/day
>12 years	2-3 µg/kg/day
Growth and puberty complete	1.7 µg/kg/day

* The dose should be adjusted based on clinical response and laboratory parameters (see PRECAUTIONS: Laboratory Tests and Pediatric Use).

PREGNANCY

Pregnancy may increase levothyroxine requirements (see PRECAUTIONS, Pregnancy Category A).

SUBCLINICAL HYPOTHYROIDISM

If this condition is treated, a lower levothyroxine sodium dose (*e.g.,* **1 µg/kg/day**) than that used for full replacement may be adequate to normalize the serum TSH level. Patients who are not treated should be monitored yearly for changes in clinical status and thyroid laboratory parameters.

TSH SUPPRESSION IN WELL-DIFFERENTIATED THYROID CANCER AND THYROID NODULES

The target level for TSH suppression in these conditions has not been established with controlled studies. In addition, the efficacy of TSH suppression for benign nodular disease is controversial. Therefore, the dose of Synthroid used for TSH suppression should be individualized based on the specific disease and the patient being treated. In the treatment of well differentiated (papillary and follicular) thyroid cancer, levothyroxine is used as an adjunct to surgery and radioiodine therapy. Generally, TSH is suppressed to <0.1 mU/L, and this usually requires a levothyroxine sodium dose of **greater than 2 µg/kg/day.** However, in patients with high-risk tumors, the target level for TSH suppression may be <0.01 mU/L.

In the treatment of benign nodules and nontoxic multinodular goiter, TSH is generally suppressed to a higher target (*e.g.,* 0.1-0.5 mU/L for nodules and 0.5-1.0 mU/L for multinodular goiter) than that used for the treatment of thyroid cancer. Levothyroxine sodium is contraindicated if the serum TSH is already suppressed due to the risk of precipitating overt thyrotoxicosis (see CONTRAINDICATIONS, WARNINGS and PRECAUTIONS).

MYXEDEMA COMA

Myxedema coma is a life-threatening emergency characterized by poor circulation and hypometabolism, and may result in unpredictable absorption of levothyroxine sodium from the gastrointestinal tract. Therefore, oral levothyroxine is not recommended to treat this condition. Intravenous levothyroxine sodium should be administered.

HOW SUPPLIED

Synthroid (levothyroxine sodium) tablets are supplied as follows:

25 µg: Orange, round, scored and debossed with "FLINT" and "25".
50 µg: White, round, scored and debossed with "FLINT" and "50".
75 µg: Violet, round, scored and debossed with "FLINT" and "75".
88 µg: Olive, round, scored and debossed with "FLINT" and "88".
100 µg: Yellow, round, scored and debossed with "FLINT" and "100".
112 µg: Rose, round, scored and debossed with "FLINT" and "112".
125 µg: Brown, round, scored and debossed with "FLINT" and "125".
150 µg: Blue, round, scored and debossed with "FLINT" and "150".
175 µg: Lilac, round, scored and debossed with "FLINT" and "175".
200 µg: Pink, round, scored and debossed with "FLINT" and "200".
300 µg: Green, round, scored and debossed with "FLINT" and "300".

Storage Conditions: Store at 25°C (77°F); excursions permitted to 15-30°C (59-86°F). Synthroid tablets should be protected from light and moisture.

PRODUCT LISTING - RATED THERAPEUTICALLY EQUIVALENT

Tablet - Oral - 0.025 mg

100's	$23.75	GENERIC, Mylan Pharmaceuticals Inc	00378-1800-01

Tablet - Oral - 0.05 mg

100's	$27.00	GENERIC, Mylan Pharmaceuticals Inc	00378-1803-01

Tablet - Oral - 0.075 mg

100's	$29.80	GENERIC, Mylan Pharmaceuticals Inc	00378-1805-01

Tablet - Oral - 0.088 mg

100's	$30.30	GENERIC, Mylan Pharmaceuticals Inc	00378-1807-01

Tablet - Oral - 0.1 mg

100's	$5.63	GENERIC, Auro Pharmaceutical	55829-0345-10
100's	$30.55	GENERIC, Mylan Pharmaceuticals Inc	00378-1809-01

Tablet - Oral - 0.112 mg

100's	$35.30	GENERIC, Mylan Pharmaceuticals Inc	00378-1811-01

Tablet - Oral - 0.125 mg

100's	$35.80	GENERIC, Mylan Pharmaceuticals Inc	00378-1813-01

Tablet - Oral - 0.15 mg

100's	$36.85	GENERIC, Mylan Pharmaceuticals Inc	00378-1815-01

Tablet - Oral - 0.175 mg

100's	$43.80	GENERIC, Mylan Pharmaceuticals Inc	00378-1817-01

Tablet - Oral - 0.2 mg

Qty	Price	Product	NDC
100's	$7.28	GENERIC, Auro Pharmaceutical	55829-0346-10
100's	$45.30	GENERIC, Mylan Pharmaceuticals Inc	00378-1819-01

Tablet - Oral - 0.3 mg

Qty	Price	Product	NDC
100's	$9.22	GENERIC, Auro Pharmaceutical	55829-0347-10
100's	$61.70	GENERIC, Mylan Pharmaceuticals Inc	00378-1821-01

PRODUCT LISTING - RATED NOT THERAPEUTICALLY EQUIVALENT

Tablet - Oral - 0.025 mg

Qty	Price	Product	NDC
100's	$22.40	GENERIC, Physicians Total Care	54868-4087-00
100's	$30.35	GENERIC, Monarch Pharmaceuticals Inc	52604-5025-01
100's	$35.20	SYNTHROID, Abbott Pharmaceutical	00074-4341-13
100's	$43.52	GENERIC, Daniels	00689-1117-05

Tablet - Oral - 0.05 mg

Qty	Price	Product	NDC
100's	$12.30	GENERIC, Physicians Total Care	54868-4092-00
100's	$34.48	GENERIC, Monarch Pharmaceuticals Inc	52604-5050-01
100's	$40.13	SYNTHROID, Abbott Pharmaceutical	00074-4552-13
100's	$42.33	SYNTHROID, Abbott Pharmaceutical	00074-4552-11
100's	$53.08	GENERIC, Daniels	00689-1118-05

Tablet - Oral - 0.075 mg

Qty	Price	Product	NDC
100's	$38.08	GENERIC, Monarch Pharmaceuticals Inc	52604-5075-01
100's	$44.30	SYNTHROID, Abbott Pharmaceutical	00074-5182-13
100's	$47.20	SYNTHROID, Abbott Pharmaceutical	00074-5182-11

Tablet - Oral - 0.088 mg

Qty	Price	Product	NDC
100's	$15.18	GENERIC, Physicians Total Care	54868-4177-00
100's	$38.75	GENERIC, Monarch Pharmaceuticals Inc	52604-5088-01
100's	$45.09	SYNTHROID, Abbott Pharmaceutical	00074-6594-13

Tablet - Oral - 0.1 mg

Qty	Price	Product	NDC
100's	$39.03	GENERIC, Monarch Pharmaceuticals Inc	52604-5100-01
100's	$45.38	SYNTHROID, Abbott Pharmaceutical	00074-6624-13
100's	$48.98	SYNTHROID, Abbott Pharmaceutical	00074-6624-11

Tablet - Oral - 0.112 mg

Qty	Price	Product	NDC
100's	$20.50	GENERIC, Physicians Total Care	54868-3849-00
100's	$45.13	GENERIC, Monarch Pharmaceuticals Inc	52604-5112-01
100's	$52.44	SYNTHROID, Abbott Pharmaceutical	00074-9296-13

Tablet - Oral - 0.125 mg

Qty	Price	Product	NDC
30's	$13.84	GENERIC, Southwood Pharmaceuticals Inc	58016-0621-30
100's	$45.75	GENERIC, Monarch Pharmaceuticals Inc	52604-5125-01
100's	$53.15	SYNTHROID, Abbott Pharmaceutical	00074-7068-13
100's	$56.93	SYNTHROID, Abbott Pharmaceutical	00074-7068-11
100's	$59.15	GENERIC, Daniels	00689-1120-05

L

Tablet - Oral - 0.137 mg

Qty	Price	Product	NDC
100's	$46.40	GENERIC, Monarch Pharmaceuticals Inc	52604-5137-01

Tablet - Oral - 0.15 mg

Qty	Price	Product	NDC
100's	$47.10	GENERIC, Monarch Pharmaceuticals Inc	52604-5150-01
100's	$54.74	SYNTHROID, Abbott Pharmaceutical	00074-7069-13
100's	$58.43	SYNTHROID, Abbott Pharmaceutical	00074-7069-11

Tablet - Oral - 0.175 mg

Qty	Price	Product	NDC
100's	$55.97	GENERIC, Monarch Pharmaceuticals Inc	52604-5175-01
100's	$65.11	SYNTHROID, Abbott Pharmaceutical	00074-7070-13

Tablet - Oral - 0.2 mg

Qty	Price	Product	NDC
100's	$57.93	GENERIC, Monarch Pharmaceuticals Inc	52604-5200-01
100's	$65.25	SYNTHROID, Abbott Pharmaceutical	00074-7148-13

Tablet - Oral - 0.3 mg

Qty	Price	Product	NDC
100's	$78.89	GENERIC, Monarch Pharmaceuticals Inc	52604-5300-01
100's	$88.80	SYNTHROID, Abbott Pharmaceutical	00074-7149-13

PRODUCT LISTING - EQUIVALENTS NOT AVAILABLE

Powder For Injection - Injectable - 0.2 mg

Qty	Price	Product	NDC
1's	$4.38	GENERIC, Bedford Laboratories	55390-0880-10
1's	$7.38	GENERIC, Chiron Therapeutics	00702-0880-10
1's	$16.50	GENERIC, Gensia Sicor Pharmaceuticals Inc	00703-5408-01
1's	$34.94	GENERIC, American Pharmaceutical Partners	63323-0247-10
1's	$51.23	SYNTHROID, Knoll Pharmaceutical Company	00048-1014-99
1's	$57.15	SYNTHROID, Abbott Pharmaceutical	00074-2327-01
1's	$62.56	LEVOTHROID, Forest Pharmaceuticals	00456-0140-88

Powder For Injection - Injectable - 0.5 mg

Qty	Price	Product	NDC
1's	$4.38	GENERIC, Bedford Laboratories	55390-0881-10
1's	$7.38	GENERIC, Chiron Therapeutics	00702-0881-10
1's	$11.88	GENERIC, Astra-Zeneca Pharmaceuticals	00186-1856-01
1's	$12.50	GENERIC, Cmc-Consolidated Midland Corporation	00223-7921-05
1's	$12.69	GENERIC, Udl Laboratories Inc	51079-0707-01
1's	$38.43	GENERIC, American Pharmaceutical Partners	63323-0248-10
1's	$56.43	SYNTHROID, Knoll Pharmaceutical Company	00048-1012-99
1's	$56.43	SYNTHROID, Abbott Pharmaceutical	00074-2326-01
1's	$89.50	LEVOTHROID, Forest Pharmaceuticals	00456-0141-88

Tablet - Oral - 0.025 mg

Qty	Price	Product	NDC
30's	$4.15	GENERIC, Prescript Pharmaceuticals	00247-0353-30
30's	$5.54	GENERIC, Pd-Rx Pharmaceuticals	55289-0076-30
50's	$13.44	SYNTHROID, Allscripts Pharmaceutical Company	54569-0934-02
100's	$4.95	GENERIC, Major Pharmaceuticals Inc	00904-7783-60
100's	$6.00	GENERIC, Prescript Pharmaceuticals	00247-0353-00
100's	$6.19	GENERIC, Physicians Total Care	54868-3388-00
100's	$9.45	GENERIC, Pd-Rx Pharmaceuticals	55289-0076-01
100's	$12.07	GENERIC, Vintage Pharmaceuticals Inc	00254-3911-28
100's	$12.35	GENERIC, Mova Pharmaceutical Corporation	55370-0125-07
100's	$12.74	GENERIC, Esi Lederle Generics	59911-5917-01
100's	$12.75	GENERIC, Caremark Inc	00339-5923-12
100's	$14.48	GENERIC, Roberts Pharmaceutical Corporation	54092-0104-01
100's	$21.94	LEVOTHROID, Forest Pharmaceuticals	00456-0320-01
100's	$26.40	GENERIC, Watson Laboratories Inc	52544-0902-01
100's	$26.88	SYNTHROID, Allscripts Pharmaceutical Company	54569-0934-00
100's	$28.55	SYNTHROID, Physicians Total Care	54868-3389-00
100's	$35.29	SYNTHROID, Knoll Pharmaceutical Company	00048-1020-03

Tablet - Oral - 0.05 mg

Qty	Price	Product	NDC
15's	$3.89	GENERIC, Southwood Pharmaceuticals Inc	58016-0249-15
20's	$5.18	GENERIC, Southwood Pharmaceuticals Inc	58016-0249-20
30's	$1.62	GENERIC, Allscripts Pharmaceutical Company	54569-3766-00
30's	$4.15	GENERIC, Prescript Pharmaceuticals	00247-0354-30
30's	$5.73	GENERIC, Heartland Healthcare Services	61392-0129-30
30's	$5.73	GENERIC, Heartland Healthcare Services	61392-0129-39
30's	$7.77	GENERIC, Southwood Pharmaceuticals Inc	58016-0249-30
30's	$9.72	SYNTHROID, Allscripts Pharmaceutical Company	54569-0908-02
30's	$11.37	SYNTHROID, Physicians Total Care	54868-1011-02
31's	$5.93	GENERIC, Heartland Healthcare Services	61392-0129-31
32's	$6.12	GENERIC, Heartland Healthcare Services	61392-0129-32
45's	$8.60	GENERIC, Heartland Healthcare Services	61392-0129-45
60's	$11.47	GENERIC, Heartland Healthcare Services	61392-0129-60
60's	$22.73	SYNTHROID, Physicians Total Care	54868-1011-00
90's	$17.20	GENERIC, Heartland Healthcare Services	61392-0129-90
90's	$18.00	SYNTHROID, Allscripts Pharmaceutical Company	54569-8573-00
100's	$5.05	GENERIC, Major Pharmaceuticals Inc	00904-7784-60
100's	$5.82	GENERIC, Physicians Total Care	54868-2131-01
100's	$5.85	GENERIC, Pd-Rx Pharmaceuticals	55289-0085-01
100's	$6.00	GENERIC, Prescript Pharmaceuticals	00247-0354-00
100's	$13.84	GENERIC, Caremark Inc	00339-5925-12
100's	$13.89	GENERIC, Mova Pharmaceutical Corporation	55370-0126-07
100's	$14.31	GENERIC, Esi Lederle Generics	59911-5918-01
100's	$14.48	GENERIC, Roberts Pharmaceutical Corporation	54092-0105-01
100's	$19.58	GENERIC, Allscripts Pharmaceutical Company	54569-3766-01
100's	$21.66	GENERIC, Vintage Pharmaceuticals Inc	00254-3912-28
100's	$24.20	LEVOTHROID, Forest Pharmaceuticals	00456-0321-01
100's	$24.20	LEVOTHROID, Forest Pharmaceuticals	00456-0321-63
100's	$25.90	GENERIC, Southwood Pharmaceuticals Inc	58016-0249-00
100's	$29.98	GENERIC, Watson Laboratories Inc	52544-0903-01
100's	$32.40	SYNTHROID, Allscripts Pharmaceutical Company	54569-0908-00
100's	$37.11	SYNTHROID, Physicians Total Care	54868-1011-01
100's	$39.19	SYNTHROID, Knoll Pharmaceutical Company	00048-1040-13
100's	$40.13	SYNTHROID, Knoll Pharmaceutical Company	00048-1040-03

Tablet - Oral - 0.075 mg

Qty	Price	Product	NDC
30's	$2.97	GENERIC, Physicians Total Care	54868-2539-00
30's	$4.15	GENERIC, Prescript Pharmaceuticals	00247-0355-30
30's	$10.85	SYNTHROID, Allscripts Pharmaceutical Company	54569-0907-01
90's	$19.94	SYNTHROID, Allscripts Pharmaceutical Company	54569-8541-00
100's	$4.74	GENERIC, Southwood Pharmaceuticals Inc	58016-0185-00
100's	$5.20	GENERIC, Major Pharmaceuticals Inc	00904-7785-60
100's	$6.00	GENERIC, Prescript Pharmaceuticals	00247-0355-00
100's	$6.12	GENERIC, Physicians Total Care	54868-2539-01
100's	$8.70	GENERIC, Pd-Rx Pharmaceuticals	55289-0082-01
100's	$14.48	GENERIC, Roberts Pharmaceutical Corporation	54092-0106-01
100's	$14.49	GENERIC, Vintage Pharmaceuticals Inc	00254-3913-28
100's	$15.43	GENERIC, Mova Pharmaceutical Corporation	55370-0127-07
100's	$15.50	GENERIC, Caremark Inc	00339-5927-12
100's	$15.90	GENERIC, Esi Lederle Generics	59911-5919-01
100's	$26.66	LEVOTHROID, Forest Pharmaceuticals	00456-0322-01
100's	$33.11	GENERIC, Watson Laboratories Inc	52544-0904-01
100's	$36.02	SYNTHROID, Physicians Total Care	54868-2005-01
100's	$43.70	SYNTHROID, Knoll Pharmaceutical Company	00048-1050-13
100's	$44.30	SYNTHROID, Knoll Pharmaceutical Company	00048-1050-03
100's	$54.81	GENERIC, Daniels	00689-1119-05

Tablet - Oral - 0.088 mg

Qty	Price	Product	NDC
30's	$9.72	SYNTHROID, Allscripts Pharmaceutical Company	54569-4993-00
100's	$14.48	GENERIC, Roberts Pharmaceutical Corporation	54092-0117-01
100's	$24.25	GENERIC, Vintage Pharmaceuticals Inc	00254-3921-28
100's	$25.82	GENERIC, Caremark Inc	00339-6546-12
100's	$27.32	LEVOTHROID, Forest Pharmaceuticals	00456-0329-01
100's	$33.70	GENERIC, Watson Laboratories Inc	52544-0905-01
100's	$36.59	SYNTHROID, Physicians Total Care	54868-2705-00
100's	$45.09	SYNTHROID, Knoll Pharmaceutical Company	00048-1060-03

Tablet - Oral - 0.1 mg

Qty	Price	Product	NDC
12's	$3.50	GENERIC, Southwood Pharmaceuticals Inc	58016-0931-12
15's	$4.37	GENERIC, Southwood Pharmaceuticals Inc	58016-0931-15

20's	$5.83	GENERIC, Southwood Pharmaceuticals Inc	58016-0931-20
30's	$1.67	GENERIC, Allscripts Pharmaceutical Company	54569-0913-01
30's	$2.15	GENERIC, Pharmaceutical Corporation Of America	51655-0091-24
30's	$2.40	GENERIC, Physicians Total Care	54868-0805-01
30's	$4.54	GENERIC, Prescript Pharmaceuticals	00247-0356-30
30's	$4.73	GENERIC, Pd-Rx Pharmaceuticals	55289-0153-30
30's	$6.24	GENERIC, Heartland Healthcare Services	61392-0014-30
30's	$6.24	GENERIC, Heartland Healthcare Services	61392-0014-39
30's	$6.86	GENERIC, Pharma Pac	52959-0089-30
30's	$8.75	GENERIC, Southwood Pharmaceuticals Inc	58016-0931-30
30's	$11.25	SYNTHROID, Allscripts Pharmaceutical Company	54569-0909-00
30's	$12.35	SYNTHROID, Physicians Total Care	54868-0376-03
31's	$6.44	GENERIC, Heartland Healthcare Services	61392-0014-31
32's	$1.58	GENERIC, Vangard Labs	00615-2522-32
32's	$6.65	GENERIC, Heartland Healthcare Services	61392-0014-32
45's	$9.36	GENERIC, Heartland Healthcare Services	61392-0014-45
50's	$14.58	GENERIC, Southwood Pharmaceuticals Inc	58016-0931-50
60's	$12.47	GENERIC, Heartland Healthcare Services	61392-0014-60
60's	$13.62	SYNTHROID, Allscripts Pharmaceutical Company	54569-8512-01
90's	$6.75	GENERIC, Pd-Rx Pharmaceuticals	55289-0153-90
90's	$6.93	GENERIC, Prescript Pharmaceuticals	00247-0356-90
90's	$18.71	GENERIC, Heartland Healthcare Services	61392-0014-90
90's	$20.43	SYNTHROID, Allscripts Pharmaceutical Company	54569-8017-00
90's	$20.43	SYNTHROID, Allscripts Pharmaceutical Company	54569-8512-00
100's	$3.05	GENERIC, Pharmaceutical Corporation Of America	51655-0091-21
100's	$6.62	GENERIC, Major Pharmaceuticals Inc	00904-2236-61
100's	$7.02	GENERIC, Physicians Total Care	54868-0805-02
100's	$7.33	GENERIC, Prescript Pharmaceuticals	00247-0356-00
100's	$9.75	GENERIC, Us Trading Corporation	56126-0468-11
100's	$9.89	GENERIC, Pd-Rx Pharmaceuticals	55289-0153-01
100's	$12.48	GENERIC, Mutual/United Research Laboratories	00677-1690-01
100's	$14.48	GENERIC, Roberts Pharmaceutical Corporation	54092-0108-01
100's	$15.80	GENERIC, Mova Pharmaceutical Corporation	55370-0129-07
100's	$16.31	GENERIC, Esi Lederle Generics	59911-5920-01
100's	$16.42	GENERIC, Caremark Inc	00339-5579-12
100's	$16.95	GENERIC, Pharma Pac	52959-0089-00
100's	$24.48	GENERIC, Vintage Pharmaceuticals Inc	00254-3914-28
100's	$25.54	GENERIC, Allscripts Pharmaceutical Company	54569-0913-00
100's	$27.60	LEVOTHROID, Forest Pharmaceuticals	00456-0323-01
100's	$27.60	LEVOTHROID, Forest Pharmaceuticals	00456-0323-63
100's	$29.15	GENERIC, Southwood Pharmaceuticals Inc	58016-0931-00
100's	$33.94	GENERIC, Watson Laboratories Inc	52544-0906-01
100's	$37.50	SYNTHROID, Allscripts Pharmaceutical Company	54569-0909-01
100's	$38.36	SYNTHROID, Physicians Total Care	54868-0376-01
100's	$45.35	SYNTHROID, Knoll Pharmaceutical Company	00048-1070-13
100's	$45.38	SYNTHROID, Knoll Pharmaceutical Company	00048-1070-03
100's	$54.69	GENERIC, Daniels	00689-1110-05

Tablet - Oral - 0.112 mg

30's	$11.32	SYNTHROID, Allscripts Pharmaceutical Company	54569-8599-01
90's	$23.67	SYNTHROID, Allscripts Pharmaceutical Company	54569-8599-00
100's	$14.48	GENERIC, Roberts Pharmaceutical Corporation	54092-0118-01
100's	$27.30	GENERIC, Caremark Inc	00339-6547-12
100's	$27.50	GENERIC, Vintage Pharmaceuticals Inc	00254-3918-28
100's	$27.50	GENERIC, Qualitest Products Inc	00603-4199-21
100's	$29.92	LEVOTHROID, Forest Pharmaceuticals	00456-0330-01
100's	$39.24	GENERIC, Watson Laboratories Inc	52544-0907-01
100's	$52.44	SYNTHROID, Knoll Pharmaceutical Company	00048-1080-03

Tablet - Oral - 0.125 mg

30's	$2.06	GENERIC, Allscripts Pharmaceutical Company	54569-3767-00
30's	$4.15	GENERIC, Prescript Pharmaceuticals	00247-0363-30
30's	$6.11	GENERIC, Pd-Rx Pharmaceuticals	55289-0858-30
30's	$12.37	SYNTHROID, Allscripts Pharmaceutical Company	54569-3369-01
90's	$23.90	SYNTHROID, Allscripts Pharmaceutical Company	54569-8520-00
100's	$5.40	GENERIC, Major Pharmaceuticals Inc	00904-7786-60
100's	$5.64	GENERIC, Southwood Pharmaceuticals Inc	58016-0644-00
100's	$6.00	GENERIC, Prescript Pharmaceuticals	00247-0363-00
100's	$7.22	GENERIC, Physicians Total Care	54868-3390-00
100's	$10.13	GENERIC, Pd-Rx Pharmaceuticals	55289-0858-01
100's	$14.48	GENERIC, Roberts Pharmaceutical Corporation	54092-0110-01
100's	$18.53	GENERIC, Mova Pharmaceutical Corporation	55370-0130-07
100's	$18.62	GENERIC, Caremark Inc	00339-5929-12
100's	$19.05	GENERIC, Mutual/United Research Laboratories	00677-1695-01
100's	$19.10	GENERIC, Esi Lederle Generics	59911-5921-01
100's	$28.71	GENERIC, Vintage Pharmaceuticals Inc	00254-3919-28
100's	$32.00	LEVOTHROID, Forest Pharmaceuticals	00456-0324-01
100's	$32.00	LEVOTHROID, Forest Pharmaceuticals	00456-0324-63
100's	$39.78	GENERIC, Watson Laboratories Inc	52544-0908-01
100's	$43.15	SYNTHROID, Physicians Total Care	54868-2638-01
100's	$43.62	SYNTHROID, Allscripts Pharmaceutical Company	54569-3369-00
100's	$52.71	SYNTHROID, Knoll Pharmaceutical Company	00048-1130-13
100's	$53.15	SYNTHROID, Knoll Pharmaceutical Company	00048-1130-03

Tablet - Oral - 0.137 mg

100's	$14.48	GENERIC, Roberts Pharmaceutical Corporation	54092-0119-01
100's	$29.25	GENERIC, Vintage Pharmaceuticals Inc	00254-3922-28
100's	$29.25	GENERIC, Qualitest Products Inc	00603-4201-21
100's	$32.56	LEVOTHROID, Forest Pharmaceuticals	00456-0331-01
100's	$54.38	SYNTHROID, Abbott Pharmaceutical	00074-3727-13

Tablet - Oral - 0.15 mg

12's	$4.16	GENERIC, Southwood Pharmaceuticals Inc	58016-0984-12
15's	$5.21	GENERIC, Southwood Pharmaceuticals Inc	58016-0984-15
20's	$6.94	GENERIC, Southwood Pharmaceuticals Inc	58016-0984-20
30's	$2.00	GENERIC, Allscripts Pharmaceutical Company	54569-1753-01
30's	$3.16	GENERIC, Physicians Total Care	54868-1093-01
30's	$4.15	GENERIC, Prescript Pharmaceuticals	00247-0357-30
30's	$10.41	GENERIC, Southwood Pharmaceuticals Inc	58016-0984-30
30's	$10.63	SYNTHROID, Southwood Pharmaceuticals Inc	58016-0962-30
30's	$13.43	SYNTHROID, Allscripts Pharmaceutical Company	54569-0910-02
50's	$4.38	GENERIC, Physicians Total Care	54868-1093-00
60's	$4.99	GENERIC, Physicians Total Care	54868-1093-05
60's	$16.38	SYNTHROID, Allscripts Pharmaceutical Company	54569-8534-01
90's	$24.57	SYNTHROID, Allscripts Pharmaceutical Company	54569-8534-00
100's	$3.15	GENERIC, Pharmaceutical Corporation Of America	51655-0209-21
100's	$6.00	GENERIC, Prescript Pharmaceuticals	00247-0357-00
100's	$7.43	GENERIC, Physicians Total Care	54868-1093-02
100's	$10.43	GENERIC, Pd-Rx Pharmaceuticals	55289-0084-01
100's	$14.48	GENERIC, Roberts Pharmaceutical Corporation	54092-0112-01
100's	$19.10	GENERIC, Mova Pharmaceutical Corporation	55370-0131-07
100's	$19.69	GENERIC, Esi Lederle Generics	59911-5922-01
100's	$20.07	GENERIC, Caremark Inc	00339-5813-12
100's	$29.52	GENERIC, Vintage Pharmaceuticals Inc	00254-3915-28
100's	$32.70	GENERIC, Allscripts Pharmaceutical Company	54569-1753-00
100's	$32.96	LEVOTHROID, Forest Pharmaceuticals	00456-0325-01
100's	$32.96	LEVOTHROID, Forest Pharmaceuticals	00456-0325-63
100's	$34.70	GENERIC, Southwood Pharmaceuticals Inc	58016-0984-00
100's	$40.18	SYNTHROID, Pharma Pac	52959-0206-00
100's	$40.95	GENERIC, Watson Laboratories Inc	52544-0909-01
100's	$42.30	SYNTHROID, Allscripts Pharmaceutical Company	54569-0910-00
100's	$44.08	SYNTHROID, Physicians Total Care	54868-1092-00
100's	$54.10	SYNTHROID, Knoll Pharmaceutical Company	00048-1090-13
100's	$54.74	SYNTHROID, Knoll Pharmaceutical Company	00048-1090-03
100's	$60.50	GENERIC, Daniels	00689-1111-05

Tablet - Oral - 0.175 mg

30's	$14.87	SYNTHROID, Allscripts Pharmaceutical Company	54569-3870-00
90's	$29.21	SYNTHROID, Allscripts Pharmaceutical Company	54569-8610-00
100's	$14.48	GENERIC, Roberts Pharmaceutical Corporation	54092-0120-01
100's	$31.25	GENERIC, Vintage Pharmaceuticals Inc	00254-3920-28
100's	$31.25	GENERIC, Qualitest Products Inc	00603-4202-21
100's	$34.06	GENERIC, Caremark Inc	00339-6548-12
100's	$37.24	LEVOTHROID, Forest Pharmaceuticals	00456-0326-01
100's	$43.52	GENERIC, Watson Laboratories Inc	52544-0881-01
100's	$48.67	GENERIC, Watson Laboratories Inc	52544-0910-01
100's	$65.11	SYNTHROID, Knoll Pharmaceutical Company	00048-1100-03
100's	$69.21	SYNTHROID, Physicians Total Care	54868-3069-00

Tablet - Oral - 0.2 mg

15's	$6.23	GENERIC, Southwood Pharmaceuticals Inc	58016-0932-15
20's	$8.30	GENERIC, Southwood Pharmaceuticals Inc	58016-0932-20
30's	$2.22	GENERIC, Allscripts Pharmaceutical Company	54569-0914-02
30's	$3.28	GENERIC, Physicians Total Care	54868-0890-01
30's	$4.54	GENERIC, Prescript Pharmaceuticals	00247-0358-30
30's	$12.45	GENERIC, Southwood Pharmaceuticals Inc	58016-0932-30
30's	$16.83	SYNTHROID, Physicians Total Care	54868-1012-03
60's	$5.23	GENERIC, Physicians Total Care	54868-0890-00
90's	$5.57	GENERIC, Pd-Rx Pharmaceuticals	55289-0154-90
90's	$6.93	GENERIC, Prescript Pharmaceuticals	00247-0358-90
90's	$29.39	SYNTHROID, Allscripts Pharmaceutical Company	54569-8575-00

100's	$3.30	GENERIC, Pharmaceutical Corporation Of America	51655-0477-01
100's	$6.30	GENERIC, Pd-Rx Pharmaceuticals	55289-0154-01
100's	$7.33	GENERIC, Prescript Pharmaceuticals	00247-0358-00
100's	$7.37	GENERIC, Major Pharmaceuticals Inc	00904-2237-61
100's	$7.84	GENERIC, Physicians Total Care	54868-0890-02
100's	$13.01	GENERIC, Us Trading Corporation	56126-0451-11
100's	$14.48	GENERIC, Roberts Pharmaceutical Corporation	54092-0113-01
100's	$19.68	GENERIC, Pharma Pac	52959-0090-00
100's	$22.87	GENERIC, Mova Pharmaceutical Corporation	55370-0132-07
100's	$23.50	GENERIC, Caremark Inc	00339-5815-12
100's	$23.58	GENERIC, Esi Lederle Generics	59911-5923-01
100's	$35.10	GENERIC, Vintage Pharmaceuticals Inc	00254-3916-28
100's	$37.44	GENERIC, Allscripts Pharmaceutical Company	54569-0914-01
100's	$40.84	LEVOTHROID, Forest Pharmaceuticals	00456-0327-01
100's	$40.84	LEVOTHROID, Forest Pharmaceuticals	00456-0327-63
100's	$41.50	GENERIC, Southwood Pharmaceuticals Inc	58016-0932-00
100's	$41.60	SYNTHROID, Pharma Pac	52959-0148-00
100's	$50.38	GENERIC, Watson Laboratories Inc	52544-0911-01
100's	$53.34	SYNTHROID, Physicians Total Care	54868-1012-00
100's	$53.76	SYNTHROID, Allscripts Pharmaceutical Company	54569-0911-01
100's	$60.17	GENERIC, Daniels	00689-1112-05
100's	$61.25	SYNTHROID, Knoll Pharmaceutical Company	00048-1140-13
100's	$65.25	SYNTHROID, Knoll Pharmaceutical Company	00048-1140-03
Tablet - Oral - 0.3 mg			
15's	$6.27	GENERIC, Southwood Pharmaceuticals Inc	58016-0769-15
20's	$8.36	GENERIC, Southwood Pharmaceuticals Inc	58016-0769-20
30's	$4.15	GENERIC, Prescript Pharmaceuticals	00247-0359-30
30's	$12.54	GENERIC, Southwood Pharmaceuticals Inc	58016-0769-30
100's	$6.00	GENERIC, Prescript Pharmaceuticals	00247-0359-00
100's	$14.48	GENERIC, Roberts Pharmaceutical Corporation	54092-0114-01
100's	$29.60	GENERIC, Vintage Pharmaceuticals Inc	00254-3917-28
100's	$30.95	GENERIC, Mova Pharmaceutical Corporation	55370-0134-07
100's	$31.90	GENERIC, Esi Lederle Generics	59911-5924-01
100's	$41.80	GENERIC, Southwood Pharmaceuticals Inc	58016-0769-00
100's	$43.34	GENERIC, Caremark Inc	00339-5817-12
100's	$54.87	GENERIC, Allscripts Pharmaceutical Company	54569-1644-00
100's	$56.78	LEVOTHROID, Forest Pharmaceuticals	00456-0328-01
100's	$56.78	LEVOTHROID, Forest Pharmaceuticals	00456-0328-63
100's	$68.59	GENERIC, Watson Laboratories Inc	52544-0912-01
100's	$88.80	SYNTHROID, Knoll Pharmaceutical Company	00048-1170-03

Lidocaine *(001638)*

Categories: Anesthesia, topical; Pregnancy Category B; FDA Approved 1951 May; WHO Formulary; Orphan Drugs

Drug Classes: Anesthetics, topical; Dermatologics

Brand Names: Alphacaine; **Xylocaine**

Foreign Brand Availability: Aeroderm (Spain); After Burn Spray (Israel); Cuivasil Spray (Israel); Dube Spray (Singapore); Dynexan (France); Esracain Jelly (Israel); Esracain Ointment (Israel); Farmacaina (Colombia); Gesicain Jelly (India); Gesicain Ointment (India); Gesicain Viscous (India); Lecasin (Korea); Leostesin Jelly (Bahrain; Cyprus; Egypt; Iran; Iraq; Jordan; Kuwait; Lebanon; Libya; Oman; Qatar; Republic-of-Yemen; Saudi-Arabia; Syria; United-Arab-Emirates); Leostesin Ointment (Bahrain; Benin; Burkina-Faso; Cyprus; Egypt; Ethiopia; Gambia; Ghana; Guinea; Iran; Iraq; Ivory-Coast; Jordan; Kenya; Kuwait; Lebanon; Liberia; Libya; Malawi; Mali; Mauritania; Mauritius; Morocco; Niger; Nigeria; Oman; Qatar; Republic-of-Yemen; Saudi-Arabia; Senegal; Seychelles; Sierra-Leone; Sudan; Syria; Tanzania; Tunia; Uganda; United-Arab-Emirates; Zambia; Zimbabwe); Lidocain Gel (Bulgaria; Finland; Germany; Hungary); Lidocain Ointment (Bulgaria); Lidocain Spray (Bulgaria; Hungary); Lidonest (Indonesia); Lignocaine Gel (Australia; New-Zealand); Ora (Taiwan); Remicaine Gel (South-Africa); Roxicaina (Colombia); Rucaina Pomada (Mexico); Xilocaina Viscosa (Portugal); Xilonest Pomada (Peru); Xilotane Gel (Portugal); Xilotane Oral (Portugal); Xylocain Aerosol (Denmark; Sweden); Xylocain Creme (Denmark; Norway); Xylocain Gargle (Finland; Sweden); Xylocain Gel (Austria; Denmark; Finland; Germany; Norway; Sweden; Switzerland); Xylocain Liniment (Denmark); Xylocain Ointment (Austria; Finland; Germany; Sweden; Switzerland); Xylocain Salve (Denmark); Xylocain Spray (Austria; Germany; Norway; Switzerland); Xylocain Viscous (Austria; Switzerland); Xylocain Viskos (Germany; Sweden); Xylocain Visks (Finland); Xylocaina Aerosol (Spain); Xylocaina Gel (Spain); Xylocaina Ointment (Italy; Mexico; Spain); Xylocaina Pomada (Peru); Xylocaina Spray (Italy; Mexico); Xylocaine Adhesive Ointment (New-Zealand); Xylocaine Aerosol (Australia; Canada; France; Hong-Kong; Netherlands); Xylocaine Gel (Bahrain; Belgium; Cyprus; Egypt; England; France; Greece; Iran; Iraq; Ireland; Jordan; Kuwait; Lebanon; Libya; Oman; Qatar; Republic-of-Yemen; Saudi-Arabia; Syria; United-Arab-Emirates); Xylocaine Heavy (Bahrain; Cyprus; Egypt; Iran; Iraq; Jordan; Kuwait; Lebanon; Libya; Oman; Qatar; Republic-of-Yemen; Saudi-Arabia; Syria; United-Arab-Emirates); Xylocaine Jelly (Benin; Burkina-Faso; Ethiopia; Gambia; Ghana; Guinea; Hong-Kong; India; Indonesia; Israel; Ivory-Coast; Kenya; Liberia; Malawi; Mali; Mauritania; Mauritius; Morocco; New-Zealand; Niger; Nigeria; Philippines; Senegal; Seychelles; Sierra-Leone; Sudan; Taiwan; Tanzania; Tunia; Uganda; Zambia; Zimbabwe); Xylocaine Ointment (Australia; Bahrain; Benin; Burkina-Faso; Cyprus; Egypt; Ethiopia; Gambia; Ghana; Greece; Guinea; India; Iran; Iraq; Israel; Ivory-Coast; Jordan; Kenya; Kuwait; Lebanon; Liberia; Libya; Malawi; Malaysia; Mali; Mauritania; Mauritius; Morocco; Netherlands; New-Zealand; Niger; Nigeria; Oman; Philippines; Qatar; Republic-of-Yemen; Saudi-Arabia; Senegal; Seychelles; Sierra-Leone; Sudan; Syria; Taiwan; Tanzania; Thailand; Tunia; Uganda; United-Arab-Emirates; Zambia; Zimbabwe); Xylocaine Solution (France); Xylocaine Spray (Belgium; Benin; Burkina-Faso; Ethiopia; France; Gambia; Ghana; Greece; Guinea; Hong-Kong; Indonesia; Israel; Ivory-Coast; Kenya; Korea; Liberia; Malawi; Malaysia; Mali; Mauritania; Mauritius; Morocco; Netherlands; New-Zealand; Niger; Nigeria; Philippines; Senegal; Seychelles; Sierra-Leone; South-Africa; Sudan; Taiwan; Tanzania; Thailand; Tunia; Uganda; Zambia; Zimbabwe); Xylocaine Topical Solution (Bahrain; Canada; Cyprus; Egypt; Iran; Iraq; Jordan; Kuwait; Lebanon; Libya; Oman; Qatar; Republic-of-Yemen; Saudi-Arabia; Syria; United-Arab-Emirates); Xylocaine Viscous (England; India; Ireland; Malaysia; Taiwan; Thailand); Xylocaine Viscous Topical Solution (Australia; Canada; England); Xylocaine Viscus (Greece); Xylocaine Viskeus Topical Solution (Netherlands); Xylocaine Visquese (France); Xylocaine Visqueuse (Belgium); Xylocard (Bahrain; Cyprus; Egypt; Iran; Iraq; Jordan; Kuwait; Lebanon; Libya; Oman; Qatar; Republic-of-Yemen; Saudi-Arabia; Syria; United-Arab-Emirates); Xyloctin (Germany)

DESCRIPTION

See INDICATIONS AND USAGE for specific uses.

5% OINTMENT

Each gram of the lain and flavored ointments contains lidocaine, 50 mg, polyethylene glycol 1500, polyethylene glycol 4000 and propylene glycol. The flavored ointment contains sodium saccharin, peppermint and spearmint oil.

Storage: Store at controlled room temperature 15-30°C (59-86°F).

10% ORAL SPRAY

WARNING: CONTENTS UNDER PRESSURE.

10% lidocaine oral spray contains a local anesthetic agent and is administered topically in the oral cavity.

Lidocaine 10% oral spray contains lidocaine, which is chemically designated as acetamide, 2-(diethylamino)-N-(2,5-dimethylphenyl)-.

Each actuation of the metered dose valve delivers a solution containing lidocaine, 10 mg, cetylpyridinium chloride, absolute alcohol, saccharin, flavor, and polyethylene glycol and as propellants: trichlorofluoromethane/dichlorodifluoromethane (65%/35%).

Storage: Store at controlled room temperature 15-30°C (59-86°F).

5% LIQUID (FLAVORED)

Each ml Contains: Lidocaine, 50 mg, propylene glycol, glycerin, saccharin, and flavor.

NOT FOR INJECTION.

Storage: Store at controlled room temperature.

4% TOPICAL SOLUTION

The 50 ml screw-cap bottle should not be autoclaved, because the closure employed cannot withstand autoclaving temperatures and pressures. Each ml contains lidocaine HCl, 40 mg, methylparaben, and sodium hydroxide and/or hydrochloric acid to adjust pH to 6.0-7.0. An aqueous solution. NOT FOR INJECTION.

Storage: Store at controlled room temperature.

2% VISCOUS SOLUTION

Each ml contains 20 mg of lidocaine HCl, flavoring, sodium saccharin, methylparaben, propylparaben and sodium carboxymethylcellulose in purified water. The pH is adjusted to 6.0-7.0 by means of sodium hydroxide and/or hydrochloric acid.

Storage: Store at controlled room temperature.

2% JELLY

Each ml contains 20 mg of lidocaine HCl. The formulation contains methylparaben, propylparaben, hydroxymethylcellulose, and sodium hydroxide and/or hydrochloric acid to adjust pH to 6.0-7.0

Storage: Store at controlled room temperature.

PATCH 5%

Lidoderm is comprised of an adhesive material containing 5% lidocaine, which is applied to a non-woven polyester felt backing and covered with a polyethylene terephthalate (PET) film release liner. The release liner is removed prior to application to the skin. The size of the patch is 10 cm × 14 cm.

Lidocaine is chemically designated as acetamide, 2-(diethylamino)-N-(2,6-dimethylphenyl), has an octanol:water partition ratio of 43 at pH 7.4.

Each adhesive patch contains 700 mg of lidocaine (50 mg per gram adhesive) in an aqueous base. It also contains the following inactive ingredients: dihydroxyaluminum aminoacetate, disodium edetate, gelatin, glycerin, kaolin, methylparaben, polyacrylic acid, polyvinyl alcohol, propylene glycol, propylparaben, sodium carboxymethylcellulose, sodium polyacrylate, D-sorbitol, tartaric acid, and urea.

KEEP ENVELOPE SEALED AT ALL TIMES WHEN NOT IN USE.

Storage: Store at 25°C (77°F); excursions permitted to 15-30°C (59-86°F).

CLINICAL PHARMACOLOGY

2% JELLY, 5% OINTMENT, 10% ORAL SPRAY, 5% LIQUID, 4% TOPICAL SOLUTION, AND 2% VISCOUS SOLUTION

Mechanism of Action

Lidocaine stabilizes the neuronal membrane by inhibiting the ionic fluxes required for the initiation and conduction of impulses, thereby effecting local anesthetic action.

Onset and Duration of Action:

- **Lidocaine 10% oral spray** acts on intact mucous membranes to produce local anesthesia. Anesthesia occurs usually within 1-2 minutes and persists for approximately 10-15 minutes.
- **Lidocaine 5% ointment** effects local, topical anesthesia. The onset of action is 3-5 minutes. It is ineffective when applied to intact skin.
- ***Lidocaine 5% liquid (flavored):*** Local anesthesia appears within 1-2 minutes after application. and persists for 15-20 minutes in soft tissue.
- ***Lidocaine 2% jelly:*** The onset of action is 3-5 minutes. It is ineffective when applied to intact skin.

Hemodynamics

Excessive blood levels may cause changes in cardiac output, total peripheral resistance, and mean arterial pressure. These changes may be attributable to a direct depressant effect of the local anesthetic agent on various components of the cardiovascular system.

Pharmacokinetics and Metabolism

Lidocaine may be absorbed following topical administration to mucous membranes, its rate of absorption and percent of dose absorbed depending upon concentration and total dose administered, the specific site of application and duration of exposure. In general, the rate of absorption of local anesthetic agents following topical application occurs most rapidly after intratracheal administration. Lidocaine is well-absorbed from the gastrointestinal tract, but little intact drug appears in the circulation because of biotransformation in the liver.

Lidocaine is metabolized rapidly by the liver, and metabolites and unchanged drug are excreted by the kidney. Biotransformation includes oxidative N-dealkylation, ring hydroxylation, cleavage of the amide linkage, and conjugation. N-dealkylation, a major pathway of biotransformation, yields the metabolites monoethylglycinexylidide and glycinexylidide. The pharmacological/toxicological actions of these metabolites are similar to, but less potent than, those of lidocaine. Approximately 90% of lidocaine administered is excreted in the form of various metabolites, and less than 10% is excreted unchanged. The primary metabolite in urine is a conjugate of 4-hydroxy-2,6-dimethylaniline.

The plasma binding of lidocaine is dependent on drug concentration, and the fraction bound decreases with increasing concentration. At concentrations of 1-4 μg of free base per ml, 60-80% of lidocaine is protein bound. Binding is also dependent on the plasma concentration of the alpha-1-acid glycoprotein.

Lidocaine crosses the blood-brain and placental barriers, presumably by passive diffusion.

Studies of lidocaine metabolism following intravenous bolus injections have shown that the elimination half-life of this agent is typically 1.5-2 hours. Because of the rapid rate at which lidocaine is metabolized, any condition that affects liver function may alter lidocaine kinetics. The half-life may be prolonged 2-fold or more in patients with liver dysfunction. Renal dysfunction does not affect lidocaine kinetics but may increase the accumulation of metabolites.

Factors such as acidosis and the use of CNS stimulants and depressants affect the CNS levels of lidocaine required to produce overt systemic effects. Objective adverse manifestations become increasingly apparent with increasing venous plasma levels above 6 μg free base per ml. In the rhesus monkey arterial blood levels of 18-21 μg/ml have been shown to be threshold for convulsive activity.

PATCH 5%

Pharmacodynamics

Lidocaine is an amide-type local anesthetic agent and is suggested to stabilize neuronal membranes by inhibiting the ionic fluxes required for the initiation and conduction of impulses. The penetration of lidocaine into intact skin after application of lidocaine patch is sufficient to produce an analgesic effect, but less than the amount necessary to produce a complete sensory block.

Pharmacokinetics

Absorption

The amount of lidocaine systemically absorbed from lidocaine patch is directly related to both the duration of application and the surface area over which it is applied. In a pharmacokinetic study, three lidocaine patches were applied over an area of 420 cm^2 of intact skin on the back of normal volunteers for 12 hours. Blood samples were withdrawn for determination of lidocaine concentration during the application and for 12 hours after removal of patches. The results are summarized in TABLE 1.

TABLE 1 *Absorption of Lidocaine from Lidocaine Patch*

Normal volunteers (n=15, 12 hour wearing time)

Lidocaine Patch	Application Site	Area (cm^2)	Dose Absorbed (mg)	C_{max} (μg/ml)	T_{max} (hours)
3 patches (2100 mg)	Back	420	64 ± 32	0.13 ± 0.06	11

When lidocaine patch is used according to the recommended dosing instructions, only 3 ± 2% of the dose applied is expected to be absorbed. At least 95% (665 mg) of lidocaine will remain in a used patch. Mean peak blood concentration of lidocaine is about 0.13 μg/ml (about 1/10 of the therapeutic concentration required to treat cardiac arrhythmias). Repeated application of three patches simultaneously for 12 hours (recommended maximum daily dose), once per day for 3 days, indicated that the lidocaine concentration does not increase with daily use.

Distribution

When lidocaine is administered intravenously to healthy volunteers, the volume of distribution is 0.7-2.7 L/kg (mean 1.5 ± 0.6 SD, n=15). At concentrations produced by application of lidocaine patch, lidocaine is approximately 70% bound to plasma proteins, primarily alpha-1-acid glycoprotein. At much higher plasma concentrations (1-4 μg/ml of free base), the plasma protein binding of lidocaine is concentration dependent. Lidocaine crosses the placental and blood brain barriers, presumably by passive diffusion.

Metabolism

It is not known if lidocaine is metabolized in the skin. Lidocaine is metabolized rapidly by the liver to a number of metabolites, including monoethylglycinexylidide (MEGX) and glycinexylidide (GX), both of which have pharmacologic activity similar to, but less potent than that of lidocaine. A minor metabolite, 2,6-xylidine, has unknown pharmacologic activity but is carcinogenic in rats. The blood concentration of this metabolite is negligible following application of lidocaine. Following intravenous administration, MEGX and GX concentrations in serum range from 11-36% and from 5-11% of lidocaine concentrations, respectively.

Excretion

Lidocaine and its metabolites are excreted by the kidneys. Less than 10% of lidocaine is excreted unchanged. The half-life of lidocaine elimination from the plasma following IV administration is 81-149 minutes (mean 107 ± 22 SD, n=15). The systemic clearance is 0.33-0.90 L/min (mean 0.64 ± 0.18 SD, n=15).

INDICATIONS AND USAGE

2% LIDOCAINE JELLY

Indicated for the prevention and control of pain in procedures involving the male and female urethra, for topical treatment of painful urethritis, and as an anesthetic lubricant for endotracheal intubation (oral and nasal).

5% LIDOCAINE LIQUID

Indicated for the symptomatic relief of painful, irritated or inflamed mucous membranes of the mouth and for anesthesia of these membranes for the performance of minor dental surgical procedures.

5% LIDOCAINE OINTMENT

Indicated for the production of anesthesia of accessible mucous membranes of the oropharynx.

10% LIDOCAINE ORAL SPRAY

Indicated for the production of topical anesthesia of the accessible mucous membranes of the mouth and oropharynx.

It is also useful as an anesthetic lubricant for intubation and for the temporary relief of pain associated with minor burns, including sunburn, abrasions of the skin, and insect bites.

THE LIDOCAINE PATCH 5%

Indicated for relief of pain associated with post-herpetic neuralgia. It should be applied only to **intact skin.**

4% LIDOCAINE TOPICAL SOLUTION

Indicated for the production of topical anesthesia of accessible mucous membranes of the oral and nasal cavities and proximal portions of the digestive tract.

2% LIDOCAINE VISCOUS SOLUTION

Indicated for the production of topical anesthesia of irritated or inflamed mucous membranes of the mouth and pharynx. It is also useful for reducing gagging during the taking of X-ray pictures and dental impressions.

CONTRAINDICATIONS

Lidocaine is contraindicated in patients with a known history of hypersensitivity to local anesthetics of the amide type or to other components of the various topical products.

WARNINGS

2% JELLY, 5% OINTMENT, 10% ORAL SPRAY, 5% LIQUID, 4% TOPICAL SOLUTION, AND 2% VISCOUS SOLUTION

EXCESSIVE DOSAGE, OR SHORT INTERVALS BETWEEN DOSES, CAN RESULT IN HIGH PLASMA LEVELS AND SERIOUS ADVERSE EFFECTS. PATIENTS SHOULD BE INSTRUCTED TO STRICTLY ADHERE TO THE RECOMMENDED DOSAGE AND ADMINISTRATION GUIDELINES AS SET FORTH IN THIS PRODUCT INFORMATION.

IN ORDER TO MANAGE POSSIBLE ADVERSE REACTIONS, RESUSCITATIVE EQUIPMENT, OXYGEN AND OTHER RESUSCITATIVE DRUGS MUST BE IMMEDIATELY AVAILABLE WHEN LOCAL ANESTHETIC AGENTS, SUCH AS LIDOCAINE, ARE ADMINISTERED TO MUCOUS MEMBRANES.

Lidocaine should be used with extreme caution if there is sepsis or extremely traumatized mucosa in the area of application, since under such conditions there is the potential for rapid systemic absorption.

Additional Information for 2% Jelly

When used for endotracheal tube lubrication care should be taken to avoid introducing the product into the lumen of the tube. Do not use the jelly to lubricate the endotracheal stylettes. If allowed into the inner lumen, the jelly may dry on the inner surface leaving a residue which tends to clump with flexion, narrowing the lumen. There have been rare reports in which this residue has caused the lumen to occlude. (See also ADVERSE REACTIONS and DOSAGE AND ADMINISTRATION.)

PATCH 5%

Accidental Exposure in Children

Even a *used* lidocaine patch contains a large amount of lidocaine (at least 665 mg). The potential exists for a small child or a pet to suffer serious adverse effects from chewing or ingesting a new or used lidocaine patch, although the risk with this formulation has not been evaluated. It is important for patients to **store and dispose of lidocaine patches out of the reach of children and pets.**

Excessive Dosing

Excessive dosing by applying lidocaine patch to larger areas or for longer than the recommended wearing time could result in increased absorption of lidocaine and high blood concentrations, leading to serious adverse effects. (See ADVERSE REACTIONS, Systemic Reactions.) Lidocaine toxicity could be expected at lidocaine blood concentrations above 5 μg/ml. The blood concentration of lidocaine is determined by the rate of systemic absorption and elimination. Longer duration of application, application of more than the recommended number of patches, smaller patients, or impaired elimination may all contribute to increasing the blood concentration of lidocaine. With recommended dosing of lidocaine patch, the average peak blood concentration is about 0.13 μg/ml, but concentrations higher than 0.25 μg/ml have been observed in some individuals.

PRECAUTIONS

GENERAL

2% Jelly, 5% Ointment, 10% Oral Spray, 5% Liquid, 4% Topical Solution, and 2% Viscous Solution

The safety and effectiveness of lidocaine depend on proper dosage, correct technique, adequate precautions, and readiness for emergencies. Resuscitative equipment, oxygen, and other resuscitative drugs should be available for immediate use. (See WARNINGS and ADVERSE REACTIONS.) The lowest dosage that results in effective anesthesia should be used to avoid high plasma levels and serious adverse effects. Repeated doses of lidocaine may cause significant increases in blood levels with each repeated dose because of slow accumulation of the drug or its metabolites. Tolerance varies with the status of the patient.

L

Debilitated, elderly patients, acutely ill patients, and children should be given reduced doses commensurate with their age and physical status. Lidocaine should also be used with caution in patients with severe shock or heart block.

Lidocaine should be used with caution in patients with known drug sensitivities. Patients allergic to para-amino-benzoic acid derivatives (procaine, tetracaine, benzocaine, etc.) have not shown cross sensitivity to lidocaine.

Many drugs used during the conduct of anesthesia are considered potential triggering agents for familiar malignant hyperthermia. Since it is not known whether amide-type local anesthetics may trigger this reaction and since the need for supplemental general anesthesia cannot be predicted in advance, it is suggested that a standard protocol for management should be available. Early unexplained signs of tachycardia, tachypnea, labile blood pressure and metabolic acidosis may precede temperature elevation. Successful outcome is dependent on early diagnosis, prompt discontinuance of the suspect triggering agents(s) and institution of treatment, including oxygen therapy, indicated supportive measures and dantrolene (consult dantrolene sodium intravenous product information before using).

Patch 5%

Hepatic Disease

Patients with severe hepatic disease are at greater risk of developing toxic blood concentrations of lidocaine, because of their inability to metabolize lidocaine normally.

Allergic Reactions

Patients allergic to para-aminobenzoic acid derivatives (procaine, tetracaine, benzocaine, etc.) have not shown cross sensitivity to lidocaine. However, lidocaine patch should be used with caution in patients with a history of drug sensitivities, especially if the etiologic agent is uncertain.

Non-Intact Skin

Application to broken or inflamed skin, although not tested, may result in higher blood concentrations of lidocaine from increased absorption. Lidocaine patch is only recommended for use on intact skin.

Eye Exposure

The contact of lidocaine patch with eyes, although not studied, should be avoided based on the findings of severe eye irritation with the use of similar products in animals. If eye contact occurs, immediately wash out the eye with water or saline and protect the eye until sensation returns.

L

INFORMATION FOR THE PATIENT

2% Jelly, 5% Ointment, 10% Oral Spray, 5% Liquid, 4% Topical Solution, and 2% Viscous Solution

When topical anesthetics are used in the mouth, the patient should be aware that the production of topical anesthesia may impair swallowing and thus enhance the danger of aspiration. For this reason, food should not be ingested for 60 minutes following use of local anesthetic preparations in the mouth or throat area. This is particularly important in children because of their frequency of eating.

Numbness of the tongue or buccal mucosa may enhance the danger of unintentional biting trauma. Food and chewing gum should not be taken while the mouth or throat area is anesthetized.

CARCINOGENESIS, MUTAGENESIS, AND IMPAIRMENT OF FERTILITY

2% Jelly, 5% Ointment, 10% Oral Spray, 5% Liquid, 4% Topical Solution, and 2% Viscous Solution

Studies of lidocaine in animals to evaluate the carcinogenic and mutagenic potential or the effect on fertility have not been conducted.

Patch 5%

Carcinogenesis

A minor metabolite, 2,6-xylidine, has been found to be carcinogenic in rats. The blood concentration of this metabolite is negligible following application of lidocaine patch.

Mutagenesis

Lidocaine HCl is not mutagenic in *Salmonella*/mammalian microsome test nor clastogenic in chromosmome aberration assay with human lymphocytes and mouse micronucleus test.

Impairment of Fertility

The effect of lidocaine patch on fertility has not been studied.

PREGNANCY, TERATOGENIC EFFECTS, PREGNANCY CATEGORY B

2% Jelly, 5% Ointment, 10% Oral Spray, 5% Liquid, 4% Topical Solution, and 2% Viscous Solution

Reproduction studies have been performed in rats at doses up to 6.6 times the human dose and have revealed no evidence of harm to the fetus caused by lidocaine. There are, however, no adequate and well-controlled studies in pregnant women. Animal reproduction studies are not always predictive of human response. General consideration should be given to this fact before administering lidocaine to women of childbearing potential, especially during early pregnancy when maximum organogenesis takes place.

Patch 5%

Lidocaine patch has not been studied in pregnancy. Reproduction studies with lidocaine have been performed in rats at doses up to 30 mg/kg subcutaneously and have revealed no evidence of harm to the fetus due to lidocaine. There are, however, no adequate and well-controlled studies in pregnant women. Because animal reproduction studies are not always predictive of human response, lidocaine patch should be used during pregnancy only if clearly needed.

LABOR AND DELIVERY

2% Jelly, 5% Ointment, 10% Oral Spray, 5% Liquid, 4% Topical Solution, and 2% Viscous Solution

Lidocaine is not contraindicated in labor and delivery. Should lidocaine be used concomitantly with other products containing lidocaine, the total dose contributed by all formulations must be kept in mind.

Patch 5%

Lidocaine patch has not been studied in labor and delivery. Lidocaine is not contraindicated in labor and delivery. Should lidocaine patch be used concomitantly with other products containing lidocaine, total doses contributed by all formulations must be considered.

NURSING MOTHERS

2% Jelly, 5% Ointment, 10% Oral Spray, 5% Liquid, 4% Topical Solution, and 2% Viscous Solution

It is not known whether this drug is excreted in human milk. Because many drugs are excreted in human milk, caution should be exercised when lidocaine is administered to a nursing woman.

Patch 5%

Lidocaine patch has not been studied in nursing mothers. Lidocaine is excreted in human milk, and the milk:plasma ratio of lidocaine is 0.4. Caution should be exercised when lidocaine patch is administered to a nursing woman.

PEDIATRIC USE

10% Oral Spray and Patch 5%

Safety and effectiveness in pediatric patients below the age of 12 years have not been established.

Other Forms

Dosages in children should be reduced, commensurate with age, body weight and physical condition. Caution must be taken to avoid overdosage when applying lidocaine ointment to large areas of injured or abraded skin, since the systemic absorption of lidocaine may be increased under such conditions. (See DOSAGE AND ADMINISTRATION.)

DRUG INTERACTIONS

Antiarrhythmic Drugs: Lidocaine patch should be used with caution in patients receiving Class I antiarrhythmic drugs (such as tocainide and mexiletine) since the toxic effects are additive and potentially synergistic.

Local Anesthetics: When lidocaine patch is used concomitantly with other products containing local anesthetic agents, the amount absorbed from all formulations must be considered.

ADVERSE REACTIONS

2% JELLY, 5% OINTMENT, 10% ORAL SPRAY, 5% LIQUID, 4% TOPICAL SOLUTION, AND 2% VISCOUS SOLUTION

Adverse experiences following the administration of lidocaine are similar in nature to those observed with other amide local anesthetic agents. These adverse experiences are, in general, dose-related and may result from high plasma levels caused by excessive dosage or rapid absorption, or may result from a hypersensitivity, idiosyncrasy or diminished tolerance on the part of the patient. Serious adverse experiences are generally systemic in nature. The following types are those most commonly reported:

Central Nervous System: CNS manifestations are excitatory and/or depressant and may be characterized by lightheadedness, nervousness, apprehension, euphoria, confusion, dizziness, drowsiness, tinnitus, blurred or double vision, vomiting, sensations of heat, cold or numbness, twitching, tremors, convulsions, unconsciousness, respiratory depression and arrest. The excitatory manifestations may be very brief or may not occur at all, in which case the first manifestation of toxicity may be drowsiness merging into unconsciousness and respiratory arrest.

Drowsiness following the administration of lidocaine is usually an early sign of a high blood level of the drug and may occur as a consequence of rapid absorption.

Cardiovascular System: Cardiovascular manifestations are usually depressant and are characterized by bradycardia, hypotension, and cardiovascular collapse, which may lead to cardiac arrest.

Allergic: Allergic reactions are characterized by cutaneous lesions, urticaria, edema or anaphylactoid reactions. Allergic reactions may occur as a result of sensitivity either to the local anesthetic agent or to other ingredients in the formulation. Allergic reactions as a result of sensitivity to lidocaine are extremely rare and, if they occur, should be managed by conventional means. The detection of sensitivity by skin testing is of doubtful value.

Additional Information for Lidocaine Jelly

There have been rare reports of endotracheal tube occlusion associated with the presence of dried jell residue in the inner lumen of the tube. (See also WARNINGS and DOSAGE AND ADMINISTRATION.)

PATCH 5%

Localized Reactions

During or immediately after treatment with lidocaine patch, the skin at the site of treatment may develop erythema or edema or may be the locus of abnormal sensation. These reactions are generally mild and transient, resolving spontaneously within a few minutes to hours. In clinical studies with lidocaine patch, there were no serious reactions reported. One (1) out of 150 subjects in a 3 week study was discontinued from treatment because of a skin reaction (erythema and hives).

Allergic Reactions

Allergic and anaphylactoid reactions associated with lidocaine, although rare, can occur. They are characterized by urticaria, angioedema, bronchospasm, and shock. If they occur, they should be managed by conventional means. The detection of sensitivity by skin testing is of doubtful value.

Systemic (Dose Related) Reactions

Systemic adverse reactions following appropriate use of lidocaine patch are unlikely, due to the small dose absorbed. (See CLINICAL PHARMACOLOGY, Pharmacokinetics.) Systemic adverse effects of lidocaine are similar in nature to those observed with other amide local anesthetic agents, including CNS excitation and/or depression (light-headedness, nervousness, apprehension, euphoria, confusion, dizziness, drowsiness, tinnitus, blurred or double vision, vomiting, sensations of heat, cold or numbness, twitching, tremors, convulsions, unconsciousness, respiratory depression and arrest). Excitatory CNS reactions may be brief or not occur at all, in which case the first manifestation may be drowsiness merging into unconsciousness. Cardiovascular manifestations may include bradycardia, hypotension and cardiovascular collapse leading to arrest.

DOSAGE AND ADMINISTRATION

When lidocaine is used concomitantly with other products containing lidocaine, the total dose contributed by all formulations must be kept in mind.

2% JELLY

The dosage varies and depends upon the area to be anesthetized, vascularity of the tissues, individual tolerance, and the technique of anesthesia. The lowest dosage needed to provide effective anesthesia should be administered. Dosages should be reduced for children and for elderly and debilitated patients. Although the incidence of adverse effects with 2% lidocaine jelly is quite low, caution should be exercised, particularly when employing large amounts, since the incidence of adverse effect is directly proportional to the total dose of local anesthetic agent administered.

For Surface Anesthesia of the Male Adult Urethra

The plastic cone is sterilized for 5 minutes in boiling water, cooled, and attached to the tube. The cone may be gas sterilized or cold sterilized, as preferred. The jelly is instilled slowly into the urethra by gently expressing the contents of the tube until the patient has a feeling of tension or until almost half the tube (15 ml, *i.e.*, 300 mg of lidocaine HCl) is emptied. A penile clamp is then applied for several minutes at the corona and then the remaining contents of the tube are instilled.

Prior to sounding or cytoscopy, a penile clamp should be applied for 5-10 minutes to obtain adequate anesthesia. The contents of 1 tube (30 ml, *i.e.*, 600 mg) are usually required to fill and dilate the male urethra.

Prior to catheterization, smaller volumes (5-10 ml, *i.e.*, 100-200 mg) are usually adequate for lubrication.

For Surface Anesthesia of the Female Adult Urethra

The plastic cone is sterilized for 5 minutes in boiling water, cooled, and attached to the tube. The cone may be gas sterilized or cold sterilized, as preferred. Three (3) to 5 ml of the jelly is instilled slowly into the urethra by gently expressing approximately 10-20% of the contents of the tube. If desired, some jelly may be deposited on a cotton swab and introduced into the urethra. In order to obtain adequate anesthesia, several minutes should be allowed prior to performing urological procedures.

Lubrication for Endotracheal Intubation

Apply a moderate amount of jelly to the external surface of the endotracheal tube shortly before use. Care should be taken to avoid introducing the product in to lumen of the tube. Do not use jelly to lubricate endotracheal stylettes. (See WARNINGS and ADVERSE REACTIONS concerning rare reports of lumen occlusion.) It is also recommended that use of endotracheal tubes with dried jelly on the external surface be avoided for lack of lubricating effect.

Maximum Dosage

No more than 1 tube (600 mg of lidocaine HCl) should be given in any 12 hour period.

Children

It is difficult to recommend a maximum dose of any drug for children since this varies as a function of age and weight. For children less than 10 years who have a normal lean body mass and a normal lean body development, the maximum dose may be determined by the application of one of the standard pediatric drug formulas (*e.g.*, Clark's rule). For example, in a child of 5 years weighing 50 lb, the dose of lidocaine HCl should not exceed 75-100 mg when calculated according to Clark's rule. In any case, the maximum amount of lidocaine administered should not exceed 4.5 mg/kg (2.0 mg/lb) of body weight.

A detachable applicator cone and a key for expressing the contents are included in each package.

5% LIQUID (FLAVORED)

Adult

The maximum recommended single adult dose of lidocaine HCl, administered parenterally, is 300 mg (equivalent to 260 mg of lidocaine.) In a 70 kg adult this dose of lidocaine equals 3.7 mg/kg or 1.7 mg/lb. Thus, a single application of 5% lidocaine liquid should not exceed a total of 5 ml for all quadrants. In general, however, much smaller volumes are adequate to produce the desired anesthesia. The maximum recommended single adult dose (5 ml) should not be exceeded within any 3 hour interval.

Pediatric

It is difficult to recommend a maximum dose of any drug for children, since this varies as a function of age and weight. For children over 3 years of age who have a normal lean body mass and normal body development, the maximum dose is determined by the child's weight and age. For example, in a child of 5 years weighing 50 lb, the dose of lidocaine should not exceed 75-100 (1.5-2.0 mg/lb).

5% OINTMENT

Adult

A single application should not exceed 5 g of lidocaine 5% ointment, containing 250 mg of lidocaine base (equivalent chemically to approximately 300 mg of lidocaine HCl). This is roughly equivalent to squeezing a 6 inch length of ointment from the tube. In a 70 kg adult this dose equals 3.6 mg/kg (1.6 mg/lb) lidocaine base. No more than one-half tube, approximately 17-20 g of ointment or 850-1000 mg lidocaine base, should be administered in any one day.

Although the incidence of adverse effects with lidocaine 5% ointment is quite low, caution should be exercised, particularly when employing large amounts, since the incidence of adverse effects is directly proportional to the total dose of local anesthetic agent administered.

Dosage for Children

It is difficult to recommend a maximum dose of any drug for children since this varies as a function of age and weight. For children less than 10 years who have a normal lean body mass and a normal lean body development, the maximum dose may be determined by the application of one of the standard pediatric drug formulas (*e.g.,* Clark's rule). For example, in a child of 5 years, weighing 50 lb, the dose of lidocaine should not exceed 75-100 mg when calculated according to clark's rule. In any case, the maximum amount of lidocaine administered should not exceed 4.5 mg/kg (2.0 mg/lb) of body weight.

10% ORAL SPRAY

Two metered doses per quadrant are recommended as the upper limit and, *under no circumstances* should one exceed three metered doses per quadrant of oral mucosa over a one-half hour period to produce the desired anesthetic effect. Experience in children is inadequate to recommend a pediatric dose at this time.

PATCH 5%

Apply lidocaine patch to intact skin to cover the most painful area. Apply up to three patches, only once for up to 12 hours within a 24 hour period. Patches may be cut into smaller sizes with scissors prior to removal of the release liner. Clothing may be worn over the area of application. Smaller areas of treatment are recommended in a debilitated patient, or a patient with impaired elimination.

If irritation or a burning sensation occurs during application, remove the patch(es) and do not reapply until the irritation subsides.

When lidocaine patch is used concomitantly with other products containing local anesthetic agents, the amount absorbed from all formulations must be considered.

Handling and Disposal

Hands should be washed after the handling of lidocaine patch, and eye contact with lidocaine patch should be avoided. The used patch should be immediately disposed of in such a way as to prevent its access by children or pets.

4% TOPICAL SOLUTION

The dosage varies and depends upon the area to be anesthetized, vascularity of the tissues, individual tolerance, and the technique of the anesthesia. The lowest dosage needed to provide effective anesthesia should be administered. Dosages should be reduced for children and for elderly and debilitated patients. The maximum dose should not exceed 4.5 mg/kg (2 mg/lb) of body weight. Although the incidence of adverse affects with 4% lidocaine topical solution is quite low, caution should be exercised, particularly when employing large volumes, since the incidence of adverse affects is directly proportional to the total dose of local anesthetic agent administered.

The dosages recommended below are for normal, healthy adults:

When used as a spray, or when applied by means of cotton applicators or packs, as when instilled into a cavity, the suggested dosage of 4% lidocaine topical solution is 1-5 ml (40-200 mg lidocaine HCl), *i.e.*, 0.6-3.0 mg/kg or 0.3-1.5 mg/lb body weight.

NOTE: The solution may be applied with a sterile swab which is discarded after a single use. When spraying, transfer the solution from the original container to an atomizer.

Maximum Recommended Dosages

Normal Healthy Adults: The maximum recommended dose of 4% lidocaine topical solution should be such that the dose of lidocaine HCl is kept below 300 mg and in any case should not exceed 4.5 mg/kg (2 mg/lb) body weight.

Children: It is difficult to recommend a maximum dose of any drug for children since this varies as a function of age and weight. For children of less than 10 years who have a normal lean body mass and normal body development, the maximum dose may be determined by the application of one of the standard pediatric drug formulas (*e.g.*, Clark's rule). For example, in a child of 5 years weighing 50 lb, the dose of lidocaine HCl should not exceed 7 mg/kg (3.2 mg/lb) of body weight. When used without epinephrine, the amount of lidocaine solution administered should be such that the dose is kept below 300 mg and in any case should not exceed 4.5 mg/kg (2.0 mg/lb) of body weight.

NOT FOR INJECTION.

2% VISCOUS SOLUTION

Adult

The maximum recommended single dose of lidocaine HCl 2% viscous solution for healthy adults should be such that the dose of lidocaine HCl does not exceed 4.5 mg/kg or 2 mg/lb body weight and does not in any case exceed a total of 300 mg.

For symptomatic treatment of irritated or inflamed mucous membranes of the mouth and pharynx, the usual adult dose is one 15 ml tablespoonful undiluted. For use in the mouth, the solution should be swished around in the mouth and spit out. For use in the pharynx, the undiluted solution should be gargled and may be swallowed. This dose should not be administered at intervals of less than 3 hours, and not more than 8 doses should be given in a 24 hour period.

This dosage should be adjusted commensurate with the patient's age, weight and physical condition. (See PRECAUTIONS.)

L

Pediatric

It is difficult to recommend a maximum dose of any drug for children since this varies as a function of age and maximum dose is determined by the child's weight or age. For example: in a child of 5 years weighing 50 lb, the dose of lidocaine HCl should not exceed 75-1000 mg (¾ to 1 teaspoonful).

For infants and in children under 3 years of age, ¼ teaspoon of the solution should be accurately measured and applied to the immediate area with a cotton-tipped applicator. This dose should not be administered at intervals of less than 3 hours. Not more than 4 doses should be given in a 12 hour period.

PRODUCT LISTING - RATED THERAPEUTICALLY EQUIVALENT

Gel with Applicator - Topical - 2%

5 gm	$187.50	GENERIC, International Medication Systems, Limited	00548-3011-00
5 gm x 10	$82.90	XYLOCAINE JELLY, Astra-Zeneca Pharmaceuticals	00186-0330-36
5 gm x 25	$179.75	GENERIC, Celltech Pharmacuetical Inc	00548-3012-00
10 gm	$69.75	XYLOCAINE JELLY, Astra-Zeneca Pharmaceuticals	00186-0330-43
10 gm x 10	$75.36	XYLOCAINE JELLY, Astra-Zeneca Pharmaceuticals	00186-0336-43
10 gm x 25	$213.13	GENERIC, Celltech Pharmacuetical Inc	00548-3013-00
15 gm	$5.44	ANESTACON, Polymedica Pharmaceuticals Usa Inc	61451-0300-01
20 gm	$86.90	XYLOCAINE JELLY, Astra-Zeneca Pharmaceuticals	00186-0330-53
20 gm x 10	$91.20	XYLOCAINE JELLY, Astra-Zeneca Pharmaceuticals	00186-0336-53
30 gm	$15.52	GENERIC, Teva Pharmaceuticals Usa	00093-9200-31
30 gm	$17.48	XYLOCAINE JELLY, Southwood Pharmaceuticals Inc	58016-3125-01
30 gm	$17.76	XYLOCAINE TOPICAL, Allscripts Pharmaceutical Company	54569-2263-00
30 gm	$19.33	XYLOCAINE TOPICAL, Physicians Total Care	54868-3503-00
30 gm	$20.13	XYLOCAINE JELLY, Astra-Zeneca Pharmaceuticals	00186-0330-01
240 gm	$21.00	ANESTACON, Polymedica Pharmaceuticals Usa Inc	61451-0300-02

Ointment - Topical - 5%

3 gm x 10	$31.40	XYLOCAINE TOPICAL, Astra-Zeneca Pharmaceuticals	00186-0350-03
35 gm	$2.50	GENERIC, Cmc-Consolidated Midland Corporation	00223-4351-35
35 gm	$13.81	GENERIC, Fougera	00168-0204-37
35 gm	$14.85	XYLOCAINE TOPICAL, Southwood Pharmaceuticals Inc	58016-3248-01
35 gm	$17.34	XYLOCAINE TOPICAL, Astra-Zeneca Pharmaceuticals	00186-0315-21
35 gm	$28.80	XYLOCAINE TOPICAL, Pharma Pac	52959-0708-35
50 gm	$2.36	GENERIC, Moore, H.L. Drug Exchange Inc	00839-5474-81
50 gm	$2.93	GENERIC, Interstate Drug Exchange Inc	00814-4410-96
50 gm	$7.86	GENERIC, Thames Pharmacal Company Inc	49158-0130-19

Solution - Mucous Membrane - 2%

5 ml x 25	$30.00	GENERIC, Cmc-Consolidated Midland Corporation	00223-7937-05
20 ml x 40	$50.40	GENERIC, Roxane Laboratories Inc	00054-8500-16
100 ml	$2.63	GENERIC, Roxane Laboratories Inc	00054-3500-49
100 ml	$4.04	GENERIC, Moore, H.L. Drug Exchange Inc	00839-6502-40
100 ml	$4.05	GENERIC, Qualitest Products Inc	00603-1392-64
100 ml	$4.62	GENERIC, Alpharma Uspd Makers Of Barre and Nmc	00472-0996-33
100 ml	$4.75	GENERIC, Major Pharmaceuticals Inc	00904-0863-04
100 ml	$5.99	GENERIC, Hi-Tech Pharmacal Company Inc	50383-0775-04
100 ml	$6.15	GENERIC, Ivax Corporation	00182-1360-70
100 ml	$6.15	GENERIC, Geneva Pharmaceuticals	00781-6190-46
100 ml	$6.29	GENERIC, Mutual/United Research Laboratories	00677-1015-27
100 ml	$6.80	GENERIC, Marlop Pharmaceuticals Inc	12939-0780-10
100 ml	$14.20	GENERIC, Morton Grove Pharmaceuticals Inc	60432-0464-00
100 ml	$21.26	XYLOCAINE VISCOUS, Astra-Zeneca Pharmaceuticals	00186-0360-01
450 ml	$71.14	XYLOCAINE VISCOUS, Astra-Zeneca Pharmaceuticals	00186-0360-11

Solution - Topical - 4%

50 ml	$10.50	GENERIC, Morton Grove Pharmaceuticals Inc	60432-0465-50
50 ml	$19.78	XYLOCAINE TOPICAL, Southwood Pharmaceuticals Inc	58016-1127-01
50 ml	$21.34	XYLOCAINE TOPICAL, Astra-Zeneca Pharmaceuticals	00186-0320-01

Spray - Mucous Membrane - 10%

30 ml x 50	$32.06	XYLOCAINE 10% ORAL, Astra-Zeneca Pharmaceuticals	00186-9035-05

PRODUCT LISTING - EQUIVALENTS NOT AVAILABLE

Cream - Topical - 0.5%

120 gm	$3.00	SOLARCAINE, Schering-Plough	41100-0044-20

Cream - Topical - 3%

30 gm	$28.50	LIDA MANTLE, Doak Dermatologics Division	10337-0700-52
90 gm	$47.64	LIDA MANTLE, Doak Dermatologics Division	10337-0700-19

Cream - Topical - 4%

5 gm x 5	$47.44	ELA-MAX, Ferndale Laboratories Inc	00496-0823-07
15 gm	$23.18	ELA-MAX, Ferndale Laboratories Inc	00496-0823-15
30 gm	$44.58	ELA-MAX, Ferndale Laboratories Inc	00496-0823-30

Cream - Topical - 5%

5 gm	$9.04	ELA-MAX, Ferndale Laboratories Inc	00496-0823-05
5 gm x 5	$44.93	ELA-MAX, Ferndale Laboratories Inc	00496-0823-06
15 gm	$25.73	ELA-MAX, Ferndale Laboratories Inc	00496-0824-15
30 gm	$52.46	ELA-MAX, Ferndale Laboratories Inc	00496-0824-30

Film - Topical - 5%

5 x 6	$142.06	LIDODERM, Southwood Pharmaceuticals Inc	58016-5611-01
5 x 6	$147.75	LIDODERM, Endo Laboratories Llc	63481-0687-06
5 x 6	$157.06	LIDODERM, Pharma Pac	52959-0694-30

Gel with Applicator - Topical - 2%

15 gm	$5.75	ANESTACON, Polymedica Pharmaceuticals Usa Inc	61451-0300-10
30 gm	$15.52	GENERIC, Allscripts Pharmaceutical Company	54569-4258-00
30 gm	$23.75	GENERIC, Physicians Total Care	54868-4195-00

Ointment - Topical - 5%

35 gm	$2.10	GENERIC, Ambix Laboratories	10038-0062-18
37.50 gm	$7.15	GENERIC, Physicians Total Care	54868-3282-00
37.50 gm	$9.54	GENERIC, Allscripts Pharmaceutical Company	54569-2943-00
454 gm	$13.21	GENERIC, Ambix Laboratories	10038-0062-16

Solution - Mucous Membrane - 2%

20 ml	$4.01	GENERIC, Prescript Pharmaceuticals	00247-0230-20
60 ml	$5.32	GENERIC, Prescript Pharmaceuticals	00247-0230-60
100 ml	$4.00	GENERIC, Raway Pharmacal Inc	00686-0996-03
100 ml	$4.02	GENERIC, Aligen Independent Laboratories Inc	00405-3150-60
100 ml	$4.75	GENERIC, Physicians Total Care	54868-1827-01
100 ml	$5.00	GENERIC, Allscripts Pharmaceutical Company	54569-1285-00
100 ml	$6.64	GENERIC, Prescript Pharmaceuticals	00247-0230-00
100 ml	$8.87	GENERIC, Pharma Pac	52959-0251-00
100 ml	$17.31	XYLOCAINE VISCOUS, Southwood Pharmaceuticals Inc	58016-9018-01

Solution - Topical - 4%

50 ml	$10.50	GENERIC, Allscripts Pharmaceutical Company	54569-1923-01

Lidocaine Hydrochloride *(001639)*

Categories: Anesthesia, infiltration; Anesthesia, local; Anesthesia, regional; Anesthesia, spinal; Anesthesia, topical; Arrhythmia, ventricular; Pregnancy Category B; FDA Approved 1948 Nov; WHO Formulary

Drug Classes: Anesthetics, local; Anesthetics, topical; Antiarrhythmics, class IB; Dermatologics

Brand Names: Alphacaine HCl; Anestacon; D-Caine; Dalcaine; Dilocaine; Duo-Trach; L-Caine; Laryng-O-Jet Kit; Lido-Storz; Lidocaine HCl Injectable; Lidocaine Hcl; Lidocaton; Lidoject; Lidomar; Lidonest; Lidopen; Lta II Kit; Mylocaine; Nervocaine; Newcaine; Norocaine; Pediatric Lta Kit; Rucaina; Shocaine; Truxacaine; Xylocaina; **Xylocaine Injectable**

Foreign Brand Availability: Dequaspray (England; Ireland); Dynexan (France)

HCFA JCODE(S): J2000 50 cc VAR

DESCRIPTION

Lidocaine HCl is chemically designated as acetamide, 2-(diethylamino)-N-(2,6-dimethylphenyl)-, monohydrochloride and has the molecular weight 270.8. The molecular formula for lidocaine HCl is $C_{14}H_{22}N_2O$·HCl.

For the solutions containing epinephrine, it is chemically designated as (-)-3,4-Dihydroxy-α-[(methylamino)methyl] benzyl alcohol and has the molecular weight 183.21. Its molecular formula is $C_9H_{13}NO_3$.

LIDOCAINE HCl STERILE SOLUTION AND LIDOCAINE HCl WITH EPINEPHRINE

See INDICATIONS AND USAGE for specific uses.

Lidocaine HCl injections are sterile, nonpyrogenic, aqueous solutions that contain a local anesthetic agent with or without epinephrine and are administered parenterally by injection.

Dosage forms listed as Xylocaine-MPF indicate solutions that are Methyl Paraben Free (MPF).

Xylocaine MPF

A sterile, nonpyrogenic, isotonic solution containing sodium chloride. *Xylocaine MPF in multiple-dose vials:* Each milliliter also contains 1 mg methylparaben as antiseptic preservative. The pH of these solutions is adjusted to approximately 6.5 (5.0-7.0) with sodium hydroxide and/or hydrochloric acid.

The chemical name for epinephrine is (-)-3,4-dihydroxy-α-[(methylamino) methyl] benzyl alcohol. It has the molecular weight 183.21. The molecular formula for epinephrine is $C_9H_{13}NO_3$.

Xylocaine MPF With Epinephrine

A sterile, nonpyrogenic, isotonic solution containing sodium chloride. Each milliliter contains lidocaine HCl and epinephrine, with 0.5 mg sodium metabisulfite as an antioxidant and 0.2 mg citric acid as a stabilizer. *Xylocaine with epinephrine in multiple dose vials:* Each milliliter also contains 1 mg methylparaben as antiseptic preservative. The pH of these solutions is adjusted to approximately 4.5 (3.3-5.5) with sodium hydroxide and/or hydrochloric acid. Filled under nitrogen.

LIDOCAINE HCl FOR VENTRICULAR ARRHYTHMIAS

Lidocaine HCl injection is a sterile aqueous solution of lidocaine, an antiarrhythmic agent, prepared with hydochloric acid. It is intended for intravenous administration by either direct injection or continuous infusion. The composition of available solutions is shown in TABLE 1.

TABLE 1 *Composition of Available Solutions*

Concentration	Lidocaine HCl (mg/ml)	Sodium Chloride (mg/ml) to Adjust Tonicity
For Direct IV Injection		
1%	10	7
2%	20	6
20% For Dilution Only		
For Preparation of Intravenous Infusions		
1 g	200	None
2 g	200	None

* pH of all solutions adjusted to 5.0-7.0 with sodium hydroxide and/or hydrochloric acid.

The medication and fluid pathway of these disposable syringes are sterile and nonpyrogenic in the original, unopened package with component caps in place. These dosage forms do not contain preservatives; once the unit is assembled and used, any remaining portion of the solution must be discarded with the entire unit.

LIDOCAINE HCl WITH DEXTROSE

Xylocaine-MPF 5% with glucose 7.5% is a sterile hyperbaric solution that contains a local anesthetic agent and is administered into the spinal subarachnoid space by injection. For specific uses see INDICATIONS AND USAGE, Lidocaine HCl With Dextrose.

Xylocaine-MPF 5% with glucose 7.5% contains lidocaine HCl, which is chemically designated as acetamide, 2-(diethylamino)-N-(2,6-dimethylphenyl)-, monohydrochloride, and dextrose (D-Glucose, anhydrous).

Xylocaine-MPF 5% with glucose 7.5% may be autoclaved at 15 lb pressure at 121°C (250°F) for 15 minutes. Since this preparation contains glucose, caramelization may occur under prolonged heating and, in some instances, prolonged storage. Therefore, this preparation should not be autoclaved more than once, according to the above instructions, and should not be permitted to remain in the autoclave any longer than necessary. The solution should not be used if it is discolored or a precipitate is present.

Each ml of Xylocaine-MPF 5% with glucose 7.5% contains lidocaine HCl, 50 mg; dextrose (D-Glucose, anhydrous), 75 mg; sodium hydroxide and/or hydrochloric acid to adjust pH to 5.5-7.0.

Specific gravity: 1.032-1.037.

LIDOCAINE HCl TOPICAL SOLUTION

Lidocaine HCl topical solution is a sterile, aqueous solution containing a local anesthetic agent and is administered topically.

Composition of Lidocaine HCl 4% Topical Solution: Each milliliter of aqueous solution contains lidocaine HCl, 40 mg, and sodium hydroxide and/or hydrocholoric acid to adjust pH to 5.0-7.0. No preservative is added since all or part of the contents of the syringe unit is administered as a single dose and the unit should not be reused.

LIDOCAINE HCl JELLY

Lidocaine HCl jelly, 2% is a sterile aqueous product that contains a local anesthetic agent and is administered topically. For specific uses see INDICATIONS AND USAGE, Lidocaine HCl Jelly.

Each milliliter contains 20 mg of lidocaine HCl, and sodium carboxymethylcellulose as a viscosity-increasing agent. Sodium hydroxide may have been added to adjust pH to 6-7. Carboxymethylcellulose sodium adjusts the resulting mixture to a suitable consistency, to enhance contact with mucosa and provide lubrication for instrumentation. This product contains no preservative and any unused portion should be discarded after initial use.

CLINICAL PHARMACOLOGY

MECHANISM OF ACTION

Lidocaine stabilizes the neuronal membrane by inhibiting the ionic fluxes required for the initiation and conduction of impulses thereby effecting local anesthetic action.

Mechanism of Action and Electrophysiology of Lidocaine HCl for Ventricular Arrhythmia

Studies of the effects of therapeutic concentrations of lidocaine on the electrophysiological properties of mammalian Purkinje fibers have shown that lidocaine attenuates phase 4 diastolic depolarization, decreases automaticity, and causes a decrease or no change in excitability and membrane responsiveness. Action potential duration and effective refractory period of Purkinje fibers are decreased, while the ratio of effective refractory period to action potential duration is increased. Action potential duration and effective refractory period of ventricular muscle are also decreased. Effective refractory period of the AV node may increase, decrease, or remain unchanged, and atrial effective refractory period is unchanged. Lidocaine raises the ventricular fibrillation threshold. No significant interactions between lidocaine and autonomic nervous system have been described and, consequently, lidocaine has little or no effect on autonomic tone.

Onset of Action

Lidocaine HCl Topical Solution

The onset of action is rapid.

Lidocaine HCl Jelly

The onset of action is 3-5 minutes. It is ineffective when applied to intact skin.

Clinical electrophysiological studies with lidocaine have demonstrated no change in sinus node recovery time or sinoatrial conduction time. AV nodal conduction time is unchanged or shortened, and His-Purkinkje conduction time is unchanged.

Onset and Duration of Anesthesia of Lidocaine HCl With Dextrose

The onset of action is rapid. The duration of perineal anesthesia provided by 1 ml (50 mg) lidocaine HCl with dextrose averages 100 minutes, with analgesia continuing for an additional 40 minutes. The duration of surgical anesthesia provided by 1.5-2 ml (75-100 mg) of this agent is approximately 2 hours.

HEMODYNAMICS

Excessive blood levels may cause changes in cardiac output, total peripheral resistance, and mean arterial pressure. With central neural blockade these changes may be attributable to block of autonomic fibers, a direct depressant effect of the local anesthetic agent on various components of the cardiovascular system, and/or the beta-adrenergic receptor stimulating action of epinephrine when present. The net effect is normally a modest hypotension when the recommended dosages are not exceeded.

Additional Information for Lidocaine HCl for Ventricular Arrhythmia

At therapeutic doses, lidocaine has minimal hemodynamic effects in normal subjects and in patients with heart disease. Lidocaine has been shown to cause no, or minimal, decrease in ventricular contractility, cardiac output, arterial pressure or heart rate.

PHARMACOKINETICS AND METABOLISM

Information derived from other formulations, concentrations and usages reveals that lidocaine is completely absorbed following parenteral administration, its rate of absorption depending, for example, upon such factors as the site of administration and the presence or absence of a vasoconstrictor agent. Lidocaine may be absorbed following topical administration to mucous membranes, its rate and extent of absorption depending upon concentration and total dose adminstered, the specific site of application and duration of exposure. In general, the rate of absorption of local anesthetic agents following topical application occurs most rapidly after intratracheal administration. Lidocaine is also well absorbed from the gastrointestinal tract, but little intact drug appears in the circulation because of biotransformation by the liver. Except for intravascular administration, the highest blood levels are obtained following intercostal nerve block and the lowest after subcutaneous administration.

Lidocaine is metabolized rapidly by the liver, and metabolites and unchanged drug are excreted by the kidneys. Biotransformation includes oxidative N-dealkylation, ring hydroxylation, cleavage of the amide linkage, and conjugation. N-dealkylation, a major pathway of biotransformation, yields the metabolites monoethylglycinexylidide and glycinexylidide. The pharmacological/toxicological actions of these metabolites are similar to, but less potent than, those of lidocaine. Approximately 90% of lidocaine administered is excreted in the form of various metabolites, and less than 10% is excreted unchanged. The primary metabolite in urine is a conjugate of 4-hydroxy-2,6-dimethylaniline.

Studies have shown that peak blood levels of lidocaine may occur as early as 5 and as late as 30 minutes after endotracheal administration of a lidocaine HCl solution.

Therapeutic effects of lidocaine are generally associated with plasma levels at 6-25 μmol/L (1.5-6.0 μg free base per ml). The blood to plasma distribution ratio is approximately 0.84. Objective adverse manifestations become increasingly apparent with increasing plasma levels above 6 μg free base per ml.

The plasma binding of lidocaine is dependent on drug concentration, and the fraction bound decreases with increasing concentration. At concentrations of 1-4 μg of free base per ml 60-80% of lidocaine is protein bound. Binding is also dependent on the plasma concentration of the alpha-1-acid glycoprotein.

Lidocaine crosses the blood-brain and placental barriers, presumably by passive diffusion.

The elimination half-life of lidocaine following an intravenous bolus injection is typically 1.5-2.0 hours. Because of the rapid rate at which lidocaine is metabolized, any condition that affects liver function may alter lidocaine kinetics. The half-life may be prolonged 2-fold or more in patients with liver dysfunction. Renal dysfunction does not affect lidocaine kinetics but may increase the accumulation of metabolites.

Factors such as acidosis and the use of CNS stimulants and depressants affect the CNS levels of lidocaine required to produce overt systemic effects. Objective adverse manifestations become increasingly apparent with increasing venous plasma levels above 6 μg free base per ml. In the rhesus monkey arterial blood levels of 18-21 μg/ml have been shown to be threshold for convulsive activity.

INDICATIONS AND USAGE

LIDOCAINE HCl AND LIDOCAINE HCl WITH EPINEPHRINE INJECTIONS

Lidocaine HCl injections are indicated for production of local or regional anesthesia by infiltration techniques such as percutaneous injection and intravenous regional anesthesia by peripheral nerve block techniques such as brachial plexus and intercostal and by central neural techniques such as lumbar and caudal epidural blocks, when the accepted procedures for these techniques as described in standard textbooks are observed.

LIDOCAINE HCl STERILE SOLUTION

Lidocaine HCl sterile solution is indicated for the production of topical anesthesia of the mucous membranes of the respiratory tract or the genito-urinary tract. It may be injected trans-tracheally to anesthetize the larynx and trachea, and it may be administered by retrobulbar injection to provide anesthesia for ophthalmic surgery.

LIDOCAINE HCl FOR VENTRICULAR ARRHYTHMIAS

Lidocaine HCl injection administered intravenously is specifically indicated in the acute management of ventricular arrhythmias such as those occurring in relation to acute myocardial infarction, or during cardiac manipulation, such as cardiac surgery.

LIDOCAINE HCl WITH DEXTROSE

Lidocaine HCl with dextrose is indicated for the production of spinal anesthesia when the accepted procedures for this technique as described in standard textbooks are observed.

LIDOCAINE HCl TOPICAL SOLUTION

Lidocaine HCl topical solution is indicated for the production of topical anesthesia of the mucous membranes of the respiratory tract.

LIDOCAINE HCl JELLY

Lidocaine HCl jelly is indicated for prevention and control of pain in procedures involving the male and female urethra for topical treatment of painful urethritis, and as an anesthetic lubricant for endotracheal intubation (oral and nasal).

CONTRAINDICATIONS

Lidocaine is contraindicated in patients with a known history of hypersensitivity to local anesthetics of the amide type or to other components of any of the forms of this drug.

LIDOCAINE HCl FOR VENTRICULAR ARRHYTHMIA

Lidocaine HCl for ventricular arrhythmia should not be used in patients with Stoke-Adams syndrome, Wolff-Parkinson-White syndrome, or with severe degrees of sinoatrial, atrioventricular, or intraventricular block in the absence of an artificial pacemaker.

LIDOCAINE HCl WITH DEXTROSE

The following conditions preclude the use of spinal anesthesia:

1. Severe hemorrhage, shock or heart block.
2. Local infection at the site of proposed puncture.
3. Septicemia.
4. Known sensitivity to the local anesthetic agent.

WARNINGS

LIDOCAINE HCl SHOULD BE EMPLOYED ONLY BY CLINICIANS WHO ARE WELL VERSED IN DIAGNOSIS AND MANAGEMENT OF DOSE-RELATED TOXICITY AND OTHER ACUTE EMERGENCIES THAT MIGHT ARISE AND THEN ONLY AFTER ENSURING THE *IMMEDIATE* AVAILABILITY OF OXYGEN, OTHER RESUSCITATIVE DRUGS, CARDIOPULMONARY EQUIPMENT AND THE PERSONNEL NEEDED FOR PROPER MANAGEMENT OF TOXIC REACTIONS AND RELATED EMERGENCIES. (See also ADVERSE REACTIONS and PRECAUTIONS.) DELAY IN PROPER MANAGEMENT OF DOSE-RELATED TOXICITY, UNDERVENTILATION FROM ANY CAUSE AND/OR ALTERED SENSITIVITY MAY LEAD TO THE DEVELOPMENT OF ACIDOSIS, CARDIAC ARREST AND, POSSIBLY, DEATH.

To avoid intravascular injection, aspiration should be performed before the local anesthetic solution is injected. The needle must be repositioned until no return of blood can be elicited by aspiration. Note, however, that the absence of blood in the syringe does not guarantee that intravascular injection has been avoided.

Local anesthetic solutions containing antimicrobial preservatives, (*e.g.,* methylparaben) should not be used for epidural or spinal anesthesia because the safety of these agents has not been established with regard to intrathecal injection, either intentional or accidental.

ADDITIONAL INFORMATION FOR LIDOCAINE HCl WITH EPINEPHRINE

Solutions contain sodium metabisulfite, a sulfite that may cause allergic-type reactions including anaphylactic symptoms and life-threatening or less severe asthmatic episodes in certain susceptible people. The overall prevalence of sulfite sensitivity in the general population is unknown and probably low. Sulfite sensitivity is seen more frequently in asthmatic than in nonasthmatic people.

ADDITIONAL INFORMATION FOR LIDOCAINE HCl WITH DEXTROSE

Spinal anesthetics should not be injected during uterine contractions since spinal fluid current may carry the drug farther cephalad than desired.

ADDITIONAL INFORMATION FOR LIDOCAINE HCl STERILE SOLUTION, TOPICAL SOLUTION, AND JELLY

Lidocaine HCl sterile solution and topical solution should be used with extreme caution if there is sepsis or severely traumatized mucosa in the area of application, since under such conditions there is the potential for rapid systemic absorption.

ADDITIONAL INFORMATION FOR LIDOCAINE HCl JELLY

EXCESSIVE DOSAGE, OR SHORT INTERVALS BETWEEN DOSES, CAN RESULT IN HIGH PLASMA LEVELS AND SERIOUS ADVERSE EFFECTS. PATIENTS SHOULD BE INSTRUCTED TO STRICTLY ADHERE TO THE RECOMMENDED DOSAGE AND ADMINISTRATION GUIDELINES AS SET FORTH IN THIS PACKAGE INSERT.

THE MANAGEMENT OF SERIOUS ADVERSE REACTIONS MAY REQUIRE THE USE OF RESUSCITATIVE EQUIPMENT, OXYGEN, AND OTHER RESUSCITATIVE DRUGS.

When used for endotracheal tube lubrication, care should be taken to avoid introducing the product into the lumen of the tube. Do not use the jelly to lubricate the endotracheal stylettes. If allowed into the inner lumen, the jelly may dry on the inner surface leaving a residue which tends to clump with flexion, narrowing the lumen. There have been rare reports in which this residue has caused the lumen to occlude. See alsoADVERSE REACTIONS and DOSAGE AND ADMINISTRATION.

ADDITIONAL INFORMATION FOR LIDOCAINE HCl FOR VENTRICULAR ARRHYTHMIAS

IN ORDER TO MANAGE POSSIBLE ADVERSE REACTIONS, RESUSCITATIVE EQUIPMENT, OXYGEN AND OTHER RESUSCITATIVE DRUGS SHOULD BE IMMEDIATELY AVAILABLE WHEN LIDOCAINE HCl INJECTION IS USED.

Systemic toxicity may result in manifestations of central nervous system depression (sedation) or irritability (twitching), which may progress to frank convulsions accompanied by respiratory depression and or arrest. Early recognition of premonitory signs, assurance of adequate oxygenation, and, where necessary, establishment of artificial airway with ventilatory support are essential to management of this problem. Should convulsions persist despite ventilatory therapy with oxygen, **small** increments of anticonvulsant drugs may be used intravenously. Examples of such agents include benzodiazepines (*e.g.,* diazepam), ultra short-acting barbiturates (*e.g.,* thiopental or thiamylal), or a short-acting barbiturate (*e.g.,* pentobarbital or secobarbital). If a patient is under anesthesia, a short-acting muscle relaxant (*e.g.,* succinylcholine) may be used. Longer-acting drugs should be used only when recurrent convulsions are evidenced.

Should circulatory depression occur, vasopressors may be used.

Constant electrocardiographic monitoring is essential to the proper administration of lidocaine HCl. Signs of excessive depression of cardiac electrical activity such as sinus node dysfunction, prolongation of the P-R interval and QRS complex or the appearance or aggravation of arrhythmias, should be followed by flow adjustment and, if necessary, prompt cessation of the intravenous infusion of this agent. Occasionally, acceleration of ventricular rate may occur when lidocaine HCl is administered to patients with atrial flutter or fibrillation.

PRECAUTIONS

GENERAL

The safety and effectiveness of lidocaine depends on proper dosage, correct technique, adequate precautions, and readiness for emergencies.

Repeated doses of lidocaine may cause significant increases in blood levels with each repeated dose because of slow accumulation of the drug or its metabolites. Tolerance to elevated blood levels varies with the physical condition of the patient. Debilitated, elderly patients, acutely ill patients, and children should be given reduced doses commensurate with their age and physical status. Lidocaine should also be used with caution in patients with severe shock or heart block.

Resuscitative equipment, oxygen, and other resuscitative drugs should be available for immediate use. (See WARNINGS and ADVERSE REACTIONS.) The lowest dosage that results in effective anesthesia should be used to avoid high plasma levels and serious adverse effects.

Local anesthetic solutions containing a vasoconstrictor should be used cautiously and in carefully circumscribed quantities in areas of the body supplied by end arteries or having otherwise compromised blood supply. Patients with peripheral vascular disease and those with hypertensive vascular disease may exhibit exaggerated vasoconstrictor response. Ischemic injury or necrosis may result. Preparations containing a vasoconstrictor should be used with caution in patients during or following the administration of potent general anesthetic agents, since cardiac arrhythmias may occur under such conditions.

Careful and constant monitoring of cardiovascular and respiratory (adequacy of ventilation) vital signs and the patient's state of consciousness should be accomplished after each local anesthetic injection. It should be kept in mind at such times that restlessness, anxiety, tinnitus, dizziness, blurred vision, tremors, depression or drowsiness may be early warning signs of central nervous system toxicity.

Since amide-type local anesthetics are metabolized by the liver, lidocaine HCl should be used with caution in patients with hepatic disease. Patients with severe hepatic disease, because of their inability to metabolize local anesthetics normally, are at greater risk of developing toxic plasma concentrations. Lidocaine HCl should also be used with caution in patients with impaired cardiovascular function since they may be less able to compensate for functional changes associated with the prolongation of AV conduction produced by these drugs.

Many drugs used during the conduct of anesthesia are considered potential triggering agents for familial malignant hyperthermia. Since it is not known whether amide-type local anesthetics may trigger this reaction and since the need for supplemental general anesthesia cannot be predicted in advance, it is suggested that a standard protocol for the management of malignant hyperthermia should be available. Early unexplained signs of tachycardia, tachypnea, labile blood pressure and metabolic acidosis may precede temperature elevation. Successful outcome is dependent on early diagnosis, prompt discontinuance of the suspect triggering agent(s) and institution of treatment, including oxygen therapy, indicated supportive measures and dantrolene (consult dantrolene sodium intravenous package insert before using).

Proper tourniquet technique, as described in publications and standard textbooks, is essential in the performance of intravenous regional anesthesia. Solutions containing epinephrine or other vasoconstrictors should not be used for this technique.

Lidocaine should be used with caution in persons with known drug sensitivities. Patients allergic to para-aminobenzoic acid derivatives (procaine, tetracaine, benzocaine, etc.) have not shown cross sensitivity to lidocaine.

Standard textbooks should be consulted for specific techniques and precautions for various regional anesthetic procedures.

Additional Information for Lidocaine HCl With Epinephrine

Syringe aspirations should be performed before and during each supplemental injection when using indwelling catheter techniques.

During the administration of epidural anesthesia, it is recommend that a test dose be administered initially and that the patient be monitored for central nervous system toxicity and cardiovascular toxicity, as well as for signs of unintended intrathecal administration, before proceeding. When clinical conditions permit, consideration should be given to employing local anesthetic solutions that contain epinephrine for the test dose because circulatory changes compatible with epinephrine may also serve as a warning sign of unintended intravascular injection. An intravascular injection is still possible even if aspirations for blood are negative. Repeated doses of lidocaine may cause significant increases in blood levels with each repeated dose because of slow accumulation of the drug or its metabolites. Tolerance to elevated blood levels varies with the status of the patient. Debilitated, elderly patients, acutely ill patients, and children should be given reduced doses commensurate with their age and physical condition. Lidocaine should also be used with caution in patients with severe shock or heart block.

Lumber and caudal epidural anesthesia should be used with extreme caution in persons with the following conditions: existing neurological disease, spinal deformities, septicemia, and severe hypertension.

Additonal Information for Lidocaine HCl With Dextrose

Neurologic deficits have been reported with the use of small bore needles and microcatheters for spinal anesthesia. It has been postulated, based on *in vitro* models, that these deficits were due to pooling and nonuniform distribution of concentrated local anesthetic within the subarachnoid space.[1] Animal studies suggest mixing 5% lidocaine HCl with an equal volume of CSF or preservative-free 0.9% saline solution may reduce the risk of nerve injury due to pooling of concentrated local anesthetic.[2] (See DOSAGE AND ADMINISTRATION.)

The following conditions may preclude the use of spinal anesthesia, depending upon the physician's ability to deal with the complications or complaints that may occur:

1. Pre-existing diseases of the central nervous system such as those attributable to poliomyelitis, pernicious anemia, paralysis from nerve injuries, and syphilis.
2. Disturbance in blood morphology and/or anticoagulant therapy. In these conditions, trauma to a blood vessel during needle puncture may result in uncontrollable hemorrhage into the epidural or subarachnoid space. Also profuse hemorrhage into the soft tissue may occur.
3. Extremes of age.
4. Chronic backache and preoperative headache.
5. Hypotension and hypertension.
6. Arthritis or spinal deformity.
7. Technical problems (persistent paresthesias, persistent bloody tap).
8. Psychotic or uncooperative patients.

CONSULT STANDARD TEXTBOOKS FOR SPECIFIC TECHNIQUES AND PRECAUTIONS FOR SPINAL ANESTHETIC PROCEDURES.

Careful and constant monitoring of cardiovascular and respiratory (adequacy of ventilation) vital signs and the patient's state of consciousness should be accomplished after each local anesthetic injection. It should be kept in mind at such times that restlessness, anxiety, tinnitus, dizziness, blurred vision, tremors, depression or drowsiness may be early warning signs of central nervous system toxicity.

Since amide-type local anesthetics are metabolized by the liver, lidocaine should be used with caution in patients with hepatic disease. Patients with severe hepatic disease, because of their inability to metabolize local anesthetics normally, are at greater risk of developing toxic plasma concentrations. Lidocaine should also be used with caution in patients with impaired cardiovascular function since they may be less able to compensate for functional changes associated with the prolongation of AV conduction produced by these drugs.

Many drugs used during the conduct of anesthesia are considered potential triggering agents for familial malignant hyperthermia. Since it is not known whether amide-type local anesthetics may trigger this reaction and since the need for supplemental general anesthesia cannot be predicted in advance, it is suggested that a standard protocol for management should be available. Early unexplained signs of tachycardia, tachypnea, labile blood pressure and metabolic acidosis may precede temperature elevation. Successful outcome is dependent on early diagnosis, prompt discontinuance of the suspect triggering agent(s) and institution of treatment, including oxygen therapy, indicated supportive measures and dantrolene (consult dantrolene sodium intravenous package insert before using).

Lidocaine should be used with caution in persons with known drug sensitivities. Patients allergic to para-aminobenzoic acid derivatives (procaine, tetracaine, benzocaine, etc.) have not shown cross sensitivity to lidocaine.

Additional Information for Lidocaine HCl Injection for Ventricular Arrhythmia

Caution should be employed in the use of lidocaine HCl in patients with severe liver or kidney disease because accumulation of the drug or metabolites may occur.

Lidocaine HCl should be used with caution in the treatment of patients with hypovolemia, severe congestive heart failure, shock, and all forms of heart block. In patients with sinus bradycardia, or incomplete heart block, the administration of lidocaine HCl intravenously for the elimination of ventricular ectopic beats, without prior acceleration in heart rate (*e.g.*, by atropine, isoproterenol or electric pacing), may promote more frequent and serious ventricular arrhythmias or complete heart block (see CONTRAINDICATIONS, Lidocaine HCl for Ventricular Arrhythmia).

Dosage should be reduced for children and for debilitated and/or elderly patients, commensurate with their age and physical status.

The safety of amide local anesthetic agents in patients with genetic predisposition to malignant hypothermia has not been fully assessed; therefore, lidocaine should be used with caution in such patients.

In hospital environments where drugs known to be triggering agents for malignant hypothermia (fulminant hypermetabolism) are administered, it is suggested that a standard protocol for management should be available.

It is not known whether lidocaine may trigger this reaction; however, large doses resulting in significant plasma concentrations, as may be achieved by intravenous infusion, pose potential risk to these individuals. Recognition of early unexplained signs of tachycardia, tachypnea, labile blood pressure and metabolic acidosis may precede temperature elevation. Successful outcome is dependent on early diagnosis, prompt discontinuance of the triggering agent and institution of treatment including oxygen therapy, supportive measures and dantrolene (for details see dantrolene prescribing information/package insert).

Use in Ophthalmic Surgery

When local anesthetic solutions are employed for retrobulbar block, lack of corneal sensation should not be relied upon to determine whether or not the patient is ready for surgery since corneal sensation usually precedes clinically acceptable external ocular muscle akinesia.

Many drugs used during the conduct of anesthesia are considered potential triggering agents for familial malignant hyperthermia. Since it is not known whether amide-type local anesthestics may trigger this reaction and since the need for supplemental general anesthesia cannot be predicted in advance, it is suggested that a standard protocol for management should be available. Early unexplained signs of tachycardia, tachypnea, labile blood pressure, and metabolic acidosis may precede temperature elevation. Successful outcome is dependent on early diagnosis, prompt discontinuance of the suspected triggering agent(s) and instituition of treatment, including oxygen therapy, indicated supportive measures, and dantrolene (consult dantrolene sodium intravenous package insert before using).

Use in the Head and Neck Area

Small doses of local anesthetics injected into the head and neck area, including retrobulbar, dental and stellate ganglion blocks, may produce adverse reactions similar to systemic toxicity seen with unintentional intravascular injections of larger doses. Confusion, convulsions, respiratory depression and/or respiratory arrest, and cardiovascular stimulation or depression have been reported. These reactions may be due to intra-arterial injection of the local anesthetic with retrograde flow to the cerebral circulation. Patients receiving these blocks should have their circulation and respiration monitored and be constantly observed. Resuscitative equipment and personnel for treating adverse reactions should be immediately available. Dosage recommendations should not be exceeded. (See DOSAGE AND ADMINISTRATION.)

INFORMATION FOR THE PATIENT

When appropriate, patients should be informed in advance that they may experience temporary loss of sensation and motor activity, usually in the lower half of the body, following proper administration of epidural anesthesia. The patient should be advised of the possible occurence of the experiences listed under ADVERSE REACTIONS.

Lidocaine HCl Sterile Solution, Topical, and Jelly

When topical anesthetics are used in the mouth, the patient should be aware that the production of topical anesthesia may impair swallowing and thus enhance the danger of aspiration. For this reason, food should not be ingested for 60 minutes following use of local anesthetic preparations in the mouth or throat area. This is particularaly important in children because of their frequency of eating.

Numbness of the tongue or buccal mucosa may enhance the danger of unintentional biting trauma. Food and chewing gum should not be taken while the mouth or throat area is anesthetized.

DRUG/LABORATORY TEST INTERACTIONS

The intramuscular injection of lidocaine may result in an increase in creatine phosphokinase levels. Thus, the use of this enzyme determination, without isoenzyme separation, as a diagnostic test for the presence of acute myocardial infarction may be compromised by the intramuscular injection of lidocaine.

CARCINOGENESIS, MUTAGENESIS, AND IMPAIRMENT OF FERTILITY

Studies of lidocaine in animals to evaluate the carcinogenic and mutagenic potential or the effect on fertility have not been conducted.

PREGNANCY, TERATOGENIC EFFECTS, PREGNANCY CATEGORY B

Reproduction studies have been performed in rats at doses up to 6.6 times the human dose and have revealed no evidence of harm to the fetus caused by lidocaine. There are, however, no adequate and well-controlled studies in pregnant women. Animal reproduction studies are not always predictive of human response. General consideration should be given to this fact before administering lidocaine to women of childbearing potential, especially during early pregnancy when maximum organogenesis takes place.

LABOR AND DELIVERY

Lidocaine is not contraindicated in labor and delivery. Should lidocaine HCl be used concomitantly with other products containing lidocaine, the total dose contributed by all formulations must be kept in mind.

Local anesthetics rapidly cross the placenta and when used for epidural, paracervical, pudendal or caudal block anesthesia, can cause varying degrees of maternal, fetal and neonatal toxicity. See CLINICAL PHARMACOLOGY, Pharmacokinetics and Metabolism.The potential for toxicity depends upon the procedure performed, the type and amount of drug used, and the technique of drug administration. Adverse reactions in the parturient, fetus and neonate involve alterations of the central nervous system, peripheral vascular tone, and cardiac function.

Maternal hypotension has resulted from regional anesthesia. Local anesthetics produce vasodilation by blocking sympathetic nerves. Elevating the patient's legs and positioning her on her left side will help prevent decreases in blood pressure. The fetal heart rate also should be monitored continuously, and electronic fetal monitoring is highly advisable.

Epidural, spinal, paracervical, or pudendal anesthesia may alter the forces of parturition through changes in uterine contractility or maternal expulsive efforts. In one study, paracervical block anesthesia was associated with a decrease in the mean duration of first stage labor and facilitation of cervical dilation. However, spinal and epidural anesthesia have also been reported to prolong the second stage of labor by removing the parturient's reflex urge to bear down or by interfering with motor function. The use of obstetrical anesthesia may increase the need for forceps assistance.

The use of some local anesthetic drug products during labor and delivery may be followed by diminished muscle strength and tone for the first day or two of life. The long-term significance of these observations is unknown. Fetal bradycardia may occur in 20-30% of patients receiving paracervical nerve block anesthesia with the amide-type local anesthetics and may be associated with fetal acidosis. Fetal heart rate should always be monitored during paracervical anesthesia. The physician should weigh the possible advantages against risks when considering a paracervical block in prematurity, toxemia of pregnancy, and fetal distress. Careful adherence to recommended dosage is of the utmost importance in obstetrical paracervical block. Failure to achieve adequate analgesia with recommended doses should arouse suspicion of intravascular or fetal intracranial injection. Cases compatible with unintended fetal intracranial injection of local anesthetic solution have been reported following intended paracervical or pudendal block or both. Babies so affected present with unexplained neonatal depression at birth, which correlates with high local anesthetic serum levels, and often manifest seizures within 6 hours. Prompt use of supportive measures com-

L

bined with forced urinary excretion of the local anesthetic has been used successfully to manage this complication.

Case reports of maternal convulsions and cardiovascular collapse following use of some local anesthetics for paracervical block in early pregnancy (as anesthesia for elective abortion) suggest that systemic absorption under these circumstances may be rapid. The recommended maximum dose of each drug should not be exceeded. Injection should be made slowly and with frequent aspiration. Allow a 5-minute interval between sides.

The effects of lidocaine HCl on the mother and the fetus, when used in the management of cardiac arrhythmias during labor and delivery, are not known.

NURSING MOTHERS

It is not known whether this drug is excreted in human milk. Because many drugs are excreted in human milk, caution should be exercised when lidocaine is administered to a nursing woman.

PEDIATRIC USE

Dosages in pediatric patients should be reduced, commensurate with age, body weight and physical condition. (See DOSAGE AND ADMINISTRATION.)

Additional Information for Lidocaine HCl With Dextrose

Safety and effectiveness in pediatric patients below the age of 16 years have not been established.

DRUG INTERACTIONS

LIDOCAINE HCl STERILE SOLUTION, LIDOCAINE HCl WITH EPINEPHRINE AND LIDOCAINE HCl WITH DEXTROSE

The administration of local anesthetic solutions containing epinephrine or norepinephrine to patients receiving monoamine oxidase inhibitors, tricyclic antidepressants, or phenothiazines may produce severe, prolonged hypotension or hypertension. Concurrent use of these agents should generally be avoided. In situations when concurrent therapy is necessary, careful patient monitoring is essential.

Concurrent administration of vasopressor drugs (for the treatment of hypotension related to obstetric blocks) and ergot-type oxytocic drugs may cause severe, persistent hypertension or cerebrovascular accidents.

Phenothiazines and butyrophenones may reduce or reverse the pressor effect of epinephrine.

L

LIDOCAINE HCl FOR VENTRICULAR ARRHYTHMIAS

Lidocaine HCl injections should be used with caution in patients with digitalis toxicity accompanied by atrioventricular block. Concomitant use of beta-blocking agents or cimetidine may reduce hepatic blood flow and thereby reduce lidocaine clearance.

Lidocaine and tocainide are pharmacodynamically similar. The concomitant use of these two agents may cause an increased incidence of adverse reactions, including central nervous system adverse reactions such as seizure.

ADVERSE REACTIONS

SYSTEMIC

Adverse experiences following the administration of lidocaine are similar in nature to those observed with other amide local anesthetic agents. These adverse experiences are, in general, dose-related and may result from high plasma levels caused by excessive dosage, rapid absorption of inadvertent intravascular injection, or may result from a hypersensitivity, idiosyncrasy or diminished to tolerance on the part of the patient. Serious adverse experiences are generally systemic in nature. The following types are those most commonly reported. The adverse experiences under Central Nervous System and Cardiovascular System are listed, in general, in a progression from mild to severe.

Additional Information for Lidocaine HCl Jelly

There have been rare reports of endotracheal tube occlusion associated with the presence of dried jelly residue in the inner lumen of the tube. (See also WARNINGS, Additional Information for Lidocaine HCl Jelly and DOSAGE AND ADMINISTRATION, Lidocaine HCl Jelly.)

CENTRAL NERVOUS SYSTEM

CNS manifestations are excitatory and/or depressant and may be characterized by lightheadedness, nervousness, apprehension, euphoria, confusion, dizziness, drowsiness, tinnitus, blurred or double vision, vomiting, sensations of heat, cold or numbness, twitching, tremors, convulsions, unconsciousness, respiratory depression and arrest. The excitatory manifestation may be very brief or may not occur at all, in which case the first manifestation of toxicity may be drowsiness merging into unconsciousness and respiratory arrest.

Drowsiness following the administration of lidocaine is usually an early sign of a high blood level of the drug and may occur as a consequence of rapid absorption.

CARDIOVASCULAR SYSTEM

Cardiovascular manifestations are usually depressant and are characterized by bradycardia, hypotension, and cardiovascular collapse, which may lead to cardiac arrest.

ALLERGIC

Allergic reactions are characterized by cutaneous lesions, urticaria, edema or anaphylactoid reactions. Allergic reactions may occur as a result of sensitivity either to local anesthetic agents or to the methylparaben used as a preservative in the multiple-dose vials. Allergic reactions as a result of sensitivity to lidocaine are extremely rare and, if they occur, should be managed by conventional means. The detection of sensitivity by skin testing is of doubtful value.

NEUROLOGIC

The incidences of adverse reactions associated with the use of local anesthetics may be related to the total dose of local anesthetic administered and are also dependent upon the particular drug used, the route of administration and the physical status of the patient.

Additional Information for Lidocaine HCl Sterile Solution

There have been reported cases of permanent injury to extraocular muscles requiring surgical repair following retrobulbar administration.

Additional Information for Lidocaine HCl With Epinephrine and Lidocaine HCl With Dextrose

In a prospective review of 10,440 patients who received lidocaine for spinal anesthesia, the incidences of adverse reactions were reported to be about 3% each for positional headaches, hypotension, and backache; 2% for shivering; and <1% each for peripheral nerve symptoms, nausea, respiratory inadequacy, and double vision. Many of these observations may be related to local anesthetic techniques, with or without a contribution from the local anesthetic.

Additional Information for Lidocaine HCl With Epinephrine

In the practice of caudal or lumbar epidural block, occasional unintentional penetration of the subarachnoid space by the catheter may occur. Subsequent adverse effects may depend partially on the amount of drug administered subdurally. These may include spinal block or varying magnitude (including total spinal block), hypotension secondary to spinal block, loss of bladder and bowel control, and loss of perineal sensation and sexual function. Persistent motor, sensory and/or autonomic (sphincter control) deficit of some lower spinal segments with slow recovery (several months) or incomplete recovery have been reported in rare instances when caudal or lumbar epidural block has been attempted. Backache and headache have also been noted following use of these anesthetic procedures.

Additional Information for Lidocaine HCl With Dextrose

Neurologic effects following spinal anesthesia may include: loss of perineal sensation and sexual function; persistent anesthesia; paresthesia; weakness and paralysis of the lower extremities; and loss of sphincter control, all of which may have slow, incomplete, or no recovery; hypotension; high or total spinal block; urinary retention; headache; backache; septic meningitis; meningismus, arachnoiditis; slowing of labor; increased incidence of forceps delivery; shivering; cranial nerve palsies due to traction on nerves from loss of cerebrospinal fluid; and fecal and urinary incontinence.

DOSAGE AND ADMINISTRATION

When lidocaine HCl is used concomitantly with other products containing lidocaine, the total dose contributed by all formulations must be kept in mind.

The dosage varies and depends upon the area to be anesthetized, vasularity of the tissues, individual tolerance and the technique of anesthesia. The lowest dosage needed to provide effective anesthesia should be administered. Dosages should be reduced for children and for elderly and debilitated patients.

Although the incidence of adverse effects with lidocaine HCl is quite low, caution should be exercised, particularly when employing large volumes and concentrations of lidocaine HCl since the incidence of adverse effects is directly proportional to the total dose of local anesthetic agent administered. For specific techniques and procedures, refer to standard textbooks.

TABLE 2 summarizes the recommended volumes and concentrations of lidocaine HCl for various types of anesthetic procedures. The dosages suggested in this table are for normal healthy adults and refer to the use of epinephrine-free solutions. When larger volumes are required, only solutions containing epinephrine should be used except in those cases where vasopressor drugs may be contraindicated.

These recommended doses serve only as a guide to the amount of anesthetic required for most routine procedures. The actual volumes and concentrations to be used depends on a number of factors such as type and extent of surgical procedure, depth of anesthesia and degree of muscular relaxation required, duration of anesthesia required, and the physical condition of the patient. In all cases the lowest concentration and smallest dose that will produce the desired result should be given. Dosages should be reduced for children and for the elderly and debilitated patients and patients with cardiac and/or liver disease.

THE ABOVE SUGGESTED CONCENTRATIONS AND VOLUMES SERVE ONLY AS A GUIDE. OTHER VOLUMES AND CONCENTRATIONS MAY BE USED PROVIDED THE TOTAL MAXIMUM RECOMMENDED DOSE IS NOT EXCEED.

For intravenous regional anesthesia, only the 50 ml single-dose vial containing lidocaine HCl 0.5% should be used.

ADDITIONAL INFORMATION FOR LIDOCAINE HCl AND LIDOCAINE HCl WITH EPINEPHRINE

Epidural Anesthesia

For epidural anesthesia, only the following dosage forms of lidocaine HCl are recommended:

1% without epinephrine; 1% with epinephrine 1:200,000.
1.5% without epinephrine; 1.5% with epinephrine 1:200,000.
2% without epinephrine; 2% with epinephrine 1:200,000.

Although these solutions are intended specifically for epidural anesthesia, they may also be used for infiltration and peripheral nerve block, provided they are employed as single-dose units. These solutions contain no bacteriostatic agent.

In epidural anesthesia, the dosage varies with the number of dermatomes to be anesthetized (generally 2-3 ml of the indicated concentration per dermatome).

Caudal and Lumbar Epidural Block

As a precaution against the adverse experience sometimes observed following unintentional penetration of the subarachnoid space, a test dose such as 2-3 ml of 1.5% lidocaine should be administered at least 5 minutes prior to injecting the total volume required for a lumbar or caudal epidural block. The test dose should be repeated if the patient is moved in a manner that may have displaced the catheter. Epinephrine, if contained in the test dose,

TABLE 2 *Recommended Dosages*

Procedure	Conc.	Vol.	Total Dose
	Lidocaine HCl		
Infiltration			
Percutaneous	0.5 or 1%	1-60 ml	5-300 mg
Intravenous regional	0.5%	10-60 ml	50-300 mg
Peripheral Nerve Blocks, *e.g.*,			
Brachial	1.5%	15-20 ml	225-300 mg
Dental	2%	1-5 ml	20-100 mg
Intercostal	1%	3 ml	30 mg
Paravertebral	1%	3-5 ml	30-50 mg
Pudendal (each side)	1%	10 ml	100 mg
Paracervical			
Obstetrical analgesia (each side)	1%	10 ml	100 mg
Sympathetic Nerve Blocks, *e.g.*,			
Cervical (stellate ganglion)	1%	5 ml	50 mg
Lumbar	1%	5-10 ml	50-100 mg
Central Neural Blocks			
Epidural*			
Thoracic	1%	20-30 ml	200-300 mg
Lumbar			
Analgesia	1%	25-30 ml	250-300 mg
Anesthesia	1.5%	15-20 ml	225-300 mg
	2%	10-15 ml	200-300 mg
Caudal			
Obstetrical analgesia	1%	20-30 ml	200-300 mg
Surgical anesthesia	1.5%	15-20 ml	225-300 mg

* Dose determined by number of dermatomes to be anesthetized (2-3 ml/dermatome).

(10-15 μg have been suggested), may serve as a warning of unintentional intravascular injection. If injected into a blood vessel, this amount of epinephrine is likely to produce a transient "epinephrine response" within 45 seconds, consisting of an increase in heart rate and systolic blood pressure, circumoral pallor, palpitations and nervousness in the unsedated patient. The sedated patient may exhibit only a pulse rate increase of 20 or more beats per minute for 15 or more seconds. Patients on beta blockers may not manifest changes in heart rate, but blood pressure monitoring can detect an evanescent rise in systolic blood pressure. Adequate time should be allowed for onset of anesthetic after administration of each test dose. The rapid injection of a large volume of lidocaine HCl through the catheter should be avoided, and, when feasible, fractional doses should be administered.

In the event of the known injection of a large volume of local anesthetic solution into the subarachnoid space, after suitable resuscitation and if the catheter is in place, consider attempting the recovery of drug by draining a moderate amount of cerebrospinal fluid (such as 10 ml) through the epidural catheter.

Maximum Recommended Dosages

Adults

For normal healthy adults, the individual maximum recommended dose of lidocaine HCl with epinephrine should not exceed 7 mg/kg (3.5 mg/lb) of body weight, and in general, it is recommended that the maximum total dose not exceed 500 mg. When used without epinephrine the maximum individual dose should be kept under 300 mg and in any case should not exceed 4.5 mg/kg (2 mg/lb) of body weight. For continuous epidural or caudal anesthesia, the maximum recommended dosage should not be administered at intervals of less than 90 minutes. When continuous lumbar or caudal epidural anesthsia is used for nonobstetrical procedures, more drug may be administered if required to produce adequate anesthesia.

The maximum recommended dose per 90 minute period of lidocaine HCl for paracervical block in obstetrical patients and nonobstetrical patients is 200 mg total. One-half of the total dose is usually administered to each side. Inject slowly, 5 minutes between sides (see also discussion of paracervical block in PRECAUTIONS, Labor and Delivery).

For intravenous regional anesthesia, the dose administered should not exceed 4 mg/kg in adults.

Children

It is difficult to recommend a maximum dose for any drug of children, since this varies as a function of age and weight. For children of less than 10 years of age who have a normal lean body mass and normal body development, the maximum dose may be determined by the application of one of the standard pediatric drug formulas (*e.g.,* Clark's rule). For example, in a child of 5 years weighing 50 lb, the dose of lidocaine HCl should not exceed 75-100 mg when calculated according to Clark's rule. In any case, the maximum dose of lidocaine HCl with epinehprine should not exceed 7 mg/kg (3.2 mg/lb) of body weight. When used without epinephrine, the amount of lidocaine HCl is kept below 300 mg and in any case should not exceed 4.5 mg/kg (2 mg/lb) of body weight.

For example, in a child of 5 years weighing 50 lb the dose of lidocaine HCl should not exceed 75-100 mg (1.5-2 mg/lb). The use of even more dilute solutions (*i.e.,* 0.25-0.5%) and total dosages not to exceed 3 mg/kg (1.4 mg/lb) are recommended for induction of intravenous regional anesthesia in children.

In order to guard against systemic toxicity, the lowest effective concentration and lowest effective dose should be used at all times. In some cases it will be necessary to dilute available concentrations with 0.9% sodium chloride injection in order to obtain the required final concentration.

ADDITIONAL INFORMATION FOR LIDOCAINE HCl FOR VENTRICULAR ARRHYTHMIAS

Adults

Single Direct Intravenous Injection (Bolus)

ONLY THE 50 mg OR 100 mg DOSAGE SIZES should be used for direct intravenous injection. The usual dose is 50-100 mg of lidocaine HCl (0.70-1.4 mg/kg; 0.32-0.63 mg/lb) administered intravenously under ECG monitoring. This dose may be administered at the rate of approximately 25-50 mg/min (0.35-0.70 mg/kg/min; 0.16-0.32 mg/lb/min). Sufficient time should be allowed to enable a slow circulation to carry the drug to the site of action. If the initial injection of 50-100 mg does not produce a desired response, a second dosage may be injected after 5 minutes. NO MORE THAN 200-300 MG OF LIDOCAINE HCl SHOULD BE ADMINISTERED DURING A 1 HOUR PERIOD.

Continuous Intravenous Infusion

Following bolus administration, intravenous infusions of lidocaine HCl may be initiated at the rate of 1-4 mg/min of lidocaine HCl (0.014-0.057 mg/kg/min; 0.006-0.026 mg/lb/min). The rate of intravenous infusions should be reassessed as soon as the patient's basic cardiac rhythm appears to be stable or at the earliest signs of toxicity. It should rarely be necessary to continue intravenous infusions of lidocaine for prolonged periods.

Solutions for intravenous infusion may be prepared by the addition of 1 g (or 2 g) of lidocaine HCl to 1 L of 5% dextrose in water using aseptic technique. Approximately a 0.1% (or 0.2%) solution will result from this procedure; that is, each milliliter will contain approximately 1 (or 2) mg of lidocaine HCl. In those cases in which fluid restriction is medically appropriate, a more concentrated solution may be prepared.

Lidocaine HCl has been found to be chemically stable for 24 hours after dilution in 5% dextrose in water. However, as with all intravenous admixtures, dilution of the solution should be made just prior to its administration.

It is very important that after adding lidocaine HCl, or any other medication, to an IV container, the contents be thoroughly mixed before beginning the infusion.

When administered by continuous IV infusion, it is advisable to use a pricision volume control IV set.

Parenteral drug products should be inspected visually for particulate matter and discoloration prior to administration whenever the solution and container permit. Do not use if solution is discolored or cloudy.

Pediatric

Although controlled clinical studies to establish pediatric dosing schedules have not been conducted, the American Heart Association's *Standards and Guidelines* recommends a bolus dose of 1 mg/kg followed by an infusion rate of 30 μg/kg/min.

Note Regarding Prolonged Infusions: There are data that indicate the half-life may be 3 hours or longer following infusions greater than 24 hours in duration.

ADDITIONAL INFORMATION FOR LIDOCAINE HCl WITH DEXTROSE

Spinal anesthesia with lidocaine HCl with dextrose may be induced in the right or left lateral recumbent or the sitting position. Since this is a hyperbaric solution, the anesthetic will tend to move in the direction in which the table is tilted. After the desired level of anesthesia is obtained and the anesthetic has become fixed, usually in 5-10 minutes with lidocaine, the patient may be positioned according to the requirement of the surgeon or obstetrician.

In clinical trials, the safety of hyperbaric lidocaine for single injection spinal anesthesia was demonstrated using 22 or 25 gauge spinal needles. In these studies, free flow of CSF was visible before injection of lidocaine.

Neurologic deficits have been reported with the use of small bore needles and microcatheters for spinal anesthesia. It has been postulated, based on *in vitro* models, that these deficits were caused by pooling and nonuniform distribution of concentrated local anesthetic within the subarachnoid space.[1] Animal studies suggest that mixing 5% lidocaine with an equal volume of CSF or preservative-free 0.9% saline solution may reduce the risk of nerve injury due to pooling of concentrated local anesthetic[2] (see PRECAUTIONS, Additonal Information for Lidocaine HCl With Dextrose).

Intrathecal distribution of anesthetic may be facilitated by using a spinal needle of sufficient gauge to insure adequate withdrawal of CSF through the needle prior to and after anesthetic administration. If the technique is properly performed and the drug is properly placed in the subarachnoid space, a separate injection is seldom necessary.

An incomplete or patchy block not responsive to patient repositioning may indicate misplacement or inadequate distribution of drug. To avoid excessive drug pooling, additional doses of lidocaine HCl should not be administered with the same needle placement.

INJECTIONS SHOULD BE MADE SLOWLY. Consult standard textbooks for specific techniques for spinal anesthetic procedures.

Recommended Dosages

Normal Healthy Adults

The following recommended dosages are for normal healthy adults and serve only as a guide to the amount of anesthetic required for most routine procedures. In all cases, the smallest dose that will produce the desired result should be given.

If the technique is properly performed, and the needle is properly placed in the subarachnoid space, it should not be necessary to administer more than one ampule (100 mg).

Obstetrical Low Spinal or "Saddle Block" Anesthesia

The dosage recommended for normal vaginal delivery is approximately 1 ml (50 mg). For Caesarean section and those deliveries requiring intrauterine manipulations, 1.5 (75 mg) is usually adequate.

Surgical Anesthesia

The dosage recommended for abdominal anesthesia is 1.5-2 ml (75-100 mg).

Children

The dosage recommendations in healthy adolescents, 16 years of age and older, is the same as for normal healthy adults. There is insufficient data in pediatric patients below the age of 16 years to make dosage recommendations (see PRECAUTIONS.)

NOTE: Parenteral drug products should be inspected visually for particulate matter and discoloration prior to administration whenever the solution and container permit. Solutions that are discolored and/or contain particulate matter should not be used.

ADDITIONAL INFORMATION FOR LIDOCAINE HCl STERILE SOLUTION

The dosages below are for normal, healthy adults.

L

Retrobulbar Injection: The suggested dose for a 70 kg person is 3-5ml (120-200 mg of lidocaine HCl), (*i.e.*, 1.7-3 mg/kg or 0.9-1.5 mg/lb body weight). A portion of this is injected retrobulbarly and the rest may be used to block the facial nerve.

Transtracheal Injection: For local anesthesia by the transtracheal route 2-3 ml should be injected through a large enough needle so that the injection can be made rapidly. By injecting during inspiration some of the drug will be carried into the bronchi and the resulting cough will distribute the rest of the drug over the vocal cords and the epiglottis.

Occasionally it may be necessary to spray the pharynx by oropharyngeal spray to achieve complete analgesia. For the combination of the injection and spray, it should rarely be necessary to utilize more than 5 ml (200 mg of lidocaine HCl), (*i.e.*, 3 mg/kg or 1.5 mg/lb body weight).

Topical Application: For laryngoscopy, bronchoscopy and endotracheal intubation, the pharynx may be sprayed with 1-5 ml (40-200 mg of lidocaine HCl) (*i.e.*, 0.6-3 mg/kg or 0.3-1.5 mg/lb body weight).

Maximum Recommended Dosages

Normal Healthy Adults: The maximum recommended dose of lidocaine HCl should be such that the dose of lidocaine HCl is kept below 300 mg and in any case should not exceed 4.5 mg/kg (2 mg/lb) body weight.

Children: It is difficult to recommend a maximum dose of any drug for children, since this varies as a function of age and weight. For children of less than 10 years of age who have a normal lean body mass and normal body development, the maximum dose may be determined by the application of one of the standard pediatric drug formulas (*e.g.*, Clark's rule). For example, in a child of 5 years weighing 50 lb, the dose of lidocaine HCl should not exceed 75-100 mg when calculated according to Clark's rule. In any case, the maximum dose of lidocaine HCl with epinehprine should not exceed 7 mg/kg (3.2 mg/lb) of body weight. When used without epinephrine, the amount of lidocaine HCl is kept below 300 mg and in any case should not exceed 4.5 mg/kg (2.0 mg/lb) of body weight.

NOTE: Parenteral drug products should be inspected visually for particulate matter and discoloration prior to administration whenever the solution and container permit. Solutions that are discolored and/or contain particulate matter should not be used.

ADDITIONAL INFORMATION FOR LIDOCAINE HCl TOPICAL SOLUTION

Topical Application: For laryngoscopy, bronchoscopy, and endotracheal intubation, the pharynx may be sprayed with 1-5 ml (40-200 mg lidocaine HCl), (*i.e.*, 0.6-3 mg/kg or 0.3-1.5 mg/lb body wieght). For local anesthesia by the transtracheal route, it may be occasionally necessary to spray the pharynx by oropharyngeal spray to achieve complete analgesia.

Maximum Recommended Dosages

Normal Healthy Adults: The maximum recommended dose of lidocaine HCl should be such that the dose of lidocaine HCl is kept below 300 mg and in any case should not exceed 4.5 mg/kg (2 mg/lb) body weight.

Children: It is difficult to recommend a maximum dose of any drug for children, since this varies as a function of age and weight. For children of less than 10 years of age who have a normal lean body mass and normal body development, the maximum dose may be determined by the application of one of the standard pediatric drug formulas (*e.g.*, Clark's rule). For example, in a child of 5 years weighing 50 lb, the dose of lidocaine HCl should not exceed 75-100 mg when calculated according to Clark's rule. The amount of lidocaine HCl topical solution administered should be such that the dose of lidocaine HCl is kept below 300 mg and in any case should not exceed 4.5 mg/kg (2.0 mg/lb) of body weight.

ADDITIONAL INFORMATION FOR LIDOCAINE HCl JELLY

For Surface Anesthesia of the Male Adult Urethra

The outer orifice is washed and disinfected. The plastic tip is introduced into the orifice, where it is firmly held in position. The jelly is instilled by an easy syringe-like action, until the patient has a feeling of tension or until about 15 ml (*i.e.*, 300 mg of lidocaine HCl) is instilled. A penile clamp is then applied for several minutes at the corona and then additional jelly (about 15 ml) is instilled. To save time, the injection is performed against the resistance of the sphincter, possibly assisted by asking the patient to strain as for defecation or to press as in voiding. The jelly will then pass into the posterior urethra. Prior to sounding or cystoscopy, a penile clamp should be applied for 5-10 minutes to obtain adequate anesthesia. If the instrument is introduced immediately, a lubricant is unnecessary. Otherwise some jelly can be expressed from the vial and applied to the insturment tip. About 30 ml (*i.e.*, 600 mg) may be required to fill and dilate the male urethra. When it is desired to anesthetize only the anterior male urethra, as prior to catheterization, considerably smaller volumes, such as the contents from a 5 ml (*i.e.*, 100 mg) or 10 ml (*i.e.*, 200 mg) size vial, are usually adequate for lubrication.

For Surface Anesthesia of the Female Adult Urethra

3-5 ml of the jelly is intilled slowly into the urethra by gently expressing the contents of the vial. If desired, some jelly may be deposited on a cotton swab and introduced into the urethra. In order to obtain adequate anesthesia, several minutes should be allowed prior to performing urological procedure.

Lubrication for Endotracheal Intubation

Apply a moderate amount of jelly to the external surface of the endotracheal tube shortly before use. Care should be taken to avoid introducing the product into the lumen of the tube. Do not use the jelly to lubricate endotracheal styletts. See WARNINGS, Additional Information for Lidocaine HCl Jelly and ADVERSE REACTIONS, Additional Information for Lidocaine HCl Jelly concerning rare reports of inner lumen occlusion. It is also recommended that use of endotracheal tubes with dried jelly on the external surface be avoided for lack of lubricating effect.

Maximum Dosage

No more than 600 mg of lidocaine HCl should be given in any 12 hour period.

Children

It is difficult to recommend a maximum dose of any drug for children, since this varies as a function of age and weight. For children of less than 10 years of age who have a normal lean body mass and normal body development, the maximum dose may be determined by the application of one of the standard pediatric drug formulas (*e.g.*, Clark's rule). For example, in a child of 5 years weighing 50 lb, the dose of lidocaine HCl should not exceed 75-100 mg when calculated according to Clark's rule. The amount of lidocaine HCl administered should not exceed 4.5 mg/kg (2.0 mg/lb) of body weight.

PRODUCT LISTING - RATED THERAPEUTICALLY EQUIVALENT

Size	Price	Product	NDC
Solution - Injectable - 0.5%			
50 ml	$3.98	XYLOCAINE HCL, Allscripts Pharmaceutical Company	54569-3917-00
50 ml	$12.96	XYLOCAINE HCL, Physicians Total Care	54868-3392-00
50 ml	$25.05	XYLOCAINE HCL, Astra-Zeneca Pharmaceuticals	00186-0135-01
50 ml	$62.05	XYLOCAINE-MPF, Astra-Zeneca Pharmaceuticals	00186-0137-01
50 ml x 25	$56.41	GENERIC, Abbott Pharmaceutical	00074-4275-01
50 ml x 25	$56.70	GENERIC, Abbott Pharmaceutical	00074-4278-01
Solution - Injectable - 1%			
2 ml x 10	$17.16	XYLOCAINE-MPF, Allscripts Pharmaceutical Company	54569-3399-00
2 ml x 10	$18.50	XYLOCAINE-MPF, Astra-Zeneca Pharmaceuticals	00186-0276-13
2 ml x 10	$19.50	XYLOCAINE-MPF, Astra-Zeneca Pharmaceuticals	00186-0210-03
2 ml x 10	$418.68	GENERIC, Abbott Pharmaceutical	00074-1986-01
2 ml x 25	$50.00	GENERIC, American Pharmaceutical Partners	63323-0201-02
2 ml x 50	$20.19	GENERIC, Abbott Pharmaceutical	00074-4713-32
2 ml x 100	$40.00	GENERIC, Abbott Pharmaceutical	00074-4713-01
5 ml	$0.65	GENERIC, Allscripts Pharmaceutical Company	54569-2356-01
5 ml x 10	$24.60	XYLOCAINE-MPF, Astra-Zeneca Pharmaceuticals	00186-0277-13
5 ml x 10	$26.40	XYLOCAINE-MPF, Astra-Zeneca Pharmaceuticals	00186-0230-03
5 ml x 10	$38.95	GENERIC, Abbott Pharmaceutical	00074-9137-05
5 ml x 10	$39.00	GENERIC, Abbott Pharmaceutical	00074-4924-15
5 ml x 10	$42.39	GENERIC, Abbott Pharmaceutical	00074-4904-34
5 ml x 10	$61.16	GENERIC, Abbott Pharmaceutical	00074-8026-01
5 ml x 10	$100.92	GENERIC, Abbott Pharmaceutical	00074-4904-01
5 ml x 10	$100.92	GENERIC, Abbott Pharmaceutical	00074-4924-01
5 ml x 10	$110.04	GENERIC, Abbott Pharmaceutical	00074-4904-23
5 ml x 10	$115.50	GENERIC, Abbott Pharmaceutical	00074-4904-15
5 ml x 25	$16.15	GENERIC, Allscripts Pharmaceutical Company	54569-2356-00
5 ml x 25	$17.52	GENERIC, Abbott Pharmaceutical	00074-4713-02
5 ml x 25	$44.50	GENERIC, Abbott Pharmaceutical	00074-2063-05
5 ml x 25	$286.20	GENERIC, Abbott Pharmaceutical	00074-4904-33
10 ml x 5	$11.30	XYLOCAINE HCL, Astra-Zeneca Pharmaceuticals	00186-0275-12
10 ml x 5	$27.55	XYLOCAINE-MPF, Astra-Zeneca Pharmaceuticals	00186-0278-12
10 ml x 5	$30.55	XYLOCAINE-MPF, Astra-Zeneca Pharmaceuticals	00186-0278-44
10 ml x 25	$40.75	GENERIC, American Pharmaceutical Partners	63323-0201-10
20 ml	$13.40	XYLOCAINE HCL, Astra-Zeneca Pharmaceuticals	00186-0110-01
20 ml	$49.70	GENERIC, Celltech Pharmacueticals Inc	00548-1078-00
20 ml	$57.80	GENERIC, Celltech Pharmacueticals Inc	00548-1080-00
20 ml x 5	$43.71	XYLOCAINE HCL, Astra-Zeneca Pharmaceuticals	00186-0278-54
20 ml x 10	$283.08	GENERIC, Abbott Pharmaceutical	00074-4786-01
20 ml x 25	$9.50	GENERIC, Abbott Pharmaceutical	00074-4276-01
30 ml	$0.60	GENERIC, Esi Lederle Generics	00641-2380-41
30 ml	$52.80	GENERIC, Celltech Pharmacueticals Inc	00548-1079-00
30 ml	$62.20	GENERIC, Celltech Pharmacueticals Inc	00548-1081-00
30 ml x 5	$48.70	XYLOCAINE-MPF, Astra-Zeneca Pharmaceuticals	00186-0112-01
30 ml x 5	$56.05	XYLOCAINE-MPF, Astra-Zeneca Pharmaceuticals	00186-0112-91
30 ml x 5	$57.15	XYLOCAINE-MPF, Astra-Zeneca Pharmaceuticals	00186-0255-02
30 ml x 25	$15.00	GENERIC, Esi Lederle Generics	00641-2380-45
30 ml x 25	$18.41	GENERIC, Abbott Pharmaceutical	00074-4279-02
30 ml x 25	$19.25	GENERIC, Baxter Pharmaceutical Products, Inc	10019-0017-56
30 ml x 25	$114.00	GENERIC, Abbott Pharmaceutical	00074-4270-01
50 ml	$2.05	GENERIC, Moore, H.L. Drug Exchange Inc	00839-5597-38
50 ml	$2.50	GENERIC, Roberts/Hauck Pharmaceutical Corporation	43797-0009-18
50 ml	$2.90	GENERIC, Mutual/United Research Laboratories	00677-0281-24
50 ml	$3.00	GENERIC, Ivax Corporation	00182-0565-67
50 ml	$3.25	GENERIC, Forest Pharmaceuticals	00456-0779-83
50 ml	$3.62	GENERIC, Hyrex Pharmaceuticals	00314-0679-50

Size	Price	Product	NDC
50 ml	$4.31	XYLOCAINE HCL, Allscripts Pharmaceutical Company	54569-1502-00
50 ml	$5.27	XYLOCAINE HCL, Physicians Total Care	54868-1795-00
50 ml	$6.60	GENERIC, Merz Pharmaceuticals	00259-0325-50
50 ml	$24.50	XYLOCAINE HCL, Astra-Zeneca Pharmaceuticals	00186-0145-01
50 ml x 25	$20.75	GENERIC, Esi Lederle Generics	00641-2390-45
50 ml x 25	$23.75	GENERIC, Abbott Pharmaceutical	00074-4276-02
50 ml x 25	$24.00	GENERIC, Baxter Pharmaceutical Products, Inc	10019-0017-57
50 ml x 25	$27.25	GENERIC, American Regent Laboratories Inc	00517-0625-25
50 ml x 25	$92.25	GENERIC, Steris Laboratories Inc	00402-0055-39

Solution - Injectable - 1.5%

Size	Price	Product	NDC
2 ml x 10	$115.90	XYLOCAINE HCL, Astra-Zeneca Pharmaceuticals	00186-0212-03
5 ml	$62.35	XYLOCAINE-MPF, Astra-Zeneca Pharmaceuticals	00186-0245-54
10 ml x 5	$35.70	XYLOCAINE-MPF, Astra-Zeneca Pharmaceuticals	00186-0244-44
20 ml x 5	$28.62	GENERIC, Abbott Pharmaceutical	00074-4056-01
20 ml x 25	$113.11	GENERIC, Abbott Pharmaceutical	00074-4776-01

Solution - Injectable - 2%

Size	Price	Product	NDC
2 ml x 10	$23.60	XYLOCAINE-MPF, Astra-Zeneca Pharmaceuticals	00186-0215-03
2 ml x 10	$26.71	XYLOCAINE-MPF, Astra-Zeneca Pharmaceuticals	00186-0241-13
2 ml x 25	$22.86	GENERIC, Abbott Pharmaceutical	00074-4282-01
2 ml x 25	$50.00	GENERIC, American Pharmaceutical Partners	63323-0202-02
5 ml x 10	$21.00	GENERIC, Abbott Pharmaceutical	00074-1323-05
5 ml x 10	$22.60	GENERIC, Abbott Pharmaceutical	00074-4903-34
5 ml x 10	$25.20	XYLOCAINE HCL, Astra-Zeneca Pharmaceuticals	00186-0611-01
5 ml x 10	$25.80	XYLOCAINE-MPF, Astra-Zeneca Pharmaceuticals	00186-0242-13
5 ml x 10	$31.30	GENERIC, International Medication Systems, Limited	00548-3390-00
5 ml x 10	$40.40	XYLOCAINE HCL, Astra-Zeneca Pharmaceuticals	00186-0232-03
5 ml x 10	$42.39	XYLOCAINE HCL, Physicians Total Care	54868-3894-00
5 ml x 10	$49.64	GENERIC, Abbott Pharmaceutical	00074-2066-05
5 ml x 10	$62.94	GENERIC, Abbott Pharmaceutical	00074-8027-01
5 ml x 10	$114.48	GENERIC, Abbott Pharmaceutical	00074-4903-23
5 ml x 10	$115.20	GENERIC, Abbott Pharmaceutical	00074-4903-15
5 ml x 10	$121.00	GENERIC, Abbott Pharmaceutical	00074-4923-15
5 ml x 25	$52.50	GENERIC, American Pharmaceutical Partners	63323-0208-05
10 ml x 5	$6.71	XYLOCAINE HCL, Physicians Total Care	54868-1798-01
10 ml x 5	$13.05	XYLOCAINE HCL, Astra-Zeneca Pharmaceuticals	00186-0243-12
10 ml x 5	$34.39	XYLOCAINE-MPF, Allscripts Pharmaceutical Company	54569-2724-00
10 ml x 5	$36.05	XYLOCAINE-MPF, Astra-Zeneca Pharmaceuticals	00186-0240-44
10 ml x 10	$59.02	GENERIC, Abbott Pharmaceutical	00074-2066-10
10 ml x 25	$28.20	GENERIC, Abbott Pharmaceutical	00074-4282-02
20 ml	$5.60	GENERIC, Morton Grove Pharmaceuticals Inc	60432-0464-20
20 ml	$15.15	XYLOCAINE HCL, Astra-Zeneca Pharmaceuticals	00186-0120-01
20 ml x 25	$9.75	GENERIC, Abbott Pharmaceutical	00074-4277-01
30 ml x 25	$16.00	GENERIC, Esi Lederle Generics	00641-2400-45
30 ml x 25	$19.75	GENERIC, Baxter Pharmaceutical Products, Inc	10019-0019-56
50 ml	$0.96	GENERIC, Esi Lederle Generics	00641-2410-41
50 ml	$2.21	GENERIC, Moore, H.L. Drug Exchange Inc	00839-5598-38
50 ml	$2.75	GENERIC, Roberts/Hauck Pharmaceutical Corporation	43797-0010-18
50 ml	$2.85	GENERIC, Major Pharmaceuticals Inc	00904-0865-50
50 ml	$3.00	GENERIC, Ivax Corporation	00182-0566-67
50 ml	$3.25	GENERIC, Forest Pharmaceuticals	00456-0782-83
50 ml	$3.62	GENERIC, Hyrex Pharmaceuticals	00314-0680-50
50 ml	$4.61	GENERIC, Watson/Schein Pharmaceuticals Inc	00364-6551-57
50 ml	$5.41	XYLOCAINE HCL, Allscripts Pharmaceutical Company	54569-1525-00
50 ml	$6.60	GENERIC, Merz Pharmaceuticals	00259-0326-50
50 ml	$25.19	XYLOCAINE HCL, Allscripts Pharmaceutical Company	54569-3922-00
50 ml x 5	$30.65	XYLOCAINE HCL, Astra-Zeneca Pharmaceuticals	00186-0155-01
50 ml x 25	$21.50	GENERIC, Esi Lederle Generics	00641-2410-45
50 ml x 25	$25.00	GENERIC, Baxter Pharmaceutical Products, Inc	10019-0019-57
50 ml x 25	$31.00	GENERIC, American Regent Laboratories Inc	00517-0626-25
50 ml x 25	$40.08	GENERIC, Abbott Pharmaceutical	00074-4277-02
50 ml x 25	$105.60	GENERIC, Abbott Pharmaceutical	00074-4903-01
50 ml x 25	$105.60	GENERIC, Abbott Pharmaceutical	00074-4923-01

Solution - Injectable - 4%

Size	Price	Product	NDC
5 ml x 10	$63.78	XYLOCAINE-MPF, Allscripts Pharmaceutical Company	54569-4491-00
5 ml x 10	$74.50	XYLOCAINE-MPF, Astra-Zeneca Pharmaceuticals	00186-0235-03
5 ml x 25	$57.59	GENERIC, Abbott Pharmaceutical	00074-4283-01
50 ml	$1.53	XYLOCAINE HCL, Allscripts Pharmaceutical Company	54569-3327-00

Solution - Injectable - 5%;0.2%

Size	Price	Product	NDC
16.72 ml	$19.21	GENERIC, B. Braun/Mcgaw Inc	00264-9592-10
500 ml x 10	$181.00	GENERIC, B. Braun/Mcgaw Inc	00264-5592-10

Solution - Injectable - 5%;0.4%

Size	Price	Product	NDC
250 ml x 12	$102.74	GENERIC, Abbott Pharmaceutical	00074-7931-32
250 ml x 24	$423.08	GENERIC, Baxter I.V. Systems Division	00338-0409-02
250 ml x 48	$481.90	GENERIC, B. Braun/Mcgaw Inc	00264-9594-20
500 ml x 12	$255.99	GENERIC, B. Braun/Mcgaw Inc	00264-9594-10
500 ml x 18	$409.32	GENERIC, Baxter I.V. Systems Division	00338-0409-03
500 ml x 24	$262.49	GENERIC, Abbott Pharmaceutical	00074-7931-24

Solution - Injectable - 5%;0.8%

Size	Price	Product	NDC
250 ml x 12	$129.25	GENERIC, Abbott Pharmaceutical	00074-7939-32
250 ml x 24	$166.23	GENERIC, Baxter I.V. Systems Division	00338-0411-02
250 ml x 48	$574.29	GENERIC, B. Braun/Mcgaw Inc	00264-9598-20
500 ml x 10	$239.00	GENERIC, B. Braun/Mcgaw Inc	00264-5598-10
500 ml x 12	$601.92	GENERIC, B. Braun/Mcgaw Inc	00264-9598-10
500 ml x 18	$167.74	GENERIC, Baxter I.V. Systems Division	00338-0411-03

Solution - Injectable - 7.5%;5%

Size	Price	Product	NDC
2 ml x 10	$105.58	XYLOCAINE HCL FOR SPINAL, Astra-Zeneca Pharmaceuticals	00186-0225-03
2 ml x 25	$67.50	GENERIC, Abbott Pharmaceutical	00074-4712-01

Solution - Injectable - 10%

Size	Price	Product	NDC
10 ml x 25	$262.50	GENERIC, Abbott Pharmaceutical	00074-6254-01

Solution - Injectable - 20%

Size	Price	Product	NDC
10 ml x 25	$144.50	GENERIC, Abbott Pharmaceutical	00074-6248-01
10 ml x 25	$239.00	GENERIC, Abbott Pharmaceutical	00074-6217-02

Solution - Oral - 2%

Size	Price	Product	NDC
100 ml	$2.78	FEDERAL UPPER LIMIT, H.C.F.A. F F P	99999-1639-01

PRODUCT LISTING - EQUIVALENTS NOT AVAILABLE

Solution - Injectable - 1%

Size	Price	Product	NDC
5 ml	$12.82	GENERIC, Allscripts Pharmaceutical Company	54569-3776-01
20 ml	$3.73	GENERIC, Prescript Pharmaceuticals	00247-0123-20
30 ml	$3.92	GENERIC, Prescript Pharmaceuticals	00247-0123-30
30 ml x 25	$25.75	GENERIC, Physicians Total Care	54868-2331-01
50 ml	$1.35	GENERIC, Vangard Labs	00615-0030-15
50 ml	$1.95	GENERIC, C.O. Truxton Inc	00463-1077-50
50 ml	$2.33	GENERIC, Interstate Drug Exchange Inc	00814-4365-48
50 ml	$2.95	GENERIC, Forest Pharmaceuticals	00785-9065-55
50 ml	$3.25	GENERIC, Physicians Total Care	54868-2331-00
50 ml	$3.43	GENERIC, Allscripts Pharmaceutical Company	54569-1415-01
50 ml	$3.56	GENERIC, Century Pharmaceuticals Inc	00436-0226-79
50 ml	$3.69	GENERIC, Allscripts Pharmaceutical Company	54569-2204-00
50 ml	$4.20	ANESTACAINE, Clint Pharmaceutical Inc	55553-0055-50
50 ml	$4.29	GENERIC, Prescript Pharmaceuticals	00247-0123-50
50 ml	$9.90	GENERIC, Legere Pharmaceuticals	25332-0026-50
50 ml x 25	$85.80	GENERIC, Allscripts Pharmaceutical Company	54569-1415-00
50's	$3.00	GENERIC, Merit Pharmaceuticals	30727-0387-90
125 ml	$30.00	GENERIC, Cmc-Consolidated Midland Corporation	00223-7936-05
750 ml	$29.25	GENERIC, Cmc-Consolidated Midland Corporation	00223-7933-30

Solution - Injectable - 2%

Size	Price	Product	NDC
5 ml	$13.66	GENERIC, Allscripts Pharmaceutical Company	54569-2354-00
5 ml x 25	$297.60	GENERIC, Abbott Pharmaceutical	00074-4903-33
50 ml	$1.41	GENERIC, Vangard Labs	00615-0031-15
50 ml	$1.80	GENERIC, Keene Pharmaceuticals Inc	00588-5957-95
50 ml	$1.95	GENERIC, C.O. Truxton Inc	00463-1078-50
50 ml	$2.00	GENERIC, Cmc-Consolidated Midland Corporation	00223-7952-00
50 ml	$2.02	GENERIC, Allscripts Pharmaceutical Company	54569-1524-00
50 ml	$2.40	GENERIC, Interstate Drug Exchange Inc	00814-4375-48
50 ml	$2.42	GENERIC, Pasadena Research Laboratories Inc	00418-1201-50
50 ml	$3.00	GENERIC, Dunhall Pharmaceuticals Inc	00217-8413-13
50 ml	$3.75	GENERIC, Primedics Laboratories	00684-0145-50
50 ml	$3.78	GENERIC, Physicians Total Care	54868-2064-00
50 ml	$4.20	ANESTACAINE, Clint Pharmaceutical Inc	55553-0056-50
50 ml	$6.50	GENERIC, Legere Pharmaceuticals	25332-0027-50
50 ml x 25	$31.73	GENERIC, Cmc-Consolidated Midland Corporation	00223-7935-30
50 ml x 25	$40.00	GENERIC, Cmc-Consolidated Midland Corporation	00223-7952-25
50 ml x 25	$50.50	GENERIC, Allscripts Pharmaceutical Company	54569-1524-01

L

Lincomycin Hydrochloride (001641)

Categories: Infection, bacterial; FDA Approved 1964 Dec; Pregnancy Category B
Drug Classes: Antibiotics, lincosamides
Brand Names: L-Mycin; **Lincocin**; Lincoject; Lincorex
Foreign Brand Availability: Albiotic (Germany); Biolincom (Indonesia); Cillimicina (Italy); Cillimycin (Bahrain; Cyprus; Egypt; Iran; Iraq; Jordan; Kuwait; Lebanon; Libya; Oman; Qatar; Republic-of-Yemen; Saudi-Arabia; Syria; United-Arab-Emirates); Frademicina (Argentina); Libiocid (Mexico); Linco ANB (Thailand); Lincobiotic (Indonesia); Lincocine (France); Lincofan (Peru); Lincomec (Indonesia); Lincomed (Bahrain; Cyprus; Egypt; Iran; Iraq; Jordan; Kuwait; Lebanon; Libya; Oman; Qatar; Republic-of-Yemen; Saudi-Arabia; Syria; United-Arab-Emirates); Lincono (Thailand); Lincophar (Indonesia); Lincoplus (Peru); Linmycin (Thailand); Lintropsin (Indonesia); Medoglycin (Hong-Kong); Princol (Mexico); Zumalin (Indonesia)
Cost of Therapy: $64.50 (Infection; Lincocin Injection; 300 mg/ml; 600 mg/day; 10 day supply)
$26.16 (Infection; Generic Injection; 300 mg/ml; 600 mg/day; 10 day supply)
HCFA JCODE(S): J2010 up to 300 mg IV

WARNING

Pseudomembranous colitis has been reported with nearly all antibacterial agents, including lincomycin, and may range in severity from mild to life-threatening. Therefore, it is important to consider this diagnosis in patients who present with diarrhea subsequent to the administration of antibacterial agents.

Because lincomycin therapy has been associated with severe colitis which may end fatally, it should be reserved for serious infections where less toxic antimicrobial agents are inappropriate, as described in INDICATIONS AND USAGE. It should not be used in patients with nonbacterial infections such as most upper respiratory tract infections. Treatment with antibacterial agents alters the normal flora of the colon and may permit overgrowth of clostridia. Studies indicate that a toxin produced by *Clostridium difficile* is one primary cause of "antibiotic-associated colitis".

After the diagnosis of pseudomembranous colitis has been established, therapeutic measures should be initiated. Mild cases of pseudomembranous colitis usually respond to drug discontinuation alone. In moderate to severe cases, consideration should be given to management with fluids and electrolytes, protein supplementation, and treatment with an antibacterial drug clinically effective against *C. difficile* colitis.

Diarrhea, colitis, and pseudomembranous colitis have been observed to begin up to several weeks following cessation of therapy with lincomycin.

L

DESCRIPTION

Lincocin capsules and sterile solution contain lincomycin hydrochloride which is the monohydrated salt of lincomycin, a substance produced by the growth of a member of the *lincolnensis* group of *Streptomyces lincolnensis* (Fam. *Streptomycetaceae*). The chemical name for lincomycin hydrochloride is Methyl 6,8-dideoxy-6-(1-methyl-trans-4-propyl-L-2-pyrolidinecarboxamido)-1-thio-D-erythro-α-D-galacto-octopyranoside monohydrochloride monohydrate. The molecular formula of lincomycin hydrochloride is $C_{18}H_{34}N_2O_6S{\cdot}HCl{\cdot}H_2O$ and the molecular weight is 461.01.

Lincomycin hydrochloride is a white or practically white, crystalline powder and is odorless or has a faint odor. Its solutions are acid and are dextrorotatory. Lincomycin hydrochloride is freely soluble in water; soluble in dimethylformamide and very slightly soluble in acetone.

Lincocin capsules contain the following inactive ingredients: FD&C blue no. 1, gelatin, lactose, magnesium stearate, talc and titanium dioxide.

CLINICAL PHARMACOLOGY

Lincomycin is rapidly absorbed after a 500 mg oral dose, reaching average peak serum levels of approximately 3 μg/ml in 2-4 hours. Following oral administration, therapeutic levels of lincomycin are maintained for 6-8 hours for most susceptible gram-positive organisms. Urinary recovery of drug in a 24 hour period ranges from 1.0-31% (mean: 4.0%) after a single oral dose of 500 mg of lincomycin. Tissue level studies indicate that bile is an important route of excretion. Significant levels have been demonstrated in the majority of body tissues. Although lincomycin appears to diffuse into cerebrospinal fluid (CSF), levels of lincomycin in the CSF appear inadequate for the treatment of meningitis.

Intramuscular administration of a single dose of 600 mg of lincomycin produces average peak serum levels of 11.6 μg/ml at 60 minutes and maintains therapeutic levels for 17-20 hours for most susceptible gram-positive organisms. Urinary excretion after this dose ranges from 1.8-24.8% (mean: 17.3%).

A 2 hour intravenous infusion of 600 mg of lincomycin achieves average peak serum levels of 15.9 μg/ml and yields therapeutic levels for 14 hours for most susceptible gram-positive organisms. Urinary excretion ranges from 4.9-30.3% (mean: 13.8%).

The biological half-life after oral, intramuscular or intravenous administration is 5.4 ± 1.0 hours. The serum half-life of lincomycin may be prolonged in patients with severe impairment of renal function compared to patients with normal renal function. In patients with abnormal hepatic function, serum half-life may be 2-fold longer than in patients with normal hepatic function. Hemodialysis and peritoneal dialysis are not effective in removing lincomycin from the serum.

MICROBIOLOGY

Lincomycin has been shown to be active against most strains of the following organisms **both *in vitro* and in clinical infections:** (see INDICATIONS AND USAGE).

Staphylococcus aureus (penicillinase- and non-penicillinase producing strains)
Streptococcus pneumoniae

The following *in vitro* data are available; **but their clinical significance is unknown.**

Lincomycin has been shown to be active *in vitro* against the following microorganisms; however, the safety and efficacy of lincomycin in treating clinical infections due to these organisms have not been established in adequate and well controlled trials.

Aerobic Gram-Positive Cocci:
Streptococcus pyogenes
Viridans group streptococci
Aerobic Gram-Positive Bacilli:
Corynebacterium diphtheriae
Anaerobic Gram-Positive Non-Sporeforming Bacilli:
Propionibacterium acnes
Anaerobic Gram-Positive Sporeforming Bacilli:
Clostridium tetani
Clostridium perfringens

This drug is not active against most strains of *Enterococcus faecalis* nor against *Neisseria gonorrhoeae, Neisseria meningitidis, Haemophilus influenzae* or other gram-negative organisms or yeasts.

Cross resistance has been demonstrated between clindamycin and lincomycin. Some cross resistance with erythromycin including a phenomenon known as dissociated cross resistance or macrolide effect has been reported.

Studies indicate that lincomycin does not share antigenicity with penicillin compounds.

INDICATIONS AND USAGE

Lincomycin HCl capsules and sterile solution are indicated in the treatment of serious infections due to susceptible strains of streptococci, pneumococci, and staphylococci. Its use should be reserved for penicillin-allergic patients or other patients for whom, in the judgment of the physician, a penicillin is inappropriate. Because of the risk of antibiotic-associated pseudomembranous colitis, as described in BOXED WARNING, before selecting lincomycin the physician should consider the nature of the infection and the suitability of less toxic alternatives (*e.g.*, erythromycin).

Bacteriologic studies should be performed to determine the causative organisms and their susceptibility to lincomycin.

Indicated surgical procedures should be performed in conjunction with antibiotic therapy.

Lincomycin has been demonstrated to be effective in the treatment of staphylococcal infections resistant to other antibiotics and susceptible to lincomycin. Staphylococcal strains resistant to lincomycin HCl have been recovered; culture and susceptibility studies should be done in conjunction with therapy with lincomycin HCl. In the case of macrolides, partial but not complete cross resistance may occur (see CLINICAL PHARMACOLOGY, Microbiology). The drug may be administered concomitantly with other antimicrobial agents when indicated.

Lincomycin is not indicated in the treatment of minor bacterial infections or viral infections.

CONTRAINDICATIONS

This drug is contraindicated in patients previously found to be hypersensitive to lincomycin or clindamycin.

WARNINGS

Pseudomembranous colitis has been reported with nearly all antibacterial agents, including lincomycin, and may range in severity from mild to life-threatening. Therefore, it is important to consider this diagnosis in patients who present with diarrhea subsequent to the administration of antibacterial agents.

Treatment with antibacterial agents alters the normal flora of the colon and may permit overgrowth of clostridia. Studies indicate that a toxin produced by *Clostridium difficile* is one primary cause of "antibiotic-associated colitis".

After the diagnosis of pseudomembranous colitis has been established, therapeutic measures should be initiated. Mild cases of pseudomembranous colitis usually respond to drug discontinuation alone. In moderate to severe cases, consideration should be given to management with fluids and electrolytes, protein supplementation, and treatment with an antibacterial drug clinically effective against *C. difficile* colitis.

Other causes of colitis should also be considered. A careful inquiry should be made concerning previous sensitivities to drugs and other allergens.

Lincomycin HCl sterile solution contains benzyl alcohol as a preservative. Benzyl alcohol has been associated with a fatal "Gasping Syndrome" in premature infants.

Usage in Meningitis: Although lincomycin appears to diffuse into cerebrospinal fluid, levels of lincomycin in the CSF may be inadequate for the treatment of meningitis.

SERIOUS ANAPHYLACTOID REACTIONS REQUIRE IMMEDIATE EMERGENCY TREATMENT WITH EPINEPHRINE. OXYGEN AND INTRAVENOUS CORTICOSTEROIDS SHOULD ALSO BE ADMINISTERED AS INDICATED. (See ADVERSE REACTIONS.)

PRECAUTIONS

GENERAL

Review of experience to date suggests that a subgroup of older patients with associated severe illness may tolerate diarrhea less well. When lincomycin HCl preparations are indicated in these patients, they should be carefully monitored for change in bowel frequency.

Lincomycin HCl should be prescribed with caution in individuals with a history of gastrointestinal disease, particularly colitis.

Lincomycin HCl should be used with caution in patients with a history of asthma or significant allergies.

Certain infections may require incision and drainage or other indicated surgical procedures in addition to antibiotic therapy.

The use of lincomycin HCl may result in overgrowth of nonsusceptible organisms—particularly yeasts. Should superinfections occur, appropriate measures should be taken as indicated by the clinical situation. When patients with pre-existing monilial infections require therapy with lincomycin HCl, concomitant antimonilial treatment should be given.

The serum half-life of lincomycin may be prolonged in patients with severe impairment of renal function compared to patients with normal renal function. In patients with abnormal hepatic function, serum half-life may be 2-fold longer than in patients with normal hepatic function.

Patients with severe impairment of renal function and/or abnormal hepatic function should be dosed with caution and serum lincomycin levels monitored during high-dose therapy. (See DOSAGE AND ADMINISTRATION.)

Lincomycin hydrochloride sterile solution should not be injected intravenously undiluted as a bolus, but should be infused over at least 60 minutes as directed in DOSAGE AND ADMINISTRATION.

LABORATORY TESTS

During prolonged therapy with lincomycin HCl, periodic liver and kidney function tests and blood counts should be performed.

CARCINOGENESIS, MUTAGENESIS, AND IMPAIRMENT OF FERTILITY

The carcinogenic potential of lincomycin has not been evaluated.

Lincomycin was not found to be mutagenic in the Ames *Salmonella* reversion assay or the V79 Chinese hamster lung cells at the HGPRT locus. It did not induce DNA strand breaks in V79 Chinese hamster lung cells as measured by alkaline elution or chromosomal abnormalities in cultured human lymphocytes. *In vivo,* lincomycin was negative in both the rat and mouse micronucleus assays and it did not induce sex-linked recessive lethal mutations in the offspring of male *Drosophila*. However lincomycin did cause unscheduled DNA syntheses in freshly isolated rat hepatocytes.

Impairment of fertility was not observed in male or female rats given oral 300 mg/kg doses of lincomycin (0.36 times the highest recommended human dose based on mg/m^2).

PREGNANCY CATEGORY C

Teratogenic Effects: There are no studies on the teratogenic potential of lincomycin in animals or adequate and well-controlled studies of pregnant women.

Nonteratogenic Effects: Reproduction studies have been performed in rats using oral doses of lincomycin up to 1000 mg/kg (1.2 times the maximum daily human dose based on mg/m^2) and have revealed no adverse effects on survival of offspring from birth to weaning.

NURSING MOTHERS

Lincomycin has been reported to appear in human milk in concentrations of 0.5-2.4 μg/ml. Because of the potential for serious adverse reactions in nursing infants from lincomycin HCl, a decision should be made whether to discontinue nursing, or to discontinue the drug, taking into account the importance of the drug to the mother.

PEDIATRIC USE

Lincomycin HCl sterile solution contains benzyl alcohol as a preservative. Benzyl alcohol has been associated with a fatal "Gasping Syndrome" in premature infants. Safety and effectiveness in pediatric patients below the age of 1 month have not been established. (See DOSAGE AND ADMINISTRATION.)

DRUG INTERACTIONS

Lincomycin has been shown to have neuromuscular blocking properties that may enhance the action of other neuromuscular blocking agents. Therefore, it should be used in caution in patients receiving such agents.

Kaolin-pectin mixtures have been shown to inhibit the absorption of orally administered lincomycin.

Antagonism between lincomycin and erythromycin *in vitro* has been demonstrated. Because of possible clinical significance, the two drugs should not be administered concurrently.

ADVERSE REACTIONS

The following reactions have been reported with the use of lincomycin:

Gastrointestinal: Glossitis, stomatitis, nausea, vomiting, antibiotic-associated diarrhea and colitis, and pruritus ani. Onset of pseudomembranous colitis symptoms may occur during or after antibiotic treatment (see WARNINGS).

Hematopoietic: Neutropenia, leukopenia, agranulocytosis and thrombocytopenic purpura have been reported. There have been rare reports of aplastic anemia and pancytopenia in which lincomycin HCl could not be ruled out as the causative agent.

Hypersensitivity Reactions: Hypersensitivity reactions such as angioneurotic edema, serum sickness and anaphylaxis have been reported. Rare instances of erythema multiforme, some resembling Stevens-Johnson syndrome, have been associated with lincomycin HCl preparations. If an allergic reaction to lincomycin HCl occurs, discontinue the drug. Serious acute hypersensitivity reactions may require treatment with epinephrine and other emergency measures, including oxygen, intravenous fluids, intravenous antihistamines, corticosteroids, pressor amines, and airway management, as clinically indicated.

Skin and Mucous Membranes: Skin rashes, urticaria and vaginitis and rare instances of exfoliative and vesiculobullous dermatitis have been reported.

Liver: Although no direct relationship of lincomycin HCl to liver dysfunction has been established, jaundice and abnormal liver function tests (particularly elevations of serum transaminase) have been observed.

Renal: Although no direct relationship of lincomycin to renal damage has been established, renal dysfunction as evidenced by azotemia, oliguria, and/or proteinuria has been observed in rare instances.

Cardiovascular: After too rapid intravenous administration, rare instances of cardiopulmonary arrest and hypotension have been reported. (See DOSAGE AND ADMINISTRATION.)

Special Senses: Tinnitus and vertigo have been reported occasionally.

Local Reactions: Patients have demonstrated excellent local tolerance to intramuscularly administered lincomycin HCl. Reports of pain following injection have been infrequent. Intravenous administration of lincomycin HCl in 250-500 ml of 5% dextrose injection or 0.9% sodium chloride injection produced no local irritation or phlebitis.

DOSAGE AND ADMINISTRATION

If significant diarrhea occurs during therapy, this antibiotic should be discontinued. (See BOXED WARNING.)

ORAL

Adults

Serious Infections: 500 mg 3 times per day (500 mg approximately every 8 hours). *More Severe Infections:* 500 mg or more 4 times per day (500 mg or more approximately every 6 hours).

Pediatric Patients Over 1 Month of Age

Serious Infections: 30 mg/kg/day (15 mg/lb/day) divided into 3 or 4 equal doses. *More Severe Infections:* 60 mg/kg/day (30 mg/lb/day) divided into 3 or 4 equal doses.

With β-hemolytic streptococcal infections, treatment should continue for at least 10 days to diminish the likelihood of subsequent rheumatic fever or glomerulonephritis.

Note: For optimal absorption it is recommended that nothing be given by mouth except water for a period of 1-2 hours before and after oral administration of lincomycin preparations.

INTRAMUSCULAR

Adults

Serious Infections: 600 mg (2 ml) intramuscularly every 24 hours. *More Severe Infections:* 600 mg (2 ml) intramuscularly every 12 hours or more often.

Pediatric Patients Over 1 Month of Age

Serious Infections: One intramuscular injection of 10 mg/kg (5 mg/lb) every 24 hours. *More Severe Infections:* One intramuscular injection of 10 mg/kg (5 mg/lb) every 12 hours or more often.

INTRAVENOUS

Adults

The intravenous dose will be determined by the severity of the infection. For serious infections doses of 600 mg of lincomycin (2 ml of lincomycin HCl) to 1 gram are given every 8-12 hours. **For more severe infections these doses may have to be increased. In life-threatening situations daily intravenous doses of as much as 8 g have been given. Intravenous doses are given on the basis of 1 g of lincomycin diluted in not less than 100 ml of appropriate solution (see Physical Compatibilities) and infused over a period of not less than 1 hour.** (See TABLE 1.)

TABLE 1

Dose	Vol. Diluent (ml)	Time (hours)
600 mg	100	1
1 g	100	1
2 g	200	2
3 g	300	3
4 g	400	4

These doses may be repeated as often as required to the limit of the maximum recommended daily dose of 8 g of lincomycin.

Pediatric Patients Over 1 Month of Age

10-20 mg/kg/day (5-10 mg/lb/day) depending on the severity of the infection may be infused in divided doses as described above for adults.

Note: Severe cardiopulmonary reactions have occurred when this drug has been given at greater than the recommended concentration and rate.

SUBCONJUNCTIVAL INJECTION

0.25 ml (75 mg) injected subconjunctivally will result in ocular fluid levels of antibiotic (lasting for at least 5 hours) with MICs sufficient for most susceptible pathogens.

PATIENTS WITH DIMINISHED RENAL FUNCTION

When therapy with lincomycin HCl is required in individuals with severe impairment of renal function, an appropriate dose is 25-30% of that recommended for patients with normally functioning kidneys.

PHYSICAL COMPATIBILITIES

Physically compatible for 24 hours at room temperature unless otherwise indicated.

Infusion Solutions

- 5% Dextrose injection
- 10% Dextrose injection
- 5% Dextrose and 0.9% sodium chloride injection
- 10% Dextrose and 0.9% sodium chloride injection
- Ringer's injection
- 1/6 M sodium lactate injection
- Travert 10%-electrolyte no. 1
- Dextran in saline 6% w/v

Vitamins in Infusion Solutions

- B-Complex
- B-Complex with ascorbic acid

Antibiotics in Infusion Solutions

- Penicillin G sodium (satisfactory for 4 hours)
- Cephalothin
- Tetracycline HCl
- Cephaloridine
- Colistimethate (satisfactory for 4 hours)
- Ampicillin

L

Methicillin
Chloramphenicol
Polymyxin B sulfate

Physically Incompatible With:

Novobiocin
Kanamycin

IT SHOULD BE EMPHASIZED THAT THE COMPATIBLE AND INCOMPATIBLE DETERMINATIONS ARE PHYSICAL OBSERVATIONS ONLY, NOT CHEMICAL DETERMINATIONS. ADEQUATE CLINICAL EVALUATION OF THE SAFETY AND EFFICACY OF THESE COMBINATIONS HAS NOT BEEN PERFORMED.

ANIMAL PHARMACOLOGY

In vivo experimental animal studies demonstrated the effectiveness of lincomycin HCl preparations in protecting animals infected with *Streptococcus viridans, β-hemolytic Streptococcus, Staphylococcus aureus, Diplococcus pneumoniae* and *Leptospira pomona.* It was ineffective in *Klebsiella, Pasteurella, Pseudomonas, Salmonella* and *Shigella* infections.

HOW SUPPLIED

LINCOCIN CAPSULES

500 mg (light blue and dark blue)

Capsules contain lincomycin hydrochloride equivalent to 500 mg of lincomycin.

Storage: Store at controlled room temperature 20-25°C (68-77°F).

LINCOCIN STERILE SOLUTION

Each ml of lincomycin HCl sterile solution contains lincomycin HCl equivalent to lincomycin 300 mg; also benzyl alcohol, 9.45 mg added as preservative.

Storage: Store at controlled room temperature 20-25°C (68-77°F).

PRODUCT LISTING - RATED THERAPEUTICALLY EQUIVALENT

Solution - Injectable - 300 mg/ml

2 ml	$9.30	LINCOCIN, Pharmacia and Upjohn	00009-0555-01
10 ml	$12.00	GENERIC, Bolan Pharmaceutical Inc	44437-0908-10
10 ml	$13.50	GENERIC, Interstate Drug Exchange Inc	00814-4415-40
10 ml	$19.88	GENERIC, General Injectables and Vaccines Inc	52584-0119-10
10 ml	$32.25	LINCOCIN, Allscripts Pharmaceutical Company	54569-1387-00
10 ml	$34.85	LINCOCIN, Pharmacia and Upjohn	00009-0555-02

L

PRODUCT LISTING - EQUIVALENTS NOT AVAILABLE

Solution - Injectable - 300 mg/ml

10 ml	$13.08	GENERIC, Moore, H.L. Drug Exchange Inc	00839-7688-30
10 ml	$14.40	BACTRAMYCIN, Clint Pharmaceutical Inc	55553-0908-10
10 ml x 25	$250.00	GENERIC, Raway Pharmacal Inc	00686-0908-10

Lindane *(001642)*

Categories: Lice, crab; Lice, head; Scabies; Pregnancy Category B; FDA Approved 1974 Dec
Drug Classes: Anti-infectives, topical; Dermatologics; Scabicides/pediculicides
Brand Names: Kwell
Foreign Brand Availability: Acaricida (Peru); Benhex Cream (New-Zealand); Bicide (Israel); Davesol (Ecuador); Delice (Taiwan); Delitex (Germany); GAB (India); Gambex (South-Africa); Herklin (Costa-Rica; Dominican-Republic; El-Salvador; Guatemala; Honduras; Nicaragua; Panama); Hexit (Canada); Jacutin (Germany); Lencid (Belgium); Linden Lotion (Korea); PMS Lindane (Canada); Quellada (Belgium; South-Africa); Quellada Cream (Australia); Quellada Creme Rinse (Australia); Quellada-H (Germany); Quellada Head Lice Treatment (Australia); Quellada Lotion (Australia); Sarconyl (Ecuador); Scabecid (France); Scabexyl (Costa-Rica; Dominican-Republic; El-Salvador; Guatemala; Honduras; Panama); Scabi (Taiwan); Scabisan (Mexico); Varsan (Japan)
Cost of Therapy: $2.30 (Head Lice; Generic Shampoo; 1%; 60 ml; 1 application; 1 day supply)
$2.10 (Head Lice; Generic Lotion; 1%; 60 ml; 1 application; 1 day supply)

DESCRIPTION

Lindane cream 1% is an ectoparasiticide and ovicide effective against Sarcoptes scabiei (scabies) and their ova. Inert ingredients: 99% in a pleasantly scented water dispersible cream containing stearic acid, glycerin, lanolin, 2-amino-2-methyl-1-propanol, perfume and purified water.

Lindane shampoo 1% is an ectoparasiticide and ovicide effective against Pediculosis capitis (head lice), Pediculosis pubis (crab lice) and their ova. In addition to the active ingredients, lindane, it contains trolamine lauryl sulfate, polysorbate 60, acetone and purified water to form a cosmetically pleasant shampoo.

Lindane is the highly purified gamma isomer of 1,2,3,4,5,6,hexachlorocyclohexane.

CLINICAL PHARMACOLOGY

Lindane exerts its parasiticidal action by being directly absorbed into the parasites and their ova. Feldmann and Maibach reported approximately 10% absorption of a lindane acetone solution applied to the forearm and left in place to 24 hours. Dale, *et al.,* reported a blood level of 290 ng/ml associated with convulsions following the accidental ingestion of a lindane containing product. Ginsburg found a mean peak blood level of 28 ng/ml 6 hours after total body application of lindane lotion to scabietic infants and children. The half-life was determined to be 18 hours.

Analysis of blood taken from subjects before and after the use of lindane shampoo showed a mean peak blood level of only 3 ng/ml which appeared at 6 hours and disappeared at 8 hours after the shampoo was applied.

INDICATIONS AND USAGE

LINDANE CREAM

Indicated for the treatment of patients infested with Sarcoptes scabiei (scabies).

LINDANE SHAMPOO

Indicated for the treatment of patients infested with Pediculus capitis (head lice), Pediculus pubis (crab lice) and their ova.

CONTRAINDICATIONS

Lindane cream is contraindicated for premature neonates because their skin may be more permeable than full term infants and their liver enzymes may not be sufficiently developed. It is also contraindicated for patients with known seizure disorders and for individuals with a known sensitivity to the product or any of its components.

WARNINGS

LINDANE PENETRATES HUMAN SKIN AND HAS THE POTENTIAL FOR CNS TOXICITY (SEE CLINICAL PHARMACOLOGY). LINDANE CREAM SHOULD BE USED ACCORDING TO RECOMMENDED DOSAGE (SEE DIRECTIONS FOR USE) ESPECIALLY ON INFANTS, PREGNANT WOMEN AND NURSING MOTHERS. ANIMAL STUDIES INDICATE THAT POTENTIAL TOXIC EFFECTS OF TOPICALLY APPLIED LINDANE ARE GREATER IN THE YOUNG. Seizures have been reported after excessive use or oral ingestion of lindane. No residual effects of Lindane treatment have been demonstrated, therefore, this product should not be used to ward off a possible infestation.

If accidental ingestion occurs prompt gastric lavage is indicated. Because oils may enhance absorption, saline rather than oily cathartics should be used. Central nervous excitation can be controlled by the administration of pentobarbital, phenobarbital or diazepam.

PRECAUTIONS

GENERAL

Care should be taken to avoid contact with the eyes. If such contact occurs, eyes should be immediately flushed with water. If irritation or sensitization occurs, the patient should be advised to consult a physician.

INFORMATION FOR THE PATIENT

Patients should be instructed on the proper use of the medication. Directions for Use should accompany the prescription.

LABORATORY TESTS

No laboratory tests are needed for the proper use of this medication.

CARCINOGENESIS

Although no studies have been conducted with Lindane cream or shampoo, numerous long term feeding studies have been conducted in mice and rats to evaluate the carcinogenic potential of the technical grade of hexachlorocyclohexane (BHC) as well as the alpha, beta, gamma lindane) and delta isomers. Both oral and topical applications have been evaluated. Nagasaki Goto and Hanada found varying amounts of benign and malignant hepatomas associated with BHC and the alpha, delta and epsilon isomers. None reported a carcinogenic potential for lindane. Tumors were found only in the animals which had received the alpha isomer. Weisse and Herbst also evaluated the carcinogenic potential of lindane in mice but could find no evidence of lindane in mice but could find no evidence of lindane carcinogenicity. The National Cancer Institute also found no evidence of carcinogenicity.

Thorpe and Walker compared beta BHC with lindane, dieldrin, DDT and hexobarbital in mice.

Despite the unusually high incidence of tumors in the control group, they concluded that 600 ppm of lindane was associated with a significant increase in the incidence of hepatoma and thus considered it a tumorigen.

Orr and Kashyap, et al evaluated the carcinogenic potential in mice of topically carcinogenic potential in mice of topically applied BHC. In neither study was there any evidence of a tumorigenic or carcinogenic potential associated with topical application of BHC.

Mutagenicity tests have been used as predictive information about the carcinogenicity of various chemical compounds. Numerous types of mutagenicity tests have been performed with lindane. The results of these tests do not indicate that lindane is mutagenic.

PREGNANCY, TERATOGENIC EFFECTS, PREGNANCY CATEGORY B

Reproduction, including multigeneration, studies have been performed in mice, rats, rabbits, pigs, and dogs at doses up to 10 times the human dose and have revealed no evidence of impaired fertility or harm to the fetus due to administered lindane. There are, however, no adequate and well controlled studies in pregnant women. Because animal reproduction studies are not always predictive of human response, the recommended dosage should not be exceeded on pregnant women. They should be treated no more than twice during a pregnancy.

NURSING MOTHERS

Lindane is secreted in human milk in low concentrations. Studies conducted in the United States as well as Europe and South America found levels of lindane in human milk ranging from 0 to 113 ppb, as the result of ingestion of foods which had been treated with lindane. There appeared to be no difference in concentrations between country and urban dwellers. Although the levels of lindane found in blood after topical application with Lindane cream and shampoo make it unlikely that amounts of lindane sufficient to cause serious adverse reactions will be excreted in the milk of nursing mothers who have used Lindane cream, if there is any concern, an alternate method of feeding may be used for 2 days.

PEDIATRIC USE

Refer to CONTRAINDICATIONS and WARNINGS.

DRUG INTERACTIONS

Oils may enhance absorption, therefore, simultaneous use of creams, ointments or oils should be avoided. If an oil-based hair dressing is used, it is recommended that the hair be shampooed, rinsed and dried before application of lindane shampoo.

ADVERSE REACTIONS

Lindane has been reported to cause central nervous stimulation ranging from dizziness to convulsions. Cases of convulsions have been reported in connection with Lindane cream therapy.

However, these incidents were almost always associated with accidental oral ingestion or misuse of the product. Eczematous eruptions due to irritation from this product have also been reported. Incidence of these adverse reactions is relatively infrequent, occurring in less than 1 in 100,000 patients.

DOSAGE AND ADMINISTRATION

CAUTION: USE ONLY AS DIRECTED. DO NOT EXCEED RECOMMENDED DOSAGE.

No residual effects of Lindane treatment have been demonstrated therefore, this product should not be used to ward off a possible infestation.

LINDANE CREAM

Pediculosis Capitis (head lice)

Kwell shampoo is the most convenient dosage form but the lotion and cream are also effective.

Apply a quantity sufficient to cover only the affected and adjacent hairy areas. The cream should be rubbed into scalp and hair and left in place for 12 hours following by thorough washing.

Retreatment is usually not necessary. Demonstrable living lice after 7 days may be evidence that retreatment is necessary.

Pediculosis Pubis (crab lice)

Apply a sufficient quantity only to cover thinly the hair and skin of the pubic area, and if infested, the thighs, trunk, and axillary regions. The material should be rubbed into the skin and hair, and left in place for 12 hours followed by a thorough washing.

Retreatment is usually not necessary. Demonstrable living lice after 7 days indicates that retreatment is necessary.

Sexual contacts should be treated simultaneously.

Scabies (Sarcoptes scabiei)

The cream should be applied to dry skin in a thin layer and rubbed in thoroughly. If crusted lesions are present, a warm bath preceding the medication is helpful. If a warm bath is used, allow the skin to dry and cool before applying the cream. Usually 1 oz is sufficient for an adult. A total body application should be made from the neck down. Scabies rarely affects the head of children or adults but may occur in infants.

The cream should be left on 8-12 hours and should then be removed by thorough washing. ONE APPLICATION IS USUALLY CURATIVE.

Many patients exhibit persistent pruritus after treatment; this is rarely a sign of treatment failure and is not an indication for retreatment, unless living mites can be demonstrated.

LINDANE LOTION

Pediculosis Capitis (head lice)

Kwell shampoo is the most convenient dosage form but the lotion and cream are also effective.

Apply a quantity sufficient to cover only the affected and adjacent hairy areas. The lotion should be rubbed into scalp and hair and left in place for 12 hours followed by thorough washing.

Retreatment is usually not necessary. Demonstrable living lice after 7 days may be evidence that retreatment is necessary.

Pediculosis Pubis (crab lice)

Apply a sufficient quantity only to cover thinly the hair and skin of the pubic area, and if infested, the thighs, trunk, and axillary regions. The material should be rubbed into the skin and hair and left in place for 12 hours followed by a thorough washing.

Retreatment is usually not necessary. Demonstrable living lice after 7 days indicates that retreatment is necessary.

Sexual contacts should be treated simultaneously.

Scabies (Sarcoptes scabiei)

The lotion should be applied to dry skin in a thin layer and rubbed in thoroughly. If crusted lesions are present, a warm bath preceding the medication is helpful. If a warm bath is used, allow the skin to dry and cool before applying the lotion. Usually 1 oz is sufficient for an adult. A total body application should be made from the neck down. Scabies rarely affects the head of children or adults but may occur in infants.

The lotion should be left on for 8-12 hours and should then be removed by through washing. ONE APPLICATION IS USUALLY CURATIVE.

Many patients exhibit persistent pruritus after treatment; this is rarely a sign of treatment failure and is not an indication for retreatment, unless living mites can be demonstrated.

HOW SUPPLIED

CREAM

Kwell Cream is supplied in 2 oz tubes and 16 oz jars.

LOTION

Kwell Lotion is supplied in bottles of 2 oz, 16 oz, and 1 gallon.

PRODUCT LISTING - RATED THERAPEUTICALLY EQUIVALENT

Size	Price	Manufacturer	NDC
Liquid - Topical - 1%			
60 ml	$6.95	GENERIC, Geneva Pharmaceuticals	00781-7160-02
480 ml	$81.29	GENERIC, Geneva Pharmaceuticals	00781-7160-16
Lotion - Topical - 1%			
59 ml	$15.45	GENERIC, Alpharma Uspd Makers Of Barre and Nmc	00472-0570-02
60 ml	$2.10	GENERIC, Stafford-Miller	55372-4670-00
60 ml	$3.35	GENERIC, Ivax Corporation	00182-1475-43
60 ml	$3.50	GENERIC, Aligen Independent Laboratories Inc	00405-3175-56
60 ml	$4.32	GENERIC, Moore, H.L. Drug Exchange Inc	00839-6571-64
60 ml	$5.95	GENERIC, Geneva Pharmaceuticals	00781-7150-02
60 ml	$6.99	GENERIC, Qualitest Products Inc	00603-1404-49
60 ml	$9.88	GENERIC, Physicians Total Care	54868-0188-02
60 ml	$14.95	GENERIC, Major Pharmaceuticals Inc	00904-0690-03
60 ml	$15.18	GENERIC, Allscripts Pharmaceutical Company	54569-1137-00
60 ml	$37.00	GENERIC, Morton Grove Pharmaceuticals Inc	60432-0546-60
480 ml	$14.68	GENERIC, Stafford-Miller	55372-4670-01
480 ml	$18.19	GENERIC, Aligen Independent Laboratories Inc	00405-3175-16
480 ml	$19.58	GENERIC, Ivax Corporation	00182-1475-40
480 ml	$24.10	GENERIC, Moore, H.L. Drug Exchange Inc	00839-6571-69
480 ml	$46.04	GENERIC, Physicians Total Care	54868-0188-00
480 ml	$71.69	GENERIC, Mutual/United Research Laboratories	00677-0808-33
480 ml	$89.99	GENERIC, Major Pharmaceuticals Inc	00904-0690-16
480 ml	$90.36	GENERIC, Morton Grove Pharmaceuticals Inc	60432-0546-16
480 ml	$90.65	GENERIC, Alpharma Uspd Makers Of Barre and Nmc	00472-0570-16
3840 ml	$97.92	GENERIC, Major Pharmaceuticals Inc	00904-0690-28
3840 ml	$543.90	GENERIC, Alpharma Uspd Makers Of Barre and Nmc	00472-0570-28
Shampoo - Topical - 1%			
60 ml	$2.29	GENERIC, Stafford-Miller	55372-4660-00
60 ml	$3.98	GENERIC, Interstate Drug Exchange Inc	00814-4417-74
60 ml	$4.00	GENERIC, Aligen Independent Laboratories Inc	00405-3200-56
60 ml	$4.05	GENERIC, Ivax Corporation	00182-1476-43
60 ml	$5.00	GENERIC, Moore, H.L. Drug Exchange Inc	00839-6572-64
60 ml	$6.50	GENERIC, Cmc-Consolidated Midland Corporation	00223-6562-02
60 ml	$6.60	GENERIC, Qualitest Products Inc	00603-1406-49
60 ml	$15.89	GENERIC, Major Pharmaceuticals Inc	00904-0692-03
60 ml	$16.12	GENERIC, Morton Grove Pharmaceuticals Inc	60432-0547-60
60 ml	$16.40	GENERIC, Alpharma Uspd Makers Of Barre and Nmc	00472-0572-02
100 ml	$2.95	GENERIC, Cmc-Consolidated Midland Corporation	00223-6562-01
100 ml	$125.00	GENERIC, Cmc-Consolidated Midland Corporation	00223-6562-03
480 ml	$15.60	GENERIC, Stafford-Miller	55372-4660-01
480 ml	$21.74	GENERIC, Interstate Drug Exchange Inc	00814-4417-82
480 ml	$22.08	GENERIC, Aligen Independent Laboratories Inc	00405-3200-16
480 ml	$22.30	GENERIC, Ivax Corporation	00182-1476-40
480 ml	$29.57	GENERIC, Moore, H.L. Drug Exchange Inc	00839-6572-69
480 ml	$37.90	GENERIC, Qualitest Products Inc	00603-1406-58
480 ml	$100.45	GENERIC, Major Pharmaceuticals Inc	00904-0692-16
480 ml	$102.44	GENERIC, Mutual/United Research Laboratories	00677-0809-33
480 ml	$102.44	GENERIC, Morton Grove Pharmaceuticals Inc	60432-0547-16
480 ml	$102.70	GENERIC, Alpharma Uspd Makers Of Barre and Nmc	00472-0572-16
3840 ml	$115.58	GENERIC, Major Pharmaceuticals Inc	00904-0692-28
3840 ml	$616.20	GENERIC, Alpharma Uspd Makers Of Barre and Nmc	00472-0572-28

PRODUCT LISTING - EQUIVALENTS NOT AVAILABLE

Size	Price	Manufacturer	NDC
Lotion - Topical - 1%			
30 ml	$5.48	GENERIC, Prescript Pharmaceuticals	00247-0151-30
60 ml	$7.61	GENERIC, Prescript Pharmaceuticals	00247-0151-60
60 ml	$10.63	GENERIC, Cardinal Pharmaceuticals	63874-0704-60
60 ml	$11.75	GENERIC, Pharma Pac	52959-1403-03
60 ml	$15.00	GENERIC, Southwood Pharmaceuticals Inc	58016-3039-01
100 ml	$16.50	GENERIC, Cmc-Consolidated Midland Corporation	00223-6546-02
100 ml	$105.00	GENERIC, Cmc-Consolidated Midland Corporation	00223-6546-03
480 ml	$17.00	GENERIC, Cmc-Consolidated Midland Corporation	00223-6546-16
3840 ml	$2.68	GENERIC, Cmc-Consolidated Midland Corporation	00223-6546-01
Shampoo - Topical - 1%			
30 ml	$5.74	GENERIC, Prescript Pharmaceuticals	00247-0152-30
60 ml	$2.61	GENERIC, Qualitest Products Inc	52446-0946-52
60 ml	$8.12	GENERIC, Prescript Pharmaceuticals	00247-0152-60
60 ml	$10.88	GENERIC, Cardinal Pharmaceuticals	63874-0705-60
60 ml	$12.56	GENERIC, Physicians Total Care	54868-0572-01
60 ml	$16.00	GENERIC, Southwood Pharmaceuticals Inc	58016-3041-01
60 ml	$16.12	GENERIC, Allscripts Pharmaceutical Company	54569-1138-00

60 ml	$16.32	GENERIC, Pharma Pac	52959-1404-03
480 ml	$22.50	GENERIC, Cmc-Consolidated Midland Corporation	00223-6562-16
480 ml	$52.77	GENERIC, Physicians Total Care	54868-0572-00

Linezolid *(003479)*

Categories: Infection, lower respiratory tract; Infection, skin and skin structures; Infection, vancomycin-resistant enterococcus; Pneumonia, community acquired; Pneumonia, nosocomial; FDA Approved 2000 Apr; Pregnancy Category C

Drug Classes: Antibiotics, oxalodinones

Foreign Brand Availability: Linox (India); Zyvox (Australia; Bahrain; Cyprus; Egypt; England; Hong-Kong; Iran; Iraq; Ireland; Israel; Jordan; Korea; Kuwait; Lebanon; Libya; New-Zealand; Oman; Qatar; Republic-of-Yemen; Saudi-Arabia; Singapore; Syria; United-Arab-Emirates); Zyvoxid (Colombia; France)

Cost of Therapy: $1192.70 (Infection; Zyvox; 600 mg; 2 tablets/day; 10 day supply)

DESCRIPTION

Zyvox IV injection, Zyvox tablets, and Zyvox for oral suspension contain linezolid, which is a synthetic antibacterial agent of the oxazolidinone class. The chemical name for linezolid is (S)-N-[[3-[3-Fluoro-4-(4-morpholinyl)phenyl]-2-oxo-5-oxazolidinyl]methyl]-acetamide.

The empirical formula is $C_{16}H_{20}FN_3O_4$. Its molecular weight is 337.35.

ZYVOX IV INJECTION

Zyvox IV injection is supplied as a ready-to-use sterile isotonic solution for intravenous infusion. Each ml contains 2 mg of linezolid. Inactive ingredients are sodium citrate, citric acid, and dextrose in an aqueous vehicle for intravenous administration. The sodium (Na^+) content is 0.38 mg/ml (5 mEq per 300 ml bag; 3.3 mEq per 200 ml bag; and 1.7 mEq per 100 ml bag).

ZYVOX TABLETS

Zyvox tablets for oral administration contain 400 or 600 mg linezolid as film-coated compressed tablets. Inactive ingredients are corn starch, microcrystalline cellulose, hydroxypropylcellulose, sodium starch glycolate, magnesium stearate, hydroxypropyl methylcellulose, polyethylene glycol, titanium dioxide, and carnauba wax. The sodium (Na^+) content is 1.95 mg per 400 mg tablet and 2.92 mg per 600 mg tablet (0.1 mEq per tablet, regardless of strength).

L

ZYVOX FOR ORAL SUSPENSION

Zyvox for oral suspension is supplied as an orange-flavored granule/powder for constitution into a suspension for oral administration. Following constitution, each 5 ml contains 100 mg of linezolid. Inactive ingredients are sucrose, citric acid, sodium citrate, microcrystalline cellulose and carboxymethylcellulose sodium, aspartame, xanthan gum, mannitol, sodium benzoate, colloidal silicon dioxide, sodium chloride, and flavors (see PRECAUTIONS,Information for the Patient). The sodium (Na^+) content is 8.52 mg per 5 ml (0.4 mEq per 5 ml).

CLINICAL PHARMACOLOGY

PHARMACOKINETICS

The mean pharmacokinetic parameters of linezolid after single and multiple oral and intravenous doses are summarized in TABLE 1A and TABLE 1B.

TABLE 1A *Mean (Standard Deviation) Pharmacokinetic Parameters of Linezolid*

Dose of Linezolid	C_{max} (μg/ml)	C_{min} (μg/ml)	T_{max} (h)
400 mg Tablet			
Single dose*	8.10 (1.83)	—	1.52 (1.01)
Every 12 hours	11.00 (4.37)	3.08 (2.25)	1.12 (0.47)
600 mg Tablet			
Single dose	12.70 (3.96)	—	1.28 (0.66)
Every 12 hours	21.20 (5.78)	6.15 (2.94)	1.03 (0.62)
600 mg IV Injection†			
Single dose	12.90 (1.60)	—	0.50 (0.10)
Every 12 hours	15.10 (2.52)	3.68 (2.36)	0.51 (0.03)
600 mg Oral Suspension			
Single dose	11.00 (2.76)	—	0.97 (0.88)

* Data dose-normalized from 375 mg.
† Data dose-normalized from 625 mg; IV dose was given as 0.5 hour infusions.
C_{max} = Maximum plasma concentration; C_{min} = Minimum plasma concentration; T_{max} = Time to C_{max}.

Absorption

Linezolid is rapidly and extensively absorbed after oral dosing. Maximum plasma concentrations are reached approximately 1-2 hours after dosing, and the absolute bioavailability is approximately 100%. Therefore, linezolid may be given orally or intravenously without dose adjustment.

Linezolid may be administered without regard to the timing of meals. The time to reach the maximum concentration is delayed from 1.5 to 2.2 hours and C_{max} is decreased by about 17% when high fat food is given with linezolid. However, the total exposure measured as AUC(0-∞) values is similar under both conditions.

Distribution

Animal and human pharmacokinetic studies have demonstrated that linezolid readily distributes to well-perfused tissues. The plasma protein binding of linezolid is approximately 31% and is concentration-independent. The volume of distribution of linezolid at steady-state averaged 40-50 liters in healthy adult volunteers.

Linezolid concentrations have been determined in various fluids from a limited number of subjects in Phase 1 volunteer studies following multiple dosing of linezolid. The ratio of linezolid in saliva relative to plasma was 1.2 to 1 and for sweat relative to plasma was 0.55 to 1.

TABLE 1B *Mean (Standard Deviation) Pharmacokinetic Parameters of Linezolid*

Dose of Linezolid	AUC* (μg·h/ml)	T½ (h)	CL (ml/min)
400 mg Tablet			
Single dose†	55.10 (25.00)	5.20 (1.50)	146 (67)
Every 12 hours	73.40 (33.50)	4.69 (1.70)	110 (49)
600 mg Tablet			
Single dose	91.40 (39.30)	4.26 (1.65)	127 (48)
Every 12 hours	138.00 (42.10)	5.40 (2.06)	80 (29)
600 mg IV Injection‡			
Single dose	80.20 (33.30)	4.40 (2.40)	138 (39)
Every 12 hours	89.70 (31.00)	4.80 (1.70)	123 (40)
600 mg Oral Suspension			
Single dose	80.80 (35.10)	4.60 (1.71)	141 (45)

* AUC for a single dose = AUC(0-∞); for multiple doses = AUC(0-τ).
† Data dose-normalized from 375 mg.
‡ Data dose-normalized from 625 mg; IV dose was given as 0.5 hour infusions.
AUC = Area under concentration-time curve; t½ = Elimination half-life; CL = Systemic clearance .

Metabolism

Linezolid is primarily metabolized by oxidation of the morpholine ring, which results in two inactive ring-opened carboxylic acid metabolites: the aminoethoxyacetic acid metabolite (A), and the hydroxyethyl glycine metabolite (B). Formation of metabolite B is mediated by a non-enzymatic chemical oxidation mechanism *in vitro*. Linezolid is not an inducer of cytochrome P450 (CYP) in rats, and it has been demonstrated from *in vitro* studies that linezolid is not detectably metabolized by human cytochrome P450 and it does not inhibit the activities of clinically significant human CYP isoforms (1A2, 2C9, 2C19, 2D6, 2E1, 3A4).

Excretion

Nonrenal clearance accounts for approximately 65% of the total clearance of linezolid. Under steady-state conditions, approximately 30% of the dose appears in the urine as linezolid, 40% as metabolite B, and 10% as metabolite A. The renal clearance of linezolid is low (average 40 ml/min) and suggests net tubular reabsorption. Virtually no linezolid appears in the feces, while approximately 6% of the dose appears in the feces as metabolite B, and 3% as metabolite A.

A small degree of nonlinearity in clearance was observed with increasing doses of linezolid, which appears to be due to lower renal and nonrenal clearance of linezolid at higher concentrations. However, the difference in clearance was small and was not reflected in the apparent elimination half-life.

SPECIAL POPULATIONS

Geriatric

The pharmacokinetics of linezolid are not significantly altered in elderly patients (65 years or older). Therefore, dose adjustment for geriatric patients is not necessary.

Pediatric

Currently, there are limited data on the pharmacokinetics of linezolid during multiple dosing in pediatric patients of all ages. No data have been collected in infants younger than 3 months of age.

Pharmacokinetic information indicates that pediatric patients dosed with 10 mg/kg IV have a similar C_{max} but a higher average clearance when corrected by body weight, and shorter apparent elimination half-life than adults receiving 625 mg of linezolid. Pediatric dosing regimens that provide a pharmacokinetic profile similar to adults have not been determined. Studies using doses higher than 10 mg/kg or dosing more frequently than every 12 hours have not been conducted in pediatric patients.

Gender

Females have a slightly lower volume of distribution of linezolid than males. Plasma concentrations are higher in females than in males, which is partly due to body weight differences. After a 600 mg dose, mean oral clearance is approximately 38% lower in females than in males. However, there are no significant gender differences in mean apparent elimination-rate constant or half-life. Thus, drug exposure in females is not expected to substantially increase beyond levels known to be well tolerated. Therefore, dose adjustment by gender does not appear to be necessary.

Renal Insufficiency

The pharmacokinetics of the parent drug, linezolid, are not altered in patients with any degree of renal insufficiency; however, the two primary metabolites of linezolid may accumulate in patients with renal insufficiency, with the amount of accumulation increasing with the severity of renal dysfunction (see TABLE 2). The clinical significance of accumulation of these two metabolites has not been determined in patients with severe renal insufficiency. Because similar plasma concentrations of linezolid are achieved regardless of renal function, no dose adjustment is recommended for patients with renal insufficiency. However, given the absence of information on the clinical significance of accumulation of the primary metabolites, use of linezolid in patients with renal insufficiency should be weighed against the potential risks of accumulation of these metabolites. Both linezolid and the two metabolites are eliminated by dialysis. No information is available on the effect of peritoneal dialysis on the pharmacokinetics of linezolid. Approximately 30% of a dose was eliminated in a 3 hour dialysis session beginning 3 hours after the dose of linezolid was administered; therefore, linezolid should be given after hemodialysis.

TABLE 2 *Mean (Standard Deviation) AUCs and Elimination Half-Lives of Linezolid and Metabolites A and B in Patients With Varying Degrees of Renal Insufficiency After a Single 600 mg Oral Dose of Linezolid*

Parameter	Healthy Subjects CLCR>80 ml/min	Renal Impairment Moderate 30<CLCR<80 ml/min	Severe 10<CLCR<30 ml/min	Hemodialysis-Dependent Off Dialysis*	On Dialysis
Linezolid					
AUC(0-∞) (μg·h/ml)	110 (22)	128 (53)	127 (66)	141 (45)	83 (23)
T½ (h)	6.4 (2.2)	6.1 (1.7)	7.1 (3.7)	8.4 (2.7)	7.0 (1.8)
Metabolite A					
AUC(0-48) (μg·h/ml)	7.6 (1.9)	11.7 (4.3)	56.5 (30.6)	185 (124)	68.8 (23.9)
T½ (hours)	6.3 (2.1)	6.6 (2.3)	9.0 (4.6)	NA	NA
Metabolite B					
AUC(0-48) (μg·h/ml)	30.5 (6.2)	51.1 (38.5)	203 (92)	467 (102)	239 (44)
T½ (h)	6.6 (2.7)	9.9 (7.4)	11.0 (3.9)	NA	NA

* Between hemodialysis sessions
NA = Not applicable

Hepatic Insufficiency

The pharmacokinetics of linezolid are not altered in patients (n=7) with mild-to-moderate hepatic insufficiency (Child-Pugh class A or B). On the basis of the available information, no dose adjustment is recommended for patients with mild-to-moderate hepatic insufficiency. The pharmacokinetics of linezolid in patients with severe hepatic insufficiency have not been evaluated.

DRUG-DRUG INTERACTIONS

Drugs Metabolized by Cytochrome P450

Linezolid is not an inducer of cytochrome P450 (CYP) in rats. It is not detectably metabolized by human cytochrome P450 and it does not inhibit the activities of clinically significant human CYP isoforms (1A2, 2C9, 2C19, 2D6, 2E1, 3A4). Therefore, no CYP450-induced drug interactions are expected with linezolid. Concurrent administration of linezolid does not substantially alter the pharmacokinetic characteristics of (S)-warfarin, which is extensively metabolized by CYP2C9. Drugs such as warfarin and phenytoin, which are CYP2C9 substrates, may be given with linezolid without changes in dosage regimen.

Antibiotics

Aztreonam: The pharmacokinetics of linezolid or aztreonam are not altered when administered together.

Gentamicin: The pharmacokinetics of linezolid or gentamicin are not altered when administered together.

Monoamine Oxidase Inhibition

Linezolid is a reversible, nonselective inhibitor of monoamine oxidase. Therefore, linezolid has the potential for interaction with adrenergic and serotonergic agents.

Adrenergic Agents

A significant pressor response has been observed in normal adult subjects receiving linezolid and tyramine doses of more than 100 mg. Therefore, patients receiving linezolid need to avoid consuming large amounts of foods or beverages with high tyramine content (see PRECAUTIONS, Information for the Patient).

A reversible enhancement of the pressor response of either pseudoephedrine HCl (PSE) or phenylpropanolamine HCl (PPA) is observed when linezolid is administered to healthy normotensive subjects (see DRUG INTERACTIONS). A similar study has not been conducted in hypertensive patients. The interaction studies conducted in normotensive subjects evaluated the blood pressure and heart rate effects of placebo, PPA or PSE alone, linezolid alone, and the combination of steady-state linezolid (600 mg q12h for 3 days) with 2 doses of PPA (25 mg) or PSE (60 mg) given 4 hours apart. Heart rate was not affected by any of the treatments. Blood pressure was increased with both combination treatments. Maximum blood pressure levels were seen 2-3 hours after the second dose of PPA or PSE, and returned to baseline 2-3 hours after peak. The results of the PPA study follow, showing the mean (and range) maximum systolic blood pressure in mm Hg: placebo = 121 (103-158); linezolid alone = 120 (107-135); PPA alone = 125 (106-139); PPA with linezolid = 147 (129-176). The results from the PSE study were similar to those in the PPA study. The mean maximum increase in systolic blood pressure over baseline was 32 mm Hg (range: 20-52 mm Hg) and 38 mm Hg (range: 18-79 mm Hg) during co-administration of linezolid with pseudoephedrine or phenylpropanolamine, respectively.

Serotonergic Agents

The potential drug-drug interaction with dextromethorphan was studied in healthy volunteers. Subjects were administered dextromethorphan (two 20 mg doses given 4 hours apart) with or without linezolid. No serotonin syndrome effects (confusion, delirium, restlessness, tremors, blushing, diaphoresis, hyperpyrexia) have been observed in normal subjects receiving linezolid and dextromethorphan. The effects of other serotonin re-uptake inhibitors have not been studied.

MICROBIOLOGY

Linezolid is a synthetic antibacterial agent of a new class of antibiotics, the oxazolidinones, which has clinical utility in the treatment of infections caused by aerobic gram-positive bacteria. The *in vitro* spectrum of activity of linezolid also includes certain gram-negative bacteria and anaerobic bacteria. Linezolid inhibits bacterial protein synthesis through a mechanism of action different from that of other antibacterial agents; therefore, cross-resistance between linezolid and other classes of antibiotics is unlikely. Linezolid binds to a site on the bacterial 23S ribosomal RNA of the 50S subunit and prevents the formation of a functional 70S initiation complex, which is an essential component of the bacterial translation process. The results of time-kill studies have shown linezolid to be bacteriostatic against enterococci and staphylococci. For streptococci, linezolid was found to be bactericidal for the majority of strains.

In clinical trials, resistance to linezolid developed in 6 patients infected with *E. faecium* (4 patients received 200 mg q12h, lower than the recommended dose, and 2 patients received 600 mg q12h). In a compassionate use program, resistance to linezolid developed in 8 patients with *E. faecium* and in 1 patient with *E. faecalis.* All patients had either unremoved prosthetic devices or undrained abscesses. Resistance to linezolid occurs *in vitro* at a frequency of 1×10^{-9} to 1×10^{-11}. *In vitro* studies have shown that point mutations in the 23S rRNA are associated with linezolid resistance. Resistance to linezolid has not been seen in clinical trials in patients infected with *Staphylococcus* spp. or *Streptococcus* spp., including *S. pneumoniae.*

In vitro studies have demonstrated additivity or indifference between linezolid and vancomycin, gentamicin, rifampin, imipenem-cilastatin, aztreonam, ampicillin, or streptomycin.

Linezolid has been shown to be active against most isolates of the following microorganisms, both *in vitro* and in clinical infections, as described in INDICATIONS AND USAGE.

Aerobic and Facultative Gram-Positive Microorganisms:

Enterococcus faecium (vancomycin-resistant strains only).
Staphylococcus aureus (including methicillin-resistant strains).
Streptococcus agalactiae.
Streptococcus pneumoniae (penicillin-susceptible strains only).
Streptococcus pyogenes.

The following *in vitro* data are available, but their clinical significance is unknown. At least 90% of the following microorganisms exhibit an *in vitro* minimum inhibitory concentration (MIC) less than or equal to the susceptible breakpoint for linezolid. However, the safety and effectiveness of linezolid in treating clinical infections due to these microorganisms have not been established in adequate and well-controlled clinical trials.

Aerobic and Facultative Gram-Positive Microorganisms:

Enterococcus faecalis (including vancomycin-resistant strains).
Enterococcus faecium (vancomycin-susceptible strains).
Staphylococcus epidermidis (including methicillin-resistant strains).
Staphylococcus haemolyticus.
Streptococcus pneumoniae (penicillin-resistant strains).
Viridans group streptococci.

Aerobic and Facultative Gram-Negative Microorganisms:

Pasteurella multocida.

Susceptibility Testing Methods

Note: Susceptibility testing by dilution methods requires the use of linezolid susceptibility powder.

When available, the results of *in vitro* susceptibility tests should be provided to the physician as periodic reports which describe the susceptibility profile of nosocomial and community-acquired pathogens. These reports should aid the physician in selecting the most effective antimicrobial.

Dilution Techniques

Quantitative methods are used to determine antimicrobial minimum inhibitory concentrations (MICs). These MICs provide estimates of the susceptibility of bacteria to antimicrobial compounds. The MICs should be determined using a standardized procedure. Standardized procedures are based on a dilution method[1,3] (broth or agar) or equivalent with standardized inoculum concentrations and standardized concentrations of linezolid powder. The MIC values should be interpreted according to criteria provided in TABLE 3.

Diffusion Techniques

Quantitative methods that require measurement of zone diameters also provide reproducible estimates of the susceptibility of bacteria to antimicrobial compounds. One such standardized procedure[2,3] requires the use of standardized inoculum concentrations. This procedure uses paper disks impregnated with 30 μg of linezolid to test the susceptibility of microorganisms to linezolid. The disk diffusion interpretive criteria are provided in TABLE 3.

A report of "Susceptible" indicates that the pathogen is likely to be inhibited if the antimicrobial compound in the blood reaches the concentrations usually achievable. A report of "Intermediate" indicates that the result should be considered equivocal, and, if the microorganism is not fully susceptible to alternative, clinically feasible drugs, the test should be repeated. This category implies possible clinical applicability in body sites where the drug is physiologically concentrated or in situations where high dosage of drug can be used. This category also provides a buffer zone which prevents small uncontrolled technical factors from causing major discrepancies in interpretation. A report of "Resistant" indicates that the pathogen is not likely to be inhibited if the antimicrobial compound in the blood reaches the concentrations usually achievable; other therapy should be selected.

Quality Control

Standardized susceptibility test procedures require the use of quality control microorganisms to control the technical aspects of the test procedures. Standard linezolid powder should provide the following range of values noted in TABLE 4. **Note:** Quality control microorganisms are specific strains of organisms with intrinsic biological properties relating to resistance mechanisms and their genetic expression within bacteria; the specific strains used for microbiological quality control are not clinically significant.

INDICATIONS AND USAGE

Linezolid formulations are indicated for the treatment of adult patients with the following infections caused by susceptible strains of the designated microorganisms (see DOSAGE AND ADMINISTRATION).

TABLE 3 *Susceptibility Interpretive Criteria for Linezolid*

	Susceptibility Interpretive Criteria					
	Minimal Inhibitory Concentrations (MIC in µg/ml)			Disk Diffusion (Zone Diameter in mm)		
Pathogen	S	I	R	S	I	R
Enterococcus spp.	≤2	4	≥8	≥23	21-22	≤20
Staphylococcus spp.*	≤4	—	—	≥21	—	—
*Streptococcus pneumoniae**	≤2†	—	—	≥21‡	—	—
Streptococcus spp. other than *S pneumoniae**	≤2†	—	—	≥21‡	—	—

* The current absence of data on resistant strains precludes defining any categories other than "Susceptible". Strains yielding test results suggestive of a "nonsusceptible" category should be retested, and if the result is confirmed, the isolate should be submitted to a reference laboratory for further testing.

† These interpretive standards for *S. pneumoniae* and *Streptococcus* spp. other than *S. pneumoniae* are applicable only to tests performed by broth microdilution using cation-adjusted Mueller-Hinton broth with 2-5% lysed horse blood inoculated with a direct colony suspension and incubated in ambient air at 35°C for 20-24 hours.

‡ These zone diameter interpretive standards are applicable only to tests performed using Mueller-Hinton agar supplemented with 5% defibrinated sheep blood inoculated with a direct colony suspension and incubated in 5% CO_2 at 35°C for 20-24 hours.

TABLE 4 *Acceptable Quality Control Ranges for Linezolid to be Used in Validation of Susceptibility Test Results*

	Acceptable Quality Control Ranges	
QC Strain	Minimum Inhibitory Concentration (MIC in µg/ml)	Disk Diffusion (Zone Diameters in mm)
Enterococcus faecalis ATCC 29212	1-4	Not applicable
Staphylococcus aureus ATCC 29213	1-4	Not applicable
Staphylococcus aureus ATCC 25923	Not applicable	27-31
Streptococcus pneumoniae ATCC 49619*	0.50-2†	28-34‡

* This organism may be used for validation of susceptibility test results when testing *Streptococcus* spp. other than *S. pneumoniae*.

† This quality control range for *S. pneumoniae* is applicable only to tests performed by broth microdilution using cation-adjusted Mueller-Hinton broth with 2-5% lysed horse blood inoculated with a direct colony suspension and incubated in ambient air at 35°C for 20-24 hours.

‡ This quality control zone diameter range is applicable only to tests performed using Mueller-Hinton agar supplemented with 5% defibrinated sheep blood inoculated with a direct colony suspension and incubated in 5% CO_2 at 35°C for 20-24 hours.

Vancomycin-Resistant *Enterococcus faecium* infections, including cases with concurrent bacteremia.

Nosocomial pneumonia caused by *Staphylococcus aureus* (methicillin-susceptible and -resistant strains), or *Streptococcus pneumoniae* (penicillin-susceptible strains only). Combination therapy may be clinically indicated if the documented or presumptive pathogens include gram-negative organisms.

Complicated skin and skin structure infections caused by *Staphylococcus aureus* (methicillin-susceptible and -resistant strains), *Streptococcus pyogenes,* or *Streptococcus agalactiae.* Linezolid has not been studied in the treatment of diabetic foot and decubitus ulcers. Combination therapy may be clinically indicated if the documented or presumptive pathogens include gram-negative organisms.

Uncomplicated skin and skin structure infections caused by *Staphylococcus aureus* (methicillin-susceptible strains only) or *Streptococcus pyogenes.*

Community-acquired pneumonia caused by *Streptococcus pneumoniae* (penicillin-susceptible strains only), including cases with concurrent bacteremia, or *Staphylococcus aureus* (methicillin-susceptible strains only).

Due to concerns about inappropriate use of antibiotics leading to an increase in resistant organisms, prescribers should carefully consider alternatives before initiating treatment with linezolid in the outpatient setting.

Appropriate specimens for bacteriological examination should be obtained in order to isolate and identify the causative organisms and to determine their susceptibility to linezolid. Therapy may be instituted empirically while awaiting the results of these tests. Once these results become available, antimicrobial therapy should be adjusted accordingly.

CONTRAINDICATIONS

Linezolid formulations are contraindicated for use in patients who have known hypersensitivity to linezolid or any of the other product components.

WARNINGS

Myelosuppression (including anemia, leukopenia, pancytopenia, and thrombocytopenia) has been reported in patients receiving linezolid. In cases where the outcome is known, when linezolid was discontinued, the affected hematologic parameters have risen toward pretreatment levels. Complete blood counts should be monitored weekly in patients who receive linezolid, particularly in those who receive linezolid for longer than 2 weeks, those with pre-existing myelosuppression, those receiving concomitant drugs and produce bone marrow suppression, or those with a chronic infection who have received previous or concomitant antibiotic therapy. Discontinuation of therapy with linezolid should be considered in patients who develop or have worsening myelosuppression.

Pseudomembranous colitis has been reported with nearly all antibacterial agents, including linezolid, and may range in severity from mild to life-threatening. Therefore, it is important to consider this diagnosis in patients who present with diarrhea subsequent to the administration of any antibacterial agent.

Treatment with antibacterial agents alters the normal flora of the colon and may permit overgrowth of clostridia. Studies indicated that a toxin produced by *Clostridium difficile* is a primary cause of "antibiotic-associated colitis".

After the diagnosis of pseudomembranous colitis has been established, appropriate therapeutic measures should be initiated. Mild cases of pseudomembranous colitis usually respond to drug discontinuation alone. In moderate to severe cases, consideration should be given to management with fluids and electrolytes, protein supplementation, and treatment with an antibacterial agent clinically effective against *Clostridium difficile*.

PRECAUTIONS

GENERAL

The use of antibiotics may promote the overgrowth of nonsusceptible organisms. Should superinfection occur during therapy, appropriate measures should be taken.

Linezolid has not been studied in patients with uncontrolled hypertension, pheochromocytoma, carcinoid syndrome, or untreated hyperthyroidism.

The safety and efficacy of linezolid formulations given for longer than 28 days have not been evaluated in controlled clinical trials.

INFORMATION FOR THE PATIENT

Patients Should Be Advised That:

- Linezolid may be taken with or without food.
- They should inform their physician if they have a history of hypertension.
- Large quantities of foods or beverages with high tyramine content should be avoided while taking linezolid. Quantities of tyramine consumed should be less than 100 mg per meal. Foods high in tyramine content include those that may have undergone protein changes by aging, fermentation, pickling, or smoking to improve flavor, such as aged cheeses (0-15 mg tyramine per ounce); fermented or air-dried meats (0.1-8 mg tyramine per ounce); sauerkraut (8 mg tyramine per 8 ounces); soy sauce (5 mg tyramine per 1 teaspoon); tap beers (4 mg tyramine per 12 ounces); red wines (0-6 mg tyramine per 8 ounces). The tyramine content of any protein-rich food may be increased if stored for long periods or improperly refrigerated.[4,5]
- They should inform their physician if taking medications containing pseudoephedrine HCl or phenylpropanolamine HCl, such as cold remedies and decongestants.
- They should inform their physician if taking serotonin re-uptake inhibitors or other antidepressants.
- *Phenylketonurics:* Each 5 ml of the 100 mg/5 ml Zyvox for oral suspension contains 20 mg phenylalanine. The other Zyvox formulations do not contain phenylalanine. Contact your physician or pharmacist.

DRUG/LABORATORY TEST INTERACTIONS

There are no reported drug-laboratory test interactions.

CARCINOGENESIS, MUTAGENESIS, AND IMPAIRMENT OF FERTILITY

Although lifetime studies in animals have not been conducted to evaluate the carcinogenic potential of linezolid, no mutagenic or clastogenic potential was found in a battery of tests, including the Ames and AS52 assays, an *in vitro* unscheduled DNA synthesis (UDS) assay, an *in vitro* chromosome aberration assay in human lymphocytes, and an *in vivo* mouse micronucleus assay.

Linezolid did not affect the fertility or reproductive performance of adult female rats. It reversibly decreased fertility and reproductive performance in adult male rats when given at doses ≥50 mg/kg/day, with exposures approximately equal to or greater than the expected human exposure level (exposure comparisons are based on AUCs). Epithelial cell hypertrophy in the epididymis may have contributed to the decreased fertility by affecting sperm maturation. Similar epididymal changes were not seen in dogs. Although the concentrations of sperm in the testes were in the normal range, the concentrations in the cauda epididymis were decreased, and sperm from the vas deferens had decreased motility.

Mildly decreased fertility occurred in juvenile male rats treated with linezolid through most of their period of sexual development (50 mg/kg/day from days 7-36 of age, and 100 mg/kg/day from days 37-55 of age, with exposures ranging from 0.4-fold to 1.2-fold that expected in humans based on AUCs). No histopathological evidence of adverse effects was observed in the male reproductive tract.

PREGNANCY, TERATOGENIC EFFECTS, PREGNANCY CATEGORY C

Linezolid was not teratogenic in mice or rats at exposure levels 4-fold (in mice) or equivalent to (in rats) the expected human exposure level, based on AUCs. However, embryo and fetal toxicities were seen (see Nonteratogenic Effects). There are no adequate and well-controlled studies in pregnant women. Linezolid should be used during pregnancy only if the potential benefit justifies the potential risk to the fetus.

NONTERATOGENIC EFFECTS

In mice, embryo and fetal toxicities were seen only at doses that caused maternal toxicity (clinical signs and reduced body weight gain). A dose of 450 mg/kg/day (4-fold the estimated human exposure level based on AUCs) correlated with increased postimplantational embryo death, including total litter loss, decreased fetal body weights, and an increased incidence of costal cartilage fusion.

In rats, mild fetal toxicity was observed at 15 and 50 mg/kg/day (exposure levels 0.13- to 0.64-fold the estimated human exposure, respectively based on AUCs). The effects consisted of decreased fetal body weights and reduced ossification of sternebrae, a finding often seen in association with decreased fetal body weights. Slight maternal toxicity, in the form of reduced body weight gain, was seen at 50 mg/kg/day.

When female rats were treated with 50 mg/kg/day (0.64-fold the estimated human exposure based on AUCs) of linezolid during pregnancy and lactation, survival of pups was decreased on postnatal days 1-4. Pups permitted to mature to reproductive age, when mated, showed an increase in preimplantation loss, with a corresponding decrease in fertility.

NURSING MOTHERS

Linezolid and its metabolites are excreted in the milk of lactating rats. Concentrations in milk were similar to those in maternal plasma. It is not known whether linezolid is excreted in human milk. Because many drugs are excreted in human milk, caution should be exercised when linezolid is administered to a nursing woman.

PEDIATRIC USE

Although it may be possible to extrapolate adult efficacy to pediatric patients, the appropriate dose and safety of linezolid have not been established in this population. Drug clearance of linezolid is increased in pediatric patients compared to adults, resulting in a shorter half-life (see CLINICAL PHARMACOLOGY, Pediatric). Pediatric dosing regimens that provide a pharmacokinetic profile similar to adults have not been determined.

GERIATRIC USE

Of the 2046 patients treated with linezolid in Phase 3 comparator-controlled clinical trials, 589 (29%) were 65 years or older and 253 (12%) were 75 years or older. No overall differences in safety or effectiveness were observed between these patients and younger patients.

DRUG INTERACTIONS

See also CLINICAL PHARMACOLOGY, Drug-Drug Interactions.

MONOAMINE OXIDASE INHIBITION

Linezolid is a reversible, nonselective inhibitor of monoamine oxidase. Therefore, linezolid has the potential for interaction with adrenergic and serotonergic agents.

Adrenergic Agents

Some individuals receiving linezolid may experience a reversible enhancement of the pressor response to indirect-acting sympathomimetic agents, vasopressor or dopaminergic agents. Commonly used drugs such as phenylpropanolamine and pseudoephedrine have been specifically studied. Initial doses of adrenergic agents, such as dopamine or epinephrine, should be reduced and titrated to achieve the desired response.

Serotonergic Agents

Co-administration of linezolid and serotonergic agents was not associated with serotonin syndrome in Phase 1, 2 or 3 studies. Since there is limited experience with concomitant administration of linezolid and serotonergic agents, physicians should be alert to the possibility of signs and symptoms of serotonin syndrome (*e.g.,* hyperpyrexia, and cognitive dysfunction) in patients receiving such concomitant therapy.

ADVERSE REACTIONS

The safety of linezolid formulations was evaluated in 2046 patients enrolled in seven Phase 3 comparator-controlled clinical trials, who were treated for up to 28 days. In these studies, 85% of the adverse events reported with linezolid were described as mild to moderate in intensity. TABLE 8 shows the incidence of adverse events reported in at least 2% of patients in these trials. The most common adverse events in patients treated with linezolid were diarrhea (incidence across studies: 2.8-11.0%), headache (incidence across studies: 0.5-11.3%), and nausea (incidence across studies: 3.4-9.6%).

TABLE 8 *Incidence (%) of Adverse Events Reported in ≥2% of Patients in Comparator-Controlled Clinical Trials With Linezolid*

Event	Linezolid (n=2046)	All Comparators* (n=2001)
Diarrhea	8.3	6.3
Headache	6.5	5.5
Nausea	6.2	4.6
Vomiting	3.7	2.0
Insomnia	2.5	1.7
Constipation	2.2	2.1
Rash	2.0	2.2
Dizziness	2.0	1.9
Fever	1.6	2.1

* Comparators included cefpodoxime proxetil 200 mg PO q12h; ceftriaxone 1 g IV q12h; clarithromycin 250 mg PO q12h; dicloxacillin 500 mg PO q6h; oxacillin 2 g IV q6h; vancomycin 1 g IV q12h.

Other adverse events reported in Phase 2 and Phase 3 studies included oral moniliasis, vaginal moniliasis, hypertension, dyspepsia, localized abdominal pain, pruritus, and tongue discoloration.

TABLE 9 shows the incidence of drug-related adverse events reported in at least 1% of patients in these trials by dose of linezolid.

LABORATORY CHANGES

Linezolid has been associated with thrombocytopenia when used in doses up to and including 600 mg every 12 hours for up to 28 days. In Phase 3 comparator-controlled trials, the percentage of patients who developed a substantially low platelet count (defined as less than 75% of lower limit of normal and/or baseline) was 2.4% (range among studies: 0.3-10.0%) with linezolid and 1.5% (range among studies: 0.4-7.0%) with a comparator. Thrombocytopenia associated with the use of linezolid appears to be dependent on duration of therapy, (generally greater than 2 weeks of treatment). The platelet counts for most patients returned to the normal range/baseline during the follow-up period. No related clinical adverse events

TABLE 9 *Incidence of Drug-Related Adverse Events Occurring in >1% of Patients Treated With Linezolid in Comparator-Controlled Clinical Trials*

	Uncomplicated Skin and Skin Structure Infection		All Other Indications	
	Linezolid	Clarithromycin	Linezolid	All Other
	400 mg PO q12h	250 mg PO q12h	600 mg PO q12h	Comparators*
Adverse Event	(n=548)	(n=537)	(n=1498)	(n=1464)
% of patients with 1 drug-related adverse event	25.4%	19.6%	20.4%	14.3%
% of patients discontinuing due to drug-related adverse events†	3.5%	2.4%	2.1%	1.7%
Diarrhea	5.3%	4.8%	4.0%	2.7%
Nausea	3.5%	3.5%	3.3%	1.8%
Headache	2.7%	2.2%	1.9%	1.0%
Taste aleration	1.8%	2.0%	0.9%	0.2%
Vaginal moniliasis	1.6%	1.3%	1.0%	0.4%
Fungal infection	1.5%	0.2%	0.1%	<0.1%
Abnormal liver function tests	0.4%	0%	1.3%	0.5%
Vomiting	0.9%	0.4%	1.2%	0.4%
Tongue discoloration	1.1%	0%	0.2%	0%
Dizziness	1.1%	1.5%	0.4%	0.3%
Oral moniliasis	0.4%	0%	1.1%	0.4%

* Comparators included cefpodoxime proxetil 200 mg PO q12h; ceftriaxone 1 g IV q12h; dicloxacillin 500 mg PO q6h; oxacillin 2 g IV q6h; vancomycin 1 g IV q12h.
† The most commonly reported drug-related adverse events leading to discontinuation in patients treated with linezolid were nausea, headache, diarrhea, and vomiting.

were identified in Phase 3 clinical trials in patients developing thrombocytopenia. Bleeding events were identified in thrombocytopenic patients in a compassionate use program for linezolid; the role of linezolid in these events cannot be determined (see WARNINGS).

Changes seen in other laboratory parameters, without regard to drug relationship, revealed no substantial differences between linezolid and the comparators. These changes were generally not clinically significant, did not lead to discontinuation of therapy, and were reversible. The incidence of patients with at least one substantially abnormal hematologic or serum chemistry value is presented in TABLE 10 and TABLE 11.

TABLE 10 *Percent of Patients Who Experienced At Least One Substantially Abnormal* Hematology Laboratory Value in Comparator-Controlled Clinical Trials With Linezolid*

	Uncomplicated Skin and Skin Structure Infections		All Other Indications	
Laboratory	Linezolid	Clarithromycin	Linezolid	All Other
Assay	400 mg q12h	250 mg q12h	600 mg q12h	Comparators†
Hemoglobin (g/dl)	0.9%	0.0%	7.1%	6.6%
Platelet count ($\times 10^3$/mm^3)	0.7%	0.8%	3.0%	1.8%
WBC ($\times 10^3$/mm^3)	0.2%	0.6%	2.2%	1.3%
Neutrophils ($\times 10^3$/mm^3)	0.0%	0.2%	1.1%	1.2%

* <75% (<50% for neutrophils) of Lower Limit of Normal (LLN) for values normal at baseline; <75% (<50% for neutrophils) of LLN and of baseline for values abnormal at baseline.
† Comparators included cefpodoxime proxetil 200 mg PO q12h; ceftriaxone 1 g IV q12h; dicloxacillin 500 mg PO q6h; oxacillin 2 g IV q6h; vancomycin 1 g IV q12h.

POSTMARKETING EXPERIENCES

Myelosuppression (including anemia, leukopenia, pancytopenia, and thrombocytopenia) has been reported during postmarketing use of linezolid (see WARNINGS). These events have been chosen for inclusion due to either their seriousness, frequency of reporting, possible causal connection to linezolid, or a combination of these factors. Because they are reported voluntarily from a population of unknown size, estimates of frequency cannot be made and a causal relationship cannot be precisely established.

DOSAGE AND ADMINISTRATION

The recommended dosage for linezolid formulations for the treatment of infections is described in TABLE 12. Doses of linezolid are administered every 12 hours (q12h).

Patients with infection due to MRSA should be treated with linezolid 600 mg q12h.

In controlled clinical trials, the protocol-defined duration of treatment for all infections ranged from 7-28 days. Total treatment duration was determined by the treating physician based on site and severity of the infection, and on the patient's clinical response.

No dose adjustment is necessary when switching from intravenous to oral administration. Patients whose therapy is started with linezolid IV injection may be switched to either linezolid tablets or oral suspension at the discretion of the physician, when clinically indicated.

INTRAVENOUS ADMINISTRATION

Linezolid IV injection is supplied in single-use, ready-to-use infusion bags (see HOW SUPPLIED for container sizes). Parenteral drug products should be inspected visually for par-

L

TABLE 11 *Percent of Patients Who Experienced At Least One Substantially Abnormal* Serum Chemistry Laboratory Value in Comparator-Controlled Clinical Trials With Linezolid*

Laboratory Assay	Uncomplicated Skin and Skin Structure Infections Linezolid 400 mg q12h	Clarithromycin 250 mg q12h	All Other Indications Linezolid 600 mg q12h	All Other Comparators†
AST (U/L)	1.7%	1.3%	5.0%	6.8%
ALT (U/L)	1.7%	1.7%	9.6%	9.3%
LDH (U/L)	0.2%	0.2%	1.8%	1.5%
Alkaline phosphatase (U/L)	0.2%	0.2%	3.5%	3.1%
Lipase (U/L)	2.8%	2.6%	4.3%	4.2%
Amalyse (U/L)	0.2%	0.2%	2.4%	2.0%
Total bilirubin (mg/dl)	0.2%	0.0%	0.9%	1.1%
BUN (mg/dl)	0.2%	0.0%	2.1%	1.5%
Creatinine (mg/dl)	0.2%	0.0%	0.2%	0.6%

* >2 × Upper Limit of Normal (ULN) for values normal at baseline; >2 × ULN and >2 × baseline for values abnormal at baseline.
† Comparators included cefpodoxime proxetil 200 mg PO q12h; ceftriaxone 1 g IV q12h; dicloxacillin 500 mg PO q6h; oxacillin 2 g IV q6h; vancomycin 1 g IV q12h.

TABLE 12 *Dosage Guidelines for Linezolid*

Infection*	Dosage and Route of Administration	Recommended Duration of Treatment (consecutive days)
Vancomycin-resistant *Enterococcus faecium* infections, including concurrent bacteremia	600 mg IV or oral† q12h	14-28
Nosocomial pneumonia		
Complicated skin and skin structure infections	600 mg IV or oral† q12h	10-14
Community-acquired pneumonia, including concurrent bacteremia		
Uncomplicated skin and skin structure infections	400 mg oral† q12h	10-14

* Due to the designated pathogens (see INDICATIONS AND USAGE).
† Oral dosing using either linezolid tablets or linezolid for oral suspension.

ticulate matter prior to administration. Check for minute leaks by firmly squeezing the bag. If leaks are detected, discard the solution, as sterility may be impaired.

Linezolid IV injection should be administered by intravenous infusion over a period of 30-120 minutes. **Do not use this intravenous infusion bag in series connections.** Additives should not be introduced into this solution. If linezolid IV injection is to be given concomitantly with another drug, each drug should be given separately in accordance with the recommended dosage and route of administration for each product. In particular, physical incompatibilities resulted when linezolid IV injection was combined with the following drugs during simulated Y-site administration: amphotericin B, chlorpromazine HCl, diazepam, pentamidine isothionate, erythromycin lactobionate, phenytoin sodium, and trimethoprim-sulfamethoxazole. Additionally, chemical incompatibility resulted when linezolid IV injection was combined with ceftriaxone sodium.

If the same intravenous line is used for sequential infusion of several drugs, the line should be flushed before and after infusion of linezolid IV injection with an infusion solution compatible with linezolid IV injection and with any other drug(s) administered via this common line (see Compatible Intravenous Solutions).

COMPATIBLE INTRAVENOUS SOLUTIONS

5% Dextrose injection
0.9% Sodium chloride injection
Lactated Ringer's injection

Keep the infusion bags in the overwrap until ready to use. Store at room temperature. Protect from freezing. Linezolid IV injection may exhibit a yellow color that can intensify over time without adversely affecting potency.

ANIMAL PHARMACOLOGY

Dose- and time-dependent myelosuppression, as evidenced by bone marrow hypocellularity, decreased hematopoiesis, and decreased levels of circulating erythrocytes, leukocytes, and platelets, has been seen in animal studies. The hematopoietic effects occurred at doses of 40 and 80 mg/kg/day in dogs and rats, respectively (at exposures approximately 0.6 times in the dog and equal in the rat to the expected human exposure based on AUC). Hematopoietic effects were reversible, although in some studies reversal was incomplete within the duration of the recovery period.

HOW SUPPLIED

INJECTION

Zyvox IV injection is available in single-use, ready-to-use flexible plastic infusion bags in a foil laminate overwrap. The infusion bags and ports are latex-free.

The infusion bags are available in the following package sizes:

100 ml bag (200 mg linezolid).
200 ml bag (400 mg linezolid).
300 ml bag (600 mg linezolid).

TABLETS

400 mg: White, oblong, film-coated tablets printed with "ZYVOX 400mg".
600 mg: White, capsule-shaped, film-coated tablets printed with "ZYVOX 600 mg".

ORAL SUSPENSION

Zyvox for oral suspension is available as a dry, white to off-white, orange-flavored granule/powder. When constituted as directed, each bottle will contain 150 ml of a suspension providing the equivalent of 100 mg of linezolid per each 5 ml.

STORAGE

Store all Zyvox formulations at 25°C (77°F); excursions permitted to 15-30°C (59-86°F). Protect from light. Keep bottles tightly closed to protect from moisture. It is recommended that the infusion bags be kept in the overwrap until ready to use. Protect infusion bags from freezing.

PRODUCT LISTING - EQUIVALENTS NOT AVAILABLE

Powder For Reconstitution - Oral - 100 mg/5 ml
150 ml $298.18 ZYVOX, Pharmacia and Upjohn 00009-5136-01
Solution - Intravenous - 2 mg/ml
100 ml $40.35 ZYVOX, Pharmacia and Upjohn 00009-5137-01
300 ml $806.90 ZYVOX, Pharmacia and Upjohn 00009-5140-01
Tablet - Oral - 600 mg
20's $1192.70 ZYVOX, Pharmacia and Upjohn 00009-5135-02
30's $1789.05 ZYVOX, Pharmacia and Upjohn 00009-5135-03

Lisinopril *(001647)*

For related information, see the comparative table section in Appendix A.

Categories: Heart failure, congestive; Hypertension, essential; Pregnancy Category C, 1st Trimester; Pregnancy Category D, 2nd & 3rd Trimesters; FDA Approved 1987 Dec
Drug Classes: Angiotensin converting enzyme inhibitors
Brand Names: Prinivil; **Zestril**
Foreign Brand Availability: Acepril (Hong-Kong); Acerbon (Germany); Alapril (Italy); Alfaken (Mexico); Carace (England; Ireland); Cipril (India); Coric (Germany); Dapril (Benin; Burkina-Faso; China; Ethiopia; Gambia; Ghana; Guinea; Ivory-Coast; Kenya; Liberia; Malawi; Mali; Mauritania; Mauritius; Morocco; Niger; Nigeria; Senegal; Seychelles; Sierra-Leone; Sudan; Tanzania; Tunia; Uganda; Zambia; Zimbabwe); ES (India); Fibsol (Australia); Inopril (Bahrain; Cyprus; Egypt; Iran; Iraq; Jordan; Kuwait; Lebanon; Libya; Oman; Qatar; Republic-of-Yemen; Saudi-Arabia; Syria; United-Arab-Emirates); Linopril (Bahrain; Cyprus; Egypt; Iran; Iraq; Jordan; Kuwait; Lebanon; Libya; Oman; Qatar; Republic-of-Yemen; Saudi-Arabia; Syria; United-Arab-Emirates); Linvas (India); Lipril (India); Lisi ABZ (Germany); Lisibeta (Germany); Lisigamma (Germany); Lisihexal (Germany); Lisipril (Colombia; Dominican-Republic); Lisodur (Australia); Lisopress (Bahamas; Barbados; Belize; Bermuda; Curacao; Guyana; Jamaica; Netherland-Antilles; Puerto-Rico; Surinam; Trinidad); Lisopril (Bahrain; Cyprus; Egypt; Iran; Iraq; Jordan; Kuwait; Lebanon; Libya; Oman; Qatar; Republic-of-Yemen; Saudi-Arabia; Syria; United-Arab-Emirates); Lisoril (India; Singapore); Lispril (Thailand); Listril (India); Noperten (Indonesia); Novatec (Belgium; Netherlands); Presiten (Dominican-Republic); Prinil (Switzerland); Sinopril (Bahrain; Cyprus; Egypt; Iran; Iraq; Jordan; Kuwait; Lebanon; Libya; Oman; Qatar; Republic-of-Yemen; Saudi-Arabia; Syria; United-Arab-Emirates); Tensopril (Israel); Tensyn (Colombia); Vivatec (Denmark; Finland; Norway; Sweden); Zestomax (South-Africa)
Cost of Therapy: $34.45 (Hypertension; Zestril; 10 mg; 1 tablet/day; 30 day supply)
$33.47 (Hypertension; Prinivil; 10 mg; 1 tablet/day; 30 day supply)
$29.51 (Hypertension; Generic Tablets; 10 mg; 1 tablet/day; 30 day supply)

WARNING

USE IN PREGNANCY

When used in pregnancy during the second and third trimesters, ACE inhibitors can cause injury and even death to the developing fetus. When pregnancy is detected, lisinopril should be discontinued as soon as possible. See WARNINGS, Fetal/Neonatal Morbidity and Mortality.

DESCRIPTION

Prinivil (lisinopril), a synthetic peptide derivative, is an oral long-acting angiotensin converting enzyme inhibitor. Lisinopril is chemically described as (*S*)-1-[N^2-(1-carboxy-3-phenylpropyl)-L-lysyl]-L-proline dihydrate. Its empirical formula is $C_{21}H_{31}N_3O_5{\cdot}2H_2O$.

Lisinopril is a white to off-white, crystalline powder, with a molecular weight of 441.52. It is soluble in water and sparingly soluble in methanol and practically insoluble in ethanol.

Prinivil is supplied as 2.5, 5, 10, 20 and 40 mg tablets for oral administration. In addition to the active ingredient lisinopril, each tablet contains the following inactive ingredients: calcium phosphate, mannitol, magnesium stearate, and starch. The 10, 20 and 40 mg tablets also contain iron oxide.

CLINICAL PHARMACOLOGY

MECHANISM OF ACTION

Lisinopril inhibits angiotensin converting enzyme (ACE) in human subjects and animals. ACE is a peptidyl dipeptidase that catalyzes the conversion of angiotensin I to the vasoconstrictor substance, angiotensin II. Angiotensin II also stimulates aldosterone secretion by the adrenal cortex. The beneficial effects of lisinopril in hypertension and heart failure appear to result primarily from suppression of the renin-angiotensin-aldosterone system. Inhibition of ACE results in decreased plasma angiotensin II which leads to decreased vasopressor activity and to decreased aldosterone secretion. The latter decrease may result in a small increase of serum potassium. In hypertensive patients with normal renal function treated with lisinopril alone for up to 24 weeks, the mean increase in serum potassium was approximately 0.1 mEq/L; however, approximately 15% of patients had increases greater than 0.5 mEq/L and approximately 6% had a decrease greater than 0.5 mEq/L. In the same study, patients treated with lisinopril and hydrochlorothiazide (HCTZ) for up to 24 weeks had a mean decrease in serum potassium of 0.1 mEq/L; approximately 4% of patients had increases greater than 0.5 mEq/L and approximately 12% had a decrease greater than 0.5

L

mEq/L. (See PRECAUTIONS.) Removal of angiotensin II negative feedback on renin secretion leads to increased plasma renin activity.

ACE is identical to kininase, an enzyme that degrades bradykinin. Whether increased levels of bradykinin, a potent vasodepressor peptide, play a role in the therapeutic effects of lisinopril remains to be elucidated.

While the mechanism through which lisinopril lowers blood pressure is believed to be primarily suppression of the renin-angiotensin-aldosterone system, lisinopril is antihypertensive even in patients with low-renin hypertension. Although lisinopril was antihypertensive in all races studied, black hypertensive patients (usually a low-renin hypertensive population) had a smaller average response to monotherapy than non-black patients.

Concomitant administration of lisinopril and HCTZ further reduced blood pressure in black and non-black patients and any racial difference in blood pressure response was no longer evident.

PHARMACOKINETICS AND METABOLISM

Following oral administration of lisinopril, peak serum concentrations of lisinopril occur within about 7 hours, although there was a trend to a small delay in time taken to reach peak serum concentrations in acute myocardial infarction patients. Declining serum concentrations exhibit a prolonged terminal phase which does not contribute to drug accumulation. This terminal phase probably represents saturable binding to ACE and is not proportional to dose. Lisinopril does not appear to be bound to other serum proteins.

Lisinopril does not undergo metabolism and is excreted unchanged entirely in the urine. Based on urinary recovery, the mean extent of absorption of lisinopril is approximately 25%, with large intersubject variability (6-60%) at all doses tested (5-80 mg). Lisinopril absorption is not influenced by the presence of food in the gastrointestinal tract. The absolute bioavailability of lisinopril is reduced to about 16% in patients with stable NYHA Class II-IV congestive heart failure, and the volume of distribution appears to be slightly smaller than that in normal subjects.

The oral bioavailability of lisinopril in patients with acute myocardial infarction is similar to that in healthy volunteers.

Upon multiple dosing, lisinopril exhibits an effective half-life of accumulation of 12 hours.

Impaired renal function decreases elimination of lisinopril, which is excreted principally through the kidneys, but this decrease becomes clinically important only when the glomerular filtration rate is below 30 ml/min. Above this glomerular filtration rate, the elimination half-life is little changed. With greater impairment, however, peak and trough lisinopril levels increase, time to peak concentration increases and time to attain steady state is prolonged. Older patients, on average, have (approximately doubled) higher blood levels and area under the plasma concentration time curve (AUC) than younger patients. (See DOSAGE AND ADMINISTRATION.) Lisinopril can be removed by hemodialysis.

Studies in rats indicate that lisinopril crosses the blood-brain barrier poorly. Multiple doses of lisinopril in rats do not result in accumulation in any tissues. Milk of lactating rats contains radioactivity following administration of ^{14}C lisinopril. By whole body autoradiography, radioactivity was found in the placenta following administration of labeled drug to pregnant rats, but none was found in the fetuses.

PHARMACODYNAMICS AND CLINICAL EFFECTS

Hypertension

Administration of lisinopril to patients with hypertension results in a reduction of supine and standing blood pressure to about the same extent with no compensatory tachycardia. Symptomatic postural hypotension is usually not observed although it can occur and should be anticipated in volume and/or salt-depleted patients. (See WARNINGS.) When given together with thiazide-type diuretics, the blood pressure lowering effects of the two drugs are approximately additive.

In most patients studied, onset of antihypertensive activity was seen at 1 hour after oral administration of an individual dose of lisinopril, with peak reduction of blood pressure achieved by 6 hours. Although an antihypertensive effect was observed 24 hours after dosing with recommended single daily doses, the effect was more consistent and the mean effect was considerably larger in some studies with doses of 20 mg or more than with lower doses. However, at all doses studied, the mean antihypertensive effect was substantially smaller 24 hours after dosing than it was 6 hours after dosing.

In some patients achievement of optimal blood pressure reduction may require 2-4 weeks of therapy.

The antihypertensive effects of lisinopril are maintained during long-term therapy. Abrupt withdrawal of lisinopril has not been associated with a rapid increase in blood pressure or a significant increase in blood pressure compared to pretreatment levels.

Two dose-response studies utilizing a once daily regimen were conducted in 438 mild to moderate hypertensive patients not on a diuretic. Blood pressure was measured 24 hours after dosing. An antihypertensive effect of lisinopril was seen with 5 mg in some patients. However, in both studies blood pressure reduction occurred sooner and was greater in patients treated with 10, 20, or 80 mg of lisinopril. In controlled clinical studies, lisinopril 20-80 mg has been compared in patients with mild to moderate hypertension to HCTZ 12.5-50 mg and with atenolol 50-500 mg; and in patients with moderate to severe hypertension to metoprolol 100-200 mg. It was superior to HCTZ in effects on systolic and diastolic blood pressure in a population that was three-fourths caucasian. Lisinopril was approximately equivalent to atenolol and metoprolol in effects on diastolic blood pressure and had somewhat greater effects on systolic blood pressure.

Lisinopril had similar effectiveness and adverse effects in younger and older (>65 years) patients. It was less effective in blacks than in caucasians.

In hemodynamic studies in patients with essential hypertension, blood pressure reduction was accompanied by a reduction in peripheral arterial resistance with little or no change in cardiac output and in heart rate. In a study in 9 hypertensive patients, following administration of lisinopril, there was an increase in mean renal blood flow that was not significant. Data from several small studies are inconsistent with respect to the effect of lisinopril on glomerular filtration rate in hypertensive patients with normal renal function, but suggest that changes, if any, are not large.

In patients with renovascular hypertension lisinopril has been shown to be well tolerated and effective in controlling blood pressure (see PRECAUTIONS).

Heart Failure

During baseline-controlled clinical trials, in patients receiving digitalis and diuretics, single doses of lisinopril resulted in decreases in pulmonary capillary wedge pressure, systemic vascular resistance and blood pressure accompanied by an increase in cardiac output and no change in heart rate.

In two placebo controlled, 12 week clinical studies, lisinopril as adjunctive therapy to digitalis and diuretics improved the following signs and symptoms due to congestive heart failure: edema, rales, paroxysmal nocturnal dyspnea and jugular venous distention. In one of the studies beneficial response was also noted for: orthopnea, presence of third heart sound and the number of patients classified as NYHA Class III and IV. Exercise tolerance was also improved in this study. The effect of lisinopril on mortality in patients with heart failure has not been evaluated.

The once daily dosage for the treatment of congestive heart failure was the only dosage regimen used during clinical trial development and was determined by the measurement of hemodynamic responses.

Acute Myocardial Infarction

The Gruppo Italiano per lo Studio della Sopravvienza nell'Infarto Miocardico (GISSI-3) study was a multicenter, controlled, randomized, unblinded clinical trial conducted in 19,394 patients with acute myocardial infarction admitted to a coronary care unit. It was designed to examine the effects of short-term (6 week) treatment with lisinopril, nitrates, their combination, or no therapy on short-term (6 week) mortality and on long-term death and markedly impaired cardiac function. Patients presenting within 24 hours of the onset of symptoms who were hemodynamically stable were randomized, in a 2×2 factorial design, to 6 weeks of either:

1. Lisinopril alone (n=4841),
2. Nitrates alone (n=4869),
3. Lisinopril plus nitrates (n=4841), or
4. Open control (n=4843).

All patients received routine therapies, including thrombolytics (72%), aspirin (84%), and a beta-blocker (31%), as appropriate, normally utilized in acute myocardial infarction (MI) patients.

The protocol excluded patients with hypotension (systolic blood pressure $\leq$100 mm Hg), severe heart failure, cardiogenic shock and renal dysfunction (serum creatinine >2 mg/dl and/or proteinuria >500 mg/24 h). Doses of lisinopril were adjusted as necessary according to protocol. (See DOSAGE AND ADMINISTRATION.)

Study treatment was withdrawn at 6 weeks except where clinical conditions indicated continuation of treatment.

The primary outcomes of the trial were the overall mortality at 6 weeks and a combined endpoint at 6 months after the myocardial infarction, consisting of the number of patients who died, had late (day 4) clinical congestive heart failure, or had extensive left ventricular damage defined as ejection fraction $\leq$35%, or an akinetic-dyskinetic [A-D] score $\geq$45%. Patients receiving lisinopril (n=9646) alone or with nitrates, had an 11% lower risk of death (2p [two-tailed] = 0.04) compared to patients receiving no lisinopril (n=9672) (6.4% vs 7.2%, respectively) at 6 weeks. Although patients randomized to receive lisinopril for up to 6 weeks also fared numerically better on the combined endpoint at 6 months, the open nature of the assessment of heart failure, substantial loss to follow-up echocardiography, and substantial excess use of lisinopril between 6 weeks and 6 months in the group randomized to 6 weeks of lisinopril, preclude any conclusion about this endpoint.

Patients with acute myocardial infarction, treated with lisinopril had a higher (9.0% vs 3.7%, respectively) incidence of persistent hypotension (systolic blood pressure <90 mm Hg for more than 1 hour) and renal dysfunction (2.4% vs 1.1%) in-hospital and at 6 weeks (increasing creatinine concentration to over 3 mg/dl or a doubling or more of the baseline serum creatinine concentration). See ADVERSE REACTIONS, Acute Myocardial Infarction.

INDICATIONS AND USAGE

HYPERTENSION

Lisinopril is indicated for the treatment of hypertension. It may be used alone as initial therapy or concomitantly with other classes of antihypertensive agents.

HEART FAILURE

Lisinopril is indicated as adjunctive therapy in the management of heart failure in patients who are not responding adequately to diuretics and digitalis.

ACUTE MYOCARDIAL INFARCTION

Lisinopril is indicated for the treatment of hemodynamically stable patients within 24 hours of acute myocardial infarction, to improve survival. Patients should receive, as appropriate, the standard recommended treatments such as thrombolytics, aspirin and beta-blockers.

In using lisinopril, consideration should be given to the fact that another angiotensin converting enzyme inhibitor, captopril, has caused agranulocytosis, particularly in patients with renal impairment or collagen vascular disease, and that available data are insufficient to show that lisinopril does not have a similar risk. (See WARNINGS.)

In considering use of lisinopril, it should be noted that in controlled clinical trials ACE inhibitors have an effect on blood pressure that is less in black patients than in non-blacks. In addition, it should be noted that black patients receiving ACE inhibitors have been reported to have a higher incidence of angioedema compared to non-blacks.

CONTRAINDICATIONS

Lisinopril is contraindicated in patients who are hypersensitive to this product and in patients with a history of angioedema related to previous treatment with an angiotensin converting enzyme inhibitor and in patients with hereditary or idiopathic angioedema.

WARNINGS

ANAPHYLACTOID AND POSSIBLY RELATED REACTIONS

Presumably because angiotensin converting enzyme inhibitors affect the metabolism of eicosanoids and polypeptides, including endogenous bradykinin, patients receiving ACE

L

inhibitors (including lisinopril) may be subject to a variety of adverse reactions, some of them serious.

Angioedema

Angioedema of the face, extremities, lips, tongue, glottis and/or larynx has been reported in patients treated with angiotensin converting enzyme inhibitors, including lisinopril. This may occur at any time during treatment. In such cases lisinopril should be promptly discontinued and appropriate therapy and monitoring should be provided until complete and sustained resolution of signs and symptoms has occurred. In instances where swelling has been confined to the face and lips the condition has generally resolved without treatment, although antihistamines have been useful in relieving symptoms. Angioedema associated with laryngeal edema may be fatal. **Where there is involvement of the tongue, glottis or larynx, likely to cause airway obstruction, appropriate therapy, *e.g.*, subcutaneous epinephrine solution 1:1000 (0.3-05 ml) and/or measures necessary to ensure a patent airway, should be promptly provided.** (See ADVERSE REACTIONS.)

Patients with a history of angioedema unrelated to ACE inhibitor therapy may be at increased risk of angioedema while receiving an ACE inhibitor (see also INDICATIONS AND USAGE and CONTRAINDICATIONS).

Anaphylactoid Reactions During Desensitization

Two patients undergoing desensitizing treatment with hymenoptera venom while receiving ACE inhibitors sustained life-threatening anaphylactoid reactions. In the same patients, these reactions were avoided when ACE inhibitors were temporarily withheld, but they reappeared upon inadvertent rechallenge.

Anaphylactoid Reactions During Membrane Exposure

Anaphylactoid reactions have been reported in patients dialyzed with high-flux membranes and treated concomitantly with an ACE inhibitor. Anaphylactoid reactions have also been reported in patients undergoing low-density lipoprotein apheresis with dextran sulfate absorption.

HYPOTENSION

Excessive hypotension is rare in patients with uncomplicated hypertension treated with lisinopril alone.

Patients with heart failure given lisinopril commonly have some reduction in blood pressure with peak blood pressure reduction occurring 6-8 hours post dose, but discontinuation of therapy because of continuing symptomatic hypotension usually is not necessary when dosing instructions are followed; caution should be observed when initiating therapy. (See DOSAGE AND ADMINISTRATION.)

Patients at risk of excessive hypotension, sometimes associated with oliguria and/or progressive azotemia, and rarely with acute renal failure and/or death, include those with the following conditions or characteristics: heart failure with systolic blood pressure below 100 mm Hg, hyponatremia, high dose diuretic therapy, recent intensive diuresis or increase in diuretic dose, renal dialysis, or severe volume and/or salt depletion of any etiology. It may be advisable to eliminate the diuretic (except in patients with heart failure), reduce the diuretic dose or increase salt intake cautiously before initiating therapy with lisinopril in patients at risk for excessive hypotension who are able to tolerate such adjustments. (See DRUG INTERACTIONS and ADVERSE REACTIONS.)

Patients with acute myocardial infarction in the GISSI-3 study had a higher (9.0% vs 3.7%) incidence of persistent hypotension (systolic blood pressure <90 mm Hg for more than 1 hour) when treated with lisinopril. Treatment with lisinopril must not be initiated in acute myocardial infarction patients at risk of further serious hemodynamic deterioration after treatment with a vasodilator (*e.g.,* systolic blood pressure of 100 mm Hg or lower) or cardiogenic shock.

In patients at risk of excessive hypotension, therapy should be started under very close medical supervision and such patients should be followed closely for the first 2 weeks of treatment and whenever the dose of lisinopril and/or diuretic is increased. Similar considerations may apply to patients with ischemic heart or cerebrovascular disease, or in patients with acute myocardial infarction, in whom an excessive fall in blood pressure could result in a myocardial infarction or cerebrovascular accident.

If excessive hypotension occurs, the patient should be placed in the supine position and, if necessary, receive an intravenous infusion of normal saline. A transient hypotensive response is not a contraindication to further doses of lisinopril which usually can be given without difficulty once the blood pressure has stabilized. If symptomatic hypotension develops, a dose reduction or discontinuation of lisinopril or concomitant diuretic may be necessary.

NEUTROPENIA/AGRANULOCYTOSIS

Another angiotensin converting enzyme inhibitor, captopril, has been shown to cause agranulocytosis and bone marrow depression, rarely in uncomplicated patients but more frequently in patients with renal impairment especially if they also have a collagen vascular disease. Available data from clinical trials of lisinopril are insufficient to show that lisinopril does not cause agranulocytosis at similar rates. Marketing experience has revealed rare cases of neutropenia and bone marrow depression in which a causal relationship to lisinopril cannot be excluded. Periodic monitoring of white blood cell counts in patients with collagen vascular disease and renal disease should be considered.

HEPATIC FAILURE

Rarely, ACE inhibitors have been associated with a syndrome that starts with cholestatic jaundice and progresses to fulminant hepatic necrosis, and (sometimes) death. The mechanism of this syndrome is not understood. Patients receiving ACE inhibitors who develop jaundice or marked elevations of hepatic enzymes should discontinue the ACE inhibitor and receive appropriate medical follow-up.

FETAL/NEONATAL MORBIDITY AND MORTALITY

ACE inhibitors can cause fetal and neonatal morbidity and death when administered to pregnant women. Several dozen cases have been reported in the world literature. When pregnancy is detected, ACE inhibitors should be discontinued as soon as possible.

The use of ACE inhibitors during the second and third trimesters of pregnancy has been associated with fetal and neonatal injury, including hypotension, neonatal skull hypoplasia, anuria, reversible or irreversible renal failure, and death. Oligohydramnios has also been reported, presumably resulting from decreased fetal renal function; oligohydramnios in this setting has been associated with fetal limb contractures, craniofacial deformation, and hypoplastic lung development. Prematurity, intrauterine growth retardation, and patent ductus arteriosus have also been reported, although it is not clear whether these occurrences were due to the ACE-inhibitor exposure.

These adverse effects do not appear to have resulted from intrauterine ACE-inhibitor exposure that has been limited to the first trimester. Mothers whose embryos and fetuses are exposed to ACE inhibitors only during the first trimester should be so informed. Nonetheless, when patients become pregnant, physicians should make every effort to discontinue the use of lisinopril as soon as possible.

Rarely (probably less often than once in every thousand pregnancies), no alternative to ACE inhibitors will be found. In these rare cases, the mothers should be apprised of the potential hazards to their fetuses, and serial ultrasound examinations should be performed to assess the intraamniotic environment.

If oligohydramnios is observed, lisinopril should be discontinued unless it is considered lifesaving for the mother. Contraction stress testing (CST), a non-stress test (NST), or biophysical profiling (BPP) may be appropriate, depending upon the week of pregnancy. Patients and physicians should be aware, however, that oligohydramnios may not appear until after the fetus has sustained irreversible injury.

Infants with histories of *in utero* exposure to ACE inhibitors should be closely observed for hypotension, oliguria, and hyperkalemia. If oliguria occurs, attention should be directed toward support of blood pressure and renal perfusion. Exchange transfusion or dialysis may be required as means of reversing hypotension and/or substituting for disordered renal function. Lisinopril, which crosses the placenta, has been removed from neonatal circulation by peritoneal dialysis with some clinical benefit, and theoretically may be removed by exchange transfusion, although there is no experience with the latter procedure.

No teratogenic effects of lisinopril were seen in studies of pregnant mice, rats and rabbits. On a body surface area basis, the doses used were 55 times, 33 times, and 0.15 times, respectively, the maximum recommended human daily dose (MRHDD).

PRECAUTIONS

GENERAL

Aortic Stenosis/Hypertrophic Cardiomyopathy

As with all vasodilators, lisinopril should be given with caution to patients with obstruction in the outflow tract of the left ventricle.

Impaired Renal Function

As a consequence of inhibiting the renin-angiotensin-aldosterone system, changes in renal function may be anticipated in susceptible individuals. In patients with severe congestive heart failure whose renal function may depend on the activity of the renin-angiotensin-aldosterone system, treatment with angiotensin converting enzyme inhibitors, including lisinopril, may be associated with oliguria and/or progressive azotemia and rarely with acute renal failure and/or death.

In hypertensive patients with unilateral or bilateral renal artery stenosis, increases in blood urea nitrogen and serum creatinine may occur. Experience with another angiotensin converting enzyme inhibitor suggests that these increases are usually reversible upon discontinuation of lisinopril and/or diuretic therapy. In such patients renal function should be monitored during the first few weeks of therapy.

Some patients with hypertension or heart failure with no apparent pre-existing renal vascular disease have developed increases in blood urea nitrogen and serum creatinine, usually minor and transient, especially when lisinopril has been given concomitantly with a diuretic. This is more likely to occur in patients with pre-existing renal impairment. Dosage reduction and/or discontinuation of the diuretic and/or lisinopril may be required.

Patients with acute myocardial infarction in the GISSI-3 study, treated with lisinopril, had a higher (2.4% vs 1.1%) incidence of renal dysfunction in-hospital and at 6 weeks (increasing creatinine concentration to over 3 mg/dl or a doubling or more of the baseline serum creatinine concentration). In acute myocardial infarction, treatment with lisinopril should be initiated with caution in patients with evidence of renal dysfunction, defined as serum creatinine concentration exceeding 2 mg/dl. If renal dysfunction develops during treatment with lisinopril (serum creatinine concentration exceeding 3 mg/dl or a doubling from the pretreatment value) then the physician should consider withdrawal of lisinopril.

Evaluation of patients with hypertension, heart failure, or myocardial infarction should always include assessment of renal function. (See DOSAGE AND ADMINISTRATION.)

Hyperkalemia

In clinical trials hyperkalemia (serum potassium greater than 5.7 mEq/L) occurred in approximately 2.2% of hypertensive patients and 4.8% of patients with heart failure. In most cases these were isolated values which resolved despite continued therapy. Hyperkalemia was a cause of discontinuation of therapy in approximately 0.1% of hypertensive patients, 0.6% of patients with heart failure and 0.1% of patients with myocardial infarction. Risk factors for the development of hyperkalemia include renal insufficiency, diabetes mellitus, and the concomitant use of potassium-sparing diuretics, potassium supplements and/or potassium-containing salt substitutes, which should be used cautiously, if at all, with lisinopril. (See DRUG INTERACTIONS.)

Cough

Presumably due to the inhibition of the degradation of endogenous bradykinin, persistent nonproductive cough has been reported with all ACE inhibitors, always resolving after discontinuation of therapy. ACE inhibitor-induced cough should be considered in the differential diagnosis of cough.

Surgery/Anesthesia

In patients undergoing major surgery or during anesthesia with agents that produce hypotension, lisinopril may block angiotensin II formation secondary to compensatory renin release. If hypotension occurs and is considered to be due to this mechanism, it can be corrected by volume expansion.

INFORMATION FOR THE PATIENT

Angioedema: Angioedema, including laryngeal edema, may occur at any time during treatment with angiotensin converting enzyme inhibitors, including lisinopril. Patients should be so advised and told to report immediately any signs or symptoms suggesting angioedema (swelling of face, extremities, eyes, lips, tongue, difficulty in swallowing or breathing) and to take no more drug until they have consulted with the prescribing physician.

Symptomatic Hypotension: Patients should be cautioned to report lightheadedness especially during the first few days of therapy. If actual syncope occurs, the patients should be told to discontinue the drug until they have consulted with the prescribing physician.

All patients should be cautioned that excessive perspiration and dehydration may lead to an excessive fall in blood pressure because of reduction in fluid volume. Other causes of volume depletion such as vomiting or diarrhea may also lead to a fall in blood pressure; patients should be advised to consult with their physician.

Hyperkalemia: Patients should be told not to use salt substitutes containing potassium without consulting their physician.

Neutropenia: Patients should be told to report promptly any indication of infection (*e.g.*, sore throat, fever) which may be a sign of neutropenia.

Pregnancy: Female patients of childbearing age should be told about the consequences of second- and third-trimester exposure to ACE inhibitors, and they should also be told that these consequences do not appear to have resulted from intrauterine ACE-inhibitor exposure that has been limited to the first trimester. These patients should be asked to report pregnancies to their physicians as soon as possible.

NOTE: As with many other drugs, certain advice to patients being treated with lisinopril is warranted. This information is intended to aid in the safe and effective use of this medication. It is not a disclosure of all possible adverse or intended effects.

CARCINOGENESIS, MUTAGENESIS, AND IMPAIRMENT OF FERTILITY

There was no evidence of a tumorigenic effect when lisinopril was administered orally for 105 weeks to male and female rats at doses up to 90 mg/kg/day or for 92 weeks to male and female mice at doses up to 135 mg/kg/day. These doses are 10 times and 7 times, respectively, the maximum recommended human daily dose (MRHDD) when compared on a body surface area basis.

Lisinopril was not mutagenic in the Ames microbial mutagen test with or without metabolic activation. It was also negative in a forward mutation assay using Chinese hamster lung cells. Lisinopril did not produce single strand DNA breaks in an *in vitro* alkaline elution rat hepatocyte assay. In addition, lisinopril did not produce increases in chromosomal aberrations in an *in vitro* test in Chinese hamster ovary cells or in an *in vivo* study in mouse bone marrow.

There were no adverse effects on reproductive performance in male and female rats treated with up to 300 mg/kg/day of lisinopril (33 times the MRHDD when compared on a body surface area basis).

PREGNANCY CATEGORIES C (FIRST TRIMESTER) AND D (SECOND AND THIRD TRIMESTERS)

See WARNINGS, Fetal/Neonatal Morbidity and Mortality.

NURSING MOTHERS

Milk of lactating rats contains radioactivity following administration of ^{14}C lisinopril. It is not known whether this drug is secreted in human milk. Because many drugs are secreted in human milk, and because of the potential for serious adverse reactions in nursing infants from ACE inhibitors, a decision should be made whether to discontinue lisinopril, taking into account the importance of the drug to the mother.

PEDIATRIC USE

Safety and effectiveness in pediatric patients have not been established.

DRUG INTERACTIONS

HYPOTENSION — PATIENTS ON DIURETIC THERAPY

Patients on diuretics, and especially those in whom diuretic therapy was recently instituted, may occasionally experience an excessive reduction of blood pressure after initiation of therapy with lisinopril. The possibility of hypotensive effects with lisinopril can be minimized by either discontinuing the diuretic or increasing the salt intake prior to initiation of treatment with lisinopril. If it is necessary to continue the diuretic, initiate therapy with lisinopril at a dose of 5 mg daily, and provide close medical supervision after the initial dose until blood pressure has stabilized. (See WARNINGS and DOSAGE AND ADMINISTRATION.) When a diuretic is added to the therapy of a patient receiving lisinopril, an additional antihypertensive effect is usually observed. Studies with ACE inhibitors in combination with diuretics indicate that the dose of the ACE inhibitor can be reduced when it is given with a diuretic. (See DOSAGE AND ADMINISTRATION.)

NON-STEROIDAL ANTI-INFLAMMATORY AGENTS

In some patients with compromised renal function who are being treated with non-steroidal anti-inflammatory drugs, the co-administration of lisinopril may result in a further deterioration of renal function. These effects are usually reversible.

Reports suggest that NSAIDs may diminish the antihypertensive effect of ACE-inhibitors, including lisinopril. This interaction should be given consideration in patients taking NSAIDs concomitantly with ACE-inhibitors.

OTHER AGENTS

Lisinopril has been used concomitantly with nitrates and/or digoxin without evidence of clinically significant adverse interactions. This included post myocardial infarction patients who were receiving intravenous or transdermal nitroglycerin. No clinically important pharmacokinetic interactions occurred when lisinopril was used concomitantly with propranolol or HCTZ. The presence of food in the stomach does not alter the bioavailability of lisinopril.

AGENTS INCREASING SERUM POTASSIUM

Lisinopril attenuates potassium loss caused by thiazide-type diuretics. Use of lisinopril with potassium-sparing diuretics (*e.g.*, spironolactone, triamterene, or amiloride), potassium supplements, or potassium-containing salt substitutes may lead to significant increases in serum potassium. Therefore, if concomitant use of these agents is indicated because of demonstrated hypokalemia, they should be used with caution and with frequent monitoring of serum potassium. Potassium sparing agents should generally not be used in patients with heart failure who are receiving lisinopril.

LITHIUM

Lithium toxicity has been reported in patients receiving lithium concomitantly with drugs which cause elimination of sodium, including ACE inhibitors. Lithium toxicity was usually reversible upon discontinuation of lithium and the ACE inhibitor. It is recommended that serum lithium levels be monitored frequently if lisinopril is administered concomitantly with lithium.

ADVERSE REACTIONS

Lisinopril has been found to be generally well tolerated in controlled clinical trials involving 1969 patients with hypertension or heart failure. For the most part, adverse experiences were mild and transient.

HYPERTENSION

In clinical trials in patients with hypertension treated with lisinopril, discontinuation of therapy due to clinical adverse experiences occurred in 5.7% of patients. The overall frequency of adverse experiences could not be related to total daily dosage within the recommended therapeutic dosage range.

For adverse experiences occurring in greater than 1% of patients with hypertension treated with lisinopril or lisinopril plus HCTZ in controlled clinical trials and more frequently with lisinopril and/or lisinopril plus HCTZ than placebo, comparative incidence data are listed in TABLE 1.

TABLE 1 *Percent of Patients in Controlled Studies*

	Incidence (Discontinuation)		
	Lisinopril (n=1349)	Lisinopril + HCTZ (n=629)	Placebo (n=207)
Body as a Whole			
Fatigue	2.5% (0.3%)	4.0% (0.5%)	1.0% (0.0%)
Asthenia	1.3% (0.5%)	2.1% (0.2%)	1.0% (0.0%)
Orthostatic effects	1.2% (0.0%)	3.5% (0.2%)	1.0% (0.0%)
Cardiovascular			
Hypotension	1.2% (0.5%)	1.6% (0.5%)	0.5% (0.5%)
Digestive			
Diarrhea	2.7% (0.2%)	2.7% (0.3%)	2.4% (0.0%)
Nausea	2.0% (0.4%)	2.5% (0.2%)	2.4% (0.0%)
Vomiting	1.1% (0.2%)	1.4% (0.1%)	0.5% (0.0%)
Dyspepsia	0.9% (0.0%)	1.9% (0.0%)	0.0% (0.0%)
Musculoskeletal			
Muscle cramps	0.5% (0.0%)	2.9% (0.8%)	0.5% (0.0%)
Nervous/Psychiatric			
Headache	5.7% (0.2%)	4.5% (0.5%)	1.9% (0.0%)
Dizziness	5.4% (0.4%)	9.2% (1.0%)	1.9% (0.0%)
Paresthesia	0.8% (0.1%)	2.1% (0.2%)	0.0% (0.0%)
Decreased libido	0.4% (0.1%)	1.3% (0.1%)	0.0% (0.0%)
Vertigo	0.2% (0.1%)	1.1% (0.2%)	0.0% (0.0%)
Respiratory			
Cough	3.5% (0.7%)	4.6% (0.8%)	1.0% (0.0%)
Upper respiratory infection	2.1% (0.1%)	2.7% (0.1%)	0.0% (0.0%)
Common cold	1.1% (0.1%)	1.3% (0.1%)	0.0% (0.0%)
Nasal congestion	0.4% (0.1%)	1.3% (0.1%)	0.0% (0.0%)
Influenza	0.3% (0.1%)	1.1% (0.1%)	0.0% (0.0%)
Skin			
Rash	1.3% (0.4%)	1.6% (0.2%)	0.5% (0.5%)
Urogenital			
Impotence	1.0% (0.4%)	1.6% (0.5%)	0.0% (0.0%)

Chest pain and back pain were also seen but were more common on placebo than lisinopril.

HEART FAILURE

In patients with heart failure treated with lisinopril for up to 4 years, discontinuation of therapy due to clinical adverse experiences occurred in 11.0% of patients. In controlled studies in patients with heart failure, therapy was discontinued in 8.1% of patients treated with lisinopril for up to 12 weeks, compared to 7.7% of patients treated with placebo for 12 weeks.

TABLE 2 lists those adverse experiences which occurred in greater than 1% of patients with heart failure treated with lisinopril or placebo for up to 12 weeks in controlled clinical trials and more frequently on lisinopril than placebo.

Also observed at >1% with lisinopril but more frequent or as frequent on placebo than lisinopril in controlled trials were asthenia, angina pectoris, nausea, dyspnea, cough and pruritus.

TABLE 2

	Incidence (Discontinuation) at 12 Weeks	
	Lisinopril (n=407)	**Placebo (n=155)**
Body as a Whole		
Chest pain	3.4% (0.2%)	1.3% (0.0%)
Abdominal pain	2.2% (0.7%)	1.9% (0.0%)
Cardiovascular		
Hypotension	4.4% (1.7%)	0.6% (0.6%)
Digestive		
Diarrhea	3.7% (0.5%)	1.9% (0.0%)
Nervous/Psychiatric		
Dizziness	11.8% (1.2%)	4.5% (1.3%)
Headache	4.4% (0.2%)	3.9% (0.0%)
Respiratory		
Upper respiratory infection	1.5% (0.0%)	1.3% (0.0%)
Skin		
Rash	1.7% (0.5%)	0.6% (0.6%)

Worsening of heart failure, anorexia, increased salivation, muscle cramps, back pain, myalgia, depression, chest sound abnormalities and pulmonary edema were also seen in controlled clinical trials, but were more common on placebo than lisinopril.

ACUTE MYOCARDIAL INFARCTION

In the GISSI-3 trial, in patients treated with lisinopril for 6 weeks following acute myocardial infarction, discontinuation of therapy occurred in 17.6% of patients.

Patients treated with lisinopril had a significantly higher incidence of hypotension and renal dysfunction compared with patients not taking lisinopril.

In the GISSI-3 trial, hypotension (9.7%), renal dysfunction (2.0%), cough (0.5%), post-infarction angina (0.3%), skin rash and generalized edema (0.01%), and angioedema (0.01%) resulted in withdrawal of treatment. In elderly patients treated with lisinopril, discontinuation due to renal dysfunction was 4.2%.

Other clinical adverse experiences occurring in 0.3-1.0% of patients with hypertension or heart failure treated with lisinopril in controlled trials and rarer, serious, possibly drug-related events reported in uncontrolled studies or marketing experience are listed below, and within each category, are in order of decreasing severity:

Body as a Whole: Anaphylactoid reactions (see WARNINGS, Anaphylactoid and Possible Related Reactions), syncope, orthostatic effects, chest discomfort, pain, pelvic pain, flank pain, edema, facial edema, virus infection, fever, chills, malaise.

Cardiovascular: Cardiac arrest; myocardial infarction or cerebrovascular accident, possibly secondary to excessive hypotension in high risk patients (see WARNINGS, Hypotension); pulmonary embolism and infarction, arrhythmias (including ventricular tachycardia, atrial tachycardia, atrial fibrillation, bradycardia and premature ventricular contractions), palpitations, transient ischemic attacks, paroxysmal nocturnal dyspnea, orthostatic hypotension, decreased blood pressure, peripheral edema, vasculitis.

Digestive: Pancreatitis, hepatitis (hepatocellular or cholestatic jaundice) (see WARNINGS, Hepatic Failure), vomiting, gastritis, dyspepsia, heartburn, gastrointestinal cramps, constipation, flatulence, dry mouth.

Hematologic: Rare cases of bone marrow depression, neutropenia, and thrombocytopenia.

Endocrine: Diabetes mellitus.

Metabolic: Weight loss, dehydration, fluid overload, gout, weight gain.

Musculoskeletal: Arthritis, arthralgia, neck pain, hip pain, low back pain, joint pain, leg pain, knee pain, shoulder pain, arm pain, lumbago.

Nervous System/Psychiatric: Stroke, ataxia, memory impairment, tremor, peripheral neuropathy (*e.g.,* dysesthesia), spasm, paresthesia, confusion, insomnia, somnolence, hypersomnia, irritability, and nervousness.

Respiratory System: Malignant lung neoplasms, hemoptysis, pulmonary infiltrates, eosinophilic pneumonitis, bronchospasm, asthma, pleural effusion, pneumonia, bronchitis, wheezing, orthopnea, painful respiration, epistaxis, laryngitis, sinusitis, pharyngeal pain, pharyngitis, rhinitis, rhinorrhea.

Skin: Urticaria, alopecia, herpes zoster, photosensitivity, skin lesions, skin infections, pemphigus, erythema, flushing, diaphoresis. Other severe skin reactions (including toxic epidermal necrolysis and Stevens-Johnson syndrome) have been reported rarely; causal relationship has not been established.

Special Senses: Visual loss, diplopia, blurred vision, tinnitus, photophobia, taste disturbances.

Urogenital System: Acute renal failure, oliguria, anuria, uremia, progressive azotemia, renal dysfunction (see PRECAUTIONS and DOSAGE AND ADMINISTRATION), pyelonephritis, dysuria, urinary tract infection, breast pain.

Miscellaneous: A symptom complex has been reported which may include a positive ANA, an elevated erythrocyte sedimentation rate, arthralgia/arthritis, myalgia, fever, vasculitis, leukocytosis, eosinophilia, photosensitivity, rash, and other dermatological manifestations.

Angioedema: Angioedema has been reported in patients receiving lisinopril with an incidence higher in black than in non-black patients. Angioedema associated with laryngeal edema may be fatal. If angioedema of the face, extremities, lips, tongue, glottis and/or larynx occurs, treatment with lisinopril should be discontinued and appropriate therapy instituted immediately. (See WARNINGS.)

Hypotension: In hypertensive patients, hypotension occurred in 1.2% and syncope occurred in 0.1% of patients. Hypotension or syncope was a cause for discontinuation of therapy in 0.5% of hypertensive patients. In patients with heart failure, hypotension occurred in 5.3% and syncope occurred in 1.8% of patients. These adverse experiences were causes for discontinuation of therapy in 1.8% of these patients. In patients treated with lisinopril for 6 weeks after acute myocardial infarction, hypotension (systolic blood pressure ≤100 mm Hg) resulted in discontinuation of therapy in 9.7% of the patients. (See WARNINGS.)

Fetal/Neonatal Morbidity and Mortality: See WARNINGS, Fetal/Neonatal Morbidity and Mortality.

Cough: See PRECAUTIONS, General, Cough.

Clinical Laboratory Test Findings

Serum Electrolytes: Hyperkalemia (see PRECAUTIONS), hyponatremia.

Creatinine, Blood Urea Nitrogen: Minor increases in blood urea nitrogen and serum creatinine, reversible upon discontinuation of therapy, were observed in about 2.0% of patients with essential hypertension treated with lisinopril alone. Increases were more common in patients receiving concomitant diuretics and in patients with renal artery stenosis. (See PRECAUTIONS.) Reversible minor increases in blood urea nitrogen and serum creatinine were observed in approximately 11.6% of patients with heart failure on concomitant diuretic therapy. Frequently, these abnormalities resolved when the dosage of the diuretic was decreased.

Hemoglobin and Hematocrit: Small decreases in hemoglobin and hematocrit (mean decreases of approximately 0.4 g percent and 1.3 vol percent, respectively) occurred frequently in patients treated with lisinopril but were rarely of clinical importance in patients without some other cause of anemia. In clinical trials, less than 0.1% of patients discontinued therapy due to anemia. Hemolytic anemia has been reported; a causal relationship to lisinopril cannot be excluded.

Liver Function Tests: Rarely, elevations of liver enzymes and/or serum bilirubin have occurred (see WARNINGS, Hepatic Failure).

In hypertensive patients, 2.0% discontinued therapy due to laboratory adverse experiences, principally elevations in blood urea nitrogen (0.6%), serum creatinine (0.5%) and serum potassium (0.4%). In the heart failure trials, 3.4% of patients discontinued therapy due to laboratory adverse experiences, 1.8% due to elevations in blood urea nitrogen and/or creatinine and 0.6% due to elevations in serum potassium. In the myocardial infarction trial, 2.0% of patients receiving lisinopril discontinued therapy due to renal dysfunction (increasing creatinine concentration to over 3 mg/dl or a doubling or more of the baseline serum creatinine concentration); less than 1.0% of patients discontinued therapy due to other laboratory adverse experiences: 0.1% with hyperkalemia and less than 0.1% with hepatic enzyme alterations.

DOSAGE AND ADMINISTRATION

HYPERTENSION

Initial Therapy

In patients with uncomplicated essential hypertension not on diuretic therapy, the recommended initial dose is 10 mg once a day. Dosage should be adjusted according to blood pressure response. The usual dosage range is 20-40 mg/day administered in a single daily dose. The antihypertensive effect may diminish toward the end of the dosing interval regardless of the administered dose, but most commonly with a dose of 10 mg daily. This can be evaluated by measuring blood pressure just prior to dosing to determine whether satisfactory control is being maintained for 24 hours. If it is not, an increase in dose should be considered. Doses up to 80 mg have been used but do not appear to give a greater effect. If blood pressure is not controlled with lisinopril alone, a low dose of a diuretic may be added. Hydrochlorothiazide 12.5 mg has been shown to provide an additive effect. After the addition of a diuretic, it may be possible to reduce the dose of lisinopril.

Diuretic Treated Patients

In hypertensive patients who are currently being treated with a diuretic, symptomatic hypotension may occur occasionally following the initial dose of lisinopril. The diuretic should be discontinued, if possible, for 2-3 days before beginning therapy with lisinopril to reduce the likelihood of hypotension. (See WARNINGS.) The dosage of lisinopril should be adjusted according to blood pressure response. If the patient's blood pressure is not controlled with lisinopril alone, diuretic therapy may be resumed as described above.

If the diuretic cannot be discontinued, an initial dose of 5 mg should be used under medical supervision for at least 2 hours and until blood pressure has stabilized for at least an additional hour. (See WARNINGS and DRUG INTERACTIONS.)

Concomitant administration of lisinopril with potassium supplements, potassium salt substitutes, or potassium-sparing diuretics may lead to increases of serum potassium (see PRECAUTIONS).

Dosage Adjustment in Renal Impairment

The usual dose of lisinopril (10 mg) is recommended for patients with a creatinine clearance >30 ml/min (serum creatinine of up to approximately 3 mg/dl). For patients with creatinine clearance ≥10 ml/min ≤30 ml/min (serum creatinine ≥3 mg/dl), the first dose is 5 mg once daily. For patients with creatinine clearance <10 ml/min (usually on hemodialysis) the recommended initial dose is 2.5 mg. The dosage may be titrated upward until blood pressure is controlled or to a maximum of 40 mg daily.

TABLE 3

Renal Status	Creatinine-Clearance	Initial Dose (mg/day)
Normal renal function to mild impairment	>30 ml/min	10 mg
Moderate to severe impairment	≥10 to ≤30 ml/min	5 mg
Dialysis patients*	<10 ml/min	2.5 mg†

* See WARNINGS, Anaphylactoid and Possibly Related Reactions, Anaphylactoid Reactions During Membrane Exposure.

† Dosage or dosing interval should be adjusted depending on the blood pressure response.

HEART FAILURE

Lisinopril is indicated as adjunctive therapy with diuretics and digitalis. The recommended starting dose is 5 mg once a day.

When initiating treatment with lisinopril in patients with heart failure, the initial dose should be administered under medical observation, especially in those patients with low blood pressure (systolic blood pressure below 100 mm Hg). The mean peak blood pressure lowering occurs 6-8 hours after dosing. Observation should continue until blood pressure is stable. The concomitant diuretic dose should be reduced, if possible, to help minimize hypovolemia which may contribute to hypotension. (See WARNINGS and DRUG INTERACTIONS.) The appearance of hypotension after the initial dose of lisinopril does not preclude subsequent careful dose titration with the drug, following effective management of the hypotension.

The usual effective dosage range is 5-20 mg/day administered as a single daily dose.

Dosage Adjustment in Patients With Heart Failure and Renal Impairment or Hyponatremia

In patients with heart failure who have hyponatremia (serum sodium <130 mEq/L) or moderate to severe renal impairment (creatinine clearance ≤30 ml/min or serum creatinine >3 mg/dl), therapy with lisinopril should be initiated at a dose of 2.5 mg once a day under close medical supervision. (See WARNINGS and DRUG INTERACTIONS.)

ACUTE MYOCARDIAL INFARCTION

In hemodynamically stable patients within 24 hours of the onset of symptoms of acute myocardial infarction, the first dose of lisinopril is 5 mg given orally, followed by 5 mg after 24 hours, 10 mg after 48 hours and then 10 mg of lisinopril once daily. Dosing should continue for 6 weeks. Patients should receive, as appropriate, the standard recommended treatments such as thrombolytics, aspirin and beta-blockers. Patients with a low systolic blood pressure (≤120 mm Hg) when treatment is started or during the first 3 days after the infarct should be given a lower 2.5 mg oral dose of lisinopril (see WARNINGS). If hypotension occurs (systolic blood pressure ≤100 mm Hg) a daily maintenance dose of 5 mg may be given with temporary reductions to 2.5 mg if needed. If prolonged hypotension occurs (systolic blood pressure <90 mm Hg for more than 1 hour) lisinopril should be withdrawn. For patients who develop symptoms of heart failure, see Heart Failure.

Dosage Adjustment in Patients With Myocardial Infarction With Renal Impairment

In acute myocardial infarction, treatment with lisinopril should be initiated with caution in patients with evidence of renal dysfunction, defined as serum creatinine concentration exceeding 2 mg/dl. No evaluation of dosage adjustment in myocardial infarction patients with severe renal impairment has been performed.

USE IN ELDERLY

In general, blood pressure response and adverse experiences were similar in younger and older patients given similar doses of lisinopril. Pharmacokinetic studies, however, indicate that maximum blood levels and area under the plasma concentration time curve (AUC) are doubled in older patients, so that dosage adjustments should be made with particular caution.

HOW SUPPLIED

Prinivil tablets are available in:

2.5 mg: White, round, flat-faced, beveled edged, compressed tablets, coded "MSD" on one side and "15" on the other.

5 mg: White, shield shaped, scored, compressed tablets, with code "MSD 19" on one side and "PRINIVIL" on the other.

10 mg: Light yellow, shield shaped, compressed tablets, with code "MSD 106" on one side and "PRINIVIL" on the other.

20 mg: Peach, shield shaped, compressed tablets, with code "MSD 207" on one side and "PRINIVIL" on the other.

40 mg: Rose red, shield shaped, compressed tablets, with code "MSD 237" on one side and "PRINIVIL" on the other.

STORAGE

Store at controlled room temperature, 15-30°C (59-86°F), and protect from moisture.

Dispense in a tight container, if product package is subdivided.

PRODUCT LISTING - RATED THERAPEUTICALLY EQUIVALENT

Tablet - Oral - 2.5 mg

30's	$21.61	PRINIVIL, Merck & Company Inc	00006-0015-31
100's	$63.55	GENERIC, Ivax Corporation	00172-3757-60
100's	$64.14	GENERIC, Teva Pharmaceuticals Usa	00093-1111-01
100's	$64.15	GENERIC, West Ward Pharmaceutical Corporation	00143-1265-01
100's	$64.20	GENERIC, Mylan Pharmaceuticals Inc	00378-2072-01
100's	$64.85	GENERIC, Eon Labs Manufacturing Inc	00185-0025-01
100's	$64.85	GENERIC, Geneva Pharmaceuticals	00781-1669-01
100's	$72.06	PRINIVIL, Merck & Company Inc	00006-0015-28
100's	$72.06	PRINIVIL, Merck & Company Inc	00006-0015-58
100's	$74.18	ZESTRIL, Astra-Zeneca Pharmaceuticals	00310-0135-10

Tablet - Oral - 5 mg

30's	$28.93	ZESTRIL, Physicians Total Care	54868-1961-01
30's	$34.14	PRINIVIL, Physicians Total Care	54868-1960-00
31 x 25	$790.81	PRINIVIL, Merck & Company Inc	00006-0019-72
60's	$53.88	PRINIVIL, Allscripts Pharmaceutical Company	54569-3300-01
90 x 12	$1057.96	PRINIVIL, Merck & Company Inc	00006-0019-94
90's	$70.76	ZESTRIL, Allscripts Pharmaceutical Company	54569-8584-00
100's	$25.51	ZESTRIL, Allscripts Pharmaceutical Company	54569-3771-00
100's	$81.00	ZESTRIL, Southwood Pharmaceuticals Inc	58016-2638-90
100's	$81.77	ZESTRIL, Astra-Zeneca Pharmaceuticals	00038-0130-10
100's	$81.77	ZESTRIL, Astra-Zeneca Pharmaceuticals	00038-0130-39
100's	$91.44	GENERIC, Udl Laboratories Inc	51079-0981-20
100's	$95.25	GENERIC, Ivax Corporation	00172-3758-60
100's	$96.16	GENERIC, Teva Pharmaceuticals Usa	00093-1112-01
100's	$96.20	GENERIC, West Ward Pharmaceutical Corporation	00143-1266-01
100's	$96.25	GENERIC, Mylan Pharmaceuticals Inc	00378-2073-01
100's	$96.78	ZESTRIL, Physicians Total Care	54868-1961-02
100's	$97.24	GENERIC, Geneva Pharmaceuticals	00781-1665-01
100's	$97.25	GENERIC, Eon Labs Manufacturing Inc	00185-5400-01
100's	$108.05	PRINIVIL, Merck & Company Inc	00006-0019-28
100's	$108.05	PRINIVIL, Merck & Company Inc	00006-0019-58
100's	$111.21	ZESTRIL, Astra-Zeneca Pharmaceuticals	00310-0130-10
100's	$111.21	ZESTRIL, Astra-Zeneca Pharmaceuticals	00310-0130-39

Tablet - Oral - 10 mg

3's	$7.76	ZESTRIL, Quality Care Pharmaceuticals Inc	60346-0871-03
8's	$11.15	PRINIVIL, Southwood Pharmaceuticals Inc	58016-0599-08
8's	$11.25	PRINIVIL, Pd-Rx Pharmaceuticals	55289-0929-08
30's	$27.72	ZESTRIL, Compumed Pharmaceuticals	00403-3029-30
30's	$28.93	PRINIVIL, Allscripts Pharmaceutical Company	54569-1752-03
30's	$29.86	ZESTRIL, Physicians Total Care	54868-1296-01
30's	$33.47	PRINIVIL, Merck & Company Inc	00006-0106-31
30's	$35.21	PRINIVIL, Physicians Total Care	54868-1970-02
30's	$37.35	ZESTRIL, Cheshire Drugs	55175-3964-03
30's	$40.54	ZESTRIL, Quality Care Pharmaceuticals Inc	60346-0871-30
31 x 25	$816.69	PRINIVIL, Merck & Company Inc	00006-0106-72
60's	$50.72	ZESTRIL, Allscripts Pharmaceutical Company	54569-1944-02
90's	$73.14	PRINIVIL, Allscripts Pharmaceutical Company	54569-8583-00
90's	$73.16	ZESTRIL, Allscripts Pharmaceutical Company	54569-8515-00
100's	$73.05	ZESTRIL, Compumed Pharmaceuticals	00403-3029-01
100's	$84.54	ZESTRIL, Astra-Zeneca Pharmaceuticals	00038-0131-10
100's	$84.54	ZESTRIL, Astra-Zeneca Pharmaceuticals	00038-0131-39
100's	$84.54	ZESTRIL, Allscripts Pharmaceutical Company	54569-1944-01
100's	$94.43	GENERIC, Udl Laboratories Inc	51079-0982-20
100's	$94.52	ZESTRIL, Physicians Total Care	54868-1296-02
100's	$98.35	GENERIC, Ivax Corporation	00172-3759-60
100's	$99.30	GENERIC, Teva Pharmaceuticals Usa	00093-1113-01
100's	$99.40	GENERIC, Mylan Pharmaceuticals Inc	00378-2074-01
100's	$99.45	GENERIC, West Ward Pharmaceutical Corporation	00143-1267-01
100's	$100.42	GENERIC, Eon Labs Manufacturing Inc	00185-0101-01
100's	$100.42	GENERIC, Geneva Pharmaceuticals	00781-1666-01
100's	$111.58	PRINIVIL, Merck & Company Inc	00006-0106-28
100's	$111.58	PRINIVIL, Merck & Company Inc	00006-0106-58
100's	$114.04	PRINIVIL, Physicians Total Care	54868-1970-01
100's	$114.84	ZESTRIL, Astra-Zeneca Pharmaceuticals	00310-0131-10
100's	$114.84	ZESTRIL, Astra-Zeneca Pharmaceuticals	00310-0131-39

Tablet - Oral - 20 mg

14's	$14.41	ZESTRIL, Southwood Pharmaceuticals Inc	58016-0363-14
21's	$21.62	ZESTRIL, Southwood Pharmaceuticals Inc	58016-0363-21
30's	$27.14	ZESTRIL, Allscripts Pharmaceutical Company	54569-2665-01
30's	$28.70	ZESTRIL, Compumed Pharmaceuticals	00403-2779-30
30's	$30.97	PRINIVIL, Allscripts Pharmaceutical Company	54569-2051-01
30's	$33.11	ZESTRIL, Physicians Total Care	54868-1001-01
30's	$35.14	PRINIVIL, Physicians Total Care	54868-1502-00
30's	$35.82	PRINIVIL, Merck & Company Inc	00006-0207-31
30's	$38.89	ZESTRIL, Southwood Pharmaceuticals Inc	58016-0363-30
30's	$39.43	ZESTRIL, Pd-Rx Pharmaceuticals	55289-0106-30
30's	$45.54	PRINIVIL, Pd-Rx Pharmaceuticals	55289-0577-30
31 x 25	$722.98	PRINIVIL, Merck & Company Inc	00006-0207-72
60's	$54.29	ZESTRIL, Allscripts Pharmaceutical Company	54569-2665-02
60's	$61.77	ZESTRIL, Southwood Pharmaceuticals Inc	58016-0363-60
60's	$61.94	PRINIVIL, Allscripts Pharmaceutical Company	54569-2051-02
90's	$78.30	ZESTRIL, Allscripts Pharmaceutical Company	54569-8527-00
90's	$107.51	PRINIVIL, Merck & Company Inc	00006-0207-54
100's	$80.95	ZESTRIL, Compumed Pharmaceuticals	00403-2779-01
100's	$90.48	ZESTRIL, Astra-Zeneca Pharmaceuticals	00038-0132-10
100's	$90.48	ZESTRIL, Astra-Zeneca Pharmaceuticals	00038-0132-39
100's	$101.10	GENERIC, Udl Laboratories Inc	51079-0983-20
100's	$102.95	ZESTRIL, Southwood Pharmaceuticals Inc	58016-0363-00
100's	$105.30	GENERIC, Ivax Corporation	00172-3760-60
100's	$106.31	GENERIC, Teva Pharmaceuticals Usa	00093-1114-01
100's	$106.40	GENERIC, Mylan Pharmaceuticals Inc	00378-2075-01
100's	$106.80	GENERIC, West Ward Pharmaceutical Corporation	00143-1268-01
100's	$107.50	GENERIC, Geneva Pharmaceuticals	00781-1667-01
100's	$107.51	GENERIC, Eon Labs Manufacturing Inc	00185-0102-01
100's	$119.45	PRINIVIL, Merck & Company Inc	00006-0207-28
100's	$119.45	PRINIVIL, Merck & Company Inc	00006-0207-58
100's	$122.94	ZESTRIL, Astra-Zeneca Pharmaceuticals	00310-0132-10
100's	$122.94	ZESTRIL, Astra-Zeneca Pharmaceuticals	00310-0132-39

Tablet - Oral - 30 mg

100's	$149.10	GENERIC, Ivax Corporation	00172-3762-60
100's	$150.60	GENERIC, Mylan Pharmaceuticals Inc	00378-2077-01
100's	$150.75	GENERIC, Geneva Pharmaceuticals	00781-1673-01
100's	$150.76	GENERIC, Teva Pharmaceuticals Usa	00093-5157-01
100's	$150.76	GENERIC, Eon Labs Manufacturing Inc	00185-0103-01
100's	$174.05	ZESTRIL, Astra-Zeneca Pharmaceuticals	00310-0133-10

Tablet - Oral - 40 mg

30's	$53.49	ZESTRIL, Quality Care Pharmaceuticals Inc	60346-0595-30
100's	$125.50	GENERIC, West Ward Pharmaceutical Corporation	00143-1270-01
100's	$132.17	ZESTRIL, Astra-Zeneca Pharmaceuticals	00038-0134-10
100's	$147.84	GENERIC, Udl Laboratories Inc	51079-0984-20
100's	$154.00	GENERIC, Ivax Corporation	00172-3761-60
100's	$155.46	GENERIC, Teva Pharmaceuticals Usa	00093-1115-01
100's	$155.60	GENERIC, Mylan Pharmaceuticals Inc	00378-2076-01
100's	$157.21	GENERIC, Eon Labs Manufacturing Inc	00185-0104-01
100's	$157.21	GENERIC, Geneva Pharmaceuticals	00781-1668-01
100's	$174.68	PRINIVIL, Merck & Company Inc	00006-0237-58
100's	$179.79	ZESTRIL, Astra-Zeneca Pharmaceuticals	00310-0134-10

PRODUCT LISTING - EQUIVALENTS NOT AVAILABLE

Tablet - Oral - 2.5 mg

100's	$63.89	GENERIC, Watson Laboratories Inc	00591-0405-01
100's	$64.24	GENERIC, Par Pharmaceutical Inc	49884-0556-01

Tablet - Oral - 5 mg

100's	$95.82	GENERIC, Watson Laboratories Inc	00591-0406-01
100's	$96.33	GENERIC, Par Pharmaceutical Inc	49884-0557-01
100's	$97.25	GENERIC, Ivax Corporation	00172-3758-10

Tablet - Oral - 10 mg

3's	$2.78	ZESTRIL, Allscripts Pharmaceutical Company	54569-1944-03
14's	$13.43	ZESTRIL, Southwood Pharmaceuticals Inc	58016-0362-14
21's	$20.15	ZESTRIL, Southwood Pharmaceuticals Inc	58016-0362-21
28's	$26.87	ZESTRIL, Southwood Pharmaceuticals Inc	58016-0362-28
30's	$28.79	ZESTRIL, Southwood Pharmaceuticals Inc	58016-0362-30
30's	$28.94	ZESTRIL, Allscripts Pharmaceutical Company	54569-1944-00
60's	$57.57	ZESTRIL, Southwood Pharmaceuticals Inc	58016-0362-60
100's	$95.95	ZESTRIL, Southwood Pharmaceuticals Inc	58016-0362-00
100's	$98.92	GENERIC, Watson Laboratories Inc	00591-0407-01
100's	$99.47	GENERIC, Par Pharmaceutical Inc	49884-0558-01
100's	$100.35	GENERIC, Ivax Corporation	00172-3759-10

Tablet - Oral - 20 mg

100's	$105.90	GENERIC, Watson Laboratories Inc	00591-0408-01
100's	$106.49	GENERIC, Par Pharmaceutical Inc	49884-0559-01

Tablet - Oral - 30 mg

100's	$149.92	GENERIC, Watson Laboratories Inc	00591-0885-01
100's	$150.75	GENERIC, Par Pharmaceutical Inc	49884-0635-01

Tablet - Oral - 40 mg

100's	$154.87	GENERIC, Watson Laboratories Inc	00591-0409-01
100's	$155.72	GENERIC, Par Pharmaceutical Inc	49884-0560-01

Lithium Carbonate (001648)

Categories: Bipolar affective disorder; Mania; FDA Approved 1970 Apr; Pregnancy Category D; WHO Formulary
Drug Classes: Antipsychotics
Brand Names: **Eskalith**; Eskalith-Cr; Lithane; Lithobid; Lithonate; Lithotabs
Foreign Brand Availability: Camcolit (Bahamas; Bahrain; Barbados; Belgium; Belize; Benin; Bermuda; Burkina-Faso; Curacao; Cyprus; Egypt; England; Ethiopia; Gambia; Ghana; Guinea; Guyana; Hong-Kong; Iran; Iraq; Ireland; Ivory-Coast; Jamaica; Jordan; Kenya; Kuwait; Lebanon; Liberia; Libya; Malawi; Mali; Mauritania; Mauritius; Morocco; Netherland-Antilles; Netherlands; Niger; Nigeria; Oman; Qatar; Republic-of-Yemen; Saudi-Arabia; Senegal; Seychelles; Sierra-Leone; Singapore; South-Africa; Sudan; Surinam; Syria; Taiwan; Tanzania; Trinidad; Tunia; Uganda; United-Arab-Emirates; Zambia; Zimbabwe); Carbolit (Colombia; Mexico); Carbolith (Canada); Ceglution (Argentina); Ceglution 300 (Ecuador); Duralith (Canada); Hynorex Retard (Germany; Switzerland); Lentolith (South-Africa); Licab (India); Licarb (Thailand); Licarbium (Israel); Lidin (Taiwan); Limas (Japan); Liskonum (Bahrain; Benin; Burkina-Faso; Cyprus; Egypt; Ethiopia; Gambia; Ghana; Guinea; Iran; Iraq; Ivory-Coast; Jordan; Kenya; Kuwait; Lebanon; Liberia; Libya; Malawi; Mali; Mauritania; Mauritius; Morocco; Niger; Nigeria; Oman; Qatar; Republic-of-Yemen; Saudi-Arabia; Senegal; Seychelles; Sierra-Leone; Sudan; Syria; Tanzania; Tunia; Uganda; United-Arab-Emirates; Zambia; Zimbabwe); Litheum 300 (Mexico); Lithicarb (Australia; Malaysia; New-Zealand); Lithionate (Taiwan); Lithocap (India); Litilent (Argentina); Litocarb (Peru); Maniprex (Belgium); Phanate (Thailand); Plenur (Spain); Priadel (Belgium; England; Netherlands; New-Zealand; Singapore); Priadel Retard (Greece; Switzerland); Quilonium-R (Philippines); Quilonorm Retardtabletten (Switzerland); Quilonum Retard (Czech-Republic; Germany; South-Africa); Quilonum SR (Australia); Teralithe (France); Theralite (Colombia)
Cost of Therapy: $18.32 (Bipolar Disorder; Eskalith; 300 mg; 3 capsules/day; 30 day supply)
$6.30 (Bipolar Disorder; Generic Capsules; 300 mg; 3 capsules/day; 30 day supply)
$8.20 (Bipolar Disorder; Generic Tablets; 300 mg; 3 tablets/day; 30 day supply)
$31.73 (Bipolar Disorder; Eskalith-CR; 450 mg; 2 tablets/day; 30 day supply)

WARNING

Note: The trade names have been used throughout this monograph for clarity.

Lithium toxicity is closely related to serum lithium levels, and can occur at doses close to therapeutic levels. Facilities for prompt and accurate serum lithium determinations should be available before initiating therapy (see DOSAGE AND ADMINISTRATION).

DESCRIPTION

Eskalith contains lithium carbonate, a white, light alkaline powder with molecular formula Li_2CO_3 and molecular weight 73.89. Lithium is an element of the alkali-metal group with atomic number 3, atomic weight 6.94 and an emission line at 671 nm on the flame photometer.

ESKALITH CAPSULES

Each capsule, with opaque gray cap and opaque yellow body, is imprinted with the product name "ESKALITH" and "SB" and contains lithium carbonate, 300 mg. Inactive ingredients consist of benzyl alcohol, cetylpyridinium chloride, D&C yellow no. 10, FD&C green no. 3, FD&C red no. 40, FD&C yellow no. 6, gelatin, lactose, magnesium stearate, povidone, sodium lauryl sulfate, titanium dioxide and trace amounts of other inactive ingredients.

ESKALITH CR CONTROLLED-RELEASE TABLETS

Each round, yellow, biconvex tablet, debossed with "SKF" and "J10" on one side and scored on the other side, contains lithium carbonate, 450 mg. Inactive ingredients consist of alginic acid, gelatin, iron oxide, magnesium stearate and sodium starch glycolate.

Eskalith CR tablets 450 mg are designed to release a portion of the dose initially and the remainder gradually; the release pattern of the controlled-release tablets reduces the variability in lithium blood levels seen with the immediate-release dosage forms.

CLINICAL PHARMACOLOGY

Preclinical studies have shown that lithium alters sodium transport in nerve and muscle cells and effects a shift toward intraneuronal metabolism of catecholamines, but the specific biochemical mechanism of lithium action in mania is unknown.

INDICATIONS AND USAGE

Eskalith (lithium carbonate) is indicated in the treatment of manic episodes of manic-depressive illness. Maintenance therapy prevents or diminishes the intensity of subsequent episodes in those manic-depressive patients with a history of mania.

Typical symptoms of mania include pressure of speech, motor hyperactivity, reduced need for sleep, flight of ideas, grandiosity, elation, poor judgment, aggressiveness and possibly hostility. When given to a patient experiencing a manic episode, Eskalith may produce a normalization of symptomatology within 1-3 weeks.

NON-FDA APPROVED INDICATIONS

Although not approved by the FDA, lithium has also been used for the treatment of cluster headaches and hyperthyroidism. One meta-analysis has concluded that with respect to efficacy, lithium augmentation of conventional antidepressants is the first choice treatment procedure for depressed patients who fail to respond to antidepressant monotherapy.

WARNINGS

Lithium should generally not be given to patients with significant renal or cardiovascular disease, severe debilitation or dehydration, or sodium depletion, since the risk of lithium toxicity is very high in such patients. If the psychiatric indication is life-threatening, and if such a patient fails to respond to other measures, lithium treatment may be undertaken with extreme caution, including daily serum lithium determinations and adjustment to the usually low doses ordinarily tolerated by these individuals. In such instances, hospitalization is a necessity.

Chronic lithium therapy may be associated with diminution of renal concentrating ability, occasionally presenting as nephrogenic diabetes insipidus, with polyuria and polydipsia. Such patients should be carefully managed to avoid dehydration with resulting lithium retention and toxicity. This condition is usually reversible when lithium is discontinued.

Morphologic changes with glomerular and interstitial fibrosis and nephron atrophy have been reported in patients on chronic lithium therapy. Morphologic changes have also been seen in manic-depressive patients never exposed to lithium. The relationship between renal functional and morphologic changes and their association with lithium therapy have not been established.

When kidney function is assessed, for baseline data prior to starting lithium therapy or thereafter, routine urinalysis and other tests may be used to evaluate tubular function (*e.g.*, urine specific gravity or osmolality following a period of water deprivation, or 24 hour urine volume) and glomerular function (*e.g.*, serum creatinine or creatinine clearance). During lithium therapy, progressive or sudden changes in renal function, even within the normal range, indicate the need for reevaluation of treatment.

An encephalopathic syndrome (characterized by weakness, lethargy, fever, tremulousness and confusion, extrapyramidal symptoms, leukocytosis, elevated serum enzymes, BUN and FBS) has occurred in a few patients treated with lithium plus a neuroleptic. In some instances, the syndrome was followed by irreversible brain damage. Because of a possible causal relationship between these events and the concomitant administration of lithium and neuroleptics, patients receiving such combined therapy should be monitored closely for early evidence of neurologic toxicity and treatment discontinued promptly if such signs appear. This encephalopathic syndrome may be similar to or the same as neuroleptic malignant syndrome (NMS).

Lithium toxicity is closely related to serum lithium levels, and can occur at doses close to therapeutic levels (see DOSAGE AND ADMINISTRATION).

Outpatients and their families should be warned that the patient must discontinue lithium carbonate therapy and contact his physician if such clinical signs of lithium toxicity as diarrhea, vomiting, tremor, mild ataxia, drowsiness or muscular weakness occur.

Lithium carbonate may impair mental and/or physical abilities. Caution patients about activities requiring alertness (*e.g.*, operating vehicles or machinery).

Lithium may prolong the effects of neuromuscular blocking agents. Therefore, neuromuscular blocking agents should be given with caution to patients receiving lithium.

USAGE IN PREGNANCY

Adverse effects on implantation in rats, embryo viability in mice and metabolism *in vitro* of rat testes and human spermatozoa have been attributed to lithium, as have teratogenicity in submammalian species and cleft palates in mice.

In humans, lithium carbonate may cause fetal harm when administered to a pregnant woman. Data from lithium birth registries suggest an increase in cardiac and other anomalies, especially Ebstein's anomaly. If this drug is used in women of childbearing potential, or during pregnancy, or if a patient becomes pregnant while taking this drug, the patient should be apprised of the potential hazard to the fetus.

USAGE IN NURSING MOTHERS

Lithium is excreted in human milk. Nursing should not be undertaken during lithium therapy except in rare and unusual circumstances where, in the view of the physician, the potential benefits to the mother outweigh possible hazards to the child.

USAGE IN PEDIATRIC PATIENTS

Since information regarding the safety and effectiveness of lithium carbonate in children under 12 years of age is not available, its use in such patients is not recommended.

There has been a report of a transient syndrome of acute dystonia and hyperreflexia occurring in a 15 kg child who ingested 300 mg of lithium carbonate.

USAGE IN THE ELDERLY

Elderly patients often require lower lithium dosages to achieve therapeutic serum levels. They may also exhibit adverse reactions at serum levels ordinarily tolerated by younger patients.

PRECAUTIONS

GENERAL

The ability to tolerate lithium is greater during the acute manic phase and decreases when manic symptoms subside (see DOSAGE AND ADMINISTRATION).

The distribution space of lithium approximates that of total body water. Lithium is primarily excreted in urine with insignificant excretion in feces. Renal excretion of lithium is proportional to its plasma concentration. The half-life of elimination of lithium is approximately 24 hours. Lithium decreases sodium reabsorption by the renal tubules which could lead to sodium depletion. Therefore, it is essential for the patient to maintain a normal diet, including salt, and an adequate fluid intake (2500-3000 ml) at least during the initial stabilization period. Decreased tolerance to lithium has been reported to ensue from protracted sweating or diarrhea and, if such occur, supplemental fluid and salt should be administered under careful medical supervision and lithium intake reduced or suspended until the condition is resolved.

In addition to sweating and diarrhea, concomitant infection with elevated temperatures may also necessitate a temporary reduction or cessation of medication.

Previously existing underlying thyroid disorders do not necessarily constitute a contraindication to lithium treatment; where hypothyroidism exists, careful monitoring of thyroid function during lithium stabilization and maintenance allows for correction of changing thyroid parameters, if any; where hypothyroidism occurs during lithium stabilization and maintenance, supplemental thyroid treatment may be used.

DRUG INTERACTIONS

Caution should be used when lithium and diuretics are used concomitantly because diuretic-induced sodium loss may reduce the renal clearance of lithium and increase serum lithium levels with risk of lithium toxicity. Patients receiving such combined therapy should have serum lithium levels monitored closely and the lithium dosage adjusted if necessary.

Lithium levels should be closely monitored when patients initiate or discontinue NSAID use. In some cases, lithium toxicity has resulted from interactions between an NSAID and lithium. Indomethacin and piroxicam have been reported to increase significantly steady-state plasma lithium concentrations. There is also evidence that other nonsteroidal anti-inflammatory agents, including the selective cyclooxygenase-2 (COX-2) inhibitors, have the same effect. In a study conducted in healthy subjects, mean steady-state lithium plasma levels increased approximately 17% in subjects receiving lithium 450 mg bid with celecoxib 200 mg bid as compared to subjects receiving lithium alone.

Concurrent use of metronidazole with lithium may provoke lithium toxicity due to reduced renal clearance. Patients receiving such combined therapy should be monitored closely.

There is evidence that angiotensin-converting enzyme inhibitors, such as enalapril and captopril, may substantially increase steady-state plasma lithium levels, sometimes resulting in lithium toxicity. When such combinations are used, lithium dosage may need to be decreased, and plasma lithium levels should be measured more often.

Concurrent use of calcium channel blocking agents with lithium may increase the risk of neurotoxicity in the form of ataxia, tremors, nausea, vomiting, diarrhea and/or tinnitus. Caution is recommended.

The concomitant administration of lithium with selective serotonin reuptake inhibitors should be undertaken with caution as this combination has been reported to result in symptoms such as diarrhea, confusion, tremor, dizziness and agitation.

The following drugs can lower serum lithium concentrations by increasing urinary lithium excretion: Acetazolamide, urea, xanthine preparations and alkalinizing agents such as sodium bicarbonate.

The following have also been shown to interact with lithium: Methyldopa, phenytoin and carbamazepine.

ADVERSE REACTIONS

The occurrence and severity of adverse reactions are generally directly related to serum lithium concentrations as well as to individual patient sensitivity to lithium, and generally occur more frequently and with greater severity at higher concentrations.

Adverse reactions may be encountered at serum lithium levels below 1.5 mEq/L. Mild to moderate adverse reactions may occur at levels from 1.5-2.5 mEq/L, and moderate to severe reactions may be seen at levels of 2.0 mEq/L and above.

Fine hand tremor, polyuria and mild thirst may occur during initial therapy for the acute manic phase, and may persist throughout treatment. Transient and mild nausea and general discomfort may also appear during the first few days of lithium administration.

These side effects usually subside with continued treatment or a temporary reduction or cessation of dosage. If persistent, cessation of lithium therapy may be required.

Diarrhea, vomiting, drowsiness, muscular weakness and lack of coordination may be early signs of lithium intoxication, and can occur at lithium levels below 2.0 mEq/L. At higher levels, ataxia, giddiness, tinnitus, blurred vision and a large output of dilute urine may be seen. Serum lithium levels above 3.0 mEq/L may produce a complex clinical picture, involving multiple organs and organ systems. Serum lithium levels should not be permitted to exceed 2.0 mEq/L during the acute treatment phase.

The following reactions have been reported and appear to be related to serum lithium levels, including levels within the therapeutic range:

Neuromuscular/Central Nervous System: Tremor, muscle hyperirritability (fasciculations, twitching, clonic movements of whole limbs), hypertonicity, ataxia, choreoathetotic movements, hyperactive deep tendon reflex, extrapyramidal symptoms including acute dystonia, cogwheel rigidity, blackout spells, epileptiform seizures, slurred speech, dizziness, vertigo, downbeat nystagmus, incontinence of urine or feces, somnolence, psychomotor retardation, restlessness, confusion, stupor, coma, tongue movements, tics, tinnitus, hallucinations, poor memory, slowed intellectual functioning, startled response, worsening of organic brain syndromes, myasthenia gravis (rarely).

Cardiovascular: Cardiac arrhythmia, hypotension, peripheral circulatory collapse, bradycardia, sinus node dysfunction with severe bradycardia (which may result in syncope).

Gastrointestinal: Anorexia, nausea, vomiting, diarrhea, gastritis, salivary gland swelling, abdominal pain, excessive salivation, flatulence, indigestion.

Genitourinary: Glycosuria, decreased creatinine clearance, albuminuria, oliguria, and symptoms of nephrogenic diabetes insipidus including polyuria, thirst and polydipsia.

Dermatologic: Drying and thinning of hair, alopecia, anesthesia of skin, acne, chronic folliculitis, xerosis cutis, psoriasis or its exacerbation, generalized pruritus with or without rash, cutaneous ulcers, angioedema.

Autonomic: Blurred vision, dry mouth, impotence/sexual dysfunction.

Thyroid Abnormalities: Euthyroid goiter and/or hypothyroidism (including myxedema) accompanied by lower T_3 and T_4. I^{131} uptake may be elevated. (See PRECAUTIONS.) Paradoxically, rare cases of hyperthyroidism have been reported.

EEG Changes: Diffuse slowing, widening of the frequency spectrum, potentiation and disorganization of background rhythm.

EKG Changes: Reversible flattening, isoelectricity or inversion of T-waves.

Miscellaneous: Fatigue, lethargy, transient scotomata, exophthalmos, dehydration, weight loss, leukocytosis, headache, transient hyperglycemia, hypercalcemia, hyperparathyroidism, excessive weight gain, edematous swelling of ankles or wrists, metallic taste, dysgeusia/taste distortion, salty taste, thirst, swollen lips, tightness in chest, swollen and/or painful joints, fever, polyarthralgia, dental caries.

Some reports of nephrogenic diabetes insipidus, hyperparathyroidism and hypothyroidism which persist after lithium discontinuation have been received.

A few reports have been received of the development of painful discoloration of fingers and toes and coldness of the extremities within one day of the starting of treatment with lithium. The mechanism through which these symptoms (resembling Raynaud's syndrome) developed is not known. Recovery followed discontinuance.

Cases of pseudotumor cerebri (increased intracranial pressure and papilledema) have been reported with lithium use. If undetected, this condition may result in enlargement of the blind spot, constriction of visual fields and eventual blindness due to optic atrophy. Lithium should be discontinued, if clinically possible, if this syndrome occurs.

DOSAGE AND ADMINISTRATION

Immediate-release capsules are usually given tid or qid. Doses of controlled-release tablets are usually given bid (approximately 12 hour intervals). When initiating therapy with immediate-release or controlled-release lithium, dosage must be individualized according to serum levels and clinical response.

When switching a patient from immediate-release capsules to Eskalith CR controlled-release tablets, give the same total daily dose when possible. Most patients on maintenance therapy are stabilized on 900 mg daily, *e.g.*, Eskalith CR 450 mg bid. When the previous dosage of immediate-release lithium is not a multiple of 450 mg, *e.g.*, 1500 mg, initiate Eskalith CR at the multiple of 450 mg nearest to, but below, the original daily dose, *i.e.*, 1350 mg. When the 2 doses are unequal, give the larger dose in the evening. In the above example, with a total daily dose of 1350 mg, generally 450 mg of Eskalith CR should be given in the morning and 900 mg of Eskalith CR in the evening. If desired, the total daily dose of 1350 mg can be given in 3 equal 450 mg doses of Eskalith CR. These patients should be monitored at 1-2 week intervals, and dosage adjusted if necessary, until stable and satisfactory serum levels and clinical state are achieved.

When patients require closer titration than that available with doses of Eskalith CR in increments of 450 mg, immediate-release capsules should be used.

ACUTE MANIA

Optimal patient response to Eskalith can usually be established and maintained with 1800 mg/day in divided doses. Such doses will normally produce the desired serum lithium level ranging between 1.0 and 1.5 mEq/L.

Dosage must be individualized according to serum levels and clinical response. Regular monitoring of the patient's clinical state and serum lithium levels is necessary. Serum levels should be determined twice per week during the acute phase, and until the serum level and clinical condition of the patient have been stabilized.

LONG-TERM CONTROL

The desirable serum lithium levels are 0.6-1.2 mEq/L. Dosage will vary from one individual to another, but usually 900-1200 mg/day in divided doses will maintain this level. Serum lithium levels in uncomplicated cases receiving maintenance therapy during remission should be monitored at least every 2 months.

Patients unusually sensitive to lithium may exhibit toxic signs at serum levels below 1.0 mEq/L.

N.B.

Blood samples for serum lithium determinations should be drawn immediately prior to the next dose when lithium concentrations are relatively stable (*i.e.*, 8-12 hours after the previous dose). Total reliance must not be placed on serum levels alone. Accurate patient evaluation requires both clinical and laboratory analysis.

Elderly patients often respond to reduced dosage, and may exhibit signs of toxicity at serum levels ordinarily tolerated by younger patients.

HOW SUPPLIED

Eskalith capsules:

300 mg: Gray and yellow, imprinted with the product name "ESKALITH" and "SB", in bottles of 100.

Eskalith CR controlled-release tablets:
450 mg: Round, yellow, biconvex, debossed with "SKF" and "J10" on one side and scored on the other side, in bottles of 100.
Storage Conditions: Store between 15 and 30°C (59 and 86°F).

PRODUCT LISTING - RATED THERAPEUTICALLY EQUIVALENT

Qty	Price	Product	NDC
Capsule - Oral - 300 mg			
30's	$3.13	GENERIC, Heartland Healthcare Services	61392-0131-30
30's	$3.13	GENERIC, Heartland Healthcare Services	61392-0131-39
31's	$3.23	GENERIC, Heartland Healthcare Services	61392-0131-31
32's	$3.33	GENERIC, Heartland Healthcare Services	61392-0131-32
45's	$4.69	GENERIC, Heartland Healthcare Services	61392-0131-45
60's	$6.25	GENERIC, Heartland Healthcare Services	61392-0131-60
90's	$5.70	GENERIC, Major Pharmaceuticals Inc	00904-2912-89
90's	$9.38	GENERIC, Heartland Healthcare Services	61392-0131-90
100's	$7.00	GENERIC, Major Pharmaceuticals Inc	00904-2912-60
100's	$7.98	GENERIC, Caremark Inc	00339-5771-12
100's	$8.48	GENERIC, Qualitest Products Inc	00603-4220-21
100's	$8.71	GENERIC, Moore, H.L. Drug Exchange Inc	00839-7149-06
100's	$13.25	GENERIC, Major Pharmaceuticals Inc	00904-2912-61
100's	$17.40	GENERIC, West Ward Pharmaceutical Corporation	00143-3189-01
100's	$17.46	GENERIC, Roxane Laboratories Inc	00054-2527-25
100's	$20.35	ESKALITH, Glaxosmithkline	00007-4007-20
100's	$20.95	GENERIC, Roxane Laboratories Inc	00054-8527-25
100's	$21.78	GENERIC, Major Pharmaceuticals Inc	00904-5568-60
100's	$22.00	GENERIC, Able Laboratories Inc	53265-0270-10
120's	$7.10	GENERIC, Major Pharmaceuticals Inc	00904-2912-18
Syrup - Oral - 300 mg/5 ml			
5 ml x 50	$25.00	GENERIC, Raway Pharmacal Inc	00686-0652-10
5 ml x 100	$72.00	GENERIC, Roxane Laboratories Inc	00054-8529-04
10 ml x 50	$30.00	GENERIC, Raway Pharmacal Inc	00686-0653-10
10 ml x 100	$84.00	GENERIC, Roxane Laboratories Inc	00054-8530-04
480 ml	$16.22	GENERIC, Ivax Corporation	00182-6148-40
480 ml	$16.22	GENERIC, Aligen Independent Laboratories Inc	00405-3223-16
480 ml	$16.25	GENERIC, Geneva Pharmaceuticals	00781-6100-16
480 ml	$17.50	GENERIC, Raway Pharmacal Inc	00686-6100-16
480 ml	$19.10	GENERIC, Major Pharmaceuticals Inc	00904-2914-16
480 ml	$19.29	GENERIC, Morton Grove Pharmaceuticals Inc	60432-0616-16
500 ml	$19.52	GENERIC, Roxane Laboratories Inc	00054-3527-63
Tablet - Oral - 300 mg			
100's	$9.11	GENERIC, Caremark Inc	00339-5773-12
100's	$19.21	GENERIC, Roxane Laboratories Inc	00054-4527-25
100's	$23.05	GENERIC, Roxane Laboratories Inc	00054-8528-25

PRODUCT LISTING - EQUIVALENTS NOT AVAILABLE

Qty	Price	Product	NDC
Capsule - Oral - 150 mg			
100's	$13.97	GENERIC, Roxane Laboratories Inc	00054-2526-25
100's	$16.76	GENERIC, Roxane Laboratories Inc	00054-8526-25
Capsule - Oral - 300 mg			
7's	$5.02	GENERIC, Prescript Pharmaceuticals	00247-0179-07
9's	$5.49	GENERIC, Prescript Pharmaceuticals	00247-0179-09
12's	$4.23	GENERIC, Pharmaceutical Corporation Of America	51655-0490-27
12's	$6.21	GENERIC, Prescript Pharmaceuticals	00247-0179-12
14's	$6.69	GENERIC, Prescript Pharmaceuticals	00247-0179-14
21's	$8.35	GENERIC, Prescript Pharmaceuticals	00247-0179-21
24's	$9.07	GENERIC, Prescript Pharmaceuticals	00247-0179-24
30's	$10.49	GENERIC, Prescript Pharmaceuticals	00247-0179-30
90's	$27.51	GENERIC, Physicians Total Care	54868-1335-03
100's	$27.18	GENERIC, Prescript Pharmaceuticals	00247-0179-00
100's	$29.75	GENERIC, Physicians Total Care	54868-1335-02
Capsule - Oral - 600 mg			
100's	$34.92	GENERIC, Roxane Laboratories Inc	00054-2531-25
100's	$41.90	GENERIC, Roxane Laboratories Inc	00054-8531-25
Tablet, Extended Release - Oral - 300 mg			
100's	$34.88	GENERIC, Barr Laboratories Inc	00555-0345-02
100's	$48.14	LITHOBID, Solvay Pharmaceuticals Inc	00032-4492-01
Tablet, Extended Release - Oral - 450 mg			
100's	$52.88	ESKALITH-CR, Physicians Total Care	54868-2557-00
100's	$56.83	ESKALITH-CR, Glaxosmithkline	00007-4010-20

Lithium Citrate (001649)

Categories: Bipolar affective disorder; Mania; FDA Approved 1980 Dec; Pregnancy Category D
Drug Classes: Antipsychotics
Brand Names: Cibalith-S
Cost of Therapy: $15.21 (Bipolar Disorder; Generic Syrup; 300 mg/5 ml; 15 ml/day; 30 day supply)

WARNING

Lithium toxicity is closely related to serum lithium levels, and can occur at doses close to therapeutic levels. Facilities for prompt and accurate serum lithium determinations should be available before initiating therapy.

DESCRIPTION

Lithium Citrate Syrup is an antimanic medication for oral administration. Lithium Carbonate is a film-coated, slow-release, 300-mg lithium carbonate tablet. This slowly dissolving, film-coated tablet is designed to give lower serum lithium peaks than obtained with conventional oral lithium dosage forms.

Lithium citrate syrup contains 8 mEq of lithium per 5 ml, equivalent to the amount in 300 mg of lithium carbonate.

Lithium citrate is prepared in solution from lithium hydroxide and citric acid in a ratio approximating dilithium citrate.

Cibalith-S: Citric acid, raspberry flavor, alcohol 0.3% v/v, purified water sodium benzoate, sodium saccharin, and sorbitol.

INDICATIONS AND USAGE

Lithium is indicated in treatment of manic episodes of manic-depressive illness. Maintenance therapy prevents or diminishes the intensity of subsequent episodes in those manic-depressive patients with a history of mania.

Typical symptoms of mania include pressure of speech, motor hyperactivity, reduced need for sleep, flight of ideas, grandiosity, elation, poor judgement, aggressiveness, and possibly hostility. When given to a patient experiencing a manic episode, lithium may produce a normalization of symptomatology within 1 to 3 weeks.

NON-FDA APPROVED INDICATIONS

Although not approved by the FDA, lithium has also been used for the treatment of cluster headaches and hyperthyroidism. One meta-analysis has concluded that with respect to efficacy, lithium augmentation of conventional antidepressants is the first choice treatment procedure for depressed patients who fail to respond to antidepressant monotherapy.

WARNINGS

Lithium should generally not be given to patients with significant renal or cardiovascular disease, severe debilitation or dehydration, or sodium depletion, and to patients receiving diuretics, since the risk of lithium toxicity is very high in such patients. If the psychiatric indication is life-threatening, and if such a patient fails to respond to other measures, lithium treatment may be undertaken with extreme caution, including daily serum lithium determinations and adjustment to the usually low doses ordinarily tolerated by these individuals. In such instances, hospitalization is a necessity.

Lithium toxicity is closely related to serum lithium levels, and can occur at doses close to therapeutic (see DOSAGE AND ADMINISTRATION.)

Lithium therapy has been reported in some cases to be associated with morphologic changes in the kidneys. The relationship between such changes and renal function has not been established.

Outpatients and their families should be warned that the patient must discontinue lithium therapy and contact his physician if such clinical signs of lithium toxicity as diarrhea, vomiting, tremor, mild ataxia, drowsiness, or muscular weakness occur.

Lithium may impair mental and/or physical abilities. Caution patients about activities requiring alertness (*e.g.*, operating vehicles or machinery).

Lithium may prolong or potentiate the effects of neuromuscular blocking agents, such as decamethonium, pancuronium, and succinylcholine. Therefore, neuromuscular blocking agents should be given with caution to patients receiving lithium.

Combined Use Of Haloperidol And Lithium: An encephalopathic syndrome (characterized by weakness; lethargy; fever; tremulousness and confusion; extrapyramidal symptoms; leukocytosis; elevated serum enzymes, BUN, and fasting blood sugar), followed by irreversible brain damage, has occurred in a few patients treated with lithium plus haloperidol. A causal relationship between these events and the concomitant administration of lithium and haloperidol has not been established. However, patients receiving such combined therapy should be monitored closely for early evidence of neurological toxicity, and treatment discontinued promptly if such signs appear. The possibility of similar adverse interactions with other antipsychotic medications exists. In addition, concurrent use of lithium with chlorpromazine and possibly other phenothiazines decreases serum chlorpromazine levels as much as 40%.

Usage in Pregnancy: Adverse effects on nidation in rats, embryo viability in mice, and metabolism in vitro of rat testis and human spermatozoa have ben attributed to lithium, as have teratogenicity in submammalian species and cleft palates in mice.

They are lithium birth registries in the United States and elsewhere; however there are at the present time insufficient data to determine the effects of lithium on human fetuses. Therefore, at this point, lithium should not be used in pregnancy, especially the first trimester, unless in the opinion of the physician, the potential benefits outweigh the possible hazards.

Usages in Nursing Mothers: Lithium is excreted in human milk. Nursing should not be undertaken during lithium therapy except in rare and unusual circumstances where, in the view of the physician, the potential benefits to the mother outweigh possible hazards to the child.

Use in Children: Since information regarding the safety and effectiveness of lithium in children under 12 years of age is not available, its use in such patients is not recommended at this time.)

PRECAUTIONS

The ability to tolerate lithium is greater during the acute manic phase and decreases when manic symptoms subside (see DOSAGE AND ADMINISTRATION.)

The distribution space of lithium approximates that of total body water. Lithium is primarily excreted in urine with insignificant excretion in feces. Renal excretion of lithium is proportional to its plasma concentration. The half-elimination time of lithium is approximately 24 hours. Lithium decreases sodium reabsorption by the renal tubules which could lead to sodium depletion. Therefore, it is essential for the patient to maintain a normal diet, including salt, and an adequate fluid intake (2500-3000 ml) at least during the initial stabilization period. Decreased tolerance to lithium has been reported to ensure from protracted sweating or diarrhea and, if such occur, supplemental fluid and salt should be administered.

In addition to sweating and diarrhea, concomitant infection with elevated temperatures may also necessitate a temporary reduction or cessation of medication.

Previously existing underlying disorders do not necessarily constitute a contraindication to lithium treatment; where hypothyroidism exists, careful monitoring of thyroid function during lithium stabilization and maintenance allows for correction of changing thyroid parameters, if any, where hypothyroidism occurs during lithium stabilization and maintenance, supplemental thyroid treatment may be used.

DRUG INTERACTIONS

Concomitant administration of carbamazepine and lithium may increase the risk of neurotoxic side effects.

Aminophylline, caffeine, dyphylline, oxtriphylline, sodium bicarbonate, or theophylline used concurrently may decrease the therapeutic effect of lithium because of its increased urinary excretion.

Concurrent use of diuretics, especially thiazides, with lithium may provoke lithium toxicity due to reduced renal clearance.

Concurrent extended use of iodide preparations, especially potassium iodide, with lithium may produce hypothyroidism.

Indomethacin and piroxicam have been reported to increase significantly steady state plasma lithium levels. In some cases, lithium toxicity has resulted from such interactions. There is also some evidence that other nonsteroidal, and-inflammatory agents may have a similar effect. When such combinations are used, increased monitoring of plasma lithium levels is recommended (see WARNINGS.)

There is evidence that angiotensin-converting enzyme inhibitors, such as enalapril and captopril, may substantially increase steady-state plasma lithium levels, sometimes resulting in lithium toxicity. When such combinations are used, lithium dosage may need to be decreased, and plasma lithium levels should be measured more often.

ADVERSE REACTIONS

Adverse reactions are seldom encountered at serum lithium levels below 1.5 mEq/l, except in the occasional patient sensitive to lithium. Mild-to-moderate toxic reactions may occur at levels from 1.5-2.5 mEq/l, and moderate-to-severe reactions may be seen at levels from 2.0-2.5 mEq/l, depending upon individual response to the drug.

Fine hand tremor, polyuria and mild thirst may occur during initial therapy for the acute manic phase, and may persist throughout treatment. Transient and mild nausea and general discomfort may also appear during the first few days of lithium administration.

These side effects are an inconvenience rather than a disabling condition, and usually subside with continued treatment or a temporary reduction or cessation of dosage. If persistent, a cessation of dosage is indicated.

Diarrhea, vomiting, drowsiness, muscular weakness and lack of coordination may be early signs of lithium intoxication, and can occur at lithium levels below 2.0 Meq/l. At higher levels, giddiness, ataxia, blurred vision, tinnitus and a large output of dilute urine may seen. Serum lithium levels above 3.0 Meq/l may produce a complex clinical picture involving multiple organs and organ systems. Serum lithium levels should not be permitted to exceed 2.0 mEq/l during thr acute treatment phase.

The following toxic reactions have been reported and appear to be related to serum lithium levels, including levels within the therapeutic range.

Neuromuscular: tremor, muscle hyperirritability (fasciculations, twitching, clonic movements of whole limbs), ataxia, choreoathetotic movements, hyperactive deep tendon reflexes.

Central Nervous System: blackout spells, epileptiform seizures, downbeat nystagmus, acute dystonia, slurred speech, dizziness, vertigo, incontinence of urine or feces, somnolence, psychomotor retardation, restlessness, confusion, stupor, coma. Cases of pseudotumor cerebri (increased intracranial pressure and papilledema) have been reported with lithium use. If undetected, this condition may result in enlargement of the blind spot, constriction of visual fields, and eventual blindness due to optic atrophy. If this syndrome occurs, lithium should be discontinued if clinically possible.

Cardiovascular: cardiac arrhythmia, hypotension, peripheral circulatory collapse.

Gastrointestinal: anorexia, nausea, vomiting, diarrhea.

Genitourinary: albuminuria, oliguria, polyuria, glycosuria.

Dermatologic: drying and thinning of hair, anesthesia of skin, chronic folliculitis, xerosis cutis, alopecia, exacerbation of psoriasis.

Autonomic Nervous System: blurred vision, dry mouth.

Miscellaneous: fatigue, lethargy, tendency to sleep, dehydration, weight loss, transient scotomata.

Thyroid Abnormalities: euthyroid goiter and/or hypothyroidism (including myxedema) accompanied by lower T_3 and T_4. I_{131} iodine uptake may be elevated (see PRECAUTIONS.) Paradoxically, rare cases of hyperthyroidism have been reported.

EEG Changes: diffuse slowing, widening of frequency spectrum, potentiation and disorganization of background rhythm.

EKG Changes: reversible flattening, isoelectricity or inversion of T-waves.

Miscellaneous reactions unrelated to dosage are: transient electroencephalographic and electrocardiographic changes, leukocytosis, headache, diffuse nontoxic goiter with or without hypothyroidism, transient hyperglycemia, generalized pruritus with or without rash, cutaneous ulcers, albuminuria, worsening or organic brain syndromes, excessive weight gain, edematous swelling of ankles or wrists, metallic taste, and thirst or polyuria, sometimes resembling diabetes insipidus.

A single report has been received of the development of painful discoloration of fingers and toes and coldness of the extremities within one day of the starting of treatment of lithium. The mechanism through which these symptoms (resembling Raynaud's Syndrome) developed is not known. Recovery followed discontinuance.

DOSAGE AND ADMINISTRATION

Acute Mania: Optimal patient response can usually be established and maintained with the following dosages: 10 ml (2 teaspoons) (16 mEq of lithium) t.i.d.

Such doses will normally produce an effective serum lithium level ranging between 1.0 and 1.5 mEq/l. Dosage must be individualized according to serum levels and clinical response. Regular monitoring of the patient's clinical state and of serum lithium levels is necessary. Serum levels should be determined twice per week during the acute phase, and until the serum level and clinical condition of the patient have been stabilized.

Long-Term Control: The desirable serum lithium levels are 0.6 to 1.2 mEq/l. Dosage will vary from one individual to another, but usually the following dosages will maintain this level: 5 ml (1 teaspoon) (8 mEq of lithium) t.i.d. or q.i.d.

Serum lithium levels in uncomplicated cases receiving maintenance therapy during remission should be monitored at least every two months. Patients abnormally sensitive to lithium may exhibit toxic signs at serum levels of 1.0 to 1.5 mEq/l. Elderly patients often respond to reduced dosage, and may exhibit signs of toxicity at serum levels ordinarily tolerated by other patients.

N.B.: Blood samples for serum lithium determinations should be drawn immediately prior to the next dose when lithium concentrations are relatively stable (*i.e.,* 8-12 hours after previous dose). Total reliance must not be placed on serum levels alone. Accurate patient evaluation requires both clinical and laboratory analysis.

Lithium Carbonate slow-release tablets must be swallowed whole and never crushed or chewed.

Store between 59 - 89° F (15 - 30° C). Protect from light.

Dispense in tight, light-resistant, child-resistant container (USP).

Lodoxamide Tromethamine *(003184)*

Categories: Conjunctivitis, vernal; Keratitis, vernal; Keratoconjunctivitis, vernal; FDA Approved 1993 Sep; Pregnancy Category B; Orphan Drugs
Drug Classes: Mast cell stabilizers; Ophthalmics
Brand Names: **Alomide**
Foreign Brand Availability: Alconmide (Philippines); Almide (France); Alomide SE (Germany); Lomide (Australia; New-Zealand)
Cost of Therapy: $51.25 (Conjunctivitis; Alomide Ophthalmic Solution; 0.1%; 10 ml; 4 drops/day; variable day supply)

DESCRIPTION

Lodoxamide tromethamin is a sterile ophthalmic solution containing the mast cell stabilizer lodoxamide tromethamine for topical administration to the eyes. Lodoxamide tromethamine is a white, crystalline, water-soluble powder with a molecular weight of 553.91.

Chemical name: N,N'-(2-chloro-5-cyano-m-phenylene)dioxamic acid tromethamine salt.

Empirical formula: $C_{19}H_{26}O_{12}N_5Cl$

Each ml of Alomide ophthalmic solution contains:

Active: 1.78 mg lodoxamide tromethamine equivalent to 1 mg lodoxamide.

Preservative: Benzalkonium chloride 0.007%.

Inactive: Mannitol, hydroxypropyl methylcellulose 2910, sodium citrate, citric acid, edetate disodium, tyloxapol, hydrochloric acid and/or sodium hydroxide (adjust pH), and purified water.

CLINICAL PHARMACOLOGY

Lodoxamide tromethamine is a mast cell stabilizer that inhibits the *in vivo* Type I immediate hypersensitivity reaction. Lodoxamide therapy inhibits the increases in cutaneous vascular permeability that are associated with reagin or IgE and antigen-mediated reactions.

In vitro studies have demonstrated the ability of lodoxamide to stabilize rodent mast cells and prevent antigen-stimulated release of histamine. In addition, lodoxamide prevents the release of other mast cell inflammatory mediators (*i.e.,* SRS-A, a slow-reacting substances of anaphylaxis, also known as the peptido-leukotrienes) and inhibits eosinophil chemotaxis. Although lodoxamide's precise mechanism of action is unknown, the drug has been reported to prevent calcium influx into mast cells upon antigen stimulation.

Lodoxamide has no intrinsic vasoconstrictor, antihistaminic, cyclooxygenase inhibition, or other anti-inflammatory activity.

The disposition of ^{14}C-lodoxamide was studied in 6 healthy adult volunteers receiving a 3 mg (50 μCi) oral dose of lodoxamide. Urinary excretion was the major route of elimination. The elimination half-life of ^{14}C-lodoxamide was 8.5 hours in the urine. In a study conducted in 12 healthy adult volunteers, topical administration of lodoxamide tromethamine ophthalmic solution 0.1%, 1 drop in each eye 4 times per day for 10 days, did not result in any measurable lodoxamide plasma levels at a detention limit of 2.5 ng/ml.

INDICATIONS AND USAGE

Lodoxamide tromethamine is indicated in the treatment of the ocular disorders referred to by the terms vernal keratoconjunctivitis, vernal conjunctivitis, and vernal keratitis.

CONTRAINDICATIONS

Hypersensitivity to any component of this product.

WARNINGS

Not for injection. As with all ophthalmic preparations containing benzalkonium chloride, patients should be instructed not to wear soft contact lenses during treatment with lodoxamide tromethamine ophthalmic solution.

PRECAUTIONS

GENERAL

Patients may experience a transient burning or stinging upon instillation of lodoxamide tromethamine ophthalmic solution. Should these symptoms persist, the patient should be advised to contact the prescribing physician.

CARCINOGENESIS, MUTAGENESIS, AND IMPAIRMENT OF FERTILITY

A long-term study with lodoxamide tromethamine in rats (2 year oral administration) showed no neoplastic or tumorigenic effects at doses 100 mg/kg/day (more than 5000 times the proposed human clinical dose). No evidence of mutagenicity or genetic damage was seen in the Ames *Salmonella* Assay, Chromosomal Aberration in CHO Cells Assay, or Mouse Forward Lymphoma Assay. In the BALB/c-3T3 Cells Transformation Assay, some increase in the number of transformation foci was seen at high concentrations (greater than

L

4000 μg/ml). No evidence of impairment of reproductive function was shown in laboratory animal studies.

PREGNANCY CATEGORY B

Reproduction studies with lodoxamide tromethamine administered orally to rats and rabbits in doses of 100 mg/kg/day (more than 5000 times the proposed human clinical dose) produced no evidence of developmental toxicity. There are, however, no adequate and well-controlled studied in pregnant women. Because animal reproduction studies are not always predictive of human response, lodoxamide tromethamine ophthalmic solution 0.1% should be used during pregnancy only if clearly needed.

NURSING MOTHERS

It is not known whether lodoxamide tromethamine is excreted in human milk. Because many drugs are excreted in human milk, caution should be exercised when lodoxamide tromethamine is administered to nursing women.

PEDIATRIC USE

Safety and effectiveness in children younger than 2 years of age have not been established.

ADVERSE REACTIONS

During clinical studies of lodoxamide tromethamine, the most frequently reported ocular adverse experiences were transient burning, stinging, or discomfort upon instillation, which occurred in approximately 15% of the subjects. Other ocular events occurring in 1-5% of the subjects included ocular itching/pruritus, blurred vision, dry eye, tearing/discharge, hyperemia, crystalline deposits, and foreign body sensation. Events that occurred in less than 1% of the subjects included corneal erosion/ulcer, scales on lid/lash, eye pain, ocular edema/swelling, ocular warming sensation, ocular fatigue, chemosis, corneal abrasion, anterior chamber cells, keratopathy/keratitis, blepharitis, allergy, sticky sensation, and epitheliopathy.

Nonocular events reported were headache (1.5%) and (at less than 1%) heat sensation, dizziness, somnolence, nausea, stomach discomfort, sneezing, dry nose, and rash.

DOSAGE AND ADMINISTRATION

The dose for adults and children greater than 2 years of age is 1-2 drops in each affected eye 4 times daily for up to 3 months.

HOW SUPPLIED

Alomide ophthalmic solution 0.1% is supplied as 10 ml in plastic ophthalmic Drop-Tainer dispenser.

Storage: Store at 15-27°C (59-80°F).

L

PRODUCT LISTING - EQUIVALENTS NOT AVAILABLE

Solution - Ophthalmic - 0.1%

10 ml	$51.25	ALOMIDE, Allscripts Pharmaceutical Company	54569-3772-00
10 ml	$67.31	ALOMIDE, Alcon Laboratories Inc	00065-0345-10

Lomefloxacin Hydrochloride *(003114)*

For related information, see the comparative table section in Appendix A.

Categories: Bronchitis, chronic, acute exacerbation; Infection, lower respiratory tract; Infection, urinary tract; Prophylaxis, surgical; Pregnancy Category C; FDA Approved 1992 Feb

Drug Classes: Antibiotics, quinolones

Brand Names: **Maxaquin**

Foreign Brand Availability: Decalogiflox (France); Lofloquin (Peru); Logiflox (France); Lomebact (Taiwan); Lomeflon (Japan); Lomflox (India; Singapore); Mahaquin (China); Okacin (Philippines; Singapore); Omniquin (Indonesia); Ontop (India); Uniquin (South-Africa)

Cost of Therapy: $72.81 (Infection; Maxaquin; 400 mg; 1 tablet/day; 10 day supply)

DESCRIPTION

Lomefloxacin hydrochloride is a synthetic broad-spectrum antimicrobial agent for oral administration. Lomefloxacin hydrochloride, a difluoroquinolone, is the monohydrochloride salt of (±)-1-ethyl-6,8-difluoro-1,4-dihydro-7-(3-methyl-1-piperazinyl)-4-oxo-3-quinolinecarboxylic acid. Its empirical formula is $C_{17}H_{19}F_2N_3O_3 \cdot HCl$.

Lomefloxacin hydrochloride is a white to pale yellow powder with a molecular weight of 387.8. It is slightly soluble in water and practically insoluble in alcohol. Lomefloxacin hydrochloride is stable to heat and moisture but is sensitive to light in dilute aqueous solution.

Maxaquin is available as a film-coated tablet formulation containing 400 mg of lomefloxacin base, present as the hydrochloride salt. The base content of the hydrochloride salt is 90.6%. The inactive ingredients are carboxymethylcellulose calcium, hydroxypropyl cellulose, hydroxypropyl methylcellulose, lactose, magnesium stearate, polyethylene glycol, polyoxyl 40 stearate, and titanium dioxide.

CLINICAL PHARMACOLOGY

PHARMACOKINETICS IN HEALTHY VOLUNTEERS

In 6 fasting healthy male volunteers, approximately 95-98% of a single oral dose of lomefloxacin was absorbed. Absorption was rapid following single doses of 200 and 400 mg (T_{max} 0.8-1.4 hours). Mean plasma concentration increased proportionally between 100 and 400 mg as shown in TABLE 1.

In 6 healthy male volunteers administered 400 mg of lomefloxacin on an empty stomach qd for 7 days, the following mean pharmacokinetic parameter values were obtained (TABLE 2).

The elimination half-life in 8 subjects with normal renal function was approximately 8 hours. At 24 hours postdose, subjects with normal renal function receiving single doses of 200 or 400 mg had mean plasma lomefloxacin concentrations of 0.10 and 0.24 μg/ml, respectively. Steady-state concentrations were achieved within 48 hours of initiating therapy with once-a-day dosing. There was no drug accumulation with single-daily dosing in patients with normal renal function.

TABLE 1

Dose	Mean Peak Plasma Concentration	Area Under Curve (AUC)
100 mg	0.8 μg/ml	5.6 μg·h/ml
200 mg	1.4 μg/ml	10.9 μg·h/ml
400 mg	3.2 μg/ml	26.1 μg·h/ml

TABLE 2

C_{max}	2.8 μg/ml
C_{min}	0.27 μg/ml
AUC(0-24) h	25.9 μg·h/ml
T_{max}	1.5 h
$T_{½}$	7.75 h

Approximately 65% of an orally administered dose was excreted in the urine as unchanged drug in patients with normal renal function. Following a 400 mg dose of lomefloxacin administered qd for 7 days, the mean urine concentration 4 hours postdose was in excess of 300 μg/ml. The mean urine concentration exceeded 35 μg/ml for at least 24 hours after dosing.

Following a single 400 mg dose, the solubility of lomefloxacin in urine usually exceeded its peak urinary concentration 2- to 6-fold. In this study, urine pH affected the solubility of lomefloxacin with solubilities ranging from 7.8 mg/ml at pH 5.2, to 2.4 mg/ml at pH 6.5, and 3.03 mg/ml at pH 8.12.

The urinary excretion of lomefloxacin was virtually complete within 72 hours after cessation of dosing, with approximately 65% of the dose being recovered as parent drug and 9% as its glucuronide metabolite. The mean renal clearance was 145 ml/min in subjects with normal renal function (GFR = 120 ml/min). This may indicate tubular secretion.

Food Effect

When lomefloxacin and food were administered concomitantly, the rate of drug absorption was delayed (T_{max} increased to 2 hours [delayed by 41%], C_{max} decreased by 18%), and the extent of absorption (AUC) was decreased by 12%.

PHARMACOKINETICS IN THE GERIATRIC POPULATION

In 16 healthy elderly volunteers (61-76 years of age) with normal renal function for their age, the half-life of lomefloxacin (mean of 8 hours) and its peak plasma concentration (mean of 4.2 μg/ml) following a single 400 mg dose were similar to those in 8 younger subjects dosed with a single 400 mg dose. Thus, drug absorption appears unaffected in the elderly. Plasma clearance was, however, reduced in this elderly population by approximately 25%, and the AUC was increased by approximately 33%. This slower elimination most likely reflects the decreased renal function normally observed in the geriatric population.

PHARMACOKINETICS IN RENALLY IMPAIRED PATIENTS

In 8 patients with creatinine clearance (CLCR) between 10 and 40 ml/min/1.73 m^2, the mean AUC after a single 400 mg dose of lomefloxacin increased 335% over the AUC demonstrated in patients with a CLCR >80 ml/min/1.73 m^2. Also, in these patients, the mean $T_{½}$ increased to 21 hours. In 8 patients with CLCR <10 ml/min/1.73 m^2, the mean AUC after a single 400 mg dose of lomefloxacin increased 700% over the AUC demonstrated in patients with a CLCR >80 ml/min/1.73 m^2. In these patients with CLCR <10 ml/min/1.73 m^2, the mean $T_{½}$ increased to 45 hours. The plasma clearance of lomefloxacin was closely correlated with creatinine clearance, ranging from 31 ml/min/1.73 m^2 when creatinine clearance was 0-271 ml/min/1.73 m^2 at a normal creatinine clearance of 110 ml/min/1.73 m^2. Peak lomefloxacin concentrations were not affected by the degree of renal function when single doses of lomefloxacin were administered. Adjustment of dosage schedules for patients with such decreases in renal function is warranted. (See DOSAGE AND ADMINISTRATION.)

PHARMACOKINETICS IN PATIENTS WITH CIRRHOSIS

In 12 patients with histologically confirmed cirrhosis, no significant changes in rate or extent of lomefloxacin exposure (C_{max}, T_{max}, $T_{½}$ or AUC) were observed when they were administered 400 mg of lomefloxacin as a single dose. No data are available in cirrhotic patients treated with multiple doses of lomefloxacin. Cirrhosis does not appear to reduce the nonrenal clearance of lomefloxacin. There does not appear to be a need for a dosage reduction in cirrhotic patients, provided adequate renal function is present.

METABOLISM AND PHARMACOKINETICS OF LOMEFLOXACIN

Lomefloxacin is minimally metabolized although 5 metabolites have been identified in human urine. The glucuronide metabolite is found in the highest concentration and accounts for approximately 9% of the administered dose. The other 4 metabolites together account for <0.5% of the dose.

Approximately 10% of an oral dose was recovered as unchanged drug in the feces.

Serum protein binding of lomefloxacin is approximately 10%.

The following are mean tissue- or fluid-to-plasma ratios of lomefloxacin following oral administration. Studies have not been conducted to assess the penetration of lomefloxacin into human cerebrospinal fluid (TABLE 3).

In two studies including 74 healthy volunteers, the minimal dose of UVA light needed to cause erythema (MED-UVA) was inversely proportional to plasma lomefloxacin concentration. The MED-UVA values (16 hours and 12 hours postdose) were significantly higher than the MED-UVA values 2 hours postdose at steady state. Increasing the interval between lomefloxacin dosing and exposure to UVA light increased the amount of light energy needed for photoreaction. In a study of 27 healthy volunteers, the steady state AUC values and C_{min} values were equivalent whether the drug was administered in the morning or in the evening.

TABLE 3

Tissue or Body Fluid	Mean Tissue- or Fluid-to-Plasma Ratio
Bronchial mucosa	2.1
Bronchial secretions	0.6
Prostatic tissue	2.0
Sputum	1.3
Urine	140.0

MICROBIOLOGY

Lomefloxacin has *in vitro* activity against a wide range of gram-negative and gram-positive microorganisms. The bactericidal action of lomefloxacin and other fluoroquinolone antimicrobials results from inhibition of bacterial topoisomerase IV and DNA gyrase (both of which are Type II topoisomerases), enzymes required for DNA replication, transcription, repair and recombination. The minimum bactericidal concentration (MBC) generally does not exceed the minimum inhibitory concentration (MIC) by more than a factor of 2, except for staphylococci, which usually have MBCs 2-4 times the MIC.

Lomefloxacin shares a number of general characteristics with other members of the quinolone class. Beta-lactamase production has no effect on the *in vitro* activity of lomefloxacin or other fluoroquinolones. Like other members of the quinolone class of antimicrobials, lomefloxacin appears slightly less active *in vitro* when tested at acidic pH, an increase in inoculum size has little effect on *in vitro* activity, and *in vitro* resistance develops slowly (multiple-step mutation). Rapid one-step development of resistance occurs only rarely (10^{-9}) *in vitro.*

Cross-resistance between lomefloxacin and other quinolone-class antimicrobial agents has been reported; however, cross-resistance between lomefloxacin and members of other classes of antimicrobial agents, such as aminoglycosides, penicillins, tetracyclines, cephalosporins, or sulfonamides has not yet been reported. Lomefloxacin is active *in vitro* against some strains of cephalosporin and aminoglycoside-resistant gram-negative bacteria.

Lomefloxacin has been shown to be active against most strains of the following microorganisms both *in vitro* and in clinical infections (see INDICATIONS AND USAGE):

Aerobic Gram-Positive Microorganisms

Staphylococcus saprophyticus (many strains are only moderately susceptible).

Aerobic Gram-Negative Microorganisms

Citrobacter (diversus) koseri, Enterobacter cloacae, Escherichia coli, Haemophilus influenzae, Klebsiella pneumoniae, Moraxella catarrhalis, Proteus mirabilis, Pseudomonas aeruginosa (urinary tract only — see INDICATIONS AND USAGE and WARNINGS).

The following *in vitro* data are available, **but their clinical significance is unknown.**

Lomefloxacin exhibits *in vitro* minimum inhibitory concentrations (MIC's) of 2 μg/ml or less against most (≥90%) strains of the following microorganisms; however, the safety and effectiveness of lomefloxacin in treating clinical infections due to these microorganisms have not been established in adequate and well-controlled trials.

Aerobic Gram-Positive Microorganisms

Staphylococcus aureus (methicillin-susceptible strains only).

Aerobic Gram-Negative Microorganisms

Aeromonas hydrophila, Enterobacter aerogenes, Haemophilus parainfluenzae, Hafnia alvei, Klebsiella oxytoca, Legionella pneumophila, Morganella morganii, Proteus vulgaris.

Most group A, B, D, and G streptococci, *Streptococcus pneumoniae, Burkholderia cepacia, Ureaplasma urealyticum, Mycoplasma hominis,* and anaerobic bacteria are resistant to lomefloxacin.

Susceptibility Tests

Dilution Techniques

Quantitative methods are used to determine antimicrobial minimum inhibitory concentrations (MICs). These MICs provide estimates of the susceptibility of bacteria to antimicrobial compounds. The MIC values should be determined using a standardized procedure. Standardized procedures are based on a dilution method[1] (broth or agar) or equivalent with standardized inoculum concentrations and standardized concentrations of lomefloxacin powder. The MIC values should be interpreted according to the following criteria (see TABLE 4 and TABLE 5).

For testing *Enterobacteriaceae, Staphylococcus* species, and *Pseudomonas aeruginosa* (see TABLE 4).

TABLE 4

MIC (μg/ml)	Interpretation
≤2	Susceptible (S)
4	Intermediate (I)
≥8	Resistant (R)

For testing *Haemophilus influenzae** (see TABLE 5).

TABLE 5

MIC (μg/ml)	Interpretation
≤2	Susceptible (S)

* This interpretive standard is applicable only to broth microdilution susceptibility testing with *Haemophilus influenzae* using *Haemophilus* Test Medium (HTM).[1]

The current absence of data on resistant strains precludes defining any results other than "Susceptible". Strains yielding MIC results suggestive of a "nonsusceptible" category should be submitted to a reference laboratory for further testing.

A report of "Susceptible" indicates that the pathogen is likely to be inhibited if the antimicrobial compound in the blood reaches the concentration usually achievable. A report of "Intermediate" indicates that the result should be considered equivocal, and if the microorganism is not fully susceptible to alternative, clinically feasible drugs, the test should be repeated. This category implies possible clinical applicability in body sites where the drug is physiologically concentrated or in situations where high dosage of drug can be used. This category also provides a buffer zone which prevents small uncontrolled technical factors from causing major discrepancies in interpretation. A report of "Resistant" indicates that the pathogen is not likely to be inhibited if the antimicrobial compound in the blood reaches the concentration usually achievable; other therapy should be selected.

Standardized susceptibility test procedures require the use of laboratory control microorganisms to control the technical aspects of the laboratory procedures. Standard lomefloxacin powder should provide the following MIC values (see TABLE 6).

TABLE 6

Microorganism	MIC Range (μg/ml)
Escherichia coli ATCC 25922	0.03-0.12
Haemophilus influenzae ATCC 49247*	0.03-0.12
Pseudomonas aeruginosa ATCC 27853	1.0-4.0
Staphylococcus aureus ATCC 29213	0.25-2.0

* This quality control range is applicable to only *H. influenzae* ATCC 49247 tested by a broth microdilution procedure using *Haemophilus* Test Medium (HTM).[1]

Diffusion Techniques

Quantitative methods that require measurement of zone diameters also provide reproducible estimates of the susceptibility of bacteria to antimicrobial compounds. One such standardized procedure[2] requires the use of standardized inoculum concentrations. This procedure uses paper disks impregnated with 10 μg lomefloxacin to test the susceptibility of microorganisms to lomefloxacin.

Reports from the laboratory providing results of the standard single-disk susceptibility test with a 10 μg lomefloxacin disk should be interpreted according to the following criteria (see TABLE 7 and TABLE 8).

For testing *Enterobacteriaceae, Staphylococcus* species, and *Pseudomonas aeruginosa* (see TABLE 7).

TABLE 7

Zone Diameter (mm)	Interpretation
≥22	Susceptible (S)
19-21	Intermediate (I)
≤18	Resistant (R)

For testing *Haemophilus influenzae** (see TABLE 8).

TABLE 8

Zone Diameter (mm)	Interpretation
≥22	Susceptible (S)

* This interpretive standard is applicable only to disk diffusion susceptibility testing with *Haemophilus influenzae* using *Haemophilus* Test Medium (HTM).[2]

The current absence of data on resistant strains precludes defining any results other than "Susceptible". Strains yielding zone diameter results suggestive of a "nonsusceptible" category should be submitted to a reference laboratory for further testing.

Interpretation should be as stated above for results using dilution techniques. Interpretation involves correlation of the diameter obtained in the disk test with the MIC for lomefloxacin.

As with standardized dilution techniques, diffusion methods require the use of laboratory control microorganisms that are used to control the technical aspects of the laboratory procedures. For the diffusion technique, the 10 μg lomefloxacin disk should provide the following zone diameters in these laboratory quality control strains (see TABLE 9).

TABLE 9

Microorganism	Zone Diameter (mm)
Escherichia coli ATCC 25922	27-33
Haemophilus influenzae ATCC 49247*	33-41
Pseudomonas aeruginosa ATCC 27853	22-28
Staphylococcus aureus ATCC 25923	23-29

* This quality control range is applicable to only *H. influenzae* ATCC 49247 tested by a disk diffusion procedure using *Haemophilus* Test Medium (HTM).[2]

INDICATIONS AND USAGE

TREATMENT

Lomefloxacin HCl film-coated tablets are indicated for the treatment of adults with mild to moderate infections caused by susceptible strains of the designated microorganisms in the conditions listed below: (See DOSAGE AND ADMINISTRATION for specific dosing recommendations.)

Lower Respiratory Tract:

Acute bacterial exacerbation of chronic bronchitis caused by *Haemophilus influenzae* or *Moraxella catarrhalis**.

Note: LOMEFLOXACIN HCl IS NOT INDICATED FOR THE EMPIRIC TREATMENT OF ACUTE BACTERIAL EXACERBATION OF CHRONIC BRONCHITIS WHEN IT IS PROBABLE THAT *S. PNEUMONIAE* IS A CAUSATIVE PATHOGEN. *S. PNEUMONIAE* EXHIBITS *IN VITRO* RESISTANCE TO LOMEFLOXACIN, AND THE SAFETY AND EFFICACY OF LOMEFLOXACIN IN

THE TREATMENT OF PATIENTS WITH ACUTE BACTERIAL EXACERBATION OF CHRONIC BRONCHITIS CAUSED BY *S. PNEUMONIAE* HAVE NOT BEEN DEMONSTRATED. IF LOMEFLOXACIN IS TO BE PRESCRIBED FOR GRAM-STAIN-GUIDED EMPIRIC THERAPY OF ACUTE BACTERIAL EXACERBATION OF CHRONIC BRONCHITIS, IT SHOULD BE USED ONLY IF SPUTUM GRAM STAIN DEMONSTRATES AN ADEQUATE QUALITY OF SPECIMEN (>25 PMNs/LPF) AND THERE IS BOTH A PREDOMINANCE OF GRAM-NEGATIVE MICROORGANISMS AND NOT A PREDOMINANCE OF GRAM-POSITIVE MICROORGANISMS.

Urinary Tract:

Uncomplicated urinary tract infections (cystitis) caused by *Escherichia coli, Klebsiella pneumoniae, Proteus mirabilis,* or *Staphylococcus saprophyticus.* (See DOSAGE AND ADMINISTRATION.)

Complicated urinary tract infections caused by *Escherichia coli, Klebsiella pneumoniae, Proteus mirabilis, Pseudomonas aeruginosa, Citrobacter diversus*,* or *Enterobacter cloacae*.*

Note: In clinical trials with patients experiencing complicated urinary tract infections (UTIs) due to *P. aeruginosa,* 12 of 16 patients had the microorganism eradicated from the urine after therapy with lomefloxacin. None of the patients had concomitant bacteremia. Serum levels of lomefloxacin do not reliably exceed the MIC of *Pseudomonas* isolates. THE SAFETY AND EFFICACY OF LOMEFLOXACIN IN TREATING PATIENTS WITH *PSEUDOMONAS* BACTEREMIA HAVE NOT BEEN ESTABLISHED.

*Although treatment of infections due to this microorganism in this organ system demonstrated a clinically acceptable overall outcome, efficacy was studied in fewer than 10 infections.

Appropriate culture and susceptibility tests should be performed before antimicrobial treatment in order to isolate and identify microorganisms causing infection and to determine their susceptibility to lomefloxacin. In patients with UTIs, therapy with lomefloxacin HCl film-coated tablets may be initiated before results of these tests are known; once these results become available, appropriate therapy should be continued. In patients with an acute bacterial exacerbation of chronic bronchitis, therapy should not be started empirically with lomefloxacin when there is a probability the causative pathogen is *S. pneumoniae.*

Beta-lactamase production should have no effect on lomefloxacin activity.

PREVENTION/PROPHYLAXIS

Lomefloxacin HCl film-coated tablets are indicated perioperatively for the prevention of infection in the following situations:

Transrectal prostate biopsy: To reduce the incidence of urinary tract infections, in the early and late postoperative periods (3-5 days and 3-4 weeks postsurgery).

Transurethral surgical procedures: To reduce the incidence of urinary tract infections in the early postoperative period (3-5 days postsurgery).

Efficacy in decreasing the incidence of infections other than urinary tract infection has not been established. Lomefloxacin HCl, like all drugs for prophylaxis of transurethral surgical procedures, usually should not be used in minor urologic procedures for which prophylaxis is not indicated (*e.g.,* simple cystoscopy or retrograde pyelography). (See DOSAGE AND ADMINISTRATION.)

L

CONTRAINDICATIONS

Lomefloxacin HCl is contraindicated in persons with a history of hypersensitivity to lomefloxacin or to any member of the quinolone group of antimicrobial agents.

WARNINGS

MODERATE TO SEVERE PHOTOTOXIC REACTIONS HAVE OCCURRED IN PATIENTS EXPOSED TO DIRECT OR INDIRECT SUNLIGHT OR TO ARTIFICIAL ULTRAVIOLET LIGHT (*e.g.,* sunlamps) DURING OR FOLLOWING TREATMENT WITH LOMEFLOXACIN. THESE REACTIONS HAVE ALSO OCCURRED IN PATIENTS EXPOSED TO SHADED OR DIFFUSE LIGHT, INCLUDING EXPOSURE THROUGH GLASS. PATIENTS SHOULD BE ADVISED TO DISCONTINUE LOMEFLOXACIN THERAPY AT THE FIRST SIGNS OR SYMPTOMS OF A PHOTOTOXICITY REACTION SUCH AS A SENSATION OF SKIN BURNING, REDNESS, SWELLING, BLISTERS, RASH, ITCHING, OR DERMATITIS.

These phototoxic reactions have occurred with and without the use of sunscreens or sunblocks. Single doses of lomefloxacin have been associated with these types of reactions. In a few cases, recovery was prolonged for several weeks. As with some other types of phototoxicity, there is the potential for exacerbation of the reaction on re-exposure to sunlight or artificial ultraviolet light prior to complete recovery from the reaction. In rare cases, reactions have recurred up to several weeks after stopping lomefloxacin therapy.

EXPOSURE TO DIRECT OR INDIRECT SUNLIGHT (EVEN WHEN USING SUNSCREENS OR SUNBLOCKS) SHOULD BE AVOIDED WHILE TAKING LOMEFLOXACIN AND FOR SEVERAL DAYS FOLLOWING THERAPY. LOMEFLOXACIN THERAPY SHOULD BE DISCONTINUED IMMEDIATELY AT THE FIRST SIGNS OR SYMPTOMS OF PHOTOTOXICITY. RISK OF PHOTOTOXICITY MAY BE REDUCED BY TAKING LOMEFLOXACIN IN THE EVENING. (See DOSAGE AND ADMINISTRATION.)

THE SAFETY AND EFFICACY OF LOMEFLOXACIN IN PEDIATRIC PATIENTS AND ADOLESCENTS (UNDER THE AGE OF 18 YEARS), PREGNANT WOMEN, AND LACTATING WOMEN HAVE NOT BEEN ESTABLISHED. (See PRECAUTIONS: Pediatric Use, Pregnancy, Teratogenic Effects, Pregnancy Category C and Nursing Mothers.) The oral administration of multiple doses of lomefloxacin to juvenile dogs at 0.3 times and to rats at 5.4 times the recommended adult human dose based on mg/m^2 (0.6 and 34 times the recommended adult human dose based on mg/kg, respectively) caused arthropathy and lameness. Histopathological examination of the weight-bearing joints of these animals revealed permanent lesions of the cartilage. Other quinolones also produce erosions of cartilage of weight-bearing joints and other signs of arthropathy in juvenile animals of various species. (See ANIMAL PHARMACOLOGY.)

Convulsions have been reported in patients receiving lomefloxacin. Whether the convulsions were directly related to lomefloxacin administration has not yet been established. However, convulsions, increased intracranial pressure, and toxic psychoses have been reported in patients receiving other quinolones. Nevertheless, lomefloxacin has been associated with a possible increased risk of seizures compared to other quinolones. Some of these may occur with a relative absence of predisposing factors. Quinolones may also cause central nervous system (CNS) stimulation, which may lead to tremors, restlessness, lightheadedness, confusion, and hallucinations. If any of these reactions occurs in patients receiving lomefloxacin, the drug should be discontinued and appropriate measures instituted. However, until more information becomes available, lomefloxacin, like all other quinolones, should be used with caution in patients with known or suspected CNS disorders, such as severe cerebral arteriosclerosis, epilepsy, or other factors that predispose to seizures. (See ADVERSE REACTIONS.) Psychiatric disturbances, agitation, anxiety, and sleep disorders may be more common with lomefloxacin than other products in the quinolone class.

The safety and efficacy of lomefloxacin in the treatment of acute bacterial exacerbation of chronic bronchitis due to *S. pneumoniae* have not been demonstrated. This product should not be used empirically in the treatment of acute bacterial exacerbation of chronic bronchitis when it is probable that *S. pneumoniae* is a causative pathogen.

In clinical trials of complicated UTIs due to *P. aeruginosa,* 12 of 16 patients had the microorganism eradicated from the urine after therapy with lomefloxacin. No patients had concomitant bacteremia. Serum levels of lomefloxacin do not reliably exceed the MIC of *Pseudomonas isolates.* THE SAFETY AND EFFICACY OF LOMEFLOXACIN IN TREATING PATIENTS WITH *PSEUDOMONAS* BACTEREMIA HAVE NOT BEEN ESTABLISHED.

Serious and occasionally fatal hypersensitivity (anaphylactoid or anaphylactic) reactions, some following the first dose, have been reported in patients receiving quinolone therapy. Some reactions were accompanied by cardiovascular collapse, loss of consciousness, tingling, pharyngeal or facial edema, dyspnea, urticaria, or itching. Only a few of these patients had a history of previous hypersensitivity reactions. Serious hypersensitivity reactions have also been reported following treatment with lomefloxacin. If an allergic reaction to lomefloxacin occurs, discontinue the drug. Serious acute hypersensitivity reactions may require immediate emergency treatment with epinephrine. Oxygen, intravenous fluids, antihistamines, corticosteroids, pressor amines, and airway management, including intubation, should be administered as indicated.

Pseudomembranous colitis has been reported with nearly all antibacterial agents, including lomefloxacin, and may range from mild to life-threatening in severity. Therefore, it is important to consider this diagnosis in patients who present with diarrhea subsequent to the administration of antibacterial agents. Treatment with antimicrobial agents alters the normal flora of the colon and may permit overgrowth of clostridia. Studies indicate that a toxin produced by *Clostridium difficile* is a primary cause of "antibiotic associated colitis". After the diagnosis of pseudomembranous colitis has been established, therapeutic measures should be initiated. Mild cases of pseudomembranous colitis usually respond to discontinuation of drug alone. In moderate to severe cases, consideration should be given to management with fluids and electrolytes, protein supplementation, and treatment with an antibacterial drug clinically effective against *C. difficile* colitis.

Ruptures of the shoulder, hand, and Achilles tendons that required surgical repair or resulted in prolonged disability have been reported with lomefloxacin. Lomefloxacin should be discontinued if the patient experiences pain, inflammation, or rupture of a tendon. Patients should rest and refrain from exercise until the diagnosis of tendinitis or tendon rupture has been confidently excluded. Tendon rupture can occur at any time during or after therapy with lomefloxacin.

PRECAUTIONS

GENERAL

Alteration of the dosage regimen is recommended for patients with impairment of renal function (CLCR <40 ml/min/1.73 m^2). (See DOSAGE AND ADMINISTRATION.)

INFORMATION FOR THE PATIENT

Patients should be advised:

To avoid to the maximum extent possible direct or indirect sunlight (including exposure through glass and exposure through sunscreens and sunblocks) and artificial ultraviolet light (*e.g.,* sunlamps) during treatment with lomefloxacin and for several days after therapy.

That they may reduce the risk of developing phototoxicity from sunlight by taking the daily dose of lomefloxacin at least 12 hours before exposure to the sun (*e.g.,* in the evening).

To discontinue lomefloxacin therapy at the first signs or symptoms of phototoxicity reaction such as a sensation of skin burning, redness, swelling, blisters, rash, itching, or dermatitis.

That a patient who has experienced a phototoxic reaction should avoid re-exposure to sunlight and artificial ultraviolet light until he has completely recovered from the reaction. In rare cases, reactions have recurred up to several weeks after stopping lomefloxacin therapy.

To drink fluids liberally.

That lomefloxacin can be taken without regard to meals.

That mineral supplements or vitamins with iron or minerals should not be taken within the 2 hour period before or after taking lomefloxacin (see DRUG INTERACTIONS).

That sucralfate or antacids containing magnesium or aluminum or didanosine chewable/buffered tablets or the pediatric powder for oral solution should not be taken within 4 hours before or 2 hours after taking lomefloxacin (see DRUG INTERACTIONS).

That lomefloxacin can cause dizziness and lightheadedness and, therefore, patients should know how they react to lomefloxacin before they operate an automobile or machinery or engage in activities requiring mental alertness and coordination.

To discontinue treatment and inform their physician if they experience pain, inflammation, or rupture of a tendon, and to rest and refrain from exercise until the diagnosis of tendinitis or tendon rupture has been confidently excluded.

That lomefloxacin may be associated with hypersensitivity reactions, even following the first dose, and to discontinue the drug at the first sign of a skin rash or other allergic reaction.

That convulsions have been reported in patients taking quinolones, including lomefloxacin, and to notify their physician before taking this drug if there is a history of this condition.

CARCINOGENESIS, MUTAGENESIS, AND IMPAIRMENT OF FERTILITY

Carcinogenesis

Hairless (Skh-1) mice were exposed to UVA light for 3.5 hours 5 times every 2 weeks for up to 52 weeks while concurrently being administered lomefloxacin. The lomefloxacin doses used in this study caused a phototoxic response. In mice treated with both UVA and lomefloxacin concomitantly, the time to development of skin tumors was 16 weeks. In mice treated concomitantly in this model with both UVA and other quinolones, the times to development of skin tumors ranged from 28-52 weeks.

Ninety-two percent (92%) of the mice treated concomitantly with both UVA and lomefloxacin developed well-differentiated squamous cell carcinomas of the skin. These squamous cell carcinomas were nonmetastatic and were endophytic in character. Two-thirds of these squamous cell carcinomas contained large central keratinous inclusion masses and were thought to arise from the vestigial hair follicles in these hairless animals.

In this model, mice treated with lomefloxacin alone did not develop skin or systemic tumors.

There are no data from similar models using pigmented mice and/or fully haired mice. The clinical significance of these findings to humans is unknown.

Mutagenesis

One *in vitro* mutagenicity test (CHO/HGPRT assay) was weakly positive at lomefloxacin concentrations of ≥226 μg/ml and negative at concentrations <226 μg/ml. Two other *in vitro* mutagenicity tests (chromosomal aberrations in Chinese hamster ovary cells, chromosomal aberrations in human lymphocytes) and two *in vivo* mouse micronucleus mutagenicity tests were all negative.

Impairment of Fertility

Lomefloxacin did not affect the fertility of male and female rats at oral doses up to 8 times the recommended human dose based on mg/m^2 (34 times the recommended human dose based on mg/kg).

PREGNANCY, TERATOGENIC EFFECTS, PREGNANCY CATEGORY C

Reproductive function studies have been performed in rats at doses up to 8 times the recommended human dose based on mg/m^2 (34 times the recommended human dose based on mg/kg), and no impaired fertility or harm to the fetus was reported due to lomefloxacin. Increased incidence of fetal loss in monkeys has been observed at approximately 3-6 times the recommended human dose based on mg/m^2 (6-12 times the recommended human dose based on mg/kg). No teratogenicity has been observed in rats and monkeys at up to 16 times the recommended human dose exposure. In the rabbit, maternal toxicity and associated fetotoxicity, decreased placental weight, and variations of the coccygeal vertebrae occurred at doses 2 times the recommended human exposure based on mg/m^2. There are, however, no adequate and well-controlled studies in pregnant women. Lomefloxacin should be used during pregnancy only if the potential benefit justifies the potential risk to the fetus.

NURSING MOTHERS

It is not known whether lomefloxacin is excreted in human milk. However, it is known that other drugs of this class are excreted in human milk and that lomefloxacin is excreted in the milk of lactating rats. Because of the potential for serious adverse reactions from lomefloxacin in nursing infants, a decision should be made whether to discontinue nursing or to discontinue the drug, taking into account the importance of the drug to the mother.

PEDIATRIC USE

The safety and effectiveness of lomefloxacin in pediatric patients and adolescents less than 18 years of age have not been established. Lomefloxacin causes arthropathy in juvenile animals of several species. (See WARNINGS and ANIMAL PHARMACOLOGY.)

GERIATRIC USE

Of the total number of subjects in clinical studies of lomefloxacin, 25% were ≥65 years and 9% were ≥75 years. No overall differences in safety or effectiveness were observed between these subjects and younger subjects, and other reported clinical experience has not identified differences in responses between the elderly and younger patients, but greater sensitivity of some older individuals cannot be ruled out.

This drug is known to be substantially excreted by the kidney, and the risk of toxic reactions to this drug may be greater in patients with impaired renal function. Because elderly patients are more likely to have decreased renal function, care should be taken in dose selection, and it may be useful to monitor renal function. (See CLINICAL PHARMACOLOGY, Pharmacokinetics in the Geriatric Population.)

DRUG INTERACTIONS

Theophylline: In three pharmacokinetic studies including 46 normal, healthy subjects, theophylline clearance and concentration were not significantly altered by the addition of lomefloxacin. In clinical studies where patients were on chronic theophylline therapy, lomefloxacin had no measurable effect on the mean distribution of theophylline concentrations or the mean estimates of theophylline clearance. Though individual theophylline levels fluctuated, there were no clinically significant symptoms of drug interaction.

Antacids and Sucralfate: Sucralfate and antacids containing magnesium or aluminum, as well as formulations containing divalent and trivalent cations such as didanosine chewable/buffered tablets or the pediatric powder for oral solution can form chelation complexes with lomefloxacin and interfere with its bioavailability. Sucralfate administered 2 hours before lomefloxacin resulted in a slower rate of absorption (mean C_{max} decreased by 30% and mean T_{max} increased by 1 hour) and a lesser extent of absorption (mean AUC decreased by approximately 25%). Magnesium- and aluminum-containing antacids, administered concomitantly with lomefloxacin, significantly decreased the bioavailability (48%) of lomefloxacin. Separating the doses of antacid and lomefloxacin minimizes this decrease in bioavailability; therefore, administration of these agents should precede lomefloxacin dosing by 4 hours or follow lomefloxacin dosing by at least 2 hours.

Caffeine: Two hundred (200) mg of caffeine (equivalent to 1-3 cups of American coffee) was administered to 16 normal, healthy volunteers who had achieved steady-state blood concentrations of lomefloxacin after being dosed at 400 mg qd. This did not result in any statistically or clinically relevant changes in the pharmacokinetic parameters of either caffeine or its major metabolite, paraxanthine. No data are available on potential interactions in individuals who consume greater than 200 mg of caffeine per day or in those, such as the geriatric population, who are generally believed to be more susceptible to the development of drug-induced CNS-related adverse effects. Other quinolones have demonstrated moderate to marked interference with metabolism of caffeine, resulting in a reduced clearance, a prolongation of plasma half-life, and an increase in symptoms that accompany high levels of caffeine.

Cimetidine: Cimetidine has been demonstrated to interfere with the elimination of other quinolones. This interference has resulted in significant increases in half-life and AUC. The interaction between lomefloxacin and cimetidine has not been studied.

Cyclosporine: Elevated serum levels of cyclosporine have been reported with concomitant use of cyclosporine with other members of the quinolone class. Interaction between lomefloxacin and cyclosporine has not been studied.

Omeprazole: No clinically significant changes in lomefloxacin pharmacokinetics (AUC, C_{max}, or T_{max}) were observed when a single dose of lomefloxacin 400 mg was given after multiple doses of omeprazole (20 mg qd) in 13 healthy volunteers. Changes in omeprazole pharmacokinetics were not studied.

Phenytoin: No significant differences were observed in mean phenytoin AUC, C_{max}, C_{min} or T_{max} (although C_{max} increased by 11%) when extended phenytoin sodium capsules (100 mg tid) were coadministered with lomefloxacin (400 mg qd) for 5 days in 15 healthy males. Lomefloxacin is unlikely to have a significant effect on phenytoin metabolism.

Probenecid: Probenecid slows the renal elimination of lomefloxacin. An increase of 63% in the mean AUC and increases of 50% and 4%, respectively, in the mean T_{max} and mean C_{max} were noted in 1 study of 6 individuals.

Terfenadine: No clinically significant changes occurred in heart rate or corrected QT intervals, or in terfenadine metabolite or lomefloxacin pharmacokinetics, during concurrent administration of lomefloxacin and terfenadine at steady-state in 28 healthy males.

Warfarin: Quinolones may enhance the effects of the oral anticoagulant, warfarin, or its derivatives. When these products are administered concomitantly, prothrombin or other suitable coagulation test should be monitored closely. However, no clinically or statistically significant differences in prothrombin time ratio or warfarin enantiomer pharmacokinetics were observed in a small study of 7 healthy males who received both warfarin and lomefloxacin under steady-state conditions.

ADVERSE REACTIONS

In clinical trials, most of the adverse events reported were mild to moderate in severity and transient in nature. During these clinical investigations, 5623 patients received lomefloxacin HCl. In 2.2% of the patients, lomefloxacin was discontinued because of adverse events, primarily involving the gastrointestinal system (0.7%), skin (0.7%), or CNS (0.5%).

ADVERSE CLINICAL EVENTS

The events with the highest incidence (≥1%) in patients, regardless of relationship to drug, were headache (3.6%), nausea (3.5%), photosensitivity (2.3%) (see WARNINGS), dizziness (2.1%), diarrhea (1.4%), and abdominal pain (1.2%).

Additional clinical events reported in <1% of patients treated with lomefloxacin HCl, regardless of relationship to drug, are listed below:

Autonomic: Increased sweating, dry mouth, flushing, syncope.

Body as a Whole: Fatigue, back pain, malaise, asthenia, chest pain, face edema, hot flashes, influenza-like symptoms, edema, chills, allergic reaction, anaphylactoid reaction, decreased heat tolerance.

Cardiovascular: Tachycardia, hypertension, hypotension, myocardial infarction, angina pectoris, cardiac failure, bradycardia, arrhythmia, phlebitis, pulmonary embolism, extrasystoles, cerebrovascular disorder, cyanosis, cardiomyopathy.

Central and Peripheral Nervous System: Tremor, vertigo, paresthesias, twitching, hypertonia, convulsions, hyperkinesia, coma.

Gastrointestinal: Dyspepsia, vomiting, flatulence, constipation, gastrointestinal bleeding, dysphagia, stomatitis, tongue discoloration, gastrointestinal inflammation.

Hearing: Earache, tinnitus.

Hematologic: Purpura, lymphadenopathy, thrombocythemia, anemia, thrombocytopenia, increased fibrinolysis.

Hepatic: Abnormal liver function.

Metabolic: Thirst, hyperglycemia, hypoglycemia, gout.

Musculoskeletal: Arthralgia, myalgia, leg cramps.

Ophthalmologic: Abnormal vision, conjunctivitis, photophobia, eye pain, abnormal lacrimation.

Psychiatric: Insomnia, nervousness, somnolence, anorexia, depression, confusion, agitation, increased appetite, depersonalization, paranoid reaction, anxiety, paroniria, abnormal thinking, concentration impairment.

Reproductive System: *Female:* Vaginal moniliasis, vaginitis, leukorrhea, menstrual disorder, perineal pain, intermenstrual bleeding. *Male:* Epididymitis, orchitis.

Resistance Mechanism: Viral infection, moniliasis, fungal infection.

Respiratory: Respiratory infection, rhinitis, pharyngitis, dyspnea, cough, epistaxis, bronchospasm, respiratory disorder, increased sputum, stridor, respiratory depression.

Skin/Allergic: Pruritus, rash, urticaria, skin exfoliation, bullous eruption, eczema, skin disorder, acne, skin discoloration, skin ulceration, angioedema. (See also Body as a Whole.)
Special Senses: Taste perversion.
Urinary: Hematuria, micturition disorder, dysuria, strangury, anuria.

ADVERSE LABORATORY EVENTS

Changes in laboratory parameters, listed as adverse events, without regard to drug relationship include:

Hematologic: Monocytosis (0.2%), eosinophilia (0.1%), leukopenia (0.1%), leukocytosis (0.1%).
Renal: Elevated BUN (0.1%), decreased potassium (0.1%), increased creatinine (0.1%).
Hepatic: Elevations of ALT (SGPT) (0.4%), AST (SGOT) (0.3%), bilirubin (0.1%), alkaline phosphatase (0.1%).

Additional laboratory changes occurring in <0.1% in the clinical studies included: Elevation of serum gamma glutamyl transferase, decrease in total protein or albumin, prolongation of prothrombin time, anemia, decrease in hemoglobin, thrombocythemia, thrombocytopenia, abnormalities of urine specific gravity or serum electrolytes, increased albumin, elevated ESR, albuminuria, macrocytosis.

QUINOLONE-CLASS ADVERSE EVENTS

Post-Marketing Adverse Events

Adverse events reported from worldwide marketing experience with lomefloxacin are: Anaphylaxis, cardiopulmonary arrest, laryngeal or pulmonary edema, ataxia, cerebral thrombosis, hallucinations, painful oral mucosa, pseudomembranous colitis, hemolytic anemia, hepatitis, tendinitis, diplopia, photophobia, phobia, exfoliative dermatitis, hyperpigmentation, Stevens-Johnson syndrome, toxic epidermal necrolysis, dysgeusia, interstitial nephritis, polyuria, renal failure, urinary retention, and vasculitis.

Quinolone-Class Adverse Events

Additional quinolone-class adverse events include: Erythema nodosum, hepatic necrosis, possible exacerbation of myasthenia gravis, dysphasia, nystagmus, intestinal perforation, manic reaction, renal calculi, acidosis and hiccough.

Laboratory adverse events include: Agranulocytosis, elevation of serum triglycerides, elevation of serum cholesterol, elevation of blood glucose, elevation of serum potassium, albuminuria, candiduria, and crystalluria.

L

DOSAGE AND ADMINISTRATION

Lomefloxacin HCl may be taken without regard to meals. Sucralfate and antacids containing magnesium or aluminum, or didanosine chewable/buffered tablets or the pediatric powder for oral solution should not be taken within 4 hours before or 2 hours after taking lomefloxacin. Risk of reaction to solar UVA light may be reduced by taking lomefloxacin HCl at least 12 hours before exposure to the sun (*e.g.*, in the evening). (See CLINICAL PHARMACOLOGY.)

See INDICATIONS AND USAGE for information on appropriate pathogens and patient populations.

TREATMENT

Patients With Normal Renal Function

The recommended daily dose of lomefloxacin HCl is described in TABLE 12.

TABLE 12

Infection	Unit Dose/ Frequency	Duration	Daily Dose
Acute bacterial exacerbation of chronic bronchitis	400 mg qd	10 days	400 mg
Uncomplicated cystitis in females caused by *E. coli*	400 mg qd	3 days	400 mg
Uncomplicated cystitis in females caused by *K. pneumoniae, P. mirabilis*, or *S. saprophyticus*	400 mg qd	10 days	400 mg
Complicated UTI	400 mg qd	14 days	400 mg

Elderly Patients

No dosage adjustment is needed for elderly patients with normal renal function (CLCR ≥40 ml/min/1.73 m^2).

Patients With Impaired Renal Function

Lomefloxacin is primarily eliminated by renal excretion. (See CLINICAL PHARMACOLOGY.) Modification of dosage is recommended in patients with renal dysfunction. In patients with a creatinine clearance >10 ml/min/1.73 m^2 but <40 ml/min/1.73 m^2, the recommended dosage is an initial loading dose of 400 mg followed by daily maintenance doses of 200 mg (½ tablet) once daily for the duration of treatment. It is suggested that serial determinations of lomefloxacin levels be performed to determine any necessary alteration in the appropriate next dosing interval.

If only the serum creatinine is known, the following formula may be used to estimate creatinine clearance.

Men: [(weight in kg) × (140 - age)] ÷ [72 × serum creatinine (mg/dl)]
Women: 0.85 × (calculated value for men)

Dialysis Patients

Hemodialysis removes only a negligible amount of lomefloxacin (3% in 4 hours). Hemodialysis patients should receive an initial loading dose of 400 mg followed by daily maintenance doses of 200 mg (½ tablet) once daily for the duration of treatment.

Patients With Cirrhosis

Cirrhosis does not reduce the nonrenal clearance of lomefloxacin. The need for a dosage reduction in this population should be based on the degree of renal function of the patient and on the plasma concentrations. (See CLINICAL PHARMACOLOGY and DOSAGE AND ADMINISTRATION, Patients With Impaired Renal Function.)

PREVENTION/PROPHYLAXIS

The recommended dose of lomefloxacin HCl is described in TABLE 13.

TABLE 13

Procedure	Dose	Oral Administration
Transrectal prostate biopsy	400 mg single dose	1-6 hours prior to procedure
Transurethral surgical procedures*	400 mg single dose	2-6 hours prior to procedure

* When preoperative prophylaxis is considered appropriate.

ANIMAL PHARMACOLOGY

Lomefloxacin and other quinolones have been shown to cause arthropathy in juvenile animals. Arthropathy, involving multiple diarthrodial joints, was observed in juvenile dogs administered lomefloxacin at doses as low as 4.5 mg/kg for 7-8 days (0.3 times the recommended human dose based on mg/m^2 or 0.6 times the recommended human dose based on mg/kg). In juvenile rats, no changes were observed in the joints with doses up to 91 mg/kg for 7 days (2 times the recommended human dose based on mg/m^2 or 11 times the recommended human dose based on mg/kg). (See WARNINGS.)

In a 13 week oral rat study, gamma globulin decreased when lomefloxacin was administered at less than the recommended human exposure. Beta globulin decreased when lomefloxacin was administered at 0.6 to 2 times the recommended human dose based on mg/m^2. The A/G ratio increased when lomefloxacin was administered at 6-20 times the human dose. Following a 4 week recovery period, beta globulins in the females and A/G ratios in the females returned to control values. Gamma globulin values in the females and beta and gamma globulins and A/G ratios in the males were still statistically significantly different from control values. No effects on globulins were seen in oral studies in dogs or monkeys in the limited number of specimens collected.

Twenty-seven NSAID's, administered concomitantly with lomefloxacin, were tested for seizure induction in mice at approximately 2 times the recommended human dose based on mg/m^2. At a dose of lomefloxacin equivalent to the recommended human exposure based on mg/m^2 (10 times the human dose based on mg/kg), only fenbufen, when co-administered, produced an increase in seizures.

Crystalluria and ocular toxicity, seen with some related quinolones, were not observed in any lomefloxacin-treated animals, either in studies designed to look for these effects specifically or in subchronic and chronic toxicity studies in rats, dogs, and monkeys.

Long-term, high-dose systemic use of other quinolones in experimental animals has caused lenticular opacities; however, this finding was not observed with lomefloxacin.

HOW SUPPLIED

Maxaquin is supplied as a scored, film-coated tablet containing the equivalent of 400 mg of lomefloxacin base present as the hydrochloride. The tablet is oval, white, and film-coated with "MAXAQUIN 400" debossed on one side and scored on the other side.

Storage: Store at 15-25°C (59-77°F).

PRODUCT LISTING - EQUIVALENTS NOT AVAILABLE

Tablet - Oral - 400 mg

20's	$138.68	MAXAQUIN, Unimed Pharmaceuticals	00051-1651-02
100's	$728.13	MAXAQUIN, Unimed Pharmaceuticals	00051-1651-32

Lomustine *(001660)*

Categories: Lymphoma, Hodgkin's; Pregnancy Category D; FDA Approved 1976 Aug
Drug Classes: Antineoplastics, alkylating agents
Brand Names: CeeNU; Lumustine
Foreign Brand Availability: Belustine (Hungary; Italy; Russia; Spain; Turkey); CCNU (Bahrain; Bulgaria; Cyprus; Egypt; England; Iran; Iraq; Jordan; Korea; Kuwait; Lebanon; Libya; Oman; Qatar; Republic-of-Yemen; Saudi-Arabia; Syria; Turkey; United-Arab-Emirates); Cecenu (Belgium; Germany; Greece); CEENU (Israel; Mexico); CiNU (Switzerland); Lomeblastin (Germany); Lomustine (India); Lucostin (Austria); Lucostine (Finland; Norway; Sweden); Lundbeck (England)

WARNING

Lomustine capsules should be administered under the supervision of a qualified physician experienced in the use of cancer chemotherapeutic agents.

Bone marrow suppression, notably thrombocytopenia and leukopenia, which may contribute to bleeding and overwhelming infections in an already compromised patient, is the most common and severe of the toxic effects of lomustine (see WARNINGS and ADVERSE REACTIONS).

Since the major toxicity is delayed bone marrow suppression, blood counts should be monitored weekly for at least 6 weeks after a dose (see ADVERSE REACTIONS). At the recommended dosage, courses of lomustine should not be given more frequently than every 6 weeks.

The bone marrow toxicity of lomustine is cumulative and therefore dosage adjustment must be considered on the basis of nadir blood counts from prior dose (see TABLE 1).

DESCRIPTION

Lomustine capsules are one of the nitrosoureas used in the treatment of certain neoplastic diseases. The chemical name for lomustine is 1-(2-chloroethyl)-3-cyclohexyl-1-nitrosourea.

It is a yellow powder with the empirical formula of $C_9H_{16}ClN_3O_2$ and a molecular weight of 233.71. Lomustine is soluble in 10% ethanol (0.05 mg per ml) and in absolute alcohol (70 mg per ml). Lomustine is relatively insoluble in water (<0.05 mg/ml).

It is relatively unionized at a physiological pH.

CeeNU is available in 10, 40, and 100 mg capsules for oral administration. *Inactive Ingredients:* Magnesium stearate and mannitol.

CLINICAL PHARMACOLOGY

Although it is generally agreed that lomustine alkylates DNA and RNA, it is not cross resistant with other alkylators. As with other nitrosoureas, it may also inhibit several key enzymatic processes by carbamoylation of amino acids in proteins.

Lomustine capsules may be given orally. Following oral administration of radioactive lomustine capsules at doses ranging from 30-100 mg/m^2 about half of the radioactivity given was excreted in the form of degradation products within 24 hours.

The serum half-life of metabolites ranges from 16 hours to 2 days. Tissue levels are comparable to plasma levels at 15 minutes after intravenous administration.

Because of the high lipid solubility and the relative lack of ionization at a physiological pH, lomustine capsules cross the blood-brain barrier quite effectively. Levels of radioactivity in the CSF are 50% or greater than those measured concurrently in plasma.

INDICATIONS AND USAGE

Lomustine capsules have been shown to be useful as a single agent in addition to other modalities, or in established combination therapy with other approved chemotherapeutic agents in the following:

Brain Tumors: Both primary and metastatic, in patients who have already received appropriate surgical and/or radiotherapeutic procedures.

Hodgkin's Disease: Secondary therapy in combination with other approved drugs in patients who relapse while being treated with primary therapy, or who fail to respond to primary therapy.

NON-FDA APPROVED INDICATIONS

Although currently, lomustine is seldom used for anything but primary brain tumors, the drug has been used without FDA approval as a part of combination chemotherapy regimens for the treatment of multiple myeloma and advanced gastrointestinal carcinoma. Advanced non-small cell lung cancer and prostate cancer are occasionally sensitive. Lomustine has also been used in the treatment of melanoma, non-Hodgkin's lymphoma, and cancers of the breast and kidney. The drug has been administered topically in the treatment of mycosis fungoides and psoriasis.

CONTRAINDICATIONS

Lomustine capsules should not be given to individuals who have demonstrated a previous hypersensitivity to it.

WARNINGS

Since the major toxicity is delayed bone marrow suppression, blood counts should be monitored weekly for at least 6 weeks after a dose (see ADVERSE REACTIONS). At the recommended dosage, courses of lomustine capsules should not be given more frequently than every 6 weeks.

The bone marrow toxicity of lomustine capsules are cumulative and therefore dosage adjustment must be considered on the basis of nadir blood counts from prior dose (see TABLE 1).

Pulmonary toxicity from lomustine capsules appear to be dose related (see ADVERSE REACTIONS).

Long term use of nitrosoureas has been reported to be possibly associated with the development of secondary malignancies.

Liver and renal function tests should be monitored periodically (see ADVERSE REACTIONS.)

PREGNANCY CATEGORY D

Lomustine capsules can cause fetal harm when administered to a pregnant woman. Lomustine capsules are embryotoxic and teratogenic in rats and embryotoxic in rabbits at dose levels equivalent to the human dose. There are no adequate and well controlled studies in pregnant women. If this drug is used during pregnancy, or if the patient becomes pregnant while taking (receiving) this drug, the patient should be apprised of the potential hazard to the fetus. Women of childbearing potential should be advised to avoid becoming pregnant.

PRECAUTIONS

GENERAL

In all instances where the use of lomustine capsules is considered for chemotherapy, the physician must evaluate the need and usefulness of the drug against the risks of toxic effects or adverse reactions. Most such adverse reactions are reversible if detected early. When such effects or reactions do occur, the drug should be reduced in dosage or discontinued and appropriate corrective measures should be taken according to the clinical judgement of the physician. Reinstitution of lomustine therapy should be carried out with caution and with adequate consideration of the further need for the drug and alertness as to possible recurrence of toxicity.

LABORATORY TESTS

Due to delayed bone marrow suppression, blood counts should be monitored weekly for at least 6 weeks after a dose.

Baseline pulmonary function studies should be conducted along with frequent pulmonary function tests during treatment. Patients with a baseline below 70% of the predicted Forced Vital Capacity (FVC) or Carbon Monoxide Diffusing Capacity (DLco) are particularly at risk.

Since lomustine capsules may cause liver dysfunction, it is recommended that liver function tests be monitored periodically.

Renal function tests should also be monitored periodically.

CARCINOGENESIS, MUTAGENESIS, AND IMPAIRMENT OF FERTILITY

Lomustine capsules are carcinogenic in rats and mice, producing a marked increase in tumor incidence in doses approximating those employed clinically. Nitrosourea therapy does have carcinogenic potential in humans (see ADVERSE REACTIONS). Lomustine also affects fertility in male rats at doses somewhat higher than the human dose.

PREGNANCY CATEGORY D

See WARNINGS, Pregnancy Category D.

NURSING MOTHERS

It is not known whether this drug is excreted in human milk. Because many drugs are excreted in human milk and because of the potential for serious adverse reactions in nursing infants from lomustine capsules, a decision should be made whether to discontinue nursing or to discontinue the drug, taking into account the importance of the drug to the mother.

PEDIATRIC USE

See ADVERSE REACTIONS, Pulmonary Toxicity and DOSAGE AND ADMINISTRATION.

INFORMATION FOR THE PATIENT

Patients receiving lomustine capsules should be given the following information and instructions by the physician.

Patients should be told that lomustine capsules are an anticancer drug and belong to the group of medicines known as alkylating agents.

In order to provide the proper dose of lomustine capsules, patients should be aware that there may be two or more different types and colors of capsules in the container dispensed by the pharmacist.

Patients should be told that lomustine capsules are given as a single oral dose and will not be repeated for at least 6 weeks.

Patients should be told that nausea and vomiting usually last less than 24 hours, although loss of appetite may last for several days.

If any of the following reactions occur, notify the physician: fever, chills, sore throat, unusual bleeding or bruising, shortness of breath, dry cough, swelling of feet or lower legs, mental confusion, or yellowing of eyes and skin.

ADVERSE REACTIONS

HEMATOLOGIC TOXICITY

The most frequent and most serious toxicity of lomustine capsules is delayed myelosuppression. It usually occurs 4-6 weeks after drug administration and is dose related. Thrombocytopenia occurs at about 4 weeks postadministration and persists for 1-2 weeks. Leukopenia occurs at 5-6 weeks after a dose of lomustine capsules and persists for 1-2 weeks. Approximately 65% of patients receiving 130 mg/m^2 develop white blood counts below 5000 wbc/mm^3. Thirty-six percent (36%) develop white blood counts below 3000 wbc/mm^3. Thrombocytopenia is generally more severe than leukopenia. However, both may be dose-limiting toxicities.

Lomustine may produce cumulative myelosuppression, manifested by more depressed indices or longer duration of suppression after repeated doses.

The occurrence of acute leukemia and bone marrow dysplasias have been reported in patients following long term nitrosourea therapy.

Anemia also occurs, but is less frequent and less severe than thrombocytopenia or leukopenia.

PULMONARY TOXICITY

Pulmonary toxicity characterized by pulmonary infiltrates and/or fibrosis has been reported rarely with lomustine capsules. Onset of toxicity has occurred after an interval of 6 months or longer from the start of therapy with cumulative doses of lomustine capsules usually greater than 1100 mg/m^2. There is one report of pulmonary toxicity at a cumulative dose of only 600 mg.

Delayed onset pulmonary fibrosis occurring up to 17 years after treatment has been reported in patients who received related nitrosoureas in childhood and early adolescence (1-16 years) combined with cranial radiotherapy for intracranial tumors. There appeared to be some late reduction of pulmonary function of all long-term survivors. This form of lung fibrosis may be slowly progressive and has resulted in death in some cases. In this long-term study of carmustine, all those initally treated at less than 5 years of age died of delayed pulmonary fibrosis.

GASTROINTESTINAL TOXICITY

Nausea and vomiting may occur 3-6 hours after an oral dose and usually lasts less than 24 hours. Prior administration of antiemetics is effective in diminishing and sometimes preventing this side effect. Nausea and vomiting can also be reduced if lomustine capsules are administered to fasting patients.

HEPATOTOXICITY

A reversible type of hepatic toxicity, manifested by increased transaminase, alkaline phosphatase, and bilirubin levels, has been reported in a small percentage of patients receiving lomustine capsules.

NEPHROTOXICITY

Renal abnormalities consisting of progressive azotemia, decrease in kidney size, and renal failure have been reported in patients who received large cumulative doses after prolonged therapy with lomustine capsules. Kidney damage has also been reported occasionally in patients receiving lower total doses.

OTHER TOXICITIES

Stomatitis, alopecia, optic atrophy, and visual disturbances such as blindness have been reported infrequently.

Neurological reactions such as disorientation, lethargy, ataxia, and dysarthria have been noted in some patients receiving lomustine capsules. However, the relationship to medication in these patients is unclear.

DOSAGE AND ADMINISTRATION

The recommended dose of lomustine capsules in adult and pediatric patients as a single agent in previously untreated patients is 130 mg/m^2 as a single oral dose every 6 weeks. In individuals with compromised bone marrow function, the dose should be reduced to 100 mg/m^2 every 6 weeks. When lomustine capsules are used in combination with other myelosuppressive drugs, the doses should be adjusted accordingly.

Doses subsequent to the initial dose should be adjusted according to the hematologic response of the patient to the preceding dose. The schedule in TABLE 1 is suggested as a guide to dosage adjustment.

TABLE 1

Nadir After Prior Dose		
Leukocytes	**Platelets**	**Percentage of Prior Dose to be Given**
>4000	>100,000	100%
3000-3999	75,000-99,999	100%
2000-2999	25,000-74,999	70%
<2000	<25,000	50%

A repeat course of lomustine capsules should not be given until circulating blood elements have returned to acceptable levels (platelets above 100,000 mm^3; leukocytes above 4000/mm^3) and this is usually in 6 weeks. Adequate number of neutrophils should be present on a peripheral blood smear. Blood counts should be monitored weekly and repeat courses should not be given before 6 weeks because the hematologic toxicity is delayed and cumulative.

HOW SUPPLIED

CeeNu capsules are available in 3 strengths, Each color-coded capsule is imprinted with the dose in milligrams:

10 mg: White/White.
40 mg: White/Green.
100 mg: Green/Green.

Storage: CeeNu capsules are stable for the lot life indicated on package labeling when stored at room temperature in well closed containers. Avoid excessive heat (over 40°C, 104°F).

Procedures for proper handling and disposal of anticancer drugs should be considered. Several guidelines on this subject have been published.[1-7] There is no general agreement that all of the procedures recommended in the guidelines are necessary or appropriate.

PRODUCT LISTING - EQUIVALENTS NOT AVAILABLE

Capsule - Oral - Triphasic			
6's	$131.57	CEENU, Bristol-Myers Squibb	00015-3034-10
Capsule - Oral - 10 mg			
20's	$152.40	CEENU, Bristol-Myers Squibb	00015-3030-20
Capsule - Oral - 40 mg			
20's	$428.90	CEENU, Bristol-Myers Squibb	00015-3031-20
Capsule - Oral - 100 mg			
20's	$872.40	CEENU, Bristol-Myers Squibb	00015-3032-20

Loperamide Hydrochloride *(001661)*

Categories: Diarrhea; Pregnancy Category B; FDA Approved 1976 Dec
Drug Classes: Antidiarrheals; Gastrointestinals
Brand Names: **Imodium**
Foreign Brand Availability: Acanol (Mexico); Amerol (Indonesia); Arestal (France); Betaperamide (South-Africa); Binaldan (Switzerland); Brek (Italy); Colifilm (Argentina); Colodium (Hong-Kong); Desitin (Peru); Diacure (Netherlands); Diadium (Indonesia); Diarlop (India); Diamide (Philippines); Diapen (Bahrain; Cyprus; Egypt; Iran; Iraq; Jordan; Kuwait; Lebanon; Libya; Oman; Qatar; Republic-of-Yemen; Saudi-Arabia; Syria; United-Arab-Emirates); Diarent (Thailand); Diarin (Philippines); Diarodil (Thailand); Diarr-Eze (Canada); Diarstop-L (Germany); Diasolv (Philippines); Dicap (New-Zealand); Dissenten (Italy); Donafan (Peru); Elcoman (Argentina); Ercestop (France); Fortasec (Spain); Gastron (South-Africa); Gastro-Stop (Australia); Glubemide (Philippines); IMD (Singapore); Imosec (Spain); Imosen (Taiwan); Imossel (France); Imotril (Bahrain; Cyprus; Egypt; Iran; Iraq; Jordan; Kuwait; Lebanon; Libya; Oman; Qatar; Republic-of-Yemen; Saudi-Arabia; Syria; United-Arab-Emirates); Lenide-T (South-Africa); Lodia (Indonesia); Lomy (Thailand); Loniper (Philippines); Lop (Germany); Lopamid (Korea); Lopamide (India); Lop-Dia (Germany); Lopedin (Taiwan); Lopemid (Italy); Lopemin (Japan); Loperacap (Canada); Loperamil (Singapore); Loperastat (South-Africa); Loperhoe (Germany); Loperid (Israel); Loperium (Bahamas; Barbados; Belize; Bermuda; Curacao; Guyana; Jamaica; Netherland-Antilles; Surinam; Trinidad); Lopermide (China; Hong-Kong); Loperol (South-Africa); Loperyl (Italy); Loridin (Ecuador); Lorpa (Singapore); Motilex (Indonesia); Nabutil (France); Nimaz (France); Oramide (Indonesia); Orulop (Spain); Pangetan NF (Colombia); Perasian (Thailand); Pramidal (Mexico); Prodium (South-Africa); Raxedin (Mexico); Regulane (Argentina); Rexamide (Israel); Sanpo (Taiwan); Seldiar (Slovenia); Stopit (Israel); Suprasec (Argentina); Tanitril (Indonesia); Tebloc (Italy); Top-Dal (Mexico); Undiarrhea (Taiwan); Vacontil (Bahrain; Benin; Burkina-Faso; Cyprus; Egypt; Ethiopia; Gambia; Ghana; Guinea; Hong-Kong; Iraq; Ivory-Coast; Jordan; Kenya; Kuwait; Lebanon; Liberia; Libya; Malawi; Malaysia; Mali; Mauritania; Mauritius; Morocco; Niger; Nigeria; Oman; Qatar; Republic-of-Yemen; Saudi-Arabia; Senegal; Seychelles; Sierra-Leone; Sudan; Syria; Tanzania; Tunia; Uganda; United-Arab-Emirates; Zambia; Zimbabwe)
Cost of Therapy: $5.60 (Diarrhea; Generic Capsules; 2 mg; 8 capsules/day; 5 day supply)

DESCRIPTION

Loperamide hydrochloride, 4-(p-chlorophenyl)-4-hydroxy-N,N-dimethyl-α,α-diphenyl-1-piperidinebutyramide monohydrochloride, is a synthetic antidiarrheal for oral use.

Imodium is available in 2 mg capsules.

The inactive ingredients are lactose, cornstarch, talc, and magnesium stearate. Imodium capsules contain FD&C yellow no. 6.

CLINICAL PHARMACOLOGY

In vitro and animal studies show that loperamide HCl acts by slowing intestinal motility and by affecting water and electrolyte movement through the bowel. Loperamide HCl inhibits peristaltic activity by a direct effect on the circular and longitudinal muscles of the intestinal wall.

In man, loperamide HCl prolongs the transit time of the intestinal contents. It reduces the daily fecal volume, increases the viscosity and bulk density, and diminishes the loss of fluid and electrolytes. Tolerance to the antidiarrheal effect has not been observed.

INDICATIONS AND USAGE

Loperamide HCl is indicated for the control and symptomatic relief of acute nonspecific diarrhea and of chronic diarrhea associated with inflammatory bowel disease. Loperamide HCl is also indicated for reducing the volume of discharge from ileostomies.

CONTRAINDICATIONS

Loperamide HCl is contraindicated in patients with known hypersensitivity to the drug and in those in whom constipation must be avoided.

WARNINGS

Loperamide HCl should not be used in the case of acute dysentery, which is characterized by blood in stools and high fever.

Fluid and electrolyte depletion often occur in patients who have diarrhea. In such cases, administration of appropriate fluid and electrolytes is very important. The use of loperamide HCl does not preclude the administration of appropriate fluid and electrolyte therapy.

In some patients with acute ulcerative colitis, and in pseudomembranous colitis associated with broad-spectrum antibiotics, agents which inhibit intestinal motility, or delay intestinal transit time have been reported to induce toxic megacolon.

Loperamide HCl therapy should be discontinued promptly if abdominal distention, constipation, or ileus occurs.

Loperamide HCl should be used with special caution in young children because of the greater variability of response in this age group. Dehydration, particularly in younger children, may further influence the variability of response to loperamide HCl.

PRECAUTIONS

GENERAL

In acute diarrhea, if clinical improvement is not observed in 48 hours, the administration of loperamide HCl should be discontinued. Patients with hepatic dysfunction should be monitored closely for signs of CNS toxicity because of the apparent large first pass biotransformation.

INFORMATION FOR THE PATIENT

Patients should be advised to check with their physician if their diarrhea does not improve after a couple of days or if they note blood in their stools or develop a fever.

CARCINOGENESIS, MUTAGENESIS, AND IMPAIRMENT OF FERTILITY

In an 18 month rat study with doses up to 133 times the maximum human dose (on a mg/kg basis), there was no evidence of carcinogenesis. Mutagenicity studies were not conducted. Reproduction studies in rats indicated that high doses (150-200 times the human dose) could cause marked female infertility and reduced male fertility.

PREGNANCY, TERATOGENIC EFFECTS, PREGNANCY CATEGORY B

Reproduction studies in rats and rabbits have revealed no evidence of impaired fertility or harm to the fetus at doses up to 30 times the human dose. Higher doses impaired the survival of mothers and nursing young. The studies offered no evidence of teratogenic activity. There are, however, no adequate and well controlled studies in pregnant women. Because animal reproduction studies are not always predictive of human response, this drug should be used during pregnancy only if clearly needed.

NURSING MOTHERS

It is not known whether this drug is excreted in human milk. Because many drugs are excreted in human milk, caution should be exercised when loperamide HCl is administered to a nursing woman.

PEDIATRIC USE

See WARNINGS for information on the greater variability of response in this age group.

DRUG INTERACTIONS

There was no evidence in clinical trials of drug interactions with concurrent medications.

ADVERSE REACTIONS

The adverse effects reported during clinical investigations of loperamide HCl are difficult to distinguish from symptoms associated with the diarrheal syndrome. Adverse experiences recorded during clinical studies with loperamide HCl were generally of a minor and self-limiting nature. They were more commonly observed during the treatment of chronic diarrhea.

The following patient complaints have been reported and are listed in decreasing order of frequency with the exception of hypersensitivity reactions which is listed first since it may be the most serious.

Hypersensitivity reactions (including skin rash) have been reported with loperamide HCl use.
Abdominal pain, distention, or discomfort.
Nausea and vomiting.
Constipation.
Tiredness.
Drowsiness or dizziness.
Dry mouth.

L

In postmarketing experiences, there have been rare reports of paralytic ileus associated with abdominal distention. Most of these reports occurred in the setting of acute dysentery, overdosage, and with very young children of less than 2 years of age.

DOSAGE AND ADMINISTRATION

(1 capsule = 2 mg)

Patients should receive appropriate fluid and electrolyte replacement as needed.

ACUTE DIARRHEA

Adults

The recommended initial dose is 4 mg (2 capsules) followed by 2 mg (1 capsule) after each unformed stool. Daily dosage should not exceed 16 mg (8 capsules). Clinical improvement is usually observed within 48 hours.

Children

Loperamide HCl use is not recommended for children under 2 years of age. In children 2-5 years of age (20 kg or less), the non-prescription liquid formulation (loperamide HCl 1 mg/5 ml) should be used; for ages 6-12, either loperamide HCl capsules or loperamide HCl liquid may be used. For children 2-12 years of age, the schedule in TABLE 1 for capsules or liquid will usually fulfill initial dosage requirements.

TABLE 1 *Recommended First Day Dosage Schedule*

Age	Dose
2-5 years (13-20 kg)	1 mg tid (3 mg daily dose)
6-8 years (20-30 kg)	2 mg bid (4 mg daily dose)
8-12 years (>30 kg)	2 mg tid (6 mg daily dose)

Recommended Subsequent Daily Dosage

Following the first treatment day, it is recommended that subsequent loperamide HCl doses (1 mg/10 kg body weight) be administered only after a loose stool. Total daily dosage should not exceed recommended dosages for the first day.

CHRONIC DIARRHEA

Children

Although loperamide HCl has been studied in a limited number of children with chronic diarrhea, the therapeutic dose for the treatment of chronic diarrhea in a pediatric population has not been established.

Adults

The recommended initial dose is 4 mg (2 capsules) followed by 2 mg (1 capsule) after each unformed stool until diarrhea is controlled, after which the dosage of loperamide HCl should be reduced to meet individual requirements. When the optimal daily dosage has been established, this amount may then be administered as a single dose or in divided doses.

The average daily maintenance dosage in clinical trials was 4-8 mg (2-4 capsules). A dosage of 16 mg (8 capsules) was rarely exceeded. If clinical improvement is not observed after treatment with 16 mg per day for at least 10 days, symptoms are unlikely to be controlled by further administration. Loperamide HCl administration may be continued if diarrhea cannot be adequately controlled with diet or specific treatment.

HOW SUPPLIED

Each Imodium capsule contains 2 mg of loperamide HCl. The capsules have a light green body and a dark green cap with "JANSSEN" imprinted on one segment and "IMODIUM" on the other segment.

Storage: Store at room temperature 15-25°C (59-77°F).

PRODUCT LISTING - RATED THERAPEUTICALLY EQUIVALENT

Capsule - Oral - 2 mg

Size	Price	Manufacturer	NDC
6's	$5.70	GENERIC, Pd-Rx Pharmaceuticals	55289-0315-06
12's	$7.18	GENERIC, Pharmaceutical Corporation Of America	51655-0547-27
12's	$7.43	GENERIC, Pd-Rx Pharmaceuticals	55289-0315-12
12's	$8.24	GENERIC, Heartland Healthcare Services	61392-0336-12
25's	$6.65	GENERIC, Udl Laboratories Inc	51079-0690-19
30's	$20.59	GENERIC, Heartland Healthcare Services	61392-0336-30
30's	$20.59	GENERIC, Heartland Healthcare Services	61392-0336-39
31 x 10	$234.91	GENERIC, Vangard Labs	00615-0362-53
31 x 10	$234.91	GENERIC, Vangard Labs	00615-0362-63
31's	$21.28	GENERIC, Heartland Healthcare Services	61392-0336-31
32's	$21.96	GENERIC, Heartland Healthcare Services	61392-0336-32
45's	$30.89	GENERIC, Heartland Healthcare Services	61392-0336-45
60's	$41.19	GENERIC, Heartland Healthcare Services	61392-0336-60
90's	$61.78	GENERIC, Heartland Healthcare Services	61392-0336-90
100's	$37.32	GENERIC, Roxane Laboratories Inc	00054-2537-25
100's	$39.02	GENERIC, Roxane Laboratories Inc	00054-8537-25
100's	$55.10	GENERIC, Major Pharmaceuticals Inc	00904-7617-60
100's	$55.67	GENERIC, Mova Pharmaceutical Corporation	55370-0169-07
100's	$55.67	GENERIC, Novopharm Usa Inc	55953-0020-40
100's	$55.75	GENERIC, Watson/Schein Pharmaceuticals Inc	00364-2481-01
100's	$57.96	GENERIC, Qualitest Products Inc	00603-4235-21
100's	$58.46	GENERIC, Moore, H.L. Drug Exchange Inc	00839-7623-06
100's	$58.60	GENERIC, Aligen Independent Laboratories Inc	00405-4592-01
100's	$61.10	GENERIC, Teva Pharmaceuticals Usa	00093-0311-01
100's	$61.10	GENERIC, Martec Pharmaceuticals Inc	52555-0519-01
100's	$61.25	GENERIC, Ivax Corporation	00182-1505-01
100's	$61.55	GENERIC, American Health Packaging	62584-0768-01
100's	$62.17	GENERIC, Novopharm Usa Inc	55953-0020-01
100's	$68.20	GENERIC, Mylan Pharmaceuticals Inc	00378-2100-01
100's	$70.25	GENERIC, Udl Laboratories Inc	51079-0690-20
200 x 5	$757.77	GENERIC, Vangard Labs	00615-0362-43

PRODUCT LISTING - EQUIVALENTS NOT AVAILABLE

Capsule - Oral - 2 mg

Size	Price	Manufacturer	NDC
2's	$3.48	GENERIC, Prescript Pharmaceuticals	00247-0136-02
4's	$3.62	GENERIC, Prescript Pharmaceuticals	00247-0136-04
5's	$3.68	GENERIC, Prescript Pharmaceuticals	00247-0136-05
6's	$3.68	GENERIC, Allscripts Pharmaceutical Company	54569-3707-02
6's	$3.75	GENERIC, Prescript Pharmaceuticals	00247-0136-06
8's	$3.88	GENERIC, Prescript Pharmaceuticals	00247-0136-08
9's	$3.95	GENERIC, Prescript Pharmaceuticals	00247-0136-09
10's	$2.56	GENERIC, Physicians Total Care	54868-2118-00
10's	$4.01	GENERIC, Prescript Pharmaceuticals	00247-0136-10
12's	$4.15	GENERIC, Prescript Pharmaceuticals	00247-0136-12
12's	$7.36	GENERIC, Allscripts Pharmaceutical Company	54569-3707-03
12's	$8.57	GENERIC, Southwood Pharmaceuticals Inc	58016-0254-12
15's	$4.34	GENERIC, Prescript Pharmaceuticals	00247-0136-15
15's	$9.20	GENERIC, Allscripts Pharmaceutical Company	54569-3707-00
15's	$10.71	GENERIC, Southwood Pharmaceuticals Inc	58016-0254-15
16's	$3.29	GENERIC, Physicians Total Care	54868-2118-03
16's	$4.41	GENERIC, Prescript Pharmaceuticals	00247-0136-16
18's	$4.54	GENERIC, Prescript Pharmaceuticals	00247-0136-18
20's	$3.78	GENERIC, Physicians Total Care	54868-2118-01
20's	$4.68	GENERIC, Prescript Pharmaceuticals	00247-0136-20
20's	$14.28	GENERIC, Southwood Pharmaceuticals Inc	58016-0254-20
30's	$5.34	GENERIC, Prescript Pharmaceuticals	00247-0136-30
30's	$21.42	GENERIC, Southwood Pharmaceuticals Inc	58016-0254-30
100's	$14.00	GENERIC, Physicians Total Care	54868-2118-04
100's	$71.39	GENERIC, Southwood Pharmaceuticals Inc	58016-0254-00

Lopinavir; Ritonavir *(003508)*

For related information, see the comparative table section in Appendix A.

Categories: Infection, human immunodeficiency virus; FDA Approved 2000 Sep; Pregnancy Category C; WHO Formulary
Drug Classes: Antivirals; Protease inhibitors
Brand Names: Kaletra
Cost of Therapy: $703.50 (HIV; Kaletra; 133.3 mg; 33.3 mg; 6 capsules/day; 30 day supply)
$659.53 (HIV; Kaletra Liquid; 400 mg; 100 mg/5 ml; 10 ml/day; 30 day supply)

DESCRIPTION

Note: The trade name has been used throughout this monograph for clarity.

Kaletra (lopinavir; ritonavir) is a co-formulation of lopinavir and ritonavir. Lopinavir is an inhibitor of the HIV protease. As co-formulated in Kaletra, ritonavir inhibits the CYP3A-mediated metabolism of lopinavir, thereby providing increased plasma levels of lopinavir.

Lopinavir is chemically designated as [1S-[1R*,(R*),3R*,4R*]]-N-[4-[[(2,6-dimethylphenoxy)acetyl]amino]-3-hydroxy-5-phenyl-1-(phenylmethyl)pentyl]tetrahydro-alpha-(1-methylethyl)-2-oxo-1(2H)-pyrimidineacetamide. Its molecular formula is $C_{37}H_{48}N_4O_5$, and its molecular weight is 628.80.

Ritonavir is chemically designated as 10-Hydroxy-2-methyl-5-(1-methylethyl)-1-[2-(1-methylethyl)-4-thiazolyl]-3,6-dioxo-8,11-bis(phenylmethyl)-2,4,7,12-tetraazatridecan-13-oic acid, 5-thiazolylmethyl ester, [5S-(5R*,8R*,10R*,11R*)]. Its molecular formula is $C_{37}H_{48}N_6O_5S_2$, and its molecular weight is 720.95.

Lopinavir is a white to light tan powder. It is freely soluble in methanol and ethanol, soluble in isopropanol and practically insoluble in water.

CAPSULES

Kaletra capsules are available for oral administration in a strength of 133.3 mg lopinavir and 33.3 mg ritonavir with the following inactive ingredients: FD&C yellow no. 6, gelatin, glycerin, oleic acid, polyoxyl 35 castor oil, propylene glycol, sorbitol special, titanium dioxide, and water.

ORAL SOLUTION

Kaletra oral solution is available for oral administration as 80 mg lopinavir and 20 mg ritonavir per milliliter with the following inactive ingredients: acesulfame potassium, alcohol, artificial cotton candy flavor, citric acid, glycerin, high fructose corn syrup, Magnasweet-110 flavor, menthol, natural & artificial vanilla flavor, peppermint oil, polyoxyl 40 hydrogenated castor oil, povidone, propylene glycol, saccharin sodium, sodium chloride, sodium citrate, and water.

Kaletra oral solution contains 42.4% alcohol (v/v).

CLINICAL PHARMACOLOGY

MICROBIOLOGY

Mechanism of Action

Lopinavir, an inhibitor of the HIV protease, prevents cleavage of the Gag-Pol polyprotein, resulting in the production of immature, non-infectious viral particles.

Antiviral Activity In Vitro

The *in vitro* antiviral activity of lopinavir against laboratory HIV strains and clinical HIV isolates was evaluated in acutely infected lymphoblastic cell lines and peripheral blood lymphocytes, respectively. In the absence of human serum, the mean 50% effective concentration (EC_{50}) of lopinavir against 5 different HIV-1 laboratory strains ranged from

10-27 nM (0.006-0.017 μg/ml, 1 μg/ml = 1.6 μM) and ranged from 4-11 nM (0.003-0.007 μg/ml) against several HIV-1 clinical isolates (n=6). In the presence of 50% human serum, the mean EC_{50} of lopinavir against these 5 laboratory strains ranged from 65-289 nM (0.04-0.18 μg/ml), representing a 7- to 11-fold attenuation. Combination drug activity studies with lopinavir and other protease inhibitors or reverse transcriptase inhibitors have not been completed.

Resistance

HIV-1 isolates with reduced susceptibility to lopinavir have been selected *in vitro*. The presence of ritonavir does not appear to influence the selection of lopinavir-resistant viruses *in vitro*.

The selection of resistance to Kaletra in antiretroviral treatment naïve patients has not yet been characterized. In a Phase 3 study of 653 antiretroviral treatment naïve patients (Study 863), plasma viral isolates from each patient on treatment with plasma HIV >400 copies/ml at Week 24, 32, 40 and/or 48 were analyzed. No evidence of resistance to Kaletra was observed in 37 evaluable Kaletra-treated patients (0%). Evidence of genotypic resistance to nelfinavir, defined as the presence of the D30N and/or L90M mutation in HIV protease, was observed in 25/76 (33%) of evaluable nelfinavir-treated patients. The selection of resistance to Kaletra in antiretroviral treatment naïve pediatric patients (Study 940) appears to be consistent with that seen in adult patients (Study 863).

Resistance to Kaletra has been noted to emerge in patients treated with other protease inhibitors prior to Kaletra therapy. In Phase 2 studies of 227 antiretroviral treatment naïve and protease inhibitor experienced patients, isolates from 4 of 23 patients with quantifiable (>400 copies/ml) viral RNA following treatment with Kaletra for 12-100 weeks displayed significantly reduced susceptibility to lopinavir compared to the corresponding baseline viral isolates. Three (3) of these patients had previously received treatment with a single protease inhibitor (nelfinavir, indinavir, or saquinavir) and 1 patient had received treatment with multiple protease inhibitors (indinavir, saquinavir and ritonavir). All 4 of these patients had at least 4 mutations associated with protease inhibitor resistance immediately prior to Kaletra therapy. Following viral rebound, isolates from these patients all contained additional mutations, some of which are recognized to be associated with protease inhibitor resistance. However, there are insufficient data at this time to identify lopinavir-associated mutational patterns in isolates from patients on Kaletra therapy. The assessment of these mutational patterns is under study.

Cross-Resistance — Preclinical Studies

Varying degrees of cross-resistance have been observed among HIV protease inhibitors. Little information is available on the cross-resistance of viruses that developed decreased susceptibility to lopinavir during Kaletra therapy.

The *in vitro* activity of lopinavir against clinical isolates from patients previously treated with a single protease inhibitor was determined. Isolates that displayed >4-fold reduced susceptibility to nelfinavir (n=13) and saquinavir (n=4), displayed <4-fold reduced susceptibility to lopinavir. Isolates with >4-fold reduced susceptibility to indinavir (n=16) and ritonavir (n=3) displayed a mean of 5.7- and 8.3-fold reduced susceptibility to lopinavir, respectively. Isolates from patients previously treated with 2 or more protease inhibitors showed greater reductions in susceptibility to lopinavir, as described in the following paragraph.

Clinical Studies — Antiviral Activity of Kaletra in Patients With Previous Protease Inhibitor Therapies

The clinical relevance of reduced *in vitro* susceptibility to lopinavir has been examined by assessing the virologic response to Kaletra therapy, with respect to baseline viral genotype and phenotype, in 56 NNRTI-naïve patients with HIV RNA >1000 copies/ml despite previous therapy with at least 2 protease inhibitors selected from nelfinavir, indinavir, saquinavir and ritonavir (Study 957). In this study, patients were initially randomized to receive 1 of 2 doses of Kaletra in combination with efavirenz and nucleoside reverse transcriptase inhibitors. The EC_{50} values of lopinavir against the 56 baseline viral isolates ranged from 0.5- to 96-fold higher than the wild-type EC_{50}. Fifty-five percent (31/56) of these baseline isolates displayed a >4-fold reduced susceptibility to lopinavir. These 31 isolates had a mean reduction in lopinavir susceptibility of 27.9-fold. TABLE 1 shows the 48 week virologic response (HIV RNA <400 and <50 copies) according to susceptibility and number of genotypic mutations at baseline in 50 evaluable patients enrolled in the study (957) described above. Because this was a select patient population and the sample size was small, the data depicted in TABLE 1 do not constitute definitive clinical susceptibility breakpoints. Additional data are needed to determine clinically significant breakpoints for Kaletra.

TABLE 1 *HIV RNA Response at Week 48 by Baseline Kaletra Susceptibility and by Number of Protease Inhibitor-Associated Mutations**

	HIV RNA <400 copies/ml	HIV RNA <50 copies/ml
Lopinavir Susceptibility† at Baseline		
<10-fold	25/27 (93%)	22/27 (81%)
>10- and <40-fold	11/15 (73%)	9/15 (60%)
≥40-fold	2/8 (25%)	2/8 (25%)
Number of Protease Inhibitor Mutations at Baseline		
Up to 5	21/23 (91%)‡	19/23 (83%)
>5	17/27 (63%)	14/27 (52%)

* Lopinavir susceptibility was determined by recombinant phenotypic technology performed by virologic; genotype also performed by virologic.
† Fold change in susceptibility from wild type.
‡ Thirteen (13) of the 23 patient isolates contained PI mutations at positions 82, 84, and/or 90.

There are insufficient data at this time to identify lopinavir-associated mutational patterns in isolates from patients on Kaletra therapy. Further studies are needed to assess the association between specific mutational patterns and virologic response rates.

PHARMACOKINETICS

The pharmacokinetic properties of lopinavir co-administered with ritonavir have been evaluated in healthy adult volunteers and in HIV-infected patients; no substantial differences were observed between the 2 groups. Lopinavir is essentially completely metabolized by CYP3A. Ritonavir inhibits the metabolism of lopinavir, thereby increasing the plasma levels of lopinavir. Across studies, administration of Kaletra 400/100 mg bid yields mean steady-state lopinavir plasma concentrations 15- to 20-fold higher than those of ritonavir in HIV-infected patients. The plasma levels of ritonavir are less than 7% of those obtained after the ritonavir dose of 600 mg bid. The *in vitro* antiviral EC_{50} of lopinavir is approximately 10-fold lower than that of ritonavir. Therefore, the antiviral activity of Kaletra is due to lopinavir.

Absorption

In a pharmacokinetic study in HIV-positive subjects (n=21) without meal restrictions, multiple dosing with 400/100 mg Kaletra bid for 3-4 weeks produced a mean ±SD lopinavir peak plasma concentration (C_{max}) of 9.6 ± 4.4 μg/ml, occurring approximately 4 hours after administration. The mean steady-state trough concentration prior to the morning dose was 5.5 ± 4.0 μg/ml. Lopinavir AUC over a 12 hour dosing interval averaged 82.8 ± 44.5 μg·h/ml. The absolute bioavailability of lopinavir co-formulated with ritonavir in humans has not been established. Under nonfasting conditions (500 kcal, 25% from fat), lopinavir concentrations were similar following administration of Kaletra co-formulated capsules and liquid. When administered under fasting conditions, both the mean AUC and C_{max} of lopinavir were 22% lower for the Kaletra liquid relative to the capsule formulation.

Effects of Food on Oral Absorption

Administration of a single 400/100 mg dose of Kaletra capsules with a moderate fat meal (500-682 kcal, 23-25% calories from fat) was associated with a mean increase of 48 and 23% in lopinavir AUC and C_{max}, respectively, relative to fasting. For Kaletra oral solution, the corresponding increases in lopinavir AUC and C_{max} were 80 and 54%, respectively. Relative to fasting, administration of Kaletra with a high fat meal (872 kcal, 56% from fat) increased lopinavir AUC and C_{max} by 97 and 43%, respectively, for capsules, and 130 and 56%, respectively, for oral solution. To enhance bioavailability and minimize pharmacokinetic variability Kaletra should be taken with food.

Distribution

At steady state, lopinavir is approximately 98-99% bound to plasma proteins. Lopinavir binds to both alpha-1-acid glycoprotein (AAG) and albumin; however, it has a higher affinity for AAG. At steady state, lopinavir protein binding remains constant over the range of observed concentrations after 400/100 mg Kaletra bid, and is similar between healthy volunteers and HIV-positive patients.

Metabolism

In vitro experiments with human hepatic microsomes indicate that lopinavir primarily undergoes oxidative metabolism. Lopinavir is extensively metabolized by the hepatic cytochrome P450 system, almost exclusively by the CYP3A isozyme. Ritonavir is a potent CYP3A inhibitor which inhibits the metabolism of lopinavir, and therefore increases plasma levels of lopinavir. A ^{14}C-lopinavir study in humans showed that 89% of the plasma radioactivity after a single 400/100 mg Kaletra dose was due to parent drug. At least 13 lopinavir oxidative metabolites have been identified in man. Ritonavir has been shown to induce metabolic enzymes, resulting in the induction of its own metabolism. Pre-dose lopinavir concentrations decline with time during multiple dosing, stabilizing after approximately 10-16 days.

Elimination

Following a 400/100 mg ^{14}C-lopinavir/ritonavir dose, approximately 10.4 ± 2.3% and 82.6 ± 2.5% of an administered dose of ^{14}C-lopinavir can be accounted for in urine and feces, respectively, after 8 days. Unchanged lopinavir accounted for approximately 2.2 and 19.8% of the administered dose in urine and feces, respectively. After multiple dosing, less than 3% of the lopinavir dose is excreted unchanged in the urine. The half-life of lopinavir over a 12 hour dosing interval averaged 5-6 hours, and the apparent oral clearance (CL/F) of lopinavir is 6-7 L/h.

Special Populations

Gender, Race and Age

Lopinavir pharmacokinetics have not been studied in elderly patients. No gender related pharmacokinetic differences have been observed in adult patients. No clinically important pharmacokinetic differences due to race have been identified.

Pediatric Patients

The pharmacokinetics of Kaletra 300/75 mg/m² bid and 230/57.5 mg/m² bid have been studied in a total of 53 pediatric patients, ranging in age from 6 months to 12 years. The 230/57.5 mg/m² bid regimen without nevirapine and the 300/75 mg/m² bid regimen with nevirapine provided lopinavir plasma concentrations similar to those obtained in adult patients receiving the 400/100 mg bid regimen (without nevirapine).

The mean steady-state lopinavir AUC, C_{max}, and C_{min} were 72.6 ± 31.1 μg·h/ml, 8.2 ± 2.9 and 3.4 ± 2.1 μg/ml, respectively after Kaletra 230/57.5 mg/m² bid without nevirapine (n=12), and were 85.8 ± 36.9 μg·h/ml, 10.0 ± 3.3 and 3.6 ± 3.5 μg/ml, respectively, after 300/75 mg/m² bid with nevirapine (n=12). The nevirapine regimen was 7 mg/kg bid (6 months to 8 years) or 4 mg/kg bid (>8 years).

Renal Insufficiency

Lopinavir pharmacokinetics have not been studied in patients with renal insufficiency; however, since the renal clearance of lopinavir is negligible, a decrease in total body clearance is not expected in patients with renal insufficiency.

Hepatic Impairment

Lopinavir is principally metabolized and eliminated by the liver. Although Kaletra has not been studied in patients with hepatic impairment, lopinavir concentrations may be increased in these patients (see PRECAUTIONS).

Drug-Drug Interactions

See also CONTRAINDICATIONS, WARNINGS and DRUG INTERACTIONS.

Kaletra is an inhibitor of the P450 isoform CYP3A *in vitro*. Co-administration of Kaletra and drugs primarily metabolized by CYP3A may result in increased plasma concentrations of the other drug, which could increase or prolong its therapeutic and adverse effects (see CONTRAINDICATIONS).

Kaletra inhibits CYP2D6 *in vitro*, but to a lesser extent than CYP3A. Clinically significant drug interactions with drugs metabolized by CYP2D6 are possible with Kaletra at the recommended dose, but the magnitude is not known. Kaletra does not inhibit CYP2C9, CYP2C19, CYP2E1, CYP2B6 or CYP1A2 at clinically relevant concentrations.

Kaletra has been shown *in vivo* to induce its own metabolism and to increase the biotransformation of some drugs metabolized by cytochrome P450 enzymes and by glucuronidation.

Kaletra is metabolized by CYP3A. Drugs that induce CYP3A activity would be expected to increase the clearance of lopinavir, resulting in lowered plasma concentrations of lopinavir. Although not noted with concurrent ketoconazole, co-administration of Kaletra and other drugs that inhibit CYP3A may increase lopinavir plasma concentrations.

Drug interaction studies were performed with Kaletra and other drugs likely to be co-administered and some drugs commonly used as probes for pharmacokinetic interactions. The effects of co-administration of Kaletra on the AUC, C_{max} and C_{min} are summarized in TABLE 2 (effect of other drugs on lopinavir) and TABLE 3 (effect of Kaletra on other drugs). The effects of other drugs on ritonavir are not shown since they generally correlate with those observed with lopinavir (if lopinavir concentrations are decreased, ritonavir concentrations are decreased) unless otherwise indicated in the table footnotes. For information regarding clinical recommendations, see DRUG INTERACTIONS, Established and Other Potentially Significant Drug Interactions.

TABLE 2 *Drug Interactions: Pharmacokinetic Parameters for Lopinavir in the Presence of the Co-Administered Drug**

Co-Administered Drug (dose in mg)	Dose of Kaletra (mg)	n	Ratio (with/without co-administered drug) of Lopinavir† C_{max}	AUC	C_{min}
Amprenavir‡					
450 or 750 bid, 5 d	400/100 bid, 22 d	12 or 10	0.89 (0.83, 0.95)	0.85 (0.81, 0.90)	0.81 (0.74, 0.89)
Atorvastatin					
20 qd, 4 d	400/100 bid, 14 d	12	0.90 (0.78, 1.06)	0.90 (0.79, 1.02)	0.92 (0.78, 1.10)
Efavirenz§					
600 qhs, 9 d	400/100 bid, 9 d	11, 7**	0.97 (0.78, 1.22)	0.81 (0.64, 1.03)	0.61 (0.38, 0.97)
Ketoconazole					
200 single dose	400/100 bid, 16 d	12	0.89 (0.80, 0.99)	0.87 (0.75, 1.00)	0.75 (0.55, 1.00)
Nevirapine					
200 bid, steady-state (>1 year)¤	400/100 bid, steady-state (>1 year)	22, 19**	0.81 (0.62, 1.05)	0.73 (0.53, 0.98)	0.49 (0.28, 0.74)
7 or 4 mg/kg qd, 2 wk; bid 1 wk¶	300/75 mg/m^2 bid, 3 wk	12, 15**	0.86 (0.64, 1.16)	0.78 (0.56, 1.09)	0.45 (0.25, 0.81)
Pravastatin					
20 qd, 4 d	400/100 bid, 14 d	12	0.98 (0.89, 1.08)	0.95 (0.85, 1.05)	0.88 (0.77, 1.02)
Rifabutin					
150 qd, 10 d	400/100 bid, 20 d	14	1.08 (0.97, 1.19)	1.17 (1.04, 1.31)	1.20 (0.96, 1.65)
Rifampin					
600 qd, 10 d	400/100 bid, 20 d	22	0.45 (0.40, 0.51)	0.25 (0.21, 0.29)	0.01 (0.01, 0.02)
Ritonavir¤					
100 bid, 3-4 wk	400/100 bid, 3-4 wk	8, 21**	1.28 (0.94, 1.76)	1.46 (1.04, 2.06)	2.16 (1.29, 3.62)

All interaction studies conducted in healthy, HIV-negative subjects unless otherwise indicated.
* See DRUG INTERACTIONS, Established and Other Potentially Significant Drug Interactions for recommended alterations in dose or regimen.
† Pharmacokinetic parameters (90% CI); No Effect = 1.00.
‡ Composite effect of amprenavir 450 and 750 mg q12h regimens on lopinavir pharmacokinetics.
§ The pharmacokinetics of ritonavir are unaffected by concurrent efavirenz.
¤ Study conducted in HIV-positive adult subjects.
¶ Study conducted in HIV-positive pediatric subjects ranging in age from 6 months to 12 years.
** Parallel group design; n for Kaletra + co-administered drug, n for Kaletra alone.

Effect of Kaletra on Other Protease Inhibitors (PIs)

The pharmacokinetics of single-dose indinavir and saquinavir, and multiple-dose amprenavir obtained in healthy subjects after at least 10 days of Kaletra 400/100 mg bid were compared to historical data in HIV-infected subjects (refer to TABLE 3 for information on study design and doses). Because of the limitations in the study design and the use of comparisons between healthy and HIV infected subjects, it is not possible to recommend definitive dosing recommendations. However, based on these comparisons, amprenavir 750 mg bid and indinavir 600 mg bid, when co-administered with Kaletra 400/100 mg bid, may produce a similar AUC, lower C_{max}, and higher C_{min} compared to their respective established clinical dosing regimens. Saquinavir 800 mg bid, when co-administered with Kaletra 400/100 mg bid, may produce a similar AUC and higher C_{min} to its respective established clinical dosing regimen (no comparative information regarding C_{max}). The clinical significance of the lower C_{max} and higher C_{min} is unknown. Appropriate doses of amprenavir, indinavir and saquinavir in combination with Kaletra with respect to safety and efficacy have not been established (see DRUG INTERACTIONS, Established and Other Potentially Significant Drug Interactions).

TABLE 3 *Drug Interactions: Pharmacokinetic Parameters for Co-Administered Drug in the Presence of Kaletra**

Co-Administered Drug (dose in mg)	Dose of Kaletra (mg)	n	Ratio (with/without Kaletra) of Co-Administered Drug† C_{max}	AUC	C_{min}
Amprenavir					
450 or 750 bid, 5 d	400/100 bid, 22 d	12 or 10	See text below for discussion of interaction.¤		
Atorvastatin					
20 qd, 4 d	400/100 bid, 14 d	12	4.67 (3.35, 6.51)	5.88 (4.69, 7.37)	2.28 (1.91, 2.71)
Efavirenz					
600 qhs, 9 d	400/100 bid, 9 d	11, 12§	0.91 (0.72, 1.15)	0.84 (0.62, 1.15)	0.84 (0.58, 1.20)
Ethinyl Estradiol					
35 μg qd, 21 d	400/100 bid, 14 d	12	0.59 (0.52, 0.66)	0.58 (0.54, 0.62)	0.42 (0.36, 0.49)
Indinavir					
600 single dose	400/100 bid, 10 d	11	See text below for discussion of interaction.¤		
Ketoconazole					
200 single dose	400/100 bid, 16 d	12	1.13 (0.91, 1.40)	3.04 (2.44, 3.79)	NA
Methadone					
5 single dose	400/100 bid, 10 d	11	0.55 (0.48, 0.64)	0.47 (0.42, 0.53)	NA
Nevirapine					
200 qd, 14 d; bid 6 d	400/100 bid, 20 d	5, 6§	1.05 (0.72, 1.52)	1.08 (0.72, 1.64)	1.15 (0.71, 1.86)
Norethindrone					
1 qd, 21 d	400/100 bid, 14 d	12	0.84 (0.75, 0.94)	0.83 (0.73, 0.94)	0.68 (0.54, 0.85)
Pravastatin					
20 qd, 4 d	400/100 bid, 14 d	12	1.26 (0.87, 1.83)	1.33 (0.91, 1.94)	NA
Rifabutin					
300 qd, 10 d; 150 qd, 10 d	400/100 bid, 10 d	12	2.12 (1.89, 2.38)	3.03 (2.79, 3.30)	4.90 (3.18, 5.76)
25-*O*-desacetyl rifabutin			23.6 (13.7, 25.3)	47.5 (29.3, 51.8)	94.9 (74.0, 122)
Rifabutin + 25-*O*-desacetyl rifabutin‡			3.46 (3.07, 3.91)	5.73 (5.08, 6.46)	9.53 (7.56, 12.01)
Saquinavir					
800 single dose	400/100 bid, 10 d	11	See text below for discussion of interaction.¤		

All interaction studies conducted in healthy, HIV-negative subjects unless otherwise indicated.
* See DRUG INTERACTIONS, Established and Other Potentially Significant Drug Interactions for recommended alterations in dose or regimen.
† Pharmacokinetic parameters (90% CI); No Effect = 1.00.
‡ Effect on the dose-normalized sum of rifabutin parent and 25-O-desacetyl rifabutin active metabolite.
§ Parallel group design; n for Kaletra + co-administered drug, n for co-administered drug alone.
¤ See Effect of Kaletra on Other Protease Inhibitors (PIs).
NA = Not available.

INDICATIONS AND USAGE

Kaletra is indicated in combination with other antiretroviral agents for the treatment of HIV-infection. This indication is based on analyses of plasma HIV RNA levels and CD4 cell counts in controlled studies of Kaletra of 48 weeks duration and in smaller uncontrolled dose-ranging studies of Kaletra of 72 weeks duration.

CONTRAINDICATIONS

Kaletra is contraindicated in patients with known hypersensitivity to any of its ingredients, including ritonavir.

Co-administration of Kaletra is contraindicated with drugs that are highly dependent on CYP3A or CYP2D6 for clearance and for which elevated plasma concentrations are associated with serious and/or life-threatening events. These drugs are listed in TABLE 7.

TABLE 7 *Drugs That Are Contraindicated With Kaletra*

Drug Class	Drugs Within Class That Are Contraindicated With Kaletra
Antiarrhythmics	Flecainide, propafenone
Antihistamines	Astemizole, terfenadine
Ergot derivatives	Dihydroergotamine, ergonovine, ergotamine, methylergonovine
GI motility agent	Cisapride
Neuroleptic	Pimozide
Sedative/hypnotics	Midazolam, triazolam

WARNINGS

ALERT: Find out about medicines that should NOT be taken with Kaletra. This statement is included on the product's bottle label.

DRUG INTERACTIONS

Kaletra is an inhibitor of the P450 isoform CYP3A. Co-administration of Kaletra and drugs primarily metabolized by CYP3A or CYP2D6 may result in increased plasma concentrations of the other drug that could increase or prolong its therapeutic and adverse effects (see CLINICAL PHARMACOLOGY, Pharmacokinetics, Special Populations, Drug-Drug Interactions; TABLE 7; TABLE 8, and DRUG INTERACTIONS, Established and Other Potentially Significant Drug Interactions).

Particular caution should be used when prescribing sildenafil in patients receiving Kaletra. Co-administration of Kaletra with sildenafil is expected to substantially increase sildenafil concentrations and may result in an increase in sildenafil-associated adverse events including hypotension, syncope, visual changes and prolonged erection (see DRUG INTERACTIONS and the complete prescribing information for sildenafil).

Concomitant use of Kaletra with lovastatin or simvastatin is not recommended. Caution should be exercised if HIV protease inhibitors, including Kaletra, are used concurrently with other HMG-CoA reductase inhibitors that are also metabolized by the CYP3A4 pathway (*e.g.*, atorvastatin). The risk of myopathy, including rhabdomyolysis may be increased when HIV protease inhibitors, including Kaletra, are used in combination with these drugs.

Concomitant use of Kaletra and St. John's wort (hypericum perforatum), or products containing St. John's wort, is not recommended. Co-administration of protease inhibitors, including Kaletra, with St. John's wort is expected to substantially decrease protease inhibitor concentrations and may result in sub-optimal levels of lopinavir and lead to loss of virologic response and possible resistance to lopinavir or to the class of protease inhibitors.

PANCREATITIS

Pancreatitis has been observed in patients receiving Kaletra therapy, including those who developed marked triglyceride elevations. In some cases, fatalities have been observed. Although a causal relationship to Kaletra has not been established, marked triglyceride elevations is a risk factor for development of pancreatitis (see PRECAUTIONS, Lipid Elevations). Patients with advanced HIV disease may be at increased risk of elevated triglycerides and pancreatitis, and patients with a history of pancreatitis may be at increased risk of recurrence during Kaletra therapy.

Pancreatitis should be considered if clinical symptoms (nausea, vomiting, abdominal pain) or abnormalities in laboratory values (such as increased serum lipase or amylase values) suggestive of pancreatitis should occur. Patients who exhibit these signs or symptoms should be evaluated and Kaletra and/or other antiretroviral therapy should be suspended as clinically appropriate.

DIABETES MELLITUS/HYPERGLYCEMIA

New onset diabetes mellitus, exacerbation of pre-existing diabetes mellitus, and hyperglycemia have been reported during postmarketing surveillance in HIV-infected patients receiving protease inhibitor therapy. Some patients required either initiation or dose adjustments of insulin or oral hypoglycemic agents for treatment of these events. In some cases, diabetic ketoacidosis has occurred. In those patients who discontinued protease inhibitor therapy, hyperglycemia persisted in some cases. Because these events have been reported voluntarily during clinical practice, estimates of frequency cannot be made and a causal relationship between protease inhibitor therapy and these events has not been established.

L

PRECAUTIONS

HEPATIC IMPAIRMENT AND TOXICITY

Kaletra is principally metabolized by the liver; therefore, caution should be exercised when administering this drug to patients with hepatic impairment, because lopinavir concentrations may be increased. Patients with underlying hepatitis B or C or marked elevations in transaminases prior to treatment may be at increased risk for developing further transaminase elevations or hepatic decompensation. There have been postmarketing reports of hepatic dysfunction, including some fatalities. These have generally occurred in patients with advanced HIV disease taking multiple concomitant medications in the setting of underlying chronic hepatitis or cirrhosis. A causal relationship with Kaletra therapy has not been established. Increased AST/ALT monitoring should be considered in these patients, especially during the first several months of Kaletra treatment.

RESISTANCE/CROSS-RESISTANCE

Various degrees of cross-resistance among protease inhibitors have been observed. The effect of Kaletra therapy on the efficacy of subsequently administered protease inhibitors is under investigation (see CLINICAL PHARMACOLOGY, Microbiology).

HEMOPHILIA

There have been reports of increased bleeding, including spontaneous skin hematomas and hemarthrosis, in patients with hemophilia type A and B treated with protease inhibitors. In some patients additional factor VIII was given. In more than half of the reported cases, treatment with protease inhibitors was continued or reintroduced. A causal relationship between protease inhibitor therapy and these events has not been established.

FAT REDISTRIBUTION

Redistribution/accumulation of body fat including central obesity, dorsocervical fat enlargement (buffalo hump), peripheral wasting, facial wasting, breast enlargement, and "cushingoid appearance" have been observed in patients receiving antiretroviral therapy. The mechanism and long-term consequences of these events are currently unknown. A causal relationship has not been established.

LIPID ELEVATIONS

Treatment with Kaletra has resulted in large increases in the concentration of total cholesterol and triglycerides (see TABLE 9A, TABLE 9B, and TABLE 9C). Triglyceride and cholesterol testing should be performed prior to initiating Kaletra therapy and at periodic intervals during therapy. Lipid disorders should be managed as clinically appropriate. See DRUG INTERACTIONS, Established and Other Potentially Significant Drug Interactions for additional information on potential drug interactions with Kaletra and HMG-CoA reductase inhibitors.

INFORMATION FOR THE PATIENT

A statement to patients and health care providers is included on the product's bottle label: **"ALERT: Find out about medicines that should NOT be taken with Kaletra."** A Patient Package Insert (PPI) for Kaletra is available for patient information.

Patients should be told that sustained decreases in plasma HIV RNA have been associated with a reduced risk of progression to AIDS and death. Patients should remain under the care of a physician while using Kaletra. Patients should be advised to take Kaletra and other concomitant antiretroviral therapy every day as prescribed. Kaletra must always be used in combination with other antiretroviral drugs. Patients should not alter the dose or discontinue therapy without consulting with their doctor. If a dose of Kaletra is missed patients should take the dose as soon as possible and then return to their normal schedule. However, if a dose is skipped the patient should not double the next dose.

Patients should be informed that Kaletra is not a cure for HIV infection and that they may continue to develop opportunistic infections and other complications associated with HIV disease. The long-term effects of Kaletra are unknown at this time. Patients should be told that there are currently no data demonstrating that therapy with Kaletra can reduce the risk of transmitting HIV to others through sexual contact.

Kaletra may interact with some drugs; therefore, patients should be advised to report to their doctor the use of any other prescription, non-prescription medication or herbal products, particularly St. John's wort.

Patients taking didanosine should take didanosine 1 hour before or 2 hours after Kaletra.

Patients receiving sildenafil should be advised that they may be at an increased risk of sildenafil-associated adverse events including hypotension, visual changes, and sustained erection, and should promptly report any symptoms to their doctor.

Patients receiving estrogen-based hormonal contraceptives should be instructed that additional or alternate contraceptive measures should be used during therapy with Kaletra.

Kaletra should be taken with food to enhance absorption.

Patients should be informed that redistribution or accumulation of body fat may occur in patients receiving antiretroviral therapy and that the cause and long-term health effects of these conditions are not known at this time.

CARCINOGENESIS, MUTAGENESIS, AND IMPAIRMENT OF FERTILITY

Long-term carcinogenicity studies of Kaletra in animal systems have not been completed.

Carcinogenicity studies in mice and rats have been carried out on ritonavir. In male mice, at levels of 50, 100 or 200 mg/kg/day, there was a dose dependent increase in the incidence of both adenomas and combined adenomas and carcinomas in the liver. Based on AUC measurements, the exposure at the high dose was approximately 4-fold for males that of the exposure in humans with the recommended therapeutic dose (400/100 mg Kaletra bid). There were no carcinogenic effects seen in females at the dosages tested. The exposure at the high dose was approximately 9-fold for the females that of the exposure in humans. In rats dosed at levels of 7, 15 or 30 mg/kg/day there were no carcinogenic effects. In this study, the exposure at the high dose was approximately 0.7-fold that of the exposure in humans with the 400/100 mg Kaletra bid regimen. Based on the exposures achieved in the animal studies, the significance of the observed effects is not known. However, neither lopinavir nor ritonavir was found to be mutagenic or clastogenic in a battery of *in vitro* and *in vivo* assays including the Ames bacterial reverse mutation assay using *S. typhimurium* and *E. coli*, the mouse lymphoma assay, the mouse micronucleus test and chromosomal aberration assays in human lymphocytes.

Lopinavir in combination with ritonavir at a 2:1 ratio produced no effects on fertility in male and female rats at levels of 10/5, 30/15 or 100/50 mg/kg/day. Based on AUC measurements, the exposures in rats at the high doses were approximately 0.7-fold for lopinavir and 1.8-fold for ritonavir of the exposures in humans at the recommended therapeutic dose (400/100 mg bid).

PREGNANCY CATEGORY C

No treatment-related malformations were observed when lopinavir in combination with ritonavir was administered to pregnant rats or rabbits. Embryonic and fetal developmental toxicities (early resorption, decreased fetal viability, decreased fetal body weight, increased incidence of skeletal variations and skeletal ossification delays) occurred in rats at a maternally toxic dosage (100/50 mg/kg/day). Based on AUC measurements, the drug exposures in rats at 100/50 mg/kg/day were approximately 0.7-fold for lopinavir and 1.8-fold for ritonavir for males and females that of the exposures in humans at the recommended therapeutic dose (400/100 mg bid). In a peri- and postnatal study in rats, a developmental toxicity (a decrease in survival in pups between birth and postnatal day 21) occurred at 40/20 mg/kg/day and greater.

No embryonic and fetal developmental toxicities were observed in rabbits at a maternally toxic dosage (80/40 mg/kg/day). Based on AUC measurements, the drug exposures in rabbits at 80/40 mg/kg/day were approximately 0.6-fold for lopinavir and 1.0-fold for ritonavir that of the exposures in humans at the recommended therapeutic dose (400/100 mg bid). There are, however, no adequate and well-controlled studies in pregnant women. Kaletra should be used during pregnancy only if the potential benefit justifies the potential risk to the fetus.

Antiretroviral Pregnancy Registry: To monitor maternal-fetal outcomes of pregnant women exposed to Kaletra, an Antiretroviral Pregnancy Registry has been established. Physicians are encouraged to register patients by calling 1-800-258-4263.

NURSING MOTHERS

The Centers for Disease Control and Prevention recommend that HIV-infected mothers not breast-feed their infants to avoid risking postnatal transmission of HIV. Studies in rats have demonstrated that lopinavir is secreted in milk. It is not known whether lopinavir is secreted in human milk. Because of both the potential for HIV transmission and the potential for serious adverse reactions in nursing infants, mothers should be instructed **not to breast-feed if they are receiving Kaletra.**

GERIATRIC USE

Clinical studies of Kaletra did not include sufficient numbers of subjects aged 65 and over to determine whether they respond differently from younger subjects. In general, appropriate caution should be exercised in the administration and monitoring of Kaletra in elderly patients reflecting the greater frequency of decreased hepatic, renal, or cardiac function, and of concomitant disease or other drug therapy.

PEDIATRIC USE

The safety and pharmacokinetic profiles of Kaletra in pediatric patients below the age of 6 months have not been established. In HIV-infected patients age 6 months to 12 years, the adverse event profile seen during a clinical trial was similar to that for adult patients. The evaluation of the antiviral activity of Kaletra in pediatric patients in clinical trials is ongoing.

Study 940 is an ongoing open-label, multicenter trial evaluating the pharmacokinetic profile, tolerability, safety and efficacy of Kaletra oral solution containing lopinavir 80 mg/ml and ritonavir 20 mg/ml in 100 antiretroviral naïve (44%) and experienced (56%) pediatric patients. All patients were non-nucleoside reverse transcriptase inhibitor naïve. Patients were randomized to either 230 mg lopinavir/57.5 mg ritonavir per m^2 or 300 mg lopinavir/75 mg ritonavir per m^2. Naïve patients also received lamivudine and stavudine. Experienced patients received nevirapine plus up to 2 nucleoside reverse transcriptase inhibitors.

Safety, efficacy and pharmacokinetic profiles of the 2 dose regimens were assessed after 3 weeks of therapy in each patient. After analysis of these data, all patients were continued on the 300 mg lopinavir/75 mg ritonavir per m^2 dose. Patients had a mean age of 5 years (range 6 months to 12 years) with 14% less than 2 years. Mean baseline CD4 cell count was 838 cells/mm^3 and mean baseline plasma HIV-1 RNA was 4.7 log_{10} copies/ml.

Through 48 weeks of therapy, the proportion of patients who achieved and sustained an HIV RNA <400 copies/ml was 80% for antiretroviral naïve patients and 71% for antiretroviral experienced patients. The mean increase from baseline in CD4 cell count was 404 cells/mm^3 for antiretroviral naïve and 284 cells/mm^3 for antiretroviral experienced patients treated through 48 weeks. At 48 weeks, 2 patients (2%) had prematurely discontinued the study. One antiretroviral naïve patient prematurely discontinued secondary to an adverse event attributed to Kaletra, while 1 antiretroviral experienced patient prematurely discontinued secondary to an HIV-related event.

Dose selection for patients 6 months to 12 years of age was based on the following results. The 230/57.5 mg/m^2 bid regimen without nevirapine and the 300/75 mg/m^2 bid regimen with nevirapine provided lopinavir plasma concentrations similar to those obtained in adult patients receiving the 400/100 mg bid regimen (without nevirapine).

DRUG INTERACTIONS

Kaletra is an inhibitor of CYP3A (cytochrome P450 3A) both *in vitro* and *in vivo*. Co-administration of Kaletra and drugs primarily metabolized by CYP3A (*e.g.*, dihydropyridine calcium channel blockers, HMG-CoA reductase inhibitors, immunosuppressants and sildenafil) may result in increased plasma concentrations of the other drugs that could increase or prolong their therapeutic and adverse effects (see Established and Other Potentially Significant Drug Interactions). Agents that are extensively metabolized by CYP3A and have high first pass metabolism appear to be the most susceptible to large increases in AUC (>3-fold) when co-administered with Kaletra.

Kaletra inhibits CYP2D6 *in vitro,* but to a lesser extent than CYP3A. Clinically significant drug interactions with drugs metabolized by CYP2D6 are possible with Kaletra at the recommended dose, but the magnitude is not known. Kaletra does not inhibit CYP2C9, CYP2C19, CYP2E1, CYP2B6 or CYP1A2 at clinically relevant concentrations.

Kaletra has been shown *in vivo* to induce its own metabolism and to increase the biotransformation of some drugs metabolized by cytochrome P450 enzymes and by glucuronidation.

Kaletra is metabolized by CYP3A. Co-administration of Kaletra and drugs that induce CYP3A may decrease lopinavir plasma concentrations and reduce its therapeutic effect (see Established and Other Potentially Significant Drug Interactions). Although not noted with concurrent ketoconazole, co-administration of Kaletra and other drugs that inhibit CYP3A may increase lopinavir plasma concentrations.

Drugs that are contraindicated and not recommended for co-administration with Kaletra are included in TABLE 8. These recommendations are based on either drug interaction studies or predicted interactions due to the expected magnitude of interaction and potential for serious events or loss of efficacy.

TABLE 8 *Drugs That Should Not Be Co-Administered With Kaletra*

Drug Class: Drug Name	Clinical Comment
Antiarrhythmics: Flecainide, propafenone	CONTRAINDICATED due to potential for serious and/or life-threatening reactions such as cardiac arrhythmias.
Antihistamines: Astemizole, terfenadine	CONTRAINDICATED due to potential for serious and/or life-threatening reactions such as cardiac arrhythmias.
Antimycobacterial: Rifampin	May lead to loss of virologic response and possible resistance to Kaletra or to the class of protease inhibitors or other co-administered antiretroviral agents.
Ergot Derivatives: Dihydroergotamine, ergonovine, ergotamine, methylergonovine	CONTRAINDICATED due to potential for serious and/or life-threatening reactions such as acute ergot toxicity characterized by peripheral vasospasm and ischemia of the extremities and other tissues.
GI Motility Agent: Cisapride	CONTRAINDICATED due to potential for serious and/or life-threatening reactions such as cardiac arrhythmias.
Herbal Products: St. John's wort (hypericum perforatum)	May lead to loss of virologic response and possible resistance to Kaletra or to the class of protease inhibitors.
HMG-CoA Reductase Inhibitors: Lovastatin, simvastatin	Potential for serious reactions such as risk of myopathy including rhabdomyolysis.
Neuroleptic: Pimozide	CONTRAINDICATED due to the potential for serious and/or life-threatening reactions such as cardiac arrhythmias.
Sedative/Hypnotics: Midazolam, triazolam	CONTRAINDICATED due to potential for serious and/or life-threatening reactions such as prolonged or increased sedation or respiratory depression.

ESTABLISHED AND OTHER POTENTIALLY SIGNIFICANT DRUG INTERACTIONS

Alteration in dose or regimen may be recommended based on drug interaction studies or predicted interaction. (See TABLE 2 and TABLE 3.)

HIV-Antiviral Agents

Non-Nucleoside Reverse Transcriptase Inhibitors

Efavirenz*, nevirapine*.

Effect: Decreases lopinavir concentration.

Clinical Comments: A dose increase of Kaletra to 533/133 mg (4 capsules or 6.5 ml) twice daily taken with food should be considered when used in combination with efavirenz or nevirapine (see DOSAGE AND ADMINISTRATION).

Note: Efavirenz and nevirapine induce the activity of CYP3A and thus have the potential to decrease plasma concentrations of other protease inhibitors when used in combination with Kaletra.

Non-Nucleoside Reverse Transcriptase Inhibitor

Delavirdine.

Effect: Increases lopinavir concentration.

Clinical Comments: Appropriate doses of the combination with respect to safety and efficacy have not been established.

Nucleoside Reverse Transcriptase Inhibitor

Didanosine.

Clinical Comments: It is recommended that didanosine be administered on an empty stomach; therefore, didanosine should be given 1 hour before or 2 hours after Kaletra (given with food).

HIV-Protease Inhibitors

Amprenavir*, indinavir*, saquinavir*.

Effect: *When co-administered with reduced doses of concomitant protease inhibitors:* Increases amprenavir concentration (similar AUC, decreases C_{max}, increases C_{min}); increases indinavir concentration (similar AUC, decreases C_{max}, increases C_{min}); increases saquinavir concentration (similar AUC, increases C_{min}).

Clinical Comments: Alterations in concentrations (*e.g.,* AUC, C_{max} and C_{min}) are noted when reduced doses of concomitant protease inhibitors are co-administered with Kaletra. Appropriate doses of the combination with respect to safety and efficacy have not been established (see TABLE 3 and CLINICAL PHARMACOLOGY, Effect of Kaletra on Other Protease Inhibitors [PIs]).

HIV-Protease Inhibitor

Ritonavir*.

Effect: Increases lopinavir concentration.

Clinical Comments: Appropriate doses of additional ritonavir in combination with Kaletra with respect to safety and efficacy have not been established.

Other Agents

Antiarrhythmics

Amiodarone, bepridil, lidocaine (systemic), and quinidine.

Effect: Increases antiarrhythmics concentration.

Clinical Comments: Caution is warranted and therapeutic concentration monitoring is recommended for antiarrhythmics when co-administered with Kaletra, if available.

Anticoagulant

Warfarin.

Clinical Comments: Concentrations of warfarin may be affected. It is recommended that INR (international normalized ratio) be monitored.

Anticonvulsants

Carbamazepine, phenobarbital, phenytoin.

Effect: Decreases lopinavir concentration.

Clinical Comments: Use with caution. Kaletra may be less effective due to decreased lopinavir plasma concentrations in patients taking these agents concomitantly.

Anti-Infective

Clarithromycin.

Effect: Increases clarithromycin concentration.

Clinical Comments: For patients with renal impairment, the following dosage adjustments should be considered:

- For patients with CLCR 30-60 ml/min the dose of clarithromycin should be reduced by 50%.
- For patients with CLCR <30 ml/min the dose of clarithromycin should be decreased by 75%.

No dose adjustment for patients with normal renal function is necessary.

Antifungals

Ketoconazole*, itraconazole.

Effect: Increases ketoconazole concentration, increases itraconazole concentration.

Clinical Comments: High doses of ketoconazole or itraconazole (>200 mg/day) are not recommended.

Antimycobacterial

Rifabutin*.

Effect: Increases rifabutin and rifabutin metabolite concentrations.

Clinical Comments: Dosage reduction of rifabutin by at least 75% of the usual dose of 300 mg/day is recommended (*i.e.,* a maximum dose of 150 mg every other day or 3 times per week). Increased monitoring for adverse events is warranted in patients receiving the combination. Further dosage reduction of rifabutin may be necessary.

Antiparasitic

Atovaquone.

Effect: Decreases atovaquone concentration.

Clinical Comments: Clinical significance is unknown; however, increase in atovaquone doses may be needed.

Calcium Channel Blockers
Dihydropyridine: *e.g.*, felodipine, nifedipine, nicardipine.
Effect: Increases dihydropyridine calcium channel blockers concentration.
Clinical Comments: Caution is warranted and clinical monitoring of patients is recommended.

Corticosteroid
Dexamethasone.
Effect: Decreases lopinavir concentration.
Clinical Comments: Use with caution. Kaletra may be less effective due to decreased lopinavir plasma concentrations in patients taking these agents concomitantly.

Disulfiram/Metronidazole
Clinical Comments: Kaletra oral solution contains alcohol, which can produce disulfiram-like reactions when co-administered with disulfiram or other drugs that produce this reaction (*e.g.*, metronidazole).

Erectile Dysfunction Agent
Sildenafil.
Effect: Increases sildenafil concentration.
Clinical Comments: Use with caution at reduced doses of 25 mg every 48 hours with increased monitoring for adverse events.

HMG-CoA Reductase Inhibitors
Atorvastatin*.
Effect: Increases atorvastatin concentration.
Clinical Comments: Use lowest possible dose of atorvastatin with careful monitoring, or consider other HMG-CoA reductase inhibitors such as pravastatin or fluvastatin in combination with Kaletra.

Immunosuppresants
Cyclosporine, tacrolimus, rapamycin.
Effect: Increases immunosuppressants concentration.
Clinical Comments: Therapeutic concentration monitoring is recommended for immunosuppressant agents when co-administered with Kaletra.

Narcotic Analgesic
Methadone*.
Effect: Decreases methadone concentration.
Clinical Comments: Dosage of methadone may need to be increased when co-administered with Kaletra.

Oral Contraceptive
Ethinyl estradiol*.
Effect: Decreases ethinyl estradiol concentration.
Clinical Comments: Alternative or additional contraceptive measures should be used when estrogen-based oral contraceptives and Kaletra are co-administered.
*See CLINICAL PHARMACOLOGY for Magnitude of Interaction, TABLE 2 and TABLE 3.

OTHER DRUGS

Drug interaction studies reveal no clinically significant interaction between Kaletra and pravastatin, stavudine or lamivudine.

Based on known metabolic profiles, clinically significant drug interactions are not expected between Kaletra and fluvastatin, dapsone, trimethoprim/sulfamethoxazole, azithromycin, erythromycin, or fluconazole.

Zidovudine and Abacavir

Kaletra induces glucuronidation; therefore, Kaletra has the potential to reduce zidovudine and abacavir plasma concentrations. The clinical significance of this potential interaction is unknown.

ADVERSE REACTIONS

ADULTS

Treatment-Emergent Adverse Events

Kaletra has been studied in 701 patients as combination therapy in Phase 1/2 and Phase 3 clinical trials. The most common adverse event associated with Kaletra therapy was diarrhea, which was generally of mild to moderate severity. Rates of discontinuation of randomized therapy due to adverse events were 5.8% in Kaletra-treated and 4.9% in nelfinavir-treated patients in Study 863.

Drug related clinical adverse events of moderate or severe intensity in ≥2% of patients treated with combination therapy for up to 48 weeks (Phase 3) and for up to 72 weeks (Phase 1/2) are presented in TABLE 9A, TABLE 9B, and TABLE 9C. For other information regarding observed or potentially serious adverse events, please see WARNINGS and PRECAUTIONS.

Treatment-emergent adverse events occurring in less than 2% of adult patients receiving Kaletra in all Phase 2/3 clinical trials and considered at least possibly related or of unknown relationship to treatment with Kaletra and of at least moderate intensity are listed below by body system.

Body as a Whole: Abdomen enlarged, allergic reaction, back pain, chest pain, chest pain substernal, cyst, drug interaction, drug level increased, face edema, flu syndrome, hypertrophy, infection bacterial, malaise, and viral infection.

Cardiovascular System: Atrial fibrillation, deep vein thrombosis, hypertension, migraine, palpitation, thrombophlebitis, varicose vein, and vasculitis.

Digestive System: Cholangitis, cholecystitis, constipation, dry mouth, enteritis, enterocolitis, eructation, esophagitis, fecal incontinence, gastritis, gastroenteritis, hemorrhagic colitis, increased appetite, jaundice, mouth ulceration, pancreatitis, sialadenitis, stomatitis, and ulcerative stomatitis.

Endocrine System: Cushing's syndrome, diabetes mellitus, and hypothyroidism.

Hemic and Lymphatic System: Anemia, leukopenia, and lymphadenopathy.

Metabolic and Nutritional Disorders: Avitaminosis, dehydration, edema, glucose tolerance decreased, lactic acidosis, obesity, peripheral edema, weight gain, and weight loss.

Musculoskeletal System: Arthralgia, arthrosis and myalgia.

Nervous System: Abnormal dreams, agitation, amnesia, anxiety, apathy, ataxia, confusion, convulsion, dizziness, dyskinesia, emotional lability, encephalopathy, facial paralysis, hypertonia, libido decreased, neuropathy, paresthesia, peripheral neuritis, somnolence, thinking abnormal, and tremor.

Respiratory System: Asthma, bronchitis, dyspnea, lung edema, pharyngitis, rhinitis, and sinusitis.

Skin and Appendages: Acne, alopecia, dry skin, eczema, exfoliative dermatitis, furunculosis, maculopapular rash, nail disorder, pruritus, seborrhea, skin benign neoplasm, skin discoloration, skin ulcer, and sweating.

Special Senses: Abnormal vision, eye disorder, otitis media, and taste perversion, and tinnitus.

Urogenital System: Abnormal ejaculation, gynecomastia, hypogonadism male, kidney calculus, and urine abnormality.

TABLE 9A *Percentage of Patients With Selected Treatment-Emergent* Adverse Events of Moderate or Severe Intensity Reported in ≥2% of Adult Patients: Study 863*

	Antiretroviral-Naïve Patients 48 Weeks	
	Kaletra 400/100 mg bid + d4T + 3TC (n=326)	Nelfinavir 750 mg tid + d4T + 3TC (n=327)
Body as a Whole		
Abdominal pain	4%	3%
Asthenia	4%	3%
Chills	0%	<1%
Fever	<1%	<1%
Headache	2%	2%
Digestive System		
Anorexia	1%	<1%
Diarrhea	16%	17%
Dyspepsia	2%	<1%
Dysphagia	0%	0%
Flatulence	2%	1%
Nausea	7%	5%
Vomiting	2%	2%
Nervous System		
Depression	1%	2%
Insomnia	2%	1%
Skin and Appendages		
Rash	1%	2%

* Includes adverse events of possible, probable or unknown relationship to study drug.

TABLE 9B *Percentage of Patients With Selected Treatment-Emergent* Adverse Events of Moderate or Severe Intensity Reported in ≥2% of Adult Patients: Study 888*

	Protease Inhibitor-Experienced Patients 48 Weeks	
	Kaletra 400/100 mg bid + NVP + NRTIs (n=148)	Investigator-Selected Protease Inhibitor(s) + NVP + NRTIs (n=140)
Body as a Whole		
Abdominal pain	2%	2%
Asthenia	3%	6%
Chills	2%	0%
Fever	2%	1%
Headache	2%	3%
Digestive System		
Anorexia	1%	3%
Diarrhea	7%	9%
Dyspepsia	1%	1%
Dysphagia	2%	1%
Flatulence	1%	2%
Nausea	7%	16%
Vomiting	4%	12%
Nervous System		
Depression	1%	2%
Insomnia	0%	2%
Skin and Appendages		
Rash	2%	1%

* Includes adverse events of possible, probable or unknown relationship to study drug.

Post-Marketing Experience

The following adverse reactions have been reported during post-marketing use of Kaletra. Because these reactions are reported voluntarily from a population of unknown size, it is not possible to reliably estimate their frequency or establish a causal relationship to Kaletra exposure.

TABLE 9C Percentage of Patients With Selected Treatment-Emergent Adverse Events of Moderate or Severe Intensity Reported in ≥2% of Adult Patients: Other Studies*

	Study 720	Study 957‡ and Study 765§
	72 Weeks	48-72 Weeks
	Kaletra bid† + d4T + 3TC	Kaletra bid + NNRTI + NRTIs
	(n=84)	(n=127)
Body as a Whole		
Abdominal pain	5%	2%
Asthenia	7%	8%
Chills	1%	0%
Fever	0%	2%
Headache	7%	2%
Digestive Systeme		
Anorexia	0%	0%
Diarrhea	24%	18%
Dyspepsia	1%	0%
Dysphagia	1%	0%
Flatulence	1%	2%
Nausea	15%	4%
Vomiting	5%	2%
Nervous System		
Depression	0%	2%
Insomnia	2%	2%
Skin and Appendages		
Rash	4%	2%

* Includes adverse events of possible, probable or unknown relationship to study drug.
† Includes adverse event data from dose group I (400/100 mg bid only [n=16]) and dose group II (400/100 mg bid [n=35] and 400/200 mg bid [n=35]). Within dosing groups, moderate to severe nausea of probable/possible rlationship to Kaletra occurred at a higher rate in the 400/200 mg dose are compared to the 400/100 mg dose arm in group II.
‡ Includes adverse event data from patients receiving 400/100 mg bid (n=29) or 533/133 mg bid (n=28) for 48 weeks. Patients received Kaletra in combination with NRTIs and efavirenz.
§ Includes adverse event data from patients receiving 400/100 mg bid (n=36) or 400/200 mg bid (n=34) for 72 weeks. Patients recieved Kaletra in combination with NRTIs and nevirapine.

Body as a Whole: Redistribution/accumulation of body fat has been reported (see PRECAUTIONS, Fat Redistribution).
Cardiovascular: Bradyarrhythmias.

Laboratory Abnormalities

The percentages of adult patients treated with combination therapy with Kaletra with Grade 3-4 laboratory abnormalities are presented in TABLE 10A, TABLE 10B, and TABLE 10C.

TABLE 10A Grade 3-4 Laboratory Abnormalities Reported in ≥2% of Adult Patients: Study 863

		Antiretroviral-Naïve Patients	
		48 Weeks	
		Kaletra 400/100 mg bid + d4T + 3 TC	Nelfinavir 750 mg tid + d4T + 3TC
Variable	Limit*	(n=326)	(n=327)
Chemistry	High		
Glucose	>250 mg/dl	2%	2%
Uric acid	>12 mg/dl	2%	2%
Total bilirubin	>3.48 mg/dl	<1%	0%
SGOT/AST	>180 U/L	2%	4%
SGPT/ALT	>215 U/L	4%	4%
GGT	>300 U/L	NA	NA
Total cholesterol	>300 mg/dl	9%	5%
Triglycerides	>750 mg/dl	9%	1%
Amylase	>2 × ULN	3%	2%
Chemistry	Low		
Inorganic phosphorus	<1.5 mg/dl	0%	0%
Hematology	Low		
Neutrophils	0.75 × 10^9/L	1%	3%

* ULN = upper limit of the normal range; NA = Not Applicable.

PEDIATRICS

Treatment-Emergent Adverse Events

Kaletra has been studied in 100 pediatric patients 6 months to 12 years of age. The adverse event profile seen during a clinical trial was similar to that for adult patients.

Taste aversion, vomiting, and diarrhea were the most commonly reported drug related adverse events of any severity in pediatric patients treated with combination therapy including Kaletra for up to 48 weeks in Study 940. A total of 8 children experienced moderate or severe adverse events at least possibly related to Kaletra. Rash (reported in 3%) was the only drug-related clinical adverse event of moderate to severe intensity in ≥2% of children enrolled.

Laboratory Abnormalities

The percentages of pediatric patients treated with combination therapy including Kaletra with Grade 3-4 laboratory abnormalities are presented in TABLE 11.

TABLE 10B Grade 3-4 Laboratory Abnormalities Reported in ≥2% of Adult Patients: Study 888

		Protease Inhibitor-Experienced Patients	
		48 Weeks	
		Kaletra 400/100 mg bid + NVP + NRTIs	Investigator-Selected Protease Inhibitor(s) + NVP + NRTIs
Variable	Limit*	(n=148)	(n=140)
Chemistry	High		
Glucose	>250 mg/dl	1%	2%
Uric acid	>12 mg/dl	0%	1%
Total bilirubin	>3.48 mg/dl	1%	3%
SGOT/AST	>180 U/L	5%	11%
SGPT/ALT	>215 U/L	6%	13%
GGT	>300 U/L	NA	NA
Total cholesterol	>300 mg/dl	20%	21%
Triglycerides	>750 mg/dl	25%	21%
Amylase	>2 × ULN	4%	8%
Chemistry	Low		
Inorganic phosphorus	<1.5 mg/dl	1%	0%
Hematology	Low		
Neutrophils	0.75 × 10^9/L	1%	2%

* ULN = upper limit of the normal range; NA = Not Applicable.

TABLE 10C Grade 3-4 Laboratory Abnormalities Reported in ≥2% of Adult Patients: Other Studies

		Study 720	Study 957‡ and Study 765§
		72 Weeks	48-72 Weeks
		Kaletra bid† + d4T + 3TC	Kaletra bid + NNRTI + NRTIs
Variable	Limit*	(n=84)	(n=127)
Chemistry	High		
Glucose	>250 mg/dl	2%	5%
Uric acid	>12 mg/dl	4%	1%
Total bilirubin	>3.48 mg/dl	1%	0%
SGOT/AST	>180 U/L	10%	6%
SGPT/ALT	>215 U/L	8%	10%
GGT	>300 U/L	4%	28%
Total cholesterol	>300 mg/dl	14%	33%
Triglycerides	>750 mg/dl	11%	32%
Amylase	>2 × ULN	5%	6%
Chemistry	Low		
Inorganic phosphorus	<1.5 mg/dl	0%	2%
Hematology	Low		
Neutrophils	0.75 × 10^9/L	2%	4%

* ULN = upper limit of the normal range; NA = Not Applicable.
† Includes clinical laboratory data from dose group I (400/100 mg bid only [n=16]) and dose group II (400/100 mg bid [n=35] and 400/200 mg bid [n=33]).
‡ Includes clinical laboratory data from patients receiving 400/100 mg bid (n=29) or 533/133 mg bid (n=28) for 48 weeks. Patients received Kaletra in combination with NRTIs and efavirenz.
§ Includes clinical laboratory data from patients receiving 400/100 mg bid (n=36) or 400/200 mg bid (n=34) for 72 weeks. Patients received Kaletra in combination with NRTIs and nevirapine.

TABLE 11 Grade 3-4 Laboratory Abnormalities Reported in ≥2% Pediatric Patients

		Kaletra bid +RTIs
Variable	Limit*	(n=100)
Chemistry	High	
Sodium	>149 mEq/L	3%
Total bilirubin	≥3.0 × ULN	3%
SGOT/AST	>180 U/L	8%
SGPT/ALT	>215 U/L	7%
Total cholesterol	>300 mg/dl	3%
Amylase	>2.5 × ULN	7%†
Chemistry	Low	
Sodium	<130 mEq/L	3%
Hematology	Low	
Platelet count	<50 × 10^9/L	4%
Neutrophils	<0.40 × 10^9/L	2%

* ULN = upper limit of the normal range.
† Subjects with Grade 3-4 amylase confirmed by elevations in pancreatic amylase.

DOSAGE AND ADMINISTRATION

ADULTS

The recommended dosage of Kaletra is 400/100 mg (3 capsules or 5.0 ml) twice daily taken with food.

Concomitant Therapy

Efavirenz or Nevirapine

A dose increase of Kaletra to 533/133 mg (4 capsules or 6.5 ml) twice daily taken with food is recommended when used in combination with efavirenz or nevirapine (see CLINICAL PHARMACOLOGY, Pharmacokinetics, Special Populations, Drug-Drug Interactions and/or DRUG INTERACTIONS, Established and Other Potentially Significant Drug Interactions).

PEDIATRIC PATIENTS

In children 6 months to 12 years of age, the recommended dosage of Kaletra oral solution is 12/3 mg/kg for those 7 to <15 kg and 10/2.5 mg/kg for those 15-40 kg (approximately equivalent to 230/57.5 mg/m^2) twice daily taken with food, up to a maximum dose of 400/100 mg in children >40 kg (5.0 ml or 3 capsules) twice daily. **It is preferred that the prescriber calculate the appropriate milligram dose for each individual child ≤12 years old and determine the corresponding volume of solution or number of capsules.** However, as an alternative, TABLE 12 contains dosing guidelines for Kaletra oral solution based on body weight. When possible, dose should be administered using a calibrated dosing syringe.

TABLE 12

Weight	Dose*	Volume of Oral Solution bid (80 mg lopinavir/20 mg ritonavir per ml)
Without Nevirapine or Efavirenz		
7 to <15 kg	12 mg/kg bid	
7 to 10 kg		1.25 ml
>10 to <15 kg		1.75 ml
15 to 40 kg	10 mg/kg bid	
15 to 20 kg		2.25 ml
>20 to 25 kg		2.75 ml
>25 to 30 kg		3.5 ml
>30 to 35 kg		4.0 ml
>35 to 40 kg		4.75 ml
>40 kg	Adult dose	5 ml (or 3 capsules)

* Dosing based on the lopinavir component of lopinavir/ritonavir solution (80 mg/20 mg per ml).
Note: Use adult dosage recommendation for children >12 years of age.

Concomitant Therapy

Efavirenz or Nevirapine

A dose increase of Kaletra oral solution to 13/3.25 mg/kg for those 7 to <15 kg and 11/2.75 mg/kg for those 15-45 kg (approximately equivalent to 300/75 mg/m^2) twice daily taken with food, up to a maximum dose of 533/133 mg in children >45 kg twice daily is recommended when used in combination with efavirenz or nevirapine. TABLE 13 contains dosing guidelines for Kaletra oral solution based on body weight, when used in combination with efavirenz or nevirapine in children (see CLINICAL PHARMACOLOGY, Pharmacokinetics, Special Populations, Drug-Drug Interactions and/or DRUG INTERACTIONS, Established and Other Potentially Significant Drug Interactions).

TABLE 13

Weight	Dose*	Volume of Oral Solution bid (80 mg lopinavir/20 mg ritonavir per ml)
With Nevirapine or Efavirenz		
7 to <15 kg	13 mg/kg bid	
7 to 10 kg		1.5 ml
>10 to <15 kg		2.0 ml
15 to 45 kg	11 mg/kg bid	
15 to 20 kg		2.5 ml
>20 to 25 kg		3.25 ml
>25 to 30 kg		4.0 ml
>30 to 35 kg		4.5 ml
>35 to 40 kg		5.0 ml (or 3 capsules)
>40 to 45 kg		5.75 ml
>45 kg	Adult dose	6.5 ml (or 4 capsules)

* Dosing based on the lopinavir component of lopinavir/ritonavir solution (80 mg/20 mg per ml).
Note: Use adult dosage recommendation for children >12 years of age.

HOW SUPPLIED

CAPSULES

Kaletra (lopinavir/ritonavir) capsules are orange soft gelatin capsules imprinted with the Abbott corporate logo and the Abbo-Code "PK". Kaletra is available as 133.3 mg lopinavir/33.3 mg ritonavir capsules.

Recommended Storage: Store Kaletra soft gelatin capsules at 2-8°C (36-46°F) until dispensed. Avoid exposure to excessive heat. For patient use, refrigerated Kaletra capsules remain stable until the expiration date printed on the label. If stored at room temperature up to 25°C (77°F), capsules should be used within 2 months.

ORAL SOLUTION

Kaletra (lopinavir/ritonavir) oral solution is a light yellow to orange colored liquid supplied in amber-colored multiple-dose bottles containing 400 mg lopinavir/100 mg ritonavir per 5 ml (80 mg lopinavir/20 mg ritonavir per ml).

Recommended Storage: Store Kaletra oral solution at 2-8°C (36-46°F) until dispensed. Avoid exposure to excessive heat. For patient use, refrigerated Kaletra oral solution remains stable until the expiration date printed on the label. If stored at room temperature up to 25°C (77°F), oral solution should be used within 2 months.

PRODUCT LISTING - EQUIVALENTS NOT AVAILABLE

Capsule - Oral - 133.3 mg;33.3 mg
180's $703.50 KALETRA, Abbott Pharmaceutical 00074-3959-77

Liquid - Oral - 400 mg;100 mg/5 ml
160 ml $351.75 KALETRA, Abbott Pharmaceutical 00074-3956-46

Loracarbef (003107)

For related information, see the comparative table section in Appendix A.

Categories: Bronchitis, chronic, acute exacerbation; Infection, ear, middle; Infection, lower respiratory tract; Infection, sinus; Infection, skin and skin structures; Infection, upper respiratory tract; Infection, urinary tract; Pharyngitis; Pyelonephritis; Tonsillitis; Pregnancy Category B; FDA Approved 1991 Dec
Drug Classes: Antibiotics, cephalosporins
Brand Names: Lorabid
Foreign Brand Availability: Carbac (Mexico); Lorafem (Germany)
Cost of Therapy: $127.58 (Infection; Lorabid; 400 mg; 2 capsules/day; 10 day supply)

DESCRIPTION

Loracarbef is a synthetic β-lactam antibiotic of the carbacephem class for oral administration. Chemically, carbacephems differ from cephalosporin-class antibiotics in the dihydrothiazine ring where a methylene group has been substituted for a sulfur atom.

The chemical name for loracarbef is: (6*R*,7*S*)-7-[(*R*)-2-amino-2-phenylacetamido]-3-chloro-8-oxo-1-azabicyclo[4.2.0]oct-2-ene-2-carboxylic acid, monohydrate. It is a white to off-white solid with a molecular weight of 367.8. The empirical formula is $C_{16}H_{16}ClN_3O_4{\cdot}H_2O$.

Lorabid pulvules and Lorabid for oral suspension are intended for oral administration only.

Each pulvule contains loracarbef equivalent to 200 mg (0.57 mmol) or 400 mg (1.14 mmol) anhydrous loracarbef activity. They also contain cornstarch, dimethicone, FD&C blue no. 2, gelatin, iron oxides, magnesium stearate, titanium dioxide, and other inactive ingredients.

After reconstitution, each 5 ml of Lorabid for oral suspension contains loracarbef equivalent to 100 mg (0.286 mmol) or 200 mg (0.57 mmol) anhydrous loracarbef activity. The suspensions also contain cellulose, FD&C red no. 40, flavors, methylparaben, propylparaben, simethicone emulsion, sodium carboxymethylcellulose, sucrose, and xanthan gum.

CLINICAL PHARMACOLOGY

Loracarbef, after oral administration, was approximately 90% absorbed from the gastrointestinal tract. When capsules were taken with food, peak plasma concentrations were 50-60% of those achieved when the drug was administered to fasting subjects and occurred from 30-60 minutes later. Total absorption, as measured by urinary recovery and area under the plasma concentration versus time curve (AUC), was unchanged. The effect of food on the rate and extent of absorption of the suspension formulation has not been studied to date.

The pharmacokinetics of loracarbef were linear over the recommended dosage range of 200-400 mg, with no accumulation of the drug noted when it was given twice daily.

Average peak plasma concentrations after administration of 200 or 400 mg single doses of loracarbef as capsules to fasting subjects were approximately 8 and 14 μg/ml, respectively, and were obtained within 1.2 hours after dosing. The average peak plasma concentration in adults following a 400 mg single dose of suspension was 17 μg/ml and was obtained within 0.8 hour after dosing (see TABLE 1).

TABLE 1

Dosage	Mean Plasma Loracarbef Concentrations: Peak C_{max}	Time to Peak T_{max}
Capsule (single dose)		
200 mg	8 μg/ml	1.2 h
400 mg	14 μg/ml	1.2 h
Suspension (single dose)		
400 mg (adult)	17 μg/ml	0.8 h
7.5 mg/kg (pediatric)	13 μg/ml	0.8 h
15 mg/kg (pediatric)	19 μg/ml	0.8 h

Following administration of 7.5 and 15 mg/kg single doses of oral suspension to children, average peak plasma concentrations were 13 and 19 μg/ml, respectively, and were obtained within 40-60 minutes.

This increased rate of absorption (suspension > capsule) should be taken into consideration if the oral suspension is to be substituted for the capsule, and capsules should not be substituted for the oral suspension in the treatment of otitis media (see DOSAGE AND ADMINISTRATION).

The elimination half-life was an average of 1.0 hour in patients with normal renal function. Concomitant administration of probenecid decreased the rate of urinary excretion and increased the half-life to 1.5 hours.

In subjects with moderate impairment of renal function (creatinine clearance 10-50 ml/min/1.73 m^2), following a single 400 mg dose, the plasma half-life was prolonged to approximately 5.6 hours. In subjects with severe renal impairment (creatinine clearance <10 ml/min/1.73 m^2), the half-life was increased to approximately 32 hours. During hemodialysis the half-life was approximately 4 hours. In patients with severe renal impairment, the C_{max} increased from 15.4 to 23 μg/ml (see PRECAUTIONS and DOSAGE AND ADMINISTRATION).

In single-dose studies, plasma half-life and AUC were not significantly altered in healthy elderly subjects with normal renal function.

There is no evidence of metabolism of loracarbef in humans.

Approximately 25% of circulating loracarbef is bound to plasma proteins.

Middle-ear fluid concentrations of loracarbef were approximately 48% of the plasma concentration 2 hours after drug administration in pediatric patients. The peak concentration of loracarbef in blister fluid was approximately half that obtained in plasma. Adequate data on CSF levels of loracarbef are not available.

MICROBIOLOGY

Loracarbef exerts its bactericidal action by binding to essential target proteins of the bacterial cell wall, leading to inhibition of cell-wall synthesis. It is stable in the presence of some bacterial β-lactamases. Loracarbef has been shown to be active against most strains of the following organisms both *in vitro* and in clinical infections (see INDICATIONS AND USAGE).

Gram-Positive Aerobes:

Staphylococcus aureus (including penicillinase-producing strains)

NOTE: Loracarbef (like most β-lactam antimicrobials) is inactive against methicillin-resistant staphylococci.

Staphylococcus saprophyticus

Streptococcus pneumoniae

Streptococcus pyogenes

Gram-Negative Aerobes:

Escherichia coli

Haemophilus influenzae (including β-lactamase-producing strains)

Moraxella (Branhamella) catarrhalis (including β-lactamase-producing strains)

The following *in vitro* data are available; however, their clinical significance is unknown.

Loracarbef exhibits *in vitro* minimum inhibitory concentrations (MIC) of 8 μg/ml or less against most strains of the following organisms; however, the safety and efficacy of loracarbef in treating clinical infections due to these organisms have not been established in adequate and well-controlled trials.

Gram-Positive Aerobes:

Staphylococcus epidermidis

Streptococcus agalactiae (group B streptococci)

Streptococcus bovis

Streptococci groups C, F, and G

Viridans group streptococci

Gram-Negative Aerobes:

Citrobacter diversus

Haemophilus parainfluenzae

Klebsiella pneumoniae

Neisseria gonorrhoeae (including penicillinase-producing strains)

Pasteurella multocida

Proteus mirabilis

Salmonella species

Shigella species

Yersinia enterocolitica

NOTE: Loracarbef is inactive against most strains of *Acinetobacter, Enterobacter, Morganella morganii, Proteus vulgaris, Providencia, Pseudomonas,* and *Serratia.*

Anaerobic Organisms:

Clostridium perfringens

Fusobacterium necrophorum

Peptococcus niger

Peptostreptococcus intermedius

Propionibacterium acnes

SUSCEPTIBILITY TESTING

Diffusion Techniques

Quantitative methods that require measurement of zone diameters give the most precise estimate of the susceptibility of bacteria to antimicrobial agents. One such standardized method[1] has been recommended for use with the 30 μg loracarbef disk. Interpretation involves the correlation of the diameter obtained in the disk test with MIC for loracarbef.

Reports from the laboratory giving results of the standard single-disk susceptibility test with a 30 μg loracarbef disk should be interpreted according to the following criteria (see TABLE 2).

TABLE 2

Zone Diameter (mm)	Interpretation
≥18	(S) Susceptible
15-17	(MS) Moderately Susceptible
≤14	(R) Resistant

A report of "susceptible" implies that the pathogen is likely to be inhibited by generally achievable blood concentrations. A report of "moderately susceptible" indicates that inhibitory concentrations of the antibiotic may be achieved if high dosage is used or if the infection is confined to tissues and fluids (*e.g.,* urine) in which high antibiotic concentrations are attained. A report of "resistant" indicates that achievable concentrations of the antibiotic are unlikely to be inhibitory and other therapy should be selected.

Standardized procedures require the use of laboratory control organisms. The 30 μg loracarbef disk should give the following zone diameters with the NCCLS approved procedure (see TABLE 3).

TABLE 3

Organism	Zone Diameter (mm)
E. coli ATCC 25922	23-29
S. aureus ATCC 25923	23-31

Dilution Techniques

Use a standardized dilution method[2] (broth, agar, or microdilution) or equivalent with loracarbef powder. The MIC values obtained should be interpreted according to the following criteria (see TABLE 4).

As with standard diffusion methods, dilution procedures require the use of laboratory control organisms. Standard loracarbef powder should give the following MIC values with the NCCLS approved procedure (see TABLE 5).

TABLE 4

MIC (μg/ml)	Interpretation
≤8	(S) Susceptible
16	(MS) Moderately Susceptible
≥32	(R) Resistant

TABLE 5

Organism	MIC Range (μg/ml)
E. coli ATCC 25922	0.5-2
S. aureus ATCC 29213	0.5-2

INDICATIONS AND USAGE

Loracarbef is indicated in the treatment of patients with mild to moderate infections caused by susceptible strains of the designated microorganisms in the conditions listed below. (As recommended dosages, durations of therapy, and applicable patient populations vary among these infections, please see DOSAGE AND ADMINISTRATION for specific recommendations.)

LOWER RESPIRATORY TRACT

Secondary Bacterial Infection of Acute Bronchitis caused by *S. pneumoniae, H. influenzae* (including β-lactamase-producing strains), or *M. catarrhalis* (including β-lactamase-producing strains).

Acute Bacterial Exacerbations of Chronic Bronchitis caused by *S. pneumoniae, H. influenzae* (including β-lactamase-producing strains), or *M. catarrhalis* (including β-lactamase-producing strains).

Pneumonia caused by *S. pneumoniae or H. influenzae* (non-β-lactamase-producing strains only). Data are insufficient at this time to establish efficacy in patients with pneumonia caused by β-lactamase-producing strains of *H. influenzae.*

UPPER RESPIRATORY TRACT

Otitis Media* caused by *S. pneumoniae, H. influenzae* (including β-lactamase-producing strains), *M. catarrhalis* (including β-lactamase-producing strains), or *S. pyogenes.*

Acute Maxillary Sinusitis* caused by *S. pneumoniae, H. influenzae* (non-β-lactamase-producing strains only), or *M. catarrhalis* (including β-lactamase-producing strains). Data are insufficient at this time to establish efficacy in patients with acute maxillary sinusitis caused by β-lactamase-producing strains of *H. influenzae.*

**NOTE:* In a patient population with significant numbers of β-lactamase-producing organisms, loracarbef's clinical cure and bacteriological eradication rates were somewhat less than those observed with a product containing a β-lactamase inhibitor. Loracarbef's decreased potential for toxicity compared to products containing β-lactamase inhibitors along with the susceptibility patterns of the common microbes in a given geographic area should be taken into account when considering the use of an antimicrobial. For information on use in pediatric patients, see PRECAUTIONS, Pediatric Use.

Pharyngitis and Tonsillitis caused by *S. pyogenes.* (The usual drug of choice in the treatment and prevention of streptococcal infections, including the prophylaxis of rheumatic fever, is penicillin administered by the intramuscular route. Loracarbef is generally effective in the eradication of *S. pyogenes* from the nasopharynx; however, data establishing the efficacy of loracarbef in the subsequent prevention of rheumatic fever are not available at present.)

SKIN AND SKIN STRUCTURE

Uncomplicated Skin and Skin Structure Infections caused by *S. aureus* (including penicillinase-producing strains) or *S. pyogenes.* Abscesses should be surgically drained as clinically indicated.

URINARY TRACT

Uncomplicated Urinary Tract Infections (cystitis) caused by *E. coli* or *S. saprophyticus**.

NOTE: In considering the use of loracarbef in the treatment of cystitis, loracarbef's lower bacterial eradication rates and lower potential for toxicity should be weighed against the increased eradication rates and increased potential for toxicity demonstrated by some other classes of approved agents.

Uncomplicated Pyelonephritis caused by *E. coli.*

*Although treatment of infections due to this organism in this organ system demonstrated a clinically acceptable overall outcome, efficacy was studied in fewer than 10 infections.

Culture and susceptibility testing should be performed when appropriate to determine the causative organism and its susceptibility to loracarbef. Therapy may be started while awaiting the results of these studies. Once these results become available, antimicrobial therapy should be adjusted accordingly.

CONTRAINDICATIONS

Loracarbef is contraindicated in patients with known allergy to loracarbef or cephalosporin-class antibiotics.

WARNINGS

BEFORE THERAPY WITH LORACARBEF IS INSTITUTED, CAREFUL INQUIRY SHOULD BE MADE TO DETERMINE WHETHER THE PATIENT HAS HAD PREVIOUS HYPERSENSITIVITY REACTIONS TO LORACARBEF, CEPHALOSPORINS, PENICILLINS, OR OTHER DRUGS. IF THIS PRODUCT IS TO BE GIVEN TO PENICILLIN-SENSITIVE PATIENTS, CAUTION SHOULD BE EXERCISED BECAUSE CROSS-HYPERSENSITIVITY AMONG β-LACTAM ANTIBIOTICS HAS

L

BEEN CLEARLY DOCUMENTED AND MAY OCCUR IN UP TO 10% OF PATIENTS WITH A HISTORY OF PENICILLIN ALLERGY. IF AN ALLERGIC REACTION TO LORACARBEF OCCURS, DISCONTINUE THE DRUG. SERIOUS ACUTE HYPERSENSITIVITY REACTIONS MAY REQUIRE THE USE OF EPINEPHRINE AND OTHER EMERGENCY MEASURES, INCLUDING OXYGEN, INTRAVENOUS FLUIDS, INTRAVENOUS ANTIHISTAMINES, CORTICOSTEROIDS, PRESSOR AMINES, AND AIRWAY MANAGEMENT, AS CLINICALLY INDICATED.

Pseudomembranous colitis has been reported with nearly all antibacterial agents and may range from mild to life-threatening. Therefore, it is important to consider this diagnosis in patients who present with diarrhea subsequent to the administration of antibacterial agents.

Treatment with broad-spectrum antibiotics alters the normal flora of the colon and may permit overgrowth of clostridia. Studies indicate that a toxin produced by *Clostridium difficile* is a primary cause of "antibiotic-associated colitis".

After the diagnosis of pseudomembranous colitis has been established, therapeutic measures should be initiated. Mild cases of pseudomembranous colitis usually respond to discontinuation of drug alone. In moderate to severe cases, consideration should be given to management with fluids and electrolytes, protein supplementation, and treatment with an antibacterial drug effective against *C. difficile*-associated colitis.

PRECAUTIONS

GENERAL

In patients with known or suspected renal impairment (see DOSAGE AND ADMINISTRATION), careful clinical observation and appropriate laboratory studies should be performed prior to and during therapy. The total daily dose of loracarbef should be reduced in these patients because high and/or prolonged plasma antibiotic concentrations can occur in such individuals administered the usual doses. Loracarbef, like cephalosporins, should be given with caution to patients receiving concurrent treatment with potent diuretics because these diuretics are suspected of adversely affecting renal function.

As with other broad-spectrum antimicrobials, prolonged use of loracarbef may result in the overgrowth of nonsusceptible organisms. Careful observation of the patient is essential. If superinfection occurs during therapy, appropriate measures should be taken.

Loracarbef, as with other broad-spectrum antimicrobials, should be prescribed with caution in individuals with a history of colitis.

INFORMATION FOR THE PATIENT

Loracarbef should be taken either at least 1 hour prior to eating or at least 2 hours after eating a meal.

L

CARCINOGENESIS, MUTAGENESIS, AND IMPAIRMENT OF FERTILITY

Although lifetime studies in animals have not been performed to evaluate carcinogenic potential, no mutagenic potential was found for loracarbef in standard tests of genotoxicity, which included bacterial mutation tests and *in vitro* and *in vivo* mammalian systems. In rats, fertility and reproductive performance were not affected by loracarbef at doses up to 33 times the maximum human exposure in mg/kg (10 times the exposure based on mg/m^2).

PREGNANCY CATEGORY B

Reproduction studies have been performed in mice, rats, and rabbits at doses up to 33 times the maximum human exposure in mg/kg (4, 10, and 4 times the exposure, respectively, based on mg/m^2) and have revealed no evidence of impaired fertility or harm to the fetus due to loracarbef. There are, however, no adequate and well-controlled studies in pregnant women. Because animal reproduction studies are not always predictive of human response, this drug should be used during pregnancy only if clearly needed.

LABOR AND DELIVERY

Loracarbef has not been studied for use during labor and delivery. Treatment should be given only if clearly needed.

NURSING MOTHERS

It is not known whether this drug is excreted in human milk. Because many drugs are excreted in human milk, caution should be exercised when loracarbef is administered to a nursing woman.

PEDIATRIC USE

The safety and efficacy of loracarbef have been established for children aged 6 months to 12 years for acute maxillary sinusitis based upon its approval in adults. Use of loracarbef in pediatric patients is supported by pharmacokinetic and safety data in adults and children, and by clinical and microbiologic data from adequate and well-controlled studies of the treatment of acute maxillary sinusitis in adults and of acute otitis media with effusion in children. It is also supported by post-marketing adverse events surveillance. (See CLINICAL PHARMACOLOGY, INDICATIONS AND USAGE, ADVERSE REACTIONS, and DOSAGE AND ADMINISTRATION).

GERIATRIC USE

Healthy geriatric volunteers (≥65 years old) with normal renal function who received a single 400 mg dose of loracarbef had no significant differences in AUC or clearance when compared to healthy adult volunteers 20-40 years of age (see CLINICAL PHARMACOLOGY). Of 3541 adult patients in controlled clinical studies of loracarbef, 705 (19.9%) were 65 years of age or older. In these controlled clinical studies, when geriatric patients received the usual recommended adult doses, clinical efficacy and safety were comparable to results in nongeriatric adult patients. Loracarbef is known to be substantially excreted by the kidney. Because significant numbers of elderly patients have decreased renal function, care should be taken in dose selection and evaluation of renal function in this population is recommended (see DOSAGE AND ADMINISTRATION).

DRUG INTERACTIONS

Probenecid: As with other β-lactam antibiotics, renal excretion of loracarbef is inhibited by probenecid and resulted in an approximate 80% increase in the AUC for loracarbef (see CLINICAL PHARMACOLOGY).

ADVERSE REACTIONS

The nature of adverse reactions to loracarbef are similar to those observed with orally administered β-lactam antimicrobials. The majority of adverse reactions observed in clinical trials were of a mild and transient nature; 1.5% of patients discontinued therapy because of drug-related adverse reactions. No one reaction requiring discontinuation accounted for >0.03% of the total patient population; however, of those reactions resulting in discontinuation, gastrointestinal events (diarrhea and abdominal pain) and skin rashes predominated.

ALL PATIENTS

The following adverse events, irrespective of relationship to drug, have been reported following the use of loracarbef in clinical trials. Incidence rates (combined for all dosing regimens and dosage forms) were less than 1% for the total patient population, except as otherwise noted:

Gastrointestinal: The most commonly observed adverse reactions were related to the gastrointestinal system. The incidence of gastrointestinal adverse reactions increased in patients treated with higher doses. Individual event rates included diarrhea, 4.1%; nausea, 1.9%; vomiting 1.4%; abdominal pain, 1.4%; and anorexia.

Hypersensitivity: Hypersensitivity reactions including, skin rashes (1.2%), urticaria, pruritus, and erythema multiforme.

Central Nervous System: Headache (2.9%), somnolence, nervousness, insomnia, and dizziness.

Hemic and Lymphatic Systems: Transient thrombocytopenia, leukopenia, and eosinophilia.

Hepatic: Transient elevations in AST (SGOT), ALT (SGPT), and alkaline phosphatase.

Renal: Transient elevations in BUN and creatinine.

Cardiovascular System: Vasodilatation.

Genitourinary: Vaginitis (1.3%), vaginal moniliasis (1.1%).

As with other β-lactam antibiotics, the following potentially severe adverse experiences have been reported rarely with loracarbef in worldwide post-marketing surveillance: anaphylaxis, hepatic dysfunction including cholestasis, prolongation of the prothrombin time with clinical bleeding in patients taking anticoagulants, and Stevens-Johnson syndrome.

PEDIATRIC PATIENTS

The incidences of several adverse events, irrespective of relationship to drug, following treatment with loracarbef were significantly different in the pediatric population and the adult population as follows inTABLE 12.

TABLE 12

Event	Pediatric	Adult
Diarrhea	5.8%	3.6%
Headache	0.9%	3.2%
Rhinitis	6.3%	1.6%
Nausea	0.0%	2.5%
Rash	2.9%	0.7%
Vomiting	3.3%	0.5%
Somnolence	2.1%	0.4%
Anorexia	2.3%	0.3%

β-LACTAM ANTIMICROBIAL CLASS LABELING

The following adverse reactions and altered laboratory test results have been reported in patients treated with β-lactam antibiotics:

Adverse Reactions

Allergic reactions, aplastic anemia, hemolytic anemia, hemorrhage, agranulocytosis, toxic epidermal necrolysis, renal dysfunction, toxic nephropathy. As with other β-lactam antibiotics, serum sickness-like reactions have been reported rarely with loracarbef.

Several β-lactam antibiotics have been implicated in triggering seizures, particularly in patients with renal impairment when the dosage was not reduced. If seizures associated with drug therapy should occur, the drug should be discontinued. Anticonvulsant therapy can be given if clinically indicated.

Altered Laboratory Tests

Increased prothrombin time, positive direct Coombs' test, elevated LDH, pancytopenia, and neutropenia.

DOSAGE AND ADMINISTRATION

Loracarbef is administered orally either at least 1 hour prior to eating or at least 2 hours after eating. The recommended dosages, durations of treatment, and applicable patient populations are described in TABLE 13.

RENAL IMPAIRMENT

Loracarbef may be administered to patients with impaired renal function. The usual dose and schedule may be employed in patients with creatinine clearance levels of 50 ml/min or greater. Patients with creatinine clearance between 10 and 49 ml/min may be given half of the recommended dose at the usual dosage interval, or the normal recommended dose at twice the usual dosage interval. Patients with creatinine clearance levels less than 10 ml/min may be treated with the recommended dose given every 3-5 days; patients on hemodialysis should receive another dose following dialysis.

TABLE 13

Population / Infection	Dosage (mg)	Duration (days)
Adults (13 years and older)		
Lower Respiratory Tract		
Secondary bacterial infection of acute bronchitis	200-400 q12h	7
Acute bacterial exacerbation of chronic bronchitis	400 q12h	7
Pneumonia	400 q12h	14
Upper Respiratory Tract		
Pharyngitis/tonsillitis	200 q12h	10*
Sinusitis‡	400 q12h	10
Skin and Skin Structure		
Uncomplicated skin and skin structure infections	200 q12h	7
Urinary Tract		
Uncomplicated cystitis‡	200 q24h	7
Uncomplicated pyelonephritis	400 q12h	14
Pediatric Patients (6 months to 12 years)		
Upper Respiratory Tract		
Acute otitis media†‡	30 mg/kg/day in divided doses q12h	10
Acute maxillary sinusitis‡	30 mg/kg/day in divided doses q12h	10
Pharyngitis/tonsillitis	15 mg/kg/day in divided doses q12h	10*
Skin and Skin Structure		
Impetigo	15 mg/kg/day in divided doses q12h	7

* In the treatment of infections due to *S. pyogenes,* loracarbef should be administered for at least 10 days.
† Otitis media should be treated with the suspension. Clinical studies of otitis media were conducted with the suspension formulation only. The suspension is more rapidly absorbed than the capsules, resulting in higher peak plasma concentrations when administered at the same dose. Therefore, the capsule should not be substituted for the suspension in the treatment of otitis media (see CLINICAL PHARMACOLOGY).
‡ See INDICATIONS AND USAGE for further information.

TABLE 14 *Pediatric Dosage Chart — Daily Dose 15 mg/kg/day — Dose Given Twice Daily*

Weight		100 mg/5 ml Suspension		200 mg/5 ml Suspension	
lb	kg	ml	tsp	ml	tsp
15	7	2.6	0.5	—	—
29	13	4.9	1.0	2.5	0.5
44	20	7.5	1.5	3.8	0.75
57	26	9.8	2.0	4.9	1.0

TABLE 15 *Pediatric Dosage Chart — Daily Dose 30 mg/kg/day — Dose Given Twice Daily*

Weight		100 mg/5 ml Suspension		200 mg/5 ml Suspension	
lb	kg	ml	tsp	ml	tsp
15	7	5.2	1.0	2.6	0.5
29	13	9.8	2.0	4.9	1.0
44	20	—	—	7.5	1.5
57	26	—	—	9.8	2.0

When only the serum creatinine is available, the following formula (based on sex, weight, and age of the patient) may be used to convert this value into creatinine clearance (CLCR, ml/min). The equation assumes the patient's renal function is stable.

Males = [(weight in kg) × (140 - age)] ÷ [72 × serum creatinine (mg/100 ml)]
Females = (0.85) × (above value)

HOW SUPPLIED

LORABID PULVULES

200 mg: Blue and gray capsules.
400 mg: Blue and pink capsules.

Storage: Keep tightly closed. Store at controlled room temperature, 15-30°C (59-86°F). Protect from heat.

LORABID ORAL SUSPENSION

Available in strawberry bubble gum flavor containing 100 or 200 mg of loracarbef per 5 ml.
Storage: After mixing, the suspension may be kept at room temperature, 15-30°C (59-86°F), for 14 days without significant loss of potency. Keep tightly closed. Discard unused portion after 14 days.

PRODUCT LISTING - EQUIVALENTS NOT AVAILABLE

Capsule - Oral - 200 mg

14's	$58.74	LORABID, Allscripts Pharmaceutical Company	54569-3659-00
15's	$68.87	LORABID, Physicians Total Care	54868-2927-00
20's	$76.41	LORABID, Prescript Pharmaceuticals	00247-0261-20
20's	$79.92	LORABID, Allscripts Pharmaceutical Company	54569-3659-01
30's	$112.94	LORABID, Prescript Pharmaceuticals	00247-0261-30
30's	$125.87	LORABID PULVULES, Lilly, Eli and Company	00002-3170-30
100's	$419.59	LORABID PULVULES, Monarch Pharmaceuticals Inc	00002-3170-02
100's	$453.15	LORABID, Monarch Pharmaceuticals Inc	61570-0170-01

Capsule - Oral - 400 mg

20's	$118.13	LORABID, Allscripts Pharmaceutical Company	54569-4219-00
30's	$177.19	LORABID, Lilly, Eli and Company	00002-3171-30
100's	$637.88	LORABID PULVULES, Monarch Pharmaceuticals Inc	00002-3171-02
100's	$637.88	LORABID, Monarch Pharmaceuticals Inc	61570-0171-01

Powder For Reconstitution - Oral - 100 mg/5 ml

50 ml	$21.20	LORABID, Lilly, Eli and Company	00002-5135-87
100 ml	$37.44	LORABID, Allscripts Pharmaceutical Company	54569-3727-00
100 ml	$47.53	LORABID, Lilly, Eli and Company	00002-5135-48
100 ml	$47.53	LORABID, Monarch Pharmaceuticals Inc	61570-0135-10

Powder For Reconstitution - Oral - 200 mg/5 ml

50 ml	$35.40	LORABID, Lilly, Eli and Company	00002-5136-87
75 ml	$47.19	LORABID, Lilly, Eli and Company	00002-5136-18
100 ml	$61.69	LORABID, Allscripts Pharmaceutical Company	54569-3729-00
100 ml	$71.85	LORABID, Lilly, Eli and Company	00002-5136-48
100 ml	$71.85	LORABID, Monarch Pharmaceuticals Inc	61570-0136-01
100 ml	$77.60	LORABID, Monarch Pharmaceuticals Inc	61570-0136-10

Loratadine *(003161)*

For related information, see the comparative table section in Appendix A.

Categories: Rhinitis, allergic; Urticaria, chronic idiopathic; Pregnancy Category B; FDA Approved 1993 Apr
Drug Classes: Antihistamines, H1
Brand Names: **Claritin**
Foreign Brand Availability: Alerfast (Peru); Alernitis (Indonesia); Alertadin (Peru); Allohex (Indonesia); Analergal (Mexico); Anhissen (Indonesia); Anlos (Indonesia); Ardin (Singapore); Bonalerg (Guatemala); Civeran (Spain); Claratyne (Australia; New-Zealand); Claritine (Bahamas; Bahrain; Barbados; Belgium; Belize; Benin; Bermuda; Burkina-Faso; Curacao; Cyprus; Czech-Republic; Egypt; Ethiopia; Gambia; Ghana; Guinea; Guyana; Hungary; Iran; Iraq; Israel; Ivory-Coast; Jamaica; Jordan; Kenya; Kuwait; Lebanon; Liberia; Libya; Malawi; Mali; Mauritania; Mauritius; Morocco; Netherland-Antilles; Netherlands; Niger; Nigeria; Oman; Portugal; Puerto-Rico; Qatar; Republic-of-Yemen; Russia; Saudi-Arabia; Senegal; Seychelles; Sierra-Leone; South-Africa; Sudan; Surinam; Switzerland; Syria; Tanzania; Trinidad; Tunia; Turkey; Uganda; United-Arab-Emirates; Zambia; Zimbabwe); Clarityn (Austria; Denmark; England; Finland; Ireland; Italy; Norway; Sweden); Clarityne (China; Colombia; Costa-Rica; Dominican-Republic; Ecuador; El-Salvador; France; Greece; Guatemala; Honduras; Hong-Kong; Korea; Malaysia; Mexico; Panama; Peru; South-Africa; Spain; Taiwan; Thailand); Cronitin (Indonesia); Cronopen (Peru); Curyken (Mexico); Demazin Anti-Allergy (South-Africa); Eclaran (Peru); Finska (Taiwan); Fristamin (Italy); Halodin (Thailand); Hislorex (Indonesia); Histalor (Singapore); Histaloran (Ecuador); Klarihist (Bahrain; Cyprus; Egypt; Iran; Iraq; Jordan; Kuwait; Lebanon; Libya; Oman; Qatar; Republic-of-Yemen; Saudi-Arabia; Syria; United-Arab-Emirates); Klinset (Indonesia); Lergia (Indonesia); Lertamine (Mexico); Lisino (Germany); Lobeta (Germany); Lodain (Korea); Lorabasics (Germany); Loracert (Colombia); Loradex (Philippines); Lora-Lich (Germany); Lorano (Germany); Loranox (Thailand); Lorastine (Israel); Lora-Tabs (New-Zealand); Loratadura (Germany); Loratrim (Israel); Loratyne (South-Africa); Lorazin (Korea); Loreen (Bahrain; Cyprus; Egypt; Iran; Iraq; Jordan; Kuwait; Lebanon; Libya; Oman; Qatar; Republic-of-Yemen; Saudi-Arabia; Syria; United-Arab-Emirates); Lorfast (Benin; Burkina-Faso; Ethiopia; Gambia; Ghana; Guinea; India; Ivory-Coast; Kenya; Liberia; Malawi; Mali; Mauritania; Mauritius; Morocco; Niger; Nigeria; Senegal; Seychelles; Sierra-Leone; Singapore; South-Africa; Sudan; Tanzania; Tunia; Uganda; Zambia; Zimbabwe); Loridin (Benin; Burkina-Faso; Ethiopia; Gambia; Ghana; Guinea; Ivory-Coast; Kenya; Liberia; Malawi; Mali; Mauritania; Mauritius; Morocco; Niger; Nigeria; Senegal; Seychelles; Sierra-Leone; Singapore; Sudan; Tanzania; Tunia; Uganda; Zambia; Zimbabwe); Lorita (Thailand); Lotadine (Hong-Kong); Lowadina (Mexico); Mosedin (Bahrain; Cyprus; Egypt; Iran; Iraq; Jordan; Kuwait; Lebanon; Libya; Oman; Qatar; Republic-of-Yemen; Saudi-Arabia; Syria; United-Arab-Emirates); Noratin (Korea); Notamin (Korea); Optimin (Spain); Polaratyne (South-Africa); Proactin (Peru); Pylor (Indonesia); Restamine (Bahrain; Cyprus; Egypt; Iran; Iraq; Jordan; Kuwait; Lebanon; Libya; Oman; Qatar; Republic-of-Yemen; Saudi-Arabia; Syria; United-Arab-Emirates); Ridamin (Singapore; Thailand); Rihest (Indonesia); Rityne (Thailand); Roletra (Singapore); Sensibit (Mexico); Sohotin (Indonesia); Tidilor (Bahrain; Cyprus; Egypt; Iran; Iraq; Jordan; Kuwait; Lebanon; Libya; Oman; Qatar; Republic-of-Yemen; Saudi-Arabia; Syria; United-Arab-Emirates); Tirlor (Thailand); Toradine (Thailand); Velodan (Spain); Zeos (Indonesia)
Cost of Therapy: $71.36 (Allergic Rhinitis; Claritin; 10 mg; 1 tablet/day; 30 day supply)
$21.54 (Allergic Rhinitis; Alavert; 10 mg; 1 tablet/day; 30 day supply)
$82.34 (Allergic Rhinitis; Claritin Reditab; 10 mg; 1 tablet/day; 30 day supply)
$24.75 (Allergic Rhinitis; Generic Tablets; 10 mg; 1 tablet/day; 30 day supply)

DESCRIPTION

Loratadine is a white to off-white powder not soluble in water, but very soluble in acetone, alcohol, and chloroform. It has a molecular weight of 382.89, and empirical formula of $C_{22}H_{23}ClN_2O_2$; its chemical name is ethyl4-(8-chloro-5,6-dihydro-11*H*-benzo[5,6]cyclohepta[1,2-*b*]pyridin-11-ylidene)-1-piperidinecarboxylate.

Claritin tablets contain 10 mg micronized loratadine, an antihistamine, to be administered orally. *They also contain the following inactive ingredients:* Corn starch, lactose, and magnesium stearate.

Claritin syrup contains 1 mg/ml micronized loratadine, an antihistamine, to be administered orally. *It also contains the following inactive ingredients:* Citric acid, artificial flavor, glycerin, propylene glycol, sodium benzoate, sugar, and water. The pH is between 2.5 and 3.1.

Claritin Reditabs (rapidly-disintegrating tablets) contain 10 mg micronized loratadine, an antihistamine, to be administered orally. It disintegrates in the mouth within seconds after placement on the tongue, allowing its contents to be subsequently swallowed with or without water. *Claritin Reditabs also contain the following inactive ingredients:* Citric acid, gelatin, mannitol, and mint flavor.

CLINICAL PHARMACOLOGY

Loratadine is a long-acting tricyclic antihistamine with selective peripheral histamine H_1-receptor antagonistic activity.

Human histamine skin wheal studies following single and repeated 10 mg oral doses of loratadine have shown that the drug exhibits an antihistaminic effect beginning within 1-3 hours, reaching a maximum at 8-12 hours, and lasting in excess of 24 hours. There was no evidence of tolerance to this effect after 28 days of dosing with loratadine.

Whole body autoradiographic studies in rats and monkeys, radiolabeled tissue distribution studies in mice and rats, and *in vivo* radioligand studies in mice have shown that neither loratadine nor its metabolites readily cross the blood-brain barrier. Radioligand binding studies with guinea pig pulmonary and brain H_1-receptors indicate that there was preferential binding to peripheral versus central nervous system H_1-receptors.

Repeated application of loratadine rapidly-disintegrating tablets to the hamster cheek pouch did not cause local irritation.

PHARMACOKINETICS

Loratadine was rapidly absorbed following oral administration of 10 mg tablets, once daily for 10 days to healthy adult volunteers with times to maximum concentration (T_{max}) of 1.3 hours for loratadine and 2.5 hours for its major active metabolite, descarboethoxyloratadine. Based on a cross-study comparison of single doses of loratadine syrup and tablets given to healthy adult volunteers, the plasma concentration profile of descarboethoxyloratadine for the two formulations is comparable. The pharmacokinetics of loratadine and descarboethoxyloratadine are independent of dose over the dose range of 10-40 mg and are not altered by the duration of treatment. In a single-dose study, food increased the systemic bioavailability (AUC) of loratadine and descarboethoxyloratadine by approximately 40% and 15%, respectively. The time to peak plasma concentration (T_{max}) of loratadine and descarboethoxyloratadine was delayed by 1 hour. Peak plasma concentrations (C_{max}) were not affected by food.

Pharmacokinetic studies showed that loratadine rapidly-disintegrating tablets provide plasma concentrations of loratadine and descarboethoxyloratadine similar to those achieved with loratadine tablets. Following administration of 10 mg loratadine once daily for 10 days with each dosage form in a randomized crossover comparison in 24 normal adult subjects, similar mean exposures (AUC) and peak plasma concentrations (C_{max}) of loratadine were observed. Loratadine rapidly-disintegrating tablets mean AUC and C_{max} were 11% and 6% greater than that of the loratadine tablet values, respectively. Descarboethoxyloratadine bioequivalence was demonstrated between the two formulations. After 10 days of dosing, mean peak plasma concentrations were attained at 1.3 hours and 2.3 hours (T_{max}) for parent and metabolite, respectively.

In a single-dose study with loratadine rapidly-disintegrating tablets, food increased the AUC of loratadine by approximately 48% and did not appreciably affect the AUC of descarboethoxyloratadine. The times to peak plasma concentration (T_{max}) of loratadine and descarboethoxyloratadine were delayed by approximately 2.4 and 3.7 hours, respectively, when food was consumed prior to loratadine rapidly-disintegrating tablets administration. Parent and metabolite peak concentrations (C_{max}) were not affected by food.

In a single-dose study with loratadine rapidly-disintegrating tablets in 24 subjects, the AUC of loratadine was increased by 26% when administered without water compared to administration with water, while C_{max} was not substantially affected. The bioavailability of descarboethoxyloratadine was not different when administered without water.

Approximately 80% of the total loratadine dose administered can be found equally distributed between urine and feces in the form of metabolic products within 10 days. In nearly all patients, exposure (AUC) to the metabolite is greater than to the parent loratadine. The mean elimination half-lives in normal adult subjects (n=54) were 8.4 hours (range = 3-20 hours) for loratadine and 28 hours (range = 8.8 to 92 hours) for descarboethoxyloratadine. Loratadine and descarboethoxyloratadine reached steady-state in most patients by approximately the fifth dosing day. There was considerable variability in the pharmacokinetic data in all studies of loratadine tablets and syrup, probably due to the extensive first-pass metabolism.

In vitro studies with human liver microsomes indicate that loratadine is metabolized to descarboethoxyloratadine predominantly by cytochrome P450 3A4 (CYP3A4) and, to a lesser extent, by cytochrome P450 2D6 (CYP2D6). In the presence of a CYP3A4 inhibitor ketoconazole, loratadine is metabolized to descarboethoxyloratadine predominantly by CYP2D6. Concurrent administration of loratadine with either ketoconazole, erythromycin (both CYP3A4 inhibitors), or cimetidine (CYP2D6 and CYP3A4 inhibitor) to healthy volunteers was associated with substantially increased plasma concentrations of loratadine (see DRUG INTERACTIONS).

The pharmacokinetic profile of loratadine in children in the 6-12 year age group is similar to that of adults. In a single-dose pharmacokinetic study of 13 pediatric volunteers (aged 8-12 years) given 10 ml of loratadine syrup containing 10 mg loratadine, the ranges of individual subject values of pharmacokinetic parameters (AUC and C_{max}) were comparable to those following administration of a 10 mg tablet or syrup to adult volunteers.

SPECIAL POPULATIONS

In a study involving twelve healthy geriatric subjects (66-78 years old), the AUC and peak plasma levels (C_{max}) of both loratadine and descarboethoxyloratadine were approximately 50% greater than those observed in studies of younger subjects. The mean elimination half-lives for the geriatric subjects were 18.2 hours (range = 6.7 to 37 hours) for loratadine and 17.5 hours (range = 11-38 hours) for descarboethoxyloratadine.

In a study involving 12 subjects with chronic renal impairment (creatinine clearance $\leq$30 ml/min) both AUC and C_{max} increased by approximately 73% for loratadine and by 120% for descarboethoxyloratadine, as compared to 6 subjects with normal renal function (creatinine clearance $\geq$80 ml/min). The mean elimination half-lives of loratadine (7.6 hours) and descarboethoxyloratadine (23.9 hours) were not substantially different from that observed in normal subjects. Hemodialysis does not have an effect on the pharmacokinetics of loratadine or descarboethoxyloratadine in subjects with chronic renal impairment.

In seven patients with chronic alcoholic liver disease, the AUC and C_{max} of loratadine were double while the pharmacokinetic profile of descarboethoxyloratadine was not substantially different from that observed in other trials enrolling normal subjects. The elimination half-lives for loratadine and descarboethoxyloratadine were 24 hours and 37 hours, respectively, and increased with increasing severity of liver disease.

INDICATIONS AND USAGE

Loratadine is indicated for the relief of nasal and non-nasal symptoms of seasonal allergic rhinitis and for the treatment of chronic idiopathic urticaria in patients 6 years of age or older.

CONTRAINDICATIONS

Loratadine is contraindicated in patients who are hypersensitive to this medication or to any of its ingredients.

PRECAUTIONS

GENERAL

Patients with liver impairment or renal insufficiency (GFR <30 ml/min) should be given a lower initial dose (10 mg every other day). (See CLINICAL PHARMACOLOGY, Special Populations.)

CARCINOGENESIS, MUTAGENESIS, AND IMPAIRMENT OF FERTILITY

In an 18-month carcinogenicity study in mice and a 2 year study in rats, loratadine was administered in the diet at doses up to 40 mg/kg (mice) and 25 mg/kg (rats). In the carcinogenicity studies, pharmacokinetic assessments were carried out to determine animal exposure to the drug. AUC data demonstrated that the exposure of mice given 40 mg/kg of loratadine was 3.6 (loratadine) and 18 (descarboethoxyloratadine) times higher than in humans given the maximum recommended daily oral dose. Exposure of rats given 25 mg/kg of loratadine was 28 (loratadine) and 67 (descarboethoxyloratadine) times higher than in humans given the maximum recommended daily oral dose. Male mice given 40 mg/kg had a significantly higher incidence of hepatocellular tumors (combined adenomas and carcinomas) than concurrent controls. In rats, a significantly higher incidence of hepatocellular tumors (combined adenomas and carcinomas) was observed in males given 10 mg/kg and males and females given 25 mg/kg. The clinical significance of these findings during long-term use of loratadine is not known.

In mutagenicity studies, there was no evidence of mutagenic potential in reverse (Ames) or forward point mutation (CHO-HGPRT) assays, or in the assay for DNA damage (rat primary hepatocyte unscheduled DNA assay) or in two assays for chromosomal aberrations (human peripheral blood lymphocyte clastogenesis assay and the mouse bone marrow erythrocyte micronucleus assay). In the mouse lymphoma assay, a positive finding occurred in the nonactivated but not the activated phase of the study.

Decreased fertility in male rats, shown by lower female conception rates, occurred at an oral dose of 64 mg/kg (approximately 50 times the maximum recommended human daily oral dose on a mg/m^2 basis) and was reversible with cessation of dosing. Loratadine had no effect on male or female fertility or reproduction in the rat at an oral dose of approximately 24 mg/kg (approximately 20 times the maximum recommended human daily oral dose on a mg/m^2 basis).

PREGNANCY CATEGORY B

There was no evidence of animal teratogenicity in studies performed in rats and rabbits at oral doses up to 96 mg/kg (approximately 75 times and 150 times, respectively, the maximum recommended human daily oral dose on a mg/m^2 basis). There are, however, no adequate and well-controlled studies in pregnant women. Because animal reproduction studies are not always predictive of human response, loratadine should be used during pregnancy only if clearly needed.

NURSING MOTHERS

Loratadine and its metabolite, descarboethoxyloratadine, pass easily into breast milk and achieve concentrations that are equivalent to plasma levels with an AUC_{milk}/AUC_{plasma} ratio of 1.17 and 0.85 for loratadine and descarboethoxyloratadine, respectively. Following a single oral dose of 40 mg, a small amount of loratadine and descarboethoxyloratadine was excreted into the breast milk (approximately 0.03% of 40 mg over 48 hours). A decision should be made whether to discontinue nursing or to discontinue the drug, taking into account the importance of the drug to the mother. Caution should be exercised when loratadine is administered to a nursing woman.

PEDIATRIC USE

The safety of loratadine syrup at a daily dose of 10 mg has been demonstrated in 188 pediatric patients 6-12 years of age in placebo-controlled 2 week trials. The effectiveness of loratadine for the treatment of seasonal allergic rhinitis and chronic idiopathic urticaria in this pediatric age group is based on an extrapolation of the demonstrated efficacy of loratadine in adults in these conditions and the likelihood that the disease course, pathophysiology, and the drug's effect are substantially similar to that of the adults. The recommended dose for the pediatric population is based on cross-study comparison of the pharmacokinetics of loratadine in adults and pediatric subjects and on the safety profile of loratadine in both adults and pediatric patients at doses equal to or higher than the recommended doses. The safety and effectiveness of loratadine in pediatric patients under 6 years of age have not been established.

DRUG INTERACTIONS

Loratadine (10 mg once daily) has been coadministered with therapeutic doses of erythromycin, cimetidine, and ketoconazole in controlled clinical pharmacology studies in adult volunteers. Although increased plasma concentrations (AUC 0-24 hrs) of loratadine and/or descarboethoxyloratadine were observed following coadministration of loratadine with each of these drugs in normal volunteers (n=24 in each study), there were no clinically relevant changes in the safety profile of loratadine, as assessed by electrocardiographic parameters, clinical laboratory tests, vital signs, and adverse events. There were no significant effects on QT_c intervals, and no reports of sedation or syncope. No effects on plasma concentrations of cimetidine or ketoconazole were observed. Plasma concentrations (AUC 0-24 hrs) of erythromycin decreased 15% with coadministration of loratadine relative to that observed with erythromycin alone. The clinical relevance of this difference is unknown. These above findings are summarized in TABLE 1.

L

TABLE 1 *Effects on Plasma Concentrations (AUC 0-24 hrs) of Loratadine and Descarboethoxyloratadine After 10 Days of Coadministration (Loratadine 10 mg) in Normal Volunteers*

	Loratadine	Descarboethoxyloratadine
Erythromycin (500 mg q8h)	+ 40%	+46%
Cimetidine (300 mg qid)	+103%	+ 6%
Ketoconazole (200 mg q12h)	+307%	+73%

There does not appear to be an increase in adverse events in subjects who received oral contraceptives and loratadine.

ADVERSE REACTIONS

LORATADINE TABLETS

Approximately 90,000 patients, aged 12 and older, received loratadine tablets 10 mg once daily in controlled and uncontrolled studies. Placebo-controlled clinical trials at the recommended dose of 10 mg once a day varied from 2 weeks' to 6 months' duration. The rate of premature withdrawal from these trials was approximately 2% in both the treated and placebo groups.

TABLE 2 *Reported Adverse Events With an Incidence of More Than 2% in Placebo-Controlled Allergic Rhinitis Clinical Trials in Patients 12 Years of Age and Older — Percent of Patients Reporting*

	Loratadine 10 mg qd n=1926	Placebo n=2545	Clemastine 1 mg bid n=536	Terfenadine 60 mg bid n=684
Headache	12%	11%	8%	8%
Somnolence	8%	6%	22%	9%
Fatigue	4%	3%	10%	2%
Dry mouth	3%	2%	4%	3%

Adverse events reported in placebo-controlled chronic idiopathic urticaria trials were similar to those reported in allergic rhinitis studies.

Adverse event rates did not appear to differ significantly based on age, sex, or race, although the number of nonwhite subjects was relatively small.

LORATADINE RAPIDLY-DISINTEGRATING TABLETS

Approximately 500 patients received loratadine rapidly-disintegrating tablets in controlled clinical trials of 2 weeks' duration. In these studies, adverse events were similar in type and frequency to those seen with loratadine tablets and placebo.

Administration of loratadine rapidly-disintegrating tablets did not result in an increased reporting frequency of mouth or tongue irritation.

LORATADINE SYRUP

Approximately 300 pediatric patients 6-12 years of age received 10 mg loratadine once daily in controlled clinical trials for a period of 8-15 days. Among these, 188 children were treated with 10 mg loratadine syrup once daily in placebo-controlled trials. Adverse events in these pediatric patients were observed to occur with type and frequency similar to those seen in the adult population. The rate of premature discontinuance due to adverse events among pediatric patients receiving loratadine 10 mg daily was less than 1%.

TABLE 3 *Adverse Events Occurring with a Frequency of ≥2% in Loratadine Syrup-Treated Patients (6-12 years old) in Placebo-Controlled Trials, and More Frequently Than in the Placebo Group — Percent of Patients Reporting*

	Loratadine 10 mg qd n=188	Placebo n=262	Chlorpheniramine 2-4 mg bid/tid n=170
Nervousness	4%	2%	2%
Wheezing	4%	2%	5%
Fatigue	3%	2%	5%
Hyperkinesia	3%	1%	1%
Abdominal pain	2%	0%	0%
Conjunctivitis	2%	<1%	1%
Dysphonia	2%	<1%	0%
Malaise	2%	0%	1%
Upper respiratory tract infection	2%	<1%	0%

In addition to those adverse events reported above (≥2%), the following adverse events have been reported in at least one patient in loratadine clinical trials in adult and pediatric patients.

Autonomic Nervous System: Altered lacrimation, altered salivation, flushing, hypoesthesia, impotence, increased sweating, thirst.

Body as a Whole: Angioneurotic edema, asthenia, back pain, blurred vision, chest pain, earache, eye pain, fever, leg cramps, malaise, rigors, tinnitus, viral infection, weight gain.

Cardiovascular System: Hypertension, hypotension, palpitations, supraventricular tachyarrhythmias, syncope, tachycardia.

Central and Peripheral Nervous System: Blepharospasm, dizziness, dysphonia, hypertonia, migraine, paresthesia, tremor, vertigo.

Gastrointestinal System: Altered taste, anorexia, constipation, diarrhea, dyspepsia, flatulence, gastritis, hiccup, increased appetite, nausea, stomatitis, toothache, vomiting.

Musculoskeletal System: Arthralgia, myalgia.

Psychiatric: Agitation, amnesia, anxiety, confusion, decreased libido, depression, impaired concentration, insomnia, irritability, paroniria.

Reproductive System: Breast pain, dysmenorrhea, menorrhagia, vaginitis.

Respiratory System: Bronchitis, bronchospasm, coughing, dyspnea, epistaxis, hemoptysis, laryngitis, nasal dryness, pharyngitis, sinusitis, sneezing.

Skin and Appendages: Dermatitis, dry hair, dry skin, photosensitivity reaction, pruritus, purpura, rash, urticaria.

Urinary System: Altered micturition, urinary discoloration, urinary incontinence, urinary retention.

In addition, the following spontaneous adverse events have been reported rarely during the marketing of loratadine: abnormal hepatic function, including jaundice, hepatitis, and hepatic necrosis; alopecia; anaphylaxis; breast enlargement; erythema multiforme; peripheral edema; and seizures.

DOSAGE AND ADMINISTRATION

Adults and Children 12 Years of Age and Over: The recommended dose of loratadine is 10 mg once daily.

Children 6-11 Years of Age: The recommended dose of loratadine is 10 mg (2 teaspoonsful) once daily.

Patients With Liver Failure or Renal Insufficiency (GFR <30 ml/min): One tablet or two teaspoonsful every other day should be the starting dose.

Administration of Loratadine Rapidly-Disintegrating Tablets: Place loratadine rapidly-disintegrating tablets on the tongue. Tablet disintegration occurs rapidly. Administer with or without water.

HOW SUPPLIED

CLARITIN TABLETS

10 mg: White to off-white compressed tablets; impressed with the product identification number "458" on one side and "CLARITIN 10" on the other.

Protect Unit-of-Use packaging and Unit Dose-Hospital Pack from excessive moisture.

Storage: Store between 2-30°C (36-86°F).

CLARITIN SYRUP

Clear, colorless to light-yellow liquid, containing 1 mg loratadine per ml; amber glass bottles of 16 fluid ounces.

Storage: Store between 2-25°C (36-77°F).

CLARITIN REDITABS

10 mg: White to off-white blister-formed tablets.

Keep Claritin Reditabs in a dry place.

Storage: Store between 2-25°C (36-77°F). Use within 6 months of opening laminated foil pouch, and immediately upon opening individual tablet blister.

L

Loratadine; Pseudoephedrine Sulfate

(003236)

For complete prescribing information, refer to the CD-ROM included with the book.

Categories: Rhinitis, seasonal allergic; Pregnancy Category B; FDA Approved 1994 Nov

Drug Classes: Antihistamines, H1; Decongestants, nasal

Brand Names: Claritin-D

Foreign Brand Availability: Airet (Colombia); Alergicol LP (Peru); Bonalerg - D (Guatemala); Chlor-Tripolon N.D. (Canada); Claratyne Cold (New-Zealand); Claratyne Decongestant (New-Zealand); Clarinase (Bahrain; Costa-Rica; Cyprus; Dominican-Republic; Egypt; El-Salvador; Guatemala; Honduras; Hong-Kong; Indonesia; Iran; Iraq; Israel; Jordan; Korea; Kuwait; Lebanon; Libya; Malaysia; Nicaragua; Oman; Panama; Philippines; Qatar; Republic-of-Yemen; Saudi-Arabia; Syria; Taiwan; Thailand; United-Arab-Emirates); Clarinase Repetabs (China); Clarinase 24 Hour Relief (Australia; New-Zealand); Clarityne-D (Greece); Clarityne D 24H (Mexico); Clarityne D Pediatrico (Mexico); Clarityne D Repetabs (Colombia; Ecuador; Mexico; Peru); Claritin Extra (Canada); Lertamine - D (Mexico); Loracert P (Colombia); Loratyne D (South-Africa); Polaratyne - D (South-Africa); Proacan D (Peru); Rhinase (Philippines); Rhinos SR (Indonesia); Rinomex (Peru); Sensibit D (Mexico); Sinease Repetab (Australia); Sinhistan D (Costa-Rica; Dominican-Republic; El-Salvador; Guatemala; Honduras; Nicaragua; Panama); Talorat D (Costa-Rica; Dominican-Republic; El-Salvador; Guatemala; Honduras; Nicaragua; Panama)

Cost of Therapy: $109.16 (Allergic Rhinitis; Claritin-D; 5 mg; 120 mg; 2 tablets/day; 30 day supply)
$109.15 (Allergic Rhinitis; Claritin-D 24 Hour; 10 mg; 240 mg; 1 tablet/day; 30 day supply)

DESCRIPTION

Loratadine is a long-acting antihistamine having the empirical formula $C_{22}H_{23}ClN_2O_2$; the chemical name ethyl 4-(8-chloro-5,6-dihydro-11*H*-benzo[5,6]cyclohepta[1,2-*b*]pyridin-11-ylidene)-1-piperidinecarboxylate.

The molecular weight of loratadine is 382.89. It is a white to off-white powder, not soluble in water, but very soluble in acetone, alcohol, and chloroform.

Pseudoephedrine sulfate is the synthetic salt of one of the naturally occurring dextrorotatory diastereomers of ephedrine and is classified as an indirect sympathomimetic amine. The empirical formula for pseudoephedrine sulfate is $(C_{10}H_{15}NO)_2 \cdot H_2SO_4$; the chemical name is α-[1-(methyl-amino) ethyl]-[*S*-(*R**,*R**)]-benzenemethanol sulfate (2:1)(salt).

The molecular weight of pseudoephedrine sulfate is 428.54. It is a white powder, freely soluble in water and methanol and sparingly soluble in chloroform.

CLARITIN-D 12 HOUR EXTENDED RELEASE TABLETS

Claritin-D 12 hour extended release tablets contain 5 mg loratadine in the tablet coating for immediate release and 120 mg pseudoephedrine sulfate equally distributed between the tablet coating for immediate release and the barrier-coated extended release core.

The inactive ingredients are acacia, butylparaben, calcium sulfate, carnauba wax, corn starch, lactose, magnesium stearate, microcrystalline cellulose, neutral soap, oleic acid, povidone, rosin, sugar, talc, titanium dioxide, white wax, and zein.

CLARITIN-D 24 HOUR EXTENDED RELEASE TABLETS

Claritin-D 24 hour extended release tablets contain 10 mg loratadine in the tablet film coating for immediate release and 240 mg pseudoephedrine sulfate in the tablet core which is released slowly allowing for once-daily administration.

The inactive ingredients for oval, biconvex Claritin-D 24 hour extended release tablets are calcium phosphate, carnauba wax, ethylcellulose, hydroxypropyl methylcellulose, magnesium stearate, polyethylene glycol, povidone, silicon dioxide, sugar, titanium dioxide, and white wax.

INDICATIONS AND USAGE

Loratadine; pseudoephedrine sulfate extended release tablets are indicated for the relief of symptoms of seasonal allergic rhinitis. Loratadine; pseudoephedrine sulfate extended release tablets should be administered when both the antihistaminic properties of loratadine and the nasal decongestant activity of pseudoephedrine are desired.

CONTRAINDICATIONS

Loratadine; pseudoephedrine sulfate extended release tablets are contraindicated in patients who are hypersensitive to this medication or to any of its ingredients.

This product, due to its pseudoephedrine component, is contraindicated in patients with narrow-angle glaucoma or urinary retention, and in patients receiving monoamine oxidase (MAO) inhibitor therapy or within 14 days of stopping such treatment. It is also contraindicated in patients with severe hypertension, severe coronary artery disease, and in those who have shown hypersensitivity or idiosyncrasy to its components, to adrenergic agents, or to other drugs of similar chemical structures. Manifestations of patient idiosyncrasy to adrenergic agents include: insomnia, dizziness, weakness, tremor, or arrhythmias.

WARNINGS

Loratadine; pseudoephedrine sulfate extended release tablets should be used with caution in patients with hypertension, diabetes mellitus, ischemic heart disease, increased intraocular pressure, hyperthyroidism, renal impairment, or prostatic hypertrophy. Central nervous system stimulation with convulsions or cardiovascular collapse with accompanying hypotension may be produced by sympathomimetic amines.

USE IN PATIENTS APPROXIMATELY 60 YEARS OF AGE AND OLDER

The safety and efficacy of loratadine; pseudoephedrine sulfate extended release tablets in patients greater than 60 years old have not been investigated in placebo-controlled clinical trials. The elderly are more likely to have adverse reactions to sympathomimetic amines.

DOSAGE AND ADMINISTRATION

ADULTS AND CHILDREN 12 YEARS OF AGE AND OVER

12 Hour Tablet: One tablet twice a day (every 12 hours); *24 Hour Tablet:* One tablet daily taken with a full glass of water. Because the doses of this fixed combination product cannot be individually titrated and hepatic insufficiency results in a reduced clearance of loratadine to a much greater extent than pseudoephedrine, loratadine; pseudoephedrine sulfate extended release tablets should generally be avoided in patients with hepatic insufficiency. Patients with renal insufficiency (GFR <30 ml/min) should be given a lower initial dose (one 12 hour tablet per day, or one 24 hour tablet every other day) because they have reduced clearance of loratadine and pseudoephedrine. Patients who have a history of difficulty in swallowing tablets or who have known upper gastrointestinal narrowing or abnormal esophageal peristalsis should not use the 24 hour tablet.

PRODUCT LISTING - EQUIVALENTS NOT AVAILABLE

Tablet, Extended Release - Oral - 5 mg;120 mg

20's $36.13 GENERIC, Pharma Pac 52959-0443-20

Lorazepam (001662)

Categories: Preanesthesia; Anxiety disorder, generalized; DEA Class CIV; FDA Approved 1977 Sep; Pregnancy Category D

Drug Classes: Anxiolytics; Benzodiazepines

Brand Names: **Ativan**

Foreign Brand Availability: Anxiedin (Taiwan); Anxira (Thailand); Anzepam (Taiwan); Aplacasse (Argentina); Apo-Lorazepam (Canada); Aripax (Greece); Azurogen (Japan); Bonatranquan (Germany); Control (Italy); Duralozam (Germany); Efasedan (Argentina); Emotion (Argentina); Emotival (Argentina); Kalmalin (Argentina); Larpose (India); Laubeel (Germany); Lonza (Thailand); Lopam (Taiwan); Lorabenz (Denmark); Loram (Slovenia); Lorans (Bahrain; Cyprus; Egypt; Hong-Kong; Iran; Iraq; Italy; Jordan; Kuwait; Lebanon; Libya; Oman; Qatar; Republic-of-Yemen; Saudi-Arabia; Syria; United-Arab-Emirates); Lorapam (New-Zealand; Thailand); Loravan (Korea); Lorax (Brazil); Lorazene (Thailand); Lorazep (Thailand); Lorazepam (Costa-Rica; Dominican-Republic; El-Salvador; Guatemala; Honduras; Nicaragua; Panama); Lorazin (Taiwan); Lorazon (Taiwan); Lorenin (Portugal); Loridem (Belgium); Lorivan (Hong-Kong; Israel); Lorsedal (Portugal); Lorzem (New-Zealand); Merlit (Austria; Russia); Nervistop L (Argentina); NIC (Argentina); Novhepar (Greece); Novo-lorazem (Canada); Orfidal (Spain); Punktyl (Germany); Renaquil (Indonesia); Rocosgen (Japan); Sedatival (Argentina); Sidenar (Argentina); Silence (Taiwan); Sinestron (Dominican-Republic; El-Salvador; Guatemala; Honduras; Nicaragua); Stapam (Taiwan); Tavor (Czech-Republic; Germany; Greece; Italy); Temesta (Austria; Belgium; Denmark; Finland; France; Netherlands; Sweden; Switzerland); Titus (Bahrain; Benin; Burkina-Faso; Cyprus; Egypt; Ethiopia; Gambia; Ghana; Greece; Guinea; Iran; Iraq; Israel; Ivory-Coast; Jordan; Kenya; Kuwait; Lebanon; Liberia; Libya; Malawi; Mali; Mauritania; Mauritius; Morocco; Niger; Nigeria; Oman; Qatar; Republic-of-Yemen; Saudi-Arabia; Senegal; Seychelles; Sierra-Leone; South-Africa; Sudan; Syria; Tanzania; Tunia; Uganda; United-Arab-Emirates; Zambia; Zimbabwe); Tranqipam (South-Africa); Trapax (Argentina); Trapex (India); Upan (Japan); Wypax (Japan)

Cost of Therapy: $70.25 (Anxiety; Ativan; 1 mg; 2 tablets/day; 30 day supply)
$2.48 (Anxiety; Generic Tablets; 1 mg; 2 tablets/day; 30 day supply)

HCFA JCODE(S): J2060 2 mg IM, IV

DESCRIPTION

Lorazepam, an antianxiety agent, has the chemical formula, 7-chloro-5-(*O*-chlorophenyl)-1,3-dihydro-3-hydroxy-2H-1,4-benzo-diazepin-2-one.

INJECTION

Lorazepam injection, a benzodiazepine with antianxiety and sedative effects, is intended for intramuscular or intravenous route of administration. Lorazepam is a nearly white powder almost insoluble in water. Each ml of sterile Ativan injection contains either 2.0 or 4.0 mg of lorazepam, 0.18 ml polyethylene glycol 400 in propylene glycol with 2.0% benzyl alcohol as preservative.

TABLETS

Lorazepam is a nearly white powder almost insoluble in water. Each Ativan tablet, to be taken orally, contains 0.5, 1, or 2 mg of lorazepam. The inactive ingredients present are lactose and other ingredients.

CLINICAL PHARMACOLOGY

INJECTION

Intravenous (IV) or intramuscular (IM) administration of the recommended dose of 2-4 mg of lorazepam injection to adult patients is followed by dose-related effects of sedation (sleepiness or drowsiness), relief of preoperative anxiety, and lack of recall of events related to the day of surgery in the majority of patients. The clinical sedation (sleepiness or drowsiness) thus noted is such that the majority of patients are able to respond to simple instructions whether they are give the appearance of being awake or asleep. The lack of recall is relative rather than absolute, as determined under conditions of careful patient questioning and testing, using props designed to enhance recall. The majority of events or recognizing props from before surgery. The lack of recall and recognition was optimum within 2 hours following IM administration and 15-20 minutes after IV injection.

The intended effects of the recommended adult dose of lorazepam injection usually last 6-8 hours. In rare instances and where patients received greater than the recommended dose, excessive sleepiness and prolonged lack of recall were noted. As with other benzodiazepines, unsteadiness, enhanced sensitivity to CNS-depressant effects of ethyl alcohol and other drugs were noted in isolated and rare cases for greater than 24 hours.

Studies in healthy adult volunteers reveal that IV lorazepam in doses up to 3.5 mg/70 kg does not alter sensitivity to the respiratory stimulating effect of carbon dioxide and does not enhance the respiratory depressant effects of doses of meperidine up to 100 mg/70 mg (also determined by carbon dioxide challenge) as long as patients remain sufficiently awake to undergo testing. Upper airway obstruction has been observed in rare instances where the patient received greater than the recommended dose and was excessively sleepy and difficult to arouse. (See WARNINGSand ADVERSE REACTIONS.)

Clinically employed doses or lorazepam injectable do not greatly affect the circulatory system in the supine position or employing a 70 degree tilt test. Doses of 8-10 mg of IV lorazepam (2 to 2.5 times the maximum recommended dosage) will produce loss of lid reflexes within 15 minutes.

Studies in 6 healthy young adults who lorazepam injection and no other drugs revealed that visual tracking (the ability to keep a moving line centered) was impaired for a mean of 8 hours following administration of 4 mg of IM lorazepam and 4 hours following administration of 2 mg intramuscularly with considerable subject variation. Similar findings were noted with pentobarbital, 150 mg and 75 mg. Although this study showed that both lorazepam and pentobarbital interfered with eye-hand coordination, the data are insufficient to predict when it would be safe to operate a motor vehicle or engage in a hazardous occupation or sport.

Pharmacokinetics

Injectable lorazepam is readily absorbed when given intramuscularly. Peak plasma concentrations occur approximately 60 to 90 minutes following administration and appear to be dose-related (*e.g.,* a 2.0 mg dose provides a level of approximately 20 ng/ml and a 4.0 mg dose approximately 40 ng/ml in plasma). The mean half-life or lorazepam is about 16 hours when given intravenously or intramuscularly. Lorazepam is rapidly conjugated at the 3-hydroxyl group into its major metabolite, lorazepam glucuronide, which is then excreted in the urine. Lorazepam glucuronide has no demonstrable CNS activity in animals. When 5 mg of IV lorazepam was administered to volunteers once a day for 4 consecutive days, a steady state of free lorazepam was achieved by the second day (approximately 52 ng/ml of plasma 3 hours after the first dose and approximately 62 ng/ml 3 hours after each subsequent dose, one day apart). At clinically relevant concentrations, lorazepam is bound 85% to plasma proteins.

TABLETS

Studies in healthy volunteers show that in single high doses lorazepam has a tranquilizing action on the central nervous system with no appreciable effect on the respiratory or cardiovascular systems.

Lorazepam is readily absorbed with an absolute bioavailability of 90%. Peak concentrations in plasma occur approximately 2 hours following administration. The peak plasma level of lorazepam from a 2 mg dose is approximately 20 ng/ml.

The mean half-life of unconjugated lorazepam in human plasma is about 12 hours and for its major metabolite, lorazepam glucuronide, about 18 hours. At clinically relevant concentrations, lorazepam is approximately 85% bound to plasma proteins. Lorazepam is rapidly conjugated at its 3-hydroxy group into lorazepam glucuronide which is then excreted in the urine. Lorazepam glucuronide has no demonstrable CNS activity in animals.

The plasma levels of lorazepam are proportional to the dose given. There is no evidence of accumulation of lorazepam on administration up to 6 months.

Studies comparing young and elderly subjects have shown that the pharmacokinetics of lorazepam remain unaltered with advancing age.

INDICATIONS AND USAGE

INJECTION

Lorazepam injection is indicated in adult patients for preanesthetic medication, producing sedation (sleepiness or drowsiness), relief of anxiety, and a decreased ability to recall events related to the day of surgery. It is most useful in those patients who are anxious about their surgical procedure and who would prefer to have diminished recall of the events of the day of surgery (see PRECAUTIONS, Information for the Patient).

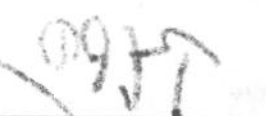

TABLETS

Lorazepam is indicated for the management of anxiety disorders or for the short-term relief of the symptoms of anxiety or anxiety associated with depressive symptoms. Anxiety or tension associated with the stress of everyday life usually does not require treatment with an anxiolytic.

The effectiveness of lorazepam in long-term use, that is, more than 4 months, has not been assessed by systematic clinical studies. The physician should periodically reassess the usefulness of the drug for the individual patient.

NON-FDA APPROVED INDICATIONS

Lorazepam has also been used for control of nausea and emesis, particularly during chemotherapy. However, this use is not approved by the FDA.

CONTRAINDICATIONS

INJECTION

Lorazepam injection is indicated in adult patients for preanesthetic medication, producing sedation (sleepiness or drowsiness), relief of anxiety, and a decreased ability to recall events related to the day of surgery. It is most useful in those patients who are anxious about their surgical procedure and who would prefer to have diminished recall of the day of surgery (PRECAUTIONS, Information for the Patient).

TABLETS

Lorazepam is contraindicated in patients with known sensitivity to the benzodiazepines or with acute narrow-angle glaucoma.

WARNINGS

INJECTION

PRIOR TO IV USE, ATIVAN INJECTION MUST BE DILUTED WITH AN EQUAL AMOUNT OF COMPATIBLE DILUENT (SEE DOSAGE AND ADMINISTRATION). IV INJECTION SHOULD BE MADE SLOWLY AND WITH REPEATED ASPIRATION. CARE SHOULD BE TAKEN TO DETERMINE THAT ANY INJECTION WILL NOT BE INTRAARTERIAL AND THAT PERIVASCULAR EXTRAVASATION WILL NOT TAKE PLACE.

PARTIAL AIRWAY OBSTRUCTION MAY OCCUR IN HEAVILY SEDATED PATIENTS. INTRAVENOUS LORAZEPAM, WHEN GIVEN ALONE IN GREATER THAN THE RECOMMENDED DOSE, OR AT THE RECOMMENDED DOSE AND ACCOMPANIED BY OTHER DRUGS USED DURING THE ADMINISTRATION OF ANESTHESIA, MAY PRODUCE HEAVY SEDATION; THEREFORE, EQUIPMENT NECESSARY TO MAINTAIN A PATENT AIRWAY AND TO SUPPORT RESPIRATION/VENTILATION SHOULD BE AVAILABLE.

There is no evidence to support the use of lorazepam injection in coma, shock or acute alcohol intoxication at this time. Since the liver os the most likely site of conjugation of lorazepam and since excretion of conjugated lorazepam (glucuronide) is a renal function, this drug is not recommended for use in patients with hepatic and/or renal failure. This does not preclude use of the drug in patients with mild-to-moderate hepatic or renal disease, the lowest effective dose should be considered since drug effect may be prolonged. Experience with other benzodiazepines and limited experience with parenteral lorazepam has demonstrated that tolerance to alcoholic beverages and other central nervous system depressants is diminished when used concomitantly.

As is true of similar CNS-acting drugs, patients receiving injectable lorazepam should not operate machinery or engage in hazardous occupations or drive a motor vehicle for a period of 24-48 hours. Impairment of performance may persist for greater intervals because of extremes of age, concomitant use of other drugs, stress of surgery, or the general condition of the patient.

Clinical trials have shown that patients over the age of 50 years may have a more profound and prolonged sedation with IV lorazepam. Ordinarily, an initial dose of 2 mg may be adequate unless a greater degree of lack of recall is desired.

As with all central nervous system depressant drugs, care should be exercised in patients given injectable lorazepam that premature ambulation may result in injury from falling.

There is no added beneficial effect to the addition of scopolamine to injectable lorazepam, and their combined effect may result in an increased incidence of sedation, hallucination, and irrational behavior.

Pregnancy

LORAZEPAM MAY CAUSE FETAL DAMAGE WHEN ADMINISTERED TO PREGNANT WOMEN. An increased risk of congenital malformations associated with the use of minor tranquilizers (chlordiazepoxide, diazepam, and meprobamate) during the first trimester of pregnancy has been suggested in several studies. In humans, blood levels obtained from umbilical cord blood indicate placental transfer of lorazepam and lorazepam glucuronide.

Lorazepam injection should not be used during pregnancy. There are insufficient date regarding obstetrical safety of parenteral lorazepam, including use in cesarean section. Such use, therefore,is not recommended.

Reproductive studies in animals were performed in mice, rats, and two strains of rabbits. Occasional anomalies (reduction of tarsals, tibia, metatarsals, malrotated limbs, gastroschisis, malformed skull, and microphthalmia) were seen in drug-related rabbits without relationship to dosage. Although all of these anomalies were not present in the concurrent control group, they have all been reported to occur randomly in historical controls. At doses of 40 mg/kg orally or 4 mg/kg intravenously and higher, there was evidence of fetal resorption and increased fetal loss in rabbits which was not seen at lower doses.

Endoscopic Procedures

The are insufficient data to support the use of lorazepam injection for outpatient endoscopic procedures. Inpatient endoscopic procedures require adequate recovery room observations.

Pharyngeal reflexes are not impaired when lorazepam injection is used for peroral endoscopic procedures; therefore, adequate topical or regional anesthesia is recommended to minimize reflex activity associated with such procedures.

TABLETS

Lorazepam is not recommended for use in patients with a primary depressive disorder or psychosis. As with all patients on CNS-acting drugs, patients receiving lorazepam should be warned not to operate dangerous machinery or motor vehicles and that their tolerance for alcohol and other CNS depressants will be diminished.

PRECAUTIONS

INJECTION

General

The additive central-nervous-system effects of other drugs, such as phenothiazines, narcotic analgesics, barbiturates, antidepressants, scopolamine, and monomine-oxidase inhibitors, should be borne in mind when these other drugs are used concomitantly with or during the period of recovery from lorazepam injection. (See CLINICAL PHARMACOLOGY and WARNINGS.)

Extreme care must be used in administering lorazepam injection to elderly patients, very ill patients, and to patients with limited pulmonary reserve because of the possibility that underventilation and/or hypoxic cardiac arrest may occur. Resuscitative equipment for ventilatory support should be readily available. (See WARNINGS and DOSAGE AND ADMINISTRATION.)

When lorazepam injection is used IV as the premedicant prior to regional or local anesthesia, the possibility of excessive sleepines or drowsiness may interfere with patient cooperation to determine levels of anesthesia. This is most likely to occur when greater than 0.05 mg/kg is given and when narcotic analgesics are used concomitantly with the recommended dose. (See ADVERSE REACTIONS.)

Information for the Patient

As appropriate, the patient should be informed of the pharmacologcal effects of the drug, such as sedation, relief of anxiety, and lack of recall, and the duration of these effects (about 8 hours), so that they may adequately perceive the risks as well as the benefits to be derived from its use.

Patients who receive lorazepam injection as a premedicant should be cautioned that driving an automobile or operating hazardous machinery, or engaging in a hazardous sport, should be delayed for 24-48 hours following the injection. Sedatives, tranquilizers, and narcotic analgesics may produce a more prolonged and profound effect when administered along with injectable lorazepam. This effect may take the form of excessive sleepiness or drowsiness and, on rare occasions, interfere with recall and recognition of events of the day of surgery and the day after.

Getting out of bed unassisted may result in falling and injury if undertaken within 8 hours of receiving lorazepam injection. Alcoholic beverages should not be consumed for at least 24-48 hours after receiving lorazepam injectable due to the additive effects on central-nervous-system depression seen with benzodiazepines in general. Elderly patients should be told that lorazepam injection may make them very sleepy for a period longer than 6 to 8 hours following surgery.

Laboratory Tests

In clinical trials no laboratory test abnormalities wre identified with either single or multiple doses of lorazepam injection. These tests included: CBC, urinalysis, SGOT, SGPT, bilirubin, alkaline phosphatase, LDH, cholesterol, uric acid, BUN, glucose, calcium, phosphorus, and total proteins.

Drug/Laboratory Test Interactions

No laboratory test abnormalities were identified when lorazepam was given alone or concomitantly with another drug, such as narcotic analgesics, inhalation anesthetics, scopolamine, atropine, and a variety of tranquilizing agents.

Carcinogenesis, Mutagenesis, and Impairment of Fertility

No evidence of carcinogenic potential emerged in rats and mice during an 18-month study with oral lorazepam. No studies regarding mutagenesis have been performed. Preimplantation study in rats was performed with oral lorazepam at a 20 mg/kg dose and showed no impairment of fertility.

Pregnancy Category D

See WARNINGS.

Labor and Delivery

There are insufficient data to support the use of lorazepam injection during labor and delivery, including cesarean section; therefore, its use in this situation is not recommended.

Nursing Mothers

Injectable lorazepam should not be administered to nursing mothers, because, like other benzodiazepines, the possibility exists that lorazepam may be excreted in human milk and sedate the infant.

Pediatric Use

There are insufficient data to support efficacy or make dosage recommendations for injectable lorazepam in patients less than 18 years of age; therefore, such use is not recommended.

TABLETS

In patients with depression accompanying anxiety, a possibility for suicide should be borne in mind.

For elderly or debilitated patients, the initial daily dosage should not exceed 2 mg in order to avoid oversedation.

Lorazepam dosage should be terminated gradually, since abrupt withdrawal of any anti-anxiety agent may result in symptoms similar to those for which patients are being treated: anxiety, agitation, irritability, tension, insomnia, and occasional convulsions.

The usual precautions for treating patients with impaired renal or hepatic function should be observed.

L

In patients where gastrointestinal or cardiovascular disorders coexist with anxiety, it should be noted that lorazepam has not been shown to be of significant benefit in treating the gastrointestinal or cardiovascular component.

Esophageal dilation occurred in rats treated with lorazepam for more than 1 year at 6 mg/kg/day. The no-effect dose was 1.25 mg/kg/day (approximately 6 times the maximum human therapeutic dose of 10 mg/day). The effect was reversible only when the treatment was withdrawn within 2 months of first observation of the phenomenon. The clinical significance of this is unknown. However, use of lorazepam for prolonged periods and in geriatric patients requires caution and there should be frequent monitoring for symptoms of upper GI disease.

Safety and effectiveness of lorazepam in children of less than 12 years have not been established.

Information for the Patient

To assure the safe and effective use of lorazepam patients should be informed that, since benzodiazepines may produce psychological and physical dependence, it is advisable that they consult with their physician before either increasing the dose or abruptly discontinuing this drug.

Essential Laboratory Tests

Some patients on lorazepam have developed leukopenia, and some have had elevations of LDH. As with other benzodiazepines, periodic blood counts and liver-function tests are recommended for patients on long-term therapy.

Carcinogenesis and Mutagenesis

No evidence of carcinogenic potential emerged in rats during an 18 month study with lorazepam. No studies regarding mutagenesis have been performed.

Pregnancy

Reproductive studies in animals were performed in mice, rats, and two strains of rabbits. Occasional anomalies (reduction of tarsals, tibia, metatarsals, malrotated limbs, gastroschisis, malformed skull, and microphthalmia) were seen in drug-treated rabbits without relationship to dosage. Although all of these anomalies were not present in the concurrent control group, they have been reported to occur randomly in historical controls. At doses of 40 mg/kg and higher, there was evidence of total resorption and increased fetal loss in rabbits which was not seen at lower doses.

The clinical significance of the above findings is not known. However, an increased risk of congenital malformations associated with the use of minor tranquilizers (chlordiazepoxide, diazepam, and meprobamate) during the first trimester of pregnancy has been suggested in several studies. Because the use of these drugs is rarely a matter of urgency, the use of lorazepam during this period should almost always be avoided. The possibility that a woman of childbearing potential may be pregnant at the time of institution of therapy should be considered. Patients should be advised that if they become pregnant, they should communicate with their physician about the desirability of discontinuing the drug.

In humans, blood levels obtained from umbilical cord blood indicate placental transfer of lorazepam and lorazepam glucuronide.

Nursing Mothers

It is not known whether oral lorazepam is excreted in human milk like the other benzodiazepine tranquilizers. As a general rule, nursing should not be undertaken while a patient is on a drug since many drugs are excreted in human milk.

DRUG INTERACTIONS

INJECTION

Lorazepam injection, like other injectable benzodiazepines, produces depression of the central nervous system when administered with ethyl alcohol, phenothiazines, barbiturates, MAO inhibitors, and other antidepressants.When scopolamine is used concomitantly with injectable lorazepam, an increased incidence of sedation, hallucinations, and irrational behavior has been observed.

TABLETS

The benzodiazepines, including lorazepam, produce CNS-depressant effects when administered with such medications as barbiturates or alcohol.

ADVERSE REACTIONS

INJECTION

Central Nervous System

The most frequent adverse effects seen with injectable lorazepam are an extension of the central-nervous-system depressant effects of the drug. The incidence varied from one study to another, depending on the dosage, route of administration, use of other central-nervous-system depressants, and the investigator's opinion concerning the degree and duration of desired sedation. Excessive sleepiness and drowsiness were the main side effects. This interfered with patient cooperation in approximately 6% (25/446) of patients undergoing regional blocks or with caudal anesthesia. Patients over 50 years of age had a higher incidence of excessive sleepiness or drowsiness when compared with those under 50 (21/106 vs 24/245) when lorazepam was given intravenously (see DOSAGE AND ADMINISTRATION). On rare occasion (3/1580) the patient was unable to give personal identification in the operating room on arrival, and 1 patient fell when attempting premature ambulation in the postoperative period.

Symptoms such as restlessness, confusion, depression, crying, sobbing, and delirium occurred in about 1.3% (20/1580). One (1) patient injured himself by picking at his incision during the immediate postoperative period.

Hallucinations were present in about 1% (14/1580) of patients and were visual and self-limiting.

An occasional patient complained of dizziness, diplopia, and/or blurred vision. Depressed hearing was infrequently reported during the peak-effect period.

An occasional patient had a prolonged recovery room stay, either because of excessive sleepiness or because of some form of inappropriate behavior. The latter was seen most commonly when scopolamine was given concomitantly as a premedicant.

Limited information derived from patients who were discharged the day after receiving injectable lorazepam showed 1 patient complained of some unsteadiness of gait and a reduced ability to perform complex mental functions. Enhanced sensitivity to alcoholic beverages has been reproted more than 24 hours after receiving injectable lorazepam, similar to experience with other benzodiazepines.

Local Effects

Intramuscular injection of lorazepam has resulted in pain at the injection site, a sensation of burning, or observed redness in the same area in a very variable incidence from one study to another. The overall incidence of pain and burning was about 17% (146/859) in the immediate postinjection period and about 1.4% (12/859) at the 24-hour observation time. Reaction at the injection site (redness) occurred in approximately 2% (17/859) in the immediate postinjection period and were present 24 hours later in about 0.8% (7/859).

Intravenous administration of lorazepam resulted in painful responses in 13/771 patients or approximately 1.6% in the immediate postinjection period, and 24 hours later 4/771 patients or about 0.5% still complained of pain. Redness did not occur immediately following IV injection but was noted in 19/771 patients at the 24-hour observation period. This incidence is similar to that observed with an IV infusion before lorazepam is given.

Cardiovascular System

Hypertension (0.1%) and hypotension (0.1%) have occasionally been observed after patients have received injectable lorazepam.

Respiratory System

Five patients (5/446) who underwent regional anesthesia were observed to have partial airway obstruction. This was believed due to excessive sleepiness at the time of the procedure and resulted in temporary underventilation. Immediate attention to the airway, employing the usual countermeasures, will usually suffice to manage this condition (see also CLINICAL PHARMACOLOGY, WARNINGS, and PRECAUTIONS).

Other Adverse Experiences

Skin rash, nausea, and vomiting have occasionally been noted in patients who have received injectable lorazepam combined with other drugs during anesthesia and surgery.

TABLETS

Adverse reactions, if they occur, are usually observed at the beginning of therapy and generally disappear on continued medication or upon decreasing the dose. In a sample of about 3500 anxious patients, the most frequent adverse reaction to lorazepam is sedation (15.9%), followed by dizziness (6.9%), weakness (4.2%), and unsteadiness (3.4%). Less frequent adverse reactions are disorientation, depression, nausea, change in appetite, headache, sleep disturbance, agitation, dermatological symptoms, eye-function disturbance, together with various gastrointestinal symptoms and autonomic manifestations. The incidence of sedation and unsteadiness increased with age.

Small decreases in blood pressure have been noted but are not clinically significant, probably being related to the relief of anxiety produced by lorazepam.

Transient amnesia or memory impairment has been reported in association with the use of benzodiazepines.

DOSAGE AND ADMINISTRATION

INJECTION

Intramuscular Injection

For the designated indications as a premedicant, the usual recommended dose of lorazepam for IM injection is 0.05 mg/kg up to a maximum of 4 mg. As with all premedicant drugs, the dose should be individualized. See also CLINICAL PHARMACOLOGY, and WARNINGS. Doses of other central nervous system depressant drugs should be ordinarily reduced. *For optimum effect, measured as lack of recall, IM lorazepam should be administered at least 2 hours before the anticipated operative procedure.* Narcotic analgesics should be administered at their usual preoperative time. There are insufficient data to support efficacy to make dosage recommendations for IM lorazepam in patients less than 18 years of age; therefore, such use is not recommended.

Intravenous Injection

For the primary purpose of sedation and relief of anxiety, the usual recommended initial dose of lorazepam for IV injection is 2 mg total, or 0.02 mg/lb (0.044 mg/kg), whichever is smaller. This dose will suffice for sedating most adult patients and should not ordinarily be exceeded in patients over 50 years of age. In those patients in whom a greater likelihood of lack of recall for perioperative events would be beneficial, larger doses as high as 0.05 mg/kg up to a total of 4 mg may be administered. (See CLINICAL PHARMACOLOGY and WARNINGS). Doses of other injectable central nervous system depressant drugs should ordinarily be reduced (see PRECAUTIONS). *For optimum effect, measured as lack of recall, IV lorazepam should be administered 15 to 20 minutes before the anticipated operative procedure.*

EQUIPMENT NECESSARY TO MAINTAIN A PATENT AIRWAY SHOULD BE IMMEDIATELY AVAILABLE PRIOR TO INTRAVENOUS ADMINISTRATION OF LORAZEPAM (see WARNINGS).

There are insufficient data to support efficacy or make dosage recommendations for IV lorazepam in patients less than 18 years of age; therefore, such use is not recommended.

Administration

When given intramuscularly, lorazepam injection, undiluted, should be injected deep in the muscle mass.

Injectable lorazepam can be used with atropine sulfate, narcotic analgesics, other parenterally used analgesics, commonly used anesthetics, and muscle relaxants.

Cozaar 25, 50 and 100 mg tablets contain potassium in the following amounts: 2.12 mg (0.054 mEq), 4.24 mg (0.108 mEq) and 8.48 mg (0.216 mEq), respectively.

CLINICAL PHARMACOLOGY

MECHANISM OF ACTION

Angiotensin II [formed from angiotensin I in a reaction catalyzed by angiotensin converting enzyme (ACE, kininase II)], is a potent vasoconstrictor, the primary vasoactive hormone of the renin-angiotensin system and an important component in the pathophysiology of hypertension. It also stimulates aldosterone secretion by the adrenal cortex. Losartan and its principal active metabolite block the vasoconstrictor and aldosterone-secreting effects of angiotensin II by selectively blocking the binding of angiotensin II to the AT_1 receptor found in many tissues, (*e.g.*, vascular smooth muscle, adrenal gland). There is also an AT_2 receptor found in many tissues but it is not known to be associated with cardiovascular homeostasis. Both losartan and its principal active metabolite do not exhibit any partial agonist activity at the AT_1 receptor and have much greater affinity (about 1000-fold) for the AT_1 receptor than for the AT_2 receptor. *In vitro* binding studies indicate that losartan is a reversible, competitive inhibitor of the AT_1 receptor. The active metabolite is 10-40 times more potent by weight than losartan and appears to be a reversible, non-competitive inhibitor of the AT_1 receptor.

Neither losartan nor its active metabolite inhibits ACE (kininase II, the enzyme that converts angiotensin I to angiotensin II and degrades bradykinin); nor do they bind to or block other hormone receptors or ion channels known to be important in cardiovascular regulation.

PHARMACOKINETICS

General

Losartan is an orally active agent that undergoes substantial first-pass metabolism by cytochrome P450 enzymes. It is converted, in part, to an active carboxylic acid metabolite that is responsible for most of the angiotensin II receptor antagonism that follows losartan treatment. The terminal half-life of losartan is about 2 hours and of the metabolite is about 6-9 hours. The pharmacokinetics of losartan and its active metabolite are linear with oral losartan doses up to 200 mg and do not change over time. Neither losartan nor its metabolite accumulate in plasma upon repeated once-daily dosing.

Following oral administration, losartan is well absorbed (based on absorption of radiolabeled losartan) and undergoes substantial first-pass metabolism; the systemic bioavailability of losartan is approximately 33%. About 14% of an orally-administered dose of losartan is converted to the active metabolite. Mean peak concentrations of losartan and its active metabolite are reached in 1 hour and in 3-4 hours, respectively. While maximum plasma concentrations of losartan and its active metabolite are approximately equal, the AUC of the metabolite is about 4 times as great as that of losartan. A meal slows absorption of losartan and decreases its C_{max} but has only minor effects on losartan AUC or on the AUC of the metabolite (about 10% decreased).

Both losartan and its active metabolite are highly bound to plasma proteins, primarily albumin, with plasma free fractions of 1.3% and 0.2%, respectively. Plasma protein binding is constant over the concentration range achieved with recommended doses. Studies in rats indicate that losartan crosses the blood-brain barrier poorly, if at all.

Losartan metabolites have been identified in human plasma and urine. In addition to the active carboxylic acid metabolite, several inactive metabolites are formed. Following oral and intravenous (IV) administration of ^{14}C-labeled losartan potassium, circulating plasma radioactivity is primarily attributed to losartan and its active metabolite. *In vitro* studies indicate that cytochrome P450 2C9 and 3A4 are involved in the biotransformation of losartan to its metabolites. Minimal conversion of losartan to the active metabolite (less than 1% of the dose compared to 14% of the dose in normal subjects) was seen in about 1% of individuals studied.

The volume of distribution of losartan is about 34 L and of the active metabolite is about 12 L. Total plasma clearance of losartan and the active metabolite is about 600 ml/min and 50 ml/min, respectively, with renal clearance of about 75 ml/min and 25 ml/min, respectively. When losartan is administered orally, about 4% of the dose is excreted unchanged in the urine and about 6% is excreted in urine as active metabolite. Biliary excretion contributes to the elimination of losartan and its metabolites. Following oral ^{14}C-labeled losartan, about 35% of radioactivity is recovered in the urine and about 60% in the feces. Following an IV dose of ^{14}C-labeled losartan, about 45% of radioactivity is recovered in the urine and 50% in the feces.

SPECIAL POPULATIONS

Pediatric

Losartan pharmacokinetics have not been investigated in patients <18 years of age.

Geriatric and Gender

Losartan pharmacokinetics have been investigated in the elderly (65-75 years) and in both genders. Plasma concentrations of losartan and its active metabolite are similar in elderly and young hypertensives. Plasma concentrations of losartan were about twice as high in female hypertensives as male hypertensives, but concentrations of the active metabolite were similar in males and females. No dosage adjustment is necessary (see DOSAGE AND ADMINISTRATION).

Race

Pharmacokinetic differences due to race have not been studied.

Renal Insufficiency

Plasma concentrations of losartan are not altered in patients with creatinine clearance above 30 ml/min. In patients with lower creatinine clearance, AUCs are about 50% greater and they are doubled in hemodialysis patients. Plasma concentrations of the active metabolite are not significantly altered in patients with renal impairment or in hemodialysis patients. Neither losartan nor its active metabolite can be removed by hemodialysis. No dosage adjustment is necessary for patients with renal impairment unless they are volume-depleted (see WARNINGS, Hypotension — Volume-Depleted Patients and DOSAGE AND ADMINISTRATION).

Hepatic Insufficiency

Following oral administration in patients with mild to moderate alcoholic cirrhosis of the liver, plasma concentrations of losartan and its active metabolite were, respectively, 5 times and about 1.7 times those in young male volunteers. Compared to normal subjects the total plasma clearance of losartan in patients with hepatic insufficiency was about 50% lower and the oral bioavailability was about 2 times higher. A lower starting dose is recommended for patients with a history of hepatic impairment (see DOSAGE AND ADMINISTRATION).

DRUG INTERACTIONS

Losartan, administered for 12 days, did not affect the pharmacokinetics or pharmacodynamics of a single dose of warfarin. Losartan did not affect the pharmacokinetics of oral or IV digoxin. Coadministration of losartan and cimetidine led to an increase of about 18% in AUC of losartan but did not affect the pharmacokinetics of its active metabolite. Coadministraion of losartan and phenobarbital led to a reduction of about 20% in the AUC of losartan and that of its active metabolite. Conversion of losartan to its active metabolite after IV administration is not affected by ketoconazole, an inhibitor of P450 3A4. There is no pharmacokinetic interaction between losartan and hydrochlorothiazide.

PHARMACODYNAMICS AND CLINICAL EFFECTS

Hypertension

Losartan inhibits the pressor effect of angiotensin II (as well as angiotensin I) infusions. A dose of 100 mg inhibits the pressor effect by about 85% at peak with 25-40% inhibition persisting for 24 hours. Removal of the negative feedback of angiotensin II causes a 2- to 3-fold rise in plasma renin activity and consequent rise in angiotensin II plasma concentration in hypertensive patients. Losartan does not affect the response to bradykinin, whereas ACE inhibitors increase the response to bradykinin. Aldosterone plasma concentrations fall following losartan administration. In spite of the effect of losartan on aldosterone secretion, very little effect on serum potassium was observed.

In a single-dose study in normal volunteers, losartan had no effects on glomerular filtration rate, renal plasma flow or filtration fraction. In multiple dose studies in hypertensive patients, there were no notable effects on systemic or renal prostaglandin concentrations, fasting triglycerides, total cholesterol or HDL-cholesterol or fasting glucose concentrations. There was a small uricosuric effect leading to a minimal decrease in serum uric acid (mean decrease <0.4 mg/dl) during chronic oral administration.

The antihypertensive effects of losartan potassium were demonstrated principally in 4 placebo-controlled 6-12 week trials of dosages from 10-150 mg/day in patients with baseline diastolic blood pressures of 95-115. The studies allowed comparisons of 2 doses (50-100 mg/day) as once-daily or twice-daily regimens, comparisons of peak and trough effects, and comparisons of response by gender, age, and race. Three additional studies examined the antihypertensive effects of losartan and hydrochlorothiazide in combination.

The 4 studies of losartan monotherapy included a total of 1075 patients randomized to several doses of losartan and 334 to placebo. The 10 and 25 mg doses produced some effect at peak (6 hours after dosing) but small and inconsistent trough (24 hour) responses. Doses of 50, 100 and 150 mg once daily gave statistically significant systolic/diastolic mean decreases in blood pressure, compared to placebo in the range of 5.5-10.5/3.5-7.5 mm Hg, with the 150 mg dose giving no greater effect than 50-100 mg. Twice-daily dosing at 50-100 mg/day gave consistently larger trough responses than once-daily dosing at the same total dose. Peak (6 hour) effects were uniformly, but moderately, larger than trough effects, with the trough-to-peak ratio for systolic and diastolic responses 50-95% and 60-90%, respectively.

Addition of a low dose of hydrochlorothiazide (12.5 mg) to losartan 50 mg once daily resulted in placebo-adjusted blood pressure reductions of 15.5/9.2 mm Hg.

Analysis of age, gender, and race subgroups of patients showed that men and women, and patients over and under 65, had generally similar responses. Losartan potassium was effective in reducing blood pressure regardless of race, although the effect was somewhat less in black patients (usually a low-renin population).

The effect of losartan is substantially present within 1 week but in some studies the maximal effect occurred in 3-6 weeks. In long-term follow-up studies (without placebo control) the effect of losartan appeared to be maintained for up to a year. There is no apparent rebound effect after abrupt withdrawal of losartan. There was essentially no change in average heart rate in losartan-treated patients in controlled trials.

Nephropathy in Type 2 Diabetic Patients

The Reduction of Endpoints in NIDDM with the Angiotensin II Receptor Antagonist Losartan (RENAAL) study was a randomized, placebo-controlled, double-blind, multicenter study conducted worldwide in 1513 patients with type 2 diabetes with nephropathy (defined as serum creatinine 1.3-3.0 mg/dl in females or males ≤60 kg and 1.5-3.0 mg/dl in males >60 kg and proteinuria [urinary albumin to creatinine ratio ≥300 mg/g]).

Patients were randomized to receive losartan potassium 50 mg once daily or placebo on a background of conventional antihypertensive therapy excluding ACE inhibitors and angiotensin II antagonists. After 1 month, investigators were instructed to titrate study drug to 100 mg once daily if the trough blood pressure goal (140/90 mm Hg) was not achieved. Overall, 72% of patients received the 100 mg daily dose more than 50% of the time they were on study drug. Because the study was designed to achieve equal blood pressure control in both groups, other antihypertensive agents (diuretics, calcium-channel blockers, alpha- or beta-blockers, and centrally acting agents) could be added as needed in both groups. Patients were followed for a mean duration of 3.4 years.

The study population was diverse with regard to race (Asian 16.7%, Black 15.2%, Hispanic 18.3%, White 48.6%). Overall, 63.2% of the patients were men, and 66.4% were under the age of 65 years. Almost all of the patients (96.6%) had a history of hypertension, and the patients entered the trial with a mean serum creatinine of 1.9 mg/dl and mean proteinuria (urinary albumin/creatinine) of 1808 mg/g at baseline.

The primary endpoint of the study was the time to first occurrence of any one of the following events: doubling of serum creatinine, end-stage renal disease (need for dialysis or transplantation), or death. Treatment with losartan potassium resulted in a 16% risk reduction in this endpoint (see TABLE 1). Treatment with losartan potassium also reduced the occurrence of sustained doubling of serum creatinine by 25% and ESRD by 29% as separate endpoints, but had no effect on overall mortality (see TABLE 1).

L

The mean baseline blood pressures were 152/82 mm Hg for losartan potassium plus conventional antihypertensive therapy and 153/82 mm Hg for placebo plus conventional antihypertensive therapy. At the end of the study, the mean blood pressures were 143/76 mm Hg for the group treated with losartan potassium and 146/77 mm Hg for the group treated with placebo.

TABLE 1 *Incidence of Primary Endpoint Events*

	Incidence				
	Losartan	Placebo	Risk Reduction	95% CI	p-Value
Primary composite endpoint	43.5%	47.1%	16.1%	2.3%-27.9%	0.022
Doubling of Serum Creatinine, ESRD and Death Occurring as a First Event					
Doubling of serum creatinine	21.6%	26.0%	-	-	-
ESRD	8.5%	8.5%	-	-	-
Death	13.4%	12.6%	-	-	-
Overall Incidence of Doubling of Serum Creatinine, ESRD and Death					
Doubling of serum creatinine	21.6%	26.0%	25.3%	7.8%-39.4%	0.006
ESRD	19.6%	25.5%	28.6%	11.5%-42.4%	0.002
Death	21.0%	20.3%	-1.7%	-26.9% to 18.6%	0.884

The secondary endpoints of the study were change in proteinuria, change in the rate of progression of renal disease, and the composite of morbidity and mortality from cardiovascular causes (hospitalization for heart failure, myocardial infarction, revascularization, stroke, hospitalization for unstable angina, or cardiovascular death). Compared with placebo, losartan potassium significantly reduced proteinuria by an average of 34%, an effect that was evident within 3 months of starting therapy, and significantly reduced the rate of decline in glomerular filtration rate during the study by 13%, as measured by the reciprocal of the serum creatinine concentration. There was no significant difference in the incidence of the composite endpoint of cardiovascular morbidity and mortality.

The favorable effects of losartan potassium were seen in patients also taking other antihypertensive medications (angiotensin II receptor antagonists and angiotensin converting enzyme inhibitors were not allowed), oral hypoglycemic agents and lipid-lowering agents.

For the primary endpoint and ESRD, the effects of losartan potassium in patient subgroups defined by age, gender and race are shown in TABLE 2A and TABLE 2B. Subgroup analyses can be difficult to interpret and it is not known whether these represent true differences or chance effects.

TABLE 2A *Efficacy Outcomes Within Demographic Subgroups*

		Primary Composite Endpoint		
	n	Losartan Potassium Event Rate	Placebo Event rate	Hazard Ratio (95% CI)
Overall Results	1513	43.5%	47.1%	0.839 (0.721, 0.977)
Age				
<65 years	1005	44.1%	49.0%	0.784 (0.653, 0.941)
≥65 years	508	42.3%	43.5%	0.978 (0.749, 1.277)
Gender				
Female	557	47.8%	54.1%	0.762 (0.603, 0.962)
Male	956	40.9%	43.3%	0.892 (0.733, 1.085)
Race				
Asian	252	41.9%	54.8%	0.655 (0.453, 0.947)
Black	230	40.0%	39.0%	0.983 (0.647, 1.495)
Hispanic	277	55.0%	54.0%	1.003 (0.728, 1.380)
White	735	40.5%	43.2%	0.809 (0.645, 1.013)

TABLE 2B *Efficacy Outcomes Within Demographic Subgroups*

		ESRD		
	n	Losartan Potassium Event Rate	Placebo Event Rate	Hazard Ratio (95% CI)
Overall Results	1513	19.6%	25.5%	0.714 (0.576, 0.885)
Age				
<65 years	1005	21.1%	28.5%	0.670 (0.521, 0.863)
≥65 years	508	16.5%	19.6%	0.847 (0.560, 1.281)
Gender				
Female	557	22.8%	32.8%	0.601 (0.436, 0.828)
Male	956	17.5%	21.5%	0.809 (0.605, 1.081)
Race				
Asian	252	18.8%	27.4%	0.625 (0.367, 1.066)
Black	230	17.6%	21.0%	0.831 (0.456, 1.516)
Hispanic	277	30.0%	28.5%	1.024 (0.661, 1.586)
White	735	16.2%	23.9%	0.596 (0.427, 0.831)

INDICATIONS AND USAGE

HYPERTENSION

Losartan potassium is indicated for the treatment of hypertension. It may be used alone or in combination with other antihypertensive agents.

NEPHROPATHY IN TYPE 2 DIABETIC PATIENTS

Losartan potassium is indicated for the treatment of diabetic nephropathy with an elevated serum creatinine and proteinuria (urinary albumin to creatinine ratio ≥300 mg/g) in patients with type 2 diabetes and a history of hypertension. In this population, losartan potassium reduces the rate of progression of nephropathy as measured by the occurrence of doubling of serum creatinine or end stage renal disease (need for dialysis or renal transplantation) (see CLINICAL PHARMACOLOGY, Pharmacodynamics and Clinical Effects).

NON-FDA APPROVED INDICATIONS

Losartan has also been studied for its effects on platelet aggregation, beneficial effects on hypoglycemic unawareness and endothelial function in patients with diabetes, antiproteinuric and uricosuric effects, treatment of post-transplant erythrocytosis, Raynaud phenomenon, scleroderma, and portal hypertension in cirrhosis. None of these uses is approved by the FDA and large, controlled clinical trials are lacking.

CONTRAINDICATIONS

Losartan potassium is contraindicated in patients who are hypersensitive to any component of this product.

WARNINGS

FETAL/NEONATAL MORBIDITY AND MORTALITY

Drugs that act directly on the renin-angiotensin system can cause fetal and neonatal morbidity and death when administered to pregnant women. Several dozen cases have been reported in the world literature in patients who were taking angiotensin converting enzyme inhibitors. When pregnancy is detected, losartan potassium should be discontinued as soon as possible.

The use of drugs that act directly on the renin-angiotensin system during the second and third trimesters of pregnancy has been associated with fetal and neonatal injury, including hypotension, neonatal skull hypoplasia, anuria, reversible or irreversible renal failure, and death. Oligohydramnios has also been reported, presumably resulting from decreased fetal renal function; oligohydramnios in this setting has been associated with fetal limb contractures, craniofacial deformation, and hypoplastic lung development. Prematurity, intrauterine growth retardation, and patent ductus arteriosus have also been reported, although it is not clear whether these occurrences were due to exposure to the drug.

These adverse effects do not appear to have resulted from intrauterine drug exposure that has been limited to the first trimester.

Mothers whose embryos and fetuses are exposed to an angiotensin II receptor antagonist only during the first trimester should be so informed. Nonetheless, when patients become pregnant, physicians should have the patient discontinue the use of losartan potassium as soon as possible.

Rarely (probably less often than once in every thousand pregnancies), no alternative to an angiotensin II receptor antagonist will be found. In these rare cases, the mothers should be apprised of the potential hazards to their fetuses, and serial ultrasound examinations should be performed to assess the intraamniotic environment.

If oligohydramnios is observed, losartan potassium should be discontinued unless it is considered life-saving for the mother. Contraction stress testing (CST), a non-stress test (NST), or biophysical profiling (BPP) may be appropriate, depending upon the week of pregnancy. Patients and physicians should be aware, however, that oligohydramnios may not appear until after the fetus has sustained irreversible injury.

Infants with histories of *in utero* exposure to an angiotensin II receptor antagonist should be closely observed for hypotension, oliguria, and hyperkalemia. If oliguria occurs, attention should be directed toward support of blood pressure and renal perfusion. Exchange transfusion or dialysis may be required as means of reversing hypotension and/or substituting for disordered renal function.

Losartan potassium has been shown to produce adverse effects in rat fetuses and neonates, including decreased body weight, delayed physical and behavioral development, mortality and renal toxicity. With the exception of neonatal weight gain (which was affected at doses as low as 10 mg/kg/day), doses associated with these effects exceeded 25 mg/kg/day (approximately 3 times the maximum recommended human dose of 100 mg on a mg/m^2 basis). These findings are attributed to drug exposure in late gestation and during lactation. Significant levels of losartan and its active metabolite were shown to be present in rat fetal plasma during late gestation and in rat milk.

HYPOTENSION — VOLUME-DEPLETED PATIENTS

In patients who are intravascularly volume-depleted (*e.g.*, those treated with diuretics), symptomatic hypotension may occur after initiation of therapy with losartan potassium. These conditions should be corrected prior to administration of losartan potassium, or a lower starting dose should be used (see DOSAGE AND ADMINISTRATION).

PRECAUTIONS

GENERAL

Hypersensitivity

Angioedema. See ADVERSE REACTIONS, Post-Marketing Experience.

IMPAIRED HEPATIC FUNCTION

Based on pharmacokinetic data which demonstrate significantly increased plasma concentrations of losartan in cirrhotic patients, a lower dose should be considered for patients with impaired liver function (see DOSAGE AND ADMINISTRATION and CLINICAL PHARMACOLOGY, Pharmacokinetics).

IMPAIRED RENAL FUNCTION

As a consequence of inhibiting the renin-angiotensin-aldosterone system, changes in renal function have been reported in susceptible individuals treated with losartan potassium; in some patients, these changes in renal function were reversible upon disconuation of therapy.

In patients whose renal function may depend on the activity of the renin-angiotensin-aldosterone system (*e.g.*, patients with severe congestive heart failure), treatment with angiotensin converting enzyme inhibitors has been associated with oliguria and/or progressive azotemia and (rarely) with acute renal failure and/or death. Similar outcomes have been reported with losartan potassium.

In studies of ACE inhibitors in patients with unilateral or bilateral renal artery stenosis, increases in serum creatinine or BUN have been reported. Similar effects have been reported with losartan potassium; in some patients, these effects were reversible upon discontinuation of therapy.

ELECTROLYTE IMBALANCE

Electrolyte imbalances are common in patients with renal impairment, with or without diabetes, and should be addressed. In a clinical study conducted in type 2 diabetic patients with proteinuria, the incidence of hyperkalemia was higher in the group treated with losartan potassium as compared to the placebo group; however, few patients discontinued therapy due to hyperkalemia (see ADVERSE REACTIONS).

INFORMATION FOR THE PATIENT

Pregnancy

Female patients of childbearing age should be told about the consequences of second- and third-trimester exposure to drugs that act on the renin-angiotensin system, and they should also be told that these consequences do not appear to have resulted from intrauterine drug exposure that has been limited to the first trimester. These patients should be asked to report pregnancies to their physicians as soon as possible.

Potassium Supplements

A patient receiving losartan potassium should be told not to use potassium supplements or salt substitutes containing potassium without consulting the prescribing physician (see DRUG INTERACTIONS).

CARCINOGENESIS, MUTAGENESIS, AND IMPAIRMENT OF FERTILITY

Losartan potassium was not carcinogenic when administered at maximally tolerated dosages to rats and mice for 105 and 92 weeks, respectively. Female rats given the highest dose (270 mg/kg/day) had a slightly higher incidence of pancreatic acinar adenoma. The maximally tolerated dosages (270 mg/kg/day in rats, 200 mg/kg/day in mice) provided systemic exposures for losartan and its pharmacologically active metabolite that were approximately 160 and 90 times (rats) and 30 and 15 times (mice) the exposure of a 50 kg human given 100 mg/day.

Losartan potassium was negative in the microbial mutagenesis and V-79 mammalian cell mutagenesis assays and in the *in vitro* alkaline elution and *in vitro* and *in vivo* chromosomal aberration assays. In addition, the active metabolite showed no evidence of genotoxicity in the microbial mutagenesis, *in vitro* alkaline elution, and *in vitro* chromosomal aberration assays.

Fertility and reproductive performance were not affected in studies with male rats given oral doses of losartan potassium up to approximately 150 mg/kg/day. The administration of toxic dosage levels in females (300/200 mg/kg/day) was associated with a significant ($p < 0.05$) decrease in the number of corpora lutea/female, implants/female, and live fetuses/female at C-section. At 100 mg/kg/day only a decrease in the number of corpora lutea/female was observed. The relationship of these findings to drug-treatment is uncertain since there was no effect at these dosage levels on implants/pregnant female, percent post-implantation loss, or live animals/litter at parturition. In nonpregnant rats dosed at 135 mg/kg/day for 7 days, systemic exposure (AUCs) for losartan and its active metabolite were approximately 66 and 26 times the exposure achieved in man at the maximum recommended human daily dosage (100 mg).

PREGNANCY CATEGORY C (FIRST TRIMESTER) AND D (SECOND AND THIRD TRIMESTERS)

See WARNINGS, Fetal/Neonatal Morbidity and Mortality.

NURSING MOTHERS

It is not known whether losartan is excreted in human milk, but significant levels of losartan and its active metabolite were shown to be present in rat milk. Because of the potential for adverse effects on the nursing infant, a decision should be made whether to discontinue nursing or discontinue the drug, taking into account the importance of the drug to the mother.

PEDIATRIC USE

Safety and effectiveness in pediatric patients have not been established.

USE IN THE ELDERLY

Of the total number of patients receiving losartan potassium in controlled clinical studies for hypertension, 391 patients (19%) were 65 years and over, while 37 patients (2%) were 75 years and over. In a controlled clinical study for renal protection in type 2 diabetic patients with proteinuria, 248 patients (33%) were 65 years and over. No overall differences in effectiveness or safety were observed between these patients and younger patients, but greater sensitivity of some older individuals cannot be ruled out.

DRUG INTERACTIONS

No significant drug-drug pharmacokinetic interactions have been found in interaction studies with hydrochlorothiazide, digoxin, warfarin, cimetidine and phenobarbital. (See CLINICAL PHARMACOLOGY, Drug Interactions.) Potent inhibitors of cytochrome P450 3A4 and 2C9 have not been studied clinically but *in vitro* studies show significant inhibition of the formation of the active metabolite by inhibitors of P450 3A4 (ketoconazole, troleandomycin, gestodene), or P450 2C9 (sulfaphenazole) and nearly complete inhibition by the combination of sulfaphenazole and ketoconazole. In humans, ketoconazole, an inhibitor of P450 3A4, did not affect the conversion of losartan to the active metabolite after IV administration of losartan. Inhibitors of cytochrome P450 2C9 have not been studied clinically. The pharmacodynamic consequences of concomitant use of losartan and inhibitors of P450 2C9 have not been examined.

As with other drugs that block angiotensin II or its effects, concomitant use of potassium-sparing diuretics (*e.g.*, spironolactone, triamterene, amiloride), potassium supplements, or salt substitutes containing potassium may lead to increases in serum potassium.

As with other antihypertensive agents, the antihypertensive effect of losartan may be blunted by the non-steroidal anti-inflammatory drug indomethacin.

ADVERSE REACTIONS

HYPERTENSION

Losartan potassium has been evaluated for safety in more than 3300 patients treated for essential hypertension and 4058 patients/subjects overall. Over 1200 patients were treated for over 6 months and more than 800 for over 1 year. In general, treatment with losartan potassium was well-tolerated. The overall incidence of adverse experiences reported with losartan potassium was similar to placebo.

In controlled clinical trials, discontinuation of therapy due to clinical adverse experiences was required in 2.3% of patients treated with losartan potassium and 3.7% of patients given placebo.

Adverse events in TABLE 3 are based on four 6-12 week placebo-controlled trials involving over 1000 patients on various doses (10-150 mg) of losartan and over 300 patients given placebo. All doses of losartan are grouped because none of the adverse events appeared to have a dose-related frequency. The adverse experiences reported in ≥1% of patients treated with losartan potassium and more commonly than placebo are shown in TABLE 3.

TABLE 3

	Incidence	
	Losartan (n=1075)	Placebo (n=334)
Musculoskeletal		
Cramp, muscle	1%	0%
Pain, back	2%	1%
Pain, leg	1%	0%
Nervous System/Psychiatric		
Dizziness	3%	2%
Respiratory		
Congestion, nasal	2%	1%
Infection, upper respiratory	8%	7%
Sinusitis	1%	0%

The following adverse events were also reported at a rate of 1% or greater in patients treated with losartan, but were as, or more frequent, in the placebo group: asthenia/fatigue, edema/swelling, abdominal pain, chest pain, nausea, headache, pharyngitis, diarrhea, dyspepsia, myalgia, insomnia, cough, sinus disorder.

Adverse events occurred at about the same rates in men and women, older and younger patients, and black and non-black patients.

A patient with known hypersensitivity to aspirin and penicillin, when treated with losartan potassium, was withdrawn from study due to swelling of the lips and eyelids and facial rash, reported as angioedema, which returned to normal 5 days after therapy was discontinued.

Superficial peeling of palms and hemolysis was reported in 1 subject.

In addition to the adverse events above, potentially important events that occurred in at least 2 patients/subjects exposed to losartan or other adverse events that occurred in <1% of patients in clinical studies are listed below. It cannot be determined whether these events were causally related to losartan:

Body as a Whole: Facial edema, fever, orthostatic effects, syncope.

Cardiovascular: Angina pectoris, second degree AV block, CVA, hypotension, myocardial infarction, arrhythmias including atrial fibrillation, palpitation, sinus bradycardia, tachycardia, ventricular tachycardia, ventricular fibrillation.

Digestive: Anorexia, constipation, dental pain, dry mouth, flatulence, gastritis, vomiting.

Hematologic: Anemia.

Metabolic: Gout.

Musculoskeletal: Arm pain, hip pain, joint swelling, knee pain, musculoskeletal pain, shoulder pain, stiffness, arthralgia, arthritis, fibromyalgia, muscle weakness.

Nervous System/Psychiatric: Anxiety, anxiety disorder, ataxia, confusion, depression, dream abnormality, hypesthesia, decreased libido, memory impairment, migraine, nervousness, paresthesia, peripheral neuropathy, panic disorder, sleep disorder, somnolence, tremor, vertigo.

Respiratory: Dyspnea, bronchitis, pharyngeal discomfort, epistaxis, rhinitis, respiratory congestion.

Skin: Alopecia, dermatitis, dry skin, ecchymosis, erythema, flushing, photosensitivity, pruritus, rash, sweating, urticaria.

Special Senses: Blurred vision, burning/stinging in the eye, conjunctivitis, taste perversion, tinnitus, decrease in visual acuity.

Urogenital: Impotence, nocturia, urinary frequency, urinary tract infection.

Persistent dry cough (with an incidence of a few percent) has been associated with ACE inhibitor use and in practice can be a cause of discontinuation of ACE inhibitor therapy. Two prospective, parallel-group, double-blind, randomized, controlled trials were conducted to assess the effects of losartan on the incidence of cough in hypertensive patients who had experienced cough while receiving ACE inhibitor therapy. Patients who had typical ACE inhibitor cough when challenged with lisinopril, whose cough disappeared on placebo, were randomized to losartan 50 mg, lisinopril 20 mg, or either placebo (one study, n=97) or 25 mg hydrochlorothiazide (n=135). The double-blind treatment period lasted up to 8 weeks. The incidence of cough is shown in TABLE 4.

These studies demonstrate that the incidence of cough associated with losartan therapy, in a population that all had cough associated with ACE inhibitor therapy, is similar to that associated with hydrochlorothiazide or placebo therapy.

Cases of cough, including positive re-challenges, have been reported with the use of losartan in post-marketing experience.

NEPHROPATHY IN TYPE 2 DIABETIC PATIENTS

In the RENAAL study involving 1513 patients treated with losartan potassium or placebo, the overall incidences of reported adverse experiences were similar for the two groups. Losartan potassium was generally well tolerated as evidenced by a similar incidence of discontinuations due to side effects compared to placebo (19% for losartan potassium, 24%

L

TABLE 4

Study 1*	HCTZ	Losartan	Lisinopril
Cough	25%	17%	69%
Study 2†	**Placebo**	**Losartan**	**Lisinopril**
Cough	35%	29%	62%

* Demographics = (89% caucasian, 64% female).
† Demographics = (90% caucasian, 51% female).

for placebo). The adverse experiences regardless of drug relationship, reported with an incidence of ≥4% of patients treated with losartan potassium and occurring more commonly than placebo, on a background of conventional antihypertensive therapy (see TABLE 5).

TABLE 5

	Conventional Antihypertensive Therapy Incidence	
	Losartan (n=751)	Placebo (n=762)
Body as a Whole		
Asthenia/fatigue	14%	10%
Chest pain	12%	8%
Fever	4%	3%
Infection	5%	4%
Influenza-like disease	10%	9%
Trauma	4%	3%
Cardiovascular		
Hypotension	7%	3%
Orthostatic hypotension	4%	1%
Digestive		
Diarrhea	15%	10%
Dyspepsia	4%	3%
Gastritis	5%	4%
Endocrine		
Diabetic neuropathy	4%	3%
Diabetic vascular disease	10%	9%
Eyes, Ears, Nose and Throat		
Cataract	7%	5%
Sinusitis	6%	5%
Hemic		
Anemia	14%	11%
Metabolic and Nutrition		
Hyperkalemia	7%	3%
Hypoglycemia	14%	10%
Weight gain	4%	3%
Musculoskeletal		
Back pain	12%	10%
Leg pain	5%	4%
Knee pain	5%	4%
Muscular weakness	7%	4%
Nervous System		
Hypesthesia	5%	4%
Respiratory		
Bronchitis	10%	9%
Cough	11%	10%
Skin		
Cellulitis	7%	6%
Urogenital		
Urinary tract infection	16%	13%

POST-MARKETING EXPERIENCE

The following additional adverse reactions have been reported in post-marketing experience:

Hypersensitivity: Angioedema, including swelling of the larynx and glottis, causing airway obstruction and/or swelling of the face, lips, pharynx, and/or tongue has been reported rarely in patients treated with losartan; some of these patients previously experienced angioedema with other drugs including ACE inhibitors. Vasculitis, including Henoch-Schöenlein purpura, has been reported. Anaphylactic reactions have been reported.

Digestive: Hepatitis (reported rarely).

Respiratory: Dry cough (see above).

Hyperkalemia and hyponatremia have been reported.

LABORATORY TEST FINDINGS

In controlled clinical trials, clinically important changes in standard laboratory parameters were rarely associated with administration of losartan potassium.

Creatinine, Blood Urea Nitrogen

Minor increases in blood urea nitrogen (BUN) or serum creatinine were observed in less than 0.1% of patients with essential hypertension treated with losartan potassium alone (see PRECAUTIONS, Impaired Renal Function).

Hemoglobin and Hematocrit

Small decreases in hemoglobin and hematocrit (mean decreases of approximately 0.11 grams percent and 0.09 volume percent, respectively) occurred frequently in patients treated with losartan potassium alone, but were rarely of clinical importance. No patients were discontinued due to anemia.

Liver Function Tests

Occasional elevations of liver enzymes and/or serum bilirubin have occurred. In patients with essential hypertension treated with losartan potassium alone, 1 patient (<0.1%) was discontinued due to these laboratory adverse experiences.

DOSAGE AND ADMINISTRATION

Losartan potassium may be administered with other antihypertensive agents, and with or without food.

HYPERTENSION

Dosing must be individualized. The usual starting dose of losartan potassium is 50 mg once daily, with 25 mg used in patients with possible depletion of intravascular volume (*e.g.*, patients treated with diuretics) (see WARNINGS, Hypotension — Volume-Depleted Patients) and patients with a history of hepatic impairment (see PRECAUTIONS, General). Losartan potassium can be administered once or twice daily with total daily doses ranging from 25-100 mg.

If the antihypertensive effect measured at trough using once-a-day dosing is inadequate, a twice-a-day regimen at the same total daily dose or an increase in dose may give a more satisfactory response. The effect of losartan is substantially present within 1 week but in some studies the maximal effect occourred in 3-6 weeks (see CLINICAL PHARMACOLOGY, Pharmacodynamics and Clinical Effects).

If blood pressure is not controlled by losartan potassium alone, a low dose of a diuretic may be added. Hydrochlorothiazide has been shown to have an additive effect (see CLINICAL PHARMACOLOGY, Pharmacodynamics and Clinical Effects).

No initial dosage adjustment is necessary for elderly patients or for patients with renal impairment, including patients on dialysis.

NEPHROPATHY IN TYPE 2 DIABETIC PATIENTS

The usual starting dose is 50 mg once daily. The dose should be increased to 100 mg once daily based on blood pressure response (see CLINICAL PHARMACOLOGY, Pharmacodynamics and Clinical Effects). Losartan potassium may be administered with insulin and other commonly used hypoglycemic agents (*e.g.*, sulfonylureas, glitazones and glucosidase inhibitors).

HOW SUPPLIED

COZAAR TABLETS

25 mg: Light green, teardrop-shaped, film-coated tablets with code "MRK" on one side and "951" on the other.

50 mg: Green, teardrop-shaped, film-coated tablets with code "MRK 952" on one side and "COZAAR" on the other.

100 mg: Dark green, teardrop-shaped, film-coated tablets with code "960" on one side and "MRK" on the other.

Storage: Store at 25°C (77°F); excursions permitted to 15-30°C (59-86°F). Keep container tightly closed. Protect from light.

PRODUCT LISTING - EQUIVALENTS NOT AVAILABLE

Tablet - Oral - 25 mg

30's	$38.99	COZAAR, Allscripts Pharmaceutical Company	54569-4437-00
90's	$142.71	COZAAR, Merck & Company Inc	00006-0951-54
100's	$158.56	COZAAR, Merck & Company Inc	00006-0951-28
100's	$158.56	COZAAR, Merck & Company Inc	00006-0951-58

Tablet - Oral - 50 mg

30's	$38.99	COZAAR, Allscripts Pharmaceutical Company	54569-4438-00
30's	$47.58	COZAAR, Merck & Company Inc	00006-0952-31
90's	$142.71	COZAAR, Merck & Company Inc	00006-0952-54
100's	$158.56	COZAAR, Merck & Company Inc	00006-0952-28
100's	$158.56	COZAAR, Merck & Company Inc	00006-0952-58

Tablet - Oral - 100 mg

30's	$64.80	COZAAR, Merck & Company Inc	00006-0960-31
100's	$194.81	COZAAR, Merck & Company Inc	00006-0960-28
100's	$215.99	COZAAR, Merck & Company Inc	00006-0960-58

Loteprednol Etabonate *(003385)*

Categories: Conjunctivitis, allergic; Cyclitis; Iritis; Keratitis; Surgery, ophthalmic, adjunct; FDA Approved 1998 Mar; Pregnancy Category C
Drug Classes: Corticosteroids, ophthalmic; Ophthalmics
Brand Names: **Lotemax; Alrex**
Cost of Therapy: $38.37 (Allergic Conjuctivitis; Alrex Ophth. Suspension; 0.2%; 5 ml; 4 drops/day; variable day supply)

DESCRIPTION

Loteprednol etabonate ophthalmic suspension contains a sterile, topical anti-inflammatory corticosteroid for ophthalmic use. Loteprednol etabonate is a white to off-white powder.

The chemical name is chloromethyl 17α-[(ethoxycarbonyl)oxy]-11β-hydroxy-3-oxoandrosta-1,4-diene-17β-carboxylate.

Each Alrex ml Contains: *Active:* Loteprednol etabonate 2 mg (0.2%); *Inactives:* Edetate disodium, glycerin, povidone, purified water and tyloxapol. Hydrochloric acid and/or sodium hydroxide may be added to adjust the pH to 5.3-5.6. The suspension is essentially isotonic with a tonicity of 250 to 310 mDsmol/kg. *Preservative Added:* Benzalkonium chloride 0.01%.

Each Lotemax ml Contains: *Active:* Loteprednol etabonate 5 mg (0.5%); *Inactives:* Edetate disodium, glycerin, povidone, purified water and tyloxapol. Hydrochloric acid and/or sodium hydroxide may be added to adjust the pH to 5.3-5.6. The suspension is essentially isotonic with a tonicity of 250 to 310 mOsmol/kg. *Preservative Added:* Benzalkonium chloride 0.01%.

CLINICAL PHARMACOLOGY

Corticosteroids inhibit the inflammatory response to a variety of inciting agents and probably delay or slow healing. They inhibit the edema, fibrin deposition, capillary dilation, leukocyte migration, capillary proliferation, fibroblast proliferation, deposition of collagen, and scar formation associated with inflammation. There is no generally accepted explanation for the mechanism of action of ocular corticosteroids. However, corticosteroids are thought to act by the induction of phospholipase A_2 inhibitory proteins, collectively called lipocortins. It is postulated that these proteins control the biosynthesis of potent mediators of inflammation such as prostaglandins and leukotrienes by inhibiting the release of their common precursor arachidonic acid. Arachidonic acid is released from membrane phospholipids by phospholipase A_2. Corticosteroids are capable of producing a rise in intraocular pressure.

Loteprednol etabonate is structurally similar to other corticosteroids. However, the number 20 position ketone group is absent. It is highly lipid soluble which enhances its penetration into cells. Loteprednol etabonate is synthesized through structural modifications of prednisolone-related compounds so that it will undergo a predictable transformation to an inactive metabolite. Based upon *in vivo* and *in vitro* preclinical metabolism studies, loteprednol etabonate undergoes extensive metabolism to inactive carboxylic acid metabolites.

Results from a bioavailability study in normal volunteers established that plasma levels of loteprednol etabonate and Δ^1 cortienic acid etabonate (PJ 91), its primary, inactive metabolite, were below the limit of quantitation (1 ng/ml) at all sampling times. The results were obtained following the ocular administration of 1 drop in each eye of 0.5% loteprednol etabonate 8 times daily for 2 days or 4 times daily for 42 days. This study suggests that limited (<1 ng/ml) systemic absorption occurs with loteprednol etabonate.

INDICATIONS AND USAGE

0.2% SUSPENSION

Loteprednol etabonate ophthalmic suspension is indicated for the temporary relief of the signs and symptoms of seasonal allergic conjunctivitis.

0.5% SUSPENSION

Loteprednol etabonate is indicated for the treatment of steroid responsive inflammatory conditions of the palpebral and bulbar conjunctiva, cornea and anterior segment of the globe such as allergic conjunctivitis, acne rosacea, superficial punctate keratitis, herpes zoster keratitis, iritis, cyclitis, selected infective conjunctivitides, when the inherent hazard of steroid use is accepted to obtain an advisable diminution in edema and inflammation.

Loteprednol etabonate is less effective than prednisolone acetate 1% in two 28 day controlled clinical studies in acute anterior uveitis, where 72% of patients treated with loteprednol etabonate experienced resolution of anterior chamber cells, compared to 87% of patients treated with prednisolone acetate 1%. The incidence of patients with clinically significant increases in IOP (≥10 mm Hg) was 1% with loteprednol etabonate and 6% with prednisolone acetate 1%. Loteprednol etabonate should not be used in patients who require a more potent corticosteroid for this indication.

Loteprednol etabonate is also indicated for the treatment of post-operative inflammation following ocular surgery.

CONTRAINDICATIONS

Loteprednol etabonate, as with other ophthalmic corticosteroids, is contraindicated in most viral diseases of the cornea and conjunctiva including epithelial herpes simplex keratitis (dendritic keratitis), vaccinia, and varicella, and also in mycobacterial infection of the eye and fungal diseases of ocular structures. Loteprednol etabonate is also contraindicated in individuals with known or suspected hypersensitivity to any of the ingredients of this preparation and to other corticosteroids.

WARNINGS

Prolonged use of corticosteroids may result in glaucoma with damage to the optic nerve, defects in visual acuity and fields of vision, and in posterior subcapsular cataract formation. Steroids should be used with caution in the presence of glaucoma.

Prolonged use of corticosteroids may suppress the host response and thus increase the hazard of secondary ocular infections. In those diseases causing thinning of the cornea or sclera, perforations have been known to occur with the use of topical steroids. In acute purulent conditions of the eye, steroids may mask infection or enhance existing infection.

Use of ocular steroids may prolong the course and may exacerbate the severity of many viral infections of the eye (including herpes simplex). Employment of a corticosteroid medication in the treatment of patients with a history of herpes simplex requires great caution. **Additional information for 0.5% suspension:** The use of steroids after cataract surgery may delay healing and increase the incidence of bleb formation.

PRECAUTIONS

GENERAL

For ophthalmic use only. The initial prescription and renewal of the medication order beyond 14 days should be made by a physician only after examination of the patient with the aid of magnification, such as slit lamp biomicroscopy and, where appropriate, fluorescein staining.

If signs and symptoms fail to improve after 2 days, the patient should be re-evaluated.

If this product is used for 10 days or longer, intraocular pressure should be monitored even though it may be difficult in children and uncooperative patients (see WARNINGS).

Fungal infections of the cornea are particularly prone to develop coincidentally with long-term local steroid application. Fungus invasion must be considered in any persistent corneal ulceration where a steroid has been used or is in use. Fungal cultures should be taken when appropriate.

INFORMATION FOR THE PATIENT

0.2% Suspension

This product is sterile when packaged. Patients should be advised not to allow the dropper tip to touch any surface, as this may contaminate the suspension. If redness or itching becomes aggravated, the patient should be advised to consult a physician.

Patients should be advised not to wear a contact lens if their eye is red. Loteprednol etabonate should not be used to treat contact lens related irritation. The preservative in loteprednol etabonate 0.2% suspension, benzalkonium chloride, may be absorbed by soft contact lenses. Patients who wear soft contact lenses **and whose eyes are not red,** should be instructed to wait at least 10 minutes after instilling loteprednol etabonate before they insert their contact lenses.

0.5% Suspension

This product is sterile when packaged. Patients should be advised not to allow the dropper tip to touch any surface, as this may contaminate the suspension. If pain develops, redness, itching or inflammation becomes aggravated, the patient should be advised to consult a physician. As with all ophthalmic preparations containing benzalkonium chloride, patients should be advised not to wear soft contact lenses when using loteprednol etabonate.

CARCINOGENESIS, MUTAGENESIS, AND IMPAIRMENT OF FERTILITY

Long-term animal studies have not been conducted to evaluate the carcinogenic potential of loteprednol etabonate. Loteprednol etabonate was not genotoxic *in vitro* in the Ames test, the mouse lymphoma tk assay, or in a chromosome aberration test in human lymphocytes, or *in vivo* in the single dose mouse micronucleus assay. Treatment of male and female rats with up to 50 mg/kg/day and 25 mg/kg/day of loteprednol etabonate, respectively, (1500 and 750 times (*0.5% Suspension:* 600 and 300 times) the maximum clinical dose, respectively) prior to and during mating did not impair fertility in either gender.

PREGNANCY, TERATOGENIC EFFECTS, PREGNANCY CATEGORY C

Loteprednol etabonate has been shown to be embryotoxic (delayed ossification) and teratogenic (increased incidence of meningocele, abnormal left common carotid artery, and limb flexures) when administered orally to rabbits during organogenesis at a dose of 3 mg/kg/day (85 times (*0.5% Suspension:* 35 times) the maximum daily clinical dose), a dose which caused no maternal toxicity. The no-observed-effect-level (NOEL) for these effects was 0.5 mg/kg/day (15 times (*0.5% Suspension:* 6 times) the maximum daily clinical dose). Oral treatment of rats during organogenesis resulted in teratogenicity (absent innominate artery at ≥5 mg/kg/day doses, and cleft palate and umbilical hernia at ≥50 mg/kg/day) and embryotoxicity (increased post-implantation losses at 100 mg/kg/day and decreased fetal body weight and skeletal ossification with ≥50 mg/kg/day). Treatment of rats with 0.5 mg/kg/day (15 times (*0.5% Suspension:* 6 times) the maximum clinical dose) during organogenesis did not result in any reproductive toxicity. Loteprednol etabonate was maternally toxic (significantly reduced body weight gain during treatment) when administered to pregnant rats during organogenesis at doses of ≥5 mg/kg/day.

Oral exposure of female rats to 50 mg/kg/day of loteprednol etabonate from the start of the fetal period through the end of lactation, a maternally toxic treatment regimen (significantly decreased body weight gain), gave rise to decreased growth and survival, and retarded development in the offspring during lactation; the NOEL for these effects was 5 mg/kg/day. Loteprednol etabonate had no effect on the duration of gestation or parturition when administered orally to pregnant rats at doses up to 50 mg/kg/day during the fetal period.

NURSING MOTHERS

It is not known whether topical ophthalmic administration of corticosteroids could result in sufficient systemic absorption to produce detectable quantities in human milk. Systemic steroids appear in human milk and could suppress growth, interfere with endogenous corticosteroid production, or cause other untoward effects. Caution should be exercised when loteprednol etabonate is administered to a nursing woman.

PEDIATRIC USE

Safety and effectiveness in pediatric patients have not been established.

ADVERSE REACTIONS

Reactions associated with ophthalmic steroids include elevated intraocular pressure, which may be associated with optic nerve damage, visual acuity and field defects, posterior subcapsular cataract formation, secondary ocular infection from pathogens including herpes simplex, and perforation of the globe where there is thinning of the cornea or sclera.

Ocular adverse reactions occurring in 5-15% of patients treated with loteprednol etabonate ophthalmic suspension (0.2%-0.5%) in clinical studies included abnormal vision/blurring, burning on instillation, chemosis, discharge, dry eyes, epiphora, foreign body sensation, itching, injection, and photophobia. Other ocular adverse reactions occurring in less than 5% of patients include conjunctivitis, corneal abnormalities, eyelid erythema, keratoconjunctivitis, ocular irritation/pain/discomfort, papillae, and uveitis. Some of these events were similar to the underlying ocular disease being studied.

Non-ocular adverse reactions occurred in less than 15% of patients. These include headache, rhinitis and pharyngitis.

In a summation of controlled, randomized studies of individuals treated for 28 days or longer with loteprednol etabonate, the incidence of significant elevation of intraocular pressure (≥10 mm Hg) was 2% (15/901) among patients receiving loteprednol etabonate, 7% (11/164) among patients receiving 1% prednisolone acetate and 0.5% (3/583) among patients receiving placebo. Among the smaller group of patients who were studied with loteprednol etabonate 0.2% suspension, the incidence of clinically significant increases in IOP (≥10 mm Hg) was 1% (1/133) with loteprednol etabonate 0.2% suspension and 1% (1/135) with placebo.

DOSAGE AND ADMINISTRATION

0.2% SUSPENSION

SHAKE VIGOROUSLY BEFORE USING.

One drop instilled into the affected eye(s) 4 times daily.

Storage: Store upright between 15-25°C (59-77°F). DO NOT FREEZE.

0.5% SUSPENSION

SHAKE VIGOROUSLY BEFORE USING.

Steroid Responsive Disease Treatment: Apply 1-2 drops of loteprednol etabonate into the conjunctival sac of the affected eye(s) 4 times daily. During the initial treatment within the first week, the dosing may be increased, up to 1 drop every hour, if necessary. Care should be taken not to discontinue therapy prematurely. If signs and symptoms fail to improve after 2 days, the patient should be re-evaluated (see PRECAUTIONS).

Post-Operative Inflammation: Apply 1-2 drops of loteprednol etabonate into the conjunctival sac of the operated eye(s) 4 times daily beginning 24 hours after surgery and continuing throughout the first 2 weeks of the postoperative period.

Storage: Store upright between 15-25°C (59-77°F). DO NOT FREEZE.

PRODUCT LISTING - EQUIVALENTS NOT AVAILABLE

Suspension - Ophthalmic - 0.2%

5 ml	$38.37	ALREX, Bausch and Lomb	24208-0353-05
10 ml	$65.06	ALREX, Bausch and Lomb	24208-0353-10

Suspension - Ophthalmic - 0.5%

2.50 ml	$10.31	LOTEMAX, Bausch and Lomb	24208-0299-25
5 ml	$29.64	LOTEMAX, Bausch and Lomb	24208-0299-05
10 ml	$48.06	LOTEMAX, Bausch and Lomb	24208-0299-10
15 ml	$72.06	LOTEMAX, Bausch and Lomb	24208-0299-15

Lovastatin (001664)

For related information, see the comparative table section in Appendix A.

Categories: Angina, unstable, prevention; Atherosclerosis; Coronary heart disease, prevention; Hypercholesterolemia; Hyperlipidemia; Myocardial infarction, prophylaxis; Pregnancy Category X; FDA Approved 1987 Aug

Drug Classes: Antihyperlipidemics; HMG CoA reductase inhibitors

Brand Names: Altocor; **Mevacor**

Foreign Brand Availability: Belvas (Indonesia); Birotin (Korea); Cholestra (Indonesia); Cysin (Taiwan); Ellanco (Hong-Kong); Elstatin (Singapore); Lipdip (India); Lipivas (Ecuador); Lipovas (Indonesia); Lofacol (Hong-Kong); Lomar (Hong-Kong); Lostatin (Singapore); Lovacel (Korea; Peru); Lovalip (Israel); Lovalord (Korea); Lovastan (Colombia); Lovasterol (Colombia); Lovastin (Taiwan); Lovatadin (Korea); Lowachol (Taiwan); Lozutin (Taiwan); Medostatin (Bahrain; Cyprus; Egypt; Iran; Iraq; Jordan; Kuwait; Lebanon; Libya; Oman; Qatar; Republic-of-Yemen; Saudi-Arabia; Singapore; Syria; United-Arab-Emirates); Meverstin (Korea); Mevinacor (Costa-Rica; El-Salvador; Germany; Guatemala; Honduras; Nicaragua; Panama; Portugal); Nergadan (Spain); Ovasta (Korea); Rodatin (Taiwan); Rovacor (India; Singapore); Taucor (Spain)

Cost of Therapy: $73.64 (Hypercholesterolemia; Mevacor; 20 mg; 1 tablet/day; 30 day supply)
$71.12 (Hypercholesterolemia; Generic Tablets; 20 mg; 1 tablet/day; 30 day supply)
$54.00 (Hypercholesterolemia; Altocor; 40; 1 tablet/day; 30 day supply)

L

DESCRIPTION

Note: The trade names have been used throughout this monograph for clarity.

MEVACOR TABLETS

Lovastatin is a cholesterol lowering agent isolated from a strain of *Aspergillus terreus.* After oral ingestion, lovastatin, which is an inactive lactone, is hydrolyzed to the corresponding β-hydroxyacid form. This is a principal metabolite and an inhibitor of 3-hydroxy-3-methylglutaryl-coenzyme A (HMG-CoA) reductase. This enzyme catalyzes the conversion of HMG-CoA to mevalonate, which is an early and rate limiting step in the biosynthesis of cholesterol.

Lovastatin is [1*S*-[1α(*R**),3α,7β,8β(2*S**,4*S**),8aβ]]-1,2,3,7,8,8a-hexahydro-3,7-dimethyl-8-[2-(tetrahydro-4-hydroxy-6-oxo-2*H*-pyran-2-yl)ethyl]-1-naphthalenyl 2-methylbutanoate. The empirical formula of lovastatin is $C_{24}H_{36}O_5$ and its molecular weight is 404.55.

Lovastatin is a white, nonhygroscopic crystalline powder that is insoluble in water and sparingly soluble in ethanol, methanol, and acetonitrile.

Mevacor tablets are supplied as 10, 20, and 40 mg tablets for oral administration. In addition to the active ingredient lovastatin, each tablet contains the following inactive ingredients: cellulose, lactose, magnesium stearate, and starch. Butylated hydroxyanisole (BHA) is added as a preservative. Mevacor tablets 10 mg also contain red ferric oxide and yellow ferric oxide. Mevacor tablets 20 mg also contain FD&C blue no. 2. Mevacor tablets 40 mg also contain D&C yellow no. 10 and FD&C blue no. 2.

ALTOCOR EXTENDED-RELEASE TABLETS

Altocor (lovastatin) extended-release tablets contain a cholesterol-lowering agent isolated from a strain of *Aspergillus terreus.* After oral ingestion, lovastatin, which is an inactive lactone, is hydrolyzed to the corresponding β-hydroxyacid form. This is a principal metabolite and inhibitor of 3-hydroxy-3-methylglutaryl-coenzyme A (HMG-CoA) reductase. This enzyme catalyzes the conversion of HMG-CoA to mevalonate, which is an early and rate limiting step in the biosynthesis of cholesterol.

Lovastatin is [1 *S*-[1α(*R**),3α,7β,8β(2*S**,4*S**),8aβ]]-1,2,3,7,8,8a-hexahydro-3,7-dimethyl-8-[2-(tetrahydro-4-hydroxy-6-oxo-2*H*-pyran-2-yl)ethyl]-1-naphthalenyl 2-methylbutanoate. The empirical formula of lovastatin is $C_{24}H_{36}O_5$ and its molecular weight is 404.55.

Lovastatin is a white, nonhygroscopic crystalline powder that is insoluble in water and sparingly soluble in ethanol, methanol, and acetonitrile.

Altocor extended-release tablets are designed for once-a-day oral administration and deliver 10, 20, 40, or 60 mg of lovastatin. In addition to the active ingredient lovastatin, each tablet contains the following inactive ingredients: acetyltributyl citrate; butylated hydroxyanisole; candellila wax; cellulose acetate; confectioner's sugar (contains corn starch); FD&C yellow no. 6; glyceryl monostearate; hydroxypropyl methylcellulose; hypromellose phthalate; lactose; methacrylic acid copolymer, type B; polyethylene glycols (PEG 400, PEG 8000); polyethylene oxides; polysorbate 80; propylene glycol; silicon dioxide; sodium chloride; sodium lauryl sulfate; synthetic black iron oxide; red iron oxide; talc; titanium dioxide and triacetin.

CLINICAL PHARMACOLOGY

MEVACOR TABLETS

The involvement of low-density lipoprotein cholesterol (LDL-C) in atherogenesis has been well-documented in clinical and pathological studies, as well as in many animal experiments. Epidemiological and clinical studies have established that high LDL-C and low high-density lipoprotein cholesterol (HDL-C) are both associated with coronary heart disease. However, the risk of developing coronary heart disease is continuous and graded over the range of cholesterol levels and many coronary events do occur in patients with total cholesterol (total-C) and LDL-C in the lower end of this range.

Mevacor has been shown to reduce both normal and elevated LDL-C concentrations. LDL is formed from very low-density lipoprotein (VLDL) and is catabolized predominantly by the high affinity LDL receptor. The mechanism of the LDL-lowering effect of Mevacor may involve both reduction of VLDL-C concentration, and induction of the LDL receptor, leading to reduced production and/or increased catabolism of LDL-C. Apolipoprotein B also falls substantially during treatment with Mevacor. Since each LDL particle contains one molecule of apolipoprotein B, and since little apolipoprotein B is found in other lipoproteins, this strongly suggests that Mevacor does not merely cause cholesterol to be lost from LDL, but also reduces the concentration of circulating LDL particles. In addition, Mevacor can produce increases of variable magnitude in HDL-C, and modestly reduces VLDL-C and plasma triglycerides (TG). The effects of Mevacor on Lp(a), fibrinogen, and certain other independent biochemical risk markers for coronary heart disease are unknown.

Mevacor is a specific inhibitor of HMG-CoA reductase, the enzyme which catalyzes the conversion of HMG-CoA to mevalonate. The conversion of HMG-CoA to mevalonate is an early step in the biosynthetic pathway for cholesterol.

Pharmacokinetics

Lovastatin is a lactone which is readily hydrolyzed *in vivo* to the corresponding β-hydroxyacid, a potent inhibitor of HMG-CoA reductase. Inhibition of HMG-CoA reductase is the basis for an assay in pharmacokinetic studies of the β-hydroxyacid metabolites (active inhibitors) and, following base hydrolysis, active plus latent inhibitors (total inhibitors) in plasma following administration of lovastatin.

Following an oral dose of ^{14}C-labeled lovastatin in man, 10% of the dose was excreted in urine and 83% in feces. The latter represents absorbed drug equivalents excreted in bile, as well as any unabsorbed drug. Plasma concentrations of total radioactivity (lovastatin plus ^{14}C-metabolites) peaked at 2 hours and declined rapidly to about 10% of peak by 24 hours postdose. Absorption of lovastatin, estimated relative to an intravenous reference dose, in each of four animal species tested, averaged about 30% of an oral dose. In animal studies, after oral dosing, lovastatin had high selectivity for the liver, where it achieved substantially higher concentrations than in non-target tissues. Lovastatin undergoes extensive first-pass extraction in the liver, its primary site of action, with subsequent excretion of drug equivalents in the bile. As a consequence of extensive hepatic extraction of lovastatin, the availability of drug to the general circulation is low and variable. In a single dose study in 4 hypercholesterolemic patients, it was estimated that less than 5% of an oral dose of lovastatin reaches the general circulation as active inhibitors. Following administration of lovastatin tablets the coefficient of variation, based on between-subject variability, was approximately 40% for the area under the curve (AUC) of total inhibitory activity in the general circulation.

Both lovastatin and its β-hydroxyacid metabolite are highly bound (>95%) to human plasma proteins. Animal studies demonstrated that lovastatin crosses the blood-brain and placental barriers.

The major active metabolites present in human plasma are the β-hydroxyacid of lovastatin, its 6′-hydroxy derivative, and two additional metabolites. Peak plasma concentrations of both active and total inhibitors were attained within 2-4 hours of dose administration. While the recommended therapeutic dose range is 10-80 mg/day, linearity of inhibitory activity in the general circulation was established by a single dose study employing lovastatin tablet dosages from 60 to as high as 120 mg. With a once-a-day dosing regimen, plasma concentrations of total inhibitors over a dosing interval achieved a steady state between the second and third days of therapy and were about 1.5 times those following a single dose. When lovastatin was given under fasting conditions, plasma concentrations of total inhibitors were on average about two-thirds those found when lovastatin was administered immediately after a standard test meal.

In a study of patients with severe renal insufficiency (creatinine clearance 10-30 ml/min), the plasma concentrations of total inhibitors after a single dose of lovastatin were approximately 2-fold higher than those in healthy volunteers.

In a study including 16 elderly patients between 70-78 years of age who received Mevacor 80 mg/day, the mean plasma level of HMG-CoA reductase inhibitory activity was increased approximately 45% compared with 18 patients between 18-30 years of age (see PRECAUTIONS, Mevacor Tablets, Geriatric Use).

The risk of myopathy is increased by high levels of HMG-CoA reductase inhibitory activity in plasma. Potent inhibitors of CYP3A4 can raise the plasma levels of HMG-CoA reductase inhibitory activity and increase the risk of myopathy (see WARNINGS, Mevacor Tablets, Myopathy/Rhabdomyolysis and DRUG INTERACTIONS).

Lovastatin is a substrate for cytochrome P450 isoform 3A4 (CYP3A4) (see DRUG INTERACTIONS, Mevacor Tablets). Grapefruit juice contains 1 or more components that inhibit CYP3A4 and can increase the plasma concentrations of drugs metabolized by CYP3A4. In one study,[1] 10 subjects consumed 200 ml of double-strength grapefruit juice (1 can of frozen concentrate diluted with 1 rather than 3 cans of water) 3 times daily for 2 days and an additional 200 ml double-strength grapefruit juice together with and 30 and 90 minutes following a single dose of 80 mg lovastatin on the third day. This regimen of grapefruit juice resulted in a mean increase in the serum concentration of lovastatin and its β-hydroxyacid metabolite (as measured by the area under the concentration-time curve) of 15-fold and 5-fold, respectively [as measured using a chemical assay — high performance liquid chromatography]. In a second study, 15 subjects consumed one 8 oz glass of single-strength grapefruit juice (1 can of frozen concentrate diluted with 3 cans of water) with breakfast for 3 consecutive days and a single dose of 40 mg lovastatin in the evening of the third day. This regimen of grapefruit juice resulted in a mean increase in the plasma concentration (as measured by the area under the concentration-time curve) of active and total HMG-CoA reductase inhibitory activity [using an enzyme inhibition assay both before (for active inhibitors) and after (for total inhibitors) base hydrolysis] of 1.34-fold and 1.36-fold, respectively, and of lovastatin and its β-hydroxyacid metabolite [measured using a chemical assay — liquid chromatography/tandem mass spectrometry — different from that used in the first[1] study] of 1.94-fold and 1.57-fold, respectively. The effect of amounts of grapefruit juice between those used in these two studies on lovastatin pharmacokinetics has not been studied.

ALTOCOR EXTENDED-RELEASE TABLETS

Mechanism of Action

Lovastatin is a lactone that is readily hydrolyzed *in vivo* to the corresponding β-hydroxyacid, a potent inhibitor of HMG-CoA reductase, the enzyme that catalyzes the conversion of HMG-CoA to mevalonate. The conversion of HMG-CoA to mevalonate is an early step in the biosynthetic pathway for cholesterol.

The involvement of low-density lipoprotein cholesterol (LDL-C) in atherogenesis has been well documented in clinical and pathological studies, as well as in many animal experiments. Epidemiological and clinical studies have established that high LDL-C and low high-density lipoprotein cholesterol (HDL-C) levels are both associated with coronary heart disease. However, the risk of developing coronary heart disease is continuous and graded over the range of cholesterol levels and many coronary events do occur in patients with total cholesterol (Total-C) and LDL-C levels in the lower end of this range.

Altocor has been shown to reduce LDL-C, and Total-C. Across all doses studied, treatment with Altocor has been shown to result in variable reductions in triglycerides (TG), and variable increases in HDL-C.

Lovastatin immediate-release tablets have been shown to reduce both normal and elevated LDL-C concentrations. LDL is formed from very low-density lipoprotein (VLDL) and is catabolized predominantly by the high-affinity LDL receptor. The mechanism of the LDL-lowering effect of lovastatin immediate-release may involve both reduction of VLDL-C concentration, and induction of the LDL receptor, leading to reduced production and/or increased catabolism of LDL-C. Apolipoprotein B (Apo B) also falls substantially during treatment with lovastatin immediate-release. Since each LDL particle contains one molecule of Apo B, and since little Apo B is found in other lipoproteins, this strongly suggests that lovastatin immediate-release does not merely cause cholesterol to be lost from LDL, but also reduces the concentration of circulating LDL particles. In addition, lovastatin immediate-release can produce increases of variable magnitude in HDL-C, and modestly reduces VLDL-C and plasma TG. The independent effect of raising HDL or lowering TG on the risk of coronary and cardiovascular morbidity and mortality has not been determined. The effects of lovastatin immediate-release on lipoprotein (a) [Lp(a)], fibrinogen, and certain other independent biochemical risk markers for coronary heart disease are unknown.

Lovastatin, as well as some of its metabolites, are pharmacologically active in humans. The liver is the primary site of action and the principal site of cholesterol synthesis and LDL clearance (see DOSAGE AND ADMINISTRATION, Altocor Extended-Release Tablets).

Pharmacokinetics and Drug Metabolism

Absorption

Altocor

The appearance of lovastatin in plasma from an Altocor extended-release tablet is slower and more prolonged compared to the lovastatin immediate-release formulation.

A pharmacokinetic study carried out with Altocor involved measurement of the systemic concentrations of lovastatin (pro-drug), lovastatin acid (active-drug) and total and active inhibitors of HMG-CoA reductase. The pharmacokinetic parameters in 12 hypercholesterolemic subjects at steady state, after 28 days of treatment, comparing Altocor 40 mg to lovastatin immediate-release 40 mg, are summarized in TABLE 1.

TABLE 1 *Altocor vs Lovastatin Immediate-Release (IR) (Steady-State Pharmacokinetic Parameters at Day 28)*

	Altocor 40 mg*	Lovastatin IR 40 mg†
C_{max}		
L	5.5 ng/ml	7.8 ng/ml
LA	5.8 ng/ml	11.9 ng/ml
TI	17.3 ng/ml	36.2 ng/ml
AI	13.4 ng/ml	26.6 ng/ml
C_{min}		
L	2.6 ng/ml	0.4 ng/ml
LA	3.1 ng/ml	0.7 ng/ml
TI	9.1 ng/ml	2.4 ng/ml
AI	4.3 ng/ml	2.1 ng/ml
T_{max}		
L	14.2 hours	3.3 hours
LA	11.8 hours	5.3 hours
AUC(0-24h)		
L	77 ng·h/ml	45 ng·h/ml
LA	87 ng·h/ml	83 ng·h/ml
TI	263 ng·h/ml	252 ng·h/ml
AI	171 ng·h/ml	186 ng·h/ml

* Administered at bedtime.
† Administered with the evening meal.
L=lovastatin, LA=lovastatin acid, TI=total inhibitors of HMG-CoA reductase, AI=active inhibitors of HMG-CoA reductase, C_{max}=highest observed plasma concentration, C_{min}=trough concentration at t=24 hours after dosing, T_{max}=time at which the C_{max} occurred, AUC(0-24h)=area under the plasma concentration-time curve from time 0-24 hours after dosing, calculated by the linear trapezoidal rule.

The extended-release properties of Altocor are characterized by a prolonged absorptive phase, which results in a longer T_{max} and lower C_{max} for lovastatin (prodrug) and its major metabolite, lovastatin acid, compared to lovastatin immediate-release.

The bioavailability of lovastatin (pro-drug) as measured by the AUC(0-24h) was greater for Altocor compared to lovastatin immediate-release (as measured by a chemical assay), while the bioavailability of total and active inhibitors of HMG-CoA reductase were equivalent to lovastatin immediate-release (as measured by an enzymatic assay).

With once-a-day dosing, mean values of AUCs of active and total inhibitors at steady state were about 1.8-1.9 times those following a single dose. Accumulation ratio of lovastatin exposure was 1.5 after multiple daily doses of Altocor compared to that of a single dose measured using a chemical assay.

Altocor appears to have dose linearity for doses from 10 up to 60 mg/day.

When Altocor was given after a meal, plasma concentrations of lovastatin and lovastatin acid were about 0.5-0.6 times those found when Altocor was administered in the fasting state, indicating that food decreases the bioavailability of Altocor. There was an association between the bioavailability of Altocor and dosing after mealtimes. Bioavailability was lowered under the following conditions, (from higher bioavailability to lower bioavailability) in the following order: under overnight fasting conditions, before bedtime, with dinner, and with a high fat breakfast. In a multicenter, randomized, parallel group study, patients were administered 40 mg of Altocor at 3 different times; before breakfast, after dinner and at bedtime. Although there was no statistical difference in the extent of lipid change between the 3 groups, there was a numerically greater reduction in LDL-C and TG and an increase in HDL-C when Altocor was administered at bedtime. Results of this study are displayed in TABLE 2.

TABLE 2 *Altocor 40 mg (Least Squares Mean % Changes From Baseline to Endpoint at 4 Weeks of Treatment*)*

	Before breakfast n=22	After dinner n=23	Before bedtime n=23
LDL-C	-32.0%	-34.1%	-36.9%
HDL-C	8.4%	7.4%	11.1%
TOTAL-C	-22.2%	-23.6%	-25.5%
TG	-10.2%	-11.2%	-19.7%

* All changes from baseline are statistically significant.

At steady state in humans, the bioavailability of lovastatin, following the administration of Altocor, was 190% compared to lovastatin immediate-release.

Lovastatin Immediate-Release

Absorption of lovastatin, estimated relative to an intravenous reference dose in each of four animal species tested, averaged about 30% of an oral dose. Following an oral dose of ^{14}C-labeled lovastatin in man, 10% of the dose was excreted in urine and 83% in feces. The latter represents absorbed drug equivalents excreted in bile, as well as any unabsorbed drug. In a single dose study in 4 hypercholesterolemic patients, it was estimated that less than 5% of an oral dose of lovastatin reaches the general circulation as active inhibitors.

Distribution

Lovastatin

Both lovastatin and its β-hydroxyacid metabolite are highly bound (>95%) to human plasma proteins. Animal studies demonstrated that lovastatin crosses the blood-brain and placental barriers.

In animal studies, after oral dosing, lovastatin had high selectivity for the liver, where it achieved substantially higher concentrations than in non-target tissues.

Lovastatin undergoes extensive first-pass extraction in the liver, its primary site of action, with subsequent excretion of drug equivalents in the bile. As a consequence of extensive hepatic extraction of lovastatin, the availability of drug to the general circulation is low and variable.

Metabolism

Metabolism studies with Altocor have not been conducted.

Lovastatin

Lovastatin is a lactone that is readily hydrolyzed *in vivo* to the corresponding β-hydroxyacid, a potent inhibitor of HMG-CoA reductase. Inhibition of HMG-CoA reductase is the basis for an assay in pharmacokinetic studies of the β-hydroxyacid metabolites (active inhibitors) and, following base hydrolysis, active plus latent inhibitors (total inhibitors) in plasma following administration of lovastatin.

The major active metabolites present in human plasma are the β-hydroxyacid of lovastatin, its 6′-hydroxy derivative, and two additional metabolites.

Lovastatin is a substrate for CYP3A4 (see DRUG INTERACTIONS, Altocor Extended-Release Tablets). Grapefruit juice contains 1 or more components that inhibit CYP3A4 and can increase the plasma concentrations of drugs metabolized by CYP3A4. In one study,[1] 10 subjects consumed 200 ml of double-strength grapefruit juice (1 can of frozen concentrate diluted with 1 rather than 3 cans of water) 3 times daily for 2 days and an additional 200 ml double-strength grapefruit juice together with and 30 and 90 minutes following a single dose of 80 mg lovastatin on the third day. This regimen of grapefruit juice resulted in mean increases in the concentration of lovastatin and its β-hydroxyacid metabolite (as measured by the area under the concentration-time curve) of 15-fold and 5-fold respectively (as measured using a chemical assay — liquid chromatography/tandem mass spectrometry). In a second study, 15 subjects consumed one 8 oz glass of single-strength grapefruit juice (1 can of frozen concentrate diluted with 3 cans of water) with breakfast for 3 consecutive days and a single dose of 40 mg lovastatin in the evening of the third day. This regimen of grapefruit juice resulted in a mean increase in the plasma concentration (as measured by the area under the concentration-time curve) of active and total HMG-CoA reductase inhibitory activity [using a validated enzyme inhibition assay different from that used in the first study, both before (for active inhibitors) and after (for total inhibitors) base hydrolysis] of 1.34-fold and 1.36-fold, respectively, and of lovastatin and its β-hydroxyacid metabolite (measured using a chemical assay - liquid chromatography/tandem mass spectrometry) of 1.94-fold and 1.57-fold, respectively. The effect of amounts of grapefruit juice between those used in these two studies on lovastatin pharmacokinetics has not been studied.

Excretion

Altocor

In a single-dose study with Altocor, the amounts of lovastatin and lovastatin acid excreted in the urine were below the lower limit of quantitation of the assay (1.0 ng/ml), indicating that negligible excretion of Altocor occurs through the kidney.

Lovastatin

Lovastatin undergoes extensive first-pass extraction in the liver, its primary site of action, with subsequent excretion of drug equivalents in the bile.

Special Populations

Geriatric

Lovastatin Immediate-Release

In a study with lovastatin immediate-release which included 16 elderly patients between 70-78 years of age who received lovastatin immediate-release 80 mg/day, the mean plasma level of HMG-CoA reductase inhibitory activity was increased approximately 45% compared with 18 patients between 18-30 years of age (see PRECAUTIONS, Altocor Extended-Release Tablets, Geriatric Use).

Pediatric

Pharmacokinetic data in the pediatric population are not available.

Gender

In a single dose pharmacokinetic study with Altocor, there were no clinically significant differences in pharmacokinetic parameters between men (n=12) and women (n=10), although exposure tended to be higher in men than women.

In clinical studies with Altocor, there was no clinically significant difference in LDL-C reduction between men and women.

Renal Insufficiency

In a study of patients with severe renal insufficiency (creatinine clearance 10-30 ml/min), the plasma concentrations of total inhibitors after a single dose of lovastatin were approximately 2-fold higher than those in healthy volunteers.

Hemodialysis

The effect of hemodialysis on plasma levels of lovastatin and its metabolites have not been studied.

Hepatic Insufficiency

No pharmacokinetic studies with Altocor have been conducted in patients with hepatic insufficiency.

INDICATIONS AND USAGE

MEVACOR TABLETS

Therapy with Mevacor should be a component of multiple risk factor intervention in those individuals with dyslipidemia at risk for atherosclerotic vascular disease. Mevacor should be used in addition to a diet restricted in saturated fat and cholesterol as part of a treatment strategy to lower total-C and LDL-C to target levels when the response to diet and other nonpharmacological measures alone has been inadequate to reduce risk.

Primary Prevention of Coronary Heart Disease

In individuals without symptomatic cardiovascular disease, average to moderately elevated total-C and LDL-C, and below average HDL-C, Mevacor is indicated to reduce the risk of:

- Myocardial infarction
- Unstable angina
- Coronary revascularization procedures

Coronary Heart Disease

Mevacor is indicated to slow the progression of coronary atherosclerosis in patients with coronary heart disease as part of a treatment strategy to lower total-C and LDL-C to target levels.

Hypercholesterolemia

Therapy with lipid-altering agents should be a component of multiple risk factor intervention in those individuals at significantly increased risk for atherosclerotic vascular disease due to hypercholesterolemia. Mevacor is indicated as an adjunct to diet for the reduction of elevated total-C and LDL-C levels in patients with primary hypercholesterolemia (Types IIa and IIb [see TABLE 10]), when the response to diet restricted in saturated fat and cholesterol and to other nonpharmacological measures alone has been inadequate.

TABLE 10 *Classification of Hyperlipoproteinemias*

Type	Lipoproteins Elevated	Lipid Elevations Major	Lipid Elevations Minor
I	Chylomicrons	TG	C*
IIa	LDL	C	
IIb	LDL, VLDL	C	TG
III (rare)	IDL	C/TG	
IV	VLDL	TG	C*
V (rare)	Chylomicrons, VLDL	TG	C*

C = cholesterol, TG = triglycerides, LDL = low-density lipoprotein, VLDL = very low-density lipoprotein, IDL = intermediate-density lipoprotein.
* Increases or no change.

Adolescent Patients With Heterozygous Familial Hypercholesterolemia

Mevacor is indicated as an adjunct to diet to reduce total-C, LDL-C and apolipoprotein B levels in adolescent boys and girls who are at least 1 year post-menarche, 10-17 years of age, with heFH if after an adequate trial of diet therapy the following findings are present:

LDL-C remains >189 mg/dl or
LDL-C remains >160 mg/dl <u>and:</u>
There is a positive family history of premature cardiovascular disease or
Two or more other CVD risk factors are present in the adolescent patient.

General Recommendations

Prior to initiating therapy with lovastatin, secondary causes for hypercholesterolemia (*e.g.*, poorly controlled diabetes mellitus, hypothyroidism, nephrotic syndrome, dysproteinemias, obstructive liver disease, other drug therapy, alcoholism) should be excluded, and a lipid profile performed to measure total-C, HDL-C, and TG.

For patients with TG less than 400 mg/dl (<4.5 mmol/L), LDL-C can be estimated using the following equation:

LDL-C = Total-C - [0.2 × (TG) + HDL-C]

For TG levels >400 mg/dl (>4.5 mmol/L), this equation is less accurate and LDL-C concentrations should be determined by ultracentrifugation. In hypertriglyceridemic patients, LDL-C may be low or normal despite elevated total-C. In such cases, Mevacor is not indicated.

The National Cholesterol Education Program (NCEP) Treatment Guidelines are summarized in TABLE 11.

TABLE 11 *NCEP Treatment Guidelines: LDL-C Goals and Cutpoints for Therapeutic Lifestyle Changes and Drug Therapy in Different Risk Categories*

Risk Category	LDL Goal	LDL Level at Which to: Initiate Therapeutic Lifestyle Changes	LDL Level at Which to: Consider Drug Therapy
CHD or CHD risk equivalents (10 year risk >20%)	<100 mg/dl	≥100 mg/dl	≥130 mg/dl (100-129: drug optional)*
2+ Risk factors (10 year risk ≤20%)	<130 mg/dl	≥130 mg/dl	10 year risk 10-20%: ≥130 mg/dl 10 year risk <10%: ≥160 mg/dl
0-1 Risk factor†	<160 mg/dl	≥160 mg/dl	≥190 mg/dl (160-189: LDL-lowering drug optional)

CHD Coronary heart disease.
* Some authorities recommend use of LDL-lowering drugs in this category if an LDL-C level of <100 mg/dl cannot be achieved by therapeutic lifestyle changes. Others prefer use of drugs that primarily modify triglycerides and HDL-C, *e.g.*, nicotinic acid or fibrate. Clinical judgment also may call for deferring drug therapy in this subcategory.
† Almost all people with 0-1 risk factor have a 10 year risk <10%; thus, 10 year risk assessment in people with 0-1 risk factor is not necessary.

After the LDL-C goal has been achieved, if the TG is still ≥200 mg/dl, non-HDL-C (total-C minus HDL-C) becomes a secondary target of therapy. Non-HDL-C goals are set 30 mg/dl higher than LDL-C goals for each risk category.

At the time of hospitalization for an acute coronary event, consideration can be given to initiating drug therapy at discharge if the LDL-C is ≥130 mg/dl (see TABLE 11).

Since the goal of treatment is to lower LDL-C, the NCEP recommends that LDL-C levels be used to initiate and assess treatment response. Only if LDL-C levels are not available, should the total-C be used to monitor therapy.

Although Mevacor may be useful to reduce elevated LDL-C levels in patients with combined hypercholesterolemia and hypertriglyceridemia where hypercholesterolemia is the major abnormality (Type IIb hyperlipoproteinemia), it has not been studied in conditions where the major abnormality is elevation of chylomicrons, VLDL or IDL (*i.e.*, hyperlipoproteinemia Types I, III, IV, or V). (See TABLE 10.)

The NCEP classification of cholesterol levels in pediatric patients with a familial history of hypercholesterolemia or premature cardiovascular disease is summarized below (see TABLE 12).

TABLE 12

Category	Total-C	LDL-C
Acceptable	<170 mg/dl	<110 mg/dl
Borderline	170-199 mg/dl	110-129 mg/dl
High	≥200 mg/dl	≥130 mg/dl

Children treated with lovastatin in adolescence should be re-evaluated in adulthood and appropriate changes made to their cholesterol-lowering regimen to achieve adult goals for LDL-C.

ALTOCOR EXTENDED-RELEASE TABLETS

Therapy with Altocor extended-release tablets should be a component of multiple risk factor intervention in those individuals with dyslipidemia who are at risk for atherosclerotic vascular disease. Altocor should be used in addition to a diet restricted in saturated fat and cholesterol as part of a treatment strategy to lower Total-C and LDL-C to target levels when the response to diet and other nonpharmacological measures alone has been inadequate to reduce risk.

Primary Prevention of Coronary Heart Disease

In individuals without symptomatic cardiovascular disease, average to moderately elevated Total-C and LDL-C, and below average HDL-C, Altocor is indicated to reduce the risk of:

- Myocardial infarction
- Unstable angina
- Coronary revascularization procedures

Coronary Heart Disease

Altocor is indicated to slow the progression of coronary atherosclerosis in patients with coronary heart disease as part of a treatment strategy to lower Total-C and LDL-C to target levels.

Hyperlipidemia

Therapy with lipid-altering agents should be a component of multiple risk factor intervention in those individuals at significantly increased risk for artherosclerotic vascular disease due to hypercholesterolemia.

Altocor is indicated as an adjunct to diet for the reduction of elevated Total-C, LDL-C, Apo B, and TG, and to increase HDL-C in patients with primary hypercholesterolemia (heterozygous familial and non-familial) and mixed dyslipidemia (Fredrickson types IIa and IIb, see TABLE 14) when the response to diet restricted in saturated fat and cholesterol and to other non-pharmacological measures alone has been inadequate.

General Recommendations

Prior to initiating therapy with Altocor, secondary causes for hypercholesterolemia (*e.g.,* poorly controlled diabetes mellitus, hypothyroidism, nephrotic syndrome, dysproteinemias, obstructive liver disease, other drug therapy, alcoholism) should be excluded, and a lipid profile performed to measure Total-C, HDL-C, and TG. For patients with TG less than 400 mg/dl (<4.5 mmol/L), LDL-C can be estimated using the following equation:

LDL-C = Total-C - [0.2 × (TG) + HDL-C]

For TG levels >400 mg/dl (>4.5 mmol/L), this equation is less accurate and LDL-C concentrations should be determined by ultracentrifugation. In hypertriglyceridemic patients, LDL-C may be low or normal despite elevated Total-C. In such cases, Altocor is not indicated.

The National Cholesterol Education Program (NCEP) Treatment Guidelines are summarized in TABLE 13.

TABLE 13 *NCEP Treatment Guidelines: LDL-C Goals and Cutpoints for Therapeutic Lifestyle Changes and Drug Therapy in Different Risk Categories*

Risk Category	LDL Goal	LDL Level at Which to: Initiate Therapeutic Lifestyle Changes	Consider Drug Therapy
CHD or CHD risk equivalents (10 year risk >20%)	<100 mg/dl	≥100 mg/dl	≥130 mg/dl (100-129: drug optional)*
2+ Risk factors (10 year risk ≤20%)	<130 mg/dl	≥130 mg/dl	10 year risk 10-20%: ≥130 mg/dl 10 year risk <10%: ≥160 mg/dl
0-1 Risk factor†	<160 mg/dl	≥160 mg/dl	≥190 mg/dl (160-189: LDL-lowering drug optional)

CHD Coronary heart disease.

* Some authorities recommend use of LDL-lowering drugs in this category if an LDL-C level of <100 mg/dl cannot be achieved by therapeutic lifestyle changes. Others prefer use of drugs that primarily modify triglycerides and HCL-C, *e.g.,* nicotinic acid or fibrate. Clinical judgment also may call for deferring drug therapy in this subcategory.

† Almost all people with 0-1 risk factor have a 10 year risk <10%; thus, 10 year risk assessment in people with 0-1 risk factor is not necessary.

After the LDL-C goal has been achieved, if the TG is still >200 mg/dl, non-HDL-C (total-C minus HDL-C) becomes a secondary target of therapy. Non-HDL-C goals are set 30 mg/dl higher than LDL-C goals for each risk category.

At the time of hospitalization for an acute coronary event, consideration can be given to initiating drug therapy at discharge if the LDL-C is ≥130 mg/dl (see TABLE 13).

Since the goal of treatment is to lower LDL-C, the NCEP recommends that LDL-C levels be used to initiate and assess treatment response. Only if LDL-C levels are not available, should the Total-C be used to monitor therapy.

Although Altocor may be useful to reduce elevated LDL-C levels in patients with combined hypercholesterolemia and hypertriglyceridemia where hypercholesterolemia is the major abnormality (Type IIb hyperlipoproteinemia), it has not been studied in conditions where the major abnormality is elevation of chylomicrons, VLDL or IDL (*i.e.,* hyperlipoproteinemia types I, III, IV, or V). (See TABLE 14.)

TABLE 14 *Classification of Hyperlipoproteinemias*

Type	Lipoproteins Elevated	Lipid Elevations: Major	Minor
I (rare)	Chylomicrons	TG	TC*
IIa	LDL	TC	—
IIb	LDL, VLDL	TC	TG
III (rare)	IDL	TC/TG	—
IV	VLDL	TG	TC*
V (rare)	Chylomicrons, VLDL	TG	TC*

TC = Total cholesterol, TG = triglycerides, LDL = low-density lipoprotein, VLDL = very low-density lipoprotein, IDL = intermediate-density lipoprotein.

* Increases or no change.

NON-FDA APPROVED INDICATIONS

While not an FDA approved indication, lovastatin may be useful in patients with hypercholesterolemia secondary to nephrotic syndrome as well as in patients with chronic renal failure.

CONTRAINDICATIONS

MEVACOR TABLETS

Hypersensitivity to any component of this medication.

Active liver disease or unexplained persistent elevations of serum transaminases (see WARNINGS, Mevacor Tablets).

Pregnancy and Lactation

Atherosclerosis is a chronic process and the discontinuation of lipid-lowering drugs during pregnancy should have little impact on the outcome of long-term therapy of primary hypercholesterolemia. Moreover, cholesterol and other products of the cholesterol biosynthesis pathway are essential components for fetal development, including synthesis of steroids and cell membranes. Because of the ability of inhibitors of HMG-CoA reductase such as Mevacor to decrease the synthesis of cholesterol and possibly other products of the cholesterol biosynthesis pathway, Mevacor is contraindicated during pregnancy and in nursing mothers. **Mevacor should be administered to women of childbearing age only when such patients are highly unlikely to conceive.** If the patient becomes pregnant while taking this drug, Mevacor should be discontinued immediately and the patient should be apprised of the potential hazard to the fetus (see PRECAUTIONS, Mevacor Tablets, Pregnancy Category X).

ALTOCOR EXTENDED-RELEASE TABLETS

Hypersensitivity to any component of this medication. Active liver disease or unexplained persistent elevations of serum transaminases (see WARNINGS, Altocor Extended-Release Tablets).

Pregnancy and Lactation

Atherosclerosis is a chronic process and the discontinuation of lipid-lowering drugs during pregnancy should have little impact on the outcome of long-term therapy of primary hypercholesterolemia. Moreover, cholesterol and other products of the cholesterol biosynthesis pathway are essential components for fetal development, including synthesis of steroids and cell membranes. Because of the ability of inhibitors of HMG-CoA reductase such as Altocor to decrease the synthesis of cholesterol and possibly other products of the cholesterol biosynthesis pathway, Altocor is contraindicated during pregnancy and in nursing mothers. **Altocor should be administered to women of childbearing age only when such patients are highly unlikely to conceive.** If the patient becomes pregnant while taking this drug, Altocor should be discontinued immediately and the patient should be apprised of the potential hazard to the fetus (see PRECAUTIONS, Altocor Extended-Release Tablets, Pregnancy Category X).

WARNINGS

MEVACOR TABLETS

Myopathy/Rhabdomyolysis

Lovastatin, like other inhibitors of HMG-CoA reductase, occasionally causes myopathy manifested as muscle pain, tenderness or weakness with creatine kinase (CK) above 10X the upper limit of normal (ULN). Myopathy sometimes takes the form of rhabdomyolysis with or without acute renal failure secondary to myoglobinuria, and rare fatalities have occurred. The risk of myopathy is increased by high levels of HMG-CoA reductase inhibitory activity in plasma.

The risk of myopathy/rhabdomyolysis is increased by concomitant use of lovastatin with the following:

Potent inhibitors of CYP3A4: **Cyclosporine, itraconazole, ketoconazole, erythromycin, clarithromycin, HIV protease inhibitors, nefazodone, or large quantities of grapefruit juice (>1 quart daily), particularly with higher doses of lovastatin** (see below; CLINICAL PHARMACOLOGY, Mevacor Tablets, Pharmacokinetics; DRUG INTERACTIONS, Mevacor Tablets, CYP3A4 Interactions).

Lipid-lowering drugs that can cause myopathy when given alone: **Gemfibrozil, other fibrates, or lipid-lowering doses (≥1 g/day) of niacin, particularly with higher doses of lovastatin** (see below; CLINICAL PHARMACOLOGY, Mevacor Tablets, Pharmacokinetics; DRUG INTERACTIONS, Mevacor Tablets, Interactions With Lipid-Lowering Drugs That Can Cause Myopathy When Given Alone).

Other drugs: The risk of myopathy/rhabdomyolysis is increased when either amiodarone or verapamil is used concomitantly with higher doses of a closely related member of the HMG-CoA reductase inhibitor class (see DRUG INTERACTIONS, Mevacor Tablets, Other Drug Interactions).

The risk of myopathy/rhabdomyolysis is dose related.

In a clinical study (EXCEL) in which patients were carefully monitored and some interacting drugs were excluded, there was 1 case of myopathy among 4933 patients randomized to lovastatin 20-40 mg daily for 48 weeks, and 4 among 1649 patients randomized to 80 mg daily.

CONSEQUENTLY:

Use of lovastatin concomitantly with itraconazole, ketoconazole, erythromycin, clarithromycin, HIV protease inhibitors, nefazodone, or large quantities of grapefruit juice (>1 quart daily) should be avoided. If treatment with itraconazole, ketoconazole, erythromycin, or clarithromycin is unavoidable, therapy with lovastatin should be suspended during the course of treatment. Concomitant use with other medicines labeled as having a potent inhibitory effect on CYP3A4 at therapeutic doses should be avoided unless the benefits of combined therapy outweigh the increased risk.

The dose of lovastatin should not exceed 20 mg daily in patients receiving concomitant medication with cyclosporine, gemfibrozil, other fibrates or lipid-lowering doses (≥1 g/day) of niacin. The combined use of lovastatin with fibrates or niacin should be avoided unless the benefit of further alteration in lipid levels is likely to outweigh the increased risk of this drug combination. Addition of these drugs to lovastatin typically provides little additional reduction in LDL-C, but further reductions of TG and further increases in HDL-C may be obtained.

The dose of lovastatin should not exceed 40 mg daily in patients receiving concomitant medication with amiodarone or verapamil. The combined use of lovastatin at doses higher than 40 mg daily with amiodarone or verapamil should be avoided unless the clinical benefit is likely to outweigh the increased risk of myopathy.

All patients starting therapy with lovastatin, or whose dose of lovastatin is being increased, should be advised of the risk of myopathy and told to report

promptly any unexplained muscle pain, tenderness or weakness. Lovastatin therapy should be discontinued immediately if myopathy is diagnosed or suspected. The presence of these symptoms, and/or a CK level >10 times the ULN indicates myopathy. In most cases, when patients were promptly discontinued from treatment, muscle symptoms and CK increases resolved. Periodic CK determinations may be considered in patients starting therapy with lovastatin or whose dose is being increased, but there is no assurance that such monitoring will prevent myopathy.

Many of the patients who have developed rhabdomyolysis on therapy with lovastatin have had complicated medical histories, including renal insufficiency usually as a consequence of long-standing diabetes mellitus. Such patients merit closer monitoring. Therapy with lovastatin should be temporarily stopped a few days prior to elective major surgery and when any major medical or surgical condition supervenes.

Liver Dysfunction

Persistent increases (to more than 3 times the upper limit of normal) in serum transaminases occurred in 1.9% of adult patients who received lovastatin for at least 1 year in early clinical trials (see ADVERSE REACTIONS, Mevacor Tablets). When the drug was interrupted or discontinued in these patients, the transaminase levels usually fell slowly to pretreatment levels. The increases usually appeared 3-12 months after the start of therapy with lovastatin, and were not associated with jaundice or other clinical signs or symptoms. There was no evidence of hypersensitivity. In the EXCEL study, the incidence of persistent increases in serum transaminases over 48 weeks was 0.1% for placebo, 0.1% at 20 mg/day, 0.9% at 40 mg/day, and 1.5% at 80 mg/day in patients on lovastatin. However, in postmarketing experience with Mevacor, symptomatic liver disease has been reported rarely at all dosages (see ADVERSE REACTIONS, Mevacor Tablets).

In AFCAPS/TexCAPS, the number of participants with consecutive elevations of either alanine aminotransferase (ALT) or aspartate aminotransferase (AST) (>3 times the upper limit of normal), over a median of 5.1 years of follow-up, was not significantly different between the Mevacor and placebo groups (18 [0.6%] vs 11 [0.3%]). The starting dose of Mevacor was 20 mg/day; 50% of the Mevacor treated participants were titrated to 40 mg/day at Week 18. Of the 18 participants on Mevacor with consecutive elevations of either ALT or AST, 11 (0.7%) elevations occurred in participants taking 20 mg/day, while 7 (0.4%) elevations occurred in participants titrated to 40 mg/day. Elevated transaminases resulted in discontinuation of 6 (0.2%) participants from therapy in the Mevacor group (n=3304) and 4 (0.1%) in the placebo group (n=3301).

L

It is recommended that liver function tests be performed before the initiation of treatment, at 6 and 12 weeks after initiation of therapy or elevation in dose, and periodically thereafter (*e.g.*, semiannually). Patients who develop increased transaminase levels should be monitored with a second liver function evaluation to confirm the finding and be followed thereafter with frequent liver function tests until the abnormality(ies) returns to normal. Should an increase in AST or ALT of 3 times the upper limit of normal or greater persist, withdrawal of therapy with Mevacor is recommended.

The drug should be used with caution in patients who consume substantial quantities of alcohol and/or have a past history of liver disease. Active liver disease or unexplained transaminase elevations are contraindications to the use of lovastatin.

As with other lipid-lowering agents, moderate (less than 3 times the upper limit of normal) elevations of serum transaminases have been reported following therapy with Mevacor (see ADVERSE REACTIONS, Mevacor Tablets). These changes appeared soon after initiation of therapy with Mevacor, were often transient, were not accompanied by any symptoms and interruption of treatment was not required.

ALTOCOR EXTENDED-RELEASE TABLETS

Skeletal Muscle

Lovastatin and other inhibitors of HMG-CoA reductase occasionally cause myopathy, which is manifested as muscle pain or weakness associated with grossly elevated creatine kinase [>10× the upper limit of normal (ULN)]. **Rhabdomyolysis, with or without acute renal failure secondary to myoglobinuria, has been reported rarely and can occur at any time.** In the EXCEL study, there was 1 case of myopathy among 4933 patients randomized to lovastatin 20-40 mg daily for 48 weeks, and 4 among 1649 patients randomized to 80 mg daily. When drug treatment was interrupted or discontinued in these patients, muscle symptoms and creatine kinase (CK) increases promptly resolved. The risk of myopathy is increased by concomitant therapy with certain drugs, some of which were excluded by the EXCEL study design.

Myopathy Caused By Drug Interactions

The incidence and severity of myopathy are increased by concomitant administration of HMG-CoA reductase inhibitors with drugs that can cause myopathy when given alone, such as gemfibrozil and other fibrates, and lipid-lowering doses (≥1 g/day) of niacin (nicotinic acid).

In addition, the risk of myopathy may be increased by high levels of lovastatin, lovastatin acid and HMG-CoA reductase inhibitory activity in plasma. Lovastatin is metabolized by the cytochrome P450 isoform 3A4 (CYP3A4). Potent inhibitors of this metabolic pathway can raise the plasma levels of lovastatin, lovastatin acid and HMG-CoA reductase inhibitory activity and may increase the risk of myopathy. These include cyclosporine, the azole antifungals (itraconazole and ketoconazole), the macrolide antibiotics (erythromycin and clarithromycin), HIV protease inhibitors, the antidepressant nefazodone; and large quantities of grapefruit juice (>1 quart daily) (see below; CLINICAL PHARMACOLOGY, Altocor Extended-Release Tablets, Pharmacokinetics and Drug Metabolism; DRUG INTERACTIONS, Altocor Extended-Release Tablets; and DOSAGE AND ADMINISTRATION, Altocor Extended-Release Tablets).

Although the data are insufficient for lovastatin, the risk of myopathy appears to be increased when verapamil is used concomitantly with a closely related HMG-CoA reductase inhibitor (see DRUG INTERACTIONS, Altocor Extended-Release Tablets).

Reducing the Risk of Myopathy

1. **General Measures: Patients starting therapy with Altocor should be advised of the risk of myopathy, and told to report promptly unexplained muscle pain, tenderness or weakness.** A creatine kinase (CK) level above 10× ULN in a patient with unexplained muscle symptoms indicates myopathy. **Altocor therapy should be discontinued if myopathy is diagnosed or suspected.** In most cases, when patients were promptly discontinued from treatment, muscle symptoms and CK increases resolved.

Of the patients with rhabdomyolysis, many had complicated medical histories. Some had preexisting renal insufficiency, usually as a consequence of long-standing diabetes. In such patients, dose escalation requires caution. Also, as there are no known adverse consequences of brief interruption of therapy, treatment with Altocor should be stopped a few days before elective major surgery and when any major acute medical or surgical condition supervenes.

2. **Measures to reduce the risk of myopathy caused by drug interactions (see above and DRUG INTERACTIONS, Altocor Extended-Release Tablets). Physicians contemplating combined therapy with Altocor and any of the interacting drugs should weigh the potential benefits and risks, and should carefully monitor patients for any signs and symptoms of muscle pain, tenderness, or weakness, particularly during the initial months of therapy and during any periods of upward dosage titration of either drug.** Periodic CK determinations may be considered in such situations, but there is no assurance that such monitoring will prevent myopathy.

The combined use of Altocor with fibrates or niacin should be avoided unless the benefit of further alteration in lipid levels is likely to outweigh the increased risk of this drug combination. Combinations of fibrates or niacin with low doses of lovastatin have been used without myopathy in small, short-term clinical trials with careful monitoring. Addition of these drugs to lovastatin typically provides little additional reduction in LDL-C, but further reductions of TG and further increases in HDL-C may be obtained. If one of these drugs must be used with lovastatin, clinical experience suggests that the risk of myopathy is less with niacin than with the fibrates.

In patients taking concomitant cyclosporine, fibrates or niacin, the dose of Altocor should generally not exceed 20 mg/day (see DOSAGE AND ADMINISTRATION, Altocor Extended-Release Tablets and DOSAGE AND ADMINISTRATION, Altocor Extended-Release Tablets, Concomitant Lipid-Lowering Therapy), as the risk of myopathy increases substantially at higher doses. Concomitant use of Altocor with itraconazole, ketoconazole, erythromycin, clarithromycin, HIV protease inhibitors, nefazodone, or large quantities of grapefruit juice (>1 quart daily) is not recommended. If no alternative to a short course of treatment with itraconazole, ketoconazole, erythromycin, or clarithromycin is available, a brief suspension of Altocor therapy during such treatment can be considered, as there are no known adverse consequences to brief interruption of long-term cholesterol-lowering therapy.

Liver Dysfunction

Persistent increases (to more than 3 times the upper limit of normal) in serum transaminases occurred in 1.9% of adult patients who received lovastatin for at least 1 year in early clinical trials (see ADVERSE REACTIONS, Altocor Extended-Release Tablets). When the drug was interrupted or discontinued in these patients, the transaminase levels usually fell slowly to pretreatment levels. The increases usually appeared 3-12 months after the start of therapy with lovastatin, and were not associated with jaundice or other clinical signs or symptoms. There was no evidence of hypersensitivity.

Altocor

In controlled clinical trials (467 patients treated with Altocor and 329 patients treated with lovastatin immediate-release) no meaningful differences in transaminase elevations between the 2 treatments were observed.

Lovastatin Immediate-Release

In the EXCEL study, the incidence of persistent increases in serum transaminases over 48 weeks was 0.1% for placebo, 0.1% at 20 mg/day, 0.9% at 40 mg/day, and 1.5% at 80 mg/day in patients on lovastatin. However, in post-marketing experience with lovastatin immediate-release, symptomatic liver disease has been reported rarely at all dosages (see ADVERSE REACTIONS, Altocor Extended-Release Tablets).

In AFCAPS/TexCAPS, the number of participants with consecutive elevations of either alanine aminotransferase (ALT) or aspartate aminotransferase (AST) (>3 times the upper limit of normal), over a median of 5.1 years of follow-up, was not significantly different between the lovastatin immediate-release and placebo groups [18 (0.6%) vs 11 (0.3%)]. The starting dose of lovastatin immediate-release was 20 mg/day; 50% of the lovastatin immediate-release treated participants were titrated to 40 mg/day at Week 18. Of the 18 participants on lovastatin immediate-release with consecutive elevations of either ALT or AST, 11 (0.7%) elevations occurred in participants taking 20 mg/day, while 7 (0.4%) elevations occurred in participants titrated to 40 mg/day. Elevated transaminases resulted in discontinuation of 6 (0.2%) participants from therapy in the lovastatin immediate-release group (n=3304) and 4 (0.1%) in the placebo group (n=3301).

It is recommended that liver function tests be performed before the initiation of treatment, at 6 and 12 weeks after initiation of therapy or elevation of dose, and periodically thereafter (*e.g.*, semiannually).

Patients who develop increased transaminase levels should be monitored with a second liver function evaluation to confirm the finding and be followed thereafter with frequent liver function tests until the abnormality(ies) return to normal. Should an increase in AST or ALT of 3 times the upper limit of normal or greater persist, withdrawal of therapy with Altocor is recommended.

The drug should be used with caution in patients who consume substantial quantities of alcohol and/or have a past history of liver disease. Active liver disease or unexplained transaminase elevations are contraindications to the use of Altocor.

As with other lipid-lowering agents, moderate (less than 3 times the upper limit of normal) elevations of serum transaminases have been reported following therapy with lovastatin (see ADVERSE REACTIONS, Altocor Extended-Release Tablets). These changes appeared soon after initiation of therapy with lovastatin, were often transient, were not accompanied by any symptoms and interruption of treatment was not required.

PRECAUTIONS

MEVACOR TABLETS

General

Lovastatin may elevate creatine phosphokinase and transaminase levels (see WARNINGS, Mevacor Tablets and ADVERSE REACTIONS, Mevacor Tablets). This should be considered in the differential diagnosis of chest pain in a patient on therapy with lovastatin.

Homozygous Familial Hypercholesterolemia

Mevacor is less effective in patients with the rare homozygous familial hypercholesterolemia, possibly because these patients have no functional LDL receptors. Mevacor appears to be more likely to raise serum transaminases (see ADVERSE REACTIONS, Mevacor Tablets) in these homozygous patients.

Information for the Patient

Patients should be advised about substances they should not take concomitantly with lovastatin and be advised to report promptly unexplained muscle pain, tenderness, or weakness (see DRUG INTERACTIONS and WARNINGS, Mevacor Tablets, Myopathy/Rhabdomyolysis). Patients should also be advised to inform other physicians prescribing a new medication that they are taking Mevacor.

Endocrine Function

HMG-CoA reductase inhibitors interfere with cholesterol synthesis and as such might theoretically blunt adrenal and/or gonadal steroid production. Results of clinical trials with drugs in this class have been inconsistent with regard to drug effects on basal and reserve steroid levels. However, clinical studies have shown that lovastatin does not reduce basal plasma cortisol concentration or impair adrenal reserve, and does not reduce basal plasma testosterone concentration. Another HMG-CoA reductase inhibitor has been shown to reduce the plasma testosterone response to HCG. In the same study, the mean testosterone response to HCG was slightly but not significantly reduced after treatment with lovastatin 40 mg daily for 16 weeks in 21 men. The effects of HMG-CoA reductase inhibitors on male fertility have not been studied in adequate numbers of male patients. The effects, if any, on the pituitary-gonadal axis in pre-menopausal women are unknown. Patients treated with lovastatin who develop clinical evidence of endocrine dysfunction should be evaluated appropriately. Caution should also be exercised if an HMG-CoA reductase inhibitor or other agent used to lower cholesterol levels is administered to patients also receiving other drugs (*e.g.*, ketoconazole, spironolactone, cimetidine) that may decrease the levels or activity of endogenous steroid hormones.

CNS Toxicity

Lovastatin produced optic nerve degeneration (Wallerian degeneration of retinogeniculate fibers) in clinically normal dogs in a dose-dependent fashion starting at 60 mg/kg/day, a dose that produced mean plasma drug levels about 30 times higher than the mean drug level in humans taking the highest recommended dose (as measured by total enzyme inhibitory activity). Vestibulocochlear Wallerian-like degeneration and retinal ganglion cell chromatolysis were also seen in dogs treated for 14 weeks at 180 mg/kg/day, a dose which resulted in a mean plasma drug level (C_{max}) similar to that seen with the 60 mg/kg/day dose.

CNS vascular lesions, characterized by perivascular hemorrhage and edema, mononuclear cell infiltration of perivascular spaces, perivascular fibrin deposits and necrosis of small vessels, were seen in dogs treated with lovastatin at a dose of 180 mg/kg/day, a dose which produced plasma drug levels (C_{max}) which were about 30 times higher than the mean values in humans taking 80 mg/day.

Similar optic nerve and CNS vascular lesions have been observed with other drugs of this class.

Cataracts were seen in dogs treated for 11 and 28 weeks at 180 mg/kg/day and 1 year at 60 mg/kg/day.

Carcinogenesis, Mutagenesis, and Impairment of Fertility

In a 21 month carcinogenic study in mice, there was a statistically significant increase in the incidence of hepatocellular carcinomas and adenomas in both males and females at 500 mg/kg/day. This dose produced a total plasma drug exposure 3-4 times that of humans given the highest recommended dose of lovastatin (drug exposure was measured as total HMG-CoA reductase inhibitory activity in extracted plasma). Tumor increases were not seen at 20 and 100 mg/kg/day, doses that produced drug exposures of 0.3 to 2 times that of humans at the 80 mg/day dose. A statistically significant increase in pulmonary adenomas was seen in female mice at approximately 4 times the human drug exposure. (Although mice were given 300 times the human dose [HD] on a mg/kg body weight basis, plasma levels of total inhibitory activity were only 4 times higher in mice than in humans given 80 mg of Mevacor.)

There was an increase in incidence of papilloma in the non-glandular mucosa of the stomach of mice beginning at exposures of 1-2 times that of humans. The glandular mucosa was not affected. The human stomach contains only glandular mucosa.

In a 24 month carcinogenicity study in rats, there was a positive dose response relationship for hepatocellular carcinogenicity in males at drug exposures between 2-7 times that of human exposure at 80 mg/day (doses in rats were 5, 30, and 180 mg/kg/day).

An increased incidence of thyroid neoplasms in rats appears to be a response that has been seen with other HMG-CoA reductase inhibitors.

A chemically similar drug in this class was administered to mice for 72 weeks at 25, 100, and 400 mg/kg body weight, which resulted in mean serum drug levels approximately 3, 15, and 33 times higher than the mean human serum drug concentration (as total inhibitory activity) after a 40 mg oral dose. Liver carcinomas were significantly increased in high dose females and mid- and high dose males, with a maximum incidence of 90% in males. The incidence of adenomas of the liver was significantly increased in mid- and high dose females. Drug treatment also significantly increased the incidence of lung adenomas in mid- and high dose males and females. Adenomas of the Harderian gland (a gland of the eye of rodents) were significantly higher in high dose mice than in controls.

No evidence of mutagenicity was observed in a microbial mutagen test using mutant strains of *Salmonella typhimurium* with or without rat or mouse liver metabolic activation. In addition, no evidence of damage to genetic material was noted in an *in vitro* alkaline elution assay using rat or mouse hepatocytes, a V-79 mammalian cell forward mutation study, an *in vitro* chromosome aberration study in CHO cells, or an *in vivo* chromosomal aberration assay in mouse bone marrow.

Drug-related testicular atrophy, decreased spermatogenesis, spermatocytic degeneration and giant cell formation were seen in dogs starting at 20 mg/kg/day. Similar findings were seen with another drug in this class. No drug-related effects on fertility were found in studies with lovastatin in rats. However, in studies with a similar drug in this class, there was decreased fertility in male rats treated for 34 weeks at 25 mg/kg body weight, although this effect was not observed in a subsequent fertility study when this same dose was administered for 11 weeks (the entire cycle of spermatogenesis, including epididymal maturation). In rats treated with this same reductase inhibitor at 180 mg/kg/day, seminiferous tubule degeneration (necrosis and loss of spermatogenic epithelium) was observed. No microscopic changes were observed in the testes from rats of either study. The clinical significance of these findings is unclear.

Pregnancy Category X

See CONTRAINDICATIONS, Mevacor Tablets.

Safety in pregnant women has not been established.

Lovastatin has been shown to produce skeletal malformations at plasma levels 40 times the human exposure (for mouse fetus) and 80 times the human exposure (for rat fetus) based on mg/m^2 surface area (doses were 800 mg/kg/day). No drug-induced changes were seen in either species at multiples of 8 times (rat) or 4 times (mouse) based on surface area. No evidence of malformations was noted in rabbits at exposures up to 3 times the human exposure (dose of 15 mg/kg/day, highest tolerated dose).

Rare reports of congenital anomalies have been received following intrauterine exposure to HMG-CoA reductase inhibitors. In a review[2] of approximately 100 prospectively followed pregnancies in women exposed to Mevacor or another structurally related HMG-CoA reductase inhibitor, the incidences of congenital anomalies, spontaneous abortions and fetal deaths/stillbirths did not exceed what would be expected in the general population. The number of cases is adequate only to exclude a 3- to 4-fold increase in congenital anomalies over the background incidence. In 89% of the prospectively followed pregnancies, drug treatment was initiated prior to pregnancy and was discontinued at some point in the first trimester when pregnancy was identified. As safety in pregnant women has not been established and there is no apparent benefit to therapy with Mevacor during pregnancy (see CONTRAINDICATIONS, Mevacor Tablets), treatment should be immediately discontinued as soon as pregnancy is recognized. Mevacor should be administered to women of childbearing potential only when such patients are highly unlikely to conceive and have been informed of the potential hazards.

Nursing Mothers

It is not known whether lovastatin is excreted in human milk. Because a small amount of another drug in this class is excreted in human breast milk and because of the potential for serious adverse reactions in nursing infants, women taking Mevacor should not nurse their infants (see CONTRAINDICATIONS, Mevacor Tablets).

Pediatric Use

Safety and effectiveness in patients 10-17 years of age with heFH have been evaluated in controlled clinical trials of 48 weeks duration in adolescent boys and controlled clinical trials of 24 weeks duration in girls who were at least 1 year post-menarche. Patients treated with lovastatin had an adverse experience profile generally similar to that of patients treated with placebo. **Doses greater than 40 mg have not been studied in this population.** In these limited controlled studies, there was no detectable effect on growth or sexual maturation in the adolescent boys or on menstrual cycle length in girls. See ADVERSE REACTIONS, Mevacor Tablets, Adolescent Patients (ages 10-17 years) and DOSAGE AND ADMINISTRATION, Mevacor Tablets, Adolescent Patients (10-17 years of age) With Heterozygous Familial Hypercholesterolemia. Adolescent females should be counseled on appropriate contraceptive methods while on lovastatin therapy (see CONTRAINDICATIONS, Mevacor Tablets and PRECAUTIONS, Mevacor Tablets, Pregnancy Category X). **Lovastatin has not been studied in pre-pubertal patients or patients younger than 10 years of age.**

Geriatric Use

A pharmacokinetic study with lovastatin showed the mean plasma level of HMG-CoA reductase inhibitory activity to be approximately 45% higher in elderly patients between 70-78 years of age compared with patients between 18-30 years of age; however, clinical study experience in the elderly indicates that dosage adjustment based on this age-related pharmacokinetic difference is not needed. In the two large clinical studies conducted with lovastatin (EXCEL and AFCAPS/TexCAPS), 21% (3,094/14,850) of patients were ≥65 years of age. Lipid-lowering efficacy with lovastatin was at least as great in elderly patients compared with younger patients, and there were no overall differences in safety over the 20-80 mg/day dosage range (see CLINICAL PHARMACOLOGY, Mevacor Tablets).

ALTOCOR EXTENDED-RELEASE TABLETS

General

Altocor may elevate creatine phosphokinase and transaminase levels (see WARNINGS, Altocor Extended-Release Tablets and ADVERSE REACTIONS, Altocor Extended-Release Tablets). This should be considered in the differential diagnosis of chest pain in a patient on therapy with Altocor.

Homozygous Familial Hypercholesterolemia

Lovastatin immediate-release was found to be less effective in patients with the rare homozygous familial hypercholesterolemia, possibly because these patients have no functional LDL receptors. Lovastatin immediate-release appears to be more likely to raise serum transaminases (see ADVERSE REACTIONS, Altocor Extended-Release Tablets) in these homozygous patients.

Information for the Patient

The Altocor extended-release tablets should be swallowed whole and not chewed or crushed.

L

Patients should be advised to report promptly unexplained muscle pain, tenderness or weakness (see WARNINGS, Altocor Extended-Release Tablets, Skeletal Muscle).

Endocrine Function

HMG-CoA reductase inhibitors interfere with cholesterol synthesis and as such might theoretically blunt adrenal and/or gonadal steroid production. Results of clinical trials with drugs in this class have been inconsistent with regard to drug effects on basal and reserve steroid levels. However, clinical studies have shown that lovastatin does not reduce basal plasma cortisol concentration or impair adrenal reserve, and does not reduce basal plasma testosterone concetration. Another HMG-CoA reductase inhibitor has been shown to reduce the plasma testosterone response to HCG. In the same study, the mean testosterone response to HCG was slightly but not significantly reduced after treatment with lovastatin 40 mg daily for 16 weeks in 21 men. The effects of HMG-CoA reductase inhibitors on male fertility have not been studied in adequate numbers of male patients. The effects, if any, on the pituitary-gonadal axis in premenopausal women are unknown. Patients treated with lovastatin who develop clinical evidence of endocrine dysfunction should be evaluated appropriately. Caution should also be exercised if an HMG-CoA reductase inhibitor or other agent used to lower cholesterol levels is administered to patients also receiving other drugs (*e.g.*, ketoconazole, spironolactone, cimetidine) that may decrease the levels or activity of endogenous steroid hormones.

CNS Toxicity

Lovastatin produced optic nerve degeneration (Wallerian degeneration of retinogeniculate fibers) in clinically normal dogs in a dose-dependent fashion starting at 60 mg/kg/day, a dose that produced mean plasma drug levels about 30 times higher than the mean drug level in humans taking the highest recommended dose (as measured by total enzyme inhibitory activity). Vestibulocochlear Wallerian-like degeneration and retinal ganglion cell chromatolysis were also seen in dogs treated for 14 weeks at 180 mg/kg/day, a dose which resulted in a mean plasma drug level (C_{max}) similar to that seen with the 60 mg/kg/day dose.

CNS vascular lesions, characterized by perivascular hemorrhage and edema, mononuclear cell infiltration of perivascular spaces, perivascular fibrin deposits and necrosis of small vessels, were seen in dogs treated with lovastatin at a dose of 180 mg/kg/day, a dose which produced plasma drug levels (C_{max}) which were about 30 times higher than the mean values in humans taking 80 mg/day.

Similar optic nerve and CNS vascular lesions have been observed with other drugs of this class. Cataracts were seen in dogs treated for 11 and 28 weeks at 180 mg/kg/day and 1 year at 60 mg/kg/day.

L

Carcinogenesis, Mutagenesis, and Impairment of Fertility

In a 21 month carcinogenic study in mice with lovastatin immediate-release, there was a statistically significant increase in the incidence of hepatocellular carcinomas and adenomas in both males and females at 500 mg/kg/day. This dose produced a total plasma drug exposure 3-4 times that of humans given the highest recommended dose of lovastatin (drug exposure was measured as total HMG-CoA reductase inhibitory activity in extracted plasma). Tumor increases were not seen at 20 and 100 mg/kg/day, doses that produced drug exposures of 0.3 to 2 times that of humans at the 80 mg/day lovastatin immediate-release dose. A statistically significant increase in pulmonary adenomas was seen in female mice at approximately 4 times the human drug exposure. [Although mice were given 300 times the human dose (HD) on a mg/kg body weight basis, plasma levels of total inhibitory activity were only 4 times higher in mice than in humans given 80 mg of lovastatin immediate-release].

There was an increase in incidence of papilloma in the non-glandular mucosa of the stomach of mice beginning at exposures of 1-2 times that of humans given lovastatin immediate-release. The glandular mucosa was not affected. The human stomach contains only glandular mucosa.

In a 24 month carcinogenicity study in rats, there was a positive dose response relationship for hepatocellular carcinogenicity in males at drug exposures between 2-7 times that of human exposure at 80 mg/day lovastatin immediate-release (doses in rats were 5, 30 and 180 mg/kg/day).

An increased incidence of thyroid neoplasms in rats appears to be a response that has been seen with other HMG-CoA reductase inhibitors.

A chemically similar drug in this class was administered to mice for 72 weeks at 25, 100, and 400 mg/kg body weight, which resulted in mean serum drug levels approximately 3, 15, and 33 times higher than the mean human serum drug concentration (as total inhibitory activity) after a 40 mg oral dose of lovastatin immediate-release. Liver carcinomas were significantly increased in high-dose females and mid- and high-dose males, with a maximum incidence of 90% in males. The incidence of adenomas of the liver was significantly increased in mid- and high-dose females. Drug treatment also significantly increased the incidence of lung adenomas in mid- and high-dose males and females. Adenomas of the Harderian gland (a gland of the eye of rodents) were significantly higher in high dose mice than in controls.

No evidence of mutagenicity was observed with lovastatin immediate-release in a microbial mutagen test using mutant strains of *Salmonella typhimurium* with or without rat or mouse liver metabolic activation. In addition, no evidence of damage to genetic material was noted in an *in vitro* alkaline elution assay using rat or mouse hepatocytes, a V-79 mammalian cell forward mutation study, an *in vitro* chromosome aberration study in CHO cells, or an *in vivo* chromosomal aberration assay in mouse bone marrow.

Drug-related testicular atrophy, decreased spermatogenesis, spermatocytic degeneration and giant cell formation were seen in dogs starting at 20 mg/kg/day with lovastatin immediate-release. Similar findings were seen with another drug in this class. No drug-related effects on fertility were found in studies with lovastatin in rats. However, in studies with a similar drug in this class, there was decreased fertility in male rats treated for 34 weeks at 25 mg/kg body weight, although this effect was not observed in a subsequent fertility study when this same dose was administered for 11 weeks (the entire cycle of spermatogenesis, including epididymal maturation). In rats treated with this same reductase inhibitor at 180 mg/kg/day, seminiferous tubule degeneration (necrosis and loss of spermatogenic epithelium) was observed. No microscopic changes were observed in the testes from rats of either study. The clinical significance of these findings is unclear.

Pregnancy Category X

See CONTRAINDICATIONS, Altocor Extended-Release Tablets.

Safety in pregnant women has not been established. Lovastatin immediate-release has been shown to produce skeletal malformations at plasma levels 40 times the human exposure (for mouse fetus) and 80 times the human exposure (for rat fetus) based on mg/m^2 surface area (doses were 800 mg/kg/day). No drug-induced changes were seen in either species at multiples of 8 times (rat) or 4 times (mouse) based on surface area. No evidence of malformations was noted in rabbits at exposures up to 3 times the human exposure (dose of 15 mg/kg/day, highest tolerated dose of lovastatin immediate-release).

Rare reports of congenital anomalies have been received following intrauterine exposure to HMG-CoA reductase inhibitors. In a review[2] of approximately 100 prospectively followed pregnancies in women exposed to lovastatin immediate-release or another structurally related HMG-CoA reductase inhibitor, the incidences of congenital anomalies, spontaneous abortions and fetal deaths/stillbirths did not exceed what would be expected in the general population. The number of cases is adequate only to exclude a 3- to 4-fold increase in congenital anomalies over the background incidence. In 89% of the prospectively followed pregnancies, drug treatment was initiated prior to pregnancy and was discontinued at some point in the first trimester when pregnancy was identified. As safety in pregnant women has not been established and there is no apparent benefit to therapy with Altocor during pregnancy (see CONTRAINDICATIONS, Altocor Extended-Release Tablets), treatment should be immediately discontinued as soon as pregnancy is recognized. Altocor should be administered to women of child-bearing potential only when such patients are highly unlikely to conceive and have been informed of the potential hazard.

Nursing Mothers

It is not known whether lovastatin is excreted in human milk. Because a small amount of another drug in this class is excreted in human breast milk and because of the potential for serious adverse reactions in nursing infants, women taking Altocor should not nurse their infants (see CONTRAINDICATIONS, Altocor Extended-Release Tablets).

Pediatric Use

Safety and effectiveness in pediatric patients have not been established. Because pediatric patients are not likely to benefit from cholesterol lowering for at least a decade and because experience with this drug is limited (no studies in subjects below the age of 20 years), treatment of pediatric patients with Altocor is not recommended at this time.

Geriatric Use

Altocor

Of the 467 patients who received Altocor in controlled clinical studies, 18% were 65 years and older. Of the 297 patients who received Altocor in uncontrolled clinical studies, 22% were 65 years and older. No overall differences in effectiveness or safety were observed between these patients and younger patients, and other reported clinical experience has not identified differences in response between the elderly and younger patients, but greater sensitivity of some older individuals cannot be ruled out.

Lovastatin Immediate-Release

In pharmacokinetic studies with lovastatin immediate-release, the mean plasma level of HMG-CoA reductase inhibitory activity was shown to be approximately 45% higher in elderly patients between 70-78 years of age compared with patients between 18-30 years of age; however, clinical study experience in the elderly indicates that dosage adjustment based on this age-related pharmacokinetic difference is not needed. In the two large clinical studies conducted with lovastatin immediate-release (EXCEL and AFCAPS/TexCAPS), 21% (3,094/14,850) of patients were ≥65 years of age. Lipid-lowering efficacy with lovastatin was at least as great in elderly patients compared with younger patients, and there were no overall differences in safety over the 20-80 mg dosage range (see CLINICAL PHARMACOLOGY, Altocor Extended-Release Tablets).

DRUG INTERACTIONS

MEVACOR TABLETS

CYP3A4 Interactions

Lovastatin is metabolized by CYP3A4 but has no CYP3A4 inhibitory activity; therefore it is not expected to affect the plasma concentrations of other drugs metabolized by CYP3A4. Potent inhibitors of CYP3A4 (below) increase the risk of myopathy by reducing the elimination of lovastatin.

See WARNINGS, Mevacor Tablets, Myopathy/Rhabdomyolysis and CLINICAL PHARMACOLOGY, Mevacor Tablets, Pharmacokinetics.

- **Itraconazole**
- **Ketoconazole**
- **Erythromycin**
- **Clarithromycin**
- **HIV protease inhibitors**
- **Nefazodone**
- **Cyclosporine**
- **Large quantities of grapefruit juice (>1 quart daily)**

Interactions With Lipid-Lowering Drugs That Can Cause Myopathy When Given Alone

The risk of myopathy is also increased by the following lipid-lowering drugs that are not potent CYP3A4 inhibitors, but which can cause myopathy when given alone.

See WARNINGS, Mevacor Tablets, Myopathy/Rhabdomyolysis.

- **Gemfibrozil**
- **Other fibrates**
- **Niacin (nicotinic acid) (≥1 g/day)**

Other Drug Interactions

Amiodarone or Verapamil

The risk of myopathy/rhabdomyolysis is increased when either amiodarone or verapamil is used concomitantly with a closely related member of the HMG-CoA reductase inhibitor class (see WARNINGS, Mevacor Tablets, Myopathy/Rhabdomyolysis).

Coumarin Anticoagulants

In a small clinical trial in which lovastatin was administered to warfarin treated patients, no effect on prothrombin time was detected. However, another HMG-CoA reductase inhibitor has been found to produce a less than 2 second increase in prothrombin time in healthy volunteers receiving low doses of warfarin. Also, bleeding and/or increased prothrombin time have been reported in a few patients taking coumarin anticoagulants concomitantly with lovastatin. It is recommended that in patients taking anticoagulants, prothrombin time be determined before starting lovastatin and frequently enough during early therapy to insure that no significant alteration of prothrombin time occurs. Once a stable prothrombin time has been documented, prothrombin times can be monitored at the intervals usually recommended for patients on coumarin anticoagulants. If the dose of lovastatin is changed, the same procedure should be repeated. Lovastatin therapy has not been associated with bleeding or with changes in prothrombin time in patients not taking anticoagulants.

Propranolol

In normal volunteers, there was no clinically significant pharmacokinetic or pharmacodynamic interaction with concomitant administration of single doses of lovastatin and propranolol.

Digoxin

In patients with hypercholesterolemia, concomitant administration of lovastatin and digoxin resulted in no effect on digoxin plasma concentrations.

Oral Hypoglycemic Agents

In pharmacokinetic studies of Mevacor in hypercholesterolemic non-insulin dependent diabetic patients, there was no drug interaction with glipizide or with chlorpropamide.

ALTOCOR EXTENDED-RELEASE TABLETS

Drug interaction studies have not been performed with Altocor. The types, frequencies and magnitude of drug interactions that may be encountered when Altocor is administered with other drugs may differ from the drug interactions encountered with the lovastatin immediate-release formulation. In addition, as the drug exposure with Altocor 60 mg is greater than that with lovastatin immediate-release 80 mg (maximum recommended dose), the severity and magnitude of drug interactions that may be encountered with Altocor 60 mg are not known. It is therefore recommended that the following precautions and recommendations for the concomitant administration of lovastatin immediate-release with other drugs be interpreted with caution, and that the monitoring of the pharmacologic effects of Altocor and/or other concomitantly administered drugs be undertaken where appropriate.

Gemfibrozil and Other Fibrates, Lipid-Lowering Doses (≥1 g/day) of Niacin (nicotinic acid)

These drugs increase the risk of myopathy when given concomitantly with lovastatin (see WARNINGS, Altocor Extended-Release Tablets, Skeletal Muscle). There has been evidence to suggest that the increased risk of myopathy may be partly due to the pharmacokinetic interactions between gemfibrozil and lovastatin.

CYP3A4 Interactions

Lovastatin has no CYP3A4 inhibitory activity; therefore, it is not expected to affect the plasma concentrations of other drugs metabolized by CYP3A4. However, lovastatin itself is a substrate for CYP3A4. Potent inhibitors of CYP3A4 may increase the risk of myopathy by increasing the plasma concentration of lovastatin, lovastatin acid and HMG-CoA reductase inhibitory activity during lovastatin therapy. These inhibitors include cyclosporine, itraconazole, ketoconazole, erythromycin, clarithromycin, HIV protease inhibitors, nefazodone and large quantities of grapefruit juice (>1 quart daily) (see CLINICAL PHARMACOLOGY, Altocor Extended-Release Tablets, Pharmacokinetics and Drug Metabolism and WARNINGS, Altocor Extended-Release Tablets, Skeletal Muscle).

Grapefruit juice contains 1 or more components that inhibit CYP3A4 and can increase the plasma concentrations of drugs metabolized by CYP3A4. Large quantities of grapefruit juice (>1 quart daily) significantly increase the serum concentrations of lovastatin and its β-hydroxyacid metabolite during lovastatin therapy and should be avoided (see CLINICAL PHARMACOLOGY, Altocor Extended-Release Tablets, Pharmacokinetics and Drug Metabolism and WARNINGS, Altocor Extended-Release Tablets, Skeletal Muscle).

Although the data are insufficient for lovastatin, the risk of myopathy appears to be increased when verapamil is used concomitantly with a closely related HMG-CoA reductase inhibitor (see WARNINGS, Altocor Extended-Release Tablets, Skeletal Muscle).

Coumarin Anticoagulants

In a small clinical trial in which lovastatin was administered to warfarin treated patients, no effect on prothrombin time was detected. However, another HMG-CoA reductase inhibitor has been found to produce a less than 2 seconds increase in prothrombin time in healthy volunteers receiving low doses of warfarin. Also, bleeding and/or increased prothrombin time has been reported in a few patients taking coumarin anticoagulants concomitantly with lovastatin. It is recommended that in patients taking anticoagulants, prothrombin time be determined before starting lovastatin and frequently enough during early therapy to ensure that no significant alteration of prothrombin time occurs. Once a stable prothrombin time has been documented, prothrombin times can be monitored at the intervals usually recommended for patients on coumarin anticoagulants. If the dose of lovastatin is changed, the same procedure should be repeated. Lovastatin therapy has not been associated with bleeding or with changes in prothrombin time in patients not taking anticoagulants.

Antipyrine

Lovastatin had no effect on the pharmacokinetics of antipyrine or its metabolites. However, since lovastatin is metabolized by the cytochrome P450 isoform 3A4, this does not preclude an interaction with other drugs metabolized by the same isoform (see WARNINGS, Altocor Extended-Release Tablets, Skeletal Muscle).

Propranolol

In normal volunteers, there was no clinically significant pharmacokinetic or pharmacodynamic interaction with concomitant administration of single doses of lovastatin and propranolol.

Digoxin

In patients with hypercholesterolemia, concomitant administration of lovastatin and digoxin resulted in no effect on digoxin plasma concentrations.

Oral Hypoglycemic Agents

In pharmacokinetic studies of lovastatin immediate-release in hypercholesterolemic non-insulin dependent diabetic patients, there was no drug interaction with glipizide or with chlorpropamide.

ADVERSE REACTIONS

MEVACOR TABLETS

Mevacor is generally well tolerated; adverse reactions usually have been mild and transient.

Phase 3 Clinical Studies

In Phase 3 controlled clinical studies involving 613 patients treated with Mevacor, the adverse experience profile was similar to that shown below for the 8245-patient EXCEL study (see Expanded Clinical Evaluation of Lovastatin [EXCEL] Study).

Persistent increases of serum transaminases have been noted (see WARNINGS, Mevacor Tablets, Liver Dysfunction). About 11% of patients had elevations of CK levels of at least twice the normal value on 1 or more occasions. The corresponding values for the control agent cholestyramine was 9%. This was attributable to the noncardiac fraction of CK. Large increases in CK have sometimes been reported (see WARNINGS, Mevacor Tablets, Myopathy/Rhabdomyolysis).

Expanded Clinical Evaluation of Lovastatin (EXCEL) Study

Mevacor was compared to placebo in 8245 patients with hypercholesterolemia (total-C 240-300 mg/dl [6.2-7.8 mmol/L]) in the randomized, double-blind, parallel, 48 week EXCEL study. Clinical adverse experiences reported as possibly, probably or definitely drug-related in ≥1% in any treatment group are shown in TABLE 15. For no event was the incidence on drug and placebo statistically different.

TABLE 15

		Mevacor			
	Placebo (n=1663)	20 mg qpm (n=1642)	40 mg qpm (n=1645)	20 mg bid (n=1646)	40 mg bid (n=1649)
Body as a Whole					
Asthenia	1.4%	1.7%	1.4%	1.5%	1.2%
Gastrointestinal					
Abdominal pain	1.6%	2.0%	2.0%	2.2%	2.5%
Constipation	1.9%	2.0%	3.2%	3.2%	3.5%
Diarrhea	2.3%	2.6%	2.4%	2.2%	2.6%
Dyspepsia	1.9%	1.3%	1.3%	1.0%	1.6%
Flatulence	4.2%	3.7%	4.3%	3.9%	4.5%
Nausea	2.5%	1.9%	2.5%	2.2%	2.2%
Musculoskeletal					
Muscle cramps	0.5%	0.6%	0.8%	1.1%	1.0%
Myalgia	1.7%	2.6%	1.8%	2.2%	3.0%
Nervous System/Psychiatric					
Dizziness	0.7%	0.7%	1.2%	0.5%	0.5%
Headache	2.7%	2.6%	2.8%	2.1%	3.2%
Skin					
Rash	0.7%	0.8%	1.0%	1.2%	1.3%
Special Senses					
Blurred vision	0.8%	1.1%	0.9%	0.9%	1.2%

Other clinical adverse experiences reported as possibly, probably or definitely drug-related in 0.5-1.0% of patients in any drug-treated group are listed below. In all these cases the incidence on drug and placebo was not statistically different.

Body as a Whole: Chest pain.

Gastrointestinal: Acid regurgitation, dry mouth, vomiting.

Musculoskeletal: Leg pain, shoulder pain, arthralgia.

Nervous System/Psychiatric: Insomnia, paresthesia.

Skin: Alopecia, pruritus.

Special Senses: Eye irritation.

In the EXCEL study, 4.6% of the patients treated up to 48 weeks were discontinued due to clinical or laboratory adverse experiences which were rated by the investigator as possibly, probably or definitely related to therapy with Mevacor. The value for the placebo group was 2.5%.

Air Force/Texas Coronary Atherosclerosis Prevention Study (AFCAPS/TexCAPS)

In AFCAPS/TexCAPS involving 6605 participants treated with 20-40 mg/day of Mevacor (n=3304) or placebo (n=3301), the safety and tolerability profile of the group treated with Mevacor was comparable to that of the group treated with placebo during a median of 5.1 years of follow-up. The adverse experiences reported in AFCAPS/TexCAPS were similar to those reported in EXCEL (see Expanded Clinical Evaluation of Lovastatin (EXCEL) Study).

Concomitant Therapy
In controlled clinical studies in which lovastatin was administered concomitantly with cholestyramine, no adverse reactions peculiar to this concomitant treatment were observed. The adverse reactions that occurred were limited to those reported previously with lovastatin or cholestyramine. Other lipid-lowering agents were not administered concomitantly with lovastatin during controlled clinical studies. Preliminary data suggests that the addition of gemfibrozil to therapy with lovastatin is not associated with greater reduction in LDL-C than that achieved with lovastatin alone. In uncontrolled clinical studies, most of the patients who have developed myopathy were receiving concomitant therapy with cyclosporine, gemfibrozil or niacin (nicotinic acid). The combined use of lovastatin at doses exceeding 20 mg/day with cyclosporine, gemfibrozil, other fibrates or lipid-lowering doses (≥1 g/day) of niacin should be avoided (see WARNINGS, Mevacor Tablets, Myopathy/Rhabdomyolysis).

The following effects have been reported with drugs in this class. Not all the effects listed below have necessarily been associated with lovastatin therapy.

Skeletal: Muscle cramps, myalgia, myopathy, rhabdomyolysis, arthralgias.

Neurological: Dysfunction of certain cranial nerves (including alteration of taste, impairment of extra-ocular movement, facial paresis), tremor, dizziness, vertigo, memory loss, paresthesia, peripheral neuropathy, peripheral nerve palsy, psychic disturbances, anxiety, insomnia, depression.

Hypersensitivity Reactions: *An apparent hypersensitivity syndrome has been reported rarely which has included 1 or more of the following features:* Anaphylaxis, angioedema, lupus erythematous-like syndrome, polymyalgia rheumatica, dermatomyositis, vasculitis, purpura, thrombocytopenia, leukopenia, hemolytic anemia, positive ANA, ESR increase, eosinophilia, arthritis, arthralgia, urticaria, asthenia, photosensitivity, fever, chills, flushing, malaise, dyspnea, toxic epidermal necrolysis, erythema multiforme, including Stevens-Johnson syndrome.

Gastrointestinal: Pancreatitis, hepatitis, including chronic active hepatitis, cholestatic jaundice, fatty change in liver; and rarely, cirrhosis, fulminant hepatic necrosis, and hepatoma; anorexia, vomiting.

Skin: Alopecia, pruritus. A variety of skin changes (*e.g.*, nodules, discoloration, dryness of skin/mucous membranes, changes to hair/nails) have been reported.

Reproductive: Gynecomastia, loss of libido, erectile dysfunction.

Eye: Progression of cataracts (lens opacities), ophthalmoplegia.

Laboratory Abnormalities: Elevated transaminases, alkaline phosphatase, γ-glutamyl transpeptidase, and bilirubin; thyroid function abnormalities.

Adolescent Patients (ages 10-17 years)
In a 48 week controlled study in adolescent boys with heFH (n=132) and a 24 week controlled study in girls who were at least 1 year post-menarche with heFH (n=54), the safety and tolerability profile of the groups treated with Mevacor (10-40 mg daily) was generally similar to that of the groups treated with placebo (see PRECAUTIONS, Mevacor Tablets, Pediatric Use).

ALTOCOR EXTENDED-RELEASE TABLETS
Altocor
Altocor Clinical Studies
In clinical studies with Altocor, adverse reactions have generally been mild and transient. In controlled studies with 467 patients who received Altocor, <3% of patients were discontinued due to adverse experiences attributable to Altocor. This was similar to the discontinuation rate in the placebo and lovastatin immediate-release treatment groups. Pooled results from clinical studies with Altocor show that the most frequently reported adverse reactions in the Altocor group were infection, headache and accidental injury. Similar incidences of these adverse reactions were seen in the lovastatin and placebo groups. The most frequent adverse events thought to be related to Altocor were nausea, abdominal pain, insomnia, dyspepsia, headache, asthenia, and myalgia. In controlled trials (*e.g.*, vs placebo and vs lovastatin immediate-release), clinical adverse experiences reported as in ≥5% in any treatment group are shown in TABLE 16.

TABLE 16 *Pooled Controlled Studies TESS by Body System and COSTART Term, Most Common (≥5% in Any Group)*

Body System / COSTART Term	Placebo n=34	Altocor n=467	Mevacor n=329
Body as a Whole			
Infection	3 (9%)	52 (11%)	52 (16%)
Accidental injury	3 (9%)	26 (6%)	12 (4%)
Asthenia	2 (6%)	12 (3%)	6 (2%)
Headache	2 (6%)	34 (7%)	26 (8%)
Back pain	1 (3%)	23 (5%)	18 (5%)
Flu syndrome	1 (3%)	24 (5%)	18 (5%)
Pain	0	14 (3%)	17 (5%)
Digestive			
Diarrhea	2 (6%)	15 (3%)	8 (2%)
Musculoskeletal			
Arthralgia	2 (6%)	24 (5%)	20 (6%)
Myalgia	5 (15%)	14 (3%)	11 (3%)
Nervous			
Dizziness	2 (6%)	10 (2%)	5 (2%)
Respiratory			
Sinusitis	1 (3%)	17 (4%)	20 (6%)
Urogenital			
Urinary tract infection	2 (6%)	8 (2%)	9 (3%)

Lovastatin Immediate-Release
Lovastatin Immediate-Release Phase 3 Clinical Studies
In Phase 3 controlled clinical studies involving 613 patients treated with lovastatin immediate-release, the adverse experience profile was similar to that shown below for the 8245 patient EXCEL study [see Expanded Clinical Evaluation of Lovastatin (EXCEL) Study]. Persistent increases of serum transaminases have been noted (see WARNINGS, Altocor Extended-Release Tablets, Liver Dysfunction). About 11% of patients had elevations of CK levels of at least twice the normal value on 1 or more occasions. The corresponding values for the control agent cholestyramine was 9 %. This was attributable to the noncardiac fraction of CK. Large increases in CK have sometimes been reported (see WARNINGS, Altocor Extended-Release Tablets, Skeletal Muscle).

Expanded Clinical Evaluation of Lovastatin (EXCEL) Study
Lovastatin immediate-release was compared to placebo in 8245 patients with hypercholesterolemia [Total-C 240-300 mg/dl (6.2-7.8 mmol/L)] in the randomized, double-blind, parallel, 48 week EXCEL study. Clinical adverse experiences reported as possibly, probably or definitely drug-related in ≥1% in any treatment group are shown in TABLE 17. For no event was the incidence on drug and placebo statistically different.

TABLE 17 *Clinical Adverse Events Reported as Possibly, Probably or Definitely Drug-Related in ≥ 1% in Any Treatment Group in the EXCEL Study*

		Lovastatin IR		Lovastatin IR	
	Placebo (n=1663)	20 mg qpm (n=1642)	40 mg qpm (n=1645)	20 mg bid (n=1646)	40 mg bid (n=1649)
Body as a Whole					
Asthenia	1.4%	1.7%	1.4%	1.5%	1.2%
Gastrointestinal					
Abdominal pain	1.6%	2.0%	2.0%	2.2%	2.5%
Constipation	1.9%	2.0%	3.2%	3.2%	3.5%
Diarrhea	2.3%	2.6%	2.4%	2.2%	2.6%
Dyspepsia	1.9%	1.3%	1.3%	1.0%	1.6%
Flatulence	4.2%	3.7%	4.3%	3.9%	4.5%
Nausea	2.5%	1.9%	2.5%	2.2%	2.2%
Musculoskeletal					
Muscle cramps	0.5%	0.6%	0.8%	1.1%	1.0%
Myalgia	1.7%	2.6%	1.8%	2.2%	3.0%
Nervous System/Psychiatric					
Dizziness	0.7%	0.7%	1.2%	0.5%	0.5%
Headache	2.7%	2.6%	2.8%	2.1%	3.2%
Skin					
Rash	0.7%	0.8%	1.0%	1.2%	1.3%
Special Senses					
Blurred vision	0.8%	1.1%	0.9%	0.9%	1.2%

Other clinical adverse experiences reported as possibly, probably or definitely drug-related in 0.5-1.0% of patients in any drug-treated group are listed below. In all these cases the incidence on drug and placebo was not statistically different.

Body as a Whole: Chest pain.

Gastrointestinal: Acid regurgitation, dry mouth, vomiting.

Musculoskeletal: Leg pain, shoulder pain, arthralgia.

Nervous System/Psychiatric: Insomnia, paresthesia.

Skin: Alopecia, pruritus.

Special Senses: Eye irritation.

In the EXCEL study, 4.6% of the patients treated up to 48 weeks were discontinued due to clinical or laboratory adverse experiences which were rated by the investigator as possibly, probably or definitely related to therapy with lovastatin immediate-release. The value for the placebo group was 2.5%.

Air Force/Texas Coronary Atherosclerosis Prevention Study (AFCAPS/TexCAPS)
In AFCAPS/TexCAPS involving 6605 participants treated with 20-40 mg/day of lovastatin immediate-release (n=3304) or placebo (n=3301), the safety and tolerability profile of the group treated with lovastatin immediate-release was comparable to that of the group treated with placebo during a median of 5.1 years of follow-up. The adverse experiences reported in AFCAPS/TexCAPS were similar to those reported in EXCEL [see ADVERSE REACTIONS, Altocor Extended-Release Tablets, Expanded Clinical Evaluation of Lovastatin (EXCEL) Study].

Concomitant Therapy
In controlled clinical studies in which lovastatin immediate-release was administered concomitantly with cholestyramine, no adverse reactions peculiar to this concomitant treatment were observed. The adverse reactions that occurred were limited to those reported previously with lovastatin or cholestyramine. Other lipid-lowering agents were not administered concomitantly with lovastatin during controlled clinical studies. Preliminary data suggests that the addition of gemfibrozil to therapy with lovastatin is not associated with greater reduction in LDL-C than that achieved with lovastatin alone. In uncontrolled clinical studies, most of the patients who have developed myopathy were receiving concomitant therapy with cyclosporine, gemfibrozil or niacin (nicotinic acid) (see WARNINGS, Altocor Extended-Release Tablets, Skeletal Muscle).

The following effects have been reported with drugs in this class. Not all the effects listed below have necessarily been associated with lovastatin therapy.

Skeletal: Muscle cramps, myalgia, myopathy, rhabdomyolysis, arthralgias.

Neurological: Dysfunction of certain cranial nerves (including alteration of taste, impairment of extra-ocular movement, facial paresis), tremor, dizziness, vertigo, memory loss, paresthesia, peripheral neuropathy, peripheral nerve palsy, psychic disturbances, anxiety, insomnia, depression.

Hypersensitivity Reactions: *An apparent hypersensitivity syndrome has been reported rarely which has included 1 or more of the following features:* Anaphylaxis, angioedema, lupus erythematous-like syndrome, polymyalgia rheumatica, vasculitis, purpura, thrombocytopenia, leukopenia, hemolytic anemia, positive ANA, ESR increase, eosinophilia, arthritis, arthralgia, urticaria, asthenia, photosensitivity, fever, chills, flushing, malaise, dyspnea, toxic epidermal necrolysis, erythema multiforme, including Stevens-Johnson syndrome.

Gastrointestinal: Pancreatitis, hepatitis, including chronic active hepatitis, cholestatic jaundice, fatty change in liver; and rarely, cirrhosis, fulminant hepatic necrosis, and hepatoma; anorexia, vomiting.

Skin: Alopecia, pruritus. A variety of skin changes (*e.g.*, nodules, discoloration, dryness of skin/mucous membranes, changes to hair/nails) have been reported.

Reproductive: Gynecomastia, loss of libido, erectile dysfunction.

Eye: Progression of cataracts (lens opacities), ophthalmoplegia.

Laboratory Abnormalities: Elevated transaminases, alkaline phosphatase, γ-glutamyl transpeptidase, and bilirubin; thyroid function abnormalities.

DOSAGE AND ADMINISTRATION

MEVACOR TABLETS

The patient should be placed on a standard cholesterol-lowering diet before receiving Mevacor and should continue on this diet during treatment with Mevacor (see TABLE 11 for details on dietary therapy). Mevacor should be given with meals.

Adult Patients

The usual recommended starting dose is 20 mg once a day given with the evening meal. The recommended dosing range is 10-80 mg/day in single or 2 divided doses; the maximum recommended dose is 80 mg/day. Doses should be individualized according to the recommended goal of therapy (see TABLE 11 and CLINICAL PHARMACOLOGY, Mevacor Tablets). Patients requiring reductions in LDL-C of 20% or more to achieve their goal (see INDICATIONS AND USAGE, Mevacor Tablets) should be started on 20 mg/day of Mevacor. A starting dose of 10 mg may be considered for patients requiring smaller reductions. Adjustments should be made at intervals of 4 weeks or more.

Cholesterol levels should be monitored periodically and consideration should be given to reducing the dosage of Mevacor if cholesterol levels fall significantly below the targeted range.

Dosage in Patients Taking Cyclosporine

In patients taking cyclosporine concomitantly with lovastatin (see WARNINGS, Mevacor Tablets, Myopathy/Rhabdomyolysis), therapy should begin with 10 mg of Mevacor and should not exceed 20 mg/day.

Dosage in Patients Taking Amiodarone or Verapamil

In patients taking amiodarone or verapamil concomitantly with Mevacor, the dose should not exceed 40 mg/day (see WARNINGS, Mevacor Tablets, Myopathy/Rhabdomyolysis and DRUG INTERACTIONS, Mevacor Tablets, Other Drug Interactions).

Adolescent Patients (10-17 years of age) With Heterozygous Familial Hypercholesterolemia

The recommended dosing range is 10-40 mg/day; the maximum recommended dose is 40 mg/day. Doses should be individualized according to the recommended goal of therapy (see NCEP Pediatric Panel Guidelines,[3] CLINICAL PHARMACOLOGY, Mevacor Tablets, and INDICATIONS AND USAGE, Mevacor Tablets). Patients requiring reductions in LDL-C of 20% or more to achieve their goal should be started on 20 mg/day of Mevacor. A starting dose of 10 mg may be considered for patients requiring smaller reductions. Adjustments should be made at intervals of 4 weeks or more.

Concomitant Lipid-Lowering Therapy

Mevacor is effective alone or when used concomitantly with bile-acid sequestrants. If Mevacor is used in combination with gemfibrozil, other fibrates or lipid-lowering doses ($\geq$1 g/day) of niacin, the dose of Mevacor should not exceed 20 mg/day (see WARNINGS, Mevacor Tablets, Myopathy/Rhabdomyolysis and DRUG INTERACTIONS, Mevacor Tablets).

Dosage in Patients With Renal Insufficiency

In patients with severe renal insufficiency (creatinine clearance $<$30 ml/min), dosage increases above 20 mg/day should be carefully considered and, if deemed necessary, implemented cautiously (see CLINICAL PHARMACOLOGY, Mevacor Tablets and WARNINGS, Mevacor Tablets, Myopathy/Rhabdomyolysis).

ALTOCOR EXTENDED-RELEASE TABLETS

The patient should be placed on a standard cholesterol-lowering diet before receiving Altocor and should continue on this diet during treatment with Altocor (see TABLE 13 for details on dietary therapy).

The usual recommended starting dose is 20, 40 or 60 mg once a day given in the evening at bedtime. The recommended dosing range is 10-60 mg/day, in single doses. Doses should be individualized according to the recommended goal of therapy (see TABLE 13 and CLINICAL PHARMACOLOGY, Altocor Extended-Release Tablets). A starting dose of 10 mg may be considered for patients requiring smaller reductions. Adjustments should be made at intervals of 4 weeks or more.

In patients taking cyclosporine concomitantly with Altocor (see WARNINGS, Altocor Extended-Release Tablets, Skeletal Muscle), therapy should begin with 10 mg of Altocor and should not exceed 20 mg/day.

Cholesterol levels should be monitored periodically and consideration should be given to reducing the dosage of Altocor if cholesterol levels fall significantly below the targeted range.

Concomitant Lipid-Lowering Therapy

Use of Altocor with fibrates or niacin should generally be avoided. However, if Altocor is used in combination with fibrates or niacin, the dose of Altocor should generally not exceed 20 mg (see WARNINGS, Altocor Extended-Release Tablets, Skeletal Muscle and DRUG INTERACTIONS, Altocor Extended-Release Tablets).

Dosage in Patients With Renal Insufficiency

In patients with severe renal insufficiency (creatinine clearance $<$30 ml/min), dosage increases above 20 mg/day should be carefully considered and, if deemed necessary, implemented cautiously (see CLINICAL PHARMACOLOGY, Altocor Extended-Release Tablets and WARNINGS, Altocor Extended-Release Tablets, Skeletal Muscle).

HOW SUPPLIED

MEVACOR TABLETS

Mevacor tablets are supplied in:

10 mg: Peach, octagonal tablets, coded "MSD 730" on one side and "MEVACOR" on the other.

20 mg: Light blue, octagonal tablets, coded "MSD 731" on one side and "MEVACOR" on the other.

40 mg: Green, octagonal tablets, coded "MSD 732" on one side and "MEVACOR" on the other.

Storage: Store between 5-30°C (41-86°F). Mevacor tablets must be protected from light and stored in a well-closed, light-resistant container.

ALTOCOR EXTENDED-RELEASE TABLETS

Altocor extended-release tablets are supplied in:

10 mg: Round, convex shaped extended-release dark orange-colored tablets imprinted with Andrx logo and "10" on one side.

20 mg: Round, convex shaped extended-release orange-colored tablets imprinted with Andrx logo and "20" on one side.

40 mg: Round, convex shaped extended-release peach-colored tablets imprinted with Andrx logo and "40" on one side.

60 mg: Round, convex shaped extended-release light peach-colored tablets imprinted with Andrx logo and "60" on one side.

Storage: Store at controlled room temperature 20-25°C (68-77°F) Avoid excessive heat and humidity.

PRODUCT LISTING - RATED THERAPEUTICALLY EQUIVALENT

Tablet - Oral - 10 mg			
60's	$80.64	GENERIC, Geneva Pharmaceuticals	00781-1323-60
60's	$80.65	GENERIC, Mylan Pharmaceuticals Inc	00378-6510-91
60's	$80.70	GENERIC, Purepac Pharmaceutical Company	00228-2633-06
60's	$80.73	GENERIC, Teva Pharmaceuticals Usa	00093-0926-06
60's	$80.73	GENERIC, Eon Labs Manufacturing Inc	00185-0070-60
100's	$134.42	GENERIC, Udl Laboratories Inc	51079-0974-20
100's	$134.54	GENERIC, Par Pharmaceutical Inc	49884-0754-01
100's	$134.55	GENERIC, Eon Labs Manufacturing Inc	00185-0070-01
Tablet - Oral - 20 mg			
60's	$142.21	GENERIC, Geneva Pharmaceuticals	00781-1210-60
60's	$142.25	GENERIC, Mylan Pharmaceuticals Inc	00378-6520-91
60's	$142.30	GENERIC, Purepac Pharmaceutical Company	00228-2634-06
60's	$142.37	GENERIC, Teva Pharmaceuticals Usa	00093-0576-06
60's	$142.37	GENERIC, Eon Labs Manufacturing Inc	00185-0072-60
100's	$237.08	GENERIC, Udl Laboratories Inc	51079-0975-20
100's	$237.28	GENERIC, Eon Labs Manufacturing Inc	00185-0072-01
100's	$241.53	GENERIC, Par Pharmaceutical Inc	49884-0755-01
Tablet - Oral - 40 mg			
60's	$256.00	GENERIC, Geneva Pharmaceuticals	00781-1213-60
60's	$256.10	GENERIC, Purepac Pharmaceutical Company	00228-2635-06
60's	$256.10	GENERIC, Mylan Pharmaceuticals Inc	00378-6540-91
60's	$256.28	GENERIC, Teva Pharmaceuticals Usa	00093-0928-06
60's	$256.28	GENERIC, Eon Labs Manufacturing Inc	00185-0074-60
100's	$426.83	GENERIC, Udl Laboratories Inc	51079-0976-20
100's	$427.11	GENERIC, Par Pharmaceutical Inc	49884-0756-01
100's	$427.14	GENERIC, Eon Labs Manufacturing Inc	00185-0074-01

PRODUCT LISTING - EQUIVALENTS NOT AVAILABLE

Tablet - Oral - 10 mg			
30's	$44.40	MEVACOR, Physicians Total Care	54868-1968-00
60's	$89.70	MEVACOR, Merck & Company Inc	00006-0730-61
Tablet - Oral - 20 mg			
3's	$6.25	MEVACOR, Allscripts Pharmaceutical Company	54569-0613-03
6's	$12.51	MEVACOR, Allscripts Pharmaceutical Company	54569-0613-04
30's	$68.70	MEVACOR, Allscripts Pharmaceutical Company	54569-0613-00
30's	$73.17	MEVACOR, Physicians Total Care	54868-0686-01
30's	$92.26	MEVACOR, Pd-Rx Pharmaceuticals	55289-0400-30
30's	$147.74	MEVACOR, Physicians Total Care	54868-0686-03
60's	$137.41	MEVACOR, Allscripts Pharmaceutical Company	54569-0613-02
60's	$144.87	MEVACOR, Cheshire Drugs	55175-5046-06
60's	$158.19	MEVACOR, Merck & Company Inc	00006-0731-61
90's	$187.58	MEVACOR, Allscripts Pharmaceutical Company	54569-8011-00
90's	$217.15	MEVACOR, Physicians Total Care	54868-0686-04
100's	$224.98	MEVACOR, Allscripts Pharmaceutical Company	54569-0613-01
100's	$245.45	MEVACOR, Physicians Total Care	54868-0686-02
100's	$268.39	MEVACOR, Merck & Company Inc	00006-0731-28
Tablet - Oral - 40 mg			
30's	$121.49	MEVACOR, Allscripts Pharmaceutical Company	54569-3256-00
30's	$130.76	MEVACOR, Physicians Total Care	54868-1087-01
30's	$218.34	MEVACOR, Pd-Rx Pharmaceuticals	55289-0548-30

60's	$242.98	MEVACOR, Allscripts Pharmaceutical Company	54569-3256-01
60's	$260.35	MEVACOR, Physicians Total Care	54868-1087-00
60's	$284.76	MEVACOR, Merck & Company Inc	00006-0732-61
90 x 12	$4698.45	MEVACOR, Merck & Company Inc	00006-0732-94
Tablet, Extended Release - Oral - 40 mg			
30's	$54.00	ALTOCOR, Andrx Pharmaceuticals	62022-0780-30
Tablet, Extended Release - Oral - 60 mg			
30's	$61.50	ALTOCOR, Andrx Pharmaceuticals	62022-0781-30

Lovastatin; Niacin *(003547)*

For related information, see the comparative table section in Appendix A.

Categories: Hypercholesterolemia; Hyperlipidemia; FDA Approved 2001 Dec; Pregnancy Category X
Drug Classes: Antihyperlipidemics; HMG CoA reductase inhibitors; Nicotinic acid derivatives
Brand Names: Advicor
Cost of Therapy: $50.02 (Hypercholesterolemia; Advicor; 20 mg; 500 mg; 1 tablet/day; 30 day supply)

DESCRIPTION

Note: The trade name has been used throughout this monograph for clarity.
Advicor contains niacin extended-release and lovastatin in combination. Niacin, a B complex vitamin, and lovastatin, an inhibitor of 3-hydroxy-3-methylglutaryl-coenzyme A (HMG-CoA) reductase, are both lipid-altering agents. Niacin is nicotinic acid, or 3-pyridinecarboxylic acid. Niacin is a white, nonhygroscopic crystalline powder that is very soluble in water, boiling ethanol and propylene glycol. It is insoluble in ethyl ether. The empirical formula of niacin is $C_6H_5NO_2$ and its molecular weight is 123.11.

Lovastatin is [1S -[1(α)(R*),3(α),7(β),8(β)(2S*,4S*),8a(β)]]-1,2,3,7,8,8a-hexahydro-3,7-dimethyl-8-[2-(tetrahydro-4-hydroxy-6-oxo-2H-pyran-2-yl)ethyl]-1-naphthalenyl 2-methylbutanoate. Lovastatin is a white, nonhygroscopic crystalline powder that is insoluble in water and sparingly soluble in ethanol, methanol, and acetonitrile. The empirical formula of lovastatin is $C_{24}H_{36}O_5$ and its molecular weight is 404.55.

Advicor tablets contain the labeled amount of niacin and lovastatin and have the following inactive ingredients: Hydroxypropyl methylcellulose, povidone, stearic acid, polyethylene glycol, titanium dioxide, polysorbate 80. The individual tablet strengths (expressed in terms of mg niacin/mg lovastatin) contain the following coloring agents: *Advicor 500 mg/20 mg:* Synthetic red and yellow iron oxides; *Advicor 750 mg/20 mg:* FD&C yellow no. 6 aluminum lake; *Advicor 1000 mg/20 mg:* Synthetic red, yellow, and black iron oxides.

L

CLINICAL PHARMACOLOGY

A variety of clinical studies have demonstrated that elevated levels of total cholesterol (TC), low-density lipoprotein cholesterol (LDL-C), and apolipoprotein B-100 (Apo B) promote human atherosclerosis. Similarly, decreased levels of high-density lipoprotein cholesterol (HDL-C) are associated with the development of atherosclerosis. Epidemiological investigations have established that cardiovascular morbidity and mortality vary directly with the level of TC and LDL-C, and inversely with the level of HDL-C.

Cholesterol-enriched triglyceride-rich lipoproteins, including very low-density lipoproteins (VLDL), intermediate-density lipoproteins (IDL), and their remnants, can also promote atherosclerosis. Elevated plasma triglycerides (TG) are frequently found in a triad with low HDL-C levels and small LDL particles, as well as in association with non-lipid metabolic risk factors for coronary heart disease (CHD). As such, total plasma TG have not consistently been shown to be an independent risk factor for CHD.

As an adjunct to diet, the efficacy of niacin and lovastatin in improving lipid profiles (either individually, or in combination with each other, or niacin in combination with other statins) for the treatment of dyslipidemia has been well documented. The effect of combined therapy with niacin and lovastatin on cardiovascular morbidity and mortality has not been determined.

EFFECTS ON LIPIDS

Advicor

Advicor reduces LDL-C, TC, and TG, and increases HDL-C due to the individual actions of niacin and lovastatin. The magnitude of individual lipid and lipoprotein responses may be influenced by the severity and type of underlying lipid abnormality.

Niacin

Niacin functions in the body after conversion to nicotinamide adenine dinucleotide (NAD) in the NAD coenzyme system. Niacin (but not nicotinamide) in gram doses reduces LDL-C, Apo B, Lp(a), TG, and TC, and increases HDL-C. The increase in HDL-C is associated with an increase in apolipoprotein A-I (Apo A-I) and a shift in the distribution of HDL subfractions. These shifts include an increase in the HDL2:HDL3 ratio, and an elevation in lipoprotein A-I (Lp A-I, an HDL-C particle containing only Apo A-I). In addition, preliminary reports suggest that niacin causes favorable LDL particle size transformations, although the clinical relevance of this effect is not yet clear.

Lovastatin

Lovastatin has been shown to reduce both normal and elevated LDL-C concentrations. Apo B also falls substantially during treatment with lovastatin. Since each LDL-C particle contains one molecule of Apo B, and since little Apo B is found in other lipoproteins, this strongly suggests that lovastatin does not merely cause cholesterol to be lost from LDL-C, but also reduces the concentration of circulating LDL particles. In addition, lovastatin can produce increases of variable magnitude in HDL-C, and modestly reduces VLDL-C and plasma TG. The effects of lovastatin on Lp(a), fibrinogen, and certain other independent biochemical risk markers for coronary heart disease are not well characterized.

MECHANISM OF ACTION

Niacin

The mechanism by which niacin alters lipid profiles is not completely understood and may involve several actions, including partial inhibition of release of free fatty acids from adipose tissue, and increased lipoprotein lipase activity (which may increase the rate of chylomicron triglyceride removal from plasma). Niacin decreases the rate of hepatic synthesis of VLDL C and LDL C, and does not appear to affect fecal excretion of fats, sterols, or bile acids.

Lovastatin

Lovastatin is a specific inhibitor of 3-hydroxy-3-methylglutaryl-coenzyme A (HMG-CoA) reductase, the enzyme that catalyzes the conversion of HMG-CoA to mevalonate. The conversion of HMG-CoA to mevalonate is an early step in the biosynthetic pathway for cholesterol. Lovastatin is a prodrug and has little, if any, activity until hydrolyzed to its active beta-hydroxyacid form, lovastatin acid. The mechanism of the LDL-lowering effect of lovastatin may involve both reduction of VLDL-C concentration and induction of the LDL receptor, leading to reduced production and/or increased catabolism of LDL-C.

PHARMACOKINETICS

Absorption and Bioavailability

Advicor

In single-dose studies of Advicor, rate and extent of niacin and lovastatin absorption were bioequivalent under fed conditions to that from extended-release niacin and lovastatin tablets, respectively. After administration of two Advicor 1000 mg/20 mg tablets, peak niacin concentrations averaged about 18 μg/ml and occurred about 5 hours after dosing; about 72% of the niacin dose was absorbed according to the urinary excretion data. Peak lovastatin concentrations averaged about 11 ng/ml and occurred about 2 hours after dosing.

The extent of niacin absorption from Advicor was increased by administration with food. The administration of two Advicor 1000 mg/20 mg tablets under low-fat or high-fat conditions resulted in a 22-30% increase in niacin bioavailability relative to dosing under fasting conditions. Lovastatin bioavailability is affected by food. Lovastatin C_{max} was increased 48% and 21% after a high- and a low-fat meal, respectively, but the lovastatin AUC was decreased 26% and 24% after a high- and a low-fat meal, respectively, compared to those under fasting conditions.

Niacin

Due to extensive and saturable first-pass metabolism, niacin concentrations in the general circulation are dose dependent and highly variable. Peak steady-state niacin concentrations were 0.6, 4.9, and 15.5 μg/ml after doses of 1000, 1500, and 2000 mg extended-release niacin once daily (given as two 500 mg, two 750 mg, and two 1000 mg tablets, respectively).

Lovastatin

Lovastatin appears to be incompletely absorbed after oral administration. Because of extensive hepatic extraction, the amount of lovastatin reaching the systemic circulation as active inhibitors after oral administration is low (<5%) and shows considerable interindividual variation. Peak concentrations of active and total inhibitors occur within 2-4 hours after lovastatin administration.

Lovastatin absorption appears to be increased by at least 30% by grapefruit juice; however, the effect is dependent on the amount of grapefruit juice consumed and the interval between grapefruit juice and lovastatin ingestion.

With a once-a-day dosing regimen, plasma concentrations of total inhibitors over a dosing interval achieved a steady-state between the second and third days of therapy and were about 1.5 times those following a single dose of lovastatin.

Distribution

Niacin

Niacin is less than 20% bound to human serum proteins and distributes into milk. Studies using radiolabeled niacin in mice show that niacin and its metabolites concentrate in the liver, kidney, and adipose tissue.

Lovastatin

Both lovastatin and its beta-hydroxyacid metabolite are highly bound (>95%) to human plasma proteins. Distribution of lovastatin or its metabolites into human milk is unknown; however, lovastatin distributes into milk in rats. In animal studies, lovastatin concentrated in the liver, and crossed the blood-brain and placental barriers.

Metabolism

Niacin

Niacin undergoes rapid and extensive first-pass metabolism that is dose-rate specific and, at the doses used to treat dyslipidemia, saturable. In humans, one pathway is through a simple conjugation step with glycine to form nicotinuric acid (NUA). NUA is then excreted, although there may be a small amount of reversible metabolism back to niacin. The other pathway results in the formation of NAD. It is unclear whether nicotinamide is formed as a precursor to, or following the synthesis of, NAD. Nicotinamide is further metabolized to at least N-methylnicotinamide (MNA) and nicotinamide-N-oxide (NNO). MNA is further metabolized to two other compounds, N-methyl-2-pyridone-5-carboxamide (2PY) and N-methyl-4-pyridone-5-carboxamide (4PY). The formation of 2PY appears to predominate over 4PY in humans.

Lovastatin

Lovastatin undergoes extensive first-pass extraction and metabolism by cytochrome P450 3A4 in the liver, its primary site of action. The major active metabolites present in human plasma are the beta-hydroxyacid of lovastatin (lovastatin acid), its 6′-hydroxy derivative, and two additional metabolites.

Elimination

Advicor

Niacin is primarily excreted in urine mainly as metabolites. After a single dose of Advicor, at least 60% of the niacin dose was recovered in urine as unchanged niacin and its metabolites. The plasma half-life for lovastatin was about 4.5 hours in single-dose studies.

Niacin

The plasma half-life for niacin is about 20-48 minutes after oral administration and dependent on dose administered. Following multiple oral doses of extended-release niacin, up to 12% of the dose was recovered in urine as unchanged niacin depending on dose administered. The ratio of metabolites recovered in the urine was also dependent on the dose administered.

Lovastatin

Lovastatin is excreted in urine and bile, based on studies of lovastatin. Following an oral dose of radiolabeled lovastatin in man, 10% of the dose was excreted in urine and 83% in feces. The latter represents absorbed drug equivalents excreted in bile, as well as any unabsorbed drug.

Special Populations

Hepatic

No pharmacokinetic studies have been conducted in patients with hepatic insufficiency for either niacin or lovastatin (see WARNINGS, Liver Dysfunction).

Renal

No information is available on the pharmacokinetics of niacin in patients with renal insufficiency.

In a study of patients with severe renal insufficiency (creatinine clearance 10-30 ml/min), the plasma concentrations of total inhibitors after a single dose of lovastatin were approximately 2-fold higher than those in healthy volunteers. In a study of patients with severe renal insufficiency (creatinine clearance 10-30 ml/min), the plasma concentrations of total inhibitors after a single dose of lovastatin were approximately 2-fold higher than those in healthy volunteers.

Advicor should be used with caution in patients with renal disease.

Gender

Plasma concentrations of niacin and metabolites after single- or multiple-dose administration of niacin are generally higher in women than in men, with the magnitude of the difference varying with dose and metabolite. Recovery of niacin and metabolites in urine, however, is generally similar for men and women, indicating similar absorption for both genders. The gender differences observed in plasma niacin and metabolite levels may be due to gender-specific differences in metabolic rate or volume of distribution. Data from clinical trials suggest that women have a greater hypolipidemic response than men at equivalent doses of extended-release niacin and Advicor.

In a multiple-dose study, plasma concentrations of active and total HMG-CoA reductase inhibitors were 20-50% higher in women than in men. In two single-dose studies with Advicor, lovastatin concentrations were about 30% higher in women than men, and total HMG-CoA reductase inhibitor concentrations were about 20-25% greater in women.

In a multi-center, randomized, double-blind, active-comparator study in patients with Type IIa and IIb hyperlipidemia, Advicor was compared to single-agent treatment (extended-release niacin and lovastatin). The treatment effects of Advicor compared to lovastatin and extended-release niacin differed for males and females with a significantly larger treatment effect seen for females. The mean percent change from baseline at endpoint for LDL-C, TG, and HDL-C by gender are shown in TABLE 1.

TABLE 1 *Mean Percent Change From Baseline at Endpoint for LDL-C, HDL-C and TG by Gender*

	Advicor 2000 mg/40 mg		Extended-Release Niacin 2000 mg		Lovastatin 40 mg	
	Women (n=22)	Men (n=30)	Women (n=28)	Men (n=28)	Women (n=21)	Men (n=38)
LDL-C	-47%	-34%	-12%	-9%	-31%	-31%
HDL-C	+33%	+24%	+22%	+15%	+3%	+7%
TG	-48%	-35%	-25%	-15%	-15%	-23%

INDICATIONS AND USAGE

Advicor is a fixed-dose combination product and is not indicated for initial therapy (see DOSAGE AND ADMINISTRATION). Therapy with lipid-altering agents should be only one component of multiple risk-factor intervention in individuals at significantly increased risk for atherosclerotic vascular disease due to hypercholesterolemia. Initial medical therapy is indicated with a single agent as an adjunct to diet when the response to a diet restricted in saturated fat and cholesterol and other nonpharmacologic measures alone has been inadequate (see also TABLE 7 and the NCEP treatment guidelines[1]).

Advicor is indicated for the treatment of primary hypercholesterolemia (heterozygous familial and nonfamilial) and mixed dyslipidemia (Frederickson Types IIa and IIb; TABLE 6) in:

Patients treated with lovastatin who require further TG-lowering or HDL-raising who may benefit from having niacin added to their regimen.

Patients treated with niacin who require further LDL-lowering who may benefit from having lovastatin added to their regimen.

GENERAL RECOMMENDATIONS

Prior to initiating therapy with a lipid-lowering agent, secondary causes for hypercholesterolemia (*e.g.*, poorly controlled diabetes mellitus, hypothyroidism, nephrotic syndrome, dysproteinemias, obstructive liver disease, other drug therapy, alcoholism) should be excluded, and a lipid profile performed to measure TC, HDL-C, and TG.

TABLE 6 *Classification of Hyperlipoproteinemias*

Type	Lipoproteins Elevated	Lipid Elevations: Major	Lipid Elevations: Minor
I (rare)	Chylomicrons	TG	TC*
IIa	LDL	TC	—
IIb	LDL, VLDL	TC	TG
III (rare)	IDL	TC/TG	—
IV	VLDL	TG	TC*
V (rare)	Chylomicrons, VLDL	TG	TC*

TC = total cholesterol; TG = triglycerides; LDL = low-density lipoprotein; VLDL = very low-density lipoprotein; IDL = intermediate-density lipoprotein.
* Increased or no change.

For patients with TG <400 mg/dl, LDL-C can be estimated using the following equation:

LDL-C = TC - [(0.20 × TG) + HDL-C]

For TG levels >400 mg/dl, this equation is less accurate and LDL-C concentrations should be determined by ultracentrifugation. Lipid determinations should be performed at intervals of no less than 4 weeks and dosage adjusted according to the patient's response to therapy. The NCEP Treatment Guidelines are summarized in TABLE 7.

TABLE 7 *NCEP Treatment Guidelines: LDL-C Goals and Cutpoints for Therapeutic Lifestyle Changes and Drug Therapy in Different Risk Categories*

Risk Category	LDL Goal (mg/dl)	LDL Level at Which to Initiate Therapeutic Lifestyle Changes (mg/dl)	LDL Level at Which to Consider Drug Therapy (mg/dl)
CHD or CHD risk equivalents (10 year risk >20%)	<100	≥100	≥130 (100-129: drug optional)*
2+ Risk factors (10 year risk ≤20%)	<130	≥130	10 year risk 10-20%: ≥130 10 year risk <10%: ≥160
0-1 Risk factor	<160	≥160	≥190 (160-189: LDL-lowering drug optional)

* Some authorities recommend use of LDL-lowering drugs in this category if an LDL-C level of <100 mg/dl cannot be achieved by theraputic lifestyle changes. Others prefer use of drugs that primarily modify triglycerides and HDC-C, *e.g.*, nicotinic acid and fibrate. Clinical judgement also may call for deferring drug therapy in this subcategory.
CHD, coronary heart disease.
Almost all people with 0-1 risk factor have 10 year risk <10%; thus, 10 year risk assessment in people with 0-1 risk factor is not necessary.

After the LDL-C goal has been achieved, if the TG is still >200 mg/dl, non-HDL-C (TC minus HDL-C) becomes a secondary target of therapy. Non-HDL-C goals are set 30 mg/dl higher than LDL-C goals for each risk category.

CONTRAINDICATIONS

Advicor is contraindicated in patients with a known hypersensitivity to niacin, lovastatin or any component of this medication, active liver disease or unexplained persistent elevations in serum transaminases (see WARNINGS), active peptic ulcer disease, or arterial bleeding.

PREGNANCY AND LACTATION

Atherosclerosis is a chronic process and the discontinuation of lipid-lowering drugs during pregnancy should have little impact on the outcome of long-term therapy of primary hypercholesterolemia. Moreover, cholesterol and other products of the cholesterol biosynthesis pathway are essential components for fetal development, including synthesis of steroids and cell membranes. Because of the ability of inhibitors of HMG-CoA reductase, such as lovastatin, to decrease the synthesis of cholesterol and possibly other products of the cholesterol biosynthesis pathway, Advicor is contraindicated in women who are pregnant and in lactating mothers. Advicor may cause fetal harm when administered to pregnant women. Advicor should be administered to women of childbearing age only when such patients are highly unlikely to conceive. If the patient becomes pregnant while taking this drug, Advicor should be discontinued immediately and the patient should be apprised of the potential hazard to the fetus (see PRECAUTIONS, Pregnancy Category X).

WARNINGS

Advicor should not be substituted for equivalent doses of immediate-release (crystalline) niacin. For patients switching from immediate-release niacin to extended-release niacin, therapy with extended-release niacin should be initiated with low doses (*i.e.*, 500 mg once daily at bedtime) and the extended-release niacin dose should then be titrated to the desired therapeutic response (see DOSAGE AND ADMINISTRATION).

LIVER DYSFUNCTION

Cases of severe hepatic toxicity, including fulminant hepatic necrosis, have occurred in patients who have substituted sustained-release (modified-release, timed-release) niacin products for immediate-release (crystalline) niacin at equivalent doses.

Advicor should be used with caution in patients who consume substantial quantities of alcohol and/or have a past history of liver disease. Active liver disease or unexplained transaminase elevations are contraindications to the use of Advicor.

Niacin preparations and lovastatin preparations have been associated with abnormal liver tests. In studies using extended-release niacin alone, 0.8% of patients were discontinued for transaminase elevations. In studies using lovastatin alone, 0.2% of patients were discontinued for transaminase elevations.[2] In three safety and efficacy studies involving titration to final daily Advicor doses ranging from 500 mg/10 mg to 2500 mg/40 mg, 10 of 1028 patients (1.0%) experienced reversible elevations in AST/ALT to more than 3 times the upper limit of normal (ULN). Three (3) of 10 elevations occurred at doses outside the recommended dosing limit of 2000 mg/40 mg; no patient receiving 1000 mg/20 mg had 3-fold elevations in AST/ALT. In clinical studies with Advicor, elevations in transaminases did not appear to be related to treatment duration; elevations in AST and ALT levels did appear to be dose related. Transaminase elevations were reversible upon discontinuation of Advicor.

Liver function tests should be performed on all patients during therapy with Advicor. Serum transaminase levels, including AST and ALT (SGOT and SGPT), should be monitored before treatment begins, every 6-12 weeks for the first 6 months, and periodically thereafter (*e.g.*, at approximately 6 month intervals). Special attention should be paid to patients who develop elevated serum transaminase levels, and in these patients, measurements should be repeated promptly and, if confirmed, then performed more frequently. If the transaminase levels show evidence of progression, particularly if they rise to 3 times ULN and are persistent, or if they are associated with symptoms of nausea, fever, and/or malaise, the drug should be discontinued.

SKELETAL MUSCLE

Lovastatin

Lovastatin and other inhibitors of HMG-CoA reductase occasionally cause myopathy, which is manifested as muscle pain or weakness associated with grossly elevated creatine kinase (>10 times ULN). Rhabdomyolysis, with or without acute renal failure secondary to myoglobinuria, has been reported rarely and can occur at any time. In a large, long-term, clinical safety and efficacy study (the EXCEL study)[3,4] with lovastatin, myopathy occurred in up to 0.2% of patients treated with lovastatin 20-80 mg for up to 2 years. When drug treatment was interrupted or discontinued in these patients, muscle symptoms and creatine kinase (CK) increases promptly resolved. The risk of myopathy is increased by concomitant therapy with certain drugs, some of which were excluded by the EXCEL study design.

The risk of myopathy appears to be increased by high levels of HMG-CoA reductase inhibitory activity in plasma. Lovastatin is metabolized by the cytochrome P450 isoform 3A4. Certain drugs which share this metabolic pathway can raise the plasma levels of lovastatin and may increase the risk of myopathy. These include cyclosporine, itraconazole, ketoconazole and other antifungal azoles, the macrolide antibiotics erythromycin and clarithromycin, HIV protease inhibitors, the antidepressant nefazodone, or large quantities of grapefruit juice (>1 quart daily).

Advicor

Myopathy and/or rhabdomyolysis have been reported when lovastatin is used in combination with lipid-altering doses (≥1 g/day) of niacin. Physicians contemplating the use of Advicor, a combination of lovastatin and niacin, should weigh the potential benefits and risks, and should carefully monitor patients for any signs and symptoms of muscle pain, tenderness, or weakness, particularly during the initial month of treatment or during any period of upward dosage titration of either drug. Periodic CK determinations may be considered in such situations, but there is no assurance that such monitoring will prevent myopathy.

In clinical studies, no cases of rhabdomyolysis and one suspected case of myopathy have been reported in 1079 patients who were treated with Advicor at doses up to 2000 mg/40 mg for periods up to 2 years.

Patients starting therapy with Advicor should be advised of the risk of myopathy, and told to report promptly unexplained muscle pain, tenderness, or weakness. A CK level above 10 times ULN in a patient with unexplained muscle symptoms indicates myopathy. Advicor therapy should be discontinued if myopathy is diagnosed or suspected.

In patients with complicated medical histories predisposing to rhabdomyolysis, such as preexisting renal insufficiency, dose escalation requires caution. Also, as there are no known adverse consequences of brief interruption of therapy, treatment with Advicor should be stopped for a few days before elective major surgery and when any major acute medical or surgical condition supervenes.

USE OF ADVICOR WITH OTHER DRUGS

The incidence and severity of myopathy may be increased by concomitant administration of Advicor with drugs that can cause myopathy when given alone, such as gemfibrozil and other fibrates. The use of Advicor in combination with fibrates should be avoided unless the benefit of further alterations in lipid levels is likely to outweigh the increased risk of this drug combination. In patients taking concomitant cyclosporine or fibrates, the dose of Advicor should generally not exceed 1000 mg/20 mg (see DOSAGE AND ADMINISTRATION), as the risk of myopathy may increase at higher doses. Interruption of Advicor therapy during a course of treatment with a systemic antifungal azole or a macrolide antibiotic should be considered.

PRECAUTIONS

GENERAL

Before instituting therapy with a lipid-altering medication, an attempt should be made to control dyslipidemia with appropriate diet, exercise, and weight reduction in obese patients, and to treat other underlying medical problems (see INDICATIONS AND USAGE).

Patients with a past history of jaundice, hepatobiliary disease, or peptic ulcer should be observed closely during Advicor therapy. Frequent monitoring of liver function tests and blood glucose should be performed to ascertain that the drug is producing no adverse effects on these organ systems.

Diabetic patients may experience a dose-related rise in fasting blood sugar (FBS). In three clinical studies, which included 1028 patients exposed to Advicor (6-22% of whom had diabetes Type 2 at baseline), increases in FBS above normal occurred in 46-65% of patients at any time during study treatment with Advicor. Fourteen patients (1.4%) were discontinued from study treatment: 3 patients for worsening diabetes, 10 patients for hyperglycemia and 1 patient for a new diagnosis of diabetes. In the studies in which lovastatin and extended-release niacin were used as active controls, 24-41% of patients receiving lovastatin and 43-58% of patients receiving extended-release niacin also had increases in FBS above normal. One patient (1.1%) receiving lovastatin was discontinued for hyperglycemia. Diabetic or potentially diabetic patients should be observed closely during treatment with Advicor, and adjustment of diet and/or hypoglycemic therapy may be necessary.

In one long-term study of 106 patients treated with Advicor, elevations in prothrombin time (PT) >3 × ULN occurred in 2 patients (2%) during study drug treatment. In a long-term study of 814 patients treated with Advicor, 7 patients were noted to have platelet counts <100,000 during study drug treatment. Four (4) of these patients were discontinued, and 1 patient with a platelet count <100,000 had prolonged bleeding after a tooth extraction. Prior studies have shown that extended-release niacin can be associated with dose-related reductions in platelet count (mean of -11% with 2000 mg) and increases of PT (mean of approximately +4%). Accordingly, patients undergoing surgery should be carefully evaluated. In controlled studies, Advicor has been associated with small but statistically significant dose-related reductions in phosphorus levels (mean of -10% with 2000 mg/40 mg). Phosphorus levels should be monitored periodically in patients at risk for hypophosphatemia. In clinical studies with Advicor, hypophosphatemia was more common in males than in females. The clinical relevance of hypophosphatemia in this population is not known.

Niacin

Caution should also be used when Advicor is used in patients with unstable angina or in the acute phase of MI, particularly when such patients are also receiving vasoactive drugs such as nitrates, calcium channel blockers, or adrenergic blocking agents.

Elevated uric acid levels have occurred with niacin therapy; therefore, in patients predisposed to gout, niacin therapy should be used with caution. Niacin is rapidly metabolized by the liver, and excreted through the kidneys. Advicor is contraindicated in patients with significant or unexplained hepatic dysfunction (see CONTRAINDICATIONS and WARNINGS) and should be used with caution in patients with renal dysfunction.

Lovastatin

Lovastatin may elevate creatine phosphokinase and transaminase levels (see WARNINGS and ADVERSE REACTIONS). This should be considered in the differential diagnosis of chest pain in a patient on therapy with lovastatin.

Endocrine Function

HMG-CoA reductase inhibitors interfere with cholesterol synthesis and as such might theoretically blunt adrenal and/or gonadal steroid production. Results of clinical studies with drugs in this class have been inconsistent with regard to drug effects on basal and reserve steroid levels. However, clinical studies have shown that lovastatin does not reduce basal plasma cortisol concentration or impair adrenal reserve, and does not reduce basal plasma testosterone concentration. Another HMG-CoA reductase inhibitor has been shown to reduce the plasma testosterone response to human chorionic gonadotropin (HCG). In the same study, the mean testosterone response to HCG was slightly but not significantly reduced after treatment with lovastatin 40 mg daily for 16 weeks in 21 men. The effects of HMG-CoA reductase inhibitors on male fertility have not been studied in adequate numbers of male patients. The effects, if any, on the pituitary-gonadal axis in premenopausal women are unknown. Patients treated with lovastatin who develop clinical evidence of endocrine dysfunction should be evaluated appropriately. Caution should also be exercised if an HMG-CoA reductase inhibitor or other agent used to lower cholesterol levels is administered to patients also receiving other drugs (*e.g.*, ketoconazole, spironolactone, cimetidine) that may decrease the levels or activity of endogenous steroid hormones.

CNS Toxicity

Lovastatin produced optic nerve degeneration (Wallerian degeneration of retinogeniculate fibers) in clinically normal dogs in a dose-dependent fashion starting at 60 mg/kg/day, a dose that produced mean plasma drug levels about 30 times higher than the mean drug level in humans taking the highest recommended dose (as measured by total enzyme inhibitory activity). Vestibulocochlear Wallerian-like degeneration and retinal ganglion cell chromatolysis were also seen in dogs treated for 14 weeks at 180 mg/kg/day, a dose which resulted in a mean plasma drug level (C_{max}) similar to that seen with the 60 mg/kg/day dose.

CNS vascular lesions, characterized by perivascular hemorrhage and edema, mononuclear cell infiltration of perivascular spaces, perivascular fibrin deposits and necrosis of small vessels, were seen in dogs treated with lovastatin at a dose of 180 mg/kg/day, a dose which produced plasma drug levels (C_{max}) which were about 30 times higher than the mean values in humans taking 80 mg/day. Similar optic nerve and CNS vascular lesions have been observed with other drugs of this class. Cataracts were seen in dogs treated with lovastatin for 11 and 28 weeks at 180 mg/kg/day and 1 year at 60 mg/kg/day.

INFORMATION FOR THE PATIENT

Patients should be advised of the following:

To report promptly unexplained muscle pain, tenderness, or weakness (see WARNINGS, Skeletal Muscle).

To take Advicor at bedtime, with a low-fat snack. Administration on an empty stomach is not recommended.

To carefully follow the prescribed dosing regimen (see DOSAGE AND ADMINISTRATION).

That flushing is a common side effect of niacin therapy that usually subsides after several weeks of consistent niacin use. Flushing may last for several hours after dosing, may vary in severity, and will, by taking Advicor at bedtime, most likely occur during sleep. If awakened by flushing, especially if taking antihypertensives, rise slowly to minimize the potential for dizziness and/or syncope.

That taking aspirin (up to approximately 30 minutes before taking Advicor) or another non-steroidal anti-inflammatory drug (*e.g.*, ibuprofen) may minimize flushing.

To avoid ingestion of alcohol or hot drinks around the time of Advicor administration, to minimize flushing.

Should not be administered with grapefruit juice.

That if Advicor therapy is discontinued for an extended length of time, their physician should be contacted prior to re-starting therapy; re-titration is recommended (see DOSAGE AND ADMINISTRATION).

To notify their physician if they are taking vitamins or other nutritional supplements containing niacin or related compounds such as nicotinamide (see DRUG INTERACTIONS).
To notify their physician if symptoms of dizziness occur.
If diabetic, to notify their physician of changes in blood glucose.
That Advicor tablets should not be broken, crushed, or chewed, but should be swallowed whole.

PEDIATRIC USE

No studies in patients under 18 years-of-age have been conducted with Advicor. Because pediatric patients are not likely to benefit from cholesterol lowering for at least a decade and because experience with this drug or its active ingredients is limited, treatment of pediatric patients with Advicor is not recommended at this time.

GERIATRIC USE

Of the 214 patients who received Advicor in double-blind clinical studies, 37.4% were 65 years-of-age and older, and of the 814 patients who received Advicor in open-label clinical studies, 36.2% were 65 years-of-age and older. Responses in LDL-C, HDL-C, and TG were similar in geriatric patients. No overall differences in the percentage of patients with adverse events were observed between older and younger patients. No overall differences were observed in selected chemistry values between the 2 groups except for amylase which was higher in older patients.

DRUG/LABORATORY TEST INTERACTIONS

Niacin may produce false elevations in some fluorometric determinations of plasma or urinary catecholamines. Niacin may also give false-positive reactions with cupric sulfate solution (Benedict's reagent) in urine glucose tests.

CARCINOGENESIS, MUTAGENESIS, AND IMPAIRMENT OF FERTILITY

No studies have been conducted with Advicor regarding carcinogenesis, mutagenesis, or impairment of fertility.

Niacin

Niacin, administered to mice for a lifetime as a 1% solution in drinking water, was not carcinogenic. The mice in this study received approximately 6-8 times a human dose of 3000 mg/day as determined on a mg/m^2 basis. Niacin was negative for mutagenicity in the Ames test. No studies on impairment of fertility have been performed.

Lovastatin

In a 21 month carcinogenic study in mice, there was a statistically significant increase in the incidence of hepatocellular carcinomas and adenomas in both males and females at 500 mg/kg/day. This dose produced a total plasma drug exposure 3-4 times that of humans given the highest recommended dose of lovastatin (drug exposure was measured as total HMG-CoA reductase inhibitory activity in extracted plasma). Tumor increases were not seen at 20 and 100 mg/kg/day, doses that produced drug exposures of 0.3 to 2 times that of humans at the 80 mg/day dose. A statistically significant increase in pulmonary adenomas was seen in female mice at approximately 4 times the human drug exposure. (Although mice were given 300 times the human dose on a mg/kg body weight basis, plasma levels of total inhibitory activity were only 4 times higher in mice than in humans given 80 mg of lovastatin.)

There was an increase in incidence of papilloma in the non-glandular mucosa of the stomach of mice beginning at exposures of 1-2 times that of humans. The glandular mucosa was not affected. The human stomach contains only glandular mucosa.

In a 24 month carcinogenicity study in rats, there was a positive dose-response relationship for hepatocellular carcinogenicity in males at drug exposures between 2-7 times that of human exposure at 80 mg/day (doses in rats were 5, 30, and 180 mg/kg/day).

An increased incidence of thyroid neoplasms in rats appears to be a response that has been seen with other HMG-CoA reductase inhibitors.

A drug in this class chemically similar to lovastatin was administered to mice for 72 weeks at 25, 100, and 400 mg/kg body weight, which resulted in mean serum drug levels approximately 3, 15, and 33 times higher than the mean human serum drug concentration (as total inhibitory activity) after a 40 mg oral dose. Liver carcinomas were significantly increased in high-dose females and mid- and high-dose males, with a maximum incidence of 90% in males. The incidence of adenomas of the liver was significantly increased in mid- and high-dose females. Drug treatment also significantly increased the incidence of lung adenomas in mid- and high-dose males and females. Adenomas of the Harderian gland (a gland of the eye of rodents) were significantly higher in high-dose mice than in controls.

No evidence of mutagenicity was observed in a microbial mutagen test using mutant strains of *Salmonella typhimurium* with or without rat or mouse liver metabolic activation. In addition, no evidence of damage to genetic material was noted in an *in vitro* alkaline elution assay using rat or mouse hepatocytes, a V-79 mammalian cell forward mutation study, an *in vitro* chromosome aberration study in CHO cells, or an *in vivo* chromosomal aberration assay in mouse bone marrow.

Drug-related testicular atrophy, decreased spermatogenesis, spermatocytic degeneration and giant cell formation were seen in dogs starting at 20 mg/kg/day. Similar findings were seen with another drug in this class. No drug-related effects on fertility were found in studies with lovastatin in rats. However, in studies with a similar drug in this class, there was decreased fertility in male rats treated for 34 weeks at 25 mg/kg body weight, although this effect was not observed in a subsequent fertility study when this same dose was administered for 11 weeks (the entire cycle of spermatogenesis, including epididymal maturation). In rats treated with this same reductase inhibitor at 180 mg/kg/day, seminiferous tubule degeneration (necrosis and loss of spermatogenic epithelium) was observed. No microscopic changes were observed in the testes from rats of either study. The clinical significance of these findings is unclear.

PREGNANCY CATEGORY X

See CONTRAINDICATIONS.

Advicor should be administered to women of childbearing potential only when such patients are highly unlikely to conceive and have been informed of the potential hazard. Safety in pregnant women has not been established and there is no apparent benefit to therapy with Advicor during pregnancy (see CONTRAINDICATIONS). Treatment should be immediately discontinued as soon as pregnancy is recognized.

Niacin

Animal reproduction studies have not been conducted with niacin or with Advicor. It is also not known whether niacin at doses typically used for lipid disorders can cause fetal harm when administered to pregnant women or whether it can affect reproductive capacity. If a woman receiving niacin or Advicor for primary hypercholesterolemia (Types IIa or IIb) becomes pregnant, the drug should be discontinued.

Lovastatin

Rare reports of congenital anomalies have been received following intrauterine exposure to HMG-CoA reductase inhibitors. In a review[5] of approximately 100 prospectively followed pregnancies in women exposed to lovastatin or another structurally related HMG-CoA reductase inhibitor, the incidences of congenital anomalies, spontaneous abortions and fetal deaths/stillbirths did not exceed what would be expected in the general population. The number of cases is adequate only to exclude a 3- to 4-fold increase in congenital anomalies over the background incidence. In 89% of the prospectively followed pregnancies, drug treatment was initiated prior to pregnancy and was discontinued at some point in the first trimester when pregnancy was identified.

Lovastatin has been shown to produce skeletal malformations at plasma levels 40 times the human exposure (for mouse fetus) and 80 times the human exposure (for rat fetus) based on mg/m^2 surface area (doses were 800 mg/kg/day). No drug-induced changes were seen in either species at multiples of 8 times (rat) or 4 times (mouse) based on surface area. No evidence of malformations was noted in rabbits at exposures up to 3 times the human exposure (dose of 15 mg/kg/day, highest tolerated dose).

LABOR AND DELIVERY

No studies have been conducted on the effect of Advicor, niacin or lovastatin on the mother or the fetus during labor or delivery, on the duration of labor or delivery, or on the growth, development, and functional maturation of the child.

NURSING MOTHERS

No studies have been conducted with Advicor in nursing mothers. Because of the potential for serious adverse reactions in nursing infants from lipid-altering doses of niacin and lovastatin (see CONTRAINDICATIONS), Advicor should not be taken while a woman is breastfeeding.

Niacin has been reported to be excreted in human milk. It is not known whether lovastatin is excreted in human milk. A small amount of another drug in this class is excreted in human breast milk.

L

DRUG INTERACTIONS

NIACIN

Antihypertensive Therapy: Niacin may potentiate the effects of ganglionic blocking agents and vasoactive drugs resulting in postural hypotension.
Aspirin: Concomitant aspirin may decrease the metabolic clearance of niacin. The clinical relevance of this finding is unclear.
Bile Acid Sequestrants: An *in vitro* study was carried out investigating the niacin-binding capacity of colestipol and cholestyramine. About 98% of available niacin was bound to colestipol, with 10-30% binding to cholestyramine. These results suggest that 4-6 hours, or as great an interval as possible, should elapse between the ingestion of bile acid-binding resins and the administration of Advicor.
Other: Concomitant alcohol or hot drinks may increase the side effects of flushing and pruritus and should be avoided around the time of Advicor ingestion. Vitamins or other nutritional supplements containing large doses of niacin or related compounds such as nicotinamide may potentiate the adverse effects of Advicor.

LOVASTATIN

Serious skeletal muscle disorders, *e.g.*, rhabdomyolysis, have been reported during concomitant therapy of lovastatin or other HMG-CoA reductase inhibitors with cyclosporine, itraconazole, ketoconazole, gemfibrozil, niacin, erythromycin, clarithromycin, nefazodone or HIV protease inhibitors. (See WARNINGS, Skeletal Muscle).

Coumarin Anticoagulants: In a small clinical study in which lovastatin was administered to warfarin-treated patients, no effect on PT was detected. However, another HMG-CoA reductase inhibitor has been found to produce a less than 2 seconds increase in PT in healthy volunteers receiving low doses of warfarin. Also, bleeding and/or increased PT have been reported in a few patients taking coumarin anticoagulants concomitantly with lovastatin. It is recommended that in patients taking anticoagulants, PT be determined before starting Advicor and frequently enough during early therapy to insure that no significant alteration of PT occurs. Once a stable PT has been documented, PT can be monitored at the intervals usually recommended for patients on coumarin anticoagulants. If the dose of Advicor is changed, the same procedure should be repeated.
Antipyrine: Lovastatin had no effect on the pharmacokinetics of antipyrine or its metabolites. However, since lovastatin is metabolized by the cytochrome P450 isoform 3A4 enzyme system, this does not preclude an interaction with other drugs metabolized by the same isoform.
Propranolol: In normal volunteers, there was no clinically significant pharmacokinetic or pharmacodynamic interaction with concomitant administration of single doses of lovastatin and propranolol.
Digoxin: In patients with hypercholesterolemia, concomitant administration of lovastatin and digoxin resulted in no effect on digoxin plasma concentrations.
Oral Hypoglycemic Agents: In pharmacokinetic studies of lovastatin in hypercholesterolemic, non-insulin-dependent diabetic patients, there was no drug interaction with glipizide or with chlorpropamide.

ADVERSE REACTIONS

OVERVIEW

In controlled clinical studies, 40/214 (19%) of patients randomized to Advicor discontinued therapy prior to study completion, 18/214 (8%) of discontinuations being due to flushing. In the same controlled studies, 9/94 (10%) of patients randomized to lovastatin and 19/92 (21%) of patients randomized to extended-release niacin also discontinued treatment prior to study completion secondary to adverse events. Flushing episodes (*i.e.*, warmth, redness, itching and/or tingling) were the most common treatment-emergent adverse events, and occurred in 53-83% of patients treated with Advicor. Spontaneous reports with extended-release niacin and clinical studies with Advicor suggest that flushing may also be accompanied by symptoms of dizziness or syncope, tachycardia, palpitations, shortness of breath, sweating, chills, and/or edema.

ADVERSE REACTIONS INFORMATION

Because clinical studies are conducted under widely varying conditions, adverse reaction rates observed in clinical studies of a drug cannot be directly compared to rates in the clinical studies of another drug and may not reflect the rates observed in clinical practice. The adverse reaction information from clinical studies does, however provide a basis for identifying the adverse events that appear to be related to drug use and for approximating rates. The data described in this section reflect the exposure to Advicor in two double-blind, controlled clinical studies of 400 patients. The population was 28-86 years of age, 54% male, 85% Caucasian, 9% Black, and 7% Other, and had mixed dyslipidemia (Frederickson Types IIa and IIb).

In addition to flushing, other adverse events occurring in 5% or greater of patients treated with Advicor are shown in TABLE 8.

TABLE 8 *Treatment-Emergent Adverse Events in ≥5% of Patients (events irrespective of causality; data from controlled, double-blind studies)*

Adverse Event	Advicor	Extended-Release Niacin	Lovastatin
Total Number of Patients	**n=214**	**n=92**	**n=94**
Cardiovascular	**163 (76%)**	**66 (72%)**	**24 (26%)**
Flushing	152 (71%)	60 (65%)	17 (18%)
Body as a Whole	**104 (49%)**	**50 (54%)**	**42 (45%)**
Asthenia	10 (5%)	6 (7%)	5 (5%)
Flu syndrome	12 (6%)	7 (8%)	4 (4%)
Headache	20 (9%)	12 (13%)	5 (5%)
Infection	43 (20%)	14 (15%)	19 (20%)
Pain	18 (8%)	3 (3%)	9 (10%)
Pain, abdominal	9 (4%)	1 (1%)	6 (6%)
Pain, back	10 (5%)	5 (5%)	5 (5%)
Digestive System	**51 (24%)**	**26 (28%)**	**16 (17%)**
Diarrhea	13 (6%)	8 (9%)	2 (2%)
Dyspepsia	6 (3%)	5 (5%)	4 (4%)
Nausea	14 (7%)	11 (12%)	2 (2%)
Vomiting	7 (3%)	5 (5%)	0
Metabolic and Nutrit. System	**37 (17%)**	**18 (20%)**	**13 (14%)**
Hyperglycemia	8 (4%)	6 (7%)	6 (6%)
Musculoskeletal System	**19 (9%)**	**9 (10%)**	**17 (18%)**
Myalgia	6 (3%)	5 (5%)	8 (9%)
Skin and Appendages	**3 (2%)**	**19 (21%)**	**11 (12%)**
Pruritus	14 (7%)	7 (8%)	3 (3%)
Rash	11 (5%)	11 (12%)	3 (3%)

Note: Percentages are calculated from the total number of patients in each column.

The following adverse events have also been reported with niacin, lovastatin, and/or other HMG-CoA reductase inhibitors, but not necessarily with Advicor, either during clinical studies or in routine patient management.

Body as a Whole: Chest pain; abdominal pain; edema; chills; malaise.

Cardiovascular: Atrial fibrillation; tachycardia; palpitation, and other cardiac arrhythmias; orthostasis; hypotension; syncope.

Eye: Toxic amblyopia; cystoid macular edema; ophthalmoplegia; eye irritation.

Gastrointestinal: Activation of peptic ulcers and peptic ulceration; dyspepsia; vomiting; anorexia; constipation; flatulence; pancreatitis; hepatitis; fatty change in liver; jaundice; and rarely, cirrhosis, fulminant hepatic necrosis, and hepatoma.

Metabolic: Gout.

Musculoskeletal: Muscle cramps; myopathy; rhabdomyolysis; arthralgia.

Nervous: Dizziness; insomnia; dry mouth; paresthesia; anxiety; tremor; vertigo; memory loss; peripheral neuropathy; psychic disturbances; dysfunction of certain cranial nerves.

Skin: Hyper-pigmentation; acanthosis nigricans; urticaria; alopecia; dry skin; sweating; and a variety of skin changes (*e.g.*, nodules, discoloration, dryness of mucous membranes, changes to hair/nails).

Respiratory: Dyspnea; rhinitis.

Urogenital: Gynecomastia; loss of libido; erectile dysfunction.

Hypersensitivity Reactions: An apparent hypersensitivity syndrome has been reported rarely, which has included one or more of the following features: anaphylaxis, angioedema, lupus erythematous-like syndrome, polymyalgia rheumatica, vasculitis, purpura, thrombocytopenia, leukopenia, hemolytic anemia, positive ANA, ESR increase, eosinophilia, arthritis, arthralgia, urticaria, asthenia, photosensitivity, fever, chills, flushing, malaise, dyspnea, toxic epidermal necrolysis, erythema multiforme, including Stevens-Johnson syndrome.

Other: Migraine.

CLINICAL LABORATORY ABNORMALITIES

Chemistry

Elevations in serum transaminases (see WARNINGS, Liver Dysfunction), CPK and fasting glucose, and reductions in phosphorus. Niacin extended-release tablets have been associated with slight elevations in LDH, uric acid, total bilirubin, and amylase. Lovastatin and/or HMG-CoA reductase inhibitors have been associated with elevations in alkaline phosphatase, γ-glutamyl transpeptidase and bilirubin, and thyroid function abnormalities.

Hematology

Niacin extended-release tablets have been associated with slight reductions in platelet counts and prolongation in PT (see WARNINGS).

DOSAGE AND ADMINISTRATION

The usual recommended starting dose for extended-release niacin is 500 mg qhs. Extended-release niacin must be titrated and the dose should not be increased by more than 500 mg every 4 weeks up to a maximum dose of 2000 mg a day, to reduce the incidence and severity of side effects. Patients already receiving a stable dose of extended-release niacin may be switched directly to a niacin-equivalent dose of Advicor.

The usual recommended starting dose of lovastatin is 20 mg once a day. Dose adjustments should be made at intervals of 4 weeks or more. Patients already receiving a stable dose of lovastatin may receive concomitant dosage titration with extended-release niacin, and switch to Advicor once a stable dose of extended-release niacin has been reached. Flushing of the skin (see ADVERSE REACTIONS) may be reduced in frequency or severity by pretreatment with aspirin (taken up to approximately 30 minutes prior to Advicor dose) or other non-steroidal anti-inflammatory drugs. Flushing, pruritus, and gastrointestinal distress are also greatly reduced by slowly increasing the dose of niacin and avoiding administration on an empty stomach. Equivalent doses of Advicor may be substituted for equivalent doses of extended-release niacin but should not be substituted for other modified-release (sustained-release or time-release) niacin preparations or immediate-release (crystalline) niacin preparations (see WARNINGS). Patients previously receiving niacin products other than extended-release niacin should be started on extended-release niacin with the recommended extended-release niacin titration schedule, and the dose should subsequently be individualized based on patient response.

Advicor should be taken at bedtime, with a low-fat snack, and the dose should be individualized according to patient response. Advicor tablets should be taken whole and should not be broken, crushed, or chewed before swallowing. The dose of Advicor should not be increased by more than 500 mg daily (based on the extended-release niacin component) every 4 weeks. The lowest dose of Advicor is 500 mg/20 mg. Doses of Advicor greater than 2000 mg/40 mg daily are not recommended. If Advicor therapy is discontinued for an extended period (>7 days), reinstitution of therapy should begin with the lowest dose of Advicor.

HOW SUPPLIED

Advicor is an unscored, capsule-shaped tablet containing 500, 750, or 1000 mgof niacin in an extended-release formulation and 20 mg of lovastatin in an immediate-release formulation. Tablets are color-coated and debossed as follows:

500 mg/20 mg: Light yellow, debossed with "KOS" on one side and "502" on the other side.

750 mg/20 mg: Light orange, , debossed with "KOS" on one side and"752" on the other side.

1000 mg/20 mg: Dark pink/light purple, , debossed with "KOS" on one side and "1002" on the other side.

Storage: Store at room temperature (20-25°C or 68-77°F).

PRODUCT LISTING - EQUIVALENTS NOT AVAILABLE

Tablet - Oral - 20 mg;500 mg
90's $150.07 ADVICOR, Kos Pharmaceuticals 60598-0006-90

Tablet - Oral - 20 mg;750 mg
90's $183.19 ADVICOR, Kos Pharmaceuticals 60598-0007-90

Tablet - Oral - 20 mg;1000 mg
90's $195.61 ADVICOR, Kos Pharmaceuticals 60598-0008-90

Loxapine Succinate *(001666)*

Categories: Psychosis; Schizophrenia; FDA Approved 1975 Feb; Pregnancy Category C
Drug Classes: Antipsychotics
Brand Names: Loxitane
Foreign Brand Availability: Desconex (Spain); Loxapac (Belgium; Canada; Denmark; England; France; Greece; India; Ireland; Netherlands; Portugal; Spain; Taiwan)
Cost of Therapy: $88.33 (Schizophrenia; Loxitane; 10 mg; 2 capsules/day; 30 day supply)
$41.67 (Schizophrenia; Generic Capsules; 10 mg; 2 capsules/day; 30 day supply)

DESCRIPTION

Loxapine, a dibenzoxazepine compound, represents a subclass of tricyclic antipsychotic agents, chemically distinct from the thioxanthenes, butyrophenones, and phenothiazines. Chemically, it is 2-chloro-11-(4-methyl-1-piperazinyl)-dibenz[*b,f*][1,4]oxazepine. It is present in capsules as the succinate salt, and in the concentrate and parenteral primarily as the hydrochloride salt.

CAPSULES

Each Loxitane capsule contains loxapine succinate equivalent to 5, 10, 25 or 50 mg of loxapine base and the following inactive ingredients: blue 1, gelatin, lactose, magnesium stearate, titanium dioxide and yellow 10. Additionally, the 5 mg capsule contains red 33 and the 10 mg capsule contains red 28 and red 33 and the 25 mg capsule contains FD&C yellow no. 6.

ORAL CONCENTRATE

Each ml of Loxitane contains loxapine hydrochloride equivalent to 25 mg of loxapine base and propylene glycol as an inactive ingredient.

Hydrochloric acid and, if necessary, sodium hydroxide are used to adjust pH to approximately 5.8 during manufacture.

INTRAMUSCULAR (STERILE)
Not for Intravenous Use.

Each ml of Loxitane contains loxapine hydrochloride equivalent to 50 mg of loxapine base. Inactive ingredients: polysorbate 80 5% w/v, propylene glycol 70% v/v, and water for injection qs ad 100% v.

Hydrochloric acid and, if necessary, sodium hydroxide are used to adjust pH to approximately 5.5 during manufacture.

CLINICAL PHARMACOLOGY

PHARMACODYNAMICS

Pharmacologically, loxapine is a tranquilizer for which the exact mode of action has not been established. However, changes in the level of excitability of subcortical inhibitory areas have been observed in several animal species in association with such manifestations of tranquilization as calming effects and suppression of aggressive behavior.

In normal human volunteers, signs of sedation were seen within 20-30 minutes after administration, were most pronounced within 1½ to 3 hours, and lasted through 12 hours. Similar timing of primary pharmacologic effects was seen in animals.

ABSORPTION, DISTRIBUTION, METABOLISM, AND EXCRETION

After administration of loxapine as an oral solution, systemic bioavailability of the parent drug was only about one-third that after an equivalent intramuscular dose (25 mg base) in male volunteers. C_{max} for the parent drug was similar for the IM and oral administrations, whereas T_{max} was significantly longer for the IM administration than the oral administration (approximately 5 vs 1 hour). The lower systemic availability of the parent drug after oral administration as compared to the IM administration may be due to first pass metabolism of the oral form.

This is supported by the finding that two metabolites found in serum (8-hydroxyloxapine and 8-hydroxydesmethylloxapine) were formed to a lesser extent after IM administration of loxapine as compared to oral administration.

The apparent half-life of loxapine after oral and IM administration is approximately 4 hours (range, 1-14 hours) and 12 hours (range, 8-23 hours) respectively. The extended half-life for the IM administration as compared to the oral administration may be explained by prolonged absorption of loxapine from the muscle during the concurrent elimination process.

Loxapine is extensively metabolized, and urinary recovery over 48 hours resulted in recoveries of approximately 30% and 40% of an IM and orally administered loxapine dose as five metabolites.

INDICATIONS AND USAGE

Loxapine is indicated for the management of the manifestations of psychotic disorders. The antipsychotic efficacy of loxapine was established in clinical studies which enrolled newly hospitalized and chronically hospitalized acutely ill schizophrenic patients as subjects.

CONTRAINDICATIONS

Loxapine is contraindicated in comatose or severe drug-induced depressed states (alcohol, barbiturates, narcotics, etc.).

Loxapine is contraindicated in individuals with known hypersensitivity to dibenzoxazepines.

WARNINGS

TARDIVE DYSKINESIA

Tardive dyskinesia, a syndrome consisting of potentially irreversible, involuntary, dyskinetic movements may develop in patients treated with neuroleptic (antipsychotic) drugs. Although the prevalence of the syndrome appears to be highest among the elderly, especially elderly women, it is impossible to rely upon prevalence estimates to predict, at the inception of neuroleptic treatment, which patients are likely to develop the syndrome. Whether neuroleptic drug products differ in their potential to cause tardive dyskinesia is unknown.

Both the risk of developing the syndrome and the likelihood that it will become irreversible are believed to increase as the duration of treatment and the total cumulative dose of neuroleptic drugs administered to the patient increase. However, the syndrome can develop, although much less commonly, after relatively brief treatment periods at low doses.

There is no known treatment for established cases of tardive dyskinesia, although the syndrome may remit, partially or completely, if neuroleptic treatment is withdrawn. Neuroleptic treatment itself, however, may suppress (or partially suppress) the signs and symptoms of the syndrome and thereby may possibly mask the underlying disease process. The effect that symptomatic suppression has upon the long-term course of the syndrome is unknown.

Given these considerations, neuroleptics should be prescribed in a manner that is most likely to minimize the occurrence of tardive dyskinesia. Chronic neuroleptic treatment should generally be reserved for patients who suffer from a chronic illness that, (1) is known to respond to neuroleptic drugs, and (2) for whom alternative, equally effective, but potentially less harmful treatments are *not* available or appropriate. In patients who do require chronic treatment, the smallest dose and the shortest duration of treatment producing a satisfactory clinical response should be sought. The need for continued treatment should be reassessed periodically.

If signs and symptoms of tardive dyskinesia appear in a patient on neuroleptics, drug discontinuation should be considered. However, some patients may require treatment despite the presence of the syndrome. (See ADVERSE REACTIONS and PRECAUTIONS, Information for the Patient.)

NEUROLEPTIC MALIGNANT SYNDROME (NMS)

A potentially fatal symptom complex sometimes referred to as Neuroleptic Malignant Syndrome (NMS) has been reported in association with antipsychotic drugs. Clinical manifestations of NMS are hyperpyrexia, muscle rigidity, altered mental status, and evidence of autonomic instability (irregular pulse or blood pressure, tachycardia, diaphoresis, and cardiac dysrhythmias).

The diagnostic evaluation of patients with this syndrome is complicated. In arriving at a diagnosis, it is important to identify cases where the clinical presentation includes both serious medical illness (*e.g.,* pneumonia, systemic infection, etc.) and untreated or inadequately treated extrapyramidal signs and symptoms (EPS). Other important considerations in the differential diagnosis include central anticholinergic toxicity, heat stroke, drug fever and primary central nervous system (CNS) pathology.

The management of NMS should include: (1) immediate discontinuation of antipsychotic drugs and other drugs not essential to concurrent therapy, (2) intensive symptomatic treatment and medical monitoring, and (3) treatment of any concomitant serious medical problems for which specific treatments are available. There is no general agreement about specific pharmacological treatment regimens for uncomplicated NMS.

If a patient requires antipsychotic drug treatment after recovery from NMS, the potential reintroduction of drug therapy should be carefully considered. The patient should be carefully monitored, since recurrences of NMS have been reported.

Loxapine, like other tranquilizers, may impair mental and/or physical abilities, especially during the first few days of therapy. Therefore, ambulatory patients should be warned about activities requiring alertness (*e.g.,* operating vehicles or machinery) and about concomitant use of alcohol and other CNS depressants.

Loxapine has not been evaluated for the management of behavioral complications in patients with mental retardation, and therefore, it cannot be recommended.

PRECAUTIONS

GENERAL

Loxapine should be used with extreme caution in patients with a history of convulsive disorders since it lowers the convulsive threshold. Seizures have been reported in patients receiving loxapine at antipsychotic dose levels, and may occur in epileptic patients even with maintenance of routine anticonvulsant drug therapy.

Loxapine has an antiemetic effect in animals. Since this effect may also occur in man, loxapine may mask signs of overdosage of toxic drugs and may obscure conditions such as intestinal obstruction and brain tumor.

Loxapine should be used with caution in patients with cardiovascular disease. Increased pulse rates have been reported in the majority of patients receiving antipsychotic doses; transient hypotension has been reported. In the presence of severe hypotension requiring vasopressor therapy, the preferred drugs may be norepinephrine or angiotensin. Usual doses of epinephrine may be ineffective because of inhibition of its vasopressor effect by loxapine.

The possibility of ocular toxicity from loxapine cannot be excluded at this time. Therefore, careful observation should be made for pigmentary retinopathy and lenticular pigmentation since these have been observed in some patients receiving certain other antipsychotic drugs for prolonged periods.

Because of possible anticholinergic action, the drug should be used cautiously in patients with glaucoma or a tendency to urinary retention, particularly with concomitant administration of anticholinergic-type antiparkinson medication.

Experience to date indicates the possibility of a slightly higher incidence of extrapyramidal effects following intramuscular administration that normally anticipated with oral formulations. The increase may be attributable to higher plasma levels following intramuscular injection.

Neuroleptic drugs elevate prolactin levels; the elevation persists during chronic administration. Tissue culture experiments indicate that approximately one-third of human breast cancers are prolactin dependent *in vitro,* a factor of potential importance if the prescription of these drugs is contemplated in a patient with a previously detected breast cancer. Although disturbances such as galactorrhea, amenorrhea, gynecomastia, and impotence have been reported, the clinical significance of elevated serum prolactin levels is unknown for most patients. An increase in mammary neoplasms has been found in rodents after chronic administration of neuroleptic drugs. Neither clinical studies nor epidemiologic studies conducted to date, however, have shown an association between chronic administration of these drugs and mammary tumorigenesis; the available evidence is considered too limited to be conclusive at this time.

INFORMATION FOR THE PATIENT

Given the likelihood that some patients exposed chronically to neuroleptics will develop tardive dyskinesia, it is advised that all patients in whom chronic use is contemplated be given, if possible, full information about this risk. The decision to inform patients and/or their guardians must obviously take into account the clinical circumstances and the competency of the patient to understand the information provided.

USAGE IN PREGNANCY

Safe use of loxapine during pregnancy or lactation has not been established; therefore, its use in pregnancy, in nursing mothers, or in women of childbearing potential requires that the benefits of treatment be weighed against the possible risks to mother and child. No embryotoxicity or teratogenicity was observed in studies in rats, rabbits or dogs although, with the exception of one rabbit study, the highest dosage was only 2 times the maximum recommended human dose and in some studies it was below this dose. Perinatal studies have shown renal papillary abnormalities in offspring of rats treated from midpregnancy with doses of 0.6 and 1.8 mg/kg, doses which approximate the usual human dose but which are considerably below the maximum recommended human dose.

NURSING MOTHERS

The extent of the excretion of loxapine or its metabolites in human milk is not known. However, loxapine and its metabolites have been shown to be transported into the milk of lactating dogs. Loxapine administration to nursing women should be avoided if clinically possible.

PEDIATRIC USE

Safety and effectiveness of loxapine in pediatric patients have not been established.

DRUG INTERACTIONS

There have been rare reports of significant respiratory depression, stupor and/or hypotension with the concomitant use of loxapine and lorazepam.

The risk of using loxapine in combination with CNS-active drugs has not been systematically evaluated. Therefore, caution is advised if the concomitant administration of loxapine and CNS-active drugs is required.

ADVERSE REACTIONS

CNS Effects: Manifestations of adverse effects on the central nervous system, other than extrapyramidal effects, have been seen infrequently. Drowsiness, usually mild, may occur at the beginning of therapy or when dosage is increased. It usually subsides with continued loxapine therapy. The incidence of sedation has been less than that of certain aliphatic phenothiazines and slightly more than the piperazine phenothiazines. Dizziness, faintness, staggering gait, shuffling gait, muscle twitching, weakness, insomnia, agitation, tension, seizures, akinesia, slurred speech, numbness, and confusional states have been reported. Neuroleptic malignant syndrome (NMS) has been reported (see WARNINGS).

Extrapyramidal Reactions: Neuromuscular (extrapyramidal) reactions during the administration of loxapine have been reported frequently, often during the first few days of treatment. In most patients, these reactions involved parkinsonian-like symptoms such as tremor, rigidity, excessive salivation, and masked facies. Akathisia (motor restlessness) also has been reported relatively frequently. These symptoms are usually not severe and can be controlled by reduction of loxapine dosage or by administration of antiparkinson drugs in usual dosage. Dystonic and dyskinetic reactions have occurred less frequently, but may be more severe. Dystonias include spasms of muscles of the neck and face, tongue protrusion, and oculogyric movement. Dyskinetic reactions have been described in the form of choreoathetoid movements. These reactions sometimes require reduction or temporary withdrawal of loxapine dosage in addition to appropriate counteractive drugs.

Persistent Tardive Dyskinesia: As with all antipsychotic agents, tardive dyskinesia may appear in some patients on long-term therapy or may appear after drug therapy has been discontinued. The risk appears to be greater in elderly patients on high-dose therapy, especially females. The symptoms are persistent and in some patients appear to be irreversible. The syndrome is characterized by rhythmical involuntary movement of the tongue, face, mouth, or jaw (*e.g.,* protrusion of tongue, puffing of cheeks, puckering of mouth, chewing movements). Sometimes these may be accompanied by involuntary movements of extremities.

There is no known effective treatment for tardive dyskinesia; antiparkinson agents usually do not alleviate the symptoms of this syndrome. It is suggested that all antipsychotic agents be discontinued if these symptoms appear. Should it be necessary to reinstitute treatment, or increase the dosage of the agent, or switch to a different antipsychotic agent, the syndrome may be masked. It has been suggested that fine vermicular movements of the tongue may be an early sign of the syndrome, and if the medication is stopped at that time the syndrome may not develop.

Cardiovascular Effects: Tachycardia, hypotension, hypertension, orthostatic hypotension, light-headedness, and syncope have been reported.

A few cases of ECG changes similar to those seen with phenothiazines have been reported. It is not known whether these were related to loxapine administration.

Hematologic: Rarely, agranulocytosis, thrombocytopenia, leukopenia.

Skin: Dermatitis, edema (puffiness of face), pruritus, rash, alopecia, and seborrhea have been reported with loxapine.

Anticholinergic Effects: Dry mouth, nasal congestion, constipation, blurred vision, urinary retention, and paralytic ileus have occurred.

Gastrointestinal: Nausea and vomiting have been reported in some patients. Hepatocellular injury (*i.e.,* SGOT/SGPT elevation) has been reported in association with loxapine administration and rarely, jaundice and/or hepatitis questionably related to loxapine treatment.

Other Adverse Reactions: Weight gain, weight loss, dyspnea, ptosis, hyperpyrexia, flushed facies, headache, paresthesia, and polydipsia have been reported in some patients. Rarely, galactorrhea, amenorrhea, gynecomastia, and menstrual irregularity of uncertain etiology have been reported.

DOSAGE AND ADMINISTRATION

Loxapine is administered, usually in divided doses, 2-4 times a day. Daily dosage (in terms of base equivalents) should be adjusted to the individual patient's needs as assessed by the severity of the symptoms and previous history of response to antipsychotic drugs.

ORAL ADMINISTRATION

Initial dosage of 10 mg twice daily is recommended, although in severely disturbed patients initial dosage up to a total of 50 mg daily may be desirable. Dosage should then be increased fairly rapidly over the first 7-10 days until there is effective control of psychotic symptoms. The usual therapeutic and maintenance range is 60-100 mg daily. However, as with other antipsychotic drugs, some patients respond to lower dosage and others require higher dosage for optimal benefit. Daily dosage higher than 250 mg is not recommended.

Loxapine C oral concentrate should be mixed with orange or grapefruit juice shortly before administration. Use only the enclosed calibrated (10, 15, 25, 50 mg) dropper for dosage.

MAINTENANCE THERAPY

For maintenance therapy, dosage should be reduced to the lowest level compatible with symptom control; many patients have been maintained satisfactorily at dosages in the range of 20-60 mg daily.

INTRAMUSCULAR ADMINISTRATION

Loxapine IM is utilized for prompt symptomatic control in the acutely agitated patient and in patients whose symptoms render oral medication temporarily impractical. During clinical trial there were only rare reports of significant local tissue reaction.

Loxapine IM is administered by intramuscular (not intravenous) injection in doses of 12.5 mg (¼ ml) to 50 mg (1 ml) at intervals of 4-6 hours or longer, both dose and interval depending on patient response. Many patients have responded satisfactorily to twice-daily dosage. As described above for oral administration, attention is directed to the necessity for dosage adjustment on an individual basis over the early days of loxapine administration.

Once the desired symptomatic control is achieved and the patient is able to take medication orally, loxapine should be administered in capsule or oral concentrate form. Usually this should occur within 5 days.

HOW SUPPLIED

LOXITANE CAPSULES

Loxitane, loxapine succinate, capsules are available in the following base equivalent strengths:

5 mg: Hard shell, opaque, dark-green capsules printed with the Watson logo over "WATSON" on one half and "LOXITANE" over "5 mg" on the other.

10 mg: Hard shell, opaque, with yellow body and a dark-green cap, printed with the Watson logo over "WATSON" on one half and "LOXITANE" over "10 mg" on the other.

25 mg: Hard shell, opaque, with a light-green body and a dark-green cap, printed with the Watson logo over "WATSON" on one half and "LOXITANE" over "25 mg" on the other.

50 mg: Hard shell, opaque, with a blue body and a dark-green cap, printed with the Watson logo over "WATSON" on one half and "LOXITANE" over "50 mg" on the other.

Storage

Store at controlled room temperature 15-30°C (59-86°F).

LOXITANE C ORAL CONCENTRATE

Each ml of Loxitane C, loxapine hydrochloride, oral concentrate contains loxapine HCl equivalent to 25 mg of loxapine base.

Storage

Store at controlled room temperature 20-25°C (68-77°F).
DO NOT FREEZE.

LOXITANE IM

Each ml of Loxitane IM, loxapine hydrochloride, for intramuscular use only, contains loxapine HCl equivalent to 50 mg of loxapine base.

Storage

Keep package closed to protect from light. Intensification of the straw color to a light amber will not alter potency of therapeutic efficacy; if noticeably discolored, ampul or vial should not be used.

Store at controlled room temperature 15-30°C (59-86°F).
DO NOT FREEZE.

PRODUCT LISTING - RATED THERAPEUTICALLY EQUIVALENT

Capsule - Oral - 5 mg			
100's	$47.25	GENERIC, Major Pharmaceuticals Inc	00904-2310-60
100's	$53.18	GENERIC, Moore, H.L. Drug Exchange Inc	00839-7495-06
100's	$54.00	GENERIC, Raway Pharmacal Inc	00686-0677-20
100's	$66.89	GENERIC, Parmed Pharmaceuticals Inc	00349-8839-01
100's	$67.20	GENERIC, Creighton Products Corporation	50752-0296-05
100's	$67.21	GENERIC, Aligen Independent Laboratories Inc	00405-5120-01
100's	$69.00	GENERIC, Ivax Corporation	00182-1305-01
100's	$69.20	GENERIC, Qualitest Products Inc	00603-4268-21
100's	$85.97	GENERIC, Watson Laboratories Inc	52544-0369-01
100's	$89.81	LOXITANE, Lederle Laboratories	00005-5359-60
100's	$121.00	GENERIC, Udl Laboratories Inc	51079-0900-20
100's	$126.59	LOXITANE, Watson Laboratories Inc	52544-0494-01
Capsule - Oral - 10 mg			
100's	$67.00	GENERIC, Raway Pharmacal Inc	00686-0678-20
100's	$69.45	GENERIC, Major Pharmaceuticals Inc	00904-2311-60
100's	$79.85	GENERIC, Moore, H.L. Drug Exchange Inc	00839-7496-06
100's	$86.80	GENERIC, Creighton Products Corporation	50752-0297-05
100's	$86.85	GENERIC, Aligen Independent Laboratories Inc	00405-5121-01
100's	$89.00	GENERIC, Qualitest Products Inc	00603-4269-21
100's	$89.53	GENERIC, Ivax Corporation	00182-1306-01
100's	$94.80	GENERIC, Dixon-Shane Inc	17236-0694-01
100's	$147.21	LOXITANE, Watson/Rugby Laboratories Inc	52544-0812-01
100's	$162.22	GENERIC, Udl Laboratories Inc	51079-0901-20
100's	$163.57	GENERIC, Watson Laboratories Inc	52544-0495-01
Capsule - Oral - 25 mg			
100's	$80.00	GENERIC, Raway Pharmacal Inc	00686-0679-20
100's	$108.90	GENERIC, Major Pharmaceuticals Inc	00904-2312-60
100's	$122.43	GENERIC, Moore, H.L. Drug Exchange Inc	00839-7497-06
100's	$131.20	GENERIC, Qualitest Products Inc	00603-4270-21
100's	$131.20	GENERIC, Creighton Products Corporation	50752-0298-05
100's	$131.23	GENERIC, Aligen Independent Laboratories Inc	00405-5122-01
100's	$135.29	GENERIC, Ivax Corporation	00182-1307-01
100's	$143.24	GENERIC, Dixon-Shane Inc	17236-0695-01
100's	$192.45	GENERIC, Watson Laboratories Inc	00591-0371-01
100's	$242.03	GENERIC, Udl Laboratories Inc	51079-0902-20
100's	$247.14	GENERIC, Watson Laboratories Inc	52544-0496-01
Capsule - Oral - 50 mg			
100's	$135.00	GENERIC, Raway Pharmacal Inc	00686-0680-20

100's	$139.95	GENERIC, Major Pharmaceuticals Inc	00904-2313-60
100's	$175.00	GENERIC, Creighton Products Corporation	50752-0299-05
100's	$175.08	GENERIC, Aligen Independent Laboratories Inc	00405-5123-01
100's	$176.30	GENERIC, Moore, H.L. Drug Exchange Inc	00839-7498-06
100's	$180.50	GENERIC, Ivax Corporation	00182-1308-01
100's	$191.10	GENERIC, Qualitest Products Inc	00603-4271-21
100's	$191.12	GENERIC, Dixon-Shane Inc	17236-0696-01
100's	$317.21	GENERIC, Udl Laboratories Inc	51079-0903-20
100's	$329.76	GENERIC, Watson Laboratories Inc	52544-0497-01

PRODUCT LISTING - EQUIVALENTS NOT AVAILABLE

Capsule - Oral - 10 mg

100's	$78.06	GENERIC, Physicians Total Care	54868-2327-00

Lymphocyte Immune Globulin (001671)

For complete prescribing information, refer to the CD-ROM included with the book.

Categories: Anemia, aplastic; Rejection, renal transplant, prophylaxis; Pregnancy Category C; FDA Pre 1938 Drugs
Drug Classes: Immune globulins; Immunosuppressives
Brand Names: Atgam

WARNING

Only physicians experienced in immunosuppressive therapy in the management of renal transplant or aplastic anemia patients should use lymphocyte immune globulin.

Patients receiving lymphocyte immune globulin should be managed in facilities equipped and staffed with adequate laboratory and supportive medical resources.

DESCRIPTION

FOR INTRAVENOUS USE ONLY

Lymphocyte immune globulin sterile solution contains lymphocyte immune globulin, anti-thymocyte globulin (equine). It is the purified, concentrated, and sterile gamma globulin, primarily monomeric IgG, from hyperimmune serum of horses immunized with human thymus lymphocytes. Lymphocyte immune globulin is a transparent to slightly opalescent aqueous protein solution. It may appear colorless to faintly pink or brown and is nearly odorless. It may develop a slight granular or flaky deposit during storage. (For information about in-line filters, see the infusion instructions in DOSAGE AND ADMINISTRATION.)

Before release for clinical use, each lot of Atgam is tested to assure its ability to inhibit rosette formation between human peripheral lymphocytes and sheep red blood cells *in vitro*. In each lot, antibody activity against human red blood cells and platelets is also measured and determined to be within acceptable limits. Only lots that test negative for antihuman serum protein antibody, antiglomerular basement membrane antibody and pyrogens are released.

Each milliliter of Atgam contains 50 mg of horse gamma globulin stabilized in 0.3 molar glycine to a pH of approximately 6.8.

INDICATIONS AND USAGE

RENAL TRANSPLANTATION

Lymphocyte immune globulin sterile solution is indicated for the management of allograft rejection in renal transplant patients. When administered with conventional therapy at the time of rejection, it increases the frequency of resolution of the acute rejection episode. The drug has also been administered as an adjunct to other immunosuppressive therapy to delay the onset of the first rejection episode. Data accumulated to date have not consistently demonstrated improvement in functional graft survival associated with therapy to delay the onset of the first rejection episode.

APLASTIC ANEMIA

Lymphocyte immune globulin is indicated for the treatment of moderate to severe aplastic anemia in patients who are unsuitable for bone marrow transplantation.

When administered with a regimen of supportive care, lymphocyte immune globulin may induce partial or complete hematologic remission. In a controlled trial, patients receiving lymphocyte immune globulin showed a statistically significant higher improvement rate compared to standard supportive care at 3 months. Improvement was defined in terms of sustained increase in peripheral blood counts and reduced transfusion needs.

Clinical trials conducted at two centers evaluated the 1-year survival rate for patients with severe and moderate to severe aplastic anemia. Seventy-four of the 83 patients enrolled were evaluable based on response to treatment. The treatment groups studied consisted of: 1) lymphocyte immune globulin and supportive care, 2) lymphocyte immune globulin administered following 3 months of supportive care alone, 3) lymphocyte immune globulin, mismatched marrow infusion, androgens, and supportive care, or 4) lymphocyte immune globulin, androgens and supportive care. There were no statistically significant differences between the treatment groups. The 1-year survival rate for the pooled treatment groups was 69%. These survival results can be compared with a historical survival rate of about 25% for patients receiving standard supportive care alone.

The usefulness of lymphocyte immune globulin has not been demonstrated in patients with aplastic anemia who are suitable candidates for bone marrow transplantation or in patients with aplastic anemia secondary to neoplastic disease, storage disease, myelofibrosis, Fanconi's syndrome, or in patients known to have been exposed to myelotoxic agents or radiation.

To date, safety and efficacy have not been established in circumstances other than renal transplantation and aplastic anemia.

SKIN TESTING

Before the first infusion of lymphocyte immune globulin, The Upjohn Company strongly recommends that patients be tested with an intradermal injection of 0.1 ml of a 1:1000 dilution (5 µg horse IgG) of lymphocyte immune globulin in sodium chloride injection and a contralateral sodium chloride injection control. Use only freshly diluted lymphocyte immune globulin for skin testing. The patient and specifically the skin test, should be observed every 15 to 20 minutes over the first hour after intradermal injection. A local reaction of 10 mm or greater with a wheal or erythema, or both, with or without pseudopod formation and itching or a marked local swelling should be considered a positive test. *Note:* The predictive value of this test has not been proven clinically. Allergic reactions such as anaphylaxis have occurred in patients whose skin test is negative. In the presence of a locally positive skin test to lymphocyte immune globulin, serious consideration to alternative forms of therapy should be given. The risk to benefit ration must be carefully weighed. If therapy with lymphocyte immune globulin is deemed appropriate following a locally positive skin test, treatment should be administered in a setting where intensive life support facilities are immediately available and with a physician familiar with the treatment of potentially life threatening allergic reactions in attendance.

A systemic reaction such as a generalized rash, tachycardia, dyspnea, hypotension, or anaphylaxis precludes any additional administration of lymphocyte immune globulin.

See WARNINGS.

CONTRAINDICATIONS

Do not administer lymphocyte immune globulin sterile solution to a patient who has had a severe systemic reaction during prior administration of lymphocyte immune globulin or any other equine gamma globulin preparation.

WARNINGS

Only physicians experienced in immunosuppressive therapy in the management of renal transplant or aplastic anemia patients should use lymphocyte immune globulin.

Patients receiving lymphocyte immune globulin should be treated in facilities equipped and staffed with adequate laboratory and supportive medical resources.

Precise methods of determining the potency of lymphocyte immune globulin have not been established, thus activity may potentially vary from lot to lot.

Discontinue Treatment With Lymphocyte Immune Globulin if Any of the Following Occurs:

1. Symptoms of anaphylaxis.
2. Severe and unremitting thrombocytopenia in renal transplant patients.
3. Severe and unremitting leukopenia in renal transplant patients.

In common with products derived from, or purified with human blood components, the possibility of transmission of infectious agents exists.

DOSAGE AND ADMINISTRATION

RENAL ALLOGRAFT RECIPIENTS

Adult renal allograft patients have received lymphocyte immune globulin sterile solution at the dosage of 10-30 mg/kg of body weight daily. The few children studied received 5-25 mg/kg daily. Lymphocyte immune globulin has been used to delay the onset of the first rejection episode[2-5] and at the time of the first rejection episode.[6-10] Most patients who received lymphocyte immune globulin for the treatment of acute rejection had not received it starting at the time of transplantation.

Usually, lymphocyte immune globulin is used concomitantly with azathioprine and corticosteroids, which are commonly used to suppress the immune response. Exercise caution during repeat courses of lymphocyte immune globulin; carefully observe patients for signs of allergic reactions.

Delaying the Onset of Allograft Rejection: Give a fixed dose of 15 mg/kg daily for 14 days, then every other day for 14 days for a total of 21 doses in 28 days. Administer the first dose within 24 hours before or after the transplant.

Treatment of Rejection: The first dose of lymphocyte immune globulin can be delayed until the diagnosis of the first rejection episode. The recommended dose is 10-15 mg/kg daily for 14 days. Additional alternate-day therapy up to a total of 21 doses can be given.

APLASTIC ANEMIA

The recommended dosage regimen is 10-20 mg/kg daily for 8-14 days. Additional alternate-day therapy up to a total of 21 doses can be administered.[11-13] Because thrombocytopenia can be associated with the administration of lymphocyte immune globulin, patients receiving it for the treatment of aplastic anemia may need prophylactic platelet transfusions to maintain platelets at clinically acceptable levels.

PREPARATION OF SOLUTION

Parenteral drug products should be inspected visually for particulate matter and discoloration prior to administration whenever solution and container permit. However, because lymphocyte immune globulin is a gamma globulin product, it can be transparent to slightly opalescent, colorless to faintly pink or brown, and may develop a slight granular or flaky deposit during storage. Lymphocyte immune globulin (diluted or undiluted) should not be shaken because excessive foaming and/or denaturation of the protein may occur.

Dilute lymphocyte immune globulin for intravenous infusion in an inverted bottle of sterile vehicle so the undiluted lymphocyte immune globulin does not contact the air inside. Add the total daily dose of lymphocyte immune globulin to the sterile vehicle (see Compatibility and Stability). The concentration should not exceed 4 mg of lymphocyte immune globulin per ml. The diluted solution should be gently rotated or swirled to effect thorough mixing.

ADMINISTRATION

The diluted lymphocyte immune globulin should be allowed to reach room temperature before infusion. Lymphocyte immune globulin is appropriately administered into a vascular shunt, arterial venous fistula, or a high-flow central vein through an in-line filter with a pore size of 0.2-1.0 micron. The in-line filter should be used with all infusions of lymphocyte immune globulin to prevent the administration of any insoluble material that may develop in the product during storage. The use of high-flow veins will minimize the occurrence of phlebitis and thrombosis. Do not infuse a dose of lymphocyte immune globulin in less than 4 hours. Always keep appropriate resuscitation equipment at the patient's bedside while lymphocyte immune globulin is being administered. Observe the patient continuously for possible allergic reactions throughout the infusions.

COMPATIBILITY AND STABILITY

Lymphocyte immune globulin, once diluted, has been shown to be physically and chemically stable for up to 24 hours at concentrations of up to 4 mg per ml in the following diluents: 0.9% sodium chloride injection, 5% dextrose and 0.225% sodium chloride injection, and 5% dextrose and 0.45% sodium chloride injection.

Adding lymphocyte immune globulin to dextrose injection is not recommended, as low salt concentrations can cause precipitation. Highly acidic infusion solutions can also contribute to physical instability over time. It is recommended that diluted lymphocyte immune globulin be stored in a refrigerator if it is prepared prior to the time of infusion. Even if it is stored in a refrigerator, the total time in dilution should not exceed 24 hours (including infusion time).

PRODUCT LISTING - EQUIVALENTS NOT AVAILABLE

Powder For Injection - Intravenous - Rabbit 25 mg

1's	$376.40	THYMOGLOBULIN, Sangstat Medical Corporation	62053-0534-25

Solution - Intravenous - Equine 50 mg/ml

5 ml	$262.24	ATGAM, Pharmacia and Upjohn	00009-0926-04
5 ml x 5	$1527.95	ATGAM, Pharmacia and Upjohn	00009-7224-02

Maprotiline Hydrochloride (001700)

For related information, see the comparative table section in Appendix A.

Categories: Depression; Pregnancy Category B; FDA Approved 1980 Dec
Drug Classes: Antidepressants, tetracyclic
Brand Names: Ludiomil
Foreign Brand Availability: Maprostad (Germany); Melodil (Israel); Mirpan (Germany); Psymion (Germany); Retinyl (Greece)
Cost of Therapy: $21.43 (Depression; Generic Tablets; 75 mg; 1 tablet/day; 30 day supply)

DESCRIPTION

Ludiomil, is a tetracyclic antidepressant, available as 25, 50, and 75 mg tablets for oral administration. The chemical name for maprotiline hydrochloride is N-methyl-9,10-ethanoanthracene-9 (10H)-propylamine hydrochloride.

Maprotiline hydrochloride is a fine, white to off-white, practically odorless crystalline powder. It is freely soluble in methanol and in chloroform, slightly soluble in water, and practically insoluble in isooctane. Its molecular weight is 313.87.

The Ludiomil inactive ingredients: are calcium phosphate, cellulose compounds, colloidal silicon dioxide, FD&C yellow no. 6 aluminum lake (25 and 50 mg tablets), lactose, magnesium stearate, povidone, shellac, starch, stearic acid, talc, and titanium dioxide.

CLINICAL PHARMACOLOGY

The mechanism of action of maprotiline HCl is not precisely known. It does not act primarily by stimulation of the central nervous system and is not a monoamine oxidase inhibitor. The postulated mechanism of maprotiline HCl is that it acts primarily by potentiation of central adrenergic synapses by blocking reuptake of norepinephrine at nerve endings. This pharmacologic action is thought to be responsible for the drug's antidepressant and anxiolytic effects.

The mean time to peak is 12 hours. The half-life of elimination averages 51 hours.

Steady-state levels measured prior to the morning dose on a one dosage regimen are summarized in TABLE 1.

TABLE 1

Regimen	Average Minimum Concentration	95% Confidence Limits
50 mg × 3 daily	238 ng/ml	181-295 ng/ml

INDICATIONS AND USAGE

Maprotiline HCl is indicated for the treatment of depressive illness in patients with depressive neurosis (dysthymic disorder) and manic-depressive illness, depressed type (major depressive disorder). Maprotiline HCl is also effective for the relief of anxiety associated with depression.

CONTRAINDICATIONS

Maprotiline HCl is contraindicated in patients hypersensitive to maprotiline and in patients with known or suspected seizure disorders. It should not be given concomitantly with monoamine oxidase (MAO) inhibitors. A minimum of 14 days should be allowed to elapse after discontinuation of MAO inhibitors before treatment with maprotiline is initiated. Effects should be monitored with gradual increase in dosage until optimum response is achieved. The drug is not recommended for use during the acute phase of myocardial infarction.

WARNINGS

Seizures have been associated with the use of maprotiline HCl. Most of the seizures have occurred in patients without a known history of seizures. However, in some of these cases, other confounding factors were present, including concomitant medications known to lower the seizure threshold, rapid escalation of the dosage of maprotiline, and dosage that exceeded the recommended therapeutic range. The incidence of direct reports is less than 1/10th of 1%. The risk of seizures may be increased when maprotiline is taken concomitantly with phenothiazines, when the dosage of benzodiazepines is rapidly tapered in patients receiving maprotiline or when the recommended dosage of maprotiline is exceeded. While a cause-and-effect relationship has not been established, the risk of seizures in patients treated with maprotiline may be reduced by (1) initiating therapy at a low dosage, (2) maintaining the initial dosage for 2 weeks before raising it gradually in small increments as necessitated by the long half-life of maprotiline (average 51 hours), and (3) keeping the dosage at the minimally effective level during maintenance therapy. (See DOSAGE AND ADMINISTRATION.)

Extreme caution should be used when this drug is given to:

- Patients with a history of myocardial infarction.
- Patients with a history of presence of cardiovascular disease because of the possibility of conduction defects, arrhythmias, myocardial infarction, strokes and tachycardia.

PRECAUTIONS

GENERAL

The possibility of suicide in seriously depressed patients is inherent in their illness and may persist until significant remission occurs. Therefore, patients must be carefully supervised during all phases of treatment with maprotiline HCl and prescriptions should be written for the smallest number of tablets consistent with good patient management.

Hypomanic or manic episodes have been known to occur in some patients taking tricyclic antidepressant drugs, particularly in patients with cyclic disorders. Such occurrences have also been noted, rarely, with maprotiline.

Prior to elective surgery, maprotiline should be discontinued for as long as clinically feasible, since little is known about the interaction between maprotiline and general anesthetics.

Maprotiline should be administered with caution in patients with increased intraocular pressure, history of urinary retention, or history of narrow-angle glaucoma because of the drug's anticholinergic properties.

INFORMATION FOR THE PATIENT

Patients should be warned of the association between seizures and the use of maprotiline. Moreover they should be informed that this association is enhanced in patients with a known history of seizures and in those patients who are taking certain other drugs. (See WARNINGS.)

Warn patients to exercise caution about potentially hazardous tasks, or operating automobiles or machinery since the drug may impair mental and/or physical abilities.

Maprotiline may enhance the response to alcohol, barbiturates, and other CNS depressants, requiring appropriate caution of administration.

LABORATORY TESTS

Maprotiline HCl should be discontinued if there is evidence of pathologic neutrophil depression. Leukocyte and differential counts should be performed in patients who develop fever and sore throat during therapy.

CARCINOGENESIS, MUTAGENESIS, AND IMPAIRMENT OF FERTILITY

Carcinogenicity and chronic toxicity studies have been conducted in laboratory rats and dogs. No drug- or dose-related occurrence of carcinogenesis was evident in rats receiving daily oral doses up to 60 mg/kg of maprotiline HCl for eighteen months or in dogs receiving daily oral doses up to 30 mg/kg of maprotiline HCl for 1 year. In addition, no evidence of mutagenic activity was found in offspring of female mice mated with males treated with up to 60 times the maximum daily human dose.

PREGNANCY CATEGORY B

Reproduction studies have been performed in female laboratory rabbits, mice, and rats at doses up to 1.3, 7, and 9 times the maximum daily human dose respectively and have revealed no evidence of impaired fertility or harm to the fetus due to maprotiline HCl. There are, however, no adequate and well-controlled studies in pregnant women. Because animal reproduction studies are not always predictive of human response, this drug should be used during pregnancy only if clearly needed.

LABOR AND DELIVERY

Although the effect of maprotiline HCl on labor and delivery is unknown, caution should be exercised as with any drug with CNS depressant action.

NURSING MOTHERS

Maprotiline is excreted in breast milk. At steady state, the concentrations in milk correspond closely to the concentrations in whole blood. Caution should be exercised when maprotiline is administered to a nursing woman.

PEDIATRIC USE

Safety and effectiveness in pediatric patients below the age of 18 have not been established.

DRUG INTERACTIONS

Close supervision and careful adjustment of dosage are required when administering maprotiline concomitantly with anticholinergic or sympathomimetic drugs because of the possibility of additive atropine-like effects.

Concurrent administration of maprotiline with electroshock therapy should be avoided because of the lack of experience in this area.

Caution should be exercised when administering maprotiline to hyperthyroid patients or those on thyroid medication because of the possibility of enhanced potential for cardiovascular toxicity of maprotiline.

Maprotiline should be used with caution in patients receiving guanethidine or similar agents since it may block the pharmacologic effects of these drugs.

The risk of seizures may be increased when maprotiline is taken concomitantly with phenothiazines or when the dosage of benzodiazepines is rapidly tapered in patients receiving maprotiline.

Because of the pharmacologic similarity of maprotiline to the tricyclic antidepressants, the plasma concentration of maprotiline may be increased when the drug is given concomitantly with hepatic enzyme inhibitors (*e.g.*, cimetidine, fluxetine) and decreased by concomitant administration with hepatic enzyme inducers (*e.g.*, barbituates, phenytoin), as has occurred with tricyclic antidepressants. Adjustment of the dosage of maprotiline may therefore be necessary in such cases. (See PRECAUTIONS, Information for the Patient.)

ADVERSE REACTIONS

The following adverse reactions have been noted with maprotiline HCl and are generally similar to those observed with tricyclic antidepressants.

Cardiovascular: Rare occurrences of hypotension, hypertension, tachycardia, palpitation, arrhythmia, heart block, and syncope have been reported with maprotiline HCl.

Psychiatric: Nervousness (6%), anxiety (3%), insomnia (2%), and agitation (2%); rarely, confusional states (especially in the elderly), hallucinations, disorientation, delusions, restlessness, nightmares, hypomania, mania, exacerbation of psychosis, decrease in memory, and feelings of unreality.

Neurological: Drowsiness (16%), dizziness (8%), tremor (3%), and, rarely, numbness, tingling, motor hyperactivity, akathisia, seizures, EEG alterations, tinnitus, extrapyramidal symptoms, ataxia, and dysarthria.

Anticholinergic: Dry mouth (22%), constipation (6%), and blurred vision (4%); rarely, accommodation disturbances, mydriasis, urinary retention, and delayed micturition.

Allergic: Rare instances of skin rash, petechiae, itching, photosensitization, edema, and drug fever.

Gastrointestinal: Nausea (2%) and, rarely, vomiting, epigastric distress, diarrhea, bitter taste, abdominal cramps and dysphagia.

Endocrine: Rare instances of increased or decreased libido, impotence, and elevation or depression of blood sugar levels.

Other: Weakness and fatigue (4%) and headache (4%); rarely, altered liver function, jaundice, weight loss or gain, excessive perspiration, flushing, urinary frequency, increased salivation, nasal congestion and alopecia.

Note: Although there have been only isolated reports of the following adverse reactions with maprotiline HCl, its pharmacologic similarity to tricyclic antidepressants requires that each reaction be considered when administering maprotiline HCl.

Bone marrow depression, including agranulocytosis, eosinophilia, purpura, and thrombocytopenia, myocardial infarction, stroke, peripheral neuropathy, sublingual adenitis, black tongue, stomatitis, paralytic ileus, gynecomastia in the male, breast enlargement and galactorrhea in the female, and testicular swelling.

POST-INTRODUCTION REPORTS

Several voluntary reports of interstitial pneumonitis, which were in some cases associated with eosinophilia and increased liver enzymes, have been received since market introduction. However, there is no clear causal relationship.

DOSAGE AND ADMINISTRATION

A single daily dose is an alternative to divided daily doses. Therapeutic effects are sometimes seen within 3-7 days, although as long as 2-3 weeks are usually necessary.

INITIAL ADULT DOSAGE

An initial dosage of 75 mg daily is suggested for outpatients with mild-to-moderate depression. However, in some patients, particularly the elderly, an initial dosage of 25 mg daily may be used. Because of the long half-life of maprotiline HCl, the initial dosage should be maintained for 2 weeks. The dosage may then be increased gradually in 25 mg increments as required and tolerated. In most outpatients a maximum dose of 150 mg daily will result in therapeutic efficacy. It is recommended that this dose not be exceeded except in the most severely depressed patients. In such patients, dosage may be gradually increased to a maximum of 225 mg.

More severely depressed, hospitalized patients should be given an initial daily dose of 100-150 mg which may be gradually increased as required and tolerated. Most hospitalized patients with moderate-to-severe depression respond to a daily dosage of 150 mg although dosages as high as 225 mg may be required in some cases. Daily dosage of 225 mg should not be exceeded.

ELDERLY PATIENTS

In general, lower dosages are recommended for patients over 60 years of age. Dosages of 50-75 mg daily are usually satisfactory as maintenance therapy for elderly patients who do not tolerate higher amounts.

MAINTENANCE

Dosage during prolonged maintenance therapy should be kept at the lowest effective level. Dosage may be reduced to levels of 75-150 mg daily during such periods, with subsequent adjustment depending on therapeutic response.

HOW SUPPLIED

Ludiomil is available in:

25 mg: Oval, dark orange, scored, coated imprinted "CIBA 110".

50 mg: Round, dark orange, scored, coated imprinted "CIBA 26".

75 mg: Oval, white, scored, coated imprinted "CIBA 135".

Storage: Do not store above 30°C (86°F). Dispense in a tight container.

PRODUCT LISTING - RATED THERAPEUTICALLY EQUIVALENT

Package	Price	Manufacturer	NDC
Tablet - Oral - 25 mg			
7's	$4.74	GENERIC, Prescript Pharmaceuticals	00247-0808-07
14's	$6.13	GENERIC, Prescript Pharmaceuticals	00247-0808-14
30's	$9.31	GENERIC, Prescript Pharmaceuticals	00247-0808-30
100's	$30.06	GENERIC, Qualitest Products Inc	00603-4294-21
100's	$30.70	GENERIC, Major Pharmaceuticals Inc	00904-3323-60
100's	$31.55	GENERIC, Major Pharmaceuticals Inc	00904-3323-61
100's	$35.95	GENERIC, Martec Pharmaceuticals Inc	52555-0355-01
100's	$37.19	GENERIC, Moore, H.L. Drug Exchange Inc	00839-7448-06
100's	$37.50	LUDIOMIL, Ivax Corporation	00182-1882-01
100's	$43.58	GENERIC, Watson Laboratories Inc	52544-0373-01
100's	$50.00	GENERIC, Mylan Pharmaceuticals Inc	00378-0060-01
Tablet - Oral - 50 mg			
7's	$5.39	GENERIC, Prescript Pharmaceuticals	00247-0809-07
14's	$7.44	GENERIC, Prescript Pharmaceuticals	00247-0809-14
30's	$12.09	GENERIC, Prescript Pharmaceuticals	00247-0809-30
100's	$36.00	GENERIC, Raway Pharmacal Inc	00686-0494-20
100's	$39.49	GENERIC, Qualitest Products Inc	00603-4295-21
100's	$47.70	GENERIC, Major Pharmaceuticals Inc	00904-3324-60
100's	$52.52	GENERIC, Moore, H.L. Drug Exchange Inc	00839-7449-06
100's	$52.80	GENERIC, Martec Pharmaceuticals Inc	52555-0356-01
100's	$55.00	GENERIC, Ivax Corporation	00182-1883-01
100's	$64.48	GENERIC, Watson Laboratories Inc	52544-0374-01
100's	$74.10	GENERIC, Mylan Pharmaceuticals Inc	00378-0087-01
Tablet - Oral - 75 mg			
7's	$6.22	GENERIC, Prescript Pharmaceuticals	00247-0810-07
14's	$9.09	GENERIC, Prescript Pharmaceuticals	00247-0810-14
30's	$15.66	GENERIC, Prescript Pharmaceuticals	00247-0810-30
100's	$71.43	GENERIC, Qualitest Products Inc	00603-4296-21
100's	$71.48	GENERIC, Moore, H.L. Drug Exchange Inc	00839-7450-06
100's	$93.00	GENERIC, Mylan Pharmaceuticals Inc	00378-0092-01
100's	$93.00	GENERIC, Watson Laboratories Inc	52544-0375-01

Measles and Rubella Virus Vaccine Live *(001702)*

For complete prescribing information, refer to the CD-ROM included with the book.

Categories: Immunization, measles; Immunization, rubella; Pregnancy Category C; FDA Pre 1938 Drugs; WHO Formulary
Drug Classes: Vaccines
Brand Names: M-R-Vax II
Foreign Brand Availability: MoRu-Viraten Berna (Canada); Rudi-Rouvax (France; Thailand)

DESCRIPTION

M-R-VAX II (Measles and Rubella Virus Vaccine Live) is a live virus vaccine for immunization against measles (rubeola) and rubella (German measles).

M-R-VAX II is a sterile lyophilized preparation of (1) Attenuvax (Measles Virus Vaccine Live), a more attenuated line of measles virus, derived from Enders' attenuated Edmonston strain and grown in cell cultures of chick embryo; and (2) Meruvax II (Rubella Virus Vaccine Live), the Wistar RA 27/3 strain of live attenuated rubella virus grown in human diploid cell (WI-38) culture.[1,2] The vaccine viruses are the same as those used in the manufacture of Attenuvax (Measles Virus Vaccine Live) and Meruvax II (Rubella Virus Vaccine Live). The two viruses are mixed before being lyophilized. The product contains no preservative.

The reconstituted vaccine is for subcutaneous administration. When reconstituted as directed, the dose for injection is 0.5 ml and contains not less than the equivalent of 1,000 $TCID_{50}$ (tissue culture infectious doses) of the U.S. Reference Measles Virus; 1,000 $TCID_{50}$ of the U.S. Reference Rubella Virus. Each dose contains approximately 25 mcg of neomycin. The product contains no preservative. Sorbitol and hydrolyzed gelatin are added as stabilizers.

INDICATIONS AND USAGE

M-R-VAX II is indicated for simultaneous immunization against measles and rubella in persons 15 months of age or older. A second dose of M-R-VAX II or monovalent measles vaccine is recommended (see Revaccination.)[17,18,19]

Infants who are less than 15 months of age may fail to respond to the measles component of the vaccine due to presence in the circulation of residual measles antibody of maternal origin; the younger the infant, the lower the likelihood of seroconversion. In geographically isolated or other relatively inaccessible populations for whom immunization programs are logistically difficult, and in population groups in which natural measles infection may occur in a significant proportion of infants before 15 months of age, it may be desirable to give the vaccine to infants at an earlier age. Infants vaccinated under these conditions at less than 12 months of age should be revaccinated after reaching 15 months of age. There is some evidence to suggest that infants immunized at less than one year of age may not develop sustained antibody levels when later reimmunized. The advantage of early protection must be weighed against the chance for failure to respond adequately on reimmunization.[20]

Previously unimmunized children of susceptible pregnant women should receive live attenuated rubella vaccine, because an immunized child will be less likely to acquire natural rubella and introduce the virus into the household.

Individuals planning travel outside the United States, if not immune, can acquire measles, mumps or rubella and import these diseases to the United States. Therefore, prior to International travel, individuals known to be susceptible to one or more of these diseases can receive either a single antigen vaccine (measles, mumps or rubella), or a combined antigen vaccine as appropriate. However, M-M-R† II (Measles, Mumps, and Rubella Virus Vaccine

Live) is preferred for persons likely to be susceptible to mumps and rubella; and if a single-antigen measles vaccine is not readily available, travelers should receive M-M-R II (Measles, Mumps, and Rubella Virus Vaccine Live) regardless of their immune status to mumps or rubella.[21,22,23]

Non-Pregnant Adolescent and Adult Females: Immunization of susceptible non-pregnant adolescent and adult females of childbearing age with live attenuated rubella virus vaccine is indicated if certain precautions are observed. Vaccinating susceptible postpubertal females confers individual protection against subsequently acquiring rubella infection during pregnancy, which in turn prevents infection of the fetus and consequent congenital rubella injury.[24]

Women of childbearing age should be advised not to become pregnant for three months after vaccination and should be informed of the reason for this precaution.*

It is recommended that rubella susceptibility be determined by serologic testing prior to immunization.** If immune, as evidenced by a specific rubella antibody titer of 1:8 or greater (hemagglutination-inhibition test), vaccination is unnecessary. Congenital malformations do occur in up to seven percent of all live births.[25] Their chance appearance after vaccination could lead to misinterpretation of the cause, particularly if the prior rubella-immune status of vaccinees is unknown.

Postpubertal females should be informed of the frequent occurrence of generally self-limited arthralgia and/or arthritis beginning 2 to 4 weeks after vaccination.

Postpartum Women: It has been found convenient in many instances to vaccinate rubella-susceptible women in the immediate postpartum period.

Revaccination: Children first vaccinated when younger than 12 months of age should be revaccinated at 15 months of age.

The American Academy of Pediatrics (AAP), the Immunization Practices Advisory Committee (ACIP), and some state and local health agencies have recommended guidelines for routine measles revaccination and to help control measles outbreaks.[26,27]***

Vaccines available for revaccination include monovalent measles vaccine (Measles Virus Vaccine Live) and polyvalent vaccines containing measles (*e.g.,* M-M-R II (Measles, Mumps, and Rubella Virus Vaccine Live) M-R-VAX II). If the prevention of sporadic measles outbreaks is the sole objective, revaccination with a monovalent measles vaccine should be considered (see appropriate product circular). If concern also exists about immune status regarding mumps or rubella, revaccination with appropriate monovalent or polyvalent vaccines should be considered after consulting the appropriate product circulars. Unnecessary doses of a vaccine are best avoided by ensuring that written documentation of vaccination is preserved and a copy given to each vaccinee's parent or guardian.

***NOTE:** The Immunization Practices Advisory Committee (ACIP) has recommended "In view of the importance of protecting this age group against rubella, reasonable precautions in a rubella immunization program include asking females if they are pregnant, excluding those who say they are, and explaining the theoretical risks to the others."[24]

****NOTE:** The Immunization Practices Advisory Committee (ACIP) has stated "When practical, and when reliable laboratory services are available, potential vaccinees of childbearing age can have serologic tests to determine susceptibility to rubella.... However, routinely performing serologic tests for all females of childbearing age to determine susceptibility so that vaccine is given only to proven susceptibles is expensive and has been ineffective in some areas. Accordingly, the ACIP believes that rubella vaccination of a woman who is not known to be pregnant and has no history of vaccination is justifiable without serologic testing."[24]

M

*****NOTE:** A primary difference among these recommendations is the timing of revaccination: the ACIP recommends routine revaccination at entry into Kindergarten or first grade, whereas the AAP recommends routine revaccination at entrance to middle school or junior high school. In addition, some public health jurisdictions mandate the age for revaccination. The complete text of applicable guidelines should be consulted.[26,27]

Use With Other Vaccines: Routine administration of DTP (diphtheria, tetanus, pertussis) and/or OPV (oral poliovirus vaccine) concomitantly with measles, mumps, and rubella vaccines is not recommended because there are insufficient data relating to the simultaneous administration of these antigens. However, the American Academy of Pediatrics has noted that in some circumstances, particularly when the patient may not return, some practitioners prefer to administer all these antigens on a single day. If done, separate sites and syringes should be used for DTP and M-R-VAX II.[28]

M-R-VAX II should not be given less than one month before or after administration of other virus vaccines.

CONTRAINDICATIONS

Do not give M-R-VAX II to pregnant females; the possible effects of the vaccine on fetal development are unknown at this time. If vaccination of postpubertal females is undertaken, pregnancy should be avoided for three months following vaccination.

Anaphylactic or anaphylactoid reactions to neomycin (each dose of reconstituted vaccine contains approximately 25 mcg of neomycin).

History of anaphylactic or anaphylactoid reactions to eggs (see HYPERSENSITIVITY TO EGGS).

Any febrile respiratory illness or other active febrile infection.

Active untreated tuberculosis.

Patients receiving immunosuppressive therapy. This contraindication does not apply to patients who are receiving corticosteroids as replacement therapy, e.g., for Addison's disease.

Individuals with blood dyscrasias, leukemia, lymphomas of any type, or other malignant neoplasms affecting the bone marrow or lymphatic systems.

Primary and acquired immunodeficiency states, including patients who are immunosuppressed in association with AIDS or other clinical manifestations of infection with human immunodeficiency viruses;[29,30] cellular immune deficiencies; and hypogammaglobulinemic and dysgammaglobulinemic states.

Individuals with a family history of congenital or hereditary immunodeficiency, until the immune competence of the potential vaccine recipient is demonstrated.[31]

HYPERSENSITIVITY TO EGGS

Live measles vaccine is produced in chick embryo cell culture. Persons with a history of anaphylactic, anaphylactoid, or other immediate reactions (*e.g.,* hives, swelling of the mouth and throat, difficulty breathing, hypotension, or shock) subsequent to egg ingestion should not be vaccinated. Evidence indicates that persons are not at increased risk if they have egg allergies that are not anaphylactic or anaphylactoid in nature. Such persons may be vaccinated in the usual manner. There is no evidence to indicate that persons with allergies to chickens or feathers are at increased risk of reaction to the vaccine.[20]

DOSAGE AND ADMINISTRATION

FOR SUBCUTANEOUS ADMINISTRATION

Do not inject intravenously

The dosage of vaccine is the same for all persons. Inject the total volume of the single dose vial (about 0.5 ml) or 0.5 ml of the multiple dose vial of reconstituted vaccine subcutaneously, preferably into the outer aspect of upper arm. *Do not give immune globulin (IG) concurrently with* M-R-VAX II.

During shipment, to insure that there is no loss of potency, the vaccine must be maintained at a temperature of 10°C (50°F) or less.

Before reconstitution, store M-R-VAX II at 2° - 8°C (36° - 46°F). *Protect from light.*

Caution: A sterile syringe free of preservatives, antiseptics, and detergents should be used for each injection and/or reconstitution of the vaccine because these substances may inactivate the live virus vaccine. A 25 gauge, 5/8" needle is recommended.

To reconstitute, use only the diluent supplied, since it is free of preservatives or other antiviral substances which might inactivate the vaccine.

Single Dose Vial: First withdraw the entire volume of diluent into the syringe to be used for reconstitution. Inject all the diluent in the syringe into the vial of lyophilized vaccine, and agitate to mix thoroughly. Withdraw the entire contents into a syringe and inject the total volume of restored vaccine subcutaneously.

It is important to use a separate sterile syringe and needle for each individual patient to prevent transmission of hepatitis B and other infectious agents from one person to another.

10 Dose Vial (available Only To Government Agencies/Institutions): Withdraw the entire contents (7 ml) of the diluent vial into the sterile syringe to be used for reconstitution, and introduce into the 10 dose vial of lyophilized vaccine. Agitate to ensure thorough mixing. The outer labeling suggests "For Jet Injector or Syringe Use". Use with separate sterile syringes is permitted for containers of 10 doses or less. The vaccine and diluent do not contain preservatives; therefore, the user must recognize the potential contamination hazards and exercise special precautions to protect the sterility and potency of the product. The use of aseptic techniques and proper storage prior to and after restoration of the vaccine and subsequent withdrawal of the individual doses is essential. Use 0.5 ml of the reconstituted vaccine for subcutaneous injection.

It is important to use a separate sterile syringe and needle for each individual patient to prevent transmission of hepatitis B and other infectious agents from one person to another.

50 Dose Vial (Available Only To Government Agencies/Institutions): Withdraw the entire contents (30 ml) of diluent vial into the sterile syringe to be used for reconstitution and introduce into the 50 dose vial of lyophilized vaccine. Agitate to ensure thorough mixing. With full aseptic precautions, attach the vial to the sterilized multidose jet injector apparatus. Use 0.5 ml of the reconstituted vaccine for subcutaneous injection.

Each dose contains not less than the equivalent of 1,000 $TCID_{50}$ of the U.S. Reference Measles Virus and 1,000 $TCID_{50}$ of the U.S. Reference Rubella Virus.

Parenteral drug products should be inspected visually for particulate matter and discoloration prior to administration. M-R-VAX II, when reconstituted, is clear yellow.

STORAGE

It is recommended that the vaccine be used as soon as possible after reconstitution. Protect vaccine from light at all times, since such exposure may inactivate the virus. Store reconstituted vaccine in the vaccine vial in a dark place at 2° - 8°C (36° - 46°F) and discard if not used within 8 hours.

Measles Virus Vaccine Live (001703)

For complete prescribing information, refer to the CD-ROM included with the book.

Categories: Immunization, measles; Pregnancy Category C; FDA Pre 1938 Drugs; WHO Formulary
Drug Classes: Vaccines
Brand Names: Attenuvax
Foreign Brand Availability: Cam-Kovac (Korea); Diplovax (South-Africa); Ervevax (Australia; Malaysia; Mexico); Lirugen Measles (Philippines); M-VAC (India); Meruvax II (Australia); Mevilin-L (Israel); Morbilvax (Taiwan; Thailand); Rimevax (Australia; Austria; Bahrain; Belgium; Bulgaria; Cyprus; Egypt; Iran; Iraq; Israel; Italy; Jordan; Kuwait; Lebanon; Libya; Malaysia; Oman; Philippines; Qatar; Republic-of-Yemen; Saudi-Arabia; South-Africa; Spain; Switzerland; Syria; Taiwan; Thailand; United-Arab-Emirates); Rouvax (Benin; Burkina-Faso; Ethiopia; France; Gambia; Ghana; Guinea; Hong-Kong; Israel; Ivory-Coast; Kenya; Liberia; Malawi; Mali; Mauritania; Mauritius; Morocco; Niger; Nigeria; Senegal; Seychelles; Sierra-Leone; South-Africa; Sudan; Taiwan; Tanzania; Thailand; Tunia; Uganda; Zambia; Zimbabwe)

DESCRIPTION

Attenuvax (Measles Virus Vaccine Live) is a live virus vaccine for immunization against measles (rubeola).

Attenuvax is a sterile lyophilized preparation of a more attenuated line of measles virus derived from Enders' attenuated Edmonston strain. The further modification of the virus in Attenuvax was achieved in the Merck Institute for Therapeutic Research by multiple passage of Edmonston strain virus in cell cultures of chick embryo at low temperature.

The reconstituted vaccine is for subcutaneous administration. When reconstituted as directed, the dose for injection is 0.5 ml and contains not less than the equivalent of 1,000 $TCID_{50}$ (tissue culture infectious doses) of the U.S. Reference Measles Virus. Each dose also contains approximately 25 mcg of neomycin. The product contains no preservative. Sorbitol and hydrolized gelatin are added as stabilizers.

INDICATIONS AND USAGE

Measles virus vaccine is indicated for immunization against measles (rubeola) in persons 15 months of age or older. A second dose of measles virus vaccine is recommended (see Revaccination).[7,8,9] Infants who are less than 15 months of age may fail to respond to the vaccine due to presence in the circulation of residual measles antibody of maternal origin; the younger the infant, the lower the likelihood of seroconversion. In geographically isolated or other relatively inaccessible populations for whom immunization programs are logistically difficult, and in population groups in which natural measles infection may occur in a significant proportion of infants before 15 months of age, it may be desirable to give the vaccine to infants at an earlier age. Infants vaccinated under these conditions at less than 12 months of age should be revaccinated after reaching 15 months of age. There is some evidence to suggest that infants immunized at less than one year of age may not develop sustained antibody levels when later reimmunized. The advantage of early protection must be weighed against the chance for failure to respond adequately on reimmunization.[10,11]

According to ACIP recommendations, most persons born in 1956 or earlier are likely to have been infected naturally and generally need not be considered susceptible. All children, adolescents, and adults born after 1956 are considered susceptible and should be vaccinated, if there are no contraindications. This includes persons who may be immune to measles but who lack adequate documentation of immunity as evidenced by: (1) physician-diagnosed measles, (2) laboratory evidence of measles immunity, or (3) adequate immunization with live measles vaccine on or after the first birthday.[12]

Measles virus vaccine given immediately after exposure to natural measles may provide some protection. If, however, the vaccine is given a few days before exposure, substantial protection may be provided.

Individuals planning travel outside the United States, if not immune, can acquire measles, mumps or rubella and import these diseases to the United States. Therefore, prior to International travel, individuals known to be susceptible to one or more of these diseases can receive either a single antigen vaccine (measles, mumps or rubella), or a combined antigen vaccine as appropriate. However, M-M-R* II (Measles, Mumps, and Rubella Virus Vaccine Live) is preferred for persons likely to be susceptible to mumps and rubella; and if single-antigen measles vaccine is not readily available, travelers should receive M-M-R II (Measles, Mumps, and Rubella Virus Vaccine Live) regardless of their immune status to mumps or rubella.[13,14,15]

Revaccination: Children first vaccinated when younger than 12 months of age should be revaccinated at 15 months of age, particularly if vaccine was administered with immune serum globulin or measles immune globulin, a standardized globulin preparation.

The American Academy of Pediatrics (AAP), the Immunization Practices Advisory Committee (ACIP), and some state and local health agencies have recommended guidelines for routine measles revaccination and to help control measles outbreaks.[16,17]*

Vaccines available for revaccination include monovalent measles vaccine and polyvalent vaccines containing measles (*e.g.,* M-M-R II (Measles, Mumps, and Rubella Virus Vaccine Live), M-R-VAX II (Measles and Rubella Virus Vaccine Live)). If the prevention of sporadic measles outbreaks is the sole objective, revaccination with a monovalent measles vaccine should be considered. If concern also exists about immune status regarding mumps or rubella, revaccination with appropriate monovalent or polyvalent vaccines should be considered after consulting the appropriate product circulars. Unnecessary doses of a vaccine are best avoided by ensuring that written documentation of vaccination is preserved and a copy given to each vaccinee's parent or guardian.

Despite the risk of reactions, persons born since 1956 who have previously been given inactivated vaccine alone or followed by live vaccine within 3 months should be revaccinated with live vaccine to reduce the risk of the severe atypical form of natural measles that may occur.[10,12]

Use with other Vaccines: Routine administration of DTP (diphtheria, tetanus, pertussis) and/or OPV (oral poliovirus vaccine) concomitantly with measles, mumps and rubella vaccines is not recommended because there are insufficient data relating to the simultaneous administration of these antigens. However, the American Academy of Pediatrics has noted that in some circumstances, particularly when the patient may not return, some practitioners prefer to administer all these antigens on a single day. If done, separate sites and syringes should be used for DTP and measles virus vaccine.[18]

Measles virus vaccine should not be given less than one month before or after administration of other virus vaccines.

CONTRAINDICATIONS

Do not give measles virus vaccine to pregnant females; the possible effects of the vaccine on fetal development are unknown at this time. If vaccination of postpubertal females is undertaken, pregnancy should be avoided for three months following vaccination.

Anaphylactic or anaphylactoid reactions to neomycin (each dose of reconstituted vaccine contains approximately 25 mcg of neomycin).

History of anaphylactic or anaphylactoid reactions to eggs (see Hypersensitivity To Eggs).

Any febrile respiratory illness or other active febrile infection.

Active untreated tuberculosis.

Patients receiving immunosuppressive therapy. This contraindication does not apply to patients who are receiving corticosteroids as replacement therapy, (*e.g.,* for Addison's disease).

Individuals with blood dyscrasias, leukemia, lymphomas of any type, or other malignant neoplasms affecting the bone marrow or lymphatic systems.

Primary and acquired immunodeficiency states, including patients who are immunosuppressed in association with AIDS or other clinical manifestations of infection with human immunodeficiency viruses;[19,20] cellular immune deficiencies; and hypogammaglobulinemic and dysgammaglobulinemic states.

Individuals with a family history of congenital or hereditary immunodeficiency, until the immune competence of the potential vaccine recipient is demonstrated.[21]

*NOTE: A primary difference among these recommendations is the timing of revaccination: the ACIP recommends routine revaccination at entry into kindergarten or first grade, whereas the AAP recommends routine revaccination at entrance to middle school or junior high school. In addition, some public health jurisdictions mandate the age for revaccination. The complete text of applicable guidelines should be consulted.[16,17]

HYPERSENSITIVITY TO EGGS

Live measles vaccine is produced in chick embryo cell culture. Persons with a history of anaphylactic, anaphylactoid or other immediate reactions (*e.g.,* hives, swelling of the mouth and throat, difficulty breathing, hypotension and shock) subsequent to egg ingestion should not be vaccinated. Evidence indicates that persons are not at increased risk if they have egg allergies that are not anaphylactic or anaphylactoid in nature. Such persons should be vaccinated in the usual manner. There is no evidence to indicate that persons with allergies to chickens or feathers are at increased risk of reaction to the vaccine.[12]

DOSAGE AND ADMINISTRATION

FOR SUBCUTANEOUS ADMINISTRATION

Do not inject intravenously

The dosage of vaccine is the same for all persons. Inject the total volume of the single dose vial (about 0.5 ml) or 0.5 ml of the multiple dose vial of reconstituted vaccine subcutaneously, preferably into the outer aspect of upper arm. *Do not give immune globulin (IG) concurrently with* measles virus vaccine.

During shipment, to insure that there is no loss of potency, the vaccine must be maintained at a temperature of 10°C (50°F) or less.

Before reconstitution, store measles virus vaccine at 2° - 8°C (36° - 46°F). *Protect from light.*

Caution: A sterile syringe free of preservatives, antiseptics, and detergents should be used for each injection and/or reconstitution of the vaccine because these substances may inactivate the live virus vaccine. A 25 gauge, 5/8" needle is recommended.

To reconstitute, use only the diluent supplied, since it is free of preservatives or other antiviral substances which might inactivate the vaccine.

Single Dose Vial: First withdraw the entire volume of diluent into the syringe to be used for reconstitution. Inject all the diluent in the syringe into the vial of lyophilized vaccine, and agitate to mix thoroughly. Withdraw the entire contents into a syringe and inject the total volume of restored vaccine subcutaneously.

It is important to use a separate sterile syringe and needle for each individual patient to prevent transmission of hepatitis B and other infectious agents from one person to another.

10 DOSE VIAL (AVAILABLE ONLY TO GOVERNMENT AGENCIES/INSTITUTIONS)

Withdraw the entire contents (7 ml) of the diluent vial into the sterile syringe to be used for reconstitution, and introduce into the 10 dose vial of lyophilized vaccine. Agitate to ensure thorough mixing. The outer labeling suggests "For Jet Injector or Syringe Use". Use with separate sterile syringes is permitted for containers of 10 doses or less. The vaccine and diluent do not contain preservatives; therefore, the user must recognize the potential contamination hazards and exercise special precautions to protect the sterility and potency of the product. The use of aseptic techniques and proper storage prior to and after restoration of the vaccine and subsequent withdrawal of the individual doses is essential. Use 0.5 ml of the reconstituted vaccine for subcutaneous injection.

It is important to use a separate sterile syringe and needle for each individual patient to prevent transmission of hepatitis B and other infectious agents from one person to another.

50 DOSE VIAL (AVAILABLE ONLY TO GOVERNMENT AGENCIES/INSTITUTIONS)

Withdraw the entire contents (30 ml) of diluent vial into the sterile syringe to be used for reconstitution and introduce into the 50 dose vial of lyophilized vaccine. Agitate to ensure thorough mixing. With full aseptic precautions, attach the vial to the sterilized multidose jet injector apparatus. Use 0.5 ml of the reconstituted vaccine for subcutaneous injection.

Each dose of measles virus vaccine contains not less than 1,000 $TCID_{50}$ (tissue culture infectious doses) of measles virus vaccine expressed in terms of the assigned titer of the U.S. Reference Measles Virus.

Parenteral drug products should be inspected visually for particulate matter and discoloration prior to administration. Measles virus vaccine, when reconstituted, is clear yellow.

STORAGE

It is recommended that the vaccine be used as soon as possible after reconstitution. Protect vaccine from light at all times, since such exposure may inactivate the virus. Store reconstituted vaccine in the vaccine vial in a dark place at 2° - 8°C (36° - 46°F) and discard if not used within 8 hours.

PRODUCT LISTING - EQUIVALENTS NOT AVAILABLE

Powder For Injection - Subcutaneous - Strength n/a

1's	$19.70	ATTENUVAX, Merck & Company Inc	00006-4709-00
10's	$158.20	ATTENUVAX, Merck & Company Inc	00006-4589-00

M

Measles, Mumps and Rubella Virus Vaccine Live (001704)

For complete prescribing information, refer to the CD-ROM included with the book.

Categories: Immunization, measles; Immunization, mumps; Immunization, rubella; Pregnancy Category C; FDA Pre 1938 Drugs; WHO Formulary
Drug Classes: Vaccines
Brand Names: **M-M-R II**
Foreign Brand Availability: MMR (Ecuador); MMR II (Hong-Kong; Philippines; Switzerland; Taiwan); M.M.R. II (Israel); M.M.R. Vaccine (Korea); M-M-R Vax (Austria; Germany); Morupar (Philippines); Mumeru Vax (Korea; Philippines); Pluserix (Bahamas; Barbados; Belize; Benin; Bermuda; Burkina-Faso; Curacao; Ethiopia; Gambia; Germany; Ghana; Guinea; Guyana; Ivory-Coast; Jamaica; Kenya; Liberia; Malawi; Mali; Mauritania; Mauritius; Morocco; Netherland-Antilles; Niger; Nigeria; Puerto-Rico; Senegal; Seychelles; Sierra-Leone; Sudan; Surinam; Tanzania; Trinidad; Tunia; Uganda; Zambia; Zimbabwe); Priorix (Australia; Israel; Korea; Philippines); R.O.R. Vax (France); Tri-Kovax (Korea); Trimovax (Bulgaria; Hong-Kong; Italy; South-Africa; Taiwan; Thailand); Triviraten Berna (Hong-Kong; Malaysia; New-Zealand; Philippines; Thailand)

DESCRIPTION

M-M-R II (Measles, Mumps, and Rubella Virus Vaccine Live) is a live virus vaccine for immunization against measles (rubeola), mumps and rubella (German measles).

M-M-R II is a sterile lyophilized preparation of (1) Attenuvax (Measles Virus Vaccine Live), a more attenuated line of measles virus, derived from Enders' attenuated Edmonston strain and grown in cell cultures of chick embryo; (2) Mumpsvax (Mumps Virus Vaccine Live), the Jeryl Lynn (B level) strain of mumps virus grown in cell cultures of chick embryo; and (3) Meruvax II (Rubella Virus Vaccine Live), the Wistar RA 27/3 strain of live attenuated rubella virus grown in human diploid cell (WI-38) culture.[1,2] The vaccine viruses are the same as those used in the manufacture of Attenuvax (Measles Virus Vaccine Live), Mumpsvax (Mumps Virus Vaccine Live) and Meruvax II (Rubella Virus Vaccine Live). The three viruses are mixed before being lyophilized. The product contains no preservative.

The reconstituted vaccine is for subcutaneous administration. When reconstituted as directed, the dose for injection is 0.5 ml and contains not less than the equivalent of 1000 $TCID_{50}$ (tissue culture infectious doses) of the US Reference Measles Virus; 20,000 $TCID_{50}$ of the US Reference Mumps Virus; and 1,000 $TCID_{50}$ of the US Reference Rubella Virus. Each dose contains approximately 25 µg of neomycin. The product contains no preservative. Sorbitol and hydrolyzed gelatin are added as stabilizers.

STORAGE

It is recommended that the vaccine be used as soon as possible after reconstitution. Protect vaccine from light at all times, since such exposure may inactivate the virus. Store reconstituted vaccine in the vaccine vial in a dark place at 2-8°C (36-46°F) and discard if not used within 8 hours.

INDICATIONS AND USAGE

M-M-R II is indicated for simultaneous immunization against measles, mumps, and rubella in persons 15 months of age or older. A second dose of M-M-R II or monovalent measles vaccine is recommended (see Revaccination).[17-19]

Infants who are less than 15 months of age may fail to respond to the measles component of the vaccine due to presence in the circulation of residual measles antibody of maternal origin, the younger the infant, the lower the likelihood of seroconversion. In geographically isolated or other relatively inaccessible populations for whom immunization programs are logistically difficult, and in population groups in which natural measles infection may occur in a significant proportion of infants before 15 months of age, it may be desirable to give the vaccine to infants at an earlier age. Infants vaccinated under these conditions at less than 12 months of age should be revaccinated after reaching 15 months of age. There is some evidence to suggest that infants immunized at less than 1 year of age may not develop sustained antibody levels when later reimmunized. The advantage of early protection must be weighed against the chance for failure to respond adequately on reimmunization.[20]

Previously unimmunized children of susceptible pregnant women should receive live attenuated rubella vaccine, because an immunized child will be less likely to acquire natural rubella and introduce the virus into the household.

Individuals planning travel outside the United States, if not immune, can acquire measles, mumps or rubella and import these diseases to the United States. Therefore, prior to international travel, individuals known to be susceptible to one or more of these diseases can receive either a single antigen vaccine (measles, mumps or rubella), or a combined antigen vaccine as appropriate. However, M-M-R II is preferred for persons likely to be susceptible to mumps and rubella; and if single-antigen measles vaccine is not readily available, travelers should receive M-M-R II regardless of their immune status to mumps or rubella.[21-23]

NON-PREGNANT ADOLESCENT AND ADULT FEMALES

Immunization of susceptible non-pregnant adolescent and adult females of childbearing age with live attenuated rubella virus vaccine is indicated if certain precautions are observed. Vaccinating susceptible postpubertal females confers individual protection against subsequently acquiring rubella infection during pregnancy, which in turn prevents infection of the fetus and consequent congenital rubella injury.[24]

Women of childbearing age should be advised not to become pregnant for 3 months after vaccination and should be informed of the reasons for this precaution.*

It is recommended that rubella susceptibility be determined by serologic testing prior to immunization.† If immune, as evidenced by a specific rubella antibody titer of 1:8 or greater (hemagglutination-inhibition test), vaccination is unnecessary. Congenital malformations do occur in up to 7% of all live births.[25] Their chance appearance after vaccination could lead to misinterpretation of the cause, particularly if the prior rubella-immune status of vaccinees is unknown.

Postpubertal females should be informed of the frequent occurrence of generally self-limited arthralgia and/or arthritis beginning 2-4 weeks after vaccination.

POSTPARTUM WOMEN

It has been found convenient in many instances to vaccinate rubella susceptible women in the immediate postpartum period.

REVACCINATION

Children first vaccinated when younger than 12 months of age should be revaccinated at 15 months of age.

The American Academy of Pediatrics (AAP), the Immunization Practices Advisory Committee (ACIP), and some state and local health agencies have recommended guidelines for routine measles revaccination and to help control measles outbreaks.[26,27]‡

*NOTE: The Immunization Practices Advisory Committee (ACIP) has recommended "In view of the importance of protecting this age group against rubella, reasonable precautions in a rubella immunization program include asking females if they are pregnant, excluding those who say they are, and explaining the theoretical risk to the others".[24]

†NOTE: The Immunization Practices Advisory Committee (ACIP)) has stated "When practical, and when reliable laboratory services are available, potential vaccinees of childbearing age can have serologic tests to determine susceptibility to rubella.... However, routinely performing serologic tests for all females of childbearing age to determine susceptibility so that vaccine is given only to proven susceptibles is expensive and has been ineffective in some areas. Accordingly, the ACIP believes that rubella vaccination of a woman who is not known to be pregnant and has no history of vaccination is justifiable without serologic testing".[24]

‡NOTE: A primary difference among these recommendations is the timing of revaccination: the ACIP recommends routine revaccination at entry into kindergarten or first grade, whereas the AAP recommends routine revaccination at entrance to middle school or junior high school. In addition, some public health jurisdictions mandate the age for revaccination. The complete text of applicable guidelines should be consulted.[26,27]

Vaccines available for revaccination include monovalent measles vaccine (Attenuvax (Measles Virus Vaccine Live)) and polyvalent vaccines containing measles (*e.g.*, M-M-R II, M-R-VAX II (Measles and Rubella Virus Vaccine Live)). If the prevention of sporadic measles outbreaks is the sole objective, revaccination with a monovalent measles vaccine should be considered (see appropriate product circular). If concern also exists about immune status regarding mumps or rubella, revaccination with appropriate monovalent or polyvalent vaccine should be considered after consulting the appropriate product circulars. Unnecessary doses of a vaccine are best avoided by ensuring that written documentation of vaccination is preserved and a copy given to each vaccinee's parent or guardian.

USE WITH OTHER VACCINES

Routine administration of DTP (diphtheria, tetanus, pertussis) and/or OPV (oral poliovirus vaccine) concomitantly with measles, mumps, and rubella vaccines is not recommended because there are limited data[28] relating to the simultaneous administration of these antigens. M-M-R II should be given 1 month before or after administration of other vaccines.

However, other schedules have been used. For example, the American Academy of Pediatrics has noted that when the patient may not return, some practitioners prefer to administer DTP, OPV, and M-M-R II on a single day. If done, separate sites and syringes should be used for DTP and M-M-R II.[29] The Immunization Practices Advisory Committee (ACIP) recommends routine simultaneous administration of M-M-R II, DTP and OPV or inactivated polio vaccine (IPV) to all children ≥15 months who are eligible to receive these vaccines on the basis that there are equivalent antibody responses and no clinically significant increases in the frequency of adverse events when DTP, M-M-R II and OPV (or IPV are administered either simultaneously at different sites or separately.* Administration of M-M-R II at 15 months followed by DTP and OPV (or IPV) at 18 months remains an acceptable alternative, especially for children with caregivers known to be generally compliant with other health-care recommendations.

*NOTE: The Immunization Practices Advisory Committee (ACIP) recommends administering M-M-R II concomitantly with the fourth dose of DTP and the third dose of OPV to children 15 months of age or older providing that 6 months have elapsed since DTP-3; or, if fewer than three DTPs have been received, at least 6 weeks have elapsed since the last dose of DTP and OPV.

CONTRAINDICATIONS

Do not give M-M-R II to pregnant females; the possible effects of the vaccine on fetal development are unknown at this time. If vaccination of postpubertal females is undertaken, pregnancy should be avoided for 3 months following vaccination.

Anaphylactic or anaphylactoid reactions to neomycin (each dose of reconstituted vaccine contains approximately 25 µg of neomycin).

History of anaphylactic or anaphylactoid reactions to eggs (see WARNINGS, Hypersensitivity to Eggs).

Any febrile respiratory illness or other active febrile infection.

Active untreated tuberculosis.

Patients receiving immunosuppressive therapy. This contraindication does not apply to patients who are receiving corticosteroids as replacement therapy, *e.g.*, for Addison's disease.

Individuals with blood dyscrasias, leukemia, lymphomas of any type, or other malignant neoplasms affecting the bone marrow or lymphatic systems.

Primary and acquired immunodeficiency states, including patients who are immunosuppressed in association with AIDS or other clinical manifestations of infection with human immunodeficiency viruses;[30,31] cellular immune deficiencies; and hypogammaglobulinemic and dysgammaglobulinemic states.

Individuals with a family history of congenital or hereditary immunodeficiency, until the immune competence of the potential vaccine recipient is demonstrated.[32]

WARNINGS

HYPERSENSITIVITY TO EGGS

Live measles vaccine and live mumps vaccine are produced in chick embryo cell culture. Persons with a history of anaphylactic, anaphylactoid, or other immediate reactions (*e.g.*, hives, swelling of the mouth and throat, difficulty breathing, hypotension, or shock) subsequent to egg ingestion should not be vaccinated. Evidence indicates that persons are not at increased risk if they have egg allergies that are not anaphylactic or anaphylactoid in nature. Such persons may be vaccinated in the usual manner. There is no evidence to indicate that persons with allergies to chickens or feathers are at increased risk of reaction to the vaccine.[20]

DOSAGE AND ADMINISTRATION

For Subcutaneous Administration.

DO NOT INJECT INTRAVENOUSLY.

The dosage of vaccine is the same for all persons. Inject the total volume of the single dose vial (about 0.5 ml) or 0.5 ml of the 10 dose vial of reconstituted vaccine subcutaneously, preferably into the outer aspect of upper arm. *Do not give immune globulin (IG) concurrently with* M-M-R II.

During shipment, to insure that there is no loss of potency, the vaccine must be maintained at a temperature of 10°C (50°F) or less.

Before reconstitution, store M-M-R II at 2-8°C (36-46°F). *Protect from light.*

Caution: A sterile syringe free of preservatives, antiseptics, and detergents should be used for each injection and/or reconstitution of the vaccine because these substances may inactivate the live virus vaccine. A 25 gauge, 5/8" needle is recommended.

To reconstitute, use only the diluent supplied, since it is free of preservatives or other antiviral substances which might inactivate the vaccine.

Parenteral drug products should be inspected visually for particulate matter and discoloration prior to administration. M-M-R II, when reconstituted, is clear yellow.

PRODUCT LISTING - EQUIVALENTS NOT AVAILABLE

Powder For Injection - Subcutaneous - Strength n/a

1's	$40.01	M-M-R II, Allscripts Pharmaceutical Company	54569-3066-00
1's	$46.17	M-M-R II, Physicians Total Care	54868-0980-00
1's	$49.21	M-M-R II, Merck & Company Inc	00006-4749-00
10's	$346.64	M-M-R II, Allscripts Pharmaceutical Company	54569-1588-00
10's	$428.45	M-M-R II, Merck & Company Inc	00006-4681-00

Mebendazole *(001705)*

Categories: Ascariasis; Hookworm; Pinworm; Trichuriasis; Pregnancy Category C; FDA Approved 1974 Jun; WHO Formulary

Drug Classes: Antihelmintics

Brand Names: **Vermox**

Foreign Brand Availability: Amycil (Mexico); Anelmin (Bahrain; Cyprus; Egypt; Iran; Iraq; Jordan; Kuwait; Lebanon; Libya; Oman; Qatar; Republic-of-Yemen; Saudi-Arabia; Syria; United-Arab-Emirates); Anthex (South-Africa); Antiox (Philippines); Bantenol (Spain); Benda (Thailand); Bestelar (Mexico); Cipex (South-Africa); Combantrin-1 (New-Zealand); Combantrin-1 with mebendazole (Australia); Conquer (Taiwan); D-Worm (South-Africa); Gamax (Colombia); Helminzole (Mexico); Lomper (Spain); Mebex (India); Mindol (New-Zealand); Noverme (Portugal); Noxworm (Thailand); Pantelmin (Austria; Colombia; Costa-Rica; Dominican-Republic; Ecuador; El-Salvador; Guatemala; Honduras; Nicaragua; Panama; Peru; Portugal); Penalcol (Peru); Pharaxis M (Colombia); Revapol (Mexico); Soltric (Mexico); Sqworm (Australia); Surfont (Germany); Thelmox (Bahamas; Barbados; Belize; Bermuda; Curacao; Guyana; Jamaica; Netherland-Antilles; Surinam; Trinidad); Toloxim (Portugal); Vagaka (Thailand); Wormin (Benin; Burkina-Faso; Ethiopia; Gambia; Ghana; Guinea; Ivory-Coast; Kenya; Liberia; Malawi; Mali; Mauritania; Mauritius; Morocco; Niger; Nigeria; Senegal; Seychelles; Sierra-Leone; Sudan; Tanzania; Tunia; Uganda; Zambia; Zimbabwe); Wormgo (South-Africa); Wormin (Bahrain; Cyprus; Egypt; India; Iran; Iraq; Jordan; Kuwait; Lebanon; Libya; Oman; Qatar; Republic-of-Yemen; Saudi-Arabia; Syria; United-Arab-Emirates); Zadomen (Malaysia); Zakor (Colombia)

Cost of Therapy: $35.45 (Helminth Infection; Vermox; 100 mg; 2 tablets/day; 3 day supply)
$31.93 (Helminth Infection; Generic Tablets; 100 mg; 2 tablets/day; 3 day supply)

DESCRIPTION

Mebendazole is a (synthetic) broad-spectrum anthelmintic available as chewable tablets, each containing 100 mg of mebendazole. Inactive ingredients are: colloidal silicon dioxide, corn starch, hydrogenated vegetable oil, magnesium stearate, microcrystalline cellulose, sodium lauryl sulfate, sodium saccharin, sodium starch glycolate, talc, tetrarome orange, and FD&C yellow No. 6.

Mebendazole is methyl 5-benzoylbenzimidazole-2-carbamate.

Mebendazole is a white to slightly yellow powder with a molecular weight of 295.29. It is less than 0.05% soluble in water, dilute mineral acid solutions, alcohol, ether and chloroform, but is soluble in formic acid.

CLINICAL PHARMACOLOGY

Following administration of 100 mg twice daily for three consecutive days, plasma levels of mebendazole and its primary metabolite, the 2-amine, do not exceed 0.03 mcg/ml and 0.09 mcg/ml, respectively. All metabolites are devoid of anthelmintic activity. In man, approximately 2% of administered mebendazole is excreted in urine and the remainder in the feces as unchanged drug or a primary metabolite.

Mode of Action: Mebendazole inhibits the formation of the worms' microtubules and causes the worms' glucose depletion.

INDICATIONS AND USAGE

Mebendazole is indicated for the treatment of *Enterobius vermicularis* (pinworm), *Trichuris trichiura* (whipworm), *Ascaris lumbricoides* (common roundworm), *Ancylostoma duodenale* (common hookworm), *Necator americanus* (American hookworm) in single or mixed infections.

Efficacy varies as a function of such factors as pre-existing diarrhea and gastrointestinal transit time, degree of infection, and helminth strains. Efficacy rates derived from various studies are shown in the table below (TABLE 1).:

TABLE 1

	Pinworm (enterobiasis)	Whipworm (trichuriasis)	Common Roundworm (ascariasis)	Hookworm
Cure rates mean	95%	68%	98%	96%
Egg reduction mean	--	93%	99%	99%

NON-FDA APPROVED INDICATIONS

Although not approved by the FDA, mebendazole therapy has been effective in the treatment of Angiostrongylus cantonensis, Onchocerca volvulus, Trichinella spiralis (trichinosis), Capillaria philippinensis, Echinococcus granulosus and multilocularis, and Wuchereri a brancrofti. It has also been used to treat gastrointestinal parasitic infections, commonly known as hookworm, giant roundworm, pinworm, capillariasis, gnathostomiasis, visceral larva migrans, angiostrongyliasis, trichinosis, whipworm, and filariasis.

Mebendazole may be used as an adjunct to surgical excision of echinococcal cysts (hydatid disease) or as primary therapy for inoperable echinococcal lesions or in patients who are not surgical candidates.

CONTRAINDICATIONS

Mebendazole is contraindicated in persons who have shown hypersensitivity to the drug.

WARNINGS

There is no evidence that mebendazole, even at high doses, is effective for hydatid disease. There have been rare reports of neutropenia and liver function elevations, including hepatitis, when mebendazole is taken for prolonged periods and at dosages substantially above those recommended.

PRECAUTIONS

Information for the Patient: Patients should be informed of the potential risk to the fetus in women taking mebendazole during pregnancy, especially during the first trimester (see Use in Pregnancy).

Patients should also be informed that cleanliness is important to prevent reinfection and transmission of the infection.

Carcinogenesis, Mutagenesis: In carcinogenicity tests of mebendazole in mice and rats, no carcinogenic effects were seen at doses as high as 40 mg/kg given daily over two years. Dominant lethal mutation tests in mice showed no mutagenicity at single doses as high as 640 mg/kg. Neither the spermatocyte test, the F_1 translocation test, not the Ames test indicated mutagenic properties.

Impairment Fertility: Doses up to 40 mg/kg in mice, given to males for 60 days and to females for 14 days prior to gestation, had no effect upon fetuses and offspring, though there was slight maternal toxicity.

Usage in Pregnancy: Pregnancy Category C. Mebendazole has shown embryotoxic and teratogenic activity in pregnant rats at single oral doses as low as 10 mg/kg. In view of these findings the use of mebendazole is not recommended in pregnant women. In humans, a post-marketing survey has been done of a limited number of women who inadvertently had consumed mebendazole during the first trimester of pregnancy. The incidence of spontaneous abortion and malformation did not exceed that in the general population. In 170 deliveries on term, no teratogenic risk of mebendazole was identified. During pregnancy, especially during the first trimester, mebendazole should be used only if the potential benefit justifies the potential risk to the fetus.

Nursing Mothers: It is not known whether mebendazole is excreted in human milk. Because many drugs are excreted in human milk, caution should be exercised when mebendazole is administered to a nursing woman.

Pediatric Use: The drug has not been extensively studied in children under two years; therefore, in the treatment of children under two years the relative benefit/risk should be considered.

ADVERSE REACTIONS

Transient symptoms of abdominal pain and diarrhea have occurred in cases of massive infection and expulsion of worms. Hypersensitivity reactions such as rash, urticaria and angioedema have been observed on rare occasions. Very rare cases of convulsions have been reported.

DOSAGE AND ADMINISTRATION

The same dosage schedule applies to children and adults. The tablet may be chewed, swallowed, or crushed and mixed with food (TABLE 2).

TABLE 2

	Pinworm (enterobiasis)	Whipworm (trichuriasis)	Common Roundworm (ascariasis)	Hookworm
Dose	1 tablet, once morning and evening for 3 consecutive days.	1 tablet morning and evening for 3 consecutive days.	1 tablet morning and evening for 3 consecutive days.	1 tablet

If the patient is not cured three weeks after treatment, a second course of treatment is advised. No special procedures, such as fasting or purging, are required.

HOW SUPPLIED

Vermox is available as chewable tablets, each containing 100 mg of mebendazole, and is supplied in boxes of twelve tablets.

Store at room temperature 15°-30°C (59°-86°F).

PRODUCT LISTING - RATED THERAPEUTICALLY EQUIVALENT

Tablet, Chewable - Oral - 100 mg

1's	$5.69	VERMOX, Allscripts Pharmaceutical Company	54569-3634-02
2's	$12.18	VERMOX, Pharma Pac	52959-0160-02
6's	$35.26	VERMOX, Pharma Pac	52959-0160-06
12's	$61.39	GENERIC, Copley	38245-0107-08
12's	$63.85	GENERIC, Teva Pharmaceuticals Usa	00093-9107-29
12's	$70.96	VERMOX, Janssen Pharmaceuticals	50458-0110-01
12's	$70.96	VERMOX, Janssen Pharmaceuticals	50580-0070-12

PRODUCT LISTING - EQUIVALENTS NOT AVAILABLE

Tablet, Chewable - Oral - 100 mg

12's	$80.76	GENERIC, Physicians Total Care	54868-3732-00

Mechlorethamine Hydrochloride *(001707)*

For complete prescribing information, refer to the CD-ROM included with the book.

Categories: Carcinoma, lung; Leukemia, chronic lymphocytic; Leukemia, chronic myelogenous; Lymphoma, Hodgkin's; Lymphosarcoma; Mycosis fungoides; Polycythemia vera; Pregnancy Category D; FDA Approved 1949 Mar
Drug Classes: Antineoplastics, alkylating agents
Brand Names: Mustargen
Foreign Brand Availability: Mustine (Belgium; Netherlands; Turkey); Mustine Hydrochloride Boots (Malaysia)
HCFA JCODE(S): J9230 10 mg IV

WARNING

Mechlorethamine HCl should be administered only under the supervision of a physician who is experienced in the use of cancer chemotherapeutic agents.

This drug is HIGHLY TOXIC and both powder and solution must be handled and administered with care. Inhalation of dust or vapors and contact with skin or mucous membranes, especially those of the eyes, must be avoided. Due to the toxic properties of mechlorethamine (*e.g.,* corrosivity, carcinogenicity, mutagenicity, teratogenicity), special handling procedures should be reviewed prior to handling and followed diligently.

Extravasation of the drug into subcutaneous tissues results in a painful inflammation. The area usually becomes indurated and and sloughing may occur. If leakage of drug is obvious, prompt infiltration of the area with sterile isotonic sodium thiosulfate (1/6 molar) and application of an ice compress for 6-12 hours may minimize the local reaction. For a 1/6 molar solution of sodium thiosulfate, use 4.14 g of sodium thiosulfate per 100 ml of sterile water for injection or 2.64 g of anhydrous sodium thiosulfate per 100 ml or dilute 4 ml of sodium thiosulfate injection (10%) with 6 ml of sterile water for injection.

M

DESCRIPTION

Mustargen, an antineoplastic nitrogen mustard also known as HN2 hydrochloride, is a nitrogen analog of sulfur mustard. It is a light yellow brown, crystalline, hygroscopic powder that is very soluble in water and also soluble in alcohol.

Mechlorethamine HCl is designated chemically as 2-chloro-*N*-(2-chlorethyl)-*N*-methylethanamine hydrochloride. The molecular weight is 192.52 and the melting point is 108-111°C. The empirical formula is $C_5H_{11}Cl_2N{\cdot}HCl$.

Trituration of Mustargen is a sterile, light yellow brown crystalline powder for injection by the intravenous or intracavitary routes after dissolution. Each vial of Mustargen contains 10 mg of mechlorethamine HCl triturated with sodium chloride qs 100 mg. When dissolved with 10 ml sterile water for injection or 0.9% sodium chloride injection, the resulting solution had a pH of 3-5 at a concentration of 1 mg mechlorethamine HCl per ml.

INDICATIONS AND USAGE

Before using mechlorethamine HCl see CONTRAINDICATIONS, WARNINGS, and DOSAGE AND ADMINISTRATION, Special Handling.

Mechlorethamine HCl, administered intravenously, is indicated for the palliative treatment of Hodgkin's disease (Stages III and IV), lymphosarcoma, chronic myelocytic or chronic lymphocytic leukemia, polycythemia vera, mycosis fungoides, and bronchogenic carcinoma.

Mechlorethamine HCl, administered intrapleurally, intraperitoneally, or intrapericardially, is indicated for the palliative treatment of metastatic carcinoma resulting in effusion.

NON-FDA APPROVED INDICATIONS

Mechlorethamine has been used without FDA approval as a solution or ointment in the treatment of cutaneous mycosis fungoides and chronic granulocytic leukemia skin lesions. The drug has also been administered by intralesional injection into heavy mycosis fungoides plaques. (A steroid and/or lidocaine may be added to the injection for patient comfort.)

CONTRAINDICATIONS

The use of mechlorethamine HCl is contraindicated in the presence of known infectious diseases and in patients who have had previous anaphylactic reactions to mechlorethamine HCl.

WARNINGS

Before using mechlorethamine HCl, an accurate histologic diagnosis of the disease, a knowledge of its natural course, and an adequate clinical history are important. The hematologic status of the patient must first be determined. It is essential to understand the hazards and therapeutic effects to be expected. Careful clinical judgement must be exercised in selecting patients. If the indication for its use is not clear, the drug should not be used.

As nitrogen mustard therapy may contribute to extensive and rapid development of amyloidosis, it should be used only if foci of acute and chronic suppurative inflammation are absent.

USE IN PREGNANCY

Mechlorethamine HCl can cause fetal harm when administered to a pregnant woman. Mechlorethamine HCl has been shown to produce fetal malformations in the rat and ferret when given as single subcutaneous injections of 1 mg/kg (2-3 times the maximum recommended human dose). There are no adequate and well-controlled studies in pregnant women. If this drug is used during pregnancy, or if the patient becomes pregnant while taking this drug, the patient should be apprised of the potential hazard to the fetus. Women of childbearing potential should be advised to avoid becoming pregnant.

DOSAGE AND ADMINISTRATION

INTRAVENOUS ADMINISTRATION

The dosage of mechlorethamine HCl varies with the clinical situation, the therapeutic response, and the magnitude of hematologic depression. A total dose of 0.4 mg/kg of body weight for each course usually is given either as a single dose or in divided doses of 0.1-0.2 mg/kg/day. Dosage should be based on ideal dry body weight. The presence of edema or ascites must be considered so that dosage will be based on actual weight unaugmented by these conditions.

The margin of safety in therapy with mechlorethamine HCl is narrow and considerable care must be exercised in the matter of dosage. Repeated examinations of blood are mandatory as a guide to subsequent therapy.

Within a few minutes after intravenous injection, mechlorethamine HCl undergoes chemical transformation, combines with reactive compounds, and is no longer present in its active form in the blood stream. Subsequent courses should not be given until the patient has recovered hematologically from the previous course; this is best determined by repeated studies of the peripheral blood elements awaiting their return to normal levels. It is often possible to give repeated courses of mechlorethamine HCl as early as 3 weeks after treatment.

PREPARATION OF SOLUTION FOR INTRAVENOUS ADMINISTRATION

This drug is **HIGHLY TOXIC** and both powder and solution must be handled and administered with care. (See BOXED WARNING and Special Handling.) Since mechlorethamine HCl is a powerful vesicant, it is intended primarily for intravenous use, and in most cases is given by this route. Inhalation of dust or vapors and contact with skin or mucous membranes, especially those of the eyes, must be avoided. Appropriate protective equipment should be worn when handling mechlorethamine HCl. Should accidental eye contact occur, copious irrigation for at least 15 minutes with water, normal saline or a balanced salt ophthalmic irrigating solution should be instituted immediately, followed by prompt ophthalmologic consultation. Should accidental skin contact occur, the affected part must be irrigated immediately with copious amounts of water, for at least 15 minutes while removing contaminated clothing and shoes, followed by 2% sodium thiosulfate solution. Medical attention should be sought immediately. Contaminated clothing should be destroyed. (See Special Handling.)

Each vial of mechlorethamine HCl contains 10 mg of mechlorethamine HCl triturated with sodium chloride qs 100 mg. In neutral or alkaline aqueous solution it undergoes rapid chemical transformation and is highly unstable. Although solutions prepared according to instructions are acidic and do not decompose as rapidly, they should be prepared immediately before each injection since they will decompose on standing. When reconstituted, mechlorethamine HCl is a clear colorless solution. *Do not use if the solution is discolored or if droplets of water are visible within the vial prior to reconstitution.*

Using a sterile 10 ml syringe, inject 10 ml of sterile water for injection or 10 ml sodium chloride injection into a vial of mechlorethamine HCl. With the needle (syringe attached) still in the rubber stopper, shake the vial several times to dissolve the drug completely. The resultant solution contains 1 mg mechlorethamine HCl per ml.

Parenteral drug products should be inspected visually for particulate matter and discoloration prior to administration whenever solution and container permit.

SPECIAL HANDLING

Animal studies have shown mechlorethamine to be corrosive to skin and eyes, a powerful vesicant, irritating to the mucous membranes of the respiratory tract, and highly toxic by the oral route. It has also been shown to be carcinogenic, mutagenic, and teratogenic. Due to the drug's toxic properties, appropriate precautions including the use of appropriate safety equipment are recommended for the preparation of mechlorethamine HCl for parenteral administration. Inhalation of dust or vapors and contact with skin or mucous membranes, especially those of the eyes, must be avoided. The National Institutes of Health presently recommends that the preparation of injectable antineoplastic drugs should be performed in a Class II laminar flow biological safety cabinet.[17] Personnel preparing drugs of this class should wear chemical resistant, impervious gloves, safety goggles, outer graments, and shoe covers. Additional body garments should be used based upon the task being performed (*e.g.,* sleevelets, apron, gauntlets, disposable suits) to avoid exposed skin surfaces and inhalation of vapors and dust. Appropriate techniques should be used to remove potentially contaminated clothing.

Several other guidelines for proper handling and disposal of antineoplastic drugs have been published and should be considered.[18-22]

ACCIDENTAL CONTACT MEASURES

Should accidental eye contact occur, copious irrigation for at least 15 minutes with water, normal saline or a balanced salt ophthalmic irrigating solution should be instituted immediately, followed by prompt ophthalmologic consultation. Should accidental skin contact occur, the affected part must be irrigated immediately with copious amounts of water, for at least 15 minutes while removing contaminated clothing and shoes, followed by 2% sodium thiosulfate solution. Medical attention should be sought immediately. Contaminated clothing should be destroyed.

TECHNIQUE FOR INTRAVENOUS ADMINISTRATION

Withdraw into the syringe the calculated volume of solution required for a single injection. *Dispose of any remaining solution after neutralization.* (See Neutralization of Equipment and Unused Solution.) Although the drug may be injected directly into any suitable vein, it is injected preferably into the rubber or plastic tubing of a flowing intravenous infusion set. This reduces the possibility of severe local reactions due to extravasation or high concentration of the drug. Injecting the drug into the tubing rather than adding it to the entire volume of the infusion fluid minimizes a chemical reactions between the drug and the solution. The rate of injection apparently is not critical provided it is completed within a few minutes.

INTRACAVITARY ADMINISTRATION

Nitrogen mustard has been used by intracavitary administration with varying success in certain malignant conditions for the control of pleural,[4-13] peritoneal,[5,6,9,11-16] and pericardial,[5,11-13] effusions caused by malignant cells.

The technique and the dose used by any of these routes varies. Therefore, if mechlorethamine HCl is given by the intracavitary route, the published articles concerning such use should be consulted. *Because of the inherent risks involved, the physician should be experienced in the appropriate injection techniques, and be thoroughly aware of the indications, dosages, hazards, and precautions as set forth in the published literature. When using mechlorethamine HCl by the intracavitary routes, the general precautions concerning this agent should be borne in mind.*

As a general guide, reference is made especially to the technics of Weisberger *et al.*[5,11-13] Intracavitary use is indicated in the presence of pleural, peritoneal, or pericardial effusion due to metastatic tumors. Local therapy with nitrogen mustard is used only when malignant cells are demonstrated in the effusion. Intracavitary injection is not recommended when the accumulated fluid is chylous in nature, since results are likely to be poor.

Paracentesis is first performed with most of the fluid being removed from the pleural or peritoneal cavity. The intracavitary use of mechlorethamine HCl may exert at least some of its effect through production of a chemical poudrage. Therefore, the removal of excess fluid allows the drug to more easily contact the peritoneal and pleural linings. For intrapleural or intrapericardial injection nitrogen mustard is introduced directly through the thoracentesis needle. For intraperitoneal injection it is given through a rubber catheter inserted into the trocar used for paracentesis or through a No. 18 gauge needle inserted at another site. This drug should be injected slowly, with frequent aspiration to insure that a free flow of fluid is present. If fluid cannot be aspirated, pain and necrosis due to injection of solution outside the cavity may occur.[5,11-13] Free flow of fluid also is necessary to prevent injection into a loculated pocket and to ensure adequate dissemination of nitrogen mustard.

The usual dose of nitrogen mustard for intracavitary injection is 0.4 mg/kg of body weight, through 0.2 mg/kg (or 10-20 mg) has been used by the intrapericardial route[5,11-13] The solution is prepared, as previously described for intravenous injection, by adding 10 ml of sterile water for injection or 10 ml of sodium chloride injection to the vial containing 10 mg of mechlorethamine HCl. (Amounts of diluent of 50-100 ml or normal saline have also been used.[4,5]) The position of the patient should be changed every 5-10 minutes for an hour after injection to obtain more uniform distribution of the drug throughout the serous cavity. The remaining fluid may be removed from the pleural or peritoneal cavity by paracentesis 24-36 hours later. The patient should be followed carefully by clinical and x-ray examination to detect reaccumulation of fluid.

Pain occurs rarely with intrapleural use; it is common with intraperitoneal injections and is often associated with nausea, vomiting, and diarrhea of 2-3 days duration. Transient cardiac irregularities may occur with intrapericardial injection. Death, possibly accelerated by nitrogen mustard, has been reported following the use of this agent by the intracavitary route.[9] Although absorption of mechlorethamine HCl when given by the intracavitary route is probably not complete because of its rapid deactivation by body fluids, the systemic effect is unpredictable. The acute side effects such as nausea and vomiting are usually mild. Bone marrow depression is generally milder than when the drug is given intravenously. Care should be taken to avoid use by the intracavitary route when other agents which may suppress bone marrow function are being used systemically.

NEUTRALIZATION OF EQUIPMENT AND UNUSED SOLUTION

To clean rubber gloves, tubing, glassware, etc., after giving mechlorethamine HCl, soak them in an aqueous solution containing equal volumes of sodium thiosulfate (5%) and sodium bicarbonate (5%) for 45 minutes. Excess reagents and reaction products are washed away easily with water. Any unused injection solution should be neutralized by mixing with an equal volume of sodium thiosulfate/sodium bicarbonate solution. Allow the mixture to stand for 45 minutes. Vials that have contained mechlorethamine HCl should be treated in the same way with thiosulfate/bicarbonate solution before disposal.

PRODUCT LISTING - EQUIVALENTS NOT AVAILABLE

Powder For Injection - Injectable - 10 mg

4's	$50.55	MUSTARGEN, Merck & Company Inc	00006-7753-31

Meclizine Hydrochloride *(001708)*

Categories: Motion sickness; Vertigo; Pregnancy Category B; FDA Approved 1973 Apr
Drug Classes: Antiemetics/antivertigo; Antihistamines, H1
Brand Names: Ancolan; **Antivert**; Duramesan; En-Vert; Meclicot; Meclizine Hcl; Meclozine; Medivert; Yonyun
Foreign Brand Availability: Bonamina (Argentina); Bonamine (Canada; Germany; Japan; Philippines; Taiwan); Chiclida (Spain); Dramine (Spain); Navicalm (Portugal); Postadoxin (Germany); Postadoxine (Philippines); Postafen (Denmark; Finland; Norway; Sweden); Postafene (Belgium; Hong-Kong); Sea-Legs (New-Zealand); Suprimal (Netherlands)
Cost of Therapy: $10.06 (Motion Sickness; Antivert; 25 mg; 1 tablet/day; 14 day supply)
$0.46 (Motion Sickness; Generic Tablets; 25 mg; 1 tablet/day; 14 day supply)

DESCRIPTION

Chemically, meclizine HCl is 1-(*p*-chloro-α-phenylbenzyl)-4-(*m*-methylbenzyl) piperazine dihydrochloride monohydrate.

Inert ingredients for the tablets are: dibasic calcium phosphate; magnesium stearate; polyethylene glycol; starch; sucrose. The 12.5 mg tablets also contain: blue no. 1. 25 mg tablets also contain: yellow no. 6 lake; yellow no. 10 lake. 50 mg tablets also contain: blue no. 1 lake; yellow no. 10 lake.

Inert ingredients for the chewable tablets are: lactose, magnesium stearate, raspberry flavor, red no. 40, saccharin sodium, siliceous earth, starch, talc.

CLINICAL PHARMACOLOGY

Meclizine HCl is an antihistamine which shows marked protective activity against nebulized histamine and lethal doses of intravenously injected histamine in guinea pigs. It has a marked effect in blocking the vasodepressor response to histamine, but only a slight blocking action against acetylcholine. Its activity is relatively weak in inhibiting the spasmogenic action of histamine on isolated guinea pig ileum.

INDICATIONS AND USAGE

Based on a review of this drug by the National Academy of Sciences-National Research Council and/or other information, FDA has classified the indications as follows:
***Effective:* Management of nausea and vomiting, and dizziness associated with motion sickness.**
***Possibly Effective:* Management of vertigo associated with diseases affecting the vestibular system.**
Final classification of the less than effective indications requires further investigation.

CONTRAINDICATIONS

Meclizine HCl is contraindicated in individuals who have shown a previous hypersensitivity to it.

WARNINGS

Since drowsiness may, on occasion, occur with use of this drug, patients should be warned of this possibility and cautioned against driving a car or operating dangerous machinery.

Patients should avoid alcoholic beverages while taking this drug. Due to its potential anticholinergic action, this drug should be used with caution in patients with asthma, glaucoma, or enlargement of the prostate gland.

USE IN CHILDREN

Clinical studies establishing safety and effectiveness in children have not been done; therefore, usage is not recommended in children under 12 years of age.

USE IN PREGNANCY, PREGNANCY CATEGORY B

Reproduction studies in rats have shown cleft palates at 25-50 times the human dose. Epidemiological studies in pregnant women, however, do not indicate that meclizine increases the risk of abnormalities when administered during pregnancy. Despite the animal findings, it would appear that the possibility of fetal harm is remote. Nevertheless, meclizine, or any other medication, should be used during pregnancy only if clearly necessary.

ADVERSE REACTIONS

Drowsiness, dry mouth and, on rare occasions, blurred vision have been reported.

DOSAGE AND ADMINISTRATION

VERTIGO

For the control of vertigo associated with diseases affecting the vestibular system, the recommended dose is 25-100 mg daily, in divided dosage, depending upon clinical response.

MOTION SICKNESS

The initial dose of 25-50 mg of meclizine HCl should be taken 1 hour prior to embarkation for protection against motion sickness. Thereafter, the dose may be repeated every 24 hours for the duration of the journey.

PRODUCT LISTING - RATED THERAPEUTICALLY EQUIVALENT

Tablet - Oral - 12.5 mg

12's	$3.00	GENERIC, Pd-Rx Pharmaceuticals	55289-0982-12
20's	$3.86	GENERIC, Pd-Rx Pharmaceuticals	55289-0982-20
25's	$5.90	GENERIC, Pd-Rx Pharmaceuticals	55289-0982-97
30's	$1.60	GENERIC, Circle Pharmaceuticals Inc	00659-3001-30
30's	$5.78	GENERIC, Pd-Rx Pharmaceuticals	55289-0982-30
30's	$6.24	GENERIC, Heartland Healthcare Services	61392-0338-30
31 x 10	$64.39	GENERIC, Vangard Labs	00615-1553-53
31 x 10	$64.39	GENERIC, Vangard Labs	00615-1553-63
100's	$0.77	GENERIC, Global Pharmaceutical Corporation	00115-3870-01
100's	$2.40	GENERIC, C.O. Truxton Inc	00463-7015-01
100's	$2.66	GENERIC, Camall Company	00147-0137-10
100's	$2.75	GENERIC, Cmc-Consolidated Midland Corporation	00223-1162-01

M

100's	$3.10	GENERIC, Major Pharmaceuticals Inc	00904-2384-60
100's	$3.75	GENERIC, Interstate Drug Exchange Inc	00814-4640-14
100's	$3.80	GENERIC, Ivax Corporation	00182-0871-01
100's	$4.60	GENERIC, Moore, H.L. Drug Exchange Inc	00839-6009-06
100's	$4.65	GENERIC, Vintage Pharmaceuticals Inc	00254-4140-28
100's	$4.65	GENERIC, Watson/Rugby Laboratories Inc	00536-3986-01
100's	$4.95	GENERIC, Vangard Labs	00615-1553-01
100's	$4.95	GENERIC, Martec Pharmaceuticals Inc	52555-0509-01
100's	$5.00	GENERIC, Aligen Independent Laboratories Inc	00405-4601-01
100's	$5.50	GENERIC, Raway Pharmacal Inc	00686-0089-20
100's	$5.84	GENERIC, Major Pharmaceuticals Inc	00904-2384-61
100's	$5.99	FEDERAL UPPER LIMIT, H.C.F.A. F F P	99999-1708-03
100's	$7.28	GENERIC, Geneva Pharmaceuticals	00781-1542-01
100's	$7.78	GENERIC, Auro Pharmaceutical	55829-0354-10
100's	$15.75	GENERIC, Udl Laboratories Inc	51079-0089-20
100's	$20.00	GENERIC, Par Pharmaceutical Inc	49884-0034-01
100's	$20.80	GENERIC, Ivax Corporation	00182-0871-89
100's	$45.46	ANTIVERT, Pfizer U.S. Pharmaceuticals	00049-2100-66
150's	$23.62	GENERIC, Sky Pharmaceuticals Packaging, Inc	63739-0162-15
200 x 5	$207.71	GENERIC, Vangard Labs	00615-1553-43

Tablet - Oral - 25 mg

8's	$6.48	GENERIC, Pd-Rx Pharmaceuticals	55289-0159-08
20's	$11.65	GENERIC, Cardinal Pharmaceuticals	63874-0014-20
20's	$11.98	GENERIC, Dhs Inc	55887-0939-20
25's	$7.15	GENERIC, Udl Laboratories Inc	51079-0090-19
25's	$9.54	GENERIC, Pd-Rx Pharmaceuticals	55289-0159-97
30's	$2.37	GENERIC, Circle Pharmaceuticals Inc	00659-3002-30
30's	$4.89	GENERIC, Heartland Healthcare Services	61392-0339-30
30's	$6.36	GENERIC, Pd-Rx Pharmaceuticals	55289-0159-30
30's	$17.31	GENERIC, Dhs Inc	55887-0939-30
30's	$17.59	GENERIC, Cardinal Pharmaceuticals	63874-0014-30
30's	$22.63	ANTIVERT, Physicians Total Care	54868-0882-02
31 x 10	$117.70	GENERIC, Vangard Labs	00615-1554-53
31 x 10	$117.70	GENERIC, Vangard Labs	00615-1554-63
32's	$2.22	GENERIC, Vangard Labs	00615-1554-32
60's	$9.78	GENERIC, Heartland Healthcare Services	61392-0339-60
90's	$14.66	GENERIC, Heartland Healthcare Services	61392-0339-90
100's	$3.25	GENERIC, Cmc-Consolidated Midland Corporation	00223-1163-01
100's	$3.56	GENERIC, Camall Company	00147-0101-10
100's	$4.13	GENERIC, Interstate Drug Exchange Inc	00814-4641-14
100's	$4.19	GENERIC, Major Pharmaceuticals Inc	00904-2350-60
100's	$5.57	GENERIC, Vangard Labs	00615-1554-01
100's	$5.75	GENERIC, Raway Pharmacal Inc	00686-0090-20
100's	$5.88	GENERIC, Vintage Pharmaceuticals Inc	00254-4141-28
100's	$5.98	GENERIC, Moore, H.L. Drug Exchange Inc	00839-6010-06
100's	$6.39	GENERIC, Major Pharmaceuticals Inc	00904-2350-61
100's	$6.45	GENERIC, Ivax Corporation	00182-0872-01
100's	$7.11	GENERIC, Aligen Independent Laboratories Inc	00405-4602-01
100's	$7.17	FEDERAL UPPER LIMIT, H.C.F.A. F F P	99999-1708-06
100's	$7.90	GENERIC, Martec Pharmaceuticals Inc	52555-0510-01
100's	$9.64	GENERIC, Auro Pharmaceutical	55829-0355-10
100's	$11.44	GENERIC, Geneva Pharmaceuticals	00781-1544-01
100's	$11.90	GENERIC, Pd-Rx Pharmaceuticals	55289-0159-01
100's	$17.50	GENERIC, Udl Laboratories Inc	51079-0090-20
100's	$17.60	GENERIC, Watson Laboratories Inc	00591-0803-01
100's	$17.60	GENERIC, Watson Laboratories Inc	52544-0803-01
100's	$18.00	GENERIC, Par Pharmaceutical Inc	49884-0035-01
100's	$38.00	GENERIC, Ivax Corporation	00182-0872-89
100's	$71.89	ANTIVERT, Pfizer U.S. Pharmaceuticals	00049-2110-66
120's	$19.55	GENERIC, Heartland Healthcare Services	61392-0339-34
150's	$26.25	GENERIC, Sky Pharmaceuticals Packaging, Inc	63739-0163-15

Tablet - Oral - 30 mg

100's	$24.65	GENERIC, Med Tek Pharmaceuticals Inc	52349-0220-10

Tablet - Oral - 50 mg

100's	$131.86	ANTIVERT, Pfizer U.S. Pharmaceuticals	00049-2140-66

Tablet, Chewable - Oral - 25 mg

100's	$1.01	GENERIC, Global Pharmaceutical Corporation	00115-3875-01
100's	$3.50	GENERIC, Cmc-Consolidated Midland Corporation	00223-1164-01

PRODUCT LISTING - EQUIVALENTS NOT AVAILABLE

Tablet - Oral - 12.5 mg

3's	$1.02	GENERIC, Allscripts Pharmaceutical Company	54569-0347-00
3's	$3.52	GENERIC, Prescript Pharmaceuticals	00247-0153-03
4's	$3.56	GENERIC, Prescript Pharmaceuticals	00247-0153-04
6's	$3.67	GENERIC, Prescript Pharmaceuticals	00247-0153-06
7's	$7.26	GENERIC, Pharma Pac	52959-0225-07
9's	$3.84	GENERIC, Prescript Pharmaceuticals	00247-0153-09
10's	$3.40	GENERIC, Allscripts Pharmaceutical Company	54569-0347-04
10's	$3.88	GENERIC, Prescript Pharmaceuticals	00247-0153-10
12's	$3.99	GENERIC, Prescript Pharmaceuticals	00247-0153-12
12's	$4.28	GENERIC, Southwood Pharmaceuticals Inc	58016-0801-12
12's	$10.24	GENERIC, Pharma Pac	52959-0225-12
14's	$4.09	GENERIC, Prescript Pharmaceuticals	00247-0153-14
15's	$4.15	GENERIC, Prescript Pharmaceuticals	00247-0153-15
15's	$5.35	GENERIC, Southwood Pharmaceuticals Inc	58016-0801-15
16's	$2.33	GENERIC, Physicians Total Care	54868-0089-03
20's	$4.41	GENERIC, Prescript Pharmaceuticals	00247-0153-20
20's	$6.80	GENERIC, Allscripts Pharmaceutical Company	54569-0347-01
20's	$7.13	GENERIC, Southwood Pharmaceuticals Inc	58016-0801-20
20's	$14.70	GENERIC, Pharma Pac	52959-0225-20
21's	$4.47	GENERIC, Prescript Pharmaceuticals	00247-0153-21
21's	$15.16	GENERIC, Pharma Pac	52959-0225-21
24's	$4.62	GENERIC, Prescript Pharmaceuticals	00247-0153-24
30's	$2.30	GENERIC, Pharmaceutical Corporation Of America	51655-0318-24
30's	$2.91	GENERIC, Physicians Total Care	54868-0089-02
30's	$4.94	GENERIC, Prescript Pharmaceuticals	00247-0153-30
30's	$10.20	GENERIC, Allscripts Pharmaceutical Company	54569-0347-03
30's	$10.70	GENERIC, Southwood Pharmaceuticals Inc	58016-0801-30
30's	$18.04	GENERIC, Pharma Pac	52959-0225-30
35's	$5.21	GENERIC, Prescript Pharmaceuticals	00247-0153-35
60's	$20.40	GENERIC, Allscripts Pharmaceutical Company	54569-0347-05
100's	$5.82	GENERIC, Physicians Total Care	54868-0089-04
100's	$34.00	GENERIC, Allscripts Pharmaceutical Company	54569-0347-02
100's	$35.65	GENERIC, Southwood Pharmaceuticals Inc	58016-0801-00
100's	$51.19	GENERIC, Pharma Pac	52959-0225-00

Tablet - Oral - 25 mg

2's	$3.44	GENERIC, Prescript Pharmaceuticals	00247-0093-02
3's	$3.47	GENERIC, Prescript Pharmaceuticals	00247-0093-03
4's	$3.52	GENERIC, Prescript Pharmaceuticals	00247-0093-04
6's	$3.59	GENERIC, Prescript Pharmaceuticals	00247-0093-06
8's	$3.67	GENERIC, Prescript Pharmaceuticals	00247-0093-08
8's	$4.51	GENERIC, Southwood Pharmaceuticals Inc	58016-0802-08
10's	$3.75	GENERIC, Prescript Pharmaceuticals	00247-0093-10
12's	$3.84	GENERIC, Prescript Pharmaceuticals	00247-0093-12
12's	$6.76	GENERIC, Southwood Pharmaceuticals Inc	58016-0802-12
15's	$2.67	GENERIC, Physicians Total Care	54868-0077-01
15's	$3.95	GENERIC, Prescript Pharmaceuticals	00247-0093-15
15's	$8.45	GENERIC, Southwood Pharmaceuticals Inc	58016-0802-15
20's	$3.52	GENERIC, Physicians Total Care	54868-0077-07
20's	$4.15	GENERIC, Prescript Pharmaceuticals	00247-0093-20
20's	$4.23	GENERIC, Pharmaceutical Corporation Of America	51655-0107-52
20's	$11.27	GENERIC, Southwood Pharmaceuticals Inc	58016-0802-20
21's	$4.19	GENERIC, Prescript Pharmaceuticals	00247-0093-21
30's	$3.68	GENERIC, Physicians Total Care	54868-0077-04
30's	$4.54	GENERIC, Prescript Pharmaceuticals	00247-0093-30
30's	$16.91	GENERIC, Southwood Pharmaceuticals Inc	58016-0802-30
35's	$4.74	GENERIC, Prescript Pharmaceuticals	00247-0093-35
40's	$4.35	GENERIC, Physicians Total Care	54868-0077-03
50's	$5.34	GENERIC, Prescript Pharmaceuticals	00247-0093-50
60's	$33.82	GENERIC, Southwood Pharmaceuticals Inc	58016-0802-60
100's	$7.33	GENERIC, Prescript Pharmaceuticals	00247-0093-00
100's	$8.38	GENERIC, Physicians Total Care	54868-0077-05
100's	$23.61	GENERIC, Seatrace Pharmaceuticals	00551-0168-01
100's	$56.36	GENERIC, Southwood Pharmaceuticals Inc	58016-0802-00

Tablet, Chewable - Oral - 25 mg

100's	$3.99	GENERIC, Amide Pharmaceutical Inc	52152-0117-02

Medroxyprogesterone Acetate *(001712)*

Categories: Amenorrhea; Carcinoma, endometrial; Carcinoma, renal; Contraception; Hemorrhage, uterine; FDA Approved 1962 Apr; Pregnancy Category X; WHO Formulary

Drug Classes: Antineoplastics, hormones/hormone modifiers; Contraceptives; Hormones/hormone modifiers; Progestins

Brand Names: Amen; Curretab; Cycrin; Depo-Provera; Depo-Provera Contraceptive; Med-Pro; **Provera**

Foreign Brand Availability: Aragest 5 (Israel); Clinofem (Germany); Depo-Prodasone (France); Farlutal (Bahrain; Belgium; China; Cyprus; Egypt; France; Iran; Iraq; Israel; Italy; Jordan; Kuwait; Lebanon; Libya; Netherlands; Oman; Qatar; Republic-of-Yemen; Saudi-Arabia; Syria; United-Arab-Emirates); GestaPolar (Germany); Gestapuran (Finland; Sweden); Manodepa (Thailand); Medrone (Taiwan); Meges (Indonesia); Meprate (India); MPA (China); MPA Gyn 5 (Germany); Perlutex (Bahamas; Barbados; Belize; Bermuda; Curacao; Denmark; Guyana; Jamaica; Netherland-Antilles; Norway; Puerto-Rico; Surinam; Trinidad); Perlutex Leo (Costa-Rica; Dominican-Republic; El-Salvador; Guatemala; Honduras; Panama); Prodafem (Austria; Switzerland); Progen (Korea); Progevera (Spain); Prothyra (Indonesia); Ralovera (Australia); Veraplex (Indonesia)

Cost of Therapy: $12.33 (Secondary Amenorrhea; Provera; 10 mg; 1 tablet/day; 10 day supply)
$1.31 (Secondary Amenorrhea; Generic Tablets; 10 mg; 1 tablet/day; 10 day supply)
$3.09 (Secondary Amenorrhea; Amen; 10 mg; 1 tablet/day; 10 day supply)

HCFA JCODE(S): J1050 100 mg IM; J1055 150 mg IM

WARNING

Medroxyprogesterone Acetate Tablets

THE USE OF MEDROXYPROGESTERONE ACETATE DURING THE FIRST 4 MONTHS OF PREGNANCY IS NOT RECOMMENDED.

Progestational agents have been used beginning with the first trimester of pregnancy in an attempt to prevent habitual abortion. There is no adequate evidence that such use is effective when such drugs are given during the first 4 months of pregnancy. Furthermore, in the vast majority of women, the cause of abortion is a defective ovum, which progestational agents could not be expected to influence. In addition, the use of progestational agents, with their uterine relaxant properties, in patients with fertilized defective ova may cause a delay in spontaneous abortion. Therefore, the use of such drugs during the first 4 months of pregnancy is not recommended.

Several reports suggest an association between intrauterine exposure to progestational drugs in the first trimester of pregnancy and genital abnormalities in male and female fetuses. The risk of hypospadias, 5-8 per 1000 male births in the general population, may be approximately doubled with exposure to these drugs. There are insufficient data to quantify the risk to exposed female fetuses, but

WARNING — Cont'd

insofar as some of these drugs induce mild virilization of the external genitalia of the female fetus, and because of the increased association of hypospadias in the male fetus, it is prudent to avoid the use of these drugs during the first trimester of pregnancy.

If the patient is exposed to medroxyprogesterone acetate during the first 4 months of pregnancy or if she becomes pregnant while taking this drug, she should be apprised of the potential risks to the fetus.

DESCRIPTION

Patients should be counseled that this product does not protect against HIV infection (AIDS) and other sexually transmitted diseases.

Medroxyprogesterone acetate is a derivative of progesterone and is active by the parenteral and oral routes of administration. It is a white to off-white, odorless crystalline powder, stable in air, melting between 200 and 210°C. It is freely soluble in chloroform, soluble in acetone and in dioxane, sparingly soluble in alcohol and in methanol, slightly soluble in ether, and insoluble in water.

The chemical name for medroxyprogesterone acetate is Pregn-4-ene-3,20-dione, 17-(acetyloxy)-6-methyl-,(6α)-.

TABLETS

Each Provera tablet for oral administration contains 2.5, 5, or 10 mg of medroxyprogesterone acetate. *Inactive ingredients:* Calcium stearate, corn starch, lactose, mineral oil, sorbic acid, sucrose, talc. The 2.5 mg tablet contain FD&C yellow no. 6.

STERILE AQUEOUS SUSPENSION

Depo-Provera sterile aqueous suspension for intramuscular injection is available as 400 mg/ml medroxyprogesterone acetate.

Each ml of the 400 mg/ml suspension contains:

Medroxyprogesterone Acetate: 400 mg.
Polyethylene Glycol 3350: 20.3 mg.
Sodium Sulfate Anhydrous: 11 mg.
Myristyl-Gamma-Picolinium Chloride (Added as a Perservative): 1.69 mg.

When necessary, pH was adjusted with sodium hydroxide and/or hydrochloric acid.

CONTRACEPTIVE INJECTION

Depo-Provera contraceptive injection for intramuscular (IM) injection is available in vials and prefilled syringes, each containing 1 ml medroxyprogesterone acetate sterile aqueous suspension 150 mg/ml.

Each ml contains:

Medroxyprogesterone Acetate: 150 mg.
Polyethylene Glycol 3350: 28.9 mg.
Polysorbate 80: 2.41 mg.
Sodium Chloride: 8.68 mg.
Methylparaben: 1.37 mg.
Propylparaben: 0.150 mg.
Water for Injection: qs.

When necessary, pH is adjusted with sodium hydroxide and/or hydrochloric acid.

CLINICAL PHARMACOLOGY

ORAL TABLETS

Medroxyprogesterone acetate, administered orally or parenterally in the recommended doses to women with adequate endogenous estrogen, transforms proliferative into secretory endometrium. Androgenic and anabolic effects have been noted, but the drug is apparently devoid of significant estrogenic activity. While parenterally administered medroxyprogesterone acetate inhibits gonadotropin production, which in turn prevents follicular maturation and ovulation, available data indicate that this does not occur when the usually recommended oral dosage is given as single daily doses.

STERILE AQUEOUS SUSPENSION

Medroxyprogesterone acetate, administered orally or parenterally in the recommended doses to women with adequate endogenous estrogen, transforms proliferative into secretory endometrium.

Medroxyprogesterone acetate inhibits (in the usual dose range) the secretion of pituitary gonadotropin which in turn, prevents follicular maturation and ovulation.

Because of its prolonged action and the resulting difficulty in predicting the time of withdrawal bleeding following injection, medroxyprogesterone acetate is not recommended in secondary amenorrhea or dysfunctional uterine bleeding. In these conditions oral therapy is recommended.

CONTRACEPTIVE INJECTION

Medroxyprogesterone acetate contraceptive injection, when administered at the recommended dose to women every 3 months, inhibits the secretion of gonadotropins which, in turn, prevents follicular maturation and ovulation and results in endometrial thinning. These actions produce its contraceptive effect.

Following a single 150 mg IM dose of medroxyprogesterone acetate contraceptive injection, measured by an extracted radioimmunoassay procedure, increase for approximately 3 weeks to reach peak plasma concentrations of 1-7 ng/ml. The levels then decrease exponentially until they become undetectable (<100 pg/ml) between 120-200 days following injection. Using an unextracted radioimmunoassay procedure for the assay of medroxyprogesterone acetate in serum, the apparent half-life for medroxyprogesterone acetate following IM administration of medroxyprogesterone acetate contraceptive injection is approximately 50 days.

Women with lower body weights conceive sooner than women with higher body weights after discontinuing medroxyprogesterone acetate contraceptive injection.

The effect of hepatic and/or renal disease on the pharmacokinetics of medroxyprogesterone acetate contraceptive injection is unknown.

INDICATIONS AND USAGE

ORAL TABLETS

Secondary amenorrhea; abnormal uterine bleeding due to hormonal imbalance in the absence of organic pathology, such as fibroids or uterine cancer.

STERILE AQUEOUS SUSPENSION

Adjunctive therapy and palliative treatment of inoperable, recurrent, and metastatic endometrial or renal carcinoma.

CONTRACEPTIVE INJECTION

Medroxyprogesterone acetate contraceptive injection is indicated only for the prevention of pregnancy. To ensure that medroxyprogesterone acetate contraceptive injection is not administered inadvertently to a pregnant woman, the first injection must be given **ONLY** during the first 5 days of a normal menstrual period; **ONLY** within the first 5-days postpartum if not breast-feeding, and if exclusively breast-feeding, **ONLY** at the sixth postpartum week. The efficacy of medroxyprogesterone acetate contraceptive injection depends on adherence to the recommended dosage schedule (see DOSAGE AND ADMINISTRATION). It is a long-term injectable contraceptive in women when administered at 3 month (13-week) intervals. Dosage does not need to be adjusted for body weight.

In five clinical studies using medroxyprogesterone acetate contraceptive injection, the 12 month failure rate for the group of women treated with medroxyprogesterone acetate contraceptive injection was zero (no pregnancies reported) to 0.7 by Life-Table method. Pregnancy rates with contraceptive measures are typically reported for only the first year of use as shown in TABLE 1. Except for intrauterine devices (IUD), implants, sterilization, and medroxyprogesterone acetate contraceptive injection, the efficacy of these contraceptive measures depends in part on the reliability of use. The effectiveness of medroxyprogesterone acetate contraceptive injection is dependent upon the patient returning every 3 months (13 weeks) for reinjection.

TABLE 1 *Lowest Expected and Typical Failure Rates* Expressed as Percent of Women Experiencing an Accidental Pregnancy in the First Year of Continuous Use*

Method	Lowest Expected	Typical
Injectable progestogen		
Medroxyprogesterone acetate contraceptive injection	0.3%	0.3%
Implants		
Norplant (6 capsules)	0.2%†	0.2%†
Female Sterilization	0.2%	0.4%
Male Sterilization	0.1%	0.15%
Pill		3%
Combined	0.1%	
Progestogen only	0.5%	
IUD		3%
Progestasert	2%	
Copper T 380A	0.8%	
Condom	2%	12%
Diaphragm	6%	18%
Cap	6%	18%
Spermicides	3%	21%
Sponge		
Parous women	9%	28%
Nulliparous women	6%	18%
Periodic abstinence	1-9%	20%
Withdrawal	4%	18%
No method	85%	85%

Source: Trussell *et al.*[5]
* Lowest expected: when used exactly as directed. Typical: includes those not following directions exactly.
† from Norplant package insert.

NON-FDA APPROVED INDICATIONS

While not FDA approved, medroxyprogesterone has been used in sexual deviancy, Pickwickian syndrome, and obstructive sleep apnea.

CONTRAINDICATIONS

ORAL TABLETS

Thrombophlebitis, thromboembolic disorders, cerebral apoplexy or patients with a past history of these conditions.
Liver dysfunction or disease.
Known or suspected malignancy of breast or genital organs.
Undiagnosed vaginal bleeding.
Missed abortion.
As a diagnostic test for pregnancy.
Known sensitivity to medroxyprogesterone acetate.

STERILE AQUEOUS SUSPENSION AND CONTRACEPTIVE INJECTION

Known or suspected pregnancy or as a diagnostic test for pregnancy.
Undiagnosed vaginal bleeding.
Known or suspected malignancy of the breast.
Active thrombophlebitis, or current or past history of thromboembolic disorders, or cerebral vascular disease.
Liver dysfunction or disease.
Known sensitivity to medroxyprogesterone acetate or any of the inactive ingredients.

WARNINGS

ORAL TABLETS

The physician should be alert to the earliest manifestations of thrombotic disorders (thrombophlebitis, cerebrovascular disorders, pulmonary embolism, and retinal thrombosis). Should any of these occur or be suspected, the drug should be discontinued immediately.

Beagle dogs treated with medroxyprogesterone acetate developed mammary nodules some of which were malignant. Although nodules occasionally appeared in control animals, they were intermittent in nature, whereas the nodules in the drug-treated animals were larger, more numerous, persistent, and there were some breast malignancies with metastases. Their significance with respect to humans has not been established.

Discontinue medication pending examination if there is sudden partial or complete loss of vision, or if there is a sudden onset of proptosis, diplopia or migraine. If examination reveals papilledema or retinal vascular lesions, medication should be withdrawn.

Detectable amounts of progestin have been identified in the milk of mothers receiving the drug. The effect of this on the nursing neonate and infant has not been determined.

Usage in pregnancy is not recommended (See BOXED WARNING).

Retrospective studies of morbidity and mortality in Great Britain and studies of morbidity in the US have shown a statistically significant association between thrombophlebitis, pulmonary embolism, and cerebral thrombosis and embolism and the use of oral contraceptives.[1-4] The estimate of the relative risk of thromboembolism in the study by Vessey and Doll[3] was about 7-fold, while Sartwell and associates[4] in the US found a relative risk of 4.4, meaning that the users are several times as likely to undergo thromboembolic disease without evident cause as nonusers. The American study also indicated that the risk did not persist after discontinuation of administration, and that it was not enhanced by long continued administration. The American study was not designed to evaluate a difference between products.

STERILE AQUEOUS SUSPENSION

Pregnancy: The use of progestational drugs during the first 4 months of pregnancy is not recommended. Progestational agents have been used beginning with the first trimester of pregnancy in attempts to prevent abortion but there is no evidence that such use is effective. Furthermore, the use of progestational agents, with their uterine-relaxant properties, in patients with fertilized defective ova may cause a delay in spontaneous abortion.

Intrauterine Exposure: Several reports suggest an association between intrauterine exposure to progestational drugs in the first trimester of pregnancy and genital abnormalities in male and female fetuses. The risk of hypospadias (5 to 8 per 1000 male births in the general population) may be approximately doubled with exposure to these drugs. There are insufficient data to quantify the risk to exposed female fetuses, but insofar as some of these drugs induce mild virilization of the external genitalia of the female fetus, and because of the increased association of hypospadias in the male fetus, it is prudent to avoid the use of these drugs during the first trimester of pregnancy. If the patient is exposed to medroxyprogesterone acetate sterile aqueous suspension during the first 4 months of pregnancy or if she becomes pregnant while taking this durg, she should be apprised of the potential risks to the fetus.

Thromboembolic Disorders: The physician should be alert to the earliest manifestations of thrombotic disorder (thrombophlebitis, cerebrovascular disorder, pulmonary embolism, and retinal thrombosis). Should any of these occur or be suspected, the drug should be discontinued immediately.

Ocular Disorders: Medication should be discontinued pending examination if there is a sudden partial or complete loss of vision, or if there is a sudden onset of proptosis, diplopia or migraine. If examination reveals papilledema or retinal vascular lesions, medication should be withdrawn.

Lactation: Detectable amounts of drug have been identified in the milk of mothers receiving progestational drugs. The effect of this on the nursing infant has not been determined.

Multi-Dose Use: Multi-dose use of medroxyprogesterone acetate sterile aqueous suspension from a single vial requires special care to avoid contamination. Although initially sterile, any multi-dose use of vials may lead to contamination unless strict aseptic technique is observed.

CONTRACEPTIVE INJECTION

Bleeding Irregularities

Most women using medroxyprogesterone acetate contraceptive injection experience disruption of menstrual bleeding patterns. Altered menstrual bleeding patterns include irregular or unpredictable bleeding or spotting, or rarely, heavy or continuous bleeding. If abnormal bleeding persists or is severe, appropriate investigation should be instituted to rule out the possibility of organic pathology, and appropriate treatment should be instituted when necessary.

As women continue using medroxyprogesterone acetate contraceptive injection, fewer experience irregular bleeding and more experience amenorrhea. By month 12 amenorrheas was reported by 55% of women, and by month 24 amenorrhea was reported by 68% of women using medroxyprogesterone acetate contraceptive injection.[5]

Bone Mineral Density Changes

Use of medroxyprogesterone acetate contraceptive injection may be considered among the risk factors for development of osteoporosis. The rate of bone loss is greatest in the early years of use and then subsequently approaches the normal rate of age related fall.

Cancer Risks

Long-term case-controlled surveillance of users of medroxyprogesterone acetate contraceptive injection found slight or no increased overall risk of breast cancer[7] and no overall increased risk of ovarian,[8] liver,[9] or cervical[10] cancer and a prolonged, protective effect of reducing the risk of endometrial[11] cancer in the population of users.

A pooled analysis[18] from two case-control studies, the World Health Organization Study[7] and the New Zealand Study,[17] reported the relative risk (RR) of breast cancer for women who had ever used medroxyprogesterone acetate contraceptive injection as 1.1 (95% confidence interval [CI] 0.97 to 1.4). Overall, there was no increase in risk with increasing duration of use of medroxyprogesterone acetate contraceptive injection. The RR of breast cancer for women of all ages who had initiated use of medroxyprogesterone acetate contraceptive injection within the previous 5 years was estimated to be 2.0 (95% CI 1.5 to 2.8).

The World Health Organization Study,[7] a component of the pooled analysis[18] described above, showed an increased RR of 2.19 (95%) CI 1.23-3.89) of breast cancer associated with use of medroxyprogesterone acetate contraceptive injection in women whose first exposure to drug was within the previous 4 years and who were under 35 years of age. However the overall RR for ever-users of medroxyprogesterone acetate contraceptive injection was only 1.2 (95% CI 0.96-1.52).

Note: A RR of 1.0 indicates neither an increased nor a decreased risk of cancer associated with the use of the drug, relative to no use of the drug. In the case of the subpopulation with a RR of 2.19, the 95% CI is fairly wide and does not include the value of 1.0, thus inferring an increased risk of breast cancer in the defined subgroup relative to nonusers. The value of 2.19 means that women whose first exposure to drug was within the previous 4 years and who are under 35 years of age have a 2.19-fold (95% C.I. 1.23- to 3.89-fold) increased risk of breast cancer relative to nonusers. The National Cancer Institute[12] reports an average annual incidence rate for breast cancer for US women, all races, age 30 to 34 years of 26.7 per 100,000. A RR of 2.19 thus, increases the possible risk from 26.7-58.5 cases per 100,000 women. The attributable risk, thus, is 31.8 per 100,000 women per year.

A statistically insignificant increase in RR estimates of invasive squamous-cell cervical cancer has been associated with the use of medroxyprogesterone acetate contraceptive injection in women who were first exposed before the age of 35 years (RR 1.22-1.28 and 95% CI 0.93-1.70). The overall, nonsignificant relative rate of invasive squamous-cell cervical cancer in women who ever used medroxyprogesterone acetate contraceptive injection was estimated to be 1.11 (95% CI 0.96 to 1.29). No trends in risk with duration of use or times since initial or most recent exposure were observed.

Thromboembolic Disorders

The physician should be alert to the earliest manifestations of thrombotic disorders (thrombophlebitis, pulmonary embolism, cerebrovascular disorders, and retinal thrombosis). Should any of these occur or be suspected, the drug should not be readministered.

Ocular Disorders

Medication should not be readministered pending examination if there is a sudden partial or complete loss of vision or if there is a sudden onset of proptosis, diplopia, or migraine. If examination reveals papilledema or retinal vascular lesions, medication should not be readministered.

Unexpected Pregnancies

To ensure that medroxyprogesterone acetate contraceptive injection is not administered inadvertently to a pregnant woman, the first injection must be given **ONLY** during the first 5 days of a normal menstrual period; **ONLY** within the first 5-days postpartum if not breastfeeding, and if exclusively breast-feeding, **ONLY** at the sixth postpartum week (see DOSAGE AND ADMINISTRATION).

Neonates from unexpected pregnancies that occur 1-2 months after injection of medroxyprogesterone acetate contraceptive injection may be at an increased risk of low birth weight, which, in turn, is associated with an increased risk of neonatal death. The attributable risk is low because such pregnancies are uncommon.[13,14]

A significant increase in incidence of polysyndactyly and chromosomal anomalies was observed among infants of users of medroxyprogesterone acetate contraceptive injection, the former being most pronounced in women under 30 years of age. The unrelated nature of these defects, the lack of confirmation from other studies, the distant preconceptual exposure to medroxyprogesterone acetate contraceptive injection, and the chance effects due to multiple statistical comparisons, make a causal association unlikely.[15]

Neonates exposed to medroxyprogesterone acetate *in utero* and followed to adolescence, showed no evidence of any adverse effects on their health including their physical, intellectual, sexual or social development.

Several reports suggest an association between intrauterine exposure to progestational drugs in the first trimester of pregnancy and genital abnormalities in male and female fetuses. The risk of hypospadia (5-8 per 1000 male births in the general population) may be approximately doubled with exposure to these drugs. There are insufficient data to quantify the risk to exposed female fetuses, but because some of these drugs induce mild virilization of the external genitalia of the female fetus and because of the increased association of hypospadia in the male fetus, it is prudent to avoid use of these drugs during the first trimester of pregnancy.

To ensure that medroxyprogesterone acetate contraceptive injection is not administered inadvertently to a pregnant woman, it is important that the first injection be given only during the first 5 days after the onset of a normal menstrual period within 5 days postpartum if not breast-feeding and if breast-feeding, at the sixth week postpartum (see DOSAGE AND ADMINISTRATION).

Ectopic Pregnancy

Health-care providers should be alert to the possibility of an ectopic pregnancy among women using medroxyprogesterone acetate contraceptive injection who become pregnant or complain of severe abdominal pain.

Lactation

Detectable amounts of drug have been identified in the milk of mothers receiving medroxyprogesterone acetatecontraceptive injection. In nursing mothers treated with medroxyprogesterone acetate contraceptive injection, milk composition, quality, and amount are not adversely affected. Neonates and infants exposed to medroxyprogesterone from breast milk have been studied for developmental and behavioral effects through puberty. No adverse effects have been noted.

Anaphylaxis and Anaphylactoid Reaction

Anaphylaxis and anaphylactoid reaction have been reported with the use of medroxyprogesterone acetate contraceptive injection. If an anaphylactic reaction occurs appropriate therapy should be instituted. Serious anaphylactic reactions require emergency medical treatment.

PRECAUTIONS

ORAL TABLETS

The pretreatment physical examination should include special reference to breast and pelvic organs, as well as Papanicolaou smear.

Because progestogens may cause some degree of fluid retention, conditions which might be influenced by this factor, such as epilepsy, migraine, asthma, cardiac or renal dysfunction, require careful observation.

In cases of breakthrough bleeding, as in all cases of irregular bleeding per vaginum, nonfunctional causes should be borne in mind. In cases of undiagnosed vaginal bleeding, adequate diagnostic measures are indicated.

Patients who have a history of psychic depression should be carefully observed and the drug discontinued if the depression recurs to a serious degree.

Any possible influence of prolonged progestin therapy on pituitary, ovarian, adrenal, hepatic or uterine functions awaits further study.

A decrease in glucose tolerance has been observed in a small percentage of patients on estrogen-progestin combination drugs. The mechanism of this decrease is obscure. For this reason, diabetic patients should be carefully observed while receiving progestin therapy.

The age of the patient constitutes no absolute limiting factor although treatment with progestins may mask the onset of the climacteric.

The pathologist should be advised of progestin therapy when relevant specimens are submitted.

Because of the occasional occurrence of thrombotic disorders, (thrombophlebitis, pulmonary embolism, retinal thrombosis, and cerebrovascular disorders) in patients taking estrogen-progestin combinations and since the mechanism is obscure, the physician should be alert to the earliest manifestation of these disorders.

Studies of the addition of a progestin product to an estrogen replacement regimen for 7 or more days of a cycle of estrogen administration have reported a lowered incidence of endometrial hyperplasia. Morphological and biochemical studies of endometrium suggest that 10-13 days of a progestin are needed to provide maximal maturation of the endometrium and to eliminate any hyperplastic changes. Whether this will provide protection from endometrial carcinoma has not been clearly established. There are possible additional risks which may be associated with the inclusion of progestin in estrogen replacement regimen. The potential risks include adverse effects on carbohydrate and lipid metabolism. The dosage used may be important in minimizing these adverse effects.

Aminoglutethimide administered concomitantly with medroxyprogesterone acetate tablets may significantly depress the bioavailability of medroxyprogesterone acetate.

Safety and effectiveness in pediatric patients below the age of 12 years have not been established.

Carcinogenesis, Mutagenesis, and Impairment of Fertility

Long-term intramuscular administration of medroxyprogesterone acetate has been shown to produce mammary tumors in beagle dogs (see WARNINGS). There was no evidence of a carcinogenic effect associated with the oral administration of medroxyprogesterone acetate to rats and mice. Medroxyprogesterone acetate was not mutagenic in a battery of *in vitro* or *in vivo* genetic toxicity assays.

Medroxyprogesterone acetate at high doses is an antifertility drug and high doses would be expected to impair fertility until the cessation of treatment.

Information for the Patient

See the Patient Instructions that are distributed with the prescription.

STERILE AQUEOUS SUSPENSION

Physical Examination

It is good medical practice for all women to have annual history and physical examinations, including women using medroxyprogesterone acetate contraceptive injection. The physical examination, however, may be deferred until after initation of medroxyprogesterone acetate sterile aqueous suspension if requested by the woman and judged appropriate by the clinician. The physical examination should include special reference to blood pressure, breasts, abdomen and pelvic organs, including cervial cytology and relevant laboratory tests. In case of undiagnosed, persistent or recurrent abnormal vaginal bleeding, appropriate measures should be conducted to rule out malignancy. Women with a strong family history of breast cancer or who have breast nodules should be monitored with particular care.

Fluid Retention

Because progestational drugs may cause some degree of fluid retention, conditions which might be influenced by this condition, such as epilepsy, migraine, asthma, cardiac or renal dysfunction, require careful observation.

Vaginal Bleeding

In cases of breakthrough bleeding, as in all cases of irregular bleeding per vaginum, nonfunctional causes should be borne in mind and adequate diagnostic measures undertaken.

Depression

Patients who have a history of psychic depression should be carefully observed and the drug discontinued if the depression recurs to a serious degree.

Masking of Climacteric

The age of the patient constitutes no absolute limiting factor although treatment with progestin may mask the onset of the climacteric.

Use with Estrogen

Studies of the addition of a progestin product to an estrogen replacement regimen for 7 or more days of a cycle of estrogen administration have reported a lowered incidence of endometrial hyperplasia. Morphological and biochemical studies of endometria suggest that 10-13 days of a progestin are needed to provide maximal maturation of the endometrium and to eliminate any hyperplastic changes. Whether this will provide protection from endometrial carcinoma has not been clearly established. There are possible risks which may be associated with the inclusion of progestin in estrogen replacement regimen, including adverse effects on carbohydrate and lipid metabolism. The dosage used may be important in minimizing these adverse effects. A decrease in glucose tolerance has been observed in a small percentage of patients on estrogen-progestin combination treatment. The mechanism of this decreas is obscure. For this reason, diabetic patients should be carefully observed while receiving such therapy.

Prolonged Use

The effect of prolonged use of medroxyprogesterone acetate sterile aqueous suspension at the recommended doses on pituitary, ovarian, adrenal, hepatic, and uterine function is not known.

Multi-Dose Use

When multi-dose vials are used, special care to prevent contamination of the contents is essential. There is some evidence that benzalkonium chloride is not an adequate antiseptic for sterilizing medroxyprogesterone acetate sterile aqueous suspension multi-dose vials. A povidone-iodine solution or similar product is recommended to cleanse the vial top prior to aspiration of contents. (See WARNINGS.)

CONTRACEPTIVE INJECTION

Physical Examination

It is good medical practice for all women to have annual history and physical examination, including women using medroxygrogesterone acetate congtraceptive injection. The physical examination, however, may be deferred until after initiation of medroxygrogesterone acetate contraceptive injection if requested by the woman and judged appropriate by the clinician. The physical examination should include special reference to blood pressure, breasts, abdomen and pelvic organs, inlcuding cervical cytology and relevant laboratory tests. In case of undiagnosed, persistent or recurrent abnormal vaginal bleeding, appropriate measures should be conducted to rule out malignancy. Women with a strong family history of breast cancer or who have breast nodules should be monitored with particular care.

Fluid Retention

Because progestational drugs may cause some degree of fluid retention, conditions that might be influenced by this condition, such as epilepsy, migraine, asthma, and cardiac or renal dysfunction, require careful observation.

Weight Changes

There is a tendency for women to gain weight while on therapy with medroxyprogesterone acetate contraceptive injection. From an initial average body weight of 136 lb, women who completed 1 year of therapy with medroxyprogesterone acetate contraceptive injection gained an average of 5.4 lb. Women who completed 2 years of therapy gained an average of 8.1 lb.

Women who completed 4 years gained an average of 13.8 lb. Women who completed 6 years gained an average of 16.5 lb. Two percent (2%) of women withdrew from a large-scale clinical trial because of excessive weight gain.

Return of Fertility

Medroxyprogesterone acetate contraceptive injection has a prolonged contraceptive effect. In a large US study of women who discontinued use of medroxyprogesterone acetate contraceptive injection to become pregnant, data are available for 61% of them. Based on Life-Table analysis of these data, it is expected that 68% of women who do become pregnant may conceive within 12 months, 83% may conceive within 15 months, and 93% may conceive within 18 months from the last injection. The median time to conception for those who do conceive is 10 months following the last injection with a range of 4 to 31 months, and is unrelated to the duration of use. No data are available for 39% of the patients who discontinued medroxyprogesterone acetate contraceptive injection to become pregnant and who were lost to follow-up or changed their mind.

CNS Disorders and Convulsions

Patients who have a history of psychic depression should be carefully observed and the drug not be readministered if the depression recurs.

There have been a few reported cases of convulsions in patients who were treated with medroxyprogesterone acetate contraceptive injection. Association with drug use or pre-existing conditions is not clear.

Carbohydrate Metabolism

A decrease in glucose tolerance has been observed in some patients on medroxyprogesterone acetate contraceptive injection treatment. The mechanism of this decrease is obscure. For this reason, diabetic patients should be carefully observed while receiving such therapy.

Liver Function

If jaundice develops, consideration should be given to not readministering the drug.

Protection Against Sexually Transmitted Diseases

Patients should be counseled that this product does not protect against HIV infection (AIDS) and other sexually transmitted diseases.

Carcinogenesis

See WARNINGS, Cancer.

Pregnancy Category X
See WARNINGS, Lactation.

Nursing Mothers
See WARNINGS, Lactation.

Pediatric Use
Safety and effectiveness in pediatric patients have not been established. See WARNINGS, Unexpected Pregnancies.

Information for the Patient
Patient labeling is included with each single-dose vial and prefilled syringe of medroxyprogesterone acetate contraceptive injection to help describe its characteristics to the patient (see the Patient Instructions that are distributed with the prescription.). It is recommended that prospective users be given this labeling and be informed about the risks and benefits associated with the use of medroxyprogesterone acetate contraceptive injection, as compared with other forms of contraception or with no contraception at all. It is recommended that physicians or other health-care providers responsible for those patients advise them at the beginning of treatment that their menstrual cycle may be disrupted and that irregular and unpredictable bleeding or spotting results, and that this usually decreases to the point of amenorrhea as treatment with medroxyprogesterone acetate contraceptive injection continues, without other therapy being required.

LABORATORY TEST INTERACTIONS
Sterile Aqueous Suspension and Contraceptive Injection
The pathologist should be advised of progestin therapy when relevant specimens are submitted.

The following laboratory tests may be affected by progestins including medroxyprogesterone acetate:

- Plasma and urinary steroid levels are decreased (*e.g.*, progesterone, estradiol, pregnanediol, testosterone, cortisol).
- Gonadotropin levels are decreased.
- Sex-hormone-binding-globulin concentrations are decreased.
- Protein-bound iodine and butanol extractable protein-bound iodine may increase. T_3 uptake values may decrease.
- Coagulation test values for prothrombin (Factor II), and Factors VII, VIII, IX, and X may increase.
- Sulfobromophthalein and other liver function test values may be increased.
- The effects of medroxyprogesterone acetate on lipid metabolism are inconsistent. Both increases and decreases in total cholesterol, triglycerides, low-density lipoprotein (LDL) cholesterol, and high-density lipoprotein (HDL) cholesterol have been observed in studies.

M

DRUG INTERACTIONS

STERILE AQUEOUS SUSPENSION AND CONTRACEPTIVE INJECTION
Aminoglutethimide administered concomitantly with the medroxyprogesterone acetate sterile aqueous suspension or contraceptive injection may significantly depress the serum concentrations of medroxyprogesterone acetate.[16] Users of medroxyprogesterone acetate should be warned of the possibility of decreased efficacy with the use of this or any related drugs.

ADVERSE REACTIONS

ORAL TABLETS

Pregnancy: See BOXED WARNING for possible adverse effects on the fetus.
Breast: Breast tenderness or galactorrhea has been reported rarely.
Skin: Sensitivity reactions consisting of urticaria, pruritus, edema and generalized rash have occurred in an occasional patient. Acne, alopecia and hirsutism have been reported in a few cases.
Thromboembolic Phenomena: Thromboembolic phenomena including thrombophlebitis and pulmonary embolism have been reported.

The following adverse reactions have been observed in women taking progestins including medroxyprogesterone acetate tablets: Breakthrough bleeding, spotting, change in menstrual flow, amenorrhea, edema, change in weight (increase or decrease), changes in cervical erosion and cervical secretions, cholestatic jaundice, anaphylactoid reactions and anaphylaxis, rash (allergic) with and without pruritus, mental depression, pyrexia, insomnia, nausea, somnolence.

A statistically significant association has been demonstrated between use of estrogen-progestin combination drugs and the following serious adverse reactions: Thrombophlebitis; pulmonary embolism and cerebral thrombosis and embolism. For this reason patients on progestin therapy should be carefully observed.

Although available evidence is suggestive of an association, such a relationship has been neither confirmed nor refuted for the following serious adverse reactions: Neuro-ocular lesions, *e.g.*, retinal thrombosis and optic neuritis.

STERILE AQUEOUS SUSPENSION
See WARNINGS for possible adverse effects on the fetus.

The following adverse reactions have been observed in women receiving injections of the sterile aqueous suspension:

Breakthrough bleeding; spotting; change in menstrual flow; amenorrhea; headache; nervousness; dizziness; edema; change in weight (increase or decrease); changes in cervial erosion and cervial secretions; cholestatic jaundice, including neonatal jaundice; breast tenderness and galactorrhea; skin sensitivity reactions consisting of urticaria, pruritus, edema and generalized rash; acne, alopecia and hirsutism; rash (allergic) with and without pruritus; anaphylactoid reactions and anaphylaxis; mental depression; pyrexia; fatigue; insomnia; nausea; somnolence.

In a few instances there have been undesirable sequelae at the first site of injection, such as residual lump, change in color of skin, or sterile abscess.

A statistically significant association has been demonstrated between use of estrogen-progestin combination durgs and pulmonary embolism and cerebral thrombosis and embolism. For this reason patients on progestin therapy should be carefully observed. There is also evidence suggestive of an associatin with neuro-ocular lesions, *e.g.*, retinal thrombosis and optic neuritis.

ORAL TABLETS AND STERILE AQUEOUS SUSPENSION
The following adverse reactions have been observed in patients receiving estrogen progestin combination drugs: Rise in blood pressure in susceptible individuals; premenstrual-like syndrome; changes in libido; changes in appetite; cystitis-like syndrome; headache; nervousness; fatigue; backache; hirsutism; loss of scalp hair; erythema multiforme; erythema nodosum; hemorrhagic eruption; itching; dizziness.
In view of these observations, patients on progestin therapy should be carefully observed.

The following laboratory results may be altered by the use of estrogen-progestin combination drugs:

- Increased sulfobromophthalein retention and other hepatic function tests.
- Coagulation tests: increase in prothrombin factors VII, VIII, IX and X.
- Metyrapone test.
- Pregnanediol determination.
- Thyroid function: increase in PBI, and butanol extractable protein bound iodine and decrease in T^3 uptake values.

CONTRACEPTIVE INJECTION
In the largest clinical trial with medroxyprogesterone acetate contraceptive injection, over 3900 women, who were treated for up to 7 years, reported the following adverse reactions, which may or may not be related to the use of medroxyprogesterone acetate contraceptive injection.

The following adverse reactions reported by more than 5% of subjects:
Menstrual irregularities (bleeding or amenorrhea, or both); abdominal pain or discomfort; weight changes; dizziness; headache; asthenia (weakness or fatigue); nervousness.

Adverse reactions reported by 1-5% of subjects:
Decreased libido or anorgasmia; pelvic pain; backache; breast pain; leg cramps; no hair growth or alopecia; depression; bloating; nausea; rash; insomnia; edema; leukorrhea; hot flashes; acne; arthralgia; vaginitis.

Events reported by fewer than 1% of subjects included: Galactorrhea, melasma, chloasma, convulsions, changes in appetite, gastrointestinal disturbances, jaundice, genitourinary infections, vaginal cysts, dyspareunia, paresthesia, chest pain, pulmonary embolus, allergic reactions, anemia, drowsiness, syncope, dyspnea and asthma, tachycardia, fever, excessive sweating and body odor, dry skin, chills, increased libido, excessive thirst, hoarseness, pain at injection site, blood dyscrasia, rectal bleeding, changes in breast size, breast lumps or nipple bleeding, axillary swelling, breast cancer, prevention of lactation, sensation of pregnancy, lack of return to fertility, paralysis, facial palsy, scleroderma, osteoporosis, uterine hyperplasia, cervical cancer, varicose veins, dysmenorrhea, hirsutism, unexpected pregnancy, thrombophlebitis, deep vein thrombosis.
In addition, voluntary reports have been received of anaphylaxis and anaphylactoid reaction with use of medroxyprogesterone acetate contraceptive injection.

DOSAGE AND ADMINISTRATION

ORAL TABLETS
Secondary Amenorrhea
Medroxyprogesterone acetate tablets may be given in dosages of 5-10 mg daily for 5-10 days. A dose for inducing an optimum secretory transformation of an endometrium that has been adequately primed with either endogenous or exogenous estrogen is 10 mg of medroxyprogesterone acetate daily for 10 days. In cases of secondary amenorrhea, therapy may be started at any time. Progestin withdrawal bleeding usually occurs within 3-7 days after discontinuing medroxyprogesterone acetate therapy.

Abnormal Uterine Bleeding Due to Hormonal Imbalance in the Absence of Organic Pathology
Beginning on the calculated 16th or 21st day of the menstrual cycle, 5-10 mg of medroxyprogesterone acetate may be given daily for 5-10 days. To produce an optimum secretory transformation of an endometrium that has been adequately primed with either endogenous or exogenous estrogen, 10 mg of medroxyprogesterone acetate daily for 10 days beginning on the 16th day of the cycle is suggested. Progestin withdrawal bleeding usually occurs within 3-7 days after discontinuing therapy with medroxyprogesterone acetate. Patients with a past history of recurrent episodes of abnormal uterine bleeding may benefit from planned menstrual cycling with medroxyprogesterone acetate.

STERILE AQUEOUS SUSPENSION
This suspension is intended for intramuscular administration only.

Endometrial or Renal Carcinoma
Doses of 400-1000 mg of medroxyprogesterone acetate sterile aqueous suspension per week are recommended initially. If improvement is noted within a few weeks or months and the disease appears stabilized, it may be possible to maintain improvement with as little as 400 mg per month. Medroxyprogesterone acetate is not recommended as primary therapy, but as adjunctive and palliative treatment in advanced inoperable cases including those with recurrent or metastatic disease.

When multi-dose vials are used, special care to prevent contamination of the contents is essential (see WARNINGS).

CONTRACEPTIVE INJECTION
Both the 1 ml vial and the 1 ml prefilled syringe of medroxyprogesterone acetate contraceptive injection should be vigorously shaken just before use to ensure that the dose being administered represents a uniform suspension.

The recommended dose is 150 mg of medroxyprogesterone acetate contraceptive injection every 3 months (13 weeks) administered by deep, IM injection in the gluteal or deltoid muscle. To ensure the patient is not pregnant at the time of the first injection, the first injection **MUST** be given **ONLY** during the first 5 days of a normal menstrual period; **ONLY** within the first 5-days postpartum if not breast-feeding; and if exclusively breast-feeding, **ONLY** at the sixth postpartum week. If the time interval between injections is greater than 13 weeks, the physician should determine that the patient is not pregnant before administering the drug. The efficacy of medroxyprogesterone acetate contracptive injection depends on adherence to the dosage schedule of administration.

HOW SUPPLIED

PROVERA TABLETS

Provera tablets are available in:

2.5 mg: Scored, round, orange.
5 mg: Scored, hexagonal, white.
10 mg: Scored, round, white.

Storage: Store at controlled room temperature 20-25°C (68-77°F).

DEPO-PROVERA CONTRACEPTIVE INJECTION

Depo-Provera contraceptive injection for intramuscular (IM) injection is available in vials and prefilled syringes, each containing 1 ml medroxyprogesterone acetate sterile aqueous suspension 150 mg/ml.

Storage: Store at controlled room temperature 20-25°C (68-77°F).

PRODUCT LISTING - RATED THERAPEUTICALLY EQUIVALENT

Tablet - Oral - 2.5 mg

Size	Price	Product	NDC
30's	$10.13	GENERIC, Pd-Rx Pharmaceuticals	55289-0816-30
30's	$13.60	PROVERA, Southwood Pharmaceuticals Inc	58016-0969-30
30's	$17.20	PROVERA, Allscripts Pharmaceutical Company	54569-1849-03
30's	$17.91	PROVERA, Pd-Rx Pharmaceuticals	55289-0121-30
30's	$19.09	PROVERA, Physicians Total Care	54868-1010-01
30's	$19.85	PROVERA, Pharmacia Corporation	00009-0064-06
40's	$25.06	PROVERA, Physicians Total Care	54868-1010-03
100's	$20.25	FEDERAL UPPER LIMIT, H.C.F.A. F F P	99999-1712-02
100's	$22.88	GENERIC, Major Pharmaceuticals Inc	00904-5227-60
100's	$29.80	GENERIC, Duramed Pharmaceuticals Inc	51285-0540-02
100's	$31.29	GENERIC, Barr Laboratories Inc	00555-0872-02
100's	$32.84	GENERIC, Watson/Rugby Laboratories Inc	00536-5905-01
100's	$46.00	PROVERA, Southwood Pharmaceuticals Inc	58016-0969-00
100's	$57.33	PROVERA, Allscripts Pharmaceutical Company	54569-1849-01
100's	$65.91	PROVERA, Pharmacia and Upjohn	00009-0064-04

Tablet - Oral - 5 mg

Size	Price	Product	NDC
30's	$13.73	GENERIC, Pd-Rx Pharmaceuticals	55289-0908-30
30's	$16.28	PROVERA, Allscripts Pharmaceutical Company	54569-8516-02
30's	$19.28	PROVERA, Pharmacia and Upjohn	00009-0286-32
90's	$48.84	PROVERA, Allscripts Pharmaceutical Company	54569-8516-00
100's	$22.50	GENERIC, Major Pharmaceuticals Inc	00904-5228-60
100's	$30.61	FEDERAL UPPER LIMIT, H.C.F.A. F F P	99999-1712-03
100's	$44.84	GENERIC, Warner Chilcott Laboratories	00047-0266-24
100's	$45.00	GENERIC, Duramed Pharmaceuticals Inc	51285-0541-02
100's	$47.25	GENERIC, Barr Laboratories Inc	00555-0873-02
100's	$49.55	GENERIC, Watson/Rugby Laboratories Inc	00536-5906-01
100's	$70.67	PROVERA, Allscripts Pharmaceutical Company	54569-1779-00
100's	$99.50	PROVERA, Pharmacia Corporation	00009-0286-03

Tablet - Oral - 10 mg

Size	Price	Product	NDC
5's	$3.48	GENERIC, Pd-Rx Pharmaceuticals	55289-0160-05
5's	$7.38	PROVERA, Physicians Total Care	54868-0290-02
7's	$3.68	GENERIC, Pd-Rx Pharmaceuticals	55289-0160-07
10's	$3.87	GENERIC, Pd-Rx Pharmaceuticals	55289-0160-10
10's	$11.24	PROVERA, Allscripts Pharmaceutical Company	54569-0816-00
10's	$14.93	PROVERA, Pd-Rx Pharmaceuticals	55289-0034-10
13's	$4.10	GENERIC, Pd-Rx Pharmaceuticals	55289-0160-13
30's	$7.23	GENERIC, Pd-Rx Pharmaceuticals	55289-0160-30
30's	$19.87	PROVERA, Allscripts Pharmaceutical Company	54569-8524-00
30's	$36.08	PROVERA, Pharmacia Corporation	00009-0050-09
30's	$38.25	PROVERA, Physicians Total Care	54868-0290-03
40's	$9.59	GENERIC, Pd-Rx Pharmaceuticals	55289-0160-40
40's	$50.59	PROVERA, Physicians Total Care	54868-0290-04
50's	$10.59	GENERIC, Pd-Rx Pharmaceuticals	55289-0160-50
90's	$59.61	PROVERA, Allscripts Pharmaceutical Company	54569-8524-01
100's	$24.88	FEDERAL UPPER LIMIT, H.C.F.A. F F P	99999-1712-04
100's	$46.71	GENERIC, Mutual/United Research Laboratories	00677-1619-01
100's	$46.75	GENERIC, Greenstone Limited	59762-3742-02
100's	$46.80	GENERIC, Duramed Pharmaceuticals Inc	51285-0542-02
100's	$49.14	GENERIC, Barr Laboratories Inc	00555-0779-02
100's	$123.25	PROVERA, Pharmacia Corporation	00009-0050-02
100's	$124.68	PROVERA, Physicians Total Care	54868-0290-00

PRODUCT LISTING - RATED NOT THERAPEUTICALLY EQUIVALENT

Tablet - Oral - 10 mg

Size	Price	Product	NDC
5's	$2.34	GENERIC, Allscripts Pharmaceutical Company	54569-0809-01
10's	$4.68	GENERIC, Allscripts Pharmaceutical Company	54569-0809-00
12's	$5.61	GENERIC, Allscripts Pharmaceutical Company	54569-0809-06
30's	$14.03	GENERIC, Allscripts Pharmaceutical Company	54569-0809-02
30's	$15.47	GENERIC, Allscripts Pharmaceutical Company	54569-8572-00
50's	$7.50	GENERIC, Major Pharmaceuticals Inc	00904-2690-51
50's	$10.11	GENERIC, Moore, H.L. Drug Exchange Inc	00839-6610-04
50's	$12.00	GENERIC, Interstate Drug Exchange Inc	00814-4660-08
50's	$12.40	GENERIC, Ivax Corporation	00182-1196-19
50's	$14.20	GENERIC, Martec Pharmaceuticals Inc	52555-0463-00
50's	$14.75	GENERIC, Qualitest Products Inc	00603-4368-19
50's	$14.75	GENERIC, Rosemont Pharmaceutical Corporation	00832-0087-26
50's	$14.82	GENERIC, Aligen Independent Laboratories Inc	00405-4618-50
50's	$18.45	AMEN, Carnrick Laboratories Inc	00086-0049-05
50's	$23.38	GENERIC, Allscripts Pharmaceutical Company	54569-0809-04
100's	$13.08	GENERIC, Moore, H.L. Drug Exchange Inc	00839-6610-06
100's	$22.01	GENERIC, Auro Pharmaceutical	55829-0356-10
100's	$28.03	GENERIC, Rosemont Pharmaceutical Corporation	00832-0087-00
100's	$30.85	AMEN, Carnrick Laboratories Inc	00086-0049-10
100's	$46.68	GENERIC, Major Pharmaceuticals Inc	00904-2690-60
100's	$59.04	GENERIC, R.I.D. Inc Distributor	54807-0550-01
250's	$29.15	GENERIC, Moore, H.L. Drug Exchange Inc	00839-6610-09
250's	$33.75	GENERIC, Major Pharmaceuticals Inc	00904-2690-70
250's	$37.50	GENERIC, Ivax Corporation	00182-1196-02
250's	$39.00	GENERIC, Interstate Drug Exchange Inc	00814-4660-22
250's	$42.75	GENERIC, Martec Pharmaceuticals Inc	52555-0463-02
250's	$57.90	GENERIC, Aligen Independent Laboratories Inc	00405-4618-04
250's	$66.48	GENERIC, Qualitest Products Inc	00603-4368-24
250's	$66.50	GENERIC, Rosemont Pharmaceutical Corporation	00832-0087-25

M

PRODUCT LISTING - EQUIVALENTS NOT AVAILABLE

Suspension - Intramuscular - 150 mg/ml

Size	Price	Product	NDC
1 ml	$50.99	DEPO-PROVERA CONTRACEPTIVE, Allscripts Pharmaceutical Company	54569-4904-00
1 ml	$56.11	DEPO-PROVERA CONTRACEPTIVE, Pharmacia and Upjohn	00009-0746-30
1 ml	$56.11	DEPO-PROVERA CONTRACEPTIVE, Pharmacia and Upjohn	00009-7376-01
1 ml x 6	$336.66	DEPO-PROVERA CONTRACEPTIVE, Pharmacia and Upjohn	00009-7376-02
1 ml x 24	$1346.64	DEPO-PROVERA CONTRACEPTIVE, Pharmacia and Upjohn	00009-7376-03
1 ml x 25	$1402.75	DEPO-PROVERA CONTRACEPTIVE, Pharmacia and Upjohn	00009-0746-35

Suspension - Intramuscular - 400 mg/ml

Size	Price	Product	NDC
2 ml	$110.39	DEPO-PROVERA, Pharmacia and Upjohn	00009-0626-01
2.50 ml	$110.39	DEPO-PROVERA, Allscripts Pharmaceutical Company	54569-3958-00
10 ml	$419.09	DEPO-PROVERA, Pharmacia and Upjohn	00009-0626-02
10 ml	$419.09	DEPO-PROVERA, Allscripts Pharmaceutical Company	54569-3957-00

Tablet - Oral - 2.5 mg

Size	Price	Product	NDC
10's	$2.98	GENERIC, Allscripts Pharmaceutical Company	54569-3806-00
30's	$7.28	GENERIC, Physicians Total Care	54868-2984-00
30's	$8.95	GENERIC, Allscripts Pharmaceutical Company	54569-3806-02
30's	$11.55	GENERIC, Pharma Pac	52959-0420-30
30's	$14.87	GENERIC, Prescript Pharmaceuticals	00247-0253-30
40's	$9.27	GENERIC, Physicians Total Care	54868-2984-02
60's	$17.90	GENERIC, Allscripts Pharmaceutical Company	54569-8570-00
90's	$26.85	GENERIC, Allscripts Pharmaceutical Company	54569-8570-01
90's	$26.85	GENERIC, Greenstone Limited	59762-3740-04
100's	$21.17	GENERIC, Physicians Total Care	54868-2984-03
100's	$29.83	GENERIC, Allscripts Pharmaceutical Company	54569-3806-01
100's	$29.83	GENERIC, Greenstone Limited	59762-3740-01

Tablet - Oral - 5 mg

Size	Price	Product	NDC
10's	$4.50	GENERIC, Allscripts Pharmaceutical Company	54569-3807-00
30's	$10.75	GENERIC, Physicians Total Care	54868-2985-00
40's	$13.89	GENERIC, Physicians Total Care	54868-2985-01
90's	$40.51	GENERIC, Allscripts Pharmaceutical Company	54569-8571-00
100's	$16.45	GENERIC, Physicians Total Care	54868-2985-02

100's	$45.01	GENERIC, Greenstone Limited	59762-3741-01
Tablet - Oral - 10 mg			
5's	$2.60	GENERIC, Physicians Total Care	54868-0109-06
5's	$3.88	GENERIC, Prescript Pharmaceuticals	00247-0178-05
7's	$4.09	GENERIC, Prescript Pharmaceuticals	00247-0178-07
10's	$3.53	GENERIC, Physicians Total Care	54868-0109-01
10's	$4.41	GENERIC, Prescript Pharmaceuticals	00247-0178-10
10's	$6.62	GENERIC, Southwood Pharmaceuticals Inc	58016-0926-10
14's	$9.27	GENERIC, Southwood Pharmaceuticals Inc	58016-0926-14
15's	$9.93	GENERIC, Southwood Pharmaceuticals Inc	58016-0926-15
20's	$13.25	GENERIC, Southwood Pharmaceuticals Inc	58016-0926-20
30's	$6.53	GENERIC, Prescript Pharmaceuticals	00247-0178-30
30's	$7.26	GENERIC, Physicians Total Care	54868-0109-02
30's	$19.87	GENERIC, Southwood Pharmaceuticals Inc	58016-0926-30
40's	$9.12	GENERIC, Physicians Total Care	54868-0109-05
40's	$26.49	GENERIC, Southwood Pharmaceuticals Inc	58016-0926-40
50's	$8.65	GENERIC, Prescript Pharmaceuticals	00247-0178-50
50's	$33.12	GENERIC, Southwood Pharmaceuticals Inc	58016-0926-50
100's	$13.94	GENERIC, Prescript Pharmaceuticals	00247-0178-00
100's	$20.31	GENERIC, Physicians Total Care	54868-0109-03
100's	$66.23	GENERIC, Southwood Pharmaceuticals Inc	58016-0926-00

Mefenamic Acid *(001714)*

For related information, see the comparative table section in Appendix A.

Categories: Dysmenorrhea; Pain, moderate; Pregnancy Category C; FDA Approved 1967 Mar

Drug Classes: Analgesics, non-narcotic; Nonsteroidal anti-inflammatory drugs

Brand Names: **Ponstel**

Foreign Brand Availability: Algastel (Philippines); Algifort (Philippines); Alpain (Indonesia); Aprostal (Philippines); Atmose (Philippines); Beafemic (Malaysia); Benostan (Indonesia); Bonabol (Japan); Dysman (England); Dyspen (Malaysia; Thailand); Ecopan (Switzerland); Eurostan (Philippines); Femen (Thailand); Fenamic (Bahrain; Cyprus; Egypt; Iran; Iraq; Jordan; Kuwait; Lebanon; Libya; Oman; Qatar; Republic-of-Yemen; Saudi-Arabia; Syria; United-Arab-Emirates); Fenamin (South-Africa); Fenamol (Bahrain; Cyprus; Egypt; Iran; Iraq; Jordan; Kuwait; Lebanon; Libya; Oman; Qatar; Republic-of-Yemen; Saudi-Arabia; Syria; United-Arab-Emirates); Gardan (Bahamas; Barbados; Belize; Bermuda; Curacao; Guyana; Jamaica; Netherland-Antilles; Puerto-Rico; Surinam; Trinidad); Hamitan (Hong-Kong); Hostan (Hong-Kong); Johnstal (Taiwan); Kemostan (Indonesia); Lysalgo (Italy); Manic (Thailand); Mecid A (Philippines); Mefac (Ireland); Mefacap (Singapore); Mefalqic (South-Africa); Mefast (Indonesia); Mefic (Australia); Metmic (Philippines); Napan (Hong-Kong); Parkemed (Austria; Germany); Passton (Taiwan); Pefamic (Thailand); Poncofen (Indonesia); Pondnadysmen (Thailand); Pondex (Indonesia); Ponstan (Australia; Bahrain; Bangladesh; Canada; Cyprus; Ecuador; Egypt; England; Finland; Ghana; Greece; Hong-Kong; India; Indonesia; Iran; Iraq; Jordan; Kenya; Kuwait; Lebanon; Libya; Malaysia; Mauritius; New-Zealand; Oman; Pakistan; Portugal; Qatar; Republic-of-Yemen; Saudi-Arabia; South-Africa; Switzerland; Syria; Taiwan; Tanzania; Thailand; Turkey; Uganda; United-Arab-Emirates; Zimbabwe); Ponstan (500 mg) (Colombia); Ponstan-500 (Mexico); Ponstan Forte (Bahrain; Cyprus; Egypt; Iran; Iraq; Jordan; Kuwait; Lebanon; Libya; Oman; Qatar; Republic-of-Yemen; Saudi-Arabia; South-Africa; Syria; United-Arab-Emirates); Ponstyl (France; Mauritius); Pontacid (Hong-Kong); Pontal (Japan; Korea); Pontyl (Singapore); Potarlon (Taiwan); Pynamic (Thailand); Ralgec (Philippines); Sefmic (Hong-Kong); Selmac (Philippines); Solasic (Indonesia); Tanston (Peru); Tropistan (Indonesia); Youfenam (Japan); Zerrmic (Philippines)

Cost of Therapy: $38.96 (Pain; Ponstel; 250 mg; 4 capsules/day; 7 day supply)

DESCRIPTION

Mefenamic acid is N-(2,3-xylyl)-anthranilic acid. It is an analgesic agent for oral administration.

It is a white powder with a melting point of 230-231°C, molecular weight 241.28, and water solubility of 0.004% at pH 7.1.

Ponstel is available in capsules containing 250 mg of mefenamic acid. Each capsule also contains lactose. The capsule shell and/or band contains citric acid; D&C yellow no. 10; FD&C blue no. 1; FD&C red no. 3; FD&C yellow no. 6; gelatin; glycerol monooleate; silicon dioxide; sodium benzoate; sodium lauryl sulfate; titanium dioxide.

CLINICAL PHARMACOLOGY

Mefenamic acid is a nonsteroidal agent with demonstrated antiinflammatory, analgesic, and antipyretic activity in laboratory animals.[1,2] The mode of action is not known. In animal studies, mefenamic acid was found to inhibit prostaglandin synthesis and to compete for binding at the prostaglandin receptor site.[3]

Pharmacologic studies show mefenamic acid did not relieve morphine abstinence signs in abstinent, morphine-habituated monkeys.[1]

Following a single 1 g oral dose, peak plasma levels of 10 µg/ml occurred in 2-4 hours with a half-life of 2 hours. Following multiple doses, plasma levels are proportional to dose with no evidence of drug accumulation. One gram (1 g) of mefenamic acid given 4 times daily produces peak blood levels of 20 µg/ml by the second day of administration.[4]

Following a single dose, 67% of the total dose is excreted in the urine as unchanged drug or as one of two metabolites. 20-25% of the dose is excreted in the feces during the first 3 days.[4]

INDICATIONS AND USAGE

Mefenamic acid is indicated for the relief of moderate pain[5] when therapy will not exceed 1 week. Mefenamic acid is also indicated for the treatment of primary dysmenorrhea.[5,6]

Studies in children under 14 years of age have been inadequate to evaluate the safety and effectiveness of mefenamic acid.

CONTRAINDICATIONS

Mefenamic acid should not be used in patients who have previously exhibited hypersensitivity to it.

Because the potential exists for cross-sensitivity to aspirin or other nonsteroidal antiinflammatory drugs, mefenamic acid should not be given to patients in whom these drugs induce symptoms of bronchospasm, allergic rhinitis, or urticaria.

Mefenamic acid is contraindicated in patients with active ulceration or chronic inflammation of either the upper or lower gastrointestinal tract.

Mefenamic acid should be avoided in patients with preexisting renal disease.

WARNINGS

If diarrhea occurs, the dosage should be reduced or temporarily suspended (see ADVERSE REACTIONS and DOSAGE AND ADMINISTRATION). Certain patients who develop diarrhea may be unable to tolerate the drug because of recurrence of the symptoms on subsequent exposure.

RISK OF GI ULCERATION, BLEEDING AND PERFORATION 7ITH NSAID THERAPY

Serious gastrointestinal toxicity such as bleeding, ulceration, and perforation, can occur at any time, with or without warning symptoms, in patients treated chronically with NSAID therapy. Although minor upper gastrointestinal problems, such as dyspepsia, are common, usually developing early in therapy, physicians should remain alert for ulceration and bleeding in patients treated chronically with NSAIDs even in the absence of previous GI tract symptoms. In patients observed in clinical trials of several months to 2 years duration, symptomatic upper GI ulcers, gross bleeding or perforation appear to occur in approximately 1% of patients treated for 3-6 months, and in about 2-4% of patients treated for 1 year. Physicians should inform patients about the signs and/or symptoms of serious GI toxicity and what steps to take if they occur.

Studies to date have not identified any subset of patients not at risk of developing peptic ulceration and bleeding. Except for a prior history of serious GI events and other risk factors known to be associated with peptic ulcer disease, such as alcoholism, smoking, etc., no risk factors (*e.g.*, age, sex) have been associated with increased risk. Elderly or debilitated patients seem to tolerate ulceration or bleeding less well than other individuals and most spontaneous reports of fatal GI events are in this population. Studies to date are inconclusive concerning the relative risk of various NSAIDs in causing such reactions. High doses of any NSAID probably carry a greater risk of these reactions, although controlled clinical trials showing this do not exist in most cases. In considering the use of relatively large doses (within the recommended dosage range), sufficient benefit should be anticipated to offset the potential increased risk of GI toxicity.

PRECAUTIONS

If rash occurs, administration of the drug should be stopped.

A false-positive reaction for urinary bile, using the diazo tablet test, may result after mefenamic acid administration. If biliuria is suspected, other diagnostic procedures, such as the Harrison spot test, should be performed.

RENAL EFFECTS

As with other nonsteroidal antiinflammatory drugs, long-term administration of mefenamic acid to animals has resulted in renal papillary necrosis and other abnormal renal pathology. In humans, there have been reports of acute interstitial nephritis with hematuria, proteinuria and occasionally nephrotic syndrome.

A second form of renal toxicity has been seen in patients with prerenal conditions leading to a reduction in renal blood flow or blood volume, where the renal prostaglandins have a supportive role in the maintenance of renal perfusion. In these patients administration of an NSAID may cause a dose-dependent reduction in prostaglandin formation and may precipitate overt renal decompensation. Patients at greatest risk of this reaction are those with impaired renal function, heart failure, liver dysfunction, those taking diuretics, and the elderly. Discontinuation of NSAID therapy is typically followed by recovery to the pretreatment state.

Since mefenamic acid is eliminated primarily by the kidneys, the drug should not be administered to patients with significantly impaired renal functions.

As with other nonsteroidal antiinflammatory drugs, borderline elevations of one or more liver tests may occur in some patients. These abnormalities may progress, may remain essentially unchanged, or may be transient with continued therapy. The SGPT (ALT) test is probably the most sensitive indicator of liver dysfunction. Meaningful (3 times the upper limit of normal) elevations of SGPT or SGOT (AST) occurred in controlled clinical trials in less than 1% of patients. A patient with symptoms and/or signs suggesting liver dysfunction, or in whom an abnormal liver test has occurred, should be evaluated for evidence of the development of more severe hepatic reaction while on therapy with mefenamic acid. Severe hepatic reactions, including jaundice and cases of fatal hepatitis, have been reported with other nonsteroidal antiinflammatory drugs. Although such reactions are rare, if abnormal liver tests persist or worsen, if clinical signs and symptoms consistent with liver disease develop, or if systemic manifestations occur (*e.g.*, eosinophilia, rash, etc.), mefenamic acid should be discontinued.

INFORMATION FOR THE PATIENT

Patients should be advised that if rash, diarrhea or other digestive problems arise, they should stop the drug and consult their physician.

Patients in whom aspirin or other nonsteroidal antiinflammatory drugs induce symptoms of bronchospasm, allergic rhinitis, or urticaria should be made aware that the potential exists for cross-sensitivity to mefenamic acid.

The long-term effects, if any, of intermittent mefenamic acid therapy for dysmenorrhea are not known. Women on such therapy should consult their physician if they should decide to become pregnant.

Mefenamic acid, like other drugs of its class, is not free of side effects. The side effects of these drugs can cause discomfort and, rarely, there are more serious side effects, such as gastrointestinal bleeding, which may result in hospitalization and even fatal outcomes.

NSAIDs (nonsteroidal antiinflammatory drugs) are often essential agents in the management of arthritis and have a major role in the treatment of pain, but they also may be commonly employed for conditions which are less serious.

Physicians may wish to discuss with their patients the potential risks (see WARNINGS, PRECAUTIONS, and ADVERSE REACTIONS) and likely benefits of NSAID treatment, particularly when the drugs are used for less serious conditions where treatment without NSAIDs may represent an acceptable alternative to both the patient and physician.

LABORATORY TESTS

Because serious GI tract ulceration and bleeding can occur without warning symptoms, physicians should follow chronically treated patients for the signs and symptoms of ulceration and bleeding and should inform them of the importance of this follow-up (see WARNINGS, Risk of GI Ulcerations, Bleeding and Perforation With NSAID Therapy).

PREGNANCY CATEGORY C

Reproduction studies have been performed in rats, rabbits and dogs. Rats given up to 10 times the human dose showed decreased fertility, delay in parturition, and a decreased rate of survival to weaning. Rabbits at 2.5 times the human dose showed an increase in the number of resorptions. There were no fetal anomalies observed in these studies nor in dogs at up to 10 times the human dose.[5]

There are no adequate and well-controlled studies in pregnant women. Because animal reproduction studies are not always predictive of human response, this drug should be used only if clearly needed.

The use of mefenamic acid in late pregnancy is not recommended because of the effects on the fetal cardiovascular system of drugs of this class.

NURSING MOTHERS

Trace amounts of mefenamic acid may be present in breast milk and transmitted to the nursing infant[7]; thus mefenamic acid should not be taken by the nursing mother because of the effects on the infant cardiovascular system of drugs of this class.

PEDIATRIC USE

Safety and effectiveness in children below the age of 14 have not been established.

DRUG INTERACTIONS

Mefenamic acid may prolong prothrombin time.[5] Therefore, when the drug is administered to patients receiving oral anticoagulant drugs, frequent monitoring of prothrombin time is necessary.

ADVERSE REACTIONS

Gastrointestinal: The most frequently reported adverse reactions associated with the use of mefenamic acid involve the gastrointestinal tract. In controlled studies for up to 8 months, the following disturbances were reported in decreasing order of frequency: diarrhea (approximately 5% of patients), nausea with or without vomiting, other gastrointestinal symptoms, and abdominal pain.

In certain patients, the diarrhea was of sufficient severity to require discontinuation of medication. The occurrence of the diarrhea is usually dose related, generally subsides on reduction of dosage, and rapidly disappears on termination of therapy.

Other gastrointestinal reactions less frequently reported were anorexia, pyrosis, flatulence, and constipation.

Gastrointestinal ulceration with and without hemorrhage has been reported.

Hematopoietic: Cases of autoimmune hemolytic anemia have been associated with the continuous administration of mefenamic acid for 12 months or longer. In such cases the Coombs test results are positive with evidence of both accelerated RBC production and RBC destruction. The process is reversible upon termination of mefenamic acid administration.

Decreases in hematocrit have been noted in 2-5% of patients and primarily in those who have received prolonged therapy. Leukopenia, eosinophilia, thrombocytopenic purpura, agranulocytosis, pancytopenia, and bone marrow hypoplasia have also been reported on occasion.

Nervous System: Drowsiness, dizziness, nervousness, headache, blurred vision, and insomnia have occurred.

Integumentary: Urticaria, rash, and facial edema have been reported.

Renal: As with other nonsteroidal anti-inflammatory agents, renal failure, including papillary necrosis, has been reported. In elderly patients, renal failure has occurred after taking mefenamic acid for 2-6 weeks. The renal damage may not be completely reversible. Hematuria and dysuria have also been reported with mefenamic acid.

Other: Eye irritation, ear pain, perspiration, mild hepatic toxicity, and increased need for insulin in a diabetic have been reported. There have been rare reports of palpitation, dyspnea, and reversible loss of color vision.

DOSAGE AND ADMINISTRATION

Administration is by the oral route, preferably with food.

The recommended regimen in acute pain for adults and children over 14 years of age is 500 mg as an initial dose followed by 250 mg every 6 hours as needed, usually not to exceed 1 week.[5]

For the treatment of primary dysmenorrhea, the recommended dosage is 500 mg as an initial dose followed by 250 mg every 6 hours, starting with the onset of bleeding and associated symptoms. Clinical studies indicate that effective treatment can be initiated with the start of menses and should not be necessary for more than 2-3 days.[6]

PRODUCT LISTING - EQUIVALENTS NOT AVAILABLE

Capsule - Oral - 250 mg

5's	$7.79	PONSTEL, Prescript Pharmaceuticals	00247-0170-05
8's	$13.98	PONSTEL, Pd-Rx Pharmaceuticals	55289-0759-08
15's	$16.66	PONSTEL, Prescript Pharmaceuticals	00247-0170-15
30's	$42.08	PONSTEL, Pd-Rx Pharmaceuticals	55289-0759-30
36's	$53.03	PONSTEL, Pd-Rx Pharmaceuticals	55289-0759-36
100's	$133.80	PONSTEL, Parke-Davis	00071-0540-24
100's	$139.15	PONSTEL, First Horizon Pharmaceutical Corporation	59630-0400-10

Mefloquine Hydrochloride *(001715)*

Categories: Malaria; Malaria, prophylaxis; Pregnancy Category C; FDA Approved 1989 May; WHO Formulary; Orphan Drugs
Drug Classes: Antiprotozoals
Brand Names: **Lariam**
Foreign Brand Availability: Laricam (Japan); Mefliam (Bahrain; Cyprus; Egypt; Iran; Iraq; Jordan; Kuwait; Lebanon; Libya; Oman; Qatar; Republic-of-Yemen; Saudi-Arabia; South-Africa; Syria; United-Arab-Emirates); Mephaquin (Colombia; Hong-Kong; Israel; Thailand); Mephaquine (Switzerland)
Cost of Therapy: $58.83 (Malaria Treatment; Lariam; 250 mg; 5 tablets; 1 day supply)

DESCRIPTION

Lariam (mefloquine hydrochloride) is an antimalarial agent available as 250 mg tablets of mefloquine hydrochloride (equivalent to 228.0 mg of the free base) for oral administration.

Mefloquine hydrochloride is a 4-quinolinemethanol derivative with the specific chemical name of (R*, S*)-(±)-α-2-piperidinyl-2,8-bis (trifluoromethyl)-4-quinolinemethanol hydrochloride. It is a 2-aryl substituted chemical structural analog of quinine. The drug is a white to almost white crystalline compound, slightly soluble in water.

Mefloquine hydrochloride has a calculated molecular weight of 414.78.

The inactive ingredients are ammonium-calcium alginate, corn starch, crospovidone, lactose, magnesium stearate, microcrystalline cellulose, poloxamer no. 331 and talc.

CLINICAL PHARMACOLOGY

Mefloquine is an antimalarial agent which acts as a blood schizonticide. Its exact mechanism of action is not known.

Pharmacokinetic studies of mefloquine in healthy male subjects showed that a significant lagtime occurred after drug administration, and the terminal elimination half-life varied widely (13-24 days) with a mean of about 3 weeks. Mefloquine is a mixture of enantiomeric molecules whose rates of release, absorption, transport, action, degradation and elimination may differ. A valid pharmacokinetic model may not exist in such a case.

Additional studies in European subjects showed slightly greater concentrations of drug for longer periods of time. The absorption half-life was 0.36 to 2 hours, and the terminal elimination half-life was 15-33 days. The primary metabolite was identified and its concentrations were found to surpass the concentrations of mefloquine.

Multiple-dose kinetic studies confirmed the long elimination half-lives previously observed. The mean metabolite to mefloquine ratio measured at steady-state was found to range between 2.3 and 8.6.

The total clearance of the drug, which is essentially all hepatic, is approximately 30 ml/min. The volume of distribution, approximately 20 L/kg, indicates extensive distribution. The drug is highly bound (98%) to plasma proteins and concentrated in blood erythrocytes, the target cells in malaria, at a relatively constant erythrocyte-to-plasma concentration ratio of about 2.

The pharmacokinetics of mefloquine in patients with compromised renal function and compromised hepatic function have not been studied.

In vitro and *in vivo* studies showed no hemolysis associated with glucose-6-phosphate dehydrogenase deficiency. (See ANIMAL PHARMACOLOGY.)

Microbiology: Strains of *Plasmodium falciparum* resistant to mefloquine have been reported.

M

INDICATIONS AND USAGE

TREATMENT OF ACUTE MALARIA INFECTIONS

Mefloquine HCl is indicated for the treatment of mild to moderate acute malaria caused by mefloquine-susceptible strains of *P. falciparum* (both chloroquine-susceptible and resistant strains) or by *Plasmodium vivax.* There are insufficient clinical data to document the effect of mefloquine in malaria caused by *P. ovale* or *P. malariae.*

Note: Patients with acute *P. vivax* malaria, treated with mefloquine HCl, are at high risk of relapse because mefloquine HCl does not eliminate exoerythrocytic (hepatic phase) parasites. To avoid relapse, after initial treatment of the acute infection with mefloquine HCl, patients should subsequently be treated with an 8-aminoquinoline (*e.g.*, primaquine).

PREVENTION OF MALARIA

Mefloquine HCl is indicated for the prophylaxis of *P. falciparum* and *P. vivax* malaria infections, including prophylaxis of chloroquine-resistant strains of*P. falciparum.*

CONTRAINDICATIONS

Use of mefloquine HCl is contraindicated in patients with a known hypersensitivity to mefloquine or related compounds (*e.g.*, quinine and quinidine). Mefloquine HCl should not be prescribed for prophylaxis in patients with active depression, a recent history of depression, generalized anxiety disorder, psychosis, or schizophrenia or other major psychiatric disorders, or with a history of convulsions.

WARNINGS

In case of life-threatening, serious or overwhelming malaria infections due to *P. falciparum,* patients should be treated with an intravenous antimalarial drug. Following completion of intravenous treatment, mefloquine HCl may be given to complete the course of therapy.

Data on the use of halofantrine subsequent to administration of mefloquine HCl suggest a significant, potentially fatal prolongation of the QTc interval of the ECG. Therefore, halofantrine must not be given simultaneously with or subsequent to mefloquine HCl. No data are available on the use of mefloquine HCl after halofantrine (see DRUG INTERACTIONS).

Mefloquine may cause psychiatric symptoms in a number of patients, ranging from anxiety, paranoia, and depression to hallucinations and psychotic behavior. On occasions, these symptoms have been reported to continue long after mefloquine has been stopped. Rare cases of suicidal ideation and suicide have been reported though no relationship to drug administration has been confirmed. To minimize the chances of

these adverse events, mefloquine should not be taken for prophylaxis in patients with active depression or with a recent history of depression, generalized anxiety disorder, psychosis, or schizophrenia or other major psychiatric disorders. Mefloquine HCl should be used with caution in patients with a previous history of depression.

During prophylactic use, if psychiatric symptoms such as acute anxiety, depression, restlessness or confusion occur, these may be considered prodomal to a more serious event. In these cases, the drug must be discontinued and an alternative medication should be substituted.

Concomitant administration of mefloquine HCl and quinine or quinidine may produce electrocardiographic abnormalities

Concomitant administration of mefloquine HCl and quinine or chloroquine may increase the risk of convulsions.

PRECAUTIONS

GENERAL

In patients with epilepsy, mefloquine HCl may increase the risk of convulsions. The drug should therefore be prescribed only for curative treatment in such patients and only if there are compelling medical reasons for its use (see DRUG INTERACTIONS).

Caution should be exercised with regard to activities requiring alertness and fine motor coordination such as driving, piloting aircraft and operating machinery, as dizziness, a loss of balance, or other disorders of the central or peripheral nervous system have been reported during and following the use of mefloquine HCl. These effects may occur after therapy is discontinued due to the long half-life of the drug. Mefloquine HCl should be used with caution in patients with psychiatric disturbances because mefloquine use has been associated with emotional disturbances. (See ADVERSE REACTIONS.)

In patients with impaired liver function the elimination of mefloquine may be prolonged, leading to higher plasma levels.

This drug has been administered for longer than 1 year. If the drug is to be administered for a prolonged period, periodic evaluations including liver function tests should be performed. Although retinal abnormalities seen in humans with long-term chloroquine use have not been observed with mefloquine use, long-term feeding of mefloquine to rats resulted in dose-related ocular lesions (retinal degeneration, retinal edema and lenticular opacity at 12.5 mg/kg/day and higher). (See ANIMAL PHARMACOLOGY.) Therefore, periodic ophthalmic examinations are recommended.

Parenteral studies in animals show that mefloquine, a myocardial depressant, possesses 20% of the antifibrillatory action of quinidine and produces 50% of the increase in the PR interval reported with quinine. The effects of mefloquine on the compromised cardiovascular system has not been evaluated. However, transitory and clinically silent ECG alterations have been reported during the use of mefloquine. Alteration included sinus bradycardia, sinus arrhythmia, first degree AV-block, prolongation of the QTc interval and abnormal T waves (see also cardiovascular effects under DRUG INTERACTIONS and ADVERSE REACTIONS). The benefits of mefloquine HCl therapy should be weighed against the possibility of adverse effects in patients with cardiac disease.

M

LABORATORY TESTS

Periodic evaluation of hepatic function should be performed during prolonged prophylaxis.

INFORMATION FOR THE PATIENT

Patients should be advised:

- That malaria can be a life-threatening infection in the traveler.
- That mefloquine HCl is being prescribed to help prevent or treat this serious infection.
- That in a small percentage of cases, patients are unable to take this medication because of side effects, and it may be necessary to change medications.
- That when used as prophylaxis, the first dose of mefloquine HCl should be taken 1 week prior to departure.
- That if the patients experience psychiatric symptoms such as acute anxiety, depression, restlessness or confusion, these may be considered prodromal to a more serious event. In these cases, the drug must be discontinued and an alternative medication should be substituted.
- That no chemoprophylactic regimen is 100% effective, and protective clothing, insect repellents, and bednets are important components of malaria prophylaxis.
- To seek medical attention for any febrile illness that occurs after return from a malarious area and inform their physician that they may have been exposed to malaria.

CARCINOGENESIS, MUTAGENESIS, AND IMPAIRMENT OF FERTILITY

Carcinogenesis

The carcinogenesis potential of mefloquine was studied in rats and mice in 2 year feeding studies at doses up to 30 mg/kg/day. No treatment-related increases in tumors of any type were noted.

Mutagenesis

The mutagenic potential of mefloquine was studied in a variety of assay systems including: Ames test, a host-mediated assay in mice, fluctuation tests and a mouse micronucleus assay. Several of these assays were performed with and without prior metabolic activation. In no instance was evidence obtained for the mutagenicity of mefloquine.

Impairment of Fertility

Fertility studies in rats at doses of 5, 20 and 50 mg/kg/day of mefloquine have demonstrated adverse effects on fertility in the male at the high dose of 50 mg/kg/day, and in the female at doses of 20 and 50 mg/kg/day. Histopathological lesions were noted in the epididymides from male rats at doses of 20 and 50 mg/kg/day. Administration of 250 mg/week of mefloquine (base) in adult males for 22 weeks failed to reveal any deleterious effects on human spermatozoa.

PREGNANCY, TERATOGENIC EFFECTS, PREGNANCY CATEGORY C

Mefloquine has been demonstrated to be teratogenic in rats and mice at a dose of 100 mg/kg/day. In rabbits, a high dose of 160 mg/kg/day was embryotoxic and teratogenic, and a dose of 80 mg/kg/day was teratogenic but not embryotoxic. There are no adequate and well-controlled studies in pregnant women. However, clinical experience with mefloquine HCl has not revealed an embryotoxic or teratogenic effect. Mefloquine should be used during pregnancy only if the potential benefit justifies the potential risk to the fetus. Women of childbearing potential who are traveling to areas where malaria is endemic should be warned against becoming pregnant. Women of childbearing potential should also be advised to practice contraception during malaria prophylaxis with mefloquine HCl.

NURSING MOTHERS

Mefloquine is excreted in human milk. Based on a study in a few subjects, low concentrations (3-4%) of mefloquine were excreted in human milk following a dose equivalent to 250 mg of the free base. Because of the potential for serious adverse reactions in nursing infants from mefloquine, a decision should be made whether to discontinue the drug, taking into account the importance of the drug to the mother.

PEDIATRIC USE

Use of mefloquine HCl to treat acute, uncomplicated *P. falciparum* malaria in pediatric patients is supported by evidence from adequate and well-controlled studies of mefloquine HCl in adults with additional data from published open-label and comparative trials using mefloquine HCl to treat malaria caused by *P. falciparum* in patients younger than 16 years of age. The safety and effectiveness of mefloquine HCl for the treatment of malaria in pediatric patients below the age of 6 months have not been established.

In several studies, the administration of mefloquine HCl for the treatment of malaria was associated with early vomiting in pediatric patients. Early vomiting was cited in some reports as a possible cause of treatment failure. If a second dose is not tolerated, the patient should be monitored closely and alternative malaria treatment considered if improvement is not observed within a reasonable period of time (see DOSAGE AND ADMINISTRATION).

DRUG INTERACTIONS

Drug-drug interactions with mefloquine HCl have not been explored in detail. There is one report of cardiopulmonary arrest, with full recovery, in a patient who was taking a beta blocker (propranolol) (see PRECAUTIONS, General). The effects of mefloquine on the compromised cardiovascular system have not been evaluated. The benefits of mefloquine HCl therapy should be weighed against the possibility of adverse effects in patients with cardiac disease.

Because of the danger of a potentially fatal prolongation of the QTc interval, halofantrine should not be given simultaneously with or subsequent to mefloquine HCl (see WARNINGS).

Concomitant administration of mefloquine HCl and other related compounds (*e.g.*, quinine, quinidine and chloroquine) may produce electrocardiographic abnormalities and increase the risk of convulsions (see WARNINGS). If these drugs are to be used in the initial treatment of severe malaria, mefloquine HCl administration should be delayed at least 12 hours after the last dose. There is evidence that the use of halofantrine after mefloquine causes a significant lengthening of the QTc interval. Clinically significant QTc prolongation has not been found with mefloquine alone.

This appears to be the only clinically relevant interaction of this kind with mefloquine HCl, although theoretically, coadministration of other drugs known to alter cardiac conduction (*e.g.*, anti-arrhythmic or beta-adrenergic blocking agents, calcium channel blockers, antihistamines or H_1-blocking agents, tricyclic antidepressants and phenothiazines) might also contribute to a prolongation of the QTc interval. There are no data that conclusively establish whether the concomitant administration of mefloquine and the above listed agents has an effect on cardiac function.

In patients taking an anticonvulsant (*e.g.*, valproic acid, carbamazepine, phenobarbital or phenytoin), the concomitant use of mefloquine HCl may reduce seizure control by lowering the plasma levels of the anticonvulsant. Therefore, patients concurrently taking antiseizure medication and mefloquine HCl should have the blood level of their antiseizure medication monitored and the dosage adjusted appropriately (see PRECAUTIONS, General).

When mefloquine HCl is taken concurrently with oral live typhoid vaccines, attenuation of immunization cannot be excluded. Vaccinations with attenuated live bacteria should therefore be completed at least 3 days before the first dose of mefloquine HCl.

No other drug interactions are known. Nevertheless, the effects of mefloquine HCl on travelers receiving comedication, particularly those on anticoagulants or antidiabetics, should be checked before departure.

In clinical trials, the concomitant administration of sulfadoxine and pyrimethamine did not alter the adverse reaction profile.

ADVERSE REACTIONS

CLINICAL

At the doses used for treatment of acute malaria infections, the symptoms possibly attributable to drug administration cannot be distinguished from those symptoms usually attributable to the disease itself.

Among subjects who received mefloquine for prophylaxis of malaria, the most frequently observed adverse experience was vomiting (3%). Dizziness, syncope, extrasystoles and other complaints affecting less than 1% were also reported.

Among subjects who received mefloquine for treatment, the most frequently observed adverse experiences included: dizziness, myalgia, nausea, fever, headache, vomiting, chills, diarrhea, skin rash, abdominal pain, fatigue, loss of appetite, and tinnitus. Those side effects occurring in less than 1% included bradycardia, hair loss, emotional problems, pruritus, asthenia, transient emotional disturbances and telogen effluvium (loss of resting hair). Seizures have also been reported.

Two serious adverse reactions were cardiopulmonary arrest in 1 patient shortly after ingesting a single prophylactic dose of mefloquine while concomitantly using propranolol (see PRECAUTIONS), and encephalopathy of unknown etiology during prophylactic mefloquine administration. The relationship of encephalopathy to drug administration could not be clearly established.

POSTMARKETING

Postmarketing surveillance indicates that the same adverse experiences are reported during prophylaxis, as well as acute treatment.

The most frequently reported adverse events are nausea, vomiting, loose stools or diarrhea, abdominal pain, dizziness or vertigo, loss of balance, and neuropsychiatric events such as headache, somnolence, and sleep disorders (insomnia, abnormal dreams). These are usually mild and may decrease despite continued use.

Occasionally, more severe neuropsychiatric disorders have been reported such as: sensory and motor neuropathies (including paresthesia, tremor and ataxia), convulsions, agitation or restlessness, anxiety, depression, mood changes, panic attacks, forgetfulness, confusion, hallucinations, aggression, psychotic or paranoid reactions and encephalopathy. Rare cases of suicidal ideation and suicide have been reported though no relationship to drug administration has been confirmed.

Other Infrequent Adverse Events Include:

Cardiovascular Disorders: Circulatory disturbances (hypotension, hypertension, flushing, syncope), chest pain, tachycardia or palpitation, bradycardia, irregular pulse, extrasystoles, A-V block, and other transient cardiac conduction alterations.

Skin Disorders: Rash, exanthema, erythema, urticaria, pruritus, edema, hair loss, erythema multiforme, and Stevens-Johnson syndrome.

Musculoskeletal Disorders: Muscle weakness, muscle cramps, myalgia, and arthralgia.

Other Symptoms: Visual disturbances, vestibular disorders including tinnitus and hearing impairment, dyspnea, asthenia, malaise, fatigue, fever, sweating, chills, dyspepsia and loss of appetite.

LABORATORY

The most frequently observed laboratory alterations which could be possibly attributable to drug administration were decreased hematocrit, transient elevation of transaminases, leukopenia and thrombocytopenia. These alterations were observed in patients with acute malaria who received treatment doses of the drug and were attributed to the disease itself.

During prophylactic administration of mefloquine to indigenous populations in malaria-endemic areas, the following occasional alterations in laboratory values were observed: transient elevation of transaminases, leukocytosis or thrombocytopenia.

Because of the long half-life of mefloquine, adverse reactions to mefloquine HCl may occur or persist up to several weeks after the last dose.

DOSAGE AND ADMINISTRATION

(See INDICATIONS AND USAGE.)

ADULT PATIENTS

Treatment of Mild to Moderate Malaria in Adults Caused by P. vivax or Mefloquine-Susceptible Strains of P. falciparum

Five tablets (1250 mg) mefloquine HCl to be given as a single oral dose. The drug should not be taken on an empty stomach and should be administered with at least 8 oz (240 ml) of water.

If a full-treatment course has been administered without clinical cure, alternative treatment should be given. Similarly, if previous prophylaxis with mefloquine has failed, mefloquine HCl should not be used for curative treatment.

Note: Patients with acute *P. vivax* malaria, treated with mefloquine HCl, are at high risk of relapse because mefloquine HCl does not eliminate exoerythrocytic (hepatic phase) parasites. To avoid relapse after initial treatment of the acute infection with mefloquine HCl, patients should subsequently be treated with an 8-aminoquinoline (*e.g.,* primaquine).

Malaria Prophylaxis

One (250 mg) mefloquine HCl tablet once weekly.

Prophylactic drug administration should begin 1 week before departure to an endemic area. Subsequent weekly doses should always be taken on the same day of the week. To reduce the risk of malaria after leaving an endemic area, prophylaxis should be continued for 4 additional weeks. Tablets should not be taken on an empty stomach and should be administered with at least 8 oz (240 ml) of water.

In certain cases, *e.g.,* when a traveler is taking other medication, it may be desirable to start prophylaxis 2-3 weeks prior to departure, in order to ensure that the combination of drugs is well tolerated.

PEDIATRIC PATIENTS

Treatment of Mild to Moderate Malaria in Pediatric Patients Caused by Mefloquine-Susceptible Strains of P. falciparum

20-50 mg/kg for non-immune patients. Splitting the total curative dose into 2 doses taken 6-8 hours apart may reduce the occurrence or severity of adverse effects. Experience with mefloquine HCl in infants less than 3 months old or weighing less than 5 kg is limited. The drug should not be taken on an empty stomach and should be administered with ample water. For very young patients, the dose may be crushed, mixed with water or sugar water and may be administered via an oral syringe.

If a full-treatment course has been administered without clinical cure, alternative treatment should be given. Similarly, if previous prophylaxis with mefloquine has failed, mefloquine HCl should not be used for curative treatment.

In pediatric patients, the administration of mefloquine HCl for the treatment of malaria has been associated with early vomiting. In some cases, early vomiting has been cited as a possible cause of treatment failure (see PRECAUTIONS). If a significant loss of drug product is observed or suspected because of vomiting, a second full dose of mefloquine HCl should be administered to patients who vomit less than 30 minutes after receiving the drug. If vomiting occurs 30-60 minutes after a dose, an additional half-dose should be given. If vomiting recurs, the patient should be monitored closely and alternative malaria treatment considered if improvement is not observed within a reasonable period of time.

The safety and effectiveness of mefloquine HCl to treat malaria in pediatric patients below the age of 6 months have not been established.

Malaria Prophylaxis

The following doses have been extrapolated from the recommended adult dose. Neither the pharmacokinetics, nor the clinical efficacy of these doses have been determined in children owing to the difficulty of acquiring this information in pediatric subjects. The recommended prophylactic dose of mefloquine HCl is 3-5 mg/kg once weekly. One 250 mg mefloquine HCl tablet should be taken once weekly in pediatric patients weighing over 45 kg. In pediatrics patients weighing less than 45 kg, the weekly dose decreases in proportion to body weight:

>30-45 kg: ¾ tablet.
>20-30 kg: ½ tablet.
Up to 20 kg: ¼ tablet.

Experience with mefloquine HCl in infants less than 3 months old or weighing less than 5 kg is limited.

ANIMAL PHARMACOLOGY

Ocular lesions were observed in rats fed mefloquine daily for 2 years. All surviving rats given 30 mg/kg/day had ocular lesions in both eyes characterized by retinal degeneration, opacity of the lens and retinal edema. Similar but less severe lesions were observed in 80% of female and 22% of male rats fed 12.5 mg/kg/day for 2 years. At doses of 5 mg/kg/day, only corneal lesions were observed. They occurred in 9% of rats studied.

HOW SUPPLIED

Lariam is available as scored, white, round tablets, containing 250 mg of mefloquine hydrochloride. Imprint on tablets is "LARIAM 250 ROCHE".

Storage: Tablets should be stored at 15-30°C (59-86°F).

PRODUCT LISTING - RATED THERAPEUTICALLY EQUIVALENT

Tablet - Oral - 250 mg

25's	$264.74	GENERIC, Geneva Pharmaceuticals	00781-5076-86

PRODUCT LISTING - EQUIVALENTS NOT AVAILABLE

Tablet - Oral - 250 mg

5's	$79.03	LARIAM, Pd-Rx Pharmaceuticals	55289-0780-05
6's	$53.26	LARIAM, Allscripts Pharmaceutical Company	54569-2965-04
8's	$71.01	LARIAM, Allscripts Pharmaceutical Company	54569-2965-03
10's	$90.54	LARIAM, Allscripts Pharmaceutical Company	54569-2965-00
25's	$198.98	LARIAM, Pharma Pac	52959-0583-00
25's	$221.92	LARIAM, Allscripts Pharmaceutical Company	54569-2965-02
25's	$230.03	LARIAM, Physicians Total Care	54868-3178-00
25's	$294.16	LARIAM, Roche Laboratories	00004-0172-02

M

Megestrol Acetate *(001716)*

Categories: AIDS, adjunct; Carcinoma, breast; Carcinoma, endometrial; Pregnancy Category D; FDA Approved 1976 Jul; Orphan Drugs
Drug Classes: Antineoplastics, hormones/hormone modifiers; Hormones/hormone modifiers; Progestins
Brand Names: Magace; **Megace**; Niagestine
Foreign Brand Availability: Endace (India); Maygace (Spain); Megace OS (Canada); Megaplex (Indonesia); Megestat (Germany); Megostat (New-Zealand); Mestrel (Mexico; Thailand)
Cost of Therapy: $155.51 (Breast Cancer; Megace; 40 mg; 4 tablets/day; 30 day supply)
$104.88 (Breast Cancer; Generic Tablets; 40 mg; 4 tablets/day; 30 day supply)

DESCRIPTION

Megestrol acetate is a white, crystalline solid chemically designated as 17α-(acetyloxy)-6-methylpregna-4,6-diene-3,20-dione. Solubility at 37°C in water is 2 μg/ml, solubility in plasma is 24 μg/ml. Its molecular weight is 384.51. The empirical formula is $C_{24}H_{32}O_4$.

ORAL SUSPENSION

Megace oral suspension contains megestrol acetate, a synthetic derivative of the naturally occurring steroid hormone, progesterone.

Megace oral suspension is supplied as an oral suspension containing 40 mg of micronized megestrol acetate per ml.

Megace oral suspension contains the following inactive ingredients: alcohol (max. 0.06% v/v from flavor), citric acid, lemon-lime flavor, polyethylene glycol, polysorbate 80, purified water, sodium benzoate, sodium citrate, sucrose and xanthan gum.

TABLETS

Megestrol acetate is a synthetic, antineoplastic and progestational drug.

Megace tablets are supplied as tablets for oral administration containing 20 and 40 mg megestrol acetate.

Megace tablets contain the following inactive ingredients: acacia, calcium phosphate, FD&C blue no. 1 aluminum lake, lactose, magnesium stearate, silicon dioxide colloidal, and starch.

CLINICAL PHARMACOLOGY

ORAL SUSPENSION

Several investigators have reported on the appetite enhancing property of megestrol acetate and its possible use in cachexia. The precise mechanism by which megestrol acetate produces effects in anorexia and cachexia is unknown at the present time.

There are several analytical methods used to estimate megestrol acetate plasma concentrations, including gas chromatography-mass fragmentography (GC-MF), high pressure liquid chromatography (HPLC) and radioimmunoassay (RIA). The GC-MF and HPLC methods are specific for megestrol acetate and yield equivalent concentrations. The RIA method reacts to megestrol acetate metabolites and is, therefore, non-specific and indicates higher concentrations than the GC-MF and HPLC methods. Plasma concentrations are dependent, not only on the method used, but also on intestinal and hepatic inactivation of the drug, which may be affected by factors such as intestinal tract motility, intestinal bacteria, antibiotics administered, body weight, diet, and liver function.

The major route of drug elimination in humans is urine. When radiolabeled megestrol acetate was administered to humans in doses of 4-90 mg, the urinary excretion within 10 days ranged from 56.5-78.4% (mean 66.4%) and fecal excretion ranged from 7.7-30.3% (mean 19.8%). The total recovered radioactivity varied between 83.1% and 94.7% (mean 86.2%). Megestrol acetate metabolites which were identified in urine constituted 5-8% of the dose administered. Respiratory excretion as labeled carbon dioxide and fat storage may have accounted for at least part of the radioactivity not found in the urine and feces.

Plasma steady state pharmacokinetics of megestrol acetate were evaluated in 10 adult, cachectic male patients with acquired immunodeficiency syndrome (AIDS) and an involuntary weight loss greater than 10% of baseline. Patients received single oral doses of 800 mg/day of megestrol acetate oral suspension for 21 days. Plasma concentration data obtained on day 21 were evaluated for up to 48 hours past the last dose.

Mean (±1SD) peak plasma concentration (C_{max}) of megestrol acetate was 753 (±539) ng/ml. Mean area under the concentration time-curve (AUC) was 10476 (±7788) ng·h/ml. Median T_{max} value was 5 hours. Seven (7) of 10 patients gained weight in 3 weeks.

Additionally, 24 adult, asymptomatic HIV seropositive male subjects were dosed once daily with 750 mg of megestrol acetate oral suspension. The treatment was administered for 14 days. Mean C_{max} and AUC values were 490 (±238) ng/ml and 6779 (±3048) ng·h/ml respectively. The median T_{max} value was 3 hours. The mean C_{min} value was 202 (±101) ng/ml. The mean percent of fluctuation value was 107 (±40).

The relative bioavailability of megestrol acetate 40 mg tablets and oral suspension has not been evaluated. The effect of food on the bioavailability of megestrol acetate oral suspension has not been evaluated.

TABLETS

While the precise mechanism by which megestrol acetate produces its antineoplastic effects against endometrial carcinoma is unknown at the present time, inhibition of pituitary gonadotropin production and resultant decrease in estrogen secretion may be factors. There is evidence to suggest a local effect as a result of the marked changes brought about by the direct instillation of progestational agents into the endometrial cavity. The antineoplastic action of megestrol acetate on carcinoma of the breast is effected by modifying the action of other steroid hormones and by exerting a direct cytotoxic effect on tumor cells. In metastatic cancer, hormone receptors may be present in some tissues but not others. The receptor mechanism is a cyclic process whereby estrogen produced by the ovaries enters the target cell, forms a complex with cytoplasmic receptor and is transported into the cell nucleus. There it induces gene transcription and leads to the alteration of normal cell functions. Pharmacologic doses of megestrol acetate not only decrease the number of hormone-dependent human breast cancer cells but also is capable of modifying and abolishing the stimulatory effects of estrogen on these cells. It has been suggested that progestins may inhibit in one of two ways: by interfering with either the stability, availability, or turnover of the estrogen receptor complex in its interaction with genes or in conjunction with the progestin receptor complex, by interacting directly with the genome to turn off specific estrogen-responsive genes.

There are several analytical methods used to estimate megestrol acetate plasma levels, including mass fragmentography, gas chromatography (GC), high pressure liquid chromatography (HPLC) and radioimmunoassay. The plasma levels by HPLC assay or radioimmunoassay methods are about one-sixth those obtained by the GC method. The plasma levels are dependent not only on the method used, but also on intestinal and hepatic inactivation of the drug, which may be affected by factors such as intestinal tract motility, intestinal bacteria, antibiotics administered, body weight, diet, and liver function.

Metabolites account for only 5-8% of the administered dose and are considered negligible. The major route of drug elimination in humans is the urine. When radiolabeled megestrol acetate was administered to humans in doses of 4-90 mg, the urinary excretion within 10 days ranged from 56.5-78.4% (mean 66.4%) and fecal excretion ranged from 7.7-30.3% (mean 19.8%). The total recovered radioactivity varied between 83.1% and 94.7% (mean 86.2%). Respiratory excretion as labeled carbon dioxide and fat storage may have accounted for at least part of the radioactivity not found in the urine and feces.

In normal male volunteers (n=23) who received 160 mg of megestrol acetate given as a 40 mg qid regimen, the oral absorption of megestrol acetate appeared to be variable. Plasma levels were assayed by a high pressure liquid chromatographic (HPLC) procedure. Peak drug levels for the first 40 mg dose ranged from 10-56 ng/ml (mean 27.6 ng/ml) and the times to peak concentrations ranged from 1.0-3.0 hours (mean 2.2 hours). Plasma elimination half-life ranged from 13.0-104.9 hours (mean 34.2 hours). The steady state plasma concentrations for a 40 mg qid regimen have not been established.

INDICATIONS AND USAGE

ORAL SUSPENSION

Megestrol acetate oral suspension is indicated for the treatment of anorexia, cachexia, or an unexplained, significant weight loss in patients with a diagnosis of acquired immunodeficiency syndrome (AIDS).

TABLETS

Megestrol acetate is indicated for the palliative treatment of advanced carcinoma of the breast or endometrium (*i.e.*, recurrent, inoperable, or metastatic disease). It should not be used in lieu of currently accepted procedures such as surgery, radiation, or chemotherapy.

NON-FDA APPROVED INDICATIONS

Megestrol has also been found to have efficacy in the treatment of hot flashes in women with a history of breast cancer and in men with a history of prostate cancer. Megestrol has been reported to be effective for the treatment of AIDS or cancer-related anorexia and cachexia. However, these uses have not been approved by the FDA and further studies are needed.

CONTRAINDICATIONS

History of hypersensitivity to megestrol acetate or any component of the formulation. For the oral suspension, known or suspected pregnancy.

WARNINGS

ORAL SUSPENSION

Megestrol acetate may cause fetal harm when administered to a pregnant woman. For animal data on fetal effects, (see PRECAUTIONS, Oral Suspension, Carcinogenesis, Mutagenesis, and Impairment of Fertility, Impairment of Fertility). There are no adequate and well-controlled studies in pregnant women. If this drug is used during pregnancy, or if the patient becomes pregnant while taking (receiving) this drug, the patient should be apprised of the potential hazard to the fetus. Women of childbearing potential should be advised to avoid becoming pregnant.

Megestrol acetate is not intended for prophylactic use to avoid weight loss. (See also PRECAUTIONS, Oral Suspension, Carcinogenesis, Mutagenesis, and Impairment of Fertility.)

The glucocorticoid activity of megestrol acetate oral suspension has not been fully evaluated. Clinical cases of new onset diabetes mellitus, exacerbation of pre-existing diabetes mellitus, and overt Cushing's syndrome have been reported in association with the chronic use of megestrol acetate. In addition, clinical cases of adrenal insufficiency have been observed in patients receiving or being withdrawn from chronic megestrol acetate therapy in the stressed and non-stressed state. Furthermore, adrenocorticotropin (ACTH) stimulation testing has revealed the frequent occurrence of asymptomatic pituitary-adrenal suppression in patients treated with chronic megestrol acetate therapy. Therefore, the possibility of adrenal insufficiency should be considered in any patient receiving or being withdrawn from chronic megestrol acetate therapy who presents with symptoms and/or signs suggestive of hypoadrenalism (*e.g.*, hypotension, nausea, vomiting, dizziness, or weakness) in either the stressed or non-stressed state. Laboratory evaluation for adrenal insufficiency and consideration of replacement or stress doses of a rapidly acting glucocorticoid are strongly recommended in such patients. Failure to recognize inhibition of the hypothalamic-pituitary-adrenal axis may result in death. Finally, in patients who are receiving or being withdrawn from chronic megestrol acetate therapy, consideration should be given to the use of empiric therapy with stress doses of a rapidly acting glucocorticoid in conditions of stress or serious intercurrent illness (*e.g.*, surgery, infection).

TABLETS

Megestrol acetate may cause fetal harm when administered to a pregnant woman. Fertility and reproduction studies with high doses of megestrol acetate have shown a reversible feminizing effect on some male rat fetuses. There are no adequate and well-controlled studies in pregnant women. If this drug is used during pregnancy, or if the patient becomes pregnant while taking (receiving) this drug, the patient should be apprised of the potential hazard to the fetus. Women of childbearing potential should be advised to avoid becoming pregnant.

The use of megestrol acetate in other types of neoplastic disease is not recommended. (See also PRECAUTIONS, Tablets,Carcinogenesis, Mutagenesis, and Impairment of Fertility.)

The glucocorticoid activity of megestrol acetate tablets has not been fully evaluated. Clinical cases of new onset diabetes mellitus, exacerbation of pre-existing diabetes mellitus, and overt Cushing's syndrome have been reported in association with the chronic use of megestrol acetate. In addition, clinical cases of adrenal insufficiency have been observed in patients receiving or being withdrawn from chronic megestrol acetate therapy in the stressed and non-stressed state. Furthermore, adrenocorticotropin (ACTH) stimulation testing has revealed the frequent occurrence of asymptomatic pituitary-adrenal suppression in patients treated with chronic megestrol acetate therapy. Therefore, the possibility of adrenal insufficiency should be considered in any patient receiving or being withdrawn from chronic megestrol acetate therapy who presents with symptoms and/or signs suggestive of hypoadrenalism (*e.g.*, hypotension, nausea, vomiting, dizziness, or weakness) in either the stressed or non-stressed state. Laboratory evaluation for adrenal insufficiency and consideration of replacement or stress doses of a rapidly acting glucocorticoid are strongly recommended in such patients. Failure to recognize inhibition of the hypothalamic-pituitary-adrenal axis may result in death. Finally, in patients who are receiving or being withdrawn from chronic megestrol acetate therapy, consideration should be given to the use of empiric therapy with stress doses of a rapidly acting glucocorticoid in conditions of stress or serious intercurrent illness (*e.g.*, surgery, infection).

PRECAUTIONS

ORAL SUSPENSION

General

Therapy with megestrol acetate oral suspension for weight loss should only be instituted after treatable causes of weight loss are sought and addressed. These treatable causes include possible malignancies, systemic infections, gastrointestinal disorders affecting absorption, endocrine disease and renal or psychiatric diseases.

Effects on HIV viral replication have not been determined.

Use with caution in patients with a history of thromboembolic disease.

Use in Diabetics

Exacerbation of pre-existing diabetes with increased insulin requirements has been reported in association with the use of megestrol acetate.

Information for the Patient

Patients using megestrol acetate should receive the following instructions:

This medication is to be used as directed by the physician.

Report any adverse reaction experiences while taking this medication.

Use contraception while taking this medication if you are a woman capable of becoming pregnant.

Notify your physician if you become pregnant while taking this medication.

Carcinogenesis, Mutagenesis, and Impairment of Fertility

Carcinogenesis

Data on carcinogenesis were obtained from studies conducted in dogs, monkeys and rats treated with megestrol acetate at doses 53.2, 26.6 and 1.3 times *lower* than the proposed dose (13.3 mg/kg/day) for humans. No males were used in the dog and monkey studies. In female beagles, megestrol acetate (0.01, 0.1 or 0.25 mg/kg/day) administered for up to 7 years induced both benign and malignant tumors of the breast. In female monkeys, no tumors were found following 10 years of treatment with 0.01, 0.1 or 0.5 mg/kg/day megestrol acetate. Pituitary tumors were observed in female rats treated with 3.9 or 10 mg/kg/day of megestrol acetate for 2 years. The relationship of these tumors in rats and dogs to humans is unknown but should be considered in assessing the risk-to-benefit ratio when prescribing megestrol acetate oral suspension and in surveillance of patients on therapy. (See WARNINGS, Oral Suspension.)

Mutagenesis

No mutagenesis data are currently available.

Impairment of Fertility

Perinatal/postnatal (segment III) toxicity studies were performed in rats at doses (0.05-12.5 mg/kg) *less* than that indicated for humans (13.3 mg/kg); in these low dose studies, the reproductive capability of male offspring of megestrol acetate-treated females was impaired. Similar results were obtained in dogs. Pregnant rats treated with megestrol acetate showed a reduction in fetal weight and number of live births, and feminization of male fetuses. No toxicity data are currently available on male reproduction (spermatogenesis).

Pregnancy Category X

See WARNINGS, Oral Suspension and PRECAUTIONS, Oral Suspension, Carcinogenesis, Mutagenesis, and Impairment of Fertility, Impairment of Fertility. No adequate animal teratology information is available at clinically relevant doses.

Nursing Mothers

Because of the potential for adverse effects on the newborn, nursing should be discontinued if megestrol acetate is required.

Use in HIV Infected Women

Although megestrol acetate has been used extensively in women for the treatment of endometrial and breast cancers, its use in HIV infected women has been limited.

All 10 women in the clinical trials reported breakthrough bleeding.

Pediatric Use

Safety and effectiveness in pediatric patients have not been established.

TABLETS

General

Close surveillance is indicated for any patient treated for recurrent or metastatic cancer. Use with caution in patients with a history of thromboembolic disease.

Use in Diabetics

Exacerbation of pre-existing diabetes with increased insulin requirements has been reported in association with the use of megestrol acetate.

Information for the Patient

Patients using megestrol acetate should receive the following instructions:

This medication is to be used as directed by the physician.

Report any adverse reaction experiences while taking this medication.

Laboratory Tests

Breast malignancies in which estrogen and/or progesterone receptors are positive are more likely to respond to megestrol acetate.

Carcinogenesis, Mutagenesis, and Impairment of Fertility

Administration of megestrol acetate to female dogs for up to 7 years is associated with an increased incidence of both benign and malignant tumors of the breast. Comparable studies in rats and studies in monkeys are not associated with an increased incidence of tumors. The relationship of the dog tumors to humans is unknown but should be considered in assessing the benefit-to-risk ratio when prescribing megestrol acetate and in surveillance of patients on therapy. (See WARNINGS, Tablets.)

Pregnancy Category D

See WARNINGS, Tablets.

Nursing Mothers

Because of the potential for adverse effects on the newborn, nursing should be discontinued if megestrol acetate is required for treatment of cancer.

Pediatric Use

Safety and effectiveness in pediatric patients have not been established.

DRUG INTERACTIONS

ORAL SUSPENSION

Pharmacokinetic studies show that there are no significant alterations in pharmacokinetic parameters of zidovudine or rifabutin to warrant dosage adjustment when megestrol acetate is administered with these drugs. The effects of zidovudine or rifabutin on the pharmacokinetics of megestrol acetate were not studied.

ADVERSE REACTIONS

ORAL SUSPENSION

Clinical Adverse Events

Adverse events which occurred in at least 5% of patients in any arm of the two clinical efficacy trials and the open trial are listed by treatment group. All patients listed had at least one post baseline visit during the 12 study weeks. These adverse events should be considered by the physician when prescribing megestrol acetate oral suspension.

TABLE 2A *Adverse Events — % of Patients Reporting: Trial 1 (n=236)*

		Megestrol Acetate mg/day		
	Placebo	**100**	**400**	**800**
	n=34	**n=68**	**n=69**	**n=65**
Diarrhea	15%	13%	8%	15%
Impotence	3%	4%	6%	14%
Rash	9%	9%	4%	12%
Flatulence	9%	0%	1%	9%
Hypertension	0%	0%	0%	8%
Asthenia	3%	2%	3%	6%
Insomnia	0%	3%	4%	6%
Nausea	9%	4%	0%	5%
Anemia	6%	3%	3%	5%
Fever	3%	6%	4%	5%
Libido decreased	3%	4%	0%	5%
Dyspepsia	0%	0%	3%	3%
Hyperglycemia	3%	0%	6%	3%
Headache	6%	10%	1%	3%
Pain	6%	0%	0%	2%
Vomiting	9%	3%	0%	2%
Pneumonia	6%	2%	0%	2%
Urinary frequency	0%	0%	1%	2%

TABLE 2B *Adverse Events — % of Patients Reporting*

	Trial 2 (n=87)		Open Label Trial
		Megestrol Acetate	**Megestrol Acetate**
	Placebo	**800 mg/day**	**1200 mg/day**
	n=38	**n=49**	**n=176**
Diarrhea	8%	6%	10%
Impotence	0%	4%	7%
Rash	3%	2%	6%
Flatulence	3%	10%	6%
Hypertension	0%	0%	4%
Asthenia	8%	4%	5%
Insomnia	0%	0%	1%
Nausea	3%	4%	5%
Anemia	0%	0%	0%
Fever	3%	2%	1%
Libido decreased	0%	2%	1%
Dyspepsia	5%	4%	2%
Hyperglycemia	0%	0%	3%
Headache	3%	0%	3%
Pain	5%	6%	4%
Vomiting	3%	6%	4%
Pneumonia	3%	0%	1%
Urinary frequency	5%	2%	1%

Adverse events which occurred in 1-3% of all patients enrolled in the two clinical efficacy trials with at least one follow-up visit during the first 12 weeks of the study are listed below by body system. Adverse events occurring less than 1% are not included. There were no significant differences between incidence of these events in patients treated with megestrol acetate and patients treated with placebo.

Body as a Whole: Abdominal pain, chest pain, infection, moniliasis and sarcoma.

Cardiovascular System: Cardiomyopathy and palpitation.

Digestive System: Constipation, dry mouth, hepatomegaly, increased salivation and oral moniliasis.

Hemic and Lymphatic System: Leukopenia.

Metabolic and Nutritional: LDH increased, edema and peripheral edema.

Nervous System: Paresthesia, confusion, convulsion, depression, neuropathy, hypesthesia and abnormal thinking.

Respiratory System: Dyspnea, cough, pharyngitis and lung disorder.

Skin and Appendages: Alopecia, herpes, pruritus, vesiculobullous rash, sweating and skin disorder.

Special Senses: Amblyopia.

Urogenital System: Albuminuria, urinary incontinence, urinary tract infection and gynecomastia.

Postmarketing

Postmarketing reports associated with megestrol acetate oral suspension include thromboembolic phenomena including thrombophlebitis, pulmonary embolism and glucose intolerance (see WARNINGS, Oral Suspension and PRECAUTIONS, Oral Suspension).

TABLETS

Weight Gain: Weight gain is a frequent side effect of megestrol acetate. This gain has been associated with increased appetite and is not necessarily associated with fluid retention.

Thromboembolic Phenomena: Thromboembolic phenomena including thrombophlebitis and pulmonary embolism (in some cases fatal) have been reported.

Glucocorticoid Effects: See WARNINGS, Tablets.

Other Adverse Reactions: Heart failure, nausea and vomiting, edema, breakthrough menstrual bleeding, dyspnea, tumor flare (with or without hypercalcemia), hyperglycemia, glucose intolerance, alopecia, hypertension, carpal tunnel syndrome, mood changes, hot flashes, malaise, asthenia, lethargy, sweating and rash.

DOSAGE AND ADMINISTRATION

ORAL SUSPENSION

The recommended adult initial dosage of megestrol acetate oral suspension is 800 mg/day (20 ml/day). Shake container well before using.

In clinical trials evaluating different dose schedules, daily doses of 400 and 800 mg/day were found to be clinically effective.

A plastic dosage cup with 10 and 20 ml markings is provided for convenience.

Special Handling

Health Hazard Data

There is no threshold limit value established by OSHA, NIOSH, or ACGIH.

Exposure or "overdose" at levels approaching recommended dosing levels could result in side effects described above (see WARNINGS, Oral Suspension and ADVERSE REACTIONS, Oral Suspension). Women at risk of pregnancy should avoid such exposure.

TABLETS

Breast Cancer: 160 mg/day (40 mg qid).

Endometrial Carcinoma: 40-320 mg/day in divided doses.

At least 2 months of continuous treatment is considered an adequate period for determining the efficacy of megestrol acetate.

Special Handling

Health Hazard Data

There is no threshold limit value established by OSHA, NIOSH, or ACGIH.

Exposure or "overdose" at levels approaching recommended dosing levels could result in side effects described above (see WARNINGS, Tablets and ADVERSE REACTIONS, Tablets). Women at risk of pregnancy should avoid such exposure.

ANIMAL PHARMACOLOGY

ORAL SUSPENSION

Long-term treatment with megestrol acetate may increase the risk of respiratory infections. A trend toward increased frequency of respiratory infections, decreased lymphocyte counts and increased neutrophil counts was observed in a 2 year chronic toxicity/carcinogenicity study of megestrol acetate conducted in rats.

HOW SUPPLIED

MEGACE ORAL SUSPENSION

Megace oral suspension is avaiable as a lemon-lime flavored oral suspension containing 40 mg of micronized megestrol acetate per ml.

Storage: Store Megace oral suspension between 15-25°C (59-77°F) and dispense in a tight container. Protect from heat.

MEGACE TABLETS

Megace is supplied as light blue scored tablets for oral administration containing 20 or 40 mg megestrol acetate.

Storage: Store at 25°C (77°F); excursions permitted to 15-30°C (59-86°F). Protect from temperatures above 40°C (104°F).

PRODUCT LISTING - RATED THERAPEUTICALLY EQUIVALENT

Suspension - Oral - 40 mg/ml

236 ml	$159.95	MEGACE, Bristol-Myers Squibb	00015-0508-42
240 ml	$135.93	MEGACE, Physicians Total Care	54868-3099-01
240 ml	$143.95	GENERIC, Roxane Laboratories Inc	00054-3542-58
240 ml	$143.95	GENERIC, Par Pharmaceutical Inc	49884-0907-38

Tablet - Oral - 20 mg

100's	$34.89	FEDERAL UPPER LIMIT, H.C.F.A. F F P	99999-1716-01
100's	$52.50	GENERIC, Major Pharmaceuticals Inc	00904-3570-60
100's	$61.95	GENERIC, Watson/Schein Pharmaceuticals Inc	00364-2235-01
100's	$63.45	GENERIC, Ivax Corporation	00182-1863-01
100's	$64.25	GENERIC, Watson/Rugby Laboratories Inc	00536-4821-01
100's	$64.25	GENERIC, Moore, H.L. Drug Exchange Inc	00839-7405-06
100's	$65.65	GENERIC, Udl Laboratories Inc	51079-0434-20
100's	$66.25	GENERIC, Ivax Corporation	00182-1863-89
100's	$66.66	MEGACE, Aligen Independent Laboratories Inc	00405-4623-01
100's	$67.12	GENERIC, Barr Laboratories Inc	00555-0606-02
100's	$69.20	GENERIC, Par Pharmaceutical Inc	49884-0289-01
100's	$69.22	GENERIC, Dixon-Shane Inc	17236-0697-01
100's	$72.03	GENERIC, Roxane Laboratories Inc	00054-8603-25
100's	$72.66	MEGACE, Bristol-Myers Squibb	00015-0595-01

Tablet - Oral - 40 mg

25's	$18.13	GENERIC, Udl Laboratories Inc	51079-0435-19
30 x 25	$784.58	GENERIC, Sky Pharmaceuticals Packaging, Inc	63739-0165-03
31 x 10	$352.00	GENERIC, Vangard Labs	00615-3570-53
31 x 10	$352.00	GENERIC, Vangard Labs	00615-3570-63
100's	$67.55	FEDERAL UPPER LIMIT, H.C.F.A. F F P	99999-1716-02
100's	$87.40	GENERIC, Major Pharmaceuticals Inc	00904-3571-60
100's	$91.87	GENERIC, Major Pharmaceuticals Inc	00904-3571-61
100's	$100.80	GENERIC, Watson/Schein Pharmaceuticals Inc	00364-2234-01
100's	$101.77	GENERIC, Aligen Independent Laboratories Inc	00405-4624-01
100's	$106.37	GENERIC, Moore, H.L. Drug Exchange Inc	00839-7406-06
100's	$106.72	GENERIC, Teva Pharmaceuticals Usa	62584-0779-01
100's	$106.95	GENERIC, Ivax Corporation	00182-1864-89
100's	$106.95	GENERIC, Udl Laboratories Inc	51079-0435-20
100's	$110.21	GENERIC, Barr Laboratories Inc	00555-0607-02
100's	$110.31	GENERIC, Ivax Corporation	00182-1864-01
100's	$110.31	GENERIC, Dixon-Shane Inc	17236-0495-01
100's	$116.63	GENERIC, Teva Pharmaceuticals Usa	00093-5138-01
100's	$123.00	GENERIC, Par Pharmaceutical Inc	49884-0290-01
100's	$123.20	GENERIC, Martec Pharmaceuticals Inc	52555-0376-01
100's	$128.48	GENERIC, Roxane Laboratories Inc	00054-8604-25
100's	$129.59	MEGACE, Bristol-Myers Squibb	00015-0596-41
250's	$192.75	GENERIC, Major Pharmaceuticals Inc	00904-3571-70
250's	$251.75	GENERIC, Aligen Independent Laboratories Inc	00405-4624-04
250's	$270.11	GENERIC, Barr Laboratories Inc	00555-0607-03
250's	$270.60	GENERIC, Par Pharmaceutical Inc	49884-0290-04

PRODUCT LISTING - EQUIVALENTS NOT AVAILABLE

Suspension - Oral - 40 mg/ml

240 ml	$143.95	GENERIC, Par Pharmaceutical Inc	49884-0907-88

Meloxicam *(003480)*

For related information, see the comparative table section in Appendix A.

Categories: Arthritis, osteoarthritis; FDA Approved 2000 Apr; Pregnancy Category C

Drug Classes: Analgesics, non-narcotic; Nonsteroidal anti-inflammatory drugs

Foreign Brand Availability: Aflamid (Mexico); Artrilox (Indonesia); Exel (Mexico); Flodin (Peru); Loxibest (Mexico); Loxicam (Colombia); Masflex (Mexico); Melocam (Colombia); Mel-OD (India); Melosteral (Mexico); Melox (Bahrain; Cyprus; Egypt; Iran; Iraq; Jordan; Kuwait; Lebanon; Libya; Oman; Qatar; Republic-of-Yemen; Saudi-Arabia; Syria; United-Arab-Emirates); Mexican (Colombia); Mexpharm (Indonesia); Mobec (Germany); Mobic (Bahamas; Bahrain; Barbados; Belize; Benin; Bermuda; Burkina-Faso; Colombia; Curacao; Cyprus; Egypt; England; Ethiopia; Gambia; Ghana; Guinea; Guyana; Hong-Kong; Iran; Iraq; Ireland; Ivory-Coast; Jamaica; Jordan; Kenya; Korea; Kuwait; Lebanon; Liberia; Libya; Malawi; Mali; Mauritania; Mauritius; Morocco; Netherland-Antilles; New-Zealand; Niger; Nigeria; Oman; Philippines; Puerto-Rico; Qatar; Republic-of-Yemen; Saudi-Arabia; Senegal; Seychelles; Sierra-Leone; Singapore; Sudan; Surinam; Syria; Taiwan; Tanzania; Thailand; Trinidad; Tunia; Uganda; United-Arab-Emirates; Zambia; Zimbabwe); Mobicox (Costa-Rica; Dominican-Republic; El-Salvador; Guatemala; Honduras; Mexico; Nicaragua; Panama); Movi-Cox (Indonesia); Mowin (Peru); Muvera (India); Rumonal (Colombia); Selektine (Bahrain; Cyprus; Egypt; Iran; Iraq; Jordan; Kuwait; Lebanon; Libya; Oman; Qatar; Republic-of-Yemen; Saudi-Arabia; Syria; United-Arab-Emirates)

Cost of Therapy: $70.73 (Osteoarthritis; Mobic; 7.5 mg; 1 tablet/day; 30 day supply)

DESCRIPTION

Meloxicam, an oxicam derivative, is a member of the enolic acid group of nonsteroidal anti-inflammatory drugs (NSAIDs). Each yellow tablet contains meloxicam 7.5 mg for oral administration. It is chemically designated as 4-hydroxy-2-methyl-*N*-(5-methyl-2-thiazolyl)-2H-1,2-benzothiazine-3-carboxamide 1, 1-dioxide. The molecular weight is 351.4. Its empirical formula is $C_{14}H_{13}N_3O_4S_2$.

Meloxicam is a yellow solid, practically insoluble in water, with higher solubility observed in strong acids and bases. It is very slightly soluble in methanol. Meloxicam has an apparent partition coefficient $(\log P)_{app} = 0.1$ in *n*-octanol/buffer pH 7.4. Meloxicam has pKa values of 1.1 and 4.2.

Mobic is available as a tablet for oral administration containing 7.5 mg meloxicam.

The inactive ingredients in Mobic include colloidal silicon dioxide, crospovidone, lactose monohydrate, magnesium stearate, microcrystalline cellulose, povidone and sodium citrate dihydrate.

CLINICAL PHARMACOLOGY

MECHANISM OF ACTION

Meloxicam is a nonsteroidal anti-inflammatory drug (NSAID) that exhibits anti-inflammatory, analgesic, and antipyretic activities in animal models. The mechanism of action of meloxicam, like that of other NSAIDs, may be related to prostaglandin synthetase (cyclooxygenase) inhibition.

PHARMACOKINETICS

Absorption

The absolute bioavailability of meloxicam capsules was 89% following a single oral dose of 30 mg compared with 30 mg IV bolus injection. Meloxicam capsules have been shown to be bioequivalent to meloxicam tablets. Following single intravenous doses, dose-proportional pharmacokinetics were shown in the range of 5-60 mg. After multiple oral doses the pharmacokinetics of meloxicam capsules were dose-proportional over the range of 7.5-15 mg. Mean C_{max} was achieved within 4-5 hours after a 7.5 mg meloxicam tablet was taken under fasted conditions, indicating a prolonged drug absorption. The rate or extent of absorption was not affected by multiple dose administration, suggesting linear pharmacokinetics. With multiple dosing, steady state conditions were reached by day 5. A second meloxicam concentration peak occurs around 12-14 hours post-dose suggesting gastrointestinal recirculation.

Food and Antacid Effects

Drug intake after a high fat breakfast (75 g of fat) did not affect extent of absorption of meloxicam capsules, but led to 22% higher C_{max} values. Mean C_{max} values were achieved between 5 and 6 hours. No pharmacokinetic interaction was detected with concomitant administration of antacids. Meloxicam tablets can be administered without regard to timing of meals and antacids.

TABLE 1A *Steady State Pharmacokinetic Parameters for Oral 7.5 and 15 mg Meloxicam (Mean and % CV)**

Pharmacokinetic Parameters (% CV)	Healthy Male Adults (Fed)† 7.5 mg tablets‡ n=18	Elderly Males (Fed)† 15 mg capsules n=5	Elderly Females (Fed)† 15 mg capsules n=8
C_{max} (μg/ml)	1.05 (20)	2.3 (59)	3.2 (24)
T_{max} (h)	4.9 (8)	5 (12)	6 (27)
$T_{½}$ (h)	20.1 (29)	21 (34)	24 (34)
CL/f (ml/min)	8.8 (29)	9.9 (76)	5.1 (22)
Vz/f§	14.7 (32)	15 (42)	10 (30)

* The parameter values in the table are from various studies.
† Not under high fat conditions.
‡ Meloxicam tablets.
§ Vz/f=Dose/(AUC·K_{el}).

TABLE 1B *Single Dose Pharmacokinetic Parameters for Oral 7.5 and 15 mg Meloxicam (Mean and % CV)**

Pharmacokinetic Parameters (% CV)	Renal Failure (Fasted) 15 mg capsules n=12	Hepatic Insufficiency (Fasted) 15 mg capsules n=12
C_{max} (μg/ml)	**0.59 (36)**	**0.84 (29)**
T_{max} (h)	4 (65)	10 (87)
$T_{½}$ (h)	18 (46)	16 (29)
CL/f (ml/min)	19 (43)	11 (44)
Vz/f§ (L)	26 (44)	14 (29)

* The parameter values in the table are from various studies.
§ Vz/f=Dose/(AUC·K_{el}).

Distribution

The mean volume of distribution (Vss) of meloxicam is approximately 10 liters. Meloxicam is ~99.4% bound to human plasma proteins (primarily albumin) within the therapeutic dose range. The fraction of protein binding is independent of drug concentration, over the clinically relevant concentration range, but decreases to ~99% in patients with renal disease. Meloxicam penetration into human red blood cells, after oral dosing, is less than 10%. Following a radiolabeled dose, over 90% of the radioactivity detected in the plasma was present as unchanged meloxicam.

Meloxicam concentrations in synovial fluid, after a single oral dose, range from 40-50% of those in plasma. The free fraction in synovial fluid is 2.5 times higher than in plasma, due to the lower albumin content in synovial fluid as compared to plasma. The significance of this penetration is unknown.

Metabolism

Meloxicam is almost completely metabolized to four pharmacologically inactive metabolites. The major metabolite, 5′-carboxy meloxicam (60% of dose), from P-450 mediated metabolism was formed by oxidation of an intermediate metabolite 5′-hydroxymethyl meloxicam which is also excreted to a lesser extent (9% of dose). *In vitro* studies indicate that cytochrome P-450 2C9 plays an important role in this metabolic pathway with a minor contribution of the CYP 3A4 isozyme. Patients' peroxidase activity is probably responsible for the other two metabolites which account for 16% and 4% of the administered dose, respectively.

Excretion

Meloxicam excretion is predominantly in the form of metabolites, and occurs to equal extents in the urine and feces. Only traces of the unchanged parent compound are excreted in the urine (0.2%) and feces (1.6%). The extent of the urinary excretion was confirmed for unlabeled multiple 7.5 mg doses: 0.5%, 6% and 13% of the dose were found in urine in the form of meloxicam, and the 5′-hydroxymethyl and 5′-carboxy metabolites, respectively. There is significant biliary and/or enteral secretion of the drug. This was demonstrated when oral administration of cholestyramine following a single IV dose of meloxicam decreased the AUC of meloxicam by 50%.

The mean elimination half-life ($T_{½}$) ranges from 15-20 hours. The elimination half-life is constant across dose levels indicating linear metabolism within the therapeutic dose range. Plasma clearance ranges from 7-9 ml/min.

SPECIAL POPULATIONS

Pediatric

The pharmacokinetics of meloxicam in pediatric patients under 18 years of age have not been investigated.

Geriatric

Elderly males (≥65 years of age) exhibited meloxicam plasma concentrations and steady state pharmacokinetics similar to young males. Elderly females (≥65 years of age) had a 47% higher AUC(ss) and 32% higher $C_{max\ ss}$ as compared to younger females (≤55 years of age) after body weight normalization. Despite the increased total concentrations in the elderly females, the adverse event profile was comparable for both elderly patient populations. A smaller free fraction was found in elderly female patients in comparison to elderly male patients.

Gender

Young females exhibited slightly lower plasma concentrations relative to young males. After single doses of 7.5 mg meloxicam, the mean elimination half-life was 19.5 hours for the female group as compared to 23.4 hours for the male group. At steady state, the data were similar (17.9 hours vs 21.4 hours). This pharmacokinetic difference due to gender is likely to be of little clinical importance. There was linearity of pharmacokinetics and no appreciable difference in the C_{max} or T_{max} across genders.

Hepatic Insufficiency

Following a single 15 mg dose of meloxicam there was no marked difference in plasma concentrations in subjects with mild (Child-Pugh Class I) and moderate (Child-Pugh Class II) hepatic impairment compared to healthy volunteers. Protein binding of meloxicam was not affected by hepatic insufficiency. No dose adjustment is necessary in mild to moderate hepatic insufficiency. Patients with severe hepatic impairment (Child-Pugh Class III) have not been adequately studied.

Renal Insufficiency

Meloxicam pharmacokinetics have been investigated in subjects with different degrees of renal insufficiency. Total drug plasma concentrations decreased with the degree of renal impairment while free AUC values were similar. Total clearance of meloxicam increased in these patients probably due to the increase in free fraction leading to an increased metabolic clearance. There is no need for dose adjustment in patients with mild to moderate renal failure (CRCL >15 ml/min). Patients with severe renal insufficiency have not been adequately studied. The use of meloxicam in subjects with severe renal impairment is not recommended (see WARNINGS, Advanced Renal Disease).

Hemodialysis

Following a single dose of meloxicam, the free C_{max} plasma concentrations were higher in patients with renal failure on chronic hemodialysis (1% free fraction) in comparison to healthy volunteers (0.3% free fraction). Hemodialysis did not lower the total drug concentration in plasma; therefore, additional doses are not necessary after hemodialysis. Meloxicam is not dialyzable.

INDICATIONS AND USAGE

Meloxicam is indicated for relief of the signs and symptoms of osteoarthritis.

NON-FDA APPROVED INDICATIONS

Unapproved uses of other oxicam derivative NSAIDs include the treatment of pain and the signs and symptoms of rheumatoid arthritis, ankylosing spondylitis and acute gout.

CONTRAINDICATIONS

Meloxicam is contraindicated in patients with known hypersensitivity to meloxicam. It should not be given to patients who have experienced asthma, urticaria, or allergic-type reactions after taking aspirin or other NSAIDs. Severe, rarely fatal, anaphylactic-like reactions to NSAIDs have been reported in such patients (see WARNINGS, Anaphylactoid Reactions, and PRECAUTIONS, Pre-Existing Asthma).

WARNINGS

GASTROINTESTINAL (GI) EFFECTS — RISK OF GI ULCERATION, BLEEDING, AND PERFORATION

Serious gastrointestinal toxicity, such as inflammation, bleeding, ulceration, and perforation of the stomach, small intestine or large intestine, can occur at any time, with or without warning symptoms, in patients treated with nonsteroidal anti-inflammatory drugs (NSAIDs). Minor upper gastrointestinal problems, such as dyspepsia, are common and may also occur at any time during NSAID therapy. Therefore, physicians and patients should remain alert for ulceration and bleeding, even in the absence of previous GI symptoms. Patients should be informed about the signs and/or symptoms of serious GI toxicity and the steps to take if they occur. The utility of periodic laboratory monitoring has not been demonstrated, nor has it been adequately assessed. Only 1 in 5 patients who develop a serious upper GI adverse event on NSAID therapy is symptomatic. It has been demonstrated that upper GI ulcers, gross bleeding or perforation, caused by NSAIDs, appear to occur in approximately 1% of the patients treated for 3-6 months, and in about 2-4% of patients treated for 1 year. These trends continue thus, increasing the likelihood of developing a serious GI event at some time during the course of therapy. However, even short-term therapy is not without risk.

NSAIDs should be prescribed with extreme caution in those with a prior history of ulcer disease or gastrointestinal bleeding. Most spontaneous reports of fatal GI events are in elderly or debilitated patients and therefore special care should be taken in treating this population. **To minimize the potential risk for an adverse GI event, the lowest effective dose should be used for the shortest possible duration.** For high-risk patients, alternate therapies that do not involve NSAIDs should be considered.

Studies have shown that patients with a *prior history of peptic ulcer disease and/or gastrointestinal bleeding* and who use NSAIDs, have a greater than 10-fold risk for developing a GI bleed than patients with neither of these risk factors. In addition to a past history of ulcer disease, pharmacoepidemiological studies have identified several other co-therapies or co-morbid conditions that may increase the risk for GI bleeding such as: treatment with oral corticosteroids, treatment with anticoagulants, longer duration of NSAID therapy, smoking, alcoholism, older age, and poor general health status.

ANAPHYLACTOID REACTIONS

As with other NSAIDs, anaphylactoid reactions have occurred in patients without known prior exposure to meloxicam. Meloxicam should not be given to patients with the aspirin triad. This symptom complex typically occurs in asthmatic patients who experience rhinitis with or without nasal polyps, or who exhibit severe, potentially fatal bronchospasm after taking aspirin or other NSAIDs (see CONTRAINDICATIONS and PRECAUTIONS, Pre-Existing Asthma). Emergency help should be sought in cases where an anaphylactoid reaction occurs.

ADVANCED RENAL DISEASE

In cases with advanced kidney disease, treatment with meloxicam is not recommended. If NSAID therapy must be initiated, close monitoring of the patient's kidney function is advisable (see PRECAUTIONS, Renal Effects).

PREGNANCY

In late pregnancy, as with other NSAIDs, meloxicam should be avoided because it may cause premature closure of the ductus arteriosus.

PRECAUTIONS

GENERAL

Meloxicam cannot be expected to substitute for corticosteroids or to treat corticosteroid insufficiency. Abrupt discontinuation of corticosteroids may lead to disease exacerbation. Patients on prolonged corticosteroid therapy should have their therapy tapered slowly if a decision is made to discontinue corticosteroids. The pharmacological activity of meloxicam in reducing inflammation and possibly fever may diminish the utility of these diagnostic signs in detecting complications of presumed noninfectious, painful conditions.

HEPATIC EFFECTS

Borderline elevations of one or more liver tests may occur in up to 15% of patients taking NSAIDs, including meloxicam. These laboratory abnormalities may progress, may remain unchanged, or may be transient with continuing therapy. Notable elevations of ALT or AST (approximately 3 or more times the upper limit of normal) have been reported in approximately 1% of patients in clinical trials with NSAIDs. In addition, rare cases of severe hepatic reactions, including jaundice and fatal fulminant hepatitis, liver necrosis and hepatic failure, some of them with fatal outcomes, have been reported with NSAIDs.

Patients with signs and/or symptoms suggesting liver dysfunction, or in whom an abnormal liver test has occurred, should be evaluated for evidence of the development of a more severe hepatic reaction while on therapy with meloxicam. If clinical signs and symptoms consistent with liver disease develop, or if systemic manifestations occur (*e.g.*, eosinophilia, rash, etc.), meloxicam should be discontinued.

RENAL EFFECTS

Caution should be used when initiating treatment with meloxicam in patients with considerable dehydration. It is advisable to rehydrate patients first and then start therapy with meloxicam. Caution is also recommended in patients with pre-existing kidney disease (see WARNINGS, Advanced Renal Disease).

Long-term administration of NSAIDs has resulted in renal papillary necrosis and other renal medullary changes. Renal toxicity has also been seen in patients in whom renal prostaglandins have a compensatory role in the maintenance of renal perfusion. In these patients, administration of NSAIDs may cause dose-dependent reduction in prostaglandin formation and, secondarily, in renal blood flow, which may precipitate overt renal decompensation. Patients at greatest risk of this reaction are those with impaired renal function, heart failure, liver dysfunction, those taking diuretics and ACE inhibitors, and the elderly. Discontinuation of NSAID therapy is usually followed by recovery to the pretreatment state.

The extent to which metabolites may accumulate in patients with renal failure has not been studied with meloxicam. Because some meloxicam metabolites are excreted by the kidney, patients with significantly impaired renal function should be more closely monitored.

HEMATOLOGICAL EFFECTS

Anemia is sometimes seen in patients receiving NSAIDs, including meloxicam. This may be due to fluid retention, GI blood loss, or an incompletely described effect upon erythropoiesis. Patients on long-term treatment with NSAIDs, including meloxicam, should have their hemoglobin or hematocrit checked if they exhibit any signs or symptoms of anemia.

Drugs which inhibit the biosynthesis of prostaglandins may interfere to some extent with platelet function and vascular responses to bleeding.

NSAIDs inhibit platelet aggregation and have been shown to prolong bleeding time in some patients. Unlike aspirin their effect on platelet function is quantitatively less, or of shorter duration, and reversible. Meloxicam does not generally affect platelet counts, prothrombin time (PT), or partial thromboplastin time (PTT). Patients receiving meloxicam who may be adversely affected by alterations in platelet function, such as those with coagulation disorders or patients receiving anticoagulants, should be carefully monitored.

FLUID RETENTION AND EDEMA

Fluid retention and edema have been observed in some patients taking NSAIDs, including meloxicam. Therefore, as with other NSAIDs, meloxicam should be used with caution in patients with fluid retention, hypertension, or heart failure.

PRE-EXISTING ASTHMA

Patients with asthma may have aspirin-sensitive asthma. The use of aspirin in patients with aspirin-sensitive asthma has been associated with severe bronchospasm which can be fatal. Since cross reactivity, including bronchospasm, between aspirin and other nonsteroidal anti-inflammatory drugs has been reported in such aspirin-sensitive patients, meloxicam should not be administered to patients with this form of aspirin sensitivity and should be used with caution in patients with pre-existing asthma.

INFORMATION FOR THE PATIENT

Meloxicam, like other drugs of its class, can cause discomfort and, rarely, more serious side effects, such as gastrointestinal bleeding, which may result in hospitalization and even fatal outcomes. Although serious GI tract ulcerations and bleeding can occur without warning symptoms, patients should be alert for the signs and symptoms of ulcerations and bleeding, and should ask for medical advice when observing any indicative signs or symptoms. Patients should be made aware of the importance of this follow-up (see WARNINGS, Gastrointestinal (GI) Effects — Risk of GI Ulceration, Bleeding, and Perforation).

Patients should report to their physicians signs or symptoms of gastrointestinal ulceration or bleeding, skin rash, weight gain, or edema.

Patients should be informed of the warning signs and symptoms of hepatotoxicity (*e.g.*, nausea, fatigue, lethargy, pruritus, jaundice, right upper quadrant tenderness, and "flu-like" symptoms). If these occur, patients should be instructed to stop therapy and seek immediate medical therapy.

Patients should also be instructed to seek immediate emergency help in the case of an anaphylactoid reaction (see WARNINGS, Anaphylactoid Reactions).

In late pregnancy, as with other NSAIDs, meloxicam should be avoided because it may cause premature closure of the ductus arteriosus.

LABORATORY TESTS

Patients on long-term treatment with NSAIDs should have their CBC and a chemistry profile checked periodically. If clinical signs and symptoms consistent with liver or renal disease develop, systemic manifestations occur (*e.g.*, eosinophilia, rash, etc.) or if abnormal liver tests persist or worsen, meloxicam should be discontinued.

CARCINOGENESIS, MUTAGENESIS, AND IMPAIRMENT OF FERTILITY

No carcinogenic effect of meloxicam was observed in rats given oral doses up to 0.8 mg/kg/day (approximately 0.4-fold the human dose at 15 mg/day for a 50 kg adult based on body surface area conversion) for 104 weeks or in mice given oral doses up to 8.0 mg/kg/day (approximately 2.2-fold the human dose, as noted above) for 99 weeks.

Meloxicam was not mutagenic in an Ames assay, or clastogenic in a chromosome aberration assay with human lymphocytes and an *in vivo* micronucleus test in mouse bone marrow.

Meloxicam did not impair male and female fertility in rats at oral doses up to 9 and 5 mg/kg/day, respectively (4.9-fold and 2.5-fold the human dose, as noted above). However, an increased incidence of embryolethality at oral doses ≥1 mg/kg/day (0.5-fold the human dose, as noted above) was observed in rats when dams were given meloxicam 2 weeks prior to mating and during early embryonic development.

PREGNANCY

Teratogenic Effects,Pregnancy Category C

Meloxicam caused an increased incidence of septal defect of the heart, a rare event, at an oral dose of 60 mg/kg/day (64.5-fold the human dose at 15 mg/day for a 50 kg adult based on body surface area conversion) and embryolethality at oral doses ≥5 mg/kg/day (5.4-fold the human dose, as noted above) when rabbits were treated throughout organogenesis. Meloxicam was not teratogenic in rats up to an oral dose of 4 mg/kg/day (approximately 2.2-fold the human dose, as noted above) throughout organogenesis. An increased incidence of stillbirths was observed when rats were given oral doses ≥1 mg/kg/day throughout organogenesis. Meloxicam crosses the placental barrier. There are no adequate and well-controlled studies in pregnant women. Meloxicam should be used during pregnancy only if the potential benefit justifies the potential risk to the fetus.

Nonteratogenic Effects

Meloxicam caused a reduction in birth index, live births, and neonatal survival at oral doses ≥0.125 mg/kg/day (approximately 0.07-fold the human dose at 15 mg/day for a 50 kg adult based on body surface area conversion) when rats were treated during the late gestation and lactation period. No studies have been conducted to evaluate the effect of meloxicam on the closure of the ductus arteriosus in humans; use of meloxicam during the third trimester of pregnancy should be avoided.

LABOR AND DELIVERY

Studies in rats with meloxicam, as with other drugs known to inhibit prostaglandin synthesis, showed an increased incidence of stillbirths, increased length of delivery time, and delayed parturition at oral dosages ≥1 mg/kg/day (approximately 0.5-fold the human dose at 15 mg/day for a 50 kg adult based on body surface area conversion), and decreased pup survival at an oral dose of 4 mg/kg/day (approximately 2.1-fold the human dose, as noted above) throughout organogenesis. Similar findings were observed in rats receiving oral dosages ≥0.125 mg/kg/day (approximately 0.07-fold the human dose, as noted above) during late gestation and the lactation period.

NURSING MOTHERS

Studies of meloxicam excretion in human milk have not been conducted; however, meloxicam was excreted in the milk of lactating rats at concentrations higher than those in plasma. Because of the potential for serious adverse reactions in nursing infants from meloxicam, a decision should be made whether to discontinue nursing or to discontinue the drug, taking into account the importance of the drug to the mother.

PEDIATRIC USE

Safety and effectiveness in pediatric patients under 18 years of age have not been established.

GERIATRIC USE

As with any NSAID, caution should be exercised in treating the elderly (65 years and older).

DRUG INTERACTIONS

ACE Inhibitors: Reports suggest that NSAIDs may diminish the antihypertensive effect of angiotensin-converting enzyme (ACE) inhibitors. This interaction should be given consideration in patients taking NSAIDs concomitantly with ACE inhibitors.

Aspirin: Concomitant administration of aspirin (1000 mg tid) to healthy volunteers tended to increase the AUC (10%) and C_{max} (24%) of meloxicam. The clinical significance of this interaction is not known; however, as with other NSAIDs, concomitant administration of meloxicam and aspirin is not generally recommended because of the potential for increased adverse effects. Concomitant administration of low-dose aspirin with meloxicam may result in an increased rate of GI ulceration or other complications, compared to use of meloxicam alone. Meloxicam is not a substitute for aspirin for cardiovascular prophylaxis.

Cholestyramine: Pretreatment for 4 days with cholestyramine significantly increased the clearance of meloxicam by 50%. This resulted in a decrease in $T_{½}$, from 19.2

hours to 12.5 hours, and a 35% reduction in AUC. This suggests the existence of a recirculation pathway for meloxicam in the gastrointestinal tract. The clinical relevance of this interaction has not been established.

Cimetidine: Concomitant administration of 200 mg cimetidine qid did not alter the single-dose pharmacokinetics of 30 mg meloxicam.

Digoxin: Meloxicam 15 mg once daily for 7 days did not alter the plasma concentration profile of digoxin after β-acetyldigoxin administration for 7 days at clinical doses. *In vitro* testing found no protein binding drug interaction between digoxin and meloxicam.

Furosemide: Clinical studies, as well as post-marketing observations, have shown that NSAIDs can reduce the natriuretic effect of furosemide and thiazide diuretics in some patients. This effect has been attributed to inhibition of renal prostaglandin synthesis. Studies with furosemide agents and meloxicam have not demonstrated a reduction in natriuretic effect. Furosemide single and multiple dose pharmacodynamics and pharmacokinetics are not affected by multiple doses of meloxicam. Nevertheless, during concomitant therapy with furosemide and meloxicam, patients should be observed closely for signs of declining renal function (see PRECAUTIONS, Renal Effects), as well as to assure diuretic efficacy.

Lithium: In clinical trials, NSAIDs have produced an elevation of plasma lithium levels and a reduction in renal lithium clearance. In a study conducted in healthy subjects, mean pre-dose lithium concentration and AUC were increased by 21% in subjects receiving lithium doses ranging from 804-1072 mg bid with meloxicam 15 mg qd as compared to subjects receiving lithium alone. These effects have been attributed to inhibition of renal prostaglandin synthesis by meloxicam. Patients on lithium treatment should be closely monitored when meloxicam is introduced or withdrawn.

Methotrexate: A study in 13 rheumatoid arthritis (RA) patients evaluated the effects of multiple doses of meloxicam on the pharmacokinetics of methotrexate taken once weekly. Meloxicam did not have a significant effect on the pharmacokinetics of single doses of methotrexate. *In vitro,* methotrexate did not displace meloxicam from its human serum binding sites.

Warfarin: Anticoagulant activity should be monitored, particularly in the first few days after initiating or changing meloxicam therapy in patients receiving warfarin or similar agents, since these patients are at an increased risk of bleeding. The effect of meloxicam on the anticoagulant effect of warfarin was studied in a group of healthy subjects receiving daily doses of warfarin that produced an INR (International Normalized Ratio) between 1.2 and 1.8. In these subjects, meloxicam did not alter warfarin pharmacokinetics and the average anticoagulant effect of warfarin as determined by prothrombin time. However, 1 subject showed an increase in INR from 1.5 to 2.1. Caution should be used when administering meloxicam with warfarin since patients on warfarin may experience changes in INR and an increased risk of bleeding complications when a new medication is introduced.

ADVERSE REACTIONS

The meloxicam Phase 2/3 clinical trial database includes 10,122 patients treated with meloxicam 7.5 mg/day and 3505 patients treated with meloxicam 15 mg/day. Meloxicam at these doses was administered to 661 patients for at least 6 months and to 312 patients for at least 1 year. Approximately 10,500 of these patients were treated in 10 placebo and/or active-controlled osteoarthritis trials. Gastrointestinal (GI) adverse events were the most frequently reported adverse events in all treatment groups across meloxicam trials.

A 12 week multicenter, double-blind, randomized trial was conducted in patients with osteoarthritis of the knee or hip to compare the efficacy and safety of meloxicam with placebo and with an active control. TABLE 2 depicts adverse events that occurred in ≥2% of the meloxicam treatment groups.

TABLE 2 *Adverse Events (%) Occurring in ≥2% of Meloxicam Patients in a 12 Week Osteoarthritis Placebo and Active-Controlled Trial*

	Daily Dose			
		Meloxicam		Diclofenac
	Placebo	7.5 mg	15 mg	100 mg
Number of Patients	157	154	156	153
Gastrointestinal	17.2%	20.1%	17.3%	28.1%
Abdominal pain	2.5%	1.9%	2.6%	1.3%
Diarrhea	3.8%	7.8%	3.2%	9.2%
Dyspepsia	4.5%	4.5%	4.5%	6.5%
Flatulence	4.5%	3.2%	3.2%	3.9%
Nausea	3.2%	3.9%	3.8%	7.2%
Body as a Whole				
Accident household	1.9%	4.5%	3.2%	2.6%
Edema*	2.5%	1.9%	4.5%	3.3%
Fall	0.6%	2.6%	0.0%	1.3%
Influenza-like symptoms	5.1%	4.5%	5.8%	2.6%
Central and Peripheral Nervous System				
Dizziness	3.2%	2.6%	3.8%	2.0%
Headache	10.2%	7.8%	8.3%	5.9%
Respiratory				
Pharyngitis	1.3%	0.6%	3.2%	1.3%
Upper respiratory tract infection	1.9%	3.2%	1.9%	3.3%
Skin				
Rash†	2.5%	2.6%	0.6%	2.0%

* WHO preferred terms edema, edema dependent, edema peripheral and edema legs combined
† WHO preferred terms rash, rash erythematous and rash maculo-papular combined

The adverse events that occurred with meloxicam in ≥2% of patients treated short-term (4-6 weeks) and long term (6 months) in active-controlled osteoarthritis trials are presented in TABLE 3.

TABLE 3 *Adverse Events (%) Occurring in ≥2% of Meloxicam Patients in 4-6 Weeks and 6 Month Active-Controlled Osteoarthritis Trials*

	Daily Dose			
	4-6 Weeks Controlled Trials		6 Month Controlled Trials	
	7.5 mg	15 mg	7.5 mg	15 mg
Number of Patients	8955	256	169	306
Gastrointestinal	11.8%	18.0%	26.6%	24.2%
Abdominal pain	2.7%	2.3%	4.7%	2.9%
Constipation	0.8%	1.2%	1.8%	2.6%
Diarrhea	1.9%	2.7%	5.9%	2.6%
Dyspepsia	3.8%	7.4%	8.9%	9.5%
Flatulence	0.5%	0.4%	3.0%	2.6%
Nausea	2.4%	4.7%	4.7%	7.2%
Vomiting	0.6%	0.8%	1.8%	2.6%
Body as a Whole				
Edema*	0.6%	2.0%	2.4%	1.6%
Pain	0.9%	2.0%	3.6%	5.2%
Central and Peripheral Nervous System				
Dizziness	1.1%	1.6%	2.4%	2.6%
Headache	2.4%	2.7%	3.6%	2.6%
Hematologic				
Anemia	0.1%	0.0%	4.1%	2.9%
Musculo-Skeletal				
Arthralgia	0.5%	0.0%	5.3%	1.3%
Back pain	0.5%	0.4%	3.0%	0.7%
Psychiatric				
Insomnia	0.4%	0.0%	3.6%	1.6%
Respiratory				
Coughing	0.2	0.8	2.4	1.0
Upper respiratory tract infection	0.2%	0.0%	8.3%	7.5%
Skin				
Pruritus	0.4%	1.2%	2.4%	0.0%
Rash†	0.3%	1.2%	3.0%	1.3%
Urinary				
Micturition frequency	0.1%	0.4%	2.4%	1.3%
Urinary tract infection	0.3%	0.4%	4.7%	6.9%

* WHO preferred terms edema, edema dependent, edema peripheral and edema legs combined.
† WHO preferred terms rash, rash erythematous and rash maculo-papular combined.

As with other NSAIDs, higher doses of meloxicam (*e.g.,* chronic daily 30 mg dose) were associated with an increased risk of serious GI events, therefore the daily dose of meloxicam should not exceed 15 mg.

The following is a list of adverse drug reactions occurring in <2% of patients receiving meloxicam in clinical trials involving approximately 15,400 patients. Adverse reactions reported only in worldwide post-marketing experience or the literature are shown in italics and are considered rare (<0.1%).

Body as a Whole: Allergic reaction, *anaphylactoid reactions including shock,* face edema, fatigue, fever, hot flushes, malaise, syncope, weight decrease, weight increase.

Cardiovascular: Angina pectoris, cardiac failure, hypertension, hypotension, myocardial infarction, vasculitis.

Central and Peripheral Nervous System: Convulsions, paresthesia, tremor, vertigo.

Gastrointestinal: Colitis, dry mouth, duodenal ulcer, eructation, esophagitis, gastric ulcer, gastritis, gastroesophageal reflux, gastrointestinal hemorrhage, hematemesis, hemorrhagic duodenal ulcer, hemorrhagic gastric ulcer, intestinal perforation, melena, pancreatitis, perforated duodenal ulcer, perforated gastric ulcer, stomatitis ulcerative.

Heart Rate and Rhythm: Arrhythmia, palpitation, tachycardia.

Hematologic: *Agranulocytosis,* leukopenia, purpura, thrombocytopenia.

Liver and Biliary System: ALT increased, AST increased, bilirubinemia, GGT increased, hepatitis, *jaundice, liver failure.*

Metabolic and Nutritional: Dehydration.

Psychiatric Disorders: Abnormal dreaming, anxiety, appetite increased, confusion, depression, nervousness, somnolence.

Respiratory: Asthma, bronchospasm, dyspnea.

Skin and Appendages: Alopecia, angioedema, bullous eruption, *erythema multiforme,* photosensitivity reaction, pruritus, *Stevens-Johnson syndrome,* sweating increased, *toxic epidermal necrolysis,* urticaria.

Special Senses: Abnormal vision, conjunctivitis, taste perversion, tinnitus.

Urinary System: Albuminuria, BUN increased, creatinine increased, hematuria, *interstitial nephritis,* renal failure.

DOSAGE AND ADMINISTRATION

The lowest dose of meloxicam should be sought for each patient. For the treatment of osteoarthritis the recommended starting and maintenance dose of meloxicam is 7.5 mg once daily. Some patients may receive additional benefit by increasing the dose to 15 mg once daily. The maximum recommended daily dose of meloxicam is 15 mg.

Meloxicam may be taken without regard to timing of meals.

HOW SUPPLIED

Mobic is available as a yellow, round, biconvex, uncoated tablet containing meloxicam 7.5 mg. The tablet is impressed with the Boehringer Ingelheim logo on one side, and on the other side, the letter "M".

STORAGE

Store at 25°C (77°F); excursions permitted to 15-30°C (59-86°F). Keep in a dry place.

Dispense in a tight container.

PRODUCT LISTING - EQUIVALENTS NOT AVAILABLE

Tablet - Oral - 7.5 mg			
14's	$30.03	MOBIC, Allscripts Pharmaceutical Company	54569-5121-00
20's	$47.15	MOBIC, Southwood Pharmaceuticals Inc	58016-0592-20
20's	$58.35	MOBIC, Pharma Pac	52959-0623-20
30's	$64.35	MOBIC, Allscripts Pharmaceutical Company	54569-5121-01
30's	$70.73	MOBIC, Southwood Pharmaceuticals Inc	58016-0592-30
30's	$77.88	MOBIC, Pharma Pac	52959-0623-30
60's	$141.46	MOBIC, Southwood Pharmaceuticals Inc	58016-0592-60
60's	$172.20	MOBIC, Pharma Pac	52959-0623-60
90's	$212.19	MOBIC, Southwood Pharmaceuticals Inc	58016-0592-90
100's	$235.77	MOBIC, Southwood Pharmaceuticals Inc	58016-0592-00
100's	$235.80	MOBIC, Pharma Pac	52959-0623-00
100's	$257.01	MOBIC, Boehringer-Ingelheim	00597-0029-01
Tablet - Oral - 15 mg			
14's	$33.07	MOBIC, Allscripts Pharmaceutical Company	54569-5179-00
30's	$70.85	MOBIC, Allscripts Pharmaceutical Company	54569-5179-01
30's	$100.34	MOBIC, Pharma Pac	52959-0663-30
100's	$298.61	MOBIC, Abbott Pharmaceutical	00597-0030-01

Melphalan *(001717)*

Categories: Myeloma, multiple; Pregnancy Category D; FDA Approved 1970 May; Orphan Drugs
Drug Classes: Antineoplastics, alkylating agents
Brand Names: **Alkeran**
Cost of Therapy: $115.05 (Multiple Myeloma; Alkeran; 2 mg; 3 tablets/day; 14 day supply)
HCFA JCODE(S): J9245 50 mg IV; J8600 2 mg ORAL

INTRAVENOUS

WARNING

Melphalan should be administered under the supervision of a qualified physician experienced in the use of cancer chemotherapeutic agents. Severe bone marrow suppression with resulting infection or bleeding may occur. Controlled trials comparing intravenous (IV) to oral melphalan have shown more myelosuppression with the IV formulation. Hypersensitivity reactions, including anaphylaxis, have occurred in approximately 2% of patients who received the IV formulation. Melphalan is leukemogenic in humans. Melphalan produces chromosomal aberrations *in vitro* and *in vivo* and, therefore, should be considered potentially mutagenic in humans.

DESCRIPTION

Melphalan, also known as L-phenylalanine mustard, phenylalanine mustard, L-PAM, or L-sarcolysin, is a phenylalanine derivative of nitrogen mustard. Melphalan is a bifunctional alkylating agent that is active against selected human neoplastic diseases. It is known chemically as 4-[bis(2-chloroethyl)amino]-*L*-phenylalanine. The molecular formula is $C_{13}H_{18}Cl_2N_2O_2$ and the molecular weight is 305.20.

Melphalan is the active L-isomer of the compound and was first synthesized in 1953 by Bergel and Stock; the D-isomer, known as medphalan, is less active against certain animal tumors, and the dose needed to produce effects on chromosomes is larger than that required with the L-isomer. The racemic (DL-) form is known as merphalan or sarcolysin.

Melphalan is practically insoluble in water and has a pKa_1 of 2.5.

Melphalan for injection is supplied as a sterile, nonpyrogenic, freeze-dried powder. Each single-use vial contains melphalan hydrochloride equivalent to 50 mg melphalan and 20 mg povidone. Alkeran for injection is reconstituted using the sterile diluent provided. Each vial of sterile diluent contains sodium citrate 0.2 g, propylene glycol 6.0 ml, ethanol (96%) 0.52 ml, and water for injection to a total of 10 ml. Alkeran for injection is administered intravenously.

CLINICAL PHARMACOLOGY

Melphalan is an alkylating agent of the bischloroethylamine type. As a result, its cytotoxicity appears to be related to the extent of its interstrand cross-linking with DNA, probably by binding at the N^7 position of guanine. Like other bifunctional alkylating agents, it is active against both resting and rapidly dividing tumor cells.

PHARMACOKINETICS

The pharmacokinetics of melphalan after IV administration has been extensively studied in adult patients. Following injection, drug plasma concentrations declined rapidly in a biexponential manner with distribution phase and terminal elimination phase half-lives of approximately 10 and 75 minutes, respectively. Estimates of average total body clearance varied among studies, but typical values of approximately 7-9 ml/min/kg (250-325 ml/min/m^2) were observed. One study has reported that on repeat dosing of 0.5 mg/kg every 6 weeks, the clearance of melphalan decreased from 8.1 ml/min/kg after the first course, to 5.5 ml/min/kg after the third course, but did not decrease appreciably after the third course. Mean ($\pm$SD) peak melphalan plasma concentrations in myeloma patients given IV melphalan at doses of 10 or 20 mg/m^2 were 1.2 $\pm$ 0.4 and 2.8 $\pm$ 1.9 µg/ml, respectively.

The steady-state volume of distribution of melphalan is 0.5 L/kg. Penetration into cerebrospinal fluid (CSF) is low. The extent of melphalan binding to plasma proteins ranges from 60-90%. Serum albumin is the major binding protein, while α_1-acid glycoprotein appears to account for about 20% of the plasma protein binding. Approximately 30% of the drug is (covalently) irreversibly bound to plasma proteins. Interactions with immunoglobulins have been found to be negligible.

Melphalan is eliminated from plasma primarily by chemical hydrolysis to monohydroxymelphalan and dihydroxymelphalan. Aside from these hydrolysis products, no other melphalan metabolites have been observed in humans. Although the contribution of renal elimination to melphalan clearance appears to be low, one study noted an increase in the occurrence of severe leukopenia in patients with elevated BUN after 10 weeks of therapy.

INDICATIONS AND USAGE

Melphalan for injection is indicated for the palliative treatment of patients with multiple myeloma for whom oral therapy is not appropriate.

NON-FDA APPROVED INDICATIONS

Melphalan has also shown efficacy in the treatment of amyloidosis (when administered along with prednisone). However, this use has not been approved by the FDA and further clinical trials are needed.

CONTRAINDICATIONS

Melphalan should not be used in patients whose disease has demonstrated prior resistance to this agent. Patients who have demonstrated hypersensitivity to melphalan should not be given the drug.

WARNINGS

Melphalan should be administered in carefully adjusted dosage by or under the supervision of experienced physicians who are familiar with the drug's actions and the possible complications of its use.

As with other nitrogen mustard drugs, excessive dosage will produce marked bone marrow suppression. Bone marrow suppression is the most significant toxicity associated with melphalan for injection in most patients. Therefore, the following tests should be performed at the start of therapy and prior to each subsequent dose of melphalan: platelet count, hemoglobin, white blood cell count, and differential. Thrombocytopenia and/or leukopenia are indications to withhold further therapy until the blood counts have sufficiently recovered. Frequent blood counts are essential to determine optimal dosage and to avoid toxicity. Dose adjustment on the basis of blood counts at the nadir and day of treatment should be considered.

Hypersensitivity reactions including anaphylaxis have occurred in approximately 2% of patients who received the IV formulation (see ADVERSE REACTIONS). These reactions usually occur after multiple courses of treatment. Treatment is symptomatic. The infusion should be terminated immediately, followed by the administration of volume expanders, pressor agents, corticosteroids, or antihistamines at the discretion of the physician. If a hypersensitivity reaction occurs, IV or oral melphalan should not be readministered since hypersensitivity reactions have also been reported with oral melphalan.

CARCINOGENESIS

Secondary malignancies, including acute nonlymphocytic leukemia, myeloproliferative syndrome, and carcinoma, have been reported in patients with cancer treated with alkylating agents (including melphalan). Some patients also received other chemotherapeutic agents or radiation therapy. Precise quantitation of the risk of acute leukemia, myeloproliferative syndrome, or carcinoma is not possible. Published reports of leukemia in patients who have received melphalan (and other alkylating agents) suggest that the risk of leukemogenesis increases with chronicity of treatment and with cumulative dose. In one study, the 10 year cumulative risk of developing acute leukemia or myeloproliferative syndrome after oral melphalan therapy was 19.5% for cumulative doses ranging from 730-9652 mg. In this same study, as well as in an additional study, the 10 year cumulative risk of developing acute leukemia or myeloproliferative syndrome after oral melphalan therapy was less than 2% for cumulative doses under 600 mg. This does not mean that there is a cumulative dose below which there is no risk of the induction of secondary malignancy. The potential benefits from melphalan therapy must be weighed on an individual basis against the possible risk of the induction of a second malignancy.

Adequate and well-controlled carcinogenicity studies have not been conducted in animals. However, intraperitoneal (IP) administration of melphalan in rats (5.4 to 10.8 mg/m^2) and in mice (2.25 to 4.5 mg/m^2) 3 times per week for 6 months followed by 12 months post-dose observation produced peritoneal sarcoma and lung tumors, respectively.

MUTAGENESIS

Melphalan has been shown to cause chromatid or chromosome damage in humans. Intramuscular administration of melphalan at 6 and 60 mg/m^2 produced structural aberrations of the chromatid and chromosomes in bone marrow cells of Wistar rats.

IMPAIRMENT OF FERTILITY

Melphalan causes suppression of ovarian function in premenopausal women, resulting in amenorrhea in a significant number of patients. Reversible and irreversible testicular suppression have also been reported.

PREGNANCY CATEGORY D

Melphalan may cause fetal harm when administered to a pregnant woman. While adequate animal studies have not been conducted with IV melphalan, oral (6-18 mg/m^2/day for 10 days) and IP (18 mg/m^2) administration in rats was embryolethal and teratogenic. Malformations resulting from melphalan included alterations of the brain (underdevelopment, deformation, meningocele, and encephalocele) and eye (anophthalmia and microphthalmos), reduction of the mandible and tail, as well as hepatocele (exomphaly). There are no adequate and well-controlled studies in pregnant women. If this drug is used during pregnancy, or if the patient becomes pregnant while taking this drug, the patient should be apprised of the potential hazard to the fetus. Women of childbearing potential should be advised to avoid becoming pregnant.

PRECAUTIONS

GENERAL

In all instances where the use of melphalan for injection is considered for chemotherapy, the physician must evaluate the need and usefulness of the drug against the risk of adverse events. Melphalan should be used with extreme caution in patients whose bone marrow reserve may have been compromised by prior irradiation or chemotherapy or whose marrow function is recovering from previous cytotoxic therapy.

Dose reduction should be considered in patients with renal insufficiency receiving IV melphalan. In one trial, increased bone marrow suppression was observed in patients with BUN levels ≥30 mg/dl. A 50% reduction in the IV melphalan dose decreased the incidence of severe bone marrow suppression in the latter portion of this study.

INFORMATION FOR THE PATIENT

Patients should be informed that the major acute toxicities of melphalan are related to bone marrow suppression, hypersensitivity reactions, gastrointestinal toxicity, and pulmonary toxicity. The major long-term toxicities are related to infertility and secondary malignancies. Patients should never be allowed to take the drug without close medical supervision and should be advised to consult their physicians if they experience skin rash, signs or symptoms of vasculitis, bleeding, fever, persistent cough, nausea, vomiting, amenorrhea, weight loss, or unusual lumps/masses. Women of childbearing potential should be advised to avoid becoming pregnant.

LABORATORY TESTS

Periodic complete blood counts with differentials should be performed during the course of treatment with melphalan. At least one determination should be obtained prior to each dose. Patients should be observed closely for consequences of bone marrow suppression, which include severe infections, bleeding, and symptomatic anemia (see WARNINGS).

CARCINOGENESIS, MUTAGENESIS, AND IMPAIRMENT OF FERTILITY

See WARNINGS.

PREGNANCY, TERATOGENIC EFFECTS, PREGNANCY CATEGORY D

See WARNINGS.

NURSING MOTHERS

It is not known whether this drug is excreted in human milk. IV melphalan should not be given to nursing mothers.

PEDIATRIC USE

The safety and effectiveness in pediatric patients have not been established.

GERIATRIC USE

Clinical experience with melphalan has not identified differences in responses between the elderly and younger patients. In general, dose selection for an elderly patient should be cautious, reflecting the greater frequency of decreased hepatic, renal, or cardiac function, and of concomitant disease or other drug therapy.

DRUG INTERACTIONS

The development of severe renal failure has been reported in patients treated with a single dose of IV melphalan followed by standard oral doses of cyclosporine. Cisplatin may affect melphalan kinetics by inducing renal dysfunction and subsequently altering melphalan clearance. IV melphalan may also reduce the threshold for BCNU lung toxicity. When nalidixic acid and IV melphalan are given simultaneously, the incidence of severe hemorrhagic necrotic enterocolitis has been reported to increase in pediatric patients.

ADVERSE REACTIONS

The following information on adverse reactions is based on data from both oral and IV administration of melphalan as a single agent, using several different dose schedules for treatment of a wide variety of malignancies.

Hematologic: The most common side effect is bone marrow suppression. White blood cell count and platelet count nadirs usually occur 2-3 weeks after treatment, with recovery in 4-5 weeks after treatment. Irreversible bone marrow failure has been reported.

Gastrointestinal: Gastrointestinal disturbances such as nausea and vomiting, diarrhea, and oral ulceration occur infrequently. Hepatic disorders ranging from abnormal liver function tests to clinical manifestations such as hepatitis and jaundice have been reported. Hepatic veno-occlusive disease has been reported.

Hypersensitivity: Acute hypersensitivity reactions including anaphylaxis were reported in 2.4% of 425 patients receiving melphalan for injection for myeloma (see WARNINGS). These reactions were characterized by urticaria, pruritus, edema, and in some patients, tachycardia, bronchospasm, dyspnea, and hypotension. These patients appeared to respond to antihistamine and corticosteroid therapy. If a hypersensitivity reaction occurs, IV or oral melphalan should not be readministered since hypersensitivity reactions have also been reported with oral melphalan.

Miscellaneous: Other reported adverse reactions include skin hypersensitivity, skin ulceration at injection site, skin necrosis rarely requiring skin grafting, vasculitis, alopecia, hemolytic anemia, allergic reaction, pulmonary fibrosis, and interstitial pneumonitis.

DOSAGE AND ADMINISTRATION

The usual IV dose is 16 mg/m^2. Dosage reduction of up to 50% should be considered in patients with renal insufficiency (BUN ≥30 mg/dl) (see PRECAUTIONS, General). The drug is administered as a single infusion over 15-20 minutes. Melphalan is administered at 2 week intervals for 4 doses, then, after adequate recovery from toxicity, at 4 week intervals. Available evidence suggests about one-third to one-half of the patients with multiple myeloma show a favorable response to the drug. Experience with oral melphalan suggests that repeated courses should be given since improvement may continue slowly over many months, and the maximum benefit may be missed if treatment is abandoned prematurely.

Dose adjustment on the basis of blood cell counts at the nadir and day of treatment should be considered.

ADMINISTRATION PRECAUTIONS

As with other toxic compounds, caution should be exercised in handling and preparing the solution of melphalan. Skin reactions associated with accidental exposure may occur. The use of gloves is recommended. If the solution of melphalan contacts the skin or mucosa, immediately wash the skin or mucosa thoroughly with soap and water.

Procedures for proper handling and disposal of anticancer drugs should be considered. Several guidelines on this subject have been published.[1-7] There is no general agreement that all of the procedures recommended in the guidelines are necessary or appropriate.

Parenteral drug products should be visually inspected for particulate matter and discoloration prior to administration whenever solution and container permit. If either occurs, do not use this product.

Preparation for Administration/Stability:

Melphalan for injection must be reconstituted by rapidly injecting 10 ml of the supplied diluent directly into the vial of lyophilized powder using a sterile needle (20 gauge or larger needle diameter) and syringe. Immediately shake vial vigorously until a clear solution is obtained. This provides a 5 mg/ml solution of melphalan. Rapid addition of the diluent followed by immediate vigorous shaking is important for proper dissolution.

Immediately dilute the dose to be administered in 0.9% sodium chloride injection to a concentration not greater than 0.45 mg/ml.

Administer the diluted product over a minimum of 15 minutes.

Complete administration within 60 minutes of reconstitution.

The time between reconstitution/dilution and administration of melphalan should be kept to a minimum because reconstituted and diluted solutions of melphalan are unstable. Over as short a time as 30 minutes, a citrate derivative of melphalan has been detected in reconstituted material from the reaction of melphalan with sterile diluent for melphalan. Upon further dilution with saline, nearly 1% label strength of melphalan hydrolyzes every 10 minutes.

A precipitate forms if the reconstituted solution is stored at 5°C. DO NOT REFRIGERATE THE RECONSTITUTED PRODUCT.

HOW SUPPLIED

Alkeran for injection is supplied in a carton containing one single-use clear glass vial of freeze-dried melphalan hydrochloride equivalent to 50 mg melphalan and one 10 ml clear glass vial of sterile diluent.

Storage: Store at controlled room temperature 15-30°C (59-86°F) and protect from light.

ORAL

> **WARNING**
>
> **Melphalan should be administered under the supervision of a qualified physician experienced in the use of cancer chemotherapeutic agents. Severe bone marrow suppression with resulting infection or bleeding may occur. Melphalan is leukemogenic in humans.**
>
> **Melphalan produces chromosomal aberrations *in vitro* and *in vivo* and, therefore, should be considered potentially mutagenic in humans.**

DESCRIPTION

Melphalan, also known as L-phenylalanine mustard, phenylalanine mustard, L-PAM, or L-sarcolysin, is a phenylalanine derivative of nitrogen mustard. Melphalan is a bifunctional alkylating agent which is active against selective human neoplastic diseases. It is known chemically as 4-[bis(2-chloroethyl)amino]-*L*-phenylalanine. The molecular formula is $C_{13}H_{18}Cl_2N_2O_2$ and the molecular weight is 305.20.

Melphalan is the active L-isomer of the compound and was first synthesized in 1953 by Bergel and Stock; the D-isomer, known as medphalan, is less active against certain animal tumors, and the dose needed to produce effects on chromosomes is larger than that required with the L-isomer. The racemic (DL-) form is known as merphalan or sarcolysin.

Melphalan is practically insoluble in water and has a pK_{a_1} of ~2.5.

Alkeran is available in tablet form for oral administration. Each film-coated tablet contains 2 mg melphalan and the inactive ingredients colloidal silicon dioxide, crospovidone, hypromellose, macrogol/PEG 400, magnesium stearate, microcrystalline cellulose, and titanium dioxide.

CLINICAL PHARMACOLOGY

Melphalan is an alkylating agent of the bischloroethylamine type. As a result, its cytotoxicity appears to be related to the extent of its interstrand cross-linking with DNA, probably by binding at the N^7 position of guanine. Like other bifunctional alkylating agents, it is active against both resting and rapidly dividing tumor cells.

PHARMACOKINETICS

The pharmacokinetics of melphalan after oral administration has been extensively studied in adult patients. Plasma melphalan levels are highly variable after oral dosing, both with respect to the time of the first appearance of melphalan in plasma (range approximately 0-6 hours) and to the peak plasma concentration (C_{max}) (range 70-4000 ng/ml, depending upon the dose) achieved. These results may be due to incomplete intestinal absorption, a variable "first pass" hepatic metabolism, or to rapid hydrolysis. Five patients were studied after both oral and intravenous (IV) dosing with 0.6 mg/kg as a single bolus dose by each route. The areas under the plasma concentration-time curves (AUC) after oral administration averaged 61% ± 26% (± standard deviation [SD]; range 25-89%) of those following IV administration. In 18 patients given a single oral dose of 0.6 mg/kg of melphalan, the terminal elimination plasma half-life ($T_{1/2}$) of parent drug was 1.5 ± 0.83 hours. The 24 hour urinary excretion of parent drug in these patients was 10% ± 4.5%, suggesting that renal clearance is not a major route of elimination of parent drug. In a separate study in 18 patients given single oral doses of 0.2 to 0.25 mg/kg of melphalan, C_{max} and AUC, when dose adjusted to a dose of 14 mg, were (mean ±SD) 212 ± 74 ng/ml and 498 ± 137 ng·h/ml, respectively. Elimination phase $T_{½}$ in these patients was approximately 1 hour and the median T_{max} was 1 hour.

One study using universally labeled ^{14}C-melphalan, found substantially less radioactivity in the urine of patients given the drug by mouth (30% of administered dose in 9 days) than in the urine of those given it intravenously (35-65% in 7 days). Following either oral or IV administration, the pattern of label recovery was similar, with the majority being recovered in the first 24 hours. Following oral administration, peak radioactivity occurred in plasma at 2 hours and then disappeared with a half-life of approximately 160 hours. In one patient where parent drug (rather than just radiolabel) was determined, the melphalan half-disappearance time was 67 minutes.

The steady-state volume of distribution of melphalan is 0.5 L/kg. Penetration into cerebrospinal fluid (CSF) is low. The extent of melphalan binding to plasma proteins ranges from 60-90%. Serum albumin is the major binding protein, while α_1-acid glycoprotein appears to account for about 20% of the plasma protein binding. Approximately 30% of melphalan is (covalently) irreversibly bound to plasma proteins. Interactions with immunoglobulins have been found to be negligible.

Melphalan is eliminated from plasma primarily by chemical hydrolysis to monohydroxymelphalan and dihydroxymelphalan. Aside from these hydrolysis products, no other melphalan metabolites have been observed in humans. Although the contribution of renal elimination to melphalan clearance appears to be low, one pharmacokinetic study showed a significant positive correlation between the elimination rate constant for melphalan and renal function and a significant negative correlation between renal function and the area under the plasma melphalan concentration/time curve.

INDICATIONS AND USAGE

Melphalan tablets are indicated for the palliative treatment of multiple myeloma and for the palliation of non-resectable epithelial carcinoma of the ovary.

NON-FDA APPROVED INDICATIONS

Melphalan has also shown efficacy in the treatment of amyloidosis (when administered along with prednisone). However, this use has not been approved by the FDA and further clinical trials are needed.

CONTRAINDICATIONS

Melphalan should not be used in patients whose disease has demonstrated a prior resistance to this agent. Patients who have demonstrated hypersensitivity to melphalan should not be given the drug.

M

WARNINGS

Melphalan should be administered in carefully adjusted dosage by or under the supervision of experienced physicians who are familiar with the drug's actions and the possible complications of its use.

As with other nitrogen mustard drugs, excessive dosage will produce marked bone marrow suppression. Bone marrow suppression is the most significant toxicity associated with melphalan in most patients. Therefore, the following tests should be performed at the start of therapy and prior to each subsequent course of melphalan: platelet count, hemoglobin, white blood cell count, and differential. Thrombocytopenia and/or leukopenia are indications to withhold further therapy until the blood counts have sufficiently recovered. Frequent blood counts are essential to determine optimal dosage and to avoid toxicity (see PRECAUTIONS, Laboratory Tests). Dose adjustment on the basis of blood counts at the nadir and day of treatment should be considered.

Hypersensitivity reactions, including anaphylaxis, have occurred rarely (see ADVERSE REACTIONS). These reactions have occurred after multiple courses of treatment and have recurred in patients who experienced a hypersensitivity reaction to IV melphalan. If a hypersensitivity reaction occurs, oral or IV melphalan should not be readministered.

CARCINOGENESIS

Secondary malignancies, including acute nonlymphocytic leukemia, myeloproliferative syndrome, and carcinoma have been reported in patients with cancer treated with alkylating agents (including melphalan). Some patients also received other chemotherapeutic agents or radiation therapy. Precise quantitation of the risk of acute leukemia, myeloproliferative syndrome, or carcinoma is not possible. Published reports of leukemia in patients who have received melphalan (and other alkylating agents) suggest that the risk of leukemogenesis increases with chronicity of treatment and with cumulative dose. In one study, the 10 year cumulative risk of developing acute leukemia or myeloproliferative syndrome after melphalan therapy was 19.5% for cumulative doses ranging from 730-9652 mg. In this same study, as well as in an additional study, the 10 year cumulative risk of developing acute leukemia or myeloproliferative syndrome after melphalan therapy was less than 2% for cumulative doses under 600 mg. This does not mean that there is a cumulative dose below which there is no risk of the induction of secondary malignancy. The potential benefits from melphalan therapy must be weighed on an individual basis against the possible risk of the induction of a second malignancy.

Adequate and well-controlled carcinogenicity studies have not been conducted in animals. However, IP administration of melphalan in rats (5.4 to 10.8 mg/m^2) and in mice (2.25 to 4.5 mg/m^2) 3 times per week for 6 months followed by 12 months post-dose observation produced peritoneal sarcoma and lung tumors, respectively.

MUTAGENESIS

Melphalan has been shown to cause chromatid or chromosome damage in humans. Intramuscular administration of melphalan at 6 and 60 mg/m^2 produced structural aberrations of the chromatid and chromosomes in bone marrow cells of Wistar rats.

IMPAIRMENT OF FERTILITY

Melphalan causes suppression of ovarian function in premenopausal women, resulting in amenorrhea in a significant number of patients. Reversible and irreversible testicular suppression have also been reported.

PREGNANCY CATEGORY D

Melphalan may cause fetal harm when administered to a pregnant woman. Melphalan was embryolethal and teratogenic in rats following oral (6-18 mg/m^2/day for 10 days) and intraperitoneal (18 mg/m^2) administration. Malformations resulting from melphalan included alterations of the brain (underdevelopment, deformation, meningocele, and encephalocele) and eye (anophthalmia and microphthalmos), reduction of the mandible and tail, as well as hepatocele (exomphaly).

There are no adequate and well-controlled studies in pregnant women. If this drug is used during pregnancy, or if the patient becomes pregnant while taking this drug, the patient should be apprised of the potential hazard to the fetus. Women of childbearing potential should be advised to avoid becoming pregnant.

PRECAUTIONS

GENERAL

In all instances where the use of melphalan is considered for chemotherapy, the physician must evaluate the need and usefulness of the drug against the risk of adverse events. Melphalan should be used with extreme caution in patients whose bone marrow reserve may have been compromised by prior irradiation or chemotherapy, or whose marrow function is recovering from previous cytotoxic therapy. If the leukocyte count falls below 3000 cells/µl, or the platelet count below 100,000 cells/µl, melphalan should be discontinued until the peripheral blood cell counts have recovered.

A recommendation as to whether or not dosage reduction should be made routinely in patients with renal insufficiency cannot be made because:

There is considerable inherent patient-to-patient variability in the systemic availability of melphalan in patients with normal renal function.

Only a small amount of the administered dose appears as parent drug in the urine of patients with normal renal function.

Patients with azotemia should be closely observed, however, in order to make dosage reductions, if required, at the earliest possible time.

INFORMATION FOR THE PATIENT

Patients should be informed that the major toxicities of melphalan are related to bone marrow suppression, hypersensitivity reactions, gastrointestinal toxicity, and pulmonary toxicity. The major long-term toxicities are related to infertility and secondary malignancies. Patients should never be allowed to take the drug without close medical supervision and should be advised to consult their physician if they experience skin rash, vasculitis, bleeding, fever, persistent cough, nausea, vomiting, amenorrhea, weight loss, or unusual lumps/masses. Women of childbearing potential should be advised to avoid becoming pregnant.

LABORATORY TESTS

Periodic complete blood counts with differentials should be performed during the course of treatment with melphalan. At least one determination should be obtained prior to each treatment course. Patients should be observed closely for consequences of bone marrow suppression, which include severe infections, bleeding, and symptomatic anemia (see WARNINGS).

CARCINOGENESIS, MUTAGENESIS, AND IMPAIRMENT OF FERTILITY

See WARNINGS.

PREGNANCY, TERATOGENIC EFFECTS, PREGNANCY CATEGORY D

See WARNINGS.

NURSING MOTHERS

It is not known whether this drug is excreted in human milk. Melphalan should not be given to nursing mothers.

PEDIATRIC USE

The safety and effectiveness of melphalan in pediatric patients have not been established.

GERIATRIC USE

Clinical experience with melphalan has not identified differences in responses between the elderly and younger patients. In general, dose selection for an elderly patient should be cautious, reflecting the greater frequency of decreased hepatic, renal, or cardiac function, and of concomitant disease or other drug therapy.

DRUG INTERACTIONS

There are no known drug/drug interactions with oral melphalan.

ADVERSE REACTIONS

Hematologic: The most common side effect is bone marrow suppression. Although bone marrow suppression frequently occurs, it is usually reversible if melphalan is withdrawn early enough. However, irreversible bone marrow failure has been reported.

Gastrointestinal: Gastrointestinal disturbances such as nausea and vomiting, diarrhea, and oral ulceration occur infrequently. Hepatic disorders ranging from abnormal liver function tests to clinical manifestations such as hepatitis and jaundice have been reported.

Miscellaneous: Other reported adverse reactions include: pulmonary fibrosis and interstitial pneumonitis, skin hypersensitivity, vasculitis, alopecia, and hemolytic anemia. Allergic reactions, including rare anaphylaxis, have occurred after multiple courses of treatment.

DOSAGE AND ADMINISTRATION

MULTIPLE MYELOMA

The usual oral dose is 6 mg (3 tablets) daily. The entire daily dose may be given at one time. The dose is adjusted, as required, on the basis of blood counts done at approximately weekly intervals. After 2-3 weeks of treatment, the drug should be discontinued for up to 4 weeks, during which time the blood count should be followed carefully. When the white blood cell and platelet counts are rising, a maintenance dose of 2 mg daily may be instituted. Because of the patient-to-patient variation in melphalan plasma levels following oral administration of the drug, several investigators have recommended that the dosage of melphalan be cautiously escalated until some myelosuppression is observed in order to assure that potentially therapeutic levels of the drug have been reached.

Other dosage regimens have been used by various investigators. Osserman and Takatsuki have used an initial course of 10 mg/day for 7-10 days. They report that maximal suppression of the leukocyte and platelet counts occurs within 3-5 weeks and recovery within 4-8 weeks. Continuous maintenance therapy with 2 mg/day is instituted when the white blood cell count is greater than 4000 cells/μl and the platelet count is greater than 100,000 cells/μl. Dosage is adjusted to between 1 and 3 mg/day depending upon the hematological response. It is desirable to try to maintain a significant degree of bone marrow depression so as to keep the leukocyte count in the range of 3000-3500 cells/μl.

Hoogstraten *et al.* have started treatment with 0.15 mg/kg/day for 7 days. This is followed by a rest period of at least 14 days, but it may be as long as 5-6 weeks. Maintenance therapy is started when the white blood cell and platelet counts are rising. The maintenance dose is 0.05 mg/kg/day or less and is adjusted according to the blood count.

Available evidence suggests that about one-third to one-half of the patients with multiple myeloma show a favorable response to oral administration of the drug.

One study by Alexanian *et al.* has shown that the use of melphalan in combination with prednisone significantly improves the percentage of patients with multiple myeloma who achieve palliation. One regimen has been to administer courses of melphalan at 0.25 mg/kg/day for 4 consecutive days (or, 0.20 mg/kg/day for 5 consecutive days) for a total dose of 1 mg/kg per course. These 4-5 day courses are then repeated every 4-6 weeks if the granulocyte count and the platelet count have returned to normal levels.

It is to be emphasized that response may be very gradual over many months; it is important that repeated courses or continuous therapy be given since improvement may continue slowly over many months, and the maximum benefit may be missed if treatment is abandoned too soon.

In patients with moderate to severe renal impairment, currently available pharmacokinetic data do not justify an absolute recommendation on dosage reduction to those patients, but it may be prudent to use a reduced dose initially.

EPITHELIAL OVARIAN CANCER

One commonly employed regimen for the treatment of ovarian carcinoma has been to administer melphalan at a dose of 0.2 mg/kg daily for 5 days as a single course. Courses are repeated every 4-5 weeks depending upon hematologic tolerance.

ADMINISTRATION PRECAUTIONS

Procedures for proper handling and disposal of anticancer drugs should be considered. Several guidelines on this subject have been published.[1-7]

There is no general agreement that all of the procedures recommended in the guidelines are necessary or appropriate.

HOW SUPPLIED

Alkeran is supplied as white, film-coated, round, biconvex tablets containing 2 mg melphalan in amber glass bottles with child-resistant closures. One side is engraved with "GX EH3" and the other side is engraved with an "A".

Storage: Store in a refrigerator, 2-8°C (36-46°F). Protect from light.

PRODUCT LISTING - EQUIVALENTS NOT AVAILABLE

Powder For Injection - Intravenous - 50 mg

1's	$460.64	ALKERAN I.V., Glaxosmithkline	00173-0130-93

Tablet - Oral - 2 mg

50's	$136.96	ALKERAN, Glaxosmithkline	00173-0045-35

Meperidine Hydrochloride (001727)

For related information, see the comparative table section in Appendix A.

Categories: Analgesia, obstetrical; Anesthesia, adjunct; Pain, moderate to severe; Pain, obstetrical; Sedation, obstetrical; DEA Class CII; FDA Approved 1942 Nov; Pregnancy Category C; WHO Formulary

Drug Classes: Analgesics, narcotic; Preanesthetics

Brand Names: **Demerol**

Foreign Brand Availability: Alodan "Gerot" (Austria); Centralgin (Switzerland); Dolantin (Germany); Dolantina (Spain); Dolantine (Belgium); Dolestine (Israel); Neomochin (Japan); Opistan (Japan); Pethidine (England; India; Korea); Pethidine Injection (Australia; New-Zealand); Pethidine Roche (South-Africa); Pethidine Tablet (New-Zealand); Petidin (Denmark; Finland; Norway; Sweden)

HCFA JCODE(S): J2175 per 100 mg IM, IV, SC

IM-IV-SC

DESCRIPTION

Warning: May be habit forming.

Meperidine hydrochloride is ethyl 1-methyl-4-phenylisonipecotate hydrochloride, a white crystalline substance with a melting point of 186-189°C. It is readily soluble in water and has a neutral reaction and a slightly bitter taste. The solution is not decomposed by a short period of boiling.

Demerol injectable is supplied in Carpuject, Carpuject with InterLink, Carpuject with Luer Lock and Carpuject with blunt cannula of 2.5% (25 mg/1 ml), 5% (50 mg/1 ml), 7.5% (75 mg/1 ml), and 10% (100 mg/1 ml). Uni-Amp unit dose pak-ampuls of 5% solution (25 mg/0.5 ml), (50 mg/1 ml), (75 mg/1.5 ml), (100 mg/2 ml), and 10% solution (100 mg/1 ml). Uni-Nest ampul pak-ampuls of 5% solution (25 mg/0.5 ml), (50 mg/1 ml), (75 mg/1.5 ml), (100 mg/2 ml), and 10% solution (100 mg/1 ml). Multiple-dose vials of 5% and 10% solutions contain metacresol 0.1% as preservative.

The pH of Demerol solutions is adjusted between 3.5 and 6 with sodium hydroxide or hydrochloric acid.

Demerol 5% solution has a specific gravity of 1.0086 at 20°C and 10% a specific gravity of 1.0165 at 20°C.

CLINICAL PHARMACOLOGY

Meperidine HCl is a narcotic analgesic with multiple actions qualitatively similar to those of morphine; the most prominent of these involve the central nervous system and organs composed of smooth muscle. The principal actions of therapeutic value are analgesia and sedation.

There is some evidence which suggests that meperidine may produce less smooth muscle spasm, constipation, and depression of the cough reflex than equianalgesic doses of morphine. Meperidine, in 60-80 mg parenteral doses, is approximately equivalent in analgesic effect to 10 mg of morphine. The onset of action is slightly more rapid than with morphine, and the duration of action is slightly shorter. Meperidine is significantly less effective by the oral than by the parenteral route, but the exact ratio of oral to parenteral effectiveness is unknown.

In clinical studies reported in the literature, changes in several pharmacokinetic parameters with increasing age have been observed. The initial volume of distribution and steady-state volume of distribution may be higher in elderly patients than in younger patients. The free fraction of meperidine in plasma may be higher in patients over 45 years than in younger patients.

INDICATIONS AND USAGE

- For the relief of moderate to severe pain.
- For preoperative medication.
- For support of anesthesia.
- For obstetrical analgesia.

NON-FDA APPROVED INDICATIONS

In addition, meperidine has been used for the symptomatic treatment of shivering, however this use is not approved by the FDA and standard dosage recommendations are not available.

Meperidine is available for administration via the oral, intramuscular, subcutaneous, and intravenous routes. Meperidine is also given by the epidural and intrathecal routes but standard dosage recommendations are not available and neither route is approved by the FDA.

CONTRAINDICATIONS

Hypersensitivity to meperidine.

Meperidine is contraindicated in patients who are receiving monoamine oxidase (MAO) inhibitors or those who have recently received such agents. Therapeutic doses of meperidine have occasionally precipitated unpredictable, severe, and occasionally fatal reactions in patients who have received such agents within 14 days. The mechanism of these reactions is unclear, but may be related to a preexisting hyperphenylalaninemia. Some have been characterized by coma, severe respiratory depression, cyanosis, and hypotension, and have resembled the syndrome of acute narcotic overdose. In other reactions the predominant manifestations have been hyperexcitability, convulsions, tachycardia, hyperpyrexia, and hypertension. Although it is not known that other narcotics are free of the risk of such reactions, virtually all of the reported reactions have occurred with meperidine. If a narcotic is needed in such patients, a sensitivity test should be performed in which repeated, small, incremental doses of morphine are administered over the course of several hours while the patient's condition and vital signs are under careful observation. (IV hydrocortisone or prednisolone have been used to treat severe reactions, with the addition of IV chlorpromazine in those cases exhibiting hypertension and hyperpyrexia. The usefulness and safety of narcotic antagonists in the treatment of these reactions is unknown.)

Solutions of meperidine HCl and barbiturates are chemically incompatible.

WARNINGS

DRUG DEPENDENCE

Meperidine can produce drug dependence of the morphine type and therefore has the potential for being abused. Psychic dependence, physical dependence, and tolerance may develop upon repeated administration of meperidine, and it should be prescribed and administered with the same degree of caution appropriate to the use of morphine. Like other narcotics, meperidine is subject to the provisions of the Federal narcotic laws.

INTERACTION WITH OTHER CENTRAL NERVOUS SYSTEM DEPRESSANTS

MEPERIDINE SHOULD BE USED WITH GREAT CAUTION AND IN REDUCED DOSAGE IN PATIENTS WHO ARE CONCURRENTLY RECEIVING OTHER NARCOTIC ANALGESICS, GENERAL ANESTHETICS, PHENOTHIAZINES, OTHER TRANQUILIZERS (SEE DOSAGE AND ADMINISTRATION), SEDATIVE-HYPNOTICS (INCLUDING BARBITURATES), TRICYCLIC ANTIDEPRESSANTS AND OTHER CNS DEPRESSANTS (INCLUDING ALCOHOL). RESPIRATORY DEPRESSION, HYPOTENSION, AND PROFOUND SEDATION OR COMA MAY RESULT.

HEAD INJURY AND INCREASED INTRACRANIAL PRESSURE

The respiratory depressant effects of meperidine and its capacity to elevate cerebrospinal fluid pressure may be markedly exaggerated in the presence of head injury, other intracranial lesions, or a preexisting increase in intracranial pressure. Furthermore, narcotics produce adverse reactions which may obscure the clinical course of patients with head injuries.

In such patients, meperidine must be used with extreme caution and only if its use is deemed essential.

INTRAVENOUS USE

If necessary, meperidine may be given intravenously, but the injection should be given very slowly, preferably in the form of a diluted solution. Rapid IV injection of narcotic analgesics, including meperidine, increases the incidence of adverse reactions; severe respiratory depression, apnea, hypotension, peripheral circulatory collapse, and cardiac arrest have occurred. Meperidine should not be administered intravenously unless a narcotic antagonist and the facilities for assisted or controlled respiration are immediately available. When meperidine is given parenterally, especially intravenously, the patient should be lying down.

ASTHMA AND OTHER RESPIRATORY CONDITIONS

Meperidine should be used with extreme caution in patients having an acute asthmatic attack, patients with chronic obstructive pulmonary disease or cor pulmonale, patients having a substantially decreased respiratory reserve, and patients with preexisting respiratory depression, hypoxia, or hypercapnia. In such patients, even usual therapeutic doses of narcotics may decrease respiratory drive while simultaneously increasing airway resistance to the point of apnea.

HYPOTENSIVE EFFECT

The administration of meperidine may result in severe hypotension in the postoperative patient or any individual whose ability to maintain blood pressure has been compromised by a depleted blood volume or the administration of drugs such as the phenothiazines or certain anesthetics.

USAGE IN AMBULATORY PATIENTS

Meperidine may impair the mental and/or physical abilities required for the performance of potentially hazardous tasks such as driving a car or operating machinery. The patient should be cautioned accordingly.

Meperidine, like other narcotics, may produce orthostatic hypotension in ambulatory patients.

USAGE IN PREGNANCY AND LACTATION

Meperidine should not be used in pregnant women prior to the labor period, unless in the judgment of the physician the potential benefits outweigh the possible hazards, because safe use in pregnancy prior to labor has not been established relative to possible adverse effects on fetal development.

When used as an obstetrical analgesic, meperidine crosses the placental barrier and can produce depression of respiration and psychophysiologic functions in the newborn. Resuscitation may be required.

Meperidine appears in the milk of nursing mothers receiving the drug.

M

PRECAUTIONS

As with all intramuscular preparations, meperidine HCl intramuscular injection should be injected well within the body of a large muscle.

SUPRAVENTRICULAR TACHYCARDIAS

Meperidine should be used with caution in patients with atrial flutter and other supraventricular tachycardias because of a possible vagolytic action which may produce a significant increase in the ventricular response rate.

CONVULSIONS

Meperidine may aggravate preexisting convulsions in patients with convulsive disorders. If dosage is escalated substantially above recommended levels because of tolerance development, convulsions may occur in individuals without a history of convulsive disorders.

ACUTE ABDOMINAL CONDITIONS

The administration of meperidine or other narcotics may obscure the diagnosis of clinical course in patients with acute abdominal conditions.

SPECIAL RISK PATIENTS

Meperidine should be given with caution and the initial dose should be reduced in certain patients such as the debilitated, and those with severe impairment of hepatic or renal function, hypothyroidism, Addison's disease, and prostatic hypertrophy or urethral stricture.

GERIATRIC USE

Clinical studies of meperidine HCl did not include sufficient numbers of subjects aged 65 and over to determine whether they respond differently from younger subjects. Other reported clinical experience has not identified differences in response between the elderly and younger patients. In general, dose selection for an elderly patient should be low, usually starting at the low end of the dosing range, reflecting the greater frequency of decreased hepatic, renal, or cardiac function, and of concomitant disease or other drug therapy. (See DOSAGE AND ADMINISTRATION.)

Sedating drugs may cause confusion and oversedation in the elderly; elderly patients generally should be started on low doses of meperidine HCl and observed closely.

This drug is known to be excreted by the kidney, and the risk of toxic reactions to this drug may be greater in patients with impaired renal function. Because elderly patients are more likely to have decreased renal function, care should be taken in dose selection, and it may be useful to monitor renal function.

Clinical studies indicate that differences in various pharmacokinetic parameters may exist between elderly and younger patients. (See CLINICAL PHARMACOLOGY.)

ADVERSE REACTIONS

The major hazards of meperidine, as with other narcotic analgesics, are respiratory depression and, to a lesser degree, circulatory depression; respiratory arrest, shock, and cardiac arrest have occurred.

The most frequently observed adverse reactions include lightheadedness, dizziness, sedation, nausea, vomiting, and sweating. These effects seem to be more prominent in ambulatory patients and in those who are not experiencing severe pain. In such individuals, lower doses are advisable. Some adverse reactions in ambulatory patients may be alleviated if the patients lies down.

Other adverse reactions include:

Nervous System: Euphoria, dysphoria, weakness, headache, agitation, tremor, uncoordinated muscle movements, severe convulsions, transient hallucinations and disorientation, visual disturbances. Inadvertent injection about a nerve trunk may result in sensory-motor paralysis which is usually, though not always, transitory.

Gastrointestinal: Dry mouth, constipation, biliary tract spasm.

Cardiovascular: Flushing of the face, tachycardia, bradycardia, palpitation, hypotension (see WARNINGS), syncope, phlebitis following IV injection.

Genitourinary: Urinary retention.

Allergic: Pruritus, urticaria, other skin rashes, wheal and flare over the vein with IV injection.

Other: Pain at injection site; local tissue irritation and induration following SC injection, particularly when repeated; antidiuretic effect.

DOSAGE AND ADMINISTRATION

FOR RELIEF OF PAIN

Dosage should be adjusted according to the severity of the pain and the response of the patient. While CS administration is suitable for occasional use, IM administration is preferred when repeated doses are required. If IV administration is required, dosage should be decreased and the injection made very slowly, preferably utilizing a diluted solution. The dose of meperidine HCl should be proportionately reduced (usually by 25-50%) when administered concomitantly with phenothiazines and many other tranquilizers since they potentiate the action of meperidine HCl.

Adults: The usual dosage is 50-150 mg intramuscularly or subcutaneously every 3 or 4 hours as necessary. Elderly patients should usually be given meperidine at the lower end of the dose range and observed closely.

Children: The usual dosage is 0.5-0.8 mg/lb intramuscularly or subcutaneously up to the adult dose, every 3 or 4 hours as necessary.

FOR PREOPERATIVE MEDICATION:

Adults: The usual dosage is 50-100 mg intramuscularly or subcutaneously, 30-90 minutes before the beginning of anesthesia. Elderly patients should usually be given meperidine at the lower end of the dose range and observed closely.

Children: The usual dosage is 0.5 to 1 mg/lb intramuscularly or subcutaneously up to the adult dose, 30-90 minutes before the beginning of anesthesia.

FOR SUPPORT OF ANESTHESIA

Repeated slow IV injections of fractional dosages (*e.g.,* 10 mg/ml) or continuous IV infusion of a more dilute solution (*e.g.,* 1 mg/ml) should be used. The dose should be titrated to the needs of the patient and will depend on the premedication and type of anesthesia being employed, the characteristics of the particular patient, and the nature and duration of the operative procedure. Elderly patients should usually be given meperidine at the lower end of the dose range and observed closely.

FOR OBSTETRICAL ANALGESIA

The usual dosage is 50-100 mg intramuscularly or subcutaneously when pain becomes regular, and may be repeated at 1-3 hour intervals.

Parenteral drug products should be inspected visually for particulate and discoloration prior to administration whenever solution and container permit.

HOW SUPPLIED

For Parenteral Use.

Solutions of Demerol for parenteral use are clear and colorless and are available as follows: Carpuject, Carpuject with InterLink system cannula, Carpuject with Luer Lock and Carpuject with blunt cannula of 2.5% (25 mg/1 ml), 5% (50 mg/1 ml), 7.5% (75 mg/1 ml), and 10% (100 mg/1 ml); Uni-Amp unit dose pak 5% (25 mg/0.5 ml), (50 mg/1 ml), (75 mg/1.5 ml), (100 mg/2 ml), and 10% solution (100 mg/1 ml); Uni-Nest ampul pak 5% (25 mg/0.5 ml), (50 mg/1 ml), (75 mg/1.5 ml), (100 mg/2 ml), and 10% solution (100 mg/1 ml); and multiple-dose vials of 5% (50 mg/ml) and 10% (100 mg/ml).

To prevent needle-stick injuries, needles should not be recapped, purposely bent, or broken by hand. Blunt cannulas should not be recapped, purposely bent or broken by hand. Demerol in the blunt cannula or InterLink configuration is not intended for IM use.

Note: The pH of Demerol solutions is adjusted between 3.5 and 6 with sodium hydroxide or hydrochloric acid. Multiple-dose vials contain metacresol 0.1% as preservative. No preservatives are added to the ampuls or Carpuject sterile cartridge units.

Storage: Store at 25°C (77°F), controlled room temperature.

ORAL

DESCRIPTION

Meperidine hydrochloride, a white crystalline substance with a melting point of 186-189°C. It is readily soluble in water and has a neutral reaction and a slightly bitter taste. The solution is not decomposed by a short period of boiling.

The syrup is a pleasant-tasting, nonalcoholic, banana-flavored solution containing 50 mg of meperidine hydrochloride per 5 ml teaspoon (25 drops contain 13 mg of meperidine hydrochloride). The tablets contain 50 or 100 mg of the analgesic.

Inactive Ingredients: *Tablets:* Calcium sulfate, dibasic calcium phosphate, starch, stearic acid, talc. *Syrup:* Benzoic acid, flavor, liquid glucose, purified water, saccharin sodium. Chemically, DEMEROL is 1-Methyl-4-phenyl-4-piperidinecarboxylic acid ethyl ester hydrochloride.

CLINICAL PHARMACOLOGY

Meperidine HCl is a narcotic analgesic with multiple actions qualitatively similar to those of morphine; the most prominent of these involve the central nervous system and organs composed of smooth muscle. The principal actions of therapeutic value are analgesia and sedation.

There is some evidence which suggests that meperidine may produce less smooth muscle spasm, constipation, and depression of the cough reflex than equianalgesic doses of morphine. Meperidine, in 60-80 mg parenteral doses, is approximately equivalent in analgesic effect to 10 mg of morphine. The onset of action is lightly more rapid than with morphine, and the duration of action is slightly shorter. Meperidine is significantly less effective by the oral than by the parenteral route, but the exact ratio of oral to parenteral effectiveness is unknown.

INDICATIONS AND USAGE

Meperidine HCl is indicated for the relief of moderate to severe pain.

NON-FDA APPROVED INDICATIONS

In addition, meperidine has been used for the symptomatic treatment of shivering, however this use is not approved by the FDA and standard dosage recommendations are not available.

Meperidine is available for administration via the oral, intramuscular, subcutaneous, and intravenous routes. Meperidine is also given by the epidural and intrathecal routes but standard dosage recommendations are not available and neither route is approved by the FDA.

CONTRAINDICATIONS

Meperidine HCl is contraindicated in patients with hypersensitivity to meperidine.

Meperidine is contraindicated in patients who are receiving monoamine oxidase (MAO) inhibitors or those who have recently received such agents. Therapeutic doses of meperidine have occasionally precipitated unpredictable, severe, and occasionally fatal reactions in patients who have received such agents within 14 days. The mechanism of these reactions is unclear, but may be related to a preexisting hyperphenylalaninemia. Some have been characterized by coma, severe respiratory depression, cyanosis, and hypotension, and have resembled the syndrome of acute narcotic overdose. In other reactions the predominant manifestations have been hyperexcitability, convulsions, tachycardia, hyperpyrexia, and hypertension. Although it is not known that other narcotics are free of the risk of such reactions, virtually all of the reported reactions have occurred with meperidine. If a narcotic is needed in such patients, a sensitivity test should be performed in which repeated, small, incremental doses of morphine are administered over the course of several hours while the patient's condition and vital signs are under careful observation. (IV hydrocortisone or prednisolone have been used to treat severe reactions, with the addition of IV chlorpromazine in those cases exhibiting hypertension and hyperpyrexia. The usefulness and safety of narcotic antagonists in the treatment of these reactions is unknown.)

WARNINGS

DRUG ABUSE AND DEPENDENCE

Meperidine can produce drug dependence of the morphine type and therefore has the potential for being abused. Psychic dependence, physical dependence, and tolerance may develop upon repeated administration of meperidine, and it should be prescribed and administered with the same degree of caution appropriate to the use of morphine.

CONTROLLED SUBSTANCE

Meperidine is classified as a Schedule C-II controlled substance by federal regulation. Like other narcotics, meperidine is subject to the provisions of the federal narcotic laws.

DRUG INTERACTIONS

MEPERIDINE SHOULD BE USED WITH GREAT CAUTION AND IN REDUCED DOSAGE IN PATIENTS WHO ARE CONCURRENTLY RECEIVING OTHER NARCOTIC ANALGESICS, GENERAL ANESTHETICS, PHENOTHIAZINES, OTHER TRANQUILIZERS (SEE DOSAGE AND ADMINISTRATION), SEDATIVE-HYPNOTICS (INCLUDING BARBITURATES), TRICYCLIC ANTIDEPRESSANTS MONOAMINDE OXIDASE (MAO) INHIBITORS (see CONTRAINDICATIONS) AND OTHER CNS DEPRESSANTS (INCLUDING ALCOHOL). RESPIRATORY DEPRESSION, HYPOTENSION, AND PROFOUND SEDATION OR COMA MAY RESULT. See also PRECAUTIONS.

HEAD INJURY AND INCREASED INTRACRANIAL PRESSURE

The respiratory depressant effects of meperidine and its capacity to elevate cerebrospinal fluid pressure may be markedly exaggerated in the presence of head injury, other intracranial lesions, or a preexisting increase in intracranial pressure. Furthermore, narcotics produce adverse reactions which may obscure the clinical course of patients with head injuries. In such patients, meperidine must be used with extreme caution and only if its use is deemed essential.

ASTHMA AND OTHER RESPIRATORY CONDITIONS

Meperidine should be used with extreme caution in patients having an acute asthmatic attack, patients with chronic obstructive pulmonary disease or cor pulmonale, patients having a substantially decreased respiratory reserve, and patients with preexisting respiratory depression, hypoxia, or hypercapnia. In such patients, even usual therapeutic doses of narcotics may decrease respiratory drive while simultaneously increasing airway resistance to the point of apnea.

HYPOTENSIVE EFFECT

The administration of meperidine may result in severe hypotension in the postoperative patient or any individual whose ability to maintain blood pressure has been compromised by a depleted blood volume or the administration of drugs such as the phenothiazines or certain anesthetics.

USAGE IN AMBULATORY PATIENTS

Meperidine may impair the mental and/or physical abilities required for the performance of potentially hazardous tasks such as driving a car or operating machinery. The patient should be cautioned accordingly.

Meperidine, like other narcotics, may produce orthostatic hypotension in ambulatory patients.

USE IN PREGNANCY

Meperidine should not be used in pregnant women prior to the labor period, unless in the judgment of the physician the potential benefits outweigh the possible risks, because safe use in pregnancy prior to labor has not been established relative to possible adverse effects on fetal development.

TERATOGENIC EFFECTS: PREGNANCY CATEGORY C

Although teratogenic effects in humans have not been documented, there are no adequate and well-controlled studies in pregnant women. Meperidine is known to cross the placental barrier.

LABOR AND DELIVERY

Meperidine crosses the placental barrier and can produce depression of respiration and psychophysiologic functions in the newborn. Resuscitation may be required.

NURSING MOTHERS

Meperidine appears in the milk of nursing mothers receiving the drug. Due to the potential for serious adverse reactions in nursing infants, a decision should be made whether to discontinue nursing or to discontinue the drug, taking into account the potential benefits of the drug to the nursing woman.

PRECAUTIONS

SUPRAVENTRICULAR TACHYCARDIAS

Meperidine should be used with caution in patients with atrial flutter and other supraventricular tachycardias because of a possible vagolytic action which may produce a significant increase in the ventricular response rate.

CONVULSIONS

Meperidine may aggravate preexisting convulsions in patients with convulsive disorders. If dosage is escalated substantially above recommended levels because of tolerance development, convulsions may occur in individuals without a history of convulsive disorders.

ACUTE ABDOMINAL CONDITIONS

The administration of meperidine or other narcotics may obscure the diagnosis of clinical course in patients with acute abdominal conditions.

SPECIAL RISK PATIENTS

Meperidine should be given with caution and the initial dose should be reduced in certain patients such as the elderly or debilitated, and those with severe impairment of hepatic or renal function, sickle cell anemia, hypothyroidism, Addison's disease, pheochromocytoma, and prostatic hypertrophy or urethral stricture. In patients with pheochromocytoma, meperidine has been reported to provoke hypertension.

USAGE IN HEPATICALLY IMPAIRED PATIENTS

Accumulation of meperidine and/or its active metabolite, normeperidine, can occur in patients with hepatic impairment. Meperidine should therefore be used with caution in patients with hepatic impairment.

USAGE IN RENALLY IMPAIRED PATIENTS

Accumulation of meperidine and/or its active metabolite, normeperidine, can also occur in patients with renal impairment. Meperidine should therefore be used with caution in patients with renal impairment.

PREGNANCY

For usage during pregnancy see WARNINGS.

LABOR AND DELIVERY

See WARNINGS.

NURSING MOTHERS

See WARNINGS.

PEDIATRIC USE

Meperidine has a slower elimination rate in neonates and young infants compared to older children and adults. Neonates and young infants may also be more susceptible to the effects, especially the respiratory depressant effects. Meperidine should therefore be used with caution in neonates and young infants, and any potential benefits of the drug weighed against the relative risk to a pediatric patient.

GERIATRIC USE

Geriatric patients have a slower elimination rate compared to young patients and they may be more susceptible to the effects of meperidine. A reduction in the total daily dose of meperidine may be required in elderly patients, and the potential benefits of the drug weighed against the relative risk to a geriatric patient.

DRUG INTERACTIONS

Also see WARNINGS.

Acyclovir: Plasma concentrations of meperidine may be increased by acyclovir, thus caution should be used with concomitant administration.

M

Cimetidine: Cimetidine reduced the clearance and volume of distribution of meperidine in healthy subjects and thus, caution should be used with concomitant administration.

Phenytoin: The hepatic metabolism of meperidine may be enhanced by phenytoin. Concomitant administration resulted in reduced half-life and bioavailability in healthy subjects, however, blood concentrations of normeperidine were increased.

Ritonavir: Plasma concentrations of meperidine may be increased by ritonavir, thus concomitant administration should be avoided.

ADVERSE REACTIONS

The major hazards of meperidine, as with other narcotic analgesics, are respiratory depression and, to a lesser degree, circulatory depression; respiratory arrest, shock, and cardiac arrest have occurred.

The most frequently observed adverse reactions include lightheadedness, dizziness, sedation, nausea, vomiting, and sweating. These effects seem to be more prominent in ambulatory patients and in those who are not experiencing severe pain. In such individuals, lower doses are advisable. Some adverse reactions in ambulatory patients may be alleviated if the patients lies down.

Other adverse reactions include:

Nervous System: Euphoria, dysphoria, weakness, headache, agitation, tremor, uncoordinated muscle movements (*e.g.*, muscle twitches, myoclonus), severe convulsions, transient hallucinations and disorientation, visual disturbances.

Gastrointestinal: Dry mouth, constipation, biliary tract spasm.

Cardiovascular: Flushing of the face, tachycardia, bradycardia, palpitation, hypotension (see WARNINGS), syncope.

Genitourinary: Urinary retention.

Allergic: Pruritus, urticaria, other skin rashes, wheal and flare over the vein with intravenous injection.

DOSAGE AND ADMINISTRATION

FOR RELIEF OF PAIN

Dosage should be adjusted according to the severity of the pain and the response of the patient. Meperidine is less effective orally than on parenteral administration. The dose of meperidine HCl should be proportionately reduced (usually by 25-50%) when administered concomitantly with phenothiazines and many other tranquilizers since they potentiate the action of meperidine HCl.

Adults: The usual dosage is 50-150 mg orally, every 3 or 4 hours as necessary.

Pediatric Patients: The usual dosage is 0.5-0.8 mg/lb orally up to the adult dose, every 3 or 4 hours as necessary.

Each dose of the syrup should be taken in one-half glass of water, since if taken undiluted, it may exert a slight topical anesthetic effect on mucous membranes.

M

HOW SUPPLIED

For Oral Use

Demerol Tablets: Tablets are white, round and convex: the 50 mg tablet is scored.

Syrup: Nonalcoholic, banana-flavored 50 mg/5 ml teaspoon.

Storage: Store at 25°C (77°F); excursions permitted to 15-30°C (59-86°F).

PRODUCT LISTING - RATED THERAPEUTICALLY EQUIVALENT

Solution - Injectable - 10 mg/ml			
30 ml x 10	$117.68	GENERIC, Abbott Pharmaceutical	00074-6030-04
Solution - Injectable - 25 mg/ml			
1 ml x 10	$5.34	DEMEROL HCL, Abbott Pharmaceutical	00074-1176-01
1 ml x 10	$5.40	GENERIC, Baxter Pharmaceutical Products, Inc	10019-0151-47
1 ml x 10	$7.48	DEMEROL HCL, Abbott Pharmaceutical	00074-1176-31
1 ml x 10	$8.10	DEMEROL HCL, Abbott Pharmaceutical	00074-1176-02
1 ml x 10	$9.50	DEMEROL HCL, Abbott Pharmaceutical	00074-1176-30
1 ml x 10	$10.57	DEMEROL HCL, Abbott Pharmaceutical	00074-1176-11
1 ml x 10	$11.28	DEMEROL HCL, Abbott Pharmaceutical	00074-1176-21
1 ml x 25	$11.07	GENERIC, Esi Lederle Generics	00641-1130-25
1 ml x 25	$11.50	GENERIC, Baxter Pharmaceutical Products, Inc	10019-0151-44
1 ml x 25	$21.50	GENERIC, Esi Lederle Generics	00641-0130-25
Solution - Injectable - 50 mg/ml			
0.50 ml x 25	$13.25	DEMEROL HCL, Abbott Pharmaceutical	00074-1203-01
0.50 ml x 25	$14.25	DEMEROL HCL, Abbott Pharmaceutical	00074-1266-01
1 ml x 10	$5.82	DEMEROL HCL, Abbott Pharmaceutical	00074-1178-01
1 ml x 10	$7.60	DEMEROL HCL, Abbott Pharmaceutical	00074-1178-31
1 ml x 10	$9.14	DEMEROL HCL, Abbott Pharmaceutical	00074-1178-02
1 ml x 10	$9.90	DEMEROL HCL, Abbott Pharmaceutical	00074-1178-30
1 ml x 10	$11.88	DEMEROL HCL, Abbott Pharmaceutical	00074-1178-11
1 ml x 10	$11.99	DEMEROL HCL, Abbott Pharmaceutical	00074-1178-21
1 ml x 10	$17.50	GENERIC, Baxter Pharmaceutical Products, Inc	10019-0152-44
1 ml x 25	$9.00	DEMEROL HCL, Abbott Pharmaceutical	00074-1253-01
1 ml x 25	$12.22	GENERIC, Esi Lederle Generics	00641-1140-25
1 ml x 25	$13.25	DEMEROL HCL, Sanofi Winthrop Pharmaceuticals	00024-0371-04
1 ml x 25	$13.32	DEMEROL HCL, Sanofi Winthrop Pharmaceuticals	00024-0361-04
1 ml x 25	$13.55	DEMEROL HCL, Abbott Pharmaceutical	00074-1267-01
1 ml x 25	$23.75	GENERIC, Esi Lederle Generics	00641-0140-25
1.50 ml x 10	$13.75	DEMEROL HCL, Abbott Pharmaceutical	00074-1269-01
1.50 ml x 25	$13.75	DEMEROL HCL, Abbott Pharmaceutical	00074-1254-01
2 ml x 25	$13.75	DEMEROL HCL, Sanofi Winthrop Pharmaceuticals	00024-0373-04
2 ml x 25	$14.00	DEMEROL HCL, Abbott Pharmaceutical	00074-1255-02
2 ml x 25	$14.00	DEMEROL HCL, Abbott Pharmaceutical	00074-1271-02
30 ml	$16.25	GENERIC, Esi Lederle Generics	00008-0258-01
30 ml	$17.65	GENERIC, Ivax Corporation	00182-9130-66
30 ml	$21.40	DEMEROL HCL, Abbott Pharmaceutical	00074-1181-30
Solution - Injectable - 75 mg/ml			
1 ml x 10	$7.13	DEMEROL HCL, Abbott Pharmaceutical	00074-1179-01
1 ml x 10	$8.43	DEMEROL HCL, Abbott Pharmaceutical	00074-1179-31
1 ml x 10	$8.60	DEMEROL HCL, Abbott Pharmaceutical	00074-1179-02
1 ml x 10	$10.30	DEMEROL HCL, Abbott Pharmaceutical	00074-1179-30
1 ml x 10	$10.70	DEMEROL HCL, Abbott Pharmaceutical	00074-1179-21
1 ml x 10	$11.99	DEMEROL HCL, Abbott Pharmaceutical	00074-1179-11
1 ml x 25	$25.25	GENERIC, Esi Lederle Generics	00641-0150-25
Solution - Injectable - 100 mg/ml			
1 ml x 10	$7.60	DEMEROL HCL, Abbott Pharmaceutical	00074-1180-01
1 ml x 10	$8.00	DEMEROL HCL, Abbott Pharmaceutical	00074-1180-02
1 ml x 10	$8.91	DEMEROL HCL, Abbott Pharmaceutical	00074-1180-31
1 ml x 10	$10.60	DEMEROL HCL, Abbott Pharmaceutical	00074-1180-69
1 ml x 10	$12.59	DEMEROL HCL, Abbott Pharmaceutical	00074-1180-11
1 ml x 10	$12.71	DEMEROL HCL, Abbott Pharmaceutical	00074-1180-21
1 ml x 25	$14.00	DEMEROL HCL, Abbott Pharmaceutical	00074-1256-01
1 ml x 25	$14.75	DEMEROL HCL, Abbott Pharmaceutical	00074-2046-01
1 ml x 25	$27.25	GENERIC, Esi Lederle Generics	00641-0160-25
1 ml x 25	$30.00	GENERIC, Baxter Pharmaceutical Products, Inc	10019-0154-44
20 ml	$21.63	GENERIC, Esi Lederle Generics	00008-0259-01
20 ml	$22.90	GENERIC, Ivax Corporation	00182-9131-65
20 ml	$28.03	DEMEROL HCL, Abbott Pharmaceutical	00074-1201-20
Syrup - Oral - 50 mg/5 ml			
5 ml x 40	$37.20	GENERIC, Roxane Laboratories Inc	00054-8545-16
473 ml	$105.85	DEMEROL HCL, Sanofi Winthrop Pharmaceuticals	00024-0332-06
500 ml	$77.06	GENERIC, Roxane Laboratories Inc	00054-3545-63
Tablet - Oral - 50 mg			
25's	$15.53	GENERIC, Roxane Laboratories Inc	00054-8595-11
25's	$23.81	DEMEROL HCL, Sanofi Winthrop Pharmaceuticals	00024-0335-02
100's	$24.70	GENERIC, Ivax Corporation	00182-9140-01
100's	$25.95	GENERIC, Major Pharmaceuticals Inc	00904-1977-60
100's	$44.75	GENERIC, Mallinckrodt Medical Inc	00406-7113-01
100's	$53.70	FEDERAL UPPER LIMIT, H.C.F.A. F F P	99999-1727-01
100's	$68.25	GENERIC, Watson Laboratories Inc	00591-0726-01
100's	$68.25	GENERIC, Watson Laboratories Inc	52544-0726-01
100's	$68.60	GENERIC, Qualitest Products Inc	00603-4415-21
100's	$68.63	GENERIC, Roxane Laboratories Inc	00054-4595-25
100's	$70.95	GENERIC, Amide Pharmaceutical Inc	52152-0158-02
100's	$104.15	DEMEROL HCL, Sanofi Winthrop Pharmaceuticals	00024-0335-04
Tablet - Oral - 100 mg			
25's	$19.03	GENERIC, Roxane Laboratories Inc	00054-8596-11
100's	$38.70	GENERIC, Major Pharmaceuticals Inc	00904-1978-60
100's	$45.85	GENERIC, Ivax Corporation	00182-9141-01
100's	$103.47	FEDERAL UPPER LIMIT, H.C.F.A. F F P	99999-1727-02
100's	$129.83	GENERIC, Watson Laboratories Inc	00591-0727-01
100's	$129.83	GENERIC, Watson Laboratories Inc	52544-0727-01
100's	$130.50	GENERIC, Qualitest Products Inc	00603-4416-21
100's	$130.55	GENERIC, Roxane Laboratories Inc	00054-4596-25
100's	$132.00	GENERIC, Mallinckrodt Medical Inc	00406-7115-01
100's	$134.95	GENERIC, Amide Pharmaceutical Inc	52152-0157-02
100's	$198.09	DEMEROL HCL, Sanofi Winthrop Pharmaceuticals	00024-0337-04

PRODUCT LISTING - RATED NOT THERAPEUTICALLY EQUIVALENT

Solution - Injectable - 10 mg/ml			
50 ml x 10	$224.50	GENERIC, Baxter I.V. Systems Division	00338-2691-75

PRODUCT LISTING - EQUIVALENTS NOT AVAILABLE

Solution - Injectable - 25 mg/ml			
1 ml x 25	$18.50	GENERIC, Baxter Pharmaceutical Products, Inc	10019-0155-68
Solution - Injectable - 50 mg/ml			
1 ml x 25	$18.75	GENERIC, Baxter Pharmaceutical Products, Inc	10019-0156-68
Solution - Injectable - 75 mg/ml			
1 ml x 25	$19.50	GENERIC, Baxter Pharmaceutical Products, Inc	10019-0157-68
Solution - Injectable - 100 mg/ml			
1 ml x 25	$20.75	GENERIC, Baxter Pharmaceutical Products, Inc	10019-0158-68

Meperidine Hydrochloride; Promethazine Hydrochloride *(001728)*

Categories: Anesthesia, adjunct; Pain, moderate; DEA Class CII; FDA Approval Pre 1982; Pregnancy Category C
Drug Classes: Analgesics, narcotic; Antiemetics/antivertigo; Antihistamines, H1; Phenothiazines; Preanesthetics
Brand Names: **Mepergan**; Meprozine
HCFA JCODE(S): J2180 up to 50 mg IM, IV

DESCRIPTION

FOR COMPLETE PRESCRIBING INFORMATION, REFER TO THE INDIVIDUAL DRUG MONOGRAPHS (MEPERIDINE HYDROCHLORIDE; PROMETHAZINE HYDROCHLORIDE).

INDICATIONS AND USAGE

CAPSULES

Affords sedation as well as analgesia for moderate pain as seen in postoperative patients, postpartum patients, and in patients with pain associated with malignancies.

INJECTION

As a preanesthetic medication when analgesia and sedation are indicated. As an adjunct to local and general anesthesia.

DOSAGE AND ADMINISTRATION

CAPSULES

The usual dosage is one capsule every 4 to 6 hours as needed for the relief of pain.

INJECTION

Parenteral drug products should be inspected visually for particulate matter and discoloration prior to administration, whenever solution and container permit.

WARNING—BARBITURATES ARE NOT CHEMICALLY COMPATIBLE IN SOLUTION WITH MEPERIDINE HCl; PROMETHAZINE HCl AND SHOULD NOT BE MIXED IN THE SAME SYRINGE.

The Tubex Sterile Cartridge-Needle Unit is designed for single-dose use. Vials should be used when required doses are fractions of a milliliter, as indicated below.

Meperidine HCl; Promethazine HCl is usually administered intramuscularly. However, in certain specific situations, the intravenous route may be employed. INADVERTENT INTRA-ARTERIAL INJECTION CAN RESULT IN GANGRENE OF THE AFFECTED EXTREMITY. SUBCUTANEOUS ADMINISTRATION IS CONTRAINDICATED, AS IT MAY RESULT IN TISSUE NECROSIS. INJECTION INTO OR NEAR PERIPHERAL NERVES MAY RESULT IN PERMANENT NEUROLOGICAL DEFICIT.

When used intravenously, the rate should not be greater than 1 ml meperidine HCl; promethazine HCl (25 mg of each component) per minute; it is preferable to inject through the tubing of an intravenous infusion set that is known to be functioning satisfactorily.

Adult Dose: 1-2 ml (25-50 mg of each component) per single injection, which can be repeated every 3-4 hours.

Children 12 Years of Age and Under: 0.5 mg of each component per pound of body weight. The dosage may be repeated every 3 to 4 hours as necessary. For preanesthetic medication the usual adult dose is 2 ml (50 mg of each component) intramuscularly with or without appropriate atropinelike drug. Atropine sulfate, 0.3-0.4 mg, or scopolamine hydrobromide, 0.25-0.4 mg, in sterile solution may be mixed in the same syringe with meperidine HCl; promethazine HCl. Repeat doses of 50 mg or less of both promethazine and meperidine may be administered by either route at 3-4 hour intervals, as necessary. As an adjunct to local or general anesthesia, the usual dose is 2 ml (50 mg each of meperidine and promethazine).

PRODUCT LISTING - EQUIVALENTS NOT AVAILABLE

Capsule - Oral - 50 mg;25 mg

100's	$36.50	GENERIC, Vintage Pharmaceuticals Inc	00254-4206-28
100's	$67.65	GENERIC, Qualitest Products Inc	00603-4424-21
100's	$67.65	GENERIC, Amide Pharmaceutical Inc	52152-0190-02
100's	$67.65	GENERIC, Ethex Corporation	58177-0027-04
100's	$75.25	MEPERGAN FORTIS, Esi Lederle Generics	00008-0261-02

Mepivacaine Hydrochloride *(001732)*

For complete prescribing information, refer to the CD-ROM included with the book.

Categories: Anesthesia, local; Anesthesia, regional; Pregnancy Category C; FDA Approved 1960 Apr
Drug Classes: Anesthetics, local
Brand Names: Arestocaine HCl; **Carbocaine**; Carbocot; Isocaine HCl; Polocaine; Scandonest Plain
Foreign Brand Availability: Carbocain (Denmark; Finland; Sweden); Carbocain Dental (Norway); Carbocaina (Italy); Carbocaine Caudal 1.5% (Australia); Carbocaine Dental (South-Africa); Isocaine 3% (Israel); Meaverin (Germany); Mepicaton 3% (Thailand); Mepihexal (Germany); Mepivastesin (Hong-Kong; Philippines); Scandicain (Austria; Germany; Switzerland); Scandicaine (Netherlands); Scandinibsa (Spain); Tevacaine (Israel)
HCFA JCODE(S): J0670 per 10 ml VAR

DESCRIPTION

THESE SOLUTIONS ARE NOT INTENDED FOR SPINAL ANESTHESIA OR DENTAL USE.

Mepivacaine hydrochloride is 2-piperidinecarboxamide,*N*-(2,6-dimethylphenyl)-1-methyl-monohydrochloride.

It is a white crystalline odorless power, soluble in water, but very resistant to both acid and alkaline hydrolysis.

Carbocaine hydrochloride is a local anesthetic available as sterile isotonic solutions in concentrations of 1%, 1.5%, and 2% for injection via local infiltration, peripheral nerve block, and caudal and lumbar epidural blocks.

Mepivacaine hydrochloride is related chemically and pharmacologically to the amide-type local anesthetics. It contains an amide linkage between the aromatic nucleus and the amino group (see TABLE 1).

STORAGE

Store at controlled room temperature between 15-30°C (59-85°F); brief exposure up to 40°C (104°F) does not adversely affect the product.

TABLE 1 *Composition of Available Solutions**

	Single-Dose			Multiple-Dose	
	1%	1.5%	2%	1%	2%
Vial Size	30 ml	30 ml	20 ml	50 ml	50 ml
Mepivacaine HCl (mg/ml)	10	15	20	10	20
Sodium chloride (mg/ml)	6.6	5.6	4.6	7	5
Potassium chloride (mg/ml)	0.3	0.3	0.3		
Calcium chloride (mg/ml)	0.33	0.33	0.33		
Methylparaben (mg/ml)				1	1

* In water for injection.
The pH of the solutions is adjusted between 4.5 and 6.8 with sodium hydroxide or hydrochloric acid.

INDICATIONS AND USAGE

Mepivacaine is indicated for production of local or regional analgesia and anesthesia by local infiltration, peripheral nerve block techniques, and central neural techniques including epidural and caudal blocks.

The routes of administration indicated concentration for mepivacaine are shown in TABLE 2.

TABLE 2

Local infiltration	0.5% (via dilution) or 1%
Peripheral nerve blocks	1% and 2%
Epidural block	1%, 1.5%, 2%
Caudal block	1%, 1.5% 2%

See DOSAGE AND ADMINISTRATION for additional information. Standard textbooks should be consulted to determine the accepted procedures and techniques for the administration of mepivacaine.

CONTRAINDICATIONS

Mepivacaine is contraindicated in patients with a known hypersensitivity to it or to any local anesthetic agent of the amide-type or to other components of solutions of mepivacaine.

WARNINGS

LOCAL ANESTHETICS SHOULD ONLY BE EMPLOYED BY CLINICIANS WHO ARE WELL VERSED IN DIAGNOSIS AND MANAGEMENT OF DOSE-RELATED TOXICITY AND OTHER ACUTE EMERGENCIES WHICH MIGHT ARISE FROM THE BLOCK TO BE EMPLOYED, AND THEN ONLY AFTER INSURING THE IMMEDIATE AVAILABILITY OF OXYGEN, OTHER RESUSCITATIVE DRUGS, CARDIOPULMONARY RESUSCITATIVE EQUIPMENT, AND THE PERSONNEL RESOURCE NEEDED FOR PROPER MANAGEMENT OF TOXIC REACTIONS AND RELATED EMERGENCIES.DELAY IN PROPER MANAGEMENT OF DOSE-RELATED TOXICITY, UNDERVENTILATION FROM ANY CAUSE, AND/OR ALTERED SENSITIVITY MAY LEAD TO THE DEVELOPMENT OF ACIDOSIS, CARDIAC ARREST, AND POSSIBLY, DEATH.

Local anesthetic solutions containing antimicrobial preservative (*i.e.,* those supplied in multiple dose vials) should not be used for epidural or caudal anesthesia because safety has not been established with regard to intrathecal injection either intentionally or inadvertently, of such preservatives.

It is essential that aspiration for blood or cerebrospinal fluid (where applicable) be done prior to injecting any local anesthetic, both the original dose and all subsequent doses, to avoid intravascular or subarachnoid injection. However, a negative aspiration does not ensure against in intravascular or subarachnoid injection.

Reactions resulting in fatality have occurred on rare occasions with the use of local anesthetics.

Mepivacaine with epinephrine or other vasopressors should not be used concomitantly with ergot-type oxytocic drugs, because a serve persistent hypertension may occur. Likewise, solutions of mepivacaine containing a vasoconstrictor, such as epinephrine, should be used with extreme caution in patients receiving monoamine oxidase inhibitors (MAOI) or antidepressants of the triptyline or imipramine types, because severe prolonged hypertension may result.

Local anesthetic procedures should be used with caution when there is inflammation and/or sepsis in the region of the proposed injection.

Mixing or the prior or intercurrent use of any local anesthetic with mepivacaine cannot be recommended because of insufficient data on the clinical use of such mixtures.

DOSAGE AND ADMINISTRATION

The dose of any local anesthetic administered varies with the anesthetic procedure, the area to be anesthetized, the vascularity of the tissues, the number of neuronal segments to be blocked, the depth of anesthesia and degree of muscle relaxation required, the duration of anesthesia desired, individual tolerance and the physician condition of the patient. The smallest dose and concentration required to produce the desired result should be administered. Dosages of mepivacaine should be reduced for elderly and debilitated patients and patients with cardiac and/or liver disease. The rapid injection of a large volume of local anesthetic solution should be avoided and fractional doses should be used when feasible.

For specific techniques and procedures, refer to standard textbooks.

The recommended single **adult** dose (or the total of series of doses given in one procedure) of mepivacaine for unseated, healthy, normal-sized individuals should not usually exceed 400 mg. The recommended dosage is based on requirements for the average adult and should be reduced for elderly or debilitated patients.

While maximum doses of 7 mg/kg (550 mg) have been administered without adverse effect, these are not recommended, except in exceptional circumstances and under no circumstances should the administration be repeated at intervals of less than 1½ hours. The

M

total dose for any 24 hour period should not exceed 1000 mg because of a slow accumulation of the anesthetic or its derivatives of slower than normal metabolic degradation or detoxification with repeat administration.

Children: Tolerate the local anesthetic as well as adults. However, the pediatric dose should be ***carefully measured*** as a percentage of the total adult dose ***based on weight,*** and should not exceed 5-6 mg/kg (2.5 to 3 mg/lb) in children, especially those weighing less than 30 lb. In children ***under 3 years of age or weighing less than 30 lb*** concentrations less than 2% (*e.g.,* 0.5-1.5%) should be employed.

Unused portions of solutions not containing preservatives, i.e. those supplied in single-dose vials, should be discarded following initial use.

This product should be inspected visually for particulate matter and discoloration prior to administration whenever solution and container permit. Solutions which are discolored or which contain particular matter should not be administered.

TABLE 3 *Recommended Concentrations and Doses of Mepivacaine*

Conc.	Total Dose ml	Total Dose mg	Comments
Cervical, Brachial, Intercostal, Pudendal Nerve Block			
1%	5-40	50-400	Pudendal block: one-half of total dose injected each side.
2%	5-20	100-400	
Transvaginal Block (paracervical plus pudendal)			
1%	up to 30 (both sides)	up to 300 (both sides)	One-half of total dose injected each side.
Paracervical Block			
1%	up to 20 (both sides)	up to 200 (both sides)	One-half of total dose injected each side. This is maximum recommended dose per 90 minute period in obstetrical patients. Inject slowly, 5 minutes between sides.
Caudal and Epidural Block			
1%	15-30	150-300	Use only single-dose vials which do not contain a preservative.
1.5%	10-25	150-375	
2%	10-20	200-400	
Infiltration			
1%	up to 40	up to 400	An equivalent amount of a 0.5% solution (prepared) by diluting the 1% solution with sodium chloride injection) may be used for large areas.
Therapeutic Block (pain management)			
1%	1-5	10-50	
2%	1-5	20-100	
Unused portions of solutions not containing preservatives should be discarded.			

PRODUCT LISTING - RATED THERAPEUTICALLY EQUIVALENT

Solution - Injectable - 1%

30 ml	$8.05	POLOCAINE-MPF, Astra-Zeneca Pharmaceuticals	00186-0412-01
30 ml	$11.54	CARBOCAINE HCL, Abbott Pharmaceutical	00074-1038-30
50 ml	$6.70	GENERIC, Ivax Corporation	00182-3053-67
50 ml	$9.96	POLOCAINE, Astra-Zeneca Pharmaceuticals	00186-0410-01
50 ml	$9.96	POLOCAINE, Allscripts Pharmaceutical Company	54569-4782-00

Solution - Injectable - 1.5%

30 ml	$10.91	POLOCAINE-MPF, Astra-Zeneca Pharmaceuticals	00186-0418-01

Solution - Injectable - 2%

20 ml	$8.94	POLOCAINE-MPF, Astra-Zeneca Pharmaceuticals	00186-0422-01
50 ml	$5.01	GENERIC, Moore, H.L. Drug Exchange Inc	00839-6798-38
50 ml	$10.25	POLOCAINE, Allscripts Pharmaceutical Company	54569-4859-00
50 ml	$11.63	POLOCAINE, Astra-Zeneca Pharmaceuticals	00186-0420-01

PRODUCT LISTING - EQUIVALENTS NOT AVAILABLE

Solution - Injectable - 1%

30 ml	$11.31	CARBOCAINE HCL, Abbott Pharmaceutical	00074-1036-30
50 ml	$14.84	GENERIC, Allscripts Pharmaceutical Company	54569-3918-00
50 ml	$16.23	CARBOCAINE HCL, Abbott Pharmaceutical	00074-1038-50

Solution - Injectable - 1.5%

30 ml	$4.94	CARBOCAINE HCL, Abbott Pharmaceutical	00074-1041-30

Solution - Injectable - 2%

20 ml	$12.69	CARBOCAINE HCL, Abbott Pharmaceutical	00074-1067-20
50 ml	$17.36	GENERIC, Allscripts Pharmaceutical Company	54569-3919-00
50 ml	$18.98	CARBOCAINE HCL, Abbott Pharmaceutical	00074-2047-50

Meprobamate *(001734)*

Categories: Anxiety disorder, generalized; DEA Class CIV; FDA Approved 1956 Nov; Pregnancy Category D

Drug Classes: Anxiolytics

Brand Names: Amosene; Atacin; Disatral; Equanil; Mepriam; Meproban-400; Meprospan; **Miltown**; Neuramate; Oasil-Simes; Probate; Procalmadiol; Sinanin; Trancot; Tranmep

Foreign Brand Availability: Ansiowas (Spain); Apo-Meprobamate (Canada); Atraxin (Japan); Distoncur (Argentina); Epikur (Austria); Harmonin (Japan); Meprin (Argentina); Mepro (Israel); Meprodil (Switzerland); Miltaun (Austria; Germany); Oasil (Belgium); Pertranquil (Austria; Belgium); Placidon (Argentina); Praol (Greece); Procalmidol (Belgium); Quanil (Italy); Restenil (Sweden); Sycropaz (Argentina); Visanon (Germany)

Cost of Therapy: $246.92 (Anxiety; Miltown; 400 mg; 3 tablets/day; 30 day supply)
$1.30 (Anxiety; Generic Tablets; 400 mg; 3 tablets/day; 30 day supply)

DESCRIPTION

TABLETS

Meprobamate is a white powder with a characteristic odor and a bitter taste. It is slightly soluble in water, freely soluble in acetone and alcohol, and sparingly soluble in ether.

Meprobamate tablets contain 200 or 400 mg meprobamate. The inactive ingredients present are lactose, methylcellulose, polacrilin potassium, and stearic acid.

SUSTAINED-RELEASE CAPSULES

Meprobamate is a white powder with a characteristic odor and a bitter taste. It is slightly soluble in water, freely soluble in acetone and alcohol, and sparingly soluble in ether.

Meprospan 400 contains 400 mg meprobamate per capsule. *Other ingredients:* Corn starch, FD&C blue no. 1, FD&C yellow no. 6, gelatin, sucrose and other ingredients.

Meprospan 200 contains 200 mg meprobamate per capsule. *Other ingredients:* Corn starch, FD&C yellow no. 6, gelatin, sucrose and other ingredients.

CLINICAL PHARMACOLOGY

Meprobamate is a carbamate derivative which has been shown (in animal and/or human studies) to have effects at multiple sites in the central nervous system, including the thalamus and limbic system.

INDICATIONS AND USAGE

Meprobamate is indicated for the management of anxiety disorders or for the short-term relief of the symptoms of anxiety. Anxiety or tension associated with the stress of everyday life usually does not require treatment with an anxiolytic.

The effectiveness of meprobamate in long-term use, that is, more than 4 months, has not been assessed by systematic clinical studies. The physician should periodically reassess the usefulness of the drug for the individual patient.

CONTRAINDICATIONS

Acute, intermittent porphyria and allergic or idiosyncratic reactions to meprobamate or related compounds, such as carisoprodol, mebutamate, tybamate or carbromal.

WARNINGS

DRUG DEPENDENCE

Physical dependence, psychological dependence, and abuse have occurred. Chronic intoxication from prolonged ingestion of, usually, greater than recommended doses is manifested by ataxia, slurred speech, and vertigo. Therefore, careful supervision of dose and amounts prescribed is advised, as well as avoidance of prolonged administration, especially for alcoholics and other patients with a known propensity for taking excessive quantities of drugs.

Sudden withdrawal of the drug after prolonged and excessive use may precipitate recurrence of preexisting symptoms such as anxiety, anorexia, or insomnia, or withdrawal reactions such as vomiting, ataxia, tremors, muscle twitching, confusional states, hallucinosis, and, rarely, convulsive seizures. Such seizures are more likely to occur in persons with central nervous system damage or preexistent or latent convulsive disorders. Onset of withdrawal symptoms occurs usually within 12-48 hours after discontinuation of meprobamate; symptoms usually cease within the next 12-48 hour period.

When excessive dosage has continued for weeks or months, dosage should be reduced gradually over a period of 1-2 weeks rather than abruptly stopped. Alternatively, a short-acting barbiturate may be substituted, then gradually withdrawn.

POTENTIALLY HAZARDOUS TASKS

Patients should be warned that meprobamate may impair the mental or physical abilities required for performance of potentially hazardous tasks, such as driving or operating machinery.

ADDITIVE EFFECTS

Since CNS-suppressant effects of meprobamate and alcohol or meprobamate and other psychotropic drugs may be additive, appropriate caution should be exercised with patients who take more than one of these agents simultaneously.

USAGE IN PREGNANCY AND LACTATION

An increased risk of congenital malformations associated with the use of minor tranquilizers (meprobamate, chlordiazepoxide, and diazepam) during the first trimester of pregnancy has been suggested in several studies. Because use of these drugs is rarely a matter of urgency, their use during this period should almost always be avoided. The possibility that a woman of childbearing potential may be pregnant at the time of institution of therapy should be considered. Patients should be advised that if they become pregnant during therapy or intend to become pregnant they should communicate with their physicians about the desirability of discontinuing the drug.

Meprobamate passes the placental barrier. It is present both in umbilical-cord blood at or near maternal plasma levels and in breast milk of lactating mothers at concentrations 2-4 times that of maternal plasma. When use of meprobamate is contemplated

in breast-feeding patients, the drug's higher concentrations in breast milk as compared to maternal plasma levels should be considered.

USE IN CHILDREN

Meprobamate should not be administered to children under 6 years of age, since there is a lack of documented evidence of safety and effectiveness.

PRECAUTIONS

The lowest effective dose should be administered, particularly to elderly and/or debilitated patients, in order to preclude oversedation.

Meprobamate is metabolized in the liver and excreted by the kidney; to avoid its excess accumulation caution should be exercised in the administration to patients with compromised liver or kidney function.

Meprobamate occasionally may precipitate seizures in epileptic patients.

The drug should be prescribed cautiously and in small quantities to patients with suicidal tendencies.

ADVERSE REACTIONS

CENTRAL NERVOUS SYSTEM

Drowsiness, ataxia, dizziness, slurred speech, headache, vertigo, weakness, paresthesias, impairment of visual accommodation, euphoria, overstimulation, paradoxical excitement, fast EEG activity.

GASTROINTESTINAL

Nausea, vomiting, diarrhea.

CARDIOVASCULAR

Palpitation, tachycardia, various forms of arrhythmia, transient ECG changes, syncope, hypotensive crisis.

ALLERGIC OR IDIOSYNCRATIC

Milder reactions are characterized by an itchy, urticarial, or erythematous maculopapular rash which may be generalized or confined to the groin.

Other reactions have included leukopenia, acute nonthrombocytopenic purpura, petechiae, ecchymoses, eosinophilia, peripheral edema, adenopathy, fever, fixed drug eruption with cross-reaction to carisoprodol, and cross-sensitivity between meprobamate/mebutamate and meprobamate/carbromal.

More severe hypersensitivity reactions, rarely reported, include hyperpyrexia, chills, angioneurotic edema, bronchospasm, oliguria, and anuria. Also, anaphylaxis, exfoliative dermatitis, stomatitis, and proctitis. Stevens-Johnson syndrome and bullous dermatitis have occurred.

HEMATOLOGIC

Also see Allergic or Idiosyncratic.

Agranulocytosis, aplastic anemia have been reported, although no causal relationship has been established, and thrombocytopenic purpura.

OTHER

Exacerbation of porphyric symptoms.

DOSAGE AND ADMINISTRATION

TABLETS

Usual adult dose is 1200-1600 mg/day in divided doses; doses greater than 2400 mg/day are not recommended. The usual dose for children, ages 6-12 years, is 100-200 mg, two or three times daily. Meprobamate is not recommended for children under 6 years.

SUSTAINED-RELEASE CAPSULES

The usual adult dosage of Meprospan (meprobamate, sustained-release capsules) is one to two 400 mg capsules in the morning and again at bedtime; doses above 2400 mg daily are not recommended. The usual dosage for children ages 6-12 is one 200 mg capsule in the morning and again at bedtime. Meprobamate is not recommended for children under age six.

PRODUCT LISTING - RATED THERAPEUTICALLY EQUIVALENT

Tablet - Oral - 200 mg

Qty	Price	Manufacturer	NDC
20's	$1.87	GENERIC, Circle Pharmaceuticals Inc	00659-3026-20
100's	$1.08	GENERIC, Global Pharmaceutical Corporation	00115-3888-01
100's	$4.50	GENERIC, Interstate Drug Exchange Inc	00814-4718-14
100's	$4.50	GENERIC, Alra	51641-0327-01
100's	$4.71	GENERIC, Moore, H.L. Drug Exchange Inc	00839-5070-06
100's	$5.35	GENERIC, Watson/Rugby Laboratories Inc	00536-4005-01
100's	$5.38	GENERIC, Aligen Independent Laboratories Inc	00405-0115-01
100's	$15.00	GENERIC, Eon Labs Manufacturing Inc	00185-0716-01
100's	$18.65	GENERIC, Major Pharmaceuticals Inc	00904-0044-60
100's	$26.32	GENERIC, Watson/Schein Pharmaceuticals Inc	00364-0160-01
100's	$26.32	GENERIC, Watson Laboratories Inc	52544-0804-01
100's	$33.25	EQUANIL, Wyeth-Ayerst Laboratories	00008-0002-03
100's	$105.28	GENERIC, Watson Laboratories Inc	00591-5239-01
100's	$202.18	MILTOWN, Wallace Laboratories	00037-1101-01

Tablet - Oral - 400 mg

Qty	Price	Manufacturer	NDC
28's	$5.21	GENERIC, Prescript Pharmaceuticals	00247-1031-28
100's	$1.44	GENERIC, Global Pharmaceutical Corporation	00115-3890-01
100's	$3.10	GENERIC, Alra	51641-0325-01
100's	$5.66	GENERIC, Vangard Labs	00615-0447-01
100's	$5.93	GENERIC, Interstate Drug Exchange Inc	00814-4720-14
100's	$7.98	GENERIC, Major Pharmaceuticals Inc	00904-0045-61
100's	$9.00	GENERIC, Watson/Rugby Laboratories Inc	00536-4006-01
100's	$9.25	GENERIC, Ivax Corporation	00182-0294-01
100's	$9.25	GENERIC, Moore, H.L. Drug Exchange Inc	00839-5004-06
100's	$9.40	GENERIC, Aligen Independent Laboratories Inc	00405-0116-01
100's	$27.12	GENERIC, Eon Labs Manufacturing Inc	00185-0717-01
100's	$33.60	GENERIC, Major Pharmaceuticals Inc	00904-0045-60
100's	$34.42	GENERIC, Watson/Schein Pharmaceuticals Inc	00364-0161-01
100's	$34.42	GENERIC, Watson/Rugby Laboratories Inc	52544-0805-01
100's	$137.68	GENERIC, Watson Laboratories Inc	00591-5238-01
100's	$274.36	MILTOWN, Wallace Laboratories	00037-1001-01

PRODUCT LISTING - EQUIVALENTS NOT AVAILABLE

Tablet - Oral - 400 mg

Qty	Price	Manufacturer	NDC
30's	$10.33	GENERIC, Allscripts Pharmaceutical Company	54569-0935-02
50's	$17.21	GENERIC, Allscripts Pharmaceutical Company	54569-0935-00

Mequinol; Tretinoin *(003462)*

Categories: Lentigines, senile; FDA Approved 1999 Dec; Pregnancy Category X
Drug Classes: Dermatologics; Retinoids
Brand Names: Solagé

DESCRIPTION

Solagé topical solution contains mequinol, 2% and tretinoin, 0.01%, by weight, in a solution base of ethyl alcohol (77.8% v/v), polyethylene glycol 400, butylated hydroxytoluene, ascorbic acid, citric acid, ascorbyl palmitate, edetate disodium and purified water.

Mequinol is 4-hydroxyanisole, the monomethyl ether of hydroquinone or 1-hydroxy-4-methoxybenzene. It has the chemical formula, $C_7H_8O_2$ and a molecular weight of 124.14.

The chemical name for tretinoin, a retinoid, is (all-*E*)-3,7-dimethyl-9-(2,6,6-trimethyl-1-cyclohexen-1-yl)-2,4,6,8-nonatetraenoic acid, also referred to as all-*trans*-retinoic acid. It has the chemical formula, $C_{20}H_{28}O_2$ and a molecular weight of 300.44.

Storage: The bottle of Solagé should be protected from light by continuing to store in the carton after opening. Store at controlled room temperature, 15-30°C (59 -86°F). **Note: FLAMMABLE. Keep away from heat and open flame.**

M

CLINICAL PHARMACOLOGY

Solar lentigines are localized, pigmented, macular lesions of the skin on the areas of the body which have been chronically exposed to sunlight.

Biopsy specimens of solar lentigines were collected in a clinical study with mequinol; tretinoin at baseline, at the end of a 24 week treatment period and at the end of a subsequent 24 week, no treatment, follow-up period. The end of treatment specimens showed a decrease in melanin pigmentation in both melanocytes and keratinocytes, and an increased lymphocytic infiltration, which may have been the result of irritation or an immunologic reaction. The end of follow-up period specimens showed repigmentation of the melanocytes and keratinocytes to a state similar to the baseline specimens. These results indicate that there is no assurance that any improvement obtained would persist upon discontinuation of drug therapy.

The mechanism of action of mequinol is unknown. Although mequinol is a substrate for the enzyme tyrosinase and acts as a competitive inhibitor of the formation of melanin precursors, the clinical significance of these findings is unknown. The mechanism of action of tretinoin as a depigmenting agent also is unknown.

PHARMACOKINETICS

The percutaneous absorption of tretinoin and the systemic exposure to tretinoin and mequinol were assessed in healthy subjects (n=8) following 2 weeks of twice daily topical treatment of mequinol; tretinoin. Approximately 0.8 ml of mequinol; tretinoin was applied to a 400 cm^2 area of the back, corresponding to a dose of 37.3 $\mu g/cm^2$ for mequinol and 0.23 $\mu g/cm^2$ for tretinoin. The percutaneous absorption of tretinoin was approximately 4.4%, and systemic concentrations did not increase over endogenous levels. The mean C_{max} for mequinol was 9.92 ng/ml (range 4.22-23.62 ng/ml) and the T_{max} was 2 hours (range 1-2 hours).

INDICATIONS AND USAGE

(To understand fully the indication for this product, please read the entire INDICATIONS AND USAGE information).

Mequinol; tretinoin topical solution is indicated for the treatment of solar lentigines.

Mequinol; tretinoin should only be used under medical supervision as an adjunct to a comprehensive skin care and sun avoidance program where the patient should primarily either avoid the sun or use protective clothing.

Neither the safety nor effectiveness of mequinol; tretinoin for the prevention or treatment of melasma or postinflammatory hyperpigmentation has been established.

The efficacy of using mequinol; tretinoin daily for greater than 24 weeks has not been established.

The local cutaneous safety of using mequinol; tretinoin in non-Caucasians has not been adequately established.

CONTRAINDICATIONS

The combination of mequinol and tretinoin may cause fetal harm when administered to a pregnant woman. Due to the known effects of these active ingredients, mequinol; tretinoin topical solution should not be used in women of childbearing potential.

In a dermal teratology study in New Zealand White rabbits, there were no statistically significant differences among treatment groups in fetal malformation data; however, marked hydrocephaly with visible doming of the head was observed in one mid-dose litter (12 and 0.06 mg/kg or 132 and 0.66 mg/m^2 of mequinol and tretinoin, respectively) and two fetuses in one high dose litter (40 and 0.2 mg/kg or 440 and 2.2 mg/m^2 of mequinol and tretinoin, respectively) of mequinol; tretinoin, and two high-dose tretinoin (0.2 mg/kg, 2.2 mg/m^2) treated litters. These malformations were considered to be treatment related and due to the known effects of tretinoin. This was further supported by coincident appearance of other malformations associated with tretinoin, such as cleft palate and appendicular skeletal defects. No effects attributed to treatment were observed in rabbits in that study treated topically with mequinol alone (dose 40 mg/kg, 440 mg/m^2). A no-observed-effect level (NOEL) for teratogenicity in rabbits was established at 4 and 0.02 mg/kg (44 and 0.22 mg/m^2 mequinol and tretinoin, respectively) for mequinol; tretinoin, which is approximately the maximum possible human daily dose, based on clinical application to 5% of total body surface area. Plasma tretinoin concentrations were not raised above endogenous levels, even at teratogenic doses. Plasma mequinol concentrations in rabbits at the NOEL at 1 hour after application were 124 ng/ml or approximately twelve times the mean peak plasma concentrations of that substance seen in human subjects in a clinical pharmacokinetic study.

In a repeated study in pregnant rabbits administered the same dose levels as the study described above, additional precautionary measures were taken to prevent ingestion, although there is no evidence to confirm that ingestion occurred in the initial study. Precautionary measures additionally limited transdermal absorption to a 6 hour exposure period, or approximately one-fourth of the human clinical daily continuous exposure time. This study did not show any significant teratogenic effects at doses up to approximately 13 times the human dose on a mg/m^2 basis. However, a concurrent tretinoin dose group (0.2 mg/kg/day) did include two litters with limb malformations.

In a published study in albino rats,[1] topical application of 5% mequinol in a cream vehicle during gestation was embryotoxic and embryolethal. Embryonic loss prior to implantation was noted in that study where animals were treated throughout gestation. Coincidentally, mean preimplantation embryonic loss was increased in the first rabbit study in all mequinol treated groups, relative to control, and in the high dose mequinol; tretinoin and tretinoin only treated groups in the second study. In those studies, dosing began at gestation day 6, when implantation is purported to occur. Increased preimplantation loss was also noted at the high combination dose in a study of early embryonic effects in rats, as was decreased body weight in male pups; these findings are consistent with the published study.

Mequinol; tretinoin was not teratogenic in Sprague-Dawley rats when given in topical doses of 80 and 0.4 mg/kg mequinol and tretinoin, respectively (480 and 2.4 mg/m^2 or 11 times the maximum human daily dose). The maximum human dose is defined as the amount of solution applied daily to 5% of the total body surface area.

With widespread use of any drug, a small number of birth defect reports associated temporally with the administration of the drug would be expected by chance alone. Thirty cases of temporally-associated congenital malformations have been reported during two decades of clinical use of another formulation of topical tretinoin. Although no definite pattern of teratogenicity and no causal association has been established from these cases, 6 of the reports describe the rare birth defect category holoprosencephaly (defects associated with incomplete midline development of the forebrain). The significance of these spontaneous reports in terms of risk to the fetus is not known.

No adequate or well-controlled trials have been conducted with mequinol; tretinoin in pregnant women.

Mequinol; tretinoin topical solution is contraindicated in individuals with a history of sensitivity reactions to any of its ingredients. It should be discontinued if hypersensitivity to any of its ingredients is noted.

WARNINGS

Mequinol; tretinoin is a dermal irritant and the results of continued irritation of the skin for greater than 52 weeks in chronic, long-term use are not known. Tretinoin has been reported to cause severe irritation on eczematous skin and should be used only with utmost caution in patients with this condition.

Safety and effectiveness of mequinol; tretinoin in individuals with moderately or heavily pigmented skin have not been established.

Mequinol; tretinoin should not be administered if the patient is also taking drugs known to be photosensitizers (*e.g.*, thiazides, tetracyclines, fluoroquinolones, phenothiazines, sulfonamides) because of the possibility of augmented phototoxicity.

Because of heightened burning susceptibility, exposure to sunlight (including sunlamps) to treated areas should be avoided or minimized during the use of mequinol; tretinoin. Patients must be advised to use protective clothing and comply with a comprehensive sun avoidance program when using mequinol; tretinoin. Data are not available to establish how or whether mequinol; tretinoin is degraded (either by sunlight or by normal interior lighting) following application to the skin. Patients with sunburn should be advised not to use mequinol; tretinoin until fully recovered. Patients who may have considerable sun exposure due to their occupation and those patients with inherent sensitivity to sunlight should exercise particular caution when using mequinol; tretinoin and ensure that the precautions outlined in the Patient Medication Guide are observed.

Mequinol; tretinoin should be kept out of the eyes, mouth, paranasal creases, and mucous membranes. Mequinol; tretinoin may cause skin irritation, erythema, burning, stinging or tingling, peeling, and pruritus. If the degree of such local irritation warrants, patients should be directed to use less medication, decrease the frequency of application, discontinue use temporarily, or discontinue use altogether. The efficacy at reduced frequencies of application has not been established.

Mequinol; tretinoin should be used with caution by patients with a history, or family history, of vitiligo. One patient in the trials, whose brother had vitiligo, experienced hypopigmentation in areas that had not been treated with study medication. Some of these areas continued to worsen for at least 1 month post treatment with mequinol; tretinoin. Six weeks later the severity of the hypopigmentation had decreased from moderate to mild and 106 days post treatment, the patient had resolution of some but not all lesions.

Application of larger amounts of medication than recommended will not lead to more rapid or better results, and marked redness, peeling, discomfort, or hypopigmentation of the skin may occur.

PRECAUTIONS

GENERAL

For external use only.

Mequinol; tretinoin should only be used as an adjunct to a comprehensive skin care and sun avoidance program. (See INDICATIONS AND USAGE.)

If a drug sensitivity, chemical irritation, or a systemic adverse reaction develops, use of mequinol; tretinoin should be discontinued.

Weather extremes, such as wind or cold, may be more irritating to patients using mequinol; tretinoin.

INFORMATION FOR THE PATIENT

Patients require detailed instruction to obtain maximal benefits and to understand all the precautions necessary to use this product with greatest safety.

CARCINOGENESIS, MUTAGENESIS, AND IMPAIRMENT OF FERTILITY

Although a dermal carcinogenicity study in CD-1 mice indicated that mequinol; tretinoin applied topically at daily doses up to 80 and 0.4 mg/kg (240 and 1.2 mg/m^2) of mequinol and tretinoin, respectively, representing approximately 5 times the maximum possible systemic human exposure was not carcinogenic, in a photocarcinogenicity study utilizing Crl:Skh-1(hr/hr BR) hairless albino mice, median time to onset of tumors decreased. Also, the number of tumors increased in all dose groups administered 1.4, 4.3, or 14 µl of mequinol; tretinoin/cm^2 of skin (24 and 0.12, 72 and 0.36, or 240 and 1.2 mg/m^2 of mequinol and tretinoin, respectively; 0.6, 1.9, or 6.5 times the daily human dose on a mg/m^2 basis) following chronic topical dosing with intercurrent exposure to ultraviolet radiation for up to 40 weeks. Similar animal studies have shown an increased tumorigenic risk with the use of retinoids when followed by ultraviolet radiation. Although the significance of these studies to human use is not clear, patients using this product should be advised to avoid or minimize exposure to either sunlight or artificial ultraviolet irradiation sources.

Mequinol was non-mutagenic in the Ames/Salmonella assay using strains TA98, TA100, TA1535, and TA1537, all of which are insensitive to mutagenic effects of structurally-related quinones. Mequinol; tretinoin was non-genotoxic in an *in vivo* dermal micronucleus assay in rats, but exposure of bone marrow to drug was not demonstrated.

A dermal reproduction study with mequinol; tretinoin in Sprague-Dawley rats at a daily dose of 80 and 0.4 mg/kg (480 and 2.4 mg/m^2) of mequinol and tretinoin, respectively, approximately 11 times the corresponding maximum possible human exposure, assuming 100% bioavailability following topical application to 5% of the total body surface area, showed no impairment of fertility.

PREGNANCY, TERATOGENIC EFFECTS, PREGNANCY CATEGORY X

Although the magnitude of the potential for teratogenicity may not be well-defined, mequinol; tretinoin is labeled as an "X" because the potential risk of the use of this drug to treat this particular indication (solar lentigines) in a pregnant woman clearly outweighs any possible benefit (see CONTRAINDICATIONS).

NURSING MOTHERS

It is not known to what extent mequinol and/or tretinoin is excreted in human milk. Because many drugs are excreted in human milk, caution should be exercised when mequinol; tretinoin is administered to a nursing woman.

PEDIATRIC USE

The safety and effectiveness of this product have not been established in pediatric patients. Mequinol; tretinoin should not be used on children.

GERIATRIC USE

Of the total number of patients in clinical studies of mequinol; tretinoin, approximately 43% were 65 and older, while approximately 8% were 75 and over. No overall differences in effectiveness or safety were observed between these patients and younger patients.

DRUG INTERACTIONS

Concomitant topical products with a strong skin drying effect, products with high concentrations of alcohol, astringents, spices or lime, medicated soaps or shampoos, permanent wave solutions, electrolysis, hair depilatories or waxes, or other preparations that might dry or irritate the skin should be used with caution in patients being treated with mequinol; tretinoin because they may increase irritation when used with mequinol; tretinoin.

Mequinol; tretinoin should not be administered if the patient is also taking drugs known to be photosensitizers (*e.g.*, thiazides, tetracyclines, fluoroquinolones, phenothiazines, sulfonamides) because of the possibility of augmented phototoxicity.

ADVERSE REACTIONS

In clinical trials, adverse reactions were primarily mild to moderate in intensity, occurring in 66% and 30% of patients, respectively. The majority of these events were limited to the skin and 64% had an onset of a skin related adverse reaction early in treatment (by week 8). The most frequent adverse reactions in patients treated with mequinol; tretinoin were erythema (49% of patients), burning, stinging or tingling (26%), desquamation (14%), pruritus (12%), and skin irritation (5%).

Some patients experienced temporary hypopigmentation of treated lesions (5%) or of the skin surrounding treated lesions (7%). Ninety-four of 106 patients (89%) had resolution of hypopigmentation upon discontinuation of treatment to the lesion, and/or reinstruction on proper application to the lesion only. Another 8% (9/106) of patients with hypopigmentation events had resolution within 120 days after the end of treatment. Three of the 106 patients (2.8%) had persistence of hypopigmentation beyond 120 days. Approximately 6% of patients discontinued study participation with mequinol; tretinoin due to adverse reactions. These discontinuations were due primarily to skin redness (erythema) or related cutaneous adverse reactions. Mequinol; tretinoin was generally well tolerated (see TABLE 2).

TABLE 2 *Adverse Events Occurring in >1% of the Population*

All Studies

Body System	Mequinol; Tretinoin	Tretinoin, 0.01%	Mequinol, 2%	Vehicle
Skin and appendages erythema	421 (49.4%)	261 (55.3%)	13 (5.1%)	8 (4.6%)
Burning/stinging/tingling	223 (26.1%)	173 (36.7%)	26 (10.2%)	20 (11.4%)
Desquamation	120 (14.1%)	93 (19.7%)	7 (2.8%)	2 (1.1%)
Pruritus	105 (12.3%)	66 (14.0%)	12 (4.7%)	3 (1.7%)
Halo hypopigmentation	60 (7.0%)	16 (3.4%)	2 (0.8%)	2 (1.1%)
Hypopigmentation	46 (5.4%)	8 (1.7%)	2 (0.8%)	0 (0.0%)
Irritation skin	45 (5.3%)	25 (5.3%)	1 (0.4%)	1 (0.6%)
Rash	27 (3.2%)	21 (4.4%)	0 (0.0%)	1 (0.6%)
Skin dry	27 (3.2%)	18 (3.8%)	3 (1.2%)	1 (0.6%)
Crusting	21 (2.5%)	18 (3.8%)	0 (0.0%)	1 (0.6%)
Rash vesicular bullae	18 (2.1%)	8 (1.7%)	0 (0.0%)	0 (0.0%)
Application site reaction*	9 (1.1%)	11 (2.3%)	1 (0.4%)	0 (0.0%)

* Events that were considered to be a contact allergic reaction.

DOSAGE AND ADMINISTRATION

Patients require detailed instruction to obtain maximal benefits and to understand all the precautions necessary to use this product with greatest safety. The physician should review the Patient Medication Guide.

Apply mequinol; tretinoin to the solar lentigines using the applicator tip while avoiding application to the surrounding skin. Use twice daily, morning and evening at least 8 hours apart, or as directed by a physician. Patients should not shower or bathe the treatment areas for at least 6 hours after application of mequinol; tretinoin. Special caution should be taken when applying mequinol; tretinoin to avoid the eyes, mouth, paranasal creases, and mucous membranes.

Application of mequinol; tretinoin may cause transitory stinging, burning or irritation.

Improvement continues gradually through the course of therapy and should be apparent by 24 weeks. Patients should avoid exposure to sunlight (including sunlamps) or wear protective clothing while using mequinol; tretinoin. Data are not available to establish how or whether mequinol; tretinoin is degraded (either by sunlight or by normal interior lighting) following application to the skin.

With discontinuation of mequinol; tretinoin therapy, a majority of patients will experience some repigmentation over time of their lesions.

Applications of larger amounts of medication or more frequently than recommended will not lead to more rapid or better results, and marked redness, peeling, irritation, or hypopigmentation (abnormal lightening) of the skin may occur.

Patients treated with mequinol; tretinoin may use cosmetics but should wait 30 minutes before applying.

Mercaptopurine *(001737)*

Categories: Leukemia, acute lymphoblastic; Leukemia, acute myelogenous; Leukemia, central nervous system; Leukemia, chronic lymphocytic; Lymphoma, Hodgkin's; Lymphoma, non-Hodgkin's; Pregnancy Category D; FDA Approved 1963 Mar; WHO Formulary

Drug Classes: Antineoplastics, antimetabolites

Brand Names: Purinethol

Foreign Brand Availability: Classen (Japan); Cystagon (Austria; Belgium; Bulgaria; Czech-Republic; Denmark; England; Finland; France; Germany; Greece; Hungary; Ireland; Italy; Netherlands; Norway; Poland; Portugal; Slovenia; Spain; Sweden; Switzerland; Turkey); Empurine (Philippines); Ismipur (Italy); Leukerin (Japan); Mercaptopurina (Spain); Puri-Nethol (Austria; Bahamas; Bahrain; Barbados; Belgium; Belize; Benin; Bermuda; Burkina-Faso; China; Curacao; Cyprus; Czech-Republic; Denmark; Egypt; England; Ethiopia; Finland; Gambia; Germany; Ghana; Guinea; Guyana; Hong-Kong; India; Indonesia; Iran; Iraq; Ireland; Israel; Ivory-Coast; Jamaica; Jordan; Kenya; Korea; Kuwait; Lebanon; Liberia; Libya; Malawi; Malaysia; Mali; Mauritania; Mauritius; Morocco; Netherland-Antilles; Niger; Nigeria; Norway; Oman; Puerto-Rico; Qatar; Republic-of-Yemen; Saudi-Arabia; Senegal; Seychelles; Sierra-Leone; South-Africa; Sudan; Surinam; Sweden; Switzerland; Syria; Taiwan; Tanzania; Thailand; Trinidad; Tunia; Uganda; United-Arab-Emirates; Zambia; Zimbabwe)

Cost of Therapy: $239.30 (Acute Lymphatic Leukemia, Maintenance; Purinethol; 50 mg; 2 tablets/day; 30 day supply)

WARNING

Mercaptopurine is a potent drug. It should not be used unless a diagnosis of acute lymphatic leukemia has been adequately established and the responsible physician is knowledgeable in assessing response to chemotherapy.

DESCRIPTION

Purinethol (mercaptopurine) was synthesized and developed by Hitchings, Elion, and associates at the Wellcome Research Laboratories.[1] It is one of a large series of purine analogues which interfere with nucleic acid biosynthesis and has been found active against human leukemias.

Mercaptopurine, known chemically as 1,7-dihydro-6*H*-purine-6-thione monohydrate, is an analogue of the purine bases adenine and hypoxanthine.

Purinethol is available in tablet form for oral administration. Each scored tablet contains 50 mg mercaptopurine and the inactive ingredients corn and potato starch, lactose, magnesium stearate, and stearic acid.

CLINICAL PHARMACOLOGY

Clinical studies have shown that the absorption of an oral dose of mercaptopurine in humans is incomplete and variable, averaging approximately 50% of the administered dose.[2] The factors influencing absorption are unknown. Intravenous (IV) administration of an investigational preparation of mercaptopurine revealed a plasma half-disappearance time of 21 minutes in pediatric patients and 47 minutes in adults. The volume of distribution usually exceeded that of the total body water.[2]

Following the oral administration of ^{35}S-6-mercaptopurine in 1 subject, a total of 46% of the dose could be accounted for in the urine (as parent drug and metabolites) in the first 24 hours. Metabolites of mercaptopurine were found in urine within the first 2 hours after administration. Radioactivity (in the form of sulfate) could be found in the urine for weeks afterwards.[3]

There is negligible entry of mercaptopurine into cerebrospinal fluid.

Plasma protein binding averages 19% over the concentration range 10-50 μg/ml (a concentration only achieved by IV administration of mercaptopurine at doses exceeding 5-10 mg/kg).[2]

Monitoring of plasma levels of mercaptopurine during therapy is of questionable value.[3] There is technical difficulty in determining plasma concentrations which are seldom greater than 1-2 μg/ml after a therapeutic oral dose. More significantly, mercaptopurine enters rapidly into the anabolic and catabolic pathways for purines, and the active intracellular metabolites have appreciably longer half-lives than the parent drug. The biochemical effects of a single dose of mercaptopurine are evident long after the parent drug has disappeared from plasma. Because of this rapid metabolism of mercaptopurine to active intracellular derivatives, hemodialysis would not be expected to appreciably reduce toxicity of the drug. There is no known pharmacologic antagonist to the biochemical actions of mercaptopurine *in vivo*.

Mercaptopurine competes with hypoxanthine and guanine for the enzyme hypoxanthine-guanine phosphoribosyltransferase (HGPRTase) and is itself converted to thioinosinic acid (TIMP). This intracellular nucleotide inhibits several reactions involving inosinic acid (IMP), including the conversion of IMP to xanthylic acid (XMP) and the conversion of IMP to adenylic acid (AMP) via adenylosuccinate (SAMP). In addition, 6-methylthioinosinate (MTIMP) is formed by the methylation of TIMP. Both TIMP and MTIMP have been reported to inhibit glutamine-5-phosphoribosylpyrophosphate amidotransferase, the first enzyme unique to the *de novo* pathway for purine ribonucleotide synthesis.[3]

Experiments indicate that radiolabeled mercaptopurine may be recovered from the DNA in the form of deoxythioguanosine.[4] Some mercaptopurine is converted to nucleotide derivatives of 6-thioguanine (6-TG) by the sequential actions of inosinate (IMP) dehydrogenase and xanthylate (XMP) aminase, converting TIMP to thioguanylic acid (TGMP).

Animal tumors that are resistant to mercaptopurine often have lost the ability to convert mercaptopurine to TIMP. However, it is clear that resistance to mercaptopurine may be acquired by other means as well, particularly in human leukemias.

It is not known exactly which of any one or more of the biochemical effects of mercaptopurine and its metabolites are directly or predominantly responsible for cell death.[5]

The catabolism of mercaptopurine and its metabolites is complex. In humans, after oral administration of ^{35}S-6-mercaptopurine, urine contains intact mercaptopurine, thiouric acid (formed by direct oxidation by xanthine oxidase, probably via 6-mercapto-8-hydroxypurine), and a number of 6-methylated thiopurines. The methylthiopurines yield appreciable amounts of inorganic sulfate.[3] The importance of the metabolism by xanthine oxidase relates to the fact that allopurinol inhibits this enzyme and retards the catabolism of mercaptopurine and its active metabolites. A significant reduction in mercaptopurine dosage is mandatory if a potent xanthine oxidase inhibitor and mercaptopurine are used simultaneously in a patient (see PRECAUTIONS).

M

INDICATIONS AND USAGE

Mercaptopurine is indicated for remission induction and maintenance therapy of acute lymphatic leukemia. The response to this agent depends upon the particular subclassification of acute lymphatic leukemia and the age of the patient (pediatric patient or adult).

ACUTE LYMPHATIC (LYMPHOCYTIC, LYMPHOBLASTIC) LEUKEMIA

Given as a single agent for remission induction, mercaptopurine induces complete remission in approximately 25% of pediatric patients and 10% of adults. However, reliance upon mercaptopurine alone is not justified for initial remission induction of acute lymphatic leukemia since combination chemotherapy with vincristine, prednisone, and L-asparaginase results in more frequent complete remission induction than with mercaptopurine alone or in combination. The duration of complete remission induced in acute lymphatic leukemia is so brief without the use of maintenance therapy that some form of drug therapy is considered essential. Mercaptopurine, as a single agent, is capable of significantly prolonging complete remission duration; however, combination therapy has produced remission duration longer than that achieved with mercaptopurine alone.

ACUTE MYELOGENOUS (AND ACUTE MYELOMONOCYTIC) LEUKEMIA

As a single agent, mercaptopurine will induce complete remission in approximately 10% of pediatric patients and adults with acute myelogenous leukemia or its subclassifications. These results are inferior to those achieved with combination chemotherapy employing optimum treatment schedules.

CENTRAL NERVOUS SYSTEM LEUKEMIA

Mercaptopurine is not effective for prophylaxis or treatment of central nervous system leukemia.

OTHER NEOPLASMS

Mercaptopurine is not effective in chronic lymphatic leukemia, the lymphomas (including Hodgkin's Disease), or solid tumors.

NON-FDA APPROVED INDICATIONS

The drug has also shown efficacy in the treatment of Crohn's disease and ulcerative colitis. However, these uses have not been approved by the FDA and further studies are needed.

CONTRAINDICATIONS

Mercaptopurine should not be used unless a diagnosis of acute lymphatic leukemia has been adequately established and the responsible physician is knowledgeable in assessing response to chemotherapy.

Mercaptopurine should not be used in patients whose disease has demonstrated prior resistance to this drug. In animals and humans, there is usually complete cross-resistance between mercaptopurine and thioguanine.

Mercaptopurine should not be used in patients who have a hypersensitivity to mercaptopurine or any component of the formulation.

WARNINGS

SINCE DRUGS USED IN CANCER CHEMOTHERAPY ARE POTENTIALLY HAZARDOUS, IT IS RECOMMENDED THAT ONLY PHYSICIANS EXPERIENCED WITH THE RISKS OF MERCAPTOPURINE AND KNOWLEDGEABLE IN THE NATURAL HISTORY OF ACUTE LEUKEMIAS ADMINISTER THIS DRUG.

BONE MARROW TOXICITY

The most consistent, dose-related toxicity is bone marrow suppression. This may be manifest by anemia, leukopenia, thrombocytopenia, or any combination of these. Any of these findings may also reflect progression of the underlying disease. Since mercaptopurine may have a delayed effect, it is important to withdraw the medication temporarily at the first sign of an abnormally large fall in any of the formed elements of the blood.

There are individuals with an inherited deficiency of the enzyme thiopurine methyltransferase (TPMT) who may be unusually sensitive to the myelosuppressive effects of mercaptopurine and prone to developing rapid bone marrow suppression following the initial treatment.[6,7] Substantial dosage reductions may be required to avoid the development of life-threatening bone marrow suppression in these patients. This toxicity may be more profound in patients treated with concomitant allopurinol (see DRUG INTERACTIONS). This problem could be exacerbated by coadministration with drugs that inhibit TPMT, such as olsalazine, mesalazine, or sulphasalazine.

HEPATOTOXICITY

Mercaptopurine is hepatotoxic in animals and humans. A small number of deaths have been reported which may have been attributed to hepatic necrosis due to administration of mercaptopurine. Hepatic injury can occur with any dosage, but seems to occur with more frequency when doses of 2.5 mg/kg/day are exceeded. The histologic pattern of mercaptopurine hepatotoxicity includes features of both intrahepatic cholestasis and parenchymal cell necrosis, either of which may predominate. It is not clear how much of the hepatic damage is due to direct toxicity from the drug and how much may be due to a hypersensitivity reaction. In some patients jaundice has cleared following withdrawal of mercaptopurine and reappeared with its reintroduction.[8]

Published reports have cited widely varying incidences of overt hepatotoxicity. In a large series of patients with various neoplastic diseases, mercaptopurine was administered orally in doses ranging from 2.5-5.0 mg/kg without any evidence of hepatotoxicity. It was noted by the authors that no definite clinical evidence of liver damage could be ascribed to the drug, although an occasional case of serum hepatitis did occur in patients receiving 6-MP who previously had transfusions.[8] In reports of smaller cohorts of adult and pediatric leukemic patients, the incidence of hepatotoxicity ranged from 0-6%.[9-11] In an isolated report by Einhorn and Davidsohn, jaundice was observed more frequently (40%), especially when doses exceeded 2.5 mg/kg.[12] Usually, clinically detectable jaundice appears early in the course of treatment (1-2 months). However, jaundice has been reported as early as 1 week and as late as 8 years after the start of treatment with mercaptopurine.[13]

Monitoring of serum transaminase levels, alkaline phosphatase, and bilirubin levels may allow early detection of hepatotoxicity. It is advisable to monitor these liver function tests at weekly intervals when first beginning therapy and at monthly intervals thereafter. Liver function tests may be advisable more frequently in patients who are receiving mercaptopurine with other hepatotoxic drugs or with known pre-existing liver disease.

The concomitant administration of mercaptopurine with other hepatotoxic agents requires especially careful clinical and biochemical monitoring of hepatic function. Combination therapy involving mercaptopurine with other drugs not felt to be hepatotoxic should nevertheless be approached with caution. The combination of mercaptopurine with doxorubicin was reported to be hepatotoxic in 19 of 20 patients undergoing remission-induction therapy for leukemia resistant to previous therapy.[14]

The hepatotoxicity has been associated in some cases with anorexia, diarrhea, jaundice, and ascites. Hepatic encephalopathy has occurred.

The onset of clinical jaundice, hepatomegaly, or anorexia with tenderness in the right hypochondrium are immediate indications for withholding mercaptopurine until the exact etiology can be identified. Likewise, any evidence of deterioration in liver function studies, toxic hepatitis, or biliary stasis should prompt discontinuation of the drug and a search for an etiology of the hepatotoxicity.

IMMUNOSUPPRESSION

Mercaptopurine recipients may manifest decreased cellular hypersensitivities and impaired allograft rejection. Induction of immunity to infectious agents or vaccines will be subnormal in these patients; the degree of immunosuppression will depend on antigen dose and temporal relationship to drug. This immunosuppressive effect should be carefully considered with regard to intercurrent infections and risk of subsequent neoplasia.

PREGNANCY CATEGORY D

Mercaptopurine can cause fetal harm when administered to a pregnant woman. Women receiving mercaptopurine in the first trimester of pregnancy have an increased incidence of abortion; the risk of malformation in offspring surviving first trimester exposure is not accurately known.[15] In a series of 28 women receiving mercaptopurine after the first trimester of pregnancy, 3 mothers died undelivered, 1 delivered a stillborn child, and 1 aborted; there were no cases of macroscopically abnormal fetuses.[16] Since such experience cannot exclude the possibility of fetal damage, mercaptopurine should be used during pregnancy only if the benefit clearly justifies the possible risk to the fetus, and particular caution should be given to the use of mercaptopurine in the first trimester of pregnancy.

There are no adequate and well-controlled studies in pregnant women. If this drug is used during pregnancy or if the patient becomes pregnant while taking the drug, the patient should be apprised of the potential hazard to the fetus. Women of childbearing potential should be advised to avoid becoming pregnant.

PRECAUTIONS

GENERAL

The safe and effective use of mercaptopurine demands a thorough knowledge of the natural history of the condition being treated. After selection of an initial dosage schedule, therapy will frequently need to be modified depending upon the patient's response and manifestations of toxicity.

The most frequent, serious, toxic effect of mercaptopurine is myelosuppression resulting in leukopenia, thrombocytopenia, and anemia. These toxic effects are often unavoidable during the induction phase of adult acute leukemia if remission induction is to be successful. Whether or not these manifestations demand modification or cessation of dosage depends both upon the response of the underlying disease and a careful consideration of supportive facilities (granulocyte and platelet transfusions) which may be available. Life-threatening infections and bleeding have been observed as a consequence of mercaptopurine-induced granulocytopenia and thrombocytopenia. Severe hematologic toxicity may require supportive therapy with platelet transfusions for bleeding, and antibiotics and granulocyte transfusions if sepsis is documented.

If it is not the intent to deliberately induce bone marrow hypoplasia, it is important to discontinue the drug temporarily at the first evidence of an abnormally large fall in white blood cell count, platelet count, or hemoglobin concentration. In many patients with severe depression of the formed elements of the blood due to mercaptopurine, the bone marrow appears hypoplastic on aspiration or biopsy, whereas in other cases it may appear normocellular. The qualitative changes in the erythroid elements toward the megaloblastic series, characteristically seen with the folic acid antagonists and some other antimetabolites, are not seen with this drug.

It is probably advisable to start with smaller dosages in patients with impaired renal function, since the latter might result in slower elimination of the drug and metabolites and a greater cumulative effect.

INFORMATION FOR THE PATIENT

Patients should be informed that the major toxicities of mercaptopurine are related to myelosuppression, hepatotoxicity, and gastrointestinal toxicity. Patients should never be allowed to take the drug without medical supervision and should be advised to consult their physician if they experience fever, sore throat, jaundice, nausea, vomiting, signs of local infection, bleeding from any site, or symptoms suggestive of anemia. Women of childbearing potential should be advised to avoid becoming pregnant.

LABORATORY TESTS

It is recommended that evaluation of the hemoglobin or hematocrit, total white blood cell count and differential count, and quantitative platelet count be obtained weekly while the patient is on therapy with mercaptopurine. In cases where the cause of fluctuations in the formed elements in the peripheral blood is obscure, bone marrow examination may be useful for the evaluation of marrow status. The decision to increase, decrease, continue, or discontinue a given dosage of mercaptopurine must be based not only on the absolute hematologic values, but also upon the rapidity with which changes are occurring. In many instances, particularly during the induction phase of acute leukemia, complete blood counts will need to be done more frequently than once weekly in order to evaluate the effect of the therapy.

CARCINOGENESIS, MUTAGENESIS, AND IMPAIRMENT OF FERTILITY

Mercaptopurine causes chromosomal aberrations in animals and humans and induces dominant-lethal mutations in male mice. In mice, surviving female offspring of mothers who received chronic low doses of mercaptopurine during pregnancy were found sterile, or if they became pregnant, had smaller litters and more dead fetuses as compared to control animals.[19] Carcinogenic potential exists in humans, but the extent of the risk is unknown.

The effect of mercaptopurine on human fertility is unknown for either males or females.

PREGNANCY, TERATOGENIC EFFECTS, PREGNANCY CATEGORY D

See WARNINGS.

NURSING MOTHERS

It is not known whether this drug is excreted in human milk. Because many drugs are excreted in human milk, and because of the potential for serious adverse reactions in nursing infants from mercaptopurine, a decision should be made whether to discontinue nursing or to discontinue the drug, taking into account the importance of the drug to the mother.

PEDIATRIC USE

See DOSAGE AND ADMINISTRATION.

DRUG INTERACTIONS

When allopurinol and mercaptopurine are administered concomitantly, it is imperative that the dose of mercaptopurine be reduced to one-third to one-quarter of the usual dose. Failure to observe this dosage reduction will result in a delayed catabolism of mercaptopurine and the strong likelihood of inducing severe toxicity.

There is usually complete cross-resistance between mercaptopurine and thioguanine.

The dosage of mercaptopurine may need to be reduced when this agent is combined with other drugs whose primary or secondary toxicity is myelosuppression. Enhanced marrow suppression has been noted in some patients also receiving trimethoprim-sulfamethoxazole.[17,18]

Inhibition of the anticoagulant effect of warfarin, when given with mercaptopurine, has been reported. As there is *in vitro* evidence that aminosalicylate derivatives (*e.g.,* olsalazine, mesalazine, or sulphasalazine) inhibit the TPMT enzyme, they should be administered with caution to patients receiving concurrent mercaptopurine therapy (see WARNINGS).

ADVERSE REACTIONS

The principal and potentially serious toxic effects of mercaptopurine are bone marrow toxicity and hepatotoxicity (see WARNINGS).

Hematologic: The most frequent adverse reaction to mercaptopurine is myelosuppression. The induction of complete remission of acute lymphatic leukemia frequently is associated with marrow hypoplasia. Maintenance of remission generally involves multiple-drug regimens whose component agents cause myelosuppression. Anemia, leukopenia, and thrombocytopenia are frequently observed. Dosages and schedules are adjusted to prevent life-threatening cytopenias.

Renal: Hyperuricemia and/or hyperuricosuria may occur in patients receiving mercaptopurine as a consequence of rapid cell lysis accompanying the antineoplastic effect. Adverse effects can be minimized by increased hydration, urine alkalinization, and the prophylactic administration of a xanthine oxidase inhibitor such as allopurinol. The dosage of mercaptopurine should be reduced to one-third to one-quarter of the usual dose if allopurinol is given concurrently.

Gastrointestinal: Intestinal ulceration has been reported.[20] Nausea, vomiting, and anorexia are uncommon during initial administration. Mild diarrhea and sprue-like symptoms have been noted occasionally, but it is difficult at present to attribute these to the medication. Oral lesions are rarely seen, and when they occur they resemble thrush rather than antifolic ulcerations.

An increased risk of pancreatitis may be associated with the investigational use of mercaptopurine in inflammatory bowel disease.[21-23]

Miscellaneous: While dermatologic reactions can occur as a consequence of disease, the administration of mercaptopurine has been associated with skin rashes and hyperpigmentation.[24] Alopecia has been reported.

Drug fever has been very rarely reported with mercaptopurine. Before attributing fever to mercaptopurine, every attempt should be made to exclude more common causes of pyrexia, such as sepsis, in patients with acute leukemia.

Transient oligospermia has been reported.

DOSAGE AND ADMINISTRATION

INDUCTION THERAPY

Mercaptopurine is administered orally. The dosage which will be tolerated and be effective varies from patient to patient, and therefore careful titration is necessary to obtain the optimum therapeutic effect without incurring excessive, unintended toxicity. The usual initial dosage for pediatric patients and adults is 2.5 mg/kg of body weight per day (100-200 mg in the average adult and 50 mg in an average 5-year-old child). Pediatric patients with acute leukemia have tolerated this dose without difficulty in most cases; it may be continued daily for several weeks or more in some patients. If, after 4 weeks at this dosage, there is no clinical improvement and no definite evidence of leukocyte or platelet depression, the dosage may be increased up to 5 mg/kg daily. A dosage of 2.5 mg/kg/day may result in a rapid fall in leukocyte count within 1-2 weeks in some adults with acute lymphatic leukemia and high total leukocyte counts.

The total daily dosage may be given at one time. It is calculated to the nearest multiple of 25 mg. Studies in pediatric patients with acute lymphoblastic leukemia suggest that the administration of mercaptopurine in the evening compared with the morning lowered the risk of relapse.

The dosage of mercaptopurine should be reduced to one-third to one-quarter of the usual dose if allopurinol is given concurrently. Because the drug may have a delayed action, it should be discontinued at the first sign of an abnormally large or rapid fall in the leukocyte or platelet count. If subsequently the leukocyte count or platelet count remains constant for 2 or 3 days, or rises, treatment may be resumed.

MAINTENANCE THERAPY

Once a complete hematologic remission is obtained, maintenance therapy is considered essential. Maintenance doses will vary from patient to patient. A usual daily maintenance dose of mercaptopurine is 1.5-2.5 mg/kg/day as a single dose. It is to be emphasized that in pediatric patients with acute lymphatic leukemia in remission, superior results have been obtained when mercaptopurine has been combined with other agents (most frequently with methotrexate) for remission maintenance. Mercaptopurine should rarely be relied upon as a single agent for the maintenance of remissions induced in acute leukemia.

Procedures for proper handling and disposal of anticancer drugs should be considered. Several guidelines on this subject have been published.[26-32]

There is no general agreement that all of the procedures recommended in the guidelines are necessary or appropriate.

DOSAGE IN RENAL IMPAIRMENT

Consideration should be given to reducing the dosage in patients with impaired renal function.

DOSAGE IN HEPATIC IMPAIRMENT

Consideration should be given to reducing the dosage in patients with impaired hepatic function.

HOW SUPPLIED

Purinethol is supplied as pale yellow to buff, scored tablets containing 50 mg mercaptopurine, imprinted with "PURINETHOL" and "04A".

Storage: Store at 15-25°C (59-77°F) in a dry place.

PRODUCT LISTING - EQUIVALENTS NOT AVAILABLE

Tablet - Oral - 50 mg

25's	$104.68	PURINETHOL, Glaxosmithkline	00173-0807-25
250's	$997.08	PURINETHOL, Glaxosmithkline	00173-0807-65

Meropenem *(003297)*

Categories: Appendicitis; Infection, intra-abdominal; Meningitis, bacterial; Peritonitis; Pregnancy Category B; FDA Approved 1996 Jul

Drug Classes: Antibiotics, carbapenems

Brand Names: **Merrem IV**

Foreign Brand Availability: Mepem (Taiwan); Meronem (Bahamas; Barbados; Belize; Benin; Bermuda; Burkina-Faso; Colombia; Curacao; Czech-Republic; Denmark; England; Ethiopia; Finland; Gambia; Germany; Ghana; Greece; Guinea; Guyana; Hong-Kong; Hungary; Indonesia; Israel; Ivory-Coast; Jamaica; Kenya; Liberia; Malawi; Mali; Mauritania; Mauritius; Morocco; Netherland-Antilles; Netherlands; Niger; Nigeria; Peru; Philippines; Puerto-Rico; Senegal; Seychelles; Sierra-Leone; South-Africa; Spain; Sudan; Surinam; Sweden; Switzerland; Tanzania; Thailand; Trinidad; Tunia; Uganda; Zambia; Zimbabwe); Meropen (Japan; Korea); Merrem (Australia; Canada; Mexico; New-Zealand)

Cost of Therapy: $1088.64 (Infection; Merrem; 1 g; 3 g/day; 7 day supply)

DESCRIPTION

Merrem IV (meropenem) is a sterile, pyrogen-free, synthetic, broad-spectrum, carbapenem antibiotic for intravenous administration. Meropenem is (4R,5S,6S)-3-[[(3S,5S)-5-(Dimethylcarbamoyl)-3-pyrrolidinyl]thio]-6-[(1R)-1-hydroxyethyl]-4-methyl-7-oxo-1-azabicyclo[3.2.0]hept-2-ene-2-carboxylic acid trihydrate. Its empirical formula is $C_{17}H_{25}N_3O_5S{\cdot}3H_2O$ with a molecular weight of 437.52.

Meropenem is a white to pale yellow crystalline powder. The solution varies from colorless to yellow depending on the concentration. The pH of freshly constituted solutions is between 7.3 and 8.3. Meropenem is soluble in 5% monobasic potassium phosphate solution, sparingly soluble in water, very slightly soluble in hydrated ethanol, and practically insoluble in acetone or ether.

When constituted as instructed, each 1 g Merrem IV vial will deliver 1 g of meropenem and 90.2 mg of sodium as sodium carbonate (3.92 mEq). Each 500 mg Merrem IV vial will deliver 500 mg meropenem and 45.1 mg of sodium as sodium carbonate (1.96 mEq).

Merrem IV in the ADD-Vantage vial is intended for intravenous use only after dilution with the appropriate volume of diluent solution in the Abbott ADD-Vantage diluent container. Merrem IV in the ADD-Vantage vial is available in two strengths. Each 1 g ADD-Vantage vial of Merrem IVwill deliver 90.2 mg of sodium as sodium carbonate (3.92 mEq), and each 500 mg ADD-Vantage vial will deliver 45.1 mg of sodium as sodium carbonate (1.96 mEq).

CLINICAL PHARMACOLOGY

At the end of a 30 minute intravenous infusion of a single dose of meropenem in normal volunteers, mean peak plasma concentrations are approximately 23 μg/ml (range 14-26) for the 500 mg dose and the 49 μg/ml (range 39-58) for the 1 g dose. A 5 minute intravenous bolus injection of meropenem in normal volunteers results in mean peak plasma concentrations of approximately 45 μg/ml (range 18-65) for the 500 mg dose and 112 μg/ml (range 83-140) for the 1 g dose.

Following intravenous doses of 500 mg, mean plasma concentrations of meropenem usually decline to approximately 1 μg/ml at 6 hours after administration.

In subjects with normal renal function, the elimination half-life of meropenem is approximately 1 hour. Approximately 70% of the intravenously administered dose is recovered as unchanged meropenem in the urine over 12 hours, after which little further urinary excretion is detectable. Urinary concentrations of meropenem in excess of 10 μg/ml are maintained for up to 5 hours after a 500 mg dose. No accumulation of meropenem in plasma or urine was observed with regimens using 500 mg administered every 8 hours or 1 g administered every 6 hours in volunteers with normal renal function.

Plasma protein binding of meropenem is approximately 2%.

There is one metabolite which is microbiologically inactive.

Meropenem penetrates well into most body fluids and tissues including cerebrospinal fluid, achieving concentrations matching or exceeding those required to inhibit most susceptible bacteria. After a single intravenous dose of meropenem, the highest mean concentrations of meropenem were found in tissues and fluids at 1 hour (0.5-1.5 hours) after the start of infusion, except where indicated in the tissues and fluids listed in TABLE 1.

TABLE 1 *Meropenem Concentrations in Selected Tissues — Highest Concentrations Reported*

Tissue	IV Dose	No. of Samples	Mean * [μg/ml or μg/(g)]	Range [μg/ml or μg/(g)]
Endometrium	0.5 g	7	4.2	1.7-10.2
Myometrium	0.5 g	15	3.8	0.4-8.1
Ovary	0.5 g	8	2.8	0.8-4.8
Cervix	0.5 g	2	7.0	5.4-8.5
Fallopian tube	0.5 g	9	1.7	0.3-3.4
Skin	0.5 g	22	3.3	0.5-12.6
Skin	1.0 g	10	5.3	1.3-16.7
Colon	1.0 g	2	2.6	2.5-2.7
Bile	1.0 g	7	14.6 (3 h)	4.0-25.7
Gall bladder	1.0 g	1	—	3.9
Interstitial fluid	1.0 g	5	26.3	20.9-37.4
Peritoneal fluid	1.0 g	9	30.2	7.4-54.6
Lung	1.0 g	2	4.8 (2 h)	1.4-8.2
Bronchial mucosa	1.0 g	7	4.5	1.3-11.1
Muscle	1.0 g	2	6.1 (2 h)	5.3-6.9
Fascia	1.0 g	9	8.8	1.5-20
Heart valves	1.0 g	7	9.7	6.4-12.1
Myocardium	1.0 g	10	15.5	5.2-25.5
CSF (inflamed)	20 mg/kg†	8	1.1 (2 h)	0.2-2.8
	40 mg/kg‡	5	3.3 (3 h)	0.9-6.5
CSF (uninflamed)	1.0 g	4	0.2 (2 h)	0.1-0.3

* At 1 hour unless otherwise noted.
† In pediatric patients of age 5 months to 8 years.
‡ In pediatric patients of age 1 month to 15 years.

M

The pharmacokinetics of meropenem in pediatric patients 2 years of age or older are essentially similar to those in adults. The elimination half-life for meropenem was approximately 1.5 hours in pediatric patients of age 3 months to 2 years. The pharmacokinetics are linear over the dose range from 10-40 mg/kg.

Pharmacokinetic studies with meropenem in patients with renal insufficiency have shown that the plasma clearance of meropenem correlates with creatnine clearance. Dosage adjustments are necessary in subjects with renal impairment. (See DOSAGE AND ADMINISTRATION, Use in Adults With Renal Impairment.) A pharmacokinetic study with meropenem in elderly patients with renal insufficiency has shown a reduction in plasma clearance of meropenem that correlates with age-associated reduction in creatnine clearance.

Meropenem is hemodialyzable. However, there is no information on the usefulness of hemodialysis to treat overdosage.

A pharmacokinetic study with meropenem in patients with hepatic impairment has shown no effects of liver disease on the pharmacokinetics of meropenem.

MICROBIOLOGY

The bactericidal activity of meropenem results from the inhibition of cell wall synthesis. Meropenem rapidly penetrates the cell wall of most gram-positive and gram-negative bacteria to reach penicillin-binding-protein (PBP) targets. Its strongest affinities are toward PBPs 2, 3, and 4 of *Escherichia coli* and *Pseudomonas aeruginosa;* and PBPs 1, 2, and 4 of *Staphyloccus aureus.* Bactericidal concentrations (defined as a 3 $\log_{10}$ reduction in cell counts within 12-24 hours) are typically 1-2 times the bacteriostatic concentrations of meropenem, with the exception of *Listeria monocytogenes,* against which lethal activity is not observed.

Meropenem has significant stability to hydrolysis by β-lactamases of most categories, both penicillinases and cephalosporinases produced by gram-positive and gram-negative bacteria, with the exception of metallo-β-lactamases. Meropenem should not be used to treat methicillin-resistant staphylococci. Cross resistance is sometimes observed with strains resistant to other carbapenems.

In vitro tests show meropenem to act synergistically with aminoglycoside antibiotics against some isolates of *Pseudomonas aeruginosa.*

Meropenem has been shown to be active against most strains of the following microorganisms, both *in vitro* and in clinical infections as described in INDICATIONS AND USAGE.

Gram-Positive Aerobes:

Streptococcus pneumoniae (excluding penicillin-resistant strains)
Viridans group streptococci
NOTE: Penicillin-resistant strains had meropenem MIC_{90} values of 1 or 2 µg/ml, which is above the 0.12 µg/ml susceptible breakpoint for this species.

Gram-Negative Aerobes:

Escherichia coli
Haemophilus influenzae (β-lactamase and non-β-lactamase-producing)
Klebsiella pneumoniae
Neisseria meningitidis
Pseudomonas aeruginosa

Anaerobes:

Bacteroides fragilis
Bacteroides thetaiotaomicron
*Peptostreptococcus*species

The following *in vitro* data are available, **but their clinical significance is unknown.**

Meropenem exhibits *in vitro* minimum inhibitory concentrations (MICs) of 0.12 µg/ml against most (≥90%) strains of *Streptococcus pneumoniae,* 0.5 µg/ml or less against most (≥90%) strains of *Haemophilus influenzae,* and 4 µg/ml or less against most (≥90%) strains of the other microorganisms in the following list; however, the safety and effectiveness of meropenem in treating clinical infections due to these microorganisms have not been established in adequate and well-controlled clinical trials.

Gram-Positive Aerobes:

Staphyloccus aureus (β-lactamase and non-β-lactamase producing)
Staphyloccus epidermidis (β-lactamase and non-β-lactamase producing)
NOTE: Staphylocci which are resistant to methicillin/oxacillin must be considered resistant to meropenem.

Gram-Negative Aerobes:

Acinetobacter species
Aeromonas hydrophila
Campylobacter jejuni
Citrobacter diversus
Citrobacter freundii
Enterobacter cloacae
Haemophilus influenzae (ampicillin-resistant, non-β-lactamase producing strains [BLNAR strains])
Hafnia alvei
Klebsiella oxytoca
Moraxella catarrhalis (β-lactamase and non-β-lactamase-producing strains)
Morganella morganii
Pasteurella multocida
Proteus mirabilis
Proteus vulgaris
Salmonella species
Serratia marcescens
Shigella species
Yersinia enterocolitica

Anaerobes:

Bacteroides distasonis
Bacteroides ovatus
Bacteroides uniformis
Bacteroides ureolyticus
Bacteroides vulgatus
Clostridium difficile
Clostridium perfringens
Eubacterium lentum
Fusobacterium species
Prevotella bivia
Prevotella intermedia
Prevotella melaninogenica
Porphyromonas asaccharolytica
Propionbacterium acnes

SUSCEPTIBILITY TESTING

Dilution Techniques

Quantitative methods are used to determine antimicrobial minimum inhibitory concentrations (MICs). These MICs provide estimates of the susceptibility of bacteria to antimicrobial compounds. The MICs should be determined using a standardized procedure. Standardized procedures are based on a dilution method[1] (broth or agar) or equivalent with standardized inoculum concentrations and standardized concentrations of meropenem powder. The MIC values should be interpreted according to the criteria shown in TABLE 2 for indicated aerobic organisms other than *Haemophilus* species and streptococci.

TABLE 2

MIC (µg/ml)	Interpretation
≤4	(S) Susceptible
8	(I) Intermediate
≥16	(R) Resistant

Haemophilus Test Media (HTM) and the interpretive criteria shown in TABLE 3 should be used when testing *Haemophilus* species.

TABLE 3

MIC (µg/ml)	Interpretation
≤0.5	(S) Susceptible

The current absence of resistant strains precludes defining any categories other than "Susceptible". Strains yielding results suggestive of a "Nonsusceptible" category should be submitted to a reference laboratory for further testing.

The criteria shown in TABLE 4 should be used when testing streptococci including *Streptococcus pneumoniae.*

TABLE 4

MIC (µg/ml)	Interpretation
When testing *Streptococcus pneumoniae*	
≤0.12	(S) Susceptible
When testing viridans group streptococci	
≤0.5	(S) Susceptible

The current absence of resistant strains precludes defining any categories other than "Susceptible". Strains yielding results suggestive of a "Nonsusceptible" category should be submitted to a reference laboratory for further testing.

A report of "Susceptible" indicates that the pathogen is likely to be inhibited if the antimicrobial compound in the blood reaches the concentrations usually achievable. A report of "Intermediate" indicates that the result should be considered equivocal, and, if the microorganism is not fully susceptible to alternative, clinically feasible drugs, the test should be repeated. This category implies possible clinical applicability in body sites where the drug is physiologically concentrated or in situations where high dosage of drug can be used. This category also provides a buffer zone which prevents small uncontrolled technical factors from causing major discrepancies in interpretation. A report of "Resistant" indicates that the pathogen is not likely to be inhibited if the antimicrobial compound in the blood reaches the concentrations usually achievable; other therapy should be selected.

Standardized susceptibility test procedures require the use of laboratory control microorganisms to control the technical aspects of the laboratory procedures. Standard meropenem powder should provide the MIC values in TABLE 5.

TABLE 5

Microorganism	ATCC	MIC (µg/ml)
Enterococcus faecalis	29212	2.0-8.0
Escherichia coli	25922	0.008-0.06
Haemophilus influenzae	49766	0.03-0.12
Pseudomonas aeruginosa	27853	0.25-1.0
Streptococcus pneumoniae	49619	0.06-0.25

Diffusion Techniques

Quantitative methods that require measurement of zone diameters also provide reproducible estimates of the susceptibility of bacteria to antimicrobial compounds. One such standardized procedure[2] requires the use of standardized inoculum concentrations. This procedure uses paper disks impregnated with 10 µg of meropenem to test the susceptibility of microorganisms to meropenem.

Reports from the laboratory providing results of the standard single-disk susceptibility test with a 10 µg disk should be interpreted according to the criteria shown in TABLE 6 for indicated aerobic organisms other than *Haemophilus* species and streptococci.

Haemophilus Test Media and the criteria shown in TABLE 7 should be used when testing *Haemophilus* species.

TABLE 6

Zone Diameter (mm)	Interpretation
≥16	(S) Susceptible
14-15	(I) Intermediate
≤13	(R) Resistant

TABLE 7

Zone Diameter (mm)	Interpretation
≥20	(S) Susceptible

The current absence of resistant strains precludes defining any categories other than "Susceptible". Strains yielding results suggestive of a "Nonsusceptible" category should be submitted to a reference laboratory for further testing.

Streptococcus pneumoniae isolates should be tested using 1 μg/ml oxacillin disk. Isolates with oxacillin zone sizes of ≥20 mm are susceptible (MIC ≤0.06 μg/ml) to peniclin and can be considered susceptible to meropenem for approved indications, and meropenem need not be tested. A meropenem MIC should be determined on isolates of *S. pneumoniae* with oxacillin zone sizes of ≤19 mm. The disk test does not distinguish penicillin intermediate strains (*i.e.*, MICs = 0.12-1.0 μg/ml) from strains that are penicillin resistant (*i.e.*, MICs ≥2 μg/ml). Viridans group streptococci should be tested for meropenem susceptibility using an MIC method. Reliable disk diffusion tests for meropenem do not yet exist for testing streptococci.

Interpretation should be as stated above for results using dilution techniques. Interpretation involves correlation of the diameter obtained in the disk test with the MIC for meropenem.

As with standardized dilution techniques, diffusion methods require the use of laboratory control microorganisms that are used to control the technical aspects of the laboratory procedures. For the diffusion technique, the 10 μg meropenem disk should provide the zone diameters shown in TABLE 8 in these laboratory test quality control strains.

TABLE 8

Microorganism	ATCC	Zone Diameter (mm)
Escherichia coli	25922	28-34
Haemophilus influenzae	49247	20-28
Pseudomonas aeruginosa	27853	27-33

Anaerobic Techniques

For anaerobic bacteria, susceptibility to meropenem as MICs can be determined by standardized test methods.[3] The MIC values obtained should be interpreted according to the criteria shown in TABLE 9.

TABLE 9

MIC (μg/ml)	Interpretation
≤4	(S) Susceptible
8	(I) Intermediate
≥16	(R) Resistant

Interpretation is identical to that stated above for results using dilution techniques.

As with other susceptibility techniques, the use of laboratory control microorganisms is required to control the technical aspects of the laboratory standardized procedures. Standardized meropenem powder should provide the MIC values in TABLE 10.

TABLE 10

Microorganism	ATCC	MIC (μg/ml)
Bacteroides fragilis	25285	0.06-0.25
Bacteroides thetaiotaomicron	29741	0.125-0.5

INDICATIONS AND USAGE

Meropenem is indicated as single agent therapy for the treatment of the following infections when caused by susceptible strains of the designated microorganisms:

Intra-Abdominal Infections: Complicated appendicitis and peritonitis caused by viridans group streptococci, *Escherichia coli, Klebsiella pneumoniae, Pseudomonas aeruginosa, Bacteroides fragilis, B. thetaiotaomicron,* and *Peptostreptococcus* species.

Bacterial Meningitis (pediatric patients ≥3 months only): Bacterial meningitis caused by *Streptococcus pneumoniae*, Haemophilus influenzae* (β-lactamase and non-β-lacatamase-producing strains), and *Neisseria meningitidis.*

*The efficacy of meropenem as monotherapy in the treatment of meningitis caused by penicillin nonsusceptible strains of *Streptococcus pneumoniae* has not been established.

Meropenem has been found to be effective in eliminating concurrent bacteremia in association with bacterial meningitis.

For information regarding use in pediatric patients (3 months of age and older) see PRECAUTIONS, Pediatric Use; ADVERSE REACTIONS; and DOSAGE AND ADMINISTRATION.

Appropriate cultures should usually be performed before initiating antimicrobial treatment in order to isolate and identify the organisms causing infection and determine their susceptibility to meropenem.

Meropenem is useful as presumptive therapy in the indicated condition (*i.e.*, intra-abdominal infections) prior to the identification of the causative organisms because of its broad spectrum of bactericidal activity.

Antimicrobial therapy should be adjusted, if appropriate, once the results of culture(s) and antimicrobial susceptibility testing are known.

NON-FDA APPROVED INDICATIONS

Although not approved by the FDA, the use of meropenem for the treatment of lower respiratory tract infections, bacteremia, skin and soft tissue infections, febrile neutropenia, pelvic infections, and urinary tract infections has been studied.

CONTRAINDICATIONS

Meropenem is contraindicated in patients with known hypersensitivity to any component of this product or to other drugs in the same class or in patients who have demonstrated anaphylactic reactions to β-lactams.

WARNINGS

SERIOUS AND OCCASIONALLY FATAL HYPERSENSITIVITY (ANAPHYLACTIC) REACTIONS HAVE BEEN REPORTED IN PATIENTS RECEIVING THERAPY WITH β-LACTAMS. THESE REACTIONS ARE MORE LIKELY TO OCCUR IN INDIVIDUALS WITH A HISTORY OF SENSITIVITY TO MULTIPLE ALLERGENS.

THERE HAVE BEEN REPORTS OF INDIVIDUALS WITH A HISTORY OF PENICILLIN HYPERSENSITIVITY WHO HAVE EXPERIENCED SEVERE HYPERSENSITIVITY REACTIONS WHEN TREATED WITH ANOTHER β-LACTAM. BEFORE INITIATING THERAPY WITH MEROPENEM, CAREFUL INQUIRY SHOULD BE MADE CONCERNING PREVIOUS HYPERSENSITIVITY REACTIONS TO PENICILLINS, CEPHALOSPORINS, OTHER β-LACTAMS, AND OTHER ALLERGENS. IF AN ALLERGIC REACTION TO MEROPENEM OCCURS, DISCONTINUE THE DRUG IMMEDIATELY. **SERIOUS ANAPHYLACTIC REACTIONS REQUIRE IMMEDIATE EMERGENCY TREATMENT WITH EPINEPHRINE, OXYGEN, INTRAVENOUS STEROIDS, AND AIRWAY MANAGEMENT, INCLUDING INTUBATION. OTHER THERAPY MAY ALSO BE ADMINISTERED AS INDICATED.**

Seizures and other CNS experiences have been reported during treatment with meropenem (see PRECAUTIONS and ADVERSE REACTIONS).

Pseudomembraneous colitis has been reported with nearly all antibacterial agents, including meropenem, and may range in severity from mild to life-threatening. Therefore, it is important to consider this diagnosis in patients who present with diarrhea subsequent to the administration of antibacterial agents.

Treatment with antibacterial agents alters the normal flora of the colon and may permit overgrowth of clostridia. Studies indicate that a toxin produced by *Clostridium difficile* is a primary cause of "antibiotic-associated colitis".

After the diagnosis of pseudomembranous colitis has been established, therapeutic measures should be initiated. Mild cases of pseudomembranous colitis usually respond to drug discontinuation alone. In moderate-to-severe cases, consideration should be given to management with fluids and electrolytes, protein supplementation, and treatment with an antibacterial drug clinically effective against *Clostridium difficile* colitis.

M

PRECAUTIONS

GENERAL

Seizures and other CNS adverse experiences have been reported during treatment with meropenem. These experiences have occurred most commonly in patients with CNS disorders (*e.g.*, brain lesions or history of seizures) or with bacterial meningitis and/or compromised renal function.

During the initial clinical investigations, 2904 immunocompetent adult patients were treated for infections outside the CNS, with the overall seizure rate being 0.7% (based on 20 patients with this adverse event). All meropenem-treated patients with seizures had preexisting contributing factors. Among these are included prior history of seizures or CNS abnormality and concomitant medications with seizure potential. Dosage adjustment is recommended in patients with advanced age and/or reduced renal function (See DOSAGE AND ADMINISTRATION, Use in Adults With Renal Impairment).

Close adherence to the recommended dosage regimens is urged, especially in patients with known factors that predispose to convulsive activity. Anticonvulsant therapy should be continued in patients with known seizure disorders. If focal tremors, myoclonus, or seizures occur, patients should be evaluated neurologically, placed on anticonvulsant therapy if not already instituted, and the dosage of meropenem re-examined to determine whether it should be decreased or the antibiotic discontinued.

In patients with renal dysfunction, thrombocytopenia has been observed but no clinical bleeding reported. (See DOSAGE AND ADMINISTRATION, Use in Adults With Renal Impairment.)

There is inadequate information regarding the use of meropenem in patients on hemodialysis.

As with other broad-spectrum antibiotics, prolonged use of meropenem may result in overgrowth of nonsusceptible organisms. Repeated evaluation of the patient is essential. If superinfection does occur during therapy, appropriate measures should be taken.

LABORATORY TESTS

While meropenem possesses the characteristic low toxicity of the β-lactam group of antibiotics, periodic assessment of organ system functions, including renal, hepatic, and hematopoietic, is advisable during prolonged therapy.

CARCINOGENESIS, MUTAGENESIS, AND IMPAIRMENT OF FERTILITY

Carcinogenesis

Carcinogenesis studies have not been performed.

Mutagenesis

Genetic toxicity studies were performed with meropenem using the bacterial reverse mutation test, the Chinese hamster ovary HGPRT assay, cultured human lymphocytes cytogenic assay, and the mouse micronucleus test. There was no evidence of mutagenic potential found in any of these tests.

Impairment of Fertility

Reproductive studies were performed with meropenem in rats at doses up to 1000 mg/kg/day, and cynomolgus monkeys at doses up to 360 mg/kg/day (on the basis of AUC comparisons, approximately 1.8 times and 3.7 times, respectively, to the human exposure at the usual dose of 1 g every 8 hours). There was no reproductive toxicity seen.

PREGNANCY CATEGORY B

Reproductive studies have been performed with meropenem in rats at doses of up to 1000 mg/kg/day, and cynomolgus monkeys at doses of up to 360 mg/kg/day (on the basis of AUC comparisons, approximately 1.8 times and 3.7 times, respectively, to the human exposure at the usual dose of 1 g every 8 hours). These studies revealed no evidence of impaired fertility or harm to the fetus due to meropenem, although there were slight changes in fetal body weight at doses of 250 mg/kg/day (on the basis of AUC comparisons, 0.4 times the human exposure at a dose of 1 g every 8 hours) and above in rats. There are, however, no adequate and well-controlled studies in pregnant women. Because animal reproduction studies are not always predictive of human response, this drug should be used in pregnancy only if clearly needed.

PEDIATRIC USE

The safety and effectiveness of meropenem have been established for pediatric patients ≥3 months of age. Use of meropenem in pediatric patients with bacterial meningitis is supported by evidence from adequate and well-controlled studies in the pediatric population. Use of meropenem in pediatric patients with intra-abdominal infections is supported by evidence from adequate and well-controlled studies with adults with additional data from pediatric pharmacokinetics studies and controlled clinical trials in pediatric patients. (See CLINICAL PHARMACOLOGY, INDICATIONS AND USAGE, ADVERSE REACTIONS, DOSAGE AND ADMINISTRATION.)

NURSING MOTHERS

It is not known whether this drug is excreted in human milk. Because many drugs are excreted in human milk, caution should be exercised when meropenem is administered to a nursing woman.

GERIATRIC USE

Of the total number of subjects in clinical studies of meropenem, approximately 1100 (30%) were 65 years of age and older, while 400 (11%) were 75 years and older. No overall differences in safety or effectiveness were observed between these subjects and younger subjects; spontaneous reports and other reported clinical experiences have not identified differences in responses between the elderly and younger patients, but greater sensitivity of some older individuals cannot be ruled out.

A pharmacokinetic study with meropenem in elderly patients with renal insufficiency has shown a reduction in plasma clearance of meropenem that correlates with age-associated reduction in creatinine clearance. (See DOSAGE AND ADMINISTRATION, Use in Adults With Renal Impairment.)

Merropenem IV is known to be substantially excreted by the kidney, and the risk of toxic reactions to this drug may be greater in patients with impaired renal function. Because elderly patients are more likely to have decreased renal function, care should be taken in dose selection, and it may be useful to monitor renal function.

DRUG INTERACTIONS

Probenecid competes with meropenem for active tubular secretion and thus inhibits the renal excretion of meropenem. This led to statistically significant increases in the elimination half-life (38%) and in the extent of systemic exposure (56%). Therefore, the coadministration of probenecid with meropenem is not recommended.

There is evidence that meropenem may reduce serum levels of valproic acid to subtherapeutic levels (therapeutic range considered to be 50-100 μg/ml total valproate).

ADVERSE REACTIONS

ADULT PATIENTS

During clinical investigations, 2904 immunocompetent adult patients were treated for infections outside the CNS with meropenem (500 or 1000 mg q8h). Deaths in 5 patients were assessed as possibly related to meropenem; 36 (1.2%) patients had meropenem discontinued because of adverse events. Many patients in these trials were severely ill and had multiple background diseases, physiological impairments and were receiving multiple other drug therapies. In the seriously ill patient population, it was not possible to determine the relationship between observed adverse events and therapy with meropenem.

The following adverse reaction frequencies were derived from the clinical trials in the 2904 patients treated with meropenem.

Local Adverse Reactions

Local adverse reactions that were reported irrespective of the relationship to therapy with meropenem were as shown in TABLE 14.

TABLE 14

Inflammation at the injection site	2.4%
Phlebitis/thrombophlebitis	0.9%
Injection site reaction	0.8%
Pain at the injection site	0.4%
Edema at the injection site	0.2%

Systemic Adverse Reactions

Systemic adverse clinical reactions that were reported irrespective of the relationship to meropenem occurring in greater than 1.0% of the patients were diarrhea (4.8%), nausea/vomiting (3.6%), headache (2.3%), rash (1.9%), sepsis (1.6%), constipation (1.4%), apnea (1.3%), shock (1.2%), and pruritus (1.2%).

Additional adverse systemic clinical reactions that were reported irrespective of relationship to therapy with meropenem and occurring in less than or equal to 1.0% but greater than 0.1% of the patients are listed below within each body system in order of decreasing frequency:

Bleeding events were seen as follows: Gastrointestinal hemorrhage (0.5%), melena (0.3%), epistaxis (0.2%), hemoperitoneum (0.2%), summing to 1.2%.

Body as a whole: Pain, abdominal pain, chest pain, fever, back pain, abdominal enlargement, chills, pelvic pain.

Cardiovascular: Heart failure, heart arrest, tachycardia, hypertension, myocardial infarction, pulmonary embolus, bradycardia, hypotension, syncope.

Digestive system: Oral moniliasis, anorexia, cholestatic jaundice/jaundice, flatulence, ileus, hepatic failure, dyspepsia, intestinal obstruction.

Hemic/lymphatic: Anemia, hypochromic anemia, hypervolemia.

Metabolic/nutritional: Peripheral edema, hypoxia.

Nervous system: Insomnia, agitation/delirium, confusion, dizziness, seizure (see PRECAUTIONS), nervousness, paresthesia, hallucinations, somnolence, anxiety, depression, asthenia.

Respiratory: Respiratory disorder, dyspnea, pleural effusion, asthma, cough increased, lung edema.

Skin and appendages: Urticaria, sweating, skin ulcer.

Urogenital system: Dysuria, kidney failure, vaginal moniliasis, urinary incontinence.

Adverse Laboratory Changes

Adverse laboratory changes that were reported irrespective of relationship to meropenem and occurring in greater than 0.2% of the patients were as follows:

Hepatic: Increased SGPT (ALT), SGOT (AST), alkaline phosphatase, LDH, and bilirubin.

Hematologic: Increased platelets, increased eosinophils, decreased platelets, decreased hemoglobin, decreased hematocrit, decreased WBC, shortened prothrombin time and shortened partial thromboplastin time, leukocytosis, hypokalemia.

Renal: Increased creatinine and increased BUN.

NOTE: For patients with varying degrees of renal impairment, the incidence of heart failure, kidney failure, seizure and shock reported irrespective of relationship to meropenem, increased in patients with moderately severe renal impairment (creatinine clearance >10 to 26 mL/min).

Urinalysis: Presence of urine red blood cells.

PEDIATRIC PATIENTS

Clinical Adverse Reactions

Meropenem was studied in 515 pediatric patients (≥3 months to <13 years of age) with serious bacterial infections (excluding meningitis. See next section.) at dosages of 10-20 mg/kg every 8 hours. The types of clinical adverse events seen in these patients are similar to the adults, with the most common adverse events reported as possibly, probably or definitely related to meropenem and their rates of occurrence are shown in TABLE 15.

TABLE 15

Diarrhea	3.5%
Rash	1.6%
Nausea and vomiting	0.8%

Meropenem was studied in 321 pediatric patients (≥3 months to <17 years of age) with meningitis at a dosage of 40 mg/kg every 8 hours. The types of clinical adverse events seen in these patients are similar to the adults, with the most common adverse events reported as possibly, probably, or definitely related to meropenem and their rates of occurrence are shown in TABLE 16.

TABLE 16

Diarrhea	4.7%
Rash (mostly diaper area moniliasis)	3.1%
Oral moniliasis	1.9%
Glossitis	1.0%

In the meningitis studies the rates of seizure activity during therapy were comparable between patients with no CNS abnormalities who received meropenem and those who received comparator agents (either cefotaxime or ceftriaxone). In the meropenem treated group, 12/15 patients with seizures had late onset seizures (defined as occurring on day 3 or later) versus 7/20 in the comparator arm.

Adverse Laboratory Changes

Laboratory abnormalities seen in the pediatric-aged patients in both the pediatric and the meningitis studies are similar to those reported in adult patients.

There is no experience in pediatric patients with renal impairment.

POST-MARKETING EXPERIENCE

Worldwide post-marketing adverse events not previously listed in the product label and reported as possibly, probably, or definitely drug related are listed within each body system in order of decreasing severity.

Hematologic: Agranulocytosis, neutropenia, and leukopenia.

Skin: Toxic epidermal necrolysis, Stevens-Johnson Syndrome, angioedema, and erythema multiforme.

DOSAGE AND ADMINISTRATION

ADULTS

One gram (1 g) by intravenous administration every 8 hours. Meropenem should be given by intravenous infusion, over approximately 15-30 minutes or as an intravenous bolus injection (5-20 ml) over approximately 3-5 minutes.

USE IN ADULTS WITH RENAL IMPAIRMENT

Dosage should be reduced in patients with creatinine clearance less than 51 ml/min. (See TABLE 17.)

TABLE 17 *Recommended Meropenem Dosage Schedule for Adults With Impaired Renal Function*

Creatinine Clearance (ml/min)	Dose (dependent on type of infection)	Dosing Interval
26-50	Recommended dose (1000 mg)	Every 12 hours
10-25	One-half recommended dose	Every 12 hours
<10	One-half recommended dose	Every 24 hours

When only serum creatinine is available, the following formula (Cockcroft and Gault equation)[4] may be used to estimate creatinine clearance:

Males: Creatinine Clearance (ml/min) = [Weight (kg) × (140 - age)] ÷ [72 × serum creatinine (mg/dl)].

Females: 0.85 × above value.

There is inadequate information regarding the use of meropenem in patients on hemodialysis.

There is no experience with peritoneal dialysis.

USE IN ADULTS WITH HEPATIC INSUFFICIENCY

No dosage adjustment is necessary in patients with impaired hepatic function.

USE IN ELDERLY PATIENTS

No dosage adjustment is required for elderly patients with creatinine clearance values above 50 ml/min.

USE IN PEDIATRIC PATIENTS

For pediatric patients from 3 months of age and older, the meropenem dose is 20 or 40 mg/kg every 8 hours (maximum dose is 2 g every 8 hours), depending on the type of infection (intra-abdominal or meningitis). (See TABLE 18.) Pediatric patients weighing over 50 kg should be administered meropenem at a dose of 1 g every 8 hours for intra-abdominal infections and 2 g every 8 hours for meningitis. Meropenem should be given as intravenous infusion over approximately 15-30 minutes or as an intravenous bolus injection (5-20 ml) over approximately 3-5 minutes.

TABLE 18 *Recommended Meropenem Dosage Schedule for Pediatrics With Normal Renal Function*

Type of Infection	Dose (mg/kg)	Dosing Interval
Intra-abdominal	20	Every 8 hours
Meningitis	40	Every 8 hours

There is no experience in pediatric patients with renal impairment.

COMPATIBILITY AND STABILITY

Compatibility of meropenem with other drugs has not been established. Meropenem should not be mixed with or physically added to solutions containing other drugs.

Freshly prepared solutions of meropenem should be used whenever possible. However, constituted solutions of meropenem maintain satisfactory potency at controlled room temperature 15-25°C (59-77°F) or under refrigeration at 4°C (39°F) as described below. Solutions of intravenous meropenem should not be frozen.

NOTE: Parenteral drug products should be inspected visually for particulate matter and discoloration prior to administration, whenever solution and container permit.

Intravenous Bolus Administration

Meropenem injection vials constituted with sterile water for injection for bolus administration (up to 50 mg/ml of meropenem) may be stored for up to 2 hours at controlled room temperature 15-25°C (59-77°F) or for up to 12 hours at 4°C (39°F).

Intravenous Infusion Administration

Stability in Infusion Vials

Meropenem infusion vials constituted with sodium chloride injection 0.9% (meropenem concentrations ranging from 2.5 to 50 mg/ml) are stable for up to 2 hours at controlled room temperature 15-25°C (55-77°F) or for up to 18 hours at 4°C (39°F). Infusion vials of meropenem constituted with dextrose injection 5% (meropenem concentrations ranging from 2.5 to 50 mg/ml) are stable for up to 1 hour at controlled room temperature 15-25°C (59-77°F) or for up to 8 hours at 4°C (39°F).

Stability in Plastic IV Bags

Solutions prepared for infusion (meropenem concentrations ranging from 1-20 mg/ml) may be stored in plastic intravenous bags with diluents as shown in TABLE 19.

Stability in Baxter Minibag Plus

Solutions of meropenem (meropenem concentrations ranging from 2.5 to 20 mg/ml) in Baxter Minibag Plus bags with sodium chloride injection 0.9% may be stored for up to 4 hours at controlled room temperatures 15-25°C (59-77°F) or for up to 24 hours at 4°C (39°F).

TABLE 19

	Number of Hours	
	Stable at Controlled Room Temperature 15-25°C (59-77°F)	Stable at 4°C (39°F)
Sodium chloride injection 0.9%	4	24
Dextrose injection 5.0%	1	4
Dextrose injection 10.0%	1	2
Dextrose and sodium chloride injection 5.0%/0.9%	1	2
Dextrose and sodium chloride injection 5.0%/0.2%	1	4
Potassium chloride in dextrose injection 0.15%/5.0%	1	6
Sodium bicarbonate in dextrose injection 0.02%/5.0%	1	6
Dextrose injection 5.0% in Normosol-M	1	8
Dextrose injection 5.0% in Ringer's lactate injection	1	4
Dextrose and sodium chloride injection 2.5%/0.45%	3	12
Mannitol injection 2.5%	2	16
Ringer's injection	4	24
Ringer's lactate injection	4	12
Sodium lactate injection 1/6 N	2	24
Sodium bicarbonate injection 5.0%	1	4

Solutions of meropenem (meropenem concentrations ranging from 2.5 to 20 mg/ml) in Baxter Minibag Plus bags with dextrose injection 5.0% may be stored up to 1 hour at controlled room temperatures 15-25°C (59-77°F) or for up to 6 hours at 4°C (39°F).

Stability in Plastic Syringes, Tubing and Intravenous Infusion Sets

Solutions of meropenem (meropenem concentrations ranging from 1-20 mg/ml) in water for injection or sodium chloride injection 0.9% (for up to 4 hours) or in dextrose injection 5.0% (for up to 2 hours) at controlled room temperatures 15-25°C (59-77°F) are stable in plastic tubing and volume control devices of common intravenous infusion sets.

Solutions of meropenem (merropenem concentrations ranging from 1-20 mg/ml) in water for injection or sodium chloride injection 0.9% (for up to 48 hours) or in dextrose injection 5% (for up to 6 hours) are stable at 4°C (39°F) in plastic syringes.

ADD-Vantage Vials

ADD-Vantage vials diluted in sodium chloride injection 0.45% (meropenem concentrations ranging from 5-20 mg/ml) may be stored for up to 6 hours at controlled room temperature 15-25°C (59-77°F) or for 24 hours at 4°C (39°F). ADD-Vantage vials diluted in sodium chloride injection 0.9% (meropenem concentrations ranging from 1-20 mg/ml) may be stored for up to 4 hours at controlled room temperature 15-25°C (59-77°F) or for 24 hours at 4°C (39°F). ADD-Vantage vials diluted with dextrose injection 5.0% (meropenem concentrations ranging from 1-20 mg/ml) may be stored for up to 1 hour at controlled room temperature 15-25°C (59-77°F) or for 8 hours at 4°C (39°F).

M

HOW SUPPLIED

Merrem IV is supplied in 20 and 30 ml injection vials containing sufficient meropenem to deliver 500 mg or 1 g for intravenous administration, respectively.

Merrem IV is supplied in 100 ml infusion vials containing sufficient meropenem to deliver 500 mg or 1 g for intravenous administration.

Merrem IV is also supplied as ADD-Vantage Vials containing sufficient meropenem to deliver 500 mg or 1 g for intravenous administration.

Storage: The dry powder should be stored at controlled room temperature 20-25°C (68-77°F).

PRODUCT LISTING - EQUIVALENTS NOT AVAILABLE

Powder For Injection - Intravenous - 1 Gm

1's	$541.20	MERREM, Astra-Zeneca Pharmaceuticals	00310-0321-11
1's	$546.30	MERREM, Astra-Zeneca Pharmaceuticals	00310-0321-15
10's	$518.40	MERREM, Astra-Zeneca Pharmaceuticals	00310-0321-30

Powder For Injection - Intravenous - 500 mg

1's	$27.41	MERREM, Astra-Zeneca Pharmaceuticals	00310-0325-11
10's	$259.20	MERREM, Astra-Zeneca Pharmaceuticals	00310-0325-20
10's	$273.40	MERREM, Astra-Zeneca Pharmaceuticals	00310-0325-15

Mesalamine (001742)

Categories: Colitis, ulcerative; Proctitis; Proctitis, ulcerative; Proctosigmoiditis; Pregnancy Category B; FDA Approved 1987 Dec
Drug Classes: Gastrointestinals; Salicylates
Brand Names: Asacol; Pentasa; **Rowasa**
Foreign Brand Availability: Asacolitin (Germany); Asacolon (Colombia); Claversal (Austria; Belgium; Czech-Republic; Germany; Italy; Portugal); Colitofalk (Belgium); Fivasa (France); Ipocol (England); Kenzomyl (Mexico); Mesacol (Benin; Burkina-Faso; Ethiopia; Gambia; Ghana; Guinea; India; Ivory-Coast; Kenya; Liberia; Malawi; Mali; Mauritania; Mauritius; Morocco; Niger; Nigeria; Senegal; Seychelles; Sierra-Leone; Sudan; Tanzania; Tunia; Uganda; Zambia; Zimbabwe); Mesalin (Korea); Mesasal (Australia; Canada; Denmark; Norway); Pentasa Enema (New-Zealand); Pentasa SR (Bahrain; Cyprus; Egypt; Iran; Iraq; Israel; Jordan; Korea; Kuwait; Lebanon; Libya; Oman; Qatar; Republic-of-Yemen; Saudi-Arabia; Syria; United-Arab-Emirates); Pentasa Tab (New-Zealand); Salofalk (Austria; Canada; Colombia; Germany; Hong-Kong; Hungary; Indonesia; Ireland; Italy; Korea; Malaysia; Netherlands; Peru; Philippines; Switzerland; Thailand)
Cost of Therapy: $194.77 (Ulcerative Colitis; Asacol; 400 mg; 6 tablets/day; 42 day supply)
$541.15 (Ulcerative Colitis; Pentasa; 250 mg; 16 tablets/day; 56 day supply)

DESCRIPTION

CONTROLLED-RELEASE CAPSULES

The controlled-release formulation of mesalamine is an aminosalicylate anti-inflammatory agent for gastrointestinal use.

Chemically, mesalamine is 5-amino-2-hydroxybenzoic acid. It has a molecular weight of 153.14.

Each Pentasa capsule contains 250 mg of mesalamine. It also contains the following inactive ingredients: acetylated monoglyceride, castor oil, colloidal silicon dioxide, ethylcellulose, hydroxypropyl, methylcellulose, starch, stearic acid, sugar, talc, and white wax. The capsule shell contains D&C yellow no. 10, FD&C blue no. 1, FD&C green no. 3, gelatin, titanium dioxide, and other ingredients.

DELAYED-RELEASE TABLETS

Each delayed-release tablet for oral administration contains 400 mg of mesalamine, an anti-inflammatory drug. The delayed-release tablets are coated with acrylic based resin, Eudragit S (methacrylic acid copolymer B), which dissolves at pH 7 or greater, releasing mesalamine in the terminal ileum and beyond for topical anti-inflammatory action in the colon. Mesalamine has the chemical name 5-amino-2-hydroxybenzoic acid.

It's molecular weight is 153.1. It's molecular formula is $C_7H_7NO_3$.

Inactive Ingredients: Each tablet contains colloidal silicon dioxide, dibutyl phthalate, edible black ink, iron oxide red, iron oxide yellow, lactose, magnesium stearate, methacrylic acid copolymer B (Eudragit S), polyethylene glycol, povidone, sodium starch glycolate, and talc.

RECTAL SUSPENSION ENEMA

M

The active ingredient is mesalamine, also known as 5-aminosalicylic acid (5-ASA). Chemically, mesalamine is 5-amino-2-hydroxybenzoic acid, and is classified as an anti-inflammatory drug.

The empirical formula is $C_7H_7NO_3$, representing a molecular weight of 153.14.

Each rectal suspension enema is a disposable (60 ml) unit and each unit contains 4 g of mesalamine. In addition to mesalamine the preparation contains the inactive ingredients potassium metabisulfite, carbomer 934P, edetate disodium, potassium acetate, water and xanthan gum. Sodium benzoate is added as a preservative. The disposable unit consists of an applicator tip protected by a polyethylene cover and lubricated with white petrolatum. The unit has a one-way valve to prevent back flow of the dispensed product.

Storage: Store at controlled room temperature 15-30°C (59-86°F).

SUPPOSITORIES

The active ingredient is mesalamine, also known as 5-aminosalicylic acid (5-ASA). Chemically, mesalamine is 5-amino-2-hydroxybenzoic acid, and is classified as an anti-inflammatory drug.

The empirical formula is $C_7H_7NO_3$, representing a molecular weight of 153.14.

Each suppository contains 500 mg of mesalamine in a base of hard fat. Each suppository is individually wrapped in foil.

Storage: Store at 19-26°C (66-79°F).

CLINICAL PHARMACOLOGY

DELAYED-RELEASE TABLETS

Mesalamine is thought to be the mThe mechanism of action of mesalamine (and sulfasalazine) is unknown, but appears to be topical rather than systemic. Mucosal production of arachidonic acid (AA) metabolites, both through the cyclooxygenase pathways, *i.e.*, prostanoids, and through the lipoxygenase pathways, *i.e.*, leukotrienes (LTs) and hydroxyeicosatetraenoic acids (HETSs), is increased in patients with chronic inflammatory bowel disease, and it is possible that mesalamine diminishes inflammation by blocking cyclooxygenase and inhibiting prostaglandin (PG) production in the colon.ajor therapeutically active part of the sulfasalazine molecule in the treatment of ulcerative colitis. Sulfasalazine is converted to equimolar amounts of sulfapyridine and mesalamine by bacterial action in the colon. The usual oral dose of sulfasalazine for active ulcerative colitis is 3-4 g daily in divided doses, which provides 1.2-1.6 g of mesalamine to the colon.

RECTAL SUSPENSION ENEMA/SUPPOSITORY

Sulfasalazine is split by bacterial action in the colon into sulfapyridine (SP) and mesalamine (5-ASA). It is thought that the mesalamine component is therapeutically active in ulcerative colitis. The usual oral doses of sulfasalazine for active ulcerative colitis in adults is 2-4 g/day in divided doses. Four (4) g of sulfasalazine provide 1.6 g of free mesalamine to the colon. Each mesalamine suspension enema delivers up to 4 g aminosalicylate of mesalamine to the left side of the colon.

Each mesalamine suppository delivers 500 mg of mesalamine to the rectum.

The mechanism of action of mesalamine (and sulfasalazine) is unknown, but appears to be topical rather than systemic. Mucosal production of arachidonic acid (AA) metabolites, both through the cyclooxygenase pathways, *i.e.*, prostanoids, and through the lipoxygenase pathways, *i.e.*, leukotrienes (LTs) and hydroxyeicosatetraenoic acids (HETEs) is increased in patients with chronic inflammatory bowel disease, and it is possible that mesalamine diminishes inflammation by blocking cyclooxygenase and inhibiting prostaglandin (PG) production in the colon.

Preclinical Toxicology

Preclinical studies have shown the kidney to be the major target organ for mesalamine toxicity. Adverse renal function changes were observed in rats after a single 600 mg/kg oral dose, but not after a 200 mg/kg dose. Gross kidney lesions, including papillary necrosis, were observed after a single oral >900 mg/kg dose, and after IV doses of >214 mg/kg. Mice responded similarly. In a 13 week oral (gavage) dose study in rats, the high dose of 640 mg/kg/day mesalamine caused deaths, probably due to renal failure, and dose-related renal lesions (papillary necrosis and/or multifocal tubular injury) were seen in most rats given the high dose (males and females) as well as in males receiving lower doses 160 mg/kg/day. Renal lesions were not observed in the 160 mg/kg/day female rats. Minimal tubular epithelial damage was seen in the 40 mg/kg/day males and was reversible. In a 6 month oral study in dogs, the no-observable dose level of mesalamine was 40 mg/kg/day and doses of 80 mg/kg/day and higher caused renal pathology similar to that described for the rat.

In a combined 52 week toxicity and 127 week carcinogenicity study in rats, degeneration in kidneys was observed at doses of 100 mg/kg/day and above admixed with diet for 52 weeks, and at 127 weeks increased incidence of kidney degeneration and hyalinization of basement membranes and Bowman's capsules was seen at 100 mg/kg/day and above. In the 12 month eye toxicity study in dogs, Keratoconjunctivitis Sicca (KCS) occurred at oral doses of 40 mg/kg/day and above. The oral preclinical studies were done with a highly bioavailable suspension where absorption throughout the gastrointestinal tract occurred. Although intrarectally administered mesalamine in humans is poorly absorbed, the potential for renal toxicity must be considered (see Pharmacokinetics and PRECAUTIONS).

PHARMACOKINETICS

Delayed-Release Tablets

Mesalamine tablets are coated with an acrylic-based resin that delays release of mesalamine until it reaches the terminal ileum and beyond. This has been demonstrated in human studies conducted with radiological and serum markers. Approximately 28% of the mesalamine in mesalamine tablets is absorbed after oral ingestion, leaving the remainder available for topical action and excretion in the feces. Absorption of mesalamine is similar in fasted and fed subjects. The absorbed mesalamine is rapidly acetylated in the gut mucosal wall and by the liver. It is excreted mainly by the kidney as N-acetyl-5-amino-salicylic acid.

Mesalamine from orally administered mesalamine tablets appears to be more extensively absorbed than the mesalamine released from sulfasalazine. Maximum plasma levels of mesalamine and N-acetyl-5-aminosalicylic acid following multiple mesalamine doses are about 1.5 to 2 times higher than those following an equivalent dose of mesalamine in the form of sulfasalazine. Combined mesalamine and N-acetyl-5-aminosalicylic acid AUC's and urine dose recoveries following multiple doses of delayed-release tablets are about 1.3-1.5 times higher than those following an equivalent dose of mesalamine in the form of sulfasalazine.

The T_{max} for mesalamine and its metabolite, N-acetyl-5-aminosalicylic acid, is usually delayed, reflecting the delayed release, and ranges from 4-12 hours. The half-lives elimination ($T_{1/2\ elm}$) for mesalamine and N-acetyl-5-aminosalicylic acid are usually about 12 hours, but are variable ranging from 2-15 hours. There is a large intersubject variability in the plasma concentrations of mesalamine and N-acetyl-5-aminosalicylic acid and in their elimination half-lives following administration of mesalamine tablets.

Rectal Suspension Enema

Mesalamine administered rectally as mesalamine suspension enema is poorly absorbed from the colon and is excreted principally in the feces during subsequent bowel movements. The extent of absorption is dependent upon the retention time of the drug product, and there is considerable individual variation. At steady state, approximately 10-30% of the daily 4 g dose can be recovered in cumulative 24 hour urine collections. Other than the kidney, the organ distribution and other bioavailability characteristics of absorbed mesalamine in man are not known. It is known that the compound undergoes acetylation but whether this process takes place at colonic or systemic sites has not been elucidated.

Whatever the metabolic site, most of the absorbed mesalamine is excreted in the urine as the N-acetyl-5-ASA metabolite. The poor colonic absorption of rectally administered mesalamine is substantiated by the low serum concentration of 5-ASA and N-acetyl-5-ASA seen in ulcerative colitis patients after dosage with mesalamine. Under clinical conditions patients demonstrated plasma levels 10-12 hours post mesalamine administration of 2 µg/ml, about two-thirds of which was the N-acetyl metabolite. While the elimination half-life of mesalamine is short (0.5-1.5 hours), the acetylated metabolite exhibits a half-life of 5-10 hours. In addition, steady state plasma levels demonstrated a lack of accumulation of either free or metabolized drug during repeated daily administrations.

Suppositories

Mesalamine administered in an enema formulation is poorly absorbed from the colon, as shown both by low recovery in urine and by low plasma levels during rectal administration. In plasma and urine, mesalamine occurs largely as its N-acetyl derivative, while the major portion recovered in feces is free mesalamine. The elimination half-life of free mesalamine is 0.5-1.5 hours and that of the 5-acetyl metabolite is 5-10 hours. Following single doses of mesalamine 500 mg suppository in normal volunteers, 24 hour urines contained (only) N-acetyl-mesalamine equivalent to 15-38% (avg. 24%) of the administered dose. This is commensurate with the finding of 3-36% (avg. 10%) in urine in a study of mesalamine 4 g rectal suspension in normals. In that study, 40-107 (avg. 75%) of the administered dose was recovered in feces. At steady state in ulcerative colitis patients (n=38) being treated with mesalamine rectal suspension, 24 hour urines contained 0-41% (avg. 0.37 µg/ml) of mesalamine equivalent (84% as N-acetyl metabolite). Multiple dose pharmacokinetic studies have not been conducted with mesalamine suppository nor have plasma levels been reported from single dose studies.

CONTROLLED-RELEASE CAPSULES

The mechanism of action of mesalamine (and sulfasalazine) is unknown, but appears to be topical rather than systemic. Mucosal production of arachidonic acid (AA) metabolites, both through the cyclooxygenase pathways, *i.e.*, prostanoids, and through the lipoxygenase pathways, *i.e.*, leukotrienes (LTs) and hydroxyeicosatetraenoic acids (HETSs), is increased in patients with chronic inflammatory bowel disease, and it is possible that mesalamine diminishes inflammation by blocking cyclooxygenase and inhibiting prostaglandin (PG) production in the colon.

Sulfasalazine is split by bacterial action in the colon into sulfapyridine (SP) and mesalamine (5-ASA). It is thought that the mesalamine component is therapeutically active in ulcerative colitis. The usual oral dose of sulfasalazine for active ulcerative colitis in adults is 2-4 g/day in divided doses. Four (4) g of sulfasalazine provide 1.6 g of free mesalamine to the colon.

Human Pharmacokinetics and Metabolism

Absorption

The ethylcellulose-coated, controlled-release formulation of mesalamine is designed to release therapeutic quantities of mesalamine throughout the gastrointestinal tract. Based on urinary excretion data, 20-30% of the mesalamine is absorbed. In contrast, when mesalamine is administered orally as an unformulated 1 g aqueous suspension, mesalamine is approximately 80% absorbed. Plasma mesalamine concentration peaked at approximately 1 μg/ml 3 hours following a 1 g mesalamine dose and declined in a biphasic manner. The literature describes a mean terminal half-life of 42 minutes for mesalamine following intravenous administration. Because of the continuous release and absorption of mesalamine throughout the gastrointestinal tract, the true elimination half-life cannot be determined after oral administration. N-acetylmesalamine, the major metabolite of mesalamine, peaked at approximately 3 hours at 1.8 μg/ml, and its concentration followed a biphasic decline. Pharmacological activities of N-acetylmesalamine are unknown, and other metabolites have not been identified. Oral mesalamine pharmacokinetics were nonlinear when mesalamine controlled-release capsules were dosed from 250 mg to 1 g four times daily, with steady-state mesalamine plasma concentrations increasing about 9 times, from 0.14 μg/ml to 1.21 μg/ml, suggesting saturable first-pass metabolism. N-acetylmesalamine pharmacokinetics were linear.

Elimination

About 130 mg free mesalamine was recovered in the feces following a single 1 g mesalamine controlled-release capsule dose, which was comparable to the 140 mg of mesalamine recovered from the molar equivalent sulfasalazine tablet dose of 2.5 g. Elimination of free mesalamine and salicylates in feces increased proportionately with a mesalamine dose. N-acetylmesalamine was the primary compound excreted in the urine (19-30%) following mesalamine dosing.

INDICATIONS AND USAGE

CONTROLLED-RELEASE CAPSULES AND DELAYED-RELEASE TABLETS

Mesalamine is indicated for the induction of remission and for the treatment of patients with mildly to moderately active ulcerative colitis.

RECTAL ENEMA/SUPPOSITORY

Mesalamine suspension enema is indicated for the treatment of active mild to moderate distal ulcerative colitis, proctosigmoiditis or proctitis.

Mesalamine suppositories are indicated for the treatment of active ulcerative proctitis.

CONTRAINDICATIONS

CONTROLLED-RELEASE CAPSULES AND DELAYED-RELEASE TABLETS

Mesalamine is contraindicated in patients who have demonstrated hypersensitivity to mesalamine, any other components of this medication, or salicylates.

RECTAL ENEMA/SUPPOSITORY

Mesalamine suspension enema is contraindicated for patients known to have hypersensitivity to the drug or any component of this medication.

Mesalamine suppositories are contraindicated for patients known to have hypersensitivity to mesalamine (5-aminosalicylic acid) or to the suppository vehicle [saturated vegetable fatty acid esters (hard fat)].

WARNINGS

RECTAL SUSPENSION ENEMA

Mesalamine suspension enema contains potassium metabisulfite, a sulfite that may cause allergic-type reactions including anaphylactic symptoms and life-threatening or less severe asthmatic episodes in certain susceptible people. The overall prevalence of sulfite sensitivity in the general population is unknown but probably low. Sulfite sensitivity is seen more frequently in asthmatic or in atopic nonasthmatic persons. Epinephrine is the preferred treatment for serious allergic or emergency situations even though epinephrine injection contains sodium or potassium metabisulfite with the above-mentioned potential liabilities. The alternatives to using epinephrine in a life-threatening situation may not be satisfactory. The presence of a sulfite(s) in epinephrine injection should not deter the administration of the drug for treatment of serious allergic or other emergency situations.

PRECAUTIONS

GENERAL

Controlled-Release Capsules

Caution should be exercised if mesalamine is administered to patients with impaired hepatic function.

Mesalamine has been associated with an acute intolerance syndrome that may be difficult to distinguish from a flare of inflammatory bowel disease. Although the exact frequency of occurrence cannot be ascertained, it has occurred in 3% of patients in controlled clinical trials of mesalamine or sulfasalazine. Symptoms include cramping, acute abdominal pain and bloody diarrhea, sometimes fever, headache, and rash. If acute intolerance syndrome is suspected, prompt withdrawal is required. If a rechallenge is performed later in order to validate the hypersensitivity, it should be carried out under close medical supervision at reduced dose and only if clearly needed.

Delayed-Release Tablets

Patients with pyloric stenosis may have prolonged gastric retention of mesalamine which could delay release of mesalamine in the colon.

Exacerbation of the symptoms of colitis, thought to have been caused by mesalamine or sulfasalazine has been reported in 3% of patients in controlled clinical trials. This acute reaction, characterized by cramping, abdominal pain, bloody diarrhea, and occasionally by fever, headache, malaise, pruritus, rash, and conjunctivitis, has been reported after the initiation of mesalamine tablets as well as other mesalamine products. Symptoms usually abate when mesalamine tablets are discontinued.

Some patients who have experienced a hypersensitivity reaction to sulfasalazine may have a similar reaction to mesalamine tablets or to other compounds which contain or are converted to mesalamine.

Rectal Suspension Enema

Mesalamine has been implicated in the production of an acute intolerance syndrome characterized by cramping, acute abdominal pain and bloody diarrhea, sometimes, fever, headache and a rash; in such cases prompt withdrawal is required. The patients's history of sulfasalazine intolerance, if any, should be re-evaluated. If a rechallenge is performed later in order to validate the hypersensitivity, it should be carried out under close supervision and only if clearly needed, given consideration to reduced dosage. In the literature, 1 patient previously sensitive to sulfasalazine was rechallenged with 400 mg oral mesalamine within 8 hours she experienced headache, fever, intensive abdominal colic, profuse diarrhea and was readmitted as an emergency. She responded poorly to steroid therapy and 2 weeks later a pancolectomy was required.

Although renal abnormalities were not noted in the clinical trials with mesalamine suspension enema, the possibility of increased absorption of mesalamine and concomitant renal tubular damage as noted in the preclinical studies must be kept in mind. Patients on mesalamine suspension enema, especially those on concurrent oral products which liberate mesalamine and those with preexisting renal disease, should be carefully monitored with urinalysis, BUN and creatinine studies.

In a clinical trial most patients who were hypersensitive to sulfasalazine were able to take mesalamine enemas without evidence of any allergic reaction. Nevertheless, caution should be exercised when mesalamine is initially used in patients known to be allergic to sulfasalazine. There patients should be instructed to discontinue therapy if signs of rash or fever become apparent.

While using mesalamine suspension enema some patients have developed pancolitis. However, extension of upper disease boundary and/or flare-ups occurred less often in the mesalamine-treated group than in the placebo-treated group.

Rare instances of pericarditis have been reported with mesalamine containing products including sulfasalazine. Cases of pericarditis have also been reported as manifestations of inflammatory bowel disease. In the cases reported with mesalamine rectal suspension enema there have been positive rechallenges with mesalamine or mesalamine containing products. In one of these cases, however, a second rechallenge with sulfasalazine was negative throughout a 2 month follow-up. Chest pain or dyspnea in patients treated with mesalamine should be investigated with this information in mind. Discontinuation of mesalamine may be warranted in some cases, but rechallenge with mesalamine can be performed under careful clinical observation should the continued therapeutic need for mesalamine be present.

Suppositories

Mesalamine has been implicated in the production of an acute intolerance syndrome characterized by cramping, acute abdominal pain and bloody diarrhea, sometimes, fever, headache and a rash; in such cases prompt withdrawal is required. The patients's history of sulfasalazine intolerance, if any, should be re-evaluated. If a rechallenge is performed later in order to validate the hypersensitivity, it should be carried out under close supervision and only if clearly needed, given consideration to reduced dosage. In the literature, 1 patient previously sensitive to sulfasalazine was rechallenged with 400 mg oral mesalamine within 8 hours she experienced headache, fever, intensive abdominal colic, profuse diarrhea and was readmitted as an emergency. She responded poorly to steroid therapy and 2 weeks later a pancolectomy was required.

The possibility of increased absorption of mesalamine and concomitant tubular damage as noted in the preclinical studies must be kept in mind. Patients of mesalamine suppositories, especially those on concurrent oral products which liberate mesalamine and those with preexisting renal disease, should be carefully monitored with urinalysis, BUN and creatinine studies.

In a clinical trial most patients who were hypersensitive to sulfasalazine were able to take mesalamine rectally without evidence of any allergic reaction.

Nevertheless, caution should be exercised when mesalamine is initially used in patients known to be allergic to sulfasalazine. These patients should be instructed to discontinue therapy if signs of rash or fever become apparent.

While using mesalamine suppositories a few patients have developed pancolitis. However, extension of upper disease boundary and/or flare-ups occurred less often in the mesalamine-treated group than in the placebo- treated group.

Rare instances of pericarditis have been reported with mesalamine containing products including sulfasalazine. Cases of pericarditis have also been reported as manifestations of inflammatory bowel disease. In the cases reported (with mesalamine enema) there have been positive rechallenges with mesalamine or mesalamine containing products. In one of these cases, however, a second rechallenge with sulfasalazine was negative throughout a 2 month follow-up. Chest pain or dyspnea in patients treated with mesalamine should be investigated with this information in mind. Discontinuation of mesalamine may be warranted in some cases, but rechallenge with mesalamine can be performed under careful observation should the continued therapeutic need for mesalamine be present.

CARCINOGENESIS, MUTAGENESIS, AND IMPAIRMENT OF FERTILITY

Controlled-Release Capsules

Long-term studies of the carcinogenic potential of mesalamine in mice and rats are ongoing. No evidence of mutagenicity was observed in an *in vitro* Ames test and in an *in vivo* mouse micronucleus test. No effects on fertility or reproductive performance were observed in male or female rats at doses up to 400 mg/kg/day (2360 mg/m^2). For a 50 kg person (1.3 m^2 body surface area), this represents 5 times the recommended clinical dose (80 mg/kg/day) on a mg/kg basis and 0.8 times the clinical dose (2960 mg/m^2) on body surface area basis.

Semen abnormalities and infertility in men, which have been reported in association with sulfasalazine, have not been seen with mesalamine controlled-release capsules during controlled clinical trials.

Delayed-Release Tablets

Long-term studies in animals have not been performed to evaluate the carcinogenicity potential of mesalamine. Mesalamine was not mutagenic in fluctuation assay in *K. pneumoniae* and Ames assay in *S. typhimurium.*. Mesalamine, at oral doses up to 480 mg/kg/day, had no adverse effect on fertility or reproductive performance of male and female rats. The oligospermia and infertility in men associated with sulfasalazine have not been reported with mesalamine delayed-release tablets.

Rectal Suspension Enema and Suppositories

Mesalamine caused no increase in the incidence of neoplastic lesions over controls in a 2 year study of Wistar rats fed up to 320 mg/kg/day of mesalamine admixed with diet. Mesalamine is not mutagenic to *Salmonella typhimurium* tester strains TA98, TA100, TA1535, TA1537, TA1538. There are no reverse mutations in an assay using *E. coli* strain WP2UVRA. There were no effects in an *in vivo* mouse moicronucleus assay at 600 mg/kg and in an *in vivi* sister chromatid exchange at doses up to 610 mg/kg. No effects on fertility were observed in rats receiving up to 320 mg/kg/day. The oligospermia and infertility in men associated with sulfasalazine have not been reported with mesalamine.

PREGNANCY, TERATOGENIC EFFECTS, PREGNANCY CATEGORY B

Controlled-Release Capsules

Reproduction studies have been performed in rats at doses up to 1000 mg/kg/day (5900 mg/m^2) and rabbits at doses of 800 mg/kg/day (6856 mg/m^2) and have revealed no evidence of teratogenic effects or harm to the fetus due to mesalamine. There are, however, no adequate and well-controlled studies in pregnant women. Because animal reproduction studies are not always predictive of human response, mesalamine should be used during pregnancy only if clearly needed. Mesalamine is known to cross the placental barrier.

Delayed-Release Tablets

Reproduction studies in rats and rabbits at oral doses up to 480 mg/kg/day have revealed no evidence of teratogenic effects or fetal toxicity due to mesalamine. There are, however, no adequate and well-controlled stuidies in pregnant women. Because animal production studies are not always predictive of human response, this drug should be used during pregnancy only if clearly needed.

Rectal Suspension Enema

Teratogenic studies have been performed in rats and rabbits at oral doses up to 5 and 8 times respectively, the maximum recommended human dose, and have revealed no evidence of harm to the embryo or fetus. There are, however, no adequate and well controlled studies in pregnant women for either sulfasalazine or 5-ASA. Because animal reproduction studies are not always predictive of human response, 5-ASA should be used during pregnancy only if clearly needed.

Suppositories

Teratologic studies have been performed in rats and rabbits at oral doses up to 10 and 16 times respectively, the maximum recommended human rectal suppository dose, and have revealed no evidence of harm to the embryo or fetus.

There are, however, no adequate and well-controlled studies in pregnant women. Because animal reproduction studies are not always predictive of human response, this drug should be used during pregnancy only if clearly needed.

NURSING MOTHERS

Controlled-Release Capsules

Minute quantities of mesalamine were distributed to breast milk and amniotic fluid of pregnant women following sulfasalazine therapy. When treated with sulfasalazine at a dose equivalent to 1.25 g/day of mesalamine, 0.02-0.08 µg/ml and trace amounts of mesalamine were measured in amniotic fluid and breast milk, respectively. N-acetylmesalamine, in quantities of 0.07- 0.77 µg/ml and 1.13-3.44 µg/ml, was identified in the same fluids, respectively. Caution should be exercised when mesalamine is administered to a nursing woman.

Delayed-Release Tablets

Low concentrations of mesalamine and higher concentrations of its N-acetyl metabolite have been detected in human breast milk. While the clinical significance of this has not been determined, caution should be exercised when mesalamine is administered to a nursing woman.

Rectal Suspension Enema and Suppositories

It is not known whether mesalamine or its metabolite(s) are excreted in human milk. As a general rule, nursing should not be undertaken while a patient is on a drug since many drugs are excreted in human milk.

PEDIATRIC USE

Safety and efficacy of mesalamine in pediatric patients have not been established.

RENAL

Controlled-Release Capsules

Caution should be exercised if mesalamine is administered to patients with impaired renal function. Single reports of nephrotic syndrome and interstitial nephritis associated with mesalamine therapy have been described in the foreign literature. There have been rare reports of interstitial nephritis in patients receiving mesalamine controlled-release capsules. In animal studies, a 13 week oral toxicity study in mice and 13 week and 52 week oral toxicity studies in rats and cynomolgus monkeys have shown the kidney to be the major target organ of mesalamine toxicity. Oral daily doses of 2400 mg/kg in mice and 1150 mg/kg in rats produced renal lesions including granular and hyaline casts, tubular degeneration, tubular dilation, renal infarct, papillary necrosis, tubular necrosis, and interstitial nephritis. In cynomolgus monkeys, oral daily doses of 250 mg/kg or higher produced nephrosis, papillary edema, and interstitial fibrosis. Patients with preexisting renal disease, increased BUN or serum creatinine, or proteinuria should be carefully monitored.

Delayed-Release Tablets

Renal impairment, including minimal change nephropathy, and acute and chronic interstitial nephritis, has been reported in patients taking mesalamine tablets as well as in patients taking other mesalamine products. In animal studies (rats, dogs), the kidneys is the principal target organ for toxicity. At doses of approximately 750-1000 mg/kg [15-20 times the administered recommended human dose (based on a 50 kg person) on a mg/kg basis and 3-4 times on a mg/m^2 basis], mesalamine causes renal papillary necrosis. **Therefore, caution should be exercised when using mesalamine or other compounds converted to mesalamine or its metabolites in patients with known renal dysfunction or history of renal disease. It is recommended that all patients have an evaluation of renal function prior to initiation of mesalamine tablets and periodically while on mesalamine therapy.**

INFORMATION FOR THE PATIENT

Delayed-Release Tablets

Patients should be instructed to swallow the mesalamine tablets whole, taking care not to break the outer coating. The outer coating is designed to remain intact to protect the active ingredient and this ensure mesalamine availability for action in the colon. In 2-3% of patients in clinical studies, intact or partially intact tablets have been reported in the stool. If this occurs repeatedly, patients should contact their physician.

DRUG INTERACTIONS

There are no known drug interactions.

ADVERSE REACTIONS

CONTROLLED-RELEASE CAPSULES

In combined domestic and foreign clinical trials, more than 2100 patients with ulcerative colitis or Crohn's disease received mesalamine controlled-release capsule therapy. Generally, mesalamine therapy was well tolerated. The most common events (*i.e.*, greater than or equal to 1%) were diarrhea (3.4%), headache (2.0%), nausea (1.8%), abdominal pain (1.7%), dyspepsia (1.6%), vomiting (1.5%), and rash (1.0%). In two domestic placebo-controlled trials involving over 600 ulcerative colitis patients, adverse events were fewer in mesalamine-treated patients than in the placebo group (mesalamine 14% vs placebo 18%) and were not dose-related. Events occurring at 1% or more are shown in TABLE 3. Of these, only nausea and vomiting were more frequent in the mesalamine group. Withdrawal from therapy due to adverse events was more common on placebo than mesalamine (7% vs 4%).

Clinical laboratory measurements showed no significant abnormal trends for any test, including measurement of hematologic, liver, and kidney function.

TABLE 3 *Adverse Events Occurring in More Than 1% of Either Placebo or Mesalamine Patients in Domestic Placebo-Controlled Ulcerative Colitis Trials*

Mesalamine Controlled-Release Comparison to Placebo

Event	Mesalamine Controlled-Release Capsules n=451	Placebo n=173
Diarrhea	16 (3.5%)	13 (7.5%)
Headache	10 (2.2%)	6 (3.5%)
Nausea	14 (3.1%)	—
Abdominal pain	5 (1.1%)	7 (4.0%)
Melena (bloody diarrhea)	4 (0.9%)	6 (3.5%)
Rash	6 (1.3%)	2 (1.2%)
Anorexia	5 (1.1%)	2 (1.2%)
Fever	4 (0.9%)	2 (1.2%)
Rectal urgency	1 (0.2%)	4 (2.3%)
Nausea and vomiting	5 (1.1%)	—
Worsening of ulcerative colitis	2 (0.4%)	2 (1.2%)
Acne	1 (0.2%)	2 (1.2%)

The following adverse events, presented by body system, were reported infrequently (*i.e.*, less than 1%) during domestic ulcerative colitis and Crohn's disease trials. In many cases, the relationship to mesalamine has not been established.

Gastrointestinal: Abdominal distention, anorexia, constipation, duodenal ulcer, dysphagia, eructation, esophageal ulcer, fecal incontinence, GGTP increase, GI bleeding, increased alkaline phosphatase, LDH increase, mouth ulcer, oral moniliases, pancreatitis, rectal bleeding, SGOT increase, SGPT increase, stool abnormalities (color or texture change), thirst.

Dermatological: Acne, alopecia, dry skin, eczema, erythema nodosum, nail disorder, photosensitivity, pruritus, sweating, urticaria.

Nervous System: Depression, dizziness, insomnia, somnolence, paresthesia.

Cardiovascular: Palpitations, pericarditis, vasodilation.

Other: Albuminuria, amenorrhea, amylase increase, arthralgia, asthenia, breast pain, conjunctivitis, ecchymosis, edema, fever, hematuria, hypomenorrhea, Kawasaki-like syndrome, leg cramps, lichen planus, lipase increase, malaise, menorrhagia, metrorrhagia, myalgia, pulmonary infiltrates, thrombocythemia, thrombocytopenia, urinary frequency.

One week after completion of an 8 week ulcerative colitis study, a 72-year-old male, with no previous history of pulmonary problems, developed dyspnea. The patient was subsequently diagnosed with interstitial pulmonary fibrosis without eosinophilia by one physician and bronchiolitis obliterans with organizing pneumonitis by a second physician. A causal relationship between this event and mesalamine therapy has not been established.

Published case reports and/or spontaneous postmarketing surveillance have described infrequent instances of pericarditis, fatal myocarditis, chest pain and T-wave abnormalities, hypersensitivity pneumonitis, pancreatitis, nephrotic syndrome, interstitial nephritis, hepatitis, aplastic anemia, pancytopenia, leukopenia, or anemia while receiving mesalamine therapy. Anemia can be a part of the clinical presentation of inflammatory bowel disease.

DELAYED-RELEASE TABLETS

Mesalamine tablets have been evaluated in about 1830 inflammatory bowel disease patients (most patients with ulcerative colitis) in controlled and open-label studies. Adverse events seen in clinical trials with mesalamine tablets have generally been mild and reversible. In two short-term (6 weeks) placebo-controlled clinical studies involving 245 patients, 155 of whom were randomized to mesalamine tablets, five (3.2%) of the mesalamine patients discontinued mesalamine therapy because of adverse events as compared to two (2.2%) of the placebo patients. Adverse reactions leading to withdrawal from mesalamine tablets included (each in 1 patient): diarrhea and colitis flare; dizziness, nausea, joint pain, and headache; rash, lethargy and constipation; dry mouth, malaise, lower back discomfort, mild disorientation, mild indigestion and cramping; headache, nausea, malaise, aching, vomiting, muscle cramps, a stuffy head, plugged ears, and fever.

Adverse events occurring at a frequency of 2% or greater in the two short-term, double-blind, placebo-controlled trials mentioned above are listed in TABLE 4. Overall, the incidence of adverse events seen with mesalamine tablets was similar to placebo.

TABLE 4 *Frequency (%) of Common Adverse Events Reported in Mesalamine or Placebo in Double-Blind Controlled Studies Ulcerative Colitis Patients Treated With Mesalamine Tablets*

Event	Placebo (n=87)	Mesalamine Tablets (n=152)
Headache	36%	35%
Abdominal pain	14%	18%
Eructation	15%	16%
Pain	8%	14%
Nausea	15%	13%
Pharyngitis	9%	11%
Dizziness	8%	8%
Asthenia	15%	7%
Diarrhea	9%	7%
Back pain	5%	7%
Fever	8%	6%
Rash	3%	6%
Dyspepsia	1%	6%
Rhinitis	5%	5%
Arthralgia	3%	5%
Vomiting	2%	5%
Constipation	1%	5%
Hypertonia	3%	5%
Flatulence	7%	3%
Flu syndrome	2%	3%
Chills	2%	3%
Colitis exacerbation	0%	3%
Chest pain	2%	3%
Peripheral edema	2%	3%
Myalgia	1%	3%
Pruritus	0%	3%
Sweating	1%	3%
Dysmenorrhea	3%	3%

Of these adverse events, only rash showed a consistently higher frequency with increasing mesalamine dose in these studies. In uncontrolled data, fever, flu syndrome, and headache also seemed dose-related.

In addition, the following adverse reactions were seen in 1-2% of the patients in the controlled studies: malaise, arthritis, increased cough, acne, and conjunctivitis.

Over 1800 patients have been treated with mesalamine tablets in clinical studies. In addition to the adverse events listed above, the following adverse events also have been reported in controlled clinical studies, open-label studies, or foreign marketing experience. The relationship of the reported events to mesalamine administration is unclear in many cases. Some complaints, including anorexia, joint pains, pyoderma gangrenosum, oral ulcers, and anemia could be part of the clinical presentation of inflammatory bowel disease.

Body as a Whole: Weakness neck pain, abdominal enlargement, facial edema, edema.

Cardiovascular: Pericarditis (rare), myocarditis (rare), vasodilation, migraine.

Digestive: Anorexia, hepatitis (rare), pancreatitis, gastroenteritis, gastritis, increased appetite, cholecystitis, dry mouth, oral ulcers, perforated peptic ulcer (rare), bloody diarrhea, tenesmus.

Hematologic: Agranulocytosis (rare), aplastic anemia (rare), thrombocytopenia, eosinophilia, leukopenia, anemia, lymphadenopathy.

Musculoskeletal: Gout.

Nervous: Anxiety, insomnia, depression, somnolence, emotional lability, hyperesthesia, vertigo, nervousness, confusion, paresthesia, tremor, peripheral neuropathy (rare), transverse myelitis (rare), Guillain-Barre syndrome (rare).

Respiratory/Pulmonary: Sinusitis, eosinophillic pneumonia, interstitial pneumonitis, asthma exacerbation.

Skin: Alopecia, psoriasis (rare), pyoderma gangrenosum (rare), dry skin, erythema nodosum, urticaria.

Special Senses: Ear pain, eye pain, taste perversion, blurred vision, tinnitus.

Urogenital: Interstitial nephritis (see also PRECAUTIONS, Renal), minimal change nephropathy (see PRECAUTIONS, Renal), dysuria, urinary urgency, hematuria, epididymitis, menorrhagia.

Laboratory Abnormalities: Elevated AST (SGPT) or ALT (SGOT), elevated alkaline phosphatase, elevated serum creatinine and BUN.

Hepatitis has been reported to occur rarely with mesalamine tablets. More commonly, asymptomatic elevations of liver enzymes have occurred which usually resolve during continued use or with discontinuation of the drug.

RECTAL SUSPENSION ENEMA

Clinical Adverse Experience

Mesalamine suspension enema is usually well tolerated. Most adverse effects have been mild and transient (see TABLE 5).

TABLE 5 *Adverse Reactions Occurring in More Than 0.1% of Mesalamine Suspension Enema-Treated Patients Comparison to Placebo*

Symptom	Mesalamine n = 815		Placebo n = 128	
Abdominal pain/cramps/discomfort	66	8.10%	10	7.81%
Headache	53	6.50%	16	12.50%
Gas/flatulence	50	6.13%	5	3.91%
Nausea	47	5.77%	12	9.38%
Flu	43	5.28%	1	0.78%
Tired/weak/malaise/fatigue	28	3.44%	8	6.25%
Fever	26	3.19%	0	0.00%
Rash/spots	23	2.82%	4	3.12%
Cold/sore throat	19	2.33%	9	7.03%
Diarrhea	17	2.09%	5	3.91%
Leg/joint pain	17	2.09%	1	0.78%
Dizziness	15	1.84%	3	2.34%
Bloating	12	1.47%	2	1.56%
Back pain	11	1.35%	1	0.78%
Pain on insertion of enema tip	11	1.35%	1	0.78%
Hemorrhoids	11	1.35%	0	0.00%
Itching	10	1.23%	1	0.78%
Rectal pain	10	1.23%	0	0.00%
Constipation	8	0.98%	4	3.12%
Hair loss	7	0.86%	0	0.00%
Peripheral edema	5	0.61%	11	8.59%
UT/urinary burning	5	0.61%	4	3.12%
Rectal pain/soreness/burning	5	0.61%	3	2.34%
Asthenia	1	0.12%	4	3.12%
Insomnia	1	0.12%	3	2.34%

In addition, the following adverse events have been associated with mesalamine and other mesalamine containing products: nephrotoxicity, pancreatitis, fibrosing, alveolitis and elevated liver enzymes. Cases of pancreatitis and fibrosing alveolitis have been reported as manifestations of inflammatory bowel disease as well.

Hair Loss

Mild hair loss characterized by "more hair in the comb" but no withdrawal from clinical trials has been observed in 7 of 815 mesalamine patients but none of the placebo-treated patients. In the literature there are at least 6 additional patients with mild hair loss who received either mesalamine or sulfasalazine. Retreatment is not always associated with repeated hair loss.

SUPPOSITORIES

Mesalamine suppository is usually well tolerated. Most adverse effects have been mild and transient (see TABLE 6).

TABLE 6 *Adverse Reactions Occurring in More Than 1% of Mesalamine Suppository Treated Patients*

Symptom	Mesalamine (n=168)		Placebo (n=84)	
Headache	11	6.5%	10	11.9%
Flatulence	6	3.6%	6	7.1%
Abdominal pain	5	3.0%	7	8.3%
Diarrhea	5	3.0%	5	6.0%
Dizziness	5	3.0%	2	2.4%
Rectal pain	3	1.8%	0	0.0%
Upper respiratory infection	3	1.8%	2	2.4%
Acne	2	1.2%	0	0.0%
Asthenia	2	1.2%	4	4.8%
Colitis	2	1.2%	0	0.0%
Fever	2	1.2%	0	0.0%
Generalized edema	2	1.2%	1	1.2%
Nausea	2	1.2%	6	7.1%
Rash	2	1.2%	0	0.0%

In addition, the following adverse events have been associated with mesalamine and other mesalamine containing products: nephrotoxicity, pancreatitis, fibrosing alveolitis and elevated liver enzymes. Cases of pancreatitis and fibrosing alveolitis have been reported as manifestations of inflammatory bowel disease as well.

DOSAGE AND ADMINISTRATION

CONTROLLED-RELEASE CAPSULES

The recommended dosage for the induction of remission and the symptomatic treatment of mildly to moderately active ulcerative colitis is 1 g (4 mesalamine controlled-release capsules) 4 times a day for a total daily dose of 4 g. Treatment duration in controlled trials was up to 8 weeks.

M

DELAYED-RELEASE TABLETS

The usual dosage in adults is two 400 mg tablets to be taken 3 times a day for a total daily dose of 2.4 g for a duration of 6 weeks.

RECTAL SUSPENSION ENEMA

The usual dosage of mesalamine suspension enema in 60 ml units is one rectal instillation (4 g) once a day, preferably at bedtime, and retained for approximately 8 hours. While the effect of Mesalamine (mesalamine) may been seen within 3-21 days, the usual course of therapy would be from 3-6 weeks depending on symptoms and sigmoidoscopic findings. Studies available to date have not assessed in mesalamine suspension enema will modify relapse rates after the 6 week short-term treatment.

Patients should be instructed to shake the bottle well to make sure the suspension is homogeneous. The patient should remove the protective sheath from the applicator tip. Holding the bottle at the neck will not cause any of the medication to be discharged. The position most often used is obtained by lying on the left side (to facilitate migration into the sigmoid colon); with the lower leg extended and the upper right leg flexed forward for balance. An alternative is the knee-chest position. The applicator tip should be gently inserted in the rectum pointing toward the umbilicus. A steady squeezing of the bottle will discharge most of the preparation. The preparation should be taken at bedtime with the objective of retaining it all night. Patient instructions are included with every seven units.

SUPPOSITORIES

The usual dosage of mesalamine suppositories 500 mg is one rectal suppository 2 times daily. The suppository should be retained for 1-3 hours or longer, if possible, to achieve the maximum benefit. While the effect of mesalamine suppositories may be seen within 3-21 days, the usual course of therapy would be from 3-6 weeks depending on symptoms and sigmoidoscopic findings. Studies available to date have not assessed if mesalamine suppositories will modify relapse rates after the 6 week short-term treatment.

HOW SUPPLIED

PENTASA CONTROLLED-RELEASE CAPSULES

Each green and blue capsule contains 250 mg of mesalamine in controlled-release beads. Pentasa controlled-release capsules are identified with a pentagonal starburst logo and the number "2010" on the green portion and "PENTASA 250 mg" on the blue portion of the capsules.

Storage: Store at controlled room temperature 15-30°C (59-86°F).

ASACOL DELAYED-RELEASE TABLETS

Asacol tablets are available as red-brown, capsul-shaped tablets containing 400 mg mesalamine and imprinted "Asacol NE" in black.

Storage: Store at controlled room temperature (15-30°C or 59-86°F).

PRODUCT LISTING - EQUIVALENTS NOT AVAILABLE

Capsule, Extended Release - Oral - 250 mg

80's	$48.13	PENTASA, Roberts Pharmaceutical Corporation	54092-0189-80
240's	$144.95	PENTASA, Roberts Pharmaceutical Corporation	54092-0189-81

Enema - Rectal - 4 Gm/60 ml

60 ml x 7	$108.78	ROWASA, Solvay Pharmaceuticals Inc	00032-1924-82

Suppository - Rectal - 500 mg

30's	$105.00	FIV-ASA, Paddock Laboratories Inc	00091-7250-03
30's	$105.00	ROWASA, Paddock Laboratories Inc	00574-7250-03
30's	$122.85	CANASA, Scandipharm Inc	58914-0500-56

Tablet, Enteric Coated - Oral - 400 mg

100's	$77.29	ASACOL, Allscripts Pharmaceutical Company	54569-4793-00
100's	$97.93	ASACOL, Procter and Gamble Pharmaceuticals	00149-0752-02

Mesoridazine Besylate (001744)

Categories: Schizophrenia; FDA Approved 1970 Feb; Pregnancy Category C
Drug Classes: Antipsychotics; Phenothiazines
Brand Names: Serentil
Foreign Brand Availability: Mesorin (Korea)
Cost of Therapy: $150.79 (Schizophrenia; Serentil; 100 mg; 3 tablets/day; 30 day supply)

WARNING

MESORIDAZINE BESYLATE HAS BEEN SHOWN TO PROLONG THE QTc INTERVAL IN A DOSE RELATED MANNER, AND DRUGS WITH THIS POTENTIAL, INCLUDING MESORIDAZINE BESYLATE, HAVE BEEN ASSOCIATED WITH TORSADE DE POINTES-TYPE ARRHYTHMIAS AND SUDDEN DEATH. DUE TO ITS POTENTIAL FOR SIGNIFICANT, POSSIBLY LIFE-THREATENING, PROARRHYTHMIC EFFECTS, MESORIDAZINE BESYLATE SHOULD BE RESERVED FOR USE IN THE TREATMENT OF SCHIZOPHRENIC PATIENTS WHO FAIL TO SHOW AN ACCEPTABLE RESPONSE TO ADEQUATE COURSES OF TREATMENT WITH OTHER ANTIPSYCHOTIC DRUGS, EITHER BECAUSE OF INSUFFICIENT EFFECTIVENESS OR THE INABILITY TO ACHIEVE AN EFFECTIVE DOSE DUE TO INTOLERABLE ADVERSE EFFECTS FROM THOSE DRUGS. (SEE WARNINGS, CONTRAINDICATIONS, AND INDICATIONS AND USAGE.)

DESCRIPTION

Serentil (mesoridazine besylate), the besylate salt of a metabolite of thioridazine, is a phenothiazine tranquilizer. Mesoridazine besylate is 10-[2(1-methyl-2-piperidyl)ethyl]-2-(methyl-sulfinyl)-phenothiazine [as the besylate].

Tablet, 10 mg for Oral Administration: *Active Ingredient:* Mesoridazine (as the besylate), 10 mg. *Inactive Ingredients:* Acacia, carnauba wax, colloidal silicon dioxide, FD&C red no. 40 aluminum lake, lactose, microcrystalline cellulose, povidone, sodium benzoate, starch, stearic acid, sucrose, synthetic black iron oxide, talc, titanium dioxide, and other ingredients.

Tablet, 25 mg for Oral Administration: *Active Ingredient:* Mesoridazine (as the besylate), 25 mg. *Inactive Ingredients:* Acacia, carnauba wax, colloidal silicon dioxide, FD&C red no. 40 aluminum lake, lactose, microcrystalline cellulose, povidone, sodium benzoate, starch, stearic acid, sucrose, synthetic black iron oxide, talc, titanium dioxide, and other ingredients.

Tablet, 50 mg for Oral Administration: *Active Ingredient:* Mesoridazine (as the besylate), 50 mg. *Inactive Ingredients:* Acacia, carnauba wax, colloidal silicon dioxide, FD&C red no. 40 aluminum lake, gelatin, lactose, microcrystalline cellulose, povidone, sodium benzoate, starch, stearic acid, sucrose, synthetic black iron oxide, talc, titanium dioxide, and other ingredients.

Tablet, 100 mg For Oral Administration: *Active Ingredient:* Mesoridazine (as the besylate), 100 mg. *Inactive Ingredients:* Acacia, carnauba wax, colloidal silicon dioxide, FD&C red no. 40 aluminum lake, gelatin, lactose, microcrystalline cellulose, povidone, sodium benzoate, starch, stearic acid, sucrose, synthetic black iron oxide, talc, titanium dioxide, and other ingredients.

Ampuls, 1 ml for Intramuscular Administration: *Active Ingredient:* Mesoridazine (as the besylate), 25 mg. *Inactive Ingredients :* Edetate disodium, 0.5 mg; sodium chloride, 7.2 mg; carbon dioxide gas (bone dry) q.s., water for injection, q.s. to 1 ml.

Concentrate for Oral Administration: *Active Ingredient:* Mesoridazine (as the besylate) 25 mg per ml. *Inactive Ingredients:* Alcohol, 0.61% by volume; citric acid, FD&C red no. 40; flavors; methylparaben; propylparaben; purified water; sodium citrate; sorbitol.

CLINICAL PHARMACOLOGY

The basic pharmacological activity of mesoridazine besylate is similar to that of other phenothiazines.

However, mesoridazine has been shown to prolong the QTc interval in a dose-dependent fashion. This effect may increase the risk of serious, potentially fatal, ventricular arrhythmias, such as torsade de pointes-type arrhythmias. Due to this risk, mesoridazine besylate is indicated only for schizophrenic patients who have not been responsive to or cannot tolerate other antipsychotic agents (see WARNINGS and CONTRAINDICATIONS).

However, the prescriber should be aware that mesoridazine besylate has not been systematically evaluated in controlled trials in treatment of refractory schizophrenic patients and its efficacy in such patients is unknown.

INDICATIONS AND USAGE

Mesoridazine besylate is indicated for the management of schizophrenic patients who fail to respond adequately to treatment with other antipsychotic drugs. Due to the risk of significant, potentially life-threatening, proarrhythmic effects with mesoridazine besylate treatment, mesoridazine besylate should be used only in patients who have failed to respond adequately to treatment with appropriate courses of other antipsychotic drugs, either because of insufficient effectiveness or the inability to achieve an effective dose due to intolerable adverse effects from those drugs. Consequently, before initiating treatment with mesoridazine besylate, it is strongly recommended that a patient be given at least two trials, each with a different antipsychotic drug product at an adequate dose, and for an adequate duration (see WARNINGS and CONTRAINDICATIONS).

However, the prescriber should be aware that mesoridazine besylate has not been systematically evaluated in controlled trials in treatment of refractory schizophrenic patients and its efficacy in such patients is unknown.

CONTRAINDICATIONS

Mesoridazine besylate use should be avoided in combination with other drugs that are known to prolong the QTc interval and in patients with congenital long QT syndrome or a history of cardiac arrhythmias (see WARNINGS and PRECAUTIONS).

As with other phenothiazines, mesoridazine besylate is contraindicated in severe central nervous system depression or comatose states from any cause including drug induced central nervous system depression (see WARNINGS).

Mesoridazine besylate is contraindicated in individuals who have previously shown hypersensitivity to the drug.

WARNINGS

POTENTIAL FOR PROARRHYTHMIC EFFECTS

DUE TO THE POTENTIAL FOR SIGNIFICANT, POSSIBLY LIFE-THREATENING, PROARRHYTHMIC EFFECTS WITH MESORIDAZINE BESYLATE TREATMENT, MESORIDAZINE BESYLATE SHOULD BE RESERVED FOR USE IN THE TREATMENT OF SCHIZOPHRENIC PATIENTS WHO FAIL TO SHOW AN ACCEPTABLE RESPONSE TO ADEQUATE COURSES OF TREATMENT WITH OTHER ANTIPSYCHOTIC DRUGS, EITHER BECAUSE OF INSUFFICIENT EFFECTIVENESS OR THE INABILITY TO ACHIEVE AN EFFECTIVE DOSE DUE TO INTOLERABLE ADVERSE EFFECTS FROM THOSE DRUGS. CONSEQUENTLY, BEFORE INITIATING TREATMENT WITH MESORIDAZINE BESYLATE, IT IS STRONGLY RECOMMENDED THAT A PATIENT BE GIVEN AT LEAST TWO TRIALS, EACH WITH A DIFFERENT ANTIPSYCHOTIC DRUG PRODUCT, AT AN ADEQUATE DOSE, AND FOR AN ADEQUATE DURATION. MESORIDAZINE BESYLATE HAS NOT BEEN SYSTEMATICALLY EVALUATED IN CONTROLLED TRIALS IN THE TREATMENT OF REFRACTORY SCHIZOPHRENIC PATIENTS AND ITS EFFICACY IN SUCH PATIENTS IS UNKNOWN.

A study in 9 chronic schizophrenic patients who were treated with mesoridazine 75 mg/day for the first week, 200 mg/day during week 2, and 300 mg/day during weeks 3 and 4, revealed evidence of a dose-related prolongation of the QT interval. All patients had a normal ECG at baseline and eight of the nine had normal ECG's 2 weeks after drug discontinuation.

Prolongation of the QTc interval has been associated with the ability to cause torsade de pointes-type arrhythmias, a potentially fatal polymorphic ventricular tachycardia, and sudden death. There are published case reports of ventricular tachycardia, in one case with a fatal outcome, in association with mesoridazine overdosage. A causal relationship between these events and mesoridazine besylate therapy has not been established but, given the ability of mesoridazine besylate to prolong the QTc interval, such a relationship is possible.

Certain circumstances may increase the risk of torsade de pointes and/or sudden death in association with the use of drugs that prolong the QTc interval, including (1) bradycardia, (2) hypokalemia, (3) concomitant use of other drugs that prolong the QTc interval, and (4) presence of congenital prolongation of the QT interval (see CONTRAINDICATIONS and PRECAUTIONS).

It is recommended that patients being considered for mesoridazine besylate treatment have a baseline ECG performed and serum potassium levels measured. Serum potassium should be normalized before initiating treatment and patients with a QTc interval greater than 450 milliseconds should not receive mesoridazine besylate treatment. It may also be useful to periodically monitor ECG's and serum potassium during mesoridazine besylate treatment especially during a period of dose adjustment. Mesoridazine besylate should be discontinued in patients who are found to have a QTc interval over 500 milliseconds.

Patients taking mesoridazine besylate who experience symptoms that may be associated with the occurrence of torsade de pointes (*e.g.*, dizziness, palpitations, or syncope) may warrant further cardiac evaluation; in particular, Holter monitoring should be considered.

TARDIVE DYSKINESIA

Tardive dyskinesia, a syndrome consisting of potentially irreversible, involuntary, dyskinetic movements may develop in patients treated with neuroleptic (antipsychotic) drugs. Although the prevalence of the syndrome appears to be highest among the elderly, especially elderly women, it is impossible to rely upon prevalence estimates to predict, at the inception of neuroleptic treatment, which patients are likely to develop the syndrome. Whether neuroleptic drug products differ in their potential to cause tardive dyskinesia is unknown.

Both the risk of developing the syndrome and the likelihood that it will become irreversible are believed to increase as the duration of treatment and the total cumulative dose of neuroleptic drugs administered to the patient increase. However, the syndrome can develop, although much less commonly, after relatively brief treatment periods at low doses.

There is no known treatment for established cases of tardive dyskinesia, although the syndrome may remit, partially or completely, if neuroleptic treatment is withdrawn. Neuroleptic treatment, itself, however, may suppress (or partially suppress) the signs and symptoms of the syndrome and thereby may possibly mask the underlying disease process. The effect that symptomatic suppression has upon the long-term course of the syndrome is unknown.

Given these considerations, neuroleptics should be prescribed in a manner that is most likely to minimize the occurrence of tardive dyskinesia. Chronic neuroleptic treatment should generally be reserved for patients who suffer from a chronic illness (1) that is known to respond to neuroleptic drugs, and, (2) for whom alternative, equally effective but potentially less harmful treatments are not available or appropriate. In the patients who do require chronic treatment, the smallest dose and the shortest duration of treatment producing a satisfactory clinical response should be sought. The need for continued treatment should be reassessed periodically.

If signs and symptoms of tardive dyskinesia appear in a patient on neuroleptics, drug discontinuation should be considered. However, some patients may require treatment despite the presence of the syndrome.

(For further information about the description of tardive dyskinesia and its clinical detection, please refer to PRECAUTIONS, Information for the Patient and ADVERSE REACTIONS.)

NEUROLEPTIC MALIGNANT SYNDROME (NMS)

A potentially fatal symptom complex sometimes referred to as Neuroleptic Malignant Syndrome (NMS) has been reported in association with antipsychotic drugs. Clinical manifestations of NMS are hyperreflexia, muscle rigidity, altered mental status and evidence of autonomic instability (irregular pulse or blood pressure, tachycardia, diaphoresis, and cardiac dysrhythmias).

The diagnostic evaluation of patients with this syndrome is complicated. In arriving at a diagnosis, it is important to identify cases where the clinical presentation includes both serious medical illness (*e.g.*, pneumonia, systemic infection, etc.) and untreated or inadequately treated extrapyramidal signs and symptoms (EPS). Other important considerations in the differential diagnosis include central anticholinergic toxicity, heat stroke, drug fever and primary central nervous system (CNS) pathology.

The management of NMS should include (1) immediate discontinuation of antipsychotic drugs and other drugs not essential to concurrent therapy, (2) intensive symptomatic treatment and medical monitoring, and (3) treatment of any concomitant serious medical problems for which specific treatments are available. There is no general agreement about specific pharmacological treatment regimens for uncomplicated NMS.

If a patient requires antipsychotic drug treatment after recovery from NMS, the potential reintroduction of drug therapy should be carefully considered. The patient should be carefully monitored, since recurrences of NMS have been reported.

Where patients are participating in activities requiring complete mental alertness (*e.g.*, driving) it is advisable to administer the phenothiazines cautiously and to increase the dosage gradually.

CENTRAL NERVOUS SYSTEM DEPRESSANTS

As in the case of other phenothiazines, mesoridazine besylate is capable of potentiating central nervous sytem depressants (*e.g.*, alcohol, anesthetics, barbiturates, narcotics, opiates, other psychoactive drugs, etc.) as well as atropine and phosphorus insecticides. Severe respiratory depression and respiratory arrest have been reported when a patient was given mesoridazine besylate and a concomitant high dose of a barbiturate.

PRECAUTIONS

While ocular changes have not to date been related to mesoridazine besylate, one should be aware that such changes have been seen with other drugs of this class.

Because of possible hypotensive effects, reserve parenteral administration for bedfast patients or for acute ambulatory cases, and keep patient lying down for at least one-half hour after injection.

Leukopenia and/or agranulocytosis have been attributed to phenothiazine therapy. A single case of transient granulocytopenia has been associated with mesoridazine besylate. Since convulsive seizures have been reported, patients receiving anticonvulsant medication should be maintained on that regimen while receiving mesoridazine besylate.

Neuroleptic drugs elevate prolactin levels; the elevation persists during chronic administration. Tissue culture experiments indicate that approximately one-third of human breast cancers are prolactin dependent *in vitro*, a factor of potential importance if the prescription of these drugs is contemplated in a patient with a previously detected breast cancer. Although disturbances such as galactorrhea, amenorrhea, gynecomastia and impotence have been reported, the clinical significance of elevated serum prolactin levels is unknown for most patients. An increase in mammary neoplasms has been found in rodents after chronic administration of neuroleptic drugs. Neither clinical studies nor epidemiologic studies conducted to date, however, have shown an association between chronic administration of these drugs and mammary tumorigenesis; the available evidence is considered too limited to be conclusive at this time.

INFORMATION FOR THE PATIENT

Patients should be informed that mesoridazine besylate has been associated with potentially fatal heart rhythm disturbances. The risk of such events may be increased when certain drugs are given together with mesoridazine besylate. Therefore, patients should inform the prescriber that they are receiving mesoridazine besylate treatment before taking any new medication.

Given the likelihood that some patients exposed chronically to neuroleptics will develop tardive dyskinesia, it is advised that all patients in whom chronic use is contemplated be given, if possible, full information about this risk.

USAGE IN PREGNANCY

The safety of this drug in pregnancy has not been established; hence, it should be given only when the anticipated benefits to be derived from treatment exceed the possible risks to mother and fetus.

PEDIATRIC USE

Safety and effectiveness in pediatric patients have not been established.

DRUG INTERACTIONS

There are no studies of the coadministration of mesoridazine and other drugs which prolong the QTc interval. However, it is expected that such coadministration would produce additive prolongation of the QTc interval and, thus, such use is contraindicated (see WARNINGS and CONTRAINDICATIONS).

M

ADVERSE REACTIONS

Drowsiness and hypotension were the most prevalent side effects encountered. Side effects tended to reach their maximum level of severity early with the exception of a few (rigidity and motoric effects) which occurred later in therapy.

With the exceptions of tremor and rigidity, adverse reactions were generally found among those patients who received relatively high doses early in treatment. Clinical data showed no tendency for the investigators to terminate treatment because of side effects.

Central Nervous System: Drowsiness, Parkinson's syndrome, dizziness, weakness, tremor, restlessness, ataxia, dystonia, rigidity, slurring, akathisia, motoric reactions (opisthotonos) have been reported.

Autonomic Nervous System: Dry mouth, nausea and vomiting, fainting, stuffy nose, photophobia, constipation and blurred vision have occurred in some instances.

Genitourinary System: Inhibition of ejaculation, impotence, enuresis, incontinence, and priapism have been reported.

Skin: Itching, rash, hypertrophic papillae of the tongue and angioneurotic edema have been reported.

Cardiovascular System: Mesoridazine besylate produces a dose related prolongation of the QTc interval, which is associated with the ability to cause torsade de pointes-type arrhythmias, a potentially fatal polymorphic ventricular tachycardia, and sudden death (see WARNINGS). Ventricular arrhythmias and death have been reported in association with mesoridazine besylate overdosage. A causal relationship between these events and mesoridazine besylate therapy has not been established but, given the ability of mesoridazine besylate to prolong the QTc interval, such a relationship is possible. Other ECG changes have been reported (see Phenothiazine Derivatives, Cardiovascular Effects).

PHENOTHIAZINE DERIVATIVES

It should be noted that efficacy, indications, and untoward effects have varied with the different phenothiazines. The physician should be aware that the following have occurred with one or more phenothiazines and should be considered whenever one of these drugs is used.

Autonomic Reactions: Miosis, obstipation, anorexia, paralytic ileus.

Cutaneous Reactions: Erythema, exfoliative dermatitis, contact dermatitis.

Blood Dyscrasias: Agranulocytosis, leukopenia, eosinophilia, thrombocytopenia, anemia, aplastic anemia, pancytopenia.

Allergic Reactions: Fever, laryngeal edema, angioneurotic edema, asthma.

Hepatotoxicity: Jaundice, biliary stasis.

Cardiovascular Effects: Changes in the terminal portion of the electrocardiogram, to include prolongation of the QT interval, depression and inversion of the T wave, and the appearance of a wave tentatively identified as a bifid T wave or a U wave have been observed in patients receiving phenothiazines, including mesoridazine besylate. To date, these appear to be due to altered repolarization, not related to myocardial damage, and appear to be reversible. Nonetheless, significant prolongation of the QT interval has been associated with serious ventricular arrhythmias and sudden death (see WARNINGS). Hypotension, rarely resulting in cardiac arrest, has been reported.

Extrapyramidal Symptoms: Akathisia, agitation, motor restlessness, dystonic reactions, trismus, torticollis, opisthotonos, oculogyric crises, tremor, muscular rigidity, akinesia.

Tardive Dyskinesia: Chronic use of neuroleptics may be associated with the development of tardive dyskinesia. The salient features of this syndrome are described in WARNINGS and below.

The syndrome is characterized by involuntary choreoathetoid movements which variously involve the tongue, face, mouth, lips, or jaw (*e.g.*, protrusion of the tongue, puffing of cheeks, puckering of the mouth, chewing movements), trunk and extremities. The severity of the syndrome and the degree of impairment produced vary widely.

The syndrome may become clinically recognizable either during treatment, upon dosage reduction, or upon withdrawal of treatment. Movements may decrease in intensity and may disappear altogether if further treatment with neuroleptics is withheld. It is generally believed that reversibility is more likely after short rather than long-term neuroleptic exposure. Consequently, early detection of tardive dyskinesia is important. To increase the likelihood of detecting the syndrome at the earliest possible time, the dosage of neuroleptic drug should be reduced periodically (if clinically possible) and the patient observed for signs of the disorder. This maneuver is critical, for neuroleptic drugs may mask the signs of the syndrome.

Endocrine Disturbances: Menstrual irregularities, altered libido, gynecomastia, lactation, weight gain, edema. False positive pregnancy tests have been reported.

Urinary Disturbances: Retention, incontinence.

Others: Hyperpyrexia. Behavioral effects suggestive of a paradoxical reaction have been reported. These include excitement, bizarre dreams, aggravation of psychoses and toxic confusional states. More recently, a peculiar skin-eye syndrome has been recognized as a side effect following long-term treatment with phenothiazines. This reactions is marked by progressive pigmentation of areas of the skin or conjunctiva and/or accompanied by discoloration of the exposed sclera and cornea. Opacities of the anterior lens and cornea described as irregular or stellate in shape have also been reported. Systemic lupus erythematous-like syndrome.

DOSAGE AND ADMINISTRATION

Since mesoridazine besylate is associated with a dose-related prolongation of the QTc interval, which is a potentially life-threatening event its use should be reserved for schizophrenia patients who fail to respond adequately to treatment with other antipsychotic drugs (see INDICATIONS AND USAGE and WARNINGS).

The dosage of mesoridazine besylate, as with most medications, should be adjusted to the needs of the individual. The lowest effective dosage should always be used. When maximum response is achieved, dosage may be reduced gradually to a maintenance dose.

Tablets and Oral Solution: For most patients, regardless of severity, a starting dose of 50 mg 3 times a day is recommended. The usual optimum total daily dose range is 100-400 mg/day.

Injectable Form: In those situations in which an intramuscular form of medication is indicated, mesoridazine besylate injectable is available. For most patients, a starting dose of 25 mg is recommended. The dose may be repeated in 30-60 minutes, if necessary. The usual optimum total daily dose range is 25-200 mg/day.

ANIMAL PHARMACOLOGY

Pharmacological studies in laboratory animals have established that mesoridazine besylate has a spectrum of pharmacodynamic actions typical of a major tranquilizer. In common with other tranquilizers it inhibits spontaneous motor activity in mice, prolongs thiopental and hexobarbital sleeping time in mice and produces spindles and block of arousal reaction in the EEG of rabbits. It is effective in blocking spinal reflexes in the cat and antagonizes d-amphetamine excitations and toxicity in grouped mice. It shows a moderate adrenergic blocking activity *in vitro* and *in vivo* and antagonizes 5-hydroxytryptamine *in vivo*. Intravenously administered, it lowers the blood pressure of anesthetized dogs. It has a weak antiacetylcholine effect *in vitro*.

The most outstanding activity of mesoridazine besylate is seen in tests developed to investigate antiemotive activity of drugs. Such tests are those in which the rat reacts to acute or chronic stress by increased defecation (emotogenic defecation) or tests in which "emotional mydriasis" is elicited in the mouse by an electric shock. In both of these tests, mesoridazine besylate is effective in reducing emotive reactions. Its ED_{50} in inhibiting emotogenic defecation in the rat is 0.053 mg/kg (subcutaneous administration). Mesoridazine besylate has a potent antiemetic action. The intravenous ED_{50} against apomorphine-induced emesis in the dog is 0.64 mg/kg. Mesoridazine besylate, in common with other phenothiazines, demonstrates antiarrhythmic activity in anesthetized dogs.

Metabolic studies in the dog and rabbit with tritium labeled mesoridazine demonstrate that the compound is well absorbed from the gastrointestinal tract. The biological half-life of mesoridazine besylate in these studies appears to be somewhere between 24-48 hours. Although significant urinary excretion was observed following the administration of mesoridazine besylate, these studies also suggest that biliary excretion is an important excretion route for mesoridazine and/or its metabolites (see TABLE 1).

TABLE 1 *Toxicity Studies*

Acute LD_{50} (mg/kg):

Route	Mouse	Rat	Rabbit	Dog
Oral	560 ± 62.5	644 ± 48	mlD = 800	mlD = 800
IM	—	509M 584F	405	
IV	26 ± 0.08	—	—	—

Chronic toxicity studies were conducted in rats and dogs. Rats were administered mesoridazine besylate orally 7 days per week for a period of 17 months in doses up to 160 mg/kg per day. Dogs were administered mesoridazine besylate orally 7 days per week for a period of 13 months. The daily dosage of the drug was increased during the period of this test such that the "top-dose" group received a daily dose of 120 mg/kg of mesoridazine for the last month of the study.

Untoward effects which occurred upon chronic administration of high dose-levels included:

Rats: Reduction of food intake, slowed weight gain, morphological changes in pituitary-supported endocrine organs, and melanin-like pigment deposition in renal tissues.

Dogs: Emesis, muscle tremors, decreased food intake and death associated with aspiration of oral-gastric contents into the respiratory system.

Increased intrauterine resorptions were seen with mesoridazine besylate in rats at 70 mg/kg and in rabbits at 125 mg/kg but not at 60 and 100 mg/kg, respectively. No drug related teratology was suggested by these reproductive studies.

Local irritation from the intramuscular injection of mesoridazine besylate was of the same order of magnitude as with other phenothiazines.

HOW SUPPLIED

SERENTIL TABLETS

Supplied in 10, 25, 50 and 100 mg mesoridazine (as the besylate) tablet sizes.

Storage: Below 86°F (30°C).

SERENTIL AMPULS

1 ml ampules containing 25 mg mesoridazine (as the besylate).

Storage: Below 86°F (30°C); protect from light.

SERENTIL CONCENTRATE

Contains 25 mg mesoridazine (as the besylate) per ml, alcohol, 0.61% by volume.

Storage: Below 77°F (25°C); protect from light; dispense in amber glass bottles only.

The concentrate may be diluted with distilled water, orange juice or grape juice. Each dose should be diluted just prior to administration. Preparation and storage of bulk dilutions is not recommended.

PRODUCT LISTING - EQUIVALENTS NOT AVAILABLE

Concentrate - Oral - 25 mg/ml

118 ml	$78.24	SERENTIL, Boehringer-Ingelheim	00597-0025-04

Solution - Injectable - 25 mg/ml

1 ml x 20	$131.98	SERENTIL, Boehringer-Ingelheim	00597-0027-02

Tablet - Oral - 10 mg

100's	$90.46	SERENTIL, Boehringer-Ingelheim	00597-0020-01

Tablet - Oral - 25 mg

100's	$121.28	SERENTIL, Boehringer-Ingelheim	00597-0021-01

Tablet - Oral - 100 mg

30's	$48.12	SERENTIL, Physicians Total Care	54868-3311-00
100's	$167.54	SERENTIL, Boehringer-Ingelheim	00597-0023-01

Metaproterenol Sulfate (001747)

For related information, see the comparative table section in Appendix A.

Categories: Asthma; Bronchitis, chronic; Chronic obstructive pulmonary disease; Emphysema; Pregnancy Category C; FDA Approved 1973 Jul

Drug Classes: Adrenergic agonists; Bronchodilators

Brand Names: **Alupent**; Arm-A-Med; Dey-Dose; Metaprel; Prometa

Foreign Brand Availability: Alotec (Japan); Nonasma (Taiwan)

Cost of Therapy: $8.78 (Asthma; Generic Tablets; 20 mg; 3 tablets/day; 30 day supply)

HCFA JCODE(S): J7670 0.4%, per 2.5 ml INH; J7672 0.6% per 2.5 ml INH; J7675 5.0%, per ml INH

DESCRIPTION

Metaproterenol sulfate 1-(3,5-dihydroxyphenyl)-2-isopropylaminoethanol sulfate, is a white, crystalline, racemic mixture of two optically active isomers. The molecular formula is $(C_{11}H_{17}NO_3)_2{\cdot}H_2SO_4$ The molecular weight is 520.59

INHALATION AEROSOL

Alupent inhalation aerosol is a bronchodilator administered by oral inhalation. The metaproterenol sulfate inhalation aerosol containing 75 mg of metaproterenol sulfate as micronized powder is sufficient medication for 100 inhalations. The metaproterenol sulfate inhalation aerosol containing 150 mg of metaproterenol sulfate as micronized powder is sufficient medication for 200 inhalations. Each metered dose delivers through the mouthpiece 0.65 mg of metaproterenol sulfate (each ml contains 15 mg). The inert ingredients are dichlorodifluoromethane, dichlorotetrafluoroethane and trichloromonofluoromethane as propellants, and sorbitan trioleate.

INHALATION SOLUTION

Alupent inhalation solution is a bronchodilator administered by oral inhalation via intermittent positive pressure breathing (IPPB) apparatus or nebulizer. It contains metaproterenol sulfate 5% in a pH-adjusted aqueous solution containing benzalkonium chloride and edetate disodium as preservatives.

It differs from isoproterenol hydrochloride by having two hydroxyl groups attached at the meta positions on the benzene ring rather than one at the meta and one at the para position.

INHALATION SOLUTION UNIT DOSE VIAL

Alupent inhalation solution unit dose vial is a bronchodilator administered by oral inhalation with the aid of an intermittent positive pressure breathing apparatus (IPPB). It contains metaproterenol sulfate 0.4% or 0.6% in a sterile pH adjusted aqueous solution with edetate disodium and sodium chloride.

It differs from isoproterenol hydrochloride by having two hydroxyl groups attached at the meta positions on the benzene ring rather than one at the meta and one at the para position.

SYRUP

Alupent syrup is an oral bronchodilator. Each teaspoonful (5 ml) of syrup contains 10 mg of metaproterenol sulfate. The inactive ingredients are edetate disodium, FD&C red no. 40, hydroxyethylcellulose, imitation black cherry flavor, methylparaben, propylparaben, saccharin and sorbitol solution.

TABLETS

Alupent in tablet form is an oral bronchodilator. Each tablet contains metaproterenol sulfate 10 or 20 mg. The inactive ingredients are colloidal silicon dioxide, corn starch, dibasic calcium phosphate, lactose, magnesium stearate.

CLINICAL PHARMACOLOGY

INHALATION AEROSOL

In vitro studies and *in vivo* pharmacologic studies have demonstrated that metaproterenol sulfate has a preferential effect on beta-2 adrenergic receptors compared with isoproterenol. While it is recognized that beta-2 adrenergic receptors are the predominant receptors in the bronchial smooth muscle, recent data indicate that there is a population of beta-2 receptors in the human heart existing in a concentration between 10-50%. The precise function of these, however, is not yet established (see WARNINGS).

The pharmacologic effects of beta adrenergic agonist drugs, including metaproterenol sulfate, are at least in part attributable to stimulation through beta adrenergic receptors of intracellular adenyl cyclase, the enzyme which catalyzes the conversion of adenosine triphosphate (ATP) to cyclic-3,5'- adenosine monophosphate (c-AMP). Increased c-AMP levels are associated with relaxation of bronchial smooth muscle and inhibition of release of mediators of immediate hypersensitivity from cells, especially from mast cells.

Pulmonary function tests performed concomitantly usually show improvement following aerosol metaproterenol sulfate administration, *e.g.*, an increase in the 1 second forced expiratory volume (FEV_1), maximum expiratory flow rate, forced vital capacity, and/or a decrease in airway resistance. The resultant decrease in airway obstruction may relieve the dyspnea associated with bronchospasm.

Controlled single- and multiple-dose studies have been performed with pulmonary function monitoring. The duration of effect of a single dose of 2-3 inhalations of metaproterenol sulfate (that is, the period of time during which there is 20% or greater increase in FEV_1) has varied from 1-5 hours.

In repetitive-dosing studies (up to qid) the duration of effect for a similar dose of metaproterenol sulfate has ranged from about 1 to 2.5 hours. Present studies are inadequate to explain the divergence in duration of the FEV_1 effect between single- and repetitive-dosing studies, respectively.

Recent studies in laboratory animals (minipigs, rodents and dogs) recorded the occurrence of cardiac arrhythmias and sudden death (with histologic evidence of myocardial necrosis) when beta agonists and methylxanthines were administered concurrently. The significance of these findings when applied to humans is currently unknown.

Pharmacokinetics

Absorption, biotransformation and excretion studies in humans following administration by inhalation have shown that approximately 3% of the actuated dose is absorbed intact through the lungs. The major metabolite, metaproterenol-3-O-sulfate, is produced in the gastrointestinal tract. metaproterenol sulfate is not metabolized by catechol-O methyltransferase nor have glucuronide conjugates been isolated to date.

INHALATION SOLUTION

The pharmacologic effects of beta adrenergic agonist drugs, including metaproterenol sulfate, are at least in part attributable to stimulation through beta adrenergic receptors of intracellular adenyl cyclase, the enzyme which catalyzes the conversion of adenosine triphosphate (ATP) to cyclic-3,5'- adenosine monophosphate (c-AMP). Increased c-AMP levels are associated with relaxation of bronchial smooth muscle and inhibition of release of mediators of immediate hypersensitivity from cells, especially from mast cells.

Recent studies in laboratory animals (minipigs, rodents and dogs) recorded the occurrence of cardiac arrhythmias and sudden death (with histologic evidence of myocardial necrosis) when beta agonists and methylxanthines were administered concurrently. The significance of these findings when applied to humans is currently unknown.

Following controlled single dose studies by an intermittent positive pressure breathing apparatus (IPPB) and by hand bulb nebulizers, significant improvement (15% or greater increase in FEV_1) occurred within 5-30 minutes and persisted for periods varying from 2-6 hours.

In these studies, the longer duration of effect occurred in the studies in which the drug was administered by IPPB, i.e., 6 hours versus 2-3 hours when administered by hand bulb nebulizer. In these studies the doses used were 0.3 ml by IPPB and 10 inhalations by hand bulb nebulizer.

In controlled repetitive dosing studies by IPPB and by hand bulb nebulizer the onset of effect occurred within 5-30 minutes and duration ranged from 4-6 hours. In these studies the doses used were 0.3 ml bid or tid when given by IPPB, and 10 inhalation qid (no more often than q4h) when given by hand bulb nebulizer. As in the single dose studies, effectiveness was measured as a sustained increase in FEV_1 of 15% or greater. In these repetitive dosing studies there was no apparent difference in duration between the two methods of delivery.

Clinical studies were conducted in which the effectiveness of metaproterenol sulfate inhalation solution was evaluated by comparison with that of isoproterenol hydrochloride over periods of 2-3 months. Both drugs continued to produce significant improvement in pulmonary function throughout this period of treatment.

In two well-controlled studies in children 6-12 years of age with acute exacerbation of asthma, 70% of patients receiving metaproterenol sulfate inhalation solution (0.1 ml-0.2 ml) showed improvement in pulmonary function as demonstrated by a 15% increase in FEV_1 above baseline.

Pharmacokinetics

Absorption, biotransformation and excretion studies following administration by inhalation have not been performed. Following oral administration of tablet and solution, an average of 40% of the drug was excreted as the unchanged drug and its major metabolite, a polar conjugate, metaproterenol-O-sulfate.

INHALATION SOLUTION UNIT DOSE VIAL

Recent studies in laboratory animals (minipigs, rodents and dogs) recorded the occurrence of cardiac arrhythmias and sudden death (with histologic evidence of myocardial necrosis) when beta agonists and methylxanthines were administered concurrently. The significance of these findings when applied to humans is currently unknown.

Following controlled single dose studies by an intermittent positive pressure breathing apparatus (IPPB) and by hand bulb nebulizers, significant improvement (15% or greater increase in FEV_1) occurred within 5-30 minutes and persisted for periods varying from 2-6 hours.

In these studies, the longer duration of effect occurred in the studies in which the drug was administered by IPPB, i.e., 6 hours versus 2-3 hours when administered by hand bulb nebulizer. In these studies the doses used were 0.3 ml by IPPB and 10 inhalations by hand bulb nebulizer.

In controlled repetitive dosing studies by IPPB and by hand bulb nebulizer the onset of effect occurred within 5-30 minutes and duration ranged from 4-6 hours. In these studies the doses used were 0.3 ml bid or tid when given by IPPB, and 10 inhalation qid (no more often than q4h) when given by hand bulb nebulizer. As in the single dose studies, effectiveness was measured as a sustained increase in FEV_1 of 15% or greater. In these repetitive dosing studies there was no apparent difference in duration between the two methods of delivery.

Clinical studies were conducted in which the effectiveness of metaproterenol sulfate inhalation solution was evaluated by comparison with that of isoproterenol hydrochloride over periods of 2-3 months. Both drugs continued to produce significant improvement in pulmonary function throughout this period of treatment.

In two well-controlled studies in children 6-12 years of age with acute exacerbation of asthma, 70% of patients receiving metaproterenol sulfate inhalation solution (0.1 ml-0.2 ml) showed improvement in pulmonary function as demonstrated by a 15% increase in FEV_1 above baseline.

Pharmacokinetics

Absorption, biotransformation and excretion studies following administration by inhalation have not been performed. Following oral administration in humans, an average of 40% of the drug is absorbed; it is not metabolized by catechol-O-methyltransferase but is excreted primarily as glucuronic acid conjugates.

SYRUP

In vitro studies and *in vivo* pharmacologic studies have demonstrated that metaproterenol sulfate has a preferential effect on beta-2 adrenergic receptors compared with isoproterenol. While it is recognized that beta-2 adrenergic receptors are the predominant receptors in the bronchial smooth muscle, recent data indicate that there is a population of beta-2 receptors in the human heart existing in a concentration between 10-50%. The precise function of these, however, is not yet established (see WARNINGS).

The pharmacologic effects of beta adrenergic agonist drugs, including metaproterenol sulfate, are at least in part attributable to stimulation through beta adrenergic receptors of intracellular adenyl cyclase, the enzyme which catalyzes the conversion of adenosine triphosphate (ATP) to cyclic-3,5'- adenosine monophosphate (c-AMP). Increased c-AMP levels are associated with relaxation of bronchial smooth muscle and inhibition of release of mediators of immediate hypersensitivity from cells, especially from mast cells.

Pulmonary function has been monitored in controlled single-and multiple-dose studies. The duration of effect of a single dose of metaproterenol sulfate syrup (that is, the period of time during which there is a 15% or greater increase in mean FEV_1) was up to 4 hours.

Recent studies in laboratory animals (minipigs, rodents and dogs) recorded the occurrence of cardiac arrhythmias and sudden death (with histologic evidence of myocardial necrosis) when beta agonists and methylxanthines were administered concurrently. The significance of these findings when applied to humans is currently unknown.

Pharmacokinetics

Absorption, biotransformation and excretion studies in humans following oral administration have indicated that an average of less than 10% of the drug is absorbed intact; it is not metabolized by catechol-O-methyltransferase nor converted to glucuronide conjugates but is excreted primarily as the polar sulfate conjugate, metaproterenol-3-0-sulfate, formed in the gut.

TABLETS

The pharmacologic effects of beta adrenergic agonist drugs, including metaproterenol sulfate, are at least in part attributable to stimulation through beta adrenergic receptors of intracellular adenyl cyclase, the enzyme which catalyzes the conversion of adenosine triphosphate (ATP) to cyclic-3,5'- adenosine monophosphate (c-AMP). Increased c-AMP levels are associated with relaxation of bronchial smooth muscle and inhibition of release of mediators of immediate hypersensitivity from cells, especially from mast cells.

Pulmonary function tests performed after the administration of metaproterenol sulfate usually show improvement, *e.g.*, an increase in the 1 second forced expiratory volume (FEV_1), maximum expiratory flow rate, peak expiratory flow rate, forced vital capacity, and/or a decrease in airway resistance. The resultant decrease in airway obstruction may relieve the dyspnea associated with bronchospasm.

In controlled single- and multiple-dose studies in which 319 patients were treated with metaproterenol sulfate tablets (89 patients with 10 mg and 230 patients with 20 mg), a majority (65%) demonstrated improvements in pulmonary function defined as an increase of at least 15% in the one- second forced expiratory volume (FEV_1). For 54% the onset was within 30 minutes. The duration of effect persisted for at least 4 hours in 51% of those patients who demonstrated a response.

Recent studies in laboratory animals (minipigs, rodents and dogs) recorded the occurrence of cardiac arrhythmias and sudden death (with histologic evidence of myocardial necrosis) when beta agonists and methylxanthines were administered concurrently. The significance of these findings when applied to humans is currently unknown.

Pharmacokinetics

Absorption, biotransformation and excretion studies in humans following oral administration have indicated that an average of less than 10% of the drug is absorbed intact; it is not metabolized by catechol-O-methyltransferase nor converted to glucuronide conjugates but is excreted primarily as the polar sulfate conjugate, metaproterenol-3-0-sulfate, formed in the gut.

INDICATIONS AND USAGE

INHALATION AEROSOL

Metaproterenol sulfate is indicated as a bronchodilator for bronchial asthma and for reversible bronchospasm which may occur in association with bronchitis and emphysema.

INHALATION SOLUTION

Metaproterenol sulfate inhalation solution is indicated as a bronchodilator in the treatment of asthma and bronchitis or emphysema when a reversible component is present in adults and for the treatment of acute asthmatic attacks in children age 6 years and older.

INHALATION SOLUTION UNIT DOSE VIAL, SYRUP, AND TABLETS

Metaproterenol sulfate inhalation solution, syrup, or tablets is indicated as a bronchodilator for bronchial asthma, and for reversible bronchospasm which may occur in association with bronchitis and emphysema.

CONTRAINDICATIONS

Use in patients with cardiac arrhythmias associated with tachycardia is contraindicated.

Although rare, immediate hypersensitivity reactions and paradoxical bronchospasm can occur. Therefore, metaproterenol sulfate is contraindicated in patients with a history of hypersensitivity to any of its components.

WARNINGS

Excessive use of adrenergic aerosols is potentially dangerous. Fatalities have been reported following excessive use of metaproterenol sulfate as with other sympathomimetic inhalation preparations, and the exact cause is unknown. Cardiac arrest was noted in several cases.

Controlled clinical studies and other clinical experience have shown that metaproterenol sulfate, like other beta-adrenergic agonists, can produce a significant cardiovascular effect in some patients, as measured by pulse rate, blood pressure, symptoms, and/or ECG changes. Paradoxical bronchospasm has been reported after the use of inhaled sympathomimetic drugs and may be life threatening. If it occurs, the preparation should be discontinued immediately and alternative therapy instituted.

Paradoxical bronchoconstriction with repeated excessive administration has been reported with sympathomimetic agents.

metaproterenol sulfate should not be used more often than prescribed. Patients should be advised to contact their physicians in the event that they do not respond to their usual dose of sympathomimetic amine aerosol.

PRECAUTIONS

GENERAL

Extreme care must be exercised with respect to the administration of additional sympathomimetic agents.

Since metaproterenol is a sympathomimetic amine, it should be used with caution in patients with cardiovascular disorders, including ischemic heart disease, hypertension or cardiac arrhythmias, in patients with hyperthyroidism or diabetes mellitus, and in patients who are unusually responsive to sympathomimetic amines or who have convulsive disorders. Significant changes in systolic and diastolic blood pressure could be expected to occur in some patients after use of any beta adrenergic bronchodilator.

Physicians should recognize that a single dose of nebulized metaproterenol sulfate inhalation solution in the treatment of acute asthma may alleviate symptoms and improve pulmonary function temporarily but fail to completely abort an attack.

INFORMATION FOR THE PATIENT

Extreme care must be exercised with respect to the administration of additional sympathomimetic agents. A sufficient interval of time should elapse prior to administration of another sympathomimetic agent.

Metaproterenol sulfate inhalation solution effects may last up to 6 hours or longer. It should not be used more often than recommended and the patient should not increase the number of inhalations or frequency of use without first consulting the physician. If symptoms of asthma get worse, adverse reactions occur, or the patient does not respond to the usual dose, the patient should be instructed to contact the physician immediately.

A single dose of nebulized metaproterenol sulfate inhalation solution in the treatment of an acute attack of asthma may not completely abort an attack.

Metaproterenol sulfate syrup or tablets should not be used more often than prescribed. If symptoms persist, patients should consult a physician promptly.

CARCINOGENESIS, MUTAGENESIS, AND IMPAIRMENT OF FERTILITY

Inhalation Aerosol

In an 18 month study in mice, metaproterenol sulfate produced an increase in benign ovarian tumors in females at doses corresponding to 320 and 640 times the maximum recommended dose (based on a 50 kg individual). In a 2 year study in rats, a non-significant incidence of benign leiomyomata of the mesovarium was noted at 640 times the maximum recommended dose. The relevance of these findings to man is not known. Mutagenic studies with metaproterenol sulfate have not been conducted. Reproduction studies in rats revealed no evidence of impaired fertility.

Syrup and Tablets

In an 18 month study in mice, metaproterenol sulfate produced a significant increase in benign hepatic adenomas in males and benign ovarian tumors in females at doses corresponding to 31 and 62 times the maximum recommended dose (based on a 50 kg individual). In a 2 year study in rats, a non-significant incidence of benign leiomyomata of the mesovarium was noted at 62 times the maximum recommended dose. The relevance of these findings to man is not known. Mutagenicity studies with metaproterenol sulfate have not been conducted. Reproduction studies in rats revealed no evidence of impaired fertility.

CARCINOGENESIS

Inhalation Solution and Inhalation Solution Unit Dose Vial

Long-term studies in mice and rats to evaluate the oral carcinogenic potential of metaproterenol sulfate have not been completed.

Studies of metaproterenol sulfate have not been conducted to determine mutagenic potential or effect on fertility.

PREGNANCY CATEGORY C

Inhalation Aerosol

Metaproterenol sulfate has been shown to be teratogenic and embryotoxic in rabbits when given in doses corresponding to 640 times the maximum recommended dose. These effects included skeletal abnormalities, hydrocephalus and skull bone separation. Results of other studies in rabbits, rats or mice have not revealed any teratogenic, embryocidal or fetotoxic effects. There are no adequate and well-controlled studies in pregnant women. metaproterenol sulfate should be used during pregnancy only if the potential benefit justifies the potential risk to the fetus.

Inhalation Solution and Inhalation Solution Unit Dose Vial

Metaproterenol sulfate has been shown to be teratogenic and embryocidal in rabbits when given orally in doses 620 times the human inhalation dose; the teratogenic effects included skeletal abnormalities and hydrocephalus with bone separation. Oral reproduction studies in mice, rats and rabbits showed no teratogenic or embryocidal effects at 50 mg/kg, corresponding or/to 310 times the human inhalation dose. There are no adequate and well-controlled studies in pregnant women. metaproterenol sulfate should be used during pregnancy only if the potential benefit justifies the potential risk to the fetus.

Syrup

Metaproterenol sulfate has been shown to be teratogenic and embryotoxic in rabbits when given in doses corresponding to 62 times the maximum recommended dose. These effects included skeletal abnormalities, hydrocephalus and skull bone separation. Results of other studies in rabbits, rats or mice have not revealed any teratogenic, embryotoxic or fetotoxic effects. There are no adequate and well-controlled studies in pregnant women. metaproterenol sulfate should be used during pregnancy only if the potential benefit justifies the potential risk to the fetus.

Tablets

Metaproterenol sulfate has been shown to be teratogenic and embryotoxic in rabbits when given orally at doses of 100 mg/kg or 62 times the maximum recommended human oral dose. These effects included skeletal abnormalities, hydrocephalus and skull bone separation.

Embryotoxicity has also been shown in mice when given orally at doses of 50 mg/kg or 31 times the maximum recommended human oral dose. Results of other oral reproduction studies in rats (40 mg/kg) and rabbits (50 mg/kg) have not revealed any teratogenic, embryotoxic or fetotoxic effects. There are no adequate and well-controlled studies in pregnant women. metaproterenol sulfate should be used during pregnancy only if the potential benefit justifies the potential risk to the fetus.

NURSING MOTHERS

It is not known whether metaproterenol sulfate is excreted in human milk; therefore, metaproterenol sulfate should be used during nursing only if the potential benefit justifies the potential risk to the newborn. Because many drugs are excreted in human milk, caution should be exercised when metaproterenol sulfate is administered to a nursing woman.

PEDIATRIC USE

Inhalation Aerosol and Inhalation Solution Unit Dose Vial

Safety and effectiveness in children below the age of 12 have not been established. Studies are currently under way in this age group.

Inhalation Solution

Metaproterenol sulfate inhalation solution may be used in the treatment of acute attacks of asthma in children 6 years and older.

Syrup

Safety and effectiveness in children below the age of 6 have been demonstrated in a limited number of patients. See DOSAGE AND ADMINISTRATIONsection.

Tablets

Metaproterenol sulfate tablets are not recommended for use in children under 6 years of age because of insufficient clinical data to establish safety and effectiveness.

DRUG INTERACTIONS

INHALATION AEROSOL AND SYRUP

Other beta adrenergic bronchodilators should not be used concomitantly with metaproterenol sulfate because they may have additive effects. Beta adrenergic agonists should be administered with caution to patients being treated with monoamine oxidase inhibitors or tricyclic antidepressants, since the action of beta adrenergic agonists on the vascular system may be potentiated.

TABLETS

Beta adrenergic agonists should be administered with caution to patients being treated with monoamine oxidase inhibitors or tricyclic antidepressants, since the action of beta adrenergic agonists on the vascular system may be potentiated.

ADVERSE REACTIONS

Adverse reactions are similar to those noted with other sympathomimetic agents.

INHALATION AEROSOL

The most frequent adverse reaction to metaproterenol sulfate administered by metered-dose inhaler among 251 patients in 90 day controlled clinical trials was nervousness. This was reported in 6.8% of patients. Less frequent adverse experiences, occurring in 1-4% of patients were headache, dizziness, palpitations, gastrointestinal distress, tremor, throat irritation, nausea, vomiting, cough and asthma exacerbation. Tachycardia occurred in less than 1% of patients.

INHALATION SOLUTION

The following (TABLE 1) summarizes the adverse experiences reported for at least 2% of the 120 patients participating in multiple-dose clinical trials of 60 and 90 day duration.

TABLE 1 *Adverse Experiences Occurring In At Least 2% of Patients In 60 and 90 Day Clinical Trials)n=120)*

Adverse Experience	No. of Patients	%
Cough	4	3.3%
Headache	4	3.3%
Nervousness	17	14.1%
Tachycardia	3	2.5%
Tremor	3	2.5%

The incidence of adverse reactions in children may be somewhat higher. In controlled clinical trials conducted in 160 pediatric patients the incidence of adverse reactions observed at the recommended doses was as follows: tachycardia in 16.6%, tremor 33%, nausea 14% and vomiting 7.7%. The corresponding incidence in placebo-treated patients was: tachycardia 7.6%, tremor 20%, nausea 7.7% and vomiting 2.5%.

In two well-controlled studies in children 6-12 years of age with acute exacerbation of asthma, metaproterenol sulfate inhalation solution was not efficacious in approximately 30% of patients, where efficacy was defined as a 15% increase in FEV_1 above baseline at two or more time points during the one-hour testing period. In 8% of patients there was a decrease in FEV_1 of 10% or more from baseline at two or more time points during the testing period. Insufficient information exists to assess the relationship of drug administration to the decline in pulmonary function observed in these patients, but paradoxical bronchospasm is one possibility.

It is important to recognize that adverse reactions from beta agonist bronchodilator solutions for nebulization may occur with the use of a new container of a product in patients who have previously tolerated that same product without adverse effect. There have been reports that indicate that such patients may subsequently tolerate replacement containers of the same product without adverse effect.

INHALATION SOLUTION UNIT DOSE VIAL

The most frequent adverse reactions to metaproterenol sulfate are nervousness and tachycardia which occur in about 1 in 7 patients, tremor which occurs in about 1 in 20 patients and nausea which occurs in about 1 in 50 patients. Less frequent adverse reactions are hypertension, palpitations, vomiting and bad taste which occur in approximately 1 in 300 patients.

SYRUP

TABLE 2 is a list of adverse experiences derived from 44 clinical trials involving 1120 patients treated with metaproterenol sulfate syrup.

TABLE 2 *Incidence of Adverse Events Occurring in at Least 1% of Patients*

Adverse Experience	No. of Patients	% Incidence
Cardiovascular		
Tachycardia	68	6.1%
Central Nervous System		
Headache	12	1.1%
Nervousness	54	4.8%
Gastrointestinal		
Nausea	15	1.3%
Musculoskeletal		
Tremor	13	1.6%

TABLETS

TABLE 3 is a list of adverse experiences derived from 26 controlled clinical trials with 496 patients treated with metaproterenol sulfate tablets.

TABLE 3 *Incidence of Adverse Events Reported Among 496 Patients Treated in 26 Controlled Clinical Trials*

Adverse Experience	Number of Patients	Incidence
Cardiovascular		
Chest pain	1	0.2%
Edema	1	0.2%
Hypertension	2	0.4%
Palpitations	19	3.8%
Tachycardia	85	17.1%
Central Nervous System		
Dizziness	12	2.4%
Drowsiness	3	0.6%
Fatigue	7	1.4%
Headache	35	7.0%
Insomnia	9	1.8%
Nervousness	100	20.2%
Sensory disturbances	1	0.2%
Syncope	2	0.4%
Weakness	1	0.2%
Dermatological		
Diaphoresis	1	0.2%
Hives	1	0.2%
Pruritus	2	0.4%
Gastrointestinal		
Appetite changes	2	0.4%
Diarrhea	6	1.2%
Gastrointestinal distress	15	3.0%
Nausea	18	3.6%
Vomiting	4	0.8%
Musculoskeletal		
Pain	1	0.2%
Spasms	1	0.2%
Tremor	84	16.9%
Ophthalmological		
Blurred vision	1	0.2%
Oro-Otolaryngeal		
Dry mouth/throat	2	0.4%
Laryngeal changes	1	0.2%
Bad taste	4	0.8%
Respiratory		
Asthma exacerbation	10	2.0%
Coughing	1	0.2%
Other		
Chatty	1	0.2%
Chills	1	0.2%
Clonus noted on flexing foot	1	0.2%
Feverish	2	0.4%
Flu symptoms	1	0.2%
Facial and finger puffiness	1	0.2%

DOSAGE AND ADMINISTRATION

INHALATION AEROSOL

The usual single dose is 2-3 inhalations. With repetitive dosing, inhalation should usually not be repeated more often than about every 3-4 hours. Total dosage per day should not exceed 12 inhalations.

Metaproterenol sulfate inhalation aerosol is not recommended for children under 12 years of age.

It is recommended that the physician titrate dosage according to each individual patient's response to therapy.

Store between 15 and 25°C (59 and 77°F). Avoid excessive humidity.

INHALATION SOLUTION

The dosage and administration are summarized in TABLE 4.

TABLE 4

Population	Method of Administration	Usual Single Dose	Range	Dilution
Adult	Hand-bulb nebulizer	10 inhalations	5-15 inhalations	No dilution
12 years and older	IPPB or nebulizer	0.3 ml	0.2-0.3 ml	Diluted in approx. 2.5 ml saline solution or other diluent
6-12 years	Nebulizer	0.1 ml	0.1-0.2 ml	Diluted in saline solution to a total volume of 3 ml

Metaproterenol sulfate inhalation solution is administered by oral inhalation via IPPB or nebulizer.

Usually, treatment need not be repeated more often than every 4 hours to relieve acute attacks of bronchospasm. metaproterenol sulfate inhalation solution may be administered 3-4 times a day for the treatment of reversible airways disease in adults. A single dose of nebulized metaproterenol sulfate in the treatment of an acute attack of asthma may not completely abort an attack.

As with all medications, the physician should begin therapy with the lowest effective dose and then titrate the dosage according to the individual patient's requirements.

Store between 15 and 25°C (59 and 77°F). Protect from light.

Do not use the solution if it is pinkish or darker than slightly yellow or contains the precipitate.

INHALATION SOLUTION UNIT DOSE VIAL

Metaproterenol sulfate inhalation solution unit dose vial is administered by oral inhalation using an IPPB device. The usual adult dose is one vial per nebulization treatment. Each vial of metaproterenol sulfate Inhalation solution 0.4% is equivalent to 0.2 ml metaproterenol sulfate Inhalation solution 5% diluted to 2.5 ml with normal saline; each vial of metaproterenol sulfate inhalation solution 0.6% is equivalent to 0.3 ml metaproterenol sulfate Inhalation solution 5% diluted to 2.5 ml with normal saline.

Usually, treatment need not be repeated more often than every 4 hours to relieve acute attacks of bronchospasm. As part of a total treatment program in chronic bronchospastic pulmonary diseases, metaproterenol sulfate inhalation solution may be administered 3-4 times a day.

M

As with all medications, the physician should begin therapy with the lowest effective dose and then titrate the dosage according to the individual patient's requirements.

metaproterenol sulfate inhalation solution is not recommended for use in children under 12 years of age.

Store between 25°C (77°F). Protect from light.

Do not use the solution if it is pinkish or darker than slightly yellow or contains a precipitate.

SYRUP

Children aged 6-9 years or weight under 60 lb: 1 teaspoonful 3 or 4 times a day.

Children over 9 years or weight over 60 lb: 2 teaspoonfuls 3 or 4 times a day. Clinical trial experience in children under the age of 6 is limited. Of 40 children treated with metaproterenol sulfate syrup for at least 1 month, daily doses of approximately 1.3-2.6 mg/kg were well tolerated.

Adults: 2 teaspoonfuls 3 or 4 times a day.

It is recommended that the physician titrate the dosage according to each individual patient's response to therapy.

Store between 15 and 30°C (59 and 86°F). Protect from light.

TABLETS

The usual dose is 20 mg three or four times a day.

Children

Aged 6-9 years or weight under 60 lb:

10 mg: 3 or 4 times a day. Over 9 years or weight over 60 lb.

20 mg: 3 or 4 times a day. Metaproterenol sulfate tablets are not recommended for use in children under 6 years at this time. (Please refer to the CLINICAL PHARMACOLOGY section for further information on clinical experience with this product.)

It is recommended that the physician titrate dosage according to each individual patient's response to therapy.

Storage for Bottles: Store between 15 and 30°C (59 and 86°F). Protect from light.

Storage for Blister Samples: Store between 15 and 25°C (59 and 77°F). Protect from light.

PRODUCT LISTING - RATED THERAPEUTICALLY EQUIVALENT

Solution - Inhalation - 0.4%

2 ml x 25	$30.75	GENERIC, Dey Laboratories	49502-0678-03
2 ml x 25	$34.40	GENERIC, Alpharma Uspd Makers Of Barre and Nmc	00472-1373-48
2 ml x 25	$34.83	GENERIC, Roxane Laboratories Inc	00054-8613-11

Solution - Inhalation - 0.6%

2 ml x 25	$29.95	GENERIC, Par Pharmaceutical Inc	49884-0361-48
2 ml x 25	$30.75	GENERIC, Dey Laboratories	49502-0676-03
2 ml x 25	$31.44	GENERIC, Moore, H.L. Drug Exchange Inc	00839-7639-07
2 ml x 25	$34.40	GENERIC, Alpharma Uspd Makers Of Barre and Nmc	00472-1377-48
2 ml x 25	$34.83	GENERIC, Roxane Laboratories Inc	00054-8614-11
2.50 ml	$54.23	ALUPENT, Pharma Pac	52959-0158-06
2.50 ml x 25	$56.42	ALUPENT, Physicians Total Care	54868-3179-00

Solution - Inhalation - 5%

10 ml	$16.37	GENERIC, Morton Grove Pharmaceuticals Inc	60432-0676-01
30 ml	$29.25	GENERIC, Major Pharmaceuticals Inc	00904-2881-30
30 ml	$45.83	GENERIC, Morton Grove Pharmaceuticals Inc	60432-0676-30

Syrup - Oral - 10 mg/5 ml

473 ml	$16.66	GENERIC, Silarx Pharmaceuticals Inc	54838-0507-80
473 ml	$18.85	GENERIC, Apotex Usa Inc	60505-5802-09
480 ml	$7.52	GENERIC, Morton Grove Pharmaceuticals Inc	60432-0650-16
480 ml	$8.50	GENERIC, Raway Pharmacal Inc	00686-6117-38
480 ml	$13.49	GENERIC, Aligen Independent Laboratories Inc	00405-3255-16
480 ml	$14.83	GENERIC, Moore, H.L. Drug Exchange Inc	00839-7442-69
480 ml	$17.25	GENERIC, Ivax Corporation	00182-6080-40
480 ml	$17.26	GENERIC, Major Pharmaceuticals Inc	00904-2880-16
480 ml	$17.30	GENERIC, Watson/Schein Pharmaceuticals Inc	00364-2417-16
480 ml	$17.90	GENERIC, Copley	38245-0138-07
480 ml	$23.70	GENERIC, Geneva Pharmaceuticals	00781-6404-16
480 ml	$31.87	GENERIC, Qualitest Products Inc	00603-1422-58

Tablet - Oral - 10 mg

8's	$7.19	GENERIC, Pd-Rx Pharmaceuticals	55289-0544-08
60's	$21.78	GENERIC, Pd-Rx Pharmaceuticals	55289-0544-60
100's	$6.75	GENERIC, Raway Pharmacal Inc	00686-2230-09
100's	$12.51	GENERIC, Qualitest Products Inc	00603-4464-21
100's	$15.70	GENERIC, Major Pharmaceuticals Inc	00904-2878-60
100's	$15.78	GENERIC, Moore, H.L. Drug Exchange Inc	00839-7485-06
100's	$16.13	GENERIC, Major Pharmaceuticals Inc	00904-2878-61
100's	$16.42	GENERIC, Aligen Independent Laboratories Inc	00405-4629-01
100's	$16.49	GENERIC, Par Pharmaceutical Inc	49884-0258-01

Tablet - Oral - 20 mg

100's	$9.75	GENERIC, Raway Pharmacal Inc	00686-2232-09
100's	$19.60	GENERIC, Major Pharmaceuticals Inc	00904-2879-60
100's	$19.90	GENERIC, Qualitest Products Inc	00603-4465-21
100's	$20.93	GENERIC, Watson/Schein Pharmaceuticals Inc	00364-2284-01
100's	$20.94	GENERIC, Major Pharmaceuticals Inc	00904-2879-61
100's	$20.99	GENERIC, Moore, H.L. Drug Exchange Inc	00839-7486-06
100's	$23.25	GENERIC, Aligen Independent Laboratories Inc	00405-4630-01
100's	$23.75	GENERIC, Par Pharmaceutical Inc	49884-0259-01

PRODUCT LISTING - EQUIVALENTS NOT AVAILABLE

Aerosol - Inhalation - 0.65 mg/Inh

14 gm	$19.38	ALUPENT, Boehringer-Ingelheim	00597-0070-18

Aerosol with Adapter - Inhalation - 0.65 mg/Inh

14 gm	$26.00	ALUPENT, Southwood Pharmaceuticals Inc	58016-6537-01
14 gm	$26.57	ALUPENT, Allscripts Pharmaceutical Company	54569-2732-00
14 gm	$28.60	ALUPENT, Physicians Total Care	54868-1043-01
14 gm	$29.25	ALUPENT, Pharma Pac	52959-0155-00
14 gm	$33.65	ALUPENT, Boehringer-Ingelheim	00597-0070-17

Syrup - Oral - 10 mg/5 ml

120 ml	$9.45	GENERIC, Pharma Pac	52959-0386-03
120 ml	$14.80	GENERIC, Southwood Pharmaceuticals Inc	58016-4021-04
120 ml	$14.80	GENERIC, Southwood Pharmaceuticals Inc	58016-4021-05
480 ml	$23.00	GENERIC, Allscripts Pharmaceutical Company	54569-2754-00

Tablet - Oral - 10 mg

12's	$4.10	GENERIC, Southwood Pharmaceuticals Inc	58016-0402-12
20's	$6.84	GENERIC, Southwood Pharmaceuticals Inc	58016-0402-20
30's	$4.58	GENERIC, Allscripts Pharmaceutical Company	54569-1967-00
30's	$10.26	GENERIC, Southwood Pharmaceuticals Inc	58016-0402-30
100's	$34.20	GENERIC, Southwood Pharmaceuticals Inc	58016-0402-00

Tablet - Oral - 20 mg

12's	$5.83	GENERIC, Southwood Pharmaceuticals Inc	58016-0403-12
15's	$7.29	GENERIC, Southwood Pharmaceuticals Inc	58016-0403-15
20's	$9.72	GENERIC, Southwood Pharmaceuticals Inc	58016-0403-20
30's	$6.53	GENERIC, Prescript Pharmaceuticals	00247-0350-30
30's	$15.31	GENERIC, Southwood Pharmaceuticals Inc	58016-0403-30
100's	$48.59	GENERIC, Southwood Pharmaceuticals Inc	58016-0403-00

Metaxalone *(001749)*

Categories: Pain, musculoskeletal; FDA Approved 1962 Aug; Pregnancy Category C
Drug Classes: Musculoskeletal agents; Relaxants, skeletal muscle
Brand Names: **Skelaxin**
Cost of Therapy: $29.94 (Musculoskeletal Pain; Skelaxin; 400 mg; 6 tablets/day; 10 day supply)

DESCRIPTION

Metaxalone has the following chemical name: 5-[(3,5-dimethylphenoxy)methyl]-2-oxazolidinone.

Skelaxin is available as a 400 mg round, pale rose tablet and an 800 mg oval, pink scored tablet.

CLINICAL PHARMACOLOGY

The mechanism of action of metaxalone in humans has not been established, but may be due to general central nervous system depression. It has no direct action on the contractile mechanism of striated muscle, the motor end plate or the nerve fiber.

PHARMACOKINETICS

In a single center randomized, two-period crossover study in 42 healthy volunteers (31 males, 11 females), a single 400 mg metaxalone tablet was administered under both fasted and fed conditions.

Under fasted conditions, mean peak plasma concentrations (C_{max}) of 865.3 ng/ml were achieved within 3.3 ± 1.2 hours (SD) after dosing (T_{max}). Metaxalone concentrations declined with a mean terminal half-life ($T_{½}$) of 9.2 ± 4.8 hours. The mean apparent oral clearance (CL/F) of metaxalone was 68 ± 34 L/h.

In the same study, following a standardized high fat meal, food statistically significantly increased the rate (C_{max}) and extent of absorption [AUC(0-t), AUC(∞)] of metaxalone from metaxalone tablets. Relative to the fasted treatment the observed increases were 177.5%, 123.5%, and 115.4%, respectively. The mean T_{max} was also increased to 4.3 ± 2.3 hours, whereas the mean $T_{½}$ was decreased to 2.4 ± 1.2 hours. This decrease in half-life over that seen in the fasted subjects is felt to be due to the more complete absorption of metaxalone in the presence of a meal resulting in a better estimate of half-life. The mean apparent oral clearance (CL/F) of metaxalone was relatively unchanged relative to fasted administration (59 ± 29 L/h). Although a higher C_{max} and AUC were observed after the administration of metaxalone with a standardized high fat meal, the clinical relevance of these effects is unknown.

In another single center, randomized four-period crossover study in 59 healthy volunteers (37 males, 22 females), the rate and extent of metaxalone absorption were determined after the administration of metaxalone tablets under both fasted and fed conditions. Under fasted conditions, the administration of 2 metaxalone 400 mg tablets produced peak plasma metaxalone concentrations (C_{max}) of 1653 ng/ml 3.0 ± 1.2 hours after dosing (T_{max}). Metaxalone concentrations declined with mean terminal half-life ($T_{½}$) of 8.0 ± 4.6 hours. The mean apparent oral clearance (CL/F) of metaxalone was 66 ± 34 L/h. Except for a 17% decrease in mean C_{max}, these values were not statistically different from those after the administration of 1 metaxalone 800 mg tablet.

In the same study, the administration of 2 metaxalone 400 mg tablets following a standardized high fat meal showed an increase in the mean C_{max}, and the area under the curve [AUC(0-∞)] of metaxalone by 194% and 142%, respectively. A high fat meal also increased the mean T_{max} to 4.9 ± 2.3 hours but decreased the mean $T_{½}$ to 4.2 ± 2.5 hours. The effect of a high fat meal on the absorption of metaxalone from 1 metaxalone 800 mg tablet was very similar to that on the absorption from 2 metaxalone 400 mg tablets in quality and quantity. The clinical relevance of these effects is unknown.

The absolute bioavailability of metaxalone from metaxalone tablets is not known. Metaxalone is metabolized by the liver and excreted in the urine as unidentified metabolites. The impact of age, gender, hepatic, and renal disease on the pharmacokinetics of metaxalone has not been determined. In the absence of such information, metaxalone should be used with caution in patients with hepatic and/or renal impairment and in the elderly.

INDICATIONS AND USAGE

Metaxalone is indicated as an adjunct to rest, physical therapy, and other measures for the relief of discomforts associated with acute, painful musculoskeletal conditions. The mode of action of this drug has not been clearly identified, but may be related to its sedative properties. Metaxalone does not directly relax tense skeletal muscles in man.

CONTRAINDICATIONS

Known hypersensitivity to any components of this product.

Known tendency to drug induced, hemolytic, or other anemias.

Significantly impaired renal or hepatic function.

WARNINGS

Metaxalone may enhance the effects of alcohol and other CNS depressants.

PRECAUTIONS

Metaxalone should be administered with great care to patients with pre-existing liver damage. Serial liver function studies should be performed in these patients.

False-positive Benedict's tests, due to an unknown reducing substance, have been noted. A glucose-specific test will differentiate findings.

INFORMATION FOR THE PATIENT

Metaxalone may impair mental and/or physical abilities required for performance of hazardous tasks, such as operating machinery or driving a motor vehicle, especially when used with alcohol or other CNS depressants.

CARCINOGENESIS, MUTAGENESIS, AND IMPAIRMENT OF FERTILITY

The carcinogenic potential of metaxalone has not been determined.

PREGNANCY

Reproduction studies in rats have not revealed evidence of impaired fertility or harm to the fetus due to metaxalone. Post marketing experience has not revealed evidence of fetal injury, but such experience cannot exclude the possibility of infrequent or subtle damage to the human fetus. Safe use of metaxalone has not been established with regard to possible adverse effects upon fetal development. Therefore, metaxalone tablets should not be used in women who are or may become pregnant and particularly during early pregnancy unless in the judgement of the physician the potential benefits outweigh the possible hazards.

NURSING MOTHERS

It is not known whether this drug is secreted in human milk. As a general rule, nursing should not be undertaken while a patient is on a drug since many drugs are excreted in human milk.

PEDIATRIC USE

Safety and effectiveness in children 12 years of age and below have not been established.

DRUG INTERACTIONS

Metaxalone may enhance the effects of alcohol, barbiturates and other CNS depressants.

ADVERSE REACTIONS

The most frequent reactions to metaxalone include:

CNS: Drowsiness, dizziness, headache, and nervousness or "irritability".
Digestive: Nausea, vomiting, gastrointestinal upset.
Immune System: Hypersensitivity reaction, rash with or without pruritus.
Hematologic: Leukopenia, hemolytic anemia.
Hepatobiliary: Jaundice.

Though rare, anaphylactoid reactions have been reported with metaxalone.

DOSAGE AND ADMINISTRATION

The recommended dose for adults and children over 12 years of age is two 400 mg tablets (800 mg) or one 800 mg tablet 3-4 times a day.

HOW SUPPLIED

Skelaxin is available as:

400 mg: Pale rose tablet, inscribed with "8662" on the scored side and "C" on the other.
800 mg: Oval, scored pink tablet inscribed with "8667" on the scored side and "S" on the other.

Storage: Store at controlled room temperature, between 15° and 30°C (59° and 86°F).

PRODUCT LISTING - EQUIVALENTS NOT AVAILABLE

Tablet - Oral - 400 mg

Qty	Price	Product	NDC
2's	$1.42	SKELAXIN, Allscripts Pharmaceutical Company	54569-4986-00
10's	$7.08	SKELAXIN, Allscripts Pharmaceutical Company	54569-0855-08
10's	$9.71	SKELAXIN, Southwood Pharmaceuticals Inc	58016-0682-10
12's	$11.66	SKELAXIN, Southwood Pharmaceuticals Inc	58016-0682-12
14's	$7.35	SKELAXIN, Southwood Pharmaceuticals Inc	58016-0682-14
14's	$22.02	SKELAXIN, Pharma Pac	52959-0410-14
15's	$10.62	SKELAXIN, Allscripts Pharmaceutical Company	54569-0855-04
15's	$14.57	SKELAXIN, Southwood Pharmaceuticals Inc	58016-0682-15
18's	$12.74	SKELAXIN, Allscripts Pharmaceutical Company	54569-0855-06
20's	$14.16	SKELAXIN, Allscripts Pharmaceutical Company	54569-0855-07
20's	$19.43	SKELAXIN, Southwood Pharmaceuticals Inc	58016-0682-20
20's	$22.70	SKELAXIN, Pd-Rx Pharmaceuticals	55289-0316-20
20's	$31.40	SKELAXIN, Pharma Pac	52959-0410-20
25's	$25.95	SKELAXIN, Pd-Rx Pharmaceuticals	55289-0316-25
28's	$27.20	SKELAXIN, Southwood Pharmaceuticals Inc	58016-0682-28
28's	$40.76	SKELAXIN, Pharma Pac	52959-0410-28
30's	$21.23	SKELAXIN, Allscripts Pharmaceutical Company	54569-0855-01
30's	$25.16	SKELAXIN, Physicians Total Care	54868-2956-03
30's	$27.34	SKELAXIN, St. Mary'S Mpp	60760-0062-30
30's	$29.14	SKELAXIN, Southwood Pharmaceuticals Inc	58016-0682-30
30's	$30.33	SKELAXIN, Pd-Rx Pharmaceuticals	55289-0316-30
30's	$43.65	SKELAXIN, Pharma Pac	52959-0410-30
40's	$28.31	SKELAXIN, Allscripts Pharmaceutical Company	54569-0855-00
40's	$38.85	SKELAXIN, Southwood Pharmaceuticals Inc	58016-0682-40
40's	$44.01	SKELAXIN, Pd-Rx Pharmaceuticals	55289-0316-40
40's	$51.04	SKELAXIN, Pharma Pac	52959-0410-40
42's	$29.73	SKELAXIN, Allscripts Pharmaceutical Company	54569-0855-05
42's	$40.80	SKELAXIN, Southwood Pharmaceuticals Inc	58016-0682-42
45's	$36.01	SKELAXIN, St. Mary'S Mpp	60760-0062-45
45's	$55.31	SKELAXIN, Pharma Pac	52959-0410-45
50's	$48.57	SKELAXIN, Southwood Pharmaceuticals Inc	58016-0682-50
50's	$59.58	SKELAXIN, Pharma Pac	52959-0410-50
60's	$42.47	SKELAXIN, Allscripts Pharmaceutical Company	54569-0855-09
60's	$49.13	SKELAXIN, Physicians Total Care	54868-2956-04
60's	$58.28	SKELAXIN, Southwood Pharmaceuticals Inc	58016-0682-60
60's	$65.37	SKELAXIN, Pd-Rx Pharmaceuticals	55289-0316-60
60's	$71.49	SKELAXIN, Pharma Pac	52959-0410-60
90's	$62.02	SKELAXIN, St. Mary'S Mpp	60760-0062-90
90's	$87.42	SKELAXIN, Southwood Pharmaceuticals Inc	58016-0682-90
90's	$107.24	SKELAXIN, Pharma Pac	52959-0410-90
100's	$49.90	SKELAXIN, Allscripts Pharmaceutical Company	54569-0855-02
100's	$80.52	SKELAXIN, Physicians Total Care	54868-2956-05
100's	$97.13	SKELAXIN, Southwood Pharmaceuticals Inc	58016-0682-00
100's	$105.88	SKELAXIN, Carnrick Laboratories Inc	00086-0062-10
180's	$205.56	SKELAXIN, Pharma Pac	52959-0410-18

Tablet - Oral - 800 mg

Qty	Price	Product	NDC
14's	$40.66	SKELAXIN, Pharma Pac	52959-0709-14
20's	$57.87	SKELAXIN, Pharma Pac	52959-0709-20
28's	$80.50	SKELAXIN, Pharma Pac	52959-0709-28
30's	$84.06	SKELAXIN, Pharma Pac	52959-0709-30
40's	$106.98	SKELAXIN, Pharma Pac	52959-0709-40
42's	$107.94	SKELAXIN, Pharma Pac	52959-0709-42
45's	$112.39	SKELAXIN, Pharma Pac	52959-0709-45
50's	$120.18	SKELAXIN, Pharma Pac	52959-0709-50
60's	$141.24	SKELAXIN, Pharma Pac	52959-0709-60
90's	$204.03	SKELAXIN, Pharma Pac	52959-0709-90
100's	$201.16	SKELAXIN, Carnrick Laboratories Inc	59075-0068-10
100's	$225.00	SKELAXIN, Pharma Pac	52959-0709-00
180's	$360.00	SKELAXIN, Pharma Pac	52959-0709-18

Metformin Hydrochloride (003204)

For related information, see the comparative table section in Appendix A.

Categories: Diabetes mellitus; Pregnancy Category C; FDA Approved 1994 Dec; WHO Formulary
Drug Classes: Antidiabetic agents; Biguanides
Brand Names: Glucophage
Foreign Brand Availability: Apophage (Israel); Benofomin (Indonesia); Dabex (Mexico); Denkaform (Philippines); Deson (Thailand); Dextin (South-Africa); Diabetformin (Peru); Diabetmin (Hong-Kong; Malaysia); Diabetmin Retard (Hong-Kong); Diabex (Australia; Indonesia); Diafat (Philippines); Diaformin (Australia; China; Hong-Kong; Taiwan); Diametin (Philippines); Diamin (Singapore); Diformin (Finland; Korea); Diformin Retard (Finland); Dimefor (Costa-Rica; El-Salvador; Guatemala; Honduras; Mexico; Nicaragua; Panama; Peru); Dybis (Korea); Eraphage (Indonesia); Espa-Formin (Germany); Formin (India); Fornidd (Philippines); Gliformin (Colombia); Glucaminol (Colombia); Glucofago (Peru); Glucomet (Australia; New-Zealand; Thailand); Glucomine (Taiwan); Glucoform (Philippines); Glucohexal (Australia); Glucoless (Thailand); Glucomin (Israel); Gluconil (Korea); Glucophage Forte (Czech-Republic; Mexico; Netherlands; Philippines; South-Africa); Glucophage-Mite (Germany); Glucophage Retard (Germany; Israel); Glucotika (Indonesia); Gludepatic (Indonesia); Glufor (Israel); Gluformin (Thailand); Glumeformin (Korea); Glumet (Hong-Kong); Glumin (Indonesia); Glupa (Korea); Glustress (Thailand); Glyciphage (India); Glycomet (Singapore); Glycon (Canada); Glycoran (Singapore); Glyformin (Taiwan); Hipoglucin (Peru); I-Max (Philippines); Juformin (Germany); Maformin (Thailand); Melbin (Japan); Metfogamma (Germany); Metforal (Italy; Singapore); Metomin (New-Zealand); Miformin (Thailand); Orabet (Austria; Denmark; England); Siamformet (Thailand); Thiabet (Germany); Walaphage (India)
Cost of Therapy: $71.43 (Diabetes Mellitus; Glucophage; 500 mg; 4 tablets/day; 30 day supply)
$84.00 (Diabetes Mellitus; Generic Tablets; 500 mg; 4 tablets/day; 30 day supply)
$82.81 (Diabetes Mellitus; Glucophage; 850 mg; 2 tablets/day; 30 day supply)
$88.74 (Diabetes Mellitus; Generic Tablets; 850 mg; 2 tablets/day; 30 day supply)
$92.09 (Diabetes Mellitus; Glucophage XR; 500 mg; 4 tablets/day; 30 day supply)

DESCRIPTION

Note: The trade name has been used throughout this monograph for clarity.

Glucophage (metformin hydrochloride tablets) and Glucophage XR (metformin hydrochloride extended-release tablets) are oral antihyperglycemic drugs used in the management of Type 2 diabetes. Metformin hydrochloride (*N,N*-dimethylimidodicarbonimidic diamide hydrochloride) is not chemically or pharmacologically related to any other classes of oral antihyperglycemic agents.

Metformin hydrochloride is a white to off-white crystalline compound with a molecular formula of $C_4H_{11}N_5 \cdot HCl$ and a molecular weight of 165.63. Metformin hydrochloride is freely soluble in water and is practically insoluble in acetone, ether, and chloroform. The pKa of metformin is 12.4. The pH of a 1% aqueous solution of metformin hydrochloride is 6.68.

GLUCOPHAGE

Glucophage tablets contain 500, 850, or 1000 mg of metformin HCl. Each tablet contains the inactive ingredients povidone and magnesium stearate. In addition, the coating for the 500 and 850 mg tablets contains hydroxypropyl methylcellulose (hypromellose) and the coating for the 1000 mg tablet contains hydroxypropyl methylcellulose and polyethylene glycol.

M

GLUCOPHAGE XR

Glucophage XR contains 500 mg of metformin HCl as the active ingredient. Each tablet contains the inactive ingredients sodium carboxymethyl cellulose, hydroxypropyl methylcellulose, microcrystalline cellulose, and magnesium stearate.

System Components and Performance

Glucophage XR tablets comprise a dual hydrophilic polymer matrix system. Metformin HCl is combined with a drug release controlling polymer to form an "inner" phase, which is then incorporated as discrete particles into an "external" phase of a second polymer. After administration, fluid from the gastrointestinal (GI) tract enters the tablet, causing the polymers to hydrate and swell. Drug is released slowly from the dosage form by a process of diffusion through the gel matrix that is essentially independent of pH. The hydrated polymer system is not rigid and is expected to be broken up by normal peristalsis in the GI tract. The biologically inert components of the tablet may occasionally remain intact during GI transit and will be eliminated in the feces as a soft, hydrated mass.

CLINICAL PHARMACOLOGY

MECHANISM OF ACTION

Metformin is an antihyperglycemic agent which improves glucose tolerance in patients with Type 2 diabetes, lowering both basal and postprandial plasma glucose. Its pharmacologic mechanisms of action are different from other classes of oral antihyperglycemic agents. Metformin decreases hepatic glucose production, decreases intestinal absorption of glucose, and improves insulin sensitivity by increasing peripheral glucose uptake and utilization. Unlike sulfonylureas, metformin does not produce hypoglycemia in either patients with Type 2 diabetes or normal subjects (except in special circumstances, see PRECAUTIONS) and does not cause hyperinsulinemia. With metformin therapy, insulin secretion remains unchanged while fasting insulin levels and day-long plasma insulin response may actually decrease.

PHARMACOKINETICS

Absorption and Bioavailability

The absolute bioavailability of a Glucophage 500 mg tablet given under fasting conditions is approximately 50-60%. Studies using single oral doses of Glucophage 500-1500 mg, and 850-2550 mg, indicate that there is a lack of dose proportionality with increasing doses, which is due to decreased absorption rather than an alteration in elimination. Food decreases the extent of and slightly delays the absorption of metformin, as shown by approximately a 40% lower mean peak plasma concentration (C_{max}), a 25% lower area under the plasma concentration versus time curve (AUC), and a 35 minute prolongation of time to peak plasma concentration (T_{max}) following administration of a single 850 mg tablet of metformin with food, compared to the same tablet strength administered fasting. The clinical relevance of these decreases is unknown.

Following a single oral dose of Glucophage XR, C_{max} is achieved with a median value of 7 hours and a range of 4-8 hours. Peak plasma levels are approximately 20% lower compared to the same dose of Glucophage, however, the extent of absorption (as measured by AUC) is similar to Glucophage.

At steady state, the AUC and C_{max} are less than dose proportional for Glucophage XR within the range of 500-2000 mg administered once daily. Peak plasma levels are approximately 0.6, 1.1, 1.4, and 1.8 μg/ml for 500, 1000, 1500, and 2000 mg once-daily doses, respectively. The extent of metformin absorption (as measured by AUC) from Glucophage XR at a 2000 mg once-daily dose is similar to the same total daily dose administered as Glucophage 1000 mg twice daily. After repeated administration of Glucophage XR, metformin did not accumulate in plasma.

Within-subject variability in C_{max} and AUC of metformin from Glucophage XR is comparable to that with metformin HCl tablets.

Although the extent of metformin absorption (as measured by AUC) from the Glucophage XR increased by approximately 50% when given with food, there was no effect of food on C_{max} and T_{max} of metformin. Both high and low fat meals had the same effect on the pharmacokinetics of Glucophage XR.

Distribution

The apparent volume of distribution (V/F) of metformin following single oral doses of Glucophage 850 mg averaged 654 ± 358 L. Metformin is negligibly bound to plasma proteins, in contrast to sulfonylureas, which are more than 90% protein bound. Metformin partitions into erythrocytes, most likely as a function of time. At usual clinical doses and dosing schedules of Glucophage, steady state plasma concentrations of metformin are reached within 24-48 hours and are generally <1 μg/ml. During controlled clinical trials of Glucophage, maximum metformin plasma levels did not exceed 5 μg/ml, even at maximum doses.

Metabolism and Elimination

Intravenous single-dose studies in normal subjects demonstrate that metformin is excreted unchanged in the urine and does not undergo hepatic metabolism (no metabolites have been identified in humans) nor biliary excretion. Renal clearance (see TABLE 1) is approximately 3.5 times greater than creatinine clearance, which indicates that tubular secretion is the major route of metformin elimination. Following oral administration, approximately 90% of the absorbed drug is eliminated via the renal route within the first 24 hours, with a plasma elimination half-life of approximately 6.2 hours. In blood, the elimination half-life is approximately 17.6 hours, suggesting that the erythrocyte mass may be a compartment of distribution.

SPECIAL POPULATIONS

Patients With Type 2 Diabetes

In the presence of normal renal function, there are no differences between single- or multiple-dose pharmacokinetics of metformin between patients with Type 2 diabetes and normal subjects (see TABLE 1), nor is there any accumulation of metformin in either group at usual clinical doses.

The pharmacokinetics of Glucophage XR in patients with Type 2 diabetes are comparable to those in healthy normal adults.

Renal Insufficiency

In patients with decreased renal function (based on measured creatinine clearance), the plasma and blood half-life of metformin is prolonged and the renal clearance is decreased in proportion to the decrease in creatinine clearance (see TABLE 1; also see WARNINGS).

Hepatic Insufficiency

No pharmacokinetic studies of metformin have been conducted in patients with hepatic insufficiency.

Geriatrics

Limited data from controlled pharmacokinetic studies of Glucophage in healthy elderly subjects suggest that total plasma clearance of metformin is decreased, the half-life is prolonged, and C_{max} is increased, compared to healthy young subjects. From these data, it appears that the change in metformin pharmacokinetics with aging is primarily accounted for by a change in renal function (see TABLE 1). Glucophage and Glucophage XR treatment should not be initiated in patients ≥80 years of age unless measurement of creatinine clearance demonstrates that renal function is not reduced. (See WARNINGS and DOSAGE AND ADMINISTRATION.)

Pediatrics

No pharmacokinetic data from studies of pediatric patients are currently available.

Gender

Metformin pharmacokinetic parameters did not differ significantly between normal subjects and patients with Type 2 diabetes when analyzed according to gender (males = 19, females = 16). Similarly, in controlled clinical studies in patients with Type 2 diabetes, the antihyperglycemic effect of Glucophage was comparable in males and females.

Race

No studies of metformin pharmacokinetic parameters according to race have been performed. In controlled clinical studies of Glucophage in patients with Type 2 diabetes, the antihyperglycemic effect was comparable in whites (n=249), blacks (n=51), and Hispanics (n=24).

INDICATIONS AND USAGE

Glucophage and Glucophage XR, as monotherapy, are indicated as an adjunct to diet and exercise to improve glycemic control in patients with Type 2 diabetes. Glucophage is indicated in patients 10 years of age and older, and Glucophage XR is indicated in patients 17 years of age and older.

TABLE 1 *Select Mean (±SD) Metformin Pharmacokinetic Parameters Following Single or Multiple Oral Doses of Glucophage*

Subject Groups: Dose* (number of subjects)	C_{max}† (µg/ml)	T_{max}‡ (h)	Renal Clearance (ml/min)
Healthy, Nondiabetic Adults:			
500 mg single dose (24)	1.03 (±0.33)	2.75 (±0.81)	600 (±132)
850 mg single dose (74)§	1.60 (±0.38)	2.64 (±0.82)	552 (±139)
850 mg 3 times daily for 19 doses¤ (9)	2.01 (±0.42)	1.79 (±0.94)	642 (±173)
Adults With Type 2 Diabetes:			
850 mg single dose (23)	1.48 (±0.5)	3.32 (±1.08)	491 (±138)
850 mg 3 times daily for 19 doses¤ (9)	1.90 (±0.62)	2.01 (±1.22)	550 (±160)
Elderly¶, Healthy Nondiabetic Adults:			
850 mg single dose (12)	2.45 (±0.70)	2.71 (±1.05)	412 (±98)
Renal-Impaired Adults: 850 mg Single Dose			
Mild (CLCR** 61-90 ml/min) (5)	1.86 (±0.52)	3.20 (±0.45)	384 (±122)
Moderate (CLCR 31-60 ml/min) (4)	4.12 (±1.83)	3.75 (±0.50)	108 (±57)
Severe (CLCR 10-30 ml/min) (6)	3.93 (±0.92)	4.01 (±1.10)	130 (±90)

* All doses given fasting except the first 18 doses of the multiple dose studies.
† Peak plasma concentration.
‡ Time to peak plasma concentration.
§ Combined results (average means) of five studies: mean age 32 years (range 23-59 years).
¤ Kinetic study done following dose 19, given fasting.
¶ Elderly subjects, mean age 71 years (range 65-81 years).
** CLCR = creatinine clearance normalized to body surface area of 1.73 m^2.

Glucophage or Glucophage XR may be used concomitantly with a sulfonylurea or insulin to improve glycemic control in adults (17 years of age and older).

CONTRAINDICATIONS

Glucophage and Glucophage XR are contraindicated in patients with:

Renal disease or renal dysfunction (*e.g.*, as suggested by serum creatinine levels ≥1.5 mg/dl [males], ≥1.4 mg/dl [females] or abnormal creatinine clearance) which may also result from conditions such as cardiovascular collapse (shock), acute myocardial infarction, and septicemia (see WARNINGS and PRECAUTIONS).

Congestive heart failure requiring pharmacologic treatment.

Known hypersensitivity to metformin HCl.

Acute or chronic metabolic acidosis, including diabetic ketoacidosis, with or without coma. Diabetic ketoacidosis should be treated with insulin.

Glucophage and Glucophage XR should be temporarily discontinued in patients undergoing radiologic studies involving intravascular administration of iodinated contrast materials, because use of such products may result in acute alteration of renal function. (See also PRECAUTIONS.)

WARNINGS

Lactic Acidosis:

Lactic acidosis is a rare, but serious, metabolic complication that can occur due to metformin accumulation during treatment with Glucophage or Glucophage XR; when it occurs, it is fatal in approximately 50% of cases. Lactic acidosis may also occur in association with a number of pathophysiologic conditions, including diabetes mellitus, and whenever there is significant tissue hypoperfusion and hypoxemia. Lactic acidosis is characterized by elevated blood lactate levels (>5 mmol/L), decreased blood pH, electrolyte disturbances with an increased anion gap, and an increased lactate/pyruvate ratio. When metformin is implicated as the cause of lactic acidosis, metformin plasma levels >5 µg/ml are generally found.

The reported incidence of lactic acidosis in patients receiving metformin HCl is very low (approximately 0.03 cases/1000 patient-years, with approximately 0.015 fatal cases/1000 patient-years). Reported cases have occurred primarily in diabetic patients with significant renal insufficiency, including both intrinsic renal disease and renal hypoperfusion, often in the setting of multiple concomitant medical/surgical problems and multiple concomitant medications. Patients with congestive heart failure requiring pharmacologic management, in particular those with unstable or acute congestive heart failure who are at risk of hypoperfusion and hypoxemia, are at increased risk of lactic acidosis. The risk of lactic acidosis increases with the degree of renal dysfunction and the patient's age. The risk of lactic acidosis may, therefore, be significantly decreased by regular monitoring of renal function in patients taking Glucophage or Glucophage XR and by use of the minimum effective dose of Glucophage or Glucophage XR. In particular, treatment of the elderly should be accompanied by careful monitoring of renal function. Glucophage or Glucophage XR treatment should not be initiated in patients ≥80 years of age unless measurement of creatinine clearance demonstrates that renal function is not reduced, as these patients are more susceptible to developing lactic acidosis. In addition, Glucophage or Glucophage XR should be promptly withheld in the presence of any condition associated with hypoxemia, dehydration, or sepsis. Because impaired hepatic function may significantly limit the ability to clear lactate, Glucophage or Glucophage XR should generally be avoided in patients with clinical or laboratory evidence of hepatic disease. Patients should be cautioned against excessive alcohol intake, either acute or chronic, when taking Glucophage or Glucophage XR, since alcohol potentiates the effects of Glucophage or Glucophage XR on lactate metabolism. In addition, Glucophage or Glucophage XR should be temporarily discontinued prior to any intravascular radiocontrast study and for any surgical procedure (see also PRECAUTIONS).

The onset of lactic acidosis often is subtle, and accompanied only by nonspecific symptoms such as malaise, myalgias, respiratory distress, increasing somnolence, and nonspecific abdominal distress. There may be associated hypothermia, hypotension, and resistant bradyarrhythmias with more marked acidosis. The patient and the patient's physician must be aware of the possible importance of such symptoms and the patient should be instructed to notify the physician immediately if they occur (see also PRECAUTIONS). Glucophage and Glucophage XR should be withdrawn until the situation is clarified. Serum electrolytes, ketones, blood glucose, and if indicated, blood pH, lactate levels, and even blood metformin levels may be useful. Once a patient is stabilized on any dose level of Glucophage and Glucophage XR, gastrointestinal symptoms, which are common during initiation of therapy, are unlikely to be drug related. Later occurrence of gastrointestinal symptoms could be due to lactic acidosis or other serious disease.

Levels of fasting venous plasma lactate above the upper limit of normal but less than 5 mmol/L in patients taking Glucophage and Glucophage XR do not necessarily indicate impending lactic acidosis and may be explainable

Cont'd

by other mechanisms, such as poorly controlled diabetes or obesity, vigorous physical activity, or technical problems in sample handling. (See also PRECAUTIONS.)

Lactic acidosis should be suspected in any diabetic patient with metabolic acidosis lacking evidence of ketoacidosis (ketonuria and ketonemia).

Lactic acidosis is a medical emergency that must be treated in a hospital setting. In a patient with lactic acidosis who is taking Glucophage and Glucophage XR, the drug should be discontinued immediately and general supportive measures promptly instituted. Because metformin HCl is dialyzable (with a clearance of up to 170 ml/min under good hemodynamic conditions), prompt hemodialysis is recommended to correct the acidosis and remove the accumulated metformin. Such management often results in prompt reversal of symptoms and recovery. (See also CONTRAINDICATIONS and PRECAUTIONS.)

PRECAUTIONS

GENERAL

Monitoring of Renal Function

Metformin is known to be substantially excreted by the kidney, and the risk of metformin accumulation and lactic acidosis increases with the degree of impairment of renal function. Thus, patients with serum creatinine levels above the upper limit of normal for their age should not receive Glucophage or Glucophage XR. In patients with advanced age, Glucophage or Glucophage XR should be carefully titrated to establish the minimum dose for adequate glycemic effect, because aging is associated with reduced renal function. In elderly patients, particularly those ≥80 years of age, renal function should be monitored regularly and, generally, Glucophage and Glucophage XR should not be titrated to the maximum dose (see WARNINGS and DOSAGE AND ADMINISTRATION).

Before initiation of Glucophage or Glucophage XR therapy and at least annually thereafter, renal function should be assessed and verified as normal. In patients in whom development of renal dysfunction is anticipated, renal function should be assessed more frequently and Glucophage or Glucophage XR discontinued if evidence of renal impairment is present.

Use of Concomitant Medications That May Affect Renal Function or Metformin Disposition

Concomitant medication(s) that may affect renal function or result in significant hemodynamic change or may interfere with the disposition of metformin, such as cationic drugs that are eliminated by renal tubular secretion (see DRUG INTERACTIONS), should be used with caution.

Radiologic Studies Involving the Use of Intravascular Iodinated Contrast Materials (for example, intravenous urogram, intravenous cholangiography, angiography, and computed tomography [CT] scans with intravascular contrast materials)

Intravascular contrast studies with iodinated materials can lead to acute alteration of renal function and have been associated with lactic acidosis in patients receiving metformin (see CONTRAINDICATIONS). Therefore, in patients in whom any such study is planned, Glucophage or Glucophage XR should be temporarily discontinued at the time of or prior to the procedure, and withheld for 48 hours subsequent to the procedure and reinstituted only after renal function has been re-evaluated and found to be normal.

Hypoxic States

Cardiovascular collapse (shock) from whatever cause, acute congestive heart failure, acute myocardial infarction and other conditions characterized by hypoxemia have been associated with lactic acidosis and may also cause prerenal azotemia. When such events occur in patients on Glucophage or Glucophage XR therapy, the drug should be promptly discontinued.

Surgical Procedures

Glucophage or Glucophage XR therapy should be temporarily suspended for any surgical procedure (except minor procedures not associated with restricted intake of food and fluids) and should not be restarted until the patient's oral intake has resumed and renal function has been evaluated as normal.

Alcohol Intake

Alcohol is known to potentiate the effect of metformin on lactate metabolism. Patients, therefore, should be warned against excessive alcohol intake, acute or chronic, while receiving Glucophage or Glucophage XR.

Impaired Hepatic Function

Since impaired hepatic function has been associated with some cases of lactic acidosis, Glucophage and Glucophage XR should generally be avoided in patients with clinical or laboratory evidence of hepatic disease.

Vitamin B_{12} Levels

In controlled clinical trials of Glucophage of 29 weeks duration, a decrease to subnormal levels of previously normal serum vitamin B_{12} levels, without clinical manifestations, was observed in approximately 7% of patients. Such decrease, possibly due to interference with B_{12} absorption from the B_{12}-intrinsic factor complex, is, however, very rarely associated with anemia and appears to be rapidly reversible with discontinuation of Glucophage or vitamin B_{12} supplementation. Measurement of hematologic parameters on an annual basis is advised in patients on Glucophage or Glucophage XR and any apparent abnormalities should be appropriately investigated and managed (see Laboratory Tests).

Certain individuals (those with inadequate vitamin B_{12} or calcium intake or absorption) appear to be predisposed to developing subnormal vitamin B_{12} levels. In these patients, routine serum vitamin B_{12} measurements at 2-3 year intervals may be useful.

Change in Clinical Status of Patients With Previously Controlled Type 2 Diabetes

A patient with Type 2 diabetes previously well controlled on Glucophage or Glucophage XR who develops laboratory abnormalities or clinical illness (especially vague and poorly defined illness) should be evaluated promptly for evidence of ketoacidosis or lactic acidosis.

Evaluation should include serum electrolytes and ketones, blood glucose and, if indicated, blood pH, lactate, pyruvate, and metformin levels. If acidosis of either form occurs, Glucophage or Glucophage XR must be stopped immediately and other appropriate corrective measures initiated (see also WARNINGS).

Hypoglycemia

Hypoglycemia does not occur in patients receiving Glucophage or Glucophage XR alone under usual circumstances of use, but could occur when caloric intake is deficient, when strenuous exercise is not compensated by caloric supplementation, or during concomitant use with other glucose-lowering agents (such as sulfonylureas and insulin) or ethanol.

Elderly, debilitated, or malnourished patients, and those with adrenal or pituitary insufficiency or alcohol intoxication are particularly susceptible to hypoglycemic effects. Hypoglycemia may be difficult to recognize in the elderly, and in people who are taking beta-adrenergic blocking drugs.

Loss of Control of Blood Glucose

When a patient stabilized on any diabetic regimen is exposed to stress such as fever, trauma, infection, or surgery, a temporary loss of glycemic control may occur. At such times, it may be necessary to withhold Glucophage or Glucophage XR and temporarily administer insulin. Glucophage or Glucophage XR may be reinstituted after the acute episode is resolved.

The effectiveness of oral antidiabetic drugs in lowering blood glucose to a targeted level decreases in many patients over a period of time. This phenomenon, which may be due to progression of the underlying disease or to diminished responsiveness to the drug, is known as secondary failure, to distinguish it from primary failure in which the drug is ineffective during initial therapy. Should secondary failure occur with either Glucophage or Glucophage XR or sulfonylurea monotherapy, combined therapy with Glucophage or Glucophage XR and sulfonylurea may result in a response. Should secondary failure occur with combined Gluphage/sulfonylurea therapy or Glucophage XR/sulfonylurea therapy, it may be necessary to consider therapeutic alternatives including initiation of insulin therapy.

INFORMATION FOR THE PATIENT

Patients should be informed of the potential risks and benefits of Glucophage or Glucophage XR and of alternative modes of therapy. They should also be informed about the importance of adherence to dietary instructions, of a regular exercise program, and of regular testing of blood glucose, glycosylated hemoglobin, renal function, and hematologic parameters.

The risks of lactic acidosis, its symptoms, and conditions that predispose to its development, as noted in WARNINGS and PRECAUTIONS, should be explained to patients. Patients should be advised to discontinue Glucophage or Glucophage XR immediately and to promptly notify their health practitioner if unexplained hyperventilation, myalgia, malaise, unusual somnolence, or other nonspecific symptoms occur. Once a patient is stabilized on any dose level of Glucophage or Glucophage XR, gastrointestinal symptoms, which are common during initiation of metformin therapy, are unlikely to be drug related. Later occurrence of gastrointestinal symptoms could be due to lactic acidosis or other serious disease.

Patients should be counselled against excessive alcohol intake, either acute or chronic, while receiving Glucophage or Glucophage XR.

Glucophage or Glucophage XR alone does not usually cause hypoglycemia, although it may occur when Glucophage or Glucophage XR is used in conjunction with oral sulfonylureas and insulin. When initiating combination therapy, the risks of hypoglycemia, its symptoms and treatment, and conditions that predispose to its development should be explained to patients and responsible family members.

Patients should be informed that Glucophage XR must be swallowed whole and not crushed or chewed, and that the inactive ingredients may occasionally be eliminated in the feces as a soft mass that may resemble the original tablet. (See patient information that is distributed with the prescription.)

LABORATORY TESTS

Response to all diabetic therapies should be monitored by periodic measurements of fasting blood glucose and glycosylated hemoglobin levels, with a goal of decreasing these levels toward the normal range. During initial dose titration, fasting glucose can be used to determine the therapeutic response. Thereafter, both glucose and glycosylated hemoglobin should be monitored. Measurements of glycosylated hemoglobin may be especially useful for evaluating long-term control (see also DOSAGE AND ADMINISTRATION).

Initial and periodic monitoring of hematologic parameters (*e.g.,* hemoglobin/hematocrit and red blood cell indices) and renal function (serum creatinine) should be performed, at least on an annual basis. While megaloblastic anemia has rarely been seen with Glucophage therapy, if this is suspected, vitamin B_{12} deficiency should be excluded.

CARCINOGENESIS, MUTAGENESIS, AND IMPAIRMENT OF FERTILITY

Long-term carcinogenicity studies have been performed in rats (dosing duration of 104 weeks) and mice (dosing duration of 91 weeks) at doses up to and including 900 mg/kg/day and 1500 mg/kg/day, respectively. These doses are both approximately 4 times the maximum recommended human daily dose of 2000 mg based on body surface area comparisons. No evidence of carcinogenicity with metformin was found in either male or female mice. Similarly, there was no tumorigenic potential observed with metformin in male rats. There was, however, an increased incidence of benign stromal uterine polyps in female rats treated with 900 mg/kg/day.

There was no evidence of a mutagenic potential of metformin in the following *in vitro* tests: Ames test (*S. typhimurium*), gene mutation test (mouse lymphoma cells), or chromosomal aberrations test (human lymphocytes). Results in the *in vivo* mouse micronucleus test were also negative.

Fertility of male or female rats was unaffected by metformin when administered at doses as high as 600 mg/kg/day, which is approximately 3 times the maximum recommended human daily dose based on body surface area comparisons.

PREGNANCY, TERATOGENIC EFFECTS, PREGNANCY CATEGORY B

Recent information strongly suggests that abnormal blood glucose levels during pregnancy are associated with a higher incidence of congenital abnormalities. Most experts recommend that insulin be used during pregnancy to maintain blood glucose levels as close to normal as possible. Because animal reproduction studies are not always predictive of human response, Glucophage and Glucophage XR should not be used during pregnancy unless clearly needed.

There are no adequate and well-controlled studies in pregnant women with Glucophage or Glucophage XR. Metformin was not teratogenic in rats and rabbits at doses up to 600 mg/kg/day. This represents an exposure of about 2 and 6 times the maximum recommended human daily dose of 2000 mg based on body surface area comparisons for rats and rabbits, respectively. Determination of fetal concentrations demonstrated a partial placental barrier to metformin.

NURSING MOTHERS

Studies in lactating rats show that metformin is excreted into milk and reaches levels comparable to those in plasma. Similar studies have not been conducted in nursing mothers. Because the potential for hypoglycemia in nursing infants may exist, a decision should be made whether to discontinue nursing or to discontinue the drug, taking into account the importance of the drug to the mother. If Glucophage or Glucophage XR is discontinued, and if diet alone is inadequate for controlling blood glucose, insulin therapy should be considered.

PEDIATRIC USE

The safety and effectiveness of metformin HCl tablets for the treatment of Type 2 diabetes have been established in pediatric patients ages 10-16 years (studies have not been conducted in pediatric patients below the age of 10 years). Use of Glucophage in this age group is supported by evidence from adequate and well-controlled studies of Glucophage in adults with additional data from a controlled clinical study in pediatric patients ages 10-16 years with Type 2 diabetes, which demonstrated a similar response in glycemic control to that seen in adults. In this study, adverse effects were similar to those described in adults. (See ADVERSE REACTIONS, Pediatric Patients.) A maximum daily dose of 2000 mg is recommended. (See DOSAGE AND ADMINISTRATION, Recommended Dosing Schedule, Pediatrics.)

Safety and effectiveness of Glucophage XR in pediatric patients have not been established.

GERIATRIC USE

Controlled clinical studies of Glucophage and Glucophage XR did not include sufficient numbers of elderly patients to determine whether they respond differently from younger patients, although other reported clinical experience has not identified differences in responses between the elderly and younger patients. Metformin is known to be substantially excreted by the kidney and because the risk of serious adverse reactions to the drug is greater in patients with impaired renal function, Glucophage and Glucophage XR should only be used in patients with normal renal function (see CONTRAINDICATIONS, WARNINGS, and CLINICAL PHARMACOLOGY, Pharmacokinetics). Because aging is associated with reduced renal function, Glucophage or Glucophage XR should be used with caution as age increases. Care should be taken in dose selection and should be based on careful and regular monitoring of renal function. Generally, elderly patients should not be titrated to the maximum dose of Glucophage or Glucophage XR (see also WARNINGS and DOSAGE AND ADMINISTRATION).

DRUG INTERACTIONS

Clinical evaluation of drug interactions done with Glucophage.

GLYBURIDE

In a single-dose interaction study in Type 2 diabetes patients, co-administration of metformin and glyburide did not result in any changes in either metformin pharmacokinetics or pharmacodynamics. Decreases in glyburide AUC and C_{max} were observed, but were highly variable. The single-dose nature of this study and the lack of correlation between glyburide blood levels and pharmacodynamic effects, makes the clinical significance of this interaction uncertain (see DOSAGE AND ADMINISTRATION, Concomitant Glucophage or Glucophage XR and Oral Sulfonylurea Therapy).

FUROSEMIDE

A single-dose, metformin-furosemide drug interaction study in healthy subjects demonstrated that pharmacokinetic parameters of both compounds were affected by co-administration. Furosemide increased the metformin plasma and blood C_{max} by 22% and blood AUC by 15%, without any significant change in metformin renal clearance. When administered with metformin, the C_{max} and AUC of furosemide were 31% and 12% smaller, respectively, than when administered alone, and the terminal half-life was decreased by 32%, without any significant change in furosemide renal clearance. No information is available about the interaction of metformin and furosemide when co-administered chronically.

NIFEDIPINE

A single-dose, metformin-nifedipine drug interaction study in normal healthy volunteers demonstrated that co-administration of nifedipine increased plasma metformin C_{max} and AUC by 20% and 9%, respectively, and increased the amount excreted in the urine. T_{max} and half-life were unaffected. Nifedipine appears to enhance the absorption of metformin. Metformin had minimal effects on nifedipine.

CATIONIC DRUGS

Cationic drugs (*e.g.,* amiloride, digoxin, morphine, procainamide, quinidine, quinine, ranitidine, triamterene, trimethoprim, or vancomycin) that are eliminated by renal tubular secretion theoretically have the potential for interaction with metformin by competing for common renal tubular transport systems. Such interaction between metformin and oral cimetidine has been observed in normal healthy volunteers in both single- and multiple-dose, metformin-cimetidine drug interaction studies, with a 60% increase in peak metformin plasma and whole blood concentrations and a 40% increase in plasma and whole blood metformin AUC. There was no change in elimination half-life in the single-dose study. Metformin had no effect on cimetidine pharmacokinetics. Although such interactions remain theoretical (except for cimetidine), careful patient monitoring and dose adjustment of Glucophage or Glucophage XR and/or the interfering drug is recommended in patients who are taking cationic medications that are excreted via the proximal renal tubular secretory system.

OTHER

Certain drugs tend to produce hyperglycemia and may lead to loss of glycemic control. These drugs include the thiazides and other diuretics, corticosteroids, phenothiazines, thyroid products, estrogens, oral contraceptives, phenytoin, nicotinic acid, sympathomimetics, calcium channel blocking drugs, and isoniazid. When such drugs are administered to a patient receiving Glucophage or Glucophage XR, the patient should be closely observed for loss of blood glucose control. When such drugs are withdrawn from a patient receiving Glucophage or Glucophage XR, the patient should be observed closely for hypoglycemia.

In healthy volunteers, the pharmacokinetics of metformin and propranolol, and metformin and ibuprofen were not affected when co-administered in single-dose interaction studies.

Metformin is negligibly bound to plasma proteins and is, therefore, less likely to interact with highly protein-bound drugs such as salicylates, sulfonamides, chloramphenicol, and probenecid, as compared to the sulfonylureas, which are extensively bound to serum proteins.

ADVERSE REACTIONS

In a US double-blind clinical study of Glucophage in patients with Type 2 diabetes, a total of 141 patients received Glucophage therapy (up to 2550 mg/day) and 145 patients received placebo. Adverse reactions reported in greater than 5% of the Glucophage patients, and that were more common in Glucophage- than placebo-treated patients, are listed in TABLE 11.

Diarrhea led to discontinuation of study medication in 6% of patients treated with Glucophage. Additionally, the following adverse reactions were reported in ≥1.0 to ≤5.0% of Glucophage patients and were more commonly reported with Glucophage tablets than placebo: abnormal stools, hypoglycemia, myalgia, lightheaded, dyspnea, nail disorder, rash, sweating increased, taste disorder, chest discomfort, chills, flu syndrome, flushing, palpitation.

TABLE 11 *Most Common Adverse Reactions (>5.0%) in a Placebo-Controlled Clinical Study of Glucophage Monotherapy**

Adverse Reaction	Glucophage Monotherapy n=141	Placebo n=145
Diarrhea	53.2%	11.7%
Nausea/vomiting	25.5%	8.3%
Flatulence	12.1%	5.5%
Asthenia	9.2%	5.5%
Indigestion	7.1%	4.1%
Abdominal discomfort	6.4%	4.8%
Headache	5.7%	4.8%

* Reactions that were more common in Glucophage- than placebo-treated patients.

In worldwide clinical trials over 900 patients with Type 2 diabetes have been treated with Glucophage XR in placebo- and active-controlled studies. In placebo-controlled trials, 781 patients were administered Glucophage XR and 195 patients received placebo. Adverse reactions reported in greater than 5% of the Glucophage XR patients, and that were more common in Glucophage XR- than placebo-treated patients, are listed in TABLE 12.

TABLE 12 *Most Common Adverse Reactions (>5.0%) in Placebo-Controlled Studies of Glucophage XR**

Adverse Reaction	Glucophage XR n=781	Placebo n=195
Diarrhea	9.6%	2.6%
Nausea/vomiting	6.5%	1.5%

* Reactions that were more common in Glucophage XR- than placebo-treated patients.

Diarrhea led to discontinuation of study medication in 0.6% of patients treated with Glucophage XR. Additionally, the following adverse reactions were reported in ≥1.0% to ≤5.0% of Glucophage XR patients and were more commonly reported with Glucophage XR than placebo: abdominal pain, constipation, distention abdomen, dyspepsia/heartburn, flatulence, dizziness, headache, upper respiratory infection, taste disturbance.

PEDIATRIC PATIENTS

In clinical trials with Glucophage in pediatric patients with Type 2 diabetes, the profile of adverse reactions was similar to that observed in adults.

DOSAGE AND ADMINISTRATION

There is no fixed dosage regimen for the management of hyperglycemia in patients with Type 2 diabetes with Glucophage or Glucophage XR or any other pharmacologic agent. Dosage of Glucophage or Glucophage XR must be individualized on the basis of both effectiveness and tolerance, while not exceeding the maximum recommended daily dose. The maximum recommended daily dose of Glucophage is 2550 mg in adults and 2000 mg in pediatric patients (10-16 years of age); the maximum recommended daily dose of Glucophage XR in adults is 2000 mg.

Glucophage should be given in divided doses with meals while Glucophage XR should generally be given once daily with the evening meal. Glucophage or Glucophage XR should be started at a low dose, with gradual dose escalation, both to reduce gastrointestinal side effects and to permit identification of the minimum dose required for adequate glycemic control of the patient.

During treatment initiation and dose titration (see Recommended Dosing Schedule), fasting plasma glucose should be used to determine the therapeutic response to Glucophage or Glucophage XR and identify the minimum effective dose for the patient. Thereafter, glycosylated hemoglobin should be measured at intervals of approximately 3 months. **The therapeutic goal should be to decrease both fasting plasma glucose and glycosylated hemoglobin levels to normal or near normal by using the lowest effective dose of Glucophage or Glucophage XR, either when used as monotherapy or in combination with sulfonylurea or insulin.**

Monitoring of blood glucose and glycosylated hemoglobin will also permit detection of primary failure, *i.e.,* inadequate lowering of blood glucose at the maximum recommended dose of medication, and secondary failure, *i.e.,* loss of an adequate blood glucose lowering response after an initial period of effectiveness.

Short-term administration of Glucophage or Glucophage XR may be sufficient during periods of transient loss of control in patients usually well-controlled on diet alone.

Glucophage XR tablets must be swallowed whole and never crushed or chewed. Occasionally, the inactive ingredients of Glucophage XR will be eliminated in the feces as a soft, hydrated mass. (See patient information that is distributed with the prescription.)

RECOMMENDED DOSING SCHEDULE

Adults

In general, clinically significant responses are not seen at doses below 1500 mg/day. However, a lower recommended starting dose and gradually increased dosage is advised to minimize gastrointestinal symptoms.

The usual starting dose of Glucophage is 500 mg twice a day or 850 mg once a day, given with meals. Dosage increases should be made in increments of 500 mg weekly or 850 mg every 2 weeks, up to a total of 2000 mg/day, given in divided doses. Patients can also be titrated from 500 mg twice a day to 850 mg twice a day after 2 weeks. For those patients requiring additional glycemic control, Glucophage may be given to a maximum daily dose of 2550 mg/day. Doses above 2000 mg may be better tolerated given 3 times a day with meals.

The usual starting dose of Glucophage XR is 500 mg once daily with the evening meal. Dosage increases should be made in increments of 500 mg weekly, up to a maximum of 2000 mg once daily with the evening meal. If glycemic control is not achieved on Glucophage XR 2000 mg once daily, a trial of Glucophage XR 1000 mg twice daily should be considered. If higher doses of metformin are required, Glucophage should be used at total daily doses up to 2550 mg administered in divided daily doses, as described above.

In a randomized trial, patients currently treated with Glucophage were switched to Glucophage XR. Results of this trial suggest that patients receiving Glucophage treatment may be safely switched to Glucophage XR once daily at the same total daily dose, up to 2000 mg once daily. Following a switch from Glucophage to Glucophage XR, glycemic control should be closely monitored and dosage adjustments made accordingly.

Pediatrics

The usual starting dose of Glucophage is 500 mg twice a day, given with meals. Dosage increases should be made in increments of 500 mg weekly up to a maximum of 2000 mg/day, given in divided doses. Safety and effectiveness of Glucophage XR in pediatric patients have not been established.

TRANSFER FROM OTHER ANTIDIABETIC THERAPY

When transferring patients from standard oral hypoglycemic agents other than chlorpropamide to Glucophage or Glucophage XR, no transition period generally is necessary. When transferring patients from chlorpropamide, care should be exercised during the first 2 weeks because of the prolonged retention of chlorpropamide in the body, leading to overlapping drug effects and possible hypoglycemia.

CONCOMITANT GLUCOPHAGE OR GLUCOPHAGE XR AND ORAL SULFONYLUREA THERAPY IN ADULT PATIENTS

If patients have not responded to 4 weeks of the maximum dose of Glucophage or Glucophage XR monotherapy, consideration should be given to gradual addition of an oral sulfonylurea while continuing Glucophage or Glucophage XR at the maximum dose, even if prior primary or secondary failure to a sulfonylurea has occurred. Clinical and pharmacokinetic drug-drug interaction data are currently available only for metformin plus glyburide (glibenclamide).

With concomitant Glucophage or Glucophage XR and sulfonylurea therapy, the desired control of blood glucose may be obtained by adjusting the dose of each drug. In a clinical trial of patients with Type 2 diabetes and prior failure on glyburide, patients started on Glucophage 500 mg and glyburide 20 mg were titrated to 1000/20 mg, 1500/20 mg, 2000/20 mg or 2500/20 mg of Glucophage and glyburide, respectively, to reach the goal of glycemic control as measured by FPG, HbA_{1c} and plasma glucose response. However, attempts should be made to identify the minimum effective dose of each drug to achieve this goal. With concomitant Glucophage or Glucophage XR and sulfonylurea therapy, the risk of hypoglycemia associated with sulfonylurea therapy continues and may be increased. Appropriate precautions should be taken. (See prescribing information of the respective sulfonylurea.)

If patients have not satisfactorily responded to 1-3 months of concomitant therapy with the maximum dose of Glucophage or Glucophage XR and the maximum dose of an oral sulfonylurea, consider therapeutic alternatives including switching to insulin with or without Glucophage or Glucophage XR.

CONCOMITANT GLUCOPHAGE OR GLUCOPHAGE XR AND INSULIN THERAPY IN ADULT PATIENTS

The current insulin dose should be continued upon initiation of Glucophage or Glucophage XR therapy. Glucophage or Glucophage XR therapy should be initiated at 500 mg once daily in patients on insulin therapy. For patients not responding adequately, the dose of Glucophage or Glucophage XR should be increased by 500 mg after approximately 1 week and by 500 mg every week thereafter until adequate glycemic control is achieved. The maximum recommended daily dose is 2500 mg for Glucophage and 2000 mg for Glucophage XR. It is recommended that the insulin dose be decreased by 10-25% when fasting

M

plasma glucose concentrations decrease to less than 120 mg/dl in patients receiving concomitant insulin and metformin HCl. Further adjustment should be individualized based on glucose-lowering response.

SPECIFIC PATIENT POPULATIONS

Glucophage or Glucophage XR are not recommended for use in pregnancy. Glucophage is not recommended in patients below the age of 10 years. Glucophage XR is not recommended in pediatric patients (below the age of 17 years).

The initial and maintenance dosing of Glucophage or Glucophage XR should be conservative in patients with advanced age, due to the potential for decreased renal function in this population. Any dosage adjustment should be based on a careful assessment of renal function. Generally, elderly, debilitated, and malnourished patients should not be titrated to the maximum dose of Glucophage or Glucophage XR.

Monitoring of renal function is necessary to aid in prevention of lactic acidosis, particularly in the elderly. (See WARNINGS.)

HOW SUPPLIED

GLUCOPHAGE

500 mg Tablets: Round, white to off-white, film coated tablets debossed with "BMS 6060" around the periphery of the tablet on one side and "500" debossed across the face of the other side.

850 mg Tablets: Round, white to off-white, film coated tablets debossed with "BMS 6070" around the periphery of the tablet on one side and "850" debossed across the face of the other side.

1000 mg Tablets: White, oval, biconvex, film coated tablets with "BMS 6071" debossed on one side and "1000" debossed on the opposite side and with a bisect line on both sides.

GLUCOPHAGE XR

500 mg Tablets: White to off-white, capsule shaped, biconvex tablets, with "BMS 6063" debossed on one side and "500" debossed across the face of the other side.

STORAGE

Store at 20-25°C (68-77°F); excursions permitted to 15-30°C (59-86°F). Dispense in light-resistant containers.

PRODUCT LISTING - RATED THERAPEUTICALLY EQUIVALENT

Tablet - Oral - 500 mg

100's	$70.00	GENERIC, Ivax Corporation	00172-4331-60
100's	$70.04	GENERIC, Watson Laboratories Inc	00591-2713-01
100's	$70.35	GENERIC, Purepac Pharmaceutical Company	00228-2657-11
100's	$70.35	GENERIC, Mylan Pharmaceuticals Inc	00378-0234-01
100's	$70.35	GENERIC, Udl Laboratories Inc	51079-0972-20
100's	$70.36	GENERIC, Geneva Pharmaceuticals	00781-5050-01
100's	$70.43	GENERIC, Teva Pharmaceuticals Usa	00093-1048-01
100's	$70.43	GENERIC, Eon Labs Manufacturing Inc	00185-0213-01
100's	$70.43	GENERIC, Barr Laboratories Inc	00555-0385-02
100's	$70.43	GENERIC, Par Pharmaceutical Inc	49884-0736-01
100's	$70.43	GENERIC, Mutual Pharmaceutical Co Inc	53489-0467-01
100's	$70.43	GENERIC, Apotex Usa Inc	60505-0190-00
100's	$70.43	GENERIC, Andrx Pharmaceuticals	62037-0674-01

Tablet - Oral - 850 mg

100's	$119.05	GENERIC, Ivax Corporation	00172-4330-60
100's	$119.06	GENERIC, Watson Laboratories Inc	00591-2775-01
100's	$119.60	GENERIC, Purepac Pharmaceutical Company	00228-2715-11
100's	$119.60	GENERIC, Geneva Pharmaceuticals	00781-5051-01
100's	$119.65	GENERIC, Mylan Pharmaceuticals Inc	00378-0240-01
100's	$119.65	GENERIC, Udl Laboratories Inc	51079-0973-20
100's	$119.69	GENERIC, Mutual Pharmaceutical Co Inc	53489-0468-01
100's	$119.72	GENERIC, Barr Laboratories Inc	00555-0386-02
100's	$119.72	GENERIC, Par Pharmaceutical Inc	49884-0737-01
100's	$119.72	GENERIC, Par Pharmaceutical Inc	49884-0740-01
100's	$119.73	GENERIC, Teva Pharmaceuticals Usa	00093-1049-01
100's	$119.73	GENERIC, Apotex Usa Inc	60505-0191-00
100's	$119.73	GENERIC, Andrx Pharmaceuticals	62037-0675-01
100's	$119.74	GENERIC, Eon Labs Manufacturing Inc	00185-0215-01
250's	$291.70	GENERIC, Watson Laboratories Inc	00591-2775-25

Tablet - Oral - 1000 mg

100's	$143.08	GENERIC, Andrx Pharmaceuticals	62037-0676-01
100's	$144.10	GENERIC, Eon Labs Manufacturing Inc	00185-0221-01
100's	$144.25	GENERIC, Ivax Corporation	00172-4432-60
100's	$144.27	GENERIC, Watson Laboratories Inc	00591-2455-01
100's	$144.90	GENERIC, Purepac Pharmaceutical Company	00228-2718-11
100's	$144.90	GENERIC, Apotex Usa Inc	60505-0192-00
100's	$144.94	GENERIC, Geneva Pharmaceuticals	00781-5052-01
100's	$144.99	GENERIC, Mutual Pharmaceutical Co Inc	53489-0469-01
100's	$145.00	GENERIC, Mylan Pharmaceuticals Inc	00378-0244-01
100's	$145.07	GENERIC, Par Pharmaceutical Inc	49884-0738-01
100's	$145.07	GENERIC, Par Pharmaceutical Inc	49884-0741-01
100's	$145.08	GENERIC, Barr Laboratories Inc	00555-0387-02

PRODUCT LISTING - EQUIVALENTS NOT AVAILABLE

Tablet - Oral - 500 mg

10's	$7.40	GLUCOPHAGE, Southwood Pharmaceuticals Inc	58016-0213-10
30's	$20.72	GLUCOPHAGE, Allscripts Pharmaceutical Company	54569-4202-02
30's	$22.19	GLUCOPHAGE, Southwood Pharmaceuticals Inc	58016-0213-30
60's	$30.04	GLUCOPHAGE, Allscripts Pharmaceutical Company	54569-4202-00
60's	$44.37	GLUCOPHAGE, Southwood Pharmaceuticals Inc	58016-0213-60
60's	$44.41	GLUCOPHAGE, Pd-Rx Pharmaceuticals	55289-0211-60
100's	$59.24	GLUCOPHAGE, Physicians Total Care	54868-3545-00
100's	$72.00	GENERIC, Ivax Corporation	00172-4331-10
100's	$73.95	GLUCOPHAGE, Southwood Pharmaceuticals Inc	58016-0213-00
100's	$81.19	GLUCOPHAGE, Bristol-Myers Squibb	00087-6060-05
120's	$76.75	GLUCOPHAGE, Physicians Total Care	54868-3545-01
120's	$82.90	GLUCOPHAGE, Allscripts Pharmaceutical Company	54569-4202-03

Tablet - Oral - 850 mg

10's	$11.90	GLUCOPHAGE, Southwood Pharmaceuticals Inc	58016-0457-10
30's	$35.23	GLUCOPHAGE, Allscripts Pharmaceutical Company	54569-4740-01
30's	$35.70	GLUCOPHAGE, Southwood Pharmaceuticals Inc	58016-0457-30
60's	$70.46	GLUCOPHAGE, Allscripts Pharmaceutical Company	54569-4740-00
60's	$71.40	GLUCOPHAGE, Southwood Pharmaceuticals Inc	58016-0457-60
100's	$100.27	GLUCOPHAGE, Physicians Total Care	54868-3546-00
100's	$119.00	GLUCOPHAGE, Southwood Pharmaceuticals Inc	58016-0457-00
100's	$121.05	GENERIC, Ivax Corporation	00172-4330-10
100's	$138.01	GLUCOPHAGE, Bristol-Myers Squibb	00087-6070-05

Tablet - Oral - 1000 mg

10's	$15.00	GLUCOPHAGE, Southwood Pharmaceuticals Inc	58016-0553-10
30's	$42.69	GLUCOPHAGE, Allscripts Pharmaceutical Company	54569-4786-00
30's	$44.99	GLUCOPHAGE, Southwood Pharmaceuticals Inc	58016-0553-30
60's	$85.38	GLUCOPHAGE, Allscripts Pharmaceutical Company	54569-4786-01
60's	$89.97	GLUCOPHAGE, Southwood Pharmaceuticals Inc	58016-0553-60
100's	$144.40	GENERIC, Udl Laboratories Inc	51079-0995-20
100's	$146.25	GENERIC, Ivax Corporation	00172-4432-10
100's	$149.95	GLUCOPHAGE, Southwood Pharmaceuticals Inc	58016-0553-00
100's	$167.24	GLUCOPHAGE, Bristol-Myers Squibb	00087-6071-11

Tablet, Extended Release - Oral - 500 mg

100's	$76.74	GLUCOPHAGE XR, Bristol-Myers Squibb	00087-6063-13

Metformin Hydrochloride; Rosiglitazone Maleate (003571)

For complete prescribing information, refer to the CD-ROM included with the book.

For related information, see the comparative table section in Appendix A.

Categories: Diabetes mellitus; Pregnancy Category C; FDA Approved 2002 Oct
Drug Classes: Antidiabetic agents; Biguanides; Thiazolidinediones
Brand Names: Avandamet
Cost of Therapy: $101.25 (Diabetes Mellitus; Avandamet; 500 mg; 2 mg; 2 tablets/day; 30 day supply)

DESCRIPTION

Note: The trade name was used throughout this monograph for clarity.

Avandamet (rosiglitazone maleate and metformin hydrochloride) tablets contains two oral antihyperglycemic drugs used in the management of Type 2 diabetes: rosiglitazone maleate and metformin hydrochloride. The combination of rosiglitazone maleate and metformin hydrochloride has been previously approved based on clinical trials in people with Type 2 diabetes mellitus inadequately controlled on metformin alone. Additional efficacy and safety information about rosiglitazone and metformin monotherapies may be found in the prescribing information for each individual drug.

Rosiglitazone maleate is an oral antidiabetic agent, which acts primarily by increasing insulin sensitivity. Rosiglitazone improves glycemic control while reducing circulating insulin levels. Pharmacologic studies in animal models indicate that rosiglitazone improves sensitivity to insulin in muscle and adipose tissue and inhibits hepatic gluconeogenesis. Rosiglitazone maleate is not chemically or functionally related to the sulfonylureas, the biguanides, or the α-glucosidase inhibitors.

Chemically, rosiglitazone maleate is (±)-5-[[4-[2-(methyl-2-pyridinylamino)ethoxy]phenyl]methyl]-2,4-thiazolidinedione, (Z)-2-butenedioate (1:1) with a molecular weight of 473.52 (357.44 free base). The molecule has a single chiral center and is present as a racemate. Due to rapid interconversion, the enantiomers are functionally indistinguishable. The molecular formula is $C_{18}H_{19}N_3O_3S{\cdot}C_4H_4O_4$. Rosiglitazone maleate is a white to off-white solid with a melting point range of 122-123°C. The pK_a values of rosiglitazone maleate are 6.8 and 6.1. It is readily soluble in ethanol and a buffered aqueous solution with pH of 2.3; solubility decreases with increasing pH in the physiological range.

Metformin hydrochloride (N,N-dimethylimidodicarbonimidic diamide hydrochloride) is not chemically or pharmacologically related to any other classes of oral antihyperglycemic agents. Metformin hydrochloride is a white to off-white crystalline compound with a molecular formula of $C_4H_{11}N_5 \cdot HCl$ and a molecular weight of 165.63. Metformin hydrochloride is freely soluble in water and is practically insoluble in acetone, ether and chloroform. The pK_a of metformin is 12.4. The pH of a 1% aqueous solution of metformin hydrochloride is 6.68.

Avandamet is available for oral administration as tablets containing rosiglitazone maleate and metformin hydrochloride equivalent to: 1 mg rosiglitazone with 500 mg metformin hydrochloride (1 mg/500 mg), 2 mg rosiglitazone with 500 mg metformin hydrochloride (2 mg/500 mg), and 4 mg rosiglitazone with 500 mg metformin hydrochloride (4 mg/500 mg). In addition, each tablet contains the following inactive ingredients: hypromellose, lactose monohydrate, magnesium stearate, microcrystalline cellulose, polyethylene glycol 400, povidone 29-32, sodium starch glycolate, titanium dioxide and 1 or more of the following: red and yellow iron oxides.

INDICATIONS AND USAGE

Avandamet is indicated as an adjunct to diet and exercise to improve glycemic control in patients with Type 2 diabetes mellitus who are already treated with combination rosiglitazone and metformin or who are not adequately controlled on metformin alone.

Management of Type 2 diabetes mellitus should include diet control. Caloric restriction, weight loss, and exercise are essential for the proper treatment of the diabetic patient because they help improve insulin sensitivity. This is important not only in the primary treatment of Type 2 diabetes, but also in maintaining the efficacy of drug therapy. Prior to initiation or escalation of oral antidiabetic therapy in patients with Type 2 diabetes mellitus, secondary causes of poor glycemic control, *e.g.*, infection, should be investigated and treated.

The safety and efficacy of Avandamet as initial pharmacologic therapy for patients with Type 2 diabetes mellitus after a trial of caloric restriction, weight loss, and exercise has not been established.

CONTRAINDICATIONS

Avandamet (rosiglitazone maleate and metformin HCl) tablets are contraindicated in patients with:

- Renal disease or renal dysfunction (*e.g.*, as suggested by serum creatinine levels ≥1.5 mg/dl [males], ≥1.4 mg/dl [females] or abnormal creatinine clearance) which may also result from conditions such as cardiovascular collapse (shock), acute myocardial infarction, and septicemia (see WARNINGS).
- Congestive heart failure requiring pharmacologic treatment.
- Known hypersensitivity to rosiglitazone maleate or metformin HCl.
- Acute or chronic metabolic acidosis, including diabetic ketoacidosis, with or without coma. Diabetic ketoacidosis should be treated with insulin.

Avandamet should be temporarily discontinued in patients undergoing radiologic studies involving intravascular administration of iodinated contrast materials, because use of such products may result in acute alteration of renal function.

WARNINGS

Metformin HCl

Lactic Acidosis

Lactic acidosis is a rare, but serious, metabolic complication that can occur due to metformin accumulation during treatment with Avandamet; when it occurs, it is fatal in approximately 50% of cases. Lactic acidosis may also occur in association with a number of pathophysiologic conditions, including diabetes mellitus, and whenever there is significant tissue hypoperfusion and hypoxemia. Lactic acidosis is characterized by elevated blood lactate levels (>5 mmol/L), decreased blood pH, electrolyte disturbances with an increased anion gap, and an increased lactate/pyruvate ratio. When metformin is implicated as the cause of lactic acidosis, metformin plasma levels >5 µg/ml are generally found.

The reported incidence of lactic acidosis in patients receiving metformin HCl is very low (approximately 0.03 cases/1000 patient-years, with approximately 0.015 fatal cases/1000 patient-years). Reported cases have occurred primarily in diabetic patients with significant renal insufficiency, including both intrinsic renal disease and renal hypoperfusion, often in the setting of multiple concomitant medical/surgical problems and multiple concomitant medications. Patients with congestive heart failure requiring pharmacologic management, in particular those with unstable or acute congestive heart failure who are at risk of hypoperfusion and hypoxemia, are at increased risk of lactic acidosis. The risk of lactic acidosis increases with the degree of renal dysfunction and the patient's age. The risk of lactic acidosis may, therefore, be significantly decreased by regular monitoring of renal function in patients taking Avandamet and by use of the minimum effective dose of Avandamet. In particular, treatment of the elderly should be accompanied by careful monitoring of renal function. Treatment with Avandamet should not be initiated in patients ≥80 years of age unless measurement of creatinine clearance demonstrates that renal function is not reduced, as these patients are more susceptible to developing lactic acidosis. In addition, Avandamet should be promptly withheld in the presence of any condition associated with hypoxemia, dehydration or sepsis. Because impaired hepatic function may significantly limit the ability to clear lactate, Avandamet should generally be avoided in patients with clinical or laboratory evidence of hepatic disease. Patients should be cautioned against excessive alcohol intake, either acute or chronic, when taking Avandamet, since alcohol potentiates the effects of metformin HCl on lactate metabolism. In addition, Avandamet should be temporarily discontinued prior to any intravascular radiocontrast study and for any surgical procedure.

The onset of lactic acidosis often is subtle, and accompanied only by nonspecific symptoms such as malaise, myalgias, respiratory distress, increasing somnolence and nonspecific abdominal distress. There may be associated hypothermia, hypotension and resistant bradyarrhythmias with more marked acidosis. The patient and the patient's physician must be aware of the possible importance of such symptoms and the patient should be instructed to notify the physician immediately if they occur. Avandamet should be withdrawn until the situation is clarified. Serum electrolytes, ketones, blood glucose and, if indicated, blood pH, lactate levels and even blood metformin levels may be useful. Once a patient is stabilized on any dose level of Avandamet, gastrointestinal symptoms, which are common during initiation of therapy, are unlikely to be drug related. Later occurrence of gastrointestinal symptoms could be due to lactic acidosis or other serious disease.

Levels of fasting venous plasma lactate above the upper limit of normal but less than 5 mmol/L in patients taking Avandamet do not necessarily indicate impending lactic acidosis and may be explainable by other mechanisms, such as poorly controlled diabetes or obesity, vigorous physical activity or technical problems in sample handling.

Lactic acidosis should be suspected in any diabetic patient with metabolic acidosis lacking evidence of ketoacidosis (ketonuria and ketonemia).

Lactic acidosis is a medical emergency that must be treated in a hospital setting. In a patient with lactic acidosis who is taking Avandamet, the drug should be discontinued immediately and general supportive measures promptly instituted. Because metformin HCl is dialyzable (with a clearance of up to 170 ml/min under good hemodynamic conditions), prompt hemodialysis is recommended to correct the acidosis and remove the accumu-

Cont'd

lated metformin. Such management often results in prompt reversal of symptoms and recovery (see also CONTRAINDICATIONS).

ROSIGLITAZONE MALEATE

Cardiac Failure and Other Cardiac Effects

Rosiglitazone, like other thiazolidinediones, can cause fluid retention, which may exacerbate or lead to heart failure. Patients should be observed for signs and symptoms of heart failure. Avandamet should be discontinued if any deterioration in cardiac status occurs.

Patients with New York Heart Association (NYHA) Class 3 and 4 cardiac status were not studied during the clinical trials with rosiglitazone maleate. In patients requiring pharmacologic treatment for congestive heart failure, Avandamet should not be used (see CONTRAINDICATIONS).

In two 26 week US trials involving 611 patients with Type 2 diabetes, rosiglitazone maleate plus insulin therapy was compared with insulin therapy alone. These trials included patients with longstanding diabetes and a high prevalence of pre-existing medical conditions, including peripheral neuropathy (34%), retinopathy (19%), ischemic heart disease (14%), vascular disease (9%), and congestive heart failure (2.5%). In these clinical studies, an increased incidence of cardiac failure and other cardiovascular adverse events were seen in patients on rosiglitazone and insulin combination therapy compared to insulin and placebo. Patients who experienced heart failure were on average older, had a longer duration of diabetes, and were mostly on the higher 8 mg daily dose of rosiglitazone. In this population, however, it was not possible to determine specific risk factors that could be used to identify all patients at risk of heart failure on combination therapy. Three (3) of 10 patients who developed cardiac failure on combination therapy during the double blind part of the studies had no known prior evidence of congestive heart failure, or pre-existing cardiac condition. **The use of rosiglitazone maleate in combination therapy with insulin is not indicated, therefore, Avandamet is not indicated for use in combination with insulin.**

DOSAGE AND ADMINISTRATION

GENERAL

The selection of the dose of Avandamet should be based on the patient's current doses of rosiglitazone and/or metformin.

The safety and efficacy of Avandamet as initial therapy for patients with Type 2 diabetes mellitus have not been established.

The following recommendations regarding the use of Avandamet in patients inadequately controlled on rosiglitazone and metformin monotherapies are based on clinical practice experience with rosiglitazone and metformin combination therapy.

- The dosage of antidiabetic therapy with Avandamet should be individualized on the basis of effectiveness and tolerability while not exceeding the maximum recommended daily dose of 8 mg/2000 mg.
- Avandamet should be given in divided doses with meals, with gradual dose escalation. This reduces GI side effects (largely due to metformin) and permits determination of the minimum effective dose for the individual patient.
- Sufficient time should be given to assess adequacy of therapeutic response. Fasting plasma glucose (FPG) should be used to determine the therapeutic response to Avandamet. After an increase in metformin dosage, dose titration is recommended if patients are not adequately controlled after 1-2 weeks. After an increase in rosiglitazone dosage, dose titration is recommended if patients are not adequately controlled after 8-12 weeks.

DOSAGE RECOMMENDATION

For Patients Inadequately Controlled on Metformin Monotherapy

The usual starting dose of Avandamet is 4 mg rosiglitazone (total daily dose) plus the dose of metformin already being taken (see TABLE 5).

For Patients Inadequately Controlled on Rosiglitazone Monotherapy

The usual starting dose of Avandamet is 1000 mg metformin (total daily dose) plus the dose of rosiglitazone already being taken (see TABLE 5).

TABLE 5 *Avandamet Starting Dose*

Prior Therapy	Usual Avandamet Starting Dose	
Total Daily Dose	Tablet Strength	Number of Tablets
Metformin HCl*		
1000 mg/day	2 mg/500 mg	1 tablet bid
2000 mg/day	1 mg/500 mg	2 tablets bid
Rosiglitazone		
4 mg/day	2 mg/500 mg	1 tablet bid
8 mg/day	4 mg/500 mg	1 tablet bid

* For patients on doses of metformin HCl between 1000 and 2000 mg/day, initiation of Avandamet requires individualization of therapy.

When Switching From Combination Therapy of Rosiglitazone Plus Metformin as Separate Tablets

The usual starting dose of Avandamet is the dose of rosiglitazone and metformin already being taken.

If Additional Glycemic Control Is Needed

The daily dose of Avandamet may be increased by increments of 4 mg rosiglitazone and/or 500 mg metformin, up to the maximum recommended total daily dose of 8 mg/2000 mg.

No studies have been performed specifically examining the safety and efficacy of Avandamet in patients previously treated with other oral hypoglycemic agents and switched to Avandamet. Any change in therapy of Type 2 diabetes should be undertaken with care and appropriate monitoring as changes in glycemic control can occur.

M

SPECIFIC PATIENT POPULATIONS

Avandamet is not recommended for use in pregnancy or for use in pediatric patients.

The initial and maintenance dosing of Avandamet should be conservative in patients with advanced age, due to the potential for decreased renal function in this population. Any dosage adjustment should be based on a careful assessment of renal function. Generally, elderly, debilitated, and malnourished patients should not be titrated to the maximum dose of Avandamet. Monitoring of renal function is necessary to aid in prevention of metformin-associated lactic acidosis, particularly in the elderly (see WARNINGS).

Therapy with Avandamet should not be initiated if the patient exhibits clinical evidence of active liver disease or increased serum transaminase levels (ALT >2.5× upper limit of normal at start of therapy). Liver enzyme monitoring is recommended in all patients prior to initiation of therapy with Avandamet and periodically thereafter.

PRODUCT LISTING - EQUIVALENTS NOT AVAILABLE

Tablet - Oral - 500 mg;1 mg

60's	$67.50	AVANDAMET, Glaxosmithkline	00007-3166-18
100's	$112.50	AVANDAMET, Glaxosmithkline	00007-3166-20

Tablet - Oral - 500 mg;2 mg

60's	$101.25	AVANDAMET, Glaxosmithkline	00007-3167-18
100's	$168.75	AVANDAMET, Glaxosmithkline	00007-3167-20

Tablet - Oral - 500 mg;4 mg

60's	$165.00	AVANDAMET, Glaxosmithkline	00007-3168-18
100's	$275.00	AVANDAMET, Glaxosmithkline	00007-3168-20

Methadone Hydrochloride *(001753)*

For related information, see the comparative table section in Appendix A.

Categories: Opiate, withdrawal; Pain, severe; DEA Class CII; FDA Approved 1947 Aug; Pregnancy Category B
Drug Classes: Analgesics, narcotic
Brand Names: **Dolophine**; Dolophine HCL; Methadone Hcl; Methadose; Tussol; Westadone
Foreign Brand Availability: Biodone (New-Zealand); Biodone Forte (New-Zealand); Biodone Extra Forte (New-Zealand); Dolmed (Finland); Eptadone (Italy); L-Polamidon (Germany); Mephenon (Belgium); Metadon (Denmark; Sweden); Metasedin (Spain); Methaddict (Germany); Methaforte Mix (New-Zealand); Pallidone (New-Zealand); Physeptone (Australia; England; Hong-Kong; South-Africa); Symoron (Netherlands)
Cost of Therapy: $8.16 (Detoxification; Generic Tablets; 10 mg; 1 tablet/day; 21 day supply)
$8.34 (Pain; Generic Injection; 10 mg/ml; 15 mg/day; 7 day supply)
HCFA JCODE(S): J1230 up to 10 mg IM, SC

M

WARNING

CONDITIONS FOR DISTRIBUTION AND USE OF METHADONE PRODUCTS:

Code of Federal Regulations, Title 21, Sec. 291.505

METHADONE PRODUCTS, WHEN USED FOR THE TREATMENT OF NARCOTIC ADDICTION IN DETOXIFICATION OR MAINTENANCE PROGRAMS, SHALL BE DISPENSED ONLY BY APPROVED HOSPITAL PHARMACIES, APPROVED COMMUNITY PHARMACIES, AND MAINTENANCE PROGRAMS APPROVED BY THE FOOD AND DRUG ADMINISTRATION AND THE DESIGNATED STATE AUTHORITY.

APPROVED MAINTENANCE PROGRAMS SHALL DISPENSE AND USE METHADONE IN ORAL FORM ONLY AND ACCORDING TO THE TREATMENT REQUIREMENTS STIPULATED IN THE FEDERAL METHADONE REGULATIONS (21 CFR 291.505).

FAILURE TO ABIDE BY THE REQUIREMENTS IN THESE REGULATIONS MAY RESULT IN CRIMINAL PROSECUTION, SEIZURE OF THE DRUG SUPPLY, REVOCATION OF THE PROGRAM APPROVAL, AND INJUNCTION PRECLUDING OPERATION OF THE PROGRAM.

A METHADONE PRODUCT, WHEN USED AS AN ANALGESIC, MAY BE DISPENSED IN ANY LICENSED PHARMACY.

DESCRIPTION

Methadone hydrochloride (3-hepatone, 6-(dimethylamino)-4,4-diphenyl-, hydrochloride) is a white crystalline material that is water soluble. Methadone hydrochloride has the empirical formula $C_{21}H_{27}NO{\cdot}HCl$, and its molecular weight is 345.91.

Each ml contains methadone hydrochloride, 10 mg (0.029 mmol) and sodium chloride 0.9%. Sodium hydroxide and/or hydrochloric acid may have been added during manufacture to adjust the pH. The 20 ml vials also contain chlorobutanol (chloroform derivative), 0.5%, as a preservative.

CLINICAL PHARMACOLOGY

Methadone HCl is a synthetic narcotic analgesic with multiple actions quantitatively similar to those of morphine, the most prominent of which involve the central nervous system and organs composed of smooth muscle. The principal actions of therapeutic value are analgesia and sedation and detoxification or temporary maintenance in narcotic addiction. The methadone abstinence syndrome, although qualitatively similar to that of morphine, differs in that the onset is slower, the course is more prolonged, and the symptoms are less severe.

A parenteral dose of 8-10 mg of methadone is approximately equivalent in analgesic effect to 10 mg of morphine. With single-dose administration, the onset and duration of analgesic action of the two drugs are similar.

When administered orally, methadone is approximately one-half as potent as when given parenterally. Oral administration results in a delay of the onset, a lowering of the peak, and an increase in the duration of analgesic effect.

INDICATIONS AND USAGE

For relief of severe pain.

For detoxification treatment of narcotic addiction.

For temporary maintenance treatment of narcotic addiction.

Note: If methadone is administered for treatment of heroin dependence for more than 3 weeks, the procedure passes from treatment of the acute withdrawal syndrome (detoxification) to maintenance therapy. Maintenance treatment is permitted to be undertaken only by approved methadone programs. This does not preclude the maintenance treatment of an addict who is hospitalized for medical conditions other than addiction and who requires temporary maintenance during the critical period of his stay or whose enrollment has been verified in a program which has approval for maintenance treatment with methadone.

CONTRAINDICATIONS

Hypersensitivity to methadone.

WARNINGS

Methadone HCl, a narcotic, is a Schedule II controlled substance under the Federal Controlled Substances Act. Appropriate security measures should be taken to safeguard stocks of methadone against diversion.

INTERACTION WITH OTHER CENTRAL-NERVOUS-SYSTEM DEPRESSANTS

Methadone should be used with caution and in reduced dosage in patients who are concurrently receiving other narcotic analgesics, general anesthetics, phenothiazines, other tranquilizers, sedative-hypnotics, tricyclic antidepressants, and other CNS depressants (including alcohol). Respiratory depression, hypotension, and profound sedation or coma may result.

ANXIETY

Since methadone, as used by tolerant subjects as a constant maintenance dosage, is not a tranquilizer, patients who are maintained on this drug will react to life problems and stresses with the same symptoms of anxiety as do other individuals. The physician should not confuse such symptoms with those of narcotic abstinence and should not attempt to treat anxiety by increasing the dosage of methadone. The action of methadone in maintenance treatment is limited to the control of narcotic symptoms and is ineffective for relief of general anxiety.

HEAD INJURY AND INCREASED INTRACRANIAL PRESSURE

The respiratory depressant effects of methadone and its capacity to elevate cerebrospinal-fluid pressure may be markedly exaggerated in the presence of increased intracranial pressure. Furthermore, narcotics produce side effects that may obscure the clinical course of patients with head injuries. In such patients, methadone must be used with caution and only if it is deemed essential.

ASTHMA AND OTHER RESPIRATORY CONDITIONS

Methadone should be used with caution in patients having an acute asthmatic attack, in those with chronic obstructive pulmonary disease or cor pulmonale, and in individuals with a substantially decreased respiratory reserve, preexisting respiratory depression, hypoxia, or hypercapnia. In such patients, even usual therapeutic doses of narcotics may decrease respiratory drive while simultaneously increasing airway resistance to the point of apnea.

HYPOTENSIVE EFFECT

The administration of methadone may result in severe hypotension in an individual whose ability to maintain his blood pressure has already been compromised by a depleted blood volume or concurrent administration of such drugs as the phenothiazines or certain anesthetics.

USE IN AMBULATORY PATIENTS

Methadone may impair the mental and/or physical abilities required for the performance of potentially hazardous tasks, such as driving a car or operating machinery. The patient should be cautioned accordingly.

Methadone, like other narcotics, may produce orthostatic hypotension in ambulatory patients.

USE IN PREGNANCY

Safe use in pregnancy has not been established in relation to possible adverse effects on fetal development. Therefore, methadone should not be used in pregnant women unless, in the judgment of the physician, the potential benefits outweigh the possible hazards.

Methadone is not recommended for obstetric analgesia because its long duration of action increased the probability of respiratory depression in the newborn.

USE IN CHILDREN

Methadone is not recommended for use as an analgesic in children, since documented clinical experience has been insufficient to establish a suitable dosage regiment for the pediatric age group.

PRECAUTIONS

SPECIAL-RISK PATIENTS

Methadone should be given with caution and the initial dose should be reduced in certain patients, such as the elderly or debilitated and those with severe impairment of hepatic or renal function, hypothyroidism, Addison's disease, prostatic hypertrophy, or urethral stricture.

ACUTE ABDOMINAL CONDITIONS

The administration of methadone or other narcotics may obscure the diagnosis or clinical course in patients with acute abdominal conditions.

DRUG INTERACTIONS

Pentazocine: **Patients who are addicted to heroin or who are on the methadone maintenance program may experience withdrawal symptoms when given pentazocine.**

Rifampin: The concurrent administration of rifampin may possibly reduce the blood concentration of methadone to a degree sufficient to produce withdrawal symptoms.

The mechanism by which rifampin may decrease blood concentrations of methadone is not fully understood, although enhanced microsomal drug-metabolized enzymes may influence drug disposition.

Monoamine Oxidase (MAO) Inhibitors: Therapeutic doses of meperidine have precipitated severe reactions in patients concurrently receiving monoamine oxidase inhibitors or those who have received such agents within 14 days. Similar reactions thus far have not been reported with methadone; but if the use of methadone is necessary in such patients, a sensitivity test should be performed in which repeated small incremental doses are administered over the course of several hours while the patient's condition and vital signs are under careful observation.

Desipramine: Blood levels of desipramine have increased with concurrent methadone therapy.

ADVERSE REACTIONS

THE MAJOR HAZARDS OF METHADONE, AS OF OTHER NARCOTIC ANALGESICS, ARE RESPIRATORY DEPRESSION AND, TO A LESSER DEGREE, CIRCULATORY DEPRESSION. RESPIRATORY ARREST, SHOCK, AND CARDIAC ARREST HAVE OCCURRED.

The most frequently observed adverse reactions include lightheadedness, dizziness, sedation, nausea, vomiting, and sweating. These effects seem to be more prominent in ambulatory patients and in those who are not suffering severe pain. In such individuals, lower doses are advisable. Some adverse reactions may be alleviated if the ambulatory patient lies down.

Other adverse reactions include the following:

Central Nervous System: Euphoria, dysphoria, weakness, headache, insomnia, agitation, disorientation, and visual disturbances.

Gastrointestinal: Dry mouth, anorexia, constipation, and biliary tract spasm.

Cardiovascular: Flushing of the face, bradycardia, palpitation, faintness, and syncope.

Genitourinary: Urinary retention or hesitancy, antidiuretic effect, and reduced libido and/or potency.

Allergic: Pruritus, urticaria, other skin rashes, edema, and rarely, hemorrhagic urticaria.

Hematologic: Reversible thrombocytopenia has been described in a narcotics addict with chronic hepatitis.

In addition, pain at injection site; local tissue irritation and induration following subcutaneous injection, particularly when repeated.

DOSAGE AND ADMINISTRATION

FOR RELIEF OF PAIN

Dosage should be adjusted according to the severity of the pain and the response of the patient. Occasionally it may be necessary to exceed the usual dosage recommended in cases of exceptionally severe pain or in those patients who have become tolerant to the analgesic effect of narcotics.

Although subcutaneous administration is suitable for occasional use, intramuscular injection is preferred when repeated doses are required.

The usual adult dosage is 2.5-10 mg intramuscularly or subcutaneously every 3-4 hours as necessary.

FOR DETOXIFICATION TREATMENT

THE DRUG SHALL BE ADMINISTERED DAILY UNDER CLOSE SUPERVISION AS FOLLOWS:

A detoxification treatment course shall not exceed 21 days and may not be repeated earlier than 4 weeks after completion of the preceding course.

The oral form of administration is preferred. However, if the patient is unable to ingest oral medication, parenteral administration may be substituted.

In detoxification, the patient may receive methadone when there are significant symptoms of withdrawal. The dosage schedules indicated below are recommended but could be varied in accordance with clinical judgment. Initially,a single oral dose of 15 to 20 mg of methadone will often be sufficient to suppress withdrawal symptoms. Additional methadone may be provided if withdrawal symptoms are not suppressed or if symptoms reappear. When patients are physically dependent on high doses, it may be necessary to exceed these levels. Forty mg/day in single or divided doses will usually constitute an adequate stabilizing dosage level. Stabilization can be continued for 2 to 3 days, and then the amount of methadone normally will be gradually decreased. The rate at which methadone is decreased will be determined separately for each patient. The dose of methadone can be decreased on a daily basis or at 2-day intervals, but the amount of intake shall always be sufficient to keep withdrawal symptoms at a tolerable level. In hospitalized patients, a daily reduction of 20% of the total daily dose may be tolerated and may cause little discomfort. In ambulatory patients, a somewhat slower schedule may be needed. If methadone is administered for more than 3 weeks, the procedure is considered to have progressed from detoxification or treatment of the acute withdrawal syndrome to maintenance treatment, even though the goal and intent may be eventual total withdrawal.

PRODUCT LISTING - RATED THERAPEUTICALLY EQUIVALENT

Concentrate - Oral - 10 mg/ml

30 ml	$22.52	GENERIC, Roxane Laboratories Inc	00054-3553-44
946 ml	$79.87	GENERIC, Roxane Laboratories Inc	00054-3553-67
946 ml	$84.67	GENERIC, Udl Laboratories Inc	51079-0694-39
1000 ml	$104.59	GENERIC, Mallinckrodt Medical Inc	00406-0527-10
1000 ml	$104.59	GENERIC, Mallinckrodt Medical Inc	00406-8725-10

Tablet - Oral - 5 mg

100's	$8.68	GENERIC, Mallinckrodt Medical Inc	00406-6974-34
100's	$8.87	GENERIC, Roxane Laboratories Inc	00054-4570-25
100's	$10.35	GENERIC, Roxane Laboratories Inc	00054-4216-25
100's	$10.35	DOLOPHINE, Roxane Laboratories Inc	00054-4218-25
100's	$34.16	GENERIC, Roxane Laboratories Inc	00054-8553-24

Tablet - Oral - 10 mg

100's	$14.10	GENERIC, Mallinckrodt Medical Inc	00406-3454-34
100's	$14.74	GENERIC, Roxane Laboratories Inc	00054-4571-25
100's	$16.81	GENERIC, Roxane Laboratories Inc	00054-4219-25
100's	$38.86	GENERIC, Roxane Laboratories Inc	00054-8554-24

Tablet - Oral - 40 mg

100's	$33.00	GENERIC, Mallinckrodt Medical Inc	00406-0540-34
100's	$36.17	GENERIC, Roxane Laboratories Inc	00054-4547-25
100's	$37.26	GENERIC, Roxane Laboratories Inc	00054-4538-25

PRODUCT LISTING - EQUIVALENTS NOT AVAILABLE

Solution - Injectable - 10 mg/ml

20 ml	$15.89	GENERIC, Roxane Laboratories Inc	00054-1218-42

Solution - Oral - 5 mg/5 ml

500 ml	$30.85	GENERIC, Roxane Laboratories Inc	00054-3555-63

Solution - Oral - 10 mg/5 ml

500 ml	$53.43	GENERIC, Roxane Laboratories Inc	00054-3556-63

Tablet - Oral - 40 mg

100's	$37.26	GENERIC, Cebert Pharmaceuticals Inc	64019-0538-25

Methimazole *(001765)*

Categories: Hyperthyroidism; Pregnancy Category D; FDA Approved 1971 Oct
Drug Classes: Antithyroid agents; Hormones/hormone modifiers
Brand Names: Tapazole
Foreign Brand Availability: Based (Taiwan); Metimazol (Finland); Strumazol (Belgium; Netherlands); Thacapzol (Sweden); Thiamazol (Austria; Germany; Russia); Thycapzol (Denmark); Thyrozol (Bulgaria; Germany; Russia); Tirodril (Germany); Unimazole (Greece)
Cost of Therapy: $48.00 (Hyperthyroidism; Tapazole; 5 mg; 3 tablets/day; 30 day supply)
$35.71 (Hyperthyroidism; Generic Tablets; 5 mg; 3 tablets/day; 30 day supply)

DESCRIPTION

Methimazole (1-methylimidazole-2-thiol) is a white crystalline substance that is freely soluble in water. It differs chemically from the drugs of the thiouracil series primarily because it has a 5- instead of a 6-membered ring.

Each Tapazole tablet contains 5 or 10 mg (43.8 or 87.6 μmol) methimazole, an orally administered antithyroid drug.

Each Tapazole tablet also contains lactose, magnesium stearate, starch, and talc.

The molecular weight is 114.16, and the empirical formula is $C_4H_6N_2S$.

CLINICAL PHARMACOLOGY

Methimazole inhibits the synthesis of thyroid hormones and thus is effective in the treatment of hyperthyroidism. The drug does not inactivate existing thyroxine and triiodothyronine that are stored in the thyroid or are circulating in the blood nor does it interfere with the effectiveness of thyroid hormones given by mouth or by injection.

The actions and use of methimazole are similar to those of propylthiouracil. On a weight basis, the drug is at least 10 times as potent as propylthiouracil, but methimazole may be less consistent in action.

Methimazole is readily absorbed from the gastrointestinal tract. It is metabolized rapidly and requires frequent administration. Methimazole is excreted in the urine.

In laboratory animals, various regimens that continuously suppress thyroid function and thereby increase TSH secretion result in thyroid tissue hypertrophy. Under such conditions, the appearance of thyroid and pituitary neoplasms have also been reported. Regimens that have been studied in this regard include antithyroid agents, as well as dietary iodine deficiency, subtotal thyroidectomy, implantation of autonomous thyrotropic hormone-secreting pituitary tumors, and administration of chemical goitrogens.

INDICATIONS AND USAGE

Methimazole is indicated in the medical treatment of hyperthyroidism. Long-term therapy may lead to remission of the disease. Methimazole may be used to ameliorate hyperthyroidism in preparation for subtotal thyroidectomy or radioactive iodine therapy. Methimazole is also used when thyroidectomy is contraindicated or not advisable.

CONTRAINDICATIONS

Methimazole is contraindicated in the presence of hypersensitivity to the drug and in nursing mothers because the drug is excreted in milk.

WARNINGS

Agranulocytosis is potentially a serious side effect. Patients should be instructed to report to their physicians any symptoms of agranulocytosis, such as fever or sore throat. Leukopenia, thrombocytopenia, and aplastic anemia (pancytopenia) may also occur. The drug should be discontinued in the presence of agranulocytosis, aplastic anemia (pancytopenia), hepatitis, or exfoliative dermatitis. The patient's bone marrow function should be monitored.

Due to the similar hepatic toxicity profiles of methimazole and propylthiouracil, attention is drawn to the severe hepatic reactions which have occurred with both drugs. There have been rare reports of fulminant hepatitis, hepatic necrosis, encephalopathy, and death. Symptoms suggestive of hepatic dysfunction (anorexia, pruritus, right upper quadrant pain, etc.) should prompt evaluation of liver function. Drug treatment should be discontinued promptly in the event of clinically significant evidence of liver abnormality including hepatic transaminase values exceeding 3 times the upper limit of normal.

Methimazole can cause fetal harm when administered to a pregnant woman. Methimazole readily crosses the placental membranes and can induce goiter and even cretinism in the developing fetus. In addition, rare instances of congenital defects: aplasia cutis, as manifested by scalp defects; esophageal atresia with tracheoesophageal fistula; and choanal atresia with absent/hypoplastic nipples, have occurred in infants born to mothers who received methimazole during pregnancy. If methimazole is used during pregnancy or if the patient becomes pregnant while taking this drug, the patient should be warned of the potential hazard to the fetus.

Since the above congenital defects have been reported in offspring of patients treated with methimazole, it may be appropriate to use other agents in pregnant women requiring treatment for hyperthyroidism.

Postpartum patients receiving methimazole should not nurse their babies.

PRECAUTIONS

GENERAL

Patients who receive methimazole should be under close surveillance and should be cautioned to report immediately any evidence of illness, particularly sore throat, skin eruptions, fever, headache, or general malaise. In such cases, white-blood-cell and differential counts should be made to determine whether agranulocytosis has developed. Particular care should be exercised with patients who are receiving additional drugs known to cause agranulocytosis.

LABORATORY TESTS

Because methimazole may cause hypoprothrombinemia and bleeding, prothrombin time should be monitored during therapy with the drug, especially before surgical procedures. (See General).

Periodic monitoring of thyroid function is warranted, and the finding of an elevated TSH warrants a decrease in the dosage of methimazole.

CARCINOGENESIS, MUTAGENESIS, AND IMPAIRMENT OF FERTILITY

In a 2 year study, rats were given methimazole at doses of 0.5, 3, and 18 mg/kg/day. These doses were 0.3, 2, and 12 times the 15 mg/day maximum human maintenance dose (when calculated on the basis of surface area). Thyroid hyperplasia, adenoma, and carcinoma developed in rats at the two higher doses. The clinical significance of these findings is unclear.

PREGNANCY CATEGORY D

See WARNINGS.

Methimazole used judiciously is an effective drug in hyperthyroidism complicated by pregnancy. In many pregnant women, the thyroid dysfunction diminishes as the pregnancy proceeds; consequently, a reduction in dosage may be possible. In some instances, use of methimazole can be discontinued 2 or 3 weeks before delivery.

NURSING MOTHERS

The drug appears in human breast milk and its use is contraindicated in nursing mothers (see WARNINGS).

PEDIATRIC USE

See DOSAGE AND ADMINISTRATION.

DRUG INTERACTIONS

ANTICOAGULANTS (ORAL)

The activity of anticoagulants may be potentiated by anti-vitamin-K activity attributed to methimazole.

BETA-ADRENERGIC BLOCKING AGENTS

Hyperthyroidism may cause an increased clearance of beta blockers with a high extraction ratio. A dose reduction of beta-adrenergic blockers may be needed when a hyperthyroid patient becomes euthyroid.

DIGITALIS GLYCOSIDES

Serum digitalis levels may be increased when hyperthyroid patients on a stable digitalis glycoside regimen become euthyroid; a reduced dosage of digitalis glycosides may be required.

THEOPHYLLINE

Theophylline clearance may decrease when hyperthyroid patients on a stable theophylline regimen become euthyroid; a reduced dose of theophylline may be needed.

ADVERSE REACTIONS

Major adverse reactions (which occur with much less frequency than the minor adverse reactions) include inhibition of myelopoiesis (agranulocytosis, granulocytopenia, and thrombocytopenia), aplastic anemia, drug fever, a lupuslike syndrome, insulin autoimmune syndrome (which can result in hypoglycemic coma), hepatitis (jaundice may persist for several weeks after discontinuation of the drug), periarteritis, and hypoprothrombinemia. Nephritis occurs very rarely.

Minor adverse reactions include skin rash, urticaria, nausea, vomiting, epigastric distress, arthralgia, paresthesia, loss of taste, abnormal loss of hair, myalgia, headache, pruritus, drowsiness, neuritis, edema, vertigo, skin pigmentation, jaundice, sialadenopathy, and lymphadenopathy.

It should be noted that about 10% of patients with untreated hyperthyroidism have leukopenia (white-blood-cell count of less than 4000/mm^3), often with relative granulopenia.

DOSAGE AND ADMINISTRATION

Methimazole is administered orally. It is usually given in 3 equal doses at approximately 8 hour intervals.

ADULT

The initial daily dosage is 15 mg for mild hyperthyroidism, 30-40 mg for moderately severe hyperthyroidism, and 60 mg for severe hyperthyroidism, divided into 3 doses at 8 hour intervals. The maintenance dosage is 5-15 mg daily.

PEDIATRIC

Initially, the daily dosage is 0.4 mg/kg of body weight divided into 3 doses and given at 8 hour intervals. The maintenance dosage is approximately ½ of the initial dose.

HOW SUPPLIED

Tapazole tablets, are available in:

5 mg: White, round, beveled, tablets scored and debossed with "J94".

10 mg: White, round, beveled, tablets scored and debossed with "J95".

Storage: Store at controlled room temperature, 15-30°C (59-86°F).

PRODUCT LISTING - RATED THERAPEUTICALLY EQUIVALENT

Tablet - Oral - 5 mg			
100's	$39.68	GENERIC, Par Pharmaceutical Inc	49884-0640-74
100's	$44.44	GENERIC, Eon Labs Manufacturing Inc	00185-0205-01
100's	$44.44	GENERIC, Par Pharmaceutical Inc	49884-0640-01
Tablet - Oral - 10 mg			
100's	$68.54	GENERIC, Par Pharmaceutical Inc	49884-0641-74
100's	$76.78	GENERIC, Eon Labs Manufacturing Inc	00185-0210-01
100's	$76.78	GENERIC, Par Pharmaceutical Inc	49884-0641-01

PRODUCT LISTING - EQUIVALENTS NOT AVAILABLE

Tablet - Oral - 5 mg			
100's	$18.38	TAPAZOLE, Southwood Pharmaceuticals Inc	58016-0958-00
100's	$53.33	TAPAZOLE, Jones Pharma Inc	52604-1094-01
Tablet - Oral - 10 mg			
100's	$92.13	TAPAZOLE, Jones Pharma Inc	52604-1095-01
Tablet - Oral - 20 mg			
30's	$54.70	GENERIC, Par Pharmaceutical Inc	49884-0689-55

Methocarbamol *(001768)*

Categories: Pain, musculoskeletal; FDA Approved 1959 Jun; Pregnancy Category C
Drug Classes: Musculoskeletal agents; Relaxants, skeletal muscle
Brand Names: Carbacot; Forbaxin; Methocarb; **Robaxin**
Foreign Brand Availability: Carbametin (Japan); Carmol (Korea); Carxin (Japan); Laxan (Thailand); Lumirelax (France); Manobaxine (Thailand); Myocin (Thailand); New-Rexan (Korea); Ortoton (Germany); Robaxin-750 (Canada; England); Robinax (India); Sinaxar (Colombia); Trolar (Greece)
Cost of Therapy: $62.53 (Musculoskeletal Pain; Robaxin; 500 mg; 8 tablets/day; 10 day supply)
$2.11 (Musculoskeletal Pain; Generic Tablets; 500 mg; 8 tablets/day; 10 day supply)
HCFA JCODE(S): J2800 up to 10 ml IV, IM

DESCRIPTION

Robaxin is available in 500 and 750 mg tablets for oral administration.

Inactive Ingredients:

500 mg Robaxin tablets: Corn starch, FD&C yellow 6 aluminum lake, hydroxypropyl cellulose, hydroxypropyl methylcellulose, magnesium stearate, polysorbate 20, povidone, propylene glycol, saccharin sodium, sodium lauryl sulfate, sodium starch glycolate, stearic acid, titanium dioxide.

750 mg Robaxin tablets: Corn starch, D&C yellow 10 aluminum lake, FD&C yellow 6 aluminum lake, hydroxypropyl cellulose, hydroxypropyl methylcellulose, magnesium stearate, polysorbate 20, povidone, propylene glycol, saccharin sodium, sodium lauryl sulfate, sodium starch glycolate, stearic acid, titanium dioxide.

CLINICAL PHARMACOLOGY

The mechanism of action of methocarbamol in humans has not been established, but may be due to general central nervous system (CNS) depression. It has no direct action on the contractile mechanism of striated muscle, the motor end plate or the nerve fiber.

PHARMACOKINETICS

Special Populations

Renally Impaired

The clearance of methocarbamol in renally impaired patients on maintenance hemodialysis was reduced about 40% compared to a normal population, although the mean elimination half-life in these two groups was similar (1.2 vs 1.1 hours, respectively).

Hepatically Impaired

In patients with cirrhosis secondary to alcohol abuse, the mean total clearance of methocarbamol was reduced approximately 70% compared to a normal population (11.9 L/hr), and the mean elimination half-life was extended to approximately 3.4 hours. The fraction of methocarbamol bound to plasma proteins was decreased to approximately 40-45% compared to 46-50% in an age- and weight-matched normal population.

INDICATIONS AND USAGE

Methocarbamol is indicated as an adjunct to rest, physical therapy, and other measures for the relief of discomforts associated with acute, painful musculoskeletal conditions. The mode of action of methocarbamol has not been clearly identified, but may be related to its sedative properties. Methocarbamol does not directly relax tense skeletal muscles in man.

NON-FDA APPROVED INDICATIONS

Methocarbamol has been reported in clinical studies to have some beneficial effect in the control of the neuromuscular manifestations of tetanus. However, methocarbamol is not recommended as a replacement for the usual procedure of debridement, tetanus antitoxin, penicillin, tracheotomy, attention to fluid balance, and supportive care.

CONTRAINDICATIONS

Methocarbamol is contraindicated in patients hypersensitive to methocarbamol or to any of the tablet components.

WARNINGS

Since methocarbamol may possess a general CNS depressant effect, patients receiving methocarbamol tablets should be cautioned about combined effects with alcohol and other CNS depressants.

Safe use of methocarbamol has not been established with regard to possible adverse effects upon fetal development. There have been very rare reports of fetal and congenital abnormalities following *in utero* exposure to methocarbamol. Therefore, methocarbamol tablets should not be used in women who are or may become pregnant and particularly during early pregnancy unless in the judgment of the physician the potential benefits outweigh the possible hazards (see PRECAUTIONS, Pregnancy, Teratogenic Effects, Pregnancy Category C).

USE IN ACTIVITIES REQUIRING MENTAL ALERTNESS

Methocarbamol may impair mental and/or physical abilities required for performance of hazardous tasks, such as operating machinery or driving a motor vehicle. Patients should be cautioned about operating machinery, including automobiles, until they are reasonably certain that methocarbamol therapy does not adversely affect their ability to engage in such activities.

PRECAUTIONS

INFORMATION FOR THE PATIENT

Patients should be cautioned that methocarbamol may cause drowsiness or dizziness, which may impair their ability to operate motor vehicles or machinery.

Because methocarbamol may possess a general CNS depressant effect, patients should be cautioned about combined effects with alcohol and other CNS depressants.

DRUG/LABORATORY TEST INTERACTIONS

Methocarbamol may cause a color interference in certain screening tests for 5-hydroxyindoleacetic acid (5-HIAA) using nitrosonaphthol reagent and in screening tests for urinary vanillylmandelic acid (VMA) using the Gitlow method.

CARCINOGENESIS, MUTAGENESIS, AND IMPAIRMENT OF FERTILITY

Long-term studies to evaluate the carcinogenic potential of methocarbamol have not been performed. No studies have been conducted to assess the effect of methocarbamol on mutagenesis or its potential to impair fertility.

PREGNANCY, TERATOGENIC EFFECTS, PREGNANCY CATEGORY C

Animal reproduction studies have not been conducted with methocarbamol. It is also not known whether methocarbamol can cause fetal harm when administered to a pregnant woman or can affect reproduction capacity. Methocarbamol should be given to a pregnant woman only if clearly needed.

Safe use of methocarbamol has not been established with regard to possible adverse effects upon fetal development. There have been very rare reports of fetal and congenital abnormalities following *in utero* exposure to methocarbamol. Therefore, methocarbamol tablets should not be used in women who are or may become pregnant and particularly during early pregnancy unless in the judgment of the physician the potential benefits outweigh the possible hazards (see WARNINGS).

NURSING MOTHERS

Methocarbamol and/or its metabolites are excreted in the milk of dogs; however, it is not known whether methocarbamol or its metabolites are excreted in human milk. Because many drugs are excreted in human milk, caution should be exercised when methocarbamol is administered to a nursing woman.

PEDIATRIC USE

Safety and effectiveness of methocarbamol in pediatric patients have not been established.

DRUG INTERACTIONS

See WARNINGS and PRECAUTIONS for interaction with CNS drugs and alcohol.

Methocarbamol may inhibit the effect of pyridostigmine bromide. Therefore, methocarbamol should be used with caution in patients with myasthenia gravis receiving anticholinesterase agents.

ADVERSE REACTIONS

Adverse reactions reported coincident with the administration of methocarbamol include:

Body as a Whole: Anaphylactic reaction, fever, headache.

Cardiovascular System: Bradycardia, flushing, hypotension, syncope.

Digestive System: Dyspepsia, jaundice (including cholestatic jaundice), nausea and vomiting.

Hemic and Lymphatic System: Leukopenia.

Nervous System: Amnesia, confusion, diplopia, dizziness or light-headedness, drowsiness, insomnia, mild muscular incoordination, nystagmus, seizures (including grand mal), vertigo.

Skin and Special Senses: Blurred vision, conjunctivitis with nasal congestion, metallic taste, pruritus, rash, urticaria.

DOSAGE AND ADMINISTRATION

Robaxin 500 mg — Adults: Initial dosage, 3 tablets qid, maintenance dosage, 2 tablets qid.
Robaxin 750 mg — Adults: Initial dosage, 2 tablets qid, maintenance dosage, 1 tablet q4h or 2 tablets tid.
Six (6) g/day are recommended for the first 48-72 hours of treatment. (For severe conditions 8 g/day may be administered). Thereafter, the dosage can usually be reduced to approximately 4 g/day.

HOW SUPPLIED

Robaxin 500 mg tablets: Light orange, round, film-coated tablets engraved with "ROBAXIN 500" on the unscored side and "SP" above the score on the other side.

Robaxin 750 mg tablets: Orange, capsule-shaped, film-coated tablets engraved with "ROBAXIN 750" on one side and "SP" on the other.
Storage: Store at controlled room temperature, between 20 and 25°C (68 and 77°F). Dispense in tight container.

PRODUCT LISTING - RATED THERAPEUTICALLY EQUIVALENT

Package	Price	Product, Manufacturer	NDC
Solution - Injectable - 100 mg/ml			
10 ml	$2.50	GENERIC, C.O. Truxton Inc	00463-1106-10
10 ml	$3.63	GENERIC, Moore, H.L. Drug Exchange Inc	00839-6359-30
10 ml x 5	$78.85	ROBAXIN, Allscripts Pharmaceutical Company	54569-2072-00
10 ml x 5	$78.90	ROBAXIN, Esi Lederle Generics	00031-7409-87
10 ml x 25	$388.75	ROBAXIN, Esi Lederle Generics	00031-7409-94
100 ml	$4.00	GENERIC, Cmc-Consolidated Midland Corporation	00223-8150-10
Tablet - Oral - 500 mg			
10's	$5.94	GENERIC, Pd-Rx Pharmaceuticals	55289-0670-10
14's	$6.89	GENERIC, Pd-Rx Pharmaceuticals	55289-0670-14
20's	$8.28	GENERIC, Pd-Rx Pharmaceuticals	55289-0670-20
20's	$9.41	GENERIC, Cardinal Pharmaceuticals	63874-0371-20
28's	$10.15	GENERIC, Pd-Rx Pharmaceuticals	55289-0670-28
30's	$41.85	GENERIC, St. Mary'S Mpp	60760-0290-30
40's	$12.96	GENERIC, Pd-Rx Pharmaceuticals	55289-0670-40
40's	$18.82	GENERIC, Cardinal Pharmaceuticals	63874-0371-40
100's	$2.64	GENERIC, Global Pharmaceutical Corporation	00115-3900-01
100's	$5.70	GENERIC, Vangard Labs	00615-0637-01
100's	$8.50	GENERIC, Cmc-Consolidated Midland Corporation	00223-1277-01
100's	$8.93	GENERIC, Interstate Drug Exchange Inc	00814-4766-14
100's	$9.57	GENERIC, Aligen Independent Laboratories Inc	00405-4635-01
100's	$9.78	GENERIC, Ivax Corporation	00182-0572-01
100's	$9.95	GENERIC, Raway Pharmacal Inc	00686-0091-20
100's	$10.56	GENERIC, Moore, H.L. Drug Exchange Inc	00839-5132-06
100's	$13.77	GENERIC, Major Pharmaceuticals Inc	00904-2364-61
100's	$18.00	GENERIC, Ivax Corporation	00182-0572-89
100's	$18.00	GENERIC, Geneva Pharmaceuticals	00781-1760-13
100's	$19.62	FEDERAL UPPER LIMIT, H.C.F.A. F F P	99999-1768-01
100's	$26.57	GENERIC, American Health Packaging	62584-0780-01
100's	$27.13	GENERIC, Pd-Rx Pharmaceuticals	55289-0670-01
100's	$34.75	GENERIC, West Ward Pharmaceutical Corporation	00143-1290-01
100's	$37.64	GENERIC, Qualitest Products Inc	00603-4487-21
100's	$37.65	GENERIC, Esi Lederle Generics	00005-3562-23
100's	$37.65	GENERIC, Watson/Schein Pharmaceuticals Inc	00364-0346-01
100's	$37.65	GENERIC, Major Pharmaceuticals Inc	00904-2364-60
100's	$37.65	GENERIC, Watson Laboratories Inc	52544-0806-01
100's	$38.03	GENERIC, Mutual/United Research Laboratories	00677-0430-01
100's	$40.20	GENERIC, Auro Pharmaceutical	55829-0372-10
100's	$47.01	GENERIC, Cardinal Pharmaceuticals	63874-0371-01
100's	$50.80	GENERIC, Geneva Pharmaceuticals	00781-1760-01
100's	$78.16	ROBAXIN, Esi Lederle Generics	00031-7429-63
Tablet - Oral - 750 mg			
10's	$6.48	GENERIC, Pd-Rx Pharmaceuticals	55289-0164-10
15's	$7.65	GENERIC, Pd-Rx Pharmaceuticals	55289-0164-15
20's	$9.00	GENERIC, Pd-Rx Pharmaceuticals	55289-0164-20
20's	$14.92	GENERIC, Dhs Inc	55887-0860-20
20's	$16.22	GENERIC, Cardinal Pharmaceuticals	63874-0372-20
20's	$25.38	ROBAXIN-750, Pd-Rx Pharmaceuticals	55289-0017-20
24's	$10.08	GENERIC, Pd-Rx Pharmaceuticals	55289-0164-24
28's	$11.16	GENERIC, Pd-Rx Pharmaceuticals	55289-0164-28
28's	$20.89	GENERIC, Dhs Inc	55887-0860-28
30's	$11.70	GENERIC, Pd-Rx Pharmaceuticals	55289-0164-30
30's	$22.39	GENERIC, Dhs Inc	55887-0860-30
30's	$24.34	GENERIC, Cardinal Pharmaceuticals	63874-0372-30
40's	$14.40	GENERIC, Pd-Rx Pharmaceuticals	55289-0164-40
40's	$23.70	GENERIC, St. Mary'S Mpp	60760-0347-40
40's	$32.30	GENERIC, Cardinal Pharmaceuticals	63874-0372-40
40's	$58.08	ROBAXIN-750, Pd-Rx Pharmaceuticals	55289-0017-40
60's	$6.10	GENERIC, Circle Pharmaceuticals Inc	00659-0414-60
60's	$19.80	GENERIC, Pd-Rx Pharmaceuticals	55289-0164-60
100's	$3.70	GENERIC, Global Pharmaceutical Corporation	00115-3902-01
100's	$7.95	GENERIC, Vangard Labs	00615-0638-01
100's	$10.78	GENERIC, Aligen Independent Laboratories Inc	00405-4636-01
100's	$11.93	GENERIC, Interstate Drug Exchange Inc	00814-4767-14
100's	$11.95	GENERIC, Cmc-Consolidated Midland Corporation	00223-1278-01
100's	$11.95	GENERIC, Raway Pharmacal Inc	00686-0092-20
100's	$12.15	GENERIC, Ivax Corporation	00182-0573-01
100's	$18.56	GENERIC, Moore, H.L. Drug Exchange Inc	00839-5101-06
100's	$22.36	FEDERAL UPPER LIMIT, H.C.F.A. F F P	99999-1768-04
100's	$25.00	GENERIC, Ivax Corporation	00182-0573-89
100's	$25.20	GENERIC, Geneva Pharmaceuticals	00781-1750-13
100's	$29.35	GENERIC, American Health Packaging	62584-0781-01
100's	$32.02	GENERIC, Pd-Rx Pharmaceuticals	55289-0164-01
100's	$46.80	GENERIC, West Ward Pharmaceutical Corporation	00143-1292-01
100's	$48.92	GENERIC, Major Pharmaceuticals Inc	00904-2365-60

100's	$49.40	GENERIC, Qualitest Products Inc	00603-4488-21
100's	$49.41	GENERIC, Esi Lederle Generics	00005-3563-23
100's	$49.41	GENERIC, Watson/Schein Pharmaceuticals Inc	00364-0347-01
100's	$49.41	GENERIC, Watson Laboratories Inc	00591-5382-01
100's	$49.41	GENERIC, Watson Laboratories Inc	52544-0807-01
100's	$49.91	GENERIC, Mutual/United Research Laboratories	00677-0431-01
100's	$72.61	GENERIC, Geneva Pharmaceuticals	00781-1750-01
100's	$81.12	GENERIC, Cardinal Pharmaceuticals	63874-0372-01
100's	$111.71	ROBAXIN-750, Esi Lederle Generics	00031-7449-63
100's	$111.71	ROBAXIN-750, Schwarz Pharma	00091-7449-63

PRODUCT LISTING - EQUIVALENTS NOT AVAILABLE

Solution - Injectable - 100 mg/ml

10 ml	$3.25	GENERIC, Roberts/Hauck Pharmaceutical Corporation	43797-0103-12

Tablet - Oral - 500 mg

3's	$3.71	GENERIC, Prescript Pharmaceuticals	00247-0180-03
4's	$1.47	GENERIC, Allscripts Pharmaceutical Company	54569-0852-09
4's	$3.84	GENERIC, Prescript Pharmaceuticals	00247-0180-04
6's	$4.07	GENERIC, Prescript Pharmaceuticals	00247-0180-06
10's	$3.69	GENERIC, Allscripts Pharmaceutical Company	54569-4614-00
10's	$4.54	GENERIC, Prescript Pharmaceuticals	00247-0180-10
12's	$4.79	GENERIC, Prescript Pharmaceuticals	00247-0180-12
12's	$7.32	GENERIC, Southwood Pharmaceuticals Inc	58016-0257-12
12's	$10.30	GENERIC, Pharma Pac	52959-0167-12
14's	$5.02	GENERIC, Prescript Pharmaceuticals	00247-0180-14
14's	$5.16	GENERIC, Allscripts Pharmaceutical Company	54569-0852-05
14's	$8.54	GENERIC, Southwood Pharmaceuticals Inc	58016-0257-14
15's	$5.14	GENERIC, Prescript Pharmaceuticals	00247-0180-15
15's	$5.19	GENERIC, Physicians Total Care	54868-0586-01
15's	$9.15	GENERIC, Southwood Pharmaceuticals Inc	58016-0257-15
15's	$12.78	GENERIC, Pharma Pac	52959-0167-15
20's	$5.74	GENERIC, Prescript Pharmaceuticals	00247-0180-20
20's	$6.48	GENERIC, Physicians Total Care	54868-0586-02
20's	$7.37	GENERIC, Allscripts Pharmaceutical Company	54569-0852-01
20's	$12.20	GENERIC, Southwood Pharmaceuticals Inc	58016-0257-20
20's	$16.79	GENERIC, Pharma Pac	52959-0167-20
21's	$5.86	GENERIC, Prescript Pharmaceuticals	00247-0180-21
21's	$17.50	GENERIC, Pharma Pac	52959-0167-21
24's	$6.21	GENERIC, Prescript Pharmaceuticals	00247-0180-24
24's	$8.84	GENERIC, Allscripts Pharmaceutical Company	54569-0852-06
24's	$14.64	GENERIC, Southwood Pharmaceuticals Inc	58016-0257-24
24's	$20.04	GENERIC, Pharma Pac	52959-0167-24
28's	$6.69	GENERIC, Prescript Pharmaceuticals	00247-0180-28
30's	$7.02	GENERIC, Heartland Healthcare Services	61392-0739-30
30's	$7.02	GENERIC, Heartland Healthcare Services	61392-0739-39
30's	$9.06	GENERIC, Physicians Total Care	54868-0586-03
30's	$11.06	GENERIC, Allscripts Pharmaceutical Company	54569-0852-04
30's	$18.30	GENERIC, Southwood Pharmaceuticals Inc	58016-0257-30
30's	$24.58	GENERIC, Pharma Pac	52959-0167-30
31's	$7.25	GENERIC, Heartland Healthcare Services	61392-0739-31
32's	$7.49	GENERIC, Heartland Healthcare Services	61392-0739-32
40's	$8.12	GENERIC, Prescript Pharmaceuticals	00247-0180-40
40's	$11.63	GENERIC, Physicians Total Care	54868-0586-05
40's	$14.74	GENERIC, Allscripts Pharmaceutical Company	54569-0852-00
40's	$16.06	GENERIC, Pharmaceutical Corporation Of America	51655-0576-51
40's	$24.40	GENERIC, Southwood Pharmaceuticals Inc	58016-0257-40
40's	$32.43	GENERIC, Pharma Pac	52959-0167-40
45's	$10.53	GENERIC, Heartland Healthcare Services	61392-0739-45
50's	$30.50	GENERIC, Southwood Pharmaceuticals Inc	58016-0257-50
60's	$10.49	GENERIC, Prescript Pharmaceuticals	00247-0180-60
60's	$14.04	GENERIC, Heartland Healthcare Services	61392-0739-60
60's	$25.59	GENERIC, Pharmaceutical Corporation Of America	51655-0576-25
60's	$47.01	GENERIC, Pharma Pac	52959-0167-60
84's	$51.24	GENERIC, Southwood Pharmaceuticals Inc	58016-0257-84
90's	$21.06	GENERIC, Heartland Healthcare Services	61392-0739-90
100's	$26.41	GENERIC, Physicians Total Care	54868-0586-06
100's	$36.85	GENERIC, Allscripts Pharmaceutical Company	54569-0852-07
100's	$37.64	GENERIC, Qualitest Products Inc	00603-4485-21
100's	$61.00	GENERIC, Southwood Pharmaceuticals Inc	58016-0257-00
100's	$66.98	GENERIC, Pharma Pac	52959-0167-00
100's	$78.16	ROBAXIN, Schwarz Pharma	00091-7429-63
120's	$32.23	GENERIC, Physicians Total Care	54868-0586-04
120's	$73.20	GENERIC, Southwood Pharmaceuticals Inc	58016-0257-02
120's	$78.75	GENERIC, Pharma Pac	52959-0167-03

Tablet - Oral - 750 mg

3's	$3.79	GENERIC, Prescript Pharmaceuticals	00247-0013-03
6's	$4.22	GENERIC, Prescript Pharmaceuticals	00247-0013-06
7's	$4.38	GENERIC, Prescript Pharmaceuticals	00247-0013-07
8's	$4.52	GENERIC, Prescript Pharmaceuticals	00247-0013-08
8's	$7.14	GENERIC, Southwood Pharmaceuticals Inc	58016-0258-08
9's	$4.66	GENERIC, Prescript Pharmaceuticals	00247-0013-09
10's	$8.93	GENERIC, Southwood Pharmaceuticals Inc	58016-0258-10
10's	$10.49	GENERIC, Pharma Pac	52959-0099-10
12's	$5.11	GENERIC, Prescript Pharmaceuticals	00247-0013-12
12's	$5.83	GENERIC, Allscripts Pharmaceutical Company	54569-0843-07
12's	$10.71	GENERIC, Southwood Pharmaceuticals Inc	58016-0258-12
14's	$12.18	GENERIC, Southwood Pharmaceuticals Inc	58016-0258-14
15's	$3.56	GENERIC, Physicians Total Care	54868-1103-08
15's	$5.54	GENERIC, Prescript Pharmaceuticals	00247-0013-15
15's	$13.39	GENERIC, Southwood Pharmaceuticals Inc	58016-0258-15
15's	$14.64	GENERIC, Pharma Pac	52959-0099-15
18's	$5.98	GENERIC, Prescript Pharmaceuticals	00247-0013-18
20's	$6.27	GENERIC, Prescript Pharmaceuticals	00247-0013-20
20's	$9.72	GENERIC, Allscripts Pharmaceutical Company	54569-0843-00
20's	$17.85	GENERIC, Southwood Pharmaceuticals Inc	58016-0258-20
20's	$18.90	GENERIC, Pharma Pac	52959-0099-20
21's	$6.41	GENERIC, Prescript Pharmaceuticals	00247-0013-21
21's	$18.74	GENERIC, Southwood Pharmaceuticals Inc	58016-0258-21
21's	$20.15	GENERIC, Pharma Pac	52959-0099-21
24's	$20.88	GENERIC, Southwood Pharmaceuticals Inc	58016-0258-24
25's	$6.99	GENERIC, Prescript Pharmaceuticals	00247-0013-25
28's	$7.44	GENERIC, Prescript Pharmaceuticals	00247-0013-28
28's	$13.61	GENERIC, Allscripts Pharmaceutical Company	54569-0843-02
28's	$24.99	GENERIC, Southwood Pharmaceuticals Inc	58016-0258-28
28's	$25.88	GENERIC, Pharma Pac	52959-0099-28
30's	$4.97	GENERIC, Physicians Total Care	54868-1103-06
30's	$7.56	GENERIC, Heartland Healthcare Services	61392-0740-30
30's	$7.56	GENERIC, Heartland Healthcare Services	61392-0740-39
30's	$7.72	GENERIC, Prescript Pharmaceuticals	00247-0013-30
30's	$14.58	GENERIC, Allscripts Pharmaceutical Company	54569-0843-03
30's	$26.78	GENERIC, Southwood Pharmaceuticals Inc	58016-0258-30
30's	$27.60	GENERIC, Pharma Pac	52959-0099-30
31's	$7.81	GENERIC, Heartland Healthcare Services	61392-0740-31
32's	$8.06	GENERIC, Heartland Healthcare Services	61392-0740-32
40's	$7.28	GENERIC, Physicians Total Care	54868-1103-03
40's	$9.18	GENERIC, Prescript Pharmaceuticals	00247-0013-40
40's	$18.82	GENERIC, Pharmaceutical Corporation Of America	51655-0141-50
40's	$19.44	GENERIC, Allscripts Pharmaceutical Company	54569-0843-01
40's	$35.70	GENERIC, Southwood Pharmaceuticals Inc	58016-0258-40
40's	$36.55	GENERIC, Pharma Pac	52959-0099-40
42's	$37.49	GENERIC, Southwood Pharmaceuticals Inc	58016-0258-42
45's	$11.34	GENERIC, Heartland Healthcare Services	61392-0740-45
45's	$40.60	GENERIC, Pharma Pac	52959-0099-45
46's	$41.06	GENERIC, Southwood Pharmaceuticals Inc	58016-0258-46
50's	$44.63	GENERIC, Southwood Pharmaceuticals Inc	58016-0258-50
50's	$47.36	GENERIC, Pharma Pac	52959-0099-50
56's	$49.98	GENERIC, Southwood Pharmaceuticals Inc	58016-0258-56
60's	$8.61	GENERIC, Physicians Total Care	54868-1103-09
60's	$12.09	GENERIC, Prescript Pharmaceuticals	00247-0013-60
60's	$15.12	GENERIC, Heartland Healthcare Services	61392-0740-60
60's	$53.55	GENERIC, Southwood Pharmaceuticals Inc	58016-0258-60
60's	$56.81	GENERIC, Pharma Pac	52959-0099-60
80's	$71.40	GENERIC, Southwood Pharmaceuticals Inc	58016-0258-80
90's	$22.68	GENERIC, Heartland Healthcare Services	61392-0740-90
90's	$80.33	GENERIC, Southwood Pharmaceuticals Inc	58016-0258-90
100's	$12.78	GENERIC, Physicians Total Care	54868-1103-07
100's	$17.92	GENERIC, Prescript Pharmaceuticals	00247-0013-00
100's	$48.60	GENERIC, Allscripts Pharmaceutical Company	54569-0843-06
100's	$49.40	GENERIC, Qualitest Products Inc	00603-4486-21
100's	$66.94	GENERIC, Pharma Pac	52959-0099-00
100's	$89.25	GENERIC, Southwood Pharmaceuticals Inc	58016-0258-00
112's	$99.96	GENERIC, Southwood Pharmaceuticals Inc	58016-0258-02
120's	$15.88	GENERIC, Physicians Total Care	54868-1103-05
120's	$78.75	GENERIC, Pharma Pac	52959-0099-03
120's	$107.10	GENERIC, Southwood Pharmaceuticals Inc	58016-0258-92

Methohexital Sodium *(001769)*

For complete prescribing information, refer to the CD-ROM included with the book.

Categories: Anesthesia, adjunct; Anesthesia, general; Insomnia; Pregnancy Category B; DEA Class CIV; FDA Approved 1960 Jun
Drug Classes: Anesthetics, general; Barbiturates
Brand Names: **Brevital Sodium**
Foreign Brand Availability: Brieta (Austria; Belgium; Bulgaria; Canada; Czech-Republic; Denmark; England; France; Hungary; Netherlands; Norway; Russia; Sweden; Switzerland; Taiwan); Brietal Sodium (Australia; Benin; Burkina-Faso; Ethiopia; Gambia; Ghana; Guinea; Ivory-Coast; Kenya; Liberia; Malawi; Mali; Mauritania; Mauritius; Morocco; Niger; Nigeria; Senegal; Seychelles; Sierra-Leone; South-Africa; Sudan; Tanzania; Tunia; Uganda; Zambia; Zimbabwe); Brevimytal (Germany); Brevital (Benin; Burkina-Faso; Ethiopia; Gambia; Ghana; Guinea; Ivory-Coast; Kenya; Liberia; Malawi; Mali; Mauritania; Mauritius; Morocco; Niger; Nigeria; Senegal; Seychelles; Sierra-Leone; Sudan; Tanzania; Tunia; Uganda; Zambia; Zimbabwe)

WARNING

This drug should be administered by persons qualified in the use of intravenous anesthetics. Cardiac life support equipment must be immediately available during use of methohexital.

DESCRIPTION

Methohexital sodium for injection is 2,4,6 (1H,3H,5H)-pyrimidinetrione, 1-methyl-5-(1-methyl-2-pentynyl)-5-(2-propenyl)-,(±)-, monosodium salt.

Methohexital sodium for injection is a freeze-dried, sterile, nonpyrogenic mixture of methohexital sodium and anhydrous sodium carbonate added as a buffer, which is prepared from an aqueous solution of methohexital, sodium hydroxide, and sodium carbonate. It contains not less than 90% and not more than 110% of the labeled amount of $C_{14}H_{17}N_2NaO_3$. This mixture is ordinarily intended to be reconstituted so as to contain 1% methohexital sodium in sterile water for injection for direct intravenous injection or 0.2% methohexital sodium in 5% dextrose injection (or 0.9% sodium chloride injection) for administration by continuous intravenous drip. The pH of the 1% solution is between 10 and 11; the pH of the 0.2% solution in 5% dextrose is between 9.5 and 10.5.

Methohexital sodium is a rapid, ultrashort-acting barbiturate anesthetic. It occurs as a white, crystalline powder that is freely soluble in water.

STORAGE

Methohexital sodium is stable in sterile water for injection at room temperature 25°C (77°F) or below for at least *6 weeks*. Solutions may be stored and used as long as they remain clear and colorless. Five percent (5%) dextrose injection or isotonic (0.9%) sodium chloride injection may be used as diluents, but the resulting solutions are not stable for much more than *24 hours*.

The vials may be stored at room temperature 77°F (below 25°C). The expiration period for the vials is 2 years.

INDICATIONS AND USAGE

Methohexital sodium can be used as follows:

- For intravenous induction of anesthesia prior to the use of other general anesthetic agents.
- For intravenous induction of anesthesia and as an adjunct to subpotent inhalational anesthetic agents (such as nitrous oxide in oxygen) for short surgical procedures; methohexital sodium may be given by infusion or intermittent injection.
- For use along with other parenteral agents, usually narcotic analgesics, to supplement subpotent inhalational anesthetic agents (such as nitrous oxide in oxygen) for longer surgical procedures.
- As intravenous anesthesia for short surgical, diagnostic, or therapeutic procedures associated with minimal painful stimuli.
- As an agent for inducing a hypnotic state.

CONTRAINDICATIONS

Methohexital sodium is contraindicated in patients in whom general anesthesia is contraindicated, in those with latent or manifest porphyria, or in patients with a known hypersensitivity to barbiturates.

WARNINGS

See BOXED WARNING.

AS WITH ALL POTENT ANESTHETIC AGENTS AND ADJUNCTS, THIS DRUG SHOULD BE ADMINISTERED ONLY BY THOSE TRAINED IN THE ADMINISTRATION OF GENERAL ANESTHESIA, THE MAINTENANCE OF A PATIENT AIRWAY AND VENTILATION, AND THE MANAGEMENT OF CARDIOVASCULAR DEPRESSION ENCOUNTERED DURING ANESTHESIA AND SURGERY.

Because the liver is involved in demethylation and oxidation of methohexital and because barbiturates may enhance preexisting circulatory depression, severe hepatic dysfunction, severe cardiovascular instability, or a shock-like condition may be reason for selecting another induction agent.

Psychomotor seizures may be elicited in susceptible individuals.[1]

Prolonged administration may result in cumulative effects, including extended somnolence, protracted unconsciousness, and respiratory and cardiovascular depression. Respiratory depression in the presence of an impaired airway may lead to hypoxia, cardiac arrest, and death.

The CNS-depressant effect of methohexital sodium may be additive with that of other CNS depressants, including ethyl alcohol and propylene glycol.

DANGER OF INTRA-ARTERIAL INJECTION

Unintended intra-arterial injection of barbiturate solutions may be followed by the production of platelet aggregates and thrombosis, starting in arterioles distal to the site of injection. The resulting necrosis may lead to gangrene, which may require amputation. The first sign in conscious patients may be a complaint of fiery burning that roughly follows the distribution path of the injected artery; if noted, the injection should be stopped immediately and the situation reevaluated. Transient blanching may or may not be noted very early; blotchy cyanosis and dark discoloration may then be the first sign in anesthetized patients. There is no established treatment other than prevention. The following should be considered prior to injection:

- The extent of injury is related to concentration. Concentrations of 1% methohexital will usually suffice; higher concentrations should ordinarily be avoided.
- Check the infusion to ensure that the catheter is in the lumen of a vein before injection. Injection through a running intravenous infusion may enhance the possibility of detecting arterial placement; however, it should be remembered that the characteristic bright-red color of arterial blood is often altered by contact with drugs. The possibility of aberrant arteries should always be considered.

Postinjury arterial injection of vasodilators and/or arterial infusion of parenteral fluids are generally regarded to be of no value in altering outcome. Animal experiments and published individual case reports concerned with a variety of arteriolar irritants, including barbiturates, suggest that one or more of the following may be of benefit in reducing the area of necrosis:

- Arterial injection of heparin at the site of injury, followed by systemic anticoagulation.
- Sympathetic blockade (or brachial plexus blockade in the arm).
- Intra-arterial glucocorticoid injection at the site of injury, followed by systemic steroids.
- A recent case report (nonbarbiturate injury) suggests that intra-arterial urokinase may promote fibrinolysis, even if administered late in treatment.

If extravasation is noted during injection of methohexital, the injection should be discontinued until the situation is remedied. Local irritation may result from extravasation; subcutaneous swelling may also serve as a sign of arterial or periarterial placement of the catheter.

DOSAGE AND ADMINISTRATION

Preanesthetic medication is generally advisable. Methohexital sodium may be used with any of the recognized preanesthetic medications, but the phenothiazines are less satisfactory than the combination of an opiate and a belladonna derivative.

Facilities for assisting respiration and administering oxygen are necessary adjuncts for intravenous anesthesia. Since cardiorespiratory arrest may occur, patients should be observed carefully during and after use of methohexital sodium. Resuscitative equipment (*i.e.,* intubation and cardioversion equipment, oxygen, suction, and a secure intravenous line) and personnel qualified in its use must be immediately available.

Solutions of methohexital sodium should be freshly prepared and used promptly. Reconstituted solutions of methohexital sodium are chemically stable at room temperature for 24 hours.

ADMINISTRATION

Methohexital sodium is administered intravenously in a concentration of no higher than 1%. Higher concentrations markedly increase the incidence of muscular movements and irregularities in respiration and blood pressure. Dosage is highly individualized; the drug should be administered only by those completely familiar with its quantitative differences from other barbiturate anesthetics.

Methohexital sodium may be dissolved in sterile water for injection, 5% dextrose injection, or sodium chloride injection. For induction of anesthesia, a 1% solution is administered at a rate of about 1 ml/5 seconds. Gaseous anesthetics and/or skeletal-muscle relaxants may be administered concomitantly. The dose required for induction may range from 50-120 mg or more but averages about 70 mg. The induction dose usually provides anesthesia for 5-7 minutes.

The usual dosage in adults ranges from 1-1.5 mg/kg. Data on dosage requirements in children are not available.

Maintenance of anesthesia may be accomplished by intermittent injections of the 1% solution or, more easily, by continuous intravenous drip of a 0.2% solution. Intermittent injections of about 20-40 mg (2-4 ml of a 1% solution) may be given as required, usually every 4-7 minutes. For continuous drip, the average rate of administration is about 3 ml of a 0.2% solution/minute (1 drop/second). The rate of flow must be individualized for each patient. For longer surgical procedures, gradual reduction in the rate of administration is recommended (see WARNINGS). Other parenteral agents, usually narcotic analgesics, are ordinarily employed along with methohexital sodium during longer procedures.

Parenteral drug products should be inspected visually for particulate matter and discoloration prior to administration, whenever solution and container permit.

COMPATIBILITY INFORMATION

Solutions of methohexital sodium should not be mixed in the same syringe or administered simultaneously during intravenous infusion through the same needle with acid solutions, such as atropine sulfate, metubine iodide (metocurine iodide injection), and succinylcholine chloride. Alteration of pH may cause free barbituric acid to be precipitated. Solubility of the soluble sodium salts of barbiturates, including methohexital sodium, is maintained only at relatively high (basic) pH.

Because of numerous requests from anesthesiologists for information regarding the chemical compatibility of these mixtures, TABLE 1 contains information obtained from compatibility studies in which a 1% solution of methohexital sodium was mixed with therapeutic amounts of agents whose solutions have a low (acid) pH.

TABLE 1

			Physical Change			
Active Ingredient	**Potency per ml**	**Vol. Used**	**Immediate**	**15 min**	**30 min**	**1 hour**
Brevital sodium	10 mg	10 ml	CONTROL			
Atropine sulfate	1/150 g	1 ml	None	Haze		
Atropine sulfate	1/100 g	1 ml	None	ppt	ppt	
Succinylcholine chloride	0.5 mg	4 ml	None	None	Haze	
Succinylcholine chloride	1 mg	4 ml	None	None	Haze	
Metocurine iodide	0.5 mg	4 ml	None	None	ppt	
Metocurine iodide	1 mg	4 ml	None	None	ppt	
Scopolamine hydrobromide	1/120 g	1 ml	None	None	None	Haze
Tubocurarine chloride	3 mg	4 ml	None	Haze		

PRODUCT LISTING - EQUIVALENTS NOT AVAILABLE

Powder For Injection - Intravenous - 2.5 Gm

1's	$55.25	BREVITAL SODIUM, Allscripts Pharmaceutical Company	54569-4474-00
25's	$1372.76	BREVITAL SODIUM, Physicians Total Care	54868-3727-00
25's	$1491.69	BREVITAL SODIUM, Jones Pharma Inc	52604-1448-05
25's	$1864.61	BREVITAL SODIUM, Monarch Pharmaceuticals Inc	61570-0096-01

Powder For Injection - Intravenous - 5 Gm

1's	$119.53	BREVITAL SODIUM, Jones Pharma Inc	52604-1445-01

Powder For Injection - Intravenous - 500 mg

1's	$32.41	BREVITAL SODIUM, Jones Pharma Inc	52604-1446-01
1's	$40.51	BREVITAL SODIUM, Monarch Pharmaceuticals Inc	61570-0095-01
25's	$810.50	BREVITAL SODIUM, Jones Pharma Inc	52604-1446-05
25's	$1012.81	BREVITAL SODIUM, Monarch Pharmaceuticals Inc	61570-0095-25

M

Methotrexate Sodium (001770)

Categories: Arthritis, rheumatoid; Carcinoma, breast; Carcinoma, lung; Carcinoma, head and neck; Chorioadenoma destruens; Choriocarcinoma; Hydatidiform mole; Leukemia, acute lymphoblastic; Leukemia, meningeal; Lymphoma, non-Hodgkin's; Lymphoma, T cell, cutaneous; Osteosarcoma; Psoriasis; FDA Approved 1953 Dec; Pregnancy Category X; Orphan Drugs; WHO Formulary

Drug Classes: Antineoplastics, antimetabolites; Disease modifying antirheumatic drugs

Brand Names: Abitrexate; Emtexate; Folex; Mexate; **Rheumatrex**; Trexall

Foreign Brand Availability: Biotrexate (India); Canceren (Korea); Emthexat (Sweden); Emthexate (Belgium; Denmark; Greece; Korea; Malaysia; Netherlands; New-Zealand; Norway; Philippines; Portugal; Spain; Switzerland; Taiwan; Thailand; Turkey); Farmitrexat (Germany; Indonesia); Farmotrex (Denmark); Ifamet (Mexico); Lantarel (Germany); Ledertrexate (Australia; Belgium; Finland; France; Mexico; Netherlands; New-Zealand; Portugal); Maxtrex (England; Philippines); Mexate (Philippines); Metex (Germany); Methoblastin (Australia; New-Zealand); Methotrexat Ebewe (Colombia); Methotrexate (Australia; Hong-Kong; Indonesia; Israel; Japan; Malaysia; Peru; Philippines; South-Africa; Taiwan; Thailand); Methotrexato (Argentina); MTX (Korea); Neotrexate (India); Novatrex (France); Texate (Mexico); Texate-T (Mexico); Texorate (Indonesia); Trexan (Finland; Hungary; Russia; Taiwan; Turkey); Trixilem (Mexico; Thailand); Xaken (Mexico); Zexate (Philippines)

Cost of Therapy: \$62.05 (Rheumatoid Arthritis; Rheumatrex Dose Pack; 2.5 mg; 3 tablets/week; 28 day supply)
\$37.64 (Rheumatoid Arthritis; Generic Tablets; 2.5 mg; 3 tablets/week; 28 day supply)

HCFA JCODE(S): J8610 2.5 mg ORAL; J9250 5 mg IV, IM, IT, IA; J9260 50 mg IV, IM, IT, IA

WARNING

METHOTREXATE SHOULD BE USED ONLY BY PHYSICIANS WHOSE KNOWLEDGE AND EXPERIENCE INCLUDE THE USE OF ANTIMETABOLITE THERAPY. BECAUSE OF THE POSSIBILITY OF SERIOUS TOXIC REACTIONS (WHICH CAN BE FATAL):

METHOTREXATE SHOULD BE USED ONLY IN LIFE THREATENING NEOPLASTIC DISEASES, OR IN PATIENTS WITH PSORIASIS OR RHEUMATOID ARTHRITIS WITH SEVERE, RECALCITRANT, DISABLING DISEASE WHICH IS NOT ADEQUATELY RESPONSIVE TO OTHER FORMS OF THERAPY.

DEATHS HAVE BEEN REPORTED WITH THE USE OF METHOTREXATE IN THE TREATMENT OF MALIGNANCY, PSORIASIS, AND RHEUMATOID ARTHRITIS.

PATIENTS SHOULD BE CLOSELY MONITORED FOR BONE MARROW, LIVER, LUNG AND KIDNEY TOXICITIES. (See PRECAUTIONS.) PATIENTS SHOULD BE INFORMED BY THEIR PHYSICIAN OF THE RISKS INVOLVED AND BE UNDER A PHYSICIAN'S CARE THROUGHOUT THERAPY.

THE USE OF METHOTREXATE HIGH DOSE REGIMENS RECOMMENDED FOR OSTEOSARCOMA REQUIRES METICULOUS CARE. (See DOSAGE AND ADMINISTRATION.) HIGH DOSE REGIMENS FOR OTHER NEOPLASTIC DISEASES ARE INVESTIGATIONAL AND A THERAPEUTIC ADVANTAGE HAS NOT BEEN ESTABLISHED.

METHOTREXATE FORMULATIONS AND DILUENTS CONTAINING PRESERVATIVES MUST NOT BE USED FOR INTRATHECAL OR HIGH DOSE METHOTREXATE THERAPY.

Methotrexate has been reported to cause fetal death and/or congenital anomalies. Therefore, it is not recommended for women of childbearing potential unless there is clear medical evidence that the benefits can be expected to outweigh the considered risks. Pregnant women with psoriasis or rheumatoid arthritis should not receive methotrexate. (See CONTRAINDICATIONS.)

Methotrexate elimination is reduced in patients with impaired renal function, ascites, or pleural effusions. Such patients require especially careful monitoring for toxicity, and require dose reduction or, in some cases, discontinuation of methotrexate administration.

Unexpectedly severe (sometimes fatal) bone marrow suppression, aplastic anemia, and gastrointestinal toxicity have been reported with concomitant administration of methotrexate (usually in high dosage) along with some non-steroidal anti-inflammatory drugs (NSAIDs). (See DRUG INTERACTIONS.)

Methotrexate causes hepatotoxicity, fibrosis and cirrhosis, but generally only after prolonged use. Acutely, liver enzyme elevations are frequently seen. These are usually transient and asymptomatic, and also do not appear predictive of subsequent hepatic disease. Liver biopsy after sustained use often shows histologic changes, and fibrosis and cirrhosis have been reported; these latter lesions may not be preceded by symptoms or abnormal liver function tests in the psoriasis population. For this reason, periodic liver biopsies are usually recommended for psoriatic patients who are under long-term treatment. Persistent abnormalities in liver function tests may precede appearance of fibrosis or cirrhosis in the rheumatoid arthritis population. (See PRECAUTIONS, Organ System Toxicity, Hepatic.)

Methotrexate-induced lung disease is a potentially dangerous lesion, which may occur acutely at any time during therapy and which has been reported at doses as low as 7.5 mg/wk. It is not always fully reversible. Pulmonary symptoms (especially a dry, nonproductive cough) may require interruption of treatment and careful investigation.

Diarrhea and ulcerative stomatitis require interruption of therapy; otherwise, hemorrhagic enteritis and death from intestinal perforation may occur.

Malignant lymphomas, which may regress following withdrawal of methotrexate, may occur in patients receiving low-dose methotrexate and, thus, may not require cytotoxic treatment. Discontinue methotrexate first and, if the lymphoma does not regress, appropriate treatment should be instituted.

Like other cytotoxic drugs, methotrexate may induce "tumor lysis syndrome" in patients with rapidly growing tumors. Appropriate supportive and pharmacologic measures may prevent or alleviate this complication.

Severe, occasionally fatal, skin reactions have been reported following single or multiple doses of methotrexate. Reactions have occurred within days of oral, intramuscular, intravenous, or intrathecal methotrexate administration. Recovery has been reported with discontinuation of therapy. (See PRECAUTIONS, Organ System Toxicity, Skin.)

Potentially fatal opportunistic infections, especially *Pneumocystis carinii* pneumonia, may occur with methotrexate therapy.

Methotrexate given concomitantly with radiotherapy may increase the risk of soft tissue necrosis and osteonecrosis.

DESCRIPTION

Methotrexate (formerly Amethopterin) is an antimetabolite used in the treatment of certain neoplastic diseases, severe psoriasis, and adult rheumatoid arthritis.

Chemically methotrexate is *N*-[4-[[(2,4-diamino-6-pteridinyl)methyl]methyl-amino] benzoyl]-L-glutamic acid. The molecular formula is $C_{20}H_{22}N_8O_5$ and the molecular weight is 454.45.

Methotrexate Sodium Tablets for oral administration are available in bottles of 100 and in a packaging system designated as the Rheumatrex Methotrexate Sodium Dose Pack for therapy with a weekly dosing schedule of 5, 7.5, 10, 12.5 and 15 mg. Methotrexate Sodium Tablets contain an amount of methotrexate sodium equivalent to 2.5 mg of methotrexate and the following inactive ingredients: lactose, magnesium stearate and pregelatinized starch. May also contain corn starch.

Methotrexate Sodium Injection and for Injection products are sterile and non-pyrogenic and may be given by the intramuscular, intravenous, intra-arterial or intrathecal route. (See DOSAGE AND ADMINISTRATION.) However, the preservative formulation contains benzyl alcohol and must not be used for intrathecal or high dose therapy.

Methotrexate Sodium Injection, Isotonic Liquid, Contains Preservative is available in 25 mg/ml, 2 ml (50 mg) and 10 ml (250 mg) vials.

Each 25 mg/ml, 2 ml and 10 ml vial contains methotrexate sodium equivalent to 50 mg and 250 mg methotrexate respectively, 0.90% w/v of benzyl alcohol as a preservative, and the following inactive ingredients: sodium chloride 0.260% w/v and water for injection qs at 100% v. Sodium hydroxide and, if necessary, hydrochloric acid are added to adjust the pH to approximately 8.5.

Methotrexate LPF Sodium (methotrexate sodium injection), Isotonic Liquid, Preservative Free, for single use only, is available in 25 mg/ml, 2 ml (50 mg), 4 ml (100 mg), and 10 ml (250 mg) vials.

Each 25 mg/ml, 2 ml, 4 ml, and 10 ml vial contains methotrexate sodium equivalent to 50 mg, 100 mg, and 250 mg methotrexate respectively, and the following inactive ingredients: sodium chloride 0.490% w/v and water for injection qs ad 100% v. sodium hydroxide and, if necessary, hydrochloric acid are added to adjust the pH to approximately 8.5. The 2 ml, 4 ml, and 10 ml solutions contain approximately 0.43 mEq, 0.86 mEq, and 2.15 mEq of Sodium per vial, respectively, and are isotonic solutions.

Methotrexate Sodium for Injection, Lyophilized, Preservative Free, for single use only, is available in 20 mg and 1 g vials.

Each 20 mg and 1 g vial of lyophilized powder contains methotrexate sodium equivalent to 20 mg and 1 g methotrexate respectively. Contains no preservative. Sodium hydroxide and, if necessary, hydrochloric acid are added during manufacture to adjust the pH. The 20 mg vial contains approximately 0.14 mEq of sodium and the 1 g vial contains approximately 7 mEq sodium.

CLINICAL PHARMACOLOGY

Methotrexate inhibits dihydrofolic acid reductase. Dihydrofolates must be reduced to tetrahydrofolates by this enzyme before they can be utilized as carriers of one-carbon groups in the synthesis of purine nucleotides and thymidylate. Therefore, methotrexate interferes with DNA synthesis, repair, and cellular replication. Actively proliferating tissues such as malignant cells, bone marrow, fetal cells, buccal and intestinal mucosa, and cells of the urinary bladder are in general more sensitive to this effect of methotrexate. When cellular proliferation in malignant tissues is greater than in most normal tissues, methotrexate may impair malignant growth without irreversible damage to normal tissues.

The mechanism of action in rheumatoid arthritis is unknown; it may affect immune function. Two reports describe *in vitro* methotrexate inhibition of DNA precursor uptake by stimulated mononuclear cells, and another describes in animal polyarthritis partial correction by methotrexate of spleen cell hyporesponsiveness and suppressed IL 2 production. Other laboratories, however, have been unable to demonstrate similar effects. Clarification of methotrexate's effect on immune activity and its relation to rheumatoid immunopathogenesis await further studies.

In patients with rheumatoid arthritis, effects of methotrexate on articular swelling and tenderness can be seen as early as 3-6 weeks. Although methotrexate clearly ameliorates symptoms of inflammation (pain, swelling, stiffness), there is no evidence that it induces remission of rheumatoid arthritis nor has a beneficial effect been demonstrated on bone erosions and other radiologic changes which result in impaired joint use, functional disability, and deformity.

Most studies of methotrexate in patients with rheumatoid arthritis are relatively short term (3-6 months). Limited data from long-term studies indicate that an initial clinical improvement is maintained for at least 2 years with continued therapy.

In psoriasis, the rate of production of epithelial cells in the skin is greatly increased over normal skin. This differential in proliferation rates is the basis for the use of methotrexate to control the psoriatic process.

Methotrexate in high doses, followed by leucovorin rescue, is used as a part of the treatment of patients with non-metastatic osteosarcoma. The original rationale for high dose methotrexate therapy was based on the concept of selective rescue of normal tissues by leucovorin. More recent evidence suggests that high dose methotrexate may also overcome methotrexate resistance caused by impaired active transport, decreased affinity of dihydrofolic acid reductase for methotrexate, increased levels of dihydrofolic acid reductase resulting from gene amplification, or decreased polyglutamation of methotrexate. The actual mechanism of action is unknown.

In a 6 month, double-blind, placebo-controlled trial of 127 pediatric patients with juvenile rheumatoid arthritis (JRA) (mean age, 10.1 years; age range 2.5 to 18 years, mean duration of disease, 5.1 years) on background non-steroidal anti-inflammatory drugs (NSAIDs) and/or prednisone, methotrexate given weekly at an oral dose of 10 mg/m^2 provided significant clinical improvement compared to placebo as measured by either the physician's global assessment, or by a patient composite (25% reduction in the articular-severity score plus improvement in parent and physician global assessments of disease activity.) Over two-thirds of the patients in this trial had polyarticular-course JRA, and the numerically greatest response was seen in this subgroup treated with 10 mg/m^2/wk methotrexate. The overwhelming majority of the remaining patients had systemic-course JRA. All patients were unresponsive to NSAIDs; approximately one-third were using low dose corticoster-

M

oids. Weekly methotrexate at a dose of 5 mg/m^2 was not significantly more effective than placebo in this trial.

Two Pediatric Oncology Group studies (one randomized and one non-randomized) demonstrated a significant improvement in relapse-free survival in patients with nonmetastatic osteosarcoma, when high dose methotrexate with leucovorin rescue was used in combination with other chemotherapeutic agents following surgical resection of the primary tumor. These studies were not designed to demonstrate the specific contribution of high dose methotrexate/leucovorin rescue therapy to the efficacy of the combination. However, a contribution can be inferred from the reports of objective responses to this therapy in patients with metastatic osteosarcoma, and from reports of extensive tumor necrosis following preoperative administration of this therapy to patients with non-metastatic osteosarcoma.

PHARMACOKINETICS

Absorption

In adults, oral absorption appears to be dose dependent. Peak serum levels are reached within 1-2 hours. At doses of 30 mg/m^2 or less, methotrexate is generally well absorbed with a mean bioavailability of about 60%. The absorption of doses greater than 80 mg/m^2 is significantly less, possibly due to a saturation effect.

In leukemic pediatric patients, oral absorption of methotrexate also appears to be dose dependent and has been reported to vary widely (23-95%). A 20-fold difference between highest and lowest peak levels (C_{max}: 0.11 to 2.3 μM after a 20 mg/m^2 dose) has been reported. Significant interindividual variability has also been noted in time to peak concentration (T_{max}: 0.67 to 4 hours after a 15 mg/m^2 dose) and fraction of dose absorbed. The absorption of doses greater than 40 mg/m^2 has been reported to be significantly less than that of lower doses. Food has been shown to delay absorption and reduce peak concentration. Methotrexate is generally completely absorbed from parenteral routes of injection. After intramuscular injection, peak serum concentrations occur in 30-60 minutes. As in leukemic pediatric patients, a wide interindividual variability in the plasma concentrations of methotrexate has been reported in pediatric patients with JRA. Following oral administration of methotrexate in doses of 6.4-11.2 mg/m^2/wk in pediatric patients with JRA, mean serum concentrations were 0.59 μM (range, 0.03-1.40) at 1 hour, 0.44 μM (range, 0.01-1.00) at 2 hours, and 0.29 μM (range 0.06-0.58) at 3 hours. In pediatric patients receiving methotrexate for acute lymphocytic leukemia (6.3 to 30 mg/m^2), or for JRA (3.75 to 26 mg/m^2), the terminal half-life has been reported to range from 0.7-5.8 hours or 0.9-2.3 hours, respectively.

Distribution

After intravenous administration, the initial volume of distribution is approximately 0.18 L/kg (18% of body weight) and steady-state volume of distribution is approximately 0.4-0.8 L/kg (40-80% of body weight). Methotrexate competes with reduced folates for active transport across cell membranes by means of a single carrier-mediated active transport process. At serum concentrations greater than 100 μM, passive diffusion becomes a major pathway by which effective intracellular concentrations can be achieved. Methotrexate in serum is approximately 50% protein bound. Laboratory studies demonstrate that it may be displaced from plasma albumin by various compounds including sulfonamides, salicylates, tetracyclines, chloramphenicol, and phenytoin.

Methotrexate does not penetrate the blood-cerebrospinal fluid barrier in therapeutic amounts when given orally or parenterally. High CSF concentrations of the drug may be attained by intrathecal administration.

In dogs, synovial fluid concentrations after oral dosing were higher in inflamed than uninflamed joints. Although salicylates did not interfere with this penetration, prior prednisone treatment reduced penetration into inflamed joints to the level of normal joints.

Metabolism

After absorption, methotrexate undergoes hepatic and intracellular metabolism to polyglutamated forms which can be converted back to methotrexate by hydrolase enzymes. These polyglutamates act as inhibitors of dihydrofolate reductase and thymidylate synthetase. Small amounts of methotrexate polyglutamates may remain in tissues for extended periods. The retention and prolonged drug action of these active metabolites vary among different cells, tissues and tumors. A small amount of metabolism to 7-hydroxymethotrexate may occur at doses commonly prescribed. Accumulation of this metabolite may become significant at the high doses used in osteogenic sarcoma. The aqueous solubility of 7-hydroxymethotrexate is 3- to 5-fold lower than the parent compound. Methotrexate is partially metabolized by intestinal flora after oral administration.

Half-Life

The terminal half-life reported for methotrexate is approximately 3-10 hours for patients receiving treatment for psoriasis, or rheumatoid arthritis or low dose antineoplastic therapy (less than 30 mg/m^2). For patients receiving high doses of methotrexate, the terminal half-life is 8-15 hours.

Excretion

Renal excretion is the primary route of elimination and is dependent upon dosage and route of administration. With IV administration, 80-90% of the administered dose is excreted unchanged in the urine within 24 hours. There is limited biliary excretion amounting to 10% or less of the administered dose. Enterohepatic recirculation of methotrexate has been proposed.

Renal excretion occurs by glomerular filtration and active tubular secretion. Nonlinear elimination due to saturation of renal tubular reabsorption has been observed in psoriatic patients at doses between 7.5 and 30 mg. Impaired renal function, as well as concurrent use of drugs such as weak organic acids that also undergo tubular secretion, can markedly increase methotrexate serum levels. Excellent correlation has been reported between methotrexate clearance and endogenous creatinine clearance.

Methotrexate clearance rates vary widely and are generally decreased at higher doses. Delayed drug clearance has been identified as one of the major factors responsible for methotrexate toxicity. It has been postulated that the toxicity of methotrexate for normal tissues is more dependent upon the duration of exposure to the drug rather than the peak level achieved. When a patient has delayed drug elimination due to compromised renal function, a third space effusion, or other causes, methotrexate serum concentrations may remain elevated for prolonged periods.

The potential for toxicity from high dose regimens or delayed excretion is reduced by the administration of leucovorin calcium during the final phase of methotrexate plasma elimination. Pharmacokinetic monitoring of methotrexate serum concentrations may help identify those patients at high risk for methotrexate toxicity and aid in proper adjustment of leucovorin dosing. Guidelines for monitoring serum methotrexate levels, and for adjustment of leucovorin dosing to reduce the risk of methotrexate toxicity, are provided below in DOSAGE AND ADMINISTRATION.

Methotrexate has been detected in human breast milk. The highest breast milk to plasma concentration ratio reached was 0.08:1.

INDICATIONS AND USAGE

NEOPLASTIC DISEASES

Methotrexate is indicated in the treatment of gestational choriocarcinoma, chorioadenoma destruens and hydatidiform mole.

In acute lymphocytic leukemia, methotrexate is indicated in the prophylaxis of meningeal leukemia and is used in maintenance therapy in combination with other chemotherapeutic agents. Methotrexate is also indicated in the treatment of meningeal leukemia.

Methotrexate is used alone or in combination with other anticancer agents in the treatment of breast cancer, epidermoid cancers of the head and neck, advanced mycosis fungoides (cutaneous T cell lymphoma), and lung cancer, particularly squamous cell and small cell types. Methotrexate is also used in combination with other chemotherapeutic agents in the treatment of advanced stage non-Hodgkin's lymphomas.

Methotrexate in high doses followed by leucovorin rescue in combination with other chemotherapeutic agents is effective in prolonging relapse-free survival in patients with non-metastatic osteosarcoma who have undergone surgical resection or amputation for the primary tumor.

PSORIASIS

Methotrexate is indicated in the symptomatic control of severe, recalcitrant, disabling psoriasis that is not adequately responsive to other forms of therapy, *but only when the diagnosis has been established, as by biopsy and/or after dermatologic consultation.* It is important to ensure that a psoriasis "flare" is not due to an undiagnosed concomitant disease affecting immune responses.

RHEUMATOID ARTHRITIS INCLUDING POLYARTICULAR-COURSE JUVENILE RHEUMATOID ARTHRITIS

Methotrexate is indicated in the management of selected adults with severe, active, rheumatoid arthritis (ACR criteria), or children with active polyarticular-course juvenile arthritis, who have had an insufficient therapeutic response to, or are intolerant of, an adequate trial of first-line therapy including full dose non-steroidal anti-inflammatory agents (NSAIDs).

Aspirin, NSAIDs, and/or low dose steroids may be continued, although the possibility of increased toxicity with concomitant use of NSAIDs including salicylates has not been fully explored. (See DRUG INTERACTIONS.) Steroids may be reduced gradually in patients who respond to methotrexate. Combined use of methotrexate with gold, penicillamine, hydroxychloroquine, sulfasalazine, or cytotoxic agents, has not been studied and may increase the incidence of adverse effects. Rest and physiotherapy as indicated should be continued.

NON-FDA APPROVED INDICATIONS

Methotrexate has been used without FDA approval for asthma, abortion induction in ectopic pregnancy, systemic lupus erythematosus, and ulcerative colitis.

CONTRAINDICATIONS

Methotrexate can cause fetal death or teratogenic effects when administered to a pregnant woman. Methotrexate is contraindicated in pregnant women with psoriasis or rheumatoid arthritis and should be used in the treatment of neoplastic diseases only when the potential benefit outweighs the risk to the fetus. Women of childbearing potential should not be started on methotrexate until pregnancy is excluded and should be fully counseled on the serious risk to the fetus (see PRECAUTIONS) should they become pregnant while undergoing treatment. Pregnancy should be avoided if either partner is receiving methotrexate; during and for a minimum of 3 months after therapy for male patients, and during and for at least one ovulatory cycle after therapy for female patients. (See BOXED WARNING.)

Because of the potential for serious adverse reactions from methotrexate in breast fed infants, it is contraindicated in nursing mothers.

Patients with psoriasis or rheumatoid arthritis with alcoholism, alcoholic liver disease or other chronic liver disease should not receive methotrexate.

Patients with psoriasis or rheumatoid arthritis who have overt or laboratory evidence of immunodeficiency syndromes should not receive methotrexate.

Patients with psoriasis or rheumatoid arthritis who have preexisting blood dyscrasias, such as bone marrow hypoplasia, leukopenia, thrombocytopenia or significant anemia, should not receive methotrexate.

Patients with a known hypersensitivity to methotrexate should not receive the drug.

WARNINGS

SEE BOXED WARNING.

Methotrexate formulations and diluents containing preservatives must not be used for intrathecal or high dose methotrexate therapy.

PRECAUTIONS

GENERAL

Methotrexate has the potential for serious toxicity. (See BOXED WARNING.) Toxic effects may be related in frequency and severity to dose or frequency of administration but have been seen at all doses. Because they can occur at any time during therapy, it is necessary to follow patients on methotrexate closely. Most adverse reactions are reversible if detected early. When such reactions do occur, the drug should be reduced in dosage or discontinued and appropriate corrective measures should be taken. If necessary, this could include the use of leucovorin calcium and/or acute, intermittent hemodialysis with a high-flux dialyzer. If methotrexate therapy is reinstituted, it should be carried out with caution, with adequate consideration of further need for the drug and with increased alertness as to possible recurrence of toxicity.

The clinical pharmacology of methotrexate has not been well studied in older individuals. Due to diminished hepatic and renal function as well as decreased folate stores in this population, relatively low doses should be considered, and these patients should be closely monitored for early signs of toxicity.

INFORMATION FOR THE PATIENT

Patients should be informed of the early signs and symptoms of toxicity, of the need to see their physician promptly if they occur, and the need for close follow-up, including periodic laboratory tests to monitor toxicity.

Both the physician and pharmacist should emphasize to the patient that the recommended dose is taken weekly in rheumatoid arthritis and psoriasis, and that mistaken daily use of the recommended dose has led to fatal toxicity. Patients should be encouraged to read the Patient Instructions sheet within the Dose Pack. Prescriptions should not be written or refilled on a prn basis.

Patients should be informed of the potential benefit and risk in the use of methotrexate. The risk of effects on reproduction should be discussed with both male and female patients taking methotrexate.

LABORATORY TESTS

Patients undergoing methotrexate therapy should be closely monitored so that toxic effects are detected promptly. Baseline assessment should include a complete blood count with differential and platelet counts, hepatic enzymes, renal function tests, and a chest X-ray. During therapy of rheumatoid arthritis and psoriasis, monitoring of these parameters is recommended: hematology at least monthly, renal function and liver function every 1-2 months. More frequent monitoring is usually indicated during antineoplastic therapy. *During initial or changing doses,* or during periods of increased risk of elevated methotrexate blood levels (*e.g.,* dehydration), more frequent monitoring may also be indicated.

Transient liver function test abnormalities are observed frequently after methotrexate administration and are usually not cause for modification of methotrexate therapy. Persistent liver function test abnormalities, and/or depression of serum albumin may be indicators of serious liver toxicity and require evaluation. (See PRECAUTIONS, Organ System Toxicity, Hepatic.)

A relationship between abnormal liver function tests and fibrosis or cirrhosis of the liver has not been established for patients with psoriasis. Persistent abnormalities in liver function tests may precede appearance of fibrosis or cirrhosis in the rheumatoid arthritis population.

Pulmonary function tests may be useful if methotrexate-induced lung disease is suspected, especially if baseline measurements are available.

M

CARCINOGENESIS, MUTAGENESIS, AND IMPAIRMENT OF FERTILITY

No controlled human data exist regarding the risk of neoplasia with methotrexate. Methotrexate has been evaluated in a number of animal studies for carcinogenic potential with inconclusive results. Although there is evidence that methotrexate causes chromosomal damage to animal somatic cells and human bone marrow cells, the clinical significance remains uncertain. Non-Hodgkin's lymphoma and other tumors have been reported in patients receiving low-dose oral methotrexate. However, there have been instances of malignant lymphoma arising during treatment with low-dose oral methotrexate, which have regressed completely following withdrawal of methotrexate, without requiring active anti-lymphoma treatment. Benefits should be weighed against the potential risks before using methotrexate alone or in combination with other drugs, especially in pediatric patients or young adults. Methotrexate causes embryotoxicity, abortion, and fetal defects in humans. It has also been reported to cause impairment of fertility, oligospermia and menstrual dysfunction in humans, during and for a short period after cessation of therapy.

PREGNANCY

Psoriasis and rheumatoid arthritis: Methotrexate is in Pregnancy Category X. See CONTRAINDICATIONS.

NURSING MOTHERS

See CONTRAINDICATIONS.

PEDIATRIC USE

Safety and effectiveness in pediatric patients have been established, only in cancer chemotherapy and in polyarticular-course juvenile rheumatoid arthritis.

Published clinical studies evaluating the use of methotrexate in children and adolescents (*i.e.,* patients 2-16 years of age) with JRA demonstrated safety comparable to that observed in adults with rheumatoid arthritis. (See CLINICAL PHARMACOLOGY, ADVERSE REACTIONS and DOSAGE AND ADMINISTRATION.)

Methotrexate Sodium for Injection contains the preservative benzyl alcohol and is not recommended for use in neonates. There have been reports of fatal 'gasping syndrome' in neonates (children less than 1 month of age) following the administrations of intravenous solutions containing the preservative benzyl alcohol. Symptoms include a striking onset of gasping respiration, hypotension, bradycardia, and cardiovascular collapse.

ORGAN SYSTEM TOXICITY

Gastrointestinal

If vomiting, diarrhea, or stomatitis occur, which may result in dehydration, methotrexate should be discontinued until recovery occurs. Methotrexate should be used with extreme caution in the presence of peptic ulcer disease or ulcerative colitis.

Hematologic

Methotrexate can suppress hematopoiesis and cause anemia, aplastic anemia, leukopenia, and/or thrombocytopenia. In patients with malignancy and preexisting hematopoietic impairment, the drug should be used with caution, if at all. In controlled clinical trials in rheumatoid arthritis (n=128), leukopenia (WBC $<3000/mm^3$) was seen in 2 patients, thrombocytopenia (platelets $<100,000/mm^3$) in 6 patients, and pancytopenia in 2 patients.

In psoriasis and rheumatoid arthritis, methotrexate should be stopped immediately if there is a significant drop in blood counts. In the treatment of neoplastic diseases, methotrexate should be continued only if the potential benefit warrants the risk of severe myelosuppression. Patients with profound granulocytopenia and fever should be evaluated immediately and usually require parenteral broad-spectrum antibiotic therapy.

Hepatic

Methotrexate has the potential for acute (elevated transaminases) and chronic (fibrosis and cirrhosis) hepatotoxicity. Chronic toxicity is potentially fatal; it generally has occurred after prolonged use (generally 2 years or more) and after a total dose of at least 1.5 g. In studies in psoriatic patients, hepatotoxicity appeared to be a function of total cumulative dose and appeared to be enhanced by alcoholism, obesity, diabetes and advanced age. An accurate incidence rate has not been determined; the rate of progression and reversibility of lesions is not known. Special caution is indicated in the presence of preexisting liver damage or impaired hepatic function.

In psoriasis, liver function tests, including serum albumin, should be performed periodically prior to dosing but are often normal in the face of developing fibrosis or cirrhosis. These lesions may be detectable only by biopsy. The usual recommendation is to obtain a liver biopsy at (1) pretherapy or shortly after initiation of therapy (2-4 months), (2) a total cumulative dose of 1.5 g, and (3) after each additional 1.0-1.5 g. Moderate fibrosis or any cirrhosis normally leads to discontinuation of the drug; mild fibrosis normally suggests a repeat biopsy in 6 months. Milder histologic findings such as fatty change and low grade portal inflammation are relatively common pretherapy. Although these mild changes are usually not a reason to avoid or discontinue methotrexate therapy, the drug should be used with caution.

In rheumatoid arthritis, age at first use of methotrexate and duration of therapy have been reported as risk factors for hepatotoxicity; other risk factors, similar to those observed in psoriasis, may be present in rheumatoid arthritis but have not been confirmed to date. Persistent abnormalities in liver function tests may precede appearance of fibrosis or cirrhosis in this population. There is a combined reported experience in 217 rheumatoid arthritis patients with liver biopsies both before and during treatment (after a cumulative dose of at least 1.5 g) and in 714 patients with a biopsy only during treatment. There are 64 (7%) cases of fibrosis and 1 (0.1%) case of cirrhosis. Of the 64 cases of fibrosis, 60 were deemed mild. The reticulin stain is more sensitive for early fibrosis and its use may increase these figures. It is unknown whether even longer use will increase these risks.

Liver function tests should be performed at baseline and at 4-8 week intervals in patients receiving methotrexate for rheumatoid arthritis. Pretreatment liver biopsy should be performed for patients with a history of excessive alcohol consumption, persistently abnormal baseline liver function test values or chronic hepatitis B or C infection. During therapy, liver biopsy should be performed if there are persistent liver function test abnormalities or there is a decrease in serum albumin below the normal range (in the setting of well controlled rheumatoid arthritis).

If the results of a liver biopsy show mild changes (Roenigk grades I, II, IIIa), methotrexate may be continued and the patient monitored as per recommendations listed above. Methotrexate should be discontinued in any patient who displays persistently abnormal liver function tests and refuses liver biopsy or in any patient whose liver biopsy shows moderate to severe changes (Roenigk grade IIIb or IV).

Infection or Immunologic States

Methotrexate should be used with extreme caution in the presence of active infection, and is usually contraindicated in patients with overt or laboratory evidence of immunodeficiency syndromes. Immunization may be ineffective when given during methotrexate therapy. Immunization with live virus vaccines is generally not recommended. There have been reports of disseminated vaccinia infections after smallpox immunization in patients receiving methotrexate therapy. Hypogammaglobulinemia has been reported rarely.

Potentially fatal opportunistic infections, especially *Pneumocystis carinii* pneumonia, may occur with methotrexate therapy. When a patient presents with pulmonary symptoms, the possibility of *Pneumocystis carinii* pneumonia should be considered.

Neurologic

There have been reports of leukoencephalopathy following intravenous administration of methotrexate to patients who have had craniospinal irradiation. Serious neurotoxicity, frequently manifested as generalized or focal seizures, has been reported with unexpectedly increased frequency among pediatric patients with acute lymphoblastic leukemia who were treated with intermediate-dose intravenous methotrexate (1 g/m^2). Symptomatic patients were commonly noted to have leukoencephalopathy and/or microangiopathic calcifications on diagnostic imaging studies. Chronic leukoencephalopathy has also been reported in patients who received repeated doses of high-dose methotrexate with leucovorin rescue even without cranial irradiation.

Discontinuation of methotrexate does not always result in complete recovery.

A transient acute neurologic syndrome has been observed in patients treated with high dosage regimens. Manifestations of this stroke-like encephalopathy may include confusion, hemiparesis, transient blindness, seizures and coma. The exact cause is unknown.

After the intrathecal use of methotrexate, the central nervous system toxicity which may occur can be classified as follows: acute chemical arachnoiditis manifested by such symptoms as headache, back pain, nuchal rigidity, and fever; sub-acute myelopathy characterized by paraparesis/paraplegia associated with involvement with one or more spinal nerve roots; chronic leukoencephalopathy manifested by confusion, irritability, somnolence, ataxia, dementia, seizures and coma. This condition can be progressive and even fatal.

Pulmonary

Pulmonary symptoms (especially a dry nonproductive cough) or a nonspecific pneumonitis occurring during methotrexate therapy may be indicative of a potentially dangerous lesion and require interruption of treatment and careful investigation. Although clinically variable, the typical patient with methotrexate induced lung disease presents with fever, cough, dyspnea, hypoxemia, and an infiltrate on chest X-ray; infection needs to be excluded. This lesion can occur at all dosages.

Renal

High doses of methotrexate used in the treatment of osteosarcoma may cause renal damage leading to acute renal failure. Nephrotoxicity is due primarily to the precipitation of methotrexate and 7-hydroxymethotrexate in the renal tubules. Close attention to renal function including adequate hydration, urine alkalinization and measurement of serum methotrexate and creatinine levels are essential for safe administration.

Skin

Severe, occasionally fatal, dermatologic reactions, including toxic epidermal necrolysis, Stevens-Johnson syndrome, exfoliative dermatitis, skin necrosis, and erythema multiforme, have been reported in children and adults, within days of oral, intramuscular, intravenous, or intrathecal methotrexate administration. Reactions were noted after single or multiple, low, intermediate or high doses of methotrexate in patients with neoplastic and non-neoplastic diseases.

Other Precautions

Methotrexate should be used with extreme caution in the presence of debility.

Methotrexate exits slowly from third space compartments (*e.g.,* pleural effusions or ascites). This results in a prolonged terminal plasma half-life and unexpected toxicity.

In patients with significant third space accumulations, it is advisable to evacuate the fluid before treatment and to monitor plasma methotrexate levels.

Lesions of psoriasis may be aggravated by concomitant exposure to ultraviolet radiation. Radiation dermatitis and sunburn may be "recalled" by the use of methotrexate.

DRUG INTERACTIONS

Non-steroidal anti-inflammatory drugs should not be administered prior to or concomitantly with the high doses of methotrexate used in the treatment of osteosarcoma. Concomitant administration of some NSAIDs with high dose methotrexate therapy has been reported to elevate and prolong serum methotrexate levels, resulting in deaths from severe hematologic and gastrointestinal toxicity.

Caution should be used when NSAIDs and salicylates are administered concomitantly with lower doses of methotrexate. These drugs have been reported to reduce the tubular secretion of methotrexate in an animal model and may enhance its toxicity.

Despite the potential interactions, studies of methotrexate in patients with rheumatoid arthritis have usually included concurrent use of constant dosage regimens of NSAIDs, without apparent problems. It should be appreciated, however, that the doses used in rheumatoid arthritis (7.5 to 15 mg/wk) are somewhat lower than those used in psoriasis and that larger doses could lead to unexpected toxicity.

Methotrexate is partially bound to serum albumin, and toxicity may be increased because of displacement by certain drugs, such as salicylates, phenylbutazone, phenytoin, and sulfonamides. Renal tubular transport is also diminished by probenecid; use of methotrexate with this drug should be carefully monitored.

In the treatment of patients with osteosarcoma, caution must be exercised if high-dose methotrexate is administered in combination with a potentially nephrotoxic chemotherapeutic agent (*e.g.,* cisplatin).

Oral antibiotics such as tetracycline, chloramphenicol, and nonabsorbable broad spectrum antibiotics, may decrease intestinal absorption of methotrexate or interfere with the enterohepatic circulation by inhibiting bowel flora and suppressing metabolism of the drug by bacteria.

Penicillins may reduce the renal clearance of methotrexate; increased serum concentrations of methotrexate with concomitant hematologic and gastrointestinal toxicity have been observed with high and low dose methotrexate. Use of methotrexate with penicillins should be carefully monitored.

The potential for increased hepatotoxicity when methotrexate is administered with other hepatotoxic agents has not been evaluated. However, hepatotoxicity has been reported in such cases. Therefore, patients receiving concomitant therapy with methotrexate and other potential hepatotoxins (*e.g.,* azathioprine, retinoids, sulfasalazine) should be closely monitored for possible increased risk of hepatotoxicity.

Methotrexate may decrease the clearance of theophylline; theophylline levels should be monitored when used concurrently with methotrexate.

Vitamin preparations containing folic acid or its derivatives may decrease responses to systemically administered methotrexate. Preliminary animal and human studies have shown that small quantities of intravenously administered leucovorin enter the CSF primarily as 5-methyltetrahydrofolate and, in humans, remain 1-3 orders of magnitude lower than the usual methotrexate concentrations following intrathecal administration. However, high doses of leucovorin may reduce the efficacy of intrathecally administered methotrexate.

Folate deficiency states may increase methotrexate toxicity. Trimethoprim/sulfamethoxazole has been reported rarely to increase bone marrow suppression in patients receiving methotrexate, probably by an additive antifolate effect.

ADVERSE REACTIONS

IN GENERAL, THE INCIDENCE AND SEVERITY OF ACUTE SIDE EFFECTS ARE RELATED TO DOSE AND FREQUENCY OF ADMINISTRATION. THE MOST SERIOUS REACTIONS ARE DISCUSSED ABOVE UNDER ORGAN SYSTEM TOXICITY IN PRECAUTIONS. THAT SECTION SHOULD ALSO BE CONSULTED WHEN LOOKING FOR INFORMATION ABOUT ADVERSE REACTIONS WITH METHOTREXATE.

The most frequently reported adverse reactions include ulcerative stomatitis, leukopenia, nausea, and abdominal distress. Other frequently reported adverse effects are malaise, undue fatigue, chills and fever, dizziness and decreased resistance to infection.

Other adverse reactions that have been reported with methotrexate are listed below by organ system. In the oncology setting, concomitant treatment and the underlying disease make specific attribution of a reaction to methotrexate difficult.

Alimentary System: Gingivitis, pharyngitis, stomatitis, anorexia, nausea, vomiting, diarrhea, hematemesis, melena, gastrointestinal ulceration and bleeding, enteritis, pancreatitis.

Blood and Lymphatic System Disorders: Suppressed hematopoiesis causing anemia, aplastic anemia, leukopenia and/or thrombocytopenia. Hypogammaglobulinemia has been reported rarely.

Cardiovascular: Pericarditis, pericardial effusion, hypotension, and thromboembolic events (including arterial thrombosis, cerebral thrombosis, deep vein thrombosis, retinal vein thrombosis, thrombophlebitis, and pulmonary embolus).

Central Nervous System: Headaches, drowsiness, blurred vision, transient blindness, speech impairment including dysarthria and aphasia, hemiparesis, paresis and convulsions have also occurred following administration of methotrexate. Following low doses, there have been occasional reports of transient subtle cognitive dysfunction, mood alteration, unusual cranial sensations, leukoencephalopathy, or encephalopathy.

Infection: There have been case reports of sometimes fatal opportunistic infections in patients receiving methotrexate therapy for neoplastic and non-neoplastic diseases. *Pneumocystis carinii* pneumonia was the most common infection. Other reported infections included sepsis, nocardiosis, histoplasmosis, cryptococcosis, *Herpes zoster, H. simplex* hepatitis, and disseminated *H. simplex.*

Musculoskeletal System: Stress fracture.

Ophthalmic: Conjunctivitis, serious visual changes of unknown etiology.

Pulmonary System: Respiratory fibrosis, respiratory failure, interstitial pneumonitis deaths have been reported, and chronic interstitial obstructive pulmonary disease has occasionally occurred.

Skin: Erythematous rashes, pruritus, urticaria, photosensitivity, pigmentary changes, alopecia, ecchymosis, telangiectasia, acne, furunculosis, erythema multiforme, toxic epidermal necrolysis, Stevens-Johnson Syndrome, skin necrosis, skin ulceration, and exfoliative dermatitis.

Urogenital System: Severe nephropathy or renal failure, azotemia, cystitis, hematuria; defective oogenesis or spermatogenesis, transient oligospermia, menstrual dysfunction, vaginal discharge, and gynecomastia; infertility, abortion, fetal defects.

Other rarer reactions related to or attributed to the use of methotrexate such as nodulosis, vasculitis, arthralgia/myalgia, loss of libido/impotence, diabetes, osteoporosis, sudden death, reversible lymphomas, tumor lysis syndrome, soft tissue necrosis and osteonecrosis. Anaphylactoid reactions have been reported.

ADVERSE REACTIONS IN DOUBLE-BLIND RHEUMATOID ARTHRITIS STUDIES

The approximate incidences of methotrexate attributed (*i.e.,* placebo rate subtracted) adverse reactions in 12-18 week double-blind studies of patients (n=128) with rheumatoid arthritis treated with low-dose oral (7.5 to 15 mg/wk) pulse methotrexate, are listed below. Virtually all of these patients were on concomitant nonsteroidal anti-inflammatory drugs and some were also taking low dosages of corticosteroids. Hepatic histology was not examined in these short-term studies. (See PRECAUTIONS.)

Incidence greater than 10%: Elevated liver function tests 15%, nausea/vomiting 10%.

Incidence 3-10%: Stomatitis, thrombocytopenia, (platelet count less than 100,000/mm^3).

Incidence 1-3%: Rash/pruritus/dermatitis, diarrhea, alopecia, leukopenia (WBC less than 3000/mm^3), pancytopenia, dizziness.

Two other controlled trails of patients (n=680) with rheumatoid arthritis on 7.5 to 15 mg/wk oral doses showed an incidence of interstitial pneumonitis of 1%. (See PRECAUTIONS.)

Other less common reactions included decreased hematocrit, headache, upper respiratory infection, anorexia, arthralgias, chest pain, coughing, dysuria, eye discomfort, epistaxis, fever, infection, sweating, tinnitus, and vaginal discharge.

ADVERSE REACTIONS IN PSORIASIS

There are no recent placebo-controlled trials in patients with psoriasis. There are two literature reports (Roenigk, 1969 and Nyfors, 1978) describing large series (n=204, 248) of psoriasis patients treated with methotrexate. Dosages ranged up to 25 mg/wk and treatment was administered for up to 4 years. With the exception of alopecia, photosensitivity, and "burning of skin lesions" (each 3-10%), the adverse reaction rates in these reports were very similar to those in the rheumatoid arthritis studies. Rarely, painful plaque erosions may appear.

ADVERSE REACTIONS IN JRA STUDIES

The approximate incidences of adverse reactions reported in pediatric patients with JRA treated with oral, weekly doses of methotrexate (5-20 mg/m^2/wk or 0.1 to 0.65 mg/kg/wk) were as follows (virtually all patients were receiving concomitant nonsteroidal anti-inflammatory drugs, and some also were taking low doses of corticosteroids): elevated liver function tests, 14%; gastrointestinal reactions (*e.g.,* nausea, vomiting, diarrhea), 11%; stomatitis, 2%, leukopenia, 2%; headache, 1.2%; alopecia, 0.5%; dizziness, 0.2%; and rash, 0.2%. Although there is experience with dosing up to 30 mg/m^2/wk in JRA, the published data for doses above 20 mg/m^2/wk are too limited to provide realiable estimates of adverse reaction rates.

DOSAGE AND ADMINISTRATION

NEOPLASTIC DISEASES

Oral administration in tablet form is often preferred when low doses are being administered since absorption is rapid and effective serum levels are obtained. Methotrexate sodium injection and for injection may be given by the intramuscular, intravenous, intra-arterial or intrathecal route. However, the preserved formulation contains benzyl alcohol and must not be used for intrathecal or high dose therapy. Parenteral drug products should be inspected visually for particulate matter and discoloration prior to administration, whenever solution and container permit.

M

Choriocarcinoma and Similar Trophoblastic Diseases

Methotrexate is administered orally or intramuscularly in doses of 15-30 mg daily for a 5 day course. Such courses are usually repeated for 3-5 times as required, with rest periods of 1 or more weeks interposed between courses, until any manifesting toxic symptoms subside. The effectiveness of therapy is ordinarily evaluated by 24 hour quantitative analysis of urinary chorionic gonadotropin (hCG), which should return to normal or less than 50 IU/24 hours usually after the third or fourth course and usually be followed by a complete resolution of measurable lesions in 4-6 weeks. One to two courses of methotrexate after normalization of hCG is usually recommended. Before each course of the drug careful clinical assessment is essential. Cyclic combination therapy of methotrexate with other antitumor drugs has been reported as being useful.

Since hydatidiform mole may precede choriocarcinoma, prophylactic chemotherapy with methotrexate has been recommended.

Chorioadenoma destruens is considered to be an invasive form of hydatidiform mole. Methotrexate is administered in these disease states in doses similar to those recommended for choriocarcinoma.

Leukemia

Acute lymphoblastic leukemia in pediatric patients and young adolescents is the most responsive to present day chemotherapy. In young adults and older patients, clinical remission is more difficult to obtain and early relapse is more common.

Methotrexate alone or in combination with steroids was used initially for induction of remission in acute lymphoblastic leukemias. More recently corticosteroid therapy, in combination with other antileukemic drugs or in cyclic combinations with methotrexate included, has appeared to produce rapid and effective remissions. When used for induction, methotrexate in doses of 3.3 mg/m^2 in combination with 60 mg/m^2 of prednisone, given daily, produced remissions in 50% of patients treated, usually within a period of 4-6 weeks. Methotrexate in combination with other agents appears to be the drug of choice for securing maintenance of drug-induced remissions. When remission is achieved and supportive care has produced general clinical improvement, maintenance therapy is initiated, as follows: Methotrexate is administered 2 times weekly either by mouth or intramuscularly in total weekly doses of 30 mg/m^2. It has also been given in doses of 2.5 mg/kg intravenously every 14 days. If and when relapse does occur, reinduction of remission can again usually be obtained by repeating the initial induction regimen.

A variety of combination chemotherapy regimens have been used for both induction and maintenance therapy in acute lymphoblastic leukemia. The physician should be familiar with the new advances in antileukemic therapy.

Meningeal Leukemia

In the treatment or prophylaxis of meningeal leukemia, methotrexate must be administered intrathecally. Preservative-free methotrexate is diluted to a concentration of 1 mg/ml in an appropriate sterile, preservative-free medium such as 0.9% sodium chloride injection.

The cerebrospinal fluid volume is dependent on age and not on body surface area. The CSF is at 40% of the adult volume at birth and reaches the adult volume in several years.

Intrathecal methotrexate administration at a dose of 12 mg/m^2 (maximum 15 mg) has been reported to result in low CSF methotrexate concentrations and reduced efficacy in pediatric patients and high concentrations and neurotoxicity in adults. The following dosage regimen is based on age instead of body surface area (see TABLE 1).

TABLE 1

Age	Dose
<1 years	6 mg
1 years	8 mg
2 years	10 mg
3 years or older	12 mg

In one study in patients under the age of 40, this dosage regimen appeared to result in more consistent CSF methotrexate concentrations and less neurotoxicity. Another study in pediatric patients with acute lymphocytic leukemia compared this regimen to a dose of 12 mg/m^2 (maximum 15 mg), a significant reduction in the rate of CNS relapse was observed in the group whose dose was based on age.

Because the CSF volume and turnover may decrease with age, a dose reduction may be indicated in elderly patients.

For the treatment of meningeal leukemia, intrathecal methotrexate may be given at intervals of 2-5 days. However, administration at intervals of less than 1 week may result in increased subacute toxicity. Methotrexate is administered until the cell count of the cerebrospinal fluid returns to normal. At this point one additional dose is advisable. For prophylaxis against meningeal leukemia, the dosage is the same as for treatment except for the intervals of administration. On this subject, it is advisable for the physician to consult the medical literature.

Untoward side effects may occur with any given intrathecal injection and are commonly neurological in character. Large doses may cause convulsions. Methotrexate given by the intrathecal route appears significantly in the systemic circulation and may cause systemic methotrexate toxicity. Therefore, systemic antileukemic therapy with the drug should be appropriately adjusted, reduced, or discontinued. Focal leukemic involvement of the central nervous system may not respond to intrathecal chemotherapy and is best treated with radiotherapy.

Lymphomas

In Burkitt's tumor, Stages I-II, methotrexate has produced prolonged remissions in some cases. Recommended dosage is 10-25 mg/day orally for 4-8 days. In Stage III, methotrexate is commonly given concomitantly with other antitumor agents. Treatment in all stages usually consists of several courses of the drug interposed with 7-10 day rest periods. Lymphosarcomas in Stage III may respond to combined drug therapy with methotrexate given in doses of 0.625 to 2.5 mg/kg daily.

Mycosis Fungoides (cutaneous T cell lymphoma)

Therapy with methotrexate as a single agent appears to produce clinical responses in up to 50% of patients treated. Dosage in early stages is usually 5-50 mg once weekly. Dose reduction or cessation is guided by patient response and hematologic monitoring. Methotrexate has also been administered twice weekly in doses ranging from 15 to 37.5 mg in patients who have responded poorly to weekly therapy. Combination chemotherapy regimens that include intravenous methotrexate administered at higher doses with leucovorin rescue have been utilized in advanced stages of the disease.

Osteosarcoma

An effective adjuvant chemotherapy regimen requires the administration of several cytotoxic chemotherapeutic agents. In addition to high-dose methotrexate with leucovorin rescue, these agents may include doxorubicin, cisplatin, and the combination of bleomycin, cyclophosphamide and dactinomycin (BCD) in the doses and schedule shown in TABLE 2. The starting dose for high dose methotrexate treatment is 12 g/m^2. If this dose is not sufficient to produce a peak serum methotrexate concentration of 1000 µM (10^{-3} mol/L) at the end of the methotrexate infusion, the dose may be escalated to 15 g/m^2 in subsequent treatments. If the patient is vomiting or is unable to tolerate oral medication, leucovorin is given IV or IM at the same dose and schedule.

TABLE 2

Drug*	Dose*	Treatment Week After Surgery
Methotrexate	12 g/m^2 IV as 4 hour infusion (starting dose)	4, 5, 6, 7, 11, 12, 15, 16, 29, 30, 44, 45
Leucovorin	15 mg orally every 6 hours for 10 doses starting at 24 hours after start of methotrexate infusion	
Doxorubicin† as a single drug	30 mg/m^2/day IV × 3 days	8, 17
Doxorubicin†	50 mg/m^2 IV	20, 23, 33, 36
Cisplatin†	100 mg/m^2 IV	20, 23, 33, 36
Bleomycin†	15 units/m^2 IV × 2 days	2, 13, 26, 39, 42
Cyclophosphamide†	600 mg/m^2 IV × 2 days	2, 13, 26, 39, 42
Dactinomycin†	0.6 mg/m^2 IV × 2 days	2, 13, 26, 39, 42

* Link MP, Goorin AM, Miser AW, *et al.:* The effect of adjuvant chemotherapy on relapse-free survival in patients with osteosarcoma of the extremity. *N Engl J of Med* 1986; 314(No.25):1600-1606.

† See each respective package insert for full prescribing information. Dosage modifications may be necessary because of drug-induced toxicity.

When these higher doses of methotrexate are to be administered, the following safety guidelines should be closely observed.

Guidelines for Methotrexate Therapy With Leucovorin Rescue

1. Administration of methotrexate should be delayed until recovery if:
   - the WBC count is less than 1500/µl
   - the neutrophil count is less than 200/µl
   - the platelet count is less than 75,000/µl
   - the serum bilirubin level is greater than 1.2 mg/dl
   - the SGPT level is greater than 450 U
   - mucositis is present, until there is evidence of healing
   - persistent pleural effusion is present; this should be drained dry prior to infusion.
2. Adequate renal function must be documented.
   a. Serum creatinine must be normal, and creatinine clearance must be greater than 60 ml/min, before initiation of therapy.
   b. Serum creatinine must be measured prior to each subsequent course of therapy. If serum creatinine has increased by 50% or more compared to a prior value, the creatinine clearance must be measured and documented to be greater than 60 ml/min (even if the serum creatinine is still within the normal range).
3. Patients must be well hydrated, and must be treated with sodium bicarbonate for urinary alkalinization.
   a. Administer 1000 ml/m^2 of intravenous fluid over 6 hours prior to initiation of the methotrexate infusion. Continue hydration at 125 ml/m^2/h (3 L/m^2/day) during the methotrexate infusion, and for 2 days after the infusion has been completed.
   b. Alkalinize urine to maintain pH above 7.0 during methotrexate infusion and leucovorin calcium therapy. This can be accomplished by the administration of sodium bicarbonate orally or by incorporation into a separate intravenous solution.
4. Repeat serum creatinine and serum methotrexate 24 hours after starting methotrexate and at least once daily until the methotrexate level is below 5×10^{-8} mol/L (0.05 µM).
5. TABLE 3 provides guidelines for leucovorin calcium dosage based upon serum methotrexate levels.

   Patients who experience delayed early methotrexate elimination are likely to develop nonreversible oliguric renal failure. In addition to appropriate leucovorin therapy, these patients require continuing hydration and urinary alkalinization, and close monitoring of fluid and electrolyte status, until the serum methotrexate level has fallen to below 0.05 µM and the renal failure has resolved. If necessary, acute, intermittent hemodialysis with a high-flux dialyzer may also be beneficial in these patients.
6. Some patients will have abnormalities in methotrexate elimination, or abnormalities in renal function following methotrexate administration, which are significant but less severe than the abnormalities described in TABLE 3. These abnormalities may or may not be associated with significant clinical toxicity. If significant clinical toxicity is observed, leucovorin rescue should be extended for an additional 24 hours (total 14 doses over 84 hours) in subsequent courses of therapy. The possibility that the patient is taking other medications which interact with methotrexate (*e.g.*, medications which may interfere

with methotrexate binding to serum albumin, or elimination) should always be reconsidered when laboratory abnormalities or clinical toxicities are observed.

CAUTION: DO NOT ADMINISTER LEUCOVORIN INTRATHECALLY.

PSORIASIS, RHEUMATOID ARTHRITIS, AND JUVENILE RHEUMATOID ARTHRITIS

Adult Rheumatoid Arthritis

Recommended starting dosage schedules:

Single oral doses of 7.5 mg once weekly.

Divided oral dosages of 2.5 mg at 12 mg at 12 hour intervals for 3 doses given as a course once weekly.

Polyarticular-Course Juvenile Rheumatoid Arthritis

The recommended starting dose is 10 mg/m^2 given once weekly.

For either adult RA or polyarticular-course JRA dosages may be adjusted gradually to achieve an optimal response. Limited experience shows a significant increase in the incidence and severity; of serious toxic reactions, especially bone marrow suppression, at doses greater than 20 mg/wk in adults. Although there is experience with doses up to 30 mg/m^2/wk in children, there are too few published data to access how doses over 20 mg/m^2/wk might affect the risk of serious toxicity in children. Experience does suggest, however that children receiving 20-30 mg/m^2/wk (0.65 to 1.0 mg/kg/wk) may have better absorption and fewer gastrointestinal side effects if methotrexate is administered either intramuscularly or subcutaneously.

Therapeutic response usually begins within 3-6 weeks and the patient may continue to improve for anther 12 weeks or more.

The optimal duration of therapy is unknown. Limited data available from long-term studies in adults indicate that the initial clinical improvement is maintained for at least 2 years with continued therapy. When methotrexate is discontinued, the arthritis usually worsens within 3-6 weeks.

The patient should be fully informed of the risks involved and should be under constant supervision of the physician. (See PRECAUTIONS, Information for the Patient.) Assessment of hematologic, hepatic, renal, and pulmonary function should be made by history, physical examination, and laboratory tests before beginning, periodically during, and before reinstituting methotrexate therapy. (See PRECAUTIONS.) Appropriate steps should be taken to avoid conception during methotrexate therapy. (See PRECAUTIONS and CONTRAINDICATIONS.)

Weekly therapy may be instituted with the Rheumatrex Methotrexate Sodium 2.5 mg Tablet Dose Packs which are designed to provide doses over a range of 5-15 mg administered as a single weekly dose. The dose packs are not recommended for administration of methotrexate in weekly doses greater than 15 mg. All schedules should be continually tailored to the individual patient. An initial test dose may be given prior to the regular dosing schedule to detect any extreme sensitivity to adverse effects. (See ADVERSE REACTIONS.) Maximal myelosuppression usually occurs in 7-10 days.

Psoriasis

Recommended starting dosage schedules:

Weekly single oral, IM or IV dose schedule: 10-25 mg/wk until adequate response is achieved.

Divided oral dose schedule: 2.5 mg at 12 hour intervals for 3 doses.

Dosages in each schedule may be gradually adjusted to achieve optimal clinical response; 30 mg/wk should not ordinarily be exceeded.

Once optimal clinical response has been achieved, each dosage schedule should be reduced to the lowest possible amount of drug and to the longest possible rest period. The use of methotrexate may permit the return to conventional topical therapy, which should be encouraged.

HANDLING AND DISPOSAL

Procedures for proper handling and disposal of anticancer drugs should be considered. Several guidelines on this subject have been published.[1-7] There is no general agreement that all of the procedures recommended in the guidelines are necessary or appropriate.

RECONSTITUTION OF LYOPHILIZED POWDERS

Reconstitute immediately prior to use.

Methotrexate sodium for injection should be reconstituted with an appropriate sterile, preservative free medium such as 5% dextrose solution, or sodium chloride injection. Reconstitute the 20 mg vial to a concentration no greater than 25 mg/ml. The 1 g vial should be reconstituted with 19.4 ml to a concentration of 50 mg/ml. When high doses of methotrexate are administered by IV infusion, the total dose is diluted in 5% dextrose solution.

For intrathecal injection, reconstitute to a concentration of 1 mg/ml with an appropriate sterile, preservative-free medium such as sodium chloride injection.

DILUTION INSTRUCTIONS FOR LIQUID METHOTREXATE SODIUM INJECTION PRODUCTS

Methotrexate Sodium Injection, Contains Preservative

If desired, the solution may be further diluted with a compatible medium such as sodium chloride injection. Storage for 24 hours at a temperature of 21-25°C results in a product which is within 90% of label potency.

Methotrexate LPF Sodium (methotrexate sodium injection), Isotonic, Preservative Free, for Single Use Only

If desired, the solution may be further diluted immediately prior to use with an appropriate sterile, preservative-free medium such as 5% dextrose solution, or sodium chloride injection.

TABLE 3 *Leucovorin Rescue Schedules Following Treatment With Higher Doses of Methotrexate*

Clinical Situation	Laboratory Findings	Leucovorin Dosage and Duration
Normal methotrexate elimination	Serum methotrexate level approximately 10 μM at 24 hours after administration, 1 μM at 48 hours, and less than 0.2 μM at 72 hours.	15 mg PO, IM or IV q6h for 60 hours (10 doses starting at 24 hours after start of methotrexate infusion).
Delayed late methotrexate elimination	Serum methotrexate level remaining above 0.2 μM at 72 hours, and more than 0.05 μM at 96 hours after administration.	Continue 15 mg PO, IM or IV q6h, until methotrexate level is less than 0.05 μM.
Delayed early methotrexate elimination and/or evidence of acute renal injury	Serum methotrexate level of 50 μM or more at 24 hours, or 5 μM or more at 48 hours after administration, OR; a 100% or greater increase in serum creatinine level at 24 hours after methotrexate administration (*e.g.*, an increase from 0.5 mg/dl to a level of 1 mg/dl or more).	150 mg IV q3h, until methotrexate level is less than 1 μM; then 15 mg IV q3h, until methotrexate level is less than 0.05 μM.

HOW SUPPLIED

PARENTERAL

Methotrexate sodium for injection, lyophilized, preservative free, for single use only:

Each 20 mg and 1 g vial of lyophilized powder contains methotrexate sodium equivalent to 20 mg and 1 g methotrexate respectively.

Methotrexate LPF sodium, isotonic liquid, preservative free, for single use only:

Each 25 mg/ml, 2 ml, 4 ml, 8 ml and 10 ml vial contains methotrexate sodium equivalent to 50 mg, 100 mg, 200 mg and 250 mg methotrexate respectively.

Methotrexate sodium injection, isotonic liquid, contains preservative:

Each 25 mg/ml, 2 ml and 10 ml vial contains methotrexate sodium equivalent to 50 mg and 250 mg methotrexate respectively.

Storage: Store at controlled room temperature, 20-25°C (68-77°F); excursions permitted to 15-30°C (59-86°F). PROTECT FROM LIGHT.

ORAL

Methotrexate Sodium Tablets contain an amount of methotrexate sodium equivalent to 2.5 mg of methotrexate and are round, convex, yellow tablets, engraved with "LL" on one side, scored in half on the other side, and engraved with "M" above the score, and "1" below.

Storage: Store at controlled room temperature 20-25°C (68-77°F); excursions permitted to 15-30°C (59-86°F). Protect from light.

PRODUCT LISTING - RATED THERAPEUTICALLY EQUIVALENT

Powder For Injection - Injectable - 1 Gm

1's	$61.39	GENERIC, American Pharmaceutical Partners	63323-0122-50
1's	$61.44	GENERIC, Immunex Corporation	58406-0671-05
1's	$61.44	GENERIC, Xanodyne Pharmacal Inc	66479-0139-29

Powder For Injection - Injectable - 20 mg

1's	$5.03	GENERIC, Immunex Corporation	58406-0671-01
1's	$5.03	GENERIC, Immunex Corporation	58406-0673-01

Powder For Injection - Injectable - 50 mg

1's	$4.75	GENERIC, Immunex Corporation	58406-0671-03

Solution - Injectable - 25 mg/ml

2 ml	$4.75	GENERIC, Immunex Corporation	58406-0681-14
2 ml	$4.75	GENERIC, Immunex Corporation	58406-0683-15
2 ml	$4.75	GENERIC, Xanodyne Pharmacal Inc	66479-0135-01
2 ml	$4.75	GENERIC, Xanodyne Pharmacal Inc	66479-0136-11
2 ml	$5.00	GENERIC, American Pharmaceutical Partners	63323-0121-02
2 ml	$5.00	GENERIC, American Pharmaceutical Partners	63323-0123-02
2 ml	$6.50	GENERIC, Baxter Pharmaceutical Products, Inc	10019-0940-01
2 ml	$6.50	GENERIC, Baxter Pharmaceutical Products, Inc	10019-0941-01
2 ml x 10	$5.00	GENERIC, Faulding Pharmaceutical Company	61703-0407-07
2 ml x 10	$6.85	GENERIC, Faulding Pharmaceutical Company	61703-0408-07
2 ml x 10	$50.00	GENERIC, Bedford Laboratories	55390-0031-10
4 ml	$7.63	GENERIC, American Pharmaceutical Partners	63323-0121-04
4 ml	$8.25	GENERIC, Baxter Pharmaceutical Products, Inc	10019-0940-02
4 ml	$8.50	GENERIC, Immunex Corporation	58406-0683-18
4 ml	$8.50	GENERIC, Xanodyne Pharmacal Inc	66479-0136-13
4 ml x 10	$8.70	GENERIC, Faulding Pharmaceutical Company	61703-0408-04
4 ml x 10	$62.50	GENERIC, Bedford Laboratories	55390-0032-10
8 ml	$10.63	GENERIC, American Pharmaceutical Partners	63323-0121-08
8 ml x 10	$17.45	GENERIC, Faulding Pharmaceutical Company	61703-0408-13
8 ml x 10	$93.70	GENERIC, Bedford Laboratories	55390-0033-10

M

Size	Price	Product	NDC
10 ml	$11.88	GENERIC, American Pharmaceutical Partners	63323-0121-10
10 ml	$11.88	GENERIC, American Pharmaceutical Partners	63323-0123-10
10 ml	$20.48	GENERIC, Immunex Corporation	58406-0681-17
10 ml	$20.48	GENERIC, Immunex Corporation	58406-0683-16
10 ml	$20.48	GENERIC, Xanodyne Pharmacal Inc	66479-0135-09
10 ml	$20.48	GENERIC, Xanodyne Pharmacal Inc	66479-0136-19
10 ml	$20.49	GENERIC, Allscripts Pharmaceutical Company	54569-4983-00
10 ml x 10	$20.48	GENERIC, Faulding Pharmaceutical Company	61703-0407-32
10 ml x 10	$26.80	GENERIC, Faulding Pharmaceutical Company	61703-0408-32
10 ml x 10	$118.80	GENERIC, Bedford Laboratories	55390-0034-10
Tablet - Oral - 2.5 mg			
8's	$23.00	GENERIC, Roxane Laboratories Inc	00054-8550-03
8's	$23.79	GENERIC, Barr Laboratories Inc	00555-0572-45
8's	$35.76	RHEUMATREX DOSE PACK, Lederle Laboratories	00005-4507-04
12's	$35.00	GENERIC, Roxane Laboratories Inc	00054-8550-05
12's	$35.43	GENERIC, Udl Laboratories Inc	51079-0670-86
12's	$35.63	GENERIC, Barr Laboratories Inc	00555-0572-46
12's	$61.99	RHEUMATREX DOSE PACK, Lederle Laboratories	00005-4507-05
16's	$49.00	GENERIC, Roxane Laboratories Inc	00054-8550-06
16's	$49.53	GENERIC, Barr Laboratories Inc	00555-0572-47
16's	$50.15	GENERIC, Udl Laboratories Inc	51079-0670-87
16's	$82.73	RHEUMATREX DOSE PACK, Lederle Laboratories	00005-4507-07
20's	$61.00	GENERIC, Roxane Laboratories Inc	00054-8550-07
20's	$61.44	GENERIC, Barr Laboratories Inc	00555-0572-48
20's	$62.72	GENERIC, Udl Laboratories Inc	51079-0670-88
20's	$78.63	GENERIC, Udl Laboratories Inc	51079-0670-05
20's	$103.45	RHEUMATREX DOSE PACK, Lederle Laboratories	00005-4507-09
24's	$72.00	GENERIC, Roxane Laboratories Inc	00054-8550-10
24's	$73.32	GENERIC, Barr Laboratories Inc	00555-0572-49
24's	$75.28	GENERIC, Udl Laboratories Inc	51079-0670-89
24's	$124.10	RHEUMATREX DOSE PACK, Lederle Laboratories	00005-4507-91
36's	$112.00	GENERIC, Aligen Independent Laboratories Inc	00405-4643-36
36's	$121.45	GENERIC, Major Pharmaceuticals Inc	00904-1749-73
36's	$130.05	GENERIC, Ivax Corporation	00182-1539-95
36's	$133.88	GENERIC, Roxane Laboratories Inc	00054-4550-15
36's	$133.88	GENERIC, Watson/Rugby Laboratories Inc	00536-3998-36
36's	$145.80	GENERIC, Barr Laboratories Inc	00555-0572-35
100's	$126.37	FEDERAL UPPER LIMIT, H.C.F.A. F F P	99999-1770-02
100's	$298.00	GENERIC, Aligen Independent Laboratories Inc	00405-4643-01
100's	$299.69	GENERIC, Moore, H.L. Drug Exchange Inc	00839-7905-06
100's	$305.16	GENERIC, Roxane Laboratories Inc	00054-4550-25
100's	$314.25	GENERIC, Geneva Pharmaceuticals	00781-1076-01
100's	$332.39	GENERIC, Ivax Corporation	00182-1539-01
100's	$349.95	GENERIC, Major Pharmaceuticals Inc	00904-1749-60
100's	$355.16	GENERIC, Roxane Laboratories Inc	00054-8550-25
100's	$356.40	GENERIC, Mylan Pharmaceuticals Inc	00378-0014-01
100's	$356.40	GENERIC, Barr Laboratories Inc	00555-0572-02
100's	$363.40	GENERIC, Mutual/United Research Laboratories	00677-1610-01
100's	$363.48	GENERIC, Esi Lederle Generics	59911-5874-01
100's	$392.48	GENERIC, Duramed Pharmaceuticals Inc	51285-0509-02
100's	$525.41	GENERIC, Lederle Laboratories	00005-4507-23
Tablet - Oral - 5 mg			
30's	$228.80	TREXALL, Barr Laboratories Inc	00555-0927-01
Tablet - Oral - 7.5 mg			
30's	$343.20	TREXALL, Barr Laboratories Inc	00555-0928-01
Tablet - Oral - 10 mg			
30's	$457.60	TREXALL, Barr Laboratories Inc	00555-0929-01
Tablet - Oral - 15 mg			
30's	$686.40	TREXALL, Barr Laboratories Inc	00555-0945-01

PRODUCT LISTING - EQUIVALENTS NOT AVAILABLE

Size	Price	Product	NDC
Powder For Injection - Injectable - 1 Gm			
1's	$73.80	GENERIC, Medisca Inc	38779-0035-06
Powder For Injection - Injectable - 20 mg			
1's	$12.85	GENERIC, Xanodyne Pharmacal Inc	66479-0137-21
Solution - Injectable - 25 mg/ml			
50 ml	$43.75	GENERIC, American Pharmaceutical Partners	63323-0121-40
Tablet - Oral - 2.5 mg			
12's	$45.80	GENERIC, Allscripts Pharmaceutical Company	54569-1818-04
16's	$61.07	GENERIC, Allscripts Pharmaceutical Company	54569-1818-05
20's	$72.59	GENERIC, Allscripts Pharmaceutical Company	54569-1818-06
28's	$106.88	GENERIC, Allscripts Pharmaceutical Company	54569-1818-07
32's	$122.14	GENERIC, Allscripts Pharmaceutical Company	54569-1818-08
60's	$229.02	GENERIC, Allscripts Pharmaceutical Company	54569-1818-00
100's	$325.55	GENERIC, Pharma Pac	52959-0244-00

M

Methyldopa (001787)

Categories: Hypertension, essential; Pregnancy Category B; FDA Approved 1962 Dec; WHO Formulary

Drug Classes: Antiadrenergics, central

Brand Names: **Aldomet**; Alfametildopa; Dimal; Elanpres; Highprepin; Hypermet; Medimet; Medomet; Methopa; Methyldopate HCl; Methyldopum; Modepres; Prodop; Scandopa

Foreign Brand Availability: Aldomet-Forte (Hong-Kong); Aldomet-M (Hong-Kong); Aldometil (Austria); Aldomin (Israel); Aldomine (Portugal); Alphadopa (India); Apo-Methyldopa (Canada); Becanta (Japan); Densul (Japan); Dopagyt (India); Dopamet (Bahrain; Cyprus; Czech-Republic; Denmark; Egypt; England; Finland; Indonesia; Iran; Iraq; Ireland; Jordan; Kuwait; Lebanon; Libya; Norway; Oman; Qatar; Republic-of-Yemen; Saudi-Arabia; Switzerland; Syria; United-Arab-Emirates); Dopasian (Thailand); Dopatens (Greece); Dopegyt (Bahamas; Bahrain; Barbados; Belize; Bermuda; Bulgaria; Curacao; Cyprus; Egypt; Guyana; Hong-Kong; Hungary; Iran; Iraq; Jamaica; Jordan; Kuwait; Lebanon; Libya; Netherland-Antilles; Oman; Qatar; Republic-of-Yemen; Saudi-Arabia; Surinam; Syria; Thailand; Trinidad; United-Arab-Emirates); Equibar (France); Grospisk (Japan); H.G. Metil Dopa (Ecuador); Hydopa (Australia); Hypolag (Bahamas; Barbados; Belize; Benin; Bermuda; Burkina-Faso; Curacao; Ethiopia; Gambia; Ghana; Guinea; Guyana; Ivory-Coast; Jamaica; Kenya; Liberia; Malawi; Mali; Mauritania; Mauritius; Morocco; Netherland-Antilles; Niger; Nigeria; Senegal; Seychelles; Sierra-Leone; Sudan; Surinam; Tanzania; Trinidad; Tunia; Uganda; Zambia; Zimbabwe); Hy-po-tone (South-Africa); Medopa (Indonesia; Japan; Thailand); Medopal (Mexico); Medopren (Italy); Meldopa (Philippines); Methoplain (Japan); Novomedopa (Canada); Nudopa (Australia); Pharmet (South-Africa); Polinal (Japan); Presilan (Peru); Presinol (Austria; Bulgaria; Germany); Presinol 500 (Austria; Germany); Prodopa (New-Zealand); Pulsoton (Mexico); Sembrina (Benin; Burkina-Faso; Ethiopia; Finland; Gambia; Ghana; Guinea; Ivory-Coast; Kenya; Liberia; Malawi; Mali; Mauritania; Mauritius; Morocco; Netherlands; Niger; Nigeria; Senegal; Seychelles; Sierra-Leone; Sudan; Tanzania; Tunia; Uganda; Zambia; Zimbabwe); Siamdopa (Thailand); Sinepress (South-Africa); Tensodopa (Peru); Tildopan (Japan)

Cost of Therapy: $26.95 (Hypertension; Aldomet; 250 mg; 2 tablets/day; 30 day supply)
$7.50 (Hypertension; Generic Tablets; 250 mg; 2 tablets/day; 30 day supply)

DESCRIPTION

Methyldopa is an antihypertensive drug.

Methyldopa, the *L*-isomer of alpha-methyldopa, is levo-3-(3,4-dihydroxyphenyl)-2-methylalanine. Its empirical formula is $C_{10}H_{13}NO_4$, with a molecular weight of 211.22.

Methyldopa is a white to yellowish white, odorless fine powder, and is soluble in water.

TABLETS

Aldomet is supplied as tablets, for oral use, in three strengths: 125, 250, or 500 mg of methyldopa per tablet. Inactive ingredients in the tablets are: calcium disodium edetate, cellulose, citric acid, colloidal silicon dioxide, D&C yellow 10, ethylcellulose, guar gum, hydroxypropyl methylcellulose, iron oxide, magnesium stearate, propylene glycol, talc, and titanium dioxide.

ORAL SUSPENSION

Aldomet oral suspension is supplied as a white to off-white preparation; each 5 ml contains 250 mg of methyldopa and alcohol 1%, with benzoic acid 0.1% and sodium bisulfite 0.2% added as preservatives. Inactive ingredients in the oral suspension are: artificial and natural flavors, cellulose, citric acid, confectioner's sugar, disodium edetate, glycerin, polysorbate, purified water, and sodium carboxymethylcellulose.

Storage: Store methyldopa oral suspension below 26°C (78°F) in tight, light-resistant container. Protect from freezing.

INJECTION

Methyldopate HCl injection is an antihypertensive agent for intravenous use. Methyldopate HCl (levo-3-(3,4-dihydroxyphenyl)-2-methylalanine, ethyl ester hydrochloride) is the ethyl ester of methyldopa, supplied as the HCl salt with a molecular weight of 275.73. Methyldopate HCl is more soluble and stable in solution than methyldopa and is the preferred form for IV use. The empirical formula for methyldopate HCl is $C_{12}H_{16}NO_4 \cdot HCl$.

Injectable ester HCl is supplied as a sterile solution in 5 ml vials each of which contains methyldopate HCl (250.0 mg). The inactive ingredients are: citric acid anhydrous (25.0 mg), disodium edetate (2.5 mg), monothioglycerol (10.0 mg), sodium hydroxide to adjust pH. Water for injection, qs to 5 ml, methylparaben 7.5 mg, propylparaben 1 mg, and sodium bisulfite 16 mg added as preservatives.

Storage: Store methyldopate HCl injection below 30°C (86°F). Protect from freezing.

CLINICAL PHARMACOLOGY

Methyldopa is an aromatic-amino-acid decarboxylase inhibitor in animals and in man. Although the mechanism of action has yet to be conclusively demonstrated, the antihypertensive effect of methyldopa probably is due to its metabolism to alpha-methylnorepinephrine, which then lowers arterial pressure by stimulation of central inhibitory alpha-adrenergic receptors, false neurotransmission, and/or reduction of plasma renin activity. Methyldopa has been shown to cause a net reduction in the tissue concentration of serotonin, dopamine, norepinephrine, and epinephrine.

Only methyldopa, the *L*-isomer of alpha-methyldopa, has the ability to inhibit dopa decarboxylase and to deplete animal tissues of norepinephrine. In man, the antihypertensive activity appears to be due solely to the *L*-isomer. About twice the dose of the racemate (*DL*-alpha-methyldopa) is required for equal antihypertensive effect.

Methyldopa has no direct effect on cardiac function and usually does not reduce glomerular filtration rate, renal blood flow, or filtration fraction. Cardiac output usually is maintained without cardiac acceleration. In some patients the heart rate is slowed.

Normal or elevated plasma renin activity may decrease in the course of methyldopa therapy.

Methyldopa reduces both supine and standing blood pressure. Methyldopa usually produces highly effective lowering of the supine pressure with infrequent symptomatic postural hypotension. Exercise hypotension and diurnal blood pressure variations rarely occur.

PHARMACOKINETICS AND METABOLISM

The maximum decrease in blood pressure occurs 4-6 hours after oral dosage. Once an effective dosage level is attained, a smooth blood pressure response occurs in most patients in 12-24 hours. After withdrawal, blood pressure usually returns to pretreatment levels within 24-48 hours.

Methyldopa is extensively metabolized. The known urinary metabolites are: α-methyldopa mono-O-sulfate; 3-O methyl-α-methyldopa; 3, 4-dihydroxyphenylacetone; α-methyldopamine; 3-O-methyl-α-methyldopamine and their conjugates.

Approximately 70% of the drug which is absorbed is excreted in the urine as methyldopa and its mono-O-sulfate conjugate. The renal clearance is about 130 ml/min in normal subjects and is diminished in renal insufficiency. The plasma half-life of methyldopa is 105 minutes. After oral doses, excretion is essentially complete in 36 hours.

Methyldopa crosses the placental barrier, appears in cord blood, and appears in breast milk.

INDICATIONS AND USAGE

Tablets And Oral Suspension: Hypertension.

Injection: Hypertension, when parenteral medication is indicated.

The treatment of hypertensive crises may be initiated with injection methyldopate ester HCl.

NON-FDA APPROVED INDICATIONS

Methyldopa has been used alone or as adjunctive treatment for congestive heart failure, hyperhidrosis, menopausal vasomotor symptoms, neuroleptic-induced tardive dyskinesia, and Raynaud's disease; however, these uses are not approved by the FDA.

CONTRAINDICATIONS

Methyldopa is contraindicated in patients:

- With active hepatic disease, such as acute hepatitis and active cirrhosis.
- With liver disorders previously associated with methyldopa therapy (see WARNINGS).
- With hypersensitivity to any component of these products, including sulfites contained in methyldopa oral suspension and methyldopate injection HCl (see WARNINGS). Methyldopa tablets do not contain sulfites.
- On therapy with monamine oxidase (MAO) inhibitors.

WARNINGS

It is important to recognize that a positive Coombs test, hemolytic anemia, and liver disorders may occur with methyldopa therapy. The rare occurrences of hemolytic anemia or liver disorders could lead to potentially fatal complications unless properly recognized and managed. Read this section carefully to understand these reactions.

With prolonged methyldopa therapy, 10-20% of patients develop a positive direct Coombs test which usually occurs between 6 and 12 months of methyldopa therapy. Lowest incidence is at daily dosage of 1 g or less. This on rare occasions may be associated with hemolytic anemia, which could lead to potentially fatal complications. One cannot predict which patients with a positive direct Coombs test may develop hemolytic anemia.

Prior existence or development of a positive direct Coombs test is not in itself a contraindication to use of methyldopa. If a positive Coombs test develops during methyldopa therapy, the physician should determine whether hemolytic anemia exists and whether the positive Coombs test may be a problem. For example, in addition to a positive direct Coombs test there is less often a positive indirect Coombs test which may interfere with cross matching of blood.

Before treatment is started, it is desirable to do a blood count (hematocrit, hemoglobin, or red cell count) for a baseline or to establish whether there is anemia. Periodic blood counts should be done during therapy to detect hemolytic anemia. It may be useful to do a direct Coombs test before therapy and at 6 and 12 months after the start of therapy.

If Coombs-positive hemolytic anemia occurs, the cause may be methyldopa and the drug should be discontinued. Usually the anemia remits promptly. If not, corticosteroids may be given and other causes of anemia should be considered. If the hemolytic anemia is related to methyldopa, the drug should not be reinstituted.

When methyldopa causes Coombs positivity alone or with hemolytic anemia, the red cell is usually coated with gamma globulin of the IgG (gamma G) class only. The positive Coombs test may not revert to normal until weeks to months after methyldopa is stopped.

Should the need for transfusion arise in a patient receiving methyldopa, both a direct and an indirect Coombs test should be performed. In the absence of hemolytic anemia, usually only the direct Coombs test will be positive. A positive direct Coombs test alone will not interfere with typing or cross matching. If the indirect Coombs test is also positive, problems may arise in the major cross match and the assistance of a hematologist or transfusion expert will be needed.

Occasionally, fever has occurred within the first 3 weeks of methyldopa therapy, associated in some cases with eosinophilia or abnormalities in one or more liver function tests, such as serum alkaline phosphatase, serum transaminases (SGOT, SGPT), bilirubin, and prothrombin time. Jaundice, with or without fever, may occur with onset usually within the first 2-3 months of therapy. In some patients the findings are consistent with those of cholestasis. In others the findings are consistent with hepatitis and hepatocellular injury.

Rarely, fatal hepatic necrosis has been reported after use of methyldopa. These hepatic changes may represent hypersensitivity reactions. Periodic determinations of hepatic function should be done particularly during the first 6-12 weeks of therapy or whenever an unexplained fever occurs. If fever, abnormalities in liver function tests, or jaundice appear, stop therapy with methyldopa. If caused by methyldopa, the temperature and abnormalities in liver function characteristically have reverted to normal when the drug was discontinued. Methyldopa should not be reinstituted in such patients.

Rarely, a reversible reduction of the white blood cell count with a primary effect on the granulocytes has been seen. The granulocyte count returned promptly to normal on discontinuance of the drug. Rare cases of granulocytopenia have been reported. In each instance, upon stopping the drug, the white cell count returned to normal. Reversible thrombocytopenia has occurred rarely.

Methyldopa oral suspension and methyldopate injection HCl (but not methyldopa tablets) contain sodium bisulfite, a sulfite that may cause allergic-type reactions including anaphylactic symptoms and life-threatening or less severe asthmatic episodes in certain susceptible people. The overall prevalence of sulfite sensitivity in the general population is unknown and probably low. Sulfite sensitivity is seen more frequently in asthmatic than in nonasthmatic people.

PRECAUTIONS

GENERAL

Methyldopa should be used with caution in patients with a history of previous liver disease or dysfunction (see WARNINGS).

Some patients taking methyldopa experience clinical edema or weight gain which may be controlled by use of a diuretic. Methyldopa should not be continued if edema progresses or signs of heart failure appear.

Hypertension has recurred occasionally after dialysis in patients given methyldopa because the drug is removed by this procedure.

Rarely involuntary choreoathetotic movements have been observed during therapy with methyldopa in patients with severe bilateral cerebrovascular disease. Should these movements occur, stop therapy.

LABORATORY TESTS

Blood count, Coombs test, and liver function tests are recommended before initiating therapy and at periodic intervals (see WARNINGS).

DRUG/LABORATORY TEST INTERACTIONS

Methyldopa may interfere with measurement of: urinary uric acid by the phosphotungstate method, serum creatinine by the alkaline picrate method, and SGOT by colorimetric methods. Interference with spectrophotometric methods for SGOT analysis has not been reported.

Since methyldopa causes fluorescence in urine samples at the same wave lengths as catecholamines, falsely high levels of urinary catecholamines may be reported. This will interfere with the diagnosis of pheochromocytoma. It is important to recognize this phenomenon before a patient with a possible pheochromocytoma is subjected to surgery. Methyldopa does not interfere with measurement of VMA (vanillylmandelic acid), a test for pheochromocytoma, by those methods which convert VMA to vanillin. Methyldopa is not recommended for the treatment of patients with pheochromocytoma. Rarely, when urine is exposed to air after voiding, it may darken because of breakdown of methyldopa or its metabolites.

CARCINOGENESIS, MUTAGENESIS, AND IMPAIRMENT OF FERTILITY

No evidence of a tumorigenic effect was seen when methyldopa was given for 2 years to mice at doses up to 1800 mg/kg/day or to rats at doses up to 240 mg/kg/day (30 and 4 times the maximum recommended human dose in mice and rats, respectively, when compared on the basis of body weight; 2.5 and 0.6 times the maximum recommended human dose in mice and rats, respectively, when compared on the basis of body surface area; calculations assume a patient weight of 50 kg).

Methyldopa was not mutagenic in the Ames Test and did not increase chromosomal aberration or sister chromatid exchanges in Chinese hamster ovary cells. These *in vitro* studies were carried out both with and without exogenous metabolic activation.

Fertility was unaffected when methyldopa was given to male and female rats at 100 mg/kg/day (1.7 times the maximum daily human dose when compared on the basis of body weight; 0.2 times the maximum daily human dose when compared on the basis of body surface area). Methyldopa decreased sperm count, sperm motility, the number of late spermatids and the male fertility index when given to male rats at 200 and 400 mg/kg/day (3.3 and 6.7 times the maximum daily human dose when compared on the basis of body weight; 0.5 and 1 times the maximum daily human dose when compared on the basis of body surface area).

Long-term studies in animals have not been performed to evaluate the carcinogenic potential of methyldopate hydrochloride; nor have evaluations of this ester's mutagenic potential or potential to affect fertility been carried.

PREGNANCY

Tablets — Pregnancy Category B

Reproduction studies performed with methyldopa at oral doses up to 1000 mg/kg/day in mice, 200 mg/kg in rabbits and 100 mg/kg in rats revealed no evidence of harm to the fetus. These doses are 16.6 times, 3.3 times and 1.7 times, respectively, the maximum daily human dose when compared on the basis of body weight; 1.4 times, 1.1 times and 0.2 times, respectively, when compared on the basis of body surface area; calculations assume a patient weight of 50 kg. There are, however, no adequate and well-controlled studies in pregnant women in the first trimester of pregnancy. Because animal reproduction studies are not always predictive of human response, methyldopa should be used during pregnancy only if clearly needed.

Published reports of the use of methyldopa during all trimesters indicate that if this drug is used during pregnancy the possibility of fetal harm appears remote. In five studies, three of which were controlled, involving 332 pregnant hypertensive women, treatment with methyldopa was associated with an improved fetal outcome. The majority of these women were in the third trimester when methyldopa therapy was begun.

In one study, women who had begun methyldopa treatment between weeks 16 and 20 of pregnancy gave birth to infants whose average head circumference was reduced by a small amount (34.2 ± 1.7 cm vs 34.6 ± 1.3 cm [mean ± 1 SD]). Long-term follow up of 195 (97.5%) of the children born to methyldopa-treated pregnant women (including those who began treatment between weeks 16 and 20) failed to uncover any significant adverse effect on the children. At 4 years of age, the developmental delay commonly seen in children born to hypertensive mothers was less evident in those whose mothers were treated with methyldopa during pregnancy than those whose mothers were untreated. The children of the treated group scored consistently higher than the children of the untreated group on five major indices of intellectual and motor development. At age 7½ developmental scores and intelligence indices showed no significant differences in children of treated or untreated hypertensive women.

Injection — Pregnancy Category C

Animal reproduction studies have not been conducted with methyldopate HCl injection. It is also not known whether methyldopate HCl injection can effect reproduction capacity or can cause fetal harm when given to a pregnant woman. Methyldopate HCl should be given to a pregnant woman only if clearly needed.

NURSING MOTHERS

Methyldopa appears in breast milk. Therefore, caution should be exercised when methyldopa is given to a nursing woman.

PEDIATRIC USE

There are not well-controlled clinical trials in pediatric patients. Information on dosing in pediatric patients is supported by evidence from published literature regarding the treatment of hypertension in pediatric patients. (See DOSAGE AND ADMINISTRATION.)

DRUG INTERACTIONS

When methyldopa is used with other antihypertensive drugs, potentiation of antihypertensive effect may occur. Patients should be followed carefully to detect side reactions on unusual manifestations of drug idiosyncrasy.

Patients may require reduced doses of anesthetics when on methyldopa. If hypotension does occur during anesthesia, it usually can be controlled by vasopressors. The adrenergic receptors remain sensitive during treatment with methyldopa.

When methyldopa and lithium are given concomitantly the patient should be carefully monitored for symptoms of lithium toxicity. Read the circular for lithium preparations.

Several studies demonstrate a decrease in the bioavailability of methyldopa when it is ingested with ferrous sulfate or ferrous gluconate. This may adversely affect blood pressure control in patients treated with methyldopa. Coadministration of methyldopa with ferrous sulfate or ferrous gluconate is not recommended.

Monoamine Oxidase (MAO) Inhibitators: See CONTRAINDICATIONS.

ADVERSE REACTIONS

Sedation, usually transient, may occur during the initial period of therapy or whenever the dose is increased. Headache, asthenia, or weakness may be noted as early and transient symptoms. However, significant adverse effects due to methyldopa have been infrequent and this agent usually is well tolerated.

The following adverse reactions have been reported and, within each category, are listed in order of decreasing severity:

Cardiovascular: Aggravation of angina pectoris, congestive heart failure, prolonged carotid sinus hypersensitivity, orthostatic hypotension (decrease daily dosage), edema or weight gain, bradycardia.

Digestive: Pancreatitis, colitis, vomiting, diarrhea, sialadenitis, sore or "black" tongue, nausea, constipation, distension, flatus, dryness of mouth.

Endocrine: Hyperprolactinemia.

Hematologic: Bone marrow depression, leukopenia, granulocytopenia, thrombocytopenia, hemolytic anemia; positive tests for antinuclear antibody, LE cells, and rheumatoid factor, positive Coombs test.

Hepatic: Liver disorders including hepatitis, jaundice, abnormal liver function tests (see WARNINGS).

Hypersensitivity: Myocarditis, pericarditis, vasculitis, lupus-like syndrome, drug-related fever, eosinophilia.

Nervous System/Psychiatric: Parkinsonism, Bell's palsy, decreased mental acuity, involuntary choreoathetotic movements, symptoms of cerebrovascular insufficiency, psychic disturbances including nightmares and reversible mild psychoses or depression, headache, sedation, asthenia or weakness, dizziness, lightheadedness, paresthesias.

Metabolic: Rise in BUN.

Musculoskeletal: Arthralgia, with or without joint swelling; myalgia.

Respiratory: Nasal stuffiness.

Skin: Toxic epidermal necrolysis, rash.

Urogenital: Amenorrhea, breast enlargement, gynecomastia, lactation, impotence, decreased libido.

DOSAGE AND ADMINISTRATION

TABLETS AND ORAL SUSPENSION

Adults

Initiation of Therapy

The usual starting dosage of methyldopa is 250 mg 2 or 3 times a day in the first 48 hours. The daily dosage then may be increased or decreased, preferably at intervals of not less than 2 days, until an adequate response is achieved. To minimize the sedation, start dosage increases in the evening. By adjustment of dosage, morning hypotension may be prevented without sacrificing control of afternoon blood pressure.

When methyldopa is given to patients on other antihypertensives, the dose of these agents may need to be adjusted to effect a smooth transition. When methyldopa is given with antihypertensives other than thiazides, the initial dosage of methyldopa should be limited to 500 mg daily in divided doses; when methyldopa is added to a thiazide, the dosage of thiazide need not be changed.

Maintenance Therapy

The usual daily dosage of methyldopa is 500 mg to 2 g in 2-4 doses. Although occasional patients have responded to higher doses, the maximum recommended daily dosage is 3 g. Once an effective dosage range is attained, a smooth blood pressure response occurs in most patients in 12-24 hours. Since methyldopa has a relatively short duration of action, withdrawal is followed by return of hypertension usually within 48 hours. This is not complicated by an overshoot of blood pressure.

Occasionally tolerance may occur, usually between the second and third month of therapy. Adding a diuretic or increasing the dosage of methyldopa frequently will restore effective control of blood pressure. A thiazide may be added at any time during methyldopa therapy and is recommended if therapy has not been started with a thiazide or if effective control of blood pressure cannot be maintained on 2 g of methyldopa daily.

Methyldopa is largely excreted by the kidney and patients with impaired renal function may respond to smaller doses. Syncope in older patients may be related to an increased sensitivity and advanced arteriosclerotic vascular disease. This may be avoided by lower doses.

Pediatric Patients

Initial dosage is based on 10 mg/kg of body weight daily in 2-4 doses. The daily dosage then is increased or decreased until an adequate response is achieved. The maximum dosage is 65 mg/kg or 3 g daily, whichever is less. (See PRECAUTIONS, Pediatric Use.)

INJECTION

Methyldopate HCl, when given intravenously in effective doses, causes a decline in blood pressure that may begin in 4-6 hours and last 10-16 hours after injection.

Add the desired dose of methyldopate injection HCl to 100 ml of 5% dextrose injection. Alternatively the desired dose may be given in 5% dextrose in water in a concentration of 100 mg/10 ml. Give this IV infusion slowly over a period of 30-60 minutes.

The vial containing methyldopate HCl should be inspected for particulate matter and discoloration before use whenever solution and container permit.

Adults

The usual adult intravenous dosage is 250-500 mg at 6 hour intervals as required. The maximum recommended IV dose is 1 g every 6 hours.

When control has been obtained, oral therapy with methyldopa tablets may be substituted for intravenous therapy, starting with the same dosage used for the parenteral route.

Since methyldopa has a relatively short duration of action, withdrawal is followed by return of hypertension usually within 48 hours. This is not complicated by an overshoot of blood pressure.

Occasionally tolerance may occur, usually between the second and the third month of therapy. Adding a diuretic or increasing the dosage of methyldopa frequently will restore effective control of blood pressure. A thiazide may be added at any time during methyldopa therapy and is recommended if therapy has not been started with a thiazide or if effective control of blood pressure cannot be maintained on 2 g of methyldopa daily.

Methyldopa is largely excreted by the kidney and patients with impaired renal function may respond to smaller doses. Syncope in older patients may be related to an increased sensitivity and advanced arteriosclerotic vascular disease. This may be avoided in lower doses.

Pediatric Patients

The recommended daily dosage is 20-40 mg/kg of body weight in divided doses every 6 hours. The maximum dosage is 65 mg/kg or 3 g daily, whichever is less. When the blood pressure is under control, continue with oral therapy using the tablet form, in the same dosage as the parenteral route.

HOW SUPPLIED

TABLETS

Aldomet tablets are available in:

125 mg: Yellow, film coated, round tablets, coded "MSD 135" on one side and "ALDOMET" on the other.

250 mg: Yellow, film coated, round tablets, coded "MSD 401" on one side and "ALDOMET" on the other.

500 mg: Yellow, film coated, round tablets, coded "MSD 516" on one side and "ALDOMET" on the other.

Storage: Store methyldopa tablets in a well-closed container at controlled room temperature [15-30°C (59-86°F)].

PRODUCT LISTING - RATED THERAPEUTICALLY EQUIVALENT

Package	Price	Manufacturer	NDC
Solution - Intravenous - 50 mg/ml			
5 ml	$12.50	GENERIC, American Regent Laboratories Inc	00517-8905-01
5 ml x 25	$31.87	GENERIC, Abbott Pharmaceutical	00074-3030-01
5 ml x 25	$42.19	GENERIC, Abbott Pharmaceutical	00074-3405-02
10 ml x 25	$49.68	GENERIC, Abbott Pharmaceutical	00074-3030-02
10 ml x 25	$58.75	GENERIC, Abbott Pharmaceutical	00074-3406-02
100 ml	$87.50	GENERIC, Dupont Pharmaceuticals	00590-5529-63
200 ml	$140.00	GENERIC, Dupont Pharmaceuticals	00590-5529-71
Suspension - Oral - 250 mg/5 ml			
5 ml	$7.71	GENERIC, Bristol-Myers Squibb	00003-2907-10
Tablet - Oral - 125 mg			
100's	$6.75	GENERIC, Us Trading Corporation	56126-0374-11
100's	$10.41	GENERIC, Qualitest Products Inc	00603-4535-21
100's	$11.75	GENERIC, Major Pharmaceuticals Inc	00904-2399-60
100's	$12.65	GENERIC, Sidmak Laboratories Inc	50111-0475-01
100's	$13.95	GENERIC, Geneva Pharmaceuticals	00781-1317-01
100's	$14.84	GENERIC, Moore, H.L. Drug Exchange Inc	00839-7217-06
Tablet - Oral - 250 mg			
25's	$8.63	GENERIC, Pd-Rx Pharmaceuticals	55289-0734-97
30's	$6.62	GENERIC, Pd-Rx Pharmaceuticals	55289-0734-30
30's	$8.12	GENERIC, Medirex Inc	57480-0349-06
100's	$7.86	GENERIC, Us Trading Corporation	56126-0343-11
100's	$12.00	GENERIC, Raway Pharmacal Inc	00686-0200-20
100's	$12.53	GENERIC, Interstate Drug Exchange Inc	00814-4777-14
100's	$13.25	GENERIC, Major Pharmaceuticals Inc	00904-2410-60
100's	$13.95	GENERIC, Moore, H.L. Drug Exchange Inc	00839-7778-06
100's	$15.40	GENERIC, Qualitest Products Inc	00603-4536-21
100's	$15.65	GENERIC, Mova Pharmaceutical Corporation	55370-0815-07

100's	$16.89	GENERIC, Major Pharmaceuticals Inc	00904-2410-61
100's	$18.97	GENERIC, Moore, H.L. Drug Exchange Inc	00839-7119-06
100's	$19.43	GENERIC, Ivax Corporation	00182-1732-89
100's	$21.22	GENERIC, Aligen Independent Laboratories Inc	00405-4652-01
100's	$24.96	GENERIC, Esi Lederle Generics	00005-3850-43
100's	$26.03	GENERIC, Auro Pharmaceutical	55829-0371-10
100's	$26.51	GENERIC, Pd-Rx Pharmaceuticals	55289-0734-01
100's	$28.75	GENERIC, Medirex Inc	57480-0349-01
100's	$29.50	GENERIC, Geneva Pharmaceuticals	00781-1320-01
100's	$31.95	GENERIC, Geneva Pharmaceuticals	00781-1320-13
100's	$33.65	GENERIC, Major Pharmaceuticals Inc	00904-2400-60
100's	$35.65	GENERIC, Ivax Corporation	00172-2931-60
100's	$35.70	GENERIC, Mylan Pharmaceuticals Inc	00378-0611-01
100's	$36.00	GENERIC, Major Pharmaceuticals Inc	00904-2400-61
100's	$36.77	GENERIC, Udl Laboratories Inc	51079-0200-20
100's	$44.92	ALDOMET, Physicians Total Care	54868-0930-01
Tablet - Oral - 500 mg			
25's	$12.50	GENERIC, Pd-Rx Pharmaceuticals	55289-0364-97
100's	$18.00	GENERIC, Raway Pharmacal Inc	00686-0201-20
100's	$18.68	GENERIC, Us Trading Corporation	56126-0344-11
100's	$20.63	GENERIC, Interstate Drug Exchange Inc	00814-4778-14
100's	$24.20	GENERIC, Major Pharmaceuticals Inc	00904-2411-60
100's	$25.95	GENERIC, Moore, H.L. Drug Exchange Inc	00839-7779-06
100's	$29.70	GENERIC, Mova Pharmaceutical Corporation	55370-0816-07
100's	$29.90	GENERIC, Major Pharmaceuticals Inc	00904-2411-61
100's	$31.40	GENERIC, Qualitest Products Inc	00603-4537-21
100's	$35.91	GENERIC, Moore, H.L. Drug Exchange Inc	00839-7120-06
100's	$36.43	GENERIC, Ivax Corporation	00182-1733-89
100's	$37.33	GENERIC, Vangard Labs	00615-2531-01
100's	$39.04	GENERIC, Vangard Labs	00615-2531-13
100's	$44.30	GENERIC, Aligen Independent Laboratories Inc	00405-4653-01
100's	$44.50	GENERIC, Esi Lederle Generics	00005-3851-43
100's	$46.05	GENERIC, Geneva Pharmaceuticals	00781-1322-13
100's	$48.25	GENERIC, Geneva Pharmaceuticals	00781-1322-01
100's	$61.55	GENERIC, Major Pharmaceuticals Inc	00904-2401-60
100's	$63.30	GENERIC, Ivax Corporation	00172-2932-60
100's	$63.30	GENERIC, Mylan Pharmaceuticals Inc	00378-0421-01
100's	$67.00	GENERIC, Major Pharmaceuticals Inc	00904-2401-61
100's	$67.26	GENERIC, Udl Laboratories Inc	51079-0201-20

PRODUCT LISTING - EQUIVALENTS NOT AVAILABLE

Solution - Intravenous - 50 mg/ml			
5 ml	$9.45	GENERIC, Raway Pharmacal Inc	00686-2501-41
10 ml	$18.00	GENERIC, Raway Pharmacal Inc	00686-2502-41
Tablet - Oral - 125 mg			
100's	$9.75	GENERIC, Consolidated Midland Corporation	00223-1584-01
Tablet - Oral - 250 mg			
30's	$6.60	GENERIC, Physicians Total Care	54868-0050-04
30's	$10.71	GENERIC, Allscripts Pharmaceutical Company	54569-0508-01
90's	$18.97	GENERIC, Physicians Total Care	54868-0050-03
100's	$12.50	GENERIC, Consolidated Midland Corporation	00223-1585-01
100's	$20.90	GENERIC, Physicians Total Care	54868-0050-02
Tablet - Oral - 500 mg			
30's	$6.94	GENERIC, Physicians Total Care	54868-1328-00
100's	$14.72	GENERIC, Physicians Total Care	54868-1328-01
100's	$22.50	GENERIC, Consolidated Midland Corporation	00223-1586-01

Methylphenidate Hydrochloride *(001790)*

Categories: Attention deficit hyperactivity disorder; Narcolepsy; DEA Class CII; FDA Approved 1956 Mar; Pregnancy Category C
Drug Classes: Stimulants, central nervous system
Brand Names: Methylphenidate Hcl; **Ritalin**; Ritalin-SR
Foreign Brand Availability: Attenta (Australia); Concerta (Colombia); Concerta XL (England; Ireland); Medikinet (Germany); Metadate E.R. (Israel); Penid (Korea); Rilatine (Belgium); Ritalina (Ecuador); Ritaline (France); Ritaphen (South-Africa); Rubifen (Costa-Rica; Dominican-Republic; El-Salvador; Guatemala; New-Zealand; Panama; Singapore; Spain; Thailand); Tranquilyn (England; Ireland)
Cost of Therapy: $43.07 (Attention Deficit Disorder; Ritalin; 10 mg; 2 tablets/day; 30 day supply)
$21.46 (Attention Deficit Disorder; Generic Tablets; 10 mg; 2 tablets/day; 30 day supply)
$69.89 (Attention Deficit Disorder; Ritalin LA; 20 mg; 1 capsule/day; 30 day supply)
$84.00 (Attention Deficit Disorder; Concerta; 18 mg; 1 tablet/day; 30 day supply)

DESCRIPTION

Note: The trade names have been used throughout this monograph for clarity.

RITALIN AND RITALIN-SR

Ritalin, methylphenidate hydrochloride, is a mild central nervous system (CNS) stimulant, available as tablets of 5, 10, and 20 mg for oral administration; Ritalin-SR is available as sustained-release tablets of 20 mg for oral administration. Methylphenidate hydrochloride is methyl α-phenyl-2-piperidineacetate hydrochloride.

Methylphenidate hydrochloride is a white, odorless, fine crystalline powder. Its solutions are acid to litmus. It is freely soluble in water and in methanol, soluble in alcohol, and slightly soluble in chloroform and in acetone. Its molecular weight is 269.77.

Inactive Ingredients:

Ritalin Tablets: D&C yellow no. 10 (5 and 20 mg tablets), FD&C green no. 3 (10 mg tablets), lactose, magnesium stearate, polyethylene glycol, starch (5 and 10 mg tablets), sucrose, talc, and tragacanth (20 mg tablets).

Ritalin-SR Tablets: Cellulose compounds, cetostearyl alcohol, lactose, magnesium stearate, mineral oil, povidone, titanium dioxide, and zein.

RITALIN LA

Ritalin LA (methylphenidate hydrochloride extended-release capsules) is an extended-release formulation of methylphenidate with a bi-modal release profile. Ritalin LA uses the proprietary SODAS (Spheroidal Oral Drug Absorption System) technology. Each bead-filled Ritalin LA capsule contains half the dose as immediate release beads and half as enteric-coated, delayed-release beads, thus providing an immediate release of methylphenidate and a second delayed release of methylphenidate. Ritalin LA 20, 30, and 40 mg capsules provide in a single dose the same amount of methylphenidate as dosages of 10, 15, or 20 mg of Ritalin tablets given bid.

Inactive ingredients in Ritalin LA: Ammonio methacrylate copolymer, black iron oxide (40 mg capsules only), gelatin, methacrylic acid copolymer, polyethylene glycol, red iron oxide (40 mg capsules only), sugar spheres, talc, titanium dioxide, triethyl citrate, and yellow iron oxide (30 and 40 mg capsules only).

CONCERTA

Concerta is available in 3 tablet strengths. Each extended-release tablet for once-a-day oral administration contains 18, 36, or 54 mg of methylphenidate HCl and is designed to have a 12 hour duration of effect.

Concerta also contains the following inert ingredients: Butylated hydroxytoluene, carnauba wax, cellulose acetate, hydroxypropyl methylcellulose, lactose, phosphoric acid, poloxamer, polyethylene glycol, polyethylene oxides, povidone, propylene glycol, sodium chloride, stearic acid, succinic acid, synthetic iron oxides, titanium dioxide, and triacetin.

System Components and Performance

Concerta uses osmotic pressure to deliver methylphenidate HCl at a controlled rate. The system, which resembles a conventional tablet in appearance, comprises an osmotically active trilayer core surrounded by a semipermeable membrane with an immediate-release drug overcoat. The trilayer core is composed of two drug layers containing the drug and excipients, and a push layer containing osmotically active components. There is a precision-laser drilled orifice on the drug-layer end of the tablet. In an aqueous environment, such as the gastrointestinal tract, the drug overcoat dissolves within 1 hour, providing an initial dose of methylphenidate. Water permeates through the membrane into the tablet core. As the osmotically active polymer excipients expand, methylphenidate is released through the orifice. The membrane controls the rate at which water enters the tablet core, which in turn controls drug delivery. The biologically inert components of the tablet remain intact during gastrointestinal transit and are eliminated in the stool as a tablet shell along with insoluble core components.

CLINICAL PHARMACOLOGY

PHARMACODYNAMICS

Ritalin and Ritalin-SR

Ritalin is a mild central nervous system stimulant.

The mode of action in man is not completely understood, but Ritalin presumably activates the brain stem arousal system and cortex to produce its stimulant effect.

There is neither specific evidence which clearly establishes the mechanism whereby Ritalin produces its mental and behavioral effects in children, nor conclusive evidence regarding how these effects relate to the condition of the central nervous system.

Ritalin LA

Methylphenidate is thought to block the reuptake of norepinephrine and dopamine into the presynaptic neuron and increase the release of these monoamines into the extraneuronal space. Methylphenidate is a racemic mixture comprised of the *d-* and *l-threo* enantiomers. The *d-threo* enantiomer is more pharmacologically active than the *l-threo* enantiomer.

PHARMACOKINETICS

Absorption

Ritalin and Ritalin-SR

Ritalin in the SR tablets is more slowly but as extensively absorbed as in the regular tablets. Relative bioavailability of the SR tablet compared to the Ritalin tablet, measured by the urinary excretion of Ritalin major metabolite (α-phenyl-2-piperidine acetic acid) was 105% (49-168%) in children and 101% (85-152%) in adults. The time to peak rate in children was 4.7 hours (1.3-8.2 hours) for the SR tablets and 1.9 hours (0.3-4.4 hours) for the tablets. An average of 67% of SR tablet dose was excreted in children as compared to 86% in adults.

In a clinical study involving adult subjects who received SR tablets, plasma concentrations of Ritalin's major metabolite appeared to be greater in females than in males. No gender differences were observed for Ritalin plasma concentration in the same subjects.

Ritalin LA

Ritalin LA produces a bi-modal plasma concentration-time profile (*i.e.,* two distinct peaks approximately 4 hours apart) when orally administered to children diagnosed with ADHD and to healthy adults. The initial rate of absorption for Ritalin LA is similar to that of Ritalin tablets as shown by the similar rate parameters between the 2 formulations, *i.e.,* initial lag time (T_{lag}), first peak concentration (C_{max1}), and time to the first peak (T_{max1}), which is reached in 1-3 hours. The mean time to the interpeak minimum (T_{minip}), and time to the second peak (T_{max2}) are also similar for Ritalin LA given once daily and Ritalin tablets given in 2 doses 4 hours apart (see TABLE 1), although the ranges observed are greater for Ritalin LA.

Ritalin LA given once daily exhibits a lower second peak concentration (C_{max2}), higher interpeak minimum concentrations (C_{minip}), and less peak and trough fluctuations than Ritalin tablets given in 2 doses given 4 hours apart. This is due to an earlier onset and more prolonged absorption from the delayed release beads (see TABLE 1).

TABLE 1 *Mean ± SD and Range of Pharmacokinetic Parameters of Methylphenidate After a Single Dose of Ritalin LA and Ritalin Given in 2 Doses 4 Hours Apart*

	Children		Adult Males	
	Ritalin 10 mg/10 mg n=21	Ritalin LA 20 mg n=18	Ritalin 10 mg/10 mg n=9	Ritalin LA 20 mg n=8
T_{lag} (hours)	0.24 ± 0.44 (0-1)	0.28 ± 0.46 (0-1)	1.0 ± 0.5 (0.7-1.3)	0.7 ± 0.2 (0.3-1.0)
T_{max1} (hours)	1.8 ± 0.6 (1-3)	2.0 ± 0.8 (1-3)	1.9 ± 0.4 (1.3-2.7)	2.0 ± 0.9 (1.3-4.0)
C_{max1} (ng/ml)	10.2 ± 4.2 (4.2-20.2)	10.3 ± 5.1 (5.5-26.6)	4.3 ± 2.3 (1.8-7.5)	5.3 ± 0.9 (3.8-6.9)
T_{minip} (hours)	4.0 ± 0.2 (4-5)	4.5 ± 1.2 (2-6)	3.8 ± 0.4 (3.3-4.3)	3.6 ± 0.6 (2.7-4.3)
C_{minip} (ng/ml)	5.8 ± 2.7 (3.1-14.4)	6.1 ± 4.1 (2.9-21.0)	1.2 ± 1.4 (0.0-3.7)	3.0 ± 0.8 (1.7-4.0)
T_{max2} (hours)	5.6 ± 0.7 (5-8)	6.6 ± 1.5 (5-11)	5.9 ± 0.5 (5.0-6.5)	5.5 ± 0.8 (4.3-6.5)
C_{max2} (ng/ml)	15.3 ± 7.0 (6.2-32.8)	10.2 ± 5.9 (4.5-31.1)	5.3 ± 1.4 (3.6-7.2)	6.2 ± 1.6 (3.9-8.3)
AUC(0-∞) (ng/ml × h-1)	102.4 ± 54.6 (40.5-261.6)	86.6 ± 64.0* (43.3-301.44)	37.8 ± 21.9 (14.3-85.3)	45.8 ± 10.0 (34.0-61.6)
T½ (hours)	2.5 ± 0.8 (1.8-5.3)	2.4 ± 0.7* (1.5-4.0)	3.5 ± 1.9 (1.3-7.7)	3.3 ± 0.4 (3.0-4.2)

* n=15.

The relative bioavailability of Ritalin LA given once daily is comparable to the same total dose of Ritalin tablets given in 2 doses 4 hours apart in both children and in adults.

Concerta

Following oral administration of Concerta to adults, plasma methylphenidate concentrations increase rapidly reaching an initial maximum at about 1-2 hours, then increase gradually over the next several hours. Peak plasma concentrations are achieved at about 6-8 hours after which a gradual decrease in plasma levels of methylphenidate begins. Concerta qd minimizes the fluctuations between peak and trough concentrations associated with immediate-release methylphenidate tid. The relative bioavailability of Concerta qd and methylphenidate tid in adults is comparable.

The mean pharmacokinetic parameters in 36 adults following the administration of Concerta 18 mg qd and methylphenidate 5 mg tid are summarized in TABLE 2.

TABLE 2 *Mean ± SD Pharmacokinetic Parameters*

Parameters	Concerta 18 mg qd (n=36)	Methylphenidate 5 mg tid (n=35)
C_{max} (ng/ml)	3.7 ± 1.0	4.2 ± 1.0
T_{max} (hours)	6.8 ± 1.8	6.5 ± 1.8
AUC(∞) (ng·h/ml)	41.8 ± 13.9	38.0 ± 11.0
T½ (hours)	3.5 ± 0.4	3.0 ± 0.5

No differences in the pharmacokinetics of Concerta were noted following single and repeated qd dosing indicating no significant drug accumulation. The AUC and T½ following repeated qd dosing are similar to those following the first dose of Concerta 18 mg.

Dose Proportionality

Ritalin LA

After oral administration of Ritalin LA 20 and 40 mg capsules to adults there is a slight upward trend in the methylphenidate area under the curve (AUC) and peak plasma concentrations (C_{max1} and C_{max2}).

Concerta

Following administration of Concerta in single doses of 18, 36, and 54 mg/day to adults, C_{max} and AUC(0-∞) of d-methylphenidate were proportional to dose, whereas l-methylphenidate C_{max} and AUC(0-∞) increased disproportionately with respect to dose. Following administration of Concerta, plasma concentrations of the l-isomer were approximately 1/40th the plasma concentrations of the d-isomer.

Distribution

Ritalin LA

Binding to plasma proteins is low (10-33%), and the apparent distribution volume at steady-state with intravenous administration has been reported to be approximately 6 L/kg.

Concerta

Plasma methylphenidate concentrations in adults decline biexponentially following oral administration. The half-life of methylphenidate in adults following oral administration of Concerta was approximately 3.5 hours.

Metabolism

Ritalin LA

The absolute oral bioavailability of methylphenidate in children has been reported to be about 30% (range 10-52%), suggesting pronounced presystemic metabolism. Biotransformation of methylphenidate is rapid and extensive leading to the main, de-esterified metabolite α-phenyl-2-piperidine acetic-acid (ritalinic acid). Only small amounts of hydroxylated metabolites (*e.g.*, hydroxymethylphenidate and hydroxyritalinic acid) are detectable in plasma. Therapeutic activity is principally due to the parent compound.

Metabolism and Excretion

Concerta

In adults the metabolism of Concerta qd as evaluated by metabolism to PPA is similar to that of methylphenidate tid. The metabolism of single and repeated qd doses of Concerta is similar.

Elimination

Ritalin LA

In studies with Ritalin LA and Ritalin tablets in adults, methylphenidate from Ritalin tablets is eliminated from plasma with an average half-life of about 3.5 hours, (range 1.3-7.7 hours). In children the average half-life is about 2.5 hours, with a range of about 1.5-5.0 hours. The rapid half-life in both children and adults may result in unmeasurable concentrations between the morning and mid-day doses with Ritalin tablets. No accumulation of methylphenidate is expected following multiple once a day oral dosing with Ritalin LA. The half-life of ritalinic acid is about 3-4 hours.

After oral administration of an immediate release formulation of methylphenidate, 78-97% of the dose is excreted in the urine and 1-3% in the feces in the form of metabolites within 48-96 hours. Only small quantities (<1%) of unchanged methylphenidate appear in the urine. Most of the dose is excreted in the urine as ritalinic acid (60-86%), the remainder being accounted for by minor metabolites.

Food Effects

Ritalin LA

Administration times relative to meals and meal composition may need to be individually titrated.

When Ritalin LA was administered with a high fat breakfast to adults, Ritalin LA had a longer lag time until absorption began and variable delays in the time until the first peak concentration, the time until the interpeak minimum, and the time until the second peak. The first peak concentration and the extent of absorption were unchanged after food relative to the fasting state, although the second peak was approximately 25% lower. The effect of a high fat lunch was not examined.

There were no differences in the pharmacokinetics of Ritalin LA when administered with applesauce, compared to administration in the fasting condition. There is no evidence of dose dumping in the presence or absence of food.

For patients unable to swallow the capsule, the contents may be sprinkled on applesauce and administered (see DOSAGE AND ADMINISTRATION, Ritalin LA).

Concerta

In patients, there were no differences in either the pharmacokinetics or the pharmacodynamic performance of Concerta when administered after a high fat breakfast. There is no evidence of dose dumping in the presence or absence of food.

Special Populations

Age

Ritalin LA

The pharmacokinetics of Ritalin LA was examined in 18 children with ADHD between 7 and 12 years of age. Fifteen (15) of these children were between 10 and 12 years of age. The time until the between peak minimum, and the time until the second peak were delayed and more variable in children compared to adults. After a 20 mg dose of Ritalin LA, concentrations in children were approximately twice the concentrations observed in 18-35 year old adults. This higher exposure is almost completely due to the smaller body size and total volume of distribution in children, as apparent clearance normalized to body weight is independent of age.

Concerta

The pharmacokinetics of Concerta has not been studied in children less than 6 years of age.

Gender

Ritalin LA

There were no apparent gender differences in the pharmacokinetics of methylphenidate between healthy male and female adults when administered Ritalin LA.

Concerta

In healthy adults, the mean dose-adjusted AUC(0-∞) values for Concerta were 36.7 ng·h/ml in men and 37.1 ng·h/ml in women, with no differences noted between the 2 groups.

Race

Concerta

In adults receiving Concerta, dose-adjusted AUC(0-∞) was consistent across ethnic groups; however, the sample size may have been insufficient to detect ethnic variations in pharmacokinetics.

Renal Insufficiency

Ritalin LA and Concerta have not been studied in renally-impaired patients. Renal insufficiency is expected to have minimal effect on the pharmacokinetics of methylphenidate since less than 1% of a radiolabeled dose is excreted in the urine as unchanged compound, and the major metabolite (ritalinic acid), has little or no pharmacologic activity.

Hepatic Insufficiency

Ritalin LA and Concerta have not been studied in patients with hepatic insufficiency. Hepatic insufficiency is expected to have minimal effect on the pharmacokinetics of methylphenidate since it is metabolized primarily to ritalinic acid by nonmicrosomal hydrolytic esterases that are widely distributed throughout the body.

INDICATIONS AND USAGE

RITALIN AND RITALIN-SR

Attention Deficit Disorders, Narcolepsy

Ritalin is indicated as an integral part of a total treatment program which typically includes other remedial measures (psychological, educational, social) for a stabilizing effect in children with a behavioral syndrome characterized by the following group of developmentally inappropriate symptoms: moderate-to-severe distractibility, short attention span, hyperactivity, emotional lability, and impulsivity. The diagnosis of this syndrome should not be made with finality when these symptoms are only of comparatively recent origin. Nonlocalizing (soft) neurological signs, learning disability, and abnormal EEG may or may not be present, and a diagnosis of central nervous system dysfunction may or may not be warranted.

RITALIN LA

Attention Deficit Hyperactivity Disorder (ADHD)

Ritalin LA is indicated for the treatment of Attention-Deficit Hyperactivity Disorder (ADHD).

The efficacy of Ritalin LA in the treatment of ADHD was established in one controlled trial of children aged 6-12 who met DSM-IV criteria for ADHD (see CLINICAL PHARMACOLOGY).

CONCERTA

Attention Deficit Hyperactivity Disorder (ADHD)

Concerta is indicated for the treatment of Attention Deficit Hyperactivity Disorder (ADHD).

The efficacy of Concerta in the treatment of ADHD was established in three controlled trials of children aged 6-12 who met DSM-IV criteria for ADHD (see CLINICAL PHARMACOLOGY).

SPECIAL DIAGNOSTIC CONSIDERATIONS

A diagnosis of Attention Deficit Hyperactivity Disorder (ADHD; DSM-IV) implies the presence of hyperactive-impulsive or inattentive symptoms that caused impairment and were present before age 7 years. The symptoms must cause clinically significant impairment, *e.g.,* in social, academic, or occupational functioning, and be present in 2 or more settings, *e.g.,* school (or work) and at home. The symptoms must not be better accounted for by another mental disorder. For the Inattentive Type, at least 6 of the following symptoms must have persisted for at least 6 months: lack of attention to details/careless mistakes; lack of sustained attention; poor listener; failure to follow through on tasks; poor organization; avoids tasks requiring sustained mental effort; loses things; easily distracted; forgetful. For the Hyperactive-Impulsive Type, at least 6 of the following symptoms must have persisted for at least 6 months: fidgeting/squirming; leaving seat; inappropriate running/climbing; difficulty with quiet activities; "on the go;" excessive talking; blurting answers; can't wait turn; intrusive. The Combined Types requires both inattentive and hyperactive-impulsive criteria to be met.

Specific etiology of this syndrome is unknown, and there is no single diagnostic test. Adequate diagnosis requires the use not only of medical but of special psychological, educational, and social resources. Learning may or may not be impaired. The diagnosis must be based upon a complete history and evaluation of the child and not solely on the presence of the required number of DSM-IV characteristics.

NEED FOR COMPREHENSIVE TREATMENT PROGRAM

Methylphenidate HCl is indicated as an integral part of a total treatment program for ADHD that may include other measures (psychological, educational, social) for patients with this syndrome. Drug treatment may not be indicated for all children with this syndrome. Stimulants are not intended for use in the child who exhibits symptoms secondary to environmental factors and/or other primary psychiatric disorders, including psychosis. Appropriate educational placement is essential and psychosocial intervention is often helpful. When remedial measures alone are insufficient, the decision to prescribe stimulant medication will depend upon the physician's assessment of the chronicity and severity of the child's symptoms.

LONG-TERM USE

Ritalin LA

The effectiveness of Ritalin LA for long-term use, *i.e.,* for more than 2 weeks, has not been systematically evaluated in controlled trials. Therefore, the physician who elects to use Ritalin LA for extended periods should periodically re-evaluate the long-term usefulness of the drug for the individual patient (see DOSAGE AND ADMINISTRATION, Ritalin LA).

Concerta

The effectiveness of Concerta for long-term use, *i.e.,* for more than 4 weeks, has not been systematically evaluated in controlled trials. Therefore, the physician who elects to use Concerta for extended periods should periodically re-evaluate the long-term usefulness of the drug for the individual patient (see DOSAGE AND ADMINISTRATION, Concerta).

CONTRAINDICATIONS

AGITATION

Methylphenidate is contraindicated in marked anxiety, tension, and agitation, since the drug may aggravate these symptoms.

HYPERSENSITIVITY TO METHYLPHENIDATE

Methylphenidate is contraindicated in patients known to be hypersensitive to methylphenidate or other components of the product.

GLAUCOMA

Methylphenidate is contraindicated in patients with glaucoma.

TICS

Methylphenidate is contraindicated in patients with motor tics or with a family history or diagnosis of Tourette's syndrome. See ADVERSE REACTIONS.

MONOAMINE OXIDASE INHIBITORS

Methylphenidate is contraindicated during treatment with monoamine oxidase inhibitors, and also within a minimum of 14 days following discontinuation of treatment with a monoamine oxidase inhibitor (hypertensive crises may result).

WARNINGS

DEPRESSION

Methylphenidate should not be used for severe depression of either exogenous or endogenous origin.

FATIGUE

Methylphenidate should not be used for the prevention or treatment of normal fatigue states.

LONG-TERM SUPPRESSION OF GROWTH

Sufficient data on the safety of long-term use of methylphenidate in children are not yet available. Although a causal relationship has not been established, suppression of growth (*i.e.,* weight gain, and/or height) has been reported with the long-term use of stimulants in children. Therefore, patients requiring long-term therapy should be carefully monitored. Patients who are not growing or gaining weight as expected should have their treatment interrupted. In the double blind placebo controlled study of Ritalin LA, the mean weight gain was greater for patients receiving placebo (+1.0 kg) than for patients receiving Ritalin LA (+0.1 kg).

PSYCHOSIS

Clinical experience suggests that in psychotic patients, administration of methylphenidate may exacerbate symptoms of behavior disturbance and thought disorder.

SEIZURES

There is some clinical evidence that methylphenidate may lower the convulsive threshold in patients with prior history of seizures, with prior EEG abnormalities in the absence of seizures, and, very rarely, in the absence of history of seizures and no prior EEG evidence of seizures. Safe concomitant use of anticonvulsants and methylphenidate has not been established. In the presence of seizures, methylphenidate should be discontinued.

HYPERTENSION AND OTHER CARDIOVASCULAR CONDITIONS

Use cautiously in patients with hypertension. Blood pressure should be monitored at appropriate intervals in patients taking methylphenidate, especially patients with hypertension. Studies of methylphenidate have shown modest increases of resting pulse and systolic and diastolic blood pressure. Therefore, caution is indicated in treating patients whose underlying medical conditions might be compromised by increases in blood pressure or heart rate, *e.g.,* those with pre-existing hypertension, heart failure, recent myocardial infarction, or hyperthyroidism.

VISUAL DISTURBANCE

Symptoms of visual disturbances have been encountered in rare cases. Difficulties with accommodation and blurring of vision have been reported with methylphenidate.

POTENTIAL FOR GASTROINTESTINAL OBSTRUCTION

Because the Concerta tablet is nondeformable and does not appreciably change in shape in the GI tract, Concerta should not ordinarily be administered to patients with preexisting severe gastrointestinal narrowing (pathologic or iatrogenic, for example: small bowel inflammatory disease, "short gut" syndrome due to adhesions or decreased transit time, past history of peritonitis, cystic fibrosis, chronic intestinal pseudoobstruction, or Meckel's diverticulum). There have been rare reports of obstructive symptoms in patients with known strictures in association with the ingestion of other drugs in nondeformable controlled-release formulations. Due to the controlled-release design of the tablet, Concerta should only be used in patients who are able to swallow the tablet whole (see PRECAUTIONS, Information for the Patient, Concerta).

USE IN CHILDREN UNDER 6 YEARS OF AGE

Methylphenidate should not be used in children under 6 years of age, since safety and efficacy in this age group have not been established.

DRUG DEPENDENCE

Methylphenidate should be given cautiously to patients with a history of drug dependence or alcoholism. Chronic abusive use can lead to marked tolerance and psychological dependence with varying degrees of abnormal behavior. Frank psychotic episodes can occur, especially with parenteral abuse. Careful supervision is required during withdrawal from abusive use, since severe depression may occur. Withdrawal following chronic therapeutic use may unmask symptoms of the underlying disorder that may require follow-up.

PRECAUTIONS

Patients with an element of agitation may react adversely; discontinue therapy if necessary.

Drug treatment is not indicated in all cases of this behavioral syndrome and should be considered only in light of the complete history and evaluation of the child. The decision to prescribe Ritalin should depend on the physician's assessment of the chronicity and severity of the child's symptoms and their appropriateness for his/her age. Prescription should not depend solely on the presence of 1 or more of the behavioral characteristics.

When these symptoms are associated with acute stress reactions, treatment with Ritalin is usually not indicated.

Hematologic Monitoring: Periodic CBC, differential, and platelet counts are advised during prolonged therapy.

INFORMATION FOR THE PATIENT

Ritalin LA

The Ritalin LA capsule may be swallowed as whole capsules or the capsule may be opened and sprinkled on a small amount of applesauce. The capsule should not be crushed or chewed or its contents divided.

To sprinkle the contents of the capsule, open the capsule carefully and sprinkle the beads over a spoonful of applesauce. The applesauce should not be warm because it could affect the modified release properties of this formulation. The mixture of drug and applesauce should be consumed immediately in its entirety. The drug and applesauce mixture should not be stored for future use.

Concerta

Patients should be informed that Concerta should be swallowed whole with the aid of liquids. Tablets should not be chewed, divided, or crushed. The medication is contained within a nonabsorbable shell designed to release the drug at a controlled rate. The tablet shell, along with insoluble core components, is eliminated from the body; patients should not be concerned if they occasionally notice in their stool something that looks like a tablet.

CARCINOGENESIS, MUTAGENESIS, AND IMPAIRMENT OF FERTILITY

In a lifetime carcinogenicity study carried out in B6C3F1 mice, methylphenidate caused an increase in hepatocellular adenomas and, in males only, an increase in hepatoblastomas, at a daily dose of approximately 60 mg/kg/day. This dose is approximately 30 times and 4 times the maximum recommended human dose on a mg/kg and mg/m^2 basis, respectively. Hepatoblastoma is a relatively rare rodent malignant tumor type. There was no increase in total malignant hepatic tumors. The mouse strain used is sensitive to the development of hepatic tumors, and the significance of these results to humans is unknown.

Methylphenidate did not cause any increases in tumors in a lifetime carcinogenicity study carried out in F344 rats; the highest dose used was approximately 45 mg/kg/day, which is approximately 22 times and 5 times the maximum recommended human dose on a mg/kg and mg/m^2 basis, respectively.

In a 24 week carcinogenicity study in the transgenic mouse strain p53+/-, which is sensitive to genotoxic carcinogens, there was no evidence of carcinogenicity. Male and female mice were fed diets containing the same concentration of methylphenidate as in the lifetime carcinogenicity study; the high-dose groups were exposed to 60-74 mg/kg/day of methylphenidate.

Methylphenidate was not mutagenic in the *in vitro* Ames reverse mutation assay or in the *in vitro* mouse lymphoma cell forward mutation assay. Sister chromatid exchanges and chromosome aberrations were increased, indicative of a weak clastogenic response, in an *in vitro* assay in cultured Chinese Hamster Ovary (CHO) cells. Methylphenidate was negative *in vivo* in males and females in the mouse bone marrow micronucleus assay.

Methylphenidate did not impair fertility in male or female mice that were fed diets containing the drug in an 18 week Continuous Breeding study. The study was conducted at doses up to 160 mg/kg/day, approximately 80-fold and 8-fold the highest recommended dose on a mg/kg and mg/m^2 basis, respectively.

PREGNANCY CATEGORY C

In studies conducted in rats and rabbits, methylphenidate was administered orally at doses of up to 75 and 200 mg/kg/day, respectively, during the period of organogenesis. Teratogenic effects (increased incidence of fetal spina bifida) were observed in rabbits at the highest dose, which is approximately 40 times the maximum recommended human dose (MRHD) on a mg/m^2 basis. The no effect level for embryo-fetal development in rabbits was 60 mg/kg/day (11 times the MRHD on a mg/m^2 basis). There was no evidence of specific teratogenic activity in rats, although increased incidences of fetal skeletal variations were seen at the highest dose level (7 times the MRHD on a mg/m^2 basis), which was also maternally toxic. The no effect level for embryo-fetal development in rats was 25 mg/kg/day (2 times the MRHD on a mg/m^2 basis). When methylphenidate was administered to rats throughout pregnancy and lactation at doses of up to 45 mg/kg/day, offspring body weight gain was decreased at the highest dose (4 times the MRHD on a mg/m^2 basis), but no other effects on postnatal development were observed. The no effect level for pre- and postnatal development in rats was 15 mg/kg/day (equal to the MRHD on a mg/m^2 basis).

Adequate and well-controlled studies in pregnant women have not been conducted. Methylphenidate should be used during pregnancy only if the potential benefit justifies the potential risk to the fetus.

NURSING MOTHERS

It is not known whether methylphenidate is excreted in human milk. Because many drugs are excreted in human milk, caution should be exercised if methylphenidate is administered to a nursing woman.

PEDIATRIC USE

Long-term effects of methylphenidate in children have not been well established. Methylphenidate should not be used in children under 6 years of age (see WARNINGS).

In a study conducted in young rats, methylphenidate was administered orally at doses of up to 100 mg/kg/day for 9 weeks, starting early in the postnatal period (Postnatal Day 7) and continuing through sexual maturity (Postnatal Week 10). When these animals were tested as adults (Postnatal Weeks 13-14), decreased spontaneous locomotor activity was observed in males and females previously treated with 50 mg/kg/day (approximately 6 times the maximum recommended human dose [MRHD] on a mg/m^2 basis) or greater, and a deficit in the acquisition of a specific learning task was seen in females exposed to the highest dose (12 times the MRHD on a mg/m^2 basis). The no effect level for juvenile neurobehavioral development in rats was 5 mg/kg/day (half the MRHD on a mg/m^2 basis). The clinical significance of the long-term behavioral effects observed in rats is unknown.

DRUG INTERACTIONS

Methylphenidate is metabolized primarily by de-esterification (nonmicrosomal hydrolytic esterases) to ritalinic acid and not through oxidative pathways.

The effects of gastrointestinal pH alterations on the absorption of methylphenidate from Ritalin LA have not been studied. Since the modified release characteristics of Ritalin LA are pH dependent, the co-administration of antacids or acid suppressants could alter the release of methylphenidate.

Methylphenidate may decrease the hypotensive effect of guanethidine. Because of possible effects on blood pressure, methylphenidate should be used cautiously with pressor agents.

Human pharmacologic studies have shown that methylphenidate may inhibit the metabolism of coumarin anticoagulants, anticonvulsants (*e.g.*, phenobarbital, phenytoin, primidone), and tricyclic drugs (*e.g.*, imipramine, clomipramine, desipramine). Downward dose adjustment of these drugs may be required when given concomitantly with methylphenidate. It may be necessary to adjust the dosage and monitor plasma drug concentrations (or, in the case of coumarin, coagulation times), when initiating or discontinuing concomitant methylphenidate.

Serious adverse events have been reported in concomitant use of methylphenidate with clonidine, although no causality for the combination has been established. The safety of using methylphenidate in combination with clonidine or other centrally acting alpha-2-agonists has not been systematically evaluated.

ADVERSE REACTIONS

Nervousness and insomnia are the most common adverse reactions reported with methylphenidate products. In children, loss of appetite, abdominal pain, weight loss during prolonged therapy, insomnia, and tachycardia may occur more frequently; however, any of the other adverse reactions listed below may also occur.

Other reactions include:

Cardiac: Angina, arrhythmia, palpitations, pulse increased or decreased, tachycardia.

Gastrointestinal: Abdominal pain, nausea.

Immune: Hypersensitivity reactions including skin rash, urticaria, fever, arthralgia, exfoliative dermatitis, erythema multiforme with histopathological findings of necrotizing vasculitis, and thrombocytopenic purpura.

Metabolism/Nutrition: Anorexia, weight loss during prolonged therapy.

Nervous System: Dizziness, drowsiness, dyskinesia, headache, rare reports of Tourette's syndrome, toxic psychosis.

Vascular: Blood pressure increased or decreased, cerebral arteritis and/or occlusion.

Although a definite causal relationship has not been established, the following have been reported in patients taking methylphenidate:

Blood/Lymphatic: Leukopenia and/or anemia.

Hepato-Biliary: Abnormal liver function, ranging from transaminase elevation to hepatic coma.

Psychiatric: Transient depressed mood.

Skin/Subcutaneous: Scalp hair loss.

Very rare reports of neuroleptic malignant syndrome (NMS) have been received, and, in most of these, patients were concurrently receiving therapies associated with NMS. In a single report, a 10-year-old boy who had been taking methylphenidate for approximately 18 months experienced an NMS-like event within 45 minutes of ingesting his first dose of venlafaxine. It is uncertain whether this case represented a drug-drug interaction, a response to either drug alone, or some other cause.

RITALIN LA

The clinical program for Ritalin LA consisted of six studies: Two controlled clinical studies conducted in children with ADHD aged 6-12 years and four clinical pharmacology studies conducted in healthy adult volunteers. These studies included a total of 256 subjects; 195 children with ADHD and 61 healthy adult volunteers. The subjects received Ritalin LA in doses of 10-40 mg/day. Safety of Ritalin LA was assessed by evaluating frequency and nature of adverse events, routine laboratory tests, vital signs, and body weight.

Adverse events during exposure were obtained primarily by general inquiry and recorded by clinical investigators using terminology of their own choosing. Consequently, it is not possible to provide a meaningful estimate of the proportion of individuals experiencing adverse events without first grouping similar types of events into a smaller number of standardized event categories. In the tables and listings that follow, MEDRA terminology has been used to classify reported adverse events. The stated frequencies of adverse events represent the proportion of individuals who experienced, at least once, a treatment-emergent adverse event of the type listed. An event was considered treatment emergent if it occurred for the first time or worsened while receiving therapy following baseline evaluation.

Adverse Events in a Double-Blind, Placebo-Controlled Clinical Trial With Ritalin LA

Treatment-Emergent Adverse Events

A placebo-controlled, double-blind, parallel-group study was conducted to evaluate the efficacy and safety of Ritalin LA in children with ADHD aged 6-12 years. All subjects received Ritalin LA for up to 4 weeks, and had their dose optimally adjusted, prior to entering the double-blind phase of the trial. In the 2 week double-blind treatment phase of this study, patients received either placebo or Ritalin LA at their individually-titrated dose (range 10-40 mg).

The prescriber should be aware that these figures cannot be used to predict the incidence of adverse events in the course of usual medical practice where patient characteristics and other factors differ from those which prevailed in the clinical trials. Similarly, the cited frequencies cannot be compared with figures obtained from other clinical investigations involving different treatments, uses, and investigators. The cited figures, however, do provide the prescribing physician with some basis for estimating the relative contribution of drug and non-drug factors to the adverse event incidence rate in the population studied.

Adverse events with an incidence >5% during the initial 4 week single-blind Ritalin LA titration period of this study were headache, insomnia, upper abdominal pain, appetite decreased, and anorexia.

Adverse Events Associated With Discontinuation of Treatment

In the 2 week double-blind treatment phase of a placebo-controlled parallel-group study in children with ADHD, only 1 Ritalin LA-treated subject (1/65, 1.5%) discontinued due to an adverse event (depression).

TABLE 3 *Treatment-Emergent Adverse Events With an Incidence >2% Among Ritalin LA-Treated Subjects, During the 2 Week Double-Blind Phase of the Clinical Study*

Preferred Term	Ritalin LA n=65	Placebo n=71
Anorexia	2 (3.1%)	0 (0.0%)
Insomnia	2 (3.1%)	0 (0.0%)

In the single-blind titration period of this study, subjects received Ritalin LA for up to 4 weeks. During this period a total of 6 subjects (6/161, 3.7%) discontinued due to adverse events. The adverse events leading to discontinuation were anger (in 2 patients), hypomania, anxiety, depressed mood, fatigue, migraine and lethargy.

CONCERTA

The premarketing development program for Concerta included exposures in a total of 755 participants in clinical trials (469 patients, 286 healthy adult subjects). These participants received Concerta 18, 36, and/or 54 mg/day. The 469 patients (ages 6-13) were evaluated in three controlled clinical studies (Studies 1, 2, and 3), two uncontrolled clinical studies (including a long-term safety study), and one clinical pharmacology study in children with ADHD. Of the 469 patients in this program, 68 Concerta-treated patients in 1 uncontrolled dose-initiation study were naïve to any pharmacologic therapy for their ADHD. Safety data on all patients are included in the discussion that follows. Adverse reactions were assessed by collecting adverse events, results of physical examinations, vital signs, weights, laboratory analyses, and ECGs.

Adverse events during exposure were obtained primarily by general inquiry and recorded by clinical investigators using terminology of their own choosing. Consequently, it is not possible to provide a meaningful estimate of the proportion of individuals experiencing adverse events without first grouping similar types of events into a smaller number of standardized event categories. In the tables and listings that follow, COSTART terminology has been used to classify reported adverse events.

The stated frequencies of adverse events represent the proportion of individuals who experienced, at least once, a treatment-emergent adverse event of the type listed. An event was considered treatment emergent if it occurred for the first time or worsened while receiving therapy following baseline evaluation.

Adverse Findings in Clinical Trials With Concerta

Adverse Events Associated With Discontinuation of Treatment

In the 4 week placebo-controlled, parallel-group trial 1 Concerta-treated patient (0.9%; 1/106) and 1 placebo-treated patient (1.0%; 1/99) discontinued due to an adverse event (sadness and increase in tics, respectively).

In uncontrolled studies up to 12 months with Concerta, 6.6% (29/441) patients discontinued for adverse events. Those events associated with discontinuation of Concerta in more than 1 patient included the following: twitching (tics, 1.8%); anorexia (loss of appetite, 0.9%); aggravation reaction (0.7%); hostility (0.7%); insomnia (0.7%); and somnolence (0.5%).

Adverse Events Occurring at an Incidence of 1% or More Among Concerta-Treated Patients

TABLE 4 enumerates, for a 4 week placebo-controlled, parallel-group trial in children with ADHD at Concerta doses of 18, 36, or 54 mg/day, the incidence of treatment-emergent adverse events. TABLE 4 includes only those events that occurred in 1% or more of patients treated with Concerta where the incidence in patients treated with Concerta was greater than the incidence in placebo-treated patients.

The prescriber should be aware that these figures cannot be used to predict the incidence of adverse events in the course of usual medical practice where patient characteristics and other factors differ from those which prevailed in the clinical trials. Similarly, the cited frequencies cannot be compared with figures obtained from other clinical investigations involving different treatments, uses, and investigators. The cited figures, however, do provide the prescribing physician with some basis for estimating the relative contribution of drug and non-drug factors to the adverse event incidence rate in the population studied.

TABLE 4 *Incidence of Treatment-Emergent Events* in a 4 week Placebo-Controlled Clinical Trial of Concerta*

Body System / Preferred Term	Concerta (n=106)	Placebo (n=99)
General		
Headache	14%	10%
Abdominal pain (stomachache)	7%	1%
Digestive		
Vomiting	4%	3%
Anorexia (loss of appetite)	4%	0%
Nervous		
Dizziness	2%	0%
Insomnia	4%	1%
Respiratory		
Upper respiratory tract infection	8%	5%
Cough increased	4%	2%
Pharyngitis	4%	3%
Sinusitis	3%	0%

* Events, regardless of causality, for which the incidence for patients treated with Concerta was at least 1% and greater than the incidence among placebo-treated patients. Incidence greater than 1% has been rounded to the nearest whole number.

Tics

In a long-term uncontrolled study (n=407 children), the cumulative incidence of new onset of tics was 8% after 10 months of treatment with Concerta.

DOSAGE AND ADMINISTRATION

RITALIN AND RITALIN-SR

Dosage should be individualized according to the needs and responses of the patient.

Adults

Tablets

Administer in divided doses 2 or 3 times daily, preferably 30-45 minutes before meals. Average dosage is 20-30 mg daily. Some patients may require 40-60 mg daily. In others, 10-15 mg daily will be adequate. Patients who are unable to sleep if medication is taken late in the day should take the last dose before 6 PM.

SR Tablets

Ritalin-SR tablets have a duration of action of approximately 8 hours. Therefore, Ritalin-SR tablets may be used in place of Ritalin tablets when the 8 hour dosage of Ritalin-SR corresponds to the titrated 8 hour dosage of Ritalin. Ritalin-SR tablets must be swallowed whole and never crushed or chewed.

Children (6 years and over)

Ritalin should be initiated in small doses, with gradual weekly increments. Daily dosage above 60 mg is not recommended.

If improvement is not observed after appropriate dosage adjustment over a 1 month period, the drug should be discontinued.

Tablets

Start with 5 mg twice daily (before breakfast and lunch) with gradual increments of 5-10 mg weekly.

SR Tablets

Ritalin-SR tablets have a duration of action of approximately 8 hours. Therefore, Ritalin-SR tablets may be used in place of Ritalin tablets when the 8 hour dosage of Ritalin-SR corresponds to the titrated 8 hour dosage of Ritalin. Ritalin-SR tablets must be swallowed whole and never crushed or chewed.

RITALIN LA

Administration of Dose

Ritalin LA is for oral administration once daily in the morning. Ritalin LA may be swallowed as whole capsules or alternatively may be administered by sprinkling the capsule contents on a small amount of applesauce (see specific instructions below). Ritalin LA and/or their contents should not be crushed, chewed, or divided.

The capsules may be carefully opened and the beads sprinkled over a spoonful of applesauce. The applesauce should not be warm because it could affect the modified release properties of this formulation. The mixture of drug and applesauce should be consumed immediately in its entirety. The drug and applesauce mixture should not be stored for future use.

Dosage Recommendation

Dosage should be individualized according to the needs and responses of the patients.

Initial Treatment

The recommended starting dose of Ritalin LA is 20 mg once daily. Dosage may be adjusted in weekly 10 mg increments to a maximum of 60 mg/day taken once daily in the morning, depending on tolerability and degree of efficacy observed. Daily dosage above 60 mg is not recommended. When in the judgement of the clinician a lower initial dose is appropriate, patients may begin treatment with an immediate-release methylphenidate product at a lower dose. After titration to 10 mg bid, these patients may be switched to Ritalin LA according to the guidelines in TABLE 5. Further titration, if necessary, may proceed as above.

Patients Currently Receiving Methylphenidate

The recommended dose of Ritalin LA for patients currently taking methylphenidate bid or sustained release (SR) is provided in TABLE 5.

TABLE 5

Previous Methylphenidate Dose	Recommended Ritalin LA Dose
10 mg Methylphenidate bid or 20 mg methylphenidate-SR	20 mg qd
15 mg Methylphenidate bid	30 mg qd
20 mg Methylphenidate bid or 40 mg of methylphenidate-SR	40 mg qd
30 mg Methylphenidate bid or 60 mg methylphenidate-SR	60 mg qd

For other methylphenidate regimens, clinical judgment should be used when selecting the starting dose. Ritalin LA dosage may be adjusted at weekly intervals in 10 mg increments.

Daily dosage above 60 mg is not recommended.

CONCERTA

Concerta is administered orally once daily in the morning.

Concerta must be swallowed whole with the aid of liquids, and must not be chewed, divided, or crushed (see PRECAUTIONS, Information for the Patient, Concerta).

Concerta may be administered with or without food and should be administered once daily in the morning.

Dosage should be individualized according to the needs and responses of the patient.

Patients New to Methylphenidate

The recommended starting dose of Concerta for patients who are not currently taking methylphenidate, or for patients who are on stimulants other than methylphenidate, is 18 mg once daily.

Dosage may be adjusted in 18 mg increments to a maximum of 54 mg/day taken once daily in the morning. In general, dosage adjustment may proceed at approximately weekly intervals.

Patients Currently Using Methylphenidate

The recommended dose of Concerta for patients who are currently taking methylphenidate bid, tid, or sustained-release (SR) at doses of 10-60 mg/day is provided in TABLE 6. Dosing recommendations are based on current dose regimen and clinical judgement.

Dosage may be adjusted in 18 mg increments to a maximum of 54 mg/day taken once daily in the morning. In general, dosage adjustment may proceed at approximately weekly intervals.

***TABLE 6** Recommended Dose Conversion From Methylphenidate Regimens to Concerta*

Previous Methylphenidate Daily Dose	Recommended Concerta Dose
5 mg methylphenidate bid or 5 mg methylphenidate tid or 20 mg methylphenidate-SR	18 mg q AM
10 mg methylphenidate bid or 10 mg methylphenidate tid or 40 mg methylphenidate-SR	36 mg q AM
15 mg methylphenidate bid or 15 mg methylphenidate tid or 60 mg methylphenidate-SR	54 mg q AM

Other Methylphenidate Regimens: Clinical judgement should be used when selecting the starting dose.

Daily dosage above 54 mg is not recommended.

MAINTENANCE/EXTENDED TREATMENT

There is no body of evidence available from controlled trials to indicate how long the patient with ADHD should be treated with methylphenidate. It is generally agreed, however, that pharmacological treatment of ADHD may be needed for extended periods. Nevertheless, the physician who elects to use methylphenidate for extended periods in patients with ADHD should periodically re-evaluate the long-term usefulness of the drug for the individual patient with trials off medication to assess the patient's functioning without pharmacotherapy. Improvement may be sustained when the drug is either temporarily or permanently discontinued.

DOSE REDUCTION AND DISCONTINUATION

If paradoxical aggravation of symptoms or other adverse events occur, the dosage should be reduced, or, if necessary, the drug should be discontinued. If improvement is not observed after appropriate dosage adjustment over a 1 month period, the drug should be discontinued.

HOW SUPPLIED

RITALIN AND RITALIN-SR

Ritalin Tablets

5 mg: Round, yellow (imprinted "CIBA 7").
10 mg: Round, pale green, scored (imprinted "CIBA 3").
20 mg: Round, pale yellow, scored (imprinted "CIBA 34").

Storage: Do not store above 30°C (86°F). Protect from light. *Dispense in tight, light-resistant container.*

Ritalin-SR Tablets

20 mg: Round, white, coated (imprinted "CIBA 16"). *Note:* SR Tablets are color-additive free.

Storage: Do not store above 30°C (86°F). Protect from moisture. *Dispense in tight, light-resistant container.*

RITALIN LA

Ritalin LA Capsules:

20 mg: White (imprinted "NVR R20").
30 mg: Yellow (imprinted "NVR R30").
40 mg: Light brown (imprinted "NVR R40").

Storage: Store at 25°C (77°F), excursions permitted 15-30°C (59-86°F). Dispense in tight container.

CONCERTA

Concerta (methylphenidate HCl) extended-release tablets are available in 18, 36, and 54 mg dosage strengths.

18 mg: Yellow tablets which are imprinted with "alza 18".
36 mg: White tablets which are imprinted with "alza 36".
54 mg: Brownish-red tablets which are imprinted with "alza 54".

Storage: Store at 25°C (77°F); excursions permitted to 15-30°C (59-86°F). Protect from humidity.

PRODUCT LISTING - RATED THERAPEUTICALLY EQUIVALENT

Tablet - Oral - 5 mg

100's $25.12 GENERIC, Aligen Independent Laboratories Inc 00405-0125-01
100's $28.09 GENERIC, Purepac Pharmaceutical Company 00228-2091-10
100's $28.98 GENERIC, Major Pharmaceuticals Inc 00904-2768-60
100's $29.61 GENERIC, Qualitest Products Inc 00603-4569-21
100's $30.20 FEDERAL UPPER LIMIT, H.C.F.A. F F P 99999-1790-01
100's $31.24 GENERIC, Md Pharmaceutical Inc 05301-4531-07
100's $33.29 GENERIC, Celltech Pharmaceuticals Inc 53014-0531-07
100's $33.39 GENERIC, Mallinckrodt Medical Inc 00406-1121-01
100's $33.40 GENERIC, Watson/Schein Pharmaceuticals Inc 00364-0561-01
100's $33.40 GENERIC, Watson/Schein Pharmaceuticals Inc 00591-5882-01
100's $34.65 GENERIC, Ivax Corporation 00182-1173-01
100's $34.85 GENERIC, Geneva Pharmaceuticals 00781-1748-01
100's $34.85 GENERIC, Geneva Pharmaceuticals 00781-8840-01
100's $34.85 GENERIC, Apothecon Inc 59772-8840-01
100's $35.00 GENERIC, Able Laboratories Inc 53265-0253-10
100's $50.35 RITALIN, Novartis Pharmaceuticals 00083-0007-30

Tablet - Oral - 10 mg

100's $35.76 GENERIC, Aligen Independent Laboratories Inc 00405-0126-01
100's $39.51 GENERIC, Purepac Pharmaceutical Company 00228-2092-10
100's $40.88 GENERIC, Major Pharmaceuticals Inc 00904-2769-60
100's $42.24 FEDERAL UPPER LIMIT, H.C.F.A. F F P 99999-1790-02
100's $42.25 GENERIC, Qualitest Products Inc 00603-4570-21
100's $44.19 GENERIC, Md Pharmaceutical Inc 05301-4530-07
100's $47.46 GENERIC, Celltech Pharmaceuticals Inc 53014-0530-07
100's $47.70 GENERIC, Watson/Schein Pharmaceuticals Inc 00364-0479-01
100's $47.70 GENERIC, Watson Laboratories Inc 00591-5883-01
100's $47.72 GENERIC, Mallinckrodt Medical Inc 00406-1122-01
100's $49.68 GENERIC, Geneva Pharmaceuticals 00781-1749-01
100's $49.68 GENERIC, Geneva Pharmaceuticals 00781-8841-01
100's $49.68 GENERIC, Apothecon Inc 59772-8841-01
100's $50.00 GENERIC, Able Laboratories Inc 53265-0254-10
100's $51.67 GENERIC, Ivax Corporation 00182-1066-01
100's $71.79 RITALIN, Novartis Pharmaceuticals 00083-0003-30

Tablet - Oral - 20 mg

100's $54.95 GENERIC, Aligen Independent Laboratories Inc 00405-0127-01
100's $56.20 GENERIC, Major Pharmaceuticals Inc 00904-2770-60
100's $60.75 GENERIC, Qualitest Products Inc 00603-4571-21
100's $61.80 FEDERAL UPPER LIMIT, H.C.F.A. F F P 99999-1790-03
100's $64.40 GENERIC, Ivax Corporation 00182-1174-01
100's $64.40 GENERIC, Md Pharmaceutical Inc 05301-4532-07
100's $64.40 GENERIC, Md Pharmaceutical Inc 05301-4562-07
100's $68.25 GENERIC, Celltech Pharmaceuticals Inc 53014-0532-07
100's $68.60 GENERIC, Watson/Schein Pharmaceuticals Inc 00364-0562-01
100's $68.60 GENERIC, Watson Laboratories Inc 00591-5884-01
100's $68.61 GENERIC, Mallinckrodt Medical Inc 00406-1124-01
100's $71.43 GENERIC, Geneva Pharmaceuticals 00781-1753-01
100's $71.43 GENERIC, Geneva Pharmaceuticals 00781-8842-01
100's $71.43 GENERIC, Apothecon Inc 59772-8842-01
100's $72.00 GENERIC, Able Laboratories Inc 53265-0255-10
100's $103.24 RITALIN, Novartis Pharmaceuticals 00083-0034-30
100's $686.10 GENERIC, Geneva Pharmaceuticals 00781-8842-10

Tablet, Extended Release - Oral - 10 mg

100's $104.22 GENERIC, Mallinckrodt Medical Inc 00406-1423-01

Tablet, Extended Release - Oral - 20 mg

100's $78.92 GENERIC, Aligen Independent Laboratories Inc 00405-0128-01
100's $84.97 GENERIC, Major Pharmaceuticals Inc 00904-2773-60
100's $88.98 GENERIC, Parmed Pharmaceuticals Inc 00349-8834-01
100's $92.95 GENERIC, Qualitest Products Inc 00603-4572-21
100's $97.28 GENERIC, Purepac Pharmaceutical Company 00228-2089-10
100's $100.80 GENERIC, Ivax Corporation 00182-9147-01
100's $105.31 METADATE ER, Celltech Pharmaceuticals Inc 53014-0594-07
100's $110.95 GENERIC, Geneva Pharmaceuticals 00781-1754-01
100's $110.95 GENERIC, Geneva Pharmaceuticals 00781-8843-01
100's $110.95 GENERIC, Apothecon Inc 59772-8843-01
100's $111.95 GENERIC, Mallinckrodt Medical Inc 00406-1451-01
100's $118.57 GENERIC, Watson Laboratories Inc 00591-3111-01
100's $152.00 GENERIC, Able Laboratories Inc 53265-0262-10
100's $160.34 RITALIN-SR, Novartis Pharmaceuticals 00083-0016-30

PRODUCT LISTING - EQUIVALENTS NOT AVAILABLE

Capsule, Extended Release - Oral - 20 mg

10 x 10 $176.88 METADATE CD, Celltech Pharmaceuticals Inc 53014-0575-72
30's $50.46 METADATE CD, Celltech Pharmaceuticals Inc 53014-0575-30
100's $168.21 METADATE CD, Celltech Pharmaceuticals Inc 53014-0575-07
100's $232.98 RITALIN LA, Novartis Pharmaceuticals 00078-0370-05

Capsule, Extended Release - Oral - 30 mg

100's $238.28 RITALIN LA, Novartis Pharmaceuticals 00078-0371-05

Capsule, Extended Release - Oral - 40 mg

100's $244.90 RITALIN LA, Novartis Pharmaceuticals 00078-0372-05

Tablet, Extended Release - Oral - 10 mg

100's $101.46 METADATE ER, Celltech Pharmaceuticals Inc 53014-0593-07

Tablet, Extended Release - Oral - 18 mg
100's $280.00 CONCERTA, Alza 17314-5850-02
Tablet, Extended Release - Oral - 27 mg
100's $287.50 CONCERTA, Alza 17314-5853-02
Tablet, Extended Release - Oral - 36 mg
100's $295.00 CONCERTA, Alza 17314-5851-02
Tablet, Extended Release - Oral - 54 mg
100's $321.25 CONCERTA, Alza 17314-5852-02

Methylprednisolone *(001791)*

For related information, see the comparative table section in Appendix A.

Categories: Adrenocortical insufficiency; Anemia, acquired hemolytic; Anemia, congenital hypoplastic; Anemia, erythroblastopenia; Ankylosing spondylitis; Arthritis, gouty; Arthritis, post-traumatic; Arthritis, psoriatic; Arthritis, rheumatoid; Asthma; Berylliosis; Bursitis; Carditis, rheumatic; Chorioretinitis; Choroiditis; Colitis, ulcerative; Conjunctivitis, allergic; Crohn's disease; Dermatitis herpetiformis, bullous; Dermatitis, atopic; Dermatitis, contact; Dermatitis, exfoliative; Dermatitis, seborrheic; Dermatomyositis, systemic; Epicondylitis; Erythema multiforme; Herpes zoster ophthalmicus; Hypercalcemia, secondary to neoplasia; Hypersensitivity reactions; Inflammation, anterior segment, ophthalmic; Inflammation, ophthalmic; Inflammatory bowel disease; Iridocyclitis; Iritis; Keratitis; Leukemia; Loffler's syndrome; Lupus erythematosus, systemic; Lymphoma; Meningitis, tuberculous; Multiple sclerosis; Mycosis fungoides; Nephrotic syndrome; Neuritis, optic; Ophthalmia, sympathetic; Pemphigus; Pneumonitis, aspiration; Polymyositis; Psoriasis; Rhinitis, perennial allergic; Rhinitis, seasonal allergic; Sarcoidosis; Serum sickness; Stevens-Johnson syndrome; Synovitis, secondary to osteoarthritis; Tenosynovitis; Thrombocytopenia, secondary; Thyroiditis, nonsuppurative; Trichinosis; Tuberculosis, disseminated; Tuberculosis, fulminating; Tuberculosis, meningitis; Ulcer, allergic corneal marginal; Uveitis; FDA Approved 1978 Apr; Pregnancy Category B

Drug Classes: Corticosteroids

Brand Names: Medlone 21; **Medrol**; Metrocort; Summicort

Foreign Brand Availability: A-Methapred (Israel); Esametone (Italy); Firmacort (Italy); Mednin (Taiwan); Medrate (Germany); Medixon (Indonesia); Medrone (England; Ireland); Metidrol (Indonesia); Metycortin (Germany); Metypred (Bahrain; Cyprus; Egypt; Iran; Iraq; Israel; Jordan; Kuwait; Lebanon; Libya; Oman; Qatar; Republic-of-Yemen; Saudi-Arabia; Syria; United-Arab-Emirates); Solomet (Finland); Urbason (Austria; Bulgaria; Czech-Republic; Germany; Netherlands; Spain; Switzerland); Urbason Retard (Belgium; Bulgaria; Germany; Italy)

Cost of Therapy: $32.40 (Asthma; Medrol; 4 mg; 1 tablet/day; 30 day supply)
$4.29 (Asthma; Generic Tablets; 4 mg; 1 tablet/day; 30 day supply)

HCFA JCODE(S): J7509 per 4 mg ORAL

DESCRIPTION

Methylprednisolone is a glucocorticoid. Glucocorticoids are adrenocortical steroids, both naturally occurring and synthetic, which are readily absorbed from the gastrointestinal tract. Methylprednisolone occurs as a white to practically white, odorless, crystalline powder. It is sparingly soluble in alcohol, in dioxane, and in methanol, slightly soluble in acetone, and in chloroform, and very slightly soluble in ether. It is practically insoluble in water.

The chemical name for methylprednisolone is pregna-1,4-diene-3,20-dione, 11,17,21-trihydroxy-6-methyl-,(6α, 11β)- and the molecular weight is 374.48.

Each Medrol tablet for oral administration contains 2, 4, 8, 16, 24, or 32 mg of methylprednisolone.

Medrol Inactive ingredients: *2 mg:* Calcium stearate, corn starch, erythrosine sodium, lactose, mineral oil, sorbic acid, sucrose. *4 and 16 mg:* Calcium stearate, corn starch, lactose, mineral oil, sorbic acid, sucrose. *8 and 32 mg:* Calcium stearate, corn starch, FD&C yellow no. 6, lactose, mineral oil, sorbic acid, sucrose. *24 mg:* Calcium stearate, corn starch, FD&C yellow no. 5, lactose, mineral oil, sorbic acid, sucrose.

CLINICAL PHARMACOLOGY

Naturally occurring glucocorticoids (hydrocortisone and cortisone), which also have salt-retaining properties, are used as replacement therapy in adrenocortical deficiency states. Their synthetic analogs are primarily used for their potent anti-inflammatory effects in disorders of many organ systems.

Glucocorticoids cause profound and varied metabolic effects. In addition, they modify the body's immune responses to diverse stimuli.

INDICATIONS AND USAGE

Methylprednisolone is indicated in the following conditions:

Endocrine Disorders: Primary or secondary adrenocortical insufficiency (hydrocortisone or cortisone is the first choice; synthetic analogs may be used in conjunction with mineralocorticoids where applicable; in infancy mineralocorticoid supplementation is of particular importance).
Congenital adrenal hyperplasia.
Nonsuppurative thyroiditis.
Hypercalcemia associated with cancer.

Rheumatic Disorders: As adjunctive therapy for short-term administration (to tide the patient over an acute episode or exacerbation) in:
Rheumatoid arthritis, including juvenile rheumatoid arthritis (selected cases may require low-dose maintenance therapy).
Ankylosing spondylitis.
Acute and subacute bursitis.
Synovitis of osteoarthritis.
Acute nonspecific tenosynovitis.
Post-traumatic osteoarthritis.
Psoriatic arthritis.
Epicondylitis.
Acute gouty arthritis.

Collagen Diseases: During an exacerbation or as maintenance therapy in selected cases of:
Systemic lupus erythematosus.
Systemic dermatomyositis (polymyositis).
Acute rheumatic carditis.

Dermatologic Diseases:
Bullous dermatitis herpetiformis.
Severe erythema multiforme (Stevens-Johnson syndrome).
Severe seborrheic dermatitis.
Exfoliative dermatitis.
Mycosis fungoides.
Pemphigus.
Severe psoriasis.

Allergic States: Control of severe or incapacitating allergic conditions intractable to adequate trials of conventional treatment:
Seasonal or perennial allergic rhinitis.
Drug hypersensitivity reactions.
Serum sickness.
Contact dermatitis.
Bronchial asthma.
Atopic dermatitis.

Ophthalmic Diseases: Severe acute and chronic allergic and inflammatory processes involving the eye and its adnexa such as:
Allergic corneal marginal ulcers.
Herpes zoster ophthalmicus.
Anterior segment inflammation.
Diffuse posterior uveitis and choroiditis.
Sympathetic ophthalmia.
Keratitis.
Optic neuritis.
Allergic conjunctivitis.
Chorioretinitis.
Iritis and iridocyclitis.

Respiratory Diseases:
Symptomatic sarcoidosis.
Berylliosis.
Loeffler's syndrome not manageable by other means.
Fulminating or disseminated pulmonary tuberculosis when used concurrently with appropriate antituberculous chemotherapy.
Aspiration pneumonitis.

Hematologic Disorders:
Idiopathic thrombocytopenic purpura in adults.
Secondary thrombocytopenia in adults.
Acquired (autoimmune) hemolytic anemia.
Erythroblastopenia (RBC anemia).
Congenital (erythroid) hypoplastic anemia.

Neoplastic Diseases: For palliative management of:
Leukemias and lymphomas in adults.
Acute leukemia of childhood.

Edematous States: To induce a diuresis or remission of proteinuria in the nephrotic syndrome, without uremia, of the idiopathic type or that due to lupus erythematosus.

Gastrointestinal Diseases: To tide the patient over a critical period of the disease in:
Ulcerative colitis.
Regional enteritis.

Nervous System: Acute exacerbations of multiple sclerosis.

Miscellaneous:
Tuberculous meningitis with subarachnoid block or impending block when used concurrently with appropriate antituberculous chemotherapy.
Trichinosis with neurologic or myocardial involvement.

CONTRAINDICATIONS

Systemic fungal infections and known hypersensitivity to components.

WARNINGS

In patients on corticosteroid therapy subjected to unusual stress, increased dosage of rapidly acting corticosteroids before, during, and after the stressful situation is indicated.

Corticosteroids may mask some signs of infection, and new infections may appear during their use. Infections with any pathogen including viral, bacterial, fungal, protozoan, or helminthic infections, in any location of the body, may be associated with the use of corticosteroids alone or in combination with other immunosuppressive agents that affect cellular immunity, humoral immunity, or neutrophil function.[1]

These infections may be mild, but can be severe and at times fatal. With increasing doses of corticosteroids, the rate of occurrence of infectious complications increases.[2] There may be decreased resistance and inability to localize infection when corticosteroids are used.

Prolonged use of corticosteroids may produce posterior subcapsular cataracts, glaucoma with possible damage to the optic nerves, and may enhance the establishment of secondary ocular infections due to fungi or viruses.

Use in Pregnancy: Since adequate human reproduction studies have not been done with corticosteroids, the use of these drugs in pregnancy, nursing mothers, or women of child-bearing potential requires that the possible benefits of the drug be weighed against the potential hazards to the mother and embryo or fetus. Infants born of mothers who have received substantial doses of corticosteroids during pregnancy should be carefully observed for signs of hypoadrenalism.

Average and large doses of hydrocortisone or cortisone can cause elevation of blood pressure, salt and water retention, and increased excretion of potassium. These effects are less likely to occur with the synthetic derivatives except when used in large doses. Dietary salt restriction and potassium supplementation may be necessary. All corticosteroids increase calcium excretion.

Administration of live or live, attenuated vaccines is contraindicated in patients receiving immunosuppressive doses of corticosteroids. Killed or inactivated vaccines may be administered to patients receiving immunosuppressive doses of corticosteroids; however, the response to such vaccines may be diminished. Indicated immunization procedures may be undertaken in patients receiving nonimmunosuppressive doses of corticosteroids.

The use of methylprednisolone tablets in active tuberculosis should be restricted to those cases of fulminating or disseminated tuberculosis in which the corticosteroid is used for the management of the disease in conjunction with an appropriate antituberculous regimen.

If corticosteroids are indicated in patients with latent tuberculosis or tuberculin reactivity, close observation is necessary as reactivation of the disease may occur. During prolonged corticosteroid therapy, these patients should receive chemoprophylaxis.

Persons who are on drugs which suppress the immune system are more susceptible to infections than healthy individuals. Chicken pox and measles, for example, can have a more serious or even fatal course in non-immune children or adults on corticosteroids. In such children or in adults who have not had these diseases, particular care should be taken to avoid exposure. How the dose, route and duration of corticosteroid administration affects the risk of developing a disseminated infection is not known. The contribution of the underlying disease and/or prior corticosteroid treatment to the risk is also not known. If exposed to chicken pox, prophylaxis with varicella zoster immune globulin (VZIG) may be indicated. If exposed to measles, prophylaxis with pooled intramuscular immunoglobulin (IG) may be indicated. (See the prescribing information for VZIG and IG.) If chicken pox develops, treatment with antiviral agents may be considered. Similarly, corticosteroids should be used with great care in patients with known or suspected Strongyloides (threadworm) infestation. In such patients, corticosteroid-induced immunosuppression may lead to Strongyloides hyperinfection and dissemination with widespread larval migration, often accompanied by severe enterocolitis and potentially fatal gram-negative septicemia.

PRECAUTIONS

GENERAL

Drug-induced secondary adrenocortical insufficiency may be minimized by gradual reduction of dosage. This type of relative insufficiency may persist for months after discontinuation of therapy; therefore, in any situation of stress occurring during that period, hormone therapy should be reinstituted. Since mineralocorticoid secretion may be impaired, salt and/or a mineralocorticoid should be administered concurrently.

There is an enhanced effect of corticosteroids on patients with hypothyroidism and in those with cirrhosis.

Corticosteroids should be used cautiously in patients with ocular herpes simplex because of possible corneal perforation.

The lowest possible dose of corticosteroid should be used to control the condition under treatment, and when reduction in dosage is possible, the reduction should be gradual.

Psychic derangements may appear when corticosteroids are used, ranging from euphoria, insomnia, mood swings, personality changes, and severe depression, to frank psychotic manifestations. Also, existing emotional instability or psychotic tendencies may be aggravated by corticosteroids.

M

Steroids should be used with caution in nonspecific ulcerative colitis, if there is a probability of impending perforation, abscess, or other pyogenic infection; diverticulitis; fresh intestinal anastomoses; active or latent peptic ulcer; renal insufficiency; hypertension; osteoporosis; and myasthenia gravis.

Growth and development of infants and children on prolonged corticosteroid therapy should be carefully observed.

Kaposi's sarcoma has been reported to occur in patients receiving corticosteroid therapy. Discontinuation of corticosteroids may result in clinical remission.

Although controlled clinical trials have shown corticosteroids to be effective in speeding the resolution of acute exacerbations of multiple sclerosis, they do not show that corticosteroids affect the ultimate outcome or natural history of the disease. The studies do show that relatively high doses of corticosteroids are necessary to demonstrate a significant effect. (See DOSAGE AND ADMINISTRATION.)

Since complications of treatment with glucocorticoids are dependent on the size of the dose and the duration of treatment, a risk/benefit decision must be made in each individual case as to dose and duration of treatment and as to whether daily or intermittent therapy should be used.

The 24 mg tablet contains FD&C yellow no. 5 (tartrazine) which may cause allergic-type reactions (including bronchial asthma) in certain susceptible individuals. Although the overall incidence of FD&C yellow no. 5 (tartrazine) sensitivity in the general population is low, it is frequently seen in patients who also have aspirin hypersensitivity.

INFORMATION FOR THE PATIENT

Patients who are on immunosuppressant doses of corticosteroids should be warned to avoid exposure to chickenpox or measles. Patients should also be advised that if they are exposed, medical advice should be sought without delay.

DRUG INTERACTIONS

The pharmacokinetic interactions listed below are potentially clinically important. Mutual inhibition of metabolism occurs with concurrent use of cyclosporin and methylprednisolone; therefore, it is possible that adverse events associated with the individual use of either drug may be more apt to occur. Convulsions have been reported with concurrent use of methylprednisolone and cyclosporin. Drugs that induce hepatic enzymes such as phenobarbital, phenytoin, and rifampin may increase the clearance of methylprednisolone and may require increases in methylprednisolone dose to achieve the desired response. Drugs such as troleandomycin and ketoconazole may inhibit the metabolism of methylprednisolone and thus decrease its clearance. Therefore, the dose of methylprednisolone should be titrated to avoid steroid toxicity.

Methylprednisolone may increase the clearance of chronic high-dose aspirin. This could lead to decreased salicylate serum levels or increase the risk of salicylate toxicity when methylprednisolone is withdrawn. Aspirin should be used cautiously in conjunction with corticosteroids in patients suffering from hypoprothrombinemia.

The effect of methylprednisolone on oral anticoagulants is variable. There are reports of enhanced as well as diminished effects of anticoagulant when given concurrently with corticosteroids. Therefore, coagulation indices should be monitored to maintain the desired anticoagulant effect.

ADVERSE REACTIONS

Fluid and Electrolyte Disturbances: Sodium retention, congestive heart failure in susceptible patients, hypertension, fluid retention, potassium loss, hypokalemic alkalosis.

Musculoskeletal: Muscle weakness; loss of muscle mass; steroid myopathy; osteoporosis; tendon rupture, particularly of the Achilles tendon; vertebral compression fractures; aseptic necrosis of femoral and humeral heads; pathologic fracture of long bones.

Gastrointestinal: (1) Peptic ulcer with possible perforation and hemorrhage; (2) pancreatitis; (3) abdominal distention; (4) ulcerative esophagitis; and (5) increases in alanine transaminase (ALT, SGPT), aspartate transaminase (AST, SGOT), and alkaline phosphatase have been observed following corticosteroid treatment. These changes are usually small, not associated with any clinical syndrome, and are reversible upon discontinuation.

Dermatologic: Impaired wound healing, petechiae and ecchymoses, may suppress reactions to skin tests, thin fragile skin, facial erythema, increased sweating.

Neurological: Increased intracranial pressure with papilledema (pseudo-tumor cerebri) usually after treatment, convulsions, vertigo, headache.

Endocrine: Development of cushingoid state; suppression of growth in children; secondary adrenocortical and pituitary unresponsiveness, particularly in times of stress, as in trauma, surgery or illness; menstrual irregularities; decreased carbohydrate tolerance; manifestations of latent diabetes mellitus; increased requirements of insulin or oral hypoglycemic agents in diabetics.

Ophthalmic: Posterior subcapsular cataracts, increased intraocular pressure, glaucoma, exophthalmos.

Metabolic: Negative nitrogen balance due to protein catabolism.

The following additional reactions have been reported following oral as well as parenteral therapy: urticaria and other allergic, anaphylactic, or hypersensitivity reactions.

DOSAGE AND ADMINISTRATION

The initial dosage of methylprednisolone may vary from 4-48 mg of methylprednisolone per day depending on the specific disease entity being treated. In situations of less severity, lower doses will generally suffice, while in selected patients higher initial doses may be required. The initial dosage should be maintained or adjusted until a satisfactory response is noted. If after a reasonable period of time there is a lack of satisfactory clinical response, methylprednisolone should be discontinued and the patient transferred to other appropriate therapy.

IT SHOULD BE EMPHASIZED THAT DOSAGE REQUIREMENTS ARE VARIABLE AND MUST BE INDIVIDUALIZED ON THE BASIS OF THE DISEASE UNDER TREATMENT AND THE RESPONSE OF THE PATIENT.

After a favorable response is noted, the proper maintenance dosage should be determined by decreasing the initial drug dosage in small decrements at appropriate time intervals until the lowest dosage which will maintain an adequate clinical response is reached. It should be kept in mind that constant monitoring is needed in regard to drug dosage. Included in the situations which may make dosage adjustments necessary are changes in clinical status secondary to remissions or exacerbations in the disease process, the patient's individual drug responsiveness, and the effect of patient exposure to stressful situations not directly related to the disease entity under treatment; in this latter situation it may be necessary to increase the dosage of methylprednisolone for a period of time consistent with the patient's condition. If after long-term therapy the drug is to be stopped, it is recommended that it be withdrawn gradually rather than abruptly.

MULTIPLE SCLEROSIS

In treatment of acute exacerbations of multiple sclerosis daily doses of 200 mg of prednisolone for a week followed by 80 mg every other day for 1 month have been shown to be effective (4 mg of methylprednisolone is equivalent to 5 mg of prednisolone).

ADT (ALTERNATE DAY THERAPY)

Alternate day therapy is a corticosteroid dosing regimen in which twice the usual daily dose of corticoid is administered every other morning. The purpose of this mode of therapy is to provide the patient requiring long-term pharmacologic dose treatment with the beneficial effects of corticoids while minimizing certain undesirable effects, including pituitary-adrenal suppression, the Cushingoid state, corticoid withdrawal symptoms, and growth suppression in children.

The rationale for this treatment schedule is based on two major premises: (a) the anti-inflammatory or therapeutic effect of corticoids persists longer that their physical presence and metabolic effects and (b) administration of the corticosteroid every other morning allows for reestablishment of more nearly normal hypothalamic-pituitary-adrenal (HPA) activity on the off-steroid day.

A brief review of the HPA physiology may be helpful in understanding this rationale. Acting primarily through the hypothalamus a fall in free cortisol stimulates the pituitary gland to produce increasing amounts of corticotropin (ACTH) while a rise in free cortisol inhibits ACTH secretion. Normally the HPA system is characterized by diurnal (circadian) rhythm. Serum levels of ACTH rise from a low point about 10 PM to a peak level about 6 AM. Increasing levels of ACTH stimulate adrenal cortical activity resulting in a rise in plasma cortisol with maximal levels occurring between 2 and 8 AM. This rise in cortisol dampens ACTH production and in turn adrenal cortical activity. There is a gradual fall in plasma corticoids during the day with lowest levels occurring about midnight.

The diurnal rhythm of the HPA axis is lost in Cushing's disease, a syndrome of adrenal cortical hyperfunction characterized by obesity with centripetal fat distribution, thinning of the skin with easy bruisability, muscle wasting with weakness, hypertension, latent diabetes, osteoporosis, electrolyte imbalance, etc. The same clinical findings of hyperadrenocorticism may be noted during long-term pharmacologic dose corticoid therapy administered in conventional daily divided doses. It would appear, then, that a disturbance in the diurnal cycle with maintenance of elevated corticoid values during the night may play a significant role in the development of undesirable corticoid effects. Escape from these constantly elevated plasma levels for even short periods of time may be instrumental in protecting against undesirable pharmacologic effects.

During conventional pharmacologic dose corticosteroid therapy, ACTH production is inhibited with subsequent suppression of cortisol production by the adrenal cortex. Recovery time for normal HPA activity is variable depending upon the dose and duration of treatment. During this time the patient is vulnerable to any stressful situation. Although it has been shown that there is considerably less adrenal suppression following a single morning dose of prednisolone (10 mg) as opposed to a quarter of that dose administered every 6 hours, there is evidence that some suppressive effect on adrenal activity may be carried over into the following day when pharmacologic doses are used. Further, it has been shown that a single dose of certain corticosteroids will produce adrenal cortical suppression for 2 or more days. Other corticoids, including methylprednisolone, hydrocortisone, prednisone, and prednisolone, are considered to be short acting (producing adrenal cortical suppression for 1¼ to 1½ days following a single dose) and thus are recommended for alternate day therapy.

The following should be kept in mind when considering alternate day therapy:

Basic principles and indications for corticosteroid therapy should apply. The benefits of ADT should not encourage the indiscriminate use of steroids.

ADT is a therapeutic technique primarily designed for patients in whom long-term pharmacologic corticoid therapy is anticipated.

In less severe disease processes in which corticoid therapy is indicated, it may be possible to initiate treatment with ADT. More severe disease states usually will require daily divided high dose therapy for initial control of the disease process. The initial suppressive dose level should be continued until satisfactory clinical response is obtained, usually 4 to 10 days in the case of many allergic and collagen diseases. It is important to keep the period of initial suppressive dose as brief as possible particularly when subsequent use of alternate day therapy is intended. Once control has been established, two courses are available: (a) change to ADT and then gradually reduce the amount of corticoid given every other day **or** (b) following control of the disease process reduce the daily dose of corticoid to the lowest effective level as rapidly as possible and then change over to an alternate day schedule. Theoretically, course (a) may be preferable.

Because of the advantages of ADT, it may be desirable to try patients on this form of therapy who have been on daily corticoids for long periods of time (*e.g.,* patients with rheumatoid arthritis). Since these patients may already have a suppressed HPA axis, establishing them on ADT may be difficult and not always successful. However, it is recommended that regular attempts be made to change them over. It may be helpful to triple or even quadruple the daily maintenance dose and administer this every other day rather than just doubling the daily dose if difficulty is encountered. Once the patient is again controlled, an attempt should be made to reduce this dose to a minimum.

As indicated above, certain corticosteroids, because of their prolonged suppressive effect on adrenal activity, are not recommended for alternate day therapy (*e.g.,* dexamethasone and betamethasone).

The maximal activity of the adrenal cortex is between 2 AM and 8 AM, and it is minimal between 4 PM and midnight. Exogenous corticosteroids suppress adrenocortical activity the least, when given at the time of maximal activity (AM).

In using ADT it is important, as in all therapeutic situations, to individualize and tailor the therapy to each patient. Complete control of symptoms will not be possible in all patients. An explanation of the benefits of ADT will help the patient to understand and tolerate the possible flare-up in symptoms which may occur in the latter part of the off-steroid day. Other symptomatic therapy may be added or increased at this time if needed.

In the event of an acute flare-up of the disease process, it may be necessary to return to a full suppressive daily divided corticoid dose for control. Once control is again established, alternate day therapy may be reinstituted.

Although many of the undesirable features of corticosteroid therapy can be minimized by ADT, as in any therapeutic situation, the physician must carefully weigh the benefit-risk ratio for each patient in whom corticoid therapy is being considered.

HOW SUPPLIED

Medrol tablets are available in:

2 mg: Pink, elliptical, scored, imprinted "MEDROL 2".
4 mg: White, elliptical, scored, imprinted "MEDROL 4".
8 mg: Peach, elliptical, scored, imprinted "MEDROL 8".
16 mg: White, elliptical, scored, imprinted "MEDROL 16".
24 mg: Yellow, elliptical, scored, imprinted "MEDROL 24".
32 mg: Peach, elliptical, scored, imprinted "MEDROL 32".

Storage: Store at controlled room temperature 20-25°C (68-77°F).

PRODUCT LISTING - RATED THERAPEUTICALLY EQUIVALENT

Tablet - Oral - 2 mg

100's	$57.08	MEDROL, Pharmacia and Upjohn	00009-0049-02

Tablet - Oral - 4 mg

21's	$6.25	GENERIC, Vangard Labs	00615-2535-21
21's	$9.98	GENERIC, Geneva Pharmaceuticals	00781-1402-07
21's	$10.65	GENERIC, Vintage Pharmaceuticals Inc	00254-4216-13
21's	$10.65	GENERIC, Lannett Company Inc	00527-1296-07
21's	$10.65	GENERIC, Qualitest Products Inc	00603-4593-15
21's	$10.89	GENERIC, Mutual/United Research Laboratories	00677-0565-13
21's	$10.99	GENERIC, Major Pharmaceuticals Inc	00904-2175-19
21's	$11.00	GENERIC, Ivax Corporation	00182-1050-03
21's	$11.00	GENERIC, Barr Laboratories Inc	00555-0301-38
21's	$11.00	GENERIC, Duramed Pharmaceuticals Inc	51285-0301-21
21's	$11.00	GENERIC, Greenstone Limited	59762-3327-01
21's	$11.20	GENERIC, Watson Laboratories Inc	00591-0790-21
21's	$11.20	GENERIC, Watson Laboratories Inc	52544-0790-21
21's	$12.00	GENERIC, Interstate Drug Exchange Inc	00814-4781-21
21's	$12.02	GENERIC, Moore, H.L. Drug Exchange Inc	00839-6224-58
21's	$13.82	GENERIC, Dhs Inc	55887-0953-21
21's	$14.09	GENERIC, Apothecon Inc	62269-0351-21
21's	$15.87	GENERIC, Aligen Independent Laboratories Inc	00405-4666-21
21's	$16.94	MEDROL, Allscripts Pharmaceutical Company	54569-0327-00
21's	$17.53	MEDROL, Prescript Pharmaceuticals	00247-0362-21
21's	$19.72	MEDROL DOSEPAK, Physicians Total Care	54868-0776-01
21's	$21.91	MEDROL DOSEPAK, Pharmacia and Upjohn	00009-0056-04
30's	$17.17	GENERIC, Heartland Healthcare Services	61392-0136-30
30's	$17.17	GENERIC, Heartland Healthcare Services	61392-0136-39
30's	$23.60	MEDROL, Prescript Pharmaceuticals	00247-0362-30
31's	$17.74	GENERIC, Heartland Healthcare Services	61392-0136-31
32's	$18.32	GENERIC, Heartland Healthcare Services	61392-0136-32
40's	$30.35	MEDROL, Prescript Pharmaceuticals	00247-0362-40
45's	$25.76	GENERIC, Heartland Healthcare Services	61392-0136-45
50's	$37.11	MEDROL, Prescript Pharmaceuticals	00247-0362-50
60's	$34.34	GENERIC, Heartland Healthcare Services	61392-0136-60
90's	$51.51	GENERIC, Heartland Healthcare Services	61392-0136-90
100's	$14.29	GENERIC, Vangard Labs	00615-2535-01
100's	$29.87	GENERIC, Us Trading Corporation	56126-0326-11
100's	$44.60	FEDERAL UPPER LIMIT, H.C.F.A. F F P	99999-1791-02
100's	$48.14	GENERIC, Geneva Pharmaceuticals	00781-1402-01
100's	$48.40	GENERIC, Vintage Pharmaceuticals Inc	00254-4216-28
100's	$48.40	GENERIC, Qualitest Products Inc	00603-4593-21
100's	$50.25	GENERIC, Major Pharmaceuticals Inc	00904-2175-60
100's	$52.25	GENERIC, Watson Laboratories Inc	00591-0790-01
100's	$52.25	GENERIC, Watson Laboratories Inc	52544-0790-01
100's	$52.50	GENERIC, Interstate Drug Exchange Inc	00814-4781-14
100's	$54.00	GENERIC, Barr Laboratories Inc	00555-0301-02
100's	$54.00	GENERIC, Mutual/United Research Laboratories	00677-0565-01
100's	$54.00	GENERIC, Mutual/United Research Laboratories	00677-1831-01
100's	$54.00	GENERIC, Duramed Pharmaceuticals Inc	51285-0301-02
100's	$54.00	GENERIC, Greenstone Limited	59762-3327-02
100's	$59.51	GENERIC, Moore, H.L. Drug Exchange Inc	00839-6224-06
100's	$69.41	GENERIC, Apothecon Inc	62269-0351-24
100's	$93.23	MEDROL, Pharmacia and Upjohn	00009-0056-05
100's	$97.51	GENERIC, Aligen Independent Laboratories Inc	00405-4666-01
100's	$107.99	MEDROL, Pharmacia and Upjohn	00009-0056-02
120's	$84.62	GENERIC, Pd-Rx Pharmaceuticals	55289-0649-98

Tablet - Oral - 8 mg

25's	$37.90	MEDROL, Pharmacia and Upjohn	00009-0022-01

Tablet - Oral - 16 mg

14's	$19.04	MEDROL, Pharmacia and Upjohn	00009-0073-02
50's	$117.11	MEDROL, Pharmacia and Upjohn	00009-0073-01

Tablet - Oral - 24 mg

25's	$65.79	MEDROL, Pharmacia and Upjohn	00009-0155-01

Tablet - Oral - 32 mg

25's	$87.20	MEDROL, Pharmacia and Upjohn	00009-0176-01

PRODUCT LISTING - EQUIVALENTS NOT AVAILABLE

Tablet - Oral - 4 mg

21's	$6.69	GENERIC, Prescript Pharmaceuticals	00247-0012-21
21's	$9.16	GENERIC, Physicians Total Care	54868-6624-01
21's	$10.65	GENERIC, Ranbaxy Laboratories	63304-0591-22
21's	$10.89	GENERIC, Mutual/United Research Laboratories	00677-1831-13
21's	$11.00	GENERIC, Allscripts Pharmaceutical Company	54569-1036-00
21's	$12.92	GENERIC, Cardinal Pharmaceuticals	63874-0413-21
21's	$15.90	GENERIC, Southwood Pharmaceuticals Inc	58016-2004-01
21's	$16.70	GENERIC, Pharma Pac	52959-0100-00
30's	$18.77	GENERIC, Physicians Total Care	54868-2913-01
100's	$36.60	GENERIC, Physicians Total Care	54868-2913-00

Methylprednisolone Acetate (001792)

For related information, see the comparative table section in Appendix A.

Categories: Adrenocortical insufficiency; Anemia, acquired hemolytic; Anemia, congenital hypoplastic; Anemia, erythroblastopenia; Ankylosing spondylitis; Arthritis, gouty; Arthritis, post-traumatic; Arthritis, psoriatic; Arthritis, rheumatoid; Asthma; Berylliosis; Bursitis; Carditis, rheumatic; Chorioretinitis; Choroiditis; Colitis, ulcerative; Conjunctivitis, allergic; Crohn's disease; Dermatitis herpetiformis, bullous; Dermatitis, atopic; Dermatitis, contact; Dermatitis, exfoliative; Dermatitis, seborrheic; Dermatomyositis, systemic; Epicondylitis; Erythema multiforme; Herpes zoster ophthalmicus; Hypercalcemia, secondary to neoplasia; Hypersensitivity reactions; Inflammation, anterior segment, ophthalmic; Inflammation, ophthalmic; Inflammatory bowel disease; Iridocyclitis; Iritis; Keratitis; Leukemia; Loffler's syndrome; Lupus erythematosus, systemic; Lymphoma; Meningitis, tuberculous; Multiple sclerosis; Mycosis fungoides; Nephrotic syndrome; Neuritis, optic; Ophthalmia, sympathetic; Pemphigus; Pneumonitis, aspiration; Polymyositis; Psoriasis; Rhinitis, perennial allergic; Rhinitis, seasonal allergic; Sarcoidosis; Serum sickness; Stevens-Johnson syndrome; Synovitis, secondary to osteoarthritis; Tenosynovitis; Thrombocytopenia, secondary; Thyroiditis, nonsuppurative; Trichinosis; Tuberculosis, disseminated; Tuberculosis, fulminating; Tuberculosis, meningitis; Ulcer, allergic corneal marginal; Uveitis; FDA Approved 1960 Jun; Pregnancy Category B

Drug Classes: Corticosteroids

Brand Names: Adlone; Deco-Plex; Depapred; Depmedalone; **Depo-Medrol**; Depo-Predate; Depoject; Depopred; Duralone; Edrol-40; M-Prednisol; Mar-Pred; Med-Jec-40; Medipred; Medralone; Medrex; Medrol Acetate; Methylcotolone; Methylone; Methylprednisolone Acetate; Predacorten; Pri-Methylate; Rep-Pred

Foreign Brand Availability: Depo-Medrate (Germany); Depo Medrol (Bahrain; Benin; Burkina-Faso; Cyprus; Egypt; Ethiopia; Gambia; Ghana; Guinea; Iran; Iraq; Israel; Ivory-Coast; Jordan; Kenya; Kuwait; Lebanon; Liberia; Libya; Malawi; Mali; Mauritania; Mauritius; Morocco; Niger; Nigeria; Oman; Qatar; Republic-of-Yemen; Saudi-Arabia; Senegal; Seychelles; Sierra-Leone; South-Africa; Sudan; Syria; Tanzania; Tunia; Uganda; United-Arab-Emirates; Zambia; Zimbabwe); Depo-Medrone (England); Depo-Moderin (Spain); Depo-Nisolone (Australia); Epizolone-Depot (Bahrain; Cyprus; Egypt; Iran; Iraq; Jordan; Kuwait; Lebanon; Libya; Oman; Qatar; Republic-of-Yemen; Saudi-Arabia; Syria; United-Arab-Emirates); Esametone (Bahrain; Cyprus; Egypt; Iran; Iraq; Jordan; Kuwait; Lebanon; Libya; Oman; Qatar; Republic-of-Yemen; Saudi-Arabia; Syria; United-Arab-Emirates); Solomet (Finland); Urbason (Austria; Czech-Republic; Germany)

HCFA JCODE(S): J1020 20 mg IM; J1030 40 mg IM; J1040 80 mg IM

DESCRIPTION

Methylprednisolone acetate is the 6-methyl derivative of prednisolone. Methylprednisolone acetate is a white or practically white, odorless, crystalline powder which melts at about 215°C with some decomposition. It is soluble in dioxane, sparingly soluble in acetone, in alcohol, in chloroform, and in methanol, and slightly soluble in ether. It is practically insoluble in water. The chemical name for methylprednisolone acetate is pregna-1,4-diene-3,20-dione,21-(acetyloxy)-11,17-dihydroxy-6-methyl-, (6α,11β) and the molecular weight is 416.51.

Methylprednisolone acetate sterile aqueous suspension is an anti-inflammatory glucocorticoid, for intramuscular, intrasynovial, soft tissue or intralesional injection.

MULTIDOSE VIAL

M

Depo-Medrol in the multidose vial is available in three strengths: 20, 40, and 80 mg/ml.

Each ml of these preparations contains the inactive ingredients shown in TABLE 1.

TABLE 1

	Methylprednisolone Acetate		
	20 mg	40 mg	80 mg
Polyethylene glycol 3350	29.5 mg	29.1 mg	28.2 mg
Polysorbate 80	1.97 mg	1.94 mg	1.88 mg
Monobasic sodium phosphate	6.9 mg	6.8 mg	6.59 mg
Dibasic sodium phosphate	1.44 mg	1.42 mg	1.37 mg
Benzyl alcohol (added as a preservative)	9.3 mg	9.16 mg	8.88 mg

Sodium chloride was added to adjust tonicity.

When necessary, pH was adjusted with sodium hydroxide and/or hydrochloric acid. The pH of the finished product remains within the USP specified range (*i.e.*, 3.5-7.0).
Storage: Store at controlled room temperature 20-25°C (68-77°F).

SINGLE-DOSE VIAL

Depo-Medrol in the single-dose vial is available in two strengths: 40 and 80 mg/ml.

Each ml of these preparations contains the inactive ingredients shown in TABLE 2.

TABLE 2

Methylprednisolone acetate	40 mg	80 mg
Polyethylene glycol 3350	29 mg	28 mg
Myristyl-gamma-picolinium chloride	0.195 mg	0.189 mg

Sodium chloride was added to adjust tonicity.
When necessary, pH was adjusted with sodium hydroxide and/or hydrochloric acid.

The pH of the finished product remains within the USP specified range; (*i.e.*, 3.5-7.0).
Storage: Store at controlled room temperature 20-25°C (68-77°F).

CLINICAL PHARMACOLOGY

Naturally occurring glucocorticoids (hydrocortisone), which also have salt retaining properties, are used in replacement therapy in adrenocortical deficiency states. Their synthetic analogs are used primarily for their potent anti-inflammatory effects in disorders of many organ systems.

Glucocorticoids cause profound and varied metabolic effects. In addition, they modify the body's immune response to diverse stimuli.

MULTIDOSE VIAL

As of November, 1990, the formulation for Depo-Medrol (methylprednisolone acetate sterile aqueous suspension) in the multidose vial was revised. In a bioavailability study with thirty subjects, the new formulation was found to be more bioavailable than the previous formulation. An increase in the extent of methylprednisolone acetate absorption was observed for the new formulation as indicated by significantly increased values for area under the serum methylprednisolone acetate concentration curve and maximum serum methylprednisolone concentration (see TABLE 3). No difference in elimination half-life ($T_{1/2}$, calculated from the mean terminal elimination rate) was observed between the two formulations. No medically meaningful differences between the two formulations were seen in relation to vital signs, safety laboratory analyses, formulation effects, local tolerance, or side effects. This increase in absorption is not considered clinically significant.

TABLE 3

	Previous Formulation	Current Formulation
AUC(0-240h) (ng·hr/ml)	1053 (47.3)* [133-2297]†	1286 (39.2) [208-2225]
C_{max}(ng/ml)	8.98 (65.9) [0-28.5]	11.8 (44.1) [3.37-23.4]
$T_{1/2}$(hours)	139 [46-990]	139 [58-866]

* Coefficient of variation (%).
† Range of values.

INDICATIONS AND USAGE

FOR INTRAMUSCULAR ADMINISTRATION

When oral therapy is not feasible and the strength, dosage form, and route of administration of the drug reasonably lend the preparation to the treatment of the condition, the intramuscular use of methylprednisolone acetate sterile aqueous suspension is indicated as follows:

Endocrine Disorders

Primary or secondary adrenocortical insufficiency (hydrocortisone or cortisone is the drug of choice; synthetic analogs may be used in conjunction with mineralocorticoids where applicable; in infancy, mineralocorticoid supplementation is of particular importance).

Acute adrenocortical insufficiency (hydrocortisone or cortisone is the drug of choice; mineralocorticoid supplementation may be necessary, particularly when synthetic analogs are used).

Preoperatively and in the event of serious trauma or illness, in patients with known adrenal insufficiency or when adrenocortical reserve is doubtful: Congenital adrenal hyperplasia, hypercalcemia associated with cancer, and nonsuppurative thyroiditis.

Rheumatic Disorders

As adjunctive therapy for short-term administration (to tide the patient over an acute episode or exacerbation) in: Post-traumatic osteoarthritis, synovitis of osteoarthritis, rheumatoid arthritis, including juvenile rheumatoid arthritis (selected cases may require low-dose maintenance therapy), acute and subacute bursitis, epicondylitis, acute nonspecific tenosynovitis, acute gouty arthritis, psoriatic arthritis, and ankylosing spondylitis.

Collagen Diseases

During an exacerbation or as maintenance therapy in selected cases of: Systemic lupus erythematosus, systemic dermatomyositis (polymyositis), acute rheumatic carditis.

Dermatologic Diseases

Pemphigus, severe erythema multiforme (Stevens-Johnson syndrome), exfoliative dermatitis, bullous dermatitis herpetiformis, severe seborrheic dermatitis, severe psoriasis, mycosis fungoides.

Allergic States

Control of severe incapacitating allergic conditions intractable to adequate trials of conventional treatment in: Bronchial asthma, contact dermatitis, atopic dermatitis, serum sickness, seasonal or perennial allergic rhinitis, drug hypersensitivity reactions, urticarial transfusion reactions, acute noninfectious laryngeal edema (epinephrine is the drug of first choice).

Ophthalmic Diseases

Severe acute and chronic allergic and inflammatory processes involving the eye, such as: Herpes zoster ophthalmicus, iritis, iridocyclitis, chorioretinitis, diffuse posterior uveitis and choroiditis, optic neuritis, sympathetic ophthalmia, anterior segment inflammation, allergic conjunctivitis, allergic corneal marginal ulcers, keratitis.

Gastrointestinal Diseases

To tide the patient over a critical period of the disease in: Ulcerative colitis (systemic therapy), regional enteritis (systemic therapy).

Respiratory Diseases

Symptomatic sarcoidosis, berylliosis, fulminating or disseminated pulmonary tuberculosis when used concurrently with appropriate antituberculous chemotherapy, Loeffler's syndrome not manageable by other means, aspiration pneumonitis.

Hematologic Disorders

Acquired (autoimmune) hemolytic anemia, secondary thrombocytopenia in adults, erythroblastopenia (RBC anemia), congenital (erythroid) hypoplastic anemia.

Neoplastic Diseases

For palliative management of: Leukemias and lymphomas in adults, acute leukemia of childhood.

Edematous States

To induce diuresis or remission of proteinuria in the nephrotic syndrome, without uremia, of the idiopathic type or that due to lupus erythematosus.

Nervous System

Acute exacerbations of multiple sclerosis.

Miscellaneous

Tuberculous meningitis with subarachnoid block or impending block when used concurrently with appropriate antituberculous chemotherapy.

Trichinosis with neurologic or myocardial involvement.

FOR INTRASYNOVIAL OR SOFT TISSUE ADMINISTRATION

See WARNINGS.

Methylprednisolone acetate sterile aqueous suspension is indicated as adjunctive therapy for short-term administration (to tide the patient over an acute episode or exacerbation) in: Synovitis of osteoarthritis, rheumatoid arthritis, acute and subacute bursitis, acute gouty arthritis, epicondylitis, acute nonspecific tenosynovitis, post-traumatic osteoarthritis.

FOR INTRALESIONAL ADMINISTRATION

Methylprednisolone acetate sterile aqueous suspension is indicated for intralesional use in the following conditions: Keloids, discoid lupus erythematosus, necrobiosis lipoidica diabeticorum, alopecia areata. Localized hypertrophic, infiltrated, inflammatory lesions of: lichen planus, psoriatic plaques, granuloma annulare, and lichen simplex chronicus (neurodermatitis).

Methylprednisolone acetate sterile aqueous suspension also may be useful in cystic tumors of an aponeurosis or tendon (ganglia).

CONTRAINDICATIONS

Methylprednisolone acetate sterile aqueous suspension is contraindicated for intrathecal administration. This formulation of methylprednisolone acetate has been associated with reports of severe medical events when administered by this route. Methylprednisolone acetate sterile aqueous suspension is also contraindicated in systemic fungal infections and patients with known hypersensitivity to the product and its constituents.

MULTIDOSE VIAL

Methylprednisolone acetate sterile aqueous suspension is contraindicated for use in premature infants because the formulation contains benzyl alcohol. Benzyl alcohol has been reported to be associated with a fatal "gasping syndrome" in premature infants.

WARNINGS

While crystals of adrenal steroids in the dermis suppress inflammatory reactions, their presence may cause disintegration of the cellular elements and physiochemical changes in the ground substance of the connective tissue. The resultant infrequently occurring dermal and/or subdermal changes may form depressions in the skin at the injection site. The degree to which this reaction occurs will vary with the amount of adrenal steroid injected. Regeneration is usually complete within a few months or after all crystals of the adrenal steroid have been absorbed.

In order to minimize the incidence of dermal and subdermal atrophy, care must be exercised not to exceed recommended doses in injections. Multiple small injections into the area of the lesion should be made whenever possible. The technique of intrasynovial and intramuscular injection should include precautions against injection or leakage into the dermis. Injection into the deltoid muscle should be avoided because of a high incidence of subcutaneous atrophy.

It is critical that, during administration of methylprednisolone acetate, appropriate technique be used and care taken to assure proper placement of drug.

MULTIDOSE VIAL

This product contains benzyl alcohol which is potentially toxic when administered locally to neural tissue.

Multidose use of methylprednisolone acetate sterile aqueous suspension from a single vial requires special care to avoid contamination. Although initially sterile, any multidose use of vials may lead to contamination unless strict aseptic technique is observed. Particular care, such as use of disposable sterile syringes and needles is necessary.

SINGLE-DOSE VIAL

This product is not suitable for multi-dose use. Following administration of the desired dose, any remaining suspension should be discarded.

In patients on corticosteroid therapy subjected to any unusual stress, increased dosage of rapidly acting corticosteroids before, during, and after the stressful situation is indicated.

Corticosteroids may mask some signs of infection, and new infections may appear during their use. There may be decreased resistance and inability to localize infection when corticosteroids are used. Infections with any pathogen including viral, bacterial, fungal, protozoan or helminthic infections, in any location of the body, may be associated with the use of corticosteroids alone or in combination with other immunosuppressive agents that affect cellular immunity, humoral immunity, or neutrophil function.[1]

These infections may be mild, but can be severe and at times fatal. With increasing doses of corticosteroids, the rate of occurrence of infectious complications increases.[2] Do not use intra-articularly, intrabursally or for intratendinous administration for *local* effect in the presence of acute infection.

Prolonged use of corticosteroids may produce posterior subcapsular cataracts, glaucoma with possible damage to the optic nerves, and may enhance the establishment of secondary ocular infections due to fungi or viruses.

Use in Pregnancy: Since adequate human reproduction studies have not been done with corticosteroids, the use of these drugs in pregnancy, nursing mothers, or women of childbearing potential requires that the possible benefits of the drug be weighed against the potential hazards to the mother and embryo or fetus. Infants born of mothers who have received substantial doses of corticosteroids during pregnancy should be carefully observed for signs of hypoadrenalism.

Average and large doses of cortisone or hydrocortisone can cause elevation of blood pressure, salt and water retention, and increased excretion of potassium. These effects are less likely to occur with the synthetic derivatives except when used in large doses. Dietary salt restriction and potassium supplementation may be necessary. All corticosteroids increase calcium excretion.

Administration of live or live, attenuated vaccines is contraindicated in patients receiving immunosuppressive doses of corticosteroids. Killed or inactivated vaccines may be administered to patients receiving immunosuppressive doses of corticosteroids; however, the response to such vaccines may be diminished. Indicated immunization procedures may be undertaken in patients receiving nonimmunosuppressive doses of corticosteroids.

The use of methylprednisolone acetate in active tuberculosis should be restricted to those cases of fulminating or disseminated tuberculosis in which the corticosteroid is used for the management of the disease in conjunction with appropriate antituberculous regimen.

If corticosteroids are indicated in patients with latent tuberculosis or tuberculin reactivity, close observation is necessary as reactivation of the disease may occur. During prolonged corticosteroid therapy, these patients should receive chemoprophylaxis.

Because rare instances of anaphylactoid reactions have occurred in patients receiving parenteral corticosteroid therapy, appropriate precautionary measures should be taken prior to administration, especially when the patient has a history of allergy to any drug.

Persons who are on drugs which suppress the immune system are more susceptible to infections than healthy individuals. Chicken pox and measles, for example, can have a more serious or even fatal course in non-immune children or adults on corticosteroids. In such children or adults who have not had these diseases, particular care should be taken to avoid exposure. How the dose, route and duration of corticosteroid administration affects the risk of developing a disseminated infection is not known. The contribution of the underlying disease and/or prior corticosteroid treatment to the risk is also not known. If exposed to chicken pox, prophylaxis with varicella zoster immune globulin (ZVIG) may be indicated. If exposed to measles, prophylaxis with pooled intramuscular immunoglobulin (IG) may be indicated. (See the respective monographs for complete VZIG and IG prescribing information.) If chicken pox develops, treatment with antiviral agents may be considered. Similarly, corticosteroids should be used with great care in patients with known or suspected Strongyloides (threadworm) infestation. In such patients, corticosteroid-induced immunosuppression may lead to Strongyloides hyperinfection and dissemination with widespread larval migration, often accompanied by severe enterocolitis and potentially fatal gram-negative septicemia.

PRECAUTIONS

GENERAL

Drug-induced secondary adrenocortical insufficiency may be minimized by gradual reduction of dosage. This type of relative insufficiency may persist for months after discontinuation of therapy; therefore, in any situation of stress occurring during that period, hormone therapy should be reinstituted. Since mineralocorticoid secretion may be impaired, salt and/or a mineralocorticoid should be administered concurrently.

There is an enhanced effect of corticosteroids in patients with hypothyroidism and in those with cirrhosis.

Corticosteroids should be used cautiously in patients with ocular herpes simplex for fear of corneal perforation.

The lowest possible dose of corticosteroid should be used to control the condition under treatment, and when reduction in dosage is possible, the reduction must be gradual.

Psychic derangements may appear when corticosteroids are used, ranging from euphoria, insomnia, mood swings, personality changes, and severe depression to frank psychotic manifestations. Also, existing emotional instability or psychotic tendencies may be aggravated by corticosteroids.

Steroids should be used with caution in nonspecific ulcerative colitis, if there is a probability of impending perforation, abscess or other pyogenic infection. Caution must also be used in diverticulitis, fresh intestinal anastomoses, active or latent peptic ulcer, renal insufficiency, hypertension, osteoporosis, and myasthenia gravis, when steroids are used as direct or adjunctive therapy.

Growth and development of infants and children on prolonged corticosteroid therapy should be carefully followed.

Kaposi's sarcoma has been reported to occur in patients receiving corticosteroid therapy. Discontinuation of corticosteroids may result in clinical remission.

Multidose Vial: When multidose vials are used, special care to prevent contamination of the contents is essential. There is some evidence that benzalkonium chloride is not an adequate antiseptic for sterilizing methylprednisolone acetate sterile aqueous suspension multidose vials. A povidone-iodine solution or similar product is recommended to cleanse the vial top prior to aspiration of contents. (See WARNINGS.)

The following additional precautions apply for parenteral corticosteroids:

Intrasynovial injection of a corticosteroid may produce systemic as well as local effects.

Appropriate examination of any joint fluid present is necessary to exclude a septic process.

A marked increase in pain accompanied by local swelling, further restriction of joint motion, fever, and malaise are suggestive of septic arthritis. If this complication occurs and the diagnosis of sepsis is confirmed, appropriate antimicrobial therapy should be instituted.

Local injection of a steroid into a previously infected joint is to be avoided.

Corticosteroids should not be injected into unstable joints.

The slower rate of absorption by intramuscular administration should be recognized.

Although controlled clinical trials have shown corticosteroids to be effective in speeding the resolution of acute exacerbations of multiple sclerosis, they do not show that corticosteroids affect the ultimate outcome or natural history of the disease. The studies do show that relatively high doses of corticosteroids are necessary to demonstrate a significant effect. (See DOSAGE AND ADMINISTRATION.)

Since complications of treatment with glucocorticoids are dependent on the size of the dose and the duration of treatment, a risk/benefit decision must be made in each individual case as to dose and duration of treatment and as to whether daily or intermittent therapy should be used.

INFORMATION FOR THE PATIENT

Patients who are on immunosuppressant doses of corticosteroids should be warned to avoid exposure to chicken pox or measles. Patients should be advised that if they are exposed, medical advice should be sought without delay.

DRUG INTERACTIONS

The pharmacokinetic interactions listed below are potentially clinically important. Mutual inhibition of metabolism occurs with concurrent use of cyclosporin and methylprednisolone; therefore, it is possible that adverse events associated with the individual use of either drug may be more apt to occur. Convulsions have been reported with concurrent use of methylprednisolone and cyclosporin. Drugs that induce hepatic enzymes such as phenobarbital, phenytoin and rifampin may increase the clearance of methylprednisolone and may require increases in methylprednisolone dose to achieve the desired response. Drugs such as troleandomycin and ketoconazole may inhibit the metabolism of methylprednisolone and thus decrease its clearance. Therefore, the dose of methylprednisolone should be titrated to avoid steroid toxicity.

Methylprednisolone may increase the clearance of chronic high dose aspirin. This could lead to decreased salicylate serum levels or increase the risk of salicylate toxicity when methyprednisolone is withdrawn. Aspirin should be used cautiously in conjunction with corticosteroids in patients suffering from hypoprothrombinemia.

The effect of methylprednisolone on oral anticoagulants is variable. There are reports of enhanced as well as diminished effects of anticoagulant when given concurrently with corticosteroids. Therefore, coagulation indices should be monitored to maintain the desired anticoagulant effect.

ADVERSE REACTIONS

Fluid and Electrolyte Disturbances: Sodium retention; fluid retention; congestive heart failure in susceptible patients; potassium loss; hypokalemic alkalosis; hypertension.

Musculoskeletal: Muscle weakness; steroid myopathy; loss of muscle mass; osteoporosis; tendon rupture, particularly of the Achilles tendon; vertebral compression fractures; aseptic necrosis of femoral and humeral heads; pathologic fracture of long bones.

Gastrointestinal: Peptic ulcer with possible subsequent perforation and hemorrhage; pancreatitis; abdominal distention; ulcerative esophagitis; increases in alanine transaminase (ALT, SGPT), aspartate transaminase (AST, SGOT), and alkaline phosphatase have been observed following corticosteroid treatment. These changes are usually small, not associated with any clinical syndrome and are reversible upon discontinuation.

Dermatologic: Impaired wound healing; thin fragile skin; petechiae and ecchymoses; facial erythema; increased sweating; may suppress reactions to skin tests.

Neurological: Convulsions; increased intracranial pressure with papilledema (pseudotumor cerebri) usually after treatment; vertigo; headache.

Endocrine: Menstrual irregularities; development of Cushingoid state; suppression of growth in children; secondary adrenocortical and pituitary unresponsiveness, particularly in times of stress, as in trauma, surgery or illness; decreased carbohydrate tolerance; manifestations of latent diabetes mellitus; increased requirements for insulin or oral hypoglycemic agents in diabetes.

Ophthalmic: Posterior subcapsular cataracts; increased intraocular pressure; glaucoma; exophthalmos.

Metabolic: Negative nitrogen balance due to protein catabolism.

The following *additional* adverse reactions are related to parenteral corticosteroid therapy: Anaphylactic reaction; allergic or hypersensitivity reactions; urticaria; hyperpigmentation or hypopigmentation; subcutaneous and cutaneous atrophy; sterile abscess; injection site infections following non-sterile administration (see WARNINGS); postinjection flare, following intrasynovial use; Charcot-like athropathy.

Adverse reactions reported with the following routes of administration:

Intrathecal/Epidural: Arachnoiditis; meningitis; paraparesis/paraplegia; sensory disturbances; bowel/bladder dysfunction; headache; seizures.

Intranasal: Temporary/permanent visual impairment including blindness; allergic reactions; rhinitis.

Ophthalmic: Temporary/permanent visual impairment including blindness; increased intraocular pressure; ocular and periocular inflammation including allergic reactions, infection, residue or slough at injection site.

Miscellaneous Injection Sites (Scalp, Tonsillar Fauces, Sphenopalatine Ganglion): Blindness.

DOSAGE AND ADMINISTRATION

Because of possible physical incompatibilities, methylprednisolone acetate sterile aqueous suspension should not be diluted or mixed with other solutions.

ADMINISTRATION FOR LOCAL EFFECT

Therapy with methylprednisolone acetate does not obviate the need for the conventional measures usually employed. Although this method of treatment will ameliorate symptoms, it is in no sense a cure and the hormone has no effect on the cause of the inflammation.

Rheumatoid and Osteoarthritis

The dose for intra-articular administration depends upon the size of the joint and varies with the severity of the condition in the individual patient. In chronic cases, injections may be repeated at intervals ranging from 1-5 or more weeks depending upon the degree of relief obtained from the initial injection. The doses in TABLE 4 are given as a general guide.

TABLE 4

Size of Joint	Examples	Range of Dosage
Large	Knees, ankles, shoulders	20-80 mg
Medium	Elbows, wrists	10-40 mg
Small	Metacarpophalangeal, interphalangeal, sternoclavicular, acromioclavicular	4-10 mg

Procedure

It is recommended that the anatomy of the joint involved be reviewed before attempting intra-articular injection. In order to obtain the full anti-inflammatory effect it is important that the injection be made into the synovial space. Employing the same sterile technique as for a lumbar puncture, a sterile 20-24 gauge needle (on a dry syringe) is quickly inserted into the synovial cavity. Procaine infiltration is elective. The aspiration of only a few drops of joint fluid proves the joint space has been entered by the needle. *The injection site for each joint is determined by that location where the synovial cavity is most superficial and most free of large vessels and nerves.* With the needle in place, the aspirating syringe is removed and replaced by a second syringe containing the desired amount of methylprednisolone acetate sterile aqueous suspension. The plunger is then pulled outward slightly to aspirate synovial fluid and to make sure the needle is still in the synovial space. After injection, the joint is moved gently a few times to aid mixing of the synovial fluid and the suspension. The site is covered with a small sterile dressing.

Suitable sites for intra-articular injection are the knee, ankle, wrist, elbow, shoulder, phalangeal, and hip joints. Since difficulty is not infrequently encountered in entering the hip joint, precautions should be taken to avoid any large blood vessels in the area. Joints not suitable for injection are those that are anatomically inaccessible such as the spinal joints and those like the sacroiliac joints that are devoid of synovial space. Treatment failures are most frequently the result of failure to enter the joint space. Little or no benefit follows injection into surrounding tissue. If failures occur when injections into the synovial spaces are certain, as determined by aspiration of fluid, repeated injections are usually futile. Local therapy does not alter the underlying disease process, and whenever possible comprehensive therapy including physiotherapy and orthopedic correction should be employed.

Following intra-articular steroid therapy, care should be taken to avoid overuse of joints in which symptomatic benefit has been obtained. Negligence in this matter may permit an increase in joint deterioration that will more than offset the beneficial effects of the steroid.

Unstable joints should not be injected. Repeated intra-articular injection may in some cases result in instability of the joint. x-ray follow-up is suggested in selected cases to detect deterioration.

If a local anesthetic is used prior to injection of methylprednisolone acetate, the anesthetic monograph should be read carefully and all the precautions observed.

Bursitis

The area around the injection site is prepared in a sterile way and a wheal at the site made with 1% procaine hydrochloride solution. A 20-24 gauge needle attached to a dry syringe is inserted into the bursa and the fluid aspirated. The needle is left in place and the aspirating syringe changed for a small syringe containing the desired dose. After injection, the needle is withdrawn and a small dressing applied.

Miscellaneous

Ganglion, Tendinitis, Epicondylitis

In the treatment of conditions such as tendinitis or tenosynovitis, care should be taken, following application of a suitable antiseptic to the overlying skin, to inject the suspension into the tendon sheath rather than into the substance of the tendon. The tendon may be readily palpated when placed on a stretch. When treating conditions such as epicondylitis, the area of greatest tenderness should be outlined carefully and the suspension infiltrated into the area. For ganglia of the tendon sheaths, the suspension is injected directly into the cyst. In many cases, a single injection causes a marked decrease in the size of the cystic tumor and may effect disappearance. The usual sterile precautions should be observed, of course, with each injection.

The dose in the treatment of the various conditions of the tendinous or bursal structures listed above varies with the condition being treated and ranges from 4-30 mg. In recurrent or chronic conditions, repeated injections may be necessary.

Injections for Local Effect in Dermatologic Conditions

Following cleansing with an appropriate antiseptic such as 70% alcohol, 20-60 mg of the suspension is injected into the lesion. It may be necessary to distribute doses ranging from 20-40 mg by repeated local injections in the case of large lesions. Care should be taken to avoid injection of sufficient material to cause blanching since this may be followed by a small slough. One (1) to 4 injections are usually employed, the intervals between injections varying with the type of lesion being treated and the duration of improvement produced by the initial injection.

When multidose vials are used, special care to prevent contamination of the contents is essential. (See WARNINGS.)

ADMINISTRATION FOR SYSTEMIC EFFECT

The intramuscular dosage will vary with the condition being treated. When employed as a temporary substitute for oral therapy, a single injection during each 24 hour period of a dose of the suspension equal to the total daily oral dose of methylprednisolone acetate tablets is usually sufficient. When a prolonged effect is desired, the weekly dose may be calculated by multiplying the daily oral dose by 7 and given as a single intramuscular injection.

Dosage must be individualized according to the severity of the disease and response of the patient. For infants and children, the recommended dosage will have to be reduced, but dosage should be governed by the severity of the condition rather than by strict adherence to the ratio indicated by age or body weight.

Hormone therapy is an adjunct to, and not a replacement for, conventional therapy. Dosage must be decreased or discontinued gradually when the drug has been administered for more than a few days. The severity, prognosis and expected duration of the disease and the reaction of the patient to medication are primary factors in determining dosage. If a period of spontaneous remission occurs in a chronic condition, treatment should be discontinued. Routine laboratory studies, such as urinalysis, 2 hour postprandial blood sugar, determination of blood pressure and body weight, and a chest X-ray should be made at regular intervals during prolonged therapy. Upper GI x-rays are desirable in patients with an ulcer history or significant dyspepsia.

In patients with the **adrenogenital syndrome**, a single intramuscular injection of 40 mg every 2 weeks may be adequate. For maintenance of patients with **rheumatoid arthritis,** the weekly intramuscular dose will vary from 40-120 mg. The usual dosage for patients with **dermatologic lesions** benefited by systemic corticoid therapy is 40-120 mg of methylprednisolone acetate administered intramuscularly at weekly intervals for 1-4 weeks. In acute severe dermatitis due to poison ivy, relief may result within 8-12 hours following intramuscular administration of a single dose of 80-120 mg. In chronic contact dermatitis repeated injections at 5-10 day intervals may be necessary. In seborrheic dermatitis, a weekly dose of 80 mg may be adequate to control the condition.

Following intramuscular administration of 80-120 mg to asthmatic patients, relief may result within 6-48 hours and persist for several days to 2 weeks. Similarly in patients with allergic rhinitis (hay fever) an intramuscular dose of 80-120 mg may be followed by relief of coryzal symptoms within 6 hours persisting for several days to 3 weeks.

If signs of stress are associated with the condition being treated, the dosage of the suspension should be increased. If a rapid hormonal effect of maximum intensity is required, the intravenous administration of highly soluble methylprednisolone sodium succinate is indicated.

MULTIPLE SCLEROSIS

In treatment of acute exacerbations of multiple sclerosis daily doses of 200 mg of prednisolone for a week followed by 80 mg every other day for 1 month have been shown to be effective (4 mg of methylprednisolone is equivalent to 5 mg of prednisolone).

PRODUCT LISTING - RATED THERAPEUTICALLY EQUIVALENT

Suspension - Injectable - 40 mg/ml

5 ml	$8.47	GENERIC, Geneva Pharmaceuticals	00781-3055-75

Suspension - Injectable - 80 mg/ml

5 ml	$15.41	GENERIC, Geneva Pharmaceuticals	00781-3050-75
5 ml	$15.41	GENERIC, Geneva Pharmaceuticals	00781-3065-75

PRODUCT LISTING - RATED NOT THERAPEUTICALLY EQUIVALENT

Suspension - Injectable - 20 mg/ml

5 ml	$14.70	DEPO-MEDROL, Pharmacia and Upjohn	00009-0274-01
10 ml	$7.50	GENERIC, Cmc-Consolidated Midland Corporation	00223-8165-10

Suspension - Injectable - 40 mg/ml

1's	$4.00	GENERIC, Cmc-Consolidated Midland Corporation	00223-8160-01
5 ml	$4.75	GENERIC, Keene Pharmaceuticals Inc	00588-5361-75
5 ml	$7.32	GENERIC, General Injectables and Vaccines Inc	52584-0196-05
5 ml	$7.50	GENERIC, Cmc-Consolidated Midland Corporation	00223-8166-05
5 ml	$7.50	GENERIC, C.O. Truxton Inc	00463-1105-05
5 ml	$8.13	GENERIC, Forest Pharmaceuticals	00785-9055-05
5 ml	$8.47	GENERIC, Geneva Pharmaceuticals	00781-3060-75
5 ml	$9.38	GENERIC, Interstate Drug Exchange Inc	00814-4780-38
5 ml	$10.67	GENERIC, Moore, H.L. Drug Exchange Inc	00839-7946-25
5 ml	$10.76	GENERIC, Hyrex Pharmaceuticals	00314-0840-75
5 ml	$11.50	GENERIC, Forest Pharmaceuticals	00456-4840-05
5 ml	$11.88	GENERIC, Pasadena Research Laboratories Inc	00418-6401-05
5 ml	$11.98	GENERIC, Forest Pharmaceuticals	00456-1071-05
10 ml	$12.95	GENERIC, Roberts/Hauck Pharmaceutical Corporation	43797-0132-12
10 ml	$14.40	GENERIC, Interstate Drug Exchange Inc	00814-4780-40
10 ml	$15.05	GENERIC, Moore, H.L. Drug Exchange Inc	00839-7946-30
10 ml	$15.75	GENERIC, Med Tek Pharmaceuticals Inc	52349-0106-10
10 ml	$16.18	GENERIC, Hyrex Pharmaceuticals	00314-0842-70
10 ml	$27.10	GENERIC, Merz Pharmaceuticals	00259-0356-10

Suspension - Injectable - 80 mg/ml

1 ml	$10.40	DEPO-MEDROL, Allscripts Pharmaceutical Company	54569-3374-00
1 ml	$13.33	DEPO-MEDROL, Pharmacia and Upjohn	00009-3475-01
1 ml x 25	$214.06	DEPO-MEDROL, Pharmacia and Upjohn	00009-3475-02
1 ml x 25	$332.95	DEPO-MEDROL, Pharmacia and Upjohn	00009-3475-03
5 ml	$9.50	GENERIC, Keene Pharmaceuticals Inc	00588-5362-75
5 ml	$12.00	GENERIC, Cmc-Consolidated Midland Corporation	00223-8167-05
5 ml	$12.41	GENERIC, Moore, H.L. Drug Exchange Inc	00839-7947-25
5 ml	$12.57	GENERIC, General Injectables and Vaccines Inc	52584-0197-05
5 ml	$12.75	GENERIC, Med Tek Pharmaceuticals Inc	52349-0107-05
5 ml	$12.81	GENERIC, Forest Pharmaceuticals	00785-0956-05
5 ml	$12.95	GENERIC, Roberts/Hauck Pharmaceutical Corporation	43797-0131-11
5 ml	$14.00	GENERIC, Bolan Pharmaceutical Inc	44437-0197-05
5 ml	$14.42	GENERIC, Moore, H.L. Drug Exchange Inc	00839-6201-25
5 ml	$14.93	GENERIC, Interstate Drug Exchange Inc	00814-4782-38
5 ml	$15.60	GENERIC, Hyrex Pharmaceuticals	00314-0841-75
5 ml	$15.70	GENERIC, Major Pharmaceuticals Inc	00904-0897-05
5 ml	$16.60	GENERIC, Pasadena Research Laboratories Inc	00418-6501-05
5 ml	$19.20	GENERIC, Ivax Corporation	00182-1068-62
5 ml	$19.20	GENERIC, Mutual/United Research Laboratories	00677-1539-20
5 ml	$20.00	GENERIC, Forest Pharmaceuticals	00456-4880-05
5 ml	$20.84	GENERIC, Forest Pharmaceuticals	00456-1072-05
5 ml	$27.10	GENERIC, Merz Pharmaceuticals	00259-0357-05
5 ml	$41.58	DEPO-MEDROL, Allscripts Pharmaceutical Company	54569-2232-00
5 ml	$45.31	DEPO-MEDROL, Pharmacia and Upjohn	00009-0306-02
5 ml x 25	$855.25	DEPO-MEDROL, Pharmacia and Upjohn	00009-0306-10
5 ml x 25	$1132.93	DEPO-MEDROL, Pharmacia and Upjohn	00009-0306-12

PRODUCT LISTING - EQUIVALENTS NOT AVAILABLE

Suspension - Injectable - 40 mg/ml

1 ml	$4.98	GENERIC, Prescript Pharmaceuticals	00247-0297-01
1 ml	$6.30	DEPO-MEDROL, Allscripts Pharmaceutical Company	54569-2213-00
1 ml	$8.06	DEPO-MEDROL, Pharmacia and Upjohn	00009-3073-01
1 ml x 25	$129.50	DEPO-MEDROL, Pharmacia and Upjohn	00009-3073-02
1 ml x 25	$157.50	DEPO-MEDROL, Allscripts Pharmaceutical Company	54569-3946-00
1 ml x 25	$201.69	DEPO-MEDROL, Pharmacia and Upjohn	00009-3073-03
5 ml	$8.98	MED-JEC-40, Hauser, A.F. Inc	52637-0756-05
5 ml	$11.49	GENERIC, Prescript Pharmaceuticals	00247-0297-05
5 ml	$14.00	METHACORT 40, Clint Pharmaceutical Inc	55553-0196-05
5 ml	$22.84	DEPO-MEDROL, Allscripts Pharmaceutical Company	54569-1901-01
5 ml	$24.89	DEPO-MEDROL, Pharmacia and Upjohn	00009-0280-02
5 ml x 25	$376.00	DEPO-MEDROL, Pharmacia and Upjohn	00009-0280-32
5 ml x 25	$622.25	DEPO-MEDROL, Pharmacia and Upjohn	00009-0280-51
10 ml	$19.64	GENERIC, Prescript Pharmaceuticals	00247-0297-10
10 ml	$41.58	DEPO-MEDROL, Allscripts Pharmaceutical Company	54569-4265-00
10 ml	$45.32	DEPO-MEDROL, Pharmacia and Upjohn	00009-0280-03
10 ml x 25	$34.20	DEPO-MEDROL, Pharmacia and Upjohn	00009-0280-33
10 ml x 25	$1132.92	DEPO-MEDROL, Pharmacia and Upjohn	00009-0280-52
10's	$12.45	GENERIC, Merit Pharmaceuticals	30727-0385-70

Suspension - Injectable - 80 mg/ml

1 ml	$10.35	GENERIC, Watson/Schein Pharmaceuticals Inc	00364-3065-51
5 ml	$15.00	METHYLCOTOLONE, Truxton Company Inc	00463-1111-05
5 ml	$21.82	GENERIC, Physicians Total Care	54868-1994-00
5 ml	$24.75	GENERIC, Clint Pharmaceutical Inc	55553-0197-05
5's	$11.55	GENERIC, Merit Pharmaceuticals	30727-0685-85

M

Methylprednisolone Sodium Succinate *(001794)*

For related information, see the comparative table section in Appendix A.

Categories: Adrenocortical insufficiency; Anemia, acquired hemolytic; Anemia, congenital hypoplastic; Anemia, erythroblastopenia; Ankylosing spondylitis; Arthritis, gouty; Arthritis, post-traumatic; Arthritis, psoriatic; Arthritis, rheumatoid; Asthma; Berylliosis; Bursitis; Carditis, rheumatic; Chorioretinitis; Choroiditis; Colitis, ulcerative; Conjunctivitis, allergic; Crohn's disease; Dermatitis herpetiformis, bullous; Dermatitis, atopic; Dermatitis, contact; Dermatitis, exfoliative; Dermatitis, seborrheic; Dermatomyositis, systemic; Epicondylitis; Erythema multiforme; Herpes zoster ophthalmicus; Hypercalcemia, secondary to neoplasia; Hypersensitivity reactions; Inflammation, anterior segment, ophthalmic; Inflammation, ophthalmic; Inflammatory bowel disease; Iridocyclitis; Iritis; Keratitis; Leukemia; Loffler's syndrome; Lupus erythematosus, systemic; Lymphoma; Meningitis, tuberculous; Multiple sclerosis; Mycosis fungoides; Nephrotic syndrome; Neuritis, optic; Ophthalmia, sympathetic; Pemphigus; Pneumonitis, aspiration; Polymyositis; Psoriasis; Rhinitis, perennial allergic; Rhinitis, seasonal allergic; Sarcoidosis; Serum sickness; Stevens-Johnson syndrome; Synovitis, secondary to osteoarthritis; Tenosynovitis; Thrombocytopenia, secondary; Thyroiditis, nonsuppurative; Trichinosis; Tuberculosis, disseminated; Tuberculosis, fulminating; Tuberculosis, meningitis; Ulcer, allergic corneal marginal; Uveitis; FDA Approved 1959 May; Pregnancy Category C

Drug Classes: Corticosteroids

Brand Names: A-Methapred; **Solu-Medrol**

Foreign Brand Availability: Cryosolona (Mexico); Medrate Solubile (Germany); Mepsolone (Korea); Solomet (Finland); Solu Medrol (Benin; Burkina-Faso; Colombia; Costa-Rica; Ecuador; El-Salvador; Ethiopia; Gambia; Ghana; Guatemala; Guinea; Honduras; Ivory-Coast; Kenya; Liberia; Malawi; Mali; Mauritania; Mauritius; Mexico; Morocco; Nicaragua; Niger; Nigeria; Panama; Senegal; Seychelles; Sierra-Leone; South-Africa; Sudan; Tanzania; Tunia; Uganda; Zambia; Zimbabwe); Solu-Medrone (England); Solu-Moderin (Spain); Urbason Solubile (Austria; Czech-Republic; Denmark; Germany); Urbason Soluble (Spain)

HCFA JCODE(S): J2920 up to 40 mg IM, IV; J2930 up to 125 mg IM, IV

DESCRIPTION

Methylprednisolone sodium succinate steril powder contains methylprednisolone sodium succinate as the active ingredient. Methylprednisolone sodium succinate occurs as a white, or nearly white, odorless hygroscopic, amorphous solid. It is very soluble in water and in alcohol; it is insoluble in chloroform and is very slightly soluble in acetone.

The chemical name for methylprednisolone sodium succinate is pregna-1,4-diene-3,20-dione,21-(3-carboxy-1-oxopropoxy)-11,17-dihydroxy-6 -methyl-monosodium salt, (6α, 11β) and the molecular weight is 496.53.

Methylprednisolone sodium succinate is so extremely soluble in water that it may be administered in a small volume of diluent and is especially well suited for intravenous use in situations in which high blood levels of methylprednisolone are required rapidly.

Methylprednisolone sodium succinate is available in several strengths and packages for intravenous or intramuscular administration.

40 mg (Single-Dose Vial): Each ml (when mixed) contains methylprednisolone sodium succinate equivalent to 40 mg methylprednisolone; also 1.6 mg monobasic sodium phosphate anhydrous; 17.46 mg dibasic sodium phosphate dried; 25 mg lactose hydrous; 8.8 mg benzyl alcohol added as preservative.

125 mg (Single-Dose Vial): Each 2 ml (when mixed) contains methylprednisolone sodium succinate equivalent to 125 mg methylprednisolone; also 1.6 mg monobasic sodium phosphate anhydrous; 17.4 mg dibasic sodium phosphate dried; 17.6 mg benzyl alcohol added as preservative.

500 mg Vial: Each 8 ml (when mixed as directed) contains methylprednisolone sodium succinate equivalent to 500 mg methylprednisolone; also 6.4 mg monobasic sodium phosphate anhydrous; 69.6 mg dibasic sodium phosphate dried.

500 mg Vial with Diluent: Each 8 ml (when mixed as directed) contains methylprednisolone sodium succinate equivalent to 500 mg methylprednisolone; also 6.4 mg monobasic sodium phosphate anhydrous; 69.6 mg dibasic sodium phosphate dried; 70.2 mg benzyl alcohol added as preservative.

500 mg (Single-Dose Vial): Each 4 ml (when mixed) contains methylprednisolone sodium succinate equivalent to 500 mg methylprednisolone; also 6.4 mg monobasic sodium phosphate anhydrous; 69.6 mg dibasic sodium phosphate dired; 33.7 mg benzyl alcohol added as preservative.

1 g Vial: Each 16 ml (when mixed as directed) contains methylprednisolone sodium succinate equivalent to 1 g methylprednisolone; also 12.8 mg monobasic sodium phosphate anhydrous; 139.2 mg dibasic sodium phosphate dried.

1 g (Single-Dose Vial): Each 8 ml (when mixed) contains methylprednisolone sodium succinate equivalent to 1 g methylprednisolone; also 12.8 mg monobasic sodium phosphate anhydrous; 139.2 mg dibasic sodium phosphate dried; 66.8 mg benzyl alcohol added as preservative.

2 g Vial: Each 30.6 ml (when mixed as directed) contains methylprednisolone sodium succinate equivalent to 2 g methylprednisolone; also 25.6 mg monobasic sodium phosphate anhydrous; 278 mg dibasic sodium phosphate dried.

2 g Vial with Diluent: Each 30.6 ml (when mixed as directed) contains methylprednisolone sodium succinate equivalent to 2 g methylprednisolone; also 25.6 mg monobasic sodium phosphate anhydrous; 278 mg dibasic sodium phosphate dried; 273 mg benzyl alcohol added as preservative.

When necessary, the pH of each formula was adjusted with sodium hydroxide so that the pH of the reconstituted solution is within the specified range of 7-8 and the tonicities are, for the 40 mg/ml solution, 0.50 osmolar; for the 125 mg per 2 ml, 500 mg per 8 ml and 1 g per 16 ml solutions, 0.40 osmolar; for the 1 g per 8 ml solution, 0.44 osmolar; for the 2 g per 30.6 ml solutions, 0.42 osmolar. (Isotonic saline = 0.28 osmolar).

IMPORTANT: Use only the accompanying diluent or bacteriostatic water for injection with benzyl alcohol when reconstituting methylprednisolone sodium succinate. **Use within 48 hours after mixing.**

STORAGE

Protect from light. Store unreconstituted product and solution at controlled room temperature 20-25°C (68-77°F).

Use solution within 48 hours after mixing.

M

CLINICAL PHARMACOLOGY

Naturally occurring glucocorticoids (hydrocortisone and cortisone), which also have salt-retaining properties, are used as replacement therapy in adrenocortical deficiency states. Their synthetic analogs are primarily used for their potent anti-inflammatory effects in disorders of many organ systems.

Glucocorticoids cause profound and varied metabolic effects. In addition, they modify the body's immune responses to diverse stimuli.

Methylprednisolone is a potent anti-inflammatory steroid synthesized in a laboratory. It has a greater anti-inflammatory potency than prednisolone and even less tendency than prednisolone to induce sodium and water retention.

Methylprednisolone sodium succinate has the same metabolic and anti-inflammatory actions as methylprednisolone. When given parenterally and in equimolar quantities, the 2 compounds are equivalent in biologic activity. The relative potency of methylprednisolone sodium succinate sterile powder and hydrocortisone sodium succinate, as indicated by depression of eosinophil count, following intravenous administration, is at least 4 to 1. This is in good agreement with the relative oral potency of methylprednisolone and hydrocortisone.

INDICATIONS AND USAGE

When oral therapy is not feasible, and the strength, dosage form and route of administration of the drug reasonably lend the preparation to the treatment of the condition, methylprednisolone sodium succinate sterile powder is indicated for intravenous or intramuscular use in the following conditions:

Endocrine Disorders:

Primary or secondary adrenocortical insufficiency (hydrocortisone or cortisone is the drug of choice; synthetic analogs may be used in conjunction with mineralocorticoids where applicable; in infancy, mineralocorticoid supplementation is of particular importance).

Acute adrenocortical insufficiency (hydrocortisone or cortisone is the drug of choice; mineralocorticoid supplementation may be necessary, particularly when synthetic analogs are used).

Preoperatively and in the event of serious trauma or illness, in patients with known adrenal insufficiency or when adrenocortical reserve is doubtful.

Shock unresponsive to conventional therapy if adrenocortical insufficiency exists or is suspected.

Congenital adrenal hyperplasia.

Nonsuppurative thyroiditis.

Hypercalcemia associated with cancer.

Rheumatic Disorders: As adjunctive therapy for short-term administration (to tide the patient over an acute episode or exacerbation) in:

Post-traumatic osteoarthritis.

Epicondylitis.

Synovitis of osteoarthritis.

Acute nonspecific tenosynovitis.

Rheumatoid arthritis, including juvenile rheumatoid arthritis (select cases may require low-dose maintenance therapy).

Acute gouty arthritis.

Psoriatic arthritis.

Ankylosing spondylitis.

Acute and subacute bursitis.

Collagen Diseases: During an exacerbation or as maintenance therapy in selected cases of:

Systemic lupus erythematosus.

Systemic dermatomyositis (polymyositis).

Acute rheumatic carditis.

Dermatologic Diseases:

Pemphigus.

Bullous dermatitis herpetiformis.

Severe erythema multiform (Stevens-Johnson syndrome).

Severe seborrheic dermatitis.

Severe psoriasis.

Exfoliative dermatitis.

Mycosis fungoides.

Allergic States: Control of severe or incapacitating allergic conditions intractable to adequate trials of conventional treatment in:

Bronchial asthma.

Drug hypersensitivity reactions.

Contact dermatitis.

Urticarial transfusion reactions.

Atopic dermatitis.

Acute noninfectious laryngeal edema (epinephrine is the drug of first choice).

Serum sickness.

Seasonal or perennial allergic rhinitis.

Ophthalmic Diseases: Severe acute and chronic allergic and inflammatory processes involving the eye, such as:

Herpes zoster ophthalmicus.

Sympathetic ophthalmia.

Iritis, iridocyclitis.

Anterior segment inflammation.

Chorioretinitis.

Allergic conjunctivitis.

Diffuse posterior uveitis and choroiditis.

Allergic corneal marginal ulcers.

Optic neuritis.

Keratitis.

Gastrointestinal Diseases: To tide the patient over a critical period of the disease in:

Ulcerative colitis (systemic therapy).

Regional enteritis (systemic therapy).

Respiratory Diseases:

Symptomatic sarcoidosis.

Loeffler's syndrome not manageable by other means.

Berylliosis.

Aspiration pneumonitis.

Fulminating or disseminated pulmonary tuberculosis when used concurrently with appropriate antituberculous chemotherapy.

Hematologic Disorders:

Acquired (autoimmune) hemolytic anemia.

Erythroblastopenia (RBC anemia).

Idiopathic thrombocytopenic purpura in adults (IV only; IM administration is contraindicated).

Congenital (erythroid) hypoplastic anemia.

Secondary thrombocytopenia in adults.

Neoplastic Disease: For palliative management of:

Leukemias and lymphomas in adults.

Acute leukemia of childhood.

Edematous States:

To induce diuresis or remission of proteinuria in the nephrotic syndrome, without uremia, of the idiopathic type or that due to lupus erythematosus.

Nervous System:

Acute exacerbations of multiple sclerosis.

Miscellaneous:

Tuberculous meningitis with subarachnoid block or impending block when used concurrently with appropriate antituberculous chemotherapy.

Trichinosis with neurologic or myocardial involvement.

CONTRAINDICATIONS

The use of methylprednisolone sodium succinate sterile powder is contraindicated in premature infants because the 40, 125, 500, 1 g, and the accompanying diluent for the 500 mg and 2 g vials contain benzyl alcohol. Benzyl alcohol has been reported to be associated with a fatal "Gasping Syndrome" in premature infants. Methylprednisolone sodium succinate sterile powder is also contraindicated in systemic fungal infections and patients with known hypersensitivity to the product and its constituents.

WARNINGS

In patients on corticosteroid therapy subjected to any unusual stress, increased dosage of rapidly acting corticosteroids before, during, and after the stressful situation is indicated.

Corticosteroids may mask some signs of infection, and new infections may appear during their use. There may be decreased resistance and inability to localize infection when corticosteroids are used. Infections with any pathogen including viral, bacterial, fungal, portozoan or helminthic infections, in any location of the body, may be associated with the use of corticosteroids alone or in combination with other immunosuppressive agents that affect cellular immunity, humoral immunity, or neutrophil function.[1]

These infections may be mild, but can be severe and at times fatal. With increasing doses of corticosteroids, the rate of occurrence of infectious complications increases.[2]

A study has failed to establish the efficacy of methylprednisolone sodium succinate in the treatment of sepsis syndrome and septic shock. The study also suggests that treatment of these conditions with methylprednisolone sodium succinate may increase the risk of mortality in certain patients (*i.e.,* patients with elevated serum creatinine levels or patients who develop secondary infections after methylprednisolone sodium succinate).

Prolonged use of corticosteroids may produce posterior subcapsular cataracts, glaucoma with possible damage to the optic nerves, and may enhance the establishment of secondary ocular infections due to fungi or viruses.

Use in Pregnancy: Since adequate human reproduction studies have not been done with corticosteroids, the use of these drugs in pregnancy, nursing mothers, or women of child-bearing potential requires that the possible benefits of the drug be weighed against the potential hazards to the mother and embryo or fetus. Infants born of mothers who have received substantial doses of corticosteroids during pregnancy should be carefully observed for signs of hypoadrenalism.

Average and large doses of cortisone or hydrocortisone can cause elevation of blood pressure, salt and water retention, and increased excretion of potassium. These effects are less likely to occur with the synthetic derivatives except when used in large doses. Dietary salt restriction and potassium supplementation may be necessary. All corticosteroids increase calcium excretion.

Administration of live or live, attenuated vaccines is contraindicated in patients receiving immunosuppressive doses of corticosteroids. Killed or inactivated vaccines may be administered to patients receiving immunosuppressive doses of corticosteroids; however, the response to such vaccines may be diminished. Indicated immunization procedures may be undertaken in patients receiving nonimmunosuppressive doses of corticosteroids.

The use of methylprednisolone sodium succinate sterile powder in active tuberculosis should be restricted to those cases of fulminating or disseminated tuberculosis in which the corticosteroid is used for the management of the disease in conjunction with appropriate antituberculous regimen.

If corticosteroids are indicated in patients with latent tuberculosis or tuberculin reactivity, close observation is necessary as reactivation of the disease may occur. During prolonged corticosteroid therapy, these patients should receive chemoprophylaxis.

Because rare instances of anaphylactic (*e.g.,* bronchospasm) reactions have occurred in patients receiving parenteral corticosteroid therapy, appropriate precautionary measures should be taken prior to administration, especially when the patient has a history of allergy to any drug.

There are reports of cardiac arrhythmias and/or circulatory collapse and/or cardiac arrest following the rapid administration of large IV doses of methylprednisolone sodium succinate (greater than 0.5 g administered over a period of less than 10 minutes). Bradycardia has been reported during or after the administration of large doses of methylprednisolone sodium succinate, and may be unrelated to the speed or duration of infusion.

Persons who are on drugs which suppress the immune system are more susceptible to infections than healthy individuals. Chicken pox and measles, for example, can have a more serious or even fatal course in non-immune children or adults on corticosteroids. In such children or adults who have not had these diseases, particular care should be taken to avoid exposure. How the dose, route and duration of corticosteroid administration affects the risk of developing a disseminated infection is not known. The contribution of the underlying disease and/or prior corticosteroid treatment to the risk is also not known. If exposed to chicken pox, prophylaxis with varicella zoster immune globulin (VZIG) may be indicated. If exposed to measles, prophylaxis with pooled intramuscular immunoglobin (IG) may be indicated. (See the respective package inserts for complete VZIG and IG prescribing information.). If chicken pox develops, treatment with antiviral agents may be considered. Similarly, corticosteroids should be used with great care in patients with known or suspected Strongyloides (threadworm) infestation. In such patients, corticosteroid-induced immunosuppression may lead to Strongyloides hyperinfection and dissemination with widespread larval migration, often accompanied by severe enterocolitis and potentially fatal g-negative septicemia.

PRECAUTIONS

GENERAL

Drug-induced secondary adrenocortical insufficiency may be minimized by gradual reduction of dosage. This type of relative insufficiency may persist for months after discontinuation of therapy; therefore, in any situation of stress occurring during that period, hormone therapy should be reinstituted. Since mineralocorticoid secretion may be impaired, salt and/or a mineralocorticoid should be administered concurrently.

There is an enhanced effect of corticosteroids on patients with hypothyroidism and in those with cirrhosis.

Corticosteroids should be used cautiously in patients with ocular herpes simplex because of possible corneal perforation.

The lowest possible dose of corticosteroid should be used to control the condition under treatment, and when reduction in dosage is possible, the reduction should be gradual.

Psychic derangements may appear when corticosteroids are used, ranging from euphoria, insomnia, mood swings, personality changes, and severe depression, to frank psychotic manifestations. Also, existing emotional instability or psychotic tendencies may be aggravated by corticosteroids.

Steroids should be used with caution in nonspecific ulcerative colitis, if there is a probability of impending perforation, abscess or other pyogenic infection; diverticulitis; fresh intestinal anastomoses; active or latent peptic ulcer; renal insufficiency; hypertension; osteoporosis; and myasthenia gravis.

Growth and development of infants and children on prolonged corticosteroid therapy should be carefully observed.

Kaposi's sarcoma has been reported to occur in patients receiving corticosteroid therapy. discontinuation of corticosteroids may result in clinical remission.

Although controlled clinical trials have shown corticosteroids to be effective in speeding the resolution of acute exacerbations of multiple sclerosis, they do not show that corticosteroids affect the ultimate outcome or natural history of the disease. The studies do show that relatively high doses of corticosteroids are necessary to demonstrate a significant effect. (See DOSAGE AND ADMINISTRATION.)

An acute myopathy has been observed with the use of high doses of corticosteroids, most often occurring in patients with disorders of neuromuscular transmission (*e.g.,* myasthenia gravis), or in patients receiving concomitant therapy with neuromuscular blocking drugs (*e.g.,* pancuronium). This acute myopathy is generalized, may involve ocular and respiratory muscles, and may result in quadriparesis. Elevations of creatine kinase may occur. Clinical imporvement or recovery after stopping corticosteroids may require weeks to years.

Since complications of treatment with glucocorticoids are dependent on the size of the dose and the duration of treatment, a risk/benefit decision must be made in each individual case as to dose and duration of treatment and as to whether daily or intermittent therapy should be used.

INFORMATION FOR THE PATIENT

Persons who are on immunosuppressant doses of corticosteroids should be warned to avoid exposure to chicken pox or measles. Patients should also be advised that if they are exposed, medical advice should be sought without delay.

DRUG INTERACTIONS

The pharmacokinetic interactions listed below are potentially clinically important. Mutual inhibition of metabolism occurs with concurrent use of cyclosporin and methlyprednisolone; therefore, it is possible that adverse events associated with the individual use of either drug may be more apt to occur. Convulsions have been reported with concurrent use of methylprednisolone and cyclosporin. Drugs that induce hepatic enzymes such as phenobarbital, phenytoin and rifampin may increase the clearance of methylprednisolone and may require increases in methylprednisolone dose to achieve the desired response. Drugs such as troleandomycin and ketoconazole may inhibit the metabolism of methylprednisolone and thus decrease its clearance. Therefore, the dose of methylprednisolone should be titrated to avoid steroid toxicity. Methylprednisolone may increase the clearance of chronic high dose aspirin. This could lead to decreased salicylate serum levels or increase the risk of salicylate toxicity when methylprednisolone is withdrawn. Aspirin should be used cautiously in conjunction with corticosteroids in patients suffering from hypoprothrombinemia. The effect of methylprednisolone on oral anticoagulants is variable. There are reports of enhanced as well as diminished effects of anticoagulant when given concurrently with corticosteroids. Therefore, coagulation indices should be monitored to maintain the desired anitcoagulant effect.

ADVERSE REACTIONS

Fluid and Electrolyte Disturbances: Sodium retention, potassium loss, fluid retention, hypokalemic alkalosis, congestive heart failure in susceptible patients, hypertension.

Musculoskeletal: Muscle weakness, aseptic necrosis of femoral and humeral heads, steroid myopathy, loss of muscle mass, pathologic fracture of long bones, severe arthralgia, osteoporosis, vertebral compression fractures, tendon rupture (particularly of the Achilles tendon).

Gastrointestinal: Peptic ulcer with possible perforation and hemorrhage, abdominal distention, ulcerative esophagitis, pancreatitis. Increases in alanine transaminase (ALT, SGPT), aspartate transaminase (AST, SGOT), and alkaline phosphatase have been observed following corticosteroid treatment. These changes are usually small, not associated with any clinical syndrome and are reversible upon discontinuation.

Dermatologic: Impaired wound healing, facial erythema, thin fragile skin, increased sweating, petechiae and ecchymoses, may suppress reactions to skin tests.

Neurological: Increased intracranial pressure with papilledema (pseudo-tumor cerebri) usually after treatment, convulsions, vertigo, headache.

Endocrine: Development of Cushingoid state, menstrual irregularities, suppression of growth in children, decreased carbohydrate tolerance, secondary adrenocortical and pituitary unresponsiveness (particularly in times of stress, as in trauma, surgery or illness), manifestations of latent diabetes mellitus, increased requirements for insulin or oral hypoglycemic agents in diabetics.

Ophthalmic: Posterior subcapsular cataracts, glaucoma, increased intraocular pressure, exophthalmos.

Metabolic: Negative nitrogen balance due to protein catabolism.

The following *additional* adverse reactions are related to parenteral corticosteroid therapy: Hyperpigmentation or hypopigmentation, subcutaneous and cutaneous atrophy, sterile abscess, anaphylactic reaction with or without circulatory collapse, cardiac arrest, bronchospasm, urticaria, nausea and vomiting, cardiac arrhythmias; hypotension or hypertension.

DOSAGE AND ADMINISTRATION

When high dose therapy is desired, the recommended dose of methylprednisolone sodium succinate sterile powder is 30 mg/kg administered intravenously over at least 30 minutes. This dose may be repeated every 4-6 hours for 48 hours.

In general, high dose corticosteroid therapy should be continued only until the patient's condition has stabilized; usually not beyond 48-72 hours.

Although adverse effects associated with high dose short-term corticoid therapy are uncommon, peptic ulceration may occur. Prophylactic antacid therapy may be indicated.

In other indications initial dosage will vary from 10-40 mg of methylprednisolone depending on the clinical problem being treated. The larger doses may be required for short-term management of severe, acute conditions. The initial dose usually should be given intravenously over a period of several minutes. Subsequent doses may be given intravenously or intramuscularly at intervals dictated by the patient's response and clinical condition. Corticoid therapy is an adjunct to, and not replacement for conventional therapy.

Dosage may be reduced for infants and children but should be governed more by the severity of the condition and response of the patient than by age or size. It should not be less than 0.5 mg/kg every 24 hours.

Dosage must be decreased or discontinued gradually when the drug has been administered for more than a few days. If a period of spontaneous remission occurs in a chronic condition, treatment should be discontinued. Routine laboratory studies, such as urinalysis, 2 hour postprandial blood sugar, determination of blood pressure and body weight, and a chest x-ray should be made at regular intervals during prolonged therapy. Upper GI x-rays are desirable in patients with an ulcer history or significant dyspepsia.

Methylprednisolone sodium succinate may be administered by intravenous or intramuscular injection or by intravenous infusion, the preferred method for initial emergency use being intravenous injection. To administer by intravenous (or intramuscular) injection, prepare solution as directed. The desired dose may be administered intravenously over a period of several minutes. If desired, the medication may be administered in diluted solutions by adding water for injection or other suitable diluent to the dilution system and withdrawing the indicated dose.

To prepare solutions for intravenous infusion, first prepare the solution for injection as directed. This solution may then be added to indicated amounts of 5% dextrose in water, isotonic saline solution or 5% dextrose in isotonic saline solution.

MULTIPLE SCLEROSIS

In treatment of acute exacerbations of multiple sclerosis, daily doses of 200 mg of prednisolone for a week followed by 80 mg every other day for 1 month have been shown to be effective (4 mg of methylprednisolone is equivalent to 5 mg of prednisolone).

PRODUCT LISTING - RATED THERAPEUTICALLY EQUIVALENT

Powder For Injection - Injectable - 1 Gm

Qty	Price	Product	NDC
1's	$9.71	A-METHAPRED, Abbott Pharmaceutical	00074-5603-44
1's	$19.83	SOLU-MEDROL, Pharmacia and Upjohn	00009-0698-01
1's	$21.16	SOLU-MEDROL, Pharmacia and Upjohn	00009-3389-01
25's	$380.30	A-METHAPRED, Abbott Pharmaceutical	00074-5631-08

Powder For Injection - Injectable - 40 mg

Qty	Price	Product	NDC
1's	$2.05	SOLU-MEDROL, Pharmacia and Upjohn	00009-0113-12
1's	$2.05	SOLU-MEDROL, Allscripts Pharmaceutical Company	54569-2136-00
1's	$3.09	SOLU-MEDROL, Physicians Total Care	54868-0768-00
1's	$5.53	SOLU-MEDROL, Prescript Pharmaceuticals	00247-0292-01
10's	$16.63	A-METHAPRED, Abbott Pharmaceutical	00074-5684-01
25's	$50.00	SOLU-MEDROL, Pharmacia and Upjohn	00009-0113-13
25's	$50.58	SOLU-MEDROL, Allscripts Pharmaceutical Company	54569-3934-00
25's	$57.75	SOLU-MEDROL, Pharmacia and Upjohn	00009-0113-19

Powder For Injection - Injectable - 125 mg

Qty	Price	Product	NDC
1's	$3.41	SOLU-MEDROL, Pharmacia and Upjohn	00009-0190-09
1's	$3.41	SOLU-MEDROL, Allscripts Pharmaceutical Company	54569-1555-00
1's	$4.55	SOLU-MEDROL, Physicians Total Care	54868-3637-00
1's	$5.31	SOLU-MEDROL, Southwood Pharmaceuticals Inc	58016-9452-01
10's	$20.19	A-METHAPRED, Abbott Pharmaceutical	00074-5685-02
25's	$93.10	SOLU-MEDROL, Pharmacia and Upjohn	00009-0190-16

Powder For Injection - Injectable - 500 mg

Qty	Price	Product	NDC
1's	$10.21	SOLU-MEDROL, Physicians Total Care	54868-3623-00
1's	$10.48	SOLU-MEDROL, Pharmacia and Upjohn	00009-0758-01
1's	$13.35	SOLU-MEDROL, Pharmacia and Upjohn	00009-0765-02
1's	$37.50	GENERIC, Cmc-Consolidated Midland Corporation	00223-8162-03
10's	$58.00	A-METHAPRED, Abbott Pharmaceutical	00074-5601-44
25's	$151.41	A-METHAPRED, Abbott Pharmaceutical	00074-5630-04

PRODUCT LISTING - EQUIVALENTS NOT AVAILABLE

Powder For Injection - Injectable - 1 Gm

Qty	Price	Product	NDC
1's	$65.00	GENERIC, Consolidated Midland Corporation	00223-8163-04

Powder For Injection - Injectable - 2 Gm

Qty	Price	Product	NDC
1's	$41.21	SOLU-MEDROL, Pharmacia and Upjohn	00009-0796-01

Powder For Injection - Injectable - 125 mg

Qty	Price	Product	NDC
1's	$7.00	GENERIC, Esi Lederle Generics	00641-2506-41
1's	$12.00	GENERIC, Cmc-Consolidated Midland Corporation	00223-8161-02
1's	$12.50	GENERIC, Cmc-Consolidated Midland Corporation	00223-8160-02

Methyltestosterone *(001795)*

Categories: Carcinoma, breast; Cryptorchidism; Hypogonadism, male, primary; Orchidectomy; Orchitis; Puberty, male, delayed; Torsion, bilateral; Pregnancy Category X; DEA Class CIII; FDA Approved 1971 Dec

Drug Classes: Androgens; Hormones/hormone modifiers

Brand Names: **Android**; Androral; Fopou; Forton; Madiol; Metandren; Metestone; Oreton Methyl; Primotest; Testo-B; Testred; Vigorex; Virilon; Virormone

Foreign Brand Availability: Enarmon (Japan); Teston (Greece); Testotonic "B" (Israel); Testovis (Italy)

Cost of Therapy: $42.92 (Male Hypogonadism; Android; 10 mg; 1 tablet/day; 30 day supply)
$1.06 (Male Hypogonadism; Generic Tableets; 10 mg; 1 tablet/day; 30 day supply)
$205.99 (Metastatic Breast Cancer (female); Android; 25 mg; 2 tablets/day; 30 day supply)
$6.18 (Metastatic Breast Cancer (female); Generic Tablets; 25 mg; 2 tablets/day; 30 day supply)

DESCRIPTION

The androgens are steroids that develop and maintain primary and secondary male sex characteristics.

Androgens are derivatives of cyclopentanoperhydrophenanthrene. Endogenous androgens are C-19 steroids with a side chain at C-17, and with two angular methyl groups. Testosterone is the primary endogenous androgen. In their active form, all drugs in the class have a 17-beta hydroxy group. 17-alpha alkylation (methyltestosterone) increases the pharmacologic activity per unit weight compared to testosterone when given orally.

Methyltestosterone, a synthetic derivative of testosterone, is an androgenic preparation given by the oral route in a capsule for. Each capsule contains 10 mg, each tablet contains 10 or 25 mg of methyltestosterone. The empirical formula $C_{20}H_{30}O_2$, and a molecular weight of 302.46.

Chemically, methyltestosterone is 17-β-hydroxy-17-methylandrost-4-en-3-one.

Each Android capsule, for oral administration, contains 10 mg of methyltestosterone. In addition, each capsule contains the following inactive ingredients: corn starch, gelatin, FD&C blue no. 1, FD&C red no., 40. 25 mg tablets also contain FD&C yellow no. 6.

CLINICAL PHARMACOLOGY

Endogenous androgens are responsible for the normal growth and development of the male sex organs and for the maintenance of secondary sex characteristics. These effects include the growth and maturation of the prostate, seminal vesicles, penis, and scrotum. The development of male hair distribution, such as beard, pubic, chest, and axillary hair; laryngeal enlargement; vocal cord thickening; alterations in body musculature; and fat distribution. Drugs in this class also cause retention of nitrogen, sodium, potassium, and phosphorus, and decreased urinary excretion of calcium. Androgens have been reported to increase protein anabolism and decrease protein catabolism. Nitrogen balance is improved only when there is sufficient intake of calories and protein.

Androgens are responsible for the growth spurt of adolescence and for the eventual termination of linear growth, which is brought about by fusion of the epiphyseal growth centers. In children, exogenous androgens accelerate linear growth rates but may cause a disproportionate advancement in bone maturation. Use over long periods may result in fusion of the epiphyseal growth centers and termination of the growth process. Androgens have been reported to stimulate the production of red blood cells by enhancing the production of erythropoietic stimulating factor.

During exogenous administration of androgens, endogenous testosterone release is inhibited through feedback inhibition of pituitary luteinizing hormone (LH). At large doses of exogenous androgens, spermatogenesis may also be suppressed through feedback inhibition of pituitary follicle-stimulating hormone (FSH).

There is a lack of substantial evidence that androgens are effective in fractures, surgery, convalescence, and functional uterine bleeding.

PHARMACOKINETICS

Testosterone given orally is metabolized by the gut and 44% is cleared by the liver of the first pass. Oral doses as high as 400 mg per day are needed to achieve clinically effective blood levels for full replacement therapy. The synthetic androgen, methyltestosterone is less extensively metabolized by the liver and has a longer half-life. It is more suitable than testosterone for oral administration.

Testosterone in plasma is 98% bound to a specific testosterone-estradiol binding globulin, and about 2% is free. Generally, the amount of this sex-hormone binding globulin in the plasma will determine the distribution of testosterone between free and bound forms, and the free testosterone concentration will determine its half-life.

About 90% of a dose of testosterone is excreted in the urine as glucuronic and sulfuric acid conjugates of testosterone and its metabolites; and 6% of a dose is excreted in the feces, mostly in the unconjugated form. Inactivation of testosterone occurs primarily in the liver. Testosterone is metabolized to various 17-keto steroids through two different pathways. There are considerable variations of the half-life of testosterone as reported in the literature, ranging from 10 to 100 minutes.

In many tissues the activity of testosterone appears to depend on reduction to dihydrotestosterone, which binds to cytosol receptor proteins. The steroid-receptor complex is transported to the nucleus where it initials transcription events and cellular changes related to androgen action.

INDICATIONS AND USAGE

MALES

Androgens are indicated for replacement therapy in conditions associated with a deficiency or absence of endogenous testosterone.

Primary hypogonadism (congenital or acquired): Testicular failure due to cryptorchidism, bilateral torsions, orchitis, vanishing testis syndrome; or orchidectomy.

Hypogonadotropic hypogonadism (congenital or acquired): Idiopathic gonadotropin or LHRH deficiency, or pituitary hypothalamic injury from tumors, trauma, or radiation. If the above, conditions occur prior to puberty, androgen replacement therapy will be needed during the adolescent years for development of secondary sexual characteristics. Prolonged androgen treatment will be required to maintain sexual characteristics in these and other males who develop testosterone deficiency after puberty.

Androgens may be used to stimulate puberty in carefully selected males with clearly delayed puberty. These patients usually have a familial pattern of delayed puberty that is not secondary to a pathological disorder; puberty is expected to occur spontaneously at a relatively late date. Brief treatment with conservative doses may occasionally be justified in these patients if they do not respond to psychological support. The potential adverse effect on maturation should be discussed with the patient and his parents prior to androgen administration. An x-ray of the hand and wrist to determine bone age should be obtained every 6 months to assess the effect of treatment on the epiphyseal centers (see WARNINGS.)

FEMALES

Androgens may be used secondarily in women with advancing inoperable metastatic (skeletal) mammary cancer who arte 1 to 5 years postmenopausal. Primary goal of therapy in these women include ablation of the ovaries. Other methods of counteracting estrogen activity are adrenalectomy, hypophysectomy, and/or antiestrogen therapy. This treatment has also been used in premenopausal women with breast cancer who have benefitted from oophorectomy and are considered to have a hormone-responsive tumor. Judgment concerning androgen therapy should be made by an oncologist with expertise in this field.

NON-FDA APPROVED INDICATIONS

Although not FDA approved, methyltestosterone has been used in combination with estrogen to enhance libido in female patients.

CONTRAINDICATIONS

Androgens are contraindicated in men with carcinoma of the breast or with known or suspected carcinomas of the prostate, and in women who are or may become pregnant. When administered to pregnant women, androgens cause virilization of the external genitalia of the female fetus. This virilization includes clitoromegaly, abnormal vaginal development, and fusion of genital folds to form a scrotal-like structure. The degree of masculinization is related to the amount of drug given and the age of the fetus, and is most likely to occur in the female fetus when the drugs are given in the first trimester. If the patient becomes pregnant while taking these drugs, she should be apprised of the potential hazard to the fetus.

WARNINGS

In patients with breast cancer, androgen therapy may cause hypercalcemia by stimulating osteolysis. In this case, the drug should be discontinued.

Prolonged use of high doses of androgens has been associated with the development of peliosis hepatis and hepatic neoplasms including hepatocellular carcinoma (see PRECAUTIONS, Carcinogenesis, Mutagenesis, and Impairment of Fertility). Peliosis hepatis can be a life, threatening or fatal complication

Cholestatic hepatitis and jaundice occur with 17 alpha-alkylandrogens at a relatively low dose. If cholestatic hepatitis with jaundice appears or if liver function tests become abnormal, the androgen should be discontinued and the etiology should be determined. Drug-induced jaundice is reversible when the medication is discontinued.

Geriatric patients treated with androgens may be at an increased risk for the development of prostatic hypertrophy and prostatic carcinoma.

Edema with or without congestive heart failure may be a serious complication in patients with preexisting cardiac, renal, or hepatic disease. In addition to discontinuation of the drug, diuretic therapy may be required.

Gynecomastia frequently develops and occasionally persists in patients being treated for hypogonadism.

Androgen therapy should be used cautiously in healthy males with delayed puberty. The effect on bone maturation should be monitored by assessing bone age of the wrist and hand every 6 months. In children, androgen treatment may accelerate bone maturation without producing compensatory gain in linear growth. This adverse effect may result in compromised adult stature. The younger the child, the greater the risk of compromising final mature height.

This drug has not been shown to be safe and effective for the enhancement of athletic performance. Because of the potential risk of serious adverse health effects, this drug should not be used for such purpose.

PRECAUTIONS

GENERAL

Women should be observed for signs of virilization (deepening of the voice, hirsutism, acne, clitoromegaly, and menstrual irregularities). Discontinuation of drug therapy at the time mild virilism becomes evident is necessary to prevent irreversible virilization. Such virilization is usual following androgen use at high doses. A decision may be made by the patient and the physician that some virilization will be tolerated during treatment for breast carcinoma.

INFORMATION FOR THE PATIENT

The physician should instruct patients to report any of the following side effects of androgens:

Adult or Adolescent Males: Too frequent or persistent erection of the penis. Any male adolescent patient receiving androgens for delayed puberty should have bone development checked every 6months.

Women: Hoarseness, acne, changes in menstrual periods, or more hair on the face.

All Patients: Any nausea, vomiting, changes in skin color, or ankle swelling.

LABORATORY TESTS

Women with disseminated breast carcinoma should have frequent determinations of urine and serum calcium levels during the coarse of androgen therapy (see WARNINGS).

Because of hematoxicity associated with the use of 17 alpha-alkylated androgens, liver function tests should be obtained periodically.

Periodic (every 6 months) X-ray examinations of bone age should be made during treatment of prepubertal males to determine the rate of bone maturation and the effects of androgen therapy on the epiphyseal centers.

Hemoglobin and hematocrit should be checked periodically for polycythemia in patients who are receiving high doses of androgens.

DRUG/LABORATORY TEST INTERFERENCES

Androgens may decrease levels of thyroxine-binding globulin, resulting in decreased total T4 serum levels and increased resin uptake of T3 and T4. Free thyroid hormone levels remain unchanged, however, and there is no clinical evidence of thyroid dysfunction.

CARCINOGENESIS, MUTAGENESIS, AND IMPAIRMENT OF FERTILITY

Animal Data

Testosterone has been tested by subcutaneous injection and implantation in mice and rats. The implant induced cervical-uterine tumors in mice, which metastasized in some cases. There is suggestive evidence that injection of testosterone in some strains of female mice increases their susceptibility to hepatoma. Testosterone is also known to decrease the degree of differentiation of chemically induced carcinomas of the liver in rats.

Human Data

There are rare reports of hepatocellular carcinoma in patients receiving long-term therapy with androgens in high doses. Withdrawal of the drugs did not lead to regression of the tumors in all cases.

Geriatric patients treated with androgens may be at an increased risk for the development of prostatic hypertrophy and prostatic carcinoma.

PREGNANCY, TERATOGENIC EFFECTS, PREGNANCY CATEGORY X

See CONTRAINDICATIONS.

NURSING MOTHERS

It is not known whether androgens are excreted in human milk. Because many drugs are excreted in human milk and because of the potential for serious adverse reactions in nursing infants from androgens, a decision should be made whether to discontinue the drug taking into account the importance of the drug to the mother.

PEDIATRIC USE

Androgen therapy should be prescribed very cautiously for use in males with clearly delayed puberty and only by specialists who are aware of the adverse effects on bone maturation. Skeletal maturation must be monitored every 6 months by an x-ray of the hand and wrist (see INDICATIONS AND USAGE and WARNINGS).

DRUG INTERACTIONS

Anticoagulants: C-17-substituted derivatives of testosterone, such as methandrostenolone, have been reported to decrease the anticoagulant requirements of patients receiving oral anticoagulants. Patients receiving oral anticoagulant therapy require close monitoring, especially when androgen therapy are started or stopped.

Oxyphenbutazone: Concurrent administration of oxyphenbutazone and androgens may result in elevated serum levels of oxyphenbutazone.

Insulin: In diabetic patients, the metabolic effects of androgens may decrease blood glucose levels and insulin requirements.

ADVERSE REACTIONS

Endocrine and Urogenital: *Female:* The most common side effects of androgen therapy are amenorrhea and other menstrual irregularities, inhibition of gonadotropin secretion, and virilization, including deepening of the voice and clitoral enlargement. The latter usually is not reversible after androgens are discontinued. When administrated to a pregnant woman, androgens cause virilization of the external genitalia of the female fetus. *Males:* Gynecomastia, and excessive frequency and duration of penile erections may occur. Oligospermia may occur at high dosages (See CLINICAL PHARMACOLOGY.)

Skin and Appendages: Hirsutism, male pattern of baldness and acne.

Fluid and Electrolyte Disturbances: Retention of sodium, chloride, water, potassium, calcium, and inorganic phosphates.

Gastrointestinal: Nausea, cholestatic jaundice, alterations in liver function tests, rarely, hepatocellular neoplasms and peliosis hepatis (see WARNINGS.)

Hematologic: Suppression of clotting factors II, V, VII, and X; bleeding in patients on concomitant anticoagulant therapy, and polycythemia.

Nervous System: Increased or decreased libido, headache, anxiety, depression, and generalized paresthesia.

Metabolic: Increased serum cholesterol.

Miscellaneous: Rarely anaphylactoid reactions.

DOSAGE AND ADMINISTRATION

Dosage must be strictly individualized. Methyltestosterone capsules are administered orally. The suggested dosage for androgens varies depending on the age, sex, and diagnosis of the individual patient. Dosage is adjusted according to the patient's response and the appearance of adverse reactions.

MALES

In the androgen-deficient male the following guideline for replacement therapy indicates the usual initial dosages:

TABLE 1 *Methyltestosterone, Dosage and Administration*

Route	Dose	Frequency
Oral	10-50 mg	Daily

Various dosage regimens have been used to induce pubertal changes in hypogonadal males; some experts have advocated lower dosages initially, gradually increasing the dose as puberty progresses with or without a decrease to maintenance levels. Other experts emphasize that higher dosages are needed to induce pubertal changes and lower dosages can be used for maintenance after puberty. The chronological and skeletal ages must be taken into consideration both in determining the initial dose and in adjusting the dose.

Doses delayed in puberty generally are in the lower range of that given above, and for a limited duration, for example 4-6 nths.

FEMALES

Women with metastatic breast carcinoma must be followed closely because androgen therapy occasionally appears to accelerate the disease. Thus, many experts prefer to use the shorter acting androgen preparations rather than those with prolonged activity for treating breast carcinoma, particularly during the early stages of androgen therapy.

TABLE 2 *Methyltestosterone, Dosage and Administration: Metastatic Breast Cancer*

Route	Dose	Frequency
Oral	50-200 mg	Daily

HOW SUPPLIED

Android Tablets, 10 mg compressed white, round tablets impressed with the ICN trademark and product identification number 311.

M

Android Tablets, 25 mg compressed peach-colored round tablets impressed with the ICN trademark and product identification number 499.

PRODUCT LISTING - RATED THERAPEUTICALLY EQUIVALENT

Capsule - Oral - 10 mg			
100's	$248.95	ANDROID, Icn Pharmaceuticals Inc	00187-0902-01
Tablet - Oral - 10 mg			
100's	$143.06	ANDROID-10, Icn Pharmaceuticals Inc	00187-0311-06
Tablet - Oral - 25 mg			
100's	$343.32	ANDROID-25, Icn Pharmaceuticals Inc	00187-0499-06

PRODUCT LISTING - RATED NOT THERAPEUTICALLY EQUIVALENT

Capsule - Oral - 10 mg			
100's	$43.00	GENERIC, Star Pharmaceuticals Inc	00076-0301-03
100's	$278.88	TESTRED, Icn Pharmaceuticals Inc	00187-0901-01
Tablet - Oral - 10 mg			
100's	$3.52	GENERIC, Global Pharmaceutical Corporation	00115-3982-01
100's	$5.95	GENERIC, Major Pharmaceuticals Inc	00904-0808-60
100's	$7.88	GENERIC, Interstate Drug Exchange Inc	00814-4788-14
100's	$7.88	GENERIC, Interstate Drug Exchange Inc	00814-4790-14
100's	$10.76	GENERIC, Allscripts Pharmaceutical Company	54569-0841-00
100's	$137.34	ORETON METHYL, Icn Pharmaceuticals Inc	00187-0311-01
100's	$171.17	GENERIC, Global Pharmaceutical Corporation	00115-3984-01
100's	$201.11	GENERIC, Global Pharmaceutical Corporation	00115-7037-01
Tablet - Oral - 25 mg			
100's	$10.30	GENERIC, Major Pharmaceuticals Inc	00904-0809-60
100's	$223.13	GENERIC, Global Pharmaceutical Corporation	00115-3986-01
100's	$223.13	GENERIC, Global Pharmaceutical Corporation	00115-7038-01

Metoclopramide Hydrochloride *(001798)*

Categories: Intubation, intestinal; Gastroparesis, diabetic; Nausea, postoperative; Nausea, secondary to cancer chemotherapy; Gastroesophageal Reflux Disease; Vomiting, postoperative; Vomiting, secondary to cancer chemotherapy; Pregnancy Category B; FDA Approved 1979 Feb; WHO Formulary

Drug Classes: Antiemetics/antivertigo; Gastrointestinals; Stimulants, gastrointestinal

Brand Names: Clopra; Maxolon; Metoclopramide HCl; **Reglan**

Foreign Brand Availability: Ametic (South-Africa); Apo-Metoclop (Canada); Aputern (Japan); Betaclopramide (South-Africa); Bondigest (Colombia); Carnotprim Primperan (Mexico); Cerucal (Germany); Clopan (Italy); Clopamon (South-Africa); Clopram (Benin; Burkina-Faso; Ethiopia; Gambia; Ghana; Guinea; Ivory-Coast; Kenya; Liberia; Malawi; Mali; Mauritania; Mauritius; Morocco; Niger; Nigeria; Senegal; Seychelles; Sierra-Leone; Sudan; Tanzania; Tunia; Uganda; Zambia; Zimbabwe); Dibertil (Belgium; Russia); Emetal (Thailand); Emitasol (Korea); Emperal (Bulgaria; Denmark); Enzimar (Colombia); Gastrobi (Korea); Gastronerton (Germany); Gastrosil (Germany; Russia; Switzerland); Gavistal (Indonesia); Gensil (Thailand); Hemesis (Peru); Imperan (Argentina); Maril (Hong-Kong; Thailand); Maxeron (India); MCP-Beta Tropfen (Germany); Meclomid (Mexico); Mepramide (Indonesia); Meramide (Thailand); Metagliz (Costa-Rica; Dominican-Republic; El-Salvador; Guatemala; Honduras; Nicaragua; Panama); Metamide (New-Zealand); Metlazel (Bahrain; Cyprus; Egypt; Iran; Iraq; Jordan; Kuwait; Lebanon; Libya; Oman; Qatar; Republic-of-Yemen; Saudi-Arabia; Syria; United-Arab-Emirates); Metoclor (Japan; Thailand); Metocobil (Italy); Metocyl (Hong-Kong); Metolon (Indonesia; Malaysia); Metopram (Finland); Metram (Hong-Kong); Nausil (Thailand); Neopramiel (Japan); Netaf (Argentina); Nilatika (Indonesia); Normastin (Indonesia); Opram (Indonesia); Perinorm (India; South-Africa); Pharmyork (Greece); Plasil (Argentina; Bahrain; Benin; Burkina-Faso; Colombia; Costa-Rica; Cyprus; Dominican-Republic; Ecuador; Egypt; El-Salvador; Ethiopia; Gambia; Ghana; Guatemala; Guinea; Honduras; Iran; Iraq; Italy; Ivory-Coast; Jordan; Kenya; Kuwait; Lebanon; Liberia; Libya; Malawi; Mali; Mauritania; Mauritius; Mexico; Morocco; Nicaragua; Niger; Nigeria; Oman; Panama; Philippines; Qatar; Republic-of-Yemen; Saudi-Arabia; Senegal; Seychelles; Sierra-Leone; Sudan; Syria; Tanzania; Thailand; Tunia; Uganda; United-Arab-Emirates; Zambia; Zimbabwe); Pramin (Australia; Israel; Taiwan); Pramotel (Mexico); Primperan (Belgium; Benin; Burkina-Faso; Colombia; Czech-Republic; Denmark; Ecuador; England; Ethiopia; Finland; France; Gambia; Ghana; Greece; Guinea; Hong-Kong; Hungary; Ivory-Coast; Japan; Kenya; Liberia; Malawi; Malaysia; Mali; Mauritania; Mauritius; Mexico; Morocco; Netherlands; Niger; Nigeria; Norway; Peru; Portugal; Senegal; Seychelles; Sierra-Leone; Spain; Sudan; Sweden; Switzerland; Taiwan; Tanzania; Tunia; Turkey; Uganda; Zambia; Zimbabwe); Primperil (Argentina); Prinparl (Japan); Prowel (Taiwan); Pulin (Singapore); Reliveran (Argentina); Setin (South-Africa); Sotatic-10 (Indonesia); Terperan (Japan); Tomid (India); Vertivom (Indonesia); Vomitrol (Indonesia); Zumatrol (Indonesia)

Cost of Therapy: $113.18 (GERD; Reglan; 10 mg; 4 tablets/day; 30 day supply)
$4.26 (GERD; Generic Tablets; 10 mg; 4 tablets/day; 30 day supply)

HCFA JCODE(S): J2765 up to 10 mg IV

DESCRIPTION

Note: The trade name has been used throughout this monograph for clarity.

Metoclopramide hydrochloride is a white crystalline, odorless substance, freely soluble in water. Chemically, it is 4-amino-5-chloro-N-[2-(diethylamino)ethyl]-2-methoxy benzamide monohydrochloride monohydrate. Its molecular formula is $C_{14}H_{22}ClN_3O_2 \cdot HCl \cdot H_2O$. Its molecular weight is 354.3.

TABLETS

For oral administration.

Each white, capsule-shaped, scored Reglan tablet contains 10 mg metoclopramide base (as the monohydrochloride monohydrate).

Inactive Ingredients: Magnesium stearate, mannitol, microcrystalline cellulose, stearic acid.

Each green, elliptical-shaped Reglan tablet contains 5 mg metoclopramide base (as the monohydrochloride monohydrate).

Inactive Ingredients: Corn starch, D&C yellow 10 lake, FD&C blue 1 aluminum lake, lactose, microcrystalline cellulose, silicon dioxide, stearic acid.

SYRUP

Reglan syrup is an orange-colored, palatable, aromatic, sugar-free liquid.

Each 5 ml (1 teaspoonful) contains 5 mg metoclopramide base (as the monohydrochloride monohydrate).

Inactive Ingredients: Citric acid, FD&C yellow 6, flavors, glycerin, methylparaben, propylparaben, sorbitol, water.

INJECTION

For parenteral administration, Reglan injectable is a clear, colorless, sterile solution with a pH of 4.5-6.5 for intravenous (IV) or intramuscular (IM) administration.

CONTAINS NO PRESERVATIVE.

This product is light sensitive. It should be inspected before use and discarded if either color or particulate is observed.

2 ml single dose vials/ampuls; 10 ml and 30 ml single dose vials.

Each 1 ml contains 5 mg metoclopramide base (as the monohydrochloride monohydrate).

Sodium chloride, 8.5 mg; water for injection, qs. pH adjusted, when necessary, with hydrochloric acid and/or sodium hydroxide.

CLINICAL PHARMACOLOGY

Metoclopramide stimulates motility of the upper gastrointestinal tract without stimulating gastric, biliary, or pancreatic secretions. Its mode of action is unclear. It seems to sensitize tissues to the action of acetylcholine. The effect of metoclopramide on motility is not dependent on intact vagal innervation, but it can be abolished by anticholinergic drugs.

Metoclopramide increases the tone and amplitude of gastric (especially antral) contractions, relaxes the pyloric sphincter and the duodenal bulb, and increases peristalsis of the duodenum and jejunum resulting in accelerated gastric emptying and intestinal transit. It increases the resting tone of the lower esophageal sphincter. It has little, if any, effect on the motility of the colon or gallbladder.

In patients with gastroesophageal reflux and low LESP (lower esophageal sphincter pressure), single oral doses of metoclopramide produce dose-related increases in LESP. Effects begin at about 5 mg and increase through 20 mg (the largest dose tested). The increase in LESP from a 5 mg dose lasts about 45 minutes and that of 20 mg lasts between 2 and 3 hours. Increased rate of stomach emptying has been observed with single oral doses of 10 mg.

The antiemetic properties of metoclopramide appear to be a result of its antagonism of central and peripheral dopamine receptors. Dopamine produces nausea and vomiting by stimulation of the medullary chemoreceptor trigger zone (CTZ), and metoclopramide blocks stimulation of the CTZ by agents like l-dopa or apomorphine which are known to increase dopamine levels or to possess dopamine-like effects. Metoclopramide also abolishes the slowing of gastric emptying caused by apomorphine.

Like the phenothiazines and related drugs, which are also dopamine antagonists, metoclopramide produces sedation and may produce extrapyramidal reactions, although these are comparatively rare (see WARNINGS). Metoclopramide inhibits the central and peripheral effects of apomorphine, induces release of prolactin and causes a transient increase in circulating aldosterone levels, which may be associated with transient fluid retention.

The onset of pharmacological action of metoclopramide is 1-3 minutes following an IV dose, 10-15 minutes following IM administration, and 30-60 minutes following an oral dose; pharmacological effects persist for 1-2 hours.

PHARMACOKINETICS

Metoclopramide is rapidly and well absorbed. Relative to an IV dose of 20 mg, the absolute oral bioavailability of metoclopramide is 80% ± 15.5% as demonstrated in a crossover study of 18 subjects. Peak plasma concentrations occur at about 1-2 hours after a single oral dose. Similar time to peak is observed after individual doses at steady state.

In a single dose study of 12 subjects, the area under the drug concentration-time curve increases linearly with doses from 20-100 mg. Peak concentrations increase linearly with dose; time to peak concentrations remains the same; whole body clearance is unchanged; and the elimination rate remains the same. The average elimination half-life in individuals with normal renal function is 5-6 hours. Linear kinetic processes adequately describe the absorption and elimination of metoclopramide.

Approximately 85% of the radioactivity of an orally administered dose appears in the urine within 72 hours. Of the 85% eliminated in the urine, about half is present as free or conjugated metoclopramide.

The drug is not extensively bound to plasma proteins (about 30%). The whole body volume of distribution is high (about 3.5 L/kg) which suggests extensive distribution of drug to the tissues.

Renal impairment affects the clearance of metoclopramide. In a study with patients with varying degrees of renal impairment, a reduction in creatinine clearance was correlated with a reduction in plasma clearance, renal clearance, non-renal clearance, and increase in elimination half-life. The kinetics of metoclopramide in the presence of renal impairment remained linear however. The reduction in clearance as a result of renal impairment suggests that adjustment downward of maintenance dosage should be done to avoid drug accumulation.

TABLE 1 *Adult Pharmacokinetic Data*

Parameter	Value
Vd	~3.5 L/kg
Plasma protein binding	~30%
T½	5-6 hours
Oral bioavailability	80% ± 15.5%

There are insufficient reliable data to conclude whether the pharmacokinetics of metoclopramide in adults and the pediatric population are similar.

Although there are insufficient data to support the efficacy of metoclopramide in pediatric patients with symptomatic gastroesophageal reflux (GER) or cancer chemotherapy-related nausea and vomiting, its pharmacokinetics have been studied in these patient populations.

In an open-label study, 6 pediatric patients (age range, 3.5 weeks to 5.4 months) with GER received metoclopramide 0.15 mg/kg oral solution every 6 hours for 10 doses. The mean peak plasma concentration of metoclopramide after the tenth dose was 2-fold (56.8 μg/L) higher compared to that observed after the first dose (29 μg/L) indicating drug accumulation with repeated dosing. After the tenth dose, the mean time to reach peak concentrations (2.2 hours), half-life (4.1 hours), clearance (0.67 L/h/kg), and volume of distribution (4.4 L/kg) of metoclopramide were similar to those observed after the first dose. In the youngest patient (age, 3.5 weeks), metoclopramide half-life after the first and the tenth dose (23.1 and 10.3 hours, respectively) was significantly longer compared to other infants due to reduced clearance. This may be attributed to immature hepatic and renal systems at birth.

Single IV doses of metoclopramide 0.22-0.46 mg/kg (mean, 0.35 mg/kg) were administered over 5 minutes to 9 pediatric cancer patients receiving chemotherapy (mean age, 11.7 years; range, 7-14 years) for prophylaxis of cytotoxic-induced vomiting. The metoclopramide plasma concentrations extrapolated to time zero ranged from 65-395 μg/L (mean, 152 μg/L). The mean elimination half-life, clearance, and volume of distribution of metoclopramide were 4.4 hours (range, 1.7-8.3 hours), 0.56 L/h/kg (range, 0.12-1.20 L/h/kg), and 3.0 L/kg (range, 1.0-4.8 L/kg), respectively.

In another study, 9 pediatric cancer patients (age range, 1-9 years) received 4-5 IV infusions (over 30 minutes) of metoclopramide at a dose of 2 mg/kg to control emesis. After the last dose, the peak serum concentrations of metoclopramide ranged from 1060-5680 μg/L. The mean elimination half-life, clearance, and volume of distribution of metoclopramide were 4.5 hours (range, 2.0-12.5 hours), 0.37 L/h/kg (range, 0.10-1.24 L/h/kg), and 1.93 L/kg (range, 0.95-5.50 L/kg), respectively.

TABLE 2 *Pediatric Pharmacokinetic Studies*

	Reference: Kearns*	Bateman†	Ford‡
Dose, route	0.15 mg/kg oral solution, multiple dose	0.35 mg/kg, IV over 5 min	2 mg/kg, 30 min IV infusion 4-5 times within 9.5 hours
T½ (h)	4.1§¤	4.4 ± 0.56	4.5¤
Cl (L/h/kg)	0.67 ± 0.14	0.56 ± 0.10	0.37¤
Vd (L/kg)	4.4 ± 0.65 (Vd_{area})	3.0 ± 0.38 ($Dose/Cp^0$)	1.93¤
C_{max} (μg/L)	1st dose = 29 ± 23 10th dose = 56.8 ± 10.5	152 ± 31	1060-5680¤

* Kearns, GL, *et al. J Pediatric Gastroenterol Nutr* 7(6):823-829, 1988.
† Bateman, DN, *et al. Br J Clin Pharmac* 15:557-559, 1983.
‡ Ford, C. *Clin Pharmac Ther* 43:196, 1988.
§ Data presented as means ±SEM.
¤ SEM not available.

INDICATIONS AND USAGE

SYMPTOMATIC GASTROESOPHAGEAL REFLUX

Reglan tablets and syrup are indicated as short-term (4-12 weeks) therapy for adults with symptomatic, documented gastroesophageal reflux who fail to respond to conventional therapy.

The principal effect of metoclopramide is on symptoms of postprandial and daytime heartburn with less observed effect on nocturnal symptoms. If symptoms are confined to particular situations, such as following the evening meal, use of metoclopramide as single doses prior to the provocative situation should be considered, rather than using the drug throughout the day. Healing of esophageal ulcers and erosions has been endoscopically demonstrated at the end of a 12 week trial using doses of 15 mg qid. As there is no documented correlation between symptoms and healing of esophageal lesions, patients with documented lesions should be monitored endoscopically.

DIABETIC GASTROPARESIS (DIABETIC GASTRIC STASIS)

Reglan is indicated for the relief of symptoms associated with acute and recurrent diabetic gastric stasis. The usual manifestations of delayed gastric emptying (*e.g.*, nausea, vomiting, heartburn, persistent fullness after meals, and anorexia) appear to respond to Reglan within different time intervals. Significant relief of nausea occurs early and continues to improve over a 3 week period. Relief of vomiting and anorexia may precede the relief of abdominal fullness by 1 week or more.

THE PREVENTION OF NAUSEA AND VOMITING ASSOCIATED WITH EMETOGENIC CANCER CHEMOTHERAPY

Reglan injectable is indicated for the prophylaxis of vomiting associated with emetogenic cancer chemotherapy.

THE PREVENTION OF POSTOPERATIVE NAUSEA AND VOMITING

Reglan injectable is indicated for the prophylaxis of postoperative nausea and vomiting in those circumstances where nasogastric suction is undesirable.

SMALL BOWEL INTUBATION

Reglan injectable may be used to facilitate small bowel intubation in adults and pediatric patients in whom the tube does not pass the pylorus with conventional maneuvers.

RADIOLOGICAL EXAMINATION

Reglan injectable may be used to stimulate gastric emptying and intestinal transit of barium in cases where delayed emptying interferes with radiological examination of the stomach and/or small intestine.

NON-FDA APPROVED INDICATIONS

Metoclopramide has also shown efficacy in the treatment of migraine headaches and intractable hiccups. However, these used have not been approved by the FDA and further studies are needed before this drug can be recommended for use for these indications.

CONTRAINDICATIONS

Metoclopramide should not be used whenever stimulation of gastrointestinal motility might be dangerous, *e.g.*, in the presence of gastrointestinal hemorrhage, mechanical obstruction, or perforation.

Metoclopramide is contraindicated in patients with pheochromocytoma because the drug may cause a hypertensive crisis, probably due to release of catecholamines from the tumor. Such hypertensive crises may be controlled by phentolamine.

Metoclopramide is contraindicated in patients with known sensitivity or intolerance to the drug.

Metoclopramide should not be used in epileptics or patients receiving other drugs which are likely to cause extrapyramidal reactions, since the frequency and severity of seizures or extrapyramidal reactions may be increased.

WARNINGS

Mental depression has occurred in patients with and without prior history of depression. Symptoms have ranged from mild to severe and have included suicidal ideation and suicide. Metoclopramide should be given to patients with a prior history of depression only if the expected benefits outweigh the potential risks.

Extrapyramidal symptoms, manifested primarily as acute dystonic reactions, occur in approximately 1 in 500 patients treated with the usual adult dosages of 30-40 mg/day of metoclopramide. These usually are seen during the first 24-48 hours of treatment with metoclopramide, occur more frequently in pediatric patients and adult patients less than 30 years of age and are even more frequent at the higher doses used in prophylaxis of vomiting due to cancer chemotherapy. These symptoms may include involuntary movements of limbs and facial grimacing, torticollis, oculogyric crisis, rhythmic protrusion of tongue, bulbar type of speech, trismus, or dystonic reactions resembling tetanus. Rarely, dystonic reactions may present as stridor and dyspnea, possibly due to laryngospasm. If these symptoms should occur, inject 50 mg diphenhydramine hydrochloride intramuscularly, and they usually will subside. Benztropine mesylate, 1-2 mg intramuscularly, may also be used to reverse these reactions.

Parkinsonian-like symptoms have occurred, more commonly within the first 6 months after beginning treatment with metoclopramide, but occasionally after longer periods. These symptoms generally subside within 2-3 months following discontinuance of metoclopramide. Patients with preexisting Parkinson's disease should be given metoclopramide cautiously, if at all, since such patients may experience exacerbation of parkinsonian symptoms when taking metoclopramide.

TARDIVE DYSKINESIA

Tardive dyskinesia, a syndrome consisting of potentially irreversible, involuntary, dyskinetic movements may develop in patients treated with metoclopramide. Although the prevalence of the syndrome appears to be highest among the elderly, especially elderly women, it is impossible to predict which patients are likely to develop the syndrome. Both the risk of developing the syndrome and the likelihood that it will become irreversible are believed to increase with the duration of treatment and the total cumulative dose.

Less commonly, the syndrome can develop after relatively brief treatment periods at low doses; in these cases, symptoms appear more likely to be reversible.

There is no known treatment for established cases of tardive dyskinesia although the syndrome may remit, partially or completely, within several weeks-to-months after metoclopramide is withdrawn. Metoclopramide itself, however, may suppress (or partially suppress) the signs of tardive dyskinesia, thereby masking the underlying disease process. The effect of this symptomatic suppression upon the long-term course of the syndrome is unknown. Therefore, the use of metoclopramide for the symptomatic control of tardive dyskinesia is not recommended.

NEUROLEPTIC MALIGNANT SYNDROME

There have been rare reports of an uncommon but potentially fatal symptom complex sometimes referred to as Neuroleptic Malignant Syndrome (NMS) associated with metoclopramide. Clinical manifestations of NMS include hyperthermia, muscle rigidity, altered consciousness, and evidence of autonomic instablility (irregular pulse or blood pressure, tachycardia, diaphoresis and cardiac arrhythmias).

The diagnostic evaluation of patients with this syndrome is complicated. In arriving at a diagnosis, it is important to identify cases where the clinical presentation includes both serious medical illness (*e.g.*, pneumonia, systemic infection, etc.) and untreated or inadequately treated extrapyramidal signs and symptoms (EPS). Other important considerations in the differential diagnosis include central anticholinergic toxicity, heat stroke, malignant hyperthermia, drug fever and primary central nervous system (CNS) pathology.

The management of NMS should include (1) immediate discontinuation of metoclopramide and other drugs not essential to concurrent therapy, (2) intensive symptomatic treatment and medical monitoring, and (3) treatment of any concomitant serious medical problems for which specific treatments are available. Bromocriptine and dantroline sodium have been used in treatment of NMS, but their effectiveness have not been established (see ADVERSE REACTIONS).

PRECAUTIONS

GENERAL

In one study in hypertensive patients, intravenously administered metoclopramide was shown to release catecholamines; hence, caution should be exercised when metoclopramide is used in patients with hypertension.

Intravenous injections of undiluted metoclopramide should be made slowly allowing 1-2 minutes for 10 mg since a transient but intense feeling of anxiety and restlessness, followed by drowsiness, may occur with rapid administration.

Because metoclopramide produces a transient increase in plasma aldosterone, certain patients, especially those with cirrhosis or congestive heart failure, may be at risk of developing fluid retention and volume overload. If this occurs within the first few weeks of metoclopramide therapy, the drug should be discontinued.

Intravenous administration of Reglan injectable diluted in a parenteral solution should be made slowly over a period of not less than 15 minutes.

Giving a promotility drug such as metoclopramide theoretically could put increased pressure on suture lines following a gut anastomosis or closure. This possibility should be considered and weighed when deciding whether to use metoclopramide or nasogastric suction in the prevention of postoperative nausea and vomiting.

INFORMATION FOR THE PATIENT

Metoclopramide may impair the mental and/or physical abilities required for the performance of hazardous tasks such as operating machinery or driving a motor vehicle. The ambulatory patient should be cautioned accordingly.

CARCINOGENESIS, MUTAGENESIS, AND IMPAIRMENT OF FERTILITY

A 77 week study was conducted in rats with oral doses up to about 40 times the maximum recommended human daily dose. Metoclopramide elevates prolactin levels and the elevation persists during chronic administration. Tissue culture experiments indicate that approximately onethird of human breast cancers are prolactin-dependent *in vitro,* a factor of potential importance if the prescription of metoclopramide is contemplated in a patient with previously detected breast cancer. Although disturbances such as galactorrhea, amenorrhea, gynecomastia, and impotence have been reported with prolactin-elevating drugs, the clinical significance of elevated serum prolactin levels is unknown for most patients. An increase in mammary neoplasms has been found in rodents after chronic administration of prolactin-stimulating neuroleptic drugs and metoclopramide. Neither clinical studies nor epidemiologic studies conducted to date, however, have shown an association between chronic administration of these drugs and mammary tumorigenesis; the available evidence is too limited to be conclusive at this time.

An Ames mutagenicity test performed on metoclopramide was negative.

PREGNANCY CATEGORY B

Reproduction studies performed in rats, mice and rabbits by the IV, IM, SC, and oral routes at maximum levels ranging from 12-250 times the human dose have demonstrated no impairment of fertility or significant harm to the fetus due to metoclopramide. There are, however, no adequate and well-controlled studies in pregnant women. Because animal reproduction studies are not always predictive of human response, this drug should be used during pregnancy only if clearly needed.

NURSING MOTHERS

Metoclopramide is excreted in human milk. Caution should be exercised when metoclopramide is administered to a nursing mother.

PEDIATRIC USE

Safety and effectiveness in pediatric patients have not been established except as stated to facilitate small bowel intubation (see DOSAGE AND ADMINISTRATION).

Care should be exercised in administering metoclopramide to neonates since prolonged clearance may produce excessive serum concentrations (see CLINICAL PHARMACOLOGY, Pharmacokinetics). In addition, neonates have reduced levels of nicotinamide adenine dinucleotidemethemoglobin reductase which, in combination with the aforementioned pharmacokinetic factors, make neonates more susceptible to methemoglobinemia.

The safety profile of metoclopramide in adults cannot be extrapolated to pediatric patients. Dystonias and other extrapyramidal reactions associated with metoclopramide are more common in the pediatric population than in adults. (See WARNINGS and ADVERSE REACTIONS; Extrapyramidal Reactions.)

DRUG INTERACTIONS

The effects of metoclopramide on gastrointestinal motility are antagonized by anticholinergic drugs and narcotic analgesics. Additive sedative effects can occur when metoclopramide is given with alcohol, sedatives, hypnotics, narcotics, or tranquilizers. The finding that metoclopramide releases catecholamines in patients with essential hypertension suggests that it should be used cautiously, if at all, in patients receiving monoamine oxidase inhibitors.

Absorption of drugs from the stomach may be diminished (*e.g.,* digoxin) by metoclopramide, whereas the rate and/or extent of absorption of drugs from the small bowel may be increased (*e.g.,* acetaminophen, tetracycline, levodopa, ethanol, cyclosporine).

Gastroparesis (gastric stasis) may be responsible for poor diabetic control in some patients. Exogenously administered insulin may begin to act before food has left the stomach and lead to hypoglycemia. Because the action of metoclopramide will influence the delivery of food to the intestines and thus the rate of absorption, insulin dosage or timing of dosage may require adjustment.

ADVERSE REACTIONS

In general, the incidence of adverse reactions correlates with the dose and duration of metoclopramide administration. The following reactions have been reported, although in most instances, data do not permit an estimate of frequency.

CNS EFFECTS

Restlessness, drowsiness, fatigue, and lassitude occur in approximately 10% of patients receiving the most commonly prescribed dosage of 10 mg qid (see PRECAUTIONS). Insomnia, headache, confusion, dizziness, or mental depression with suicidal ideation (see WARNINGS) occur less frequently. In cancer chemotherapy patients being treated with 1-2 mg/kg per dose, incidence of drowsiness is about 70%. There are isolated reports of convulsive seizures without clearcut relationship to metoclopramide. Rarely, hallucinations have been reported.

EXTRAPYRAMIDAL REACTIONS (EPS)

Acute dystonic reactions, the most common type of EPS associated with metoclopramide, occur in approximately 0.2% of patients (1 in 500) treated with 30-40 mg of metoclopramide per day. In cancer chemotherapy patients receiving 1-2 mg/kg per dose, the incidence is 2% in patients over the ages of 30-35, and 25% or higher in pediatric patients and adult patients less than 30 years of age who have not had prophylactic administration of diphenhydramine. Symptoms include involuntary movements of limbs, facial grimacing, torticollis, oculogyric crisis, rhythmic protrusion of tongue, bulbar type of speech, trismus, opisthotonus (tetanus-like reactions), and, rarely, stridor and dyspnea possibly due to laryngospasm; ordinarily these symptoms are readily reversed by diphenhydramine (see WARNINGS).

Parkinsonian-like symptoms may include bradykinesia, tremor, cogwheel rigidity, mask-like facies (see WARNINGS).

Tardive dyskinesia most frequently is characterized by involuntary movements of the tongue, face, mouth, or jaw, and sometimes by involuntary movements of the trunk and/or extremities; movements may be choreoathetotic in appearance (see WARNINGS).

Motor restlessness (akathisia) may consist of feelings of anxiety, agitation, jitteriness, and insomnia, as well as inability to sit still, pacing, foot tapping. These symptoms may disappear spontaneously or respond to a reduction in dosage.

NEUROLEPTIC MALIGNANT SYNDROME

Rare occurrences of neuroleptic malignant syndrome (NMS) have been reported. This potentially fatal syndrome is comprised of the symptom complex of hyperthermia, altered consciousness, muscular rigidity, and autonomic dysfunction (see WARNINGS).

ENDOCRINE DISTURBANCES

Galactorrhea, amenorrhea, gynecomastia, impotence secondary to hyperprolactinemia (see PRECAUTIONS). Fluid retention secondary to transient elevation of aldosterone (see CLINICAL PHARMACOLOGY).

CARDIOVASCULAR

Hypotension, hypertension, supraventricular tachycardia, bradycardia, fluid retention, acute congestive heart failure and possible AV block (see CONTRAINDICATIONS and PRECAUTIONS).

GASTROINTESTINAL

Nausea and bowel disturbances, primarily diarrhea.

HEPATIC

Rarely, cases of hepatotoxicity, characterized by such findings as jaundice and altered liver function tests, when metoclopramide was administered with other drugs with known hepatotoxic potential.

RENAL

Urinary frequency and incontinence.

HEMATOLOGIC

A few cases of neutropenia, leukopenia, or agranulocytosis, generally without clearcut relationship to metoclopramide. Methemoglobinemia, especially with overdosage in neonates. Sulfhemoglobinemia in adults.

ALLERGIC REACTIONS

A few cases of rash, urticaria, or bronchospasm, especially in patients with a history of asthma. Rarely, angioneurotic edema, including glossal or laryngeal edema.

MISCELLANEOUS

Visual disturbances. Porphyria.

Transient flushing of the face and upper body, without alterations in vital signs, following high doses intravenously.

DOSAGE AND ADMINISTRATION

FOR THE RELIEF OF SYMPTOMATIC GASTROESOPHAGEAL REFLUX

Administer from 10-15 mg Reglan orally up to qid 30 minutes before each meal and at bedtime, depending upon symptoms being treated and clinical response (see CLINICAL PHARMACOLOGY and INDICATIONS AND USAGE). If symptoms occur only intermittently or at specific times of the day, use of metoclopramide in single doses up to 20 mg prior to the provoking situation may be preferred rather than continuous treatment. Occasionally, patients (such as elderly patients) who are more sensitive to the therapeutic or adverse effects of metoclopramide will require only 5 mg per dose.

Experience with esophageal erosions and ulcerations is limited, but healing has thus far been documented in one controlled trial using qid therapy at 15 mg/dose, and this regimen should be used when lesions are present, so long as it is tolerated (see ADVERSE REACTIONS). Because of the poor correlation between symptoms and endoscopic appearance of the esophagus, therapy directed at esophageal lesions is best guided by endoscopic evaluation.

Therapy longer than 12 weeks has not been evaluated and cannot be recommended.

FOR THE RELIEF OF SYMPTOMS ASSOCIATED WITH DIABETIC GASTROPARESIS (DIABETIC GASTRIC STASIS)

Administer 10 mg of metoclopramide 30 minutes before each meal and at bedtime for 2-8 weeks, depending upon response and the likelihood of continued well-being upon drug discontinuation.

The initial route of administration should be determined by the severity of the presenting symptoms. If only the earliest manifestations of diabetic gastric stasis are present, oral administration of Reglan may be initiated. However, if severe symptoms are present, therapy should begin with Reglan injectable (IM or IV). Doses of 10 mg may be administered slowly by the IV route over a 1-2 minute period.

Administration of Reglan injectable up to 10 days may be required before symptoms subside, at which time oral administration may be instituted. Since diabetic gastric stasis is frequently recurrent, Reglan therapy should be reinstituted at the earliest manifestation.

FOR THE PREVENTION OF NAUSEA AND VOMITING ASSOCIATED WITH EMETOGENIC CANCER CHEMOTHERAPY

For doses in excess of 10 mg, Reglan injectable should be diluted in 50 ml of a parenteral solution.

The preferred parenteral solution is sodium chloride injection (normal saline), which when combined with Reglan injectable, can be stored frozen for up to 4 weeks. Reglan injectable is degraded when admixed and frozen with dextrose 5% in water. Reglan injectable diluted in sodium chloride injection, dextrose 5% in water, dextrose 5% in 0.45% sodium chloride, Ringer's injection, or lactated Ringer's injection may be stored up to 48 hours (without freezing) after preparation if protected from light. All dilutions may be stored unprotected from light under normal light conditions up to 24 hours after preparation.

Intravenous infusions should be made slowly over a period of not less than 15 minutes, 30 minutes before beginning cancer chemotherapy and repeated every 2 hours for two doses, then every 3 hours for three doses.

The initial two doses should be 2 mg/kg if highly emetogenic drugs such as cisplatin or dacarbazine are used alone or in combination. For less emetogenic regimens, 1 mg/kg per dose may be adequate.

If extrapyramidal symptoms should occur, inject 50 mg diphenhydramine hydrochloride intramuscularly, and EPS usually will subside.

FOR THE PREVENTION OF POSTOPERATIVE NAUSEA AND VOMITING

Reglan injectable should be given intramuscularly near the end of surgery. The usual adult dose is 10 mg; however, doses of 20 mg may be used.

TO FACILITATE SMALL BOWEL INTUBATION

If the tube has not passed the pylorus with conventional maneuvers in 10 minutes, a single dose (undiluted) may be administered slowly by the IV route over a 1-2 minute period.

The recommended single dose is:

Above 14 years of age and adults: 10 mg metoclopramide base.

6-14 years of age: 2.5 to 5 mg metoclopramide base.

Under 6 years of age: 0.1 mg/kg metoclopramide base.

TO AID IN RADIOLOGICAL EXAMINATIONS

In patients where delayed gastric emptying interferes with radiological examination of the stomach and/or small intestine, a single dose may be administered slowly by the IV route over a 1-2 minute period.

For dosage, see intubation above.

USE IN PATIENTS WITH RENAL OR HEPATIC IMPAIRMENT

Since metoclopramide is excreted principally through the kidneys, in those patients whose creatinine clearance is below 40 ml/min, therapy should be initiated at approximately one-half the recommended dosage. Depending upon clinical efficacy and safety considerations, the dosage may be increased or decreased as appropriate.

Metoclopramide undergoes minimal hepatic metabolism, except for simple conjugation. Its safe use has been described in patients with advanced liver disease whose renal function was normal.

NOTE: Parenteral drug products should be inspected visually for particulate matter and discoloration prior to administration, whenever solution and container permit.

ADMIXTURE COMPATIBILITIES

Reglan injectable is compatible for mixing and injection with the following dosage forms to the extent indicated below:

Physically and chemically compatible up to 48 hours: Cimetidine hydrochloride (SK&F), mannitol (Abbott), potassium acetate (Invenex), potassium phosphate (Invenex).

Physically compatible up to 48 hours: Ascorbic acid (Abbott), benztropine mesylate (MS&D), cytarabine (Upjohn), dexamethasone sodium phosphate (ESI, MS&D), diphenhydramine hydrochloride (Parke-Davis), doxorubicin hydrochloride (Adria), heparin sodium (ESI), hydrocortisone sodium phosphate (MS&D), lidocaine hydrochloride (ESI), multi-vitamin infusion (must be refrigerated-USV), vitamin B complex with ascorbic acid (Roche).

Physically compatible up to 24 hours (Do not use if precipitation occurs): Clindamycin phosphate (Upjohn), cyclophosphamide (Mead-Johnson), insulin (Lilly).

Conditionally compatible (Use within 1 hour after mixing or may be infused directly into the same running IV line): Ampicillin sodium (Bristol), cisplatin (Bristol), erythromycin lactobionate (Abbott), methotrexate sodium (Lederle), penicillin G potassium (Squibb), tetracycline hydrochloride (Lederle).

Incompatible (Do not mix): Cephalothin sodium (Lilly), chloramphenicol sodium (Parke-Davis), sodium bicarbonate (Abbott).

HOW SUPPLIED

TABLET

Reglan tablets are available in:

5 mg: Green, elliptical-shaped tablets engraved "Reglan 5" on one side and "AHR" on the opposite side.

10 mg: White, scored, capsule-shaped tablets engraved "Reglan" on one side and "AHR 10" on the opposite side.

Storage

Store at controlled room temperature, between 20 and 25°C (68 and 77°F). Dispense in tight, light-resistant container.

SYRUP

Reglan syrup, 5 mg metoclopramide base (as the monohydrochloride monohydrate) per 5 ml, available in pints.

Storage

Store at controlled room temperature, between 20 and 25°C (68 and 77°F). Dispense in tight, light-resistant container.

INJECTION

Reglan injectable 5 mg metoclopramide base (as the monohydrochloride monohydrate) per ml; available in 2 ml single dose vials in cartons of 25, 10 ml single dose vials in cartons of 25, 30 ml single dose vials in cartons of 25, 2 ml ampuls in cartons of 25.

Reglan injectable is available in:

2 ml single dose vials/ampuls for IV or IM administration.

10 ml and 30 ml single dose vials. Dilute before using.

Each 1 ml contains 5 mg metoclopramide base (as the monohydrochloride monohydrate).

Storage

Store vials and ampuls in carton until used. Do not store open single dose vials or ampuls for later use, as they contain no preservative.

This product is light sensitive. It should be inspected before use and discarded if either color or particulate is observed.

Dilutions may be stored unprotected from light under normal light conditions up to 24 hours after preparation.

Store at controlled room temperature, between 20 and 25°C (68 and 77°F).

PRODUCT LISTING - RATED THERAPEUTICALLY EQUIVALENT

Solution - Injectable - 5 mg/ml			
2 ml	$58.75	REGLAN, Esi Lederle Generics	00031-6709-72
2 ml x 5	$11.09	REGLAN, Esi Lederle Generics	00031-6709-90
2 ml x 10	$8.91	GENERIC, Abbott Pharmaceutical	00074-2173-02
2 ml x 10	$9.40	GENERIC, Abbott Pharmaceutical	00074-2173-32
2 ml x 25	$22.00	GENERIC, Gensia Sicor Pharmaceuticals Inc	00703-4502-04
2 ml x 25	$22.00	GENERIC, Baxter Pharmaceutical Products, Inc	10019-0450-02
2 ml x 25	$49.75	GENERIC, Faulding Pharmaceutical Company	61703-0210-07
2 ml x 25	$92.63	GENERIC, Abbott Pharmaceutical	00074-3414-01
2 ml x 25	$101.00	GENERIC, Abbott Pharmaceutical	00074-3413-01
10 ml x 25	$186.75	GENERIC, Faulding Pharmaceutical Company	61703-0210-11
10 ml x 25	$227.25	REGLAN, Esi Lederle Generics	00031-6709-78
20 ml x 10	$141.80	GENERIC, Faulding Pharmaceutical Company	61703-0210-21
30 ml x 10	$203.00	GENERIC, Faulding Pharmaceutical Company	61703-0210-31
30 ml x 25	$613.00	REGLAN, Esi Lederle Generics	00031-6709-24
50 ml	$41.56	GENERIC, Dupont Pharmaceuticals	00590-5709-57
200 ml	$118.14	GENERIC, Dupont Pharmaceuticals	00590-5709-77
250 ml	$164.05	GENERIC, Dupont Pharmaceuticals	00590-5709-73
300 ml	$174.99	GENERIC, Dupont Pharmaceuticals	00590-5709-85
Solution - Oral - 5 mg/5 ml			
480 ml	$7.44	FEDERAL UPPER LIMIT, H.C.F.A. F F P	99999-1798-07
Syrup - Oral - 5 mg/5 ml			
10 ml x 50	$40.50	GENERIC, Udl Laboratories Inc	51079-0590-10
10 ml x 50	$54.00	GENERIC, Xactdose Inc	50962-0425-60
10 ml x 100	$48.60	GENERIC, Pharmaceutical Assoc Inc Div Beach Products	00121-0576-10
10 ml x 100	$62.00	GENERIC, Roxane Laboratories Inc	00054-8563-04
10 ml x 100	$85.00	GENERIC, Xactdose Inc	50962-0425-10
120 ml x 100	$10.89	GENERIC, Roxane Laboratories Inc	00054-3563-50
473 ml	$12.72	GENERIC, Silarx Pharmaceuticals Inc	54838-0508-80
480 ml	$6.25	GENERIC, Pharmaceutical Assoc Inc Div Beach Products	00121-0576-16
480 ml	$14.00	GENERIC, Ivax Corporation	00182-6082-40
480 ml	$14.00	GENERIC, Raway Pharmacal Inc	00686-6105-38
480 ml	$16.03	GENERIC, Moore, H.L. Drug Exchange Inc	00839-7359-69
480 ml	$16.69	GENERIC, Alpharma Uspd Makers Of Barre and Nmc	00472-0454-16
480 ml	$16.70	GENERIC, Qualitest Products Inc	00603-1435-58
480 ml	$18.26	GENERIC, Geneva Pharmaceuticals	00781-6031-16
480 ml	$18.26	GENERIC, Geneva Pharmaceuticals	00781-6301-16
480 ml	$19.25	GENERIC, Major Pharmaceuticals Inc	00904-1073-16
480 ml	$19.25	GENERIC, Morton Grove Pharmaceuticals Inc	60432-0622-16
480 ml	$22.37	GENERIC, Aligen Independent Laboratories Inc	00405-3260-16
480 ml	$62.04	REGLAN, Esi Lederle Generics	00031-6706-25
500 ml	$21.24	GENERIC, Roxane Laboratories Inc	00054-3563-63
3840 ml	$117.89	GENERIC, Major Pharmaceuticals Inc	00904-1073-28
Tablet - Oral - 5 mg			
12's	$3.37	GENERIC, Allscripts Pharmaceutical Company	54569-3851-00
30 x 25	$315.60	GENERIC, Sky Pharmaceuticals Packaging, Inc	63739-0171-03
30's	$12.76	GENERIC, Heartland Healthcare Services	61392-0137-30
30's	$12.76	GENERIC, Heartland Healthcare Services	61392-0137-39
30's	$15.75	GENERIC, Medirex Inc	57480-0475-06
31 x 10	$131.84	GENERIC, Vangard Labs	00615-3546-53
31 x 10	$131.84	GENERIC, Vangard Labs	00615-3546-63
31's	$13.18	GENERIC, Heartland Healthcare Services	61392-0137-31
32's	$13.61	GENERIC, Heartland Healthcare Services	61392-0137-32
45's	$19.14	GENERIC, Heartland Healthcare Services	61392-0137-45
60's	$25.52	GENERIC, Heartland Healthcare Services	61392-0137-60
90's	$38.28	GENERIC, Heartland Healthcare Services	61392-0137-90
100's	$5.25	GENERIC, Us Trading Corporation	56126-0408-11

Qty	Price	Manufacturer	NDC
100's	$18.42	FEDERAL UPPER LIMIT, H.C.F.A. F F P	99999-1798-09
100's	$27.16	GENERIC, Duramed Pharmaceuticals Inc	51285-0585-02
100's	$27.16	GENERIC, Duramed Pharmaceuticals Inc	51285-0834-02
100's	$27.16	GENERIC, Invamed Inc	52189-0227-24
100's	$27.16	GENERIC, Invamed Inc	52189-0263-24
100's	$28.41	GENERIC, Caremark Inc	00339-5232-12
100's	$29.25	GENERIC, Martec Pharmaceuticals Inc	52555-0523-01
100's	$31.02	GENERIC, Aligen Independent Laboratories Inc	00405-4671-01
100's	$31.04	GENERIC, Moore, H.L. Drug Exchange Inc	00839-7530-06
100's	$32.00	GENERIC, Sidmak Laboratories Inc	50111-0517-01
100's	$32.20	GENERIC, Esi Lederle Generics	59911-5814-01
100's	$32.35	GENERIC, Martec Pharmaceuticals Inc	52555-0657-01
100's	$33.20	GENERIC, Watson/Rugby Laboratories Inc	00536-5902-01
100's	$33.25	GENERIC, Teva Pharmaceuticals Usa	00093-2204-01
100's	$39.35	GENERIC, Major Pharmaceuticals Inc	00904-1069-60
100's	$39.70	GENERIC, Geneva Pharmaceuticals	00781-5030-01
100's	$39.75	GENERIC, Qualitest Products Inc	00603-4616-21
100's	$39.75	GENERIC, Mutual/United Research Laboratories	00677-1323-01
100's	$39.75	GENERIC, Mutual Pharmaceutical Co Inc	53489-0384-01
100's	$40.40	GENERIC, Udl Laboratories Inc	51079-0629-20
100's	$41.11	GENERIC, Teva Pharmaceuticals Usa	62584-0785-01
100's	$42.53	GENERIC, Ivax Corporation	00182-1898-89
100's	$52.12	GENERIC, Major Pharmaceuticals Inc	00904-1069-61
100's	$63.61	REGLAN, Esi Lederle Generics	00031-6705-63

Tablet - Oral - 10 mg

Qty	Price	Manufacturer	NDC
25's	$7.15	GENERIC, Udl Laboratories Inc	51079-0283-19
30 x 25	$221.33	GENERIC, Sky Pharmaceuticals Packaging, Inc	63739-0172-01
30 x 25	$221.33	GENERIC, Sky Pharmaceuticals Packaging, Inc	63739-0172-03
30's	$8.92	GENERIC, Heartland Healthcare Services	61392-0558-30
30's	$8.92	GENERIC, Heartland Healthcare Services	61392-0558-39
30's	$18.96	GENERIC, Pharma Pac	52959-0480-30
30's	$22.41	REGLAN, Pd-Rx Pharmaceuticals	55289-0975-30
30's	$29.30	REGLAN, Physicians Total Care	54868-0513-00
31 x 10	$102.92	GENERIC, Vangard Labs	00615-2536-53
31 x 10	$102.92	GENERIC, Vangard Labs	00615-2536-63
31's	$9.21	GENERIC, Heartland Healthcare Services	61392-0558-31
32's	$9.51	GENERIC, Heartland Healthcare Services	61392-0558-32
45's	$13.37	GENERIC, Heartland Healthcare Services	61392-0558-45
60's	$17.83	GENERIC, Heartland Healthcare Services	61392-0558-60
90's	$26.75	GENERIC, Heartland Healthcare Services	61392-0558-90
100's	$3.55	GENERIC, Raway Pharmacal Inc	00686-2203-09
100's	$4.13	GENERIC, Interstate Drug Exchange Inc	00814-4806-14
100's	$4.35	GENERIC, Us Trading Corporation	56126-0328-11
100's	$5.75	GENERIC, Raway Pharmacal Inc	00686-0283-20
100's	$9.45	GENERIC, Invamed Inc	52189-0207-24
100's	$9.45	GENERIC, Invamed Inc	52189-0264-24
100's	$10.95	FEDERAL UPPER LIMIT, H.C.F.A. F F P	99999-1798-08
100's	$16.51	GENERIC, Caremark Inc	00339-5233-12
100's	$17.21	GENERIC, Moore, H.L. Drug Exchange Inc	00839-7127-06
100's	$19.82	GENERIC, Aligen Independent Laboratories Inc	00405-4672-01
100's	$22.00	GENERIC, Martec Pharmaceuticals Inc	52555-0120-01
100's	$25.40	GENERIC, Martec Pharmaceuticals Inc	52555-0658-01
100's	$25.87	GENERIC, Auro Pharmaceutical	55829-0378-10
100's	$26.05	GENERIC, Mutual/United Research Laboratories	00677-1039-01
100's	$26.05	GENERIC, Mutual/United Research Laboratories	00677-1746-01
100's	$27.25	GENERIC, Major Pharmaceuticals Inc	00904-1070-60
100's	$27.44	GENERIC, Esi Lederle Generics	59911-5815-01
100's	$27.50	GENERIC, Sidmak Laboratories Inc	50111-0430-01
100's	$27.75	GENERIC, Teva Pharmaceuticals Usa	00093-2203-01
100's	$27.75	GENERIC, Purepac Pharmaceutical Company	00228-2269-10
100's	$28.54	GENERIC, Udl Laboratories Inc	51079-0283-20
100's	$31.32	GENERIC, Ivax Corporation	00182-1789-89
100's	$31.33	GENERIC, Geneva Pharmaceuticals	00781-1301-13
100's	$35.70	GENERIC, Major Pharmaceuticals Inc	00904-1070-61
100's	$94.32	REGLAN, Physicians Total Care	54868-0513-01
100's	$100.29	REGLAN, Esi Lederle Generics	00031-6701-63

PRODUCT LISTING - EQUIVALENTS NOT AVAILABLE

Concentrate - Oral - 10 mg/ml

Qty	Price	Manufacturer	NDC
30 ml	$19.49	GENERIC, Roxane Laboratories Inc	00054-3564-44

Solution - Injectable - 5 mg/ml

Qty	Price	Manufacturer	NDC
2 ml x 25	$21.59	GENERIC, Physicians Total Care	54868-4167-00

Syrup - Oral - 5 mg/5 ml

Qty	Price	Manufacturer	NDC
120 ml	$10.39	GENERIC, Southwood Pharmaceuticals Inc	58016-0650-24
480 ml	$9.53	GENERIC, Physicians Total Care	54868-3485-00
480 ml	$15.98	GENERIC, Liquipharm Inc	54198-0128-16

Tablet - Oral - 5 mg

Qty	Price	Manufacturer	NDC
12's	$4.74	GENERIC, Southwood Pharmaceuticals Inc	58016-0729-12
15's	$5.93	GENERIC, Southwood Pharmaceuticals Inc	58016-0729-15
20's	$7.91	GENERIC, Southwood Pharmaceuticals Inc	58016-0729-20
21's	$6.49	GENERIC, Allscripts Pharmaceutical Company	54569-3851-01
30's	$9.28	GENERIC, Allscripts Pharmaceutical Company	54569-3851-02
30's	$11.86	GENERIC, Southwood Pharmaceuticals Inc	58016-0729-30
100's	$33.20	GENERIC, Watson/Rugby Laboratories Inc	00536-4038-01
100's	$39.53	GENERIC, Southwood Pharmaceuticals Inc	58016-0729-00

Tablet - Oral - 10 mg

Qty	Price	Manufacturer	NDC
4's	$1.11	GENERIC, Allscripts Pharmaceutical Company	54569-0434-06
6's	$1.67	GENERIC, Allscripts Pharmaceutical Company	54569-0434-07
12's	$7.41	GENERIC, Southwood Pharmaceuticals Inc	58016-0733-12
15's	$9.26	GENERIC, Southwood Pharmaceuticals Inc	58016-0733-15
20's	$12.35	GENERIC, Southwood Pharmaceuticals Inc	58016-0733-20
30's	$2.81	GENERIC, Physicians Total Care	54868-0034-04
30's	$8.33	GENERIC, Allscripts Pharmaceutical Company	54569-0434-00
30's	$18.53	GENERIC, Southwood Pharmaceuticals Inc	58016-0733-30
40's	$3.19	GENERIC, Physicians Total Care	54868-0034-07
50's	$3.58	GENERIC, Physicians Total Care	54868-0034-05
60's	$3.96	GENERIC, Physicians Total Care	54868-0034-02
60's	$19.52	GENERIC, Allscripts Pharmaceutical Company	54569-0434-05
60's	$37.06	GENERIC, Southwood Pharmaceuticals Inc	58016-0733-60
100's	$5.49	GENERIC, Physicians Total Care	54868-0034-03
100's	$27.75	GENERIC, Allscripts Pharmaceutical Company	54569-0434-02
100's	$61.76	GENERIC, Southwood Pharmaceuticals Inc	58016-0733-00
120's	$33.30	GENERIC, Allscripts Pharmaceutical Company	54569-0434-04

Metolazone *(001800)*

Categories: Edema; Hypertension, essential; Pregnancy Category B; FDA Approved 1973 Nov
Drug Classes: Diuretics, thiazide and derivatives
Brand Names: Mykrox; Zaroxolyn
Foreign Brand Availability: Barolyn (Finland); Diondel (Spain); Diulo (Hong-Kong; Portugal); Metenix 5 (England); Normelan (Japan); Xuret (England; Ireland)
Cost of Therapy: $12.86 (Hypertension; Zaroxolyn; 2.5 mg; 1 tablet/day; 30 day supply)
$15.96 (Edematous States; Zaroxolyn; 5 mg; 1 tablet/day; 30 day supply)
$37.21 (Hypertension; Mykrox; 0.5 mg; 1 tablet/day; 30 day supply)

WARNING

ZAROXOLYN:

DO NOT INTERCHANGE ZAROXOLYN TABLETS AND OTHER FORMULATIONS OF METOLAZONE THAT SHARE ITS SLOW AND INCOMPLETE BIOAVAILABILITY AND ARE NOT THERAPEUTICALLY EQUIVALENT AT THE SAME DOSES TO MYKROX TABLETS, A MORE RAPIDLY AVAILABLE AND COMPLETELY BIOAVAILABLE METOLAZONE PRODUCT. FORMULATIONS BIOEQUIVALENT TO ZAROXOLYN AND FORMULATIONS BIOEQUIVALENT TO MYKROX SHOULD NOT BE INTERCHANGED FOR ONE ANOTHER.

MYKROX:

DO NOT INTERCHANGE MYKROX TABLETS ARE A RAPIDLY AVAILABLE FORMULATION OF METOLAZONE FOR ORAL ADMINISTRATION. MYKROX TABLETS AND OTHER FORMULATIONS OF METOLAZONE THAT SHARE ITS MORE RAPID AND COMPLETE BIOAVAILABILITY ARE NOT THERAPEUTICALLY EQUIVALENT TO ZAROXOLYN TABLETS AND OTHER FORMULATIONS OF METOLAZONE THAT SHARE ITS SLOW AND INCOMPLETE BIOAVAILABILITY. FORMULATIONS BIOEQUIVALENT TO MYKROX AND FORMULATIONS BIOEQUIVALENT TO ZAROXOLYN SHOULD NOT BE INTERCHANGED FOR ONE ANOTHER.

DESCRIPTION

Metolazone is a diuretic/saluretic/antihypertensive drug of the quinazoline class, it has the molecular formula $C_{16}H_{16}ClN_3O_3S$, the chemical name 7-chloro-1,2,3,4-tetrahydro-2-methyl-3-(2-methylphenyl)-4-oxo-6-quinazolinesulfonamide, and a molecular weight of 365.83.

Metolazone is only sparingly soluble in water, but more soluble in plasma, blood, alkali, and organic solvents.

ZAROXOLYN TABLETS

Zaroxolyn tablets for oral administration contain 2½, 5, or 10 mg of metolazone. The inactive ingredients are magnesium stearate, microcrystalline cellulose and dye: *2½ mg:* D&C red no. 33; *5 mg:* FD&C blue no. 2; *10 mg:* D&C yellow no. 10 and FD&C yellow no. 6.

MYKROX TABLETS

Mykrox tablets for oral administration contain ½ mg of metolazone. The inactive ingredients are dibasic calcium phosphate, magnesium stearate, microcrystalline cellulose, pregelatinized starch, sodium starch glycolate.

CLINICAL PHARMACOLOGY

Metolazone is a quinazoline diuretic, with properties generally similar to the thiazide diuretics. The actions of metolazone result from interference with the renal tubular mechanism of electrolyte reabsorption. Metolazone acts primarily to inhibit sodium reabsorption at the cortical dilution site and to a lesser extent in the proximal convoluted tubule. Sodium and chloride ions are excreted in approximately equivalent amounts. The increased delivery of sodium to the distal tubular exchange site results in increased potassium excretion. Metolazone does not inhibit carbonic anhydrase. A proximal action of metolazone has been shown in humans by increased excretion of phosphate and magnesium ions and by a markedly increased fractional excretion of sodium in patients with severely compromised glomerular filtration. This action has been demonstrated in animals by micropuncture studies.

ZAROXOLYN

When Zaroxolyn tablets are given, diuresis and saluresis usually begin within 1 hour and may persist for 24 hours or more. For most patients, the duration of effect can be varied by adjusting the daily dose. High doses may prolong the effect. A single daily dose is recommended. When a desired therapeutic effect has been obtained, it may be possible to reduce dosage to a lower maintenance level.

The diuretic potency of Zaroxolyn at maximum therapeutic dosage is approximately equal to thiazide diuretics. However, unlike thiazides, Zaroxolyn may produce diuresis in patients with glomerular filtration rates below 20 ml/min.

Zaroxolyn and furosemide administered concurrently have produced marked diuresis in some patients where edema or ascites was refractory to treatment with maximum recommended doses of these or other diuretics administered alone. The mechanism of this interaction is unknown (see DRUG INTERACTIONS and WARNINGS).

Maximum blood levels of metolazone are found approximately 8 hours after dosing. A small fraction of metolazone is metabolized. Most of the drug is excreted in the unconverted form in the urine.

MYKROX

The antihypertensive mechanism of action of metolazone is not fully understood but is presumed to be related to its saluretic and diuretic properties.

In two double-blind, controlled clinical trials of Mykrox tablets, the maximum effect on mean blood pressure was achieved within 2 weeks of treatment and showed some evidence of an increased response at 1 mg compared to ½ mg. There was no indication of an increased response with 2 mg.

After 6 weeks of treatment, the mean fall in serum potassium was 0.42 mEq/L at ½ mg, 0.66 mEq/L at 1 mg, and 0.7 mEq/L at 2 mg. Serum uric acid increased by 1.1 to 1.4 mg/dl at increasing doses. There were small falls in serum sodium and chloride and a 1.3-2.1 mg/dl increase in BUN at increasing doses.

The rate and extent of absorption of metolazone from Mykrox tablets were equivalent to those from an oral solution of metolazone. Peak blood levels are obtained within 2-4 hours of oral administration with an elimination half-life of approximately 14 hours. Mykrox tablets have been shown to produce blood levels that are dose proportional between ½ and 2 mg. Steady state blood levels are usually reached in 4-5 days.

In contrast, other formulations of metolazone produce peak blood concentrations approximately 8 hours following oral administration; absorption continues for an additional 12 hours.

INDICATIONS AND USAGE

ZAROXOLYN

Zaroxolyn is indicated for the treatment of salt and water retention including:

- Edema accompanying congestive heart failure.
- Edema accompanying renal diseases, including the nephrotic syndrome and states of diminished renal function.

Zaroxolyn is also indicated for the treatment of hypertension, alone or in combination with other antihypertensive drugs of a different class. Mykrox tablets, a more rapidly available form of metolazone, are intended for the treatment of new patients with mild to moderate hypertension. A dose titration is necessary if Mykrox tablets are to be substituted for Zaroxolyn in the treatment of hypertension.

Usage in Pregnancy

The routine use of diuretics in an otherwise healthy woman is inappropriate and exposes mother and fetus to unnecessary hazard. Diuretics do not prevent development of toxemia of pregnancy, and there is no evidence that they are useful in the treatment of developed toxemia.

Edema during pregnancy may arise from pathologic causes or from the physiologic and mechanical consequences of pregnancy. Zaroxolyn is indicated in pregnancy when edema is due to pathologic causes, just as it is in the absence of pregnancy (see PRECAUTIONS). Dependent edema in pregnancy resulting from restriction of venous return by the expanded uterus is properly treated through elevation of the lower extremities and use of support hose; use of diuretics to lower intravascular volume in this case is illogical and unnecessary. There is hypervolemia during normal pregnancy which is harmful to neither the fetus nor the mother (in the absence of cardiovascular disease), but which is associated with edema, including generalized edema, in the majority of pregnant women. If this edema produces discomfort, increased recumbency will often provide relief. In rare instances, this edema may cause extreme discomfort which is not relieved by rest. In these cases, a short course of diuretics may be appropriate.

MYKROX

Mykrox tablets are indicated for the treatment of hypertension, alone or in combination with other antihypertensive drugs of a different class.

MYKROX TABLETS HAVE NOT BEEN EVALUATED FOR THE TREATMENT OF CONGESTIVE HEART FAILURE OR FLUID RETENTION DUE TO RENAL OR HEPATIC DISEASE AND THE CORRECT DOSAGE FOR THESE CONDITIONS AND OTHER EDEMA STATES HAS NOT BEEN ESTABLISHED.

SINCE A SAFE AND EFFECTIVE DIURETIC DOSE HAS NOT BEEN ESTABLISHED, MYKROX TABLETS SHOULD NOT BE USED WHEN DIURESIS IS DESIRED.

Usage in Pregnancy

The routine use of diuretics in an otherwise healthy woman is inappropriate and exposes mother and fetus to unnecessary hazard. Diuretics do not prevent development of toxemia of pregnancy, and there is no evidence that they are useful in the treatment of developed toxemia (see PRECAUTIONS).

Edema during pregnancy may arise from pathologic causes or from the physiologic and mechanical consequences of pregnancy. Mykrox is not indicated for the treatment of edema in pregnancy. Dependent edema in pregnancy resulting from restriction of venous return by the expanded uterus is properly treated through elevation of the lower extremities and use of support hose; use of diuretics to lower intravascular volume in this case is illogical and unnecessary. There is hypervolemia during normal pregnancy which is harmful to neither the fetus nor the mother (in the absence of cardiovascular disease), but which is associated with edema, including generalized edema, in the majority of pregnant women. If this edema produces discomfort, increased recumbency will often provide relief. In rare instances, this edema may cause extreme discomfort which is not relieved by rest. In these cases, a short course of diuretics may be appropriate.

CONTRAINDICATIONS

Anuria, hepatic coma or precoma, known allergy or hypersensitivity to metolazone.

WARNINGS

RAPID ONSET HYPONATREMIA

Rarely, the rapid onset of severe hyponatremia and/or hypokalemia has been reported following initial doses of thiazide and non-thiazide diuretics. When symptoms consistent with severe electrolyte imbalance appear rapidly, drug should be discontinued and supportive measures should be initiated immediately. Parenteral electrolytes may be required. Appropriateness of therapy with this class of drugs should be carefully reevaluated.

HYPOKALEMIA

Hypokalemia may occur with consequent weakness, cramps, and cardiac dysrhythmias. Serum potassium should be determined at regular intervals, and dose reduction, potassium supplementation or addition of a potassium-sparing diuretic instituted whenever indicated. Hypokalemia is a particular hazard in patients who are digitalized or who have or have had a ventricular arrhythmia; dangerous or fatal arrhythmias may be precipitated. Hypokalemia is dose related.

CONCOMITANT THERAPY

Lithium: In general, diuretics should not be given concomitantly with lithium because they reduce its renal clearance and add a high risk of lithium toxicity. Read prescribing information for lithium preparations before use of such concomitant therapy.

Furosemide: Unusually large or prolonged losses of fluids and electrolytes may result when metolazone is administered concomitantly to patients receiving furosemide (see PRECAUTIONS and DRUG INTERACTIONS).

Other Antihypertensive Drugs: When metolazone is used with other antihypertensive drugs, particular care must be taken to avoid excessive reduction of blood pressure, especially during initial therapy.

Cross-Allergy: Cross-allergy, while not reported to date, theoretically may occur when metolazone is given to patients known to be allergic to sulfonamide-derived drugs, thiazides, or quinethazone.

Sensitivity Reactions: Sensitivity reactions (*e.g.,* angioedema, bronchospasm) may occur with or without a history of allergy or bronchial asthma and may occur with the first dose of metolazone.

MYKROX

In controlled clinical trials, 1.5% of patients taking ½ mg and 3.1% of patients taking 1 mg of Mykrox daily developed clinical hypokalemia (defined as hypokalemia accompanied by signs or symptoms); 21% of the patients taking ½ mg and 30% of the patients taking 1 mg of Mykrox daily developed hypokalemia (defined as a serum potassium concentration below 3.5 mEq/L); in another controlled clinical trial in which the patients started therapy with a serum potassium level greater than 4.0 mEq/L, 8% of patients taking ½ mg of Mykrox daily developed hypokalemia (defined as a serum potassium concentration below 3.5 mEq/L).

PRECAUTIONS

See BOXED WARNING.

GENERAL

Fluid and Electrolytes

All patients receiving therapy with metolazone should have serum electrolyte measurements done at appropriate intervals and be observed for clinical signs of fluid and/or electrolyte imbalance: namely, hyponatremia, hypochloremic alkalosis, and hypokalemia. In patients with severe edema accompanying cardiac failure or renal disease, a low-salt syndrome may be produced, especially with hot weather and a low-salt diet. Serum and urine electrolyte determinations are particularly important when the patient has protracted vomiting, severe diarrhea, or in receiving parenteral fluids. Warning signs of imbalance are: dryness of mouth, thirst, weakness, lethargy, drowsiness, restlessness, muscle pains or cramps, muscle fatigue, hypotension, oliguria, tachycardia, and gastrointestinal disturbances such as nausea and vomiting. Hyponatremia may occur at any time during long term therapy and, on rare occasions, may be life threatening.

The risk of hypokalemia is increased when larger doses are used, when diuresis is rapid, when severe liver disease is present, when corticosteroids are given concomitantly, when oral intake is inadequate or when excess potassium is being lost extrarenally, such as with vomiting or diarrhea.

Thiazide-like diuretics have been shown to increase the urinary excretion of magnesium; this may result in hypomagnesemia.

Glucose Tolerance

Metolazone may raise blood glucose concentrations possibly causing hyperglycemia and glycosuria in patients with diabetes or latent diabetes.

Hyperuricemia

Metolazone regularly causes an increase in serum uric acid and can occasionally precipitate gouty attacks even in patients without a prior history of them.

M

Azotemia

Azotemia, presumably prerenal azotemia, may be precipitated during the administration of metolazone. If azotemia and oliguria worsen during treatment of patients with severe renal disease, metolazone should be discontinued.

Renal Impairment

Use caution when administering metolazone to patients with severely impaired renal function. As most of the drug is excreted by the renal route, accumulation may occur.

Orthostatic Hypotension

Orthostatic hypotension may occur; this may be potentiated by alcohol, barbiturates, narcotics, or concurrent therapy with other antihypertensive drugs.
Mykrox: In controlled clinical trials, 1.4% of patients treated with Mykrox tablets (½ mg) had orthostatic hypotension; this effect was not reported in the placebo group.

Hypercalcemia

Hypercalcemia may infrequently occur with metolazone, especially in patients taking high doses of vitamin D or with high bone turnover states, and may signify hidden hyperparathyroidism. Metolazone should be discontinued before tests for parathyroid function are performed.

Systemic Lupus Erythematosus

Thiazide diuretics have exacerbated or activated systemic lupus erythematosus and this possibility should be considered with metolazone.

INFORMATION FOR THE PATIENT

Patients should be informed of possible adverse effects, advised to take the medication as directed, and promptly report any possible adverse reactions to the treating physician.

DRUG/LABORATORY TEST INTERACTIONS

None reported.

CARCINOGENESIS, MUTAGENESIS, AND IMPAIRMENT OF FERTILITY

Mice and rats administered metolazone 5 days/week for up to 18 and 24 months, respectively, at daily doses of 2, 10, and 50 mg/kg, exhibited no evidence of a tumorigenic effect of the drug. The small number of animals examined histologically and poor survival in the mice limit the conclusions that can be reached from these studies.

Metolazone was not mutagenic *in vitro* in the Ames Test using *Salmonella typhimurium* strains TA-97, TA-98, TA-100, TA-102, and TA- 1535.

Reproductive performance has been evaluated in mice and rats. There is no evidence that metolazone possesses the potential for altering reproductive capacity in mice. In a rat study, in which males were treated orally with metolazone at doses of 2, 10, and 50 mg/kg for 127 days prior to mating with untreated females, an increased number of resorption sites was observed in dams mated with males from the 50 mg/kg group. In addition, the birth weight of offspring was decreased and the pregnancy rate was reduced in dams mated with males from the 10 and 50 mg/kg groups.

M

PREGNANCY CATEGORY B

Teratogenic Effects

Reproduction studies performed in mice, rabbits, and rats treated during the appropriate period of gestation at doses up to 50 mg/kg/day have revealed no evidence of harm to the fetus due to metolazone. There are, however, no adequate and well-controlled studies in pregnant women. Because animal reproduction studies are not always predictive of human response, metolazone should be used during pregnancy only if clearly needed. Metolazone crosses the placental barrier and appears in cord blood.

Nonteratogenic Effects

The use of metolazone in pregnant women requires that the anticipated benefit be weighed against possible hazards to the fetus. These hazards include fetal or neonatal jaundice, thrombocytopenia, and possibly other adverse reactions which have occurred in the adult. It is not known what effect the use of the drug during pregnancy has on the later growth, development, and functional maturation of the child. No such effects have been reported with metolazone.

LABOR AND DELIVERY

Based on clinical studies in which women received metolazone in late pregnancy until the time of delivery, there is no evidence that the drug has any adverse effects on the normal course of labor or delivery.

NURSING MOTHERS

Metolazone appears in breast milk. Because of the potential for serious adverse reactions in nursing infants from metolazone, a decision should be made whether to discontinue nursing or to discontinue the drug, taking into account the importance of the drug to the mother.

PEDIATRIC USE

Safety and effectiveness in children have not been established and such use is not recommended.

DRUG INTERACTIONS

Diuretics: Furosemide and probably other loop diuretics given concomitantly with metolazone can cause unusually large or prolonged losses of fluid and electrolytes (see WARNINGS).

Other Antihypertensives: When metolazone is used with other antihypertensive drugs, care must be taken, especially during initial therapy. Dosage adjustments of other antihypertensives may be necessary.

Alcohol, Barbiturates, and Narcotics: The hypotensive effects of these drugs may be potentiated by the volume contraction that may be associated with metolazone therapy.

Digitalis Glycosides: Diuretic-induced hypokalemia can increase the sensitivity of the myocardium to digitalis. Serious arrhythmias can result.

Corticosteroids or ACTH: May increase the risk of hypokalemia and increase salt and water retention.

Lithium: Serum lithium levels may increase (see WARNINGS.)

Curariform Drugs: Diuretic-induced hypokalemia may enhance neuromuscular blocking effects of curariform drugs (such as tubocurarine)—the most serious effect would be respiratory depression which could proceed to apnea. Accordingly, it may be advisable to discontinue metolazone 3 days before elective surgery.

Salicylates and Other Non-Steroidal Anti-Inflammatory Drugs: May decrease the antihypertensive effects of metolazone.

Sympathomimetics: Metolazone may decrease arterial responsiveness to norepinephrine, but this diminution is not sufficient to preclude effectiveness of the pressor agent for therapeutic use.

Insulin and Oral Antidiabetic Agents: See PRECAUTIONS, General, Glucose Tolerance

Methenamine: Efficacy may be decreased due to urinary alkalizing effect of metolazone.

Anticoagulants: Metolazone, as well as other thiazide-like diuretics, may affect the hypoprothrombinemic response to anticoagulants; dosage adjustments may be necessary.

ADVERSE REACTIONS

ZAROXOLYN

Zaroxolyn is usually well tolerated, and most reported adverse reactions have been mild and transient. Many Zaroxolyn related adverse reactions represent extensions of its expected pharmacologic activity and can be attributed to either its antihypertensive action or its renal/metabolic actions. The following adverse reactions have been reported. Several are single or comparably rare occurrences. Adverse reactions are listed in decreasing order of severity within body systems.

Cardiovascular: Chest pain/discomfort, orthostatic hypotension, excessive volume depletion, hemoconcentration, venous thrombosis, palpitations.

Central and Peripheral Nervous System: Syncope, neuropathy, vertigo, paresthesias, psychotic depression, impotence, dizziness/lightheadedness, drowsiness, fatigue, weakness, restlessness (sometimes resulting in insomnia), headache.

Dermatologic/Hypersensitivity: Necrotizing angitis (cutaneous vasculitis), purpura, dermatitis (photosensitivity), urticaria, and skin rashes.

Gastrointestinal: Hepatitis, intrahepatic cholestatic jaundice, pancreatitis, vomiting, nausea, epigastric distress, diarrhea, constipation, anorexia, abdominal bloating.

Hematologic: Aplastic/hypoplastic anemia, agranulocytosis, leukopenia.

Metabolic: Hypokalemia, hyponatremia, hyperuricemia, hypochloremia, hypochloremic alkalosis, hyperglycemia, glycosuria, increase in serum urea nitrogen (BUN) or creatinine, hypophosphatemia, hypomagnesemia, hypercalcemia.

Musculoskeletal: Joint pain, acute gouty attacks, muscle cramps or spasm.

Other: Transient blurred vision, chills.

In addition, adverse reactions reported with similar antihypertensive-diuretics, but which have not been reported to date for Zaroxolyn include: bitter taste, dry mouth, sialadenitis, xanthopsia, respiratory distress (including pneumonitis), thrombocytopenia, and anaphylactic reactions. These reactions should be considered as possible occurrences with clinical usage of Zaroxolyn.

Whenever adverse reactions are moderate or severe, Zaroxolyn dosage should be reduced or therapy withdrawn.

MYKROX

Adverse experience information is available from more than 14 years of accumulated marketing experience with other formulations of metolazone for which reliable quantitative information is lacking and from controlled clinical trials with Mykrox from which incidences can be calculated.

In controlled clinical trials with Mykrox, adverse experiences resulted in discontinuation of therapy in 6.7-6.8% of patients given ½ to 1 mg of Mykrox.

Adverse experiences occurring in controlled clinical trials with Mykrox with an incidence of >2%, whether or not considered drug-related, are summarized in TABLE 1.

TABLE 1 *Incidence of Adverse Experiences Volunteered or Elicited (by Patient in Percent)**

	Mykrox† (n = 226)
Dizziness (lightheadedness)	10.2%
Headaches	9.3%
Muscle cramps	5.8%
Fatigue (malaise, lethargy, lassitude)	4.4%
Joint pain, swelling	3.1%
Chest pain (precordial discomfort)	2.7%

* Percent of patients reporting an adverse experience one or more times.
† All doses combined (Glucose Tolerance, 1, and 2 mg).

Some of the adverse effects reported in association with Mykrox also occur frequently in untreated hypertensive patients, such as headache and dizziness, which occurred in 14.8 and 7.4% of patients in a smaller parallel placebo group.

The following adverse effects were reported in less than 2% of the mykrox treated patients:

Cardiovascular: Cold extremities, edema, orthostatic hypotension, palpitations.

Central and Peripheral Nervous System: Anxiety, depression, dry mouth, impotence, nervousness, neuropathy, weakness, "weird" feeling

Dermatological: Pruritus, rash, skin dryness.

Eyes, Ears, Nose, Throat: Cough, epistaxis, eye itching, sinus congestion, sore throat, tinnitus.

Gastrointestinal: Abdominal discomfort (pain, bloating), bitter taste, constipation, diarrhea, nausea, vomiting.
Genitourinary: Nocturia.
Musculoskeletal: Back Pain.

Other Adverse Experiences

Adverse experiences reported with other marketed metolazone formulations and most thiazide diuretics, for which quantitative data are not available, are listed in decreasing order of severity within body systems. Several are single or rare occurrences.

Cardiovascular: Excessive volume depletion, hemoconcentration, venous thrombosis.
Central and Peripheral Nervous System: Syncope, paresthesias, drowsiness, restlessness (sometimes resulting in insomnia).
Dermatologic/Hypersensitivity: Necrotizing angitis (cutaneous vasculitis), purpura, dermatitis, photosensitivity, urticaria.
Gastrointestinal: Hepatitis, intrahepatic cholestatic jaundice, pancreatitis, anorexia.
Hematologic: aplastic (hypoplastic) anemia, agranulocytosis, leukopenia.
Metabolic: Hypokalemia (see WARNINGS, Hypokalemia), hyponatremia, hyperuricemia, hypochloremia, hypochloremic alkalosis, hyperglycemia, glycosuria, increase in serum urea nitrogen (BUN) or creatinine, hypophosphatemia, hypomagnesemia, hypercalcemia.
Musculoskeletal: Acute gouty attacks.
Other: Transient blurred vision, chills.

In addition, rare adverse experiences reported in association with similar antihypertensive-diuretics but not reported to date for metolazone include: sialadenitis, xanthopsia, respiratory distress (including pneumonitis), thrombocytopenia, and anaphylactic reactions. These experiences could occur with clinical use of metolazone.

DOSAGE AND ADMINISTRATION

ZAROXOLYN

Effective dosage of Zaroxolyn should be individualized according to indication and patient response. A single daily dose is recommended. Therapy with Zaroxolyn should be titrated to gain an initial therapeutic response and to determine the minimal dose possible to maintain the desired therapeutic response.

Usual Single Daily Dosage Schedules

Suitable initial dosages will usually fall in the ranges given.

Edema of Cardiac Failure: Zaroxolyn 5-20 mg once daily.
Edema of Renal Disease: Zaroxolyn 5-20 mg once daily.
Mild to Moderate Essential Hypertension: Zaroxolyn 2.5-5 mg once daily.

New Patients

Mykrox tablets. If considered desirable to switch patients currently on Zaroxolyn to Mykrox, the dose should be determined by titration starting at 1 tablet (½ mg) once daily and increasing to 2 tablets (1 mg) once daily if needed.

Treatment of Edematous States

The time interval required for the initial dosage to produce an effect may vary. Diuresis and saluresis usually begin within 1 hour and persist for 24 hours or longer. When a desired therapeutic effect has been obtained, it may be advisable to reduce the dose if possible. The daily dose depends on the severity of the patient's condition, sodium intake, and responsiveness. A decision to change the daily dose should be based on the results of thorough clinical and laboratory evaluations. If antihypertensive drugs or diuretics are given concurrently with Zaroxolyn, more careful dosage adjustment may be necessary. For patients who tend to experience paroxysmal nocturnal dyspnea, it may be advisable to employ a larger dose to ensure prolongation of diuresis and saluresis for a full 24 hour period.

Treatment of Hypertension

The time interval required for the initial dosage regimen to show effect may vary from 3 or 4 days to 3-6 weeks in the treatment of elevated blood pressure. Doses should be adjusted at appropriate intervals to achieve maximum therapeutic effect.

MYKROX

Therapy should be individualized according to patient response.

For initial treatment of mild to moderate hypertension, the recommended dose is 1 Mykrox tablet (½ mg) once daily, usually in the morning. If patients are inadequately controlled with one ½ mg tablet, the dose can be increased to 2 Mykrox tablets (1 mg) once a day. An increase in hypokalemia may occur. Doses larger than 1 mg do not give increased effectiveness.

The same dose titration is necessary if Mykrox tablets are to be substituted for other dosage forms of metolazone in the treatment of hypertension.

If blood pressure is not adequately controlled with 2 Mykrox tablets alone, the dose should not be increased; rather, another antihypertensive agent with a different mechanism of action should be added to therapy with Mykrox tablets.

HOW SUPPLIED

ZAROXOLYN

Zaroxolyn tablets are shallow biconvex, round tablets, and are available in three strengths:

2½ mg: Pink, debossed "Zaroxolyn" on one side, and "2½" on reverse side.
5 mg: Blue, debossed "Zaroxolyn" on one side, and "5" on reverse side.
10 mg: Yellow, debossed "Zaroxolyn" on one side, and "10" on reverse side.

Storage: Store at room temperature. Dispense in a tight, light-resistant container. Keep out of the reach of children.

MYKROX

Mykrox tablets, ½ mg are white, flat-faced, round tablets, debossed "Mykrox" on one side, and "½" on reverse side.

Storage: Store at room temperature. Dispense in a tight, light-resistant container. Keep out of the reach of children.

PRODUCT LISTING - RATED THERAPEUTICALLY EQUIVALENT

Tablet - Oral - 2.5 mg

100's	$42.86	ZAROXOLYN, Celltech Pharmacueticals Inc	00585-0975-71

PRODUCT LISTING - EQUIVALENTS NOT AVAILABLE

Tablet - Oral - 0.5 mg			
100's	$124.04	GENERIC, Celltech Pharmacueticals Inc	53014-0847-71
Tablet - Oral - 2.5 mg			
100's	$55.64	ZAROXOLYN, Celltech Pharmacueticals Inc	00585-0975-72
100's	$108.91	ZAROXOLYN, Celltech Pharmacueticals Inc	53014-0975-71
100's	$129.43	ZAROXOLYN, Celltech Pharmacueticals Inc	53014-0975-72
Tablet - Oral - 5 mg			
25's	$23.81	ZAROXOLYN, Pd-Rx Pharmaceuticals	55289-0132-97
60's	$52.95	ZAROXOLYN, Physicians Total Care	54868-0476-01
100's	$53.21	ZAROXOLYN, Celltech Pharmacueticals Inc	00585-0850-71
100's	$61.94	ZAROXOLYN, Celltech Pharmacueticals Inc	00585-0850-72
100's	$86.87	ZAROXOLYN, Physicians Total Care	54868-0476-02
100's	$123.77	ZAROXOLYN, Celltech Pharmacueticals Inc	53014-0850-71
100's	$144.11	ZAROXOLYN, Celltech Pharmacueticals Inc	53014-0850-72
Tablet - Oral - 10 mg			
100's	$119.83	ZAROXOLYN, Celltech Pharmacueticals Inc	53014-0835-72
100's	$148.19	ZAROXOLYN, Celltech Pharmacueticals Inc	53014-0835-71

Metoprolol (001801)

For related information, see the comparative table section in Appendix A.

Categories: Angina pectoris; Hypertension, essential; Myocardial infarction; Heart failure, congestive; Pregnancy Category C; FDA Approved 1978 Aug

Drug Classes: Antiadrenergics, beta blocking

Brand Names: **Lopressor**; Toprol XL

Foreign Brand Availability: Apo-Metoprolol (Canada); Beloc (Austria; Colombia; Germany); Beloc Duriles (Austria); Beloc Zok (Switzerland); Betaloc (Australia; Canada; China; England; Hong-Kong; Hungary; India; Ireland; Korea; Malaysia; Philippines; Russia; Taiwan; Thailand); Betaloc CR (New-Zealand); Betaloc Zok (Hong-Kong; Singapore; Taiwan); Betazok (Philippines); Betoprolol (Colombia); Cardeloc (Thailand); Cardiosel (Indonesia; Philippines); Cardiostat (Philippines); Denex (Hong-Kong; Thailand); Jutabloc (Germany); Kenaprol (Mexico); Lofarbil (Greece); Lopresor (Australia; Austria; Bahamas; Bahrain; Barbados; Belgium; Belize; Benin; Bermuda; Bulgaria; Burkina-Faso; Canada; Colombia; Curacao; Cyprus; Czech-Republic; Egypt; England; Ethiopia; Gambia; Germany; Ghana; Greece; Guinea; Guyana; Indonesia; Iran; Iraq; Ireland; Israel; Italy; Ivory-Coast; Jamaica; Japan; Jordan; Kenya; Kuwait; Lebanon; Liberia; Libya; Malawi; Mali; Mauritania; Mauritius; Mexico; Morocco; Netherland-Antilles; Netherlands; New-Zealand; Niger; Nigeria; Oman; Portugal; Puerto-Rico; Qatar; Republic-of-Yemen; Russia; Saudi-Arabia; Senegal; Seychelles; Sierra-Leone; South-Africa; Spain; Sudan; Surinam; Syria; Tanzania; Trinidad; Tunia; Turkey; Uganda; United-Arab-Emirates; Zambia; Zimbabwe); Lopresor Oros (Taiwan); Lopresor Retard (Austria; Bulgaria; Greece; Italy; Portugal; Switzerland); Lopresor SR (England); Meto-Hennig (Germany); Metohexal (Australia); Metolol (Australia; Thailand); Metopress Retard (Israel); Metoprim (Philippines); Metoprogamma (Germany); Minax (Australia; Hong-Kong; New-Zealand; Taiwan); Montebloc (Philippines); Neobloc (Israel); Prolaken (Mexico); Ritmolol (Mexico); Sefloc (Hong-Kong); Selokeen (Netherlands); Seloken (Belgium; Denmark; Finland; France; Indonesia; Italy; Japan; Mexico; Norway; Spain; Sweden); Seloken Retard (Austria; Italy); Seloken Zoc (Finland; Mexico; Sweden); Selopral (Finland); Selozok (Belgium); Selo-zok (Denmark; Norway); Slow-Lopresor (New-Zealand); Vasocardin (China)

Cost of Therapy: $56.92 (Hypertension; Lopressor; 50 mg; 2 tablets/day; 30 day supply)
$5.60 (Hypertension; Generic Tablets; 50 mg; 2 tablets/day; 30 day supply)
$56.92 (Angina Pectoris; Lopressor; 50 mg; 2 tablets/day; 30 day supply)
$85.46 (Myocardial Infarction; Lopressor; 100 mg; 2 tablets/day; 30 day supply)
$37.65 (Myocardial Infarction; Generic Tablets; 100 mg; 2 tablets/day; 30 day supply)
$22.76 (Hypertension; Toprol-XL; 50 mg; 1 tablet/day; 30 day supply)
$34.20 (Angina Pectoris; Toprol-XL; 100 mg; 1 tablet/day; 30 day supply)

DESCRIPTION

Note: The trade names have been used throughout this monograph for clarity.

LOPRESSOR

Lopressor, metoprolol tartrate, is a selective $beta_1$-adrenoreceptor blocking agent, available as 50 and 100 mg tablets for oral administration and in 5 ml ampuls for intravenous (IV) administration. Each ampul contains a sterile solution of metoprolol tartrate, 5 mg, and sodium chloride, 45 mg. Metoprolol tartrate is (±)-1-(isopropylamino)-3-[*p*-(2-methoxyethyl)phenoxy]-2-propanol (2:1) *dextro*-tartrate salt.

Metoprolol tartrate is a white, practically odorless, crystalline powder with a molecular weight of 684.82. It is very soluble in water; freely soluble in methylene chloride, in chloroform, and in alcohol; slightly soluble in acetone; and insoluble in ether.

Inactive Ingredients: Tablets contain cellulose compounds, colloidal silicon dioxide, D&C red no. 30 aluminum lake (50 mg tablets), FD&C blue no. 2 aluminum lake (100 mg tablets), lactose, magnesium stearate, polyethylene glycol, propylene glycol, povidone, sodium starch glycolate, talc, and titanium dioxide.

TOPROL-XL

Toprol-XL, metoprolol succinate, is a $beta_1$-selective (cardioselective) adrenoceptor blocking agent, for oral administration, available as extended release tablets. Toprol-XL has been formulated to provide a controlled and predictable release of metoprolol for once daily administration. The tablets comprise a multiple unit system containing metoprolol succinate in a multitude of controlled release pellets. Each pellet acts as a separate drug delivery unit and is designed to deliver metoprolol continuously over the dosage interval. The tablets contain 23.75, 47.5, 95 and 190 mg of metoprolol succinate equivalent to 25, 50, 100 and 200 mg of metoprolol tartrate, respectively. Its chemical name is (±)1-(isopropylamino)-3-[p-(2-methoxyethyl) phenoxy]-2-propanol succinate (2:1) (salt).

Metoprolol succinate is a white crystalline powder with a molecular weight of 652.8. It is freely soluble in water; soluble in methanol; sparingly soluble in ethanol; slightly soluble in dichloromethane and 2-propanol; practically insoluble in ethylacetate, acetone, diethylether and heptane. Inactive ingredients: silicon dioxide, cellulose compounds, sodium stearyl fumarate, polyethylene glycol, titanium dioxide, paraffin.

CLINICAL PHARMACOLOGY

LOPRESSOR

Lopressor is a beta-adrenergic receptor blocking agent. *In vitro* and *in vivo* animal studies have shown that it has a preferential effect on $beta_1$ adrenoreceptors, chiefly located in cardiac muscle. This preferential effect is not absolute, however, and at higher doses, Lopressor also inhibits $beta_2$ adrenoreceptors, chiefly located in the bronchial and vascular musculature.

Clinical pharmacology studies have confirmed the beta-blocking activity of metoprolol in man, as shown by (1) reduction in heart rate and cardiac output at rest and upon exercise, (2) reduction of systolic blood pressure upon exercise, (3) inhibition of isoproterenol-induced tachycardia, and (4) reduction of reflex orthostatic tachycardia.

Relative $beta_1$ selectivity has been confirmed by the following: (1) In normal subjects, Lopressor is unable to reverse the $beta_2$-mediated vasodilating effects of epinephrine. This contrasts with the effect of nonselective ($beta_1$ plus $beta_2$) beta blockers, which completely reverse the vasodilating effects of epinephrine. (2) In asthmatic patients, Lopressor reduces FEV_1 and FVC significantly less than a nonselective beta blocker, propranolol, at equivalent $beta_1$-receptor blocking doses.

Lopressor has no intrinsic sympathomimetic activity, and membrane-stabilizing activity is detectable only at doses much greater than required for beta blockade. Lopressor crosses the blood-brain barrier and has been reported in the CSF in a concentration 78% of the simultaneous plasma concentration. Animal and human experiments indicate that Lopressor slows the sinus rate and decreases AV nodal conduction.

In controlled clinical studies, Lopressor has been shown to be an effective antihypertensive agent when used alone or as concomitant therapy with thiazide-type diuretics, at dosages of 100-450 mg daily. In controlled, comparative, clinical studies, Lopressor has been shown to be as effective an antihypertensive agent as propranolol, methyldopa, and thiazide-type diuretics, and to be equally effective in supine and standing positions.

The mechanism of the antihypertensive effects of beta-blocking agents has not been elucidated. However, several possible mechanisms have been proposed: (1) competitive antagonism of catecholamines at peripheral (especially cardiac) adrenergic neuron sites, leading to decreased cardiac output; (2) a central effect leading to reduced sympathetic outflow to the periphery; and (3) suppression of renin activity.

M

By blocking catecholamine-induced increases in heart rate, in velocity and extent of myocardial contraction, and in blood pressure, Lopressor reduces the oxygen requirements of the heart at any given level of effort, thus making it useful in the long-term management of angina pectoris. However, in patients with heart failure, beta-adrenergic blockade may increase oxygen requirements by increasing left ventricular fiber length and end-diastolic pressure.

Although beta-adrenergic receptor blockade is useful in the treatment of angina and hypertension, there are situations in which sympathetic stimulation is vital. In patients with severely damaged hearts, adequate ventricular function may depend on sympathetic drive. In the presence of AV block, beta blockade may prevent the necessary facilitating effect of sympathetic activity on conduction. $Beta_2$-adrenergic blockade results in passive bronchial constriction by interfering with endogenous adrenergic bronchodilator activity in patients subject to bronchospasm and may also interfere with exogenous bronchodilators in such patients.

In controlled clinical trials, Lopressor, administered 2 or 4 times daily, has been shown to be an effective antianginal agent, reducing the number of angina attacks and increasing exercise tolerance. The dosage used in these studies ranged from 100-400 mg daily. A controlled, comparative, clinical trial showed that Lopressor was indistinguishable from propranolol in the treatment of angina pectoris.

In a large (1395 patients randomized), double-blind, placebo-controlled clinical study, Lopressor was shown to reduce 3 month mortality by 36% in patients with suspected or definite myocardial infarction.

Patients were randomized and treated as soon as possible after their arrival in the hospital, once their clinical condition had stabilized and their hemodynamic status had been carefully evaluated. Subjects were ineligible if they had hypotension, bradycardia, peripheral signs of shock, and/or more than minimal basal rales as signs of congestive heart failure. Initial treatment consisted of IV followed by oral administration of Lopressor or placebo, given in a coronary care or comparable unit. Oral maintenance therapy with Lopressor or placebo was then continued for 3 months. After this double-blind period, all patients were given Lopressor and followed up to 1 year.

The median delay from the onset of symptoms to the initiation of therapy was 8 hours in both the Lopressor and placebo treatment groups. Among patients treated with Lopressor, there were comparable reductions in 3 month mortality for those treated early (≤8 hours) and those in whom treatment was started later. Significant reductions in the incidence of ventricular fibrillation and in chest pain following initial IV therapy were also observed with Lopressor and were independent of the interval between onset of symptoms and initiation of therapy.

The precise mechanism of action of Lopressor in patients with suspected or definite myocardial infarction is not known.

In this study, patients treated with metoprolol received the drug both very early (intravenously) and during a subsequent 3 month period, while placebo patients received no beta-blocker treatment for this period. The study thus was able to show a benefit from the overall metoprolol regimen but cannot separate the benefit of very early IV treatment from the benefit of later beta-blocker therapy. Nonetheless, because the overall regimen showed a clear beneficial effect on survival without evidence of an early adverse effect on survival, one acceptable dosage regimen is the precise regimen used in the trial. Because the specific benefit of very early treatment remains to be defined however, it is also reasonable to administer the drug orally to patients at a later time as is recommended for certain other beta blockers.

Pharmacokinetics

In man, absorption of Lopressor is rapid and complete. Plasma levels following oral administration, however, approximate 50% of levels following IV administration, indicating about 50% first-pass metabolism.

Plasma levels achieved are highly variable after oral administration. Only a small fraction of the drug (about 12%) is bound to human serum albumin. Elimination is mainly by biotransformation in the liver, and the plasma half-life ranges from approximately 3-7 hours. Less than 5% of an oral dose of Lopressor is recovered unchanged in the urine; the rest is excreted by the kidneys as metabolites that appear to have no clinical significance. The systemic availability and half-life of Lopressor in patients with renal failure do not differ to a clinically significant degree from those in normal subjects. Consequently, no reduction in dosage is usually needed in patients with chronic renal failure.

Significant beta-blocking effect (as measured by reduction of exercise heart rate) occurs within 1 hour after oral administration, and its duration is dose-related. For example, a 50% reduction of the maximum registered effect after single oral doses of 20, 50, and 100 mg occurred at 3.3, 5.0, and 6.4 hours, respectively, in normal subjects. After repeated oral dosages of 100 mg twice daily, a significant reduction in exercise systolic blood pressure was evident at 12 hours.

Following IV administration of Lopressor, the urinary recovery of unchanged drug is approximately 10%. When the drug was infused over a 10 minute period, in normal volunteers, maximum beta blockade was achieved at approximately 20 minutes. Doses of 5 mg and 15 mg yielded a maximal reduction in exercise-induced heart rate of approximately 10% and 15%, respectively. The effect on exercise heart rate decreased linearly with time at the same rate for both doses, and disappeared at approximately 5 hours and 8 hours for the 5 mg and 15 mg doses, respectively.

Equivalent maximal beta-blocking effect is achieved with oral and IV doses in the ratio of approximately 2.5:1.

There is a linear relationship between the log of plasma levels and reduction of exercise heart rate. However, antihypertensive activity does not appear to be related to plasma levels. Because of variable plasma levels attained with a given dose and lack of a consistent relationship of antihypertensive activity to dose, selection of proper dosage requires individual titration.

In several studies of patients with acute myocardial infarction, IV followed by oral administration of Lopressor caused a reduction in heart rate, systolic blood pressure, and cardiac output. Stroke volume, diastolic blood pressure, and pulmonary artery end diastolic pressure remained unchanged.

In patients with angina pectoris, plasma concentration measured at 1 hour is linearly related to the oral dose within the range of 50-400 mg. Exercise heart rate and systolic blood pressure are reduced in relation to the logarithm of the oral dose of metoprolol. The increase in exercise capacity and the reduction in left ventricular ischemia are also significantly related to the logarithm of the oral dose.

TOPROL-XL

General

Metoprolol is a $beta_1$-selective (cardioselective) adrenergic receptor blocking agent. This preferential effect is not absolute, however, and at higher plasma concentrations, metoprolol also inhibits $beta_2$-adrenoreceptors, chiefly located in the bronchial and vascular musculature. Metoprolol has no intrinsic sympathomimetic activity, and membrane-stabilizing activity is detectable only at plasma concentrations much greater than required for beta-blockade. Animal and human experiments indicate that metoprolol slows the sinus rate and decreases AV nodal conduction.

Clinical pharmacology studies have confirmed the beta-blocking activity of metoprolol in man, as shown by (1) reduction in heart rate and cardiac output at rest and upon exercise, (2) reduction of systolic blood pressure upon exercise, (3) inhibition of isoproterenol-induced tachycardia, and (4) reduction of reflex orthostatic tachycardia.

The relative $beta_1$-selectivity of metoprolol has been confirmed by the following: (1) In normal subjects, metoprolol is unable to reverse the $beta_2$-mediated vasodilating effects of epinephrine. This contrasts with the effect of nonselective beta-blockers, which completely reverse the vasodilating effects of epinephrine. (2) In asthmatic patients, metoprolol reduces FEV_1 and FVC significantly less than a nonselective beta-blocker, propranolol, at equivalent $beta_1$-receptor blocking doses.

In five controlled studies in normal healthy subjects, the same daily doses of Toprol-XL and immediate release metoprolol were compared in terms of the extent and duration of $beta_1$-blockade produced. Both formulations were given in a dose range equivalent to 100-400 mg of immediate release metoprolol per day. In these studies, Toprol-XL was administered once a day and immediate release metoprolol was administered once to 4 times a day. A sixth controlled study compared the $beta_1$-blocking effects of a 50 mg daily dose of the 2 formulations. In each study, $beta_1$-blockade was expressed as the percent change from baseline in exercise heart rate following standardized submaximal exercise tolerance tests at steady-state. Toprol-XL administered once a day, and immediate release metoprolol administered once to 4 times a day, provided comparable total $beta_1$- blockade over 24 hours (area under the $beta_1$-blockade versus time curve) in the dose range 100-400 mg. At a dosage of 50 mg once daily, Toprol-XL produced significantly higher total $beta_1$-blockade over 24 hours than immediate release metoprolol. For Toprol-XL, the percent reduction in exercise heart rate was relatively stable throughout the entire dosage interval and the level of $beta_1$-blockade increased with increasing doses from 50-300 mg daily. The effects at peak/trough (*i.e.,* at 24 hours post dosing) were; 14/9, 16/10, 24/14, 27/22 and 27/20% reduction in exercise heart rate for doses of 50, 100, 200, 300 and 400 mg Toprol-XL once a day, respectively. In contrast to Toprol-XL, immediate release metoprolol given at a dose of 50-100 mg once a day produced a significantly larger peak effect on exercise tachycardia, but the effect was not evident at 24 hours. To match the peak to trough ratio obtained with

Toprol-XL over the dosing range of 200-400 mg, a tid to qid divided dosing regimen was required for immediate release metoprolol. A controlled cross-over study in heart failure patients compared the plasma concentrations and beta$_1$-blocking effects of 50 mg immediate release metoprolol administered tid, 100 and 200 mg Toprol-XL once daily. A 50 mg dose of immediate release metoprolol tid produced a peak plasma level of metoprolol similar to the peak level observed with 200 mg of Toprol-XL. A 200 mg dose of Toprol-XL produced a larger effect on suppression of exercise-induced and Holter-monitored heart rate over 24 hours compared to 50 mg tid of immediate release metoprolol.

The relationship between plasma metoprolol levels and reduction in exercise heart rate is independent of the pharmaceutical formulation. Using the E_{max} model, the maximal beta$_1$-blocking effect has been estimated to produce a 30% reduction in exercise heart rate. Beta$_1$-blocking effects in the range of 30-80% of the maximal effect (corresponding to approximately 8-23% reduction in exercise heart rate) are expected to occur at metoprolol plasma concentrations ranging from 30-540 nmol/L. The concentration-effect curve begins reaching a plateau between 200-300 nmol/L, and higher plasma levels produce little additional beta^1-blocking effect. The relative beta$_1$-selectivity of metoprolol diminishes and blockade of beta$_2$-adrenoceptors increases at higher plasma concentrations.

Although beta-adrenergic receptor blockade is useful in the treatment of angina, hypertension, and heart failure there are situations in which sympathetic stimulation is vital. In patients with severely damaged hearts, adequate ventricular function may depend on sympathetic drive. In the presence of AV block, beta-blockade may prevent the necessary facilitating effect of sympathetic activity on conduction. Beta$_2$-adrenergic blockade results in passive bronchial constriction by interfering with endogenous adrenergic bronchodilator activity in patients subject to bronchospasm and may also interfere with exogenous bronchodilators in such patients.

In other studies, treatment with Toprol-XL produced an improvement in left ventricular ejection fraction. Toprol-XL was also shown to delay the increase in left ventricular end-systolic and end-diastolic volumes after 6 months of treatment.

Hypertension

The mechanism of the antihypertensive effects of beta-blocking agents has not been elucidated. However, several possible mechanisms have been proposed: (1) competitive antagonism of catecholamines at peripheral (especially cardiac) adrenergic neuron sites, leading to decreased cardiac output; (2) a central effect leading to reduced sympathetic outflow to the periphery; and (3) suppression of renin activity.

Clinical Trials

In controlled clinical studies, an immediate release dosage form of metoprolol has been shown to be an effective antihypertensive agent when used alone or as concomitant therapy with thiazide-type diuretics at dosages of 100-450 mg daily. Toprol-XL, in dosages of 100-400 mg once daily, has been shown to possess comparable β_1-blockade as conventional metoprolol tablets administered 2-4 times daily. In addition, Toprol-XL administered at a dose of 50 mg once daily has been shown to lower blood pressure 24 hours post dosing in placebo-controlled studies. In controlled, comparative, clinical studies, immediate release metoprolol appeared comparable as an antihypertensive agent to propranolol, methyldopa, and thiazide-type diuretics, and affected both supine and standing blood pressure. Because of variable plasma levels attained with a given dose and lack of consistent relationship of antihypertensive activity to drug plasma concentration, selection of proper dosage requires individual titration.

Angina Pectoris

By blocking catecholamine-induced increases in heart rate, in velocity and extent of myocardial contraction, and in blood pressure, metoprolol reduces the oxygen requirements of the heart at any given level of effort, thus making it useful in the long-term management of angina pectoris.

Clinical Trials

In controlled clinical trials, an immediate release formulation of metoprolol has been shown to be an effective antianginal agent, reducing the number of angina attacks and increasing exercise tolerance. The dosage used in these studies ranged from 100-400 mg daily. Toprol-XL, in dosages of 100-400 mg once daily, has been shown to possess beta-blockade similar to conventional metoprolol tablets administered 2-4 times daily.

Heart Failure

The precise mechanism for the beneficial effects of beta-blockers in heart failure has not been elucidated.

Clinical Trials

MERIT-HF was a double-blind, placebo-controlled study of Toprol-XL conducted in 14 countries including the US. It randomized 3991 patients (1990 to Toprol-XL) with ejection fraction ≤0.40 and NYHA Class II-IV heart failure attributable to ischemia, hypertension, or cardiomyopathy. The protocol excluded patients with contraindications to beta-blocker use, those expected to undergo heart surgery, and those within 28 days of myocardial infarction or unstable angina. The primary endpoints of the trial were (1) all-cause mortality plus all-cause hospitalization (time to first event) and (2) all-cause mortality. Patients were stabilized on optimal concomitant therapy for heart failure, including diuretics, ACE inhibitors, cardiac glycosides, and nitrates. At randomization, 41% of patients were NYHA Class II, 55% NYHA Class III; 65% of patients had heart failure attributed to ischemic heart disease; 44% had a history of hypertension; 25% had diabetes mellitus; 48% had a history of myocardial infarction. Among patients in the trial, 90% were on diuretics, 89% were on ACE inhibitors, 64% were on digitalis, 27% were on a lipid-lowering agent, 37% were on an oral anticoagulant, and the mean ejection fraction was 0.28. The mean duration of follow-up was 1 year. At the end of the study, the mean daily dose of Toprol-XL was 159 mg.

The trial was terminated early for a statistically significant reduction in all-cause mortality (34%, nominal p=0.00009). The risk of all-cause mortality plus all-cause hospitalization was reduced by 19% (p=0.00012). The trial also showed improvements in heart failure-related mortality and heart failure-related hospitalizations, and NYHA functional class.

TABLE 1 shows the principal results for the overall study population. The combined endpoints of all-cause mortality plus all-cause hospitalization and of mortality plus heart failure hospitalization showed consistent effects in the overall study population and the subgroups, including women and the US population. However, in the US subgroup (n=1071) and women (n=898), overall mortality and cardiovascular mortality appeared less affected. Analyses of female and US patients were carried out because they each represented about 25% of the overall population. Nonetheless, subgroup analyses can be difficult to interpret and it is not known whether these represent true differences or chance effects.

TABLE 1 *Clinical Endpoints in the MERIT-HF Study*

Clinical Endpoint	Placebo n=2001	Toprol-XL n=1990	Relative Risk (95% CI)	Risk Reduction With Toprol-XL	Nominal P-value
All-cause mortality plus all-cause hospitalization*	767	641	0.81 (0.73-0.90)	19%	0.00012
All-cause mortality	217	145	0.66 (0.53-0.81)	34%	0.00009
All-cause mortality plus heart failure hospitalization*	439	311	0.69 (0.60-0.80)	31%	0.0000008
Cardiovascular mortality	203	128	0.62 (0.50-0.78)	38%	0.000022
Sudden death	132	79	0.59 (0.45-0.78)	41%	0.0002
Death due to worsening heart failure	58	30	0.51 (0.33-0.79)	49%	0.0023
Hospitalizations due to worsening heart failure†	451	317	N/A	N/A	0.0000076
Cardiovascular hospitalization†	773	649	N/A	N/A	0.00028

* Time to first event.
† Comparison of treatment groups examines the number of hospitalizations (Wilcoxon test); relative risk and risk reduction are not applicable.

Pharmacokinetics

In man, absorption of metoprolol is rapid and complete. Plasma levels following oral administration of conventional metoprolol tablets, however, approximate 50% of levels following intravenous (IV) administration, indicating about 50% first-pass metabolism. Metoprolol crosses the blood-brain barrier and has been reported in the CSF in a concentration 78% of the simultaneous plasma concentration.

Plasma levels achieved are highly variable after oral administration. Only a small fraction of the drug (about 12%) is bound to human serum albumin. Metoprolol is a racemic mixture of R- and S-enantiomers, and is primarily metabolized by CYP2D6. When administered orally, it exhibits stereoselective metabolism that is dependent on oxidation phenotype. Elimination is mainly by biotransformation in the liver, and the plasma half-life ranges from approximately 3-7 hours. Less than 5% of an oral dose of metoprolol is recovered unchanged in the urine; the rest is excreted by the kidneys as metabolites that appear to have no beta-blocking activity. Following IV administration of metoprolol, the urinary recovery of unchanged drug is approximately 10%. The systemic availability and half-life of metoprolol in patients with renal failure do not differ to a clinically significant degree from those in normal subjects. Consequently, no reduction in dosage is usually needed in patients with chronic renal failure.

Metoprolol is metabolized predominantly by CYP2D6, an enzyme that is absent in about 8% of Caucasians (poor metabolizers) and about 2% of most other populations. CYP2D6 can be inhibited by a number of drugs. Concomitant use of inhibiting drugs in poor metabolizers will increase blood levels of metoprolol several-fold, decreasing metoprolol's cardioselectivity. (See DRUG INTERACTIONS, Toprol-XL.)

In comparison to conventional metoprolol, the plasma metoprolol levels following administration of Toprol-XL are characterized by lower peaks, longer time to peak and significantly lower peak to trough variation. The peak plasma levels following once daily administration of Toprol-XL average one-fourth to one-half the peak plasma levels obtained following a corresponding dose of conventional metoprolol, administered once daily or in divided doses. At steady-state the average bioavailability of metoprolol following administration of Toprol-XL, across the dosage range of 50-400 mg once daily, was 77% relative to the corresponding single or divided doses of conventional metoprolol. Nevertheless, over the 24 hour dosing interval, β_1-blockade is comparable and dose-related (see CLINICAL PHARMACOLOGY, Toprol-XL). The bioavailability of metoprolol shows a dose-related, although not directly proportional, increase with dose and is not significantly affected by food following Toprol-XL administration.

INDICATIONS AND USAGE

LOPRESSOR

Hypertension

Lopressor tablets are indicated for the treatment of hypertension. They may be used alone or in combination with other antihypertensive agents.

Angina Pectoris

Lopressor is indicated in the long-term treatment of angina pectoris.

Myocardial Infarction

Lopressor ampuls and tablets are indicated in the treatment of hemodynamically stable patients with definite or suspected acute myocardial infarction to reduce cardiovascular mortality. Treatment with IV Lopressor can be initiated as soon as the patient's clinical condition allows (see DOSAGE AND ADMINISTRATION, Lopressor; CONTRAINDI-

CATIONS, Lopressor; and WARNINGS, Lopressor). Alternatively, treatment can begin within 3-10 days of the acute event (see DOSAGE AND ADMINISTRATION, Lopressor).

TOPROL-XL

Hypertension

Toprol-XL is indicated for the treatment of hypertension. They may be used alone or in combination with other antihypertensive agents.

Angina Pectoris

Toprol-XL is indicated in the long-term treatment of angina pectoris.

Heart Failure

Toprol-XL is indicated for the treatment of stable, symptomatic (NYHA Class II or III) heart failure of ischemic, hypertensive, or cardiomyopathic origin. It was studied in patients already receiving ACE inhibitors, diuretics, and, in the majority of cases, digitalis. In this population, Toprol-XL decreased the rate of mortality plus hospitalization, largely through a reduction in cardiovascular mortality and hospitalizations for heart failure.

CONTRAINDICATIONS

LOPRESSOR

Hypertension and Angina

Lopressor is contraindicated in sinus bradycardia, heart block greater than first degree, cardiogenic shock, and overt cardiac failure (see WARNINGS, Lopressor).

Myocardial Infarction

Lopressor is contraindicated in patients with a heart rate <45 beats/min; second- and third-degree heart block; significant first-degree heart block (P-R interval ≥0.24 seconds); systolic blood pressure <100 mm Hg; or moderate-to-severe cardiac failure (see WARNINGS, Lopressor).

TOPROL-XL

Toprol-XL is contraindicated in severe bradycardia, heart block greater than first degree, cardiogenic shock, decompensated cardiac failure, sick sinus syndrome (unless a permanent pacemaker is in place) (see WARNINGS, Toprol-XL) and in patients who are hypersensitive to any component of this product.

WARNINGS

LOPRESSOR

Hypertension and Angina

Cardiac Failure

Sympathetic stimulation is a vital component supporting circulatory function in congestive heart failure, and beta blockade carries the potential hazard of further depressing myocardial contractility and precipitating more severe failure. In hypertensive and angina patients who have congestive heart failure controlled by digitalis and diuretics, Lopressor should be administered cautiously. Both digitalis and Lopressor slow AV conduction.

In Patients Without a History of Cardiac Failure

Continued depression of the myocardium with beta-blocking agents over a period of time can, in some cases, lead to cardiac failure. At the first sign or symptom of impending cardiac failure, patients should be fully digitalized and/or given a diuretic. The response should be observed closely. If cardiac failure continues, despite adequate digitalization and diuretic therapy, Lopressor should be withdrawn.

Ischemic Heart Disease

Following abrupt cessation of therapy with certain beta-blocking agents, exacerbations of angina pectoris and, in some cases, myocardial infarction have occurred. When discontinuing chronically administered Lopressor, particularly in patients with ischemic heart disease, the dosage should be gradually reduced over a period of 1-2 weeks and the patient should be carefully monitored. If angina markedly worsens or acute coronary insufficiency develops, Lopressor administration should be reinstated promptly, at least temporarily, and other measures appropriate for the management of unstable angina should be taken. Patients should be warned against interruption or discontinuation of therapy without the physician's advice. Because coronary artery disease is common and may be unrecognized, it may be prudent not to discontinue Lopressor therapy abruptly even in patients treated only for hypertension.

Bronchospastic Diseases

PATIENTS WITH BRONCHOSPASTIC DISEASES SHOULD, IN GENERAL, NOT RECEIVE BETA BLOCKERS. Because of its relative $beta_1$ selectivity, however, Lopressor may be used with caution in patients with bronchospastic disease who do not respond to, or cannot tolerate, other antihypertensive treatment. Since $beta_1$ selectivity is not absolute, a $beta_2$-stimulating agent should be administered concomitantly, and the lowest possible dose of Lopressor should be used. In these circumstances it would be prudent initially to administer Lopressor in smaller doses 3 times daily, instead of larger doses 2 times daily, to avoid the higher plasma levels associated with the longer dosing interval. (See DOSAGE AND ADMINISTRATION, Lopressor.)

Major Surgery

The necessity or desirability of withdrawing beta-blocking therapy prior to major surgery is controversial; the impaired ability of the heart to respond to reflex adrenergic stimuli may augment the risks of general anesthesia and surgical procedures.

Lopressor, like other beta blockers, is a competitive inhibitor of beta-receptor agonists, and its effects can be reversed by administration of such agents, *e.g.*, dobutamine or isoproterenol. However, such patients may be subject to protracted severe hypotension. Difficulty in restarting and maintaining the heart beat has also been reported with beta blockers.

Diabetes and Hypoglycemia

Lopressor should be used with caution in diabetic patients if a beta-blocking agent is required. Beta blockers may mask tachycardia occurring with hypoglycemia, but other manifestations such as dizziness and sweating may not be significantly affected.

Thyrotoxicosis

Beta-adrenergic blockade may mask certain clinical signs (*e.g.*, tachycardia) of hyperthyroidism. Patients suspected of developing thyrotoxicosis should be managed carefully to avoid abrupt withdrawal of beta blockade, which might precipitate a thyroid storm.

Myocardial Infarction

Cardiac Failure

Sympathetic stimulation is a vital component supporting circulatory function, and beta blockade carries the potential hazard of depressing myocardial contractility and precipitating or exacerbating minimal cardiac failure.

During treatment with Lopressor, the hemodynamic status of the patient should be carefully monitored. If heart failure occurs or persists despite appropriate treatment, Lopressor should be discontinued.

Bradycardia

Lopressor produces a decrease in sinus heart rate in most patients; this decrease is greatest among patients with high initial heart rates and least among patients with low initial heart rates. Acute myocardial infarction (particularly inferior infarction) may in itself produce significant lowering of the sinus rate. If the sinus rate decreases to <40 beats/min, particularly if associated with evidence of lowered cardiac output, atropine (0.25-0.5 mg) should be administered intravenously. If treatment with atropine is not successful, Lopressor should be discontinued, and cautious administration of isoproterenol or installation of a cardiac pacemaker should be considered.

AV Block

Lopressor slows AV conduction and may produce significant first- (P-R interval ≥0.26 seconds), second-, or third-degree heart block. Acute myocardial infarction also produces heart block.

If heart block occurs, Lopressor should be discontinued and atropine (0.25-0.5 mg) should be administered intravenously. If treatment with atropine is not successful, cautious administration of isoproterenol or installation of a cardiac pacemaker should be considered.

Hypotension

If hypotension (systolic blood pressure ≤90 mm Hg) occurs, Lopressor should be discontinued, and the hemodynamic status of the patient and the extent of myocardial damage carefully assessed. Invasive monitoring of central venous, pulmonary capillary wedge, and arterial pressures may be required. Appropriate therapy with fluids, positive inotropic agents, balloon counterpulsation, or other treatment modalities should be instituted. If hypotension is associated with sinus bradycardia or AV block, treatment should be directed at reversing these (see above).

Bronchospastic Diseases

PATIENTS WITH BRONCHOSPASTIC DISEASES SHOULD, IN GENERAL, NOT RECEIVE BETA BLOCKERS. Because of its relative $beta_1$ selectivity, Lopressor may be used with extreme caution in patients with bronchospastic disease. Because it is unknown to what extent $beta_2$-stimulating agents may exacerbate myocardial ischemia and the extent of infarction, these agents should not be used prophylactically. If bronchospasm not related to congestive heart failure occurs, Lopressor should be discontinued. A theophylline derivative or a $beta_2$ agonist may be administered cautiously, depending on the clinical condition of the patient. Both theophylline derivatives and $beta_2$ agonists may produce serious cardiac arrhythmias.

TOPROL-XL

Ischemic Heart Disease

Following abrupt cessation of therapy with certain beta-blocking agents, exacerbations of angina pectoris and, in some cases, myocardial infarction have occurred. When discontinuing chronically administered Toprol-XL, particularly in patients with ischemic heart disease, the dosage should be gradually reduced over a period of 1-2 weeks and the patient should be carefully monitored. If angina markedly worsens or acute coronary insufficiency develops, Toprol-XL administration should be reinstated promptly, at least temporarily, and other measures appropriate for the management of unstable angina should be taken. Patients should be warned against interruption or discontinuation of therapy without the physician's advice. Because coronary artery disease is common and may be unrecognized, it may be prudent not to discontinue Toprol-XL therapy abruptly even in patients treated only for hypertension.

Bronchospastic Diseases

PATIENTS WITH BRONCHOSPASTIC DISEASES SHOULD, IN GENERAL, NOT RECEIVE BETA-BLOCKERS. Because of its relative $beta_1$-selectivity, however, Toprol-XL may be used with caution in patients with bronchospastic disease who do not respond to, or cannot tolerate, other antihypertensive treatment. Since $beta_1$- selectivity is not absolute, a $beta_2$-stimulating agent should be administered concomitantly, and the lowest possible dose of Toprol-XL should be used (see DOSAGE AND ADMINISTRATION, Toprol-XL).

Major Surgery

The necessity or desirability of withdrawing beta-blocking therapy prior to major surgery is controversial; the impaired ability of the heart to respond to reflex adrenergic stimuli may augment the risks of general anesthesia and surgical procedures.

Toprol-XL, like other beta-blockers, is a competitive inhibitor of beta-receptor agonists, and its effects can be reversed by administration of such agents, *e.g.*, dobutamine or isoproterenol. However, such patients may be subject to protracted severe hypotension. Difficulty in restarting and maintaining the heart beat has also been reported with beta-blockers.

M

Diabetes and Hypoglycemia

Toprol-XL should be used with caution in diabetic patients if a beta-blocking agent is required. Beta-blockers may mask tachycardia occurring with hypoglycemia, but other manifestations such as dizziness and sweating may not be significantly affected.

Thyrotoxicosis

Beta-adrenergic blockade may mask certain clinical signs (*e.g.,* tachycardia) of hyperthyroidism. Patients suspected of developing thyrotoxicosis should be managed carefully to avoid abrupt withdrawal of beta-blockade, which might precipitate a thyroid storm.

Peripheral Vascular Disease

Beta-blockers can precipitate or aggravate symptoms of arterial insufficiency in patients with peripheral vascular disease. Caution should be exercised in such individuals.

Calcium Channel Blockers

Because of significant inotropic and chronotropic effects in patients treated with beta-blockers and calcium channel blockers of the verapamil and diltiazem type, caution should be exercised in patients treated with these agents concomitantly.

PRECAUTIONS

LOPRESSOR

General

Lopressor should be used with caution in patients with impaired hepatic function.

Information for the Patient

Patients should be advised to take Lopressor regularly and continuously, as directed, with or immediately following meals. If a dose should be missed, the patient should take only the next scheduled dose (without doubling it). Patients should not discontinue Lopressor without consulting the physician.

Patients should be advised (1) to avoid operating automobiles and machinery or engaging in other tasks requiring alertness until the patient's response to therapy with Lopressor has been determined; (2) to contact the physician if any difficulty in breathing occurs; (3) to inform the physician or dentist before any type of surgery that he or she is taking Lopressor.

Carcinogenesis, Mutagenesis, and Impairment of Fertility

Long-term studies in animals have been conducted to evaluate carcinogenic potential. In a 2 year study in rats at three oral dosage levels of up to 800 mg/kg/day, there was no increase in the development of spontaneously occurring benign or malignant neoplasms of any type. The only histologic changes that appeared to be drug related were an increased incidence of generally mild focal accumulation of foamy macrophages in pulmonary alveoli and a slight increase in biliary hyperplasia. In a 21 month study in Swiss albino mice at three oral dosage levels of up to 750 mg/kg/day, benign lung tumors (small adenomas) occurred more frequently in female mice receiving the highest dose than in untreated control animals. There was no increase in malignant or total (benign plus malignant) lung tumors, nor in the overall incidence of tumors or malignant tumors. This 21 month study was repeated in CD-1 mice, and no statistically or biologically significant differences were observed between treated and control mice of either sex for any type of tumor.

All mutagenicity tests performed (a dominant lethal study in mice, chromosome studies in somatic cells, a *Salmonella*/mammalian-microsome mutagenicity test, and a nucleus anomaly test in somatic interphase nuclei) were negative.

No evidence of impaired fertility due to Lopressor was observed in a study performed in rats at doses up to 55.5 times the maximum daily human dose of 450 mg.

Pregnancy Category C

Lopressor has been shown to increase postimplantation loss and decrease neonatal survival in rats at doses up to 55.5 times the maximum daily human dose of 450 mg. Distribution studies in mice confirm exposure of the fetus when Lopressor is administered to the pregnant animal. These studies have revealed no evidence of impaired fertility or teratogenicity. There are no adequate and well-controlled studies in pregnant women. Because animal reproduction studies are not always predictive of human response, this drug should be used during pregnancy only if clearly needed.

Nursing Mothers

Lopressor is excreted in breast milk in a very small quantity. An infant consuming 1 liter of breast milk daily would receive a dose of less than 1 mg of the drug. Caution should be exercised when Lopressor is administered to a nursing woman.

Pediatric Use

Safety and effectiveness in pediatric patients have not been established.

TOPROL-XL

General

Toprol-XL should be used with caution in patients with impaired hepatic function. In patients with pheochromocytoma, an alpha-blocking agent should be initiated prior to the use of any beta-blocking agent.

Worsening cardiac failure may occur during up-titration of Toprol-XL. If such symptoms occur, diuretics should be increased and the dose of Toprol-XL should not be advanced until clinical stability is restored (see DOSAGE AND ADMINISTRATION, Toprol-XL). It may be necessary to lower the dose of Toprol-XL or temporarily discontinue it. Such episodes do not preclude subsequent successful titration of Toprol-XL.

Information for the Patient

Patients should be advised to take Toprol-XL regularly and continuously, as directed, preferably with or immediately following meals. If a dose should be missed, the patient should take only the next scheduled dose (without doubling it). Patients should not interrupt or discontinue Toprol-XL without consulting the physician.

Patients should be advised (1) to avoid operating automobiles and machinery or engaging in other tasks requiring alertness until the patient's response to therapy with Toprol-XL has been determined; (2) to contact the physician if any difficulty in breathing occurs; (3) to inform the physician or dentist before any type of surgery that he or she is taking Toprol-XL.

Heart failure patients should be advised to consult their physician if they experience signs or symptoms of worsening heart failure such as weight gain or increasing shortness of breath.

Laboratory Tests

Clinical laboratory findings may include elevated levels of serum transaminase, alkaline phosphatase, and lactate dehydrogenase.

Carcinogenesis, Mutagenesis, and Impairment of Fertility

Long-term studies in animals have been conducted to evaluate the carcinogenic potential of metoprolol tartrate. In 2 year studies in rats at 3 oral dosage levels of up to 800 mg/kg/day (41 times, on a mg/m^2 basis, the daily dose of 200 mg for a 60 kg patient), there was no increase in the development of spontaneously occurring benign or malignant neoplasms of any type. The only histologic changes that appeared to be drug related were an increased incidence of generally mild focal accumulation of foamy macrophages in pulmonary alveoli and a slight increase in biliary hyperplasia. In a 21 month study in Swiss albino mice at 3 oral dosage levels of up to 750 mg/kg/day (18 times, on a mg/m^2 basis, the daily dose of 200 mg for 60 kg patient), benign lung tumors (small adenomas) occurred more frequently in female mice receiving the highest dose than in untreated control animals. There was no increase in malignant or total (benign plus malignant) lung tumors, nor in the overall incidence of tumors or malignant tumors. This 21 month study was repeated in CD-1 mice, and no statistically or biologically significant differences were observed between treated and control mice of either sex for any type of tumor.

All genotoxicity tests performed on metoprolol tartrate (a dominant lethal study in mice, chromosome studies in somatic cells, a *Salmonella*/mammalian-microsome mutagenicity test, and a nucleus anomaly test in somatic interphase nuclei) and metoprolol succinate (a *Salmonella*/mammalian-microsome mutagenicity test) were negative.

No evidence of impaired fertility due to metoprolol tartrate was observed in a study performed in rats at doses up to 22 times, on a mg/m^2 basis, the daily dose of 200 mg in a 60 kg patient.

Pregnancy Category C

Metoprolol tartrate has been shown to increase post-implantation loss and decrease neonatal survival in rats at doses up to 22 times, on a mg/m^2 basis, the daily dose of 200 mg in a 60 kg patient. Distribution studies in mice confirm exposure of the fetus when metoprolol tartrate is administered to the pregnant animal. These studies have revealed no evidence of impaired fertility or teratogenicity. There are no adequate and well-controlled studies in pregnant women. Because animal reproduction studies are not always predictive of human response, this drug should be used during pregnancy only if clearly needed.

Nursing Mothers

Metoprolol is excreted in breast milk in very small quantities. An infant consuming 1 L of breast milk daily would receive a dose of less than 1 mg of the drug. Caution should be exercised when Toprol-XL is administered to a nursing woman.

Pediatric Use

Safety and effectiveness in pediatric patients have not been established.

Geriatric Use

Clinical studies of Toprol-XL in hypertension did not include sufficient numbers of subjects aged 65 and over to determine whether they respond differently from younger subjects. Other reported clinical experience in hypertensive patients has not identified differences in responses between elderly and younger patients.

Of the 1990 patients with heart failure randomized to Toprol-XL in the MERIT-HF trial, 50% (990) were 65 years of age and older and 12% (238) were 75 years of age and older. There were no notable differences in efficacy or the rate of adverse events between older and younger patients.

In general, dose selection for an elderly patient should be cautious, usually starting at the low end of the dosing range, reflecting greater frequency of decreased hepatic, renal, or cardiac function, and of concomitant disease or other drug therapy.

Risk of Anaphylactic Reactions

While taking beta-blockers, patients with a history of severe anaphylactic reactions to a variety of allergens may be more reactive to repeated challenge, either accidental, diagnostic or therapeutic. Such patients may be unresponsive to the usual doses of epinephrine used to treat allergic reaction.

DRUG INTERACTIONS

LOPRESSOR

Catecholamine-depleting drugs (*e.g.,* reserpine) may have an additive effect when given with beta-blocking agents. Patients treated with Lopressor plus a catecholamine depletor should therefore be closely observed for evidence of hypotension or marked bradycardia, which may produce vertigo, syncope, or postural hypotension.

Risk of Anaphylactic Reaction

While taking beta blockers, patients with a history of severe anaphylactic reaction to a variety of allergens may be more reactive to repeated challenge, either accidental, diagnostic, or therapeutic. Such patients may be unresponsive to the usual doses of epinephrine used to treat allergic reaction.

TOPROL-XL

Catecholamine-depleting drugs (*e.g.,* reserpine, mono amine oxidase (MAO) inhibitors) may have an additive effect when given with beta-blocking agents. Patients treated with

M

Toprol-XL plus a catecholamine depletor should therefore be closely observed for evidence of hypotension or marked bradycardia, which may produce vertigo, syncope, or postural hypotension.

Drugs that inhibit CYP2D6 such as quinidine, fluoxetine, paroxetine, and propafenone are likely to increase metoprolol concentration. In healthy subjects with CYP2D6 extensive metabolizer phenotype, coadministration of quinidine 100 mg and immediate release metoprolol 200 mg tripled the concentration of S-metoprolol and doubled the metoprolol elimination half-life. In 4 patients with cardiovascular disease, coadministration of propafenone 150 mg tid with immediate release metoprolol 50 mg tid resulted in 2- to 5-fold increases in the steady-state concentration of metoprolol. These increases in plasma concentration would decrease the cardioselectivity of metoprolol.

Beta-blockers may exacerbate the rebound hypertension which can follow the withdrawal of clonidine. If the 2 drugs are coadministered, the beta blocker should be withdrawn several days before the gradual withdrawal of clonidine. If replacing clonidine by beta-blocker therapy, the introduction of beta-blockers should be delayed for several days after clonidine administration has stopped.

ADVERSE REACTIONS

LOPRESSOR

Hypertension and Angina

Most adverse effects have been mild and transient.

Central Nervous System: Tiredness and dizziness have occurred in about 10 of 100 patients. Depression has been reported in about 5 of 100 patients. Mental confusion and short-term memory loss have been reported. Headache, nightmares, and insomnia have also been reported.

Cardiovascular: Shortness of breath and bradycardia have occurred in approximately 3 of 100 patients. Cold extremities; arterial insufficiency, usually of the Raynaud type; palpitations; congestive heart failure; peripheral edema; and hypotension have been reported in about 1 of 100 patients. (See CONTRAINDICATIONS, Lopressor; WARNINGS, Lopressor; and PRECAUTIONS, Lopressor.)

Respiratory: Wheezing (bronchospasm) and dyspnea have been reported in about 1 of 100 patients (see WARNINGS, Lopressor).

Gastrointestinal: Diarrhea has occurred in about 5 of 100 patients. Nausea, dry mouth, gastric pain, constipation, flatulence, and heartburn have been reported in about 1 of 100 patients. Post-marketing experience reveals very rare reports of hepatitis, jaundice and non-specific hepatic dysfunction. Isolated cases of transaminase, alkaline phosphatase, and lactic dehydrogenase elevations have also been reported.

Hypersensitive Reactions: Pruritus or rash have occurred in about 5 of 100 patients. Worsening of psoriasis has also been reported.

Miscellaneous: Peyronie's disease has been reported in fewer than 1 of 100,000 patients. Musculoskeletal pain, blurred vision, and tinnitus have also been reported.

M

There have been rare reports of reversible alopecia, agranulocytosis, and dry eyes. Discontinuation of the drug should be considered if any such reaction is not otherwise explicable.

The oculomucocutaneous syndrome associated with the beta blocker practolol has not been reported with Lopressor.

Myocardial Infarction

Central Nervous System: Tiredness has been reported in about 1 of 100 patients. Vertigo, sleep disturbances, hallucinations, headache, dizziness, visual disturbances, confusion, and reduced libido have also been reported, but a drug relationship is not clear.

Cardiovascular: In the randomized comparison of Lopressor and placebo described in CLINICAL PHARMACOLOGY, the adverse reactions found in TABLE 2 were reported.

Respiratory: Dyspnea of pulmonary origin has been reported in fewer than 1 of 100 patients.

Gastrointestinal: Nausea and abdominal pain have been reported in fewer than 1 of 100 patients.

Dermatologic: Rash and worsened psoriasis have been reported, but a drug relationship is not clear.

Miscellaneous: Unstable diabetes and claudication have been reported, but a drug relationship is not clear.

TABLE 2

	Lopressor	Placebo
Hypotension (systolic BP <90 mm Hg)	27.4%	23.2%
Bradycardia (heart rate <40 beats/min)	15.9%	6.7%
Second- or third-degree heart block	4.7%	4.7%
First-degree heart block (P-R ≥0.26 seconds)	5.3%	1.9%
Heart failure	27.5%	29.6%

Potential Adverse Reactions

A variety of adverse reactions not listed above have been reported with other beta-adrenergic blocking agents and should be considered potential adverse reactions to Lopressor.

Central Nervous System: Reversible mental depression progressing to catatonia; an acute reversible syndrome characterized by disorientation for time and place, short-term memory loss, emotional lability, slightly clouded sensorium, and decreased performance on neuropsychometrics.

Cardiovascular: Intensification of AV block (see CONTRAINDICATIONS, Lopressor).

Hematologic: Agranulocytosis, nonthrombocytopenic purpura, thrombocytopenic purpura.

Hypersensitive Reactions: Fever combined with aching and sore throat, laryngospasm, and respiratory distress.

TOPROL-XL

Hypertension and Angina

Most adverse effects have been mild and transient. The following adverse reactions have been reported for immediate release metoprolol tartrate.

Central Nervous System: Tiredness and dizziness have occurred in about 10 of 100 patients. Depression has been reported in about 5 of 100 patients. Mental confusion and short-term memory loss have been reported. Headache, somnolence, nightmares, and insomnia have also been reported.

Cardiovascular: Shortness of breath and bradycardia have occurred in approximately 3 of 100 patients. Cold extremities; arterial insufficiency, usually of the Raynaud type; palpitations; congestive heart failure; peripheral edema; syncope; chest pain; and hypotension have been reported in about 1 of 100 patients (see CONTRAINDICATIONS, Toprol-XL; WARNINGS, Toprol-XL; and PRECAUTIONS, Toprol-XL).

Respiratory: Wheezing (bronchospasm) and dyspnea have been reported in about 1 of 100 patients (see WARNINGS, Toprol-XL).

Gastrointestinal: Diarrhea has occurred in about 5 of 100 patients. Nausea, dry mouth, gastric pain, constipation, flatulence, digestive tract disorders, and heartburn have been reported in about 1 of 100 patients.

Hypersensitive Reactions: Pruritus or rash have occurred in about 5 of 100 patients. Worsening or psoriasis has also been reported.

Miscellaneous: Peyronie's disease has been reported in fewer than 1 of 100,000 patients. Musculoskeletal pain, blurred vision, decreased libido and tinnitus have also been reported.

There have been rare reports of reversible alopecia, agranulocytosis, and dry eyes. Discontinuation of the drug should be considered if any such reaction is not otherwise explicable. The oculomucocutaneous syndrome associated with the beta-blocker practolol has not been reported with metoprolol.

Potential Adverse Reactions

A variety of adverse reactions not listed above have been reported with other beta-adrenergic blocking agents and should be considered potential adverse reactions to Toprol-XL.

Central Nervous System: Reversible mental depression progressing to catatonia; an acute reversible syndrome characterized by disorientation for time and place, short-term memory loss, emotional lability, slightly clouded sensorium, and decreased performance on neuropsychometrics.

Cardiovascular: Intensification of AV block (see CONTRAINDICATIONS, Toprol-XL).

Hematologic: Agranulocytosis, nonthrombocytopenic purpura, thrombocytopenic purpura.

Hypersensitive Reactions: Fever combined with aching and sore throat, laryngospasm, and respiratory distress.

Heart Failure

In the MERIT-HF study, serious adverse events and adverse events leading to discontinuation of study medication were systematically collected. In the MERIT-HF study comparing Toprol-XL in daily doses up to 200 mg (mean dose 159 mg once daily) (n=1990) to placebo (n=2001), 10.3% of Toprol-XL patients discontinued for adverse events versus 12.2% of placebo patients.

TABLE 3 lists adverse events in the MERIT-HF study that occurred at an incidence of equal to or greater than 1% in the Toprol-XL group and greater than placebo by more than 0.5%, regardless of the assessment of causality.

TABLE 3 *Adverse Events Occurring in the MERIT-HF Study at an Incidence ≥1% in the Toprol-XL Group and Greater Than Placebo by More Than 0.5%*

	Toprol-XL n=1990	Placebo n=2001
Dizziness/vertigo	1.8%	1.0%
Bradycardia	1.5%	0.4%
Accident and/or injury	1.4%	0.8%

Other adverse events with an incidence of >1% on Toprol-XL and as common on placebo (within 0.5%) included myocardial infarction, pneumonia, cerebrovascular disorder, chest pain, dyspnea/dyspnea aggravated, syncope, coronary artery disorder, ventricular tachycardia/arrhythmia aggravated, hypotension, diabetes mellitus/ diabetes mellitus aggravated, abdominal pain, and fatigue.

Post-Marketing Experience

The following adverse reactions have been reported with Toprol-XL in worldwide post-marketing use, regardless of causality:

Cardiovascular: 2nd and 3rd degree heart block

Gastrointestinal: Hepatitis, vomiting

Hematologic: Thrombocytopenia

Musculoskeletal: Arthralgia

Nervous System/Psychiatric: Anxiety/nervousness, hallucinations, paresthesia

Reproductive, Male: Impotence

Skin: Increased sweating, photosensitivity

Special Sense Organs: Taste disturbances

DOSAGE AND ADMINISTRATION

LOPRESSOR

Hypertension

The dosage of Lopressor should be individualized. Lopressor should be taken with or immediately following meals.

The usual initial dosage is 100 mg daily in single or divided doses, whether used alone or added to a diuretic. The dosage may be increased at weekly (or longer) intervals until optimum blood pressure reduction is achieved. In general, the maximum effect of any given dosage level will be apparent after 1 week of therapy. The effective dosage range is 100-450 mg/day. Dosages above 450 mg/day have not been studied. While once-daily dosing is effective and can maintain a reduction in blood pressure throughout the day, lower doses (especially 100 mg) may not maintain a full effect at the end of the 24 hour period, and larger or more frequent daily doses may be required. This can be evaluated by measuring blood pressure near the end of the dosing interval to determine whether satisfactory control is being maintained throughout the day. $Beta_1$ selectivity diminishes as the dose of Lopressor is increased.

Angina Pectoris

The dosage of Lopressor should be individualized. Lopressor should be taken with or immediately following meals.

The usual initial dosage is 100 mg daily, given in two divided doses. The dosage may be gradually increased at weekly intervals until optimum clinical response has been obtained or there is pronounced slowing of the heart rate. The effective dosage range is 100-400 mg/day. Dosages above 400 mg/day have not been studied. If treatment is to be discontinued, the dosage should be reduced gradually over a period of 1-2 weeks (see WARNINGS, Lopressor).

Myocardial Infarction

Early Treatment

During the early phase of definite or suspected acute myocardial infarction, treatment with Lopressor can be initiated as soon as possible after the patient's arrival in the hospital. Such treatment should be initiated in a coronary care or similar unit immediately after the patient's hemodynamic condition has stabilized.

Treatment in this early phase should begin with the IV administration of three bolus injections of 5 mg of Lopressor each; the injections should be given at approximately 2 minute intervals. During the IV administration of Lopressor, blood pressure, heart rate, and electrocardiogram should be carefully monitored.

In patients who tolerate the full IV dose (15 mg), Lopressor tablets, 50 mg every 6 hours, should be initiated 15 minutes after the last IV dose and continued for 48 hours. Thereafter, patients should receive a maintenance dosage of 100 mg twice daily (see Late Treatment).

Patients who appear not to tolerate the full IV dose should be started on Lopressor tablets either 25 or 50 mg every 6 hours (depending on the degree of intolerance) 15 minutes after the last IV dose or as soon as their clinical condition allows. In patients with severe intolerance, treatment with Lopressor should be discontinued (see WARNINGS, Lopressor).

Late Treatment

Patients with contraindications to treatment during the early phase of suspected or definite myocardial infarction, patients who appear not to tolerate the full early treatment, and patients in whom the physician wishes to delay therapy for any other reason should be started on Lopressor tablets, 100 mg twice daily, as soon as their clinical condition allows. Therapy should be continued for at least 3 months. Although the efficacy of Lopressor beyond 3 months has not been conclusively established, data from studies with other beta blockers suggest that treatment should be continued for 1-3 years.

Note: Parenteral drug products should be inspected visually for particulate matter and discoloration prior to administration, whenever solution and container permit.

TOPROL-XL

Toprol-XL is an extended release tablet intended for once a day administration. When switching from immediate release metoprolol tablet to Toprol-XL, the same total daily dose of Toprol-XL should be used.

As with immediate release metoprolol, dosages of Toprol-XL should be individualized and titration may be needed in some patients.

Toprol-XL tablets are scored and can be divided; however, the whole or half tablet should be swallowed whole and not chewed or crushed.

Hypertension

The usual initial dosage is 50-100 mg daily in a single dose, whether used alone or added to a diuretic. The dosage may be increased at weekly (or longer) intervals until optimum blood pressure reduction is achieved. In general, the maximum effect of any given dosage level will be apparent after 1 week of therapy. Dosages above 400 mg/day have not been studied.

Angina Pectoris

The dosage of Toprol-XL should be individualized. The usual initial dosage is 100 mg daily, given in a single dose. The dosage may be gradually increased at weekly intervals until optimum clinical response has been obtained or there is a pronounced slowing of the heart rate. Dosages above 400 mg/day have not been studied. If treatment is to be discontinued, the dosage should be reduced gradually over a period of 1-2 weeks (see WARNINGS, Toprol-XL).

Heart Failure

Dosage must be individualized and closely monitored during up-titration. Prior to initiation of Toprol-XL, the dosing of diuretics, ACE inhibitors, and digitalis (if used) should be stabilized. The recommended starting dose of Toprol-XL is 25 mg once daily for 2 weeks in patients with NYHA Class II heart failure and 12.5 mg once daily in patients with more severe heart failure. The dose should then be doubled every 2 weeks to the highest dosage level tolerated by the patient or up to 200 mg of Toprol-XL. If transient worsening of heart failure occurs, it may be treated with increased doses of diuretics, and it may also be necessary to lower the dose of Toprol-XL or temporarily discontinue it. The dose of Toprol-XL should not be increased until symptoms of worsening heart failure have been stabilized. Initial difficulty with titration should not preclude later attempts to introduce Toprol-XL. If heart failure patients experience symptomatic bradycardia, the dose of Toprol-XL should be reduced.

HOW SUPPLIED

LOPRESSOR

Lopressor Tablets

Lopressor (metoprolol tartrate) tablets are available in:

50 mg: Capsule-shaped, biconvex, pink, scored (imprinted "GEIGY" on one side and "51" twice on the scored side).

100 mg: Capsule-shaped, biconvex, light blue, scored (imprinted "GEIGY" on one side and "71" twice on the scored side).

Storage: Store between 15-30°C (59-86°F). Protect from moisture. Dispense in tight, light-resistant container.

Lopressor Injection

Lopressor (metoprolol tartrate) injection is available in:

Ampuls 5 ml: Each containing 5 mg of metoprolol tartrate.

Storage: Do not store above 30°C (86°F). Protect from light.

TOPROL-XL TABLETS

25 mg: Contain 23.75 mg of metoprolol succinate equivalent to 25 mg of metoprolol tartrate. They are white, biconvex, oval and film-coated. They are engraved "A β" on one side and scored on both sides.

50 mg: Contain 47.5 mg of metoprolol succinate equivalent to 50 mg of metoprolol tartrate. They are white, biconvex, round and film-coated. They are engraved "A mo" on one side and scored on the other.

100 mg: Contain 95 mg of metoprolol succinate equivalent to 100 mg of metoprolol tartrate. They are white, biconvex, round and film-coated. They are engraved "A ms" on one side and scored on the other.

200 mg: Contain 190 mg of metoprolol succinate equivalent to 200 mg of metoprolol tartrate. They are white, biconvex, oval and film-coated. They are engraved "A my" and scored on one side.

Storage: Store at 25°C (77°F). Excursions permitted to 15-30°C (59-86°F).

PRODUCT LISTING - RATED THERAPEUTICALLY EQUIVALENT

Package	Price	Product	NDC
Solution - Injectable - 1 mg/ml			
5 ml x 3	$13.75	GENERIC, Abbott Pharmaceutical	00074-1778-35
5 ml x 3	$13.93	GENERIC, Abbott Pharmaceutical	00074-1778-25
5 ml x 12	$41.28	GENERIC, Abbott Pharmaceutical	00074-2285-05
5 ml x 12	$54.96	GENERIC, Geneva Pharmaceuticals	00781-3070-75
5 ml x 12	$121.20	LOPRESSOR, Novartis Pharmaceuticals	00028-4201-33
Tablet - Oral - 50 mg			
3's	$1.67	GENERIC, Allscripts Pharmaceutical Company	54569-3787-02
25's	$12.42	GENERIC, Udl Laboratories Inc	51079-0801-19
25's	$13.86	GENERIC, Pd-Rx Pharmaceuticals	55289-0413-97
30 x 25	$371.85	GENERIC, Sky Pharmaceuticals Packaging, Inc	63739-0173-03
30's	$8.70	GENERIC, Pd-Rx Pharmaceuticals	55289-0413-30
30's	$13.42	GENERIC, Heartland Healthcare Services	61392-0286-30
30's	$13.42	GENERIC, Heartland Healthcare Services	61392-0286-39
30's	$14.03	GENERIC, Allscripts Pharmaceutical Company	54569-3787-00
30's	$16.04	GENERIC, Golden State Medical	60429-0126-30
30's	$25.80	LOPRESSOR, Physicians Total Care	54868-0685-01
30's	$31.52	LOPRESSOR, Pd-Rx Pharmaceuticals	55289-0627-30
31 x 10	$172.08	GENERIC, Vangard Labs	00615-3552-53
31 x 10	$172.08	GENERIC, Vangard Labs	00615-3552-63
31's	$13.87	GENERIC, Heartland Healthcare Services	61392-0286-31
32's	$14.31	GENERIC, Heartland Healthcare Services	61392-0286-32
45's	$20.13	GENERIC, Heartland Healthcare Services	61392-0286-45
60's	$26.84	GENERIC, Heartland Healthcare Services	61392-0286-60
60's	$31.49	GENERIC, Golden State Medical	60429-0126-60
60's	$33.30	GENERIC, Allscripts Pharmaceutical Company	54569-3787-01
90's	$40.26	GENERIC, Heartland Healthcare Services	61392-0286-90
90's	$42.08	GENERIC, Allscripts Pharmaceutical Company	54569-8574-00
90's	$46.85	LOPRESSOR, Allscripts Pharmaceutical Company	54569-8543-00
100's	$7.03	FEDERAL UPPER LIMIT, H.C.F.A. F F P	99999-1801-01
100's	$13.32	GENERIC, Pd-Rx Pharmaceuticals	55289-0413-01
100's	$41.75	GENERIC, Novopharm Usa Inc	55953-0727-40
100's	$41.75	GENERIC, Warrick Pharmaceuticals Corporation	59930-1795-01
100's	$43.00	GENERIC, Ivax Corporation	00182-1966-01
100's	$43.00	GENERIC, Copley	38245-0136-10
100's	$43.50	GENERIC, Major Pharmaceuticals Inc	00904-7772-60
100's	$43.50	GENERIC, Major Pharmaceuticals Inc	00904-7820-60
100's	$43.50	GENERIC, Major Pharmaceuticals Inc	00904-7946-60
100's	$44.51	GENERIC, Qualitest Products Inc	00603-4627-21
100's	$45.35	GENERIC, Purepac Pharmaceutical Company	00228-2554-10
100's	$45.35	GENERIC, Mova Pharmaceutical Corporation	55370-0820-07
100's	$45.90	GENERIC, Brightstone Pharma	62939-2211-01
100's	$46.31	GENERIC, Ivax Corporation	00182-1987-01
100's	$46.80	GENERIC, Creighton Products Corporation	50752-0308-05
100's	$47.23	GENERIC, Aligen Independent Laboratories Inc	00405-5673-01
100's	$47.90	GENERIC, Mutual Pharmaceutical Co Inc	53489-0366-01
100's	$47.91	GENERIC, Moore, H.L. Drug Exchange Inc	00839-7809-06

Qty	Price	Product	NDC
100's	$47.91	GENERIC, Moore, H.L. Drug Exchange Inc	00839-7841-06
100's	$47.91	GENERIC, Watson Laboratories Inc	52544-0462-01
100's	$49.00	GENERIC, Vangard Labs	00615-3552-13
100's	$49.91	GENERIC, American Health Packaging	62584-0788-01
100's	$51.15	GENERIC, Caraco Pharmaceutical Laboratories	57664-0166-08
100's	$52.93	GENERIC, Par Pharmaceutical Inc	49884-0412-01
100's	$55.50	GENERIC, Teva Pharmaceuticals Usa	00093-0733-01
100's	$55.50	GENERIC, Mylan Pharmaceuticals Inc	00378-0032-01
100's	$55.50	GENERIC, Watson Laboratories Inc	00591-0462-01
100's	$55.50	GENERIC, Geneva Pharmaceuticals	00781-1223-01
100's	$55.56	GENERIC, Geneva Pharmaceuticals	00781-1223-13
100's	$55.56	GENERIC, Geneva Pharmaceuticals	00781-1371-13
100's	$56.00	GENERIC, Major Pharmaceuticals Inc	00904-7772-61
100's	$57.17	GENERIC, Udl Laboratories Inc	51079-0801-20
100's	$90.96	LOPRESSOR, Novartis Pharmaceuticals	00028-0051-61
100's	$94.86	LOPRESSOR, Novartis Pharmaceuticals	00028-0051-01

Tablet - Oral - 100 mg

Qty	Price	Product	NDC
25's	$23.44	GENERIC, Udl Laboratories Inc	51079-0802-19
25's	$23.45	GENERIC, Pd-Rx Pharmaceuticals	55289-0093-97
30's	$6.53	GENERIC, Pd-Rx Pharmaceuticals	55289-0093-30
30's	$20.03	GENERIC, Heartland Healthcare Services	61392-0280-30
30's	$20.03	GENERIC, Heartland Healthcare Services	61392-0280-39
30's	$21.08	GENERIC, Allscripts Pharmaceutical Company	54569-3788-00
30's	$23.79	GENERIC, Golden State Medical	60429-0127-30
30's	$32.39	LOPRESSOR, Pd-Rx Pharmaceuticals	55289-0171-30
30's	$38.15	LOPRESSOR, Physicians Total Care	54868-1063-01
31's	$20.70	GENERIC, Heartland Healthcare Services	61392-0280-31
32's	$21.37	GENERIC, Heartland Healthcare Services	61392-0280-32
45's	$30.05	GENERIC, Heartland Healthcare Services	61392-0280-45
60's	$40.07	GENERIC, Heartland Healthcare Services	61392-0280-60
60's	$42.75	GENERIC, Golden State Medical	60429-0127-60
60's	$43.18	GENERIC, Allscripts Pharmaceutical Company	54569-3788-01
90's	$60.10	GENERIC, Heartland Healthcare Services	61392-0280-90
90's	$70.39	LOPRESSOR, Allscripts Pharmaceutical Company	54569-8545-01
100's	$9.14	FEDERAL UPPER LIMIT, H.C.F.A. F F P	99999-1801-04
100's	$39.75	GENERIC, Geneva Pharmaceuticals	00781-1372-13
100's	$62.75	GENERIC, Novopharm Usa Inc	55953-0734-40
100's	$62.75	GENERIC, Warrick Pharmaceuticals Corporation	59930-1797-01
100's	$64.60	GENERIC, Ivax Corporation	00182-1967-01
100's	$64.65	GENERIC, Copley	38245-0417-10
100's	$65.40	GENERIC, Major Pharmaceuticals Inc	00904-7773-60
100's	$65.40	GENERIC, Major Pharmaceuticals Inc	00904-7821-60
100's	$65.40	GENERIC, Major Pharmaceuticals Inc	00904-7947-60
100's	$65.41	GENERIC, Moore, H.L. Drug Exchange Inc	00839-7810-06
100's	$65.41	GENERIC, Moore, H.L. Drug Exchange Inc	00839-7842-06
100's	$67.41	GENERIC, Purepac Pharmaceutical Company	00228-2555-10
100's	$67.41	GENERIC, Mova Pharmaceutical Corporation	55370-0821-07
100's	$67.86	GENERIC, Qualitest Products Inc	00603-4628-21
100's	$67.95	GENERIC, Par Pharmaceutical Inc	49884-0413-01
100's	$68.32	GENERIC, Brightstone Pharma	62939-2221-01
100's	$70.30	GENERIC, Creighton Products Corporation	50752-0309-05
100's	$70.82	GENERIC, Aligen Independent Laboratories Inc	00405-4674-01
100's	$71.68	GENERIC, Major Pharmaceuticals Inc	00904-7773-61
100's	$73.85	GENERIC, Caraco Pharmaceutical Laboratories	57664-0167-08
100's	$73.99	GENERIC, Watson/Rugby Laboratories Inc	00536-5639-01
100's	$73.99	GENERIC, Geneva Pharmaceuticals	00781-1228-01
100's	$73.99	GENERIC, Watson Laboratories Inc	52544-0463-01
100's	$80.10	GENERIC, Teva Pharmaceuticals Usa	00093-0734-01
100's	$80.10	GENERIC, Mylan Pharmaceuticals Inc	00378-0047-01
100's	$80.10	GENERIC, Watson Laboratories Inc	00591-0463-01
100's	$80.10	GENERIC, Mutual Pharmaceutical Co Inc	53489-0367-01
100's	$80.65	GENERIC, Geneva Pharmaceuticals	00781-1228-13
100's	$82.50	GENERIC, Udl Laboratories Inc	51079-0802-20
100's	$142.44	LOPRESSOR, Novartis Pharmaceuticals	00028-0071-01
180's	$140.78	LOPRESSOR, Allscripts Pharmaceutical Company	54569-8545-00

PRODUCT LISTING - EQUIVALENTS NOT AVAILABLE

Tablet - Oral - 50 mg

Qty	Price	Product	NDC
30's	$2.90	GENERIC, Physicians Total Care	54868-2989-02
30's	$13.05	GENERIC, Southwood Pharmaceuticals Inc	58016-0467-30
60's	$5.59	GENERIC, Physicians Total Care	54868-2989-03
100's	$9.34	GENERIC, Physicians Total Care	54868-2989-00
100's	$43.53	GENERIC, Apothecon Inc	59772-3692-02
100's	$43.53	GENERIC, Apothecon Inc	59772-3692-20

Tablet - Oral - 100 mg

Qty	Price	Product	NDC
30's	$3.91	GENERIC, Physicians Total Care	54868-2990-00
100's	$9.93	GENERIC, Physicians Total Care	54868-2990-02
100's	$65.40	GENERIC, Apothecon Inc	59772-3693-02
100's	$73.86	GENERIC, Boca Pharmacal Inc	64376-0503-01

Tablet, Extended Release - Oral - 25 mg

Qty	Price	Product	NDC
100's	$75.86	TOPROL XL, Astra-Zeneca Pharmaceuticals	00186-1088-05
100's	$75.86	TOPROL XL, Astra-Zeneca Pharmaceuticals	00186-1088-39

Tablet, Extended Release - Oral - 50 mg

Qty	Price	Product	NDC
30's	$18.19	TOPROL XL, Allscripts Pharmaceutical Company	54569-4441-00
30's	$21.16	TOPROL XL, Physicians Total Care	54868-3587-01
50's	$36.84	TOPROL XL, Physicians Total Care	54868-3587-00
100's	$75.86	TOPROL XL, Astra-Zeneca Pharmaceuticals	00186-1090-05
100's	$75.86	TOPROL XL, Astra-Zeneca Pharmaceuticals	00186-1090-39

Tablet, Extended Release - Oral - 100 mg

Qty	Price	Product	NDC
30's	$27.33	TOPROL XL, Allscripts Pharmaceutical Company	54569-4442-00
100's	$113.99	TOPROL XL, Astra-Zeneca Pharmaceuticals	00186-1092-05
100's	$113.99	TOPROL XL, Astra-Zeneca Pharmaceuticals	00186-1092-39

Tablet, Extended Release - Oral - 200 mg

Qty	Price	Product	NDC
100's	$195.89	TOPROL XL, Astra-Zeneca Pharmaceuticals	00186-1094-05

Metronidazole *(001803)*

Categories: Abscess, brain; Abscess, intra-abdominal; Abscess, liver; Abscess, lung; Abscess, tubo-ovarian; Acne rosacea; Amebiasis; Empyema; Endocarditis; Endometritis; Endomyometritis; Infection, anaerobic bacterial; Infection, bone; Infection, central nervous system; Infection, gynecologic; Infection, intra-abdominal; Infection, joint; Infection, lower respiratory tract; Infection, skin and skin structures; Infection, vaginal cuff; Meningitis; Peritonitis; Pneumonia; Prophylaxis, perioperative; Septicemia; Trichomoniasis; Pregnancy Category B; FDA Approved 1980 Feb; WHO Formulary; Orphan Drugs

Drug Classes: Antibiotics, miscellaneous; Anti-infectives, topical; Antiprotozoals; Dermatologics

Brand Names: **Flagyl**; Flagyl 375; Metizol; Metro IV; Metrocream; Metrogel; Metromidol; Metryl; Noritate; Protostat; Satric

Foreign Brand Availability: Acea Gel (England; Ireland); Acromona (Ecuador); Amevan (Ecuador); Amiyodazol (Mexico); Anaerobex (Austria); Anerobia (Philippines); Apo-Metronidazole (Canada); Arcazol (Taiwan); Arilin (Germany; Switzerland); Ariline (Austria); Asiazole (Thailand); Asuzol (Japan); Biotazol (Mexico); Camezol (Benin; Burkina-Faso; Ethiopia; Gambia; Ghana; Guinea; Ivory-Coast; Kenya; Liberia; Malawi; Mali; Mauritania; Mauritius; Morocco; Niger; Nigeria; Senegal; Seychelles; Sierra-Leone; Sudan; Tanzania; Tunia; Uganda; Zambia; Zimbabwe); Clont (Germany); Debetrol (Argentina); Deflamon (Italy); Dumozol (Indonesia); Elyzol (Bahrain; Cyprus; Denmark; Egypt; Finland; Iran; Iraq; Jordan; Kuwait; Lebanon; Libya; Norway; Oman; Qatar; Republic-of-Yemen; Saudi-Arabia; Sweden; Switzerland; Syria; United-Arab-Emirates); Endazole (Philippines); Epaq (Mexico); Farnat (Indonesia); Fladex (Indonesia; Singapore); Flagenase (Mexico); Flagizole (Bahrain; Cyprus; Egypt; Iran; Iraq; Jordan; Kuwait; Lebanon; Libya; Oman; Qatar; Republic-of-Yemen; Saudi-Arabia; Syria; United-Arab-Emirates); Flasinyl (Korea); Flazol (Bahrain; Cyprus; Egypt; Iran; Iraq; Jordan; Kuwait; Lebanon; Libya; Oman; Qatar; Republic-of-Yemen; Saudi-Arabia; Syria; United-Arab-Emirates); Frotin (Taiwan); Gynoplix (Hong-Kong); Ivemetro (Republic-Of-Yemen); Metrogyl (Australia; Greece); Metrolag (Bahamas; Bahrain; Barbados; Belize; Benin; Bermuda; Burkina-Faso; Curacao; Cyprus; Egypt; Ethiopia; Gambia; Ghana; Guinea; Guyana; Iran; Iraq; Ivory-Coast; Jamaica; Jordan; Kenya; Kuwait; Lebanon; Liberia; Libya; Malawi; Mali; Mauritania; Mauritius; Morocco; Netherland-Antilles; Niger; Nigeria; Oman; Qatar; Republic-of-Yemen; Saudi-Arabia; Senegal; Seychelles; Sierra-Leone; Sudan; Surinam; Switzerland; Syria; Taiwan; Tanzania; Trinidad; Tunia; Uganda; United-Arab-Emirates; Zambia; Zimbabwe); Metrolex (Thailand); Metronidazole IV (Australia; New-Zealand); Metronidazol McKesson (Costa-Rica; Dominican-Republic; El-Salvador; Guatemala; Honduras; Nicaragua; Panama); Metronide (Australia); Metrozin (Colombia); Metrozine (Indonesia); Nalox (Argentina); Nida (Japan); Nor-Metrogel (Dominican-Republic; El-Salvador; Guatemala; Panama); Novazole (Benin; Burkina-Faso; Ethiopia; Gambia; Ghana; Guinea; Ivory-Coast; Kenya; Liberia; Malawi; Mali; Mauritania; Mauritius; Morocco; Niger; Nigeria; Senegal; Seychelles; Sierra-Leone; Sudan; Tanzania; Tunia; Uganda; Zambia; Zimbabwe); Novonidazole (Canada); Otrozol (Colombia); Protozol (Benin; Burkina-Faso; Ethiopia; Gambia; Ghana; Guinea; Ivory-Coast; Kenya; Liberia; Malawi; Mali; Mauritania; Mauritius; Morocco; Niger; Nigeria; Senegal; Seychelles; Sierra-Leone; Sudan; Tanzania; Tunia; Uganda; Zambia; Zimbabwe); Robaz (Philippines); Rosaced Gel (France); Rozacreme (France); Rozagel (France); Rozex (Australia; Belgium; England; France; Hong-Kong; New-Zealand; South-Africa; Switzerland); Rozex Gel (Israel; Netherlands; Peru); Sharizole (Bahrain; Cyprus; Egypt; Iran; Iraq; Jordan; Kuwait; Lebanon; Libya; Oman; Qatar; Republic-of-Yemen; Saudi-Arabia; Syria; United-Arab-Emirates); Supplin (Bahrain; Cyprus; Egypt; Iran; Iraq; Jordan; Kuwait; Lebanon; Libya; Oman; Qatar; Republic-of-Yemen; Saudi-Arabia; Syria; United-Arab-Emirates); Takimetol (Japan); Trichex (Austria); Trichozole (New-Zealand); Tricowas B (Spain); Trikacide (Indonesia); Trogiar (Indonesia); Unigo (Hong-Kong); Zadstat (England); Zidoval Gel (Israel); Zol (Philippines)

Cost of Therapy: $49.37 (Trichomoniasis; Flagyl tablets; 250 mg; 3 tablets/day; 7 day supply)
$1.25 (Trichomoniasis; Generic tablets; 250 mg; 3 tablets/day; 7 day supply)
$119.92 (Anaerobic Infections; Flagyl tablets; 500 mg; 4 tablets/day; 7 day supply)
$3.51 (Anaerobic Infections; Generic tablets; 500 mg; 4 tablets/day; 7 day supply)

WARNING

Metronidazole has been shown to be carcinogenic in mice and rats (see PRECAUTIONS). Unnecessary use of the drug should be avoided. Its use should be reserved for the conditions described in INDICATIONS AND USAGE.

DESCRIPTION

INJECTION

Metronidazole hydrochloride sterile IV and metronidazole sterile IV, are parenteral dosage forms of the synthetic antibacterial agents 1-(β-hydroxyethyl)-2-methyl-5-nitroimidazole hydrochloride and 1-(β-hydroxyethyl)-methyl-5-nitroimidazole, respectively.

Each single-dose vial of lyophilized Metronidazole IV contains sterile, nonpyrogenic Metronidazole hydrochloride, equivalent to 500 mg metronidazole, and 415 mg mannitol.

Each metronidazole IV RTU (Ready-To-Use) 100 ml single-dose plastic container contains a sterile, nonpyrogenic, isotonic, buffered solution of 500 mg metronidazole, 47.6 mg sodium phosphate, 22.9 mg citric acid, and 790 mg sodium chloride in water for injection. Metronidazole IV RTU has a tonicity of 310 mOsm/L and a pH of 5-7. Each container contains 14 mEq of sodium.

The plastic container is fabricated from a specially formulated polyvinyl chloride plastic. Water can permeate from inside the container into the overwrap in amounts insufficient to affect the solution significantly. Solutions in contact with the plastic container can leach out certain of its chemical components in very small amounts within the expiration period, *e.g.*, di 2-ethyhexyl phthalate (DEHP), up to 5 parts per million. However, the safety of the plastic has been confirmed in tests in animal according to USP biological tests for plastic containers as well as by tissue culture toxicity studies.

M

TABLETS

Metronidazole is an oral synthetic antiprotozoal and antibacterial agent, 1-(β-hydroxyethyl)-2-methyl-5-nitroimidazole.

Metronidazole tablets contain 250 or 500 mg of metronidazole. Inactive ingredients include cellulose, FD&C blue no. 2 lake, hydroxypropyl cellulose, hydroxypropyl methylcellulose, polyethylene glycol, stearic acid, and titanium dioxide.

TOPICAL

Metronidazole gel contains metronidazole at a concentration of 7.5 mg/g (0.75%) in a gelled, purified water solution, containing methyl and propyl parabens, propylene glycol, carbomer 940, and edetate disodium. Metronidazole is classified therapeutically as an antiprotozoal and antibacterial agent. Chemically, metronidazole is named 2-methyl-5-nitro-1*H*-imidazole-1-ethanol.

CLINICAL PHARMACOLOGY

Disposition of metronidazole in the body is similar for both oral and intravenous dosage forms, with an average elimination half-life in healthy humans of 8 hours.

The major route of elimination of metronidazole and its metabolites is via the urine (60-80% of the dose), with fecal excretion accounting for 6-15% of the dose. The metabolites that appear in the urine result primarily from side-chain oxidation (1-(β-hydroxyethyl)-2-hydroxymethyl-5-nitroimidazole and 2-methyl-5-nitroimidazole-1-yl-acetic acid) and glucuronide conjugation, with unchanged metronidazole accounting for approximately 20% of the total. Renal clearance of metronidazole is approximately 10 ml/min/1.73 m^2.

Metronidazole is the major component appearing in the plasma, with lesser quantities of the 2-hydroxymethyl metabolite also being present. Less than 20% of the circulating metronidazole is bound to plasma proteins. Both the parent compound and the metabolite possess *in vitro* bactericidal activity against most strains of anaerobic bacteria and *in vitro* trichomonacidal activity.

Metronidazole appears in cerebrospinal fluid, saliva, and breast milk in concentrations similar to those found in plasma. Bactericidal concentrations of metronidazole have also been detected in pus from hepatic abscesses.

Following oral administration metronidazole is well absorbed with peak plasma concentrations occurring between 1 and 2 hours after administration. Plasma concentrations of metronidazole are proportional to the administered dose. Oral administration of 250, 500, or 2000 mg produced peak plasma concentrations of 6, 12, and 40 µg/ml, respectively. Studies reveal no significant bioavailability differences between males and females; however, because of weight differences, the resulting plasma levels in males are generally lower.

Decreased renal function dose not alter the single-dose pharmacokinetics of metronidazole. However, plasma clearance of metronidazole is decreased in patients with decreased liver function.

MICROBIOLOGY

Trichomonas vaginalis, Entamoeba histolytica

Metronidazole possesses direct trichomonacidal and amebicidal activity against *T. vaginalis* and *E. histolytica.* The *in vitro* minimal inhibitory concentration (MIC) for most strains of these organisms is 1 µg/ml or less.

Anaerobic Bacteria

Metronidazole is active *in vitro* against most obligate anaerobes, but does not appear to possess any clinically relevant activity against facultative anaerobes or obligate aerobes. Against susceptible organisms, metronidazole is generally bactericidal at concentrations equal to or slightly higher than the minimal inhibitory concentrations. Metronidazole has been shown to have*in vitro* and clinical activity against the following organisms:

Anaerobic Gram-Negative Bacilli, Including:

Bacteroides species including the *Bacteroides fragilis* group (*B. fragilis, B. distasonis, B. ovatus, B. thetaiotaomicron, B vulgatus*) and *Fusobacterium* species.

Anaerobic Gram-Positive Bacilli, Including:

Clostridium species and susceptible strains of *Eubacterium.*

Anaerobic Gram-Positive Cocci, Including:

Peptococcus species and Peptostreptococcus species.

Susceptibility Testing

Bacteriologic studies should be performed to determine the causative organisms and their susceptibility to metronidazole; however, the rapid, routine susceptibility testing of individual isolates of anaerobic bacteria is not always practical, and therapy may be started while awaiting these results.

Quantitative methods give the most precise estimates of susceptibility to antibacterial drugs. A standardized agar dilution method and a broth microdilution method are recommended.[1]

Control strains are recommended for standardized susceptibility testing. Each time the test is performed, one or more of the following strains should be included: *Clostridium perfringens* ATCC 13124, *Bacteroides fragilis* ATCC 25285, and *Bacteroides thetaiotamicron* ATCC 29741. The mode metronidazole MICs for those three strains are reported to be 0.25, 0.25, and 0.5 µg/ml, respectively.

A clinical laboratory is considered under acceptable control if the results of the control strains are within one doubling dilution of the mode MICs reported for metronidazole.

A bacterial isolate may be considered susceptible if the MIC value for metronidazole is not more than 16 µg/ml. An organism is considered resistant if the MIC is greater than 16 µg/ml. A report of "resistant" from the laboratory indicates that the infecting organism is not likely to respond to therapy.

TOPICAL

Bioavailability studies on the administration of 1 g of metronidazole topical gel to the face, (7.5 mg of metronidazole) of rosacea patients showed a maximum serum concentration of 66 ng/ml in 1 patient. This concentration is approximately 100 times less than concentrations afforded by a single 250 mg oral tablet. The serum metronidazole concentrations were below the detectable limits of the assay at the majority of time points in all patients. Three (3) of the patients had no detectable serum concentrations of metronidazole at any time point. The mean dose of gel applied during clinical studies was 600 mg which represents 4.5 mg of metronidazole per application. Therefore, under normal usage levels, the formulation affords minimal serum concentrations of metronidazole.

The mechanisms by which metronidazole topical gel acts in reducing inflammatory lesions of rosacea are unknown, but may include an antibacterial and/or an anti-inflammatory effect.

INDICATIONS AND USAGE

TABLETS

Symptomatic Trichomoniasis

Metronidazole is indicated for the treatment of symptomatic trichomoniasis in females and males when the presence of the trichomonad has been confirmed by appropriate laboratory procedures (wet smears and/or cultures).

Asymptomatic Trichomoniasis

Metronidazole is indicated in the treatment of asymptomatic females when the organism is associated with endocervicitis, cervicitis, or cervical erosion. Since there is evidence that presence of the trichomonad can interfere with accurate assessment of abnormal cytological smears, additional smears should be performed after eradication of the parasite.

Treatment of Asymptomatic Consorts

T. vaginalis infection is a venereal disease. Therefore, asymptomatic sexual partners of treated patients should be treated simultaneously if the organism has been found to be present, in the order to prevent reinfection of the partner. The decision as to whether to treat an asymptomatic male partner who has a negative culture or one for whom no culture has been attempted is an individual one. In making this decision, it should be noted that there is evidence that a woman may become reinfected if her consort is not treated. Also, since there can be considerable difficulty in isolating the organism from the asymptomatic male carrier, negative smears and cultures cannot be relied upon in this regard. In any event, the consort should be treated with metronidazole in cases of reinfection.

Amebiasis

Metronidazole is indicated in the treatment of acute intestinal amebiasis (amebic dysentery and amebic liver abscess.

In amebic liver abscess. Metronidazole therapy does not obviate the need for aspiration or drainage of pus.

Anaerobic Bacterial Infections

Metronidazole is indicated in the treatment of serious infections caused by susceptible anaerobic bacteria. Indicated surgical procedures should be performed in conjunction with metronidazole therapy. In a mixed aerobic and anaerobic infection, antibiotics appropriate for the treatment of the aerobic infection should be used in addition to metronidazole.

In the treatment of most serious anaerobic infections, metronidazole IV RTU (metronidazole) is usually administered initially. This may be followed by oral therapy with metronidazole at the discretion of the physician.

Intra-Abdominal Infections: Including peritonitis, intra-abdominal abscess, and liver abscess, caused by Bacteroides species including the *B. fragilis* group (*B. fragilis, B. distasonis, B. ovatus, B. thetaiotaomicron, B. vulgatus*), Clostridium species, Eubacterium species, Peptococcus species, and Peptostreptococcus species.

Skin and Skin Structure Infections: Caused by Bacteroides species including the *B. fragilis* group, Clostridium species, Peptococcus species, Peptostreptococcus species, and Fusobacterium species.

Gynecological Infections: Including endometritis, endomyometritis, tubo-ovarian abscess, and postsurgical vaginal cuff infection, caused by Bacteroides species including the *B. fragilis* group, Clostridium species, Peptococcus species, and Peptostreptococcus species.

Bacterial Septicemia: Caused by Bacteroides species including the *B. fragilis* group, and *Clostridium* species.

Bone and Joint Infections: As adjunctive therapy, caused by Bacteroides species including the *B. fragilis* group.

Central Nervous System (CNS) Infections: Including meningitis and brain abscess, caused by Bacteroides species including the *B. fragilis* group.

Lower Respiratory Tract Infections: Including pneumonia, empyema, and lung abscess, caused by Bacteroides species including the *B. fragilis* group.

Endocarditis: Caused by Bacteroides species including the *B. fragilis* group.

INJECTION

Treatment of Anaerobic Infections

Metronidazole IV is indicated in the treatment of serious infections caused by susceptible anaerobic bacteria. Indicated surgical procedures should be performed in conjunction with metronidazole IV therapy. In a mixed aerobic and anaerobic infection, antibiotics appropriate for the treatment of the aerobic infection should be used in addition to metronidazole IV.

Metronidazole IV is effective in *Bacteroides fragilis* infections resistant to clindamycin, chloramphenicol, and penicillin.

Intra-Abdominal Infections: Including peritonitis, intra-abdominal abscess, and liver abscess, caused by Bacteroides species including the *B. fragilis* group (*B. fragilis, B. distasonis, B. ovatus, B. thetaiotaomicron, B. vulgatus*), Clostridium species, Eubacterium species, Peptococcus species, and Peptostreptococcus species.

Skin and Skin Structure Infections: Caused by Bacteroides species including the *B. fragilis* group, Clostridium species, Peptococcus species, Peptostreptococcus species, and Fusobacterium species.

Gynecological Infections: Including endometritis, endomyometritis, tubo-ovarian abscess, and postsurgical vaginal cuff infection, caused by Bacteroides species including the *B. fragilis* group, Clostridium species, Peptococcus species, and Peptostreptococcus species.

M

Bacterial Septicemia: Caused by Bacteroides species including the *B. fragilis* group, and Clostridium species.

Bone and Joint Infection: As adjunctive therapy, caused by Bacteroides species including the *B. fragilis* group.

Central Nervous System (CNS) Infections: Including meningitis and brain abscess, caused by Bacteroides species including the *B. fragilis* group.

Lower Respiratory Tract Infections: Including pneumonia, empyema, and lung abscess, caused by Bacteroides species including the *B. fragilis* group.

Endocarditis: Caused by the Bacteroides species, including the *B. fragilis* group.

PROPHYLAXIS

The prophylactic administration of metronidazole IV preoperatively, intraoperatively, and postoperatively may reduce the incidence of postoperative infection in patients undergoing elective colorectal surgery which is classified as contaminated or potentially contaminated.

Prophylactic use of metronidazole IV should be discontinued within 12 hours after surgery. If there are signs of infection, specimens for cultures should be obtained for the identification of the causative organism(s) so that appropriate therapy may be given (see DOSAGE AND ADMINISTRATION).

TOPICAL

Metronidazole topical gel is indicated for topical application in the treatment of inflammatory papules, pustules, and erythema of rosacea.

NON-FDA APPROVED INDICATIONS

Metronidazole has been investigated for the treatment of generalized idiopathic lichen planus, Crohn's disease, and granulomatous cheilitis. It is also used in the treatment of giardiasis, although this is not an FDA-approved use.

CONTRAINDICATIONS

INJECTION

Metronidazole is contraindicated in patients with a prior history of hypersensitivity to metronidazole or other nitroimidazole derivatives.

TABLETS

Metronidazole is contraindicated in patients with a prior history of hypersensitivity to metronidazole or other nitroimidazole derivatives.

In patients with trichomoniasis, metronidazole is contraindicated during the first trimester of pregnancy (see WARNINGS).

TOPICAL

Metronidazole topical gel is contraindicated in individuals with a history of hypersensitivity to metronidazole, parabens, or other ingredients of the formulations.

M

WARNINGS

CONVULSIVE SEIZURES AND PERIPHERAL NEUROPATHY

Convulsive seizures and peripheral neuropathy, the latter characterized mainly by numbness or paresthesia of an extremity, have been reported in patients treated with metronidazole. The appearance of abnormal neurologic signs demands the prompt discontinuation of metronidazole therapy. Metronidazole should be administered with caution to patients with central nervous system diseases.

PRECAUTIONS

GENERAL

Injection/Tablets

Patients with severe hepatic disease metabolize metronidazole slowly, with resultant accumulation of metronidazole and its metabolites in the plasma. Accordingly, for such patients, doses below those usually recommended should be administered cautiously.

Known or previously unrecognized candidiasis may present more prominent symptoms during therapy with metronidazole and requires treatment with a candicidal agent.

Additional information for injection: Administration of solutions containing sodium ions may result in sodium retention. Care should be taken when administering metronidazole IV RTU to patients receiving corticosteroids or to patients presdisposed to edema.

Topical

Because of the minimal absorption of metronidazole and consequently its insignificant plasma concentration after topical administration, the adverse experiences reported with the oral form of the drug have not been reported with metronidazole topical gel. Metronidazole topical gel has been reported to cause tearing of the eyes. Therefore, contact with the eyes should be avoided. If a reaction suggesting local irritation occurs, patients should be directed to use the medication less frequently, discontinue use temporarily, or discontinue use until further instructions. Metronidazole is a nitroimidazole and should be used with care in patients with evidence of, or history of, blood dyscrasia.

INFORMATION FOR THE PATIENT

Alcoholic beverages should be avoided while taking metronidazole and for at least one day afterward. (See DRUG INTERACTIONS.)

Topical

This medication is to be used as directed by the physician. It is for external use only. Avoid contact with the eyes.

LABORATORY TESTS

Injection/Tablets

Metronidazole is a nitroimidazole and should be used with care in patients with evidence of or history of blood dyscrasia. A mild leukopenia has been observed during its administration; however, no persistent hematologic abnormalities attributable to metronidazole have been observed in clinical studies. Total and differential leukocyte counts are recommended before and after therapy for trichomoniasis and amebiasis, especially if a second course of therapy is necessary, and before and after therapy for anaerobic infection.

DRUG/LABORATORY TEST INTERACTIONS

Injection/Tablets

Metronidazole may interfere with certain types of determinations of serum chemistry values, such as aspartate aminotransferase (AST, SGOT), alanine aminotransferase (ALT, SGPT), lactate dehydrogenase (LDH), triglycerides, and hexokinase glucose. Values of zero may be observed. All of the assays in which interference has been reported involve enzymatic coupling of the assay to oxidation-reduction of nicotine adenine dinucleotide ($NAD^+ \leftrightarrow NADH$). Interference is due to the similarity in absorbance peaks of NADH (340 nm) and metronidazole (322 nm) at pH 7.

CARCINOGENESIS, MUTAGENESIS, AND IMPAIRMENT OF FERTILITY

Tumorigenicity Studies in Rodents

Metronidazole has shown evidence of carcinogenic activity in a number of studies involving chronic, oral administration in mice and rats.

Prominent among the effects in the mouse was pulmonary tumorigenesis. This has been observed in all 6 reported studies in that species, including one study in which the animals were dosed on an intermittent schedule (administration during every fourth week only). At very high dose levels (approx. 500 mg/kg/day) there was statistically significant increase in the incidence of malignant liver tumors in males. Also, the published results of one of the mouse studies indicate an increase in the incidence of malignant lymphomas as well as pulmonary neoplasms associated with lifetime feeding of the drug. All these effects are statistically significant.

Several long-term, oral-dosing studies in the rat have been completed. There were statistically significant increase in the incidence of various neoplasms, particularly in mammary and hepatic tumors, among female rats administered metronidazole over those noted in the concurrent female control groups.

Two lifetime tumorigenicity studies in hamsters have been performed and reported to be negative.

Mutagenicity Studies

Although metronidazole has shown mutagenic activity in a number of *in vitro* assay systems, studies in mammals (*in vivo*) have failed to demonstrate a potential for genetic damage.

PREGNANCY, TERATOGENIC EFFECTS, PREGNANCY CATEGORY B

Metronidazole crosses the placental barrier and enters the fetal circulation rapidly. Reproduction studies have been performed in rats at doses up to 5 times the human dose and have revealed no evidence of impaired fertility or harm to the fetus due to metronidazole. Metronidazole administered intraperitoneally to pregnant mice at approximately the human dose caused fetotoxicity; administered orally to pregnant mice, no fetotoxicity was observed. There are, however, no adequate and well-controlled studies in pregnant women. Because animal reproduction studies are not always predictive of human response, and because metronidazole is a carcinogen in rodents, this drug should be used during pregnancy only if clearly needed (see CONTRAINDICATIONS).

Use of metronidazole for trichomoniasis in the second and third trimesters should be restricted to those in whom local palliative treatment has been inadequate to control symptoms.

NURSING MOTHERS

Tablets

Because of the potential for tumorigenicity shown for metronidazole in mouse and rat studies, a decision should be made whether to discontinue nursing or to discontinue the drug, taking into account the importance of the drug to the mother. Metronidazole is secreted in breast milk in concentrations similar to those found in plasma.

Topical

Even though metronidazole topical gel blood levels are significantly lower than those achieved after oral metronidazole, a decision should be made whether to discontinue nursing or to discontinue the drug, taking into account the importance of the drug to the mother.

PEDIATRIC USE

Safety and effectiveness in children have not been established, except for the treatment of amebiasis.

Topical: Safety and effectiveness in children have not been established.

DRUG INTERACTIONS

TABLETS

Metronidazole has been reported to potentiate the anticoagulant effect of warfarin and other oral coumarin anticoagulants, resulting in a prolongation of prothrombin time. This possible drug interaction should be considered when metronidazole is prescribed for patients on this type of anticoagulant, therapy.

The simultaneous administration of drugs that induce microsomal liver enzymes, such as phenytoin or phenobarbital, may accelerate the elimination of metronidazole, resulting in reduced plasma levels; impaired clearance of phenytoin has also been reported.

The simultaneous administration of drugs that decrease microsomal liver enzyme activity, such as cimetidine, may prolong the half-life and decrease plasma clearance of metronidazole. In patients stabilized on relatively high doses of lithium, short-term metronidazole therapy has been associated with elevation of serum lithium and, in a few cases, signs of lithium toxicity. Serum lithium and serum creatinine levels should be obtained several days after beginning metronidazole to detect any increase that may precede clinical symptoms of lithium intoxication.

Alcoholic beverages should not be consumed during metronidazole therapy and for at least one day afterward because abdominal cramps, nausea, vomiting, headaches, and flushing may occur.

Psychotic reactions have been reported in alcoholic patients who are using metronidazole and disulfiram concurrently. Metronidazole should not be given to patients who have taken disulfiram within the last 2 weeks.

TOPICAL

Drug interactions are less likely with topical administration but should be kept in mind when metronidazole topical gel is prescribed for patients who are receiving anticoagulant treatment. Oral metronidazole has been reported to potentiate the anticoagulant effect of coumarin and warfarin resulting in a prolongation of prothrombin time.

ADVERSE REACTIONS

Two serious adverse reactions reported in patients treated with metronidazole have been convulsive seizures and peripheral neuropathy, the latter characterized mainly by numbness or paresthesia of an extremity. Since persistent peripheral neuropathy has been reported in some patients receiving prolonged administration of metronidazole, patients should be specifically warned about these reactions and should be told to stop the drug and report immediately to their physicians if any neurologic symptoms occur.

The most common adverse reactions reported have been referable to the gastrointestinal tract, particularly nausea reported by about 12% of patients, sometimes accompanied by headache, anorexia, and occasionally vomiting; diarrhea; epigastric distress, and abdominal cramping. Constipation has been reported.

The following reactions have also been reported during treatment with metronidazole:

Mouth: A sharp, unpleasant metallic taste is not unusual. Furry tongue, glossitis, and stomatitis have occurred; these may be associated with a sudden overgrowth of *Candida* which may occur during effective therapy.

Hematopoietic: Reversible neutropenia (leukopenia); rarely, reversible thrombocytopenia.

Cardiovascular: Flattening of the T-wave may be seen in electrocardiographic tracings.

Central Nervous System: Convulsive seizures, peripheral neuropathy, dizziness, vertigo, incoordination, ataxia, confusion, irritability, depression, weakness, and insomnia.

Hypersensitivity: Urticaria, erythematous rash, flushing, nasal congestion, dryness of the mouth (or vagina or vulva), and fever.

Renal: Dysuria, cystitis, polyuria, incontinence, and a sense of pelvic pressure. Instances of darkened urine have been reported by approximately 1 patient in 100,000. Although the pigment which is which is probably responsible for this phenomenon has not been positively identified, it is almost certainly a metabolite of metronidazole and seems to have no clinical significance.

Other: Proliferation of *Candida* in the vagina, dyspareunia, decrease of libido, proctitis, and fleeting joint pains sometimes resembling "serum sickness." If patients receiving metronidazole drink alcoholic beverages, they may experience abdominal distress, nausea, vomiting, flushing, or headache. A modification of the taste of alcoholic beverages has also been reported. Rare cases of pancreatitis, which abated on withdrawal of the drug, have been reported.

Crohn's disease patients are known to have an increased incidence of gastrointestinal and certain extraintestinal cancers. There have been some reports in the medical literature of breast and colon cancer in Crohn's disease patients who have been treated with metronidazole at high doses for extended periods of time. A cause and effect relationship has not been established. Crohn's disease is not an approved indication for metronidazole.

TOPICAL

Adverse conditions reported include watery (tearing) eyes if the gel is applied too closely to this area, transient redness, and mild dryness, burning and skin irritation. None of the side effects exceeded an incidence of 2% of patients.

DOSAGE AND ADMINISTRATION

INJECTION

In elderly patients the pharmacokinetics of metronidazole may be altered and therefore monitoring of serum levels may be necessary to adjust the metronidazole dosage accordingly.

Treatment of Anaerobic Infections

The recommended dosage schedule for *Adults* is:

Loading Dose: 15 mg/kg infused over 1 hour (approximately 1 g for a 70 kg adult).

Maintenance Dose: 7.5 mg/kg infused over 1 hour every 6 hours (approximately 500 mg for a 70 kg adult). The first maintenance dose should be instituted 6 hours following the initiation of the loading dose.

Parenteral therapy may be changed to oral metronidazole when conditions warrant, based upon the severity of the disease and the response of the patient to metronidazole IV treatment. The usual adult oral dosage is 7.5 mg/kg every 6 hours.

A maximum of 4 g should not be exceeded during a 24 hour period.

Patients with severe hepatic disease metabolize metronidazole slowly, with resultant accumulation of metronidazole and its metabolites in the plasma. Accordingly, for such patients, doses below those usually recommended should be administered cautiously. Close monitoring of plasma metronidazole levels[1] and toxicity is recommended.

In patients receiving metronidazole in whom gastric secretions are continuously removed by nasogastric aspiration, sufficient metronidazole may be removed in the aspirate to cause a reduction in serum levels.

The dose of metronidazole should not be specifically rescued in anuric patients since accumulated metabolites may be rapidly removed by dialysis.

The usual duration of therapy is 7-10 days; however, infections of the bone and joint, lower respiratory tract, and endocardium may require longer treatment.

Prophylaxis

For surgical; prophylactic use, to prevent postoperative infection in contaminated or potentially contaminated colorectal surgery, the recommended dosage schedule for adults is:

15 mg/kg infused over 30-60 minutes and completed approximately 1 hour before surgery; followed by

7.5 mg/kg infused over 30-60 minutes at 6 and 12 hours after the initial dose.

It is important that (1) administration of the initial preoperative dose be completed approximately 1 hour before surgery so that adequate drug levels are present in the serum and tissues at the time of initial incision, and (2) metronidazole IV be administered, if necessary, at 6 hours intervals to maintain effective drug levels. Prophylactic use of metronidazole IV should be limited to the day of surgery only, following the above guidelines.

CAUTION: Metronidazole IV is to be administered by slow intravenous drip infusion only, either as a continuous or intermittent infusion. IV admixtures containing metronidazole and other drugs should be avoided. Additives should not be introduced into the metronidazole IV RTU solution. If used with a primary intravenous fluid system, the primary solution should be discontinued during metronidazole infusion. DO NOT USE EQUIPMENT CONTAINING ALUMINUM (*e.g.,* NEEDLES, CANNULAE) THAT WOULD COME IN CONTACT WITH THE DRUG SOLUTION.

TABLETS

In elderly patients the pharmacokinetics of metronidazole may be altered and therefore monitoring of serum levels may be necessary to adjust the metronidazole dosage accordingly.

Trichomoniasis

In the Female

1 day treatment: 2 g of metronidazole, given either as a single dose or in two divided doses of 1 g each given in the same day.

7 day course of treatment: 250 mg 3 times daily for 7 consecutive days. There is some indication from controlled comparative studies that cure rates as determined by vaginal smears, signs and symptoms, may be higher after a 7 day course of treatment than after a 1 day treatment regimen.

The dosage regimen should be individualized. Single-dose treatment can assure compliance, especially if administered under supervision, in those patients who cannot be relied on to continue the 7 day regimen. A 7 day course of treatment may minimize reinfection of the female long enough to treat sexual contacts. Further, some patients may tolerate one course of therapy better than the other.

Pregnant patients should not be treated during the first trimester with either regimen. If treated during the second or third trimester, the 1 day course of therapy should not be used, as it results in higher serum levels which reach the fetal circulation. (See CONTRAINDICATIONS and PRECAUTIONS.)

When repeat courses of the drug are required, it is recommended that an interval of 4-6 weeks elapse between courses and that the presence of the trichomonad be reconfirmed by appropriate laboratory measures. Total and differential leukocyte counts should be made before and after re-treatment.

In the Male

Treatment should be individualized as for the female.

Amebiasis

Adults

For acute intestinal amebiasis (acute amebic dysentery): 750 mg orally 3 times daily for 5-10 days.

For amebic liver abscess: 500 mg or 750 mg orally 3 times daily for 5-10 days.

Children

36-50 mg/kg/24 hours, divided into 3 doses, orally for 10 days.

Anaerobic Bacterial Infections

In the treatment of most serious anaerobic infections, metronidazole HCl IV or metronidazole IV RTU is usually administered initially.

The usual adult *oral* dosage is 7.5 mg/kg every 6 hours (approx. 500 mg for a 70 kg adult). A maximum of 4 g should not be exceeded during a 24 hours period.

The usual duration of therapy is 7-10 days; however, infections of the bone and joint, lower respiratory tract, and endocardium may require longer treatment.

Patients with severe hepatic disease metabolize metronidazole slowly, with resultant accumulation of metronidazole and its metabolites in the plasma. Accordingly, for such patients, doses below those usually recommended should be administered cautiously. Close monitoring of plasma metronidazole levels[2] and toxicity is recommended.

The dose of metronidazole should not be specifically reduced in anuric patients since accumulated metabolites may be rapidly removed by dialysis.

TOPICAL

Apply and rub in a thin film of metronidazole topical solution twice daily, morning and evening, to entire affected areas after washing. Significant therapeutic results should be noticed within 3 weeks. Clinical studies have demonstrated continuing improvement through 9 weeks of therapy.

Area to be treated should be cleansed before application of metronidazole topical gel. Patients may use cosmetics after application of metronidazole topical gel.

PRODUCT LISTING - RATED THERAPEUTICALLY EQUIVALENT

Solution - Intravenous - 500 mg/100 ml

100 ml x 24	$68.16	GENERIC, Abbott Pharmaceutical	00074-7811-24
100 ml x 24	$368.16	GENERIC, Baxter I.V. Systems Division	00338-1055-48
100 ml x 24	$732.00	GENERIC, B. Braun/Mcgaw Inc	00264-5535-32
100 ml x 80	$196.00	GENERIC, Abbott Pharmaceutical	00074-7811-37

Tablet - Oral - 250 mg

8's	$2.87	GENERIC, Pd-Rx Pharmaceuticals	55289-0172-08

21's	$2.71	GENERIC, Vangard Labs	00615-1576-22
21's	$3.42	GENERIC, Circle Pharmaceuticals Inc	00659-0117-21
21's	$3.78	GENERIC, Pd-Rx Pharmaceuticals	55289-0172-21
25's	$7.60	GENERIC, Pd-Rx Pharmaceuticals	55289-0172-97
25's	$13.86	GENERIC, Udl Laboratories Inc	51079-0122-19
28's	$2.99	GENERIC, Dixon-Shane Inc	17236-0303-28
28's	$3.85	GENERIC, Vangard Labs	00615-1576-28
28's	$3.90	GENERIC, Pd-Rx Pharmaceuticals	58864-0354-28
28's	$5.03	GENERIC, Pd-Rx Pharmaceuticals	55289-0172-28
28's	$8.44	GENERIC, Physicians Total Care	60429-0128-28
30's	$5.37	GENERIC, Pd-Rx Pharmaceuticals	55289-0172-30
30's	$22.59	GENERIC, Heartland Healthcare Services	61392-0745-30
30's	$22.59	GENERIC, Heartland Healthcare Services	61392-0745-39
31's	$23.34	GENERIC, Heartland Healthcare Services	61392-0745-31
32's	$24.10	GENERIC, Heartland Healthcare Services	61392-0745-32
45's	$33.89	GENERIC, Heartland Healthcare Services	61392-0745-45
50's	$122.20	FLAGYL, Searle	00025-1831-50
56's	$10.02	GENERIC, Pd-Rx Pharmaceuticals	55289-0172-56
60's	$45.18	GENERIC, Heartland Healthcare Services	61392-0745-60
90's	$67.77	GENERIC, Heartland Healthcare Services	61392-0745-90
100's	$5.52	GENERIC, Us Trading Corporation	56126-0095-11
100's	$5.63	FEDERAL UPPER LIMIT, H.C.F.A. F F P	99999-1803-03
100's	$5.93	GENERIC, Interstate Drug Exchange Inc	00814-4810-14
100's	$7.00	GENERIC, Raway Pharmacal Inc	00686-0122-20
100's	$8.15	GENERIC, Pd-Rx Pharmaceuticals	55289-0172-01
100's	$8.75	GENERIC, Major Pharmaceuticals Inc	00904-1453-60
100's	$15.00	GENERIC, Eon Labs Manufacturing Inc	00185-0551-01
100's	$18.75	GENERIC, Moore, H.L. Drug Exchange Inc	00839-6415-06
100's	$19.10	GENERIC, Par Pharmaceutical Inc	49884-0095-01
100's	$20.19	GENERIC, Vangard Labs	00615-1576-01
100's	$20.39	GENERIC, Purepac Pharmaceutical Company	00228-2258-10
100's	$21.50	GENERIC, Geneva Pharmaceuticals	00781-1742-01
100's	$21.50	GENERIC, Martec Pharmaceuticals Inc	52555-0095-01
100's	$21.55	GENERIC, Qualitest Products Inc	00603-4640-21
100's	$21.82	GENERIC, Aligen Independent Laboratories Inc	00405-4677-01
100's	$28.92	GENERIC, Major Pharmaceuticals Inc	00904-1453-61
100's	$30.00	GENERIC, Marin Pharmaceutical	12539-0551-01
100's	$41.20	GENERIC, Martec Pharmaceuticals Inc	52555-0725-01
100's	$41.20	GENERIC, Mutual Pharmaceutical Co Inc	53489-0135-01
100's	$41.25	GENERIC, Watson/Schein Pharmaceuticals Inc	00364-0595-01
100's	$43.39	GENERIC, Sidmak Laboratories Inc	50111-0333-01
100's	$43.46	GENERIC, Teva Pharmaceuticals Usa	00093-0851-01
100's	$43.46	GENERIC, Ivax Corporation	00172-2971-60
100's	$54.22	GENERIC, Vangard Labs	00615-1576-13
100's	$55.45	GENERIC, Udl Laboratories Inc	51079-0122-20
100's	$62.63	GENERIC, Ivax Corporation	00182-1330-89
100's	$70.06	GENERIC, Auro Pharmaceutical	55829-0364-10
100's	$75.30	GENERIC, Geneva Pharmaceuticals	00781-1742-13
100's	$122.46	GENERIC, Janssen Pharmaceuticals	00062-1570-01
100's	$235.09	FLAGYL, Searle	00025-1831-31
250's	$12.75	GENERIC, Interstate Drug Exchange Inc	00814-4810-22
250's	$16.95	GENERIC, Major Pharmaceuticals Inc	00904-1453-70
250's	$20.20	GENERIC, Vangard Labs	00615-1576-15
250's	$35.50	GENERIC, Eon Labs Manufacturing Inc	00185-0551-52
250's	$39.95	GENERIC, Moore, H.L. Drug Exchange Inc	00839-6415-09
250's	$43.50	GENERIC, Aligen Independent Laboratories Inc	00405-4677-04
250's	$43.95	GENERIC, Qualitest Products Inc	00603-4640-24
250's	$43.95	GENERIC, Geneva Pharmaceuticals	00781-1742-25
250's	$45.50	GENERIC, Martec Pharmaceuticals Inc	52555-0095-02
250's	$45.75	GENERIC, Par Pharmaceutical Inc	49884-0095-04
250's	$83.80	GENERIC, Mutual Pharmaceutical Co Inc	53489-0135-03
250's	$83.85	GENERIC, Watson/Schein Pharmaceuticals Inc	00364-0595-04
250's	$83.85	GENERIC, Watson/Schein Pharmaceuticals Inc	00591-5540-25
250's	$105.22	GENERIC, Teva Pharmaceuticals Usa	00093-0851-52
250's	$105.22	GENERIC, Sidmak Laboratories Inc	50111-0333-06
280's	$19.93	GENERIC, Major Pharmaceuticals Inc	00904-1453-23

Tablet - Oral - 500 mg

4's	$1.99	GENERIC, Dixon-Shane Inc	17236-0304-04
4's	$5.88	GENERIC, Pd-Rx Pharmaceuticals	55289-0521-04
8's	$3.38	GENERIC, Pd-Rx Pharmaceuticals	55289-0521-08
10's	$3.98	GENERIC, Pd-Rx Pharmaceuticals	55289-0521-10
14's	$2.75	GENERIC, Dixon-Shane Inc	17236-0304-14
14's	$4.92	GENERIC, Pd-Rx Pharmaceuticals	55289-0521-14
21's	$6.75	GENERIC, Pd-Rx Pharmaceuticals	55289-0521-21
21's	$8.45	GENERIC, Circle Pharmaceuticals Inc	00659-0118-21
25's	$6.56	GENERIC, Udl Laboratories Inc	51079-0126-19
28's	$4.20	GENERIC, Pd-Rx Pharmaceuticals	58864-0355-28
28's	$8.19	GENERIC, Pd-Rx Pharmaceuticals	55289-0521-28
30's	$8.78	GENERIC, Pd-Rx Pharmaceuticals	55289-0521-30
30's	$40.55	GENERIC, Heartland Healthcare Services	61392-0746-30
30's	$40.55	GENERIC, Heartland Healthcare Services	61392-0746-39
31's	$41.90	GENERIC, Heartland Healthcare Services	61392-0746-31
32's	$43.25	GENERIC, Heartland Healthcare Services	61392-0746-32
40's	$11.63	GENERIC, Pd-Rx Pharmaceuticals	55289-0521-40
45's	$60.82	GENERIC, Heartland Healthcare Services	61392-0746-45
50's	$17.95	GENERIC, Moore, H.L. Drug Exchange Inc	00839-6620-04
50's	$18.75	GENERIC, Par Pharmaceutical Inc	49884-0114-03
50's	$30.00	GENERIC, Marin Pharmaceutical	12539-0500-53
50's	$35.75	GENERIC, Teva Pharmaceuticals Usa	00093-0852-53
50's	$35.77	GENERIC, Watson/Schein Pharmaceuticals Inc	00364-0687-50
50's	$35.77	GENERIC, Watson Laboratories Inc	00591-5552-50
50's	$38.27	GENERIC, Ivax Corporation	00172-3007-48
50's	$111.84	GENERIC, Janssen Pharmaceuticals	00062-1571-01
50's	$218.29	FLAGYL, Searle	00025-1821-50
60's	$81.09	GENERIC, Heartland Healthcare Services	61392-0746-60
90's	$121.64	GENERIC, Heartland Healthcare Services	61392-0746-90
100's	$12.00	GENERIC, Raway Pharmacal Inc	00686-0126-20
100's	$12.53	GENERIC, Interstate Drug Exchange Inc	00814-4815-14
100's	$14.79	FEDERAL UPPER LIMIT, H.C.F.A. F F P	99999-1803-09
100's	$21.75	GENERIC, Pd-Rx Pharmaceuticals	55289-0521-17
100's	$30.98	GENERIC, Moore, H.L. Drug Exchange Inc	00839-6620-06
100's	$31.79	GENERIC, Geneva Pharmaceuticals	00781-1747-01
100's	$31.82	GENERIC, Aligen Independent Laboratories Inc	00405-4678-01
100's	$33.15	GENERIC, Major Pharmaceuticals Inc	00904-2694-60
100's	$34.75	GENERIC, Eon Labs Manufacturing Inc	00185-0555-01
100's	$39.96	GENERIC, Major Pharmaceuticals Inc	00904-2694-61
100's	$46.49	GENERIC, Qualitest Products Inc	00603-4641-21
100's	$46.50	GENERIC, Martec Pharmaceuticals Inc	52555-0114-01
100's	$46.75	GENERIC, Par Pharmaceutical Inc	49884-0114-01
100's	$67.82	GENERIC, Martec Pharmaceuticals Inc	52555-0726-01
100's	$67.82	GENERIC, Mutual Pharmaceutical Co Inc	53489-0136-01
100's	$72.79	GENERIC, Sidmak Laboratories Inc	50111-0334-01
100's	$72.88	GENERIC, Ivax Corporation	00172-3007-60
100's	$82.94	GENERIC, Udl Laboratories Inc	51079-0126-20
100's	$85.02	GENERIC, Vangard Labs	00615-1577-13
100's	$98.03	GENERIC, Auro Pharmaceutical	55829-0365-10
100's	$114.01	GENERIC, Ivax Corporation	00182-1517-89
100's	$130.00	GENERIC, Medirex Inc	57480-0433-01
100's	$135.15	GENERIC, Geneva Pharmaceuticals	00781-1747-13
100's	$428.28	FLAGYL, Searle	00025-1821-31
140's	$56.10	GENERIC, Golden State Medical	60429-0129-14
250's	$24.75	GENERIC, Interstate Drug Exchange Inc	00814-4815-22
250's	$80.38	GENERIC, Par Pharmaceutical Inc	49884-0114-04

PRODUCT LISTING - EQUIVALENTS NOT AVAILABLE

Capsule - Oral - 375 mg

50's	$177.51	FLAGYL 375, Pharmacia Corporation	00025-1942-50
100's	$264.20	FLAGYL 375, Pharmacia Corporation	00025-1942-34

Cream - Topical - 0.75%

45 gm	$44.69	METROCREAM, Allscripts Pharmaceutical Company	54569-4638-00
45 gm	$51.07	METROCREAM, Physicians Total Care	54868-3825-00
45 gm	$63.69	METROCREAM, Galderma Laboratories Inc	00299-3836-45

Cream - Topical - 1%

30 gm	$43.21	NORITATE, Allscripts Pharmaceutical Company	54569-4795-00
30 gm	$52.49	NORITATE, Aventis Pharmaceuticals	00066-9850-30

Gel - Topical - 0.75%

28 gm	$39.25	METROGEL, Galderma Laboratories Inc	00299-3835-28
28.40 gm	$31.94	METROGEL, Allscripts Pharmaceutical Company	54569-2604-00
30 gm	$27.43	METROGEL, Southwood Pharmaceuticals Inc	58016-3197-01
30 gm	$36.66	METROGEL, Physicians Total Care	54868-0943-00
45 gm	$44.69	METROGEL, Allscripts Pharmaceutical Company	54569-4639-00
45 gm	$63.69	METROGEL, Galderma Laboratories Inc	00299-3835-45

Gel with Applicator - Vaginal - 0.75%

70 gm	$30.42	METROGEL-VAGINAL, Southwood Pharmaceuticals Inc	58016-3517-00
70 gm	$30.42	METROGEL-VAGINAL, Southwood Pharmaceuticals Inc	58016-3517-70
70 gm	$41.04	METROGEL-VAGINAL, Allscripts Pharmaceutical Company	54569-3660-00
70 gm	$41.95	METROGEL-VAGINAL, Southwood Pharmaceuticals Inc	58016-3517-01
70 gm	$48.87	METROGEL-VAGINAL, Physicians Total Care	54868-3110-00
70 gm	$54.44	METROGEL-VAGINAL, 3M Pharmaceuticals	00089-0200-25

Lotion - Topical - 0.75%

60 ml	$68.25	METROLOTION, Galderma Laboratories Inc	00299-3838-02

Powder For Injection - Intravenous - 500 mg

10's	$244.03	FLAGYL I.V., Scs Pharmaceuticals	00905-1804-10

Solution - Intravenous - 500 mg/100 ml

100 ml x 24	$370.49	FLAGYL I.V. RTU, Scs Pharmaceuticals	00905-1847-24

Tablet - Oral - 250 mg

2's	$3.44	GENERIC, Prescript Pharmaceuticals	00247-0098-02
3's	$3.47	GENERIC, Prescript Pharmaceuticals	00247-0098-03
4's	$3.52	GENERIC, Prescript Pharmaceuticals	00247-0098-04
5's	$3.55	GENERIC, Prescript Pharmaceuticals	00247-0098-05
5's	$6.53	GENERIC, Southwood Pharmaceuticals Inc	58016-0129-05
6's	$3.59	GENERIC, Prescript Pharmaceuticals	00247-0098-06
8's	$2.59	GENERIC, Allscripts Pharmaceutical Company	54569-0965-06
8's	$3.67	GENERIC, Prescript Pharmaceuticals	00247-0098-08
8's	$10.45	GENERIC, Southwood Pharmaceuticals Inc	58016-0129-08
9's	$3.71	GENERIC, Prescript Pharmaceuticals	00247-0098-09
9's	$11.75	GENERIC, Southwood Pharmaceuticals Inc	58016-0129-09
10's	$2.62	GENERIC, Physicians Total Care	54868-0108-02

10's	$13.05	GENERIC, Southwood Pharmaceuticals Inc	58016-0129-10
12's	$15.67	GENERIC, Southwood Pharmaceuticals Inc	58016-0129-12
14's	$3.91	GENERIC, Prescript Pharmaceuticals	00247-0098-14
14's	$18.28	GENERIC, Southwood Pharmaceuticals Inc	58016-0129-14
15's	$3.95	GENERIC, Prescript Pharmaceuticals	00247-0098-15
15's	$4.80	GENERIC, Pharma Pac	52959-0400-15
20's	$3.58	GENERIC, Physicians Total Care	54868-0108-03
20's	$26.12	GENERIC, Southwood Pharmaceuticals Inc	58016-0129-20
21's	$4.19	GENERIC, Prescript Pharmaceuticals	00247-0098-21
21's	$6.75	GENERIC, Pharma Pac	52959-0400-21
21's	$6.80	GENERIC, Allscripts Pharmaceutical Company	54569-0965-00
21's	$27.42	GENERIC, Southwood Pharmaceuticals Inc	58016-0129-21
24's	$4.31	GENERIC, Prescript Pharmaceuticals	00247-0098-24
25's	$32.65	GENERIC, Southwood Pharmaceuticals Inc	58016-0129-25
28's	$4.47	GENERIC, Prescript Pharmaceuticals	00247-0098-28
28's	$6.40	GENERIC, Pharmaceutical Corporation Of America	51655-0123-29
28's	$9.06	GENERIC, Allscripts Pharmaceutical Company	54569-0965-01
28's	$36.56	GENERIC, Southwood Pharmaceuticals Inc	58016-0129-28
30's	$4.54	GENERIC, Prescript Pharmaceuticals	00247-0098-30
30's	$4.54	GENERIC, Physicians Total Care	54868-0108-06
30's	$8.29	GENERIC, Pharma Pac	52959-0400-30
30's	$9.71	GENERIC, Allscripts Pharmaceutical Company	54569-0965-02
30's	$39.17	GENERIC, Southwood Pharmaceuticals Inc	58016-0129-30
40's	$4.94	GENERIC, Prescript Pharmaceuticals	00247-0098-40
40's	$12.95	GENERIC, Allscripts Pharmaceutical Company	54569-0965-03
42's	$5.02	GENERIC, Prescript Pharmaceuticals	00247-0098-42
56's	$13.61	GENERIC, Pharma Pac	52959-0400-56
56's	$18.13	GENERIC, Allscripts Pharmaceutical Company	54569-0965-07
100's	$7.33	GENERIC, Prescript Pharmaceuticals	00247-0098-00
100's	$11.23	GENERIC, Physicians Total Care	54868-0108-07
100's	$130.58	GENERIC, Southwood Pharmaceuticals Inc	58016-0129-00
Tablet - Oral - 500 mg			
4's	$1.78	GENERIC, Allscripts Pharmaceutical Company	54569-0967-00
4's	$2.24	GENERIC, Physicians Total Care	54868-0158-02
4's	$3.73	GENERIC, Prescript Pharmaceuticals	00247-0132-04
4's	$4.20	GENERIC, Pharma Pac	52959-0102-04
4's	$9.48	GENERIC, Southwood Pharmaceuticals Inc	58016-0725-04
7's	$16.55	GENERIC, Southwood Pharmaceuticals Inc	58016-0725-07
8's	$2.81	GENERIC, Physicians Total Care	54868-0158-04
8's	$3.56	GENERIC, Allscripts Pharmaceutical Company	54569-0967-01
8's	$4.09	GENERIC, Prescript Pharmaceuticals	00247-0132-08
8's	$5.00	GENERIC, Pharma Pac	52959-0102-08
8's	$18.92	GENERIC, Southwood Pharmaceuticals Inc	58016-0725-08
9's	$21.29	GENERIC, Southwood Pharmaceuticals Inc	58016-0725-09
10's	$3.09	GENERIC, Physicians Total Care	54868-0158-03
10's	$23.65	GENERIC, Southwood Pharmaceuticals Inc	58016-0725-10
12's	$4.47	GENERIC, Prescript Pharmaceuticals	00247-0132-12
12's	$28.38	GENERIC, Southwood Pharmaceuticals Inc	58016-0725-12
14's	$3.67	GENERIC, Physicians Total Care	54868-0158-01
14's	$4.65	GENERIC, Prescript Pharmaceuticals	00247-0132-14
14's	$5.90	GENERIC, Pharma Pac	52959-0102-14
14's	$6.22	GENERIC, Allscripts Pharmaceutical Company	54569-0967-03
14's	$33.10	GENERIC, Southwood Pharmaceuticals Inc	58016-0725-14
15's	$6.30	GENERIC, Pharma Pac	52959-0102-15
15's	$35.48	GENERIC, Southwood Pharmaceuticals Inc	58016-0725-15
18's	$42.57	GENERIC, Southwood Pharmaceuticals Inc	58016-0725-18
20's	$4.52	GENERIC, Physicians Total Care	54868-0158-05
20's	$5.21	GENERIC, Prescript Pharmaceuticals	00247-0132-20
20's	$7.60	GENERIC, Pharma Pac	52959-0102-20
20's	$8.89	GENERIC, Allscripts Pharmaceutical Company	54569-0967-09
20's	$47.30	GENERIC, Southwood Pharmaceuticals Inc	58016-0725-20
21's	$5.29	GENERIC, Prescript Pharmaceuticals	00247-0132-21
21's	$9.33	GENERIC, Allscripts Pharmaceutical Company	54569-0967-04
21's	$49.67	GENERIC, Southwood Pharmaceuticals Inc	58016-0725-21
24's	$56.76	GENERIC, Southwood Pharmaceuticals Inc	58016-0725-24
28's	$5.95	GENERIC, Prescript Pharmaceuticals	00247-0132-28
28's	$10.29	GENERIC, Pharma Pac	52959-0102-28
28's	$12.44	GENERIC, Allscripts Pharmaceutical Company	54569-0967-06
28's	$66.20	GENERIC, Southwood Pharmaceuticals Inc	58016-0725-28
30's	$5.95	GENERIC, Physicians Total Care	54868-0158-08
30's	$6.13	GENERIC, Prescript Pharmaceuticals	00247-0132-30
30's	$70.95	GENERIC, Southwood Pharmaceuticals Inc	58016-0725-30
40's	$7.06	GENERIC, Prescript Pharmaceuticals	00247-0132-40
40's	$7.38	GENERIC, Physicians Total Care	54868-0158-06
40's	$17.78	GENERIC, Allscripts Pharmaceutical Company	54569-0967-08
42's	$7.25	GENERIC, Prescript Pharmaceuticals	00247-0132-42
42's	$13.02	GENERIC, Pharma Pac	52959-0102-42
100's	$107.68	GENERIC, Allscripts Pharmaceutical Company	54569-3951-00
100's	$236.50	GENERIC, Southwood Pharmaceuticals Inc	58016-0725-00
250's	$26.52	GENERIC, Prescript Pharmaceuticals	00247-0132-69
Tablet, Extended Release - Oral - 750 mg			
30's	$258.94	FLAGYL ER, Searle	00025-1961-30

Mexiletine Hydrochloride *(001806)*

Categories: Arrhythmia, ventricular; Pregnancy Category C; FDA Approved 1985 Dec
Drug Classes: Antiarrhythmics, class IB
Brand Names: Mexitil
Foreign Brand Availability: Mexihexal (Germany); Mexitec (Indonesia); Mugadine (Taiwan)
Cost of Therapy: $135.03 (Arrhythmia; Mexitil; 200 mg; 3 capsules/day; 30 day supply)
$74.00 (Arrhythmia; Generic Capsules; 200 mg; 3 capsules/day; 30 day supply)

DESCRIPTION

Mexiletine hydrochloride is an orally active antiarrhythmic agent available as 150, 200, and 250 mg capsules. 100 mg of mexiletine hydrochloride is equivalent to 83.31 mg of mexiletine base. It is a white to off-white crystalline powder with slightly bitter taste, freely soluble in water and in alcohol. Mexiletine hydrochloride has a pKa of 9.2.

Chemically, mexiletine hydrochloride is 1-methyl-2-(2, 6-xylyloxy)ethylamine hydrochloride.

Mexitil capsules contain the following inactive ingredients: colloidal silicon dioxide, corn starch, magnesium stearate, titanium dioxide, gelatin, FD&C red no. 40, D&C red no. 28 and FD&C blue no. 1; the Mexitil 150 and 250 mg capsule also contain FD&C yellow no. 10. Mexitil capsules may contain one or more of the following components: sodium lauryl sulfate, sodium propionate, edetate calcium disodium, benzyl alcohol, carboxymethylcellulose sodium, glycerin, butylparaben, propyl paraben, methylparaben, pharmaceutical glaze, ethylene glycol monoethylether, soya lecithin, dimethylpolysiloxane, refined shellac (food grade) and other inactive ingredients.

CLINICAL PHARMACOLOGY

MECHANISM OF ACTION

Mexiletine HCl is a local anesthetic, antiarrhythmic agent, structurally similar to lidocaine, but orally active. In animal studies, mexiletine HCl has been to be effective in the suppression of induced ventricular arrhythmias, including those induced by glycoside toxicity and coronary artery ligation. Mexiletine HCl,like lidocaine, inhibits the inward sodium current, thus reducing the rate of rise of the action potential, Phase O. Mexiletine HCl decreased the effective refractory period (ERP) in Purkinje fibers. The decrease in ERP was of lesser magnitude than the decrease in action potential duration (APD), with a resulting increase in the ERP/APD ratio.

ELECTROPHYSIOLOGY IN MAN

Mexiletine is a Class 1B antiarrhythmic compound with electrophysiologic properties in man similar to those of lidocaine, but dissimilar from quinidine, procainamide, and disopyramide.

In patients with normal conduction systems, mexiletine HCl has a minimal effect on cardiac impulse generation and propagation. In clinical trials, no development of second-degree or third-degree AV block was observed. Mexiletine HCl did not prolong ventricular depolarization (QRS duration) or repolarization (QT intervals) as measured by electrocardiography. Theoretically, therefore, mexiletine HCl may be useful in the treatment of ventricular arrhythmias associated with a prolonged QT interval.

In patients with pre-existing conduction defects, depression of the sinus rate, prolongation of sinus nod recovery time, decreased conduction velocity and increased effective refractory period of the intraventricular conduction system have occasionally been observed.

The antiarrhythmic effect of mexiletine HCl has been established in controlled comparative trials against placebo, quinidine, procainamide and disopyramide. Mexiletine HCl, at doses of 200-400 mg q8h, produced a significant reduction of ventricular premature beats, paired beats, and episodes of non-sustained ventricular tachycardia compared to placebo and was similar in effectiveness to the active agents. Among all patients entered into the studies, about 30% in each treatment group had a 70% or greater reduction in PVC count and about 40% failed to complete the 3 month studies because of adverse effects. Follow-up of patients from the controlled trials has demonstrated continued effectiveness of mexiletine HCl in long-term use.

HEMODYNAMICS

Hemodynamic studies in a limited number of patients, with normal or abnormal myocardial function, following oral administration of mexiletine HCl, have shown small, usually not statistically significant, decreases in cardiac output and increased in systemic vascular resistance, but no significant negative inotropic effect. Blood pressure and pulse rate remain essentially unchanged. Mild depression of myocardial function, similar to that produced by lidocaine, has occasionally been observed following intravenous mexiletine HCl therapy in patients with cardiac disease.

PHARMACOKINETICS

Mexiletine HCl is well absorbed (~90%) from the gastrointestinal tract. Unlike lidocaine, its first-pass metabolism is low. Peak blood levels are reached in 2-3 hours. In normal subjects, the plasma elimination half-life of mexiletine HCl is approximately 10-12 hours. It is 50-60% bound to plasma protein, with a volume of distribution of 5-7 L/kg. Mexiletine HCl is metabolized in the liver. Approximately 10% is excreted unchanged by the kidney. While urinary pH does not normally have much influence on elimination, marked changes in the urinary pH influence the rate of excretion; acidification accelerates excretion, while alkalinization retards it.

Several metabolites of mexiletine have shown minimal antiarrhythmic activity in animal models. The most active is the minor metabolite N-methylmexiletine, which is less than 20% as potent as mexiletine. The urinary excretion of N-methylmexiletine in man is less than 0.5% Thus the therapeutic activity of mexiletine HCl is due to the parent compound.

Hepatic impairment prolongs the elimination half-life of mexiletine HCl. In 8 patients with moderate to severe liver disease, the mean half-life was approximately 25 hours.

Consistent with the limited renal elimination of mexiletine HCl, little change in the half-life has been detected in patients with reduced renal function. In 8 patients with creatinine clearance less than 10 ml/min, the mean plasma elimination half-life was 15.7 hours; in 7 patients with creatinine clearance between 11-40 ml/min, the mean half-life was 13.4 hours.

The absorption rate of mexiletine HCl is reduced in clinical situations such as acute myocardial infarction in which gastric emptying time is increased. Narcotics, atropine and magnesium-aluminum hydroxide have also been reported to slow the absorption of mexiletine HCl. Metoclopramide has been reported to accelerate absorption.

Mexiletine plasma levels of at least 0.5 μg/ml are generally required for therapeutic response. An increase in the frequency of central nervous system adverse effects has been observed when plasma levels exceed 2.0 μg/ml. Thus the therapeutic range is approximately 0.5-2.0 μg/ml. Plasma levels within the therapeutic range can be attained with either 3 times daily or twice daily dosing but peak to trough differences are greater with the latter regimen, creating the possibility of adverse effects at peak and antiarrhythmic escape at trough. Nevertheless, some patients may be transferred successfully to the twice daily regimen. (See DOSAGE AND ADMINISTRATION.)

INDICATIONS AND USAGE

Mexiletine HCl is indicated for the treatment of documented ventricular arrhythmias, such as sustained ventricular tachycardia, that, in the judgement of the physicians, are life-threatening. Because of the proarrhythmic effects of mexiletine HCl, its use with lesser arrhythmias is generally not recommended. Treatment of patients with asymptomatic ventricular premature contractions should be avoided.

Initiation of mexiletine HCl treatment, as with other antiarrhythmic agents used to treat life-threatening arrhythmias, should be carried out in the hospital.

Antiarrhythmic drugs have not been shown to enhance survival in patients with ventricular arrhythmias.

NON-FDA APPROVED INDICATIONS

Although not FDA approved, mexiletine has been used in the treatment of chronic neuropathic pain.

CONTRAINDICATIONS

Mexiletine HCl is contraindicated in the presence of cardiogenic shock or pre-existing second- or third-degree AV block (if no pacemaker is present).

WARNINGS

MORTALITY

In the National Heart, Lung and Blood Institute's Cardiac Arrhythmia Suppression Trial (CAST), a long-term, multi-centered, randomized, double-bind study in patients with asymptomatic non-life-threatening ventricular arrhythmias who had had myocardial infarctions more than 6 days but less than 2 years previously, and excessive mortality or non-fatal cardiac arrest rate was seen in patients treated with encainide or flecainide (56/730) compared with that seen in patients assigned to matched placebo-treated groups (22/725). The average duration of treatment with encainide or flecainide in this study was 10 months.

The applicability of these results to other populations (*e.g.,* those without recent myocardial infarction) or to other antiarrhythmic drugs is uncertain, but at present it is prudent to consider any antiarrhythmic agent to have a significant risk in patients with structural heart disease.

ACUTE LIVER INJURY

In postmarketing experience abnormal liver function tests have been reported, some in the first few weeks of therapy with mexiletine HCl. Most of these have been observed in the setting of congestive heart failure or ischemia and their relationship to mexiletine HCl has not been established.

PRECAUTIONS

GENERAL

If a ventricular pacemaker is operative, patients with second or third degree heart block may be treated with mexiletine HCl if continuously monitored. A limited number of patients (45 of 475 in controlled clinical trials) with pre-existing first degree AV block were treated with mexiletine HCl; none of these patients developed second or third degree AV block. Caution should be exercised when it is used in such patients or in patients with pre-existing sinus node dysfunction or intraventricular conduction abnormalities.

Like other antiarrhythmics Mexiletine HCl can cause worsening of arrhythmias. This has been uncommon in patients with less serious arrhythmias (Frequent premature beats or non-sustained ventricular tachycardia; see ADVERSE REACTIONS), but is of greater concern in patients with life-threatening arrhythmias such as sustained ventricular tachycardia. In patients with such arrhythmias subjected to programmed electrical stimulation or to exercise provocation, 10-15% of patients had exacerbation of the arrhythmia, a rate not greater than that of other agents.

Mexiletine HCl should be used with caution in patients with hypotension and severe congestive heart failure because of the potential for aggravating these conditions.

Since mexiletine HCl is metabolized in the liver, and hepatic impairment has been reported to prolong the elimination half-life of mexiletine HCl, patients with liver disease should be followed carefully while receiving mexiletine HCl. The same caution should be observed in patients with hepatic dysfunction secondary to decongestive heart failure.

Concurrent drug therapy or dietary regimens which may markedly after urinary pH should avoided during mexiletine HCl therapy. The minor fluctuations in urinary pH associated with normal diet do not affect the excretion of mexiletine HCl.

SGOT Elevation and Liver Injury

In 3 month controlled trials, elevations of SGOT greater than 3 times the upper limit of normal occurred in about 1% of both mexiletine-treated and control patients. Approximately 2% of patients in the mexiletine compassionate use program had elevations of SGOT greater than or equal to 3 times the upper limit of normal. These elevations frequently occurred in association with identifiable clinical events and therapeutic measures such as congestive heart failure, acute myocardial infarction, blood transfusions and other medications. These elevations were often asymptomatic and transient, usually not associated with elevated bilirubin levels and usually did not require discontinuation of therapy. Marked elevations of SGOT (> 1000 U/L) were seen before death in 4 patients with end-stage cardiac disease (severe congestive heart failure, cardiogenic shock).

Rare instances of severe liver injury, including hepatic necrosis, have been reported in association with mexiletine HCl treatment. It is recommended that patients in whom an abnormal liver test has occurred, or who have signs or symptoms suggesting liver dysfunction, be carefully evaluated. If persistent or worsening elevation of hepatic enzymes is detected, consideration should be given to discontinuing therapy.

Blood Dyscrasias

Among 10,867 patients treated with mexiletine in the compassionate use program, marked leukopenia (neutrophils less than 1000/mm^3) or agranulocytosis were seen in 0.06% and milder depressions of leukocytes were seen in 0.08%, and thrombocytopenia was observed in 0.16%. Many of these patients were seriously ill and receiving concomitant medications with known hematologic adverse effects. Rechallenge with mexiletine in several cases was negative. Marked leukopenia or agranulocytosis did not occur in any patient receiving mexiletine HCl alone; 5 of the 6 cases of agranulocytosis were associated with procainamide (sustained release preparations in 4) and 1 with vinblastine. If significant hematologic changes are observed the patient should be carefully evaluated, and, if warranted, mexiletine HCl should be discontinued. Blood counts usually return to normal within 1 month of discontinuation. (See ADVERSE REACTIONS.)

Convulsions (seizures) did not occur in mexiletine HCl controlled clinical trials. In the compassionate use program, convulsions were reported in about 2 of 1000 patients. Twenty-eight percent (28%) of these patients discontinued therapy. Convulsions were reported in patients with and without a prior history of seizures. Mexiletine should be used with caution in patients with known seizure disorder.

CARCINOGENESIS, MUTAGENESIS, AND IMPAIRMENT OF FERTILITY

Studies of carcinogenesis in rats (24 months) and mice (18 months) did not demonstrate any tumorigenic potential. Mexiletine HCl was found to be non-mutagenic in the Ames test. Mexiletine HCl did not impair fertility in the rat.

PREGNANCY, TERATOGENIC EFFECTS, PREGNANCY CATEGORY C

Reproduction studies performed with mexiletine HCl in rats, mice and rabbits at doses up to 4 times the maximum human oral dose (24 mg/kg in a 50 kg patient) revealed no evidence of teratogenicity or impaired fertility but did show an increase in fetal resorption. There are no adequate and well-controlled studies in pregnant women; this drug should be used in pregnancy only if the potential benefit justifies the potential risk to the fetus.

NURSING MOTHERS

Mexiletine HCl appears in human milk in concentrations similar to those observed in plasma. Therefore, if the use of mexiletine HCl is deemed essential, an alternative method of infant feeding should be considered.

PEDIATRIC USE

Safety and effectiveness in children have not been established.

DRUG INTERACTIONS

In a large compassionate use program mexiletine HCl has been used concurrently with commonly employed antianginal, antihypertensive, and anticoagulant drugs without observed interactions. A variety of antiarrhythmics such as quinidine or propanolol were also added, sometimes with improved control of ventricular ectopy. When phenytoin or other hepatic enzyme inducers such as rifampin and phenobarbital have been taken concurrently with mexiletine HCl, lowered mexiletine HCl plasma levels gave been reported. Monitoring of mexiletine HCl plasma levels is recommended during such concurrent use to avoid ineffective therapy.

In a formal study, benzodiazepine were shown not to effect mexiletine HCl plasma concentration. ECG intervals (PR, QRS, and QT) were not effected by concurrent mexiletine HCl and digoxin, diuretics, or propanolol.

Concurrent administration of cimetidine and mexiletine HCl has been reported to increase, decrease, or leave unchanged mexiletine HCl plasma levels; Therefore patients should be followed carefully during concurrent therapy.

Mexiletine HCl does not alter serum digoxin levels but magnesium-aluminum hydroxide, when used to treat gastrointestinal symptoms due to mexiletine HCl, has been reported to lower serum digoxin levels.

Concurrent use of mexiletine HCl and theophylline may lead to increased plasma theophylline levels. One controlled study in 8 normal subjects showed a 72% mean increase (range 35-136%) in plasma theophylline levels. This increase was observed at the first test point which was the second day after starting mexiletine HCl. Theophylline plasma levels returns to pre-mexiletine HCl values within 48 hours after discontinuing mexiletine HCl. If mexiletine HCl and theophylline are to be used concurrently,theophylline blood levels should be monitored, particularly when the mexiletine HCl dose is changed. An appropriate adjustment in the theophylline dose should be considered.

Additionally, in one controlled study in 5 normal subjects and 7 patients, the clearance if caffeine was decreased 50% following the administration of mexiletine HCl.

ADVERSE REACTIONS

Mexiletine HCl commonly produces reversible gastrointestinal and nervous system adverse reactions but is otherwise well-tolerated. Mexiletine HCl has been evaluated in 483 patients in 1 month ad 3 month controlled studies and in over 10,000 patients in a large compassionate use program. Dosages in the controlled studies ranged from 600-1200 mg/day: some patients (8%) in the compassionate use program were treated with higher daily doses (1600-3200 mg/day). In the 3 month controlled trials comparing mexiletine HCl to quinidine, procainamide and disopyramide, the most frequent adverse reactions were upper gastrointestinal distress (41%), lightheadedness (10.5%), tremor (12.6%) and coordination difficulties (10.2%). Similar frequency and incidence were observed in the 1 month placebo-controlled trial. Although these reactions were generally not serious, and were dose-related and reversible with a reduction in dosage, by taking the drug with food or antacid or by therapy discontinuation, they led to therapy discontinuation in 40% of patients in the controlled trials. A tabulation of the adverse events reported in the 1 month placebo controlled trial follows (see TABLE 1).

TABLE 1 *Mexiletine Hydrochloride, Adverse Reactions*

Comparative incidence (%) of adverse events among patients treated with mexiletine and placebo in the 4 week, double-blind crossover trial

	Mexiletine (n=53)	Placebo (n=49)
Cardiovascular		
Palpitations	7.5%	10.2%
Chest pain	7.5%	4.1%
Increased ventricular arrhythmias/PVCs	1.9%	—
Digestive		
Nausea/vomiting/heartburn	39.6%	6.1%
Central Nervous System		
Dizziness/lightheadedness	26.4%	14.3%
Tremor	13.2%	—
Nervousness	11.3%	6.1%
Coordination difficulties	9.4%	—
Changes in sleep habits	7.5%	16.3%
Paresthesias/numbness	3.8%	2.0%
Weakness	1.9%	4.1%
Fatigue	1.9%	2.0%
Tinnitus	1.9%	4.1%
Confusion/clouded sensorium	1.9%	2.0%
Other		
Headache	7.5%	6.1%
Blurred vision/visual disturbances	7.5%	2.0%
Dyspnea	5.7%	10.2%
Rash	3.8%	2.0%
Non-specific edema	3.8%	—

A tabulation of adverse reactions occurring in 1% or more of patients in the 3 month controlled studies follows (see TABLE 2).

TABLE 2 *Mexiletine Hydrochloride, Adverse Reactions*

Comparative incidence (%) of adverse events among patients treated with mexiletine or control drugs in the 12 week double-blind trials

	Mexiletine (n=430)	Quinidine (n=262)	Procainamide (n=78)	Disopyramide (n=69)
Cardiovascular				
Palpitations	4.3%	4.6%	1.3%	5.8%
Chest pain	2.6%	3.4%	1.3%	2.9%
Angina/angina-like pain	1.7%	1.9%	2.6%	2.9%
Increased ventricular arrhythmias/ PVCs	1.0%	2.7%	2.7%	—
Digestive				
Nausea/vomiting/heartburn	39.3%	21.4%	33.3%	14.5%
Diarrhea	5.2%	33.2%	2.6%	8.7%
Constipation	4.0%	—	6.4%	11.6%
Changes in appetite	2.6%	1.9%	—	—
Abdominal pain/cramps/discomfort	1.2%	1.5%	—	1.4%
Central Nervous System				
Dizziness/lightheadedness	18.9%	14.1%	14.1%	2.9%
Tremor	13.2%	2.3%	3.8%	1.4%
Coordination difficulties	9.7%	1.1%	1.3%	—
Changes in sleep habits	7.1%	2.7%	11.5%	8.7%
Weakness	5.0%	5.3%	7.7%	2.9%
Nervousness	5.0%	1.9%	6.4%	5.8%
Fatigue	3.8%	5.7%	5.1%	1.4%
Speech difficulties	2.6%	0.4%	—	—
Confusion/clouded sensorium	2.6%	—	3.8%	—
Paresthesias/numbness	2.4%	2.3%	2.6%	—
Tinnitus	2.4%	1.5%	—	—
Depression	2.4%	1.1%	1.3%	1.4%
Other				
Blurred vision/visual disturbances	5.7%	3.1%	5.1%	7.2%
Headache	5.7%	6.9%	7.7%	4.3%
Rash	4.2%	3.8%	10.3%	1.4%
Dyspnea/respiratory	3.3%	3.1%	5.1%	2.9%
Dry mouth	2.8%	1.9%	5.1%	14.5%
Arthralgia	1.7%	2.3%	5.1%	1.4%
Fever	1.2%	3.1%	2.6%	—

Less than 1%: Syncope, edema, hot flashes, hypertension, short-term memory loss, loss of consciousness, other physiological changes, diaphoresis, urinary hesitancy/retention, malaise, impotence/decreased libido, pharyngitis, congestive heart failure.

An additional group of over 10,000 patients has been treated in a program allowing administration of Mexiletine HCl under compassionate use circumstances. These patients were seriously ill with the large majority on multiple drug therapy. Twenty-four percent (24%) of the patients continued in the program for 1 year or longer. Adverse reactions leading to therapy, discontinuation occurred in 15% of patients (usually upper gastrointestinal system or nervous system effects). In general, the more common adverse reactions were similar to those in the controlled trials. Less common adverse events related to mexiletine HCl use include.

Cardiovascular System: Syncope and hypotension, each about 6 in 1000; bradycardia, about 4 in 1000; angina/angina-like pain, about 3 in 1000; edema, atrioventricular block.conduction disturbances and hot flashes, each about 2 in 1000; atrial arrhythmias. hypertension and cardiogenic shock, each about 1 in 1000.

Central Nervous System: Short-term memory loss, about 9 in 1000 patients; hallucinations and other psychological changes, each about 3 in 1000; psychosis and convulsions/seizures, each about 2 in 1000, loss of consciousness, about 6 in 10,000.

Digestive: Dysphagia, about 2 in 1000; peptic ulcer, about 8 in 10,000; upper gastrointestinal bleeding, about 7 in 10,000; esophageal ulceration, about 1 in 10,00. Rare cases of severe hepatitis/acute hepatic necrosis.

Skin: Rare cases of exfoliative dermatitis and Stevens-Johnson Syndrome with Mexiletine HCl treatment have been reported.

Laboratory: Abnormal liver function tests, about 5 in 100 patients, positive ANA and thrombocytopenia, each about 2 in 1000; leukopenia (including neutropenia and agranulocytosis), about 1 in 1000; myelofibrosis, about 2 in 10,000 patients.

Other: Diaphoresis, about 6 in 1000; altered taste, about 5 in 1000; salivary changes, hair loss and impotence/decreased libido, each about 4 in 1000; malaise, about 3 in 100; urinary hesitancy/retention, each about 2 in 1000; hiccups, dry skin, laryngeal and pharyngeal changes and changes in oral mucous membranes, each about 1 in 1000; SLE syndrome about 4 in 10,000.

Hematology: Blood dyscrasias were not seen in the controlled clinical trials but did occur among 10,867 patients treated with mexiletine in the compassionate use program (see PRECAUTIONS).

Myelofibrosis was reported in 2 patients in the compassionate use program; 1 was receiving long-term thiotepa therapy and the other had pretreatment myeloid abnormalities.

In postmarketing experience, there have been isolated, spontaneous reports of pulmonary changes including pulmonary fibrosis during mexiletine HCl therapy with or without other drugs or diseases that are known to produce pulmonary toxicity. A causal relationship to mexiletine HCl therapy has not been established. In addition, there have been isolated reports of exacerbation of congestive heart failure in patients with pre-existing compromised ventricular function.

DOSAGE AND ADMINISTRATION

The dosage of mexiletine HCl must be individualized on the basis of response and tolerance, both of which are dose-related. Administration with food or antacid is recommended. Initiate mexiletine HCl therapy with 200 mg every 8 hours when rapid control of arrhythmia is not essential. A minimum of 2-3 days between dose adjustments is recommended. Dose may be adjusted in 50 or 100 mg increments up or down.

As with any antiarrhythmic drug, clinical and electrocardiographic evaluation (including Holter monitoring if necessary for evaluation) are needed to determine whether the desired antiarrhythmic effect has been obtained and to guide titration and dose adjustment.

Satisfactory control can be achieved in most patients by 200-300 mg given every 8 hours with food or antacid. If satisfactory response had not been achieved at 300 mg q8h, and the patient tolerates mexiletine HCl well, a dose of 400 mg q8h may be tried. As the severity of CNS side effects increases with total daily dose, the dose should not exceed 1200 mg/day.

In general, patients with renal failure will require the usual doses of mexiletine HCl. Patients with severe liver disease, however, may require lower doses and must be monitored closely. Similarly, marked right-sided congestive heart failure can reduce hepatic metabolism and reduce the needed dose. Plasma level may also be affected by certain concomitant drugs (see DRUG INTERACTIONS).

Loading Dose: When rapid control of ventricular arrhythmia is essential, an initial loading dose of 400 mg of mexiletine HCl may be administered, followed by a 200 mg dose in 8 hours. Onset of therapeutic effect is usually observed within 30 minutes to 2 hours.

q12h Dosage Schedule: Some patients responding to mexiletine HCl may be transferee to a 12 hour dosage schedule to improve convenience and compliance. If adequate suppression is achieved on a mexiletine HCl dose of 300 mg or less every 8 hours, the same total daily dose may be given in divided doses every 12 hours while carefully monitoring the degree of suppression of ventricular ectopy. This dose may be adjusted up to a maximum of 450 mg every 12 hours to achieve the desired response.

TRANSFERRING TO MEXILETINE HCl

The following dosage schedule, based on theoretical considerations rather than experimental data, is suggested for transferring patients from other Class I oral antiarrhythmic agents to mexiletine HCl: mexiletine HCl treatment may be initiated with a 200 mg dose, and titrated to response as described above, 6-12 hours after the last dose of quinidine sulfate, 3-6 hours after the last dose of procainamide, 6-12 hours after the last dose of disopyramide or 8-12 hours after the last dose of tocainide.

In patients in whom withdrawal of the previous antiarrhythmic agent is likely to produce life-threatening arrhythmias, hospitalization of the patient is recommended.

When transferring from lidocaine to mexiletine HCl, the lidocaine infusion should be stopped when the first oral dose of mexiletine HCl is administered. The infusion line should be left open until suppression of the arrhythmias appears to be satisfactorily maintained. Consideration should be given to the similarity of the adverse effects of lidocaine and mexiletine HCl and the possibility that they may be additive.

HOW SUPPLIED

Mexitil is supplied in hard gelatin capsules containing 150, 200, or 250 mg of mexiletine hydrochloride:

Mexitil 150 mg capsules are red and caramel with the marking "Bl 66".
Mexitil 200 mg capsules are red with the marking "Bl 67".
Mexitil 250 mg capsules are red and aqua green with the marking "Bl 68".

Storage: Store below 86°F (30°C).

PRODUCT LISTING - RATED THERAPEUTICALLY EQUIVALENT

Capsule - Oral - 150 mg

31 x 10	$223.08	GENERIC, Vangard Labs	00615-1326-53
100's	$69.05	GENERIC, Moore, H.L. Drug Exchange Inc	00839-8005-06
100's	$69.13	GENERIC, Brightstone Pharma	62939-2312-01

M

100's	$69.91	GENERIC, Geneva Pharmaceuticals	00781-2130-01
100's	$90.49	GENERIC, Teva Pharmaceuticals Usa	00093-8739-01
100's	$90.49	GENERIC, Watson Laboratories Inc	52544-0491-01
100's	$126.05	MEXITIL, Boehringer-Ingelheim	00597-0066-01
Capsule - Oral - 200 mg			
100's	$82.22	GENERIC, Warrick Pharmaceuticals Corporation	59930-1686-01
100's	$82.22	GENERIC, Brightstone Pharma	62939-2322-01
100's	$82.28	GENERIC, Moore, H.L. Drug Exchange Inc	00839-8006-06
100's	$82.42	GENERIC, Geneva Pharmaceuticals	00781-2131-01
100's	$97.12	FEDERAL UPPER LIMIT, H.C.F.A. F F P	99999-1806-02
100's	$107.15	GENERIC, Teva Pharmaceuticals Usa	00093-8740-01
100's	$107.15	GENERIC, Watson Laboratories Inc	52544-0492-01
100's	$150.03	MEXITIL, Boehringer-Ingelheim	00597-0067-01
Capsule - Oral - 250 mg			
100's	$95.25	GENERIC, Watson Laboratories Inc	52544-0493-01
100's	$95.65	GENERIC, Moore, H.L. Drug Exchange Inc	00839-8007-06
100's	$95.66	GENERIC, Brightstone Pharma	62939-2332-01
100's	$96.75	GENERIC, Geneva Pharmaceuticals	00781-2132-01
100's	$123.83	GENERIC, Teva Pharmaceuticals Usa	00093-8741-01
100's	$172.84	MEXITIL, Boehringer-Ingelheim	00597-0068-01

PRODUCT LISTING - EQUIVALENTS NOT AVAILABLE

Capsule - Oral - 150 mg			
90's	$62.47	GENERIC, Allscripts Pharmaceutical Company	54569-4732-00
100's	$35.95	GENERIC, Physicians Total Care	54868-3776-00
100's	$69.06	GENERIC, Roxane Laboratories Inc	00054-2616-25
100's	$72.60	GENERIC, Roxane Laboratories Inc	00054-8616-25
Capsule - Oral - 200 mg			
90's	$74.07	GENERIC, Allscripts Pharmaceutical Company	54569-4789-00
100's	$82.24	GENERIC, Roxane Laboratories Inc	00054-2617-25
100's	$86.35	GENERIC, Roxane Laboratories Inc	00054-8617-25
Capsule - Oral - 250 mg			
100's	$95.66	GENERIC, Roxane Laboratories Inc	00054-2618-25

Miconazole (001809)

Categories: Candidiasis; Coccidioidomycosis; Cryptococcosis; Infection, urinary tract, fungal; Meningitis, fungal; Monilia; Paracoccidioidomycosis; Pseudoallerscheriosis; Tinea corporis; Tinea cruris; Tinea pedis; Tinea versicolor; FDA Approval Pre 1982; Pregnancy Category C; WHO Formulary

Drug Classes: Antifungals; Antifungals, topical; Dermatologics

Brand Names: Fungoid; **Monistat**; Ony-Clear Nail

Foreign Brand Availability: Acromizol (Ecuador); Aflorix (Argentina); Albistat (Belgium); Aloid (Mexico); Amykon (Germany); Andergin (Italy); Antifungal (Taiwan); Brentan (Denmark); Candiplas (Taiwan); Candizol (Bahrain; Cyprus; Egypt; Iran; Iraq; Jordan; Kuwait; Lebanon; Libya; Oman; Qatar; Republic-of-Yemen; Saudi-Arabia; Syria; United-Arab-Emirates); Candizol oral (Bahrain; Cyprus; Egypt; Iran; Iraq; Jordan; Kuwait; Lebanon; Libya; Oman; Qatar; Republic-of-Yemen; Saudi-Arabia; Syria; United-Arab-Emirates); Covarex (South-Africa); Daktar (Germany; Norway; Sweden; Switzerland); Daktarin (Argentina; Australia; Austria; Bangladesh; Belgium; Benin; Bulgaria; Burkina-Faso; Colombia; Costa-Rica; Czech-Republic; Dominican-Republic; Ecuador; El-Salvador; England; Ethiopia; Finland; France; Gambia; Ghana; Greece; Guatemala; Guinea; Honduras; Hong-Kong; India; Indonesia; Ireland; Israel; Italy; Ivory-Coast; Kenya; Korea; Liberia; Malawi; Malaysia; Mali; Mauritania; Mauritius; Mexico; Morocco; Netherlands; New-Zealand; Nicaragua; Niger; Nigeria; Pakistan; Panama; Peru; Philippines; Portugal; Russia; Senegal; Seychelles; Sierra-Leone; South-Africa; Spain; Sudan; Switzerland; Tanzania; Thailand; Tunia; Uganda; Zambia; Zimbabwe); Decozol (Singapore); Deralbine (Argentina); Derma-Mycotral (Germany); Dermonistat (Bahrain; Cyprus; Egypt; Iran; Iraq; Jordan; Kuwait; Lebanon; Libya; Oman; Qatar; Republic-of-Yemen; Saudi-Arabia; Syria; United-Arab-Emirates); Epi-Monistat (Germany); Escortin (Indonesia); Florid (Japan); Florid D (Japan); Funcort (Thailand); Funga (Hong-Kong); Fungares (Indonesia); Fungi-M (Thailand); Fungiquim (Mexico); Fungo (Hong-Kong; Singapore); Fungo Powder (Australia; New-Zealand); Fungo Vaginal Cream (New-Zealand); Fungtopic (Philippines); Gyno-Daktar (Germany); Gyno-Daktarin (Argentina; Austria; Bahrain; Bangladesh; Belgium; Bulgaria; Colombia; Costa-Rica; Cyprus; Czech-Republic; Dominican-Republic; Ecuador; Egypt; El-Salvador; England; Finland; France; Guatemala; Honduras; Hong-Kong; India; Indonesia; Iran; Iraq; Israel; Jordan; Korea; Kuwait; Lebanon; Libya; Malaysia; Mexico; Nicaragua; Oman; Pakistan; Panama; Portugal; Qatar; Republic-of-Yemen; Russia; Saudi-Arabia; South-Africa; Syria; United-Arab-Emirates); Gyno-Monistat (Germany); Gynospor (South-Africa); Hairscience Antidandruff Shampoo (Singapore); Liconar (Thailand); Medacter (Greece); Micatin (Canada; Ecuador); Micoffen (Mexico); Miconal (Italy); Micotar Mundgel (Germany); Micotef (Italy); Micozole (Canada); Micreme (New-Zealand); Minaza (Thailand); Miracol (Colombia); Monazole 7 (Canada); Monistat Derm (Australia); Monistat-7 (Australia; Canada); Mycoheal Cream (Bahrain; Cyprus; Egypt; Iran; Iraq; Jordan; Kuwait; Lebanon; Libya; Oman; Qatar; Republic-of-Yemen; Saudi-Arabia; Syria; United-Arab-Emirates); Mycoheal Oral Gel (Bahrain; Cyprus; Egypt; Iran; Iraq; Jordan; Kuwait; Lebanon; Libya; Oman; Qatar; Republic-of-Yemen; Saudi-Arabia; Syria; United-Arab-Emirates); Mycorine (Indonesia); Mykoderm (Germany); Mysocort (Thailand); Nazoderm (Indonesia); Neomicol (Mexico); Nilozanoc (Indonesia); Noxraxin (Thailand); Pitrion (Israel); Ranozol (Thailand); Shinaderm (Philippines); Skindure (Thailand); Tara (Thailand); Tinazol (Malaysia); Zarin (Malaysia); Zolagel (Indonesia); Zole (India)

Cost of Therapy: $17.92 (Moniliasis; Monistat 3 Suppository; 200 mg; 1 suppository/day; 3 day supply)
$7.98 (Moniliasis; Monistat 7 Suppository; 100 mg; 1 suppository/day; 7 day supply)

DESCRIPTION

Derm Cream: Monistat-Derm cream contains miconazole nitrate 2%, formulated into a water-miscible base consisting of pegoxol 7 stearate, peglicol 5 oleate, mineral oil, benzoic acid, butylated hydroxyanisole and purified water. Miconazole nitrate is 1-[2,4-Dichloro-β-[(2,4-dichlorobenzyl)oxy]phenethyl]-imidazole mononitrate.

External Vulvar Cream: Monistat external vulvar cream is a white to off-white oil-in-water emulsion base that contains miconazole nitrate, 1-[2,4-Dichloro-β-[(2,4-dichlorobenzyl) oxy]phenethyl]-imidazole mononitrate, 2%, purified water, propylene glycol, stearyl alcohol, cetyl alcohol, polysorbate 60, isopropyl myristate, benzoic acid, and potassium hydroxide.

Intravenous Infusion: Monistat IV, 1[2-(2,4 dichlorophenyl)-2-[(2,4-dichlorophenyl)methoxy]ethyl]-1H-imidazole, is a synthetic antifungal agent supplied as a sterile solution for intravenous infusion. Each ml of this solution contains 10 mg of miconazole with 0.115 ml PEG 35 castor oil, 1.0 mg lactic acid, 0.5 mg methylparaben, 0.05 mg propylparaben in water for injection. Miconazole IV is a clear, colorless to slightly yellow solution having a pH of 3.7 to 5.7.

Soft Gel Vaginal Inserts: Monistat soft gel vaginal insert is an off-white soft gelatin capsule containing the antifungal agent, miconazole nitrate, 1-[2,4-Dichloro-β-[(2,4-dichlorobenzyl) oxy]phenethyl]-imidazole mononitrate, 1200 mg, in a petrolatum base containing liquid paraffin, white petrolatum, and lecithin.

Suppositories: Monistat 3 vaginal suppositories are white to off-white suppositories, each containing the antifungal agent, miconazole nitrate, 1-[2,4-Dichloro-β-[(2,4-dichlorobenzyl)oxy]phenethyl]-imidazole mononitrate, 200 mg, in a hydrogenated vegetable oil base. Miconazole nitrate for vaginal use is also available as Monistat 7 vaginal cream and Monistat 7 vaginal suppositories.

CLINICAL PHARMACOLOGY

DERM CREAM

Miconazole nitrate is a synthetic antifungal agent which inhibits the growth of the common dermatophytes, *Trichophyton rubrum, Trichophyton mentagrophytes* and *Epidermophyton floccusum,* the yeast-like fungus, *Candida albicans,* and the organism responsible for tinea versicolor (*Malassezia furfur*).

EXTERNAL VULVAR CREAM AND SOFT GEL VAGINAL INSERTS

Following intravaginal administration of a single miconazole nitrate soft gel vaginal insert in 10 healthy females, plasma miconazole concentrations were detectable at 4 hours and peaked at 12-24 hours, with an average T_{max} at 18.4 hours. The mean (range) plasma miconazole concentrations at 24, 48, 72, and 96 hours are summarized in TABLE 1.

TABLE 1

	Hours Post-Dose			
	24	48	72	96
Mean Conc. (ng/ml)	9.22	4.51	2.95	1.84
Range	4.53-16.78	1.25-10.06	0.57-7.78	0.29-6.31

The average (range) peak plasma concentration, C_{max}, was 10.71 (5.78-18.33) ng/ml while the AUC(0-96) was 477.3 (244.8-774.8) ng·h/ml. These results demonstrated that overall systemic exposure to miconazole nitrate is similar between miconazole nitrate 4% vaginal cream and miconazole nitrate soft gel vaginal insert.

Microbiology

Mechanism of Action

Miconazole nitrate inhibits the biosynthesis of ergosterol, an essential component of the fungal cell wall. Miconazole nitrate has also been shown to interact with the synthesis of triglycerides and fatty acids, and to inhibit fungal oxidative and peroxidase enzymes.

In Vitro and In Vivo Activity

In vitro miconazole nitrate is active against a variety of yeasts and moulds. Miconazole nitrate has demonstrated *in vitro* and *in vivo* activity against susceptible strains of *Candida albicans* and the dermatophytes including *Trichophyton* spp., *Microsporum* spp. and *Epidermophyton* spp.

Susceptibility Testing

Miconazole nitrate susceptibility testing has been performed using numerous testing methods. Minor modifications to laboratory test conditions can alter the minimum inhibitory concentration (MIC) for azole antifungals. In one study where the National Committee for Clinical Laboratory Standards (NCCLS) antifungal susceptibility testing methodology M27-T was employed, 177 *Candida* isolates obtained from 50 patients with recurrent vulvovaginal candidiasis were tested. Most strains of *Candida albicans* exhibited miconazole MICs of <0.01 μg/ml.[1] Breakpoints to determine whether clinical isolates of *Candida albicans* or other *Candida* spp. are susceptible or resistant to miconazole nitrate have not been established using the National Committee for Clinical Laboratory Standards (NCCLS) antifungal susceptibility testing methodology M27-A.[2]

Data from clinical isolates have shown that the more common non-*albicans* strains of *Candida* producing vulvovaginal candidiasis have substantially higher MICs for the antifungal azoles, including miconazole, than *C. albicans* strains, suggesting that these pathogens may be more difficult to treat. However, the relevance of miconazole *in vitro* susceptibility data to clinical outcome remains to be defined.

Resistance

In vitro studies have shown that some *Candida* strains that demonstrate reduced susceptibility to one antifungal azole may also exhibit reduced susceptibility to other azole compounds, including miconazole. Clinical cases have shown that *Candida albicans* strains can develop antifungal azole resistance. Cross-resistance between azole compounds has been observed. The finding of cross-resistance is dependent upon a number of factors including the species evaluated, its clinical history, the particular azole compounds compared, and the type of susceptibility test that is performed. The exact mechanism of action producing azole resistance and cross-resistance to other antifungal azoles, including miconazole, is not fully understood at this time.

INTRAVENOUS INFUSION

Miconazole IV is rapidly metabolized in the liver and about 14-22% of the administered dose is excreted in the urine, mainly as inactive metabolites. The pharmacokinetic profile fits a three compartment open model with the following biologic half life: 0.4, 2.1, and 24.1 hours for each phase respectively. The pharmacokinetic profile of miconazole IV is unaltered in patients with renal insufficiency, including those patients on hemodialysis. The *in vitro* antifungal activity of miconazole IV is very broad. Clinical efficacy has been demonstrated in patients with the following species of fungi: *Coccidioides immitis, Candida albicans, Cryptococcus neoformans, Pseudallescheria boydii* (*Petriellidium boydii; Allescheria boydii*), and *Paracoccidioides brasiliensis.*

Recommended doses of miconazole IV produce serum concentrations of drug which exceed the *in vitro* minimum inhibitory concentration (MIC) values listed in TABLE 2.

TABLE 2 *Median Minimal Inhibitory Concentrations of Miconazole in μg/ml*

Clinical Isolates	Median	Range
Coccidioides immitis	0.4	0.1-1.6
Candida albicans	0.2	0.1-0.8
Cryptococcus neoformans	0.8	0.4-1.3
Paracoccidioides brasiliensis	0.24	0.16-0.31
Pseudallescheria boydii (*Petriellidium boydii*)	1.0	0.16-10

Doses above 9 mg/kg of miconazole IV produce peak blood levels above 1 μg/ml in most cases. The drug penetrates into joints.

SUPPOSITORIES

Miconazole nitrate exhibits fungicidal activity *in vitro* against species of the genus *Candida*. The pharmacologic mode of action is unknown. Following intravaginal administration of miconazole nitrate, small amounts are absorbed. Administration of a single dose of miconazole nitrate suppositories (100 mg) to healthy subjects resulted in a total recovery from the urine and feces of 0.85% (± 0.43%) of the administered dose.

Animal studies indicate that the drug crossed the placenta and doses above those used in humans result in embryo- and fetotoxicity (80 mg/kg, orally), although this has not been reported in human subjects (see PRECAUTIONS).

In multi-center clinical trials in 440 women with vulvovaginal candidiasis, the efficacy of treatment with the Monistat 3 vaginal suppository for 3 days was compared with treatment for 7 days with Monistat 7 vaginal cream. The clinical cure rates (free of microbiological evidence and clinical signs and symptoms of candidiasis at 8-10 days and 30-35 days post-therapy) were numerically lower, although not statistically different, with the 3-Day suppository when compared with the 7-Day cream.

INDICATIONS AND USAGE

DERM CREAM

For topical application in the treatment of tinea pedis (athlete's foot), tinea cruris, and tinea corporis caused by *Trichophyton rubrum* and *Epidermophyton floccosum* in the treatment of cutaneous candidiasis (moniliasis), and in the treatment of tinea versicolor.

EXTERNAL VULVAR CREAM

Miconazole nitrate external vulvar cream is indicated for the relief of external vulvar itching and irritation associated with a yeast infection.

INTRAVENOUS INFUSION

Miconazole IV is indicated for the treatment of the following severe systemic fungal infections, based on data derived from open clinical trials: coccidioidomycosis (n=52*), candidiasis (n=151), cryptococcosis (n=13), pseudoallescheriosis (petriellidiosis; allescheriosis) (n=12), paracoccidioidomycosis (n=12), and for the treatment of chronic mucocutaneous candidiasis (n=16).

*Represents treatment courses, as some patients were treated more than once.

However, in the treatment of fungal meningitis and *Candida* urinary bladder infections an intravenous infusion alone is inadequate. It must be supplemented with intrathecal administration or bladder irrigation. Appropriate diagnostic procedures should be performed and MIC's should be measured to determine if the organism is susceptible to miconazole.

Miconazole IV should only be used to treat severe systemic fungal disease.

SOFT GEL VAGINAL INSERTS

One miconazole nitrate soft gel vaginal insert is indicated for the topical treatment of vulvovaginal candidiasis (moniliasis). As miconazole nitrate is effective only for candidal vulvovaginitis, the diagnosis should be confirmed by KOH smear and/or cultures. Other pathogens commonly associated with vulvovaginitis (*Trichomonas vaginalis* and *Haemophilus vaginalis*) should be ruled out by appropriate laboratory methods.

SUPPOSITORIES

Monistat 3 vaginal suppositories are indicated for the local treatment of vulvovaginal candidiasis (moniliasis). Effectiveness in pregnancy and in diabetic patients has not been established. As miconazole nitrate is effective only for candidal vulvovaginitis, the diagnosis should be confirmed by KOH smear and/or cultures. Other pathogens commonly associated with vulvovaginitis (*Trichomonas* and *Haemophilus vaginalis* [*Gardnerella*]) should be ruled out by appropriate laboratory methods.

CONTRAINDICATIONS

DERM CREAM

No known contraindications.

EXTERNAL VULVAR CREAM AND SOFT GEL VAGINAL INSERTS

Patients known to be hypersensitive to miconazole nitrate or any component of the soft gel vaginal insert or external vulvar cream. There is limited information regarding cross-hypersensitivity between miconazole and other azole antifungal agents. Caution should be used in prescribing miconazole nitrate soft gel vaginal insert and external vulvar cream to patients with hypersensitivity to other azoles.

INTRAVENOUS INFUSION AND SUPPOSITORIES

Patients known to be hypersensitive to this drug, or its components.

WARNINGS

EXTERNAL VULVAR CREAM AND SOFT GEL VAGINAL INSERTS

The base contained in the soft gel vaginal insert and the external vulvar cream may interact with certain latex products, such as those used in vaginal contraceptive diaphragms or condoms. Therefore, condoms and diaphragms should not be relied upon to prevent sexually transmitted diseases or pregnancy until 3 days after last use of the vaginal insert and the external vulvar cream.

Tampons, douches or spermicides may remove the product from the vagina. Therefore, use of tampons, douches or spermicides should not be resumed until 7 days after last use of the soft gel vaginal insert and external vaginal cream.

INTRAVENOUS INFUSION

There have been several reports of cardiorespiratory arrest and/or anaphylaxis in patients receiving miconazole IV Excessively rapid administration of the drug may have been responsible in some cases. Rapid injection of undiluted miconazole IV may produce transient tachycardia or dysrhythmia (see DOSAGE AND ADMINISTRATION).

Miconazole IV should be used only to treat severe systemic fungal diseases.

PRECAUTIONS

DERM CREAM

If a reaction suggesting sensitivity or chemical irritation should occur, use of the medication should be discontinued.

For external use only. Avoid introduction of cream into the eyes.

INTRAVENOUS INFUSION

General

Before a treatment course of miconazole IV is started, the physician should ascertain insofar as possible that the patient is not hypersensitive to the drug product. Miconazole IV should be given by intravenous infusion. The treatment should be started under stringent conditions of hospitalization but subsequently may be administered to suitable patients under ambulatory conditions with close clinical monitoring. It is recommended that an initial dose of 200 mg be administered with the physician in attendance. It is also recommended that clinical laboratory monitoring including hemoglobin, hematocrit, electrolytes and lipids be performed.

It should be borne in mind that systemic fungal mycoses may be complications of chronic underlying conditions which in themselves may require appropriate measures.

Since *Pseudoallescheria boydii* is difficult to distinguish histologically from species of *Aspergillus*, it is strongly recommended that cultures be planted.

Pregnancy Category C

Reproduction studies using miconazole IV were performed in rats and rabbits. At intravenous doses of 40 mg/kg in the rat and 20 mg/kg in the rabbit, no evidence of impaired fertility or harm to the fetus appeared. There are no adequate and well-controlled studies using miconazole IV in pregnant women. Miconazole IV should be given to a pregnant woman only if clearly needed.

Pediatric Use

The safety of miconazole IV in children under 1 year has not been extensively studied. However, reports in the literature describe the treatment of 21 neonates for periods ranging from 1-56 days at doses ranging from 3-50 mg/kg/day in 3 or 4 divided doses. No unanticipated adverse events occurred in children who received these doses. The majority of use was a daily dose in the 15-30 mg/kg range. Seven (7) of the 11 evaluable children recovered or improved.

SOFT GEL VAGINAL INSERTS AND EXTERNAL VULVAR CREAM

General

Discontinue drug if sensitization or irritation is reported during use.

Carcinogenesis

Studies to determine the carcinogenic potential of miconazole nitrate have not been performed.

Mutagenesis

Miconazole nitrate was not genotoxic when tested *in vitro* for induction of microbial point mutations (Ames test) or *in vivo* for dominant lethal mutation in mouse germ cells or structural chromosome aberrations in mouse or rat bone marrow cells following high oral or intraperitoneal doses (equivalent to a human dose of 52 mg/kg based on body surface area conversions).

Impairment of Fertility

No impairment of fertility occurred when female rats were administered miconazole nitrate orally at doses equivalent to a human dose of 53 mg/kg/day based on body surface area conversions.

Pregnancy Category C

There are no adequate and well-controlled studies of miconazole nitrate soft gel vaginal inserts and external vulvar cream in pregnant women. Intravaginal administration of miconazole nitrate in rabbits 1 hour prior to mating did not affect reproductive performance or the offspring of these dams. Miconazole crosses the placenta and produces maternal and fetotoxicity when administered orally to rats and rabbits. Decreased food consumption and decreased pup survival were observed in rats and rabbits at or above doses equivalent to oral human doses of 13 mg/kg/day (rats) or 26 mg/kg/day (rabbits) based on body surface area conversions. Oral administration of miconazole nitrate has been reported to produce prolonged gestation in rats but not rabbits.

Nursing Mothers

It is not known whether miconazole nitrate is excreted in human milk. Because many drugs are excreted in human milk, caution should be exercised when miconazole nitrate is administered to a nursing woman.

Pediatric Use
The safety and efficacy of miconazole nitrate soft gel vaginal inserts and external vulvar cream in the treatment of vulvovaginal candidiasis in post-menarchal females have been established based on the extrapolation of clinical trial data from adult women. When a post-menarchal adolescent presents to a health professional with vulvovaginal symptoms, a careful evaluation for sexually transmitted diseases and other risk factors for vulvovaginal candidiasis should be considered. The safety and efficacy of miconazole nitrate soft gel vaginal inserts and external vulvar cream in pre-menarchal females have not been established.

Geriatric Use
Clinical studies of miconazole nitrate soft gel vaginal inserts and external vulvar cream did not include sufficient numbers of subjects aged 65 and over to determine whether they respond differently from younger subjects.

SUPPOSITORIES
General
Discontinue drug if sensitization or irritation is reported during use. The base contained in the suppository formulation may interact with certain latex products, such as the used in vaginal contraceptive diaphragms. Concurrent use is not recommended. Monistat 7 vaginal cream may be considered for use under these conditions.

Laboratory Tests
If there is a lack of response to Monistat 3 vaginal suppositories, appropriate microbiological studies (standard KOH smear and/or cultures) should be repeated to confirm the diagnosis and rule out other pathogens.

Carcinogenesis, Mutagenesis, and Impairment of Fertility
Long-term animal studies to determine carcinogenic potential have not been performed.

Fertility (Reproduction)
Oral administration of miconazole nitrate in rats has been reported to produce prolonged gestation. However, this effect was not observed in oral rabbit studies. In addition, signs of fetal and embryo toxicity were reported in rat and rabbit studies, and dystocia was reported in rat studies after oral doses at and above 80 mg/kg. Intravaginal administration did into produce these effects in rats.

Pregnancy
Since imidazoles are absorbed in small amounts from the human vagina, they should not be used in the first trimester of pregnancy unless the physician considers it essential to the welfare of the patient.

Clinical studies, during which miconazole nitrate vaginal cream and suppositories were used for up to 14 days, were reported to include 514 pregnant patients. Follow-up reports available in 471 of these patients reveal no adverse effects or complications attributable to miconazole nitrate therapy in infants born to these women.

Nursing Mothers
It is not known whether miconazole nitrate is excreted in human milk. Because many drugs are excreted in human milk, caution should be exercised when miconazole nitrate is administered to a nursing woman.

DRUG INTERACTIONS

INTRAVENOUS INFUSION
Drugs containing cremophor type vehicles are known to cause electrophoretic abnormalities of the lipoprotein; for example, the values and/or patterns may be altered. These effects are reversible upon discontinuation of treatment but are usually not an indication that treatment should be discontinued.

Interaction with oral and IV anticoagulant drugs, resulting in an enhancement of the anticoagulant effect, may occur. However, this has only been reported with oral (coumarin) administration. In cases of simultaneous treatment with miconazole IV and anticoagulant drugs, the anticoagulant effect should be carefully titrated since reductions of the anticoagulant doses may be indicated.

Interactions between oral miconazole and oral hypoglycemic agents leading to severe hypoglycemia have been reported.

Since concomitant administration of rifampin and ketoconazole (an imidazole) reduces the blood levels of the latter, the concurrent administration of miconazole IV (an imidazole) and rifampin should be avoided.

Ketoconazole (an imidazole) increases the blood level of cyclosporine; therefore there is the possibility of a similar drug interaction involving cyclosporine and miconazole IV (an imidazole). Blood levels of cyclosporine should be monitored if the two drugs must be given concurrently.

Concomitant administration of miconazole with CNS-active drugs such as carbamazepine or phenytoin may alter the metabolism of one or both of the drugs. Therefore, consideration should be given to the advisability of monitoring plasma levels of these drugs. It is not known whether miconazole may affect the metabolism of other CNS-active drugs.

ADVERSE REACTIONS

DERM CREAM
There have been isolated reports of irritation, burning, maceration, and allergic contact dermatitis with the application of miconazole nitrate.

INTRAVENOUS INFUSION
Adverse reactions which have been observed with miconazole IV therapy include phlebitis, pruritus, rash, nausea, vomiting, febrile reactions, drowsiness, diarrhea, anorexia and flushes. In the US studies, 29% of 209 patients studied had phlebitis, 21% pruritus, 18% nausea, 10% fever and chills, 9% rash, and 7% emesis. Transient decreases in hematocrit and serum sodium values have been observed following infusion of miconazole IV.

In rare cases, anaphylaxis has occurred.

Thrombocytopenia has also been reported. No serious renal or hepatic toxicity has been reported. If pruritus and skin rashes are severe, discontinuation of treatment may be necessary. Nausea and vomiting can be lessened with antihistaminic or antiemetic drugs given prior to miconazole IV infusion, or by reducing the dose, slowing the rate of infusion, or avoiding administration with foods.

Aggregation of erythrocytes or rouleau formation on blood smears has been reported. Hyperlipemia has occurred in patients and is reported to be due to the vehicle, Cremophor EL (PEG 35 castor oil).

EXTERNAL VULVAR CREAM AND SOFT GEL VAGINAL INSERTS
In controlled clinical studies, 272 patients with vulvovaginal candidiasis were treated with miconazole nitrate soft gel vaginal inserts and external vulvar cream. Miconazole nitrate soft gel vaginal inserts and external vulvar cream reactions most frequently involved the genital area (see TABLE 3).

TABLE 3 *Drug-Related Adverse Reactions (Frequency ≥1%) in Clinical Studies*

Adverse Experience	Miconazole Nitrate External Vulvar Cream and Soft Gel Vaginal Inserts (n=272)		Monistat 7 Vaginal Cream (n=265)	
Genital Reproductive System				
Burning, female genitalia	48	18%	49	18%
Irritation, female genitalia	33	12%	29	11%
Pruritus, external female genitalia	32	12%	45	17%
Discharge, female genitalia	11	4%	2	1%
Edema, female genitalia	3	1%	3	1%
Pain, female genitalia	3	1%	1	<1%
Gastrointestinal System				
Cramps, GI	5	2%	0	0%
Nausea	3	1%	0	0%
Nervous System				
Headache	4	1%	1	<1%

Miconazole soft gel vaginal inserts and external vulvar cream drug-related adverse events with a frequency <1% in clinical trials included: genital erythema, vaginal tenderness, dysuria, allergic reaction, dry mouth, flatulence, perianal burning, pelvic cramping, rash, urticaria, skin irritation, periorbital edema, and conjunctival pruritus.

The drug-related adverse event dropout rate was 1% in the miconazole soft gel vaginal inserts and external vulvar cream treatment group and 2% in the comparator arm. The adverse experiences most frequently causing study discontinuation were vulvovaginal burning and irritation for both the miconazole soft gel vaginal inserts and external vulvar cream and the comparator agent.

SUPPOSITORIES
During clinical studies with the Monistat 3 vaginal suppository (200 mg) 301 patients were treated. The incidence of vulvovaginal burning, itching or irritation was 2%. Complaints of cramping (2%) and headaches (1.3%) were also reported. Other complaints (hives, skin rash) occurred with less than a 0.5% incidence. The therapy-related dropout rate was 0.3%.

DOSAGE AND ADMINISTRATION

DERM CREAM
Sufficient miconazole nitrate cream should be applied to cover affected areas twice daily (morning and evening) in patients with tinea pedis, tinea cruris, tinea corporis, and cutaneous candidiasis, and once daily in patients with tinea versicolor. If miconazole nitrate cream is used in intertriginous areas, it should be applied sparingly and smoothed in well to avoid maceration effects.

Early relief of symptoms (2-3 days) is experienced by the majority of patients and clinical improvement may be seen fairly soon after treatment is begun; however *Candida* infections and tinea cruris and corporis should be treated for 2 weeks and tinea pedis for 1 month in order to reduce the possibility of recurrence. If a patient shows no clinical improvement after a month of treatment, the diagnosis should be redetermined. Patients with tinea versicolor usually exhibit clinical and mycological clearing after 2 weeks of treatment.

INTRAVENOUS INFUSION
Dosage
Adults
Doses may vary from 200-1200 mg per infusion depending on severity of infection and sensitivity of the organism. The following daily doses, which may be divided over 3 infusions, are recommended (see TABLE 4).

TABLE 4

Organism	Dosage Range*	Duration of Successful Therapy
Candidiasis	600-1800 mg/day	1 to >20 weeks
Cryptococcosis	1200-2400 mg/day	3 to >12 weeks
Coccidioidomycosis	1800-3600 mg/day	3 to >20 weeks
Pseudoallescheriosis (Petriellidosis, Allescheriosis)	600-3000 mg/day	5 to >20 weeks
Paracoccidioidomycosis	200 to 1200 mg/day	2 to >16 weeks

* May be divided over 3 infusions

Repeated courses may be necessitated by relapse or reinfection.

Children

Children Under 1 Year: Total daily doses of 15-30 mg/kg have been used (see PRECAUTIONS, Intravenous Infusion, Pediatric Use).

Children 1 to 12 Years

Total daily doses of 20-40 mg/kg have generally been adequate.

However, a dose of 15 mg/kg body weight per infusion should not be exceeded.

Administration

For daily doses of up to 2400 mg, miconazole IV should be diluted in at least 200 ml of diluent per ampoule and should be administered at a rate of approximately 2 hours per ampoule. For daily doses higher than 2400 mg adjust the rate of infusion and the diluent in terms of patient tolerability (see WARNINGS).

It is recommended that 0.9% sodium chloride injection be used as the diluent to minimize the possibility of transient hyponatremia following an infusion of miconazole IV. Alternatively, if clinically indicated, 5% Dextrose-Injection may used.

Generally, treatment should be continued until all clinical and laboratory tests no longer indicate that active fungal infection is present. Inadequate periods of treatment may yield poor response an lead to early recurrence of clinical symptoms. The dosing intervals and sites and the duration of treatment vary from patient and depend on the causative organism.

Other Modes of Administration:

Intrathecal: Administration of the undiluted injectable solution of miconazole IV by the various intrathecal routes (20 mg/dose) is indicated as an adjunct to intravenous treatment in fungal meningitis. Succeeding intrathecal injections may be alternated between lumbar, cervical, and cisternal punctures every 3-7 days.

Bladder Instillation: 200 mg of miconazole in a diluted solution is indicated in the treatment of *Candida* of the urinary bladder.

EXTERNAL VULVAR CREAM

Sufficient external vulvar cream should be applied to cover affected areas twice daily (morning and evening) for up to 7 days as needed.

SOFT GEL VAGINAL INSERTS

One insert (1200 mg) is inserted intravaginally once at bedtime. Before prescribing another course of therapy, the diagnosis should be reconfirmed by smears and/or cultures to rule out other pathogens.

SUPPOSITORIES

Monistat 3 Vaginal Suppositories: One suppository (miconazole nitrate, 200 mg) is inserted intravaginally once daily at bedtime for 3 consecutive days. Before prescribing another course of therapy, the diagnosis should be reconfirmed by smears and/or cultures to rule out other pathogens.

PRODUCT LISTING - EQUIVALENTS NOT AVAILABLE

Cream with Applicator - Vaginal - 4%			
15 gm	$14.38	MONISTAT 3, Mcneil Consumer Healthcare	00062-5402-01
25 gm	$13.20	MONISTAT 3, Mcneil Consumer Healthcare	00062-5401-01
Kit - Vaginal - 1200 mg;2%			
1's	$28.74	MONISTAT-1 DUAL PACK, Ortho Mcneil Pharmaceutical	08004-5410-05
1's	$32.35	MONISTAT-1 DUAL PACK, Prescript Pharmaceuticals	00247-0351-01
Tampon - Vaginal - 100 mg			
5's	$15.96	MONISTAT 5, Johnson and Johnson/Merck	00062-5436-01

Midazolam Hydrochloride *(001810)*

Categories: Anesthesia, adjunct; Sedation; Pregnancy Category D; DEA Class CIV; FDA Approved 1985 Dec
Drug Classes: Benzodiazepines; Preanesthetics; Sedatives/hypnotics
Brand Names: **Versed**
Foreign Brand Availability: Dormicum (Austria; Bahamas; Bahrain; Bangladesh; Barbados; Belgium; Belize; Benin; Bermuda; Bulgaria; Burkina-Faso; Curacao; Cyprus; Czech-Republic; Denmark; Ecuador; Egypt; Ethiopia; Finland; Gambia; Germany; Ghana; Greece; Guinea; Guyana; Hong-Kong; Hungary; Indonesia; Iran; Iraq; Israel; Ivory-Coast; Jamaica; Japan; Jordan; Kenya; Korea; Kuwait; Lebanon; Liberia; Libya; Malawi; Malaysia; Mali; Mauritania; Mauritius; Morocco; Netherland-Antilles; Netherlands; Niger; Nigeria; Norway; Oman; Pakistan; Philippines; Portugal; Puerto-Rico; Qatar; Republic-of-Yemen; Saudi-Arabia; Senegal; Seychelles; Sierra-Leone; South-Africa; Spain; Sudan; Surinam; Sweden; Switzerland; Syria; Taiwan; Tanzania; Thailand; Trinidad; Tunia; Turkey; Uganda; United-Arab-Emirates; Zambia; Zimbabwe); Dormonid (Peru); Fulsed (India; Singapore); Hypnovel (Australia; Belgium; Colombia; Costa-Rica; Dominican-Republic; El-Salvador; England; France; Guatemala; Honduras; Ireland; Mexico; New-Zealand; Nicaragua; Panama); Ipnovel (Italy); Midazol (Israel; Thailand); Midolam (Israel)
HCFA JCODE(S): J2250 per 1 mg IM, IV

IM-IV

WARNING

Adults and Pediatrics: Intravenous midazolam HCl has been associated with respiratory depression and respiratory arrest, especially when used for sedation in noncritical care settings. In some cases, where this was not recognized promptly and treated effectively, death or hypoxic encephalopathy has resulted. Intravenous midazolam HCl should be used only in hospital or ambulatory care settings, including physicians' and dental offices, that provide for continuous monitoring of respiratory and cardiac function, *i.e.,* pulse oximetry. Immediate availability of resuscitative drugs and age- and size-appropriate equipment for bag/valve/mask ventilation and intubation, and personnel trained in their

WARNING — Cont'd

use and skilled in airway management should be assured (see WARNINGS). For deeply sedated pediatric patients, a dedicated individual, other than the practitioner performing the procedure, should monitor the patient throughout the procedure.

The initial intravenous dose for sedation in adult patients may be as little as 1 mg, but should not exceed 2.5 mg in a normal healthy adult. Lower doses are necessary for older (over 60 years) or debilitated patients and in patients receiving concomitant narcotics or other central nervous system (CNS) depressants. The initial dose and all subsequent doses should always be titrated slowly; administer over at least 2 minutes and allow an additional 2 or more minutes to fully evaluate the sedative effect. The use of the 1 mg/ml formulation or dilution of the 1 mg/ml or 5 mg/ml formulation is recommended to facilitate slower injection. Doses of sedative medications in pediatric patients must be calculated on a mg/kg basis, and initial doses and all subsequent doses should always be titrated slowly. The initial pediatric dose of midazolam HCl for sedation/anxiolysis/amnesia is age, procedure, and route dependent (see DOSAGE AND ADMINISTRATION).

Neonates: Midazolam HCl should not be administered by rapid injection in the neonatal population. Severe hypotension and seizures have been reported following rapid IV administration, particularly with concomitant use of fentanyl (see DOSAGE AND ADMINISTRATION).

DESCRIPTION

Versed is a water-soluble benzodiazepine available as a sterile, nonpyrogenic parenteral dosage form for intravenous or intramuscular injection. Each ml contains midazolam hydrochloride equivalent to 1 or 5 mg midazolam compounded with 0.8% sodium chloride and 0.01% edetate disodium, with 1% benzyl alcohol as preservative; the pH is adjusted to approximately 3 with hydrochloric acid and, if necessary, sodium hydroxide.

Midazolam is a white to light yellow crystalline compound, insoluble in water. The hydrochloride salt of midazolam, which is formed *in situ,* is soluble in aqueous solutions. Chemically, midazolam HCl is: 8-chloro-6-(2-fluorophenyl)-1-methyl-4*H*-imidazo[1,5-a][1,4]benzodiazepine hydrochloride. Midazolam hydrochloride has the empirical formula $C_{18}H_{13}ClFN_3 \cdot HCl$, and a calculated molecular weight of 362.25.

Under the acidic conditions required to solubilize midazolam in the product, midazolam is present as an equilibrium mixture of the closed ring form and an open-ring structure formed by the acid-catalyzed ring opening of the 4,5-double bond of the diazepine ring. The amount of open-ring form is dependent upon the pH of the solution. At the specified pH of the product, the solution may contain up to about 25% of the open-ring compound. At the physiologic conditions under which the product is absorbed (pH of 5-8) into the systemic circulation, any open-ring form present reverts to the physiologically active, lipophilic, closed-ring form (midazolam) and is absorbed as such.

CLINICAL PHARMACOLOGY

Midazolam HCl is a short-acting benzodiazepine central nervous system (CNS) depressant.

The effects of midazolam HCl on the CNS are dependent on the dose administered, the route of administration, and the presence or absence of other medications. Onset time of sedative effects after IM administration in adults is 15 minutes, with peak sedation occurring 30-60 minutes following injection. In one adult study, when tested the following day, 73% of the patients who received midazolam HCl intramuscularly had no recall of memory cards shown 30 minutes following drug administration; 40% had no recall of the memory cards shown 60 minutes following drug administration. Onset time of sedative effects in the pediatric population begins within 5 minutes and peaks at 15-30 minutes depending upon the dose administered. In pediatric patients, up to 85% had no recall of pictures shown after receiving intramuscular midazolam HCl compared with 5% of the placebo controls.

Sedation in adult and pediatric patients is achieved within 3-5 minutes after intravenous (IV) injection; the time of onset is affected by total dose administered and the concurrent administration of narcotic premedication. Seventy-one percent (71%) of the adult patients in endoscopy studies had no recall of introduction of the endoscope; 82% of the patients had no recall of withdrawal of the endoscope. In one study of pediatric patients undergoing lumbar puncture or bone marrow aspiration, 88% of patients had impaired recall vs 9% of the placebo controls. In another pediatric oncology study, 91% of midazolam HCl treated patients were amnestic compared with 35% of patients who had received fentanyl alone.

When midazolam HCl is given IV as an anesthetic induction agent, induction of anesthesia occurs in approximately 1.5 minutes when narcotic premedication has been administered and in 2-2.5 minutes without narcotic premedication or other sedative premedication. Some impairment in a test of memory was noted in 90% of the patients studied. A dose response study of pediatric patients premedicated with 1.0 mg/kg intramuscular (IM) meperidine found that only 4 out of 6 pediatric patients who received 600 μg/kg IV midazolam HCl lost consciousness, with eye closing at 108 ± 140 seconds. This group was compared with pediatric patients who were given thiopental 5 mg/kg IV; 6 out of 6 closed their eyes at 20 ± 3.2 seconds. Midazolam HCl did not dependably induce anesthesia at this dose despite concomitant opioid administration in pediatric patients.

Midazolam HCl, used as directed, does not delay awakening from general anesthesia in adults. Gross tests of recovery after awakening (orientation, ability to stand and walk, suitability for discharge from the recovery room, return to baseline Trieger competency) usually indicate recovery within 2 hours but recovery may take up to 6 hours in some cases. When compared with patients who received thiopental, patients who received midazolam generally recovered at a slightly slower rate. Recovery from anesthesia or sedation for procedures in pediatric patients depends on the dose of midazolam HCl administered, coadministration of other medications causing CNS depression and duration of the procedure.

In patients without intracranial lesions, induction of general anesthesia with IV midazolam HCl is associated with a moderate decrease in cerebrospinal fluid pressure (lumbar puncture measurements), similar to that observed following IV thiopental. Preliminary data in neurosurgical patients with normal intracranial pressure but decreased compliance (subarachnoid screw measurements) show comparable elevations of intracranial pressure with midazolam HCl and with thiopental during intubation. No similar studies have been reported in pediatric patients.

The usual recommended intramuscular premedicating doses of midazolam HCl do not depress the ventilatory response to carbon dioxide stimulation to a clinically significant extent in adults. Intravenous induction doses of midazolam HCl depress the ventilatory response to carbon dioxide stimulation for 15 minutes or more beyond the duration of ventilatory depression following administration of thiopental in adults. Impairment of ventilatory response to carbon dioxide is more marked in adult patients with chronic obstructive pulmonary disease (COPD). Sedation with IV midazolam HCl does not adversely affect the mechanics of respiration (resistance, static recoil, most lung volume measurements); total lung capacity and peak expiratory flow decrease significantly but static compliance and maximum expiratory flow at 50% of awake total lung capacity (V_{max}) increase. In one study of pediatric patients under general anesthesia, intramuscular midazolam HCl (100 or 200 µg/kg) was shown to depress the response to carbon dioxide in a dose-related manner.

In cardiac hemodynamic studies in adults, IV induction of general anesthesia with midazolam HCl was associated with a slight to moderate decrease in mean arterial pressure, cardiac output, stroke volume and systemic vascular resistance. Slow heart rates (less than 65/min), particularly in patients taking propranolol for angina, tended to rise slightly; faster heart rates (*e.g.*, 85/min) tended to slow slightly. In pediatric patients, a comparison of IV midazolam HCl (500 µg/kg) with propofol (2.5 mg/kg) revealed a mean 15% decrease in systolic blood pressure in patients who had received IV midazolam HCl versus a mean 25% decrease in systolic blood pressure following propofol.

PHARMACOKINETICS

Midazolam's activity is primarily due to the parent drug. Elimination of the parent drug takes place via hepatic metabolism of midazolam to hydroxylated metabolites that are conjugated and excreted in the urine. Six single-dose pharmacokinetic studies involving healthy adults yield pharmacokinetic parameters for midazolam in the following ranges: volume of distribution (Vd), 1.0-3.1 L/kg; elimination half-life, 1.8-6.4 hours (mean approximately 3 hours); total clearance (Cl), 0.25-0.54 L/hr/kg. In a parallel group study, there was no difference in the clearance, in subjects administered 0.15 mg/kg (n=4) and 0.30 mg/kg (n=4) IV doses indicating linear kinetics. The clearance was successively reduced by approximately 30% at doses of 0.45 mg/kg (n=4) and 0.6 mg/kg (n=5) indicating non-linear kinetics in this dose range.

Absorption

The absolute bioavailability of the intramuscular route was greater than 90% in a crossover study in which healthy subjects (n=17) were administered a 7.5 mg IV or IM dose. The mean peak concentration (C_{max}) and time to peak (T_{max}) following the IM dose was 90 ng/ml (20% CV) and 0.5 hour (50% CV). C_{max} for the 1-hydroxy metabolite following the IM dose was 8 ng/ml (T_{max}=1.0 h).

Following IM administration, C_{max} for midazolam and its 1-hydroxy metabolite were approximately one-half of those achieved after intravenous injection.

M

Distribution

The volume of distribution (Vd) determined from 6 single-dose pharmacokinetic studies involving healthy adults ranged from 1.0-3.1 L/kg. Female gender, old age, and obesity are associated with increased values of midazolam Vd. In humans, midazolam has been shown to cross the placenta and enter into fetal circulation and has been detected in human milk and CSF (see Special Populations).

In adults and pediatric patients older than 1 year, midazolam is approximately 97% bound to plasma protein, principally albumin.

Metabolism

In vitro studies with human liver microsomes indicate that the biotransformation of midazolam is mediated by cytochrome P450 3A4. This cytochrome also appears to be present in gastrointestinal tract mucosa as well as liver. Sixty percent (60%) to 70% of the biotransformation products is 1-hydroxy-midazolam (also termed alpha-hydroxy-midazolam) while 4-hydroxy-midazolam constitutes 5% or less. Small amounts of a dihydroxy derivative have also been detected but not quantified. The principal urinary excretion products are glucuronide conjugates of the hydroxylated derivatives.

Drugs that inhibit the activity of cytochrome P450 3A4 may inhibit midazolam clearance and elevate steady-state midazolam concentrations.

Studies of the intravenous administration of 1-hydroxy-midazolam in humans suggest that 1-hydroxy-midazolam is at least as potent as the parent compound and may contribute to the net pharmacologic activity of midazolam. *In vitro* studies have demonstrated that the affinities of 1- and 4-hydroxy-midazolam for the benzodiazepine receptor are approximately 20% and 7%, respectively, relative to midazolam.

Excretion

Clearance of midazolam is reduced in association with old age, congestive heart failure, liver disease (cirrhosis) or conditions which diminish cardiac output and hepatic blood flow.

The principal urinary excretion product is 1-hydroxy-midazolam in the form of a glucuronide conjugate; smaller amounts of the glucuronide conjugates of 4-hydroxy- and dihydroxy-midazolam are detected as well. The amount of midazolam excreted unchanged in the urine after a single IV dose is less than 0.5% (n=5). Following a single IV infusion in 5 healthy volunteers, 45–57% of the dose was excreted in the urine as 1-hydroxymethyl midazolam conjugate.

Pharmacokinetics — Continuous Infusion

The pharmacokinetic profile of midazolam following continuous infusion, based on 282 adult subjects, has been shown to be similar to that following single-dose administration for subjects of comparable age, gender, body habitus and health status. However, midazolam can accumulate in peripheral tissues with continuous infusion. The effects of accumulation are greater after long-term infusions than after short-term infusions. The effects of accumulation can be reduced by maintaining the lowest midazolam infusion rate that produces satisfactory sedation.

Infrequent hypotensive episodes have occurred during continuous infusion; however, neither the time to onset nor the duration of the episode appeared to be related to plasma concentrations of midazolam or alpha-hydroxy-midazolam. Further, there does not appear to be an increased chance of occurrence of a hypotensive episode with increased loading doses.

Patients with renal impairment may have longer elimination half-lives for midazolam (see Special Populations, Renal Failure).

SPECIAL POPULATIONS

Changes in the pharmacokinetic profile of midazolam due to drug interactions, physiological variables, etc., may result in changes in the plasma concentration-time profile and pharmacological response to midazolam in these patients. For example, patients with acute renal failure appear to have a longer elimination half-life for midazolam and may experience delayed recovery (see Special Populations, Renal Failure). In other groups, the relationship between prolonged half-life and duration of effect has not been established.

Pediatrics and Neonates

In pediatric patients aged 1 year and older, the pharmacokinetic properties following a single dose of midazolam HCl reported in 10 separate studies of midazolam are similar to those in adults. Weight-normalized clearance is similar or higher (0.19-0.80 L/hr/kg) than in adults and the terminal elimination half-life (0.78-3.3 hours) is similar to or shorter than in adults. The pharmacokinetic properties during and following continuous intravenous infusion in pediatric patients in the operating room as an adjunct to general anesthesia and in the intensive care environment are similar to those in adults.

In seriously ill neonates, however, the terminal elimination half-life of midazolam is substantially prolonged (6.5-12.0 hours) and the clearance reduced (0.07-0.12 L/hr/kg) compared to healthy adults or other groups of pediatric patients. It cannot be determined if these differences are due to age, immature organ function or metabolic pathways, underlying illness or debility.

Obese

In a study comparing normals (n=20) and obese patients (n=20) the mean half-life was greater in the obese group (5.9 vs 2.3 hours). This was due to an increase of approximately 50% in the Vd corrected for total body weight. The clearance was not significantly different between groups.

Geriatric

In three parallel group studies, the pharmacokinetics of midazolam administered IV or IM were compared in young (mean age 29, n=52) and healthy elderly subjects (mean age 73, n=53). Plasma half-life was approximately 2-fold higher in the elderly. The mean Vd based on total body weight increased consistently between 15–100% in the elderly. The mean Cl decreased approximately 25% in the elderly in two studies and was similar to that of the younger patients in the other.

Congestive Heart Failure

In patients suffering from congestive heart failure, there appeared to be a 2-fold increase in the elimination half-life, a 25% decrease in the plasma clearance and a 40% increase in the volume of distribution of midazolam.

Hepatic Insufficiency

Midazolam pharmacokinetics were studied after an IV single dose (0.075 mg/kg) was administered to 7 patients with biopsy proven alcoholic cirrhosis and 8 control patients. The mean half-life of midazolam increased 2.5-fold in the alcoholic patients. Clearance was reduced by 50% and the Vd increased by 20%. In another study in 21 male patients with cirrhosis, without ascites and with normal kidney function as determined by creatinine clearance, no changes in the pharmacokinetics of midazolam or 1-hydroxy-midazolam were observed when compared to healthy individuals.

Renal Failure

Patients with renal impairment may have longer elimination half-lives for midazolam and its metabolites which may result in slower recovery.

Midazolam and 1-hydroxy-midazolam pharmacokinetics in 6 ICU patients who developed acute renal failure (ARF) were compared with a normal renal function control group. Midazolam was administered as an infusion (5-15 mg/hr). Midazolam clearance was reduced (1.9 vs 2.8 ml/min/kg) and the half-life was prolonged (7.6 vs 13 hours) in the ARF patients. The renal clearance of the 1-hydroxy-midazolam glucuronide was prolonged in the ARF group (4 vs 136 ml/min) and the half-life was prolonged (12 vs >25 hours). Plasma levels accumulated in all ARF patients to about 10 times that of the parent drug. The relationship between accumulating metabolite levels and prolonged sedation is unclear.

In a study of chronic renal failure patients (n=15) receiving a single IV dose, there was a 2-fold increase in the clearance and volume of distribution but the half-life remained unchanged. Metabolite levels were not studied.

Plasma Concentration-Effect Relationship

Concentration-effect relationships (after an IV dose) have been demonstrated for a variety of pharmacodynamic measures (*e.g.*, reaction time, eye movement, sedation) and are associated with extensive intersubject variability. Logistic regression analysis of sedation scores and steady-state plasma concentration indicated that at plasma concentrations greater than 100 ng/ml there was at least a 50% probability that patients would be sedated, but respond to verbal commands (sedation score = 3). At 200 ng/ml there was at least a 50% probability that patients would be asleep, but respond to glabellar tap (sedation score = 4).

Drug Interactions

For information concerning pharmacokinetic drug interactions with midazolam HCl (see DRUG INTERACTIONS).

INDICATIONS AND USAGE

Injectable Midazolam HCl Is Indicated:

- Intramuscularly or intravenously for preoperative sedation/anxiolysis/amnesia.
- Intravenously as an agent for sedation/anxiolysis/amnesia prior to or during diagnostic, therapeutic or endoscopic procedures, such as bronchoscopy, gastroscopy, cystoscopy,

coronary angiography, cardiac catheterization, oncology procedures, radiologic procedures, suture of lacerations and other procedures either alone or in combination with other CNS depressants.

- Intravenously for induction of general anesthesia, before administration of other anesthetic agents. With the use of narcotic premedication, induction of anesthesia can be attained within a relatively narrow dose range and in a short period of time. Intravenous midazolam HCl can also be used as a component of intravenous supplementation of nitrous oxide and oxygen (balanced anesthesia).
- Continuous intravenous infusion for sedation of intubated and mechanically ventilated patients as a component of anesthesia or during treatment in a critical care setting.

Midazolam HCl is associated with a high incidence of partial or complete impairment of recall for the next several hours (see CLINICAL PHARMACOLOGY).

NON-FDA APPROVED INDICATIONS

Midazolam has also been used to achieve a variety of clinical objectives including decreased agitation in ventilator-dependent patients. In addition, midazolam has been used in the treatment of insomnia and status epilepticus.

CONTRAINDICATIONS

Injectable midazolam HCl is contraindicated in patients with a known hypersensitivity to the drug. Benzodiazepines are contraindicated in patients with acute narrow-angle glaucoma. Benzodiazepines may be used in patients with open-angle glaucoma only if they are receiving appropriate therapy. Measurements of intraocular pressure in patients without eye disease show a moderate lowering following induction with midazolam HCl; patients with glaucoma have not been studied.

Midazolam HCl is not intended for intrathecal or epidural administration due to the presence of the preservative benzyl alcohol in the dosage form.

WARNINGS

Midazolam HCl must never be used without individualization of dosage particularly when used with other medications capable of producing central nervous system depression. Prior to the intravenous administration of midazolam HCl in any dose, the immediate availability of oxygen, resuscitative drugs, age- and size-appropriate equipment for bag/valve/mask ventilation and intubation, and skilled personnel for the maintenance of a patent airway and support of ventilation should be ensured. Patients should be continuously monitored with some means of detection for early signs of hypoventilation, airway obstruction, or apnea, *i.e.,* pulse oximetry. Hypoventilation, airway obstruction, and apnea can lead to hypoxia and/or cardiac arrest unless effective countermeasures are taken immediately. The immediate availability of specific reversal agents (flumazenil) is highly recommended. Vital signs should continue to be monitored during the recovery period. Because intravenous midazolam HCl depresses respiration (see CLINICAL PHARMACOLOGY) and because opioid agonists and other sedatives can add to this depression, midazolam HCl should be administered as an induction agent only by a person trained in general anesthesia and should be used for sedation/anxiolysis/amnesia only in the presence of personnel skilled in early detection of hypoventilation, maintaining a patent airway and supporting ventilation. **When used for sedation/anxiolysis/amnesia, midazolam HCl should always be titrated slowly in adult or pediatric patients.** Adverse hemodynamic events have been reported in pediatric patients with cardiovascular instability; rapid intravenous administration should also be avoided in this population (see DOSAGE AND ADMINISTRATION).

Serious cardiorespiratory adverse events have occurred after administration of midazolam HCl. These have included respiratory depression, airway obstruction, oxygen desaturation, apnea, respiratory arrest and/or cardiac arrest, sometimes resulting in death or permanent neurologic injury. There have also been rare reports of hypotensive episodes requiring treatment during or after diagnostic or surgical manipulations particularly in adult or pediatric patients with hemodynamic instability. Hypotension occurred more frequently in the sedation studies in patients premedicated with a narcotic.

Reactions such as agitation, involuntary movements (including tonic/clonic movements and muscle tremor), hyperactivity and combativeness have been reported in both adult and pediatric patients. These reactions may be due to inadequate or excessive dosing or improper administration of midazolam HCl; however, consideration should be given to the possibility of cerebral hypoxia or true paradoxical reactions. Should such reactions occur, the response to each dose of midazolam HCl and all other drugs, including local anesthetics, should be evaluated before proceeding. Reversal of such responses with flumazenil has been reported in pediatric patients.

Concomitant use of barbiturates, alcohol or other central nervous system depressants may increase the risk of hypoventilation, airway obstruction, desaturation, or apnea and may contribute to profound and/or prolonged drug effect. Narcotic premedication also depresses the ventilatory response to carbon dioxide stimulation.

Higher risk adult and pediatric surgical patients, elderly patients and debilitated adult and pediatric patients require lower dosages, whether or not concomitant sedating medications have been administered. Adult or pediatric patients with COPD are unusually sensitive to the respiratory depressant effect of midazolam HCl. Pediatric and adult patients undergoing procedures involving the upper airway such as upper endoscopy or dental care, are particularly vulnerable to episodes of desaturation and hypoventilation due to partial airway obstruction. Adult and pediatric patients with chronic renal failure and patients with congestive heart failure eliminate midazolam more slowly (see CLINICAL PHARMACOLOGY). Because elderly patients frequently have inefficient function of 1 or more organ systems and because dosage requirements have been shown to decrease with age, reduced initial dosage of midazolam HCl is recommended, and the possibility of profound and/or prolonged effect should be considered.

Injectable midazolam HCl should not be administered to adult or pediatric patients in shock or coma, or in acute alcohol intoxication with depression of vital signs. Particular care should be exercised in the use of intravenous midazolam HCl in adult or pediatric patients with uncompensated acute illnesses, such as severe fluid or electrolyte disturbances.

There have been limited reports of intra-arterial injection of midazolam HCl. Adverse events have included local reactions, as well as isolated reports of seizure activity in which no clear causal relationship was established. Precautions against unintended intra-arterial injection should be taken. Extravasation should also be avoided.

The safety and efficacy of midazolam HCl following nonintravenous and nonintramuscular routes of administration have not been established. Midazolam HCl should only be administered intramuscularly or intravenously.

The decision as to when patients who have received injectable midazolam HCl, particularly on an outpatient basis, may again engage in activities requiring complete mental alertness, operate hazardous machinery or drive a motor vehicle must be individualized. Gross tests of recovery from the effects of midazolam HCl (see CLINICAL PHARMACOLOGY) cannot be relied upon to predict reaction time under stress. It is recommended that no patient operate hazardous machinery or a motor vehicle until the effects of the drug, such as drowsiness, have subsided or until 1 full day after anesthesia and surgery, whichever is longer. For pediatric patients, particular care should be taken to assure safe ambulation.

USE IN PREGNANCY

An increased risk of congenital malformations associated with the use of benzodiazepine drugs (diazepam and chlordiazepoxide) has been suggested in several studies. If this drug is used during pregnancy, the patient should be apprised of the potential hazard to the fetus.

Withdrawal symptoms of the barbiturate type have occurred after the discontinuation of benzodiazepines.

USAGE IN PRETERM INFANTS AND NEONATES

Rapid injection should be avoided in the neonatal population. Midazolam HCl administered rapidly as an intravenous injection (less than 2 minutes) has been associated with severe hypotension in neonates, particularly when the patient has also received fentanyl. Likewise, severe hypotension has been observed in neonates receiving a continuous infusion of midazolam who then receive a rapid intravenous injection of fentanyl. Seizures have been reported in several neonates following rapid intravenous administration.

The neonate also has reduced and/or immature organ function and is also vulnerable to profound and/or prolonged respiratory effects of midazolam HCl.

Exposure to excessive amounts of benzyl alcohol has been associated with toxicity (hypotension, metabolic acidosis), particularly in neonates, and an increased incidence of kernicterus, particularly in small preterm infants. There have been rare reports of deaths, primarily in preterm infants, associated with exposure to excessive amounts of benzyl alcohol. The amount of benzyl alcohol from medications is usually considered negligible compared to that received in flush solutions containing benzyl alcohol. Administration of high dosages of medications (including midazolam HCl) containing this preservative must take into account the total amount of benzyl alcohol administered. The recommended dosage range of midazolam HCl for preterm and term infants includes amounts of benzyl alcohol well below that associated with toxicity; however, the amount of benzyl alcohol at which toxicity may occur is not known. If the patient requires more than the recommended dosages or other medications containing this preservative, the practitioner must consider the daily metabolic load of benzyl alcohol from these combined sources.

PRECAUTIONS

GENERAL

Intravenous doses of midazolam HCl should be decreased for elderly and for debilitated patients (see WARNINGS and DOSAGE AND ADMINISTRATION). These patients will also probably take longer to recover completely after midazolam HCl administration for the induction of anesthesia.

Midazolam HCl does not protect against the increase in intracranial pressure or against the heart rate rise and/or blood pressure rise associated with endotracheal intubation under light general anesthesia.

USE WITH OTHER CNS DEPRESSANTS

The efficacy and safety of midazolam HCl in clinical use are functions of the dose administered, the clinical status of the individual patient, and the use of concomitant medications capable of depressing the CNS. Anticipated effects range from mild sedation to deep levels of sedation virtually equivalent to a state of general anesthesia where the patient may require external support of vital functions. Care must be taken to individualize and carefully titrate the dose of midazolam HCl to the patient's underlying medical/surgical conditions, administer to the desired effect being certain to wait an adequate time for peak CNS effects of both midazolam HCl and concomitant medications, and have the personnel and size-appropriate equipment and facilities available for monitoring and intervention (see BOXED WARNING, WARNINGS and DOSAGE AND ADMINISTRATION). Practitioners administering midazolam HCl must have the skills necessary to manage reasonably foreseeable adverse effects, particularly skills in airway management.

INFORMATION FOR THE PATIENT

To assure safe and effective use of benzodiazepines, the following information and instructions should be communicated to the patient when appropriate:

1. Inform your physician about any alcohol consumption and medicine you are now taking, especially blood pressure medication and antibiotics, including drugs you buy without a prescription. Alcohol has an increased effect when consumed with benzodiazepines; therefore, caution should be exercised regarding simultaneous ingestion of alcohol during benzodiazepine treatment.
2. Inform your physician if you are pregnant or are planning to become pregnant.
3. Inform your physician if you are nursing.
4. Patients should be informed of the pharmacological effects of midazolam HCl, such as sedation and amnesia, which in some patients may be profound. The decision as to when patients who have received injectable midazolam HCl, particularly on an outpatient basis, may again engage in activities requiring complete mental alertness, operate hazardous machinery or drive a motor vehicle must be individualized.
5. Patients receiving continuous infusion of midazolam in critical care settings over an extended period of time, may experience symptoms of withdrawal following abrupt discontinuation.

DRUG/LABORATORY TEST INTERACTIONS

Midazolam has not been shown to interfere with results obtained in clinical laboratory tests.

CARCINOGENESIS, MUTAGENESIS, AND IMPAIRMENT OF FERTILITY

Carcinogenesis

Midazolam maleate was administered with diet in mice and rats for 2 years at dosages of 1, 9 and 80 mg/kg/day. In female mice in the highest dose group there was a marked increase in the incidence of hepatic tumors. In high-dose male rats there was a small but statistically significant increase in benign thyroid follicular cell tumors. Dosages of 9 mg/kg/day of midazolam maleate (25 times a human dose of 0.35 mg/kg) do not increase the incidence of tumors. The pathogenesis of induction of these tumors is not known. These tumors were found after chronic administration, whereas human use will ordinarily be of single or several doses.

Mutagenesis

Midazolam did not have mutagenic activity in *Salmonella typhimurium* (5 bacterial strains), Chinese hamster lung cells (V79), human lymphocytes or in the micronucleus test in mice.

Impairment of Fertility

A reproduction study in male and female rats did not show any impairment of fertility at dosages up to 10 times the human IV dose of 0.35 mg/kg.

PREGNANCY, TERATOGENIC EFFECTS, PREGNANCY CATEGORY D

See WARNINGS.

Segment II teratology studies, performed with midazolam maleate injectable in rabbits and rats at 5 and 10 times the human dose of 0.35 mg/kg, did not show evidence of teratogenicity.

Nonteratogenic Effects: Studies in rats showed no adverse effects on reproductive parameters during gestation and lactation. Dosages tested were approximately 10 times the human dose of 0.35 mg/kg.

LABOR AND DELIVERY

In humans, measurable levels of midazolam were found in maternal venous serum, umbilical venous and arterial serum and amniotic fluid, indicating placental transfer of the drug. Following intramuscular administration of 0.05 mg/kg of midazolam, both the venous and the umbilical arterial serum concentrations were lower than maternal concentrations.

The use of injectable midazolam HCl in obstetrics has not been evaluated in clinical studies. Because midazolam is transferred transplacentally and because other benzodiazepines given in the last weeks of pregnancy have resulted in neonatal CNS depression, midazolam HCl is not recommended for obstetrical use.

NURSING MOTHERS

Midazolam is excreted in human milk. Caution should be exercised when midazolam HCl is administered to a nursing woman.

PEDIATRIC USE

The safety and efficacy of midazolam HCl for sedation/anxiolysis/amnesia following single dose intramuscular administration, intravenously by intermittent injections and continuous infusion have been established in pediatric and neonatal patients. For specific safety monitoring and dosage guidelines (see BOXED WARNING, CLINICAL PHARMACOLOGY, INDICATIONS AND USAGE, WARNINGS, ADVERSE REACTIONS and DOSAGE AND ADMINISTRATION). UNLIKE ADULT PATIENTS, PEDIATRIC PATIENTS GENERALLY RECEIVE INCREMENTS OF MIDAZOLAM HCl ON A MG/KG BASIS. As a group, pediatric patients generally require higher dosages of midazolam HCl (mg/kg) than do adults. Younger (less than 6 years) pediatric patients may require higher dosages (mg/kg) than older pediatric patients, and may require closer monitoring. In obese PEDIATRIC PATIENTS, the dose should be calculated based on ideal body weight. When midazolam HCl is given in conjunction with opioids or other sedatives, the potential for respiratory depression, airway obstruction, or hypoventilation is increased. The health care practitioner who uses this medication in pediatric patients should be aware of and follow accepted professional guidelines for pediatric sedation appropriate to their situation.

Midazolam HCl should not be administered by rapid injection in the neonatal population. Severe hypotension and seizures have been reported following rapid IV administration, particularly, with concomitant use of fentanyl.

GERIATRIC USE

Because geriatric patients may have altered drug distribution and diminished hepatic and/or renal function, reduced doses of midazolam HCl are recommended: Intravenous and intramuscular doses of midazolam HCl should be decreased for elderly and for debilitated patients (see WARNINGS and DOSAGE AND ADMINISTRATION) and subjects over 70 years of age may be particularly sensitive. These patients will also probably take longer to recover completely after midazolam HCl administration for the induction of anesthesia. Administration of IM and IV midazolam HCl to elderly and/or high-risk surgical patients has been associated with rare reports of death under circumstances compatible with cardiorespiratory depression. In most of these cases, the patients also received other central nervous system depressants capable of depressing respiration, especially narcotics (see DOSAGE AND ADMINISTRATION).

Specific dosing and monitoring guidelines for geriatric patients are provided in DOSAGE AND ADMINISTRATION for premedicated patients for sedation/anxiolysis/amnesia following IV and IM administration, for induction of anesthesia following IV administration and for continuous infusion.

DRUG INTERACTIONS

The sedative effect of intravenous midazolam HCl is accentuated by any concomitantly administered medication, which depresses the central nervous system, particularly narcotics (*e.g.*, morphine, meperidine and fentanyl) and also secobarbital and droperidol. Consequently, the dosage of midazolam HCl should be adjusted according to the type and amount of concomitant medications administered and the desired clinical response (see DOSAGE AND ADMINISTRATION).

Caution is advised when midazolam is administered concomitantly with drugs that are known to inhibit the P450 3A4 enzyme system such as cimetidine (not ranitidine), erythromycin, diltiazem, verapamil, ketoconazole and itraconazole. These drug interactions may result in prolonged sedation due to a decrease in plasma clearance of midazolam.

The effect of single oral doses of 800 mg cimetidine and 300 mg ranitidine on steady-state concentrations of midazolam was examined in a randomized crossover study (n=8). Cimetidine increased the mean midazolam steady-state concentration from 57 to 71 ng/ml. Ranitidine increased the mean steady-state concentration to 62 ng/ml. No change in choice reaction time or sedation index was detected after dosing with the H2 receptor antagonists.

In a placebo-controlled study, erythromycin administered as a 500 mg dose, tid, for 1 week (n=6), reduced the clearance of midazolam following a single 0.5 mg/kg IV dose. The half-life was approximately doubled.

Caution is advised when midazolam is administered to patients receiving erythromycin since this may result in a decrease in the plasma clearance of midazolam.

The effects of diltiazem (60 mg tid) and verapamil (80 mg tid) on the pharmacokinetics and pharmacodynamics of midazolam were investigated in a three-way cross-over study (n=9). The half-life of midazolam increased from 5 to 7 hours when midazolam was taken in conjunction with verapamil or diltiazem. No interaction was observed in healthy subjects between midazolam and nifedipine.

In a placebo-controlled study, saquinavir administered as a 1200 mg dose, tid, for 5 days (n=12), a 56% reduction in the clearance of midazolam following a single 0.05 mg/kg IV dose was observed. The half-life was approximately doubled.

A moderate reduction in induction dosage requirements of thiopental (about 15%) has been noted following use of intramuscular midazolam HCl for premedication in adults.

The intravenous administration of midazolam HCl decreases the minimum alveolar concentration (MAC) of halothane required for general anesthesia. This decrease correlates with the dose of midazolam HCl administered; no similar studies have been carried out in pediatric patients but there is no scientific reason to expect that pediatric patients would respond differently than adults.

Although the possibility of minor interactive effects has not been fully studied, midazolam HCl and pancuronium have been used together in patients without noting clinically significant changes in dosage, onset or duration in adults. Midazolam HCl does not protect against the characteristic circulatory changes noted after administration of succinylcholine or pancuronium and does not protect against the increased intracranial pressure noted following administration of succinylcholine. Midazolam HCl does not cause a clinically significant change in dosage, onset or duration of a single intubating dose of succinylcholine; no similar studies have been carried out in pediatric patients but there is no scientific reason to expect that pediatric patients would respond differently than adults.

No significant adverse interactions with commonly used premedications or drugs used during anesthesia and surgery (including atropine, scopolamine, glycopyrrolate, diazepam, hydroxyzine, d-tubocurarine, succinylcholine and other nondepolarizing muscle relaxants) or topical local anesthetics (including lidocaine, dyclonine HCl and Cetacaine) have been observed in adults or pediatric patients. In neonates, however, severe hypotension has been reported with concomitant administration of fentanyl. This effect has been observed in neonates on an infusion of midazolam who received a rapid injection of fentanyl and in patients on an infusion of fentanyl who have received a rapid injection of midazolam.

ADVERSE REACTIONS

See WARNINGS concerning serious cardiorespiratory events and possible paradoxical reactions. Fluctuations in vital signs were the most frequently seen findings following parenteral administration of midazolam HCl in adults and included decreased tidal volume and/or respiratory rate decrease (23.3% of patients following IV and 10.8% of patients following IM administration) and apnea (15.4% of patients following IV administration), as well as variations in blood pressure and pulse rate. The majority of serious adverse effects, particularly those associated with oxygenation and ventilation, have been reported when midazolam HCl is administered with other medications capable of depressing the central nervous system. **The incidence of such events is higher in patients undergoing procedures involving the airway without the protective effect of an endotracheal tube (*e.g.*, upper endoscopy and dental procedures).**

ADULTS

The following additional adverse reactions were reported after intramuscular administration:

Headache (1.3%).

Local effects at IM injection site:

Pain (3.7%).
Induration (0.5%).
Redness (0.5%).
Muscle stiffness (0.3%).

Administration of IM midazolam HCl to elderly and/or higher risk surgical patients has been associated with rare reports of death under circumstances compatible with cardiorespiratory depression. In most of these cases, the patients also received other central nervous system depressants capable of depressing respiration, especially narcotics (see DOSAGE AND ADMINISTRATION).

The following additional adverse reactions were reported subsequent to intravenous administration as a single sedative/anxiolytic/amnestic agent in adult patients:

Hiccoughs (3.9%).
Nausea (2.8%).
Vomiting (2.6%).
Coughing (1.3%).
"Oversedation" (1.6%).
Headache (1.5%).
Drowsiness (1.2%).

Local effects at the IV site:
Tenderness (5.6%).
Pain during injection (5.0%).
Redness (2.6%).
Induration (1.7%).
Phlebitis (0.4%).

PEDIATRIC PATIENTS

The following adverse events related to the use of IV midazolam HCl in pediatric patients were reported in the medical literature:
Desaturation 4.6%.
Apnea 2.8%.
Hypotension 2.7%.
Paradoxical reactions 2.0%.
Hiccough 1.2%.
Seizure-like activity 1.1%.
Nystagmus 1.1%.

The majority of airway-related events occurred in patients receiving other CNS depressing medications and in patients where midazolam HCl was not used as a single sedating agent.

NEONATES

For information concerning hypotensive episodes and seizures following the administration of midazolam HCl to neonates (see BOXED WARNING, CONTRAINDICATIONS, WARNINGS and PRECAUTIONS).

Other adverse experiences, observed mainly following IV injection as a single sedative/anxiolytic/amnesia agent and occurring at an incidence of <1.0% in adult and pediatric patients, are as follows:

Respiratory: Laryngospasm, bronchospasm, dyspnea, hyperventilation, wheezing, shallow respirations, airway obstruction, tachypnea.

Cardiovascular: Bigeminy, premature ventricular contractions, vasovagal episode, bradycardia, tachycardia, nodal rhythm.

Gastrointestinal: Acid taste, excessive salivation, retching.

CNS/Neuromuscular: Retrograde amnesia, euphoria, hallucination, confusion, argumentativeness, nervousness, anxiety, grogginess, restlessness, emergence delirium or agitation, prolonged emergence from anesthesia, dreaming during emergence, sleep disturbance, insomnia, nightmares, athetoid movements, seizure-like activity, ataxia, dizziness, dysphoria, slurred speech, dysphonia, paresthesia.

Special Senses: Blurred vision, diplopia, nystagmus, pinpoint pupils, cyclic movements of eyelids, visual disturbance, difficulty focusing eyes, ears blocked, loss of balance, light-headedness.

Integumentary: Hive-like elevation at injection site, swelling or feeling of burning, warmth or coldness at injection site.

Hypersensitivity: Allergic reactions including anaphylactoid reactions, hives, rash, pruritus.

Miscellaneous: Yawning, lethargy, chills, weakness, toothache, faint feeling, hematoma.

DOSAGE AND ADMINISTRATION

Midazolam HCl is a potent sedative agent that requires slow administration and individualization of dosage. Clinical experience has shown midazolam HCl to be 3-4 times as potent per mg as diazepam. BECAUSE SERIOUS AND LIFE-THREATENING CARDIORESPIRATORY ADVERSE EVENTS HAVE BEEN REPORTED, PROVISION FOR MONITORING, DETECTION AND CORRECTION OF THESE REACTIONS MUST BE MADE FOR EVERY PATIENT TO WHOM MIDAZOLAM HCl INJECTION IS ADMINISTERED, REGARDLESS OF AGE OR HEALTH STATUS. Excessive single doses or rapid intravenous administration may result in respiratory depression, airway obstruction and/or arrest. The potential for these latter effects is increased in debilitated patients, those receiving concomitant medications capable of depressing the CNS, and patients without an endotracheal tube but undergoing a procedure involving the upper airway such as endoscopy or dental (see BOXED WARNING and WARNINGS).

Reactions such as agitation, involuntary movements, hyperactivity and combativeness have been reported in adult and pediatric patients. Should such reactions occur, caution should be exercised before continuing administration of midazolam HCl (see WARNINGS).

Midazolam HCl should only be administered IM or IV (see WARNINGS).

Care should be taken to avoid intra-arterial injection or extravasation (see WARNINGS).

Midazolam HCl injection may be mixed in the same syringe with the following frequently used premedications:
Morphine sulfate
Meperidine
Atropine sulfate
Scopolamine

Midazolam HCl, at a concentration of 0.5 mg/ml, is compatible with 5% dextrose in water and 0.9% sodium chloride for up to 24 hours and with lactated Ringer's solution for up to 4 hours. Both the 1 mg/ml and 5 mg/ml formulations of midazolam HCl may be diluted with 0.9% sodium chloride or 5% dextrose in water.

MONITORING

Patient response to sedative agents, and resultant respiratory status, is variable. Regardless of the intended level of sedation or route of administration, sedation is a continuum; a patient may move easily from light to deep sedation, with potential loss of protective reflexes. This is especially true in pediatric patients. Sedative doses should be individually titrated, taking into account patient age, clinical status and concomitant use of other CNS depressants. Continuous monitoring of respiratory and cardiac function is required (*i.e.,* pulse oximetry).

Adults and Pediatrics

Sedation guidelines recommend a careful presedation history to determine how a patient's underlying medical conditions or concomitant medications might affect their response to sedation/analgesia as well as a physical examination including a focused examination of the airway for abnormalities. Further recommendations include appropriate presedation fasting.

Titration to effect with multiple small doses is essential for safe administration. It should be noted that adequate time to achieve peak central nervous system effect (3-5 minutes) for midazolam should be allowed between doses to minimize the potential for oversedation. Sufficient time must elapse between doses of concomitant sedative medications to allow the effect of each dose to be assessed before subsequent drug administration. This is an important consideration for all patients who receive intravenous midazolam HCl.

Immediate availability of resuscitative drugs and *age- and size-appropriate* equipment and personnel trained in their use and skilled in airway management should be assured (see WARNINGS).

Pediatrics

For deeply sedated pediatric patients a dedicated individual, other than the practitioner performing the procedure, should monitor the patient throughout the procedure.

Intravenous access is not thought to be necessary for all pediatric patients sedated for a diagnostic or therapeutic procedure because in some cases the difficulty of gaining IV access would defeat the purpose of sedating the child; rather, emphasis should be placed upon having the intravenous equipment available and a practitioner skilled in establishing vascular access in pediatric patients immediately available.

USUAL ADULT DOSE — INTRAMUSCULAR ADMINISTRATION

Preoperative Sedation/Anxiolysis/Amnesia

For preoperative sedation/anxiolysis/amnesia (induction of sleepiness or drowsiness and relief of apprehension and to impair memory of perioperative events).

Note: For intramuscular use, midazolam HCl should be injected deep in a large muscle mass.

Use

The recommended premedication dose of midazolam HCl for good risk (ASA Physical Status I & II) adult patients below the age of 60 years is 0.07-0.08 mg/kg IM (approximately 5 mg IM) administered up to 1 hour before surgery.

The dose must be individualized and reduced when IM midazolam HCl is administered to patients with chronic obstructive pulmonary disease, other higher risk surgical patients, patients 60 or more years of age, and patients who have received concomitant narcotics or other CNS depressants (see ADVERSE REACTIONS). In a study of patients 60 years or older, who did not receive concomitant administration of narcotics, 2-3 mg (0.02-0.05 mg/kg) of midazolam HCl produced adequate sedation during the preoperative period. The dose of 1 mg IM midazolam HCl may suffice for some older patients if the anticipated intensity and duration of sedation is less critical. As with any potential respiratory depressant, these patients require observation for signs of cardiorespiratory depression after receiving IM midazolam HCl.

Onset is within 15 minutes, peaking at 30-60 minutes. It can be administered concomitantly with atropine sulfate or scopolamine hydrochloride and reduced doses of narcotics.

USUAL ADULT DOSE — INTRAVENOUS ADMINISTRATION

Sedation/Anxiolysis/Amnesia for Procedures

See INDICATIONS AND USAGE.

Narcotic premedication results in less variability in patient response and a reduction in dosage of midazolam HCl. For peroral procedures, the use of an appropriate topical anesthetic is recommended. For bronchoscopic procedures, the use of narcotic premedication is recommended.

Note: Midazolam HCl 1 mg/ml formulation is recommended for sedation/anxiolysis/amnesia for procedures to facilitate slower injection. Both the 1 mg/ml and the 5 mg/ml formulations may be diluted with 0.9% sodium chloride or 5% dextrose in water.

Use

When used for sedation/anxiolysis/amnesia for a procedure, dosage must be individualized and titrated. Midazolam HCl should always be titrated slowly; administer over at least 2 minutes and allow an additional 2 or more minutes to fully evaluate the sedative effect. Individual response will vary with age, physical status and concomitant medications, but may also vary independent of these factors (see WARNINGS concerning cardiac/respiratory arrest/airway obstruction/hypoventilation).

Healthy Adults Below the Age of 60

Titrate slowly to the desired effect (*e.g.,* the initiation of slurred speech). Some patients may respond to as little as 1 mg. No more than 2.5 mg should be given over a period of at least 2 minutes. Wait an additional 2 or more minutes to fully evaluate the sedative effect. If further titration is necessary, continue to titrate, using small increments, to the appropriate level of sedation. Wait an additional 2 or more minutes after each increment to fully evaluate the sedative effect. A total dose greater than 5 mg is not usually necessary to reach the desired endpoint.

If narcotic premedication or other CNS depressants are used, patients will require approximately 30% less midazolam HCl than unpremedicated patients.

Patients Age 60 or Older, and Debilitated or Chronically Ill Patients

Because the danger of hypoventilation, airway obstruction, or apnea is greater in elderly patients and those with chronic disease states or decreased pulmonary reserve, and because the peak effect may take longer in these patients, increments should be smaller and the rate of injection slower.

Titrate slowly to the desired effect (*e.g.,* the initiation of slurred speech). Some patients may respond to as little as 1 mg. No more than 1.5 mg should be given over a period of no less than 2 minutes. Wait an additional 2 or more minutes to fully evaluate the sedative effect. If additional titration is necessary, it should be given at a rate of no more than 1 mg

M

over a period of 2 minutes, waiting an additional 2 or more minutes each time to fully evaluate the sedative effect. Total doses greater than 3.5 mg are not usually necessary.

If concomitant CNS depressant premedications are used in these patients, they will require at least 50% less midazolam HCl than healthy young unpremedicated patients.

Maintenance Dose

Additional doses to maintain the desired level of sedation may be given in increments of 25% of the dose used to first reach the sedative endpoint, but again only by slow titration, especially in the elderly and chronically ill or debilitated patient. These additional doses should be given only after a thorough clinical evaluation clearly indicates the need for additional sedation.

Induction of Anesthesia

For induction of general anesthesia, before administration of other anesthetic agents.

Note: Injectable midazolam HCl can also be used during maintenance of anesthesia, for surgical procedures, as a component of balanced anesthesia. Effective narcotic premedication is especially recommended in such cases.

Use

Individual response to the drug is variable, particularly when a narcotic premedication is not used. The dosage should be titrated to the desired effect according to the patient's age and clinical status.

When midazolam HCl is used before other intravenous agents for induction of anesthesia, the initial dose of each agent may be significantly reduced, at times to as low as 25% of the usual initial dose of the individual agents.

Unpremedicated Patients

In the absence of premedication, an average adult under the age of 55 years will usually require an initial dose of 0.3-0.35 mg/kg for induction, administered over 20-30 seconds and allowing 2 minutes for effect. If needed to complete induction, increments of approximately 25% of the patient's initial dose may be used; induction may instead be completed with inhalational anesthetics. In resistant cases, up to 0.6 mg/kg total dose may be used for induction, but such larger doses may prolong recovery.

Unpremedicated patients over the age of 55 years usually require less midazolam HCl for induction; an initial dose of 0.3 mg/kg is recommended. Unpremedicated patients with severe systemic disease or other debilitation usually require less midazolam HCl for induction. An initial dose of 0.2-0.25 mg/kg will usually suffice; in some cases, as little as 0.15 mg/kg may suffice.

Premedicated Patients

When the patient has received sedative or narcotic premedication, particularly narcotic premedication, the range of recommended doses is 0.15-0.35 mg/kg.

In average adults below the age of 55 years, a dose of 0.25 mg/kg, administered over 20-30 seconds and allowing 2 minutes for effect, will usually suffice.

The initial dose of 0.2 mg/kg is recommended for good risk (ASA I & II) surgical patients over the age of 55 years.

In some patients with severe systemic disease or debilitation, as little as 0.15 mg/kg may suffice.

Narcotic premedication frequently used during clinical trials included fentanyl (1.5-2 μg/kg IV, administered 5 minutes before induction), morphine (dosage individualized, up to 0.15 mg/kg IM), and meperidine (dosage individualized, up to 1 mg/kg IM). Sedative premedications were hydroxyzine pamoate (100 mg orally) and sodium secobarbital (200 mg orally). Except for intravenous fentanyl, administered 5 minutes before induction, all other premedications should be administered approximately 1 hour prior to the time anticipated for midazolam HCl induction.

Incremental injections of approximately 25% of the induction dose should be given in response to signs of lightening of anesthesia and repeated as necessary.

USUAL ADULT DOSE — CONTINUOUS INFUSION

Note: For continuous infusion, midazolam HCl 5 mg/ml formulation is recommended diluted to a concentration of 0.5 mg/ml with 0.9% sodium chloride or 5% dextrose in water.

Use

Usual Adult Dose

If a loading dose is necessary to rapidly initiate sedation, 0.01-0.05 mg/kg (approximately 0.5-4.0 mg for a typical adult) may be given slowly or infused over several minutes. This dose may be repeated at 10-15 minute intervals until adequate sedation is achieved. For maintenance of sedation, the usual initial infusion rate is 0.02-0.10 mg/kg/h (1-7 mg/h). Higher loading or maintenance infusion rates may occasionally be required in some patients. The lowest recommended doses should be used in patients with residual effects from anesthetic drugs, or in those concurrently receiving other sedatives or opioids.

Individual response to midazolam HCl is variable. The infusion rate should be titrated to the desired level of sedation, taking into account the patient's age, clinical status and current medications. In general, midazolam HCl should be infused at the lowest rate that produces the desired level of sedation. Assessment of sedation should be performed at regular intervals and the midazolam HCl infusion rate adjusted up or down by 25–50% of the initial infusion rate so as to assure adequate titration of sedation level. Larger adjustments or even a small incremental dose may be necessary if rapid changes in the level of sedation are indicated. In addition, the infusion rate should be decreased by 10–25% every few hours to find the minimum effective infusion rate. Finding the minimum effective infusion rate decreases the potential accumulation of midazolam and provides for the most rapid recovery once the infusion is terminated. Patients who exhibit agitation, hypertension, or tachycardia in response to noxious stimulation, but who are otherwise adequately sedated, may benefit from concurrent administration of an opioid analgesic. Addition of an opioid will generally reduce the minimum effective midazolam HCl infusion rate.

PEDIATRIC PATIENTS

UNLIKE ADULT PATIENTS, PEDIATRIC PATIENTS GENERALLY RECEIVE INCREMENTS OF MIDAZOLAM HCl ON A MG/KG BASIS. As a group, pediatric patients generally require higher dosages of midazolam HCl (mg/kg) than do adults. Younger (less than 6 years) pediatric patients may require higher dosages (mg/kg) than older pediatric patients, and may require close monitoring (see TABLE 1 and TABLE 2). In obese PEDIATRIC PATIENTS, the dose should be calculated based on ideal body weight. When midazolam HCl is given in conjunction with opioids or other sedatives, the potential for respiratory depression, airway obstruction, or hypoventilation is increased. For appropriate patient monitoring see BOXED WARNING, WARNINGS, and DOSAGE AND ADMINISTRATION, Monitoring. The health care practitioner who uses this medication in pediatric patients should be aware of and follow accepted professional guidelines for pediatric sedation appropriate to their situation.

TABLE 1 *Observer's Assessment of Alertness/Sedation (OAA/S)*

Assessment Categories				
Responsiveness	**Speech**	**Facial Expression**	**Eyes**	**Composite Score**
Responds readily to name spoken in normal tone	Normal	Normal	Clear, no ptosis	5 (alert)
Lethargic response to name spoken in normal tone	Mild slowing or thickening	Mild relaxation	Glazed or mild ptosis (less than half the eye)	4
Responds only after name is called loudly and/or repeatedly	Slurring or prominent slowing	Marked relaxation (slack jaw)	Glazed and marked ptosis (half the eye or more)	3
Responds only after mild prodding or shaking	Few recognizable words	—	—	2
Does not respond to mild prodding or shaking	—	—	—	1 (deep sleep)

TABLE 2 *Frequency of Observer's Assessment of Alertness/Sedation Composite Scores in One Study of Children Undergoing Procedures With Intravenous Midazolam for Sedation*

		OAA/S Score				
Age Range (years)	**n**	**1 (Deep Sleep)**	**2**	**3**	**4**	**5 (Alert)**
1–2	16	6 (38%)	4 (25%)	3 (19%)	3 (19%)	0
>2–5	22	9 (41%)	5 (23%)	8 (36%)	0	0
>5–12	34	1 (3%)	6 (18%)	22 (65%)	5 (15%)	0
>12–17	18	0	4 (22%)	14 (78%)	0	0
Total (1–17)	90	16 (18%)	19 (21%)	47 (52%)	8 (9%)	0

Intramuscularly

For sedation/anxiolysis/amnesia prior to anesthesia or for procedures, intramuscular midazolam HCl can be used to sedate pediatric patients to facilitate less traumatic insertion of an intravenous catheter for titration of additional medication.

Usual Pediatric Dose (Non-Neonatal)

Sedation after intramuscular midazolam HCl is age and dose dependent. Higher doses may result in deeper and more prolonged sedation. Doses of 0.1-0.15 mg/kg are usually effective and do not prolong emergence from general anesthesia. For more anxious patients, doses up to 0.5 mg/kg have been used. Although not systematically studied, the total dose usually does not exceed 10 mg. If midazolam HCl is given with an opioid, the initial dose of each must be reduced.

Intravenously by Intermittent Injection

For sedation/anxiolysis/amnesia prior to and during procedures or prior to anesthesia.

Usual Pediatric Dose (Non-Neonatal)

It should be recognized that the depth of sedation/anxiolysis needed for pediatric patients depends on the type of procedure to be performed. For example, simple light sedation/anxiolysis in the preoperative period is quite different from the deep sedation and analgesia required for an endoscopic procedure in a child. For this reason, there is a broad range of dosage. For all pediatric patients, regardless of the indications for sedation/anxiolysis, it is vital to titrate midazolam HCl and other concomitant medications slowly to the desired clinical effect. The initial dose of midazolam HCl should be administered over 2-3 minutes. Since midazolam HCl is water soluble, it takes approximately three times longer than diazepam to achieve peak EEG effects, therefore one must wait an additional 2–3 minutes to fully evaluate the sedative effect before initiating a procedure or repeating a dose. If further sedation is necessary, continue to titrate with small increments until the appropriate level of sedation is achieved. If other medications capable of depressing the CNS are coadministered, the peak effect of those concomitant medications must be considered and the dose of midazolam HCl adjusted. The importance of drug titration to effect is vital to the safe sedation/anxiolysis of the pediatric patient. The total dose of midazolam HCl will depend on patient response, the type and duration of the procedure, as well as the type and dose of concomitant medications.

Pediatric Patients Less Than 6 Months of Age
Limited information is available in non-intubated pediatric patients less than 6 months of age. It is uncertain when the patient transfers from neonatal physiology to pediatric physiology, therefore the dosing recommendations are unclear. Pediatric patients less than 6 months of age are particularly vulnerable to airway obstruction and hypoventilation, therefore titration with small increments to clinical effect and careful monitoring are essential.

Pediatric Patients 6 Months to 5 Years of Age
Initial dose 0.05-0.1 mg/kg; total dose up to 0.6 mg/kg may be necessary to reach the desired endpoint but usually does not exceed 6 mg. Prolonged sedation and risk of hypoventilation may be associated with the higher doses.

Pediatric Patients 6-12 Years of Age
Initial dose 0.025-0.05 mg/kg; total dose up to 0.4 mg/kg may be needed to reach the desired endpoint but usually does not exceed 10 mg. Prolonged sedation and risk of hypoventilation may be associated with the higher doses.

Pediatric Patients 12-16 Years of Age
Should be dosed as adults. Prolonged sedation may be associated with higher doses; some patients in this age range will require higher than recommended adult doses but the total dose usually does not exceed 10 mg.

The dose of midazolam HCl must be reduced in patients premedicated with opioid or other sedative agents including midazolam HCl. Higher risk or debilitated patients may require lower dosages whether or not concomitant sedating medications have been administered (see WARNINGS).

Continuous Intravenous Infusion
For sedation/anxiolysis/amnesia in critical care settings.

Usual Pediatric Dose (Non-Neonatal)
To initiate sedation, an intravenous loading dose of 0.05-0.2 mg/kg administered over at least 2-3 minutes can be used to establish the desired clinical effect IN PATIENTS WHOSE TRACHEA IS INTUBATED. (Midazolam HCl should not be administered as a rapid intravenous dose.) This loading dose may be followed by a continuous intravenous infusion to maintain the effect. An infusion of midazolam HCl has been used in patients whose trachea was intubated but who were allowed to breathe spontaneously. Assisted ventilation is recommended for pediatric patients who are receiving other central nervous system depressant medications such as opioids. Based on pharmacokinetic parameters and reported clinical experience, continuous intravenous infusions of midazolam HCl should be initiated at a rate of 0.06-0.12 mg/kg/h (1-2 μg/kg/min). The rate of infusion can be increased or decreased (generally by 25% of the initial or subsequent infusion rate) as required, or supplemental intravenous doses of midazolam HCl can be administered to increase or maintain the desired effect. Frequent assessment at regular intervals using standard pain/sedation scales is recommended. Drug elimination may be delayed in patients receiving erythromycin and/or other P450 3A4 enzyme inhibitors (see DRUG INTERACTIONS) and in patients with liver dysfunction, low cardiac output (especially those requiring inotropic support), and in neonates. Hypotension may be observed in patients who are critically ill, particularly those receiving opioids and/or when midazolam HCl is rapidly administered.

When initiating an infusion with midazolam HCl in hemodynamically compromised patients, the usual loading dose of midazolam HCl should be titrated in small increments and the patient monitored for hemodynamic instability (*e.g.,* hypotension). These patients are also vulnerable to the respiratory depressant effects of midazolam HCl and require careful monitoring of respiratory rate and oxygen saturation.

Continuous Intravenous Infusion
For sedation in critical care settings.

Usual Neonatal Dose
Based on pharmacokinetic parameters and reported clinical experience in preterm and term neonates WHOSE TRACHEA WAS INTUBATED, continuous intravenous infusions of midazolam HCl should be initiated at a rate of 0.03 mg/kg/h (0.5 μg/kg/min) in neonates <32 weeks and 0.06 mg/kg/h (1 μg/kg/min) in neonates >32 weeks. Intravenous loading doses should not be used in neonates, rather the infusion may be run more rapidly for the first several hours to establish therapeutic plasma levels. The rate of infusion should be carefully and frequently reassessed, particularly after the first 24 hours so as to administer the lowest possible effective dose and reduce the potential for drug accumulation. This is particularly important because of the potential for adverse effects related to metabolism of the benzyl alcohol (see WARNINGS, Usage in Preterm Infants and Neonates). Hypotension may be observed in patients who are critically ill and in preterm and term infants, particularly those receiving fentanyl and/or when midazolam HCl is administered rapidly. Due to an increased risk of apnea, extreme caution is advised when sedating preterm and former preterm patients whose trachea is not intubated.

Note: Parenteral drug products should be inspected visually for particulate matter and discoloration prior to administration, whenever solution and container permit.

HOW SUPPLIED

Package configurations containing midazolam HCl equivalent to **5 mg** midazolam/**ml**:

- ***1 ml Vials:*** (5 mg)
- ***2 ml Vials:*** (10 mg)
- ***5 ml Vials:*** (25 mg)
- ***10 ml Vials:*** (50 mg)
- ***2 ml Tel-E-Ject Disposable Syringes:*** (10 mg)

Package configurations containing midazolam HCl equivalent to **1 mg** midazolam/**ml**:

- ***2 ml vials:*** (2 mg)
- ***5 ml vials:*** (5 mg)
- ***10 ml vials:*** (10 mg)

Storage: Store at 59–86°F (15–30°C).

ORAL

WARNING

Midazolam HCl syrup has been associated with respiratory depression and respiratory arrest, especially when used for sedation in noncritical care settings. Midazolam HCl syrup has been associated with reports of respiratory depression, airway obstruction, desaturation, hypoxia, and apnea, most often when used concomitantly with other central nervous system depressants (*e.g.,* opioids). Midazolam HCl syrup should be used only in hospital or ambulatory care settings, including physicians' and dentists' offices, THAT CAN PROVIDE FOR CONTINUOUS MONITORING OF RESPIRATORY AND CARDIAC FUNCTION. IMMEDIATE AVAILABILITY OF RESUSCITATIVE DRUGS AND AGE- AND SIZE-APPROPRIATE EQUIPMENT FOR VENTILATION AND INTUBATION, AND PERSONNEL TRAINED IN THEIR USE AND SKILLED IN AIRWAY MANAGEMENT SHOULD BE ASSURED (see WARNINGS). For deeply sedated patients, a dedicated individual, other than the practitioner performing the procedure, should monitor the patient throughout the procedure.

DESCRIPTION

Midazolam is a benzodiazepine available as Versed syrup for oral administration. Midazolam, a white to light yellow crystalline compound, is insoluble in water, but can be solubilized in aqueous solutions by formation of the hydrochloride salt *in situ* under acidic conditions. Chemically, midazolam HCl is 8-chloro-6-(2-fluorophenyl)-1-methyl-4*H*-imidazo[1,5-a][1,4]benzodiazepine hydrochloride. Midazolam hydrochloride has the empirical formula $C_{18}H_{13}ClFN_3{\cdot}HCl$, and a calculated molecular weight of 362.25.

Each ml of the syrup contains midazolam hydrochloride equivalent to 2 mg midazolam compounded with sorbitol, glycerin, citric acid anhydrous, sodium citrate, sodium benzoate, sodium saccharin, edetate di sodium, FD&C red no. 33, artificial cough syrup flavor, artificial bitterness modifier and water; the pH is adjusted to approximately 3 with hydrochloric acid.

Under the acidic conditions required to solubilize midazolam in the syrup, midazolam is present as an equilibrium mixture of the closed ring form and an open-ring structure formed by the acid-catalyzed ring opening of the 4,5-double bond of the diazepine ring. The amount of open-ring form is dependent upon the pH of the solution. At the specified pH of the syrup, the solution may contain up to about 40% of the open-ring compound. At the physiologic conditions under which the product is absorbed (pH of 5-8) into the systemic circulation, any open-ring form present reverts to the physiologically active, lipophilic, closed-ring form (midazolam) and is absorbed as such.

CLINICAL PHARMACOLOGY

Midazolam is a short-acting benzodiazepine central nervous system (CNS) depressant.

PHARMACODYNAMICS

Pharmacodynamic properties of midazolam and its metabolites, which are similar to those of other benzodiazepines, include sedative, anxiolytic, amnesic and hypnotic activities. Benzodia zepine pharmacologic effects appear to result from reversible interactions with the gamma-amino butyric acid (GABA) benzodiazepine receptor in the CNS, the major inhibitory neurotransmitter in the central nervous system. The action of midazolam is readily reversed by the benzodiazepine receptor antagonist, flumazenil.

Data from published reports of studies in pediatric patients clearly demonstrate that oral midazolam provides safe and effective sedation and anxiolysis prior to surgical procedures that require anesthesia as well as before other procedures that require sedation but may not require anesthesia. The most commonly reported effective doses range from 0.25-1.0 mg/kg in children (6 months to <16 years). The single most commonly reported effective dose is 0.5 mg/kg. Time to onset of effect is most frequently reported as 10-20 minutes.

The effects of midazolam on the CNS are dependent on the dose administered, the route of administration, and the presence or absence of other medications.

Following premedication with oral midazolam, time to recovery has been assessed in pediatric patients using various measures, such as time to eye opening, time to extubation, time in the recovery room, and time to discharge from the hospital. Most placebo-controlled trials (8 total) have shown little effect of oral midazolam on recovery time from general anesthesia; however, a number of other placebo-controlled studies (5 total) have demonstrated some prolongation in recovery time following premedication with oral midazolam. Prolonged recovery may be related to duration of the surgical procedure and/or use of other medications with central nervous system depressant properties.

Partial or complete impairment of recall following oral midazolam has been demonstrated in several studies. Amnesia for the surgical experience was greater after oral midazolam when used as a premedicant than after placebo and was generally considered a benefit. In one study, 69% of midazolam patients did not remember mask application versus 6% of placebo patients.

Episodes of oxygen desaturation, respiratory depression, apnea, and airway obstruction have been reported in <1% of pediatric patients following premedication (*e.g.,* sedation prior to induction of anesthesia) with midazolam HCl syrup; the potential for such adverse events are markedly increased when oral midazolam is combined with other central nervous system depressing agents and in patients with abnormal airway anatomy, patients with cyanotic congenital heart disease, or patients with sepsis or severe pulmonary disease (see WARNINGS).

Concomitant use of barbiturates or other central nervous system depressants may increase the risk of hypoventilation, airway obstruction, desaturation or apnea, and may contribute to profound and/or prolonged drug effect. In one study of pediatric patients undergoing elective repair of congenital cardiac defects, premedication regimens (oral dose of 0.75 mg/kg midazolam or IM morphine plus scopolamine) increased transcutaneous carbon dioxide ($PtcCO_2$), decreased SpO_2 (as measured by pulse oximetry), and decreased respiratory rates preferentially in patients with pulmonary hypertension. This suggests that hypercarbia or hypoxia following premedication might pose a risk to children with congenital heart disease and pulmonary hypertension. In a study of an adult population 65 years and older, the pre-induction administration of oral midazolam 7.5 mg resulted in a 60% incidence of hypox-

M

emia (paO2 <90% for over 30 seconds) at some time during the operative procedure versus 15% for the nonpremedicated group.

PHARMACOKINETICS

Absorption

Midazolam is rapidly absorbed after oral administration and is subject to substantial intestinal and hepatic first-pass metabolism. The pharmacokinetics of midazolam and its major metabolite, alpha-hydroxymidazolam, and the absolute bioavailability of midazolam HCl syrup were studied in pediatric patients of different ages (6 months to <16 years old) over a 0.25-1.0 mg/kg dose range. Pharmacokinetic parameters from this study are presented in TABLE 3. The mean T_{max} values across dose groups (0.25, 0.5, and 1.0 mg/kg) range from 0.17-2.65 hours. Midazolam exhibits linear pharmacokinetics between oral doses of 0.25-1.0 mg/kg (up to a maximum dose of 40 mg) across the age groups ranging from 6 months to <16 years. Linearity was also demonstrated across the doses within the age group of 2 years to <12 years having 18 patients at each of the 3 doses. The absolute bioavailability of the midazolam syrup in pediatric patients is about 36%, which is not affected by pediatric age or weight. The AUC(0-∞) ratio of alpha-hydroxymidazolam to midazolam for the oral dose in pediatric patients is higher than for an IV dose (0.38-0.75 vs 0.21-0.39 across the age group of 6 months to <16 years), and the AUC(0-∞) ratio of alpha-hydroxymidazolam to midazolam for the oral dose is higher in pediatric patients than in adults (0.38-0.75 vs 0.40-0.56).

Food effect has not been tested using midazolam HCl syrup. When a 15 mg oral tablet of midazolam was administered with food to adults, the absorption and disposition of midazolam was not affected. Feeding is generally contraindicated prior to sedation of pediatric patients for procedures.

TABLE 3 *Pharmacokinetics of Midazolam Following Single Dose Administration of Midazolam HCl Syrup*

Number of Subjects	Dose (mg/kg)	T_{max} (h)	C_{max} (ng/ml)	T½ (h)	AUC(0-∞) (ng·h/ml)
		6 Months to <2 Years Old			
1	0.25	0.17	28.0	5.82	67.6
1	0.50	0.35	66.0	2.22	152
1	1.00	0.17	61.2	2.97	224
		2 to <12 Years Old			
18	0.25	0.72 ± 0.44	63.0 ± 30.0	3.16 ± 1.50	138 ± 89.5
18	0.50	0.95 ± 0.53	126 ± 75.8	2.71 ± 1.09	306 ± 196
18	1.00	0.88 ± 0.99	201 ± 101	2.37 ± 0.96	743 ± 642
		12 to <16 Years Old			
4	0.25	2.09 ± 1.35	29.1 ± 8.2	6.83 ± 3.84	155 ± 84.6
4	0.50	2.65 ± 1.58	118 ± 81.2	4.35 ± 3.31	821 ± 568
2	1.00	0.55 ± 0.28	191 ± 47.4	2.51 ± 0.18	566 ± 15.7

M

Distribution

The extent of plasma protein binding of midazolam is moderately high and concentration independent. In adults and pediatric patients older than 1 year, midazolam is approximately 97% bound to plasma protein, principally albumin. In healthy volunteers, alpha-hydroxymidazolam is bound to the extent of 89%. In pediatric patients (6 months to <16 years) receiving 0.15 mg/kg IV midazolam, the mean steady-state volume of distribution ranged from 1.24-2.02 L/kg.

Metabolism

Midazolam is primarily metabolized in the liver and gut by human cytochrome P450 3A4 (CYP3A4) to its pharmacologic active metabolite, alpha-hydroxymidazolam, followed by glucuronidation of the alpha-hydroxyl metabolite which is present in unconjugated and conjugated forms in human plasma. The alpha-hydroxymidazolam glucuronide is then excreted in urine. In a study in which adult volunteers were administered intravenous midazolam (0.1 mg/kg) and alpha-hydroxymidazolam (0.15 mg/kg), the pharmacodynamic parameter values of the maximum effect (E_{max}) and concentration eliciting half-maximal effect (EC_{50}) were similar for both compounds. The effects studied were reaction time and errors in tracing tests. The results indicate that alpha-hydroxymidazolam is equipotent and equally effective as unchanged midazolam on a total plasma concentration basis. After oral or intravenous administration, 63–80% of midazolam is recovered in urine as alpha-hydroxymidazolam glucuronide. No significant amount of parent drug or metabolites is extractable from urine before beta-glucuronidase and sulfatase deconjugation, indicating that the urinary metabolites are excreted mainly as conjugates.

Midazolam is also metabolized to two other minor metabolites: 4-hydroxy metabolite (about 3% of the dose) and 1,4-dihydroxy metabolite (about 1% of the dose) are excreted in small amounts in the urine as conjugates.

Elimination

The mean elimination half-life of midazolam ranged from 2.2-6.8 hours following single oral doses of 0.25, 0.5, and 1.0 mg/kg of midazolam (midazolam HCl syrup). Similar results (ranged from 2.9-4.5 hours) for the mean elimination half-life were observed following IV administration of 0.15 mg/kg of midazolam to pediatric patients (6 months to <16 years old). In the same group of patients receiving the 0.15 mg/kg IV dose, the mean total clearance ranged from 9.3-11.0 ml/min/kg.

Pharmacokinetics—Pharmacodynamics Relationships

The relationship between plasma concentration and sedation and anxiolysis scores of oral midazolam syrup (single oral doses of 0.25, 0.5, or 1.0 mg/kg) was investigated in three age groups of pediatric patients (6 months to <2 years, 2 to <12 years, and 12 to <16 years old). In this study, the patient's sedation scores were recorded at baseline and at 10 minute intervals up to 30 minutes after oral dosing until satisfactory sedation ("drowsy" or "asleep but responsive to mild shaking" or "asleep and not responsive to mild shaking") was achieved. Anxiolysis scores were measured at the time when the patient was separated from his/her parents and at mask induction. The results of the analyses showed that the mean midazolam plasma concentration as well as the mean of midazolam plus alpha-hydroxymidazolam for those patients with a sedation score of 4 (asleep but responsive to mild shaking) is significantly different than the mean concentrations for those patients with a sedation score of 3 (drowsy), which is significantly different than the mean concentrations for patients with a sedation score of 2 (awake/calm). The statistical analysis indicates that the greater the midazolam, or midazolam plus alpha-hydroxymidazolam concentration, the greater the maximum sedation score for pediatric patients. No such trend was observed between anxiolysis scores and the mean midazolam concentration or mean of midazolam plus alpha-hydroxymidazolam concentration; however, anxiolysis is a more variable surrogate measurement of clinical response.

Special Populations

Renal Impairment

Although the pharmacokinetics of intravenous midazolam in adult patients with chronic renal failure differed from those of subjects with normal renal function, there were no alterations in the distribution, elimination, or clearance of unbound drug in the renal failure patients. However, the effects of renal impairment on the active metabolite alpha-hydroxymidazolam are unknown.

Hepatic Dysfunction

Chronic hepatic disease alters the pharmacokinetics of midazolam. Following oral administration of 15 mg of midazolam, C_{max} and bioavailability values were 43% and 100% higher, respectively, in adult patients with hepatic cirrhosis than adult subjects with normal liver function. In the same patients with hepatic cirrhosis, following IV administration of 7.5 mg of midazolam, the clearance of midazolam was reduced by about 40% and the elimination half-life was increased by about 90% compared with subjects with normal liver function. Midazolam should be titrated for the desired effect in patients with chronic hepatic disease.

Congestive Heart Failure

Following oral administration of 7.5 mg of midazolam, elimination half-life values were 43% higher in adult patients with congestive heart failure than in control subjects.

Neonates

Midazolam HCl syrup has not been studied in pediatric patients less than 6 months of age.

Drug-Drug Interactions

See DRUG INTERACTIONS.

Inhibitors of CYP3A4 Isozymes

TABLE 4 summarizes the changes in the C_{max} and AUC of midazolam when drugs known to inhibit CYP3A4 were concurrently administered with oral midazolam in adult subjects.

TABLE 4

Interacting Drug	Adult Doses Studied	% Increase in C_{max} of Oral Midazolam	% Increase in AUC of Oral Midazolam
Erythromycin	500 mg tid	170–171	281–341
Cimetidine	800–1200 mg up to qid in divided doses	6–138	10–102
Diltiazem	60 mg tid	105	275
Fluconazole	200 mg qd	150	250
Grapefruit juice	200 ml	56	52
Itraconazole	100–200 mg qd	80–240	240–980
Ketoconazole	400 mg qd	309	1490
Ranitidine	150 mg bid or tid; 300 mg qd	15–67	9–66
Roxithromycin	300 mg qd	37	47
Verapamil	80 mg tid	97	192

Other drugs known to inhibit the effects of CYP3A4 would be expected to have similar effects on these midazolam pharmacokinetic parameters.

Inducers of CYP3A4 Isozymes

TABLE 5 summarizes the changes in the C_{max} and AUC of midazolam when drugs known to induce CYP3A4 were concurrently administered with oral midazolam in adult subjects. The clinical significance of these changes is unclear.

TABLE 5

Interacting Drug	Adult Doses Studied	% Decrease in C_{max} of Oral Midazolam	% Decrease in AUC of Oral Midazolam
Carbamazepine	Therapeutic doses	93	94
Phenytoin	Therapeutic doses	93	94
Rifampin	500 mg/day	94	96

Although not tested, phenobarbital, rifabutin and other drugs known to induce the effects of CYP3A4 would be expected to have similar effects on these midazolam pharmacokinetic parameters.

Drugs that did not affect midazolam pharmacokinetics are presented in TABLE 6.

INDICATIONS AND USAGE

Midazolam HCl syrup is indicated for use in pediatric patients for sedation, anxiolysis and amnesia prior to diagnostic, therapeutic or endoscopic procedures or before induction of anesthesia.

Midazolam HCl syrup is intended for use in monitored settings only and not for chronic or home use (see WARNINGS). **MIDAZOLAM HCl SYRUP MUST BE USED AS SPECIFIED IN THE LABEL.**

TABLE 6

Interacting Drug	Adult Doses Studies
Azithromycin	500 mg/day
Magnesium	Not available
Nitrendipine	20 mg
Terbinafine	200 mg/day

Midazolam is associated with a high incidence of partial or complete impairment of recall for the next several hours (see CLINICAL PHARMACOLOGY).

NON-FDA APPROVED INDICATIONS

Midazolam has also been used to achieve a variety of clinical objectives including decreased agitation in ventilator-dependent patients. In addition, midazolam has been used in the treatment of insomnia and status epilepticus.

CONTRAINDICATIONS

Midazolam HCl syrup is contraindicated in patients with a known hypersensitivity to the drug or allergies to cherries or formulation excipients. Benzodiazepines are contraindicated in patients with acute narrow-angle glaucoma. Benzodiazepines may be used in patients with open-angle glaucoma only if they are receiving appropriate therapy. Measurements of intraocular pressure in patients without eye disease show a moderate lowering following induction of general anesthesia with injectable midazolam HCl; patients with glaucoma have not been studied.

WARNINGS

Serious respiratory adverse events have occurred after administration of oral midazolam HCl, most often when midazolam HCl was used in combination with other central nervous system depressants. These adverse events have included respiratory depression, airway obstruction, oxygen desaturation, apnea, and rarely, respiratory and/or cardiac arrest (see BOXED WARNING). When oral midazolam is administered as the sole agent at recommended doses respiratory depression, airway obstruction, oxygen desaturation, and apnea occur infrequently (see DOSAGE AND ADMINISTRATION).

Prior to the administration of midazolam HCl in any dose, the immediate availability of oxygen, resuscitative drugs, age- and size-appropriate equipment for bag/valve/mask ventilation and intubation, and skilled personnel for the maintenance of a patent airway and support of ventilation should be ensured. Midazolam HCl syrup must never be used without individualization of dosage, particularly when used with other medications capable of producing central nervous system depression.

Midazolam HCl syrup should be used only in hospital or ambulatory care settings, including physicians' and dentists' offices, that are equipped to provide continuous monitoring of respiratory and cardiac function. Midazolam HCl syrup must only be administered to patients if they will be monitored by direct visual observation by a health care professional. If midazolam HCl syrup will be administered in combination with other anesthetic drugs or drugs which depress the central nervous system, patients must be monitored by persons specifically trained in the use of these drugs and, in particular, in the management of respiratory effects of these drugs, including respiratory and cardiac resuscitation of patients in the age group being treated.

For deeply sedated patients, a dedicated individual whose sole responsibility is to observe the patient, other than the practitioner performing the procedure, should monitor the patient throughout the procedure.

Patients should be continuously monitored for early signs of hypoventilation, airway obstruction, or apnea with means for detection readily available (*e.g.*, pulse oximetry). Hypoventilation, airway obstruction, and apnea can lead to hypoxia and/or cardiac arrest unless effective countermeasures are taken immediately. The immediate availability of specific reversal agents (flumazenil) is highly recommended. Vital signs should continue to be monitored during the recovery period. Because midazolam HCl can depress respiration (see CLINICAL PHARMACOLOGY), especially when used concomitantly with opioid agonists and other sedatives (see DOSAGE AND ADMINISTRATION), it should be used for sedation/anxiolysis/amnesia only in the presence of personnel skilled in early detection of hypoventilation, maintaining a patent airway, and supporting ventilation.

Episodes of oxygen desaturation, respiratory depression, apnea, and airway obstruction have been occasionally reported following premedication (sedation prior to induction of anesthesia) with oral midazolam; such events are markedly increased when oral midazolam is combined with other central nervous system depressing agents and in patients with abnormal airway anatomy, patients with cyanotic congenital heart disease, or patients with sepsis or severe pulmonary disease.

Reactions such as agitation, involuntary movements (including tonic/clonic movements and muscle tremor), hyperactivity and combativeness have been reported in both adult and pediatric patients. Consideration should be given to the possibility of paradoxical reaction. Should such reactions occur, the response to each dose of midazolam HCl and all other drugs, including local anesthetics, should be evaluated before proceeding. Reversal of such responses with flumazenil has been reported in pediatric and adult patients.

Concomitant use of barbiturates, alcohol or other central nervous system depressants may increase the risk of hypoventilation, airway obstruction, desaturation, or apnea and may contribute to profound and/or prolonged drug effect. Narcotic premedication also depresses the ventilatory response to carbon dioxide stimulation.

Coadministration of oral midazolam in patients who are taking ketoconazole and itraconazole has been shown to result in large increases in C_{max} and AUC of midazolam due to a decrease in plasma clearance of midazolam (see CLINICAL PHARMACOLOGY, Pharmacokinetics, Special Populations, Drug-Drug Interactions and PRECAUTIONS). Due to the potential for intense and prolonged sedation and respiratory depression, midazolam HCl syrup should only be coadministered with these medications if absolutely necessary and with appropriate equipment and personnel available to respond to respiratory insufficiency.

Higher risk pediatric surgical patients may require lower doses, whether or not concomitant sedating medications have been administered. Pediatric patients with cardiac or respiratory compromise may be unusually sensitive to the respiratory depressant effect of midazolam HCl. Pediatric patients undergoing procedures involving the upper airway such as upper endoscopy or dental care, are particularly vulnerable to episodes of desaturation and hypoventilation due to partial airway obstruction. Patients with chronic renal failure and patients with congestive heart failure eliminate midazolam more slowly (see CLINICAL PHARMACOLOGY).

The decision as to when patients who have received midazolam HCl syrup, particularly on an outpatient basis, may again engage in activities requiring complete mental alertness, operate hazardous machinery or drive a motor vehicle must be individualized. Gross tests of recovery from the effects of midazolam HCl syrup (see CLINICAL PHARMACOLOGY) cannot be relied upon to predict reaction time under stress. It is recommended that no patient operate hazardous machinery or a motor vehicle until the effects of the drug, such as drowsiness, have subsided or until 1 full day after anesthesia and surgery, whichever is longer. Particular care should be taken to assure safe ambulation.

USE IN PREGNANCY

Although midazolam HCl syrup has not been studied in pregnant patients, an increased risk of congenital malformations associated with the use of benzodiazepine drugs (diazepam and chlordiazepoxide) have been suggested in several studies. If this drug is used during pregnancy, the patient should be apprised of the potential hazard to the fetus.

USAGE IN PRETERM INFANTS AND NEONATES

Midazolam HCl syrup has not been studied in patients less than 6 months of age.

PRECAUTIONS

USE WITH OTHER CNS DEPRESSANTS

The efficacy and safety of midazolam HCl in clinical use are functions of the dose administered, the clinical status of the individual patient, and the use of concomitant medications capable of depressing the CNS. Anticipated effects may range from mild sedation to deep levels of sedation with a potential loss of protective reflexes, particularly when coadministered with anesthetic agents or other CNS depressants. Care must be taken to individualize the dose of midazolam HCl based on the patient's age, underlying medical/surgical conditions, concomitant medications, and to have the personnel, age- and size-appropriate equipment and facilities available for monitoring and intervention. Practitioners administering midazolam HCl must have the skills necessary to manage reasonably foreseeable adverse effects, particularly skills in airway management.

USE WITH INHIBITORS OF CYP3A4 ISOZYMES

Oral midazolam should be used with caution in patients treated with drugs known to inhibit CYP3A4 because inhibition of metabolism may lead to more intense and prolonged sedation (see CLINICAL PHARMACOLOGY, Pharmacokinetics, Special Populations, Drug-Drug Interactions). Patients being treated with medications known to inhibit CYP3A4 isozymes should be treated with lower than recommended doses of midazolam HCl syrup and the clinician should expect a more intense and prolonged effect.

INFORMATION FOR THE PATIENT

To assure safe and effective use of midazolam HCl syrup, the following information and instructions should be communicated to the patient when appropriate:

1. Inform your physician about any alcohol consumption and medicine you are now taking, especially blood pressure medication and antibiotics, including drugs you buy without a prescription. Alcohol has an increased effect when consumed with benzodiazepines; therefore, caution should be exercised regarding simultaneous ingestion of alcohol during benzodiazepine treatment.
2. Inform your physician if you are pregnant or are planning to become pregnant.
3. Inform your physician if you are nursing.
4. Patients should be informed of the pharmacological effects of midazolam HCl syrup, such as sedation and amnesia, which in some patients may be profound. The decision as to when patients who have received midazolam HCl syrup, particularly on an outpatient basis, may again engage in activities requiring complete mental alertness, operate hazardous machinery or drive a motor vehicle must be individualized.
5. Midazolam HCl syrup should not be taken in conjunction with grapefruit juice.
6. For pediatric patients, particular care should be taken to assure safe ambulation.

DRUG/LABORATORY TEST INTERACTIONS

Midazolam has not been shown to interfere with results obtained in clinical laboratory tests.

CARCINOGENESIS, MUTAGENESIS, AND IMPAIRMENT OF FERTILITY

Carcinogenesis

Midazolam maleate was administered with diet in mice and rats for 2 years at dosages of 1, 9, and 80 mg/kg/day. In female mice in the highest dose (10 times the highest oral dose of 1.0 mg/kg for a pediatric patient, on a mg/m^2 basis) group there was a marked increase in the incidence of hepatic tumors. In high-dose (19 times the pediatric dose) male rats there was a small but statistically significant increase in benign thyroid follicular cell tumors. Dosages of 9 mg/kg/day of midazolam maleate (1-2 times the pediatric dose) did not increase the incidence of tumors in mice or rats. The pathogenesis of induction of these tumors is not known. These tumors were found after chronic administration, whereas human use will ordinarily be single or intermittent doses.

Mutagenesis

Midazolam did not have mutagenic activity in *Salmonella typhimurium* (5 bacterial strains), Chinese hamster lung cells (V79), human lymphocytes or in the micronucleus test in mice.

Impairment of Fertility

A reproduction study in male and female rats did not show any impairment of fertility at dosages up to 16 mg/kg/day PO (3 times the human dose of 1.0 mg/kg, on a mg/m^2 basis).

M

PREGNANCY, TERATOGENIC EFFECTS, PREGNANCY CATEGORY D

See WARNINGS.

Embryo-fetal development studies, performed with midazolam maleate in mice (at up to 120 mg/kg/day PO, 10 times the human dose of 1.0 mg/kg on a mg/m^2 basis), rats (at up to 4 mg/kg/day IV, 8 times the human IV dose of 5 mg) and rabbits (at up to 100 mg/kg/day PO, 32 times the human oral dose of 1.0 mg/kg on a mg/m^2 basis), did not show evidence of teratogenicity.

Nonteratogenic Effects: Studies in rats showed no adverse effects on reproductive parameters during gestation and lactation. Dosages tested (4 mg/kg IV and 50 mg/kg PO) were approximately 8 times each of the human doses on a mg/m^2 basis.

LABOR AND DELIVERY

In humans, measurable levels of midazolam were found in maternal venous serum, umbilical venous and arterial serum and amniotic fluid, indicating placental transfer of the drug.

The use of midazolam HCl syrup in obstetrics has not been evaluated in clinical studies. Because midazolam is transferred transplacentally and because other benzodiazepines given in the last weeks of pregnancy have resulted in neonatal CNS depression, midazolam HCl syrup is not recommended for obstetrical use.

NURSING MOTHERS

Midazolam is excreted in human milk. Caution should be exercised when midazolam HCl syrup is administered to a nursing woman.

GERIATRIC USE

The safety and efficacy of this product have not been fully studied in geriatric patients. Therefore, there are no available data on a safe dosing regimen. One study in geriatric subjects, using midazolam 7.5 mg as a premedicant prior to general anesthesia, noted a 60% incidence of hypoxemia (pO_2 <90% for over 30 seconds) at sometime during the operative procedure versus 15% for the nonpremedicated group. Until further information is available it is recommended that this product should not be used in geriatric patients.

USE IN PATIENTS WITH HEART DISEASE

Following oral administration of 7.5 mg of midazolam to adult patients with congestive heart failure, the half-life of midazolam was 43% higher than in control subjects. One study suggests that hypercarbia or hypoxia following premedication with oral midazolam might pose a risk to children with congenital heart disease and pulmonary hypertension, although there are no known reports of pulmonary hypertensive crises that had been triggered by premedication. In the study, 22 children were premedicated with oral midazolam (0.75 mg/kg) or IM morphine plus scopolamine prior to elective repair of congenital cardiac defects. Both premedication regimens increased $PtcCO_2$ and decreased SpO_2 and respiratory rates preferentially in patients with pulmonary hypertension.

M

DRUG INTERACTIONS

INHIBITORS OF CYP3A4 ISOZYMES

Caution is advised when midazolam is administered concomitantly with drugs that are known to inhibit the cytochrome P450 3A4 enzyme system (*i.e.*, some drugs in the drug classes of azole antimycotics, protease inhibitors, calcium channel antagonists, and macrolide antibiotics). Drugs such as erythromycin, diltiazem, verapamil, ketoconazole, fluconazole and itraconazole were shown to significantly increase the C_{max} and AUC of orally administered midazolam. These drug interactions may result in increased and prolonged sedation due to a decrease in plasma clearance of midazolam. Although not studied, the potent cytochrome P450 3A4 inhibitors ritonavir and nelfinavir may cause intense and prolonged sedation and respiratory depression due to a decrease in plasma clearance of midazolam. Caution is advised when midazolam HCl syrup is used concomitantly with these drugs. Dose adjustments should be considered and possible prolongation and intensity of effect should be anticipated (see CLINICAL PHARMACOLOGY, Pharmacokinetics, Special Populations, Drug-Drug Interactions).

INDUCERS OF CYP3A4 ISOZYMES

Cytochrome P450 inducers, such as rifampin, carbamazepine, and phenytoin, induce metabolism and caused a markedly decreased C_{max} and AUC of oral midazolam in adult studies. Although clinical studies have not been performed, phenobarbital is expected to have the same effect. Caution is advised when administering midazolam HCl syrup to patients receiving these medications and if necessary dose adjustments should be considered.

CNS DEPRESSANTS

One case was reported of inadequate sedation with chloral hydrate and later with oral midazolam due to a possible interaction with methylphenidate administered chronically in a 2-year-old boy with a history of Williams syndrome. The difficulty in achieving adequate sedation may have been the result of decreased absorption of the sedatives due to both the gastrointestinal effects and stimulant effects of methylphenidate.

The sedative effect of midazolam HCl syrup is accentuated by any concomitantly administered medication which depresses the central nervous system, particularly narcotics (*e.g.*, morphine, meperidine and fentanyl), propofol, ketamine, nitrous oxide, secobarbital and droperidol. Consequently, the dose of midazolam HCl syrup should be adjusted according to the type and amount of concomitant medications administered and the desired clinical response (see DOSAGE AND ADMINISTRATION).

No significant adverse interactions with common premedications (such as atropine, scopolamine, glycopyrrolate, diazepam, hydroxyzine, and other muscle relaxants) or local anesthetics have been observed.

ADVERSE REACTIONS

The distribution of adverse events occurring in patients evaluated in a randomized, double-blind, parallel-group trial are presented in TABLE 7 and TABLE 8 by body system in order of decreasing frequency: for the premedication period (*e.g.*, sedation period prior to induction of anesthesia) alone, see TABLE 7; for over the entire monitoring period including premedication, anesthesia and recovery, see TABLE 8.

The distribution of adverse events occurring during the premedication period, before induction of anesthesia, is presented in TABLE 7. Emesis, which occurred in 31/397 (8%) patients over the entire monitoring period, occurred in 3/397 (0.8%) of patients during the premedication period (from midazolam administration to mask induction). Nausea, which occurred in 14/397 (4%) patients over the entire monitoring period (premedication, anesthesia and recovery), occurred in 2/397 (0.5%) patients during the premedication period.

This distribution of all adverse events occurring in ≥1% of patients over the entire monitoring period are presented in TABLE 8. For the entire monitoring period (premedication, anesthesia and recovery), adverse events were reported by 82/397 (21%) patients who received midazolam overall. The most frequently reported adverse events were emesis occurring in 31/397 (8%) patients and nausea occurring in 14/397 (4%) patients. Most of these gastrointestinal events occurred after the administration of other anesthetic agents.

For the respiratory system overall, adverse events (hypoxia, laryngospasm, rhonchi, coughing, respiratory depression, airway obstruction, upper-airway congestion, shallow respirations), occurred during the entire monitoring period in 31/397 (8%) patients and increased in frequency as dosage was increased: 7/132 (5%) patients in the 0.25 mg/kg dose group, 9/132 (7%) patients in the 0.5 mg/kg dose group, and 15/133 (11%) patients in the 1.0 mg/kg dose group.

Most of the respiratory adverse events occurred during induction, general anesthesia or recovery. One patient (0.25%) experienced a respiratory system adverse event (laryngospasm) during the premedication period. This adverse event occurred precisely at the time of induction. Although many of the respiratory complications occurred in settings of upper airway procedures or concurrently administered opioids, a number of these events occurred outside of these settings as well. In this study, administration of midazolam HCl syrup was generally accompanied by a slight decrease in both systolic and diastolic blood pressures, as well as a slight increase in heart rate.

***TABLE 7** Adverse Events Occurring During the Premedication Period Before Mask Induction in the Randomized, Double-Blind, Parallel-Group Trial*

	Treatment Regimen			Overall
	0.25 mg/kg	0.50 mg/kg	1.0 mg/kg	
	(n=132)	(n=132)	(n=133)	(n=397)
Body System	**No. (%)**	**No. (%)**	**No. (%)**	**No. (%)**
Gastrointestinal System Disorders				
Emesis	1 (0.76%)	1 (0.76%)	1 (0.75%)	3 (0.76%)
Nausea			2 (1.5%)	2 (0.50%)
Respiratory System Disorders				
Laryngospasm			1* (0.75%)	1 (0.25%)
Sneezing/Rhinorrhea			1 (0.75%)	1 (0.25%)
All Body Systems	1 (0.76%)	1 (0.76%)	5 (3.8%)	1 (1.8%)

* This adverse event occurred precisely at the time of induction.

***TABLE 8** Adverse Events (≥1%) From the Randomized, Double-Blind, Parallel-Group Trial on Entire Monitoring Period*

(Premedication, Anesthesia, Recovery)

	Treatment Regimen			Overall
	0.25 mg/kg	0.50 mg/kg	1.0 mg/kg	
	(n=132)	(n=132)	(n=133)	(n=397)
Body System	**No. (%)**	**No. (%)**	**No. (%)**	**No. (%)**
Gastrointestinal System Disorders				
Emesis	11 (8%)	5 (4%)	15 (11%)	31 (8%)
Nausea	6 (5%)	2 (2%)	6 (5%)	14 (4%)
Overall	16 (12%)	8 (6%)	16 (12%)	40 (10%)
Respiratory System Disorders				
Hypoxia	0	5 (4%)	4 (3%)	9 (2%)
Laryngospasm	0	1 (<1%)	5 (4%)	6 (2%)
Respiratory depression	2 (2%)	1 (<1%)	2 (2%)	5 (1%)
Rhonchi	2 (2%)	1 (<1%)	2 (2%)	5 (1%)
Airway obstruction	2 (2%)	2 (2%)	0	4 (1%)
Upper airway congestion	2 (2%)	0	2 (2%)	4 (1%)
Overall	7 (5%)	9 (7%)	15 (11%)	31 (8%)
Psychiatric Disorders				
Agitated	1 (<1%)	2 (2%)	3 (2%)	6 (2%)
Overall	1 (<1%)	3 (2%)	4 (3%)	8 (2%)
Heart Rate, Rhythm Disorders				
Bradycardia	1 (<1%)	3 (2%)	0	4 (1%)
Bigeminy	2 (2%)	0	0	2 (<1%)
Overall	3 (2%)	3 (2%)	1 (<1%)	7 (2%)
Central & Peripheral Nervous System Disorders				
Prolonged sedation	0	0	2 (2%)	2 (<1%)
Overall	2 (2%)	0	3 (2%)	5 (1%)
Skin and Appendages Disorders				
Rash	2 (2%)	0	0	2 (<1%)
Overall	2 (2%)	2 (2%)	0	4 (1%)
All Body Systems	26 (20%)	23 (17%)	33 (25%)	82 (21%)

There were no deaths during the study and no patient withdrew from the study due to adverse events. Serious adverse events (both respiratory disorders) were experienced post-operatively by 2 patients: one case of airway obstruction and desaturation (SpO_2 of 33%) in a patient given midazolam HCl syrup 0.25 mg/kg, and one case of upper airway obstruction and respiratory depression following 0.5 mg/kg. Both patients had received intravenous morphine sulfate (1.5 mg total for both patients).

Other adverse events that have been reported in the literature with the oral administration of midazolam (not necessarily midazolam HCl syrup), are listed below.

The incidence rate for these events was generally <1%.

Respiratory: Apnea, hypercarbia, desaturation, stridor.

Cardiovascular: Decreased systolic and diastolic blood pressure, increased heart rate.

Gastrointestinal: Nausea, vomiting, hiccoughs, gagging, salivation, drooling.

Central Nervous System: Dysphoria, disinhibition, excitation, aggression, mood swings, hallucinations, adverse behavior, agitation, dizziness, confusion, ataxia, vertigo, dysarthria.

Special Senses: Diplopia, strabismus, loss of balance, blurred vision.

DOSAGE AND ADMINISTRATION

Syrup is indicated for use as a single dose (0.25-1.0 mg/kg with a maximum dose of 20 mg) for preprocedural sedation and anxiolysis in pediatric patients. Midazolam HCl syrup is not intended for chronic administration.

MONITORING

Midazolam HCl syrup should only be used in hospital or ambulatory care settings, including physicians' and dentists' offices, that can provide for continuous monitoring of respiratory and cardiac function. Immediate availability of resuscitative drugs and age- and size-appropriate equipment for bag/valve/mask ventilation and intubation, and personnel trained in their use and skilled in airway management should be assured (see WARNINGS). For deeply sedated patients, a dedicated individual whose sole responsibility it is to observe the patient, other than the practitioner performing the procedure, should monitor the patient throughout the procedure. Continuous monitoring of respiratory and cardiac function is required.

Midazolam HCl syrup must be given only to patients if they will be monitored by direct visual observation by a health care professional. Midazolam HCl syrup should only be administered by persons specifically trained in the use of anesthetic drugs and the management of respiratory effects of anesthetic drugs, including respiratory and cardiac resuscitation of patients in the age group being treated.

Patient response to sedative agents, and resultant respiratory status, is variable. Regardless of the intended level of sedation or route of administration, sedation is a continuum; a patient may move easily from light to deep sedation, with potential loss of protective reflexes, particularly when coadministered with anesthetic agents and other CNS depressants. This is especially true in pediatric patients. The health care practitioner who uses this medication in pediatric patients should be aware of and follow accepted professional guidelines for pediatric sedation appropriate to their situation.

Sedation guidelines recommend a careful presedation history to determine how a patient's underlying medical conditions or concomitant medications might affect their response to sedation/analgesia as well as a physical examination including a focused examination of the airway for abnormalities. Further recommendations include appropriate presedation fasting.

Intravenous access is not thought to be necessary for all pediatric patients sedated for a diagnostic or therapeutic procedure because in some cases the difficulty of gaining IV access would defeat the purpose of sedating the child; rather, emphasis should be placed upon having the intravenous equipment available and a practitioner skilled in establishing vascular access in pediatric patients immediately available.

Midazolam HCl syrup must never be used without individualization of dosage, particularly when used with other medications capable of producing CNS depression. Younger (<6 years of age) pediatric patients may require higher dosages (mg/kg) than older pediatric patients, and may require close monitoring.

When midazolam HCl syrup is given in conjunction with opioids or other sedatives, the potential for respiratory depression, airway obstruction, or hypoventilation is increased. For appropriate patient monitoring, see WARNINGS and DOSAGE AND ADMINISTRATION, Monitoring. The health care practitioner who uses this medication in pediatric patients should be aware of and follow accepted professional guidelines for pediatric sedation appropriate to their situation.

The recommended dose for pediatric patients is a single dose of 0.25–0.5 mg/kg, depending on the status of the patient and desired effect, up to a maximum dose of 20 mg. In general, it is recommended that the dose be individualized and modified based on patient age, level of anxiety, and medical need. The younger (6 months to <6 years of age) and less cooperative patients may require a higher than usual dose up to 1.0 mg/kg. A dose of 0.25 mg/kg may suffice for older (6 to <16 years of age) or cooperative patients, especially if the anticipated intensity and duration of sedation is less critical. For all pediatric patients, a dose of 0.25 mg/kg should be considered when midazolam HCl syrup is administered to patients with cardiac or respiratory compromise, other higher risk surgical patients, and patients who have received concomitant narcotics or other CNS depressants. As with any potential respiratory depressant, these patients must be monitored for signs of cardiorespiratory depression after receiving midazolam HCl syrup. In obese pediatric patients, the dose should be calculated based on ideal body weight. Midazolam HCl syrup has not been studied, nor is it intended for chronic use.

DISPOSAL OF MIDAZOLAM HCl SYRUP

The disposal of Schedule IV controlled substances must be consistent with State and Federal Regulations.

HOW SUPPLIED

Versed syrup is supplied as a clear, red to purplish-red, cherry-flavored syrup containing midazolam hydrochloride equivalent to 2 mg of midazolam/ml.

Storage: Store at 25°C (77°F); excursions permitted to 15–30°C (59–86°F).

PRODUCT LISTING - RATED THERAPEUTICALLY EQUIVALENT

Size	Price	Product, Manufacturer	NDC
Solution - Injectable - 1 mg/ml			
2 ml	$4.50	GENERIC, Watson/Schein Pharmaceuticals Inc	00364-2913-47
2 ml x 10	$6.90	GENERIC, Abbott Pharmaceutical	00074-2587-02
2 ml x 10	$7.50	GENERIC, Bedford Laboratories	55390-0137-02
2 ml x 10	$14.00	GENERIC, Baxter Pharmaceutical Products, Inc	10019-0028-02
2 ml x 10	$39.19	GENERIC, Abbott Pharmaceutical	00074-2295-32
2 ml x 10	$55.50	GENERIC, Faulding Pharmaceutical Company	61703-0320-07
2 ml x 25	$35.75	GENERIC, American Pharmaceutical Partners	63323-0411-12
2 ml x 25	$93.75	GENERIC, Esi Lederle Generics	59911-5911-02
5 ml	$9.90	GENERIC, Watson/Schein Pharmaceuticals Inc	00364-2914-31
5 ml x 10	$15.50	GENERIC, Abbott Pharmaceutical	00074-2587-03
5 ml x 10	$35.00	GENERIC, Baxter Pharmaceutical Products, Inc	10019-0028-05
5 ml x 10	$35.50	GENERIC, American Pharmaceutical Partners	63323-0411-05
5 ml x 10	$63.13	GENERIC, Bedford Laboratories	55390-0137-05
5 ml x 10	$82.50	GENERIC, Esi Lederle Generics	59911-5912-02
5 ml x 10	$83.72	GENERIC, Abbott Pharmaceutical	00074-2295-35
5 ml x 10	$121.95	GENERIC, Faulding Pharmaceutical Company	61703-0320-53
10 ml	$17.69	GENERIC, Watson/Schein Pharmaceuticals Inc	00364-2915-33
10 ml x 10	$37.50	GENERIC, Bedford Laboratories	55390-0125-10
10 ml x 10	$43.80	GENERIC, Abbott Pharmaceutical	00074-2587-05
10 ml x 10	$61.20	GENERIC, Baxter Pharmaceutical Products, Inc	10019-0028-10
10 ml x 10	$71.30	GENERIC, American Pharmaceutical Partners	63323-0411-10
10 ml x 10	$147.50	GENERIC, Esi Lederle Generics	59911-5913-02
10 ml x 10	$218.05	GENERIC, Faulding Pharmaceutical Company	61703-0320-32
Solution - Injectable - 5 mg/ml			
1 ml	$9.90	GENERIC, Watson/Schein Pharmaceuticals Inc	00364-2916-45
1 ml x 10	$15.10	GENERIC, Abbott Pharmaceutical	00074-2596-01
1 ml x 10	$35.00	GENERIC, Baxter Pharmaceutical Products, Inc	10019-0027-01
1 ml x 10	$35.80	GENERIC, American Pharmaceutical Partners	63323-0412-01
1 ml x 10	$63.13	GENERIC, Bedford Laboratories	55390-0138-01
1 ml x 10	$83.72	GENERIC, Abbott Pharmaceutical	00074-2296-31
1 ml x 10	$121.95	GENERIC, Faulding Pharmaceutical Company	61703-0321-42
1 ml x 25	$206.25	GENERIC, Esi Lederle Generics	59911-5914-02
2 ml	$11.01	GENERIC, Baxter Pharmaceutical Products, Inc	10019-0127-08
2 ml	$17.67	GENERIC, Watson/Schein Pharmaceuticals Inc	00364-2917-47
2 ml	$21.75	GENERIC, Faulding Pharmaceutical Company	61703-0321-73
2 ml	$22.22	GENERIC, Watson/Schein Pharmaceuticals Inc	00364-2928-89
2 ml	$41.76	GENERIC, Watson/Schein Pharmaceuticals Inc	00364-2918-31
2 ml x 10	$37.50	GENERIC, Bedford Laboratories	55390-0138-02
2 ml x 10	$40.14	GENERIC, Abbott Pharmaceutical	00074-2596-02
2 ml x 10	$63.80	GENERIC, Baxter Pharmaceutical Products, Inc	10019-0027-02
2 ml x 10	$70.50	GENERIC, American Pharmaceutical Partners	63323-0412-02
2 ml x 10	$147.96	GENERIC, Abbott Pharmaceutical	00074-2296-32
2 ml x 10	$163.75	GENERIC, Bedford Laboratories	55390-0141-02
2 ml x 10	$273.95	GENERIC, Faulding Pharmaceutical Company	61703-0321-07
2 ml x 25	$368.75	GENERIC, Esi Lederle Generics	59911-5915-02
5 ml x 10	$107.11	GENERIC, Abbott Pharmaceutical	00074-2596-03
5 ml x 10	$150.00	GENERIC, Baxter Pharmaceutical Products, Inc	10019-0027-05
5 ml x 10	$174.00	GENERIC, American Pharmaceutical Partners	63323-0412-05
5 ml x 10	$315.63	GENERIC, Bedford Laboratories	55390-0126-05
5 ml x 10	$514.85	GENERIC, Faulding Pharmaceutical Company	61703-0321-53
10 ml	$77.79	GENERIC, Watson/Schein Pharmaceuticals Inc	00364-2919-33
10 ml x 10	$135.90	GENERIC, Abbott Pharmaceutical	00074-2596-05
10 ml x 10	$281.30	GENERIC, Baxter Pharmaceutical Products, Inc	10019-0027-10
10 ml x 10	$346.50	GENERIC, American Pharmaceutical Partners	63323-0412-10
10 ml x 10	$606.00	GENERIC, Bedford Laboratories	55390-0126-10
10 ml x 10	$648.10	GENERIC, Esi Lederle Generics	59911-5916-02
10 ml x 10	$959.00	GENERIC, Faulding Pharmaceutical Company	61703-0321-32
Syrup - Oral - 2 mg/ml			
118 ml	$127.15	GENERIC, Roxane Laboratories Inc	00054-3566-99

PRODUCT LISTING - EQUIVALENTS NOT AVAILABLE

Size	Price	Product, Manufacturer	NDC
Solution - Injectable - 1 mg/ml			
2 ml	$7.40	VERSED, Prescript Pharmaceuticals	00247-0295-02
2 ml x 10	$18.80	VERSED, Roche Laboratories	00004-1998-06
5 ml	$13.48	VERSED, Prescript Pharmaceuticals	00247-0295-05
5 ml x 10	$41.20	VERSED, Roche Laboratories	00004-1999-01
10 ml x 10	$235.90	VERSED, Roche Laboratories	00004-2000-06
Solution - Injectable - 5 mg/ml			
1 ml x 10	$41.20	VERSED, Roche Laboratories	00004-1974-01

M

2 ml x 10	$73.70	VERSED, Roche Laboratories	00004-1973-01
2 ml x 10	$296.30	VERSED, Roche Laboratories	00004-1947-01
5 ml x 10	$556.80	VERSED, Roche Laboratories	00004-1975-01
10 ml x 10	$311.16	VERSED, Roche Laboratories	00004-1946-01
Syrup - Oral - 2 mg/ml			
118 ml	$147.16	VERSED, Roche Laboratories	00004-0168-51

Mifepristone *(003083)*

Categories: Abortion; FDA Approved 2000 Sep
Drug Classes: Abortifacients; Stimulants, uterine
Brand Names: **Mifeprex**; RU-486
Foreign Brand Availability: Mifegest (India); Mifegyne (England; France; Israel; Sweden)

WARNING

If mifepristone results in incomplete abortion, surgical intervention may be necessary. Prescribers should determine in advance whether they will provide such care themselves or through other providers. Prescribers should also give patients clear instructions on whom to call and what to do in the event of an emergency following administration of mifepristone.

Prescribers should make sure that patients receive and have an opportunity to discuss the Medication Guide and the Patient Agreement.

DESCRIPTION

Mifeprex tablets each contain 200 mg of mifepristone, a synthetic steroid with antiprogestational effects. The tablets are light yellow in color, cylindrical and biconvex, and are intended for oral administration only. The tablets include the inactive ingredients colloidal silica anhydrous, corn starch, povidone, microcrystalline cellulose, and magnesium stearate.

Mifepristone is a substituted 19-nor steroid compound chemically designated as 11β-[*p*-(Dimethylamino)phenyl]-17β-hydroxy-17-(1-propynyl)estra-4,9-dien-3-one. Its empirical formula is $C_{29}H_{35}NO_2$.

The compound is a yellow powder with a molecular weight of 429.6 and a melting point of 191-196°C. It is very soluble in methanol, chloroform and acetone and poorly soluble in water, hexane and isopropyl ether.

M

CLINICAL PHARMACOLOGY

PHARMACODYNAMIC ACTIVITY

The anti-progestational activity of mifepristone results from competitive interaction with progesterone at progesterone-receptor sites. Based on studies with various oral doses in several animal species (mouse, rat, rabbit and monkey), the compound inhibits the activity of endogenous or exogenous progesterone. The termination of pregnancy results.

Doses of 1 mg/kg or greater of mifepristone have been shown to antagonize the endometrial and myometrial effects of progesterone in women. During pregnancy, the compound sensitizes the myometrium to the contraction-inducing activity of prostaglandins.

Mifepristone also exhibits antiglucocorticoid and weak antiandrogenic activity. The activity of the glucocorticoid dexamethasone in rats was inhibited following doses of 10-25 mg/kg of mifepristone. Doses of 4.5 mg/kg or greater in human beings resulted in a compensatory elevation of adrenocorticotropic hormone (ACTH) and cortisol. Antiandrogenic activity was observed in rats following repeated administration of doses from 10-100 mg/kg.

PHARMACOKINETICS AND METABOLISM

Absorption

Following oral administration of a single dose of 600 mg, mifepristone is rapidly absorbed, with a peak plasma concentration of 1.98 mg/L occurring approximately 90 minutes after ingestion. The absolute bioavailability of a 20 mg oral dose is 69%.

Distribution

Mifepristone is 98% bound to plasma proteins, albumin and α_1-acid glycoprotein. Binding to the latter protein is saturable, and the drug displays nonlinear kinetics with respect to plasma concentration and clearance. Following a distribution phase, elimination of mifepristone is slow at first (50% eliminated between 12 and 72 hours) and then becomes more rapid with a terminal elimination half-life of 18 hours.

Metabolism

Metabolism of mifepristone is primarily via pathways involving N-demethylation and terminal hydroxylation of the 17-propynyl chain. *In vitro* studies have shown that CYP450 3A4 is primarily responsible for the metabolism. The three major metabolites identified in humans are: (1) RU 42 633, the most widely found in plasma, is the N-monodemethylated metabolite; (2) RU 42 848, which results from the loss of two methyl groups from the 4-dimethylaminophenyl in position 11β; and (3) RU 42 698, which results from terminal hydroxylation of the 17-propynyl chain.

Excretion

By 11 days after a 600 mg dose of tritiated compound, 83% of the drug has been accounted for by the feces and 9% by the urine. Serum levels are undetectable by 11 days.

Special Populations

The effects of age, hepatic disease and renal disease on the safety, efficacy and pharmacokinetics of mifepristone have not been investigated.

INDICATIONS AND USAGE

Mifepristone is indicated for the medical termination of intrauterine pregnancy through 49 days' pregnancy. For purposes of this treatment, pregnancy is dated from the first day of the last menstrual period in a presumed 28 day cycle with ovulation occurring at mid-cycle. The duration of pregnancy may be determined from menstrual history and by clinical examination. Ultrasonographic scan should be used if the duration of pregnancy is uncertain, or if ectopic pregnancy is suspected.

Any intrauterine device ("IUD") should be removed before treatment with mifepristone begins.

Patients taking mifepristone must take 400 μg of misoprostol 2 days after taking mifepristone unless a complete abortion has already been confirmed before that time (see DOSAGE AND ADMINISTRATION).

Pregnancy termination by surgery is recommended in cases when mifepristone and misoprostol fail to cause termination of intrauterine pregnancy (see PRECAUTIONS).

CONTRAINDICATIONS

Administration of mifepristone and misoprostol for the termination of pregnancy (the "treatment procedure") is contraindicated in patients with any one of the following conditions:

- Confirmed or suspected ectopic pregnancy or undiagnosed adnexal mass (the treatment procedure will not be effective to terminate an ectopic pregnancy).
- IUD in place (see INDICATIONS AND USAGE).
- Chronic adrenal failure.
- Concurrent long-term corticosteroid therapy.
- History of allergy to mifepristone, misoprostol or other prostaglandin.
- Hemorrhagic disorders or concurrent anticoagulant therapy.
- Inherited porphyrias.

Because it is important to have access to appropriate medical care if an emergency develops, the treatment procedure is contraindicated if a patient does not have adequate access to medical facilities equipped to provide emergency treatment of incomplete abortion, blood transfusions, and emergency resuscitation during the period from the first visit until discharged by the administering physician.

Mifepristone also should not be used by any patient who may be unable to understand the effects of the treatment procedure or to comply with its regimen. Patients should be instructed to review the Medication Guide and the Patient Agreement provided with mifepristone carefully and should be given a copy of the product label for their review. Patients should discuss their understanding of these materials with their health care providers, and retain the Medication Guide for later reference (see PRECAUTIONS).

WARNINGS

See CONTRAINDICATIONS.

BLEEDING

Vaginal bleeding occurs in almost all patients during the treatment procedure. According to data from the US and French trials, women should expect to experience bleeding or spotting for an average of 9-16 days, while up to 8% of all subjects may experience some type of bleeding for 30 days or more. Bleeding was reported to last for 69 days in 1 patient in the French trials. In general the duration of bleeding and spotting increased as the duration of the pregnancy increased.

In some cases, excessive bleeding may require treatment by vasoconstrictor drugs, curettage, administration of saline infusions, and/or blood transfusions. In the US trials, 4.8% of subjects received administration of uterotonic medications and 9 women (1.0%) received intravenous fluids. Vasoconstrictor drugs were used in 4.3% of all subjects in the French trials, and in 5.5% of women there was a decrease in hemoglobin of more than 2 g/dl. Blood transfusions were administered in 1 of 859 subjects in the US trials and in 2 of 1800 subjects in the French trials. Since heavy bleeding requiring curettage occurs in about 1% of patients, special care should be given to patients with hemostatic disorders, hypocoagulability, or severe anemia.

CONFIRMATION OF PREGNANCY TERMINATION

Patients should be scheduled for and return for a follow-up visit at approximately 14 days after administration of mifepristone to confirm that the pregnancy is completely terminated and to assess the degree of bleeding. Vaginal bleeding is not evidence of the termination of pregnancy. Termination can be confirmed by clinical examination or ultrasonographic scan. Lack of bleeding following treatment, however, usually indicates failure. Medical abortion failures should be managed with surgical termination.

PRECAUTIONS

GENERAL

Mifepristone is available only in single dose packaging. Administration must be under the supervision of a qualified physician (see DOSAGE AND ADMINISTRATION).

The use of mifepristone is assumed to require the same preventive measures as those taken prior to and during surgical abortion to prevent rhesus immunization.

There are no data on the safety and efficacy of mifepristone in women with chronic medical conditions such as cardiovascular, hypertensive, hepatic, respiratory or renal disease; insulin-dependent diabetes mellitus; severe anemia or heavy smoking. Women who are more than 35 years of age and who also smoke 10 or more cigarettes per day should be treated with caution because such patients were generally excluded from clinical trials of mifepristone.

Although there is no clinical evidence, the effectiveness of mifepristone may be lower if misoprostol is administered more than 2 days after mifepristone administration.

INFORMATION FOR THE PATIENT

Patients should be fully advised of the treatment procedure and its effects. Patients should be given a copy of the Medication Guide and the Patient Agreement. (Additional copies of the Medication Guide and the Patient Agreement are available by contacting Danco Laboratories at 1-877-4 Early Option) (1-877-432-7596). Patients should be advised to review both the Medication Guide and the Patient Agreement, and should be given the opportunity to discuss them and obtain answers to any questions they may have. Each patient must understand:

The necessity of completing the treatment schedule, including a follow-up visit approximately 14 days after taking mifepristone.
That vaginal bleeding and uterine cramping probably will occur.
That prolonged or heavy vaginal bleeding is not proof of a complete expulsion.
That if the treatment fails, there is a risk of fetal malformation.
That medical abortion treatment failures are managed by surgical termination.
The steps to take in an emergency situation, including precise instructions and a telephone number that she can call if she has any problems or concerns.

Another pregnancy can occur following termination of pregnancy and before resumption of normal menses. Contraception can be initiated as soon as the termination of the pregnancy has been confirmed, or before the woman resumes sexual intercourse.

Patient information is included with each package of mifepristone.

LABORATORY TESTS

Clinical examination is necessary to confirm the complete termination of pregnancy after the treatment procedure. Changes in quantitative human Chorionic Gonadotropin (hCG) levels will not be decisive until at least 10 days after the administration of mifepristone. A continuing pregnancy can be confirmed by ultrasonographic scan.

The existence of debris in the uterus following the treatment procedure will not necessarily require surgery for its removal.

Decreases in hemoglobin concentration, hematocrit and red blood cell count occur in some women who bleed heavily. Hemoglobin decreases of more than 2 g/dl occurred in 5.5% of subjects during the French clinical trials of mifepristone and misoprostol.

Clinically significant changes in serum enzyme (serum glutamic oxaloacetic transaminase (SGOT), serum glutamic pyruvic transaminase (SGPT), alkaline phosphatase, gamma-glutamyltransferase (GT)) activities were rarely reported.

CARCINOGENESIS, MUTAGENESIS, AND IMPAIRMENT OF FERTILITY

No long-term studies to evaluate the carcinogenic potential of mifepristone have been performed. Results from studies conducted *in vitro* and in animals have revealed no genotoxic potential for mifepristone. Among the tests carried out were: Ames test with and without metabolic activation; gene conversion test in *Saccharomyces cerevisiae* D4 cells; forward mutation in *Schizosaccharomyces pompe* P1 cells; induction of unscheduled DNA synthesis in cultured HeLa cells; induction of chromosome aberrations in CHO cells; *in vitro* test for gene mutation in V79 Chinese hamster lung cells; and micronucleus test in mice.

The pharmacological activity of mifepristone disrupts the estrus cycle of animals, precluding studies designed to assess effects on fertility during drug administration. Three studies have been performed in rats to determine whether there were residual effects on reproductive function after termination of the drug exposure.

In rats, administration of the lowest oral dose of 0.3 mg/kg/day caused severe disruption of the estrus cycles for the 3 weeks of the treatment period. Following resumption of the estrus cycle, animals were mated and no effect on reproductive performance was observed. In a neonatal exposure study in rats, the administration of a subcutaneous dose of mifepristone up to 100 mg/kg on the first day after birth had no adverse effect on future reproductive function in males or females. The onset of puberty was observed to be slightly premature in female rats neonatally exposed to mifepristone. In a separate study in rats, oviduct and ovary malformations in female rats, delayed male puberty, deficient male sexual behavior, reduced testicular size, and lowered ejaculation frequency were noted after exposure to mifepristone (1 mg every other day) as neonates.

PREGNANCY

Mifepristone is indicated for use in the termination of pregnancy (through 49 days' pregnancy) and has no other approved indication for use during pregnancy.

Teratogenic Effects

Human Data

Over 620,000 women in Europe have taken mifepristone in combination with a prostaglandin to terminate pregnancy. Among these 620,000 women, about 415,000 have received mifepristone together with misoprostol. As of May 2000 a total of 82 cases have been reported in which women with on-going pregnancies after using mifepristone alone or mifepristone followed by misoprostol declined to have a surgical procedure at that time. These cases are summarized in TABLE 2.

TABLE 2 *Reported Cases (as of May 2000) of On-going Pregnancies Not Terminated by Surgical Abortion at the End of Treatment with Mifepristone Alone or With Mifepristone-Misoprostol*

	Mifepristone Alone	Mifepristone-Misoprostol	Total
Subsequently had surgical abortion	**3**	**7**	**10**
No abnormalites detected	2	7	9
Abnormalitites detected (sirenomelia, cleft palate)	1	0	1
Subsequently resulted in live birth	**13**	**13**	**26**
No abnormalities detected at birth	13	13	26
Abnormalities detected at birth	0	0	0
Other/Unknown	**26**	**20**	**43**
Total	**42**	**40**	**82**

Several reports in the literature indicate that prostaglandins, including misoprostol, may have teratogenic effects in human beings. Skull defects, cranial nerve palsies, delayed growth and psychomotor development, facial malformation and limb defects have all been reported after exposure during the first trimester.

Animal Data

Teratology studies in mice, rats and rabbits at doses of 0.25-4.0 mg/kg (less than 1/100 to approximately 1/3 the human exposure level based on body surface area) were carried out. Because of the antiprogestational activity of mifepristone, fetal losses were much higher than in control animals. Skull deformities were detected in rabbit studies at approximately 1/6 the human exposure, although no teratogenic effects of mifepristone have been observed to date in rats or mice. These deformities were most likely due to the mechanical effects of uterine contractions resulting from decreased progesterone levels.

Nonteratogenic Effects

The indication for use of mifepristone in conjunction with misoprostol is for the termination of pregnancy through 49 days' duration of pregnancy (as dated from the first day of the last menstrual period). These drugs together disrupt pregnancy by causing decidual necrosis, myometrial contractions and cervical softening, leading to the expulsion of the products of conception.

NURSING MOTHERS

It is not known whether mifepristone is excreted in human milk. Many hormones with a similar chemical structure, however, are excreted in breast milk. Since the effects of mifepristone on infants are unknown, breast-feeding women should consult with their health care provider to decide if they should discard their breast milk for a few days following administration of the medications.

PEDIATRIC USE

Safety and effectiveness in pediatric patients have not been established.

DRUG INTERACTIONS

Although specific drug or food interactions with mifepristone have not been studied, on the basis of this drug's metabolism by CYP 3A4, it is possible that ketoconazole, itraconazole, erythromycin, and grapefruit juice may inhibit its metabolism (increasing serum levels of mifepristone). Furthermore, rifampin, dexamethasone, St. John's Wort, and certain anticonvulsants (phenytoin, phenobarbital, carbamazepine) may induce mifepristone metabolism (lowering serum levels of mifepristone).

Based on *in vitro* inhibition information, coadministration of mifepristone may lead to an increase in serum levels of drugs that are CYP 3A4 substrates. Due to the slow elimination of mifepristone from the body, such interaction may be observed for a prolonged period after its administration. Therefore, caution should be exercised when mifepristone is administered with drugs that are CYP 3A4 substrates and have narrow therapeutic range, including some agents used during general anesthesia.

ADVERSE REACTIONS

The treatment procedure is designed to induce the vaginal bleeding and uterine cramping necessary to produce an abortion. Nearly all of the women who receive mifepristone and misoprostol will report adverse reactions, and many can be expected to report more than one such reaction. About 90% of patients report adverse reactions following administration of misoprostol on day 3 of the treatment procedure. Those adverse events that occurred with a frequency greater than 1% in the US and French trials are shown in TABLE 3.

Bleeding and cramping are expected consequences of the action of mifepristone as used in the treatment procedure. Following administration of mifepristone and misoprostol in the French clinical studies, 80-90% of women reported bleeding more heavily than they do during a heavy menstrual period (see WARNINGS, Bleeding). Women also typically experience abdominal pain, including uterine cramping. Other commonly reported side effects were nausea, vomiting and diarrhea. Pelvic pain, fainting, headache, dizziness, and asthenia occurred rarely. Some adverse reactions reported during the 4 hours following administration of misoprostol were judged by women as being more severe than others: the percentage of women who considered any particular adverse event as severe ranged from 2-35% in the US and French trials. After the third day of the treatment procedure, the number of reports of adverse reactions declined progressively in the French trials, so that by day 14, reports were rare except for reports of bleeding and spotting.

DOSAGE AND ADMINISTRATION

Treatment with mifepristone and misoprostol for the termination of pregnancy requires 3 office visits by the patient. Mifepristone should be prescribed only by physicians who have read and understood the prescribing information. Mifepristone may be administered only in a clinic, medical office, or hospital, by or under the supervision of a physician, able to assess the gestational age of an embryo and to diagnose ectopic pregnancies. Physicians must also be able to provide surgical intervention in cases of incomplete abortion or severe bleeding, or have made plans to provide such care through others, and be able to assure patient access to medical facilities equipped to provide blood transfusions and resuscitation, if necessary.

DAY 1: MIFEPRISTONE ADMINISTRATION

Patients must read the Medication Guide and read and sign the Patient Agreement before mifepristone is administered.

Three 200 mg tablets (600 mg) of mifepristone are taken in a single oral dose.

DAY 3: MISOPROSTOL ADMINISTRATION

The patient returns to the healthcare provider 2 days after ingesting mifepristone. Unless abortion has occurred and has been confirmed by clinical examination or ultrasonographic scan, the patient takes two 200 μg tablets (400 μg) of misoprostol orally.

During the period immediately following the administration of misoprostol, the patient may need medication for cramps or gastrointestinal symptoms (see ADVERSE REACTIONS). The patient should be given instructions on what to do if significant discomfort, excessive bleeding or other adverse reactions occur and should be given a phone number to call if she has questions following the administration of the misoprostol. In addition, the name and phone number of the physician who will be handling emergencies should be provided to the patient.

TABLE 3 *Type of Reported Adverse Events Following Administration of Mifepristone and Misoprostol in the US and French Trials* (percentages)*

	US Trials	French Trials
Abdominal pain (cramping)	96	NA
Uterine cramping	NA	83
Nausea	61	43
Headache	31	2
Vomiting	26	18
Diarrhea	20	12
Dizziness	12	1
Fatigue	10	NA
Back pain	9	NA
Uterine hemorrhage	5	NA
Fever	4	NA
Viral infections	4	NA
Vaginitis	3	NA
Rigors (chills/shaking)	3	NA
Dyspepsia	3	NA
Insomnia	3	NA
Asthenia	2	1
Leg pain	2	NA
Anxiety	2	NA
Anemia	2	NA
Leukorrhea	2	NA
Sinusitus	2	NA
Syncope	1	NA
Decrease in hemoglobin greater than 2 g/dl	NA	6
Pelvic pain	NA	2
Fainting	NA	2

* Only adverse reactions with incidence >1% are included.

DAY 14: POST-TREATMENT EXAMINATION

Patients will return for a follow-up visit approximately 14 days after the administration of mifepristone. This visit is very important to confirm by clinical examination or ultrasonographic scan that a complete termination of pregnancy has occurred.

According to data from the US and French studies, women should expect to experience bleeding or spotting for an average of 9-16 days. Up to 8% of women may experience some type of bleeding for more than 30 days. Persistence of heavy or moderate vaginal bleeding at this visit, however, could indicate an incomplete abortion.

Patients who have an ongoing pregnancy at this visit have a risk of fetal malformation resulting from the treatment. Surgical termination is recommended to manage medical abortion treatment failures (see PRECAUTIONS, Pregnancy).

Adverse events, such as hospitalization, blood transfusion, ongoing pregnancy, or other major complications following the use of mifepristone and misoprostol must be reported to Danco Laboratories. Please provide a brief clinical and administrative synopsis of any such adverse events in writing to: Medical Director, Danco Laboratories, LLC, P.O. Box 4816, New York, NY 10185 1-877-4-Early Option (1-877-432-7596).

For immediate consultation 24 hours a day, 7 days a week with an expert in mifepristone, call Danco Laboratories at 1-877-4 Early Option (1-877-432-7596).

HOW SUPPLIED

Mifepristone will be supplied only to licensed physicians who sign and return a Prescriber's Agreement. Distribution of mifepristone will be subject to specific requirements imposed by the distributor, including procedures for storage, dosage tracking, damaged product returns and other matters. Mifepristone is a prescription drug, although it will not be available to the public through licensed pharmacies.

Mifeprex is supplied as light yellow, cylindrical, bi-convex tablets imprinted on one side with "MF." Each tablet contains 200 mg of mifepristone.

Storage: Store at 25°C (77°F); excursions permitted to 15-30°C (59-86°F).

PRODUCT LISTING - EQUIVALENTS NOT AVAILABLE

Tablet - Oral - 200 mg

3's $250.00 MIFEPREX, Danco Laboratories 64875-0001-03

Miglitol (003310)

For related information, see the comparative table section in Appendix A.

Categories: Diabetes mellitus; Pregnancy Category B; FDA Approved 1996 Dec
Drug Classes: Alpha glucosidase inhibitors; Antidiabetic agents
Brand Names: Glyset
Foreign Brand Availability: Diastabol (France; Germany)
Cost of Therapy: $67.62 (Diabetes Mellitus; Glyset; 50 mg; 3 tablets/day; 30 day supply)

DESCRIPTION

Miglitol is an oral alpha-glucosidase inhibitor for use in the management of non-insulin dependent diabetes mellitus (NIDDM). Miglitol is a desoxynojirimycin derivative, and is chemically known as 3,4,5-piperidinetriol, 1-(2-hydroxyethyl)-2-(hydroxymethyl)-,[2R-(2α,3β, 4α, 5β)]-. It is a white to pale-yellow powder with a molecular weight of 207.2. Miglitol is soluble in water and has a pKa of 5.9. Its empirical formula is $C_8H_{17}NO_5$.

Glyset tablets are available as 25, 50, and 100 mg tablets for oral use. *Inactive Ingredients:* Starch, microcrystalline cellulose, magnesium stearate, hydroxypropyl methylcellulose, polyethylene glycol, titanium dioxide, and polysorbate 80.

CLINICAL PHARMACOLOGY

Miglitol is a desoxynojirimycin derivative that delays the digestion of ingested carbohydrates, thereby resulting in a smaller rise in blood glucose concentration following meals. As a consequence of plasma glucose reduction, miglitol reduces levels of glycosylated hemoglobin in patients with Type II (non-insulin-dependent) diabetes mellitus. Systemic nonenzymatic protein glycosylation, as reflected by levels of glycosylated hemoglobin, is a function of average blood glucose concentration over time.

MECHANISM OF ACTION

In contrast to sulfonylureas, miglitol does not enhance insulin secretion. The antihyperglycemic action of miglitol results from a reversible inhibition of membrane-bound intestinal α-glucoside hydrolase enzymes. Membrane-bound intestinal α-glucosidases hydrolyze oligosaccharides and disaccharides to glucose and other monosaccharides in the brush border of the small intestine. In diabetic patients, this enzyme inhibition results in delayed glucose absorption and lowering of postprandial hyperglycemia.

Because its mechanism of action is different, the effect of miglitol to enhance glycemic control is additive to that of sulfonylureas when used in combination. In addition, miglitol diminishes the insulinotropic and weight-increasing effects of sulfonylureas.

Miglitol has minor inhibitory activity against lactase and consequently, at the recommended doses, would not be expected to induce lactose intolerance.

PHARMACOKINETICS

Absorption

Absorption of miglitol is saturable at high doses; a dose of 25 mg is completely absorbed, whereas a dose of 100 mg is only 50-70% absorbed. For all doses, peak concentrations are reached in 2-3 hours. There is no evidence that systemic absorption of miglitol contributes to its therapeutic effect.

Distribution

The protein binding of miglitol is negligible (<4.0%). Miglitol has a volume of distribution of 0.18 L/kg, consistent with distribution primarily into the extracellular fluid.

Metabolism

Miglitol is not metabolized in man or in any animal species studied. No metabolites have been detected in plasma, urine, or feces, indicating a lack of either systemic or pre-systemic metabolism.

Elimination

Miglitol is eliminated by renal excretion as unchanged drug. Thus, following a 25 mg dose, over 95% of the dose is recovered in the urine within 24 hours. At higher doses, the cumulative recovery of drug from urine is somewhat lower due to the incomplete bioavailability. The elimination half-life from plasma is approximately 2 hours.

Special Populations

Renal Impairment

Because miglitol is excreted primarily by the kidneys, accumulation of miglitol is expected in patients with renal impairment. Patients with creatinine clearance <25 ml/min taking 25 mg three times daily exhibited a greater than 2-fold increase in miglitol plasma levels as compared to subjects with creatinine clearance >60 ml/min. Dosage adjustment to correct the increased plasma concentrations is not feasible because miglitol acts locally. Little information is available on the safety of miglitol in patients with creatinine clearance <25 ml/min.

Hepatic Impairment

Miglitol pharmacokinetics were not altered in cirrhotic patients relative to healthy control subjects. Since miglitol is not metabolized, no influence of hepatic function on the kinetics of miglitol is expected.

Elderly

The pharmacokinetics of miglitol were studied in elderly and young males (n=8 per group). At a dosage of 100 mg three times daily for 3 days, no differences between the two groups were found.

Gender

No significant difference in the pharmacokinetics of miglitol was observed between elderly men and women when body weight was taken into account.

Race

Several pharmacokinetic studies were conducted in Japanese volunteers, with results similar to those observed in caucasians. A study comparing the pharmacodynamic response to a single 50 mg dose in black and caucasian healthy volunteers indicated similar glucose and insulin responses in both populations.

INDICATIONS AND USAGE

Miglitol tablets, as monotherapy, are indicated as an adjunct to diet to improve glycemic control in patients with non-insulin dependent diabetes mellitus (NIDDM) whose hyperglycemia cannot be managed with diet alone. Miglitol may also be used in combination with a sulfonylurea when diet plus either miglitol or a sulfonylurea alone do not result in adequate glycemic control. The effect of miglitol to enhance glycemic control is additive to that of sulfonylureas when used in combination, presumably because its mechanism of action is different.

In initiating treatment for NIDDM, diet should be emphasized as the primary form of treatment. Caloric restriction and weight loss are essential in the obese diabetic patient. Proper dietary management alone may be effective in controlling blood glucose and symptoms of hyperglycemia. The importance of regular physical activity when appropriate should also be stressed. If this treatment program fails to result in adequate glycemic control, the use of miglitol should be considered. The use of miglitol must be viewed by both the physician and patient as a treatment in addition to diet and not as a substitute for diet or as a convenient mechanism for avoiding dietary restraint.

CONTRAINDICATIONS

Miglitol is contraindicated in patients with:

- Diabetic ketoacidosis.
- Inflammatory bowel disease, colonic ulceration, or partial intestinal obstruction, and in patients predisposed to intestinal obstruction.
- Chronic intestinal disease associated with marked disorders of digestion or absorption, or with conditions that may deteriorate as a result of increased gas formation in the intestine.
- Hypersensitivity to the drug or any of its components.

PRECAUTIONS

GENERAL

Hypoglycemia

Because of the mechanism of action, miglitol when administered alone should not cause hypoglycemia in the fasted or postprandial state. Sulfonylurea agents may cause hypoglycemia. Because miglitol given in combination with a sulfonylurea will cause a further lowering of blood glucose, it may increase the hypoglycemic potential of the sulfonylurea, although this was not observed in clinical trials. Oral glucose (dextrose), whose absorption is not delayed by miglitol, should be used instead of sucrose (cane sugar) in the treatment of mild-to-moderate hypoglycemia. Sucrose, whose hydrolysis to glucose and fructose is inhibited by miglitol, is unsuitable for the rapid correction of hypoglycemia. Severe hypoglycemia may require the use of either intravenous glucose infusion or glucagon injection.

Loss of Control of Blood Glucose

When diabetic patients are exposed to stress such as fever, trauma, infection, or surgery, a temporary loss of control of blood glucose may occur. At such times, temporary insulin therapy may be necessary.

Renal Impairment

Plasma concentrations of miglitol in renally impaired volunteers were proportionally increased relative to the degree of renal dysfunction. Long-term clinical trials in diabetic patients with significant renal dysfunction (serum creatinine >2.0 mg/dl) have not been conducted. Therefore, treatment of these patients with miglitol is not recommended.

INFORMATION FOR THE PATIENT

The following information should be provided to patients:

- Miglitol should be taken orally 3 times a day at the start (with the first bite) of each main meal. It is important to continue to adhere to dietary instructions, a regular exercise program, and regular testing of urine and/or blood glucose.
- Miglitol itself does not cause hypoglycemia even when administered to patients in the fasted state. Sulfonylurea drugs and insulin, however, can lower blood sugar levels enough to cause symptoms or sometimes life-threatening hypoglycemia. Because miglitol given in combination with a sulfonylurea or insulin will cause a further lowering of blood sugar, it may increase the hypoglycemic potential of these agents. The risk of hypoglycemia, its symptoms and treatment, and conditions that predispose to its development should be well understood by patients and responsible family members. Because miglitol prevents the breakdown of table sugar, a source of glucose (dextrose, D-glucose) should be readily available to treat symptoms of low blood sugar when taking miglitol in combination with a sulfonylurea or insulin.
- If side effects occur with miglitol, they usually develop during the first few weeks of therapy. They are most commonly mild-to-moderate dose-related gastrointestinal effects, such as flatulence, soft stools, diarrhea, or abdominal discomfort, and they generally diminish in frequency and intensity with time. Discontinuation of drug usually results in rapid resolution of the gastrointestinal symptoms.

LABORATORY TESTS

Therapeutic response to miglitol may be monitored by periodic blood glucose tests. Measurement of glycosylated hemoglobin levels is recommended for the monitoring of long-term glycemic control.

CARCINOGENESIS, MUTAGENESIS, AND IMPAIRMENT OF FERTILITY

Miglitol was administered to mice by the dietary route at doses as high as approximately 500 mg/kg body weight (corresponding to greater than 5 times the exposure in humans based on AUC) for 21 months. In a 2 year rat study, miglitol was administered in the diet at exposures comparable to the maximum human exposures based on AUC. There was no evidence of carcinogenicity resulting from dietary treatment with miglitol.

In vitro, miglitol was found to be non-mutagenic in the bacterial mutagenesis (Ames) assay and the eukaryotic forward mutation assay (CHO/HGPRT). Miglitol did not have any clastogenic effects *in vivo* in the mouse micronucleus test. There were no heritable mutations detected in dominant lethal assay.

A combined male and female fertility study in Wistar rats treated orally with miglitol at dose levels of 300 mg/kg body weight (approximately 8 times the maximum human exposure based on body surface area) produced no untoward effect on reproductive performance or capability to reproduce. In addition, survival, growth, development, and fertility of the offspring were not compromised.

PREGNANCY, TERATOGENIC EFFECTS, PREGNANCY CATEGORY B

The safety of miglitol in pregnant women has not been established. Developmental toxicology studies have been performed in rats at doses of 50, 150 and 450 mg/kg, corresponding to levels of approximately 1.5, 4, and 12 times the maximum recommended human exposure based on body surface area. In rabbits, doses of 10, 45, and 200 mg/kg corresponding to levels of approximately 0.5, 3, and 10 times the human exposure were examined. These studies revealed no evidence of fetal malformations attributable to miglitol. Doses of miglitol up to 4 and 3 times the human dose (based on body surface area) for rats and rabbits, respectively, did not reveal evidence of impaired fertility or harm to the fetus. The highest doses tested in these studies, 450 mg/kg in the rat and 200 mg/kg in the rabbit promoted maternal and/or fetal toxicity. Fetotoxicity was indicated by a slight but significant reduction in fetal weight in the rat study and slight reduction in fetal weight, delayed ossification of the fetal skeleton and increase in the percentage of non-viable fetuses in the rabbit study. In the peri-postnatal study in rats, the NOAEL (No Observed Adverse Effect Level) was 100 mg/kg (corresponding to approximately 4 times the exposure to humans, based on the body surface area). An increase in stillborn progeny was noted at the high dose (300 mg/kg) in the rat peri-postnatal study, but not at the high dose (450 mg/kg) in the delivery segment of the rat developmental toxicity study. Otherwise, there was no adverse effect on survival, growth, development, behavior, or fertility in either the rat development toxicity or peri-postnatal studies. There are, however, no adequate and well-controlled studies in pregnant women. Because animal reproduction studies are not always predictive of human response, this drug should be used during pregnancy only if clearly needed.

NURSING MOTHERS

Miglitol has been shown to be excreted in human milk to a very small degree. Total excretion into milk accounted for 0.02% of a 100 mg maternal dose. The estimated exposure to a nursing infant is approximately 0.4% of the maternal dose. Although the levels of miglitol reached in human milk are exceedingly low, it is recommended that miglitol not be administered to a nursing woman.

PEDIATRIC USE

Safety and effectiveness of miglitol in pediatric patients have not been established.

GERIATRIC USE

Of the total number of subjects in clinical studies of miglitol in the US, patients valid for safety analyses included 24% over 65, and 3% over 75. No overall differences in safety and effectiveness were observed between these subjects and younger subjects. The pharmacokinetics of miglitol were studied in elderly and young males (n=8 per group). At the dosage of 100 mg three times daily for 3 days, no differences between the two groups were found.

DRUG INTERACTIONS

Several studies investigated the possible interaction between miglitol and glyburide. In 6 healthy volunteers given a single dose of 5 mg glyburide on a background of 6 days treatment with miglitol (50 mg three times daily for 4 days followed by 100 mg three times daily for 2 days) or placebo, the mean C_{max} and AUC values for glyburide were 17% and 25% lower, respectively, when glyburide was given with miglitol. In a study in diabetic patients in which the effects of adding miglitol 100 mg three times daily × 7 days or placebo to a background regimen of 3.5 mg glyburide daily were investigated, the mean AUC value for glyburide was 18% lower in the miglitol-treated group, although this difference was not statistically significant. Further information on a potential interaction with glyburide was obtained from one of the large US clinical trials (Study 7) in which patients were dosed with either miglitol or placebo on a background of glyburide 10 mg twice daily. At the 6 month and 1 year clinic visits, patients taking concomitant miglitol 100 mg three times daily exhibited mean C_{max} values for glyburide that were 16% and 8% lower, respectively, compared to patients taking glyburide alone. However, these differences were not statistically significant. Thus, although there was a trend toward lower AUC and C_{max} values for glyburide when co-administered with miglitol, no definitive statement regarding a potential interaction can be made based on the foregoing 3 studies.

The effect of miglitol (100 mg three times daily × 7 days) on the pharmacokinetics of a single 1000 mg dose of metformin was investigated in healthy volunteers. Mean AUC and C_{max} values for metformin were 12-13% lower when the volunteers were given miglitol as compared with placebo, but this difference was not statistically significant.

In a healthy volunteer study, co-administration of either 50 mg or 100 mg miglitol 3 times daily together with digoxin reduced the average plasma concentrations of digoxin by 19% and 28%, respectively. However, in diabetic patients under treatment with digoxin, plasma digoxin concentrations were not altered by co-administration of miglitol 100 mg three times daily × 14 days.

Other healthy volunteer studies have demonstrated that miglitol may significantly reduce the bioavailability or ranitidine and propranolol by 60% and 40%, respectively. No effect of miglitol was observed on the pharmacokinetics or pharmacodynamics of either warfarin or nifedipine.

Intestinal absorbents (*e.g.,* charcoal) and digestive enzyme preparations containing carbohydrate-splitting enzymes (*e.g.,* amylase, pancreatin) may reduce the effect of miglitol and should not be taken concomitantly.

In 12 healthy males, concomitantly administered antacid did not influence the pharmacokinetics of miglitol.

ADVERSE REACTIONS

GASTROINTESTINAL

Gastrointestinal symptoms are the most common reactions to miglitol. In US placebo-controlled trials, the incidences of abdominal pain, diarrhea, and flatulence were 11.7%, 28.7%, and 41.5%, respectively in 962 patients treated with miglitol 25-100 mg three times daily, whereas the corresponding incidences were 4.7%, 10.0%, and 12.0% in 603 placebo-treated patients. The incidence of diarrhea and abdominal pain tended to diminish considerably with continued treatment.

DERMATOLOGIC

Skin rash was reported in 4.3% of patients treated with miglitol compared to 2.4% of placebo-treated patients. Rashes were generally transient and most were assessed as unrelated to miglitol by physician-investigators.

ABNORMAL LABORATORY FINDINGS

Low serum iron occurred more often in patients treated with miglitol (9.2%) than in placebo-treated patients (4.2%) but did not persist in the majority of cases and was not associated with reductions in hemoglobin or changes in other hematological indices.

M

DOSAGE AND ADMINISTRATION

There is no fixed dosage regimen for the management of diabetes mellitus with miglitol or any other pharmacologic agent. Dosage of miglitol must be individualized on the basis of both effectiveness and tolerance while not exceeding the maximum recommended dosage of 100 mg three times daily. Miglitol should be taken 3 times daily at the start (with the first bite) of each main meal. Miglitol should be started at 25 mg, and the dosage gradually increased as described below, both to reduce gastrointestinal adverse effects and to permit identification of the minimum dose required for adequate glycemic control of the patient.

During treatment initiation and dose titration, 1 hour postprandial plasma glucose may be used to determine the therapeutic response to miglitol and identify the minimum effective dose for the patient. Thereafter, glycosylated hemoglobin should be measured at intervals of approximately 3 months. The therapeutic goal should be to decrease both postprandial plasma glucose and glycosylated hemoglobin levels to normal or near normal by using the lowest effective dose of miglitol, either as monotherapy or in combination with a sulfonylurea.

INITIAL DOSAGE

The recommended starting dose of miglitol is 25 mg, given orally 3 times daily at the start (with the first bite) of each main meal. However, some patients may benefit by starting at 25 mg once daily to minimize gastrointestinal adverse effects, and gradually increasing the frequency of administration to 3 times daily.

MAINTENANCE

The usual maintenance dose of miglitol is 50 mg three times daily, although some patients may benefit from increasing the dose to 100 mg three times daily. In order to allow adaptation to potential gastrointestinal adverse effects, it is recommended that miglitol therapy be initiated at a dosage of 25 mg three times daily, the lowest effective dosage, and then gradually titrated upward to allow adaptation. After 4-8 weeks of the 25 mg three times daily regimen, the dosage should be increased to 50 mg three times daily for approximately 3 months, following which a glycosylated hemoglobin level should be measured to assess therapeutic response. If, at that time, the glycosylated hemoglobin level is not satisfactory, the dosage may be further increased to 100 mg three times daily, the maximum recommended dosage. Pooled data from controlled studies suggest a dose-response for both HbA1c and 1 hour postprandial plasma glucose throughout the recommended dosage range. However, no single study has examined the effect on glycemic control of titrating patients' doses upwards within the same study. If no further reduction in postprandial glucose or glycosylated hemoglobin levels is observed with titration to 100 mg three times daily, consideration should be given to lowering the dose. Once an effective and tolerated dosage is established, it should be maintained.

M

MAXIMUM DOSAGE

The maximum recommended dosage of miglitol is 100 mg three times daily. In one clinical trial, 200 mg three times daily gave additional improved glycemic control but increased the incidence of the gastrointestinal symptoms described in ADVERSE REACTIONS.

PATIENTS RECEIVING SULFONYLUREAS

Sulfonylurea agents may cause hypoglycemia. There was no increased incidence of hypoglycemia in patients who took miglitol in combination with sulfonylurea agents compared to the incidence of hypoglycemia in patients receiving sulfonylureas alone in any clinical trial. However, miglitol given in combination with a sulfonylurea will cause a further lowering of blood glucose and may increase the risk of hypoglycemia due to the additive effects of the two agents. If hypoglycemia occurs, appropriate adjustments in the dosage of these agents should be made.

HOW SUPPLIED

Glyset tablets are available as 25, 50, and 100 mg white, round, film-coated tablets. The tablets are debossed with the word "Glyset" on one side and the strength on the other side. **Storage:** Store at 25°C; excursions permitted to 15-30°C (59-86°F).

PRODUCT LISTING - EQUIVALENTS NOT AVAILABLE

Tablet - Oral - 25 mg

100's	$68.31	GLYSET, Pharmacia and Upjohn	00009-5012-01

Tablet - Oral - 50 mg

100's	$75.13	GLYSET, Pharmacia and Upjohn	00009-5013-01

Tablet - Oral - 100 mg

100's	$88.61	GLYSET, Pharmacia and Upjohn	00009-5014-01

Minocycline Hydrochloride *(001818)*

Categories: Acne vulgaris; Actinomycosis; Amebiasis, adjunct; Anthrax; Bartonellosis; Brucellosis; Chancroid; Cholera; Conjunctivitis, inclusion; Gonorrhea; Granuloma inguinale; Infection, genital tract; Infection, lower respiratory tract; Infection, skin and skin structures; Infection, upper respiratory tract; Infection, urinary tract; Listeriosis; Lymphogranuloma venereum; Meningococcal carrier state; Plague; Periodontitis; Psittacosis; Q fever; Relapsing fever; Rickettsialpox; Rocky mountain spotted fever; Syphilis; Tick fevers; Trachoma; Tularemia; Typhus fever; Infection, Vincent's; Yaws; Pregnancy Category D; FDA Approved 1972 Oct

Drug Classes: Antibiotics, tetracyclines

Brand Names: Dynacin; **Minocin**

Foreign Brand Availability: Akamin (Australia); Borymycin (Philippines; Singapore; Taiwan); Cyclimycin (South-Africa); Cynomycin (India); Klinomycin (Germany); Lederderm (Germany); Mestacine (France); Micromycin (Mexico); Minaxen (Hong-Kong); Mino-50 (Belgium); Minocin G (Taiwan); Minocin MR (Hong-Kong); Minoclin (Israel); Minoclir 50 (Germany); Minocyclin 50 Stada (Germany); Minogalen (Germany); Minoline (Taiwan); Minomycin (Australia; Japan; New-Zealand; South-Africa); Minotab 50 (New-Zealand; South-Africa); Mino-Wolff (Germany); Mynocine (France); Romin (South-Africa); Skinocyclin (Germany); Spicline (France)

Cost of Therapy: $54.40 (Infection; Minocin; 100 mg; 2 capsules/day; 7 day supply)
$26.87 (Infection; Generic Capsule; 100 mg; 2 capsules/day; 7 day supply)

DENTAL

DESCRIPTION

Note: The trade name has been used throughout this monograph for clarity.

Arestin (minocycline hydrochloride) Microspheres is a subgingival sustained-release product containing the antibiotic minocycline hydrochloride incorporated into a bioresorbable polymer, Poly (glycolide-co-dl-lactide) or PGLA, for professional subgingival administration into periodontal pockets. Each unit-dose cartridge delivers minocycline hydrochloride equivalent to 1 mg of minocycline free base.

The molecular formula of minocycline hydrochloride is $C_{23}H_{27}N_3O_7 \cdot HCl$ and the molecular weight is 493.94.

INDICATIONS AND USAGE

Arestin is indicated as an adjunct to scaling and root planing procedures for reduction of pocket depth in patients with adult periodontitis. Arestin may be used as part of a periodontal maintenance program which includes good oral hygiene, and scaling and root planing.

CONTRAINDICATIONS

Arestin should not be used in any patient who has a known sensitivity to minocycline or tetracyclines.

WARNINGS

THE USE OF DRUGS OF THE TETRACYCLINE CLASS DURING TOOTH DEVELOPMENT (LAST HALF OF PREGNANCY, INFANCY, AND CHILDHOOD TO THE AGE OF 8 YEARS) MAY CAUSE PERMANENT DISCOLORATION OF THE TEETH (YELLOW-GRAY BROWN). This adverse reaction is more common during long-term use of the drugs, but has been observed following repeated short-term courses. Enamel hypoplasia has also been reported. TETRACYCLINE DRUGS, THEREFORE, SHOULD NOT BE USED IN THIS AGE GROUP, OR IN PREGNANT OR NURSING WOMEN, UNLESS THE POTENTIAL BENEFITS ARE CONSIDERED TO OUTWEIGH THE POTENTIAL RISKS. Results of animal studies indicate that tetracyclines cross the placenta, are found in fetal tissues, and can have toxic effects on the developing fetus (often related to retardation of skeletal development). Evidence of embryotoxicity has also been noted in animals treated early in pregnancy. If any tetracyclines are used during pregnancy, or if the patient becomes pregnant while taking this drug, the patient should be apprised of the potential hazard to the fetus. Photosensitivity manifested by an exaggerated sunburn reaction has been observed in some individuals taking tetracyclines. Patients apt to be exposed to direct sunlight or ultraviolet light should be advised that this reaction can occur with tetracycline drugs, and treatment should be discontinued at the first evidence of skin erythema.

PRECAUTIONS

The use of Arestin in an acutely abscessed periodontal pocket has not been studied and is not recommended.

While no overgrowth by opportunistic microorganisms, such as yeast, were noted during clinical studies, as with other antimicrobials the use of Arestin may result in overgrowth of nonsusceptible microorganisms including fungi. The effects of treatment for greater than 6 months has not been studied.

Arestin should be used with caution in patients having a history of predisposition to oral candidiasis. The safety and effectiveness of Arestin has not been established for the treatment of periodontitis in patients with coexistent oral candidiasis.

Arestin has not been clinically tested in immunocompromised patients (such as those immunocompromised by diabetes, chemotherapy, radiation therapy, or infection with HIV).

If superinfection is suspected, appropriate measures should be taken.

Arestin has not been clinically tested in pregnant women.

Arestin has not been clinically tested for use in the regeneration of alveolar bone, either in preparation for or in conjunction with the placement of endosseous (dental) implants or in the treatment of failing implants.

INFORMATION FOR THE PATIENT

After treatment, patients should avoid eating hard, crunchy, or sticky foods for 1 week and postpone brushing for a 12 hour period, as well as avoid touching treated areas. Patients should also postpone the use of interproximal cleaning devices for 10 days after administration of Arestin. Patients should be advised that although some mild to moderate sensitivity is expected during the first week after SRP and administration of Arestin, they should notify the dentist promptly if pain, swelling, or other problems occur.

CARCINOGENESIS, MUTAGENESIS, AND IMPAIRMENT OF FERTILITY

Dietary administration of minocycline in long-term tumorigenicity studies in rats resulted in evidence of thyroid tumor production. Minocycline has also been found to produce thyroid hyperplasia in rats and dogs. In addition, there has been evidence of oncogenic activity in rats in studies with a related antibiotic, oxytetracycline (*i.e.,* adrenal and pituitary tumors). Minocycline demonstrated no potential to cause genetic toxicity in a battery of assays which included a bacterial reverse mutation assay (Ames test), an *in vitro* mammalian cell gene mutation test (L5178Y/TK$^{+/-}$ mouse lymphoma assay), an *in vitro* mammalian chromosome aberration test, and an *in vivo* micronucleus assay conducted in ICR mice.

Fertility and general reproduction studies have provided evidence that minocycline impairs fertility in male rats.

PREGNANCY, TERATOGENIC EFFECTS, PREGNANCY CATEGORY D

See WARNINGS.

LABOR AND DELIVERY

The effects of tetracyclines on labor and delivery are unknown.

NURSING MOTHERS

Tetracyclines are excreted in human milk. Because of the potential for serious adverse reactions in nursing infants from the tetracyclines, a decision should be made whether to discontinue nursing or discontinue the drug, taking into account the importance of the drug to the mother. (See WARNINGS.)

PEDIATRIC USE

Since adult periodontitis does not affect children, the safety and effectiveness of Arestin in pediatric patients cannot be established.

ADVERSE REACTIONS

The most frequently reported nondental treatment-emergent adverse events in the 3 multicenter US trials were headache, infection, flu syndrome, and pain.

TABLE 5 *Adverse Events (AEs) Reported in ≥3% of the Combined Clinical Trial Population of 3 Multicenter US Trials by Treatment Group*

	SRP Alone	SRP + Vehicle	SRP + Arestin
	n=250	n=249	n=423
Number (%) of Patients Treatment-Emergent AEs	62.4%	71.9%	68.1%
Total Number of AEs	543	589	987
Periodontitis	25.6%	28.1%	16.3%
Tooth disorder	12.0%	13.7%	12.3%
Tooth caries	9.2%	11.2%	9.9%
Dental pain	8.8%	8.8%	9.9%
Gingivitis	7.2%	8.8%	9.2%
Headache	7.2%	11.6%	9.0%
Infection	8.0%	9.6%	7.6%
Stomatitis	8.4%	6.8%	6.4%
Mouth ulceration	1.6%	3.2%	5.0%
Flu syndrome	3.2%	6.4%	5.0%
Pharyngitis	3.2%	1.6%	4.3%
Pain	4.0%	1.2%	4.3%
Dyspepsia	2.0%	0%	4.0%
Infection dental	4.0%	3.6%	3.8%
Mucous membrane disorder	2.4%	0.8%	3.3%

The change in clinical attachment levels was similar across all study arms, suggesting that neither the vehicle nor Arestin compromise clinical attachment.

DOSAGE AND ADMINISTRATION

Arestin is provided as a dry powder, packaged in a unit-dose cartridge, which is inserted into a cartridge handle to administer the product. The oral health care professional removes the disposable cartridge from its pouch and connects the cartridge to the handle mechanism. Arestin is a variable dose product, dependent on the size, shape, and number of pockets being treated. In US clinical trials, up to 121 unit-dose cartridges were used in a single visit and up to 3 treatments, at 3 month intervals, were administered in pockets with pocket depth of 5 mm or greater.

The administration of Arestin does not require local anesthesia. Professional subgingival administration is accomplished by inserting the unit-dose cartridge to the base of the periodontal pocket and then pressing the thumb ring in the handle mechanism to expel the powder while gradually withdrawing the tip from the base of the pocket. The handle mechanism should be sterilized between patients. Arestin does not have to be removed, as it is bioresorbable, nor is an adhesive or dressing required.

HOW SUPPLIED

Arestin Microspheres, 1 mg is supplied in unit doses of 12 cartridges in one tray packaged with desiccant in a heat-sealed foil laminated resealable pouch. Each unit-dose cartridge contains the product identifier "OP-1".

Storage Conditions: Store at 20-25°C (68-77°F)/60% RH: excursions permitted to 15-30°C (59-86°F). Avoid exposure to excessive heat.

INTRAVENOUS

DESCRIPTION

Minocycline hydrochloride, a semisynthetic derivative of tetracycline, is named [4*S*-(4(alpha),4a(alpha),5a(alpha),12a(alpha))]-4,7-bis(dimethylamino)-1,4,4a,5,5a,6,11,12a-octahydro-3,10,12,12a-tetrahydroxy-1,11-dioxo-2-naphthacenecarboxamide monohydrochloride.

Each vial of Minicin, dried by cryodesiccation, contains sterile minocycline hydrochloride equivalent to 100 mg minocycline. When reconstituted with 5 ml of sterile water for injection, the pH ranges from 2.0-2.8.

CLINICAL PHARMACOLOGY

MICROBIOLOGY

The tetracyclines are primarily bacteriostatic and are thought to exert their antimicrobial effect by the inhibition of protein synthesis. Minocycline HCl is a tetracycline with antibacterial activity comparable to other tetracyclines with activity against a wide range of gram-negative and gram-positive organisms.

Tube Dilution Testing

Microorganisms may be considered susceptible (likely to respond to minocycline therapy) if the minimum inhibitory concentration (MIC) is not more than 4 µg/ml. Microorganisms may be considered intermediate (harboring partial resistance) if the MIC is 4 to 12.5 µg/ml and resistant (not likely to respond to minocycline therapy) if the MIC is greater than 12.5 µg/ml.

Susceptibility Plate Testing

If the Kirby-Bauer method of susceptibility testing (using a 30 µg tetracycline disc) gives a zone of 18 mm or greater, the bacterial strain is considered to be susceptible to any tetracycline. Minocycline shows moderate *in vitro* activity against certain strains of staphylococci which have been found resistant to other tetracyclines. For such strains, minocycline susceptibility powder may be used for additional susceptibility testing.

HUMAN PHARMACOLOGY

Following a single dose of 200 mg administered intravenously to 10 healthy male volunteers, serum levels ranged from 2.52-6.63 µg/ml (average 4.18), after 12 hours they ranged from 0.82-2.64 µg/ml (average 1.38). In a group of 5 healthy male volunteers, serum levels of 1.4-1.8 µg/ml were maintained at 12 and 24 hours with doses of 100 mg every 12 hours for 3 days. When given 200 mg once daily for 3 days, the serum levels had fallen to approximately 1 µg/ml at 24 hours. The serum half-life following IV doses of 100 mg every 12 hours or 200 mg once daily did not differ significantly and ranged from 15-23 hours. The serum half-life following a single 200 mg oral dose in 12 essentially normal volunteers ranged from 11-17 hours, in 7 patients with hepatic dysfunction ranged from 11-16 hours, and in 5 patients with renal dysfunction from 18-69 hours.

Intravenously administered minocycline appears similar to oral doses in excretion. The urinary and fecal recovery of oral minocycline when administered to 12 normal volunteers is one-half to one-third that of other tetracyclines.

INDICATIONS AND USAGE

Minocin is indicated in infections caused by the following microorganisms:

Rickettsia: (Rocky Mountain spotted fever, typhus fever and the typhus group, Q fever, rickettsialpox, tick fevers.)

Mycoplasma pneumoniae (PPLO, Eaton agent).

Agents of psittacosis and ornithosis.

Agents of lymphogranuloma venereum and granuloma inguinale.

The spirochetal agent of relapsing fever (Borrelia recurrentis).

The following gram-negative microorganisms:

Haemophilus ducreyi (chancroid), Yersinia pestis and Francisella tularensis, formerly Pasteurella pestis and Pasteurella tularensis, Bartonella bacilliformis, Bacteroides species, Vibrio comma and Vibrio fetus, Brucella species (in conjunction with streptomycin).

Because many strains of the following groups of microorganisms have been shown to be resistant to tetracyclines, culture and susceptibility testing are recommended.

Minocin is indicated for treatment of infections caused by the following gram-negative microorganisms when bacteriologic testing indicates appropriate susceptibility to the drug:

Escherichia coli, Enterobacter aerogenes (formerly Aerobacter aerogenes), Shigella species, Mima species and Herellea species, Haemophilus influenzae (respiratory infections), Klebsiella species (respiratory and urinary infections).

Minocin is indicated for treatment of infections caused by the following gram-positive microorganisms when bacteriologic testing indicates appropriate susceptibility to the drug:

Streptococcus species:

Up to 44% of strains of Streptococcus pyogenes and 74% of Streptococcus faecalis have been found to be resistant to tetracycline drugs. Therefore, tetracyclines should not be used for streptococcal disease unless the organism has been demonstrated to be sensitive.

For upper respiratory infections due to Group A beta-hemolytic streptococci, penicillin is the usual drug of choice, including prophylaxis of rheumatic fever.

Streptococcus pneumoniae.

Staphylococcus aureus, *skin and soft tissue infections.*

Tetracyclines are not the drugs of choice in the treatment of any type of staphylococcal infection.

When penicillin is contraindicated, tetracyclines are alternative drugs in the treatment of infections due to:

Neisseria gonorrhoeae, and Neisseria meningitidis, Treponema pallidum and Treponema pertenue (syphilis and yaws), Listeria monocytogenes, Clostridium species, Bacillus anthracis, Fusobacterium fusiforme (Vincent's infection), Actinomyces species.

In acute intestinal amebiasis, the tetracyclines may be a useful adjunct to amebicides.

Minocin is indicated in the treatment of trachoma, although the infectious agent is not always eliminated, as judged by immunofluorescence.

Inclusion conjunctivitis may be treated with oral tetracyclines or with a combination of oral and topical agents.

NON-FDA APPROVED INDICATIONS

Due to its anti-collagenase, immunosuppressive and immunomodulating effects, minocycline has also been investigated for the management of rheumatoid arthritis. A dosage of 200

M

mg/day has been shown to be effective in some patients, although this use has not been approved by the FDA.

CONTRAINDICATIONS

This drug is contraindicated in persons who have shown hypersensitivity to any of the tetracyclines.

WARNINGS

In the presence of renal dysfunction, particularly in pregnancy, IV tetracycline therapy in daily doses exceeding 2 g has been associated with deaths through liver failure.

When the need for intensive treatment outweighs its potential dangers (mostly during pregnancy or in individuals with known or suspected renal or liver impairment), it is advisable to perform renal and liver function tests before and during therapy. Also, tetracycline serum concentrations should be followed.

If renal impairment exists, even usual oral or parenteral doses may lead to excessive systemic accumulation of the drug and possible liver toxicity. Under such conditions, lower than usual total doses are indicated, and if therapy is prolonged, serum level determinations of the drug may be advisable. This hazard is of particular importance in the parenteral administration of tetracyclines to pregnant or postpartum patients with pyelonephritis. When used under these circumstances, the blood level should not exceed 15 μg/ml and liver function tests should be made at frequent intervals. Other potentially hepatotoxic drugs should not be prescribed concomitantly.

THE USE OF TETRACYCLINES DURING TOOTH DEVELOPMENT (LAST HALF OF PREGNANCY, INFANCY, AND CHILDHOOD TO THE AGE OF 8 YEARS) MAY CAUSE PERMANENT DISCOLORATION OF THE TEETH (YELLOW-GRAY-BROWN). This adverse reaction is more common during long-term use of the drugs but has been observed following repeated short-term courses. Enamel hypoplasia has also been reported. TETRACYCLINES, THEREFORE, SHOULD NOT BE USED IN THIS AGE GROUP UNLESS OTHER DRUGS ARE NOT LIKELY TO BE EFFECTIVE OR ARE CONTRAINDICATED.

Photosensitivity manifested by an exaggerated sunburn reaction has been observed in some individuals taking tetracyclines. Patients apt to be exposed to direct sunlight or ultraviolet light should be advised that this reaction can occur with tetracycline drugs, and treatment should be discontinued at the first evidence of skin erythema. Studies to date indicate that photosensitivity is rarely reported with Minocin.

The anti-anabolic action of the tetracyclines may cause an increase in BUN. While this is not a problem in those with normal renal function, in patients with significantly impaired function, higher serum levels of tetracycline may lead to azotemia, hyperphosphatemia, and acidosis.

CNS side effects including light-headedness, dizziness or vertigo have been reported. Patients who experience these symptoms should be cautioned about driving vehicles or using hazardous machinery while on minocycline therapy. These symptoms may disappear during therapy and usually disappear rapidly when the drug is discontinued.

M

USAGE IN PREGNANCY

See above WARNINGS about use during tooth development.

Results of animal studies indicate that tetracyclines cross the placenta, are found in fetal tissues and can have toxic effects on the developing fetus (often related to retardation of skeletal development). Evidence of embryotoxicity has also been noted in animals treated early in pregnancy.

The safety of Minocin for use during pregnancy has not been established.

USAGE IN NEWBORNS, INFANTS, AND CHILDREN

See above WARNINGS about use during tooth development.

All tetracyclines form a stable calcium complex in any bone-forming tissue. A decrease in the fibula growth rate has been observed in prematures given oral tetracycline in doses of 25 mg/kg every 6 hours. This reaction was shown to be reversible when the drug was discontinued.

Tetracyclines are present in the milk of lactating women who are taking a drug in this class.

PRECAUTIONS

GENERAL

Pseudotumor cerebri (benign intracranial hypertension) in adults has been associated with the use of tetracyclines. The usual clinical manifestations are headache and blurred vision. Bulging fontanels have been associated with the use of tetracyclines in infants. While both of these conditions and related symptoms usually resolve soon after discontinuation of the tetracycline, the possibility for permanent sequelae exists.

As with other antibiotic preparations, use of this drug may result in overgrowth of nonsusceptible organisms, including fungi. If superinfection occurs, the antibiotic should be discontinued and appropriate therapy should be instituted.

In venereal diseases when coexistent syphilis is suspected, darkfield examination should be done before treatment is started and the blood serology repeated monthly for at least 4 months.

In long-term therapy, periodic laboratory evaluation of organ systems, including hematopoietic, renal, and hepatic studies should be performed.

All infections due to Group A beta-hemolytic streptococci should be treated for at least 10 days.

DRUG INTERACTIONS

Because tetracyclines have been shown to depress plasma prothrombin activity, patients who are on anticoagulant therapy may require downward adjustment of their anticoagulant dosage.

Since bacteriostatic drugs may interfere with the bactericidal action of penicillin, it is advisable to avoid giving tetracycline in conjunction with penicillin.

Concurrent use of tetracyclines with oral contraceptives may render oral contraceptives less effective.

ADVERSE REACTIONS

GASTROINTESTINAL

Anorexia, nausea, vomiting, diarrhea, glossitis, dysphagia, enterocolitis, pancreatitis, inflammatory lesions (with monilial overgrowth) in the anogenital region, and increases in liver enzymes. Rarely, hepatitis and liver failure have been reported.

These reactions have been caused by both the oral and parenteral administration of tetracyclines.

SKIN

Maculopapular and erythematous rashes. Exfoliative dermatitis has been reported but is uncommon. Fixed drug eruptions, including balanitis, have been rarely reported. Erythema multiforme and rarely Stevens-Johnson syndrome have been reported. Photosensitivity is discussed above. (See WARNINGS.)

Pigmentation of the skin and mucous membranes has been reported.

Tooth discoloration has been reported, rarely, in adults.

RENAL TOXICITY

Rise in BUN has been reported and is apparently dose related. (See WARNINGS.) Reversible acute renal failure has been rarely reported.

HYPERSENSITIVITY REACTIONS

Urticaria, angioneurotic edema, polyarthralgia, anaphylaxis, anaphylactoid purpura, pericarditis, exacerbation of systemic lupus erythematosus, and rarely, pulmonary infiltrates with eosinophilia have been reported. A transient lupus-like syndrome has also been reported.

BLOOD

Hemolytic anemia, thrombocytopenia, neutropenia, and eosinophilia have been reported.

CNS

(See WARNINGS.) Pseudotumor cerebri (benign intracranial hypertension) in adults and bulging fontanels in infants. (See PRECAUTIONS, General.) Headache has also been reported.

OTHER

When given over prolonged periods, tetracyclines have been reported to produce brown-black microscopic discoloration of the thyroid glands. Very rare cases of abnormal thyroid function have been reported.

Decreased hearing has been rarely reported in patients on Minocin.

DOSAGE AND ADMINISTRATION

Note: Rapid administration is to be avoided. Parenteral therapy is indicated only when oral therapy is not adequate or tolerated. Oral therapy should be instituted as soon as possible. If IV therapy is given over prolonged periods of time, thrombophlebitis may result.

Adults: *Usual adult dose:* 200 mg followed by 100 mg every 12 hours and should not exceed 400 mg in 24 hours. The cryodesiccated powder should be reconstituted with 5 ml sterile water for injection and immediately further diluted to 500-1000 ml with sodium chloride injection, dextrose injection, dextrose and sodium chloride injection, Ringer's injection, or lactated Ringer's injection, but not other solutions containing calcium because a precipitate may form. When further diluted in 500-1000 ml compatible solutions (except lactated Ringer's), the pH usually ranges from 2.5-4.0. The pH of Minocin IV 100 mg in lactated Ringer's 500-1000 ml usually ranges from 4.5-6.0.

Final dilutions (500-1000 ml) should be administered immediately but product and diluents are compatible at room temperature for 24 hours without a significant loss of potency. Any unused portions must be discarded after that period.

For children above 8 years of age: *Usual pediatric dose:* 4 mg/kg followed by 2 mg/kg every 12 hours.

In patients with renal impairment: See WARNINGS.

Total dosage should be decreased by reduction of recommended individual doses and/or by extending time intervals between doses.

Parenteral drug products should be inspected visually for particulate matter and discoloration prior to administration, whenever solution and container permit.

HOW SUPPLIED

Minocin IV is supplied as 100 mg vials of sterile cryodesiccated powder.

Storage: Store at controlled room temperature 15-30°C (59-86°F).

ORAL

DESCRIPTION

CAPSULES

Minocycline hydrochloride, a semisynthetic derivative of tetracycline, is [4S-(4(alpha),4a(alpha),5a(alpha),12a(alpha))]-4,7-bis(dimethylamino)-1,4,4a,5,5a,6,11,12a-octahydro-3,10,12,12a-tetrahydroxy-1,11-dioxo-2-naphthacenecarboxamide monohydrochloride.

Minocin pellet-filled capsules for oral administration contain pellets of minocycline hydrochloride equivalent to 50 or 100 mg of minocycline in microcrystalline cellulose.

The capsule shells contain the following inactive ingredients: Blue 1, gelatin, titanium dioxide and yellow 10. The 50 mg capsule shells also contain black and yellow iron oxides.

ORAL SUSPENSION

Minocycline hydrochloride, a semisynthetic derivative of tetracycline, is named [4S-(4(alpha),4a(alpha),5a(alpha),12a(alpha))]-4,7-bis(dimethylamino)-1,4,4a,5,5a,6,11,12a-octahydro-3,10,12,12a-tetrahydroxy-1,11-dioxo-2- naphthacenecarboxamide monohydrochloride.

The empirical formula is $C_{23}H_{27}N_3O_7$·HCl and the molecular weight is 493.94.

Minocin oral suspension contains minocycline hydrochloride equivalent to 50 mg of minocycline per 5 ml (10 mg/ml) and the following inactive ingredients: alcohol, butylparaben, calcium hydroxide, cellulose, decaglyceryl tetraoleate, edetate calcium disodium, glycol, guar gum, polysorbate 80, propylparaben, propylene glycol, sodium saccharin, sodium sulfite (see WARNINGS) and sorbitol.

CLINICAL PHARMACOLOGY

CAPSULES

Minocin pellet-filled capsules are rapidly absorbed from the gastrointestinal tract following oral administration. Following a single dose of two 100 mg pellet-filled capsules of Minocin administered to 18 normal fasting adult volunteers, maximum serum concentrations were attained in 1-4 hours (average 2.1 hours) and ranged from 2.1-5.1 µg/ml (average 3.5 µg/ml). The serum half-life in the normal volunteers ranged from 11.1-22.1 hours (average 15.5 hours).

When Minocin pellet-filled capsules were given concomitantly with a meal which included dairy products, the extent of absorption of Minocin pellet-filled capsules was not noticeably influenced. The peak plasma concentrations were slightly decreased (11.2%) and delayed by 1 hour when administered with food, compared to dosing under fasting conditions.

In previous studies with other minocycline dosage forms, the minocycline serum half-life ranged from 11-16 hours in 7 patients with hepatic dysfunction, and from 18-69 hours in 5 patients with renal dysfunction. The urinary and fecal recovery of minocycline when administered to 12 normal volunteers is one-half to one-third that of other tetracyclines.

Microbiology

The tetracyclines are primarily bacteriostatic and are thought to exert their antimicrobial effect by the inhibition of protein synthesis. The tetracyclines, including minocycline, have similar antimicrobial spectra of activity against a wide range of gram-positive and gram-negative organisms. Cross-resistance of these organisms to tetracyclines is common.

While *in vitro* studies have demonstrated the susceptibility of most strains of the following microorganisms, clinical efficacy for infections other than those included in the INDICATIONS AND USAGE section has not been documented.

Gram-Negative Bacteria:

Bartonella bacilliformis, Brucella species, *Calymmatobacterium granulomatis, Campylobacter fetus, Francisella tularensis, Haemophilus ducreyi, Haemophilus influenzae, Listeria monocytogenes, Neisseria gonorrhoeae, Vibrio cholerae, Yersinia pestis.*

Because many strains of the following groups of gram-negative microorganisms have been shown to be resistant to tetracyclines, culture and susceptibility tests are especially recommended:

Acinetobacter species, *Bacteroides* species, *Enterobacter aerogenes, Escherichia coli, Klebsiella* species, *Shigella* species.

Gram-Positive Bacteria:

Because many strains of the following groups of gram-positive microorganisms have been shown to be resistant to tetracyclines, culture and susceptibility testing are especially recommended. Up to 44% of *Streptococcus pyogenes* strains have been found to be resistant to tetracycline drugs. Therefore, tetracyclines should not be used for streptococcal disease unless the organism has been demonstrated to be susceptible.

Enterococcus group [*Enterococcus faecalis* (formerly *Streptococcus faecalis*) and *Enterococcus faecium* (formerly *Streptococcus faecium*)], *Streptococcus pneumoniae, Streptococcus pyogenes,* Viridans group streptococci.

Other Microorganisms:

Actinomyces species, *Bacillus anthracis, Balantidium coli, Borrelia recurrentis, Chlamydia psittaci, Chlamydia trachomatis, Clostridium* species, *Entamoeba* species, *Fusobacterium fusiforme, Mycoplasma pneumoniae, Propionibacterium acnes, Rickettsia, Treponema pallidum, Treponema pertenue, Ureaplasma urealyticum.*

Susceptibility Testing

Diffusion Techniques

The use of antibiotic disk susceptibility test methods which measure zone diameter gives an accurate estimation of susceptibility of microorganisms to Minocin. One such standard procedure[1] has been recommended for use with disks for testing antimicrobials. Either the 30 µg tetracycline-class disk or the 30 µg minocycline disk should be used for the determination of the susceptibility of microorganisms to minocycline.

With this type of procedure a report of "susceptible" from the laboratory indicates that the infecting organism is likely to respond to therapy. A report of "intermediate susceptibility" suggests that the organism would be susceptible if a high dosage is used or if the infection is confined to tissues and fluids (*e.g.,* urine) in which high antibiotic levels are attained. A report of "resistant" indicates that the infecting organism is not likely to respond to therapy. With either the tetracycline-class disk or the minocycline disk, zone sizes of 19 mm or greater indicate susceptibility, zone sizes of 14 mm or less indicate resistance, and zone sizes of 15-18 mm indicate intermediate susceptibility.

Standardized procedures require the use of laboratory control organisms. The 30 µg tetracycline disk should give zone diameters between 19 and 28 mm for *Staphylococcus aureus* ATCC 25923 and between 18 and 25 mm for *Escherichia coli* ATCC 25922. The 30 µg minocycline disk should give zone diameters between 25 and 30 mm for *S. aureus* ATCC 25923 and between 19 and 25 mm for *E. coli* ATCC 25922.

Dilution Techniques

When using the NCCLS agar dilution or broth dilution (including microdilution) method[2] or equivalent, a bacterial isolate may be considered susceptible if the MIC (minimal inhibitory concentration) of minocycline is 4 µg/ml or less. Organisms are considered resistant if the MIC is 16 µg/ml or greater. Organisms with an MIC value of less than 16 µg/ml but greater than 4 µg/ml are expected to be susceptible if a high dosage is used or if the infection is confined to tissues and fluids (*e.g.,* urine) in which high antibiotic levels are attained.

As with standard diffusion methods, dilution procedures require the use of laboratory control organisms. Standard tetracycline or minocycline powder should give MIC values of 0.25–1.0 µg/ml for *S. aureus* ATCC 25923, and 1.0–4.0 µg/ml for *E. coli* ATCC 25922.

ORAL SUSPENSION

Microbiology

The tetracyclines are primarily bacteriostatic and are thought to exert their antimicrobial effect by the inhibition of protein synthesis. Minocycline HCl is a tetracycline with antibacterial activity comparable to other tetracyclines with activity against a wide range of gram-negative and gram-positive organisms.

Tube Dilution Testing

Microorganisms may be considered susceptible (likely to respond to minocycline therapy) if the minimum inhibitory concentration (MIC) is not more than 4 µg/ml. Microorganisms may be considered intermediate (harboring partial resistance) if the MIC is 4 to 12.5 µg/ml and resistant (not likely to respond to minocycline therapy) if the MIC is greater than 12.5 µg/ml.

Susceptibility Plate Testing

If the Kirby-Bauer method of susceptibility testing (using a 30 µg tetracycline disc) gives a zone of 18 mm or greater, the bacterial strain is considered to be susceptible to any tetracycline. Minocycline shows moderate *in vitro* activity against certain strains of staphylococci which have been found resistant to other tetracyclines. For such strains minocycline susceptibility powder may be used for additional susceptibility testing.

Human Pharmacology

Following a single dose of two 100 mg minocycline HCl capsules administered to 10 normal adult volunteers, serum levels ranged from 0.74-4.45 µg/ml in 1 hour (average 2.24), after 12 hours, they ranged from 0.34-2.36 µg/ml (average 1.25). The serum half-life following a single 200 mg dose in 12 essentially normal volunteers ranged from 11-17 hours. In 7 patients with hepatic dysfunction it ranged from 11-16 hours, and in 5 patients with renal dysfunction from 18-69 hours. The urinary and fecal recovery of minocycline when administered to 12 normal volunteers is one-half to one-third that of other tetracyclines.

INDICATIONS AND USAGE

CAPSULES

Minocin pellet-filled capsules are indicated in the treatment of the following infections due to susceptible strains of the designated microorganisms:

Rocky Mountain spotted fever, typhus fever and the typhus group, Q fever, rickettsialpox and tick fevers caused by *Rickettsia.*
Respiratory tract infections caused by *Mycoplasm pneumoniae.*
Lymphogranuloma venereum caused by *Chlamydia trachomatis.*
Psittacosis (Ornithosis) due to *Chlamydia psittaci.*
Trachoma caused by *Chlamydia trachomatis,* although the infectious agent is not always eliminated, as judged by immunofluorescence.
Inclusion conjunctivitis caused by *Chlamydia trachomatis.*
Nongonococcal urethritis in adults caused by *Ureaplasma urealyticum* or *Chlamydia trachomatis.*
Relapsing fever due to *Borrelia recurrentis.*
Chancroid caused by *Haemophilus ducreyi.*
Plague due to *Yersinia pestis.*
Tularemia due to *Francisella tularensis.*
Cholera caused by *Vibrio cholerae.*
Campylobacter fetus infections caused by *Campylobacter fetus.*
Brucellosis due to *Brucella* species (in conjunction with streptomycin).
Bartonellosis due to *Bartonella bacilliformis.*
Granuloma inguinale caused by *Calymmatobacterium granulomatis.*

Minocycline is indicated for treatment of infections caused by the following gram-negative microorganisms, when bacteriologic testing indicates appropriate susceptibility to the drug:

Escherichia coli.
Enterobacter aerogenes.
Shigella species.
Acinetobacter species.
Respiratory tract infections caused by *Haemophilus influenzae.*
Respiratory tract and urinary tract infections caused by *Klebsiella* species.

Minocin pellet-filled capsules are indicated for the treatment of infections caused by the following gram-positive microorganisms when bacteriologic testing indicates appropriate susceptibility to the drug:

Upper respiratory tract infections caused by *Streptococcus pneumoniae.*
Skin and skin structure infections caused by *Staphylococcus aureus.* (*Note:* Minocycline is not the drug of choice in the treatment of any type of staphylococcal infection.)
Uncomplicated urethritis in men due to *Neisseria gonorrhoeae* and for the treatment of other gonococcal infections when penicillin is contraindicated.

When penicillin is contraindicated, minocycline is an alternative drug in the treatment of the following infections:

Infections in women caused by *Neisseria gonorrhoeae.*
Syphilis caused by *Treponema pallidum.*
Yaws caused by *Treponema pertenue.*
Listeriosis due to *Listeria monocytogenes.*
Anthrax due to *Bacillus anthracis.*
Vincent's infection caused by *Fusobacterium fusiforme.*
Actinomycosis caused by *Actinomyces israelii.*
Infections caused by *Clostridium species.*

In *acute intestinal amebiasis,* minocycline may be a useful adjunct to amebicides.

In severe *acne,* minocycline may be useful adjunctive therapy.

Oral minocycline is indicated in the treatment of asymptomatic carriers of *Neisseria meningitidis* to eliminate meningococci from the nasopharynx. In order to preserve the usefulness of minocycline in the treatment of asymptomatic meningococcal carrier, diagnostic laboratory procedures, including serotyping and susceptibility testing, should be performed to establish the carrier state and the correct treatment. It is recommended that the prophylactic use of minocycline be reserved for situations in which the risk of meningococcal meningitis is high.

Oral minocycline is not indicated for the treatment of meningococcal infection.

Although no controlled clinical efficacy studies have been conducted, limited clinical data show that oral minocycline hydrochloride has been used successfully in the treatment of infections caused by *Mycobacterium marinum.*

ORAL SUSPENSION

Minocin is indicated in infections caused by the following microorganisms:

Rickettsia: (Rocky Mountain spotted fever, typhus fever and the typhus group, Q fever, rickettsialpox, tick fevers.)

Mycoplasma pneumoniae (PPLO, Eaton agent).

Agents of psittacosis and ornithosis.

Agents of lymphogranuloma venereum and granuloma inguinale.

The spirochetal agent of relapsing fever (Borrelia recurrentis).

The following gram-negative microorganisms:

Haemophilus ducreyi (chancroid), Yersinia pestis and Francisella tularensis (formerly Pasteurella pestis and Pasteurella tularensis), Bartonella bacilliformis, Bacteroides species, Vibrio comma and Vibrio fetus, Brucella species (in conjunction with streptomycin).

Because many strains of the following groups of microorganisms have been shown to be resistant to tetracyclines, culture and susceptibility testing are recommended.

Minocin is indicated for treatment of infections caused by the following gram-negative microorganisms when bacteriologic testing indicates appropriate susceptibility to the drug:

Escherichia coli, Enterobacter aerogenes (formerly Aerobacter aerogenes), Shigella species, Acinetobacter calcoaceticus (formerly Herellea, Mima), Haemophilus influenzae (respiratory infections), Klebsiella species (respiratory and urinary infections).

Minocin is indicated for treatment of infections caused by the following gram-positive microorganisms when bacteriologic testing indicates appropriate susceptibility to the drug:

Streptococcus species:

Up to 44% of strains of Streptococcus pyogenes and 74% of Streptococcus faecalis have been found to be resistant to tetracycline drugs. Therefore, tetracyclines should not be used for streptococcal disease unless the organism has been demonstrated to be sensitive.

For upper respiratory infections due to Group A beta-hemolytic streptococci, penicillin is the usual drug of choice, including prophylaxis of rheumatic fever.

***Streptococcus pneumoniae** (formerly Diplococcus pneumoniae).*

***Staphylococcus aureus,** skin and soft tissue infections.*

Tetracyclines are not the drugs of choice in the treatment of any type of staphylococcal infection.

Minocin is indicated for the treatment of uncomplicated gonococcal urethritis in men due to Neisseria gonorrhoeae.

When penicillin is contraindicated, tetracyclines are alternative drugs in the treatment of infections due to:

Neisseria gonorrhoeae (in women), Treponema pallidum and Treponema pertenue (syphilis and yaws), Listeria monocytogenes, Clostridium species, Bacillus anthracis, Fusobacterium fusiforme (Vincent's infection), Actinomyces species.

In acute intestinal amebiasis, the tetracyclines may be a useful adjunct to amebicides.

In severe acne, the tetracyclines may be useful adjunctive therapy.

Minocin is indicated in the treatment of trachoma, although the infectious agent is not always eliminated, as judged by immunofluorescence.

Minocin is indicated for the treatment of uncomplicated urethral, endocervical or rectal infections in adults caused by Chlamydia trachomatis or Ureaplasma urealyticum.[1]

Inclusion conjunctivitis may be treated with oral tetracyclines or with a combination of oral and topical agents.

Minocin is indicated in the treatment of asymptomatic carriers of Neisseria meningitidis to eliminate meningococci from the nasopharynx.

In order to preserve the usefulness of Minocin in the treatment of asymptomatic meningococcal carriers, diagnostic laboratory procedures, including serotyping and susceptibility testing, should be performed to establish the carrier state and the correct treatment. It is recommended that the drug be reserved for situations in which the risk of meningococcal meningitis is high.

Minocin by oral administration is not indicated for the treatment of meningococcal infection.

Although no controlled clinical efficacy studies have been conducted, limited clinical data show that oral Minocin has been used successfully in the treatment of infections caused by Mycobacterium marinum.

NON-FDA APPROVED INDICATIONS

Due to its anti-collagenase, immunosuppressive and immunomodulating effects, minocycline has also been investigated for the management of rheumatoid arthritis. A dosage of 200 mg/day has been shown to be effective in some patients, although this use has not been approved by the FDA.

CONTRAINDICATIONS

Minocin pellet-filled capsules and oral suspension are contraindicated in persons who have shown hypersensitivity to any of the tetracyclines.

WARNINGS

CAPSULES

MINOCIN PELLET-FILLED CAPSULES, LIKE OTHER TETRACYCLINE-CLASS ANTIBIOTICS, CAN CAUSE FETAL HARM WHEN ADMINISTERED TO A PREGNANT WOMAN. IF ANY TETRACYCLINE IS USED DURING PREGNANCY OR IF THE PATIENT BECOMES PREGNANT WHILE TAKING THESE DRUGS, THE PATIENT SHOULD BE APPRISED OF THE POTENTIAL HAZARD TO THE FETUS. THE USE OF DRUGS OF THE TETRACYCLINE CLASS DURING TOOTH DEVELOPMENT (LAST HALF OF PREGNANCY, INFANCY, AND CHILDHOOD TO THE AGE OF 8 YEARS) MAY CAUSE PERMANENT DISCOLORATION OF THE TEETH (YELLOW-GRAY-BROWN).

This adverse reaction is more common during long-term use of the drug but has been observed following repeated short-term courses. Enamel hypoplasia has also been reported. TETRACYCLINE DRUGS, THEREFORE, SHOULD NOT BE USED DURING TOOTH DEVELOPMENT UNLESS OTHER DRUGS ARE NOT LIKELY TO BE EFFECTIVE OR ARE CONTRAINDICATED.

All tetracyclines form a stable calcium complex in any bone-forming tissue. A decrease in fibula growth rate has been observed in premature human infants given oral tetracycline in doses of 25 mg/kg every 6 hours. This reaction was shown to be reversible when the drug was discontinued.

Results of animal studies indicate that tetracyclines cross the placenta, are found in fetal tissues, and can have toxic effects on the developing fetus (often related to retardation of skeletal development). Evidence of embryotoxicity has been noted in animals treated early in pregnancy.

The anti-anabolic action of the tetracyclines may cause an increase in BUN. While this is not a problem in those with normal renal function, in patients with significantly impaired function, higher serum levels of tetracycline may lead to azotemia, hyperphosphatemia, and acidosis. If renal impairment exists, even usual oral or parenteral doses may lead to excessive systemic accumulations of the drug and possible liver toxicity. Under such conditions, lower than usual total doses are indicated, and if therapy is prolonged, serum level determinations of the drug may be advisable.

Photosensitivity manifested by an exaggerated sunburn reaction has been observed in some individuals taking tetracyclines. This has been reported rarely with minocycline.

Central nervous system side effects including lightheadedness, dizziness, or vertigo have been reported with minocycline therapy. Patients who experience these symptoms should be cautioned about driving vehicles or using hazardous machinery while on minocycline therapy. These symptoms may disappear during therapy and usually disappear rapidly when the drug is discontinued.

ORAL SUSPENSION

THE USE OF DRUGS OF THE TETRACYCLINE CLASS DURING TOOTH DEVELOPMENT (LAST HALF OF PREGNANCY, INFANCY, AND CHILDHOOD TO THE AGE OF 8 YEARS) MAY CAUSE PERMANENT DISCOLORATION OF THE TEETH (YELLOW-GRAY-BROWN). This adverse reaction is more common during long-term use of the drugs but has been observed following repeated short-term courses. Enamel hypoplasia has also been reported. TETRACYCLINE DRUGS, THEREFORE, SHOULD NOT BE USED IN THIS AGE GROUP UNLESS OTHER DRUGS ARE NOT LIKELY TO BE EFFECTIVE OR ARE CONTRAINDICATED.

If renal impairment exists, even usual oral or parenteral doses may lead to excessive systemic accumulations of the drug and possible liver toxicity. Under such conditions, lower than usual total doses are indicated, and if therapy is prolonged, serum level determinations of the drug may be advisable.

Photosensitivity manifested by an exaggerated sunburn reaction has been observed in some individuals taking tetracyclines. Patients apt to be exposed to direct sunlight or ultraviolet light should be advised that this reaction can occur with tetracycline drugs, and treatment should be discontinued at the first evidence of skin erythema. Studies to date indicate that photosensitivity is rarely reported with Minocin.

The anti-anabolic action of the tetracyclines may cause an increase in BUN. While this is not a problem in those with normal renal function, in patients with significantly impaired function, higher serum levels of tetracycline may lead to azotemia, hyperphosphatemia, and acidosis.

CNS side effects including light-headedness, dizziness, or vertigo have been reported. Patients who experience these symptoms should be cautioned about driving vehicles or using hazardous machinery while on minocycline therapy. These symptoms may disappear during therapy and usually disappear rapidly when the drug is discontinued.

Minocin oral suspension contains sodium sulfite, a sulfite that may cause allergic-type reactions including anaphylactic symptoms and life-threatening or less severe asthmatic episodes in certain susceptible people. The overall prevalence of sulfite sensitivity in the general population is unknown and probably low. Sulfite sensitivity is seen more frequently in asthmatic than in nonasthmatic people.

Usage in Pregnancy

See above WARNINGS about use during tooth development.

Results of animal studies indicate that tetracyclines cross the placenta, are found in fetal tissues and can have toxic effects on the developing fetus (often related to retardation of skeletal development). Evidence of embryotoxicity has also been noted in animals treated early in pregnancy.

The safety of Minocin for use during pregnancy has not been established.

Usage in Newborns, Infants, and Children

See above WARNINGS about use during tooth development.

All tetracyclines form a stable calcium complex in any bone forming tissue. A decrease in the fibula growth rate has been observed in prematures given oral tetracycline in doses of 25 mg/kg every 6 hours. This reaction was shown to be reversible when the drug was discontinued.

Tetracyclines are present in the milk of lactating women who are taking a drug in this class.

PRECAUTIONS

CAPSULES

General

As with other antibiotic preparations, use of this drug may result in overgrowth of nonsusceptible organisms, including fungi. If superinfection occurs, the antibiotic should be discontinued and appropriate therapy instituted.

Pseudotumor cerebri (benign intracranial hypertension) in adults has been associated with the use of tetracyclines. The usual clinical manifestations are headache and blurred vision. Bulging fontanels have been associated with the use of tetracyclines in infants. While both of these conditions and related symptoms usually resolve after discontinuation of the tetracycline, the possibility for permanent sequelae exists.

Incision and drainage or other surgical procedures should be performed in conjunction with antibiotic therapy when indicated.

Information for the Patient

Photosensitivity manifested by an exaggerated sunburn reaction has been observed in some individuals taking tetracyclines. Patients apt to be exposed to direct sunlight or ultraviolet light should be advised that this reaction can occur with tetracycline drugs, and treatment should be discontinued at the first evidence of skin erythema. This reaction has been reported rarely with use of minocycline.

Patients who experience central nervous system symptoms (see WARNINGS) should be cautioned about driving vehicles or using hazardous machinery while on minocycline therapy.

Concurrent use of tetracycline may render oral contraceptives less effective (see DRUG INTERACTIONS).

Laboratory Tests

In venereal disease when coexistent syphilis is suspected, a dark-field examination should be done before treatment is started and the blood serology repeated monthly for at least 4 months.

In long-term therapy, periodic laboratory evaluations of organ systems, including hematopoietic, renal, and hepatic studies, should be performed.

Drug/Laboratory Test Interactions

False elevations of urinary catecholamine levels may occur due to interference with the fluorescence test.

Carcinogenesis, Mutagenesis, and Impairment of Fertility

Dietary administration of minocycline in long term tumorigenicity studies in rats resulted in evidence of thyroid tumor production. Minocycline has also been found to produce thyroid hyperplasia in rats and dogs. In addition, there has been evidence of oncogenic activity in rats in studies with a related antibiotic, oxytetracycline (*i.e.,* adrenal and pituitary tumors). Likewise, although mutagenicity studies of minocycline have not been conducted, positive results in *in vitro* mammalian cell assays (*i.e.,* mouse lymphoma and Chinese hamster lung cells) have been reported for related antibiotics (tetracycline hydrochloride and oxytetracycline). Segment I (fertility and general reproduction) studies have provided evidence that minocycline impairs fertility in male rats.

Pregnancy, Teratogenic Effects, Pregnancy Category D

See WARNINGS.

Nonteratogenic Effects: See WARNINGS.

Labor and Delivery

The effect of tetracyclines on labor and delivery is unknown.

Nursing Mothers

Tetracyclines are excreted in human milk. Because of the potential for serious adverse reactions in nursing infants from the tetracyclines, a decision should be made whether to discontinue nursing or discontinue the drug, taking into account the importance of the drug to the mother (see WARNINGS).

Pediatric Use

See WARNINGS.

ORAL SUSPENSION

General

Pseudotumor cerebri (benign intracranial hypertension) in adults has been associated with the use of tetracyclines. The usual clinical manifestations are headache and blurred vision. Bulging fontanels have been associated with the use of tetracyclines in infants. While both of these conditions and related symptoms usually resolve soon after discontinuation of the tetracycline, the possibility for permanent sequelae exists.

As with other antibiotic preparations, use of this drug may result in overgrowth of nonsusceptible organisms, including fungi. If superinfection occurs, the antibiotic should be discontinued and appropriate therapy should be instituted.

In venereal diseases when coexistent syphilis is suspected, darkfield examination should be done before treatment is started and the blood serology repeated monthly for at least 4 months.

In long-term therapy, periodic laboratory evaluation of organ systems, including hematopoietic, renal and hepatic studies should be performed.

All infections due to Group A beta-hemolytic streptococci should be treated for at least 10 days.

DRUG INTERACTIONS

CAPSULES

Because tetracyclines have been shown to depress plasma prothrombin activity, patients who are on anticoagulant therapy may require downward adjustment of their anticoagulant dosage.

Since bacteriostatic drugs may interfere with the bactericidal action of penicillin, it is advisable to avoid giving tetracycline-class drugs in conjunction with penicillin.

Absorption of tetracyclines is impaired by antacids containing aluminum, calcium or magnesium, and iron-containing preparations.

The concurrent use of tetracycline and methoxyflurane has been reported to result in fatal renal toxicity.

Concurrent use of tetracyclines with oral contraceptives may render oral contraceptives less effective.

ORAL SUSPENSION

Because tetracyclines have been shown to depress plasma prothrombin activity, patients who are on anticoagulant therapy may require downward adjustment of their anticoagulant dosage.

Since bacteriostatic drugs may interfere with the bactericidal action of penicillin, it is advisable to avoid giving tetracycline in conjunction with penicillin.

Concurrent use of tetracyclines with oral contraceptives may render oral contraceptives less effective.

ADVERSE REACTIONS

CAPSULES

Due to oral minocycline's virtually complete absorption, side effects to the lower bowel, particularly diarrhea, have been infrequent. The following adverse reactions have been observed in patients receiving tetracyclines.

Gastrointestinal: Anorexia, nausea, vomiting, diarrhea, glossitis, dysphagia, enterocolitis, pancreatitis, inflammatory lesions (with monilial overgrowth) in the anogenital region, and increases in liver enzymes. Rarely, hepatitis and liver failure have been reported. Rare instances of esophagitis and esophageal ulcerations have been reported in patients taking the tetracycline-class antibiotics in capsule and tablet form. Most of these patients took the medication immediately before going to bed (see DOSAGE AND ADMINISTRATION).

Skin: Maculopapular and erythematous rashes. Exfoliative dermatitis has been reported but is uncommon. Fixed drug eruptions have been rarely reported. Lesions occurring on the glans penis have caused balanitis. Erythema multiforme and rarely Stevens-Johnson syndrome have been reported. Photosensitivity is discussed above (see WARNINGS). Pigmentation of the skin and mucous membranes has been reported.

Renal Toxicity: Elevations in BUN have been reported and are apparently dose related (see WARNINGS). Reversible acute renal failure has been rarely reported.

Hypersensitivity Reactions: Urticaria, angioneurotic edema, polyarthralgia, anaphylaxis, anaphylactoid purpura, pericarditis, exacerbation of systemic lupus erythematosus and rarely pulmonary infiltrates with eosinophilia have been reported. A transient lupus-like syndrome has also been reported.

Blood: Hemolytic anemia, thrombocytopenia, neutropenia, and eosinophilia have been reported.

Central Nervous System: Bulging fontanels in infants and benign intracranial hypertension (Pseudotumor cerebri) in adults (see PRECAUTIONS, General) have been reported. Headache has also been reported.

Other: When given over prolonged periods, tetracyclines have been reported to produce brown-black microscopic discoloration of the thyroid glands. Very rare cases of abnormal thyroid function have been reported.

Decreased hearing has been rarely reported in patients on Minocin.

Tooth discoloration in children less than 8 years of age (see WARNINGS) and also, rarely, in adults has been reported.

M

ORAL SUSPENSION

Gastrointestinal

Anorexia, nausea, vomiting, diarrhea, glossitis, dysphagia, enterocolitis, pancreatitis, inflammatory lesions (with monilial overgrowth) in the anogenital region and increases in liver enzymes. Rarely, hepatitis and liver failure have been reported.

These reactions have been caused by both the oral and parenteral administration of tetracyclines.

Skin

Maculopapular and erythematous rashes. Exfoliative dermatitis has been reported but is uncommon. Fixed drug eruptions, including balanitis, have been rarely reported. Erythema multiforme and rarely Stevens-Johnson syndrome have been reported. Photosensitivity is discussed above. (See WARNINGS.)

Pigmentation of the skin and mucous membranes has been reported.

Tooth discoloration has been reported rarely in adults.

Renal Toxicity

Rise in BUN has been reported and is apparently dose related. (See WARNINGS.) Reversible acute renal failure has been rarely reported.

Hypersensitivity Reactions

Urticaria, angioneurotic edema, polyarthralgia, anaphylaxis, anaphylactoid purpura, pericarditis, exacerbation of systemic lupus erythematosus and rarely pulmonary infiltrates with eosinophilia have been reported. A transient lupus-like syndrome has also been reported.

Blood

Hemolytic anemia, thrombocytopenia, neutropenia and eosinophilia have been reported.

CNS

(See WARNINGS.) Pseudotumor cerebri (benign intracranial hypertension) in adults and bulging fontanels in infants. (See PRECAUTIONS, General.) Headache has also been reported.

Other

When given over prolonged periods, tetracyclines have been reported to produce brown-black microscopic discoloration of the thyroid glands. Very rare cases of abnormal thyroid function have been reported.

Decreased hearing has been rarely reported in patients on Minocin.

DOSAGE AND ADMINISTRATION

CAPSULES

THE USUAL DOSAGE AND FREQUENCY OF ADMINISTRATION OF MINOCYCLINE DIFFERS FROM THAT OF THE OTHER TETRACYCLINES. EXCEEDING THE RECOMMENDED DOSAGE MAY RESULT IN AN INCREASED INCIDENCE OF SIDE EFFECTS.

Minocin pellet-filled capsules may be taken with or without food (see CLINICAL PHARMACOLOGY).

Adults: The usual dosage of Minocin pellet-filled capsules is 200 mg initially followed by 100 mg every 12 hours. Alternatively, if more frequent doses are preferred, two or four 50 mg pellet-filled capsules may be given initially followed by one 50 mg capsule 4 times daily.

For children above 8 years of age: The usual dosage of Minocin pellet-filled capsules is 4 mg/kg initially followed by 2 mg/kg every 12 hours.

Uncomplicated gonococcal infections other than urethritis and anorectal infections in men: 200 mg initially, followed by 100 mg every 12 hours for a minimum of 4 days, with post-therapy cultures within 2-3 days.

In the treatment of uncomplicated gonococcal urethritis in men, 100 mg every 12 hours for 5 days is recommended.

For the treatment of syphilis, the usual dosage of Minocin pellet-filled capsules should be administered over a period of 10-15 days. Close follow-up, including laboratory tests, is recommended.

In the treatment of meningococcal carrier state, the recommended dosage is 100 mg every 12 hours for 5 days.

Mycobacterium marinum **infections:** Although optimal doses have not been established, 100 mg every 12 hours for 6-8 weeks have been used successfully in a limited number of cases.

Uncomplicated nongonococcal urethral infection in adults caused by ***Chlamydia trachomatis*** **or** ***Ureaplasma urealyticum*:** 100 mg orally, every 12 hours for at least 7 days.

Ingestion of adequate amounts of fluids along with capsule and tablet forms of drugs in the tetracycline-class is recommended to reduce the risk of esophageal irritation and ulceration.

In patients with renal impairment (see WARNINGS), the total dosage should be decreased by either reducing the recommended individual doses and/or by extending the time intervals between doses.

ORAL SUSPENSION

Therapy should be continued for at least 24-48 hours after symptoms and fever have subsided.

Concomitant therapy: Antacids containing aluminum, calcium, or magnesium impair absorption and should not be given to patients taking oral tetracycline.

Studies to date have indicated that the absorption of Minocin is not notably influenced by foods and dairy products.

In patients with renal impairment: (See WARNINGS.) Total dosage should be decreased by reduction of recommended individual doses and/or extending time intervals between doses.

In the treatment of streptococcal infections, a therapeutic dose of tetracycline should be administered for at least 10 days.

Adults: The usual dosage of Minocin is 200 mg initially followed by 100 mg every 12 hours.

For children above 8 years of age: The usual dosage of Minocin is 4 mg/kg initially followed by 2 mg/kg every 12 hours.

For treatment of syphilis, the usual dosage of Minocin should be administered over a period of 10-15 days. Close follow up, including laboratory tests, is recommended.

Gonorrhea patients sensitive to penicillin may be treated with Minocin, administered as 200 mg initially followed by 100 mg every 12 hours for a minimum of 4 days, with post-therapy cultures within 2-3 days.

In the treatment of meningococcal carrier state, recommended dosage is 100 mg every 12 hours for 5 days.

Mycobacterium marinum **infections:** Although optimal doses have not been established, 100 mg twice a day for 6-8 weeks have been used successfully in a limited number of cases.

Uncomplicated urethral, endocervical, or rectal infection in adults caused by ***Chlamydia trachomatis*** **or** ***Ureaplasma urealyticum*:** 100 mg, by mouth, 2 times a day for at least 7 days.[1]

In the treatment of uncomplicated gonococcal urethritis in men, 100 mg twice a day orally for 5 days is recommended.

ANIMAL PHARMACOLOGY

CAPSULES

Minocin has been observed to cause a dark discoloration of the thyroid in experimental animals (rats, minipigs, dogs, and monkeys). In the rat, chronic treatment with Minocin has resulted in goiter accompanied by elevated radioactive iodine uptake and evidence of thyroid tumor production. Minocin has also been found to produce thyroid hyperplasia in rats and dogs.

ORAL SUSPENSION

Minocin has been found to produce high blood concentrations following oral dosage to various animal species and to be extensively distributed to all tissues examined in ^{14}C-labeled drug studies in dogs. Minocin has been found experimentally to produce discoloration of the thyroid glands. This finding has been observed in rats and dogs. Changes in thyroid function have also been found in these animal species. However, no change in thyroid function has been observed in humans.

HOW SUPPLIED

CAPSULES

Minocin pellet-filled capsules are supplied as capsules containing minocycline hydrochloride equivalent to 50 and 100 mg minocycline.

100 mg, two-piece, hard-shell capsule with an opaque light green cap and a transparent green body, printed in white ink with "Lederle" over "M46" on one half and "Lederle" over "100 mg" on the other half. Each capsule contains pellets of minocycline HCl equivalent to 100 mg of minocycline.

50 mg, two-piece, hard-shell capsule with an opaque yellow cap and a transparent green body, printed in black ink with "Lederle" over "M45" on one half and "Lederle" over "50 mg" on the other half. Each capsule contains pellets of minocycline HCl equivalent to 50 mg of minocycline.

Storage

Store at controlled room temperature 20-25°C (68-77°F).

Protect from light, moisture and excessive heat.

ORAL SUSPENSION

Minocin oral suspension contains minocycline hydrochloride equivalent to 50 mg minocycline per teaspoonful (5 ml). Preserved with propylparaben 0.10% and butylparaben 0.06% with alcohol 5% v/v, custard-flavored.

Storage

Store at controlled room temperature, between 20 and 25°C (68 and 77°F).

DO NOT FREEZE.

PRODUCT LISTING - RATED THERAPEUTICALLY EQUIVALENT

Capsule - Oral - 50 mg			
30's	$20.25	GENERIC, Pd-Rx Pharmaceuticals	55289-0202-30
100's	$39.36	FEDERAL UPPER LIMIT, H.C.F.A. F F P	99999-1818-07
100's	$107.99	GENERIC, Moore, H.L. Drug Exchange Inc	00839-7649-06
100's	$118.40	GENERIC, Geneva Pharmaceuticals	00781-2333-01
100's	$119.86	GENERIC, Qualitest Products Inc	00603-4678-21
100's	$120.00	GENERIC, Aligen Independent Laboratories Inc	00405-4680-01
100's	$120.36	GENERIC, Major Pharmaceuticals Inc	00904-2413-61
100's	$120.55	GENERIC, Major Pharmaceuticals Inc	00904-2413-60
100's	$120.55	GENERIC, Major Pharmaceuticals Inc	00904-7682-60
100's	$125.00	GENERIC, Watson/Rugby Laboratories Inc	00536-1482-01
100's	$125.00	GENERIC, Esi Lederle Generics	59911-5869-01
100's	$144.45	GENERIC, Teva Pharmaceuticals Usa	00093-3165-01
100's	$144.50	GENERIC, Global Pharmaceutical Corporation	00115-7017-01
100's	$144.50	GENERIC, Watson/Schein Pharmaceuticals Inc	00364-2497-01
100's	$144.50	GENERIC, Watson Laboratories Inc	00591-5694-01
100's	$144.50	GENERIC, Par Pharmaceutical Inc	49884-0643-01
100's	$144.50	GENERIC, Ranbaxy Laboratories	63304-0694-01
100's	$157.36	GENERIC, Warner Chilcott Laboratories	00047-0687-24
100's	$233.28	MINOCIN, Lederle Laboratories	00005-5343-23
Capsule - Oral - 75 mg			
100's	$197.96	GENERIC, Watson Laboratories Inc	00591-3153-01
100's	$197.96	GENERIC, Ranbaxy Laboratories	63304-0695-01
100's	$210.22	GENERIC, Esi Lederle Generics	59911-5883-04
100's	$248.04	GENERIC, Global Pharmaceutical Corporation	00115-7054-01
Capsule - Oral - 100 mg			
30's	$37.13	GENERIC, Pd-Rx Pharmaceuticals	55289-0201-30
50's	$39.38	FEDERAL UPPER LIMIT, H.C.F.A. F F P	99999-1818-06
50's	$39.81	GENERIC, Esi Lederle Generics	59911-5870-01
50's	$95.95	GENERIC, Breckenridge Inc	51991-0034-52
50's	$97.45	GENERIC, Major Pharmaceuticals Inc	00904-2414-51
50's	$97.45	GENERIC, Major Pharmaceuticals Inc	00904-7683-51
50's	$97.80	GENERIC, Geneva Pharmaceuticals	00781-2341-50
50's	$98.00	GENERIC, Qualitest Products Inc	00603-4679-19
50's	$98.20	GENERIC, Aligen Independent Laboratories Inc	00405-4681-50
50's	$100.56	GENERIC, Moore, H.L. Drug Exchange Inc	00839-7650-04
50's	$111.25	GENERIC, Watson/Rugby Laboratories Inc	00536-1492-06
50's	$121.79	GENERIC, Major Pharmaceuticals Inc	00904-5480-51
50's	$122.95	GENERIC, Teva Pharmaceuticals Usa	00093-3167-53
50's	$123.00	GENERIC, Global Pharmaceutical Corporation	00115-7018-06
50's	$123.00	GENERIC, Watson/Schein Pharmaceuticals Inc	00364-2498-50
50's	$123.00	GENERIC, Watson Laboratories Inc	00591-5695-50
50's	$123.00	GENERIC, Par Pharmaceutical Inc	49884-0644-03
50's	$123.00	GENERIC, Ranbaxy Laboratories	63304-0696-50
50's	$135.65	GENERIC, Warner Chilcott Laboratories	00047-0688-19
50's	$194.30	MINOCIN, Lederle Laboratories	00005-5344-18
100's	$196.25	GENERIC, Major Pharmaceuticals Inc	00904-2414-61

PRODUCT LISTING - EQUIVALENTS NOT AVAILABLE

Capsule - Oral - 50 mg			
1's	$43.35	GENERIC, Allscripts Pharmaceutical Company	54569-4712-01
15's	$21.40	GENERIC, Southwood Pharmaceuticals Inc	58016-0873-15
20's	$32.90	GENERIC, Southwood Pharmaceuticals Inc	58016-0873-20
30's	$42.25	GENERIC, Southwood Pharmaceuticals Inc	58016-0873-30
60's	$85.34	GENERIC, Allscripts Pharmaceutical Company	54569-4712-00

100's	$163.35	GENERIC, Southwood Pharmaceuticals Inc	58016-0873-00
100's	$266.53	DYNACIN, Medicis Dermatologics Inc	99207-0497-10
Capsule - Oral - 75 mg			
100's	$391.28	DYNACIN, Medicis Dermatologics Inc	99207-0499-10
Capsule - Oral - 100 mg			
15's	$40.80	GENERIC, Southwood Pharmaceuticals Inc	58016-0284-15
20's	$54.40	GENERIC, Southwood Pharmaceuticals Inc	58016-0284-20
30's	$32.83	GENERIC, Physicians Total Care	54868-2391-02
30's	$81.60	GENERIC, Southwood Pharmaceuticals Inc	58016-0284-30
50's	$136.06	GENERIC, Southwood Pharmaceuticals Inc	58016-0284-50
50's	$233.56	DYNACIN, Medicis Dermatologics Inc	99207-0498-50
60's	$64.34	GENERIC, Physicians Total Care	54868-2391-01
60's	$147.60	GENERIC, Allscripts Pharmaceutical Company	54569-4713-00
Granule, Extended Release - Mucous Membrane - 1 mg			
12 x 1	$141.93	ARESTIN, Orapharma Inc	65976-0100-24
Powder For Injection - Intravenous - 100 mg			
1's	$46.38	MINOCIN, Lederle Laboratories	00205-5305-94
Suspension - Oral - 50 mg/5 ml			
60 ml	$39.01	MINOCIN, Lederle Laboratories	00005-5313-56

Minoxidil *(001819)*

Categories: Hypertension, essential; Pregnancy Category C; FDA Approved 1979 Oct
Drug Classes: Vasodilators
Brand Names: Alostil; Loniten
Foreign Brand Availability: Alopexy (France); Alopexyl (France); Crecisan (Spain); Hairgaine (Israel); Hairgrow (Hong-Kong); Headway (New-Zealand); Hebald (India); Kapodin (Spain); Locion EPC (Dominican-Republic); Lonnoten (Belgium; Finland; Netherlands); Lonolox (Germany); Lonoten (France); Minona (Finland); Minoxidil Isac (Philippines); Minoxidil MK (Colombia); Minoximen (Italy); Minoxitrim (Singapore); Minoxyl (Korea); Multigain (India); Moxidil (Korea); Neocapil (Switzerland); Neoxidil (Hong-Kong; Israel; Singapore); Nuhair (Thailand); Regaine (Australia; Austria; Bahrain; Belgium; Bulgaria; Cyprus; Denmark; Egypt; England; Finland; France; Germany; Greece; Hong-Kong; Hungary; Indonesia; Iran; Iraq; Ireland; Italy; Jordan; Kuwait; Lebanon; Libya; Malaysia; Mexico; Netherlands; New-Zealand; Norway; Oman; Peru; Portugal; Qatar; Republic-of-Yemen; Russia; Saudi-Arabia; South-Africa; Spain; Sweden; Switzerland; Syria; Taiwan; Thailand; United-Arab-Emirates); Regroe (Philippines); Regrou (Indonesia); Regrowth (Thailand); Rehair (Indonesia); Tiazolin (Colombia)
Cost of Therapy: $54.68 (Hypertension; Loniten; 2.5 mg; 2 tablets/day; 30 day supply)
$13.21 (Hypertension; Generic Tablets; 2.5 mg; 2 tablets/day; 30 day supply)

WARNING

Minoxidil may produce serious adverse effects. It can cause pericardial effusion, occasionally progressing to tamponade, and angina pectoris may be exacerbated. Minoxidil should be reserved for hypertensive patients who do not respond adequately to maximum therapeutic doses of a diuretic and two other antihypertensive agents.

In experimental animals, minoxidil caused several kinds of myocardial lesions as well as other adverse cardiac effects (see CLINICAL PHARMACOLOGY, Cardiac Lesions in Animals).

Minoxidil must be administered under close supervision, usually concomitantly with therapeutic doses of a beta-adrenergic blocking agent to prevent tachycardia and increased myocardial workload. It must also usually be given with a diuretic, frequently one acting in the ascending limb of the loop of Henle, to prevent serious fluid accumulation. Patients with malignant hypertension and those already receiving guanethidine (see WARNINGS) should be hospitalized when minoxidil is first administered so that they can be monitored to avoid too rapid, or large orthostatic, decreases in blood pressure.

DESCRIPTION

Loniten tablets contain minoxidil, an antihypertensive peripheral vasodilator. Minoxidil occurs as a white or off-white, odorless, crystalline solid that is soluble in water to the extent of approximately 2 mg/ml, is readily soluble in propylene glycol or ethanol, and is almost insoluble in acetone, chloroform or ethyl acetate. The chemical name for minoxidil is 2,4-pyrimidinediamine, 6-(1-piperidinyl)-, 3-oxide. The molecular weight is 209.25.

Loniten tablets for oral administration contain either 2.5 mg or 10 mg of minoxidil. *Inactive Ingredients:* Cellulose, corn starch, lactose, magnesium stearate, silicon dioxide.

CLINICAL PHARMACOLOGY

GENERAL PHARMACOLOGIC PROPERTIES

Minoxidil is an orally effective direct acting peripheral vasodilator that reduces elevated systolic and diastolic blood pressure by decreasing peripheral vascular resistance. Microcirculatory blood flow in animals is enhanced or maintained in all systemic vascular beds. In man, forearm and renal vascular resistance decline; forearm blood flow increases while renal blood flow and glomerular filtration rate are preserved.

Because it causes peripheral vasodilation, minoxidil elicits a number of predictable reactions. Reduction of peripheral arteriolar resistance and the associated fall in blood pressure trigger sympathetic, vagal inhibitory, and renal homeostatic mechanisms, including an increase in renin secretion, that lead to increased cardiac rate and output and salt and water retention. These adverse effects can usually be minimized by concomitant administration of a diuretic and a beta-adrenergic blocking agent or other sympathetic nervous system suppressant.

Minoxidil does not interfere with vasomotor reflexes and therefore does not produce orthostatic hypotension. The drug does not enter the central nervous system in experimental animals in significant amounts, and it does not affect CNS function in man.

EFFECTS ON BLOOD PRESSURE AND TARGET ORGANS

The extent and time-course of blood pressure reduction by minoxidil do not correspond closely to its concentration in plasma. After an effective single oral dose, blood pressure usually starts to decline within one-half hour, reaches a minimum between 2 and 3 hours and recovers at an arithmetically linear rate of about 30% per day. The total duration of effect is approximately 75 hours. When minoxidil is administered chronically, once or twice a day, the time required to achieve maximum effect on blood pressure with a given daily dose is inversely related to the size of the dose. Thus, maximum effect is achieved on 10 mg/day within 7 days, on 20 mg/day within 5 days, and on 40 mg/day within 3 days.

The blood pressure response to minoxidil is linearly related to the logarithm of the dose administered. The slope of this log-linear dose-response relationship is proportional to the extent of hypertension and approaches zero at a supine diastolic blood pressure of approximately 85 mm Hg.

When used in severely hypertensive patients resistant to other therapy, frequently with an accompanying diuretic and beta-blocker, minoxidil tablets usually decreased the blood pressure and reversed encephalopathy and retinopathy.

ABSORPTION AND METABOLISM

Minoxidil is at least 90% absorbed from the GI tract in experimental animals and man. Plasma levels of the parent drug reach maximum within the first hour and decline rapidly thereafter. The average plasma half-life in man is 4.2 hours. Approximately 90% of the administered drug is metabolized, predominantly by conjugation with glucuronic acid at the N-oxide position in the pyrimidine ring, but also by conversion to more polar products. Known metabolites exert much less pharmacologic effect than minoxidil itself; all are excreted principally in the urine. Minoxidil does not bind to plasma proteins, and its renal clearance corresponds to the glomerular filtration rate. In the absence of functional renal tissue, minoxidil and its metabolites can be removed by hemodialysis.

CARDIAC LESIONS IN ANIMALS

Minoxidil produces several cardiac lesions in animals. Some are characteristic of agents that cause tachycardia and diastolic hypotension (beta-agonists like isoproterenol, arterial dilators like hydralazine) while others are produced by a narrower range of agents with arterial dilation properties. The significance of these lesions for humans is not clear, as they have not been recognized in patients treated with oral minoxidil at systemically active doses, despite formal review of over 150 autopsies of treated patients.

Papillary Muscle/Subendocardial Necrosis

The most characteristic lesion of minoxidil, seen in rat, dog, and minipig (but not monkeys) is focal necrosis of the papillary muscle and subendocardial areas of the left ventricle. These lesions appear rapidly, within a few days of treatment with doses of 0.5 to 10 mg/kg/day in the dog and minipig, and are not progressive, although they leave residual scars. They are similar to lesions produced by other peripheral arterial dilators, by theobromine, and by beta-adrenergic receptor agonists such as isoproterenol, epinephrine, and albuterol. The lesions are thought to reflect ischemia provoked by increased oxygen demand (tachycardia, increased cardiac ouptut) and relative decrease in coronary flow (decreased diastolic pressure and decreased time in diastole) caused by the vasodilatiory effects of these agents coupled with reflex or directly induced tachycardia.

Hemorrhagic Lesions

After acute oral minoxidil treatment (0.5-10 mg/kg/day) in dogs and minipigs, hemorrhagic lesions are seen in many parts of the heart, mainly in the epicardium, endocardium, and walls of small coronary arteries and arterioles. In minipigs the lesions occur primarily in the left atrium while in dogs they are most prominent in the right atrium, frequently appearing as grossly visible hemorrhagic lesions. With exposure of 1-20 mg/kg/day in the dog for 30 days or longer, there is replacement of myocardial cells by porliferating fibroblasts and angioblasts, hemorrhage and hemosiderin accumulation. These lesions can be produced by topical minoxidil administration that gives systemic absorption of 0.5 to 1 mg/kg/day. Other peripheral dilators, including an experimental agent, nicorandil, and theobromine, have produced similar lesions.

Epicarditis

A less fully studied lesion is focal epicarditis, seen in dogs after 2 days of oral minoxidil. More recently, chronic proliferative epicarditis was observed in dogs treated topically twice a day for 90 days. In a 1 year oral dog study, serosanguinous pericardial fluid was seen.

Hypertrophy and Dilation

Oral and topical studies in rats, dogs, monkeys (oral only), and rabbits (dermal only) show cardiac hypertrophy and dilation. This is presumed to represent the consequences of prolonged fluid overload; there is preliminary evidence in monkeys that diuretics partly reverse these effects.

Autopsies of over 150 patients who died of various causes after receiving minoxidil for hypertension have not revelated the characteristic hemorrhagic (especially atrial) lesions seen in dogs and minipigs. While areas of papillary muscle and subendocardial necrosis were occasionally seen, they occurred in the presence of known pre-existing coronary artery disease and were also seen in patients never exposed to minoxidl in another series using similar, but not identical, autopsy methods.

INDICATIONS AND USAGE

Because of the potential for serious adverse effects, minoxidil tablets are indicated only in the treatment of hypertension that is symptomatic or associated with target organ damage and is not manageable with maximum therapeutic doses of a diuretic plus two other antihypertensive drugs. At the present time use in milder degrees of hypertension is not recommended because the benefit-risk relationship in such patients has not been defined.

Minoxidil reduced supine diastolic blood pressure by 20 mm Hg or to 90 mm Hg or less in approximately 75% of patients, most of whom had hypertension that could not be controlled by other drugs.

CONTRAINDICATIONS

Minoxidil tablets are contraindicated in pheochromocytoma, because it may stimulate secretion of catecholamines from the tumor through its antihypertensive action. Minoxidil is contraindicated in those patients with a history of hypersensitivity to any of the components of the preparation.

WARNINGS

SALT AND WATER RETENTION

Congestive Heart Failure

Concomitant use of an adequate diuretic is required—minoxidil tablets must usually be administered concomitantly with a diuretic adequate to prevent fluid retention and possible congestive heart failure; a high ceiling (loop) diuretic is *almost always* required. Body weight should be monitored closely. If minoxidil is used without a diuretic, retention of several hundred milli-equivalents of salt and corresponding volumes of water can occur within a few days, leading to increased plasma and interstitial fluid volume and local or generalized edema. Diuretic treatment alone, or in combination with restricted salt intake, will usually minimize fluid retention, although reversible edema did develop in approximately 10% of non-dialysis patients so treated. Ascites has also been reported. Diuretic effectiveness was limited mostly by disease-related impaired renal function. The condition of patients with pre-existing congestive heart failure occasionally deteriorated in association with fluid retention although because of the fall in blood pressure (reduction of afterload), more than twice as many improved than worsened. Rarely, refractory fluid retention may require discontinuation of minoxidil. Provided that the patient is under close medical supervision, it may be possible to resolve refractory salt retention by discontinuing minoxidil for 1 or 2 days and then resuming treatment in conjunction with vigorous diuretic therapy.

CONCOMITANT TREATMENT TO PREVENT TACHYCARDIA IS USUALLY REQUIRED

Minoxidil increases the heart rate. Angina may worsen or appear for the first time during minoxidil treatment, probably because of the increased oxygen demands associated with increased heart rate and cardiac output. The increase in rate and the occurrence of angina generally can be prevented by the concomitant administration of a beta-adrenergic blocking drug or other sympathetic nervous system suppressant. The ability of beta-adrenergic blocking agents to minimize papillary muscle lesions in animals is further reason to utilize such an agent concomitantly. Round-the-clock effectiveness of the sympathetic suppressant should be ensured.

PERICARDITIS, PERICARDIAL EFFUSION, AND TAMPONADE

There have been reports of pericarditis occurring in association with the use of minoxidil. The relationship of this association to renal status is uncertain. Pericardial effusion, occasionally with tamponade, has been observed in about 3% of treated patients not on dialysis, especially those with inadequate or compromised renal function. Although in many cases, the pericardial effusion was associated with a connective tissue disease, the uremic syndrome, congestive heart failure, or marked fluid retention, there have been instances in which these potential causes of effusion were not present. Patients should be observed closely for any suggestion of a pericardial disorder, and echocardiographic studies should be carried out if suspicion arises. More vigorous diuretic therapy, dialysis, pericardiocentesis, or surgery may be required. If the effusion persists, withdrawal of minoxidil should be considered in light of other means of controlling the hypertension and the patient's clinical status.

M

INTERACTION WITH GUANETHIDINE

Although minoxidil does not itself cause orthostatic hypotension, its administration to patients already receiving guanethidine can result in profound orthostatic effects. If at all possible, guanethidine should be discontinued well before minoxidil is begun. Where this is not possible, minoxidil therapy should be started in the hospital and the patient should remain institutionalized until severe orthostatic effects are no longer present or the patient has learned to avoid activities that provoke them.

HAZARD OF RAPID CONTROL OF BLOOD PRESSURE

In patients with very severe blood pressure elevation, too rapid control of blood pressure, especially with intravenous agents, can precipitate syncope, cerebrovascular accidents, myocardial infarction and ischemia of special sense organs with resulting decrease or loss of vision or hearing. Patients with compromised circulation or cryoglobulinemia may also suffer ischemic episodes of the affected organs. Although such events have not been unequivocally associated with minoxidil use, total experience is limited at present.

Any patient with malignant hypertension should have initial treatment with minoxidil carried out in a hospital setting, both to assure that blood pressure is falling and to assure that it is not falling more rapidly than intended.

PRECAUTIONS

GENERAL

Monitor fluid and electrolyte balance and body weight: See WARNINGS, Salt and Water Retention.

Observe patients for signs and symptoms of pericardial effusion: See WARNINGS, Pericarditis, Pericardial Effusion, and Tamponade.

Use after myocardial infarction: Minoxidil tablets have not been used in patients who have had a myocardial infarction within the preceding month. It is possible that a reduction of arterial pressure with minoxidil might further limit blood flow to the myocardium, although this might be compensated by decreased oxygen demand because of lower blood pressure.

Hypersensitivity: Possible hypersensitivity to minoxidil, manifested as a skin rash, has been seen in less than 1% of patients; whether the drug should be discontinued when this occurs depends on treatment alternatives.

Renal failure or dialysis: Patients may require smaller doses of minoxidil and should have close medical supervision to prevent exacerbation of renal failure or precipitation of cardiac failure.

INFORMATION FOR THE PATIENT

The patient should be fully aware of the importance of continuing all of his antihypertensive medications and of the nature of symptoms that would suggest fluid overload. A patient brochure has been prepared and is included with each minoxidil package.

LABORATORY TESTS

Those laboratory tests which are abnormal at the time of initiation of minoxidil therapy, such as urinalysis, renal function tests, EKG, chest x-ray, echocardiogram, etc., should be repeated at intervals to ascertain whether improvement or deterioration is occurring under minoxidil therapy. Initially such tests should be performed frequently *e.g.,* 1-3 month intervals; later as stabilization occurs, at intervals of 6-12 months.

CARCINOGENESIS, MUTAGENESIS, AND IMPAIRMENT OF FERTILITY

Two year carcinogenicity studies of minoxidil have been conducted by the dermal and oral (dietary) routes of administration in mice and rats. There were no positive finding with the oral (dietary) route of administration in mice and rats. There were no positive findings with the oral (dietary) route of administration in rats.

In the 2 year dermal study in mice, an increased incidence of mammary adenomas and adenocarcinomas in the females at all dose levels (8, 25, and 80 mg/kg/day) was attributed to increased prolactin activity. Hyperprolactinemia is a well-known mechanism in the enhancement of mouse mammary tumors, but has not been associated with mammary tumorigenesis in women. Additionally, topical minoxidil has not been shown to cause hyperprolactinemia in women on clinical trials. Absorption of minoxidil through rodent skin is greater than would be experience by patients treated topically with minoxidil for hair loss. Dietary administration of minoxidil to mice for up to 2 years was associated with an increased incidence of malignant lymphomas in females at all dose levels (10, 25, and 63 mg/kg/day) and an increased incidence of hepatic nodules in males (63 mg/kg/day). There was no effect of dietary monoxidil on the incidence of malignant liver tumors.

In the 2 year dermal study in rats there were significant increases in incidence of pheochromocytomas in males and females and preputial gland adenomas in males. Changes in incidence of neoplasms found to be increased in the dermal or oral carcinogenicity studies were typical of those expected in rodents treated with other hypotensive agents (adrenal pheochromocytomas in rats), treatment-related hormonal alterations (mammary carcinomas in female mice; preputial gland adenomas in male rats) or representative of normal variations within the range of historical incidence for rodent neoplasms (malignant lymphomas, liver nodules/adenomas in mice). Based on differences in absorption of minoxidil and mechanisms of tumorigenesis in these rodent species, none of these changes were considered to be relevant to the safety of patients treated topically with minoxidil for hair loss.

There was no evidence of epithelial hyperplasia or tumorigenesis at the sites of topical application of minoxidil in either species in the 2 year dermal carcinogenesis studies. No evidence of carcinogenicity was detected in rats or rabbits treated topically with minoxidil for 1 year. Topical minoxidil (2% and 5%) did not significantly ($p < 0.05$) reduce the latency period of UV light-initiated skin tumors in hairless mice, as compared to controls, in a 12 month photocarcinogenicity study.

Minoxidil was not mutagenic in *Salmonella* (Ames) test, the DNA damage alkaline elution assay, the *in vitro* rat hepatocyte unscheduled DNA synthesis (UDS) assay, the rat bone marrow micronucleus assay, or the mouse bone marrow micronucleus assay. An equivocal result was recorded in an *in vitro* cytogenetic assay using Chinese hamster cells at long exposure times, but a similar assay using human lymphocytes was negative.

In a study in which male and female rats received 1 or 5 times the maximum recommended human oral antihypertensive dose of minoxidil (multiples based on a 50 kg patient) there was a dose-dependent reduction in conception rate.

PREGNANCY, TERATOGENIC EFFECTS, PREGNANCY CATEGORY C

Oral administration of minoxidil has been associated with evidence of increased fetal resorption in rabbits, but not rats, when administered at 5 times the maximum recommended oral antihypertensive human dose. There was no evidence of teratogenic effects in rats and rabbits. Subcutaneous administration of minoxidil to pregnant rats at 80 mg/kg/day was maternally toxic but not teratogenic. Higher subcutaneous doses produced evidence of developmental toxicity. There are no adequate and well controlled studies in pregnant women. Minoxidil should be used during pregnancy only if the potential benefit justifies the potential risk to the fetus.

LABOR AND DELIVERY

The effects on labor and delivery are unknown.

NURSING MOTHERS

There has been one report of minoxidil excretion in the breast milk of a woman treated with 5 mg oral minoxidil twice daily for hypertension. Because of the potential for adverse effects in nursing infants from minoxidil absorption, minoxidil should not be administered to a nursing woman.

PEDIATRIC USE

Use in pediatric patients has been limited to date, particularly in infants. The recommendations under DOSAGE AND ADMINISTRATION can be considered only a rough guide at present and a careful titration is essential.

UNAPPROVED USE

Use of minoxidil tablets, in any formulation, to promote hair growth is not an approved indication. While clinical trials with minoxidil topical solution 2% demonstrated that formulation and dosage were safe and effective, the effects of extemporaneous formulations and dosages have not been shown to safe or effective. Because systemic absorption of topically applied drug may occur and is dependent on vehicle and/or method of use, extemporaneous topical formulations made from minoxidil should be considered to share in the full range of CONTRAINDICATIONS, WARNINGS, PRECAUTIONS, and ADVERSE REACTIONS. In addition, skin intolerance to drug and/or vehicle may occur.

DRUG INTERACTIONS

See WARNINGS, Interaction With Guanethidine.

ADVERSE REACTIONS

SALT AND WATER RETENTION

See WARNINGS, Concomitant Treatment to Prevent Tachycardia is Usually Required. Temporary edema developed in 7% of patients who were not edematous at the start of therapy.

PERICARDITIS, PERICARDIAL EFFUSION, AND TAMPONADE

See WARNINGS.

DERMATOLOGIC

Hypertrichosis

Elongation, thickening, and enhanced pigmentation of fine body hair are seen in about 80% of patients taking minoxidil tablets. This develops within 3-6 weeks after starting therapy. It is usually first noticed on the temples, between the eyebrows, between the hairline and the eyebrows, or in the side-burn area of the upper lateral cheek, later extending to the back, arms, legs, and scalp. Upon discontinuation of minoxidil, new hair growth stops, but 1-6 months may be required for restoration to pretreatment appearance. No endocrine abnormalities have been found to explain the abnormal hair growth; thus, it is hypertrichosis without virilism. Hair growth is especially disturbing to children and women and such patients should be thoroughly informed about this effect before therapy with minoxidil is begun.

Allergic

Rashes have been reported, including rare reports of bullous eruptions, and Stevens-Johnson Syndrome.

HEMATOLOGIC

Thrombocytopenia and leukopenia (WBC <3000/mm^3) have rarely been reported.

GASTROINTESTINAL

Nausea and/or vomiting has been reported. In clinical trials the incidence of nausea and vomiting associated with the underlying disease has shown a decrease from pretrial levels.

MISCELLANEOUS

Breast tenderness developed in less than 1% of patients.

ALTERED LABORATORY FINDINGS

ECG Changes

Changes in direction and magnitude of the ECG T-waves occur in approximately 60% of patients treated with minoxidil. In rare instances a large negative amplitude of the T-wave may encroach upon the S-T segment, but the S-T segment is not independently altered. These changes usually disappear with continuance of treatment and revert to the pretreatment state if minoxidil is discontinued. No symptoms have been associated with these changes, nor have there been alterations in blood cell counts or in plasma enzyme concentrations that would suggest myocardial damage. Long-term treatment of patients manifesting such changes has provided no evidence of deteriorating cardiac function. At present the changes appear to be nonspecific and without identifiable clinical significance.

Effects of Hemodilution

Hematocrit, hemoglobin, and erythrocyte count usually fall about 7% initially and then recover to pretreatment levels.

Other

Alkaline phosphatase increased varyingly without other evidence of liver or bone abnormality. Serum creatinine increased an average of 6% and BUN slightly more, but later declined to pretreatment levels.

DOSAGE AND ADMINISTRATION

Patients over 12 years of age: The recommended initial dosage of minoxidil tablets is 5 mg of minoxidil given as a single daily dose. Daily dosage can be increased to 10, 20, and then to 40 mg in single or divided doses if required for optimum blood pressure control. The effective dosage range is usually 10-40 mg/day. The maximum recommended dosage is 100 mg/day.

Patients under 12 years of age: The initial dosage is 0.2 mg/kg minoxidil as a single daily dose. The dosage may be increased in 50-100% increments until optimum blood pressure control is achieved. The effective dosage range is usually 0.25-1.0 mg/kg/day. The maximum recommended dosage is 50 mg daily (see PRECAUTIONS, Pediatric Use).

DOSE FREQUENCY

The magnitude of within-day fluctuation of arterial pressure during therapy with minoxidil is directly proportional to the extent of pressure reduction. If supine diastolic pressure has been reduced less than 30 mmHg, the drug need be administered only once a day; if supine diastolic pressure has been reduced more than 30 mm Hg, the daily dosage should be divided into two equal parts.

FREQUENCY OF DOSAGE ADJUSTMENT

Dosage must be titrated carefully according to individual response. Intervals between dosage adjustments normally should be at least 3 days since the full response to given dose is not obtained for at least that amount of time. **Where a more rapid management of hypertension is required, dose adjustments can be made every 6 hours if the patient is carefully monitored.**

CONCOMITANT THERAPY

Diuretic and beta-blocker or other sympathetic nervous system suppressant.

Diuretics

Minoxidil must be used in conjunction with a diuretic in conjunction with a diuretic in patients relying on renal function for maintaining salt and water balance. Diuretics have been used at the following dosages when starting therapy with minoxidil: hydrochlorothiazide (50 mg, bid) or other thiazides at equieffective dosage; chlorthalidone (50-100 mg, once daily); furosemide (40 mg, bid). If excessive salt and water retention results in a weight gain of more than 5 pounds, diuretic therapy should be changed to furosemide; if the patient is already taking furosemide, dosage should be increased in accordance with the patient's requirements.

Beta-Blocker or Other Sympathetic Nervous System Suppressants:

When therapy with minoxidil is begun, the dosage of a beta-adrenergic receptor blocking drug should be the equivalent of 80 to 160 mg of propranolol per day in divided doses.

If beta-blockers are contraindicated, methyldopa (250-750 mg, bid) may be used instead. Methyldopa must be given for at least 24 hours before starting therapy with minoxidil because of the delay in the onset of methyldopa's action. Limited clinical experience indicates that clonidine may also be used to prevent tachycardia induced by minoxidil; the usual dosage is 0.1-0.2 mg twice daily.

Sympathetic nervous system suppressant may not completely prevent an increase in heart rate due to minoxidil but usually do prevent tachycardia. Typically, patients receiving a beta-blocker prior to initiation of therapy with minoxidil have a bradycardia and can be expected to have an increase in heart rate toward normal when minoxidil is added. When treatment with minoxidil and beta-blocker or other sympathetic nervous system suppressant are begun simultaneously, their opposing cardiac effects usually nullify each other, leading to little change in heart rate.

HOW SUPPLIED

Loniten tablets are available as follows:

2.5 mg: White, round, scored, and imprinted "U/121" and "2½".

10 mg: White, round, scored, and imprinted "LONITEN 10".

Storage: Store at controlled room temperature 20-25°C (68-77°F).

PRODUCT LISTING - RATED THERAPEUTICALLY EQUIVALENT

Tablet - Oral - 2.5 mg			
100's	$22.01	GENERIC, Qualitest Products Inc	00603-4687-21
100's	$31.70	FEDERAL UPPER LIMIT, H.C.F.A. F F P	99999-1819-01
100's	$33.64	GENERIC, Ivax Corporation	00182-1602-01
100's	$45.00	GENERIC, Aligen Independent Laboratories Inc	00405-4683-01
100's	$45.00	GENERIC, Martec Pharmaceuticals Inc	52555-0444-01
100's	$47.25	GENERIC, Moore, H.L. Drug Exchange Inc	00839-7353-06
100's	$58.18	GENERIC, Major Pharmaceuticals Inc	00904-1279-60
100's	$58.78	GENERIC, Watson/Schein Pharmaceuticals Inc	00364-2172-01
100's	$58.78	GENERIC, Watson Laboratories Inc	00591-5642-01
100's	$58.78	GENERIC, Mutual Pharmaceutical Co Inc	53489-0386-01
100's	$78.17	GENERIC, Par Pharmaceutical Inc	49884-0256-01
100's	$91.13	LONITEN, Pharmacia and Upjohn	00009-0121-01
Tablet - Oral - 10 mg			
100's	$25.43	GENERIC, Interstate Drug Exchange Inc	00814-4850-14
100's	$53.50	GENERIC, Major Pharmaceuticals Inc	00904-1280-60
100's	$54.00	GENERIC, Ivax Corporation	00182-1280-01
100's	$54.00	GENERIC, Aligen Independent Laboratories Inc	00405-4684-01
100's	$55.10	GENERIC, Martec Pharmaceuticals Inc	52555-0445-01
100's	$56.70	GENERIC, Moore, H.L. Drug Exchange Inc	00839-7342-06
100's	$69.65	FEDERAL UPPER LIMIT, H.C.F.A. F F P	99999-1819-03
100's	$129.09	GENERIC, Mutual Pharmaceutical Co Inc	53489-0387-01
100's	$129.14	GENERIC, Watson/Schein Pharmaceuticals Inc	00364-2173-01
100's	$129.14	GENERIC, Watson Laboratories Inc	00591-5643-01
100's	$168.75	GENERIC, Par Pharmaceutical Inc	49884-0257-01
100's	$200.20	LONITEN, Pharmacia and Upjohn	00009-0137-01

PRODUCT LISTING - EQUIVALENTS NOT AVAILABLE

Tablet - Oral - 2.5 mg			
30's	$11.10	GENERIC, Southwood Pharmaceuticals Inc	58016-0915-30
Tablet - Oral - 10 mg			
30's	$9.63	GENERIC, Southwood Pharmaceuticals Inc	58016-0914-30

Mirtazapine (003274)

For related information, see the comparative table section in Appendix A.

Categories: Depression; Pregnancy Category C; FDA Approved 1996 Apr
Drug Classes: Antidepressants, tetracyclic
Brand Names: Remeron
Foreign Brand Availability: Avanza (Australia); Norset (France); Remergil (Germany)
Cost of Therapy: $90.51 (Depression; Remeron; 15 mg; 1 tablet/day; 30 day supply)
$81.46 (Depression; Generic Tablets; 15 mg; 1 tablet/day; 30 day supply)
$69.00 (Depression; Remeron SolTab; 15 mg; 1 tablet/day; 30 day supply)

DESCRIPTION

Mirtazapine tablets and orally disintegrating tablets are an orally administrered drug. Mertazapine has a tetracyclic chemical structure and belongs to the piperazino-azepine group of compounds. Mirtazapine belongs to the piperazino-azepine group of compounds. It is designated 1,2,3,4,10,14b-hexahydro-2-methylpyrazino [2,1-a]pyrido[2,3-c] benzazepine and has the empirical formula of $C_{17}H_{19}N_3$. Its molecular weight is 265.36.

Mirtazapine is a white to creamy white crystalline powder which is slightly soluble in water.

REMERON TABLETS

Remeron tablets are supplied for oral administration as scored film-coated tablets containing 15 or 30 mg of mirtazapine, and unscored film-coated tablets containing 45 mg of mirtazapine. Each tablet also contains corn starch, hydroxypropyl cellulose, magnesium stearate, colloidal silicon dioxide, lactose and other inactive ingredients.

REMERON SOLTAB ORALLY DISINTEGRATING TABLETS

Remeron SolTab orally disintegrating tablets are available for oral administration as an orally disintegrating tablet containing 15, 30, or 45 mg of mirtazapine. It disintegrates in the mouth within seconds after placement on the tongue allowing its contents to be subsequently swallowed with or without water. *Remeron SolTab also contains the following inactive ingrediants:* Aspartame, citric acid, crospovidone, hydroxypropyl methylcellulose, magnesium stearate, mannitol, microcrystalline cellulose, natural and artificial orange flavor, polymethacrylate, povidone, sodium bicarbonate, starch, sucrose.

CLINICAL PHARMACOLOGY

PHARMACODYNAMICS

The mechanism of action of mirtazapine tablets and orally disintegrating tablets, as with other drugs effective in the treatment of major depressive disorder, is unknown.

Evidence gathered in preclinical studies suggests that mirtazapine enhances central noradrenergic and serotonergic activity. These studies have shown that mirtazapine acts as an antagonist at central presynaptic α_2 adrenergic inhibitory autoreceptors and heteroreceptors, an action that is postulated to result in an increase in central noradrenergic and serotonergic activity.

Mirtazapine is a potent antagonist of $5\text{-}HT_2$and $5\text{-}HT_3$ receptors. Mirtazapine has no significant affinity for the $5\text{-}HT_{1A}$ and $5\text{-}HT_{1B}$ receptors.

Mirtazapine is a potent antagonist histamine (H_1) receptors, a property that may explain its prominent sedative effects.

Mirtazapine is a moderate peripheral α_1 adrenergic antagonist, a property that may explain the occasional orthostatic hypotension reported in association with its use.

Mirtazapine is a moderate antagonist at muscarinic receptors, a property that may explain the relatively low incidence of anticholinergic side effects associated with its use.

PHARMACOKINETICS

Mirtazapine tablets and orally disintegrating tablets are rapidly and completely absorbed following oral administration and have a half-life of about 20-40 hours. Peak plasma concentrations are reached within about 2 hours following an oral dose. The presence of food in the stomach has a minimal effect on both the rate and extent of absorption and does not require a dosage adjustment.

Mirtazapine is extensively metabolized after oral administration. Major pathways of biotransformation are demethylation and hydroxylation followed by glucuronide conjugation. *In vitro* data from human liver microsomes indicate that cytochrome 2D6 and 1A2 are involved in the formation of the 8-hydroxy metabolite of mirtazapine, whereas cytochrome 3A is considered to be responsible for the formation of the N-desmethyl and N-oxide metabolite. Mirtazapine has an absolute bioavailability of about 50%. It is eliminated predominantly via urine (75%) with 15% in feces. Several unconjugated metabolites possess pharmacological activity but are present in the plasma at very low levels. The (-) enantiomer has an elimination half-life that is approximately twice as long as the (+) enantiomer and therefore achieves plasma levels that are about 3 times as high as that of the (+) enantiomer.

Plasma levels are linearly related to dose over a dose range of 15-80 mg. The mean elimination half-life of mirtazapine after oral administration ranges from approximately 20-40 hours across age and gender subgroups, with females of all ages exhibiting significantly longer elimination half-lives than males (mean half-life of 37 hours for females vs 26 hours for males). Steady state plasma levels of mirtazapine are attained within 5 days, with about 50% accumulation (accumulation ratio = 1.5).

Mirtazapine is approximately 85% bound to plasma proteins over a concentration range of 0.01 to 10 μg/ml.

Mirtazapine orally disintegrating tablets are bioequivalent to mirtazapine tablets.

Special Populations

Geriatric

Following oral administration of mirtazapine tablets 20 mg/day for 7 days to subjects of varying ages (range, 25-74), oral clearance of mirtazapine was reduced in the elderly compared to the younger subjects. The differences were most striking in males, with a 40% lower clearance in elderly males compared to younger males, while the clearance in elderly females was only 10% lower compared to younger females. Caution is indicated in administering mirtazapine to elderly patients (see PRECAUTIONS and DOSAGE AND ADMINISTRATION).

Pediatrics

Safety and effectiveness of mirtazapine in the pediatric population have not been established (see PRECAUTIONS).

Gender

The mean elimination half-life of mirtazapine after oral administration ranges from approximately 20-40 hours across age and gender subgroups, with females of all ages exhibiting significantly longer elimination half-lives than males (mean half-life of 37 hours for females vs 26 hours for males) (see Pharmacokinetics).

Race

There have been no clinical studies to evaluate the effect of race on the pharmacokinetics of mirtazapine.

Renal Insufficiency

The disposition of mirtazapine was studied in patients with varying degrees of renal function. Elimination of mirtazapine is correlated with creatinine clearance. Total body clearance of mirtazapine was reduced approximately 30% in patients with moderate (CLCR = 11-39 ml/min/1.73 m^2) and approximately 50% in patients with severe (CLCR = <10 ml/min/1.73 m^2) renal impairment when compared to normal subjects. Caution is indicated in administering mirtazapine to patients with compromised renal function (see PRECAUTIONS and DOSAGE AND ADMINISTRATION).

Hepatic Insufficiency

Following a single 15 mg oral dose of mirtazapine, the oral clearance of mirtazapine was decreased by approximately 30% in hepatically impaired patients compared to subjects with normal hepatic function. Caution is indicated in administering mirtazapine to patients with compromised hepatic function (see PRECAUTIONS and DOSAGE AND ADMINISTRATION).

INDICATIONS AND USAGE

Mirtazapine tablets and orally disintegrating tablets are indicated for the treatment of major depressive disorder.

The efficacy of the mirtazapine in the treatment of major depressive disorder was established in 6 week controlled trials of outpatients whose diagnoses corresponded most closely to the Diagnostic and Statistical Manual of Mental Disorders — 3rd edition (DSM-III) category of major depressive disorder (see CLINICAL PHARMACOLOGY).

A major depressive episode (DSM-IV) implies a prominent and relatively persistent (nearly every day for at least 2 weeks) depressed or dysphoric mood that usually interferes with daily functioning, and includes at least 5 of the following 9 symptoms:

Depressed mood.
Loss of interest in usual activities.
Significant change in weight and/or appetite.
Insomnia or hypersomnia.
Psychomotor agitation or retardation.
Increased fatigue.
Feelings of guilt or worthlessness.
Slowed thinking or impaired concentration.
Suicide attempt or suicidal ideation.

The effectiveness of mirtazapine in hospitalized depressed patients has not been adequately studied.

The efficacy of mirtazapine in maintaining a response in patients with major depressive disorder for up to 40 weeks following 8-12 weeks of initial open-label treatment was demonstrated in a placebo-controlled trial. Nevertheless, the physician who elects to use mirtazapine for extended periods should periodically re-evaluate the long-term usefulness of the drug for the individual patient (see CLINICAL PHARMACOLOGY).

The effectiveness of mirtazapine orally disintegrating tablets in long-term use, that is, for more than 6 weeks, has not been systematically evaluated in controlled trials. Therefore, the physician who elects to use mirtazapine orally disintigrating tablets for extended periods should periodically evaluate the long-term usefulness of the drug for the individual patient.

NON-FDA APPROVED INDICATIONS

Limited data have reported that mirtazapine may have beneficial anxiolytic and sedative effects. However, these uses have not been approved by the FDA.

CONTRAINDICATIONS

Mirtazapine tablets and orally disintegrating tablets are contraindicated in patients with a known hypersensitivity to mirtazapine.

WARNINGS

AGRANULOCYTOSIS

In premarketing clinical trials, 2 (1 with Sjögren's Syndrome) out of 2796 patients treated with mirtazapine tablets developed agranulocytosis [absolute neutrophil count (ANC) <500/mm^3 with associated signs and symptoms, *e.g.,* fever, infection, etc.] and a third patient developed severe neutropenia (ANC <500/mm^3 without any associated symptoms). For these 3 patients, onset of severe neutropenia was detected on days 61, 9, and 14 of treatment, respectively. All 3 patients recovered after mirtazapine was stopped. These three cases yield a crude incidence of severe neutropenia (with or without associated infection) of approximately 1.1 per 1000 patients exposed, with a very wide 95% confidence interval, *i.e.,* 2.2 cases per 10,000 to 3.1 cases per 1000. If a patient develops a sore throat, fever, stomatitis or other signs of infection, along with a low WBC count, treatment with mirtazapine should be discontinued and the patient should be closely monitored.

MAO INHIBITORS

In patients receiving other drugs for major depressive disorder in combination with a monoamine oxidase inhibitor (MAOI) and in patients who have recently discontinued a drug for major depressive disorder and then are started on an MAOI, there have been reports of serious, and sometimes fatal, reactions, *e.g.,* including nausea, vomiting, flushing, dizziness, tremor, myoclonus, rigidity, diaphoresis, hyperthermia, autonomic instability with rapid fluctuations of vital signs, seizures, and mental status changes ranging from agitation to coma. Although there are no human data pertinent to such an interaction with mirtazapine tablets and orally disintegrating tablets, it is recommended that mirtazapine tablets and orally disintegrating tablets not be used in combination with an MAOI, or within 14 days of initiating or discontinuing therapy with an MAOI.

PRECAUTIONS

GENERAL

Somnolence

In US controlled studies, somnolence was reported in 54% of patients treated with mirtazapine tablets, compared to 18% for placebo and 60% for amitriptyline. In these studies, somnolence resulted in discontinuation for 10.4% of mirtazapine-treated patients, compared to 2.2% for placebo. It is unclear whether or not tolerance develops to the somnolent effects of mirtazapine. Because of mirtazapine's potentially significant effects on impairment of performance, patients should be cautioned about engaging in activities requiring alertness until they have been able to assess the drug's effect on their own psychomotor performance (see Information for the Patient).

Dizziness

In US controlled studies, dizziness was reported in 7% of patients treated with mirtazapine, compared to 3% for placebo and 14% for amitriptyline. It is unclear whether or not tolerance develops to the dizziness observed in association with the use of mirtazapine.

Increased Appetite/Weight Gain

In US controlled studies, appetite increase was reported in 17% of patients treated with mirtazapine, compared to 2% for placebo and 6% for amitriptyline. In these same trials, weight gain of ≥7% of body weight was reported in 7.5% of patients treated with mirtazapine, compared to 0% for placebo and 5.9% for amitriptyline. In a pool of premarketing US studies, including many patients for long-term, open label treatment, 8% of patients receiving mirtazapine discontinued for weight gain.

Cholesterol/Triglycerides

In US controlled studies, nonfasting cholesterol increases to ≥20% above the upper limits of normal were observed in 15% of patients treated with mirtazapine, compared to 7% for placebo and 8% for amitriptyline. In these same studies, nonfasting triglyceride increases to ≥500 mg/dl were observed in 6% of patients treated with mirtazapine, compared to 3% for placebo and 3% for amitriptyline.

Transaminase Elevations

Clinically significant ALT (SGPT) elevations (≥3 times the upper limit of the normal range) were observed in 2.0% (8/424) of patients exposed to mirtazapine in a pool of short-term US controlled trials, compared to 0.3% (1/328) of placebo patients and 2.0% (3/181) of amitriptyline patients. Most of these patients with ALT increases did not develop signs or symptoms associated with compromised liver function. While some patients were discontinued for the ALT increases, in other cases, the enzyme levels returned to normal despite continued mirtazapine treatment. Mirtazapine tablets and orally disintegrating tablets should be used with caution in patients with impaired hepatic function (see CLINICAL PHARMACOLOGY and DOSAGE AND ADMINISTRATION).

Activation of Mania/Hypomania

Mania/hypomania occurred in approximately 0.2% (3/1299 patients) of mirtazapine-treated patients in US studies. Although the incidence of mania/hypomania was very low during treatment with mirtazapine, it should be used carefully in patients with a history of mania/hypomania.

Seizure

In premarketing clinical trials only one seizure was reported among the 2796 US and non-US patients treated with mirtazapine. However, no controlled studies have been carried out in patients with a history of seizures. Therefore, care should be exercised when mirtazapine is used in these patients.

Suicide

Suicidal ideation is inherent in major depressive disorder and may persist until significant remission occurs. As with any patient receiving drugs effective in the treatment of major depressive disorder, high-risk patients should be closely supervised during initial drug therapy. Prescriptions of mirtazapine tablets and orally disintegrating tablets should be written for the smallest quantity consistent with good patient management, in order to reduce the risk of overdose.

Use in Patients With Concomitant Illness

Clinical experience with mirtazapine in patients with concomitant systemic illness is limited. Accordingly, care is advisable in prescribing mirtazapine for patients with diseases or conditions that affect metabolism or hemodynamic responses.

Mirtazapine tablets and orally disintegrating tablets have not been systemically evaluated or used to any appreciable extent in patients with a recent history of myocardial infarction or other significant heart disease. Mirtazapine was associated with significant orthostatic hypotension in early clinical pharmacology trials with normal volunteers. Orthostatic hypotension was infrequently observed in clinical trials with depressed patients. Mirtazapine tablets and orally disintegrating tablets should be used with caution in patients with known cardiovascular or cerebrovascular disease that could be exacerbated by hypotension (history of myocardial infarction, angina, or ischemic stroke) and conditions that would predispose patients to hypotension (dehydration, hypovolemia, and treatment with antihypertensive medication).

Mirtazapine clearance is decreased in patients with moderate [glomerular filtration rate (GFR) = 11-39 ml/min/1.73 m^2] and severe [GFR <10 ml/min/1.73 m^2] renal impairment, and also in patients with hepatic impairment. Caution is indicated in administering mirtazapine tablets and orally disintegrating tablets to such patients (see CLINICAL PHARMACOLOGY and DOSAGE AND ADMINISTRATION).

INFORMATION FOR THE PATIENT

Physicians are advised to discuss the following issues with patients for whom they prescribe mirtazapine tablets and orally disintegrating tablets:

Agranulocytosis: Patients who are to receive mirtazapine should be warned about the risk of developing agranulocytosis. Patients should be advised to contact their physician if they experience any indication of infection such as fever, chills, sore throat, mucous membrane ulceration or other possible signs of infection. Particular attention should be paid to any flu-like complaints or other symptoms that might suggest infection.

Interference with cognitive and motor performance: Mirtazapine tablets and orally disintegrating tablets may impair judgement, thinking, and particularly, motor skills, because of its prominent sedative effect. The drowsiness associated with mirtazapine use may impair a patient's ability to drive, use machines or perform tasks that require alertness. Thus, patients should be cautioned about engaging in hazardous activities until they are reasonably certain that mirtazapine tablets and orally disintegrating tablets therapy does not adversely affect their ability to engage in such activities.

Completing course of therapy: While patients may notice improvement with mirtazapine tablets and orally disintegrating tablets therapy in 1-4 weeks, they should be advised to continue therapy as directed.

Concomitant medication: Patients should be advised to inform their physician if they are taking, or intend to take, any prescription or over-the-counter drugs since there is a potential for mirtazapine tablets and orally disintegrating tablets to interact with other drugs.

Alcohol: The impairment of cognitive and motor skills produced by mirtazapine has been shown to be additive with those produced by alcohol. Accordingly, patients should be advised to avoid alcohol while taking mirtazapine.

Phenylketonurics: Phenylketonuric patients should be informed that Remeron SolTab contains phenylalanine 2.6 mg per 15 mg tablet, 5.2 mg per 30 mg tablet, and 7.8 mg per 45 mg tablet.

Pregnancy: Patients should be advised to notify their physician if they become pregnant or intend to become pregnant during mirtazapine tablets and orally disintegrating tablets therapy.

Nursing: Patients should be advised to notify their physician if they are breast-feeding an infant.

LABORATORY TESTS

There are no routine laboratory tests recommended.

CARCINOGENESIS, MUTAGENESIS, AND IMPAIRMENT OF FERTILITY

Carcinogenesis

Carcinogenicity studies were conducted with mirtazapine given in the diet at doses of 2, 20, and 200 mg/kg/day to mice and 2, 20, and 60 mg/kg/day to rats. The highest doses used are approximately 20 and 12 times the maximum recommended human dose (MRHD) of 45 mg/day on a mg/m^2 basis in mice and rats, respectively. There was an increased incidence of hepatocellular adenoma and carcinoma in male mice at the high dose. In rats, there was an increase in hepatocellular adenoma in females at the mid- and high doses and in hepatocellular tumors and thyroid follicular adenoma/cystadenoma and carcinoma in males at the high dose. The data suggest that the above effects could possibly be mediated by non-genotoxic mechanisms, the relevance of which to humans is not known.

The doses used in the mouse study may not have been high enough to fully characterize the carcinogenic potential of mirtazapine tablets.

Mutagenesis

Mirtazapine was not mutagenic or clastogenic and did not induce general DNA damage as determined in several genotoxicity tests: Ames test, *in vitro* gene mutation assay in Chinese hamster V 79 cells, *in vitro* sister chromatid exchange assay in cultured rabbit lymphocytes, *in vivo* bone marrow micronucleus test in rats, and unscheduled DNA synthesis assay in HeLa cells.

Impairment of Fertility

In a fertility study in rats, mirtazapine was given at doses up to 100 mg/kg (20 times the maximum recommended human dose (MRHD) on a mg/m^2 basis). Mating and conception were not affected by the drug, but estrous cycling was disrupted at doses that were 3 or more times the MRHD and pre-implantation losses occurred at 20 times the MRHD.

PREGNANCY, TERATOGENIC EFFECTS, PREGNANCY CATEGORY C

Reproduction studies in pregnant rats and rabbits at doses up to 100 mg/kg and 40 mg/kg, respectively [20 and 17 times the maximum recommended human dose (MRHD) on a mg/m^2 basis, respectively], have revealed no evidence of teratogenic effects. However, in rats, there was an increase in post-implantation losses in dams treated with mirtazapine. There was an increase in pup deaths during the first 3 days of lactation and a decrease in pup birth weights. The cause of these deaths is not known. These effects occurred at doses that were 20 times the MRHD, but not at 3 times the MRHD, on a mg/m^2 basis. There are no adequate and well-controlled studies in pregnant women. Because animal reproduction studies are not always predictive of human response, this drug should be used during pregnancy only if clearly needed.

NURSING MOTHERS

It is not known whether mirtazapine is excreted in human milk. Because many drugs are excreted in human milk, caution should be exercised when mirtazapine tablets and orally disintegrating tablets are administered to nursing women.

PEDIATRIC USE

Safety and effectiveness in children have not been established.

GERIATRIC USE

Approximately 190 elderly individuals (≥65 years of age) participated in clinical studies with mirtazapine tablets. This drug is known to be substantially excreted by the kidney (75%), and the risk of decreased clearance of this drug is greater in patients with impaired renal function. Because elderly patients are more likely to have decreased renal function, care should be taken in dose selection. Sedating drugs may cause confusion and over-sedation in the elderly. No unusual adverse age-related phenomena were identified in this

M

group. Pharmacokinetic studies revealed a decreased clearance in the elderly. Caution is indicated in administering mirtazapine tablets and orally disintegrating tablets to elderly patients (see CLINICAL PHARMACOLOGY and DOSAGE AND ADMINISTRATION).

DRUG INTERACTIONS

As with other drugs, the potential for interaction by a variety of mechanisms (*e.g.*, pharmacodynamic, pharmacokinetic inhibition or enhancement, etc.) is a possibility (see CLINICAL PHARMACOLOGY).

DRUGS AFFECTING HEPATIC METABOLISM

The metabolism and pharmacokinetics of mirtazapine tablets and orally disintegrating tablets may be affected by the induction or inhibition of drug-metabolizing enzymes.

DRUGS THAT ARE METABOLIZED BY AND/OR INHIBIT CYTOCHROME P450 ENZYMES

Many drugs are metabolized by and/or inhibit various cytochrome P450 enzymes, *e.g.*, 2D6, 1A2, 3A4, etc. *In vitro* studies have shown that mirtazapine is a substrate for several of these enzymes, including 2D6, 1A2, and 3A4. While *in vitro* studies have shown that mirtazapine is not a potent inhibitor of any of these enzymes, an indication that mirtazapine is not likely to have a clinically significant inhibitory effect on the metabolism of other drugs that are substrates for these cytochrome P450 enzymes, the concomitant use of mirtazapine tablets and orally disintegrating tablets with most other drugs metabolized by these enzymes has not been formally studied. Consequently, it is not possible to make any definitive statements about the risks of coadministration of mirtazapine tablets and orally disintegrating tablets with such drugs.

ALCOHOL

Concomitant administration of alcohol (equivalent to 60 g) had a minimal effect on plasma levels of mirtazapine (15 mg) in 6 healthy male subjects. However, the impairment of cognitive and motor skills produced by mirtazapine were shown to be additive with those produced by alcohol. Accordingly, patients should be advised to avoid alcohol while taking mirtazapine tablets and orally disintegrating tablets.

DIAZEPAM

Concomitant administration of diazepam (15 mg) had a minimal effect on plasma levels of mirtazapine (15 mg) in 12 healthy subjects. However, the impairment of motor skills produced by mirtazapine has been shown to be additive with those caused by diazepam. Accordingly, patients should be advised to avoid diazepam and other similar drugs while taking mirtazapine tablets and orally disintegrating tablets.

ADVERSE REACTIONS

ASSOCIATED WITH DISCONTINUATION OF TREATMENT

M

Approximately 16% of the 453 patients who received mirtazapine tablets in US 6 week controlled clinical trials discontinued treatment due to an adverse experience, compared to 7% of 361 placebo-treated patients in those studies. The most common events (≥1%) associated with discontinuation and considered to be drug related (*i.e.*, those events associated with dropout at a rate at least twice that of placebo) are shown in TABLE 1.

TABLE 1 *Common Adverse Events Associated With Discontinuation of Treatment in 6 Week US Mirtazapine Trials*

	Percentage of Patients Discontinuing With Adverse Event	
	Mirtazapine	Placebo
Adverse Event	(n=453)	(n=361)
Somnolence	10.4%	2.2%
Nausea	1.5%	0%

COMMONLY OBSERVED ADVERSE EVENTS IN US CONTROLLED CLINICAL TRIALS

The most commonly observed adverse events associated with the use of mirtazapine tablets (incidence of 5% or greater) and not observed at an equivalent incidence among placebo-treated patients (mirtazapine incidence at least twice that for placebo) are shown in TABLE 2.

TABLE 2 *Common Treatment-Emergent Adverse Events Associated With the Use of Mirtazapine in 6 Week US Trials*

	Percentage of Patients Reporting Adverse Event	
	Mirtazapine	Placebo
Adverse Event	(n=453)	(n=361)
Somnolence	54%	18%
Increased appetite	17%	2%
Weight gain	12%	2%
Dizziness	7%	3%

ADVERSE EVENTS OCCURRING AT AN INCIDENCE OF 1% OR MORE AMONG MIRTAZAPINE-TREATED PATIENTS

TABLE 3 enumerates adverse events that occurred at an incidence of 1% or more, and were more frequent than in the placebo group, among mirtazapine tablets-treated patients who participated in short-term US placebo-controlled trials in which patients were dosed in a range of 5-60 mg/day. TABLE 3 shows the percentage of patients in each group who had at least one episode of an event at some time during their treatment. Reported adverse events were classified using a standard COSTART-based dictionary terminology.

The prescriber should be aware that these figures cannot be used to predict the incidence of side effects in the course of usual medical practice where patient characteristics and other factors differ from those which prevailed in the clinical trials. Similarly, the cited frequencies cannot be compared with figures obtained from other investigations involving different treatments, uses and investigators. The cited figures, however, do provide the prescribing physician with some basis for estimating the relative contribution of drug and non-drug factors to the side effect incidence rate in the population studied.

TABLE 3 *Incidence of Adverse Clinical Experiences* (≥1%) in Short-Term US Controlled Studies*

Body System Adverse Clinical Experience	Mirtazapine (n=453)	Placebo (n=361)
Body as a Whole		
Asthenia	8%	5%
Flu syndrome	5%	3%
Back pain	2%	1%
Digestive System		
Dry mouth	25%	15%
Increased appetite	17%	2%
Constipation	13%	7%
Metabolic and Nutritional Disorders		
Weight gain	12%	2%
Peripheral edema	2%	1%
Edema	1%	0%
Musculoskeletal System		
Myalgia	2%	1%
Nervous System		
Somnolence	54%	18%
Dizziness	7%	3%
Abnormal dreams	4%	1%
Thinking abnormal	3%	1%
Tremor	2%	1%
Confusion	2%	0%
Respiratory System		
Dyspnea	1%	0%
Urogenital System		
Urinary frequency	2%	1%

* Events reported by at least 1% of patients treated with mirtazapine are included, except the following events which had an incidence on placebo ≥mirtazapine: headache, infection, pain, chest pain, palpitation, tachycardia, postural hypotension, nausea, dyspepsia, diarrhea, flatulence, insomnia, nervousness, libido decreased, hypertonia, pharyngitis, rhinitis, sweating, amblyopia, tinnitus, taste perversion.

ECG CHANGES

The electrocardiograms for 338 patients who received mirtazapine and 261 patients who received placebo in 6 week, placebo-controlled trials were analyzed. Prolongation in QTc ≥500 milliseconds was not observed among mirtazapine-treated patients; mean change in QTc was +1.6 milliseconds for mirtazapine and -3.1 milliseconds for placebo. Mirtazapine was associated with a mean increase in heart rate of 3.4 bpm, compared to 0.8 bpm for placebo. The clinical significance of these changes is unknown.

OTHER ADVERSE EVENTS OBSERVED DURING THE PREMARKETING EVALUATION OF MIRTAZAPINE

During its premarketing assessment, multiple doses of mirtazapine tablets were administered to 2796 patients in clinical studies. The conditions and duration of exposure to mirtazapine varied greatly, and included (in overlapping categories) open and double-blind studies, uncontrolled and controlled studies, inpatient and outpatient studies, fixed dose and titration studies. Untoward events associated with this exposure were recorded by clinical investigators using terminology of their own choosing. Consequently, it is not possible to provide a meaningful estimate of the proportion of individuals experiencing adverse events without first grouping similar types of untoward events into a smaller number of standardized event categories.

In the tabulations that follow, reported adverse events were classified using a standard COSTART-based dictionary terminology. The frequencies presented, therefore, represent the proportion of the 2796 patients exposed to multiple doses of mirtazapine who experienced an event of the type cited on at least one occasion while receiving mirtazapine. All reported events are included except those already listed in TABLE 3, those adverse experiences subsumed under COSTART terms that are either overly general or excessively specific so as to be uninformative, and those events for which a drug cause was very remote.

It is important to emphasize that, although the events reported occurred during treatment with mirtazapine, they were not necessarily caused by it.

Events are further categorized by body system and listed in order of decreasing frequency according to the following definitions: *Frequent* adverse events are those occurring on one or more occasions in at least 1/100 patients. *Infrequent* adverse events are those occurring in 1/100 to 1/1000 patients. *Rare* events are those occurring in fewer than 1/1000 patients. Only those events not already listed in TABLE 3 appear in this listing. Events of major clinical importance are also described in WARNINGS and PRECAUTIONS.

Body as a Whole: *Frequent:* Malaise, abdominal pain, abdominal syndrome acute; *Infrequent:* Chills, fever, face edema, ulcer, photosensitivity reaction, neck rigidity, neck pain, abdomen enlarged; *Rare:* Cellulitis, chest pain substernal.

Cardiovascular System: *Frequent:* Hypertension, vasodilatation; *Infrequent:* Angina pectoris, myocardial infarction, bradycardia, ventricular extrasystoles, syncope, migraine, hypotension; *Rare:* Atrial arrhythmia, bigeminy, vascular headache, pulmonary embolus, cerebral ischemia, cardiomegaly, phlebitis, left heart failure.

Digestive System: *Frequent:* Vomiting, anorexia; *Infrequent:* Eructation, glossitis, cholecystitis, nausea and vomiting, gum hemorrhage, stomatitis, colitis, liver function tests abnormal; *Rare:* Tongue discoloration, ulcerative stomatitis, salivary gland enlargement, increased salivation, intestinal obstruction, pancreatitis, aphthous stomatitis, cirrhosis of liver, gastritis, gastroenteritis, oral moniliasis, tongue edema.

Endocrine System: *Rare:* Goiter, hypothyroidism.

Hemic and Lymphatic System: *Rare:* Lymphadenopathy, leukopenia, petechia, anemia, thrombocytopenia, lymphocytosis, pancytopenia.

Metabolic and Nutritional Disorders: *Frequent:* Thirst; *Infrequent:* Dehydration, weight loss; *Rare:* Gout, SGOT increased, healing abnormal, acid phosphatase increased, SGPT increased, diabetes mellitus.

Musculoskeletal System: *Frequent:* Myasthenia, arthralgia; *Infrequent:* Arthritis, tenosynovitis; *Rare:* Pathological fracture, osteoporosis fracture, bone pain, myositis, tendon rupture, arthrosis, bursitis.

Nervous System: *Frequent:* Hypesthesia, apathy, depression, hypokinesia, vertigo, twitching, agitation, anxiety, amnesia, hyperkinesia, paresthesia; *Infrequent:* Ataxia, delirium, delusions, depersonalization, dyskinesia, extrapyramidal syndrome, libido increased, coordination abnormal, dysarthria, hallucinations, manic reaction, neurosis, dystonia, hostility, reflexes increased, emotional lability, euphoria, paranoid reaction; *Rare:* Aphasia, nystagmus, akathisia, stupor, dementia, diplopia, drug dependence, paralysis, grand mal convulsion, hypotonia, myoclonus, psychotic depression, withdrawal syndrome.

Respiratory System: *Frequent:* Cough increased, sinusitis; *Infrequent:* Epistaxis, bronchitis, asthma, pneumonia; *Rare:* Asphyxia, laryngitis, pneumothorax, hiccup.

Skin and Appendages: *Frequent:* Pruritus, rash; *Infrequent:* Acne exfoliative dermatitis, dry skin, herpes simplex, alopecia; *Rare:* Urticarial, herpes zoster, skin hypertrophy, seborrhea, skin ulcer.

Special Senses: *Infrequent:* Eye pain, abnormality of accommodation, conjunctivitis, deafness, keratoconjunctivitis, lacrimation disorder, glaucoma, hyperacusis, ear pain; *Rare:* Blepharitis, partial transitory deafness, otitis media, taste loss, parosmia.

Urogenital System: *Frequent:* Urinary tract infection; *Infrequent:* Kidney calculus, cystitis, dysuria, urinary incontinence, urinary retention, vaginitis, hematuria, breast pain, amenorrhea, dysmenorrhea, leukorrhea, impotence; *Rare:* Polyuria, urethritis, metrorrhagia, menorrhagia, abnormal ejaculation, breast engorgement, breast enlargement, urinary urgency.

OTHER ADVERSE EVENTS OBSERVED DURING POSTMARKETING EVALUATION OF MIRTAZAPINE

Adverse events reported since market introduction, which were temporally (but not necessarily causally) related to mirtazapine therapy, include 4 cases of the ventricular arrhythmia torsades de pointes. In 3 of the 4 cases, however, concomitant drugs were implicated. All patients recovered.

DOSAGE AND ADMINISTRATION

INITIAL TREATMENT

The recommended starting dose for mirtazapine is 15 mg/day, administered in a single dose, preferably in the evening prior to sleep. In the controlled clinical trials establishing the antidepressant efficacy of mirtazapine in the treatment of major depressive disorder, the effective dose range was generally 15-45 mg/day. While the relationship between dose and satisfactory response in the treatment of major depressive disorder for mirtazapine has not been adequately explored, patients not responding to the initial 15 mg dose may benefit from dose increases up to a maximum of 45 mg/day. Mirtazapine has an elimination half-life of approximately 20-40 hours; therefore, dose changes should not be made at intervals of less than 1-2 weeks in order to allow sufficient time for evaluation of the therapeutic response to a given dose.

ADMINISTRATION OF MIRTAZAPINE ORALLY DISINTEGRATING TABLETS

Patients should be instructed to open tablet blister pack with dry hands and place the tablet on the tongue. The tablet should be used immediately after removal from its blister; once removed, it cannot be stored. Mirtazapine orally disintegrating tablets will disintegrate rapidly on the tongue and can be swallowed with saliva. No water is needed for taking the tablet. Patients should not attempt to split the tablet.

ELDERLY AND PATIENTS WITH RENAL OR HEPATIC IMPAIRMENT

The clearance of mirtazapine is reduced in elderly patients and in patients with moderate to severe renal or hepatic impairment. Consequently, the prescriber should be aware that plasma mirtazapine levels may be increased in these patient groups, compared to levels observed in younger adults without renal or hepatic impairment (see PRECAUTIONS and CLINICAL PHARMACOLOGY).

MAINTENANCE/EXTENDED TREATMENT

It is generally agreed that acute episodes of depression require several months or longer of sustained pharmacological therapy beyond response to the acute episode. Systematic evaluation of mirtazapine tablets has demonstrated that its efficacy in major depressive disorder is maintained for periods of up to 40 weeks following 8-12 weeks of initial treatment at a dose of 15-45 mg/day (see CLINICAL PHARMACOLOGY). Based on these limited data, it is unknown whether or not the dose of mirtazapine needed for maintenance treatment is identical to the dose needed to achieve an initial response. Patients should be periodically reassessed to determine the need for maintenance treatment and the appropriate dose for such treatment.

There is no body of evidence available from controlled trials to indicate how long the depressed patient should be treated with mirtazapine tablets and orally disintegrating tablets. It is generally agreed, however, that pharmacological treatment for acute episodes of depression should continue for up to 6 months or longer. Whether the dose of antidepressant needed to induce remission is identical to the dose needed to maintain euthymia is unknown.

SWITCHING PATIENTS TO OR FROM A MONOAMINE OXIDASE INHIBITOR

At least 14 days should elapse between discontinuation of an MAOI and initiation of therapy with mirtazapine tablets and orally disintegrating tablets. In addition, at least 14 days should be allowed after stopping mirtazapine tablets and orally disintegrating tablets before starting an MAOI.

HOW SUPPLIED

REMERON TABLETS

Remeron Tablets Are Supplied as:

15 mg: Oval, scored, yellow, coated, with "Organon" debossed on one side and with the letters T and Z above the number 3 on the other side.

30 mg: Oval, scored, red-brown, coated, with "Organon" debossed on one side and with the letters T and Z above the number 5 on the other side.

45 mg: Oval, white, coated, with "Organon" debossed on one side and with the letters T and Z above the number 7 on the other side.

Storage: Store at 25°C (77°F); excursions permitted to 15-30°C (59-86°F). Protect from light and moisture.

REMERON SOLTAB ORALLY DISINTEGRATING TABLETS

Remeron SolTab Orally Disintegrating Tablets Are Supplied as:

15 mg: Round, white, with the letters T and Z above the number 1 debossed on one side.

30 mg: Round, white, with the letters T and Z above the number 2 debossed on one side.

45 mg: Round, white, with the letters T and Z above the number 4 debossed on one side.

Storage: Store at 25°C (77°F); excursions permitted to 15-30°C (59-86°F). Protect from light and moisture. Use immediately upon opening individual tablet blister.

PRODUCT LISTING - EQUIVALENTS NOT AVAILABLE

Tablet - Oral - 15 mg			
10 x 10	$301.68	REMERON, Organon	00052-0105-90
30 each	$81.46	GENERIC, Teva Pharmaceuticals Usa	00093-7206-56
30's	$90.51	REMERON, Organon	00052-0105-30
Tablet - Oral - 30 mg			
10 x 10	$310.83	REMERON, Organon	00052-0107-90
30's	$83.91	GENERIC, Teva Pharmaceuticals Usa	00093-7207-56
30's	$93.23	REMERON, Organon	00052-0107-30
Tablet - Oral - 45 mg			
30's	$95.03	REMERON, Organon	00052-0109-30
Tablet, Disintegrating - Oral - 15 mg			
30's	$75.33	REMERON SOLTAB, Organon	00052-0106-30
30's	$75.33	REMERON SOLTAB, Organon	00052-0106-93
90's	$207.00	REMERON SOLTAB, Organon	00052-0106-90
Tablet, Disintegrating - Oral - 30 mg			
30's	$77.61	REMERON SOLTAB, Organon	00052-0108-30
30's	$77.61	REMERON SOLTAB, Organon	00052-0108-93
90's	$213.19	REMERON SOLTAB, Organon	00052-0108-90
Tablet, Disintegrating - Oral - 45 mg			
30's	$82.69	REMERON SOLTAB, Organon	00052-0110-30
90's	$227.14	REMERON SOLTAB, Organon	00052-0110-90

Misoprostol *(001820)*

M

Categories: Ulcer, NSAID-associated, prophylaxis; Pregnancy Category X; FDA Approved 1988 Dec
Drug Classes: Abortifacients; Gastrointestinals; Oxytocics; Prostaglandins; Stimulants, uterine
Brand Names: Cytotec
Foreign Brand Availability: Cityl (Colombia); Cyprostol (Austria); Cytolog (India); Gastotec (Korea); Gastrul (Indonesia); Misel (Korea); U-Miso (Taiwan)
Cost of Therapy: $107.03 (Prevention of NSAID-induced ulcers; Cytotec; 200 µg; 4 tablets/day; 30 day supply)

WARNING

MISOPROSTOL ADMINISTRATION TO WOMEN WHO ARE PREGNANT CAN CAUSE ABORTION, PREMATURE BIRTH, OR BIRTH DEFECTS. UTERINE RUPTURE HAS BEEN REPORTED WHEN MISOPROSTOL WAS ADMINISTERED IN PREGNANT WOMEN TO INDUCE LABOR OR TO INDUCE ABORTION BEYOND THE EIGHTH WEEK OF PREGNANCY (see also PRECAUTIONS; and PRECAUTIONS, Labor and Delivery). MISOPROSTOL SHOULD NOT BE TAKEN BY PREGNANT WOMEN TO REDUCE THE RISK OF ULCERS INDUCED BY NON-STEROIDAL ANTI-INFLAMMATORY DRUGS (NSAIDS) (see CONTRAINDICATIONS, WARNINGS and PRECAUTIONS).

PATIENTS MUST BE ADVISED OF THE ABORTIFACIENT PROPERTY AND WARNED NOT TO GIVE THE DRUG TO OTHERS.

Misoprostol should not be used for reducing the risk of NSAID-induced ulcers in women of childbearing potential unless the patient is at high risk of complications from gastric ulcers associated with use of the NSAID, or is at high risk of developing gastric ulceration. In such patients, misoprostol may be prescribed if the patient:

Has had a negative serum pregnancy test within 2 weeks prior to beginning therapy.

Is capable of complying with effective contraceptive measures.

Has received both oral and written warnings of the hazards of misoprostol, the risk of possible contraception failure, and the danger to other women of childbearing potential should the drug be taken by mistake.

Will begin misoprostol only on the second or third day of the next normal menstrual period.

DESCRIPTION

Cytotec oral tablets contain either 100 or 200 µg of misoprostol, a synthetic prostaglandin E_1 analog.

Misoprostol contains approximately equal amounts of the two diastereomers presented below with their enantiomers indicated by (±):

Misoprostol contains approximately equal amounts of the two diastereomers presented below with their enantiomers indicated by (±):

$C_{22}H_{38}O_5$

Molecular weight = 382.5

(±)methyl 11α,16-dihydroxy-16-methyl-9-oxoprost-13E-en-1-oate

Misoprostol is a water-soluble, viscous liquid.

Inactive ingredients of Cytotec tablets are hydrogenated castor oil, hydroxypropyl methylcellulose, microcrystalline cellulose, and sodium starch glycolate.

CLINICAL PHARMACOLOGY

PHARMACOKINETICS

Misoprostol is extensively absorbed, and undergoes rapid de-esterification to its free acid, which is responsible for its clinical activity and, unlike the parent compound, is detectable in plasma. The alpha side chain undergoes beta oxidation and the beta side chain undergoes omega oxidation followed by reduction of the ketone to give prostaglandin F analogs.

In normal volunteers, misoprostol is rapidly absorbed after oral administration with a T_{max} of misoprostol acid of 12 ± 3 minutes and a terminal half-life of 20-40 minutes.

There is high variability of plasma levels of misoprostol acid between and within studies but mean values after single doses show a linear relationship with dose over the range of 200-400 μg. No accumulation of misoprostol acid was noted in multiple dose studies; plasma steady state was achieved within 2 days.

Maximum plasma concentrations of misoprostol acid are diminished when the dose is taken with food and total availability of misoprostol acid is reduced by use of concomitant antacid. Clinical trials were conducted with concomitant antacid, however, so this effect does not appear to be clinically important (TABLE 1).

TABLE 1

Mean ±SD	C_{max} (pg/ml)	AUC(0-4) (pg·h/ml)	T_{max} (min)
Fasting	811 ± 317	417 ± 135	14 ± 8
With antacid	689 ± 315	349 ± 108*	20 ± 14
With high fat breakfast	303 ± 176*	373 ± 111	64 ± 79*

* Comparisons with fasting results statistically significant, $p < 0.05$.

After oral administration of radiolabeled misoprostol, about 80% of detected radioactivity appears in urine. Pharmacokinetic studies in patients with varying degrees of renal impairment showed an approximate doubling of $T_{½}$, C_{max}, and AUC compared to normals, but no clear correlation between the degree of impairment and AUC. In subjects over 64 years of age, the AUC for misoprostol acid is increased. No routine dosage adjustment is recommended in older patients or patients with renal impairment, but dosage may need to be reduced if the usual dose is not tolerated.

Misoprostol does not affect the hepatic mixed function oxidase (cytochrome P-450) enzyme systems in animals.

Drug interaction studies between misoprostol and several nonsteroidal anti-inflammatory drugs showed no effect on the kinetics of ibuprofen or diclofenac, and a 20% decrease in aspirin AUC, not thought to be clinically significant.

Pharmacokinetic studies also showed a lack of drug interaction with antipyrine and propranolol when these drugs were given with misoprostol. Misoprostol given for 1 week had no effect on the steady state pharmacokinetics of diazepam when the two drugs were administered 2 hours apart.

The serum protein binding of misoprostol acid is less than 90% and is concentration-independent in the therapeutic range.

PHARMACODYNAMICS

Misoprostol has both antisecretory (inhibiting gastric acid secretion) and (in animals) mucosal protective properties. NSAIDs inhibit prostaglandin synthesis, and a deficiency of prostaglandins within the gastric mucosa may lead to diminishing bicarbonate and mucus secretion and may contribute to the mucosal damage caused by these agents. Misoprostol can increase bicarbonate and mucus production, but in man this has been shown at doses 200 μg and above that are also antisecretory. It is therefore not possible to tell whether the ability of misoprostol to reduce the risk of gastric ulcer is the result of its antisecretory effect, its mucosal protective effect, or both.

In vitro studies on canine parietal cells using tritiated misoprostol acid as the ligand have led to the identification and characterization of specific prostaglandin receptors. Receptor binding is saturable, reversible, and stereospecific. The sites have a high affinity for misoprostol, for its acid metabolite, and for other E type prostaglandins, but not for F or I prostaglandins and other unrelated compounds, such as histamine or cimetidine. Receptor-site affinity for misoprostol correlates well with an indirect index of antisecretory activity. It is likely that these specific receptors allow misoprostol taken with food to be effective topically, despite the lower serum concentrations attained.

Misoprostol produces a moderate decrease in pepsin concentration during basal conditions, but not during histamine stimulation. It has no significant effect on fasting or postprandial gastrin nor on intrinsic factor output.

EFFECTS ON GASTRIC ACID SECRETION

Misoprostol, over the range of 50-200 μg, inhibits basal and nocturnal gastric acid secretion, and acid secretion in response to a variety of stimuli, including meals, histamine, pentagastrin, and coffee. Activity is apparent 30 minutes after oral administration and persists for at least 3 hours. In general, the effects of 50 μg were modest and shorter lived, and only the 200 μg dose had substantial effects on nocturnal secretion or on histamine and meal-stimulated secretion.

UTERINE EFFECTS

Misoprostol has been shown to produce uterine contractions that may endanger pregnancy. (See BOXED WARNING.)

OTHER PHARMACOLOGIC EFFECTS

Misoprostol does not produce clinically significant effects on serum levels of prolactin, gonadotropins, thyroid-stimulating hormone, growth hormone, thyroxine, cortisol, gastrointestinal hormones (somatostatin, gastrin, vasoactive intestinal polypeptide, and motilin), creatinine, or uric acid. Gastric emptying, immunologic competence, platelet aggregation, pulmonary function, or the cardiovascular system are not modified by recommended doses of misoprostol.

INDICATIONS AND USAGE

Misoprostol is indicated for reducing the risk of NSAID (nonsteroidal anti-inflammatory drugs, including aspirin)-induced gastric ulcers in patients at high risk of complications from gastric ulcer, *e.g.*, the elderly and patients with concomitant debilitating disease, as well as patients at high risk of developing gastric ulceration, such as patients with a history of ulcer. Misoprostol has not been shown to reduce the risk of duodenal ulcers in patients taking NSAIDs. Misoprostol should be taken for the duration of NSAID therapy. Misoprostol has been shown to reduce the risk of gastric ulcers in controlled studies of 3 months' duration. It had no effect, compared to placebo, on gastrointestinal pain or discomfort associated with NSAID use.

NON-FDA APPROVED INDICATIONS

While not FDA-approved indications, misoprostol is also used for the treatment of duodenal and gastric ulcers. In addition, intravaginal misoprostol has been used as an abortifacient in women with intrauterine fetal death or other medical reasons for the termination of pregnancy. Finally, vaginal misoprostol has been used to induce labor in healthy women at term.

CONTRAINDICATIONS

See BOXED WARNING. **Misoprostol should not be taken by pregnant women to reduce the risk of ulcers induced by non-steroidal anti-inflammatory drugs (NSAIDs).**

Misoprostol should not be taken by anyone with a history of allergy to prostaglandins.

WARNINGS

See BOXED WARNING.

PRECAUTIONS

INFORMATION FOR THE PATIENT

Women of childbearing potential using misoprostol to decrease the risk of NSAID induced ulcers should be told that they must not be pregnant when misoprostol therapy is initiated, and they must use an effective contraception method while taking misoprostol.

See BOXED WARNING.

Misoprostol is intended for administration along with nonsteroidal anti-inflammatory drugs (NSAIDs), including aspirin, to decrease the chance of developing an NSAID-induced gastric ulcer.

Misoprostol should be taken only according to the directions given by a physician.

If the patient has questions about or problems with misoprostol, the physician should be contacted promptly.

THE PATIENT SHOULD NOT GIVE MISOPROSTOL TO ANYONE ELSE. Misoprostol has been prescribed for the patient's specific condition, may not be the correct treatment for another person, and may be dangerous to the other person if she is or were to become pregnant.

The misoprostol package the patient receives from the pharmacist will include a leaflet containing patient information. The patient should read the leaflet before taking misoprostol and each time the prescription is renewed because the leaflet may have been revised.

Keep misoprostol out of the reach of children.

SPECIAL NOTE FOR WOMEN: Misoprostol may cause abortion (sometimes incomplete), premature labor, or birth defects if given to pregnant women.

Misoprostol is available only as a unit-of-use package that includes a leaflet containing patient information. See the Patient Information that is distributed with the prescription.

CARCINOGENESIS, MUTAGENESIS, AND IMPAIRMENT OF FERTILITY

There was no evidence of an effect of misoprostol on tumor occurrence or incidence in rats receiving daily doses up to 150 times the human dose for 24 months. Similarly, there was no effect of misoprostol on tumor occurrence or incidence in mice receiving daily doses up to 1000 times the human dose for 21 months. The mutagenic potential of misoprostol was tested in several *in vitro* assays, all of which were negative.

Misoprostol, when administered to breeding male and female rats at doses 6.25 to 625 times the maximum recommended human therapeutic dose, produced dose-related pre- and post-implantation losses and a significant decrease in the number of live pups born at the highest dose. These findings suggest the possibility of a general adverse effect on fertility in males and females.

PREGNANCY CATEGORY X

Teratogenic Effects

See BOXED WARNING. Congenital anomalies sometimes associated with fetal death have been reported subsequent to the unsuccessful use of misoprostol as an abortifacient but the drug's teratogenic mechanism has not been demonstrated. Several reports in the literature associate the use of misoprostol during the first trimester of pregnancy with skull defects, cranial nerve palsies, facial malformations, and limb defects.

Misoprostol in not fetotoxic or teratogenic in rats and rabbits at doses 625 and 63 times the human dose, respectively.

Nonteratogenic Effects

See BOXED WARNING. Misoprostol may endanger pregnancy (may cause abortion) and thereby cause harm to the fetus when administered to a pregnant woman. Misoprostol may produce uterine contractions, uterine bleeding, and expulsion of the products of conception. Abortions caused by misoprostol may be incomplete. If a woman is or becomes pregnant while taking this drug to reduce the risk of NSAID induced ulcers, the drug should be discontinued and the patient apprised of the potential hazard to the fetus.

LABOR AND DELIVERY

Misoprostol can induce or augment uterine contractions. Vaginal administration of misoprostol, outside of its approved indication, has been used as a cervical ripening agent, for the induction of labor and for treatment of serious postpartum hemorrhage in the presence of uterine atony. A major adverse effect of the obstetrical use of misoprostol is hyperstimulation of the uterus which may progress to uterine tetany with marked impairment of uteroplacental blood flow, uterine rupture (requiring surgical repair, hysterectomy, and/or salpingo-oophorectomy), or amniotic fluid embolism. Pelvic pain, retained placenta, severe genital bleeding, shock, fetal bradycardia, and fetal and maternal death have been reported.

There may be an increased risk of uterine tachysystole, uterine rupture, meconium passage, meconium staining of amniotic fluid, and Cesarean delivery due to uterine hyperstimulation with the use of higher doses of misoprostol; including the manufactured 100 μg tablet. The risk of uterine rupture increases with advancing gestational ages and with prior uterine surgery, including Cesarean delivery. Grand multiparity also appears to be a risk factor for uterine rupture.

The effect of misoprostol on the later growth, development, and functional maturation of the child when misoprostol is used for cervical ripening or induction of labor have not been established. Information on misoprostol's effect on the need for forceps delivery or other intervention is unknown.

NURSING MOTHERS

It is unlikely that misoprostol is excreted in human milk since it is rapidly metabolized throughout the body. However, it is not known if the active metabolite (misoprostol acid) is excreted in human milk. Therefore, misoprostol should not be administered to nursing mothers because the potential excretion of misoprostol acid could cause significant diarrhea in nursing infants.

PEDIATRIC USE

Safety and effectiveness of misoprostol in pediatric patients have not been established.

DRUG INTERACTIONS

See CLINICAL PHARMACOLOGY. Misoprostol has not been shown to interfere with the beneficial effects of aspirin on signs and symptoms of rheumatoid arthritis. Misoprostol does not exert clinically significant effects on the absorption, blood levels, and antiplatelet effects of therapeutic doses of aspirin. Misoprostol has no clinically significant effect on the kinetics of diclofenac or ibuprofen.

ADVERSE REACTIONS

The following have been reported as adverse events in subjects receiving misoprostol:

Gastrointestinal: In subjects receiving misoprostol 400 or 800 μg daily in clinical trials, the most frequent gastrointestinal adverse events were diarrhea and abdominal pain. The incidence of diarrhea at 800 μg in controlled trials in patients on NSAIDs ranged from 14-40% and in all studies (over 5000 patients) averaged 13%. Abdominal pain occurred in 13-20% of patients in NSAID trials and about 7% in all studies, but there was no consistent difference from placebo.

Diarrhea was dose related and usually developed early in the course of therapy (after 13 days), usually was self-limiting (often resolving after 8 days), but sometimes required discontinuation of misoprostol (2% of the patients). Rare instances of profound diarrhea leading to severe dehydration have been reported. Patients with an underlying condition such as inflammatory bowel disease, or those in whom dehydration, were it to occur, would be dangerous, should be monitored carefully if misoprostol is prescribed. The incidence of diarrhea can be minimized by administering after meals and at bedtime, and by avoiding coadministration of misoprostol with magnesium-containing antacids.

Gynecological: *Women who received misoprostol during clinical trials reported the following gynecological disorders:* Spotting (0.7%), cramps (0.6%), hypermenorrhea (0.5%), menstrual disorder (0.3%) and dysmenorrhea (0.1%). Postmenopausal vaginal bleeding may be related to misoprostol administration. If it occurs, diagnostic workup should be undertaken to rule out gynecological pathology. (See BOXED WARNING.)

Elderly: There were no significant differences in the safety profile of misoprostol in approximately 500 ulcer patients who were 65 years of age or older compared with younger patients.

Additional adverse events which were reported are categorized as follows:

Incidence greater than 1%: In clinical trials, the following adverse reactions were reported by more than 1% of the subjects receiving misoprostol and may be causally related to the drug: nausea (3.2%), flatulence (2.9%), headache (2.4%), dyspepsia (2.0%), vomiting (1.3%), and constipation (1.1%). However, there were no significant differences between the incidences of these events for misoprostol and placebo.

Causal relationship unknown: The following adverse events were infrequently reported. Causal relationships between misoprostol and these events have not been established but cannot be excluded:

Body as a Whole: Aches/pains, asthenia, fatigue, fever, rigors, weight changes.

Skin: Rash, dermatitis, alopecia, pallor, breast pain.

Special Senses: Abnormal taste, abnormal vision, conjunctivitis, deafness, tinnitus, earache.

Respiratory: Upper respiratory tract infection, bronchitis, bronchospasm, dyspnea, pneumonia, epistaxis.

Cardiovascular: Chest pain, edema, diaphoresis, hypotension, hypertension, arrhythmia, phlebitis, increased cardiac enzymes, syncope.

Gastrointestinal: GI bleeding, GI inflammation/infection, rectal disorder, abnormal hepatobiliary function, gingivitis, reflux, dysphagia, amylase increase.

Hypersensitivity: Anaphylaxis.

Metabolic: Glycosuria, gout, increased nitrogen, increased alkaline phosphatase.

Genitourinary: Polyuria, dysuria, hematuria, urinary tract infection.

Nervous System/Psychiatric: Anxiety, change in appetite, depression, drowsiness, dizziness, thirst, impotence, loss of libido, sweating increase, neuropathy, neurosis, confusion.

Musculoskeletal: Arthralgia, myalgia, muscle cramps, stiffness, back pain.

Blood/Coagulation: Anemia, abnormal differential, thrombocytopenia, purpura, ESR increased.

DOSAGE AND ADMINISTRATION

The recommended adult oral dose of misoprostol for reducing the risk of NSAID-induced gastric ulcers is 200 μg four times daily with food. If this dose cannot be tolerated, a dose of 100 μg can be used. Misoprostol should be taken for the duration of NSAID therapy as prescribed by the physician. Misoprostol should be taken with a meal, and the last dose of the day should be at bedtime.

RENAL IMPAIRMENT

Adjustment of the dosing schedule in renally impaired patients is not routinely needed, but dosage can be reduced if the 200 μg dose is not tolerated. (See CLINICAL PHARMACOLOGY.)

ANIMAL PHARMACOLOGY

A reversible increase in the number of normal surface gastric epithelial cells occurred in the dog, rat, and mouse. No such increase has been observed in humans administered misoprostol for up to 1 year.

An apparent response of the female mouse to misoprostol in long-term studies at 100-1000 times the human dose was hyperostosis, mainly of the medulla of sternebrae. Hyperostosis did not occur in long-term studies in the dog and rat and has not been seen in humans treated with misoprostol.

HOW SUPPLIED

Cytotec tablets are available in:

100 μg: White, round, with "SEARLE" debossed on one side and "1451" on the other side.

200 μg: White, hexagonal, with "SEARLE" debossed above and "1461" debossed below the line on one side and a double stomach debossed on the other side.

Storage: Store at or below 25°C (77°F) in a dry area.

PRODUCT LISTING - RATED THERAPEUTICALLY EQUIVALENT

Tablet - Oral - 100 mcg

Qty	Price	Product	NDC
60's	$49.45	GENERIC, Ivax Corporation	00172-4430-49
120's	$98.85	GENERIC, Ivax Corporation	00172-4430-59

Tablet - Oral - 200 mcg

Qty	Price	Product	NDC
60's	$71.95	GENERIC, Ivax Corporation	00172-4431-49
100's	$119.95	GENERIC, Ivax Corporation	00172-4431-60

PRODUCT LISTING - EQUIVALENTS NOT AVAILABLE

Tablet - Oral - 100 mcg

Qty	Price	Product	NDC
10's	$11.20	CYTOTEC, Southwood Pharmaceuticals Inc	58016-0347-10
12's	$11.92	CYTOTEC, Southwood Pharmaceuticals Inc	58016-0347-12
12's	$17.00	GENERIC, Pharma Pac	52959-0369-12
12's	$17.00	GENERIC, Pharma Pac	52959-0369-22
12's	$19.90	CYTOTEC, Pharma Pac	52959-0353-12
14's	$13.88	CYTOTEC, Southwood Pharmaceuticals Inc	58016-0347-14
15's	$14.87	CYTOTEC, Southwood Pharmaceuticals Inc	58016-0347-15
16's	$15.75	CYTOTEC, Southwood Pharmaceuticals Inc	58016-0347-16
20's	$16.40	CYTOTEC, Southwood Pharmaceuticals Inc	58016-0347-20
21's	$17.61	CYTOTEC, Southwood Pharmaceuticals Inc	58016-0347-21
24's	$18.84	CYTOTEC, Southwood Pharmaceuticals Inc	58016-0347-24
28's	$21.84	CYTOTEC, Southwood Pharmaceuticals Inc	58016-0347-28
28's	$28.00	CYTOTEC, Pharma Pac	52959-0353-28
28's	$32.40	GENERIC, Pharma Pac	52959-0369-28
30's	$23.40	CYTOTEC, Southwood Pharmaceuticals Inc	58016-0347-30
30's	$29.55	CYTOTEC, Pharma Pac	52959-0353-30
30's	$34.50	GENERIC, Pharma Pac	52959-0369-30
40's	$31.20	CYTOTEC, Southwood Pharmaceuticals Inc	58016-0347-40
40's	$38.55	CYTOTEC, Pharma Pac	52959-0353-40
40's	$44.12	GENERIC, Pharma Pac	52959-0369-40
60's	$41.93	CYTOTEC, Allscripts Pharmaceutical Company	54569-3426-01
60's	$46.80	CYTOTEC, Southwood Pharmaceuticals Inc	58016-0347-60
60's	$49.45	GENERIC, Greenstone Limited	59762-5007-01
60's	$55.25	CYTOTEC, Searle	00025-1451-60
60's	$58.00	CYTOTEC, Pharma Pac	52959-0353-60
60's	$60.12	GENERIC, Pharma Pac	52959-0369-60
100's	$96.61	CYTOTEC, Searle	00025-1451-34
120's	$58.20	CYTOTEC, Southwood Pharmaceuticals Inc	58016-0347-00
120's	$98.85	GENERIC, Greenstone Limited	59762-5007-02
120's	$110.48	CYTOTEC, Searle	00025-1451-20

Tablet - Oral - 200 mcg

Qty	Price	Product	NDC
10's	$8.92	CYTOTEC, Southwood Pharmaceuticals Inc	58016-0190-10
12's	$10.70	CYTOTEC, Southwood Pharmaceuticals Inc	58016-0190-12
12's	$19.25	GENERIC, Pharma Pac	52959-0693-12
12's	$22.90	CYTOTEC, Pharma Pac	52959-0354-12
14's	$12.49	CYTOTEC, Southwood Pharmaceuticals Inc	58016-0190-14

15's	$13.38	CYTOTEC, Southwood Pharmaceuticals Inc	58016-0190-15
16's	$24.35	GENERIC, Pharma Pac	52959-0693-16
20's	$17.84	CYTOTEC, Southwood Pharmaceuticals Inc	58016-0190-20
20's	$30.25	GENERIC, Pharma Pac	52959-0693-20
28's	$37.12	GENERIC, Pharma Pac	52959-0693-28
30's	$26.76	CYTOTEC, Southwood Pharmaceuticals Inc	58016-0190-30
30's	$33.39	CYTOTEC, Pd-Rx Pharmaceuticals	55289-0698-30
30's	$38.85	GENERIC, Pharma Pac	52959-0693-30
30's	$46.65	CYTOTEC, Pharma Pac	52959-0354-30
40's	$49.80	GENERIC, Pharma Pac	52959-0693-40
40's	$60.20	CYTOTEC, Pharma Pac	52959-0354-40
60's	$53.51	CYTOTEC, Southwood Pharmaceuticals Inc	58016-0190-60
60's	$71.95	GENERIC, Greenstone Limited	59762-5008-01
60's	$80.46	CYTOTEC, Searle	00025-1461-60
100's	$89.19	CYTOTEC, Southwood Pharmaceuticals Inc	58016-0190-00
100's	$119.95	GENERIC, Greenstone Limited	59762-5008-02
100's	$134.05	CYTOTEC, Searle	00025-1461-31
100's	$140.75	CYTOTEC, Searle	00025-1461-34
120's	$106.80	CYTOTEC, Southwood Pharmaceuticals Inc	58016-0190-02
120's	$164.50	CYTOTEC, Pharma Pac	52959-0354-01

Mitomycin *(001821)*

Categories: Carcinoma, pancreatic; Carcinoma, gastric; FDA Approved 1981 Aug; Pregnancy Category C
Drug Classes: Antineoplastics, antibiotics
Brand Names: Mutamycin
Foreign Brand Availability: Ametycine (France); Mitomicina-C (Portugal); Mitomycin (Denmark; Germany; Malaysia; Sweden); Mitomycin C (Hong-Kong; India; Israel); Mitomycin-C (Austria; Bulgaria; Greece; Hungary; Indonesia; Italy; Netherlands; Philippines; Russia; Spain; Switzerland; Taiwan; Thailand; Turkey); Mitomycin-C Kyowa (Australia; Czech-Republic; England); Mitomycine (Belgium); Mixandex (Mexico)
HCFA JCODE(S): J9280 5 mg IV; J9291 40 mg IV

WARNING

Mitomycin should be administered under the supervision of qualified physician experienced in the use of cancer chemotherapeutic agents. Appropriate management of therapy and complications is possible only when adequate diagnostic and treatment facilities are readily available.

Bone marrow suppression, notably thrombocytopenia and leukopenia, which may contribute to overwhelming infections in an already compromised patient, is the most common and severe of the toxic effects of mitomycin (see WARNINGS and ADVERSE REACTIONS).

Hemolytic Uremic Syndrome (HUS) a serious complication of chemotherapy, consisting primarily of microangiopathic hemolytic anemia, thrombocytopenia, and irreversible renal failure has been reported in patients receiving systemic mitomycin. The syndrome may occur at any time during systemic therapy with mitomycin as a single agent or in combination with other cytotoxic drugs, however, most cases occur at doses ≥60 mg of mitomycin. Blood product transfusion may exacerbate the symptoms associated with this syndrome.

The incidence of the syndrome has not been defined.

DESCRIPTION

Mitomycin is an antibiotic isolated from the broth of *Streptomyces caespitosus* which has been shown to have antitumor activity. The compound is heat stable, has a high melting point, and is freely soluble in organic solvents.

CLINICAL PHARMACOLOGY

Mitomycin selectively inhibits the synthesis of deoxyribonucleic and (DNA). The guanine and cytosine content correlates with the degree of mitomycin-induced cross-linking. At high concentrations of the drug, cellular RNA and protein synthesis are also suppressed.

In humans, mitomycin is rapidly cleared from the serum after intravenous administration. Time required to reduce the serum concentration by 50% after a 30 mg bolus injection is 17 minutes. After injection of 30 mg, 20 mg, or 10 mg IV, the maximal serum concentrations were 2.4 μg/ml, 1.7 μg/ml, and 0.52 μg/ml, respectively. Clearance is effected primarily by metabolism in the liver, but metabolism occurs in other tissues as well. The rate of clearance is inversely proportional to the maximal serum concentration because, it is thought, of saturation of the degradative pathways.

Approximately 10% of a dose of mitomycin is excreted unchanged in the urine. Since metabolic pathways are saturated at relatively low doses, the percent of a dose excreted in urine increases with increasing dose. In children, excretion of intravenously administered mitomycin is similar.

INDICATIONS AND USAGE

Mitomycin is not recommended as single-agent, primary therapy. It has been shown to be useful in the therapy of disseminated adenocarcinoma of the stomach or pancreas in proven combinations with other approved chemotherapeutic agents and as palliative treatment when other modalities have failed. Mitomycin is not recommended to replace appropriate surgery and/or radiotherapy.

NON-FDA APPROVED INDICATIONS

The drug has been used for bladder cancer and as a part of combination therapy for squamous cell cancer of the anus. However, these uses have not been approved by the FDA.

CONTRAINDICATIONS

Mitomycin is contraindicated in patients who have demonstrated a hypersensitive or idiosyncratic reaction to it in the past.

Mitomycin is contraindicated in patients with thrombocytopenia, coagulation disorder, or an increase in bleeding tendency due to other causes.

WARNINGS

Patients being treated with mitomycin must be observed carefully and frequently during and after therapy.

The use of mitomycin results in a high incidence of bone marrow suppression, particularly thrombocytopenia and leukopenia. Therefore, the following studies should be obtained repeatedly during therapy and for at least 8 weeks following therapy: platelet count, white blood cell count, differential, and hemoglobin. The occurrence of a platelet count below $100{,}000/mm^3$ or a WBC below $4000/mm^3$ or a progressive decline in either is an indication to withhold further therapy until blood counts have recovered above these levels.

Patients should be advised of the potential toxicity of this drug, particularly bone marrow suppression. Deaths have been reported due to septicemia as a result of leukopenia due to the drug.

Patients receiving mitomycin should be observed for evidence of renal toxicity. Mitomycin should not be given to patients with a serum creatinine greater than 1.7 mg percent.

USAGE IN PREGNANCY

Safe use of mitomycin in pregnant women has not been established. Teratological changes have been noted in animal studies. The effect of mitomycin on fertility is unknown.

PRECAUTIONS

Acute shortness of breath and severe bronchospasm have been reported following the administration of vinca alkaloids in patients who had previously or simultaneously received mitomycin. The onset of this acute respiratory distress occurred within minutes to hours after the vinca alkaloid injection. The total number of doses for each drug have varied considerably. Bronchodilators, steroids and/or oxygen have produced symptomatic relief.

A few cases of adult respiratory distress syndrome have been reported in patients receiving mitomycin in combination with other chemotherapy and maintained at FIO_2 concentrations greater than 50% perioperatively. Therefore, caution should be exercised using only enough oxygen to provide adequate arterial saturation since oxygen itself is toxic to the lungs. Careful attention should be paid to fluid balance and overhydration should be avoided.

ADVERSE REACTIONS

BONE MARROW TOXICITY

This was the most common and most serious toxicity, occurring in 605 of 937 patients (64.4%). Thrombocytopenia and/or leukopenia may occur anytime within 8 weeks after onset of therapy with an average time of 4 weeks. Recovery after cessation of therapy was within 10 weeks. About 25% of the leukopenic or thrombocytopenic episodes did not recover. Mitomycin produces cumulative myelosuppression.

INTEGUMENT AND MUCUS MEMBRANE TOXICITY

This has occurred in approximately 4% of patients treated with mitomycin. Cellulitis at the injection site has been reported and is occasionally severe. Stomatitis and alopecia also occur frequently. Rashes are rarely reported. The most important dermatological problem with this drug, however, is the necrosis and consequent sloughing of tissue which results if the drug is extravasated during injection. Extravasation may occur with or without an accompanying stinging or burning sensation and even if there is adequate blood return when the injection needle is aspirated. There have been reports of delayed erythema and/or ulceration occurring either at or distant from the injection site, weeks to months after mitomycin, even when no obvious evidence of extravasation was observed during administration. Skin grafting has been required in some of the cases.

RENAL TOXICITY

2% of 1281 patients demonstrated a statistically significant rise in creatinine. There appeared to be no correlation between total dose administered or duration of therapy and the degree of renal impairment.

PULMONARY TOXICITY

This has occurred infrequently but can be severe and may be life threatening. Dyspnea with a nonproductive cough and radiographic evidence of pulmonary infiltrates may be indicative of mitomycin-induced pulmonary toxicity. If other etiologies are eliminated, mitomycin therapy should be discontinued. Steroids have been employed as treatment of this toxicity, but the therapeutic value has not been determined. A few cases of adult respiratory distress syndrome have been reported in patients receiving mitomycin in combination with other chemotherapy and maintained at FIO_2 concentrations greater than 50% perioperatively.

HEMOLYTIC UREMIC SYNDROME (HUS)

This serious complication of chemotherapy, consisting primarily of microangiopathic hemolytic anemia (hematocrit ≤25%, thrombocytopenia ($\leq 100{,}000/mm^3$), and irreversible renal failure (serum creatinine ≥1.6 mg/dl) has been reported in patients receiving systemic mitomycin. Microangiopathic hemolysis with fragmented red blood cells on peripheral blood smears has occurred in 98% of patients with the syndrome. Other less frequent complications of the syndrome may include pulmonary edema (65%), neurologic abnormalities (16%), and hypertension. Exacerbation of the symptoms associated with HUS has been reported in some patients receiving blood product transfusions. A high mortality rate (52%) has been associated with this syndrome.

The syndrome may occur at any time during systemic therapy with mitomycin as a single agent or in combination with other cytotoxic drugs. Less frequently, HUS has also been reported in patients receiving combinations of cytotoxic drugs not including mitomycin. Of 83 patients studied, 72 developed the syndrome at total dose exceeding 60 mg of mitomycin. Consequently, patients receiving ≥ 60 mg of mitomycin should be monitored closely for unexplained anemia with fragmented cells on peripheral blood smear, thrombocytopenia, and decreased renal function.

The incidence of the syndrome has not been defined.

Therapy for the syndrome is investigational.

CARDIAC TOXICITY

Congestive heart failure, often treated effectively with diuretics and cardiac glycosides, has rarely been reported. Almost all patients who experienced this side effect had received prior doxorubicin therapy.

Acute side effects due to mitomycin were fever, anorexia, nausea, and vomiting. They occurred in about 14% of 1281 patients.

Other undesirable side effects that have been reported during mitomycin therapy have been headache, blurring of vision, confusion, drowsiness syncope, fatigue, edema, thrombophlebitis, hematemesis, diarrhea, and pain. These did not appear to be dose related and were not unequivocally drug related. They may have been due to the primary or metastatic disease processes.

DOSAGE AND ADMINISTRATION

Mitomycin should be given intravenously only, using care to avoid extravasation of the compound. If extravasation occurs, cellulitis, ulceration, and slough may result.

Each vial contains either mitomycin 5 mg and mannitol 10 mg, mitomycin 20 mg and mannitol 40 mg, or mitomycin 40 mg and mannitol 80 mg. To administer, add sterile water for injection, 10 ml, 40 ml, or 80 ml respectively. Shake to dissolve. If product does not dissolve immediately, allow to stand at room temperature until solution is obtained.

After full hematological recovery (see TABLE 1) from any previous chemotherapy, the following dosage schedule may be used at 6-8 week intervals:

20 mg/m^2 intravenously as a single dose via a functioning intravenous catheter.

Because of cumulative myelosuppression, patients should be fully reevaluated after each course of mitomycin, and the dose reduced if the patient has experienced any toxicities. Doses greater than 20 mg/m^2 have not been shown to be more effective, and are more toxic than lower doses.

TABLE 1 is suggested as a guide to dosage adjustment.

TABLE 1 *Mitomycin, Dosage and Administration*

Nadir After Prior Dose		
Leukocytes/mm^3	**Platelets/mm^3**	**Percentage of Prior Dose to be given**
>4000	>100,000	100%
3000-3999	75,000-99,999	100%
2000-2999	25,000-74,999	70%
<2000	<25,000	50%

No repeat dosage should be given until leukocyte count has returned to 4000/mm^3 and platelet count to 100,000/mm^3.

When mitomycin is used in combination with other myelosuppressive agents, the doses should be adjusted accordingly. If the disease continues to progress after two courses of mitomycin, the drug should be stopped since chances of response are minimal.

STABILITY

Unreconstituted mitomycin stored at room temperature is stable for the lot life indicated on the package. Avoid excessive heat (over 40°C).

Reconstituted with sterile water for injection to a concentration of 0.5 mg/ml, mitomycin is stable for 14 days refrigerated or 7 days at room temperature.

Diluted in various IV fluids at room temperature, to a concentration of 20-40 μg/ml (see TABLE 2).

The combination of mitomycin (5-15 mg) and heparin (1000-10,000 units) in 30 ml of 0.9% sodium chloride injection is stable for 48 hours at room temperature.

TABLE 2

IV Fluid	Stability
5% Dextrose injection	3 hours
0.9% Sodium chloride injection	12 hours
Sodium lactate injection	24 hours

Procedures for proper handling and disposal of anticancer drugs should be considered. Several guidelines on this subject have been published.[1-7]

There is no general agreement that all of the procedures recommended in the guidelines are necessary of appropriate.

ANIMAL PHARMACOLOGY

Mitomycin has been found to be carcinogenic in rats and mice. At doses approximating the recommended clinical dose in man, it produces a greater than 100% increase in tumor incidence in male Sprague-Dawley rats, and a greater than 50% increase in tumor incidence in female Swiss mice.

PRODUCT LISTING - RATED THERAPEUTICALLY EQUIVALENT

Powder For Injection - Intravenous - 5 mg

1's	$70.00	GENERIC, Bedford Laboratories	55390-0251-01
1's	$128.77	MUTAMYCIN, Bristol-Myers Squibb	00015-3001-20
1's	$134.11	GENERIC, Supergen Inc	62701-0010-01

Powder For Injection - Intravenous - 20 mg

1's	$227.50	GENERIC, Bedford Laboratories	55390-0252-01
1's	$434.60	GENERIC, Bedford Laboratories	55390-0452-01
1's	$452.91	MUTAMYCIN, Bristol-Myers Squibb	00015-3002-20
1's	$452.91	MUTAMYCIN, Bristol-Myers Squibb	00015-3002-22
1's	$452.91	GENERIC, Supergen Inc	62701-0011-01
10's	$435.49	GENERIC, Faulding Pharmaceutical Company	61703-0306-50

Powder For Injection - Intravenous - 40 mg

1's	$915.00	GENERIC, Bedford Laboratories	55390-0253-01
1's	$915.00	GENERIC, Bedford Laboratories	55390-0453-01

PRODUCT LISTING - EQUIVALENTS NOT AVAILABLE

Powder For Injection - Intravenous - 40 mg

1's	$915.09	MUTAMYCIN, Bristol-Myers Squibb	00015-3059-20

Mitotane *(001822)*

Categories: Carcinoma, adrenal cortex; Pregnancy Category C; FDA Approved 1970 Jul
Drug Classes: Antineoplastics, miscellaneous
Brand Names: Lysodren
Foreign Brand Availability: Opeprim (Japan)
Cost of Therapy: $1328.15 (Adrenal Cancer; Lysodren; 500 mg; 12 tablets/day; 30 day supply)

WARNING

Mitotane should be administered under the supervision of a qualified physician experienced in the uses of cancer chemotherapeutic agents. Mitotane should be temporarily discontinued immediately following shock or severe trauma since adrenal suppression is its prime action. Exogenous steroids should be administered in such circumstances, since the depressed adrenal may not immediately start to secret steroids.

DESCRIPTION

Mitotane is an oral chemotherapeutic agent. It is best known by its trivial name, o,p'-DDD, and is chemically, 1,1-dichloro-2-(0-chlorophenyl)-2-(p-chlorophenyl) ethane.

Mitotane is a white granular solid composed of clear colorless crystals. It is tasteless and has a slight pleasant aromatic odor. It is soluble in ethanol, isoctane and carbon tetrachloride. It has a molecular weight of 320.05.

Inactive ingredients in Lysodren tablets are: avicel, Polyethylene Glycol 4000, silicon dioxide, and starch.

Lysodren is available as 500 mg scored tablets for oral administration.

CLINICAL PHARMACOLOGY

Mitotane can best be described as an adrenal cytotoxic agent, although it can cause adrenal inhibition, apparently without cellular destruction. Its biochemical mechanism of action is unknown. Data are available to suggest that the drug modifies the peripheral metabolism of steroids as well as directly suppressing the adrenal cortex. The administration of mitotane alters the extra-adrenal metabolism of cortisol in man; leading to a reduction in measurable 17-hydroxy corticosteroids, even though plasma levels of corticosteroids do not fall. The drug apparently causes increased formation of 6-B-hydroxyl cortisol.

Data in adrenal carcinoma patients indicate that about 40% of oral mitotane is absorbed and approximately 10% of administered dose is recovered in the urine as water-soluble metabolite. A variable amount of metabolite (1 to 17%) is excreted in the bile and the balance is apparently stored in the tissues.

Following discontinuation of mitotane, the plasma terminal half life has ranged from 18 to 159 days. In most patients blood levels become undetectable after six to nine weeks. Autopsy data have provided evidence that mitotane is found in most tissues of the body; however, fat tissues are the primary site of storage. Mitotane us converted to a water-soluble metabolite.

No unchanged mitotane has been found in urine or bile.

INDICATIONS AND USAGE

Mitotane is indicated in the treatment of inoperable adrenal cortical carcinoma of both functional and non-functional types.

NON-FDA APPROVED INDICATIONS

Mitotane has successfully been used without FDA approval for the treatment of inoperable Cushing's disease.

CONTRAINDICATIONS

Mitotane should not be given to individuals who have demonstrated a previous hypersensitivity to it.

WARNINGS

Mitotane should be temporarily discontinued immediately following shock or severe trauma, since adrenal suppression is its prime action. Exogenous steroids should be administered in such circumstances, since the depressed adrenal may not immediately start to secrete steroids.

Mitotane should be administered with care to patients with liver disease other than metastatic lesions from the adrenal cortex, since the metabolism of mitotane may be interfered with and the drug may accumulate.

All possible tumor tissues should be surgically removed from large metastatic masses before mitotane administration is instituted. This is necessary to minimize the possibility of infarction and hemorrhage in the tumor due to a rapid cytotoxic effect of the drug.

Long-term continuous administration f high doses of mitotane may lead to brain damage and impairment of function. Behavioral and neurological assessments should be made at regular intervals when continuous mitotane treatment exceeds two years.

A substantial percentage of the patients treated show signs of adrenal insufficiency. It therefore appears necessary too watch for and institute steroid replacement in those patients.

M

However, some investigators have recommended that steroid replacement therapy be administered concomitantly with mitotane. It has been shown that the metabolism of exogenous steroids is modified and consequently somewhat higher doses than normal replacement therapy may be required.

PRECAUTIONS

General: Adrenal insufficiency may develop in patients treated with Mitotane, and adrenal steroid replacement should be considered for these patients.

Since sedation, lethargy, vertigo, and other CNS side effect can occur, ambulatory patients should be cautioned about driving, operating machinery, and other hazardous pursuits requiring mental and physical alertness.

Carcinogenesis, Mutagenesis, and Impairment of Fertility: The carcinogenic and mutagenic potential of mitotane are unknown. However, the mechanism of action of this compound suggests that it probably has less carcinogenic potential than other cytotoxic chemotherapeutic drugs.

Pregnancy Category C: Animal reproduction studies have not been conducted with mitotane. It is also not known whether mitotane can cause fetal harm when administered to a pregnant women or can affect reproduction capacity. Mitotane should be given to a pregnant woman only if clearly needed.

Nursing Mothers: It is not known whether this drug is excreted in human milk. Because many drugs are excreted in human milk and because of the potential for adverse reactions in nursing infants from mitotane, a decision should be made whether to discontinue nursing or to discontinue the drug, taking into account the importance of the drug to the mother.

DRUG INTERACTIONS

Mitotane has been reported to accelerate the metabolism of warfarin by the mechanism of hepatic microsomal enzyme induction, leading to an increase in dosage requirements for warfarin. Therefore, physicians should closely monitor patients for a change in anticoagulant dosage requirements when administering Mitotane to patients on coumarin-type anticoagulants. In addition, mitotane should be given with caution to patients receiving other drugs susceptible to the influence of hepatic enzyme induction.

ADVERSE REACTIONS

A very high percentage of patients treated with mitotane have shown at least one type off side effects. The main types of adverse reactions consist of the following:

1. Gastrointestinal disturbances, which consist of anorexia, nausea or vomiting, and in some cases diarrhea, occur in about 80% of the patients.
2. Central nervous system side effects occur in 40% of the patients. These consist primarily of depression as manifested by lethargy and somnolence (25%), and dizziness or vertigo (15%).
3. Skin toxicity has been observed in about 15% of the cases. These skin changes consist primarily of transient skin rashes which do not seem to be dose-related. In some instances, this side effect subsided while the patients were maintained on the drug without a change of dose.

M

Infrequently occurring side effects involve the eye (visual blurring, diplopia, lens opacity, toxic retinopathy); the genitourinary system (hematuria, hemorrhagic cystitis, and albuminuria); cardiovascular system (hypertension, orthostatic hypotension, and flushing); and some miscellaneous effect including generalized aching, hyperpyrexia, and lowered protein bound iodine (PBI).

DOSAGE AND ADMINISTRATION

The recommended treatment schedule is to start the patient at 2 to 6 g of Mitotane per day in divided doses, either three or four times a day. Doses are usually increased incrementally to 9 to 10 g per day. If severe side effects appear, the dose should be reduced until the maximum tolerated dose is achieved. If the patient can tolerate higher doses and improved clinical response appears possible, the dose should be increased until adverse reactions interfere. Experience has shown that the maximum tolerated dose (MTD) will very from 2 to 16 g per day, but has usually been 9 to 10 g per day. The highest doses used in the studies to date were 18 to 19 g per day.

Treatment should be instituted in the hospital until a stable dosage regimen is achieved.

Treatment should be continued as long as clinical benefits are observed. Maintenance of clinical status or slowing of growth of metastatic lesions can be considered clinical benefits if they can clearly be shown to have occurred.

If no clinical benefits are observed after three months at the maximum tolerated dose, the case would generally be considered a clinical failure. However, 10% of the patients who showed a measurable response required more than three months at the MTD. Early diagnosis and prompt institution of treatment improve the probability of a positive clinical response. Clinical effectiveness can be shown by reduction in tumor mass, reduction in pain, weakness or anorexia and reduction of symptoms and signs due to excessive steroid production.

A number of patients have been treated intermittently with treatment being restarted when severe symptoms have reappeared. Patients often do not respond after the third or fourth such course. Experience accumulated to date suggests that continuous treatment with the maximum possible dosage of Mitotane is the best approach.

Procedure for proper handling and disposal of anti-cancer drugs should be considered. Several guideline on this subject have been published.[1-6] There is no general agreement that all of the procedures recommended in the guidelines are necessary or appropriate.

PRODUCT LISTING - EQUIVALENTS NOT AVAILABLE

Tablet - Oral - 500 mg

100's $368.93 LYSODREN, Bristol-Myers Squibb 00015-3080-60

Mitoxantrone Hydrochloride *(001823)*

For complete prescribing information, refer to the CD-ROM included with the book.

Categories: Carcinoma, prostate; Multiple sclerosis; Leukemia, acute erythroid; Leukemia, acute monocytic; Leukemia, acute myelogenous; Leukemia, acute nonlymphocytic; Leukemia, acute promyelocytic; Pregnancy Category D; FDA Approved 1987 Dec; Orphan Drugs

Drug Classes: Antineoplastics, miscellaneous

Brand Names: **Novantrone**

Foreign Brand Availability: Formyxan (Mexico); Mitoxantrona (Peru); Mitroxone (Mexico); Norexan (Indonesia); Novantron (Austria; Germany; Switzerland); Oncotron (India); Onkotrone (Australia)

HCFA JCODE(S): J9293 per 5 mg IV

WARNING

Mitoxantrone for injection concentrate should be administered under the supervision of a physician experienced in the use of cytotoxic chemotherapy agents.

Mitoxantrone should be given slowly into a freely flowing intravenous infusion. It must *never* be given subcutaneously, intramuscularly, or intra-arterially. Severe local tissue damage may occur if there is extravasation during administration.

NOT FOR INTRATHECAL USE. Severe injury with permanent sequelae can result from intrathecal administration. (See WARNINGS, General.)

Except for the treatment of acute nonlymphocytic leukemia, mitoxantrone therapy generally should not be given to patients with baseline neutrophil counts of less than 1500 cells/mm^3. In order to monitor the occurrence of bone marrow suppression, primarily neutropenia, which may be severe and result in infection, it is recommended that frequent peripheral blood cell counts be performed on all patients receiving mitoxantrone.

Myocardial toxicity, manifested in its most severe form by potentially fatal congestive heart failure (CHF), may occur either during therapy with mitoxantrone or months to years after termination of therapy. Use of mitoxantrone has been associated with cardiotoxicity; this risk increases with cumulative dose. In cancer patients, the risk of symptomatic congestive heart failure (CHF) was estimated to be 2.6% for patients receiving up to a cumulative dose of 140 mg/m^2. For this reason, patients should be monitored for evidence of cardiac toxicity and questioned about symptoms of heart failure prior to initiation of treatment. Patients with multiple sclerosis who reach a cumulative dose of 100 mg/m^2 should be monitored for evidence of cardiac toxicity prior to each subsequent dose. Ordinarily, patients with multiple sclerosis should not receive a cumulative dose greater than 140 mg/m^2. Active or dormant cardiovascular disease, prior or concomitant radiotherapy to the mediastinal/pericardial area, previous therapy with other anthracyclines or anthracenediones, or concomitant use of other cardiotoxic drugs may increase the risk of cardiac toxicity. Cardiac toxicity with mitoxantrone may occur at lower cumulative doses whether or not cardiac risk factors are present. For additional information, see WARNINGS, Cardiac Effects, and DOSAGE AND ADMINISTRATION.

Secondary acute myelogenous leukemia (AML) has been reported in cancer patients treated with anthracyclines. Mitoxantrone is an anthracenedione, a related drug. The occurrence of refractory secondary leukemia is more common when anthracyclines are given in combination with DNA-damaging antineoplastic agents, when patients have been heavily pretreated with cytotoxic drugs, or when doses of anthracyclines have been escalated. The cumulative risk of developing treatment-related AML, in 1774 patients with breast cancer who received mitoxantrone concomitantly with other cytotoxic agents and radiotherapy, was estimated as 1.1% and 1.6% at 5 and 10 years, respectively (see WARNINGS).

DESCRIPTION

Novantrone (mitoxantrone hydrochloride) is a synthetic antineoplastic anthracenedione for intravenous use. The molecular formula is $C_{22}H_{28}N_4O_6 \cdot 2HCl$ and the molecular weight is 517.41. It is supplied as a concentrate that MUST BE DILUTED PRIOR TO INJECTION. The concentrate is a sterile, nonpyrogenic, dark blue aqueous solution containing mitoxantrone hydrochloride equivalent to 2 mg/ml mitoxantrone free base, with sodium chloride (0.80% w/v), sodium acetate (0.005% w/v), and acetic acid (0.046% w/v) as inactive ingredients. The solution has a pH of 3.0-4.5 and contains 0.14 mEq of sodium per ml. The product does not contain preservatives. The chemical name is 1,4-dihydroxy-5,8-bis[[2-[(2-hydroxyethyl)amino]ethyl]amino]-9,10-anthracenedione dihydrochloride.

INDICATIONS AND USAGE

Mitoxantrone is indicated for reducing neurologic disability and/or the frequency of clinical relapses in patients with secondary (chronic) progressive, progressive relapsing, or worsening relapsing-remitting multiple sclerosis (*i.e.,* patients whose neurologic status is significantly abnormal between relapses). Mitoxantrone is not indicated in the treatment of patients with primary progressive multiple sclerosis.

The clinical patterns of multiple sclerosis in the studies were characterized as follows: secondary progressive and progressive relapsing disease were characterized by gradual increasing disability with or without superimposed clinical relapses, and worsening relapsing-remitting disease was characterized by clinical relapses resulting in a step-wise worsening of disability.

Mitoxantrone in combination with corticosteroids is indicated as initial chemotherapy for the treatment of patients with pain related to advanced hormone-refractory prostate cancer.

Mitoxantrone in combination with other approved drug(s) is indicated in the initial therapy of acute nonlymphocytic leukemia (ANLL) in adults. This category includes myelogenous, promyelocytic, monocytic, and erythroid acute leukemias.

NON-FDA APPROVED INDICATIONS

Mitoxantrone has been used without FDA approval for the treatment of breast and ovarian cancer, lymphoma (Hodgkin's and non-Hodgkin's), and chronic myelocytic leukemia in blast phase. Additional studies are needed regarding these indications.

CONTRAINDICATIONS

Mitoxantrone is contraindicated in patients who have demonstrated prior hypersensitivity to it.

WARNINGS

WHEN MITOXANTRONE IS USED IN HIGH DOSES (>14 mg/m²/d × 3 days) SUCH AS INDICATED FOR THE TREATMENT OF LEUKEMIA, SEVERE MYELOSUPPRESSION WILL OCCUR. THEREFORE, IT IS RECOMMENDED THAT MITOXANTRONE BE ADMINISTERED ONLY BY PHYSICIANS EXPERIENCED IN THE CHEMOTHERAPY OF THIS DISEASE. LABORATORY AND SUPPORTIVE SERVICES MUST BE AVAILABLE FOR HEMATOLOGIC AND CHEMISTRY MONITORING AND ADJUNCTIVE THERAPIES, INCLUDING ANTIBIOTICS. BLOOD AND BLOOD PRODUCTS MUST BE AVAILABLE TO SUPPORT PATIENTS DURING THE EXPECTED PERIOD OF MEDULLARY HYPOPLASIA AND SEVERE MYELOSUPPRESSION. PARTICULAR CARE SHOULD BE GIVEN TO ASSURING FULL HEMATOLOGIC RECOVERY BEFORE UNDERTAKING CONSOLIDATION THERAPY (IF THIS TREATMENT IS USED) AND PATIENTS SHOULD BE MONITORED CLOSELY DURING THIS PHASE. MITOXANTRONE ADMINISTERED AT ANY DOSE CAN CAUSE MYELOSUPPRESSION.

GENERAL

Patients with preexisting myelosuppression as the result of prior drug therapy should not receive mitoxantrone unless it is felt that the possible benefit from such treatment warrants the risk of further medullary suppression.

The safety of mitoxantrone (mitoxantrone for injection concentrate) in patients with hepatic insufficiency is not established.

Safety for use by routes other than intravenous administration has not been established.

Mitoxantrone is not indicated for subcutaneous, intramuscular, or intra-arterial injection. There have been reports of local/regional neuropathy, some irreversible, following intra-arterial injection.

Mitoxantrone must not be given by intrathecal injection. There have been reports of neuropathy and neurotoxicity, both central and peripheral, following intrathecal injection. These reports have included seizures leading to coma and severe neurologic sequelae, and paralysis with bowel and bladder dysfunction.

Topoisomerase II inhibitors, including mitoxantrone, in combination with other antineoplastic agents, have been associated with the development of acute leukemia and myelodysplasia.

CARDIAC EFFECTS

Because of the possible danger of cardiac effects in patients previously treated with daunorubicin or doxorubicin, the benefit-to-risk ratio of mitoxantrone therapy in such patients should be determined before starting therapy.

Functional cardiac changes including decreases in left ventricular ejection fraction (LVEF) and irreversible congestive heart failure can occur with mitoxantrone. Cardiac toxicity may be more common in patients with prior treatment with anthracyclines, prior mediastinal radiotherapy, or with preexisting cardiovascular disease. Such patients should have regular cardiac monitoring of LVEF from the initiation of therapy. Cancer patients who received cumulative doses of 140 mg/m² either alone or in combination with other chemotherapeutic agents had a cumulative 2.6% probability of clinical congestive heart failure. In comparative oncology trials, the overall cumulative probability rate of moderate or severe decreases in LVEF at this dose was 13%.

Multiple Sclerosis

Functional cardiac changes may occur in patients with multiple sclerosis treated with mitoxantrone. In one controlled trial, 2 patients (2%) of 127 receiving mitoxantrone, one receiving a 5 mg/m² dose and the other receiving the 12 mg/m² dose, had LVEF values that decreased to below 50%. An additional patient receiving 12 mg/m², who did not have LVEF measured, had a decrease in another echocardiographic measurement of ventricular function (fractional shortening) that led to discontinuation from the trial. There were no reports of congestive heart failure in either controlled trial.

Evaluation of LVEF (by echocardiogram or MUGA) is recommended prior to administration of the initial dose of mitoxantrone. Ordinarily, multiple sclerosis patients with a baseline LVEF of <50% should not be treated with mitoxantrone. Subsequent LVEF evaluations are recommended if signs or symptoms of congestive heart failure develop, and prior to all doses administered to patients who have received a cumulative dose of ≥100 mg/m². Mitoxantrone should not ordinarily be administered to multiple sclerosis patients who have received a cumulative lifetime dose of ≥140 mg/m², or those with either LVEF of <50% or a clinically significant reduction in LVEF.

Leukemia

Acute congestive heart failure may occasionally occur in patients treated with mitoxantrone for ANLL. In first-line comparative trials of mitoxantrone + cytarabine vs daunorubicin + cytarabine in adult patients with previously untreated ANLL, therapy was associated with congestive heart failure in 6.5% of patients on each arm. A causal relationship between drug therapy and cardiac effects is difficult to establish in this setting since myocardial function is frequently depressed by the anemia, fever and infection, and hemorrhage that often accompany the underlying disease.

Hormone-Refractory Prostate Cancer

Functional cardiac changes such as decreases in LVEF and congestive heart failure may occur in patients with hormone-refractory prostate cancer treated with mitoxantrone. In a randomized comparative trial of mitoxantrone plus low-dose prednisone versus low-dose prednisone, 7 of 128 patients (5.5%) treated with mitoxantrone had a cardiac event defined as any decrease in LVEF below the normal range, congestive heart failure (n=3), or myocardial ischemia. Two patients had a prior history of cardiac disease. The total mitoxantrone dose administered to patients with cardiac effects ranged from >48 to 212 mg/m².

Among 112 patients evaluable for safety on the mitoxantrone + hydrocortisone arm of the CALGB trial, 18 patients (19%) had a reduction in cardiac function, 5 patients (5%) had cardiac ischemia, and 2 patients (2%) experienced pulmonary edema. The range of total mitoxantrone doses administered to these patients is not available.

PREGNANCY

Mitoxantrone may cause fetal harm when administered to a pregnant woman. Women of childbearing potential should be advised to avoid becoming pregnant. Mitoxantrone is considered a potential human teratogen because of its mechanism of action and the developmental effects demonstrated by related agents. Treatment of pregnant rats during the organogenesis period of gestation was associated with fetal growth retardation at doses ≥0.1 mg/kg/day (0.01 times the recommended human dose on a mg/m² basis). When pregnant rabbits were treated during organogenesis, an increased incidence of premature delivery was observed at doses ≥0.1 mg/kg/day (0.01 times the recommended human dose on a mg/m² basis). No teratogenic effects were observed in these studies, but the maximum doses tested were well below the recommended human dose (0.02 and 0.05 times in rats and rabbits, respectively, on a mg/m² basis). There are no adequate and well-controlled studies in pregnant women. Women with multiple sclerosis who are biologically capable of becoming pregnant should have a pregnancy test prior to each dose, and the results should be known prior to administration of the drug. If this drug is used during pregnancy or if the patient becomes pregnant while taking this drug, the patient should be apprised of the potential risk to the fetus.

SECONDARY LEUKEMIA

Secondary leukemia has been reported in cancer patients treated with mitoxantrone concomitantly with other cytotoxic agents and/or radiotherapy. The largest published report[5] involved 1774 patients with breast cancer treated with mitoxantrone in combination with methotrexate with or without mitomycin. In this study, the cumulative probability of developing secondary leukemia was estimated to be 1.1% and 1.6% at 5 and 10 years, respectively. The second largest report[6] involved 449 patients with breast cancer treated with mitoxantrone, usually in combination with radiotherapy and/or other cytotoxic agents. In this study, the cumulative probability of developing secondary leukemia was estimated to be 2.2% at 4 years.

There are insufficient long-term follow-up data to estimate the risk of leukemia or myelodysplasia in patients with multiple sclerosis treated with mitoxantrone.

DOSAGE AND ADMINISTRATION

See also WARNINGS.

MULTIPLE SCLEROSIS

The recommended dosage of mitoxantrone is 12 mg/m² given as a short (approximately 5-15 minutes) intravenous infusion every 3 months.

Evaluation of LVEF (by echocardiogram or MUGA) is recommended prior to administration of the initial dose of mitoxantrone. Subsequent LVEF evaluations are recommended if signs or symptoms of congestive heart failure develop, and prior to all doses administered to patients who have received a cumulative dose of ≥100 mg/m². Mitoxantrone should not ordinarily be administered to multiple sclerosis patients who have received a cumulative lifetime dose of ≥140 mg/m², or those with either LVEF of <50% or a clinically-significant reduction in LVEF.

Complete blood counts, including platelets, should be monitored prior to each course of mitoxantrone and in the event that signs or symptoms of infection develop. Mitoxantrone generally should not be administered to multiple sclerosis patients with neutrophil counts less than 1500 cells/mm³. Liver function tests should also be monitored prior to each course. Mitoxantrone therapy in multiple sclerosis patients with abnormal liver function tests is not recommended because mitoxantrone clearance is reduced by hepatic impairment and no laboratory measurement can predict drug clearance and dose adjustments.

Women with multiple sclerosis who are biologically capable of becoming pregnant, even if they are using birth control, should have a pregnancy test, and the results should be known, before receiving each dose of mitoxantrone (see WARNINGS, Pregnancy).

HORMONE-REFRACTORY PROSTATE CANCER

Based on data from two Phase 3 comparative trials of mitoxantrone plus corticosteroids versus corticosteroids alone, the recommended dosage of mitoxantrone is 12-14 mg/m² given as a short intravenous infusion every 21 days.

COMBINATION INITIAL THERAPY FOR ANLL IN ADULTS

For induction, the recommended dosage is 12 mg/m² of mitoxantrone daily on days 1-3 given as an intravenous infusion, and 100 mg/m² of cytarabine for 7 days given as a continuous 24 hour infusion on days 1-7.

Most complete remissions will occur following the initial course of induction therapy. In the event of an incomplete antileukemic response, a second induction course may be given. Mitoxantrone should be given for 2 days and cytarabine for 5 days using the same daily dosage levels.

If severe or life-threatening nonhematologic toxicity is observed during the first induction course, the second induction course should be withheld until toxicity resolves.

Consolidation therapy which was used in two large randomized multicenter trials consisted of mitoxantrone, 12 mg/m² given by intravenous infusion daily on days 1 and 2 and cytarabine, 100 mg/m² for 5 days given as a continuous 24 hour infusion on days 1-5. The first course was given approximately 6 weeks after the final induction course, the second was generally administered 4 weeks after the first. Severe myelosuppression occurred.

HEPATIC IMPAIRMENT

For patients with hepatic impairment, there is at present no laboratory measurement that allows for dose adjustment recommendations.

PREPARATION AND ADMINISTRATION PRECAUTIONS

MITOXANTRONE CONCENTRATE MUST BE DILUTED PRIOR TO USE.

Parenteral drug products should be inspected visually for particulate matter and discoloration prior to administration whenever solution and container permit.

The dose of mitoxantrone should be diluted to at least 50 ml with either 0.9% sodium chloride injection or 5% dextrose injection. Mitoxantrone may be further diluted into dextrose 5% in water, normal saline or dextrose 5% with normal saline and used immediately. DO NOT FREEZE.

Mitoxantrone should not be mixed in the same infusion as heparin since a precipitate may form. Because specific compatibility data are not available, it is recommended that mitoxantrone not be mixed in the same infusion with other drugs. The diluted solution should be introduced slowly into the tubing as a freely running intravenous infusion of 0.9% sodium chloride injection or 5% dextrose injection over a period of not less than 3 minutes. Unused infusion solutions should be discarded immediately in an appropriate fashion. In the case of multidose use, after penetration of the stopper, the remaining portion of the undiluted mitoxantrone concentrate should be stored not longer than 7 days between 15-25°C (59-77°F) or 14 days under refrigeration. DO NOT FREEZE. CONTAINS NO PRESERVATIVE.

If extravasation occurs, the administration should be stopped immediately and restarted in another vein. The extravasation site should be carefully monitored for signs of necrosis and/or phlebitis that may require further medical attention. Care should be taken to avoid extravasation at the infusion site and to avoid contact of mitoxantrone with the skin, mucous membranes or eyes. MITOXANTRONE SHOULD NOT BE ADMINISTERED SUBCUTANEOUSLY.

Skin accidentally exposed to mitoxantrone should be rinsed copiously with warm water and if the eyes are involved, standard irrigation techniques should be used immediately. The use of goggles, gloves, and protective gowns is recommended during preparation and administration of the drug.

Procedures for proper handling and disposal of anticancer drugs should be considered. Several guidelines on this subject have been published.[7-13] There is no general agreement that all of the procedures recommended in the guidelines are necessary or appropriate.

PRODUCT LISTING - EQUIVALENTS NOT AVAILABLE

Solution - Intravenous - 2 mg/ml

10 ml	$1120.79	NOVANTRONE, Immunex Corporation	58406-0640-03
12.50 ml	$1891.29	NOVANTRONE, Immunex Corporation	58406-0640-05
15 ml	$2269.59	NOVANTRONE, Immunex Corporation	58406-0640-07

Modafinil (003404)

Categories: Narcolepsy; FDA Approved 1998 Dec; Pregnancy Category C; Orphan Drugs
Drug Classes: Analeptics; Stimulants, central nervous system
Brand Names: Provigil
Foreign Brand Availability: Alertec (Canada); Modavigil (New-Zealand); Modiodal (France); Vigil (Germany)
Cost of Therapy: $179.10 (Narcolepsy; Provigil; 200 mg; 1 tablet/day; 30 day supply)

M

DESCRIPTION

Provigil is a wakefulness-promoting agent for oral administration. Provigil is a racemic compound. The chemical name for modafinil is 2-[(diphenylmethyl)sulfinyl]acetamide. The molecular formula is $C_{15}H_{15}NO_2S$ and the molecular weight is 273.36.

Modafinil is a white to off-white, crystalline powder that is practically insoluble in water and cyclohexane. It is sparingly to slightly soluble in methanol and acetone. Provigil tablets contain 100 or 200 mg of modafinil and the following inactive ingredients; lactose, corn starch, magnesium silicate, croscarmellose sodium, povidone, magnesium stearate, and talc.

CLINICAL PHARMACOLOGY

MECHANISM OF ACTION AND PHARMACOLOGY

The precise mechanism(s) through which modafinil promotes wakefulness is unknown. Modafinil has wake-promoting actions like sympathomimetic agents including amphetamine and methylphenidate, although the pharmacologic profile is not identical to that of sympathomimetic amines.

At pharmacologically relevant concentrations, modafinil does not bind to most potentially relevant receptors for sleep/wake regulation, including those for norepinephrine, serotonin, dopamine, GABA, adenosine, histamine-3, melatonin, or benzodiazepines. Modafinil also does not inhibit the activities of MAO-B or phosphodiesterases II-V.

Modafinil is not a direct- or indirect-acting dopamine receptor agonist and is inactive in several *in vivo* preclinical models capable of detecting enhanced dopaminergic activity. *In vitro,* modafinil binds to the dopamine reuptake site and causes an increase in extracellular dopamine, but no increase in dopamine release. In a preclinical model, the wakefulness induced by amphetamine, but not modafinil, is antagonized by the dopamine receptor antagonist haloperidol.

Modafinil does not appear to be a direct or indirect α_1-adrenergic agonist. Although modafinil-induced wakefulness can be attenuated by the α_1-adrenergic receptor antagonist, prazosin, in assay systems known to be responsive to α-adrenergic agonists, modafinil has no activity. Modafinil does not display sympathomimetic activity in the rat vas deferens preparations (agonist-stimulated or electrically stimulated) nor does it increase the formation of the adrenergic receptor-mediated second messenger phosphatidyl inositol in *in vitro* models. Unlike sympathomimetic agents, modafinil does not reduce cataplexy in narcoleptic canines and has minimal effects on cardiovascular and hemodynamic parameters.

In the cat, equal wakefulness-promoting doses of methylphenidate and amphetamine increased neuronal activation throughout the brain. Modafinil at an equivalent wakefulness-promoting dose selectively and prominently increased neuronal activation in more discrete regions of the brain. The relationship of this finding in cats to the effects of modafinil in humans is unknown.

In addition to its wakefulness-promoting effects and increased locomotor activity in animals, in humans, modafinil produces psychoactive and euphoric effects, alterations in mood, perception, thinking, and feelings typical of other CNS stimulants. Modafinil is reinforcing, as evidenced by its self-administration in monkeys previously trained to self-administer cocaine; modafinil was also partially discriminated as stimulant-like.

The optical enantiomers of modafinil have similar pharmacological actions in animals. The enantiomers have not been individually studied in humans. Two major metabolites of modafinil, modafinil acid and modafinil sulfone, do not appear to contribute to the CNS-activating properties of modafinil.

PHARMACOKINETICS

Modafinil is a racemic compound, whose enantiomers have different pharmacokinetics (*e.g.,* the half-life of the *l*-isomer is approximately 3 times that of the *d*-isomer in humans). The enantiomers do not interconvert. At steady state, total exposure to the *l*-isomer is approximately 3 times that for the *d*-isomer. The trough concentration (C_{minss}) of circulating modafinil after once daily dosing consists of 90% of the *l*-isomer and 10% of the *d*-isomer. The effective elimination half-life of modafinil after multiple doses is about 15 hours. The enantiomers of modafinil exhibit linear kinetics upon multiple dosing of 200-600 mg/day once daily in healthy volunteers. Apparent steady states of total modafinil and *l*-(-)-modafinil are reached after 2-4 days of dosing.

Absorption and Distribution

Absorption of modafinil tablets is rapid, with peak plasma concentrations occurring at 2-4 hours. The bioavailability of modafinil tablets is approximately equal to that of an aqueous suspension. The absolute oral bioavailability was not determined due to the aqueous insolubility (<1 mg/ml) of modafinil, which precluded intravenous administration. Food has no effect on overall modafinil bioavailability; however, its absorption (T_{max}) may be delayed by approximately 1 hour if taken with food.

Modafinil is well distributed in body tissue with an apparent volume of distribution (~0.9 L/kg) larger than the volume of total body water (0.6 L/kg). In human plasma, *in vitro,* modafinil is moderately bound to plasma protein (~60%, mainly to albumin). At serum concentrations obtained at steady state after doses of 200 mg/day, modafinil exhibits no displacement of protein binding of warfarin, diazepam, or propranolol. Even at much larger concentrations (1000 μM; >25 times the C_{max} of 40μM at steady state at 400 mg/day), modafinil has no effect on warfarin binding. Modafinil acid at concentrations >500μM decreases the extent of warfarin binding, but these concentrations are >35 times those achieved therapeutically.

Metabolism and Elimination

The major route of elimination (~90%) is metabolism, primarily by the liver, with subsequent renal elimination of the metabolites. Urine alkalinization has no effect on the elimination of modafinil.

Metabolism occurs through hydrolytic deamidation, S-oxidation, aromatic ring hydroxylation, and glucuronide conjugation. Less than 10% of an administered dose is excreted as the parent compound. In a clinical study using radiolabeled modafinil, a total of 81% of the administered radioactivity was recovered in 11 days post-dose; predominantly in the urine (80% vs 1.0% in the feces). The largest fraction of the drug in urine was modafinil acid, but at least six other metabolites were present in lower concentrations. Only two metabolites reach appreciable concentrations in plasma, *i.e.,* modafinil acid and modafinil sulfone. In preclinical models, modafinil acid, modafinil sulfone, 2-[(diphenylmethyl)sulfonyl]acetic acid and 4-hydroxy modafinil, were inactive or did not appear to mediate the arousal effects of modafinil.

In humans, modafinil shows a possible induction effect on its own metabolism after chronic administration of doses ≥ 400 mg/day. Induction of hepatic metabolizing enzymes, most importantly cytochrome P-450 (CYP) 3A4, has also been observed *in vitro* after incubation of primary cultures of human hepatocytes with modafinil. (For further discussion of the effects of modafinil on CYP enzyme activities see DRUG INTERACTIONS.)

Drug-Drug Interactions

Because modafinil is a reversible inhibitor of the drug-metabolizing enzyme CYP2C19, co-administration of modafinil with drugs such as diazepam, phenytoin and propranolol, which are largely eliminated via that pathway, may increase the circulating levels of those compounds. In addition, in individuals deficient in the enzyme CYP2D6 (*i.e.,* 7-10% of the Caucasian population; similar or lower in other populations), the levels of CYP2D6 substrates such as tricyclic antidepressants and selective serotonin reuptake inhibitors, which have ancillary routes of elimination through CYP2C19, may be increased by co-administration of modafinil. Dose adjustments may be necessary for patients being treated with these and similar medications (see DRUG INTERACTIONS).

Chronic administration of modafinil may also cause modest induction of the metabolizing enzyme CYP3A4, thus reducing the levels of co-administered substrates for that enzyme system, such as steroidal contraceptives, cyclosporine and, to a lesser degree, theophylline. Dose adjustments may be necessary for patients being treated with these and similar medications (see DRUG INTERACTIONS).

An apparent concentration-related suppression of CYP2C9 activity was observed in human hepatocytes after exposure to modafinil *in vitro.* Although no other indication of CYP2C9 suppression has been observed, the *in vitro* results suggest that there is potential for metabolic interaction between modafinil and CYP2C9 substrates, such as warfarin or phenytoin (see DRUG INTERACTIONS).

SPECIAL POPULATIONS

Gender Effect

The pharmacokinetics of modafinil are not affected by gender.

Age Effect

A slight decrease (-20%) in the oral clearance (CL/F) of modafinil was observed in a single dose study at 200 mg in 12 subjects with a mean age of 63 years (range 53-72 years), but the change was considered unlikely to be clinically significant. In a multiple dose study (300 mg/day) in 12 patients with a mean age of 82 years (range 67-87 years), the mean levels of modafinil in plasma were approximately 2 times those historically obtained in matched younger subjects. Due to potential effects from the multiple concomitant medications with which most of the patients were being treated, the apparent difference in modafinil pharmacokinetics may not be attributable solely to the effects of aging. However, the results suggest that the clearance of modafinil may be reduced in the elderly (see DOSAGE AND ADMINISTRATION).

Race Effect
The influence of race on the pharmacokinetics of modafinil has not been studied.

Renal Impairment
In a single dose 200 mg modafinil study, severe chronic renal failure (creatinine clearance ≤20 ml/min) did not significantly influence the pharmacokinetics of modafinil, but exposure to modafinil acid (an inactive metabolite) was increased 9-fold (see PRECAUTIONS).

Hepatic Impairment
Pharmacokinetics and metabolism were examined in patients with cirrhosis of the liver (6 M and 3 F). Three patients had stage B or B+ cirrhosis (per the Child criteria) and 6 patients had stage C or C+ cirrhosis. Clinically 8 of 9 patients were icteric and all had ascites. In these patients, the oral clearance of modafinil was decreased by about 60% and the steady state concentration was doubled compared to normal patients. The dose of modafinil should be reduced in patients with severe hepatic impairment (see PRECAUTIONS and DOSAGE AND ADMINISTRATION).

INDICATIONS AND USAGE

Modafinil is indicated to improve wakefulness in patients with excessive daytime sleepiness associated with narcolepsy.

NON-FDA APPROVED INDICATIONS
Modafinil may also have clinical utility for the treatment of idiopathic hypersomnolence, and excessive daytime sleepiness associated with closed-head brain injury and with sedating drugs. However, these uses have not been specifically approved by the FDA.

CONTRAINDICATIONS

Modafinil is contraindicated in patients with known hypersensitivity to modafinil.

PRECAUTIONS

GENERAL
Although modafinil has not been shown to produce functional impairment, any drug affecting the CNS may alter judgment, thinking or motor skills. Patients should be cautioned about operating an automobile or other hazardous machinery until they are reasonably certain that modafinil therapy will not adversely affect their ability to engage in such activities.

CARDIOVASCULAR SYSTEM
In clinical studies of modafinil, signs and symptoms including chest pain, palpitations, dyspnea and transient ischemic T-wave changes on ECG were observed in 3 subjects in association with mitral valve prolapse or left ventricular hypertrophy. It is recommended that modafinil tablets not be used in patients with a history of left ventricular hypertrophy or ischemic ECG changes, chest pain, arrhythmia or other clinically significant manifestations of mitral valve prolapse in association with CNS stimulant use.

Modafinil has not been evaluated or used to any appreciable extent in patients with a recent history of myocardial infarction or unstable angina, and such patients should be treated with caution.

Modafinil has not been systematically evaluated in patients with hypertension. Periodic monitoring of hypertensive patients may be appropriate.

CENTRAL NERVOUS SYSTEM
One healthy male volunteer developed ideas of reference, paranoid delusions, and auditory hallucinations in association with multiple daily 600 mg doses of modafinil and sleep deprivation. There was no evidence of psychosis 36 hours after drug discontinuation. Caution should be exercised when modafinil is given to patients with a history of psychosis.

PATIENTS WITH SEVERE RENAL IMPAIRMENT
In patients with severe renal impairment (mean creatinine clearance = 16.6 ml/min), a 200 mg single dose of modafinil did not lead to increased exposure to modafinil but resulted in much higher exposure to the inactive metabolite, modafinil acid, than is seen in subjects with normal renal function. There is little information available about the safety of such levels of this metabolite (see CLINICAL PHARMACOLOGY).

PATIENTS WITH SEVERE HEPATIC IMPAIRMENT
In patients with severe hepatic impairment, with or without cirrhosis (see CLINICAL PHARMACOLOGY), modafinil should be administered at a reduced dose as the clearance of modafinil was decreased compared to that in normal subjects (see DOSAGE AND ADMINISTRATION).

ELDERLY PATIENTS
To the extent that elderly patients may have diminished renal and/or hepatic function, dosage reductions should be considered (see DOSAGE AND ADMINISTRATION).

PATIENTS USING CONTRACEPTIVES
The effectiveness of steroidal contraceptives may be reduced when used with modafinil tablets and for 1 month after discontinuation of therapy (see Potential Interactions with Drugs That Inhibit, Induce, or are Metabolized by Cytochrome P-450 Isoenzymes and Other Hepatic Enzymes). Alternative or concomitant methods of contraception are recommended for patients treated with modafinil tablets, and for 1 month after discontinuation of modafinil.

INFORMATION FOR THE PATIENT
Physicians are advised to discuss the following issues with patients for whom they prescribe modafinil tablets.

Pregnancy
Animal studies to assess the effects of modafinil on reproduction and the developing fetus were not conducted at adequately high doses or according to guidelines which would ensure a comprehensive evaluation of the potential of modafinil to adversely affect fertility, or cause embryolethality or teratogenicity (see Impairment of Fertility and Pregnancy Category C).

Patients should be advised to notify their physician if they become pregnant or intend to become pregnant during therapy. Patients should be cautioned regarding the potential increased risk of pregnancy when using steroidal contraceptives (including depot or implantable contraceptives) with modafinil tablets and for 1 month after discontinuation of therapy.

Nursing
Patients should be advised to notify their physician if they are breast feeding an infant.

Concomitant Medication
Patients should be advised to inform their physician if they are taking, or plan to take, any prescription or over-the-counter drugs, because of the potential for interactions between modafinil tablets and other drugs.

Alcohol
Patients should be advised that the use of modafinil in combination with alcohol has not been studied. Patients should be advised that it is prudent to avoid alcohol while taking modafinil tablets.

Allergic Reactions
Patients should be advised to notify their physician if they develop a rash, hives, or a related allergic phenomenon.

CARCINOGENESIS, MUTAGENESIS, AND IMPAIRMENT OF FERTILITY

Carcinogenesis
Carcinogenicity studies were conducted in which modafinil was administered in the diet to mice for 78 weeks and to rats for 104 weeks at doses of 6, 30 and 60 mg/kg/day. The highest dose studied represents 1.5 times (mouse) or 3 times (rat) greater than the maximum recommended human daily dose of 200 mg on a mg/m^2 basis. There was no evidence of tumorigenesis associated with modafinil administration in these studies, but because the mouse study used an inadequate high dose that was not representative of a maximum tolerated dose, the carcinogenic potential of modafinil has not been fully evaluated.

Mutagenesis
There was no evidence of mutagenic or clastogenic potential of modafinil in a series of assays. It was not mutagenic in the *in vitro* Ames bacterial reverse mutation test, the *in vitro* mouse lymphoma/TK locus assay in the presence or absence of metabolic activation; and it was not clastogenic in the *in vitro* human lymphocyte chromosomal aberration assay in the presence or absence of metabolic activation, or in two *in vivo* mouse bone marrow micronucleus assays. Modafinil did not increase unscheduled DNA synthesis in rat hepatocytes. In a cell transformation assay in BALB/3T3 mouse embryo cells, modafinil did not cause an increase in the frequency of transformed foci in the presence or absence of metabolic activation.

Impairment of Fertility
When modafinil was administered orally to male and female rats prior to and throughout mating and gestation at doses up to 100 mg/kg/day (4.8 times the maximum recommended daily dose of 200 mg on a mg/m^2 basis) no effects on fertility were seen. The study to evaluate these effects, however, did not use sufficiently high doses or large enough sample size to adequately assess effects on fertility.

PREGNANCY CATEGORY C
Embryotoxicity was observed in the absence of maternal toxicity when rats received oral modafinil throughout the period of organogenesis. At a dose of 200 mg/kg/day (10 times the maximum recommended daily human dose of 200 mg on a mg/m^2 basis) there was an increase in resorption, hydronephrosis, and skeletal variations. The no-effect dose for these effects was 100 mg/kg/day (5 times the maximum recommended daily human dose on a mg/m^2 basis). When rabbits received oral modafinil throughout organogenesis at doses up to 100 mg/kg/day (10 times the maximum recommended daily human dose on a mg/m^2 basis), no embryotoxicity was seen. Neither of these studies, however, used optimal doses for the evaluation of embryotoxicity. Although a threshold dose for embryotoxicity has been identified, the full spectrum of potential toxic effects on the fetus has not been characterized. When rats were dosed throughout gestation and lactation at doses up to 200 mg/kg/day, no developmental toxicity was noted post-natally in the offspring. There are no adequate and well-controlled trials with modafinil in pregnant women and this drug should be used during pregnancy only if the potential benefit outweighs the potential risk.

LABOR AND DELIVERY
The effect of modafinil on labor and delivery in humans has not been systematically investigated. Seven normal births occurred in patients who had received modafinil during pregnancy. One patient gave birth 3 weeks earlier than the expected range of delivery dates (estimated using ultrasound) to a healthy male infant. One woman with a history of spontaneous abortions suffered a spontaneous abortion while being treated with modafinil.

NURSING MOTHERS
It is not known whether modafinil or its metabolites are excreted in human milk. Because many drugs are excreted in human milk, caution should be exercised when modafinil tablets are administered to a nursing woman.

PEDIATRIC USE
Safety and effectiveness in individuals below 16 years of age have not been established.

GERIATRIC USE

Safety and effectiveness in individuals above 65 years of age have not been established. Experience in a limited number of patients (15) who were greater than 65 years of age in US clinical trials showed an incidence of adverse experiences similar to other age groups.

DRUG INTERACTIONS

CNS ACTIVE DRUGS

Methylphenidate: In a single-dose study in healthy volunteers, coadministration of modafinil (200 mg) with methylphenidate (40 mg) did not cause any significant alterations in the pharmacokinetics of either drug. However, the absorption of modafinil may be delayed by approximately 1 hour when coadministered with methylphenidate.

Clomipramine: The coadministration of a single dose of clomipramine (50 mg) on the first of 3 days of treatment with modafinil (200 mg/day) in healthy volunteers did not show an effect on the pharmacokinetics of either drug. However, one incident of increased levels of clomipramine and its active metabolite desmethylclomipramine has been reported in a patient with narcolepsy during treatment with modafinil (see Potential Interactions with Drugs That Inhibit, Induce, or are Metabolized by Cytochrome P-450 Isoenzymes and Other Hepatic Enzymes).

Triazolam: In a single-dose pharmacodynamic study with modafinil in healthy volunteers (50, 100 or 200 mg) and triazolam (0.25 mg), no clinically important alterations in the safety profile of modafinil or triazolam were noted.

Monoamine Oxidase (MAO) Inhibitors: Interaction studies with monoamine oxidase inhibitors have not been performed. Therefore, caution should be used when concomitantly administering MAO inhibitors and modafinil.

POTENTIAL INTERACTIONS WITH DRUGS THAT INHIBIT, INDUCE, OR ARE METABOLIZED BY CYTOCHROME P-450 ISOENZYMES AND OTHER HEPATIC ENZYMES

In a controlled study in patients with narcolepsy, chronic dosing of modafinil at 400 mg/day once daily resulted in a -20% mean decrease in modafinil plasma trough concentrations by week 9, relative to those at week 3, suggesting that chronic administration of modafinil might have caused induction of its metabolism. In addition, coadministration of potent inducers of CYP3A4 (*e.g.*, carbamazepine, phenobarbital, rifampin) or inhibitors of CYP3A4 (*e.g.*, ketoconazole, itraconazole) could alter the levels of modafinil due to the partial involvement of that enzyme in the metabolic elimination of the compound.

In *in vitro* studies using primary human hepatocyte cultures, modafinil was shown to slightly induce CYP1A2, CYP2B6 and CYP3A4 in a concentration-dependent manner. Although induction results based on *in vitro* experiments are not necessarily predictive of response *in vivo*, caution needs to be exercised when modafinil is coadministered with drugs that depend on these three enzymes for their clearance. Specifically, lower blood levels of such drugs could result. In the case of CYP1A2 and CYP2B6, no other evidence of enzyme induction has been observed. A modest induction of CYP3A4 by modafinil has been indicated by other results, hence the clearance of CYP3A4 substrates such as cyclosporine, steroidal contraceptives and, to a lesser degree, theophylline, may be increased. One case of an interaction between modafinil and cyclosporine has been reported in a 41 year old woman who had undergone an organ transplant. After 1 month of administration of 200 mg/day of modafinil, cyclosporine blood levels were decreased by 50%. The interaction was postulated to be due to the increased metabolism of cyclosporine, since no other factor expected to affect the disposition of the drug had changed.

The exposure of human hepatocytes to modafinil *in vitro* produced an apparent concentration-related suppression of expression of CYP2C9 activity. The clinical relevance of this finding is unclear, since no other indication of CYP2C9 suppression has been observed. However, monitoring of prothrombin times is suggested as a precaution for the first several months of coadministration of modafinil and warfarin, a CYP2C9 substrate, and thereafter whenever modafinil dosing is changed. In addition, patients receiving modafinil and phenytoin, a CYP2C9 substrate, concomitantly should be monitored for signs of phenytoin toxicity.

In vitro studies using human liver microsomes showed that modafinil has little or no capacity to inhibit the major CYP enzymes except for CYP2C19, which is reversibly inhibited at pharmacologically relevant concentrations of modafinil. Drugs that are largely eliminated via CYP2C19 metabolism, such as diazepam, propranolol, phenytoin or S-mephenytoin may have prolonged elimination upon coadministration with modafinil and may require dosage reduction.

In addition, CYP2C19 provides an ancillary pathway for the metabolism of certain tricyclic antidepressants (*e.g.*, clomipramine and desipramine) that are primarily metabolized by CYP2D6. In tricyclic-treated patients deficient in CYP2D6 (*i.e.*, those who are poor metabolizers of debrisoquine; 7-10% of the Caucasian population; similar or lower in other populations), the amount of metabolism by CYP2C19 may be substantially increased. Modafinil may cause elevation of the levels of the tricyclics in this subset of patients. Physicians should be aware that a reduction in the dose of tricyclic agents might be needed in these patients.

ADVERSE REACTIONS

Modafinil has been evaluated for safety in over 2200 subjects, of whom more than 900 subjects with narcolepsy or narcolepsy/hypersomnia were given at least one dose of modafinil. Modafinil has been found to be generally well-tolerated. In controlled clinical trials, most adverse experiences were mild to moderate.

The most commonly observed adverse events (≥5%) associated with the use of modafinil more frequently than placebo-treated patients in controlled US and foreign studies were headache, infection, nausea, nervousness, anxiety, and insomnia.

In US placebo-controlled Phase 3 clinical trials, 5% of the 369 patients who received modafinil discontinued due to an adverse experience. The most frequent (≥1%) reasons for discontinuation that occurred at a higher rate for modafinil than placebo patients were headache (1%), nausea (1%), depression (1%) and nervousness (1%). In foreign, controlled clinical trials, reasons for discontinuation were similar to those in US trials. In a Canadian clinical trial, a 35 year old obese narcoleptic male with a prior history of syncopal episodes experienced a 9-second episode of asystole after 27 days of modafinil treatment (300 mg/day in divided doses).

INCIDENCE IN CONTROLLED TRIALS

TABLE 3 presents the adverse experiences that occurred in narcolepsy patients at a rate of 1% or more and were more frequent in patients treated with modafinil than in placebo patients in US placebo-controlled clinical trials.

The prescriber should be aware that the figures provided below cannot be used to predict the frequency of adverse experiences in the course of usual medical practice, where patient characteristics and other factors may differ from those occurring during clinical studies. Similarly, the cited frequencies cannot be directly compared with figures obtained from other clinical investigations involving different treatments, uses, or investigators. Review of these frequencies, however, provides prescribers with a basis to estimate the relative con-

***TABLE 3** Incidence of Treatment-Emergent Adverse Experiences in US 9 Week Placebo-Controlled Clinical Trials* with Modafinil (200 and 400 mg) Daily*

Body System Preferred Term	Modafinil (n=369)	Placebo (n=185)
Body as a Whole		
Headache	50%	40%
Chest pain	2%	1%
Neck pain	2%	1%
Chills	2%	0%
Rigid neck	1%	0%
Fever/chills	1%	0%
Digestive		
Nausea	13%	4%
Diarrhea	8%	4%
Dry mouth	5%	1%
Anorexia	5%	1%
Abnormal liver function†	3%	2%
Vomiting	2%	1%
Mouth ulcer	1%	0%
Gingivitis	1%	0%
Thirst	1%	0%
Respiratory System		
Rhinitis	11%	8%
Pharyngitis	6%	3%
Lung disorder	4%	2%
Dyspnea	2%	1%
Asthma	1%	0%
Epistaxis	1%	0%
Nervous System		
Nervousness	8%	6%
Dizziness	5%	4%
Depression	4%	3%
Anxiety	4%	1%
Cataplexy	3%	2%
Insomnia	3%	1%
Paresthesia	3%	1%
Dyskinesia‡	2%	0%
Hypertonia	2%	0%
Confusion	1%	0%
Amnesia	1%	0%
Emotional lability	1%	0%
Ataxia	1%	0%
Tremor	1%	0%
Cardiovascular		
Hypotension	2%	1%
Hypertension	2%	0%
Vasodilation	1%	0%
Arrhythmia	1%	0%
Syncope	1%	0%
Hemic/Lymphatic		
Eosinophilia	2%	0%
Special Senses		
Amblyopia	2%	1%
Abnormal vision	2%	0%
Metabolic/Nutritional		
Hyperglycemia	1%	0%
Albuminuria	1%	0%
Musculoskeletal		
Joint disorder	1%	0%
Skin/Appendages		
Herpes simplex	1%	0%
Dry skin	1%	0%
Urogenital		
Abnormal urine	1%	0%
Urinary retention	1%	0%
Abnormal ejaculation§	1%	0%

* Events reported by at least 1% of patients treated with modafinil that were more frequent than in the placebo group are included; incidence is rounded to the nearest 1%. The adverse experience terminology is coded using a standard modified COSTART Dictionary.

† Elevated liver enzymes.

‡ Oro-facial dyskinesias.

§ Incidence adjusted for gender.

Events for which the modafinil incidence was at least 1%, but equal to or less than placebo are not listed in the table. These events included the following: infection, back pain, pain, hypothermia, abdominal pain, flu syndrome, allergic reaction, fever, asthenia, accidental injury, general edema, tachycardia, palpitations, migraine, ventricular extrasystole, bradycardia, dyspepsia, tooth disorder, constipation, flatulence, increased appetite, gastroenteritis, GI disorder, ecchymosis, anemia, leukocytosis, peripheral edema, increased weight, increased SGOT, myalgia, arthritis, arthralgia, somnolence, thinking abnormality, leg cramps, sleep disorder, hallucinations, hyperkinesia, decreased libido, increased cough, sinusitis, bronchitis, pneumonia, rash, sweating, pruritus, skin disorder, psoriasis, ear pain, eye pain, ear disorder, taste perversion, dysmenorrhea§, urinary tract infection, pyuria, hematuria, cystitis, and disturbed menses.§

tribution of drug and non-drug factors to the incidence of adverse events in the population studied.

DOSE DEPENDENCY OF ADVERSE EVENTS

In the US Phase 3 clinical trials, the only adverse experience that was more frequent (≥5% difference) in the modafinil dose group of 400 mg/day than in the modafinil dose group of 200 mg/day and placebo was headache.

VITAL SIGN CHANGES

There were no consistent effects or patterns of change in vital signs for patients treated with modafinil enrolled in the US Phase 3 clinical trials.

WEIGHT CHANGES

There were no clinically significant differences in body weight change in patients treated with modafinil compared to placebo-treated patients.

LABORATORY CHANGES

Clinical chemistry, hematology, and urinalysis parameters were monitored in US Phase 1, 2 and 3 studies. In these studies, mean plasma levels of gamma-glutamyl transferase (GGT) were found to be higher following administration of modafinil, but not placebo. Few subjects (1%), however, had GGT elevations outside of the normal range. Shift to higher, but not clinically significantly abnormal, GGT values appeared to increase with time in the population treated with modafinil in the 9 week US Phase 3 clinical trials. No differences were apparent in alkaline phosphatase, alanine aminotransferase, aspartate aminotransferase, total protein, albumin, or total bilirubin.

Although there were more abnormal eosinophil counts following modafinil administration than placebo in US Phase 1 and 2 studies, the difference does not appear to be clinically significant. Observed shifts were from normal to high.

ECG CHANGES

No treatment-emergent pattern of ECG abnormalities was found in US Phase 1, 2, and 3 studies following administration of modafinil.

DOSAGE AND ADMINISTRATION

The dose of modafinil is 200 mg/day, given as a single dose in the morning.

Doses of 400 mg/day, given as a single dose, have been well tolerated, but there is no consistent evidence that this dose confers additional benefit beyond that of the 200 mg dose.

In patients with severe hepatic impairment, the dose of modafinil should be reduced to one-half of that recommended for patients with normal hepatic function (see CLINICAL PHARMACOLOGY and PRECAUTIONS).

There is inadequate information to determine safety and efficacy of dosing in patients with severe renal impairment (see CLINICAL PHARMACOLOGY and PRECAUTIONS).

In elderly patients, elimination of modafinil and its metabolites may be reduced as a consequence of aging. Therefore, consideration should be given to the use of lower doses in this population (see CLINICAL PHARMACOLOGY and PRECAUTIONS).

HOW SUPPLIED

Provigil tablets are available in:

100 mg: Each capsule-shaped, white, uncoated tablet is debossed with "PROVIGIL" on one side and "100 MG" on the other.

200 mg: Each capsule-shaped, white, scored, uncoated tablet is debossed with "PROVIGIL" on one side and "200 MG" on the other.

Storage: Store at 20-25°C (68-77°F).

PRODUCT LISTING - EQUIVALENTS NOT AVAILABLE

Tablet - Oral - 100 mg

100's	$432.00	PROVIGIL, Cephalon, Inc	63459-0100-01

Tablet - Oral - 200 mg

100's	$597.00	PROVIGIL, Cephalon, Inc	63459-0200-01

Moexipril Hydrochloride *(003261)*

For related information, see the comparative table section in Appendix A.

Categories: Hypertension, essential; FDA Approved 1995 May; Pregnancy Category C, 1st Trimester; Pregnancy Category D, 2nd & 3rd Trimesters
Drug Classes: Angiotensin converting enzyme inhibitors
Brand Names: Fampress; **Univasc**
Foreign Brand Availability: Fempres (Peru); Fempress (Germany); Moex (France; Hong-Kong; Israel)
Cost of Therapy: $29.31 (Hypertension; Univasc; 7.5 mg; 1 tablet/day; 30 day supply)

WARNING

Use in Pregnancy

When used in pregnancy during the second and third trimesters, ACE inhibitors can cause injury and even death to the developing fetus. When pregnancy is detected, moexipril HCl should be discontinued as soon as possible. See WARNINGS, Fetal/Neonatal Morbidity and Mortality.

DESCRIPTION

Univasc (moexipril hydrochloride), the hydrochloride of moexipril, has the empirical formula $C_{27}H_{34}N_2O_7 \cdot HCl$ and a molecular weight of 535.04. It is chemically described as [3S-[2[R*(R*)],3R*]]-2-[2-[[1-(ethoxycarbonyl)-3-phenylpropyl]amino]-1-oxopropyl]-1,2,3,4-tetrahydro-6,7-dimethoxy-3-isoquinolinecarboxylic acid, monohydrochloride. It is a nonsulfhydryl containing precursor of the active angiotensin-converting enzyme (ACE) inhibitor moexiprilat.

Moexipril hydrochloride is a fine white to off-white powder. It is soluble (about 10% weight-to-volume) in distilled water at room temperature.

Univasc is supplied as scored, coated tablets containing 7.5 and 15 mg of moexipril hydrochloride for oral administration. In addition to the active ingredient, moexipril hydrochloride, the tablet core contains the following inactive ingredients: lactose, magnesium oxide, crospovidone, magnesium stearate, and gelatin. The film coating contains hydroxypropyl methylcellulose, hydroxypropyl cellulose, polyethylene glycol 6000, magnesium stearate, titanium dioxide, and ferric oxide.

CLINICAL PHARMACOLOGY

MECHANISM OF ACTION

Moexipril HCl is a prodrug for moexiprilat, which inhibits ACE in humans and animals. The mechanism through which moexiprilat lowers blood pressure is believed to be primarily inhibition of ACE activity. ACE is a peptidyl dipeptidase that catalyzes the conversion of the inactive decapeptide angiotensin I to the vasoconstrictor substance angiotensin II. Angiotensin II is a potent peripheral vasoconstrictor that also stimulates aldosterone secretion by the adrenal cortex and provides negative feedback on renin secretion. ACE is identical to kininase II, an enzyme that degrades bradykinin, an endothelium-dependent vasodilator. Moexiprilat is about 1000 times as potent as moexipril in inhibiting ACE and kininase II. Inhibition of ACE results in decreased angiotensin II formation, leading to decreased vasoconstriction, increased plasma renin activity, and decreased aldosterone secretion. The latter results in diuresis and natriuresis and a small increase in serum potassium concentration (mean increases of about 0.25 mEq/L were seen when moexipril was used alone, see PRECAUTIONS).

Whether increased levels of bradykinin, a potent vasodepressor peptide, play a role in the therapeutic effects of moexipril remains to be elucidated. Although the principal mechanism of moexipril in blood pressure reduction is believed to be through the renin-angiotensin-aldosterone system, ACE inhibitors have some effect on blood pressure even in apparent low-renin hypertension. As is the case with other ACE inhibitors, however, the antihypertensive effect of moexipril is considerably smaller in black patients, a predominantly low-renin population, than in non-black hypertensive patients.

PHARMACOKINETICS AND METABOLISM

Pharmacokinetics

Moexipril's antihypertensive activity is almost entirely due to its deesterified metabolite, moexiprilat. Bioavailability of oral moexipril is about 13% compared to intravenous (IV) moexipril (both measuring the metabolite moexiprilat), and is markedly affected by food, which reduces the peak plasma level (C_{max}) and AUC (see Absorption). Moexipril should therefore be taken in a fasting state. The time of peak plasma concentration (T_{max}) of moexiprilat is about 1½ hours and elimination half-life (T½) is estimated at 2-9 hours in various studies, the variability reflecting a complex elimination pattern that is not simply exponential. Like all ACE inhibitors, moexiprilat has a prolonged terminal elimination phase, presumably reflecting slow release of drug bound to the ACE. Accumulation of moexiprilat with repeated dosing is minimal, about 30%, compatible with a functional elimination T½ of about 12 hours. Over the dose range of 7.5 to 30 mg, pharmacokinetics are approximately dose proportional.

Absorption

Moexipril is incompletely absorbed, with bioavailability as moexiprilat of about 13%. Bioavailability varies with formulation and food intake which reduces C_{max} and AUC by about 70% and 40% respectively after the ingestion of a low-fat breakfast or by 80% and 50% respectively after the ingestion of a high-fat breakfast.

Distribution

The clearance (CL) for moexipril is 441 ml/min and for moexiprilat 232 ml/min with a T½ of 1.3 and 9.8 hours, respectively. Moexiprilat is about 50% protein bound. The volume of distribution of moexiprilat is about 183 liters.

Metabolism and Excretion

Moexipril is relatively rapidly converted to its active metabolite moexiprilat, but persists longer than some other ACE inhibitor prodrugs, such that its half-life is over 1 hour and it has a significant AUC. Both moexipril and moexiprilat are converted to diketopiperazine derivatives and unidentified metabolites. After IV administration of moexipril, about 40% of the dose appears in urine as moexiprilat, about 26% as moexipril, with small amounts of the metabolites; about 20% of the IV dose appears in feces, principally as moexiprilat. After oral administration, only about 7% of the dose appears in urine as moexiprilat, about 1% as moexipril, with about 5% as other metabolites. Fifty-two percent (52%) of the dose is recovered in feces as moexiprilat and 1% as moexipril.

Special Populations

Decreased Renal Function

The effective elimination of T½ and AUC of both moexipril and moexiprilat are increased with decreasing renal function. There is insufficient information available to characterize this relationship fully, but at creatinine clearances in the range of 10-40 ml/min, the T½ of moexiprilat is increased by a factor of 3-4.

Decreased Hepatic Function

In patients with mild to moderate cirrhosis given single 15 mg doses of moexipril, the C_{max} of moexipril was increased by about 50% and the AUC increased by about 120%, while the C_{max} for moexiprilat was decreased by about 50% and the AUC increased by almost 300%.

Elderly Patients

In elderly male subjects (65-80 years old) with clinically normal renal and hepatic function, the AUC and C_{max} of moexiprilat is about 30% greater than those of younger subjects (19-42 years old).

Pharmacokinetic Interactions With Other Drugs
No clinically important pharmacokinetic interactions occurred when moexipril HCl was administered concomitantly with hydrochlorothiazide, digoxin, or cimetidine.

PHARMACODYNAMICS AND CLINICAL EFFECT

Single and multiple doses of 15 mg or more of moexipril HCl give a sustained inhibition of plasma ACE activity of 80-90%, beginning within 2 hours and lasting 24 hours (80%).

In controlled trials, the peak effects of orally administered moexipril increased with the dose administered over a dose range of 7.5 to 60 mg, given once a day. Antihypertensive effects were first detectable about 1 hour after dosing, with a peak effect between 3 and 6 hours after dosing. Just before dosing (*i.e.,* at trough), the antihypertensive effects were less prominently related to dose and the antihypertensive effect tended to diminish during the 24 hour dosing interval when the drug was administered once a day.

In multiple dose studies in the dose range of 7.5 to 30 mg once a day, moexipril HCl lowered sitting diastolic and systolic blood pressure effects at trough by 3-6 mm Hg and 4-11 mm Hg, more than placebo, respectively. There was a tendency toward increased response with higher doses over this range. These effects are typical of ACE inhibitors but, to date, there are no trials of adequate size comparing moexipril with other antihypertensive agents.

The trough diastolic blood pressure effects of moexipril were approximately 3-6 mm Hg in various studies. Generally, higher doses of moexipril leave a greater fraction of the peak blood pressure effect still present at trough. During dose titration, any decision as to the adequacy of a dosing regimen should be based on trough blood pressure measurements. If diastolic blood pressure control is not adequate at the end of the dosing interval, the dose can be increased or given as a divided (bid) regimen.

During chronic therapy, the antihypertensive effect of any dose of moexipril HCl is generally evident within 2 weeks of treatment, with maximal reduction after 4 weeks. The antihypertensive effects of moexipril HCl have been proven to continue during therapy for up to 24 months.

Moexipril HCl, like other ACE inhibitors, is less effective in decreasing trough blood pressures in blacks than in non-blacks. Placebo-corrected trough group mean diastolic blood pressure effects in blacks in the proposed dose range varied between +1 to -3 mm Hg compared with responses in non-blacks of -4 to -6 mm Hg.

The effectiveness of moexipril HCl was not significantly influenced by patient age, gender, or weight. Moexipril HCl has been shown to have antihypertensive activity in both pre- and postmenopausal women who have participated in placebo-controlled clinical trials.

Formal interaction studies with moexipril have not been carried out with antihypertensive agents other than thiazide diuretics. In these studies, the added effect of moexipril was similar to its effect as monotherapy. In general, ACE inhibitors have less than additive effects with beta-adrenergic blockers, presumably because both work by inhibiting the renin-angiotensin system.

M

INDICATIONS AND USAGE

Moexipril HCl is indicated for treatment of patients with hypertension. It may be used alone or in combination with thiazide diuretics.

In using moexipril HCl, consideration should be given to the fact that another ACE inhibitor, captopril, has caused agranulocytosis, particularly in patients with renal impairment or collagen-vascular disease. Available data are insufficient to show that moexipril HCl does not have a similar risk (see WARNINGS).

In considering use of moexipril HCl, it should be noted that in controlled trials ACE inhibitors have an effect on blood pressure that is less in black patients than in non-blacks. In addition, ACE inhibitors (for which adequate data are available) cause a higher rate of angioedema in black than in non-black patients (see WARNINGS, Anaphylactoid and Possibly Related Reactions, Angioedema).

NON-FDA APPROVED INDICATIONS

ACE inhibitors are also used for the treatment of heart failure, left ventricular dysfunction following myocardial infarction (MI), and diabetic nephropathy (> 500 mg/day proteinuria) in patients with diabetes mellitus and retinopathy. Recent data have shown that some ACE inhibitors improve survival and exercise tolerance and reduce the incidence of overt heart failure and subsequent hospitalizations in patients with recent MI. Data have also shown that ACE inhibitors reduce the 3-year incidence of heart failure and related hospitalization in patients with asymptomatic left ventricular dysfunction. A trend toward reduced mortality associated with the use of ACE inhibitors in these patients has not been statistically significant. There are no data on the use, efficacy, safety, or dose-ranging of moexipril for the treatment of any condition except hypertension.

CONTRAINDICATIONS

Moexipril HCl is contraindicated in patients who are hypersensitive to this product and in patients with a history of angioedema related to previous treatment with an ACE inhibitor.

WARNINGS

ANAPHYLACTOID AND POSSIBLY RELATED REACTIONS

Presumably because angiotensin-converting enzyme inhibitors affect the metabolism of eicosanoids and polypeptides, including endogenous bradykinin, patients receiving ACE inhibitors, including moexipril HCl, may be subject to a variety of adverse reactions, some of them serious.

Angioedema
Angioedema involving the face, extremities, lips, tongue, glottis, and/or larynx has been reported in patients treated with ACE inhibitors, including moexipril HCl. Symptoms suggestive of angioedema or facial edema occurred in <0.5% of moexipril-treated patients in placebo-controlled trials. None of the cases were considered life-threatening and all resolved either without treatment or with medication (antihistamines or glucocorticoids). One (1) patient treated with hydrochlorothiazide alone experienced laryngeal edema. No instances of angioedema were reported in placebo-treated patients.

In cases of angioedema, treatment should be promptly discontinued and the patient carefully observed until the swelling disappears. In instances where swelling has been confined to the face and lips, the condition has generally resolved without treatment, although antihistamines have been useful in relieving symptoms.

Angioedema associated with involvement of the tongue, glottis, or larynx, may be fatal due to airway obstruction. Appropriate therapy, *e.g.*, subcutaneous epinephrine solution 1:1000 (0.3-0.5 ml) and/or measures to ensure a patent airway, should be promptly provided (see ADVERSE REACTIONS).

Anaphylactoid Reactions During Desensitization
Two (2) patients undergoing desensitizing treatment with hymenoptera venom while receiving ACE inhibitors sustained life-threatening anaphylactoid reactions. In the same patients, these reactions did not occur when ACE inhibitors were temporarily withheld, but they reappeared when the ACE inhibitors were inadvertently readministered.

Anaphylactoid Reactions During Membrane Exposure
Anaphylactoid reactions have been reported in patients dialyzed with high-flux membranes and treated concomitantly with an ACE inhibitor. Anaphylactoid reactions have also been reported in patients undergoing low-density lipoprotein apheresis with dextran sulfate absorption.

HYPOTENSION

Moexipril HCl can cause symptomatic hypotension, although, as with other ACE inhibitors, this is unusual in uncomplicated hypertensive patients treated with moexipril HCl alone. Symptomatic hypotension was seen in 0.5% of patients given moexipril and led to discontinuation of therapy in about 0.25%. Symptomatic hypotension is most likely to occur in patients who have been salt- and volume-depleted as a result of prolonged diuretic therapy, dietary salt restriction, dialysis, diarrhea, or vomiting. Volume- and salt-depletion should be corrected and, in general, diuretics stopped, before initiating therapy with moexipril HCl (see DRUG INTERACTIONS and ADVERSE REACTIONS).

In patients with congestive heart failure, with or without associated renal insufficiency, ACE inhibitor therapy may cause excessive hypotension, which may be associated with oliguria or progressive azotemia, and rarely, with acute renal failure and death. In these patients, moexipril HCl therapy should be started under close medical supervision, and patients should be followed closely for the first 2 weeks of treatment and whenever the dose of moexipril or an accompanying diuretic is increased. Care in avoiding hypotension should also be taken in patients with ischemic heart disease, aortic stenosis, or cerebrovascular disease, in whom an excessive decrease in blood pressure could result in a myocardial infarction or a cerebrovascular accident.

If hypotension occurs, the patient should be placed in a supine position and, if necessary, treated with an IV infusion of normal saline. Moexipril HCl treatment usually can be continued following restoration of blood pressure and volume.

NEUTROPENIA/AGRANULOCYTOSIS

Another ACE inhibitor, captopril, has been shown to cause agranulocytosis and bone marrow depression, rarely in patients with uncomplicated hypertension, but more frequently in hypertensive patients with renal impairment, especially if they also have a collagen-vascular disease such as systemic lupus erythematosus or scleroderma. Although there were no instances of severe neutropenia (absolute neutrophil count <500/mm^3) among patients given moexipril HCl, as with other ACE inhibitors, monitoring of white blood cell counts should be considered for patients who have collagen-vascular disease, especially if the disease is associated with impaired renal function. Available data from clinical trials of moexipril HCl are insufficient to show that moexipril HCl does not cause agranulocytosis at rates similar to captopril.

FETAL/NEONATAL MORBIDITY AND MORTALITY

ACE inhibitors can cause fetal and neonatal morbidity and death when administered to pregnant women. Several dozen cases have been reported in the world literature. When pregnancy is detected, ACE inhibitors should be discontinued as soon as possible.

The use of ACE inhibitors during the second and third trimesters of pregnancy has been associated with fetal and neonatal injury, including hypotension, neonatal skull hypoplasia, anuria, reversible or irreversible renal failure, and death. Oligohydramnios has also been reported, presumably resulting from decreased fetal renal function; oligohydramnios in this setting has been associated with fetal limb contractures, craniofacial deformation, and hypoplastic lung development. Prematurity, intrauterine growth retardation, and patent ductus arteriosus have also been reported, although it is not clear whether these were caused by the ACE inhibitor exposure.

Fetal and neonatal morbidity do not appear to have resulted from intrauterine ACE inhibitor exposure limited to the first trimester. Mothers who have used ACE inhibitors only during the first trimester should be informed of this. Nonetheless, when patients become pregnant, physicians should make every effort to discontinue the use of moexipril as soon as possible. Rarely (probably less often than once in every 1000 pregnancies), no alternative to ACE inhibitors will be found. In these rare cases, the mothers should be apprised of the potential hazards to their fetuses, and serial ultrasound examinations should be performed to assess the intraamniotic environment.

If oligohydramnios is observed, moexipril should be discontinued unless it is considered life-saving for the mother. Contraction stress (CST), a non-stress test (NST), or biophysical profiling (BPP) may be appropriate, depending upon the week of pregnancy. Patients and physicians should be aware, however, that oligohydramnios may not be detected until after the fetus has sustained irreversible injury.

Infants with histories of *in utero* exposure to ACE inhibitors should be closely observed for hypotension, oliguria, and hyperkalemia. If oliguria occurs, attention should be directed toward support of blood pressure and renal perfusion. Exchange transfusion or peritoneal dialysis may be required as means of reversing hypotension and/or substituting for disordered renal function.

Theoretically, the ACE inhibitor could be removed from the neonatal circulation by exchange transfusion, but no experience with this procedure has been reported.

No embryotoxic, fetotoxic, or teratogenic effects were seen in rats or in rabbits treated with up to 90.9 and 0.7 times, respectively, the Maximum Recommended Human Dose (MRHD) on a mg/m^2 basis.

HEPATIC FAILURE

Rarely, ACE inhibitors have been associated with a syndrome that starts with cholestatic jaundice and progresses to fulminant hepatic necrosis and sometimes death. The mechanism of this syndrome is not understood. Patients receiving ACE inhibitors who develop jaundice or marked elevations of hepatic enzymes should discontinue the ACE inhibitor and receive appropriate medical follow-up.

PRECAUTIONS

GENERAL

Impaired Renal Function

As a consequence of inhibition of the renin-angiotensin-aldosterone system, changes in renal function may be anticipated in susceptible individuals. There is no clinical experience of moexipril HCl in the treatment of hypertension in patients with renal failure.

Some hypertensive patients with no apparent preexisting renal vascular disease have developed increases in blood urea nitrogen and serum creatinine, usually minor and transient, especially when moexipril HCl has been given concomitantly with a thiazide diuretic. This is more likely to occur in patients with preexisting renal impairment. There may be a need for dose adjustment of moexipril HCl and/or the discontinuation of the thiazide diuretic.

Evaluation of hypertensive patients should always include assessment of renal function (see DOSAGE AND ADMINISTRATION).

Hypertensive Patients With Congestive Heart Failure

In hypertensive patients with severe congestive heart failure, whose renal function may depend on the activity of the renin-angiotensin-aldosterone system, treatment with ACE inhibitors, including moexipril HCl, may be associated with oliguria and/or progressive azotemia and, rarely, acute renal failure and/or death.

Hypertensive Patients With Renal Artery Stenosis

In hypertensive patients with unilateral or bilateral renal artery stenosis, increases in blood urea nitrogen and serum creatinine have been observed in some patients following ACE inhibitor therapy. These increases were almost always reversible upon discontinuation of the ACE inhibitor and/or diuretic therapy. In such patients, renal function should be monitored during the first few weeks of therapy.

Hyperkalemia

In clinical trials, persistent hyperkalemia (serum potassium above 5.4 mEq/L) occurred in approximately 1.3% of hypertensive patients receiving moexipril HCl. Risk factors for the development of hyperkalemia with ACE inhibitors include renal insufficiency, diabetes mellitus, and the concomitant use of potassium-sparing diuretics, potassium supplements, and/or potassium-containing salt substitutes, which should be used cautiously, if at all, with moexipril HCl (see DRUG INTERACTIONS).

Surgery/Anesthesia

In patients undergoing major surgery or during anesthesia with agents that produce hypotension, moexipril may block the effects of compensatory renin release. If hypotension occurs in this setting and is considered to be due to this mechanism, it can be corrected by volume expansion.

Cough

Presumably due to the inhibition of the degradation of endogenous bradykinin, persistent nonproductive cough has been reported with all ACE inhibitors, always resolving after discontinuation of therapy. ACE inhibitor-induced cough should be considered in the differential diagnosis of cough. In controlled trials with moexipril, cough was present in 6.1% of moexipril patients and 2.2% of patients given placebo.

INFORMATION FOR THE PATIENT

Food

Patients should be advised to take moexipril 1 hour before meals (see CLINICAL PHARMACOLOGY and DOSAGE AND ADMINISTRATION).

Angioedema

Angioedema, including laryngeal edema, may occur with treatment with ACE inhibitors, usually occurring early in therapy (within the first month). Patients should be so advised and told to report immediately any signs or symptoms suggesting angioedema (swelling of the face, extremities, eyes, lips, tongue, difficulty in breathing) and to take no more moexipril HCl until they have consulted with the prescribing physician.

Symptomatic Hypotension

Patients should be cautioned that lightheadedness can occur with moexipril HCl, especially during the first few days of therapy. If fainting occurs, the patient should stop taking moexipril HCl and consult the prescribing physician.

All patients should be cautioned that excessive perspiration and dehydration may lead to an excessive fall in blood pressure because of reduction in fluid volume. Other causes of volume depletion such as vomiting or diarrhea may also lead to a fall in blood pressure; patients should be advised to consult their physician if they develop these conditions.

Hyperkalemia

Patients should be told not to use potassium supplements or salt substitutes containing potassium without consulting their physician.

Neutropenia

Patients should be told to report promptly any indication of infection (*e.g.*, sore throat, fever) that could be a sign of neutropenia.

Pregnancy

Female patients of childbearing age should be told about the consequences of second- and third-trimester exposure to ACE inhibitors and should also be told that these consequences do not appear to have resulted from intrauterine ACE inhibitor exposure that has been limited to the first trimester. Patients should be asked to report pregnancies to their physicians as soon as possible.

CARCINOGENESIS, MUTAGENESIS, AND IMPAIRMENT OF FERTILITY

No evidence of carcinogenicity was detected on long-term studies in mice and rats at doses up to 14 or 27.3 times the MRHD on a mg/m^2 basis.

No mutagenicity was detected in the Ames test and microbial reverse mutation assay, with and without metabolic activation, or in an *in vivo* nucleus anomaly test. However, increased chromosomal aberration frequency in Chinese hamster ovary cells was detected under metabolic activation conditions at a 20 hour harvest time.

Reproduction studies have been performed in rabbits at oral doses up to 0.7 times the MRHD on a mg/m^2 basis, and in rats up to 90.9 times the MRHD on a mg/m^2 basis. No indication of impaired fertility, reproductive toxicity, or teratogenicity was observed.

PREGNANCY CATEGORIES C (FIRST TRIMESTER) AND D (SECOND AND THIRD TRIMESTERS)

See WARNINGS, Fetal/Neonatal Morbidity and Mortality.

NURSING MOTHERS

It is not known whether moexipril HCl is excreted in human milk. Because many drugs are excreted in human milk, caution should be exercised when moexipril HCl is given to a nursing mother.

PEDIATRIC USE

Safety and effectiveness of moexipril HCl in pediatric patients have not been established.

GERIATRIC USE

Clinical studies of moexipril HCl did not include sufficient numbers of subjects aged 65 and over to determine whether they respond differently from younger subjects. Other reported clinical experience has not identified differences in responses between the elderly and younger patients. In general, dose selection for an elderly patient should be cautious, usually starting at the low end of the dosing range, reflecting the greater frequency of decreased hepatic, renal, or cardiac function, and of concomitant disease or other drug therapy.

DRUG INTERACTIONS

DIURETICS

Excessive reductions in blood pressure may occur in patients on diuretic therapy when ACE inhibitors are started. The possibility of hypotensive effects with moexipril HCl can be minimized by discontinuing diuretic therapy for several days or cautiously increasing salt intake before initiation of treatment with moexipril HCl. If this is not possible, the starting dose of moexipril should be reduced. (See WARNINGS and DOSAGE AND ADMINISTRATION.)

POTASSIUM SUPPLEMENTS AND POTASSIUM-SPARING DIURETICS

Moexipril HCl can increase serum potassium because it decreases aldosterone secretion. Use of potassium-sparing diuretics (spironolactone, triamterene, amiloride) or potassium supplements concomitantly with ACE inhibitors can increase the risk of hyperkalemia. Therefore, if concomitant use of such agents is indicated, they should be given with caution and the patient's serum potassium should be monitored.

ORAL ANTICOAGULANTS

Interaction studies with warfarin failed to identify any clinically important effect on the serum concentrations of the anticoagulant or on its anticoagulant effect.

LITHIUM

Increased serum lithium levels and symptoms of lithium toxicity have been reported in patients receiving ACE inhibitors during therapy with lithium. These drugs should be coadministered with caution, and frequent monitoring of serum lithium levels is recommended. If a diuretic is also used, the risk of lithium toxicity may be increased.

OTHER AGENTS

No clinically important pharmacokinetic interactions occurred when moexipril HCl was administered concomitantly with hydrochlorothiazide, digoxin, or cimetidine.

Moexipril HCl has been used in clinical trials concomitantly with calcium-channel-blocking agents, diuretics, H_2 blockers, digoxin, oral hypoglycemic agents, and cholesterol-lowering agents. There was no evidence of clinically important adverse interactions.

ADVERSE REACTIONS

Moexipril HCl has been evaluated for safety in more than 2500 patients with hypertension; more than 250 of these patients were treated for approximately 1 year. The overall incidence of reported adverse events was only slightly greater in patients treated with moexipril HCl than patients treated with placebo.

Reported adverse experiences were usually mild and transient, and there were no differences in adverse reaction rates related to gender, race, age, duration of therapy, or total daily dosage within the range of 3.75 to 60 mg. Discontinuation of therapy because of adverse experiences was required in 3.4% of patients treated with moexipril HCl and in 1.8% of patients treated with placebo. The most common reasons for discontinuation in patients treated with moexipril HCl were cough (0.7%) and dizziness (0.4%).

All adverse experiences considered at least possibly related to treatment that occurred at any dose in placebo-controlled trials of once-daily dosing in more than 1% of patients treated with moexipril HCl alone and that were at least as frequent in the moexipril HCl group as in the placebo group are shown in TABLE 1.

M

TABLE 1 *Adverse Events in Placebo-Controlled Studies*

Adverse Event	Moexipril HCl (n=674)	Placebo (n=226)
Cough increased	41 (6.1%)	5 (2.2%)
Dizziness	29 (4.3%)	5 (2.2%)
Diarrhea	21 (3.1%)	5 (2.2%)
Flu syndrome	21 (3.1%)	0 (0%)
Fatigue	16 (2.4%)	4 (1.8%)
Pharyngitis	12 (1.8%)	2 (0.9%)
Flushing	11 (1.6%)	0 (0%)
Rash	11 (1.6%)	2 (0.9%)
Myalgia	9 (1.3%)	0 (0%)

Other adverse events occurring in more than 1% of patients on moexipril that were at least as frequent on placebo include: Headache, upper respiratory infection, pain, rhinitis, dyspepsia, nausea, peripheral edema, sinusitis, chest pain, and urinary frequency. See WARNINGS and PRECAUTIONS for discussion of anaphylactoid reactions, angioedema, hypotension, neutropenia/agranulocytosis, second and third trimester fetal/neonatal morbidity and mortality, hyperkalemia, and cough.

Other potentially important adverse experiences reported in controlled or uncontrolled clinical trials in less than 1% of moexipril patients or that have been attributed to other ACE inhibitors include the following:

Cardiovascular: Symptomatic hypotension, postural hypotension, or syncope were seen in 9/1750 (0.51%) patients; these reactions led to discontinuation of therapy in controlled trials in 3/1254 (0.24%) patients who had received moexipril HCl monotherapy and in 1/344 (0.3%) patients who had received moexipril HCl with hydrochlorothiazide (see PRECAUTIONS and WARNINGS). Other adverse events included angina/myocardial infarction, palpitations, rhythm disturbances, and cerebrovascular accident.

Renal: Of hypertensive patients with no apparent preexisting renal disease, 1% of patients receiving moexipril HCl alone and 2% of patients receiving moexipril HCl with hydrochlorothiazide experienced increases in serum creatinine to at least 140% of their baseline values (see PRECAUTIONS and DOSAGE AND ADMINISTRATION).

Gastrointestinal: Abdominal pain, constipation, vomiting, appetite/weight change, dry mouth, pancreatitis, hepatitis.

Respiratory: Bronchospasm, dyspnea, eosinophilic pneumonitis.

Urogenital: Renal insufficiency, oliguria.

Dermatologic: Apparent hypersensitivity reactions manifested by urticaria, rash, pemphigus, pruritus, photosensitivity, alopecia.

Neurological and Psychiatric: Drowsiness, sleep disturbances, nervousness, mood changes, anxiety.

Other: Angioedema (see WARNINGS), taste disturbances, tinnitus, sweating, malaise, arthralgia, hemolytic anemia.

M

CLINICAL LABORATORY TEST FINDINGS

Serum Electrolytes

Hyperkalemia (see PRECAUTIONS), hyponatremia.

Creatinine and Blood Urea Nitrogen

As with other ACE inhibitors, minor increases in blood urea nitrogen or serum creatinine, reversible upon discontinuation of therapy, were observed in approximately 1% of patients with essential hypertension who were treated with moexipril HCl. Increases are more likely to occur in patients receiving concomitant diuretics and in patients with compromised renal function (see PRECAUTIONS, General).

Other (causal relationship unknown)

Clinically important changes in standard laboratory tests were rarely associated with moexipril HCl administration.

Elevations of liver enzymes and uric acid have been reported. In trials, less than 1% of moexipril-treated patients discontinued moexipril HCl treatment because of laboratory abnormalities. The incidence of abnormal laboratory values with moexipril was similar to that in the placebo-treated group.

DOSAGE AND ADMINISTRATION

HYPERTENSION

The recommended initial dose of moexipril HCl in patients not receiving diuretics is 7.5 mg, 1 hour prior to meals, once daily. Dosage should be adjusted according to blood pressure response. The antihypertensive effect of moexipril HCl may diminish towards the end of the dosing interval. Blood pressure should, therefore, be measured just prior to dosing to determine whether satisfactory blood pressure control is obtained. If control is not adequate, increased dose or divided dosing can be tried. The recommended dose range is 7.5 to 30 mg daily, administered in 1 or 2 divided doses 1 hour before meals. Total daily doses above 60 mg/day have not been studied in hypertensive patients.

In patients who are currently being treated with a diuretic, symptomatic hypotension may occasionally occur following the initial dose of moexipril HCl. The diuretic should, if possible, be discontinued for 2-3 days before therapy with moexipril HCl is begun, to reduce the likelihood of hypotension (see WARNINGS). If the patient's blood pressure is not controlled with moexipril HCl alone, diuretic therapy may then be reinstituted. If diuretic therapy cannot be discontinued, an initial dose of 3.75 mg of moexipril HCl should be used with medical supervision until blood pressure has stabilized (see WARNINGS and DRUG INTERACTIONS).

DOSE ADJUSTMENT IN RENAL IMPAIRMENT

For patients with a creatinine clearance ≤40 ml/min/1.73 m^2, an initial dose of 3.75 mg once daily should be given cautiously. Doses may be titrated upward to a maximum daily dose of 15 mg.

HOW SUPPLIED

Univasc is available in:

7.5 mg tablets: Pink colored, biconvex, film-coated and scored with engraved code "707" on the unscored side and "SP" above and "7.5" below the score.

15 mg tablets: Salmon colored, biconvex, film-coated and scored with engraved code "715" on the unscored side and "SP" above and "15" below the score.

STORAGE

Store, tightly closed, at controlled room temperature. Protect from excessive moisture.

If product package is subdivided, dispense in tight containers.

PRODUCT LISTING - EQUIVALENTS NOT AVAILABLE

Tablet - Oral - 7.5 mg

30's	$18.64	UNIVASC, Allscripts Pharmaceutical Company	54569-4990-00
90's	$87.93	UNIVASC, Schwarz Pharma	00091-3707-09
100's	$97.71	UNIVASC, Schwarz Pharma	00091-3707-01

Tablet - Oral - 15 mg

30's	$20.91	UNIVASC, Allscripts Pharmaceutical Company	54569-4276-00
30's	$28.13	UNIVASC, Physicians Total Care	54868-4088-00
90's	$74.01	UNIVASC, Schwarz Pharma	00091-3715-09
100's	$97.71	UNIVASC, Schwarz Pharma	00091-3715-01

Molindone Hydrochloride *(001826)*

Categories: Schizophrenia; FDA Approved 1974 Jul; Pregnancy Category C
Drug Classes: Antipsychotics
Brand Names: **Moban**
Cost of Therapy: $108.26 (Schizophrenia; Moban; 50 mg; 1 tablet/day; 30 day supply)

DESCRIPTION

Molindone hydrochloride is a dihydroindolone compound which is not structurally related to the phenothiazines, the butyrophenones or the thioxanthenes.

Molindone hydrochloride is 3-ethyl-6,7-dihydro-2-methyl-5-(morpholinomethyl)indol-4(5H)-one hydrochloride. It is a white to off-white crystalline powder, freely soluble in water and alcohol and has a molecular weight of 312.67.

Moban tablets also contain:

All strengths: Calcium sulfate, lactose, magnesium stearate, microcrystalline cellulose and povidone.

5 mg: Alginic acid, colloidal silicon dioxide and FD&C yellow 6.

10 mg: Alginic acid, colloidal silicon dioxide, FD&C blue 2 and FD&C red 40.

25 mg: Alginic acid, colloidal silicon dioxide, D&C yellow 10, FD&C blue 2, and FD&C yellow 6.

50 mg: FD&C blue 2 and sodium starch glycolate.

100 mg: FD&C blue 2, FD&C yellow 6 and sodium starch glycolate.

Moban concentrate contains: Alcohol, artificial cherry flavor, artificial cover flavor, edetate disodium, glycerin, liquid sugar, methylparaben, propylparaben, sodium metabisulfite, sorbitol solution, and hydrochloric acid reagent grade for pH adjustment.

CLINICAL PHARMACOLOGY

Molindone HCl has a pharmacological profile in laboratory animals which predominantly resembles that of other antipsychotic agents causing reduction of spontaneous locomotion and aggressiveness, suppression of a conditioned response and antagonism of the bizarre stereotyped behavior and hyperactivity induced by amphetamines. In addition, molindone HCl antagonizes the depression caused by the tranquilizing agent tetrabenazine.

In human clinical studies an antipsychotic effect is achieved in the absence of muscle relaxing or incoordinating effects. Based on EEG studies, molindone HCl exerts its effect on the ascending reticular activating system.

Human metabolic studies show molindone HCl to be rapidly absorbed and metabolized when given orally. Unmetabolized drug reached a peak blood level at 1.5 hours. Pharmacological effect from a single oral dose persists for 24-36 hours. There are 36 recognized metabolites with less than 2-3% unmetabolized molindone HCl being excreted in urine and feces.

INDICATIONS AND USAGE

Molindone HCl is indicated in the management of schizophrenia. The efficacy of molindone HCl in schizophrenia was established in clinical studies which enrolled newly hospitalized and chronically hospitalized, acutely ill, schizophrenic patients as subjects.

CONTRAINDICATIONS

Molindone HCl is contraindicated in severe central nervous system depression (alcohol, barbiturates, narcotics, etc.) or comatose states, and in patients with known hypersensitivity to the drug.

WARNINGS

TARDIVE DYSKINESIA

Tardive dyskinesia, a syndrome consisting of potentially irreversible, involuntary, dyskinetic movements, may develop in patients treated with antipsychotic drugs. Although the prevalence of the syndrome appears to be highest among the elderly, especially elderly women, it is impossible to rely upon prevalence estimates to predict, at the inception of antipsychotic treatment, which patients are likely to develop the syndrome. Whether antipsychotic drug products differ in their potential to cause tardive dyskinesia is unknown.

Both the risk of developing the syndrome and the likelihood that will become irreversible are believed to increase as the duration of treatment and the total cumulative dose of antipsychotic drugs administered to the patient increase. However, the syndrome can develop, although much less commonly, after relatively brief treatment periods at low doses.

There is no known treatment for established cases of tardive dyskinesia, although the syndrome may remit, partially or completely, if antipsychotic treatment is withdrawn. Antipsychotic treatment, itself, however, may suppress (or partially suppress) the signs and symptoms of the syndrome and thereby may possibly mask the underlying disease process. The effect that symptomatic suppression has upon the long-term course of the syndrome is unknown.

Given these considerations, antipsychotics should be prescribed in a manner that is most likely to minimize the occurrence of tardive dyskinesia. Chronic antipsychotic treatment should generally be reserved for patients who suffer from chronic illness that, (1) is known to respond to antipsychotic drugs, and (2) for whom alternative, equally effective, but potentially less harmful treatments are not available or appropriate. In patients who do require chronic treatment, the smallest dose and the shortest duration of treatment producing a satisfactory clinical response should be sought. The need for continued treatment should be reassessed periodically.

If signs and symptoms of tardive dyskinesia appear in a patient on antipsychotics, drug discontinuation should be considered. However, some patients may require treatment despite the presence of the syndrome.

(For further information about the description of tardive dyskinesia and its clinical detection, please refer to the section on ADVERSE REACTIONS.)

NEUROLEPTIC MALIGNANT SYNDROME (NMS)

A potentially fatal symptom complex sometimes referred to as Neuroleptic Malignant Syndrome (NMS) has been reported in association with antipsychotic drugs. Clinical manifestations of NMS are hyperpyrexia, muscle rigidity, altered mental status and evidence of autonomic instability (irregular pulse or blood pressure, tachycardia, diaphoresis, and cardiac dysrhythmias).

The diagnostic evaluation of patients with this syndrome is complicated. In arriving at a diagnosis, it is important to identify cases where the clinical presentation includes both serious medical illness (*e.g.*, pneumonia, systemic infection, etc.) and untreated or inadequately treated extrapyramidal signs and symptoms (EPS). Other important considerations in the differential diagnosis include central and anticholinergic toxicity, heat stroke, drug fever and primary central nervous system (CNS) pathology.

The management of NMS should include, (1) immediate discontinuation of antipsychotic drugs and other drugs not essential to concurrent therapy, (2) intensive symptomatic treatment and medical monitoring, and (3) treatment of any concomitant serious medical problems for which specific treatments are available. There is no general agreement about specific pharmacological treatment regimens for uncomplicated NMS.

If a patient requires antipsychotic drug treatment after recovery from NMS, the potential reintroduction of drug therapy should be carefully considered. The patient should be carefully monitored, since recurrences or NMS have been reported.

PREGNANCY

Studies in pregnant patients have not been carried out. Reproduction studies have been performed in the following animals (see TABLE 1).

TABLE 1

Pregnant Rats Oral Dose:	
No adverse effect	20 mg/kg/day for 10 days
No adverse effect	40 mg/kg/day for 10 days
Pregnant Mice Oral Dose:	
Slight increase resorptions	20 mg/kg/day for 10 days
Slight increase resorptions	40 mg/kg/day for 10 days
Pregnant Rabbits Oral Dose:	
No adverse effect	5 mg/kg/day for 12 days
No adverse effect	10 mg/kg/day for 12 days
No adverse effect	20 mg/kg/day for 12 days

Animal reproductive studies have not demonstrated a teratogenic potential. The anticipated benefits must be weighed against the unknown risks to the fetus if used in pregnant patients.

NURSING MOTHERS

Data are not available on the content of molindone HCl in the milk of nursing mothers.

PEDIATRIC USE

Use of molindone HCl in children below the age of 12 years is not recommended because safe and effective conditions for its usage have not been established.

Molindone HCl has not been shown effective in the management of behavioral complications in patients with mental retardation.

SULFITES SENSITIVITY

Molindone HCl concentrate contains sodium metabisulfite, a sulfite that may cause allergic-type reactions including anaphylactic symptoms and life-threatening or less severe asthmatic episodes in certain susceptible people. The overall prevalence of sulfite sensitivity in the general population is unknown and probably low. Sulfite sensitivity is seen more frequently in asthmatic than in nonasthmatic people.

PRECAUTIONS

GENERAL

Some patients receiving molindone HCl may note drowsiness initially and they should be advised against activities requiring mental alertness until their response to the drug has been established.

Increased activity has been noted in patients receiving molindone HCl. Caution should be exercised where increased activity may be harmful.

Molindone HCl does not lower the seizure threshold in experimental animals to the degree noted with more sedating antipsychotic drugs. However, in humans, convulsive seizures have been reported in a few instances.

The physician should be aware that this tablet preparation contains calcium sulfate as an excipient and that calcium ions may interfere with the absorption of preparations containing phenytoin sodium and tetracyclines.

Molindone HCl has an antiemetic effect in animals. A similar effect may occur in humans and may obscure signs of intestinal obstruction or brain tumor.

Antipsychotic drugs elevate prolactin levels; the elevation persists during chronic administration. Tissue culture experiments indicate that approximately one-third of human breast cancers are prolactin dependent *in vitro*, a factor of potential importance if the prescription of these drugs is contemplated in a patient with a previously detected breast cancer. Although disturbances such as galactorrhea, amenorrhea, gynecomastia, and impotence have been reported, the clinical significance of elevated serum prolactin levels is unknown for most patients. An increase in mammary neoplasms has been found in rodents after chronic administration of antipsychotic drugs. Neither clinical studies nor epidemiologic studies conducted to date, however, have shown an association between chronic administration of these drugs and mammary tumorigenesis; the available evidence is considered too limited to be conclusive at this time.

DRUG INTERACTIONS

Potentiation of drugs administered concurrently with molindone HCl has not been reported. Additionally, animal studies have not shown increased toxicity when molindone HCl is given concurrently with representative members of three classes of drugs (*i.e.*, barbiturates, chloral hydrate and antiparkinson drugs).

ADVERSE REACTIONS

CNS EFFECTS

The most frequently occurring effect is initial drowsiness that generally subsides with continued usage of the drug or lowering of the dose.

Noted less frequently were depression, hyperactivity and euphoria.

NEUROLOGICAL

Extrapyramidal Reactions

Extrapyramidal reactions noted below may occur in susceptible individuals and are usually reversible with appropriate management.

Akathisia

Motor restlessness may occur early.

Parkinson Syndrome

Akinesia, characterized by rigidity, immobility and reduction of voluntary movements and tremor, have been observed. Occurrence is less frequent than akathisia.

Dystonic Syndrome

Prolonged abnormal contractions of muscle groups occur infrequently. These symptoms may be managed by the addition of a synthetic antiparkinson agent (other than L-dopa), small doses of sedative drugs, and/or reduction in dosage.

Tardive Dyskinesia

Antipsychotic drugs are known to cause a syndrome of dyskinetic movements commonly referred to as tardive dyskinesia. The movements may appear during treatment or upon withdrawal of treatment and may be either reversible or irreversible (*i.e.*, persistent) upon cessation of further antipsychotic administration.

The syndrome is known to have a variable latency for development and the duration of the latency cannot be determined reliably. It is thus wise to assume that any antipsychotic agent has the capacity to induce the syndrome and act accordingly until sufficient data have been collected to settle the issue definitively for a specific drug product. In the case of antipsychotics known to produce the irreversible syndrome, the following has been observed.

Tardive dyskinesia has appeared in some patients on long-term therapy and has also appeared after drug therapy has been discontinued. The risk appears to be greater in elderly patients on high-dose therapy, especially females. The symptoms are persistent and in some patients appear to be irreversible. The syndrome is characterized by rhythmical involuntary movements of the tongue, face, mouth or jaw (*e.g.*, protrusion of the tongue, puffing of cheeks, puckering of mouth, chewing movements). There may be involuntary movements of the extremities.

There is no known effective treatment of tardive dyskinesia; antiparkinsonism agents usually do not alleviate the symptoms of this syndrome. It is suggested that all antipsychotic agents be discontinued if these symptoms appear. Should it be necessary to reinstitute treatment, or increase the dosage of the agent, or switch to a different antipsychotic agent, the syndrome may be masked. It has been reported that fine vermicular movements of the tongue may be an early sign of the syndrome and if the medication is stopped at that time the syndrome may not develop (see WARNINGS).

Autonomic Nervous System

Occasionally blurring of vision, tachycardia, nausea, dry mouth and salivation have been reported. Urinary retention and constipation may occur particularly if anticholinergic drugs are used to treat extrapyramidal symptoms. One patient being treated with molindone HCl experienced priapism which required surgical intervention, apparently resulting in residual impairment of erectile function.

LABORATORY TESTS

There have been rare reports of leukopenia and leukocytosis. If such reactions occur, treatment with molindone HCl may continue if clinical symptoms are absent. Alterations of blood glucose, BUN, and red blood cells have not been considered clinically significant.

METABOLIC AND ENDOCRINE EFFECTS
Alteration of thyroid function has not been significant. Amenorrhea has been reported infrequently. Resumption of menses in previously amenorrheic women has been reported. Initially heavy menses may occur. Galactorrhea and gynecomastia have been reported infrequently. Increase in libido has been noted in some patients. Impotence has not been reported. Although both weight gain and weight loss has been in the direction of normal or ideal weight, excessive weight gain has not occurred with molindone HCl.

HEPATIC EFFECTS
There have been rare reports of clinically significant alterations in liver function in association with molindone HCl use.

CARDIOVASCULAR
Rare, transient, non-specific T wave changes have been reported on EKG. Association with a clinical syndrome has not been established. Rarely has significant hypotension been reported.

OPHTHALMOLOGICAL
Lens opacities and pigmentary retinopathy have not been reported where patients have received molindone HCl. In some patients, phenothiazine induced lenticular opacities have resolved following discontinuation of the phenothiazine while continuing therapy with molindone HCl.

SKIN
Early, non-specific skin rash, probably of allergic origin, has occasionally been reported. Skin pigmentation has not been seen with molindone HCl usage alone.

Molindone HCl has certain pharmacological similarities to other antipsychotic agents. Because adverse reactions are often extensions of the pharmacological activity of a drug, all of the known pharmacological effects associated with other antipsychotic drugs should be kept in mind when molindone HCl is used. Upon abrupt withdrawal after prolonged high dosage an abstinence syndrome has not been noted.

DOSAGE AND ADMINISTRATION

Initial and maintenance doses of molindone HCl should be individualized.

INITIAL DOSAGE SCHEDULE
The usual starting dosage is 50-75 mg/day.

- Increase to 100 mg/day in 3 or 4 days.
- Based on severity of symptomatology, dosage may be titrated up or down depending on individual patient response.
- An increase to 225 mg/day may be required in patients with severe symptomatology.

Elderly and debilitated patients should be started on lower dosage.

MAINTENANCE DOSAGE SCHEDULE
Mild: 5-15 mg three or four times a day.
Moderate: 10-25 mg three or four times a day.
Severe: 225 mg/day may be required.

HOW SUPPLIED

Moban tablets are available in the following dosage strengths:

5 mg: Orange, round, biconvex tablet, one face inscribed with "Moban 5", and the other face plain.

10 mg: Lavender, round, biconvex tablet, one face inscribed with "Moban 10", and the other face plain.

25 mg: Green, round, biconvex tablet, one face scored inscribed with "Moban 25", and the other face plain with partial bisect.

50 mg: Blue, round, biconvex tablet, one face scored and inscribed with "Moban 50", and the other face plain.

100 mg: Tan, round, biconvex tablet, one face scored and inscribed with "Moban 100", and the other face plain.

As a concentrate (clear, colorless to straw-yellow syrup) containing 20 mg molindone HCl per ml.

Storage: Store at controlled room temperature 15-30°C (59-86°F). Protect from light.

PRODUCT LISTING - EQUIVALENTS NOT AVAILABLE

Concentrate - Oral - 20 mg/ml
120 ml $254.81 MOBAN, Endo Laboratories Llc 63481-0460-04
Tablet - Oral - 5 mg
100's $126.00 MOBAN, Endo Laboratories Llc 63481-0072-70
Tablet - Oral - 10 mg
100's $181.13 MOBAN, Endo Laboratories Llc 63481-0073-70
Tablet - Oral - 25 mg
100's $270.19 MOBAN, Endo Laboratories Llc 63481-0074-70
Tablet - Oral - 50 mg
100's $360.88 MOBAN, Endo Laboratories Llc 63481-0076-70
Tablet - Oral - 100 mg
100's $459.06 MOBAN, Endo Laboratories Llc 63481-0077-70

Mometasone Furoate *(001828)*

For related information, see the comparative table section in Appendix A.

Categories: Dermatosis, corticosteroid responsive; Rhinitis, allergic; Pregnancy Category C; FDA Approved 1987 Apr
Drug Classes: Corticosteroids, inhalation; Corticosteroids, topical; Dermatologics
Brand Names: Elocon
Foreign Brand Availability: Allermax Aqueous (Australia); Asmanex Twisthaler (England); Ecotone (Japan); Ecural (Germany); Elica (Mexico; Philippines); Elocom (Bahrain; Belgium; Benin; Burkina-Faso; Canada; Colombia; Costa-Rica; Cyprus; Czech-Republic; Dominican-Republic; Egypt; El-Salvador; Ethiopia; Gambia; Ghana; Guatemala; Guinea; Honduras; Hungary; Iran; Iraq; Israel; Ivory-Coast; Jordan; Kenya; Kuwait; Lebanon; Liberia; Libya; Malawi; Mali; Mauritania; Mauritius; Morocco; Nicaragua; Niger; Nigeria; Oman; Panama; Peru; Qatar; Republic-of-Yemen; Russia; Saudi-Arabia; Senegal; Seychelles; Sierra-Leone; South-Africa; Spain; Sudan; Switzerland; Syria; Tanzania; Tunia; Uganda; United-Arab-Emirates; Zambia; Zimbabwe); Elocon Cream (Australia; New-Zealand); Elocon Ointment (Australia; New-Zealand); Elocyn (Korea); Elomet (Ecuador; Hong-Kong; Malaysia; Mexico; Taiwan; Thailand); Eloson (China); Elox (Indonesia); Flumeta (Japan); Metaspray (India); Monovel (Bahrain; Colombia; Cyprus; Egypt; Iran; Iraq; Israel; Jordan; Kuwait; Lebanon; Libya; Oman; Qatar; Republic-of-Yemen; Saudi-Arabia; Syria; United-Arab-Emirates); Motaderm (Indonesia); Nasonex Nasal Spray (Australia; England; Germany; Hong-Kong; Indonesia; Ireland; Korea; Peru; Philippines; Singapore); Novasone Cream (Australia); Novasone Lotion (Australia); Novasone Ointment (Australia); Rinelon (Mexico; South-Africa; Thailand); Rivelon (Philippines); Uniclar (Colombia; Mexico)
Cost of Therapy: $51.71 (Allergic Rhinitis; Nasonex Spray; 50 µg/inh; 17 g; 4 sprays/day; 30 day supply)

INTRANASAL

DESCRIPTION

FOR INTRANASAL USE ONLY.

Mometasone furoate monohydrate, the active component of Nasonex nasal spray, 50 µg, is an anti-inflammatory corticosteroid having the chemical name, 9,21-dichloro-11β,17-dihydroxy-16α-methylpregna-1,4-diene-3,20-dione 17-(2 furoate) monohydrate.

Mometasone furoate monohydrate is a white powder, with an empirical formula of $C_{27}H_{30}Cl_2O_6 \cdot H_2O$, and a molecular weight of 539.45. It is practically insoluble in water; slightly soluble in methanol, ethanol, and isopropanol; soluble in acetone and chloroform; and freely soluble in tetrahydrofuran. Its partition coefficient between octanol and water is greater than 5000.

Nasonex nasal spray, 50 µg is a metered-dose, manual pump spray unit containing an aqueous suspension of mometasone furoate monohydrate equivalent to 0.05% w/w mometasone furoate calculated on the anhydrous basis; in an aqueous medium containing glycerin, microcrystalline cellulose and carboxymethylcellulose sodium, sodium citrate, 0.25% w/w phenylethyl alcohol, citric acid, benzalkonium chloride, and polysorbate 80. The pH is between 4.3 and 4.9.

After initial priming (10 actuations), each actuation of the pump delivers a metered spray containing 100 mg of suspension containing mometasone furoate monohydrate equivalent to 50 µg of mometasone furoate calculated on the anhydrous basis. Each bottle of Nasonex nasal spray, 50 µg provides 120 sprays.

CLINICAL PHARMACOLOGY

Mometasone furoate nasal spray, 50 µg is a corticosteroid demonstrating anti-inflammatory properties. The precise mechanism of corticosteroid action on allergic rhinitis is not known. Corticosteroids have been shown to have a wide range of effects on multiple cell types (*e.g.*, mast cells, eosinophils, neutrophils, macrophages, and lymphocytes) and mediators (*e.g.*, histamine, eicosanoids, leukotrienes, and cytokines) involved in inflammation.

In two clinical studies utilizing nasal antigen challenge, mometasone furoate nasal spray, 50 µg decreased some markers of the early- and late-phase allergic response. These observations included decreases (versus placebo) in histamine and eosinophil cationic protein levels, and reductions (versus baseline) in eosinophils, neutrophils, and epithelial cell adhesion proteins. The clinical significance of these findings is not known.

The effect of mometasone furoate nasal spray, 50 µg on nasal mucosa following 12 months of treatment was examined in 46 patients with allergic rhinitis. There was no evidence of atrophy and there was a marked reduction in intraepithelial eosinophilia and inflammatory cell infiltration (*e.g.*, eosinophils, lymphocytes, monocytes, neutrophils, and plasma cells).

PHARMACOKINETICS

Absorption
Mometasone furoate monohydrate administered as a nasal spray is virtually undetectable in plasma from adult and pediatric subjects despite the use of a sensitive assay with a lower quantitation limit (LOQ) of 50 pcg/ml.

Distribution
The *in vitro* protein binding for mometasone furoate was reported to be 98-99% in concentration range of 5-500 ng/ml.

Metabolism
Studies have shown that any portion of a mometasone furoate dose which is swallowed and absorbed undergoes extensive metabolism to multiple metabolites. There are no major metabolites detectable in plasma. Upon *in vitro* incubation, one of the minor metabolites formed is 6β-hydroxy-mometasone furoate. In human liver microsomes, the formation of the metabolite is regulated by cytochrome P-450 3A4 (CYP3A4).

Elimination
Following intravenous administration, the effective plasma elimination half-life of mometasone furoate is 5.8 hours. Any absorbed drug is excreted as metabolites mostly via the bile, and to a limited extent, into the urine.

Special Populations
The effects of renal impairment, hepatic impairment, age, or gender on mometasone furoate pharmacokinetics have not been adequately investigated.

PHARMACODYNAMICS

Three clinical pharmacology studies have been conducted in humans to assess the effect of mometasone furoate nasal spray, 50 μg at various doses on adrenal function. In one study, daily doses of 200 and 400 μg of mometasone furoate nasal spray, 50 μg and 10 mg of prednisone were compared to placebo in 64 patients with allergic rhinitis. Adrenal function before and after 36 consecutive days of treatment was assessed by measuring plasma cortisol levels following a 6 hour Cortrosyn (ACTH) infusion and by measuring 24 hour urinary-free cortisol levels. Mometasone furoate nasal spray, 50 μg, at both the 200 and 400 μg dose, was not associated with a statistically significant decrease in mean plasma cortisol levels post-Cortrosyn infusion or a statistically significant decrease in the 24 hour urinary-free cortisol levels compared to placebo. A statistically significant decrease in the mean plasma cortisol levels post-Cortrosyn infusion and 24 hour urinary-free cortisol levels was detected in the prednisone treatment group compared to placebo.

A second study assessed adrenal response to mometasone furoate nasal spray, 50 μg (400 and 1600 μg/day), prednisone (10 mg/day), and placebo, administered for 29 days in 48 male volunteers. The 24 hour plasma cortisol area under the curve [AUC(0-24)], during and after an 8 hour Cortrosyn infusion and 24 hour urinary-free cortisol levels were determined at baseline and after 29 days of treatment. No statistically significant differences of adrenal function were observed with mometasone furoate nasal spray, 50 μg compared to placebo.

A third study evaluated single, rising doses of mometasone furoate nasal spray, 50 μg (1000, 2000, and 4000 μg/day), orally administered mometasone furoate (2000, 4000, and 8000 μg/day), orally administered dexamethasone (200, 400, and 800 μg/day), and placebo (administered at the end of each series of doses) in 24 male volunteers. Dose administrations were separated by at least 72 hours. Determination of serial plasma cortisol levels at 8 AM and for the 24 hour period following each treatment were used to calculate the plasma cortisol area under the curve [AUC(0-24)]. In addition, 24 hour urinary-free cortisol levels were collected prior to initial treatment administration and during the period immediately following each dose. No statistically significant decreases in the plasma cortisol AUC, 8 AM cortisol levels, or 24 hour urinary-free cortisol levels were observed in volunteers treated with either mometasone furoate nasal spray, 50 μg or oral mometasone, as compared with placebo treatment. Conversely, nearly all volunteers treated with the 3 doses of dexamethasone demonstrated abnormal 8 AM cortisol levels (defined as a cortisol level <10 μg/dl), reduced 24 hour plasma AUC values, and decreased 24 hour urinary-free cortisol levels, as compared to placebo treatment.

Three clinical pharmacology studies have been conducted in pediatric patients to assess the effect of mometasone furoate nasal spray, on the adrenal function at daily doses of 50, 100, and 200 μg vs placebo. In one study, adrenal function before and after 7 consecutive days of treatment was assessed in 48 pediatric patients with allergic rhinitis (ages 6-11 years) by measuring morning plasma cortisol and 24 hour urinary-free cortisol levels. Mometasone furoate nasal spray, at all 3 doses, was not associated with a statistically significant decrease in mean plasma cortisol levels or a statistically significant decrease in the 24 hour urinary-free cortisol levels compared to placebo. In the second study, adrenal function before and after 14 consecutive days of treatment was assessed in 48 pediatric patients (ages 3-5 years) with allergic rhinitis by measuring plasma cortisol levels following a 30 minute Cortrosyn infusion. Mometasone furoate nasal spray, 50 μg, at all 3 doses (50, 100, and 200 μg/day), was not associated with a statistically significant decrease in mean plasma cortisol levels post-Cortrosyn infusion compared to placebo. All patients had a normal response to Cortrosyn. In the third study, adrenal function before and after up to 42 consecutive days of once-daily treatment was assessed in 52 patients with allergic rhinitis (ages 2-5 years), 28 of whom received mometasone furoate nasal spray, 50 μg per nostril (total daily dose 100 μg), by measuring morning plasma cortisol and 24 hour urinary-free cortisol levels. Mometasone furoate nasal spray was not associated with a statistically significant decrease in mean plasma cortisol levels or a statistically significant decrease in the 24 hour urinary-free cortisol levels compared to placebo.

INDICATIONS AND USAGE

Mometasone furoate nasal spray, 50 μg is indicated for the treatment of the nasal symptoms of seasonal allergic and perennial allergic rhinitis, in adults and pediatric patients 2 years of age and older. Mometasone furoate nasal spray, 50 μg is indicated for the prophylaxis of the nasal symptoms of seasonal allergic rhinitis in adult and adolescent patients 12 years and older. In patients with a known seasonal allergen that precipitates nasal symptoms of seasonal allergic rhinitis, initiation of prophylaxis with mometasone furoate nasal spray, 50 μg is recommended 2-4 weeks prior to the anticipated start of the pollen season. Safety and effectiveness of mometasone furoate nasal spray, 50 μg in pediatric patients less than 2 years of age have not been established.

CONTRAINDICATIONS

Hypersensitivity to any of the ingredients of this preparation contraindicates its use.

WARNINGS

The replacement of a systemic corticosteroid with a topical corticosteroid can be accompanied by signs of adrenal insufficiency and, in addition, some patients may experience symptoms of withdrawal; *i.e.*, joint and/or muscular pain, lassitude, and depression. Careful attention must be given when patients previously treated for prolonged periods with systemic corticosteroids are transferred to topical corticosteroids, with careful monitoring for acute adrenal insufficiency in response to stress. This is particularly important in those patients who have associated asthma or other clinical conditions where too rapid a decrease in systemic corticosteroid dosing may cause a severe exacerbation of their symptoms.

If recommended doses of intranasal corticosteroids are exceeded or if individuals are particularly sensitive or predisposed by virtue of recent systemic steroid therapy, symptoms of hypercorticism may occur, including very rare cases of menstrual irregularities, acneiform lesions, and cushingoid features. If such changes occur, topical corticosteroids should be discontinued slowly, consistent with accepted procedures for discontinuing oral steroid therapy.

Persons who are on drugs which suppress the immune system are more susceptible to infections than healthy individuals. Chickenpox and measles, for example, can have a more serious or even fatal course in nonimmune children or adults on corticosteroids. In such children or adults who have not had these diseases, particular care should be taken to avoid exposure. How the dose, route, and duration of corticosteroid administration affects the risk of developing a disseminated infection is not known. The contribution of the underlying disease and/or prior corticosteroid treatment to the risk is also not known. If exposed to chickenpox, prophylaxis with varicella zoster immune globin (VZIG) may be indicated. If exposed to measles, prophylaxis with pooled intramuscular immunoglobulin (IG) may be indicated. (See the respective prescribing information for complete VZIG and IG information.) If chickenpox develops, treatment with antiviral agents may be considered.

PRECAUTIONS

GENERAL

Intranasal corticosteroids may cause a reduction in growth velocity when administered to pediatric patients (see Pediatric Use). In clinical studies with mometasone furoate nasal spray, 50 μg, the development of localized infections of the nose and pharynx with *Candida albicans* has occurred only rarely. When such an infection develops, use of mometasone furoate nasal spray, 50 μg should be discontinued and appropriate local or systemic therapy instituted, if needed.

Nasal corticosteroids should be used with caution, if at all, in patients with active or quiescent tuberculous infection of the respiratory tract, or in untreated fungal, bacterial, systemic viral infections, or ocular herpes simplex.

Rarely, immediate hypersensitivity reactions may occur after the intranasal administration of mometasone furoate monohydrate. Extreme rare instances of wheezing have been reported.

Rare instances of nasal septum perforation and increased intraocular pressure have also been reported following the intranasal application of aerosolized corticosteroids. As with any long-term topical treatment of the nasal cavity, patients using mometasone furoate nasal spray, 50 μg over several months or longer should be examined periodically for possible changes in the nasal mucosa.

Because of the inhibitory effect of corticosteroids on wound healing, patients who have experienced recent nasal septum ulcers, nasal surgery, or nasal trauma should not use a nasal corticosteroid until healing has occurred.

Glaucoma and cataract formation was evaluated in one controlled study of 12 weeks' duration and one uncontrolled study of 12 months' duration in patients treated with mometasone furoate nasal spray, 50 μg at 200 μg/day, using intraocular pressure measurements and slit lamp examination. No significant change from baseline was noted in the mean intraocular pressure measurements for the 141 mometasone furoate-treated patients in the 12 week study, as compared with 141 placebo-treated patients. No individual mometasone furoate-treated patient was noted to have developed a significant elevation in intraocular pressure or cataracts in this 12 week study. Likewise, no significant change from baseline was noted in the mean intraocular pressure measurements for the 139 mometasone furoate-treated patients in the 12 month study and again, no cataracts were detected in these patients. Nonetheless, nasal and inhaled corticosteroids have been associated with the development of glaucoma and/or cataracts. Therefore, close follow-up is warranted in patients with a change in vision and with a history of glaucoma and/or cataracts.

When nasal corticosteroids are used at excessive doses, systemic corticosteroid effects such as hypercorticism and adrenal suppression may appear. If such changes occur, mometasone furoate nasal spray, 50 μg should be discontinued slowly, consistent with accepted procedures for discontinuing oral steroid therapy.

INFORMATION FOR THE PATIENT

Patients being treated with mometasone furoate nasal spray, 50 μg should be given the following information and instructions. This information is intended to aid in the safe and effective use of this medication. It is not a disclosure of all intended or possible adverse effects. Patients should use mometasone furoate nasal spray, 50 μg at regular intervals (once daily) since its effectiveness depends on regular use. Improvement in nasal symptoms of allergic rhinitis has been shown to occur within 11 hours after the first dose based on one single-dose, parallel-group study of patients in an outdoor "park" setting (park study) and one environmental exposure unit (EEU) study and within 2 days after the first dose in two randomized, double-blind, placebo-controlled, parallel-group seasonal allergic rhinitis studies. Maximum benefit is usually achieved within 1-2 weeks after initiation of dosing. Patients should take the medication as directed and should not increase the prescribed dosage by using it more than once a day in an attempt to increase its effectiveness. Patients should contact their physician if symptoms do not improve, or if the condition worsens. To assure proper use of this nasal spray, and to attain maximum benefit, patients should read and follow the accompanying Patient's Instructions for Use carefully. Administration to young children should be aided by an adult.

Patients should be cautioned not to spray mometasone furoate nasal spray, 50 μg into the eyes or directly onto the nasal septum.

Persons who are on immunosuppressant doses of corticosteroids should be warned to avoid exposure to chickenpox or measles, and patients should also be advised that if they are exposed, medical advice should be sought without delay.

CARCINOGENESIS, MUTAGENESIS, AND IMPAIRMENT OF FERTILITY

In a 2 year carcinogenicity study of Sprague Dawley rats, mometasone furoate demonstrated no statistically significant increase in the incidence of tumors at inhalation doses up to 67 μg/kg (approximately 3 and 2 times the maximum recommended daily intranasal dose in adults and children, respectively, on a μg/m^2 basis). In a 19 month carcinogenicity study of Swiss CD-1 mice, mometasone furoate demonstrated no statistically significant increase in the incidence of tumors at inhalation doses up to 160 μg/kg (approximately 3 and 2 times the maximum recommended daily intranasal dose in adults and children, respectively, on a μg/m^2 basis).

Mometasone furoate increased chromosomal aberrations in an *in vitro* Chinese hamster ovary-cell assay, but did not increase chromosomal aberrations in an *in vitro* Chinese hamster lung cell assay. Mometasone furoate was not mutagenic in the Ames test or mouse-lymphoma assay, and was not clastogenic in an *in vivo* mouse micronucleus assay and a rat bone marrow chromosomal aberration assay or a mouse male germ-cell chromosomal aberration assay. Mometasone furoate also, did not induce unscheduled DNA synthesis *in vivo* in rat hepatocytes.

In reproductive studies in rats, impairment of fertility was not produced by subcutaneous doses up to 15 μg/kg (less than the maximum recommended daily intranasal dose in adults on a μg/m^2 basis).

PREGNANCY CATEGORY C

Teratogenic Effects

When administered to pregnant mice, rats and rabbits, mometasone furoate increased fetal malformations. The doses that produced malformations also decreased fetal growth, as measured by lower fetal weights and/or delayed ossification. Mometasone furoate also caused dystocia and related complications when administered to rats during the end of pregnancy.

In mice, mometasone furoate caused cleft palate at subcutaneous doses of 60 μg/kg and above (approximately equivalent to the maximum recommended daily intranasal dose in adults on a μg/m^2 basis). Fetal survival was reduced at 180 μg/kg (approximately 4 times the maximum recommended daily intranasal dose in adults on a μg/m^2 basis). No toxicity was observed at 20 μg/kg (less than the maximum recommended daily intranasal dose in adults on a μg/m^2 basis).

In rats, mometasone furoate produced umbilical hernia at topical dermal doses of 600 μg/kg and above (approximately 25 times the maximum recommended daily intranasal dose in adults on a μg/m^2 basis). A dose of 300 μg/kg (approximately 10 times the maximum recommended daily intranasal dose in adults on a μg/m^2 basis) produced delays in ossification, but no malformations.

In rabbits, mometasone furoate caused multiple malformations (*e.g.,* flexed front paws, gallbladder agenesis, umbilical hernia, hydrocephaly) at topical dermal doses of 150 μg/kg and above (approximately 10 times the maximum recommended daily intranasal dose in adults on a μg/m^2 basis). In an oral study, mometasone furoate increased resorptions and caused cleft palate and/or head malformations (hydrocephaly or domed head) at 700 μg/kg (approximately 55 times the maximum recommended daily intranasal dose in adults on a μg/m^2 basis). At 2800 μg/kg (approximately 230 times the maximum recommended daily intranasal dose in adults on a μg/m^2 basis), most litters were aborted or resorbed. No toxicity was observed at 140 μg/kg (approximately 10 times the maximum recommended daily intranasal dose in adults on a μg/m^2 basis).

When rats received subcutaneous doses of mometasone furoate throughout pregnancy or during the later stages of pregnancy, 15 μg/kg (less than the maximum recommended daily intranasal dose in adults on a μg/m^2 basis) caused prolonged and difficult labor and reduced the number of live births, birth weight and early pup survival. Similar effects were not observed at 7.5 μg/kg (less than the maximum recommended daily intranasal dose in adults on a μg/m^2 basis).

There are no adequate and well-controlled studies in pregnant women. Mometasone furoate nasal spray, 50 μg, like other corticosteroids, should be used during pregnancy only if the potential benefits justify the potential risk to the fetus. Experience with oral corticosteroids since their introduction in pharmacologic, as opposed to physiologic, doses suggests that rodents are more prone to teratogenic effects from corticosteroids than humans. In addition, because there is a natural increase in corticosteroid production during pregnancy, most women will require a lower exogenous corticosteroid dose and many will not need corticosteroid treatment during pregnancy.

Nonteratogenic Effects

Hypoadrenalism may occur in infants born to women receiving corticosteroids during pregnancy. Such infants should be carefully monitored.

NURSING MOTHERS

It is not known if mometasone furoate is excreted in human milk. Because other corticosteroids are excreted in human milk, caution should be used when mometasone furoate nasal spray, 50 μg is administered to nursing women.

PEDIATRIC USE

Controlled clinical studies have shown intranasal corticosteroids may cause a reduction in growth velocity in pediatric patients. This effect has been observed in the absence of laboratory evidence of hypothalamic-pituitary-adrenal (HPA) axis suppression, suggesting that growth velocity is a more sensitive indicator of systemic corticosteroid exposure in pediatric patients than some commonly used tests of HPA axis function. The long-term effects of this reduction in growth velocity associated with intranasal corticosteroids, including the impact on final adult height, are unknown. The potential for "catch up" growth following discontinuation of treatment with intranasal corticosteroids has not been adequately studied. The growth of pediatric patients receiving intranasal corticosteroids, including mometasone furoate nasal spray, 50 μg should be monitored routinely (*e.g.,* via stadiometry). The potential growth effects of prolonged treatment should be weighed against clinical benefits obtained and the availability of safe and effective noncorticosteroid treatment alternatives. To minimize the systemic effects of intranasal corticosteroids, including mometasone furoate nasal spray, 50 μg, each patient should be titrated to his/her lowest effective dose.

Seven hundred and twenty (720) patients 3-11 years of age were treated with mometasone furoate nasal spray, 50 μg (100 μg total daily dose) in controlled clinical trials. Twenty-eight (28) patients 2-5 years of age were treated with mometasone furoate nasal spray, 50 μg (100 μg total daily dose) in a controlled trial to evaluate safety (see CLINICAL PHARMACOLOGY, Pharmacokinetics). Safety and effectiveness in children less than 2 years of age have not been established.

A clinical study has been conducted for 1 year in pediatric patients (ages 3-9 years) to assess the effect of mometasone furoate nasal spray, 50 μg (100 μg total daily dose) on growth velocity. No statistically significant effect on growth velocity was observed for mometasone furoate nasal spray, 50 μg compared to placebo. No evidence of clinically relevant HPA axis suppression was observed following a 30 minute Cosyntropin infusion.

The potential of mometasone furoate nasal spray, 50 μg to cause growth suppression in susceptible patients or when given at higher doses cannot be ruled out.

GERIATRIC USE

A total of 203 patients above 64 years of age (age range 64-85 years) have been treated with mometasone furoate nasal spray, 50 μg for up to 3 months. The adverse reactions reported in this population were similar in type and incidence to those reported by younger patients.

ADVERSE REACTIONS

In controlled US and international clinical studies, a total of 3210 adult and adolescent patients aged 12 years and older received treatment with mometasone furoate nasal spray, 50 μg at doses of 50-800 μg/day. The majority of patients (n=2103) were treated with 200 μg/day. In controlled US and international studies, a total of 990 pediatric patients (ages 3-11 years) received treatment with mometasone furoate, 50 μg, at doses of 25-200 μg/day. The majority of pediatric patients (720) were treated with 100 μg/day. A total of 513 adult, adolescent, and pediatric patients have been treated for 1 year or longer. The overall incidence of adverse events for patients treated with mometasone furoate nasal spray, 50 μg was comparable to patients treated with the vehicle placebo. Also, adverse events did not differ significantly based on age, sex, or race. Three percent (3%) or less of patients in clinical trials discontinued treatment because of adverse events; this rate was similar for the vehicle and active comparators.

All adverse events (regardless of relationship to treatment) reported by 5% or more of adult and adolescent patients ages 12 years and older who received mometasone furoate nasal spray, 50 μg, 200 μg/day and by pediatric patients ages 3-11 years who received mometasone furoate nasal spray, 50 μg, 100 μg/day in clinical trials versus placebo and that were more common with mometasone furoate nasal spray, 50 μg than placebo, are displayed in TABLE 1.

***TABLE 1** Adverse Events From Controlled Clinical Trials in Seasonal Allergic and Perennial Allergic Rhinitis (Percent of Patients Reporting)*

	Adult and Adolescent Patients*		Pediatric Patients†	
	Mometasone Furoate 200 μg	Vehicle Placebo	Mometasone Furoate 100 μg	Vehicle Placebo
	(n=2103)	(n=1671)	(n=374)	(n=376)
Headache	26%	22%	17%	18%
Viral infection	14%	11%	8%	9%
Pharyngitis	12%	10%	10%	10%
Epistaxis/blood-tinged mucus	11%	6%	8%	9%
Coughing	7%	6%	13%	15%
Upper respiratory tract infection	6%	2%	5%	4%
Dysmenorrhea	5%	3%	1%	0%
Musculoskeletal pain	5%	3%	1%	1%
Sinusitis	5%	3%	4%	4%
Vomiting	1%	1%	5%	4%

* 12 years of age and older.
† Ages 3-11 years.

Other adverse events which occurred in less than 5% but greater than or equal to 2% of mometasone furoate adult and adolescent patients (aged 12 years and older) treated with 200 μg doses (regardless of relationship to treatment), and more frequently than in the placebo group included: arthralgia, asthma, bronchitis, chest pain, conjunctivitis, diarrhea, dyspepsia, earache, flu-like symptoms, myalgia, nausea, and rhinitis.

Other adverse events which occurred in less than 5% but greater or equal to 2% of mometasone furoate pediatric patients aged 3-11 years treated with 100 μg doses versus placebo (regardless of relationship to treatment) and more frequently than in the placebo group included: diarrhea, nasal irritation, otitis media, and wheezing.

The adverse event (regardless of relationship to treatment) reported by 5% of pediatric patients ages 2-5 years who received mometasone furoate nasal spray, 50 μg, 100 μg/day in a clinical trial versus placebo including 56 subjects (28 each mometasone furoate and placebo) and that was more common with mometasone furoate nasal spray, 50 μg than placebo, included: upper respiratory tract infection (7% vs 0%, respectively). The other adverse event which occurred in less than 5% but greater than or equal to 2% of mometasone furoate pediatric patients ages 2-5 years treated with 100 μg doses versus placebo (regardless of relationship to treatment) and more frequently than in the placebo group included: skin trauma.

Rare cases of nasal ulcers and nasal and oral candidiasis were also reported in patients treated with mometasone furoate nasal spray, 50 μg, primarily in patients treated for longer than 4 weeks.

In postmarketing surveillance of this product, cases of nasal burning and irritation, anaphylaxis and angioedema, and rare cases of nasal septal perforation have been reported.

DOSAGE AND ADMINISTRATION

ADULTS AND CHILDREN 12 YEARS OF AGE AND OLDER

The usual recommended dose for prophylaxis and treatment of the nasal symptoms of seasonal allergic rhinitis and treatment of the nasal symptoms of perennial allergic rhinitis is 2 sprays (50 μg of mometasone furoate in each spray) in each nostril once daily (total daily dose of 200 μg).

In patients with a known seasonal allergen that precipitates nasal symptoms of seasonal allergic rhinitis, prophylaxis with mometasone furoate nasal spray, 50 μg (200 μg/day) is recommended 2-4 weeks prior to the anticipated start of the pollen season.

CHILDREN 2-11 YEARS OF AGE

The usual recommended dose for treatment of the nasal symptoms of seasonal allergic and perennial allergic rhinitis is 1 spray (50 μg of mometasone furoate in each spray) in each nostril once daily (total daily dose of 100 μg).

Improvement in nasal symptoms of allergic rhinitis has been shown to occur within 11 hours after the first dose based on one single-dose, parallel-group study of patients in an outdoor "park" setting (park study) and one environmental exposure unit (EEU) study and within 2 days after the first dose in two randomized, double-blind, placebo-controlled, parallel-group seasonal allergic rhinitis studies. Maximum benefit is usually achieved within 1-2 weeks. Patients should use mometasone furoate nasal spray, 50 μg only once daily at a regular interval.

Prior to initial use of mometasone furoate nasal spray, 50 µg, the pump must be primed by actuating 10 times or until a fine spray appears. The pump may be stored unused for up to 1 week without repriming. If unused for more than 1 week, reprime by actuating 2 times, or until a fine spray appears.

DIRECTIONS FOR USE

Illustrated Patient's Instructions for Use accompany each package of mometasone furoate nasal spray, 50 µg.

HOW SUPPLIED

Nasonex (mometasone furoate monohydrate) nasal spray, 50 µg is supplied in a white, high-density, polyethylene bottle fitted with a white metered-dose, manual spray pump, and teal-green cap. It contains 17 g of product formulation, 120 sprays, each delivering 50 µg of mometasone furoate per actuation. Supplied with Patient's Instructions for Use.

STORAGE

Store between 2 and 25°C (36 and 77°F). Protect from light.

When Nasonex nasal spray, 50 µg is removed from its cardboard container, prolonged exposure of the product to direct light should be avoided. Brief exposure to light, as with normal use, is acceptable.

SHAKE WELL BEFORE EACH USE.

TOPICAL

DESCRIPTION

For Dermatologic Use Only.

Not for Ophthalmic Use.

Elocon products contain mometasone furoate for dermatologic use. Mometasone furoate is a synthetic corticosteroid with anti-inflammatory activity.

Chemically, mometasone furoate is 9α,21-dichloro-11β,17-dihydroxy-16α-methylpregna-1,4-diene-3,20-dione 17-(2-furoate), with the empirical formula $C_{27}H_{30}Cl_2O_6$, and a molecular weight of 521.4.

Mometasone furoate is a white to off-white powder practically insoluble in water, slightly soluble in octanol, and moderately soluble in ethyl alcohol.

Each gram of Elocon cream 0.1% contains: 1 mg mometasone furoate in a cream base of hexylene glycol, phosphoric acid, propylene glycol stearate (55% monoester), stearyl alcohol and ceteareth-20, titanium dioxide, aluminum starch ocetenylsuccinate (Gamma irradiated), white wax, white petrolatum, and purified water.

Each gram of Elocon ointment 0.1% contains: 1 mg mometasone furoate in an ointment base of hexylene glycol, phosphoric acid, propylene glycol stearate (55% monester), white wax, white petrolatum, and purified water.

Each gram of Elocon lotion 0.1% contains: 1 mg of mometasone furoate in a lotion base of isopropyl alcohol (40%), propylene glycol, hydroxypropylcellulose, sodium phosphate monobasic monohydrate and water. May also contain phosphoric acid used to adjust the pH to approximately 4.5.

CLINICAL PHARMACOLOGY

Like other topical corticosteroids, mometasone furoate has anti-inflammatory, anti-pruritic, and vasoconstrictive properties. The mechanism of the anti-inflammatory activity of the topical steroids, in general, is unclear. However, corticosteroids are thought to act by the induction of phospholipase A_2 inhibitory proteins, collectively called lipocortins. It is postulated that these proteins control the biosynthesis of potent mediators of inflammation such as prostaglandins and leukotrienes by inhibiting the release of their common precursor arachidonic acid. Arachidonic acid is released from membrane phospholipids by phospholipase A_2.

PHARMACOKINETICS

Cream and Ointment

The extent of percutaneous absorption of topical corticosteroids is determined by many factors including the vehicle and the integrity of the epidermal barrier. Occlusive dressings with hydrocortisone for up to 24 hours have not been demonstrated to increase penetration; however, occlusion of hydrocortisone for 96 hours markedly enhances penetration. Studies in humans indicate that approximately 0.4% of the applied dose of mometasone furoate cream 0.1% and 0.7% of the applied dose of mometasone furoate ointment 0.1% enters the circulation after 8 hours of contact on normal skin without occlusion. Inflammation and/or other disease processes in the skin may increase percutaneous absorption.

Studies performed with mometasone furoate cream and ointment indicate that it is in the medium range of potency as compared with other topical corticosteroids.

In a study evaluating the effects of mometasone furoate cream and ointment on the hypothalamic-pituitary-adrenal (HPA) axis, 15 g were applied twice daily for 7 days to 6 adult patients with psoriasis or atopic dermatitis. The cream and ointment were applied without occlusion to at least 30% of the body surface. The results show that the drug caused a slight lowering of adrenal corticosteroid secretion.

In a pediatric trial, 24 atopic dermatitis patients, of which 19 patients were age 2-12 years, were treated with mometasone furoate cream 0.1% once daily. The majority of patients cleared within 3 weeks.

Cream

Ninety-seven (97) pediatric patients ages 6-23 months, with atopic dermatitis, were enrolled in an open-label, hypothalamic-pituitary-adrenal (HPA) axis safety study. Mometasone furoate cream was applied once daily for approximately 3 weeks over a mean body surface area of 41% (range 15-94%). In approximately 16% of patients who showed normal adrenal function by Cortrosyn test before starting treatment, adrenal suppression was observed at the end of treatment with mometasone furoate cream. The criteria for suppression were: basal cortisol level of ≤5 µg/dl, 30 minute post-stimulation level of ≤18 µg/dl, or an increase of <7 µg/dl. Follow-up testing 2-4 weeks after stopping treatment, available for 5 of the patients, demonstrated suppressed HPA axis function in 1 patient, using these same criteria.

Ointment

Sixty-three (63) pediatric patients ages 6-23 months, with atopic dermatitis, were enrolled in an open-label, hypothalamic-pituitary-adrenal (HPA) axis safety study. Mometasone furoate ointment was applied once daily for approximately 3 weeks over a mean body surface area of 39% (range 15-99%). In approximately 27% of patients who showed normal adrenal function by Cortrosyn test before starting treatment, adrenal suppression was observed at the end of treatment with mometasone furoate ointment. The criteria for suppression were: basal cortisol level of ≤5 µg/dl, 30 minute post-stimulation level of ≤18 µg/dl, or an increase of <7 µg/dl. Follow-up testing 2-4 weeks after stopping treatment, available for 8 of the patients, demonstrated suppressed HPA axis function in 3 patients, using these same criteria.

Lotion

The extent of percutaneous absorption of topical corticosteroids is determined by many factors including the vehicle and the integrity of the epidermal barrier. Occlusive dressings with hydrocortisone for up to 24 hours have not been demonstrated to increase penetration; however, occlusion of hydrocortisone for 96 hours markedly enhances penetration. Studies in humans indicate that approximately 0.7% of the applied dose of mometasone furoate ointment, 0.1%, enters the circulation after 8 hours of contact on normal skin without occlusion. A similar minimal degree of absorption of the corticosteroid from the lotion formulation would be anticipated. Inflammation and/or other disease processes in the skin may increase percutaneous absorption.

Studies performed with mometasone furoate lotion indicate that it is in the medium range of potency as compared with other topical corticosteroids.

In a study evaluating the effects of mometasone furoate lotion on the hypothalamic-pituitary-adrenal (HPA) axis, 15 ml were applied without occlusion twice daily (30 ml/day) for 7 days to 4 adult patients with scalp and body psoriasis. At the end of treatment, the plasma cortisol levels for each of the 4 patients remained within the normal range and changed little from baseline.

Sixty-five (65) pediatric patients ages 6-23 months, with atopic dermatitis, were enrolled in an open-label, hypothalamic-pituitary-adrenal (HPA) axis safety study. Mometasone furoate lotion was applied once daily for approximately 3 weeks over a mean body surface area of 40% (range 16-90%). In approximately 29% of patients who showed normal adrenal function by Cortrosyn test before starting treatment, adrenal suppression was observed at the end of treatment with mometasone furoate lotion. The criteria for suppression were: basal cortisol level of ≤5 µg/dl, 30 minute post-stimulation level of ≤18 µg/dl, or an increase of <7 µg/dl. Follow-up testing 2-4 weeks after stopping treatment, available for 8 of the patients, demonstrated suppressed HPA axis function in 1 patient, using these same criteria.

INDICATIONS AND USAGE

CREAM AND OINTMENT

Mometasone furoate cream and ointment 0.1% are a medium potency corticosteroid indicated for the relief of the inflammatory and pruritic manifestations of corticosteroid-responsive dermatoses.

Mometasone furoate cream and ointment 0.1% may be used in pediatric patients 2 years of age or older, although the safety and efficacy of drug use for longer than 3 weeks have not been established (see PRECAUTIONS, Pediatric Use). Since safety and efficacy of mometasone furoate cream and ointment have not been adequately established in pediatric patients below 2 years of age, its use in this age group is not recommended.

LOTION

Mometasone furoate lotion, 0.1%, is a medium potency corticosteroid indicated for the relief of the inflammatory and pruritic manifestations of corticosteroid-responsive dermatoses. Since safety and efficacy of mometasone furoate lotion have not been established in pediatric patients below 12 years of age, its use in this age group is not recommended (see PRECAUTIONS, Pediatric Use).

CONTRAINDICATIONS

Mometasone furoate cream, ointment, and lotion are contraindicated in those patients with a history of hypersensitivity to any of the components in the preparation.

PRECAUTIONS

GENERAL

Cream and Ointment

Systemic absorption of topical corticosteroids can produce reversible hypothalamic-pituitary-adrenal (HPA) axis suppression with the potential for glucocorticosteroid insufficiency after withdrawal of treatment. Manifestations of Cushing's syndrome, hyperglycemia, and glucosuria can also be produced in some patients by systemic absorption of topical corticosteroids while on treatment.

Patients applying a topical steroid to a large surface area or areas under occlusion should be evaluated periodically for evidence of HPA axis suppression. This may be done by using the ACTH stimulation, AM plasma cortisol, and urinary free cortisol tests.

In a study evaluating the effects of mometasone furoate cream and ointment on the hypothalamic-pituitary-adrenal (HPA) axis, 15 g were applied twice daily for 7 days to 6 adult patients with psoriasis or atopic dermatitis. The cream and ointment were each applied without occlusion to at least 30% of the body surface. The results show that the drug caused a slight lowering of adrenal corticosteroid secretion.

If HPA axis suppression is noted, an attempt should be made to withdraw the drug, to reduce the frequency of application, or to substitute a less potent corticosteroid. Recovery of HPA axis function is generally prompt upon discontinuation of topical corticosteroids. Infrequently, signs and symptoms of glucocorticosteroid insufficiency may occur requiring supplemental systemic corticosteroids. For information on systemic supplementation, see the prescribing information for those products.

Pediatric patients may be more susceptible to systemic toxicity from equivalent doses due to their larger skin surface to body mass ratios (see Pediatric Use).

If irritation develops, mometasone furoate cream and ointment should be discontinued and appropriate therapy instituted. Allergic contact dermatitis with corticosteroids is usually diagnosed by observing a failure to heal rather than noting a clinical exacerbation as with most topical products not containing corticosteroids. Such an observation should be corroborated with appropriate diagnostic patch testing.

If concomitant skin infections are present or develop, an appropriate antifungal or antibacterial agent should be used. If a favorable response does not occur promptly, use of mometasone furoate cream and ointment should be discontinued until the infection has been adequately controlled.

Lotion

Systemic absorption of topical corticosteroids can produce reversible hypothalamic-pituitary-adrenal (HPA) axis suppression with the potential for glucocorticosteroid insufficiency after withdrawal of treatment. Manifestations of Cushing's syndrome, hyperglycemia, and glucosuria can also be produced in some patients by systemic absorption of topical corticosteroids while on treatment.

Patients applying a topical steroid to a large surface area or areas under occlusion should be evaluated periodically for evidence of HPA axis suppression. This may be done by using the ACTH stimulation, AM plasma cortisol, and urinary free cortisol tests.

In a study evaluating the effects of mometasone furoate lotion on the hypothalamic-pituitary-adrenal (HPA) axis, 15 ml were applied without occlusion twice daily (30 ml/day) for 7 days to 4 adult patients with scalp and body psoriasis. At the end of treatment, the plasma cortisol levels for each of the 4 patients remained within the normal range and changed little from baseline.

If HPA axis suppression is noted, an attempt should be made to withdraw the drug, to reduce the frequency of application, or to substitute a less potent corticosteroid. Recovery of HPA axis function is generally prompt upon discontinuation of topical corticosteroids. Infrequently, signs and symptoms of glucocorticosteroid insufficiency may occur requiring supplemental systemic corticosteroids. For information on systemic supplementation, see the prescribing information for those products.

Pediatric patients may be more susceptible to systemic toxicity from equivalent doses due to their larger skin surface to body mass ratios (see Pediatric Use).

If irritation develops, mometasone furoate lotion should be discontinued and appropriate therapy instituted. Allergic contact dermatitis with corticosteroids is usually diagnosed by observing failure to heal rather than noting a clinical exacerbation as with most topical products not containing corticosteroids. Such an observation should be corroborated with appropriate diagnostic patch testing.

If concomitant skin infections are present or develop, an appropriate antifungal or antibacterial agent should be used. If a favorable response does not occur promptly, use of mometasone furoate lotion should be discontinued until the infection has been adequately controlled.

INFORMATION FOR THE PATIENT

Patients using topical corticosteroids should receive the following information and instructions:

- This medication is to be used as directed by the physician. It is for external use only. Avoid contact with the eyes.
- This medication should not be used for any disorder other than that for which it was prescribed.
- The treated skin area should not be bandaged or otherwise covered or wrapped so as to be occlusive unless directed by the physician.
- Patients should report to their physician any signs of local adverse reactions.
- Parents of pediatric patients should be advised not to use mometasone furoate cream, ointment, or lotion in the treatment of diaper dermatitis. Mometasone furoate cream, ointment, and lotion should not be applied in the diaper area as diapers or plastic pants may constitute occlusive dressing (see DOSAGE AND ADMINISTRATION).
- This medication should not be used on the face, underarms, or groin areas unless directed by the physician.
- As with other corticosteroids, therapy should be discontinued when control is achieved. If no improvement is seen within 2 weeks, contact the physician.
- Other corticosteroid-containing products should not be used with mometasone furoate cream, ointment, or lotion without first consulting with the physician.

LABORATORY TESTS

The following tests may be helpful in evaluating HPA axis suppression:

- ACTH stimulation test.
- AM plasma cortisol test.
- Urinary free cortisol test.

CARCINOGENESIS, MUTAGENESIS, AND IMPAIRMENT OF FERTILITY

Long-term animal studies have not been performed to evaluate the carcinogenic potential of mometasone furoate cream, ointment, or lotion. Long-term carcinogenicity studies of mometasone furoate were conducted by the inhalation route in rats and mice. In a 2 year carcinogenicity study in Sprague-Dawley rats, mometasone furoate demonstrated no statistically significant increase of tumors at inhalation doses up to 67 μg/kg (approximately 0.04 times the estimated maximum clinical topical dose from mometasone furoate cream, ointment, and lotion on a μg/m² basis). In a 19 month carcinogenicity study in Swiss CD-1 mice, mometasone furoate demonstrated no statistically significant increase in the incidence of tumors at inhalation doses up to 160 μg/kg (approximately 0.05 times the estimated maximum clinical topical dose from mometasone furoate cream, ointment, and lotion on a μg/m² basis).

Mometasone furoate increased chromosomal aberrations in an *in vitro* Chinese hamster ovary cell assay, but did not increase chromosomal aberrations in an *in vitro* Chinese hamster lung cell assay. Mometasone furoate was not mutagenic in the Ames test or mouse lymphoma assay, and was not clastogenic in an *in vivo* mouse micronucleus assay, a rat bone marrow chromosomal aberration assay, or a mouse male germ-cell chromosomal aberration assay. Mometasone furoate also did not induce unscheduled DNA synthesis *in vivo* in rat hepatocytes.

In reproductive studies in rats, impairment of fertility was not produced in male or female rats by subcutaneous doses up to 15 μg/kg (approximately 0.01 times the estimated maximum clinical topical dose from mometasone furoate cream, ointment, and lotion on a μg/m² basis).

PREGNANCY, TERATOGENIC EFFECTS, PREGNANCY CATEGORY C

Corticosteroids have been shown to be teratogenic in laboratory animals when administered systemically at relatively low dosage levels. Some corticosteroids have been shown to be teratogenic after dermal application in laboratory animals.

When administered to pregnant rats, rabbits, and mice, mometasone furoate increased fetal malformations. The doses that produced malformations also decreased fetal growth, as measured by lower fetal weights and/or delayed ossification. Mometasone furoate also caused dystocia and related complications when administered to rats during the end of pregnancy.

In mice, mometasone furoate caused cleft palate at subcutaneous doses of 60 μg/kg and above. Fetal survival was reduced at 180 μg/kg. No toxicity was observed at 20 μg/kg. (Doses of 20, 60 and 180 μg/kg in the mouse are approximately 0.01, 0.02 and 0.05 times the estimated maximum clinical topical dose from mometasone furoate cream, ointment, and lotion on a μg/m² basis.)

In rats, mometasone furoate produced umbilical hernias at topical doses of 600 μg/kg and above. A dose of 300 μg/kg produced delays in ossification, but no malformations. (Doses of 300 and 600 μg/kg in the rat are approximately 0.2 and 0.4 times the estimated maximum clinical topical dose from mometasone furoate cream, ointment, and lotion on a μg/m² basis.)

In rabbits, mometasone furoate caused multiple malformations (*e.g.,* flexed front paws, gallbladder agenesis, umbilical hernia, hydrocephaly) at topical doses of 150 μg/kg and above (approximately 0.2 times the estimated maximum clinical topical dose from mometasone furoate cream, ointment, and lotion on a μg/m² basis). In an oral study, mometasone furoate increased resorptions and caused cleft palate and/or head malformations (hydrocephaly and domed head) at 700 μg/kg. At 2800 μg/kg most litters were aborted or resorbed. No toxicity was observed at 140 μg/kg. (Doses of 140, 700 and 2800 μg/kg in the rabbit are approximately 0.2, 0.9 and 3.6 times the estimated maximum clinical topical dose from mometasone furoate cream, ointment, and lotion on a μg/m² basis.)

When rats received subcutaneous doses of mometasone furoate throughout pregnancy or during the later stages of pregnancy, 15 μg/kg caused prolonged and difficult labor and reduced the number of live births, birth weight and early pup survival. Similar effects were not observed at 7.5 μg/kg. (Doses of 7.5 and 15 μg/kg in the rat are approximately 0.005 and 0.01 times the estimated maximum clinical topical dose from mometasone furoate cream, ointment, and lotion on a μg/m² basis.)

There are no adequate and well-controlled studies of teratogenic effects from topically applied corticosteroids in pregnant women. Therefore, topical corticosteroids should be used during pregnancy only if the potential benefit justifies the potential risk to the fetus.

NURSING MOTHERS

Systemically administered corticosteroids appear in human milk and could suppress growth, interfere with endogenous corticosteroid production, or cause other untoward effects. It is not known whether topical administration of corticosteroids could result in sufficient systemic absorption to produce detectable quantities in human milk. Because many drugs are excreted in human milk, caution should be exercised when mometasone furoate cream, ointment, and lotion are administered to a nursing woman.

PEDIATRIC USE

Cream and Ointment

Mometasone furoate cream and ointment may be used with caution in pediatric patients 2 years of age or older, although the safety and efficacy of drug use for longer than 3 weeks have not been established. Use of mometasone furoate cream and ointment is supported by results from adequate and well-controlled studies in pediatric patients with corticosteroid-responsive dermatoses. Since safety and efficacy of mometasone furoate cream and ointment have not been adequately established in pediatric patients below 2 years of age, its use in this age group is not recommended.

Mometasone furoate cream and ointment caused HPA axis suppression in approximately 16% and 27%, respectively, of pediatric patients ages 6-23 months, who showed normal adrenal function by Cortrosyn test before starting treatment, and were treated for approximately 3 weeks over a mean body surface area of 41% and 39%, respectively, (range 15–94% and 15-99%, respectively). The criteria for suppression were: basal cortisol level of ≤5 μg/dl, 30 minute post-stimulation level of ≤18 μg/dl, or an increase of <7 μg/dl. Follow-up testing 2-4 weeks after stopping treatment or study completion , available for 5 of the patients using cream and for 8 of the patients using ointment, demonstrated suppressed HPA axis function in 1 patient using cream and in 3 patients using ointment, using these same criteria. Long-term use of topical corticosteroids has not been studied in this population (see CLINICAL PHARMACOLOGY, Pharmacokinetics).

Because of a higher ratio of skin surface area to body mass, pediatric patients are at a greater risk than adults of HPA axis suppression and Cushing's syndrome when they are treated with topical corticosteroids. They are, therefore, also at greater risk of glucocorticosteroid insufficiency during and/or after withdrawal of treatment. Pediatric patients may be more susceptible than adults to skin atrophy, including striae, when they are treated with topical corticosteroids. Pediatric patients applying topical corticosteroids to greater than 20% of body surface are at higher risk of HPA axis suppression.

HPA axis suppression, Cushing's syndrome, linear growth retardation, delayed weight gain, and intracranial hypertension have been reported in pediatric patients receiving topical corticosteroids. Manifestations of adrenal suppression in children include low plasma cortisol levels, and absence of response to ACTH stimulation. Manifestations of intracranial hypertension include bulging fontanelles, headaches, and bilateral papilledema.

Mometasone furoate cream and ointment 0.1% should not be used in the treatment of diaper dermatitis.

Lotion

Since safety and efficacy of mometasone furoate lotion have not been established in pediatric patients below 12 years of age, its use in this age group is not recommended.

Mometasone furoate lotion caused HPA axis suppression in approximately 29% of pediatric patients ages 6-23 months who showed normal adrenal function by Cortrosyn test before starting treatment, and were treated for approximately 3 weeks over a mean body surface area of 40% (range 16-90%). The criteria for suppression were: basal cortisol level of ≤5 μg/dl, 30 minute post-stimulation level of ≤18 μg/dl, or an increase of <7 μg/dl. Follow-up testing 2-4 weeks after stopping treatment, available for 8 of the patients, demonstrated suppressed HPA axis function in 1 patient, using these same criteria. Long-term use of topical corticosteroids has not been studied in this population (see CLINICAL PHARMACOLOGY, Pharmacokinetics).

Because of a higher ratio of skin surface area to body mass, pediatric patients are at a greater risk than adults of HPA axis suppression and Cushing's syndrome when they are treated with topical corticosteroids. They are, therefore, also at greater risk of glucocorticosteroid insufficiency during and/or after withdrawal of treatment. Pediatric patients may be more susceptible than adults to skin atrophy, including striae, when they are treated with topical corticosteroids. Pediatric patients applying topical corticosteroids to greater than 20% of body surface are at higher risk of HPA axis suppression.

HPA axis suppression, Cushing's syndrome, linear growth retardation, delayed weight gain and intracranial hypertension have been reported in pediatric patients receiving topical corticosteroids. Manifestations of adrenal suppression in children include low plasma cortisol levels and absence of response to ACTH stimulation. Manifestations of intracranial hypertension include bulging fontanelles, headaches, and bilateral papilledema.

Mometasone furoate lotion should not be used in the treatment of diaper dermatitis.

GERIATRIC USE

Cream

Clinical studies of mometasone furoate cream included 190 subjects who were 65 years of age and over and 39 subjects who were 75 years of age and over. No overall differences in safety or effectiveness were observed between these subjects and younger subjects, and other reported clinical experience has not identified differences in responses between the elderly and younger patients. However, greater sensitivity of some older individuals cannot be ruled out.

Ointment

Clinical studies of mometasone furoate ointment included 310 subjects who were 65 years of age and over and 57 subjects who were 75 years of age and over. No overall differences in safety or effectiveness were observed between these subjects and younger subjects, and other reported clinical experience has not identified differences in responses between the elderly and younger patients. However, greater sensitivity of some older individuals cannot be ruled out.

Lotion

Clinical studies of mometasone furoate lotion did not include sufficient number of subjects aged 65 and over to determine whether they respond differently from younger subjects. Other reported clinical experience has not identified differences in responses between the elderly and younger patients. In general, dose selection for an elderly patient should be cautious.

ADVERSE REACTIONS

CREAM

In controlled clinical studies involving 319 patients, the incidence of adverse reactions associated with the use of mometasone furoate cream was 1.6%. Reported reactions included burning, pruritus, and skin atrophy. Reports of rosacea associated with the use of mometasone furoate cream have also been received. In controlled clinical studies (n=74) involving pediatric patients 2-12 years of age, the incidence of adverse experiences associated with the use of mometasone furoate cream was approximately 7%. Reported reactions included stinging, pruritus, and furunculosis.

The following adverse reactions were reported to be possibly or probably related to treatment with mometasone furoate cream during clinical studies in 4% of 182 pediatric patients 6 months to 2 years of age: decreased glucocorticoid levels, 2; paresthesia, 2; folliculitis, 1; moniliasis, 1; bacterial infection, 1; skin depigmentation, 1. The following signs of skin atrophy were also observed among 97 patients treated with mometasone furoate cream in a clinical study: shininess 4, telangiectasia 1, loss of elasticity 4, loss of normal skin markings 4, thinness 1, and bruising 1. Striae were not observed in this study.

The following additional local adverse reactions have been reported infrequently with topical corticosteroids, but may occur more frequently with the use of occlusive dressings. These reactions are listed in an approximate decreasing order of occurrence: irritation, dryness, folliculitis, hypertrichosis, acneiform eruptions, hypopigmentation, perioral dermatitis, allergic contact dermatitis, secondary infection, striae, and miliaria.

OINTMENT

In controlled clinical studies involving 812 patients, the incidence of adverse reactions associated with the use of mometasone furoate ointment was 4.8%. Reported reactions included burning, pruritus, skin atrophy, tingling/stinging, and furunculosis. Reports of rosacea associated with the use of mometasone furoate ointment have been received. In controlled clinical studies (n=74) involving pediatric patients 2-12 years of age, the incidence of adverse experiences associated with the use of mometasone furoate cream is approximately 7%. Reported reactions included stinging, pruritus, and furunculosis.

The following adverse reactions were reported to be possibly or probably related to treatment with mometasone furoate ointment during a clinical study, in 5% of 63 pediatric patients 6 months to 2 years of age: decreased glucocorticoid levels, 1; an unspecified skin disorder, 1; and a bacterial skin infection, 1. The following signs of skin atrophy were also observed among 63 patients treated with mometasone furoate ointment in a clinical study: shininess 4, telangiectasia 1, loss of elasticity 4, loss of normal skin markings 4, thinness 1. Striae and bruising were not observed in this study.

The following additional local adverse reactions have been reported infrequently with topical corticosteroids, but may occur more frequently with the use of occlusive dressings. These reactions are listed in an approximate decreasing order of occurrence: irritation, dryness, folliculitis, hypertrichosis, acneiform eruptions, hypopigmentation, perioral dermatitis, allergic contact dermatitis, secondary infection, striae, and miliaria.

LOTION

In clinical studies involving 209 patients, the incidence of adverse reactions associated with the use of mometasone furoate lotion was 3%. Reported reactions included acneiform reaction, 2; burning, 4; and itching, 1. In an irritation/sensitization study involving 156 normal subjects, the incidence of folliculitis was 3% (4 subjects).

The following adverse reactions were reported to be possibly or probably related to treatment with mometasone furoate lotion during a clinical study, in 14% of 65 pediatric patients 6 months to 2 years of age: decreased glucocorticoid levels, 4; paresthesia, 2; dry mouth, 1; an unspecified endocrine disorder, 1; pruritus, 1; and an unspecified skin disorder, 1. The following signs of skin atrophy were also observed among 65 patients treated with mometasone furoate lotion in a clinical study: shininess 4, telangiectasia 2, loss of elasticity 2, and loss of normal skin markings 3. Striae, thinness and bruising were not observed in this study.

The following additional local adverse reactions have been reported infrequently with topical corticosteroids, but may occur more frequently with the use of occlusive dressings. These reactions are listed in an approximate decreasing order of occurrence: irritation, dryness, hypertrichosis, hypopigmentation, perioral dermatitis, allergic contact dermatitis, secondary infection, skin atrophy, striae, and miliaria.

DOSAGE AND ADMINISTRATION

CREAM AND OINTMENT

Apply a thin film of mometasone furoate cream or ointment to the affected skin areas once daily. Mometasone furoate cream and ointment may be used in pediatric patients 2 years of age or older. Since safety and efficacy of mometasone furoate cream and ointment have not been adequately established in pediatric patients below 2 years of age, its use in this age group is not recommended (see PRECAUTIONS, Pediatric Use).

As with other corticosteroids, therapy should be discontinued when control is achieved. If no improvement is seen within 2 weeks, reassessment of diagnosis may be necessary. Safety and efficacy of mometasone furoate cream and ointment in pediatric patients for more than 3 weeks have not been established.

Mometasone furoate cream and ointment should not be used with occlusive dressings unless directed by a physician. Mometasone furoate cream and ointment should not be applied in the diaper area if the child still requires diapers or plastic pants as these garments may constitute occlusive dressing.

LOTION

Apply a few drops of mometasone furoate lotion to the affected areas once daily and massage lightly until it disappears. For the most effective and economical use, hold the nozzle of the bottle very close to the affected areas and gently squeeze. Since safety and efficacy of mometasone furoate lotion have not been established in pediatric patients below 12 years of age, its use in this age group is not recommended. (see PRECAUTIONS, Pediatric Use).

As with other corticosteroids, therapy should be discontinued when control is achieved. If no improvement is seen within 2 weeks, reassessment of diagnosis may be necessary.

Mometasone furoate lotion should not be used with occlusive dressings unless directed by a physician. Mometasone furoate lotion should not be applied in the diaper area if the patient requires diapers or plastic pants as these garments may constitute occlusive dressing.

HOW SUPPLIED

CREAM

Elocon cream, 0.1% is supplied in 15 and 45 g tubes.

Storage: Store Elocon cream between 2 and 25°C (36 and 77°F).

OINTMENT

Elocon ointment, 0.1% is supplied in 15 and 45 g tubes.

Storage: Store Elocon ointment between 2 and 30°C (36 and 86°F).

LOTION

Elocon lotion, 0.1%, is supplied in 30 and 60 ml bottles.

Storage: Store Elocon lotion between 2 and 30°C (36 and 86°F).

PRODUCT LISTING - RATED THERAPEUTICALLY EQUIVALENT

Ointment - Topical - 0.1%

Size	Price	Product, Manufacturer	NDC
15 gm	$20.19	GENERIC, Clay-Park Laboratories Inc	45802-0119-37
45 gm	$36.98	GENERIC, Clay-Park Laboratories Inc	45802-0119-42

PRODUCT LISTING - EQUIVALENTS NOT AVAILABLE

Size	Price	Product, Manufacturer	NDC
Cream - Topical - 0.1%			
15 gm	$20.72	ELOCON, Allscripts Pharmaceutical Company	54569-2011-00
15 gm	$21.95	ELOCON, Southwood Pharmaceuticals Inc	58016-3241-01
15 gm	$24.04	ELOCON, Dhs Inc	55887-0735-15
15 gm	$26.13	ELOCON, Schering Corporation	00085-0567-01
30 gm	$38.25	ELOCON, Dhs Inc	55887-0735-45
45 gm	$37.96	ELOCON, Allscripts Pharmaceutical Company	54569-2619-00
45 gm	$41.08	ELOCON, Southwood Pharmaceuticals Inc	58016-5605-01
45 gm	$47.84	ELOCON, Schering Corporation	00085-0567-02
Lotion - Topical - 0.1%			
30 ml	$28.33	ELOCON, Schering Corporation	00085-0854-01
60 ml	$54.09	ELOCON, Schering Corporation	00085-0854-02
Ointment - Topical - 0.1%			
15 gm	$26.13	ELOCON, Schering Corporation	00085-0370-01

M

45 gm $47.84 ELOCON, Schering Corporation 00085-0370-02
Spray - Nasal - 50 mcg/Inh
17 gm $51.17 NASONEX, Schering Corporation 54569-4601-00
17 gm $62.60 NASONEX, Physicians Total Care 54868-4174-00
17 gm $72.16 NASONEX, Schering Corporation 00085-1197-01

Montelukast Sodium *(003383)*

Categories: Asthma; Pregnancy Category B; FDA Approved 1998 Feb
Drug Classes: Leucotriene antagonists/inhibitors
Brand Names: Singulair
Foreign Brand Availability: Kipres (Japan); Montair (India); Singulair Chew (Korea)
Cost of Therapy: $91.61 (Asthma; Singulair; 10 mg; 1 tablet/day; 30 day supply)

DESCRIPTION

Montelukast sodium is a selective and orally active leukotriene receptor antagonist that inhibits the cysteinyl leukotriene $CysLT_1$ receptor.

Montelukast sodium is described chemically as [R-(E)]-1-[[[1-[3-[2-(7-chloro-2-quinolinyl)ethenyl]phenyl]-3-[2-(1-hydroxy-1-methylethyl)phenyl]propyl]thio]methyl]cyclopropaneacetic acid, monosodium salt.

The empirical formula is $C_{35}H_{35}ClNNaO_3S$, and its molecular weight is 608.18.

Montelukast sodium is a hygroscopic, optically active, white to off-white powder. Montelukast sodium is freely soluble in ethanol, methanol, and water and practically insoluble in acetonitrile.

Each 10 mg film-coated Singulair tablet contains 10.4 mg montelukast sodium, which is equivalent to 10 mg of montelukast, and the following inactive ingredients: microcrystalline cellulose, lactose monohydrate, croscarmellose sodium, hydroxypropyl cellulose, and magnesium stearate. The film coating consists of: hydroxypropyl methylcellulose, hydroxypropyl cellulose, titanium dioxide, red ferric oxide, yellow ferric oxide, and carnauba wax.

Each 4 and 5 mg chewable Singulair tablet contains 4.2 and 5.2 mg montelukast sodium, respectively, which are equivalent to 4 and 5 mg of montelukast, respectively. Both chewable tablets contain the following inactive ingredients: mannitol, microcrystalline cellulose, hydroxypropyl cellulose, red ferric oxide, croscarmellose sodium, cherry flavor, aspartame, and magnesium stearate.

Each packet of Singulair 4 mg oral granules contains 4.2 mg montelukast sodium, which is equivalent to 4 mg of montelukast. The oral granule formulation contains the following inactive ingredients: mannitol, hydroxypropyl cellulose, and magnesium stearate.

M

CLINICAL PHARMACOLOGY

MECHANISM OF ACTION

The cysteinyl leukotrienes (LTC_4, LTD_4, LTE_4) are products of arachidonic acid metabolism and are released from various cells, including mast cells and eosinophils. These eicosanoids bind to cysteinyl leukotriene receptors (CysLT) found in the human airway. Cysteinyl leukotrienes and leukotriene receptor occupation have been correlated with the pathophysiology of asthma, including airway edema, smooth muscle contraction, and altered cellular activity associated with the inflammatory process, which contribute to the signs and symptoms of asthma.

Montelukast is an orally active compound that binds with high affinity and selectivity to the $CysLT_1$ receptor (in preference to other pharmacologically important airway receptors, such as the prostanoid, cholinergic, or β-adrenergic receptor). Montelukast inhibits physiologic actions of LTD_4 at the $CysLT_1$ receptor without any agonist activity.

PHARMACOKINETICS

Absorption

Montelukast is rapidly absorbed following oral administration. After administration of the 10 mg film-coated tablet to fasted adults, the mean peak montelukast plasma concentration (C_{max}) is achieved in 3-4 hours (T_{max}). The mean oral bioavailability is 64%. The oral bioavailability and C_{max} are not influenced by a standard meal in the morning.

For the 5 mg chewable tablet, the mean C_{max} is achieved in 2 to 2.5 hours after administration to adults in the fasted state. The mean oral bioavailability is 73% in the fasted state versus 63% when administered with a standard meal in the morning.

For the 4 mg chewable tablet, the mean C_{max} is achieved 2 hours after administration in pediatric patients 2-5 years of age in the fasted state.

The 4 mg oral granule formulation is bioequivalent to the 4 mg chewable tablet when administered to adults in the fasted state. The coadministration of the oral granule formulation with applesauce did not have a clinically significant effect on the pharmacokinetics of montelukast. A high fat meal in the morning did not affect the AUC of montelukast oral granules, however, the meal decreased C_{max} by 35% and prolonged T_{max} from 2.3 ± 1.0 hours to 6.4 ± 2.9 hours.

The safety and efficacy of montelukast sodium were demonstrated in clinical trials in which the 10 mg film-coated tablet and 5 mg chewable tablet formulations were administered in the evening without regard to the time of food ingestion. The safety of montelukast sodium was also demonstrated in clinical trials in which the 4 mg chewable tablet and 4 mg oral granule formulations were administered in the evening without regard to the time of food ingestion.

The comparative pharmacokinetics of montelukast when administered as two 5 mg chewable tablets versus one 10 mg film-coated tablet have not been evaluated.

Distribution

Montelukast is more than 99% bound to plasma proteins. The steady-state volume of distribution of montelukast averages 8-11 L. Studies in rats with radiolabeled montelukast indicate minimal distribution across the blood-brain barrier. In addition, concentrations of radiolabeled material at 24 hours postdose were minimal in all other tissues.

Metabolism

Montelukast is extensively metabolized. In studies with therapeutic doses, plasma concentrations of metabolites of montelukast are undetectable at steady state in adults and pediatric patients.

In vitro studies using human liver microsomes indicate that cytochromes P450 3A4 and 2C9 are involved in the metabolism of montelukast. Clinical studies investigating the effect of known inhibitors of cytochromes P450 3A4 (*e.g.,* ketoconazole, erythromycin) or 2C9 (*e.g.,* fluconazole) on montelukast pharmacokinetics have not been conducted. Based on further *in vitro* results in human liver microsomes, therapeutic plasma concentrations of montelukast do not inhibit cytochromes P450 3A4, 2C9, 1A2, 2A6, 2C19, or 2D6 (see DRUG INTERACTIONS).

Elimination

The plasma clearance of montelukast averages 45 ml/min in healthy adults. Following an oral dose of radiolabeled montelukast, 86% of the radioactivity was recovered in 5 day fecal collections and <0.2% was recovered in urine. Coupled with estimates of montelukast oral bioavailability, this indicates that montelukast and its metabolites are excreted almost exclusively via the bile.

In several studies, the mean plasma half-life of montelukast ranged from 2.7-5.5 hours in healthy young adults. The pharmacokinetics of montelukast are nearly linear for oral doses up to 50 mg. During once-daily dosing with 10 mg montelukast, there is little accumulation of the parent drug in plasma (14%).

Special Populations

Gender

The pharmacokinetics of montelukast are similar in males and females.

Elderly

The pharmacokinetic profile and the oral bioavailability of a single 10 mg oral dose of montelukast are similar in elderly and younger adults. The plasma half-life of montelukast is slightly longer in the elderly. No dosage adjustment in the elderly is required.

Race

Pharmacokinetic differences due to race have not been studied.

Hepatic Insufficiency

Patients with mild-to-moderate hepatic insufficiency and clinical evidence of cirrhosis had evidence of decreased metabolism of montelukast resulting in 41% (90% CI=7%, 85%) higher mean montelukast area under the plasma concentration curve (AUC) following a single 10 mg dose. The elimination of montelukast was slightly prolonged compared with that in healthy subjects (mean half-life, 7.4 hours). No dosage adjustment is required in patients with mild-to-moderate hepatic insufficiency. The pharmacokinetics of montelukast sodium in patients with more severe hepatic impairment or with hepatitis have not been evaluated.

Renal Insufficiency

Since montelukast and its metabolites are not excreted in the urine, the pharmacokinetics of montelukast were not evaluated in patients with renal insufficiency. No dosage adjustment is recommended in these patients.

Adolescents and Pediatric Patients

Pharmacokinetic studies evaluated the systemic exposure of the 4 mg oral granule formulation in pediatric patients 6-23 months of age, the 4 mg chewable tablets in pediatric patients 2-5 years of age, the 5 mg chewable tablets in pediatric patients 6-14 years of age, and the 10 mg film-coated tablets in young adults and adolescents ≥15 years of age.

The plasma concentration profile of montelukast following administration of the 10 mg film-coated tablet is similar in adolescents ≥15 years of age and young adults. The 10 mg film-coated tablet is recommended for use in patients ≥15 years of age.

The mean systemic exposure of the 4 mg chewable tablet in pediatric patients 2-5 years of age and the 5 mg chewable tablets in pediatric patients 6-14 years of age is similar to the mean systemic exposure of the 10 mg film-coated tablet in adults. The 5 mg chewable tablet should be used in pediatric patients 6-14 years of age and the 4 mg chewable tablet should be used in pediatric patients 2-5 years of age.

In children 6-11 months of age, the systemic exposure to montelukast and the variability of plasma montelukast concentrations were higher than those observed in adults. Based on population analyses, the mean AUC (4296 ng·h/ml [range 1200-7153]) was 60% higher and the mean C_{max} (667 ng/ml [range 201-1058]) was 89% higher than those observed in adults (mean AUC 2689 ng·h/ml [range 1521-4595]) and mean C_{max} (353 ng/ml [range 180-548]). The systemic exposure in children 12-23 months of age was less variable, but was still higher than that observed in adults. The mean AUC (3574 ng·h/ml [range 2229-5408]) was 33% higher and the mean C_{max} (562 ng/ml [range 296-814]) was 60% higher than those observed in adults. Safety and tolerability of montelukast in a single-dose pharmacokinetic study in 26 children 6-23 months of age were similar to that of patients 2 years and above (see ADVERSE REACTIONS). The 4 mg oral granule formulation should be used for pediatric patients 12-23 months of age. Since the 4 mg oral granule formulation is bioequivalent to the 4 mg chewable tablet, it can also be used as an alternative formulation to the 4 mg chewable tablet in pediatric patients 2-5 years of age.

Drug Interactions

Montelukast at a dose of 10 mg once daily dosed to pharmacokinetic steady state:

- Did not cause clinically significant changes in the kinetics of a single intravenous dose of theophylline (predominantly a cytochrome P450 1A2 substrate).
- Did not change the pharmacokinetic profile of warfarin (a substrate of cytochromes P450 2A6 and 2C9) or influence the effect of a single 30 mg oral dose of warfarin on prothrombin time or the INR (International Normalized Ratio).
- Did not change the pharmacokinetic profile or urinary excretion of immunoreactive digoxin.

- Did not change the plasma concentration profile of terfenadine (a substrate of cytochrome P450 3A4) or fexofenadine, its carboxylated metabolite, and did not prolong the QTc interval following co-administration with terfenadine 60 mg twice daily.

Montelukast at doses of ≥100 mg daily dosed to pharmacokinetic steady state:

Did not significantly alter the plasma concentrations of either component of an oral contraceptive containing norethindrone 1 mg/ethinyl estradiol 35 μg.

Did not cause any clinically significant change in plasma profiles of prednisone or prednisolone following administration of either oral prednisone or intravenous prednisolone.

Phenobarbital, which induces hepatic metabolism, decreased the AUC of montelukast approximately 40% following a single 10 mg dose of montelukast. No dosage adjustment for montelukast sodium is recommended. It is reasonable to employ appropriate clinical monitoring when potent cytochrome P450 enzyme inducers, such as phenobarbital or rifampin, are co-administered with montelukast sodium.

PHARMACODYNAMICS

Montelukast causes inhibition of airway cysteinyl leukotriene receptors as demonstrated by the ability to inhibit bronchoconstriction due to inhaled LTD_4 in asthmatics. Doses as low as 5 mg cause substantial blockage of LTD_4-induced bronchoconstriction. In a placebo-controlled, crossover study (n=12), montelukast sodium inhibited early- and late-phase bronchoconstriction due to antigen challenge by 75% and 57%, respectively.

The effect of montelukast sodium on eosinophils in the peripheral blood was examined in clinical trials in adults and pediatric asthmatic patients. A decrease in mean peripheral blood eosinophil counts ranging from 9-15% was noted in patients receiving montelukast sodium, compared with placebo over the double-blind treatment periods in clinical trials conducted in patients 2 years of age and above. The relationship between this observation and the clinical benefits noted in the clinical trials is not known.

INDICATIONS AND USAGE

Montelukast sodium is indicated for the prophylaxis and chronic treatment of asthma in adults and pediatric patients 12 months of age and older.

CONTRAINDICATIONS

Hypersensitivity to any component of this product.

PRECAUTIONS

GENERAL

Montelukast sodium is not indicated for use in the reversal of bronchospasm in acute asthma attacks, including status asthmaticus.

Patients should be advised to have appropriate rescue medication available. Therapy with montelukast sodium can be continued during acute exacerbations of asthma.

While the dose of inhaled corticosteroid may be reduced gradually under medical supervision, montelukast sodium should not be abruptly substituted for inhaled or oral corticosteroids.

Montelukast sodium should not be used as monotherapy for the treatment and management of exercise-induced bronchospasm. Patients who have exacerbations of asthma after exercise should continue to use their usual regimen of inhaled β-agonists as prophylaxis and have available for rescue a short-acting inhaled β-agonist.

Patients with known aspirin sensitivity should continue avoidance of aspirin or non-steroidal anti-inflammatory agents while taking montelukast sodium. Although montelukast sodium is effective in improving airway function in asthmatics with documented aspirin sensitivity, it has not been shown to truncate bronchoconstrictor response to aspirin and other non-steroidal anti-inflammatory drugs in aspirin-sensitive asthmatic patients.

EOSINOPHILIC CONDITIONS

In rare cases, patients on therapy with montelukast sodium may present with systemic eosinophilia, sometimes presenting with clinical features of vasculitis consistent with Churg-Strauss syndrome, a condition which is often treated with systemic corticosteroid therapy. These events usually, but not always, have been associated with the reduction of oral corticosteroid therapy. Physicians should be alert to eosinophilia, vasculitic rash, worsening pulmonary symptoms, cardiac complications, and/or neuropathy presenting in their patients. A causal association between montelukast sodium and these underlying conditions has not been established (see ADVERSE REACTIONS).

INFORMATION FOR THE PATIENT

- Patients should be advised to take montelukast sodium daily as prescribed, even when they are asymptomatic, as well as during periods of worsening asthma, and to contact their physicians if their asthma is not well controlled.
- Patients should be advised that oral tablets of montelukast sodium are not for the treatment of acute asthma attacks. They should have appropriate short-acting inhaled β-agonist medication available to treat asthma exacerbations.
- Patients should be advised that, while using montelukast sodium, medical attention should be sought if short-acting inhaled bronchodilators are needed more often than usual, or if more than the maximum number of inhalations of short-acting bronchodilator treatment prescribed for 24 hour period are needed.
- Patients receiving montelukast sodium should be instructed not to decrease the dose or stop taking any other anti-asthma medications unless instructed by a physician.
- Patients who have exacerbations of asthma after exercise should be instructed to continue to use their usual regimen of inhaled β-agonists as prophylaxis unless otherwise instructed by their physician. All patients should have available for rescue a short-acting inhaled β-agonist.
- Patients with known aspirin sensitivity should be advised to continue avoidance of aspirin or non-steroidal anti-inflammatory agents while taking montelukast sodium.

CHEWABLE TABLETS

Phenylketonurics: Phenylketonuric patients should be informed that the 4 mg and 5 mg chewable tablets contain phenylalanine (a component of aspartame), 0.674 and 0.842 mg per 4 mg and 5 mg chewable tablet, respectively.

CARCINOGENESIS, MUTAGENESIS, AND IMPAIRMENT OF FERTILITY

No evidence of tumorigenicity was seen in either a 2-year carcinogenicity study in Sprague-Dawley rats at oral gavage doses up to 200 mg/kg/day (estimated exposure was approximately 90 times the area under the plasma concentration versus time curve (AUC) for adults and children at the maximum recommended daily oral dose) or in a 92 week carcinogenicity study in mice at oral gavage doses up to 100 mg/kg/day (estimated exposure was approximately 30 times the AUC for adults and children at the maximum recommended daily oral dose).

Montelukast demonstrated no evidence of mutagenic or clastogenic activity in the following assays: the microbial mutagenesis assay, the V-79 mammalian cell mutagenesis assay, the alkaline elution assay in rat hepatocytes, the chromosomal aberration assay in Chinese hamster ovary cells, and in the *in vivo* mouse bone marrow chromosomal aberration assay.

In fertility studies in female rats, montelukast produced reductions in fertility and fecundity indices at an oral dose of 200 mg/kg (estimated exposure was approximately 70 times the AUC for adults at the maximum recommended daily oral dose). No effects on female fertility or fecundity were observed at an oral dose of 100 mg/kg (estimated exposure was approximately 20 times the AUC for adults at the maximum recommended daily oral dose). Montelukast had no effects on fertility in male rats at oral doses up to 800 mg/kg (estimated exposure was approximately 160 times the AUC for adults at the maximum recommended daily oral dose).

PREGNANCY, TERATOGENIC EFFECTS, PREGNANCY CATEGORY B

No teratogenicity was observed in rats at oral doses up to 400 mg/kg/day (estimated exposure was approximately 100 times the AUC for adults at the maximum recommended daily oral dose) and in rabbits at oral doses up to 300 mg/kg/day (estimated exposure was approximately 110 times the AUC for adults at the maximum recommended daily oral dose). Montelukast crosses the placenta following oral dosing in rats and rabbits. There are, however, no adequate and well-controlled studies in pregnant women. Because animal reproduction studies are not always predictive of human response, montelukast sodium should be used during pregnancy only if clearly needed.

Merck & Co., Inc. maintains a registry to monitor the pregnancy outcomes of women exposed to montelukast sodium while pregnant. Healthcare providers are encouraged to report any prenatal exposure to montelukast sodium by calling the Pregnancy Registry at (800) 986-8999.

NURSING MOTHERS

Studies in rats have shown that montelukast is excreted in milk. It is not known if montelukast is excreted in human milk. Because many drugs are excreted in human milk, caution should be exercised when montelukast sodium is given to a nursing mother.

PEDIATRIC USE

Safety and efficacy of montelukast sodium have been established in adequate and well-controlled studies in pediatric patients 6-14 years of age. Safety and efficacy profiles in this age group are similar to those seen in adults. (See ADVERSE REACTIONS.)

The safety of montelukast sodium 4 mg chewable tablets in pediatric patients 2-5 years of age has been demonstrated by adequate and well-controlled data (see ADVERSE REACTIONS). Efficacy of montelukast sodium in this age group is extrapolated from the demonstrated efficacy in patients 6 years of age and older with asthma and is based on similar pharmacokinetic data, as well as the assumption that the disease course, pathophysiology and the drug's effect are substantially similar among these populations. Efficacy in this age group is supported by exploratory efficacy assessments from a large, well-controlled safety study conducted in patients 2-5 years of age.

The safety of montelukast sodium 4 mg oral granules in pediatric patients 12-23 months of age has been demonstrated in an analysis of 172 pediatric patients, 124 of whom were treated with montelukast sodium, in a 6 week, double-blind, placebo-controlled study (see ADVERSE REACTIONS). Efficacy of montelukast sodium in this age group is extrapolated from the demonstrated efficacy in patients 6 years of age and older with asthma based on similar mean systemic exposure (AUC), and that the disease course, pathophysiology and the drug's effect are substantially similar among these populations, supported by efficacy data from a safety trial in which efficacy was an exploratory assessment.

The safety and effectiveness in pediatric patients below the age of 12 months have not been established. Long-term trials evaluating the effect of chronic administration of montelukast sodium on linear growth in pediatric patients have not been conducted.

GERIATRIC USE

Of the total number of subjects in clinical studies of montelukast, 3.5% were 65 years of age and over and 0.4% were 75 years of age and over. No overall differences in safety or effectiveness were observed between these subjects and younger subjects, and other reported clinical experience has not identified differences in responses between the elderly and younger patients, but greater sensitivity of some older individuals cannot be ruled out.

DRUG INTERACTIONS

Montelukast sodium has been administered with other therapies routinely used in the prophylaxis and chronic treatment of asthma with no apparent increase in adverse reactions. In drug-interaction studies, the recommended clinical dose of montelukast did not have clinically important effects on the pharmacokinetics of the following drugs: theophylline, prednisone, prednisolone, oral contraceptives (norethindrone 1 mg/ethinyl estradiol 35 μg), terfenadine, digoxin, and warfarin.

Although additional specific interaction studies were not performed, montelukast sodium was used concomitantly with a wide range of commonly prescribed drugs in clinical studies without evidence of clinical adverse interactions. These medications included thyroid hormones, sedative hypnotics, non-steroidal anti-inflammatory agents, benzodiazepines, and decongestants.

Phenobarbital, which induces hepatic metabolism, decreased the AUC of montelukast approximately 40% following a single 10 mg dose of montelukast. No dosage adjustment for montelukast sodium is recommended. It is reasonable to employ appropriate clinical monitoring when potent cytochrome P450 enzyme inducers, such as phenobarbital or rifampin, are co-administered with montelukast sodium.

ADVERSE REACTIONS

ADULTS AND ADOLESCENTS 15 YEARS OF AGE AND OLDER

Montelukast sodium has been evaluated for safety in approximately 2600 adult and adolescent patients 15 years of age and older in clinical trials. In placebo-controlled clinical trials, the adverse experiences listed in TABLE 3 reported with montelukast sodium occurred in greater than or equal to 1% of patients and at an incidence greater than that in patients treated with placebo, regardless of causality assessment.

TABLE 3 *Adverse Experiences Occurring in ≥1% of Patients With an Incidence Greater Than That in Patients Treated With Placebo, Regardless of Causality Assessment*

	Montelukast Sodium 10 mg/day (n=1955)	Placebo (n=1180)
Body as a Whole		
Asthenia/fatigue	1.8%	1.2%
Fever	1.5%	0.9%
Pain, abdominal	2.9%	2.5%
Trauma	1.0%	0.8%
Digestive System Disorders		
Dyspepsia	2.1%	1.1%
Gastroenteritis, infectious	1.5%	0.5%
Pain, dental	1.7%	1.0%
Nervous System/Psychiatric		
Dizziness	1.9%	1.4%
Headache	18.4%	18.1%
Respiratory System Disorders		
Congestion, nasal	1.6%	1.3%
Cough	2.7%	2.4%
Influenza	4.2%	3.9%
Skin/Skin Appendages Disorder		
Rash	1.6%	1.2%
Laboratory Adverse Experiences*		
ALT increased	2.1%	2.0%
AST increased	1.6%	1.2%
Pyuria	1.0%	0.9%

* Number of patients tested (montelukast sodium and placebo, respectively): ALT and AST, 1935, 1170; pyuria, 1924, 1159.

The frequency of less common adverse events was comparable between montelukast sodium and placebo.

Cumulatively, 569 patients were treated with montelukast sodium for at least 6 months, 480 for 1 year, and 49 for 2 years in clinical trials. With prolonged treatment, the adverse experience profile did not significantly change.

PEDIATRIC PATIENTS 6-14 YEARS OF AGE

Montelukast sodium has been evaluated for safety in 321 pediatric patients 6-14 years of age. Cumulatively, 169 pediatric patients were treated with montelukast sodium for at least 6 months, and 121 for 1 year or longer in clinical trials. The safety profile of montelukast sodium in the 8 week, double-blind, pediatric efficacy trial was generally similar to the adult safety profile. In pediatric patients 6-14 years of age receiving montelukast sodium, the following events occurred with a frequency ≥2% and more frequently than in pediatric patients who received placebo, regardless of causality assessment: pharyngitis, influenza, fever, sinusitis, nausea, diarrhea, dyspepsia, otitis, viral infection, and laryngitis. The frequency of less common adverse events was comparable between montelukast sodium and placebo. With prolonged treatment, the adverse experience profile did not significantly change.

PEDIATRIC PATIENTS 2-5 YEARS OF AGE

Montelukast sodium has been evaluated for safety in 573 pediatric patients 2-5 years of age in single and multiple dose studies. Cumulatively, 426 pediatric patients 2-5 years of age were treated with montelukast sodium for at least 3 months, 230 for 6 months or longer, and 63 patients for 1 year or longer in clinical trials. Montelukast sodium 4 mg administered once daily at bedtime was generally well tolerated in clinical trials. In pediatric patients 2-5 years of age receiving montelukast sodium, the following events occurred with a frequency ≥2% and more frequently than in pediatric patients who received placebo, regardless of causality assessment: fever, cough, abdominal pain, diarrhea, headache, rhinorrhea, sinusitis, otitis, influenza, rash, ear pain, gastroenteritis, eczema, urticaria, varicella, pneumonia, dermatitis, and conjunctivitis.

PEDIATRIC PATIENTS 12-23 MONTHS AGE

Montelukast sodium has been evaluated for safety in 124 pediatric patients 12-23 months of age. The safety profile of montelukast sodium in a 6 week, double-blind, placebo-controlled clinical study was generally similar to the safety profile in adults and pediatric patients 2-14 years of age. Montelukast sodium administered once daily at bedtime was generally well tolerated. In pediatric patients 12-23 months of age receiving montelukast sodium, the following events occurred with a frequency ≥2% and more frequently than in pediatric patients who received placebo, regardless of causality assessment: upper respiratory infection, wheezing; otitis media; pharyngitis, tonsillitis, cough; and rhinitis. The frequency of less common adverse events was comparable between montelukast sodium and placebo.

POST-MARKETING EXPERIENCE

The following additional adverse reactions have been reported in post-marketing use: Hypersensitivity reactions (including anaphylaxis, angioedema, pruritus, urticaria, and very rarely, hepatic eosinophilic infiltration); dream abnormalities and hallucinations, drowsiness, irritability, restlessness, insomnia, and very rarely seizures; nausea, vomiting, dyspepsia, diarrhea, and very rarely pancreatitis; myalgia including muscle cramps; increased bleeding tendency, bruising; and edema.

In rare cases, patients on therapy with montelukast sodium may present with systemic eosinophilia, sometimes presenting with clinical features of vasculitis consistent with Churg-Strauss syndrome, a condition which is often treated with systemic corticosteroid therapy. These events usually, but not always, have been associated with the reduction of oral corticosteroid therapy. Physicians should be alert to eosinophilia, vasculitic rash, worsening pulmonary symptoms, cardiac complications, and/or neuropathy presenting in their patients. A causal association between montelukast sodium and these underlying conditions has not been established (see PRECAUTIONS, Eosinophilic Conditions).

DOSAGE AND ADMINISTRATION

GENERAL INFORMATION

The safety and efficacy of montelukast sodium was demonstrated in clinical trials where it was administered in the evening without regard to the time of food ingestion. There have been no clinical trials evaluating the relative efficacy of morning versus evening dosing.

Adults and adolescents 15 years of age and older: The dosage for adults and adolescents 15 years of age and older is one 10 mg tablet daily to be taken in the evening.

Pediatric patients 6-14 years of age: The dosage for pediatric patients 6-14 years of age is one 5 mg chewable tablet daily to be taken in the evening. No dosage adjustment within this age group is necessary.

Pediatric patients 2-5 years of age: The dosage for pediatric patients 2-5 years of age is one 4 mg chewable tablet or 1 packet of 4 mg oral granules daily to be taken in the evening.

Pediatric patients 12-23 months of age: The dosage for pediatric patients 12-23 months of age is 1 packet of 4 mg oral granules daily to be taken in the evening. Safety and effectiveness in pediatric patients younger than 12 months of age have not been established.

ADMINISTRATION OF MONTELUKAST SODIUM ORAL GRANULES

Montelukast sodium 4 mg oral granules can be administered either directly in the mouth, or mixed with a spoonful of cold or room temperature soft foods; based on stability studies, only applesauce, carrots, rice or ice cream should be used. The packet should not be opened until ready to use. After opening the packet, the full dose (with or without mixing with food) must be administered within 15 minutes. If mixed with food, montelukast sodium oral granules must not be stored for future use. Discard any unused portion. Montelukast sodium oral granules are not intended to be dissolved in liquid for administration. However, liquids may be taken subsequent to administration. Montelukast sodium oral granules can be administered without regard to the time of meals.

HOW SUPPLIED

CHEWABLE TABLETS

4 mg Chewable Tablets: Pink, oval, bi-convex-shaped chewable tablets, with code "MRK 711" on 1 side and "SINGULAIR" on the other.

5 mg Chewable Tablets: Pink, round, bi-convex-shaped chewable tablets, with code "MRK 275" on 1 side and "SINGULAIR" on the other.

TABLETS

10 mg Tablets: Beige, rounded square-shaped, film-coated tablets, with code "MRK 117" on 1 side and "SINGULAIR" on the other.

ORAL GRANULES

4 mg Oral Granules: White granules with 500 mg net weight, packed in a child-resistant foil packet.

STORAGE

Store Singulair 4 mg chewable tablets, 5 mg chewable tablets, 10 mg film-coated tablets, and the 4 mg oral granules at 25°C (77°F), excursions permitted to 15-30°C (59-86°F). Protect from moisture and light. Store in original package.

PRODUCT LISTING - EQUIVALENTS NOT AVAILABLE

Tablet - Oral - 10 mg

30's	$78.71	SINGULAIR, Allscripts Pharmaceutical Company	54569-4605-00
30's	$91.61	SINGULAIR, Merck & Company Inc	00006-0117-31
90's	$274.84	SINGULAIR, Merck & Company Inc	00006-0117-54
100's	$305.38	SINGULAIR, Merck & Company Inc	00006-0117-28

Tablet, Chewable - Oral - 4 mg

30's	$91.61	SINGULAIR, Merck & Company Inc	00006-0711-31
90's	$274.84	SINGULAIR, Merck & Company Inc	00006-0711-54
100's	$251.88	SINGULAIR, Merck & Company Inc	00006-0711-28

Tablet, Chewable - Oral - 5 mg

30's	$78.71	SINGULAIR, Allscripts Pharmaceutical Company	54569-4736-00
30's	$91.61	SINGULAIR, Merck & Company Inc	00006-0275-31
90's	$274.84	SINGULAIR, Merck & Company Inc	00006-0275-54
100's	$251.67	SINGULAIR, Merck & Company Inc	00006-0275-28

Moricizine Hydrochloride *(001832)*

Categories: Arrhythmia, ventricular; Tachycardia, ventricular; Pregnancy Category B; FDA Approved 1990 Jun
Drug Classes: Antiarrhythmics, class IA
Brand Names: Ethmozine
Cost of Therapy: $98.36 (Arrhythmia; Ethmozine; 300 mg; 2 tablets/day; 30 day supply)

DESCRIPTION

Ethmozine (moricizine hydrochloride) is an orally active antiarrhythmic drug available for administration in tablets containing 200, 250, and 300 mg of moricizine hydrochloride. The chemical name of moricizine hydrochloride is 10-(3-morpholinopropionyl)phenothiazine-2-carbamic acid ethyl ester hydrochloride.

Moricizine hydrochloride is a white to tan crystalline powder, freely soluble in water and has a pKa of 6.4 (weak base). Ethmozine tablets contain: lactose, microcrystalline cellulose, sodium starch glycolate, magnesium stearate and dyes [FD&C blue 1, D&C yellow 10 and FD&C yellow 6 (200 mg tablet); FD&C yellow 6 and FD&C red 40 (250 mg tablet); FD&C blue 1 (300 mg tablet)].

CLINICAL PHARMACOLOGY

MECHANISM OF ACTION

Moricizine HCl is a Class 1 antiarrhythmic agent with potent local anesthetic activity and myocardial membrane stabilizing effects. Moricizine HCl reduces the fast inward current carried by sodium ions.

In isolated dog Purkinje fibers, moricizine HCl shortens Phase II and III repolarization, resulting in a decreased action potential duration and effective refractory period. A dose-related decrease in the maximum rate of Phase O depolarization (V_{max}) occurs without effect on maximum diastolic potential or action potential amplitude. The sinus node and atrial tissue of the dog are not affected.

ELECTROPHYSIOLOGY

Electrophysiology studies in patients with ventricular tachycardia have shown that moricizine HCl, at daily doses of 750 mg and 900 mg, prolongs atrioventricular conduction. Both AV nodal conduction time (AH interval) and His-Purkinje conduction time (HV interval) are prolonged by 10-13% and 21-26%, respectively. The PR interval is prolonged by 16-20% and the QRS by 7-18%. Prolongations of 2-5% in the corrected QT interval result from widening of the QRS interval, but there is shortening of the JT interval, indicating an absence of significant effect on ventricular repolarization. Intra-atrial conduction or atrial effective refractory periods are not consistently affected. In patients without sinus node dysfunction, moricizine HCl has minimal effects on sinus cycle length and sinus node recovery time. These effects may be significant in patients with sinus node dysfunction (see PRECAUTIONS, General, Electrocardiographic Changes/Conduction Abnormalities).

HEMODYNAMICS

In patients with impaired left ventricular function, moricizine HCl has minimal effects on measurements of cardiac performance such as cardiac index, stroke volume index, pulmonary capillary wedge pressure, systemic or pulmonary vascular resistance or ejection fraction, either at rest or during exercise. Moricizine HCl is associated with a small, but consistent increase in resting blood pressure and heart rate. Exercise tolerance in patients with ventricular arrhythmias is unaffected. In patients with a history of congestive heart failure or angina pectoris, exercise duration and rate-pressure product at maximal exercise are unchanged during moricizine HCl administration. Nonetheless, in some cases worsened heart failure in patients with severe underlying heart disease has been attributed to moricizine HCl.

OTHER PHARMACOLOGIC EFFECTS

Although moricizine HCl is chemically related to the neuroleptic phenothiazines, it has no demonstrated central or peripheral dopaminergic activity in animals. Moreover, in patients on chronic moricizine HCl, serum prolactin levels did not increase.

PHARMACOKINETICS AND PHARMACODYNAMICS

The antiarrhythmic and electrophysiologic effects of moricizine HCl are not related in time course or intensity to plasma moricizine concentrations or to the concentrations of any identified metabolite, all of which have short (2-3 hours) half-lives. Following single doses of moricizine HCl, there is a prompt prolongation of the PR interval, which becomes normal within 2 hours, consistent with the rapid fall of plasma moricizine. JT interval shortening, however, peaks at about 6 hours and persists for at least 10 hours. Although an effect on VPD rates is seen within 2 hours after dosing, the full effect is seen after 10-14 hours and persists in full, when therapy is terminated, for more than 10 hours, after which the effect decays slowly, and is still substantial at 24 hours. This suggests either an unidentified, active, long half-life metabolite or a structural or functional "deep compartment" with slow entry from, and release to, the plasma. The following description of parent compound pharmacokinetics is therefore of uncertain relevance to clinical actions.

Following oral administration, moricizine HCl undergoes significant first-past metabolism resulting in an absolute bio-availability of approximately 38%. Peak plasma concentrations of moricizine HCl are usually reached within 0.5-2 hours. Administration 30 minutes after a meal delays the rate of absorption, resulting in lower peak plasma concentrations, but the extent of absorption is not altered. Moricizine HCl plasma levels are proportional to dose over the recommended therapeutic dose range.

The apparent volume of distribution after oral administration is very large (≥300 L) and is not significantly related to body weight. Moricizine HCl is approximately 95% bound to human plasma proteins. This binding interaction is independent of moricizine HCl plasma concentration.

Moricizine HCl undergoes extensive biotransformation. Less than 1% of orally administered moricizine HCl is excreted unchanged in the urine. There are at least 26 metabolites, but no single metabolite has been found to represent as much as 1% of the administered dose, and as stated above, antiarrhythmic response has relatively slow onset and offset. Two metabolites are pharmacologically active in at least one animal model: moricizine sulfoxide and phenothiazine-2-carbamic acid ethyl ester sulfoxide. Each of these metabolites represents a small percentage of the administered dose (<0.6%), is present in lower concentrations in the plasma than the parent drug, and has a plasma elimination half-life of approximately 3 hours.

Moricizine HCl has been shown to induce its own metabolism. Average moricizine HCl plasma concentrations in patients decrease with multiple dosing. This decrease in plasma levels of parent drug does not appear to affect clinical outcome for patients receiving chronic moricizine HCl therapy.

The plasma half-life of moricizine HCl is 1.5-3.5 hours (most values about 2 hours) following single or multiple oral doses in patients with ventricular ectopy. Approximately 56% of the administered dose is excreted in the feces and 39% is excreted in the urine. Some moricizine HCl is also recycled through enterohepatic circulation.

CLINICAL ACTIONS

Moricizine HCl at daily doses of 600-900 mg produces a dose-related reduction in the occurrence of frequent ventricular premature depolarizations (VPDs) and reduces the incidence of nonsustained and sustained ventricular tachycardia (VT). In controlled clinical trials, moricizine HCl has been shown to have antiarrhythmic activity that is generally similar to that of disopyramide, propranolol and quinidine at the doses studied. In controlled and compassionate use programmed electrical stimulation studies (PES), moricizine HCl prevented the induction of sustained ventricular tachycardia in approximately 25% (19/75) of patients. In a post-marketing randomized comparative PES study, moricizine HCl had a response rate of approximately 12% (7/59). Activity of moricizine HCl is maintained during long-term use.

Moricizine HCl is effective in treating ventricular arrhythmias in patients with and without organic heart disease. Moricizine HCl may be effective in patients in whom other antiarrhythmic agents are ineffective, not tolerated and/or contraindicated.

Arrhythmia exacerbation or "rebound" is not noted following discontinuation of moricizine HCl therapy.

INDICATIONS AND USAGE

Moricizine HCl is indicated for the treatment of documented ventricular arrhythmias, such as sustained ventricular tachycardia, that, in the judgement of the physician are life-threatening. Because of the proarrhythmic effects of moricizine HCl, its use with lesser arrhythmias is generally not recommended. Treatment of patients with asymptomatic ventricular premature contractions should be avoided.

Initiation of moricizine HCl treatment, as with other antiarrhythmic agents used to treat life-threatening arrhythmias, should be carried out in the hospital.

Antiarrhythmic drugs have not been shown to enhance survival in patients with ventricular arrhythmias.

CONTRAINDICATIONS

Moricizine HCl is contraindicated in patients with pre-existing second- or third-degree AV block and in patients with right bundle branch block when associated with left hemiblock (bifascicular block) unless a pacemaker is present. Moricizine HCl is also contraindicated in the presence of cardiogenic shock or known hypersensitivity to the drug.

WARNINGS

Mortality moricizine HCl was one of three antiarrhythmic drugs included in the National Heart Lung and Blood Institute's Cardiac Arrhythmia Suppression Trial (CAST I), a long-term multicenter, randomized, double-blind study in patients with asymptomatic non-life-threatening ventricular arrhythmias who had a myocardial infarction more than 6 days, but less than 2 years, previously. An excessive mortality or nonfatal cardiac arrest rate was seen in patients treated with both of the Class IC agents included in the trial, which led to discontinuation of those 2 arms of the trial. The average duration of treatment with these agents was 10 months.

The moricizine HCl and placebo arms of the trial were continued in the NHLBI sponsored CAST II. In this randomized, double-blind trial, patients with asymptomatic non-life-threatening arrhythmias who had a myocardial infarction within 4 to 90 days and left ventricular ejection fraction ≤0.40 prior to enrollment were evaluated. The average duration of treatment with moricizine HCl in this study was 18 months. The study was discontinued because there was no possibility of demonstrating a benefit toward improved survival with moricizine HCl and because of an evolving adverse trend after long-term treatment.

The applicability of the CAST results to other populations (*e.g.,* those without recent myocardial infarction) is uncertain. Considering the known proarrhythmic properties of moricizine HCl and the lack of evidence of improved survival for any antiarrhythmic drug in patients without life-threatening arrhythmias, the use of moricizine HCl, as well as other antiarrhythmic agents, should be reserved for patients with life-threatening ventricular arrhythmias.

PROARRHYTHMIA

Like other antiarrhythmic drugs, moricizine HCl can provoke new rhythm disturbances or make existing arrhythmias worse. These proarrhythmic effects can range from an increase in the frequency of VPDs to the development of new or more severe ventricular tachycardia, e.g., tachycardia that is more sustained or more resistant to conversion to sinus rhythm, with potentially fatal consequences. It is often not possible to distinguish a proarrhythmic effect from the patient's underlying rhythm disorder, so that the occurrence rates given below must be considered approximations. Note also that drug-induced arrhythmias can generally be identified only when they occur early after starting the drug and when the rhythm can be identified, usually because the patient is being monitored. It is clear from the NIH sponsored CAST (Cardiac Arrhythmia Suppression Trial) that some antiarrhythmic drugs can cause increased sudden death mortality, presumably due to new arrhythmias or asystole that do not appear early after treatment but that represent a sustained increased risk.

Domestic pre-marketing trials included 1072 patients given moricizine HCl; 397 had baseline lethal arrhythmias (sustained VT or VF and non-sustained VT with hemodynamic symptoms) and 576 had potentially lethal arrhythmias (increased VPDs or NSVT in patients

M

with known structural heart disease, active ischemia, congestive heart failure or an LVEF <40% and/or CI <2.0 L/min/m^2). In this population there were 40 (3.7%) identified proarrhythmic events, 26 (2.5%) of which were serious, either fatal (6), new hemodynamically significant sustained VT or VF (4), new sustained VT that was not hemodynamically significant (11) or sustained VT that became syncopal/presyncopal when it had not been before (5). Proarrhythmic effects described as incessant ventricular tachycardia were observed in the post-marketing PES study and in post-marketing adverse event reports.

In general, serious proarrhythmic effects in the domestic pre-marketing trials were equally common in patients with more and less severe arrhythmias, 2.5% in the patients with baseline lethal arrhythmias vs 2.8% in patients with potentially lethal arrhythmias, although the patients with serious effects were more likely to have a history of sustained VT (38% vs 23%). In post-marketing comparative PES study, patients treated with moricizine HCl (250-300 mg tid) had a proarrhythmia rate of 14% (8/59).

Five (5) of the 6 fatal proarrhythmic events were in patients with baseline lethal arrhythmias; 4 had prior cardiac arrests. Rates and severity of proarrhythmic events were similar in patients given 600-900 mg of moricizine HCl per day and those given higher doses. Patients with proarrhythmic events were more likely than the overall population to have coronary artery disease (85% vs 67%), history of acute myocardial infarction (75% vs 53%), congestive heart failure (60% vs 43%), and cardiomegaly (55% vs 33%). All of the 6 proarrhythmic deaths were in patients with coronary artery disease; 5/6 each had documented acute myocardial infarction, congestive heart failure, and cardiomegaly.

ELECTROLYTE DISTURBANCES

Hypokalemia, hyperkalemia or hypomagnesemia may alter the effects of Class I antiarrhythmic drugs. Electrolyte imbalances should be corrected before administration of moricizine HCl.

SICK SINUS SYNDROME

Moricizine HCl should be used only with extreme caution in patients with sick sinus syndrome, as it may cause sinus bradycardia, sinus pause or sinus arrest.

PRECAUTIONS

GENERAL

Electrocardiographic Changes/Conduction Abnormalities

Moricizine HCl slows AV nodal and intraventricular conduction, producing dose-related increases in the PR and QRS intervals. In clinical trials, the average increase in the PR interval was 12% and the QRS interval was 14%. Although the QTC interval is increased, this is wholly because of QRS prolongation; the JT interval is shortened, indicating the absence of significant slowing of ventricular repolarization. The degree of lengthening of PR and QRS intervals does not predict efficacy.

In controlled clinical trials and in open studies, the overall incidence of delayed ventricular conduction, including new bundle branch block pattern, was approximately 9.4%. In patients without baseline conduction abnormalities, the frequency of second-degree AV block was 0.2% and third-degree AV block did not occur. In patients with baseline conduction abnormalities, the frequencies of second-degree AV block and third-degree AV block were 0.9% and 1.4%, respectively.

Moricizine HCl therapy was discontinued in 1.6% of patients due to electrocardiographic changes (0.6% due to sinus pause or asystole, 0.2% to AV block, 0.2% to junctional rhythm, 0.4% to intraventricular conduction delay, and 0.2% to wide QRS and/or PR interval).

In patients with pre-existing conduction abnormalities, moricizine HCl therapy should be initiated cautiously. If second- or third-degree AV block occurs, moricizine HCl therapy should be discontinued unless a ventricular pacemaker is in place. When changing the dose of moricizine HCl or adding concomitant medications which may also affect cardiac conduction, patients should be monitored electrocardiographically.

Hepatic Impairment

Patients with significant liver dysfunction have reduced plasma clearance and an increased half-life of moricizine HCl. Although the precise relationship of moricizine HCl levels to effect is not clear, patients with hepatic disease should be treated with lower doses and closely monitored for excessive pharmacological effects, including effects on ECG intervals, before dosage adjustment. Patients with severe liver disease should be administered moricizine HCl with particular care, if at all. (See DOSAGE AND ADMINISTRATION.

Renal Impairment

Plasma levels of intact moricizine HCl are unchanged in hemodialysis patients, but a significant portion (39%) of moricizine HCl is metabolized and excreted in the urine. Although no identified active metabolite is known to increase in people with renal failure, metabolites of unrecognized importance could be affected. For this reason, moricizine HCl should be administered cautiously in patients with impaired renal function. Patients with significant renal dysfunction should be started on lower doses and monitored for excessive pharmacologic effects, including ECG intervals, before dosage adjustment. (See DOSAGE AND ADMINISTRATION.)

Congestive Heart Failure

Most patients with congestive heart failure have tolerated the recommended moricizine HCl daily doses without unusual toxicity or change in effect. Pharmacokinetic differences between moricizine HCl patients with and without congestive heart failure were not apparent (see Hepatic Impairment). In some cases, worsened heart failure has been attributed to moricizine HCl. Patients with pre-existing heart failure should be monitored carefully when moricizine HCl is initiated.

Effects on Pacemaker Threshold

The effect of moricizine HCl on the sensing and pacing thresholds of artificial pacemakers has not been sufficiently studied. In such patients, pacing parameters must be monitored, if moricizine HCl is used.

CARCINOGENESIS, MUTAGENESIS, AND IMPAIRMENT OF FERTILITY

In a 24 month mouse study in which moricizine HCl was administered in the feed at concentrations calculated to provide doses ranging up to 320 mg/kg/day, ovarian tubular adenomas and granulosa cell tumors were limited in occurrence to moricizine HCl treated animals. Although the findings were of borderline statistical significance, or not statistically significant, historical control data indicate that both of these tumors are uncommon in the strain of mouse studied.

In a 24 month study in which moricizine HCl was administered by gavage to rats at doses of 25, 50 and 100 mg/kg/day, Zymbal's Gland Carcinoma was observed in one mid-dose and two high dose males. This tumor appears to be uncommon in the strain of rat studied. Rats of both sexes showed a dose-related increase in hepatocellular cholangioma (also described as bile ductile cystadenoma or cystic hyperplasia) along with fatty metamorphosis, possibly due to disruption of hepatic choline utilization for phospholipid biosynthesis. The rat is known to be uniquely sensitive to alteration in choline metabolism.

Moricizine HCl was not mutagenic when assayed for genotoxicity in *in vitro* bacterial (Ames test) and mammalian (Chinese hamster ovary/hypoxanthine-guanine phosphoribosyl transferase and sister chromatid exchange) cell systems or in *in vivo* mammalian systems (rat bone cytogenicity and mouse micronucleus).

A general reproduction and fertility study was conducted in rats at dose levels up to 6.7 times the maximum recommended human dose of 900 mg/day (based upon 50 kg human body weight) and revealed no evidence of impaired male or female fertility.

PREGNANCY CATEGORY B

Teratogenic Effects

Teratology studies have been performed with moricizine HCl in rats and in rabbits at doses up to 6.7 and 4.7 times the maximum recommended human daily dose, respectively, and have revealed no evidence of harm to the fetus. There are, however, no adequate and well-controlled studies in pregnant women. Because animal reproduction studies are not always predictive of human response, moricizine HCl should be used during pregnancy only if clearly needed.

Nonteratogenic Effects

in a study in which rats were dosed with moricizine hcl prior to mating, during mating and throughout gestation and lactation, dose levels 3.4 and 6.7 times the maximum recommended human daily dose produced a dose-related decrease in pup and maternal weight gain, possibly related to a larger litter size. In a study in which dosing was begun on day 15 of gestation, moricizine hcl, at a level 6.7 times the maximum recommended human daily dose, produced a retardation in maternal weight gain but no effect on pup growth.

NURSING MOTHERS

Moricizine HCl is secreted in the milk of laboratory animals and has been reported to be present in human milk. Because of the potential for serious adverse reactions in nursing infants from moricizine HCl, a decision should be made whether to discontinue the drug, taking into account the importance of the drug to the mother.

PEDIATRIC USE

The safety and effectiveness of moricizine HCl in children less than 18 years of age have not been established.

DRUG INTERACTIONS

No significant changes in serum digoxin levels or pharmacokinetics have been observed in patients or healthy subjects receiving concomitant moricizine HCl therapy. Concomitant use was associated with additive prolongation of the PR interval, but not with a significant increase in the rate of second- or third-degree AV block.

Concomitant administration of cimetidine resulted in a decrease in moricizine HCl clearance of 49% and a 1.4-fold increase in plasma levels in healthy subjects. During clinical trials, no significant changes in the efficacy or tolerance of moricizine HCl have been observed in patients receiving concomitant cimetidine therapy. Patients on cimetidine should have moricizine HCl therapy initiated at relatively low doses, not more than 600 mg/day. Patients should be monitored when concomitant cimetidine therapy is instituted or discontinued or when the moricizine HCl dose is changed.

Concomitant administration of beta blocker therapy did not reveal significant changes in overall electrocardiographic intervals in patients. In one controlled study, moricizine HCl and propranolol administered concomitantly produced a small additive increase in the PR interval.

Theophylline clearance and plasma half-life were significantly affected by multiple dose moricizine HCl administration when both conventional and sustained release theophylline were given to healthy subjects (clearance increased 44-66% and plasma half-life decreased 19-33%). Plasma theophylline levels should be monitored when concomitant moricizine HCl is initiated or discontinued.

Because of possible additive pharmacologic effects, caution is indicated when moricizine HCl is used with any drug that affects cardiac electrophysiology. Uncontrolled experience in patients indicates no serious adverse interaction during the concomitant use of moricizine HCl and diuretics, vasodilators, antihypertensive drugs, calcium channel blockers, beta-blockers, angiotensin-converting enzyme inhibitors, or warfarin. Plasma warfarin levels, warfarin pharmacokinetics, and prothrombin times were unaffected during multiple dose moricizine HCl administration to young, healthy male subjects in a controlled study. However, there are isolated reports of the need to either increase or decrease warfarin doses after initiation of moricizine HCl. Some patients who were taking warfarin with a stable prothrombin time experienced excessive prolongation of the prothrombin time following the initiation of moricizine HCl. In some cases, liver enzymes also were elevated. Bleeding or bruising may occur. When moricizine HCl is started or stopped in a patient stabilized on warfarin, more frequent prothrombin time monitoring is advisable.

Results from *in vitro* studies do not suggest alterations in moricizine HCl plasma protein binding in the presence of other highly plasma protein bound drugs.

ADVERSE REACTIONS

The most serious adverse reaction reported for moricizine HCl is proarrhythmia (see WARNINGS). This occurred in 3.7% of 1072 patients with ventricular arrhythmias who received a wide range of doses under a variety of circumstances.

In addition to discontinuations because of proarrhythmias, in controlled clinical trials and in open studies, adverse reactions led to discontinuation of moricizine HCl in 7% of 1105 patients with ventricular and supraventricular arrhythmias, including 3.2% due to nausea, 1.6% due to ECG abnormalities (principally conduction defects, sinus pause, junctional rhythm, or AV block), 1% due to congestive heart failure, and 0.3-0.4% due to dizziness, anxiety, drug fever, urinary retention, blurred vision, gastrointestinal upset, rash, and laboratory abnormalities.

The most frequently occurring adverse reactions in the 1072 patients (including all adverse experiences whether or not considered moricizine HCl-related by the investigator) were dizziness (15.1%), nausea (9.6%), headache (8.0%), fatigue (5.9%), palpitations (5.8%) and dyspnea (5.7%). Dizziness appears to be related to the size of each dose. In a comparison of 900 mg/day given at 450 mg bid or 300 mg tid, more than 20% of patients experienced dizziness on the bid regimen vs 12% on the tid regimen.

Adverse reactions reported by less than 5%, but in 2% or greater of the patients were: sustained ventricular tachycardia, hypesthesias, abdominal pain, dyspepsia, vomiting, sweating, cardiac chest pain, asthenia, nervousness, paresthesias, congestive heart failure, musculoskeletal pain, diarrhea, dry mouth, cardiac death, sleep disorders, and blurred vision.

Adverse reactions infrequently reported (in less than 2% of the patients) were:

Cardiovascular: Hypotension, hypertension, syncope, supraventricular arrhythmias (including atrial fibrillation/flutter), cardiac arrest, bradycardia, pulmonary embolism, myocardial infarction, vasodilation, cerebrovascular events, thrombophlebitis;

Nervous System: Tremor, anxiety, depression, euphoria, confusion, somnolence, agitation, seizure, coma, abnormal gait, hallucinations, nystagmus, diplopia, speech disorder, akathisia, loss of memory, ataxia, abnormal coordination, dyskinesia, vertigo, tinnitus;

Genitourinary: Urinary retention or frequency, dysuria, urinary incontinence, kidney pain, impotence, decreased libido;

Respiratory: Hyperventilation, apnea, asthma, pharyngitis, cough, sinusitis;

Gastrointestinal: Anorexia, bitter taste, dysphagia, flatulence, ileus;

Other: Drug fever, hypothermia, temperature intolerance, eye pain, rash, pruritus, dry skin, urticaria, swelling of the lips and tongue, periorbital edema.

During moricizine HCl therapy, 2 patients developed thrombocytopenia that may have been drug-related. Clinically significant elevations in liver function tests (bilirubin, serum transaminases) and jaundice consistent with hepatitis were rarely reported. Although a cause and effect relationship has not been established, caution is advised in patients who develop unexplained signs of hepatic dysfunction, and consideration should be given to discontinuing therapy.

Three (3) patients developed rechallenge-confirmed drug fever, with 1 patient experiencing an elevation above 103°F (to 105°F, with rigors). Fevers occurred at about 2 weeks in 2 cases, and after 21 weeks in the third. Fevers resolved within 48 hours of discontinuation of moricizine.

Adverse reactions were generally similar in patients over 65 (n=375) and under 65 (n=697), although discontinuation of therapy for reasons other than proarrhythmia was more common in older patients (13.9% vs 7.7%). Overall mortality was greater in older patients (9.3% vs 3.9%), but those were not deaths attributed to treatment and the older patients had more serious underlying heart disease.

TABLE 1 compares the most common (occurrence in more than 2% of the patients) noncardiac adverse reactions (*i.e.*, drug-related or of unknown relationship) in controlled clinical trials during the first 1-2 weeks of therapy with moricizine HCl, quinidine, placebo, disopyramide, or propranolol in patients with ventricular arrhythmias.

TABLE 1 *Incidence (%) of the Most Common Adverse Reactions*

(Therapy Duration = 1-14 Days)

Adverse Reactions	Moricizine n=1072	Placebo n=618	Quinidine n=110	Disopyramide n=31	Propranolol n=24
Dizziness	121 (11.3%)	33 (5.3%)	8 (7.3%)	—	2 (8.3%)
Nausea	74 (6.9%)	18 (2.9%)	7 (6.4%)	3 (9.7%)	—
Headache	62 (5.8%)	27 (4.4%)	—	—	4 (16.7%)
Pain	41 (3.8%)	31 (5.0%)	6 (5.5%)	2 (6.5%)	—
Dyspnea	41 (3.8%)	22 (3.6%)	—	—	—
Hypesthesia	40 (3.7%)	—	3 (2.7%)	—	—
Fatigue	33 (3.1%)	16 (2.6%)	6 (5.5%)	2 (6.5%)	3 (12.5%)
Vomiting	22 (2.1%)	—	—	—	—
Dry mouth	—	—	—	11 (35.5%)	—
Nervousness	—	—	—	3 (9.7%)	—
Blurred vision	—	—	3 (2.7%)	2 (6.5%)	3 (12.5%)
Diarrhea	—	—	25 (22.7%)	—	—
Constipation	—	—	—	2 (6.5%)	—
Somnolence	—	—	—	—	2 (8.3%)
Urinary Retention	—	—	—	4 (12.9%)	—

DOSAGE AND ADMINISTRATION

The dosage of moricizine HCl must be individualized on the basis of antiarrhythmic response and tolerance. Clinical, cardiac rhythm monitoring, electrocardiogram intervals, exercise testing, and/or programmed electrical stimulation testing may be used to guide antiarrhythmic response and dosage adjustment. In general, the patients will be at high risk and should be hospitalized for the initiation of therapy (see INDICATIONS AND USAGE).

The usual adult dosage is between 600 and 900 mg/day, given every 8 hours in 3 equally divided doses. Within this range, the dosage can be adjusted as tolerated, in increments of 150 mg/day at 3 day intervals, until the desired effect is obtained. Patients with life-threatening arrhythmias who exhibit a beneficial response as judged by objective criteria (Holter monitoring, programmed electrical stimulation, exercise testing, etc.) can be maintained on chronic moricizine HCl therapy. As the antiarrhythmic effect of moricizine HCl persists for more than 12 hours, some patients whose arrhythmias are well-controlled on a q8h regimen may be given the same total daily dose in a q12h regimen to increase convenience and help assure compliance. When higher doses are used, patients may experience more dizziness and nausea on the q12h regimen.

PATIENTS WITH HEPATIC IMPAIRMENT

Patients with hepatic disease should be started at 600 mg/day or lower and monitored closely, including measurement of ECG intervals, before dosage adjustment.

PATIENTS WITH RENAL IMPAIRMENT:

Patients with significant renal dysfunction should be started at 600 mg/day or lower and monitored closely, including measurement of ECG intervals, before dosage adjustment.

TRANSFER TO MORICIZINE HCl:

Recommendations for transferring patients from another antiarrhythmic to moricizine HCl can be given based on theoretical considerations. Previous antiarrhythmic therapy should be withdrawn for 1-2 plasma half-lives before starting moricizine HCl at the recommended dosages. In patients in whom withdrawal of a previous antiarrhythmic is likely to produce life-threatening arrhythmias, hospitalization is recommended (see TABLE 2).

TABLE 2

Transferred From:	Start Moricizine HCl
Quinidine, Disopyramide	6-12 hours after last dose
Procainamide	3-6 hours after last dose
Encainide, Propafenone,	8-12 hours after last dose
Tocainide, or Mexiletine Flecainide	12-24 hours after last dose

HOW SUPPLIED

Ethmozine is available as follows:

200 mg: Light green oval, convex, film-coated tablets.

250 mg: Light orange oval, convex, film-coated tablets.

300 mg: Light blue oval, convex, film-coated tablets.

Storage: Store at controlled room temperature: 15-30°C (59-86°F) in a tightly-closed, light resistant container. Protect from light.

PRODUCT LISTING - RATED THERAPEUTICALLY EQUIVALENT

Tablet - Oral - 250 mg

100's	$137.14	ETHMOZINE, Roberts Pharmaceutical Corporation	54092-0047-01
100's	$137.14	ETHMOZINE, Roberts Pharmaceutical Corporation	54092-0047-52

Tablet - Oral - 300 mg

100's	$145.92	ETHMOZINE, Roberts Pharmaceutical Corporation	54092-0048-52
100's	$163.94	ETHMOZINE, Roberts Pharmaceutical Corporation	54092-0048-01

PRODUCT LISTING - EQUIVALENTS NOT AVAILABLE

Tablet - Oral - 200 mg

100's	$120.61	ETHMOZINE, Roberts Pharmaceutical Corporation	54092-0046-01

Morphine Sulfate *(001833)*

For related information, see the comparative table section in Appendix A.

Categories: Anesthesia, adjunct; Pain, moderate to severe; Pregnancy Category C; DEA Class CII; FDA Approved 1984 Sep; WHO Formulary; Orphan Drugs

Drug Classes: Analgesics, narcotic

Brand Names: Astramorph-Pf; **Duramorph**; Infumorph; Kadian; MS Contin; MSIR; OMS; Oramorph SR; RMS; Roxanol

Foreign Brand Availability: Actiskenan (France); Anafil - L.C. (Mexico); Anafil - S.T. (Mexico); Anamorph (Australia); Contalgin (Denmark); Continue DR (Korea); Dolcontin (Finland; Sweden); Dolcontin Depottab (Norway); Duralmor (Mexico); Duromorph (England); Graten (Mexico); Kapanol (Australia); Kapanol LP (France); La Morph (New-Zealand); Longphine SR (Korea); M-Long (Germany); MCR (Israel); M.Elson (Hong-Kong); M-Eslon (Canada); Meslon (Colombia); M.I.R. (Israel); M S Contin (Canada); MS-Contin (Korea); MSI (Germany); MS Mono (Australia); MSP (Israel); MST 10 Mundipharma (Germany); MST 30 Mundipharma (Germany); MST 60 Mundipharma (Germany); MST 100 Mundipharma (Germany); MST 200 Mundipharma (Germany); MST Continus (Bahamas; Bahrain; Barbados; Belize; Benin; Bermuda; Burkina-Faso; Curacao; Cyprus; Czech-Republic; Egypt; England; Ethiopia; Gambia; Ghana; Guinea; Guyana; Hungary; Indonesia; Iran; Iraq; Ireland; Ivory-Coast; Jamaica; Jordan; Kenya; Kuwait; Lebanon; Liberia; Libya; Malawi; Malaysia; Mali; Mauritania; Mauritius; Mexico; Morocco; Netherland-Antilles; New-Zealand; Niger; Nigeria; Oman; Philippines; Qatar; Republic-of-Yemen; Saudi-Arabia; Senegal; Seychelles; Sierra-Leone; South-Africa; Spain; Sudan; Surinam; Syria; Taiwan; Tanzania; Trinidad; Tunia; Uganda; United-Arab-Emirates; Zambia; Zimbabwe); MST Continus Retard (Switzerland); Morcontin Continus (India); Morficontin (Greece); Morphine Mixtures (Australia); Moscontin (France); Mundidol Retard (Austria); Oramorph (England); Ra-Morph (New-Zealand); Relimal (Philippines); Sevredol (New-Zealand); SRM-Rotard (Singapore); Statex (Canada; Singapore)

Cost of Therapy: $13.02 (Pain; MSIR; 15 mg; 6 tablets/day; 10 day supply)
$7.29 (Pain; Generic Tablets; 15 mg; 6 tablets/day; 10 day supply)
$37.87 (Pain; MS Contin; 30 mg; 2 tablets/day; 10 day supply)
$14.17 (Pain; Generic Extended Release Tablets; 30 mg; 2 tablets/day; 10 day supply)

HCFA JCODE(S): J2270 up to 10 mg IM, IV, SC; J2271 100 mg IM, IV, SC; J2275 per 10 mg IM, IV, SC

DESCRIPTION

Morphine sulfate occurs as odorless, white, feathery, silky crystals, cubical masses of crystals, or white crystalline powder. It has a solubility of 1 in 21 parts of water and 1 in 1000 parts of alcohol, but is practically insoluble in chloroform or ether. The octal:water partition

M

coefficient of morphine is 1.42 at physiologic pH and the pKb is 7.9 for the tertiary nitrogen (mostly ionized at pH 7.4).

The chemical name for morphine sulfate is 7,8-didehydro-4,5α-epoxy-17-methylmorphinan-3,6α-diol sulfate (2:1) (salt), pentahydrate.

The empirical formula is $(C_{17}H_{19}NO_3)_2 \cdot H_2SO_4 \cdot 5H_2O$. Its molecular weight is 758.83.

Immediate-Release Capsules: Each morphine sulfate immediate-release capsule for oral administration contains 15 or 30 mg of morphine sulfate. *Inactive Ingredients:* FD&C blue no. 1, FD&C blue no. 2, FD&C red no. 40, FD&C yellow no. 6, gelatin, hydroxypropyl methylcellulose, lactose, polyethylene glycol, polysorbate 80, polyvinylpyrrolidone, starch, sucrose, titanium dioxide, and other ingredients. In addition, the 30 mg capsule contains black iron oxide and D&C red no. 28.

Immediate-Release Tablets: Each morphine sulfate immediate-release tablet for oral administration contains 15 or 30 mg of morphine sulfate. *Inactive Ingredients:* Corn starch, lactose, magnesium stearate, and talc.

Injection: The injectable form is a sterile solution of morphine sulfate in water for injection. Each ml of morphine sulfate injection contains 15 mg (20 µg/mol) morphine sulfate, with 0.5% chlorobutanol (chloroform derivative) and not more than 0.1% sodium bisulfate.

Oral Solution: Each 5 ml of morphine sulfate immediate-release oral solution contains 10 or 20 mg of morphine sulfate.

Oral Solution Concentrate: Each 1 ml of morphine sulfate immediate-release oral solution concentrate contains 20 mg of morphine sulfate.

Kadian Controlled-Release Capsules: Each Kadian controlled-release capsule contains either 20, 50 or 100 mg of morphine sulfate and the following ingredients common to all strengths: hydroxypropyl methylcellulose, ethylcellulose, methacrylic acid copolymer, polyethylene glycol, diethyl phthalate, talc, black ink sw, corn starch and sucrose.

MS Contin Controlled-Release Tablets: Each MS Contin controlled-release tablet contains either 15, 30, 60, or 100 mg morphine sulfate. *Inactive Ingredients:* Cetostearyl alcohol, hydroxyethyl cellulose, hydroxypropyl methylcellulose, lactose, magnesium stearate, talc, titanium dioxide and other ingredients and may contain FD&C blue no.1, FD&C blue no. 2, FD&C red no. 40, FD&C yellow no. 6.

Suppositories: Each Roxanol suppository for rectal administration contains: morphine sulfate: 5, 10, 20, or 30 mg. Each suppository contains morphine sulfate, butylated hydroxyanisole, colloidal silicon dioxide, and hydrogenated suppository base, for rectal administration. Morphine sulfate acts as a narcotic analgesic.

CLINICAL PHARMACOLOGY

PHARMACOKINETICS

General

Injection

Morphine sulfate is a potent, centrally active analgesic. Other actions include respiratory depression; depression of the cough center;-release of antidiuretic hormone; activation of the vomiting center; pupillary constriction; a decrease in gastric, pancreatic, and biliary secretion; a reduction in intestinal motility; an increase in biliary tract pressure; and an increased amplitude of ureteral contractions.

Onset of analgesia following intramuscular or subcutaneous administration occurs within 10-30 minutes. The effect persists for 4-5 hours.

Approximately 90% of a parenteral dose of morphine appears in the urine within 24 hours as the product of glucuronide conjugation. Most of the remainder is excreted in the bile and eliminated in the feces.

Oral Forms

Following oral administration of a given dose of morphine controlled-release tablets, the amount ultimately absorbed is essentially the same whether the source is morphine sulfate controlled-release or a conventional formulation. Morphine is-released from morphine sulfate controlled-release somewhat more slowly than from conventional oral preparations. Because of pre-systemic elimination (*i.e.*, metabolism in the gut wall and liver) only about 40% of the administered dose reaches the central compartment.

Morphine is a natural product that is the prototype for the class of natural and synthetic opioid analgesics. Opioids produce a wide spectrum of pharmacologic effects including analgesia, dysphoria, euphoria, somnolence, respiratory depression, diminished gastrointestinal motility, altered circulatory dynamics, histamine-release and physical dependence.

Morphine produces both its therapeutic and its adverse effects by interaction with one or more classes of specific opioid receptors located throughout the body. Morphine acts as a pure agonist, binding with and activating opioid receptors at sites in the peri-aqueductal and peri-ventricular grey matter, the ventro-medial medulla and the spinal cord to produce analgesia.

Suppositories

Morphine sulfate given as a rectal suppository can produce analgesic effects and duration similar to that of oral administration at similar dose levels. Analgesic effects are commonly seen 20-60 minutes after administration.

Central Nervous System

The principal actions of therapeutic value of morphine are analgesia, sedation, and alterations of mood. Opioids of this class do not usually eliminate pain, but they do reduce the perception of pain by the central nervous system.

The precise mechanism of analgesic action is unknown. However, specific CNS opiate receptors and endogenous compounds with morphine-like activity have been identified throughout the brain and spinal cord and are likely to play a role in the expression of analgesic effects.

Morphine produces respiratory depression by direct action on brain stem respiratory centers. The mechanism of respiratory depression involves a reduction in the responsiveness of the brain stem respiratory centers to increases in carbon dioxide tension, and to electrical stimulation.

Morphine depresses the cough reflex by direct effect on the cough center in the medulla. Antitussive effects may occur with doses lower than those usually required for analgesia.

Morphine causes miosis, even in total darkness, and little tolerance develops to this effect. Pinpoint pupils are a sign of opioid overdose but are not pathognomonic (*e.g.*, pontine lesions of hemorrhagic or ischemic origins may produce similar findings). Marked mydriasis rather than miosis may be seen due to severe hypoxia in overdose situations.

Gastrointestinal Tract and Other Smooth Muscle

Gastric, biliary and pancreatic secretions are decreased by morphine. Morphine causes a reduction in motility associated with an increase in tone in the antrum of the stomach and duodenum. Digestion of food in the small intestine is delayed and propulsive contractions are decreased. Propulsive peristaltic waves in the colon are decreased, while tone is increased to the point of spasm. The end result is constipation. Morphine can cause a marked increase in biliary tract pressure as a result of spasm of the sphincter of Oddi.

Cardiovascular System

Morphine produces peripheral vasodilation which may result in orthostatic hypotension or syncope.-Release of histamine can occur and may be induced by morphine and can contribute to opioid-induced hypotension. Manifestations of histamine-release and/or peripheral vasodilation may include pruritus, flushing, red eyes and sweating.

Distribution

Once absorbed, morphine is distributed to skeletal muscle, kidneys, liver, intestinal tract, lungs, spleen and brain. The volume of distribution of morphine is approximately 3-4 L/kg. Morphine is 30-35% reversibly bound to plasma proteins. Although the primary site of action of morphine is in the CNS, only small quantities pass the blood-brain barrier. Morphine also crosses the placental membranes (see PRECAUTIONS, Pregnancy Category C) and has been found in breast milk (see PRECAUTIONS, Nursing Mothers).

Metabolism

The major pathway of the detoxification of morphine is conjugation, either with D-glucuronic acid in the liver to produce glucuronides or with sulfuric acid to give morphine-3-etheral sulfate. Although a small fraction (less than 5%) of morphine is demethylated, for all practical purposes, virtually all morphine is converted to glucuronide metabolites including morphine-3-glucuronide, M3G (about 50%) and morphine-6-glucuronide, M6G (about 5-15%). Studies in healthy subjects and cancer patients have shown that the glucuronide metabolite to morphine mean molar ratios (based on AUC) are similar after both single doses and at steady state for morphine sulfate controlled-release capsules, 12 hour tablets and morphine sulfate solution.

M3G has no significant analgesic activity. M6G has shown to have opioid agonist and analgesic activity in humans.

The glucuronide system has a very high capacity and is not easily saturated, even in disease. Therefore, the rate of delivery of morphine to the gut and liver does not influence the total and/or the relative quantities of the various metabolites formed. Moreover, even if rate affected the relative amounts of each metabolite formed, it should be unimportant clinically because morphine's metabolites are ordinarily inactive.

The following pharmacokinetic parameters show considerable inter-subject variation but are representative of average values reported in the literature. The volume of distribution (Vd) for morphine is 4 L/kg, and its terminal elimination half-life is approximately 2-4 hours.

Following the administration of conventional oral morphine products, approximately 50% of the morphine that will reach the central compartment intact reaches it within 30 minutes. Following the administration of an equal amount of morphine sulfate controlled-release to normal volunteers, however, this extent of absorption occurs, on average, after 1.5 hours.

Variation in the physical/mechanical properties of a formulation of an oral morphine drug product can affect both its absolute bioavailability and its absorption rate constant (Ka). The formulation employed in morphine sulfate extended-release tablets has not been show to affect morphine's bioavailability, but does decrease its apparent Ka. The basic pharmacokinetic parameters (*e.g.*, volume of distribution [Vd], elimination rate constant [Ke], clearance [Cl]) are fundamental properties of morphine in the organism. However, in chronic use, the possibility that shifts in metabolite to parent drug ratios may occur cannot be excluded.

When immediate-release oral morphine is given on a fixed dosing regimen, steady state is achieved in about a day.

For a given dose and dosing interval, the AUC and average blood concentration of morphine at steady state (Css) will be independent of the specific type of oral formulation administered so long as the formulations have the same absolute bioavailability. The absorption rate of a formulation will, however, affect the maximum (C_{max}) and minimum (C_{min}) blood levels and the times of their occurrence.

While there is no predictable relationship between morphine blood levels and analgesic response, effective analgesia will not occur below some minimum blood level in a given patient. The minimum effective blood level for analgesia will vary among patients, especially among patients who have been previously treated with potent mu (µ) agonist opioids. Similarly, there is no predictable relationship between blood morphine concentration and untoward clinical responses; again, however, higher concentration are more likely to be toxic than lower ones.

Excretion

Approximately 10% of morphine dose is excreted unchanged in the urine. Most of the dose is excreted in the urine as M3G and M6G. A small amount of the glucuronide metabolites is excreted in the bile and there is some minor enterohepatic cycling. Seven (7) to 10% of administered morphine is excreted in the feces.

The mean adult plasma clearance is about 20-30 ml/minute/kg. The effective terminal half-life of morphine after IV administration is reported to be approximately 2.0 hours. Longer plasma sampling in some studies suggests a longer terminal half-life of morphine of about 15 hours.

Controlled-Release Capsules

Controlled-release capsules contain polymer coated sustained-release pellets of morphine sulfate that-release morphine significantly more slowly than form morphine sulfate tablets and shorter-acting controlled-release oral morphine sulfate preparations. Controlled-release capsules activity is primarily due to morphine. One metabolite, morphine-6-glucuronide, has been shown to have analgesic activity, but poorly crosses the blood-brain barrier.

The single-dose pharmacokinetics of Kadian are linear over the dosage range of 30-100 mg. The single dose and multiple dose pharmacokinetic parameters of the controlled-release capsules in normal volunteers are summarized in TABLE 1.

TABLE 1 *Mean Pharmacokinetic Parameters (%Coefficient Variation) Resulting From a Fasting Single Dose Study in Normal Volunteers and a Multiple Dose Study in Patients with Cancer Pain*

	AUC * † (ng·h/ml)	C_{max} † (ng/ml)	T_{max} (h)	C_{min} † (ng/ml)	Fluctuation‡
Single Dose (n=24)					
Kadian capsule	271.0 (19.4)	15.6 (24.4)	8.6 (41.1)	na§	na
Controlled-release tablet	304.3 (19.1)	30.5 (32.1)	2.5 (52.6)	na	na
Morphine solution	362.4 (42.6)	64.4 (38.2)	0.9 (55.8)	na	na
Multiple Dose (n=24)					
Kadian capsule q24h	500.9 (38.6)	37.3 (37.7)	10.3 (32.2)	9.9 (52.3)	3.0 (45.5)
Controlled-release tablet q12h	457.3 (40.2)	36.9 (42.0)	4.4 (53.0)	7.6 (60.3)	4.1 (51.5)

* For single dose AUC=AUC(0-48h), for multiple dose AUC=AUC(0-24h), at steady state.
† For single dose parameter normalized to 100 mg, for multiple dose parameter normalized to 100 mg per 24 hours.
‡ Steady-state fluctuation in plasma concentrations=C_{max}-C_{min}/C_{min}.
§ Not applicable.

Immediate and Controlled-Release Oral Forms

The elimination of morphine occurs primarily as renal excretion of 3-morphine glucuronide. A small amount of the glucuronide conjugate is excreted in the bile, and there is some minor enterohepatic recycling.

The elimination half-life of morphine is reported to vary between 2-4 hours, however, a longer term half-life of about 15 hours has been reported in studies where blood has been sampled up to 48 hours. Thus, steady state is probably achieved on most regimens within a day. Because morphine is primarily metabolized to inactive metabolites, the effects of renal disease on morphine's elimination are not likely to be pronounced. However, as with any drug, caution should be taken to guard against unanticipated accumulation if renal and/or hepatic function is seriously impaired.

Individual differences in the metabolism of morphine suggest that morphine sulfate immediate-release oral solutions, tablets and capsules be dosed conservatively according to the dosing initiation and titration recommendations in DOSAGE AND ADMINISTRATION.

SPECIAL POPULATIONS

Geriatric

The elderly may have increased sensitivity to morphine and may achieve higher and more variable serum levels than younger patients. In adults, the duration of analgesia increases progessively with age, though the degree of analgesia remains unchanged. Morphine sulfate pharmacokinetics have not been investigated in elderly patients (>65 years) although such patients were included in the clinical studies.

Nursing Mothers

Morphine is excreted in the maternal milk, and the milk to plasma morphine AUC ratio is about 2.5:1. The amount of morphine received by the infant depends on the maternal plasma concentration, amount of milk ingested by the infant, and the extent of first pass metabolism.

Pediatric

Infants under 1 month of age have a prolonged elimination half-life and decreased clearance relative to older infants and children. The clearance of morphine and its elimination half-life begin to approach adult values by the second month of life. Children old enough to take capsules should have pharmacokinetic parameters similar to adults, dosed on a per kilogram basis (see PRECAUTIONS, Pediatric Use).

Gender

No meaningful differences between male and female patients were demonstrated in the analysis of the pharmacokinetic data from clinical studies.

Race

Pharmacokinetic differences due to race may exist. Chinese subjects given intravenous morphine in one study had a higher clearance when compared to caucasian subjects (1852 ± 116 ml/min versus 1495 ± 80 ml/min).

Hepatic Failure

The pharmacokinetics of morphine were found to be significantly altered in individuals with alcoholic cirrhosis. The clearance was found to decrease with a corresponding increase in half-life. The M3G and M6G to morphine plasma AUC ratios also decreased in these patients indicating a decrease in metabolic activity.

Renal Insufficiency

The pharmacokinetics of morphine are altered in renal failure patients. AUC is increased and clearance is decreased. The metabolites, M3G and M6G accumulate several fold in renal failure patients compared with healthy subjects.

PHARMACODYNAMICS

The relationship between the blood level of morphine and the analgesic response will depend on the patient's age, state of health, medical condition, and the extent of previous opioid treatment.

A minimum effective concentration (MEC) of morphine for pain relief has been reported as 27.2 ± 14.5 ng/ml (mean ±SD) in cancer patients treated with morphine solution. These results compare with the MEC for plasma morphine reported as 14.7 ± 4.8 ng/ml (mean ±SD) in patients with postoperative pain. The high degree of variation is of clinical significance as it may result in either under-dosing or over-dosing if the dosage is not adjusted to the patient's clinical status and analgesic response (see PRECAUTIONS and DOSAGE AND ADMINISTRATION).

For opioid-tolerant patients the situation is much more complex. Some patients will become rapidly tolerant to the analgesic effects of morphine, and will require high daily oral morphine doses for adequate pain control. Since the development of tolerance to both the therapeutic and adverse effects of opioids is highly individualized, the dose of morphine should be individualized to the patient's condition and should not be based on an arbitrary choice of a dose or blood level to be achieved.

Plasma Level-Analgesia Relationships

In any particular patient, both analgesic effects and plasma morphine concentrations are related to the morphine dose. In non-tolerant individuals, plasma morphine concentration-efficacy relationships have been demonstrated and suggest that opiate receptors occupy effector compartments, leading to a lag-time, or hysteresis, between rapid changes in plasma morphine concentrations and the effects of such changes. The most direct and predictable concentration-effect relationships can, therefore, be expected at distribution equilibrium and/or steady state conditions. In general, the minimum effective analgesic concentration in the plasma of non-tolerant patients ranges from approximately 5-20 ng/ml.

While plasma morphine-efficacy relationships can be demonstrated in non-tolerant individuals, they are influenced by a wide variety of factors and are not generally useful as a guide to the clinical use of morphine. The effective dose in opiod-toerlant patients may be 10-50 times as great (or greater) than the appropriate dose for opioid-naive individuals. Dosages of morphine should be chosen and must be titrated on the bases of clinical evaluation of the patient and the balance between therapeutic and adverse effects.

For any fixed dose and dosing interval, morphine sulfate extended-release tablets will have at steady state, a lower C_{max} and a higher C_{min} than conventional morphine. This is a potential advantage; a reduced fluctuation in morphine concentration during the dosing interval should keep morphine blood levels more centered within the theoretical "therapeutic window". (Fluctuation for a dosing interval is defined as [C_{max}-C_{min}]/Css average].) On the other hand, the degree of fluctuation in serum morphine concentration might conceivably affect other phenomena. For example, reduced fluctuations in blood morphine concentrations might influence the rate of tolerance induction.

The elimination of morphine occurs primarily as renal excretion of 3-morphine glucuronide. A small amount of the glucuronide conjugate is excreted in the bile, and there is some minor enterohepatic recycling. Because morphine is primarily metabolized to inactive metabolites, the effects of renal disease on morphine's elimination are not likely pronounced. However, as with any drug, caution should be taken to guard against unanticipated accumulation if and/or hepatic function is seriously impaired.

CONTROLLED-RELEASE

Absorption

Following the administration of oral morphine solution, approximately 50% of the morphine absorbed reached the systemic circulation within 30 minutes. However, following the administration of an equal amount of morphine sulfate controlled-release to healthy volunteers, this occurs, on average, after 8 hours. As with most forms of oral morphine, because of presystemic elimination, only about 20-40% of the administered dose reaches the systemic circulation.

Food Effects

While concurrent administration of food slows the rate of absorption of morphine sulfate controlled-release, the extent of absorption is not affected and morphine sulfate controlled-release can be administered without regard to meals. However, data from at least one study suggests that concurrent administration of morphine sulfate extended-release tablets with a fatty meal may cause a slight decrease in peak plasma concentration.

Steady State

When morphine sulfate is given on a fixed dosing regimen to patients with chronic pain due to malignancy, steady state is achieved in about 2 days. At steady state, morphine sulfate controlled-release capsules will have significantly lower C_{max} and a higher C_{min} than equivalent doses of oral morphine solution and some other controlled-release preparations.

When given once-daily (every 24 hours) to 24 patients with malignancy, Kadian (morphine sulfate controlled-release capsules) had a similar C_{max} and higher C_{min} at steady state in clinical usage, when compared to twice-daily (every 12 hours) MS Contin (morphine sulfate controlled-release tablets), given at an equivalent total daily dosage. Drug-disease interactions are frequently seen in the older and more gravely ill patients, and may result in both altered absorption and reduced clearance as compared to normal volunteers (see Geriatric, Hepatic Failure, and Renal Insufficiency).

DRUG-DRUG INTERACTIONS

The known drug interactions involving morphine are pharmacodynamic, not pharmacokinetic (see DRUG INTERACTIONS).

M

INDICATIONS AND USAGE

CONTROLLED-RELEASE ORAL FORMS

Morphine sulfate controlled-release capsules and tablets are indicated for the management of moderate to severe pain where treatment with an opioid analgesic is indicated for more than a few days (see CLINICAL PHARMACOLOGY).

Morphine sulfate controlled-release capsules were developed for use in patients with chronic pain who require repeated dosing with a potent opioid analgesic, and has been tested in patients with pain due to malignant conditions. Morphine sulfate controlled-release capsules has not been tested as an analgesic for the treatment of acute pain or in the postoperative setting and is not recommended for such use.

IMMEDIATE-RELEASE ORAL FORMS

Morphine sulfate immediate-release oral solutions, tablets, capsules are indicated for the relief of moderate to severe pain.

INJECTION

Morphine sulfate is a potent analgesic used for the relief of moderate to severe pain. It is also used preoperatively to sedate the patient and allay apprehension, facilitate induction of anesthesia, and reduce anesthetic dosage.

SUPPOSITORIES

Morphine sulfate suppositories are indicated for the relief of moderate to severe chronic pain, and severe acute pain.

NON-FDA APPROVED INDICATIONS

Several case reports have suggested that nebulized morphine may have clinical utility in decreasing dyspnea, although no standard dosage recommendations are available for this route of administration.

CONTRAINDICATIONS

INJECTION

Hypersensitivity to morphine. Because of its stimulating effect on the spinal cord, morphine should not be used in convulsive states, such as those occurring in status epilepticus, tetanus, and strychnine poisoning.

ORAL FORMS

Morphine sulfate oral products are contraindicated in patients with known hypersensitivity to morphine, morphine salts, or any component of the dose form; in patients with respiratory depression in the absence of resuscitative equipment, and in patients with acute or severe bronchial asthma.

Morphine sulfate oral products are contraindicated in any patient who has or is suspected of having paralytic ileus.

M

SUPPOSITORIES

Hypersensitivity to morphine; respiratory insufficiency or depression; severe CNS depression; attack of bronchial asthma; heart failure secondary to chronic lung disease; cardiac arrhythmias; increased intracranial or cerebrospinal fluid pressure; head injuries; brain tumor; acute alcoholism; delirium tremens; convulsive disorders; after biliary tract surgery; suspected surgical abdomen; surgical anastomosis; concomitantly with MAO inhibitors or within 14 days of such treatment.

WARNINGS

INJECTION ONLY

Morphine sulfate injection contains sodium bisulfite, which may cause allergic-type reactions including anaphylactic symptoms and life-threatening or less severe asthmatic episodes in certain susceptible people. The overall prevalence of sulfite sensitivity in the general population is unknown and probably low. Sulfite sensitivity is seen more frequently in asthmatic than in nonasthmatic people.

ALL FORMS

See also CLINICAL PHARMACOLOGY.

Impaired Respiration

Respiratory depression is the chief hazard of all morphine preparations. Respiratory depression occurs more frequently in elderly and debilitated patients, and those suffering from conditions accompanied by hypoxia, hypercapnia, or upper airway obstruction (when even moderate therapeutic doses may dangerously decrease pulmonary ventilation).

Morphine should be used with extreme caution in patients with chronic obstructive pulmonary disease or cor pulmonale, and in patients having a substantially decreased respiratory reserve (*e.g.*, severe kyphoscoliosis), hypoxia, hypercapnia, or pre-existing respiratory depression. In such patients, even usual therapeutic doses of morphine may increase respiratory airway resistance and decrease respiratory drive to the point of apnea.

Head Injury and Increased Intracranial Pressure

The respiratory depressant effects of morphine with carbon dioxide retention and secondary elevation of cerebrospinal fluid pressure may be markedly exaggerated in the presence of head injury, other intracranial lesions, or pre-existing increase in intracranial pressure. Morphine produces effects which may obscure neurologic signs of further increase in pressure in patients with head injuries. Morphine should only be administered under such circumstances when considered essential and then with extreme care.

Hypotensive Effects

All opioid analgesics may cause severe hypotension in an individual whose ability to maintain blood pressure has already been compromised by a depleted blood volume, or a concurrent administration of drugs such as phenothiazines, or general anesthetics. (See DRUG INTERACTIONS.) Morphine may produce orthostatic hypotension in ambulatory patients.

Morphine sulfate, like all opioid analgesics, should be administered with caution to patients in circulatory shock, since vasodilation produced by the drug may further reduce cardiac output and blood pressure.

Gastrointestinal Obstruction

Morphine sulfate controlled-release capsules should not be given to patients with gastrointestinal obstruction, particularly paralytic ileus, as there is a risk of the product remaining in the stomach for an extended period and the subsequent-release of a bolus of morphine when normal gut motility is restored. As with other solid morphine formulations diarrhea may reduce morphine absorption.

Acute Abdominal Conditions

The administration of morphine or other narcotics may obscure the diagnosis or clinical course in patients with acute abdominal conditions.

Special Risk Groups

Morphine sulfate controlled-release capsules should be administered with caution, and in reduced dosages in elderly or debilitated patients; patients with severe renal or hepatic insufficiency; patients with Addison's disease; myxedema; hypothyroidism; prostatic hypertrophy or urethral stricture.

Caution should also be exercised in the administration of morphine sulfate to patients with CNS depression, toxic psychosis, acute alcoholism and delirium tremens, and convulsive disorders.

Morphine sulfate should be used with extreme caution in patients with disorders characterized by hypoxia, since even usual therapeutic doses of narcotics may decrease respiratory drive to the point of apnea while simultaneously increasing airway resistance.

Cordotomy

Patients taking morphine sulfate who are scheduled for cordotomy or other interruption of pain transmission pathways should have morphine sulfate controlled-release capsules ceased 24 hours prior to the procedure and the pain controlled by parenteral short-acting opioids. In addition, the post-procedure titration of analgesics for such patients should be individualized to avoid either oversedation or withdrawl syndromes.

Use in Pancreatic/Biliary Tract Disease

Morphine sulfate may cause spasm of the sphincter of Oddi and should be used with caution in patients with biliary tract disease, including acute pancreatitis. Opioids may cause increases in the serum amylase level.

Driving and Operating Machinery

Morphine may impair the mental and/or physical abilities needed to perform potentially hazardous activities such as driving a care or operating machinery. Patients must be cautioned accordingly. Patients should also be warned about the potential combined effects of morphine with other CNS depressants, including other opioids, phenothiazines, sedative/hypnotics and alcohol (see DRUG INTERACTIONS).

PRECAUTIONS

GENERAL

See CLINICAL PHARMACOLOGY.

Injection Only

Supraventricular Tachycardias: Because of a possible vagolytic action that may produce a significant increase in the ventricular response rate, morphine sulfate should be used with caution in patients with atrial flutter and other supraventricular tachycardias.

Convulsions: Morphine sulfate may aggravate preexisting convulsions in patients with convulsive disorders. If dosage is escalated substantially above recommended levels because of tolerance development, convulsions may occur in individuals without a history of convulsive disorders.

Kidney or Liver Dysfunction: Morphine sulfate may have a prolonged duration and cumulative effect in patients with kidney or liver dysfunction.

Oral Forms

See CLINICAL PHARMACOLOGY.

Morphine sulfate oral solutions, tablets and capsules are intended for use in patients who require a potent opioid analgesic for analgesic relief of moderate to severe pain.

Selection of patients for treatment with morphine sulfate oral products should be governed by the same principles that apply to the use of morphine and other potent opioid analgesics. Specifically, the increased risks associated with its use in the following populations should be considered: the elderly or debilitated and those with severe impairment of hepatic, pulmonary or renal function; myxedema or hypothyroidism; adrenocortical insufficiency (*e.g.*, Addison's Disease); CNS depression or coma; toxic psychoses; prostatic hypertrophy or urethral stricture; acute alcoholism; delirium tremens; kyphoscoliosis, or inability to swallow.

The administration of morphine, like all opioid analgesics, may obscure the diagnosis or clinical course in patients with acute abdominal conditions.

Morphine may aggravate preexisting convulsions in patients with convulsive disorders.

Morphine should be used with caution in patients about to undergo surgery of the biliary tract, since it may cause spasm of the sphincter of Oddi. Similarly, morphine should be used with caution in patients with acute pancreatitis secondary to biliary tract disease.

Controlled-Release Oral Forms

Special Precautions Regarding Morphine Sulfate Controlled-Release 200 Tablets: Morphine sulfate controlled-release 200 mg tablets are for use only in opioid tolerant patients requiring daily morphine equivalent dosages of 400 mg or more. Care should be taken in its prescription and patients should be instructed against use by individuals

other than the patient for whom it was prescribed, as this may have severe medical consequences for that individual.

General

Morphine sulfate controlled-release is intended for use in patients who require continuous treatment with a potent opioid analgesic.

The controlled-release nature of the formulation allows it to be administered on a more convenient schedule than conventional immediate-release oral morphine products (See CLINICAL PHARMACOLOGY). However, morphine sulfate controlled-release does not-release morphine continuously over the course of a dosing interval. The administration of single doses of morphine sulfate controlled-release on a every 12 hour dosing schedule will result in higher peak and lower trough plasma levels than those that occur when an identical daily dose of morphine is administered using conventional oral formulations on a every 4 hour regimen. The clinical significance of greater fluctuations in morphine plasma level has not been systematically evaluated. (See DOSAGE AND ADMINISTRATION.)

As with any potent opioid, it is critical to adjust the dosing regimen for each patient individually, taking into account the patient's prior analgesic treatment experience. Although it is clearly impossible to enumerate every consideration that is important to the selection of the initial dose and dosing interval of morphine sulfate extended-release tablets, attention should be given to 1) the daily dose, potency, and characteristics of the opoid the patient has been taking previously (*e.g.,* whether it is pure agonist or mixed agonist/antagonist), 2) the reliability of the relative potency estimate used to calculate the dose of morphine needed (N.B. potency estimates may vary with the route of administration), 3) the degree of opioid tolerance, if any, and 4) the general condition and medical status of the patient. (See DOSAGE AND ADMINISTRATION.)

INFORMATION FOR THE PATIENT

If clinically advisable, patients receiving morphine sulfate controlled-release capsules should be given the following instructions by the physician:

- While psychological dependence ("addiction") to morphine used in the treatment of pain is very rare, morphine is one of a class of drugs known to be abused and should be handled accordingly.
- The dose of the drug should not be adjusted without consulting a physician.
- Morphine may impair mental and/or physical ability required for the performance of potentially hazardous tasks (*e.g.,* driving, operating machinery). Patients started on morphine sulfate extended-release tablets or whose dose has been changed should refrain from dangerous activity until it is established that they are not adversly affected.
- Morphine should not be taken with alcohol or other CNS depressants (sleep aids, tranquilizers) because additive effects including CNS depression may occur. A physician should be consulted if other prescription medications are currently being used or are prescribed for future use.
- For women of childbearing potential who become or are planning to become pregnant, a physician should be consulted regarding analgesics and other drug use.
- Upon completion of therapy, it may be appropriate to taper morphine dose, rather than abruptly discontinue it.
- The morphine sulfate controlled-release 200 mg tablet is for use only in opioid tolerant patients requiring daily morphine equivalent dosages of 400 mg or more. Special care must be taken to avoid accidental ingestion or the use by individuals (including children) other than the patient for whom it was originally prescribed, as such unsupervised use may have severe, even fatal, consequences.
- Morphine sulfate controlled-release capsules should NOT be opened, chewed, crushed or dissolved. The pellets in the controlled-release capsules should NOT be chewed or dissolved.
- As with other opioids, patients taking morphine sulfate should be advised that severe constipation could occur and appropriate laxatives, stool softeners and other appropriate treatments should be initiated from the beginning of opioid therapy.

CARCINOGENESIS, MUTAGENESIS, AND IMPAIRMENT OF FERTILITY

Injection and Suppositories

Morphine has no known carcinogenic or mutagenic potential. However, no long-term animal studies are available to support this observation.

Oral Forms

Studies of morphine sulfate in animals to evaluate the drug's carcinogenic and mutagenic potential or the effect on fertility have not been conducted. There are no reports of carcinogenic effects in humans.

In vitro studies have reported that morphine is non-mutagenic in the Ames test with *Salmonella,* and induces chromosomal aberrations in human leukocytes and lethal mutation induction in *Drosophila.* Morphine was found to be mutagenic *in vitro* in human T-cells, increasing the DNA fragmentation. *In vivo,* morphine was mutagenic in the mouse micronucleus test and induced chromosomal aberrations in spermatids and murine lymphocytes.

Chronic opioid abusers (*e.g.,* heroin abusers) and their offspring display higher rates of chromosomal damage. However, the rates of chromosomal abnormalities were similar in nonexposed individuals and in heroin users enrolled in long term opioid maintenance programs.

PREGNANCY CATEGORY C

On the basis of the historical use of morphine sulfate during all stages if pregnancy, there is no known risk of fetal abnormality at usual therapeutic dosages. Morphine sulfate should be given to a pregnant woman only if clearly needed.

Teratogenic Effects

Teratogenic effects of morphine have been reported in the animal literature. High parental doses during the second trimester were teratogenic in neurological, soft and skeletal tissue. The abnormalities included encephalopathy and axial skeletal fusions. These doses were often maternally toxic and were 0.3- to 3-fold the maximum recommended human dose (MRHD) on a mg/m^2 basis. The relative contribution of morphine-induced maternal hypoxia and malnutrition, each of which can be teratogenic, has not been clearly defined. Treatment of male rats with approximately 3-fold the MRHD for 10 days prior to mating decreased litter size and viability.

Adequate animal studies on reproduction have not been performed to determine whether morphine affects fertility in males or females. There are no well-controlled studies in women, but marketing experience does not include any evidence of adverse effects on the fetus following routine (short-term) clinical use of morphine sulfate products. Reproductive effects have been observed in mice treated on gestation days 8 and/or 9 with doses ranging from 100-500 mg/kg morphine sulfate. Although there is no clearly defined risk, such experience cannot exclude the possibility of infrequent or subtle damage to the human fetus. Morphine sulfate should be used in pregnant women only when clearly needed. See Labor and Delivery.

Nonteratogenic Effects

Morphine given subcutaneously, at non-maternally toxic doses, to rats during the third trimester with approximately 0.15-fold the MRHD caused reversible reductions in brain and spinal cord volume, and testes size and body weight in the offspring, and decreased fertility in female offspring. The offspring of rats and hamsters treated orally or intraperitoneally throughout pregnancy with 0.04- to 0.3-fold the MRHD of morphine have demonstrated delayed growth, motor and sexual maturation and decreased male fertility. Chronic morphine exposure of fetal animals resulted in mild withdrawal, altered reflex and motor skill development, and altered responsivenes to morphine that persisted into adulthood.

There are no well-controlled studies of chronic *in utero* exposure to morphine sulfate in human subjects. However, uncontrolled retrospective studies of human neonates chronically exposed to other opioids *in utero,* demonstrated reduced brain volume which normalized over the first month of life. Infants born to opioid-abusing mothers are more often small for gestational age, have a decreased ventilatory response to CO_2 and increased risk of sudden infant death syndrome.

Infants born from mothers who have been taking morphine chronically may exhibit withdrawal symptoms.

Morphine should only be used during pregnancy if the need for strong opioid analgesia justifies the potential risk to the fetus.

LABOR AND DELIVERY

Morphine sulfate oral products are not recommended for use in women during and immediately prior to labor, where shorter acting analgesics or other analgesic techniques are more appropriate. Occasionally, opioid analgesics may prolong labor through actions which temporarily reduce the strength, duration and frequency of uterine contractions. However, this effect is not consistent and may be offset by an increased rate of cervical dilation which tends to shorten labor.

Morphine readily crosses the placental barrier and should be used with caution in women delivering premature infants since respiratory depression in the neonate may occur. Neonates whose mothers received morphine sulfate during labor should be observed closely for signs of respiratory depression. A specific narcotic antagonist, naloxone, is available for reversal of narcotic-induced respiratory depression in the neonate.

NEONATAL WITHDRAWAL SYNDROME

Chronic maternal use of opiates or opioids during pregnancy coexposes the fetus. The newborn may experience subsequent neonatal withdrawal syndrome (NWS). Manifestations of NWS include irritability, hyperactivity, abnormal sleep pattern, high-pitched cry, tremor, vomiting, diarrhea, weight loss, and failure to gain weight. The onset, duration, and severity of the disorder differ based on such factors as the addictive drug used, time and amount of mother's last dose, and rate of elimination of the drug from the newborn. Approaches to the treatment of this syndrome have included supportive care and, when indicated, drugs such as paragoric or phenobarbital.

NURSING MOTHERS

Low levels of morphine have been detected in human milk. Withdrawal symptoms can occur in breast-feeding infants when maternal administration of morphine sulfate is stopped. Nursing should not be undertaken while a patient is receiving morphine sulfate oral products since morphine may be excreted in the milk. Because of the potential for adverse reactions in nursing infants from morphine sulfate, a decision should be made whether to discontinue nursing or discontinue the drug, taking into account the importance of the drug to the mother.

PEDIATRIC USE

There are studies from the literature reporting the safe and effective use of both immediate and controlled-release oral morphine preparations for analgesia in children who were dosed on a per kilogram basis. The safety of morphine sulfate controlled-release has not been directly investigated in patients below the age of 18 years and both the dosage form and range of doses available are suitable for the treatment of very small children or those who are not old enough to take capsules safely.

DRUG INTERACTIONS

CNS DEPRESSANTS

Morphine should be used with great caution and in reduced dosage in patients who are concurrently receiving other central nervous system (CNS) depressants including sedatives, hypnotics, general anesthetics, antiemetics, phenothiazines, other tranquilizers and alcohol because of the risk of respiratory depression, hypotension and profound sedation or coma. When such combined therapy is contemplated, the initial dose of one or both agents should be reduced by at least 50%.

Opioid analgesics, including morphine sulfate oral products, may enhance the neuromuscular blocking action of skeletal muscle relaxants and produce an increased degree of respiratory depression.

See WARNINGS.

M

MUSCLE RELAXANTS

Morphine may enhance the neuromuscular blocking action of skeletal relaxants and produce an increased degree of respiratory depression.

MIXED AGONIST/ANTAGONIST OPIOID ANALGESICS

From a theoretical perspective, mixed agonist/antagonist analgesics (*i.e.,* petazocine, nalbupine and butorphanol) should NOT be administered to patients who have received or are receiving a course of therapy with pure opioid agonist analgesic. In these patients, mixed agonist/antagonist analgesics may reduce the analgesic effect and/or may precipitate withdrawal symptoms.

MONOAMINE OXIDASE INHIBITORS (MAOIS)

MAOIs have been reported to intensify the effects of at least one opioid drug causing anxiety, confusion and significant depression of respiration or coma. We do not recommend the use of morphine sulfate in patients taking MAOIs or within 14 days of stopping such treatment.

CIMETIDINE

There is an isolated report of confusion and sever respiratory depression when a hemodialysis patient was concurrently administered morphine and cimetidine.

DIURETICS

Morphine can reduce the efficacy of diuretics by inducing the-release of antidiuretic hormone. Morphine may also lead to acute retention of urine by causing spasm of the sphincter of the bladder, particularly in men with prostatism.

FOOD

The bioavailability of morphine sulfate controlled-release capsules is not significantly affected by food. Capsules should be swallowed whole. The capsules, as well as the pellets contained in the capsules, however, must not be crushed, chewed, or mixed with food due to risk of overdose (see DOSAGE AND ADMINISTRATION and PRECAUTIONS, Information for the Patient).

Generally, the effects of morphine may be potentiated by alkalizing agents and antagonized by acidifying agents. Analgesic effect of morphine is potentiated by chlorpromazine and methocarbamol. CNS depressants such as anesthetics, hypnotics, barbiturates, phenothiazines, chloral hydrate, glutethimide, sedatives, MAO inhibitors (including procarbazine hydrochloride), antihistamines, β-blockers (propranolol), alcohol, furazolidone and other narcotics may enhance the depressant effects of morphine. Morphine may increase anticoagulant activity of coumarin and other anticoagulants.

ADVERSE REACTIONS

The adverse reactions caused by morphine are essentially the same as those observed with other opioid analgesics. They include the following major hazards: respiratory depression, apnea, circulatory depression; respiratory arrest, shock, hypotension and cardiac arrest. (See WARNINGS.)

MOST FREQUENTLY OBSERVED

Constipation, lightheadedness, dizziness, drowsiness, sedation, nausea, vomiting, sweating, dysphoria and euphoria.

Some of these effects seem to be more prominent in ambulatory patients and in those not experiencing severe pain. Some adverse reactions in ambulatory patients may be alleviated if the patient lies down.

The less severe adverse events seen on initiation of therapy with morphine sulfate are also typical opioid side effects. These events are dose dependent, and their frequency depends on the clinical setting, the patient's level of opioid tolerance, and host factors specific to the individual. They should be expected and managed as a part of opioid analgesia. The most frequent of these include drowsiness, dizziness, constipation and nausea. In many cases, the frequency of these events during initiation of therapy may be minimized by careful individualization of starting dosage, slow titration, and the avoidance of large rapid swings in plasma concentrations of the opioid. Many of these adverse events, will cease or decrease as morphine sulfate therapy is continued and some degree of tolerance is developed, but others may be expected to remain troublesome throughout therapy.

LESS FREQUENTLY OBSERVED REACTIONS

Body as a Whole: Asthenia, accidental injury, fever, pain, chest pain, headache, diaphoresis, chills, flu syndrome, back pain, malaise and withdrawal syndrome, antidiuretic effect, paresthesia, muscle tremor, blurred vision, nystagmus, diplopia and miosis.

Cardiovascular: Tachycardia, atrial fibrillation, hypotension, hypertension, pallor, facial flushing, palpitations, bradycardia, syncope and faintness.

Central Nervous System: Confusion, dry mouth, anxiety, abnormal thinking, abnormal dreams, lethargy, depression, tremor, loss of concentration, insomnia, amnesia, paresthesia, agitation, vertigo, foot drop, ataxia, hypethesia, slurred speech, hallucinations, vasodilation, euphoria, apathy, seizures, myoclonus, weakness, uncoordinated muscle movements, alterations of mood (nervousness, apprehension, depression, floating feelings), muscle rigidity, transient hallucinations and disorientation, visual disturbances, insomnia and increased intracranial pressure.

Endocrine: Hypoatremia due to inappropriate ADH secretion, gynecomastia.

Gastrointestinal: Vomiting, anorexia, dysphagia, dyspepsia, diarrhea, abdominal pain, stomach atony disorder, gastro-esophageal reflux, delayed gastric emptying, biliary colic, biliary tract spasm, laryngospasm, cramps and taste alterations.

Hemic and Lymphatic: Anemia, leukopenia, thrombocytopenia.

Metabolic and Nutritional: Peripheral edema, hyponatremia, edema.

Musculoskeletal: Back pain, bone pain, arthralgia.

Respiratory: Hiccup, rhinitis, atelectasis, asthma, hypoxia, dyspnea, respiratory insufficiency, voice alteration, depressed cough reflex, non-cardiogenic pulmonary edema.

Skin and Appendages: Rash, decubitis ulcer, pruitis, skin flush, urticaria, edema and diaphoresis.

Special Senses: Amblyopia, conjunctivitis, miosis, blurred vision, nystagmus, diplopia.

Urogenital: Urinary abnormality, amenorrhea, urinary retention, urinary hesitance, reduced libido, reduced potency, prolonged labor.

MANAGEMENT OF EXCESSIVE DROWSINESS

Most patients receiving morphine will experience initial drowsiness. This usually within 3-5 days and is not a cause of concern unless it is excessive, or accompanied by unsteadiness or confusion. Dizziness and unsteadiness may be associated with postural hypotension, particularly in elderly or debilitated patients, and has been associated with syncope and falls in non-tolerant patients started on opiods.

Excessive or persistent sedation should be investigated. Factors to be considered should include: concurrent sedative medications, the presence of hepatic or renal insufficiency, hypoxia or hypercapnia due to exacerbated respiratory failure, intolerance to the dose used (especially in older patients), disease severity and the patient's general condition.

The dosage should be adjusted accordingly to individual needs, but additional care should be used in the selection of initial doses for the elderly patient, the cachectic or gravely ill patient, or in patients not already familiar with opioid analgesic medications to prevent excessive sedation at the onset of treatment.

MANAGEMENT OF NAUSEA AND VOMITING

Nausea and vomiting is common after single doses of morphine or as an early undesirable effect of chronic opioid therapy. The prescription of a suitable antiemetic should be considered, with the awareness that sedation may result (see DRUG INTERACTIONS). The frequency of nausea and vomiting decreases within a week or so but may persist due to opioid-induced gastric stasis. Metoclopramide is often useful in such patients.

MANAGEMENT OF CONSTIPATION

Virtually all patients suffer from constipation while taking opioids on a chronic basis. Some patients, particularly elderly, debilitated or bedridden patients may become impacted. Tolerance does not usually develop for the constipating effects of opiods. Patients must be cautioned accordingly and laxatives, softeners and other appropriate treatments should be used prophylactically from the beginning of the opioid therapy.

DOSAGE AND ADMINISTRATION

INJECTION

Dosage should be adjusted according to the severity of the pain and the response of the patient.

Morphine sulfate injection may be administered subcutaneously, intramuscularly, or intravenously but not intrathecally or epidurally.

For Analgesia

Intravenous Route: *Adults:* 2.5-15 mg in 4-5 ml of water for injection, injected slowly over a period of 4-5 minutes.

Subcutaneous or Intramuscular Route: *Adults:* 10 mg/70 kg of body weight (range, 5-20 mg), depending on the cause of the pain and the individual patient; *Children:* (subcutaneous route) 0.1-0.2 mg/kg (maximum dose, 15 mg).

For Preanesthetic Medication

The following doses are given 45-60 minutes before anesthesia:

Subcutaneous or Intramuscular Route: *Adults:* 10 mg/70 kg of body weight (range, 5-20 mg); *Children, 1 year of age and over:* 0.1 (maximum dose, 10 mg).

Note: Morphine sulfate solutions may darken with age. Do not use if the solution is darker than pale yellow, is discolored in any other way, or contains a precipitate.

IMMEDIATE-RELEASE ORAL FORMS

Dosage of morphine is a patient-dependent variable, which must be individualized according to patient metabolism, age and disease state, and also response to morphine. Each patient should be maintained at the lowest dosage level that will produce acceptable analgesia. As the patient's well-being improved after successful relief of moderate to severe pain, periodic reduction of dosage and/or extension of dosing interval should be attempted to minimize exposure to morphine.

Usual Adult Oral Dose

5-30 mg every 4 hours or as directed by physician, administered either as morphine sulfate immediate-release oral solutions, morphine sulfate immediate-release oral tablets or morphine sulfate immediate-release oral capsules. For control of pain in terminal illness, it is recommended that the appropriate dose of morphine sulfate oral products be given on a regularly scheduled basis every 4 hours at the minimum dose to achieve acceptable analgesia. If converting a patient from another narcotic to morphine sulfate on the basis of standard equivalence tables, a 1-3 ratio of parenteral to oral morphine equivalence is suggested. This ratio is conservative and may underestimate the amount of morphine required. If this is the case, the dose of morphine sulfate oral products should be gradually increased to achieve acceptable analgesia and tolerable side effects.

SPRINKLING CONTENTS OF CAPSULE ON FOOD OR LIQUIDS

Morphine sulfate immediate-release oral capsules may be carefully opened and the entire beaded contents added to a small amount of cool, soft food, such as applesauce or pudding, or a liquid, such as water or orange juice. The bead-food mixture should be swallowed immediately and not stored for future use.

CONTROLLED-RELEASE ORAL TABLETS

WARNING

MORPHINE SULFATE CONTROLLED-RELEASE TABLETS ARE TO BE TAKEN WHOLE, AND ARE NOT TO BE BROKEN, CHEWED OR CRUSHED.

Cont'd

TAKING BROKEN, CHEWED OR CRUSHED MORPHINE SULFATE CONTROLLED-RELEASE TABLETS COULD LEAD TO THE RAPID RELEASE AND ABSORPTION OF A POTENTIALLY TOXIC DOSE OF MORPHINE.

Morphine sulfate controlled-release is intended for use in patients who require more than several days continuous treatment with a potent opioid analgesic. The controlled-release nature of the formulation allows it to be administered on a more convenient schedule than conventional immediate-release oral morphine products. (See CLINICAL PHARMACOLOGY.) However, morphine sulfate controlled-release does not-release morphine continuously over the course of a dosing interval. The administration of single doses of morphine sulfate controlled-release on an every 12 hour dosing schedule will result in higher peak and lower trough plasma levels than those that occur when an identical daily dose of morphine is administered using conventional oral formulations on an every 4 hour regimen. The clinical significance of greater fluctuations in morphine plasma level has not been systematically evaluated.

As with any potent opioid drug product, it is critical to adjust the dosing regimen for each patient individually, taking into account the patient's prior analgesic treatment experience. Although it is clearly impossible to enumerate every consideration that is important to the selection of initial dose and dosing interval of morphine sulfate controlled-release, attention should be given to:

The daily dose, potency and precise characteristics of the opioid the patient has been taking previously (*e.g.,* whether it is a pure agonist or mixed agonist-antagonist).

The reliability of the relative potency estimate used to calculate the dose of morphine needed [N.B. potency estimates may vary with the route of administration].

The degree of opioid tolerance, if any.

The general condition and medical status of the patient.

Concurrent medication.

The type and severity of the patient's pain.

The following dosing recommendations, therefore, can only be considered suggested approaches to what is actually a series of clinical decisions in the management of the pain of an individual patient.

Conversion from Conventional Oral Morphine to Morphine Sulfate Controlled-Release

A patient's daily morphine requirement is established using immediate-release oral morphine (dosing every 4-6 hours). The patient is then converted to morphine sulfate controlled-release in either of two ways:

Kadian or MS Contin: By administering one-half of the patient's 24 hour requirement as morphine sulfate controlled-release on an every 12 hour schedule; or,

Note: Kadian should not be given more frequently than every 12 hours.

MS Contin Only: By administering one-third of the patient's daily requirement as morphine sulfate controlled-release on an every 8 hour schedule.

With either method, dose and dosing interval is then adjusted as needed. The MS Contin 15 mg tablet should be used for initial conversion for patients whose total daily requirement is expected to be less than 60 mg. The 30 mg tablet strength is recommended for patients with a daily morphine requirement of 60-120 mg. When the total daily dose is expected to be greater than 120 mg, the appropriate combination of tablet strengths should be employed.

Conversion from Parenteral Morphine or Other Opioids (Parenteral or Oral) to Morphine Sulfate Controlled-Release

Morphine sulfate controlled-release can be administered as the initial oral morphine drug product; in this case, however, particular care must be exercised in the conversion process. Because of uncertainty about, and intersubject variation in, relative estimates of opioid potency and cross tolerance, initial dosing regimens should be conservative; that is, an underestimation of the 24 hour oral morphine requirement is preferred to an overestimate. To this end, initial individual doses of morphine sulfate controlled-release should be estimated conservatively. In patients whose daily morphine requirements are expected to be less than or equal to 120 mg/day, the MS Contin 30 mg tablet strength is recommended for the initial titration period. Once a stable dose regimen is reached, the patient can be converted to the 60 mg or 100 mg tablet strength, or appropriate combination of tablet strengths, if desired.

Estimates of the relative potency of opioids are only approximate and are influenced by route of administration, individual patient differences, and possibly, by an individual's medical condition. Consequently, it is difficult to recommend any fixed rule for converting a patient to morphine sulfate controlled-release directly. The following general points should be considered however.

Parenteral to oral morphine ratio: Estimates of the oral to parenteral potency of morphine vary. Some authorities suggest that a dose of oral morphine only 3 times the daily parenteral morphine requirement may be sufficient in chronic use settings.

Other parenteral or oral opioids to oral Morphine: Because there is lack of systemic evidence bearing on these type of analgesic substitutions, specific recommendations are not possible. Physicians are advised to refer to published relative potency data, keeping in mind that such ratios are only approximate. In general, it is safer to underestimate the daily dose of morphine sulfate extended-release tablets required and rely upon ad hoc supplementation to deal with inadequate analgesia. See discussion that follows.

The first dose of morphine sulfate controlled-release may be taken with the last dose of any immediate-release (short-acting) opioid medication due to the long delay until the peak effect after administration.

Use of Morphine Sulfate Controlled-Release as the First Opioid Analgesic

There has been no systematic evaluation of morphine sulfate controlled-release as an initial opioid analgesic in the management of pain. Because it may be more difficult to titrate a patient using a controlled-release morphine, it is ordinarily advisable to begin treatment using an immediate-release formulation.

Individualization Of Dosage

The best use of opioid analgesics in the management of chronic malignant and non-malignant pain is challenging, and is well described in materials published by the World Health Organization and the Agency for Health Care Policy and Research which are available from Zeneca Pharmaceuticals upon request. Morphine sulfate controlled-release capsules is a third step drug which is most useful when the patient requires a constant level of opioid analgesia as a "floor" or "platform" from which to manage breakthrough pain. When a patient has reached the point where comfort cannot be provided with a combination of non-opioid medications (NSAIDs and acetaminophen) and intermittent use of moderate or strong opioids, the patient's total opioid therapy should be converted into a 24 hour oral morphine equivalent.

Morphine sulfate controlled-release capsules should be started by administering one-half of the estimated total daily oral morphine dose every 12 hours (twice-a-day) or by administering the total daily oral morphine dose every 24 hours (once-a-day). The dose should be titrated no more frequently than every-other-day to allow the patients to stabilize before escalating the dose. If breakthrough pain occurs, the dose may be supplemented with a small dose (less than 20% of the total daily dose) of a short-acting analgesic. Patients who are excessively sedated after a once-a-day dose or who regularly experience inadequate analgesia before the next dose should be switched to twice-a-day dosing.

Patients who do not have a proven tolerance to opioids should be started only on the 20 mg strength, and usually should be increased at a rate not greater than 20 mg every-other-day. Most patients will rapidly develop some degree of tolerance, requiring dosage adjustment until they have achieved their individual best balance between baseline analgesia and opioid side effects such as confusion, sedation and constipation. No guidance can be given as to the recommended maximal dose, especially in patients with chronic pain of malignancy. In such cases the total dose of morphine sulfate controlled-release capsules should be advanced until the desired therapeutic endpoint is reached or clinically significant opioid-related adverse reactions intervene.

Considerations in the Adjustment of Dosing Regimens

Whatever the approach, if signs of excessive opioid effects are observed early in a dosing interval, the next dose should be reduced. If this adjustment leads to inadequate analgesia, that is, "breakthrough" pain occurs late in the dosing interval, the dosing interval may be shortened. Alternatively, a supplemental dose of a short-acting analgesic may be given. As experience is gained, adjustments can be made to obtain an appropriate balance between pain relief, opioid side effects, and the convenience of the dosing schedule.

In adjusting dosing requirements, it is recommended that the dosing interval never be extended beyond 12 hours because the administration of very large single doses may lead to acute overdose. (N.B. this product is a controlled-release formulation; it does not-release morphine continuously over the dosing interval.)

For patients with low daily morphine requirements, the 15 mg tablet should be used.

SPECIAL INSTRUCTIONS FOR MORPHINE SULFATE CONTROLLED-RELEASE 200 MG TABLETS

(For use in opioid tolerant patients only.)

The morphine sulfate controlled-release 200 mg tablet is for use only in opioid tolerant patients requiring daily morphine equivalent dosages of 400 mg or more. It is recommended that this strength be reserved for patients that have already been titrated to a stable analgesic regimen using lower strengths of morphine sulfate controlled-release or other opioid.

CONVERSION FROM KADIAN TO OTHER CONTROLLED-RELEASE ORAL MORPHINE FORMULATIONS

Kadian is not bioequivalent to other controlled-release morphine preparations. Although for a given dose the same total amount of morphine is available from Kadian as from morphine solution or controlled-release morphine tablets, the slow-release of morphine from Kadian results in reduced maximum and increased minimum plasma morphine concentrations than with shorter acting morphine products. Conversion from Kadian to the same total daily dose of controlled-release morphine preparations may lead to either excessive sedation at peak or inadequate analgesia at trough and close observation and appropriate dosage adjustments are recommended.

CONVERSION FROM MS CONTIN TO PARENTERAL OPIOIDS

When converting a patient from morphine sulfate controlled-release to parenteral opioids, it is best to calculate an equivalent parenteral dose, and then initiate treatment at half of this calculated value. For example, to estimate the required 24 hour dose of parenteral morphine for a patient taking Kadian, one would take the 24 hour Kadian dose, divide by and oral to parenteral conversion ration of 3, divide the estimated 24 hour parenteral dose into six divided doses (for a 4 hour dosing interval), then halve this dose as an initial trial.

For example, to estimate the required parenteral morphine dose for a patient taking 360 mg of Kadian a day, divide the 360 mg daily oral morphine dose by a conversion ration of 1 mg of parenteral morphine for every 3 mg of oral morphine. The estimated 120 mg daily parenteral requirement is then divided into six 20 mg doses, and half of this, or 10 mg, is then given every 4 hours as an initial trial dose.

This approach is likely to require a dosage increase in the first 24 hours for many patients, but is recommended because it is less likely to cause overdose than trying to establish an equivalent dose without titration.

Opioid analgesic agents may not effectively relieve dysesthetic pain, post-herpetic neuralgia, stabbing pains, activity-related pain, and some forms of headache. This does not mean that patients suffering from these types of pain should not be given an adequate trial of opioid analgesics. However, such patients may need to be promptly evaluated for other types of pain therapy.

SUPPOSITORIES

Rectal Administration

Dosage should be adjusted according to the severity of the pain and the response of the patient. Morphine sulfate suppositories are to be administered rectally.

Usual Adult Dose: 10-20 mg every 4 hours or as directed by a physician.

Dosage is a patient dependent variable, therefore, increased dosage may be required to achieve adequate analgesia.

For control of severe chronic pain in patients with certain terminal diseases, this drug should be administered on a regularly scheduled basis, every 4 hours, at the lowest dosage level that will achieve adequate analgesia.

Note: Medication may suppress respiration in the elderly, the very ill, and those patients with respiratory problems, therefore lower doses may be required.

Morphine Dosage Reduction

During the first 2-3 days of effective pain relief, the patient may sleep for many hours. This can be misinterpreted as the effect of excessive analgesic dosing rather than the first sign of relief in a pain exhausted patient. The dose, therefore, should be maintained for at least 3 days before reduction, if respiratory activity and other vital signs are adequate.

Following successful relief of severe pain, periodic attempts to reduce the narcotic dose should be made. Smaller doses or complete discontinuation of the narcotic analgesic may become feasible due to a physiologic change or the improved mental state of the patient.

SAFETY AND HANDLING

The morphine sulfate controlled-release 200 mg tablet strength is for use only in opioid tolerant patients requiring daily morphine equivalent dosages of 400 mg or more. This strength is potentially toxic if accidentally ingested and patients and their families should be instructed to take special care to avoid accidental or intentional ingestion by individuals other than those for whom the medication was originally prescribed.

HOW SUPPLIED

IMMEDIATE-RELEASE ORAL SOLUTION

Immediate-release oral solution (pleasantly flavored) is dispensed in 10 mg per 5 ml and 20 mg per 5 ml high density, polyethylene plastic, bottles of 120 ml with child-resistant closure.

Storage: Store at controlled room temperature 15-30°C (59-86°F). Dispense in tight, light-resistant container with a child-resistant closure.

IMMEDIATE-RELEASE ORAL SOLUTION CONCENTRATE

Immediate-release oral solution concentrate (unflavored) is dispensed in 20 mg per 1 ml high density, polyethylene plastic, child-resistant closure bottles with child-resistant droppers in 30 ml and 120 mL sizes. Discard opened bottle of oral solution after 90 days. Protect from light.

Storage: Store at controlled room temperature 15-30°C (59-86°F). Dispense in tight, light-resistant container with a child-resistant closure.

IMMEDIATE-RELEASE TABLETS

Immediate-release tablets are dispensed as 15 mg round, white scored tablets and 30 mg capsule-shaped, white scored tablets in opaque plastic bottles containing 100 tablets. The 15 mg tablets bear the symbol PF on the scored side and MI 15 on the other side. 30 mg tablets bear the symbol PF on the scored side and MI 30 on the other side.

Storage: Store at controlled room temperature 15-30°C (59-86°F). Dispense in tight, light-resistant container with a child-resistant closure.

IMMEDIATE-RELEASE CAPSULES

Immediate-release capsules are dispense as 15 mg white opaque capsule body with blue cap in opaque plastic bottles containing 50 capsules. Each capsule bears the symbols PF MSIR 15 and "This End Up".

Storage: Store controlled room temperature 15-30°C (59-86°F). Dispense in tight, light-resistant container with a child-resistant closure.

MS CONTIN CONTROLLED-RELEASE TABLETS

MS Contin controlled-release tablets are available in:

- ***15 mg:*** Round, blue-colored and bear the symbol "PF" on one side and "M15" on the other side.
- ***30 mg:*** Round, lavender-colored and bear the symbol "PF" on one side and "M30" on the other side.
- ***60 mg:*** Round orange-colored and bear the symbol "PF" on one side and "M60" on the other side.
- ***100 mg:*** Round, gray-colored and bear the symbol "PF" on one side and "M100" on the other side.
- ***200 mg:*** Capsule-shaped, green-colored and bear the symbol "PF" on one side and "200" on the other side.

KADIAN SUSTAINED-RELEASE CAPSULES

Kadian sustained-release capsules are available in:

- ***20 mg:*** The size 4 capsule has a clear cap imprinted "KADIAN" and clear body imprinted "20 mg".
- ***50 mg:*** The size 2 capsule has a clear cap imprinted "KADIAN" and clear body imprinted "50 mg".
- ***100 mg:*** The size 0 capsule has a clear cap imprinted "KADIAN" and clear body imprinted "100 mg".

ROXANOL SUPPOSITORIES

The 5, 10, 20, and 30 mg suppositories are supplied in 12 foil packets per carton.

PRODUCT LISTING - RATED THERAPEUTICALLY EQUIVALENT

Package	Price	Product, Manufacturer	NDC
Solution - Injectable - 0.5 mg/ml Preservative;Free			
2 ml x 10	$95.00	ASTRAMORPH PF, Astra-Zeneca Pharmaceuticals	00186-1159-03
10 ml x 5	$12.65	GENERIC, Abbott Pharmaceutical	00074-4057-12
10 ml x 5	$34.75	ASTRAMORPH PF, Astra-Zeneca Pharmaceuticals	00186-1150-02
10 ml x 5	$42.39	GENERIC, Abbott Pharmaceutical	00074-3814-12
10 ml x 10	$86.00	GENERIC, Esi Lederle Generics	00641-1112-33
30 ml x 10	$138.70	GENERIC, Abbott Pharmaceutical	00074-2028-02
Solution - Injectable - 1 mg/ml			
10 ml x 10	$92.20	GENERIC, Baxter Pharmaceutical Products, Inc	10019-0007-73
10 ml x 25	$191.00	GENERIC, Celltech Pharmaceuticals Inc	00548-2901-25
30 ml x 10	$125.28	GENERIC, Abbott Pharmaceutical	00074-6023-04
50 ml	$269.50	GENERIC, Baxter I.V. Systems Division	00338-2689-75
Solution - Injectable - 1 mg/ml Preservative;Free			
2 ml x 10	$104.60	ASTRAMORPH PF, Astra-Zeneca Pharmaceuticals	00186-1160-03
10 ml x 5	$37.55	GENERIC, Abbott Pharmaceutical	00074-4058-12
10 ml x 5	$44.18	GENERIC, Abbott Pharmaceutical	00074-3815-12
10 ml x 5	$55.45	ASTRAMORPH PF, Astra-Zeneca Pharmaceuticals	00186-1151-02
10 ml x 10	$92.30	GENERIC, Esi Lederle Generics	00641-1114-33
30 ml x 10	$176.34	GENERIC, Abbott Pharmaceutical	00074-2029-02
Solution - Injectable - 5 mg/ml			
30 ml x 10	$169.93	GENERIC, Abbott Pharmaceutical	00074-6028-04
50 ml	$400.00	GENERIC, Baxter I.V. Systems Division	00338-2690-75
Solution - Injectable - 8 mg/ml			
1 ml x 10	$7.90	GENERIC, Baxter Pharmaceutical Products, Inc	10019-0177-47
1 ml x 25	$22.00	GENERIC, Baxter Healthcare Corporation	10019-0177-44
Solution - Injectable - 10 mg/ml Preservative;Free			
20 ml	$156.00	GENERIC, Esi Lederle Generics	00641-1131-31
Solution - Injectable - 15 mg/ml			
1 ml x 10	$9.03	GENERIC, Abbott Pharmaceutical	00074-1262-01
20 ml	$13.73	GENERIC, Steris Laboratories Inc	00402-0913-20
20 ml x 5	$56.80	GENERIC, Abbott Pharmaceutical	00074-3819-12
Solution - Injectable - 25 mg/ml			
4 ml x 5	$18.70	GENERIC, Abbott Pharmaceutical	00074-1133-21
4 ml x 10	$125.52	GENERIC, Abbott Pharmaceutical	00074-6177-14
10 ml x 5	$26.18	GENERIC, Abbott Pharmaceutical	00074-1133-22
10 ml x 10	$141.31	GENERIC, Abbott Pharmaceutical	00074-6179-14
20 ml	$7.67	GENERIC, Abbott Pharmaceutical	00074-1133-03
40 ml	$15.06	GENERIC, Abbott Pharmaceutical	00074-1133-04
Solution - Injectable - 25 mg/ml Preservative;Free			
4 ml	$6.64	GENERIC, Abbott Pharmaceutical	00074-1135-01
10 ml	$30.28	GENERIC, Abbott Pharmaceutical	00074-1135-02
20 ml	$59.38	GENERIC, Abbott Pharmaceutical	00074-1135-03
20 ml	$281.00	GENERIC, Esi Lederle Generics	00641-1132-31
40 ml	$118.81	GENERIC, Abbott Pharmaceutical	00074-1135-04
Solution - Injectable - 50 mg/ml			
10 ml	$42.98	GENERIC, King Pharmaceuticals Inc	60793-0095-10
10 ml	$286.62	GENERIC, International Medication Systems, Limited	00548-6358-00
40 ml	$64.00	GENERIC, King Pharmaceuticals Inc	60793-0096-40
Solution - Intravenous - 5%;20 mg/100 ml			
250 ml	$8.28	GENERIC, Abbott Pharmaceutical	00074-6063-02
500 ml	$10.11	GENERIC, Abbott Pharmaceutical	00074-6063-03
Solution - Intravenous - 5%;100 mg/100 ml			
100 ml	$10.11	GENERIC, Abbott Pharmaceutical	00074-6062-11
250 ml	$13.89	GENERIC, Abbott Pharmaceutical	00074-6062-02
500 ml	$19.52	GENERIC, Abbott Pharmaceutical	00074-6062-03
Tablet, Extended Release - Oral - 15 mg			
25's	$27.08	MS CONTIN, Purdue Frederick Company	00034-0514-25
100's	$89.17	GENERIC, Endo Laboratories Llc	60951-0652-70
100's	$90.95	GENERIC, Ab Generics	60999-0900-10
100's	$99.63	MS CONTIN, Purdue Frederick Company	00034-0514-10
120's	$119.55	MS CONTIN, Purdue Frederick Company	00034-0514-12
Tablet, Extended Release - Oral - 30 mg			
25's	$54.09	MS CONTIN, Purdue Frederick Company	00034-0515-25
50's	$99.63	MS CONTIN, Purdue Frederick Company	00034-0515-50
100's	$169.46	GENERIC, Endo Laboratories Llc	60951-0653-70
100's	$189.34	MS CONTIN, Purdue Frederick Company	00034-0515-10
120's	$227.20	MS CONTIN, Purdue Frederick Company	00034-0515-12
250's	$459.04	MS CONTIN, Purdue Frederick Company	00034-0515-45
Tablet, Extended Release - Oral - 60 mg			
25's	$108.15	MS CONTIN, Purdue Frederick Company	00034-0516-25
100's	$330.61	GENERIC, Endo Laboratories Llc	60951-0655-70
100's	$337.32	GENERIC, Ab Generics	60999-0902-10
100's	$369.44	MS CONTIN, Purdue Frederick Company	00034-0516-10
120's	$443.33	MS CONTIN, Purdue Frederick Company	00034-0516-12
Tablet, Extended Release - Oral - 100 mg			
25's	$164.51	MS CONTIN, Purdue Frederick Company	00034-0517-25
100's	$489.56	GENERIC, Watson Laboratories Inc	00591-0617-01
100's	$489.56	GENERIC, Endo Laboratories Llc	60951-0658-70
100's	$546.99	MS CONTIN, Purdue Frederick Company	00034-0517-10
120's	$656.39	MS CONTIN, Purdue Frederick Company	00034-0517-12
Tablet, Extended Release - Oral - 200 mg			
100's	$896.53	GENERIC, Endo Laboratories Llc	60951-0659-70
100's	$1001.71	MS CONTIN, Purdue Frederick Company	00034-0513-10
120's	$1202.05	MS CONTIN, Purdue Frederick Company	00034-0513-12

PRODUCT LISTING - RATED NOT THERAPEUTICALLY EQUIVALENT

Package	Price	Product, Manufacturer	NDC
Tablet, Extended Release - Oral - 15 mg			
100's	$90.03	ORAMORPH SR, Roxane Laboratories Inc	00054-4790-25
100's	$97.89	ORAMORPH SR, Roxane Laboratories Inc	00054-8790-24
Tablet, Extended Release - Oral - 30 mg			
50's	$84.45	ORAMORPH SR, Roxane Laboratories Inc	00054-4805-19
100's	$171.09	ORAMORPH SR, Roxane Laboratories Inc	00054-4805-25
100's	$195.53	ORAMORPH SR, Roxane Laboratories Inc	00054-8805-24
250's	$414.78	ORAMORPH SR, Roxane Laboratories Inc	00054-4805-27
Tablet, Extended Release - Oral - 60 mg			
25's	$97.71	ORAMORPH SR, Roxane Laboratories Inc	00054-8792-11
100's	$333.83	ORAMORPH SR, Roxane Laboratories Inc	00054-4792-25
100's	$337.32	GENERIC, Ab Generics	60999-0103-10

Tablet, Extended Release - Oral - 100 mg

25's	$153.69	ORAMORPH SR, Roxane Laboratories Inc	00054-8793-11
100's	$511.24	ORAMORPH SR, Roxane Laboratories Inc	00054-4793-25

PRODUCT LISTING - EQUIVALENTS NOT AVAILABLE

Capsule - Oral - 15 mg			
100's	$37.19	MSIR, Purdue Frederick Company	00034-1025-10
Capsule - Oral - 30 mg			
100's	$69.40	MSIR, Purdue Frederick Company	00034-1026-10
Capsule, Extended Release - Oral - 20 mg			
60's	$68.85	KADIAN, Astra-Zeneca Pharmaceuticals	00310-0342-60
60's	$130.34	KADIAN, Faulding Pharmaceutical Company	63857-0322-06
100's	$109.04	KADIAN, Astra-Zeneca Pharmaceuticals	00310-0342-10
100's	$124.61	KADIAN, Astra-Zeneca Pharmaceuticals	00310-0342-39
Capsule, Extended Release - Oral - 30 mg			
60's	$130.34	KADIAN, Faulding Pharmaceutical Company	63857-0325-06
Capsule, Extended Release - Oral - 30 mg/24 Hours			
100's	$231.00	AVINZA, Ligand Pharmaceuticals	64365-0505-03
Capsule, Extended Release - Oral - 50 mg			
60's	$167.92	KADIAN, Astra-Zeneca Pharmaceuticals	00310-0345-60
60's	$248.25	KADIAN, Faulding Pharmaceutical Company	63857-0323-06
100's	$265.94	KADIAN, Astra-Zeneca Pharmaceuticals	00310-0345-10
100's	$311.44	KADIAN, Astra-Zeneca Pharmaceuticals	00310-0345-39
Capsule, Extended Release - Oral - 60 mg			
60's	$248.25	KADIAN, Faulding Pharmaceutical Company	63857-0326-06
Capsule, Extended Release - Oral - 60 mg/24 Hours			
100's	$445.00	AVINZA, Ligand Pharmaceuticals	64365-0506-03
Capsule, Extended Release - Oral - 90 mg/24 Hours			
100's	$675.00	AVINZA, Ligand Pharmaceuticals	64365-0507-02
Capsule, Extended Release - Oral - 100 mg			
60's	$298.34	KADIAN, Astra-Zeneca Pharmaceuticals	00310-0341-60
60's	$431.24	KADIAN, Faulding Pharmaceutical Company	63857-0324-06
100's	$472.50	KADIAN, Astra-Zeneca Pharmaceuticals	00310-0341-10
100's	$568.44	KADIAN, Astra-Zeneca Pharmaceuticals	00310-0341-39
Capsule, Extended Release - Oral - 120 mg/24 Hours			
100's	$790.00	AVINZA, Ligand Pharmaceuticals	64365-0508-02
Concentrate - Oral - 20 mg/ml			
30 ml	$18.62	GENERIC, Ethex Corporation	58177-0886-01
30 ml	$20.76	ROXANOL, Elan Pharmaceuticals	00054-3751-44
30 ml	$20.76	ROXANOL-T, Roxane Laboratories Inc	00054-3774-44
30 ml	$20.76	GENERIC, Endo Laboratories Llc	60951-0648-74
30 ml	$21.80	MSIR, Purdue Frederick Company	00034-0523-01
30 ml	$122.52	GENERIC, Apotex Usa Inc	60999-0132-01
120 ml	$56.70	GENERIC, Liquipharm Inc	54198-0145-04
120 ml	$59.50	GENERIC, Apotex Usa Inc	60999-0132-02
120 ml	$69.95	GENERIC, Ethex Corporation	58177-0886-03
120 ml	$77.96	ROXANOL, Elan Pharmaceuticals	00054-3751-50
120 ml	$77.96	ROXANOL-T, Roxane Laboratories Inc	00054-3774-50
120 ml	$77.96	GENERIC, Endo Laboratories Llc	60951-0648-80
120 ml	$81.90	MSIR, Purdue Frederick Company	00034-0523-02
240 ml	$131.22	ROXANOL, Roxane Laboratories Inc	00054-3751-58
240 ml	$131.22	GENERIC, Ethex Corporation	58177-0886-05
240 ml	$131.22	GENERIC, Endo Laboratories Llc	60951-0648-91
Solution - Injectable - 1 mg/ml			
10 ml x 10	$23.01	GENERIC, Faulding Pharmaceutical Company	61703-0219-80
10 ml x 10	$50.00	GENERIC, International Medication Systems, Limited	00548-3391-10
30 ml x 10	$18.75	GENERIC, Faulding Pharmaceutical Company	61703-0219-75
30 ml x 10	$18.75	GENERIC, Faulding Pharmaceutical Company	61703-0219-85
30 ml x 10	$125.00	GENERIC, International Medication Systems, Limited	00548-1933-10
30 ml x 10	$150.00	GENERIC, Celltech Pharmacueticals Inc	00548-1931-10
30 ml x 25	$375.00	GENERIC, Celltech Pharmacueticals Inc	00548-1911-25
60 ml	$8.94	GENERIC, Baxter Pharmaceutical Products, Inc	10019-0175-80
250 ml	$229.13	GENERIC, Celltech Pharmacueticals Inc	00548-2901-00
300 ml	$180.00	GENERIC, Celltech Pharmacuetical Inc	00548-1931-00
Solution - Injectable - 2 mg/ml			
1 ml x 10	$7.24	GENERIC, Abbott Pharmaceutical	00074-1762-01
1 ml x 10	$9.10	GENERIC, Esi Lederle Generics	00008-0649-01
1 ml x 10	$9.14	GENERIC, Abbott Pharmaceutical	00074-1762-31
1 ml x 10	$10.09	GENERIC, Abbott Pharmaceutical	00074-1762-02
1 ml x 10	$11.00	GENERIC, Abbott Pharmaceutical	00074-1762-30
1 ml x 10	$11.70	GENERIC, Esi Lederle Generics	00008-0649-50
1 ml x 10	$12.35	GENERIC, Abbott Pharmaceutical	00074-1762-11
1 ml x 10	$12.35	GENERIC, Abbott Pharmaceutical	00074-1762-21
30 ml x 10	$165.18	GENERIC, Abbott Pharmaceutical	00074-6022-02
Solution - Injectable - 4 mg/ml			
1 ml x 10	$7.00	GENERIC, Abbott Pharmaceutical	00074-1258-01
1 ml x 10	$8.40	GENERIC, Abbott Pharmaceutical	00074-1258-31
1 ml x 10	$9.10	GENERIC, Esi Lederle Generics	00008-0653-01
1 ml x 10	$10.33	GENERIC, Abbott Pharmaceutical	00074-1258-02
1 ml x 10	$11.30	GENERIC, Abbott Pharmaceutical	00074-1258-30
1 ml x 10	$12.35	GENERIC, Abbott Pharmaceutical	00074-1258-21
1 ml x 10	$12.94	GENERIC, Abbott Pharmaceutical	00074-1258-11
Solution - Injectable - 5 mg/ml			
1 ml x 25	$24.75	GENERIC, Esi Lederle Generics	00641-0168-25
30 ml x 10	$25.29	GENERIC, Faulding Pharmaceutical Company	61703-0221-75
30 ml x 10	$25.29	GENERIC, Faulding Pharmaceutical Company	61703-0221-85
Solution - Injectable - 8 mg/ml			
1 ml x 10	$7.30	GENERIC, Abbott Pharmaceutical	00074-1259-01
1 ml x 10	$8.08	GENERIC, Abbott Pharmaceutical	00074-1260-01
1 ml x 10	$9.38	GENERIC, Abbott Pharmaceutical	00074-1260-31
1 ml x 10	$9.70	GENERIC, Esi Lederle Generics	00008-0655-03
1 ml x 10	$9.80	GENERIC, Abbott Pharmaceutical	00074-1259-60
1 ml x 10	$11.10	GENERIC, Abbott Pharmaceutical	00074-1260-69
1 ml x 10	$12.40	GENERIC, Abbott Pharmaceutical	00074-1260-21
1 ml x 25	$19.80	GENERIC, Esi Lederle Generics	00641-1170-35
1 ml x 25	$22.30	GENERIC, Esi Lederle Generics	00641-0170-25
Solution - Injectable - 10 mg/ml			
1 ml x 10	$6.60	GENERIC, Abbott Pharmaceutical	00074-1261-01
1 ml x 10	$7.80	GENERIC, Abbott Pharmaceutical	00074-1263-01
1 ml x 10	$9.30	GENERIC, Esi Lederle Generics	00008-0656-01
1 ml x 10	$10.00	GENERIC, Abbott Pharmaceutical	00074-1261-02
1 ml x 10	$10.21	GENERIC, Abbott Pharmaceutical	00074-1261-31
1 ml x 10	$11.90	GENERIC, Abbott Pharmaceutical	00074-1261-30
1 ml x 10	$12.35	GENERIC, Abbott Pharmaceutical	00074-1263-21
1 ml x 10	$12.80	GENERIC, Esi Lederle Generics	00008-0656-50
1 ml x 10	$12.94	GENERIC, Abbott Pharmaceutical	00074-1263-11
1 ml x 25	$16.75	GENERIC, Baxter Pharmaceutical Products, Inc	10019-0178-44
1 ml x 25	$17.00	GENERIC, Esi Lederle Generics	00641-1180-35
1 ml x 25	$18.50	GENERIC, Baxter Pharmaceutical Products, Inc	10019-0178-68
1 ml x 25	$21.50	GENERIC, Esi Lederle Generics	00641-0180-25
3 ml x 10	$93.75	GENERIC, Abbott Pharmaceutical	00074-6176-14
10 ml	$11.65	GENERIC, Esi Lederle Generics	00641-2343-41
10 ml	$11.65	GENERIC, Baxter Pharmaceutical Products, Inc	10019-0178-62
10 ml x 5	$51.30	GENERIC, Abbott Pharmaceutical	00074-3817-12
Solution - Injectable - 10 mg/ml Preservative;Free			
30 ml	$23.16	GENERIC, Faulding Pharmaceutical Company	61703-0232-86
Solution - Injectable - 15 mg/ml			
1 ml x 10	$9.67	GENERIC, Sanofi Winthrop Pharmaceuticals	00024-1264-20
1 ml x 10	$10.40	GENERIC, Abbott Pharmaceutical	00074-1264-31
1 ml x 10	$11.07	GENERIC, Esi Lederle Generics	00008-0657-01
1 ml x 25	$18.00	GENERIC, Esi Lederle Generics	00641-1190-35
1 ml x 25	$20.25	GENERIC, Baxter Pharmaceutical Products, Inc	10019-0179-44
1 ml x 25	$22.50	GENERIC, Esi Lederle Generics	00641-0190-25
20 ml	$12.38	GENERIC, Esi Lederle Generics	00641-2345-41
20 ml	$12.38	GENERIC, Baxter Pharmaceutical Products, Inc	10019-0179-63
20 ml	$14.50	GENERIC, Ivax Corporation	00182-9139-65
Solution - Injectable - 25 mg/ml			
4 ml x 25	$283.13	GENERIC, International Medication Systems, Limited	00548-6045-25
10 ml	$21.26	GENERIC, King Pharmaceuticals Inc	60793-0090-10
10 ml x 25	$265.75	GENERIC, International Medication Systems, Limited	00548-6042-25
20 ml	$36.17	GENERIC, King Pharmaceuticals Inc	60793-0092-20
20 ml x 10	$365.50	GENERIC, Faulding Pharmaceutical Company	61703-0223-21
20 ml x 25	$904.13	GENERIC, International Medication Systems, Limited	00548-6043-25
40 ml	$77.82	GENERIC, King Pharmaceuticals Inc	60793-0093-40
40 ml x 10	$825.90	GENERIC, Faulding Pharmaceutical Company	61703-0223-43
40 ml x 10	$829.30	GENERIC, Marsam Pharmaceuticals Inc	00209-6858-22
50 ml	$2553.75	GENERIC, Celltech Pharmacuetical Inc	00548-6038-00
Solution - Injectable - 25 mg/ml Preservative;Free			
4 ml	$27.00	GENERIC, Faulding Pharmaceutical Company	61703-0224-71
10 ml	$108.50	GENERIC, Faulding Pharmaceutical Company	61703-0224-80
20 ml	$190.50	GENERIC, Faulding Pharmaceutical Company	61703-0224-72
30 ml	$202.50	GENERIC, Faulding Pharmaceutical Company	61703-0224-86
50 ml	$457.50	GENERIC, Faulding Pharmaceutical Company	61703-0224-76
Solution - Injectable - 50 mg/ml			
10 ml	$112.50	GENERIC, Faulding Pharmaceutical Company	61703-0226-80
10 ml x 5	$56.11	GENERIC, Abbott Pharmaceutical	00074-1134-22
20 ml	$10.49	GENERIC, Abbott Pharmaceutical	00074-1134-03
20 ml	$80.00	GENERIC, Watson/Schein Pharmaceuticals Inc	00364-3067-55
20 ml	$86.03	GENERIC, Apotex Usa Inc	60505-0656-00
20 ml	$86.03	GENERIC, King Pharmaceuticals Inc	60793-0091-20
20 ml x 10	$225.00	GENERIC, Faulding Pharmaceutical Company	61703-0226-72
20 ml x 10	$890.20	GENERIC, Faulding Pharmaceutical Company	61703-0225-21
40 ml	$160.00	GENERIC, Watson/Schein Pharmaceuticals Inc	00364-3067-18
40 ml	$172.05	GENERIC, Apotex Usa Inc	60505-0656-01
40 ml x 10	$1775.50	GENERIC, Faulding Pharmaceutical Company	61703-0225-43

M

40 ml x 25	$1363.25	GENERIC, International Medication Systems, Limited	00548-6041-25
50 ml	$21.46	GENERIC, Abbott Pharmaceutical	00074-1134-05
50 ml	$215.05	GENERIC, Apotex Usa Inc	60505-0656-02
50 ml	$215.05	GENERIC, King Pharmaceuticals Inc	60793-0097-50
50 ml x 25	$1704.06	GENERIC, International Medication Systems, Limited	00548-6223-25
Solution - Injectable - 50 mg/ml Preservative;Free			
30 ml	$337.01	GENERIC, Faulding Pharmaceutical Company	61703-0226-86
50 ml	$562.50	GENERIC, Faulding Pharmaceutical Company	61703-0226-76
Solution - Oral - 10 mg/5 ml			
5 ml x 40	$24.80	GENERIC, Roxane Laboratories Inc	00054-8585-16
10 ml x 40	$37.60	GENERIC, Roxane Laboratories Inc	00054-8586-16
100 ml	$9.04	GENERIC, Roxane Laboratories Inc	00054-3785-49
100 ml	$10.00	GENERIC, Morton Grove Pharmaceuticals Inc	60432-0122-00
120 ml	$8.33	GENERIC, Apotex Usa Inc	60999-0130-01
120 ml	$11.46	MSIR, Purdue Frederick Company	00034-0521-02
500 ml	$20.00	GENERIC, Liquipharm Inc	54198-0144-50
500 ml	$30.00	GENERIC, Morton Grove Pharmaceuticals Inc	60432-0122-17
500 ml	$31.20	GENERIC, Roxane Laboratories Inc	00054-3785-63
Solution - Oral - 20 mg/5 ml			
100 ml	$12.88	GENERIC, Roxane Laboratories Inc	00054-3786-49
100 ml	$13.00	GENERIC, Morton Grove Pharmaceuticals Inc	60432-0123-00
120 ml	$12.08	GENERIC, Apotex Usa Inc	60999-0131-01
120 ml	$15.71	MSIR, Purdue Frederick Company	00034-0522-02
500 ml	$40.00	GENERIC, Morton Grove Pharmaceuticals Inc	60432-0123-17
500 ml	$52.61	GENERIC, Roxane Laboratories Inc	00054-3786-63
Suppository - Rectal - 5 mg			
12's	$14.35	GENERIC, Upsher-Smith Laboratories Inc	00245-0160-12
12's	$15.10	GENERIC, Paddock Laboratories Inc	00574-7110-12
Suppository - Rectal - 10 mg			
12's	$14.39	ROXANOL, Roxane Laboratories Inc	00054-8776-05
12's	$16.95	GENERIC, Upsher-Smith Laboratories Inc	00245-0161-12
12's	$17.75	GENERIC, Paddock Laboratories Inc	00574-7112-12
Suppository - Rectal - 20 mg			
12's	$17.02	ROXANOL, Roxane Laboratories Inc	00054-8777-05
12's	$20.56	GENERIC, Upsher-Smith Laboratories Inc	00245-0162-12
12's	$21.06	GENERIC, G and W Laboratories Inc	00713-0195-12
12's	$21.60	GENERIC, Paddock Laboratories Inc	00574-7114-12
Suppository - Rectal - 30 mg			
12's	$21.87	ROXANOL, Roxane Laboratories Inc	00054-8778-05
12's	$25.37	GENERIC, Shire Richwood Pharmaceutical Company Inc	58521-0030-12
12's	$28.71	GENERIC, Upsher-Smith Laboratories Inc	00245-0163-12
12's	$29.44	GENERIC, G and W Laboratories Inc	00713-0196-12
12's	$29.80	GENERIC, Paddock Laboratories Inc	00574-7116-12
Tablet - Oral - 10 mg			
100's	$25.79	GENERIC, Lilly, Eli and Company	00002-2549-02
100's	$33.26	GENERIC, Ddn/Obergfel	63304-0706-01
Tablet - Oral - 15 mg			
100's	$12.15	GENERIC, Apotex Usa Inc	60999-0120-10
100's	$18.32	GENERIC, Roxane Laboratories Inc	00054-4582-25
100's	$19.31	GENERIC, Ethex Corporation	58177-0313-04
100's	$21.70	MSIR, Purdue Frederick Company	00034-0518-10
100's	$26.12	GENERIC, Roxane Laboratories Inc	00054-8582-24
100's	$32.72	GENERIC, Lilly, Eli and Company	00002-2550-02
100's	$42.21	GENERIC, Ddn/Obergfel	63304-0707-01
Tablet - Oral - 30 mg			
100's	$23.08	GENERIC, Apotex Usa Inc	60999-0121-10
100's	$31.22	GENERIC, Roxane Laboratories Inc	00054-4583-25
100's	$32.63	GENERIC, Ethex Corporation	58177-0314-04
100's	$36.67	MSIR, Purdue Frederick Company	00034-0519-10
100's	$44.34	GENERIC, Roxane Laboratories Inc	00054-8583-24
100's	$54.91	GENERIC, Lilly, Eli and Company	00002-2551-02
Tablet, Extended Release - Oral - 30 mg			
100's	$70.84	GENERIC, Ddn/Obergfel	63304-0708-01

Moxifloxacin Hydrochloride *(003461)*

For related information, see the comparative table section in Appendix A.

Categories: Bronchitis, chronic, acute exacerbation; Conjunctivitis, bacterial; Infection, lower respiratory tract; Infection, upper respiratory tract; Infection, skin and skin structures; Pneumonia; Infection, sinus; FDA Approved 1999 Dec; Pregnancy Category C
Drug Classes: Antibiotics, quinolones; Anti-infectives, ophthalmic; Ophthalmics
Foreign Brand Availability: Avalox (Bahrain; Cyprus; Egypt; Germany; Iran; Iraq; Jordan; Kuwait; Lebanon; Libya; Oman; Qatar; Republic-of-Yemen; Saudi-Arabia; Syria; United-Arab-Emirates); Avelon (South-Africa); Avelox (Australia; Bahamas; Barbados; Belize; Benin; Bermuda; Burkina-Faso; Colombia; Curacao; Ethiopia; Gambia; Ghana; Guinea; Guyana; Hong-Kong; Indonesia; Ivory-Coast; Jamaica; Kenya; Korea; Liberia; Malawi; Mali; Mauritania; Mauritius; Mexico; Morocco; Netherland-Antilles; New-Zealand; Niger; Nigeria; Peru; Philippines; Puerto-Rico; Senegal; Seychelles; Sierra-Leone; Singapore; Sudan; Surinam; Tanzania; Thailand; Trinidad; Tunia; Uganda; Zambia; Zimbabwe); Bacterol (Colombia); Izilox (France); Megaxin (Israel); Moxif (India); Vigamox (Us)
Cost of Therapy: $98.00 (Community Acquired Pneumonia; Avelox; 400 mg; 1 tablet/day; 10 day supply)

DESCRIPTION

TABLETS AND IV

Avelox (moxifloxacin hydrochloride) is a synthetic broad spectrum antibacterial agent and is available as Avelox tablets for oral administration and as Avelox IV for intravenous (IV) administration. Moxifloxacin hydrochloride, a fluoroquinolone, is available as the monohydrochloride salt of 1-cyclopropyl-7-[(S,S)-2,8-diazabicyclo[4.3.0]non-8-yl]-6-fluoro-8-methoxy-1,4-dihydro-4-oxo-3-quinoline carboxylic acid. It is a slightly yellow to yellow crystalline substance with a molecular weight of 437.9. Its empirical formula is $C_{21}H_{24}FN_3O_4{\cdot}HCl$.

Avelox tablets are available as film-coated tablets containing moxifloxacin hydrochloride (equivalent to 400 mg moxifloxacin). The inactive ingredients are microcrystalline cellulose, lactose monohydrate, croscarmellose sodium, magnesium stearate, hydroxypropyl methylcellulose, titanium dioxide, polyethylene glycol and ferric oxide.

Avelox IV is available in ready-to-use 250 ml latex-free flexibags as a sterile, preservative free, 0.8% sodium chloride aqueous solution of moxifloxacin HCl (containing 400 mg moxifloxacin) with pH ranging from 4.1-4.6. The appearance of the IV solution is yellow. The color does not affect, nor is it indicative of, product stability. The inactive ingredients are sodium chloride, water for injection, and may include hydrochloric acid and/or sodium hydroxide for pH adjustment.

OPHTHALMIC SOLUTION

Vigamox (moxifloxacin HCl ophthalmic solution) 0.5% is a sterile ophthalmic solution. It is an 8-methoxy fluoroquinolone anti-infective for topical ophthalmic use.

The empirical formula is $C_{21}H_{24}FN_3O_4{\cdot}HCl$ and the molecular weight 437.9.

Chemical Name

1-Cyclopropyl-6-fluoro-1,4-dihydro-8-methoxy-7-[(4aS,7aS)-octahydro-6Hpyrrolol[3,4-b]pyridin-6-yl]-4-oxo-3-quinolinecarboxylic acid, monohydrochloride.

Moxifloxacin hydrochloride is a slightly yellow to yellow crystalline powder. Each milliliter of moxifloxacin HCl ophthalmic solution contains 5.45 mg moxifloxacin hydrochloride equivalent to 5 mg moxifloxacin base.

Contains: *Active:* Moxifloxacin 0.5% (5 mg/ml); *Inactives:* Boric acid, sodium chloride, and purified water. May also contain hydrochloric acid/sodium hydroxide to adjust pH to approximately 6.8.

Moxifloxacin HCl ophthalmic solution is an isotonic solution with an osmolality of approximately 290 mOsm/kg.

CLINICAL PHARMACOLOGY

TABLETS AND IV

Absorption

Moxifloxacin, given as an oral tablet, is well absorbed from the gastrointestinal tract. The absolute bioavailability of moxifloxacin is approximately 90%. Coadministration with a high fat meal (*i.e.,* 500 calories from fat) does not affect the absorption of moxifloxacin.

Consumption of 1 cup of yogurt with moxifloxacin does not significantly affect the extent or rate of systemic absorption (AUC).

The mean (±SD) C_{max} and AUC values following single and multiple doses of 400 mg moxifloxacin given orally are summarized in TABLE 1.

TABLE 1

	C_{max} (mg/L)	AUC (mg·h/L)	Half-Life (hour)
Single Dose Oral			
Healthy (n=372)	3.1 ± 1.0	36.1 ± 9.1	11.5-15.6*
Multiple Dose Oral			
Healthy young male/female (n=15)	4.5 ± 0.5	48.0 ± 2.7	12.7 ± 1.9
Healthy elderly male (n=8)	3.8 ± 0.3	51.8 ± 6.7	
Healthy elderly female (n=8)	4.6 ± 0.6	54.6 ± 6.7	
Healthy young male (n=8)	3.6 ± 0.5	48.2 ± 9.0	
Healthy young female (n=9)	4.2 ± 0.5	49.3 ± 9.5	

* Range of means from different studies.

The mean (±SD) C_{max} and AUC values following single and multiple doses of 400 mg moxifloxacin given by 1 hour IV infusion are summarized in TABLE 2.

Plasma concentrations increase proportionately with dose up to the highest dose tested (1200 mg single oral dose). The mean (±SD) elimination half-life from plasma is 12 ± 1.3 hours; steady-state is achieved after at least 3 days with a 400 mg once daily regimen.

Distribution

Moxifloxacin is approximately 50% bound to serum proteins, independent of drug concentration. The volume of distribution of moxifloxacin ranges from 1.7-2.7 L/kg. Moxifloxacin is widely distributed throughout the body, with tissue concentrations often exceeding plasma concentrations. Moxifloxacin has been detected in the saliva, nasal and bronchial secretions, mucosa of the sinuses, skin blister fluid, and subcutaneous (SC) tissue, and skeletal muscle following oral or IV administration of 400 mg. Concentrations measured at 3 hours post-dose are summarized in TABLE 3. The rates of elimination of moxifloxacin from tissues generally parallel the elimination from plasma.

Metabolism

Moxifloxacin is metabolized via glucuronide and sulfate conjugation. The cytochrome P450 system is not involved in moxifloxacin metabolism, and is not affected by moxifloxacin. The sulfate conjugate (M1) accounts for approximately 38% of the dose, and is eliminated primarily in the feces. Approximately 14% of an oral or IV dose is converted to a glucuronide conjugate (M2), which is excreted exclusively in the urine. Peak plasma concentrations of M2 are approximately 40% those of the parent drug, while plasma concentrations of M1 are generally <10% those of moxifloxacin.

TABLE 2

	C_{max} (mg/L)	AUC (mg·h/L)	Half-Life (hour)
Single Dose IV			
Healthy young male/ female (n=56)	3.9 ± 0.9	39.3 ± 8.6	8.2-15.4*
Patients (n=118)			
Male (n=64)	4.4 ± 3.7		
Female (n=54)	4.5 ± 2.0		
<65 years (n=58)	4.6 ± 4.2		
≥65 years (n=60)	4.3 ± 1.3		
Multiple Dose IV			
Healthy young male (n=8)	4.2 ± 0.8	38.0 ± 4.7	14.8 ± 2.2
Healthy elderly (n=12; 8 male, 4 female)	6.1 ± 1.3	48.2 ± 0.9	10.1 ± 1.6
Patients† (n=107)			
Male (n=58)	4.2 ± 2.6		
Female (n=49)	4.6 ± 1.5		
<65 years (n=52)	4.1 ± 1.4		
≥65 years (n=55)	4.7 ± 2.7		

* Range of means from different studies.
† Expected C_{max} (concentration obtained around the time of the end of the infusion).

TABLE 3 *Moxifloxacin HCl Concentrations (Mean ±SD) After Oral Dosing in Plasma and Tissues Measured 3 Hours After Dosing With 400 mg**

Tissue or Fluid	n	Plasma Concentration (µg/ml)	Tissue or Fluid Concentration (µg/ml or µg/g)	Tissue Plasma Ratio:
Respiratory				
Alveolar macrophages	5	3.3 ± 0.7	61.8 ± 27.3	21.2 ± 10.0
Bronchial mucosa	8	3.3 ± 0.7	5.5 ± 1.3	1.7 ± 0.3
Epithelial lining fluid	5	3.3 ± 0.7	24.4 ± 14.7	8.7 ± 6.1
Sinus				
Maxillary sinus mucosa	4	3.7 ± 1.1†	7.6 ± 1.7	2.0 ± 0.3
Anterior ethmoid mucosa	3	3.7 ± 1.1†	8.8 ± 4.3	2.2 ± 0.6
Nasal polyps	4	3.7 ± 1.1†	9.8 ± 4.5	2.6 ± 0.6

* All moxifloxacin HCl concentrations were measured after a single 400 mg dose, except the sinus concentrations which were measured after 5 days of dosing.
† n=5.

In vitro studies with cytochrome (CYP) P450 enzymes indicate that moxifloxacin does not inhibit CYP3A4, CYP2D6, CYP2C9, CYP2C19, or CYP1A2, suggesting that moxifloxacin is unlikely to alter the pharmacokinetics of drugs metabolized by these enzymes.

Excretion

Approximately 45% of an oral or IV dose of moxifloxacin is excreted as unchanged drug (~20% in urine and ~25% in feces). A total of 96% ± 4% of an oral dose is excreted as either unchanged drug or known metabolites. The mean (±SD) apparent total body clearance and renal clearance are 12 ± 2.0 L/h and 2.6 ± 0.5 L/h, respectively.

Special Populations

Geriatric

Following oral administration of 400 mg moxifloxacin for 10 days in 16 elderly (8 male; 8 female) and 16 young (8 male; 8 female) healthy volunteers, there were no age-related changes in moxifloxacin pharmacokinetics. In 16 healthy elderly male and female volunteers (66-81 years of age) given a single 200 mg dose of oral moxifloxacin, the extent of systemic exposure (AUC and C_{max}) was not statistically different between young and elderly males and elimination half-life was unchanged. No dosage adjustment is necessary based on age. In large Phase 3 studies, the concentrations around the time of the end of the infusion in elderly patients following IV infusion of 400 mg were similar to those observed in young patients.

Pediatric

The pharmacokinetics of moxifloxacin in pediatric subjects have not been studied.

Gender

Following oral administration of 400 mg moxifloxacin daily for 10 days to 23 healthy males (19-75 years) and 24 healthy females (19-70 years), the mean AUC and C_{max} were 8% and 16% higher, respectively, in females compared to males. There are no significant differences in moxifloxacin pharmacokinetics between male and female subjects when differences in body weight are taken into consideration.

A 400 mg single dose study was conducted in 18 young males and females. The comparison of moxifloxacin pharmacokinetics in this study (9 young females and 9 young males) showed no differences in AUC or C_{max} due to gender. Dosage adjustments based on gender are not necessary.

Race

Steady-state moxifloxacin pharmacokinetics in male Japanese subjects were similar to those determined in Caucasians, with a mean C_{max} of 4.1 µg/ml, an AUC(24) of 47 µg·h/ml, and an elimination half-life of 14 hours, following 400 mg PO daily.

Renal Insufficiency

The pharmacokinetic parameters of moxifloxacin are not significantly altered by mild, moderate, or severe renal impairment. No dosage adjustment is necessary in patients with renal impairment.

In a single oral dose study of 24 patients with varying degrees of renal function from normal to severely impaired, the mean peak concentrations (C_{max}) of moxifloxacin were reduced by 22% and 21% in the patients with moderate (CLCR ≥30 and ≤60 ml/min) and severe (CLCR <30 ml/min) renal impairment, respectively. The mean systemic exposure (AUC) in these patients was increased by 13%. In the moderate and severe renally impaired patients, the mean AUC for the sulfate conjugate (M1) increased by 1.7-fold (ranging up to 2.8-fold) and mean AUC and C_{max} for the glucuronide conjugate (M2) increased by 2.8-fold (ranging up to 4.8-fold) and 1.4-fold (ranging up to 2.5-fold), respectively. The sulfate and glucuronide conjugates are not microbiologically active, and the clinical implication of increased exposure to these metabolites in patients with renal impairment has not been studied.

The effect of hemodialysis or continuous ambulatory peritoneal dialysis (CAPD) on the pharmacokinetics of moxifloxacin has not been studied.

Hepatic Insufficiency

In 400 mg single oral dose studies in 6 patients with mild (Child Pugh Class A), and 10 patients with moderate (Child Pugh Class B), hepatic insufficiency, moxifloxacin mean systemic exposure (AUC) was 78% and 102%, respectively, of 18 healthy controls and mean peak concentration (C_{max}) was 79% and 84% of controls.

The mean AUC of the sulfate conjugate of moxifloxacin (M1) increased by 3.9-fold (ranging up to 5.9-fold) and 5.7-fold (ranging up to 8.0-fold) in the mild and moderate groups, respectively. The mean C_{max} of M1 increased by approximately 3-fold in both groups (ranging up to 4.7- and 3.9-fold). The mean AUC of the glucuronide conjugate of moxifloxacin (M2) increased by 1.5-fold (ranging up to 2.5-fold) in both groups. The mean C_{max} of M2 increased by 1.6- and 1.3-fold (ranging up to 2.7- and 2.1-fold), respectively. The clinical significance of increased exposure to the sulfate and glucuronide conjugates has not been studied. No dosage adjustment is recommended for mild or moderate hepatic insufficiency (Child Pugh Classes A and B). The pharmacokinetics of moxifloxacin in severe hepatic insufficiency (Child Pugh Class C) have not been studied. (See DOSAGE AND ADMINISTRATION, Tablets and IV.)

Photosensitivity Potential

A study of the skin response to ultraviolet (UVA and UVB) and visible radiation conducted in 32 healthy volunteers (8/group) demonstrated that moxifloxacin does not show phototoxicity in comparison to placebo. The minimum erythematous dose (MED) was measured before and after treatment with moxifloxacin (200 or 400 mg once daily), lomefloxacin (400 mg once daily), or placebo. In this study, the MED measured for both doses of moxifloxacin were not significantly different from placebo, while lomefloxacin significantly lowered the MED. (See PRECAUTIONS, Tablets and IV, Information for the Patient.)

Drug-Drug Interactions

The potential for pharmacokinetic drug interactions between moxifloxacin and itraconazole, theophylline, warfarin, digoxin, probenecid, morphine, oral contraceptive, ranitidine, glyburide, calcium, iron, and antacids has been evaluated. There was no clinically significant effect of moxifloxacin on itraconazole, theophylline, warfarin, digoxin, oral contraceptives, or glyburide kinetics. Itraconazole, theophylline, warfarin, digoxin, probenecid, morphine, ranitidine, and calcium did not significantly affect the pharmacokinetics of moxifloxacin. These results and the data from *in vitro* studies suggests that moxifloxacin is unlikely to significantly alter the metabolic clearance of drugs metabolized by CYP3A4, CYP2D6, CYP2C9, CYP2C19 or CYP1A2 enzymes.

As with all other quinolones, iron and antacids significantly reduced bioavailability of moxifloxacin.

Itraconazole: In a study involving 11 healthy volunteers, there was no significant effect of itraconazole (200 mg once daily for 9 days), a potent inhibitor of cytochrome P4503A4, on the pharmacokinetics of moxifloxacin (a single 400 mg dose given on the 7th day of itraconazole dosing). In addition, moxifloxacin was shown not to affect the pharmacokinetics of itraconazole.

Theophylline: No significant effect of moxifloxacin (200 mg every 12 hours for 3 days) on the pharmacokinetics of theophylline (400 mg every 12 hours for 3 days) was detected in a study involving 12 healthy volunteers. In addition, theophylline was not shown to affect the pharmacokinetics of moxifloxacin. The effect of coadministration of a 400 mg dose of moxifloxacin with theophylline has not been studied, but it is not expected to be clinically significant based on *in vitro* metabolic data showing that moxifloxacin does not inhibit the CYP1A2 isoenzyme.

Warfarin: No significant effect of moxifloxacin (400 mg once daily for 8 days) on the pharmacokinetics of R- and S-warfarin (25 mg single dose of warfarin sodium on the fifth day) was detected in a study involving 24 healthy volunteers. No significant change in prothrombin time was observed. (See DRUG INTERACTIONS, Tablets and IV.)

Digoxin: No significant effect of moxifloxacin (400 mg once daily for 2 days) on digoxin (0.6 mg as a single dose) AUC was detected in a study involving 12 healthy volunteers. The mean digoxin C_{max} increased by about 50% during the distribution phase of digoxin. This transient increase in digoxin C_{max} is not viewed to be clinically significant. Moxifloxacin pharmacokinetics were similar in the presence or absence of digoxin. No dosage adjustment for moxifloxacin or digoxin is required when these drugs are administered concomitantly.

Morphine: No significant effect of morphine sulfate (a single 10 mg intramuscular dose) on the mean AUC and C_{max} of moxifloxacin (400 mg single dose) was observed in a study of 20 healthy male and female volunteers.

Oral Contraceptives: A placebo-controlled study in 29 healthy female subjects showed that moxifloxacin 400 mg daily for 7 days did not interfere with the hormonal suppression of oral contraception with 0.15 mg levonorgestrel/0.03 mg ethinylestradiol (as measured by serum progesterone, FSH, estradiol, and LH), or with the pharmacokinetics of the administered contraceptive agents.

Probenecid: Probenecid (500 mg twice daily for 2 days) did not alter the renal clearance and total amount of moxifloxacin (400 mg single dose) excreted renally in a study of 12 healthy volunteers.

Ranitidine: No significant effect of ranitidine (150 mg twice daily for 3 days as pretreatment) on the pharmacokinetics of moxifloxacin (400 mg single dose) was detected in a study involving 10 healthy volunteers.

Antidiabetic Agents: In diabetics, glyburide (2.5 mg once daily for 2 weeks pretreatment and for 5 days concurrently) mean AUC and C_{max} were 12% and 21% lower, respectively, when taken with moxifloxacin (400 mg once daily for 5 days) in comparison to placebo. Nonetheless, blood glucose levels were decreased slightly in patients taking glyburide and moxifloxacin in comparison to those taking glyburide alone, suggesting no interference by moxifloxacin on the activity of glyburide. These interaction results are not viewed as clinically significant.

Calcium: Twelve (12) healthy volunteers were administered concomitant moxifloxacin (single 400 mg dose) and calcium (single dose of 500 mg Ca^{++} dietary supplement) followed by an additional 2 doses of calcium 12 and 24 hours after moxifloxacin administration. Calcium had no significant effect on the mean AUC of moxifloxacin. The mean C_{max} was slightly reduced and the time to maximum plasma concentration was prolonged when moxifloxacin was given with calcium compared to when moxifloxacin was given alone (2.5 vs 0.9 hours). These differences are not considered to be clinically significant.

Antacids: When moxifloxacin (single 400 mg tablet dose) was administered 2 hours before, concomitantly, or 4 hours after an aluminum/magnesium-containing antacid (900 mg aluminum hydroxide and 600 mg magnesium hydroxide as a single oral dose) to 12 healthy volunteers there was a 26%, 60% and 23% reduction in the mean AUC of moxifloxacin, respectively. Moxifloxacin should be taken at least 4 hours before or 8 hours after antacids containing magnesium or aluminum, as well as sucralfate, metal cations such as iron, and multivitamin preparations with zinc, or didanosine chewable/buffered tablets or the pediatric powder for oral solution. (See DRUG INTERACTIONS, Tablets and IV and DOSAGE AND ADMINISTRATION, Tablets and IV.)

Iron: When moxifloxacin tablets were administered concomitantly with iron (ferrous sulfate 100 mg once daily for 2 days), the mean AUC and C_{max} of moxifloxacin was reduced by 39% and 59%, respectively. Moxifloxacin should only be taken more than 4 hours before or 8 hours after iron products. (See DRUG INTERACTIONS, Tablets and IV and DOSAGE AND ADMINISTRATION, Tablets and IV.)

Electrocardiogram

Prolongation of the QT interval in the ECG has been observed in some patients receiving moxifloxacin. Following oral dosing with 400 mg of moxifloxacin the mean (±SD) change in QTc from the pre-dose value at the time of maximum drug concentration was 6 milliseconds (±26) (n=787). Following a course of daily IV dosing (400 mg; 1 hour infusion each day) the mean change in QTc from the Day 1 pre-dose value was 9 milliseconds (±24) on Day 1 (n=69) and 3 milliseconds (±29) on Day 3 (n=290). (See WARNINGS, Tablets and IV.)

There is limited information available on the potential for a pharmacodynamic interaction in humans between moxifloxacin and other drugs that prolong the QTc interval of the electrocardiogram. Sotalol, a Class III antiarrhythmic, has been shown to further increase the QTc interval when combined with high doses of IV moxifloxacin in dogs. Therefore, moxifloxacin should be avoided with Class IA and Class III antiarrhythmics. (See ANIMAL PHARMACOLOGY, Tablets and IV; WARNINGS, Tablets and IV; and PRECAUTIONS, Tablets and IV.)

Microbiology

Moxifloxacin has *in vitro* activity against a wide range of gram-positive and gram-negative microorganisms. The bactericidal action of moxifloxacin results from inhibition of the topoisomerase II (DNA gyrase) and topoisomerase IV required for bacterial DNA replication, transcription, repair, and recombination. It appears that the C8-methoxy moiety contributes to enhanced activity and lower selection of resistant mutants of gram-positive bacteria compared to the C8-H moiety. The presence of the bulky bicycloamine substituent at the C-7 position prevents active efflux, associated with the *NorA* or *pmrA* genes seen in certain gram-positive bacteria.

The mechanism of action for quinolones, including moxifloxacin, is different from that of macrolides, beta-lactams, aminoglycosides, or tetracyclines; therefore, microorganisms resistant to these classes of drugs may be susceptible to moxifloxacin and other quinolones. There is no known cross-resistance between moxifloxacin and other classes of antimicrobials.

In vitro resistance to moxifloxacin develops slowly via multiple-step mutations. Resistance to moxifloxacin occurs *in vitro* at a general frequency of between 1.8×10^{-9} to $<1 \times 10^{-11}$ for gram-positive bacteria.

Cross-resistance has been observed between moxifloxacin and other fluoroquinolones against gram-negative bacteria. Gram-positive bacteria resistant to other fluoroquinolones may, however, still be susceptible to moxifloxacin.

Moxifloxacin has been shown to be active against most strains of the following microorganisms, both *in vitro* and in clinical infections as described in INDICATIONS AND USAGE.

Aerobic Gram-Positive Microorganisms:

Staphylococcus aureus (methicillin-susceptible strains only), *Streptococcus pneumoniae* (including penicillin-resistant strains*), *Streptococcus pyogenes.*

**Note:* Penicillin-resistant *S. pneumoniae* are those strains with a penicillin MIC value of ≥2 µg/ml.

Aerobic Gram-Negative Microorganisms:

Haemophilus influenzae, Haemophilus parainfluenzae, Klebsiella pneumoniae, Moraxella catarrhalis.

Other Microorganisms:

Chlamydia pneumoniae, Mycoplasma pneumoniae.

The following *in vitro* data are available, **but their clinical significance is unknown.**

Moxifloxacin exhibits *in vitro* minimum inhibitory concentrations (MICs) of 2 µg/ml or less against most (≥90%) strains of the following microorganisms; however, the safety and effectiveness of moxifloxacin in treating clinical infections due to these microorganisms have not been established in adequate and well-controlled clinical trials.

Aerobic Gram-Positive Microorganisms:

Staphylococcus epidermidis (methicillin-susceptible strains only), *Streptococcus agalactiae, Streptococcus* viridans group.

Aerobic Gram-Negative Microorganisms:

Citrobacter freundii, Enterobacter cloacae, Escherichia coli, Klebsiella oxytoca, Legionella pneumophila, Proteus mirabilis.

Anaerobic Microorganisms:

Fusobacterium species, *Peptostreptococcus* species, *Prevotella* species.

Susceptibility Testing

Dilution Techniques

Quantitative methods are used to determine antimicrobial minimum inhibitory concentrations (MICs). These MICs provide estimates of the susceptibility of bacteria to antimicrobial compounds. The MICs should be determined using a standardized procedure. Standardized procedures are based on a dilution method[1] (broth or agar) or equivalent with standardized inoculum concentrations and standardized concentrations of moxifloxacin powder. The MIC values should be interpreted according to the following criteria:

For testing Enterobacteriaceae and *Staphylococcus* species (see TABLE 4).

TABLE 4

MIC	Interpretation
≤2.0 µg/ml	Susceptible (S)
4.0 µg/ml	Intermediate (I)
≥8.0 µg/ml	Resistant (R)

For testing *Haemophilus influenzae* and *Haemophilus parainfluenzae** (see TABLE 5).

TABLE 5

MIC	Interpretation
≤1.0 µg/ml	Susceptible (S)

* This interpretive standard is applicable only to broth microdilution susceptibility tests with *Haemophilus influenzae* and *Haemophilus parainfluenzae* using *Haemophilus* Test Medium.[1]

The current absence of data on resistant strains precludes defining any results other than "Susceptible". Strains yielding MIC results suggestive of a "nonsusceptible" category should be submitted to a reference laboratory for further testing.

For testing *Streptococcus* species including *Streptococcus pneumoniae** (see TABLE 6).

TABLE 6

MIC	Interpretation
≤1.0 µg/ml	Susceptible (S)
2.0 µg/ml	Intermediate (I)
≥4.0 µg/ml	Resistant (R)

* This interpretive standard is applicable only to broth microdilution susceptibility tests using cation-adjusted Mueller-Hinton broth with 2-5% lysed horse blood.

A report of "Susceptible" indicates that the pathogen is likely to be inhibited if the antimicrobial compound in the blood reaches the concentrations usually achievable. A report of "Intermediate" indicates that the result should be considered equivocal, and, if the microorganism is not fully susceptible to alternative, clinically feasible drugs, the test should be repeated. This category implies possible clinical applicability in body sites where the drug is physiologically concentrated or in situations where a high dosage of drug can be used. This category also provides a buffer zone which prevents small uncontrolled technical factors from causing major discrepancies in interpretation. A report of "Resistant" indicates that the pathogen is not likely to be inhibited if the antimicrobial compound in the blood reaches the concentrations usually achievable; other therapy should be selected.

Standardized susceptibility test procedures require the use of laboratory control microorganisms to control the technical aspects of the laboratory procedures. Standard moxifloxacin powder should provide the MIC values in TABLE 7.

TABLE 7

Microorganism		MIC
Enterococcus faecalis	ATCC 29212	0.06-0.5 µg/ml
Escherichia coli	ATCC 25922	0.008-0.06 µg/ml
Haemophilus influenzae	ATCC 49247*	0.008-0.03 µg/ml
Staphylococcus aureus	ATCC 29213	0.015-0.06 µg/ml
Streptococcus pneumoniae	ATCC 49619†	0.06-0.25 µg/ml

* This quality control range is applicable to only *H. influenzae* ATCC 49247 tested by a broth microdilution procedure using *Haemophilus* Test Medium (HTM).[1]

† This quality control range is applicable to only *S. pneumoniae* ATCC 49619 tested by a broth microdilution procedure using cation-adjusted Mueller-Hinton broth with 2-5% lysed horse blood.

Diffusion Techniques

Quantitative methods that require measurement of zone diameters also provide reproducible estimates of the susceptibility of bacteria to antimicrobial compounds. One such standardized procedure[2] requires the use of standardized inoculum concentrations. This procedure

M

uses paper disks impregnated with 5 μg moxifloxacin to test the susceptibility of microorganisms to moxifloxacin.

Reports from the laboratory providing results of the standard single-disk susceptibility test with a 5 μg moxifloxacin disk should be interpreted according to the following criteria:

The zone diameter interpretive criteria as summarized in TABLE 8 should be used for testing *Enterobacteriaceae* and *Staphylococcus* species.

TABLE 8

Zone Diameter	Interpretation
≥19 mm	Susceptible (S)
16-18 mm	Intermediate (I)
≤15 mm	Resistant (R)

For testing *Haemophilus influenzae* and *Haemophilus parainfluenzae** (see TABLE 9).

TABLE 9

Zone Diameter	Interpretation
≥18 mm	Susceptible (S)

* This zone diameter standard is applicable only to tests with *Haemophilus influenzae* and *Haemophilus parainfluenzae* using *Haemophilus* Test Medium (HTM).[2]

The current absence of data on resistant strains precludes defining any results other than "Susceptible". Strains yielding zone diameter results suggestive of a "nonsusceptible" category should be submitted to a reference laboratory for further testing.

For testing *Streptococcus* species including *Streptococcus pneumoniae** (see TABLE 10).

TABLE 10

Zone Diameter	Interpretation
≥18 mm	Susceptible (S)
15-17 mm	Intermediate (I)
≤14 mm	Resistant (R)

* These interpretive standards are applicable only to disk diffusion tests using Mueller-Hinton agar supplemented with 5% sheep blood incubated in 5% CO_2.

Interpretation should be as stated above for results using dilution techniques. Interpretation involves correlation of the diameter obtained in the disk test with the MIC for moxifloxacin.

As with standardized dilution techniques, diffusion methods require the use of laboratory control microorganisms that are used to control the technical aspects of the laboratory procedures. For the diffusion technique, the 5 μg moxifloxacin disk should provide the following zone diameters in these laboratory test quality control strains (see TABLE 11).

TABLE 11

Microorganism		Zone Diameter
Escherichia coli	ATCC 25922	28-35 mm
Haemophilus influenzae	ATCC 49247*	31-39 mm
Staphylococcus aureus	ATCC 25923	28-35 mm
Streptococcus pneumoniae	ATCC 49619†	25-31 mm

* These quality control limits are applicable to only *H. influenzae* ATCC 49247 testing using *Haemophilus* Test Medium (HTM).[2]

† These quality control limits are applicable only to tests conducted with *S. pneumoniae* ATCC 49619 performed by disk diffusion using Mueller-Hinton agar supplemented with 5% defibrinated sheep blood.

OPHTHALMIC SOLUTION

Pharmacokinetics

Plasma concentrations of moxifloxacin were measured in healthy adult male and female subjects who received bilateral topical ocular doses of moxifloxacin HCl ophthalmic solution 3 times a day. The mean steady-state C_{max} (2.7 ng/ml) and estimated daily exposure AUC (45 ng·h/ml) values were 1600 and 1000 times lower than the mean C_{max} and AUC reported after therapeutic 400 mg oral doses of moxifloxacin. The plasma half-life of moxifloxacin was estimated to be 13 hours.

Microbiology

Moxifloxacin is an 8-methoxy fluoroquinolone with a diazabicyclononyl ring at the C7 position. The antibacterial action of moxifloxacin results from inhibition of the topoisomerase II (DNA gyrase) and topoisomerase IV. DNA gyrase is an essential enzyme that is involved in the replication, transcription and repair of bacterial DNA. Topoisomerase IV is an enzyme known to play a key role in the partitioning of the chromosomal DNA during bacterial cell division.

The mechanism of action for quinolones, including moxifloxacin, is different from that of macrolides, aminoglycosides, or tetracyclines. Therefore, moxifloxacin may be active against pathogens that are resistant to these antibiotics and these antibiotics may be active against pathogens that are resistant to moxifloxacin. There is no cross-resistance between moxifloxacin and the aforementioned classes of antibiotics. Cross resistance has been observed between systemic moxifloxacin and some other quinolones.

In vitro resistance to moxifloxacin develops via multiple-step mutations. Resistance to moxifloxacin occurs *in vitro* at a general frequency of between 1.8×10^{-9} to $<1 \times 10^{-11}$ for gram-positive bacteria.

Moxifloxacin has been shown to be active against most strains of the following microorganisms, both *in vitro* and in clinical infections as described in INDICATIONS AND USAGE, Ophthalmic Solution.

Aerobic Gram-Positive Microorganisms:

Corynebacterium species*, *Micrococcus luteus**, *Staphylococcus aureus, Staphylococcus epidermidis, Staphylococcus haemolyticus, Staphylococcus hominis, Staphylococcus warneri**, *Streptococcus pneumoniae, Streptococcus* viridans group.

Aerobic Gram-Negative Microorganisms:

*Acinetobacter lwoffii**, *Haemophilus influenzae, Haemophilus parainfluenzae**.

Other Microorganisms:

Chlamydia trachomatis.

*Efficacy for this organism was studied in fewer than 10 infections.

The following *in vitro* data are also available, **but their clinical significance in ophthalmic infections is unknown.** The safety and effectiveness of moxifloxacin HCl ophthalmic solution in treating ophthalmological infections due to these microorganisms have not been established in adequate and well-controlled trials.

The following organisms are considered susceptible when evaluated using systemic breakpoints. However, a correlation between the *in vitro* systemic breakpoint and ophthalmological efficacy has not been established. The list of organisms is provided as guidance only in assessing the potential treatment of conjunctival infections. Moxifloxacin exhibits *in vitro* minimal inhibitory concentrations (MICs) of 2 μg/ml or less (systemic susceptible breakpoint) against most (≥90%) of strains of the following ocular pathogens.

Aerobic Gram-Positive Microorganisms:

Streptococcus pyogenes.

Aerobic Gram-Negative Microorganisms:

Escherichia coli, Klebsiella oxytoca, Klebsiella pneumoniae, Moraxella catarrhalis, Proteus mirabilis.

Anaerobic Microorganisms:

Fusobacterium species, *Prevotella* species.

INDICATIONS AND USAGE

TABLETS AND IV

Moxifloxacin HCl tablets and IV are indicated for the treatment of adults (≥18 years of age) with infections caused by susceptible strains of the designated microorganisms in the conditions listed below. (See DOSAGE AND ADMINISTRATION, Tablets and IV for specific recommendations. In addition, for IV use see PRECAUTIONS, Tablets and IV, Geriatric Use.)

Acute bacterial sinusitis caused by *Streptococcus pneumoniae, Haemophilus influenzae,* or *Moraxella catarrhalis.*

Acute bacterial exacerbation of chronic bronchitis caused by *Streptococcus pneumoniae, Haemophilus influenzae, Haemophilus parainfluenzae, Klebsiella pneumoniae, Staphylococcus aureus,* or *Moraxella catarrhalis.*

Community acquired pneumonia caused by *Streptococcus pneumoniae* (including penicillin-resistant strains, MIC value for penicillin ≥2 μg/ml), *Haemophilus influenzae, Moraxella catarrhalis, Staphylococcus aureus, Klebsiella pneumoniae, Mycoplasma pneumoniae,* or *Chlamydia pneumoniae.*

Uncomplicated skin and skin structure infections caused by *Staphylococcus aureus* or *Streptococcus pyogenes.*

Appropriate culture and susceptibility tests should be performed before treatment in order to isolate and identify organisms causing infection and to determine their susceptibility to moxifloxacin. Therapy with moxifloxacin HCl may be initiated before results of these tests are known; once results become available, appropriate therapy should be continued.

OPHTHALMIC SOLUTION

Moxifloxacin HCl ophthalmic solution is indicated for the treatment of bacterial conjunctivitis caused by susceptible strains of the following organisms:

Aerobic Gram-Positive Microorganisms:

Corynebacterium species*, *Micrococcus luteus**, *Staphylococcus aureus, Staphylococcus epidermidis, Staphylococcus haemolyticus, Staphylococcus hominis, Staphylococcus warneri**, *Streptococcus pneumoniae, Streptococcus* viridans group.

Aerobic Gram-Negative Microorganisms:

*Acinetobacter lwoffii**, *Haemophilus influenzae, Haemophilus parainfluenzae**.

Other Microorganisms:

Chlamydia trachomatis.

*Efficacy for this organism was studied in fewer than 10 infections.

CONTRAINDICATIONS

TABLETS AND IV

Moxifloxacin is contraindicated in persons with a history of hypersensitivity to moxifloxacin or any member of the quinolone class of antimicrobial agents.

OPHTHALMIC SOLUTION

Moxifloxacin HCl ophthalmic solution is contraindicated in patients with a history of hypersensitivity to moxifloxacin, to other quinolones, or to any of the components in this medication.

WARNINGS

TABLETS AND IV

THE SAFETY AND EFFECTIVENESS OF MOXIFLOXACIN IN PEDIATRIC PATIENTS, ADOLESCENTS (<18 YEARS OF AGE), PREGNANT WOMEN, AND LACTATING WOMEN HAVE NOT BEEN ESTABLISHED. (SEE PRECAUTIONS, Tablets and IV: Pediatric Use, Pregnancy, Teratogenic Effects, Pregnancy Category C AND Nursing Mothers.)

Moxifloxacin has been shown to prolong the QT interval of the electrocardiogram in some patients. The drug should be avoided in patients with known prolongation of the QT interval, patients with uncorrected hypokalemia and patients receiving Class IA

M

(*e.g.*, quinidine, procainamide) or Class III (*e.g.*, amiodarone, sotalol) antiarrhythmic agents, due to the lack of clinical experience with the drug in these patient populations.

Pharmacokinetic studies between moxifloxacin and other drugs that prolong the QT interval such as cisapride, erythromycin, antipsychotics, and tricyclic antidepressants have not been performed. An additive effect of moxifloxacin and these drugs cannot be excluded, therefore caution should be exercised when moxifloxacin is given concurrently with these drugs. In premarketing clinical trials, the rate of cardiovascular adverse events was similar in 798 moxifloxacin and 702 comparator treated patients who received concomitant therapy with drugs known to prolong the QTc interval.

Because of limited clinical experience, moxifloxacin should be used with caution in patients with ongoing proarrhythmic conditions, such as clinically significant bradycardia, acute myocardial ischemia. The magnitude of QT prolongation may increase with increasing concentrations of the drug or increasing rates of infusion of the IV formulation. Therefore the recommended dose or infusion rate should not be exceeded. QT prolongation may lead to an increased risk for ventricular arrhythmias including torsade de pointes. No cardiovascular morbidity or mortality attributable to QTc prolongation occurred with moxifloxacin treatment in over 7900 patients in controlled clinical studies, including 223 patients who were hypokalemic at the start of treatment, and there was no increase in mortality in over 18,000 moxifloxacin tablet treated patients in a post-marketing observational study in which ECGs were not performed. (See CLINICAL PHARMACOLOGY, Tablets and IV, Drug-Drug Interactions, Electrocardiogram. For IV use see DOSAGE AND ADMINISTRATION, Tablets and IV and PRECAUTIONS, Tablets and IV, Geriatric Use.)

The oral administration of moxifloxacin caused lameness in immature dogs. Histopathological examination of the weight-bearing joints of these dogs revealed permanent lesions of the cartilage. Related quinolone-class drugs also produce erosions of cartilage of weight-bearing joints and other signs of arthropathy in immature animals of various species. (See ANIMAL PHARMACOLOGY, Tablets and IV.)

Convulsions have been reported in patients receiving quinolones. Quinolones may also cause central nervous system (CNS) events including: dizziness, confusion, tremors, hallucinations, depression, and, rarely, suicidal thoughts or acts. These reactions may occur following the first dose. If these reactions occur in patients receiving moxifloxacin, the drug should be discontinued and appropriate measures instituted. As with all quinolones, moxifloxacin should be used with caution in patients with known or suspected CNS disorders (*e.g.*, severe cerebral arteriosclerosis, epilepsy) or in the presence of other risk factors that may predispose to seizures or lower the seizure threshold. (See PRECAUTIONS, Tablets and IV: General and Information for the Patient; and ADVERSE REACTIONS, Tablets and IV.)

Serious anaphylactic reactions, some following the first dose, have been reported in patients receiving quinolone therapy, including moxifloxacin. Some reactions were accompanied by cardiovascular collapse, loss of consciousness, tingling, pharyngeal or facial edema, dyspnea, urticaria, and itching. Serious anaphylactic reactions require immediate emergency treatment with epinephrine. Moxifloxacin should be discontinued at the first appearance of a skin rash or any other sign of hypersensitivity. Oxygen, IV steroids, and airway management, including intubation, may be administered as indicated.

M

Severe and sometimes fatal events, some due to hypersensitivity, and some of uncertain etiology, have been reported in patients receiving therapy with all antibiotics. These events may be severe and generally occur following the administration of multiple doses. Clinical manifestations may include 1 or more of the following: rash, fever, eosinophilia, jaundice, and hepatic necrosis.

Pseudomembranous colitis has been reported with nearly all antibacterial agents and may range in severity from mild to life-threatening. Therefore, it is important to consider this diagnosis in patients who present with diarrhea subsequent to the administration of antibacterial agents.

Treatment with antibacterial agents alters the normal flora of the colon and may permit overgrowth of clostridia. Studies indicate that a toxin produced by *Clostridium difficile* is one primary cause of "antibiotic-associated colitis".

After the diagnosis of pseudomembranous colitis has been established, therapeutic measures should be initiated. Mild cases of pseudomembranous colitis usually respond to drug discontinuation alone. In moderate to severe cases, consideration should be given to management with fluids and electrolytes, protein supplementation, and treatment with an antibacterial drug clinically effective against *C. difficile* colitis.

Achilles and other tendon ruptures that required surgical repair or resulted in prolonged disability have been reported with quinolones, including moxifloxacin. Post-marketing surveillance reports indicate that the risk may be increased in patients receiving concomitant corticosteroids, especially in the elderly. Moxifloxacin should be discontinued if the patient experiences pain, inflammation, or rupture of a tendon.

OPHTHALMIC SOLUTION

NOT FOR INJECTION.

Moxifloxacin HCl ophthalmic solution should not be injected subconjunctivally, nor should it be introduced directly into the anterior chamber of the eye.

In patients receiving systemically administered quinolones, including moxifloxacin, serious and occasionally fatal hypersensitivity (anaphylactic) reactions have been reported, some following the first dose. Some reactions were accompanied by cardiovascular collapse, loss of consciousness, angioedema (including laryngeal, pharyngeal or facial edema), airway obstruction, dyspnea, urticaria, and itching. If an allergic reaction to moxifloxacin occurs, discontinue use of the drug. Serious acute hypersensitivity reactions may require immediate emergency treatment. Oxygen and airway management should be administered as clinically indicated.

PRECAUTIONS

TABLETS AND IV

General

Quinolones may cause CNS events, including: nervousness, agitation, insomnia, anxiety, nightmares or paranoia. (See WARNINGS, Tablets and IV and Information for the Patient.)

Information for the Patient

To assure safe and effective use of moxifloxacin, the following information and instructions should be communicated to the patient when appropriate:

Patients should be advised:

- That moxifloxacin may produce changes in the electrocardiogram (QTc interval prolongation).
- That moxifloxacin should be avoided in patients receiving Class IA (*e.g.*, quinidine, procainamide) or Class III (*e.g.*, amiodarone, sotalol) antiarrhythmic agents.
- That moxifloxacin may add to the QTc prolonging effects of other drugs such as cisapride, erythromycin, antipsychotics, and tricyclic antidepressants.
- To inform their physician of any personal or family history of QTc prolongation or proarrhythmic conditions such as recent hypokalemia, significant bradycardia, acute myocardial ischemia.
- To inform their physician of any other medications when taken concurrently with moxifloxacin, including over-the-counter medications.
- To contact their physician if they experience palpitations or fainting spells while taking moxifloxacin.
- That moxifloxacin tablets may be taken with or without meals, and to drink fluids liberally.
- That moxifloxacin tablets should be taken at least 4 hours before or 8 hours after multivitamins (containing iron or zinc), antacids (containing magnesium or aluminum), sucralfate or (didanosine) chewable/buffered tablets or the pediatric powder for oral solution. (See CLINICAL PHARMACOLOGY, Tablets and IV, Drug-Drug Interactions and DRUG INTERACTIONS, Tablets and IV.)
- That moxifloxacin may be associated with hypersensitivity reactions, including anaphylactic reactions, even following a single dose, and to discontinue the drug at the first sign of a skin rash or other signs of an allergic reaction.
- To discontinue treatment; rest and refrain from exercise; and inform their physician if they experience pain, inflammation, or rupture of a tendon.
- That moxifloxacin may cause dizziness and lightheadedness; therefore, patients should know how they react to this drug before they operate an automobile or machinery or engage in activities requiring mental alertness or coordination.
- That phototoxicity has been reported in patients receiving certain quinolones. There was no phototoxicity seen with moxifloxacin at the recommended dose. In keeping with good medical practice, avoid excessive sunlight or artificial ultraviolet light (*e.g.*, tanning beds). If sunburn-like reaction or skin eruptions occur, contact your physician. (See CLINICAL PHARMACOLOGY, Tablets and IV, Photosensitivity Potential.)
- That convulsions have been reported in patients receiving quinolones, and they should notify their physician before taking this drug if there is a history of this condition.

Carcinogenesis, Mutagenesis, and Impairment of Fertility

Long term studies in animals to determine the carcinogenic potential of moxifloxacin have not been performed.

Moxifloxacin was not mutagenic in 4 bacterial strains (TA 98, TA 100, TA 1535, TA 1537) used in the Ames *Salmonella* reversion assay. As with other quinolones, the positive response observed with moxifloxacin in strain TA 102 using the same assay may be due to the inhibition of DNA gyrase. Moxifloxacin was not mutagenic in the CHO/HGPRT mammalian cell gene mutation assay. An equivocal result was obtained in the same assay when v79 cells were used. Moxifloxacin was clastogenic in the v79 chromosome aberration assay, but it did not induce unscheduled DNA synthesis in cultured rat hepatocytes. There was no evidence of genotoxicity *in vivo* in a micronucleus test or a dominant lethal test in mice.

Moxifloxacin had no effect on fertility in male and female rats at oral doses as high as 500 mg/kg/day, approximately 12 times the maximum recommended human dose based on body surface area (mg/m^2), or at IV doses as high as 45 mg/kg/day, approximately equal to the maximum recommended human dose based on body surface area (mg/m^2). At 500 mg/kg orally there were slight effects on sperm morphology (head-tail separation) in male rats and on the estrous cycle in female rats.

Pregnancy, Teratogenic Effects, Pregnancy Category C

Moxifloxacin was not teratogenic when administered to pregnant rats during organogenesis at oral doses as high as 500 mg/kg/day or 0.24 times the maximum recommended human dose based on systemic exposure (AUC), but decreased fetal body weights and slightly delayed fetal skeletal development (indicative of fetotoxicity) were observed. Intravenous administration of 80 mg/kg/day [approximately 2 times the maximum recommended human dose based on body surface area (mg/m^2)] to pregnant rats resulted in maternal toxicity and a marginal effect on fetal and placental weights and the appearance of the placenta. There was no evidence of teratogenicity at IV doses as high as 80 mg/kg/day. Intravenous administration of 20 mg/kg/day (approximately equal to the maximum recommended human oral dose based upon systemic exposure) to pregnant rabbits during organogenesis resulted in decreased fetal body weights and delayed fetal skeletal ossification. When rib and vertebral malformations were combined, there was an increased fetal and litter incidence of these effects. Signs of maternal toxicity in rabbits at this dose included mortality, abortions, marked reduction of food consumption, decreased water intake, body weight loss and hypoactivity. There was no evidence of teratogenicity when pregnant Cynomolgus monkeys were given oral doses as high as 100 mg/kg/day (2.5 times the maximum recommended human dose based upon systemic exposure). An increased incidence of smaller fetuses was observed at 100 mg/kg/day. In an oral pre- and postnatal development study conducted in rats, effects observed at 500 mg/kg/day included slight increases in duration of pregnancy and prenatal loss, reduced pup birth weight and decreased neonatal survival. Treatment-related maternal mortality occurred during gestation at 500 mg/kg/day in this study.

Since there are no adequate or well-controlled studies in pregnant women, moxifloxacin should be used during pregnancy only if the potential benefit justifies the potential risk to the fetus.

Nursing Mothers

Moxifloxacin is excreted in the breast milk of rats. Moxifloxacin may also be excreted in human milk. Because of the potential for serious adverse reactions in infants nursing from mothers taking moxifloxacin, a decision should be made whether to discontinue nursing or to discontinue the drug, taking into account the importance of the drug to the mother.

Pediatric Use

Safety and effectiveness in pediatric patients and adolescents <18 years of age have not been established. Moxifloxacin causes arthropathy in juvenile animals. (See WARNINGS.)

Geriatric Use

In controlled multiple-dose clinical trials, 23% of patients receiving oral moxifloxacin were ≥65 years of age and 9% were ≥75 years of age. The clinical trial data demonstrate that there is no difference in the safety and efficacy of oral moxifloxacin in patients aged 65 or older compared to younger adults.

In IV trials in community acquired pneumonia, 45% of moxifloxacin patients were ≥65 years of age, and 24% were ≥75 years of age. In the pool of 491 elderly (≥65 years) patients, the following ECG abnormalities were reported in moxifloxacin versus comparator patients: ST-T wave changes (2 events vs 0 events), QT prolongation (2 vs 0), ventricular tachycardia (1 vs 0), atrial flutter (1 vs 0), tachycardia (2 vs 1), atrial fibrillation (1 vs 0), supraventricular tachycardia (1 vs 0), ventricular extrasystoles (2 vs 0), and arrhythmia (0 vs 1). None of the abnormalities was associated with a fatal outcome and a majority of these patients completed a full course of therapy.

OPHTHALMIC SOLUTION

General

As with other anti-infectives, prolonged use may result in overgrowth of non-susceptible organisms, including fungi. If superinfection occurs, discontinue use and institute alternative therapy. Whenever clinical judgment dictates, the patient should be examined with the aid of magnification, such as slit-lamp biomicroscopy, and, where appropriate, fluorescein staining.

Patients should be advised not to wear contact lenses if they have signs and symptoms of bacterial conjunctivitis.

Information for the Patient

Avoid contaminating the applicator tip with material from the eye, fingers or other source.

Systemically administered quinolones including moxifloxacin have been associated with hypersensitivity reactions, even following a single dose. Discontinue use immediately and contact your physician at the first sign of a rash or allergic reaction.

Carcinogenesis, Mutagenesis, and Impairment of Fertility

Long term studies in animals to determine the carcinogenic potential of moxifloxacin have not been performed. However, in an accelerated study with initiators and promoters, moxifloxacin was not carcinogenic in rats following up to 38 weeks of oral dosing at 500 mg/kg/day (approximately 21,700 times the highest recommended total daily human ophthalmic dose for a 50 kg person, on a mg/kg basis).

Moxifloxacin was not mutagenic in 4 bacterial strains used in the Ames *Salmonella* reversion assay. As with other quinolones, the positive response observed with moxifloxacin in strain TA 102 using the same assay may be due to the inhibition of DNA gyrase. Moxifloxacin was not mutagenic in the CHO/HGPRT mammalian cell gene mutation assay. An equivocal result was obtained in the same assay when v79 cells were used. Moxifloxacin was clastogenic in the v79 chromosome aberration assay, but it did not induce unscheduled DNA synthesis in cultured rat hepatocytes. There was no evidence of genotoxicity *in vivo* in a micronucleus test or a dominant lethal test in mice.

Moxifloxacin had no effect on fertility in male and female rats at oral doses as high as 500 mg/kg/day, approximately 21,700 times the highest recommended total daily human ophthalmic dose. At 500 mg/kg orally there were slight effects on sperm morphology (head-tail separation) in male rats and on the estrous cycle in female rats.

Pregnancy, Teratogenic Effects, Pregnancy Category C

Moxifloxacin was not teratogenic when administered to pregnant rats during organogenesis at oral doses as high as 500 mg/kg/day (approximately 21,700 times the highest recommended total daily human ophthalmic dose); however, decreased fetal body weights and slightly delayed fetal skeletal development were observed. There was no evidence of teratogenicity when pregnant Cynomolgus monkeys were given oral doses as high as 100 mg/kg/day (approximately 4,300 times the highest recommended total daily human ophthalmic dose). An increased incidence of smaller fetuses was observed at 100 mg/kg/day.

Since there are no adequate and well-controlled studies in pregnant women, moxifloxacin HCl ophthalmic solution should be used during pregnancy only if the potential benefit justifies the potential risk to the fetus.

Nursing Mothers

Moxifloxacin has not been measured in human milk, although it can be presumed to be excreted in human milk. Caution should be exercised when moxifloxacin HCl ophthalmic solution is administered to a nursing mother.

Pediatric Use

The safety and effectiveness of moxifloxacin HCl ophthalmic solution in infants below 1 year of age have not been established.

There is no evidence that the ophthalmic administration of moxifloxacin HCl ophthalmic solution has any effect on weight bearing joints, even though oral administration of some quinolones has been shown to cause arthropathy in immature animals.

Geriatric Use

No overall differences in safety and effectiveness have been observed between elderly and younger patients.

DRUG INTERACTIONS

TABLETS AND IV

Antacids, Sucralfate, Metal Cations, Multivitamins

Quinolones form chelates with alkaline earth and transition metal cations. Oral administration of quinolones with antacids containing aluminum magnesium or with sucralfate, with metal cations such as iron, or with multivitamins containing iron or zinc, or with formulations containing divalent and trivalent cations such as (didanosine) chewable/buffered tablets or the pediatric powder for oral solution, may substantially interfere with the absorption of quinolones, resulting in systemic concentrations considerably lower than desired. Therefore, moxifloxacin should be taken at least 4 hours before or 8 hours after these agents. (See CLINICAL PHARMACOLOGY, Tablets and IV, Drug-Drug Interactions and DOSAGE AND ADMINISTRATION, Tablets and IV.)

No clinically significant drug-drug interactions between itraconazole, theophylline, warfarin, digoxin, oral contraceptives or glyburide have been observed with moxifloxacin. Itraconazole, theophylline, digoxin, probenecid, morphine, ranitidine, and calcium have been shown not to significantly alter the pharmacokinetics of moxifloxacin. (See CLINICAL PHARMACOLOGY, Tablets and IV.)

Warfarin

No significant effect of moxifloxacin on R- and S-warfarin was detected in a clinical study involving 24 healthy volunteers. No significant changes in prothrombin time were noted in the presence of moxifloxacin. Quinolones, including moxifloxacin, have been reported to enhance the anticoagulant effects of warfarin or its derivatives in the patient population. In addition, infectious disease and its accompanying inflammatory process, age, and general status of the patient are risk factors for increased anticoagulant activity. Therefore the prothrombin time, International Normalized Ratio (INR), or other suitable anticoagulation tests should be closely monitored if a quinolone is administered concomitantly with warfarin or its derivatives.

Drugs Metabolized by Cytochrome P450 Enzymes

In vitro studies with cytochrome P450 isoenzymes (CYP) indicate that moxifloxacin does not inhibit CYP3A4, CYP2D6, CYP2C9, CYP2C19, or CYP1A2, suggesting that moxifloxacin is unlikely to alter the pharmacokinetics of drugs metabolized by these enzymes (*e.g.,* midazolam, cyclosporine, warfarin, theophylline).

Nonsteroidal Anti-Inflammatory Drugs (NSAIDs)

Although not observed with moxifloxacin in preclinical and clinical trials, the concomitant administration of a nonsteroidal anti-inflammatory drug with a quinolone may increase the risks of CNS stimulation and convulsions. (See WARNINGS, Tablets and IV.)

OPHTHALMIC SOLUTION

Drug-drug interaction studies have not been conducted with moxifloxacin HCl ophthalmic solution. *In vitro* studies indicate that moxifloxacin does not inhibit CYP3A4, CYP2D6, CYP2C9, CYP2C19, or CYP1A2 indicating that moxifloxacin is unlikely to alter the pharmacokinetics of drugs metabolized by these cytochrome P450 isozymes.

ADVERSE REACTIONS

TABLETS AND IV

Clinical efficacy trials enrolled over 7900 moxifloxacin orally and intravenously treated patients, of whom over 6700 patients received the 400 mg dose. Most adverse events reported in moxifloxacin trials were described as mild to moderate in severity and required no treatment. Moxifloxacin was discontinued due to adverse reactions thought to be drug-related in 3.6% of orally treated patients and 5.7% of sequentially (IV followed by oral) treated patients. The latter studies were conducted in community acquired pneumonia with, in general, a sicker patient population compared to the tablet studies.

Adverse reactions, judged by investigators to be at least possibly drug-related, occurring in ≥3% of moxifloxacin treated patients were: nausea (7%), diarrhea (6%), dizziness (3%).

Additionally relevant uncommon events, judged by investigators to be at least possibly drug-related, that occurred in ≥0.1% and <3% of moxifloxacin treated patients were:

Body as a Whole: Headache, abdominal pain, injection site reaction, asthenia, moniliasis, pain, malaise, lab test abnormal (not specified), allergic reaction, leg pain, back pain, chest pain.

Cardiovascular: Palpitation, tachycardia, hypertension, peripheral edema, QT interval prolonged.

Central Nervous System: Insomnia, nervousness, anxiety, confusion, somnolence, tremor, vertigo, paresthesia.

Digestive: Vomiting, abnormal liver function test, dyspepsia, dry mouth, constipation, oral moniliasis, anorexia, stomatitis, glossitis, flatulence, gastrointestinal disorder, GGTP increased.

Hemic and Lymphatic: Prothrombin decrease, thrombocythemia, thrombocytopenia, eosinophilia, leukopenia.

Metabolic and Nutritional: Amylase increased, lactic dehydrogenase increased.

Musculoskeletal: Arthralgia, myalgia.

Respiratory: Dyspnea.

Skin/Appendages: Rash (maculopapular, purpuric, pustular), pruritus, sweating.

Special Senses: Taste perversion.

Urogenital: Vaginal moniliasis, vaginitis.

Additional clinically relevant rare events, judged by investigators to be at least possibly drug-related, that occurred in <0.1% of moxifloxacin treated patients were: abnormal dreams, abnormal vision, agitation, amblyopia, amnesia, anemia, aphasia, arthritis, asthma, atrial fibrillation, convulsions, depersonalization, depression, diarrhea *(Clostridium difficile)*, dysphagia, ECG abnormal, emotional lability, face edema, gastritis, hallucinations, hyperglycemia, hyperlipidemia, hypertonia, hyperuricemia, hypesthesia, hypotension, incoordination, jaundice (predominantly cholestatic), kidney function abnormal, parosmia, pelvic pain, prothrombin increase, sleep disorders, speech disorders, supraventricular tachycardia, taste loss, tendon disorder, thinking abnormal, thromboplastin decrease, tinnitus, tongue discoloration, urticaria, vasodilatation, ventricular tachycardia.

M

Post-Marketing Adverse Event Reports

Additional adverse events reported from worldwide post-marketing experience with moxifloxacin include anaphylactic reaction, anaphylactic shock, hepatitis (predominantly cholestatic), pseudomembranous colitis, psychotic reaction, Stevens-Johnson syndrome, syncope, and tendon rupture.

Laboratory Changes

Changes in laboratory parameters, without regard to drug relationship, which are not listed above and which occurred in ≥2% of patients and at an incidence greater than in controls included: increases in MCH, neutrophils, WBCs, PT ratio, ionized calcium, chloride, albumin, globulin, bilirubin; decreases in hemoglobin, RBCs, neutrophils, eosinophils, basophils, PT ratio, glucose, pO_2, bilirubin and amylase. It cannot be determined if any of the above laboratory abnormalities were caused by the drug or the underlying condition being treated.

OPHTHALMIC SOLUTION

The most frequently reported ocular adverse events were conjunctivitis, decreased visual acuity, dry eye, keratitis, ocular discomfort, ocular hyperemia, ocular pain, ocular pruritus, subconjunctival hemorrhage, and tearing. These events occurred in approximately 1-6% of patients.

Nonocular adverse events reported at a rate of 1-4% were fever, increased cough, infection, otitis media, pharyngitis, rash, and rhinitis.

DOSAGE AND ADMINISTRATION

TABLETS AND IV

The dose of moxifloxacin HCl is 400 mg (orally or as an IV infusion) once every 24 hours. The duration of therapy depends on the type of infection as described in TABLE 14.

TABLE 14

Infection*	Daily Dose	Duration
Acute bacterial sinusitis	400 mg	10 days
Acute bacterial exacerbation of chronic bronchitis	400 mg	5 days
Community acquired pneumonia	400 mg	7-14 days
Uncomplicated skin and skin structure infections	400 mg	7 days

* Due to the designated pathogens. (See INDICATIONS AND USAGE.) For IV use see PRECAUTIONS, Tablets and IV, Geriatric Use.

Oral doses of moxifloxacin should be administered at least 4 hours before or 8 hours after antacids containing magnesium or aluminum, as well as sucralfate, metal cations such as iron, and multivitamin preparations with zinc, or didanosine chewable/buffered tablets or the pediatric powder for oral solution. (See CLINICAL PHARMACOLOGY, Tablets and IV, Drug-Drug Interactions and DRUG INTERACTIONS, Tablets and IV.)

Impaired Renal Function

No dosage adjustment is required in renally impaired patients. Moxifloxacin has not been studied in patients on hemodialysis or continuous ambulatory peritoneal dialysis (CAPD).

Impaired Hepatic Function

No dosage adjustment is required in patients with mild or moderate hepatic insufficiency (Child Pugh Classes A and B). The pharmacokinetics of moxifloxacin in patients with severe hepatic insufficiency (Child Pugh Class C) have not been studied. (See CLINICAL PHARMACOLOGY, Tablets and IV, Special Populations, Hepatic Insufficiency.)

When switching from IV to oral dosage administration, no dosage adjustment is necessary. Patients whose therapy is started with moxifloxacin HCl IV may be switched to moxifloxacin HCl tablets when clinically indicated at the discretion of the physician.

Moxifloxacin HCl IV should be administered by IV infusion only. It is not intended for intramuscular, intrathecal, intraperitoneal, or SC administration.

Moxifloxacin HCl IV should be administered by IV infusion over a period of 60 minutes by direct infusion or through a Y-type IV infusion set which may already be in place. CAUTION: RAPID OR BOLUS IV INFUSION MUST BE AVOIDED.

Since only limited data are available on the compatibility of moxifloxacin IV injection with other IV substances, additives or other medications should not be added to moxifloxacin IV or infused simultaneously through the same IV line. If the same IV line or a Y-type line is used for sequential infusion of other drugs, or if the "piggyback" method of administration is used, the line should be flushed before and after infusion of moxifloxacin IV with an infusion solution compatible with moxifloxacin IV as well as with other drug(s) administered via this common line.

Moxifloxacin HCl IV is Compatible With the Following IV Solutions at Ratios From 1:10 to 10:1

0.9% Sodium chloride injection, sterile water for injection, 1M sodium chloride injection, 10% dextrose for injection, 5% dextrose injection, lactated Ringer's for injection.

OPHTHALMIC SOLUTION

Instill 1 drop in the affected eye 3 times a day for 7 days.

ANIMAL PHARMACOLOGY

TABLETS AND IV

Quinolones have been shown to cause arthropathy in immature animals. In studies in juvenile dogs oral doses of moxifloxacin ≥30 mg/kg/day (approximately 1.5 times the maximum recommended human dose based upon systemic exposure) for 28 days resulted in arthropathy. There was no evidence of arthropathy in mature monkeys and rats at oral doses up to 135 and 500 mg/kg, respectively.

Unlike some other members of the quinolone class, crystalluria was not observed in 6 month repeat dose studies in rats and monkeys with moxifloxacin.

No ocular toxicity was observed in a 13 week oral repeat dose study in dogs with a moxifloxacin dose of 60 mg/kg. Ocular toxicity was not observed in 6 month repeat dose studies in rats and monkeys (daily oral doses up to 500 mg/kg and 135 mg/kg, respectively). In beagle dogs, electroretinographic (ERG) changes were observed in a 2 week study at oral doses of 60 and 90 mg/kg. Histopathological changes were observed in the retina from 1 of 4 dogs at 90 mg/kg, a dose associated with mortality in this study.

Some quinolones have been reported to have proconvulsant activity that is exacerbated with concomitant use of non-steroidal anti-inflammatory drugs (NSAIDs). Moxifloxacin at an oral dose of 300 mg/kg did not show an increase in acute toxicity or potential for CNS toxicity (*e.g.,* seizures) in mice when used in combination with NSAIDs such as diclofenac, ibuprofen, or fenbufen.

In dog studies, at plasma concentrations about 5 times the human therapeutic level, a QT-prolonging effect of moxifloxacin was found. Electrophysiological *in vitro* studies suggested an inhibition of the rapid activating component of the delayed rectifier potassium current (I_{Kr}) as an underlying mechanism. In dogs, the combined infusion of sotalol, a Class III antiarrhythmic agent, with moxifloxacin induced a higher degree of QTc prolongation than that induced by the same dose (30 mg/kg) of moxifloxacin alone.

HOW SUPPLIED

TABLETS

Avelox tablets are available as oblong, dull red film-coated tablets containing 400 mg moxifloxacin. The tablet is coded with the word "BAYER" on one side and "M400" on the reverse side.

Storage: Store at 25°C (77°F); Excursions permitted to 15-30°C (59-86°F). Avoid high humidity.

IV SOLUTION — PREMIX BAGS

Avelox IV is available in ready-to-use 250 ml latex-free flexible bags containing 400 mg of moxifloxacin in 0.8% saline. NO FURTHER DILUTION OF THIS PREPARATION IS NECESSARY.

Parenteral drug products should be inspected visually for particulate matter prior to administration. Samples containing visible particulates should not be used.

Since the premix flexible containers are for single-use only, any unused portion should be discarded.

Storage: Store at 25°C (77°F); Excursions permitted to 15-30°C (59-86°F). **DO NOT REFRIGERATE — PRODUCT PRECIPITATES UPON REFRIGERATION.**

OPHTHALMIC SOLUTION

Vigamox 0.5% is supplied as a sterile ophthalmic solution in Alcon's DROP-TAINER dispensing system consisting of a natural low density polyethylene bottle and dispensing plug and tan polypropylene closure. Tamper evidence is provided with a shrink band around the closure and neck area of the package.

Storage: Store at 2-25°C (36-77°F).

PRODUCT LISTING - EQUIVALENTS NOT AVAILABLE

Solution - Intravenous - 400 mg/250 ml

250 ml	$525.00	AVELOX I.V., Bayer	00026-8582-31

Tablet - Oral - 400 mg

5's	$43.56	AVELOX, Allscripts Pharmaceutical Company	54569-4922-00
5's	$49.00	AVELOX, Bayer	00026-8581-41
10's	$87.13	AVELOX, Allscripts Pharmaceutical Company	54569-4922-01
30's	$294.01	AVELOX, Bayer	00026-8581-69
50's	$490.10	AVELOX, Bayer	00026-8581-88

Mumps and Rubella Virus Vaccine Live (002195)

For complete prescribing information, refer to the CD-ROM included with the book.

Categories: Immunization, mumps; Immunization, rubella; Pregnancy Category C; FDA Pre 1938 Drugs
Drug Classes: Vaccines
Brand Names: Biavax II

DESCRIPTION

Biavax II (Rubella and Mumps Virus Vaccine Live) is a live virus vaccine for immunization against rubella (German measles) and mumps.

Biavax II is a sterile lyophilized preparation of the Wistar RA 27/3 strain of live attenuated rubella virus grown in human diploid cell (WI-38) culture;[1,2] and the Jeryl Lynn (B level) strain of mumps virus grown in cell cultures of chick embryo. The vaccine viruses are the same as those used in the manufacture of Meruvax II (Rubella Virus Vaccine Live) and Mumpsvax (Mumps Virus Vaccine Live). The two viruses are mixed before being lyophilized.

The reconstituted vaccine is for subcutaneous administration. When reconstituted as directed, the dose for injection is 0.5 ml and contains not less than the equivalent of 1,000 $TCID_{50}$ of the U.S. Reference Rubella Virus and 20,000 $TCID_{50}$ of the U.S. Reference Mumps Virus. Each dose contains approximately 25 mcg of neomycin. The product contains no preservative. Sorbitol and hydrolyzed gelatin are added as stabilizers.

INDICATIONS AND USAGE

Biavax II is indicated for simultaneous immunization against rubella and mumps in persons 12 months of age or older. A booster is not needed.

The vaccine is not recommended for infants younger than 12 months because they may retain maternal rubella and mumps neutralizing antibodies which may interfere with the immune response.

Previously unimmunized children of susceptible pregnant women should receive live attenuated rubella vaccine, because an immunized child will be less likely to acquire natural rubella and introduce the virus into the household.

Individuals planning travel outside the United States, if not immune, can acquire measles, mumps or rubella and import these diseases to the United States. Therefore, prior to International travel, individuals known to be susceptible to one or more of these diseases can receive either a single antigen vaccine (measles, mumps, or rubella), or a combined antigen vaccine as appropriate. However, M-M-R* II (Measles, Mumps, and Rubella Virus Vaccine Live) is preferred for persons likely to be susceptible to mumps and rubella; and if a single-antigen measles vaccine is not readily available, travelers should receive M-M-R II (Measles, Mumps, and Rubella Virus Vaccine Live) regardless of their immune status to mumps or rubella.[18,19,20]

NON-PREGNANT ADOLESCENT AND ADULT FEMALES

Immunization of susceptible non-pregnant adolescent and adult females of childbearing age with live attenuated rubella virus vaccine is indicated if certain precautions are observed (see below). Vaccinating susceptible postpubertal females confers individual protection against subsequently acquiring rubella infection during pregnancy, which in turn prevents infection of the fetus and consequent congenital rubella injury.[21]

Women of childbearing age should be advised not to become pregnant for three months after vaccination and should be informed of the reasons for this precaution.*

It is recommended that rubella susceptibility be determined by serologic testing prior to immunization.** If immune, as evidenced by a specific rubella antibody titer of 1:8 or greater (hemagglutination-inhibition test), vaccination is unnecessary. Congenital malformations do occur in up to seven percent of all live births.[22] Their chance appearance after vaccination could lead to misinterpretation of the cause, particularly if the prior rubella-immune status of vaccinees is unknown.

Postpubertal females should be informed of the frequent occurrence of generally self-limited arthralgia and/or arthritis beginning 2 to 4 weeks after vaccination.

POSTPARTUM WOMEN

It has been found convenient in many instances to vaccinate rubella-susceptible women in the immediate postpartum period.

Revaccination: Children vaccinated when younger than 12 months of age should be revaccinated. Based on available evidence, there is no reason to routinely revaccinate persons who were vaccinated originally when 12 months of age or older. However, persons should be revaccinated if there is evidence to suggest that initial immunization was ineffective.

USE WITH OTHER VACCINES

Routine administration of DTP (diphtheria, tetanus, pertussis) and/or OPV (oral poliovirus vaccine) concomitantly with measles, mumps and rubella vaccines is not recommended because there are insufficient data relating to the simultaneous administration of these antigens. However, the American Academy of Pediatrics has noted that in some circumstances, particularly when the patient may not return, some practitioners prefer to administer all these antigens on a single day. If done, separate sites and syringes should be used for DTP and Biavax II.[23]

Biavax II should not be given less than one month before or after administration of other virus vaccines.

CONTRAINDICATIONS

Do not give Biavax II to pregnant females; the possible effects of the vaccine on fetal development are unknown at this time. If vaccination of postpubertal females is undertaken, pregnancy should be avoided for three months following vaccination.

Anaphylactic or anaphylactoid reactions to neomycin (each dose of reconstituted vaccine contains approximately 25 mcg of neomycin).

History of anaphylactic or anaphylactoid reactions to eggs (see Hypersensitivity To Eggs.)

Any febrile respiratory illness or other active febrile infection.

Active untreated tuberculosis.

Patients receiving immunosuppressive therapy. This contraindication does not apply to patients who are receiving corticosteroids as replacement therapy, e.g., for Addison's disease.

Individuals with blood dyscrasias, leukemia, lymphomas of any type, or other malignant neoplasms affecting the bone marrow or lymphatic systems.

Primary and acquired immunodeficiency states, including patients who are immunosuppressed in association with AIDS or other clinical manifestations of infection with human immunodeficiency viruses;[24,25] cellular immune deficiencies; and hypogammaglobulinemic and dysgammaglobulinemic states.

Individuals with a family history of congenital or hereditary immunodeficiency, until the immune competence of the potential vaccine recipient is demonstrated.[26]

*NOTE: The Immunization Practices Advisory Committee (ACIP) has recommended "In view of the importance of protecting this age group against rubella, reasonable precautions in a rubella immunization program include asking females if they are pregnant, excluding those who say they are, and explaining the theoretical risks to the others."[21]

**NOTE: The Immunization Practices Advisory Committee (ACIP) has stated "When practical, and when reliable laboratory services are available, potential vaccinees of childbearing age can have serologic tests to determine susceptibility to rubella.... However, routinely performing serologic tests for all females of childbearing age to determine susceptibility so that vaccine is given only to proven susceptibles is expensive and has been ineffective in some areas. Accordingly, the ACIP believes that rubella vaccination of a woman who is not known to be pregnant and has no history of vaccination is justifiable without serologic testing."[21]

HYPERSENSITIVITY TO EGGS

Live mumps vaccine is produced in chick embryo cell culture. Persons with a history of anaphylactic, anaphylactoid, or other immediate reactions (*e.g.,* hives, swelling of the mouth and throat, difficulty breathing, hypotension, or shock) subsequent to egg ingestion should not be vaccinated. Evidence indicates that persons are not at increased risk if they have egg allergies that are not anaphylactic or anaphylactoid in nature. Such persons may be vaccinated in the usual manner. There is no evidence to indicate that persons with allergies to chickens or feathers are at increased risk of reaction to the vaccine.[21]

DOSAGE AND ADMINISTRATION

FOR SUBCUTANEOUS ADMINISTRATION

Do not inject intravenously.

The dosage of vaccine is the same for all persons. Inject the total volume (about 0.5 ml) of reconstituted vaccine subcutaneously, preferably into the outer aspect of upper arm. *Do not give immune globulin (IG) concurrently with* Biavax II.

During shipment, to insure that there is no loss of potency, the vaccine must be maintained at a temperature of 10°C (50°F) or less.

Before reconstitution, store Biavax II at 2 - 8°C (36 - 46°F). *Protect from light.*

CAUTION: A sterile syringe free of preservatives, antiseptics, and detergents should be used for each injection of the vaccine because these substances may inactivate the live virus vaccine. A 25 gauge, 5/8" needle is recommended.

To reconstitute, use only the diluent supplied, since it is free of preservatives or other antiviral substances which might inactivate the vaccine. First withdraw the entire volume of diluent into the syringe to be used for reconstitution. Inject all the diluent in the syringe into the vial of lyophilized vaccine, and agitate to mix thoroughly. Withdraw the entire contents into a syringe and inject the total volume of restored vaccine subcutaneously.

It is important to use a separate sterile syringe and needle for each individual patient to prevent transmission of hepatitis B virus and other infectious agents from one person to another.

Each dose of Biavax II contains not less than the equivalent of 1,000 $TCID_{50}$ of the U.S. Reference Rubella Virus and 20,000 $TCID_{50}$ of the U.S. Reference Mumps Virus.

Parenteral drug products should be inspected visually for particulate matter and discoloration prior to administration. Biavax II, when reconstituted, is clear yellow.

STORAGE

It is recommended that the vaccine be used as soon as possible after reconstitution. Protect the vaccine from light at all times, since such exposure may inactivate the virus. Store reconstituted vaccine in the vaccine vial in a dark place at 2 - 8°C (36 - 46°F) and discard if not used within eight hours.

PRODUCT LISTING - EQUIVALENTS NOT AVAILABLE

Powder For Injection - Subcutaneous - Strength n/a

1's	$30.61	BIAVAX II, Merck & Company Inc	00006-4746-00
10's	$276.20	BIAVAX II, Merck & Company Inc	00006-4669-00

Mumps Virus Vaccine Live (001842)

For complete prescribing information, refer to the CD-ROM included with the book.

Categories: Immunization, mumps; Pregnancy Category C; FDA Pre 1938 Drugs
Drug Classes: Vaccines
Brand Names: Mumpsvax
Foreign Brand Availability: Pariorix (Benin; Burkina-Faso; Ethiopia; Gambia; Ghana; Guinea; Israel; Ivory-Coast; Kenya; Liberia; Malawi; Mali; Mauritania; Mauritius; Morocco; Niger; Nigeria; Senegal; Seychelles; Sierra-Leone; Sudan; Tanzania; Tunia; Uganda; Zambia; Zimbabwe)

DESCRIPTION

Mumpsvax (Mumps Virus Vaccine Live) is a live virus vaccine for immunization against mumps.

Mumpsvax is a sterile lyophilized preparation of the Jeryl Lynn (B level strain of mumps virus.[1] The virus was adapted to and propagated in cell cultures of chick embryo free of avian leukosis virus and other adventitious agents.

The reconstituted vaccine is for subcutaneous administration. When reconstituted as directed, the dose for injection is 0.5 ml and contains not less than the equivalent of 20,000 $TCID_{50}$ (tissue culture infectious doses) of the U.S. Reference Mumps Virus. Each dose contains approximately 25 mcg of neomycin. The product contains no preservative. Sorbitol and hydrolyzed gelatin are added as stabilizers.

INDICATIONS AND USAGE

Mumpsvax is indicated for immunization against mumps in persons 12 months of age or older. Most adults are likely to have been infected naturally and generally may be considered immune, even if they did not have clinically recognizable disease.[3] A booster is not needed. It is not recommended for infants younger than 12 months because they may retain maternal mumps neutralizing antibodies which may interfere with the immune response.

Evidence indicates that the vaccine will not offer protection when given after exposure to natural mumps.[3] Passively acquired antibody can interfere with the response to live, attenuated-virus vaccines. Therefore, administration of mumps virus vaccine should be deferred until approximately three months after passive immunization.[3]

Individuals planning travel outside the United States, if not immune, can acquire measles, mumps or rubella and import these diseases to the United States. Therefore, prior to International travel, individuals known to be susceptible to one or more of these diseases can receive either a single antigen vaccine (measles, mumps or rubella), or a combined antigen vaccine as appropriate. However, M-M-R*II (Measles, Mumps, and Rubella Virus Vaccine Live) is preferred for persons likely to be susceptible to mumps and rubella; and if single-antigen measles vaccine is not readily available, travelers should receive M-M-R II

(Measles, Mumps, and Rubella Virus Vaccine Live) regardless of their immune status to mumps or rubella.[19,20,21]

Revaccination: Children vaccinated when younger than 12 months of age should be revaccinated. Based on available evidence, there is no reason to routinely revaccinate persons who were vaccinated originally when 12 months of age or older. However, persons should be revaccinated if there is evidence to suggest that initial immunization was ineffective.

USE WITH OTHER VACCINES

Routine administration of DTP (diphtheria, tetanus, pertussis) and/or OPV (oral poliovirus vaccine) concomitantly with measles, mumps and rubella vaccines is not recommended because there are insufficient data relating to the simultaneous administration of these antigens. However, the American Academy of Pediatrics has noted that in some circumstances, particularly when the patient may not return, some practitioners prefer to administer all these antigens on a single day. If done, separate sites and syringes should be used for DTP and Mumpsvax.[22]

Mumpsvax should not be given less than one month before or after administration of other virus vaccines.

CONTRAINDICATIONS

Do not give Mumpsvax to pregnant females; the possible effects of the vaccine on fetal development are unknown at this time. If vaccination of postpubertal females is undertaken, pregnancy should be avoided for three months following vaccination.

Anaphylactic or anaphylactoid reactions to neomycin (each dose of reconstituted vaccine contains approximately 25 mcg of neomycin).

History of anaphylactic or anaphylactoid reactions to eggs see WARNINGS, HYPERSENSITIVITY TO EGGS.

Any febrile respiratory illness or other active febrile infection.

Active untreated tuberculosis.

Patients receiving immunosuppressive therapy. This contraindication does not apply to patients who are receiving corticosteroids as replacement therapy, e.g., for Addison's disease.

Individuals with blood dyscrasias, leukemia, lymphomas of any type or other malignant neoplasms affecting the bone marrow or lymphatic systems.

Primary and acquired immunodeficiency states, including patients who are immunosuppressed in association with AIDS or other clinical manifestations of infection with human immunodeficiency viruses;[23,24]cellular immune deficiencies; and hypogammaglobulinemic and dysgammaglobulinemic states.

Individuals with a family history of congenital or hereditary immunodeficiency, until the immune competence of the potential vaccine recipient is demonstrated.[25]

M

WARNINGS

HYPERSENSITIVITY TO EGGS

Live mumps vaccine is produced in chick embryo cell culture. Persons with a history of anaphylactic, anaphylactoid, or other immediate reactions (*e.g.,* hives, swelling of the mouth and throat, difficulty breathing hypotension, or shock) subsequent to egg ingestion should be vaccinated only with extreme caution. Evidence indicates that persons are not at increased risk if they have egg allergies that are not anaphylactic or anaphylactoid in nature. Such persons may be vaccinated in the usual manner. There is no evidence to indicate that persons with, allergies to chickens or feathers are at increased risk of reaction to the vaccine.[3]

DOSAGE AND ADMINISTRATION

FOR SUBCUTANEOUS ADMINISTRATION

Do not inject intravenously

The dosage of vaccine is the same for all persons. Inject the total volume (about 0.5 ml) of reconstituted vaccine subcutaneously, preferably into the outer aspect of upper arm. *Do not give immune serum globulin (ISG) concurrently with Mumpsvax.*

During shipment, to insure that there is no loss of potency, the vaccine must be maintained at a temperature of 10°C (50°F) or less.

Before reconstitution, store Mumpsvax at 2 - 8°C (36 - 46°F). *Protect from light.*

CAUTION: A sterile syringe free of preservatives, antiseptics, and detergents should be used for each injection and/or reconstitution of the vaccine because these substances may inactivate the live virus vaccine. A 25 gauge, 5/8″ needle is recommended.

To reconstitute, use only the diluent supplied, since it is free of preservatives or other antiviral substances which might inactivate the vaccine.

Single Dose Vial—First withdraw the entire volume of diluent into the syringe to be used for reconstitution. Inject all the diluent in the syringe into the vial of lyophilized vaccine, and agitate to mix thoroughly. Withdraw the entire contents into a syringe and inject the total volume of restored vaccine subcutaneously.

It is important to use a separate sterile syringe and needle for each individual patient to prevent transmission of hepatitis B and other infectious agents from one person to another.

10 Dose Vial (available only to government agencies/institutions)— Withdraw the entire contents (7 ml) of the diluent vial into the sterile syringe to be used for reconstitution, and introduce into the 10 dose vial of lyophilized vaccine. Agitate to ensure thorough mixing. The outer labeling suggests ″For Jet Injector or Syringe Use″. Use with separate sterile syringes is permitted for containers of 10 doses or less. The vaccine and diluent do not contain preservatives; therefore, the user must recognize the potential contamination hazards and exercise special precautions to protect the sterility and potency of the product. The use of aseptic techniques and proper storage prior to and after restoration of the vaccine and subsequent withdrawal of the individual doses is essential. Use 0.5 ml of the reconstituted vaccine for subcutaneous injection.

It is important to use a separate sterile syringe and needle for each individual patient to prevent transmission of hepatitis B and other infectious agents from one person to another.

50 Dose Vial (available only to government agencies/institutions)— Withdraw the entire contents (30 ml) of the diluent vial into the sterile syringe to be used for reconstitution and introduce into the 50 dose vial of lyophilized vaccine. Agitate to ensure thorough mixing. With full aseptic precautions, attach the vial to the sterilized multidose jet injector apparatus. Use 0.5 ml of the reconstituted vaccine for subcutaneous injection.

Each dose of Mumpsvax contains not less than the equivalent of 20,000 $TCID_{50}$ of the U.S. Reference Mumps Virus.

Parenteral drug products should be inspected visually for particulate matter and discoloration prior to administration. Mumpsvax, when reconstituted, is clear yellow.

STORAGE

It is recommended that the vaccine be used as soon as possible after reconstitution. Protect vaccine from light at all times, since such exposure may inactivate the virus. Store reconstituted vaccine in the vaccine vial in a dark place at 2 - 8°C (36 - 46°F) and discard if not used within 8 hours.

PRODUCT LISTING - EQUIVALENTS NOT AVAILABLE

Powder For Injection - Subcutaneous - Strength n/a

1's	$22.73	MUMPSVAX, Merck & Company Inc	00006-4753-00
10's	$204.49	MUMPSVAX, Merck & Company Inc	00006-4584-00

Mupirocin (001843)

Categories: Impetigo; Infection, skin lesions; Infection, prophylaxis; Pregnancy Category B; FDA Approved 1987 Dec
Drug Classes: Anti-infectives, topical; Dermatologics
Brand Names: **Bactroban**
Foreign Brand Availability: Bactoderm (Indonesia; Israel); Eismycin (Germany); Mupiderm (France)
Cost of Therapy: $31.48 (Impetigo; Bactroban Ointment; 2%; 15 g; 3 applications/day; variable day supply)

TOPICAL

DESCRIPTION

For Dermatologic Use.

BACTROBAN CALCIUM CREAM, 2%

Bactroban Cream (mupirocin calcium cream), 2% contains the dihydrate crystalline calcium hemi-salt of the antibiotic mupirocin. Chemically, it is (α*E,2S,3R,4R,5S*)-5-[(*2S,3S,4S,5S*)-2,3-Epoxy-5-hydroxy-4-methylhexyl]tetrahydro-3,4-dihydroxy-β-methyl-2*H*-pyran-2-crotonic acid, ester with 9-hydroxynonanoic acid, calcium salt (2:1), dihydrate.

The molecular formula of mupirocin calcium is $(C_{26}H_{43}O_9)_2Ca{\cdot}2H_2O$, and the molecular weight is 1075.3. The molecular weight of mupirocin free acid is 500.6.

Bactroban Cream is a white cream that contains 2.15% w/w mupirocin calcium (equivalent to 2.0% mupirocin free acid) in an oil and water-based emulsion. The inactive ingredients are benzyl alcohol, cetomacrogol 1000, cetyl alcohol, mineral oil, phenoxyethanol, purified water, stearyl alcohol, and xanthan gum.

BACTROBAN OINTMENT, 2%

Each gram of Bactroban Ointment (mupirocin ointment), 2% contains 20 mg mupirocin in a bland water miscible ointment base (polyethylene glycol ointment) consisting of polyethylene glycol 400 and polyethylene glycol 3350. Mupirocin is a naturally occurring antibiotic. The chemical name is (*E*)-(*2S,3R,4R,5S*)-5-[(*2S,3S,4S,5S*)-2,3-Epoxy-5-hydroxy-4-methylhexyl]tetrahydro-3,4-dihydroxy-β-methyl-2*H*-pyran-2-crotonic acid, ester with 9-hydroxynonanoic acid. The molecular formula of mupirocin is $C_{26}H_{44}O_9$ and the molecular weight is 500.63.

CLINICAL PHARMACOLOGY

MUPIROCIN CALCIUM CREAM, 2%

Pharmacokinetics

Systemic absorption of mupirocin through intact human skin is minimal. The systemic absorption of mupirocin was studied following application of mupirocin calcium cream, 2% three times a day for 5 days to various skin lesions (greater than 10 cm in length or 100 cm^2 in area) in 16 adults (aged 29-60 years) and 10 children (aged 3-12 years). Some systemic absorption was observed as evidenced by the detection of the metabolite, monic acid, in urine. Data from this study indicated more frequent occurrence of percutaneous absorption in children (90% of patients) compared to adults (44% of patients). However, the observed urinary concentrations in children [0.07-1.3 μg/ml (1 pediatric patient had no detectable level)] are within the observed range [0.08-10.03 μg/ml (9 adults had no detectable level)] in the adult population. In general, the degree of percutaneous absorption following multiple dosing appears to be minimal in adults and children. Any mupirocin reaching the systemic circulation is rapidly metabolized, predominantly to inactive monic acid, which is eliminated by renal excretion.

Microbiology

Mupirocin is an antibacterial agent produced by fermentation using the organism *Psuedomonas fluorescens.* It is active against a wide range of gram-positive bacteria including methicillin-resistant *Staphylococcus aureus* (MRSA). It is also active against certain gram-negative bacteria. Mupirocin inhibits bacterial protein synthesis by reversibly and specifically binding to bacterial isoleucyl transfer-RNA synthetase. Due to this unique mode of action, mupirocin demonstrates no *in vitro* cross-resistance with other classes of antimicrobial agents.

Resistance occurs rarely. However, when mupirocin resistance does occur, it appears to result from the production of a modified isoleucyl-tRNA synthetase. High-level plasmid-mediated resistance (MIC >1024 μg/ml) has been reported in some strains of *S. aureus* and coagulase-negative staphylococci.

Mupirocin is bactericidal at concentrations achieved by topical application. However, the minimum bactericidal concentration (MBC) against relevant pathogens is generally 8- to 30-fold higher than the minimum inhibitory concentration (MIC). In addition, mupirocin is highly protein bound (>97%), and the effect of wound secretions on the MICs of mupirocin has not been determined.

Mupirocin has been shown to be active against most strains of *Staphylococcus aureus* and *Streptococcus pyogenes,* both *in vitro* and in clinical studies. (See INDICATIONS AND USAGE.) The following *in vitro* data are available, BUT THEIR CLINICAL SIGNIFICANCE IS UNKNOWN. Mupirocin is active against most strains of *Staphylococcus epidermidis* and *Staphylococcus saprophyticus.*

MUPIROCIN OINTMENT, 2%

Application of ^{14}C-labeled mupirocin ointment to the lower arm of normal male subjects followed by occlusion for 24 hours showed no measurable systemic absorption (<1.1 ng mupirocin per ml of whole blood). Measurable radioactivity was present in the stratum corneum of these subjects 72 hours after application.

Following intravenous (IV) or oral administration, mupirocin is rapidly metabolized. The principal metabolite, monic acid, is eliminated by renal excretion, and demonstrates no antibacterial activity. In a study conducted in 7 healthy adult male subjects, the elimination half-life after IV administration of mupirocin was 20-40 mins for mupirocin and 30-80 mins for monic acid. The pharmacokinetics of mupirocin has not been studied in individuals with renal insufficiency.

Microbiology

Mupirocin is an antibacterial agent produced by fermentation using the organism *Pseudomonas fluorescens.* It is active against a wide range of gram-positive bacteria including methicillin-resistant *Staphylococcus aureus* (MRSA). It is also active against certain gram-negative bacteria. Mupirocin inhibits bacterial protein synthesis by reversibly and specifically binding to bacterial isoleucyl transfer-RNA synthetase. Due to this unique mode of action, mupirocin demonstrates no *in vitro* cross-resistance with other classes of antimicrobial agents.

Resistance occurs rarely. However, when mupirocin resistance does occur, it appears to result from the production of a modified isoleucyl-tRNA synthetase. High-level plasmid-mediated resistance (MIC >1024 μg/ml) has been reported in some strains of *S. aureus* and coagulase-negative staphylococci.

Mupirocin is bactericidal at concentrations achieved by topical administration. However, the minimum bactericidal concentration (MBC) against relevant pathogens is generally 8- to 30-fold higher than the minimum inhibitory concentration (MIC). In addition, mupirocin is highly protein bound (>97%), and the effect of wound secretions on the MICs of mupirocin has not been determined.

Mupirocin has been shown to be active against most strains of *Staphylococcus aureus* and *Streptococcus pyogenes,* both *in vitro* and in clinical studies. (See INDICATIONS AND USAGE.) The following *in vitro* data are available, BUT THEIR CLINICAL SIGNIFICANCE IS UNKNOWN. Mupirocin is active against most strains of *Staphylococcus epidermidis* and *Staphylococcus saprophyticus.*

INDICATIONS AND USAGE

Mupirocin calcium cream, 2% is indicated for the treatment of secondarily infected traumatic skin lesions (up to 10 cm in length or 100 cm^2 in area) due to susceptible strains of *Staphylococcus aureus* and *Streptococcus pyogenes.*

Mupirocin ointment, 2% is indicated for the topical treatment of impetigo due to: *Staphylococcus aureus* and *Streptococcus pyogenes.*

CONTRAINDICATIONS

Mupirocin calcium cream, 2% and mupirocin ointment, 2% are contraindicated in individuals with a history of sensitivity reactons to any of its components.

WARNINGS

Avoid contact with the eyes.

In the event of a sensitization or severe local irritation from mupirocin calcium cream, 2%, usage should be discontinued, and appropriate alternative therapy for the infection instituted.

Mupirocin ointment is not for ophthalmic use.

PRECAUTIONS

MUPIROCIN CALCIUM CREAM, 2%

General

As with other antibacterial products, prolonged use may result in overgrowth of nonsusceptible microorganisms, including fungi. (See DOSAGE AND ADMINISTRATION.)

Mupirocin calcium cream, 2% is not formulated for use on mucosal surfaces.

Information for the Patient

- Use this medication only as directed by your healthcare provider. It is for external use only. Avoid contact with the eyes.
- The treated area may be covered by gauze dressing if desired.
- Report to your healthcare provider any signs of local adverse reactions. The medication should be stopped and your healthcare provider contacted if irritation, severe itching or rash occurs.
- If no improvement is seen in 3-5 days, contact your healthcare provider.

Carcinogenesis, Mutagenesis, and Impairment of Fertility

Long-term studies in animals to evaluate carcinogenic potential of mupirocin calcium have not been conducted.

Results of the following studies performed with mupirocin calcium or mupirocin sodium *in vitro* and *in vivo* did not indicate a potential for mutagenicity: Rat primary hepatocyte unscheduled DNA synthesis, sediment analysis for DNA strand breaks, *Salmonella* reversion test (Ames), *Escherichia coli* mutation assay, metaphase analysis of human lymphocytes, mouse lymphoma assay, and bone marrow micronuclei assay in mice.

Fertility studies were performed in rats with mupirocin administered subcutaneously at doses up to 49 times a human topical dose of 1 g/day (approximately 20 mg mupirocin per day) on a mg/m^2 basis and revealed no evidence of impaired fertility from mupirocin sodium.

Pregnancy, Teratogenic Effects, Pregnancy Category B

Teratology studies have been performed in rats and rabbits with mupirocin administered subcutaneously at doses up to 78 and 154 times, respectively, a human topical dose of 1 g/day (approximately 20 mg mupirocin per day) on a mg/m^2 basis and revealed no evidence of harm to the fetus due to mupirocin. There are, however, no adequate and well-controlled studies in pregnant women. Because animal reproduction studies are not always predictive of human response, this drug should be used during pregnancy only if clearly needed.

Nursing Mothers

It is not known whether this drug is excreted in human milk. Because many drugs are excreted in human milk, caution should be exercised when mupirocin calcium cream, 2% is administered to a nursing woman.

Pediatric Use

The safety and effectiveness of mupirocin calcium cream, 2% have been established in the age groups 3 months to 16 years. Use of mupirocin calcium cream, 2% in these age groups is supported by evidence from adequate and well-controlled studies of mupirocin calcium cream, 2% in adults with additional data from 93 pediatric patients studied as part of the pivotal trials in adults.

Geriatric Use

In two well-controlled studies, 30 patients over 65 years old were treated with mupirocin calcium cream, 2%. No overall difference in the efficacy or safety of mupirocin calcium cream, 2% was observed in this patient population when compared to that observed in younger patients.

MUPIROCIN OINTMENT, 2%

If a reaction suggesting sensitivity of chemical irritation should occur with the use of mupirocin ointment, 2%, treatment should be discontinued and appropriate alternative therapy for the infection instituted.

As with other antibacterial products, prolonged use may result in overgrowth of nonsusceptible organisms, including fungi.

Mupirocin ointment, 2% is not formulated for use on mucosal surfaces. Intranasal use has been associated with isolated reports of stinging and drying. A paraffin-based formulation — mupirocin calcium ointment, 2% — is available for intranasal use.

Polyethylene glycol can be absorbed from open wounds and damaged skin and is excreted by the kidneys. In common with other polyethylene glycol-based ointments, mupirocin ointment, 2% should not be used in conditions where absorption of large quantities of polyethylene glycol is possible, especially if there is evidence of moderate or severe renal impairment.

Information for the Patient

Use this medication only as directed by your healthcare provider. It is for external use only. Avoid contact with the eyes. The medication should be stopped and your healthcare practitioner contacted if irritation, severe itching, or rash occurs.

If impetigo has not improved in 3-5 days, contact your healthcare practitioner.

Carcinogenesis, Mutagenesis, and Impairment of Fertility

Long-term studies in animals to evaluate carcinogenic potential of mupirocin have not been conducted.

Results of the following studies performed with mupirocin calcium or mupirocin sodium *in vitro* and *in vivo* did not indicate a potential for genotoxicity: Rat primary hepatocyte unscheduled DNA synthesis, sediment analysis for DNA strand breaks, *Salmonella* reversion test (Ames), *Escherichia coli* mutation assay, metaphase analysis of human lymphocytes, mouse lymphoma assay, and bone marrow micronuclei assay in mice.

Reproduction studies were performed in male and female rats with mupirocin administered subcutaneously at doses up to 14 times a human topical dose (approximately 60 mg mupirocin per day) on a mg/m^2 basis and revealed no evidence of impaired fertility and reproductive performance from mupirocin.

Pregnancy, Teratogenic Effects, Pregnancy Category B

Reproduction studies have been performed in rats and rabbits with mupirocin administered subcutaneously at doses up to 22 and 43 times, respectively, the human topical dose (approximately 60 mg mupirocin per day) on a mg/m^2 basis and revealed no evidence of harm to the fetus due to mupirocin. There are, however, no adequate and well-controlled studies in pregnant women. Because animal studies are not always predictive of human response, this drug should be used during pregnancy only if clearly needed.

Nursing Mothers

It is not known whether this drug is excreted in human milk. Because many drugs are excreted in human milk, caution should be exercised when mupirocin ointment, 2% is administered to a nursing woman.

Pediatric Use

The safety and effectiveness of mupirocin ointment, 2% have been established in the age range of 2 months to 16 years. Use of mupirocin ointment, 2% in these age groups is supported by evidence from adequate and well-controlled studies of mupirocin ointment, 2% in impetigo in pediatric patients studied as a part of the pivotal clinical trials.

DRUG INTERACTIONS

The effect of the concurrent application of topical mupirocin calcium cream, mupirocin ointment, and other drug products has not been studied.

M

ADVERSE REACTIONS

MUPIROCIN CALCIUM CREAM, 2%

In two randomized, double-blind, double-dummy trials, 339 patients were treated with topical mupirocin calcium cream, 2% plus oral placebo. Adverse events thought to be possibly or probably drug-related occurred in 28 (8.3%) patients. *The incidence of those events that were reported in at least 1% of patients enrolled in these trials were:* Headache (1.7%), rash and nausea (1.1% each).

Other adverse events thought to be possibly or probably drug-related which occurred in less than 1% of patients were: Abdominal pain, burning at application site, cellulitis, dermatitis, dizziness, pruritus, secondary wound infection, and ulcerative stomatitis.

In a supportive study in the treatment of secondarily infected eczema, 82 patients were treated with mupirocin calcium cream, 2%. *The incidence of adverse events thought to be possibly or probably drug-related was as follows:* Nausea (4.9%), headache and burning at application site (3.6% each), pruritus (2.4%) and 1 report each of abdominal pain, bleeding secondary to eczema, pain secondary to eczema, hives, dry skin, and rash.

MUPIROCIN OINTMENT, 2%

The following local adverse reactions have been reported in connection with the use of mupirocin ointment, 2%: Burning, stinging, or pain in 1.5% of patients; itching in 1% of patients; rash, nausea, erythema, dry skin, tenderness, swelling, contact dermatitis, and increased exudate in less than 1% in patients. Systemic reactions to mupirocin oinment, 2% have occurred rarely.

DOSAGE AND ADMINISTRATION

A small amount of mupirocin calcium cream, 2% or mupirocin ointment, 2% should be applied to the affected area 3 times daily for 10 days. The area treated may be covered with a gauze dressing if desired. Patients not showing a clinical response within 3-5 days should be re-evaluated.

HOW SUPPLIED

BACTROBAN CREAM, 2%

Bactroban Cream, 2% is supplied in 15 and 30 g tubes.
Storage: Store at or below 25°C (77°F). Do not freeze.

BACTROBAN OINTMENT, 2%

Bactroban Ointment, 2% is supplied in 22 g tubes.
Storage: Store at controlled room temperature 20-25°C (68-77°F).

INTRANASAL

M

DESCRIPTION

For Intranasal Use Only.

Bactroban Nasal (mupirocin calcium ointment), 2% contains the dihydrate crystalline calcium hemi-salt of the antibiotic mupirocin. Chemically, it is (αE,2S,3R,4R,5S)-5-[(2S,3S,4S,5S)-2,3-Epoxy-5-hydroxy-4-methylhexyl]tetra-hydro-3,4-dihydroxy-β-methyl-2H-pyran-2-crotonic acid, ester with 9-hydroxynonanoic acid, calcium salt (2:1), dihydrate.

The molecular formula of mupirocin calcium is $(C_{26}H_{43}O_9)_2Ca \cdot 2H_2O$, and the molecular weight is 1075.3. The molecular weight of mupirocin free acid is 500.6.

Bactroban Nasal is a white to off-white ointment that contains 2.15% w/w mupirocin calcium (equivalent to 2.0% pure mupirocin free acid) in a soft white ointment base. The inactive ingredients are paraffin and a mixture of glycerin esters.

CLINICAL PHARMACOLOGY

PHARMACOKINETICS

Following single or repeated intranasal applications of 0.2 g of intranasal mupirocin calcium ointment, 2% tid for 3 days to 5 healthy **adult** male subjects, no evidence of systemic absorption of mupirocin was demonstrated. The dosage regimen use in this study was for pharmacokinetic characterization only. (See DOSAGE AND ADMINISTRATION for proper clinical dosing information.)

In this study, the concentrations of mupirocin in urine and of monic acid in urine and serum were below the limit of determination of the assay for up to 72 hours after the applications. The lowest levels of determination of the assay used were 50 ng/ml of mupirocin in urine, 75 ng/ml of monic acid in urine, and 10 ng/ml of monic acid in serum. Based on the detectable limit of the urine assay for monic acid, one can extrapolate that a mean of 3.3% (range: 1.2-5.1%) of the applied dose could be systemically absorbed from the nasal mucosa of **adults.**

Data from a report of a pharmacokinetic study in neonates and premature infants indicate that, unlike in adults, significant systemic absorption occurred following intranasal administration of intranasal mupirocin calcium ointment, 2% in this population. **At this time, the pharmacokinetic properties of mupirocin following intranasal application of intranasal mupirocin calcium ointment, 2% have not been adequately characterized in neonates or other children less than 12 years of age, and in addition, the safety of the product in children less than 12 years of age has not been established.**

The effect of the concurrent application of intranasal mupirocin calcium ointment, 2% with other intranasal products has not been studied. (See DRUG INTERACTIONS.)

Following IV or oral administration, mupirocin is rapidly metabolized. The principal metabolite, monic acid, demonstrates no antibacterial activity. In a study conducted in 7 healthy adult male subjects, the elimination half-life after IV administration of mupirocin was 20-40 mins for mupirocin and 30-80 mins for monic acid. Monic acid is predominantly eliminated by renal excretion. The pharmacokinetics of mupirocin has not been studied in individuals with renal insufficiency.

MICROBIOLOGY

Mupirocin is an antibacterial agent produced by fermentation using the organism *Pseudomonas fluorescens.* Mupirocin inhibits bacterial protein synthesis by reversibly and specifically binding to bacterial isoleucyl transfer-RNA synthetsae. Due to this mode of action, mupirocin demonstrates no *in vitro* cross-resistance with other classes of antimicrobial agents.

When mupirocin resistance does occur, it appears to result from the production of a modified isoleucyl-tRNA synthetase. High-level plasmid-mediated resistance (MIC >1024 μg/ml) has been reported in some strains of *S. aureus* and coagulase-negative staphylococci.

Mupirocin is bactericidal at concentrations achieved topically by intranasal administration. However, the minimum bactericidal concentration (MBC) against relevant intranasal pathogens is generally 8- to 30-fold higher than the minimum inhibitory concentration (MIC). In addition, mupirocin is highly protein bound (>97%), and the effect of nasal secretions on the MICs of intranasally applied mupirocin has not been determined.

Mupirocin has been shown to be active against most strains of methicillin-resistant *S. aureus,* both *in vitro* and in clinical studies of the eradication of nasal colonization. Intranasal mupirocin calcium ointment, 2% only has established clinical utility in nasal eradication as part of a comprehensive program to curtail institutional outbreaks of infections with methicillin-resistant *S. aureus.* (See INDICATIONS AND USAGE.)

The following *in vitro* data are available, **but their clinical significance is unknown.** Mupirocin exhibits *in vitro* MICs of 1 μg/ml or less against most (>90%) strains of methicillin-susceptible *S. aureus;* however, the safety and effectiveness of mupirocin calcium in eradicating nasal colonization of and preventing subsequent infections due to methicillin-susceptible *S. aureus* have not been established.

INDICATIONS AND USAGE

Intranasal mupirocin calcium ointment, 2% is indicated for the eradication of nasal colonization with methicillin-resistant *Staphylococcus aureus* in adult patients and health care workers as part of a comprehensive infection control program to reduce the risk of infection among patients at high risk of methicillin-resistant *S. aureus* infection during institutional outbreaks of infections with this pathogen.

Note:

- There are insufficient data at this time to establish that this product is safe and effective as part of an intervention program to prevent autoinfection of high-risk patients from their own nasal colonization with *S. aureus.*
- There are insufficient data at this time to recommend use of intranasal mupirocin calcium ointment, 2% for general prophylaxis of any infection in any patient population.
- Greater than 90% of subjects/patients in clinical trials had eradication of nasal colonization 2-4 days after therapy was completed. Approximately 30% recolonization was reported in one domestic study within 4 weeks after completion of therapy. These eradication rates were clinically and statistically superior to those reported in subjects/patients in the vehicle-treated arms of the adequate and well-controlled studies. Those treated with vehicle had eradication rates of 5-30% at 2-4 days post-therapy with 85-100% recolonization within 4 weeks.

All adequate and well-controlled trials of this product were vehicle-controlled; therefore, no data from direct, head-to-head comparisons with other products are available at this time.

CONTRAINDICATIONS

Intranasal mupirocin calcium ointment, 2% is contraindicated in patients with known hypersensitivity to any of the constituents of the product.

WARNINGS

AVOID CONTACT WITH THE EYES.

Application of intranasal mupirocin calcium ointment, 2% to the eye under testing conditions has caused severe symptoms such as burning and tearing. These symptoms resolved within days to weeks after discontinuation of the ointment.

In the event of a sensitization or severe local irritation from intranasal mupirocin calcium ointment, 2%, usage should be discontinued.

PRECAUTIONS

GENERAL

As with other antibacterial products, prolonged use may result in overgrowth of nonsusceptible microorganisms, including fungi. (See DOSAGE AND ADMINISTRATION.)

INFORMATION FOR THE PATIENT

Patients should be given the following instructions:

Apply approximately one-half of the ointment form the single-use tube directly into 1 nostril and the other half into the other nostril.

Avoid contact of the medication with the eyes.

Discard the tube after using, do not re-use.

Press the sides of the nose together and gently massage after application to spread the ointment throughout the inside of the nostrils.

Discontinue usage of the medication and call your health care practitioner if sensitization or severe local irritation occurs.

CARCINOGENESIS, MUTAGENESIS, AND IMPAIRMENT OF FERTILITY

Long-term studies in animals to evaluate carcinogenic potential of mupirocin calcium have not been conducted.

Results of the following studies performed with mupirocin calcium or mupirocin sodium *in vitro* and *in vivo* did not indicate a potential for mutagenicity: Rat primary hepatocyte unscheduled DNA synthesis, sediment analysis for DNA strand breaks. *Salmonella* reversion test (Ames), *Escherichia coli* mutation assay, metaphase analysis of human lymphocytes, mouse lymphoma assay, and bone marrow micronuclei assay in mice.

Reproduction studies were performed in rats with mupirocin administered subcutaneously at doses up to **40** times the human intranasal dose (approximately 20 mg mupirocin per day) on a mg/m^2 basis and revealed no evidence of impaired fertility from mupirocin sodium.

PREGNANCY, TERATOGENIC EFFECTS, PREGNANCY CATEGORY B

Reproduction studies have been performed in rats and rabbits with mupirocin administered subcutaneously at doses up to 65 and 130 times, respectively, the human intranasal dose (approximately 20 mg mupirocin per day) on a mg/m^2 basis and revealed no evidence of harm to the fetus due to mupirocin. There are, however, no adequate and well-controlled studies in pregnant women. Because animal reproduction studies are not always predictive of human response, this drug should be used during pregnancy only if clearly needed.

NURSING MOTHERS

It is not known whether this drug is excreted in human milk. Because many drugs are excreted in human milk, caution should be exercised when intranasal mupirocin calcium ointment, 2% is administered to a nursing woman.

PEDIATRIC USE

Safety in children under the age of 12 years has not been established. (See CLINICAL PHARMACOLOGY.)

DRUG INTERACTIONS

The effect of the concurrent application of intranasal mupirocin calcium and other intranasal products has not been studied. Until further information is known, mupirocin calcium ointment, 2% should not be applied concurrently with any other intranasal products.

ADVERSE REACTIONS

CLINICAL TRIALS

In clinical trials, 210 domestic and 2130 foreign adult subjects/patients received intranasal mupirocin calcium ointment, 2%. Less than 1% of domestic or foreign subjects and patients in clinical trials were withdrawn due to adverse events.

The most frequently reported adverse events in foreign clinical trials were as follows: Rhinitis (1.0%), taste perversion (0.8%), pharyngitis (0.5%).

In domestic clinical trials, 17% (36/210) of adults treated with intranasal mupirocin calcium ointment, 2% reported adverse events thought to be at least possibly drug-related. The incidence of adverse events that were reported in at least 1% of adults enrolled in domestic clinical trials is shown in TABLE 1.

TABLE 1 *Adverse Events (≥1% Incidence) With Intranasal Mupirocin Calcium Ointment, 2% — Adults in US Trials*

	Subjects/Patients Experiencing Event (n=210)
Headache	9%
Rhinitis	6%
Respiratory disorder, including upper respiratory tract congestion	5%
Pharyngitis	4%
Taste Perversion	3%
Burning/Stinging	2%
Cough	2%
Pruritus	1%

The following events thought possibly drug-related were reported in less than 1% of adults enrolled in domestic clinical trials: Blepharitis, diarrhea, dry mouth, ear pain, epistaxis, nausea, and rash.

All adequate and well-controlled clinical trials have been performed using intranasal mupirocin calcium ointment, 2% in one arm and the vehicle ointment in the other arm of the study. No adequate and well-controlled safety data are available from direct, head-to-head comparative studies of this product and other products for this indication.

DOSAGE AND ADMINISTRATION

See INDICATIONS AND USAGE.

ADULTS (12 YEARS OF AGE AND OLDER)

Approximately one-half of the ointment from the single-use tube should be applied into 1 nostril and the other half into the other nostril twice daily (morning and evening) for 5 days.

After application, the nostrils should be closed by pressing together and releasing the sides of the nose repetitively for approximately 1 min. This will spread the ointment throughout the nares.

The single-use 1.0 g tube will deliver a total of approximately 0.5 g of the ointment (approximately 0.25 g/nostril).

The tube should be discarded after usage; it should not be re-used.

The safety and effectiveness of applications of this medication for greater than 5 days have not been established. There are no human clinical or pre-clinical animal data to support the use of this product in a chronic manner or in manners other than those described in this package insert.

Until further information is known, intranasal mupirocin calcium ointment, 2% should not be applied concurrently with any other intranasal products.

HOW SUPPLIED

Bactroban Nasal, 2% is supplied in 1.0 g tubes.

Storage: Store at or below 25°C (77°F).

PRODUCT LISTING - EQUIVALENTS NOT AVAILABLE

Cream - Topical - 2%			
15 gm	$31.48	BACTROBAN, Glaxosmithkline	00029-1527-22
30 gm	$53.36	BACTROBAN, Glaxosmithkline	00029-1527-25
Ointment - Topical - 2%			
15 gm	$16.55	BACTROBAN, Compumed Pharmaceuticals	00403-2647-18
15 gm	$17.35	BACTROBAN, Allscripts Pharmaceutical Company	54569-2004-00
15 gm	$19.22	BACTROBAN, Physicians Total Care	54868-0202-01
15 gm	$20.48	BACTROBAN, Cheshire Drugs	55175-2200-05
15 gm	$20.95	BACTROBAN, Pharma Pac	52959-1014-00
15 gm	$22.00	BACTROBAN, Southwood Pharmaceuticals Inc	58016-3154-00
15 gm	$22.00	BACTROBAN, Southwood Pharmaceuticals Inc	58016-3154-15
15 gm	$24.95	BACTROBAN, Southwood Pharmaceuticals Inc	58016-3154-01
22 gm	$36.85	BACTROBAN, Allscripts Pharmaceutical Company	54569-4960-00
22 gm	$41.43	BACTROBAN, Southwood Pharmaceuticals Inc	58016-5571-01
22 gm	$51.59	BACTROBAN, Pharma Pac	52959-1014-22
22.50 gm	$45.68	BACTROBAN, Glaxosmithkline	00029-1525-44
22.50 gm	$51.06	BACTROBAN, Prescript Pharmaceuticals	00247-0284-22
30 gm	$28.65	BACTROBAN, Southwood Pharmaceuticals Inc	58016-3267-00
30 gm	$32.75	BACTROBAN, Allscripts Pharmaceutical Company	54569-4052-00
30 gm	$35.78	BACTROBAN, Physicians Total Care	54868-0202-02
Ointment W/Applicator - Nasal - 2%			
1 gm x 10	$56.38	BACTROBAN, Physicians Total Care	54868-4325-00
1 gm x 10	$58.90	BACTROBAN, Glaxosmithkline	00029-1526-11

Muromonab-CD3 *(001845)*

Categories: Rejection, heart transplant; Rejection, liver transplant; Rejection, renal transplant; Pregnancy Category C; Recombinant DNA Origin; FDA Approved 1986 Jun

Drug Classes: Immunosuppressives; Monoclonal antibodies

Brand Names: **Orthoclone OKT-3**

Cost of Therapy: $8182.20 (Transplant Rejection; Orthoclone OKT-3 Injection; 1 mg/ml; 5 ml; 5 mg/day; 10 day supply)

WARNING

Only physicians experienced in immunosuppressive therapy and management of solid organ transplant patients should use muromonab-CD3. Patients treated with muromonab-CD3 must be managed in a facility equipped and staffed for cardiopulmonary resuscitation and where the patient can be closely monitored for an appropriate period based on his or her health status.

Anaphylactic and anaphylactoid reactions may occur following administration of any dose or course of muromonab-CD3. In addition, serious, occasionally life-threatening or lethal, systemic, cardiovascular, and central nervous system reactions have been reported following administration of muromonab-CD3. These have included: pulmonary edema, especially in patients with volume overload; shock, cardiovascular collapse, cardiac or respiratory arrest, seizures, coma, cerebral edema, herniation, blindness, and paralysis. Fluid status should be carefully monitored prior to and during muromonab-CD3 administration. Pretreatment with methylprednisolone is recommended to minimize symptoms of Cytokine Release Syndrome. (See WARNINGS, Cytokine Release Syndrome, WARNINGS, Central Nervous System Events, WARNINGS, Anaphylactic Reactions and DOSAGE AND ADMINISTRATION.)

DESCRIPTION

Orthoclone OKT3 sterile solution is a murine monoclonal antibody to the CD3 antigen of human T cells which functions as an immunosuppressant. It is for intravenous use only. The antibody is a biochemically purified IgG_{2a} immunoglobulin with a heavy chain of approximately 50,000 daltons and a light chain of approximately 25,000 daltons. It is directed to a glycoprotein with a molecular weight of 20,000 in the human T cell surface which is essential for T cell functions. Because it is a monoclonal antibody preparation, Orthoclone OKT3 sterile solution is a homogeneous, reproducible antibody product with consistent, measurable reactivity to human T cells.

Each 5 ml ampule of Orthoclone OKT3 sterile solution contains 5 mg (1 mg/ml) of muromonab-CD3 in a clear colorless solution which may contain a few fine translucent protein particles. Each ampule contains a buffered solution (pH 7.0 ± 0.5) of monobasic sodium phosphate (2.25 mg), dibasic sodium phosphate (9.0 mg), sodium chloride (43 mg), and polysorbate 80 (1.0 mg) in water for injection.

The proper name, muromonab-CD3, is derived from the descriptive term murine monoclonal antibody. The CD3 designation identifies the specificity of the antibody as the Cell Differentiation (CD) cluster 3 defined by the First International Workshop on Human Leukocyte Differentiation Antigens.

CLINICAL PHARMACOLOGY

Muromonab-CD3 reverses graft rejection, probably by blocking the function of T cells which play a major role in acute allograft rejection. Muromonab-CD3 reacts with and blocks the function of a 20,000 dalton molecule (CD3) in the membrane of human T cells that has been associated *in vitro* with the antigen recognition structure of T cells and is essential for signal transduction. In *in vitro* cytolytic assays, muromonab-CD3 blocks both the generation and function of effector cells. Binding of muromonab-CD3 to T lymphocytes results in early activation of T cells, which leads to cytokine release, followed by blocking T cell functions. After termination of muromonab-CD3 therapy, T cell function usually returns to normal within 1 week.

In vivo, muromonab-CD3 reacts with most peripheral blood T cells and T cells in body tissues, but has not been found to react with other hematopoietic elements or other tissues of the body.

A rapid and concomitant decrease in the number of circulating CD3 positive cells, including those that are CD2, CD4, or CD8 positive has been observed in patients studied within minutes after the administration of muromonab-CD3. This decrease in the number of CD3 positive T cells results from the specific interaction between muromonab-CD3 and the CD3 antigen on the surface of all T lymphocytes. T cell activation results in the release of numerous cytokines/lymphokines, which are felt to be responsible for many of the acute clinical manifestations seen following muromonab-CD3 administration. (See WARNINGS, Cytokine Release Syndrome, WARNINGS, Central Nervous System Events.)

While CD3 positive cells are not detectable between days 2 and 7, increasing numbers of circulating CD2, CD4, and CD8 positive cells have been observed. The presence of these CD2, CD4, and CD8 positive cells has not been shown to affect reversal of rejection. After termination of muromonab-CD3 therapy, CD3 positive cells reappear rapidly and reach pre-treatment levels within a week. In some patients however, increasing numbers of CD3 positive cells have been observed prior to termination of muromonab-CD3 therapy. This reappearance of CD3 positive cells has been attributed to the development of neutralizing antibodies to muromonab-CD3, which in turn block its ability to bind to the CD3 antigen on T lymphocytes. (See PRECAUTIONS, General, Sensitization.)

Pediatric patients are known to have higher CD3 lymphocyte counts than adults. Pediatric patients receiving muromonab-CD3 therapy often require progressively higher doses of muromonab-CD3 to achieve depletion of CD3 positive cells (<25 cells/mm^3) and ensure therapeutic muromonab-CD3 serum concentrations (>800 ng/ml). (See DOSAGE AND ADMINISTRATION and PRECAUTIONS, Laboratory Tests.)

Serum levels of muromonab-CD3 are measurable using an enzyme-linked immunosorbent assay (ELISA). During the initial clinical trials in renal allograft rejection, in patients treated with 5 mg per day for 14 days, mean serum trough levels of the drug rose over the first 3 days and then averaged 900 ng/ml on days 3-14. Serum concentrations measured daily during treatment with muromonab-CD3 in renal, hepatic, and cardiac allograft recipients revealed that pediatric patients less than 10 years of age have higher levels than patients 10-50 years of age. Subsequent clinical experience has demonstrated that serum levels greater than or equal to 800 ng/ml of muromonab-CD3 blocks the function of cytotoxic T cells *in vitro* and *in vivo.* Reduced T cell clearance or low plasma muromonab-CD3 levels provide a basis for adjusting muromonab-CD3 dosage or for discontinuing therapy. (See WARNINGS, Anaphylactic Reactions; PRECAUTIONS, Laboratory Tests; ADVERSE REACTIONS, Hypersensitivity Reactions and DOSAGE AND ADMINISTRATION.)

Following administration of muromonab-CD3 *in vivo,* leukocytes have been observed in cerebrospinal and peritoneal fluids. The mechanism for this effect is not completely understood, but probably is related to cytokines altering membrane permeability, rather than an active inflammatory process. (See WARNINGS, Cytokine Release Syndrome, WARNINGS, Central Nervous System Events.)

INDICATIONS AND USAGE

Muromonab-CD3 is indicated for the treatment of acute allograft rejection in renal transplant patients.

Muromonab-CD3 is indicated for the treatment of steroid-resistant acute allograft rejection in cardiac and hepatic transplant patients.

The dosage of other immunosuppressive agents used in conjunction with muromonab-CD3 should be reduced to the lowest level compatible with an effective therapeutic response. (See WARNINGS and ADVERSE REACTIONS, Infections, ADVERSE REACTIONS, Neoplasia and DOSAGE AND ADMINISTRATION.)

M

NON-FDA APPROVED INDICATIONS

While not an FDA approved indication, muromonab CD3 has also been used for prophylaxis of allograft rejection.

CONTRAINDICATIONS

Muromonab-CD3 should not be given to patients who:

- Are hypersensitive to this or any other product of murine origin.
- Have anti-mouse antibody titers ≥1:1000.
- Are in (uncompensated) heart failure or in fluid overload, as evidenced by chest x-ray or a greater than 3% weight gain within the week prior to planned muromonab-CD3 administration.
- Have uncontrolled hypertension.
- Have a history of seizures, or are predisposed to seizures.
- Are determined or suspected to be pregnant, or who are breast-feeding. (See PRECAUTIONS, Pregnancy Category C, PRECAUTIONS, Nursing Mothers.)

WARNINGS

SEE BOXED WARNING.

CYTOKINE RELEASE SYNDROME

Most patients develop an acute clinical syndrome [*i.e.,* Cytokine Release Syndrome (CRS)] that has been attributed to the release of cytokines by activated lymphocytes or monocytes and is temporally associated with the administration of the first few doses of muromonab-CD3 (particularly, the first 2-3 doses).

This clinical syndrome has ranged from a more frequently reported mild, self-limited, "flu-like" illness to a less frequently reported severe, life-threatening shock-like reaction, which may include serious cardiovascular and central nervous system manifestations.

The syndrome typically begins approximately 30-60 minutes after administration of a dose of muromonab-CD3 (but may occur later) and may persist for several hours. The frequency and severity of this symptom complex is usually greatest with the first dose. With each successive dose of muromonab-CD3, both the frequency and severity of the Cytokine Release Syndrome tends to diminish.

Increasing the amount of muromonab-CD3 or resuming treatment after a hiatus may result in a reappearance of the CRS.

Common clinical manifestations of CRS may include: High fever (often spiking, up to 107°F), chills/rigors, headache, tremor, nausea/vomiting, diarrhea, abdominal pain, malaise, muscle/joint aches and pains, and generalized weakness. *Less frequently reported adverse experiences include:* Minor dermatologic reactions (*e.g.,* rash, pruritus, etc.) and a spectrum of often serious, occasionally fatal, cardiorespiratory and central nervous system adverse experiences.

Cardiorespiratory findings may include: Dyspnea, shortness of breath, bronchospasm/wheezing, tachypnea, respiratory arrest/failure/distress, cardiovascular collapse, cardiac arrest, angina/myocardial infarction, chest pain/tightness, tachycardia (including ventricular), hypertension, hemodynamic instability, hypotension including profound shock, heart failure, pulmonary edema (cardiogenic and non-cardiogenic), adult respiratory distress syndrome, hypoxemia, apnea, and arrhythmias. (See BOXED WARNING; PRECAUTIONS and ADVERSE REACTIONS.)

In the initial studies of renal allograft rejection, potentially fatal, severe pulmonary edema occurred in 5% of the initial 107 patients. Fluid overload was present before treatment in all of these cases. It occurred in none of the subsequent 311 patients treated with first-dose volume/weight restrictions. In subsequent trials and in post-marketing experience, severe pulmonary edema has occurred in patients who appeared to be euvolemic. The pathogenesis of pulmonary edema may involve all or some of the following: volume overload; increased pulmonary vascular permeability; and/or reduced left ventricular compliance/contractility. During the first 1-3 days of muromonab-CD3 therapy, some patients have experienced an acute and transient decline in the glomerular filtration rate (GFR) and diminished urine output with a resulting increase in the level of serum creatinine. Massive release of cytokines appears to lead to reversible renal functional impairment and/or delayed renal allograft function. Similarly, transient elevations in hepatic transaminases have been reported following administration of the first few doses of muromonab-CD3.

Patients at risk for more serious complications of CRS may include those with the following conditions: Unstable angina; recent myocardial infarction or symptomatic ischemic heart disease; heart failure of any etiology; pulmonary edema of any etiology; any form of chronic obstructive pulmonary disease; intravascular volume overload or depletion of any etiology (*e.g.,* excessive dialysis, recent intensive diuresis, blood loss, etc.); cerebrovascular disease; patients with advanced symptomatic vascular disease or neuropathy; a history of seizures; and septic shock. Efforts should be made to correct or stabilize background conditions prior to the initiation of therapy. (See PRECAUTIONS.)

Prior to administration of muromonab-CD3, the patient's volume (fluid) status and a chest x-ray should be assessed to rule out volume overload, uncontrolled hypertension, or uncompensated heart failure. Patients should not weigh >3% above their minimum weight during the week prior to injection.

The Cytokine Release Syndrome is associated with increased serum levels of cytokines (*e.g.,* TNF-α, IL-2, IL-6, IFN-γ) that peak between 1 and 4 hours following administration of muromonab-CD3. The serum levels of cytokines and the manifestations of CRS may be reduced by pretreatment with 8 mg/kg of methylprednisolone (*i.e.,* high-dose steroids), given 1-4 hours prior to administration of the first dose of muromonab-CD3, and by closely following recommendations for dosage and treatment duration. (See DOSAGE AND ADMINISTRATION.) It is not known if corticosteroid pretreatment decreases organ damage and sequelae associated with CRS. For example, increased intracranial pressure and cerebral herniation have occurred despite pretreatment with currently recommended doses and schedules of methylprednisolone.

If any of the more serious presentations of the Cytokine Release Syndrome occur, intensive treatment including oxygen, intravenous fluids, corticosteroids, pressor amines, antihistamines, intubation, etc., may be required.

CENTRAL NERVOUS SYSTEM EVENTS

Seizures, encephalopathy, cerebral edema, aseptic meningitis, and headache have been reported, even following the first dose, during therapy with muromonab-CD3. Seizures, some accompanied by loss of consciousness or cardiorespiratory arrest, or death, have occurred independently or in conjunction with any of the neurologic syndromes described below.

A few cases of fatal cerebral herniations subsequent to cerebral edema have been reported. All patients, particularly pediatric patients, must be carefully evaluated for fluid retention and hypertension before the initiation of muromonab-CD3 therapy. Close monitoring for neurologic symptoms must be performed during the first 24 hours following each of the first few doses of muromonab-CD3 injection.

Patients should be closely monitored for convulsions and manifestations of encephalopathy, including: Impaired cognition, confusion, obtundation, altered mental status, disorientation, auditory/visual hallucinations, psychosis (delirium, paranoia), mood changes (*e.g.,* mania, agitation, combativeness, etc.), diffuse hypotonus, hyperreflexia, myoclonus, tremor, asterixis, involuntary movements, major motor seizures, lethargy/stupor/coma, and diffuse weakness. Approximately one-third of patients with a diagnosis of encephalopathy may have had coexisting aseptic meningitis syndrome.

Signs and symptoms of the aseptic meningitis syndrome described in association with the use of muromonab-CD3 have included: Fever, headache, meningismus (stiff neck), and photophobia. Diagnosis is confirmed by cerebrospinal fluid (CSF) analysis demonstrating leukocytosis with pleocytosis, elevated protein and normal or decreased glucose, with negative viral, bacterial, and fungal cultures. The possibility of infection should be evaluated in any immunosuppressed transplant patient with clinical findings suggesting meningitis. Approximately one-third of the patients with a diagnosis of aseptic meningitis had coexisting signs and symptoms of encephalopathy. Most patients with the aseptic meningitis syndrome had a benign course and recovered without any permanent sequelae during therapy or subsequent to its completion or discontinuation. However, because meningitis is a frequent infection encountered in pediatric allograft recipients, and the immunosuppression associated with transplantation increases the risk of opportunistic infection, pediatric patients with signs or symptoms suggestive of meningeal irritation while receiving muromonab-CD3 should have lumbar punctures performed to rule out an infectious etiology. (See PRECAUTIONS, Pediatric Use.)

Signs or symptoms of encephalopathy, meningitis, seizures, and cerebral edema, with or without headache, typically have been reversible. Headache, aseptic meningitis, seizures, and less severe forms of encephalopathy resolved in most patients despite continued treatment with muromonab-CD3. However, some events resulted in permanent neurologic impairment.

The following additional central nervous system events have each been reported: Irreversible blindness, impaired vision, quadri- or paraparesis/plegia, cerebrovascular accident (hemiparesis/plegia), aphasia, transient ischemic attack, subarachnoid hemorrhage, palsy of the VI cranial nerve, hearing decrease, and deafness.

Patients who may be at greater risk for CNS adverse experiences include those: With known or suspected CNS disorders (*e.g.,* history of seizure disorder, etc.); with cerebrovascular disease (small or large vessel); with conditions having associated neurologic problems (*e.g.*, head trauma, uremia, infection, fluid and electrolyte disturbance, etc.); with underlying vascular diseases; or who are receiving a medication concomitantly that may, by itself, affect the central nervous system. (See WARNINGS; PRECAUTIONS and ADVERSE REACTIONS, Cytokine Release Syndrome.)

ANAPHYLACTIC REACTIONS

Serious and occasionally fatal, immediate (usually within 10 minutes) hypersensitivity (anaphylactic) reactions have been reported in patients treated with muromonab-CD3. **Manifestations of anaphylaxis may appear similar to manifestations of the Cytokine Release Syndrome (described above). It may be impossible to determine the mechanism responsible for any systemic reaction(s).** Reactions attributed to hypersensitivity have been reported less frequently than those attributed to cytokine release. Acute hypersensitivity reactions may be characterized by: cardiovascular collapse, cardiorespiratory arrest, loss of consciousness, hypotension/shock, tachycardia, tingling, angioedema (including laryngeal, pharyngeal, or facial edema), airway obstruction, bronchospasm, dyspnea, urticaria, and pruritus.

Serious allergic events, including anaphylactic or anaphylactoid reactions, have been reported in patients re-exposed to muromonab-CD3 subsequent to their initial course of therapy. Pretreatment with antihistamines and/or steroids may not reliably prevent anaphylaxis in this setting.

Possible allergic hazards of retreatment should be weighed against expected therapeutic benefits and alternatives. If a patient is retreated with muromonab-CD3, it is particularly important that epinephrine and other emergency life-support equipment should be immediately available.

If hypersensitivity is suspected, discontinue the drug immediately; do not resume therapy or re-expose the patient to muromonab-CD3. Serious acute hypersensitivity reactions may require emergency treatment with 0.3-0.5 ml aqueous epinephrine (1:1000 dilution) subcutaneously and other resuscitative measures including oxygen, intravenous fluids, antihistamines, corticosteroids, pressor amines, and airway management, as clinically indicated. (See PRECAUTIONS, General, Severe Cytokine Release Syndrome Versus Anaphylactic Reactions and ADVERSE REACTIONS, Hypersensitivity Reactions.)

CONSEQUENCES OF IMMUNOSUPPRESSION

Serious and sometimes fatal infections and neoplasias have been reported in association with all immunosuppressive therapies, including those regimens containing muromonab-CD3.

Infections

Muromonab-CD3 is usually added to immunosuppressive therapeutic regimens, thereby augmenting the degree of immunosuppression. This increase in the total amount of immunosuppression may alter the spectrum of infections observed and increase the risk, the severity, and the morbidity of infectious complications. During the first month post-transplant, patients are at greatest risk for the following infections: (1) those present prior to transplant, perhaps exacerbated by post-transplant immunosuppression; (2) infection conveyed by the donor organ; and (3) the usual post-operative urinary tract, intravenous line related, wound, or pulmonary infections due to bacterial pathogens. (See ADVERSE REACTIONS, Infections.)

Approximately 1-6 months post-transplant, patients are at risk for viral infections [*e.g.*, cytomegalovirus (CMV), Epstein-Barr virus (EBV), herpes simplex virus (HSV), etc.] which produce serious systemic disease and which also increase the overall state of immunosuppression.

Reactivation (1-4 months post-transplant) of EBV and CMV has been reported. When administration of an anti-lymphocyte antibody, including muromonab-CD3, is followed by an immunosuppressive regimen including cyclosporine, there is an increased risk of reactivating CMV and impaired ability to limit its proliferation, resulting in symptomatic and disseminated disease.

EBV infection, either primary or reactivated, may play an important role in the development of post-transplant lymphoproliferative disorders. (See WARNINGS and ADVERSE REACTIONS, Neoplasia.) In the pediatric transplant population, viral infections often include pathogens uncommon in adults, such as varicella zoster virus (VZV), adenovirus, and respiratory syncytial virus (RSV). A large proportion of pediatric patients have not been infected with the herpes viruses prior to transplantation and, therefore, are susceptible to developing primary infections from the grafted organ and/or blood products.

Anti-infective prophylaxis may reduce the morbidity associated with certain potential pathogens and should be considered for pediatric and other high-risk patients. Judicious use of immunosuppressive drugs, including type, dosage, and duration, may limit the risk and seriousness of some opportunistic infections. It is also possible to reduce the risk of serious CMV or EBV infection by avoiding transplantation of a CMV-seropositive (donor) and/or EBV-seropositive (donor) organ into a seronegative patient.

Neoplasia

As a result of depressed cell-mediated immunity from immunosuppressive agents, organ transplant patients have an increased risk of developing malignancies. This risk is evidenced almost exclusively by the occurrence of lymphoproliferative disorders, squamous cell carcinomas of the skin and lip, and sarcomas. In immunosuppressed patients, T cell cytotoxicity is impaired allowing for transformation and proliferation of EBV-infected B lymphocytes. Transformed B lymphocytes are thought to initiate oncogenesis, which ultimately culminates in the development of most post-transplant lymphoproliferative disorders. Patients, especially pediatric patients, with primary EBV infection may be at a higher risk for the development of EBV-associated lymphoproliferative disorders. Data support an association between the development of lymphoproliferative disorders at the time of active EBV infection and muromonab-CD3 administration in pediatric liver allograft recipients. (See ADVERSE REACTIONS, Infections and ADVERSE REACTIONS, Neoplasia.)

Following the initiation of muromonab-CD3 therapy, patients should be continuously monitored for evidence of lymphoproliferative disorders through physical examination and histological evaluation of any suspect lymphoid tissue. Close surveillance is advised, since early detection with subsequent reduction of total immunosuppression may result in regression of some of these lymphoproliferative disorders. Since the potential for the development of lymphoproliferative disorders is related to the duration and extent (intensity) of total immunosuppression, physicians are advised: to adhere to the recommended dosage and duration of muromonab-CD3 therapy; to limit the number of courses of muromonab-CD3 and other anti-T lymphocyte antibody preparations administered within a short period of time; and, if appropriate, to reduce the dosage(s) of immunosuppressive drugs used concomitantly to the lowest level compatible with an effective therapeutic response. (See DOSAGE AND ADMINISTRATION.)

A recent study examined the incidence of non-Hodgkin's lymphoma (NHL) among 45,000 kidney transplant recipients and over 7500 heart transplant recipients. This study suggested that all transplant patients, regardless of the immunosuppressive regimen employed, are at increased risk of NHL over the general population. The relative risk was highest among those receiving the most aggressive regimens.

The long-term risk of neoplastic events in patients being treated with muromonab-CD3 has not been determined.

PRECAUTIONS

GENERAL

When using combinations of immunosuppressive agents, the dose of each agent, including muromonab-CD3, should be reduced to the lowest level compatible with an effective therapeutic response so as to reduce the potential for and severity of infections and malignant transformations.

Fever

If the temperature of the patient exceeds 37.8°C (100°F), it should be lowered by antipyretics before administration of each dose of muromonab-CD3. The possibility of infection should be evaluated.

Severe Cytokine Release Syndrome Versus Anaphylactic Reactions

It may not be possible to distinguish between an acute hypersensitivity reaction (*e.g.*, anaphylaxis, angioedema, etc.) and the Cytokine Release Syndrome.

Potentially serious signs and symptoms having an immediate onset (usually within 10 minutes) following administration of muromonab-CD3 are probably due to acute hypersensitivity. If hypersensitivity is suspected, discontinue the drug immediately; do not resume therapy or re-expose the patient to muromonab-CD3. Clinical manifestations beginning approximately 30-60 minutes (or later) following administration of muromonab-CD3 are more likely cytokine-mediated. (See WARNINGS, Cytokine Release Syndrome and WARNINGS, Anaphylactic Reactions.)

Central Nervous System Events

Since some seizures (and other serious central nervous system events) following muromonab-CD3 administration have been life-threatening, anti-seizure precautions (*e.g.*, an airway ready for use, if needed) should be taken. (See WARNINGS and ADVERSE REACTIONS.)

Infection/Viral-Induced Lymphoproliferative Disorders

If infection or a viral induced lymphoproliferative disorder occurs, culture or biopsy as soon as possible, promptly institute appropriate anti-infective therapy, and (if possible) reduce/discontinue immunosuppressive therapy. (See WARNINGS and ADVERSE REACTIONS.)

Low Protein-Binding Filter

Use a low protein-binding 0.2 or 0.22 micrometer (μm) filter to prepare the injections. (See DOSAGE AND ADMINISTRATION, Administration Instructions.)

Sensitization

Muromonab-CD3 is a mouse (immunoglobulin) protein that can induce human anti-mouse antibody production (*i.e.*, sensitization) in some patients following exposure; a titer ≥1:1000 is a contraindication for use. (See WARNINGS and ADVERSE REACTIONS.)

In the initial clinical trials using low doses of prednisone and azathioprine during muromonab-CD3 therapy for renal allograft rejection, antibodies to muromonab-CD3 were observed with an incidence of 21% (n=43) for IgM, 86% (n=43) for IgG and 29% (n=35) for IgE. The mean time of appearance of IgG antibodies was 20 ± 2 days (mean ±SD). Early IgG antibodies appeared towards the end of the second week of treatment in 3% (n=86) of the patients.

Subsequent clinical experience has shown that the dose, duration, and type of immunosuppressive medications used in combination with muromonab-CD3 may affect both the incidence and magnitude of the host antibody response. Furthermore, immunosuppressive agents used concomitantly with muromonab-CD3 (*i.e.*, steroids, azathioprine, prednisone, or cyclosporine) have altered the time course of anti-mouse antibody development and the specificity of the antibodies formed (*i.e.*, idiotypic, isotypic, allotypic).

Thrombosis

As with other immunosuppressive therapies, arterial, venous, and capillary thromboses of allografts and other vascular beds (*e.g.*, heart, lungs, brain, bowel, etc.) have been reported in patients treated with muromonab-CD3. In addition, microangiopathic changes (*e.g.*, platelet microthrombi) in the renal allograft associated in some patients with microangiopathic hemolytic anemia have been reported. This was observed in 5 of 93 (5%) patients receiving doses above the recommended dose.

The relationship to dose remains uncertain; however, the relative risk appears to be greater with doses above the recommended dose. Patients with a history of thrombosis or underlying vascular disease should be given muromonab-CD3 only when the potential benefits clearly outweigh the increased risks of therapy.

M

INFORMATION FOR THE PATIENT

Patients should be advised:

- Of the signs and symptoms associated with the Cytokine Release Syndrome and the potentially serious nature of this syndrome (*e.g.,* systemic, cardiovascular, central nervous system events).
- To seek medical attention for skin rash, urticaria, rapid heart beat, respiratory distress, dysphagia, or any swelling suggesting an allergic reaction or angioedema.
- That muromonab-CD3 may impair mental alertness and coordination and may effect the ability to operate an automobile or machinery.
- Of other risks associated with the use of muromonab-CD3. (See BOXED WARNING; WARNINGS; PRECAUTIONS and ADVERSE REACTIONS.)

LABORATORY TESTS

The following tests should be monitored prior to and during muromonab-CD3 therapy:

Renal: BUN, serum creatinine, etc.;

Hepatic: Transaminases, alkaline phosphatase, bilirubin;

Hematopoietic: WBCs and differential, platelet count, etc.;

Chest x-ray within 24 hours before initiating muromonab-CD3 treatment to rule out heart failure or fluid overload.

Blood Tests: Periodic assessment of organ system functions (renal, hepatic, and hematopoietic) should be performed.

During therapy with muromonab-CD3: In adults, periodic monitoring to ensure plasma muromonab-CD3 levels (≥800 ng/ml) or T cell clearance (CD3 positive T cells <25 cells/mm^3) is recommended. In pediatric patients, both plasma muromonab-CD3 levels (≥800 ng/ml) and T cell clearance (CD3 positive T cells <25 cells/mm^3) should be monitored daily. (See CLINICAL PHARMACOLOGY.)

CARCINOGENESIS

Long-term studies have not been performed in laboratory animals to evaluate the carcinogenic potential of muromonab-CD3; however, neoplasia has been reported in patients receiving this product. (See WARNINGS and ADVERSE REACTIONS, Neoplasia.)

PREGNANCY CATEGORY C

Animal reproductive studies have not been conducted with muromonab-CD3. It is also not known whether muromonab-CD3 can cause fetal harm when administered to a pregnant woman or can affect reproduction capacity. However, muromonab-CD3 is an IgG antibody and may cross the human placenta. The effect on the fetus of the release of cytokines and/or immunosuppression after treatment with muromonab-CD3 is not known. Muromonab-CD3 should be given to a pregnant woman only if clearly needed. If this drug is used during pregnancy, or the patient becomes pregnant while taking this drug, the patient should be apprised of the potential hazard to the fetus. (See CONTRAINDICATIONS; WARNINGS and ADVERSE REACTIONS.)

NURSING MOTHERS

It is not known whether muromonab-CD3 is excreted in human milk. Because many drugs are excreted in human milk and because of the potential for serious adverse events/oncogenesis shown for muromonab-CD3 in human studies, a decision should be made to discontinue nursing or to discontinue the drug, taking into account the importance of the drug to the mother. (See CONTRAINDICATIONS.)

PEDIATRIC USE

Safety and effectiveness have been established in infants (1 month up to 2 years); children (2 years up to 12 years); and adolescents (12 years up to 16 years). Use of muromonab-CD3 in these age groups is supported by clinical studies that included adults and pediatric patients. In those studies, the safety and efficacy of muromonab-CD3 in pediatric patients receiving renal or hepatic transplants was similar to that in the overall cohort. There were insufficient data to compare the safety and efficacy of muromonab-CD3 in pediatric patients in a study of patients receiving cardiac transplants. Additional pharmacokinetic, pharmacodynamic, and clinical studies in infants, children, and adolescents have been reported in published literature.

Pediatric patients are known to have higher CD3 lymphocyte counts than adults; therefore, progressively higher doses of muromonab-CD3 are often required to achieve therapeutic levels of lymphocyte clearance. (See DOSAGE AND ADMINISTRATION.)

Specific Safety Concerns in Pediatric Patients

Deaths Due to Cerebral Herniation

The postmarketing data base indicates that pediatric patients may be at increased risk of developing cerebral edema with or without herniation compared to adults. In the period between 1986 and 1996, twenty-five cases (6 in pediatric patients) of cerebral edema were identified with subsequent cerebral herniation and death in 5 cases (4 in pediatric patients). Herniation in the pediatric patients and one 19 year old subject occurred within a few hours to 1 day after the first dose (2.5 or 5 mg) of muromonab-CD3 administered in the investigational setting for prophylaxis of renal allograft rejection. All pediatric patients and especially those receiving a renal allograft must be carefully evaluated for fluid retention and hypertension before the initiation of muromonab-CD3 therapy. (See WARNINGS, Cytokine Release Syndrome and DOSAGE AND ADMINISTRATION, General.) Patients should be closely monitored for neurologic symptoms during the first 24 hours following each of the first few doses of muromonab-CD3 injection.

Other Serious Central Nervous System Adverse Events

Other significant neurologic complications reported in pediatric transplant recipients receiving muromonab-CD3 include status epilepticus, cerebral edema, diffuse encephalopathy, cerebritis, seizures, cortical dysfunction, and intracranial hemorrhage. Permanent neurologic impairments (*e.g.,* blindness, deafness, paralysis) have been reported rarely. Because meningitis is a frequent infection encountered in pediatric allograft recipients, and the immunosuppression associated with transplantation increases the risk of opportunistic infection, patients with meningeal irritation following treatment with muromonab-CD3 therapy should be evaluated with lumbar puncture as early as possible to rule out an infectious etiology.

Viral Infection

The overall incidence of infections appeared to be similar in pediatric patients compared to the overall population studied. In the pediatric population, viral infections often include pathogens uncommon in adults, such as varicella zoster virus (VZV), adenovirus, enterovirus, parainfluenza virus, and respiratory syncytial virus (RSV). In addition, many viral diseases often manifest differently in pediatric patients than they do in adults.

Because a large proportion of pediatric patients have not been infected by herpes viruses (*e.g.,* EBV, HSV, CMV) prior to transplantation they may be more susceptible to acquiring primary infections from the grafted organ and/or blood products when immunosuppressed. Antiviral prophylactic therapy may be particularly useful in these high risk pediatric patients. (See ADVERSE REACTIONS, Infections.)

Neoplasia

Patients with primary EBV infection may be at higher risk for the development of EBV-associated lymphoproliferative disorders.

There are data to support an association between the development of lymphoproliferative disorders at the time of active EBV infection and muromonab-CD3 administration in pediatric liver allograft recipients. Antiviral prophylactic therapy may be particularly useful in these high risk pediatric patients.

Gastrointestinal Fluid Losses

Parenteral hydration may be required for gastrointestinal fluid loss secondary to diarrhea and/or vomiting resulting from the "Cytokine Release Syndrome".

Thrombosis

Pediatric patients may be at an increased risk of thrombosis. Pediatric patients weighing less than 15 kg are at high-risk for hepatic artery thrombosis. Thrombosis has been reported in pediatric transplant recipients treated with muromonab-CD3. A number of factors, including surgical technique, the presence of a hypercoagulable state, and the absence of prior dialysis experience may be relevant to the pathophysiology of the increased risk of thrombosis. (See BOXED WARNING; WARNINGS; PRECAUTIONS; ADVERSE REACTIONS and DOSAGE AND ADMINISTRATION.)

ADVERSE REACTIONS

CYTOKINE RELEASE SYNDROME

In controlled clinical trials for treatment of acute renal allograft rejection, patients treated with muromonab-CD3 plus concomitant low-dose immunosuppressive therapy (primarily azathioprine and corticosteroids) were observed to have an increased incidence of adverse experiences during the first 2 days of treatment, as compared with the group of patients receiving azathioprine and high-dose steroid therapy. During this period the majority of patients experienced pyrexia (90%), of which 19% were 40.0°C (104°F) or above, and chills (59%). In addition, other adverse experiences occurring in 8% or more of the patients during the first 2 days of muromonab-CD3 therapy included: dyspnea (21%), nausea (19%), vomiting (19%), chest pain (14%), diarrhea (14%), tremor (13%), wheezing (13%), headache (11%), tachycardia (10%), rigor (8%), and hypertension (8%). A similar spectrum of clinical manifestations has been observed in open clinical studies and in post-marketing experience involving patients treated with muromonab-CD3 for rejection following renal, cardiac, and hepatic transplantation.

Additional serious and occasionally fatal cardiorespiratory manifestations have been reported following any of the first few doses. (See WARNINGS, Cytokine Release Syndrome and ADVERSE REACTIONS.)

In the acute renal allograft rejection trials, potentially fatal pulmonary edema had been reported following the first two doses in less than 2% of the patients treated with muromonab-CD3. Pulmonary edema was usually associated with fluid overload. However, post-marketing experience revealed that pulmonary edema has occurred in patients who appeared to be euvolemic, presumably as a consequence of cytokine-mediated increased vascular permeability ("leaky capillaries") and/or reduced myocardial contractility/compliance (*i.e.,* left ventricular dysfunction). (See WARNINGS, Cytokine Release Syndrome and DOSAGE AND ADMINISTRATION.)

INFECTIONS

In the controlled randomized renal allograft rejection trial conducted before cyclosporine was marketed, the most common infections during the first 45 days of muromonab-CD3 therapy were due to herpes simplex virus (27%) and cytomegalovirus (19%). Other severe and life-threatening infections were *Staphylococcus epidermidis* (5%), *Pneumocystis carinii* (3%), *Legionella* (2%), *Cryptococcus* (2%), *Serratia* (2%) and gram-negative bacteria (2%). The incidence of infections was similar in patients treated with muromonab-CD3 and in patients treated with high-dose steroids.

In a clinical trial of acute hepatic allograft rejection, refractory to conventional treatment, the most common infections reported in patients treated with muromonab-CD3 during the first 45 days of the study were cytomegalovirus (16% of patients, of which 43% of infections were severe), fungal infections (15% of patients, of which 30% were severe), and herpes simplex virus (8% of patients, of which 10% were severe). Other severe and life-threatening infections were gram-positive infections (9% of patients), gram-negative infections (8% of patients), viral infections (2% of patients), and *Legionella* (1% of patients). In another trial studying the use of muromonab-CD3 in patients with hepatic allografts, the incidence of fungal infections was 34% and infections with the herpes simplex virus was 31%.

In a clinical trial studying the use of muromonab-CD3 in patients with acute cardiac rejection refractory to conventional treatment, the most common infections in the muromonab-CD3 group reported during the first 45 days of the study were herpes simplex virus (5% of patients, of which 20% were severe), fungal infections (4% of patients, of which 75% were severe), and cytomegalovirus (3% of patients, of which 33% were severe). No other severe or life-threatening infections were reported during this period.

In a retrospective analysis of pediatric patients treated for acute hepatic rejection, the most common infections reported in patients treated with muromonab-CD3 therapy were due to bacterial infections (47%), fungal infections (21%), cytomegalovirus (19%), herpes simplex virus (15%), adenovirus (8%), and Epstein-Barr virus (8%). The overall rates of viral, fungal, and bacterial infections were similar in patients treated with muromonab-CD3 (n=53) and in patients whose rejection was treated with steroids alone (n=27). In another study of 149 pediatric liver allograft patients where 59 episodes of steroid-resistant rejection were treated with muromonab-CD3, the incidence of invasive cytomegalovirus infection was higher in patients receiving muromonab-CD3 than in those receiving steroids alone.

Clinically significant infections (*e.g.*, pneumonia, sepsis, etc.) due to the following pathogens have been reported:

Bacterial: *Clostridium* species (including *perfringens*), *Corynebacterium,* Enterococcus, *Enterobacter aerogenes, Escherichia coli, Klebsiella* species, *Lactobacillus, Legionella, Listeria monocytogenes, Mycobacteria* species, *Nocardia asteroides, Proteus* species, *Providencia* species, *Pseudomonas aeruginosa, Serratia* species, *Staphylococcus* species, *Streptococcus* species, *Yersinia enterocolitica,* and other gram-negative bacteria.

Fungal*: *Aspergillus, Candida, Cryptococcus, Dermatophytes.*

Protozoa: *Neumocystis carinii, Toxoplasma gondii.*

Viral: Cytomegalovirus* (CMV), Epstein-Barr virus* (EBV), herpes simplex virus* (HSV), hepatitis viruses, varicella zoster virus (VZV), adenovirus, enterovirus, respiratory syncytial virus (RSV), parainfluenza virus.

As a consequence of being a potent immunosuppressive, the incidence and severity of infections with designated (*) pathogens, especially the herpes family of viruses, may be increased. (See WARNINGS, Consequences of Immunosuppression, Infections.)

NEOPLASIA

In patients treated with muromonab-CD3, post-transplant lymphoproliferative disorders have ranged from lymphadenopathy or benign polyclonal B cell hyperplasias to malignant and often fatal monoclonal B cell lymphomas. In post-marketing experience, approximately one-third of the lymphoproliferations reported were benign and two-thirds were malignant. Lymphoma types included: B cell, large cell, polyclonal, non-Hodgkin's, lymphocytic, T cell, Burkitt's. The majority were not histologically classified. Malignant lymphomas appear to develop early after transplantation, the majority within the first 4 months post-treatment. Many of these have been rapidly progressive. Some were fulminant, involving the allografted organ and were widely disseminated at the time of diagnosis. Carcinomas of the skin included: basal cell, squamous cell, sarcoma, melanoma, and keratoacanthoma. Other neoplasms infrequently reported include: multiple myeloma, leukemia, carcinoma of the breast, adenocarcinoma, cholangiocarcinoma, and recurrencesof pre-existing hepatoma and renal cell carcinoma. (See WARNINGS, Consequences of Immunosuppression, Neoplasia.)

HYPERSENSITIVITY REACTIONS

Reported adverse reactions resulting from the formation of antibodies to muromonab-CD3 have included antigen-antibody (immune complex) mediated syndromes and IgE-mediated reactions. Hypersensitivity reactions have ranged from a mild, self-limited rash or pruritus to severe, life-threatening anaphylactic reactions/shock or angioedema (including: swelling of lips, eyelids, laryngeal spasm and airway obstruction with hypoxia). (See WARNINGS, Anaphylactic Reactions.)

Other hypersensitivity reactions have included: Ineffectiveness of treatment, serum sickness, arthritis, allergic interstitial nephritis, immune complex deposition resulting in glomerulonephritis, vasculitis (including temporal and retinal), and eosinophilia.

ADVERSE REACTIONS BY BODY SYSTEM

Adverse events reported in greater than or equal to 1% of clinical trial patients treated with muromonab-CD3 (n=393) are shown in TABLE 1.

TABLE 1 *Adverse Events Reported in Clinical Trials*

(≥1% Incidence, n=393)

Body System	Incidence
Autonomic Nervous System Disorders	
Diaphoresis	7%
Vasodilation	7%
Body as a Whole, General Disorders	
Anorexia	4%
Asthenia	10%
Chills	43%
Fatigue	9%
Lethargy	6%
Malaise	5%
Pain, trunk	6%
Pyrexia	77%
Cardiovascular Disorders, General	
Arrhythmia	4%
Bradycardia	4%
Hypertension	19%
Hypotension	25%
Pain, chest	9%
Tachycardia	26%
Vascular occlusion	2%
Central & Peripheral Nervous System Disorders	
Convulsions	1%
Dizziness	6%
Headache	28%
Meningitis	1%
Tremor	14%
Gastrointestinal System Disorders	
Diarrhea	37%
Nausea	32%
Pain, abdominal	6%
Pain, GI	7%
Vomiting	25%
Hematopoietic Disorders	
Anemia	2%
Leukocytosis	1%
Thrombocytopenia	2%
Metabolic and Nutritional Disorders	
Edema	12%
Musculoskeletal System Disorders	
Arthralgia	7%
Myalgia	1%
Psychiatric Disorders	
Confusion	6%
Depression	3%
Nervousness	5%
Somnolence	2%
Renal Disorders	
Renal dysfunction	3%
Respiratory System Disorders	
Abnormal chest sounds	10%
Dyspnea	16%
Hyperventilation	7%
Hypoxia	1%
Pneumonia	1%
Pulmonary edema	2%
Respiratory congestion	4%
Wheezing	6%
Skin and Appendages Disorders	
Pruritus	7%
Rash	14%
Rash erythematous	2%
Special Senses	
Photophobia	1%
Tinnitus	1%
White Cell & Reticuloendothelial System Disorders	
Leukopenia	7%

Selected Adverse Events Reported In Clinical Trials (<1% incidence, n=393):

Cardiovascular Disorders, General: Angina, cardiac arrest, fluctuation in blood pressure, heart failure, myocardial infarction, shock, thrombosis.

Central & Peripheral Nervous System Disorders: Coma, encephalopathy, epilepsy, hypotonia.

Gastrointestinal Disorders: Gastrointestinal hemorrhage.

Hemapoietic Disorders: Coagulation disorder, lymphadenopathy, lymphopenia.

Hepatobiliary: Hepatitis, SGOT increased, SGPT increased.

Psychiatric Disorders: Hallucinations, mood changes, paranoia, psychosis.

Renal Disorders: Anuria, oliguria.

Respiratory System Disorders: Apnea, pneumonitis.

Special Senses: Conjunctivitis, hearing decrease.

Worldwide Postmarketing Experience — Body Systems/Events Listed Alphabetically:

Body as a Whole, General Disorders: Fever (including spiking temperatures as high as 107°F), flu-like syndrome.

Cardiovascular Disorders: Cardiovascular collapse, hemodynamic instability, left ventricular dysfunction.

Central & Peripheral Nervous System Disorders: Agitation, aphasia, asterixis, cerebritis, cerebral edema, cerebral herniation, cerebrovascular accident, CNS infection, CNS malignancy, cranial nerve VI palsy, encephalitis, hyperreflexia, involuntary movements, intracranial hemorrhage, impaired cognition, myoclonus, obnubilation, paresis/plegia including quadriparesis/plegia, status epilepticus, stupor, transient ischemic attack, vertigo.

In a post-marketing survey involving 214 renal transplant patients, the incidence of aseptic meningitis syndrome was 6%.

Fever (89%), headache (44%), neck stiffness (14%), and photophobia (10%) were the most commonly reported symptoms; a combination of these four symptoms occurred in 5% of patients.

Between 1987 and 1992, 75 post-marketing reports have described seizures, averaging about 12 per year, and including 23 fatalities. More than two-thirds of these reports (53) were of domestic spontaneous origin, and their age and sex distributions were broad. Post-licensure reports generally provide insufficient data to allow accurate estimation of risk or of incidence.

Gastrointestinal Disorders: Bowel infarction.

Hematopoietic Disorders: Aplastic anemia, arterial, venous and capillary thrombosis of allografts and other vascular beds *e.g.*, heart, lung, brain and bowel etc., disseminated intravascular coagulation, microangiopathic changes (*e.g.*, platelet microthrombi), microangiopathic hemolytic anemia, neutropenia, pancytopenia.

Hepatobiliary: Hepatitis or hepato/splenomegaly, usually secondary to viral infection or lymphoma.

Musculoskeletal Disorders: Arthritis, stiffness/aches/pains.

Renal Disorders: Azotemia, abnormal urinary cytology including exfoliation of damaged lymphocytes, collecting duct cells and cellular casts, delayed graft function, renal insufficiency/renal failure, usually transient and reversible and occasionally in association with Cytokine Release Syndrome.

Respiratory System Disorders: Adult respiratory distress syndrome, respiratory arrest, respiratory failure.

Skin and Appendages: Erythema, flushing, Stevens-Johnson syndrome, urticaria.

Special Senses: Blindness, blurred vision, deafness, diplopia, otitis media, nasal and ear stuffiness, papilledema.

M

DOSAGE AND ADMINISTRATION

ADULTS

The recommended dose of muromonab-CD3 for the treatment of acute renal, steroid-resistant cardiac, or steroid-resistant hepatic allograft rejection is 5 mg/day in a single (bolus) intravenous injection in less than 1 minute for 10-14 days. For acute renal rejection, treatment should begin upon diagnosis. For steroid-resistant cardiac or hepatic allograft rejection, treatment should begin when the treating physician deems a rejection has not been reversed by an adequate course of corticosteroid therapy. (See CLINICAL PHARMACOLOGY; PRECAUTIONS, General, Sensitization and PRECAUTIONS, Laboratory Tests.)

PEDIATRIC PATIENTS

The initial recommended dose is 2.5 mg/day in pediatric patients weighing less than or equal to 30 kg and 5 mg/day in pediatric patients weighing greater than 30 kg in a single (bolus) intravenous injection in less than 1 minute for 10-14 days. Daily increases in muromonab-CD3 doses (*i.e.,* 2.5 mg increments) may be required to achieve depletion of CD3 positive cells (<25 cells/mm^3) and ensure therapeutic muromonab-CD3 serum concentrations (>800 ng/ml). Pediatric patients may require augmentation of the muromonab-CD3 dose. For acute renal rejection, treatment should begin upon diagnosis. For steroid-resistant cardiac or hepatic allograft rejection, treatment should begin when the treating physician deems a rejection has not been reversed by an adequate course of corticosteroid therapy. (See CLINICAL PHARMACOLOGY; PRECAUTIONS, Laboratory Tests and PRECAUTIONS, Pediatric Use.)

GENERAL

For the first few doses, patients should be monitored in a facility equipped and staffed for cardiopulmonary resuscitation (CPR). Patients receiving subsequent doses of muromonab-CD3, should also be monitored in a facility equipped and staffed for CPR. Vital signs should be monitored frequently. Patients receiving muromonab-CD3 should also be carefully monitored for signs and symptoms of Cytokine Release Syndrome, particularly after the first few doses but also after a treatment hiatus with resumption of therapy. The patient's temperature should be lowered to <37.8°C (100°F) before the administration of any dose of muromonab-CD3.

Prior to administration of muromonab-CD3, the patient's volume status should be assessed carefully. It is imperative, especially prior to the first few doses, that there be no clinical evidence of volume overload, uncontrolled hypertension, or uncompensated heart failure. Patients should have a clear chest x-ray and should not weigh more than 3% above their minimum weight during the week prior to injection.

To decrease the incidence and severity of Cytokine Release Syndrome, associated with the first dose of muromonab-CD3, it is strongly recommended that methylprednisolone sodium succinate 8.0 mg/kg be administered intravenously 1-4 hours prior to the initial dose of muromonab-CD3. Acetaminophen and antihistamines given concomitantly with muromonab-CD3 may also help to reduce some early reactions. (See WARNINGS and ADVERSE REACTIONS, Cytokine Release Syndrome.)

When using concomitant immunosuppressive drugs, the dose of each should be reduced to the lowest level compatible with an effective therapeutic response in order to reduce the potential for malignancy and infections. Maintenance immunosuppression should be resumed approximately 3 days prior to the cessation of muromonab-CD3 therapy. (See WARNINGS; ADVERSE REACTIONS, Infection and ADVERSE REACTIONS, Neoplasia.)

Reduced T cell clearance or low plasma muromonab-CD3 levels provide a basis for adjusting muromonab-CD3 dosage or for discontinuing therapy. (See WARNINGS, Anaphylactic Reactions; PRECAUTIONS, Laboratory Tests and ADVERSE REACTIONS, Hypersensitivity Reactions.)

ADMINISTRATION INSTRUCTIONS

1. Before administration, muromonab-CD3 should be inspected for particulate matter and discoloration. Because muromonab-CD3 is a protein solution, it may develop fine translucent particles (shown not to affect potency).
2. No bacteriostatic agent is present in this product. Adherence to aseptic technique is advised. Once the ampule is opened, use immediately and discard the unused portion.
3. Prepare muromonab-CD3 for injection by drawing solution into a syringe through a low protein-binding 0.2 or 0.22 micrometer (μm) filter. Detach filter and attach a new needle for a single intravenous (bolus) injection.
4. Because no data is available on compatibility of muromonab-CD3 with other intravenous substances or additives, other medications/substances should not be added or infused simultaneously through the same intravenous line. If the same intravenous line is used for sequential infusion of several different drugs, the line should be flushed with saline before and after injection of muromonab-CD3.
5. Administer muromonab-CD3 as a single intravenous (bolus) injection in less than 1 minute. Do not administer by intravenous infusion or in conjunction with other drug solutions.

HOW SUPPLIED

Orthoclone OKT3 is supplied as a sterile solution in packages of 5 ampules. Each 5 ml ampule contains 5 mg of muromonab-CD3.

Storage: Store in a refrigerator at 2-8°C (36-46°F).

DO NOT FREEZE OR SHAKE.

PRODUCT LISTING - EQUIVALENTS NOT AVAILABLE

Solution - Intravenous - 1 mg/ml

5 ml $818.22 ORTHOCLONE OKT3, Ortho Biotech Inc 59676-0101-01

Mycophenolate Mofetil *(003256)*

Categories: Rejection, heart transplant, prophylaxis; Rejection, liver transplant, prophylaxis; Rejection, renal transplant, prophylaxis; FDA Approved 1995 May; Pregnancy Category C

Drug Classes: Immunosuppressives

Brand Names: Cellcept

Cost of Therapy: $704.44 (Transplant Rejection; Cellcept; 500 mg; 4 tablets/day; 30 day supply)
$704.52 (Transplant Rejection; Cellcept; 250 mg; 8 tablets/day; 30 day supply)

WARNING

Increased susceptibility to infection and the possible development of lymphoma may result from immunosuppression. Only physicians experienced in immunosuppressive therapy and management of renal, cardiac or hepatic transplant patients should use mycophenolate mofetil. Patients receiving the drug should be managed in facilities equipped and staffed with adequate laboratory and supportive medical resources. The physician responsible for maintenance therapy should have complete information requisite for the follow-up of the patient.

DESCRIPTION

Mycophenolate mofetil is the 2-morpholinoethyl ester of mycophenolic acid (MPA), an immunosuppressive agent; inosine monophosphate dehydrogenase (IMPDH) inhibitor.

The chemical name for mycophenolate mofetil (MMF) is 2-morpholinoethyl (E)-6-(1,3-dihydro-4-hydroxy-6-methoxy-7-methyl-3-oxo-5-isobenzofuranyl)-4-methyl-4-hexenoate. It has an empirical formula of $C_{23}H_{31}NO_7$, and a molecular weight of 433.50.

Mycophenolate mofetil is a white to off-white crystalline powder. It is slightly soluble in water (43 μg/ml at pH 7.4); the solubility increases in acidic medium (4.27 mg/ml at pH 3.6). It is freely soluble in acetone, soluble in methanol, and sparingly soluble in ethanol. The apparent partition coefficient in 1-octanol/water (pH 7.4) buffer solution is 238. The pKa values for mycophenolate mofetil are 5.6 for the morpholino group and 8.5 for the phenolic group.

Mycophenolate mofetil hydrochloride has a solubility of 65.8 mg/ml in 5% dextrose injection (D5W). The pH of the reconstituted solution is 2.4-4.1.

CellCept is available for oral administration as capsules containing 250 mg of mycophenolate mofetil, tablets containing 500 mg of mycophenolate mofetil, and as a powder for oral suspension, which when constituted contains 200 mg/ml mycophenolate mofetil.

Inactive ingredients in CellCept 250 mg capsules include croscarmellose sodium, magnesium stearate, povidone (K-90) and pregelatinized starch. The capsule shells contain black iron oxide, FD&C blue no. 2, gelatin, red iron oxide, silicon dioxide, sodium lauryl sulfate, titanium dioxide, and yellow iron oxide.

Inactive ingredients in CellCept 500 mg tablets include black iron oxide, croscarmellose sodium, FD&C blue no. 2 aluminum lake, hydroxypropyl cellulose, hydroxypropyl methylcellulose, magnesium stearate, microcrystalline cellulose, polyethylene glycol 400, povidone (K-90), red iron oxide, talc, and titanium dioxide; may also contain ammonium hydroxide, ethyl alcohol, methyl alcohol, n-butyl alcohol, propylene glycol, and shellac.

Inactive ingredients in CellCept oral suspension include aspartame, citric acid anhydrous, colloidal silicon dioxide, methylparaben, mixed fruit flavor, sodium citrate dihydrate, sorbitol, soybean lecithin, and xanthan gum.

CellCept intravenous is the hydrochloride salt of mycophenolate mofetil. The chemical name for the hydrochloride salt of mycophenolate mofetil is 2-morpholinoethyl (E)-6-(1,3-dihydro-4-hydroxy-6-methoxy-7-methyl-3-oxo-5-isobenzofuranyl)-4-methyl-4-hexenoate hydrochloride. It has an empirical formula of $C_{23}H_{31}NO_7HCl$ and a molecular weight of 469.96.

CellCept intravenous is available as a sterile white to off-white lyophilized powder in vials containing mycophenolate mofetil hydrochloride for administration by intravenous infusion only. Each vial of CellCept intravenous contains the equivalent of 500 mg mycophenolate mofetil as the hydrochloride salt. The inactive ingredients are polysorbate 80, 25 mg, and citric acid, 5 mg. Sodium hydroxide may have been used in the manufacture of CellCept intravenous to adjust the pH. Reconstitution and dilution with 5% dextrose injection yields a slightly yellow solution of mycophenolate mofetil, 6 mg/ml. (For detailed method of preparation, refer to the Patient Instructions that are distributed with the prescription for complete instructions.)

CLINICAL PHARMACOLOGY

MECHANISM OF ACTION

Mycophenolate mofetil has been demonstrated in experimental animal models to prolong the survival of allogeneic transplants (kidney, heart, liver, intestine, limb, small bowel, pancreatic islets, and bone marrow).

Mycophenolate mofetil has also been shown to reverse ongoing acute rejection in the canine renal and rat cardiac allograft models. Mycophenolate mofetil also inhibited proliferative arteriopathy in experimental models of aortic and heart allografts in rats, as well as in primate cardiac xenografts. Mycophenolate mofetil was used alone or in combination with other immunosuppressive agents in these studies. Mycophenolate mofetil has been demonstrated to inhibit immunologically mediated inflammatory responses in animal models and to inhibit tumor development and prolong survival in murine tumor transplant models.

Mycophenolate mofetil is rapidly absorbed following oral administration and hydrolyzed to form MPA, which is the active metabolite. MPA is a potent, selective, uncompetitive, and reversible inhibitor of inosine monophosphate dehydrogenase (IMPDH), and therefore inhibits the *de novo* pathway of guanosine nucleotide synthesis without incorporation into DNA. Because T- and B-lymphocytes are critically dependent for their proliferation on *de novo* synthesis of purines, whereas other cell types can utilize salvage pathways, MPA has potent cytostatic effects on lymphocytes. MPA inhibits proliferative responses of T- and B-lymphocytes to both mitogenic and allospecific stimulation. Addition of guanosine or deoxyguanosine reverses the cytostatic effects of MPA on lymphocytes. MPA also suppresses antibody formation by B-lymphocytes. MPA prevents the glycosylation of lymphocyte and monocyte glycoproteins that are involved in intercellular adhesion to endothelial cells and may inhibit recruitment of leukocytes into sites of inflammation and graft rejection. Mycophenolate mofetil did not inhibit early events in the activation of human peripheral blood mononuclear cells, such as the production of interleukin-1 (IL-1) and interleukin-2 (IL-2), but did block the coupling of these events to DNA synthesis and proliferation.

PHARMACOKINETICS

Following oral and intravenous (IV) administration, mycophenolate mofetil undergoes rapid and complete metabolism to MPA, the active metabolite. Oral absorption of the drug is rapid and essentially complete. MPA is metabolized to form the phenolic glucuronide of MPA (MPAG) which is not pharmacologically active. The parent drug, mycophenolate mofetil, can be measured systemically during the IV infusion; however, shortly (about 5 minutes) after the infusion is stopped or after oral administration, MMF concentration is below the limit of quantitation (0.4 µg/ml).

Absorption

In 12 healthy volunteers, the mean absolute bioavailability of oral mycophenolate mofetil relative to IV mycophenolate mofetil (based on MPA AUC) was 94%. The area under the plasma-concentration time curve (AUC) for MPA appears to increase in a dose-proportional fashion in renal transplant patients receiving multiple doses of mycophenolate mofetil up to a daily dose of 3 g (see TABLE 1 on pharmacokinetic parameters).

Food (27 g fat, 650 calories) had no effect on the extent of absorption (MPA AUC) of mycophenolate mofetil when administered at doses of 1.5 g bid to renal transplant patients. However, MPA C_{max} was decreased by 40% in the presence of food (see DOSAGE AND ADMINISTRATION).

Distribution

The mean (±SD) apparent volume of distribution of MPA in 12 healthy volunteers is approximately 3.6 (±1.5) and 4.0 (±1.2) L/kg following IV and oral administration, respectively. MPA, at clinically relevant concentrations, is 97% bound to plasma albumin. MPAG is 82% bound to plasma albumin at MPAG concentration ranges that are normally seen in stable renal transplant patients; however, at higher MPAG concentrations (observed in patients with renal impairment or delayed graft function), the binding of MPA may be reduced as a result of competition between MPAG and MPA for protein binding. Mean blood to plasma ratio of radioactivity concentrations was approximately 0.6 indicating that MPA and MPAG do not extensively distribute into the cellular fractions of blood.

In vitro studies to evaluate the effect of other agents on the binding of MPA to human serum albumin (HSA) or plasma proteins showed that salicylate (at 25 mg/dl with HSA) and MPAG (at ≥460 µg/ml with plasma proteins) increased the free fraction of MPA. At concentrations that exceeded what is encountered clinically, cyclosporine, digoxin, naproxen, prednisone, propranolol, tacrolimus, theophylline, tolbutamide, and warfarin did not increase the free fraction of MPA. MPA at concentrations as high as 100 µg/ml had little effect on the binding of warfarin, digoxin or propranolol, but decreased the binding of theophylline from 53% to 45% and phenytoin from 90% to 87%.

Metabolism

Following oral and IV dosing, mycophenolate mofetil undergoes complete metabolism to MPA, the active metabolite. Metabolism to MPA occurs presystemically after oral dosing. MPA is metabolized principally by glucuronyl transferase to form the phenolic glucuronide of MPA (MPAG) which is not pharmacologically active. *In vivo,* MPAG is converted to MPA via enterohepatic recirculation. The following metabolites of the 2-hydroxyethyl-morpholino moiety are also recovered in the urine following oral administration of mycophenolate mofetil to healthy subjects: N-(2-carboxymethyl)-morpholine, N-(2-hydroxyethyl)-morpholine, and the N-oxide of N-(2-hydroxyethyl)-morpholine.

Secondary peaks in the plasma MPA concentration-time profile are usually observed 6-12 hours postdose. The coadministration of cholestyramine (4 g tid) resulted in approximately a 40% decrease in the MPA AUC (largely as a consequence of lower concentrations in the terminal portion of the profile). These observations suggest that enterohepatic recirculation contributes to MPA plasma concentrations.

Increased plasma concentrations of mycophenolate mofetil metabolites (MPA 50% increase and MPAG about a 3- to 6-fold increase) are observed in patients with renal insufficiency (see CLINICAL PHARMACOLOGY, Special Populations).

Excretion

Negligible amount of drug is excreted as MPA (<1% of dose) in the urine. Orally administered radiolabeled mycophenolate mofetil resulted in complete recovery of the administered dose, with 93% of the administered dose recovered in the urine and 6% recovered in feces. Most (about 87%) of the administered dose is excreted in the urine as MPAG. At clinically encountered concentrations, MPA and MPAG are usually not removed by hemodialysis. However, at high MPAG plasma concentrations (>100 µg/ml), small amounts of MPAG are removed. Bile acid sequestrants, such as cholestyramine, reduce MPA AUC by interfering with enterohepatic circulation of the drug.

Mean (±SD) apparent half-life and plasma clearance of MPA are 17.9 (±6.5) hours and 193 (±48) ml/min following oral administration and 16.6 (±5.8) hours and 177 (±31) ml/min following IV administration, respectively.

Pharmacokinetics in Healthy Volunteers, Renal, Cardiac, and Hepatic Transplant Patients

Shown in TABLE 1 are the mean (±SD) pharmacokinetic parameters for MPA following the administration of mycophenolate mofetil given as single doses to healthy volunteers and multiple doses to renal, cardiac, and hepatic transplant patients. In the early posttransplant period (<40 days posttransplant), renal, cardiac, and hepatic transplant patients had mean MPA AUCs approximately 20-41% lower and mean C_{max} approximately 32-44% lower compared to the late transplant period (3-6 months posttransplant).

Mean MPA AUC values following administration of 1 g bid IV mycophenolate mofetil over 2 hours to renal transplant patients for 5 days were about 24% higher than those observed after oral administration of a similar dose in the immediate posttransplant phase. In hepatic transplant patients, administration of 1 g bid IV mycophenolate mofetil followed by 1.5 g bid oral mycophenolate mofetil resulted in mean MPA AUC values similar to those found in renal transplant patients administered 1 g mycophenolate mofetil bid.

TABLE 1 *Pharmacokinetic Parameters for MPA [Mean (±SD)] Following Administration of Mycophenolate Mofetil to Healthy Volunteers (Single Dose), Renal, Cardiac, and Hepatic Transplant Patients (Multiple Doses)*

Time After Transplantation	Dose/Route	T_{max} (h)	C_{max} (µg/ml)	AUC (µg·h/ml)
Healthy Volunteers (single dose)*				
	1 g/oral	0.80 (±0.36) (n=129)	24.5 (±9.5) (n=129)	63.9 (±16.2) (n=117)
Renal Transplant Patients (bid dosing)†				
5 days	1 g/IV	1.58 (±0.46) (n=31)	12.0 (±3.82) (n=31)	40.8 (±11.4) (n=31)
6 days	1 g/oral	1.33 (±1.05) (n=31)	10.7 (±4.83) (n=31)	32.9 (±15.0) (n=31)
Early (<40 days)	1 g/oral	1.31 (±0.76) (n=25)	8.16 (±4.50) (n=25)	27.3 (±10.9) (n=25)
Early (<40 days)	1.5 g/oral	1.21 (±0.81) (n=27)	13.5 (±8.18) (n=27)	38.4 (±15.4) (n=27)
Late (>3 months)	1.5 g/oral	0.90 (±0.24) (n=23)	24.1 (±12.1) (n=23)	65.3 (±35.4) (n=23)
Cardiac Transplant Patients (bid dosing)†				
Early (day before discharge	1.5 g/oral	1.8 (±1.3) (n=11)	11.5 (±6.8) (n=11)	43.3 (±20.8) (n=9)
Late (>6 months)	1.5 g/oral	1.1 (±0.7) (n=52)	20.0 (±9.4) (n=52)	54.1‡ (±20.4) (n=49)
Hepatic Transplant Patients (bid dosing)†				
4-9 days	1 g/IV	1.50 (±0.517) (n=22)	17.0 (±12.7) (n=22)	34.0 (±17.4) (n=22)
Early (5-8 days)	1.5 g/oral	1.15 (±0.432) (n=20)	13.1 (±6.76) (n=20)	29.2 (±11.9) (n=20)
Late (>6 months)	1.5 g/oral	1.54 (±0.51) (n=6)	19.3 (±11.7) (n=6)	49.3 (±14.8) (n=6)

* Total AUC.
† Interdosing interval AUC(0-12h).
‡ AUC(0-12h) values quoted are extrapolated from data from samples collected over 4 hours.

Two 500 mg tablets have been shown to be bioequivalent to four 250 mg capsules. Five (5) ml of the 200 mg/ml constituted oral suspension have been shown to be bioequivalent to four 250 mg capsules.

Special Populations

Shown in TABLE 2A and TABLE 2B are the mean (±SD) pharmacokinetic parameters for MPA following the administration of oral mycophenolate mofetil given as single doses to non-transplant subjects with renal or hepatic impairment.

TABLE 2A *Pharmacokinetic Parameters for MPA [Mean (±SD)] Following Single (1 g) Doses of Mycophenolate Mofetil Capsules in Chronic Renal Impairment*

	n	T_{max} (h)	C_{max} (µg/ml)	AUC(0-96h) (µg·h/ml)
Healthy Volunteers				
GFR >80 ml/min/1.73 m^2	6	0.75 (±0.27)	25.3 (±7.99)	45.0 (±22.6)
Mild Renal Impairment				
GFR 50-80 ml/min/1.73 m^2	6	0.75 (±0.27)	26.0 (±3.82)	59.9 (±12.9)
Moderate Renal Impairment				
GFR 25-49 ml/min/1.73 m^2	6	0.75 (±0.27)	19.0 (±13.2)	52.9 (±25.5)
Severe Renal Impairment				
GFR <25 ml/min/1.73 m^2	7	1.00 (±0.41)	16.3 (±10.8)	78.6 (±46.4)

TABLE 2B *Pharmacokinetic Parameters for MPA [Mean (±SD)] Following Single (1 g) Doses of Mycophenolate Mofetil Capsules in Chronic Hepatic Impairment*

	n	T_{max} (h)	C_{max} (µg/ml)	AUC(0-48h) (µg·h/ml)
Healthy volunteers	6	0.63 (±0.14)	24.3 (±5.73)	29.0 (±5.78)
Alcoholic cirrhosis	18	0.85 (±0.58)	22.4 (±10.1)	29.8 (±10.7)

Renal Insufficiency

In a single-dose study, MMF was administered as capsule or IV infusion over 40 minutes. Plasma MPA AUC observed after oral dosing to volunteers with severe chronic renal impairment [glomerular filtration rate (GFR) <25 ml/min/1.73 m^2] was about 75% higher relative to that observed in healthy volunteers (GFR >80 ml/min/1.73 m^2). In addition, the single-dose plasma MPAG AUC was 3- to 6-fold higher in volunteers with severe renal impairment than in volunteers with mild renal impairment or healthy volunteers, consistent with the known renal elimination of MPAG. No data are available on the safety of long-term exposure to this level of MPAG.

Plasma MPA AUC observed after single-dose (1 g) IV dosing to volunteers (n=4) with severe chronic renal impairment (GFR <25 ml/min/1.73 m^2) was 62.4 µg·h/ml (±19.3). Multiple dosing of mycophenolate mofetil in patients with severe chronic renal impairment has not been studied (see PRECAUTIONS, General and DOSAGE AND ADMINISTRATION).

In patients with delayed renal graft function posttransplant, mean MPA AUC(0-12h) was comparable to that seen in posttransplant patients without delayed graft function. There is a potential for a transient increase in the free fraction and concentration of plasma MPA in patients with delayed renal graft function. However, dose adjustment does not appear to be necessary in patients with delayed renal graft function. Mean plasma MPAG AUC(0-12h) was 2- to 3-fold higher than in posttransplant patients without delayed renal graft function (see PRECAUTIONS, General and DOSAGE AND ADMINISTRATION).

In 8 patients with primary non-function of the organ following renal transplantation, plasma concentrations of MPAG accumulated about 6- to 8-fold after multiple dosing for 28 days. Accumulation of MPA was about 1- to 2-fold.

The pharmacokinetics of mycophenolate mofetil are not altered by hemodialysis. Hemodialysis usually does not remove MPA or MPAG. At high concentrations of MPAG (>100 μg/ml), hemodialysis removes only small amounts of MPAG.

Hepatic Insufficiency

In a single-dose (1 g oral) study of 18 volunteers with alcoholic cirrhosis and 6 healthy volunteers, hepatic MPA glucuronidation processes appeared to be relatively unaffected by hepatic parenchymal disease when pharmacokinetic parameters of healthy volunteers and alcoholic cirrhosis patients within this study were compared. However, it should be noted that for unexplained reasons, the healthy volunteers in this study had about a 50% lower AUC as compared to healthy volunteers in other studies, thus making comparisons between volunteers with alcoholic cirrhosis and healthy volunteers difficult. Effects of hepatic disease on this process probably depend on the particular disease. Hepatic disease with other etiologies, such as primary biliary cirrhosis, may show a different effect. In a single-dose (1 g IV) study of 6 volunteers with severe hepatic impairment (aminopyrine breath test less than 0.2% of dose) due to alcoholic cirrhosis, MMF was rapidly converted to MPA. MPA AUC was 44.1 μg·h/ml (±15.5).

Pediatrics

The pharmacokinetic parameters of MPA and MPAG have been evaluated in 55 pediatric patients (ranging from 1-18 years of age) receiving mycophenolate mofetil oral suspension at a dose of 600 mg/m^2 bid (up to a maximum of 1 g bid) after allogeneic renal transplantation. The pharmacokinetic data for MPA is provided in TABLE 3.

TABLE 3 *Mean (±SD) Computed Pharmacokinetic Parameters for MPA by Age and Time After Allogeneic Renal Transplantation*

Age Group	n	T_{max} (h)	C_{max}* (μg/ml)	AUC(0-12)* (μg·h/ml)
Early (Day 7)				
1 to <2 y	6§	3.03 (4.70)	10.3 (5.80)	22.5 (6.66)
1 to <6 y	17	1.63 (2.85)	13.2 (7.16)	27.4 (9.54)
6 to <12 y	16	0.940 (0.546)	13.1 (6.30)	33.2 (12.1)
12-18 y	21	1.16 (0.830)	11.7 (10.7)	26.3 (9.14)†
Late (Month 3)				
1 to <2 y	4§	0.725 (0.276)	23.8 (13.4)	47.4 (14.7)
1 to <6 y	15	0.989 (0.511)	22.7 (10.1)	49.7 (18.2)
6 to <12 y	14	1.21 (0.532)	27.8 (14.3)	61.9 (19.6)
12-18 y	17	0.978 (0.484)	17.9 (9.57)	53.6 (20.3)‡
Late (Month 9)				
1 to <2 y	4§	0.604 (0.208)	25.6 (4.25)	55.8 (11.6)
1 to <6 y	12	0.869 (0.479)	30.4 (9.16)	61.0 (10.7)
6 to <12 y	11	1.12 (0.462)	29.2 (12.6)	66.8 (21.2)
12-18 y	14	1.09 (0.518)	18.1 (7.29)	56.7 (14.0)

* Dose Adjusted — adjusted to a dose of 600 mg/m^2.
† n=20.
‡ n=16.
§ A subset of 1 to <6 y.

The mycophenolate mofetil oral suspension dose of 600 mg/m^2 bid (up to a maximum of 1 g bid) achieved mean MPA AUC values in pediatric patients similar to those seen in adult renal transplant patients receiving mycophenolate mofetil capsules at a dose of 1 g bid in the early posttransplant period. There was wide variability in the data. As observed in adults, early posttransplant MPA AUC values were approximately 45-53% lower than those observed in the later posttransplant period (>3 months). MPA AUC values were similar in the early and late posttransplant period across the 1-18 year age range.

Gender

Data obtained from several studies were pooled to look at any gender-related differences in the pharmacokinetics of MPA (data were adjusted to 1 g oral dose). Mean (±SD) MPA AUC(0-12h) for males (n=79) was 32.0 (±14.5) and for females (n=41) was 36.5 (±18.8) μg·h/ml while mean (±SD) MPA C_{max} was 9.96 (±6.19) in the males and 10.6 (±5.64) μg/ml in the females. These differences are not of clinical significance.

Geriatrics

Pharmacokinetics in the elderly have not been studied.

INDICATIONS AND USAGE

RENAL, CARDIAC, AND HEPATIC TRANSPLANT

Mycophenolate mofetil is indicated for the prophylaxis of organ rejection in patients receiving allogeneic renal, cardiac or hepatic transplants. Mycophenolate mofetil should be used concomitantly with cyclosporine and corticosteroids.

Mycophenolate mofetil IV is an alternative dosage form to mycophenolate mofetil capsules, tablets and oral suspension. Mycophenolate mofetil IV should be administered within 24 hours following transplantation. Mycophenolate mofetil IV can be administered for up to 14 days; patients should be switched to oral mycophenolate mofetil as soon as they can tolerate oral medication.

NON-FDA APPROVED INDICATIONS

Mycophenolate has shown efficacy as a monotherapy maintenance regimen in renal transplant patients. The drug has also been reported to be effective in the treatment of rheumatoid arthritis, Crohn's disease, ulcerative colitis, resistant membranous nephropathy, and inflammatory skin disorders including atopic eczema (in a very small study) and atopic dermatitis. However, these uses are not approved by the FDA and further clinical trials may be necessary.

CONTRAINDICATIONS

Allergic reactions to mycophenolate mofetil have been observed; therefore, mycophenolate mofetil is contraindicated in patients with a hypersensitivity to mycophenolate mofetil, mycophenolic acid or any component of the drug product. Mycophenolate mofetil IV is contraindicated in patients who are allergic to polysorbate 80 (TWEEN).

WARNINGS

See BOXED WARNING.

Patients receiving immunosuppressive regimens involving combinations of drugs, including mycophenolate mofetil, as part of an immunosuppressive regimen are at increased risk of developing lymphomas and other malignancies, particularly of the skin. The risk appears to be related to the intensity and duration of immunosuppression rather than to the use of any specific agent. Oversuppression of the immune system can also increase susceptibility to infection, including opportunistic infections, fatal infections, and sepsis.

As usual for patients with increased risk for skin cancer, exposure to sunlight and UV light should be limited by wearing protective clothing and using a sunscreen with a high protection factor.

Mycophenolate mofetil has been administered in combination with the following agents in clinical trials: antithymocyte globulin (ATGAM), OKT3, cyclosporine and corticosteroids. The efficacy and safety of the use of mycophenolate mofetil in combination with other immunosuppressive agents have not been determined.

Lymphoproliferative disease or lymphoma developed in 0.4 to 1% of patients receiving mycophenolate mofetil (2 or 3 g) with other immunosuppressive agents in controlled clinical trials of renal, cardiac, and hepatic transplant patients (see ADVERSE REACTIONS).

In pediatric patients, no other malignancies besides lymphoproliferative disorder (2/148 patients) have been observed (see ADVERSE REACTIONS).

Adverse effects on fetal development (including malformations) occurred when pregnant rats and rabbits were dosed during organogenesis. These responses occurred at doses lower than those associated with maternal toxicity, and at doses below the recommended clinical dose for renal, cardiac or hepatic transplantation. There are no adequate and well-controlled studies in pregnant women. However, as mycophenolate mofetil has been shown to have teratogenic effects in animals, it may cause fetal harm when administered to a pregnant woman. Therefore, mycophenolate mofetil should not be used in pregnant women unless the potential benefit justifies the potential risk to the fetus.

Women of childbearing potential should have a negative serum or urine pregnancy test with a sensitivity of at least 50 mIU/ml within 1 week prior to beginning therapy. It is recommended that mycophenolate mofetil therapy should not be initiated by the physician until a report of a negative pregnancy test has been obtained.

Effective contraception must be used before beginning mycophenolate mofetil therapy, during therapy, and for 6 weeks following discontinuation of therapy, even where there has been a history of infertility, unless due to hysterectomy. Two reliable forms of contraception must be used simultaneously unless abstinence is the chosen method (see DRUG INTERACTIONS). If pregnancy does occur during treatment, the physician and patient should discuss the desirability of continuing the pregnancy (see PRECAUTIONS: Pregnancy Category C and Information for the Patient).

In patients receiving mycophenolate mofetil (2 or 3 g) in controlled studies for prevention of renal, cardiac or hepatic rejection, fatal infection/sepsis occurred in approximately 2% of renal and cardiac patients and in 5% of hepatic patients (see ADVERSE REACTIONS).

Severe neutropenia [absolute neutrophil count (ANC) <0.5 × 10^3/μl] developed in up to 2.0% of renal, up to 2.8% of cardiac, and up to 3.6% of hepatic transplant patients receiving mycophenolate mofetil 3 g daily (see ADVERSE REACTIONS). Patients receiving mycophenolate mofetil should be monitored for neutropenia (see PRECAUTIONS, Laboratory Tests). The development of neutropenia may be related to mycophenolate mofetil itself, concomitant medications, viral infections, or some combination of these causes. If neutropenia develops (ANC <1.3 × 10^3/μl), dosing with mycophenolate mofetil should be interrupted or the dose reduced, appropriate diagnostic tests performed, and the patient managed appropriately (see DOSAGE AND ADMINISTRATION). Neutropenia has been observed most frequently in the period from 31-180 days posttransplant in patients treated for prevention of renal, cardiac, and hepatic rejection.

Patients receiving mycophenolate mofetil should be instructed to report immediately any evidence of infection, unexpected bruising, bleeding or any other manifestation of bone marrow depression.

CAUTION: MYCOPHENOLATE MOFETIL IV SOLUTION SHOULD NEVER BE ADMINISTERED BY RAPID OR BOLUS IV INJECTION.

PRECAUTIONS

GENERAL

Gastrointestinal bleeding (requiring hospitalization) has been observed in approximately 3% of renal, in 1.7% of cardiac, and in 5.4% of hepatic transplant patients treated with mycophenolate mofetil 3 g daily. In pediatric renal transplant patients, 5/148 cases of gastrointestinal bleeding (requiring hospitalization) were observed.

Gastrointestinal perforations have rarely been observed. Most patients receiving mycophenolate mofetil were also receiving other drugs known to be associated with these complications. Patients with active peptic ulcer disease were excluded from enrollment in studies with mycophenolate mofetil. Because mycophenolate mofetil has been associated with an increased incidence of digestive system adverse events, including infrequent cases of gastrointestinal tract ulceration, hemorrhage, and perforation, mycophenolate mofetil should be administered with caution in patients with active serious digestive system disease.

Subjects with severe chronic renal impairment (GFR <25 ml/min/1.73 m^2) who have received single doses of mycophenolate mofetil showed higher plasma MPA and MPAG AUCs relative to subjects with lesser degrees of renal impairment or normal healthy volunteers. No data are available on the safety of long-term exposure to these levels of MPAG. Doses of mycophenolate mofetil greater than 1 g administered twice a day to renal transplant patients should be avoided and they should be carefully observed (see CLINICAL PHARMACOLOGY, Pharmacokinetics and DOSAGE AND ADMINISTRATION).

No data are available for cardiac or hepatic transplant patients with severe chronic renal impairment. Mycophenolate mofetil may be used for cardiac or hepatic transplant patients with severe chronic renal impairment if the potential benefits outweigh the potential risks.

In patients with delayed renal graft function posttransplant, mean MPA AUC(0-12h) was comparable, but MPAG AUC(0-12h) was 2- to 3-fold higher, compared to that seen in posttransplant patients without delayed renal graft function. In the three controlled studies of prevention of renal rejection, there were 298 of 1483 patients (20%) with delayed graft function. Although patients with delayed graft function have a higher incidence of certain adverse events (anemia, thrombocytopenia, hyperkalemia) than patients without delayed graft function, these events were not more frequent in patients receiving mycophenolate mofetil than azathioprine or placebo. No dose adjustment is recommended for these patients; however, they should be carefully observed (see CLINICAL PHARMACOLOGY, Pharmacokinetics and DOSAGE AND ADMINISTRATION).

In cardiac transplant patients, the overall incidence of opportunistic infections was approximately 10% higher in patients treated with mycophenolate mofetil than in those receiving azathioprine therapy, but this difference was not associated with excess mortality due to infection/sepsis among patients treated with mycophenolate mofetil (see ADVERSE REACTIONS).

There were more herpes virus (H. simplex, H. zoster, and cytomegalovirus) infections in cardiac transplant patients treated with mycophenolate mofetil compared to those treated with azathioprine (see ADVERSE REACTIONS).

It is recommended that mycophenolate mofetil not be administered concomitantly with azathioprine because both have the potential to cause bone marrow suppression and such concomitant administration has not been studied clinically.

In view of the significant reduction in the AUC of MPA by cholestyramine, caution should be used in the concomitant administration of mycophenolate mofetil with drugs that interfere with enterohepatic recirculation because of the potential to reduce the efficacy of mycophenolate mofetil (see DRUG INTERACTIONS).

On theoretical grounds, because mycophenolate mofetil is an IMPDH (inosine monophosphate dehydrogenase) inhibitor, it should be avoided in patients with rare hereditary deficiency of hypoxanthine-guanine phosphoribosyl-transferase (HGPRT) such as Lesch-Nyhan and Kelley-Seegmiller syndrome.

During treatment with mycophenolate mofetil, the use of live attenuated vaccines should be avoided and patients should be advised that vaccinations may be less effective (see DRUG INTERACTIONS, Live Vaccines).

PHENYLKETONURICS

Mycophenolate mofetil oral suspension contains aspartame, a source of phenylalanine (0.56 mg phenylalanine/ml suspension). Therefore, care should be taken if mycophenolate mofetil oral suspension is administered to patients with phenylketonuria.

INFORMATION FOR THE PATIENT

Patients should be informed of the need for repeated appropriate laboratory tests while they are receiving mycophenolate mofetil. Patients should be given complete dosage instructions and informed of the increased risk of lymphoproliferative disease and certain other malignancies. Women of childbearing potential should be instructed of the potential risks during pregnancy, and that they should use effective contraception before beginning mycophenolate mofetil therapy, during therapy, and for 6 weeks after mycophenolate mofetil has been stopped (see WARNINGS and Pregnancy Category C).

LABORATORY TESTS

Complete blood counts should be performed weekly during the first month, twice monthly for the second and third months of treatment, then monthly through the first year (see WARNINGS, ADVERSE REACTIONS and DOSAGE AND ADMINISTRATION).

CARCINOGENESIS, MUTAGENESIS, AND IMPAIRMENT OF FERTILITY

In a 104 week oral carcinogenicity study in mice, mycophenolate mofetil in daily doses up to 180 mg/kg was not tumorigenic. The highest dose tested was 0.5 times the recommended clinical dose (2 g/day) in renal transplant patients and 0.3 times the recommended clinical dose (3 g/day) in cardiac transplant patients when corrected for differences in body surface area (BSA). In a 104 week oral carcinogenicity study in rats, mycophenolate mofetil in daily doses up to 15 mg/kg was not tumorigenic. The highest dose was 0.08 times the recommended clinical dose in renal transplant patients and 0.05 times the recommended clinical dose in cardiac transplant patients when corrected for BSA. While these animal doses were lower than those given to patients, they were maximal in those species and were considered adequate to evaluate the potential for human risk (see WARNINGS).

The genotoxic potential of mycophenolate mofetil was determined in 5 assays. Mycophenolate mofetil was genotoxic in the mouse lymphoma/thymidine kinase assay and the *in vivo* mouse micronucleus assay. Mycophenolate mofetil was not genotoxic in the bacterial mutation assay, the yeast mitotic gene conversion assay or the Chinese hamster ovary cell chromosomal aberration assay.

Mycophenolate mofetil had no effect on fertility of male rats at oral doses up to 20 mg/kg/day. This dose represents 0.1 times the recommended clinical dose in renal transplant patients and 0.07 times the recommended clinical dose in cardiac transplant patients when corrected for BSA. In a female fertility and reproduction study conducted in rats, oral doses of 4.5 mg/kg/day caused malformations (principally of the head and eyes) in the first generation offspring in the absence of maternal toxicity. This dose was 0.02 times the recommended clinical dose in renal transplant patients and 0.01 times the recommended clinical dose in cardiac transplant patients when corrected for BSA. No effects on fertility or reproductive parameters were evident in the dams or in the subsequent generation.

PREGNANCY CATEGORY C

In teratology studies in rats and rabbits, fetal resorptions and malformations occurred in rats at 6 mg/kg/day and in rabbits at 90 mg/kg/day, in the absence of maternal toxicity. These levels are equivalent to 0.03-0.92 times the recommended clinical dose in renal transplant patients and 0.02-0.61 times the recommended clinical dose in cardiac transplant patients on a BSA basis. In a female fertility and reproduction study conducted in rats, oral doses of 4.5 mg/kg/day caused malformations (principally of the head and eyes) in the first generation offspring in the absence of maternal toxicity. This dose was 0.02 times the recommended clinical dose in renal transplant patients and 0.01 times the recommended clinical dose in cardiac transplant patients when corrected for BSA.

There are no adequate and well-controlled studies in pregnant women. Mycophenolate mofetil should not be used in pregnant women unless the potential benefit justifies the potential risk to the fetus. Effective contraception must be used before beginning mycophenolate mofetil therapy, during therapy and for 6 weeks after mycophenolate mofetil has been stopped (see WARNINGS and Information for the Patient).

NURSING MOTHERS

Studies in rats treated with mycophenolate mofetil have shown mycophenolic acid to be excreted in milk. It is not known whether this drug is excreted in human milk. Because many drugs are excreted in human milk, and because of the potential for serious adverse reactions in nursing infants from mycophenolate mofetil, a decision should be made whether to discontinue nursing or to discontinue the drug, taking into account the importance of the drug to the mother.

PEDIATRIC USE

Based on pharmacokinetic and safety data in pediatric patients after renal transplantation, the recommended dose of mycophenolate mofetil oral suspension is 600 mg/m^2 bid (up to maximum of 1 g bid). Also see CLINICAL PHARMACOLOGY, ADVERSE REACTIONS, and DOSAGE AND ADMINISTRATION.

Safety and effectiveness in pediatric patients receiving allogeneic cardiac or hepatic transplants have not been established.

GERIATRIC USE

Clinical studies of mycophenolate mofetil did not include sufficient numbers of subjects aged 65 and over to determine whether they respond differently from younger subjects. Other reported clinical experience has not identified differences in responses between the elderly and younger patients. In general dose selection for an elderly patient should be cautious, reflecting the greater frequency of decreased hepatic, renal or cardiac function and of concomitant or other drug therapy. Elderly patients may be at an increased risk of adverse reactions compared with younger individuals (see ADVERSE REACTIONS).

DRUG INTERACTIONS

Drug interaction studies with mycophenolate mofetil have been conducted with acyclovir, antacids, cholestyramine, cyclosporine, ganciclovir, oral contraceptives, and trimethoprim/sulfamethoxazole. Drug interaction studies have not been conducted with other drugs that may be commonly administered to renal, cardiac or hepatic transplant patients. Mycophenolate mofetil has not been administered concomitantly with azathioprine.

ACYCLOVIR

Coadministration of mycophenolate mofetil (1 g) and acyclovir (800 mg) to 12 healthy volunteers resulted in no significant change in MPA AUC and C_{max}. However, MPAG and acyclovir plasma AUCs were increased 10.6% and 21.9%, respectively. Because MPAG plasma concentrations are increased in the presence of renal impairment, as are acyclovir concentrations, the potential exists for the 2 drugs to compete for tubular secretion, further increasing the concentrations of both drugs.

ANTACIDS WITH MAGNESIUM AND ALUMINUM HYDROXIDES

Absorption of a single dose of mycophenolate mofetil (2 g) was decreased when administered to 10 rheumatoid arthritis patients also taking Maalox TC (10 ml qid). The C_{max} and AUC(0-24h) for MPA were 33% and 17% lower, respectively, than when mycophenolate mofetil was administered alone under fasting conditions. Mycophenolate mofetil may be administered to patients who are also taking antacids containing magnesium and aluminum hydroxides; however, it is recommended that mycophenolate mofetil and the antacid not be administered simultaneously.

CHOLESTYRAMINE

Following single-dose administration of 1.5 g mycophenolate mofetil to 12 healthy volunteers pretreated with 4 g tid of cholestyramine for 4 days, MPA AUC decreased approximately 40%. This decrease is consistent with interruption of enterohepatic recirculation which may be due to binding of recirculating MPAG with cholestyramine in the intestine. Some degree of enterohepatic recirculation is also anticipated following IV administration of mycophenolate mofetil. Therefore, mycophenolate mofetil is not recommended to be given with cholestyramine or other agents that may interfere with enterohepatic recirculation.

CYCLOSPORINE

Cyclosporine pharmacokinetics (at doses of 275-415 mg/day) were unaffected by single and multiple doses of 1.5 g bid of mycophenolate mofetil in 10 stable renal transplant patients. The mean (±SD) AUC(0-12h) and C_{max} of cyclosporine after 14 days of multiple doses of mycophenolate mofetil were 3290 (±822) ng·h/ml and 753 (±161) ng/ml, respectively, compared to 3245 (±1088) ng·h/ml and 700 (±246) ng/ml, respectively, 1 week before administration of mycophenolate mofetil. The effect of cyclosporine on mycophenolate mofetil pharmacokinetics could not be evaluated in this study; however, plasma concentrations of MPA were similar to that for healthy volunteers.

GANCICLOVIR

Following single-dose administration to 12 stable renal transplant patients, no pharmacokinetic interaction was observed between mycophenolate mofetil (1.5 g) and IV ganciclovir

M

(5 mg/kg). Mean (±SD) ganciclovir AUC and C_{max} (n=10) were 54.3 (±19.0) μg·h/ml and 11.5 (±1.8) μg/ml, respectively, after coadministration of the 2 drugs, compared to 51.0 (±17.0) μg·h/ml and 10.6 (±2.0) μg/ml, respectively, after administration of IV ganciclovir alone. The mean (±SD) AUC and C_{max} of MPA (n=12) after coadministration were 80.9 (±21.6) μg·h/ml and 27.8 (±13.9) μg/ml, respectively, compared to values of 80.3 (±16.4) μg·h/ml and 30.9 (±11.2) μg/ml, respectively, after administration of mycophenolate mofetil alone. Because MPAG plasma concentrations are increased in the presence of renal impairment, as are ganciclovir concentrations, the 2 drugs will compete for tubular secretion and thus further increases in concentrations of both drugs may occur. In patients with renal impairment in which MMF and ganciclovir are coadministered, patients should be monitored carefully.

ORAL CONTRACEPTIVES

A study of coadministration of mycophenolate mofetil (1 g bid) and combined oral contraceptives containing ethinylestradiol (0.02-0.04 mg) and levonorgestrel (0.05-0.20 mg), desogestrel (0.15 mg) or gestodene (0.05-0.10 mg) was conducted in 18 women with psoriasis over 3 consecutive menstrual cycles. Mean AUC(0-24h) was similar for ethinylestradiol and 3-keto desogestrel; however, mean levonorgestrel AUC(0-24h) significantly decreased by about 15%. There was large inter-patient variability (%CV in the range of 60-70%) in the data, especially for ethinylestradiol. Mean serum levels of LH, FSH and progesterone were not significantly affected. Mycophenolate mofetil may not have any influence on the ovulation-suppressing action of the studied oral contraceptives. However, it is recommended that oral contraceptives are coadministered with mycophenolate mofetil with caution and additional birth control methods be considered (see PRECAUTIONS, Pregnancy Category C).

TRIMETHOPRIM/SULFAMETHOXAZOLE

Following single-dose administration of mycophenolate mofetil (1.5 g) to 12 healthy male volunteers on Day 8 of a 10 day course of trimethoprim 160 mg/sulfamethoxazole 800 mg administered bid, no effect on the bioavailability of MPA was observed. The mean (±SD) AUC and C_{max} of MPA after concomitant administration were 75.2 (±19.8) μg·h/ml and 34.0 (±6.6) μg/ml, respectively, compared to 79.2 (±27.9) μg·h/ml and 34.2 (±10.7) μg/ml, respectively, after administration of mycophenolate mofetil alone.

OTHER INTERACTIONS

The measured value for renal clearance of MPAG indicates removal occurs by renal tubular secretion as well as glomerular filtration. Consistent with this, coadministration of probenecid, a known inhibitor of tubular secretion, with mycophenolate mofetil in monkeys results in a 3-fold increase in plasma MPAG AUC and a 2-fold increase in plasma MPA AUC. Thus, other drugs known to undergo renal tubular secretion may compete with MPAG and thereby raise plasma concentrations of MPAG or the other drug undergoing tubular secretion.

Drugs that alter the gastrointestinal flora may interact with mycophenolate mofetil by disrupting enterohepatic recirculation. Interference of MPAG hydrolysis may lead to less MPA available for absorption.

LIVE VACCINES

During treatment with mycophenolate mofetil, the use of live attenuated vaccines should be avoided and patients should be advised that vaccinations may be less effective (see PRECAUTIONS, General). Influenza vaccination may be of value. Prescribers should refer to national guidelines for influenza vaccination.

ADVERSE REACTIONS

The principal adverse reactions associated with the administration of mycophenolate mofetil include diarrhea, leukopenia, sepsis, vomiting, and there is evidence of a higher frequency of certain types of infections *e.g.*, opportunistic infection (see WARNINGS). The adverse event profile associated with the administration of mycophenolate mofetil IV has been shown to be similar to that observed after administration of oral dosage forms of mycophenolate mofetil.

MYCOPHENOLATE MOFETIL ORAL

The incidence of adverse events for mycophenolate mofetil was determined in randomized, comparative, double-blind trials in prevention of rejection in renal (2 active, 1 placebo-controlled trials), cardiac (1 active-controlled trial), and hepatic (1 active-controlled trial) transplant patients.

Elderly patients (≥65 years), particularly those who are receiving mycophenolate mofetil as part of a combination immunosuppressive regimen, may be at increased risk of certain infections [including cytomegalovirus (CMV) tissue invasive disease] and possibly gastrointestinal hemorrhage and pulmonary edema, compared to younger individuals (see PRECAUTIONS).

Safety data are summarized in TABLE 8A, TABLE 8B, and TABLE 8C for all active-controlled trials in renal (2 trials), cardiac (1 trial), and hepatic (1 trial) transplant patients. Approximately 53% of the renal patients, 65% of the cardiac patients, and 48% of the hepatic patients have been treated for more than 1 year. Adverse events reported in ≥20% of patients in the mycophenolate mofetil treatment groups are presented in TABLE 8A, TABLE 8B, and TABLE 8C.

The placebo-controlled renal transplant study generally showed fewer adverse events occurring in ≥20% of patients. In addition, those that occurred were not only qualitatively similar to the azathioprine-controlled renal transplant studies, but also occurred at lower rates, particularly for infection, leukopenia, hypertension, diarrhea and respiratory infection.

The above data demonstrate that in three controlled trials for prevention of renal rejection, patients receiving 2 g/day of mycophenolate mofetil had an overall better safety profile than did patients receiving 3 g/day of mycophenolate mofetil.

The above data demonstrate that the types of adverse events observed in multicenter controlled trials in renal, cardiac, and hepatic transplant patients are qualitatively similar except for those that are unique to the specific organ involved.

Sepsis, which was generally CMV viremia, was slightly more common in renal transplant patients treated with mycophenolate mofetil compared to patients treated with azathioprine.

TABLE 8A *Adverse Events in Controlled Studies in Prevention of Renal Allograft Rejection — Reported in ≥20% of Patients in the Mycophenolate Mofetil Group*

	Mycophenolate Mofetil		Azathioprine
	2 g/day	3 g/day	1-2 mg/kg/day or 100-150 mg/day
	n=336	n=330	n=326
Body as a Whole			
Pain	33.0%	31.2%	32.2%
Abdominal pain	24.7%	27.6%	23.0%
Fever	21.4%	23.3%	23.3%
Headache	21.1%	16.1%	21.2%
Infection	18.2%	20.9%	19.9%
Hemic and Lymphatic			
Anemia	25.6%	25.8%	23.6%
Leukopenia	23.2%	34.5%	24.8%
Urogenital			
Urinary tract infection	37.2%	37.0%	33.7%
Cardiovascular			
Hypertension	32.4%	28.2%	32.2%
Metabolic and Nutritional			
Peripheral edema	28.6%	27.0%	28.2%
Digestive			
Diarrhea	31.0%	36.1%	20.9%
Constipation	22.9%	18.5%	22.4%
Nausea	19.9%	23.6%	24.5%
Respiratory			
Infection	22.0%	23.9%	19.6%

TABLE 8B *Adverse Events in Controlled Studies in Prevention of Cardiac Allograft Rejection — Reported in ≥20% of Patients in the Mycophenolate Mofetil Group*

	Mycophenolate Mofetil	Azathioprine
	3 g/day	1.5 to 3 mg/kg/day
	n=289	n=289
Body as a Whole		
Pain	75.8%	74.7%
Abdominal pain	33.9%	33.2%
Fever	47.4%	46.4%
Headache	54.3%	51.9%
Infection	25.6%	19.4%
Asthenia	43.3%	36.3%
Chest pain	26.3%	26.0%
Back pain	34.6%	28.4%
Hemic and Lymphatic		
Anemia	42.9%	43.9%
Leukopenia	30.4%	39.1%
Thrombocytopenia	23.5%	27.0%
Hypochromic anemia	24.6%	23.5%
Leukocytosis	40.5%	35.6%
Urogenital		
Kidney function abnormal	21.8%	26.3%
Cardiovascular		
Hypertension	77.5%	72.3%
Hypotension	32.5%	36.0%
Cardiovascular disorder	25.6%	24.2%
Tachycardia	20.1%	18.0%
Metabolic and Nutritional		
Peripheral edema	64.0%	53.3%
Hypercholesteremia	41.2%	38.4%
Edema	26.6%	25.6%
Hypokalemia	31.8%	25.6%
Hyperglycemia	46.7%	52.6%
Creatinine increased	39.4%	36.0%
BUN increased	34.6%	32.5%
Lactic dehydrogenase increased	23.2%	17.0%
Digestive		
Diarrhea	45.3%	34.3%
Constipation	41.2%	37.7%
Nausea	54.0%	54.3%
Vomiting	33.9%	28.4%
Respiratory		
Infection	37.0%	35.3%
Dyspnea	36.7%	36.3%
Cough increased	31.1%	25.6%
Lung disorder	30.1%	29.1%
Sinusitis	26.0%	19.0%
Skin and Appendages		
Rash	22.1%	18.0%
Nervous System		
Tremor	24.2%	23.9%
Insomnia	40.8%	37.7%
Dizziness	28.7%	27.7%
Anxiety	28.4%	23.9%
Paresthesia	20.8%	18.0%

The incidence of sepsis was comparable in mycophenolate mofetil and in azathioprine-treated patients in cardiac and hepatic studies.

In the digestive system, diarrhea was increased in renal and cardiac transplant patients receiving mycophenolate mofetil compared to patients receiving azathioprine, but was comparable in hepatic transplant patients treated with mycophenolate mofetil or azathioprine.

Patients receiving mycophenolate mofetil alone or as part of an immunosuppressive regimen are at increased risk of developing lymphomas and other malignancies, particularly of the skin (see WARNINGS). The incidence of malignancies among the 1483 patients treated

TABLE 8C *Adverse Events in Controlled Studies in Prevention of Hepatic Allograft Rejection — Reported in ≥20% of Patients in the Mycophenolate Mofetil Group*

	Mycophenolate Mofetil 3 g/day n=277	Azathioprine 1-2 mg/kg/day n=287
Body as a Whole		
Pain	74.0%	77.7%
Abdominal pain	62.5%	51.2%
Fever	52.3%	56.1%
Headache	53.8%	49.1%
Infection	27.1%	25.1%
Sepsis	27.4%	26.5%
Asthenia	35.4%	33.8%
Back pain	46.6%	47.4%
Ascites	24.2%	22.6%
Hemic and Lymphatic		
Anemia	43.0%	53.0%
Leukopenia	45.8%	39.0%
Thrombocytopenia	38.3%	42.2%
Leukocytosis	22.4%	21.3%
Urogenital		
Kidney function abnormal	25.6%	28.9%
Cardiovascular		
Hypertension	62.1%	59.6%
Tachycardia	22.0%	15.7%
Metabolic and Nutritional		
Peripheral edema	48.4%	47.7%
Edema	28.2%	28.2%
Hypokalemia	37.2%	41.1%
Hyperkalemia	22.0%	23.7%
Hyperglycemia	43.7%	48.8%
Hypomagnesemia	39.0%	37.6%
Hypocalcemia	30.0%	30.0%
Digestive		
Diarrhea	51.3%	49.8%
Constipation	37.9%	38.3%
Nausea	54.5%	51.2%
Dyspepsia	22.4%	20.9%
Vomiting	32.9%	33.4%
Anorexia	25.3%	17.1%
Liver function tests abnormal	24.9%	19.2%
Respiratory		
Dyspnea	31.0%	30.3%
Lung disorder	22.0%	18.8%
Pleural effusion	34.3%	35.9%
Nervous System		
Tremor	33.9%	35.5%
Insomnia	52.3%	47.0%

in controlled trials for the prevention of renal allograft rejection who were followed for ≥1 year was similar to the incidence reported in the literature for renal allograft recipients.

Lymphoproliferative disease or lymphoma developed in 0.4 to 1% of patients receiving mycophenolate mofetil (2 or 3 g daily) with other immunosuppressive agents in controlled clinical trials of renal, cardiac, and hepatic transplant patients followed for at least 1 year (see WARNINGS). Non-melanoma skin carcinomas occurred in 1.6-4.2% of patients, other types of malignancy in 0.7-2.1% of patients. Three year safety data in renal and cardiac transplant patients did not reveal any unexpected changes in incidence of malignancy compared to the 1 year data.

In pediatric patients, no other malignancies besides lymphoproliferative disorder (2/148 patients) have been observed.

Severe neutropenia (ANC $<0.5 \times 10^3/\mu l$) developed in up to 2.0% of renal transplant patients, up to 2.8% of cardiac transplant patients and up to 3.6% of hepatic transplant patients receiving mycophenolate mofetil 3 g daily (see WARNINGS; PRECAUTIONS, Laboratory Tests; and DOSAGE AND ADMINISTRATION).

All transplant patients are at increased risk of opportunistic infections. The risk increases with total immunosuppressive load (see WARNINGS). TABLE 9A, TABLE 9B, and TABLE 9C show the incidence of opportunistic infections that occurred in the renal, cardiac, and hepatic transplant populations in the azathioprine-controlled prevention trials.

TABLE 9A *Viral and Fungal Infections in Controlled Studies in Prevention of Renal Transplant Rejection*

	Mycophenolate Mofetil 2 g/day (n=336)	Mycophenolate Mofetil 3 g/day (n=330)	Azathioprine 1-2 mg/kg/day or 100-150 mg/day (n=326)
Herpes Simplex	16.7%	20.0%	19.0%
CMV			
Viremia/syndrome	13.4%	12.4%	13.8%
Tissue invasive disease	8.3%	11.5%	6.1%
Herpes Zoster	6.0%	7.6%	5.8%
Cutaneous disease	6.0%	7.3%	5.5%
Candida	17.0%	17.3%	18.1%
Mucocutaneous	15.5%	16.4%	15.3%

The following other opportunistic infections occurred with an incidence of less than 4% in mycophenolate mofetil patients in the above azathioprine-controlled studies: Herpes zoster, visceral disease; *Candida,* urinary tract infection, fungemia/disseminated disease, tissue invasive disease; cryptococcosis; *Aspergillus/Mucor; Pneumocystis carinii.*

TABLE 9B *Viral and Fungal Infections in Controlled Studies in Prevention of Cardiac Transplant Rejection*

	Mycophenolate Mofetil 3 g/day (n=289)	Azathioprine 1.5 to 3 mg/kg/day (n=289)
Herpes Simplex	20.8%	14.5%
CMV		
Viremia/syndrome	12.1%	10.0%
Tissue invasive disease	11.4%	8.7%
Herpes Zoster	10.7%	5.9%
Cutaneous disease	10.0%	5.5%
Candida	18.7%	17.6%
Mucocutaneous	18.0%	17.3%

TABLE 9C *Viral and Fungal Infections in Controlled Studies in Prevention of Hepatic Transplant Rejection*

	Mycophenolate Mofetil 3 g/day (n=277)	Azathioprine 1-2 mg/kg/day (n=287)
Herpes Simplex	10.1%	5.9%
CMV		
Viremia/syndrome	14.1%	12.2%
Tissue invasive disease	5.8%	8.0%
Herpes Zoster	4.3%	4.9%
Cutaneous disease	4.3%	4.9%
Candida	22.4%	24.4%
Mucocutaneous	18.4%	17.4%

In the placebo-controlled renal transplant study, the same pattern of opportunistic infection was observed compared to the azathioprine-controlled renal studies, with a notably lower incidence of the following: Herpes simplex and CMV tissue-invasive disease.

In patients receiving mycophenolate mofetil (2 or 3 g) in controlled studies for prevention of renal, cardiac or hepatic rejection, fatal infection/sepsis occurred in approximately 2% of renal and cardiac patients and in 5% of hepatic patients (see WARNINGS).

In cardiac transplant patients, the overall incidence of opportunistic infections was approximately 10% higher in patients treated with mycophenolate mofetil than in those receiving azathioprine, but this difference was not associated with excess mortality due to infection/sepsis among patients treated with mycophenolate mofetil.

The following adverse events were reported with 3 to <20% incidence in renal, cardiac, and hepatic transplant patients treated with mycophenolate mofetil, in combination with cyclosporine and corticosteroids.

Adverse Events Reported in 3% to <20% of Patients Treated With Mycophenolate Mofetil in Combination With Cyclosporine and Corticosteroids

Body as a Whole: Abdomen enlarged, abscess, accidental injury, cellulitis, chills occurring with fever, cyst, face edema, flu syndrome, hemorrhage, hernia, lab test abnormal, malaise, neck pain, pelvic pain, peritonitis.

Hemic and Lymphatic System: Coagulation disorder, ecchymosis, pancytopenia, petechia, polycythemia, prothrombin time increased, thromboplastin time increased.

Urogenital System: Acute kidney failure, albuminuria, dysuria, hydronephrosis, hematuria, impotence, kidney failure, kidney tubular necrosis nocturia, oliguria, pain, prostatic disorder, pyelonephritis, scrotal edema, urine abnormality, urinary frequency, urinary incontinence, urinary retention, urinary tract disorder.

Cardiovascular System: Angina pectoris, arrhythmia, arterial thrombosis, atrial fibrillation, atrial flutter, bradycardia, cardiovascular disorder, congestive heart failure, extrasystole, heart arrest, heart failure, hypotension, pallor, palpitation, pericardial effusion, peripheral vascular disorder, postural hypotension, pulmonary hypertension, supraventricular tachycardia, supraventricular extrasystoles, syncope, tachycardia, thrombosis, vasodilatation, vasospasm, ventricular extrasystole, ventricular tachycardia, venous pressure increased.

Metabolic and Nutritional System: Abnormal healing, acidosis, alkaline phosphatase increased, alkalosis, bilirubinemia, creatinine increased, dehydration, gamma glutamyl transpeptidase increased, generalized edema, gout, hypercalcemia, hypercholesteremia, hyperlipemia, hyperphosphatemia, hyperuricemia, hypervolemia, hypocalcemia, hypochloremia, hypoglycemia, hyponatremia, hypophosphatemia, hypoproteinemia, hypovolemia, hypoxia, lactic dehydrogenase increased, respiratory acidosis, SGOT increased, SGPT increased, thirst, weight gain, weight loss.

Digestive System: Anorexia, cholangitis, cholestatic jaundice, dysphagia, esophagitis, flatulence, gastritis, gastroenteritis, gastrointestinal disorder, gastrointestinal hemorrhage, gastrointestinal moniliasis, gingivitis, gum hyperplasia, hepatitis, ileus, infection, jaundice, liver damage, liver function tests abnormal, melena, mouth ulceration, nausea and vomiting, oral moniliasis, rectal disorder, stomach ulcer, stomatitis.

Respiratory System: Apnea, asthma, atelectasis, bronchitis, epistaxis, hemoptysis, hiccup, hyperventilation, lung edema, lung disorder, neoplasm, pain, pharyngitis, pleural effusion, pneumonia, pneumothorax, respiratory disorder, respiratory moniliasis, rhinitis, sinusitis, sputum increased, voice alteration.

Skin and Appendages: Acne, alopecia, fungal dermatitis, hemorrhage, hirsutism, pruritus, rash, skin benign neoplasm, skin carcinoma, skin disorder, skin hypertrophy, skin ulcer, sweating, vesiculobullous rash.

Nervous System: Agitation, anxiety, confusion, convulsion, delirium, depression, dry mouth, emotional lability, hallucinations, hypertonia, hypesthesia, nervousness, neuropathy, paresthesia, psychosis, somnolence, thinking abnormal, vertigo.

Endocrine System: Cushing's syndrome, diabetes mellitus, hypothyroidism, parathyroid disorder.
Musculoskeletal System: Arthralgia, joint disorder, leg cramps, myalgia, myasthenia, osteoporosis.
Special Senses: Abnormal vision, amblyopia, cataract (not specified), conjunctivitis, deafness, ear disorder, ear pain, eye hemorrhage, tinnitus, lacrimation disorder.

Pediatrics

The type and frequency of adverse events in a clinical study in 100 pediatric patients 3 months to 18 years of age dosed with mycophenolate mofetil oral suspension 600 mg/m^2 bid (up to 1 g bid) were generally similar to those observed in adult patients dosed with mycophenolate mofetil capsules at a dose of 1 g bid with the exception of abdominal pain, fever, infection, pain, sepsis, diarrhea, vomiting, pharyngitis, respiratory tract infection, hypertension, and anemia, which were observed in a higher proportion in pediatric patients.

MYCOPHENOLATE MOFETIL IV

The adverse event profile of mycophenolate mofetil IV was determined from a single, double-blind, controlled comparative study of the safety of 2 g/day of IV and oral mycophenolate mofetil in renal transplant patients in the immediate posttransplant period (administered for the first 5 days). The potential venous irritation of mycophenolate mofetil IV was evaluated by comparing the adverse events attributable to peripheral venous infusion of mycophenolate mofetil IV with those observed in the IV placebo group; patients in this group received active medication by the oral route.

Adverse events attributable to peripheral venous infusion were phlebitis and thrombosis, both observed at 4% in patients treated with mycophenolate mofetil IV.

In the active controlled study in hepatic transplant patients, 2 g/day of mycophenolate mofetil IV were administered in the immediate posttransplant period (up to 14 days). The safety profile of IV mycophenolate mofetil was similar to that of IV azathioprine.

POSTMARKETING EXPERIENCE

Digestive: Colitis (sometimes caused by cytomegalovirus), pancreatitis, isolated cases of intestinal villous atrophy.

Resistance Mechanism Disorders: Serious life-threatening infections such as meningitis and infectious endocarditis have been reported occasionally and there is evidence of a higher frequency of certain types of serious infections such as tuberculosis and atypical mycobacterial infection.

Respiratory: Interstitial lung disorders, including fatal pulmonary fibrosis, have been reported rarely and should be considered in the differential diagnosis of pulmonary symptoms ranging from dyspnea to respiratory failure in posttransplant patients receiving mycophenolate mofetil.

M

DOSAGE AND ADMINISTRATION

RENAL TRANSPLANTATION

Adults

A dose of 1 g administered orally or intravenously (over NO LESS THAN 2 HOURS) twice a day (daily dose of 2 g) is recommended for use in renal transplant patients. Although a dose of 1.5 g administered twice daily (daily dose of 3 g) was used in clinical trials and was shown to be safe and effective, no efficacy advantage could be established for renal transplant patients. Patients receiving 2 g/day of mycophenolate mofetil demonstrated an overall better safety profile than did patients receiving 3 g/day of mycophenolate mofetil.

Pediatrics

The recommended dose of mycophenolate mofetil oral suspension is 600 mg/m^2 administered twice daily (up to a maximum daily dose of 2 g/10 ml oral suspension). Patients with a body surface area of 1.25-1.5 m^2 may be dosed with mycophenolate mofetil capsules at a dose of 750 mg twice daily (1.5 g daily dose). Patients with a body surface area >1.5 m^2 may be dosed with mycophenolate mofetil capsules or tablets at a dose of 1 g twice daily (2 g daily dose).

CARDIAC TRANSPLANTATION

A dose of 1.5 g bid administered intravenously (over NO LESS THAN 2 HOURS) or 1.5 g bid oral (daily dose of 3 g) is recommended for use in adult cardiac transplant patients.

HEPATIC TRANSPLANTATION

A dose of 1 g bid administered intravenously (over NO LESS THAN 2 HOURS) or 1.5 g bid oral (daily dose of 3 g) is recommended for use in adult hepatic transplant patients.

MYCOPHENOLATE MOFETIL CAPSULES, TABLETS, AND ORAL SUSPENSION

The initial oral dose of mycophenolate mofetil should be given as soon as possible following renal, cardiac or hepatic transplantation. Food had no effect on MPA AUC, but has been shown to decrease MPA C_{max} by 40%. Therefore, it is recommended that mycophenolate mofetil be administered on an empty stomach. However, in stable renal transplant patients, mycophenolate mofetil may be administered with food if necessary.

Note: If required, mycophenolate mofetil oral suspension can be administered via a nasogastric tube with a minimum size of 8 French (minimum 1.7 mm interior diameter).

Patients With Hepatic Impairment

No dose adjustments are recommended for renal patients with severe hepatic parenchymal disease. However, it is not known whether dose adjustments are needed for hepatic disease with other etiologies (see CLINICAL PHARMACOLOGY, Pharmacokinetics).

No data are available for cardiac transplant patients with severe hepatic parenchymal disease.

Geriatrics

The recommended dose of 1 g bid for renal transplant patients, 1.5 g bid for cardiac transplant patients, and 1 g bid administered intravenously or 1.5 g bid administered orally in hepatic transplant patients is appropriate for elderly patients (see PRECAUTIONS, Geriatric Use).

MYCOPHENOLATE MOFETIL IV

Mycophenolate mofetil IV is an alternative dosage form to mycophenolate mofetil capsules, tablets and oral suspension recommended for patients unable to take oral mycophenolate mofetil. Mycophenolate mofetil IV should be administered within 24 hours following transplantation. Mycophenolate mofetil IV can be administered for up to 14 days; patients should be switched to oral mycophenolate mofetil as soon as they can tolerate oral medication.

Mycophenolate mofetil IV must be reconstituted and diluted to a concentration of 6 mg/ml using 5% dextrose injection. Mycophenolate mofetil IV is incompatible with other IV infusion solutions. Following reconstitution, mycophenolate mofetil IV must be administered by slow IV infusion over a period of NO LESS THAN 2 HOURS by either peripheral or central vein.

CAUTION: MYCOPHENOLATE MOFETIL IV SOLUTION SHOULD NEVER BE ADMINISTERED BY RAPID OR BOLUS IV INJECTION (SEE WARNINGS).

DOSE ADJUSTMENT

In renal transplant patients with severe chronic renal impairment (GFR <25 ml/min/1.73 m^2) outside the immediate posttransplant period, doses of mycophenolate mofetil greater than 1 g administered twice a day should be avoided. These patients should also be carefully observed. No dose adjustments are needed in renal transplant patients experiencing delayed graft function postoperatively (see CLINICAL PHARMACOLOGY, Pharmacokinetics and PRECAUTIONS, General).

No data are available for cardiac or hepatic transplant patients with severe chronic renal impairment. Mycophenolate mofetil may be used for cardiac or hepatic transplant patients with severe chronic renal impairment if the potential benefits outweigh the potential risks.

If neutropenia develops (ANC $<1.3 \times 10^3/\mu l$), dosing with mycophenolate mofetil should be interrupted or the dose reduced, appropriate diagnostic tests performed, and the patient managed appropriately (see WARNINGS, ADVERSE REACTIONS, and PRECAUTIONS, Laboratory Tests).

HANDLING AND DISPOSAL

Mycophenolate mofetil has demonstrated teratogenic effects in rats and rabbits (see PRECAUTIONS, Pregnancy Category C). Mycophenolate mofetil tablets should not be crushed and mycophenolate mofetil capsules should not be opened or crushed. Avoid inhalation or direct contact with skin or mucous membranes of the powder contained in mycophenolate mofetil capsules and mycophenolate mofetil oral suspension (before or after constitution). If such contact occurs, wash thoroughly with soap and water; rinse eyes with plain water. Should a spill occur, wipe up using paper towels wetted with water to remove spilled powder or suspension. Caution should be exercised in the handling and preparation of solutions of mycophenolate mofetil IV. Avoid direct contact of the prepared solution of mycophenolate mofetil IV with skin or mucous membranes. If such contact occurs, wash thoroughly with soap and water; rinse eyes with plain water.

HOW SUPPLIED

CELLCEPT CAPSULES, 250 MG

CellCept 250 mg capsules are blue-brown, 2-piece hard gelatin capsules, printed in black with "CellCept 250" on the blue cap and "Roche" on the brown body.

Storage: Store at 25°C (77°F); excursions permitted to 15-30°C (59-86°F).

CELLCEPT TABLETS, 500 MG

CellCept 500 mg tablets are lavender-colored, caplet-shaped, film-coated tablets printed in black with "CellCept 500" on one side and "Roche" on the other.

Storage and Dispensing Information: Store at 25°C (77°F); excursions permitted to 15-30°C (59-86°F). Dispense in light-resistant containers, such as the manufacturer's original container.

CELLCEPT ORAL SUSPENSION

CellCept oral suspension is supplied as a white to off-white powder blend for constitution to a white to off-white mixed-fruit flavor suspension.

Storage: Store dry powder at 25°C (77°F); excursions permitted to 15-30°C (59-86°F). Store constituted suspension at 25°C (77°F); excursions permitted to 15-30°C (59-86°F) for up to 60 days. Storage in a refrigerator at 2-8°C (36-46°F) is acceptable. Do not freeze.

CELLCEPT IV

CellCept IV is supplied in a 20 ml, sterile vial containing the equivalent of 500 mg mycophenolate mofetil as the hydrochloride salt.

Storage: Store powder and reconstituted/infusion solutions at 25°C (77°F); excursions permitted to 15-30°C (59-86°F).

PRODUCT LISTING - EQUIVALENTS NOT AVAILABLE

Capsule - Oral - 250 mg

100's	$293.55	CELLCEPT, Roche Laboratories	00004-0259-01
120's	$319.02	CELLCEPT, Roche Laboratories	00004-0259-05

Injection - Intravenous - 500 mg

4's	$139.48	CELLCEPT, Roche Laboratories	00004-0298-09

Suspension - Oral - 200 mg/ml

175 ml	$410.93	CELLCEPT, Roche Laboratories	00004-0261-29

Tablet - Oral - 500 mg

100's	$587.03	CELLCEPT, Roche Laboratories	00004-0260-01

Nabumetone (003108)

For related information, see the comparative table section in Appendix A.

Categories: Arthritis, osteoarthritis; Arthritis, rheumatoid; Pregnancy Category C; FDA Approved 1991 Dec
Drug Classes: Analgesics, non-narcotic; Nonsteroidal anti-inflammatory drugs
Brand Names: Relafen
Foreign Brand Availability: Arthaxan (Germany); Consolan (Denmark); Deku (Taiwan); Nabone (Thailand); Nabonet (Thailand); Nabuco (Israel); Naburen (Colombia); Nabuser (Italy); Nacton (Korea); Nadorex (Colombia); Naflex (Thailand); Nametone (Thailand); No-Ton (Taiwan); Goflex (Bahrain; Cyprus; Egypt; Indonesia; Iran; Iraq; Israel; Jordan; Kuwait; Lebanon; Libya; Oman; Qatar; Republic-of-Yemen; Saudi-Arabia; Syria; United-Arab-Emirates); Prodac (Korea); Relif (Spain); Relifen (Japan; South-Africa); Relifex (Bahamas; Bahrain; Barbados; Belize; Benin; Bermuda; Bulgaria; Burkina-Faso; Costa-Rica; Curacao; Cyprus; Czech-Republic; Denmark; Dominican-Republic; Ecuador; Egypt; El-Salvador; England; Ethiopia; Finland; Gambia; Ghana; Greece; Guatemala; Guinea; Guyana; Honduras; Hong-Kong; Hungary; Iran; Iraq; Ireland; Israel; Italy; Ivory-Coast; Jamaica; Jordan; Kenya; Kuwait; Lebanon; Liberia; Libya; Malawi; Mali; Mauritania; Mauritius; Mexico; Morocco; Netherland-Antilles; Nicaragua; Niger; Nigeria; Oman; Panama; Philippines; Puerto-Rico; Qatar; Republic-of-Yemen; Saudi-Arabia; Senegal; Seychelles; Sierra-Leone; South-Africa; Sudan; Surinam; Sweden; Syria; Taiwan; Tanzania; Thailand; Trinidad; Tunia; Turkey; Uganda; United-Arab-Emirates; Zambia; Zimbabwe); Relisan (South-Africa); Relitone (South-Africa); Tanleeg (Taiwan); Unimetone (Korea)
Cost of Therapy: $91.73 (Osteoarthritis; Relafen; 500 mg; 2 tablets/day; 30 day supply)
$77.82 (Osteoarthritis; Generic Tablets; 500 mg; 2 tablets/day; 30 day supply)

DESCRIPTION

Relafen (nabumetone) is a naphthylalkanone designated chemically as 4-(6-methoxy-2-naphthalenyl)-2-butanone.

Nabumetone is a white to off-white crystalline substance with a molecular weight of 228.3. It is non-acidic and practically insoluble in water, but soluble in alcohol and most organic solvents. It has an n-octanol:phosphate buffer partition coefficient of 2400 at pH 7.4.

Tablets for oral administration: Each oval-shaped, film-coated tablet contains 500 or 750 mg of nabumetone. Inactive ingredients consist of hydroxypropyl methylcellulose, microcrystalline cellulose, polyethylene glycol, polysorbate 80, sodium lauryl sulfate, sodium starch glycolate and titanium dioxide. The 750 mg tablets also contain iron oxides.

CLINICAL PHARMACOLOGY

Nabumetone is a nonsteroidal anti-inflammatory drug (NSAID) that exhibits anti-inflammatory, analgesic and antipyretic properties in pharmacologic studies. As with other nonsteroidal anti-inflammatory agents, its mode of action is not known. However, the ability to inhibit prostaglandin synthesis may be involved in the anti-inflammatory effect.

The parent compound is a prodrug, which undergoes hepatic biotransformation to the active component, 6-methoxy-2-naphthylacetic acid (6MNA), that is a potent inhibitor of prostaglandin synthesis.

It is acidic and has an n-octanol:phosphate buffer partition coefficient of 0.5 at pH 7.4.

PHARMACOKINETICS

After oral administration, approximately 80% of a radiolabelled dose of nabumetone is found in the urine, indicating that nabumetone is well absorbed from the gastrointestinal tract. Nabumetone itself is not detected in the plasma because, after absorption, it undergoes rapid biotransformation to the principal active metabolite, 6-methoxy-2-naphthylacetic acid (6MNA). Approximately 35% of a 1000 mg oral dose of nabumetone is converted to 6MNA and 50% is converted into unidentified metabolites which are subsequently excreted in the urine. Following oral administration of nabumetone, 6MNA exhibits pharmacokinetic characteristics that generally follow a one-compartment model with first order input and first order elimination.

6MNA is more than 99% bound to plasma proteins. The free fraction is dependent on total concentration of 6MNA and is proportional to dose over the range of 1000-2000 mg. It is 0.2-0.3% at concentrations typically achieved following administration of nabumetone 1000 mg and is approximately 0.6-0.8% of the total concentrations at steady state following daily administration of 2000 mg.

Steady-state plasma concentrations of 6MNA are slightly lower than predicted from single-dose data. This may result from the higher fraction of unbound 6MNA which undergoes greater hepatic clearance.

Coadministration of food increases the rate of absorption and subsequent appearance of 6MNA in the plasma but does not affect the extent of conversion of nabumetone into 6MNA. Peak plasma concentrations of 6MNA are increased by approximately one-third.

Coadministration with an aluminum-containing antacid had no significant effect on the bioavailability of 6MNA.

TABLE 1 *Mean Pharmacokinetic Parameters of Nabumetone Active Metabolite (6MNA) at Steady State Following Oral Administration of 1000 or 2000 mg Doses of Nabumetone*

Abbreviations (units)	Young Adults* 1000 mg n=31	Young Adults* 2000 mg n=12	Elderly* 1000 mg n=27
T_{max} (h)	3.0 (1.0-12.0)	2.5 (1.0-8.0)	4.0 (1.0-10.0)
T½ (h)	22.5 ± 3.7	26.2 ± 3.7	29.8 ± 8.1
CLss/F (ml/min)	26.1 ± 17.3	21.0 ± 4.0	18.6 ± 13.4
Vdss/F (L)	55.4 ± 26.4	53.4 ± 11.3	50.2 ± 25.3

* Mean ±SD.

6MNA undergoes biotransformation in the liver, producing inactive metabolites that are eliminated as both free metabolites and conjugates. None of the known metabolites of 6MNA has been detected in plasma. Preliminary *in vivo* and *in vitro* studies suggest that unlike other NSAIDs, there is no evidence of enterohepatic recirculation of the active metabolite. Approximately 75% of a radiolabelled dose was recovered in urine in 48 hours. Approximately 80% was recovered in 168 hours. A further 9% appeared in the feces. In the first 48 hours, metabolites consisted of those listed in TABLE 2.

TABLE 2

Nabumetone, unchanged	Not detectable
6-methoxy-2-naphthylacetic acid (6MNA), unchanged	<1%
6MNA, conjugated	11%
6-hydroxy-2-naphthylacetic acid (6HNA), unchanged	5%
6HNA, conjugated	7%
4-(6-hydroxy-2-naphthyl)-butan-2-ol, conjugated	9%
O-desmethyl-nabumetone, conjugated	7%
Unidentified minor metabolites	34%
Total % Dose:	**73%**

Following oral administration of dosages of 1000-2000 mg to steady state, the mean plasma clearance of 6MNA is 20-30 ml/min and the elimination half-life is approximately 24 hours.

Elderly Patients

Steady-state plasma concentrations in elderly patients were generally higher than in young healthy subjects. (See TABLE 1 for summary of pharmacokinetic parameters.)

Renal Insufficiency

In studies of patients with renal insufficiency, the mean terminal half-life of 6MNA was increased in patients with severe renal dysfunction (creatinine clearance <30 ml/min/1.73 m^2). In patients undergoing hemodialysis, steady-state plasma concentrations of the active metabolite were similar to those observed in healthy subjects. Due to extensive protein-binding, 6MNA is not dialyzable.

Hepatic Impairment

Data in patients with severe hepatic impairment are limited. Biotransformation of nabumetone to 6MNA and the further metabolism of 6MNA to inactive metabolites is dependent on hepatic function and could be reduced in patients with severe hepatic impairment (history of or biopsy-proven cirrhosis).

SPECIAL STUDIES

Gastrointestinal

Nabumetone was compared to aspirin in inducing gastrointestinal blood loss. Food intake was not monitored. Studies utilizing ^{51}Cr-tagged red blood cells in healthy males showed no difference in fecal blood loss after 3 or 4 weeks' administration of nabumetone 1000 or 2000 mg daily when compared to either placebo-treated or non-treated subjects. In contrast, aspirin 3600 mg daily produced an increase in fecal blood loss when compared to the nabumetone-treated, placebo-treated or non-treated subjects. The clinical relevance of the data is unknown.

The following endoscopy trials entered patients who had been previously treated with NSAIDs. These patients had varying baseline scores and different courses of treatment. The trials were not designed to correlate symptoms and endoscopy scores. The clinical relevance of these endoscopy trials, *i.e.,* either GI symptoms or serious GI events, is not known.

Ten (10) endoscopy studies were conducted in 488 patients who had baseline and post-treatment endoscopy. In 5 clinical trials that compared a total of 194 patients on nabumetone 1000 mg daily or naproxen 250 or 500 mg twice daily for 3-12 weeks, nabumetone treatment resulted in fewer patients with endoscopically detected lesions (>3 mm). In 2 trials a total of 101 patients on nabumetone 1000 or 2000 mg daily or piroxicam 10-20 mg for 7-10 days, there were fewer nabumetone patients with endoscopically detected lesions. In 3 trials of a total of 47 patients on nabumetone 1000 mg daily or indomethacin 100-150 mg daily for 3-4 weeks, the endoscopy scores were higher with indomethacin. Another 12 week trial in a total of 171 patients compared the results of treatment with nabumetone 1000 mg/day to ibuprofen 2400 mg/day and ibuprofen 2400 mg/day plus misoprostol 800 μg/day. The results showed that patients treated with nabumetone had a lower number of endoscopically detected lesions (>5 mm) than patients treated with ibuprofen alone but comparable to the combination of ibuprofen plus misoprostol. The results did not correlate with abdominal pain.

Other

In 1 week repeat-dose studies in healthy volunteers, nabumetone 1000 mg daily had little effect on collagen-induced platelet aggregation and no effect on bleeding time. In comparison, naproxen 500 mg daily suppressed collagen-induced platelet aggregation and significantly increased bleeding time.

INDICATIONS AND USAGE

Nabumetone is indicated for acute and chronic treatment of signs and symptoms of osteoarthritis and rheumatoid arthritis.

CONTRAINDICATIONS

Nabumetone is contraindicated in patients who have previously exhibited hypersensitivity to it.

Nabumetone is contraindicated in patients in whom nabumetone, aspirin or other NSAIDs induce asthma, urticaria or other allergic-type reactions. Fatal asthmatic reactions have been reported in such patients receiving NSAIDs.

WARNINGS

RISK OF GI ULCERATION, BLEEDING AND PERFORATION WITH NSAID THERAPY

Serious gastrointestinal toxicity such as bleeding, ulceration and perforation can occur at any time, with or without warning symptoms, in patients treated chronically with NSAID therapy. Although minor upper gastrointestinal problems, such as dyspepsia, are common, usually developing early in therapy, physicians should remain alert for ulceration and bleed-

N

ing in patients treated chronically with NSAIDs even in the absence of previous GI tract symptoms.

In controlled clinical trials involving 1677 patients treated with nabumetone (1140 followed for 1 year and 927 for 2 years), the cumulative incidence of peptic ulcers was 0.3% (95% CI; 0%, 0.6%) at 3-6 months, 0.5% (95% CI; 0.1%, 0.9%) at 1 year and 0.8% (95% CI; 0.3%, 1.3%) at 2 years. Physicians should inform patients about the signs and symptoms of serious GI toxicity and what steps to take if they occur. In patients with active peptic ulcer, physicians must weigh the benefits of nabumetone therapy against possible hazards, institute an appropriate ulcer treatment regimen and monitor the patients' progress carefully.

Studies to date have not identified any subset of patients not at risk of developing peptic ulceration and bleeding. Except for a prior history of serious GI events and other risk factors known to be associated with peptic ulcer disease, such as alcoholism, smoking, etc., no risk factors (*e.g.*, age, sex) have been associated with increased risk. Elderly or debilitated patients seem to tolerate ulceration or bleeding less well than other individuals and most spontaneous reports of fatal GI events are in this population.

High doses of any NSAID probably carry a greater risk of these reactions, although controlled clinical trials showing this do not exist in most cases. In considering the use of relatively large doses (within the recommended dosage range), sufficient benefit should be anticipated to offset the potential increased risk of GI toxicity.

PRECAUTIONS

GENERAL

Renal Effects

As a class, NSAIDs have been associated with renal papillary necrosis and other abnormal renal pathology during long-term administration to animals.

A second form of renal toxicity often associated with NSAIDs is seen in patients with conditions leading to a reduction in renal blood flow or blood volume, where renal prostaglandins have a supportive role in the maintenance of renal perfusion. In these patients, administration of an NSAID results in a dose-dependent decrease in prostaglandin synthesis and, secondarily, in a reduction of renal blood flow, which may precipitate overt renal decompensation. Patients at greatest risk of this reaction are those with impaired renal function, heart failure, liver dysfunction, those taking diuretics, and the elderly. Discontinuation of NSAID therapy is typically followed by recovery to the pretreatment state.

Because nabumetone undergoes extensive hepatic metabolism, no adjustment of nabumetone dosage is generally necessary in patients with renal insufficiency. However, as with all NSAIDs, patients with impaired renal function should be monitored more closely than patients with normal renal function (see CLINICAL PHARMACOLOGY, Pharmacokinetics, Renal Insufficiency). In patients with severe renal impairment (creatinine clearance ≤30 ml/min), laboratory tests should be performed at baseline and within weeks of starting therapy. Further tests should be carried out as necessary; if the impairment worsens, discontinuation of therapy may be warranted. The oxidized and conjugated metabolites of 6MNA are eliminated primarily by the kidneys. The extent to which these largely inactive metabolites may accumulate in patients with renal failure has not been studied. As with other drugs whose metabolites are excreted by the kidneys, the possibility that adverse reactions (not listed in ADVERSE REACTIONS) may be attributable to these metabolites should be considered.

N

Hepatic Function

As with other NSAIDs, borderline elevations of 1 or more liver function tests may occur in up to 15% of patients. These abnormalities may progress, may remain essentially unchanged, or may return to normal with continued therapy. The ALT (SGPT) test is probably the most sensitive indicator of liver dysfunction. Meaningful (3 times the upper limit of normal) elevations of ALT (SGPT) or AST (SGOT) have occurred in controlled clinical trials of nabumetone in less than 1% of patients. A patient with symptoms and/or signs suggesting liver dysfunction, or in whom an abnormal liver test has occurred, should be evaluated for evidence of the development of a more severe hepatic reaction while on nabumetone therapy. Severe hepatic reactions, including jaundice and fatal hepatitis, have been reported with nabumetone and other NSAIDs. Although such reactions are rare, if abnormal liver tests persist or worsen, if clinical signs and symptoms consistent with liver disease develop, or if systemic manifestations occur (*e.g.*, eosinophilia, rash, etc.), nabumetone should be discontinued. Because nabumetone's biotransformation to 6MNA is dependent upon hepatic function, the biotransformation could be decreased in patients with severe hepatic dysfunction. Therefore, nabumetone should be used with caution in patients with severe hepatic impairment (see CLINICAL PHARMACOLOGY, Pharmacokinetics, Hepatic Impairment).

Fluid Retention and Edema

Fluid retention and edema have been observed in some patients taking nabumetone. Therefore, as with other NSAIDs, nabumetone should be used cautiously in patients with a history of congestive heart failure, hypertension or other conditions predisposing to fluid retention.

Photosensitivity

Based on UV light photosensitivity testing, nabumetone may be associated with more reactions to sun exposure than might be expected based on skin tanning types.

INFORMATION FOR THE PATIENT

Nabumetone, like other drugs of its class, is not free of side effects. The side effects of these drugs can cause discomfort and, rarely, there are more serious side effects, such as gastrointestinal bleeding, which may result in hospitalization and even fatal outcome.

NSAIDs are often essential agents in the management of arthritis, but they also may be commonly employed for conditions which are less serious. Physicians may wish to discuss with their patients the potential risks (see WARNINGS, PRECAUTIONS and ADVERSE REACTIONS) and likely benefits of NSAID treatment, particularly when the drugs are used for less serious conditions where treatment without NSAIDs may represent an acceptable alternative to both the patient and the physician.

LABORATORY TESTS

Because severe GI tract ulceration and bleeding can occur without warning symptoms, physicians should follow chronically treated patients for signs and symptoms of ulceration and bleeding, and should inform them of the importance of this follow-up (see WARNINGS, Risk of GI Ulceration, Bleeding and Perforation With NSAID Therapy).

CARCINOGENESIS, MUTAGENESIS

In 2 year studies conducted in mice and rats, nabumetone had no statistically significant tumorigenic effect. Nabumetone did not show mutagenic potential in the Ames test and mouse micronucleus test *in vivo*. However, nabumetone- and 6MNA-treated lymphocytes in culture showed chromosomal aberrations at 80 μg/ml and higher concentrations (equal to the average human exposure to nabumetone at the maximum recommended dose).

IMPAIRMENT OF FERTILITY

Nabumetone did not impair fertility of male or female rats treated orally at doses of 320 mg/kg/day (1888 mg/m^2) before mating.

PREGNANCY, TERATOGENIC EFFECTS, PREGNANCY CATEGORY C

Nabumetone did not cause any teratogenic effect in rats given up to 400 mg/kg (2360 mg/m^2) and in rabbits up to 300 mg/kg (3540 mg/m^2) orally. However, increased post-implantation loss was observed in rats at 100 mg/kg (590 mg/m^2) orally and at higher doses (equal to the average human exposure to 6MNA at the maximum recommended human dose). There are no adequate, well-controlled studies in pregnant women. This drug should be used during pregnancy only if clearly needed.

Because of the known effect of prostaglandin-synthesis-inhibiting drugs on the human fetal cardiovascular system (closure of ductus arteriosus), use of nabumetone during the third trimester of pregnancy is not recommended.

LABOR AND DELIVERY

The effects of nabumetone on labor and delivery in women are not known. As with other drugs known to inhibit prostaglandin synthesis, an increased incidence of dystocia and delayed parturition occurred in rats treated throughout pregnancy.

NURSING MOTHERS

Nabumetone is not recommended for use in nursing mothers because of the possible adverse effects of prostaglandin-synthesis-inhibiting drugs on neonates. It is not known whether nabumetone or its metabolites are excreted in human milk; however, 6MNA is excreted in the milk of lactating rats.

PEDIATRIC USE

Safety and effectiveness in pediatric patients have not been established.

GERIATRIC USE

Of the 1677 patients in US clinical studies who were treated with nabumetone, 411 patients (24%) were 65 years of age or older; 22 patients (1%) were 75 years of age or older. No overall differences in efficacy or safety were observed between these older patients and younger ones. Similar results were observed in a 1 year, non-US postmarketing surveillance study of 10,800 nabumetone patients, of whom 4,577 patients (42%) were 65 years of age or older.

DRUG INTERACTIONS

In vitro studies have shown that, because of its affinity for protein, 6MNA may displace other protein-bound drugs from their binding site. Caution should be exercised when administering nabumetone with warfarin since interactions have been seen with other NSAIDs.

Concomitant administration of an aluminum-containing antacid had no significant effect on the bioavailability of 6MNA. When administered with food or milk, there is more rapid absorption; however, the total amount of 6MNA in the plasma is unchanged (see CLINICAL PHARMACOLOGY, Pharmacokinetics).

ADVERSE REACTIONS

Adverse reaction information was derived from blinded- controlled and open-labelled clinical trials and from worldwide marketing experience. In the description below, rates of the more common events (greater than 1%) and many of the less common events (less than 1%) represent results of US clinical studies.

Of the 1677 patients who received nabumetone during US clinical trials, 1524 were treated for at least 1 month, 1327 for at least 3 months, 929 for at least a year and 750 for at least 2 years. Over 300 patients have been treated for 5 years or longer.

The most frequently reported adverse reactions were related to the gastrointestinal tract. They were diarrhea, dyspepsia and abdominal pain.

Incidence ≥1% — Probably Causally Related:

Gastrointestinal: Diarrhea (14%), dyspepsia (13%), abdominal pain (12%), constipation*, flatulence*, nausea*, positive stool guaiac*, dry mouth, gastritis, stomatitis, vomiting.

Central Nervous System: Dizziness*, headache*, fatigue, increased sweating, insomnia, nervousness, somnolence.

Dermatologic: Pruritus*, rash*.

Special Senses: Tinnitus*.

Miscellaneous: Edema*.

*Incidence of reported reaction between 3% and 9%. Reactions occurring in 1-3% of the patients are unmarked.

Incidence ≤1% — Probably Causally Related†:

Gastrointestinal: Anorexia, jaundice, duodenal ulcer, dysphagia, gastric ulcer, gastroenteritis, gastrointestinal bleeding, increased appetite, liver function abnormalities, melena, *hepatic failure.*

Central Nervous System: Asthenia, agitation, anxiety, confusion, depression, malaise, paresthesia, tremor, vertigo.

Dermatologic: Bullous eruptions, photosensitivity, urticaria, pseudoporphyria cutanea tarda, *toxic epidermal necrolysis, erythema multiforme, Stevens-Johnson Syndrome.*
Cardiovascular: Vasculitis.
Metabolic: Weight gain.
Respiratory: Dyspnea, *eosinophilic pneumonia, hypersensitivity pneumonitis, idiopathic interstitial pneumonitis.*
Genitourinary: Albuminuria, azotemia, *hyperuricemia, interstitial nephritis, nephrotic syndrome, vaginal bleeding, renal failure.*
Special Senses: Abnormal vision.
Hematologic/Lymphatic: *Thrombocytopenia.*
Hypersensitivity: *Anaphylactoid reaction, anaphylaxis,* angioneurotic edema.
†Adverse reactions reported only in worldwide postmarketing experience or in the literature, not seen in clinical trials, are considered rarer and are italicized.

Incidence ≤1% — Causal Relationship Unknown:
Gastrointestinal: Bilirubinuria, duodenitis, eructation, gallstones, gingivitis, glossitis, pancreatitis, rectal bleeding.
Central Nervous System: Nightmares.
Dermatologic: Acne, alopecia.
Cardiovascular: Angina, arrhythmia, hypertension, myocardial infarction, palpitations, syncope, thrombophlebitis.
Respiratory: Asthma, cough.
Genitourinary: Dysuria, hematuria, impotence, renal stones.
Special Senses: Taste disorder.
Body as a Whole: Fever, chills.
Hematologic/Lymphatic: Anemia, leukopenia, granulocytopenia.
Metabolic/Nutritional: Hyperglycemia, hypokalemia, weight loss.

DOSAGE AND ADMINISTRATION

OSTEOARTHRITIS AND RHEUMATOID ARTHRITIS

The recommended starting dose is 1000 mg taken as a single dose with or without food. Some patients may obtain more symptomatic relief from 1500-2000 mg/day. Nabumetone can be given in either a single or twice-daily dose. Dosages over 2000 mg/day have not been studied. The lowest effective dose should be used for chronic treatment.

HOW SUPPLIED

Relafen tablets are available in:

500 mg: White, oval-shaped, film-coated tablets, imprinted with the product name "RELAFEN" and "500".

750 mg: Beige, oval-shaped, film-coated tablets, imprinted with the product name "RELAFEN" and "750".

Storage: Store at 25°C (77°F); excursions permitted to 15-30°C (59-86°F) in well-closed container; dispense in light-resistant container.

PRODUCT LISTING - RATED THERAPEUTICALLY EQUIVALENT

Tablet - Oral - 500 mg

10's	$16.74	RELAFEN, Pd-Rx Pharmaceuticals	55289-0015-10
10's	$17.78	RELAFEN, Prescript Pharmaceuticals	00247-0087-10
14's	$16.16	RELAFEN, Allscripts Pharmaceutical Company	54569-3535-04
14's	$17.65	RELAFEN, Compumed Pharmaceuticals	00403-4143-14
14's	$23.55	RELAFEN, Prescript Pharmaceuticals	00247-0087-14
14's	$24.15	RELAFEN, Pd-Rx Pharmaceuticals	55289-0015-14
14's	$25.42	RELAFEN, Dhs Inc	55887-0744-14
14's	$27.49	RELAFEN, Pharma Pac	52959-0227-14
15's	$17.32	RELAFEN, Allscripts Pharmaceutical Company	54569-3535-01
15's	$18.05	RELAFEN, Compumed Pharmaceuticals	00403-4143-15
15's	$24.99	RELAFEN, Prescript Pharmaceuticals	00247-0087-15
15's	$29.45	RELAFEN, Pharma Pac	52959-0227-15
20's	$23.09	RELAFEN, Allscripts Pharmaceutical Company	54569-3535-05
20's	$24.05	RELAFEN, Compumed Pharmaceuticals	00403-4143-20
20's	$32.21	RELAFEN, Prescript Pharmaceuticals	00247-0087-20
20's	$32.65	RELAFEN, Physicians Total Care	54868-2014-00
20's	$33.79	RELAFEN, Pd-Rx Pharmaceuticals	55289-0015-20
20's	$38.90	RELAFEN, Pharma Pac	52959-0227-20
20's	$43.89	RELAFEN, Dhs Inc	55887-0744-20
21's	$26.68	RELAFEN, Allscripts Pharmaceutical Company	54569-3535-06
28's	$32.33	RELAFEN, Allscripts Pharmaceutical Company	54569-3535-02
28's	$43.75	RELAFEN, Prescript Pharmaceuticals	00247-0087-28
28's	$46.62	RELAFEN, Pd-Rx Pharmaceuticals	55289-0015-28
28's	$48.96	RELAFEN, Dhs Inc	55887-0744-28
28's	$56.43	RELAFEN, Pharma Pac	52959-0227-28
30's	$36.10	RELAFEN, Compumed Pharmaceuticals	00403-4143-30
30's	$38.12	RELAFEN, Allscripts Pharmaceutical Company	54569-3535-07
30's	$46.64	RELAFEN, Prescript Pharmaceuticals	00247-0087-30
30's	$48.38	RELAFEN, Physicians Total Care	54868-2014-02
30's	$50.01	RELAFEN, Pd-Rx Pharmaceuticals	55289-0015-30
30's	$56.71	RELAFEN, Pharma Pac	52959-0227-30
40's	$64.10	RELAFEN, Physicians Total Care	54868-2014-04
40's	$68.76	RELAFEN, Pd-Rx Pharmaceuticals	55289-0015-40
40's	$73.45	RELAFEN, Pharma Pac	52959-0227-40
42's	$48.49	RELAFEN, Allscripts Pharmaceutical Company	54569-3535-03
42's	$63.94	RELAFEN, Prescript Pharmaceuticals	00247-0087-42
50's	$75.48	RELAFEN, Prescript Pharmaceuticals	00247-0087-50
60's	$59.75	RELAFEN, Compumed Pharmaceuticals	00403-4143-71
60's	$69.27	RELAFEN, Allscripts Pharmaceutical Company	54569-3535-00
60's	$89.92	RELAFEN, Prescript Pharmaceuticals	00247-0087-60
60's	$95.55	RELAFEN, Physicians Total Care	54868-2014-03
60's	$103.13	RELAFEN, Pd-Rx Pharmaceuticals	55289-0015-60
60's	$103.67	RELAFEN, Pharma Pac	52959-0227-60
100's	$129.49	GENERIC, Udl Laboratories Inc	51079-0989-20
100's	$129.70	GENERIC, Teva Pharmaceuticals Usa	00093-1015-01
100's	$129.70	GENERIC, Eon Labs Manufacturing Inc	00185-0145-01
100's	$129.70	GENERIC, Geneva Pharmaceuticals	00781-1306-01
100's	$152.88	RELAFEN, Glaxosmithkline	00029-4851-20
100's	$152.88	RELAFEN, Glaxosmithkline	00029-4851-21
180's	$183.96	RELAFEN, Allscripts Pharmaceutical Company	54569-8535-00

Tablet - Oral - 750 mg

14's	$21.01	RELAFEN, Allscripts Pharmaceutical Company	54569-3845-01
14's	$36.60	RELAFEN, Compumed Pharmaceuticals	00403-4845-14
20's	$30.01	RELAFEN, Allscripts Pharmaceutical Company	54569-3845-02
20's	$38.90	RELAFEN, Pharma Pac	52959-0373-20
20's	$44.15	RELAFEN, Pd-Rx Pharmaceuticals	55289-0721-20
28's	$54.41	RELAFEN, Pharma Pac	52959-0373-28
30's	$40.91	RELAFEN, Allscripts Pharmaceutical Company	54569-3845-00
30's	$52.02	RELAFEN, Physicians Total Care	54868-3208-01
30's	$57.50	RELAFEN, Pharma Pac	52959-0373-30
30's	$65.45	RELAFEN, Pd-Rx Pharmaceuticals	55289-0721-30
40's	$76.13	RELAFEN, Pharma Pac	52959-0373-40
60's	$112.62	RELAFEN, Physicians Total Care	54868-3208-00
100's	$117.25	RELAFEN, Compumed Pharmaceuticals	00403-4845-01
100's	$153.17	GENERIC, Teva Pharmaceuticals Usa	00093-1016-01
100's	$153.17	GENERIC, Eon Labs Manufacturing Inc	00185-0146-01
100's	$153.17	GENERIC, Geneva Pharmaceuticals	00781-1308-01
100's	$180.54	RELAFEN, Glaxosmithkline	00029-4852-20

PRODUCT LISTING - EQUIVALENTS NOT AVAILABLE

Tablet - Oral - 500 mg

6's	$8.64	GENERIC, Southwood Pharmaceuticals Inc	58016-0619-06
10's	$14.40	GENERIC, Southwood Pharmaceuticals Inc	58016-0619-10
12's	$17.28	GENERIC, Southwood Pharmaceuticals Inc	58016-0619-12
14's	$20.16	GENERIC, Southwood Pharmaceuticals Inc	58016-0619-14
14's	$20.25	GENERIC, Pharma Pac	52959-0650-14
15's	$21.60	GENERIC, Southwood Pharmaceuticals Inc	58016-0619-15
20's	$28.80	GENERIC, Southwood Pharmaceuticals Inc	58016-0619-20
20's	$29.15	GENERIC, Pharma Pac	52959-0650-20
24's	$34.56	GENERIC, Southwood Pharmaceuticals Inc	58016-0619-24
28's	$40.32	GENERIC, Southwood Pharmaceuticals Inc	58016-0619-28
30's	$43.20	GENERIC, Southwood Pharmaceuticals Inc	58016-0619-30
30's	$43.50	GENERIC, Pharma Pac	52959-0650-30
40's	$57.60	GENERIC, Southwood Pharmaceuticals Inc	58016-0619-40
50's	$72.00	GENERIC, Southwood Pharmaceuticals Inc	58016-0619-50
60's	$86.40	GENERIC, Southwood Pharmaceuticals Inc	58016-0619-60
100's	$144.00	GENERIC, Southwood Pharmaceuticals Inc	58016-0619-00

Tablet - Oral - 750 mg

30's	$39.25	RELAFEN, Compumed Pharmaceuticals	00403-4845-30
30's	$48.90	GENERIC, Southwood Pharmaceuticals Inc	58016-0628-30
30's	$49.50	GENERIC, Pharma Pac	52959-0656-30
60's	$97.80	GENERIC, Southwood Pharmaceuticals Inc	58016-0628-60
90's	$146.70	GENERIC, Southwood Pharmaceuticals Inc	58016-0628-90

Nadolol *(001849)*

For related information, see the comparative table section in Appendix A.

Categories: Angina pectoris; Hypertension, essential; Pregnancy Category C; FDA Approved 1979 Dec
Drug Classes: Antiadrenergics, beta blocking
Brand Names: **Corgard**
Foreign Brand Availability: Apo-Nadol (Hong-Kong); Apo-Nadolol (New-Zealand); Farmagard (Indonesia); Nadic (Japan); Solgol (Austria; Germany; Spain)
Cost of Therapy: $57.39 (Angina; Corgard; 40 mg; 1 tablet/day; 30 day supply)
$12.01 (Angina; Generic Tablets; 40 mg; 1 tablet/day; 30 day supply)

DESCRIPTION

Nadolol is a synthetic nonselective beta-adrenergic receptor blocking agent designated chemically as 1-(*tert*-butylamino)-3-((5,6,7,8-tetrahydro-*cis*-6,7-dihydroxy-1-naphthyl)oxy)-2-propanol.

Its molecular formula is $C_{17}H_{27}NO_4$, with a molecular weight of 309.41.

Nadolol is a white crystalline powder. It is freely soluble in ethanol, soluble in hydrochloric acid, slightly soluble in water and in chloroform, and very slightly soluble in sodium hydroxide.

Each tablet for oral administration contains 20, 40, or 80 mg of nadolol and the following inactive ingredients: croscarmellose sodium, lactose (anhydrous), magnesium stearate, microcrystalline cellulose, sodium lauryl sulfate, and D&C yellow no. 10 aluminum lake.

CLINICAL PHARMACOLOGY

Nadolol is a nonselective beta-adrenergic receptor blocking agent. Clinical pharmacology studies have demonstrated beta-blocking activity by showing (1) reduction in heart rate and cardiac output at rest and on exercise; (2) reduction of systolic and diastolic blood pressure at rest and on exercise; (3) inhibition of isoproterenol-induced tachycardia; and (4) reduction of reflex orthostatic tachycardia.

Nadolol specifically competes with beta-adrenergic receptor agonists for available beta receptor sites; it inhibits both the $beta_1$, receptors located chiefly in cardiac muscle and the

$beta_2$ receptors located chiefly in the bronchial and vascular musculature, inhibiting the chronotropic, inotropic, and vasodilator responses to beta-adrenergic stimulation proportionately. Nadolol has no intrinsic sympathomimetic activity and, unlike some other beta-adrenergic blocking agents, nadolol has little direct myocardial depressant activity and does not have an anesthetic-like membrane-stabilizing action. Animal and human studies show that nadolol slows the sinus rate and depresses AV conduction. In dogs, only minimal amounts of nadolol were detected in the brain relative to amounts in blood and other organs and tissues. Nadolol has low lipophilicity as determined by octanol/water partition coefficient, a characteristic of certain beta-blocking agents that has been correlated with the limited extent to which these agents cross the blood-brain barrier, their low concentration in the brain, and low incidence of CNS-related side effects.

In controlled clinical studies, nadolol at doses of 40-320 mg/day has been shown to decrease both standing and supine blood pressure, the effect persisting for approximately 24 hours after dosing.

The mechanism of the antihypertensive effects of beta-adrenergic receptor blocking agents has not been established; however, factors that may be involved include (1) competitive antagonism of catecholamines at peripheral (non-CNS) adrenergic neuron sites (especially cardiac) leading to decreased cardiac output; (2) a central effect leading to reduced tonic-sympathetic nerve outflow to the periphery; and (3) suppression of renin secretion by blockade of the beta-adrenergic receptors responsible for renin release from the kidneys.

While cardiac output and arterial pressure are reduced by nadolol therapy, renal hemodynamics are stable, with preservation of renal blood flow and glomerular filtration rate.

By blocking catecholamine-induced increases in heart rate, velocity and extent of myocardial contraction, and blood pressure, nadolol generally reduces the oxygen requirements of the heart at any given level of effort, making it useful for many patients in the long-term management of angina pectoris. On the other hand, nadolol can increase oxygen requirements by increasing left ventricular fiber length and end diastolic pressure, particularly in patients with heart failure.

Although beta-adrenergic receptor blockade is useful in treatment of angina and hypertension, there are also situations in which sympathetic stimulation is vital. For example, in patients with severely damaged hearts, adequate ventricular function may depend on sympathetic drive. Beta-adrenergic blockade may worsen AV block by preventing the necessary facilitating effects of sympathetic activity on conduction. $Beta_2$-adrenergic blockade results in passive bronchial constriction by interfering with endogenous adrenergic bronchodilator activity in patients subject to bronchospasm and may also interfere with exogenous bronchodilators in such patients.

Absorption of nadolol after oral dosing is variable, averaging about 30%. Peak serum concentrations of nadolol usually occur in 3-4 hours after oral administration and the presence of food in the gastrointestinal tract does not affect the rate or extent of nadolol absorption. Approximately 30% of the nadolol present in serum is reversibly bound to plasma protein.

Unlike many other beta-adrenergic blocking agents, nadolol is not metabolized by the liver and is excreted unchanged, principally by the kidneys.

The half-life of therapeutic doses of nadolol is about 20-24 hours, permitting once-daily dosage. Because nadolol is excreted predominantly in the urine, its half-life increases in renal failure (see PRECAUTIONS and DOSAGE AND ADMINISTRATION). Steady state serum concentrations of nadolol are attained in 6-9 days with once-daily dosage in persons with normal renal function. Because of variable absorption and different individual responsiveness, the proper dosage must be determined by titration.

Exacerbation of angina and, in some cases, myocardial infarction and ventricular dysrhythmia have been reported after abrupt discontinuation of therapy with beta-adrenergic blocking agents in patients with coronary artery disease. Abrupt withdrawal of these agents in patients without coronary artery disease has resulted in transient symptoms, including tremulousness, sweating, palpitation, headache, and malaise. Several mechanisms have been proposed to explain these phenomena, among them increased sensitivity to catecholamines because of increased numbers of beta receptors.

INDICATIONS AND USAGE

ANGINA PECTORIS

Nadolol tablets are indicated for the long-term management of patients with angina pectoris.

HYPERTENSION

Nadolol tablets are indicated in the management of hypertension; it may be used alone or in combination with other antihypertensive agents, especially thiazide-type diuretics.

NON-FDA APPROVED INDICATIONS

Non-FDA-approved uses include management of parkinsonian, essential, and lithium-induced tremors, migraine prophylaxis, prevention of esophageal variceal hemorrhage, anxiety, ventricular tachyarrhythmias, and reduction of intraocular pressure in glaucoma.

CONTRAINDICATIONS

Nadolol is contraindicated in bronchial asthma, sinus bradycardia and greater than first-degree conduction block, cardiogenic shock, and overt cardiac failure (see WARNINGS).

WARNINGS

CARDIAC FAILURE

Sympathetic stimulation may be a vital component supporting circulatory function in patients with congestive heart failure, and its inhibition by beta-blockade may precipitate more severe failure. Although beta blockers should be avoided in overt congestive heart failure, if necessary, they can be used with caution in patients with a history of failure who are well compensated, usually with digitalis and diuretics. Beta-adrenergic blocking agents do not abolish the inotropic action of digitalis on heart muscle.

In patients without a history of heart failure, continued use of beta blockers can, in some cases, lead to cardiac failure. Therefore, at the first sign or symptom of heart failure, the patient should be digitalized and/or treated with diuretics, and the response observed closely, or nadolol should be discontinued (gradually, if possible).

Exacerbation of Ischemic Heart Disease Following Abrupt Withdrawal

Hypersensitivity to catecholamines has been observed in patients withdrawn from beta blocker therapy; exacerbation of angina and, in some cases, myocardial infarction have occurred after abrupt discontinuation of such therapy. When discontinuing chronically administered nadolol, particularly in patients with ischemic heart disease, the dosage should be gradually reduced over a period of 1-2 weeks and the patient should be carefully monitored. If angina markedly worsens or acute coronary insufficiency develops, nadolol administration should be reinstituted promptly, at least temporarily, and other measures appropriate for the management of unstable angina should be taken. Patients should be warned against interruption or discontinuation of therapy without the physician's advice. Because coronary artery disease is common and may be unrecognized, it may be prudent not to discontinue nadolol therapy abruptly even in patients treated only for hypertension.

NONALLERGIC BRONCHOSPASM (E.G., CHRONIC BRONCHITIS, EMPHYSEMA)

Patients with bronchospastic diseases should in general not receive beta blockers. Nadolol should be administered with caution since it may block bronchodilation produced by endogenous or exogenous catecholamine stimulation of $beta_2$ receptors.

MAJOR SURGERY

Because beta-blockade impairs the ability of the heart to respond to reflex stimuli and may increase the risks of general anesthesia and surgical procedures, resulting in protracted hypotension or low cardiac output, it has generally been suggested that such therapy should be withdrawn several days prior to surgery. Recognition of the increased sensitivity to catecholamines of patients recently withdrawn from beta blocker therapy, however, has made this recommendation controversial. If possible, beta blockers should be withdrawn well before surgery takes place. In the event of emergency surgery, the anesthesiologist should be informed that the patient is on beta blocker therapy. The effects of nadolol can be reversed by administration of beta-receptor agonists such as isoproterenol, dopamine, dobutamine, or norepinephrine. Difficulty in restarting and maintaining the heartbeat has also been reported with beta-adrenergic receptor blocking agents.

DIABETES AND HYPOGLYCEMIA

Beta-adrenergic blockade may prevent the appearance of premonitory signs and symptoms (*e.g.,* tachycardia and blood pressure changes) of acute hypoglycemia. This is especially important with labile diabetics. Beta blockade also reduces the release of insulin in response to hyperglycemia; therefore, it may be necessary to adjust the dose of antidiabetic drugs.

THYROTOXICOSIS

Beta-adrenergic blockade may mask certain clinical signs (*e.g.,* tachycardia) of hyperthyroidism. Patients suspected of developing thyrotoxicosis should be managed carefully to avoid abrupt withdrawal of beta-adrenergic blockade which might precipitate a thyroid storm.

PRECAUTIONS

IMPAIRED RENAL FUNCTION

Nadolol should be used with caution in patients with impaired renal function (see DOSAGE AND ADMINISTRATION).

INFORMATION FOR THE PATIENT

Patients, especially those with evidence of coronary artery insufficiency, should be warned against interruption or discontinuation of nadolol therapy without the physician's advice. Although cardiac failure rarely occurs in properly selected patients, patients being treated with beta-adrenergic blocking agents should be advised to consult the physician at the first sign or symptom of impending failure. The patient should also be advised of a proper course in the event of an inadvertently missed dose.

RESPONSE TO TREATMENT FOR ANAPHYLACTIC REACTION

While taking beta blockers, patients with a history of severe anaphylactic reaction to a variety of allergens may be more reactive to repeated challenge, either accidental, diagnostic, or therapeutic. Such patients may be unresponsive to the usual doses of epinephrine used to treat allergic reaction.

CARCINOGENESIS, MUTAGENESIS, AND IMPAIRMENT OF FERTILITY

In chronic oral toxicologic studies (1-2 years) in mice, rats, and dogs, nadolol did not produce any significant toxic effects. In 2-year oral carcinogenic studies in rats and mice, nadolol did not produce any neoplastic, preneoplastic, or non-neoplastic pathologic lesions. In fertility and general reproductive performance studies in rats, nadolol caused no adverse effects.

PREGNANCY CATEGORY C

In animal reproduction studies with nadolol, evidence of embryo and fetotoxicity was found in rabbits, but not in rats or hamsters, at doses 5-10 times greater (on a mg/kg basis) than the maximum indicated human dose. No teratogenic potential was observed in any of these species.

There are no adequate and well-controlled studies in pregnant women. Nadolol should be used during pregnancy only if the potential benefit justifies the potential risk to the fetus. Neonates whose mothers are receiving nadolol at parturition have exhibited bradycardia, hypoglycemia, and associated symptoms.

NURSING MOTHERS

Nadolol is excreted in human milk. Because of the potential for adverse effects in nursing infants, a decision should be made whether to discontinue nursing or to discontinue therapy taking into account the importance of nadolol to the mother.

PEDIATRIC USE

Safety and effectiveness in children have not been established.

DRUG INTERACTIONS

When administered concurrently, the following drugs may interact with beta-adrenergic receptor blocking agents:

Anesthetics, General: Exaggeration of the hypotension induced by general anesthetics (see WARNINGS, Major Surgery).

Antidiabetic Drugs (oral agents and insulin): Hypoglycemia or hyperglycemia; adjust dosage of antidiabetic drug accordingly (see WARNINGS, Diabetes and Hypoglycemia).

Catecholamine-Depleting Drugs (e.g., reserpine): Additive effect; monitor closely for evidence of hypotension and/or excessive bradycardia (*e.g.,* vertigo, syncope, postural hypotension).

ADVERSE REACTIONS

Most adverse effects have been mild and transient and have rarely required withdrawal of therapy.

Cardiovascular: Bradycardia with heart rates of less than 60 beats/min occurs commonly, and heart rates below 40 beats/min and/or symptomatic bradycardia were seen in about 2 of 100 patients. Symptoms of peripheral vascular insufficiency, usually of the Raynaud type, have occurred in approximately 2 of 100 patients. Cardiac failure, hypotension, and rhythm/conduction disturbances have each occurred in about 1 of 100 patients. Single instances of first- and third-degree heart block have been reported; intensification of AV block is a known effect of beta blockers (see also CONTRAINDICATIONS, WARNINGS, and PRECAUTIONS).

Central Nervous System: Dizziness or fatigue have been reported in approximately 2 of 100 patients; paresthesias, sedation, and change in behavior have each been reported in approximately 6 of 1000 patients.

Respiratory: Bronchospasm has been reported in approximately 1 of 1000 patients (see CONTRAINDICATIONS, and WARNINGS).

Gastrointestinal: Nausea, diarrhea, abdominal discomfort, constipation, vomiting, indigestion, anorexia, bloating, and flatulence have been reported in 1-5 of 1000 patients.

Miscellaneous: *Each of the following has been reported in 1-5 of 1000 patients:* Rash; pruritus; headache; dry mouth, eyes, or skin; impotence or decreased libido; facial swelling; weight gain; slurred speech; cough; nasal stuffiness; sweating; tinnitus; blurred vision. Reversible alopecia has been reported infrequently.

The following adverse reactions have been reported in patients taking nadolol and/or other beta-adrenergic blocking agents, but no causal relationship to nadolol has been established:

Central Nervous System:

Reversible mental depression progressing to catatonia.

Visual disturbances.

Hallucinations.

An acute reversible syndrome characterized by disorientation for time and place, short-term memory loss, emotional lability with slightly clouded sensorium, and decreased performance on neuropsychometrics.

Hematologic:

Agranulocytosis.

Thrombocytopenic or nonthrombocytopenic purpura.

Allergic:

Fever combined with aching and sore throat.

Laryngospasm.

Respiratory distress.

Miscellaneous:

Pemphigoid rash.

Hypertensive reaction in patients with pheochromocytoma.

Sleep disturbances.

Peyronie's disease.

The oculomucocutaneous syndrome associated with the beta blocker practolol has not been reported with nadolol.

DOSAGE AND ADMINISTRATION

Dosage must be individualized. nadolol may be administered without regard to meals.

ANGINA PECTORIS

The usual initial dose is 40 mg nadolol once daily. Dosage may be gradually increased in 40-80 mg increments at 3-7 day intervals until optimum clinical response is obtained or there is pronounced slowing of the heart rate. The usual maintenance dose is 40 or 80 mg administered once daily. Doses of up to 160 or 240 mg administered once daily may be needed.

The usefulness and safety in angina pectoris of dosage exceeding 240 mg/day have not been established. If treatment is to be discontinued, reduce the dosage gradually over a period of 1-2 weeks (see WARNINGS).

HYPERTENSION

The usual initial dose is 40 mg nadolol once daily, whether it is used alone or in addition to diuretic therapy. Dosage may be gradually increased in 40-80 mg increments until optimum blood pressure reduction is achieved. The usual maintenance dose is 40-80 mg administered once daily. Doses of up to 240 or 320 mg administered once daily may be needed.

DOSAGE ADJUSTMENT IN RENAL FAILURE

Absorbed nadolol is excreted principally by the kidneys and, although nonrenal elimination does occur, dosage adjustments are necessary in patients with renal impairment. The dose intervals are recommended (see TABLE 1).

TABLE 1

Creatinine Clearance (ml/min/1.73 m^2)	Dosage Interval (hours)
>50	24
31-50	24-36
10-30	24-48
<10	40-60

HOW SUPPLIED

Nadolol tablets are available in:

20 mg: Yellow, round, scored tablets marked with "M28".

40 mg: Yellow, round, scored tablets marked with "M171".

80 mg: Yellow, round, scored tablets marked with "M132".

STORAGE

Store at controlled room temperature 15-30°C (59-86°F). Avoid excessive heat. Protect from light. Keep bottle tightly closed.

Dispense in a tight, light-resistant container using a child-resistant closure.

PRODUCT LISTING - RATED THERAPEUTICALLY EQUIVALENT

Tablet - Oral - 20 mg

30's	$25.60	GENERIC, Allscripts Pharmaceutical Company	54569-3789-00
50's	$36.45	GENERIC, Pd-Rx Pharmaceuticals	55289-0096-50
100's	$46.50	FEDERAL UPPER LIMIT, H.C.F.A. F F P	99999-1849-01
100's	$72.40	GENERIC, Invamed Inc	52189-0236-24
100's	$73.60	GENERIC, Major Pharmaceuticals Inc	00904-7816-60
100's	$82.95	GENERIC, Major Pharmaceuticals Inc	00904-5069-60
100's	$84.11	GENERIC, Geneva Pharmaceuticals	00781-1181-01
100's	$85.50	GENERIC, Mylan Pharmaceuticals Inc	00378-0028-01
100's	$87.80	GENERIC, Ivax Corporation	00172-4235-60
100's	$92.49	GENERIC, Udl Laboratories Inc	51079-0812-20

Tablet - Oral - 40 mg

30's	$25.70	GENERIC, Pd-Rx Pharmaceuticals	55289-0097-30
30's	$30.00	GENERIC, Allscripts Pharmaceutical Company	54569-3790-00
30's	$30.66	GENERIC, Heartland Healthcare Services	61392-0069-30
30's	$30.66	GENERIC, Heartland Healthcare Services	61392-0069-39
31's	$31.68	GENERIC, Heartland Healthcare Services	61392-0069-31
32's	$32.70	GENERIC, Heartland Healthcare Services	61392-0069-32
45's	$45.99	GENERIC, Heartland Healthcare Services	61392-0069-45
60's	$61.32	GENERIC, Heartland Healthcare Services	61392-0069-60
90's	$90.00	GENERIC, Allscripts Pharmaceutical Company	54569-8591-00
90's	$91.98	GENERIC, Heartland Healthcare Services	61392-0069-90
90's	$98.60	CORGARD, Allscripts Pharmaceutical Company	54569-8532-00
100's	$42.89	FEDERAL UPPER LIMIT, H.C.F.A. F F P	99999-1849-02
100's	$84.00	GENERIC, Invamed Inc	52189-0237-24
100's	$86.25	GENERIC, Major Pharmaceuticals Inc	00904-7817-60
100's	$93.95	GENERIC, Major Pharmaceuticals Inc	00904-5070-60
100's	$96.59	GENERIC, Moore, H.L. Drug Exchange Inc	00839-7870-06
100's	$98.60	GENERIC, Geneva Pharmaceuticals	00781-1182-01
100's	$99.99	GENERIC, Mylan Pharmaceuticals Inc	00378-1171-01
100's	$101.00	GENERIC, Ivax Corporation	00172-4236-60
100's	$108.15	GENERIC, Udl Laboratories Inc	51079-0813-20
100's	$191.30	CORGARD, Bristol-Myers Squibb	00003-0207-50

Tablet - Oral - 80 mg

30's	$41.14	GENERIC, Allscripts Pharmaceutical Company	54569-3791-00
100's	$80.25	FEDERAL UPPER LIMIT, H.C.F.A. F F P	99999-1849-04
100's	$111.90	GENERIC, Invamed Inc	52189-0238-24
100's	$118.30	GENERIC, Major Pharmaceuticals Inc	00904-7818-60
100's	$127.95	GENERIC, Major Pharmaceuticals Inc	00904-5071-60
100's	$129.82	GENERIC, Watson/Rugby Laboratories Inc	00536-4247-01
100's	$132.41	GENERIC, Moore, H.L. Drug Exchange Inc	00839-7871-06
100's	$135.20	GENERIC, Geneva Pharmaceuticals	00781-1183-01
100's	$135.50	GENERIC, Mylan Pharmaceuticals Inc	00378-1132-01
100's	$139.30	GENERIC, Ivax Corporation	00172-4237-60
100's	$146.57	GENERIC, Udl Laboratories Inc	51079-0814-20

Tablet - Oral - 120 mg

100's	$176.65	GENERIC, Ivax Corporation	00172-4238-60

Tablet - Oral - 160 mg

100's	$196.45	GENERIC, Ivax Corporation	00172-4239-60
100's	$380.96	CORGARD, Monarch Pharmaceuticals Inc	61570-0204-01

PRODUCT LISTING - EQUIVALENTS NOT AVAILABLE

Tablet - Oral - 20 mg

100's	$89.75	GENERIC, Apothecon Inc	59772-2461-01
100's	$163.50	CORGARD, Bristol-Myers Squibb	00003-0232-50
100's	$163.50	CORGARD, Monarch Pharmaceuticals Inc	61570-0200-01

Tablet - Oral - 40 mg

100's	$40.04	GENERIC, Physicians Total Care	54868-3257-01
100's	$103.75	GENERIC, Apothecon Inc	59772-2462-01
100's	$191.30	CORGARD, Monarch Pharmaceuticals Inc	61570-0201-01

Tablet - Oral - 80 mg

100's	$116.09	GENERIC, Qualitest Products Inc	00603-4742-21
100's	$141.70	GENERIC, Apothecon Inc	59772-2463-01
100's	$262.81	CORGARD, Bristol-Myers Squibb	00003-0241-50

Tablet - Oral - 120 mg

100's	$185.48	GENERIC, Apothecon Inc	59772-2464-01
100's	$342.54	CORGARD, Bristol-Myers Squibb	00003-0208-50
100's	$342.54	CORGARD, Monarch Pharmaceuticals Inc	61570-0203-01

Tablet - Oral - 160 mg

100's	$206.27	GENERIC, Apothecon Inc	59772-2465-01
100's	$380.96	CORGARD, Bristol-Myers Squibb	00003-0246-49

Nafarelin Acetate (001850)

For complete prescribing information, refer to the CD-ROM included with the book.

Categories: Endometriosis; Puberty, precocious; Pregnancy Category X; FDA Approved 1990 Feb; Orphan Drugs
Drug Classes: Hormones/hormone modifiers
Brand Names: Synarel
Foreign Brand Availability: Nasanyl (Japan); Nasarel (India); Synarela (Denmark; Finland; Germany; Norway; Sweden)
Cost of Therapy: $587.75 (Endometriosis; Synarel; 0.2 mg/inh; 8 ml; 2 inhalations/day; 30 day supply)

DESCRIPTION

NOTE: This monograph contains information for two distinct indications of nafarelin acetate: **Endometriosis** and **Central Precocious Puberty**.

Nafarelin acetate nasal solution is intended for administration as a spray to the nasal mucosa. Nafarelin acetate, the active component of nafarelin nasal solution, is a decapeptide with the chemical name: 5-oxo-L-prolyl-L-histidyl-L-tryptophyl-L-seryl-L-tyrosyl-3-(2-naphthyl)-D-alanyl-L-leucyl-L-arginyl-L-prolyl-glycinamide acetate. Nafarelin acetate is a synthetic analog of the naturally occurring gonadotropin-releasing hormone (GnRH).

Nafarelin nasal solution contains nafarelin acetate (2 mg/ml, content expressed as nafarelin base) in a solution of benzalkonium chloride, glacial acetic acid, sodium hydroxide or hydrochloric acid (to adjust pH), sorbitol, and purified water.

After priming the pump unit for nafarelin, each actuation of the unit delivers approximately 100 µL of the spray containing approximately 200 mcg nafarelin base. The contents of one spray bottle are intended to deliver at least 60 sprays.

INDICATIONS AND USAGE

ENDOMETRIOSIS

Nafarelin is indicated for management of endometriosis, including pain relief and reduction of endometriotic lesions. Experience with nafarelin for the management of endometriosis has been limited to women 18 years of age and older treated for 6 months.

CENTRAL PRECOCIOUS PUBERTY

Nafarelin is indicated for the treatment of **central precocious puberty (CPP)** (gonadotropin-dependent precocious puberty) in children of both sexes.

The diagnosis of **central precocious puberty (CPP)** is suspected when premature development of secondary sexual characteristics occurs at or before the age of 8 years in girls and 9 years in boys, and is accompanied by significant advancement of bone age and/or a poor adult height prediction. The diagnosis should be confirmed by pubertal gonadal sex steroid levels and a pubertal LH response to stimulation by native GnRH. Pelvic ultrasound assessment in girls usually reveals enlarged uterus and ovaries, the latter often with multiple cystic formations. Magnetic resonance imaging or CT-scanning of the brain is recommended to detect hypothalamic or pituitary tumors, or anatomical changes associated with increased intracranial pressure. Other causes of sexual precocity, such as congenital adrenal hyperplasia, testotoxicosis, testicular tumors and/or other autonomous feminizing or masculinizing disorders must be excluded by proper clinical hormonal and diagnostic imaging examinations.

N

CONTRAINDICATIONS

1. Hypersensitivity to GnRH, GnRH agonist analogs or any of the excipients in nafarelin.
2. Undiagnosed abnormal vaginal bleeding.
3. Use in pregnancy or in women who may become pregnant while receiving the drug. Nafarelin may cause fetal harm when administered to a pregnant woman. Major fetal abnormalities were observed in rats, but not in mice or rabbits after administration of nafarelin throughout gestation. There was a dose-related increase in fetal mortality and a decrease in fetal weight in rats. The effects on rat fetal mortality are expected consequences of the alterations in hormonal levels brought about by the drug. If this drug is used during pregnancy or if the patient becomes pregnant while taking this drug, she should be apprised of the potential hazard to the fetus.
4. Use in women who are breast feeding.

WARNINGS

ENDOMETRIOSIS

Safe use of nafarelin acetate in pregnancy has not been established clinically. Before starting treatment with nafarelin, pregnancy must be excluded.

When used regularly at the recommended dose, nafarelin usually inhibits ovulation and stops menstruation. Contraception is not ensured, however, by taking nafarelin, particularly if patients miss successive doses. Therefore, patients should use nonhormonal methods of contraception. Patients should be advised to see their physician if they believe they may be pregnant. If a patient becomes pregnant during treatment, the drug must be discontinued and the patient must be apprised of the potential risk to the fetus.

CENTRAL PRECOCIOUS PUBERTY

The diagnosis of central precocious puberty (CPP) must be established before treatment is initiated. Regular monitoring of CPP patients is needed to assess both patient response as well as compliance. This is particularly important during the first 6 to 8 weeks of treatment to assure that suppression of pituitary-gonadal function is rapid. Testing may include LH response to GnRH stimulation and circulating gonadal sex steroid levels. Assessment of growth velocity and bone age velocity should begin within 3 to 6 months of treatment initiation.

Some patients may not show suppression of the pituitary-gonadal axis by clinical and/or biochemical parameters. This may be due to lack of compliance with the recommended treatment regimen and may be rectified by recommending that the dosing be done by caregivers. If compliance problems are excluded, the possibility of gonadotropin-independent sexual precocity should be reconsidered and appropriate examinations should be conducted. If compliance problems are excluded and if gonadotropin-independent sexual precocity is not present, the dose of nafarelin may be increased to 1800 mcg/day administered as 600 mcg t.i.d.

DOSAGE AND ADMINISTRATION

ENDOMETRIOSIS

For the management of endometriosis, the recommended daily dose of nafarelin is 400 mcg. This is achieved by one spray (200 mcg) into one nostril in the morning and one spray into the other nostril in the evening. Treatment should be started between days 2 and 4 of the menstrual cycle.

In an occasional patient, the 400 mcg daily dose may not produce amenorrhea. For these patients with persistent regular menstruation after 2 months of treatment, the dose of nafarelin may be increased to 800 mcg daily. The 800 mcg dose is administered as one spray into each nostril in the morning (a total of two sprays) and again in the evening.

The recommended duration of administration is six months. Retreatment cannot be recommended since safety data for retreatment are not available. If the symptoms of endometriosis recur after a course of therapy, and further treatment with nafarelin is contemplated, it is recommended that bone density be assessed before retreatment begins to ensure that values are within normal limits.

There appeared to be no significant effect of rhinitis, *i.e.,* nasal congestion, on the systemic bioavailability of nafarelin; however, if the use of a topical nasal decongestant is necessary during treatment with nafarelin, the decongestant should not be used until at least 2 hours following dosing with nafarelin .

Sneezing during or immediately after dosing with nafarelin should be avoided, if possible, since this may impair drug absorption.

At 400 mcg/day, a bottle of nafarelin provides a 30-day (about 60 sprays) supply. If the daily dose is increased, increase the supply to the patient to ensure uninterrupted treatment for the recommended duration of therapy.

CENTRAL PRECOCIOUS PUBERTY (CPP)

For the treatment of **central precocious puberty (CPP)**, the recommended daily dose of nafarelin is 1600 mcg. The dose can be increased to 1800 mcg daily if adequate suppression cannot be achieved at 1600 mcg/day.

The 1600 mcg dose is achieved by two sprays (400 mcg) into each nostril in the morning (4 sprays) and two sprays into each nostril in the evening (4 sprays), a total of 8 sprays per day. The 1800 mcg dose is achieved by 3 sprays (600 mcg) into alternating nostrils three times a day, a total of 9 sprays per day. The patient's head should be tilted back slightly, and 30 seconds should elapse between sprays.

If the prescribed therapy has been well tolerated by the patient, treatment of CPP with nafarelin should continue until resumption of puberty is desired.

There appeared to be no significant effect of rhinitis, *i.e.,* nasal congestion, on the systemic bioavailability of nafarelin; however, if the use of a nasal decongestant for rhinitis is necessary during treatment with nafarelin, the decongestant should not be used until at least 2 hours following dosing with nafarelin .

Sneezing during or immediately after dosing with nafarelin should be avoided, if possible, since this may impair drug absorption.

At 1600 mcg/day, a bottle of nafarelin provides about a 7-day supply (about 56 sprays). If the daily dose is increased, increase the supply to the patient to ensure uninterrupted treatment for the duration of therapy.

Store upright at room temperature. Avoid heat above 30°C (86°F). Protect from light. Protect from freezing.

PRODUCT LISTING - EQUIVALENTS NOT AVAILABLE

Spray - Nasal - 0.2 mg/Inh

8 ml $587.75 SYNAREL, Searle 00025-0166-08

Nafcillin Sodium (001851)

For related information, see the comparative table section in Appendix A.

Categories: Infection, staphylococcal, penicillinase-producing; FDA Approved 1970 Apr; Pregnancy Category B
Drug Classes: Antibiotics, penicillins
Brand Names: Nafcil; Nallpen; **Unipen**
Foreign Brand Availability: Vigopen (Philippines)
Cost of Therapy: $13.20 (Infection; Generic Injection; 0.5 g; 3 g/day; 10 day supply)

DESCRIPTION

Nafcillin sodium for injection is a semisynthetic penicillin derived from the penicillin nucleus, 6-aminopenicillanic acid. Chemically, nafcillin sodium is 6-(2-ethoxy-1-naphthamido)-penicillanic acid monohydrate. It is resistant to inactivation by the enzyme penicillinase (betalactamase).

Each gram of nafcillin is buffered with sodium citrate and contains approximately 2.9 mEq of sodium.

Its molecular formula is $C_{21}H_{21}N_2NaO_5S{\cdot}H_2O$ and the molecular weight is 454.47. [CAS-7177-50-6] Monosodium (*2S,5R,6R*)-6-(2-ethoxy-1-naphthamido)-3,3- dimethyl-7-oxo-4-thia-1-azabicyclo[3.2.0]heptane-2-carboxylate monohydrate.

Nafcillin sodium, equivalent to 500 mg, 1 gram or 2 grams of nafcillin, is a sterile mixture of nafcillin sodium monohydrate and sodium citrate intended for intravenous or intramuscular administration after reconstitution.

CLINICAL PHARMACOLOGY

PHARMACOKINETICS

In a study of 5 healthy adults administered a single 500 mg dose of nafcillin by intravenous injection over 7 minutes, the mean plasma concentration of the drug was approximately 30 µg/ml at 5 minutes after injection. The mean area under the plasma concentration-versus-time curve (AUC) for nafcillin in this study was 18.06 µg·h/ml.

The serum half-life of nafcillin administered by the intravenous route ranged from 33 to 61 minutes as measured in three separate studies. In contrast to the other penicillinase-resistant penicillins, only about 30% of nafcillin is excreted as unchanged drug in the urine of normal volunteers, and most within the first 6 hours. Nafcillin is primarily eliminated by nonrenal routes, namely hepatic inactivation and excretion in the bile.

Nafcillin binds to serum proteins, mainly albumin. The degree of protein binding reported for nafcillin is 89.9 ± 1.5%. Reported values vary with the method of study and the investigator.

The concurrent administration of probenecid with nafcillin increases and prolongs plasma concentration of nafcillin. Probenecid significantly reduces the total body of nafcillin with renal clearance being decreased to a greater extent than nonrenal clearance.

The penicillinase-resistant penicillins are widely distributed in various body fluids, including bile, pleural, amniotic and synovial fluids. With normal doses insignificant concentrations are found in the aqueous humor of the eye. High nafcillin CSF levels have been obtained in the presence of inflamed meninges.

Renal failure does not appreciably affect the serum half-life of nafcillin; therefore, no modification of the usual nafcillin dosage is necessary in renal failure with or without hemodialysis. Hemodialysis does not accelerate the rate of clearance of nafcillin from the blood.

A study which assessed the effects of cirrhosis and extrahepatic biliary obstruction in man demonstrated that the plasma clearance of nafcillin was significantly decreased in patients with hepatic dysfunction. In these patients with cirrhosis and extrahepatic obstruction, nafcillin excretion in the urine was significantly increased from about 30% to 50% of the administered dose, suggesting that renal disease superimposed on hepatic disease could further decrease nafcillin clearance.

MICROBIOLOGY

Penicillinase-resistant penicillins exert a bactericidal action against penicillin-susceptible microorganisms during the state of active multiplication. All penicillins inhibit the biosynthesis of the bacterial cell wall.

The drugs in this class are highly resistant to inactivation by staphylococcal penicillinase and are active against penicillinase-producing and nonpenicillinase-producing strains of *Staphylococcus aureus*. The penicillinase-resistant penicillins are active *in vitro* against a variety of other bacteria.

SUSCEPTIBILITY TESTING

Diffusion Techniques

Quantitative methods of susceptibility testing that require measurements of zone diameters or minimal inhibitory concentrations (MICs) give the most precise estimates of antibiotic susceptibility. One such procedure has been recommended for use with discs to test susceptibility to this class of drugs. Interpretations correlate diameters on the disc test with MIC values.

A penicillinase-resistant class disc may be used to determine microbial susceptibility to nafcillin.

TABLE 1 shows the interpretation of test results for penicillinase-resistant penicillins using the FDA Standard Disc Test Method (formerly Bauer-Kirby-Sherris-Turck method) of disc bacteriological susceptibility testing for staphylococci with a disc containing 5 µg of methicillin sodium. With this procedure, a report from a laboratory of "susceptible" indicates that the infecting organism is likely to respond to therapy. A report of "resistant" indicates that the infecting organism is not likely to respond to therapy. A report of "intermediate" susceptibility suggests that the organism might be susceptible if high doses of the antibiotic are used, or if the infection is confined to tissues and fluids (*e.g.,* urine) in which high antibiotic levels are attained.

In general, all staphylococci should be tested against the penicillin G disc and the methicillin disc. Routine methods of antibiotic susceptibility testing may fail to detect strains of organisms resistant to the penicillinase-resistant penicillins. For this reason, the use of large inocula and 48 hour incubation periods may be necessary to obtain accurate susceptibility studies with these antibiotics. Bacterial strains which are resistant to one of the penicillinase-resistant penicillins should be considered resistant to all of the drugs in the class.

TABLE 1 *Standardized Disc Test Method of Bacteriological Susceptibility Testing Using a Class Disc Containing 5 µg of Methicillin Sodium.*

	Zone Diameter (mm)
Susceptible	At least 14 mm
Intermediate	10-13 mm
Resistant	Less than 10 mm

INDICATIONS AND USAGE

Nafcillin sodium is indicated in the treatment of infections caused by penicillinase-producing staphylococci which have demonstrated susceptibility to the drug. Culture and susceptibility tests should be performed initially to determine the causative organism and its sensitivity to the drug (see CLINICAL PHARMACOLOGY, Susceptibility Testing).

Nafcillin sodium may be used to initiate therapy in suspected cases of resistant staphylococcal infections prior to the availability of laboratory test results. Nafcillin sodium should not be used in infections caused by organisms susceptible to penicillin G. If the susceptibility tests indicate that the infection is due to an organism other than a resistant staphylococcus, therapy should not be continued with nafcillin sodium.

CONTRAINDICATIONS

A history of a hypersensitivity (anaphylactic) reaction to any penicillin is a contraindication.

WARNINGS

SERIOUS AND OCCASIONALLY FATAL HYPERSENSITIVITY (ANAPHYLACTIC) REACTIONS HAVE BEEN REPORTED IN PATIENTS ON PENICILLIN THERAPY. THESE REACTIONS ARE MORE LIKELY TO OCCUR IN INDIVIDUALS WITH A HISTORY OF PENICILLIN HYPERSENSITIVITY AND/OR A HISTORY OF SENSITIVITY TO MULTIPLE ALLERGENS. THERE HAVE BEEN REPORTS OF INDIVIDUALS WITH A HISTORY OF PENICILLIN HYPERSENSITIVITY WHO HAVE EXPERIENCED SEVERE REACTIONS WHEN TREATED WITH CEPHALOSPORINS. BEFORE INITIATING THERAPY WITH NAFCILLIN SODIUM, CAREFUL INQUIRY SHOULD BE MADE CONCERNING PREVIOUS HYPERSENSITIVITY REACTIONS TO PENICILLINS, CEPHALOSPORINS OR OTHER ALLERGENS. IF AN ALLERGIC REACTION OCCURS, NAFCILLIN SODIUM SHOULD BE DISCONTINUED AND APPROPRIATE THERAPY INSTITUTED. **SERIOUS ANAPHYLACTIC REACTIONS REQUIRE IMMEDIATE EMERGENCY TREATMENT WITH EPINEPHRINE, OXYGEN, INTRAVENOUS STEROIDS AND AIRWAY MANAGEMENT, INCLUDING INTUBATION, SHOULD ALSO BE ADMINISTERED AS INDICATED. Pseudomembranous colitis has been reported with nearly all antibacterial agents, including nafcillin, and may range in severity from mild to life-threatening. Therefore, it is important to consider this diagnosis in patients who present with diarrhea subsequent to the administration of antibacterial agents.**

Treatment with antibacterial agents alters the normal flora of the colon and may permit overgrowth of clostridia. Studies indicate that a toxin produced by *Clostridium difficile* is one primary cause of "antibiotic-associated colitis."

After a diagnosis of pseudomembranous colitis has been established, therapeutic measures should be initiated. Mild cases of pseudomembranous colitis usually respond to drug discontinuation alone. In moderate to severe cases, consideration should be given to management with fluids and electrolytes, protein supplementation and treatment with an antibacterial drug clinically effective against *C. difficile* colitis.

PRECAUTIONS

GENERAL

Nafcillin sodium generally should not be administered to patients with a history of sensitivity to any penicillin.

Penicillin should be used with caution in individuals with histories of significant allergies and/or asthma. Whenever allergic reactions occur, penicillin should be withdrawn unless, in the opinion of the physician, the condition being treated is life-threatening and amenable only to penicillin therapy.

The use of antibiotics may result in overgrowth of nonsusceptible organisms. If new infections due to bacteria or fungi occur, the drug should be discontinued and appropriate measures taken.

The liver/biliary tract is the primary route of nafcillin clearance. Caution should be exercised when patients with concomitant hepatic insufficiency and renal dysfunction are treated with nafcillin. Serum levels should be measured and the dosage adjusted appropriately to avoid possible neurotoxin reactions associated with very high concentrations (see DOSAGE AND ADMINISTRATION).

LABORATORY TESTS

Bacteriologic studies to determine the causative organisms and their susceptibility to nafcillin should be performed (see CLINICAL PHARMACOLOGY, Microbiology). In the treatment of suspected staphylococcal infections, therapy should be changed to another active agent if culture tests fail to demonstrate the presence of staphylococci.

Periodic assessment of organ system function including renal, hepatic and hematopoietic should be made during prolonged therapy with nafcillin. White blood cells and differential cell counts should be obtained prior to initiation of therapy and periodically during therapy with nafcillin. Periodic urinalysis, blood urea nitrogen and creatinine determinations should be performed during therapy with nafcillin.

SGOT and SGPT values should be obtained periodically during therapy to monitor for possible liver function abnormalities.

DRUG/LABORATORY TEST INTERACTIONS

Nafcillin in the urine can cause a false-positive urine reaction for protein when the sulfosalicylic acid test is used, but not with the dipstick.

CARCINOGENESIS, MUTAGENESIS, AND IMPAIRMENT OF FERTILITY

No long animal studies have been conducted with nafcillin.

Studies on reproduction in rats and rabbits reveal no fetal or material abnormalities before conception and continuously during weaning (one generation).

PREGNANCY, TERATOGENIC EFFECTS, PREGNANCY CATEGORY B

Reproduction studies have been performed in the mouse with oral doses up to 20 times the human dose and orally in the rat at doses up to 40 times the human dose and have revealed no evidence of impaired fertility or harm to the rodent fetus due to nafcillin sodium. There are, however, no adequate or well-controlled studies in pregnant women. Because animal reproduction studies are not always predictive of human response, this drug should be used during pregnancy only if clearly needed.

NURSING MOTHERS

Penicillins are excreted in human milk. Caution should be exercised when penicillins are administered to a nursing woman.

PEDIATRIC USE

The liver/biliary tract is the principal route of nafcillin elimination. Because of immature hepatic and renal function in newborns, nafcillin excretion may be impaired with abnormally high serum levels resulting. Serum levels should be monitored and the dosage adjusted appropriately.[1,2] There are no approved neonatal or pediatric dosage regimens for intravenous nafcillin.

DRUG INTERACTIONS

Tetracycline, a bacteriostatic antibiotic, may antagonize the bactericidal effect of penicillin and concurrent use of these drugs should be avoided. Nafcillin in high dosage regimens, *i.e.*, 2 g every 4 hours, has been reported to decrease the effects of warfarin. When nafcillin and warfarin are used concomitantly, the prothrombin time should be closely monitored and the dose of warfarin adjusted as necessary. This effect may persist for up to 30 days after nafcillin has been discontinued.

Nafcillin when administered concomitantly with cyclosporine has been reported to result in subtherapeutic cyclosporine levels. The nafcillin-cyclosporine interaction was documented in a patient during two separate courses of therapy. When cyclosporine and nafcillin are used concomitantly in organ transplant patients, the cyclosporine levels should be monitored.

ADVERSE REACTIONS

BODY AS A WHOLE

The reported incidence of allergic reactions to penicillin ranges from 0.7-10% (see WARNINGS). Sensitization is usually the result of treatment but some individuals have had immediate reactions to penicillin when first treated. In such cases,it is thought that the patients may have had prior exposure to the drug via trace amounts present in milk or vaccines.

Two types of allergic reactions to penicillins are noted clinically, immediately and delayed.

Immediate reactions usually occur within 20 minutes of administration and range in severity from urticaria and pruritus to angioneurotic edema, laryngospasm, bronchospasm, hypotension, vascular collapse and death. Such immediate anaphylactic reactions are very rare (see WARNINGS) and usually occur after parenteral therapy but have occurred in patients receiving oral therapy. Another type of immediate reaction, an accelerated reaction, may occur between 20 minutes and 48 hours after administration and may include urticaria, pruritus and fever. Although laryngeal edema, laryngospasm and hypotension occasionally occur, fatality is uncommon.

Delayed allergic reactions to penicillin therapy usually occur after 48 hours and sometimes as late as 2-4 weeks after initiation of therapy. Manifestations of this type of reaction include serum-sickness-like symptoms (*i.e.*, fever, malaise, urticaria, myalgia, arthralgia, abdominal pain) and various skin rashes. Nausea, vomiting, diarrhea, stomatitis, black or hairy tongue, and other symptoms of gastrointestinal irritation may occur, especially during oral penicillin therapy.

LOCAL REACTIONS

Pain, swelling and inflammation at the injection site and phlebitis or thrombophlebitis have occurred with intravenous administration of nafcillin (see DOSAGE AND ADMINISTRATION).

NERVOUS SYSTEM REACTIONS

Neurotoxic reactions similar to those observed with penicillin G could occur with large intravenous doses of nafcillin, especially in patients with concomitant hepatic insufficiency and renal dysfunction (see PRECAUTIONS).

UROGENITAL REACTIONS

Renal tubular damage and interstitial nephritis have been associated infrequently with the administration of nafcillin. Manifestations of this reaction may include rash, fever, eosinophilia, hematuria, proteinuria and renal insufficiency.

GASTROINTESTINAL REACTIONS

Pseudomembranous colitis has been reported with the use of nafcillin. The onset of pseudomembranous colitis symptoms may occur during or after antibiotic treatment (see WARNINGS).

METABOLIC REACTIONS

Agranulocytosis, neutropenia and bone marrow depression have been associated with the use of nafcillin.

DOSAGE AND ADMINISTRATION

The usual IV dosage for adults is 500 mg every 4 hours. For severe infections, 1 g every 4 hours is recommended (see TABLE 2).

Administered slowly over at least 30-60 minutes to minimize the risk of vein irritation.

Bacteriologic studies to determine the causative organisms and their sensitivity to nafcillin should always be performed. Duration of therapy varies with the type and severity of infection as well as the overall condition of the patient; therefore, it should be determined by the clinical and bacteriologic responses of the patient. In severe staphylococcal infections, therapy with Nafcillin sodium for Injection should be continued for at least 14 days. Therapy should be continued for at least 48 hours after the patient has become afebrile, asymptomatic and cultures are negative. The treatment of endocarditis and osteomyelitis may require a longer term of therapy.

Concurrent administration of nafcillin and probenecid increases and prolongs serum penicillin levels. Probenecid decreases the apparent volume of distribution and slows the rate of excretion by competitively inhibiting renal tubular secretion of penicillin. Penicillin-probenecid therapy is generally limited to those infections where very high serum levels of penicillin are necessary. For intramuscular gluteal injections, care should be taken to avoid sciatic nerve injury. With intravenous administration, particularly in elderly patients, care should be taken because of the possibility of thrombophlebitis.

Dosage alterations are necessary for patients with renal dysfunction, including those on hemodialysis. Hemodialysis does not accelerate nafcillin clearance from the blood.

For patients with hepatic insufficiency and renal failure, measurement of nafcillin serum levels should be performed and the dosage adjusted accordingly.

Parenteral drug products should be inspected visually for particulate matter and discoloration prior to administration whenever solution and container permit.

Do not add supplementary medication to nafcillin sodium for injection.

TABLE 2 *Recommended Dosages for Nafcillin Sodium*

Adult	Infants and Children <40 kg (88 lbs)	Neonates
500 mg IM every 4-6 Hours IV every 4 hours 1 g IM or IV every 4 hours (severe infections)	25 mg/kg IM twice daily	10 mg/kg IM twice daily

PRODUCT LISTING - RATED THERAPEUTICALLY EQUIVALENT

Powder For Injection - Injectable - 1 Gm

1's	$3.84	GENERIC, Glaxosmithkline	00029-6372-40
1's	$6.10	UNIPEN, Wyeth-Ayerst Laboratories	00008-0751-02
1's	$6.55	UNIPEN, Wyeth-Ayerst Laboratories	00008-0751-15
1's	$31.60	GENERIC, Bristol-Myers Squibb	00015-7195-28
10's	$22.70	GENERIC, Bristol-Myers Squibb	00015-7225-20
10's	$26.00	GENERIC, Glaxosmithkline	00029-6372-22
10's	$26.80	GENERIC, Bristol-Myers Squibb	00015-7225-18
10's	$28.30	GENERIC, Bristol-Myers Squibb	00015-7225-99
10's	$31.56	GENERIC, Bristol-Myers Squibb	00015-7195-95
10's	$33.50	GENERIC, Bristol-Myers Squibb	00015-7225-89
10's	$36.22	GENERIC, Glaxosmithkline	00029-6372-07
10's	$63.03	GENERIC, Geneva Pharmaceuticals	00781-3744-46
10's	$82.70	GENERIC, Bristol-Myers Squibb	00015-7225-22
10's	$115.00	GENERIC, Bristol-Myers Squibb	00015-7225-21

Powder For Injection - Injectable - 2 Gm

1's	$11.83	UNIPEN, Wyeth-Ayerst Laboratories	00008-0751-03
1's	$12.28	UNIPEN, Wyeth-Ayerst Laboratories	00008-0751-13
1's	$44.00	GENERIC, Bristol-Myers Squibb	00015-7226-20
1's	$45.00	GENERIC, Bristol-Myers Squibb	00015-7226-18
1's	$56.00	GENERIC, Glaxosmithkline	00029-6374-40
1's	$66.00	GENERIC, Bristol-Myers Squibb	00015-7196-28
10's	$6.68	GENERIC, Glaxosmithkline	00029-6374-27
10's	$6.96	GENERIC, Glaxosmithkline	00029-6374-21
10's	$55.10	GENERIC, Bristol-Myers Squibb	00015-7226-99
10's	$56.30	GENERIC, Bristol-Myers Squibb	00015-7226-89
10's	$66.00	GENERIC, Bristol-Myers Squibb	00015-7196-95
10's	$66.50	GENERIC, Glaxosmithkline	00029-6374-07
10's	$160.20	GENERIC, Bristol-Myers Squibb	00015-7226-22
10's	$192.40	GENERIC, Bristol-Myers Squibb	00015-7226-21

Powder For Injection - Injectable - 10 Gm

1's	$141.70	GENERIC, Bristol-Myers Squibb	00015-7101-28
10's	$177.10	GENERIC, Bristol-Myers Squibb	00015-7101-98
10's	$275.28	GENERIC, Glaxosmithkline	00029-6376-21

Powder For Injection - Injectable - 500 mg

10's	$2.20	GENERIC, Glaxosmithkline	00029-6370-25
10's	$12.00	GENERIC, Bristol-Myers Squibb	00015-7224-99

PRODUCT LISTING - EQUIVALENTS NOT AVAILABLE

Solution - Intravenous - 1 Gm/50 ml

50 ml x 24	$541.75	GENERIC, Baxter I.V. Systems Division	00338-1017-41
100 ml x 12	$389.85	GENERIC, Baxter I.V. Systems Division	00338-1019-48

Naftifine Hydrochloride *(001852)*

Categories: Tinea corporis; Tinea cruris; Tinea pedis; Pregnancy Category B; FDA Approved 1988 Feb
Drug Classes: Antifungals, topical; Dermatologics
Brand Names: **Naftin**
Foreign Brand Availability: Exoderil (Austria; Bahrain; Bulgaria; Costa-Rica; Cyprus; Dominican-Republic; Egypt; El-Salvador; Germany; Greece; Guatemala; Honduras; Hong-Kong; Indonesia; Iran; Iraq; Israel; Jordan; Kuwait; Lebanon; Libya; Nicaragua; Oman; Panama; Qatar; Republic-of-Yemen; Russia; Saudi-Arabia; Syria; Taiwan; Turkey; United-Arab-Emirates)
Cost of Therapy: $24.95 (Tinea Pedis; Naftin Cream; 1%; 15 g; 1 application/day; variable day supply)

DESCRIPTION

Naftinine HCl cream 1% and gel 1% contains the synthetic, broad-spectrum, antifungal agent naftifine hydrochloride. Naftinine HCl cream 1% and gel 1% are for topical use only.
Chemical Name: (E)-N-Cinnamyl-N-methyl-1-naphthalenemethylamine hydrochloride.
Naftifine hydrochloride has an empirical formula of $C_{21}H_{21}N{\cdot}HCl$ and a molecular weight of 323.86.
Active Ingredient: Naftifine hydrochloride 1%.
Naftin Inactive Ingredients: *Cream:* benzyl alcohol, cetyl alcohol, cetyl esters wax, isopropyl myristate, polysorbate 60, purified water, sodium hydroxide, sorbitan monostearate, and stearyl alcohol. Hydrochloric acid may be added to adjust the pH. *Gel:* polysorbate 80, carbomer 934P, diisopropanolamine, edetate disodium, alcohol (52% v/v), and purified water.

CLINICAL PHARMACOLOGY

Naftifine hydrochloride is a synthetic, allylamine derivative. The following *in vitro* data are available, but their clinical significance is unknown. Naftifine hydrochloride has been shown to exhibit fungicidal activity *in vitro* against a broad spectrum of organisms including *Trichophyton rubrum, Trichophyton mentagrophytes, Trichophyton tonsurans, Epidermophyton floccosum,Microsporum canis, Microsporum audouini,* and *Microsporum gypseum;* and fungistatic activity against *Candida* species, including *Candida albicans*. Naftinine HCl cream 1% and gel 1% have only been shown to be clinically effective against the disease entities listed in INDICATIONS AND USAGE.

Although the exact mechanism of action against fungi is not known, naftifine hydrochloride appears to interfere with sterol biosynthesis by inhibiting the enzyme squalene 2,

3-epoxidase. This inhibition of enzyme activity results in decreased amounts of sterols, especially ergosterol, and a corresponding accumulation of squalene in the cells.

PHARMACOKINETICS

In vitro and *in vivo* bioavailability studies have demonstrated that naftifine penetrates the stratum corneum in sufficient concentration to inhibit the growth of dermatophytes.

Cream: Following a single topical application of 1% naftifine cream to the skin of healthy subjects, systemic absorption of naftifine was approximately 6% of the applied dose. Naftifine and/or its metabolites are excreted via the urine and feces with a half-life of approximately two to three days.

Gel: Following single topical applications of ^{3}H- labeled naftifine gel 1% to the skin of healthy subjects, up to 4.2% of the applied dose was absorbed. Naftifine and/or its metabolites are excreted via the urine and feces with a half-life of approximately two to three days.

INDICATIONS AND USAGE

Naftinine HCl cream 1% and gel 1% are indicated for the topical application of tinea pedis, tinea cruris and tinea corporis caused by the organisms *Trichophyton rubrum, Trichophyton mentagrophytes, Trichophyton tonsurans** and *Epidermophytonfloccosum.**

*Efficacy for this organism in this organ system was studied in fewer than 10 infections.

CONTRAINDICATIONS

Naftinine HCl cream 1% and gel 1% are contraindicated in individuals who have shown hypersensitivity to any of its components.

WARNINGS

Naftinine HCl cream 1% and gel 1% are for topical use only and not for ophthalmic use.

PRECAUTIONS

General: Naftinine HCl are for external use only. If irritation or sensitivity develops with the use of naftinine HCl cream 1% or gel 1%, treatment should be discontinued and appropriate therapy instituted. Diagnosis of the disease should be confirmed either by direct microscopic examination of a mounting of infected tissue in a solution of potassium hydroxide or by culture on an appropriate medium.

Information for the Patient: The patient should be told to:

1. Avoid the use of occlusive dressings or wrappings unless otherwise directed by the physician.
2. Keep Naftinine HCl cream 1% and gel 1% away from the eyes, nose, mouth and other mucous membranes.

Carcinogenesis, Mutagenesis, and Impairment of Fertility: Long-term studies to evaluate the carcinogenic potential of naftinine HCl cream 1% and gel 1% have not been performed. *In vitro* and animal studies have not demonstrated any mutagenic effect or effect on fertility.

Pregnancy, Teratogenic Effects, Pregnancy Category B Reproduction studies have not been performed in rats and rabbits (via oral administration) at doses 150 times or more the topical human dose and have revealed no evidence of impaired fertility or harm to the fetus due to naftifine. There are, however, no adequate and well-controlled studies in pregnant women. Because animal reproduction studies are not always predictive of human response, the drug should be used during pregnancy only if clearly needed.

Nursing Mothers: It is not known whether this drug is excreted in human milk. Because many drugs are excreted in human milk, caution should be exercised when naftinine HCl cream 1% and gel 1% is administered to a nursing woman.

Pediatric Use: Safety and effectiveness in children have not been established.

ADVERSE REACTIONS

Cream: During clinical trials with naftin cream 1%, the incidence of adverse reactions was as follows: burning/stinging (6%), dryness (3%), erythema (2%), itching (2%), local irritation (2%).

Gel: During clinical trials with naftinine gel 1%, the incidence of adverse reactions was as follows: burning/stinging (5.0%), itching (1.0%), erythema (0.5%), rash (0.5%), skin tenderness (0.5%).

DOSAGE AND ADMINISTRATION

Cream: A sufficient quantity of naftinine cream 1% should be gently massaged into the affected and surrounding skin areas once a day. The hands should be washed after application.

If no clinical improvement is seen after four weeks of treatment with naftinine cream 1%, the patient should be re-evaluated.

Note: Store below 30°C (86°F).

Gel: A sufficient quantity of naftinine gel 1% should be gently massaged into the affected and surrounding skin areas twice a day, in the morning and evening. The hands should be washed after application.

If no clinical improvement is seen after four weeks of treatment with naftinine gel 1%, the patient should be re-evaluated.

Note: Store at room temperature.

PRODUCT LISTING - EQUIVALENTS NOT AVAILABLE

Cream - Topical - 1%			
15 gm	$24.95	NAFTIN, Merz Pharmaceuticals	00259-4126-15
15 gm x 4	$65.60	NAFTIN, Merz Pharmaceuticals	00259-4126-04
30 gm	$29.36	NAFTIN, Southwood Pharmaceuticals Inc	58016-3288-01
30 gm	$41.62	NAFTIN, Merz Pharmaceuticals	00259-4126-30
60 gm	$61.43	NAFTIN, Merz Pharmaceuticals	00259-4126-60
Gel - Topical - 1%			
20 gm	$33.31	NAFTIN, Merz Pharmaceuticals	00259-4770-20
40 gm	$57.12	NAFTIN, Merz Pharmaceuticals	00259-4770-40
60 gm	$66.92	NAFTIN, Merz Pharmaceuticals	00259-4770-60

Nalbuphine Hydrochloride *(001853)*

For related information, see the comparative table section in Appendix A.

Categories: Anesthesia, adjunct; Pain, moderate to severe; Pain, obstetrical; Pregnancy Category B; FDA Approved 1979 May
Drug Classes: Analgesics, narcotic agonist-antagonist
Brand Names: Nubain
Foreign Brand Availability: Bufigen (Mexico); Nalcryn SP (Mexico); Nubain SP (Mexico)
Cost of Therapy: $42.53 (Pain; Nubain Injection; 10 mg/ml; 1 ml; 4 injections/day; 7 day supply)
$31.92 (Pain; Generic Injection; 10 mg/ml; 1 ml; 4 injections/day; 7 day supply)
HCFA JCODE(S): J2300 per 10 mg IM, IV, SC

DESCRIPTION

Nalbuphine hydrochloride is a synthetic opioid agonist-antagonist analgesic of the phenanthrene series. It is chemically related to both the widely used opioid antagonist, naloxone, and the potent opioid analgesic, oxymorphone.

Nalbuphine hydrochloride is (-)-17-(cyclobutylmethyl)-4,5α-epoxymorphinan-3,6α, 14-triol hydrochloride.

Nubain is a sterile solution suitable for subcutaneous, intramuscular, or intravenous injection. Nalbuphine hydrochloride injection is available in two concentrations, 10 and 20 mg of nalbuphine hydrochloride per milliliter. Both strengths in 10 ml vials contain 0.94% odium citrate hydrous, 1.26% citric acid anhydrous, and 0.2% of a 9:1 mixture of methylparaben and propylparaben as preservatives; pH is adjusted, if necessary, to 3.5-3.7 with hydrochloric acid. The 10 mg/ml strength also contains 0.2% sodium chloride.

Nubain is also available in ampuls in a sterile, paraben-free formulation in two concentrations, 10 mg and 20 mg of nalbuphine hydrochloride per milliliter. One ml of each strength contains 0.94% sodium citrate hydrous, and 1.26% citric acid anhydrous; pH is adjusted, if necessary, to 3.5-3.7 with hydrochloric acid. The 10 mg/ml strength contains 0.2% sodium chloride.

CLINICAL PHARMACOLOGY

Nalbuphine HCl is a potent analgesic. Its analgesic potency is essentially equivalent to that of morphine on a milligram basis. Receptor studies show that nalbuphine HCl binds to mu, kappa, and delta receptors, but not to sigma receptors. Nalbuphine HCl is primarily a kappa agonist/partial mu antagonist analgesic.

The onset of action of nalbuphine HCl occurs within 2-3 minutes after IV administration, and in less than 15 minutes following SC or IM injection. The plasma half-life of nalbuphine is 5 hours and in clinical studies the duration of analgesic activity has been reported to range from 3-6 hours.

The opioid antagonist activity of nalbuphine is one-fourth as potent as nalorphine and 10 times that of pentazocine.

Nalbuphine HCl may produce the same degree of respiratory depression as equianalgesic doses of morphine. However, nalbuphine HCl exhibits a ceiling effect such that increases in dose greater than 30 mg do not produce further respiratory depression.

Nalbuphine HCl by itself has potent opioid antagonist activity at doses equal to or lower than its analgesic dose. When administered following or concurrent with mu agonist opioid analgesics (*e.g.*, morphine, oxymorphone, fentanyl), nalbuphine HCl may partially reverse or block opioid-induced respiratory depression from the mu agonist analgesic. Nalbuphine HCl may precipitate withdrawal in patients dependent on opioid drugs. Nalbuphine HCl should be used with caution in patients who have been receiving mu opioid analgesics on a regular basis.

INDICATIONS AND USAGE

Nalbuphine HCl is indicated for the relief of moderate to severe pain. Nalbuphine HCl can also be used as a supplement to balanced anesthesia, for preoperative and postoperative analgesia, and for obstetrical analgesia during labor and delivery.

CONTRAINDICATIONS

Nubain should not be administered to patients who are hypersensitive to nalbuphine HCl, or to any of the other ingredients in Nubain.

WARNINGS

Nalbuphine HCl should be administered as a supplement to general anesthesia only by persons specifically trained in the use of intravenous anesthetics and management of the respiratory effects of potent opioids.

Naloxone, resuscitative and intubation equipment and oxygen should be readily available.

DRUG ABUSE

Caution should be observed in prescribing nalbuphine HCl for emotionally unstable patients, or for individuals with a history of opioid abuse. Such patients should be closely supervised when long-term therapy is contemplated.

USE IN AMBULATORY PATIENTS

Nalbuphine HCl may impair the mental or physical abilities required for the performance of potentially dangerous tasks such as driving a car or operating machinery. Therefore, nalbuphine HCl should be administered with caution to ambulatory patients who should be warned to avoid such hazards.

USE IN EMERGENCY PROCEDURES

Maintain patient under observation until recovered from nalbuphine HCl effects that would affect driving or other potentially dangerous tasks.

USE IN PREGNANCY (OTHER THAN LABOR)

Safe use of nalbuphine HCl in pregnancy has not been established. Although animal reproductive studies have not revealed teratogenic or embryotoxic effects, nalbuphine should be administered to pregnant women only if clearly needed.

USE DURING LABOR AND DELIVERY

The placental transfer of nalbuphine is high, rapid, and variable with a maternal to fetal ratio ranging from 1:0.37 to 1:6. Fetal and neonatal adverse effects that have been reported following the administration of nalbuphine to the mother during labor include fetal bradycardia, respiratory depression at birth, apnea, cyanosis and hypotonia. Maternal administration of naloxone during labor has normalized these effects in some cases. Severe and prolonged fetal bradycardia has been reported. Permanent neurological damage attributed to fetal bradycardia has occurred. A sinusoidal fetal heart rate pattern associated with the use of nalbuphine has also been reported. Nalbuphine HCl should be used with caution in women during labor and delivery, and newborns should be monitored for respiratory depression, apnea, bradycardia, and arrhythmias if nalbuphine HCl has been used.

HEAD INJURY AND INCREASED INTRACRANIAL PRESSURE

The possible respiratory depressant effects and the potential of potent analgesics to elevate cerebrospinal fluid pressure (resulting from vasodilation following CO_2 retention) may be markedly exaggerated in the presence of head injury, intracranial lesions or a pre-existing increase in intracranial pressure. Furthermore, potent analgesics can produce effects which may obscure the clinical course of patients with head injuries. Therefore, nalbuphine HCl injection should be used in these circumstances only when essential, and then should be administered with extreme caution.

INTERACTION WITH OTHER CENTRAL NERVOUS SYSTEM DEPRESSANTS

Although nalbuphine HCl possesses opioid antagonist activity, there is evidence that in nondependent patients it will not antagonize an opioid analgesic administered just before, concurrently, or just after an injection of nalbuphine HCl. Therefore, patients receiving an opioid analgesic, general anesthetics, phenothiazines, or other tranquilizers, sedatives, hypnotics, or other CNS depressants (including alcohol) concomitantly with nalbuphine HCl may exhibit an additive effect. When such combined therapy is contemplated, the dose of one or both agents should be reduced.

PRECAUTIONS

GENERAL

Impaired Respiration

At the usual adult dose of 10 mg/70 kg, nalbuphine HCl causes some respiratory depression approximately equal to that produced by equal doses of morphine. However, in contrast to morphine, respiratory depression is not appreciably increased with higher doses of nalbuphine HCl. Respiratory depression induced by nalbuphine HCl can be reversed by naloxone HCl when indicated. Nalbuphine HCl should be administered with caution at low doses to patients with impaired respiration (*e.g.*, from other medication, uremia, bronchial asthma, severe infection, cyanosis or respiratory obstructions).

Impaired Renal or Hepatic Function

Because nalbuphine HCl is metabolized in the liver and excreted by the kidneys, nalbuphine HCl should be used with caution in patients with renal or liver dysfunction and administered in reduced amounts.

Myocardial Infarction

As with all potent analgesics, nalbuphine HCl should be used with caution in patients with myocardial infarction who have nausea or vomiting.

Biliary Tract Surgery

As with all opioid analgesics, nalbuphine HCl should be used with caution in patients about to undergo surgery of the biliary tract since it may cause spasm of the sphincter of Oddi.

Cardiovascular System

During evaluation of nalbuphine HCl in anesthesia, a higher incidence of bradycardia has been reported in patients who did not receive atropine pre-operatively.

INFORMATION FOR THE PATIENT

Patients should be advised of the following information:

- Nalbuphine HCl is associated with sedation and may impair mental and physical abilities required for the performance of potentially dangerous tasks such as driving a car or operating machinery.
- Nalbuphine HCl is to be used as prescribed by a physician. Dose or frequency should not be increased without first consulting with a physician since nalbuphine HCl may cause psychological or physical dependence.
- The use of nalbuphine HCl with other opioids can cause signs and symptoms of withdrawal.
- Abrupt discontinuation of nalbuphine HCl after prolonged usage may cause signs and symptoms of withdrawal.

LABORATORY TESTS

Nalbuphine HCl may interfere with enzymatic methods for the detection of opioids depending on the specificity/sensitivity of the test. Please consult the test manufacturer for specific details.

CARCINOGENESIS, MUTAGENESIS, AND IMPAIRMENT OF FERTILITY

No evidence of carcinogenicity was found in a 24 month carcinogenicity study in rats and an 18 month carcinogenicity study in mice at oral doses as high as the equivalent of approximately 3 times the maximum recommended therapeutic dose.

No evidence of a mutagenic/genotoxic potential to nalbuphine HCl was found in the Ames, Chinese Hamster Ovary HGPRT, and Sister Chromatid Exchange, mouse micronucleus, and rat bone marrow cytogenicity assays. Nalbuphine induced an increased frequency of mutation in mouse lymphoma cells.

PREGNANCY CATEGORY B

Teratogenic Effects

Reproduction studies have been performed in rabbits and in rats at dosages as high as approximately 14 and 31 times respectively the maximum recommended daily dose and revealed no evidence of impaired fertility or harm to the fetus due to nalbuphine HCl. There are, however, no adequate and well-controlled studies in pregnant women. Because animal reproduction studies are not always predictive of human response, this drug should be used during pregnancy only if clearly needed (see WARNINGS).

Nonteratogenic Effects

Neonatal body weight and survival was reduced when nalbuphine HCl was subcutaneously administered to female rats prior to mating and throughout gestation and lactation or to pregnant rats during the last third of gestation and throughout lactation at doses approximately 8-17 times the maximum recommended therapeutic dose. The clinical significance of this effect is unknown.

USE DURING LABOR AND DELIVERY

See WARNINGS.

NURSING MOTHERS

Limited data suggest that nalbuphine HCl is excreted in maternal milk but only in a small amount (less than 1% of the administered dose) and with a clinically insignificant effect. Caution should be exercised when nalbuphine HCl is administered to a nursing woman.

PEDIATRIC USE

Safety and effectiveness in pediatric patients below the age of 18 years have not been established.

ADVERSE REACTIONS

The most frequent adverse reaction in 1066 patients treated with nalbuphine HCl was sedation 381 (36%).

Less frequent reactions were: sweaty/clammy 99 (9%), nausea/vomiting 68 (6%), dizziness/vertigo 58 (5%), dry mouth 44 (4%), and headache 27 (3%).

Other adverse reactions which occurred (reported incidence of 1% or less) were:

CNS Effects: Nervousness, depression, restlessness, crying, euphoria, floating, hostility, unusual dreams, confusion, faintness, hallucinations, dysphoria, feeling of heaviness, numbness, tingling, unreality. The incidence of psychotomimetic effects, such as unreality, depersonalization, delusions, dysphoria and hallucinations has been shown to be less than that which occurs with pentazocine.

Cardiovascular: Hypertension, hypotension, bradycardia, tachycardia.

Gastrointestinal: Cramps, dyspepsia, bitter taste.

Respiration: Depression, dyspnea, asthma.

Dermatologic: Itching, burning, urticaria.

Miscellaneous: Speech difficulty, urinary urgency, blurred vision, flushing and warmth.

Allergic Reactions: Anaphylactic/anaphylactoid and other serious hypersensitivity reactions have been reported following the use of nalbuphine and may require immediate, supportive medical treatment. These reactions may include shock, respiratory distress, respiratory arrest, bradycardia, cardiac arrest, hypotension, or laryngeal edema. Other allergic-type reactions reported include stridor, bronchospasm, wheezing, edema, rash, pruritus, nausea, vomiting, diaphoresis, weakness, and shakiness.

Post-Marketing: Other reports include pulmonary edema, agitation and injection site reactions such as pain, swelling, redness, burning, and hot sensations.

DOSAGE AND ADMINISTRATION

The usual recommended adult dose is 10 mg for a 70 kg individual, administered subcutaneously, intramuscularly or intravenously; this dose may be repeated every 3-6 hours as necessary. Dosage should be adjusted according to the severity of the pain, physical status of the patient, and other medications which the patient may be receiving. (See WARNINGS, Interaction With Other Central Nervous System Depressants.) In non-tolerant individuals, the recommended single maximum dose is 20 mg, with a maximum total daily dose of 160 mg.

The use of nalbuphine HCl as a supplement to balanced anesthesia requires larger doses than those recommended for analgesia. Induction doses of nalbuphine HCl range from 0.3 to 3.0 mg/kg intravenously to be administered over a 10-15 minute period with maintenance doses of 0.25-0.50 mg/kg in single intravenous administrations as required. The use of nalbuphine HCl may be followed by respiratory depression which can be reversed with the opioid antagonist naloxone HCl.

Nalbuphine HCl is physically incompatible with nafcillin and keterolac.

PATIENTS DEPENDENT ON OPIOIDS

Patients who have been taking opioids chronically may experience withdrawal symptoms upon the administration of nalbuphine HCl. If unduly troublesome, opioid withdrawal symptoms can be controlled by the slow IV administration of small increments of morphine, until relief occurs. If the previous analgesic was morphine, meperidine, codeine, or other opioid with similar duration of activity, one-fourth of the anticipated dose of nalbuphine HCl can be administered initially and the patient observed for signs of withdrawal, *i.e.*, abdominal cramps, nausea and vomiting, lacrimation, rhinorrhea, anxiety, restlessness, elevation of temperature or piloerection. If untoward symptoms do not occur, progressively larger doses may be tried at appropriate intervals until the desired level of analgesia is obtained with nalbuphine HCl.

HOW SUPPLIED

Nubain injection for IM, SC, or IV use is a sterile solution available in:

Sulfite-free 10 mg/ml, 10 ml multiple dose vials.

Sulfite/paraben-free 10 mg/ml, 1 ml ampuls.

Sulfite-free 20 mg/ml, 10 ml multiple dose vials.
Sulfite/paraben-free 20 mg/ml, 1 ml ampuls.

STORAGE

Store at 25°C (77°F); excursions permitted to 15-30°C (59-86°F). Protect from excessive light. Store in carton until contents have been used.

Parenteral drug products should be inspected visually for particulate matter and discoloration prior to administration whenever solution and container permit.

PRODUCT LISTING - RATED THERAPEUTICALLY EQUIVALENT

Solution - Injectable - 10 mg/ml			
1 ml	$2.30	NUBAIN, Physicians Total Care	54868-3686-01
1 ml x 10	$11.40	GENERIC, Abbott Pharmaceutical	00074-1463-01
1 ml x 10	$15.19	NUBAIN, Dupont Pharmaceuticals	54569-2101-00
1 ml x 10	$15.20	NUBAIN, Dupont Pharmaceuticals	00590-0432-10
1 ml x 10	$16.00	NUBAIN, Dupont Pharmaceuticals	63481-0432-10
1 ml x 10	$17.74	NUBAIN, Physicians Total Care	54868-3686-00
10 ml	$24.31	NUBAIN, Dupont Pharmaceuticals	54569-3080-00
10 ml	$25.50	NUBAIN, Endo Laboratories Llc	63481-0508-05
10 ml	$28.05	NUBAIN, Physicians Total Care	54868-3471-00
10 ml x 25	$196.53	GENERIC, Abbott Pharmaceutical	00074-1464-01
Solution - Injectable - 20 mg/ml			
1 ml x 10	$14.61	GENERIC, Abbott Pharmaceutical	00074-1465-01
1 ml x 10	$22.80	NUBAIN, Dupont Pharmaceuticals	00590-0433-10
1 ml x 10	$22.81	NUBAIN, Allscripts Pharmaceutical Company	54569-4819-00
1 ml x 10	$24.00	NUBAIN, Endo Laboratories Llc	63481-0433-10
10 ml	$39.69	NUBAIN, Endo Laboratories Llc	63481-0509-05
10 ml x 25	$317.95	GENERIC, Abbott Pharmaceutical	00074-1467-01

PRODUCT LISTING - EQUIVALENTS NOT AVAILABLE

Solution - Injectable - 10 mg/ml			
10 ml	$14.43	GENERIC, Moore, H.L. Drug Exchange Inc	00839-7536-30
10 ml	$20.40	GENERIC, Southwood Pharmaceuticals Inc	58016-9384-01
Solution - Injectable - 20 mg/ml			
10 ml	$19.16	GENERIC, Moore, H.L. Drug Exchange Inc	00839-7537-30

Naloxone Hydrochloride (001855)

Categories: Diagnosis, opiate intoxication; Overdose, opiate; Poisoning, opiate; Pregnancy Category B; FDA Approved 1971 Apr; WHO Formulary
Drug Classes: Antagonists, narcotic; Antidotes
Brand Names: Narcan
Foreign Brand Availability: Mapin (Hong-Kong); Nalone (France); Naloxon (Germany); Narcan Neonatal (France); Narcanti (Austria; Bulgaria; Czech-Republic; Denmark; Finland; Germany; Hungary; Mexico; Norway; Sweden); Narcotan (India); Naxone (Bahrain; Cyprus; Egypt; Iran; Iraq; Jordan; Kuwait; Lebanon; Libya; Oman; Qatar; Republic-of-Yemen; Saudi-Arabia; Syria; United-Arab-Emirates); Zynox (South-Africa)
HCFA JCODE(S): J2310 per 1 mg IM, IV, SC

DESCRIPTION

Naloxone hydrochloride, a narcotic antagonist, is a synthetic congener of oxymorphone. In structure it differs from oxymorphone in that the methyl group on the nitrogen atom is replaced by an allyl group.

The molecular formula is $C_{19}H_{21}NO_4 \cdot HCl$.

The chemical name is (-)-17-allyl-4-5α-epoxy-3,14 - dihydroxymorphinan-6-one-hydrochloride.

Naloxone hydrochloride occurs as a white to slightly off-white powder, and is soluble in water, in dilute acids, and in strong alkali; slightly soluble in alcohol; practically insoluble in ether and in chloroform.

Naloxone hydrochloride injection is available as a sterile solution for intravenous, intramuscular, subcutaneous administration in three concentrations, 0.02, 0.4, and 1.0 mg of naloxone hydrochloride per ml. One ml of the 0.02 and 0.4 mg strengths contains 8.6 mg of sodium chloride. One ml of the 1.0 mg strength contains 8.35 mg of sodium chloride. One ml of the 0.4 and 1.0 mg strengths also contains 2.0 mg of methylparaben and propylparaben as preservatives in a ratio of 9:1. pH is adjusted to 3.5 ± 0.5 with hydrochloric acid.

Naloxone hydrochloride injection is also available in a paraben-free formulation in three concentrations; 0.02, 0.4, and 1.0 mg of naloxone hydrochloride per ml. One ml of each strength contains 9.0 mg of sodium chloride. pH is adjusted to 3.5 ± 0.5 with hydrochloric acid.

STORAGE

Protect from light. Store at controlled room temperature 15-30°C (59-86°F).

CLINICAL PHARMACOLOGY

Naloxone HCl prevents or reverses the effects of opioids including respiratory depression, sedation and hypotension. Also, it can reverse the psychotomimetic and dysphoric effects of agonist-antagonists such as pentazocine.

Naloxone HCl is an essentially pure narcotic antagonist, *i.e.*, it does not possess the "agonistic" or morphine-like properties characteristic of other narcotic antagonists; naloxone HCl does not produce respiratory depression, psychotomimetic effects or pupillary constriction. In the absence of narcotics or agonistic effects of other narcotic antagonists, it exhibits essentially no pharmacologic activity.

Naloxone HCl has not been shown to produce tolerance nor to cause physical or psychological dependence.

In the presence of physical dependence on narcotics, naloxone will produce withdrawal symptoms.

MECHANISM OF ACTION

While the mechanism of action of naloxone is not fully understood, the preponderance of evidence suggests that naloxone antagonizes the opioid effects by competing for the same receptor sites.

When naloxone HCl injection is administered intravenously, the onset of action is generally apparent within 2 minutes; the onset of action is only slightly less rapid when it is administered subcutaneously or intramuscularly. The duration of action is dependent upon the dose and route of administration of naloxone HCl. Intramuscular administration produces a more prolonged effect than intravenous administration. The requirement for repeat doses of naloxone HCl, however, will also be dependent upon the amount, type and route of administration of the narcotic being antagonized.

Following parenteral administration, naloxone HCl is rapidly distributed in the body. It is metabolized in the liver, primarily by glucuronide conjugation and excreted in urine. In one study, the serum half-life in adults ranged from 30-81 minutes (mean 64 ± 12 minutes). In a neonatal study, the mean plasma half-life was observed to be 3.1 ± 0.5 hours.

INDICATIONS AND USAGE

Naloxone HCl injection is indicated for the complete or partial reversal of narcotic depression, including respiratory depression, induced by opioids including natural and synthetic narcotics, propoxyphene, methadone and the narcotic-antagonist analgesics: nalbuphine, pentazocine and butorphanol. Naloxone HCl Injection is also indicated for the diagnosis of suspected acute opioid overdosage.

NON-FDA APPROVED INDICATIONS

Although not FDA approved, naloxone may be useful as adjunctive therapy to increase blood pressure in the management of septic shock. This pressor response lasts for up to several hours but has not been shown to improve survival. Patients who responded received naloxone early in the course of treatment. Optimal dosages have not been established. Naloxone has also been used for relief of cholestatic pruritus, in senile dementia to improve cognitive functions, hemorrhagic shock, hemiplegic migraine, Tourette's syndrome, and to improve neurologic function in stroke and spinal cord injury victims. Some study data suggest that naloxone has antipsychotic properties and may be useful in treatment of non-opiate overdoses such as clonidine, nitrous oxide, valproic acid, benzodiazepines, phenothiazines, barbiturates and ethanol. Results, however, have been mixed or negative.

CONTRAINDICATIONS

Naloxone HCl injection is contraindicated in patients known to be hypersensitive to it.

WARNINGS

Naloxone HCl injection should be administered cautiously to persons including newborns of mothers who are known or suspected to be physically dependent on opioids. In such cases, an abrupt and complete reversal of narcotic effects may precipitate an acute abstinence syndrome.

The patient who has satisfactorily responded to naloxone should be kept under continued surveillance and repeated doses should be administered, as necessary, since the duration of action of some narcotics may exceed that of naloxone.

Naloxone is not effective against respiratory depression due to non-opioid drugs. Reversal of buprenorpinephrine-induced respiratory depression may be incomplete. If an incomplete response occurs, respirations should be mechanically assisted.

PRECAUTIONS

In addition to naloxone HCl injection, other resuscitative measures, such as maintenance of a free airway, artificial ventilation, cardiac massage and vasopressor agents should be available and employed, when necessary, to counteract acute narcotic poisoning.

Several instances of hypotension, hypertension, ventricular tachycardia and fibrillation, and pulmonary edema have been reported. These have occurred in postoperative patients most of whom had pre-existing cardiovascular disorders or received other drugs which may have similar adverse cardiovascular effects. Although a direct cause and effect relationship has not been established, naloxone HCl injection should be used with caution in patients with pre-existing cardiac disease or patients who have received potentially cardiotoxic drugs.

CARCINOGENESIS, MUTAGENESIS, AND IMPAIRMENT OF FERTILITY

Carcinogenicity and mutagenicity studies have not been performed with naloxone HCl. Reproductive studies in mice and rats demonstrated no impairment of fertility.

PREGNANCY CATEGORY B

Reproduction studies have been performed in mice and rats at doses up to 1000 times the human dose and have revealed no evidence of impaired fertility or harm to the fetus due to naloxone HCl. There are, however, no adequate and well-controlled studies in pregnant women. Because animal reproduction studies are not always predictive of human response, this drug should be used during pregnancy only if clearly needed.

NURSING MOTHERS

It is not known whether this drug is excreted in human milk. Because many drugs are excreted in human milk, caution should be exercised when naloxone HCl injection is administered to a nursing woman.

ADVERSE REACTIONS

Abrupt reversal of narcotic depression may result in nausea, vomiting, sweating, tachycardia, increased blood pressure and tremulousness. In postoperative patients, larger than necessary dosage of naloxone HCl may result in significant reversal of analgesia, and in excitement. Hypotension, hypertension, ventricular tachycardia and fibrillation, and pulmonary edema have been associated with the use of naloxone HCl postoperatively (see PRECAUTIONS and DOSAGE AND ADMINISTRATION, Usage in Adults, Postoperative Narcotic Depression).

DOSAGE AND ADMINISTRATION

Naloxone HCl injection may be administered intravenously, intramuscularly, or subcutaneously. The most rapid onset of action is achieved by intravenous administration, and this route is recommended in emergency situations.

Since the duration of action of some narcotics may exceed that of naloxone, the patient should be kept under continued surveillance and repeated doses of naloxone HCl should be administered, as necessary.

INTRAVENOUS INFUSION

Naloxone HCl injection may be diluted for intravenous infusion in 0.9% sodium chloride injection or 5% dextrose injection. The addition of 2 mg of naloxone HCl in 500 ml of either solution provides a concentration of 0.004 mg/ml. Mixtures should be used within 24 hours. After 24 hours, the remaining unused solution must be discarded. The rate of administration should be titrated in accordance with the patient's response.

Parenteral drug products should be inspected visually for particulate matter and discoloration prior to administration whenever solution and container permit. Naloxone HCl injection should not be mixed with preparations containing bisulfite, metabisulfite, long-chain or high molecular weight anions, or any solution having an alkaline pH. No drug or chemical agent should be added to naloxone HCl injection unless its effect on the chemical and physical stability of the solution has first been established.

USAGE IN ADULTS

Narcotic Overdose — Known or Suspected

An initial dose of 0.4 mg to 2 mg of naloxone HCl may be administered intravenously. If the desired degree of counteraction and improvement in respiratory functions is not obtained, it may be repeated at 2 to 3 minute intervals. If no response is observed after 10 mg of naloxone HCl have been administered, the diagnosis of narcotic induced or partial narcotic induced toxicity should be questioned. Intramuscular or subcutaneous administration may be necessary if the intravenous route is not available.

Postoperative Narcotic Depression

For the partial reversal of narcotic depression following the use of narcotics during surgery, smaller doses of naloxone HCl are usually sufficient. The dose of naloxone HCl should be titrated according to the patient's response. For the initial reversal of respiratory depression, naloxone HCl injection should be injected in increments of 0.1-0.2 mg intravenously at 2-3 minute intervals to the desired degree of reversal, *i.e.,* adequate ventilation and alertness without significant pain or discomfort. Larger than necessary dosage of naloxone HCl may result in significant reversal of analgesia and increase in blood pressure. Similarly, too rapid reversal may induce nausea, vomiting, sweating or circulatory stress.

Repeat doses of naloxone HCl may be required within 1-2 hour intervals depending upon the amount, type (*i.e.,* short or long acting) and time interval since last administration of narcotic. Supplemental intramuscular doses have been shown to produce a longer lasting effect.

USAGE IN CHILDREN

Narcotic Overdose — Known or Suspected

The usual initial dose in children is 0.01 mg/kg body weight given intravenously. If this dose does not result in the desired degree of clinical improvement, a subsequent dose of 0.1 mg/kg body weight may be administered. If an intravenous route of administration is not available, naloxone HCl injection may be administered intramuscularly or subcutaneously in divided doses. If necessary, naloxone HCl injection can be diluted with sterile water for injection.

Postoperative Narcotic Depression

Follow the recommendations and cautions under Usage in Adults; Postoperative Narcotic Depression. For the initial reversal of respiratory depression, naloxone HCl should be injected in increments of 0.005 mg to 0.01 mg intravenously at 2-3 minute intervals to the desired degree of reversal.

USAGE IN NEONATES

Narcotic Induced Depression

The usual initial dose is 0.01 mg/kg body weight administered IV, IM or SC. This dose may be repeated in accordance with adult administration guidelines for postoperative narcotic depression.

When using naloxone HCl injection in neonates, a product containing 0.02 mg/ml should be used.

PRODUCT LISTING - RATED THERAPEUTICALLY EQUIVALENT

Solution - Injectable - 0.02 mg/ml

Size	Price	Product	NDC
2 ml x 10	$11.38	GENERIC, Abbott Pharmaceutical	00074-1216-01
2 ml x 10	$14.01	GENERIC, Abbott Pharmaceutical	00074-1211-01
2 ml x 10	$16.88	GENERIC, Astra-Zeneca Pharmaceuticals	00186-1252-13
2 ml x 10	$20.50	NARCAN, Endo Laboratories Llc	63481-0359-10
2 ml x 10	$26.93	GENERIC, Abbott Pharmaceutical	00074-1790-02
2 ml x 10	$29.20	GENERIC, Sanofi Winthrop Pharmaceuticals	00024-1314-27

Solution - Injectable - 0.4 mg/ml

Size	Price	Product	NDC
1 ml x 10	$5.00	GENERIC, Baxter Pharmaceutical Products, Inc	10019-0039-68
1 ml x 10	$13.30	GENERIC, Abbott Pharmaceutical	00074-1212-01
1 ml x 10	$14.49	GENERIC, Abbott Pharmaceutical	00074-1215-01
1 ml x 10	$15.32	GENERIC, Abbott Pharmaceutical	00074-1782-01
1 ml x 10	$17.46	GENERIC, Abbott Pharmaceutical	00074-1782-21
1 ml x 10	$22.43	GENERIC, Physicians Total Care	54868-2062-00
1 ml x 10	$32.50	NARCAN, Dupont Pharmaceuticals	00590-0358-10
1 ml x 10	$34.10	NARCAN, Endo Laboratories Llc	63481-0358-10
1 ml x 10	$37.19	NARCAN, Physicians Total Care	54868-0114-00
1 ml x 25	$75.00	GENERIC, Abbott Pharmaceutical	00074-1213-01
10 ml	$41.88	NARCAN, Endo Laboratories Llc	63481-0365-05
10 ml x 5	$17.35	GENERIC, Astra-Zeneca Pharmaceuticals	00186-1254-12
10 ml x 25	$86.09	GENERIC, Abbott Pharmaceutical	00074-1219-01

Solution - Injectable - 1 mg/ml

Size	Price	Product	NDC
1 ml x 10	$34.10	GENERIC, Astra-Zeneca Pharmaceuticals	00186-1251-13
2 ml	$529.75	GENERIC, Celltech Pharmaceuticals Inc	00548-1469-00
2 ml x 10	$47.50	NARCAN, Dupont Pharmaceuticals	00590-0377-10
2 ml x 10	$49.90	NARCAN, Endo Laboratories Llc	63481-0377-10
2 ml x 10	$150.00	GENERIC, International Medication Systems, Limited	00548-3369-00
5 ml x 5	$64.00	GENERIC, Astra-Zeneca Pharmaceuticals	00186-1253-13
10 ml	$46.44	NARCAN, Endo Laboratories Llc	63481-0368-05
10 ml x 5	$107.10	GENERIC, Astra-Zeneca Pharmaceuticals	00186-1255-12

PRODUCT LISTING - EQUIVALENTS NOT AVAILABLE

Solution - Injectable - 0.4 mg/ml

Size	Price	Product	NDC
1 ml x 50	$55.00	GENERIC, Raway Pharmacal Inc	00686-1910-00
10 ml	$30.00	GENERIC, Truxton Company Inc	00463-1045-10
10 ml	$45.00	GENERIC, Allscripts Pharmaceutical Company	54569-3385-00

Solution - Injectable - 1 mg/ml

Size	Price	Product	NDC
2 ml x 10	$30.57	GENERIC, International Medication Systems, Limited	00482-0158-06

Naltrexone Hydrochloride *(001857)*

Categories: Alcohol, dependence; Opiate, dependence; Pregnancy Category C; FDA Approved 1984 Nov; Orphan Drugs
Drug Classes: Antagonists, narcotic; Antidotes
Brand Names: Naltrexone HCl; Revia; **Trexan**
Foreign Brand Availability: Antaxone (Italy; Spain); Celupan (Spain); Nalerona (Peru); Nalorex (England; France; Ireland; Netherlands); Nemexin (Austria; Denmark; Finland; Germany; Switzerland); Phaltrexia (Indonesia); Re-Via (Mexico)
Cost of Therapy: $152.45 (Alcohol Dependence; Revia; 50 mg; 1 tablet/day; 30 day supply)
$128.25 (Alcohol Dependence; Generic Tablets; 50 mg; 1 tablet/day; 30 day supply)

DESCRIPTION

Naltrexone hydrochloride, an opioid antagonist, is a synthetic congener of oxymorphone with no opioid agonist properties. Naltrexone differs in structure from oxymorphone in that the methyl group on the nitrogen atom is replaced by a cyclopropylmethyl group. Naltrexone hydrochloride is also related to the potent opioid antagonist, naloxone, or n-allylnoroxymorphone.

Naltrexone hydrochloride is a white, crystalline compound. The hydrochloride salt is soluble in water to the extent of about 100 mg/ml. Revia is available in scored tablets containing 50 mg of naltrexone hydrochloride.

Revia tablets also contain: lactose, microcrystalline cellulose, crospovidone, colloidal silicon dioxide, magnesium stearate, hydroxypropyl methylcellulose, titanium dioxide, polyethylene glycol, polysorbate 80, yellow iron oxide and red iron oxide.

CLINICAL PHARMACOLOGY

PHARMACODYNAMIC ACTIONS

Naltrexone HCl is a pure opioid antagonist. It markedly attenuates or completely blocks, reversibly, the subjective effects of IV administered opioids.

When co-administered with morphine, on a chronic basis, naltrexone HCl blocks the physical dependence to morphine, heroin and other opioids.

Naltrexone HCl has few, if any, intrinsic actions besides its opioid blocking properties. However, it does produce some pupillary constriction, by an unknown mechanism.

The administration of naltrexone HCl is not associated with the development of tolerance or dependence. In subjects physically dependent on opioids, naltrexone HCl will precipitate withdrawal symptomatology.

Clinical studies indicate that 50 mg of naltrexone HCl will block the pharmacologic effects of 25 mg of intravenously administered heroin for periods as long as 24 hours. Other data suggest that doubling the dose of naltrexone HCl provides blockade for 48 hours, and tripling the dose of naltrexone HCl provides blockade for about 72 hours.

Naltrexone HCl blocks the effects of opioids by competitive binding (*i.e.,* analogous to competitive inhibition of enzymes) at opioid receptors. This makes the blockade produced potentially surmountable, but overcoming full naltrexone blockade by administration of very high doses of opiates has resulted in excessive symptoms of histamine release in experimental subjects.

The mechanism of action of naltrexone HCl in alcoholism is not understood; however, involvement of the endogenous opioid system is suggested by preclinical data. Naltrexone HCl, an opioid receptor antagonist, competitively binds to such receptors and may block the effects of endogenous opioids. Opioid antagonists have been shown to reduce alcohol consumption by animals, and naltrexone HCl has been shown to reduce alcohol consumption in clinical studies.

Naltrexone HCl is not aversive therapy and does not cause a disulfiram-like reaction wither as a result of opiate use or ethanol ingestion.

PHARMACOKINETICS

Naltrexone HCl is a pure opioid receptor antagonist. Although well absorbed orally, naltrexone is subject to significant first pass metabolism with oral bioavailability estimates ranging from 5-40%. The activity of naltrexone is believed to be due to both parent and the 6-β-naltrexol metabolite. Both parent drug and metabolites are excreted primarily by the kidney (53-79% of the dose), however, urinary excretion of unchanged naltrexone accounts for less than 2% of an oral dose and fecal excretion is a minor elimination pathway. The mean elimination half-life ($T_{1/2}$) values for naltrexone and 6-β-naltrexol are 4 hours and 13 hours respectively. Naltrexone and 6-β-naltrexol are dose proportional in terms of AUC and C_{max} over the range of 50-200 mg and do not accumulate after 100 mg daily doses.

Absorption

Following oral administration, naltrexone undergoes rapid and nearly complete absorption with approximately 96% of the dose absorbed from the gastrointestinal tract. Peak plasma levels of both naltrexone and 6-β-naltrexol occur within 1 hour of dosing.

Distribution

The volume of distribution for naltrexone following IV administration is estimated to be 1350 liters. *In vitro* tests with human plasma show naltrexone to be 21% bound to plasma proteins over the therapeutic dose range.

Metabolism

The systemic clearance (after IV administration) of naltrexone is ~3.5 L/min, which exceeds liver blood flow (~1.2 L/min). This suggests both that naltrexone is a highly extracted drug (>98% metabolized) and that extra-hepatic sites of drug metabolism exist. The major metabolite of naltrexone is 6-β-naltrexol. Two other minor metabolites are 2-hydroxy-3-methoxy-6-β-naltrexol and 2-hydroxy-3-methyl-naltrexone. Naltrexone and its metabolites are also conjugated to form additional metabolic products.

Elimination

The renal clearance for naltrexone ranges from 30-127 ml/min and suggests that renal elimination is primarily by glomerular filtration. In comparison the renal clearance for 6-β-naltrexol ranges from 230-369 ml/min, suggesting an additional renal tubular secretory mechanism. The urinary excretion of unchanged naltrexone accounts for less than 2% of an oral dose; urinary excretion of unchanged and conjugated 6-β-naltrexol accounts for 43% of an oral dose. The pharmacokinetic profile of naltrexone suggests that naltrexone and its metabolites may undergo enterohepatic recycling.

Hepatic and Renal Impairment

Naltrexone appears to have extra-hepatic sites of drug metabolism and its major metabolite undergoes active tubular secretion (see Metabolism). Adequate studies of naltrexone in patients with severe hepatic or renal impairment have not been conducted.

INDICATIONS AND USAGE

Naltrexone HCl is indicated in the treatment of alcohol dependence and for the blockade of the effects of exogenously administered opioids.

Naltrexone HCl has not been shown to provide any therapeutic benefit except as part of an appropriate plan of management for the addictions.

NON-FDA APPROVED INDICATIONS

Unapproved and/or investigational uses of naltrexone have included treatment of schizophrenia, self-injurious behavior, uremia, kleptomania, and to improve behavior and attention in autistic children.

CONTRAINDICATIONS

Naltrexone HCl is contraindicated in:

- Patients receiving opioid analgesics.
- Patients currently dependent on opioids, including those currently maintained on opiate agonists [*e.g.*, methadone or LAAM (levo-alpha-acetyl-methadol)].
- Patients in acute opioid withdrawal (see WARNINGS).
- Any individual who has failed the naloxone challenge test or who has a positive urine screen for opioids.
- Any individual with a history of sensitivity to naltrexone HCl or any other components of this product. It is not known if there is any cross-sensitivity with naloxone or the phenanthrene containing opioids.
- Any individual with acute hepatitis or liver failure.

WARNINGS

HEPATOTOXICITY

Naltrexone HCl has the capacity to cause dose related hepatocellular injury when given in excessive doses.

Naltrexone HCl is contraindicated in acute hepatitis or liver failure, and its use in patients with active liver disease must be carefully considered in light of its hepatotoxic effects.

The margin of separation between the apparently safe dose of naltrexone HCl and the dose causing hepatic injury appears to be only 5-fold or less. Naltrexone HCl does not appear to be hepatotoxin at the recommended doses.

Patients should be warned of risk of the risk of hepatic injury and advised to stop the use of naltrexone HCl and seek medical attention if they experience symptoms of acute hepatitis.

Evidence of the hepatotoxic potential of naltrexone HCl is derived primarily from a placebo controlled study in which naltrexone HCl was administered to obese subjects at a dose approximately 5-fold that recommended for the blockade of opiate receptors (300 mg/day). In the study, 5 of 26 naltrexone HCl recipients developed elevations or serum transaminase (*i.e.*, peak ALT values ranging from a low of 121 to a high of 532; or 3 to 19 times their baseline values) after 3-8 weeks of treatment. Although the patients involved were generally clinically asymptomatic and the transaminase levels of all patients on whom follow-up was obtained returned to (or toward) baseline values in a matter of weeks, the lack of any transaminase elevations of similar magnitude in any of the 24 placebo patients in the same study is persuasive evidence that naltrexone HCl is a direct (*i.e.*, not an idiosyncratic) hepatotoxin.

This conclusion is also supported by evidence from other placebo controlled studies in which exposure to naltrexone HCl at doses above the amount recommended for the treatment of alcoholism or opiate blockade (50 mg/day) consistently produced more numerous and more significant elevations of serum transaminases than did placebo. Transaminase elevations in 3 of 9 patients with Alzheimer's Disease who received naltrexone HCl (at doses up to 300 mg/day) for 5-8 weeks in open clinical trial have been reported.

Although no cases of hepatic failure due to naltrexone HCl administration have ever been reported, physicians are advised to consider this as a possible risk of treatment and to use the same care in prescribing naltrexone HCl as they would other drugs with the potential for causing hepatic injury.

UNINTENDED PRECIPITATION OF ABSTINENCE

To prevent occurrence of an acute abstinence syndrome, or exacerbation of a pre-existing sub-clinical abstinence syndrome, patients must be opioid-free for a minimum of 7-10 days before starting naltrexone HCl. Since the absence of an opioid drug in the urine is often not sufficient proof that a patient is opioid-free, a naloxone challenge should be employed if the prescribing physician feels there is a risk of precipitating a withdrawal reaction following administration of naltrexone HCl. The naloxone challenge test is described in DOSAGE AND ADMINISTRATION.

ATTEMPT TO OVERCOME BLOCKADE

While naltrexone HCl is a potent antagonist with a prolonged pharmacologic effect (24-72 hours), the blockade produced by naltrexone HCl is surmountable. This is useful in patients who may require analgesia, but poses a potential risk to individuals who attempt, on their own, to overcome the blockade by administering large amounts of exogenous opioids. Indeed, any attempt by a patient to overcome the antagonism by taking opioids is very dangerous and may lead to a fatal overdose. Injury may arise because the plasma concentration of exogenous opioids attained immediately following their acute administration may be sufficient to overcome the competitive receptor blockade. As a consequence, the patient may be in immediate danger of suffering life endangering opioid intoxication (*e.g.*, respiratory arrest, circulatory collapse). Patients should be told of the serious consequences of trying to overcome the opiate blockade (see PRECAUTIONS, Information for the Patient).

There is also the possibility that a patient who had been treated with naltrexone will respond to lower doses of opioids than previously used, particularly if taken in such a manner that high plasma concentrations remain in the body beyond the time that naltrexone exerts its therapeutic effects. This could result in potentially life-threatening opioid intoxication (respiratory compromise or arrest, circulatory collapse, etc.). Patients should be aware that they may be more sensitive to lower doses of opioids after naltrexone treatment is discontinued.

ULTRA RAPID OPIOID WITHDRAWAL

Safe use of naltrexone HCl in ultra rapid opiate detoxification programs has not been established (see ADVERSE REACTIONS).

PRECAUTIONS

GENERAL

When Reversal of Naltrexone HCl Blockade Is Required

In an emergency situation in patients receiving fully blocking doses of naltrexone HCl, a suggested plan of management is regional analgesia, conscious sedation with a benzodiazepine, use of non-opioid analgesics or general anesthesia.

In a situation requiring opioid analgesia, the amount of opioid required may be greater than usual, and the resulting respiratory depression may be deeper and more prolonged.

A rapidly acting opioid analgesic which minimizes the duration of respiratory depression is preferred. The amounts of analgesic administered should be titrated to the needs of the patient. Non-receptor mediated actions may occur and should be expected (*e.g.*, facial swelling, itching, generalized erythema, or bronchoconstriction) presumably due to histamine release.

Irrespective of the drug chosen to reverse naltrexone HCl blockade, the patient should be monitored closely by appropriately trained personnel in a setting equipped and staffed for cardiopulmonary resuscitation.

Accidentally Precipitated Withdrawal

Severe opioid withdrawal syndromes precipitated by the accidental ingestion of naltrexone HCl have been reported in opioid-dependent individuals. Symptoms of withdrawal have usually appeared within 5 minutes of injection of naltrexone HCl and have lasted for up to 48 hours. Mental status changes including confusion, somnolence and visual hallucinations have occurred. Significant fluid losses from vomiting and diarrhea have required IV fluid administration. In all cases patients were closely monitored and therapy with non-opioid medications was tailored to meet individual requirements.

Use of naltrexone HCl does not eliminate or diminish withdrawal symptoms. If naltrexone HCl is initiated early in the abstinence process, it will not preclude the patient's experience of the full range of signs and symptoms that would be experienced if naltrexone HCl had not been started. Numerous adverse events are known to be associated with withdrawal.

Special Risk Patients

Renal Impairment

Naltrexone HCl and its primary metabolite are excreted primarily in the urine, and caution is recommended in administering the drug to patients with renal impairment.

Hepatic Impairment

Caution should be exercised when naltrexone HCl is administered to patients with liver disease. An increase in naltrexone AUC of approximately 5- and 10-fold in patients with compensated and decompensated liver cirrhosis, respectively, compared with subjects with normal liver function has been reported. These data also suggest that alterations in naltrexone bioavailability are related to liver disease severity.

Suicide

The risk of suicide is known to be increased in patients with substance abuse with or without concomitant depression. This risk is not abated by treatment with naltrexone HCl (see ADVERSE REACTIONS).

INFORMATION FOR THE PATIENT

It is recommended that the prescribing physician relate the following information to patients being treated with naltrexone HCl:

You have been prescribed naltrexone HCl as part of the comprehensive treatment for your alcoholism or drug dependence. You should carry identification to alert medical personnel to the fact that you are taking naltrexone HCl. A naltrexone HCl medication card may be obtained from your physician and can be used for this purpose.

Carrying this identification card should help to ensure you that you can obtain adequate treatment in an emergency. If you require medical treatment, be sure to tell the treating physician that you are receiving naltrexone HCl therapy.

You should take naltrexone HCl as directed by your physician. If you attempt to self-administer heroin or any other opiate drug, in small doses while on naltrexone HCl, you will not perceive any effect. Most important, however, if you attempt to self-administer large doses of heroin or any other opioid (including methadone or LAAM) while on naltrexone HCl, you may die or sustain serious injury, including coma.

Naltrexone HCl is well-tolerated in the recommended doses, but may cause liver injury when taken in excess or in people who develop liver disease from other causes. If you develop abdominal pain lasting more than a few days, white bowel movements, dark urine, or yellowing of your eyes, you should stop taking naltrexone HCl immediately and see your doctor as soon as possible.

LABORATORY TESTS

A high index of suspicion for drug-related hepatic injury is critical of the occurrence of liver damage induced by naltrexone HCl is to be detected at the earliest possible time. Evaluations, using appropriate batteries of tests to detect liver injury are recommended at a frequency appropriate to the clinical situation and dose of naltrexone HCl.

Naltrexone HCl does not interfere with thin-layer, gas-liquid, and high pressure liquid chromatographic methods which may be used for the separation and detection of morphine, methadone or quinine in the urine. Naltrexone HCl may or may not interfere with enzymatic methods for the detection of opioids depending on the specificity of the test. Please consult the test manufacturer for specific details.

CARCINOGENESIS, MUTAGENESIS, AND IMPAIRMENT OF FERTILITY

The following statements are based on the results of experiments in mice and rats. The potential carcinogenic, mutagenic and fertility effects of the metabolite 6-β-naltrexol are unknown.

In a 2 year carcinogenicity study in rats, there were small increases in the numbers of testicular mesotheliomas in males and tumors of vascular origin in males and females. The incidence of mesothelioma in males given naltrexone at a dietary dose of 100 mg/kg/day (600 mg/m^2/day; 16 times the recommended therapeutic dose, based on body surface area) was 6%, compared with a maximum historical incidence of 4%. The incidence of vascular tumors in males and females given dietary doses of 100 mg/kg/day (600 mg/m^2/day) was 4%, but only the incidence in females was increased compared with a maximum historical control incidence of 2%. There was no evidence of carcinogenicity in a 2 year dietary study with naltrexone in male and female mice.

There was limited evidence of a weak genotoxic effect of naltrexone in one gene mutation assay in a mammalian cell line, in the *Drosophila* recessive lethal assay, and in non-specific DNA repair tests with *E. coli.* However, no evidence of genotoxic potential was observed in a range of other *in vitro* tests, including assays for gene mutation in bacteria, yeast, or in a second mammalian cell line, a chromosomal aberration assay, and an assay for DNA damage in human cells. Naltrexone did not exhibit clastogenicity in an *in vivo* mouse micronucleus assay.

N

Naltrexone (100 mg/kg/day [600 mg/m^2/day] po; 16 times the recommended therapeutic dose, based on body surface area) caused a significant increase in pseudopregnancy in the rat. A decrease in the pregnancy rate of mated female rats also occurred. There was no effect on male fertility at this dose level. The relevance of these observations to human fertility is not known.

PREGNANCY CATEGORY C

Naltrexone has been shown to increase the incidence of early fetal loss when given to rats at doses ≥30 mg/kg/day (180 mg/m^2/day; 5 times the recommended therapeutic dose, based on body surface area) and to rabbits at oral doses ≥60 mg/kg/day (720 mg/m^2/day; 18 times the recommended therapeutic dose, based on body surface area). There was no evidence of teratogenicity when naltrexone was administered orally to rats and rabbits during the period of major organogenesis at doses up to 200 mg/kg/day (32 and 65 times the recommended therapeutic dose, respectively, based on body surface area).

Rats do not form appreciable quantities of the major human metabolite, 6-β-naltrexol; therefore, the potential reproductive toxicity of the metabolite in rats is not known.

There are no adequate and well-controlled studies in pregnant women. Naltrexone HCl should be used during pregnancy only if the potential benefit justifies the potential risk to the fetus.

LABOR AND DELIVERY

Whether or not naltrexone HCl affects the duration of labor and delivery is unknown.

NURSING MOTHERS

In animal studies, naltrexone and 6-β-naltrexol were excreted in the milk of lactating rats dosed orally with naltrexone. Whether or not naltrexone HCl is excreted in human milk is unknown. Because many drugs are excreted in human milk, caution should be exercised when naltrexone HCl is administered to a nursing woman.

PEDIATRIC USE

The safe use of naltrexone HCl in subjects younger than 18 years old has not been established.

DRUG INTERACTIONS

Studies to evaluate possible interactions between naltrexone HCl and drugs other than opiates have not been performed. Consequently, caution is advised if the concomitant administration of naltrexone HCl and other drugs is required.

The safety and efficacy of concomitant use of naltrexone HCl and disulfiram is unknown, and the concomitant use of two potentially hepatotoxic medications is not ordinarily recommended unless the probable benefits outweigh the known risks.

Lethargy and somnolence have not been reported following doses of naltrexone HCl and thioridazine.

Patients taking naltrexone HCl may not benefit from opioid containing medicines, such as cough and cold preparations, antidiarrheal preparations, and opioid analgesia must be administered to a patient receiving naltrexone HCl, the amount of opioid required may be greater than usual, and the resulting respiratory depression may be deeper and more prolonged. (See PRECAUTIONS.)

ADVERSE REACTIONS

During two randomized, double-blind placebo-controlled 12 week trials to evaluate the efficacy of naltrexone HCl as an adjunctive treatment of alcohol dependence, most patients tolerated naltrexone HCl well. In these studies, a total of 93 patients received naltrexone HCl at a dose of 50 mg once daily. Five (5) of these patients discontinued naltrexone HCl because of nausea. No serious adverse events were reported during these two trials.

While extensive clinical studies evaluating the use of naltrexone HCl in detoxified, formerly opioid-dependent individuals failed to identify any single, serious untoward risk of naltrexone HCl use, placebo-controlled studies employing up to 5-fold higher doses of naltrexone HCl (up to 300 mg/day) than that recommended for use in opiate receptor blockade have shown that naltrexone HCl causes hepatocellular injury in a substantial proportion of patients exposed at higher doses (see WARNINGS and PRECAUTIONS, Laboratory Tests).

Aside from this finding, and the risk of precipitated opioid withdrawal, available evidence does not incriminate naltrexone HCl, used at any dose, as a cause of any other serious adverse reaction for the patient who is "opioid free". It is critical to recognize that naltrexone HCl can precipitate or exacerbate abstinence signs and symptoms in any individual who is not completely free of exogenous opioids.

Patients with addictive disorders, especially narcotic addiction, are risk for multiple numerous adverse events and abnormal laboratory findings, including liver function abnormalities. Data from both controlled and observational studies suggest that these abnormalities, other than the dose-related hepatotoxicity described above, are not related to the use of naltrexone HCl.

Among opioid free individuals, naltrexone HCl administration at the recommended dose has not been associated with a predictable profile of serious adverse or untoward events. However, as mentioned above, among individuals using opioids, naltrexone HCl may cause serious withdrawal reactions (see CONTRAINDICATIONS, WARNINGS, and DOSAGE AND ADMINISTRATION).

REPORTED ADVERSE EVENTS

Naltrexone HCl has not been shown to cause significant increases in complaints in placebo-controlled trials in patients known to be free of opioids for more than 7-10 days. Studies in alcoholic populations and in volunteers in clinical pharmacology studies have suggested that a small fraction of patients may experience an opioid withdrawal-like symptom complex consisting of tearfulness, mild nausea, abdominal cramps, restlessness, bone or joint pain, myalgia, and nasal symptoms. This may represent the unmasking of occult opioid use, or it may represent symptoms attributable to naltrexone. A number of alternative dosing patterns have been recommended to try to reduce the frequency of these complaints.

ALCOHOLISM

In an open label safety study with approximately 570 individuals with alcoholism receiving naltrexone HCl, the following new-onset adverse reactions occurred in 2% or more of the patients: nausea (10%), headache (7%), dizziness (4%), nervousness (4%), fatigue (4%), insomnia (3%), vomiting (3%), anxiety (2%) and somnolence (2%).

Depression, suicidal ideation, and suicidal attempts have been reported in all groups when comparing naltrexone, placebo, or controls undergoing treatment for alcoholism.

TABLE 1 *Rate Ranges of New Onset Events*

	Naltrexone	Placebo
Depression	0-15%	0-17%
Suicide attempt/ideation	0-1%	0-3%

Although no causal relationship with naltrexone HCl is suspected, physicians should be aware that treatment with naltrexone HCl does not reduce the risk of suicide in these patients (see PRECAUTIONS).

OPIOID ADDICTION

The following adverse reactions have been reported both at baseline and during the naltrexone HCl clinical trials in opioid addiction:

At an incidence rate of more than 10%: Difficulty sleeping, anxiety, nervousness, abdominal pain/cramps, nausea and/or vomiting, low energy, joint and muscle pain, and headache.

The incidence was less than 10% for: Loss of appetite, diarrhea, constipation, increased thirst, increased energy, feeling down, irritability, dizziness, skin rash, delayed ejaculation, decreased potency and chills.

The following events occurred in less than 1% of subjects:

Respiratory: Nasal congestion, itching, rhinorrhea, sneezing, sore throat, excess mucus or phlegm, sinus trouble, heavy breathing, hoarseness, cough, shortness of breath.

Cardiovascular: Nose bleeds, phlebitis, edema, increased blood pressure, non-specific ECG changes, palpitations, tachycardia.

Gastrointestinal: Excessive gas, hemorrhoids, diarrhea, ulcer.

Musculoskeletal: Painful shoulders, legs or knees; tremors, twitching.

Genitourinary: Increased frequency of, or discomfort during, urination; increased or decreased sexual interest.

Dermatologic: Oily skin, pruritus, acne, athlete's foot, cold sores, alopecia.

Psychiatric: Depression, paranoia, fatigue, restlessness, confusion, disorientation, hallucinations, nightmares, bad dreams.

Special Senses: *Eyes:* Blurred, burning, light sensitive, swollen, aching, strained; *Ears:* "Clogged", aching, tinnitus.

General: Increased appetite, weight loss, weight gain, yawning, somnolence, fever, dry mouth, head "pounding", inguinal pain, swollen glands, "side" pains, cold feet, "hot spells".

POST-MARKETING EXPERIENCE

Data collected from post-marketing use of naltrexone HCl show that most events usually occur early in the course of drug therapy and are transient. It is not always possible to distinguish these occurrences from those signs and symptoms that may result from a withdrawal syndrome. Events that have been reported include anorexia, asthenia, chest pain, fatigue, headache, hot flushes, malaise, changes in blood pressure, agitation, dizziness, hyperkinesia, nausea, vomiting, tremor, abdominal pain, diarrhea, elevations in liver enzymes or bilirubin, hepatic function abnormalities or hepatitis, palpitations, myalgia, anxiety, confusion, euphoria, hallucinations, insomnia, nervousness, somnolence, abnormal thinking, dyspnea, rash, increased sweating, and vision abnormalities.

Depression, suicide, attempted suicide and suicidal ideation have been reported in the post-marketing experience with naltrexone HCl used in the treatment of opioid dependence. No causal relationship has been demonstrated. In the literature, endogenous opioids have been theorized to contribute to a variety of conditions. In some individuals the use of opioid antagonists has been associated with a change in baseline levels of some hypothalamic, pituitary, adrenal, or gonadal hormones. The clinical significance of such changes is not fully understood.

Adverse events, including withdrawal symptoms and death, have been reported with the use of naltrexone HCl in ultra rapid opiate detoxification programs. The cause of death in these cases is not known (see WARNINGS).

LABORATORY TESTS

With the exception of liver test abnormalities (see WARNINGS and PRECAUTIONS) results of laboratory tests, like adverse reaction reports have not shown consistent patterns of abnormalities that can be attributed to treatment with naltrexone HCl.

Idiopathic thrombocytopenia purpura was reported in 1 patient who may have been sensitized to naltrexone HCl in a previous course of treatment with naltrexone HCl. The condition cleared without sequelae after discontinuation of naltrexone HCl and corticosteroid treatment.

DOSAGE AND ADMINISTRATION

IF THERE IS ANY QUESTION OF OCCULT OPIOID DEPENDENCE, PERFORM A NALOXONE CHALLENGE TEST AND DO NOT INITIATE NALTREXONE HCL THERAPY UNTIL THE NALOXONE CHALLENGE IS NEGATIVE.

TREATMENT OF ALCOHOLISM

A dose of 50 mg once daily is recommended for most patients. The placebo-controlled studies that demonstrated the efficacy of naltrexone HCl as an adjunctive treatment of alcoholism used a dose regimen of naltrexone HCl 50 mg once daily for up to 12 weeks. Other dose regimens or durations of therapy were not evaluated in these trials.

A patient is a candidate for treatment with naltrexone HCl if:

- The patient is willing to take a medicine to help with alcohol dependence.
- The patient is opioid free for 7-10 days.
- The patient does not have severe or active liver or kidney problems (Typical guidelines suggest liver function tests no greater than 3 times the upper limits of normal, and bilirubin normal.).
- The patient is not allergic to naltrexone HCl, and no other contraindications are present.

Refer to CONTRAINDICATIONS, WARNINGS, and PRECAUTIONS for additional information.

Naltrexone HCl should be considered as only one of many factors determining the success of treatment of alcoholism. Factors associated with a good outcome in the clinical trials with naltrexone HCl were the type, intensity, and duration of treatment; appropriate management of comorbid conditions; use of community-based support groups; and good medication compliance. To achieve the best possible treatment outcome, appropriate compliance-enhancing techniques should be implemented for all components of the treatment program, especially medication compliance.

TREATMENT OF OPIOID DEPENDENCE

Initiate treatment with naltrexone HCl using the following guidelines:

Treatment should not be attempted unless the patient has remained opioid-free for at least 7-10 days. Self-reporting of abstinence from opioids in narcotic addicts should be verified by analysis of the patient's urine for absence of opioids. The patient should not be manifesting withdrawal signs or reporting withdrawal symptoms.

If there is any question of occult opioid dependence, perform a naloxone challenge test. If signs of opioid withdrawal are still observed following naloxone challenge, treatment with naltrexone HCl should not be attempted. The naloxone challenge can be repeated in 24 hours.

Treatment should be initiated carefully, with an initial dose of 25 mg of naltrexone HCl. If no withdrawal signs occur, the patient may be started on 50 mg a day thereafter.

NALOXONE CHALLENGE TEST

The naloxone challenge test should not be performed in a patient showing clinical signs or symptoms of opioid withdrawal, or in a patient whose urine contains opioids. The naloxone challenge test may be administered by either the intravenous or subcutaneous routes.

Intravenous:

Inject 0.2 mg naloxone.
Observe for 30 seconds for signs or symptoms of withdrawal.
If no evidence of withdrawal, inject 0.6 mg of naloxone.
Observe for an additional 20 minutes.

Subcutaneous:

Administer 0.8 mg naloxone.
Observe for 20 minutes for signs or symptoms of withdrawal.

Note: Individual patients, especially those with opioid dependence, may respond to lower doses of naloxone. In some cases, 0.1 mg IV naloxone has produced a diagnostic response.

Interpretation of the Challenge

Monitor vital signs and observe the patient for signs and symptoms of opioid withdrawal. These may include, but are not limited to: nausea, vomiting, dysphoria, yawning, sweating, tearing, rhinorrhea, stuffy nose, craving for opioids, poor appetite, abdominal cramps, sense of fear, skin erythema, disrupted sleep patterns, fidgeting, uneasiness, poor ability to focus, mental lapses, muscle aches or cramps, pupillary dilation, piloerection, fever, changes in blood pressure, pulse or temperature, anxiety, depression, irritability, back ache, bone or joint pains, tremors, sensations of skin crawling or fasciculations. If signs or symptoms of withdrawal appear, the test is positive and no additional naloxone should be administered.

Warning: If the test is positive, do NOT initiate naltrexone HCl therapy. Repeat the challenge in 24 hours. If the test is negative, naltrexone HCl therapy may be started if no other contraindications are present. If there is any doubt about the result of the test, hold naltrexone HCl and repeat the challenge in 24 hours.

ALTERNATIVE DOSING SCHEDULES

Once the patient has been started on naltrexone HCl, 50 mg every 24 hours will produce adequate clinical blockade of the actions of parenterally administered opioids (*i.e.,* this dose will block the effects of a 25 mg IV heroin challenge). A flexible approach to a dosing regimen may need to be employed in cases of supervised administration. Thus, patients may receive 50 mg of naltrexone HCl every weekday with a 100 mg dose on Saturday, 100 mg every other day, or 150 mg every third day. The degree of blockade produced by naltrexone HCl may be reduced by these extended dosing intervals.

There may be a higher risk of hepatocellular injury with single doses above 50 mg, and use of higher doses and extended dosing intervals should balance the possible risks against the probable benefits (see WARNINGS).

PATIENT COMPLIANCE

Naltrexone HCl should be considered as only one of many factors determining the success of treatment. To achieve the best possible treatment outcome, appropriate compliance-enhancing techniques should be implemented for all components of the treatment program, including medication compliance.

HOW SUPPLIED

Revia tablets are available in pale yellow 50 mg capsule-shaped film-coated tablets, scored and imprinted with "DuPont" on one side and "11" on the other.

Storage: Store at 25°C (77°F); excursions permitted to 15-30°C (59-86°F).

PRODUCT LISTING - RATED THERAPEUTICALLY EQUIVALENT

Tablet - Oral - 50 mg

30's	$128.25	GENERIC, Mallinckrodt Medical Inc	00406-1170-03
30's	$128.25	GENERIC, Barr Laboratories Inc	00555-0902-01
30's	$137.05	GENERIC, Amide Pharmaceutical Inc	52152-0105-30
30's	$137.21	GENERIC, Eon Labs Manufacturing Inc	00185-0039-30
100's	$404.00	FEDERAL UPPER LIMIT, H.C.F.A. F F P	99999-1857-01
100's	$427.51	GENERIC, Mallinckrodt Medical Inc	00406-1170-01
100's	$427.51	GENERIC, Barr Laboratories Inc	00555-0902-02
100's	$456.83	GENERIC, Amide Pharmaceutical Inc	52152-0105-02
100's	$457.34	GENERIC, Eon Labs Manufacturing Inc	00185-0039-01

PRODUCT LISTING - EQUIVALENTS NOT AVAILABLE

Tablet - Oral - 50 mg

30's	$152.45	REVIA, Dupont Pharmaceuticals	00056-0011-30
100's	$508.16	REVIA, Dupont Pharmaceuticals	00056-0011-70

Naproxen *(001864)*

For related information, see the comparative table section in Appendix A.

Categories: Ankylosing spondylitis; Arthritis, gouty; Arthritis, juvenile; Arthritis, osteoarthritis; Arthritis, rheumatoid; Bursitis; Dysmenorrhea; Pain, mild to moderate; Tendonitis; Pregnancy Category B; FDA Approved 1982 Apr

Drug Classes: Analgesics, non-narcotic; Nonsteroidal anti-inflammatory drugs

Brand Names: EC-Naprosyn; Ec-Naprosyn; **Naprosyn**

Foreign Brand Availability: Acusprain (South-Africa); Aflamax (Peru); Alpron (Philippines); Anexopen (Greece); Antalgin (Spain); Apo-Naproxen (Canada); Apranax (Bulgaria; France; Russia); Artagen (India); Artron (Mexico); Artroxen (Italy); Bipronyl (Singapore); Bonyl (Denmark); Complement (Peru); Congex (Argentina); Crysanal (Australia); Daprox (Denmark); Diocodal (Argentina); Dysmenalgit (Germany); Femex (Netherlands); Flanax (Brazil); Floginax (Italy); Fuxen (Mexico); Gibixen (Italy); Headlon (Japan); Inza (Australia; Hong-Kong; Malaysia); Laraflex (England); Laser (Italy); Leniartil (Italy); Nafasol (South-Africa); Naixan (Japan); Napolon (Korea); Naposin (Taiwan); Naprium (Bahrain; Benin; Burkina-Faso; Cyprus; Egypt; Ethiopia; Gambia; Ghana; Guinea; Iran; Iraq; Israel; Ivory-Coast; Jordan; Kenya; Kuwait; Lebanon; Liberia; Libya; Malawi; Mali; Mauritania; Mauritius; Morocco; Niger; Nigeria; Oman; Qatar; Republic-of-Yemen; Saudi-Arabia; Senegal; Seychelles; Sierra-Leone; South-Africa; Sudan; Syria; Tanzania; Tunia; Uganda; United-Arab-Emirates; Zambia; Zimbabwe); Naprius (Italy); Naproflam (Germany); Naprong (Korea); Naprontag (Argentina); Naprorex (Bahrain; Cyprus; Egypt; Hong-Kong; Iran; Iraq; Israel; Jordan; Kuwait; Lebanon; Libya; Oman; Qatar; Republic-of-Yemen; Saudi-Arabia; Syria; United-Arab-Emirates); Naprosyn LLE (Philippines); Naprosyn LLE Forte (Philippines); Naprosyne (Belgium; France; Netherlands); Naproxi 250 (Israel); Naproxi 500 (Israel); Naprux (Argentina); Napxen (Thailand); Narma (Japan); Naxen (Canada; Indonesia; Mexico; South-Africa); Naxen F (Korea); Naxen-F CR (Korea); Naxopren (Finland); Naxyn 250 (Israel); Naxyn 500 (Israel); Norswel (Benin; Burkina-Faso; Ethiopia; Gambia; Ghana; Guinea; Ivory-Coast; Kenya; Liberia; Malawi; Mali; Mauritania; Mauritius; Morocco; Niger; Nigeria; Senegal; Seychelles; Sierra-Leone; South-Africa; Sudan; Tanzania; Tunia; Uganda; Zambia; Zimbabwe); Novonaprox (Canada); Nuprafem (Singapore); Nycopren (Austria; Denmark; Finland); Prexan (Italy); Priaxen (Bahamas; Barbados; Belize; Benin; Bermuda; Burkina-Faso; Curacao; Ethiopia; Gambia; Ghana; Guinea; Guyana; Ivory-Coast; Jamaica; Kenya; Liberia; Malawi; Mali; Mauritania; Mauritius; Morocco; Netherland-Antilles; Niger; Nigeria; Puerto-Rico; Senegal; Seychelles; Sierra-Leone; South-Africa; Sudan; Surinam; Tanzania; Trinidad; Tunia; Uganda; Zambia; Zimbabwe); Primeral (Italy); Prodexin (Bahrain; Cyprus; Egypt; Iran; Iraq; Israel; Jordan; Kuwait; Lebanon; Libya; Oman; Qatar; Republic-of-Yemen; Saudi-Arabia; Syria; United-Arab-Emirates); Pronaxen (Malaysia; Sweden); Proxen (Austria; Bahrain; Cyprus; Egypt; Germany; Iran; Iraq; Israel; Jordan; Kuwait; Lebanon; Libya; Oman; Qatar; Republic-of-Yemen; Saudi-Arabia; Spain; Switzerland; Syria; United-Arab-Emirates); Proxen LLE (Taiwan); Rahsen (Japan); Roxen (Thailand); Saritilron (Japan); Shiprosyn (Philippines); Sutolin (Taiwan); Synflex (England; Hong-Kong); Tohexen (Japan); U-Ritis (Taiwan); Velsay (Mexico); Veradol (Argentina); Vinsen (Thailand); Wintrex (Peru); Xenar (Italy)

Cost of Therapy: $50.16 (Osteoarthritis; Naprosyn; 250 mg; 2 tablets/day; 30 day supply)
$5.58 (Osteoarthritis; Generic Tablets; 250 mg; 2 tablets/day; 30 day supply)

DESCRIPTION

Naproxen tablets for oral administration each contain 250, 375, or 500 mg of naproxen. Naproxen suspension for oral administration contains 125 mg/5 ml of naproxen. Naproxen is a member of the arylacetic acid group of nonsteroidal anti-inflammatory drugs.

The chemical name for naproxen is 2-naphthaleneacetic acid, 5 methoxy- α-methyl-,(+).

Naproxen is an odorless, white to off-white crystalline substance. It is lipid soluble, practically insoluble in water at low pH and freely soluble in water at high pH.

Naproxen suspension for oral administration contains 125 mg/5 ml of naproxen, the active ingredient, in a vehicle of FD&C yellow no. 6, fumaric acid, imitation orange flavor, imitation pineapple flavor, magnesium aluminum silicate, methyl paraben, purified water, sodium chloride, sorbitol solution and sucrose.

STORAGE

Store Naprosyn suspension at room temperature; avoid excessive heat, above 40°C (104°F). Dispense in light-resistant container.

Store Naprosyn tablets at room temperature and in well-closed containers; dispense in light-resistant container.

CLINICAL PHARMACOLOGY

Naproxen is a nonsteroidal anti-inflammatory drug with analgesic and antipyretic properties. Naproxen sodium, the sodium slat of naproxen, has been developed as an analgesic because it is more rapidly adsorbed. The naproxen anion inhibits prostaglandin synthesis but this its mode of action is unknown.

Naproxen is rapidly and completely absorbed from the gastrointestinal tract. After administration of naproxen, peak plasma levels of naproxen anion are attained in 2-4 hours, with steady-state conditions normally achieved after 4-5 doses. The mean biological half-life of the anion in humans is approximately 13 hours, and at therapeutic levels it is greater than 99% albumin bound. Approximately 95% of the dose is excreted in the urine, primarily as naproxen, 6-O-desmethyl naproxen or their conjugates. The rate of excretion has been found to coincide closely with the rate of drug disappearance from the plasma. The drug does not induce metabolizing enzymes.

In children of 5-16 years of age with arthritis, plasma naproxen levels following a 5 mg/kg single dose of suspension were found to be similar to those found in normal adults following a 500 mg dose. The terminal half-life appears to be similar in children and adults. Pharmacokinetic studies of naproxen were not performed in children of less than 5 years of age.

The drug was studied in patients with rheumatoid arthritis, osteoarthritis, juvenile arthritis, ankylosing spondylitis, tendinitis and bursitis, and acute gout. It is not a corticosteroid. Improvement in patients treated for rheumatoid arthritis has been demonstrated by a reduction in joint swelling, a reduction in pain, a reduction in direction of morning stiffness, a reduction in disease activity as assesses by both the investigator and the patient, and increased mobility as demonstrated by a reduction in walking time.

In patients with osteoarthritis, the therapeutic action of the drug has been shown by a reduction in joint pain or tenderness, and increase in range of motion in knee joints, increased mobility as demonstrated by a reduction in walking time, and improvement in capacity to perform activities of daily living impaired by the disease.

In clinical studies in patients with rheumatoid arthritis, osteoarthritis, and juvenile arthritis, the drug has been shown to be comparable to aspirin and indomethacin in controlling the aforementioned measures of disease activity, but the frequency and severity if the milder gastrointestinal adverse effects (nausea, dyspepsia, heartburn) and nervous system adverse effects (tinnitus, dizziness, lightheadedness) were less than in both the aspirin- and indomethacin-treated patients. It is not known whether the drug causes less peptic ulceration than aspirin.

In patients with ankylosing spondylitis, the drug has been shown to decrease night pain, morning stiffness and pain at rest. In double-blind studies the drug was shown to be as effective as aspirin, but with fewer side effects.

In patients with acute gout, a favorable response to the drug was shown by significant clearing of inflammatory changes (*e.g.*, decrease in swelling, heat) within 24-48 hours, as well as by relief of pain and tenderness.

This drug may be used safely in combination with gold salts and/or corticosteroids; however, in controlled clinical trials, when added to the regimen of patients receiving corticosteroids it did not appear to cause greater improvement over that seen with corticosteroids alone. Whether the drug could be used in conjunction with partially effective doses of corticosteroids for a "steroid-sparing" effect has not been adequately studied. When added to the regimen of patients receiving gold salts the drug did result in greater improvement. Its use in combination with salicylates is not recommended because data are inadequate to demonstrate that the drug produces greater improvement over that achieved with aspirin alone. Further, there is some evidence that aspirin increases the rate of excretion of the drug.

Generally, improvement due to the drug has not been found to be dependent on age, sex, severity or duration of disease.

In clinical trials in patients with osteoarthritis and rheumatoid arthritis comparing treatments of 750 mg/day with 1500 mg/day, there were trends toward increased efficacy with the higher dose and a more clear-cut increase in adverse reactions, particularly gastrointestinal reactions severe enough to cause the patient to leave the trial, which approximately doubled.

The drug was studied in patients with mild to moderate pain, and pain relief was obtained within 1 hour. It is not a narcotic and is not a CNS-acting drug. Controlled double-blind studies have demonstrated the analgesic properties of the drug in, for example, post-operative, post-partum, orthopedic and uterine contraction pain and dysmenorrhea. In dysmenorrheic patients, the drug reduces the level of prostaglandins in the uterus, which correlates with a reduction in the frequency and severity of uterine contractions. Analgesic action has been shown by such measures as a reduction of pain intensity scores, increase in pain relief scores, decrease in numbers of patients requiring additional analgesic medication, and in time for required remedication. The analgesic effect has been found to last for up to 7 hours.

In ^{51}Cr blood loss and gastroscopy studies with normal volunteers, daily administration of 1000 mg of the drug has been demonstrated to cause statistically significantly less gastric bleeding and erosion than 3250 mg of aspirin.

INDICATIONS AND USAGE

Naproxen is indicated for the treatment of rheumatoid arthritis, osteoarthritis, juvenile arthritis, ankylosing spondylitis, tendinitis and bursitis, and acute gout. It is also indicated in the relief of mild to moderate pain, and for the treatment of primary dysmenorrhea.

NON-FDA APPROVED INDICATIONS

Naproxen has also been reported to have efficacy in the prevention of migraine headaches. However, this use has not been approved by the FDA and additional studies are needed before the drug can be recommended for this indication.

CONTRAINDICATIONS

The drug is contraindicated in patients who have had allergic reactions to naproxen. It is also contraindicated in patients in whom aspirin or other nonsteroidal anti-inflammatory/analgesic drugs induce the syndrome of asthma, rhinitis, and nasal polyps. Both types of reactions have the potential of being fatal. Anaphylactoid reactions to naproxen whether of the true allergic type ot the pharmacologic idiosyncratic (*e.g.*, aspirin syndrome) type, usually but not always occur in patients with a known history of such reactions. Therefore, careful questioning of patients for such things as asthma, nasal polyps, urticaria, and hypotension associated with nonsteroidal anti-inflammatory drugs before starting therapy is important. In addition, if such symptoms occur during therapy, treatment should be discontinued.

WARNINGS

RISK OF GI ULCERATION, BLEEDING AND PERFORATION WITH NSAID THERAPY

Serious gastrointestinal toxicity such as bleeding, ulceration, and perforation, can occur at any time, with or without warning symptoms, in patients treated chronically with NSAID therapy. Although minor upper gastrointestinal problems, such as dyspepsia, are common, usually developing early in therapy, physicians should remain alert for ulceration and bleeding in patients treated chronically with NSAIDs even in the absence of previous GI tract symptoms. In patients observed in clinical trials of several months to 2 years duration, symptomatic upper GI ulcers, gross bleeding or perforation appear to occur in approximately 1% of patients treated for 3-6 months, and in about 2-4% of patients treated for 1 year. Physicians should inform patients about the signs and/or symptoms of serious GI toxicity and what steps to take if they occur.

Studies to date have not identified any subset of patients not at risk of developing peptic ulceration and bleeding. Except for a prior history of serious GI events and other risk factors known to be associated with peptic ulcer disease, such as alcoholism, smoking, etc., no risk factors (*e.g.*, age, sex) have been associated with increased risk. Elderly or debilitated patients seem to tolerate ulceration or bleeding less well than other individuals and most spontaneous reports of fatal GI events are in this population. Studies to date are inconclusive concerning the relative risk of various NSAIDs in causing such reactions. High doses of any NSAID probably carry a greater risk of these reactions, although controlled clinical trials showing this do not exist in most cases. In considering the use of relatively large doses (within the recommended dosage range), sufficient benefit should be anticipated to offset the potential increased risk of GI toxicity.

PRECAUTIONS

GENERAL

NAPROXEN SHOULD NOT BE USED CONCOMITANTLY WITH THE RELATED DRUG *ANAPROX* OR *ANAPROX DS* (NAPROXEN SODIUM) SINCE THEY BOTH CIRCULATE IN PLASMA AS THE NAPROXEN ANION.

Renal Effects: As with other nonsteroidal anti-inflammatory drugs, long-term administration of naproxen to animals has resulted in renal papillary necrosis and other abnormal renal pathology. In humans, there have been reports of acute interstitial nephritis with hematuria, proteinuria, and occasionally nephrotic syndrome.

A second form of renal toxicity has been seen in patients with prerenal conditions leading to a reduction in renal blood flow or blood volume, where the renal prostaglandins have a supportive role in the maintenance of renal perfusion. In these patients, administration of a nonsteroidal anti-inflammatory drug may cause a dose-dependent reduction in prostaglandin formation and may precipitate overt renal decompensation. Patients at greatest risk of this reaction are those with impaired renal function, heart failure, liver dysfunction, those taking diuretics, and the elderly. Discontinuation of nonsteroidal anti-inflammatory therapy is typically followed by recovery to the pretreatment state.

Naproxen and its metabolites are eliminated primarily by the kidneys, therefore, the drug should be used with great caution in patients with significantly impaired renal function and the monitoring of serum creatinine and/or creatinine clearance is advised in these patients. Caution should be used if the drug is given to patients with creatinine clearance of less than 20 ml/minute because accumulation of naproxen metabolites has been seen in patients.

Chronic alcoholic liver disease and probably other forms of cirrhosis reduce the total plasma concentration of naproxen, but the plasma concentration of unbound naproxen is increased. It is prudent to use the lowest effective dose.

One study indicates that, although total plasma concentration of naproxen is unchanged, the unbound plasma fraction of naproxen is increased in the elderly. As with other drugs used in the elderly, it is prudent to use the lowest effective dose.

As with other nonsteroidal anti-inflammatory drugs, borderline elevations of one or more liver tests may occur in up to 15% of patients. These abnormalities may progress, may remain essentially unchanged, or may be transient with continued therapy. The SGPT (ALT) test is probably the most sensitive indicator of liver dysfunction. Meaningful (3 times the upper limit of normal) elevations of SGPT or SGOT (AST) occurred in controlled clinical trials in less than 1% of patients. A patient with symptoms and/or signs suggesting liver dysfunction, or in whom an abnormal liver test has occurred, should be evaluated for evidence of the development of more severe hepatic reaction while on therapy with this drug. Severe hepatic reactions, including jaundice and cases of fatal hepatitis, have been reported with this drug as with other nonsteroidal anti-inflammatory drugs. Although such reactions are rare, if abnormal liver tests persist or worsen, if clinical signs and symptoms consistent with liver disease develop, or if systemic manifestations occur (*e.g.,* eosinophilia, rash, etc.), this drug should be discontinued.

If steroid dosage is reduced or eliminated during therapy, the steroid dosage should be reduced slowly and the patients must be observed closely for any evidence of adverse effects, including adrenal insufficiency and exacerbation of symptoms of arthritis.

Patients with initial hemoglobin values of 10 g or less who are to receive long-term therapy should have hemoglobin values determined periodically.

Peripheral edema has been observed in some patients. For this reason, the drug should be used with caution in patients with retention, hypertension or heart failure.

Naproxen suspension contains 8 mg/ml of sodium. This should be considered in patients whose overall intake of sodium must be restricted.

The antipyretic and anti-inflammatory activities of the drug may reduce fever and inflammation, thus diminishing their utility as diagnostic signs in detecting complications of presumed non-infectious, non-inflammatory painful conditions.

Because of adverse eye findings in animal studies with drugs of this class, it is recommended that ophthalmic studies be carried out if any change or disturbance in vision occurs.

INFORMATION FOR THE PATIENT

Naproxen, like other drugs of its class, is not free of side effects. The side effects of these drugs can cause discomfort and, rarely, there are more serious side effects, such as gastrointestinal bleeding, which may result in hospitalization and even fatal outcomes.

NSAIDs are often essential agents in the management of arthritis and have a major role in the treatment of pain, but they also may be commonly employed for conditions which are less serious.

Physicians may wish to discuss with their patients the potential risks (see WARNINGS and ADVERSE REACTIONS) and likely benefits of NSAID treatment, particularly when the drugs are used for less serious conditions where treatment without NSAIDs may represent an acceptable alternative to both the patient and physician.

Caution should be exercised by patients whose activities require alertness if they experience drowsiness, dizziness, vertigo or depression during therapy with the drug.

LABORATORY TESTS

Because serious GI tract ulceration and bleeding can occur without warning symptoms, physicians should follow chronically treated patients for the signs and symptoms of ulceration and bleeding and should inform them of the importance of this follow-up (see WARNINGS, Risk of GI Ulceration, Bleeding and Perforation With NSAID Therapy.)

DRUG/LABORATORY TEST INTERACTIONS

The drug may decrease platelet aggregation and prolong bleeding time. This effect should be kept in mind when bleeding times are determined.

The administration of the drug may result in increased urinary values for 17-ketogenic steroids because of an interaction between the drug and/or its metabolites with m-dinitrobenzene used in this assay. Although 17 hydroxy-corticosteroid measurements (Porter-Silber test) do not appear to be artifactually altered, it is suggested that therapy with the drug be temporarily discontinued 72 hours before adrenal function tests are performed.

The drug may interfere with some urinary assays of 5-hydroxy indoleacetic acid (5HIAA).

CARCINOGENESIS

A 2 year study was performed in rats to evaluate the carcinogenic potential of the drug. No evidence of carcinogenicity was found.

PREGNANCY CATEGORY B

Teratogenic Effects

Reproduction studies have been performed in rats, rabbits, and mice at doses up to 6 times the human dose and have revealed no evidence of impaired fertility or harm to the fetus due to the drug. There are, however, no adequate and well-controlled studies in pregnant women. Because animal reproduction studies are not always predictive of human response, the drug should not be used during pregnancy unless clearly needed. Because of the known effect of drugs of this class on the human fetal cardiovascular system (closure of ductus arteriosus), use during late pregnancy should be avoided.

Nonteratogenic Effects

As with other drugs known to inhibit prostaglandin synthesis, an increased incidence of dystocia and delayed parturition occurred in rats.

NURSING MOTHERS

The naproxen anion has been found in the milk of lactating women at a concentration of approximately 1% of that found in the plasma. Because of the possible adverse effects of prostaglandin-inhibiting drugs on neonates, use in nursing mothers should be avoided.

PEDIATRIC USE

Safety and effectiveness in children below the age of 2 years have not been established. Pediatric dosing recommendations for juvenile arthritis are based on well-controlled studies (see DOSAGE AND ADMINISTRATION). There are no adequate effectiveness or dose-response data for other pediatric conditions, but the experience in juvenile arthritis and other use experience have established that single doses of 2.5-5 mg/kg, with a total daily dose not exceeding 15 mg/kg/day, are safe in children over 2 years of age.

DRUG INTERACTIONS

In vitro studies have shown that naproxen anion, because of its affinity for protein, may displace from their binding sites other drugs which are also albumin-bound. Theoretically, the naproxen anion itself could likewise be displaced. Short-term controlled studies failed to show that taking the drug significantly affects prothrombin times when administered to individuals on coumarin-type anticoagulants. Caution is advised nonetheless, since interactions have been seen with other nonsteroidal agents of this class. Similarly, patients receiving the drug and a hydantoin, sulfonamide or sulfonylurea should be observed for signs of toxicity to these drugs.

The natriuretic effect of the furosemide has been reported to be inhibited by some drugs of this class. Inhibition of renal lithium clearance leading to increases in plasma lithium concentrations has also been reported.

This and other nonsteroidal anti-inflammatory drugs can reduce the antihypertensive effect of propanolol and other beta-blockers.

Probenecid given concurrently increases naproxen anion plasma levels and extends is plasma half-life significantly.

Caution should be used if this drug is administered concomitantly with methotrexate. Naproxen and other nonsteroidal anti-inflammatory drugs have been reported to reduce the tubular secretion of methotrexate in an animal model, possibly enhancing the toxicity of that drug.

ADVERSE REACTIONS

The following adverse reactions are divided into 3 parts based on frequency and likelihood of causal relationship to naproxen.

INCIDENCE GREATER THAN 1%:

Possible Causal Relationship: Adverse reactions reported in controlled clinical trials in 960 patients treated for rheumatoid arthritis or osteoarthritis are listed below. In general, these reactions were reported 2 to 10 times more frequently than they were in studies in the 962 patients treated for mild to moderate pain or for dysmenorrhea.

A clinical study found gastrointestinal reactions to more frequent and more severe in rheumatoid arthritis patients taking 1500 mg naproxen daily compared to those taking 750 mg daily. (See CLINICAL PHARMACOLOGY.)

In controlled clinical trials with about 80 children and in well-monitored open studies with about 400 children with juvenile arthritis, the incidences of rash and prolonged bleeding times were increased, the incidences of gastrointestinal and central nervous system reactions were about the same, and the incidences of other reactions were lower in children than in adults.

Gastrointestinal: The most frequent complaints reported related to the gastrointestinal tract. They were: constipation*, heartburn*, abdominal pain*, nausea*, dyspepsia, diarrhea, stomatitis.

Central Nervous System: Headache*, dizziness*, drowsiness*, lightheadedness, vertigo.

Dermatologic: Itching (pruritus)*, skin eruption*, ecchymoses*, sweating, purpura.

Special Senses: Tinnitus*, hearing disturbances, visual disturbances.

Cardiovascular: Edema*, dyspnea*, palpitations.

General: Thirst

* Incidence of reported reaction between 3% and 9%. Those reactions occurring in less than 3% of the patients are unmarked.

INCIDENCE LESS THAN 1%

Probable Causal Relationship

The following adverse reactions were reported less frequently than 1% during controlled clinical trial and through voluntary reports since marketing. The probability of a causal relationship exists between the drug and these adverse reactions:

Gastrointestinal: Abnormal liver function tests, gastrointestinal bleeding and/or perforation, hematemesis, jaundice, melena, peptic ulceration with bleeding and/or perforation, vomiting.

Renal: Glomerular nephritis, hematuria, interstitial nephritis, nephrotic syndrome, renal disease, renal failure, renal papillary necrosis.

Hematologic: Eosinophilia, granulocytopenia, leukopenia, thrombocytopenia.
Central Nervous System: Depression, dream abnormalities, inability to concentrate, insomnia, malaise, myalgia and muscle weakness.
Dermatologic: Alopecia, photosensitive dermatitis, skin rashes.
Special Senses: Hearing impairment.
Cardiovascular: Congestive heart failure.
Respiratory: Eosinophilic pneumonitis.
General: Anaphylactoid reactions, menstrual disorders, pyrexia (chills and fever).

Causal Relationship Unknown

Other reactions have been reported in circumstances in which a causal relationship could not be established. However, in these rarely reported events, the possibility cannot be excluded. Therefore, these observations are being listed to serve as alerting information to the physicians:

Hematologic: Aplastic anemia, hemolytic anemia.
Central Nervous System: Aseptic meningitis, cognitive dysfunction.
Dermatologic: Epidermal necrolysis, erythema multiforme, photosensitivity reactions resembling porphyria cutanea tarda and epidermolysis bullosa, Stevens-Johnson syndrome, urticaria.
Gastrointestinal: Non-peptic gastrointestinal ulceration, ulcerative stomatitis.
Cardiovascular: Vasculitis.
General: Angioneurotic edema, hyperglycemia, hypoglycemia.

DOSAGE AND ADMINISTRATION

A measuring cup marked in ½ teaspoon and 2.5 ml increments is provided with the suspension. This cup or a teaspoon may be used to measure the appropriate dose.

FOR RHEUMATOID ARTHRITIS, OSTEOARTHRITIS, AND ANKYLOSING SPONDYLITIS

The recommended dose of naproxen in adults is 250 mg (10 ml or 2 tsp of suspension), 375 mg (15 ml or 3 tsp), or 500 mg (20 ml or 4 tsp) twice daily (morning and evening). During long-term administration, the dose may be adjusted up or down depending on the clinical response of the patient. A lower daily dose may suffice for long-term administration. The morning and evening doses do not have to be equal in size and the administration of the drug more frequently than twice daily is not necessary. In patients who tolerate lower doses well, the dose may be increased to 1500 mg/day for limited periods when a higher level of anti-inflammatory/analgesic activity is required. When treating such patients with the 1500 mg/day dose, the physician should observe sufficient increased clinical benefits to offset the potential increased risk (see CLINICAL PHARMACOLOGY).

Symptomatic improvement in arthritis usually begins with 2 weeks. However, if improvement is not seen within this period, a trial for an additional 2 weeks should be considered.

FOR JUVENILE ARTHRITIS

The recommended total daily dose of naproxen is approximately 10 mg/kg given in 2 divided doses. One-half of the 250 mg tablet may be used to approximate this dose. The following table may be used as a guide for suspension (see TABLE 1).

TABLE 1

Child's Weight	Dose
13 kg (29 lb)	2.5 ml (½ tsp) bid
25 kg (55 lb)	5 ml (1 tsp) bid
38 kg (84 lb)	7.5 ml (1-½ tsp) bid

FOR ACUTE GOUT

The recommended starting dose of naproxen is 750 mg (30 ml or 6 tsp), followed by 250 mg (10 ml or 2 tsp) every 8 hours until the attack has subsided.

FOR MILD TO MODERATE PAIN, PRIMARY DYSMENORRHEA AND ACUTE TENDINITIS AND BURSITIS

The recommended starting dose of naproxen is 500 mg (20 ml or 4 tsp), followed by 250 mg (10 ml or 2 tsp) every 6 to 8 hours as required. The total daily dose should not exceed 1250 mg (50 ml or 10 tsp).

PRODUCT LISTING - RATED THERAPEUTICALLY EQUIVALENT

Suspension - Oral - 125 mg/5 ml			
15 ml x 25	$50.00	GENERIC, Roxane Laboratories Inc	00054-8632-11
20 ml x 25	$66.65	GENERIC, Roxane Laboratories Inc	00054-8633-11
480 ml	$56.10	NAPROSYN, Roche Laboratories	00004-0028-28
500 ml	$38.23	GENERIC, Roxane Laboratories Inc	00054-3630-63
Tablet - Oral - 250 mg			
10 x 10	$87.60	GENERIC, Major Pharmaceuticals Inc	00904-5535-61
14's	$13.13	GENERIC, Heartland Healthcare Services	61392-0289-14
15's	$4.45	GENERIC, Pd-Rx Pharmaceuticals	58864-0445-15
20's	$13.85	GENERIC, Allscripts Pharmaceutical Company	54569-3758-00
20's	$16.75	GENERIC, Golden State Medical	60429-0133-20
20's	$22.50	NAPROSYN, Pharma Pac	52959-0110-20
25's	$18.20	GENERIC, Udl Laboratories Inc	51079-0793-19
28's	$19.39	GENERIC, Allscripts Pharmaceutical Company	54569-3758-02
30's	$23.31	GENERIC, Allscripts Pharmaceutical Company	54569-3758-04
30's	$25.12	GENERIC, Golden State Medical	60429-0133-30
30's	$26.87	GENERIC, Pd-Rx Pharmaceuticals	55289-0445-30
30's	$28.14	GENERIC, Heartland Healthcare Services	61392-0289-30
30's	$28.14	GENERIC, Heartland Healthcare Services	61392-0289-39
30's	$28.90	NAPROSYN, Pharma Pac	52959-0110-30
31's	$29.08	GENERIC, Heartland Healthcare Services	61392-0289-31
32's	$30.02	GENERIC, Heartland Healthcare Services	61392-0289-32
45's	$42.21	GENERIC, Heartland Healthcare Services	61392-0289-45
60's	$9.60	GENERIC, Pd-Rx Pharmaceuticals	58864-0359-60
60's	$41.55	GENERIC, Allscripts Pharmaceutical Company	54569-3758-01
60's	$49.53	GENERIC, Golden State Medical	60429-0133-60
60's	$56.28	GENERIC, Heartland Healthcare Services	61392-0289-60
90's	$84.43	GENERIC, Heartland Healthcare Services	61392-0289-90
100's	$9.30	GENERIC, Pd-Rx Pharmaceuticals	58864-0356-01
100's	$10.44	FEDERAL UPPER LIMIT, H.C.F.A. F F P	99999-1864-01
100's	$66.10	GENERIC, Roxane Laboratories Inc	00054-4641-25
100's	$67.05	GENERIC, Qualitest Products Inc	00603-4730-21
100's	$67.05	GENERIC, Major Pharmaceuticals Inc	00904-7745-60
100's	$67.05	GENERIC, West Point Pharma	59591-0253-68
100's	$67.07	GENERIC, Purepac Pharmaceutical Company	00228-2521-10
100's	$67.08	GENERIC, Moore, H.L. Drug Exchange Inc	00839-7881-06
100's	$67.10	GENERIC, Mova Pharmaceutical Corporation	55370-0521-07
100's	$71.02	GENERIC, Dixon-Shane Inc	17236-0076-01
100's	$71.75	GENERIC, Martec Pharmaceuticals Inc	52555-0488-01
100's	$71.75	GENERIC, Martec Pharmaceuticals Inc	52555-0625-01
100's	$72.45	GENERIC, Ivax Corporation	00172-4107-60
100's	$72.45	GENERIC, Ivax Corporation	00182-1971-01
100's	$73.50	GENERIC, Brightstone Pharma	62939-8311-01
100's	$73.96	GENERIC, Mylan Pharmaceuticals Inc	00378-0377-01
100's	$73.96	GENERIC, Watson/Rugby Laboratories Inc	00536-4842-01
100's	$73.96	GENERIC, Geneva Pharmaceuticals	00781-1163-01
100's	$75.23	GENERIC, Geneva Pharmaceuticals	00781-1163-13
100's	$76.22	GENERIC, Aligen Independent Laboratories Inc	00405-4693-01
100's	$77.65	GENERIC, Mova Pharmaceutical Corporation	55370-0139-07
100's	$77.70	GENERIC, Teva Pharmaceuticals Usa	00093-0147-01
100's	$77.70	GENERIC, Watson Laboratories Inc	00591-0821-01
100's	$77.70	GENERIC, Teva Pharmaceuticals Usa	38245-0146-10
100's	$77.70	GENERIC, Watson/Rugby Laboratories Inc	52544-0821-01
100's	$80.03	GENERIC, Udl Laboratories Inc	51079-0793-20
100's	$83.60	NAPROSYN, Syntex Laboratories Inc	18393-0272-53
100's	$110.54	GENERIC, Roche Laboratories	00004-6312-01
100's	$116.97	NAPROSYN, Pd-Rx Pharmaceuticals	55289-0977-17
120's	$67.00	GENERIC, Golden State Medical	60429-0133-12
180's	$100.50	GENERIC, Golden State Medical	60429-0133-18
Tablet - Oral - 375 mg			
10 x 10	$111.50	GENERIC, Major Pharmaceuticals Inc	00904-5536-61
10's	$8.71	GENERIC, Allscripts Pharmaceutical Company	54569-3759-00
10's	$14.15	NAPROSYN, Pharma Pac	52959-0192-10
10's	$20.48	GENERIC, Pd-Rx Pharmaceuticals	55289-0297-10
14's	$11.72	GENERIC, Heartland Healthcare Services	61392-0292-14
14's	$12.20	GENERIC, Allscripts Pharmaceutical Company	54569-3759-03
14's	$20.32	NAPROSYN, Pharma Pac	52959-0192-14
14's	$24.57	GENERIC, Pd-Rx Pharmaceuticals	55289-0297-14
15's	$13.07	GENERIC, Allscripts Pharmaceutical Company	54569-3759-05
15's	$24.03	NAPROSYN, Pd-Rx Pharmaceuticals	55289-0435-15
15's	$25.88	GENERIC, Pd-Rx Pharmaceuticals	55289-0297-15
20's	$17.43	GENERIC, Allscripts Pharmaceutical Company	54569-3759-04
20's	$22.38	GENERIC, St. Mary'S Mpp	60760-0140-20
20's	$29.76	NAPROSYN, Pharma Pac	52959-0192-20
20's	$30.83	GENERIC, Pd-Rx Pharmaceuticals	55289-0297-20
20's	$32.09	NAPROSYN, Pd-Rx Pharmaceuticals	55289-0435-20
21's	$18.30	GENERIC, Allscripts Pharmaceutical Company	54569-3759-01
21's	$24.10	NAPROSYN, Allscripts Pharmaceutical Company	54569-0293-01
21's	$32.36	GENERIC, Pd-Rx Pharmaceuticals	55289-0297-21
21's	$33.45	NAPROSYN, Pd-Rx Pharmaceuticals	55289-0435-21
24's	$32.40	GENERIC, Pd-Rx Pharmaceuticals	55289-0297-24
28's	$41.43	NAPROSYN, Pharma Pac	52959-0192-28
30's	$25.12	GENERIC, Heartland Healthcare Services	61392-0292-30
30's	$25.13	GENERIC, Heartland Healthcare Services	61392-0292-39
30's	$26.14	GENERIC, Allscripts Pharmaceutical Company	54569-3759-02
30's	$34.43	NAPROSYN, Allscripts Pharmaceutical Company	54569-0293-02
30's	$34.43	GENERIC, Pd-Rx Pharmaceuticals	55289-0297-30
30's	$44.13	NAPROSYN, Pharma Pac	52959-0192-30
30's	$52.61	NAPROSYN, Pd-Rx Pharmaceuticals	55289-0435-30
31's	$25.96	GENERIC, Heartland Healthcare Services	61392-0292-31
32's	$26.80	GENERIC, Heartland Healthcare Services	61392-0292-32
40's	$34.85	GENERIC, Allscripts Pharmaceutical Company	54569-3759-07
40's	$58.70	NAPROSYN, Pharma Pac	52959-0192-40
40's	$67.23	NAPROSYN, Pd-Rx Pharmaceuticals	55289-0435-40
42's	$38.25	GENERIC, Pd-Rx Pharmaceuticals	55289-0297-42
42's	$42.55	GENERIC, Allscripts Pharmaceutical Company	54569-3759-09
45's	$37.69	GENERIC, Heartland Healthcare Services	61392-0292-45
45's	$39.21	GENERIC, Allscripts Pharmaceutical Company	54569-3759-06
60's	$41.40	GENERIC, Pd-Rx Pharmaceuticals	55289-0297-60
60's	$50.25	GENERIC, Heartland Healthcare Services	61392-0292-60
60's	$63.14	GENERIC, St. Mary'S Mpp	60760-0140-60
60's	$63.40	GENERIC, Golden State Medical	60429-0134-60

90's	$75.37	GENERIC, Heartland Healthcare Services	61392-0292-90
100's	$13.83	FEDERAL UPPER LIMIT, H.C.F.A. F F P	99999-1864-04
100's	$73.12	GENERIC, Ivax Corporation	00172-4108-60
100's	$86.20	GENERIC, Qualitest Products Inc	00603-4731-21
100's	$86.20	GENERIC, Major Pharmaceuticals Inc	00904-7746-60
100's	$86.20	GENERIC, West Point Pharma	59591-0254-68
100's	$86.21	GENERIC, Purepac Pharmaceutical Company	00228-2522-10
100's	$86.25	GENERIC, Mova Pharmaceutical Corporation	55370-0522-07
100's	$87.92	GENERIC, Aligen Independent Laboratories Inc	00405-4694-01
100's	$90.82	GENERIC, Dixon-Shane Inc	17236-0077-01
100's	$92.56	GENERIC, Martec Pharmaceuticals Inc	52555-0489-01
100's	$94.84	GENERIC, Moore, H.L. Drug Exchange Inc	00839-7833-06
100's	$94.99	GENERIC, Geneva Pharmaceuticals	00781-1164-01
100's	$95.00	GENERIC, Brightstone Pharma	62939-8321-01
100's	$95.03	GENERIC, Esi Lederle Generics	00005-3301-43
100's	$95.03	GENERIC, Watson/Rugby Laboratories Inc	00536-4843-01
100's	$95.97	GENERIC, Geneva Pharmaceuticals	00781-1164-13
100's	$101.31	GENERIC, Allscripts Pharmaceutical Company	54569-3759-08
100's	$101.35	GENERIC, Mylan Pharmaceuticals Inc	00378-0555-01
100's	$106.35	GENERIC, Mova Pharmaceutical Corporation	55370-0140-07
100's	$106.40	GENERIC, Teva Pharmaceuticals Usa	00093-0148-01
100's	$106.40	GENERIC, Watson Laboratories Inc	00591-0822-01
100's	$106.40	GENERIC, Teva Pharmaceuticals Usa	38245-0443-10
100's	$106.40	GENERIC, Watson/Rugby Laboratories Inc	52544-0822-01
100's	$106.40	GENERIC, Novopharm Usa Inc	55953-0518-40
100's	$109.59	GENERIC, Udl Laboratories Inc	51079-0794-20
100's	$142.06	NAPROSYN, Roche Laboratories	00004-6311-01
100's	$142.06	NAPROSYN, Roche Laboratories	00004-6314-01
180's	$156.83	GENERIC, Allscripts Pharmaceutical Company	54569-8547-00
180's	$188.79	GENERIC, Golden State Medical	60429-0134-18

Tablet - Oral - 500 mg

2's	$2.50	GENERIC, Allscripts Pharmaceutical Company	54569-4762-00
6's	$20.93	GENERIC, Pd-Rx Pharmaceuticals	55289-0298-06
9's	$11.25	GENERIC, Allscripts Pharmaceutical Company	54569-3760-08
10 x 10	$135.50	GENERIC, Major Pharmaceuticals Inc	00904-5537-61
10's	$10.76	GENERIC, Allscripts Pharmaceutical Company	54569-3760-03
10's	$20.18	NAPROSYN, Pd-Rx Pharmaceuticals	55289-0420-10
12's	$20.09	GENERIC, Dhs Inc	55887-0959-12
14's	$15.06	GENERIC, Allscripts Pharmaceutical Company	54569-3760-04
14's	$19.63	NAPROSYN, Allscripts Pharmaceutical Company	54569-0294-06
14's	$23.41	GENERIC, Dhs Inc	55887-0959-14
14's	$26.70	NAPROSYN, Pharma Pac	52959-0111-14
14's	$28.19	NAPROSYN, Pd-Rx Pharmaceuticals	55289-0420-14
14's	$28.26	GENERIC, Pd-Rx Pharmaceuticals	55289-0298-14
15's	$16.14	GENERIC, Allscripts Pharmaceutical Company	54569-3760-00
15's	$24.01	GENERIC, Dhs Inc	55887-0959-15
15's	$29.70	GENERIC, Pd-Rx Pharmaceuticals	55289-0298-15
15's	$34.02	NAPROSYN, Pd-Rx Pharmaceuticals	55289-0420-15
20's	$20.55	GENERIC, Heartland Healthcare Services	61392-0295-20
20's	$21.52	GENERIC, Allscripts Pharmaceutical Company	54569-3760-01
20's	$24.23	GENERIC, Golden State Medical	60429-0135-20
20's	$28.04	NAPROSYN, Allscripts Pharmaceutical Company	54569-0294-01
20's	$28.85	GENERIC, St. Mary'S Mpp	60760-0460-20
20's	$33.38	NAPROSYN, Physicians Total Care	54868-0300-04
20's	$37.13	GENERIC, Pd-Rx Pharmaceuticals	55289-0298-20
20's	$38.00	NAPROSYN, Pharma Pac	52959-0111-20
20's	$39.35	NAPROSYN, Pd-Rx Pharmaceuticals	55289-0420-20
21's	$26.24	GENERIC, Allscripts Pharmaceutical Company	54569-4255-00
24's	$40.14	GENERIC, Pd-Rx Pharmaceuticals	55289-0298-24
25's	$33.45	GENERIC, Udl Laboratories Inc	51079-0795-19
25's	$79.43	GENERIC, Pd-Rx Pharmaceuticals	55289-0298-97
28's	$35.91	GENERIC, Pd-Rx Pharmaceuticals	55289-0298-28
28's	$41.11	GENERIC, Dhs Inc	55887-0959-28
28's	$53.00	NAPROSYN, Pharma Pac	52959-0111-28
30's	$30.82	GENERIC, Heartland Healthcare Services	61392-0295-30
30's	$30.82	GENERIC, Heartland Healthcare Services	61392-0295-39
30's	$32.28	GENERIC, Allscripts Pharmaceutical Company	54569-3760-02
30's	$40.18	GENERIC, St. Mary'S Mpp	60760-0460-30
30's	$42.06	NAPROSYN, Allscripts Pharmaceutical Company	54569-0294-02
30's	$42.75	GENERIC, Pd-Rx Pharmaceuticals	55289-0298-30
30's	$49.46	NAPROSYN, Physicians Total Care	54868-0300-00
30's	$56.00	NAPROSYN, Pharma Pac	52959-0111-30
30's	$58.22	GENERIC, Dhs Inc	55887-0959-30
30's	$59.03	NAPROSYN, Pd-Rx Pharmaceuticals	55289-0420-30
31 x 10	$353.40	GENERIC, Vangard Labs	00615-3563-43
31 x 10	$353.40	GENERIC, Vangard Labs	00615-3563-53
31 x 10	$353.40	GENERIC, Vangard Labs	00615-3563-63
31's	$31.85	GENERIC, Heartland Healthcare Services	61392-0295-31
32's	$32.88	GENERIC, Heartland Healthcare Services	61392-0295-32
40's	$43.04	GENERIC, Allscripts Pharmaceutical Company	54569-3760-05
40's	$47.88	GENERIC, Pd-Rx Pharmaceuticals	55289-0298-40
40's	$58.22	GENERIC, Dhs Inc	55887-0959-40
40's	$74.00	NAPROSYN, Pharma Pac	52959-0111-40
40's	$87.35	NAPROSYN, Pd-Rx Pharmaceuticals	55289-0420-40
45's	$46.23	GENERIC, Heartland Healthcare Services	61392-0295-45
60's	$54.09	GENERIC, Pd-Rx Pharmaceuticals	55289-0298-60
60's	$61.64	GENERIC, Heartland Healthcare Services	61392-0295-60
60's	$72.70	GENERIC, Golden State Medical	60429-0135-60
60's	$74.97	GENERIC, Allscripts Pharmaceutical Company	54569-3760-07
60's	$90.00	NAPROSYN, Pharma Pac	52959-0111-60
90's	$92.46	GENERIC, Heartland Healthcare Services	61392-0295-90
100's	$17.92	FEDERAL UPPER LIMIT, H.C.F.A. F F P	99999-1864-07
100's	$105.30	GENERIC, Purepac Pharmaceutical Company	00228-2523-10
100's	$105.30	GENERIC, Qualitest Products Inc	00603-4732-21
100's	$105.30	GENERIC, Moore, H.L. Drug Exchange Inc	00839-7883-06
100's	$105.30	GENERIC, Major Pharmaceuticals Inc	00904-7747-60
100's	$105.30	GENERIC, West Point Pharma	59591-0255-68
100's	$107.54	GENERIC, Aligen Independent Laboratories Inc	00405-4695-01
100's	$111.66	GENERIC, Dixon-Shane Inc	17236-0078-01
100's	$112.35	GENERIC, Martec Pharmaceuticals Inc	52555-0490-01
100's	$113.74	GENERIC, Ivax Corporation	00172-4109-60
100's	$115.50	GENERIC, Brightstone Pharma	62939-8331-01
100's	$115.99	GENERIC, Geneva Pharmaceuticals	00781-1165-01
100's	$116.04	GENERIC, Esi Lederle Generics	00005-3302-43
100's	$116.04	GENERIC, Watson/Rugby Laboratories Inc	00536-4844-01
100's	$117.23	GENERIC, Geneva Pharmaceuticals	00781-1165-13
100's	$123.75	GENERIC, Mylan Pharmaceuticals Inc	00378-0451-01
100's	$124.95	GENERIC, Allscripts Pharmaceutical Company	54569-3760-06
100's	$129.00	GENERIC, Watson Laboratories Inc	52544-0791-01
100's	$129.85	GENERIC, Mova Pharmaceutical Corporation	55370-0141-07
100's	$129.90	GENERIC, Teva Pharmaceuticals Usa	00093-0149-01
100's	$130.24	NAPROSYN, Syntex Laboratories Inc	18393-0277-53
100's	$133.80	GENERIC, Udl Laboratories Inc	51079-0795-20
100's	$173.53	NAPROSYN, Roche Laboratories	00004-6310-01
100's	$173.53	NAPROSYN, Roche Laboratories	00004-6316-01
120's	$183.52	NAPROSYN, Physicians Total Care	54868-0300-08
180's	$193.66	GENERIC, Allscripts Pharmaceutical Company	54569-8582-00
180's	$218.10	GENERIC, Golden State Medical	60429-0135-18
180's	$227.59	NAPROSYN, Allscripts Pharmaceutical Company	54569-8529-00

Tablet, Delayed Release - Oral - 375 mg

100's	$67.50	FEDERAL UPPER LIMIT, H.C.F.A. F F P	99999-1864-10

Tablet, Enteric Coated - Oral - 375 mg

14's	$15.76	EC NAPROSYN, Allscripts Pharmaceutical Company	54569-3981-00
100's	$98.85	GENERIC, Apothecon Inc	62269-0289-24
100's	$101.21	GENERIC, Geneva Pharmaceuticals	00781-1646-01
100's	$101.31	GENERIC, Purepac Pharmaceutical Company	00228-2617-11
100's	$101.31	GENERIC, Purepac Pharmaceutical Company	00228-2745-11
100's	$101.31	GENERIC, Ethex Corporation	58177-0302-04
100's	$106.40	GENERIC, Teva Pharmaceuticals Usa	00093-1005-01

Tablet, Enteric Coated - Oral - 500 mg

15's	$21.66	EC NAPROSYN, Allscripts Pharmaceutical Company	54569-3982-00
15's	$73.08	GENERIC, Pd-Rx Pharmaceuticals	55289-0307-15
20's	$33.75	GENERIC, St. Mary'S Mpp	60760-0618-20
24's	$85.95	GENERIC, Pd-Rx Pharmaceuticals	55289-0307-24
30's	$43.31	EC NAPROSYN, Allscripts Pharmaceutical Company	54569-3982-01
30's	$68.58	EC NAPROSYN, Pharma Pac	52959-0456-30
30's	$108.00	GENERIC, Pd-Rx Pharmaceuticals	55289-0307-30
40's	$87.59	EC NAPROSYN, Pharma Pac	52959-0456-40
60's	$119.88	EC NAPROSYN, Pharma Pac	52959-0456-60
100's	$120.74	GENERIC, Apothecon Inc	62269-0290-24
100's	$125.20	GENERIC, Purepac Pharmaceutical Company	00228-2618-11
100's	$125.20	GENERIC, Purepac Pharmaceutical Company	00228-2746-10
100's	$125.20	GENERIC, Ethex Corporation	58177-0303-04
100's	$129.90	GENERIC, Teva Pharmaceuticals Usa	00093-1006-01

PRODUCT LISTING - EQUIVALENTS NOT AVAILABLE

Tablet - Oral - 250 mg

2's	$3.67	GENERIC, Prescript Pharmaceuticals	00247-0334-02
3's	$3.84	GENERIC, Prescript Pharmaceuticals	00247-0334-03
4's	$3.99	GENERIC, Prescript Pharmaceuticals	00247-0334-04
5's	$4.15	GENERIC, Prescript Pharmaceuticals	00247-0334-05
6's	$4.31	GENERIC, Prescript Pharmaceuticals	00247-0334-06
10's	$4.94	GENERIC, Prescript Pharmaceuticals	00247-0334-10
10's	$8.05	GENERIC, Southwood Pharmaceuticals Inc	58016-0314-10
12's	$10.71	GENERIC, Southwood Pharmaceuticals Inc	58016-0314-12
14's	$12.50	GENERIC, Southwood Pharmaceuticals Inc	58016-0314-14
15's	$5.74	GENERIC, Prescript Pharmaceuticals	00247-0334-15
15's	$12.08	GENERIC, Southwood Pharmaceuticals Inc	58016-0314-15

20's	$4.30	GENERIC, Physicians Total Care	54868-2964-03
20's	$6.53	GENERIC, Prescript Pharmaceuticals	00247-0334-20
20's	$16.09	GENERIC, Southwood Pharmaceuticals Inc	58016-0314-20
20's	$16.64	GENERIC, Cardinal Pharmaceuticals	63874-0301-20
20's	$19.90	GENERIC, Pharma Pac	52959-0190-20
21's	$6.69	GENERIC, Prescript Pharmaceuticals	00247-0334-21
21's	$17.16	GENERIC, Cardinal Pharmaceuticals	63874-0301-21
21's	$18.74	GENERIC, Southwood Pharmaceuticals Inc	58016-0314-21
24's	$7.16	GENERIC, Prescript Pharmaceuticals	00247-0334-24
24's	$24.99	GENERIC, Southwood Pharmaceuticals Inc	58016-0314-24
28's	$7.80	GENERIC, Prescript Pharmaceuticals	00247-0334-28
28's	$23.57	GENERIC, Pharma Pac	52959-0190-28
28's	$24.99	GENERIC, Southwood Pharmaceuticals Inc	58016-0314-28
30's	$5.79	GENERIC, Physicians Total Care	54868-2964-01
30's	$8.12	GENERIC, Prescript Pharmaceuticals	00247-0334-30
30's	$22.64	GENERIC, Pharmaceutical Corporation Of America	51655-0685-24
30's	$24.16	GENERIC, Southwood Pharmaceuticals Inc	58016-0314-30
30's	$27.17	GENERIC, Pharma Pac	52959-0190-30
40's	$35.70	GENERIC, Southwood Pharmaceuticals Inc	58016-0314-40
40's	$39.88	GENERIC, Pharma Pac	52959-0190-40
60's	$10.24	GENERIC, Physicians Total Care	54868-2964-02
60's	$12.88	GENERIC, Prescript Pharmaceuticals	00247-0334-60
60's	$53.55	GENERIC, Southwood Pharmaceuticals Inc	58016-0314-60
60's	$59.62	GENERIC, Pharma Pac	52959-0190-60
100's	$80.54	GENERIC, Southwood Pharmaceuticals Inc	58016-0314-00
100's	$83.72	GENERIC, Cardinal Pharmaceuticals	63874-0301-01

Tablet - Oral - 375 mg

2's	$3.54	GENERIC, Prescript Pharmaceuticals	00247-0052-02
3's	$3.64	GENERIC, Prescript Pharmaceuticals	00247-0052-03
4's	$3.73	GENERIC, Prescript Pharmaceuticals	00247-0052-04
10's	$4.28	GENERIC, Prescript Pharmaceuticals	00247-0052-10
10's	$12.49	GENERIC, Southwood Pharmaceuticals Inc	58016-0267-10
10's	$13.94	GENERIC, Pharma Pac	52959-0191-10
12's	$14.98	GENERIC, Southwood Pharmaceuticals Inc	58016-0267-12
14's	$4.65	GENERIC, Prescript Pharmaceuticals	00247-0052-14
14's	$14.56	GENERIC, Cardinal Pharmaceuticals	63874-0325-14
14's	$17.33	GENERIC, Pharma Pac	52959-0191-14
14's	$17.48	GENERIC, Southwood Pharmaceuticals Inc	58016-0267-14
15's	$4.74	GENERIC, Prescript Pharmaceuticals	00247-0052-15
15's	$18.73	GENERIC, Southwood Pharmaceuticals Inc	58016-0267-15
15's	$19.64	GENERIC, Pharma Pac	52959-0191-15
15's	$20.84	GENERIC, Cardinal Pharmaceuticals	63874-0325-15
18's	$5.02	GENERIC, Prescript Pharmaceuticals	00247-0052-18
20's	$4.60	GENERIC, Physicians Total Care	54868-2965-06
20's	$5.21	GENERIC, Prescript Pharmaceuticals	00247-0052-20
20's	$19.45	GENERIC, Pharmaceutical Corporation Of America	51655-0625-52
20's	$22.15	GENERIC, Cardinal Pharmaceuticals	63874-0325-20
20's	$24.97	GENERIC, Southwood Pharmaceuticals Inc	58016-0267-20
20's	$27.33	GENERIC, Pharma Pac	52959-0191-20
21's	$5.29	GENERIC, Prescript Pharmaceuticals	00247-0052-21
21's	$26.22	GENERIC, Southwood Pharmaceuticals Inc	58016-0267-21
21's	$26.31	GENERIC, Cardinal Pharmaceuticals	63874-0325-21
24's	$29.97	GENERIC, Southwood Pharmaceuticals Inc	58016-0267-24
28's	$5.95	GENERIC, Prescript Pharmaceuticals	00247-0052-28
28's	$34.96	GENERIC, Southwood Pharmaceuticals Inc	58016-0267-28
28's	$36.02	GENERIC, Pharma Pac	52959-0191-28
30's	$6.13	GENERIC, Prescript Pharmaceuticals	00247-0052-30
30's	$6.23	GENERIC, Physicians Total Care	54868-2965-02
30's	$33.23	GENERIC, Cardinal Pharmaceuticals	63874-0325-30
30's	$37.46	GENERIC, Southwood Pharmaceuticals Inc	58016-0267-30
30's	$39.29	GENERIC, Pharma Pac	52959-0191-30
40's	$7.06	GENERIC, Prescript Pharmaceuticals	00247-0052-40
40's	$7.86	GENERIC, Physicians Total Care	54868-2965-03
40's	$49.18	GENERIC, Pharma Pac	52959-0191-40
40's	$49.94	GENERIC, Southwood Pharmaceuticals Inc	58016-0267-40
42's	$51.12	GENERIC, Pharma Pac	52959-0191-42
42's	$52.44	GENERIC, Southwood Pharmaceuticals Inc	58016-0267-42
50's	$9.50	GENERIC, Physicians Total Care	54868-2965-01
60's	$8.92	GENERIC, Prescript Pharmaceuticals	00247-0052-60
60's	$11.13	GENERIC, Physicians Total Care	54868-2965-04
60's	$56.35	GENERIC, Pharmaceutical Corporation Of America	51655-0625-25
60's	$74.92	GENERIC, Southwood Pharmaceuticals Inc	58016-0267-60
90's	$11.69	GENERIC, Prescript Pharmaceuticals	00247-0052-90
90's	$118.37	GENERIC, Southwood Pharmaceuticals Inc	58016-0267-90
100's	$12.62	GENERIC, Prescript Pharmaceuticals	00247-0052-00
100's	$16.99	GENERIC, Physicians Total Care	54868-2965-05
100's	$110.76	GENERIC, Cardinal Pharmaceuticals	63874-0325-01
100's	$124.86	GENERIC, Southwood Pharmaceuticals Inc	58016-0267-00

Tablet - Oral - 500 mg

2's	$3.54	GENERIC, Prescript Pharmaceuticals	00247-0053-02
3's	$3.64	GENERIC, Prescript Pharmaceuticals	00247-0053-03
4's	$3.73	GENERIC, Prescript Pharmaceuticals	00247-0053-04
6's	$3.91	GENERIC, Prescript Pharmaceuticals	00247-0053-06
10's	$4.28	GENERIC, Prescript Pharmaceuticals	00247-0053-10
10's	$12.26	GENERIC, Pharmaceutical Corporation Of America	51655-0626-53
10's	$15.26	GENERIC, Southwood Pharmaceuticals Inc	58016-0289-10
12's	$4.47	GENERIC, Prescript Pharmaceuticals	00247-0053-12
12's	$18.31	GENERIC, Southwood Pharmaceuticals Inc	58016-0289-12
14's	$4.65	GENERIC, Prescript Pharmaceuticals	00247-0053-14
14's	$18.96	GENERIC, Cardinal Pharmaceuticals	63874-0326-14
14's	$21.36	GENERIC, Southwood Pharmaceuticals Inc	58016-0289-14
14's	$23.22	GENERIC, Pharma Pac	52959-0193-14
15's	$4.07	GENERIC, Physicians Total Care	54868-2966-07
15's	$4.74	GENERIC, Prescript Pharmaceuticals	00247-0053-15
15's	$22.89	GENERIC, Southwood Pharmaceuticals Inc	58016-0289-15
15's	$24.44	GENERIC, Cardinal Pharmaceuticals	63874-0326-15
15's	$24.73	GENERIC, Pharma Pac	52959-0193-15
18's	$27.46	GENERIC, Southwood Pharmaceuticals Inc	58016-0289-18
20's	$5.21	GENERIC, Prescript Pharmaceuticals	00247-0053-20
20's	$5.46	GENERIC, Physicians Total Care	54868-2966-06
20's	$25.80	GENERIC, Pharmaceutical Corporation Of America	51655-0626-52
20's	$27.04	GENERIC, Cardinal Pharmaceuticals	63874-0326-20
20's	$30.51	GENERIC, Southwood Pharmaceuticals Inc	58016-0289-20
20's	$32.95	GENERIC, Pharma Pac	52959-0193-20
21's	$5.29	GENERIC, Prescript Pharmaceuticals	00247-0053-21
21's	$32.04	GENERIC, Southwood Pharmaceuticals Inc	58016-0289-21
21's	$34.40	GENERIC, Pharma Pac	52959-0193-21
24's	$36.62	GENERIC, Southwood Pharmaceuticals Inc	58016-0289-24
24's	$39.28	GENERIC, Pharma Pac	52959-0193-24
28's	$5.95	GENERIC, Prescript Pharmaceuticals	00247-0053-28
28's	$42.72	GENERIC, Southwood Pharmaceuticals Inc	58016-0289-28
28's	$45.74	GENERIC, Pharma Pac	52959-0193-28
30's	$6.13	GENERIC, Prescript Pharmaceuticals	00247-0053-30
30's	$7.52	GENERIC, Physicians Total Care	54868-2966-04
30's	$40.56	GENERIC, Cardinal Pharmaceuticals	63874-0326-30
30's	$45.77	GENERIC, Southwood Pharmaceuticals Inc	58016-0289-30
30's	$48.04	GENERIC, Pharma Pac	52959-0193-30
35's	$49.67	GENERIC, Pharma Pac	52959-0193-35
40's	$7.06	GENERIC, Prescript Pharmaceuticals	00247-0053-40
40's	$9.59	GENERIC, Physicians Total Care	54868-2966-03
40's	$52.00	GENERIC, Cardinal Pharmaceuticals	63874-0326-40
40's	$56.54	GENERIC, Pharma Pac	52959-0193-40
40's	$61.03	GENERIC, Southwood Pharmaceuticals Inc	58016-0289-40
42's	$64.08	GENERIC, Southwood Pharmaceuticals Inc	58016-0289-42
50's	$7.99	GENERIC, Prescript Pharmaceuticals	00247-0053-50
50's	$76.29	GENERIC, Southwood Pharmaceuticals Inc	58016-0289-50
56's	$85.44	GENERIC, Southwood Pharmaceuticals Inc	58016-0289-56
60's	$8.92	GENERIC, Prescript Pharmaceuticals	00247-0053-60
60's	$13.71	GENERIC, Physicians Total Care	54868-2966-02
60's	$75.40	GENERIC, Pharmaceutical Corporation Of America	51655-0626-25
60's	$80.56	GENERIC, Pharma Pac	52959-0193-60
60's	$91.54	GENERIC, Southwood Pharmaceuticals Inc	58016-0289-60
90's	$11.69	GENERIC, Prescript Pharmaceuticals	00247-0053-90
90's	$137.31	GENERIC, Southwood Pharmaceuticals Inc	58016-0289-90
100's	$12.62	GENERIC, Prescript Pharmaceuticals	00247-0053-00
100's	$135.20	GENERIC, Cardinal Pharmaceuticals	63874-0326-01
100's	$152.57	GENERIC, Southwood Pharmaceuticals Inc	58016-0289-00
120's	$183.07	GENERIC, Southwood Pharmaceuticals Inc	58016-0289-02
150's	$228.86	GENERIC, Southwood Pharmaceuticals Inc	58016-0289-03

Tablet, Enteric Coated - Oral - 375 mg

14's	$14.20	GENERIC, Allscripts Pharmaceutical Company	54569-4523-00
15's	$27.62	GENERIC, Pd-Rx Pharmaceuticals	55289-0267-15
24's	$42.51	GENERIC, Pd-Rx Pharmaceuticals	55289-0267-24
100's	$101.41	GENERIC, Allscripts Pharmaceutical Company	54569-4523-01

Tablet, Enteric Coated - Oral - 500 mg

10's	$19.50	GENERIC, Pharma Pac	52959-0516-10
14's	$27.02	GENERIC, Pharma Pac	52959-0516-14
15's	$18.70	GENERIC, Allscripts Pharmaceutical Company	54569-4520-00
20's	$37.15	GENERIC, Pharma Pac	52959-0516-20
30's	$37.40	GENERIC, Allscripts Pharmaceutical Company	54569-4520-01
30's	$55.19	GENERIC, Pharma Pac	52959-0516-30
40's	$72.80	GENERIC, Pharma Pac	52959-0516-40
60's	$107.99	GENERIC, Pharma Pac	52959-0516-60
84's	$132.19	GENERIC, Southwood Pharmaceuticals Inc	58016-0372-84
100's	$124.67	GENERIC, Allscripts Pharmaceutical Company	54569-4520-02
120's	$148.08	GENERIC, Pharma Pac	52959-0516-02

Naproxen Sodium *(001865)*

For related information, see the comparative table section in Appendix A.

Categories: Ankylosing spondylitis; Arthritis, gouty; Arthritis, juvenile; Arthritis, osteoarthritis; Arthritis, rheumatoid; Bursitis; Dysmenorrhea; Pain, mild to moderate; Tendonitis; Pregnancy Category B; FDA Approved 1987 Sep

Drug Classes: Analgesics, non-narcotic; Nonsteroidal anti-inflammatory drugs

Brand Names: **Anaprox**; Anaprox DS; Naprelan

Foreign Brand Availability: Agilxen (Colombia); Anax (Korea); Apranax (Bahrain; Belgium; Cyprus; Czech-Republic; Egypt; France; Germany; Iran; Iraq; Jordan; Kuwait; Lebanon; Libya; Oman; Qatar; Republic-of-Yemen; Russia; Saudi-Arabia; Switzerland; Syria; United-Arab-Emirates); Apraxin (Turkey); Apronax (Colombia; Ecuador; Peru); Babel (Korea); Dafloxen (Mexico); Deflamox (Mexico); Diferbest (Mexico); Flanax (Costa-Rica; Dominican-Republic; El-Salvador; Guatemala; Honduras; Nicaragua; Panama; Philippines); Flanax Forte (Peru); Flonax (Peru); Iraxen (Peru); Lefaine (Philippines); Licorax (Korea); Naprogesic (Australia; New-Zealand); Naprosyn (Turkey); Narocin (Israel); Proxidol (Bahrain; Cyprus; Egypt; Iran; Iraq; Jordan; Kuwait; Lebanon; Libya; Oman; Qatar; Republic-of-Yemen; Saudi-Arabia; Syria; United-Arab-Emirates); Sanomed (Philippines); Sutolin (Taiwan); Synflex (Hong-Kong; Indonesia; Malaysia; New-Zealand); Uniflam (Peru); Xenobid (India)

Cost of Therapy: $47.70 (Osteoarthritis; Anaprox; 275 mg; 2 tablets/day; 30 day supply)
$6.68 (Osteoarthritis; Generic Tablets; 275 mg; 2 tablets/day; 30 day supply)

DESCRIPTION

Naproxen sodium filmcoated tablets for oral administration each contain 275 mg of naproxen, which is equivalent to 250 mg naproxen with 25 mg (about 1 mEq) sodium. Naproxen sodium filmcoated tablets for oral administration each contain 550 mg of

N

naproxen sodium, which is equivalent to 500 mg naproxen with 50 mg (about 2 mEq) sodium. Naproxen sodium is a member of arylacetic acid group of nonsteroidal anti-inflammatory drugs.

The chemical name of naproxen sodium is 2-naphthaleneacetic acid, 6-methoxy-α-methyl-, sodium salt, (-).

Naproxen sodium is a white to creamy white, crystalline solid, freely soluble in water.

Each naproxen sodium 275 mg tablet contains naproxen sodium, the active ingredient, with lactose, magnesium stearate, and microcrystalline cellulose. The coating suspension may contain hydroxypropyl methylcellulose 2910, Opaspray K-1-4210A, polyethylene glycol 8000 or Opadry YS-1-4215. Each naproxen sodium DS 550 mg tablet contains naproxen sodium, the active ingredient, with magnesium stearate, microcrystalline cellulose, povidone, and talc. The coating suspension may contain hydroxypropyl methylcellulose 2910, Opaspray K-1-4227, polyethylene glycol 8000 or Opadry YS-1-4216.

CLINICAL PHARMACOLOGY

The sodium salt of naproxen has been developed as an analgesic because it is more rapidly absorbed. Naproxen is a nonsteroidal anti-inflammatory drug with analgesic and antipyretic properties. Naproxen anion inhibits prostaglandin synthesis but beyond this its mode of action is unknown.

Naproxen sodium is rapidly and completely absorbed from the gastrointestinal tract. After administration of naproxen sodium, peak plasma levels of naproxen anion are attained at 1-2 hours with steady-state conditions normally achieved after 4-5 doses. The mean biological half-life of the anion in humans is approximately 13 hours, and at therapeutic levels it is greater than 99% albumin bound. Approximately 95% of the dose is excreted in the urine, primarily as naproxen, 6-O-desmethyl naproxen or their conjugates. The rate of excretion had been found to coincide closely with the rate of drug disappearance from the plasma. The drug does not induce the metabolizing enzymes.

In children of 5 to 16 years of age with arthritis, plasma naproxen levels following a 5 mg/kg single dose of naproxen suspension (see DOSAGE AND ADMINISTRATION) were found to be similar to those found in normal adults following a 500 mg dose. The terminal half-life appears to be similar in children and adults. Pharmacokinetic studies of naproxen were not performed in children less than 5 years of age.

The drug was studied in patients with mild to moderate pain, and pain relief was obtained within 1 hour. It is not a narcotic and is not a CNS-acting drug. Controlled double-blind studies have demonstrated the analgesic properties of the drug in, for example, post-operative, post-partum, orthopedic and uterine contraction pain and dysmenorrhea. In dysmenorrheic patients, the drug reduces the level of prostaglandins in the uterus, which correlates with a reduction in the frequency and severity of uterine contractions. Analgesic action has been shown by such measures as reduction of pain intensity scores, increase in pain relief scores, decrease in numbers of patients requiring additional analgesic medication and delay in time for required remedication. The analgesic effect has been found to last for up to 7 hours.

The drug was studied in patients with rheumatoid arthritis, osteoarthritis, ankylosing spondylitis, tendinitis and bursitis, and acute gout. It is not a corticosteroid. Improvement in patients treated for rheumatoid arthritis has been demonstrated by a reduction in joint swelling, a reduction in pain, a reduction in duration for morning stiffness, a reduction in disease activity as assessed by both the investigator and patient, and by increased mobility as demonstrated by a reduction in walking time.

In patients with osteoarthritis, the therapeutic action of the drug has been shown by a reduction in joint pain or tenderness, an increase in range of motion in knee joints, increased mobility as demonstrated by a reduction in walking time, and improvement in capacity to perform activities of daily living impaired by the disease.

In clinical studies in patients rheumatoid arthritis, osteoarthritis, and juvenile arthritis, the drug has been shown to be comparable to aspirin and indomethacin in controlling the aforementioned measures of disease activity, but the frequency and severity of the milder gastrointestinal adverse effects (nausea, dyspepsia, heartburn) and nervous system adverse effects (tinnitus, dizziness, lightheadedness) were less than in both the aspirin- and indomethacin-treated patients. It is not known whether the drug causes less peptic ulceration than aspirin.

In patients with ankylosing spondylitis, the drug has been shown to decrease night pain, morning stiffness and pain at rest. In double-blind studies the drug was shown to as effective as aspirin, but with fewer side effects.

In patients with acute gout, a favorable response to the drug was shown by significant clearing of inflammatory changes (*e.g.*, decrease in swelling, heat) within 24-48 hours, as well as by relief of pain and tenderness.

The drug may be used in combination with gold salts and/or corticosteroids; however, in controlled clinical trials, when added to the regimen of patients receiving corticosteroids it did not appear to cause greater improvement over that seen with corticosteroids alone. Whether the drug could be used in conjunction with partially effective doses of corticosteroid for a "steroid-sparing" effect has not been adequately studied. When added to the regimen of patients receiving gold salts,the drug did result in greater improvement. Its use in combination with salicylates is not recommended because data are inadequate to demonstrate that the drug produces greater improvement over that achieved with aspirin alone. Further, there is some evidence that aspirin increases the rate of excretion of the drug.

Generally, improvement due to the drug has not been found to be dependent on age, sex, severity or duration of disease.

In clinical trials in patients with osteoarthritis and rheumatoid arthritis comparing treatments of 825 mg/day with 1650 mg/day, there were trends toward increased efficacy with the higher dose and a more clearcut increase in adverse reactions, particularly gastrointestinal reactions severe enough to cause the patient to leave the trial, which approximately doubled.

In ^{51}Cr blood loss and gastroscopy studies with normal volunteers, daily administration of 1100 mg of naproxen sodium has been demonstrated to cause statistically significantly less gastric bleeding and erosion than 3250 mg of aspirin.

INDICATIONS AND USAGE

Naproxen sodium is indicate in the relief of mild to moderate pain and for the treatment of primary dysmenorrhea.

It is also indicated for the treatment of rheumatoid arthritis, osteoarthritis, juvenile arthritis, ankylosing spondylitis, tendinitis and bursitis and acute gout.

CONTRAINDICATIONS

The drug is contraindicated in patients who have had allergic reactions to naproxen sodium or to naproxen. It is also contraindicated in patients in whom aspirin or other nonsteroidal anti-inflammatory/analgesic drugs induce the syndrome of asthma, rhinitis, and nasal polyps. Both these types of reactions have the potential of being fatal. Anaphylactoid reactions to naproxen sodium or naproxen, whether of the true allergic type or the pharmacologic idiosyncratic (*e.g.*, aspirin syndrome) type, usually but not always occur in patients with a known history of such reactions. Therefore, careful questioning of patients for such things as asthma, nasal polyps, urticaria, and hypotension associated with nonsteroidal anti-inflammatory drugs before starting therapy is important. In addition, if such symptoms occur during therapy, treatment should be discontinued.

WARNINGS

RISK OF GI ULCERATION, BLEEDING AND PERFORATION WITH NSAID THERAPY

Serious gastrointestinal toxicity such as bleeding, ulceration, and perforation, can occur at any time, with or without warning symptoms, in patients treated chronically with NSAID therapy. Although minor upper gastrointestinal problems, such as dyspepsia, are common, usually developing early in therapy, physicians should remain alert for ulceration and bleeding in patients treated chronically with NSAIDs even in the absence of previous GI tract symptoms. In patients observed in clinical trials of several months to 2 years duration, symptomatic upper GI ulcers, gross bleeding or perforation appear to occur in approximately 1% of patients treated for 3-6 months, and in about 2-4% of patients treated for 1 year. Physicians should inform patients about the signs and/or symptoms of serious toxicity and what steps to take if they occur.

Studies to date have not identified any subset of patients not at risk of developing peptic ulceration and bleeding. Except for a prior history of serious GI events and other risk factors known to be associated with peptic ulcer disease, such as alcoholism, smoking, etc., no risk factors (*e.g.*, age, sex) have been associated with increased risk. Elderly or debilitated patients seem to tolerate ulceration or bleeding less well than other individuals and most spontaneous reports of fatal GI events are in this population. Studies to date are inconclusive concerning the relative risk of various NSAIDs in causing such reactions. High doses of any NSAID probably carry a greater risk of these reactions, although controlled clinical trials showing this do not exist in most cases. In considering the use of relatively large doses (within the recommended dosage range), sufficient benefit should be anticipated to offset the potential increased risk of GI toxicity.

PRECAUTIONS

GENERAL

NAPROXEN SODIUM SHOULD NOT BE USED CONCOMITANTLY WITH THE RELATED DRUG NAPROXEN SINCE THEY BOTH CIRCULATE IN PLASMA AS THE NAPROXEN ANION.

Renal Effects: As with other nonsteroidal anti-inflammatory drugs, long-term administration of naproxen to animals has resulted in renal papillary necrosis and other abnormal renal pathology. In humans, there have been reports of acute interstitial nephritis with hematuria, proteinuria, and occasionally nephrotic syndrome.

A second form of renal toxicity has been seen in patients with prerenal conditions leading to a reduction in renal blood flow or blood volume, where the renal prostaglandins have a supportive role in the maintenance of renal perfusion. In these patients, administration of a nonsteroidal anti-inflammatory drug may cause a dose-dependent reduction in prostaglandin formation and may precipitate overt renal decompensation. Patients at greatest risk of this reduction are those with impaired renal function, heart failure, liver dysfunction, those taking diuretics, and the elderly. Discontinuation of nonsteroidal anti-inflammatory therapy is typically followed by recovery to the pretreatment state.

Naproxen sodium and its metabolites are eliminated primarily by the kidneys, therefore the drug should be used with great caution in patients with significantly impaired renal function and the monitoring of serum creatinine and/or creatinine clearance is advised in these patients. Caution should be used if the drug is given to patients with creatinine clearance of less than 20 ml/minute because accumulation of naproxen metabolites has been seen in such patients.

Chronic alcoholic liver disease and probably other forms of cirrhosis reduce the total plasma concentration of naproxen, but the plasma concentration of unbound naproxen is increased. Caution is advised when high doses are required and some adjustment of dosage may be required in elderly patients. As with other drugs used in the elderly, it is prudent to use the lowest effective dose.

Studies indicate that although total plasma concentration of naproxen is unchanged, the unbound plasma fraction of naproxen is increased in the elderly. Caution is advised when high doses are required and some adjustment of dosage may be required in elderly patients. As with other drugs used in the elderly, it is prudent to use the lowest effective dose.

As with other nonsteroidal anti-inflammatory drugs, borderline elevations of one or more liver function tests may occur in up to 15% of patients. These abnormalities may progress, may remain essentially unchanged, or may be transient with continued therapy. The SGPT (ALT) test is probably the most sensitive indicator of liver dysfunction. Meaningful (3 times the upper limit of normal) elevations of SGPT or SGOT (AST) occurred in controlled clinical trials in less than 1% of patients. A patient with symptoms and/or signs suggesting liver dysfunction, or in whom an abnormal liver test has occurred, should be evaluated for evidence of the development of more severe hepatic reactions while on therapy with this drug. Severe hepatic reactions, including jaundice and cases of fatal hepatitis, have been reported with this drug as with other nonsteroidal anti-inflammatory drugs. Although such reactions are rare, if abnormal liver tests persist or worsen, if clinical signs and symptoms consistent with liver disease develop, or if systemic manifestations occur (*e.g.*, eosinophilia, rash, etc.), this drug should be discontinued.

If steroid dosage is reduced or eliminated during therapy, the steroid dosage should be reduced slowly and the patients must be observed closely for any evidence of adverse effects, including adrenal insufficiency and exacerbation of symptoms of arthritis.

Patients with initial hemoglobin values of 10 grams or less who are to receive long-term therapy should have hemoglobin values determined periodically.

Peripheral edema has been observed in some patients. Since each naproxen sodium tablet contains approximately 25 mg (about 1 or 2 mEq) of sodium, this should be considered in patients whose overall intake of sodium must be markedly restricted. For these reasons, the drug should be used with caution in patients with fluid retention, hypertension or heart failure.

The antipyretic and anti-inflammatory activities of the drug may reduce fever and inflammation, thus diminishing their utility as diagnostic signs in detecting complications of presumed non-infectious, non-inflammatory painful conditions.

Because of adverse eye findings in animal studies with drugs of this class it is recommended that ophthalmic studies be carried out if any change or disturbance in vision occurs.

INFORMATION FOR THE PATIENT

Naproxen sodium, like other drugs of its class, is not free of side effects. The side effects of these drugs can cause discomfort and, rarely, there are more serious side effects, such as gastrointestinal bleeding, which may result in hospitalization and even fatal outcomes.

NSAIDs are often essential agents in the management of arthritis and have a major role in the treatment of pain, but they also may be commonly employed for conditions which are less serious.

Physicians may wish to discuss with their patients the potential risks (see WARNINGS and ADVERSE REACTIONS) and likely benefits of NSAID treatment, particularly when the drugs are used for less serious conditions where treatment without NSAIDs may represent an acceptable alternative to both the patient and physician.

Caution should be exercised by patients whose activities require alertness if they experience drowsiness, dizziness, vertigo or depression during therapy with the drug.

LABORATORY TESTS

Because serious GI tract ulceration and bleeding can occur without warning symptoms, physicians should follow chronically treated patients for the signs and symptoms of ulceration and bleeding and should inform them of the importance of this follow-up (see WARNINGS, Risk of GI Ulcerations, Bleeding and Perforation With NSAID Therapy).

DRUG/LABORATORY TEST INTERACTIONS

The drug may decrease platelet aggregation and prolong bleeding time. This effect should be kept in mind when bleeding times are determined.

The administration of the drug may result in increased urinary values for 17-keratogenic steroids because of an interaction between the drug and/or its metabolites with m-dinitrobenzene used in this assay. Although 17 hydroxy-corticosteroid measurements (Porter-Silber test) do not appear to be artifactually altered, it is suggested that therapy with the drug be temporarily discontinued 72 hours before adrenal function tests are performed.

The drug may interfere with some urinary assays of 5-hydroxy indoleacetic acid (5HIAA).

CARCINOGENESIS

N

A 2 year study was performed in rats to evaluate the carcinogenic potential of the drug. No evidence of carcinogenicity was found.

PREGNANCY CATEGORY B

Teratogenic Effects

Reproduction studies have been performed in rats, rabbits, and mice at doses up to 6 times the human dose and have revealed no evidence of impaired fertility or harm to the fetus due to the drug. There are, however, no adequate and well- controlled studies in pregnant women. Because animal reproduction studies are not always predictive of human response, the drug should not be used during pregnancy unless clearly needed. Because of the known effect of drugs of this class on the human fetal cardiovascular system (closure of ductus arteriosus), use during late pregnancy should be avoided.

Nonteratogenic Effects

As with other drugs known to inhibit prostaglandin synthesis, an increased incidence of dystocia and delayed parturition occurred in rats.

NURSING MOTHERS

The naproxen anion has been found in the milk of lactating women at a concentration of approximately 1% of that found in the plasma. Because of the possible adverse effects of prostaglandin-inhibiting drugs on neonates, use in nursing mothers should be avoided.

PEDIATRIC USE

Safety and effectiveness in children below the age of 2 years have not been established. Pediatric dosing recommendations for juvenile arthritis are based on well-controlled studies. There are no adequate effectiveness or dose-responsive data for other pediatric conditions, but the experience in juvenile arthritis and other use experience have established that single doses of 2.5-5 mg/kg (as naproxen suspension, see DOSAGE AND ADMINISTRATION), with total daily dose not exceeding 15 mg/kg/day, are safe in children over 2 years of age.

DRUG INTERACTIONS

In vitro studies have shown that naproxen anion, because if its affinity for protein, may displace from their binding sites other drugs which are also albumin-bound. Theoretically, the naproxen anion itself could likewise be displaced. Short-term controlled studies failed to show that taking the drug significantly affects prothrombin times when administered to individuals on coumarin-type anticoagulants. Caution is advised nonetheless, since interactions have been seen with other nonsteroidal agents of this class. Similarly, patients receiving the drug and a hydantoin, sulfonamide or sulfonylurea should be observed for signs of toxicity to these drugs.

The natriuretic effect of furosemide has been reported to be inhibited by some drugs of this class. Inhibition of renal lithium clearance leading to increases in plasma lithium concentrations has also been reported.

This and other nonsteroidal anti-inflammatory drugs can reduce the antihypertensive effect of propranolol and other beta-blockers.

Probenecid given concurrently increases naproxen anion plasma levels and extends its plasma half-life significantly.

Caution should be used if this drug is administered concomitantly with methotrexate. Naproxen and other nonsteroidal anti-inflammatory drugs have been reported to reduce the tubular secretion of methotrexate in an animal model, possibly enhancing the toxicity of that drug.

ADVERSE REACTIONS

The following adverse reactions are divided into three parts based on frequency and likelihood o causal relationship to naproxen sodium.

INCIDENCE GREATER THAN 1%

Probable Causal Relationship

Adverse reactions reported in controlled clinical trials in 960 patients treated for rheumatoid arthritis or osteoarthritis are listed below. In general, these reactions were reported 2-10 times more frequently than they were in studies in the 962 patients treated for mild to moderate pain or for dysmenorrhea.

A clinical study found gastrointestinal reactions to be more frequent and more severe in rheumatoid arthritis patients taking 1650 mg naproxen sodium daily compared to those taking 825 mg daily (see CLINICAL PHARMACOLOGY).

In controlled clinical trials with about 80 children and in well monitored open studies with about 400 children with juvenile arthritis, the incidences of rash and prolonged bleeding times were increased, the incidences of gastrointestinal and central nervous system reactions were about the same, and the incidences of other reactions were lower in children than adults.

Gastrointestinal: The most frequent complaints reported related to the gastrointestinal tract. They were: constipation*, heartburn*, abdominal pain*, nausea*, dyspepsia, diarrhea, stomatitis.

Central Nervous System: Headache*, dizziness*, Drowsiness*, lightheadedness, vertigo.

Dermatologic: Itching (pruritus)*,skin eruption*, ecchymoses*, sweating, purpura.

Special Senses: Tinnitus*, hearing disturbances, visual disturbances.

Cardiovascular: Edema*, dyspnea*, palpitations.

General: Thirst.

* Incidence of reported reaction between 3% and 9%. Those reactions occurring in less than 3% of the patients are unmarked.

INCIDENCE LESS THAN 1%

Probable Causal Relationship

The following adverse reactions were reported less frequently than 1% during controlled clinical trials and through voluntary reports since marketing. The probability of a causal relationship exists between the drug and these adverse reactions.

Gastrointestinal: Abnormal liver function tests, gastrointestinal bleeding, hematemesis, jaundice, melena, peptic ulceration with bleeding and/or perforation, vomiting.

Renal: Glomerular nephritis, hematuria, intestinal nephritis, nephrotic syndrome, renal disease, renal failure, renal papillary necrosis.

Hematologic: Agranulocytosis, eosinophilia, granulocytopenia, leukopenia, thrombocytopenia.

Central Nervous System: Depression, dream abnormalities, inability to concentrate, insomnia, malaise, myalgia and muscle weakness.

Dermatologic: Alopecia, photosensitive dermatitis, skin rashes.

Special Senses: Hearing impairment.

Cardiovascular: Congestive heart failure.

General: Anaphylactoid reactions, menstrual disorders, pyrexia (chills and fever).

Causal Relationship Unknown

Other reactions have been reported in circumstances in which a causal relationship could not be established. However, in these rarely reported events, the possibility cannot be excluded. Therefore these observations are being listed to serve as alerting information to the physicians.

Hematologic: Aplastic anemia, hemolytic anemia.

Dermatologic: Epidermal necrolysis, erythema multiforme, photosensitivity reactions resembling porphyria cutanea tarda and epidermolysis bullosa, Stevens-Johnson syndrome, urticaria.

Gastrointestinal: Non-peptic gastrointestinal ulceration, ulcerative stomatitis.

Cardiovascular: Vasculitis.

General: Angioneurotic edema, hyperglycemia, hypoglycemia.

DOSAGE AND ADMINISTRATION

FOR MILD TO MODERATE PAIN, PRIMARY DYSMENORRHEA, AND ACUTE TENDINITIS AND BURSITIS

The recommended starting dose is 550 mg, followed by 275 mg every 6-8 hours, as required. The total daily dose should not exceed 5 tablets (1375 mg).

FOR RHEUMATOID ARTHRITIS, OSTEOARTHRITIS, AND ANKYLOSING SPONDYLITIS

The recommended dose in adults is 275 or 550 mg twice daily (morning and evening). During long-term administration, the dose may be adjusted up or down depending on the clinical response of the patient. A lower daily dose may suffice for long-term administration. The morning and evening doses do not have to be equal in size and the administration of the drug more frequently than twice daily is not necessary.

In patients who tolerate lower doses well, the dose may be increased to 1650 mg/day for limited periods when a higher level of anti- inflammatory/analgesic activity is required. When treating such patients with the 1650 mg/day dose, the physician should observe sufficient increased clinical benefits to offset the potential increased risk (see CLINICAL PHARMACOLOGY).

Symptomatic improvement in arthritis usually begins within 2 weeks. However, if improvement is not seen within this period, a trial for an additional 2 weeks should be considered.

FOR ACUTE

The recommended starting dose is 825 mg, followed by 275 mg every 8 hours until the attack has subsided.

FOR JUVENILE ARTHRITIS

The recommended total daily dose is approximately 10 mg/kg given in two divided doses. The 275 mg naproxen sodium tablet is not well suited to this dosage so use of the related drug naproxen as the 250 mg scored tablet or the 125 mg/5 ml suspension is recommended for this indication.

PRODUCT LISTING - RATED THERAPEUTICALLY EQUIVALENT

Tablet - Oral - Sodium 275 mg

Qty	Price	Product	NDC
6's	$14.40	GENERIC, Pd-Rx Pharmaceuticals	55289-0467-06
10's	$17.78	GENERIC, Pd-Rx Pharmaceuticals	55289-0467-10
10's	$34.89	ANAPROX, Pd-Rx Pharmaceuticals	55289-0837-10
12's	$9.83	ANAPROX, Allscripts Pharmaceutical Company	54569-0264-04
14's	$10.32	GENERIC, Allscripts Pharmaceutical Company	54569-3761-04
16's	$12.72	ANAPROX, Allscripts Pharmaceutical Company	54569-0264-02
20's	$13.44	GENERIC, Allscripts Pharmaceutical Company	54569-3761-00
20's	$15.90	ANAPROX, Allscripts Pharmaceutical Company	54569-0264-06
20's	$60.51	ANAPROX, Pd-Rx Pharmaceuticals	55289-0837-20
21's	$14.11	GENERIC, Allscripts Pharmaceutical Company	54569-3761-01
21's	$17.20	ANAPROX, Allscripts Pharmaceutical Company	54569-0264-00
21's	$29.25	GENERIC, Pd-Rx Pharmaceuticals	55289-0467-21
28's	$22.26	ANAPROX, Allscripts Pharmaceutical Company	54569-0264-07
30's	$18.80	GENERIC, Heartland Healthcare Services	61392-0298-30
30's	$18.80	GENERIC, Heartland Healthcare Services	61392-0298-39
30's	$20.16	GENERIC, Allscripts Pharmaceutical Company	54569-3761-02
30's	$24.57	ANAPROX, Allscripts Pharmaceutical Company	54569-0264-01
30's	$27.61	ANAPROX, Physicians Total Care	54868-1872-01
30's	$30.99	ANAPROX, Pharma Pac	52959-0015-30
30's	$35.33	GENERIC, Pd-Rx Pharmaceuticals	55289-0467-30
31's	$19.42	GENERIC, Heartland Healthcare Services	61392-0298-31
32's	$20.05	GENERIC, Heartland Healthcare Services	61392-0298-32
45's	$28.20	GENERIC, Heartland Healthcare Services	61392-0298-45
60's	$37.59	GENERIC, Heartland Healthcare Services	61392-0298-60
90's	$56.39	GENERIC, Heartland Healthcare Services	61392-0298-90
100's	$11.13	GENERIC, Purepac Pharmaceutical Company	00228-2547-10
100's	$60.00	GENERIC, Roxane Laboratories Inc	00054-4638-25
100's	$60.00	GENERIC, Roxane Laboratories Inc	00054-8638-25
100's	$66.85	GENERIC, Major Pharmaceuticals Inc	00904-7802-60
100's	$66.86	GENERIC, Invamed Inc	52189-0286-24
100's	$66.90	GENERIC, Qualitest Products Inc	00603-4733-21
100's	$66.90	GENERIC, West Point Pharma	59591-0256-68
100's	$66.92	GENERIC, Aligen Independent Laboratories Inc	00405-4711-01
100's	$67.90	GENERIC, Martec Pharmaceuticals Inc	52555-0587-01
100's	$68.70	GENERIC, Vangard Labs	00615-3579-13
100's	$69.93	GENERIC, Moore, H.L. Drug Exchange Inc	00839-7889-06
100's	$69.95	GENERIC, Dixon-Shane Inc	17236-0083-01
100's	$71.50	GENERIC, Brightstone Pharma	62939-8431-01
100's	$71.51	GENERIC, Ivax Corporation	00172-4116-60
100's	$71.51	GENERIC, Ivax Corporation	00182-1974-01
100's	$71.51	GENERIC, Watson/Rugby Laboratories Inc	00536-4841-01
100's	$71.51	GENERIC, Geneva Pharmaceuticals	00781-1187-01
100's	$73.75	GENERIC, Mylan Pharmaceuticals Inc	00378-0537-01
100's	$79.50	ANAPROX, Allscripts Pharmaceutical Company	54569-0264-03
100's	$84.55	GENERIC, Teva Pharmaceuticals Usa	00093-0536-01
100's	$89.30	GENERIC, Watson Laboratories Inc	00591-0792-01
100's	$105.10	ANAPROX, Roche Laboratories	00004-6202-01

Tablet - Oral - Sodium 550 mg

Qty	Price	Product	NDC
6's	$19.58	GENERIC, Pd-Rx Pharmaceuticals	55289-0367-06
6's	$27.90	ANAPROX-DS, Pd-Rx Pharmaceuticals	55289-0332-06
9's	$16.60	ANAPROX-DS, Cheshire Drugs	55175-1793-09
10's	$10.44	GENERIC, Allscripts Pharmaceutical Company	54569-3762-00
10's	$12.38	ANAPROX-DS, Allscripts Pharmaceutical Company	54569-1763-00
10's	$13.00	GENERIC, Dhs Inc	55887-0923-10
10's	$22.86	GENERIC, Pd-Rx Pharmaceuticals	55289-0367-10
12's	$12.53	GENERIC, Allscripts Pharmaceutical Company	54569-3762-01
12's	$14.85	ANAPROX-DS, Allscripts Pharmaceutical Company	54569-1763-07
14's	$14.62	GENERIC, Allscripts Pharmaceutical Company	54569-3762-07
14's	$18.82	GENERIC, Dhs Inc	55887-0923-14
14's	$22.86	GENERIC, Pd-Rx Pharmaceuticals	55289-0367-14
15's	$20.39	ANAPROX-DS, Physicians Total Care	54868-0197-02
15's	$25.74	GENERIC, Pd-Rx Pharmaceuticals	55289-0367-15
15's	$54.75	ANAPROX-DS, Pd-Rx Pharmaceuticals	55289-0332-15
16's	$16.71	GENERIC, Allscripts Pharmaceutical Company	54569-3762-02
16's	$19.80	ANAPROX-DS, Allscripts Pharmaceutical Company	54569-1763-02
20's	$20.89	GENERIC, Allscripts Pharmaceutical Company	54569-3762-03
20's	$24.76	ANAPROX-DS, Allscripts Pharmaceutical Company	54569-1763-05
20's	$26.81	ANAPROX-DS, Physicians Total Care	54868-0197-03
20's	$27.12	GENERIC, St. Mary'S Mpp	60760-0537-20
20's	$32.13	GENERIC, Pd-Rx Pharmaceuticals	55289-0367-20
20's	$35.49	ANAPROX-DS, Pharma Pac	52959-0016-20
20's	$74.52	ANAPROX-DS, Pd-Rx Pharmaceuticals	55289-0332-20
21's	$21.93	GENERIC, Allscripts Pharmaceutical Company	54569-3762-04
21's	$25.99	ANAPROX-DS, Allscripts Pharmaceutical Company	54569-1763-01
21's	$28.35	GENERIC, Dhs Inc	55887-0923-21
28's	$27.77	GENERIC, Pd-Rx Pharmaceuticals	55289-0367-28
28's	$34.66	ANAPROX-DS, Allscripts Pharmaceutical Company	54569-1763-06
30's	$28.59	GENERIC, Heartland Healthcare Services	61392-0301-30
30's	$28.59	GENERIC, Heartland Healthcare Services	61392-0301-39
30's	$31.33	GENERIC, Allscripts Pharmaceutical Company	54569-3762-05
30's	$37.13	ANAPROX-DS, Allscripts Pharmaceutical Company	54569-1763-03
30's	$39.69	GENERIC, Pd-Rx Pharmaceuticals	55289-0367-30
30's	$40.32	GENERIC, Dhs Inc	55887-0923-30
30's	$42.39	ANAPROX-DS, Physicians Total Care	54868-0197-04
30's	$52.20	ANAPROX-DS, Pharma Pac	52959-0016-30
30's	$112.23	ANAPROX-DS, Pd-Rx Pharmaceuticals	55289-0332-30
31's	$29.55	GENERIC, Heartland Healthcare Services	61392-0301-31
32's	$30.50	GENERIC, Heartland Healthcare Services	61392-0301-32
42's	$69.03	GENERIC, Pd-Rx Pharmaceuticals	55289-0367-42
45's	$42.89	GENERIC, Heartland Healthcare Services	61392-0301-45
45's	$51.64	GENERIC, Allscripts Pharmaceutical Company	54569-3762-09
60's	$57.19	GENERIC, Heartland Healthcare Services	61392-0301-60
60's	$62.66	GENERIC, Allscripts Pharmaceutical Company	54569-3762-06
60's	$71.35	GENERIC, St. Mary'S Mpp	60760-0537-60
60's	$74.27	ANAPROX-DS, Allscripts Pharmaceutical Company	54569-1763-04
90's	$85.78	GENERIC, Heartland Healthcare Services	61392-0301-90
100's	$90.00	GENERIC, Roxane Laboratories Inc	00054-4639-25
100's	$103.00	GENERIC, West Ward Pharmaceutical Corporation	00143-9908-01
100's	$104.05	GENERIC, Major Pharmaceuticals Inc	00904-7803-60
100's	$104.09	GENERIC, Invamed Inc	52189-0287-24
100's	$104.10	GENERIC, West Point Pharma	59591-0258-68
100's	$104.15	GENERIC, Mova Pharmaceutical Corporation	55370-0526-07
100's	$104.23	GENERIC, Aligen Independent Laboratories Inc	00405-4712-01
100's	$105.45	GENERIC, Vangard Labs	00615-3580-13
100's	$105.70	GENERIC, Martec Pharmaceuticals Inc	52555-0588-01
100's	$108.68	GENERIC, Dixon-Shane Inc	17236-0084-01
100's	$109.28	GENERIC, Moore, H.L. Drug Exchange Inc	00839-7890-06
100's	$110.16	GENERIC, Purepac Pharmaceutical Company	00228-2548-10
100's	$111.34	GENERIC, Ivax Corporation	00172-4275-60
100's	$111.34	GENERIC, Ivax Corporation	00182-1975-01
100's	$111.34	GENERIC, Watson/Rugby Laboratories Inc	00536-4848-01
100's	$111.34	GENERIC, Geneva Pharmaceuticals	00781-1188-01
100's	$113.50	GENERIC, Major Pharmaceuticals Inc	00904-5431-60
100's	$114.75	GENERIC, Mylan Pharmaceuticals Inc	00378-0733-01
100's	$114.75	GENERIC, Allscripts Pharmaceutical Company	54569-3762-08
100's	$116.05	GENERIC, Geneva Pharmaceuticals	00781-1188-13
100's	$120.50	GENERIC, Teva Pharmaceuticals Usa	55953-0533-40
100's	$131.64	GENERIC, Teva Pharmaceuticals Usa	00093-0537-01
100's	$139.02	GENERIC, Watson Laboratories Inc	00591-0793-01
100's	$139.02	GENERIC, Watson/Rugby Laboratories Inc	52544-0793-01
100's	$157.08	ANAPROX-DS, Roche Laboratories	00004-6200-01
100's	$163.63	ANAPROX-DS, Roche Laboratories	00004-6203-01

Tablet, Extended Release - Oral - Sodium 550 mg

Qty	Price	Product	NDC
75's	$110.59	GENERIC, Andrx Pharmaceuticals	62037-0826-75

PRODUCT LISTING - EQUIVALENTS NOT AVAILABLE

Tablet - Oral - Sodium 275 mg

Qty	Price	Product	NDC
4's	$4.36	GENERIC, Prescript Pharmaceuticals	00247-0166-04
6's	$4.86	GENERIC, Prescript Pharmaceuticals	00247-0166-06
8's	$5.36	GENERIC, Prescript Pharmaceuticals	00247-0166-08
9's	$5.61	GENERIC, Prescript Pharmaceuticals	00247-0166-09
10's	$5.87	GENERIC, Prescript Pharmaceuticals	00247-0166-10
12's	$6.38	GENERIC, Prescript Pharmaceuticals	00247-0166-12
12's	$9.43	GENERIC, Southwood Pharmaceuticals Inc	58016-0694-12
14's	$6.87	GENERIC, Prescript Pharmaceuticals	00247-0166-14
14's	$11.00	GENERIC, Southwood Pharmaceuticals Inc	58016-0694-14
15's	$7.13	GENERIC, Prescript Pharmaceuticals	00247-0166-15

N

16's	$7.38	GENERIC, Prescript Pharmaceuticals	00247-0166-16
18's	$7.88	GENERIC, Prescript Pharmaceuticals	00247-0166-18
20's	$8.39	GENERIC, Prescript Pharmaceuticals	00247-0166-20
20's	$14.80	GENERIC, Pharmaceutical Corporation Of America	51655-0629-52
20's	$15.70	GENERIC, Southwood Pharmaceuticals Inc	58016-0694-20
21's	$8.64	GENERIC, Prescript Pharmaceuticals	00247-0166-21
21's	$20.03	GENERIC, Pharma Pac	52959-0357-21
26's	$9.89	GENERIC, Prescript Pharmaceuticals	00247-0166-26
30's	$5.52	GENERIC, Physicians Total Care	54868-3359-00
30's	$10.89	GENERIC, Prescript Pharmaceuticals	00247-0166-30
30's	$23.50	GENERIC, Southwood Pharmaceuticals Inc	58016-0694-30
30's	$27.60	GENERIC, Pharma Pac	52959-0357-30
32's	$11.40	GENERIC, Prescript Pharmaceuticals	00247-0166-32
100's	$78.60	GENERIC, Southwood Pharmaceuticals Inc	58016-0694-00
100's	$105.10	ANAPROX, Roche Laboratories	00004-6201-01
Tablet - Oral - Sodium 550 mg			
2's	$3.65	GENERIC, Prescript Pharmaceuticals	00247-0074-02
3's	$3.79	GENERIC, Prescript Pharmaceuticals	00247-0074-03
6's	$4.22	GENERIC, Prescript Pharmaceuticals	00247-0074-06
9's	$4.66	GENERIC, Prescript Pharmaceuticals	00247-0074-09
10's	$4.81	GENERIC, Prescript Pharmaceuticals	00247-0074-10
10's	$15.70	GENERIC, Southwood Pharmaceuticals Inc	58016-0321-10
12's	$5.11	GENERIC, Prescript Pharmaceuticals	00247-0074-12
12's	$18.83	GENERIC, Southwood Pharmaceuticals Inc	58016-0321-12
14's	$5.39	GENERIC, Prescript Pharmaceuticals	00247-0074-14
14's	$21.97	GENERIC, Southwood Pharmaceuticals Inc	58016-0321-14
14's	$29.90	GENERIC, Pharma Pac	52959-0271-14
15's	$5.54	GENERIC, Prescript Pharmaceuticals	00247-0074-15
15's	$6.59	GENERIC, Physicians Total Care	54868-3043-01
15's	$23.54	GENERIC, Southwood Pharmaceuticals Inc	58016-0321-15
15's	$31.86	GENERIC, Pharma Pac	52959-0271-15
16's	$5.68	GENERIC, Prescript Pharmaceuticals	00247-0074-16
20's	$6.27	GENERIC, Prescript Pharmaceuticals	00247-0074-20
20's	$6.67	GENERIC, Physicians Total Care	54868-3043-03
20's	$23.00	GENERIC, Pharmaceutical Corporation Of America	51655-0627-52
20's	$27.04	GENERIC, Cardinal Pharmaceuticals	63874-0339-20
20's	$31.39	GENERIC, Southwood Pharmaceuticals Inc	58016-0321-20
20's	$41.73	GENERIC, Pharma Pac	52959-0271-20
21's	$6.41	GENERIC, Prescript Pharmaceuticals	00247-0074-21
24's	$37.67	GENERIC, Southwood Pharmaceuticals Inc	58016-0321-24
28's	$43.95	GENERIC, Southwood Pharmaceuticals Inc	58016-0321-28
30's	$7.72	GENERIC, Prescript Pharmaceuticals	00247-0074-30
30's	$9.21	GENERIC, Physicians Total Care	54868-3043-02
30's	$40.56	GENERIC, Cardinal Pharmaceuticals	63874-0339-30
30's	$47.09	GENERIC, Southwood Pharmaceuticals Inc	58016-0321-30
30's	$61.59	GENERIC, Pharma Pac	52959-0271-30
40's	$9.18	GENERIC, Prescript Pharmaceuticals	00247-0074-40
40's	$62.78	GENERIC, Southwood Pharmaceuticals Inc	58016-0321-40
40's	$80.64	GENERIC, Pharma Pac	52959-0271-40
42's	$9.47	GENERIC, Prescript Pharmaceuticals	00247-0074-42
42's	$65.94	GENERIC, Southwood Pharmaceuticals Inc	58016-0321-42
50's	$10.64	GENERIC, Prescript Pharmaceuticals	00247-0074-50
56's	$87.89	GENERIC, Southwood Pharmaceuticals Inc	58016-0321-56
60's	$12.09	GENERIC, Prescript Pharmaceuticals	00247-0074-60
60's	$17.09	GENERIC, Physicians Total Care	54868-3043-05
60's	$94.17	GENERIC, Southwood Pharmaceuticals Inc	58016-0321-60
60's	$118.78	GENERIC, Pharma Pac	52959-0271-60
90's	$141.26	GENERIC, Southwood Pharmaceuticals Inc	58016-0321-90
100's	$95.77	GENERIC, International Ethical Laboratories Inc	11584-0465-01
100's	$110.50	GENERIC, Brightstone Pharma	62939-8441-01
100's	$128.95	ANAPROX-DS, Syntex Laboratories Inc	18393-0276-53
100's	$135.20	GENERIC, Cardinal Pharmaceuticals	63874-0339-01
100's	$156.95	GENERIC, Southwood Pharmaceuticals Inc	58016-0321-00
120's	$25.43	GENERIC, Physicians Total Care	54868-3043-06
Tablet, Extended Release - Oral - Sodium 412.5 mg			
30's	$44.53	NAPRELAN '375', Physicians Total Care	54868-3974-00
100's	$134.34	NAPRELAN '375', Elan Pharmaceuticals	00086-0090-10
Tablet, Extended Release - Oral - Sodium 550 mg			
10's	$16.26	NAPRELAN '500', Southwood Pharmaceuticals Inc	58016-0388-10
14's	$33.21	NAPRELAN '500', Pd-Rx Pharmaceuticals	55289-0304-14
20's	$32.52	NAPRELAN '500', Southwood Pharmaceuticals Inc	58016-0388-20
30's	$48.78	NAPRELAN '500', Southwood Pharmaceuticals Inc	58016-0388-30
30's	$56.69	NAPRELAN '500', Physicians Total Care	54868-3973-00
30's	$75.00	NAPRELAN '500', Pd-Rx Pharmaceuticals	55289-0304-30
40's	$65.04	NAPRELAN '500', Southwood Pharmaceuticals Inc	58016-0388-40
40's	$75.19	NAPRELAN '500', Physicians Total Care	54868-3973-01
60's	$97.56	NAPRELAN '500', Southwood Pharmaceuticals Inc	58016-0388-60
60's	$112.20	NAPRELAN '500', Physicians Total Care	54868-3973-02
75's	$117.02	NAPRELAN '500', Elan Pharmaceuticals	00860-0091-75
75's	$121.95	NAPRELAN '500', Southwood Pharmaceuticals Inc	58016-0388-75
90's	$104.40	NAPRELAN '500', Southwood Pharmaceuticals Inc	58016-0388-90

Naratriptan Hydrochloride *(003386)*

For related information, see the comparative table section in Appendix A.

Categories: Headache, migraine; Pregnancy Category C; FDA Approved 1998 Feb
Drug Classes: Serotonin receptor agonists
Brand Names: Amerge
Foreign Brand Availability: Naramig (Australia; Bahrain; Colombia; Cyprus; Egypt; England; France; Germany; Iran; Iraq; Ireland; Israel; Jordan; Kuwait; Lebanon; Libya; Mexico; Oman; Peru; Qatar; Republic-of-Yemen; Saudi-Arabia; Singapore; South-Africa; Syria; Thailand; United-Arab-Emirates)
Cost of Therapy: $20.80 (Migraine Headache; Amerge; 1 mg; 1 tablet/day; 1 day supply)

DESCRIPTION

Amerge tablets contain naratriptan as the hydrochloride, which is a selective 5-hydroxytryptamine$_1$ receptor subtype agonist. Naratriptan HCl is chemically designated as N-methyl-3-(1-methyl-4-piperidinyl)-1H-indole-5-ethanesulfonamide monohydrochloride.

The empirical formula is $C_{17}H_{25}N_3O_2S{\cdot}HCl$, representing a molecular weight of 371.93. Naratriptan HCl is a white to pale yellow powder that is readily soluble in water. Each Amerge tablet for oral administration contains 1.11 or 2.78 mg of naratriptan HCl equivalent to 1 or 2.5 mg of naratriptan, respectively. Each tablet also contains the inactive ingredients croscarmellose sodium; hydroxypropyl methylcellulose; lactose; magnesium stearate; microcrystalline cellulose; triacetin; and titanium dioxide, iron oxide yellow, and indigo carmine aluminum lake (FD&C blue no. 2) for coloring.

CLINICAL PHARMACOLOGY

MECHANISM OF ACTION

Naratriptan binds with high affinity to 5-HT_{1D} and 5-HT_{1B} receptors and has no significant affinity or pharmacological activity at 5-HT_{2-4} receptor subtypes or at adrenergic α_1, α_2, or β; dopaminergic D_1 or D_2; muscarinic; or benzodiazepine receptors.

The therapeutic activity of naratriptan in migraine is generally attributed to its agonist activity at 5-$HT_{1D/1B}$ receptors. Two current theories have been proposed to explain the efficacy of 5-$HT_{1D/1B}$ receptor agonists in migraine. One theory suggests that activation of 5-$HT_{1D/1B}$ receptors located on intracranial blood vessels, including those on the arteriovenous anastomoses, leads to vasoconstriction, which is correlated with the relief of migraine headache. The other hypothesis suggests that activation of 5-$HT_{1D/1B}$ receptors on sensory nerve endings in the trigeminal system results in the inhibition of pro-inflammatory neuropeptide release.

In the anesthetized dog, naratriptan has been shown to reduce the carotid arterial blood flow with little or no effect on arterial blood pressure or total peripheral resistance. While the effect on blood flow was selective for the carotid arterial bed, increases in vascular resistance of up to 30% were seen in the coronary arterial bed. Naratriptan has also been shown to inhibit trigeminal nerve activity in rat and cat. In 10 human subjects with suspected coronary artery disease (CAD) undergoing coronary artery catheterization, there was a 1-10% reduction in coronary artery diameter following subcutaneous (SC) injection of 1.5 mg of naratriptan.

PHARMACOKINETICS

Naratriptan tablets are well absorbed, with about 70% oral bioavailability. Following administration of a 2.5 mg tablet orally, the peak concentrations are obtained in 2-3 hours. After administration of 1 or 2.5 mg tablets, the C_{max} is somewhat (about 50%) higher in women (not corrected for mg/kg dose) than in men. During a migraine attack, absorption was slower, with a T_{max} of 3-4 hours. Food does not affect the pharmacokinetics of naratriptan. Naratriptan displays linear kinetics over the therapeutic dose range.

The steady-state volume of distribution of naratriptan is 170 L. Plasma protein binding is 28-31% over the concentration range of 50-1000 ng/ml.

Naratriptan is predominantly eliminated in urine, with 50% of the dose recovered unchanged and 30% as metabolites in urine. *In vitro*, naratriptan is metabolized by a wide range of cytochrome P450 isoenzymes into a number of inactive metabolites.

The mean elimination half-life of naratriptan is 6 hours. The systemic clearance of naratriptan is 6.6 ml/min/kg. The renal clearance (220 ml/min) exceeds glomerular filtration rate, indicating active tubular secretion. Repeat administration of naratriptan tablets does not result in drug accumulation.

SPECIAL POPULATIONS

Age

A small decrease in clearance (approximately 26%) was observed in healthy elderly subjects (65-77 years) compared to younger patients, resulting in slightly higher exposure (see PRECAUTIONS).

Race

The effect of race on the pharmacokinetics of naratriptan has not been examined.

Renal Impairment

Clearance of naratriptan was reduced by 50% in patients with moderate renal impairment (creatinine clearance: 18-39 ml/min) compared to the normal group. Decrease in clearances resulted in an increase of mean half-life from 6 hours (healthy) to 11 hours (range: 7-20 hours). The mean C_{max} increased by approximately 40%. The effects of severe renal impairment (creatinine clearance $\leq$15 ml/min) on the pharmacokinetics of naratriptan has not been assessed (see CONTRAINDICATIONS and DOSAGE AND ADMINISTRATION).

Hepatic Impairment

Clearance of naratriptan was decreased by 30% in patients with moderate hepatic impairment (Child-Pugh Grade A or B). This resulted in an approximately 40% increase in the half-life (range: 8-16 hours). The effects of severe hepatic impairment (Child-Pugh Grade

C) on the pharmacokinetics of naratriptan have not been assessed (see CONTRAINDICATIONS and DOSAGE AND ADMINISTRATION).

DRUG INTERACTIONS

In normal volunteers, coadministration of single doses of naratriptan tablets and alcohol did not result in substantial modification of naratriptan pharmacokinetic parameters.

From population pharmacokinetic analyses, coadministration of naratriptan and fluoxetine, beta-blockers, or tricyclic antidepressants did not affect the clearance of naratriptan.

Naratriptan does not inhibit monoamine oxidase (MAO) enzymes and is a poor inhibitor of P450; metabolic interactions between naratriptan and drugs metabolized by P450 or MAO are therefore unlikely.

Oral Contraceptives: Oral contraceptives reduced clearance by 32% and volume of distribution by 22%, resulting in slightly higher concentrations of naratriptan. Hormone replacement therapy had no effect on pharmacokinetics in older female patients.

Smoking increased the clearance of naratriptan by 30%.

INDICATIONS AND USAGE

Naratriptan tablets are indicated for the acute treatment of migraine attacks with or without aura in adults.

Naratriptan tablets are not intended for the prophylactic therapy of migraine or for use in the management of hemiplegic or basilar migraine (see CONTRAINDICATIONS). Safety and effectiveness of naratriptan tablets have not been established for cluster headache, which is present in an older, predominantly male population.

CONTRAINDICATIONS

Naratriptan tablets should not be given to patients with history, symptoms, or signs of ischemic cardiac, cerebrovascular, or peripheral vascular syndromes. In addition, patients with other significant underlying cardiovascular diseases should not receive naratriptan tablets. Ischemic cardiac syndromes include, but are not limited to, angina pectoris of any type (*e.g.,* stable angina of effort and vasospastic forms of angina such as the Prinzmetal variant), all forms of myocardial infarction, and silent myocardial ischemia. Cerebrovascular syndromes include, but are not limited to, strokes of any type as well as transient ischemic attacks. Peripheral vascular disease includes, but is not limited to, ischemic bowel disease (see WARNINGS).

Because naratriptan tablets may increase blood pressure, they should not be given to patients with uncontrolled hypertension (see WARNINGS).

Naratriptan tablets are contraindicated in patients with severe renal impairment (creatinine clearance, <15 ml/min) (see CLINICAL PHARMACOLOGY and DOSAGE AND ADMINISTRATION).

Naratriptan tablets are contraindicated in patients with severe hepatic impairment (Child-Pugh Grade C) (see CLINICAL PHARMACOLOGY and DOSAGE AND ADMINISTRATION).

Naratriptan tablets should not be administered to patients with hemiplegic or basilar migraine.

Naratriptan tablets should not be used within 24 hours of treatment with another 5-HT$_1$ agonist, an ergotamine-containing or ergot-type medication like dihydroergotamine or methysergide.

Naratriptan tablets are contraindicated in patients with hypersensitivity to naratriptan or any of the components.

WARNINGS

Naratriptan tablets should only be used where a clear diagnosis of migraine has been established.

RISK OF MYOCARDIAL ISCHEMIA AND/OR INFARCTION AND OTHER ADVERSE CARDIAC EVENTS

Because of the potential of this class of compounds (5-HT$_{1B/1D}$ agonists) to cause coronary vasospasm, naratriptan should not be given to patients with documented ischemic or vasospastic coronary artery disease (CAD) (see CONTRAINDICATIONS). It is strongly recommended that 5-HT$_1$ agonists (including naratriptan) not be given to patients in whom unrecognized CAD is predicted by the presence of risk factors (*e.g.,* hypertension, hypercholesterolemia, smoker, obesity, diabetes, strong family history of CAD, female with surgical or physiological menopause, or male over 40 years of age) unless a cardiovascular evaluation provides satisfactory clinical evidence that the patient is reasonably free of coronary artery and ischemic myocardial disease or other significant underlying cardiovascular disease. The sensitivity of cardiac diagnostic procedures to detect cardiovascular disease or predisposition to coronary artery vasospasm is modest, at best. If, during the cardiovascular evaluation, the patient's medical history, electrocardiographic, or other investigations reveal findings indicative of, or consistent with, coronary artery vasospasm or myocardial ischemia, naratriptan should not be administered (see CONTRAINDICATIONS).

For patients with risk factors predictive of CAD, who are determined to have a satisfactory cardiovascular evaluation, it is strongly recommended that administration of the first dose of naratriptan take place in the setting of a physician's office or similar medically staffed and equipped facility. Because cardiac ischemia can occur in the absence of clinical symptoms, consideration should be given to obtaining on the first occasion of use an electrocardiogram (ECG) during the interval immediately following administration of naratriptan tablets, in these patients with risk factors.

It is recommended that patients who are intermittent long-term users of 5-HT$_1$ agonists, including naratriptan tablets, and who have or acquire risk factors predictive of CAD, as described above, undergo periodic cardiovascular evaluation as they continue to use naratriptan tablets.

The systematic approach described above is intended to reduce the likelihood that patients with unrecognized cardiovascular disease will be inadvertently exposed to naratriptan.

CARDIAC EVENTS AND FATALITIES ASSOCIATED WITH 5-HT$_1$ AGONISTS

Naratriptan can cause coronary artery vasospasm (see CLINICAL PHARMACOLOGY). Serious adverse cardiac events, including acute myocardial infarction, life-threatening disturbances of cardiac rhythm, and death have been reported within a few hours following the administration of 5-HT$_1$ agonists. Considering the extent of use of 5-HT$_1$ agonists in patients with migraine, the incidence of these events is extremely low.

PREMARKETING EXPERIENCE WITH NARATRIPTAN TABLETS

Among approximately 3500 patients with migraine who participated in premarketing clinical trials of naratriptan tablets, 4 patients treated with single oral doses of naratriptan ranging from 1-10 mg experienced asymptomatic ischemic ECG changes with at least 1, who took 7.5 mg, likely due to coronary vasospasm.

CEREBROVASCULAR EVENTS AND FATALITIES WITH 5-HT$_1$ AGONISTS

Cerebral hemorrhage, subarachnoid hemorrhage, stroke, and other cerebrovascular events have been reported in patients treated with 5-HT$_1$ agonists, and some have resulted in fatalities. In a number of cases, it appears possible that the cerebrovascular events were primary, the agonist having been administered in the incorrect belief that the symptoms experienced were a consequence of migraine, when they were not. It should be noted that patients with migraine may be at increased risk of certain cerebrovascular events (*e.g.,* stroke, hemorrhage, transient ischemic attack).

OTHER VASOSPASM-RELATED EVENTS

5-HT$_1$ agonists may cause vasospastic reactions other than coronary artery spasm. Both peripheral vascular ischemia and colonic ischemia with abdominal pain and bloody diarrhea have been reported with 5-HT$_1$ agonists.

INCREASE IN BLOOD PRESSURE

In healthy volunteers, dose-related increases in systemic blood pressure have been observed after administration of up to 20 mg of oral naratriptan. At the recommended doses, the elevations are generally small, although an increase of systolic pressure of 32 mm Hg was seen in 1 patient following a single 2.5 mg dose. The effect may be more pronounced in the elderly and hypertensive patients. A patient who was mildly hypertensive (the baseline blood pressure was 150/98) experienced a significant increase in blood pressure to 204/144 mm Hg 225 minutes after administration of a 10 mg oral dose. Significant elevation in blood pressure, including hypertensive crisis, has been reported on rare occasions in patients receiving 5-HT$_1$ agonists with and without a history of hypertension. Naratriptan is contraindicated in patients with uncontrolled hypertension (see CONTRAINDICATIONS).

An 18% increase in mean pulmonary artery pressure and an 8% increase in mean aortic pressure was seen following dosing with 1.5 mg of subcutaneous naratriptan in a study evaluating 10 subjects with suspected CAD undergoing cardiac catheterization.

HYPERSENSITIVITY

Hypersensitivity (anaphylaxis/anaphylactoid) reactions may occur in patients receiving naratriptan. Such reactions can be life threatening or fatal. In general, hypersensitivity reactions to drugs are more likely to occur in individuals with a history of sensitivity to multiple allergens (see CONTRAINDICATIONS).

PRECAUTIONS

GENERAL

Chest discomfort (including pain, pressure, heaviness, tightness) has been reported after administration of 5-HT$_1$ agonists, including naratriptan tablets. These events have not been associated with arrhythmias or ischemic ECG changes in clinical trials with naratriptan tablets. Because naratriptan may cause coronary artery vasospasm, patients who experience signs or symptoms suggestive of angina following naratriptan should be evaluated for the presence of CAD or a predisposition to Prinzmetal's variant angina before receiving additional doses of naratriptan, and should be monitored electrocardiographically if dosing is resumed and similar symptoms recur. Similarly, patients who experience other symptoms or signs suggestive of decreased arterial flow, such as ischemic bowel syndrome or Raynaud's syndrome following naratriptan administration should be evaluated for atherosclerosis or predisposition to vasospasm (see CONTRAINDICATIONS and WARNINGS).

Naratriptan tablets should also be administered with caution to patients with diseases that may alter the absorption, metabolism, or excretion of drugs, such as impaired renal or hepatic function (see CLINICAL PHARMACOLOGY, CONTRAINDICATIONS, and DOSAGE AND ADMINISTRATION).

Care should be taken to exclude other potentially serious neurological conditions before treating headache in patients not previously diagnosed with migraine or who experience a headache that is atypical for them. There have been rare reports where patients received 5-HT$_1$ agonists for severe headaches that were subsequently shown to have been secondary to an evolving neurologic lesion (see WARNINGS).

For a given attack, if a patient has no response to the first dose of naratriptan, the diagnosis of migraine should be reconsidered before administration of a second dose.

Binding to Melanin-Containing Tissues

In rats treated with a single oral dose (10 mg/kg) of radiolabeled naratriptan, the elimination half-life of radioactivity from the eye was 90 days, suggesting that naratriptan and/or its metabolites may bind to the melanin of the eye. Because there could be accumulation in melanin-rich tissues over time, this raises the possibility that naratriptan could cause toxicity in these tissues after extended use. Although no systematic monitoring of ophthalmologic function was undertaken in clinical trials, and no specific recommendations for ophthalmologic monitoring are offered, prescribers should be aware of the possibility of long-term ophthalmologic effects.

Changes in the Precorneal Tear Film

Dogs receiving oral naratriptan showed transient changes in the precorneal tear film. Corneal stippling was seen at the lowest dose tested, 1 mg/kg/day, and occurred intermittently from Day 1 throughout the first 2-3 weeks of treatment. Although a no-effect dose was not

N

established, the exposure at the lowest dose tested was approximately 5 times the human exposure after a 5 mg oral dose.

INFORMATION FOR THE PATIENT

See the Patient Instructions that are distributed with the prescription.

LABORATORY TESTS

No specific laboratory tests are recommended for monitoring patients prior to and/or after treatment with naratriptan tablets.

DRUG/LABORATORY TEST INTERACTIONS

Naratriptan tablets are not known to interfere with commonly employed clinical laboratory tests.

CARCINOGENESIS, MUTAGENESIS, AND IMPAIRMENT OF FERTILITY

Carcinogenesis

Lifetime carcinogenicity studies, 104 weeks in duration, were carried out in mice and rats by oral gavage. There was no evidence of an increase in tumors related to naratriptan administration in mice receiving up to 200 mg/kg/day. That dose was associated with a plasma AUC exposure that was 110 times the exposure in humans receiving the maximum recommended daily dose of 5 mg. Two rat studies were conducted, one using a standard diet and the other a nitrite-supplemented diet (naratriptan can be nitrosated *in vitro* to form a mutagenic product that has been detected in the stomachs of rats fed a high nitrite diet). Doses of 5, 20, and 90 mg/kg were associated with Week 13 AUC exposures that in the standard diet study were 7, 40, and 236 times, and in the nitrite-supplemented diet study were 7, 29, and 180 times, the exposure attained in humans given the maximum recommended daily dose of 5 mg. In both studies, there was an increase in the incidence of thyroid follicular hyperplasia in high-dose males and females and in thyroid follicular adenomas in high-dose males. In the standard diet study only, there was also an increase in the incidence of benign c-cell adenomas in the thyroid of high-dose males and females. The exposures achieved at the no-effect dose for thyroid tumors were 40 (standard diet) and 29 (nitrite-supplemented diet) times the exposure achieved in humans receiving the maximum recommended daily dose of 5 mg. In the nitrite-supplemented diet study only, the incidence of benign lymphocytic thymoma was increased in all treated groups of females. It was not determined if the nitrosated product is systemically absorbed. However, no changes were seen in the stomachs of rats in that study.

Mutagenesis

Naratriptan was not mutagenic when tested in 2 gene mutation assays, the Ames test and the *in vitro* thymidine locus mouse lymphoma assay. It was not clastogenic in 2 cytogenetics assays, the *in vitro* human lymphocyte assay and the *in vivo* mouse micronucleus assay. Naratriptan can be nitrosated *in vitro* to form a mutagenic product (WHO nitrosation assay) that has been detected in the stomachs of rats fed a nitrite-supplemented diet.

Impairment of Fertility

In a reproductive toxicity study in which male and female rats were dosed prior to and throughout the mating period with 10, 60, 170, or 340 mg/kg/day [plasma exposures (AUC) approximately 11, 70, 230, and 470 times, respectively, the human exposure at the maximum recommended daily dose (MRDD) of 5 mg], there was a treatment-related decrease in the number of females exhibiting normal estrous cycles at doses of 170 mg/kg/day or greater and an increase in pre-implantation loss at 60 mg/kg/day or greater. In high-dose group males, testicular/epididymal atrophy accompanied by spermatozoa depletion reduced mating success and may have contributed to the observed preimplantation loss. The exposures achieved at the no-effect doses for preimplantation loss, anestrus, and testicular effects were approximately 11, 70, and 230 times, respectively, the exposures in humans receiving the MRDD.

In a study in which rats were dosed orally with 10, 60, or 340 mg/kg/day for 6 months, changes in the female reproductive tract including atrophic or cystic ovaries and anestrus were seen at the high dose. The exposure at the no-effect dose of 60 mg/kg was approximately 85 times the exposure in humans receiving the MRDD.

PREGNANCY CATEGORY C

There are no adequate and well-controlled studies in pregnant women; therefore, naratriptan should be used during pregnancy only if the potential benefit justifies the potential risk to the fetus.

To monitor fetal outcomes of pregnant women exposed to naratriptan, GlaxoSmithKline maintains a Naratriptan Pregnancy Registry. Healthcare providers are encouraged to register patients by calling (800) 336-2176.

In reproductive toxicity studies in rats and rabbits, oral administration of naratriptan was associated with developmental toxicity (embryolethality, fetal abnormalities, pup mortality, offspring growth retardation) at doses producing maternal plasma drug exposures as low as 11 and 2.5 times, respectively, the exposure in humans receiving the MRDD of 5 mg.

When pregnant rats were administered naratriptan during the period of organogenesis at doses of 10, 60, or 340 mg/kg/day, there was a dose-related increase in embryonic death, with a statistically significant difference at the highest dose, and incidences of fetal structural variations (incomplete/irregular ossification of skull bones, sternebrae, ribs) were increased at all doses. The maternal plasma exposures (AUC) at these doses were approximately 11, 70, and 470 times the exposure in humans at the MRDD. The high dose was maternally toxic, as evidenced by decreased maternal body weight gain during gestation. A no-effect dose for developmental toxicity in rats exposed during organogenesis was not established.

When doses of 1, 5, or 30 mg/kg/day were given to pregnant Dutch rabbits throughout organogenesis, the incidence of a specific fetal skeletal malformation (fused sternebrae) was increased at the high dose, and increased incidences of embryonic death and fetal variations (major blood vessel variations, supernumerary ribs, incomplete skeletal ossification) were observed at all doses (4, 20, and 120 times, respectively, the MRDD on a body surface area basis). Maternal toxicity (decreased body weight gain) was evident at the high dose in this study. In a similar study in New Zealand White rabbits (1, 5, or 30 mg/kg/day throughout organogenesis), decreased fetal weights and increased incidences of fetal skeletal variations were observed at all doses (maternal exposures equivalent to 2.5, 19, and 140 times exposure in humans receiving the MRDD), while maternal body weight gain was reduced at 5 mg/kg or greater. A no-effect dose for developmental toxicity in rabbits exposed during organogenesis was not established.

When female rats were treated with 10, 60, or 340 mg/kg/day during late gestation and lactation, offspring behavioral impairment (tremors) and decreased offspring viability and growth were observed at doses of 60 mg/kg or greater, while maternal toxicity occurred only at the highest dose. Maternal exposures at the no-effect dose for developmental effects in this study were approximately 11 times the exposure in humans receiving the MRDD.

NURSING MOTHERS

Naratriptan-related material is excreted in the milk of rats. Therefore, caution should be exercised when considering the administration of naratriptan tablets to a nursing woman.

PEDIATRIC USE

Safety and effectiveness of naratriptan tablets in pediatric patients (younger than 18 year) have not been established.

One randomized, placebo-controlled clinical trial evaluating oral naratriptan (0.25-2.5 mg) in pediatric patients aged 12-17 years evaluated a total of 300 adolescent migraineurs. This study did not establish the efficacy of oral naratriptan compared to placebo in the treatment of migraine in adolescents. Adverse events observed in this clinical trial were similar in nature to those reported in clinical trials in adults.

GERIATRIC USE

The use of naratriptan tablets in elderly patients is not recommended.

Naratriptan is known to be substantially excreted by the kidney, and the risk of adverse reactions to this drug may be greater in elderly patients who have reduced renal function. In addition, elderly patients are more likely to have decreased hepatic function; they are at higher risk for CAD; and blood pressure increases may be more pronounced in the elderly. Clinical studies of naratriptan tablets did not include patients over 65 years of age.

DRUG INTERACTIONS

Ergot-containing drugs have been reported to cause prolonged vasospastic reactions. Because there is a theoretical basis that these effects may be additive, use of ergotamine-containing or ergot-type medications (like dihydroergotamine or methysergide) and naratriptan within 24 hours is contraindicated (see CONTRAINDICATIONS).

The administration of naratriptan with other 5-HT_1 agonists has not been evaluated in migraine patients. Because their vasospastic effects may be additive, coadministration of naratriptan and other 5-HT_1 agonists within 24 hours of each other is not recommended (see CONTRAINDICATIONS).

Selective serotonin reuptake inhibitors (SSRIs) (*e.g.,* fluoxetine, fluvoxamine, paroxetine, sertraline) have been reported, rarely, to cause weakness, hyperreflexia, and incoordination when coadministered with 5-HT_1 agonists. If concomitant treatment with naratriptan and an SSRI is clinically warranted, appropriate observation of the patient is advised.

ADVERSE REACTIONS

Serious cardiac events, including some that have been fatal, have occurred following the use of 5-HT_1 agonists. These events are extremely rare and most have been reported in patients with risk factors predictive of CAD. Events reported have included coronary artery vasospasm, transient myocardial ischemia, myocardial infarction, ventricular tachycardia, and ventricular fibrillation (see CONTRAINDICATIONS, WARNINGS, and PRECAUTIONS).

INCIDENCE IN CONTROLLED CLINICAL TRIALS

The most common adverse events were paresthesias, dizziness, drowsiness, malaise/fatigue, and throat/neck symptoms, which occurred at a rate of 2% and at least 2 times placebo rate. Since patients treated only 1-3 headaches in the controlled clinical trials, the opportunity for discontinuation of therapy in response to an adverse event was limited. In a long-term, open label study where patients were allowed to treat multiple migraine attacks for up to 1 year, 15 patients (3.6%) discontinued treatment due to adverse events.

TABLE 2 lists adverse events that occurred in 5 placebo-controlled clinical trials of approximately 1752 exposures to placebo and naratriptan tablets in adult migraine patients. The events cited reflect experience gained under closely monitored conditions of clinical trials in a highly selected patient population. In actual clinical practice or in other clinical trials, these frequency estimates may not apply, as the conditions of use, reporting behavior, and the kinds of patients treated may differ. Only events that occurred at a frequency of 2% or more in the group treated with naratriptan tablets 2.5 mg treatment group and were more frequent in that group than in the placebo group are included in TABLE 2. From this table, it appears that many of these adverse events are dose related.

TABLE 2 *Treatment-Emergent Adverse Events Reported by at Least 2% of Patients in Placebo-Controlled Migraine Trials*

		Naratriptan	
	Placebo	1 mg	2.5 mg
Adverse Event Type	**(n=498)**	**(n=627)**	**(n=627)**
Atypical Sensation	1%	2%	4%
Paresthesias (all types)	<1%	1%	2%
Gastrointestinal	5%	6%	7%
Nausea	4%	4%	5%
Neurological	3%	4%	7%
Dizziness	1%	1%	2%
Drowsiness	<1%	1%	2%
Malaise/fatigue	1%	2%	2%
Pain and Pressure Sensation	2%	2%	4%
Throat/neck symptoms	1%	1%	2%

One event (vomiting) present in more than 1% of patients receiving naratriptan tablets (vomiting) occurred more frequently on placebo than on naratriptan 2.5 mg.

Naratriptan tablets are generally well tolerated. Most adverse reactions were mild and transient.

The incidence of adverse events in placebo-controlled clinical trials was not affected by age or weight of the patients, duration of headache prior to treatment, presence of aura, use of prophylactic medications, or tobacco use. There was insufficient data to assess the impact of race on the incidence of adverse events.

OTHER EVENTS OBSERVED IN ASSOCIATION WITH THE ADMINISTRATION OF NARATRIPTAN TABLETS

In the paragraphs that follow, the frequencies of less commonly reported adverse clinical events are presented. Because the reports include events observed in open and uncontrolled studies, the role of naratriptan tablets in their causation cannot be reliably determined. Furthermore, variability associated with adverse event reporting, the terminology used to describe adverse events, etc. limit the value of the quantitative frequency estimates provided. Event frequencies are calculated as the number of patients reporting an event divided by the total number of patients (n=3557) exposed to oral naratriptan doses up to 10 mg. All reported events are included except those already listed in TABLE 2, those too general to be informative, and those not reasonably associated with the use of the drug. Events are further classified within body system categories and enumerated in order of decreasing frequency using the following definitions: *frequent* adverse events are those occurring in at least 1/100 patients, *infrequent* adverse events are those occurring in 1/100 to 1/1000 patients, and *rare* adverse events are those occurring in fewer than 1/1000 patients.

Atypical Sensations: *Frequent:* Warm/cold temperature sensations. *Infrequent:* Feeling strange and burning/stinging sensation.

Cardiovascular: *Infrequent:* Palpitations, increased blood pressure, tachyarrhythmias, and abnormal ECG (PR prolongation, QTc prolongation, ST/T wave abnormalities, premature ventricular contractions, atrial flutter, or atrial fibrillation), and syncope. *Rare:* Bradycardia, varicosities, hypotension, and heart murmurs.

Ear, Nose, and Throat: *Frequent:* Ear, nose, and throat infections. *Infrequent:* Phonophobia, sinusitis, upper respiratory inflammation, and tinnitus. *Rare:* Allergic rhinitis; labyrinthitis; ear, nose, and throat hemorrhage; and hearing difficulty.

Endocrine and Metabolic: *Infrequent:* Thirst and polydipsia, dehydration, and fluid retention. *Rare:* Hyperlipidemia, hypercholesterolemia, hypothyroidism, hyperglycemia, glycosuria and ketonuria, and parathyroid neoplasm.

Eye: *Frequent:* Photophobia. *Infrequent:* Blurred vision. *Rare:* Eye pain and discomfort, sensation of eye pressure, eye hemorrhage, dry eyes, difficulty focusing, and scotoma.

Gastrointestinal: *Frequent:* Hyposalivation and vomiting. *Infrequent:* Dyspeptic symptoms, diarrhea, gastrointestinal discomfort and pain, gastroenteritis, and constipation. *Rare:* Abnormal liver function tests, abnormal bilirubin levels, hemorrhoids, gastritis, esophagitis, salivary gland inflammation, oral itching and irritation, regurgitation and reflux, and gastric ulcers.

Hematological Disorders: *Infrequent:* Increased white cells. *Rare:* Thrombocytopenia, quantitative red cell or hemoglobin defects, anemia, and purpura.

Lower Respiratory Tract: *Infrequent:* Bronchitis, cough, and pneumonia. *Rare:* Tracheitis, asthma, pleuritis, and airway constriction and obstruction.

Musculoskeletal: *Infrequent:* Muscle pain, arthralgia and articular rheumatism, muscle cramps and spasms, joint and muscle stiffness, tightness, and rigidity. *Rare:* Bone and skeletal pain.

Neurological: *Frequent:* Vertigo. *Infrequent:* Tremors, cognitive function disorders, sleep disorders, and disorders of equilibrium. *Rare:* Compressed nerve syndromes, confusion, sedation, hyperesthesia, coordination disorders, paralysis of cranial nerves, decreased consciousness, dreams, altered sense of taste, neuralgia, neuritis, aphasia, hypoesthesia, motor retardation, muscle twitching and fasciculation, psychomotor restlessness, and convulsions.

Non-Site Specific: *Infrequent:* Chills and/or fever, descriptions of odor or taste, edema and swelling, allergies, and allergic reactions. *Rare:* Spasms and mobility disorders.

Pain and Pressure Sensations: *Frequent:* Pressure/tightness/heaviness sensations.

Psychiatry: *Infrequent:* Anxiety, depressive disorders, and detachment. *Rare:* Aggression and hostility, agitation, hallucinations, panic, and hyperactivity.

Reproduction: *Rare:* Lumps of female reproductive tract, breast inflammation, inflammation of vagina, inflammation of fallopian tube, breast discharge, endometrium disorders, decreased libido, and lumps of breast.

Skin: *Infrequent:* Sweating, skin rashes, pruritus, and urticaria. *Rare:* Skin erythema, dermatitis and dermatosis, hair loss and alopecia, pruritic skin rashes, acne and folliculitis, allergic skin reactions, macular skin/rashes, skin photosensitivity, photodermatitis, skin flakiness, and dry skin.

Urology: *Infrequent:* Bladder inflammation and polyuria and diuresis. *Rare:* Urinary tract hemorrhage, urinary urgency, pyelitis, and urinary incontinence.

OBSERVED DURING CLINICAL PRACTICE

The following list enumerates potentially important adverse events that have occurred in clinical practice and that have been reported spontaneously to various surveillance systems. The events enumberated represent reports arising from both domestic and nondomestic use of naratriptan. These events do not include those already listed above. Because the reports cite events reported spontaneously from worldwide postmarketing experience, frequency of events and the role of naratriptan in their causation cannot be reliably determined.

Cardiovascular: Angina, myocardial infarction (see WARNINGS).

Gastrointestinal: Colonic ischemia (see WARNINGS).

Lower Respiratory: Dyspnea.

Neurologic: Cerebral vascular accident, including transient ischemic attack, subarachnoid hemorrhage, and cerebral infarction (see WARNINGS).

General: Hypersensitivity, including anaphylaxis/anaphylactoid reactions, in some cases severe (*e.g.*, circulatory collapse) (see WARNINGS).

DOSAGE AND ADMINISTRATION

In controlled clinical trials, single doses of 1 and 2.5 mg of naratriptan tablets taken with fluid were effective for the acute treatment of migraines in adults. A greater proportion of patients had headache response following a 2.5 mg dose than following a 1 mg dose. Individuals may vary in response to doses of naratriptan tablets. The choice of dose should therefore be made on an individual basis, weighing the possible benefit of the 2.5 mg dose with the potential for a greater risk of adverse events. If the headache returns or if the patient has only partial response, the dose may be repeated once after 4 hours, for a maximum dose of 5 mg in a 24 hour period. There is evidence that doses of 5 mg do not provide a greater effect than 2.5 mg.

The safety of treating, on average, more than 4 headaches in a 30 day period has not been established.

RENAL IMPAIRMENT

The use of naratriptan is contraindicated in patients with severe renal impairment (creatinine clearance <15 ml/min) because of decreased clearance of the drug (see CONTRAINDICATIONS and CLINICAL PHARMACOLOGY). In patients with mild to moderate renal impairment, the maximum daily dose should not exceed 2.5 mg over a 24 hour period and a lower starting dose should be considered.

HEPATIC IMPAIRMENT

The use of naratriptan is contraindicated in patients with severe hepatic impairment (Child-Pugh Grade C) because of decreased clearance (see CONTRAINDICATIONS and CLINICAL PHARMACOLOGY). In patients with mild or moderate hepatic impairment, the maximum daily dose should not exceed 2.5 mg over a 24 hour period and a lower starting dose should be considered (see CLINICAL PHARMACOLOGY).

HOW SUPPLIED

Amerge tablets 1 and 2.5 mg of naratriptan (base) as the hydrochloride.

1 mg: White, D-shaped, film-coated tablets debossed with "GX CE3" on one side.

2.5 mg: Green, D-shaped, film-coated tablets debossed with "GX CE5" on one side.

Storage: Store at controlled room temperature, 20-25°C (68-77°F).

PRODUCT LISTING - EQUIVALENTS NOT AVAILABLE

Tablet - Oral - 1 mg

9's $187.19 AMERGE, Glaxosmithkline 00173-0561-00

Tablet - Oral - 2.5 mg

9's $187.19 AMERGE, Glaxosmithkline 00173-0562-00

Nateglinide *(003516)*

For related information, see the comparative table section in Appendix A.

Categories: Diabetes mellitus; FDA Approved 2000 Dec; Pregnancy Category C
Drug Classes: Antidiabetic agents; Meglitinides
Brand Names: Starlix
Foreign Brand Availability: Glinate (India); Trazec (Austria; Belgium; Bulgaria; Czech-Republic; Denmark; England; Finland; France; Germany; Greece; Hungary; Ireland; Italy; Netherlands; Norway; Poland; Portugal; Slovenia; Spain; Sweden; Switzerland; Turkey)
Cost of Therapy: $102.02 (Diabetes mellitus; Starlix; 120 mg; 3 tablets/day; 30 day supply)

DESCRIPTION

Starlix (nateglinide) is an oral antidiabetic agent used in the management of Type 2 diabetes mellitus [also known as non-insulin dependent diabetes mellitus (NIDDM) or adult-onset diabetes]. Starlix, (-)-N-[(trans-4-isopropylcyclohexane)carbonyl]-D-phenylalanine, is structurally unrelated to the oral sulfonylurea insulin secretagogues.

Nateglinide is a white powder with a molecular weight of 317.43. It is freely soluble in methanol, ethanol, and chloroform, soluble in ether, sparingly soluble in acetonitrile and octanol, and practically insoluble in water. Starlix biconvex tablets contain 60 or 120 mg of nateglinide for oral administration.

Inactive ingredients: Colloidal silicon dioxide, croscarmellose sodium, hydroxypropyl methylcellulose, iron oxides (red or yellow), lactose monohydrate, magnesium stearate, microcrystalline cellulose, polyethylene glycol, povidone, talc, and titanium dioxide.

CLINICAL PHARMACOLOGY

MECHANISM OF ACTION

Nateglinide is an amino-acid derivative that lowers blood glucose levels by stimulating insulin secretion from the pancreas. This action is dependent upon functioning beta-cells in the pancreatic islets. Nateglinide interacts with the ATP-sensitive potassium ($K+_{ATP}$) channel on pancreatic beta-cells. The subsequent depolarization of the beta cell opens the calcium channel, producing calcium influx and insulin secretion. The extent of insulin release is glucose dependent and diminishes at low glucose levels. Nateglinide is highly tissue selective with low affinity for heart and skeletal muscle.

PHARMACOKINETICS

Absorption

Following oral administration immediately prior to a meal, nateglinide is rapidly absorbed with mean peak plasma drug concentrations (C_{max}) generally occurring within 1 hour (T_{max}) after dosing. When administered to patients with Type 2 diabetes over the dosage range 60-240 mg three times a day for 1 week, nateglinide demonstrated linear pharmacokinetics for both AUC (area under the time/plasma concentration curve) and C_{max}. T_{max} was also found to be independent of dose in this patient population. Absolute bioavailability is estimated to be approximately 73%. When given with or after meals, the extent of nateglinide absorption (AUC) remains unaffected. However, there is a delay in the rate of absorption characterized by a decrease in C_{max} and a delay in time to peak plasma

N

concentration (T_{max}). Plasma profiles are characterized by multiple plasma concentration peaks when nateglinide is administered under fasting conditions. This effect is diminished when nateglinide is taken prior to a meal.

Distribution

Based on data following intravenous (IV) administration of nateglinide, the steady-state volume of distribution of nateglinide is estimated to be approximately 10 L in healthy subjects. Nateglinide is extensively bound (98%) to serum proteins, primarily serum albumin, and to a lesser extent α^1-acid glycoprotein. The extent of serum protein binding is independent of drug concentration over the test range of 0.1-10 µg/ml.

Metabolism

Nateglinide is metabolized by the mixed-function oxidase system prior to elimination. The major routes of metabolism are hydroxylation followed by glucuronide conjugation. The major metabolites are less potent antidiabetic agents than nateglinide. The isoprene minor metabolite possesses potency similar to that of the parent compound nateglinide.

In vitro data demonstrate that nateglinide is predominantly metabolized by cytochrome P450 isoenzymes CYP2C9 (70%) and CYP3A4 (30%).

Excretion

Nateglinide and its metabolites are rapidly and completely eliminated following oral administration. Within 6 hours after dosing, approximately 75% of the administered ^{14}C-nateglinide was recovered in the urine. Eighty-three percent (83%) of the ^{14}C-nateglinide was excreted in the urine with an additional 10% eliminated in the feces. Approximately 16% of the ^{14}C-nateglinide was excreted in the urine as parent compound. In all studies of healthy volunteers and patients with Type 2 diabetes, nateglinide plasma concentrations declined rapidly with an average elimination half-life of approximately 1.5 hours. Consistent with this short elimination half-life, there was no apparent accumulation of nateglinide upon multiple dosing of up to 240 mg three times daily for 7 days.

SPECIAL POPULATIONS

Geriatric: Age did not influence the pharmacokinetic properties of nateglinide. Therefore no dose adjustments are necessary for elderly patients.

Gender: No clinically significant differences in nateglinide pharmacokinetics were observed between men and women. Therefore, no dose adjustment based on gender is necessary.

Race: Results of a population pharmacokinetic analysis including subjects of Caucasian, Black, and other ethnic origins suggest that race has little influence on the pharmacokinetics of nateglinide.

Renal Impairment: Compared to healthy matched subjects, patients with Type 2 diabetes and moderate-to-severe renal insufficiency (CRCL 15-50 ml/min) not on dialysis displayed similar apparent clearance, AUC and C_{max}. Patients with Type 2 diabetes and renal failure on dialysis exhibited reduced overall drug exposure. However, hemodialysis patients also experienced reductions in plasma protein binding compared to the matched healthy volunteers.

Hepatic Impairment: The peak and total exposure of nateglinide in non-diabetic subjects with mild hepatic insufficiency were increased by 30% compared to matched healthy subjects. Nateglinide should be used with caution in patients with chronic liver disease. (See PRECAUTIONS, Hepatic Impairment.)

PHARMACODYNAMICS

Nateglinide is rapidly absorbed and stimulates pancreatic insulin secretion within 20 minutes of oral administration. When nateglinide is dosed 3 times daily before meals there is a rapid rise in plasma insulin, with peak levels approximately 1 hour after dosing and a fall to baseline by 4 hours after dosing.

In a double-blind, controlled clinical trial in which nateglinide was administered before each of 3 meals, plasma glucose levels were determined over a 12 hour, daytime period after 7 weeks of treatment. Nateglinide was administered 10 minutes before meals. The meals were based on standard diabetic weight maintenance menus with the total caloric content based on each subject's height. Nateglinide produced statistically significant decreases in fasting and post-prandial glycemia compared to placebo.

INDICATIONS AND USAGE

Nateglinide is indicated as monotherapy to lower blood glucose in patients with Type 2 diabetes (non-insulin dependent diabetes mellitus, NIDDM) whose hyperglycemia cannot be adequately controlled by diet and physical exercise and who have not been chronically treated with other antidiabetic agents.

Nateglinide is also indicated for use in combination with metformin. In patients whose hyperglycemia is inadequately controlled with metformin, nateglinide may be added to, but not substituted for, metformin.

Patients whose hyperglycemia is not adequately controlled with glyburide or other insulin secretagogues should not be switched to nateglinide, nor should nateglinide be added to their treatment regimen.

CONTRAINDICATIONS

Nateglinide is contraindicated in patients with:

Known hypersensitivity to the drug or its inactive ingredients.

Type 1 diabetes.

Diabetic ketoacidosis. This condition should be treated with insulin.

PRECAUTIONS

HYPOGLYCEMIA

All oral blood glucose lowering drugs that are absorbed systemically are capable of producing hypoglycemia. The frequency of hypoglycemia is related to the severity of the diabetes, the level of glycemic control, and other patient characteristics. Geriatric patients, malnourished patients, and those with adrenal or pituitary insufficiency are more susceptible to the glucose lowering effect of these treatments. The risk of hypoglycemia may be increased by strenuous physical exercise, ingestion of alcohol, insufficient caloric intake on an acute or chronic basis, or combinations with other oral antidiabetic agents. Hypoglycemia may be difficult to recognize in patients with autonomic neuropathy and/or those who use beta-blockers. Nateglinide should be administered prior to meals to reduce the risk of hypoglycemia. Patients who skip meals should also skip their scheduled dose of nateglinide to reduce the risk of hypoglycemia.

HEPATIC IMPAIRMENT

Nateglinide should be used with caution in patients with moderate-to-severe liver disease because such patients have not been studied.

LOSS OF GLYCEMIC CONTROL

Transient loss of glycemic control may occur with fever, infection, trauma, or surgery. Insulin therapy may be needed instead of nateglinide therapy at such times. Secondary failure, or reduced effectiveness of nateglinide over a period of time, may occur.

INFORMATION FOR THE PATIENT

Patients should be informed of the potential risks and benefits of nateglinide and of alternative modes of therapy. The risks and management of hypoglycemia should be explained. Patients should be instructed to take nateglinide 1-30 minutes before ingesting a meal, but to skip their scheduled dose if they skip the meal so that the risk of hypoglycemia will be reduced. Drug interactions should be discussed with patients. Patients should be informed of potential drug-drug interactions with nateglinide.

LABORATORY TESTS

Response to therapies should be periodically assessed with glucose values and HbA_{1C} levels.

DRUG/FOOD INTERACTIONS

The pharmacokinetics of nateglinide were not affected by the composition of a meal (high protein, fat, or carbohydrate). However, peak plasma levels were significantly reduced when nateglinide was administered 10 minutes prior to a liquid meal. Nateglinide did not have any effect on gastric emptying in healthy subjects as assessed by acetaminophen testing.

CARCINOGENESIS, MUTAGENESIS, AND IMPAIRMENT OF FERTILITY

Carcinogenesis: A 2 year carcinogenicity study in Sprague Dawley rats was performed with oral doses of nateglinide up to 900 mg/kg/day, which produced AUC exposures in male and female rats approximately 30 and 40 times the human therapeutic exposure respectively with a recommended nateglinide dose of 120 mg, three times daily before meals. A 2 year carcinogenicity study in B6C3F1 mice was performed with oral doses of nateglinide up to 400 mg/kg/day, which produced AUC exposures in male and female mice approximately 10 and 30 times the human therapeutic exposure with a recommended nateglinide dose of 120 mg, three times daily before meals. No evidence of a tumorigenic response was found in either rats or mice.

Mutagenesis: Nateglinide was not genotoxic in the *in vitro* Ames test, mouse lymphoma assay, chromosome aberration assay in Chinese hamster lung cells, or in the *in vivo* mouse micronucleus test.

Impairment of Fertility: Fertility was unaffected by administration of nateglinide to rats at doses up to 600 mg/kg (approximately 16 times the human therapeutic exposure with a recommended nateglinide dose of 120 mg three times daily before meals).

PREGNANCY CATEGORY C

Nateglinide was not teratogenic in rats at doses up to 1000 mg/kg (approximately 60 times the human therapeutic exposure with a recommended nateglinide dose of 120 mg, three times daily before meals). In the rabbit, embryonic development was adversely affected and the incidence of gallbladder agenesis or small gallbladder was increased at a dose of 500 mg/kg (approximately 40 times the human therapeutic exposure with a recommended nateglinide dose of 120 mg, three times daily before meals). There are no adequate and well-controlled studies in pregnant women. Nateglinide should not be used during pregnancy.

LABOR AND DELIVERY

The effect of nateglinide on labor and delivery in humans is not known.

NURSING MOTHERS

Studies in lactating rats showed that nateglinide is excreted in the milk; the AUC(0-48h) ratio in milk to plasma was approximately 1:4. During the peri- and postnatal period body weights were lower in offspring of rats administered nateglinide at 1000 mg/kg (approximately 60 times the human therapeutic exposure with a recommended nateglinide dose of 120 mg, three times daily before meals). It is not known whether nateglinide is excreted in human milk. Because many drugs are excreted in human milk, nateglinide should not be administered to a nursing woman.

PEDIATRIC USE

The safety and effectiveness of nateglinide in pediatric patients have not been established.

GERIATRIC USE

No differences were observed in safety or efficacy of nateglinide between patients age 65 and over, and those under age 65. However, greater sensitivity of some older individuals to nateglinide therapy cannot be ruled out.

DRUG INTERACTIONS

In vitro drug metabolism studies indicate that nateglinide is predominantly metabolized by the cytochrome P450 isozyme CYP2C9 (70%) and to a lesser extent CYP3A4 (30%). Nateglinide is a potential inhibitor of the CYP2C9 isoenzyme *in vivo* as indicated by its ability to inhibit the *in vitro* metabolism of tolbutamide. Inhibition of CYP 3A4 metabolic reactions was not detected in *in vitro* experiments.

Glyburide: In a randomized, multiple-dose crossover study, patients with Type 2 diabetes were administered 120 mg nateglinide 3 times a day before meals for 1 day in combination with glyburide 10 mg daily. There were no clinically relevant alterations in the pharmacokinetics of either agent.

Metformin: When nateglinide 120 mg three times daily before meals was administered in combination with metformin 500 mg three times daily to patients with Type 2 diabetes, there were no clinically relevant changes in the pharmacokinetics of either agent.

Digoxin: When nateglinide 120 mg before meals was administered in combination with a single 1 mg dose of digoxin to healthy volunteers there were no clinically relevant changes in the pharmacokinetics of either agent.

Warfarin: When healthy subjects were administered nateglinide 120 mg three times daily before meals for 4 days in combination with a single dose of warfarin 30 mg on Day 2, there were no alterations in the pharmacokinetics of either agent. Prothrombin time was not affected.

Diclofenac: Administration of morning and lunch doses of nateglinide 120 mg in combination with a single 75 mg dose of diclofenac in healthy volunteers resulted in no significant changes to the pharmacokinetics of either agent.

Nateglinide is highly bound to plasma proteins (98%), mainly albumin. *In vitro* displacement studies with highly protein-bound drugs such as furosemide, propranolol, captopril, nicardipine, pravastatin, glyburide, warfarin, phenytoin, acetylsalicylic acid, tolbutamide, and metformin showed no influence on the extent of nateglinide protein binding. Similarly, nateglinide had no influence on the serum protein binding of propranolol, glyburide, nicardipine, warfarin, phenytoin, acetylsalicylic acid, and tolbutamide *in vitro*. However, prudent evaluation of individual cases is warranted in the clinical setting.

Certain drugs, including nonsteroidal anti-inflammatory agents (NSAIDs), salicylates, monoamine oxidase inhibitors, and non-selective beta-adrenergic-blocking agents may potentiate the hypoglycemic action of nateglinide and other oral antidiabetic drugs.

Certain drugs including thiazides, corticosteroids, thyroid products, and sympathomimetics may reduce the hypoglycemic action of nateglinide and other oral antidiabetic drugs.

When these drugs are administered to or withdrawn from patients receiving nateglinide, the patient should be observed closely for changes in glycemic control.

ADVERSE REACTIONS

In clinical trials, approximately 2400 patients with Type 2 diabetes were treated with nateglinide. Of these, approximately 1200 patients were treated for 6 months or longer and approximately 190 patients for 1 year or longer.

Hypoglycemia was relatively uncommon in all treatment arms of the clinical trials. Only 0.3% of nateglinide patients discontinued due to hypoglycemia. Gastrointestinal symptoms, especially diarrhea and nausea, were no more common in patients using the combination of nateglinide and metformin than in patients receiving metformin alone. TABLE 3 lists events that occurred more frequently in nateglinide patients than placebo patients in controlled clinical trials.

***TABLE 3** Common Adverse Events (≥2% in Nateglinide Patients) in Nateglinide Monotherapy Trials (% of Patients)*

Preferred Term	Placebo n=458	Nateglinide n=1441
Upper respiratory infection	8.1%	10.5%
Back pain	3.7%	4.0%
Flu symptoms	2.6%	3.6%
Dizziness	2.2%	3.6%
Arthropathy	2.2%	3.3%
Diarrhea	3.1%	3.2%
Accidental trauma	1.7%	2.9%
Bronchitis	2.6%	2.7%
Coughing	2.2%	2.4%
Hypoglycemia	0.4%	2.4%

During postmarketing experience, rare cases of hypersensitivity reactions such as rash, itching and uticaria have been reported.

LABORATORY ABNORMALITIES

Uric Acid: There were increases in mean uric acid levels for patients treated with nateglinide alone, nateglinide in combination with metformin, metformin alone, and glyburide alone. The respective differences from placebo were 0.29 mg/dl, 0.45 mg/dl, 0.28 mg/dl, and 0.19 mg/dl. The clinical significance of these findings is unknown.

DOSAGE AND ADMINISTRATION

Nateglinide should be taken 1-30 minutes prior to meals.

MONOTHERAPY AND COMBINATION WITH METFORMIN

The recommended starting and maintenance dose of nateglinide, alone or in combination with metformin, is 120 mg three times daily before meals.

The 60 mg dose of nateglinide, either alone or in combination with metformin, may be used in patients who are near goal HbA_{1C} when treatment is initiated.

DOSAGE IN GERIATRIC PATIENTS

No special dose adjustments are usually necessary. However, greater sensitivity of some individuals to nateglinide therapy cannot be ruled out.

DOSAGE IN RENAL AND HEPATIC IMPAIRMENT

No dosage adjustment is necessary in patients with mild-to-severe renal insufficiency or in patients with mild hepatic insufficiency. Dosing of patients with moderate-to-severe hepatic dysfunction has not been studied. Therefore, nateglinide should be used with caution in patients with moderate-to-severe liver disease (see PRECAUTIONS, Hepatic Impairment).

HOW SUPPLIED

Starlix tablets are available in the following dosage strengths:

60 mg: Pink, round, beveled edge tablet with "STARLIX" debossed on one side and "60" on the other.

120 mg: Yellow, ovaloid tablet with "STARLIX" debossed on one side and "120" on the other.

Storage: Store at 25°C (77°F), excursions permitted to 15-30°C (59-86°F). Dispense in a tight container.

PRODUCT LISTING - EQUIVALENTS NOT AVAILABLE

Tablet - Oral - 60 mg
100's $109.11 STARLIX, Novartis Pharmaceuticals 00078-0351-05
Tablet - Oral - 120 mg
100's $113.36 STARLIX, Novartis Pharmaceuticals 00078-0352-05

Nedocromil Sodium (003084)

For related information, see the comparative table section in Appendix A.

Categories: Asthma; Conjunctivitis, allergic; Pregnancy Category B; FDA Approved 1992 Dec
Drug Classes: Mast cell stabilizers
Brand Names: Alocril; **Tilade**
Foreign Brand Availability: Telavist (France; Israel)
Cost of Therapy: $46.58 (Asthma; Tilade Inhaler; 1.75 mg/inh; 16 g; 8 inhalations/day; 13 day supply)
$64.01 (Allergic Conjunctivitis; Alocril Ophthalmic Solution; 2%; 5 ml; 2 drops/day; variable day supply)

INHALATION

DESCRIPTION

Note: The trade names have been used throughout this monograph for clarity.

Tilade (nedocromil sodium) is an inhaled anti-inflammatory agent for the preventive management of asthma. Nedocromil sodium is a pyranoquinoline with the chemical name 4*H*-Pyrano[3,2-g]quinoline-2,8-dicarboxylic acid,9-ethyl-6,9-dihydro-4,6-dioxo-10-propyl-, disodium salt, and it has a molecular weight of 415.3. The empirical formula is $C_{19}H_{15}NNa_2O_7$. Nedocromil sodium, a yellow powder, is soluble in water.

Tilade Inhaler (nedocromil sodium inhalation aerosol) is a pressurized metered-dose aerosol suspension for oral inhalation containing micronized nedocromil sodium and sorbitan trioleate, as well as dichlorotetrafluoroethane and dichlorodifluoromethane as propellants. Each Tilade canister contains 210 mg nedocromil sodium. Each actuation meters 2.00 mg nedocromil sodium from the valve and delivers 1.75 mg nedocromil sodium from the mouthpiece. Each 16.2 g canister provides at least 104 metered actuations. **After 104 metered actuations, the amount delivered per actuation may not be consistent and the unit should be discarded.** Each Tilade Inhaler canister must be primed with 3 actuations prior to the first use. If a canister remains unused for more than 7 days, then it should be reprimed with 3 actuations.

N

CLINICAL PHARMACOLOGY

GENERAL

Nedocromil sodium has been shown to inhibit the *in vitro* activation of, and mediator release from, a variety of inflammatory cell types associated with asthma, including eosinophils, neutrophils, macrophages, mast cells, monocytes, and platelets. *In vitro* studies on cells obtained by bronchoalveolar lavage from antigen-sensitized macaque monkeys show that nedocromil sodium inhibits the release of mediators including histamine, leukotriene C_4, and prostaglandin D_2. Similar studies with human bronchoalveolar cells showed inhibition of histamine release from mast cells and beta-glucuronidase release from macrophages.

Nedocromil sodium has been tested in experimental models of asthma using allergic animals and shown to inhibit the development of early and late bronchoconstriction responses to inhaled antigen. The development of airway hyper-responsiveness to nonspecific bronchoconstrictors was also inhibited. Nedocromil sodium reduced antigen-induced increases in airway microvasculature leakage when administered intravenously in a model system.

In humans, nedocromil sodium has been shown to inhibit acutely the bronchoconstrictor response to several kinds of challenge. Pretreatment with single doses of nedocromil sodium inhibited the bronchoconstriction caused by sulfur dioxide, inhaled neurokinin A, various antigens, exercise, cold air, fog, and adenosine monophosphate.

Nedocromil sodium has no bronchodilator, antihistamine, or corticosteroid activity.

Nedocromil sodium, when delivered by inhalation at the recommended dose, has no known systemic activity.

PHARMACOKINETICS AND BIOAVAILABILITY

Systemic bioavailability of nedocromil sodium administered as an inhaled aerosol is low. In a single dose study involving 20 healthy adult subjects who were administered a 3.5 mg dose of nedocromil sodium (2 actuations of 1.75 mg each), the mean AUC was 5.0 ng·h/ml and the mean C_{max} was 1.6 ng/ml attained about 28 minutes after dosing. The mean half-life was 3.3 hours. Urinary excretion over 12 hours averaged 3.4% of the administered dose, of which approximately 75% was excreted in the first 6 hours of dosing.

In a multiple dose study, 6 healthy adult volunteers (3 males and 3 females) received a 3.5 mg single dose followed by 3.5 mg four times a day for 7 consecutive days. Accumulation of the drug was not observed. Following single and multiple dose inhalations, urinary excretion of nedocromil accounted for 5.6% and 12% of the drug administered, respectively. After intravenous (IV) administration to healthy adults, urinary excretion of nedocromil was approximately 70%. The absolute bioavailability of nedocromil was thus 8% (5.6/70) for single and 17% (12/70) for multiple inhaled doses.

Similarly, in a multiple dose study of 12 asthmatic adult patients, each given a 3.5 mg single dose followed by 3.5 mg four times a day for 1 month, both single dose and multiple dose inhalations gave a mean high plasma concentration of 2.8 ng/ml between 5 and 90 minutes, mean AUC of 5.6 ng·h/ml, and a mean terminal half-life of 1.5 hours. The mean 24 hour urinary excretion after either single or multiple dose administration represented approximately 5% of the administered dose.

Studies involving very high oral doses of nedocromil (600 mg single dose, and subsequently 200 mg three times a day for 7 days) showed an absolute bioavailability of less than 2%. In a radiolabeled (^{14}C) nedocromil IV study involving 2 healthy adult males, urinary excretion accounted for 64% of the dose, fecal excretion for 36%.

Although minimal pharmacokinetic data are available in children between the ages of 6-11 years, the nedocromil sodium levels obtained at 1 hour after chronic dosing in this age group appear to be similar to those observed in adults.

Protein Binding

Nedocromil is approximately 89% protein bound in human plasma over a concentration range of 0.5 to 50 μg/ml. This binding is reversible.

Metabolism

Nedocromil is not metabolized after IV administration and is excreted unchanged.

INDICATIONS AND USAGE

Tilade Inhaler is indicated for maintenance therapy in the management of adult and pediatric patients 6 years and older with mild to moderate asthma.

Tilade is not indicated for the reversal of acute bronchospasm.

NON-FDA APPROVED INDICATIONS

Although not approved by the FDA, nedocromil is effective in preventing exercise-induced bronchospasm.

CONTRAINDICATIONS

Tilade Inhaler is contraindicated in patients who have shown hypersensitivity to nedocromil sodium or other ingredients in this preparation.

WARNINGS

Tilade Inhaler is not a bronchodilator and, therefore, should not be used for the reversal of acute bronchospasm, particularly status asthmaticus. Tilade should ordinarily be continued during acute exacerbations, unless the patient becomes intolerant to the use of inhaled dosage forms.

As with other inhaled asthma medications, bronchospasm, which can be life-threatening, may occur immediately after administration. If this occurs, Tilade should be discontinued and alternative therapy instituted.

PRECAUTIONS

GENERAL

The role of Tilade as a corticosteroid-sparing agent in patients receiving oral or inhaled corticosteroids remains to be defined. If systemic or inhaled corticosteroid therapy is reduced in patients receiving Tilade, careful monitoring is necessary.

INFORMATION FOR THE PATIENT

Patients should be told that:

Tilade must be taken regularly to achieve benefit, even during symptom-free periods.

Tilade is not meant to relieve acute asthma symptoms. If symptoms do not improve or the patient's condition worsens, the patient should not increase the dosage but should notify the physician immediately.

They should not decrease the dose without the physician's knowledge. The recommended dose should not be exceeded.

The full therapeutic effect of Tilade may not be obtained for 1 week or longer after initiating treatment.

Because the therapeutic effect depends upon local delivery to the lungs, it is essential that patients be properly instructed in the correct method of use (see Patient Instructions for use that is distributed with the prescription).

An illustrated leaflet for the patient is included in each Tilade Inhaler pack.

CARCINOGENESIS, MUTAGENESIS, AND IMPAIRMENT OF FERTILITY

A 2 year inhalation carcinogenicity study of nedocromil sodium at a dose of 24 mg/kg/day (approximately 8 times the maximum recommended human daily inhalation dose on a mg/m^2 basis) in Wistar rats showed no carcinogenic potential. A 21 month oral dietary carcinogenicity study of nedocromil sodium performed in B6C3F1 mice with doses up to 180 mg/kg/day (approximately 30 times the maximum recommended human daily inhalation dose on a mg/m^2 basis) showed no carcinogenic potential.

Nedocromil sodium showed no mutagenic potential in the Ames *Salmonella*/microsome plate assay, mitotic gene conversion in *Saccharomyces cerevisiae*, mouse lymphoma forward mutation, and mouse micronucleus assays.

Reproduction and fertility studies in mice and rats showed no effects on male and female fertility at a subcutaneous (SC) dose of 100 mg/kg/day (approximately 30 times and 60 times, respectively, the maximum recommended human daily inhalation dose on a mg/m^2 basis).

PREGNANCY CATEGORY B

Reproduction studies performed in mice, rats, and rabbits using a SC dose of 100 mg/kg/day (approximately 30 times, 60 times, and 116 times, respectively, the maximum recommended human daily inhalation dose on a mg/m^2 basis) revealed no evidence of teratogenicity or harm to the fetus due to nedocromil sodium. There are, however, no adequate and well-controlled studies in pregnant women. Because animal reproduction studies are not always predictive of human response, this drug should be used during pregnancy only if clearly needed.

NURSING MOTHERS

It is not known whether this drug is excreted in human milk. Because many drugs are excreted in human milk, caution should be exercised when Tilade is administered to a nursing woman.

PEDIATRIC USE

Safety data in normal volunteers and asthmatic patients between the ages of 6 and 11 years are available on a total of 311 children from US clinical trials and 192 children from foreign clinical trials (total = 503) of 4-12 weeks duration. An additional 225 children received Tilade for 40 weeks and 24 received Tilade for 52 weeks.

The safety and effectiveness of Tilade in children ages 6-11 have been established in adequate and well-controlled clinical trials. Use of Tilade in children ages 6-11 years is also supported by evidence from adequate and well-controlled studies of Tilade in adults.

The safety and effectiveness of Tilade in patients below the age of 6 years have not been established.

DRUG INTERACTIONS

In clinical studies, Tilade has been coadministered with other anti-asthma medications, including inhaled and oral bronchodilators, and inhaled corticosteroids, with no evidence of increased frequency of adverse events or laboratory abnormalities. No formal drug-drug interaction studies, however, have been conducted.

ADVERSE REACTIONS

Tilade is generally well tolerated. Adverse event information was derived from 6469 patients receiving Tilade in controlled and open-label clinical trials of 1-52 weeks in duration. A total of 4400 patients received 2 inhalations 4 times a day. An additional 2069 patients received 2 inhalations twice daily or another dose regimen. Seventy-seven percent (77%) of patients were treated with Tilade for 8 weeks or longer.

Of the 4400 patients who received 2 inhalations of Tilade 4 times a day, 2632 were in placebo-controlled, parallel trials and of these 6.0% withdrew from the trials due to adverse events, compared to 5.7% of the 2446 patients who received placebo.

The reasons for withdrawal were generally similar in the Tilade and placebo-treated groups, except that patients withdrew due to bad taste statistically more frequently on Tilade than on placebo. Headache reported as severe or very severe, some with nausea and ill feeling, was experienced by 1.0% of Tilade patients and 0.7% of placebo patients.

The events reported with a frequency of 1% or greater across all placebo-controlled studies are displayed for all patients ages 6 years and older who received Tilade or placebo at 2 inhalations 4 times daily.

The adverse event profile observed in children ages 6-11 was similar to that observed in adults.

See TABLE 4.

TABLE 4

Adverse Event (AE)	% Experienceing AE Tilade (n=2632)	% Experienceing AE Placebo (n=2402)	% Withdrawing Tilade	% Withdrawing Placebo
Special Senses				
Unpleasant taste*	11.6%	3.1%	1.6%	0.0%
Respiratory System Disorders				
Coughing	8.9%	10.2%	1.1%	1.2%
Pharyngitis	7.6%	7.5%	0.5%	0.4%
Rhinitis*	7.3%	6.0%	0.1%	0.1%
Upper respiratory infection	6.7%	6.3%	0.1%	0.2%
Sputum increased	1.5%	1.4%	0.1%	0.2%
Bronchitis	1.1%	1.5%	0.1%	0.1%
Dyspnea	2.5%	3.3%	0.8%	1.0%
Bronchospasm†	8.4%	11.8%	1.4%	2.0%
Sinusitis	3.3%	4.1%	1.1%	0.0%
Respiratory disorder	0.8%	1.1%	0.0%	0.0%
Gastrointestinal Tract				
Nausea*	3.9%	2.3%	1.1%	0.5%
Vomiting*	2.5%	1.6%	0.2%	0.3%
Dyspepsia	1.5%	1.1%	0.1%	0.1%
Diarrhea	1.3%	1.2%	0.1%	0.0%
Abdominal pain	1.9%	1.3%	0.2%	0.1%
Central and Peripheral Nervous System				
Dizziness	0.8%	1.3%	0.1%	0.2%
Body as a Whole				
Headache	8.1%	7.5%	0.4%	0.2%
Chest pain	3.6%	3.8%	0.7%	0.5%
Fatigue	1.0%	0.8%	0.2%	0.0%
Fever	3.1%	3.7%	0.1%	0.1%
Resistance Mechanism Disorders				
Infection viral	2.4%	3.2%	0.1%	0.1%
Vision Disorders				
Conjunctivitis	1.1%	0.7%	0.0%	0.1%
Skin and Appendages Disorders				
Rash†	0.5%	1.2%	0.1%	0.0%

* Statistically significant higher frequency on Tilade $p < 0.05$.
† Statistically significant higher frequency on placebo $p < 0.05$.

Other adverse events present at less than the 1% level of occurrence, but that might be related to Tilade administration, include arthritis, tremor, and a sensation of warmth. In clinical trials with 2632 patients receiving Tilade, 2 patients (0.08%) developed neutropenia and 3 patients (0.11%) developed leukopenia. Although it is unclear if these reactions were caused by Tilade, in several cases these abnormal laboratory tests returned to normal when Tilade was discontinued.

There have been reports of clinically significant elevation of hepatic transaminases (ALT and AST greater than 10 times the upper limit of the normal reference range in 1 patient) associated with the administration of Tilade. It is unclear if these abnormal laboratory tests in asymptomatic patients were caused by Tilade.

Cases of bronchospasm immediately following dosing with Tilade have been reported from postmarketing experience. (See WARNINGS.) Isolated cases of pneumonitis with eosinophilia (PIE syndrome) and anaphylaxis have also been reported in which a relationship to drug is undetermined.

DOSAGE AND ADMINISTRATION

The recommended dosage for adult and pediatric patients 6 years of age and older is 2 inhalations 4 times a day at regular intervals, which provides a dose of 14 mg/day. In patients whose asthma is well controlled on this dosage (*e.g.,* patients who only need occasional inhaled or oral $beta_2$-agonists and who are not experiencing serious exacerbations), less frequent administration may be effective.

Each Tilade Inhaler canister must be primed with 3 actuations prior to the first use. If a canister remains unused for more than 7 days, then it should be reprimed with 3 actuations.

Tilade Inhaler may be added to the patient's existing treatment regimen (*e.g.,* bronchodilators). When a clinical response to Tilade Inhaler is evident and if the patient's asthma is under good control, an attempt may be made to decrease concomitant medication usage gradually.

Proper inhalational technique is essential (see Patient Instructions for use that is distributed with the prescription).

Patients should be advised that the optimal effect of Tilade therapy depends upon its administration at regular intervals, even during symptom-free periods.

HOW SUPPLIED

Tilade Inhaler is available in 16.2 g canisters providing at least 104 metered inhalations. Each Tilade canister contains 210 mg nedocromil sodium. Each pack is supplied with patient instructions, a tan-colored rubber valve cover, and white plastic mouthpiece and cover, bearing the Tilade logo. The Tilade canister is to be used only with the Tilade Inhaler mouthpiece. The Tilade mouthpiece should not be used with other aerosol medications and should not be used with other mouthpieces. Each actuation meters 2.00 mg nedocromil sodium from the valve and delivers 1.75 mg nedocromil sodium from the mouthpiece.

The canister should be discarded after the labeled number of actuations have been used. The amount of medication in each actuation cannot be assured after this point.

Storage: Store between 2-30°C (36-86°F). Do not freeze. **Avoid spraying in eyes.** Contents under pressure. Do not puncture, incinerate, place near sources of heat, or use with other mouthpieces. Exposure to temperatures above 120°F may cause bursting. Never throw canister into fire or incinerator. **Keep out of the reach of children.** For best results, the canister should be at room temperature before use. Shake well before using.

Note: The indented statement below is required by the Federal government's Clean Air Act for all products containing or manufactured with chlorofluorocarbons (CFCs).

> *WARNING:* Contains CFC-12 and CFC-114, substances which harm public health and the environment by destroying ozone in the upper atmosphere.

A notice similar to the above WARNING has been placed in the "Information For The Patient" leaflet that is distributed with the prescription under the Environmental Protection Agency's (EPA's) regulations. The patient's warning states that the patient should consult his or her physician if there are questions about alternatives.

OPHTHALMIC

DESCRIPTION

Note: The trade names have been used throughout this monograph for clarity.

Alocril (nedocromil sodium ophthalmic solution) 2% is a clear, yellow, sterile solution for topical ophthalmic use.

Nedocromil sodium has the chemical formula $C_{19}H_{15}NNa_2O_7$, and a molecular weight of 415.30.

Chemical Name: 4H-Pyrano[3,2-g]quinoline-2,8-dicarboxylic acid, 9-ethyl-6,9-dihydro-4,6-dioxo-10-propyl-, disodium salt.

Each ml Contains:

Active: Nedocromil sodium 20 mg (2%); *Preservative:* Benzalkonium chloride 0.01%; *Inactives:* Edetate disodium 0.05%; purified water; and sodium chloride 0.5%. It has a pH of 4.0-5.5 and osmolality range of 270-330 mOsm/kg.

CLINICAL PHARMACOLOGY

Nedocromil sodium is a mast cell stabilizer. Nedocromil sodium inhibits the release of mediators from cells involved in hypersensitivity reactions. Decreased chemotaxis and decreased activation of eosinophils have also been demonstrated.

In vitro studies with adult human bronchoalveolar cells showed that nedocromil sodium inhibits histamine release from a population of mast cells having been defined as belonging to the mucosal subtype and beta-glucuronidase release from macrophages.

PHARMACOKINETICS AND BIOAVAILABILITY

Nedocromil sodium exhibits low systemic absorption. When administered as a 2% ophthalmic solution in adult human volunteers, less than 4% of the total dose was systemically absorbed following multiple dosing. Absorption is mainly through the nasolacrimal duct rather than through the conjunctiva. It is not metabolized and is eliminated primarily unchanged in urine (70%) and feces (30%).

INDICATIONS AND USAGE

Alocril ophthalmic solution is indicated for the treatment of itching associated with allergic conjunctivitis.

CONTRAINDICATIONS

Alocril ophthalmic solution is contraindicated in those patients who have shown hypersensitivity to nedocromil sodium or to any of the other ingredients.

PRECAUTIONS

INFORMATION FOR THE PATIENT

Patients should be advised to follow the patient instructions listed on the Information for Patients sheet that is distributed with the prescription.

Users of contact lenses should refrain from wearing lenses while exhibiting the signs and symptoms of allergic conjunctivitis.

Patients should be instructed to avoid allowing the tip of the dispensing container to contact the eye, surrounding structures, fingers, or any other surface in order to avoid contamination of the solution by common bacteria known to cause ocular infections. Serious damage to the eye and subsequent loss of vision may result from using contaminated solutions.

CARCINOGENESIS, MUTAGENESIS, AND IMPAIRMENT OF FERTILITY

A 2 year inhalation carcinogenicity study of nedocromil sodium at a dose of 24 mg/kg/day (approximately 400 times the maximum recommended human daily ocular dose on a mg/kg basis) in Wistar rats showed no carcinogenic potential.

Nedocromil sodium showed no mutagenic potential in the Ames *Salmonella*/ microsome plate assay, mitotic gene conversion in *Saccharomyces cerevisiae,* mouse lymphoma forward mutation and mouse micronucleus assays.

Reproduction and fertility studies in mice and rats showed no effects on male and female fertility at a SC dose of 100 mg/kg/day (more than 1600 times the maximum recommended human daily ocular dose).

PREGNANCY, TERATOGENIC EFFECTS, PREGNANCY CATEGORY B

Reproduction studies performed in mice, rats and rabbits using a SC dose of 100 mg/kg/day (more than 1600 times the maximum human daily ocular dose on a mg/kg basis) revealed no evidence of teratogenicity or harm to the fetus due to nedocromil sodium. There are, however, no adequate and well-controlled studies in pregnant women. Because animal reproduction studies are not always predictive of human response, Alocril ophthalmic solution should be used during pregnancy only if clearly needed.

NURSING MOTHERS

After IV administration to lactating rats, nedocromil was excreted in milk. It is not known whether this drug is excreted in human milk. Because many drugs are excreted in human milk, caution should be exercised when Alocril is administered to a nursing woman.

PEDIATRIC USE

Safety and effectiveness in children below the age of 3 years have not been established.

GERIATRIC USE

No overall differences in safety or effectiveness have been observed between elderly and younger patients.

ADVERSE REACTIONS

The most frequently reported adverse experience was headache (~40%).

Ocular burning, irritation and stinging, unpleasant taste, and nasal congestion have been reported to occur in 10-30% of patients. Other events occurring between 1-10% included asthma, conjunctivitis, eye redness, photophobia,and rhinitis.

Some of these events were similar to the underlying ocular disease being studied.

DOSAGE AND ADMINISTRATION

The recommended dosage is 1 or 2 drops in each eye twice a day.

Alocril ophthalmic solution should be used at regular intervals.

Treatment should be continued throughout the period of exposure (*i.e.,* until the pollen season is over or until exposure to the offending allergen is terminated), even when symptoms are absent.

HOW SUPPLIED

Alocril (nedocromil sodium ophthalmic solution) 2% is supplied sterile in opaque white LDPE plastic bottles with dropper tips and white high impact polystyrene (HIPS) caps as 5 ml in 8 ml bottle.

Storage: Store between 2-25°C (36-77°F). Keep bottle tightly closed and out of the reach of children.

PRODUCT LISTING - EQUIVALENTS NOT AVAILABLE

Aerosol with Adapter - Inhalation - 1.75 mg/Inh

16 gm	$46.58	TILADE, Aventis Pharmaceuticals	00585-0685-02

Solution - Ophthalmic - 2%

5 ml	$64.01	ALOCRIL, Allergan Inc	00023-8842-05
5 ml	$64.01	ALOCRIL, Allergan Inc	00238-8420-50

Nefazodone Hydrochloride (003237)

For related information, see the comparative table section in Appendix A.

Categories: Depression; FDA Approved 1994 Dec; Pregnancy Category C
Drug Classes: Antidepressants, miscellaneous
Brand Names: Serzone
Foreign Brand Availability: Nefadar (Germany); Serzonil (Israel)
Cost of Therapy: $74.12 (Depression; Serzone; 150 mg; 2 tablets/day; 30 day supply)

WARNING

Before prescribing nefazodone hydrochloride (HCl), the physician should be thoroughly familiar with the details of this prescribing information.

WARNING — Cont'd

Cases of life-threatening hepatic failure have been reported in patients treated with nefazodone HCl.

The reported rate in the US is about 1 case of liver failure resulting in death or transplant per 250,000-300,000 patient-years of nefazodone HCl treatment. The total patient-years is a summation of each patient's duration of exposure expressed in years. For example, 1 patient-year is equal to 2 patients each treated for 6 months, 3 patients each treated for 4 months, etc. (See WARNINGS.)

Ordinarily, treatment with nefazodone HCl should not be initiated in individuals with active liver disease or with elevated baseline serum transaminases. There is no evidence that pre-existing liver disease increases the likelihood of developing liver failure, however, baseline abnormalities can complicate patient monitoring.

Patients should be advised to be alert for signs and symptoms of liver dysfunction (jaundice, anorexia, gastrointestinal complaints, malaise, etc.) and to report them to their doctor immediately if they occur.

Nefazodone HCl should be discontinued if clinical signs or symptoms suggest liver failure (see PRECAUTIONS, Information for the Patient). Patients who develop evidence of hepatocellular injury such as increased serum AST or serum ALT levels ≥3 times the upper limit of NORMAL, while on nefazodone HCl should be withdrawn from the drug. These patients should be presumed to be at increased risk for liver injury if nefazodone HCl is reintroduced. Accordingly, such patients should not be considered for re-treatment.

DESCRIPTION

Nefazodone hydrochloride (HCl) is an antidepressant for oral administration with a chemical structure unrelated to selective serotonin reuptake inhibitors, tricyclics, tetracyclics, or monoamine oxidase inhibitors (MAOI).

Nefazodone HCl is a synthetically derived phenylpiperazine antidepressant. The chemical name for nefazodone HCl is 2-[3-[4-(3-chlorophenyl)-1-piperazinyl]propyl]-5-ethyl-2,4-dihydro-4-(2-phenoxyethyl)-3H-1,2,4-triazol-3-one monohydrochloride. The molecular formula is $C_{25}H_{32}ClN_5O_2$·HCl, which corresponds to a molecular weight of 506.5.

Nefazodone HCl is a nonhygroscopic, white crystalline solid. It is freely soluble in chloroform, soluble in propylene glycol, and slightly soluble in polyethylene glycol and water.

Serzone is supplied as hexagonal tablets containing 50, 100, 150, 200, or 250 mg of nefazodone HCl and the following inactive ingredients: microcrystalline cellulose, povidone, sodium starch glycolate, colloidal silicon dioxide, magnesium stearate, and iron oxides (red and/or yellow) as colorants.

CLINICAL PHARMACOLOGY

PHARMACODYNAMICS

The mechanism of action of nefazodone, as with other antidepressants, is unknown.

Preclinical studies have shown that nefazodone inhibits neuronal uptake of serotonin and norepinephrine.

N

Nefazodone occupies central $5\text{-}HT_2$ receptors at nanomolar concentrations, and acts as an antagonist at this receptor. Nefazodone was shown to antagonize $alpha_1$-adrenergic receptors, a property which may be associated with postural hypotension. *In vitro* binding studies showed that nefazodone had no significant affinity for the following receptors: $alpha_2$ and beta adrenergic, $5\text{-}HT_{1A}$, cholinergic, dopaminergic, or benzodiazepine.

PHARMACOKINETICS

Nefazodone HCl is rapidly and completely absorbed but is subject to extensive metabolism, so that its absolute bioavailability is low, about 20%, and variable. Peak plasma concentrations occur at about 1 hour and the half-life of nefazodone is 2-4 hours.

Both nefazodone and its pharmacologically similar metabolite, hydroxynefazodone, exhibit nonlinear kinetics for both dose and time, with AUC and C_{max} increasing more than proportionally with dose increases and more than expected upon multiple dosing over time, compared to single dosing. For example, in a multiple-dose study involving bid dosing with 50, 100, and 200 mg, the AUC for nefazodone and hydroxynefazodone increased by about 4-fold with an increase in dose from 200-400 mg/day; C_{max} increased by about 3-fold with the same dose increase. In a multiple-dose study involving bid dosing with 25, 50, 100, and 150 mg, the accumulation ratios for nefazodone and hydroxynefazodone AUC, after 5 days of bid dosing relative to the first dose, ranged from approximately 3-4 at the lower doses (50-100 mg/day) and from 5-7 at the higher doses (200-300 mg/day); there were also approximately 2- to 4-fold increases in C_{max} after 5 days of bid dosing relative to the first dose, suggesting extensive and greater than predicted accumulation of nefazodone and its hydroxy metabolite with multiple dosing. Steady-state plasma nefazodone and metabolite concentrations are attained within 4-5 days of initiation of bid dosing or upon dose increase or decrease.

Nefazodone is extensively metabolized after oral administration by n-dealkylation and aliphatic and aromatic hydroxylation, and less than 1% of administered nefazodone is excreted unchanged in urine. Attempts to characterize three metabolites identified in plasma, hydroxynefazodone (HO-NEF), meta-chlorophenylpiperazine (mCPP), and a triazole-dione metabolite, have been carried out. The AUC (expressed as a multiple of the AUC for nefazodone dosed at 100 mg bid) and elimination half-lives for these three metabolites were as shown in TABLE 1.

TABLE 1 *AUC Multiples and T½ for Three Metabolites of Nefazodone (100 mg bid)*

Metabolite	AUC Multiple	T½
HO-NEF	0.4	1.5-4 hours
mCPP	0.07	4-8 hours
Triazole-dione	4.0	18 hours

HO-NEF possesses a pharmacological profile qualitatively and quantitatively similar to that of nefazodone. mCPP has some similarities to nefazodone, but also has agonist activity at some serotonergic receptor subtypes. The pharmacological profile of the triazole-dione metabolite has not yet been well characterized. In addition to the above compounds, several other metabolites were present in plasma but have not been tested for pharmacological activity.

After oral administration of radiolabeled nefazodone, the mean half-life of total label ranged between 11 and 24 hours. Approximately 55% of the administered radioactivity was detected in urine and about 20-30% in feces.

Distribution

Nefazodone is widely distributed in body tissues, including the central nervous system (CNS). In humans the volume of distribution of nefazodone ranges from 0.22-0.87 L/kg.

Protein Binding

At concentrations of 25-2500 ng/ml nefazodone is extensively (>99%) bound to human plasma proteins *in vitro*. The administration of 200 mg bid of nefazodone for 1 week did not increase the fraction of unbound warfarin in subjects whose prothrombin times had been prolonged by warfarin therapy to 120-150% of the laboratory control (see DRUG INTERACTIONS). While nefazodone did not alter the *in vitro* protein binding of chlorpromazine, desipramine, diazepam, diphenylhydantoin, lidocaine, prazosin, propranolol, or verapamil, it is unknown whether displacement of either nefazodone or these drugs occurs *in vivo*. There was a 5% decrease in the protein binding of haloperidol; this is probably of no clinical significance.

Effect of Food

Food delays the absorption of nefazodone and decreases the bioavailability of nefazodone by approximately 20%.

Renal Disease

In studies involving 29 renally impaired patients, renal impairment (creatinine clearances ranging from 7-60 ml/min/1.73 m^2) had no effect on steady-state nefazodone plasma concentrations.

Liver Disease

In a multiple-dose study of patients with liver cirrhosis, the AUC values for nefazodone and HO-NEF at steady state were approximately 25% greater than those observed in normal volunteers.

Age/Gender Effects

After single doses of 300 mg to younger (18-45 years) and older patients (>65 years), C_{max} and AUC for nefazodone and hydroxynefazodone were up to twice as high in the older patients. With multiple doses, however, differences were much smaller, 10-20%. A similar result was seen for gender, with a higher C_{max} and AUC in women after single doses but no difference after multiple doses.

Treatment with nefazodone HCl should be initiated at half the usual dose in elderly patients, especially women (see DOSAGE AND ADMINISTRATION), but the therapeutic dose range is similar in younger and older patients.

INDICATIONS AND USAGE

Nefazodone HCl is indicated for the treatment of depression.

The efficacy of nefazodone HCl in the treatment of depression was established in 6-8 week controlled trials of outpatients and in a 6 week controlled trial of depressed inpatients whose diagnoses corresponded most closely to the DSM-III or DSM-IIIR category of major depressive disorder (see CLINICAL PHARMACOLOGY).

A major depressive episode implies a prominent and relatively persistent depressed or dysphoric mood that usually interferes with daily functioning (nearly every day for at least 2 weeks). It must include either depressed mood or loss of interest or pleasure and at least five of the following nine symptoms: depressed mood, loss of interest in usual activities, significant change in weight and/or appetite, insomnia or hypersomnia, psychomotor agitation or retardation, increased fatigue, feelings of guilt or worthlessness, slowed thinking or impaired concentration, a suicide attempt or suicidal ideation.

The efficacy of nefazodone HCl in reducing relapse in patients with major depression who were judged to have had a satisfactory clinical response to 16 weeks of open-label nefazodone HCl treatment for an acute depressive episode has been demonstrated in a randomized placebo-controlled trial (see CLINICAL PHARMACOLOGY). Although remitted patients were followed for as long as 36 weeks in the study cited (*i.e.*, 52 weeks total), the physician who elects to use nefazodone HCl for extended periods should periodically re-evaluate the long-term usefulness of the drug for the individual patient.

NON-FDA APPROVED INDICATIONS

Nefazodone may also have clinical utility for the treatment of a number of other conditions including panic disorder, post-traumatic stress disorder, and social phobia, although none of these uses is approved by the FDA and comparative efficacy trials for these uses have not yet been performed.

CONTRAINDICATIONS

Coadministration of terfenadine, astemizole, cisapride, pimozide, or carbamazepine with nefazodone HCl is contraindicated (see WARNINGS and PRECAUTIONS).

Nefazodone HCl tablets are contraindicated in patients who were withdrawn from nefazodone HCl because of evidence of liver injury (see BOXED WARNING). Nefazodone HCl tablets are also contraindicated in patients who have demonstrated hypersensitivity to nefazodone HCl, its inactive ingredients, or other phenylpiperazine antidepressants.

The coadministration of triazolam and nefazodone causes a significant increase in the plasma level of triazolam (see WARNINGS and PRECAUTIONS), and a 75% reduction in the initial triazolam dosage is recommended if the 2 drugs are to be given together. Because not all commercially available dosage forms of triazolam permit a sufficient dosage reduction, the coadministration of triazolam and nefazodone HCl should be avoided for most patients, including the elderly.

WARNINGS

HEPATOTOXICITY

See BOXED WARNING.

Cases of life-threatening hepatic failure have been reported in patients treated with nefazodone HCl.

The reported rate in the US is about 1 case of liver failure resulting in death or transplant per 250,000-300,000 patient-years of use. This represents a rate of about 3-4 times the estimated background rate of liver failure. This rate is an underestimate because of under reporting, and the true risk could be considerably greater than this. A large cohort study of antidepressant users found no cases of liver failure leading to death or transplant among nefazodone HCl users in about 30,000 patient-years of exposure. The spontaneous report data and the cohort study results provide estimates of the upper and lower limits of the risk of liver failure in nefazodone-treated patients, but are not capable of providing a precise risk estimate.

The time to liver injury for the reported liver failure cases resulting in death or transplant generally ranged from 2 weeks to 6 months on nefazodone HCl therapy. Although some reports described dark urine and nonspecific prodromal symptoms (*e.g.*, anorexia, malaise, and gastrointestinal symptoms), other reports did not describe the onset of clear prodromal symptoms prior to the onset of jaundice.

The physician may consider the value of liver function testing. Periodic serum transaminase testing has not been proven to prevent serious injury but it is generally believed that early detection of drug-induced hepatic injury along with immediate withdrawal of the suspect drug enhances the likelihood for recovery.

Patients should be advised to be alert for signs and symptoms of liver dysfunction (jaundice, anorexia, gastrointestinal complaints, malaise, etc.) and to report them to their doctor immediately if they occur. Ongoing clinical assessment of patients should govern physician interventions, including diagnostic evaluations and treatment.

Nefazodone HCl should be discontinued if clinical signs or symptoms suggest liver failure (see PRECAUTIONS, Information for the Patient). Patients who develop evidence of hepatocellular injury such as increased serum AST or serum ALT levels ≥3 times the upper limit of NORMAL, while on nefazodone HCl should be withdrawn from the drug. These patients should be presumed to be at increased risk for liver injury if nefazodone HCl is reintroduced. Accordingly, such patients should not be considered for re-treatment.

POTENTIAL FOR INTERACTION WITH MONOAMINE OXIDASE INHIBITORS

In patients receiving antidepressants with pharmacological properties similar to nefazodone in combination with a monoamine oxidase inhibitor (MAOI), there have been reports of serious, sometimes fatal, reactions. For a selective serotonin reuptake inhibitor (SSRI), these reactions have included hyperthermia, rigidity, myoclonus, autonomic instability with possible rapid fluctuations of vital signs, and mental status changes that include extreme agitation progressing to delirium and coma. These reactions have also been reported in patients who have recently discontinued that drug and have been started on an MAOI. Some cases presented with features resembling neuroleptic malignant syndrome. Severe hyperthermia and seizures, sometimes fatal, have been reported in association with the combined use of tricyclic antidepressants and MAOIs. These reactions have also been reported in patients who have recently discontinued these drugs and have been started on an MAOI.

Although the effects of combined use of nefazodone and MAOI have not been evaluated in humans or animals, because nefazodone is an inhibitor of both serotonin and norepinephrine reuptake, it is recommended that nefazodone not be used in combination with an MAOI, or within 14 days of discontinuing treatment with an MAOI. At least 1 week should be allowed after stopping nefazodone before starting an MAOI.

INTERACTION WITH TRIAZOLOBENZODIAZEPINES

Interaction studies of nefazodone with two triazolobenzodiazepines, *i.e.*, triazolam and alprazolam, metabolized by cytochrome P450 3A4, have revealed substantial and clinically important increases in plasma concentrations of these compounds when administered concomitantly with nefazodone.

Triazolam

When a single oral 0.25 mg dose of triazolam was coadministered with nefazodone (200 mg bid) at steady state, triazolam half-life and AUC increased 4-fold and peak concentrations increased 1.7-fold. Nefazodone plasma concentrations were unaffected by triazolam. ***Coadministration of nefazodone potentiated the effects of triazolam on psychomotor performance tests.*** If triazolam is coadministered with nefazodone HCl, a 75% reduction in the initial triazolam dosage is recommended. Because not all commercially available dosage forms of triazolam permit sufficient dosage reduction, coadministration of triazolam with nefazodone HCl should be avoided for most patients, including the elderly. In the exceptional case where coadministration of triazolam with nefazodone HCl may be considered appropriate, only the lowest possible dose of triazolam should be used (see CONTRAINDICATIONS and PRECAUTIONS).

Alprazolam

When alprazolam (1 mg bid) and nefazodone (200 mg bid) were coadministered, steady-state peak concentrations, AUC and half-life values for alprazolam increased by approximately 2-fold. Nefazodone plasma concentrations were unaffected by alprazolam. If alprazolam is coadministered with nefazodone HCl, a 50% reduction in the initial alprazolam dosage is recommended. No dosage adjustment is required for nefazodone HCl.

POTENTIAL TERFENADINE, ASTEMIZOLE, CISAPRIDE, AND PIMOZIDE INTERACTIONS

Terfenadine, astemizole, cisapride, and pimozide are all metabolized by the cytochrome P450 3A4 (CYP3A4) isozyme, and it has been demonstrated that ketoconazole, erythromycin, and other inhibitors of CYP3A4 can block the metabolism of these drugs, which can result in increased plasma concentrations of parent drug. Increased plasma concentrations of terfenadine, astemizole, cisapride, and pimozide are associated with QT prolongation and with rare cases of serious cardiovascular adverse events, including death, due principally to ventricular tachycardia of the torsades de pointes type. Nefazodone has been shown *in vitro* to be an inhibitor of CYP3A4. Consequently, it is recommended that nefazodone not be used in combination with either terfenadine, astemizole, cisapride, or pimozide (see CONTRAINDICATIONS and PRECAUTIONS).

INTERACTION WITH CARBAMAZEPINE

The coadministration of carbamazepine 200 mg bid with nefazodone 200 mg bid, at steady state for both drugs, resulted in almost 95% reductions in AUCs for nefazodone and hydroxynefazodone, likely resulting in insufficient plasma nefazodone and hydroxynefazodone concentrations for achieving an antidepressant effect for nefazodone HCl. Consequently, it is recommended that nefazodone HCl not be used in combination with carbamazepine (see CONTRAINDICATIONS and PRECAUTIONS).

PRECAUTIONS

GENERAL

Hepatotoxicity

See BOXED WARNING.

Postural Hypotension

A pooled analysis of the vital signs monitored during placebo-controlled premarketing studies revealed that 5.1% of nefazodone patients compared to 2.5% of placebo patients (p ≤0.01) met criteria for a potentially important decrease in blood pressure at some time during treatment (systolic blood pressure ≤90 mm Hg *and* a change from baseline of ≥20 mm Hg). While there was no difference in the proportion of nefazodone and placebo patients having adverse events characterized as 'syncope' (nefazodone, 0.2%; placebo, 0.3%), the rates for adverse events characterized as 'postural hypotension' were as follows: nefazodone (2.8%), tricyclic antidepressants (10.9%), SSRI (1.1%), and placebo (0.8%). Thus, the prescriber should be aware that there is some risk of postural hypotension in association with nefazodone use. Nefazodone HCl should be used with caution in patients with known cardiovascular or cerebrovascular disease that could be exacerbated by hypotension (history of myocardial infarction, angina, or ischemic stroke) and conditions that would predispose patients to hypotension (dehydration, hypovolemia, and treatment with antihypertensive medication).

Activation of Mania/Hypomania

During premarketing testing, hypomania or mania occurred in 0.3% of nefazodone-treated unipolar patients, compared to 0.3% of tricyclic- and 0.4% of placebo-treated patients. In patients classified as bipolar the rate of manic episodes was 1.6% for nefazodone, 5.1% for the combined tricyclic-treated groups, and 0% for placebo-treated patients. Activation of mania/hypomania is a known risk in a small proportion of patients with major affective disorder treated with other marketed antidepressants. As with all antidepressants, nefazodone HCl should be used cautiously in patients with a history of mania.

Suicide

The possibility of a suicide attempt is inherent in depression and may persist until significant remission occurs. Close supervision of high-risk patients should accompany initial drug therapy. Prescriptions for nefazodone HCl should be written for the smallest quantity of tablets consistent with good patient management in order to reduce the risk of overdose.

Seizures

During premarketing testing, a recurrence of a petit mal seizure was observed in a patient receiving nefazodone who had a history of such seizures. In addition, 1 nonstudy participant reportedly experienced a convulsion (type not documented) following a multiple-drug overdose. Rare occurrences of convulsions (including grand mal seizures) following nefazodone administration have been reported since market introduction. A causal relationship to nefazodone has not been established (see ADVERSE REACTIONS).

Priapism

While priapism did not occur during premarketing experience with nefazodone, rare reports of priapism have been received since market introduction. A causal relationship to nefazodone has not been established (see ADVERSE REACTIONS). If patients present with prolonged or inappropriate erections, they should discontinue therapy immediately and consult their physicians. If the condition persists for more than 24 hours, a urologist should be consulted to determine appropriate management.

Use in Patients With Concomitant Illness

Nefazodone HCl has not been evaluated or used to any appreciable extent in patients with a recent history of myocardial infarction or unstable heart disease. Patients with these diagnoses were systematically excluded from clinical studies during the product's premarketing testing. Evaluation of electrocardiograms of 1153 patients who received nefazodone in 6-8 week, double-blind, placebo-controlled trials did not indicate that nefazodone is associated with the development of clinically important ECG abnormalities. However, sinus bradycardia, defined as heart rate ≤50 bpm and a decrease of at least 15 bpm from baseline, was observed in 1.5% of nefazodone-treated patients compared to 0.4% of placebo-treated patients (p ≤0.05). Because patients with a recent history of myocardial infarction or unstable heart disease were excluded from clinical trials, such patients should be treated with caution.

In patients with cirrhosis of the liver, the AUC values of nefazodone and HO-NEF were increased by approximately 25%.

INFORMATION FOR THE PATIENT

See the Patient Information that is distributed with the prescription.

N

Physicians are advised to discuss the following issues with patients for whom they prescribe nefazodone HCl:

Hepatotoxicity: Patients should be informed that nefazodone HCl therapy has been associated with liver abnormalities ranging from asymptomatic reversible serum transaminase increases to cases of liver failure resulting in transplant and/or death. At present, there is no way to predict who is likely to develop liver failure. Ordinarily, patients with active liver disease should not be treated with nefazodone HCl. Patients should be advised to be alert for signs of liver dysfunction (jaundice, anorexia, gastrointestinal complaints, malaise, etc.) and to report them to their doctor immediately if they occur.

Time to response/continuation: As with all antidepressants, several weeks on treatment may be required to obtain the full antidepressant effect. Once improvement is noted, it is important for patients to continue drug treatment as directed by their physician.

Interference with cognitive and motor performance: Since any psychoactive drug may impair judgment, thinking, or motor skills, patients should be cautioned about operating hazardous machinery, including automobiles, until they are reasonably certain that nefazodone HCl therapy does not adversely affect their ability to engage in such activities.

Pregnancy: Patients should be advised to notify their physician if they become pregnant or intend to become pregnant during therapy.

Nursing: Patients should be advised to notify their physician if they are breast-feeding an infant (see Nursing Mothers).

Concomitant medication: Patients should be advised to inform their physicians if they are taking, or plan to take, any prescription or over-the-counter drugs, since there is a potential for interactions. Significant caution is indicated if nefazodone HCl is to be used in combination with alprazolam, concomitant use with triazolam should be avoided for most patients including the elderly, and concomitant use with terfenadine, astemizole, cisapride, pimozide, or carbamazepine is contraindicated (see CONTRAINDICATIONS and WARNINGS).

Alcohol: Patients should be advised to avoid alcohol while taking nefazodone HCl.

Allergic reactions: Patients should be advised to notify their physician if they develop a rash, hives, or a related allergic phenomenon.

Visual disturbances: There have been reports of visual disturbances associated with the use of nefazodone, including blurred vision, scotoma, and visual trails. Patients should be advised to notify their physician if they develop visual disturbances. (See ADVERSE REACTIONS.)

LABORATORY TESTS

There are no specific laboratory tests recommended.

CARCINOGENESIS, MUTAGENESIS, AND IMPAIRMENT OF FERTILITY

Carcinogenesis

There is no evidence of carcinogenicity with nefazodone. The dietary administration of nefazodone to rats and mice for 2 years at daily doses of up to 200 mg/kg and 800 mg/kg, respectively, which are approximately 3 and 6 times, respectively, the maximum human daily dose on a mg/m^2 basis, produced no increase in tumors.

Mutagenesis

Nefazodone has been shown to have no genotoxic effects based on the following assays: bacterial mutation assays, a DNA repair assay in cultured rat hepatocytes, a mammalian mutation assay in Chinese hamster ovary cells, an *in vivo* cytogenetics assay in rat bone marrow cells, and a rat dominant lethal study.

Impairment of Fertility

A fertility study in rats showed a slight decrease in fertility at 200 mg/kg/day (approximately 3 times the maximum human daily dose on a mg/m^2 basis) but not at 100 mg/kg/day (approximately 1.5 times the maximum human daily dose on a mg/m^2 basis).

PREGNANCY, TERATOGENIC EFFECTS, PREGNANCY CATEGORY C

Reproduction studies have been performed in pregnant rabbits and rats at daily doses up to 200 and 300 mg/kg, respectively (approximately 6 and 5 times, respectively, the maximum human daily dose on a mg/m^2 basis). No malformations were observed in the offspring as a result of nefazodone treatment. However, increased early pup mortality was seen in rats at a dose approximately 5 times the maximum human dose, and decreased pup weights were seen at this and lower doses, when dosing began during pregnancy and continued until weaning. The cause of these deaths is not known. The no-effect dose for rat pup mortality was 1.3 times the human dose on a mg/m^2 basis. There are no adequate and well-controlled studies in pregnant women. Nefazodone should be used during pregnancy only if the potential benefit justifies the potential risk to the fetus.

LABOR AND DELIVERY

The effect of nefazodone HCl on labor and delivery in humans is unknown.

NURSING MOTHERS

It is not known whether nefazodone HCl or its metabolites are excreted in human milk. Because many drugs are excreted in human milk, caution should be exercised when nefazodone HCl is administered to a nursing woman.

PEDIATRIC USE

Safety and effectiveness in individuals below 18 years of age have not been established.

GERIATRIC USE

Of the approximately 7000 patients in clinical studies who received nefazodone HCl for the treatment of depression, 18% were 65 years and older, while 5% were 75 years and older. Based on monitoring of adverse events, vital signs, electrocardiograms, and results of laboratory tests, no overall differences in safety between elderly and younger patients were observed in clinical studies. Efficacy in the elderly has not been demonstrated in placebo-controlled trials. Other reported clinical experience has not identified differences in responses between elderly and younger patients, but greater sensitivity of some older individuals cannot be ruled out.

Due to the increased systemic exposure to nefazodone seen in single-dose studies in elderly patients (see CLINICAL PHARMACOLOGY, Pharmacokinetics), treatment should be initiated at half the usual dose, but titration upward should take place over the same range as in younger patients (see DOSAGE AND ADMINISTRATION). The usual precautions should be observed in elderly patients who have concomitant medical illnesses or who are receiving concomitant drugs.

DRUG INTERACTIONS

DRUGS HIGHLY BOUND TO PLASMA PROTEIN

Because nefazodone is highly bound to plasma protein (see CLINICAL PHARMACOLOGY, Pharmacokinetics), administration of nefazodone HCl to a patient taking another drug that is highly protein bound may cause increased free concentrations of the other drug, potentially resulting in adverse events. Conversely, adverse effects could result from displacement of nefazodone by other highly bound drugs.

Warfarin

There were no effects on the prothrombin or bleeding times or upon the pharmacokinetics of R-warfarin when nefazodone (200 mg bid) was administered for 1 week to subjects who had been pretreated for 2 weeks with warfarin. Although the coadministration of nefazodone did decrease the subjects' exposure to S-warfarin by 12%, the lack of effects on the prothrombin and bleeding times indicates this modest change is not clinically significant. Although these results suggest no adjustments in warfarin dosage are required when nefazodone is administered to patients stabilized on warfarin, such patients should be monitored as required by standard medical practices.

CNS-ACTIVE DRUGS

Monoamine Oxidase Inhibitors

See WARNINGS.

Haloperidol

When a single oral 5 mg dose of haloperidol was coadministered with nefazodone (200 mg bid) at steady state, haloperidol apparent clearance decreased by 35% with no significant increase in peak haloperidol plasma concentrations or time of peak. This change is of unknown clinical significance. Pharmacodynamic effects of haloperidol were generally not altered significantly. There were no changes in the pharmacokinetic parameters for nefazodone. Dosage adjustment of haloperidol may be necessary when coadministered with nefazodone.

Lorazepam

When lorazepam (2 mg bid) and nefazodone (200 mg bid) were coadministered to steady state, there was no change in any pharmacokinetic parameter for either drug compared to each drug administered alone. Therefore, dosage adjustment is not necessary for either drug when coadministered.

Triazolam/Alprazolam

See CONTRAINDICATIONS and WARNINGS.

Alcohol

Although nefazodone did not potentiate the cognitive and psychomotor effects of alcohol in experiments with normal subjects, the concomitant use of nefazodone HCl and alcohol in depressed patients is not advised.

Buspirone

In a study of steady-state pharmacokinetics in healthy volunteers, coadministration of buspirone (2.5 or 5 mg bid) with nefazodone (250 mg bid) resulted in marked increases in plasma buspirone concentrations (increases up to 20-fold in C_{max} and up to 50-fold in AUC) and statistically significant decreases (about 50%) in plasma concentrations of the buspirone metabolite 1-pyrimidinylpiperazine. With 5 mg bid doses of buspirone, slight increases in AUC were observed for nefazodone (23%) and its metabolites hydroxynefazodone (17%) and mCPP (9%). Subjects receiving nefazodone 250 mg bid and buspirone 5 mg bid experienced lightheadedness, asthenia, dizziness, and somnolence, adverse events also observed with either drug alone. If the 2 drugs are to be used in combination, a low dose of buspirone (*e.g.*, 2.5 mg qd) is recommended. Subsequent dose adjustment of either drug should be based on clinical assessment.

Pimozide

See CONTRAINDICATIONS, WARNINGS, and DRUG INTERACTIONS, Pharmacokinetics of Nefazodone in 'Poor Metabolizers' and Potential Interaction With Drugs That Inhibit and/or Are Metabolized by Cytochrome P450 Isozymes.

Fluoxetine

When fluoxetine (20 mg qd) and nefazodone (200 mg bid) were administered at steady state there were no changes in the pharmacokinetic parameters for fluoxetine or its metabolite, norfluoxetine. Similarly, there were no changes in the pharmacokinetic parameters of nefazodone or HO-NEF; however, the mean AUC levels of the nefazodone metabolites mCPP and triazole-dione increased by 3- to 6-fold and 1.3-fold, respectively. When a 200 mg dose of nefazodone was administered to subjects who had been receiving fluoxetine for 1 week, there was an increased incidence of transient adverse events such as headache, lightheadedness, nausea, or paresthesia, possibly due to the elevated mCPP levels. Patients who are switched from fluoxetine to nefazodone without an adequate washout period may experience similar transient adverse events. The possibility of this happening can be minimized by allowing a washout period before initiating nefazodone therapy and by reducing the initial dose of nefazodone. Because of the long half-life of fluoxetine and its metabolites, this washout period may range from 1 to several weeks depending on the dose of fluoxetine and other individual patient variables.

Phenytoin

Pretreatment for 7 days with 200 mg bid of nefazodone had no effect on the pharmacokinetics of a single 300 mg oral dose of phenytoin. However, due to the nonlinear pharmacokinetics of phenytoin, the failure to observe a significant effect on the single-dose pharmacokinetics of phenytoin does not preclude the possibility of a clinically significant interaction with nefazodone when phenytoin is dosed chronically. However, no change in the initial dosage of phenytoin is considered necessary and any subsequent adjustment of phenytoin dosage should be guided by usual clinical practices.

Desipramine

When nefazodone (150 mg bid) and desipramine (75 mg qd) were administered together there were no changes in the pharmacokinetics of desipramine or its metabolite, 2-hydroxy desipramine. There were also no changes in the pharmacokinetics of nefazodone or its triazole-dione metabolite, but the AUC and C_{max} of mCPP increased by 44% and 48%, respectively, while the AUC of HO-NEF decreased by 19%. No changes in doses of either nefazodone or desipramine are necessary when the 2 drugs are given concomitantly. Subsequent dose adjustments should be made on the basis of clinical response.

Lithium

In 13 healthy subjects the coadministration of nefazodone (200 mg bid) with lithium (500 mg bid) for 5 days (steady-state conditions) was found to be well tolerated. When the 2 drugs were coadministered, there were no changes in the steady-state pharmacokinetics of either lithium, nefazodone, or its metabolite HO-NEF; however, there were small decreases in the steady-state plasma concentrations of two nefazodone metabolites, mCPP and triazole-dione, which are considered not to be of clinical significance. Therefore, no dosage adjustment of either lithium or nefazodone is required when they are coadministered.

Carbamazepine

The coadministration of nefazodone (200 mg bid) for 5 days to 12 healthy subjects on carbamazepine who had achieved steady state (200 mg bid) was found to be well tolerated. Steady-state conditions for carbamazepine, nefazodone, and several of their metabolites were achieved by Day 5 of coadministration. With coadministration of the 2 drugs there were significant increases in the steady-state C_{max} and AUC of carbamazepine (23% and 23%, respectively), while the steady-state C_{max} and the AUC of the carbamazepine metabolite, 10,11 epoxycarbamazepine, decreased by 21% and 20%, respectively. The coadministration of the 2 drugs significantly reduced the steady-state C_{max} and AUC of nefazodone by 86% and 93%, respectively. Similar reductions in the C_{max} and AUC of HO-NEF were also observed (85% and 94%), while the reductions in C_{max} and AUC of mCPP and triazole-dione were more modest (13% and 44% for the former and 28% and 57% for the latter). Due to the potential for coadministration of carbamazepine to result in insufficient plasma nefazodone and hydroxynefazodone concentrations for achieving an antidepressant effect for nefazodone HCl, it is recommended that nefazodone HCl not be used in combination with carbamazepine (see CONTRAINDICATIONS and WARNINGS).

General Anesthetics

Little is known about the potential for interaction between nefazodone and general anesthetics; therefore, prior to elective surgery, nefazodone HCl should be discontinued for as long as clinically feasible.

Other CNS-Active Drugs

The use of nefazodone in combination with other CNS-active drugs has not been systematically evaluated. Consequently, caution is advised if concomitant administration of nefazodone HCl and such drugs is required.

CIMETIDINE

When nefazodone (200 mg bid) and cimetidine (300 mg qid) were coadministered for 1 week, no change in the steady-state pharmacokinetics of either nefazodone or cimetidine was observed compared to each dosed alone. Therefore, dosage adjustment is not necessary for either drug when coadministered.

THEOPHYLLINE

When nefazodone (200 mg bid) was given to patients being treated with theophylline (600-1200 mg/day) for chronic obstructive pulmonary disease, there was no change in the steady-state pharmacokinetics of either nefazodone or theophylline. FEV_1 measurements taken when theophylline and nefazodone were coadministered did not differ from baseline dosage (*i.e.,* when theophylline was administered alone). Therefore, dosage adjustment is not necessary for either drug when coadministered.

CARDIOVASCULAR-ACTIVE DRUGS

Digoxin

When nefazodone (200 mg bid) and digoxin (0.2 mg qd) were coadministered for 9 days to healthy male volunteers (n=18) who were phenotyped as CYP2D6 extensive metabolizers, C_{max}, C_{min}, and AUC of digoxin were increased by 29%, 27%, and 15%, respectively. Digoxin had no effects on the pharmacokinetics of nefazodone and its active metabolites. Because of the narrow therapeutic index of digoxin, caution should be exercised when nefazodone and digoxin are coadministered; plasma level monitoring for digoxin is recommended.

Propranolol

The coadministration of nefazodone (200 mg bid) and propranolol (40 mg bid) for 5.5 days to healthy male volunteers (n=18), including 3 poor and 15 extensive CYP2D6 metabolizers, resulted in 30% and 14% reductions in C_{max} and AUC of propranolol, respectively, and a 14% reduction in C_{max} for the metabolite, 4-hydroxypropranolol. The kinetics of nefazodone, hydroxynefazodone, and triazole-dione were not affected by coadministration of propranolol. However, C_{max}, C_{min}, and AUC of m-chlorophenylpiperazine were increased by 23%, 54%, and 28%, respectively. No change in initial dose of either drug is necessary and dose adjustments should be made on the basis of clinical response.

HMG-CoA Reductase Inhibitors

When single 40 mg doses of simvastatin or atorvastatin, both substrates of CYP3A4, were given to healthy adult volunteers who had received nefazodone HCl 200 mg bid for 6 days, approximately 20-fold increases in plasma concentrations of simvastatin and simvastatin acid and 3- to 4-fold increases in plasma concentrations of atorvastatin and atorvastatin lactone were seen. These effects appear to be due to the inhibition of CYP3A4 by nefazodone HCl because, in the same study, nefazodone HCl had no significant effect on the plasma concentrations of pravastatin, which is not metabolized by CYP3A4 to a clinically significant extent.

There have been rare reports of rhabdomyolysis involving patients receiving the combination of nefazodone HCl and either simvastatin or lovastatin, also a substrate of CYP3A4 (see ADVERSE REACTIONS, Postintroduction Clinical Experience). Rhabdomyolysis has been observed in patients receiving HMG-CoA reductase inhibitors administered alone (at recommended dosages) and in particular, for certain drugs in this class, when given in combination with inhibitors of the CYP3A4 isozyme.

Caution should be used if nefazodone HCl is administered in combination with HMG-CoA reductase inhibitors that are metabolized by CYP3A4, such as simvastatin, atorvastatin, and lovastatin, and dosage adjustments of these HMG-CoA reductase inhibitors are recommended. Since metabolic interactions are unlikely between nefazodone HCl and HMG-CoA reductase inhibitors that undergo little or no metabolism by the CYP3A4 isozyme, such as pravastatin or fluvastatin, dosage adjustments should not be necessary.

IMMUNOSUPPRESSIVE AGENTS

There have been reports of increased blood concentrations of cyclosporine and tacrolimus into toxic ranges when patients received these drugs concomitantly with nefazodone HCl. Both cyclosporine and tacrolimus are substrates of CYP3A4, and nefazodone is known to inhibit this enzyme. If either cyclosporine or tacrolimus is administered with nefazodone HCl, blood concentrations of the immunosuppressive agent should be monitored and dosage adjusted accordingly.

PHARMACOKINETICS OF NEFAZODONE IN 'POOR METABOLIZERS' AND POTENTIAL INTERACTION WITH DRUGS THAT INHIBIT AND/OR ARE METABOLIZED BY CYTOCHROME P450 ISOZYMES

CYP3A4 Isozyme

Nefazodone has been shown *in vitro* to be an inhibitor of CYP3A4. This is consistent with the interactions observed between nefazodone and triazolam, alprazolam, buspirone, atorvastatin, and simvastatin, drugs metabolized by this isozyme. Consequently, caution is indicated in the combined use of nefazodone with any drugs known to be metabolized by CYP3A4. In particular, the combined use of nefazodone with triazolam should be avoided for most patients, including the elderly. The combined use of nefazodone with terfenadine, astemizole, cisapride, or pimozide is contraindicated (see CONTRAINDICATIONS and WARNINGS).

CYP2D6 Isozyme

A subset (3-10%) of the population has reduced activity of the drug-metabolizing enzyme CYP2D6. Such individuals are referred to commonly as "poor metabolizers" of drugs such as debrisoquin, dextromethorphan, and the tricyclic antidepressants. The pharmacokinetics of nefazodone and its major metabolites are not altered in these "poor metabolizers". Plasma concentrations of one minor metabolite (mCPP) are increased in this population; the adjustment of nefazodone HCl dosage is not required when administered to "poor metabolizers". Nefazodone and its metabolites have been shown *in vitro* to be extremely weak inhibitors of CYP2D6. Thus, it is not likely that nefazodone will decrease the metabolic clearance of drugs metabolized by this isozyme.

CYP1A2 Isozyme

Nefazodone and its metabolites have been shown *in vitro* not to inhibit CYP1A2. Thus, metabolic interactions between nefazodone and drugs metabolized by this isozyme are unlikely.

ELECTROCONVULSIVE THERAPY (ECT)

There are no clinical studies of the combined use of ECT and nefazodone.

ADVERSE REACTIONS

ASSOCIATED WITH DISCONTINUATION OF TREATMENT

Approximately 16% of the 3496 patients who received nefazodone HCl in worldwide premarketing clinical trials discontinued treatment due to an adverse experience. The more common (≥1%) events in clinical trials associated with discontinuation and considered to be drug related (*i.e.,* those events associated with dropout at a rate approximately twice or greater for nefazodone HCl compared to placebo) included: nausea (3.5%), dizziness (1.9%), insomnia (1.5%), asthenia (1.3%), and agitation (1.2%).

INCIDENCE IN CONTROLLED TRIALS

Commonly Observed Adverse Events in Controlled Clinical Trials

The most commonly observed adverse events associated with the use of nefazodone HCl (incidence of 5% or greater) and not seen at an equivalent incidence among placebo-treated patients (*i.e.,* significantly higher incidence for nefazodone HCl compared to placebo, $p \leq 0.05$), derived from TABLE 2, were: somnolence, dry mouth, nausea, dizziness, constipation, asthenia, lightheadedness, blurred vision, confusion, and abnormal vision.

Adverse Events Occurring at an Incidence of 1% or More Among Nefazodone HCl-Treated Patients

TABLE 2 enumerates adverse events that occurred at an incidence of 1% or more, and were more frequent than in the placebo group, among nefazodone HCl-treated patients who participated in short-term (6-8 week) placebo-controlled trials in which patients were dosed with nefazodone HCl to ranges of 300-600 mg/day. TABLE 2 shows the percentage of patients in each group who had at least one episode of an event at some time during their

N

treatment. Reported adverse events were classified using standard COSTART-based Dictionary terminology.

The prescriber should be aware that these figures cannot be used to predict the incidence of side effects in the course of usual medical practice where patient characteristics and other factors differ from those which prevailed in the clinical trials. Similarly, the cited frequencies cannot be compared with figures obtained from other clinical investigations involving different treatments, uses, and investigators. The cited figures, however, do provide the prescribing physician with some basis for estimating the relative contribution of drug and non-drug factors to the side-effect incidence rate in the population studied.

TABLE 2 *Treatment-Emergent Adverse Experience Incidence in 6-8 Week Placebo-Controlled Clinical Trials,* Nefazodone 300-600 mg/day Dose Range*

Body System Preferred Term	Nefazodone HCl (n=393)	Placebo (n=394)
Body as a Whole		
Headache	36%	33%
Asthenia	11%	5%
Infection	8%	6%
Flu syndrome	3%	2%
Chills	2%	1%
Fever	2%	1%
Neck rigidity	1%	0%
Cardiovascular		
Postural hypotension	4%	1%
Hypotension	2%	1%
Dermatologic		
Pruritus	2%	1%
Rash	2%	1%
Gastrointestinal		
Dry mouth	25%	13%
Nausea	22%	12%
Constipation	14%	8%
Dyspepsia	9%	7%
Diarrhea	8%	7%
Increased appetite	5%	3%
Nausea & vomiting	2%	1%
Metabolic		
Peripheral edema	3%	2%
Thirst	1%	<1%
Musculoskeletal		
Arthralgia	1%	<1%
Nervous		
Somnolence	25%	14%
Dizziness	17%	5%
Insomnia	11%	9%
Lightheadedness	10%	3%
Confusion	7%	2%
Memory impairment	4%	2%
Paresthesia	4%	2%
Vasodilatation†	4%	2%
Abnormal dreams	3%	2%
Concentration decreased	3%	1%
Ataxia	2%	0%
Incoordination	2%	1%
Psychomotor retardation	2%	1%
Tremor	2%	1%
Hypertonia	1%	0%
Libido decreased	1%	<1%
Respiratory		
Pharyngitis	6%	5%
Cough increased	3%	1%
Special Senses		
Blurred vision	9%	3%
Abnormal vision‡	7%	1%
Tinnitus	2%	1%
Taste perversion	2%	1%
Visual field defect	2%	0%
Urogenital		
Urinary frequency	2%	1%
Urinary tract infection	2%	1%
Urinary retention	2%	1%
Vaginitis§	2%	1%
Breast pain§	1%	<1%

* Events reported by at least 1% of patients treated with nefazodone HCl and more frequent than the placebo group are included; incidence is rounded to the nearest 1% (<1% indicates an incidence less than 0.5%). Events for which the nefazodone HCl incidence was equal to or less than placebo are not listed in the table, but included the following: abdominal pain, pain, back pain, accidental injury, chest pain, neck pain, palpitation, migraine, sweating, flatulence, vomiting, anorexia, tooth disorder, weight gain, edema, myalgia, cramp, agitation, anxiety, depression, hypesthesia, CNS stimulation, dysphoria, emotional lability, sinusitis, rhinitis, dysmenorrhea§, dysuria.

† Vasodilatation: flushing, feeling warm.

‡ Abnormal vision: scotoma, visual trails.

§ Incidence adjusted for gender.

Dose Dependency of Adverse Events

TABLE 3 enumerates adverse events that were more frequent in the nefazodone HCl dose range of 300-600 mg/day than in the nefazodone HCl dose range of up to 300 mg/day. TABLE 3 shows only those adverse events for which there was a statistically significant difference ($p \leq 0.05$) in incidence between the nefazodone HCl dose ranges as well as a difference between the high dose range and placebo.

Visual Disturbances

In controlled clinical trials, blurred vision occurred in 9% of nefazodone-treated patients compared to 3% of placebo-treated patients. In these same trials abnormal vision, including scotomata and visual trails, occurred in 7% of nefazodone-treated patients compared to 1% of placebo-treated (see TABLE 2). Dose-dependendency was observed for these events in

TABLE 3 *Dose Dependency of Adverse Events in Placebo-Controlled Trials**

Body System Preferred Term	Nefazodone HCl 300-600 mg/day (n=209)	Nefazodone HCl ≤300 mg/day (n=211)	Placebo (n=212)
Gastrointestinal			
Nausea	23%	14%	12%
Constipation	17%	10%	9%
			Nervous
Somnolence	28%	16%	13%
Dizziness	22%	11%	4%
Confusion	8%	2%	1%
Special Senses			
Abnormal vision	10%	0%	2%
Blurred vision	9%	3%	2%
Tinnitus	3%	0%	1%

* Events for which there was a statistically significant difference ($p \leq 0.05$) between the nefazodone dose groups.

these trials, with none of the scotomata and visual trails at doses below 300 mg/day. However, scotomata and visual trails observed at doses below 300 mg/day have been reported in postmarketing experience with nefazodone HCl. (See PRECAUTIONS, Information for the Patient.)

Vital Sign Changes

See PRECAUTIONS, General, Postural Hypotension.

Weight Changes

In a pooled analysis of placebo-controlled premarketing studies, there were no differences between nefazodone and placebo groups in the proportions of patients meeting criteria for potentially important increases or decreases in body weight (a change of ≥7%).

Laboratory Changes

Of the serum chemistry, serum hematology, and urinalysis parameters monitored during placebo-controlled premarketing studies with nefazodone, a pooled analysis revealed a statistical trend between nefazodone and placebo for hematocrit, *i.e.*, 2.8% of nefazodone patients met criteria for a potentially important decrease in hematocrit (≤37% male or ≤32% female) compared to 1.5% of placebo patients ($0.05 < p \leq 0.10$). Decreases in hematocrit, presumably dilutional, have been reported with many other drugs that block $alpha_1$-adrenergic receptors. There was no apparent clinical significance of the observed changes in the few patients meeting these criteria.

ECG Changes

Of the ECG parameters monitored during placebo-controlled premarketing studies with nefazodone, a pooled analysis revealed a statistically significant difference between nefazodone and placebo for sinus bradycardia, *i.e.*, 1.5% of nefazodone patients met criteria for a potentially important decrease in heart rate (≤50 bpm and a decrease of ≥15 bpm) compared to 0.4% of placebo patients ($p < 0.05$). There was no obvious clinical significance of the observed changes in the few patients meeting these criteria.

OTHER EVENTS OBSERVED DURING THE PREMARKETING EVALUATION OF NEFAZODONE HCl

During its premarketing assessment, multiple doses of nefazodone HCl were administered to 3496 patients in clinical studies, including more than 250 patients treated for at least 1 year. The conditions and duration of exposure to nefazodone HCl varied greatly, and included (in overlapping categories) open and double-blind studies, uncontrolled and controlled studies, inpatient and outpatient studies, fixed-dose and titration studies. Untoward events associated with this exposure were recorded by clinical investigators using terminology of their own choosing. Consequently, it is not possible to provide a meaningful estimate of the proportion of individuals experiencing adverse events without first grouping similar types of untoward events into a smaller number of standardized event categories.

In the tabulations that follow, reported adverse events were classified using standard COSTART-based Dictionary terminology. The frequencies presented, therefore, represent the proportion of the 3496 patients exposed to multiple doses of nefazodone HCl who experienced an event of the type cited on at least one occasion while receiving nefazodone HCl. All reported events are included except those already listed in TABLE 2, those events listed in other safety-related sections of this insert, those adverse experiences subsumed under COSTART terms that are either overly general or excessively specific so as to be uninformative, those events for which a drug cause was very remote, and those events which were not serious and occurred in fewer than 2 patients.

It is important to emphasize that, although the events reported occurred during treatment with nefazodone HCl, they were not necessarily caused by it.

Events are further categorized by body system and listed in order of decreasing frequency according to the following definitions: *frequent* adverse events are those occurring on one or more occasions in at least 1/100 patients (only those not already listed in the tabulated results from placebo-controlled trials appear in this listing); *infrequent* adverse events are those occurring in 1/100 to 1/1000 patients; *rare* events are those occurring in fewer than 1/1000 patients.

Body as a Whole: *Infrequent:* Allergic reaction, malaise, photosensitivity reaction, face edema, hangover effect, abdomen enlarged, hernia, pelvic pain, and halitosis. *Rare:* Cellulitis.

Cardiovascular System: *Infrequent:* Tachycardia, hypertension, syncope, ventricular extrasystoles, and angina pectoris. *Rare:* AV block, congestive heart failure, hemorrhage, pallor, and varicose vein.

Dermatologic System: *Infrequent:* Dry skin, acne, alopecia, urticaria, maculopapular rash, vesiculobullous rash, and eczema.

Gastrointestinal System: *Frequent:* Gastroenteritis. *Infrequent:* Eructation, periodontal abscess, abnormal liver function tests, gingivitis, colitis, gastritis, mouth ulceration, stomatitis, esophagitis, peptic ulcer, and rectal hemorrhage. *Rare:* Glossitis, hepatitis, dysphagia, gastrointestinal hemorrhage, oral moniliasis, and ulcerative colitis.

Hemic and Lymphatic System: *Infrequent:* Ecchymosis, anemia, leukopenia, and lymphadenopathy.

Metabolic and Nutritional System: *Infrequent:* Weight loss, gout, dehydration, lactic dehydrogenase increased, SGOT increased, and SGPT increased. *Rare:* Hypercholesteremia and hypoglycemia.

Musculoskeletal System: *Infrequent:* Arthritis, tenosynovitis, muscle stiffness, and bursitis. *Rare:* Tendinous contracture.

Nervous System: *Infrequent:* Vertigo, twitching, depersonalization, hallucinations, suicide attempt, apathy, euphoria, hostility, suicidal thoughts, abnormal gait, thinking abnormal, attention decreased, derealization, neuralgia, paranoid reaction, dysarthria, increased libido, suicide, and myoclonus. *Rare:* Hyperkinesia, increased salivation, cerebrovascular accident, hyperesthesia, hypotonia, ptosis, and neuroleptic malignant syndrome.

Respiratory System: *Frequent:* Dyspnea and bronchitis. *Infrequent:* Asthma, pneumonia, laryngitis, voice alteration, epistaxis, hiccup. *Rare:* Hyperventilation and yawn.

Special Senses: *Frequent:* Eye pain. *Infrequent:* Dry eye, ear pain, abnormality of accommodation, diplopia, conjunctivitis, mydriasis, keratoconjunctivitis, hyperacusis, and photophobia. *Rare:* Deafness, glaucoma, night blindness, and taste loss.

Urogenital System: *Frequent:* Impotence*. *Infrequent:* Cystitis, urinary urgency, metrorrhagia*, amenorrhea*, polyuria, vaginal hemorrhage*, breast enlargement*, menorrhagia*, urinary incontinence, abnormal ejaculation*, hematuria, nocturia, and kidney calculus. *Rare:* Uterine fibroids enlarged*, uterine hemorrhage*, anorgasmia, and oliguria.

*Adjusted for gender.

POSTINTRODUCTION CLINICAL EXPERIENCE

Postmarketing experience with nefazodone HCl has shown an adverse experience profile similar to that seen during the premarketing evaluation of nefazodone. Voluntary reports of adverse events temporally associated with nefazodone HCl have been received since market introduction that are not listed above and for which a causal relationship has not been established. These include:

Anaphylactic reactions; angioedema; convulsions (including grand mal seizures); galactorrhea; gynecomastia (male); hyponatremia; liver necrosis and liver failure, in some cases leading to liver transplantation and/or death (see WARNINGS); priapism (see PRECAUTIONS); prolactin increased; rhabdomyolysis involving patients receiving the combination of nefazodone HCl and lovastatin or simvastatin (see PRECAUTIONS); serotonin syndrome; and Stevens-Johnson syndrome; and thrombocytopenia.

DOSAGE AND ADMINISTRATION

INITIAL TREATMENT

The recommended starting dose for nefazodone HCl is 200 mg/day, administered in 2 divided doses (bid). In the controlled clinical trials establishing the antidepressant efficacy of nefazodone HCl, the effective dose range was generally 300-600 mg/day. Consequently, most patients, depending on tolerability and the need for further clinical effect, should have their dose increased. Dose increases should occur in increments of 100-200 mg/day, again on a bid schedule, at intervals of no less than 1 week. As with all antidepressants, several weeks on treatment may be required to obtain a full antidepressant response.

DOSAGE FOR ELDERLY OR DEBILITATED PATIENTS

The recommended initial dose for elderly or debilitated patients is 100 mg/day, administered in 2 divided doses (bid). These patients often have reduced nefazodone clearance and/or increased sensitivity to the side effects of CNS-active drugs. It may also be appropriate to modify the rate of subsequent dose titration. As steady-state plasma levels do not change with age, the final target dose based on a careful assessment of the patient's clinical response may be similar in healthy younger and older patients.

MAINTENANCE/CONTINUATION/EXTENDED TREATMENT

There is no body of evidence available from controlled trials to indicate how long the depressed patient should be treated with nefazodone HCl. It is generally agreed, however, that pharmacological treatment for acute episodes of depression should continue for up to 6 months or longer. Whether the dose of antidepressant needed to induce remission is identical to the dose needed to maintain euthymia is unknown. Systematic evaluation of the efficacy of nefazodone HCl has shown that efficacy is maintained for periods of up to 36 weeks following 16 weeks of open-label acute treatment (treated for 52 weeks total) at dosages that averaged 438 mg/day. For most patients, their maintenance dose was that associated with response during acute treatment. (See CLINICAL PHARMACOLOGY.) The safety of nefazodone HCl in long-term use is supported by data from both double-blind and open-label trials involving more than 250 patients treated for at least 1 year.

SWITCHING PATIENTS TO OR FROM A MONOAMINE OXIDASE INHIBITOR

At least 14 days should elapse between discontinuation of an MAOI and initiation of therapy with nefazodone HCl. In addition, at least 7 days should be allowed after stopping nefazodone HCl before starting an MAOI.

HOW SUPPLIED

Serzone tablets are available in:

50 mg: Light pink hexagonal tablet imprinted with "BMS" and "50 mg" on one side and "31" on the other.

100 mg: White hexagonal bisect scored tablet imprinted with "BMS" and "100 mg" on one side and "32" on the other.

150 mg: Peach hexagonal bisect scored tablet imprinted with "BMS" and "150 mg" on one side and "39" on the other.

200 mg: Light yellow hexagonal tablet imprinted with "BMS" and "200 mg" on one side and "33" on the other.

250 mg: White hexagonal tablet imprinted with "BMS" and "250 mg" on one side and "41" on the other.

Storage: Store at room temperature, below 40°C (104°F) and dispense in a tight container.

PRODUCT LISTING - EQUIVALENTS NOT AVAILABLE

Tablet - Oral - 50 mg			
60's	$95.41	SERZONE, Bristol-Myers Squibb	00087-0031-47
Tablet - Oral - 100 mg			
60's	$87.79	SERZONE, Physicians Total Care	54868-3707-00
60's	$97.71	SERZONE, Bristol-Myers Squibb	00087-0032-31
90's	$137.70	SERZONE, Pharma Pac	52959-0645-90
Tablet - Oral - 150 mg			
30's	$37.06	SERZONE, Allscripts Pharmaceutical Company	54569-4127-01
60's	$74.12	SERZONE, Allscripts Pharmaceutical Company	54569-4127-00
60's	$87.79	SERZONE, Physicians Total Care	54868-3708-00
60's	$99.55	SERZONE, Bristol-Myers Squibb	00087-0039-31
Tablet - Oral - 200 mg			
30's	$37.06	SERZONE, Almay	54569-4195-01
60's	$101.43	SERZONE, Bristol-Myers Squibb	00087-0033-31
Tablet - Oral - 250 mg			
30's	$37.06	SERZONE, Allscripts Pharmaceutical Company	54569-4594-00
30's	$48.28	SERZONE, Southwood Pharmaceuticals Inc	58016-0516-30
60's	$96.55	SERZONE, Southwood Pharmaceuticals Inc	58016-0516-60
60's	$103.31	SERZONE, Bristol-Myers Squibb	00087-0041-31

Nelfinavir Mesylate *(003329)*

For related information, see the comparative table section in Appendix A.

Categories: Infection, human immunodeficiency virus; FDA Approved 1997 Mar; Pregnancy Category B; Patent Expiration 2013 Oct; WHO Formulary
Drug Classes: Antivirals; Protease inhibitors
Brand Names: **Viracept**
Cost of Therapy: $609.12 (HIV; Viracept; 250 mg; 9 tablets/day; 30 day supply)

DESCRIPTION

Nelfinavir mesylate is an inhibitor of the human immunodeficiency virus (HIV) protease.

Viracept Tablets: Available for oral administration as a light blue, capsule-shaped tablet with a clear film coating in a 250 mg strength (as nelfinavir free base). Each tablet also contains the following inactive ingredients: calcium silicate, crospovidone, magnesium stearate, FD&C blue no. 2 powder, hydroxypropyl methylcellulose and triacetin.

Viracept Oral Powder: Available for oral administration in a 50 mg/g strength (as nelfinavir free base) in bottles. The oral powder also contains the following inactive ingredients: microcrystalline cellulose, maltodextrin, dibasic potassium phosphate, crospovidone, hydroxypropyl methylcellulose, aspartame, sucrose palmitate, and natural and artificial flavor.

The chemical name for nelfinavir mesylate is [3*S*-[2(2*S**,3*S**),3α,4aβ,8aβ]]-*N*-(1,1-dimethylethyl)decahydro-2-[2-hydroxy-3-[(3-hydroxy-2-methylbenzoyl)amino]-4-(phenylthio)butyl]-3-isoquinolinecarboxamide mono-methanesulfonate (salt) and the molecular weight is 663.90 (567.79 as the free base).

Nelfinavir mesylate is a white to off-white amorphous powder, slightly soluble in water at pH ≤4 and freely soluble in methanol, ethanol, isopropanol and propylene glycol.

CLINICAL PHARMACOLOGY

MICROBIOLOGY

Mechanism of Action

Nelfinavir is an inhibitor of the HIV-1 protease. Inhibition of the viral protease prevents cleavage of the gag-pol polyprotein resulting in the production of immature, non-infectious virus.

Antiviral Activity In Vitro

The antiviral activity of nelfinavir *in vitro* has been demonstrated in both acute and/or chronic HIV infections in lymphoblastoid cell lines, peripheral blood lymphocytes and monocytes/macrophages. Nelfinavir was found to be active against several laboratory strains of HIV-1 and several clinical isolates of HIV-1 and the HIV-2 strain ROD. The EC_{95} (95% effective concentration) of nelfinavir ranged from 7-196 nM. In combination with reverse transcriptase inhibitors, nelfinavir demonstrated additive (didanosine or stavudine) to synergistic (zidovudine, lamivudine or zalcitabine) antiviral activity *in vitro* without enhanced cytotoxicity. Drug combination studies with protease inhibitors (ritonavir, saquinavir or indinavir) showed variable results ranging from antagonistic to synergistic.

Drug Resistance

HIV-1 isolates with reduced susceptibility to nelfinavir have been selected *in vitro*. HIV isolates from selected patients treated with nelfinavir alone or in combination with reverse transcriptase inhibitors were monitored for phenotypic (n=19) and genotypic (n=195, 157 of which were evaluable) changes in clinical trials over a period of 2-82 weeks. One or more virus protease mutations at amino acid positions 30, 35, 36, 46, 71, 77 and 88 were detected in >10% of patients with evaluable isolates. Of 19 patients for which both phenotypic and genotypic analyses were performed on clinical isolates, 9 showed reduced susceptibility (5- to 93-fold) to nelfinavir *in vitro*. All 9 patients possessed one or more mutations in the virus protease gene. Amino acid position 30 appeared to be the most frequent mutation site.

The overall incidence of the D30N mutation in the virus protease of evaluable patients (n=157) receiving nelfinavir monotherapy or nelfinavir in combination with zidovudine and lamivudine or stavudine was 54.8%. The overall incidence of other mutations associated with primary protease inhibitor resistance was 9.6% for the L90M substitution whereas substitutions at 48, 82, or 84 were not observed.

Cross-Resistance

Preclinical Studies

HIV isolates obtained from 5 patients during nelfinavir therapy showed a 5- to 93-fold decrease in nelfinavir susceptibility *in vitro* when compared to matched baseline isolates, but did not demonstrate a concordant decrease in susceptibility to indinavir, ritonavir, saquinavir or amprenavir, *in vitro*. Conversely, following ritonavir therapy 6 of 7 clinical isolates with decreased ritonavir susceptibility (8- to 113-fold) *in vitro* compared to baseline also exhibited decreased susceptibility to nelfinavir *in vitro* (5- to 40-fold). An HIV isolate obtained from a patient receiving saquinavir therapy showed decreased susceptibility to saquinavir (7-fold), but did not demonstrate a concordant decrease in susceptibility to nelfinavir. Cross-resistance between nelfinavir and reverse transcriptase inhibitors is unlikely because different enzyme targets are involved. Clinical isolates (n=5) with decreased susceptibility to zidovudine, lamivudine, or nevirapine remain fully susceptible to nelfinavir *in vitro*.

Clinical Studies

There have been no controlled or comparative studies evaluating the virologic response to subsequent protease inhibitor-containing regimens in patients who have demonstrated loss of virologic response to a nelfinavir-containing regimen. However, virologic response was evaluated in a single-arm prospective study of 26 patients with extensive prior antiretroviral experience with reverse transcriptase inhibitors (mean 2.9) who had received nelfinavir mesylate for a mean duration of 59.7 weeks and were switched to a ritonavir (400 mg bid)/saquinavir hard-gel (400 mg bid) containing regimen after a prolonged period of nelfinavir mesylate failure (median 48 weeks). Sequence analysis of HIV-1 isolates prior to switch demonstrated a D30N or an L90M substitution in 18 and 6 patients, respectively. Subjects remained on therapy for a mean of 48 weeks (range 40-56 weeks) where 17 of 26 (65%) subjects and 13 of 26 (50%) subjects were treatment responders with HIV RNA below the assay limit of detection (Chiron bDNA) at 24 and 48 weeks, respectively.

PHARMACOKINETICS

The pharmacokinetic properties of nelfinavir were evaluated in healthy volunteers and HIV-infected patients; no substantial differences were observed between the 2 groups.

Absorption

In a pharmacokinetic study in HIV-positive patients, multiple dosing with 750 mg (three 250 mg tablets) three times daily (tid) for 28 days (11 patients) achieved peak plasma concentrations (C_{max}) of 3.0 ± 1.6 mg/L and morning and afternoon trough concentrations of 1.4 ± 0.6 mg/L and 1.0 ± 0.5 mg/L, respectively. In the same study, multiple dosing with 1250 mg (five 250 mg tablets) twice daily (bid) for 28 days (10 patients) achieved C_{max} of 4.0 ± 0.8 mg/L and morning and evening trough concentrations of 2.2 ± 1.3 mg/L and 0.7 ± 0.4 mg/L, respectively. The difference between morning and afternoon or evening trough concentrations for the tid and bid regimens was also observed in healthy volunteers who were dosed at precise 8 or 12 hour intervals.

Effect of Food on Oral Absorption

Maximum plasma concentrations and area under the plasma concentration-time curve (AUC) were 2- to 3-fold higher under fed conditions compared to fasting. The effect of food on nelfinavir absorption was evaluated in two studies (n=14, total). The meals evaluated contained 517-759 Kcal, with 153-313 Kcal derived from fat.

Distribution

The apparent volume of distribution following oral administration of nelfinavir was 2-7 L/kg. Nelfinavir in serum is extensively protein-bound (>98%).

Metabolism

Unchanged nelfinavir comprised 82-86% of the total plasma radioactivity after a single oral 750 mg dose of ^{14}C-nelfinavir. *In vitro*, multiple cytochrome P-450 isoforms including CYP3A are responsible for metabolism of nelfinavir. One major and several minor oxidative metabolites were found in plasma. The major oxidative metabolite has *in vitro* antiviral activity comparable to the parent drug.

Elimination

The terminal half-life in plasma was typically 3.5 to 5 hours. The majority (87%) of an oral 750 mg dose containing ^{14}C-nelfinavir was recovered in the feces; fecal radioactivity consisted of numerous oxidative metabolites (78%) and unchanged nelfinavir (22%). Only 1-2% of the dose was recovered in urine, of which unchanged nelfinavir was the major component.

SPECIAL POPULATIONS

Hepatic Insufficiency

The multi-dose pharmacokinetics of nelfinavir have not been studied in HIV-positive patients with hepatic insufficiency.

Renal Insufficiency

The pharmacokinetics of nelfinavir have not been studied in patients with renal insufficiency; however, less than 2% of nelfinavir is excreted in the urine, so the impact of renal impairment on nelfinavir elimination should be minimal.

Gender and Race

No significant pharmacokinetic differences have been detected between males and females. Pharmacokinetic differences due to race have not been evaluated.

Pediatrics

See PRECAUTIONS, Pediatric Use.

Geriatric Patients

The pharmacokinetics of nelfinavir have not been studied in patients over 65 years of age.

DRUG INTERACTIONS

Also see CONTRAINDICATIONS, WARNINGS, andDRUG INTERACTIONS.

The potential ability of nelfinavir to inhibit the major human cytochrome P450 isoforms (CYP3A, CYP2C19, CYP2D6, CYP2C9, CYP1A2 and CYP2E1) has been investigated *in vitro*. Only CYP3A was inhibited at concentrations in the therapeutic range.

Specific drug interaction studies were performed with nelfinavir and a number of drugs. TABLE 1 summarizes the effects of nelfinavir on the geometric mean AUC, C_{max} and C_{min} of coadministered drugs. TABLE 2 shows the effects of coadministered drugs on the geometric mean AUC, C_{max} and C_{min} of nelfinavir.

For information regarding clinical recommendations, see CONTRAINDICATIONS, WARNINGS, and DRUG INTERACTIONS.

INDICATIONS AND USAGE

Nelfinavir mesylate in combination with other antiretroviral agents is indicated for the treatment of HIV infection.

CONTRAINDICATIONS

Nelfinavir mesylate is contraindicated in patients with clinically significant hypersensitivity to any of its components.

Coadministration of nelfinavir mesylate is contraindicated with drugs that are highly dependent on CYP3A for clearance and for which elevated plasma concentrations are associated with serious and/or life-threatening events. These drugs are listed in TABLE 4.

WARNINGS

ALERT: Find out about medicines that should not be taken with nelfinavir mesylate. This statement is included on the product's bottle label.

DRUG INTERACTIONS

Also see PRECAUTIONS.

Nelfinavir is an inhibitor of the P450 isoform CYP3A. Coadministration of nelfinavir mesylate and drugs primarily metabolized by CYP3A may result in increased plasma concentrations of the other drug that could increase or prolong its therapeutic and adverse effects. Nelfinavir is metabolized in part by CYP3A. Coadministration of nelfinavir mesylate and drugs that induce CYP3A may decrease nelfinavir plasma concentrations and reduce its therapeutic effect. Coadministration of nelfinavir mesylate and drugs that inhibit CYP3A may increase nelfinavir plasma concentrations. (Also see TABLE 5.)

Concomitant use of nelfinavir mesylate with lovastatin or simvastatin is not recommended. Caution should be exercised if HIV protease inhibitors, including nelfinavir mesylate, are used concurrently with other HMG-CoA reductase inhibitors that are also metabolized by the CYP3A4 pathway (*e.g.*, atorvastatin). Also see TABLE 1 and TABLE 2. The risk of myopathy including rhabdomyolysis may be increased when protease inhibitors, including nelfinavir mesylate, are used in combination with these drugs.

Particular caution should be used when prescribing sildenafil in patients receiving protease inhibitors, including nelfinavir mesylate. Coadministration of a protease inhibitor with sildenafil is expected to substantially increase sildenafil concentrations and may result in an increase in sildenafil-associated adverse events, including hypotension, visual changes, and priapism. (See DRUG INTERACTIONS and PRECAUTIONS, Information for the Patient, and the complete prescribing information for sildenafil.)

Concomitant use of St. John's wort (hypericum perforatum) or St. John's wort containing products and nelfinavir mesylate is not recommended. Coadministration of St. John's wort with protease inhibitors, including nelfinavir mesylate, is expected to substantially decrease protease inhibitor concentrations and may result in sub-optimal levels of nelfinavir mesylate and lead to loss of virologic response and possible resistance to nelfinavir mesylate or to the class of protease inhibitors.

PATIENTS WITH PHENYLKETONURIA

Nelfinavir mesylate oral powder contains 11.2 mg phenylalanine per gram of powder.

DIABETES MELLITUS/HYPERGLYCEMIA

New onset diabetes mellitus, exacerbation of pre-existing diabetes mellitus and hyperglycemia have been reported during post-marketing surveillance in HIV-infected patients receiving protease inhibitor therapy. Some patients required either initiation or dose adjustments of insulin or oral hypoglycemic agents for treatment of these events. In some cases diabetic ketoacidosis has occurred. In those patients who discontinued protease inhibitor therapy, hyperglycemia persisted in some cases. Because these events have been reported voluntarily during clinical practice, estimates of frequency cannot be made and a causal relationship between protease inhibitor therapy and these events has not been established.

PRECAUTIONS

GENERAL

Nelfinavir is principally metabolized by the liver. Therefore, caution should be exercised when administering this drug to patients with hepatic impairment.

RESISTANCE/CROSS-RESISTANCE

HIV cross-resistance between protease inhibitors has been observed (see CLINICAL PHARMACOLOGY, Microbiology).

TABLE 1 *Drug Interactions: Changes in Pharmacokinetic Parameters for Coadministered Drug in the Presence of Nelfinavir Mesylate*

Coadministered Drug	Nelfinavir Dose	n	% Change of Coadministered Drug Pharmacokinetic Parameters (90% CI) AUC	C_{max}	C_{min}
HIV-Protease Inhibitors					
Indinavir 800 mg SD	750 mg q8h × 7 days	6	inc 51% (inc 29-inc 77%)	dec 10% (dec 28-inc 13%)	NA
Ritonavir 500 mg SD	750 mg q8h × 5 doses	10	NC	NC	NA
Saquinavir 1200 mg SD*	750 mg tid × 4 days	14	inc 392% (inc 291-inc 521%)	inc 179% (inc 117-inc 259%)	NA
Amprenavir 800 mg tid × 14 days	750 mg tid × 14 days	6	NC	dec 14% (dec 38-inc 20%)	inc 189% (inc 52-inc 448%)
Nucleoside Reverse Transcriptase Inhibitors					
Lamivudine 150 mg SD	750 mg q8h × 7-10 days	11	inc 10% (inc 2-inc 18%)	inc 31% (inc 9-inc 56%)	NA
Stavudine 30-40 mg†	750 mg tid × 56 days	8		See footnote‡	
Zidovudine 200 mg SD	750 mg q8h × 7-10 days	11	dec 35% (dec 29-dec 40%)	dec 31% (dec 13-dec 46%)	NA
Non-Nucleoside Reverse Transcriptase Inhibitors					
Efavirenz 600 mg qd × 7 days	750 mg q8h × 7 days	10	dec 12% (dec 31-inc 12%)	dec 12% (dec 29-inc 8%)	dec 22% (dec 54-inc 32%)
Nevirapine 200 mg qd × 14 days‡ followed by 200 mg bid × 14 days	750 mg tid × 36 days	23		See footnote‡	
Delavirdine 400 mg q8h × 14 days	750 mg q8h × 7 days	7	dec 31% (dec 57-inc 10%)	dec 27% (dec 49-inc 4%)	dec 33% (dec 70-inc 49%)
Anti-infective Agents					
Rifabutin 150 mg qd × 8 days§	750 mg q8h × 7-8 days¤	12	inc 83% (inc 72-inc 96%)	inc 19% (inc 11-inc 28%)	inc 177% (inc 144-inc 215%)
Rifabutin 300 mg qd × 8 days	750 mg q8h × 7-8 days	10	inc 207% (inc 161-inc 263%)	inc 146% (inc 118-inc 178%)	inc 305% (inc 245-inc 375%)
Azithromycin 1200 mg SD	750 mg tid × 11 days	12	inc 112% (inc 80-inc 150%)	inc 136% (inc 77-inc 215%)	NA
HMG-CoA Reductase Inhibitors					
Atorvastatin 10 mg qd × 28 days	1250 mg bid × 14 days	15	inc 74% (inc 41-inc 116%)	inc 122% (inc 68-inc 193%)	inc 39% (dec 21-inc 145%)
Simvastatin 20 mg qd × 28 days	1250 mg bid × 14 days	16	inc 505% (inc 393-inc 643%)	inc 517% (inc 367-inc 715%)	ND
Other Agents					
Ethinyl estradiol 35 μg qd × 15 days	750 mg q8h × 7 days	12	dec 47% (dec 42-dec 52%)	dec 28% (dec 16-dec 37%)	dec 62% (dec 57-dec 67%)
Norethindrone 0.4 mg qd × 15 days	750 mg q8h × 7 days	12	dec 18% (dec 13-dec 23%)	NC	dec 46% (dec 38-dec 53%)
Methadone 80 mg ±21 mg qd¶ >1 month	1250 mg bid × 8 days	13	dec 47% (dec 42-dec 51%)	dec 46% (dec 42-dec 49%)	dec 53% (dec 49-dec 57%)
Phenytoin 300 mg qd × 14 days**	1250 mg bid × 7 days	12	dec 29% (dec 17-dec 39%)	dec 21% (dec 12-dec 29%)	dec 39% (dec 27-dec 49%)

inc: Indicates increase; dec: indicates decrease; NC: indicates no change (geometric mean exposure increased or decreased <10%); NA: not relevant for single-dose treatment; ND: cannot be determined; SD: single dose.
* Using the soft-gelatin capsule formulation of saquinavir 1200 mg.
† bid × 56 days.
‡ Based on non-definitive cross-study comparison, drug plasma concentrations appeared to be unaffected by coadministration.
§ Rifabutin 150 mg qd changes are relative to rifabutin 300 mg qd × 8 days without coadministration with nelfinavir.
¤ Comparable changes in rifabutin concentrations were observed with nelfinavir mesylate 1250 mg q12h × 7 days.
¶ Changes are reported for total plasma methadone; changes for the individual R-enantiomer and S-enantiomer were similar.
** Phenytoin exposure measures are reported for total phenytoin exposure. The effect of nelfinavir on unbound phenytoin was similar.

HEMOPHILIA

There have been reports of increased bleeding, including spontaneous skin hematomas and hemarthrosis, in patients with hemophilia Type A and B treated with protease inhibitors. In some patients, additional factor VIII was given. In more than half of the reported cases, treatment with protease inhibitors was continued or reintroduced. A causal relationship has not been established.

FAT REDISTRIBUTION

Redistribution/accumulation of body fat including central obesity, dorsocervical fat enlargement (buffalo hump), peripheral wasting, facial wasting, breast enlargement, and "cushingoid appearance" have been observed in patients receiving antiretroviral therapy. The mechanism and long-term consequences of these events are currently unknown. A causal relationship has not been established.

TABLE 2 *Drug Interactions: Changes in Pharmacokinetic Parameters for Nelfinavir in the Presence of the Coadministered Drug*

Coadministered Drug	Nelfinavir Dose	n	% Change of Nelfinavir Pharmacokinetic Parameters (90% CI) AUC	C_{max}	C_{min}
HIV-Protease Inhibitors					
Indinavir 800 mg q8h × 7 days	750 mg SD	6	inc 83% (inc 42-inc 137%)	inc 31% (inc 16-inc 48%)	NA
Ritonavir 500 mg q12h × 3 doses	750 mg SD	10	inc 152% (inc 96-inc 224%)	inc 44% (inc 28-inc 63%)	NA
Saquinavir 1200 mg tid × 4 days*	750 mg SD	14	inc 18% (inc 7-inc 30%)	NC	NA
Amprenavir 800 mg tid × 14 days	750 mg tid × 14 days	6		See footnote†	
Nucleoside Reverse Transcriptase Inhibitors					
Didanosine 200 mg SD	750 mg SD	9	NC	NC	NA
Zidovudine 200 mg + lamivudine 150 mg SD	750 mg q8h × 7-10 days	11	NC	NC	NC
Non-Nucleoside Reverse Transcriptase Inhibitors					
Efavirenz 600 mg qd × 7 days	750 mg q8h × 7 days	7	inc 20% (inc 8-inc 34%)	inc 21% (inc 10-inc 33%)	NC
Nevirapine 200 mg qd × 14 days followed by 200 mg bid × 14 days	750 mg tid × 36 days	23	NC	NC	dec 32% (dec 50-inc 5%)
Delavirdine 400 mg q8h × 7 days	750 mg q8h × 14 days	12	inc 107% (inc 83-inc 135%)	inc 88% (inc 66-inc 113%)	inc 136% (inc 103-inc 175%)
Anti-Infective Agents					
Ketoconazole 400 mg qd × 7 days	500 mg q8h × 5-6 days	12	inc 35% (inc 24-inc 46%)	inc 25% (inc 11-inc 40%)	inc 14% (dec 23-inc 69%)
Rifabutin 150 mg qd × 8 days	750 mg q8h × 7-8 days	11	dec 23% (dec 14-dec 31%)	dec 18% (dec 8-dec 27%)	dec 25% (dec 23-dec 39%)
	1250 mg q12h × 7-8 days	11	NC	NC	dec 15% (dec 43-inc 27%)
Rifabutin 300 mg qd × 8 days	750 mg q8h × 7-8 days	10	dec 32% (dec 15-dec 46%)	dec 24% (dec 10-dec 36%)	dec 53% (dec 15-dec 73%)
Rifampin 600 mg qd × 7 days	750 mg q8h × 5-6 days	12	dec 83% (dec 79-dec 86%)	dec 76% (dec 69-dec 82%)	dec 92% (dec 86-dec 95%)
Azithromycin 1200 mg SD	750 mg tid × 9 days	12	dec 15% (dec 7-dec 22%)	dec 10% (dec 19-inc 1%)	dec 29% (dec 19-dec 38%)
HMG-CoA Reductase Inhibitors					
Atorvastatin 10 mg qd × 28 days	1250 mg bid × 14 days	15		See footnote†	
Simvastatin 20 mg qd × 28 days	1250 mg bid × 14 days	16		See footnote†	
Other Agents					
Methadone 80 mg ±21 mg qd >1 month	1250 mg bid × 8 days	13		See footnote†	
Phenytoin 300 mg qd × 7 days	1250 mg bid × 14 days	15	NC	NC	dec 18% (dec 45-inc 23%)

inc: Indicates increase; dec: indicates decrease; NA = not relevant for single-dose treatment; NC = indicates no change (geometric mean exposure increased or decreased <10%); SD = single dose.
* Using the soft-gelatin capsule formulation of saquinavir 1200 mg.
† Based on non-definitive cross-study comparison, nelfinavir plasma concentrations appeared to be unaffected by coadministration.

TABLE 4 *Drugs That Are Contraindicated With Nelfinavir Mesylate*

Drug Class	Drugs Within Class That Are Contraindicated With Nelfinavir Mesylate
Antiarrhythmics	Amiodarone, quinidine
Ergot derivatives	Dihydroergotamine, ergonovine, ergotamine, methylergonovine
Neuroleptic	Pimozide
Sedative/hypnotics	Midazolam, triazolam
HMG-CoA reductase inhibitors	Lovastatin, simvastatin

INFORMATION FOR THE PATIENT

"A statement to patients and health care providers is included on the product's bottle label: **ALERT: Find out about medicines that should NOT be taken with nelfinavir mesylate.** A Patient Package Insert (PPI) for nelfinavir mesylate is available for patient information."

For optimal absorption, patients should be advised to take nelfinavir mesylate with food (see CLINICAL PHARMACOLOGY, Pharmacokinetics and DOSAGE AND ADMINISTRATION).

Patients should be informed that nelfinavir mesylate is not a cure for HIV infection and that they may continue to acquire illnesses associated with advanced HIV infection, including opportunistic infections.

Patients should be told that there is currently no data demonstrating that nelfinavir mesylate therapy can reduce the risk of transmitting HIV to others through sexual contact or blood contamination.

Patients should be told that sustained decreases in plasma HIV RNA have been associated with a reduced risk of progression to AIDS and death. Patients should be advised to take nelfinavir mesylate and other concomitant antiretroviral therapy every day as prescribed. Patients should not alter the dose or discontinue therapy without consulting with their doctor. If a dose of nelfinavir mesylate is missed, patients should take the dose as soon as possible and then return to their normal schedule. However, if a dose is skipped, the patient should not double the next dose.

Patients should be informed that nelfinavir mesylate tablets are film-coated and that this film-coating is intended to make the tablets easier to swallow.

The most frequent adverse event associated with nelfinavir mesylate is diarrhea, which can usually be controlled with non-prescription drugs, such as loperamide, which slow gastrointestinal motility.

Patients should be informed that redistribution or accumulation of body fat may occur in patients receiving antiretroviral therapy and that the cause and long term health effects of these conditions are not known at this time.

Nelfinavir mesylate may interact with some drugs, therefore, patients should be advised to report to their doctor the use of any other prescription, non-prescription medication or herbal products, particularly St. John's wort.

Patients receiving oral contraceptives should be instructed that alternate or additional contraceptive measures should be used during therapy with nelfinavir mesylate.

Patients receiving sildenafil and nelfinavir should be advised that they may be at an increased risk of sildenafil-associated adverse events including hypotension, visual changes, and prolonged penile erection, and should promptly report any symptoms to their doctor.

CARCINOGENESIS, MUTAGENESIS, AND IMPAIRMENT OF FERTILITY

Long-term carcinogenicity studies in rats have been conducted with nelfinavir at doses of 0, 100, 300, and 1000 mg/kg/day via oral gavage. Thyroid follicular cell adenomas and carcinomas were increased in male rats at 300 mg/kg/day and higher and in female rats at 1000 mg/kg/day. The systemic exposures (C_{max}) at 300 and 1000 mg/kg/day were 1- to 3-fold, respectively, of those measured in humans at the recommended therapeutic dose (750 mg tid or 1250 mg bid). The mechanism of nelfinavir-induced tumorogenesis in rats is unknown. However, nelfinavir showed no evidence of mutagenic or clastogenic activity in a battery of *in vitro* and *in vivo* genetic toxicology assays. These studies included bacterial mutation assays in *S. typhimurium* and *E. coli,* a mouse lymphoma tyrosine kinase assay, a chromosomal aberration assay in human lymphocytes, and an *in vivo* mouse bone marrow micronucleus assay. Given the lack of genotoxic activity of nelfinavir, the relevance to humans of neoplasms in nelfinavir-treated rats is not known.

N

Nelfinavir produced no effects on either male or female mating and fertility or embryo survival in rats at systemic exposures comparable to the human therapeutic exposure.

PREGNANCY CATEGORY B

There were no effects on fetal development or maternal toxicity when nelfinavir was administered to pregnant rats at systemic exposures (AUC) comparable to human exposure. Administration of nelfinavir to pregnant rabbits resulted in no fetal development effects up to a dose at which a slight decrease in maternal body weight was observed; however, even at the highest dose evaluated, systemic exposure in rabbits was significantly lower than human exposure. Additional studies in rats indicated that exposure to nelfinavir in females from mid-pregnancy through lactation had no effect on the survival, growth, and development of the offspring to weaning. Subsequent reproductive performance of these offspring was also not affected by maternal exposure to nelfinavir. However, there are no adequate and well-controlled studies in pregnant women taking nelfinavir mesylate. Because animal reproduction studies are not always predictive of human response, nelfinavir mesylate should be used during pregnancy only if clearly needed.

Antiretroviral Pregnancy Registry: To monitor maternal-fetal outcomes of pregnant women exposed to nelfinavir mesylate and other antiretroviral agents, an Antiretroviral Pregnancy Registry has been established. Physicians are encouraged to register patients by calling (800) 258-4263.

NURSING MOTHERS

The Centers for Disease Control and Prevention recommends that HIV-infected mothers not breast-feed their infants to avoid risking postnatal transmission of HIV. Studies in lactating rats have demonstrated that nelfinavir is excreted in milk. Because of both the potential for HIV transmission and the potential for serious adverse reactions in nursing infants, **mothers should be instructed not to breast-feed if they are receiving nelfinavir mesylate.**

PEDIATRIC USE

Nelfinavir was studied in one open-label, uncontrolled trial in 38 pediatric patients ranging in age from 2-13 years. In order to achieve plasma concentrations in pediatric patients which approximate those observed in adults, the recommended pediatric dose is 20-30 mg/kg given three times daily with a meal, not to exceed 750 mg three times a day (see DOSAGE AND ADMINISTRATION).

A similar adverse event profile was seen during the pediatric clinical trial as in adult patients. The evaluation of the antiviral activity of nelfinavir in pediatric patients is ongoing. The evaluation of the safety, effectiveness and pharmacokinetics of nelfinavir in pediatric patients below the age of 2 years is ongoing.

GERIATRIC USE

Clinical studies of nelfinavir mesylate did not include sufficient numbers of subjects aged 65 and over to determine whether they respond differently from younger subjects.

DRUG INTERACTIONS

Also see CONTRAINDICATIONS; WARNINGS; and CLINICAL PHARMACOLOGY, Drug Interactions.

Nelfinavir is an inhibitor of CYP3A (cytochrome P450 3A). Coadministration of nelfinavir mesylate and drugs primarily metabolized by CYP3A (*e.g.,* dihydropyridine calcium channel blockers, HMG-CoA reductase inhibitors, immunosuppressants and sildenafil) may result in increased plasma concentrations of the other drug that could increase or prolong both its therapeutic and adverse effects, see TABLE 5. Nelfinavir is metabolized in part by CYP3A. Coadministration of nelfinavir mesylate and drugs that induce CYP3A, such as rifampin, may decrease nelfinavir plasma concentrations and reduce its therapeutic effect. Coadministration of nelfinavir mesylate and drugs that inhibit CYP3A may increase nelfinavir plasma concentrations.

Drug interaction studies reveal no clinically significant drug interactions between nelfinavir and didanosine, lamivudine, stavudine, zidovudine, efavirenz, nevirapine, or ketoconazole and no dose adjustments are needed. In the case of didanosine, it is recommended that didanosine be administered on an empty stomach; therefore, nelfinavir should be administered with food 1 hour after or more than 2 hours before didanosine.

Based on known metabolic profiles, clinically significant drug interactions are not expected between nelfinavir mesylate and dapsone, trimethoprim/sulfamethoxazole, clarithromycin, erythromycin, itraconazole or fluconazole.

TABLE 5 *Drugs That Should Not Be Coadministered With Nelfinavir Mesylate Drug*

Drug Class: Drug Name	Clinical Comment
Antiarrhythmics: amiodarone, quinidine	CONTRAINDICATED due to potential for serious and/or life threatening reactions such as cardiac arrhymias.
Antimycobacterial: rifampin	May lead to loss of virologic response and possible resistance to nelfinavir mesylate or other coadministered antiretroviral agents.
Ergot derivatives: dihydroergotamine, ergonovine, ergotamine, methylergonovine	CONTRAINDICATED due to potential for serious and/or life threatening reactions such as acute ergot toxicity characterized by peripheral vasospasm and ischemia of the extremities and other tissues.
Herbal products: St. John's wort (hypericum perforatum)	May lead to loss of virologic response and possible resistance to nelfinavir mesylate or other coadministered antiretroviral agents.
HMG-CoA reductase inhibitors: lovastatin, simvastatin	CONTRAINDICATED due to potential for serious reactions such as risk of myopathy including rhabdomyolysis.
Neuroleptic: pimozide	CONTRAINDICATED due to potential for serious and/or life threatening reactions such as cardiac arrhythmias.
Sedative/hypnotics: midazolam, triazolam	CONTRAINDICATED due to potential for serious and/or life threatening reactions such as prolonged or increased sedation or respiratory depression.

ESTABLISHED AND OTHER POTENTIALLY SIGNIFICANT DRUG INTERACTIONS

Alteration in dose or regimen may be recommended based on drug interaction studies. (See TABLE 1 and TABLE 2.)

HIV-Antiviral Agents

Protease Inhibitors:

Indinavir: Increases nelfinavir and indinavir concentrations.

Ritonavir: Increases nelfinavir concentration.

Saquinavir: Increases saquinavir concentration.

Clinical Comment: Appropriate doses for these combinations, with respect to safety and efficacy, have not been established.

Nonnucleoside Reverse Transcriptase Inhibitors:

Delavirdine: Increases nelfinavir and decreases delavirdine concentrations.

Nevirapine: Decreases nelfinavir (C_{min}) concentration.

Clinical Comment: Appropriate doses for these combinations, with respect to safety and efficacy, have not been established.

Nucleoside Reverse Transcriptase Inhibitor:

Didanosine.

Clinical Comment: It is recommended that didanosine be administered on an empty stomach; therefore, didanosine should be given 1 hour before or 2 hours after nelfinavir mesylate (given with food).

Other Agents

Anti-Convulsants:

Carbamazepine.

Phenobarbital.

Clinical Comment: May decrease nelfinavir plasma concentrations. Nelfinavir mesylate may not be effective due to decreased nelfinavir plasma concentrations in patients taking these agents concomitantly.

Anti-Convulsant:

Phenytoin: Decreases phenytoin concentration.

Clinical Comment: Phenytoin plasma/serum concentrations should be monitored; phenytoin dose may require adjustment to compensate for altered phenytoin concentration.

Anti-Mycobacterial:

Rifabutin: Increases rifabutin, decreases nelfinavir (750 mg tid) and no change to nelfinavir (1250 mg bid) concentrations.

Clinical Comment: It is recommended that the dose of rifabutin be reduced to one-half the usual dose when administered with nelfinavir mesylate; 1250 mg bid is the preferred dose of nelfinavir mesylate when coadministered with rifabutin.

Erectile Dysfunction Agent:

Sildenafil: Increases sildenafil concentration.

Clinical Comment: Sildenafil should not exceed a maximum single dose of 25 mg in a 48 hour period.

HMG-CoA Reductase Inhibitor:

Atorvastatin: Increases atorvastatin concentration.

Clinical Comment: Use lowest possible dose of atorvastatin with careful monitoring, or consider other HMG-CoA reductase inhibitors such as pravastatin or fluvastatin in combination with nelfinavir mesylate.

Immuno-Suppressants:

Cyclosporine, tacrolimus, sirolimus: Increases immuno-suppressants.

Clinical Comment: Plasma concentrations may be increased by nelfinavir mesylate.

Narcotic Analgesic:

Methadone: Decreases methadone concentation.

Clinical Comment: Dosage of methadone may need to be increased when coadministered with nelfinavir mesylate.

Oral Contraceptive:

Ethinyl estradiol: Decreases ethinyl estradiol concentation.

Clinical Comment: Alternative or additional contraceptive measures should be used when oral contraceptives and nelfinavir mesylate are coadministered.

Macrolide Antibiotic:

Azithromycin: Increases azithromycin concentation.

Clinical Comment: Dose adjustment of azithromycin is not recommended, but close monitoring for known side effects such as liver enzyme abnormalities and hearing impairment is warranted.

ADVERSE REACTIONS

The safety of nelfinavir mesylate was studied in over 5000 patients who received drug either alone or in combination with nucleoside analogues. The majority of adverse events were of mild intensity. The most frequently reported adverse event among patients receiving nelfinavir mesylate was diarrhea, which was generally of mild to moderate intensity.

Drug-related clinical adverse experiences of moderate or severe intensity in ≥2% of patients treated with nelfinavir mesylate coadministered with d4T and 3TC (Study 542) for up to 48 weeks or with ZDV plus 3TC (Study 511) for up to 24 weeks are presented in TABLE 7.

TABLE 7 *Percentage of Patients With Treatment-Emergent* Adverse Events of Moderate or Severe Intensity Reported in ≥2% of Patients*

	Study 511 (24 Weeks)			Study 542 (48 Weeks)	
	Placebo + ZDV/3TC	500 mg tid Viracept + ZDV/3TC	750 mg tid Viracept + ZDV/3TC	1250 mg bid Viracept + d4T/3TC	750 mg tid Viracept + d4T/3TC
Adverse Events	(n=101)	(n=97)	(n=100)	(n=344)	(n=210)
Digestive System					
Diarrhea	3%	14%	20%	20%	15%
Nausea	4%	3%	7%	3%	3%
Flatulence	0%	5%	2%	1%	1%
Skin/Appendages					
Rash	1%	1%	3%	2%	1%

* Includes those adverse events at least possibly related to study drug or of unknown relationship and excludes concurrent HIV conditions.

Adverse events occurring in less than 2% of patients receiving nelfinavir mesylate in all Phase 2/3 clinical trials and considered at least possibly related or of unknown relationship to treatment and of at least moderate severity are listed below.

Body as a Whole: Abdominal pain, accidental injury, allergic reaction, asthenia, back pain, fever, headache, malaise, pain, and redistribution/accumulation of body fat (see PRECAUTIONS, Fat Redistribution).

Digestive System: Anorexia, dyspepsia, epigastric pain, gastrointestinal bleeding, hepatitis, mouth ulceration, pancreatitis and vomiting.

Hemic/Lymphatic System: Anemia, leukopenia and thrombocytopenia.

Metabolic/Nutritional System: Increases in alkaline phosphate, amylase, creatine phosphokinase, lactic dehydrogenase, SGOT, SGPT and gamma glutamyl transpeptidase; hyperlipemia, hyperuricemia, hyperglycemia, hypoglycemia, dehydration, and liver function tests abnormal.

Musculoskeletal System: Arthralgia, arthritis, cramps, myalgia, myasthenia and myopathy.

Nervous System: Anxiety, depression, dizziness, emotional lability, hyperkinesia, insomnia, migraine, paresthesia, seizures, sleep disorder, somnolence and suicide ideation.

Respiratory System: Dyspnea, pharyngitis, rhinitis, and sinusitis.

Skin/Appendages: Dermatitis, folliculitis, fungal dermatitis, maculopapular rash, pruritus, sweating, and urticaria.

Special Senses: Acute iritis and eye disorder.

Urogenital System: Kidney calculus, sexual dysfunction and urine abnormality.

POST-MARKETING EXPERIENCE

The following additional adverse experiences have been reported from post-marketing surveillance as at least possibly related or of unknown relationship to nelfinavir mesylate:

Body as a Whole: Hypersensitivity reactions (including bronchospasm, moderate to severe rash, fever and edema).

Digestive System: Jaundice.

Metabolic/Nutritional System: Bilirubinemia, metabolic acidosis.

LABORATORY ABNORMALITIES

The percentage of patients with marked laboratory abnormalities in Studies 542 and 511 are presented in TABLE 8. Marked laboratory abnormalities are defined as a Grade 3 or 4 abnormality in a patient with a normal baseline value or a Grade 4 abnormality in a patient with a Grade 1 abnormality at baseline.

TABLE 8 *Percentage of Patients by Treatment Group With Marked Laboratory Abnormalities* in >2% of Patients*

	Study 511			Study 542	
	Placebo + ZDV/3TC	500 mg tid Viracept + ZDV/3TC	750 mg tid Viracept + ZDV/3TC	1250 mg bid Viracept + d4T/3TC	750 mg tid Viracept + d4T/3TC
	(n=101)	(n=97)	(n=100)	(n=344)	(n=210)
Hematology					
Hemoglobin	6%	3%	2%	0%	0%
Neutrophils	4%	3%	5%	2%	1%
Lymphocytes	1%	6%	1%	1%	0%
Chemistry					
ALT (SGPT)	6%	1%	1%	2%	1%
AST (SGOT)	4%	1%	0%	2%	1%
Creatine kinase	7%	2%	2%	NA	NA

* Marked laboratory abnormalities are defined as a shift from Grade 0 at baseline to at least Grade 3 or from Grade 1 to Grade 4.

DOSAGE AND ADMINISTRATION

ADULTS

The recommended dose is 1250 mg (five 250 mg tablets) twice daily or 750 mg (three 250 mg tablets) three times daily. Nelfinavir mesylate should be taken with a meal. It is recommended that nelfinavir mesylate be used in combination with nucleoside analogues. Patients unable to swallow tablets may place whole tablets or crushed tablets in a small amount of water to dissolve before ingestion or they may mix crushed tablets in a small amount of food. Once mixed with food or dissolved in water, the entire contents must be consumed in order to obtain the full dose. If the mixture is not consumed immediately, it must be stored under refrigeration, but storage must not exceed 6 hours.

PEDIATRIC PATIENTS (2-13 YEARS)

The recommended oral dose of nelfinavir mesylate for pediatric patients 2-13 years of age is 20-30 mg/kg/dose, three times daily with a meal. The pharmacokinetics of twice daily dosing of nelfinavir mesylate in pediatric patients has not been established. For children unable to take tablets, nelfinavir mesylate oral powder may be administered. The oral powder may be mixed with a small amount of water, milk, formula, soy formula, soy milk or dietary supplements; once mixed, the entire contents must be consumed in order to obtain the full dose. If the mixture is not consumed immediately, it must be stored under refrigeration, but storage must not exceed 6 hours. Acidic food or juice (*e.g.,* orange juice, apple juice or apple sauce) are not recommended to be used in combination with nelfinavir mesylate, because the combination may result in a bitter taste. Nelfinavir mesylate oral powder should not be reconstituted with water in its original container. The recommended pediatric dose of nelfinavir mesylate to be administered 3 times daily is described in TABLE 9.

TABLE 9 *Pediatric Dose to be Administered 3 Times Daily*

Body Weight		Number of Level		Number of
kg	lb	1 g Scoops	Teaspoons	Tablets
7 to <8.5	15.5 to <18.5	4	1	—
8.5 to <10.5	18.5 to <23	5	1¼	—
10.5 to <12	23 to <26.5	6	1½	—
12 to <14	26.5 to <31	7	1¾	—
14 to <16	31 to <35	8	2	—
16 to <18	35 to <39.5	9	2¼	—
18 to <23	39.5 to <50.5	10	2½	2
≥23	≥50.5	15	3¾	3

HOW SUPPLIED

Viracept Tablets:

250 mg: Light blue, capsule-shaped tablets with a clear film coating engraved with "VIRACEPT" on one side and "250 mg" on the other.

Viracept Oral Powder:

50 mg/g: Off-white powder containing 50 mg (as nelfinavir free base) in each level scoopful (1 g).

STORAGE

Viracept tablets and oral powder should be stored at 15-30°C (59-86°F).

Keep container tightly closed. Dispense in original container.

PRODUCT LISTING - EQUIVALENTS NOT AVAILABLE

Powder For Reconstitution - Oral - 50 mg/Gm

144 gm	$66.48	VIRACEPT, Agouron Pharma Inc	63010-0011-90

Tablet - Oral - 250 mg

18's	$51.88	VIRACEPT, St. Mary'S Mpp	60760-0010-18
27's	$97.47	VIRACEPT, Pd-Rx Pharmaceuticals	55289-0477-27

30's	$67.68	VIRACEPT, Allscripts Pharmaceutical Company	54569-4543-02
63's	$156.88	VIRACEPT, St. Mary'S Mpp	60760-0010-63
270's	$609.12	VIRACEPT, Allscripts Pharmaceutical Company	54569-4543-04
270's	$658.08	VIRACEPT, Physicians Total Care	54868-3947-00

Nesiritide *(003527)*

Categories: Heart failure, congestive; FDA Approved 2001 Aug; Pregnancy Category C
Drug Classes: Natriuretic peptide, human B-type
Brand Names: **Natrecor**

DESCRIPTION

FOR INTRAVENOUS INFUSION ONLY.

Natrecor (nesiritide) is a sterile, purified preparation of a new drug class, human B-type natriuretic peptide (hBNP), and is manufactured from *E. coli* using recombinant DNA technology. Nesiritide has a molecular weight of 3464 g/mol and an empirical formula of $C_{143}H_{244}N_{50}O_{42}S_4$. Nesiritide has the same 32 amino acid sequence as the endogenous peptide, which is produced by the ventricular myocardium.

Natrecor is formulated as the citrate salt of rhBNP, and is provided in a sterile, single-use vial. Each 1.5 mg vial contains a white- to off-white lyophilized powder for intravenous (IV) administration after reconstitution. The quantitative composition of the lyophilized drug per vial is: nesiritide 1.58 mg, mannitol 20.0 mg, citric acid monohydrate 2.1 mg, and sodium citrate dihydrate 2.94 mg.

CLINICAL PHARMACOLOGY

MECHANISM OF ACTION

Human BNP binds to the particulate guanylate cyclase receptor of vascular smooth muscle and endothelial cells, leading to increased intracellular concentrations of guanosine 3′5′-cyclic monophosphate (cGMP) and smooth muscle cell relaxation. Cyclic GMP serves as a second messenger to dilate veins and arteries. Nesiritide has been shown to relax isolated human arterial and venous tissue preparations that were precontracted with either endothelin-1 or the alpha-adrenergic agonist, phenylephrine.

In human studies, nesiritide produced dose-dependent reductions in pulmonary capillary wedge pressure (PCWP) and systemic arterial pressure in patients with heart failure.

In animals, nesiritide had no effects on cardiac contractility or on measures of cardiac electrophysiology such as atrial and ventricular effective refractory times or atrioventricular node conduction.

Naturally occurring atrial natriuretic peptide (ANP), a related peptide, increases vascular permeability in animals and humans and may reduce intravascular volume. The effect of nesiritide on vascular permeability has not been studied.

PHARMACOKINETICS

In patients with congestive heart failure (CHF), nesiritide administered intravenously by infusion or bolus exhibits biphasic disposition from the plasma. The mean terminal elimination half-life ($T_{1/2}$) of nesiritide is approximately 18 minutes and was associated with approximately 2/3 of the area-under-the-curve (AUC). The mean initial elimination phase was estimated to be approximately 2 minutes. In these patients, the mean volume of distribution of the central compartment (Vc) of nesiritide was estimated to be 0.073 L/kg, the mean steady-state volume of distribution (Vss) was 0.19 L/kg, and the mean clearance (CL) was approximately 9.2 ml/min/kg. At steady state, plasma BNP levels increase from baseline endogenous levels by approximately 3- to 6-fold with nesiritide infusion doses ranging from 0.01-0.03 μg/kg/min.

ELIMINATION

Human BNP is cleared from the circulation via the following three independent mechanisms, in order of decreasing importance: (1) binding to cell surface clearance receptors with subsequent cellular internalization and lysosomal proteolysis; (2) proteolytic cleavage of the peptide by endopeptidases, such as neutral endopeptidase, which are present on the vascular lumenal surface; and (3) renal filtration.

SPECIAL POPULATIONS

Although nesiritide is eliminated, in part, through renal clearance, clinical data suggest that dose adjustment is not required in patients with renal insufficiency. The effects of nesiritide on PCWP, cardiac index (CI), and systolic blood pressure (SBP) were not significantly different in patients with chronic renal insufficiency (baseline serum creatinine ranging from 2 to 4.3 mg/dl), and patients with normal renal function. The population pharmacokinetic (PK) analyses carried out to determine the effects of demographics and clinical variables on PK parameters showed that clearance of nesiritide is proportional to body weight, supporting the administration of weight-adjusted dosing of nesiritide (*i.e.*, administration on a μg/kg/min basis). Clearance was not influenced significantly by age, gender, race/ethnicity, baseline endogenous hBNP concentration, severity of CHF (as indicated by baseline PCWP, baseline CL, or New York Heart Association [NYHA] classification), or concomitant administration of an ACE inhibitor.

EFFECTS OF CONCOMITANT MEDICATIONS

The coadministration of nesiritide with enalapril did not have significant effects on the PK of nesiritide. The PK effect of coadministration of nesiritide with other IV vasodilators such as nitroglycerin, nitroprusside, milrinone, or IV ACE inhibitors has not been evaluated. During clinical studies, nesiritide was administered concomitantly with other medications, including: diuretics, digoxin, oral ACE inhibitors, anticoagulants, oral nitrates, statins, Class III antiarrhythmic agents, beta-blockers, dobutamine, calcium channel blockers, angiotensin II receptor antagonists, and dopamine. Although no PK interactions were specifically assessed, there did not appear to be evidence suggesting any clinically significant PK interaction.

PHARMACODYNAMICS

The recommended dosing regimen of nesiritide is a 2 μg/kg IV bolus followed by an IV infusion dose of 0.01 μg/kg/min. With this dosing regimen, 60% of the 3 hour effect on PCWP reduction is achieved within 15 minutes after the bolus, reaching 95% of the 3 hour effect within 1 hour. Approximately 70% of the 3 hour effect on SBP reduction is reached within 15 minutes. The pharmacodynamic (PD) half-life of the onset and offset of the hemodynamic effect of nesiritide is longer than what the PK half-life of 18 minutes would predict. For example, in patients who developed symptomatic hypotension in the VMAC (Vasodilation in the Management of Acute Congestive Heart Failure) trial, half of the recovery of SBP toward the baseline value after discontinuation or reduction of the dose of nesiritide was observed in about 60 minutes. When higher doses of nesiritide were infused, the duration of hypotension was sometimes several hours.

INDICATIONS AND USAGE

Nesiritide is indicated for the intravenous treatment of patients with acutely decompensated congestive heart failure who have dyspnea at rest or with minimal activity. In this population, the use of nesiritide reduced pulmonary capillary wedge pressure and improved dyspnea.

CONTRAINDICATIONS

Nesiritide is contraindicated in patients who are hypersensitive to any of its components. Nesiritide should not be used as primary therapy for patients with cardiogenic shock or in patients with a systolic blood pressure <90 mm Hg.

WARNINGS

Administration of nesiritide should be avoided in patients suspected of having, or known to have, low cardiac filling pressures.

PRECAUTIONS

GENERAL

Parenteral administration of protein pharmaceuticals or *E. coli*-derived products should be attended by appropriate precautions in case of an allergic or untoward reaction. No serious allergic or anaphylactic reactions have been reported with nesiritide.

Nesiritide is not recommended for patients for whom vasodilating agents are not appropriate, such as patients with significant valvular stenosis, restrictive or obstructive cardiomyopathy, constrictive pericarditis, pericardial tamponade, or other conditions in which cardiac output is dependent upon venous return, or for patients suspected to have low cardiac filling pressures. (See CONTRAINDICATIONS.)

RENAL

Nesiritide may affect renal function in susceptible individuals. In patients with severe heart failure whose renal function may depend on the activity of the renin-angiotensin-aldosterone system, treatment with nesiritide may be associated with azotemia. When nesiritide was initiated at doses higher than 0.01 μg/kg/min (0.015 and 0.030 μg/kg/min), there was an increased rate of elevated serum creatinine over baseline compared with standard therapies, although the rate of acute renal failure and need for dialysis was not increased. In the 30 day follow-up period in the VMAC trial, 5 patients in the nitroglycerin group (2%) and 9 patients in the nesiritide group (3%) required first-time dialysis.

CARDIOVASCULAR

Nesiritide may cause hypotension. In the VMAC trial, in patients given the recommended dose (2 μg/kg bolus followed by a 0.01 μg/kg/min infusion) or the adjustable dose, the incidence of symptomatic hypotension in the first 24 hours was similar for nesiritide (4%) and IV nitroglycerin (5%). When hypotension occurred, however, the duration of symptomatic hypotension was longer with nesiritide (mean duration was 2.2 hours) than with nitroglycerin (mean duration was 0.7 hours). In earlier trials, when nesiritide was initiated at doses higher than the 2 μg/kg bolus followed by a 0.01 μg/kg/min infusion (*i.e.*, 0.015 and 0.030 μg/kg/min preceded by a small bolus), there were more hypotensive episodes and these episodes were of greater intensity and duration. They were also more often symptomatic and/or more likely to require medical intervention (see ADVERSE REACTIONS). Nesiritide should be administered only in settings where blood pressure can be monitored closely, and the dose of nesiritide should be reduced or the drug discontinued in patients who develop hypotension (see DOSAGE AND ADMINISTRATION, Dosing Instructions). The rate of symptomatic hypotension may be increased in patients with a blood pressure <100 mm Hg at baseline, and nesiritide should be used cautiously in these patients. The potential for hypotension may be increased by combining nesiritide with other drugs that may cause hypotension. For example, in the VMAC trial in patients treated with either nesiritide or nitroglycerin therapy, the frequency of symptomatic hypotension in patients who received an oral ACE inhibitor was 6%, compared to a frequency of symptomatic hypotension of 1% in patients who did not receive an oral ACE inhibitor.

CARCINOGENESIS, MUTAGENESIS, AND IMPAIRMENT OF FERTILITY

Long-term studies in animals have not been performed to evaluate the carcinogenic potential or the effect on fertility of nesiritide.

Nesiritide did not increase the frequency of mutations when used in an *in vitro* bacterial cell assay (Ames test). No other genotoxicity studies were performed.

PREGNANCY CATEGORY C

Animal reproductive studies have not been conducted with nesiritide. It is also not known whether nesiritide can cause fetal harm when administered to pregnant women or can affect reproductive capacity. Nesiritide should be used during pregnancy only if the potential benefit justifies any possible risk to the fetus.

NURSING MOTHERS

It is not known whether this drug is excreted in human milk. Therefore, caution should be exercised when nesiritide is administered to a nursing woman.

PEDIATRIC USE

The safety and effectiveness of nesiritide in pediatric patients has not been established.

GERIATRIC USE

Of the total number of subjects in clinical trials treated with nesiritide (n=941), 38% were 65 years or older and 16% were 75 years or older. No overall differences in effectiveness were observed between these subjects and younger subjects, and other reported clinical experience has not identified differences in responses between the elderly and younger patients. Some older individuals may be more sensitive to the effect of nesiritide than younger individuals.

DRUG INTERACTIONS

No trials specifically examining potential drug interactions with nesiritide were conducted, although many concomitant drugs were used in clinical trials. No drug interactions were detected except for an increase in symptomatic hypotension in patients receiving oral ACE inhibitors (see PRECAUTIONS, Cardiovascular).

The coadministration of nesiritide with IV vasodilators such as nitroglycerin, nitroprusside, milrinone, or IV ACE inhibitors has not been evaluated (these drugs were not coadministered with nesiritide in clinical trials).

ADVERSE REACTIONS

Adverse events that occurred with at least a 3% frequency during the first 24 hours of nesiritide infusion are shown in TABLE 2A and TABLE 2B.

TABLE 2A *VMAC Trial*

Adverse Event	Nitroglycerin (n=216)	Nesiritide* (n=273)
Cardiovascular		
Hypotension	25 (12%)	31 (11%)
Symptomatic hypotension	10 (5%)	12 (4%)
Asymptomatic hypotension	17 (8%)	23 (8%)
Ventricular tachycardia (VT)	11 (5%)	9 (3%)
Non-sustained VT	11 (5%)	9 (3%)
Ventricular extrasystoles	2 (1%)	7 (3%)
Angina pectoris	5 (2%)	5 (2%)
Bradycardia	1 (<1%)	3 (1%)
Body as a Whole		
Headache	44 (20%)	21 (8%)
Abdominal pain	11 (5%)	4 (1%)
Back pain	7 (3%)	10 (4%)
Nervous		
Insomnia	9 (4%)	6 (2%)
Dizziness	4 (2%)	7 (3%)
Anxiety	6 (3%)	8 (3%)
Digestive		
Nausea	13 (6%)	10 (4%)
Vomiting	4 (2%)	4 (1%)

* Recommended dose.

TABLE 2B *Other Long-Term Infusion Trials*

		Nesiritide μg/kg/min	
Adverse Event	Control* (n=256)	0.015 (n=253)	0.03 (n=246)
Cardiovascular			
Hypotension	20 (8%)	56 (22%)	87 (35%)
Symptomatic hypotension	8 (3%)	28 (11%)	42 (17%)
Asymptomatic hypotension	13 (5%)	31 (12%)	49 (20%)
Ventricular tachycardia (VT)	25 (10%)	25 (10%)	10 (4%)
Non-sustained VT	23 (9%)	24 (9%)	9 (4%)
Ventricular extrasystoles	15 (6%)	10 (4%)	9 (4%)
Angina pectoris	6 (2%)	14 (6%)	6 (2%)
Bradycardia	1 (<1%)	8 (3%)	13 (5%)
Body as a Whole			
Headache	23 (9%)	23 (9%)	17 (7%)
Abdominal pain	10 (4%)	6 (2%)	8 (3%)
Back pain	4 (2%)	5 (2%)	3 (1%)
Nervous			
Insomnia	7 (3%)	15 (6%)	15 (6%)
Dizziness	7 (3%)	16 (6%)	12 (5%)
Anxiety	2 (1%)	8 (3%)	4 (2%)
Digestive			
Nausea	12 (5%)	24 (9%)	33 (13%)
Vomiting	2 (1%)	6 (2%)	10 (4%)

* Includes dobutamine, milrinone, nitroglycerin, placebo, dopamine, nitroprusside, or amrinone.

Adverse events that are not listed in TABLE 2A and TABLE 2B that occurred in at least 1% of patients who received any of the above nesiritide doses included: Tachycardia, atrial fibrillation, AV node conduction abnormalities, catheter pain, fever, injection site reaction, confusion, paresthesia, somnolence, tremor, increased cough, hemoptysis, apnea, increased creatinine, sweating, pruritus, rash, leg cramps, amblyopia, anemia. All reported events (at least 1%) are included except those already listed, those too general to be informative, and those not reasonably associated with the use of the drug because they were associated with the condition being treated or are very common in the treated population.

In placebo and active-controlled clinical trials, nesiritide has not been associated with an increase in atrial or ventricular tachyarrhythmias. In placebo-controlled trials, the incidence of VT in both nesiritide and placebo patients was 2%. In the *PRECEDENT (Prospective Randomized Evaluation of Cardiac Ectopy with Dobutamine or Natrecor Therapy)* trial, the effects of nesiritide (n=163) and dobutamine (n=83) on the provocation or aggravation of existing ventricular arrhythmias in patients with decompensated CHF was compared using Holter monitoring. Treatment with nesiritide (0.015 and 0.03 μg/kg/min without an initial bolus) for 24 hours did not aggravate pre-existing VT or the frequency of premature ventricular beats, compared to a baseline 24 hour Holter tape.

CLINICAL LABORATORY

In the PRECEDENT trial, the incidence of elevations in serum creatinine to >0.5 mg/dl above baseline through day 14 was higher in the nesiritide 0.015 μg/kg/min group (17%) and the nesiritide 0.03 μg/kg/min group (19%) than with standard therapy (11%). In the VMAC trial, through day 30, the incidence of elevations in creatinine to >0.5 mg/dl above baseline was 28% and 21% in the nesiritide (2 μg/kg bolus followed by 0.010 μg/kg/min) and nitroglycerin groups, respectively.

EFFECT ON MORTALITY

In the VMAC trial, the mortality rates at 6 months in the patients receiving nesiritide and nitroglycerin were 25.1% (95% confidence interval, 20.0-30.5%) and 20.8% (95% confidence interval, 15.5-26.5%), respectively. In all controlled trials combined, the mortality rates for nesiritide and active control (including nitroglycerin, dobutamine, nitroprusside, milrinone, amrinone, and dopamine) patients were 21.5% and 21.7%, respectively.

DOSAGE AND ADMINISTRATION

Nesiritide is for intravenous use only. There is limited experience with administering nesiritide for longer than 48 hours. Blood pressure should be monitored closely during nesiritide administration.

If hypotension occurs during the administration of nesiritide, the dose should be reduced or discontinued and other measures to support blood pressure should be started (IV fluids, changes in body position). In the VMAC trial, when symptomatic hypotension occurred, nesiritide was discontinued and subsequently could be restarted at a dose that was reduced by 30% (with no bolus administration) once the patient was stabilized. Because hypotension caused by nesiritide may be prolonged (up to hours), a period of observation may be necessary before restarting the drug.

DOSING INSTRUCTIONS

The recommended dose of nesiritide is an IV bolus of 2 μg/kg followed by a continuous infusion at a dose of 0.01 μg/kg/min. Nesiritide should not be initiated at a dose that is above the recommended dose.

Prime the IV tubing with an infusion of 25 ml prior to connecting to the patient's vascular access port and prior to administering the bolus or starting the infusion.

Bolus Followed by Infusion

Withdraw the bolus volume from the nesiritide infusion bag, and administer it over approximately 60 seconds through an IV port in the tubing. Immediately following the administration of the bolus, infuse nesiritide at a flow rate of 0.1 ml/kg/h. This will deliver a nesiritide infusion dose of 0.01 μg/kg/min.

To calculate the appropriate bolus volume and infusion flow rate to deliver a 0.01 μg/kg/min dose, use the following formulas:

Bolus Volume (ml): 0.33 × Patient Weight (kg)
Infusion Flow Rate (ml/h): 0.1 × Patient Weight (kg)

Dose Adjustment

The dose-limiting side effect of nesiritide is hypotension. Do not initiate nesiritide at a dose that is higher than the recommended dose of a 2 μg/kg bolus followed by an infusion of 0.01 μg/kg/min. In the VMAC trial there was limited experience with increasing the dose of nesiritide above the recommended dose (23 patients, all of whom had central hemodynamic monitoring). In those patients, the infusion dose of nesiritide was increased by 0.005 μg/kg/min (preceded by a bolus of 1 μg/kg), no more frequently than every 3 hours up to a maximum dose of 0.03 μg/kg/min. Nesiritide should not be titrated at frequent intervals as is done with other IV agents that have a shorter half-life.

CHEMICAL/PHYSICAL INTERACTIONS

Nesiritide is physically and/or chemically incompatible with injectable formulations of heparin, insulin, ethacrynate sodium, bumetamide, enalaprilat, hydralazine, and furosemide. These drugs should not be coadministered as infusions with nesiritide through the same IV catheter. The preservative sodium metabisulfite is incompatible with nesiritide. Injectable drugs that contain sodium metabisulfite should not be administered in the same infusion line as nesiritide. The catheter must be flushed between administration of nesiritide and incompatible drugs.

Nesiritide binds to heparin and therefore could bind to the heparin lining of a heparin-coated catheter, decreasing the amount of nesiritide delivered to the patient for some period of time. Therefore, nesiritide must not be administered through a central heparin-coated catheter. Concomitant administration of a heparin infusion through a separate catheter is acceptable.

HOW SUPPLIED

Natrecor is provided as a sterile lyophilized powder in 1.5 mg, single-use vials.

Storage: Store Natrecor at controlled room temperature (20-25°C; 68-77°F); excursions permitted to 15-30°C (59-86°F); or refrigerated (2-8°C; 36-46°F). Keep in carton until time of use.

PRODUCT LISTING - EQUIVALENTS NOT AVAILABLE

Powder For Injection - Intravenous - 1.5 mg

1's $456.00 NATRECOR, Scios Inc 65847-0205-25

Nevirapine (003290)

For related information, see the comparative table section in Appendix A.

Categories: Infection, human immunodeficiency virus; Pregnancy Category C; FDA Approved 1996 Jun; WHO Formulary
Drug Classes: Antivirals; Non-nucleoside reverse transcriptase inhibitors
Brand Names: Viramune
Foreign Brand Availability: Ciplanevimune (Colombia); Nevimune (India)
Cost of Therapy: $283.55 (HIV; Viramune; 200 mg; 2 tablets/day; 30 day supply)

WARNING

Severe, life-threatening, and in some cases fatal hepatotoxicity, including fulminant and cholestatic hepatitis, hepatic necrosis and hepatic failure, has been reported in patients treated with nevirapine. In some cases, patients presented with nonspecific prodromal signs or symptoms of hepatitis and progressed to hepatic failure. Patients with signs or symptoms of hepatitis must seek medical evaluation immediately and should be advised to discontinue nevirapine. (See WARNINGS.)

Severe, life-threatening skin reactions, including fatal cases, have occurred in patients treated with nevirapine. These have included cases of Stevens-Johnson syndrome, toxic epidermal necrolysis, and hypersensitivity reactions characterized by rash, constitutional findings, and organ dysfunction. Patients developing signs or symptoms of severe skin reactions or hypersensitivity reactions must discontinue nevirapine as soon as possible. (See WARNINGS.)

It is essential that patients be monitored intensively during the first 12-16 weeks of therapy with nevirapine to detect potentially life-threatening hepatotoxicity or skin reactions. However, the risk continues past this period and monitoring should continue at frequent intervals. Nevirapine should not be restarted following severe hepatic, skin or hypersensitivity reactions. In addition, the 14 day lead-in period with nevirapine 200 mg daily dosing must be strictly followed. (See WARNINGS.)

DESCRIPTION

Nevirapine (NVP) is a non-nucleoside reverse transcriptase inhibitor with activity against Human Immunodeficiency Virus Type 1 (HIV-1). Nevirapine is structurally a member of the dipyridodiazepinone chemical class of compounds.

Viramune tablets are for oral administration. Each tablet contains 200 mg of nevirapine and the inactive ingredients microcrystalline cellulose, lactose monohydrate, povidone, sodium starch glycolate, colloidal silicon dioxide, and magnesium stearate.

Viramune oral suspension is for oral administration. Each 5 ml of Viramune suspension contains 50 mg of nevirapine (as nevirapine hemihydrate). The suspension also contains the following excipients: carbomer 934P, methylparaben, propylparaben, sorbitol, sucrose, polysorbate 80, sodium hydroxide, and water.

The chemical name of nevirapine is 11-cyclopropyl-5,11-dihydro-4-methyl-6H-dipyrido[3,2-b:2′,3′-][1,4]diazepin-6-one. Nevirapine is a white to off-white crystalline powder with the molecular weight of 266.3 and the molecular formula $C_{15}H_{14}N_4O$.

N

CLINICAL PHARMACOLOGY

MICROBIOLOGY

Mechanism of Action

Nevirapine is a non-nucleoside reverse transcriptase inhibitor (NNRTI) of HIV-1. Nevirapine binds directly to reverse transcriptase (RT) and blocks the RNA-dependent and DNA-dependent DNA polymerase activities by causing a disruption of the enzyme's catalytic site. The activity of nevirapine does not compete with template or nucleoside triphosphates. HIV-2 RT and eukaryotic DNA polymerases (such as human DNA polymerases α, β, γ, or δ) are not inhibited by nevirapine.

In Vitro HIV Susceptibility

The *in vitro* antiviral activity of nevirapine was measured in peripheral blood mononuclear cells, monocyte derived macrophages, and lymphoblastoid cell lines. IC_{50} values (50% inhibitory concentration) ranged from 10-100 nM against laboratory and clinical isolates of HIV-1. In cell culture, nevirapine demonstrated additive to synergistic activity against HIV-1 in drug combination regimens with zidovudine (ZDV), didanosine (ddI), stavudine (d4T), lamivudine (3TC), saquinavir, and indinavir. The relationship between *in vitro* susceptibility of HIV-1 to nevirapine and the inhibition of HIV-1 replication in humans has not been established.

Resistance

HIV-1 isolates with reduced susceptibility (100- to 250-fold) to nevirapine emerge *in vitro.* Genotypic analysis showed mutations in the HIV-1 RT gene Y181C and/or V106A depending upon the virus strain and cell line employed. Time to emergence of nevirapine resistance *in vitro* was not altered when selection included nevirapine in combination with several other NNRTIs.

Phenotypic and genotypic changes in HIV-1 isolates from patients treated with either nevirapine (n=24) or nevirapine and ZDV (n=14) were monitored in Phase 1 and 2 trials over 1 to ≥12 weeks. After 1 week of nevirapine monotherapy, isolates from 3/3 patients had decreased susceptibility to nevirapine *in vitro;* one or more of the RT mutations K103N, V106A, V108I, Y181C, Y188C and G190A were detected in HIV-1 isolates from some patients as early as 2 weeks after therapy initiation. By Week 8 of nevirapine monotherapy, 100% of the patients tested (n=24) had HIV-1 isolates with a >100-fold decrease in susceptibility to nevirapine *in vitro* compared to baseline, and had one or more of the nevirapine-associated RT resistance mutations; 19 of 24 patients (80%) had isolates with Y181C mutations regardless of dose. Nevirapine + ZDV combination therapy did not alter the emergence rate of nevirapine-resistant virus or the magnitude of nevirapine resistance *in vitro.* The clinical relevance of phenotypic and genotypic changes associated with nevirapine therapy has not been established.

Cross-Resistance

Rapid emergence of HIV-1 strains which are cross-resistant to NNRTIs has been observed *in vitro.* Nevirapine-resistant HIV-1 isolates were cross-resistant to the NNRTIs efavirenz and delavirdine. However, nevirapine-resistant isolates were susceptible to the nucleoside analogues ZDV and ddI. Similarly, ZDV-resistant isolates were susceptible to nevirapine *in vitro.*

PHARMACOKINETICS IN ADULTS

Absorption and Bioavailability

Nevirapine is readily absorbed (>90%) after oral administration in healthy volunteers and in adults with HIV-1 infection. Absolute bioavailability in 12 healthy adults following single-dose administration was 93 ± 9% (mean ±SD) for a 50 mg tablet and 91 ± 8% for an oral solution. Peak plasma nevirapine concentrations of 2 ± 0.4 μg/ml (7.5 μM) were attained by 4 hours following a single 200 mg dose. Following multiple doses, nevirapine peak concentrations appear to increase linearly in the dose range of 200-400 mg/day. Steady-state trough nevirapine concentration of 4.5 ± 1.9 μg/ml (17 ± 7 μM), (n=242) were attained at 400 mg/day. Nevirapine tablets and suspension have been shown to be comparably bioavailable and interchangeable at doses up to 200 mg. When nevirapine (200 mg) was administered to 24 healthy adults (12 female, 12 male), with either a high-fat breakfast (857 kcal, 50 g fat, 53% of calories from fat) or antacid (Maalox 30 ml), the extent of nevirapine absorption (AUC) was comparable to that observed under fasting conditions. In a separate study in HIV-1-infected patients (n=6), nevirapine steady-state systemic exposure (AUC_T) was not significantly altered by ddI, which is formulated with an alkaline buffering agent. Nevirapine may be administered with or without food, antacid or ddI.

Distribution

Nevirapine is highly lipophilic and is essentially nonionized at physiologic pH. Following intravenous administration to healthy adults, the apparent volume of distribution (Vdss) of nevirapine was 1.21 ± 0.09 L/kg, suggesting that nevirapine is widely distributed in humans. Nevirapine readily crosses the placenta and is also found in breast milk. (See PRECAUTIONS, Nursing Mothers.) Nevirapine is about 60% bound to plasma proteins in the plasma concentration range of 1-10 μg/ml. Nevirapine concentrations in human cerebrospinal fluid (n=6) were 45% (±5%) of the concentrations in plasma; this ratio is approximately equal to the fraction not bound to plasma protein.

Metabolism/Elimination

In vivo studies in humans and *in vitro* studies with human liver microsomes have shown that nevirapine is extensively biotransformed via cytochrome P450 (oxidative) metabolism to several hydroxylated metabolites. *In vitro* studies with human liver microsomes suggest that oxidative metabolism of nevirapine is mediated primarily by cytochrome P450 isozymes from the CYP3A family, although other isozymes may have a secondary role. In a mass balance/excretion study in 8 healthy male volunteers dosed to steady-state with nevirapine 200 mg given twice daily followed by a single 50 mg dose of ^{14}C-nevirapine, approximately 91.4 ± 10.5% of the radiolabeled dose was recovered, with urine (81.3 ± 11.1%) representing the primary route of excretion compared to feces (10.1 ± 1.5%). Greater than 80% of the radioactivity in urine was made up of glucuronide conjugates of hydroxylated metabolites. Thus cytochrome P450 metabolism, glucuronide conjugation, and urinary excretion of glucuronidated metabolites represent the primary route of nevirapine biotransformation and elimination in humans. Only a small fraction (<5%) of the radioactivity in urine (representing <3% of the total dose) was made up of parent compound; therefore, renal excretion plays a minor role in elimination of the parent compound.

Nevirapine has been shown to be an inducer of hepatic cytochrome P450 metabolic enzymes. The pharmacokinetics of autoinduction are characterized by an approximately 1.5- to 2-fold increase in the apparent oral clearance of nevirapine as treatment continues from a single dose to 2-4 weeks of dosing with 200-400 mg/day. Autoinduction also results in a corresponding decrease in the terminal phase half-life of nevirapine in plasma from approximately 45 hours (single dose) to approximately 25-30 hours following multiple dosing with 200-400 mg/day.

PHARMACOKINETICS IN SPECIAL POPULATIONS

Renal/Hepatic Dysfunction

The pharmacokinetics of nevirapine have not been evaluated in patients with either renal or hepatic dysfunction.

Gender

In one Phase 1 study in healthy volunteers (15 females, 15 males), the weight-adjusted apparent volume of distribution (Vdss/F) of nevirapine was higher in the female subjects (1.54 L/kg) compared to the males (1.38 L/kg), suggesting that nevirapine was distributed more extensively in the female subjects. However, this difference was offset by a slightly shorter terminal-phase half-life in the females resulting in no significant gender difference in nevirapine oral clearance (24.6 ± 7.7 ml/kg/h in females versus 19.9 ± 3.9 ml/kg/h in males after single dose) or plasma concentrations following either single- or multiple-dose administration(s).

Race

An evaluation of nevirapine plasma concentrations (pooled data from several clinical trials) from HIV-1-infected patients (27 Black, 24 Hispanic, 189 Caucasian) revealed no marked difference in nevirapine steady-state trough concentrations (median C_{minss} = 4.7 μg/ml Black, 3.8 μg/ml Hispanic, 4.3 μg/ml Caucasian) with long-term nevirapine treatment at 400 mg/day. However, the pharmacokinetics of nevirapine have not been evaluated specifically for the effects of ethnicity.

Geriatric Patients

Nevirapine pharmacokinetics in HIV-1-infected adults do not appear to change with age (range 18-68 years); however, nevirapine has not been extensively evaluated in patients beyond the age of 55 years.

Pediatric Patients

The pharmacokinetics of nevirapine have been studied in two open-label studies in children with HIV-1 infection. In one study (BI 853; ACTG 165), 9 HIV-1-infected children ranging in age from 9 months to 14 years were administered a single dose (7.5, 30, or 120 mg/m^2; n=3 per dose) of nevirapine suspension after an overnight fast. The mean nevirapine apparent clearance adjusted for body weight was greater in children compared to adults.

In a multiple dose study (BI 882; ACTG 180), nevirapine suspension or tablets (240 or 400 mg/m^2/day) were administered as monotherapy or in combination with ZDV or ZDV + ddI to 37 HIV-1-infected pediatric patients with the following demographics: male (54%), racial minority groups (73%), median age of 11 months (range: 2 months-15 years). The majority of these patients received 120 mg/m^2/day of nevirapine for approximately 4 weeks followed by 120 mg/m^2/bid (patients >9 years of age) or 200 mg/m^2/bid (patients ≤9 years of age). Nevirapine apparent clearance adjusted for body weight reached maximum values by age 1 to 2 years and then decreased with increasing age. Nevirapine apparent clearance adjusted for body weight was at least 2-fold greater in children younger than 8 years compared to adults. The pediatric dosing regimens were selected in order to achieve steady-state plasma concentrations in pediatric patients that approximate those in adults. (See DOSAGE AND ADMINISTRATION, Pediatric Patients.)

Drug Interactions

Nucleoside Analogues

No dosage adjustments are required when nevirapine is taken in combination with ZDV, ddI, or zalcitabine (ddC). Results from studies in HIV-1-infected patients who were administered nevirapine with different combinations of ddI or ddC, on a background of ZDV therapy, indicated that no clinically significant pharmacokinetic interactions occurred when the nucleoside analogues were administered in combination with nevirapine.

Protease Inhibitors

In the following three studies, nevirapine was given 200 mg once daily for 2 weeks followed by 200 mg twice daily for 28 days:

Ritonavir: No dosage adjustments are required when nevirapine is taken in combination with ritonavir. Results from a 49 day study in HIV-infected patients (n=14) administered nevirapine and ritonavir (600 mg bid [using a gradual dose escalation regimen]) indicated that their coadministration did not affect ritonavir AUC or C_{max}. Comparison of nevirapine pharmacokinetics from this study to historical data suggested that coadministration did not affect the pharmacokinetics of nevirapine.

Indinavir: Results from a 36 day study in HIV-infected patients (n=19) administered nevirapine and indinavir (800 mg q8h) indicated that their coadministration led to a 28% mean decrease (95% CI -39, -16) in indinavir AUC and an 11% mean decrease (95% CI -49, +59) in indinavir C_{max}. The clinical significance of this interaction is not known. Comparison of nevirapine pharmacokinetics from this study to historical data suggested that coadministration did not affect the pharmacokinetics of nevirapine.

Saquinavir: Results from a 42 day study in HIV-infected patients (n=23) administered nevirapine and saquinavir (hard gelatin capsules, 600 mg tid) indicated that their coadministration led to a 24% mean decrease (95% CI -42, -1) in saquinavir AUC and a 28% mean decrease (95% CI -47, -1) in saquinavir C_{max}. The clinical significance of this interaction is not known. Coadministration did not affect the pharmacokinetics of nevirapine.

In Vitro

Studies using human liver microsomes indicated that the formation of nevirapine hydroxylated metabolites was not affected by the presence of dapsone, rifabutin, rifampin, and trimethoprim/sulfamethoxazole. Ketoconazole significantly inhibited the formation of nevirapine hydroxylated metabolites.

In Vivo

Ketoconazole

Nevirapine and ketoconazole should not be administered concomitantly. Ketoconazole AUC and C_{max} decreased by a median 63% (95% CI -95, +33) and 40% (95% CI -52, +11), respectively, in HIV-infected patients (n=22) who were given nevirapine 200 mg once daily for 2 weeks followed by 200 mg twice daily for 2 weeks along with ketoconazole 400 mg daily. (See DRUG INTERACTIONS.) Comparison of the pharmacokinetics from this study to historical data suggested that coadministration with ketoconazole may result in a 15-30% increase in nevirapine plasma concentrations. The clinical significance of this observation is not known.

Monitoring of nevirapine plasma concentrations in patients who received long-term nevirapine treatment indicate that steady-state nevirapine trough plasma concentrations were elevated in patients who received cimetidine (+21%, n=11) and macrolides (+12%, n=24), known inhibitors of CYP3A.

Steady-state nevirapine trough concentrations were reduced in patients who received rifabutin (-16%, n=19) and rifampin (-37%, n=3), known inducers of CYP3A. Nevirapine is an inducer of CYP3A, with maximal induction occurring within 2-4 weeks of initiating multiple-dose therapy. Other compounds that are substrates of CYP3A may have decreased plasma concentrations when coadministered with nevirapine. Therefore, careful monitoring of the therapeutic effectiveness of CYP3A-metabolized drugs is recommended when taken in combination with nevirapine. (See DRUG INTERACTIONS for recommendations regarding rifampin, rifabutin, oral contraceptives, and methadone.)

INDICATIONS AND USAGE

Nevirapine is indicated for use in combination with other antiretroviral agents for the treatment of HIV-1 infection. This indication is based on one principal clinical trial that demonstrated prolonged suppression of HIV-RNA and two smaller supportive studies.

NON-FDA APPROVED INDICATIONS

Nevirapine has been investigated for use in pregnant women to prevent vertical transmission of HIV. Interim data from a study sponsored by the National Institute of Allergy and Infectious Diseases (NIAID) demonstrate that a single oral dose of nevirapine given to infected women (200 mg at the onset of labor) and their babies (2 mg/kg within 3 days of birth) reduces the transmission rate by 47% compared to a similar short course of AZT. These results show promise for potential widespread use of nevirapine in developing countries where effective, practical and affordable antiretroviral regimens are needed to curtail the high prevalence of HIV infection and perinatal transmission. In industrialized countries, nevirapine may offer a prevention option to women who do not know their HIV status until they begin labor.

CONTRAINDICATIONS

Nevirapine is contraindicated in patients with clinically significant hypersensitivity to any of the components contained in the tablet or the oral suspension.

WARNINGS

GENERAL

The first 12-16 weeks of therapy with nevirapine are a critical period during which intensive monitoring of patients is required to detect potentially life-threatening hepatic events and skin reactions. The optimal frequency of monitoring during this time period has not been established. Some experts recommend clinical and laboratory monitoring more often than once per month, and in particular, would include monitoring of liver function tests at baseline, prior to dose escalation and at 2 weeks post-dose escalation. After the initial 12-16 week period, frequent clinical and laboratory monitoring should continue throughout nevirapine treatment. In addition, the 14 day lead-in period with nevirapine 200 mg daily dosing has been demonstrated to reduce the frequency of rash.

Resistant virus emerges rapidly and uniformly when nevirapine is administered as monotherapy. Therefore, nevirapine should always be administered in combination with other antiretroviral agents for the treatment of HIV-1 infection.

HEPATIC EVENTS

Severe, life-threatening, and in some cases fatal hepatotoxicity, including fulminant and cholestatic hepatitis, hepatic necrosis and hepatic failure, have been reported in patients treated with nevirapine. Serious hepatic events occur most frequently during the first 12-16 weeks of nevirapine therapy, and have been reported to occur as early as within the first few weeks of therapy. However, these events may occur at any time during treatment. In some cases, patients presented with non-specific, prodromal signs or symptoms of fatigue, malaise, anorexia, nausea, jaundice, liver tenderness or hepatomegaly, with or without initially abnormal serum transaminase levels. These events progressed to hepatic failure with transaminase elevation, with or without hyperbilirubinemia, prolonged partial thromboplastin time, or eosinophilia. Rash and fever accompanied some of these hepatic events. Patients with signs or symptoms of hepatitis must immediately seek medical evaluation, have liver function tests performed, and be advised to discontinue nevirapine as soon as possible.

In addition, serious hepatotoxicity (including liver failure requiring transplantation in 1 instance) has been reported in HIV-uninfected individuals receiving multiple doses of nevirapine in the setting of post-exposure prophylaxis, an unapproved use.

Increased AST or ALT levels and/or co-infection with hepatitis B and C infection and CD4+ cell count >350 cells/mm^3 prior to the start of antiretroviral therapy are associated with a greater risk of hepatic adverse events. It appears that women may be at higher risk for nevirapine-associated hepatic events.

Intensive clinical and laboratory monitoring, including liver function tests, is essential at baseline and during the first 12-16 weeks of treatment. (See WARNINGS, General.) Monitoring should continue at frequent intervals thereafter, depending on the patient's clinical status. Liver function tests should be performed if a patient experiences signs or symptoms suggestive of hepatitis and/or hypersensitivity reaction. Physicians and patients should be vigilant for the appearance of signs or symptoms of hepatitis, such as fatigue, malaise, anorexia, nausea, jaundice, bilirubinuria, acholic stools, liver tenderness or hepatomegaly. The diagnosis of hepatotoxicity should be considered in this setting, even if liver function tests are initially normal or alternative diagnoses are possible. (See PRECAUTIONS, Information for the Patient; ADVERSE REACTIONS; and DOSAGE AND ADMINISTRATION.)

If clinical hepatitis occurs, nevirapine should be permanently discontinued and not restarted after recovery.

SKIN REACTIONS

Severe, life-threatening skin reactions, including fatal cases, have been reported with nevirapine treatment, occurring most frequently during the first 6 weeks of therapy. These have included cases of Stevens-Johnson syndrome, toxic epidermal necrolysis, and hypersensitivity reactions characterized by rash, constitutional findings, and organ dysfunction. Patients developing signs or symptoms of severe skin reactions or hypersensitivity reactions (including, but not limited to, severe rash or rash accompanied by fever, general malaise, fatigue, muscle or joint aches, blisters, oral lesions, conjunctivitis, facial edema, and/or hepatitis, eosinophilia, granulocytopenia, lymphadenopathy, and renal dysfunction) must permanently discontinue nevirapine and seek medical evaluation immediately. (See PRECAUTIONS, Information for the Patient and ADVERSE REACTIONS.) Nevirapine should not be restarted following severe skin rash or hypersensitivity reaction. Some of the risk factors for developing serious cutaneous reactions include failure to follow the initial dosing of 200 mg daily during the 14 day lead-in period and delay in stopping the nevirapine treatment after the onset of the initial symptoms.

Therapy with nevirapine must be initiated with a 14 day lead-in period of 200 mg/day (4 mg/kg/day in pediatric patients), which has been shown to reduce the frequency of rash. If rash is observed during this lead-in period, dose escalation should not occur until the rash has resolved. (See DOSAGE AND ADMINISTRATION.) Patients should be monitored closely if isolated rash of any severity occurs.

Women appear to be at higher risk than men of developing rash with nevirapine.

In a clinical trial, concomitant prednisone use (40 mg/day for the first 14 days of nevirapine administration) was associated with an increase in incidence and severity of rash during the first 6 weeks of nevirapine therapy. Therefore, use of prednisone to prevent nevirapine-associated rash is not recommended.

N

ST. JOHN'S WORT

Concomitant use of St. John's wort (hypericum perforatum) or St. John's wort-containing products and nevirapine is not recommended. Coadministration of non-nucleoside reverse transcriptase inhibitors (NNRTIs), including nevirapine, with St. John's wort is expected to substantially decrease NNRTI concentrations and may result in sub-optimal levels of nevirapine and lead to loss of virologic response and possible resistance to nevirapine or to the class of NNRTIs.

PRECAUTIONS

GENERAL

Nevirapine is extensively metabolized by the liver and nevirapine metabolites are extensively eliminated by the kidney. However, the pharmacokinetics of nevirapine have not been evaluated in patients with either hepatic or renal dysfunction. Therefore, nevirapine should be used with caution in these patient populations.

The duration of clinical benefit from antiretroviral therapy may be limited. Patients receiving nevirapine or any other antiretroviral therapy may continue to develop opportunistic infections and other complications of HIV infection, and therefore should remain under close clinical observation by physicians experienced in the treatment of patients with associated HIV diseases.

When administering nevirapine as part of an antiretroviral regimen, the complete product information for each therapeutic component should be consulted before initiation of treatment.

FAT REDISTRIBUTION

Redistribution/accumulation of body fat including central obesity, dorsocervical fat enlargement (buffalo hump), peripheral wasting, facial wasting, breast enlargement, and "cushingoid appearance" have been observed in patients receiving antiretroviral therapy. The mechanism and long-term consequences of these events are currently unknown. A causal relationship has not been established.

INFORMATION FOR THE PATIENT

Patients should be informed of the possibility of severe liver disease or skin reactions associated with nevirapine that may result in death. Patients developing signs or symptoms of liver disease or skin reactions should be instructed to seek medical attention immediately, including performance of laboratory monitoring. Symptoms of liver disease include fatigue, malaise, anorexia, nausea, jaundice, acholic stools, liver tenderness or hepatomegaly. Symptoms of severe skin or hypersensitivity reactions include rash accompanied by fever, general malaise, fatigue, muscle or joint aches, blisters, oral lesions, conjunctivitis, facial edema and/or hepatitis.

Severe liver disease occurs most frequently during the first 12 weeks of therapy. Intensive clinical and laboratory monitoring, including liver function tests, is essential during this period. However, liver disease can occur after this period, therefore monitoring should continue at frequent intervals throughout nevirapine treatment. Patients with signs and symptoms of hepatitis should seek medical evaluation immediately. If nevirapine is discontinued due to hepatitis it should not be restarted. Patients should be advised that co-infection with hepatitis B or C infection, increased liver function tests and increased CD4+ cell count (>350 cells/mm^3) prior to the start of antiretroviral therapy are associated with a greater risk of hepatic events with nevirapine. Women may be at higher risk for development of nevirapine associated hepatic events.

The majority of rashes associated with nevirapine occur within the first 6 weeks of initiation of therapy. Patients should be instructed that if any rash occurs during the 2 week lead-in period, the nevirapine dose should not be escalated until the rash resolves. Any patient experiencing severe rash or hypersensitivity reactions should discontinue nevirapine and consult a physician. Nevirapine should not be restarted following severe skin rash or hypersensitivity reaction. Women tend to be at higher risk for development of nevirapine associated rash.

Oral contraceptives and other hormonal methods of birth control should not be used as a method of contraception in women taking nevirapine. (See DRUG INTERACTIONS.)

Patients should be informed that nevirapine therapy has not been shown to reduce the risk of transmission of HIV-1 to others through sexual contact or blood contamination. The long-term effects of nevirapine are unknown at this time.

Nevirapine is not a cure for HIV-1 infection; patients may continue to experience illnesses associated with advanced HIV-1 infection, including opportunistic infections. Patients should be advised to remain under the care of a physician when using nevirapine.

Patients should be informed to take nevirapine every day as prescribed. Patients should not alter the dose without consulting their doctor. If a dose is missed, patients should take the next dose as soon as possible. However, if a dose is skipped, the patient should not double the next dose. Patients should be advised to report to their doctor the use of any other medications. Based on the known metabolism of methadone, nevirapine may decrease plasma concentrations of methadone by increasing its hepatic metabolism. Narcotic withdrawal syndrome has been reported in patients treated with nevirapine and methadone concomitantly. Methadone-maintained patients beginning nevirapine therapy should be monitored for evidence of withdrawal and methadone dose should be adjusted accordingly.

Nevirapine may interact with some drugs, therefore, patients should be advised to report to their doctor the use of any other prescription, nonprescription medication or herbal products, particularly St. John's wort.

Patients should be informed that redistribution or accumulation of body fat may occur in patients receiving antiretroviral therapy and that the cause and long term health effects of these conditions are not known at this time.

Prescribing information provides written information for the patient, and should be dispensed with each new prescription and refill.

CARCINOGENESIS, MUTAGENESIS, AND IMPAIRMENT OF FERTILITY

Long-term carcinogenicity studies in mice and rats were carried out with nevirapine. Mice were dosed with 0, 50, 375 or 750 mg/kg/day for 2 years. Hepatocellular adenomas and carcinomas were increased at all doses in males and at the two high doses in females. In studies in which rats were administered nevirapine at doses of 0, 3.5, 17.5 or 35 mg/kg/day for 2 years, an increase in hepatocellular adenomas was seen in males at all doses and in females at the high dose. The systemic exposure (based on AUCs) at all doses in the two animal studies were lower than that measured in humans at the 200 mg bid dose. The mechanism of the carcinogenic potential is unknown. However, in genetic toxicology assays, nevirapine showed no evidence of mutagenic or clastogenic activity in a battery of *in vitro* and *in vivo* studies. These included microbial assays for gene mutation (Ames: Salmonella strains and *E. coli*), mammalian cell gene mutation assay (CHO/HGPRT), cytogenetic assays using a Chinese hamster ovary cell line and a mouse bone marrow micronucleus assay following oral administration. Given the lack of genotoxic activity of nevirapine, the relevance to humans of hepatocellular neoplasms in nevirapine treated mice and rats is not known. In reproductive toxicology studies, evidence of impaired fertility was seen in female rats at doses providing systemic exposure, based on AUC, approximately equivalent to that provided with the recommended clinical dose of nevirapine.

PREGNANCY CATEGORY C

No observable teratogenicity was detected in reproductive studies performed in pregnant rats and rabbits. In rats, a significant decrease in fetal body weight occurred at doses providing systemic exposure approximately 50% higher, based on AUC, than that seen at the recommended human clinical dose.

The maternal and developmental no-observable-effect level dosages in rats and rabbits produced systemic exposures approximately equivalent to or approximately 50% higher, respectively, than those seen at the recommended daily human dose, based on AUC. There are no adequate and well-controlled studies in pregnant women. Nevirapine should be used during pregnancy only if the potential benefit justifies the potential risk to the fetus.

Antiretroviral Pregnancy Registry: To monitor maternal-fetal outcomes of pregnant women exposed to nevirapine, an Antiretroviral Pregnancy Registry has been established. Physicians are encouraged to register patients by calling 800-258-4263.

NURSING MOTHERS

The Centers for Disease Control and Prevention recommend that HIV-infected mothers not breast-feed their infants to avoid risking postnatal transmission of HIV. Nevirapine is excreted in breast milk. Because of both the potential for HIV transmission and the potential for serious adverse reactions in nursing infants, mothers should be instructed not to breast-feed if they are receiving nevirapine.

PEDIATRIC USE

The pharmacokinetics of nevirapine have been studied in two open-label studies in children with HIV-1 infection. (See CLINICAL PHARMACOLOGY, Pharmacokinetics in Special Populations.) For dose recommendations for pediatric patients see DOSAGE AND ADMINISTRATION. The most frequently reported adverse events related to nevirapine in pediatric patients were similar to those observed in adults, with the exception of granulocytopenia, which was more commonly observed in children. (See ADVERSE REACTIONS, Pediatric Patients.) The evaluation of the antiviral activity of nevirapine in pediatric patients is ongoing.

DRUG INTERACTIONS

The induction of CYP3A by nevirapine may result in lower plasma concentrations of other concomitantly administered drugs that are extensively metabolized by CYP3A. (See CLINICAL PHARMACOLOGY.) Thus, if a patient has been stabilized on a dosage regimen for a drug metabolized by CYP3A, and begins treatment with nevirapine, dose adjustments may be necessary.

Rifampin/Rifabutin: There are insufficient data to assess whether dose adjustments are necessary when nevirapine and rifampin or rifabutin are coadministered. Therefore, these drugs should only be used in combination if clearly indicated and with careful monitoring.

Ketoconazole: Nevirapine and ketoconazole should not be administered concomitantly. Coadministration of nevirapine and ketoconazole resulted in a significant reduction in ketoconazole plasma concentrations. (See CLINICAL PHARMACOLOGY, Drug Interactions.)

Oral Contraceptives: There are no clinical data on the effects of nevirapine on the pharmacokinetics of oral contraceptives. Nevirapine may decrease plasma concentrations of oral contraceptives (also other hormonal contraceptives); therefore, these drugs should not be administered concomitantly with nevirapine.

Methadone: Based on the known metabolism of methadone, nevirapine may decrease plasma concentrations of methadone by increasing its hepatic metabolism. Narcotic withdrawal syndrome has been reported in patients treated with nevirapine and methadone concomitantly. Methadone-maintained patients beginning nevirapine therapy should be monitored for evidence of withdrawal and methadone dose should be adjusted accordingly.

ADVERSE REACTIONS

ADULTS

Clinical trials and clinical practice has shown that the most serious adverse reactions associated with nevirapine are clinical hepatitis/hepatic failure, Stevens-Johnson syndrome, toxic epidermal necrolysis, and hypersensitivity reactions. Clinical hepatitis/hepatic failure may be isolated or associated with signs of hypersensitivity which may include severe rash or rash accompanied by fever, general malaise, fatigue, muscle or joint aches, blisters, oral lesions, conjunctivitis, facial edema, and/or hepatitis, eosinophilia, granulocytopenia, lymphadenopathy, and renal dysfunction.

Severe and life-threatening hepatotoxicity, and fatal fulminant hepatitis have been reported in patients treated with nevirapine. Hepatic adverse events have been reported to occur more frequently during the first 12-16 weeks of treatment, but such events may occur at any time during treatment.

In clinical trials, the risk of clinical hepatic events with nevirapine at 1 year was approximately 2-fold that of placebo. Approximately one-half of these events occurred within the first 12-16 weeks of treatment. Increased AST or ALT levels and/or seropositivity for hepatitis B and/or C, and CD4+ cell count >350 cells/mm^3, were associated with a greater risk of hepatic adverse events for both nevirapine and control groups. The risk of hepatic events at 1 year of nevirapine treatment was less than 2% among patients who were hepatitis B and/or C negative. (See TABLE 2.) It appears that women may be at higher risk for nevirapine-associated hepatic events.

TABLE 2 *Risk of Hepatic Events by 1 Year in Adult Placebo-Controlled Trials*

	Trial 1090*		Trials 1037, 1038, 1046†	
	Nevirapine	Placebo	Nevirapine	Placebo
	n=1121	n=1128	n=253	n=203
Median CD4+ cells/mm^3	93	98	363	359
Risk of Hepatitis or Related Hepatic Events‡	3.4%	2.2%	8.1%	3.0%
Risk when hepatitis B or C positive at baseline	7.8% (of 294)	5.2% (of 326)	ND	ND
Risk when hepatitis B or C negative at baseline	1.8% (of 814)	0.9% (of 795)	ND	ND
Risk when ALT or AST > Grade 1 at baseline	4.8% (of 358)	4.0% (of 363)	12.2% (of 53)	0% (of 48)
Risk when ALT or AST < Grade 1 at baseline	2.7% (of 745)	1.3% (of 748)	7.2% (of 199)	4.2% (of 155)
Risk of Grade 2 ALT or AST Elevations	25.6%	25.4%	32.3%	15.7%
Risk of Grade 3/4 ALT or AST Elevations	8.3%	7.8%	19.3%	11.0%
Risk of Fatal Hepatic Events	0.2%	0.3%	0%	0%

* Background therapy included 3TC for all patients and combinations of NRTIs and PIs.
† Background therapy included ZDV and ZDV + ddI; nevirapine monotherapy was administered in some patients.
‡ Includes hepatitis, cholestatic hepatitis, infectious hepatitis, hepatic failure and LFT abnormalities with concurrent clinical symptoms.
ND = serologies not done.

The most common clinical toxicity of nevirapine is rash. Severe or life-threatening rash occurred in approximately 2% of nevirapine-treated patients, most frequently within the first 6 weeks of therapy. (See TABLE 3.) Rashes are usually mild to moderate, maculopapular erythematous cutaneous eruptions, with or without pruritus, located on the trunk, face and extremities. Women tend to be at higher risk for development of nevirapine associated rash.

TABLE 3 *Risk of Rash (%) in Adult Placebo Controlled Trials* — Regardless of Causality*

		Nevirapine	Placebo
		n=1374	n=1331
Through 6 Weeks of Treatment†			
Rash Events of All Grades‡		14.8%	5.9%
Grade 1	Erythema, pruritus	8.5%	4.2%
Grade 2	Diffuse maculopapular rash, dry desquamation	4.8%	1.6%
Grade 3 or 4	Grade 3: Vesiculation, moist desquamation, ulceration; Grade 4: erythema multiforme, Stevens Johnson syndrome, toxic epidermal necrolysis, necrosis requiring surgery, exfoliative dermatitis	1.5%	0.1%
Through 52 Weeks of Treatment†			
Rash Events of All Grades‡		24.0%	14.8%
Grade 1	See above	15.5%	10.8%
Grade 2	See above	7.1%	3.9%
Grade 3 or 4	See above	1.7%	0.2%
Proportion of Patients Who Discontinued Treatment Due to Rash		4.3%	1.2%

* Trials 1037, 1038, 1046 and 1090.
† % based on Kaplan-Meier probability estimates.
‡ NCI grading system.

Treatment related, adverse experiences of moderate or severe intensity observed in >2% of patients receiving nevirapine in placebo-controlled trials are shown in TABLE 4.

Laboratory Abnormalities

Liver function test abnormalities (AST, ALT) were observed more frequently in patients receiving nevirapine than in controls (TABLE 2). Asymptomatic elevations in GGT occur frequently but are not a contraindication to continue nevirapine therapy in the absence of elevations in other liver function tests. Other laboratory abnormalities (bilirubin, anemia, neutropenia, thrombocytopenia) were observed with similar frequencies in clinical trials comparing nevirapine and control regimens. (See TABLE 5.)

Because clinical hepatitis has been reported in nevirapine-treated patients, intensive clinical and laboratory monitoring, including liver function tests, is essential at baseline and during the first 12-16 weeks of treatment. Monitoring should continue at frequent intervals thereafter, depending on the patient's clinical status. (See WARNINGS.)

Postmarketing Surveillance

In addition to the adverse events identified during clinical trials, the following events have been reported with the use of nevirapine in clinical practice:

Body as a Whole: Fever, somnolence, drug withdrawal (see DRUG INTERACTIONS), redistribution/accumulation of body fat (see PRECAUTIONS, Fat Redistribution).

Gastrointestinal: Vomiting.

Liver and Biliary: Jaundice, fulminant and cholestatic hepatitis, hepatic necrosis, hepatic failure.

TABLE 4 *Percentage of Patients With Moderate or Severe Drug Related Events in Adult Placebo Controlled Trials*

	Trial 1090*		Trials 1037, 1038, 1046†	
	Nevirapine	Placebo	Nevirapine	Placebo
	n=1121	n=1128	n=253	n=203
Median exposure (weeks)	58	52	28	28
Any adverse event	14.5%	11.1%	31.6%	13.3%
Rash	5.1%	1.8%	6.7%	1.5%
Abnormal LFTs	1.2%	0.9%	6.7%	1.5%
Nausea	0.5%	1.1%	8.7%	3.9%
Granulocytopenia	1.8%	2.8%	0.4%	0%
Headache	0.7%	0.4%	3.6%	0.5%
Fatigue	0.2%	0.3%	4.7%	3.9%
Diarrhea	0.2%	0.8%	2.0%	0.5%
Abdominal pain	0.1%	0.4%	2.0%	0%
Myalgia	0.2%	0%	1.2%	2.0%

* Background therapy included 3TC for all patients and combinations of NRTIs and PIs. Patients had CD4+ cell counts <200 cells/mm^3.
† Background therapy included ZDV and ZDV + ddI; nevirapine monotherapy was administered in some patients. Patients had CD4+ cell count ≥200 cells/mm^3.

TABLE 5 *Percentage of Adult Patients With Laboratory Abnormalities*

	Trial 1090*		Trials 1037, 1038, 1046†	
	Nevirapine	Placebo	Nevirapine	Placebo
Laboratory Abnormality	n=1121	n=1128	n=253	n=203
Blood Chemistry				
SGPT (ALT) >250 U/L	5.3%	4.4%	14.0%	4.0%
SGOT (AST) >250 U/L	3.7%	2.5%	7.6%	1.5%
Bilirubin >2.5 mg/dl	1.7%	2.2%	1.7%	1.5%
Hematology				
Hemoglobin <8.0 g/dl	3.2%	4.1%	0%	0%
Platelets <50,000/mm^3	1.3%	1.0%	0.4%	1.5%
Neutrophils <750/mm^3	13.3%	13.5%	3.6%	1.0%

* Background therapy included 3TC for all patients and combinations of NRTIs and PIs. Patients had CD4+ cell counts <200 cells/mm^3.
† Background therapy included ZDV and ZDV + ddI; nevirapine monotherapy was administered in some patients. Patients had CD4+ cell count >200 cells/mm^3.

Hematology: Eosinophilia, neutropenia.

Musculoskeletal: Arthralgia.

Neurologic: Paraesthesia.

Skin and Appendages: Allergic reactions including anaphylaxis, angioedema, bullous eruptions, ulcerative stomatitis and urticaria have all been reported. In addition, hypersensitivity reactions with rash associated with constitutional findings such as fever, blistering, oral lesions, conjunctivitis, facial edema, muscle or joint aches, general malaise, fatigue or significant hepatic abnormalities (see WARNINGS) plus one or more of the following: hepatitis, eosinophiia, granulocytopenia, lymphadenopathy and/or renal dysfunction have been reported with the use of nevirapine.

PEDIATRIC PATIENTS

Safety was assessed in trial BI 882 in which patients were followed for a mean duration of 33.9 months (range: 6.8 months to 5.3 years, including long-term follow-up in 29 of these patients in trial BI 892). The most frequently reported adverse events related to nevirapine in pediatric patients were similar to those observed in adults, with the exception of granulocytopenia which was more commonly observed in children. Serious adverse events were assessed in ACTG 245, a double-blind, placebo-controlled trial of nevirapine (n=305) in which pediatric patients received combination treatment with nevirapine. In this trial 2 patients were reported to experience Stevens-Johnson syndrome or Stevens-Johnson/toxic epidermal necrolysis transition syndrome. Cases of allergic reaction, including one case of anaphylaxis, were also reported.

TABLE 6 summarizes the marked laboratory abnormalities occurring in pediatric patients in Trial BI 882 and in follow-up Trial BI 892.

TABLE 6 *Number of Pediatric Patients (%) With Laboratory Abnormalities in Trials BI 882 and BI 892 Combined*

	No. (%) of Patients
	n=37
Blood Chemistry	
Increased ALT (>250 U/L)	4 (11%)
Increased AST (>250 U/L)	5 (14%)
Increased GGT (>450 U/L)	4 (11%)
Increased total bilirubin (>2.5 mg/dl)	1 (3%)
Increased alkaline phosphatase (>2 × ULN)	19 (51%)
Increased amylase (>2 × ULN)	6 (16%)
Hematology	
Decreased Hg (<8.0 g/dl)	7 (19%)
Decreased platelets (<50,000/mm^3)	4 (11%)
Decreased neutrophils (<750/mm^3)	14 (38%)
Increased MCV (>100 F/L)	13 (35%)

DOSAGE AND ADMINISTRATION

ADULTS

The recommended dose for nevirapine is one 200 mg tablet daily for the first 14 days (**this lead-in period should be used because it has been found to lessen the frequency of**

N

rash), followed by one 200 mg tablet twice daily, in combination with antiretroviral agents. For concomitantly administered antiretroviral therapy, the manufacturer's recommended dosage and monitoring should be followed.

PEDIATRIC PATIENTS

The recommended oral dose of nevirapine for pediatric patients 2 months up to 8 years of age is 4 mg/kg once daily for the first 14 days followed by 7 mg/kg twice daily thereafter. For patients 8 years and older the recommended dose is 4 mg/kg once daily for 2 weeks followed by 4 mg/kg twice daily thereafter. The total daily dose should not exceed 400 mg for any patient.

Nevirapine suspension should be shaken gently prior to administration. It is important to administer the entire measured dose of suspension by using an oral dosing syringe or dosing cup. An oral dosing syringe is recommended, particularly for volumes of 5 ml or less. If a dosing cup is used, it should be thoroughly rinsed with water and the rinse should also be administered to the patient.

MONITORING OF PATIENTS

Intensive clinical and laboratory monitoring, including liver function tests, is essential at baseline and during the first 12-16 weeks of treatment with nevirapine. The optimal frequency of monitoring during this period has not been established. Some experts recommend clinical and laboratory monitoring more often than once per month, and in particular, would include monitoring of liver function tests at baseline, prior to dose escalation, and at 2 weeks post dose escalation. After the initial 12-16 week period, frequent clinical and laboratory monitoring should continue throughout nevirapine treatment. (See WARNINGS.)

DOSE ADJUSTMENT

Nevirapine should be discontinued if patients experience severe rash or a rash accompanied by constitutional findings. (See WARNINGS.) Patients experiencing rash during the 14 day lead-in period of 200 mg/day (4 mg/kg/day in pediatric patients) should not have their nevirapine dose increased until the rash has resolved. (See PRECAUTIONS, Information for the Patient.)

If clinical hepatitis occurs, nevirapine should be permanently discontinued and not restarted after recovery.

Patients who interrupt nevirapine dosing for more than 7 days should restart the recommended dosing, using one 200 mg tablet daily (4 mg/kg/day in pediatric patients) for the first 14 days (lead-in) followed by one 200 mg tablet twice daily (4 or 7 mg/kg twice daily, according to age, for pediatric patients).

No data are available to recommend a dosage of nevirapine in patients with hepatic dysfunction, renal insufficiency, or undergoing dialysis.

ANIMAL PHARMACOLOGY

Animal studies have shown that nevirapine is widely distributed to nearly all tissues and readily crosses the blood-brain barrier.

HOW SUPPLIED

Viramune is available as follows:

Viramune Tablets, 200 mg: White, oval, biconvex tablets, 9.3 mm × 19.1 mm. One side is embossed with "54 193", with a single bisect separating the "54" and "193". The opposite side has a single bisect.

Viramune Oral Suspension: White to off-white preserved suspension containing 50 mg nevirapine (as nevirapine hemihydrate) in each 5 ml.

Storage: Viramune tablets and oral suspension should be stored at 15-30°C (59-86°F).

PRODUCT LISTING - EQUIVALENTS NOT AVAILABLE

Suspension - Oral - 50 mg/5 ml

240 ml	$69.05	VIRAMUNE, Roxane Laboratories Inc	00054-3905-58
240 ml	$82.78	VIRAMUNE, Boehringer-Ingelheim	00597-0047-24

Tablet - Oral - 200 mg

3's	$14.61	VIRAMUNE, Allscripts Pharmaceutical Company	54569-4561-01
3's	$18.82	VIRAMUNE, Pd-Rx Pharmaceuticals	55289-0392-63
60's	$292.29	VIRAMUNE, Allscripts Pharmaceutical Company	54569-4561-00
60's	$318.86	VIRAMUNE, Roxane Laboratories Inc	00054-4647-21
60's	$382.19	VIRAMUNE, Boehringer-Ingelheim	00597-0046-60
100's	$472.59	VIRAMUNE, Physicians Total Care	54868-3844-00
100's	$540.36	VIRAMUNE, Roxane Laboratories Inc	00054-8647-25
100's	$560.12	VIRAMUNE, Boehringer-Ingelheim	00597-0046-01
100's	$647.74	VIRAMUNE, Boehringer-Ingelheim	00597-0046-61

Niacin *(001876)*

For related information, see the comparative table section in Appendix A.

Categories: Hypercholesterolemia; Hyperlipoproteinemia; Hypertriglyceridemia; Pregnancy Category C; FDA Approved 1973 Nov; WHO Formulary

Drug Classes: Antihyperlipidemics; Nicotinic acid derivatives; Vitamins/minerals

Brand Names: Acido Nicotino; Akotin; Niaspan; **Nicolar**; Niconacid; Nicotinic Acid; Nikacid; Nikotime; Novoniacin; Slo-Niacin; Span Niacin; Vitaplex; Wampocap

Foreign Brand Availability: Acido Nicotinico (Colombia); Akotin 250 (Argentina); Apo-Nicotinic Acid (New-Zealand); Natinate (Thailand); Nicangin (Sweden); Nicobid (Hong-Kong); Nyclin (Japan; Taiwan); Pepevit (Mexico)

Cost of Therapy: $59.66 (Hyperlipidemia; Niaspan ER; 500 mg; 2 tablets/day; 30 day supply)
$2.39 (Hyperlipidemia; Generic Tablets; 500 mg; 4 tablets/day; 30 day supply)

DESCRIPTION

Niacin or nicotinic acid, a water-soluble B complex vitamin and antihyperlipidemic agent, is 3-pyridinecarboxylic acid. It is a white, crystalline powder, sparingly soluble in water. It has the following structural formula: $C_6H_5NO_2$ with a molecular weight of 123.11.

Each Nicolar tablet, for oral administration, is a scored yellow-colored tablet containing 500 mg of nicotinic acid. In addition, each tablet contains the following inactive ingredients: microcrystalline cellulose, FD&C yellow no. 5 (tartrazine) (see PRECAUTIONS), magnesium stearate, povidone, and colloidal silica.

CLINICAL PHARMACOLOGY

The role of low-density lipoprotein (LDL) cholesterol in atherogenesis is supported by pathological observations, clinical studies, and many animal experiments. Observational epidemiological studies have clearly established that high total or LDL (low-density lipoprotein) cholesterol and low HDL (high-density lipoprotein) cholesterol are risk factors for coronary heart disease. The Coronary Drug Project,[1] compared in 1975, was designed to assess the safety and efficacy of nicotinic acid and other lipid-altering drugs in men 30-64 years old with a history of myocardial infarction. Over an observation period of 5 years, nicotinic acid showed a statistically significant benefit in decreasing nonfatal, recurrent myocardial infarctions. The incidence of definite, non-fatal MI was 8.9% for the 1119 patients randomized to nicotinic acid versus 12.2% for the 2789 patients who received placebo ($p < 0.004$). Though total mortality was similar in the two groups at 5 years (24.4% with nicotinic acid versus 25.4% with placebo; p=NS), in a 15 year cumulative follow-up there were 11% (69) fewer deaths in the nicotinic acid group compared to the placebo cohort (52.% vs 58.2%; p=0004).[2]

The Cholesterol-Lowering Atherosclerosis Study (CLAS) was a randomized, placebo-controlled, angiographic trial testing combined colestipol and nicotinic acid therapy in 162 non-smoking males with previous coronary bypass surgery.[3] The primary, per subject cardiac endpoint was global coronary artery change score. After 2 years, 61% of patients in the placebo cohort showed disease progression by global change score (n=82), compared with only 38.8% of drug-treated subjects (n=80), when both native arteries and grafts were considered ($p < 0.005$). In a follow- up to this trial in a subgroup of 103 patients treated for 4 years, again, significantly fewer patients in the drug-treated group demonstrated progression than in the placebo cohort (48% vs 85%, respectively; $p < 0.0001$).[4]

The Familial Atherosclerosis Treatment Study (FATS) in 146 men ages 62 and younger with apolipoprotein B levels ≥125 mg/dl, established coronary artery disease, and family histories of vascular disease, assessed change in severity of disease in the proximal coronary arteries by quantitative arteriography.[5] Patients were given dietary counselling and randomized to treatment with either conventional therapy with double placebo (or placebo plus colestipol if the LDL-cholesterol was elevated); lovastatin plus colestipol; or nicotinic acid plus colestipol. In the conventional therapy group, 46% of patients had disease progression (and no regression) in at least 1 of 9 proximal coronary segments. In contrast, progression (as the only change) was seen in only 25% in the nicotinic acid plus colestipol group. Though not an original endpoint of the trial, clinical events (death, myocardial infarction, or revascularization for worsening angina) occurred in 10 of 52 patients who received conventional therapy, compared with 2 of 48 who received nicotinic acid plus colestipol.

Nicotinic acid (but not nicotinamide) in gram doses produces an average 10-20% reduction in total and LDL-cholesterol, a 30-70% reduction in triglycerides, and an average 20-35% increase in HDL-cholesterol. The magnitude of individual lipid and lipoprotein responses may be influenced by the severity and type of underlying lipid abnormality. The increase in total HDL is associated with a shift in the distribution of HDL subfractions (as defined by ultra-centrifugation) with an increase in the HDL_2:HDL_3 ratio; and an increase in apolipoprotein Al content. The mechanism by which nicotinic acid exerts these effects is not entirely understood, but may involve several actions, including a decrease in esterification of hepatic triglycerides. Nicotinic acid treatment also decreases the serum levels of apolipoprotein B-100 (apo B), the major protein component of the VLDL and LDL fractions, and of lipoprotein, Lp(a), a variant form of LDL independently associated with coronary risk. The effect of nicotinic acid-induced changes in lipids/lipoproteins on cardiovascular morbidity or mortality in individuals without pre-existing coronary disease has not been established.

PHARMACOKINETICS

Following an oral dose, the pharmacokinetic profile of nicotinic acid is characterized by rapid absorption from the gastrointestinal tract and a short plasma elimination half-life. At a 1 g dose, peak plasma concentrations of 15-30 µg/ml are reached within 30-60 minutes. Approximately 88% of an oral pharmacologic dose is eliminated by the kidneys as unchanged drug and nicotinuric acid, its primary metabolite. The plasma elimination half-life of nicotinic acid ranges from 20-45 minutes.

INDICATIONS AND USAGE

- Therapy with lipid-altering agents should be only one component of multiple risk factor intervention in those individuals at significantly increased risk for atherosclerotic vascular disease due to hypercholesterolemia. Nicotinic acid, alone or in combination with a bile-acid binding resin, is indicated as an adjunct to diet for the reduction of elevated total and LDL cholesterol levels in patients with primary hypercholesterolemia (Types IIa and IIb), (see TABLE 1) when the response to a diet restricted in saturated fat and cholesterol and other nonpharmacologic measures alone has been inadequate (see also the NCEP treatment guidelines[6]). Prior to initiating therapy with nicotinic acid, secondary causes for hypercholesterolemia (*e.g.*, poorly controlled diabetes mellitus, hypothyroidism, nephrotic syndrome, dysproteinemias, obstructive liver disease, other drug therapy, alcoholism) should be excluded, and a lipid profile performed to measure total cholesterol, HDL-cholesterol, and triglycerides.

- Nicotinic acid is also indicated as adjunctive therapy for the treatment of adult patients with very high serum triglyceride levels (Types IV and V hyperlipidemia)† who present a risk of pancreatitis and who do not respond adequately to a determined dietary effort to control them. Such patients typically have serum triglyceride levels over 2000 mg/dl and have elevations of VLDL-cholesterol as well as fasting chylomicrons (Type V hyperlipidemia).† Subjects who consistently have total serum or plasma triglycerides below 1000 mg/dl are unlikely to develop pancreatitis. Therapy with nicotinic acid may be considered for those subjects with triglyceride elevations between 1000 and 2000 mg/dl who have a history of pancreatitis or of recurrent abdominal pain typical of pancreatitis. Some Type IV patients with triglycerides under 1000 mg/dl may, through dietary or alcoholic indiscretion, convert to a Type V pattern with massive triglyceride elevations accompanying fasting chylomicronemia, but the influence of nicotinic acid therapy on the risk of pancreatitis in such situations has not been adequately studied. Drug therapy is not indicated for patients with Type I hyperlipoproteinemia, who have elevations of chylomicrons and plasma triglycerides, but who have normal levels of very low density lipoprotein (VLDL). Inspection of plasma refrigerated for 14 hours is helpful in distinguishing Types I, IV, and V hyperlipoproteinemia.[7]

TABLE 1 *Classification of Hyperlipoproteinemias*

Type	Lipoproteins Elevated	Lipid Elevations: Major	Lipid Elevations: Minor
I (rare)	chylomicrons	TG	C*
IIa	LDL	C	-
IIb	LDL, VLDL	C	TG
III (rare)	IDL	C/TG	-
IV	VLDL	TG	C*
V (rare)	chylomicrons, VLDL	TG	C*

* Increases or no change.
C = cholesterol, TG = triglycerides, LDL = low-density lipoprotein, VLDL = very-low-density lipoprotein, IDL = intermediate-density lipoprotein.

CONTRAINDICATIONS

Nicotinic acid is contraindicated in patients with a known hypersensitivity to any component of this medication; significant or unexplained hepatic dysfunction; active peptic ulcer disease; or arterial bleeding.

WARNINGS

LIVER DYSFUNCTION

Cases of severe hepatic toxicity, including fulminant hepatic necrosis have occurred in patients who have substituted sustained-release (modified-release, timed-release) nicotinic acid products for immediate-release (crystalline) nicotinic acid at equivalent doses.

Liver function tests should be performed on all patients during therapy with nicotinic acid. Serum transaminase levels, including ALT (SGPT), should be monitored before treatment begins, every 6-12 weeks for the first year, and periodically thereafter (*e.g.*, at approximately 6 month intervals). Special attention should be paid to patients who develop elevated serum transaminase levels, and in these patients, measurements should be repeated promptly and then performed more frequently. If the transaminase levels show evidence of progression, particularly if they rise to 3 times the upper limit of normal and are persistent, the drug should be discontinued. Liver biopsy should be considered if elevation persist beyond discontinuation of the drug.

Nicotinic acid should be used with caution in patients who consume substantial quantities of alcohol and/or have a past history of liver disease. Active liver diseases or unexplained transaminase elevations are contraindication to the use of nicotinic acid.

SKELETAL MUSCLE

Rare cases of rhabdomyolysis have been associated with concomitant administration of lipid-altering doses ($\geq$ 1 g/day) of nicotinic acid and HMG-CoA reductase inhibitors. Physicians contemplating combined therapy with HMG-CoA reductase inhibitors and nicotinic acid should carefully weigh the potential benefits and risks and should carefully monitor patients for any signs and symptoms of muscle pain, tenderness, or weakness, particularly during the initial months of therapy and during any periods of upward dosage titration of either drug. Periodic serum creatine phosphokinase (CPK) and potassium determinations should be considered in such situations, but there is no assurance that such monitoring will prevent the occurrence of severe myopathy.

PRECAUTIONS

GENERAL

Before instituting therapy with nicotinic acid, an attempt should be made to control hyperlipidemia with appropriate diet, exercise, and weight reduction in obese patients, and to treat other underlying medical problems (see INDICATIONS AND USAGE).

Patients with a past history of jaundice, hepatobiliary disease, or peptic ulcer should be observed closely during nicotinic acid therapy. Frequent monitoring of liver function tests and blood glucose should be performed to ascertain that the drug is producing no adverse effects on these organ systems. Diabetic patients may experience a dose-related rise in glucose intolerance, the clinical significance of which is unclear. Diabetic or potentially diabetic patients should be observed closely. Adjustment of diet and/or hypoglycemic therapy may be necessary.

Caution should also be used when nicotinic acid is used in patients with unstable angina or in the acute phase of myocardial infarction, particularly when such patients are also receiving vasoactive drugs such as nitrates, calcium channel blockers, or adrenergic blocking agents.

Elevated uric acid levels have occurred with nicotinic acid therapy, therefore use with caution in patients predisposed to gout.

This product contains FD&C yellow no. 5 (tartrazine) which may cause allergic-type reactions (including bronchial asthma) in certain susceptible persons. Although the overall incidence of FD&C yellow no. 5 (tartrazine) sensitivity in the general population is low, it is frequently seen in patients who also have aspirin hypersensitivity.

CARCINOGENESIS, MUTAGENESIS, AND IMPAIRMENT OF FERTILITY

Nicotinic acid administered to mice for a lifetime as a 1% solution in drinking water was not carcinogenic. The mice in this study received approximately 6-8 times a human dose of 3000 mg/day as determined on a mg/m^2 basis. Nicotinic acid was negative for mutagenicity in the Ames test. No studies on impairment of fertility have been performed.

PREGNANCY CATEGORY C

Animal reproduction studies have not been conducted with nicotinic acid. It is also not known whether nicotinic acid at doses typically used for lipid disorders can cause fetal harm when administered to pregnant women or whether it can affect reproductive capacity. If a woman receiving nicotinic acid for primary hypercholesterolemia (Types IIa or IIb) becomes pregnant, the drug should be discontinued. If a woman being treated with nicotinic acid for hypertriglyceridemia (Types IV and V) conceives, the benefits and risks of continued drug therapy should be assessed on an individual basis.

NURSING MOTHERS

It is not known whether this drug is excreted in human milk. Because many drugs are excreted in human milk and because of the potential for serious adverse reactions in nursing infants from lipid-altering doses of nicotinic acid, a decision should be made whether to discontinue nursing or to discontinue the drug, taking into account the importance of the drug to the mother.

PEDIATRIC USE

Safety and effectiveness in children and adolescents have not been established.

DRUG INTERACTIONS

HMG-CoA Reductase Inhibitors: Skeletal muscle.

Antihypertensive Therapy: Nicotinic acid may potentiate the effects of ganglionic blocking agents and vasoactive drugs resulting in postural hypotension.

Aspirin: Concomitant aspirin may decrease the metabolic clearance of nicotinic acid. The clinical relevance of this finding is unclear.

Other: Concomitant alcohol or hot drinks may increase the side effects of flushing and pruritus and should be avoided at the time of drug ingestion.

ADVERSE REACTIONS

Cardiovascular: Atrial fibrillation and other cardiac arrhythmias; orthostasis; hypotension.

Gastrointestinal: Dyspepsia; vomiting; diarrhea; peptic ulceration; jaundice; abnormal liver function tests.

Skin: Mild to severe cutaneous flushing; pruritus; hyperpigmentation; acanthosis nigricans; dry skin.

Metabolic: Decreased glucose tolerance; hyperuricemia; gout.

Eye: Toxic amblyopia; cystoid macular edema.

Nervous System/Psychiatric: Headache.

DOSAGE AND ADMINISTRATION

The usual adult dosage of nicotinic acid is 1-2 g 2-3 times a day. Doses should be individualized according to the patient's response. Start with one-half tablet (250 mg) as a single daily dose following the evening meal. The frequency of dosing and total daily dose can be increased every 4-7 days until the desired LDL-cholesterol and/or triglyceride level is achieved or the first-level therapeutic dose of 1.5 to 2 g/day is reached. If the patient's hyperlipidemia is not adequately controlled after 2 months at this level, the dosage can then be increased at 2-4 week intervals to 3 g/day (1 g three times per day). In patients with marked lipid abnormalities, a higher dose is occasionally required, but generally should not exceed 6 g/day.

Flushing of the skin appears frequently and can be minimized by pretreatment with aspirin or non-steroidal anti-inflammatory drugs. Tolerance to this flushing develops rapidly over the course of several weeks. Flushing, pruritus, and gastrointestinal distress are also greatly reduced by slowly increasing the dose of nicotinic acid and avoiding administration on an empty stomach.

Sustained-release (modified-release, timed-release) nicotinic acid preparations should **not** be substituted for equivalent doses of immediate-release (crystalline) nicotinic acid.

HOW SUPPLIED

Nicolar Tablets are scored, yellow-colored, oval-shaped 500 mg tablets.

Storage: Dispense in a tight container. Store at controlled room temperature, 15-30°C (59-86°F).

PRODUCT LISTING - RATED THERAPEUTICALLY EQUIVALENT

Tablet - Oral - 500 mg

100's $3.90 FEDERAL UPPER LIMIT, H.C.F.A. F F P 99999-1876-01

N

PRODUCT LISTING - EQUIVALENTS NOT AVAILABLE

Tablet - Oral - 50 mg
100's $36.80 GENERIC, West Ward Pharmaceutical Corporation 00143-1345-25
Tablet, Extended Release - Oral - 500 mg
100's $99.44 NIASPAN ER, Kos Pharmaceuticals 60598-0001-01

Nicardipine Hydrochloride (001882)

For related information, see the comparative table section in Appendix A.

Categories: Angina, chronic stable; Hypertension, essential; Pregnancy Category C; FDA Approved 1988 Dec
Drug Classes: Calcium channel blockers
Brand Names: **Cardene**; Cardene SR
Foreign Brand Availability: Antagonil (Germany); Cardepine (Philippines); Cardibloc (Singapore); Cardipene (Thailand); Convertal (Peru); Dacarel (Ecuador); Dagan (Spain); Flusemide (Spain); Lincil (Costa-Rica; Dominican-Republic; El-Salvador; Guatemala; Honduras; Nicaragua; Panama; Spain); Loxen (France; Indonesia); Nicardal (Italy); Nicodel (Japan); Nimicor (Italy); Perdipina (Italy); Perdipine (China; Japan; Korea; Taiwan); Perdipine LA (China; Japan); Ranvil (Italy); Ridene (Mexico); Rycarden (Denmark; Sweden); Rydene (Belgium); Saf Card (Indonesia); Vasodin (Thailand)
Cost of Therapy: $52.30 (Angina; Cardene; 20 mg; 3 capsules/day; 30 day supply)
$35.33 (Angina; Generic Capsules; 20 mg; 3 capsules/day; 30 day supply)
$54.49 (Angina; Cardene SR; 30 mg; 2 capsules/day; 30 day supply)

DESCRIPTION

Nicardipine hydrochloride capsules for oral administration each contain 20 or 30 mg of nicardipine hydrochloride. Nicardipine HCl is a calcium ion flux inhibitor (slow channel blocker or calcium channel blocker).

Nicardipine hydrochloride is a dihydropyridine structure with the chemical name 2-(benzyl-methyl amino)ethylmethyl 1,4-dihydro-2,6-dimethyl-4-(*m*-nitrophenyl)-3,5-pyridinedicarboxylate monohydrochloride.

Nicardipine hydrochloride is a greenish-yellow, odorless, crystalline powder that melts at about 169°C. It is freely soluble in chloroform, methanol, and glacial acetic acid, sparingly soluble in anhydrous ethanol, slightly soluble in n-butanol, water, 0.01 M potassium dihydrogen phosphate, acetone, and dioxane, very slightly soluble in ethyl acetate, and practically insoluble in benzene, ether and hexane. It has a molecular weight of 515.99.

Nicardipine hydrochloride is available in hard gelatin capsules containing 20 or 30 mg nicardipine hydrochloride with magnesium stearate and pregelatinized starch as the inactive ingredients. The 20 mg strength is provided in opaque white-white capsules with a brilliant blue band while the 30 mg capsules are opaque light blue-powder blue with a brilliant blue band. The colorants used in the 20 mg capsules are titanium dioxide, D&C red no. 7 calcium lake and FD&C blue no. 1 and the 30 mg capsules use titanium dioxide, FD&C blue no. 1, D&C yellow no. 10 aluminum lake, D&C red no. 7 calcium lake and FD&C blue no. 2.

STORAGE

Store bottles at room temperature and dispense in light resistant containers.

Store blister packages at room temperature and protect from excessive humidity and light. To protect from light, product should remain in manufacturer's package until consumed.

CLINICAL PHARMACOLOGY

MECHANISM OF ACTION

Nicardipine HCl is a calcium entry blocker (slow channel blocker or calcium ion antagonist) which inhibits the transmembrane influx of calcium ions into cardiac muscle and smooth muscle without changing serum calcium concentrations. The contractile processes of cardiac muscle and vascular smooth muscle are dependent upon the movement of extracellular calcium ions into these cells through specific ion channels. The effects of nicardipine HCl are more selective to vascular smooth muscle than cardiac muscle. In animal models, nicardipine HCl produces relaxation of coronary vascular smooth muscle at drug levels which cause little or no negative inotropic effect.

PHARMACOKINETICS AND METABOLISM

Nicardipine HCl is completely absorbed following oral doses administered as capsules. Plasma levels are detectable as early as 20 minutes following an oral dose and maximal plasma levels are observed within 30 minutes to 2 hours (mean T_{max}=1 hour). While nicardipine HCl is completely absorbed, it is subject to saturable first pass metabolism and the systemic bioavailability is about 35% following a 30 mg oral dose at steady state.

When nicardipine HCl was administered 1 or 3 hours after a high fat meal, the mean C_{max} and mean AUC were lower (20-30%) than when nicardipine HCl was given to fasting subjects. These decreases in plasma observed following a meal may be significant but the clinical trials establishing the efficacy and safety of nicardipine HCl were done in patients without regard to the timing of meals. Thus the results of these trials reflect the effects of meal-induced variability.

The pharmacokinetics of nicardipine HCl are nonlinear due to saturable hepatic first pass metabolism. Following oral administration, increasing doses result in a disproportionate increase in plasma levels. Steady state C_{max} values following 20, 30, and 40 mg doses every 8 hours averaged 36, 88, and 133 ng/ml, respectively. Hence, increasing the dose from 20 to 30 mg every 8 hours more than doubled C_{max} and increasing the dose from 20 to 40 mg every 8 hours increased C_{max} more than 3-fold. A similar disproportionate increase in AUC with dose was observed. Considerable inter-subject variability in plasma levels was also observed.

Post-absorption kinetics of nicardipine HCl are also non-linear, although there is a reproducible terminal plasma half-life that averaged 8.6 hours following 30 and 40 mg doses at steady state (tid). The terminal half-life represents the elimination of less than 5% of the absorbed drug (measured by plasma concentrations). Elimination over the first 8 hours after dosing is much faster with a half-life of 3-4 hours. Steady state plasma levels are achieved after 2-3 days of tid dosing (every 8 hours) and are 2-fold higher than after a single dose.

Nicardipine HCl is highly protein bound (>95%) in human plasma over a wide concentration range.

Nicardipine HCl is metabolized extensively by the liver; less than 1% of intact drug is detected in the urine. Following a radioactive oral dose in solution, 60% of the radioactivity was recovered in the urine and 35% in feces. Most of the dose (over 90%) was recovered within 48 hours of dosing. Nicardipine HCl does not induce its own metabolism and does not induce hepatic microsomal enzymes.

The steady-state pharmacokinetics of nicardipine HCl in elderly hypertensive patients (≥65 years) are similar to those obtained in young normal adults. After 1 week of nicardipine HCl dosing at 20 mg three times a day, the C_{max}, T_{max}, AUC, terminal plasma half-life, and the extent of protein binding of nicardipine HCl observed in healthy elderly hypertensive patients did not differ significantly from those observed in young normal volunteers.

Nicardipine HCl plasma levels were higher in patients with mild renal impairment (baseline serum creatinine concentration ranged from 1.2 to 5.5 mg/dl) than in normal subjects. After 30 mg nicardipine HCl tid at steady state, C_{max} and AUC were approximately 2-fold higher in these patients.

Because nicardipine HCl is extensively metabolized by the liver, the plasma levels of the drug are influenced by changes in hepatic function. Nicardipine HCl plasma levels were higher in patients with severe liver disease (hepatic cirrhosis confirmed by liver biopsy or presence of endoscopically confirmed esophageal varices) than in normal subjects. After 20 mg nicardipine HCl bid at steady state, C_{max} and AUC were 1.8- and 4-fold higher, and the terminal half-life was prolonged to 19 hours in these patients.

HEMODYNAMICS

In man, nicardipine HCl produces a significant decrease in systemic vascular resistance. The degree of vasodilation and the resultant hypotensive effects are more prominent in hypertensive patients. In hypertensive patients, nicardipine reduces the blood pressure at rest and during isometric and dynamic exercise. In normotensive patients, a small decrease of about 9 mmg Hg in systolic and 7 mmg Hg in diastolic blood pressure may accompany this fall in peripheral resistance. An increase in heart rate may occur in response to the vasodilation and decrease in blood pressure, and in a few patients this heart rate may be pronounced. In clinical studies mean heart rate at time of peak plasma levels was usually increased by 5-10 beats per minute compared to placebo, with the greater increases at higher doses, while there was no difference from placebo at the end of the dosing interval. Hemodynamic studies following intravenous dosing in patients with coronary artery disease and normal or moderately abnormal left ventricular function have shown significant increases in ejection fraction and cardiac output with no significant change, or a small decrease, in left ventricular end-diastolic pressure (LVEDP). Although there is evidence that nicardipine HCl increases coronary blood flow, there is no evidence that this property plays any role in its effectiveness in stable angina. In patients with coronary artery disease, intracoronary administration of nicardipine caused no direct myocardial depression. Nicardipine HCl does, however, have a negative inotropic effect in some patients with severe left ventricular dysfunction and could, in patients with very impaired function, lead to worsened failure.

"Coronary Steal", the detrimental redistribution of coronary blood flow in patients with coronary artery disease (diversion of blood from underperfused areas toward better perfused areas), has not been observed during nicardipine treatment. On the contrary, nicardipine has been shown to improve systolic shortening in normal and hypokinetic segments of myocardial muscle, and radio-nuclide angiography has confirmed that wall motion remained improved during an increase in oxygen demand. Nonetheless, occasional patients have developed increased angina upon receiving nicardipine. Whether this represents steal in those patients, or is the result of increased heart rate and decreased diastolic pressure, is not clear.

In patients with coronary artery disease nicardipine improved LV diastolic distensibility during the early filling phase, probably due to a faster rate of myocardial relaxation in previously underperfused areas. There is little or no effect on normal myocardium, suggesting the improvement is mainly by indirect mechanisms such as afterload reduction, and reduced ischemia. Nicardipine has no negative effect on myocardial relaxation at therapeutic doses. The clinical consequences of these properties are as yet undemonstrated.

ELECTROPHYSIOLOGIC EFFECTS

In general, no detrimental effects on the cardiac conduction system were seen with the use of nicardipine HCl.

Nicardipine HCl increased the heart rate when given intravenously during acute electrophysiologic studies, and prolonged the corrected QT interval to a minor degree. The sinus node recovery times and SA conduction times were not affected by the drug. The PA, AH and HV intervals* and the functional and effective refractory periods of the atrium were not prolonged by nicardipine HCl and the relative and effective refractory periods of the His-Purkinje system were slightly shortened after intravenous nicardipine HCl.

* PA = conduction time from high to low right atrium, AH = conduction time from low right atrium to His bundle deflection, or AV nodal conduction time, HV = conduction time through the His bundle and the bundle branch-Purkinje system.

RENAL FUNCTION

There is a transient increase in electrolyte excretion, including sodium. Nicardipine HCl does not cause generalized fluid retention, as measured by weight changes, though 7-8% of patients experience pedal edema.

EFFECTS IN ANGINA PECTORIS

In controlled clinical trials of up to 12 weeks duration in patients with chronic stable angina, nicardipine HCl increased exercise tolerance and reduced nitroglycerin consumption and the frequency of anginal attacks. The antianginal efficacy of nicardipine HCl (20-40 mg) has been demonstrated in four placebo-controlled studies involving 258 patients with chronic stable angina. In exercise tolerance testing, nicardipine HCl significantly increased time to angina, total exercise duration and time to 1 mm ST segment depression. Included among these four studies was a dose-definition in which dose-related improvements in exercise tolerance at 1 and 4 hours post-dosing and reduced frequency of anginal attacks were seen at doses of 10, 20 and 30 mg tid. Effectiveness at 10 mg tid was, however, marginal. In a fifth placebo-controlled study, the antianginal efficacy of nicardipine HCl was demonstrated at 8 hours post-dose (trough). The sustained efficacy of nicardipine HCl has been demonstrated over long-term dosing. Blood pressure fell in patients with angina by about 10/8 mmg Hg at peak blood levels and was little different from placebo at trough blood levels.

EFFECTS IN HYPERTENSION

Nicardipine HCl produced dose-related decreases in both systolic and diastolic blood pressure in clinical trials. The antihypertensive efficacy of nicardipine HCl administered 3 times daily has been demonstrated in three placebo-controlled studies involving 517 patients with mild to moderate hypertension. The blood pressure responses in the three studies were statistically significant from placebo at peak (1 hour post-dosing) and trough (8 hours post-dosing) although it is apparent that well over half of the antihypertensive effect is lost by the end of the dosing interval. The results from placebo controlled studies of nicardipine HCl given 3 times daily are shown in TABLE 1 and TABLE 2.

TABLE 1 *Systolic BP (mmg Hg)*

Dose	Number of Patients	Mean Peak Response	Mean Trough Response	Trough/Peak
20 mg				
	50	-10.3	-4.9	48%
	52	-17.6	-7.9	45%
30 mg				
	45	-14.5	-7.2	50%
	44	-14.6	-7.5	51%
40 mg				
	50	-16.3	-9.5	58%
	38	-15.9	-6.0	38%

TABLE 2 *Diastolic BP (mm Hg)*

Dose	Number of Patients	Mean Peak Response	Mean Trough Response	Trough/Peak
20 mg				
	50	-10.6	-4.6	43%
	52	-9.0	-2.9	32%
30 mg				
	45	-12.8	-4.9	38%
	44	-14.2	-4.3	30%
40 mg				
	50	-15.4	-5.9	38%
	38	-14.8	-3.7	25%

The responses are shown as differences from the concurrent placebo control group. The large changes between peak and trough effects were not accompanied by observed side effects at peak response times. In a study using 24 hour intra-arterial blood pressure monitoring, the circadian variation in blood pressure remained unaltered, but the systolic and diastolic blood pressures were reduced throughout the whole 24 hours.

When added to beta-blocker therapy, nicardipine HCl further lowers both systolic and diastolic blood pressure.

INDICATIONS AND USAGE

STABLE ANGINA

Nicardipine HCl is indicated for the management of patients with chronic stable angina (effort-associated angina). Nicardipine HCl may be used alone or in combination with beta-blockers.

HYPERTENSION

Nicardipine HCl is indicated for the treatment of hypertension. Nicardipine HCl may be used alone or in combination with other anti hypertensive drugs. In administering nicardipine it is important to be aware of the relatively large peak to trough differences in blood pressure effect. (See DOSAGE AND ADMINISTRATION.)

NON-FDA APPROVED INDICATIONS

Unapproved uses of nicardipine include treatment of migraine headaches, Raynaud's phenomenon, and congestive heart failure.

CONTRAINDICATIONS

Nicardipine HCl is contraindicated in patients with hypersensitivity to the drug.

Because part of the effect of nicardipine HCl is secondary to reduced afterload, the drug is also contraindicated in patients with advanced aortic stenosis. Reduction of diastolic pressure in these patients may worsen rather than improve myocardial oxygen balance.

WARNINGS

INCREASED ANGINA

About 7% of patients in short-term placebo-controlled angina trials have developed increased frequency, duration or severity of angina on starting nicardipine HCl or at the time of dosage increases, compared with 4% of patients on placebo. Comparisons with beta-blockers also show a greater frequency of increased angina, 4% vs 1%. The mechanism of this effect has not been established. (See ADVERSE REACTIONS.)

USE IN PATIENTS WITH CONGESTIVE HEART FAILURE

Although preliminary hemodynamic studies in patients with congestive heart failure have shown that nicardipine HCl reduced afterload without impairing myocardial contractility, it has a negative inotropic effect *in vitro* and in some patients. Caution should be exercised when using the drug in congestive heart failure patients, particularly in combination with a beta-blocker.

BETA-BLOCKER WITHDRAWAL

Nicardipine HCl is not a beta blocker and therefore gives no protection against the dangers of abrupt beta-blocker withdrawal; any such withdrawal should be by gradual reduction of the dose of beta-blocker, preferably over 8-10 days.

PRECAUTIONS

GENERAL

Blood Pressure

Because nicardipine HCl decreases peripheral resistance, careful monitoring of blood pressure during the initial administration and titration of nicardipine HCl is suggested. Nicardipine HCl, like other calcium channel blockers, may occasionally produce symptomatic hypotension. Caution is advised to avoid systemic hypotension when administering the drug to patients who have sustained an acute cerebral infarction or hemorrhage. Because of prominent effects at the time of peak blood levels, initial titration should be performed with measurements of blood pressure at peak effect (1-2 hours after dosing) and just before the next dose.

Use in Patients With Impaired Hepatic Function

Since the liver is the major site of biotransformation and since nicardipine HCl is subject to first pass metabolism, the drug should be used with caution in patients having impaired liver function or reduced hepatic blood flow. Patients with severe liver disease developed elevated blood levels (4-fold increase in AUC) and prolonged half-life (19 hours) of nicardipine HCl. (See DOSAGE AND ADMINISTRATION.)

Use in Patients With Impaired Renal Function

When nicardipine HCl 20 or 30 mg tid was given to hypertensive patients with mild renal impairment, mean plasma concentrations, AUC, and C_{max} were approximately 2-fold higher in renally impaired patients than in healthy controls. Doses in these patients must be adjusted. (See CLINICAL PHARMACOLOGY and DOSAGE AND ADMINISTRATION).

CARCINOGENESIS, MUTAGENESIS, AND IMPAIRMENT OF FERTILITY

Rats treated with nicardipine in the diet (at concentrations calculated to provide daily dosage levels of 5, 15 or 45 mg/kg/day) for 2 years showed a dose-dependent increase in thyroid hyperplasia and neoplasia (follicular adenoma/carcinoma). One (1) and 3 month studies in the rat have suggested that these results are linked to a nicardipine-induced reduction in plasma thyroxine (T4) levels with a consequent increase in plasma levels of thyroid stimulating hormone (TSH). Chronic elevation of TSH is known to cause hyperstimulation of the thyroid. in rats on an iodine deficient diet, nicardipine administration for 1 month was associated with thyroid hyperplasia that was prevented by T4 supplementation. Mice treated with nicardipine in the diet (at concentrations calculated to provide daily dosage levels of up to 100 mg/kg/day) for up to 18 months showed no evidence of neoplasia of any tissue and no evidence of thyroid changes. There was no evidence of thyroid pathology in dogs treated with up to 25 mg nicardipine/kg/day for 1 year and no evidence of effects of nicardipine on thyroid function (plasma T4 and TSH) in man.

There was no evidence of a mutagenic potential of nicardipine in a battery of genotoxicity in tests conducted on microbial indicator organisms, in micronucleus tests in mice and hamsters, or in a sister chromatid exchange study in hamsters.

No impairment of fertility was seen in male or female rats administered nicardipine at oral doses as high as 100 mg/kg/day (50 times the 40 mg tid maximum recommended antianginal or antihypertensive dose in man, assuming a patient weight of 60 kg).

PREGNANCY CATEGORY C

Nicardipine was embryocidal when administered orally to pregnant Japanese White rabbits, during organogenesis, at 150 mg/kg/day (a dose associated with marked body weight gain suppression in the treated doe) but not at 50 mg/kg/day (25 times the maximum recommended antianginal or antihypertensive dose in man). No adverse effects on the fetus were observed when New Zealand albino rabbits were treated, during organogenesis, with up to 100 mg nicardipine/kg/day (a dose associated with significant mortality in the treated doe). In pregnant rats administered nicardipine orally at up to 100 mg/kg/day (50 times the maximum recommended human dose) there was no evidence of embryolethality or teratogenicity. However, dystocia, reduced birth weights, reduced neonatal survival and reduced neonatal weight gain were noted. There are no adequate and well-controlled studies in pregnant women. Nicardipine HCl should be used during pregnancy only if the potential benefit justifies the potential risk to the fetus.

NURSING MOTHERS

Studies in rats have shown significant concentrations of nicardipine HCl in maternal milk following oral administration. For this reason it is recommended that women who wish to breast-feed should not take this drug.

PEDIATRIC USE

Safety and efficacy in patients under the age of 18 have not been established.

GERIATRIC USE

Pharmacokinetic parameters did not differ between elderly hypertensive patients (≥65 years) and healthy controls after 1 week of nicardipine HCl treatment at 20 mg tid. Plasma nicardipine HCl concentrations in elderly hypertensive patients were similar to plasma concentrations in healthy young adult subjects when nicardipine HCl was administered at doses of 10, 200 and 30 mg tid, suggesting that the pharmacokinetics of nicardipine HCl are similar in young and elderly hypertensive patients. No significant differences in responses to nicardipine HCl have been observed in elderly patients and the general adult population of patients who participated in clinical studies.

DRUG INTERACTIONS

BETA-BLOCKERS

In controlled clinical studies, adrenergic beta-receptor blockers have been frequently administered concomitantly with nicardipine HCl. The combination is well tolerated.

N

CIMETIDINE

Cimetidine increases nicardipine HCl plasma levels. Patients receiving the two drugs concomitantly should be carefully monitored.

DIGOXIN

Some calcium blockers may increase the concentration of digitalis preparations in the blood. Nicardipine HCl usually does not alter the plasma levels of digoxin, however, serum digoxin levels should be evaluated after concomitant therapy with nicardipine HCl is initiated.

MAALOX

Co-administration of Maalox TC had no effect on nicardipine HCl absorption.

FENTANYL ANESTHESIA

Severe hypotension has been reported during fentanyl anesthesia with concomitant use of a beta-blocker and a calcium channel blocker. Even though such interactions were not seen during clinical studies with nicardipine HCl, an increased volume of circulating fluids might be required if such an interaction were to occur.

CYCLOSPORINE

Concomitant administration of nicardipine and cyclosporine levels. Plasma concentrations of cyclosporine should therefore be closely monitored, and its dosage reduced accordingly, in patients treated with nicardipine.

When therapeutic concentrations of *furosemide, propranolol, dipyridamole, warfarin, quinidine,* or *naproxen* were added to human plasma *(in vitro),* the plasma protein binding of nicardipine HCl was not altered.

ADVERSE REACTIONS

In multiple-dose US and foreign controlled short-term (up to 3 months) studies 1910 patients received nicardipine HCl alone or in combination with other drugs. in these studies adverse events were reported spontaneously; adverse experiences were generally not serious but occasionally required dosage adjustment and about 10% of patients left the studies prematurely because of them. Peak responses were not observed to be associated with adverse effects during clinical trials, but physicians should be aware that adverse effects associated with decreases in blood pressure (tachycardia, hypotension, etc.) could occur around the time of the peak effect. Most adverse effects were expected consequences of the vasodilator effects of nicardipine HCl.

ANGINA

The incidence rates of adverse effects in anginal patients were derived from multicenter, controlled clinical trials. Following are the rates of adverse effects for nicardipine HCl (n=520) and placebo (n=310), respectively, that occurred in 0.4% of patients or more. These represent events considered probably drug-related by the investigator (except for certain cardiovascular events which were recorded in a different category). Where the frequency of adverse effects for nicardipine HCl and placebo is similar, causal relationship is uncertain. The only dose-related effects were pedal edema and increased angina.

N

TABLE 3 *Percent of Patients With Adverse Effects in Controlled Studies (Incidence of discontinuations shown in parentheses)*

Adverse Experience	Nicardipine HCl (n=520)	Placebo (n=310)
Pedal edema	7.1% (0%)	0.3% (0%)
Dizziness	6.9% (1.2%)	0.6% (0%)
Headache	6.4% (0.6%)	2.6% (0%)
Asthenia	5.8% (0.4%)	2.6% (0%)
Flushing	5.6% (3.5%)	1.0% (0%)
Increased angina	5.6% (3.5%)	4.2% (1.9%)
Palpitations	3.3% (0.4%)	0.0% (0%)
Nausea	1.9% (0%)	0.3% (0%)
Dyspepsia	1.5% (0.6%)	0.6% (0.3%)
Dry mouth	1.4% (0%)	0.3% (0%)
Somnolence	1.4% (0%)	1.0% (0%)
Rash	1.2% (0.2%)	0.3% (0%)
Tachycardia	1.2% (0.2%)	0.6% (0%)
Myalgia	1.0% (0%)	0.0% (0%)
Other edema	1.0% (0%)	0.0% (0%)
Paresthesia	1.0% (0.2%)	0.3% (0%)
Sustained tachycardia	0.8% (0.6%)	0.0% (0%)
Syncope	0.8% (0.2%)	0.0% (0%)
Constipation	0.6% (0.2%)	0.6% (0%)
Dyspnea	0.6% (0%)	0.0% (0%)
Abnormal ECG	0.6% (0.6%)	0.0% (0%)
Malaise	0.6% (0%)	0.0% (0%)
Nervousness	0.6% (0%)	0.3% (0%)
Tremor	0.6% (0%)	0.0% (0%)

In addition, adverse events were observed which are not readily distinguishable from the natural history of the atherosclerotic vascular disease in these patients. Adverse events in this category each occurred in <0.4% of patients receiving nicardipine HCl and included myocardial infarction, atrial fibrillation, exertional hypotension, pericarditis, heart block, cerebral ischemia and ventricular tachycardia. it is possible that some of these events were drug-related.

HYPERTENSION

The incidence rates of adverse effects in hypertensive patients were derived from multicenter, controlled clinical trials. Following are the rates of adverse effects for nicardipine HCl (n=1390) and placebo (n=211), respectively, that occurred in 0.4% of patients or more. These represent events considered probably drug-related by the investigator. Where the frequency of adverse effects for nicardipine HCl and placebo is similar, causal relationship is uncertain. The only dose-related effect was pedal edema.

TABLE 4 *Percent of Patients with Adverse Effects in Controlled Studies (Incidence of discontinuations shown in parentheses)*

Adverse Experience	Nicardipine HCl (n=1390)	Placebo (n=211)
Flushing	9.7% (2.1%)	2.8% (0%)
Headache	8.2% (2.6%)	4.7% (0%)
Pedal edema	8.0% (1.8%)	0.9% (0%)
Asthenia	4.2% (1.7%)	0.5% (0%)
Palpitations	4.1% (1.0%)	0.0% (0%)
Dizziness	4.0% (1.8%)	0.0% (0%)
Tachycardia	3.4% (1.2%)	0.5% (0%)
Nausea	2.2% (0.9%)	0.9% (0%)
Somnolence	1.1% (0.1%)	0.0% (0%)
Dyspepsia	0.8% (0.3%)	0.5% (0%)
Insomnia	0.6% (0.1%)	0.0% (0%)
Malaise	0.6% (0.1%)	0.0% (0%)
Other edema	0.6% (0.3%)	1.4% (0%)
Abnormal dreams	0.4% (0%)	0.0% (0%)
Dry mouth	0.4% (0.1%)	0.0% (0%)
Nocturia	0.4% (0%)	0.0% (0%)
Rash	0.4% (0.4%)	0.0% (0%)
Vomiting	0.4% (0.4%)	0.0% (0%)

RARE EVENTS

The following rare adverse events have been reported in clinical trials or the literature:

Body as a Whole: Infection, allergic reaction.

Cardiovascular: Hypotension, postural hypotension, atypical chest pain, peripheral vascular disorder, ventricular extrasystoles, ventricular tachycardia.

Digestive: Sore throat, abnormal liver chemistries.

Musculoskeletal: Arthralgia.

Nervous: Hot flashes, vertigo, hyperkinesia, impotence, depression, confusion, anxiety.

Respiratory: Rhinitis, sinusitis.

Special Senses: Tinnitus, abnormal vision, blurred vision.

Urogenital: Increased urinary frequency.

DOSAGE AND ADMINISTRATION

ANGINA

The dose should be individually titrated for each patient beginning with 20-40 mg three times daily. Doses in the range of 20-40 mg three times a day have been shown to be effective. At least 3 days should be allowed before increasing the nicardipine HCl dose to ensure achievement of steady state plasma drug concentrations.

CONCOMITANT USE WITH OTHER ANTIHYPERTENSIVE AGENTS

Sublingual NTG: May be taken as required to abort acute anginal attacks during nicardipine HCl therapy.

Prophylactic Nitrate Therapy: Nicardipine HCl may be safely coadministered with short- and long-acting nitrates.

Beta-blockers: Nicardipine HCl may be safely coadministered with beta-blockers. (See DRUG INTERACTIONS.)

HYPERTENSION

The dose of nicardipine HCl should be individually adjusted according to the blood pressure response beginning with 20 mg three times daily. The effective doses in clinical trials have ranged from 20-40 mg three times daily. The maximum blood pressure lowering effect occurs approximately 1-2 hours after dosing. **To assess the adequacy of blood pressure response, the blood pressure should be measured at trough (8 hours after dosing). Because of the prominent peak effects of nicardipine, blood pressure should be measured 1-2 hours after dosing, particularly during initiation of therapy.** (See PRECAUTIONS, General, Blood Pressure, INDICATIONS AND USAGE and CLINICAL PHARMACOLOGY.) At least 3 days should be allowed before increasing the nicardipine HCl dose to ensure achievement of steady state plasma drug concentrations.

CONCOMITANT USE WITH OTHER ANTIHYPERTENSIVE AGENTS

Diuretics: Nicardipine HCl may be safely coadministered with thiazide diuretics.

Beta-blockers: Nicardipine HCl may be safely coadministered with beta-blockers. (See DRUG INTERACTIONS.)

SPECIAL PATIENT POPULATIONS

Renal Insufficiency: Although there is no evidence that nicardipine HCl impairs renal function, careful dose titration beginning with 20 mg tid is advised. (See PRECAUTIONS.)

Hepatic Insufficiency: Nicardipine HCl should be administered cautiously in,patients with severely impaired hepatic function. A suggested starting dose of 20 mg twice a day is advised with individual titration based on clinical findings maintaining the twice a day schedule. (See PRECAUTIONS.)

Congestive Heart Failure: Caution is advised when titrating nicardipine HCl dosage in patients with congestive heart failure. (See WARNINGS.)

PRODUCT LISTING - RATED THERAPEUTICALLY EQUIVALENT

Capsule - Oral - 20 mg

90's	$39.25	GENERIC, Mylan Pharmaceuticals Inc	00378-1020-77
100's	$33.75	FEDERAL UPPER LIMIT, H.C.F.A. F F P	99999-1882-01
100's	$39.25	GENERIC, Ivax Corporation	00172-4288-60
100's	$39.25	GENERIC, Par Pharmaceutical Inc	49884-0498-01
100's	$45.77	GENERIC, Teva Pharmaceuticals Usa	00093-0793-01

Capsule - Oral - 30 mg

90's	$56.17	GENERIC, Mylan Pharmaceuticals Inc	00378-1430-77
100's	$40.50	FEDERAL UPPER LIMIT, H.C.F.A. F F P	99999-1882-02

100's	$62.42	GENERIC, Ivax Corporation	00172-4289-60
100's	$62.42	GENERIC, Par Pharmaceutical Inc	49884-0499-01
100's	$65.55	GENERIC, Teva Pharmaceuticals Usa	00093-0794-01

PRODUCT LISTING - EQUIVALENTS NOT AVAILABLE

Capsule - Oral - 20 mg

100's	$58.11	CARDENE, Roche Laboratories	00004-0183-01

Capsule - Oral - 30 mg

100's	$92.40	CARDENE, Roche Laboratories	00004-0184-01

Capsule, Extended Release - Oral - 30 mg

50's	$42.27	CARDENE SR, Physicians Total Care	54868-3817-00
60's	$54.49	CARDENE SR, Roche Laboratories	00004-0180-22
200's	$181.48	CARDENE SR, Roche Laboratories	00004-0180-91

Capsule, Extended Release - Oral - 45 mg

60's	$86.51	CARDENE SR, Roche Laboratories	00004-0181-22
200's	$288.24	CARDENE SR, Roche Laboratories	00004-0181-91

Capsule, Extended Release - Oral - 60 mg

60's	$103.55	CARDENE SR, Roche Laboratories	00004-0182-22
200's	$265.60	CARDENE SR, Roche Laboratories	00004-0182-91

Solution - Injectable - 2.5 mg/ml

10 ml x 10	$669.40	CARDENE IV, Wyeth-Ayerst Laboratories	00008-0812-02

Nicotine *(003109)*

Categories: Smoking cessation; Pregnancy Category D; FDA Approved 1991 Nov
Drug Classes: Stimulants, central nervous system
Brand Names: Habitrol; **Nicoderm**; Nicotrol; Prostep
Foreign Brand Availability: Nicabate (Australia); Nicabate TTS (New-Zealand); Nicobate CQ Clear (Australia); Nicolan (Denmark; Mexico); Nicolan Light (Denmark); Nicopatch (France); Nicorest (France); Nicorette (Australia; Austria; Bahrain; Belgium; Benin; Burkina-Faso; Canada; China; Colombia; Cyprus; Denmark; Egypt; Ethiopia; Finland; France; Gambia; Germany; Ghana; Greece; Guinea; Hong-Kong; Hungary; Iran; Iraq; Israel; Italy; Ivory-Coast; Jordan; Kenya; Korea; Kuwait; Lebanon; Liberia; Libya; Malawi; Mali; Mauritania; Mauritius; Mexico; Morocco; Netherlands; Niger; Nigeria; Norway; Oman; Poland; Qatar; Republic-of-Yemen; Saudi-Arabia; Senegal; Seychelles; Sierra-Leone; South-Africa; Spain; Sudan; Sweden; Switzerland; Syria; Taiwan; Tanzania; Thailand; Tunia; Uganda; United-Arab-Emirates; Zambia; Zimbabwe); Nicorette Fruit (France); Nicorette Inhaler (Australia); Nicorette Menthe (Bahrain; Cyprus; Egypt; France; Iran; Iraq; Israel; Jordan; Kuwait; Lebanon; Libya; Oman; Qatar; Republic-of-Yemen; Saudi-Arabia; Syria; United-Arab-Emirates); Nicorette Orange (France); Nicorette Orange sans sucre (France); Nicostop (Portugal); Nicotinell (Australia; Austria; Belgium; Denmark; England; Finland; France; Germany; Greece; Hungary; Ireland; Italy; Netherlands; Norway; Portugal; Sweden; Switzerland); Nicotinell Chewing Gum (Hong-Kong); Nicotinell Fruit sans sucre (France); Nicotinell Lozenge (Hong-Kong); Nicotinell Menthe sans sucre (France); Nicotinell Mint Lozenge (Singapore); Nicotinell TTS (Bahamas; Bahrain; Barbados; Belize; Benin; Bermuda; Burkina-Faso; Curacao; Cyprus; Egypt; Ethiopia; France; Gambia; Ghana; Guinea; Guyana; Hong-Kong; Iran; Iraq; Israel; Ivory-Coast; Jamaica; Jordan; Kenya; Kuwait; Lebanon; Liberia; Libya; Malawi; Malaysia; Mali; Mauritania; Mauritius; Mexico; Morocco; Netherland-Antilles; New-Zealand; Niger; Nigeria; Oman; Qatar; Republic-of-Yemen; Saudi-Arabia; Senegal; Seychelles; Sierra-Leone; Sudan; Surinam; Syria; Taiwan; Tanzania; Thailand; Trinidad; Tunia; Uganda; United-Arab-Emirates; Zambia; Zimbabwe); Nicotrans (Italy); Nikofrenon (Germany); Niquitin (France; Mexico); Niquitin CQ (Israel); Niquitin-clear (France); Niquitin sans sucre (France); Quit Spray (South-Africa)

INHALATION

DESCRIPTION

Note: The trade names have been used throughout this monograph for clarity.

NICOTROL INHALER

Nicotrol Inhaler (nicotine inhalation system) consists of a mouthpiece and a plastic cartridge delivering 4 mg of nicotine from a porous plug containing 10 mg nicotine. The cartridge is inserted into the mouthpiece prior to use. Nicotine is a tertiary amine composed of a pyridine and a pyrrolidine ring. It is a colorless to pale yellow, freely water-soluble, strongly alkaline, oily, volatile, hygroscopic liquid obtained from the tobacco plant. Nicotine has a characteristic pungent odor and turns brown on exposure to air or light. Of its two stereoisomers, S(-)nicotine is the more active. It is the prevalent form in tobacco, and is the form in the Nicotrol Inhaler. The free alkaloid is absorbed rapidly through skin, mucous membranes, and the respiratory tract.

Chemical Name: S-3-(1-methyl-2-pyrrolidinyl)pyridine
Molecular Formula: $C_{10}H_{14}N_2$
Molecular Weight: 162.23
Ionization Constants: pKa1 = 7.84, pKa2 = 3.04 at 15°C
Octanol-Water Partition Coefficient: 15:1 at pH 7

Nicotine is the active ingredient; inactive components of the product are menthol and a porous plug which are pharmacologically inactive. Nicotine is released when air is inhaled through the Inhaler.

NICOTROL NS

Nicotrol NS (nicotine nasal spray) is an aqueous solution of nicotine intended for administration as a metered spray to the nasal mucosa.

Nicotine is a tertiary amine composed of pyridine and a pyrrolidine ring. It is a colorless to pale yellow, freely water-soluble, strongly alkaline, oily, volatile, hygroscopic liquid obtained from the tobacco plant. Nicotine has a characteristic pungent odor and turns brown on exposure to air or light. Of its two stereoisomers, S(-)nicotine is the more active. It is the prevalent form in tobacco, and is the form in Nicotrol NS. The free alkaloid is absorbed rapidly through skin, mucous membranes, and the respiratory tract.

Chemical Name: S-3-(1-methyl-2-pyrrolidinyl)pyridine
Molecular Formula: $C_{10}H_{14}N_2$
Molecular Weight: 162.23
Ionization Constants: pKa1 = 7.84, pKa2 = 3.04 at 15°C
Octanol-Water Partition Coefficient: 15:1 at pH 7

Each 10 ml spray bottle contains 100 mg nicotine (10 mg/ml) in an inactive vehicle containing disodium phosphate, sodium dihydrogen phosphate, citric acid, methylparaben, propylparaben, edetate disodium, sodium chloride, polysorbate 80, aroma and water. The solution is isotonic with a pH of 7. It contains no chlorofluorocarbons.

After priming the delivery system for Nicotrol NS, each actuation of the unit delivers a metered dose spray containing approximately 0.5 mg of nicotine. The size of the droplets produced by the unit is in excess of 8 microns. One Nicotrol NS unit delivers approximately 200 applications.

CLINICAL PHARMACOLOGY

NICOTROL INHALER

Pharmacologic Action

Nicotine, the chief alkaloid in tobacco products, binds stereo-selectively to nicotinic-cholinergic receptors at the autonomic ganglia, in the adrenal medulla, at neuromuscular junctions, and in the brain. Two types of central nervous system effects are believed to be the basis of nicotine's positively reinforcing properties. A stimulating effect is exerted mainly in the cortex via the locus ceruleus and a reward effect is exerted in the limbic system. At low doses the stimulant effects predominate while at high doses the reward effects predominate. Intermittent intravenous administration of nicotine activates neurohormonal pathways, releasing acetylcholine, norepinephrine, dopamine, serotonin, vasopressin, beta-endorphin, growth hormone, and ACTH.

Pharmacodynamics

The cardiovascular effects of nicotine include peripheral vasoconstriction, tachycardia, and elevated blood pressure. Acute and chronic tolerance to nicotine develops from smoking tobacco or ingesting nicotine preparations. Acute tolerance (a reduction in response for a given dose) develops rapidly (less than 1 hour), but not at the same rate for different physiologic effects (skin temperature, heart rate, subjective effects). Withdrawal symptoms such as cigarette craving can be reduced in most individuals by plasma nicotine levels lower than those from smoking. Withdrawal from nicotine in addicted individuals can be characterized by craving, nervousness, restlessness, irritability, mood lability, anxiety, drowsiness, sleep disturbances, impaired concentration, increased appetite, minor somatic complaints (headache, myalgia, constipation, fatigue), and weight gain. Nicotine toxicity is characterized by nausea, abdominal pain, vomiting, diarrhea, diaphoresis, flushing, dizziness, disturbed hearing and vision, confusion, weakness, palpitations, altered respiration and hypotension. Both smoking and nicotine can increase circulating cortisol and catecholamines, and tolerance does not develop to the catecholamine-releasing effects of nicotine. Changes in the response to a concomitantly administered adrenergic agonist or antagonist should be watched for when nicotine intake is altered during Nicotrol Inhaler therapy and/or smoking cessation (see DRUG INTERACTIONS, Nicotrol Inhaler).

Pharmacokinetics

Absorption

Most of the nicotine released from the Nicotrol Inhaler is deposited in the mouth. Only a fraction of the dose released, less than 5%, reaches the lower respiratory tract. An intensive inhalation regimen (80 deep inhalations over 20 minutes) releases on the average 4 mg of the nicotine content of each cartridge of which about 2 mg is systemically absorbed. Peak plasma concentrations are typically reached within 15 minutes of the end of inhalation.

Absorption of nicotine through the buccal mucosa is relatively slow and the high and rapid rise followed by the decline in nicotine arterial plasma concentrations seen with cigarette smoking are not achieved with the Inhaler. After use of the single Inhaler the arterial nicotine concentrations rise slowly to an average of 6 ng/ml in contrast to those of a cigarette, which increase rapidly and reach a mean C_{max} of approximately 49 ng/ml within 5 minutes.

The temperature dependency of nicotine release from the Nicotrol Inhaler was studied between 68°F and 104°F in 18 patients. Average achievable steady state plasma levels after 20 minutes of an intensive in-halation regimen each hour at ambient room temperature are on the order of 23 ng/ml. The corresponding nicotine plasma levels achievable at 86°F and 104°F are on the order of 30 and 34 ng/ml. Nicotine peak plasma concentration (C_{max}) at steady-state, after 20 minutes of an intensive inhalation regimen per hour, for 10 hours. (See TABLE 1.)

TABLE 1

	C_{max} (ng/ml)		
	20°C/68°F	30°C/86°F	40°C/104°F
	n=18	n=18	n=18
Mean	22.5	29.7	34.0
SD	7.7	8.3	6.9
Min	11.1	17.6	24.1
Max	40.4	47.2	48.6

Ad libitum use of the Nicotrol Inhaler typically produces nicotine plasma levels of 6-8 ng/ml, corresponding to about 1/3 of those achieved with cigarette smoking.

Distribution

The volume of distribution following IV administration of nicotine is approximately 2-3 L/kg. Plasma protein binding of nicotine is <5%. Therefore, changes in nicotine binding from use of concomitant drugs or alterations of plasma proteins by disease states would not be expected to have significant effects on nicotine kinetics.

Metabolism

More than 20 metabolites of nicotine have been identified, all of which are less active than the parent compound. The primary urinary metabolites are cotinine (15% of the dose) and trans-3-hydroxycotinine (45% of the dose). Cotinine has a half-life of 15-20 hours and concentrations that exceed nicotine by 10-fold. The major site for the metabolism of nicotine is the liver. The kidney and lung are also sites of nicotine metabolism.

N

Elimination
About 10% of the nicotine absorbed is excreted unchanged in the urine. This may be increased to up to 30% with high urine flow rates and urinary acidification below pH 5. The average plasma clearance is about 1.2 L/min in a healthy adult smoker. The apparent elimination half-life of nicotine is 1-2 hours.

Gender Differences
Intersubject variability coefficients of variation (CV) for the pharma-cokinetic parameters (AUC and C_{max}) were approximately 40% and 30% respectively, for males and females. There were no medically significant differences between females and males in the kinetics of Nicotrol Inhaler.

NICOTROL NS
Pharmacologic Action
Nicotine, the chief alkaloid in tobacco products, binds stereo-selectively to nicotinic-cholinergic receptors at the autonomic ganglia, in the adrenal medulla, at neuromuscular junctions, and in the brain. Two types of central nervous system effects are believed to be the basis of nicotine's positively reinforcing properties. A stimulating effect is exerted mainly in the cortex via the locus ceruleus and a reward effect is exerted in the limbic system. At low doses, the stimulant effects predominate while at high doses the reward effects predominate. Intermittent intravenous administration of nicotine activates neurohormonal pathways, releasing acetylcholine, norepinephrine, dopamine, serotonin, vasopressin, beta-endorphin, growth hormone, and ACTH.

Pharmacodynamics
The cardiovascular effects of nicotine include peripheral vasoconstriction, tachycardia, and elevated blood pressure. Acute and chronic tolerance to nicotine develops from smoking tobacco or ingesting nicotine preparations. Acute tolerance (a reduction in response for a given dose) develops rapidly (less than 1 hour), but not at the same rate for different physiologic effects (skin temperature, heart rate, subjective effects). Withdrawal symptoms such as cigarette craving can be reduced in most individuals by plasma nicotine levels lower than those from smoking.

Withdrawal from nicotine in addicted individuals can be characterized by craving, nervousness, restlessness, irritability, mood lability, anxiety, drowsiness, sleep disturbances, impaired concentration, increased appetite, minor somatic complaints (headache, myalgia, constipation, fatigue), and weight gain. Nicotine toxicity is characterized by nausea, abdominal pain, vomiting, diarrhea, diaphoresis, flushing, dizziness, disturbed hearing and vision, confusion, weakness, palpitations, altered respiration and hypotension.

Both smoking and nicotine can increase circulating cortisol and catecholamines, and tolerance does not develop to the catecholamine-releasing effects of nicotine. Changes in the response to a concomitantly administered adrenergic agonist or antagonist should be watched for when nicotine intake is altered during Nicotrol NS therapy and/or smoking cessation (see DRUG INTERACTIONS, Nicotrol NS).

Pharmacokinetics
Each actuation of Nicotrol NS delivers a metered 50 µl spray containing approximately 0.5 mg of nicotine. One dose is considered 1 mg of nicotine (2 sprays, one in each nostril).

Absorption
Following administration of 2 sprays of Nicotrol NS approximately 53% ± 16% (Mean ±SD) enters the systemic circulation. No significant difference in rate or extent of absorption could be seen due to the deposition of nicotine on different parts of the nasal mucosa. Plasma concentrations of nicotine obtained from 1 dose (1 mg nicotine) of Nicotrol NS rise rapidly, reaching maximum venous concentrations of 2-12 ng/ml in 4-15 minutes. The apparent absorption half-life of nicotine is approximately 3 minutes. There is wide variation among subjects in their plasma nicotine concentrations from the spray. As a result, after a 1 mg dose of spray approximately 20% of the subjects reached peak nicotine concentrations similar to those seen after smoking one cigarette (7-17 ng/ml).

TABLE 2 *Trough Plasma Nicotine Concentrations After 11 hours of Dosing With 1, 2 and 3 mg of Nicotrol NS per Hour (n=16)*

Dose	Mean (ng/ml) ±SD	(Range)
1 mg every 60 minutes (1 mg/h)	6 ± 3	(1.7-12)
1 mg every 30 minutes (2 mg/h)	14 ± 6	(1.5-24)
1 mg every 20 minutes (3 mg/h)	18 ± 10	(1.2-35)

The data from TABLE 2 is derived from a three-way cross-over study of repeated applications of Nicotrol NS in 16 smokers (8 male, 8 female) ranging in age from 18-48 years.

Sixteen smokers (7 males and 9 females) ranging in age from 22-44 years were dosed with 1 mg of Nicotrol NS every hour for 10 hours. The pharmacokinetic parameters that were obtained are presented in TABLE 3.

TABLE 3 *Nicotine Pharmacokinetic Parameters at Steady-State for 1 mg/h of Nicotrol NS Administered Hourly for 10 Hours (Mean ±SD and Range) (n=16)*

Parameter	1 mg (2 sprays)	(Range)
C_{avg} (ng/ml)	8 ± 3	(2.5-12)
C_{max} (ng/ml)	9 ± 3	(3.1-14)
T_{max} (minutes)	13 ± 5	(10-20)

C_{avg}: Average plasma nicotine concentration for the dosing interval of 10-11 hours.
C_{max}: Maximum measured plasma concentration after last dose administration.
T_{max}: Time of maximum plasma concentration after last dose administration.

Distribution
The volume of distribution following IV administration of nicotine is approximately 2-3 L/kg. Plasma protein binding of nicotine is 5%. Therefore, changes in nicotine binding from use of concomitant drugs or alterations of plasma proteins by disease states would not be expected to have significant effects on nicotine kinetics.

Metabolism
More than 20 metabolites of nicotine have been identified, all of which are less active than the parent compound. The primary urinary metabolites are cotinine (15% of the dose) and trans-3-hydroxycotinine (45% of the dose). Cotinine has a half-life of 15-20 hours and concentrations that exceed nicotine by 10-fold. The major site for the metabolism of nicotine is the liver. The kidney and lung are also sites of nicotine metabolism.

Elimination
About 10% of the nicotine absorbed is excreted unchanged in the urine. This may be increased to up to 30% with high urine flow rates and urinary acidification below pH 5. The average plasma clearance is about 1.2 L/min in a healthy adult smoker. The apparent elimination half-life of nicotine from Nicotrol NS is 1-2 hours.

Pharmacokinetic Model
The data were well described by a two-compartment model with first-order input. Based on individual fits (n=18) the following parameters were derived after the administration of a 1 mg dose: Absorption rate constant (Ka) = 14.4 ± 7.3 h^{-1} (Mean ±SD), Elimination rate constant (Ke) = 0.60 ± 0.53 h^{-1}, Distribution rate constants (K12) = 4.84 ± 2.57 h^{-1}, (K21) = 4.35 ± 2.30 h^{-1}, Volume of distribution over fraction absorbed (V/F) = 2.73 ± 0.82 L/kg in 8 female and 10 male adults weighing 76 ± 15 kg.

Gender Differences
Intersubject variability (50% coefficient of variation) among the pharmacokinetic parameters (AUC, C_{max} and Clearance/kg) were observed for both genders. There were no differences between females or males in the kinetics of Nicotrol NS.

Drug/Drug Interactions
The extent of absorption is slightly reduced (approximately 10%) in patients with the common cold/rhinitis. In patients with rhinitis the peak plasma concentration is reduced by approximately 20% (concentrations are lower by 1.5 ng/ml on average) and the time to peak concentration prolonged by approximately 30% (delayed by 7 minutes on average). The use of a nasal vasoconstrictor such as xylometazoline in patients with rhinitis will further prolong the time to peak by approximately 40% (delayed by 15 minutes on average), but the peak plasma concentration remains on average the same as those with rhinitis.

INDICATIONS AND USAGE

NICOTROL INHALER
Nicotrol Inhaler is indicated as an aid to smoking cessation for the relief of nicotine withdrawal symptoms. Nicotrol Inhaler therapy is recommended for use as part of a comprehensive behavioral smoking cessation program.

NICOTROL NS
Nicotrol NS is indicated as an aid to smoking cessation for the relief of nicotine withdrawal symptoms. Nicotrol NS therapy should be used as a part of a comprehensive behavioral smoking cessation program.

The safety and efficacy of the continued use of Nicotrol NS for periods longer than 6 months have not been adequately studied and such use is not recommended.

CONTRAINDICATIONS

NICOTROL INHALER
Use of Nicotrol Inhaler therapy is contraindicated in patients with known hypersensitivity or allergy to nicotine or to menthol.

NICOTROL NS
Use of Nicotrol NS therapy is contraindicated in patients with known hypersensitivity or allergy to nicotine or to any component of the product.

WARNINGS

NICOTROL INHALER
Nicotine from any source can be toxic and addictive. Smoking causes lung disease, cancer and heart disease, and may adversely affect pregnant women or the fetus. For any smoker, with or without concomitant disease or pregnancy, the risk of nicotine replacement in a smoking cessation program should be weighed against the hazard of continued smoking, and the likelihood of achieving cessation of smoking without nicotine replacement.

Pregnancy, Warning
Tobacco smoke, which has been shown to be harmful to the fetus, contains nicotine, hydrogen cyanide, and carbon monoxide. The Nicotrol Inhaler does not deliver hydrogen cyanide and carbon monoxide. However, nicotine has been shown in animal studies to cause fetal harm. It is therefore presumed that Nicotrol Inhaler can cause fetal harm when administered to a pregnant woman. The effect of nicotine delivery by Nicotrol Inhaler has not been examined in pregnancy (see PRECAUTIONS, Nicotrol Inhaler). Therefore, pregnant smokers should be encouraged to attempt cessation using educational and behavioral interventions before using pharmacological approaches. If Nicotrol Inhaler is used during pregnancy, or if the patient becomes pregnant while using it, the patient should be apprised of the potential hazard to the fetus.

Safety Note Concerning Children
This product contains nicotine and should be kept out of the reach of children and pets. The amounts of nicotine that are tolerated by adult smokers can produce symptoms of poisoning and could prove fatal if the nicotine from the Nicotrol Inhaler is inhaled, ingested, or buc-

cally absorbed by children or pets. A cartridge contains about 60% of its initial drug content when it is discarded, which is about 6 mg. Patients should be cautioned to keep both the used and unused cartridges of Nicotrol Inhaler out of the reach of children and pets.

All components of the Nicotrol Inhaler system should also be kept out of the reach of children and pets to avoid accidental swallowing and choking.

NICOTROL NS

Nicotine from any source can be toxic and addictive. Smoking causes lung disease, cancer and heart disease, and may adversely affect pregnant women or the fetus. For any smoker, with or without concomitant disease or pregnancy, the risk of nicotine replacement in a smoking cessation program should be weighed against the hazard of continued smoking, and the likelihood of achieving cessation of smoking without nicotine replacement.

Pregnancy, Warning

Tobacco smoke, which has been shown to be harmful to the fetus, contains nicotine, hydrogen cyanide, and carbon monoxide. The Nicotrol NS does not deliver hydrogen cyanide and carbon monoxide. However, nicotine has been shown in animal studies to cause fetal harm. It is therefore presumed that Nicotrol NS can cause fetal harm when administered to a pregnant woman. The effect of nicotine delivery by Nicotrol NS has not been examined in pregnancy (see PRECAUTIONS, Nicotrol NS). Therefore, pregnant smokers should be encouraged to attempt cessation using educational and behavioral interventions before using pharmacological approaches. If Nicotrol NS is used during pregnancy, or if the patient becomes pregnant while using it, the patient should be apprised of the potential hazard to the fetus.

Safety Note Concerning Children

This product contains nicotine and should be kept out of the reach of children and pets. The amounts of nicotine that are tolerated by adult smokers can produce symptoms of poisoning and could prove fatal if the nicotine from the Nicotrol NS is inhaled, ingested, or buccally absorbed by children or pets. A cartridge contains about 60% of its initial drug content when it is discarded, which is about 6 mg. Patients should be cautioned to keep both the used and unused cartridges of Nicotrol Nasal Spray out of the reach of children and pets.

All components of the Nicotrol NS system should also be kept out of the reach of children and pets to avoid accidental swallowing and choking.

PRECAUTIONS

NICOTROL INHALER

General

The patient should be urged to stop smoking completely when initiating Nicotrol Inhaler therapy (see DOSAGE AND ADMINISTRATION, Nicotrol Inhaler). Patients should be informed that if they continue to smoke while using the product, they may experience adverse effects due to peak nicotine levels higher than those experienced from smoking alone. If there is a clinically significant increase in cardiovascular or other effects attributable to nicotine, the treatment should be discontinued (see WARNINGS, Nicotrol Inhaler). Physicians should anticipate that concomitant medications may need dosage adjustment (see DRUG INTERACTIONS, Nicotrol Inhaler). Sustained use (beyond 6 months) of Nicotrol Inhaler by patients who stop smoking has not been studied and is not recommended.

Bronchospastic Disease

Nicotrol Inhaler has not been specifically studied in asthma or chronic pulmonary disease. Nicotine is an airway irritant and might cause bronchospasm. Nicotrol Inhaler should be used with caution in patients with bronchospastic disease. Other forms of nicotine replacement might be preferable in patients with severe bronchospastic airway disease.

Cardiovascular or Peripheral Vascular Diseases

The risks of nicotine replacement in patients with cardiovascular and peripheral vascular diseases should be weighed against the benefits of including nicotine replacement in a smoking cessation program for them. Specifically, patients with coronary heart disease (history of myocardial infarction and/or angina pectoris), serious cardiac arrhythmias, or vasospastic diseases (Buerger's disease, Prinzmetal's variant angina and Raynaud's phenomena) should be evaluated carefully before nicotine replacement is prescribed. Tachycardia and palpitations have been reported occasionally with the use of Nicotrol Inhaler as well as with other nicotine replacement therapies. No serious cardiovascular events were reported in clinical studies with Nicotrol Inhaler, but if such symptoms occur, its use should be discontinued. Nicotrol Inhaler generally should not be used in patients during the immediate post-myocardial infarction period, nor in patients with serious arrhythmias, or with severe or worsening angina.

Renal or Hepatic Insufficiency

The pharmacokinetics of nicotine have not been studied in the elderly or in patients with renal or hepatic impairment. However, given that nicotine is extensively metabolized and that its total system clearance is dependent on liver blood flow, some influence of hepatic impairment on drug kinetics (reduced clearance) should be anticipated. Only severe renal impairment would be expected to affect the clearance of nicotine or its metabolites from the circulation (see CLINICAL PHARMACOLOGY, Pharmacokinetics, Nicotrol Inhaler).

Endocrine Diseases

Nicotrol Inhaler therapy should be used with caution in patients with hyperthyroidism, pheochromocytoma or insulin-dependent diabetes, since nicotine causes the release of catecholamines by the adrenal medulla.

Peptic Ulcer Disease

Nicotine delays healing in peptic ulcer disease; therefore, Nicotrol Inhaler therapy should be used with caution in patients with active peptic ulcers and only when the benefits of including nicotine replacement in a smoking cessation program outweigh the risks.

Accelerated Hypertension

Nicotine therapy constitutes a risk factor for development of malignant hypertension in patients with accelerated hypertension; therefore, Nicotrol Inhaler therapy should be used with caution in these patients and only when the benefits of including nicotine replacement in a smoking cessation program outweigh the risks.

Information for the Patient

A patient information sheet is included in the package of Nicotrol Inhaler cartridges dispensed to the patient. Patients should be encouraged to read the information sheet carefully and to ask their physician and pharmacist about the proper use of the product (see DOSAGE AND ADMINISTRATION, Nicotrol Inhaler). Patients must be advised to keep both used and unused cartridges out of the reach of children and pets.

Carcinogenesis, Mutagenesis, and Impairment of Fertility

Nicotine itself does not appear to be a carcinogen in laboratory animals. However, nicotine and its metabolites increased the incidences of tumors in the cheek pouches of hamsters and forestomach of F344 rats, respectively when given in combination with tumor-initiators. One study, which could not be replicated, suggested that cotinine, the primary metabolite of nicotine, may cause lymphoreticular sarcoma in the large intestine of rats.

Neither nicotine nor cotinine was mutagenic in the Ames *Salmonella* test. Nicotine induced reparable DNA damage in an *E. coli* test system. Nicotine was shown to be genotoxic in a test system using Chinese hamster ovary cells. In rats and rabbits, implantation can be delayed or inhibited by a reduction in DNA synthesis that appears to be caused by nicotine. Studies have shown a decrease in litter size in rats treated with nicotine during gestation.

Pregnancy Category D

See WARNINGS, Nicotrol Inhaler.

The harmful effects of cigarette smoking on maternal and fetal health are clearly established. These include low birth weight, an increased risk of spontaneous abortion, and increased perinatal mortality. The specific effects of Nicotrol Inhaler therapy on fetal development are unknown. Therefore pregnant smokers should be encouraged to attempt cessation using educational and behavioral interventions before using pharmacological approaches.

Spontaneous abortion during nicotine replacement therapy has been reported; as with smoking, nicotine as a contributing factor cannot be excluded.

Nicotrol Inhaler therapy should be used during pregnancy only if the likelihood of smoking cessation justifies the potential risk of using it by the pregnant patient, who might continue to smoke.

Teratogenicity

Animal Studies

Nicotine was shown to produce skeletal abnormalities in the offspring of mice when toxic doses were given to the dams (25 mg/kg IP or SC).

Human Studies

Nicotine teratogenicity has not been studied in humans except as a component of cigarette smoke (each cigarette smoked delivers about 1 mg of nicotine). It has not been possible to conclude whether cigarette smoking is teratogenic to humans.

Other Effects

Animal Studies

A nicotine bolus (up to 2 mg/kg) to pregnant rhesus monkeys caused acidosis, hypercarbia, and hypotension (fetal and maternal concentrations were about 20 times those achieved after smoking one cigarette in 5 minutes). Fetal breathing movements were reduced in the fetal lamb after intravenous injection of 0.25 mg/kg nicotine to the ewe (equivalent to smoking 1 cigarette every 20 seconds for 5 minutes). Uterine blood flow was reduced about 30% after infusion of 0.1 μg/kg/min nicotine to pregnant rhesus monkeys (equivalent to smoking about 6 cigarettes every minute for 20 minutes).

Human Experience

Cigarette smoking during pregnancy is associated with an increased risk of spontaneous abortion, low birth weight infants and perinatal mortality. Nicotine and carbon monoxide are considered the most likely mediators of these outcomes. The effects of cigarette smoking on fetal cardiovascular parameters have been studied near term. Cigarettes increased fetal aortic blood flow and heart rate and decreased uterine blood flow and fetal breathing movements. Nicotrol Inhaler therapy has not been studied in pregnant women.

Labor and Delivery

Nicotrol Inhaler is not recommended for use during labor and delivery. The effect of nicotine on a mother or the fetus during labor is unknown.

Use in Nursing Mothers

Caution should be exercised when the Nicotrol Inhaler is administered to nursing mothers. The safety of Nicotrol Inhaler therapy in nursing infants has not been examined. Nicotine passes freely into breast milk; the milk to plasma ratio averages 2.9. Nicotine is absorbed orally. An infant has the ability to clear nicotine by hepatic first-pass clearance; however, the efficiency of removal is probably lowest at birth. Nicotine concentrations in milk can be expected to be lower with Nicotrol Inhaler when used as recommended than with cigarette smoking, as maternal plasma nicotine concentrations are generally reduced with nicotine replacement. The risk of exposure of the infant to nicotine from Nicotrol Inhaler therapy should be weighed against the risks associated with the infant's exposure to nicotine from continued smoking by the mother (passive smoke exposure and contamination of breast milk with other components of tobacco smoke) and from the Nicotrol Inhaler alone, or in combination with continued smoking.

Pediatric Use

Safety and effectiveness in pediatric and adolescent patients below the age of 18 years have not been established for any nicotine replacement product. However, no specific medical

N

risk is known or expected in nicotine dependent adolescents. Nicotrol Inhaler should be used for the treatment of tobacco dependence in the older adolescent only if the potential benefit justifies the potential risk.

Geriatric Use

One hundred and thirty-two (132) patients aged 60 or more participated in clinical trials of Nicotrol Inhaler. Nicotrol Inhaler appeared to be as effective in this age group as in younger smokers. Because medical conditions that are precautions to nicotine use are more common in the elderly, physicians should use care in prescribing this product to these patients.

NICOTROL NS

General

The patient should be urged to stop smoking completely when initiating Nicotrol NS therapy (see DOSAGE AND ADMINISTRATION, Nicotrol NS). Patients should be informed that if they continue to smoke while using the product, they may experience adverse effects due to peak nicotine levels higher than those experienced from smoking alone. If there is a clinically significant increase in cardiovascular or other effects attributable to nicotine, the treatment should be discontinued (see WARNINGS, Nicotrol NS). Physicians should anticipate that concomitant medications may need dosage adjustment.

Sustained use (beyond 6 months) of Nicotrol NS by patients who stop smoking is not recommended and should be discouraged.

Use of Nicotrol NS is not recommended in patients with known chronic nasal disorders (*e.g.*, allergy, rhinitis, nasal polyps and sinusitis) since such use has not been adequately studied.

Asthma, Bronchospasm and Reactive Airway Disease

Exacerbation of bronchospasm in patients with pre-existing asthma has been reported. Use of Nicotrol NS in patients with severe reactive airway disease is not recommended.

Effect of Nicotrol NS on the Nasal Mucosa

Topical application of either nicotine or tobacco products is irritating to the nasal mucosa and physicians should consider both the risks and benefits to the patient before initiating or continuing Nicotrol NS therapy.

The effect of Nicotrol NS on the nasal mucosa was studied in 39 cigarette smokers who used Nicotrol NS for 1 month. When compared to baseline, random biopsies taken after 4 weeks of treatment revealed 1 patient with persistence of pre-existing dysplasia and 1 patient with a newly found dysplasia. In both, dysplasia was not seen after a recovery period of 8 weeks.

Forty-two (42) patients who used Nicotrol NS for more than 6 months underwent follow-up ear, nose and throat examinations 1-3 months after discontinuing the use of the spray. Many reported local irritant effects of the spray during spray use, but none showed persistent mucosal injury that the examining physician could attribute to use of the product.

The clinical significance of these findings is not known, but extended use of the product beyond 6 months is not recommended.

Cardiovascular or Peripheral Vascular Diseases

The risks of nicotine replacement in patients with cardiovascular and peripheral vascular diseases should be weighed against the benefits of including nicotine replacement in a smoking cessation program for them. Specifically, patients with coronary heart disease (history of myocardial infarction and/or angina pectoris), serious cardiac arrhythmias, or vasospastic diseases (Buerger's disease, Prinzmetal's variant angina and Raynaud's phenomena) should be evaluated carefully before nicotine replacement is prescribed.

Tachycardia occurring in association with nicotine replacement therapy has been reported. No serious cardiovascular events were reported in clinical studies with Nicotrol NS, but if symptoms occur, its use should be discontinued.

Nicotrol NS generally should not be used in patients during the immediate post-myocardial infarction period, nor in patients with serious arrhythmias, or with severe or worsening angina.

Renal or Hepatic Insufficiency

The pharmacokinetics of nicotine have not been studied in the elderly or in patients with renal or hepatic impairment. However, given that nicotine is extensively metabolized and that its total system clearance is dependent on liver blood flow, some influence of hepatic impairment on drug kinetics (reduced clearance) should be anticipated. Only severe renal impairment would be expected to affect the clearance of nicotine or its metabolites from the circulation (see CLINICAL PHARMACOLOGY, Pharmacokinetics, Nicotrol NS).

Endocrine Diseases

Nicotrol NS therapy should be used with caution in patients with hyperthyroidism, pheochromocytoma or insulin-dependent diabetes, since nicotine causes the release of catecholamines by the adrenal medulla.

Peptic Ulcer Disease

Nicotine delays healing in peptic ulcer disease; therefore, Nicotrol NS therapy should be used with caution in patients with active peptic ulcers and only when the benefits of including nicotine replacement in a smoking cessation program outweigh the risks.

Accelerated Hypertension

Nicotine therapy constitutes a risk factor for development of malignant hypertension in patients with accelerated hypertension; therefore, Nicotrol NS therapy should be used with caution in these patients and only when the benefits of including nicotine replacement in a smoking cessation program outweigh the risks.

Information for the Patient

A patient instruction sheet is included in the package of Nicotrol NS dispensed to the patient. Patients should be encouraged to read the instruction sheet carefully and to ask their physician and pharmacist about the proper use of the product (see DOSAGE AND ADMINISTRATION, Nicotrol NS).

It should be explained to patients that they are likely to experience nasal irritation, which may become less bothersome with continued use.

Patients must be advised to keep both used and unused containers out of the reach of children and pets.

Carcinogenesis, Mutagenesis, and Impairment of Fertility

Nicotine itself does not appear to be a carcinogen in laboratory animals. However, nicotine and its metabolites increased the incidences of tumors in the cheek pouches of hamsters and forestomach of F344 rats, respectively, when given in combination with tumor-initiators. One study, which could not be replicated, suggested that cotinine, the primary metabolite of nicotine, may cause lymphoreticular sarcoma in the large intestine of rats.

Neither nicotine nor cotinine were mutagenic in the Ames *Salmonella* test. Nicotine induced repairable DNA damage in an *E. coli* test system. Nicotine was shown to be genotoxic in a test system using Chinese hamster ovary cells. In rats and rabbits, implantation can be delayed or inhibited by a reduction in DNA synthesis that appears to be caused by nicotine. Studies have shown a decrease in litter size in rats treated with nicotine during gestation.

Pregnancy Category D

See WARNINGS, Nicotrol NS.

The harmful effects of cigarette smoking on maternal and fetal health are clearly established. These include low birth weight, an increased risk of spontaneous abortion, and increased perinatal mortality. The specific effects of Nicotrol NS on fetal development are unknown. Therefore pregnant smokers should be encouraged to attempt cessation using educational and behavioral interventions before using pharmacological approaches.

Spontaneous abortion during nicotine replacement therapy has been reported; as with smoking, nicotine as a contributing factor cannot be excluded.

Nicotrol NS should be used during pregnancy only if the likelihood of smoking cessation justifies the potential risk of using it by the pregnant patient, who might continue to smoke.

Teratogenicity

Animal Studies

Nicotine was shown to produce skeletal abnormalities in the offspring of mice when toxic doses were given to the dams (25 mg/kg IP or SC).

Human Studies

Nicotine teratogenicity has not been studied in humans except as a component of cigarette smoke (each cigarette smoked delivers about 1 mg of nicotine). It has not been possible to conclude whether cigarette smoking is teratogenic to humans.

Other Effects

Animal Studies

A nicotine bolus (up to 2 mg/kg) to pregnant rhesus monkeys caused acidosis, hypercarbia, and hypotension (fetal and maternal concentrations were about 20 times those achieved after smoking one cigarette in 5 minutes). Fetal breathing movements were reduced in the fetal lamb after intravenous injection of 0.25 mg/kg nicotine to the ewe (equivalent to smoking 1 cigarette every 20 seconds for 5 minutes). Uterine blood flow was reduced about 30% after infusion of 0.1 μg/kg/min nicotine to pregnant rhesus monkeys (equivalent to smoking about 6 cigarettes every minute for 20 minutes).

Human Experience

Cigarette smoking during pregnancy is associated with an increased risk of spontaneous abortion, low birth weight infants and perinatal mortality. Nicotine and carbon monoxide are considered the most likely mediators of these outcomes. The effects of cigarette smoking on fetal cardiovascular parameters have been studied near term. Cigarettes increased fetal aortic blood flow and heart rate and decreased uterine blood flow and fetal breathing movements. Nicotrol NS has not been studied in pregnant women.

Labor and Delivery

Nicotrol NS is not recommended for use during labor and delivery. The effect of nicotine on a mother or the fetus during labor is unknown.

Use in Nursing Mothers

Caution should be exercised when Nicotrol NS is administered to nursing mothers. The safety of Nicotrol NS therapy in nursing infants has not been examined. Nicotine passes freely into breast milk; the milk to plasma ratio averages 2.9. Nicotine is absorbed orally. An infant has the ability to clear nicotine by hepatic first-pass clearance; however, the efficiency of removal is probably lowest at birth. Nicotine concentrations in milk can be expected to be lower with Nicotrol NS when used as recommended than with cigarette smoking, as maternal plasma nicotine concentrations are generally reduced with nicotine replacement. The risk of exposure of the infant to nicotine from Nicotrol NS therapy should be weighed against the risks associated with the infant's exposure to nicotine from continued smoking by the mother (passive smoke exposure and contamination of breast milk with other components of tobacco smoke) and from Nicotrol NS alone, or in combination with continued smoking.

Pediatric Use

Nicotrol NS therapy is not recommended for use in the pediatric population because its safety and effectiveness in children and adolescents who smoke have not been evaluated.

Geriatric Use

Clinical studies of Nicotrol NS did not include sufficient numbers of subjects age 65 and over to determine whether they respond differently from younger subjects. Other reports on clinical experience have not identified differences between older and younger patients. In general, dosage selection for an elderly patient should be cautious, usually starting at the low end of the dosage range reflecting the greater frequency of decreased hepatic, renal, or cardiac function, and of concomitant disease.

N

DRUG INTERACTIONS

NICOTROL INHALER

Physiological changes resulting from smoking cessation, with or without nicotine replacement, may alter the pharmacokinetics of certain concomitant medications, such as tricyclic antidepressants and theophylline. Doses of these and perhaps other medications may need to be adjusted in patients who successfully quit smoking.

NICOTROL NS

The extent of absorption and peak plasma concentration is slightly reduced in patients with the common cold/rhinitis. In addition, the time to peak concentration is prolonged. The use of a nasal vasoconstrictor such as xylometazoline in patients with rhinitis will further prolong the time to peak (see CLINICAL PHARMACOLOGY, Pharmacokinetics, Nicotrol NS). Smoking cessation, with or without nicotine replacement, may alter the pharmacokinetics of certain concomitant medications. (See TABLE 6.)

TABLE 6

May Require a Decrease in Dose at Cessation of Smoking	Possible Mechanism
Acetaminophen, caffeine, imipramine, oxazepam, pentazocine, propranolol, or other beta-blockers, theophylline.	Deinduction of hepatic enzymes on smoking cessation.
Insulin.	Increase in subcutaneous insulin absorption with smoking cessation.
Adrenergic antagonists (*e.g.*, prazosin, labetalol).	Decrease in circulating catecholamines with smoking cessation.
May Require an Increase in Dose at Cessation of Smoking	**Possible Mechanism**
Adrenergic agonists (*e.g.*, isoproterenol, phenylephrine).	Decrease in circulating catecholamines with smoking cessation.

ADVERSE REACTIONS

NICOTROL INHALER

Assessment of adverse events in the 1439 patients (730 on active drug) who participated in controlled clinical trials (including three dose finding studies) is complicated by the occurrence of signs and symptoms of nicotine withdrawal in some patients and nicotine excess in others. The incidence of adverse events is confounded by: (1) the many minor complaints that smokers commonly have, (2) continued smoking by many patients and (3) the local irritation from both the active drug and the placebo.

Local Irritation

Nicotrol Inhaler and the placebo were both associated with local irritant side effects. Local irritation in mouth and throat was reported by 40% of patients on active drug as compared to 18% of patients on placebo. Irritant effects were higher in the two pivotal trials with higher doses being 66% on active drug and 42% on placebo. Coughing (32% active vs 12% placebo) and rhinitis (23% active vs 16% placebo) were also higher on active drug. The majority of patients rated these symptoms as mild. The frequency of cough, and mouth and throat irritation declined with continued use of Nicotrol Inhaler. Other adverse events that occurred in over 3% of patients on active drug in placebo controlled pivotal trials considered possibly related to the local irritant effects of the Nicotrol Inhaler are taste comments, pain in jaw and neck, tooth disorders and sinusitis.

Withdrawal

Symptoms of withdrawal were common in both active and placebo groups. Common withdrawal symptoms seen in over 3% of patients on active drug included: dizziness, anxiety, sleep disorder, depression, withdrawal symdrome, drug dependence, fatigue and myalgia.

Nicotine-Related Adverse Events

The most common nicotine-related adverse event was dyspepsia. This was present in 18% of patients in the active group compared to 9% of patients in the placebo group. Other nicotine related events present in greater than 3% of patients on active drug include nausea, diarrhea, and hiccup.

Smoking Related Adverse Events

Smoking related adverse events present in greater than 3% of patients on active drug include chest discomfort, bronchitis, and hypertension.

Other Adverse Events

Adverse events of unknown relationship to nicotine occurring in greater than 3% of patients on active drug include headache (26% of patients on active and 15% of patients on placebo), influenza-like symptoms, pain, back-pain, allergy, paresthesias, flatulence and fever.

NICOTROL NS

Assessment of adverse events in the 730 patients who participated in controlled clinical trials is complicated by the occurrence of signs and symptoms of nicotine withdrawal in some patients and nicotine excess in others. The incidence of adverse events is confounded by the many minor complaints that smokers commonly have, by continued smoking by many patients and the local irritation from both active drug and the pepper placebo. No serious adverse events were reported during the trials.

Common Smoker's Complaints

Common complaints experienced by the smokers in the study (users of both active and placebo spray) include: chest tightness, dyspepsia, paraesthesia (tingling) in limbs, constipation, and stomatitis.

Tobacco Withdrawal

Symptoms of tobacco withdrawal were frequent in users of both active and placebo sprays. Common withdrawal symptoms seen in over 5% of patients included: anxiety, irritability, restlessness, cravings, dizziness, impaired concentration, weight increase, emotional lability, somnolence and fatigue, increased sweating, and insomnia. Less frequently seen probable withdrawal symptoms (under 5%) included: confusion, depression, apathy, tremor, increased appetite, incoordination and increased dreaming.

Anxiety, irritability, restlessness and tobacco cravings occurred about equally in both groups, while other symptoms tended to be slightly more common on placebo spray.

Effects of the Spray

Nicotrol NS and the pepper-containing placebo were both associated with irritant side effects on the nasopharyngeal and ocular tissues. During the first 2 days of treatment, nasal irritation was reported by nearly all (94%) of the patients, the majority of whom rated it as either moderate or severe. Both the frequency and severity of nasal irritation declined with continued use of Nicotrol NS but was still experienced by most (81%) of the patients after 3 weeks of treatment, with most patients rating it as moderate or mild.

Other common side-effects for both active and placebo groups were: runny nose, throat irritation, watering eyes, sneezing, and cough.

The following local events were reported somewhat more commonly for active than for placebo spray: Nasal congestion, subjective comments related to the taste or use of the dosage form, sinus irritation, transient epistaxis, eye irritation, transient changes in sense of smell, pharyngitis, paraesthesias of the nose, mouth or head, numbness of the nose, or mouth, burning of the nose or eyes, earache, facial flushing, transient changes in sense of taste, hoarseness, nasal ulcer or blister.

Effects of Nicotine

Feelings of dependence on the spray were reported by more patients on active spray than placebo. Drug-like effects such as calming were also more frequent on active spray.

Other Adverse Effects

Adverse events which could not be classified and listed above and which were reported by >1% of patients on active spray are listed in TABLE 7.

TABLE 7 *Adverse Events Not Attributable to Intercurrent Illness*

Adverse Event	Active	Placebo
Headache	18%	15%
Back pain	6%	4%
Dyspnea	5%	6%
Nausea	5%	5%
Arthralgia	5%	1%
Menstrual disorder	4%	4%
Palpitation	4%	4%
Flatulence	4%	3%
Tooth disorder	4%	1%
Gum problems	4%	1%
Myalgia	3%	4%
Abdominal pain	3%	3%
Confusion	3%	3%
Acne	3%	1%
Dysmenorrhea	3%	0%
Pruritus	2%	3%

Adverse events reported with a frequency of <1% among active spray users are listed below:

Body as a Whole: Edema peripheral, pain, numbness, allergy.
Gastrointestinal: Dry mouth, hiccup, diarrhea.
Hematologic: Purpura.
Neurological: Aphasia, amnesia, migraine, numbness.
Respiratory: Bronchitis, bronchospasm, sputum increased.
Skin and Appendages: Rash, purpura.
Special Senses: Vision abnormal.

DOSAGE AND ADMINISTRATION

NICOTROL INHALER

Patients must desire to stop smoking and should be instructed to stop smoking completely as they begin using Nicotrol Inhaler. It is important that patients understand the instructions, and have their questions answered. They should clearly understand the directions for using the Nicotrol Inhaler and safely disposing of the used cartridges.

The initial dosage of Nicotrol Inhaler is individualized. Patients may self-titrate to the level of nicotine they require. Most successful patients in the clinical trials used between 6 and 16 cartridges a day. Best effect was achieved by frequent continuous puffing (20 minutes). The recommended duration of treatment is 3 months, after which patients may be weaned from the Nicotrol Inhaler by gradual reduction of the daily dose over the following 6-12 weeks. The safety and efficacy of the continued use of Nicotrol Inhaler for periods longer than 6 months have not been studied and such use is not recommended.

Dosing recommendations are summarized in TABLE 8.

TABLE 8

	Duration	Recommended Cartridges/day
INITIAL TREATMENT	Up to 12 weeks	6-16
Gradual Reduction (if needed)	6-12 weeks	No tapering strategy has been shown to be superior to any other in clinical studies.

Initial Treatment (Up to 12 Weeks)

For best results, patients should be encouraged to use at least 6 cartridges per day at least for the first 3-6 weeks of treatment. In clinical trials, the average daily dose was >6 (range 3-18) cartridges for patients who successfully quit smoking. Additional doses may be needed to control the urge to smoke with a maximum of 16 cartridges daily for up to 12 weeks. Regular use of Nicotrol Inhaler during the first week of treatment may help patients adapt to the irritant effects of the product. Some patients may exhibit signs or symptoms of nicotine withdrawal or excess which will require an adjustment of the dosage (see Individualization Of Dosage).

Gradual Reduction of Dose (Up to 12 Weeks)

Most patients will need to gradually discontinue the use of Nicotrol Inhaler after the initial treatment period. Gradual reduction of dose may begin after 12 weeks of initial treatment and may last for up to 12 weeks. Recommended strategies for discontinuing use include suggesting to patients that they use the product less frequently, keep a tally of daily usage, try to meet a steadily reducing target or set a planned quit date for stopping use of the product.

Individualization Of Dosage

The Nicotrol Inhaler provides the smoker with adequate amounts of nicotine to reduce the urge to smoke, and may provide some degree of comfort by providing a hand-to-mouth ritual similar to smoking, although the importance of such effect in smoking cessation is, as yet, unknown.

The success or failure of smoking cessation is influenced by the quality, intensity and frequency of supportive care. Patients are more likely to quit smoking if they are seen frequently and participate in formal smoking cessation programs.

The goal of Nicotrol Inhaler therapy is complete abstinence. If a patient is unable to stop smoking by the fourth week of therapy, treatment should probably be discontinued.

Patients who fail to quit on any attempt may benefit from interventions to improve their chances for success on subsequent attempts. Patients who were unsuccessful should be counseled and should then probably be given a therapeutic holiday before the next attempt. A new quit attempt should be encouraged when conditions are more favorable.

Based on the clinical trials, a reasonable approach to assisting patients in their attempt to quit smoking is to begin initial treatment, using the recommended dosage (see DOSAGE AND ADMINISTRATION, Nicotrol Inhaler). Dosage can then be adjusted in those patients with signs or symptoms of nicotine withdrawal or excess. Patients who are successfully abstinent on Nicotrol Inhaler should be treated at the selected dosage for up to 12 weeks, after which use of the Inhaler should be gradually reduced over the next 6-12 weeks. Some patients may not require gradual reduction of dosage and may abruptly stop treatment successfully. The safe use of this product for longer than 6 months has not been established.

The symptoms of nicotine withdrawal overlap those of nicotine excess (see CLINICAL PHARMACOLOGY, Pharmacodynamics, Nicotrol Inhaler and ADVERSE REACTIONS, Nicotrol Inhaler). Since patients using Nicotrol Inhaler may also smoke intermittently, it is sometimes difficult to determine if they are experiencing nicotine withdrawal or nicotine excess. Controlled clinical trials of nicotine products suggest that palpitations, nausea and sweating are more often symptoms of nicotine excess, whereas anxiety, nervousness and irritability are more often symptoms of nicotine withdrawal.

N

Safety and Handling

Disposal

See patient information sheet for instructions on handling and disposal. After using the Nicotrol Inhaler, carefully separate the mouthpiece, remove the used cartridge and throw it away, out of the reach of children and pets. Store the mouthpiece in the plastic storage case for further use. The mouthpiece is reusable and should be cleaned regularly with soap and water. The Nicotrol Inhaler cartridges can be detected on a radiogram.

NICOTROL NS

It is important that patients understand the instructions for use of Nicotrol NS, and have their questions answered. They should clearly understand the directions for using Nicotrol NS and safely disposing of the used container. They should be instructed to stop smoking completely when they begin using the product.

Patients should be instructed not to sniff, swallow or inhale through the nose as the spray is being administered. They should also be advised to administer the spray with the head tilted back slightly.

The dose of Nicotrol NS, should be individualized on the basis of each patient's nicotine dependence and the occurrence of symptoms of nicotine excess (see Individualization Of Dosage).

Each actuation of Nicotrol NS delivers a metered 50 µl spray containing 0.5 mg of nicotine. One dose is 1 mg of nicotine (2 sprays, 1 in each nostril).

Patients should be started with 1 or 2 doses per hour, which may be increased up to a maximum recommended dose of 40 mg (80 sprays, somewhat less than ½ bottle) per day. For best results, patients should be encouraged to use at least the recommended minimum of 8 doses per day, as less is unlikely to be effective. In clinical trials, the patients who successfully quit smoking used the product heavily when nicotine withdrawal was at its peak, sometimes up to the recommended maximum of 40 doses per day (in heavier smokers). Dosing recommendations are summarized in TABLE 9.

TABLE 9

Maximum recommended duration of treatment	3 months
Recommended doses per hour	1-2*
Maximum doses per hour	5
Maximum doses per day	40

* One dose = 2 sprays (1 in each nostril). One dose delivers 1 mg of nicotine to the nasal mucosa.

No tapering strategy has been shown to be optimal in clinical studies. Many patients simply stopped using the spray at their last clinic visit.

Recommended strategies for discontinuation of use include suggesting that patients: use only ½ a dose (1 spray) at a time, use the spray less frequently, keep a tally of daily usage, try to meet a steadily reducing usage target, skip a dose by not medicating every hour, or set a planned "quit date" for stopping use of the spray.

Individualization Of Dosage

The success or failure of smoking cessation is influenced by the quality, intensity and frequency of supportive care. Patients are more likely to quit smoking if they are seen frequently and participate in formal smoking cessation programs.

The goal of Nicotrol NS therapy is complete abstinence. If a patient is unable to stop smoking by the fourth week of therapy, treatment should probably be discontinued.

Patients who fail to quit on any attempt may benefit from interventions to improve their chances for success on subsequent attempts. Patients who were unsuccessful should be counseled and should then probably be given a "therapy holiday" before the next attempt. A new quit attempt should be encouraged when conditions are more favorable.

Based on the clinical trials, a reasonable approach to assisting patients in their attempt to quit smoking is to begin initial treatment, using the recommended dosage (see DOSAGE AND ADMINISTRATION, Nicotrol NS). Regular use of the spray during the first week of treatment may help patients adapt to the irritant effects of the spray. Dosage can then be adjusted in those subjects with signs or symptoms of nicotine withdrawal or excess. Patients who are successfully abstinent on Nicotrol NS should be treated at the selected dosage for up to 8 weeks, following which use of the spray should be discontinued over the next 4-6 weeks. Some patients may not require gradual reduction of dosage and may abruptly stop treatment successfully. Treatment with Nicotrol NS for longer periods has not been shown to improve outcome, and the safety of use for periods longer than 6 months has not been established.

The symptoms of nicotine withdrawal overlap those of nicotine excess (see CLINICAL PHARMACOLOGY, Pharmacodynamics, Nicotrol NS). Since patients using Nicotrol NS may also smoke intermittently, it is sometimes difficult to determine if patients are experiencing nicotine withdrawal or nicotine excess. Controlled clinical trials of nicotine products suggest that palpitations, nausea and sweating are more often symptoms of nicotine excess, whereas anxiety, nervousness and irritability are more often symptoms of nicotine withdrawal.

Safety and Handling

As with all medicines, especially ones in liquid form, care should be taken in handling Nicotrol NS during periods of opening and closing the container (see WARNINGS, Nicotrol NS). If it is dropped it may break. If this occurs, the spill should be cleaned up immediately with an absorbent cloth/paper towel. Care should be taken to avoid contact of the solution with the skin. Broken glass should be picked up carefully, using a broom. The area of the spill should be washed several times. Absorbent material may be disposed of as any other household waste. Should even a small amount of Nicotrol NS come in contact with the skin, lips, mouth, eyes or ears, the affected area(s) should be immediately rinsed with water only.

Disposal

Used bottles of Nicotrol NS should be disposed of with their child-resistant caps in place. Used bottles should be disposed of in such a way as to prevent access by children or pets. See patient information for further information on handling and disposal.

HOW SUPPLIED

NICOTROL INHALER

Nicotrol Inhaler (nicotine inhalation system) is supplied as 42 cartridges each containing 10 mg (4 mg is delivered) nicotine. Each unit consists of 1 mouthpiece, 7 storage trays each containing 6 cartridges and 1 plastic storage case. A patient information leaflet is enclosed with the package.

Storage: Store at room temperature not to exceed 30°C (86°F). Protect cartridges from light.

NICOTROL NS

Nicotrol NS (nicotine nasal spray) 10 mg/ml, is supplied in individual 10 ml bottles. Each unit consists of a glass container, mounted with a metered spray pump. A patient information leaflet is enclosed with the package.

Storage: Store at room temperature not to exceed 30°C (86°F). Protect cartridges from light.

TRANSDERMAL

DESCRIPTION

Note: The trade names have been used throughout this monograph for clarity.

Nicotrol (nicotine transdermal system) is a multilayered, rectangular, thin film laminated unit containing nicotine as the active ingredient. Nicotrol Patch provides systemic delivery of 15 mg of nicotine over 16 hours. Nicotrol Patch is for people who smoke over 10 cigarettes a day.

Inactive Ingredients: Polyisobutylenes, polybutene non-woven polyester, pigmented aluminized and clear polyesters.

CLINICAL PHARMACOLOGY

Nicotrol (nicotine transdermal system) Patch helps smokers quit by reducing nicotine withdrawal symptoms. Many Nicotrol Patch users will be able to stop smoking for a few days but often will start smoking again. Most smokers have to try to quit several times before they completely stop.

Your own chances of quitting smoking depend on how much you want to quit, how strongly you are addicted to nicotine and how closely you follow a quitting program like the PATHWAYS TO CHANGE Program that comes with the Nicotrol Patch.

If you find you cannot stop or if you start smoking again after using Nicotrol Patch, please talk to a health care professional who can help you find a program that may work better for you. Remember that breaking this addiction doesn't happen overnight.

Because the Nicotrol Patch provides some nicotine, the Nicotrol Patch will help you stop smoking by reducing nicotine withdrawal symptoms such as nicotine cravings, nervousness and irritability.

INDICATIONS AND USAGE

To reduce withdrawal symptoms, including nicotine craving, associated with quitting smoking.

NON-FDA APPROVED INDICATIONS

Nicotine therapy has also be used without FDA approval in the treatment of ulcerative colitis, Parkinson's disease, Alzheimer's disease and Tourette's syndrome. However, further clinical trials are needed.

WARNINGS

Keep this and all medication out of reach of children and pets. Even used patches have enough nicotine to poison children and pets. Be sure to fold sticky ends together and throw away out of reach of children and pets. In case of accidental overdose, seek professional assistance or contact a poison control center immediately.

Nicotine can increase your baby's heart rate. First try to stop smoking without the nicotine patch. As with any drug, if you are pregnant or nursing a baby, seek the advice of a health professional before using this product.

Do not smoke even when you are not wearing the patch. The nicotine in your skin will still be entering your bloodstream for several hours after you take the patch off.

If you forget to remove the patch at bedtime you may have vivid dreams or other sleep disruptions.

Do not use if you:

Continue to smoke, chew tobacco, use snuff, or use a nicotine gum or other nicotine containing products.

Ask your doctor before use if you:

Are under 18 years of age.

Have heart disease, recent heart attack or irregular heartbeat. Nicotine can increase your heart rate.

Have high blood pressure not controlled with medication — Nicotine can increase blood pressure.

Take prescription medicine for depression or asthma — Your prescription dose may need to be adjusted.

Are allergic to adhesive tape or have skin problems, because you are more likely to get rashes.

Stop use and see your doctor if you have:

Skin redness caused by the patch that does not go away after 4 days, or if your skin swells or you get a rash.

Irregular heartbeat or palpitations.

Symptoms of nicotine overdose such as nausea, vomiting, dizziness, weakness and rapid heartbeat.

DOSAGE AND ADMINISTRATION

Stop smoking completely when you begin using the Nicotrol Patch.

Refer to enclosed patient information leaflet before using this product.

Use one Nicotrol Patch every day for 6 weeks. Remove backing from the patch and immediately press onto clean dry hairless skin. Hold for 10 seconds. Wash hands.

The Nicotrol Patch should be worn during awake hours and removed prior to sleep.

For best results in quitting smoking:

Firmly commit to quitting smoking.

Use enclosed support materials.

Use the Nicotrol Patches for 6 weeks.

Stop using Nicotrol Patches at the end of week 6. If you still feel the need for Nicotrol Patches talk to your doctor.

HOW SUPPLIED

Starter Kit-7, Refill Kit-7. DO NOT USE IF POUCH IS DAMAGED OR OPEN. Do not store above 30°C (86°F).

Not for sale to those under 18 years of age.

Proof of age required.

Not for sale in vending machines or from any source where proof of age cannot be verified.

PRODUCT LISTING - RATED THERAPEUTICALLY EQUIVALENT

Film, Extended Release - Transdermal - 7 mg/24 Hr

30's	$98.64	GENERIC, Par Pharmaceutical Inc	49884-0058-72
30's	$188.37	GENERIC, Watson/Schein Pharmaceuticals Inc	00364-2890-30

Film, Extended Release - Transdermal - 14 mg/24 Hr

30's	$104.13	GENERIC, Par Pharmaceutical Inc	49884-0059-72
30's	$188.72	GENERIC, Watson/Schein Pharmaceuticals Inc	00364-2893-30

Film, Extended Release - Transdermal - 21 mg/24 Hr

30's	$109.58	GENERIC, Par Pharmaceutical Inc	49884-0063-72
30's	$198.58	GENERIC, Watson/Schein Pharmaceuticals Inc	00364-2901-30

PRODUCT LISTING - EQUIVALENTS NOT AVAILABLE

Device - Inhalation - 10 mg/ml

42's	$42.50	NICOTROL INHALER, Pharmacia and Upjohn	00009-5195-01
168's	$138.75	NICOTROL INHALER, Pharmacia and Upjohn	00009-5195-08

Film, Extended Release - Transdermal - 5 mg/16 Hr

14's	$46.16	NICOTROL, Pharmacia and Upjohn	00009-5269-01

Film, Extended Release - Transdermal - 7 mg/24 Hr

7's	$24.21	NICODERM C-Q, Glaxosmithkline Healthcare	00135-0147-01
14's	$41.72	NICODERM C-Q, Glaxosmithkline Healthcare	00135-0147-02
14's	$41.72	NICODERM C-Q CLEAR, Glaxosmithkline Healthcare	00135-0196-03

Film, Extended Release - Transdermal - 10 mg/16 Hr

14's	$46.16	NICOTROL, Pharmacia and Upjohn	00009-5270-01

Film, Extended Release - Transdermal - 14 mg/24 Hr

7's	$24.21	NICODERM C-Q, Glaxosmithkline Healthcare	00135-0146-01
14's	$41.72	NICODERM C-Q, Glaxosmithkline Healthcare	00135-0146-02
14's	$41.72	NICODERM C-Q CLEAR, Glaxosmithkline Healthcare	00135-0195-03

Film, Extended Release - Transdermal - 21 mg/24 Hr

7's	$24.21	NICODERM C-Q, Glaxosmithkline Healthcare	00135-0145-01
14's	$41.72	NICODERM C-Q, Glaxosmithkline Healthcare	00135-0145-02
14's	$41.72	NICODERM C-Q CLEAR, Glaxosmithkline Healthcare	00135-0194-03

Nifedipine

(001886)

For related information, see the comparative table section in Appendix A.

Categories: Angina, chronic stable; Angina, variant; Hypertension, essential; Pregnancy Category C; FDA Approved 1986 Jul; WHO Formulary

Drug Classes: Calcium channel blockers

Brand Names: Adalat; Adalat CC; **Procardia**; Procardia XL

Foreign Brand Availability: Adalat 5 (Australia); Adalat 10 (Australia); Adalat 20 (Australia); Adalat CR (Greece; Japan; Switzerland; Thailand); Adalat Crono (Italy); Adalat FT (Canada); Adalat GITS (Hong-Kong); Adalat GITS 30 (Philippines); Adalat L (Japan); Adalat LA (England; Malaysia); Adalat LP (France); Adalat Oros (Australia; Bahamas; Barbados; Belize; Bermuda; Costa-Rica; Curacao; Denmark; Dominican-Republic; El-Salvador; Finland; Guatemala; Guyana; Honduras; Indonesia; Jamaica; Korea; Mexico; Netherland-Antilles; Netherlands; New-Zealand; Nicaragua; Norway; Panama; Puerto-Rico; Spain; Surinam; Sweden; Taiwan; Trinidad); Adalat P.A. (Canada); Adalat Retard (Austria; Bahrain; Benin; Burkina-Faso; Costa-Rica; Cyprus; Dominican-Republic; Egypt; El-Salvador; England; Ethiopia; Gambia; Germany; Ghana; Greece; Guatemala; Guinea; Honduras; Hong-Kong; Indonesia; Iran; Iraq; Israel; Ivory-Coast; Jordan; Kenya; Kuwait; Lebanon; Liberia; Libya; Malawi; Malaysia; Mali; Mauritania; Mauritius; Mexico; Morocco; Netherlands; New-Zealand; Nicaragua; Niger; Nigeria; Oman; Panama; Peru; Philippines; Qatar; Republic-of-Yemen; Saudi-Arabia; Senegal; Seychelles; Sierra-Leone; South-Africa; Spain; Sudan; Syria; Tanzania; Thailand; Tunia; Uganda; United-Arab-Emirates; Zambia; Zimbabwe); Adalate (France); Alat (Taiwan); Alonix-S (Taiwan); Alpha-Nifedipine Retard (New-Zealand); Angipec (Peru); Antiblut (Peru); Apo-Nifed (Canada); Aprical (Germany); Calcheck (Philippines); Calcibloc (Philippines); Calcibloc OD (Philippines); Calcigard (India; Thailand); Calcigard Retard (China); Calcilat (England); Cardifen (South-Africa); Cardilat (South-Africa); Cardionorm (Philippines); Chronadalate LP (France); Cipilat (South-Africa); Citilat (Italy); Coracten (Bahrain; Cyprus; Egypt; England; Germany; Hong-Kong; Iran; Iraq; Israel; Jordan; Kuwait; Lebanon; Libya; Oman; Qatar; Republic-of-Yemen; Saudi-Arabia; Syria; United-Arab-Emirates); Coral (Italy); Cordalat (Indonesia); Cordipen (Singapore); Cordipin (Slovenia); Corotrend (Germany; Israel); Denkifed (Philippines); Depin (India); Dignokonstant (Germany); Dilafed (Mexico); Dilcor (Spain); Dipinkor (Indonesia); Duranifin (Germany); Ecodipin (China; Switzerland); Fedcor (Philippines); Fedipin (Indonesia); Fenamon (Bahrain; Benin; Burkina-Faso; Cyprus; Egypt; Ethiopia; Gambia; Ghana; Guinea; Hong-Kong; Iran; Iraq; Israel; Ivory-Coast; Jordan; Kenya; Kuwait; Lebanon; Liberia; Libya; Malawi; Malaysia; Mali; Mauritania; Mauritius; Morocco; Niger; Nigeria; Oman; Qatar; Republic-of-Yemen; Saudi-Arabia; Senegal; Seychelles; Sierra-Leone; South-Africa; Sudan; Syria; Taiwan; Tanzania; Thailand; Tunia; Uganda; United-Arab-Emirates; Zambia; Zimbabwe); Fenamon SR (Thailand); Glopir (Greece); Hadipine S.R. (Korea); Hexadilat (Denmark); Jutadilat (Germany); Kemolat (Indonesia); Megalat (Israel); Myogard (India); Nadipine (Korea); Nedipin (Taiwan); Nelapine (Philippines); Nelapine Retard (Philippines); Nifangin (Finland); Nifar (Benin; Burkina-Faso; Ethiopia; Gambia; Ghana; Guinea; Ivory-Coast; Kenya; Liberia; Malawi; Mali; Mauritania; Mauritius; Morocco; Niger; Nigeria; Senegal; Seychelles; Sierra-Leone; Sudan; Tanzania; Tunia; Uganda; Zambia; Zimbabwe); Nifdemin (Finland); Nifebene (Austria); Nifecard (Austria; Hong-Kong); Nifecor (Germany); Nifedepat (Germany); Nifedicor (Italy); NIfedilat (South-Africa); Nifedin (Italy); Nifedine (India); Nifedipres (Mexico); Nifedirex LP (France); Nifehexal (Australia); Nifelat (Argentina; Bahamas; Barbados; Belize; Bermuda; Curacao; Guyana; Jamaica; Netherland-Antilles; Puerto-Rico; Surinam; Thailand; Trinidad); Nifelat-Q (Thailand); Nifensar (Peru); Nifensar Retard (Peru); Nifestad (Philippines); Nificard (Bahrain; Cyprus; Egypt; Iran; Iraq; Israel; Jordan; Kuwait; Lebanon; Libya; Oman; Qatar; Republic-of-Yemen; Saudi-Arabia; Syria; Thailand; United-Arab-Emirates); Nifidine (South-Africa); Nifipen (Bahrain; Cyprus; Egypt; Iran; Iraq; Israel; Jordan; Kuwait; Lebanon; Libya; Oman; Qatar; Republic-of-Yemen; Saudi-Arabia; Syria; United-Arab-Emirates); Nipine (Korea); Normadil (Philippines); Novo Nifedin (Canada); Nyefax (Australia; New-Zealand); Nyefax Retard (New-Zealand); Odipin (Philippines); Orix (Greece); Osmo-Adalat (Israel); Pidilat (Germany); Sepamit (Japan); Tibricol (Argentina); Unidipine XL (China); Vascard (South-Africa); Vasdalat (Indonesia; Singapore); Zenusin (Bahrain; Benin; Burkina-Faso; Costa-Rica; Cyprus; Dominican-Republic; Ecuador; Egypt; El-Salvador; Ethiopia; Gambia; Ghana; Guatemala; Guinea; Honduras; Iran; Iraq; Israel; Ivory-Coast; Jordan; Kenya; Kuwait; Lebanon; Liberia; Libya; Malawi; Malaysia; Mali; Mauritania; Mauritius; Morocco; Nicaragua; Niger; Nigeria; Oman; Panama; Qatar; Republic-of-Yemen; Saudi-Arabia; Senegal; Seychelles; Sierra-Leone; Sudan; Syria; Tanzania; Tunia; Uganda; United-Arab-Emirates; Zambia; Zimbabwe)

Cost of Therapy: $7.09 (Angina; Generic Capsules; 10 mg; 3 capsules/day; 30 day supply)
$42.80 (Hypertension; Procardia XL; 30 mg; 1 tablet/day; 30 day supply)
$37.85 (Hypertension; Adalat CC; 30 mg; 1 tablet/day; 30 day supply)
$32.44 (Hypertension; Generic Extended Release Tablets; 30 mg; 1 tablet/day; 30 day supply)

DESCRIPTION

IMMEDIATE-RELEASE CAPSULES AND EXTENDED-RELEASE TABLETS

Nifedipine is an antianginal drug belonging to a class of pharmacological agents, the calcium channel blockers. Nifedipine is 3,5-pyridinedicarboxylic acid, 1,4-dihydro-2,6-dimethyl-4-(2-nitrophenyl)-,dimethyl ester, and its molecular formula is $C_{17}H_{18}N_2O_6$.

Nifedipine is a yellow crystalline substance, practically insoluble in water but soluble in ethanol. It has a molecular weight of 346.3.

IMMEDIATE-RELEASE CAPSULES

Procardia capsules are formulated as soft gelatin capsules for oral administration each containing 10 or 20 mg nifedipine.

Inert Ingredients: Glycerin; peppermint oil; polyethylene glycol; soft gelatin capsules (which contain yellow 6, and may contain red ferric oxide and other inert ingredients), and water. The 10 mg capsules also contain saccharin sodium.

EXTENDED-RELEASE TABLETS

Procardia XL is a trademark for nifedipine GITS. Nifedipine GITS (Gastrointestinal Therapeutic System) tablet is formulated as a once-a-day controlled-release tablet for oral administration designed to deliver 30, 60, or 90 mg of nifedipine.

Inert Ingredients in the Formulations

Cellulose acetate; hydroxypropyl cellulose; hydroxypropyl methylcellulose; magnesium stearate; polyethylene glycol; polyethylene oxide; red ferric oxide; sodium chloride; titanium dioxide.

System Components and Performance

Procardia XL extended-release tablet is similar in appearance to a conventional tablet. It consists, however, of a semipermeable membrane surrounding an osmotically active drug core. The core itself is divided into two layers: an "active" layer containing the drug, and a "push" layer containing pharmacologically inert (but osmotically active) components. As water from the gastrointestinal tract enters the tablet, pressure increases in the osmotic layer and "pushes" against the drug layer, releasing drug through the precision laser-drilled tablet orifice in the active layer.

Procardia XL extended-release tablet is designed to provide nifedipine at an approximately constant rate over 24 hours. This controlled rate of drug delivery into the gastrointestinal lumen is independent of pH or gastrointestinal motility. Procardia XL depends for its action on the existence of an osmotic gradient between the contents of the bi-layer core and fluid in the GI tract. Drug delivery is essentially constant as long as the osmotic gradient remains constant, and then gradually falls to zero. Upon swallowing, the biologically inert components of the tablet remain intact during GI transit and are eliminated in the feces as an insoluble shell.

CLINICAL PHARMACOLOGY

Nifedipine is a calcium ion influx inhibitor (slow-channel blocker or calcium ion antagonist) and inhibits the transmembrane influx of calcium ions into cardiac muscle and smooth muscle. The contractile processes of cardiac muscle and vascular smooth muscle are dependent upon the movement of extracellular calcium ions into these cells through specific ion channels. Nifedipine selectively inhibits calcium ion influx across the cell membrane of cardiac muscle and vascular smooth muscle without changing serum calcium concentrations.

MECHANISM OF ACTION

The precise means by which this inhibition relieves angina has not been fully determined, but includes at least the following two mechanisms:

RELAXATION AND PREVENTION OF CORONARY ARTERY SPASM

Nifedipine dilates the main coronary arteries and coronary arterioles, both in normal and ischemic regions, and is a potent inhibitor of coronary artery spasm, whether spontaneous or ergonovine-induced. This property increases myocardial oxygen delivery in patients with coronary artery spasm, and is responsible for the effectiveness of nifedipine in vasospastic (Prinzmetal's or variant) angina. Whether this effect plays any role in classical angina is not clear, but studies of exercise tolerance have not shown an increase in the maximum exercise rate-pressure product, a widely accepted measure of oxygen utilization. This suggests that, in general, relief of spasm or dilation of coronary arteries is not an important factor in classical angina.

REDUCTION OF OXYGEN UTILIZATION

Nifedipine regularly reduces arterial pressure at rest and at a given level of exercise by dilating peripheral arterioles and reducing the total peripheral resistance (afterload) against which the heart works. This unloading of the heart reduces myocardial energy consumption and oxygen requirements, and probably accounts for the effectiveness of nifedipine in chronic stable angina.

ELECTROPHYSIOLOGIC EFFECTS

Although, like other members of its class, nifedipine decreases sinoatrial node function and atrioventricular conduction in isolated myocardial preparations, such effects have not been seen in studies in intact animals or in man. In formal electrophysiologic studies, predominantly in patients with normal conduction systems, nifedipine has had no tendency to prolong atrioventricular conduction, prolong sinus node recovery time, or slow sinus rate.

ADDITIONAL INFORMATION FOR IMMEDIATE-RELEASE CAPSULES

Hemodynamics

Like other slow-channel blockers, nifedipine exerts a negative inotropic effect on isolated myocardial tissue. This is rarely, if ever, seen in intact animals or man, probably because of reflex responses to its vasodilating effects. In man, nifedipine causes decreased peripheral vascular resistance and a fall in systolic and diastolic pressure, usually modest (5-10 mm Hg systolic), but sometimes larger. There is usually a small increase in heart rate, a reflex response to vasodilation. Measurements of cardiac function in patients with normal ventricular function have generally found a small increase in cardiac index without major effects on ejection fraction, left ventricular end diastolic pressure (LVEDP) or volume (LVEDV). In patients with impaired ventricular function, most acute studies have shown some increase in ejection fraction and reduction in left ventricular filling pressure.

Pharmacokinetics and Metabolism

Nifedipine is rapidly and fully absorbed after oral administration. The drug is detectable in serum 10 minutes after oral administration, and peak blood levels occur in approximately 30 minutes. Bioavailability is proportional to dose from 10- 30 mg; half-life does not change significantly with dose. There is little difference in relative bioavailability when nifedipine capsules are given orally and either swallowed whole, bitten and swallowed, or, bitten and held sublingually. However, biting through the capsule prior to swallowing does result in slightly earlier plasma concentrations (27 ng/ml 10 minutes after 10 mg) than if capsules are swallowed intact. It is highly bound by serum proteins. Nifedipine is extensively converted to inactive metabolites and approximately 80% of nifedipine and metabolites are eliminated via the kidneys. The half-life of nifedipine in plasma is approximately 2 hours. Since hepatic biotransformation is the predominant route for the disposition of nifedipine, the pharmacokinetics may be altered in patients with chronic liver disease. Patients with hepatic impairment (liver cirrhosis) have a longer disposition half-life and higher bioavailability of nifedipine than healthy volunteers. The degree of serum protein binding of nifedipine is high (92-98%). Protein binding may be greatly reduced in patients with renal or hepatic impairment.

ADDITIONAL INFORMATION FOR EXTENDED-RELEASE TABLETS

Hypertension

The mechanism by which nifedipine reduces arterial blood pressure involves peripheral arterial vasodilation and the resulting reduction in peripheral vascular resistance. The increased peripheral vascular resistance that is an underlying cause of hypertension results from an increase in active tension in the vascular smooth muscle. Studies have demonstrated that the increase in active tension reflects an increase in cytosolic free calcium.

Nifedipine is a peripheral arterial vasodilator which acts directly on vascular smooth muscle. The binding of nifedipine to voltage-dependent and possibly receptor-operated channels in vascular smooth muscle results in an inhibition of calcium influx through these channels. Stores of intracellular calcium in vascular smooth muscle are limited and thus dependent upon the influx of extracellular calcium for contraction to occur. The reduction in calcium influx by nifedipine causes arterial vasodilation and decreased peripheral vascular resistance which results in reduced arterial blood pressure.

Pharmacokinetics and Metabolism

Nifedipine is completely absorbed after oral administration. Plasma drug concentrations rise at a gradual, controlled rate after a nifedipine extended-release tablet dose and reach a plateau at approximately 6 hours after the first dose. For subsequent doses, relatively constant plasma concentrations at the plateau are maintained with minimal fluctuations over the 24 hour dosing interval. About a 4-fold higher fluctuation index (ratio of peak to trough plasma concentration) was observed with the conventional immediate-release nifedipine capsule at tid dosing than once daily nifedipine extended-release tablet. At steady-state the bioavailability of nifedipine extended-release tablets is 86% relative to nifedipine capsules. Administration of the nifedipine extended-release tablets in the presence of food slightly alters the early rate of drug absorption, but does not influence the extent of drug bioavailability. Markedly reduced GI retention time over prolonged periods (*i.e.,* short bowel syndrome), however, may influence the pharmacokinetic profile of the drug which could potentially result in lower plasma concentration. Pharmacokinetics of nifedipine extended-release tablets are linear over the dose range of 30-180 mg in that plasma drug concentrations are proportional to dose administered. There was no evidence of dose dumping either in the presence or absence of food for over 150 subjects in pharmacokinetic studies.

Nifedipine is extensively metabolized to highly water-soluble, inactive metabolites accounting for 60-80% of the dose excreted in the urine. The elimination half-life of nifedipine is approximately 2 hours. Only traces (less than 0.1% of the dose) of unchanged form can be detected in the urine. The remainder is excreted in the feces in metabolized form, most likely as a result of biliary excretion. Thus, the pharmacokinetics of nifedipine are not significantly influenced by the degree of renal impairment. Patients in hemodialysis or chronic ambulatory peritoneal dialysis have not reported significantly altered pharmacokinetics of nifedipine. Since hepatic biotransformation is the predominant route for the disposition of nifedipine, the pharmacokinetics may be altered in patients with chronic liver disease. Patients with hepatic impairment (liver cirrhosis) have a longer disposition half-life and higher bioavailability of nifedipine than healthy volunteers. The degree of serum protein binding of nifedipine is high (92-98%). Protein binding may be greatly reduced in patients with renal or hepatic impairments.

Hemodynamics

Like other slow-channel blockers, nifedipine exerts a negative inotropic effect on isolated myocardial tissue. This is rarely, if ever, seen in intact animals or man, probably because of reflex responses to its vasodilating effects. In man, nifedipine decreases peripheral vascular resistance which leads to a fall in systolic and diastolic pressures, usually minimal in normotensive volunteers (less than 5-10 mm Hg systolic), but sometimes larger. With nifedipine extended-release tablets, these decreases in blood pressure are not accompanied by any significant change in heart rate. Hemodynamic studies in patients with normal ventricular function have generally found a small increase in cardiac index without major effects on ejection fraction LVEDP or LVEDV. In patients with impaired ventricular function, most acute studies have shown some increase in ejection fraction and reduction in left ventricular filling pressure.

INDICATIONS AND USAGE

VASOSPASTIC ANGINA

Nifedipine is indicated for the management of vasospastic angina confirmed by any of the following criteria: (1) classical pattern of angina at rest accompanied by ST segment elevation, (2) angina or coronary artery spasm provoked by ergonovine, or (3) angiographically demonstrated coronary artery spasm. In those patients who have had angiography, the presence of significant fixed obstructive disease is not incompatible with the diagnosis of vasospastic angina, provided that the above criteria are satisfied. Nifedipine may also be used where the clinical presentation suggests a possible vasospastic component but where vasospasm has not been confirmed, *e.g.,* where pain has a variable threshold on exertion (or, in the extended-release tablets, in unstable angina where electrocardiographic findings are compatible with intermittent vasospasm), or when angina is refractory to nitrates and/or adequate doses of beta blockers.

CHRONIC STABLE ANGINA

Classical Effort-Associated Angina

Nifedipine is indicated for the management of chronic stable angina (effort-associated angina) without evidence of vasospasm in patients who remain symptomatic despite adequate doses of beta blockers and/or organic nitrates or who cannot tolerate those agents.

In chronic stable angina (effort-associated angina) nifedipine has been effective in controlled trials of up to 8 weeks duration in reducing angina frequency and increasing exercise tolerance, but confirmation of sustained effectiveness and evaluation of long-term safety in these patients are incomplete.

Controlled studies in small numbers of patients suggest concomitant use of nifedipine and beta-blocking agents may be beneficial in patients with chronic stable angina, but available information is not sufficient to predict with confidence the effects of concurrent treatment, especially in patients with compromised left ventricular function or cardiac conduction abnormalities. When introducing such concomitant therapy, care must be taken to monitor blood pressure closely since severe hypotension can occur from the combined effects of the drugs. (See WARNINGS.)

ADDITIONAL INFORMATION FOR EXTENDED-RELEASE TABLETS

Hypertension

Nifedipine is also indicated for the treatment of hypertension. It may be used alone or in combination with other antihypertensive agents.

NON-FDA APPROVED INDICATIONS

Use of nifedipine to treat heart failure, aortic regurgitation, or to prevent labor or migraine headaches is not approved by the FDA.

CONTRAINDICATIONS

Known hypersensitivity reaction to nifedipine.

WARNINGS

EXCESSIVE HYPOTENSION

Although, in most patients, the hypotensive effect of nifedipine is modest and well tolerated, occasional patients have had excessive and poorly tolerated hypotension. These responses have usually occurred during initial titration or at the time of subsequent upward dosage adjustment, and with the extended-release tablets, may be more likely in patients on concomitant beta blockers.

Severe hypotension and/or increased fluid volume requirements have been reported in patients receiving nifedipine together with a beta blocking agent who underwent coronary artery bypass surgery using high dose fentanyl anesthesia. The interaction with high dose fentanyl appears to be due to the combination of nifedipine and a beta blocker, but the possibility that it may occur with nifedipine alone, with low doses of fentanyl, in other surgical procedures, or with other narcotic analgesics cannot be ruled out. In nifedipine treated patients where surgery using high dose fentanyl anesthesia is contemplated, the physician should be aware of these potential problems and, if the patient's condition permits, sufficient time (at least 36 hours) should be allowed for nifedipine to be washed out of the body prior to surgery.

Additional Information for Immediate-Release Capsules

Although patients have rarely experienced excessive hypotension on nifedipine alone, this may be more common in patients on concomitant beta-blocker therapy. Although not approved for this purpose, nifedipine and other immediate-release nifedipine capsules have been used (orally and sublingually) for acute reduction of blood pressure. Several well-documented reports describe cases of profound hypotension, myocardial infarction, and death when immediate-release nifedipine was used in this way. Nifedipine capsules should not be used for the acute reduction of blood pressure.

Nifedipine and other immediate-release nifedipine capsules have also been used for the long-term control of essential hypertension, although no properly-controlled studies have been conducted to define an appropriate dose or dose interval for such treatment. Nifedipine capsules should not be used for the control of essential hypertension.

Several well-controlled, randomized trials studied the use of immediate-release nifedipine in patients who had just sustained myocardial infarctions. In none of these trials did immediate-release nifedipine appear to provide any benefit. In some of the trials, patients who received immediate-release nifedipine had significantly worse outcomes than patients who received placebo. Nifedipine capsules should not be administered within the first week or two after myocardial infarction, and they should also be avoided in the setting of acute coronary syndrome (when infarction may be imminent).

The following information should be taken into account in those patients who are being treated for hypertension as well as angina:

Increased angina and/or myocardial infarction: Rarely, patients, particularly those who have severe obstructive coronary artery disease, have developed well documented increased frequency, duration and/or severity of angina or acute myocardial infarction on starting nifedipine or at the time of dosage increase. The mechanism of this effect is not established.

Beta blocker withdrawal: Patients recently withdrawn from beta blockers may develop a withdrawal syndrome with increased angina, probably related to increased sensitivity to catecholamines. Initiation of nifedipine treatment will not prevent this occurrence and might be expected to exacerbate it by provoking reflex catecholamine release. *Additional information for immediate-release capsules:* There have been occasional reports of increased angina in a setting of beta blocker withdrawal and nifedipine initiation. It is important to taper beta blockers if possible, rather than stopping them abruptly before beginning nifedipine. *Additional information for extended-release tablets:* It is important to taper beta blockers if possible, rather than stopping them abruptly before beginning nifedipine.

Congestive heart failure: Rarely, patients usually receiving a beta blocker, have developed heart failure after beginning nifedipine. Patients with tight aortic stenosis may be at greater risk for such an event, as the unloading effect of nifedipine would be expected to be of less benefit to these patients, owing to their fixed impedance to flow across the aortic valve.

PRECAUTIONS

GENERAL

Hypotension

Because nifedipine decreases peripheral vascular resistance, careful monitoring of blood pressure during the initial administration and titration of nifedipine is suggested. Close observation is especially recommended for patients already taking medications that are known to lower blood pressure. (See WARNINGS.)

Peripheral Edema

Immediate-Release Capsules

Mild to moderate peripheral edema, typically associated with arterial vasodilation and not due to left ventricular dysfunction, occurs in about 1 in 10 patients treated with nifedipine. This edema occurs primarily in the lower extremities and usually responds to diuretic therapy. With patients whose angina is complicated by congestive heart failure, care should be taken to differentiate this peripheral edema from the effects of increasing left ventricular dysfunction.

Extended-Release Tablets

Mild to moderate peripheral edema occurs in a dose dependent manner with an incidence ranging from approximately 10% to about 30% at the highest dose studied (180 mg). It is a localized phenomenon thought to be associated with vasodilation of dependent arterioles and small blood vessels and not due to left ventricular dysfunction or generalized fluid retention. With patients whose angina or hypertension is complicated by congestive heart failure, care should be taken to differentiate this peripheral edema from the effects of increasing left ventricular dysfunction.

Additional Information for Extended-Release Tablets

As with any other non-deformable material, caution should be used when administering nifedipine in patients with preexisting severe gastrointestinal narrowing (pathologic or iatrogenic). There have been rare reports of obstructive symptoms in patients with known strictures in association with the ingestion of nifedipine.

INFORMATION FOR THE PATIENT

Extended-Release Tablets

Nifedipine extended-release tablets should be swallowed whole. Do not chew, divide or crush tablets. Do not be concerned if you occasionally notice in you stool something that looks like a tablet. In nifedipine, the medication is contained within a nonabsorbable shell that has been specially designed to slowly release the drug for your body to absorb. When this process is completed, the empty tablet is eliminated from your body.

Adalat CC should be taken on an empty stomach. It should not be administered with food.

LABORATORY TESTS

Nifedipine, like other calcium channel blockers, decreases platelet aggregation *in vitro*. Limited clinical studies have demonstrated a moderate but statistically significant decrease in platelet aggregation and an increase in bleeding time in some nifedipine patients. This is thought to be a function of inhibition of calcium transport across the platelet membrane. No clinical significance for these findings has been demonstrated.

Positive direct Coombs test with/without hemolytic anemia has been reported but a causal relationship between nifedipine administration and positivity of this laboratory test, including hemolysis, could not be determined.

Although nifedipine has been used safely in patients with renal dysfunction and has been reported to exert a beneficial effect, in certain cases, rare, reversible elevations in BUN and serum creatinine have been reported in patients with pre-existing chronic renal insufficiency. The relationship to nifedipine therapy is uncertain in most cases but probable in some.

Additional Information for Immediate-Release Capsules

Rare, usually transient, but occasionally significant elevations of enzymes such as alkaline phosphatase, CPK, LDH, SGOT, and SGPT have been noted. The relationship to nifedipine therapy is uncertain in most cases, but probable in some. These laboratory abnormalities have rarely been associated with clinical symptoms,; however, cholestasis with or without jaundice has been reported. Rare instances of allergic hepatitis have been reported.

Additional Information for Extended-Release Tablets

Rare, usually transient, but occasionally significant elevations of enzymes such as alkaline phosphatase, CPK, LDH, SGOT, and SGPT have been noted. The relationship to nifedipine therapy is uncertain in most case, but probable in some. These laboratory abnormalities have rarely been associated with clinical symptoms; however, cholestasis with or without jaundice has been reported. A small (5.4%) increase in mean alkaline phosphatase was noted in patients treated with nifedipine. This was an isolated finding not associated with clinical symptoms and it rarely resulted in values which fell outside the normal range. Rare instances of allergic hepatitis have been reported. In controlled studies, nifedipine did not adversely affect serum uric acid, glucose, or cholesterol. Serum potassium was unchanged in patients receiving nifedipine in the absence of concomitant diuretic therapy, and slightly decreased in patients receiving concomitant diuretics.

CARCINOGENESIS, MUTAGENESIS, AND IMPAIRMENT OF FERTILITY

Nifedipine was administered orally to rats for 2 years and was not shown to be carcinogenic. When given to rats prior to mating, nifedipine caused reduced fertility at a dose approximately 30 times the maximum recommended human dose. There is a literature report of reversible reduction in the ability of human sperm obtained from a limited number of infertile men taking recommended doses of nifedipine to bind to and fertilize an ovum *in vitro*. *In vivo* mutagenicity studies were negative.

PREGNANCY CATEGORY C

Nifedipine has been shown to produce teratogenic findings in rats and rabbits, including digital anomalies similar to those reported for phenytoin. Digital anomalies have been reported to occur with other members of the dihydropyridine class and are possibly a result of compromised uterine blood flow. Nifedipine administration was associated with a variety of

N

embryotoxic, placentotoxic, and fetotoxic effects, including stunted fetuses (rats, mice, rabbits), rib deformities (mice), cleft palate (mice), small placentas and underdeveloped chorionic villi (monkeys), embryonic and fetal deaths (rats, mice, rabbits), and prolonged pregnancy/decreased neonatal survival (rats; not evaluated in other species). On a mg/kg basis, all of the doses associated with the teratogenic embryotoxic or fetotoxic effects in animals were higher (3.5-42 times) than the maximum recommended human dose of 120 mg/day. On a mg/m^2 basis, some doses were higher and some were lower than the maximum recommended human dose but all are within an order of magnitude of it. The doses associated with placentotoxic effects in monkeys were equivalent to or lower than the maximum recommended human dose on a mg/m^2 basis.

There are no adequate and well-controlled studies in pregnant women. Nifedipine should be used during pregnancy only if the potential benefit justifies the potential risk to the fetus.

PEDIATRIC USE

Safety and effectiveness in pediatric patients have not been established. *Immediate-Release Capsules:* Use in pediatric population is not recommended.

DRUG INTERACTIONS

Beta-Adrenergic Blocking Agents: See INDICATIONS AND USAGE and WARNINGS. Experience in over 1400 patients in a non-comparative clinical trial has shown that concomitant administration of nifedipine and beta-blocking agents is usually well tolerated, but there have been occasional literature reports suggesting that the combination may increase the likelihood of congestive heart failure, severe hypotension or exacerbation of angina.

Long Acting Nitrates: Nifedipine may be safely co-administered with nitrates, but there have been no controlled studies to evaluate the antianginal effectiveness of this combination.

Digitalis: *Immediate-Release Capsules:* Since there have been isolated reports of patients with elevated digoxin levels, and there is a possible interaction between digoxin and nifedipine, it is recommended that digoxin levels be monitored when initiating, adjusting, and discontinuing nifedipine to avoid possible over- or under-digitalization. *Extended-Release Tablets:* Administration of nifedipine with digoxin increased digoxin levels in 9 of 12 normal volunteers. The average increase was 45%. Another investigator found no increase in digoxin levels in 13 patients with coronary artery disease. In an uncontrolled study of over 200 patients with congestive heart failure during which digoxin blood levels were not measured, digitalis toxicity was not observed. Since there have been isolated reports of patients with elevated digoxin levels, it is recommended that digoxin levels be monitored when initiating, adjusting, and discontinuing nifedipine to avoid possible over- or under-digitalization.

Quinidine: *Immediate-Release Capsules:* There have been rare reports of an interaction between quinidine and nifedipine (with a decreased plasma level of quinidine).

Coumarin Anticoagulants: There have been rare reports of increased prothrombin time in patients taking coumarin anticoagulants to whom nifedipine was administered. However, the relationship to nifedipine therapy is uncertain.

Cimetidine: A study in 6 healthy volunteers has shown a significant increase in peak nifedipine plasma levels (80%) and area-under-the-curve (74%) after a 1 week course of cimetidine at 1000 mg/day and nifedipine at 40 mg/day. Ranitidine produced smaller, non-significant increases. The effect may be mediated by the known inhibition of cimetidine on hepatic cytochrome P-450, the enzyme system probably responsible for the first-pass metabolism of nifedipine. If nifedipine therapy is initiated in a patient currently receiving cimetidine, cautious titration is advised.

ADVERSE REACTIONS

IMMEDIATE-RELEASE CAPSULES

In multiple-dose US and foreign controlled studies in which adverse reactions were reported spontaneously, adverse effects were frequent but generally not serious and rarely required discontinuation of therapy or dosage adjustment. Most were expected consequences of the vasodilator effects of nifedipine. (See TABLE 1.)

TABLE 1

Adverse Effect	Nifedipine (n=226)	Placebo (n=235)
Dizziness, lightheadedness, giddiness	27%	15%
Flushing, heat sensation	25%	8%
Headache	23%	20%
Weakness	12%	10%
Nausea, heartburn	11%	8%
Muscle cramps, tremor	8%	3%
Peripheral edema	7%	1%
Nervousness, mood changes	7%	4%
Palpitation	7%	5%
Dyspnea, cough, wheezing	6%	3%
Nasal congestion, sore throat	6%	8%

There is also a large uncontrolled experience in over 2100 patients in the US. Most of the patients had vasospastic or resistant angina pectoris, and about half had concomitant treatment with beta-adrenergic blocking agents. The most common adverse events were:

Incidence approximately 10%:
- *Cardiovascular:* Peripheral edema.
- *Central Nervous System:* Dizziness or lightheadedness.
- *Gastrointestinal:* Nausea.
- *Systemic:* Headache and flushing, weakness.

Incidence approximately 5%:
- *Cardiovascular:* Transient hypotension.

Incidence 2% or less:
- *Cardiovascular:* Palpitation.
- *Respiratory:* Nasal and chest congestion, shortness of breath.
- *Gastrointestinal:* Diarrhea, constipation, cramps, flatulence.
- *Musculoskeletal:* Inflammation, joint stiffness, muscle cramps.
- *Central Nervous System:* Shakiness, nervousness, jitteriness, sleep disturbances, blurred vision, difficulties in balance.
- *Other:* Dermatitis, pruritus, urticaria, fever, sweating, chills, sexual difficulties.

Incidence approximately 0.5%:
- *Cardiovascular:* Syncope (mostly with initial dosing and/or an increase in dose), erythromelalgia.

Incidence less than 0.5%:
- *Hematologic:* Thrombocytopenia, anemia, leukopenia, purpura.
- *Gastrointestinal:* Allergic hepatitis.
- *Face and Throat:* Angioedema (mostly oropharyngeal edema with breathing difficulty in a few patients), gingival hyperplasia.
- *CNS:* Depression, paranoid syndrome.
- *Special Senses:* Transient blindness at the peak of plasma level, tinnitus.
- *Urogenital:* Nocturia, polyuria.
- *Other:* Arthritis with ANA (+), exfoliative dermatitis, gynecomastia.
- *Musculoskeletal:* Myalgia.

Several of these side effects appear to be dose related. Peripheral edema occurred in about 1 in 25 patients at doses less than 60 mg/day and in about 1 patient in 8 at 120 mg/day or more. Transient hypotension, generally of mild to moderate severity and seldom requiring discontinuation of therapy, occurred in 1 of 50 patients at less than 60 mg/day and in 1 of 20 patients at 120 mg/day or more.

Very rarely, introduction of nifedipine therapy was associated with an increase in anginal pain, possibly due to associated hypotension. Transient unilateral loss of vision has also occurred.

In addition, more serious adverse events were observed, not readily distinguishable from the natural history of the disease in these patients. It remains possible, however, that some or many of these events were drug related. Myocardial infarction occurred in about 4% of patients and congestive heart failure or pulmonary edema in about 2%. Ventricular arrhythmias or conduction disturbances each occurred in fewer than 0.5% of patients.

In a subgroup of over 1000 patients receiving nifedipine with concomitant beta blocker therapy, the pattern and incidence of adverse experiences was not different from that of the entire group of nifedipine treated patients. (See PRECAUTIONS.)

In a subgroup of approximately 250 patients with a diagnosis of congestive heart failure as well as angina pectoris (about 10% of the total patient population), dizziness or lightheadedness, peripheral edema, headache or flushing each occurred in 1 in 8 patients. Hypotension occurred in about 1 in 20 patients. Syncope occurred in approximately 1 patient in 250. Myocardial infarction or symptoms of congestive heart failure each occurred in about 1 patient in 15. Atrial or ventricular dysrhythmias each occurred in about 1 patient in 150.

In post-marketing experience, there have been rare reports of exfoliative dermatitis caused by nifedipine. There have been rare reports of exfoliative or bullous skin adverse events (such as exfoliative dermatitis, erythema multiforme, Stevens-Johnson Syndrome, and toxic epidermal necrolysis) and photosensitivity reactions.

EXTENDED-RELEASE TABLETS

Over 1000 patients from both controlled and open trials with nifedipine extended-release tablets in hypertension and angina were included in the evaluation of adverse experiences. All side effects reported during nifedipine extended-release tablet therapy were tabulated independent of their causal relation to medication. The most common side effect reported with nifedipine was edema which was dose related and ranged in frequency from approximately 10% to about 30% at the highest dose studied (180 mg). Other common adverse experiences reported in placebo-controlled trials include those shown in TABLE 2.

TABLE 2

Adverse Effect	Nifedipine Extended Release Tablets (n=707)	Placebo (n=266)
Headache	15.8%	9.8%
Fatigue	5.9%	4.1%
Dizziness	4.1%	4.5%
Constipation	3.3%	2.3%
Nausea	3.3%	1.9%

Of these, only edema and headache were more common in nifedipine patients than placebo patients.

The following adverse reactions occurred with an incidence of less than 3.0%. With the exception of leg cramps, the incidence of these side effects was similar to that of placebo alone.

- *Body as a Whole/Systemic:* Asthenia, flushing, pain.
- *Cardiovascular:* Palpitations.
- *Central Nervous System:* Insomnia, nervousness, paresthesia, somnolence.
- *Dermatologic:* Pruritus, rash.
- *Gastrointestinal:* Abdominal pain, diarrhea, dry mouth, dyspepsia, flatulence.
- *Musculoskeletal:* Arthralgia, leg cramps.
- *Respiratory:* Chest pain (nonspecific), dyspnea.
- *Urogenital:* Impotence, polyuria.

Other adverse reactions were reported sporadically with an incidence of 1.0% or less. These include:

- *Body as a Whole/System:* Face edema, fever, hot flashes, malaise, periorbital edema, rigors.
- *Cardiovascular:* Arrhythmia, hypotension, increased angina, tachycardia, syncope.

N

Central Nervous System: Anxiety, ataxia, decreased libido, depression, hypertonia, hypoesthesia, migraine, paroniria, tremor, vertigo.
Dermatologic: Alopecia, increased sweating, urticaria, purpura.
Gastrointestinal: Eructation, gastroesophageal reflux, gum hyperplasia, melena, vomiting, weight increase.
Musculoskeletal: Back pain, gout, myalgias.
Respiratory: Coughing, epistaxis, upper respiratory tract infection, respiratory disorder, sinusitis.
Special Senses: Abnormal lacrimation, abnormal vision, taste perversion, tinnitus.
Urogenital/Reproductive: Breast pain, dysuria, hematuria, nocturia.

Adverse experiences which occurred in less than 1 in 1000 patients cannot be distinguished from concurrent disease states or medications.

The following adverse experiences, reported in less than 1% of patients, occurred under conditions (*e.g.,* open trials, marketing experience) where a causal relationship is uncertain: gastrointestinal irritation, gastrointestinal bleeding, gynecomastia.

There is also a large uncontrolled experience in over 2100 patients in the US. Most of the patients had vasospastic or resistant angina pectoris, and about half had concomitant treatment with beta-adrenergic blocking agents. The relatively common adverse events were similar in nature to those seen with nifedipine.

In addition, more serious adverse events were observed, not readily distinguishable from the natural history of the disease in these patients. It remains possible, however, that some or many of these events were drug related. Myocardial infarction occurred in about 4% of patients and congestive heart failure or pulmonary edema in about 2%. Ventricular arrhythmias or conduction disturbances each occurred in fewer than 0.5% of patients.

In a subgroup of over 1000 patients receiving nifedipine with concomitant beta blocker therapy, the pattern and incidence of adverse experiences were not different from that of the entire group of nifedipine treated patients. (See PRECAUTIONS.)

In a subgroup of approximately 250 patients with a diagnosis of congestive heart failure as well as angina, dizziness or lightheadedness, peripheral edema, headache or flushing each occurred in 1 in 8 patients. Hypotension occurred in about 1 in 20 patients. Syncope occurred in approximately 1 patient in 250. Myocardial infarction or symptoms of congestive heart failure each occurred in about 1 patient in 15. Atrial or ventricular dysrhythmias each occurred in about 1 patient in 150.

In post-marketing experience, there have been rare reports of exfoliative dermatitis caused by nifedipine. There have been rare reports of exfoliative or bullous skin adverse events (such as exfoliative dermatitis, erythema multiforme, Stevens-Johnson Syndrome, and toxic epidermal necrolysis) and photosensitivity reactions.

DOSAGE AND ADMINISTRATION

IMMEDIATE-RELEASE CAPSULES

The dosage of nifedipine needed to suppress angina and that can be tolerated by the patient must be established by titration. Excessive doses can result in hypotension.

Therapy should be initiated with the 10 mg capsule. The starting dose is one 10 mg capsule, swallowed whole, 3 tid. The usual effective dose range is 10-20 mg 3 tid. Some patients, especially those with evidence of coronary artery spasm, respond only to higher doses, more frequent administration, or both. In such patients, doses of 20-30 mg 3 or 4 times daily may be effective. Doses above 120 mg daily are rarely necessary. More than 180 mg/day is not recommended.

In most cases, nifedipine titration should proceed over a 7-14 day period so that the physician can assess the response to each dose level and monitor the blood pressure before proceeding to higher doses.

If symptoms so warrant, titration may proceed more rapidly provided that the patient is assessed frequently. Based on the patient's physical activity level, attack frequency, and sublingual nitroglycerin consumption, the dose of nifedipine may be increased from 10 mg tid to 20 mg tid and then to 30 mg tid over a 3 day period.

In hospitalized patients under close observation, the dose may be increased in 10 mg increments over 4-6 hour periods as required to control pain and arrhythmias due to ischemia. A single dose should rarely exceed 30 mg.

No "rebound effect" has been observed upon discontinuation of nifedipine. However, if discontinuation of nifedipine is necessary, sound clinical practice suggests that the dosage should be decreased gradually with close physician supervision.

Coadministration With Other Antianginal Drugs

Sublingual nitroglycerin may be taken as required for the control of acute manifestations of angina, particularly during nifedipine titration. See DRUG INTERACTIONS for information on co-administration of nifedipine with beta blockers or long-acting nitrates.

EXTENDED-RELEASE TABLETS

Dosage must be adjusted according to each patient's needs. Therapy for either hypertension or angina should be initiated with 30 or 60 mg once daily. Nifedipine extended-release tablets should be swallowed whole and should not be bitten or divided. In general, titration should proceed over a 7-14 day period so that the physician can fully assess the response to each dose level and monitor blood pressure before proceeding to higher doses. Since steady-state plasma levels are achieved on the second day of dosing, if symptoms so warrant, titration may proceed more rapidly provided the patient is assessed frequently. Titration to doses above 120 mg are not recommended.

Angina patients controlled on nifedipine capsules alone or in combination with other antianginal medications may be safety switched to nifedipine extended-release tablets at the nearest equivalent total daily dose (*e.g.,* 30 mg tid of nifedipine capsules may be changed to 90 mg once daily of nifedipine extended-release tablets). Subsequent titration to higher or lower doses may be necessary and should be initiated as clinically warranted. Experience with dose greater than 90 mg in patients with angina is limited. Therefore, doses greater than 90 mg should be used with caution and only when clinically warranted.

No "rebound effect" has been observed upon discontinuation of nifedipine extended-release tablets. However, if discontinuation of nifedipine is necessary, sound clinical practice suggests that the dosage should be decreased gradually with close physician supervision.

Care should be taken when dispensing nifedipine to assure that the extended-release dosage form has been prescribed.

Coadministration With Other Antianginal Drugs

Sublingual nitroglycerin may be taken as required for the control of acute manifestations of angina, particularly during nifedipine titration. See DRUG INTERACTIONS for information on co-administration of nifedipine with beta blockers or long-acting nitrates.

HOW SUPPLIED

PROCARDIA IMMEDIATE-RELEASE CAPSULES

Procardia soft gelatin capsules are supplied as:

10 mg: Orange #260.
20 mg: Orange and light brown #261.

Storage: The capsules should be protected from light and moisture and stored at controlled room temperature 15-25°C (59-77°F) in the manufacturer's original container.

PROCARDIA XL EXTENDED-RELEASE TABLETS

Procardia XL extended-release tablets are supplied as 30, 60, and 90 mg round biconvex, rose-pink, film-coated tablets.

Storage: Stored below 30°C (86°F). Protect from moisture and humidity.

PRODUCT LISTING - RATED THERAPEUTICALLY EQUIVALENT

Capsule - Oral - 10 mg			
8's	$3.60	GENERIC, Pd-Rx Pharmaceuticals	55289-0907-08
15's	$6.95	GENERIC, Heartland Healthcare Services	61392-0356-15
25's	$6.84	GENERIC, Pd-Rx Pharmaceuticals	55289-0907-97
30 x 25	$397.13	GENERIC, Sky Pharmaceuticals Packaging, Inc	63739-0185-03
30's	$7.35	GENERIC, Pd-Rx Pharmaceuticals	55289-0907-30
30's	$13.91	GENERIC, Heartland Healthcare Services	61392-0356-30
30's	$13.91	GENERIC, Heartland Healthcare Services	61392-0356-39
30's	$274.60	GENERIC, Medirex Inc	57480-0389-06
31 x 10	$161.01	GENERIC, Vangard Labs	00615-0360-53
31 x 10	$161.01	GENERIC, Vangard Labs	00615-0360-63
31's	$14.37	GENERIC, Heartland Healthcare Services	61392-0356-31
32's	$14.83	GENERIC, Heartland Healthcare Services	61392-0356-32
45's	$20.86	GENERIC, Heartland Healthcare Services	61392-0356-45
60's	$27.81	GENERIC, Heartland Healthcare Services	61392-0356-60
90's	$41.72	GENERIC, Heartland Healthcare Services	61392-0356-90
100's	$12.37	FEDERAL UPPER LIMIT, H.C.F.A. F F P	99999-1886-01
100's	$19.00	GENERIC, Raway Pharmacal Inc	00686-0664-20
100's	$36.75	GENERIC, Interstate Drug Exchange Inc	00814-5333-14
100's	$39.39	GENERIC, Us Trading Corporation	56126-0449-11
100's	$40.42	GENERIC, Dixon-Shane Inc	17236-0923-11
100's	$42.50	GENERIC, Chase Laboratories Inc	54429-3227-01
100's	$43.25	GENERIC, Major Pharmaceuticals Inc	00904-7685-60
100's	$43.45	GENERIC, Major Pharmaceuticals Inc	00904-0407-60
100's	$43.45	GENERIC, Major Pharmaceuticals Inc	00904-0409-60
100's	$43.45	GENERIC, Major Pharmaceuticals Inc	00904-7950-60
100's	$44.05	GENERIC, Mova Pharmaceutical Corporation	55370-0156-07
100's	$44.51	GENERIC, Caremark Inc	00339-5717-12
100's	$44.51	GENERIC, Aligen Independent Laboratories Inc	00405-4696-01
100's	$45.86	GENERIC, Major Pharmaceuticals Inc	00904-0407-61
100's	$48.00	GENERIC, Geneva Pharmaceuticals	00781-2504-01
100's	$48.09	GENERIC, Moore, H.L. Drug Exchange Inc	00839-7564-06
100's	$49.50	GENERIC, Ivax Corporation	00182-1547-01
100's	$49.75	GENERIC, Teva Pharmaceuticals Usa	00093-8171-01
100's	$51.00	GENERIC, Watson/Schein Pharmaceuticals Inc	00364-2376-90
100's	$51.95	GENERIC, Ivax Corporation	00182-1547-89
100's	$59.95	GENERIC, Purepac Pharmaceutical Company	00228-2497-10
100's	$66.61	GENERIC, Major Pharmaceuticals Inc	00904-0409-61
100's	$77.28	PROCARDIA, Pfizer U.S. Pharmaceuticals	00069-2600-66
200 x 5	$519.39	GENERIC, Vangard Labs	00615-0360-43
Capsule - Oral - 20 mg			
30's	$27.11	GENERIC, Heartland Healthcare Services	61392-0353-30
30's	$27.11	GENERIC, Heartland Healthcare Services	61392-0353-39
31 x 10	$311.17	GENERIC, Vangard Labs	00615-0359-53
31 x 10	$311.17	GENERIC, Vangard Labs	00615-0359-63
31's	$28.01	GENERIC, Heartland Healthcare Services	61392-0353-31
32's	$28.91	GENERIC, Heartland Healthcare Services	61392-0353-32
45's	$40.66	GENERIC, Heartland Healthcare Services	61392-0353-45
60's	$54.21	GENERIC, Heartland Healthcare Services	61392-0353-60
90's	$81.32	GENERIC, Heartland Healthcare Services	61392-0353-90
100's	$38.00	GENERIC, Raway Pharmacal Inc	00686-0665-20
100's	$69.00	GENERIC, Interstate Drug Exchange Inc	00814-5335-14
100's	$71.00	GENERIC, Chase Laboratories Inc	54429-3453-01
100's	$77.70	GENERIC, Us Trading Corporation	56126-0453-11
100's	$80.04	GENERIC, Aligen Independent Laboratories Inc	00405-4697-01
100's	$80.18	GENERIC, Moore, H.L. Drug Exchange Inc	00839-7565-06
100's	$80.18	GENERIC, Moore, H.L. Drug Exchange Inc	00839-7717-06
100's	$81.65	GENERIC, Major Pharmaceuticals Inc	00904-0408-61
100's	$81.82	GENERIC, Caremark Inc	00339-5718-12
100's	$83.10	GENERIC, Mova Pharmaceutical Corporation	55370-0157-07
100's	$84.90	GENERIC, Major Pharmaceuticals Inc	00904-0408-60
100's	$84.90	GENERIC, Major Pharmaceuticals Inc	00904-7699-60

100's	$84.90	GENERIC, Major Pharmaceuticals Inc	00904-7951-60
100's	$86.50	GENERIC, Ivax Corporation	00182-1548-01
100's	$86.50	GENERIC, Geneva Pharmaceuticals	00781-2506-01
100's	$90.00	GENERIC, Vangard Labs	00615-0359-13
100's	$100.39	GENERIC, Ivax Corporation	00182-1548-89
100's	$101.00	GENERIC, Purepac Pharmaceutical Company	00228-2530-10
100's	$134.20	PROCARDIA, Pfizer U.S. Pharmaceuticals	00069-2610-66
120's	$108.42	GENERIC, Heartland Healthcare Services	61392-0353-34
180's	$162.63	GENERIC, Heartland Healthcare Services	61392-0353-36

Tablet, Extended Release - Oral - 60 mg

100's	$224.07	GENERIC, Watson Laboratories Inc	00591-0661-01

Tablet, Extended Release - Oral - 90 mg

100's	$256.54	GENERIC, Teva Pharmaceuticals Usa	00093-1023-01

PRODUCT LISTING - RATED NOT THERAPEUTICALLY EQUIVALENT

Tablet, Extended Release - Oral - 30 mg

10's	$14.27	PROCARDIA XL, Allscripts Pharmaceutical Company	54569-2780-03
30's	$39.93	ADALAT CC, Allscripts Pharmaceutical Company	54569-3891-00
30's	$42.80	PROCARDIA XL, Allscripts Pharmaceutical Company	54569-2780-00
30's	$45.19	ADALAT CC, Physicians Total Care	54868-2868-01
30's	$49.51	PROCARDIA XL, Physicians Total Care	54868-1006-02
30's	$53.46	PROCARDIA XL, Pd-Rx Pharmaceuticals	55289-0323-30
60's	$85.59	PROCARDIA XL, Allscripts Pharmaceutical Company	54569-2780-02
60's	$89.18	ADALAT CC, Physicians Total Care	54868-2868-00
90's	$110.87	PROCARDIA XL, Allscripts Pharmaceutical Company	54569-8504-00
100's	$115.35	GENERIC, Teva Pharmaceuticals Usa	00093-1021-01
100's	$126.16	ADALAT CC, Allscripts Pharmaceutical Company	54569-3891-01
100's	$132.45	GENERIC, Mylan Pharmaceuticals Inc	00378-3475-01
100's	$136.47	GENERIC, Teva Pharmaceuticals Usa	00093-0819-01
100's	$139.09	ADALAT CC, Physicians Total Care	54868-2868-02
100's	$142.65	PROCARDIA XL, Allscripts Pharmaceutical Company	54569-2780-01
100's	$143.36	ADALAT CC, Bayer	00026-8841-51
100's	$150.51	ADALAT CC, Bayer	00026-8841-48
100's	$152.75	PROCARDIA XL, Physicians Total Care	54868-1006-03
100's	$156.94	PROCARDIA XL, Pfizer U.S. Pharmaceuticals	00069-2650-66
100's	$182.54	PROCARDIA XL, Pd-Rx Pharmaceuticals	55289-0323-01

Tablet, Extended Release - Oral - 60 mg

10's	$29.06	PROCARDIA XL, Physicians Total Care	54868-1008-00
30's	$71.13	ADALAT CC, Allscripts Pharmaceutical Company	54569-3892-00
30's	$74.06	PROCARDIA XL, Allscripts Pharmaceutical Company	54569-2781-00
30's	$79.56	ADALAT CC, Physicians Total Care	54868-2869-03
30's	$84.82	PROCARDIA XL, Physicians Total Care	54868-1008-01
30's	$92.66	ADALAT CC, Pd-Rx Pharmaceuticals	55289-0543-30
30's	$94.41	PROCARDIA XL, Pd-Rx Pharmaceuticals	55289-0357-30
60's	$149.21	ADALAT CC, Physicians Total Care	54868-2869-00
90's	$191.84	PROCARDIA XL, Allscripts Pharmaceutical Company	54569-8509-00
100's	$216.79	GENERIC, Teva Pharmaceuticals Usa	00093-1022-01
100's	$229.15	GENERIC, Mylan Pharmaceuticals Inc	00378-3482-01
100's	$236.17	GENERIC, Teva Pharmaceuticals Usa	00093-5173-01
100's	$246.86	PROCARDIA XL, Allscripts Pharmaceutical Company	54569-2781-01
100's	$247.88	ADALAT CC, Physicians Total Care	54868-2869-01
100's	$255.38	ADALAT CC, Bayer	00026-8851-51
100's	$263.91	PROCARDIA XL, Physicians Total Care	54868-1008-02
100's	$268.13	ADALAT CC, Bayer	00026-8851-48
100's	$271.59	PROCARDIA XL, Pfizer U.S. Pharmaceuticals	00069-2660-66
100's	$302.61	PROCARDIA XL, Pfizer U.S. Pharmaceuticals	00069-2660-41
100's	$321.57	PROCARDIA XL, Pd-Rx Pharmaceuticals	55289-0357-01

Tablet, Extended Release - Oral - 90 mg

30's	$85.45	PROCARDIA XL, Allscripts Pharmaceutical Company	54569-3055-02
30's	$86.02	ADALAT CC, Allscripts Pharmaceutical Company	54569-3893-00
30's	$92.65	ADALAT CC, Physicians Total Care	54868-2870-00
30's	$97.68	PROCARDIA XL, Physicians Total Care	54868-1443-03
30's	$113.03	ADALAT CC, Pd-Rx Pharmaceuticals	55289-0545-30
60's	$170.90	PROCARDIA XL, Allscripts Pharmaceutical Company	54569-3055-00
100's	$256.15	GENERIC, Mylan Pharmaceuticals Inc	00378-3495-01
100's	$299.29	ADALAT CC, Bayer	00026-8861-51
100's	$313.35	PROCARDIA XL, Pfizer U.S. Pharmaceuticals	00069-2670-66
100's	$314.29	ADALAT CC, Bayer	00026-8861-48
100's	$337.25	PROCARDIA XL, Pfizer U.S. Pharmaceuticals	00069-2670-41

PRODUCT LISTING - EQUIVALENTS NOT AVAILABLE

Capsule - Oral - 10 mg

1's	$3.42	GENERIC, Prescript Pharmaceuticals	00247-0206-01
2's	$3.48	GENERIC, Prescript Pharmaceuticals	00247-0206-02
3's	$3.55	GENERIC, Prescript Pharmaceuticals	00247-0206-03
5's	$3.68	GENERIC, Prescript Pharmaceuticals	00247-0206-05
8's	$5.03	GENERIC, Southwood Pharmaceuticals Inc	58016-0622-08
8's	$7.12	GENERIC, Pharma Pac	52959-0273-08
9's	$3.95	GENERIC, Prescript Pharmaceuticals	00247-0206-09
10's	$4.01	GENERIC, Prescript Pharmaceuticals	00247-0206-10
10's	$8.25	GENERIC, Pharma Pac	52959-0273-10
12's	$4.15	GENERIC, Prescript Pharmaceuticals	00247-0206-12
12's	$7.27	GENERIC, Southwood Pharmaceuticals Inc	58016-0622-12
14's	$4.28	GENERIC, Prescript Pharmaceuticals	00247-0206-14
15's	$4.34	GENERIC, Prescript Pharmaceuticals	00247-0206-15
15's	$8.99	GENERIC, Allscripts Pharmaceutical Company	54569-3121-04
15's	$9.09	GENERIC, Southwood Pharmaceuticals Inc	58016-0622-15
20's	$4.68	GENERIC, Prescript Pharmaceuticals	00247-0206-20
20's	$12.12	GENERIC, Southwood Pharmaceuticals Inc	58016-0622-20
20's	$13.95	GENERIC, Pharma Pac	52959-0273-20
21's	$12.59	GENERIC, Allscripts Pharmaceutical Company	54569-3121-05
30's	$5.34	GENERIC, Prescript Pharmaceuticals	00247-0206-30
30's	$14.42	GENERIC, Allscripts Pharmaceutical Company	54569-3121-00
30's	$18.17	GENERIC, Southwood Pharmaceuticals Inc	58016-0622-30
30's	$20.00	GENERIC, Pharma Pac	52959-0273-30
40's	$6.00	GENERIC, Prescript Pharmaceuticals	00247-0206-40
40's	$25.85	GENERIC, Pharma Pac	52959-0273-40
50's	$30.29	GENERIC, Southwood Pharmaceuticals Inc	58016-0622-50
50's	$31.95	GENERIC, Pharma Pac	52959-0273-50
60's	$7.33	GENERIC, Prescript Pharmaceuticals	00247-0206-60
60's	$35.97	GENERIC, Allscripts Pharmaceutical Company	54569-3121-01
60's	$36.35	GENERIC, Southwood Pharmaceuticals Inc	58016-0622-60
60's	$37.95	GENERIC, Pharma Pac	52959-0273-60
80's	$49.25	GENERIC, Pharma Pac	52959-0273-80
90's	$9.31	GENERIC, Prescript Pharmaceuticals	00247-0206-90
90's	$53.96	GENERIC, Allscripts Pharmaceutical Company	54569-3121-02
90's	$54.52	GENERIC, Southwood Pharmaceuticals Inc	58016-0622-90
100's	$7.88	GENERIC, Physicians Total Care	54868-1326-02
100's	$9.98	GENERIC, Prescript Pharmaceuticals	00247-0206-00
100's	$59.95	GENERIC, Allscripts Pharmaceutical Company	54569-3121-03
100's	$60.58	GENERIC, Southwood Pharmaceuticals Inc	58016-0622-00
100's	$60.75	GENERIC, Pharma Pac	52959-0273-00
120's	$72.00	GENERIC, Pharma Pac	52959-0273-01

Capsule - Oral - 20 mg

12's	$13.08	GENERIC, Southwood Pharmaceuticals Inc	58016-0620-12
15's	$16.35	GENERIC, Southwood Pharmaceuticals Inc	58016-0620-15
20's	$21.80	GENERIC, Southwood Pharmaceuticals Inc	58016-0620-20
30's	$5.35	GENERIC, Physicians Total Care	54868-1521-02
30's	$19.86	GENERIC, Pharma Pac	52959-0488-30
30's	$32.70	GENERIC, Southwood Pharmaceuticals Inc	58016-0620-30
60's	$9.19	GENERIC, Physicians Total Care	54868-1521-00
90's	$82.30	GENERIC, Allscripts Pharmaceutical Company	54569-3122-02
90's	$98.10	GENERIC, Southwood Pharmaceuticals Inc	58016-0620-90
100's	$109.01	GENERIC, Southwood Pharmaceuticals Inc	58016-0620-00

Tablet, Extended Release - Oral - 30 mg

30's	$38.49	GENERIC, American Health Packaging	62584-0992-30
90's	$97.33	GENERIC, American Health Packaging	62584-0992-90
100's	$108.14	GENERIC, Caremark Inc	00339-6549-12
100's	$125.79	GENERIC, Watson Laboratories Inc	00591-0660-01
100's	$128.35	GENERIC, Mylan Pharmaceuticals Inc	00378-0474-01
100's	$132.45	GENERIC, Udl Laboratories Inc	51079-0940-20

Tablet, Extended Release - Oral - 60 mg

30's	$66.62	GENERIC, American Health Packaging	62584-0991-30
90's	$199.84	GENERIC, American Health Packaging	62584-0991-90
100's	$229.15	GENERIC, Udl Laboratories Inc	51079-0968-20

Tablet, Extended Release - Oral - 90 mg

30's	$76.85	GENERIC, American Health Packaging	62584-0999-30
90's	$199.84	GENERIC, American Health Packaging	62584-0999-90
100's	$256.15	GENERIC, Udl Laboratories Inc	51079-0969-20

Nilutamide *(003247)*

Categories: Carcinoma, prostate; Pregnancy Category C; FDA Approved 1996 Sep
Drug Classes: Antineoplastics, antiandrogens; Hormones/hormone modifiers
Brand Names: **Nilandron**
Foreign Brand Availability: Anandron (Canada; Costa-Rica; Czech-Republic; Dominican-Republic; El-Salvador; Finland; France; Guatemala; Honduras; Japan; Mexico; Netherlands; New-Zealand; Nicaragua; Norway; Panama; Peru; Portugal; Sweden)
Cost of Therapy: $525.48 (Prostate Cancer; Nilandron; 50 mg; 6 tablets/day; 30 day supply)
$604.30 (Prostate Cancer; Nilandron; 150 mg; 2 tablets/day; 30 day supply)
$344.33 (Prostate Cancer; Nilandron; 150 mg; 1 tablets/day; 30 day supply)

DESCRIPTION

Nilandron tablets contain nilutamide, a nonsteroidal, orally active antiandrogen having the chemical name 5,5-dimethyl 3-[4-nitro3-(trifluoromethyl) phenyl]2,4-imidazolidinedione.

Nilutamide is a microcrystalline, white to practically white powder with a molecular weight of 317.25.

It is freely soluble in ethyl acetate, acetone, chloroform, ethyl alcohol, dichloromethane, and methanol. It is slightly soluble in water [<0.1% W/V at 25°C (77°F)]. It melts between 153°C and 156°C (307.4°F and 312.8°F).

Each Nilandron tablet contains 50 mg nilutamide. Other ingredients in Nilandron tablets are corn starch, lactose, providone, docusate sodium, magnesium stearate, and talc.

CLINICAL PHARMACOLOGY

MECHANISM OF ACTION

Prostate cancer is known to be androgen sensitive and responds to androgen ablation. In animal studies, nilutamide has demonstrated antiandrogenic activity without other hormonal (estrogen, progesterone, mineralocorticoid, and glucocorticoid) effects. *In vitro*, nilutamide blocks the effects of testosterone at the androgen receptor level. *In vivo*, nilutamide interacts with the androgen receptor and prevents the normal androgenic response.

PHARMACOKINETICS

Absorption: Analysis of blood, urine, and feces samples following a single oral 150 mg dose of [^{14}C]-nilutamide in patients with metastatic prostate cancer showed that the drug is rapidly and completely absorbed and that it yields high and persistent plasma concentrations.

Distribution: After absorption of the drug, there is a detectable distribution phase. There is moderate binding of the drug to plasma proteins and low binding to erythrocytes. The binding is nonsaturable except in the case of alpha-1-glycoprotein, which makes a minor contribution to the total concentration of proteins in the plasma. The results of binding studies do not indicate any effects that would cause nonlinear pharmacokinetics.

Metabolism: The results of a human metabolism study using ^{14}C radiolabelled tablets show that nilutamide is extensively metabolized and less than 2% of the drug is excreted unchanged in urine after 5 days. Five metabolites have been isolated from human urine. Two metabolites display an asymmetric center, due to oxidation of a methyl group, resulting in the formation of D- and L-isomers. One of the metabolites was shown *in vitro*, to possess 25 to 50% of the pharmacological activity of the parent drug, and the D-isomer of the active metabolite showed equal or greater potency compared to the L-isomer. However, the pharmacokinetics and the pharmacodynamics of the metabolites have not been fully investigated.

Elimination: The majority (62%) of orally administered [^{14}C]-nilutamide is eliminated in the urine during the first 120 hours after a single 150 mg dose. Fecal elimination is negligible, ranging from 1.4% to 7% of the dose after 4 to 5 days. Excretion of radioactivity in urine likely continues beyond 5 days. The mean elimination half-life of nilutamide determined in studies in which subject received a single dose of 100-300 mg ranged from 38.0 to 59.1 hours with most values between 41 and 49 hours. The elimination of at least one metabolite is generally longer than that of unchanged nilutamide (59-126 hours). During multiple dosing of 3 x 50 mg twice a day, steady state was reached within 2 to 4 weeks for most patients, and mean steady state $AUC_{0-\infty}$ was 110% higher than the $AUC_{0-\infty}$ obtained from the first dose of 3 x 50 mg. These data and *in vitro* metabolism data suggest that upon multiple dosing metabolic enzyme inhibition may occur for this drug.

INDICATIONS AND USAGE

Metastatic Prostate Cancer: Nilutamide tablets are indicated for use in combination with surgical castration for the treatment of metastatic prostate cancer (Stage D_2). For maximum benefit, Nilutamide treatment must begin on the same day as or on the day after surgical castration.

CONTRAINDICATIONS

Nilutamide Tablets are Contraindicated in Patients:

- with severe hepatic impairment (baseline hepatic enzymes should be evaluated prior to treatment)
- with severe respiratory insufficiency
- with hypersensitivity to nilutamide or any component of this preparation.

WARNINGS

Interstitial Pneumonitis: Interstitial Pneumonitis has been reported in 2% of patients in controlled clinical trials in patients exposed to nilutamide. Patients typically presented with progressive exertional dyspnea, and possibly with cough, chest pain, and fever. X-rays showed interstitial or alveolo- interstitial changes. The suggestive signs of pneumonitis most often occurred within the first three months of nilutamide treatment. A routine chest x-ray should be performed before treatment, and patients should be told to report immediately any dyspnea or aggravation of pre-existing dyspnea.

At the onset of dyspnea or worsening of pre-existing dyspnea at any time during treatment, nilutamide should be interrupted until it can be determined if respiratory symptoms are drug related. A chest x-ray should be obtained, and if there are findings suggestive of interstitial pneumonitis, treatment with nilutamide should be discontinued. The pneumonitis is almost always reversible when treatment is discontinued.

If the chest x-ray appears normal. pulmonary function tests including DL_{CO} (diffusing capability of the lung for carbon monoxide) should be performed. If a significant decrease of DL_{CO} and/or a restrictive pattern is observed on pulmonary function testing, nilutamide treatment should be terminated. In the absence of chest x-ray and pulmonary function test findings consistent with interstitial pneumonitis, treatment with nilutamide can be restarted under close monitoring of pulmonary symptoms.

Because interstitial pneurnonltis was reported in 8 of 47 patients (17%) in a small study performed in Japan, specific caution should be observed in the treatment of Asian patients.

Hepatitis: Hepatitis or marked increases in liver enzymes leading to drug discontinuation occurred in 1% of nilutamide patients in controlled clinical trials;

Serum hepatic enzyme levels should be measured at baseline and at regular intervals (3 months); if transaminases increase over 2-3 times the upper limit of normal, treatment should be discontinued.

Appropriate laboratory testing should be done at the first symptom/sign of liver injury (*e.g.*, jaundice, dark urine, fatigue, abdominal pain, or unexplained gastrointestinal symptoms) and nilutamide treatment must be discontinued immediately if transaminases exceed 3 times the upper limit of normal.

There has been a report of elevated hepatic enzymes followed by death in a 65-year-old patient being treated with nilutamide.

Other: Foreign post marketing surveillance has revealed isolated cases of aplastic anemia in which a causal relationship with nilutamide could not be ascertained.

PRECAUTIONS

Information for the Patient: Patients should be informed that nilutamide tablets should be started on the day of, or on the day after, surgical castration. They should also be informed that they should not interrupt their dosing of nilutamide or stop taking this medication without consulting their physician. Because of the possibility of interstitial pneumonitis, patients should also be told to report immediately any dyspnea or aggravation of pre-existing dyspnea.

Because of the possibility of hepatitis, patients should be told to consult with their physician should nausea, vomiting, abdominal pain, or jaundice occur.

Because of the possibility of an intolerance to alcohol (facial flushes, malaise, hypotension) following ingestion of nilutamide, it is recommended that intake of alcoholic beverages be avoided by patients who experience this reaction. This effect has been reported in about 5% of patients treated with nilutamide.

In clinical trials 13% to 57% of patients receiving nilutamide reported a delay in adaptation to dark, ranging from seconds to a few minutes, when passing from a lighted area to a dark area. This effect sometimes does not abate as drug treatment is continued. Patients who experience this effect should be cautioned about driving at night or through tunnels. This effect can be alleviated by the wearing of tinted glasses.

Carcinogenesis, Mutagenesis, and Impairment of Fertility: Administration of nilutamide to rats for 18 months at doses of 0, 5, 15, or 45 mg/kg/day produced benign Leydig cell tumors in 35% of the high-dose male rats (AUC exposure in high-dose rats were approximately 1-2 times human AUC exposures with therapeutic doses). The increased incidence of Leydig cell tumors is secondary to elevated luteinizing hormone (LH) concentrations resulting from loss of feedback inhibition at the pituitary. Elevated LH and testosterone concentrations are not observed in castrated men receiving nilutamide. Nilutamide had no effect on the incidence, size, or time of onset of any spontaneous tumor in rats.

Nilutamide displayed no mutagenic effects in a variety of *in vitro* and *in vivo* tests (Ames test, mouse micronucleus test, and two chromosomal aberration tests).

In reproduction studies in rats, nilutamide had no effect on the reproductive function of males and females, and no lethal, teratogenic or growth-suppressive effects on fetuses were found. The maximal dose at which nilutamide did not affect reproductive function in either sex or have an effect on fetuses was estimated to be 45 mg/kg orally (AUC exposures in rats approximately 1-2 times human therapeutic AUC exposures).

Pregnancy Category C: Animal reproduction studies have not been conducted with nilutamide. It is also not known whether nilutamide can cause fetal harm when administered to a pregnant woman or can affect reproductive capacity. Nilutamide should be given to a pregnant woman only if clearly needed.

Pediatric Use: Safety and effectiveness in pediatric patients have not been determined.

DRUG INTERACTIONS

In vitro, nilutamide has been shown to inhibit the activity of liver cytochrome P-450 isoenzymes and, therefore, may reduce the metabolism of compounds requiring these systems.

Consequently, drugs with a low therapeutic margin, such as vitamin K antagonists, phenytoin and theophylline, could have a delayed elimination and increases in their serum half-life leading to a toxic level. The dosage of these drugs or others with a similar metabolism may need to be modified if they are administered concomitantly with nilutamide. For example, when vitamin K antagonists are administered concomitantly with nilutamide, prothrombin time should be carefully monitored and, if necessary, the dosage of vitamin K antagonists should be reduced.

ADVERSE REACTIONS

The following adverse experiences were reported during a multicenter clinical trial comparing nilutamide + surgical castration versus placebo + surgical castration. The most frequently reported (greater than 5%) adverse experiences during treatment with nilutamide tablets in combination with surgical castration are listed in TABLE 2. For comparison, adverse experiences seen with surgical castration and placebo are also listed.

TABLE 2

Adverse Experience	Nilutamide + Surgical Castration (N=225) % All	Placebo + Surgical Castration (N=232) % All
Cardiovascular System		
Hypertension	5.3	2.6
Digestive System		
Nausea	9.8	6.0
Constipation	7.1	3.9
Endocrine System		
Hot Flushes	28.4	22.4
Metabolic and Nutritional System		
Increased AST	8.0	3.9
Increased ALT	7.6	4.3
Nervous System		
Dizziness	7.1	3.4
Respiratory System		
Dyspnea	6.2	7.3
Special Senses		
Impaired Adaption to Dark	12.9	1.3
Abnormal Vision	6.7	1.7
Urogenital System		
Urinary Tracy Infection	8.0	9.1

The overall incidence of adverse experiences was 86% (194/225) for the nilutamide group and 81% (188/ 232) for the placebo group. The following adverse experiences were reported during a multicenter clinical trial comparing nilutamide + leuprolide versus placebo + leuprolide. The most frequently reported (greater than 5%) adverse experiences during treatment with nilutamide tablets in combination with leuprolide are listed in TABLE 3. For comparison, adverse experiences seen with leuprolide and placebo are also listed.

TABLE 3

Adverse Experience	Nilutamide + Leuprolide (N=209) % All	Placebo + Leuprolide (N=202) % All
Body as a Whole		
Pain	26.6	27.7
Headache	13.9	10.4
Asthenia	19.1	20.8
Back Pain	11.5	16.8
Abdominal pain	10.0	5.4
Chest pain	7.2	4.5
Flu syndrome	7.2	3.0
Fever	5.3	6.4
Cardiovascular System		
Hypertension	9.1	9.9
Digestive System		
Nausea	23.9	8.4
Constipation	19.6	16.8
Anorexia	11.0	6.4
Dyspepsia	6.7	4.5
Vomiting	5.7	4.0
Endocrine System		
Hot flushes	66.5	59.4
Impotence	11.0	12.9
Libido decreased	11.0	4.5
Hemic and Lymphatic System		
Anemia	7.2	6.4
Metabolic and Nutritional System		
Increased AST	12.9	13.9
Peripheral edema	12.4	17.3
Increased ALT	9.1	8.9
Musculo-Skeletal System		
Bone pain	6.2	5.0
Nervous System		
Insomnia	16.3	15.8
Dizziness	10.0	11.4
Depression	8.6	7.4
Hypesthesia	5.3	2.0
Respiratory System		
Dyspnea	10.5	7.4
Upper respiratory infection	8.1	10.9
Pneumonia	5.3	3.5
Skin and Appendages		
Sweating	6.2	3.0
Body hair loss	5.7	0.5
Dry skin	5.3	2.5
Rash	5.3	4.0
Special Senses		
Impaired adaption to dark	56.9	5.4
Chromatopsia	8.6	0.0
Impaired adaption to light	7.7	1.0
Abnormal Vision	6.2	4.5
Urogenital System		
Testicular atrophy	16.3	12.4
Gynecomastia	10.5	11.9
Urinary tract infection	8.6	21.3
Hematuria	8.1	7.9
Urinary tract disorder	7.2	10.4
Nocturia	6.7	6.4

The overall incidence of adverse experiences is 99.5% (208/209) for the nilutamide group and 98.5% (199/202) for the placebo group. Some frequently occurring adverse experiences, for example hot flushes, impotence, and decreased libido, are known to be associated with low serum androgen levels and known to occur with medical or surgical castration alone. Notable was the higher incidence of visual disturbances (variously described as impaired adaptation to darkness, abnormal vision, and colored vision), which led to treatment discontinuation in 1% to 2% of patients.

Interstitial pneumonitis occurred in one (<1%) patient receiving nilutamide in combination with surgical castration and in seven patients (3%) receiving nilutamide in combination with leuprolide and one patient receiving placebo in combination with leuprolide. Overall, it has been reported in 2% of patients receiving nilutamide. This included a report of interstitial pneumonitis in 8 of 47 patients (17%) in a small study performed in Japan.

In addition, the following adverse experiences were reported in 2 to 5% of patients treated with nilutamide in combination with leuprolide or orchiectomy.

Body as a Whole: Malaise (2%).

Cardiovascular System: Angina (2%), heart failure (3%), syncope (2%).

Digestive System: Diarrhea (2%), gastrointestinal disorder (2%), gastrointestinal hemorrhage (2%), melena (2%).

Metabolic and Nutritional System: Alcohol Intolerance (5%), edema (2%), weight loss (2%).

Musculoskeletal System: Arthritis (2%).

Nervous System: Dry mouth (2%), nervousness (2%), paresthesia (3%).

Respiratory System Cough increased (2%), interstitial lung disease (2%), lung disorder (4%), rhinitis (2%).

Skin and Appendages: Pruritus (2%).

Special Senses Cataract (2%), photophobia (2%).

Laboratory Values: Haptoglobin increased (2%), leukopenia (3%), alkaline phosphatase increased (3%), BUN increased (2%), creatinine increased (2%), hyperglycemia (4%).

DOSAGE AND ADMINISTRATION

The recommended dosage is six tablets (50 mg each) once a day for a total daily dose of 300 mg for 30 days followed thereafter by three tablets (50 mg each) once a day for a total daily dosage of 150 mg. Nilutamide tablets can be taken with or without food.

ANIMAL PHARMACOLOGY

Administration of nilutamide to beagle dogs resulted in drug-related deaths at dose levels that produce AUC exposures in dogs much lower than the AUC exposures of men receiving the therapeutic doses of 150 and 300 mg/day. Nilutamide-induced toxicity in dogs was cumulative with progressively lower doses producing death when given for longer durations. Nilutamide given to dogs at 60 mg/kg/day (1-2 times human AUC exposure) for 1 month produced 100% mortality. Administration of 20 and 30 mg/kg/day nliutamide (½ -1 times human AUC exposure) for 6 months resulted in 20% and 70% mortality in treated dogs. Administration to dogs of 3, 6, and 12 mg/kg/day nilutamide (1/10-1/2 human AUC exposure) for 1 year resulted in 8%, 33%, and 50% mortality, respectively. **A "no-effect level" for nilutamide-induced mortality in dogs was not identified.** Pathology data from the one-year oral toxicity study suggest that the deaths in dogs were secondary to liver toxicity. Marked-to-massive hepatocellular swelling and vacuolization were observed in affected dogs. Liver toxicity in dogs was not consistently associated with elevations of liver enzymes.

Administration of nilutamide to rats at a dose level of 45 mg/kg/day (AUC exposure in rats 1-2 times human therapeutic AUC exposures) for 18 months increased the incidence of lung pathology (granulomatous inflammation and chronic alveolitis).

The hepatic and pulmonary adverse effects observed in nilutamide-treated animals and men are similar to effects observed with another nitroaromatic compound, nitrofurantoin. Nilutamide and nitrofurantoin are both metabolized *in vitro* to nitroanion free-radicals by microsomal NADPH-cytochrome P450 reductase in the lungs and liver of rats and humans.

HOW SUPPLIED

White, biconvex (with a triangular logo on one face and an internal reference number [168] on the other), cylindrical (about 7 mm in diameter) NILANDRON tablets contain 50 mg of nilutamide

Storage: Store at room temperature between 15°C and 30°C (59°F and 86°F). Protect from light.

PRODUCT LISTING - EQUIVALENTS NOT AVAILABLE

Tablet - Oral - 50 mg

90's $262.74 NILANDRON, Aventis Pharmaceuticals 00088-1110-35

Tablet - Oral - 150 mg

30's $344.33 NILANDRON, Aventis Pharmaceuticals 00088-1111-14

Nimodipine *(001888)*

For related information, see the comparative table section in Appendix A.

Categories: Aneurysm, berry; Hemorrhage, subarachnoid; Pregnancy Category C; FDA Approved 1988 Dec
Drug Classes: Calcium channel blockers
Brand Names: **Nimotop**
Foreign Brand Availability: Admon (Spain); Eugerial (Peru); Irrigor (Peru); Nidip (Colombia); Periplum (Italy); Tropocer (Colombia); Vasotop (India)
Cost of Therapy: $2015.85 (Subarachnoid Hemorrhage; Nimotop; 30 mg; 12 capsules/day; 21 day supply)

DESCRIPTION

For Oral Use

Nimodipine belongs to the class of pharmacological agents known as calcium channel blockers. Nimodipine is isopropyl 2-methoxyethyl 1,4-dihydro-2,6-dimethyl-4-(m-nitrophenyl)-3,5-pyridinedicarboxylate. It has a molecular weight of 418.5 and a molecular formula of $C_{21}H_{26}N_2O_7$.

Nimodipine is a yellow crystalline substance, practically insoluble in water.

Nimotop capsules are formulated as soft gelatin capsules for oral administration. Each liquid filled capsule contains 30 mg of nimodipine in a vehicle of glycerin, peppermint oil, purified water and polyethylene glycol 400. The soft gelatin capsule shell contains gelatin, glycerin, purified water and titanium dioxide.

CLINICAL PHARMACOLOGY

MECHANISM OF ACTION

Nimodipine is a calcium channel blocker. The contractile processes of smooth muscle cells are dependent upon calcium ions, which enter these cells during depolarization as slow ionic transmembrane currents. Nimodipine inhibits calcium ion transfer into these cells and thus inhibits contractions of vascular smooth muscle. In animal experiments, nimodipine had a greater effect on cerebral arteries than on arteries elsewhere in the body perhaps because it is highly lipophilic, allowing it to cross the blood-brain barrier; concentrations of nimodipine as high as 12.5 ng/ml have been detected in the cerebrospinal fluid of nimodipine-treated subarachnoid hemorrhage (SAH) patients.

The precise mechanism of action of nimodipine in humans is unknown. Although the clinical studies demonstrate a favorable effect of nimodipine on the severity of neurological deficits caused by cerebral vasospasm following SAH, there is no arteriographic evidence that the drug either prevents or relieves the spasm of these arteries. However, whether or not the arteriographic methodology utilized was adequate to detect a clinically meaningful effect, if any, on vasospasm is unknown.

PHARMACOKINETICS AND METABOLISM

In man, nimodipine is rapidly absorbed after oral administration, and peak concentrations are generally attained within 1 hour. The terminal elimination half-life is approximately 8-9 hours but earlier elimination rates are much more rapid, equivalent to a half-life of 1-2 hours; a consequence is the need for frequent (every 4 hours) dosing. There were no signs of accumulation when nimodipine was given 3 times a day for 7 days. Nimodipine is over 95% bound to plasma proteins. The binding was concentration independent over the range of 10 ng/ml to 10 μg/ml. Nimodipine is eliminated almost exclusively in the form of metabolites and less than 1% is recovered in the urine as unchanged drug. Numerous metabolites, all of which are either inactive or considerably less active than the parent compound, have been identified. Because of a high first-pass metabolism, the bioavailability of nimodipine averages 13% after oral administration. The bioavailability is significantly increased in patients with hepatic cirrhosis, with C_{max} approximately double that in normals which necessitates lowering the dose in this group of patients (see DOSAGE AND ADMINISTRATION). In a study of 24 healthy male volunteers, administration of nimodipine capsules following a standard breakfast resulted in a 68% lower peak plasma concentration and 38% lower bioavailability relative to dosing under fasted conditions.

In a single parallel-group study involving 24 elderly subjects (aged 59-79) and 24 younger subjects (aged 22-40), the observed AUC and C_{max} of nimodipine was approximately 2-fold higher in the elderly population compared to the younger study subjects following oral administration (given as a single dose of 30 mg and dosed to steady-state with 30 mg tid for 6 days). The clinical response to these age-related pharmacokinetic differences, however, was not considered significant. (See PRECAUTIONS, Geriatric Use.)

INDICATIONS AND USAGE

Nimodipine is indicated for the improvement of neurological outcome by reducing the incidence and severity of ischemic deficits in patients with subarachnoid hemorrhage from ruptured intracranial berry aneurysms regardless of their post-ictus neurological condition (*i.e.*, Hunt and Hess Grades I-V).

NON-FDA APPROVED INDICATIONS

Nimodipine has also been used in the treatment of ischemic stroke and the prophylaxis of migraine headaches.

CONTRAINDICATIONS

None known.

PRECAUTIONS

GENERAL

Blood Pressure

Nimodipine has the hemodynamic effects expected of a calcium channel blocker, although they are generally not marked. However, intravenous administration of the contents of nimodipine capsules has resulted in serious adverse consequences including hypotension, cardiovascular collapse, and cardiac arrest. In patients with subarachnoid hemorrhage given nimodipine in clinical studies, about 5% were reported to have had lowering of the blood pressure and about 1% left the study because of this (not all could be attributed to nimodipine). Nevertheless, blood pressure should be carefully monitored during treatment with nimodipine based on its known pharmacology and the known effects of calcium channel blockers.

Hepatic Disease

The metabolism of nimodipine is decreased in patients with impaired hepatic function. Such patients should have their blood pressure and pulse rate monitored closely and should be given a lower dose (see DOSAGE AND ADMINISTRATION.) Intestinal pseudo-obstruction and ileus have been reported rarely in patients treated with nimodipine. A causal relationship has not been established. The condition has responded to conservative management.

LABORATORY TEST INTERACTIONS

None known.

CARCINOGENESIS, MUTAGENESIS, AND IMPAIRMENT OF FERTILITY

In a 2 year study, higher incidences of adenocarcinoma of the uterus and Leydig-cell adenoma of the testes were observed in rats given a diet containing 1800 ppm nimodipine (equivalent to 91-121 mg/kg/day nimodipine) than in placebo controls. The differences were not statistically significant, however, and the higher rates were well within historical control range for these tumors in the Wistar strain. Nimodipine was found not to be carcinogenic in a 91 week mouse study but the high dose of 1800 ppm nimodipine-in-feed (546-774 mg/kg/day) shortened the life expectancy of the animals. Mutagenicity studies, including the Ames, micronucleus and dominant lethal tests were negative.

Nimodipine did not impair the fertility and general reproductive performance of male and female Wistar rats following oral doses of up to 30 mg/kg/day when administered daily for more than 10 weeks in the males and 3 weeks in the females prior to mating and continued to day 7 of pregnancy. This dose in a rat is about 4 times the equivalent clinical dose of 60 mg q4h in a 50 kg patient.

PREGNANCY CATEGORY C

Nimodipine has been shown to have a teratogenic effect in Himalayan rabbits. Incidences of malformations and stunted fetuses were increased at oral doses of 1 and 10 mg/kg/day administered (by gavage) from day 6 through day 18 of pregnancy but not at 3.0 mg/kg/day in one of two identical rabbit studies. In the second study an increased incidence of stunted fetuses was seen at 1.0 mg/kg/day but not at higher doses. Nimodipine was embryotoxic, causing resorption and stunted growth of fetuses, in Long Evans rats at 100 mg/kg/day administered by gavage from day 6 through day 15 of pregnancy. In two other rat studies, doses of 30 mg/kg/day nimodipine administered by gavage from day 16 of gestation and continued until sacrifice (day 20 of pregnancy or day 21 post partum) were associated with higher incidences of skeletal variation, stunted fetuses and stillbirths but no malformations. There are no adequate and well controlled studies in pregnant women to directly assess the effect on human fetuses. Nimodipine should be used during pregnancy only if the potential benefit justifies the potential risk to the fetus.

NURSING MOTHERS

Nimodipine and/or its metabolites have been shown to appear in rat milk at concentrations much higher than in maternal plasma. It is not known whether the drug is excreted in human milk. Because many drugs are excreted in human milk, nursing mothers are advised not to breast feed their babies when taking the drug.

PEDIATRIC USE

Safety and effectiveness in children have not been established.

GERIATRIC USE

Clinical studies of nimodipine did not include sufficient numbers of subjects aged 65 and over to determine whether they respond differently from younger subjects. Other reported clinical experience has not identified differences in responses between the elderly and younger patients. In general, dosing in elderly patients should be cautious, reflecting the greater frequency of decreased hepatic, renal or cardiac function, and of concomitant disease or other drug therapy.

DRUG INTERACTIONS

It is possible that the cardiovascular action of other calcium channel blockers could be enhanced by the addition of nimodipine.

In Europe, nimodipine was observed to occasionally intensify the effect of antihypertensive compounds taken concomitantly by patients suffering from hypertension; this phenomenon was not observed in North American clinical trials.

A study in 8 healthy volunteers has shown a 50% increase in mean peak nimodipine plasma concentrations and a 90% increase in mean area under the curve, after a 1 week course of cimetidine at 1000 mg/day and nimodipine at 90 mg/day. This effect may be mediated by the known inhibition of hepatic cytochrome P-450 by cimetidine, which could decrease first-pass metabolism of nimodipine.

ADVERSE REACTIONS

Adverse experiences were reported by 92 of 823 patients with subarachnoid hemorrhage (11.2%) who were given nimodipine. The most frequently reported adverse experience was decreased blood pressure in 4.4% of these patients. Twenty-nine of 479 (6.1%) placebo treated patients also reported adverse experiences. The events reported with a frequency greater than 1% are displayed inTABLE 5A and TABLE 5B by dose.

TABLE 5A

	Dose q4h Number of Patients Nimodipine		
	0.35 mg/kg	30 mg	60 mg
Sign/Symptom	(n=82)	(n=71)	(n=494)
Decreased blood pressure	1 (1.2%)	0	19 (3.8%)
Abnormal liver function test	1 (1.2%)	0	2 (0.4%)
Edema	0	0	2 (0.4%)
Diarrhea	0	3 (4.2%)	0
Rash	2 (2.4%)	0	3 (0.6%)
Headache	0	1 (1.4%)	6 (1.2%)
Gastrointestinal symptoms	2 (2.4%)	0	0
Nausea	1 (1.2%)	1 (1.4%)	6 (1.2%)
Dyspnea	1 (1.2%)	0	0
EKG abnormalities	0	1 (1.4%)	0
Tachycardia	0	1 (1.4%)	0
Bradycardia	0	0	5 (1.0%)
Muscle pain/cramp	0	1 (1.4%)	1 (0.2%)
Acne	0	1 (1.4%)	0
Depression	0	1 (1.4%)	0

TABLE 5B

	Dose q4h Number of Patients		
	Nimodipine		
	90 mg	120 mg	Placebo
Sign/Symptom	(n=172)	(n=4)	(n=479)
Decreased blood pressure	14 (8.1%)	2 (50.0%)	6 (1.2%)
Abnormal liver function test	1 (0.6%)	0	7 (1.5%)
Edema	2 (1.2%)	0	3 (0.6%)
Diarrhea	3 (1.7%)	0	3 (0.6%)
Rash	2 (1.2%)	0	3 (0.6%)
Headache	0	0	1 (0.2%)
Gastrointestinal symptoms	2 (1.2%)	0	0
Nausea	1 (0.6%)	0	0
Dyspnea	0	0	0
EKG abnormalities	1 (0.6%)	0	0
Tachycardia	0	0	0
Bradycardia	1 (0.6%)	0	0
Muscle pain/cramp	1 (0.6%)	0	0
Acne	0	0	0
Depression	0	0	0

There were no other adverse experiences reported by the patients who were given 0.35 mg/kg q4h, 30 mg q4h or 120 mg q4h. Adverse experiences with an incidence rate of less than 1% in the 60 mg q4h dose group were: hepatitis; itching; gastrointestinal hemorrhage; thrombocytopenia; anemia; palpitations; vomiting; flushing; diaphoresis; wheezing; phenytoin toxicity; lightheadedness; dizziness; rebound vasospasm; jaundice; hypertension; hematoma.

Adverse experiences with an incidence rate less than 1% in the 90 mg q4h dose group were: Itching, gastrointestinal hemorrhage; thrombocytopenia; neurological deterioration; vomiting; diaphoresis; congestive heart failure; hyponatremia; decreasing platelet count; disseminated intravascular coagulation; deep vein thrombosis.

As can be seen from TABLE 5A and TABLE 5B, side effects that appear related to nimodipine use based on increased incidence with higher dose or a higher rate compared to

N

placebo control, included decreased blood pressure, edema and headaches which are known pharmacologic actions of calcium channel blockers. It must be noted, however, that SAH is frequently accompanied by alterations in consciousness which lead to an under reporting of adverse experiences. Patients who received nimodipine in clinical trials for other indications reported flushing (2.1%), headache (4.1%) and fluid retention (0.3%), typical responses to calcium channel blockers. As a calcium channel blocker, nimodipine may have the potential to exacerbate heart failure in susceptible patients or to interfere with A-V conduction, but these events were not observed.

No clinically significant effects on hematologic factors, renal or hepatic function or carbohydrate metabolism have been causally associated with oral nimodipine. Isolated cases of non-fasting elevated serum glucose levels (0.8%), elevated LDH levels (0.4%), decreased platelet counts (0.3%), elevated alkaline phosphatase levels (0.2%) and elevated SGPT levels (0.2%) have been reported rarely.

DOSAGE AND ADMINISTRATION

Nimodipine is given orally in the form of ivory colored, soft gelatin 30 mg capsules for subarachnoid hemorrhage.

The oral dose is 60 mg (two 30 mg capsules) every 4 hours for 21 consecutive days, preferably not less than 1 hour before or 2 hours after meals. Oral nimodipine therapy should commence within 96 hours of the subarachnoid hemorrhage.

If the capsule cannot be swallowed, *e.g.,* at the time of surgery, or if the patient is unconscious, a hole should be made in both ends of the capsule with an 18 gauge needle, and the contents of the capsule extracted into a syringe. The contents should then be emptied into the patient's *in situ* naso-gastric tube and washed down the tube with 30 ml of normal saline (0.9%).

The contents of nimodipine capsules must not be administered by intravenous injection or other parenteral routs.

Patients with hepatic cirrhosis have substantially reduced clearance and approximately doubled C_{max}. Dosage should be reduced to 30 mg every 4 hours, with close monitoring of blood pressure and heart rate.

HOW SUPPLIED

Each ivory colored, soft gelatin Nimotop capsule is imprinted with the word "Nimotop" and contains 30 mg of nimodipine.

Storage: The capsules should be stored in the manufacturer's original foil package at 25°C (77°F), excursions permitted to 15-30°C (59-86°F). Capsules should be protected from light and freezing.

PRODUCT LISTING - EQUIVALENTS NOT AVAILABLE

Capsule - Oral - 30 mg

30's	$251.16	NIMOTOP, Bayer	00026-2855-70
100's	$799.94	NIMOTOP, Bayer	00026-2855-48

Nisoldipine *(003246)*

For related information, see the comparative table section in Appendix A.

Categories: Hypertension, essential; FDA Approved 1995 Feb; Pregnancy Category C
Drug Classes: Calcium channel blockers
Brand Names: **Sular**
Foreign Brand Availability: Baymycard (Germany; Japan); Nisoldin (Korea); Syscor (Austria; Belgium; Costa-Rica; Dominican-Republic; El-Salvador; Finland; Greece; Guatemala; Honduras; Italy; Netherlands; Nicaragua; Panama; Spain; Switzerland; Taiwan); Syscor CC (Bahamas; Barbados; Belize; Bermuda; Curacao; Guyana; Jamaica; Netherland-Antilles; Peru; Puerto-Rico; Surinam; Trinidad)
Cost of Therapy: $36.09 (Hypertension; Sular; 20 mg; 1 tablet/day; 30 day supply)

DESCRIPTION

Nisoldipine is an extended release tablet dosage form of the dihydropyridine calcium channel blocker nisoldipine. Nisoldipine is 3,5-pyridinadicarboxylic acid,1,4-dihydro-2,6-dimethyl-4-(2-nitrophenyl)-,methyl,2-methylpropyl estar, $C_{20}H_{24}N_2O_6$.

Nisoldipine is a yellow crystalline substance, practically insoluble in water but soluble in ethanol. It has a molecular weight of 388.4.

Sular tablets consist of an external coat and an internal core. Both coat and core contain nisoldipine, the coat as a slow release formulation and the core as a fast release formulation. SULAR tablets contain either 10, 20, 30, or 40 mg of nisoldipine for once-a-day oral administration.

Sular Inert ingredients in the formulation are: hydroxypropylcellulose, lactose, corn starch, crospovidone, microcrystalline cellulose, sodium lauryl sulfate, povidone and magnesium stearate. The inert ingredients in the film coating are: hydroxypropylmethylcellulose, polyethylene glycol, ferric oxide, and titanium dioxide.

CLINICAL PHARMACOLOGY

MECHANISMS OF ACTION

Nisoldipine is a member of the dihydropyridine class of calcium channel antagonists (calcium ion antagonists or slow channel blockers) that inhibit the transmembrane influx of calcium into vascular smooth muscle and cardiac muscle. It reversibly competes with other dihydropyridines for binding to the calcium channel. Because the contratife process of vascular smoothe muscle is dependent upon the movement of extracellular calcium into the muscle through specific ion channels, inhibition of the calcium channel results in dilation of the arterioles. *In vitro* studies show that the effects of nisoldipine on contractile processes are selective, with greater potency on vascular smooth muscle than on cardiac muscle. Although, like other dihydropyridine calcium channel blockers, nisoldipine has negative inotropic effects *in vitro,* studies conducted in intact anesthetized animals have shown that the vasodilating effect occurs at doses lower than those that affect cardiac contractibility.

The effect of nisoldipine on blood pressure is principally a consequence of a dose-related decrease of peripheral vascular resistance. While nisoldipine, like other dihydropyridines, exhibits a mild diuretic effect, most of the antihypertensive activity is attributed to its effect on peripheral vascular resistance.

PHARMACOKINETICS AND METABOLISM

Nisoldipine pharmacokinetics are independent of the dose in the range of 20-60 mg, with plasma concentrations proportional to dose. Nisoldipine accumulation during multiple dosing is predictable from a single dose.

Nisoldipine is relatively well absorbed into the systemic circulation with 87% of the radio labeled drug recovered in urine and feces. The absolute bioavailability of nisoldipine is about 5%. Nisoldipine's low bioavailability is due, in part, to pre-systemic metabolism in the gut wall, and this metabolism decreases from the proximal to the distal parts of the intestine. Food with a high fat content has a pronounced effect on the release of nisoldipine from the coat to core formulation and results in a significant increase in peak concentration (C_{max}) by up to 300%. Total exposure, however, is decreased about 25%, presumably because more of the drug is released proximally. This effect appears to be specific for nisoldipine in the controlled release formulation, as a less pronounced food effect was seen with the immediate release tablet. Concomitant intake of a high fat meat with nisoldipine should be avoided.

Maximal plasma concentrations of nisoldipine are reached 6-12 hours after dosing. The terminal elimination half-life (reflecting post absorption clearance of nisoldipine) ranges from 7-12 hours. C_{max} and AUC increase by factors of approximately 1.3 and 1.5, respectively, from first dose-steady state. After oral administration, the concentration of (+) nisoldipine, the active enantiomer, is about 6 times higher than the (-) inactive enantiomer. The plasma protein binding of nisoldipine is very high, with less than 1% unbound over the plasma concentration range of 100 ng/ml to 10 μg/ml.

Nisoldipine is highly metabolized; 5 major urinary metabolites have been identified. Although 60-80% of an oral dose undergoes urinary excretion, only traces of unchanged nisoldipine are found in urine. The major biotransformation pathway appears to be the hydroxylation of the isobutyl ester. A hydroxylated derivative of the side chain, present in plasma at concentrations approximately equal to the parent compound, appears to be the only active metabolites, and has about 10% of the activity of the parent compound. Cytochrome P_{450} enzymes are believed to play a major role in the metabolism of nisoldipine. The particular isoenzyme system responsible for its metabolism has not been identified, but other dihydropyridines are metabolized by cytochrome P_{450}IIIA4. Nisoldipine should not be administered with grapefruit juice as this has been shown, in a study of 12 subjects, to interfere with nisoldipine metabolism, resulting in a mean increase in C_{max} of about 3-fold (ranging up-about 7-fold) and AUC of almost 2-fold (ranging up to about 5-fold). A similar phenomenon has been seen with several other dihydropyridine calcium channel blockers.

PHARMACODYNAMICS

Hemodynamic Effects

Administration of a single dose of nisoldipine leads to decreased systemic vascular resistance and blood pressure with a transient increase in heart rate. The change in heart rate is greater with immediate release nisoldipine preparations. The effect on blood pressure is directly related to the initial degree of elevation above normal. Chronic administration of nisoldipine results in a sustained decrease in vascular resistance and small increases in stroke index and left ventricular ejection fraction. A study of the immediate release formulation showed no effect of nisoldipine on the renin to angiotensin to aldosterone system or on plasma norepinephrine concentration in normals. Changes in blood pressure in hypertensive patients given nisoldipine were dose related over the range of 10-60 mg/day.

Nisoldipine does not appear to have significant negative inotropic activity in intact animals or humans, and did not lead to worsening of clinical heart failure in three small studies of patients with asymptomatic and symptomatic left ventricular dysfunction. There is little information, however, in patients with severe congestive heart failure, and all calcium channel blockers should be used with caution in any patient with heart failure.

Electrophysiologic Effects

Nisoldipine has no clinically important chronotropic effects. Except for mild shortening of sinus cycle, SA conduction time and AH intervals, single oral doses up to 20 mg of immediate release nisoldipine did not significantly change other conduction parameters. Similar electrophysiologic effects were seen with single IV doses, which could be blunted in patients pre-treated with beta-blockers. Dose and plasma level related flattening or inversion of T-waves have been observed in a few small studies. Such reports were concentrated in patients receiving rapidly increased high doses in one study; the phenomenon has not been a cause of safety concern in large clinical trials.

SPECIAL POPULATIONS

Renal Dysfunction

Because renal elimination is not an important pathway, bioavaliability and pharmacokinetics of nisoldipine were not significantly different in patients with various degrees of renal impairment. Dosing adjustments in patients with mild to moderate renal impairment are not necessary.

Geriatrics

Elderly patients have been found to have 2- to 3-fold higher plasma concentrations (C_{max} and AUC) than young subjects. This should be reflected in more cautious dosing (see DOSAGE AND ADMINISTRATION).

Hepatic Insufficiency

In patients with liver cirrhosis given 10 mg nisoldipine, plasma concentrations of the parent compound were 4-5 times higher than those in healthy young subjects. Lower starting and maintenance doses should be used in cirrhotic patients (see DOSAGE AND ADMINISTRATION).

Gender and Race

The effect of gender or race on the pharmacokinetics of nisoldipine has not been investigated.

Disease States

Hypertension does not significantly alter the pharmacokinetics of nisoldipine.

INDICATIONS AND USAGE

Nisoldipine is indicated for the treatment of hypertension. It may be used alone or in combination with other antihypertensive agents.

NON-FDA APPROVED INDICATIONS

Nisoldipine has been used without FDA approval for the prevention of angina pectoris.

CONTRAINDICATIONS

Nisoldipine is contraindicated in patients with known hypersensitivity to dihydropyridine calcium channel blockers.

WARNINGS

INCREASED ANGINA AND/OR MYOCARDIAL INFARCTION IN PATIENTS WITH CORONARY ARTERY DISEASE

Rarely, patients, particularly those with severe obstructive coronary artery disease, have developed increased frequency, duration and/or severity of angina, or acute myocardial infarction on starting calcium channel blocker therapy or at the time of dosage increase. The mechanism of this effect has not been established. In controlled studies of nisoldipine in patients with angina this was seen about 1.5% of the time in patients given nisoldipine, compared with 0.9% in patients given placebo.

PRECAUTIONS

GENERAL

Hypotension

Because nisoldipine, like other vasodilators, decreases peripheral vascular resistance, careful monitoring of blood pressure during the initial administration and titration of nisoldipine is recommended. Close observation is especially important for patients already taking medications that are known to lower blood pressure. Although in most patients the hypotensive effect of nisoldipine is modest and well tolerated, occasional patients have had excessive and poorly tolerated hypotension. These responses have usually occurred during initial titration or at the time of subsequent upward dosage adjustment.

Congestive Heart Failure

Although acute hemodynamic studies of nisoldipine in patients with NYHA Class II to IV heart failure have not demonstrated negative inotropic effects, safety of nisoldipine in patients with heart failure has not been established. Caution therefore should be exercised when using nisoldipine in patients with heart failure or compromised ventricular function, particularly in combination with a beta-blocker.

Patients With Hepatic Impairment

Because nisoldipine is extensively metabolized by the liver and, in patients with cirrhosis, it reaches blood concentrations about 5 times those in normals, nisoldipine should be administered cautiously in patients with severe hepatic dysfunction (see DOSAGE AND ADMINISTRATION).

LABORATORY TESTS

Nisoldipine is not known to interfere with the interpretation of laboratory tests.

CARCINOGENESIS, MUTAGENESIS, AND IMPAIRMENT OF FERTILITY

Dietary administration of nisoldipine to male and female rats for up to 24 months (mean doses up to 82 and 111 mg/kg/day, 15 and 19 times the maximum recommended human dose (MRHD) on a mg/m^2 basis, respectively) and female mice for up to 21 months (mean doses of up to 217 mg/kg/day, 20 times the MRHD on a mg/m^2 basis) revealed no evidence of tumorigenic effect of nisoldipine. In male mice receiving a mean dose of 163 mg nisoldipine/kg/day (16 times the MRHD of 60 mg/day on a mg/m^2 basis), an increased frequency of stomach papilloma, but still within the historical range, was observed. No evidence of stomach neoplasia was observed at lower doses (up to 58 mg/kg/day). Nisoldipine was negative when tested in a battery of genotoxicity assays including the Ames test and the CHO/HGRPT assay for mutagenicity and the *in vivo* mouse micronucleus test and *in vitro* CHO cell test for clastogenicity.

When administered to male and female rats at doses of up to 30 mg/kg/day (about 5 times the MRHD on a mg/m^2 basis) nisoldipine had no effect on fertility.

PREGNANCY CATEGORY C

Nisoldipine was neither teratogenic nor fetotoxic at doses that were maternally toxic. Nisoldipine was fetotoxic but not teratogenic in rats and rabbits at doses resulting in maternal toxicity (reduced maternal body weight gain). In pregnant rats, increased fetal resorption (post-implantation loss) was observed at 100 mg/kg/day and decreased fetal weight was observed at both 30 and 100 mg/kg/day. These doses are, respectively, about 5 and 16 times the MRHD when compared on a mg/m^2. In a study in which pregnant rabbits, decreased fetal and placental weights were observed at a dose of 30 mg/kg/day, about 10 times the MRHD when compared on a mg/m^2 basis. In a study in which pregnant monkeys (both treated and control) had high rates of abortion and mortality, the only surviving fetus from a group exposed to a maternal dose of 100 mg nisoldipine/kg/day (about 30 times the MRHD when compared on a mg/m^2 basis) presented with forelimb and vertebral abnormalities not previously seen in control monkey of the same strain. There are no adequate and well controlled studies in pregnant women. Nisoldipine should be used in pregnancy only if the potential benefit justifies the potential risk to the fetus.

NURSING MOTHERS

It is not known whether nisoldipine is excreted in human milk. Because many drugs are excreted in human milk, a decision should be made to discontinue nursing, or to discontinue nisoldipine, taking into account the importance of the drug to the mother.

DRUG INTERACTIONS

A 30-45% increase in AUC and C_{max} of nisoldipine was observed with concomitant administration of cimetidine 400 mg twice daily. Ranitidine 150 mg twice daily did not interact significantly with nisoldipine (AUC was decreased by 15-20%). No pharmacodynamic effects of either H_2 antihistamine were observed.

Pharmacokinetic interactions between nisoldipine and beta-blockers (atenolol, propranolol) were variable and not significant. Propranolol attenuated the heart rate increase following administration of immediate release nisoldipine. The blood pressure effect of nisoldipine tended to be greater in patients on atenolol than in patients on no other antihypertensive therapy.

Quinidine at 648 mg bid decreased the bioavailability (AUC) of nisoldipine by 26%, but not the peak concentration. The immediate release, but not the coat to core formulation of nisoldipine increased plasma quinidine concentrations by about 20%. This interaction was not accompanied by ECG changes and its clinical significance is not known.

No significant interactions were found between nisoldipine and warfarin or digoxin.

ADVERSE REACTIONS

More than 6000 patients world-wide have received nisoldipine in clinical trials for the treatment of hypertension, either as the immediate release or the nisoldipine extended release formulation. Of about 1,500 patients who received nisoldipine in hypertension studies about 55% were exposed for at least 2 months and about one-third were exposed for over 6 months, the great majority at doses of 20-60 mg daily.

Nisoldipine is generally well-tolerated. In the US clinical trials of nisoldipine in hypertension, 10.9% of the 921 nisoldipine patients discontinued treatment due to adverse events compared with 2.9% of 280 placebo patients. The frequency discontinuations due to adverse experiences was related to dose, with a 5.4% discontinuation rate at 10 mg daily and a 10.9% discontinuation rate at 60 mg daily.

The most frequently occurring adverse experiences with nisoldipine are those related to its vasodilator properties; these are generally mild and only occasionally lead to patient withdrawal from treatment. In TABLE 2, from US placebo-controlled parallel dose response trials of nisoldipine using doses from 10-60 mg once daily in patients with hypertension, lists all of the adverse events, regardless of the causal relationship to nisoldipine, which the overall incidence on nisoldipine was both > 1% and greater with nisoldipine than with placebo.

TABLE 2

Adverse Event	Nisoldipine (n=663)	Placebo (n=280)
Peripheral edema	22%	10%
Headache	22%	15%
Dizziness	5%	4%
Pharyngitis	5%	4%
Vasodilation	4%	2%
Sinusitis	3%	2%
Palpitation	3%	1%
Chest pain	2%	1%
Nausea	2%	1%
Flash	2%	1%

Only peripheral edema and possibly dizziness appear to be dose related.

TABLE 3

		Nisoldipine (mg)				
	Placebo	10	20	30	40	60
Adverse Event	n=280	n=30	n=170	n=105	n=139	n=137
Peripheral edema	10%	7%	15%	20%	27%	29%
Dizziness	4%	7%	3%	3%	4%	10%

The common adverse events occurred at about the same rate in men as in women, and at a similar rate in patients over age 65 as in those under that age, except that headache was much less common in older patients. Except for peripheral edema and vasodilation, which were more common in whites, adverse event rates were similar in blacks and whites.

The following adverse events occurred in ≤1% of all patients treated for hypertension in US and foreign clinical trials, or with unspecified incidence in other studies. Although a causal relationship of nisoldipine to these events cannot be established, they are listed to alert the physician to a possible relationship with nisoldipine treatment.

Body as a Whole: Cellulitis, chills, facial edema, fever, flu syndrome, malaise.

Cardiovascular: Atrial fibrillation, cerebrovascular accident, congestive heart failure, first degree AV block, hypertension, hypotension, jugular venous distension, migraine, myocardial infarction, postural hypotension, ventricular extrasystoles, supraventricular tachycardia, syncope, systolic ejection murmur, T wave abnormalities on ECG (flattening, inversion, nonspecific changes), venous insufficiency.

Digestive: Abnormal liver function tests, anorexia, colitis, diarrhea, dry mouth, dyspepsia, dysphagia, flatulence, gastritis, gastrointestinal hemorrhage, gingival hyperplasia, glossitis, heptomegaly, increased appetite, melea, mouth ulceration.

Endocrine: Diabetes mellitus, thyroiditis.

Hemic and Lymphatic: Anemia, ecchymoses, leukopenia, petechiae.

Metabolic and Nutritional: Gout, hypokalemia, increased serum creatinine kinase, increased nonprotein nitrogen, weight gain, weight loss.

Musculoskeletal: Arthralgia, arthritis, leg cramps, myalgia, myasthenia, myositis, tenosynovitis.
Nervous: Abnormal dreams, abnormal thinking and confusion, amnesia, anxiety, ataxia, cerebral ischemia, decreased libido, depression, hypesthesia, hypertonia, insomnia, nervousness, paresthesia, somnolence, tremor, vertigo.
Respiratory: Asthma, dyspnea, and inspiratory wheeze and fine rales, epistaxis, increased cough, laryngitis, pharyngitis, pleural effusion, rhinitis, sinusitis.
Skin and Appendages: Acne, alopecia, dry skin, exfoliative dermatitis, fungal dermatitis, herpes simplex, herpes zoster, maculopapular rash, pruritus, pustular rash, skin discoloration, skin ulcer, sweating, urticaria.
Special Senses: Abnormal vision, amblyopia, blepharitis, conjunctivitis, ear pain, glaucoma, itchy eyes, keratoconjunctivitis, otitis media, retinal detachment, tinnitus, watery eyes, taste disturbance, temporary unilateral loss of vision, vitreous floater, watery eyes.
Urogenital: Dysuria, hematuria, impotence, nocturia, urinary frequency, increased BUN and serum creatinine, vaginal hemorrhage, vaginitis.

In addition to experience with nisoldipine, there is extensive experience with the immediate release formulation of nisoldipine. Adverse events were generally similar to those seen with nisoldipine. Unusual events observed with immediate release nisoldipine but not observed with nisoldipine, were 1 case each of angioedema and photosensitivity. Spontaneous reports from postmarketing experience with the immediate release formulation of nisoldipine have not revealed any additional adverse events not identified in the above listings.

DOSAGE AND ADMINISTRATION

The dosage of nisoldipine must be adjusted to each patient's needs. Therapy usually should be initiated with 20 mg orally once daily, then increased by 10 mg per week or longer intervals, to attain adequate control of blood pressure. Usual maintenance dosage is 20-40 mg once daily. Blood pressure response increases over the 10-60 mg daily dose range but adverse event rates also increase. Doses beyond 60 mg once daily are not recommended. Nisoldipine has been used safely with diuretics, ACE inhibitors, and beta-blocking agents.

Patients over age 65, or patients with impaired liver function are expected to develop higher plasma concentrations of nisoldipine. Their blood pressure should be monitored closely during any dosage adjustment. A starting dose not exceeding 10 mg daily is recommended in these patient groups.

Nisoldipine tablets should be administered orally once daily. Administration with a high fat meal can lead to excessive peak drug concentration and should be avoided. Grapefruit products should be avoided before and after dosing. Nisoldipine is an extended release dosage form and tablets should be swallowed whole, not bitten or divided.

HOW SUPPLIED

Sular extended release tablets are supplied as 10, 20, 30, and 40 mg round film coated tablets.

Storage: The tablets should be protected from light and moisture and store below 30°C (86°F). Dispense in tight, light-resistant containers.

N

PRODUCT LISTING - EQUIVALENTS NOT AVAILABLE

Tablet, Extended Release - Oral - 10 mg

30's	$28.91	SULAR, Allscripts Pharmaceutical Company	54569-4991-00
100's	$120.30	SULAR, Astra-Zeneca Pharmaceuticals	00310-0891-10
100's	$120.30	SULAR, Astra-Zeneca Pharmaceuticals	00310-0891-39

Tablet, Extended Release - Oral - 20 mg

100's	$115.67	SULAR, Astra-Zeneca Pharmaceuticals	00310-0892-39
100's	$120.30	SULAR, Astra-Zeneca Pharmaceuticals	00310-0892-10

Tablet, Extended Release - Oral - 30 mg

100's	$92.68	SULAR, Astra-Zeneca Pharmaceuticals	00310-0893-39
100's	$120.30	SULAR, Astra-Zeneca Pharmaceuticals	00310-0893-10

Tablet, Extended Release - Oral - 40 mg

30's	$28.91	SULAR, Allscripts Pharmaceutical Company	54569-4992-00
100's	$120.30	SULAR, Astra-Zeneca Pharmaceuticals	00310-0894-10

Nitazoxanide *(003576)*

Categories: Cryptosporidiosis; Diarrhea, infectious; Giardiasis; Pregnancy Category B; FDA Approved 2002 Nov; Orphan Drugs
Drug Classes: Antiprotozoals
Brand Names: Alinia
Foreign Brand Availability: Colufase (Peru); Daxon (Mexico)
Cost of Therapy: $60.00 (Diarrhea, infectious; Alinia; 100 mg/5 ml; 20 ml/day; 3 day supply)

DESCRIPTION

Alinia for oral suspension contains the active ingredient, nitazoxanide, a synthetic antiprotozoal agent for oral administration. Nitazoxanide is a light yellow crystalline powder. It is poorly soluble in ethanol and practically insoluble in water. Chemically, nitazoxanide is 2-acetyloxy-*N*-(5-nitro-2-thiazolyl)benzamide. The molecular formula is $C_{12}H_9N_3O_5S$ and the molecular weight is 307.3.

Alinia for oral suspension, after reconstitution, contains 100 mg nitazoxanide/5 ml and the following inactive ingredients: sodium benzoate, sucrose, xanthan gum, microcrystalline cellulose and carboxymethylcellulose sodium, anhydrous citric acid, sodium citrate dihydrate, acacia gum, sugar syrup, FD&C red no. 40 and natural strawberry flavoring.

CLINICAL PHARMACOLOGY

ABSORPTION

Following oral administration of nitazoxanide for oral suspension, maximum plasma concentrations of the active metabolites tizoxanide and tizoxanide glucuronide are observed within 1-4 hours. The parent nitazoxanide is not detected in plasma. Pharmacokinetic parameters of tizoxanide and tizoxanide glucuronide are shown in TABLE 1.

TABLE 1 *Mean (±SD) Plasma Pharmacokinetic Parameter Values Following Administration of a Single Dose of Nitazoxanide for Oral Suspension With Food to Pediatric Subjects*

Age	Dose*	C_{max} µg/ml	T_{max}† h	AUC(inf) µg·h/ml
		Tizoxanide		
12-47 Months	100 mg	3.11 (2.0)	3.5 (2-4)	11.7 (4.46)
4-11 Years	200 mg	3.00 (0.99)	2.0 (1-4)	13.5 (3.3)
		Tizoxanide Glucuronide		
12-47 Months	100 mg	3.64 (1.16)	4.0 (3-4)	19.0 (5.03)
4-11 Years	200 mg	2.84 (0.97)	4.0 (2-4)	16.9 (5.00)

* Dose: 100 mg/5 ml nitazoxanide, 200 mg/10 ml nitazoxanide.
† T_{max} is given as mean (range).

No studies have been conducted to determine if the pharmacokinetics of tizoxanide and tizoxanide glucuronide differ in fasted versus fed subjects following administration of nitazoxanide for oral suspension.

DISTRIBUTION

In plasma, more than 99% of tizoxanide is bound to proteins.

METABOLISM

Following oral administration in humans, nitazoxanide is rapidly hydrolyzed to an active metabolite, tizoxanide (desacetyl-nitazoxanide). Tizoxanide then undergoes conjugation, primarily by glucuronidation.

ELIMINATION

Tizoxanide is excreted in the urine, bile and feces, and tizoxanide glucuronide is excreted in urine and bile.

SPECIAL POPULATIONS

Patients With Impaired Hepatic and/or Renal Function

The pharmacokinetics of nitazoxanide in patients with impaired hepatic and/or renal function has not been studied.

Pediatric Patients

The pharmacokinetics of nitazoxanide in pediatric patients less than 1 year of age has not been studied.

MICROBIOLOGY

Mechanism of Action

The antiprotozoal activity of nitazoxanide is believed to be due to interference with the pyruvate:ferredoxin oxidoreductase (PFOR) enzyme-dependent electron transfer reaction which is essential to anaerobic energy metabolism. Studies have shown that the PFOR enzyme from *Giardia lamblia* directly reduces nitazoxanide by transfer of electrons in the absence of ferredoxin. The DNA-derived PFOR protein sequence of *Cryptosporidium parvum* appears to be similar to that of *Giardia lamblia.* Interference with the PFOR enzyme-dependent electron transfer reaction may not be the only pathway by which nitazoxanide exhibits antiprotozoal activity.

Activity in Vitro and in Vivo

Nitazoxanide and its metabolite, tizoxanide, are active *in vitro* in inhibiting the growth of (i) sporozoites and oocysts of *Cryptosporidium parvum* and (ii) trophozoites of *Giardia lamblia.*

Nitazoxanide for oral suspension is effective in pediatric patients with *Cryptosporidium parvum* or *Giardia lamblia* infection (see INDICATIONS AND USAGE).

Drug Resistance

A potential for development of resistance by *Cryptosporidium parvum* or *Giardia lamblia* to nitazoxanide has not been examined.

Susceptibility Testing

For protozoa such as *Cryptosporidium parvum* and*Giardia lamblia,* standardized tests for use in clinical microbiology laboratories are not available.

INDICATIONS AND USAGE

Nitazoxanide for oral suspension is indicated for the treatment of diarrhea caused by *Cryptosporidium parvum* and *Giardia lamblia* in pediatric patients 1 through 11 years of age. Safety and effectiveness of nitazoxanide for oral suspension have not been established in HIV positive patients or patients with immunodeficiency. Safety and effectiveness of nitazoxanide for oral suspension in pediatric patients less than 1 year of age, pediatric patients greater than 11 years of age and adults have not been studied.

CONTRAINDICATIONS

Nitazoxanide is contraindicated in patients with a prior hypersensitivity to nitazoxanide.

PRECAUTIONS

GENERAL

The pharmacokinetics of nitazoxanide in patients with compromised renal or hepatic function have not been studied. Therefore, nitazoxanide must be administered with caution to patients with hepatic and biliary disease, to patients with renal disease and to patients with combined renal and hepatic disease.

Information for the Patient

Nitazoxanide for oral suspension should be taken with food.

Diabetic patients and caregivers should be aware that the oral suspension contains 1.48 g of sucrose/5 ml.

CARCINOGENESIS, MUTAGENESIS, AND IMPAIRMENT OF FERTILITY

Long-term carcinogenicity studies have not been conducted.

Nitazoxanide was not genotoxic in the Chinese hamster ovary (CHO) cell chromosomal aberration assay or the mouse micronucleus assay. Nitazoxanide was genotoxic in one tester strain (TA 100) in the Ames bacterial mutagenicity assay.

Nitazoxanide did not adversely affect male or female fertility in the rat at 2400 mg/kg/day (approximately 66 times the recommended dose for patients 11 years of age, adjusted for body surface area).

PREGNANCY, TERATOGENIC EFFECTS, PREGNANCY CATEGORY B

Reproduction studies have been performed at doses up to 3200 mg/kg/day in rats (approximately 48 times the clinical dose adjusted for body surface area) and 100 mg/kg/day in rabbits (approximately 3 times the clinical dose adjusted for body surface area) and have revealed no evidence of impaired fertility or harm to the fetus due to nitazoxanide. There are, however, no adequate and well-controlled studies in pregnant women.

NURSING MOTHERS

It is not known whether nitazoxanide is excreted in human milk. Because many drugs are excreted in human milk, caution should be exercised when nitazoxanide is administered to a nursing woman.

PEDIATRIC USE

Safety and effectiveness of nitazoxanide for oral suspension in pediatric patients less than 1 year of age or greater than 11 years of age have not been studied.

ADULTS AND GERIATRICS

Safety and effectiveness of nitazoxanide for oral suspension in adult and geriatric patients have not been studied.

HIV POSITIVE PATIENTS

Safety and effectiveness of nitazoxanide for oral suspension HIV positive patients have not been established.

IMMUNODEFICIENT PATIENTS

Safety and effectiveness of nitazoxanide for oral suspension in immunodeficient patients have not been established.

DRUG INTERACTIONS

Tizoxanide is highly bound to plasma protein (>99.9%). Therefore, caution should be used when administering nitazoxanide concurrently with other highly plasma protein-bound drugs with narrow therapeutic indices, as competition for binding sites may occur.

No interactions with other medicinal products have been reported by patients using nitazoxanide. However, no clinical studies have been conducted to specifically exclude the possibility of interactions between nitazoxanide and other medicinal products.

ADVERSE REACTIONS

In controlled and uncontrolled clinical studies of 613 HIV-negative pediatric patients who received nitazoxanide for oral suspension, the most frequent adverse events reported regardless of causality assessment were: abdominal pain (7.8%), diarrhea (2.1%), vomiting (1.1%) and headache (1.1%). These were typically mild and transient in nature. In placebo-controlled clinical trials, the rates of occurrence of these events did not differ significantly from those of the placebo. None of the 613 pediatric patients discontinued therapy because of adverse events.

Adverse events occurring in less than 1% of the patients participating in clinical trials are listed below:

Digestive System: Nausea, anorexia, flatulence, appetite increase, enlarged salivary glands.

Body as a Whole: Fever, infection, malaise.

Metabolic & Nutrition: Increased creatinine, increased SGPT.

Skin: Pruritus, sweat.

Special Senses: Eye discoloration (pale yellow).

Respiratory System: Rhinitis.

Nervous System: Dizziness.

Urogenital System: Discolored urine.

DOSAGE AND ADMINISTRATION

Age 12-47 months: 5 ml (100 mg nitazoxanide) every 12 hours for 3 days.

Age 4-11 years: 10 ml (200 mg nitazoxanide) every 12 hours for 3 days.

The oral suspension should be taken with food.

HOW SUPPLIED

Alinia for oral suspension is a pink-colored powder formulation that, when reconstituted as directed, contains 100 mg nitazoxanide/5 ml. The reconstituted suspension has a pink color and strawberry flavor.

STORAGE AND STABILITY

Store the unsuspended powder and the reconstituted oral suspension at 25°C (77°F); excursions permitted to 15-30°C (59-86°F).

The container should be kept tightly closed, and the suspension should be shaken well before each administration. The suspension may be stored for 7 days, after which any unused portion must be discarded.

PRODUCT LISTING - EQUIVALENTS NOT AVAILABLE

Powder For Reconstitution - Oral - 100 mg/5 ml

60 ml $60.00 ALINIA, Romark Laboratories L.C. 67546-0212-21

Nitric Oxide (003465)

For complete prescribing information, refer to the CD-ROM included with the book.

Categories: Hypertension, pulmonary; FDA Approved 1999 Dec; Pregnancy Category C; Orphan Drugs
Drug Classes: Vasodilators, pulmonary
Brand Names: INOmax

DESCRIPTION

Nitric oxide gas is a drug administered by inhalation. Nitric oxide, the active substance in INOmax, is a pulmonary vasodilator. INOmax is a gaseous blend of nitric oxide (0.8%) and nitrogen (99.2%). INOmax is supplied in aluminum cylinders as a compressed gas under high pressure (2000 pounds per square inch gauge [psig]).

INDICATIONS AND USAGE

Nitric oxide, in conjunction with ventilatory support and other appropriate agents, is indicated for the treatment of term and near-term (>34 weeks) neonates with hypoxic respiratory failure associated with clinical or echocardiographic evidence of pulmonary hypertension, where it improves oxygenation and reduces the need for extracorporeal membrane oxygenation.

CONTRAINDICATIONS

Nitric oxide should not be used in the treatment of neonates known to be dependent on right-to-left shunting of blood.

DOSAGE AND ADMINISTRATION

DOSAGE

The recommended dose of nitric oxide is 20 ppm. Treatment should be maintained up to 14 days or until the underlying oxygen desaturation has resolved and the neonate is ready to be weaned from nitric oxide therapy.

An initial dose of 20 ppm was used in the NINOS and CINRGI trials. In CINRGI, patients whose oxygenation improved with 20 ppm were dose-reduced to 5 ppm as tolerated at the end of 4 hours of treatment. In the NINOS trial, patients who oxygenation failed to improve on 20 ppm could be increased to 80 ppm, but those patients did not then improve on the higher dose. As the risk of methemoglobinemia and elevated NO_2 levels increases significantly when nitric oxide is administered at doses >20 ppm, doses above this level ordinarily should not be used.

ADMINISTRATION

Additional therapies should be used to maximize oxygen delivery. In patients with collapsed alveoli, additional therapies might include surfactant and high frequency oscillatory ventilation.

The safety and effectiveness of inhaled nitric oxide have been established in a population receiving other therapies for hypoxic respiratory failure, including vasodilators, intravenous fluids, bicarbonate therapy, and mechanical ventilation. Different dose regimens for nitric oxide were used in the clinical studies.

Nitric oxide should be administered with monitoring for PaO_2, methemoglobin, and NO_2.

The nitric oxide delivery systems used in the clinical trials provided operator-determined concentrations of nitric oxide in the breathing gas, and the concentration was constant throughout the respiratory cycle. Nitric oxide must be delivered through a system with these characteristics and which does not cause generation of excessive inhaled nitrogen dioxide. The INOvent system and other systems meeting these criteria were used in the clinical trials. In the ventilated neonate, precise monitoring of inspired nitric oxide and NO_2 should be instituted, using a properly calibrated analysis device with alarms. This system should be calibrated using a precisely defined calibration mixture of nitric oxide and nitrogen dioxide, such as INOcal. Sample gas for analysis should be drawn before the Y-piece, proximal to the patient. Oxygen levels should also be measured.

In the event of a system failure or a wall-outlet power failure, a backup battery power supply and reserve nitric oxide delivery system should be available.

The nitric oxide dose should not be discontinued abruptly as it may result in an increase in pulmonary artery pressure and/or worsening of blood oxygenation (PaO_2). Deterioration in oxygenation and elevation in PAP may also occur in children with no apparent response to nitric oxide. Discontinue/wean cautiously.

N

Nitrofurantoin (001890)

Categories: Infection, urinary tract; Pregnancy Category B; FDA Approved 1953 Dec; WHO Formulary
Drug Classes: Antibiotics, nitrofurans
Brand Names: Furadantin
Foreign Brand Availability: Furadantin Suspension (Australia; New-Zealand); Furadantina (Mexico); Furadoine (France); Furantoina (Costa-Rica; Dominican-Republic; El-Salvador; Guatemala; Honduras; Nicaragua; Panama); Furobactina (Spain); Infurin (Peru); Urantin (South-Africa); Urofuran (Finland)

DESCRIPTION

Nitrofurantoin, a synthetic chemical, is a stable, yellow, crystalline compound. Nitrofurantoin is an antibacterial agent for specific urinary tract infections. Nitrofurantoin is available in 50-mg and 100-mg tablets and in 5-mg/ml liquid suspension for oral administration.

1-(((5-nitro-2-furanyl)methylene)amino)-2,4-imidazolidinedione

Furadantin Inactive Ingredients: Nitrofurantoin tablets contain calcium pyrophosphate, magnesium stearate, starch, and sucrose. Nitrofurantoin Oral Suspension contains carboxymethylcellulose sodium, citric acid, flavors, glycerin, magnesium aluminum silicate, methylparaben, propylparaben, purified water, saccharin, sodium citrate, and sorbitol.

CLINICAL PHARMACOLOGY

Orally administered nitrofurantoin is readily absorbed and rapidly excreted in urine. Blood concentrations at therapeutic dosage are usually low. It is highly soluble in urine, to which it may impart a brown color. Following a dose regimen of 100 mg q.i.d. for 7 days, average urinary drug recoveries (0-24 hours) on day 1 and day 7 were 42.7% and 43.6%.

Unlike many drugs, the presence of food or agents delaying gastric emptying can increase the bioavailability of nitrofurantoin, presumably by allowing better dissolution in gastric juices.

Microbiology: Nitrofurantoin, *in vitro*, is bacteriostatic in low concentrations (5-10 mcg/ml) and is considered bactericidal in higher concentrations. Its mode of action is presumed to be interference with several bacterial enzyme systems. Bacteria develop only a limited resistance to furan derivatives.

While *in vitro* studies have demonstrated the susceptibility of most strains of the following organisms, clinical efficacy for infections other than those included in the INDICATIONS AND USAGE section has not been documented: *Escherichia Coli*, Enterococci (*e.g., Streptococcus Faecalis*), *Staphylococcus Aureus,Staphylococcus Epidermis*.

NOTE: Some strains of *Enterobacter* species and *Klebsiella* species are resistant to nitrofurantoin. It is not active against most strains of *Proteus* and *Serratia* species. It has no activity against *Pseudomonas* species.

Antagonism has been demonstrated between nitrofurantoin and both nalidixic acid and oxolinic acid *in vitro*.

Susceptibility Tests: Quantitative methods that require measurement of zone diameters give the most precise estimates of antimicrobial susceptibility. One recommended procedure, (NCCLS, ASM-2)*, uses a disc containing 300 micrograms for testing susceptibility; interpretations correlate zone diameters of this disc test with MIC values for nitrofurantoin. Reports from the laboratory should be interpreted according to the following criteria:

Susceptible organisms produce zones of 17 mm or greater, indicating that the tested organism is likely to respond to therapy.

Organisms of intermediate susceptibility produce zones of 15 to 16 mm, indicating that the tested organism would be susceptible if high dosage is used.

Resistant organisms produce zones of 14 mm or less, indicating that other therapy should be selected.

A bacterial isolate may be considered susceptible if the MIC value for nitrofurantoin is 25 micrograms per ml or less. Organisms are considered resistant if the MIC is 100 micrograms per ml or more.

NOTE: Specimens for culture and susceptibility testing should be obtained prior to and during drug administration.

INDICATIONS AND USAGE

Nitrofurantoin is specifically indicated for the treatment of urinary tract infections when due to susceptible strains of *E. coli*, enterococci, *S. aureus* (it is not indicated for the treatment or associated renal cortical or perinephric abscesses), and certain susceptible strains of *Klebsiella, Enterobacter,* and *Proteus species.*

CONTRAINDICATIONS

Anuria, oliguria, or significant impairment of renal function (creatinine clearance under 40 ml per minute) are contraindications. Treatment of this type of patient carries an increased risk of toxicity and is much less effective because of impaired excretion of the drug.

The drug is contraindicated in pregnant patients at term (during labor and delivery) as well as in infants under one month of age because of the possibility of hemolytic anemia in the fetus or in the newborn infant due to immature erythrocyte enzyme systems (glutathione instability).

Nitrofurantoin is also contraindicated in those patients with known hypersensitivity to nitrofurantoin.

WARNINGS

ACUTE, SUBACUTE OR CHRONIC PULMONARY REACTIONS HAVE BEEN OBSERVED IN PATIENTS TREATED WITH NITROFURANTOIN. IF THESE REACTIONS OCCUR, NITROFURANTOIN SHOULD BE DISCONTINUED AND APPROPRIATE MEASURES TAKEN. REPORTS HAVE CITED PULMONARY REACTIONS AS A CONTRIBUTING CAUSE OF DEATH.

CHRONIC PULMONARY REACTIONS (DIFFUSE INTERSTITIAL PNEUMONITIS OR PULMONARY FIBROSIS, OR BOTH) CAN DEVELOP INSIDIOUSLY. THESE REACTIONS OCCUR RARELY AND GENERALLY IN PATIENTS RECEIVING THERAPY FOR SIX MONTHS OR LONGER. CLOSE MONITORING OF THE PULMONARY CONDITION OF PATIENTS RECEIVING LONG-TERM THERAPY IS WARRANTED AND REQUIRES THAT THE BENEFITS OF THERAPY BE WEIGHED AGAINST POTENTIAL RISKS. (SEE RESPIRATORY REACTIONS.)

Hepatitis, including chronic active hepatitis, occurs rarely. Fatalities have been reported. The onset of chronic active hepatitis may be insidious, and patients receiving long-term therapy should be monitored periodically for changes in liver function. If hepatitis occurs, the drug should be withdrawn immediately and appropriate measures taken.

Peripheral neuropathy, which may become severe or irreversible, has occurred. Fatalities have been reported. Conditions such as renal impairment (creatinine clearance under 40 ml per minute), anemia, diabetes mellitus, electrolyte imbalance, vitamin B deficiency, and debilitating disease may enhance the occurrence of peripheral neuropathy.

Cases of hemolytic anemia of the primaquine sensitivity type have been induced by nitrofurantoin. Hemolysis appears to be linked to a glucose-6-phosphate dehydrogenase deficiency in the red blood cells of the affected patients. This deficiency is found in 10 percent of Negroes and a small percentage of ethnic groups of Mediterranean and Near-Eastern origin. Hemolysis is an indication for discontinuing nitrofurantoin; hemolysis ceases when the drug is withdrawn.

PRECAUTIONS

Carcinogenesis, Mutagenesis, and Impairment of Fertility: Nitrofurantoin, when fed to female Holtzman rats at levels of 0.3% in a commercial diet for up to 44.5 weeks, was not carcinogenic. Nitrofurantoin was not carcinogenic when female Sprague-Dawley rats were fed a commercial diet with nitrofurantoin levels at 0.1% to 0.187% (total cumulative, 9.25g) for 75 weeks. Further studies of the effects of chronic administration to rodents are in progress.

Results of microbial in vitro tests using *Escherichia Coli*, *Salmonella Typhimurium*, and *Aspergillus Nidulans* suggest that nitrofurantoin is a weak mutagen. Results of a dominant lethal assay in the mouse were negative.

Impairment of Fertility: The administration of high doses of nitrofurantoin to rats causes temporary spermatogenic arrest; this is reversible on discontinuing the drug. Doses of 10 mg/kg or greater in healthy human males may, in certain unpredictable instances, produce slight to moderate spermatogenic arrest with a decrease in sperm count.

Pregnancy: The safety of nitrofurantoin during pregnancy and lactation has not been established. Use of this drug in women of childbearing potential requires that the anticipated benefit be weighed against the possible risks.

Labor and Delivery: See CONTRAINDICATIONS.

Nursing Mothers: Nitrofurantoin has been detected in breast milk, in trace amounts. Caution should be exercised when nitrofurantoin is administered to a nursing woman, especially if the infant is known or suspected to have a glucose-6-phosphate dehydrogenase deficiency.

Pediatric Use: Contraindicated in infants under one month of age.(See CONTRAINDICATIONS.)

DRUG INTERACTIONS

Magnesium trisilicate, when administered concomitantly with nitrofurantoin, reduces both the rate and extent of absorption. The mechanism for this interaction probably is adsorption of drug onto the surface of magnesium trisilicate.

Uricosuric drugs such as probenecid and sulfinpyrazone may inhibit renal tubular secretion of nitrofurantoin. The resulting increase in serum levels may increase toxicity and the decreased urinary levels could lessen its efficacy as a urinary tract antibacterial.

ADVERSE REACTIONS

Respiratory: CHRONIC, SUBACUTE, OR ACUTE PULMONARY HYPERSENSITIVITY REACTIONS MAY OCCUR.

CHRONIC PULMONARY REACTIONS OCCUR GENERALLY IN PATIENTS WHO HAVE RECEIVED CONTINUOUS TREATMENT FOR SIX MONTHS OR LONGER. MALAISE, DYSPNEA ON EXERTION, COUGH, AND ALTERED PULMONARY FUNCTION ARE COMMON MANIFESTATIONS WHICH CAN OCCUR INSIDIOUSLY. RADIOLOGIC AND HISTOLOGIC FINDINGS OF DIFFUSE INTERSTITIAL PNEUMONITIS OR FIBROSIS, OR BOTH, ARE ALSO COMMON MANIFESTATIONS OF THE CHRONIC PULMONARY REACTION. FEVER IS RARELY PROMINENT.

THE SEVERITY OF CHRONIC PULMONARY REACTIONS AND THEIR DEGREE OF RESOLUTION APPEAR TO BE RELATED TO THE DURATION OF THERAPY AFTER THE FIRST CLINICAL SIGNS APPEAR. PULMONARY FUNCTION MAY BE IMPAIRED PERMANENTLY, EVEN AFTER CESSATION OF THERAPY. THE RISK IS GREATER WHEN CHRONIC PULMONARY REACTIONS ARE NOT RECOGNIZED EARLY.

In subacute pulmonary reactions, fever and eosinophilia occur less often than in the acute form. Upon cessation of therapy, recovery may require several months. If the symptoms are not recognized as being drug-related and nitrofurantoin therapy is not stopped, the symptoms may become more severe.

Acute pulmonary reactions are commonly manifested by fever, chills, cough, chest pain, dyspnea, pulmonary infiltration with consolidation or pleural effusion on x-ray, and eosinophilia. Acute reactions usually occur within the first week of treatment and are reversible with cessation of therapy. Resolution often is dramatic. (See WARNINGS.)

Gastrointestinal: Hepatitis, including chronic active hepatitis, and cholestatic jaundice occur rarely.

Nausea, emesis, and anorexia occur most often. Abdominal pain and diarrhea are less common gastrointestinal reactions. These dose-related reactions can be minimized by reduction of dosage.

Neurologic: Peripheral neuropathy, which may become severe or irreversible, has occurred. Fatalities have been reported. Conditions such as renal impairment (creatinine clearance under 40 ml per minute), anemia, diabetes mellitus, electrolyte imbalance, vitamin B deficiency, and debilitating diseases may increase the possibility of peripheral neuropathy.

Less frequent reactions, of unknown causal relationship, are nystagmus, vertigo, dizziness, asthenia, headache, and drowsiness.

Dermatologic: Exfoliative dermatitis and erythema multiforme (including Stevens-Johnson Syndrome) have been reported rarely. Transient alopecia also has been reported.

Allergic Reactions: Lupus-like syndrome associated with pulmonary reaction to nitrofurantoin has been reported. Also, angioedema, maculopapular, erythematous or eczematous eruptions, urticaria, rash, and pruritus have occurred. Anaphylaxis, sialoadenitis, pancreatitis, arthralgia, myalgia, drug fever, and chills or chills and fever have been reported.

Hematologic: Agranulocytosis, leukopenia, granulocytopenia, hemolytic anemia, thrombocytopenia, glucose-6-phosphate dehydrogenase deficiency anemia, megaloblastic anemia, and eosinophilia have occurred. Cessation of therapy has returned the blood picture to normal. Aplastic anemia has been reported rarely.

Miscellaneous: As with other antimicrobial agents, superinfections by resistant organisms, *e.g.,* pseudomonas, may occur. However, these are limited to the genitourinary tract because suppression of normal bacterial flora does not occur elsewhere in the body.

DOSAGE AND ADMINISTRATION

Nitrofurantoin should be given with food to improve drug absorption and, in some patients, tolerance.

Adults: 50-100 mg four times a day - the lower dosage level is recommended for uncomplicated urinary tract infections.

Children: 5-7 mg/kg of body weight per 24 hours, given in four divided doses (contraindicated under one month of age). The following table can be used to calculate an average dose of nitrofurantoin oral suspension (5 mg/ml) for children (one 5-ml teaspoon of nitrofurantoin oral suspension contains 25 mg of nitrofurantoin).

TABLE 1

Body Weight		No. Teaspoonfuls
Pounds	Kilograms	4 Times Daily
15 to 26	7 to 11	1/2 (2.5 ml)
27 to 46	12 to 21	1 (5 ml)
47 to 68	22 to 30	1-1/2 (7.5 ml)
69 to 91	31 to 41	2 (10 ml)

Therapy should be continued for one week or for at least 3 days after sterility of the urine is obtained. Continued infection indicates the need for reevaluation.

For long-term suppressive therapy in adults, a reduction of dosage to 50-100 mg at bedtime may be adequate. For long-term suppressive therapy in children, doses as low as 1 mg/kg per 24 hours, given in a single dose or in two divided doses, may be adequate. See WARNINGS regarding risks associated with long-term therapy.

Avoid exposure to strong light which may darken the drug. It is stable in storage. It should be dispensed in amber bottles.

PRODUCT LISTING - RATED THERAPEUTICALLY EQUIVALENT

Capsule - Oral - Macrocrystals 25 mg

100's	$90.83	MACRODANTIN, Procter and Gamble Pharmaceuticals	00149-0007-05

Capsule - Oral - Macrocrystals 50 mg

10's	$12.51	MACRODANTIN, Prescript Pharmaceuticals	00247-0159-10
12's	$11.65	GENERIC, Pd-Rx Pharmaceuticals	55289-0186-12
12's	$14.79	MACRODANTIN, Pd-Rx Pharmaceuticals	55289-0179-12
14's	$12.16	GENERIC, Pd-Rx Pharmaceuticals	55289-0186-14
14's	$16.16	MACRODANTIN, Prescript Pharmaceuticals	00247-0159-14
20's	$17.65	GENERIC, Pd-Rx Pharmaceuticals	55289-0186-20
20's	$21.66	MACRODANTIN, Prescript Pharmaceuticals	00247-0159-20
21's	$18.21	GENERIC, Pd-Rx Pharmaceuticals	55289-0186-21
21's	$22.58	MACRODANTIN, Prescript Pharmaceuticals	00247-0159-21
28's	$24.74	GENERIC, Pd-Rx Pharmaceuticals	55289-0186-28
28's	$28.99	MACRODANTIN, Prescript Pharmaceuticals	00247-0159-28
28's	$34.28	MACRODANTIN, Pd-Rx Pharmaceuticals	55289-0179-28
30's	$21.75	GENERIC, Heartland Healthcare Services	61392-0169-30
30's	$21.75	GENERIC, Heartland Healthcare Services	61392-0169-39
30's	$30.81	MACRODANTIN, Prescript Pharmaceuticals	00247-0159-30
30's	$383.35	GENERIC, Medirex Inc	57480-0816-06
31's	$22.48	GENERIC, Heartland Healthcare Services	61392-0169-31
32's	$23.20	GENERIC, Heartland Healthcare Services	61392-0169-32
40's	$35.33	GENERIC, Pd-Rx Pharmaceuticals	55289-0186-40
40's	$39.96	MACRODANTIN, Prescript Pharmaceuticals	00247-0159-40
40's	$46.23	MACRODANTIN, Pd-Rx Pharmaceuticals	54868-0429-03
40's	$51.00	MACRODANTIN, Pd-Rx Pharmaceuticals	55289-0179-40
45's	$32.63	GENERIC, Heartland Healthcare Services	61392-0169-45
60's	$43.51	GENERIC, Heartland Healthcare Services	61392-0169-60
90's	$65.26	GENERIC, Heartland Healthcare Services	61392-0169-90
100's	$58.20	GENERIC, Qualitest Products Inc	00603-4776-21
100's	$66.10	GENERIC, Aligen Independent Laboratories Inc	00405-4699-01
100's	$66.50	GENERIC, Watson/Rugby Laboratories Inc	00536-5618-01
100's	$66.75	GENERIC, Major Pharmaceuticals Inc	00904-7721-60
100's	$66.85	GENERIC, Martec Pharmaceuticals Inc	52555-0476-01
100's	$66.95	GENERIC, Geneva Pharmaceuticals	00781-2502-01
100's	$67.49	GENERIC, Moore, H.L. Drug Exchange Inc	00839-7518-06
100's	$70.20	GENERIC, Vangard Labs	00615-1308-13
100's	$71.20	GENERIC, Mylan Pharmaceuticals Inc	00378-1650-01
100's	$89.78	MACRODANTIN, Procter and Gamble Pharmaceuticals	00149-0008-77
100's	$109.44	GENERIC, Ivax Corporation	00172-2130-60
100's	$110.50	GENERIC, Ivax Corporation	00182-1944-89
100's	$119.60	MACRODANTIN, Procter and Gamble Pharmaceuticals	00149-0008-05

Capsule - Oral - Macrocrystals 100 mg

12's	$17.51	GENERIC, Pd-Rx Pharmaceuticals	55289-0203-12
12's	$26.78	MACRODANTIN, Pd-Rx Pharmaceuticals	55289-0914-12
14's	$21.37	GENERIC, Pd-Rx Pharmaceuticals	55289-0203-14
14's	$29.42	MACRODANTIN, Pd-Rx Pharmaceuticals	55289-0914-14
15's	$32.04	MACRODANTIN, Pd-Rx Pharmaceuticals	55289-0914-15
20's	$27.93	GENERIC, Pd-Rx Pharmaceuticals	55289-0203-20
28's	$41.87	GENERIC, Pd-Rx Pharmaceuticals	55289-0203-28
28's	$56.33	MACRODANTIN, Pd-Rx Pharmaceuticals	55289-0914-28
30's	$38.50	GENERIC, Heartland Healthcare Services	61392-0168-30
30's	$38.50	GENERIC, Heartland Healthcare Services	61392-0168-39
30's	$47.52	GENERIC, Pd-Rx Pharmaceuticals	55289-0203-30
30's	$60.35	MACRODANTIN, Pd-Rx Pharmaceuticals	55289-0914-30
30's	$638.91	GENERIC, Medirex Inc	57480-0817-06
31's	$39.78	GENERIC, Heartland Healthcare Services	61392-0168-31
32's	$41.07	GENERIC, Heartland Healthcare Services	61392-0168-32
40's	$63.14	GENERIC, Pd-Rx Pharmaceuticals	55289-0203-40
40's	$80.46	MACRODANTIN, Pd-Rx Pharmaceuticals	55289-0914-40
45's	$57.75	GENERIC, Heartland Healthcare Services	61392-0168-45
60's	$77.00	GENERIC, Heartland Healthcare Services	61392-0168-60
90's	$115.50	GENERIC, Heartland Healthcare Services	61392-0168-90
100's	$98.50	GENERIC, Qualitest Products Inc	00603-4777-21
100's	$105.95	GENERIC, Medirex Inc	57480-0817-01
100's	$108.75	GENERIC, Aligen Independent Laboratories Inc	00405-4700-01
100's	$108.75	GENERIC, Major Pharmaceuticals Inc	00904-7722-60
100's	$113.65	GENERIC, Geneva Pharmaceuticals	00781-2503-01
100's	$114.00	GENERIC, Martec Pharmaceuticals Inc	52555-0477-01
100's	$114.74	GENERIC, Moore, H.L. Drug Exchange Inc	00839-7519-06
100's	$114.89	GENERIC, Watson/Rugby Laboratories Inc	00536-5619-01
100's	$121.80	GENERIC, Mylan Pharmaceuticals Inc	00378-1700-01
100's	$125.32	GENERIC, Ivax Corporation	62584-0808-01
100's	$156.80	MACRODANTIN, Procter and Gamble Pharmaceuticals	00149-0009-77
100's	$185.87	GENERIC, Ivax Corporation	00172-2131-60
100's	$186.37	GENERIC, Ivax Corporation	00182-1945-89
100's	$203.13	MACRODANTIN, Procter and Gamble Pharmaceuticals	00149-0009-05

PRODUCT LISTING - EQUIVALENTS NOT AVAILABLE

Capsule - Oral - Macrocrystals 50 mg

2's	$4.26	GENERIC, Prescript Pharmaceuticals	00247-0137-02
4's	$5.15	GENERIC, Prescript Pharmaceuticals	00247-0137-04
10's	$7.15	GENERIC, Southwood Pharmaceuticals Inc	58016-0142-10
10's	$7.86	GENERIC, Prescript Pharmaceuticals	00247-0137-10
12's	$8.58	GENERIC, Southwood Pharmaceuticals Inc	58016-0142-12
12's	$8.75	GENERIC, Prescript Pharmaceuticals	00247-0137-12
14's	$9.66	GENERIC, Prescript Pharmaceuticals	00247-0137-14
14's	$10.01	GENERIC, Southwood Pharmaceuticals Inc	58016-0142-14
15's	$10.73	GENERIC, Southwood Pharmaceuticals Inc	58016-0142-15
20's	$10.87	GENERIC, Physicians Total Care	54868-0107-06
20's	$12.35	GENERIC, Prescript Pharmaceuticals	00247-0137-20
20's	$14.24	GENERIC, Allscripts Pharmaceutical Company	54569-0181-04
20's	$14.31	GENERIC, Southwood Pharmaceuticals Inc	58016-0142-20
21's	$12.80	GENERIC, Prescript Pharmaceuticals	00247-0137-21
24's	$17.17	GENERIC, Southwood Pharmaceuticals Inc	58016-0142-24
28's	$15.95	GENERIC, Prescript Pharmaceuticals	00247-0137-28
28's	$19.94	GENERIC, Allscripts Pharmaceutical Company	54569-0181-00
28's	$20.03	GENERIC, Southwood Pharmaceuticals Inc	58016-0142-28
30's	$16.86	GENERIC, Prescript Pharmaceuticals	00247-0137-30
30's	$21.36	GENERIC, Allscripts Pharmaceutical Company	54569-0181-01
30's	$21.46	GENERIC, Southwood Pharmaceuticals Inc	58016-0142-30
30's	$33.50	GENERIC, Pharma Pac	52959-0406-30
40's	$21.35	GENERIC, Prescript Pharmaceuticals	00247-0137-40
40's	$28.48	GENERIC, Allscripts Pharmaceutical Company	54569-0181-02
40's	$29.76	GENERIC, Southwood Pharmaceuticals Inc	58016-0142-40
100's	$71.53	GENERIC, Southwood Pharmaceuticals Inc	58016-0142-00
100's	$73.34	GENERIC, Udl Laboratories Inc	51079-0584-20

Capsule - Oral - Macrocrystals 100 mg

2's	$4.18	GENERIC, Prescript Pharmaceuticals	00247-0258-47
4's	$4.68	GENERIC, Prescript Pharmaceuticals	00247-0258-04
6's	$5.34	GENERIC, Prescript Pharmaceuticals	00247-0258-06
10's	$6.66	GENERIC, Prescript Pharmaceuticals	00247-0258-10
10's	$12.14	GENERIC, Southwood Pharmaceuticals Inc	58016-0141-10
12's	$14.57	GENERIC, Southwood Pharmaceuticals Inc	58016-0141-12
14's	$7.99	GENERIC, Prescript Pharmaceuticals	00247-0258-14
14's	$10.23	GENERIC, Physicians Total Care	54868-0473-01
14's	$17.00	GENERIC, Southwood Pharmaceuticals Inc	58016-0141-14
14's	$19.05	GENERIC, Pharma Pac	52959-0405-14
15's	$18.21	GENERIC, Southwood Pharmaceuticals Inc	58016-0141-15
20's	$9.98	GENERIC, Prescript Pharmaceuticals	00247-0258-20
20's	$15.56	GENERIC, Physicians Total Care	54868-0473-02
20's	$23.08	GENERIC, Allscripts Pharmaceutical Company	54569-1969-02
20's	$24.28	GENERIC, Southwood Pharmaceuticals Inc	58016-0141-20
20's	$25.50	GENERIC, Pharma Pac	52959-0405-20
21's	$25.50	GENERIC, Southwood Pharmaceuticals Inc	58016-0141-21
21's	$27.20	GENERIC, Pharma Pac	52959-0405-21
24's	$29.14	GENERIC, Southwood Pharmaceuticals Inc	58016-0141-24
28's	$12.62	GENERIC, Prescript Pharmaceuticals	00247-0258-28
28's	$34.00	GENERIC, Southwood Pharmaceuticals Inc	58016-0141-28
28's	$34.10	GENERIC, Allscripts Pharmaceutical Company	54569-1969-00
30's	$13.28	GENERIC, Prescript Pharmaceuticals	00247-0258-30
30's	$36.43	GENERIC, Southwood Pharmaceuticals Inc	58016-0141-30
40's	$16.59	GENERIC, Prescript Pharmaceuticals	00247-0258-40
40's	$23.09	GENERIC, Physicians Total Care	54868-0473-00
40's	$46.15	GENERIC, Allscripts Pharmaceutical Company	54569-1969-01
90's	$33.13	GENERIC, Prescript Pharmaceuticals	00247-0258-90
100's	$121.42	GENERIC, Southwood Pharmaceuticals Inc	58016-0141-00
100's	$125.45	GENERIC, Udl Laboratories Inc	51079-0585-20

Capsule - Oral - Macrocrystals;Monohydrate 100 mg

2's	$7.35	MACROBID, Prescript Pharmaceuticals	00247-0164-02
6's	$9.64	MACROBID, Allscripts Pharmaceutical Company	54569-3544-03

6's	$15.34	MACROBID, Prescript Pharmaceuticals	00247-0164-06
6's	$15.47	MACROBID, Pd-Rx Pharmaceuticals	55289-0031-06
10's	$16.07	MACROBID, Allscripts Pharmaceutical Company	54569-3544-02
10's	$20.08	MACROBID, Physicians Total Care	54868-2366-01
10's	$23.34	MACROBID, Prescript Pharmaceuticals	00247-0164-10
10's	$26.34	MACROBID, Pd-Rx Pharmaceuticals	55289-0031-10
14's	$22.50	MACROBID, Allscripts Pharmaceutical Company	54569-3544-01
14's	$29.16	MACROBID, Pharma Pac	52959-0404-14
14's	$31.33	MACROBID, Prescript Pharmaceuticals	00247-0164-14
14's	$31.88	MACROBID, Pd-Rx Pharmaceuticals	55289-0031-14
14's	$40.76	MACROBID, Pd-Rx Pharmaceuticals	58864-0323-14
20's	$32.79	MACROBID, Allscripts Pharmaceutical Company	54569-3544-00
20's	$43.33	MACROBID, Prescript Pharmaceuticals	00247-0164-20
20's	$43.68	MACROBID, Pd-Rx Pharmaceuticals	55289-0031-20
21's	$45.32	MACROBID, Prescript Pharmaceuticals	00247-0164-21
60's	$96.43	MACROBID, Allscripts Pharmaceutical Company	54569-3544-04
60's	$114.62	MACROBID, Physicians Total Care	54868-2366-00
90's	$183.22	MACROBID, Prescript Pharmaceuticals	00247-0164-90
100's	$205.71	MACROBID, Procter and Gamble Pharmaceuticals	00149-0710-01
Suspension - Oral - 25 mg/5 ml			
60 ml	$21.76	FURADANTIN, Procter and Gamble Pharmaceuticals	00149-0735-15
60 ml	$34.30	FURADANTIN, Dura Pharmaceuticals	51479-0029-06
470 ml	$84.22	FURADANTIN, Procter and Gamble Pharmaceuticals	00149-0735-61
470 ml	$134.68	FURADANTIN, Dura Pharmaceuticals	51479-0029-47

Nitrofurantoin, Macrocrystalline *(001891)*

Categories: Infection, urinary tract; FDA Approved 1968 Apr; Pregnancy Category B
Drug Classes: Antibiotics, nitrofurans
Brand Names: Macpac; **Macrodantin**; Ro-Antoin; Uvamin-E Retard
Foreign Brand Availability: Biofurin (Mexico); Furadantin Retard (Switzerland); Furadantina (Mexico); Furadantina MC (Costa-Rica; Dominican-Republic; El-Salvador; Guatemala; Honduras; Nicaragua; Panama); Furadantine (France); Furadantine-MC (Netherlands); Macrobid (England); Macrodantina (Colombia; Mexico; Peru); Macrofuran (Indonesia); Macrofurin (Mexico); Ralodantin (Australia); Uro-Tablinen (Germany); Uvamin (Israel); Uvamin Retard (Costa-Rica; Dominican-Republic; Ecuador; El-Salvador; Guatemala; Honduras; Nicaragua; Panama; Switzerland)
Cost of Therapy: $33.49 (Urinary Tract Infections; Macrodantin; 50 mg; 4 capsules/day; 7 day supply)
$16.30 (Urinary Tract Infections; Generic Capsules; 50 mg; 4 capsules/day; 7 day supply)

N

DESCRIPTION

Macrodantin (nitrofurantoin macrocrystals) is a synthetic chemical of controlled crystal size. It is a stable, yellow, crystalline compound. Macrodantin is an antibacterial agent for specific urinary tract infections. It is available in 25, 50, and 100 mg capsules for oral administration. 1-[[(5-nitro-2-furanyl)methylene]amino]-2,4-imidazolidinedione.

Macrodantin inactive ingredients: Each capsule contains edible black ink, gelatin, lactose, starch, talc, titanium dioxide, and may contain FD&C yellow no. 6 and D&C yellow no. 10.

CLINICAL PHARMACOLOGY

Macrodantin is a larger crystal form of Furadantin (nitrofurantoin). The absorption of Macrodantin is slower and its excretion somewhat less when compared to Furadantin. Blood concentrations at therapeutic dosage are usually low. It is highly soluble in urine, to which it may impart a brown color.

Following a dose regimen of 100 mg qid for 7 days, average urinary drug recoveries (0-24 hours) on day 1 and day 7 were 37.9% and 35.0%.

Unlike many drugs, the presence of food or agents delaying gastric emptying can increase the bioavailability of nitrofurantoin, presumably by allowing better dissolution in gastric juices.

MICROBIOLOGY

Nitrofurantoin is bactericidal in urine at therapeutic doses. The mechanism of the antimicrobial action of nitrofurantoin is unusual among antibacterials. Nitrofurantoin is reduced by bacterial flavoproteins to reactive intermediates which inactivate or alter bacterial ribosomal proteins and other macromolecules. As a result of such inactivations, the vial biochemical processes of protein synthesis, aerobic energy metabolism, DNA synthesis, RNA synthesis, and cell wall synthesis are inhibited. The broad-based nature of this mode of action may explain the lack of acquired bacterial resistance to nitrofurantoin, as the necessary multiple and simultaneous mutations of the target macromolecules would likely be lethal to the bacteria. Development of resistance to nitrofurantoin has not been a significant problem since its introduction in 1953. Cross-resistance with antibiotics and sulfonamides has not been observed, and transferable resistance is, at most, a very rare phenomenon.

Nitrofurantoin, in the form of Macrodantin, has been shown to be active against most strains of the following bacteria both *in vitro* and in clinical infections: (See INDICATIONS AND USAGE.)

Gram-Positive Aerobes: *Staphylococcus aureus; Enterococci (e.g., Enterococcus faecalis)*

Gram-Negative Aerobes: *Escherichia coli*

Note: Some strains of *Enterobacter* species and *Klebsiella* species are resistant to nitrofurantoin.

Nitrofurantoin also demonstrates *in vitro* activity against the following microorganisms, although the clinical significance of these data with respect to treatment with nitrofurantoin is unknown:

Gram-Positive Aerobes: *Coagulase-negative staphylococci (including Staphylococcus epidermidis and Staphylococcus saprophyticus); Streptococcus agalactiae; Group D streptococci; Viridans group streptococci*

Gram-Negative Aerobes: *Citrobacter amalonaticus; Citrobacter diversus; Citrobacter freundii; Klebsiella oxytoca; Klebsiella ozaenae*

Nitrofurantoin is not active against most strains of *Proteus* species or *Serratia* species. It has no activity against *Pseudomonas* species.

Antagonism has been demonstrated *in vitro* between nitrofurantoin and quinolone antimicrobial agents. The clinical significance of this finding is unknown.

SUSCEPTIBILITY TESTS

Diffusion Techniques

Quantitative methods that require measurement of zone diameters give the most precise estimate of the susceptibility of bacteria to antimicrobial agents. One such standardized procedure,[1] which has been recommended for use with disks to test susceptibility of organisms to nitrofurantoin, uses the 300 mcg nitrofurantoin disk. Interpretation involves the correlation of the diameter obtained in the disk test with the minimum inhibitory concentration (MIC) for nitrofurantoin.

Reports from the laboratory giving results of the standard single-disk susceptibility test with a 300 mcg nitrofurantoin disk should be interpreted according to the following criteria (see TABLE 1).

TABLE 1

Zone Diameter (mm)	Interpretation
≥17	Susceptible
15-16	Intermediate
≤14	Resistant

A report of "susceptible" indicates that the pathogen is likely to be inhibited by generally achievable urinary levels. A report of "intermediate" indicates that the result be considered equivocal and, if the organism is not fully susceptible to alternative clinically feasible drugs, the test should be repeated. This category provides a buffer zone which prevents small uncontrolled technical factors from causing major discrepancies in interpretations. A report of "resistant" indicates that achievable concentrations are unlikely to be inhibitory, and other therapy should be selected.

Standardized procedures require the use of laboratory control organisms. The 300 mcg nitrofurantoin disk should give the following zone diameters (see TABLE 2).

TABLE 2

Organism	Zone Diameter (mm)
E. coli ATCC 25922	20-25
S. aureus ATCC 25923	18-22

Dilution Techniques

Use a standardized dilution method[2] (broth, agar, microdilution) or equivalent with nitrofurantoin powder. The MIC values obtained should be interpreted according to the following criteria (see TABLE 3).

TABLE 3

MIC (mcg/ml)	Interpretation
≤32	Susceptible
64	Intermediate
≥128	Resistant

As with standard diffusion techniques, dilution methods require the use of laboratory control organisms. Standard nitrofurantoin powder should provide the following MIC values:

TABLE 4

Organism	MIC (mcg/ml)
E. coli ATCC 25922	4-16
S. aureus ATCC 29213	8-32
E. faecalis ATCC 29212	4-16

INDICATIONS AND USAGE

Nitrofurantoin is specifically indicated for the treatment of urinary tract infections when due to susceptible strains of *Escherichia coli*, enterococci, *Staphylococcus aureus*, and certain susceptible strains of *Klebsiella* and *Enterobacter* species.

Nitrofurantoin is not indicated for the treatment of pyelonephritis or perinephric abscesses.

Nitrofurantoins lack the broader tissue distribution of other therapeutic agents approved for urinary tract infections. Consequently, many patients who are treated with nitrofurantoin are predisposed to persistence or reappearance of bacteriuria. Urine specimens for culture and susceptibility testing should be obtained before and after completion of therapy. If persistence or reappearance of bacteriuria occurs after treatment with nitrofurantoin, other therapeutic agents with broader tissue distribution should be selected. In considering the use of nitrofurantoin, lower eradication rates should be balanced against the increased potential for systemic toxicity and for the development of antimicrobial resistance when agents with broader tissue distribution are utilized.

CONTRAINDICATIONS

Anuria, oliguria, or significant impairment of renal function (creatinine clearance under 60 ml per minute or clinically significant elevated serum creatinine) are contraindications.

Treatment of this type of patient carries an increased risk of toxicity because of impaired excretion of the drug.

Because of the possibility of hemolytic anemia due to immature erythrocyte enzyme systems (glutathione instability), the drug is contraindicated in pregnant patients at term (38-42 weeks gestation), during labor and delivery, or when the onset of labor is imminent. For the same reason, the drug is contraindicated in neonates under 1 month of age.

Nitrofurantoin is also contraindicated in those patients with known hypersensitivity to nitrofurantoin.

WARNINGS

ACUTE, SUBACUTE, OR CHRONIC PULMONARY REACTIONS HAVE BEEN OBSERVED IN PATIENTS TREATED WITH NITROFURANTOIN. IF THESE REACTIONS OCCUR, MACRODANTIN SHOULD BE DISCONTINUED AND APPROPRIATE MEASURES TAKEN. REPORTS HAVE CITED PULMONARY REACTIONS AS A CONTRIBUTING CAUSE OF DEATH.

CHRONIC PULMONARY REACTIONS (DIFFUSE INTERSTITIAL PNEUMONITIS OR PULMONARY FIBROSIS, OR BOTH) CAN DEVELOP INSIDIOUSLY. THESE REACTIONS OCCUR RARELY AND GENERALLY IN PATIENTS RECEIVING THERAPY FOR 6 MONTHS OR LONGER. CLOSE MONITORING OF THE PULMONARY CONDITION OF PATIENTS RECEIVING LONG-TERM THERAPY IS WARRANTED AND REQUIRES THAT THE BENEFITS OF THERAPY BE WEIGHED AGAINST POTENTIAL RISKS. (SEE RESPIRATORY REACTIONS.)

Hepatic reactions, including hepatitis, cholestatic jaundice, chronic active hepatitis, and hepatic necrosis, occur rarely. Fatalities have been reported. The onset of chronic active hepatitis may be insidious, and patients should be monitored periodically for changes in liver function. If hepatitis occurs, the drug should be withdrawn immediately and appropriate measures should be taken.

Peripheral neuropathy (including optic neuritis), which may become severe or irreversible, has occurred. Fatalities have been reported. Conditions such as renal impairment (creatinine clearance under 60 ml per minute or clinically significant elevated serum creatinine), anemia, diabetes mellitus, electrolyte imbalance, vitamin B deficiency, and debilitating disease may enhance the occurrence of peripheral neuropathy. Patients receiving long-term therapy should be monitored periodically for changes in renal function.

Cases of hemolytic anemia of the primaquine-sensitivity type have been induced by nitrofurantoin. Hemolysis appears to be linked to a glucose-6-phosphate dehydrogenase deficiency in the red blood cells of the affected patients. This deficiency is found in 10% of Blacks and a small percentage of ethnic groups of Mediterranean and Near-Eastern origin. Hemolysis is an indication for discontinuing Nitrofurantoin; hemolysis ceases when the drug is withdrawn.

PRECAUTIONS

INFORMATION FOR THE PATIENT

Patients should be advised to take nitrofurantoin with food to further enhance tolerance and improve drug absorption. Patients should be instructed to complete the full course of therapy; however, they should be advised to contact their physician if any unusual symptoms occur during therapy.

Many patients who cannot tolerate microcrystalline nitrofurantoin are able to take nitrofurantoin without nausea.

Patients should be advised not to use antacid preparations containing magnesium trisilicate while taking nitrofurantoin.

DRUG/LABORATORY TEST INTERACTIONS

As a result of the presence of nitrofurantoin, a false-positive reaction for glucose in the urine may occur. This has been observed with Benedict's and Fehling's solutions but not with the glucose enzymatic test.

CARCINOGENESIS, MUTAGENESIS, AND IMPAIRMENT OF FERTILITY

Nitrofurantoin was not carcinogenic when fed to female Holtzman rats for 44.5 weeks or to female Sprague-Dawley rats for 75 weeks. Two chronic rodent bioassays utilizing male and female Sprague-Dawley rats and two chronic bioassays in Swiss mice and in BDF_1 mice revealed no evidence of carcinogenicity.

Nitrofurantoin presented evidence of carcinogenic activity in female $B6C3F_1$ mice as shown by increased incidences of tubular adenomas, benign mixed tumors, and granulosa cell tumors of the ovary. In male F344/N rats, there were increased incidences of uncommon kidney tubular cell neoplasms, osteosarcomas of the bone, and neoplasms of the subcutaneous tissue. In one study involving subcutaneous administration of 75 mg/kg nitrofurantoin to pregnant female mice, lung papillary adenomas of unknown significance were observed in the F1 generation.

Nitrofurantoin has been shown to induce point mutations in certain strains of *Salmonella typhimurium* and forward mutations in L5178Y mouse lymphoma cells. Nitrofurantoin induced increased numbers of sister chromatid exchanges and chromosomal aberrations in Chinese hamster ovary cells but not in human cells in culture. Results of the sex-linked recessive lethal assay in *Drosophila* were negative after administration of nitrofurantoin by feeding or by injection. Nitrofurantoin did not induce heritable mutation in the rodent models examined.

The significance of the carcinogenicity and mutagenicity findings relative to the therapeutic use of nitrofurantoin in humans is unknown.

The administration of high doses of nitrofurantoin to rats causes temporary spermatogenic arrest; this is reversible on discontinuing the drug. Doses of 10 mg/kg/day or greater in healthy human males may, in certain unpredictable instances, produce a slight to moderate spermatogenic arrest with a decrease in sperm count.

PREGNANCY CATEGORY B

Teratogenic Effects

Several reproduction studies have been performed in rabbits and rats at doses up to 6 times the human dose and have revealed no evidence of impaired fertility or harm to the fetus due to nitrofurantoin. In a single published study conducted in mice at 68 times the human dose (based on mg/kg administered to the dam), growth retardation and a low incidence of minor and common malformations were observed. However, at 25 times the human dose, fetal malformations were not observed; the relevance of these findings to humans is uncertain. There are, however, no adequate and well-controlled studies in pregnant women. Because animal reproduction studies are not always predictive of human response, this drug should be used during pregnancy only if clearly needed.

Nonteratogenic Effects

Nitrofurantoin has been shown in one published transplacental carcinogenicity study to induce lung papillary adenomas in the F1 generation mice at doses 19 times the human dose on a mg/kg basis. The relationship of this finding to potential human carcinogenesis is presently unknown. Because of the uncertainty regarding the human implications of these animal data, this drug should be used during pregnancy only if clearly needed.

LABOR AND DELIVERY

See CONTRAINDICATIONS.

NURSING MOTHERS

Nitrofurantoin has been detected in breast milk in trace amounts. Because of the potential for serious adverse reactions from nitrofurantoin in nursing infants under 1 month of age, a decision should be made whether to discontinue nursing or to discontinue the drug, taking into account the importance of the drug to the mother. (See CONTRAINDICATIONS.)

PEDIATRIC USE

Nitrofurantoin is contraindicated in infants below the age of 1 month. (See CONTRAINDICATIONS.)

DRUG INTERACTIONS

Antacids containing magnesium trisilicate, when administered concomitantly with nitrofurantoin, reduce both the rate and extent of absorption. The mechanism for this interaction probably is adsorption of nitrofurantoin onto the surface of magnesium trisilicate.

Uricosuric drugs, such as probenecid and sulfinpyrazone, can inhibit renal tubular secretion of nitrofurantoin. The resulting increase in nitrofurantoin serum levels may increase toxicity, and the decreased urinary levels could lessen its efficacy as a urinary tract antibacterial.

ADVERSE REACTIONS

RESPIRATORY

CHRONIC, SUBACUTE, OR ACUTE PULMONARY HYPERSENSITIVITY REACTIONS MAY OCCUR.

CHRONIC PULMONARY REACTIONS OCCUR GENERALLY IN PATIENTS WHO HAVE RECEIVED CONTINUOUS TREATMENT FOR 6 MONTHS OR LONGER. MALAISE, DYSPNEA ON EXERTION, COUGH, AND ALTERED PULMONARY FUNCTION ARE COMMON MANIFESTATIONS WHICH CAN OCCUR INSIDIOUSLY. RADIOLOGIC AND HISTOLOGIC FINDINGS OF DIFFUSE INTERSTITIAL PNEUMONITIS OR FIBROSIS, OR BOTH, ARE ALSO COMMON MANIFESTATIONS OF THE CHRONIC PULMONARY REACTION. FEVER IS RARELY PROMINENT.

THE SEVERITY OF CHRONIC PULMONARY REACTIONS AND THEIR DEGREE OF RESOLUTION APPEAR TO BE RELATED TO THE DURATION OF THERAPY AFTER THE FIRST CLINICAL SIGNS APPEAR. PULMONARY FUNCTION MAY BE IMPAIRED PERMANENTLY, EVEN AFTER CESSATION OF THERAPY. THE RISK IS GREATER WHEN CHRONIC PULMONARY REACTIONS ARE NOT RECOGNIZED EARLY.

In subacute pulmonary reactions, fever and eosinophilia occur less often than in the acute form. Upon cessation of therapy, recovery may require several months. If the symptoms are not recognized as being drug-related and nitrofurantoin therapy is not stopped, the symptoms may become more severe.

Acute pulmonary reactions are commonly manifested by fever, chills, cough, chest pain, dyspnea, pulmonary infiltration with consolidation or pleural effusion on x-ray, and eosinophilia. Acute reactions usually occur within the first week of treatment and are reversible with cessation of therapy. Resolution often is dramatic. (See WARNINGS.)

Changes in EKG may occur associated with pulmonary reactions.

Collapse and cyanosis have seldom been reported.

CHRONIC, SUBACUTE, OR ACUTE PULMONARY HYPERSENSITIVITY REACTIONS MAY OCCUR.

CHRONIC PULMONARY REACTIONS OCCUR GENERALLY IN PATIENTS WHO HAVE RECEIVED CONTINUOUS TREATMENT FOR 6 MONTHS OR LONGER. MALAISE, DYSPNEA ON EXERTION, COUGH, AND ALTERED PULMONARY FUNCTION ARE COMMON MANIFESTATIONS WHICH CAN OCCUR INSIDIOUSLY. RADIOLOGIC AND HISTOLOGIC FINDINGS OF DIFFUSE INTERSTITIAL PNEUMONITIS OR FIBROSIS, OR BOTH, ARE ALSO COMMON MANIFESTATIONS OF THE CHRONIC PULMONARY REACTION. FEVER IS RARELY PROMINENT.

THE SEVERITY OF CHRONIC PULMONARY REACTIONS AND THEIR DEGREE OF RESOLUTION APPEAR TO BE RELATED TO THE DURATION OF THERAPY AFTER THE FIRST CLINICAL SIGNS APPEAR. PULMONARY FUNCTION MAY BE IMPAIRED PERMANENTLY, EVEN AFTER CESSATION OF THERAPY. THE RISK IS GREATER WHEN CHRONIC PULMONARY REACTIONS ARE NOT RECOGNIZED EARLY.

In subacute pulmonary reactions, fever and eosinophilia occur less often than in the acute form. Upon cessation of therapy, recovery may require several months. If the symptoms are not recognized as being drug-related and nitrofurantoin therapy is not stopped, the symptoms may become more severe.

Acute pulmonary reactions are commonly manifested by fever, chills, cough, chest pain, dyspnea, pulmonary infiltration with consolidation or pleural effusion on x-ray, and eosinophilia. Acute reactions usually occur within the first week of treatment and are reversible with cessation of therapy. Resolution often is dramatic. (See WARNINGS.)

Changes in EKG may occur associated with pulmonary reactions.

Collapse and cyanosis have seldom been reported.

HEPATIC

Hepatic reactions, including hepatitis, cholestatic jaundice, chronic active hepatitis, and hepatic necrosis, occur rarely. (See WARNINGS.)

NEUROLOGIC

Peripheral neuropathy (including optic neuritis), which may become severe or irreversible, has occurred. Fatalities have been reported. Conditions such as renal impairment (creatinine clearance under 60 ml per minute or clinically significant elevated serum creatinine), anemia, diabetes mellitus, electrolyte imbalance, vitamin B deficiency, and debilitating diseases may increase the possibility of peripheral neuropathy. (See WARNINGS.)

Asthenia, vertigo, nystagmus, dizziness, headache, and drowsiness have also been reported with the use of nitrofurantoin.

Benign intracranial hypertension has seldom been reported.

Confusion, depression, euphoria, and psychotic reactions have been reported rarely.

DERMATOLOGIC

Exfoliative dermatitis and erythema multiforme (including Stevens-Johnson syndrome) have been reported rarely. Transient alopecia also has been reported.

ALLERGIC

A lupus-like syndrome associated with pulmonary reactions to nitrofurantoin has been reported. Also, angioedema; maculopapular, erythematous, or eczematous eruptions; pruritus; urticaria; anaphylaxis; arthralgia; myalgia; drug fever; and chills have been reported.

GASTROINTESTINAL

Nausea, emesis, and anorexia occur most often. Abdominal pain and diarrhea are less common gastrointestinal reactions. These dose-related reactions can be minimized by reduction of dosage. Sialadenitis and pancreatitis have been reported.

MISCELLANEOUS

As with other antimicrobial agents, superinfections caused by resistant organisms, *e.g.*, *Pseudomonas* species, or *Candida* species, can occur. There are sporadic reports of *Clostridium difficile* superinfections, or pseudomembranous colitis, with the use of nitrofurantoin.

LABORATORY ADVERSE EVENTS

The following laboratory adverse events have been reported with the use of nitrofurantoin: increased AST (SGOT), increased ALT (SGPT), decreased hemoglobin, increased serum phosphorus, eosinophilia, glucose-6-phosphate dehydrogenase deficiency anemia (see WARNINGS), agranulocytosis, leukopenia, granulocytopenia, hemolytic anemia, thrombocytopenia, megaloblastic anemia. In most cases, these hematologic abnormalities resolved following cessation of therapy. Aplastic anemia has been reported rarely.

DOSAGE AND ADMINISTRATION

Nitrofurantoin should be given with food to improve drug absorption and, in some patients, tolerance.

Adults: 50-100 mg four times a day — the lower dosage level is recommended for uncomplicated urinary tract infections.

Children: 5-7 mg/kg of body weight per 24 hours, given in four divided doses (contraindicated under 1 month of age).

Therapy should be continued for 1 week or for at least 3 days after sterility of the urine is obtained. Continued infection indicates the need for reevaluation.

For long-term suppressive therapy in adults, a reduction of dosage to 50-100 mg at bedtime may be adequate. For long-term suppressive therapy in children, doses as low as 1 mg/kg per 24 hours, given in a single dose or in two divided doses, may be adequate. **SEE WARNINGS REGARDING RISKS ASSOCIATED WITH LONG-TERM THERAPY.**

HOW SUPPLIED

Macrodantin is available as follows:

25 mg: Opaque, white capsule imprinted with one black line encircling the capsule and coded "Macrodantin 25 mg" and "0149-0007".

50 mg: Opaque, yellow and white capsule imprinted with two black lines encircling the capsule and coded "Macrodantin 50 mg" and "0149-0008".

100 mg: Opaque, yellow capsule imprinted with three black lines encircling the capsule and coded "Macrodantin 100 mg" and "0149-0009".

Nitrofurantoin; Nitrofurantoin, Macrocrystalline *(003110)*

Categories: Infection, urinary tract; Pregnancy Category B; FDA Approved 1991 Dec

Drug Classes: Antibiotics, nitrofurans

Brand Names: Macrobid

Cost of Therapy: $28.80 (Urinary Tract Infection; Macrobid; 100 mg; 2 capsules/day; 7 day supply)

DESCRIPTION

FOR COMPLETE PRESCRIBING INFORMATION, REFER TO THE INDIVIDUAL DRUG MONOGRAPHS (NITROFURANTOIN, NITROFURANTOIN MACROCRYSTALLINE).

INDICATIONS AND USAGE

This drug combination is indicated only for the treatment of acute uncomplicated urinary tract infections (acute cystitis) caused by susceptible strains of *Escherichia coli* or *Staphylococcus saprophyticus.*

Nitrofurantoin is not indicated for the treatment of pyelonephritis or perinephric abscesses.

Nitrofurantoins lack the broader tissue distribution of other therapeutic agents approved for urinary tract infections. Consequently, many patients who are treated with this drug combination are predisposed to persistence or reappearance of bacteriuria. Urine specimens for culture and susceptibility testing should be obtained before and after completion of therapy. If persistence or reappearance of bacteriuria occurs after treatment with this drug combination, other therapeutic agents with broader tissue distribution should be selected. In considering the use of this drug combination, lower eradication rates should be balanced against the increased potential for systemic toxicity and for the development of antimicrobial resistance when agents with broader tissue distribution are utilized.

DOSAGE AND ADMINISTRATION

Capsules of this drug combination should be taken with food.

Adults and Children Over 12 Years: One 100-mg capsule every 12 hours for seven days.

HOW SUPPLIED

Macrobid is available as 100-mg opaque black and yellow capsules imprinted "Macrobid" on the black portion and "Norwich Eaton" on the yellow portion.

Store at controlled room temperature (59 to 86°F or 15 to 30°C).

Nitroglycerin *(001893)*

Categories: Angina pectoris; Heart failure associated with myocardial infarction; Hypertension, perioperative; Surgery, adjunct; Pregnancy Category C; FDA Approved 1981 Oct; WHO Formulary

Drug Classes: Vasodilators

Brand Names: Deponit; Mi-Trates; Minitran; Nitrek; Nitro; Nitro-Bid; Nitrocap T.D.; Nitrocine; Nitrocot; Nitro-Dur; Nitro-Par; Nitro-Time; Nitrodisc; Nitrogard; Nitroglyn; Nitrol; Nitrolin; Nitrolingual; Nitronal; Nitrong; Nitrorex; Nitrospan; Nitrostat; NTS; NTG; **Transderm-Nitro**; Tridil

Foreign Brand Availability: Anginine (Australia; New-Zealand); Anglix (Mexico); Cardinit (Mexico); Coro-Nitro (Germany); Deponit-5 (Korea; Thailand); Deponit NT (Hong-Kong; Israel); Deponit TTS 5 (Israel); Deponit TTS 10 (Israel); Gilustenon (Germany); Glytrin Spray (New-Zealand); Lenitral (France; Hong-Kong); Millsrol (Japan); Myovin (India); Niong Retard (Switzerland); Nitradisc (Australia; Denmark; Germany; Hong-Kong; Indonesia; Mexico; Norway; Peru; Portugal; Spain); Nitradisc Pad (New-Zealand); Nitradisc TTS (Greece); Nit-Ret (Czech-Republic); Nitriderm TTS (France; Germany); Nitro Retard (Bulgaria; Norway; Sweden); Nitrobaat (Belgium; Netherlands); Nitrobid (Japan); Nitrobid Oint (New-Zealand); Nitrocerin (Greece); Nitrocine 5 (Bahrain; Cyprus; Egypt; Iran; Iraq; Israel; Jordan; Kuwait; Lebanon; Libya; Oman; Qatar; Republic-of-Yemen; Saudi-Arabia; Syria; United-Arab-Emirates); Nitrocontin (Benin; Burkina-Faso; Ethiopia; Gambia; Ghana; Guinea; Ireland; Ivory-Coast; Kenya; Liberia; Malawi; Mali; Mauritania; Mauritius; Morocco; Niger; Nigeria; Senegal; Seychelles; Sierra-Leone; South-Africa; Sudan; Tanzania; Tunia; Uganda; Zambia; Zimbabwe); Nitrocontin Continus (Bahrain; Cyprus; Egypt; England; India; Iran; Iraq; Israel; Jordan; Kuwait; Lebanon; Libya; Oman; Qatar; Republic-of-Yemen; Saudi-Arabia; Syria; United-Arab-Emirates); Nitrocor (Italy; Portugal); NitroCor (New-Zealand); Nitroderm TTS (Austria; Bahamas; Bahrain; Barbados; Belgium; Belize; Benin; Bermuda; Bulgaria; Burkina-Faso; China; Curacao; Cyprus; Ecuador; Egypt; Ethiopia; Gambia; Germany; Ghana; Guinea; Guyana; Hong-Kong; India; Iran; Iraq; Israel; Italy; Ivory-Coast; Jamaica; Jordan; Kenya; Kuwait; Lebanon; Liberia; Libya; Malawi; Malaysia; Mali; Mauritania; Mauritius; Morocco; Netherland-Antilles; New-Zealand; Niger; Nigeria; Oman; Portugal; Puerto-Rico; Qatar; Republic-of-Yemen; Saudi-Arabia; Senegal; Seychelles; Sierra-Leone; South-Africa; Spain; Sudan; Surinam; Switzerland; Syria; Taiwan; Tanzania; Thailand; Trinidad; Tunia; Uganda; United-Arab-Emirates; Zambia; Zimbabwe); Nitroderm TTS Ext (Czech-Republic); Nitro-Dur 10 (Israel); Nitro Dur TTS (Switzerland); Nitrodyl (Greece); Nitrodyl TTS (Greece); Nitro-Gesanit Retard (Germany); Nitrogesic (India); Nitro-M-Bid (Belgium); Nitro Mack (China); Nitro Mack Retard (Austria; Bahrain; Costa-Rica; Cyprus; Czech-Republic; Dominican-Republic; Egypt; El-Salvador; Germany; Greece; Honduras; Iran; Iraq; Israel; Jordan; Kuwait; Lebanon; Libya; Malaysia; Oman; Panama; Qatar; Republic-of-Yemen; Saudi-Arabia; Switzerland; Syria; United-Arab-Emirates); Nitromack Retard (Hong-Kong; Indonesia); Nitro-Mack Retard (Thailand); Nitromex (Denmark; Finland; Norway; Sweden); Nitromint (Hungary; Switzerland); Nitromint Aerosol (Benin; Burkina-Faso; Ethiopia; Gambia; Ghana; Guinea; Ivory-Coast; Kenya; Liberia; Malawi; Mali; Mauritania; Mauritius; Morocco; Niger; Nigeria; Senegal; Seychelles; Sierra-Leone; South-Africa; Sudan; Tanzania; Tunia; Uganda; Zambia; Zimbabwe); Nitromint Retard (Bahamas; Bahrain; Barbados; Belize; Bermuda; Curacao; Cyprus; Egypt; Guyana; Iran; Iraq; Israel; Jamaica; Jordan; Kuwait; Lebanon; Libya; Netherland-Antilles; Oman; Puerto-Rico; Qatar; Republic-of-Yemen; Saudi-Arabia; Surinam; Syria; Trinidad; United-Arab-Emirates); Nitroprol (Belgium); Nitroderm TTS-5 (Colombia; Mexico); Nitro-Pflaster (Germany); Nitroglin (Germany); Nitrolingual Spray (Korea; New-Zealand); Nitrolong (Switzerland); Nitrong Retard (Austria; Greece); Nitrong-SR (Canada); Nitropen (Japan); Nitroplast (Spain); Nitropront (Finland); Nitroprontan (Argentina); Nitrorectal (Germany); Nitro Rorer (Germany); Nitrozell Retard (Austria; Netherlands); Nysconitrine (Belgium); Percutol (Ireland); Percutol Oint. (England); Perlinganit (Korea); Ratiopharm (Germany); Rectogesic (Australia); Suscard (England); Sustac (Bahamas; Bahrain; Barbados; Belize; Bermuda; Curacao; Cyprus; Egypt; England; Guyana; Iran; Iraq; Israel; Jamaica; Jordan; Kuwait; Lebanon; Libya; Netherland-Antilles; Oman; Puerto-Rico; Qatar; Republic-of-Yemen; Saudi-Arabia; Surinam; Syria; Trinidad; United-Arab-Emirates); Transiderm Nitro (Australia; Denmark; Finland; Netherlands; Norway; Sweden); Trinipatch (Israel); Vasolator (Japan); Venitrin (Italy)

Cost of Therapy: $39.00 (Angina; Nitrogard; 3 mg; 3 tablets/day; 30 day supply)

DESCRIPTION

Nitroglycerin, an organic nitrate, is a vasodilator which has effects on both arteries and veins. The chemical name for nitroglycerin is 1,2,3-propanetriol trinitrate ($C_3H_5N_3O_9$). The compound has a molecular weight of 227.09.

NITROGLYCERIN INJECTION

FOR INTRAVENOUS USE ONLY:

NOT FOR DIRECT INTRAVENOUS INJECTION (MUST BE DILUTED), NITROGLYCERIN MUST BE DILUTED IN DEXTROSE 5% INJECTION OR SODIUM CHLORIDE (0.9%) INJECTION BEFORE INTRAVENOUS ADMINISTRATION. THE ADMINISTRATION SET USED FOR INFUSION MAY AFFECT THE AMOUNT OF NITROGLYCERIN DELIVERED TO THE PATIENT. (See WARNINGS and DOSAGE AND ADMINISTRATION.)

CAUTION:

SEVERAL PREPARATIONS OF NITROGLYCERIN INJECTION ARE AVAILABLE. THEY DIFFER IN CONCENTRATION AND/OR VOLUME PER VIAL. WHEN SWITCHING FROM ONE PRODUCT TO ANOTHER, ATTENTION MUST BE PAID TO THE DILUTION AND DOSAGE AND ADMINISTRATION INSTRUCTIONS.

Nitro-Bid IV is a clear, practically colorless additive solution for intravenous infusion after dilution. The solution is sterile, nonpyrogenic, and nonexplosive. Each milliliter contains 5 mg nitroglycerin and 45 mg propylene glycol.
Storage: Store at controlled room temperature 20-25°C (68-77°F). Protect from freezing. Protect from light.

NITROGLYCERIN SUBLINGUAL TABLETS

Nitrostat is a stablilized sublingual tablet manufactured by a patented process which prevents the migration of nitroglycerin by adding the nonvolatile fixing agent polyethylene glycol 3350. This stabilized formulation has been shown to be more stable and more uniform than conventional molded tablets. Nitrostat sublingual tablets contain 0.3 mg (1/200 grain), 0.4 mg (1/150 grain) and 0.6 (1/100 grain) nitroglycerin. *Inactive Ingredients:* Lactose, polyethylene glycol 3350, and sucrose.
Storage: Store at controlled room temperature between 15-30°C (59-86°F).

NITROGLYCERIN EXTENDED-RELEASE ORAL TABLETS

Each Nitrong 2.6 mg tablet for oral administration contains 2.6 mg nitroglycerin in extended-release form with light green granules containing corn-starch, D&C yellow no. 10 lake and iron oxide. Each Nitrong 6.5 mg tablet for oral administration contains 6.5 mg nitroglycerin in extended-release form with light orange granules containing cornstarch, D&C yellow no. 10 lake, FD&C yellow no. 6 lake, iron oxide and povidone.
Storage: Store at controlled room temperature between 15-30°C (59-86°F).

NITROGLYCERIN LINGUAL AEROSOL SPRAY

Nitrolingual spray is a metered dose aerosol containing nitroglycerin in propellants (dichlorodifluoromethane and dichlorotetrafluoroethane). Each metered dose delivers 0.4 mg of nitroglycerin per spray emission. This product delivers nitroglycerin in the form of spray droplets onto or under the tongue. *Inactive Ingredients:* Caprylic/capric/diglycereryl succinate, ether, and flavors.
Storage: Store at room temperature. Do not expose to temperatures exceeding 50°C (122°F).

NITROGLYCERIN OINTMENT

Nitro-Bid ointment contains 2% nitroglycerin and lactose in a base of lanolin and white petrolatum. Each inch (2.5 cm), as squeezed from the tube, contains approximately 15 mg nitroglycerin.

NITROGLYCERIN TRANSDERMAL DELIVERY SYSTEM

The Transderm-Nitro transdermal system is a flat unit designed to provide continuous controlled release of nitroglycerin through intact skin. The rate of release of nitroglycerin is linearly dependent upon the area of the applied system; each cm^2 of applied system delivers approximately 0.02 mg of nitroglycerin per hour. Thus, 5, 10, 20, and 30 cm^2 system delivers approximately 0.1, 0.2, 0.4, and 0.6 mg of nitroglycerin per hour, respectively.

The remainder of nitroglycerin in each system serves as a reservoir and is not delivered in normal use. After 12 hours, for example, each system has delivered approximately 10% of its original content of nitroglycerin.

The Transderm-Nitro system comprises 4 layers. Proceeding from the visible surface towards the surface attached to the skin, these layers are:

1. A tan-colored backing layer (aluminized plastic) that is impermeable to nitroglycerin.
2. A drug reservoir containing nitroglycerin adsorbed on lactose, colloidal silicon dioxide, and silicone medical fluid.
3. An ethylene vinyl acetate copolymer membrane that is permeable to nitroglycerin.
4. A layer of hypoallergenic silicone adhesive. Prior to use, a protective peel strip is removed from the adhesive surface.

Storage: Store at controlled room temperature between 15-30°C (59-86°F). Extremes of temperature and/or humidity should be avoided.

CLINICAL PHARMACOLOGY

The principal pharmacologic action of nitroglycerin is relaxation of vascular smooth muscle, producing a vasodilator effect on both peripheral arteries and veins with more prominent effects on the latter. Dilation of the postcapillary vessels, including large veins, promotes peripheral pooling of blood and decreases venous return to the heart, thereby reducing left ventricular end-diastolic pressure (preload). Arteriolar relaxation reduces systemic vascular resistance and arterial pressure (afterload).

The mechanism by which nitroglycerin relieves angina pectoris is not fully understood. Myocardial oxygen consumption or demand (as measured by the pressure-rate product, tension-time index, and stroke-work index) is decreased by both the arterial and venous effects of nitroglycerin, and a more favorable supply-demand ratio can be achieved.

While large epicardial coronary arteries are also dilated by nitroglycerin, the extent to which this action contributes to relief of exertional angina is unclear.

Therapeutic doses of nitroglycerin reduce systolic, diastolic, and mean arterial blood pressures. Effective coronary perfusion pressure is usually maintained, but can be compromised if blood pressure falls excessively or increased heart rate decreases diastolic filling time.

Elevated central venous and pulmonary capillary wedge pressures, pulmonary vascular resistance, and systemic vascular resistance are also reduced by nitroglycerin therapy. Heart rate is usually slightly increased, presumably a reflex response to the fall in blood pressure. Cardiac index may be increased, decreased, or unchanged. Patients with elevated left ventricular filling pressure and systemic vascular resistance values in conjunction with a depressed cardiac index are likely to experience an improvement in cardiac index. On the other hand, when filling pressures and cardiac index are normal, cardiac index may be slightly reduced by intravenous nitroglycerin.

Nitroglycerin is widely distributed in the body with an apparent volume of distribution of approximately 200 liters in adult male subjects, and is rapidly metabolized to dinitrates and mononitrates, with a short half-life, estimated at 1-4 minutes. This results in a low plasma concentration after intravenous infusion. At plasma concentrations of between 50 and 500 ng/ml, the binding of nitroglycerin to plasma proteins is approximately 60%, while that of 1,2 dinitroglycerin and 1,3 dinitroglycerin is 60% and 30%, respectively. The activity and half-life of the nitroglycerin metabolites are not well characterized. The mononitrate is not active.

PHARMACOKINETICS

The volume of distribution of nitroglycerin is about 3 L/kg, and nitroglycerin is cleared from this volume at extremely rapid rates, with a resulting serum half-life of about 3 minutes. The observed clearance rates (close to 1 L/kg/min) greatly exceed hepatic blood flow; known sites of extrahepatic metabolism include red blood cells and vascular walls.

Nitroglycerin is rapidly metabolized *in vivo,* with a liver reductase enzyme having primary importance in the formation of glycerol nitrate metabolites and inorganic nitrate. The first products in the metabolism of nitroglycerin are inorganic nitrate and two active major metabolites, 1,2- and 1,3-dinitroglycerols, the products of hydrolysis, although less potent as vasodilators, have longer plasma half-lives than the parent compound. Their net contribution to the overall effect of chronic nitroglycerin regimes is not known. The dinitrates are further metabolized to (nonvasoactive) mononitrates and, ultimately, to glycerol and carbon dioxide.

To avoid development of tolerance to nitroglycerin, drug-free intervals of 10-12 hours are known to be sufficient; shorter intervals have not been well studied. In one well controlled clinical trial, subjects receiving nitroglycerin appeared to exhibit a rebound or withdrawal effect, so that their exercise tolerance at the end of the daily drug-free interval was *less* than that exhibited by the parallel group receiving placebo.

Additional Information for Nitroglycerin Lingual Aerosol Spray

A pharmacokinetic study in 13 healty men showed no statistically significant difference between the mean values for maximum plasma concentration and time to achieve maximum plasma level with equal doses (0.8 mg) of nitroglycerin sublingual spray and sublingual nitroglycerin tablets. Peak plasma concentration after 0.8 mg of nitroglycerin sublingual spray occurred within 4 minutes and the apparent plasma half-life was approximately 5 minutes. In a randomized, double-blind study in patients with exertional angina pectoris dose-related increases in exercise tolerance were seen following doses of 0.2, 0.4, and 0.8 mg delivered by metered spray.

Additional Information for Nitroglycerin Ointment

Reliable assay techniques for plasma nitroglycerin levels have only recently become available, and studies using these techniques to define the pharmacokinetics of nitroglycerin ointment have not been reported. Published studies using older techniques provide results that often differ, in similar experimental settings, by an order of magnitude. The data are consistent, however, in suggesting that nitroglycerin levels rise to a steady state within an hour or so of application of ointment, and that after removal of nitroglycerin ointment, levels wane with a half-life of about half an hour.

The onset of action of transdermal nitroglycerin is not sufficiently rapid for this product to be useful in aborting an acute anginal episode.

The maximal achievable daily duration of antianginal activity provided by nitroglycerin ointment therapy has not been studied. Recent studies of other formulations of nitroglycerin suggest that the maximal achievable daily duration of anti-anginal effect from nigroglycerin ointment will be about 12 hours.

It is reasonable to believe that the rate and extent of nitroglycerin absorption from ointment may vary with the site and square measure of the skin over which a given dose of ointment is spread, but these relationships have not been adequately studied.

Additional Information for Nitroglycerin Transdermal Delivery System

In healthy volunteers, steady-state plasma concentrations of nitroglycerin are reached by about 2 hours after application of a patch and are maintained for the duration of wearing the system (observations have been limited to 24 hours). Upon removal of the patch, the plasma concentration declines with a half-life of about an hour.

INDICATIONS AND USAGE

NITROGLYCERIN INJECTION

Nitroglycerin injection is indicated for:

- Control of blood pressure in perioperative hypertension, *i.e.,* hypertension associated with surgical procedures, especially cardiovascular procedures, such as the hypertension seen during intratracheal intubation, anesthesia, skin incision, sternotomy, cardiac bypass, and in the immediate postsurgical period.
- Congestive heart failure associated with acute myocardial infarction.
- Treatment of angina pectoris in patients who have not responded to recommended doses of organic nitrates and/or a beta-blocker.
- Production of controlled hypotension during surgical procedures.

NITROGLYCERIN SUBLINGUAL TABLETS

Indicated for the prophylaxis, treatment and management of patients with angina pectoris.

NITROGLYCERIN EXTENDED-RELEASE ORAL TABLETS

Indicated for the prevention of angina pectoris due to coronary artery disease. The onset of action is not sufficiently rapid for this form to be useful in aborting an acute anginal episode.

NITROGLYCERIN LINGUAL AEROSOL SPRAY

Indicated for acute relief of an attack or prophylaxis of angina pectoris due to coronary artery disease.

NITROGLYCERIN OINTMENT

Indicated for the prevention of angina pectoris due to coronary artery disease. Controlled clinical trials have demonstrated that this form of nitroglycerin is effective in improving exercise tolerance in patients with exertional angina pectoris. Double-blind, placebo-controlled trials have shown significant improvement in exercise time until chest pain for up to 6 hours after single application of various doses of nitroglycerin ointment (mean doses ranged from 5-36 mg) to a 36 square inch area of trunk.

N

NITROGLYCERIN TRANSDERMAL DELIVERY SYSTEM

Indicated for the prevention of angina pectoris due to coronary artery disease. The onset of action of transdermal nitroglycerin is not sufficiently rapid for this product to be useful in aborting an acute attack. Tolerance to the anti-anginal effects of nitrates (measured by exercise stress testing) has been shown to be a major factor limiting efficacy when transdermal nitrates are used continuously for longer than 12 hours each day. The development of tolerance can be altered (prevented or attenuated) by use of a noncontinuous (intermittent) dosing schedule with a nitrate-free interval of 10-12 hours.

Controlled clinical trial data suggest that the intermittent use of nitrates is associated with decreased exercise tolerance, on comparison to placebo, during the last part of the nitrate-free interval; the clinical relevance of this observation is unknown, but the possibility of increased frequency of severity of angina during the nitrate-free interval should be considered. Further investigations of the tolerance phenomenon and best regimen are ongoing. A final evaluation of the effectiveness of the product will be announced by the FDA.

NON-FDA APPROVED INDICATIONS

Unlabelled uses include the reduction of cardiac work in acute MI and in CHF (sublingual, topical, and oral forms), Raynaud's disease (topical ointment), peripheral vascular disease (oral form often combined with prostaglandin E1), and hypertensive crisis (IV form). Although not approved by the FDA for MI, meta-analysis of the use of nitroglycerin in patients with MI has shown decreased mortality. Other unapproved uses include reduction of variceal pressure in patients with hepatic cirrhosis and esophageal varices.

CONTRAINDICATIONS

Allergic reactions to organic nitrates are extremely rare, but they do occur. Nitroglycerin should not be administered to individuals with a known hypersensitivity or idiosyncrasy reaction to nitroglycerin, other organic nitrates, or nitrites.

ADDITIONAL INFORMATION FOR NITROGLYCERIN INJECTION

Nitroglycerin injection should not be administered to individuals with:

- Hypotension or uncorrected hypovolemia, as the use of nitroglycerin in such states could produce severe hypotension or shock.
- Increased intracranial pressure (*e.g.,* head trauma or cerebral hemorrhage).
- Inadequate cerebral circulation.
- Constrictive pericarditis and pericardial tamponade.

ADDITIONAL INFORMATION FOR NITROGLYCERIN SUBLINGUAL TABLETS

Sublingual nitroglycerin therapy is contraindicated in patients with early myocardial infarction, severe anemia, and increased intracranial pressure.

ADDITIONAL INFORMATION FOR NITROGLYCERIN TRANSDERMAL DELIVERY SYSTEM

Allergy to the adhesives used in nitroglycerin patches have been reported, and therefore constitute a contraindication to the use of this product.

N

WARNINGS

Amplification of the vasodilatory effects of nitroglycerin by sildenafil can result in severe hypotension. The time course and dose dependence of this interaction have not been studied. Appropriate supportive care has not been studied, but it seems reasonable to treat this as a nitrate overdose, with elevation of the extremities and with central volume expansion.

The use of any form of nitroglycerin during the early days of acute myocardial infarction requires particular attention to hemodynamic monitoring and clinical status to avoid the hazards of hypothension and tachycardia.

ADDITIONAL INFORMATION FOR NITROGLYCERIN INJECTION

Nitroglycerin readily migrates into many plastics. To avoid absorption of nitroglycerin into plastic parenteral solution containers, the dilution of nitroglycerin injection should be made only in glass parenteral solution bottles.

Some filters absorb nitroglycerin; they should be avoided.

Forty percent (40%) to 80% of the total amount of nitroglycerin in the final diluted solution for infusion is absorbed by the polyvinyl chloride (PVC) tubing of the intravenous administration sets currently in general use. The higher rates of absorption occur when flow rates are low, nitroglycerin concentrations are high, and tubing is long. Although the rate of loss is highest during the early phase of administration (when flow rates are lowest), the loss is neither constant nor self-limiting; consequently, no simple calculation or correction can be performed to convert the theoretical infusion rate (based on the concentration of the infusion solution) to the actual delivery rate. Because of this problem, Marion Laboratories recommends the use of the least absorptive infusion tubing available (*i.e.,* non-PVC tubing) for infusions of nitroglycerin injection. DOSING INSTRUCTIONS MUST BE FOLLOWED WITH CARE. IT SHOULD BE NOTED THAT WHEN THE APPROPRIATE INFUSION SETS ARE USED, THE CALCULATED DOSE WILL BE DELIVERED TO THE PATIENT BECAUSE THE LOSS OF NITROGLYCERIN DUE TO ABSORPTION IN STANDARD PVC TUBING WILL BE KEPT TO A MINIMUM. NOTE THAT THE DOSAGES COMMONLY USED IN PUBLISHED STUDIES UTILIZED GENERAL-USE PVC INFUSION SETS, AND RECOMMENDED DOSES BASED ON THIS EXPERIENCE ARE TOO HIGH IF THE LOW ABSORBING INFUSION SETS ARE USED.

A potential safety problem exists with the combined use of some infusion pumps and some non-PVC infusion sets. Because the special tubing required to prevent the absorption of nitroglycerin tends to be less pliable than the conventional PVC tubing normally used with such infusion pumps, the pumps may fail to occlude the infusion sets completely. The results may be excessive flow at low infusion rate settings, causing alarms, or unregulated gravity flow when the infusion pump is stopped; this could lead to over-infusion of nitroglycerin. All infusion pumps should be tested with the infusion sets to ensure their ability to deliver nitroglycerin accurately at low flow rates, and to occlude the infusion sets properly when the infusion is stopped.

ADDITIONAL INFORMATION FOR NITROGLYCERIN EXTENDED-RELEASE ORAL TABLETS

The benefits of transdermal nitroglycerin in patients with acute myocardial infarction or congestive heart failure have not been established. If one elects to use nitroglycerin in these conditions, careful clinical or hemodynamic monitoring must be used to avoid the hazards of hypotension and tachycardia. Because the effects of tablets are so difficult to terminate rapidly, tablets are not recommended in these settings.

ADDITIONAL INFORMATION FOR NITROGLYCERIN TRANSDERMAL DELIVERY SYSTEM AND NITROGLYCERIN OINTMENT

The benefits of transdermal nitroglycerin in patients with acute myocardial infarction or congestive heart failure have not been established. If one elects to use nitroglycerin in these conditions, careful clinical or hemodynamic monitoring must be used to avoid the hazards of hypotension and tachycardia.

A cardioverter/defibrillator should not be discharged through a paddle electrode that overlies a nitroglycerin transdermal system patch. The arcing that may be seen in this situation is harmless in itself, but it may be associated with local current concentration that can cause damage to the paddles and burns to the patient.

PRECAUTIONS

GENERAL

Severe hypotension, particularly with upright posture, may occur even with small doses of nitroglycerin. The drug, therefore, should be used with caution in subjects who may have volume depletion from diuretic therapy or in patients who have low systolic blood pressure (*e.g.,* below 90 mm Hg). Paradoxical bradycardia and increased angina pectoris may accompany nitroglycerin-induced hypotension. Nitrate therapy may aggravate the angina caused by hypertrophic cardiomyopathy. Tolerance to this drug and cross-tolerance to other nitrates and nitrites may occur.

Tolerance to the vascular and anti-anginal effects of nitrates has been demonstrated in clinical trials, experience through occupational exposure, and in isolated tissue experiments in the laboratory.

In industrial workers who have had long-term exposure to unknown (presumably high) doses of organic nitrates, tolerance clearly occurs. Chest pain, acute myocardial infarction, and even sudden death have occurred during temporary withdrawal of nitroglycerin from the workers demonstrating the existence of true physical dependence. In various clinical trials in angina patients, there are reports of anginal attacks being more easily provoked and of rebound in the hemodynamic effects soon after nitrate withdrawal. The relative importance of these observations to the routine, clinical use of nitroglycerin is not known.

Several clinical trials in patients with angina pectoris have evaluated nitroglycerin regimens which incorporated a 10-12 hour nitrate-free interval. In some of these trials, an increase in the frequency of anginal attacks during the nitrate-free interval was observed in a small number of patients. In one trial, patients had decreased exercise tolerance at the end of the nitrate-free interval. Hemodynamic rebound has been observed only rarely; on the other hand, few studies were so designed that rebound, if it had occurred, would have been detected. The importance of these observations to the routine, clinical use of nitroglycerin is unknown.

Additional Information for Nitroglycerin Injection

Nitroglycerin injection should be used with caution in patients who have severe hepatic or renal disease.

Excessive hypotension, especially for prolonged periods of time, must be avoided because of possible deleterious effects on the brain, heart, liver, and kidney from poor perfusion and the attendant risk of ischemia, thrombosis, and altered function of these organs. Paradoxical bradycardia and increased angina pectoris may accompany nitroglycerin-induced hypotension. Patients with normal or low pulmonary capillary wedge pressure are especially sensitive to the hypotensive effects of nitroglycerin injection. If pulmonary capillary wedge pressure is being monitored, it will be noted that a fall in wedge pressure precedes the onset of arterial hypotension, and the pulmonary capillary wedge pressure is thus a useful guide to safe titration of the drug.

Nitroglycerin contains alcohol and propylene glycol; safety for intracoronary injection has not been shown.

Additional Information for Nitroglycerin Sublingual Tablets

Only the smallest dose required for effective relief of the acute anginal attack should be used. Excessive use may lead to the development of tolerance. Nitroglycerin sublingual tablets are intended for sublingual or buccal administration and should not be swallowed. The drug should be discontinued if blurring of vision or drying of the mouth occurs. Excessive dosage of nitroglycerin may produce severe headaches.

INFORMATION FOR THE PATIENT

Daily headaches sometime accompany treatment with nitroglycerin. In patients who get these headaches, the headaches may be a marker of the activity of the drug. Patients should resist the temptation to avoid headaches by altering the schedule of their treatment with nitroglycerin, since loss of headache may be associated with simultaneious loss of antianginal efficacy.

Treatment with nitroglycerin may be associated with light-headedness on standing. Especially just after rising from a recumbent or seated position. This effect may be more frequent in patients who have also consumed alcohol.

Physicians should discuss with patients the contraindication of nitroglycerin with concurrent sildenafil.

Additional Information for Nitroglycerin Transdermal Delivery System

After normal use, there is enough residual nitroglycerin in discard patches that they are a potentiona hazard to children and pets.

CARCINOGENESIS, MUTAGENESIS, AND IMPAIRMENT OF FERTILITY

Animal carcinogenesis studies with nitroglycerin have not been performed. Rats receiving up to 434 mg/kg/day of dietary nitroglycerin for 2 years developed dose-related fibrotic and neoplastic changes in liver, including carcinomas, and interstitial cell tumors in testes. At high dose, the incidences of hepatocellular carcinomas in both sexes were 52% vs 0% in controls, and incidences of testicular tumors were 52% vs 8% in controls. Lifetime dietary administration of up to 1058 mg/kg/day of nitroglycerin was not tumorigenic in mice.

Nitroglycerin was weakly mutagenic in Ames tests performed in two different laboratories. Nevertheless, there was no evidence of mutagenicity in an *in vivo* dominant letal assay with male rats treated with doses up to about 363 mg/kg/day, po, or *in vitro* cytogenic tests in rat and dog tissues.

In a three generation reproduction study, rats received dietary nitroglycerin at doses up to about 434 mg/kg/day for 6 months prior to mating of the F_0 generation with treatment continuing through successive F_1 and F_2 generations. The high-dose was associated with decreased feed intake and body weight gain in both sexes at all matings. No specific effect on the fertility of the F_0 generation was seen. Infertility noted in subsequent generations, however, was attributed to increased interstitial cell tissue and aspermatogenesis in the high dose males. In this three generation study there was no clear evidence of teratogenicity.

PREGNANCY CATEGORY C

Animal reproduction studies have not been conducted with nitroglycerin spray, transdermal delivery system, or tablets. Teratology studies in rats and rabbits, however, were conducted with topically applied nitroglycerin ointment at doses up to 80 mg/kg/day and 240 mg/kg/day, respectively. No toxic effects on dams or fetuses were seen at any dose tested. There are no adequate and well-controlled studies in pregnant women. Nitroglycerin should be given to a pregnant woman only if clearly needed.

NURSING MOTHERS

It is not known whether nitroglycerin is excreted in human milk. Because many drugs are excreted in human milk, caution should be exercised when nitroglycerin is administered to a nursing woman.

PEDIATRIC USE

The safety and effectiveness of nitroglycerin in children have not been established.

DRUG INTERACTIONS

Alcohol may enhance sensitivity to the hypotensive effects of nitrates and the vasodilating effects of nitroglycerin may be additive with those of other vasodilators. Nitroglycerin acts directly on vascular muscle as the final common path can be expected to have decreased or increased effect depending upon the agent. Marked symptomatic orthostatic hypotension has been reported when calcium channel blockers and organic nitrates were used in combination. Dose adjustments of either class of agents may be necessary.

ADVERSE REACTIONS

Adverse reactions to nitroglycerin's activity are generally dose-related, and almost all of these reactions are the result of nitroglycerin's activity as a vasodilator. Headache, which may be severe, is the most commonly reported side effect. Headache may be recurrent with each daily dose, especially at higher doses. Transient episodes of light-headedness, occasionally related to blood pressure changes, may also occur. Hypotension occurs infrequently, but in some patients it may be severe enough to warrant discontinuation of therapy. Syncope, crescendo angina, and rebound hypertension have been reported but are uncommon.

Allergic reactions to nitroglycerin are also uncommon, and the great majority of those reported have been cases of contact dermatitis or fixed drug eruptions in patients receiving nitroglycerin in ointments or patches. There have been a few reports of genuine anaphylactoid reactions, and these reactions can probably occur in patients receiving nitroglycerin by any route.

Extremely rarely, ordinary doses of organic nitrates have caused methemoglobineamia in normal-seeming patients. Methemoglobinemia is so infrequent at these doses that futher discussion of its diagnosis and treatment is deferred.

Other adverse reactions occurring in less than 1% of patients are the following: Tachycardia, nausea, vomiting, apprehension, restlessness, muscle twitching, retrosternal discomfort, palpitations, dizziness, and abdominal pain.

DOSAGE AND ADMINISTRATION

NITROGLYCERIN INJECTION

(NOT FOR DIRECT INTRAVENOUS INJECTION) NITROGLYCERIN INJECTION IS A CONCENTRATED, POTENT DRUG WHICH MUST BE DILUTED IN DEXTROSE 5% INJECTION OR SODIUM CHLORIDE (0.9%) INJECTION PRIOR TO ITS INFUSION. NITROGLYCERIN SHOULD NOT BE MIXED WITH OTHER DRUGS.

Initial Dilution

Aseptically transfer 25 or 50 mg of nitroglycerin (see TABLE 1) into a 500 ml *glass* bottle containing the proper volume of either 5% dextrose injection or 0.9% sodium chloride injection for dilution. This yields a final concentration of 50 or 100 µg/ml (see TABLE 1). Invert the glass parenteral bottle several times to assure uniform dilution of nitroglycerin injection.

Maintenance Dilution

It is important to consider the fluid requirements of the patient as well as the expected duration of infusion in selecting the appropriate dilution of nitroglycerin.

After the initial dosage titration, the concentration of the solution may be increased, if necessary, to limit fluids given to the patient. The nitroglycerin concentration should not exceed 400 µg/ml.

If the concentration is adjusted, it is imperative to flush or replace the infusion set before a new concentration is utilized. If the set were not flushed, or replaced, it could take minutes to hours, depending upon the flow rate and the dead space of the set, for the new concentration to reach the patient.

TABLE 1A *Dilution Table*

Diluent Volume	Quantity of Nitroglycerin (5 mg/ml)	Approximate Final Concentration
100 ml	10 mg (2 ml)	100 µg/ml
100 ml	20 mg (4 ml)	200 µg/ml
100 ml	40 mg (8 ml)	400 µg/ml
250 ml	25 mg (5 ml)	100 µg/ml
250 ml	50 mg (10 ml)	200 µg/ml
250 ml	100 mg (20 ml)	400 µg/ml
500 ml	50 mg (10 ml)	100 µg/ml
500 ml	100 mg (20 ml)	200 µg/ml
500 ml	200 mg (40 ml)	400 µg/ml

TABLE 1B *Administration Table (60 microdrops = 1 milliliter)*

Concentration (µg/ml)	Flow Rate (microdrops/min = ml/h)		
Dose (µg/min)	100	200	400
5	3	—	—
10	6	3	—
15	9	—	—
20	12	6	3
30	18	9	—
40	24	12	6
60	36	18	9
80	48	24	12
120	72	36	18
160	96	48	24
240	—	72	36
320	—	96	48
480	—	—	72
640	—	—	96

Dosage

Dosage is affected by the type of infusion set used (see WARNINGS, Additional Information for Nitroglycerin Injection). Although the usual starting adult dose range reported in clinical studies was 25 µg/min or more, those studies used PVC TUBING. **The use of non-absorbing tubing will result in the need to use reduced doses.**

When using a nonabsorbing infusion set, initial dosage should be 5 µg/min delivered through an infusion pump capable of exact and constant delivery of the drug. Subsequent titration must be adjusted to the clinical situation, with dose increments becoming more cautious as partial response is seen. Initial titration should be in 5 µg/min increments, with increases every 3-5 minutes until some response is noted. If no response is seen at 20 µg/min, increments of 10 and later 20 µg/min can be used. Once a partial blood pressure response is observed, the dose increase should be reduced and the interval between increments should be lengthened. Patients with normal or low left ventricular filling pressure or pulmonary capillary wedge pressure (*e.g.*, angina patients without other complications) may be hypersensitive to the effects of nitroglycerin and may respond fully to doses as small as 5 µg/min. These patients require especially careful titration and monitoring.

There is no fixed optimum dose of nitroglycerin. Due to variations in the responsiveness of individual patients to the drug, each patient must be titrated to the desired level of hemodynamic function. Therefore, continuous monitoring of physiologic parameters (*i.e.*, blood pressure, heart rate, and pulmonary capillary wedge pressure) MUST be performed to achieve the correct dose. Adequate systemic blood pressure and coronary perfusion pressure must be maintained.

As with all parenteral drug products, nitroglycerin injection should be inspected visually for particulate matter and discoloration prior to administration, whenever solution and container permit.

NITROGLYCERIN SUBLINGUAL TABLETS

One tablet should be dissolved under the tongue or in the buccal pouch at the first sign of an acute anginal attack. The dose may be repeated approximately every 5 minutes until relief is obtained. If the pain persists after a total of 3 tablets in a 15 minute period, the physician should be notified. These tablets may be used prophylactically 5-10 minutes prior to engaging in activities which might precipitate an acute attack.

NITROGLYCERIN EXTENDED-RELEASE ORAL TABLETS

Careful studies with other formulations of nitroglycerin have shown that maintenance of continuous 24 hour plasma levels of nitroglycerin results in tolerance (*i.e.*, loss of clinical response). Every dosing regimen should provide a daily nitrate-free interval to avoid the development of this tolerance. The minimum necessary length of such an interval has not yet been defined, but studies with other nitroglycerin formulations have shown that 10-12 hours is sufficient. Large controlled studies with other formulations of nitroglycerin show that no dosing regimen with these tablets should be expected to provide more than about 12 hours of continuous antianginal efficacy per day.

The pharmacokinetics of extended-release nitroglycerin tablets, and the clinical effects of multiple-dose regimens, have not been well studied, In clinical trials, the initial regimen of nitroglycerin tablets has been 2.6-.5 mg 3 times a day, with subsequent upward dose adjustment guided by symptoms and side effects. In 1 trial, 5 of the 18 subjects were titrated up to a dose of 26 mg 4 times a day.

NITROGLYCERIN LINGUAL AEROSOL SPRAY

At the onset of an attack, 1 or 2 metered doses should be sprayed onto or under the tongue. No more than 3 metered doses are recommended within a 15 minute period. If the chest pain persists, prompt medical attention is recommended. Nitroglycerin Spray may be used pro-

N

phylactically 5-10 minutes prior to engaging in activities which might precipitate an acute attack.

During application the patient should rest, ideally in the sitting position. The canister should be held vertically with the valve head uppermost and the spray orifice as close to the mouth as possible. The dose should be preferably sprayed onto the tongue by pressing the button firmly and the mouth should be closed immediately after each dose. THE SPRAY SHOULD NOT BE INHALED. Patients should be instructed to familiarize themselves with the position of the spray orifice, which can be identified by the finger rest on top of the valve, in order to facilitate orientation for administration at night.

NITROGLYCERIN OINTMENT

When applying the ointment, place the dose-determining applicator supplied with the package printed-side down and squeeze the necessary amount of ointment from the tube onto the applicator. Then place the applicator with the ointment-side down onto the desired area of skin, usually the chest or back. Several studies suggest that absorption of nitroglycerin through the skin varies with the site of the application of the drug. Application of the drug to the skin of the chest is reported to give higher blood levels of nitroglycerin and greater hemodynamic effects than the application of extremities.

The amount of nitroglycerin entering the circulation varies directly with the size of the skin area exposed to the drug and the amount of ointment applied. Although in major clinical trials the dose was often applied to a 6 × 6-inch (150 × 150-mm) area of skin, in clinical practice the dose is usually applied to a smaller area. The ointment should be applied in a thin, uniform layer and the dose-to-area ratio kept reasonably constant. For example: 1 inch on a 2 × 3 inch area; 2 inches on a 3 × 4 inch area; 3 inches on a 4 × 5 inch area. When doubling the dose, the surface area over which the ointment is placed should be doubled.

As with all nitrates, clinical studies suggest that clinical response is variable. A suggested starting dose is ½ inch (7.5 mg) applied to a 1 × 3 area every 8 hours. Response to treatment should be assessed over the next several days. If angina occurs after ointment has been in place for several hours, the frequency of dosing should be increased (*e.g.,* every 6 hours). Administer the smallest effective dose 3-4 times daily, unless clinical response suggests a different regimen. An initiation of therapy or change in dosage, blood pressure (patient standing) should be monitored. Controlled trials have been carried out for up to 7 hours after dosing; therefore, it is not known whether the drug is effective in prevention of exertional angina beyond several hours after dosing. The effectiveness of repetitive applications of nitroglycerin ointment for the chronic management of angina pectoris has not been established. Nitroglycerin ointment is not intended for the immediate relief of anginal attacks.

NITROGLYCERIN TRANSDERMAL DELIVERY SYSTEM

The suggested starting dose is between 0.2 and 0.4 mg/h*. Doses between 0.4 and 0.8 mg/h* have shown continued effectiveness for 10-12 hours daily for at least 1 month (the longest period studied) of intermittent administration. Although the minimum nitrate-free interval has not yet been defined, data show that a nitrate-free interval of 10-12 hours is sufficient (see CLINICAL PHARMACOLOGY). Thus, an appropriate dosing schedule for nitroglycerin patches would include a daily patch-on period of 12-14 hours and a patch-off period of 10-12 hours.

Although some well-controlled clinical trials using exercise tolerance testing have shown maintenance of effectiveness when patches are worn continuously, the large majority of such controlled trials have shown the development of tolerance (*i.e.,* complete loss of effect) within the first 24 hours after therapy was initiated. Dose adjustment, even to levels much higher than generally used, did not restore efficacy.

*Release rates for formerly described in terms of drug delivered per 24 hours. In these terms, the supplied systems would be rated at 2.5 mg/24 h (0.1 mg/h), 5 mg/24 h (0.2 mg/h), 10 mg/24 h (0.4 mg/h), and 15 mg/24 h (0.6 mg/h).

PRODUCT LISTING - RATED THERAPEUTICALLY EQUIVALENT

Capsule, Extended Release - Oral - 2.5 mg

100's	$10.20	GENERIC, Auro Pharmaceutical	55829-0685-10

Solution - Intravenous - 5 mg/ml

1 ml x 10	$36.88	NITRO-BID IV, Aventis Pharmaceuticals	00088-1800-31
5 ml x 10	$88.88	NITRO-BID IV, Aventis Pharmaceuticals	00088-1800-32
5 ml x 10	$90.60	GENERIC, American Regent Laboratories Inc	00517-4805-10
5 ml x 20	$159.27	GENERIC, Faulding Pharmaceutical Company	61703-0213-09
5 ml x 25	$40.08	GENERIC, Abbott Pharmaceutical	00074-4107-01
10 ml x 5	$79.20	NITRO-BID IV, Aventis Pharmaceuticals	00088-1800-33
10 ml x 10	$140.60	GENERIC, American Regent Laboratories Inc	00517-4810-10
10 ml x 20	$22.50	GENERIC, Faulding Pharmaceutical Company	61703-0212-10
10 ml x 20	$254.40	GENERIC, Faulding Pharmaceutical Company	61703-0213-11
10 ml x 25	$48.69	GENERIC, Abbott Pharmaceutical	00074-4104-01
20 ml x 25	$347.88	GENERIC, Faulding Pharmaceutical Company	61703-0213-21
100 ml	$118.75	GENERIC, Dupont Pharmaceuticals	00590-0085-05
100 ml	$150.00	GENERIC, Dupont Pharmaceuticals	00590-0085-86
200 ml	$212.50	GENERIC, Dupont Pharmaceuticals	00590-0090-10
200 ml	$225.00	GENERIC, Dupont Pharmaceuticals	00590-0090-66
400 ml	$300.00	GENERIC, Dupont Pharmaceuticals	00590-0095-79

Solution - Intravenous - 5%;10 mg/100 ml

250 ml x 12	$82.51	GENERIC, Abbott Pharmaceutical	00074-1483-02
250 ml x 12	$192.00	GENERIC, Baxter I.V. Systems Division	00338-1047-02
500 ml x 12	$89.63	GENERIC, Abbott Pharmaceutical	00074-1483-03

Solution - Intravenous - 5%;20 mg/100 ml

250 ml x 12	$83.52	GENERIC, Abbott Pharmaceutical	00074-1482-02
250 ml x 12	$196.08	GENERIC, Baxter I.V. Systems Division	00338-1049-02

Solution - Intravenous - 5%;40 mg/100 ml

250 ml x 12	$87.45	GENERIC, Baxter I.V. Systems Division	00338-1051-02
250 ml x 12	$96.00	GENERIC, Abbott Pharmaceutical	00074-1484-02
500 ml x 12	$112.01	GENERIC, Abbott Pharmaceutical	00074-1484-03

PRODUCT LISTING - RATED NOT THERAPEUTICALLY EQUIVALENT

Film, Extended Release - Transdermal - 0.1 mg/Hr

30's	$45.10	GENERIC, Mylan Pharmaceuticals Inc	00378-9102-93
30's	$48.15	TRANSDERM-NITRO, Summit Pharmaceuticals	57267-0902-42
30's	$50.63	NITROGLYCERIN TRANSDERMAL SYSTEM, 3M Pharmaceuticals	00089-1301-30
30's	$53.32	NITRO-DUR, Physicians Total Care	54868-3633-00
30's	$58.99	NITRO-DUR, Schering Corporation	00085-3305-35
30's	$61.81	MINITRAN, 3M Pharmaceuticals	00089-0301-02
30's	$67.05	NITRO-DUR, Schering Corporation	00085-3305-30
100's	$160.49	TRANSDERM-NITRO, Summit Pharmaceuticals	57267-0902-30

Film, Extended Release - Transdermal - 0.2 mg/Hr

30's	$33.06	GENERIC, Hercon Laboratories	49730-0001-30
30's	$44.35	GENERIC, Hercon Laboratories	49730-0111-30
30's	$46.15	GENERIC, Mylan Pharmaceuticals Inc	00378-9104-93
30's	$48.50	GENERIC, Major Pharmaceuticals Inc	00904-5495-46
30's	$49.29	TRANSDERM-NITRO, Summit Pharmaceuticals	57267-0905-42
30's	$51.25	NITREK, Bertek Pharmaceuticals Inc	62794-0202-93
30's	$56.71	MINITRAN, Physicians Total Care	54868-2716-01
30's	$59.88	NITRO-DUR, Schering Corporation	00085-3310-35
30's	$60.74	NITRO-DUR, Physicians Total Care	54868-1289-01
30's	$62.75	MINITRAN, 3M Pharmaceuticals	00089-0302-02
30's	$68.08	NITRO-DUR, Schering Corporation	00085-3310-30
30's	$69.51	NITROGLYCERIN TRANSDERMAL SYSTEM, 3M Pharmaceuticals	00089-1302-30
100's	$164.26	TRANSDERM-NITRO, Summit Pharmaceuticals	57267-0905-30

Film, Extended Release - Transdermal - 0.4 mg/Hr

30's	$50.75	GENERIC, Hercon Laboratories	49730-0112-30
30's	$52.75	GENERIC, Mylan Pharmaceuticals Inc	00378-9112-93
30's	$55.40	GENERIC, Major Pharmaceuticals Inc	00904-5496-46
30's	$58.45	NITREK, Bertek Pharmaceuticals Inc	62794-0204-93
30's	$60.11	NITROGLYCERIN TRANSDERMAL SYSTEM, 3M Pharmaceuticals	00089-1303-30
30's	$67.08	NITRO-DUR, Schering Corporation	00085-3320-35
30's	$70.31	MINITRAN, 3M Pharmaceuticals	00089-0303-02
30's	$76.26	NITRO-DUR, Schering Corporation	00085-3320-30

Film, Extended Release - Transdermal - 0.6 mg/Hr

30's	$51.30	GENERIC, Hercon Laboratories	49730-0002-30
30's	$55.80	GENERIC, Hercon Laboratories	49730-0113-30
30's	$58.15	GENERIC, Mylan Pharmaceuticals Inc	00378-9116-93
30's	$61.10	GENERIC, Major Pharmaceuticals Inc	00904-5497-46
30's	$62.08	TRANSDERM-NITRO, Summit Pharmaceuticals	57267-0915-42
30's	$64.55	NITREK, Bertek Pharmaceuticals Inc	62794-0206-93
30's	$65.22	NITROGLYCERIN TRANSDERMAL SYSTEM, 3M Pharmaceuticals	00089-1304-30
30's	$72.77	NITRO-DUR, Schering Corporation	00085-3330-35
30's	$76.25	MINITRAN, 3M Pharmaceuticals	00089-0304-02
30's	$82.71	NITRO-DUR, Schering Corporation	00085-3330-30

Film, Extended Release - Transdermal - 0.8 mg/Hr

30's	$72.77	NITRO-DUR, Schering Corporation	00085-0819-35
30's	$82.71	NITRO-DUR, Schering Corporation	00085-0819-30

PRODUCT LISTING - EQUIVALENTS NOT AVAILABLE

Capsule, Extended Release - Oral - 2.5 mg

60's	$3.71	GENERIC, Moore, H.L. Drug Exchange Inc	00839-5146-05
60's	$4.16	GENERIC, Marlex Pharmaceuticals	10135-0194-60
60's	$5.40	GENERIC, Geneva Pharmaceuticals	00781-2718-60
60's	$5.95	GENERIC, Major Pharmaceuticals Inc	00904-0643-52
60's	$5.95	GENERIC, Time Cap Laboratories Inc	49483-0221-06
60's	$12.80	GENERIC, Ethex Corporation	58177-0004-03
60's	$12.82	GENERIC, Eon Labs Manufacturing Inc	00185-5174-60
100's	$3.95	GENERIC, Veratex Corporation	17022-5971-02
100's	$5.00	GENERIC, C.O. Truxton Inc	00463-3010-01
100's	$5.53	GENERIC, Physicians Total Care	54868-1554-00
100's	$6.19	GENERIC, Marlex Pharmaceuticals	10135-0194-01
100's	$6.20	GENERIC, Moore, H.L. Drug Exchange Inc	00839-5146-06
100's	$6.68	GENERIC, Interstate Drug Exchange Inc	00814-5365-14
100's	$6.70	GENERIC, Major Pharmaceuticals Inc	00904-0643-60
100's	$6.99	GENERIC, Aligen Independent Laboratories Inc	00405-4702-01
100's	$8.25	GENERIC, Geneva Pharmaceuticals	00781-2718-01
100's	$8.25	GENERIC, Allscripts Pharmaceutical Company	54569-0456-00
100's	$9.10	GENERIC, Watson/Rugby Laboratories Inc	00536-4083-01
100's	$9.10	GENERIC, Time Cap Laboratories Inc	49483-0221-10
100's	$9.11	GENERIC, Bradley Pharmaceuticals Inc	00482-1025-01
100's	$11.45	GENERIC, Southwood Pharmaceuticals Inc	58016-0300-00
100's	$11.68	GENERIC, Geneva Pharmaceuticals	00781-2718-13
100's	$13.01	GENERIC, Mutual/United Research Laboratories	00677-0485-01
100's	$14.20	GENERIC, Qualitest Products Inc	00603-4782-21
100's	$14.95	GENERIC, Major Pharmaceuticals Inc	00904-0643-61
100's	$17.43	GENERIC, Ethex Corporation	58177-0004-04
100's	$17.45	GENERIC, Eon Labs Manufacturing Inc	00185-5174-01
100's	$17.90	GENERIC, Ivax Corporation	00182-0702-89

Capsule, Extended Release - Oral - 6.5 mg

60's	$5.22	GENERIC, Marlex Pharmaceuticals	10135-0195-60
60's	$5.47	GENERIC, Moore, H.L. Drug Exchange Inc	00839-5978-05
60's	$6.25	GENERIC, Geneva Pharmaceuticals	00781-2786-60
60's	$6.95	GENERIC, Major Pharmaceuticals Inc	00904-0644-52
60's	$7.99	GENERIC, Time Cap Laboratories Inc	49483-0222-06
60's	$13.89	GENERIC, Ethex Corporation	58177-0005-03
60's	$13.91	GENERIC, Eon Labs Manufacturing Inc	00185-1235-60
100's	$3.95	GENERIC, Veratex Corporation	17022-5992-02
100's	$6.74	GENERIC, Moore, H.L. Drug Exchange Inc	00839-5978-06
100's	$7.28	GENERIC, Interstate Drug Exchange Inc	00814-5366-14
100's	$7.46	GENERIC, Physicians Total Care	54868-0689-01
100's	$7.51	GENERIC, Marlex Pharmaceuticals	10135-0195-01
100's	$9.15	GENERIC, Geneva Pharmaceuticals	00781-2786-01
100's	$9.70	GENERIC, Allscripts Pharmaceutical Company	54569-0459-00
100's	$12.16	GENERIC, Auro Pharmaceutical	55829-0686-10
100's	$13.90	GENERIC, Time Cap Laboratories Inc	49483-0222-10
100's	$13.92	GENERIC, Aligen Independent Laboratories Inc	00405-4703-01
100's	$14.65	GENERIC, Kenwood Laboratories	00482-1065-01
100's	$17.45	GENERIC, Major Pharmaceuticals Inc	00904-0644-61
100's	$17.95	GENERIC, Geneva Pharmaceuticals	00781-2786-13
100's	$18.25	GENERIC, Qualitest Products Inc	00603-4783-21
100's	$18.25	GENERIC, Mutual/United Research Laboratories	00677-0486-01
100's	$19.26	GENERIC, Major Pharmaceuticals Inc	00904-0644-60
100's	$19.34	GENERIC, Ethex Corporation	58177-0005-04
100's	$19.36	GENERIC, Eon Labs Manufacturing Inc	00185-1235-01
100's	$22.05	GENERIC, Ivax Corporation	00182-0703-89

Capsule, Extended Release - Oral - 9 mg

60's	$6.33	GENERIC, Marlex Pharmaceuticals	10135-0196-60
60's	$7.55	GENERIC, Moore, H.L. Drug Exchange Inc	00839-6724-05
60's	$9.41	GENERIC, Qualitest Products Inc	00603-4784-20
60's	$9.72	GENERIC, Aligen Independent Laboratories Inc	00405-4704-31
60's	$9.99	GENERIC, Ivax Corporation	00182-1670-26
60's	$10.25	GENERIC, Time Cap Laboratories Inc	49483-0223-06
60's	$10.55	GENERIC, Geneva Pharmaceuticals	00781-2798-60
60's	$10.55	GENERIC, Allscripts Pharmaceutical Company	54569-3317-00
60's	$10.95	GENERIC, Watson/Rugby Laboratories Inc	00536-4090-08
60's	$10.95	GENERIC, Major Pharmaceuticals Inc	00904-0647-52
60's	$14.96	GENERIC, Mutual/United Research Laboratories	00677-0967-06
60's	$29.90	GENERIC, Ethex Corporation	58177-0006-03
60's	$29.92	GENERIC, Eon Labs Manufacturing Inc	00185-1217-60
100's	$8.25	GENERIC, Major Pharmaceuticals Inc	00904-0647-60
100's	$8.59	GENERIC, Marlex Pharmaceuticals	10135-0196-01
100's	$14.97	GENERIC, Geneva Pharmaceuticals	00781-2798-01
100's	$15.60	GENERIC, Time Cap Laboratories Inc	49483-0223-10
100's	$17.95	GENERIC, Major Pharmaceuticals Inc	00904-0647-61
100's	$19.90	GENERIC, Auro Pharmaceutical	55829-0687-10
100's	$20.75	GENERIC, Ivax Corporation	00182-1670-89
100's	$49.78	GENERIC, Ethex Corporation	58177-0006-04
100's	$49.80	GENERIC, Eon Labs Manufacturing Inc	00185-1217-01

Film, Extended Release - Transdermal - 0.2 mg/Hr

30's	$32.18	GENERIC, Physicians Total Care	54868-2183-01
30's	$33.06	GENERIC, Circa Pharmaceuticals Inc	49470-0001-30
30's	$36.46	GENERIC, Allscripts Pharmaceutical Company	54569-3208-00
30's	$37.60	GENERIC, Moore, H.L. Drug Exchange Inc	00839-7790-19
30's	$41.95	GENERIC, Major Pharmaceuticals Inc	00904-0652-46
30's	$42.64	GENERIC, Mylan Pharmaceuticals Inc	00378-9004-93
30's	$61.84	NITRODISC, Roberts Pharmaceutical Corporation	54092-0342-30
100's	$173.93	NITRODISC, Roberts Pharmaceutical Corporation	54092-0342-01

Film, Extended Release - Transdermal - 0.3 mg/Hr

30's	$57.29	NITRO-DUR, Allscripts Pharmaceutical Company	54569-2690-00
30's	$65.18	NITRODISC, Roberts Pharmaceutical Corporation	54092-0343-30
30's	$67.08	NITRO-DUR, Schering Corporation	00085-3315-35
30's	$76.26	NITRO-DUR, Schering Corporation	00085-3315-30
100's	$183.32	NITRODISC, Roberts Pharmaceutical Corporation	54092-0343-01

Film, Extended Release - Transdermal - 0.4 mg/Hr

30's	$38.49	GENERIC, Physicians Total Care	54868-1992-01
30's	$39.33	GENERIC, Circa Pharmaceuticals Inc	49470-0004-30
30's	$39.33	GENERIC, Hercon Laboratories	49730-0004-30
30's	$41.26	GENERIC, Moore, H.L. Drug Exchange Inc	00839-7791-19
30's	$43.15	GENERIC, Allscripts Pharmaceutical Company	54569-3209-00
30's	$49.95	GENERIC, Mylan Pharmaceuticals Inc	00378-9012-93
30's	$68.52	NITRODISC, Roberts Pharmaceutical Corporation	54092-0344-30
100's	$192.62	NITRODISC, Roberts Pharmaceutical Corporation	54092-0344-01

Film, Extended Release - Transdermal - 0.6 mg/Hr

30's	$49.98	GENERIC, Physicians Total Care	54868-2744-00
30's	$50.50	GENERIC, Qualitest Products Inc	00603-4727-16
30's	$51.30	GENERIC, Circa Pharmaceuticals Inc	49470-0002-30
30's	$59.25	GENERIC, Major Pharmaceuticals Inc	00904-0654-46
30's	$59.50	GENERIC, Mylan Pharmaceuticals Inc	00378-9016-93

Ointment - Topical - 2%

1 gm x 48	$30.72	NITRO-BID, Fougera	00168-0326-08
3 gm x 50	$50.56	NITROL APPLI-KIT, Savage Laboratories	00281-5804-48
3 gm x 50	$53.99	NITROL APPLI-KIT, Savage Laboratories	00281-5804-59
30 gm	$3.84	NITRO-BID, Aventis Pharmaceuticals	00088-1552-20
30 gm	$5.87	GENERIC, Allscripts Pharmaceutical Company	54569-3360-00
30 gm	$6.95	GENERIC, Fougera	00168-0038-30
30 gm	$8.88	NITROL APPLI-KIT, Savage Laboratories	00281-5804-46
30 gm	$9.20	NITRO-BID, Fougera	00168-0326-30
60 gm	$6.48	GENERIC, Fougera	00168-0038-60
60 gm	$7.26	NITRO-BID, Aventis Pharmaceuticals	00088-1552-60
60 gm	$8.50	GENERIC, Watson/Rugby Laboratories Inc	00536-2558-25
60 gm	$10.40	NITROL APPLI-KIT, Savage Laboratories	00281-5804-56
60 gm	$15.80	NITRO-BID, Fougera	00168-0326-60
60 gm	$16.33	NITROL APPLI-KIT, Savage Laboratories	00281-5804-47

Spray - Sublingual - 0.4 mg

12 gm	$32.79	NITROLINGUAL, Allscripts Pharmaceutical Company	54569-4974-00
12 gm	$39.67	NITROLINGUAL, First Horizon Pharmaceutical Corporation	59630-0300-20
14.49 ml	$31.22	NITROLINGUAL, First Horizon Pharmaceutical Corporation	59630-0305-20

Tablet - Sublingual - 0.3 mg

100's	$6.76	NITROSTAT, Southwood Pharmaceuticals Inc	58016-5108-00
100's	$7.36	GENERIC, Mutual/United Research Laboratories	00677-1777-01
100's	$7.42	GENERIC, Able Laboratories Inc	53265-0249-10
100's	$7.42	GENERIC, Teva Pharmaceuticals Usa	55953-0294-40
100's	$7.78	GENERIC, Ethex Corporation	58177-0323-04
100's	$7.79	GENERIC, Endo Laboratories Llc	60951-0692-70
100's	$8.67	NITROSTAT, Allscripts Pharmaceutical Company	54569-1866-02
100's	$10.01	NITROSTAT, Parke-Davis	00071-0417-24
100's	$10.78	NITROSTAT, Physicians Total Care	54868-1538-01

Tablet - Sublingual - 0.4 mg

25 x 4	$16.98	GENERIC, Ethex Corporation	58177-0324-18
25 x 4	$16.99	GENERIC, Endo Laboratories Llc	60951-0718-62
25 x 4	$18.25	GENERIC, Able Laboratories Inc	53265-0250-04
25 x 4	$21.84	NITROSTAT, Parke-Davis	00071-0418-13
25's	$4.72	NITROSTAT, Allscripts Pharmaceutical Company	54569-2140-00
25's	$5.93	NITROSTAT, Physicians Total Care	54868-0691-00
25's	$16.18	GENERIC, Southwood Pharmaceuticals Inc	58016-0297-25
100's	$7.36	GENERIC, Mutual/United Research Laboratories	00677-1778-01
100's	$7.42	GENERIC, Able Laboratories Inc	53265-0250-10
100's	$7.78	GENERIC, Allscripts Pharmaceutical Company	54569-4631-00
100's	$7.78	GENERIC, Ethex Corporation	58177-0324-04
100's	$7.79	GENERIC, Endo Laboratories Llc	60951-0718-70
100's	$8.67	NITROSTAT, Allscripts Pharmaceutical Company	54569-0461-00
100's	$8.69	NITROSTAT, Southwood Pharmaceuticals Inc	58016-5006-00
100's	$8.69	NITROSTAT, Southwood Pharmaceuticals Inc	58016-5006-01
100's	$10.01	NITROSTAT, Parke-Davis	00071-0418-24
100's	$11.08	NITROSTAT, Physicians Total Care	54868-0691-01
100's	$16.06	GENERIC, Mutual/United Research Laboratories	00677-1778-76

Tablet - Sublingual - 0.6 mg

100's	$7.36	GENERIC, Mutual/United Research Laboratories	00677-1779-01
100's	$7.42	GENERIC, Able Laboratories Inc	53265-0251-10
100's	$7.42	GENERIC, Teva Pharmaceuticals Usa	55953-0296-40
100's	$7.78	GENERIC, Ethex Corporation	58177-0325-04
100's	$7.79	GENERIC, Endo Laboratories Llc	60951-0726-70
100's	$8.69	NITROSTAT, Southwood Pharmaceuticals Inc	58016-5009-01
100's	$10.01	NITROSTAT, Parke-Davis	00071-0419-24
100's	$11.36	NITROSTAT, Physicians Total Care	54868-1508-01

Tablet, Extended Release - Oral Transmucosal - 1 mg

100's	$37.87	NITROGARD, Forest Pharmaceuticals	00456-0686-01

Tablet, Extended Release - Oral Transmucosal - 2.6 mg

100's	$33.54	NITRONG, Aventis Pharmaceuticals	00075-0221-20

Tablet, Extended Release - Oral Transmucosal - 3 mg

100's	$43.33	NITROGARD, Forest Pharmaceuticals	00456-0683-01

Tablet, Extended Release - Oral Transmucosal - 6.5 mg

100's	$41.98	NITRONG, Aventis Pharmaceuticals	00075-0274-20

Nitroprusside, Sodium (002254)

Categories: Hypertension, essential; Surgery, adjunct; Pregnancy Category C; FDA Approval Pre 1982; WHO Formulary
Drug Classes: Vasodilators
Brand Names: **Nipride**; Nitropress; Nitroprusside Sodium
Foreign Brand Availability: Nitan (Mexico); Nitroprusiato de sodio-ecar (Colombia)

WARNING

After reconstitution, sodium nitroprusside is not suitable for direct injection. THE RECONSTITUTED SOLUTION MUST BE FURTHER DILUTED IN STERILE 5% DEXTROSE INJECTION BEFORE INFUSION (SEE DOSAGE AND ADMINISTRATION).

Sodium nitroprusside can cause PRECIPITOUS DECREASES IN BLOOD PRESSURE (SEE DOSAGE AND ADMINISTRATION). In patients not properly monitored, these decreases can lead to IRREVERSIBLE ISCHEMIC INJURIES OR DEATH. Sodium nitroprusside should be used only when available equipment and personnel allow blood pressure to be continuously monitored.

Except when used briefly or at low (<2 μg/kg/min) infusion rates, sodium nitroprusside injection gives rise to important quantities of cyanide ion, which can reach TOXIC, POTENTIALLY LETHAL LEVELS (SEE WARNINGS). The usual dose rate is 0.5 to 10 μg/kg/min, but INFUSION AT THE MAXIMUM DOSE RATE SHOULD NEVER LAST MORE THAN 10 MINUTES. If blood pressure has not been adequately controlled after 10 minutes of infusion at the maximum rate, administration of sodium nitroprusside should be terminated immediately.

Although acid-base balance and venous oxygen concentration should be monitored and may indicate cyanide toxicity, these laboratory tests provide imperfect guidance.

This package insert should be thoroughly reviewed before administration of sodium nitroprusside infusion.

DESCRIPTION

Sodium nitroprusside is disodium pentacyanonitrosylferrate(2-)dihydrate, an inorganic hypotensive agent whose molecular formula is $Na_2(Fe(CN)_5NO) \cdot 2H_2O$, and whose molecular weight is 297.95. Dry sodium nitroprusside is a reddish-brown powder, soluble in water. In an aqueous solution infused intravenously, sodium nitroprusside is rapid-acting vasodilator, active on both arteries and veins.

Sodium nitroprusside solution is rapidly degraded by trace contaminants, often with resulting color changes (see DOSAGE AND ADMINISTRATION). The solution is also sensitive to certain wavelengths of light, and it must be protected from light in clinical use.

Each 5 ml vial contains the equivalent of 50 mg sodium nitroprusside dihydrate.

Storage: Store the 5 ml amber-colored vials at 59-86°F.

CLINICAL PHARMACOLOGY

N

The principal pharmacological action of sodium nitroprusside is relaxation of vascular smooth muscle and consequent dilatation of peripheral arteries and veins. Other smooth muscle (*e.g.*, uterus, duodenum) is not affected. Sodium nitroprusside is more active on veins than on arteries, but this selectivity is much less marked than that of nitroglycerin. Dilatation of the veins promotes peripheral pooling of blood and decreases venous return to the heart, thereby reducing left ventricular end-diastolic pressure and pulmonary capillary wedge pressure (preload). Arteriolar relaxation reduces systemic vascular resistance, systolic arterial pressure and mean arterial pressure (afterload). Dilatation of the coronary arteries also occurs.

In association with the decrease in blood pressure, sodium nitroprusside administered intravenously to hypertensive and normotensive patients produces slight increases in heart rate and a variable effect on cardiac output. In hypertensive patients, moderate doses induce renal vasodilatation roughly proportional to the decrease in systemic blood pressure, so there is no appreciable change in renal blood flow or glomerular filtration rate.

In normotensive subjects, acute reduction of mean arterial pressure to 60-75 mm Hg by infusion of sodium nitroprusside caused a significant increase in renin activity. In the same study, ten renovascular-hypertensive patients given sodium nitroprusside had significant increases in renin release from the involved kidney at mean arterial pressures of 90-137 mm Hg.

The hypotensive effect of sodium nitroprusside is seen within a minute or two after the start of an adequate infusion, and it dissipates almost as rapidly after an infusion is discontinued. The effect is augmented by ganglionic blocking agents and inhaled anesthetics.

PHARMACOKINETICS AND METABOLISM

Infused sodium nitroprusside is rapidly distributed to a volume that is approximately coextensive with the extracellular space. The drug is cleared from this volume by intraerythrocytic reaction with hemoglobin (Hgb), and sodium nitroprusside's resulting circulatory half-life is about 2 minutes.

The products of the nitroprusside/hemoglobin reaction are cyanmethemoglobin (cyanmetHgb) and cyanide ion (CN^-). Safe use of sodium nitroprusside injection must be guided by knowledge of the further metabolism of these products.

The essential features of nitroprusside metabolism are:

- One molecule of sodium nitroprusside is metabolized by combination with hemoglobin to produce one molecule of cyanmethemoglobin and four CN^- ions;
- Methemoglobin, obtained from hemoglobin, can sequester cyanide as cyanmethemoglobin;
- Thiosulfate reacts with cyanide to produce thiocyanate;
- Thiocyanate is eliminated in the urine;
- Cyanide not otherwise removed binds to cytochromes; and
- Cyanide is much more toxic than methemoglobin or thiocyanate.

Cyanide ion is normally found in serum; it is derived from dietary substrates and from tobacco smoke. Cyanide binds avidly (but reversibly) to ferric ion (Fe^{+++}), most body stores of which are found in erythrocyte methemoglobin (metHgb) and in mitochondrial cytochromes. When CN^- is infused or generated within the bloodstream, essentially all of it is bound to methemoglobin until intraerythrocytic methemoglobin has been saturated.

When the Fe^{+++} of cytochromes is bound to cyanide, the cytochromes are unable to participate in oxidative metabolism. In this situation, cells may be able to provide for their energy needs by utilizing anaerobic pathways, but they thereby generate an increasing body burden of lactic acid. Other cells may be unable to utilize these alternate pathways, and they may die hypoxic deaths.

CN^- levels in packed erythrocytes are typically less than 1 μmol/L (less than 25 μg/L); levels are roughly doubled in heavy smokers.

At healthy steady-state, most people have less than 1% of their hemoglobin in the form of methemoglobin. Nitroprusside metabolism can lead to methemoglobin formation (a) through dissociation of cyanmethemoglobin formed in the original reaction of sodium nitroprusside with Hgb and (b) by direct oxidation of Hgb by the released nitroso group. Relatively large quantities of sodium nitroprusside, however, are required to produce significant methemoglobinemia.

At physiologic methemoglobin levels, the CN^- binding capacity of packed red cells is a little less than 200 μmol/L (5 mg/L). Cytochrome toxicity is seen at levels only slightly higher, and death has been reported at levels from 300-3000 μmol/L (8-80 mg/L). Put another way, a patient with a normal red-cell mass (35 ml/kg) and normal methemoglobin levels can buffer about 175 μg/kg of CN^-, corresponding to a little less than 500 μg/kg of infused sodium nitroprusside.

Some cyanide is eliminated from the body as expired hydrogen cyanide, but most is enzymatically converted to thiocyanate (SCN^-) by thiosulfate-cyanide sulfur transferase (rhodanese, EC 2.8.1.1), a mitochondrial enzyme. The enzyme is normally present in great excess, so the reaction is rate-limited by the availability of sulfur donors, especially thiosulfate, cystine and cysteine.

Thiosulfate is a normal constituent of serum, produced from cysteine by way of β-mercaptopyruvate. Physiological levels of thiosulfate are typically about 0.1 mmol/L (11 mg/L), but they are approximately twice this level in children and in adults who are not eating. Infused thiosulfate is cleared from the body (primarily by the kidneys) with a $T_{1/2}$ of about 20 minutes.

When thiosulfate is being supplied only by normal physiologic mechanisms, conversion of CN^- to SCN^- generally proceeds at about 1 μg/kg/min. This rate of CN^- clearance corresponds to steady-state processing of a sodium nitroprusside infusion of slightly more than 2 μg/kg/min. CN^- begins to accumulate when sodium nitroprusside infusions exceed this rate.

Thiocyanate (SCN^-) is also a normal physiological constituent of serum, with normal levels typically in the range of 50-250 μmol/L (3-15 mg/L). Clearance of SCN^- is primarily renal, with a $T_{1/2}$ of about 3 days. In renal failure, the $T_{1/2}$ can be doubled or tripled.

INDICATIONS AND USAGE

Sodium nitroprusside is indicated for the immediate reduction of blood pressure of patients in hypertensive crises. Concomitant longer-acting antihypertensive medication should be administered so that the duration of treatment with sodium nitroprusside can be minimized.

sodium nitroprusside is also indicated for producing controlled hypotension in order to reduce bleeding during surgery.

NON-FDA APPROVED INDICATIONS

Nitroprusside is commonly used without FDA approval for the treatment of advanced, decompensated congestive heart failure.

CONTRAINDICATIONS

Sodium nitroprusside should not be used in the treatment of compensatory hypertension, where the primary hemodynamic lesion is aortic coarctation or arteriovenous shunting.

Sodium nitroprusside should not be used to produce hypotension during surgery in patients with known inadequate cerebral circulation or in moribund patients (A.S.A. Class 5E) coming to emergency surgery.

Patients with congenital (Leber's) optic atrophy or with tobacco amblyopia have unusually high cyanide/thiocyanate ratios. These rare conditions are probably associated with defective or absent rhodanese, and sodium nitroprusside use should be avoided in these patients.

WARNINGS

See BOXED WARNING.

The principal hazards of sodium nitroprusside administration are excessive hypotension and excessive accumulation of cyanide (see DOSAGE AND ADMINISTRATION).

EXCESSIVE HYPOTENSION

Small transient excesses in the infusion rate of sodium nitroprusside can result in excessive hypotension, sometimes to levels so low as to compromise the perfusion of vital organs. These hemodynamic changes may lead to a variety of associated symptoms: (see ADVERSE REACTIONS). Nitroprusside-induced hypotension will be self-limited within 1-10 minutes after discontinuation of the nitroprusside infusion; during these few minutes, it may be helpful to put the patient into a head-down (Trendelenburg) position to maximize venous return. **If hypotension persists more than a few minutes after discontinuation of the infusion of sodium nitroprusside, sodium nitroprusside is not the cause, and the true cause must be sought.**

CYANIDE TOXICITY

As described in CLINICAL PHARMACOLOGY, sodium nitroprusside infusions at rates above 2 μg/kg/min generate cyanide ion (CN^-) faster than the body can normally dispose of it. (When sodium thiosulfate is given, as described under DOSAGE AND ADMINISTRATION, the body's capacity for CN^- elimination is greatly increased.) Methemoglobin normally present in the body can buffer a certain amount of CN^-, but the capacity of this system is exhausted by the CN^- produced from about 500 μg/kg of sodium nitroprusside. This amount of sodium nitroprusside is administered in less than an hour when the drug is administered at 10 μg/kg/min (the maximum recommended rate). Thereafter, the toxic effects of CN^- may be rapid, serious and even lethal.

The true rates of clinically important cyanide toxicity cannot be assessed from spontaneous reports or published data. Most patients reported to have experienced such toxicity have received relatively prolonged infusions, and the only patients whose deaths have been unequivocally attributed to nitroprusside-induced cyanide toxicity have been patients who had received nitroprusside infusions at rates (30-120 µg/kg/min) much greater than those now recommended. Elevated cyanide levels, metabolic acidosis, and marked clinical deterioration, however, have occasionally been reported in patients who received infusions at recommended rates for only a few hours and even, in one case, for only 35 minutes. In some of these cases, infusion of sodium thiosulfate caused dramatic clinical improvement, supporting the diagnosis of cyanide toxicity.

Cyanide toxicity may manifest itself as venous hyperoxemia with bright red venous blood, as cells become unable to extract the oxygen delivered to them; metabolic (lactic) acidosis; air hunger; confusion; and death. Cyanide toxicity due to causes other than nitroprusside has been associated with angina pectoris and myocardial infarction; ataxia, seizures and stroke; and other diffuse ischemic damage.

Hypertensive patients, and patients concomitantly receiving other antihypertensive medications, may be more sensitive to the effects of sodium nitroprusside than normal subjects.

PRECAUTIONS

GENERAL

Like other vasodilators, sodium nitroprusside can cause increases in intracranial pressure. In patients whose intracranial pressure is already elevated, sodium nitroprusside should be used only with extreme caution.

HEPATIC

Use caution when administering sodium nitroprusside to patients with hepatic insufficiency.

USE IN ANESTHESIA

When sodium nitroprusside (or any other vasodilator) is used for controlled hypotension during anesthesia, the patient's capacity to compensate for anemia and hypovolemia may be diminished. If possible, pre-existing anemia and hypovolemia should be corrected prior to administration of sodium nitroprusside.

Hypotensive anesthetic techniques may also cause abnormalities of the pulmonary ventilation/perfusion ratio. Patients intolerant of these abnormalities may require a higher fraction of inspired oxygen.

Extreme caution should be exercised in patients who are especially poor surgical risks (A.S.A. Classes 4 and 4E).

LABORATORY TESTS

The cyanide-level assay is technically difficult, and cyanide levels in body fluids other than packed red blood cells are difficult to interpret. Cyanide toxicity will lead to lactic acidosis and venous hyperoxemia, but these findings may not be present until an hour or more after the cyanide capacity of the body's red-cell mass has been exhausted.

CARCINOGENESIS, MUTAGENESIS, AND IMPAIRMENT OF FERTILITY

sodium nitroprusside has not undergone adequate carcinogenicity testing in animals. The mutagenic potential of sodium nitroprusside has not been assessed. Sodium nitroprusside has not been tested for effects on fertility.

PREGNANCY, TERATOGENIC EFFECTS, PREGNANCY CATEGORY C

There are no adequate or well-controlled studies of sodium nitroprusside in either laboratory animals or pregnant women. It is not known whether sodium nitroprusside can cause fetal harm when administered to a pregnant woman or can affect reproductive capacity. Sodium nitroprusside should be given to a pregnant woman only if clearly needed.

NONTERATOGENIC EFFECTS

In three studies in pregnant ewes, nitroprusside was shown to cross the placental barrier. Fetal cyanide levels were shown to be dose-related to maternal levels of nitroprusside. The metabolic transformation of sodium nitroprusside given to pregnant ewes led to fatal levels of cyanide in the fetuses. The infusion of 25 µg/kg/min of sodium nitroprusside for 1 hour in pregnant ewes resulted in the death of all fetuses. Pregnant ewes infused with 1 µg/kg/min of sodium nitroprusside for one hour delivered normal lambs.

The effects of administering sodium thiosulfate in pregnancy, either by itself or as a co-infusion with sodium nitroprusside, are completely unknown.

NURSING MOTHERS

It is not known whether sodium nitroprusside and its metabolites are excreted in human milk. Because many drugs are excreted in human milk and because of the potential for serious adverse reactions in nursing infants from sodium nitroprusside, a decision should be made whether to discontinue nursing or to discontinue the drug, taking into account the importance of the drug to the mother.

PEDIATRIC USE

See DOSAGE AND ADMINISTRATION.

DRUG INTERACTIONS

The hypotensive effect of sodium nitroprusside is augmented by that of most other hypotensive drugs, including ganglionic blocking agents, negative inotropic agents and inhaled anesthetics.

ADVERSE REACTIONS

The most important adverse reactions to sodium nitroprusside are the avoidable ones of excessive hypotension and cyanide toxicity, described above under WARNINGS. The adverse reactions described in this section develop less rapidly and, as it happens, less commonly.

METHEMOGLOBINEMIA

As described in CLINICAL PHARMACOLOGY, sodium nitroprusside infusions can cause sequestration of hemoglobin as methemoglobin. The back-conversion process is normally rapid, and clinically significant methemoglobinemia (>10%) is seen only rarely in patients receiving sodium nitroprusside. Even patients congenitally incapable of back-converting methemoglobin should demonstrate 10% methemoglobinemia only after they have received about 10 mg/kg of sodium nitroprusside, and a patient receiving sodium nitroprusside at the maximum recommended rate (10 µg/kg/min) would take over 16 hours to reach this total accumulated dose.

Methemoglobin levels can be measured by most clinical laboratories. The diagnosis should be suspected in patients who have received >10 mg/kg of sodium nitroprusside and who exhibit signs of impaired oxygen delivery despite adequate cardiac output and adequate arterial pO_2. Classically, methemoglobinemic blood is described as chocolate brown, without color change on exposure to air.

When methemoglobinemia is diagnosed, the treatment of choice is 1-2 mg/kg of methylene blue, administered intravenously over several minutes. In patients likely to have substantial amounts of cyanide bound to methemoglobin as cyanmethemoglobin, treatment of methemoglobinemia with methylene blue must be undertaken with extreme caution.

THIOCYANATE TOXICITY

As described in CLINICAL PHARMACOLOGY, most of the cyanide produced during metabolism of sodium nitroprusside is eliminated in the form of thiocyanate. When cyanide elimination is accelerated by the co-infusion of thiosulfate, thiocyanate production is increased.

Thiocyanate is mildly neurotoxic (tinnitus, miosis, hyperreflexia) at serum levels of 1 mmol/L (60 mg/L). Thiocyanate toxicity is life-threatening when levels are 3 or 4 times higher (200 mg/L).

The steady-state thiocyanate level after prolonged infusions of sodium nitroprusside is increased with increased infusion rate, and the half-time of accumulation is 3-4 days. To keep the steady-state thiocyanate level below 1 mmol/L, a prolonged infusion of sodium nitroprusside should not be more rapid than 3 µg/kg/min; in anuric patients, the corresponding limit is just 1 µg/kg/min. When prolonged infusions are more rapid than these, thiocyanate levels should be measured daily.

Physiologic maneuvers (*e.g.*, those that alter the pH of the urine) are not known to increase the elimination of thiocyanate. Thiocyanate clearance rates during dialysis, on the other hand, can approach the blood flow rate of the dialyzer.

Thiocyanate interferes with iodine uptake by the thyroid.

Abdominal pain, apprehension, diaphoresis, "dizziness", headache, muscle twitching, nausea, palpitations, restlessness, retching, and retrosternal discomfort have been noted when the blood pressure was too rapidly reduced. These symptoms quickly disappeared when the infusion was slowed or discontinued, and they did not reappear with a continued (or resumed) slower infusion.

Other adverse reactions reported are:

Cardiovascular: Bradycardia, electrocardiographic changes, tachycardia.
Dermatologic: Rash.
Endocrine: Hypothyroidism.
Gastrointestinal: Ileus
Hematologic: Decreased platelet aggregation, methemoglobinemia.
Neurologic: Increased intracranial pressure.
Miscellaneous: Flushing, venous streaking, irritation at the infusion site.

DOSAGE AND ADMINISTRATION

SOLUTION OF THE POWDER

The contents of a 50 mg sodium nitroprusside vial should be dissolved in 2-3 ml of dextrose in water. No other diluent should be used.

DILUTION TO PROPER STRENGTH FOR INFUSION

Depending on the desired concentration, the initially reconstituted solution containing 50 mg of sodium nitroprusside must be further diluted in 250-1000 ml of sterile 5% dextrose injection. The diluted solution should be protected from light by promptly wrapping with aluminum foil or other opaque material. It is not necessary to cover the infusion drip chamber or the tubing.

VERIFICATION OF THE CHEMICAL INTEGRITY OF THE PRODUCT

Sodium nitroprusside solution can be inactivated by reactions with trace contaminants. The products of these reactions are often blue, green or red, much brighter than the faint brownish color of unreacted sodium nitroprusside. Discolored solutions, or solutions in which particulate matter is visible, should not be used. If properly protected from light, the freshly reconstituted and diluted solution is stable for 24 hours.

No other drugs should be administered in the same solution with sodium nitroprusside.

AVOIDANCE OF EXCESSIVE HYPOTENSION

While the average effective rate in adults and children is about 3 µg/kg/min, some patients will become dangerously hypotensive when they receive sodium nitroprusside at this rate. Infusion of sodium nitroprusside should therefore be started at a very low rate (0.3 µg/kg/min), with gradual upward titration every few minutes until the desired effect is achieved or the maximum recommended infusion rate (10 µg/kg/min) has been reached.

Because sodium nitroprusside's hypotensive effect is very rapid in onset and in dissipation, small variations in infusion rate can lead to wide, undesirable variations in blood pressure. **Sodium nitroprusside should not be infused through ordinary IV apparatus regulated only by gravity and mechanical clamps. Only an infusion pump, preferably a volumetric pump, should be used.**

Because sodium nitroprusside can induce essentially unlimited blood-pressure reduction, **the blood pressure of a patient receiving this drug must be continuously monitored,** using either a continually reinflated sphygmomanometer or (preferably) an intra-arterial

N

pressure sensor. Special caution should be used in elderly patients, since they may be more sensitive to the hypotensive effects of the drug.

TABLE 1 shows the infusion rates for adults and children of various weights corresponding to the recommended initial and maximal doses (0.3 μg/kg/min and 10 μg/kg/min, respectively). Some of the listed infusion rates are so slow or so rapid as to be impractical, and these practicalities must be considered when the concentration to be used is selected. Note that when the concentration used in a given patient is changed, the tubing is still filled with a solution at the previous concentration.

AVOIDANCE OF CYANIDE TOXICITY

As described in CLINICAL PHARMACOLOGY, when more than 500 μg/kg of sodium nitroprusside is administered faster than 2 μg/kg/min, cyanide is generated faster than the unaided patient can eliminate it. Administration of sodium thiosulfate has been shown to increase the rate of cyanide processing, reducing the hazard of cyanide toxicity. Although toxic reactions to sodium thiosulfate have not been reported, the co-infusion regimen has not been extensively studied and it cannot be recommended without reservation. In one study, sodium thiosulfate appeared to potentiate the hypotensive effects of sodium nitroprusside.

TABLE 1 *Infusion Rates (ml/h) to Achieve Initial (0.3 μg/kg/min) and Maximal (10 μg/kg/min) Dosing of Sodium Nitroprusside*

Volume sodium nitroprusside concentration pt weight		250 ml 50 mg 200 μg/ml		500 ml 50 mg 100 μg/ml		1000 ml 50 mg 50 μg/ml	
kg	lbs	init	max	init	max	init	max
10	22	1	30	2	60	4	120
20	44	2	60	4	120	7	240
30	66	3	90	5	180	11	360
40	88	4	120	7	240	14	480
50	110	5	150	9	300	18	600
60	132	5	180	11	360	22	720
70	154	6	210	13	420	25	840
80	176	7	240	14	480	29	960
90	198	8	270	16	540	32	1080
100	220	9	300	18	600	36	1200

Co-infusions of sodium thiosulfate have been administered at rates of 5-10 times that of sodium nitroprusside. Care must be taken to avoid the indiscriminate use of prolonged or high doses of sodium nitroprusside with sodium thiosulfate as this may result in thiocyanate toxicity and hypovolemia. In cautious administration of sodium nitroprusside must still be avoided, and all of the precautions concerning sodium nitroprusside administration must still be observed.

CONSIDERATION OF METHEMOGLOBINEMIA AND THIOCYANATE TOXICITY

Rare patients receiving more than 10 mg/kg of sodium nitroprusside will develop methemoglobinemia; other patients, especially those with impaired renal function, will predictably develop thiocyanate toxicity after prolonged, rapid infusions. In accordance with the descriptions in ADVERSE REACTIONS, patients with suggestive findings should be tested for these toxicities.

PRODUCT LISTING - RATED THERAPEUTICALLY EQUIVALENT

Powder For Injection - Intravenous - 50 mg

1's	$1.75	NITROPRESS, Abbott Pharmaceutical	00074-3024-01
1's	$3.90	NITROPRESS, Abbott Pharmaceutical	00074-3034-44
1's	$5.00	NITROPRESS, Physicians Total Care	54868-3582-00
10's	$124.80	NITROPRESS, Abbott Pharmaceutical	00074-3250-01

Solution - Intravenous - 25 mg/ml

2 ml	$1.88	GENERIC, Baxter Pharmaceutical Products, Inc	10019-0082-02
2 ml	$4.80	GENERIC, Gensia Sicor Pharmaceuticals Inc	00703-1802-01

Nizatidine *(001894)*

For related information, see the comparative table section in Appendix A.

Categories: Esophagitis, erosive; Gastroesophageal Reflux Disease; Ulcer, duodenal; Ulcer, gastric; FDA Approved 1988 Apr; Pregnancy Category B

Drug Classes: Antihistamines, H2; Gastrointestinals

Brand Names: **Axid**

Foreign Brand Availability: Acinon (Japan); Antizid (South-Africa); Axadine (Korea); Calmaxid (Belgium; Switzerland); Cronizat (Italy); Distaxid (Spain); Gastrax (Germany); Nacid (Korea); Naxidine (Netherlands); Nex (Korea); Nizax (Denmark; Finland; Germany; Italy); Nizaxid (France; Korea; Portugal); Panaxid (Belgium); Tazac (Australia; Taiwan); Tinza (Korea); Zanitin (Korea); Zanizal (Italy); Zinga (England)

Cost of Therapy: $220.30 (GERD; Axid; 150 mg; 2 capsules/day; 60 day supply)
$171.59 (GERD; Generic Capsules; 150 mg; 2 capsules/day; 60 day supply)
$179.93 (Duodenal Ulcer; Axid; 300 mg; 1 capsules/day; 30 day supply)
$140.80 (Duodenal Ulcer; Generic Capsules; 300 mg; 1 capsules/day; 30 day supply)

DESCRIPTION

Nizatidine is a histamine H_2-receptor antagonist. Chemically, it is N-[2-[[[2-[(dimethylamino)methyl]-4-thiazolyl]methyl]thio]ethyl]-N′-methyl-2-nitro-1,1-ethenediamine.

Nizatidine has the empirical formula $C_{12}H_{21}N_5O_2S_2$ representing a molecular weight of 331.47. It is an off-white to buff crystalline solid that is soluble in water. Nizatidine has a bitter taste and mild sulfur-like odor. Each Axid Pulvule (capsule) contains for oral administration gelatin, pregelatinized starch, dimethicone, starch, titanium dioxide, yellow iron oxide, 150 mg (0.45 mmol) or 300 mg (0.91 mmol) of nizatidine, and other inactive ingredients. The 150 mg Pulvule also contains magnesium stearate, and the 300 mg Pulvule also contains croscarmellose sodium, povidone, red iron oxide, and talc.

CLINICAL PHARMACOLOGY

Nizatidine is a competitive, reversible inhibitor of histamine at the histamine H_2-receptors, particularly those in the gastric parietal cells.

ANTISECRETORY ACTIVITY

Effects on Acid Secretion

Nizatidine significantly inhibited nocturnal gastric acid secretion for up to 12 hours. Nizatidine also significantly inhibited gastric acid secretion stimulated by food, caffeine, betazole, and pentagastrin (TABLE 1).

TABLE 1 *Effect of Oral Nizatidine on Gastric Acid Secretion*

	Time After Dose (hours)	% Inhibition of Gastric Acid Output by Dose (mg) 20-50	75	100	150	300
Nocturnal	Up to 10	57%		73%		90%
Betazole	Up to 3		93%		100%	99%
Pentagastrin	Up to 6		25%		64%	67%
Meal	Up to 4	41%	64%		98%	97%
Caffeine	Up to 3		73%		85%	96%

Effects on Other Gastrointestinal Secretions

Pepsin: Oral administration of 75-300 mg of nizatidine did not affect pepsin activity in gastric secretions. Total pepsin output was reduced in proportion to the reduced volume of gastric secretions.

Intrinsic Factor: Oral administration of 75-300 mg of nizatidine increased betazole-stimulated secretion of intrinsic factor.

Serum Gastrin: Nizatidine had no effect on basal serum gastrin. No rebound of gastrin secretion was observed when food was ingested 12 hours after administration of nizatidine.

Other Pharmacologic Actions

Hormones: Nizatidine was not shown to affect the serum concentrations of gonadotropins, prolactin, growth hormone, antidiuretic hormone, cortisol, triiodothyronine, thyroxin, testosterone, 5α-dihydrotestosterone, androstenedione, or estradiol.

Nizatidine had no demonstrable antiandrogenic action.

Pharmacokinetics

The absolute oral bioavailability of nizatidine exceeds 70%. Peak plasma concentrations (700-1800 μg/L for a 150 mg dose and 1400-3600 μg/L for a 300 mg dose) occur from 0.5 to 3 hours following the dose. A concentration of 1000 μg/L is equivalent to 3 μmol/L; a dose of 300 mg is equivalent to 905 μmoles. Plasma concentrations 12 hours after administration are less than 10 μg/L. The elimination half-life is 1-2 hours, plasma clearance is 40-60 L/h, and the volume of distribution is 0.8-1.5 L/kg. Because of the short half-life and rapid clearance of nizatidine, accumulation of the drug would not be expected in individuals with normal renal function who take either 300 mg once daily at bedtime or 150 mg twice daily. Nizatidine exhibits dose proportionality over the recommended dose range.

The oral bioavailability of nizatidine is unaffected by concomitant ingestion of propantheline. Antacids consisting of aluminum and magnesium hydroxides with simethicone decrease the absorption of nizatidine by about 10%. With food, the AUC and C_{max} increase by approximately 10%.

In humans, less than 7% of an oral dose is metabolized as N2-monodesmethylnizatidine, an H_2-receptor antagonist, which is the principal metabolite excreted in the urine. Other likely metabolites are the N2-oxide (less than 5% of the dose) and the S-oxide (less than 6% of the dose).

More than 90% of an oral dose of nizatidine is excreted in the urine within 12 hours. About 60% of an oral dose is excreted as unchanged drug. Renal clearance is about 500 ml/min, which indicates excretion by active tubular secretion. Less than 6% of an administered dose is eliminated in the feces.

Moderate to severe renal impairment significantly prolongs the half-life and decreases the clearance of nizatidine. In individuals who are functionally anephric, the half-life is 3.5 to 11 hours, and the plasma clearance is 7-14 L/h. To avoid accumulation of the drug in individuals with clinically significant renal impairment, the amount and/or frequency of doses of nizatidine should be reduced in proportion to the severity of dysfunction (see DOSAGE AND ADMINISTRATION).

Approximately 35% of nizatidine is bound to plasma protein, mainly to α_1-acid glycoprotein. Warfarin, diazepam, acetaminophen, propantheline, phenobarbital, and propranolol did not affect plasma protein binding of nizatidine *in vitro*.

INDICATIONS AND USAGE

Nizatidine is indicated for up to 8 weeks for the treatment of active duodenal ulcer. In most patients, the ulcer will heal within 4 weeks.

Nizatidine is indicated for maintenance therapy for duodenal ulcer patients, at a reduced dosage of 150 mg hs after healing of an active duodenal ulcer. The consequences of continuous therapy with nizatidine for longer than 1 year are not known.

Nizatidine is indicated for up to 12 weeks for the treatment of endoscopically diagnosed esophagitis, including erosive and ulcerative esophagitis, and associated heartburn due to GERD.

Nizatidine is indicated for up to 8 weeks for the treatment of active benign gastric ulcer. Before initiating therapy, care should be taken to exclude the possibility of malignant gastric ulceration.

CONTRAINDICATIONS

Nizatidine is contraindicated in patients with known hypersensitivity to the drug. Because cross sensitivity in this class of compounds has been observed, H_2-receptor antagonists, including nizatidine, should not be administered to patients with a history of hypersensitivity to other H_2-receptor antagonists.

PRECAUTIONS

GENERAL

1. Symptomatic response to nizatidine therapy does not preclude the presence of gastric malignancy.
2. Because nizatidine is excreted primarily by the kidney, dosage should be reduced in patients with moderate to severe renal insufficiency (see DOSAGE AND ADMINISTRATION).
3. Pharmacokinetic studies in patients with hepatorenal syndrome have not been done. Part of the dose of nizatidine is metabolized in the liver. In patients with normal renal function and uncomplicated hepatic dysfunction, the disposition of nizatidine is similar to that in normal subjects.

LABORATORY TESTS

False-positive tests for urobilinogen with Multistix may occur during therapy with nizatidine.

CARCINOGENESIS, MUTAGENESIS, AND IMPAIRMENT OF FERTILITY

A 2 year oral carcinogenicity study in rats with doses as high as 500 mg/kg/day (about 80 times the recommended daily therapeutic dose) showed no evidence of a carcinogenic effect. There was a dose-related increase in the density of enterochromaffin-like (ECL) cells in the gastric oxyntic mucosa. In a 2 year study in mice, there was no evidence of a carcinogenic effect in male mice; although hyperplastic nodules of the liver were increased in the high-dose males as compared with placebo. Female mice given the high dose of nizatidine (2000 mg/kg/day, about 330 times the human dose) showed marginally statistically significant increases in hepatic carcinoma and hepatic nodular hyperplasia with no numerical increase seen in any of the other dose groups. The rate of hepatic carcinoma in the high-dose animals was within the historical control limits seen for the strain of mice used. The female mice were given a dose larger than the maximum tolerated dose, as indicated by excessive (30%) weight decrement as compared with concurrent controls and evidence of mild liver injury (transaminase elevations). The occurrence of a marginal finding at high dose only in animals given an excessive and somewhat hepatotoxic dose, with no evidence of a carcinogenic effect in rats, male mice, and female mice (given up to 360 mg/kg/day, about 60 times the human dose), and a negative mutagenicity battery are not considered evidence of a carcinogenic potential for nizatidine.

Nizatidine was not mutagenic in a battery of tests performed to evaluate its potential genetic toxicity, including bacterial mutation tests, unscheduled DNA synthesis, sister chromatid exchange, mouse lymphoma assay, chromosome aberration tests, and a micronucleus test.

In a 2-generation, perinatal and postnatal fertility study in rats, doses of nizatidine up to 650 mg/kg/day produced no adverse effects on the reproductive performance of parental animals or their progeny.

PREGNANCY, TERATOGENIC EFFECTS, PREGNANCY CATEGORY B

Oral reproduction studies in pregnant rats at doses up to 1500 mg/kg/day (9000 mg/m^2/day, 40.5 times the recommended human dose based on body surface area) and in pregnant rabbits at doses up to 275 mg/kg/day (3245 mg/m^2/day, 14.6 times the recommended human dose based on body surface area) have revealed no evidence of impaired fertility or harm to the fetus due to nizatidine. There are, however, no adequate and well-controlled studies in pregnant women. Because animal reproduction studies are not always predictive of human response, this drug should be used during pregnancy only if clearly needed.

NURSING MOTHERS

Studies conducted in lactating women have shown that 0 .1% of the administered oral dose of nizatidine is secreted in human milk in proportion to plasma concentrations. Because of the growth depression in pups reared by lactating rats treated with nizatidine, a decision should be made whether to discontinue nursing or discontinue the drug, taking into account the importance of the drug to the mother.

PEDIATRIC USE

Safety and effectiveness in pediatric patients have not been established.

GERIATRIC USE

Of the 955 patients in clinical studies who were treated with nizatidine, 337 (35.3%) were 65 and older. No overall differences in safety or effectiveness were observed between these and younger subjects. Other reported clinical experience has not identified differences in responses between the elderly and younger patients, but greater sensitivity of some older individuals cannot be ruled out.

This drug is known to be substantially excreted by the kidney, and the risk of toxic reactions to this drug may be greater in patients with impaired renal function. Because elderly patients are more likely to have decreased renal function, care should be taken in dose selection, and it may be useful to monitor renal function (see DOSAGE AND ADMINISTRATION).

DRUG INTERACTIONS

No interactions have been observed between nizatidine and theophylline, chlordiazepoxide, lorazepam, lidocaine, phenytoin, and warfarin. Nizatidine does not inhibit the cytochrome P-450-linked drug-metabolizing enzyme system; therefore, drug interactions mediated by inhibition of hepatic metabolism are not expected to occur. In patients given very high doses (3900 mg) of aspirin daily, increases in serum salicylate levels were seen when nizatidine, 150 mg bid, was administered concurrently.

ADVERSE REACTIONS

Worldwide, controlled clinical trials of nizatidine included over 6000 patients given nizatidine in studies of varying durations. Placebo-controlled trials in the US and Canada included over 2600 patients given nizatidine and over 1700 given placebo. Among the adverse events in these placebo-controlled trials, anemia (0.2% vs 0%) and urticaria (0.5% vs 0.1%) were significantly more common in the nizatidine group.

INCIDENCE IN PLACEBO-CONTROLLED CLINICAL TRIALS IN THE US AND CANADA

TABLE 5 lists adverse events that occurred at a frequency of 1% or more among nizatidine-treated patients who participated in placebo-controlled trials. The cited figures provide some basis for estimating the relative contribution of drug and nondrug factors to the side effect incidence rate in the population studied.

TABLE 5 *Incidence of Treatment-Emergent Adverse Events in Placebo-Controlled Clinical Studies in the US and Canada*

Body System / Adverse Event*	Percentage of Patients Reporting Event: Nizatidine (n=2694)	Placebo (n=1729)
Body as a Whole		
Headache	16.6%	15.6%
Abdominal pain	7.5%	12.5%
Pain	4.2%	3.8%
Asthenia	3.1%	2.9%
Back pain	2.4%	2.6%
Chest pain	2.3%	2.1%
Infection	1.7%	1.1%
Fever	1.6%	2.3%
Surgical procedure	1.4%	1.5%
Injury, accident	1.2%	0.9%
Digestive		
Diarrhea	7.2%	6.9%
Nausea	5.4%	7.4%
Flatulence	4.9%	5.4%
Vomiting	3.6%	5.6%
Dyspepsia	3.6%	4.4%
Constipation	2.5%	3.8%
Dry mouth	1.4%	1.3%
Nausea and vomiting	1.2%	1.9%
Anorexia	1.2%	1.6%
Gastrointestinal disorder	1.1%	1.2%
Tooth disorder	1.0%	0.8%
Musculoskeletal		
Myalgia	1.7%	1.5%
Nervous		
Dizziness	4.6%	3.8%
Insomnia	2.7%	3.4%
Abnormal dreams	1.9%	1.9%
Somnolence	1.9%	1.6%
Anxiety	1.6%	1.4%
Nervousness	1.1%	0.8%
Respiratory		
Rhinitis	9.8%	9.6%
Pharyngitis	3.3%	3.1%
Sinusitis	2.4%	2.1%
Cough, increased	2.0%	2.0%
Skin and Appendages		
Rash	1.9%	2.1%
Pruritus	1.7%	1.3%
Special Senses		
Amblyopia	1.0%	0.9%

* Events reported by at least 1% of nizatidine-treated patients are included.

A variety of less common events were also reported; it was not possible to determine whether these were caused by nizatidine.

Hepatic: Hepatocellular injury, evidenced by elevated liver enzyme tests (SGOT [AST], SGPT [ALT], or alkaline phosphatase), occurred in some patients and was possibly or probably related to nizatidine. In some cases there was marked elevation of SGOT, SGPT enzymes (greater than 500 IU/L) and, in a single instance, SGPT was greater than 2000 IU/L. The overall rate of occurrences of elevated liver enzymes and elevations to 3 times the upper limit of normal, however, did not significantly differ from the rate of liver enzyme abnormalities in placebo-treated patients. All abnormalities were reversible after discontinuation of nizatidine. Since market introduction, hepatitis and jaundice have been reported. Rare cases of cholestatic or mixed hepatocellular and cholestatic injury with jaundice have been reported with reversal of the abnormalities after discontinuation of nizatidine.

Cardiovascular: In clinical pharmacology studies, short episodes of asymptomatic ventricular tachycardia occurred in 2 individuals administered nizatidine and in 3 untreated subjects.

CNS: Rare cases of reversible mental confusion have been reported.

Endocrine: Clinical pharmacology studies and controlled clinical trials showed no evidence of antiandrogenic activity due to nizatidine. Impotence and decreased libido were reported with similar frequency by patients who received nizatidine and by those given placebo. Rare reports of gynecomastia occurred.

Hematologic: Anemia was reported significantly more frequently in nizatidine- than in placebo-treated patients. Fatal thrombocytopenia was reported in a patient who was treated with nizatidine and another H_2-receptor antagonist. On previous occasions, this patient had experienced thrombocytopenia while taking other drugs. Rare cases of thrombocytopenic purpura have been reported.

Integumental: Sweating and urticaria were reported significantly more frequently in nizatidine- than in placebo-treated patients. Rash and exfoliative dermatitis were also reported. Vasculitis has been reported rarely.

Hypersensitivity: As with other H_2-receptor antagonists, rare cases of anaphylaxis following administration of nizatidine have been reported. Rare episodes of hypersensitivity reactions (*e.g.*, bronchospasm, laryngeal edema, rash, and eosinophilia) have been reported.

Body as a Whole: Serum sickness-like reactions have occurred rarely in conjunction with nizatidine use.

Genitourinary: Reports of impotence have occurred.

Other: Hyperuricemia unassociated with gout or nephrolithiasis was reported. Eosinophilia, fever, and nausea related to nizatidine administration have been reported.

DOSAGE AND ADMINISTRATION

ACTIVE DUODENAL ULCER

The recommended oral dosage for adults is 300 mg once daily at bedtime. An alternative dosage regimen is 150 mg twice daily.

MAINTENANCE OF HEALED DUODENAL ULCER

The recommended oral dosage for adults is 150 mg once daily at bedtime.

GASTROESOPHAGEAL REFLUX DISEASE

The recommended oral dosage in adults for the treatment of erosions, ulcerations, and associated heartburn is 150 mg twice daily.

ACTIVE BENIGN GASTRIC ULCER

The recommended oral dosage is 300 mg given either as 150 mg twice daily or 300 mg once daily at bedtime. Prior to treatment, care should be taken to exclude the possibility of malignant gastric ulceration.

DOSAGE ADJUSTMENT FOR PATIENTS WITH MODERATE TO SEVERE RENAL INSUFFICIENCY

The dose for patients with renal dysfunction should be reduced as follows:

TABLE 6

Ccr	Dose
Active Duodenal Ulcer, GERD and Benign Gastric Ulcer	
20-50 ml/min	150 mg daily
<20 ml/min	150 mg every other day
Maintenance Therapy	
20-50 ml/min	150 mg every other day
<20 ml/min	150 mg every 3 days

Some elderly patients may have creatinine clearances of less than 50 ml/min, and, based on pharmacokinetic data in patients with renal impairment, the dose for such patients should be reduced accordingly. The clinical effects of this dosage reduction in patients with renal failure have not been evaluated.

HOW SUPPLIED

Axid Pulvules are available in:

150 mg: The 150 mg Axid Pulvules are imprinted with script "Lilly" and "3144" on the opaque dark yellow cap and "AXID 150 mg" on the opaque pale yellow body, using black ink.

300 mg: The 300 mg Axid Pulvules are imprinted with script "Lilly" and "3145" on the opaque brown cap and "AXID 300 mg" on the opaque pale yellow body, using black ink.

Storage: Store at controlled room temperature 20-25°C (68-77°F) in a tightly closed container.

PRODUCT LISTING - RATED THERAPEUTICALLY EQUIVALENT

Capsule - Oral - 150 mg

60's	$143.65	GENERIC, Mylan Pharmaceuticals Inc	00378-5150-91
60's	$143.79	GENERIC, Eon Labs Manufacturing Inc	00185-0150-60
100's	$238.30	GENERIC, Ivax Corporation	00172-5623-60

Capsule - Oral - 300 mg

30's	$140.80	GENERIC, Mylan Pharmaceuticals Inc	00378-5300-93
30's	$140.94	GENERIC, Eon Labs Manufacturing Inc	00185-0300-30
100's	$467.15	GENERIC, Ivax Corporation	00172-5624-60
100's	$469.80	GENERIC, Eon Labs Manufacturing Inc	00185-0300-01

PRODUCT LISTING - EQUIVALENTS NOT AVAILABLE

Capsule - Oral - 150 mg

1's	$1.63	AXID PULVULES, Lilly, Eli and Company	00002-3144-01
20's	$46.50	AXID PULVULES, Pd-Rx Pharmaceuticals	55289-0637-20
30's	$46.56	AXID PULVULES, Heartland Healthcare Services	61392-0357-30
30's	$58.91	AXID PULVULES, Allscripts Pharmaceutical Company	54569-2605-01
30's	$75.10	AXID PULVULES, Pharma Pac	52959-0366-30
31's	$50.42	AXID PULVULES, Lilly, Eli and Company	00002-3144-81
50's	$114.80	AXID PULVULES, Pharma Pac	52959-0366-50
60's	$93.12	AXID PULVULES, Heartland Healthcare Services	61392-0357-60
60's	$120.15	AXID PULVULES, Pharma Pac	52959-0366-60
60's	$122.42	AXID PULVULES, Physicians Total Care	54868-1130-01
60's	$132.29	AXID PULVULES, Lilly, Eli and Company	00002-3144-60
60's	$142.99	GENERIC, Watson Laboratories Inc	00591-3137-60
60's	$183.58	AXID PULVULES, Reliant Pharmaceuticals, Llc.	65726-0144-15
90's	$139.68	AXID PULVULES, Heartland Healthcare Services	61392-0357-90
100's	$245.05	GENERIC, Ivax Corporation	00172-5623-10
100's	$273.85	AXID PULVULES, Reliant Pharmaceuticals, Llc.	65726-0144-90
100's	$314.65	AXID PULVULES, Lilly, Eli and Company	00002-3144-33
120's	$243.65	AXID PULVULES, Physicians Total Care	54868-1130-02

Capsule - Oral - 300 mg

30's	$88.86	AXID PULVULES, Heartland Healthcare Services	61392-0358-30
30's	$125.37	AXID PULVULES, Physicians Total Care	54868-1131-01
30's	$142.99	GENERIC, Watson Laboratories Inc	00591-3138-30
30's	$179.93	AXID PULVULES, Lilly, Eli and Company	00002-3145-30
30's	$179.93	AXID PULVULES, Reliant Pharmaceuticals, Llc.	65726-0145-10
60's	$177.72	AXID PULVULES, Heartland Healthcare Services	61392-0358-60
90's	$266.58	AXID PULVULES, Heartland Healthcare Services	61392-0358-90
100's	$539.76	GENERIC, Par Pharmaceutical Inc	49884-0767-01

Norepinephrine Bitartrate *(001898)*

Categories: Cardiac arrest, adjunct; Hypotension; Shock; Pregnancy Category C; FDA Approved 1950 Jul
Drug Classes: Adrenergic agonists; Inotropes
Brand Names: Lavarterenol; **Levophed**
Foreign Brand Availability: Adrenor (India); Norpin (Korea)

DESCRIPTION

Norepinephrine (sometimes referred to as *l-arterenol/Levarterenol* or *l-norepinephrine*) is a sympathomimetic amine which differs from epinephrine by the absence of a methyl group on the nitrogen atom.

Norepinephrine bitartrate is (-)-α-(aminomethyl)-3,4-dihydroxybenzyl alcohol tartrate (1:1)(salt) monohydrate.

Levophed is supplied in sterile aqueous solution in the form of the bitartrate salt to be administered by intravenous infusion following dilution. Norepinephrine is sparingly soluble in water, very slightly soluble in alcohol and ether, and readily soluble in acids. Each ml of Levophed injection contains the equivalent of 1 mg base of norepinephrine bitartrate, sodium chloride for isotonicity, and not more than 2 mg of sodium metabisulfite as an antioxidant. It has a pH of 3-4.5. The air in the ampuls has been displaced by nitrogen gas.

CLINICAL PHARMACOLOGY

Norepinephrine bitartrate functions as a peripheral vasoconstrictor (alpha-adrenergic action) and as an inotropic stimulator of the heart and dilator of coronary arteries (beta-adrenergic action).

INDICATIONS AND USAGE

For blood pressure control in certain acute hypotensive states (*e.g.*, pheochromocytomectomy, sympathectomy, poliomyelitis, spinal anesthesia, myocardial infarction, septicemia, blood transfusion, and drug reactions).

As an adjunct in the treatment of cardiac arrest and profound hypotension.

CONTRAINDICATIONS

Norepinephrine bitartrate should not be given to patients who are hypotensive from blood volume deficits except as an emergency measure to maintain coronary and cerebral artery perfusion until blood volume replacement therapy can be completed. If norepinephrine bitartrate is continuously administered to maintain blood pressure in the absence of blood volume replacement, the following may occur: severe peripheral and visceral vasoconstriction, decreased renal perfusion and urine output, poor systemic blood flow despite "normal" blood pressure, tissue hypoxia, and lactate acidosis.

Norepinephrine bitartrate should also not be given to patients with mesenteric or peripheral vascular thrombosis (because of the risk of increasing ischemia and extending the area of infarction) unless, in the opinion of the attending physician, the administration of norepinephrine bitartrate is necessary as a life-saving procedure.

Cyclopropane and halothane anesthetics increase cardiac autonomic irritability and therefore seem to sensitize the myocardium to the action of intravenously administered epinephrine or norepinephrine. Hence, the use of norepinephrine bitartrate during cyclopropane and halothane anesthesia is generally considered contraindicated because of the risk of producing ventricular tachycardia or fibrillation.

The same type of cardiac arrhythmias may result from the use of norepinephrine bitartrate in patients with profound hypoxia or hypercarbia.

WARNINGS

Norepinephrine bitartrate should be used with extreme caution in patients receiving monoamine oxidase inhibitors (MAOI) or antidepressants of the triptyline or imipramine types, because severe, prolonged hypertension may result.

Norepinephrine bitartrate injection contains sodium metabisulfite, a sulfite that may cause allergic-type reactions including anaphylactic symptoms and life-threatening or less severe asthmatic episodes in certain susceptible people. The overall prevalence of sulfite sensitivity in the general population is unknown. Sulfite sensitivity is seen more frequently in asthmatic than in nonasthmatic people.

PRECAUTIONS

GENERAL

Avoid Hypertension

Because of the potency of norepinephrine bitartrate and because of varying response to pressor substances, the possibility always exists that dangerously high blood pressure may be produced with overdoses of this pressor agent. It is desirable, therefore, to record the blood pressure every 2 minutes from the time administration is started until the desired blood pressure is obtained, then every 5 minutes if administration is to be continued.

The rate of flow must be watched constantly, and the patient should never be left unattended while receiving norepinephrine bitartrate. Headache may be a symptom of hypertension due to overdosage.

Site of Infusion

Whenever possible, infusions of norepinephrine bitartrate should be given into a large vein, particularly an antecubital vein because, when administered into this vein, the risk of necrosis of the overlying skin from prolonged vasoconstriction is apparently very slight. Some authors have indicated that the femoral vein is also an acceptable route of administration. A catheter tie-in technique should be avoided, if possible, since the obstruction to blood flow around the tubing may cause stasis and increased local concentration of the drug. Occlusive vascular diseases (for example, atherosclerosis, arteriosclerosis, diabetic endarteritis, Buerger's disease) are more likely to occur in the lower than in the upper extremity. Therefore, one should avoid the veins of the leg in elderly patients or in those suffering from such disorders. Gangrene has been reported in a lower extremity when infusions of norepinephrine bitartrate were given in an ankle vein.

Extravasation

The infusion site should be checked frequently for free flow. Care should be taken to avoid extravasation of norepinephrine bitartrate into the tissues, as local necrosis might ensue due to the vasoconstrictive action of the drug. Blanching along the course of the infused vein, sometimes without obvious extravasation, has been attributed to vasa vasorum constriction with increased permeability of the vein wall, permitting some leakage.

This also may progress on rare occasions to superficial slough, particularly during infusion into leg veins in elderly patients or in those suffering from obliterative vascular disease. Hence, if blanching occurs, consideration should be given to the advisability of changing the infusion site at intervals to allow the effects of local vasoconstriction to subside.

IMPORTANT — ANTIDOTE FOR EXTRAVASATION ISCHEMIA:

To prevent sloughing and necrosis in areas in which extravasation has taken place, the area should be infiltrated as soon as possible with 10-15 ml of saline solution containing from 5-10 mg of phentolamine, an adrenergic blocking agent. A syringe with a fine hypodermic needle should be used, with the solution being infiltrated liberally throughout the area, which is easily identified by its cold, hard, and pallid appearance. Sympathetic blockade with phentolamine causes immediate and conspicuous local hyperemic changes if the area is infiltrated within 12 hours. Therefore, phentolamine should be given as soon as possible after the extravasation is noted.

CARCINOGENESIS, MUTAGENESIS, AND IMPAIRMENT OF FERTILITY

Studies have not been performed.

PREGNANCY CATEGORY C

Animal reproduction studies have not been conducted with norepinephrine bitartrate. It is also not known whether norepinephrine bitartrate can cause fetal harm when administered to a pregnant woman or can affect reproduction capacity. Norepinephrine bitartrate should be given to a pregnant woman only if clearly needed.

NURSING MOTHERS

It is not known whether this drug is excreted in human milk. Because many drugs are excreted in human milk, caution should be exercised when norepinephrine bitartrate is administered to a nursing woman.

PEDIATRIC USE

Safety and effectiveness in children has not been established.

DRUG INTERACTIONS

Cyclopropane and halothane anesthetics increase cardiac automatic irritability and therefore seem to sensitize the myocardium to the action of intravenously administered epinephrine or norepinephrine. Hence, the use of norepinephrine bitartrate during cyclopropane and halothane anesthesia is generally considered contraindicated because of the risk of producing ventricular tachycardia or fibrillation. The same type of cardiac arrhythmias may result from the use of norepinephrine bitartrate in patients with profound hypoxia or hypercarbia.

Norepinephrine bitartrate should be used with extreme caution in patients receiving monoamine oxidase inhibitors (MAOI) or antidepressants of the triptyline or imipramine types, because severe, prolonged hypertension may result.

ADVERSE REACTIONS

The following reactions can occur:

Body as a Whole: Ischemic injury due to potent vasoconstrictor action tissue hypoxia.
Cardiovascular System: Bradycardia, probably as a reflex result of a rise in blood pressure, arrhythmias.
Nervous System: Anxiety, transient headache.
Respiratory System: Respiratory difficulty.
Skin and Appendages: Extravasation necrosis at injection site.

Prolonged administration of any potent vasopressor may result in plasma volume depletion which should be continuously corrected by appropriate fluid and electrolyte replacement therapy. If plasma volumes are not corrected, hypotension may recur when norepinephrine bitartrate is discontinued, or blood pressure may be maintained at the risk of severe peripheral and visceral vasoconstriction (*e.g.,* decreased renal perfusion) with diminution in blood flow and tissue perfusion with subsequent tissue hypoxia and lactic acidosis and possible ischemic injury. Gangrene of extremities has been rarely reported.

Overdoses or conventional doses in hypersensitive persons (*e.g.,* hyperthyroid patients) cause severe hypertension with violent headache, photophobia, stabbing retrosternal pain, pallor, intense sweating, and vomiting.

DOSAGE AND ADMINISTRATION

Norepinephrine bitartrate injection is a concentrated, potent drug which must be diluted in dextrose containing solutions prior to infusion. An infusion of norepinephrine bitartrate should be given into a large vein. (See PRECAUTIONS.)

RESTORATION OF BLOOD PRESSURE IN ACUTE HYPOTENSIVE STATE

Blood volume depletion should always be corrected as fully as possible before any vasopressor is administered. When, as an emergency measure, intraaortic pressures must be maintained to prevent cerebral or coronary artery ischemia, norepinephrine bitartrate can be administered before and concurrently with blood volume replacement.

DILUENT

Norepinephrine bitartrate should be diluted in 5% dextrose injection or 5% dextrose and sodium chloride injections. These dextrose containing fluids are protection against significant loss of potency due to oxidation. **Administration in saline solution alone is not recommended.** Whole blood or plasma, if indicated to increase blood volume, should be administered separately (for example, by use of a Y-tube and individual containers if given simultaneously).

AVERAGE DOSAGE

Add a 4 ml ampul (4 mg) of norepinephrine bitartrate to 1000 ml of a 5% dextrose containing solution. Each 1 ml of this dilution contains 4 μg of the base of norepinephrine bitartrate. Give this solution by intravenous infusion. Insert a plastic intravenous catheter through a suitable bore needle well advanced centrally into the vein and securely fixed with adhesive tape, avoiding, if possible, a catheter tie-in technique as this promotes stasis. An IV drip chamber or other suitable metering device is essential to permit an accurate estimation of the rate of flow in drops per minute. After observing the response to an initial dose of 2-3 ml (from 8-12 μg of base) per minute, adjust the rate of flow to establish and maintain a low normal blood pressure (usually 80-100 mm Hg systolic) sufficient to maintain the circulation to vital organs. In previously hypertensive patients, it is recommended that the blood pressure should be raised no higher than 40 mm Hg below the preexisting systolic pressure. The average maintenance dose ranges from 0.5-1 ml per minute (from 2-4 μg of base).

HIGH DOSAGE

Great individual variation occurs in the dose required to attain and maintain an adequate blood pressure. In all cases, dosage of norepinephrine bitartrate should be titrated according to the response of the patient. Occasionally much larger or even enormous daily doses (as high as 68 mg base or 17 ampuls) may be necessary if the patient remains hypotensive, but occult blood volume depletion should always be suspected and corrected when present. Central venous pressure monitoring is usually helpful in detecting and treating this situation.

FLUID INTAKE

The degree of dilution depends on clinical fluid volume requirements. If large volumes of fluid (dextrose) are needed at a flow rate that would involve an excessive dose of the pressor agent per unit of time, a solution more dilute than 4 μg/ml should be used. On the other hand, when large volumes of fluid are clinically undesirable, a concentration greater than 4 μg/ml may be necessary.

DURATION OF THERAPY

The infusion should be continued until adequate blood pressure and tissue perfusion are maintained without therapy. Infusions of norepinephrine bitartrate should be reduced gradually, avoiding abrupt withdrawal. In some of the reported cases of vascular collapse due to acute myocardial infarction, treatment was required for up to 6 days.

ADJUNCTIVE TREATMENT IN CARDIAC ARREST

Infusions of norepinephrine bitartrate are usually administered intravenously during cardiac resuscitation to restore and maintain an adequate blood pressure after an effective heartbeat and ventilation have been established by other means. (Norepinephrine bitartrate's powerful beta-adrenergic stimulating action is also thought to increase the strength and effectiveness of systolic contractions once they occur.)

AVERAGE DOSAGE

To maintain systemic blood pressure during the management of cardiac arrest, norepinephrine bitartrate is used in the same manner as described under Restoration of Blood Pressure in Acute Hypotensive States.

Parenteral drug products should be inspected visually for particulate matter and discoloration prior to use, whenever solution and container permit.

PRODUCT LISTING - RATED THERAPEUTICALLY EQUIVALENT

Solution - Intravenous - 1 mg/ml

4 ml x 10	$109.84	GENERIC, Abbott Pharmaceutical	00074-7041-01

PRODUCT LISTING - EQUIVALENTS NOT AVAILABLE

Solution - Intravenous - 1 mg/ml

4 ml x 10	$130.80	GENERIC, Abbott Pharmaceutical	00074-1443-04

Norethindrone (001899)

Categories: Contraception; Pregnancy Category X; FDA Approved 1973 Jan; WHO Formulary
Drug Classes: Contraceptives; Hormones/hormone modifiers; Progestins
Brand Names: Dianor; Micronor; Nor-QD; Norethisterone; **Norlutin**; Primulut
Foreign Brand Availability: Aminor (Bahrain; Cyprus; Egypt; Iran; Iraq; Jordan; Kuwait; Lebanon; Libya; Oman; Qatar; Republic-of-Yemen; Saudi-Arabia; Syria; United-Arab-Emirates); Menzol (England); Micro-Novom (South-Africa); Micronovum (Austria; Germany; Switzerland); Nor-Ethis (Malaysia); Norcolut (Bahamas; Barbados; Belize; Bermuda; Curacao; Guyana; Hong-Kong; Jamaica; Malaysia; Netherland-Antilles; Surinam; Trinidad); Norelut (Indonesia); Noriday (Australia; Benin; Burkina-Faso; England; Ethiopia; Gambia; Ghana; Guinea; Ivory-Coast; Kenya; Liberia; Malawi; Mali; Mauritania; Mauritius; Morocco; Niger; Nigeria; Senegal; Seychelles; Sierra-Leone; Sudan; Tanzania; Tunia; Uganda; Zambia; Zimbabwe); Noriday 28 (New-Zealand); Norluten (France); Primolut N (Bahamas; Bahrain; Bangladesh; Barbados; Belize; Benin; Bermuda; Burkina-Faso; Curacao; Cyprus; Egypt; England; Ethiopia; Finland; Gambia; Ghana; Guinea; Guyana; Hong-Kong; India; Indonesia; Iran; Iraq; Ireland; Ivory-Coast; Jamaica; Japan; Jordan; Kenya; Kuwait; Lebanon; Liberia; Libya; Malawi; Malaysia; Mali; Mauritania; Mauritius; Morocco; Netherland-Antilles; Netherlands; Niger; Nigeria; Norway; Oman; Pakistan; Philippines; Qatar; Republic-of-Yemen; Saudi-Arabia; Senegal; Seychelles; Sierra-Leone; South-Africa; Sudan; Surinam; Switzerland; Syria; Tanzania; Thailand; Trinidad; Tunia; Uganda; United-Arab-Emirates; Zambia; Zimbabwe); Primolut-N (Korea); Shiton (Taiwan); Steron (Thailand); Styptin 5 (India); Sunolut (Malaysia); Utovlan (England)
Cost of Therapy: $44.05 (Contraception; Micronor; 0.35 mg; 1 tablet/day; 28 day supply)
$36.92 (Contraception; Nor-QD; 0.35 mg; 1 tablet/day; 28 day supply)

DESCRIPTION

Patients should be counseled that this product does not protect against HIV infection (AIDS) and other sexually transmitted diseases.

Micronor 28 Day Regimen: Each tablet contains 0.35 mg norethindrone. Inactive ingredients include D&C green no. 5, D&C yellow no. 10, lactose, magnesium stearate, povidone and starch.

CLINICAL PHARMACOLOGY

MODE OF ACTION

Norethindrone progestin-only oral contraceptives prevent conception by suppressing ovulation in approximately half of users, thickening the cervical mucus to inhibit sperm penetration, lowering the midcycle LH and FSH peaks, slowing the movement of the ovum through the fallopian tubes, and altering the endometrium.

PHARMACOKINETICS

Serum progestin levels peak about 2 hours after oral administration, followed by rapid distribution and elimination. By 24 hours after drug ingestion, serum levels are near baseline, making efficacy dependent upon rigid adherence to the dosing schedule. There are large variations in serum levels among individual users. Progestin-only administration results in lower steady-state serum progestin levels and a shorter elimination half-life than concomitant administration with estrogens.

INDICATIONS AND USAGE

INDICATIONS

Progestin-only oral contraceptives are indicated for the prevention of pregnancy.

EFFICACY

If used perfectly, the first-year failure rate for progestin-only oral contraceptives is 0.5%. However, the typical failure rate is estimated to be closer to 5%, due to late or omitted pills. TABLE 1 lists the pregnancy rates for users of all major methods of contraception.

TABLE 1 *Percentage of Women Experiencing an Unintended Pregnancy During the First Year of Typical Use and the First Year of Perfect Use of Contraception and the Percentage Continuing Use at the End of the First Year*

United States

Method (1)	% of Women Experiencing an Unintended Pregnancy Within the First Year of Use: Typical Use† (2)	Perfect Use‡ (3)	% of Women Continuing Use at 1 Year* (4)
Chance§	85%	85%	
Spermicides¤	26%	6%	40%
Periodic abstinence	25%		63%
Calendar		9%	
Ovulation method		3%	
Sympto-thermal¶		2%	
Post-ovulation		1%	
Withdrawal	19%	4%	
Cap**			
Parous women	40%	26%	42%
Nulliparous women	20%	9%	56%
Sponge			
Parous women	40%	20%	42%
Nulliparous women	20%	9%	56%
Diaphragm**	20%	6%	56%
Condom††			
Female	21%	5%	56%
Male	14%	3%	61%
Pill	5%		71%
Progestin only		0.5%	
Combined		0.1%	
IUD			
Progesterone T	2.0%	1.5%	81%
Copper T380A	0.8%	0.6%	78%
LNg 20	0.1%	0.1%	81%
Depo-Provera	0.3%	0.3%	70%
Norplant & Norplant-2	0.05%	0.05%	88%
Female sterilization	0.5%	0.5%	100%
Male sterilization	0.15%	0.10%	100%

Adapted from Trussel J. Contraceptive efficacy. In Hatcher RA, Trussel J, Stewart F, Cates W, Stewart GK, Kowal D, Guest F, Contraceptive Technology: Seventeenth Revised Edition. New York NY: Irvington Publishers, 1998, in press.
† Among *typical* couples who initiate use of a method (not necessarily for the first time), the percentage who experience an accidental pregnancy during the first year if they do not stop use for any other reason.
‡ Among couples who initiate use of a method (not necessarily for the first time) and who use it *perfectly* (both consistently and correctly), the percentage who experience an accidental pregnancy during the first year if they do not stop use for any other reason.
* Among couples attempting to avoid pregnancy, the percentage who continue to use a method for 1 year.
§ The percents becoming pregnant in columns (2) and (3) are based on data from populations where contraception is not used and from women who cease using contraception in order to become pregnant. Among such populations, about 89% become pregnant within 1 year. This estimate was lowered slightly (to 85%) to represent the percent who would become pregnant within 1 year among women now relying on reversible methods of contraception if they abandoned contraception altogether.
¤ Foams, creams, gels, vaginal suppositories, and vaginal film.
¶ Cervical mucus (ovulation) method supplemented by calendar in the pre-ovulatory and basal body temperature in the post-ovulatory phases.
** With spermicidal cream or jelly.
†† Without spermicides.

CONTRAINDICATIONS

Progestin-only oral contraceptives (POPs) should not be used by women who currently have the following conditions:

- Known or suspected pregnancy.
- Known or suspected carcinoma of the breast.
- Undiagnosed abnormal genital bleeding.
- Hypersensitivity to any component of this product.
- Benign or malignant liver tumors.
- Acute liver disease.

WARNINGS

Cigarette smoking increases the risk of serious cardiovascular disease. Women who use oral contraceptives should be strongly advised not to smoke.

Norethindrone does not contain estrogen and, therefore, this insert does not discuss the serious health risks that have been associated with the estrogen component of combined oral contraceptives (COCs). The health care provider is referred to the prescribing information of combined oral contraceptives for a discussion of those risks. The relationship between progestin-only oral contraceptives and these risks is not fully defined. The physician should remain alert to the earliest manifestation of symptoms of any serious disease and discontinue oral contraceptive therapy when appropriate.

ECTOPIC PREGNANCY

The incidence of ectopic pregnancies for progestin-only oral contraceptive users is 5 per 1000 woman-years. Up to 10% of pregnancies reported in clinical studies of progestin-only oral contraceptive users are extrauterine. Although symptoms of ectopic pregnancy should be watched for, a history of ectopic pregnancy need not be considered a contraindication to use of this contraceptive method. Health providers should be alert to the possibility of an ectopic pregnancy in women who become pregnant or complain of lower abdominal pain while on progestin-only oral contraceptives.

DELAYED FOLLICULAR ATRESIA/OVARIAN CYSTS

If follicular development occurs, atresia of the follicle is sometimes delayed and the follicle may continue to grow beyond the size it would attain in a normal cycle. Generally these enlarged follicles disappear spontaneously. Often they are asymptomatic; in some cases they are associated with mild abdominal pain. Rarely they may twist or rupture, requiring surgical intervention.

IRREGULAR GENITAL BLEEDING

Irregular menstrual patterns are common among women using progestin-only oral contraceptives. If genital bleeding is suggestive of infection, malignancy or other abnormal conditions, such nonpharmacologic causes should be ruled out. If prolonged amenorrhea occurs, the possibility of pregnancy should be evaluated.

CARCINOMA OF THE BREAST AND REPRODUCTIVE ORGANS

Some epidemiological studies of oral contraceptive users have reported an increased relative risk of developing breast cancer, particularly at a younger age and apparently related to duration of use. These studies have predominantly involved combined oral contraceptives and there is insufficient data to determine whether the use of POPs similarly increases the risk.

A meta-analysis of 54 studies found a small increase in the frequency of having breast cancer diagnosed for women who were currently using combined oral contraceptives or had used them within the past 10 years. This increase in the frequency of breast cancer diagnosis, within 10 years of stopping use, was generally accounted for by cancers localized to the breast. There was no increase in the frequency of having breast cancer diagnosed 10 or more years after cessation of use.

Women with breast cancer should not use oral contraceptives because the role of female hormones in breast cancer has not been fully determined.

Some studies suggest that oral contraceptive use has been associated with an increase in the risk of cervical intraepithealial neoplasia in some populations of women. However, there continues to be controversy about the extent to which such findings may be due to differences in sexual behavior and other factors. There is insufficient data to determine whether the use of POPs increases the risk of developing cervical intraepithelial neoplasia.

HEPATIC NEOPLASIA

Benign hepatic adenomas are associated with combined oral contraceptive use, although the incidence of benign tumors is rare in the US. Rupture of benign, hepatic adenomas may cause death through intraabdominal hemorrhage.

Studies have shown an increased risk of developing hepatocellular carcinoma in combined oral contraceptive users. However, these cancers are rare in the US. There is insufficient data to determine whether POPs increase the risk of developing hepatic neoplasia.

PRECAUTIONS

GENERAL

Patients should be counseled that this product does not protect against HIV infection (AIDS) and other sexually transmitted diseases.

PHYSICAL EXAMINATION AND FOLLOW-UP

It is considered good medical practice for sexually active women using oral contraceptives to have annual history and physical examinations. The physical examination may be deferred until after initiation of oral contraceptives if requested by the woman and judged appropriate by the clinician.

CARBOHYDRATE AND LIPID METABOLISM

Some users may experience slight deterioration in glucose tolerance, with increases in plasma insulin but women with diabetes mellitus who use progestin-only oral contraceptives do not generally experience changes in their insulin requirements. Nonetheless, prediabetic and diabetic women in particular should be carefully monitored while taking POPs.

Lipid metabolism is occasionally affected in that HDL, HDL2, and apolipoprotein A-I and A-II may be decreased; hepatic lipase may be increased. There is usually no effect on total cholesterol, HDL_3, LDL, or VLDL.

INTERACTIONS WITH LABORATORY TESTS

The following endocrine tests may be affected by progestin-only oral contraceptive use:

- Sex hormone-binding globulin (SHBG) concentrations may be decreased.
- Thyroxine concentrations may be decreased, due to a decrease in thyroid binding globulin (TBG).

CARCINOGENESIS

See WARNINGS.

PREGNANCY

Many studies have found no effects on fetal development associated with long-term use of contraceptive doses of oral progestins. The few studies of infant growth and development that have been conducted have not demonstrated significant adverse effects. It is nonetheless prudent to rule out suspected pregnancy before initiating any hormonal contraceptive use.

NURSING MOTHERS

No adverse effects have been found on breastfeeding performance or on the health, growth or development of the infant. Small amounts of progestin pass into the breast milk, resulting in steroid levels in infant plasma of 1-6% of the levels of maternal plasma.

PEDIATRIC USE

Safety and efficacy of norethindrone tablets have been established in women of reproductive age. Safety and efficacy are expected to be the same for postpubertal adolescents under the age of 16 and for users 16 years and older. Use of this product before menarche is not indicated.

FERTILITY FOLLOWING DISCONTINUATION

The limited available data indicate a rapid return of normal ovulation and fertility following discontinuation of progestin-only oral contraceptives.

HEADACHE

The onset or exacerbation of migraine or development of severe headache with focal neurological symptoms which is recurrent or persistent requires discontinuation of progestin-only contraceptives and evaluation of the cause.

INFORMATION FOR THE PATIENT

See the Detailed Patient Labeling which will be given with the prescription for detailed instruction.

Counseling Issues

The following points should be discussed with prospective users before prescribing progestin-only oral contraceptives:

- The necessity of taking pills at the same time every day, including throughout all bleeding episodes.
- The need to use a backup method such as condoms and spermicides for the next 48 hours whenever a progestin-only oral contraceptive is taken 3 or more hours late.
- The potential side effects of progestin-only oral contraceptives, particularly menstrual irregularities.
- The need to inform the clinician of prolonged episodes of bleeding, amenorrhea or severe abdominal pain.
- The importance of using a barrier method in addition to progestin-only oral contraceptives if a woman is at risk of contracting or transmitting STDs/HIV.

DRUG INTERACTIONS

The effectiveness of progestin-only pills is reduced by hepatic enzyme-inducing drugs such as the anticonvulsants phenytoin, carbamazepine, and barbiturates, and the antituberculosis drug rifampin. No significant interaction has been found with broad-spectrum antibiotics.

ADVERSE REACTIONS

Adverse reactions reported with the use of POPs include:

- Menstrual irregularity is the most frequently reported side effect.
- Frequent and irregular bleeding are common, while long duration of bleeding episodes and amenorrhea are less likely.
- Headache, breast tenderness, nausea, and dizziness are increased among progestin-only oral contraceptive users in some studies.
- Androgenic side effects such as acne, hirsutism, and weight gain occur rarely.

DOSAGE AND ADMINISTRATION

To achieve maximum contraceptive effectiveness, norethindrone must be taken exactly as directed.

One tablet is taken every day, at the same time. Administration is continuous, with no interruption between pill packs.

See the Detailed Patient Labeling which will be given with the prescription for detailed instruction.

HOW SUPPLIED

Micronor Tablets are available in a Dialpak Tablet Dispenser containing 28 green tablets (0.35 mg norethindrone).

Storage: Store at controlled room temperature (15-30°C; 59-86°F).

PRODUCT LISTING - RATED THERAPEUTICALLY EQUIVALENT

Tablet - Oral - 0.35 mg			
28 x 6	$221.52	GENERIC, Barr Laboratories Inc	00555-0344-58
Tablet - Oral - 5 mg			
50's	$75.85	GENERIC, Barr Laboratories Inc	00555-0211-10
50's	$84.28	AYGESTIN, Wyeth-Ayerst Laboratories	00046-0894-01
50's	$84.28	AYGESTIN, Esi Lederle Generics	59911-5894-01

PRODUCT LISTING - EQUIVALENTS NOT AVAILABLE

Tablet - Oral - 0.35 mg			
28 x 6	$221.52	GENERIC, Barr Laboratories Inc	00555-0715-58
28 x 6	$221.52	GENERIC, Watson Laboratories Inc	52544-0629-28
28 x 6	$264.30	ORTHO MICRONOR, Ortho Pharmaceutical Corporation-Advanced Care	00062-1411-16
28 x 6	$264.30	NOR-QD, Watson/Rugby Laboratories Inc	52544-0235-28
28's	$36.53	ORTHO MICRONOR, Allscripts Pharmaceutical Company	54569-4984-00
28's	$39.65	ORTHO MICRONOR, Janssen Pharmaceuticals	00062-1411-01

Norfloxacin *(001901)*

For related information, see the comparative table section in Appendix A.

Categories: Conjunctivitis, infectious; Gonorrhea; Infection, urinary tract; Prostatitis; Pregnancy Category C; FDA Approved 1986 Oct

Drug Classes: Antibiotics, quinolones; Anti-infectives, ophthalmic; Ophthalmics

Brand Names: Chibroxin; **Noroxin**

Foreign Brand Availability: Ambigram (Colombia); Amicrobin (Spain); Ampliron (Peru); Anquin (Israel); Apirol (Israel); Baccidal (Japan; Spain; Taiwan); Barazan (Germany); Bexinor (Singapore); B.G.B. Norflox (Thailand); Biofloxin (India); Chibroxine (France); Chibroxol (Netherlands; Switzerland); Effectsal (Singapore); Euroflox (Bahrain; Cyprus; Egypt; Iran; Iraq; Israel; Jordan; Kuwait; Lebanon; Libya; Oman; Philippines; Qatar; Republic-of-Yemen; Saudi-Arabia; Syria; United-Arab-Emirates); Floxacin (Mexico); Fluseminal (Greece); Foxinon (Thailand); Fulgram (Italy); Gonorcin (Thailand); Grenis (Peru); Gyrablock (Bahrain; Cyprus; Egypt; Iran; Iraq; Jordan; Kuwait; Lebanon; Libya; Oman; Qatar; Republic-of-Yemen; Saudi-Arabia; Singapore; Syria; United-Arab-Emirates); Hurusfec (Korea); Insensye (Australia); Janacin (Hong-Kong; Malaysia; Thailand); Lexinor (Bangladesh; Finland; Hong-Kong; India; Indonesia; Japan; Malaysia; Pakistan; Philippines; Sweden; Taiwan); Manoflox (Thailand); N-Flox (Peru); Noprose (Colombia); Norbactin (Benin; Burkina-Faso; Ethiopia; Gambia; Ghana; Guinea; Ivory-Coast; Kenya; Liberia; Malawi; Malaysia; Mali; Mauritania; Mauritius; Morocco; Niger; Nigeria; Philippines; Senegal; Seychelles; Sierra-Leone; Sudan; Tanzania; Thailand; Tunia; Uganda; Zambia; Zimbabwe); Norbactin Eye Drops (Benin; Burkina-Faso; Ethiopia; Gambia; Ghana; Guinea; India; Ivory-Coast; Kenya; Liberia; Malawi; Mali; Mauritania; Mauritius; Morocco; Niger; Nigeria; Senegal; Seychelles; Sierra-Leone; Sudan; Tanzania; Tunia; Uganda; Zambia; Zimbabwe); Norbiotic (Peru); Norflox (India); Norflox-AZU (Germany); Norflox Eye (India); Noritacin (Peru); Normax Eye Ear Drops (India); Norocin (Greece); Noroxin Oftalmico (Mexico); Noroxin Ophthalmic (Canada); Noroxine (France); Norpurisine (Korea); Oranor (Mexico); Orsanac (Ecuador); Proxinor (Thailand); Sefnor (Singapore); Snoffocin (Thailand); Sofasin (Greece); Trizolin (Malaysia); Urekacin (Korea); Urinex (Colombia); Urisold (Greece); Uritracin (Thailand); Urobacid (Indonesia; Philippines; Singapore); Uroctal (Bahrain; Costa-Rica; Cyprus; Dominican-Republic; Egypt; El-Salvador; Guatemala; Honduras; Hong-Kong; Iran; Iraq; Jordan; Kuwait; Lebanon; Libya; Oman; Panama; Qatar; Republic-of-Yemen; Saudi-Arabia; Syria; United-Arab-Emirates); Uroflox (India; Peru; Republic-Of-Yemen); Uroxacin (Argentina); UT-in (Slovenia); Utinor (England); Xacin (Thailand); Zoroxin (Austria; Belgium; Costa-Rica; Denmark; El-Salvador; Guatemala; Honduras; Nicaragua; Panama)

Cost of Therapy: $55.91 (Urinary Tract Infections; Noroxin; 400 mg; 2 tablets/day; 7 day supply)
$7.99 (Uncomplicated Gonorrhea; Noroxin; 400 mg; 2 tablets/day; 1 day supply)

OPHTHALMIC

DESCRIPTION

Chibroxin (norfloxacin ophthalmic solution) is a synthetic broad-spectrum antibacterial agent supplied as a sterile isotonic solution for topical ophthalmic use. Norfloxacin, a fluoroquinolone, is 1-ethyl-6-fluoro-1,4-dihydro-4-oxo-7-(1-piperazinyl)-3-quinolinecarboxylic acid. Its empirical formula is $C_{16}H_{18}FN_3O_3$.

Norfloxacin is a white to pale yellow crystalline powder with a molecular weight of 319.34 and a melting point of about 221°C. It is freely soluble in glacial acetic acid and very slightly soluble in ethanol, methanol and water.

Chibroxin ophthalmic solution 0.3% is supplied as a sterile isotonic solution. Each ml contains 3 mg norfloxacin. *Inactive Ingredients:* Disodium edetate, sodium acetate, sodium chloride, hydrochloric acid (to adjust pH) and water for injection. Benzalkonium chloride 0.0025% is added as preservative. The pH of Chibroxin is approximately 5.2 and the osmolarity is approximately 285 mOsmol/liter.

Norfloxacin, a fluoroquinolone, differs from quinolones by having a fluorine atom at the 6 position and a piperazine moiety at the 7 position.

CLINICAL PHARMACOLOGY

MICROBIOLOGY

Norfloxacin has *in vitro* activity against a broad spectrum of gram-positive and gram-negative aerobic bacteria. The fluorine atom at the 6 position provides increased potency against gram-negative organisms and the piperazine moiety at the 7 position is responsible for anti-pseudomonal activity.

Norfloxacin inhibits bacterial deoxyribonucleic acid synthesis and is bactericidal. At the molecular level three specific events are attributed to norfloxacin in *E. coli* cells:

1. Inhibition of the ATP-dependent DNA supercoiling reaction catalyzed by DNA gyrase.
2. Inhibition of the relaxation of supercoiled DNA.
3. Promotion of double-stranded DNA breakage.

There is generally no cross-resistance between norfloxacin and other classes of antibacterial agents.

Therefore, norfloxacin generally demonstrates activity against indicated organisms resistant to some other antimicrobial agents. When such cross-resistance does occur, it is probably due to decreased entry of the drugs into the bacterial cells. Antagonism has been demonstrated *in vitro* between norfloxacin and nitrofurantoin.

Norfloxacin has been shown to be active against most strains of the following organisms both *in vitro* and clinically in ophthalmic infections (see INDICATIONS AND USAGE):

Gram-Positive Bacteria Including: *Staphylococcus aureus, Staphylococcus epidermidis, Staphylococcus warnerii,* and *Streptococcus pneumoniae.*

Gram-Negative Bacteria Including: *Acinetobacter calcoaceticus, Aeromonas hydrophila, Haemophilus influenzae, Proteus mirabilis, Pseudomonas aeruginosa,* and *Serratia marcescens.*

Norfloxacin has been shown to be active *in vitro* against most strains of the following organisms; however, *the clinical significance of these data in ophthalmic infections is unknown.*

Gram-Positive Bacteria: *Bacillus cereus, Enterococcus faecalis* (formerly *Streptococcus faecalis*) and *Staphylococcus saprophyticus.*

Gram-Negative Bacteria: *Citrobacter diversus, Citrobacter freundii, Edwardsiella tarda, Enterobacter aerogenes, Enterobacter cloacae, Escherichia coli, Hafnia alvei, Haemophilus aegyptius (Koch-Weeks bacillus), Klebsiella oxytoca, Klebsiella pneumoniae, Klebsiella rhinoscleromatis, Morganella morganii, Neisseria gonorrhoeae, Proteus vulgaris, Providencia alcalifaciens, Providencia rettgeri, Providencia stuartii, Salmonella typhi, Vibrio cholerae, Vibrio parahemolyticus,* and *Yersinia enterocolitica.*

Other: *Ureaplasma urealyticum.*

Norfloxacin is not active against obligate anaerobes.

INDICATIONS AND USAGE

Norfloxacin ophthalmic solution is indicated for the treatment of conjunctivitis when caused by susceptible strains of the following bacteria:

Acinetobacter calcoaceticus, Aeromonas hydrophila*, Haemophilus influenzae, Proteus mirabilis*, Pseudomonas aeruginosa*, Serratia marcescens*, Staphylococcus aureus, Staphylococcus epidermidis, Staphylococcus warnerii*,* and *Streptococcus pneumoniae.*

*Efficacy for this organism was studied in fewer than 10 infections.

Appropriate monitoring of bacterial response to topical antibiotic therapy should accompany the use of norfloxacin ophthalmic solution.

CONTRAINDICATIONS

Norfloxacin ophthalmic solution is contraindicated in patients with a history of hypersensitivity to norfloxacin, or the other members of the quinolone group of antibacterial agents or any other component of this medication.

WARNINGS

NOT FOR INJECTION INTO THE EYE.

Serious and occasionally fatal hypersensitivity (anaphylactoid or anaphylactic) reactions, some following the first dose, have been reported in patients receiving systemic quinolone therapy. Some reactions were accompanied by cardiovascular collapse, loss of consciousness, tingling, pharyngeal or facial edema, dyspnea, urticaria, and itching. Only a few patients had a history of hypersensitivity reactions. Serious anaphylactoid or anaphylactic reactions require immediate emergency treatment with epinephrine. Oxygen, intravenous steroids and airway management, including intubation, should be administered as indicated.

PRECAUTIONS

GENERAL

As with other antibiotic preparations, prolonged use may result in overgrowth of nonsusceptible organisms, including fungi. If superinfection occurs, appropriate measures should be initiated. Whenever clinical judgment dictates, the patient should be examined with the aid of magnification, such as slit lamp biomicroscopy and, where appropriate, fluorescein staining.

There have been reports of bacterial keratitis associated with the use of multiple dose containers of topical ophthalmic products. These containers have been inadvertently contaminated by patients who, in most cases, had a concurrent corneal disease or a disruption of the ocular epithelial surface. (See Information for the Patient.)

INFORMATION FOR THE PATIENT

Patients should be instructed to avoid allowing the tip of the dispensing container to contact the eye or surrounding structures.

Patients should also be instructed that ocular preparations, if handled improperly or if the tip of the dispensing container contacts the eye or surrounding structures, can become contaminated by common bacteria known to cause ocular infections. Serious damage to the eye and subsequent loss of vision may result from using contaminated preparations (see General). If redness, irritation, swelling or pain persists or becomes aggravated, the patient should be advised to consult a physician.

Patients should also be advised that if they have ocular surgery or develop an intercurrent ocular condition (*e.g.*, trauma or infection), they should immediately seek their physician's advice concerning the continued use of the present multidose container.

Patients should be advised that norfloxacin may be associated with hypersensitivity reactions, even following a single dose, and to discontinue the drug at the first sign of a skin rash or other allergic reaction.

Patients should be advised not to wear contact lenses if they have signs and symptoms of bacterial conjunctivitis.

CARCINOGENESIS, MUTAGENESIS, AND IMPAIRMENT OF FERTILITY

No increase in neoplastic changes was observed with norfloxacin as compared to controls in a study in rats, lasting up to 96 weeks at doses 8-9 times the usual human oral dose [based on a standard patient weight of 50 kg. The usual oral dose of norfloxacin is 800 mg daily. One (1) drop of norfloxacin ophthalmic solution 0.3% contains about 1/6666 of this dose (0.12 mg).].

Norfloxacin was tested for mutagenic activity in a number of *in vivo* and *in vitro* tests. Norfloxacin had no mutagenic effect in the dominant lethal test in mice and did not cause chromosomal aberrations in hamsters or rats at doses 30-60 times the usual oral dose [based on a standard patient weight of 50 kg. The usual oral dose of norfloxacin is 800 mg daily. One (1) drop of norfloxacin ophthalmic solution 0.3% contains about 1/6666 of this dose (0.12 mg).]. Norfloxacin had no mutagenic activity *in vitro* in the Ames microbial mutagen test, Chinese hamster fibroblasts and V-79 mammalian cell assay. Although norfloxacin was weakly positive in the Rec-assay for DNA repair, all other mutagenic assays were negative including a more sensitive test (V-79).

Norfloxacin did not adversely affect the fertility of male and female mice at oral doses up to 33 times the usual human oral dose [based on a standard patient weight of 50 kg. The usual oral dose of norfloxacin is 800 mg daily. One (1) drop of norfloxacin ophthalmic solution 0.3% contains about 1/6666 of this dose (0.12 mg)].

PREGNANCY, TERATOGENIC EFFECTS, PREGNANCY CATEGORY C

Norfloxacin has been shown to produce embryonic loss in monkeys when given in doses 10 times the maximum human oral dose (400 mg bid) [based on a standard patient weight of 50 kg. The usual oral dose of norfloxacin is 800 mg daily. One (1) drop of norfloxacin ophthalmic solution 0.3% contains about 1/6666 of this dose (0.12 mg).], with peak plasma levels that are 2-3 times those obtained in humans. There has been no evidence of a teratogenic effect in any of the animal species tested (rat, rabbit, mouse, monkey) at 6-50 times the human oral dose. There are no adequate and well-controlled studies in pregnant women. Norfloxacin ophthalmic solution should be used during pregnancy only if the potential benefit justifies the potential risk to the fetus.

NURSING MOTHERS

It is not known whether norfloxacin is excreted in human milk following ocular administration. Because many drugs are excreted in human milk, and because of the potential for serious adverse reactions in nursing infants from norfloxacin, a decision should be made to discontinue nursing or to discontinue the drug, taking into account the importance of the drug to the mother (see ANIMAL PHARMACOLOGY).

PEDIATRIC USE

Safety and effectiveness in infants below the age of 1 year have not been established.

Although quinolones including norfloxacin have been shown to cause arthropathy in immature animals after oral administration, topical ocular administration of other quinolones to immature animals has not shown any arthropathy and there is no evidence that the ophthalmic dosage form of those quinolones has any effects on the weight-bearing joints.

GERIATRIC USE

No overall differences in safety or effectiveness have been observed between elderly and young patients.

DRUG INTERACTIONS

Specific drug interaction studies have not been conducted with norfloxacin ophthalmic solution. However, the systemic administration of some quinolones has been shown to elevate plasma concentrations of theophylline, interfere with the metabolism of caffeine, and enhance the effects of the oral anticoagulant warfarin and its derivatives. Elevated serum levels of cyclosporine have been reported with concomitant use of cyclosporine with norfloxacin. Therefore, cyclosporine serum levels should be monitored and appropriate cyclosporine dosage adjustments made when these drugs are used concomitantly.

ADVERSE REACTIONS

In clinical trials, the most frequently reported drug-related adverse reaction was local burning or discomfort. Other drug-related adverse reactions were conjunctival hyperemia, chemosis, corneal deposits, photophobia and a bitter taste following instillation.

ADDITIONAL CAUTIONARY INFORMATION

Norfloxacin is available as an oral dosage form in addition to the ophthalmic dosage form. The following adverse effects, while they have not been reported with the ophthalmic dosage form, have been reported with the oral dosage form. However, it should be noted that the usual dosage of oral norfloxacin (800 mg/day) contains 6666 times the amount in 1 drop of norfloxacin ophthalmic solution 0.3% (0.12 mg).

Convulsions have been reported in patients receiving oral norfloxacin. Convulsions, increased intracranial pressure, and toxic psychoses have been reported with other drugs in this class. Orally administered quinolones may also cause central nervous system (CNS) stimulation which may lead to tremors, restlessness, lightheadedness, confusion and hallucinations. If these reactions occur in patients receiving norfloxacin, the drug should be discontinued and appropriate measures instituted.

The effects of norfloxacin on brain function or on the electrical activity of the brain have not been tested. Therefore, as with the oral formulation, norfloxacin should be used with caution in patients with known or suspected CNS disorders, such as severe cerebral arteriosclerosis, epilepsy, and other factors which predispose to seizures.

The following adverse effects have been reported with norfloxacin tablets:

Hypersensitivity Reactions: Hypersensitivity reactions including anaphylactoid reactions, angioedema, arthralgia, arthritis, dyspnea, myalgia, urticaria, vasculitis.

Gastrointestinal: Hepatitis, jaundice, including cholestatic jaundice, pancreatitis, pseudomembranous colitis.

Hematologic: Hemolytic anemia, sometimes associated with glucose-6-phosphate dehydrogenase deficiency, leukopenia, neutropenia, thrombocytopenia.

Musculoskeletal: Possible exacerbation of myasthenia gravis, tendinitis, tendon rupture.

Nervous System/Psychiatric: Ataxia, CNS effects characterized as generalized seizures and myoclonus. Guillain-Barre syndrome, paresthesia, peripheral neuropathy, psychic disturbances including confusion, depression, psychotic reactions.

Renal: Interstitial nephritis, renal failure.

Skin: Erythema multiforme and Stevens-Johnson syndrome, exfoliative dermatitis, photosensitivity, rash, toxic epidermal necrolysis.

Special Senses: Diplopia, tinnitus, transient hearing loss.

Abnormal laboratory values observed with oral norfloxacin included elevation of ALT (SGPT) and AST (SGOT), alkaline phosphatase, BUN, serum creatinine, and LDH.

Please consult the norfloxacin tablets prescribing information for additional information concerning these and other adverse effects and other cautionary information.

DOSAGE AND ADMINISTRATION

The recommended dose in adults and pediatric patients (1 year and older) is 1 or 2 drops of norfloxacin ophthalmic solution applied topically to the affected eye(s) 4 times daily for up to 7 days. Depending on the severity of the infection, the dosage for the first day of therapy may be 1 or 2 drops every 2 hours during the waking hours.

ANIMAL PHARMACOLOGY

The oral administration of single doses of norfloxacin, 6 times the recommended human oral dose [based on a standard patient weight of 50 kg. The usual oral dose of norfloxacin is 800 mg daily. One (1) drop of norfloxacin ophthalmic solution 0.3% contains about 1/6666 of this dose (0.12 mg).], caused lameness in immature dogs. Histologic examination of the weight-bearing joints of these dogs revealed permanent lesions of the cartilage. Related drugs also produced erosions of the cartilage in weight-bearing joints and other signs of arthropathy in immature animals of various species.

HOW SUPPLIED

Chibroxin ophthalmic solution is a clear, colorless to light yellow solution.

Chibroxin ophthalmic solution 0.3% is supplied in a white, opaque, plastic Ocumeter ophthalmic dispenser with a controlled drop tip in bottles of 5 ml.

Storage: Store Chibroxin ophthalmic solution at room temperature, 15-30°C (59-86°F). Protect from light.

ORAL

DESCRIPTION

Noroxin (norfloxacin) is a synthetic, broad-spectrum antibacterial agent for oral administration. Norfloxacin, a fluoroquinolone, is 1-ethyl-6-fluoro-1,4-dihydro-4-oxo-7-(1-piperazinyl)-3-quinolinecarboxylic acid. Its empirical formula is $C_{16}H_{18}FN_3O_3$.

Norfloxacin is a white to pale yellow crystalline powder with a molecular weight of 319.34 and a melting point of about 221°C. It is freely soluble in glacial acetic acid, and very slightly soluble in ethanol, methanol and water.

Noroxin is available in 400 mg tablets. Each tablet contains the following inactive ingredients: cellulose, croscarmellose sodium, hydroxypropyl cellulose, hydroxypropyl methylcellulose, iron oxide, magnesium stearate, and titanium dioxide.

Norfloxacin, a fluoroquinolone, differs from non-fluorinated quinolones by having a fluorine atom at the 6 position and a piperazine moiety at the 7 position.

CLINICAL PHARMACOLOGY

In fasting healthy volunteers, at least 30-40% of an oral dose of norfloxacin is absorbed. Absorption is rapid following single doses of 200, 400 and 800 mg. At the respective doses, mean peak serum and plasma concentrations of 0.8, 1.5 and 2.4 µg/ml are attained approximately 1 hour after dosing. The presence of food and/or dairy products may decrease absorption. The effective half-life of norfloxacin in serum and plasma is 3-4 hours. Steady-state concentrations of norfloxacin will be attained within 2 days of dosing.

In healthy elderly volunteers (65-75 years of age with normal renal function for their age), norfloxacin is eliminated more slowly because of their slightly decreased renal function. Drug absorption appears unaffected. However, the effective half-life of norfloxacin in these elderly subjects is 4 hours.

The disposition of norfloxacin in patients with creatinine clearance rates greater than 30 ml/min/1.73 m^2 is similar to that in healthy volunteers. In patients with creatinine clearance rates equal to or less than 30 ml/min/1.73 m^2, the renal elimination of norfloxacin decreases so that the effective serum half-life is 6.5 hours. In these patients, alteration of dosage is necessary (see DOSAGE AND ADMINISTRATION). Drug absorption appears unaffected by decreasing renal function.

Norfloxacin is eliminated through metabolism, biliary excretion, and renal excretion. After a single 400 mg dose of norfloxacin, mean antimicrobial activities equivalent to 278, 773, and 82 µg of norfloxacin/g of feces were obtained at 12, 24, and 48 hours, respectively. Renal excretion occurs by both glomerular filtration and tubular secretion as evidenced by the high rate of renal clearance (approximately 275 ml/min). Within 24 hours of drug administration, 26-32% of the administered dose is recovered in the urine as norfloxacin with an additional 5-8% being recovered in the urine as six active metabolites of lesser antimicrobial potency. Only a small percentage (less than 1%) of the dose is recovered thereafter. Fecal recovery accounts for another 30% of the administered dose.

Two (2) to 3 hours after a single 400 mg dose, urinary concentrations of 200 µg/ml or more are attained in the urine. In healthy volunteers, mean urinary concentrations of norfloxacin remain above 30 µg/ml for at least 12 hours following a 400 mg dose. The urinary pH may affect the solubility of norfloxacin. Norfloxacin is least soluble at urinary pH of 7.5 with greater solubility occurring at pHs above and below this value. The serum protein binding of norfloxacin is between 10 and 15%.

The mean concentrations of norfloxacin in various fluids and tissues measured 1-4 hours post-dose after two 400 mg doses, unless otherwise indicated are listed in TABLE 1.

TABLE 1

Renal parenchyma	7.3 µg/g
Prostate	2.5 µg/g
Seminal fluid	2.7 µg/ml
Testicle	1.6 µg/g
Uterus/Cervix	3.0 µg/g
Vagina	4.3 µg/g
Fallopian tube	1.9 µg/g
Bile	6.9 µg/ml (after two 200 mg doses)

MICROBIOLOGY

Norfloxacin has *in vitro* activity against a broad range of gram-positive and gram-negative aerobic bacteria. The fluorine atom at the 6 position provides increased potency against gram-negative organisms, and the piperazine moiety at the 7 position is responsible for antipseudomonal activity.

Norfloxacin inhibits bacterial deoxyribonucleic acid synthesis and is bactericidal. At the molecular level, three specific events are attributed to norfloxacin in *E. coli* cells:

1. Inhibition of the ATP-dependent DNA supercoiling reaction catalyzed by DNA gyrase.
2. Inhibition of the relaxation of supercoiled DNA.
3. Promotion of double-stranded DNA breakage.

Resistance to norfloxacin due to spontaneous mutation *in vitro* is a rare occurrence (range: 10^{-9} to 10^{-12} cells). Resistant organisms have emerged during therapy with norfloxacin in less than 1% of patients treated. Organisms in which development of resistance is greatest are the following:

Pseudomonas aeruginosa, Klebsiella pneumoniae, Acinetobacter spp., and *Enterococcus* spp.

For this reason, when there is a lack of satisfactory clinical response, repeat culture and susceptibility testing should be done. Nalidixic acid-resistant organisms are generally susceptible to norfloxacin *in vitro;* however, these organisms may have higher minimum inhibitory concentrations (MICs) to norfloxacin than nalidixic acid-susceptible strains. There is generally no cross-resistance between norfloxacin and other classes of antibacterial agents. Therefore, norfloxacin may demonstrate activity against indicated organisms resistant to some other antimicrobial agents including the aminoglycosides, penicillins, cephalosporins, tetracyclines, macrolides, and sulfonamides, including combinations of sulfamethoxazole and trimethoprim. Antagonism has been demonstrated *in vitro* between norfloxacin and nitrofurantoin.

Norfloxacin has been shown to be active against most strains of the following microorganisms both *in vitro* and in clinical infections as described in INDICATIONS AND USAGE.

Gram-Positive Aerobes: *Enterococcus faecalis, Staphylococcus aureus, Staphylococcus epidermidis, Staphylococcus saprophyticus,* and *Streptococcus agalactiae.*

Gram-Negative Aerobes: *Citrobacter freundii, Enterobacter aerogenes, Enterobacter cloacae, Escherichia coli, Klebsiella pneumoniae, Neisseria gonorrhoeae, Proteus mirabilis, Proteus vulgaris, Pseudomonas aeruginosa,* and *Serratia marcescens.*

The following *in vitro* data are available, but their clinical significance is unknown.

Norfloxacin exhibits *in vitro* minimal inhibitory concentrations (MICs) of ≤4 µg/ml against most (≥90%) strains of the following microorganisms; however, the safety and effectiveness of norfloxacin in treating clinical infections due to these microorganisms have not been established in adequate and well-controlled clinical trials.

Gram-Negative Aerobes: *Citrobacter diversus, Edwardsiella tarda, Enterobacter agglomerans, Haemophilus ducreyi, Klebsiella oxytoca, Morganella morganii, Providencia alcalifaciens, Providencia rettgeri, Providencia stuartii, Pseudomonas fluorescens,* and *Pseudomonas stutzeri.*

Other: *Ureaplasma urealyticum.*

Norfloxacin is not generally active against obligate anaerobes.

Norfloxacin has not been shown to be active against *Treponema pallidum.* (See WARNINGS.)

Susceptibility Tests

Dilution Techniques

Quantitative methods are used to determine antimicrobial minimal inhibitory concentrations (MICs). These MICs provide estimates of the susceptibility of bacteria to antimicrobial compounds. The MICs should be determined using a standardized procedure. Standardized procedures are based on a dilution method[1] (broth, agar, or microdilution) or equivalent with standardized inoculum concentrations and standardized concentrations of norfloxacin powder. The MIC values should be interpreted according to the following criteria (see TABLE 2).

TABLE 2*

MIC (µg/ml)	Interpretation
≤4	Susceptible (S)
8	Intermediate (I)
≥16	Resistant (R)

* These interpretative criteria apply only to isolates from urinary tract infections. There are no established norfloxacin interpretive criteria for *Neisseria gonorrhoeae* or organisms isolated from other infection sites.

A report of "Susceptible" indicates that the pathogen is likely to be inhibited if the antimicrobial compound in the blood reaches the concentrations usually achievable. A report of "Intermediate" indicates that the result should be considered equivocal, and, if the microorganism is not fully susceptible to alternative, clinically feasible drugs, the test should be repeated. This category implies possible clinical applicability in body sites where the drug is physiologically concentrated or in situations where high dosage of drug can be used. This category also provides a buffer zone which prevents small uncontrolled technical factors from causing major discrepancies in interpretation. A report of "Resistant" indicates that the pathogen is not likely to be inhibited if the antimicrobial compound in the blood reaches the concentrations usually achievable; other therapy should be selected.

Standardized susceptibility test procedures require the use of laboratory control microorganisms to control the technical aspects of the laboratory procedures. Standard norfloxacin powder should provide the following MIC values (see TABLE 3).

TABLE 3

Organism	MIC range (µg/ml)
E. coli ATCC 25922	0.03-0.12
E. faecalis ATCC 29212	2-8
P. aeruginosa ATCC 27853	1-4
S. aureus ATCC 29213	0.5-2

Diffusion Techniques

Quantitative methods that require measurement of zone diameters also provide reproducible estimates of the susceptibility of bacteria to antimicrobial compounds. One such standardized procedure[2] requires the use of standardized inoculum concentrations. This procedure uses paper disks impregnated with 10 µg norfloxacin to test the susceptibility of microorganisms to norfloxacin. Reports from the laboratory providing results of the standard single-disk susceptibility test with a 10 µg norfloxacin disk should be interpreted according to the following criteria (see TABLE 4).

TABLE 4*

Zone Diameter (mm)	Interpretation
≥17	Susceptible (S)
13-16	Intermediate (I)
≤12	Resistant (R)

* These interpretative criteria apply only to isolates from urinary tract infections. There are no established norfloxacin interpretive criteria for *Neisseria gonorrhoeae* or organisms isolated from other infection sites.

Interpretation should be as stated above for results using dilution techniques. Interpretation involves correlation of the diameter obtained in the disk test with the MIC for norfloxacin.

As with standard dilution techniques, diffusion methods require the use of laboratory control microorganisms that are used to control the technical aspects of the laboratory procedures. For the diffusion techniques, the 10 µg norfloxacin disk should provide the following zone diameters in these laboratory test quality control strains (see TABLE 5).

TABLE 5

Organism	Zone Diameter (mm)
E. coli ATCC 25922	28-35
P. aeruginosa ATCC 27853	22-29
S. aureus ATCC 25923	17-28

INDICATIONS AND USAGE

Norfloxacin is indicated for the treatment of adults with the following infections caused by susceptible strains of the designated microorganisms:

Urinary Tract Infections:

Uncomplicated urinary tract infections (including cystitis) due to *Enterococcus faecalis, Escherichia coli, Klebsiella pneumoniae, Proteus mirabilis, Pseudomonas aeruginosa, Staphylococcus epidermidis, Staphylococcus saprophyticus, Citrobacter freundii**, *Enterobacter aerogenes**, *Enterobacter cloacae**, *Proteus vulgaris**, *Staphylococcus aureus**, or *Streptococcus agalactiae**.

Complicated urinary tract infections due to *Enterococcus faecalis, Escherichia coli, Klebsiella pneumoniae, Proteus mirabilis, Pseudomonas aeruginosa*, or *Serratia marcescens**.

Sexually Transmitted Diseases: (See WARNINGS.) Uncomplicated urethral and cervical gonorrhea due to *Neisseria gonorrhoeae*.

Prostatitis: Prostatitis due to *Escherichia coli*.

*Efficacy for this organism in this organ system was studied in fewer than 10 infections.

(See DOSAGE AND ADMINISTRATION for appropriate dosing instructions.)

Penicillinase production should have no effect on norfloxacin activity.

Appropriate culture and susceptibility tests should be performed before treatment in order to isolate and identify organisms causing the infection and to determine their susceptibility to norfloxacin. Therapy with norfloxacin may be initiated before results of these tests are known; once results become available, appropriate therapy should be given. Repeat culture and susceptibility testing performed periodically during therapy will provide information not only on the therapeutic effect of the antimicrobial agents but also on the possible emergence of bacterial resistance.

CONTRAINDICATIONS

Norfloxacin is contraindicated in persons with a history of hypersensitivity, tendinitis, or tendon rupture associated with the use of norfloxacin or any member of the quinolone group of antimicrobial agents.

WARNINGS

THE SAFETY AND EFFICACY OF ORAL NORFLOXACIN IN PEDIATRIC PATIENTS, ADOLESCENTS (UNDER THE AGE OF 18), PREGNANT WOMEN, AND NURSING MOTHERS HAVE NOT BEEN ESTABLISHED. (See PRECAUTIONS: Pediatric Use; Pregnancy, Teratogenic Effects, Pregnancy Category C; and Nursing Mothers.) The oral administration of single doses of norfloxacin, 6 times, based on a patient weight of 50 kg, the recommended human clinical dose (on a mg/kg basis), caused lameness in immature dogs. Histologic examination of the weight-bearing joints of these dogs revealed permanent lesions of the cartilage. Other quinolones also produced erosions of the cartilage in weight-bearing joints and other signs of arthropathy in immature animals of various species. (See ANIMAL PHARMACOLOGY.)

Convulsions have been reported in patients receiving norfloxacin. Convulsions, increased intracranial pressure, and toxic psychoses have been reported in patients receiving drugs in this class. Quinolones may also cause central nervous system (CNS) stimulation which may lead to tremors, restlessness, lightheadedness, confusion, and hallucinations. If these reactions occur in patients receiving norfloxacin, the drug should be discontinued and appropriate measures instituted.

The effects of norfloxacin on brain function or on the electrical activity of the brain have not been tested. Therefore, until more information becomes available, norfloxacin, like all other quinolones, should be used with caution in patients with known or suspected CNS disorders, such as severe cerebral arteriosclerosis, epilepsy, and other factors which predispose to seizures. (See ADVERSE REACTIONS.)

Serious and occasionally fatal hypersensitivity (anaphylactoid or anaphylactic) reactions, some following the first dose, have been reported in patients receiving quinolone therapy. Some reactions were accompanied by cardiovascular collapse, loss of consciousness, tingling, pharyngeal or facial edema, dyspnea, urticaria and itching. Only a few patients had a history of hypersensitivity reactions. If an allergic reaction to norfloxacin occurs, discontinue the drug. Serious acute hypersensitivity reactions may require immediate emergency treatment with epinephrine. Oxygen, intravenous fluids, antihistamines, corticosteroids, pressor amines, and airway management, including intubation, should be administered as indicated.

Pseudomembranous colitis has been reported with nearly all antibacterial agents, including norfloxacin, and may range in severity from mild to life-threatening. Therefore, it is important to consider this diagnosis in patients who present with diarrhea subsequent to the administration of antibacterial agents.

Treatment with antibacterial agents alters the normal flora of the colon and may permit overgrowth of clostridia. Studies indicate that a toxin produced by *Clostridium difficile* is one primary cause of "antibiotic-associated colitis".

After the diagnosis of pseudomembranous colitis has been established, therapeutic measures should be initiated. Mild cases of pseudomembranous colitis usually respond to drug discontinuation alone. In moderate to severe cases, consideration should be given to management with fluids and electrolytes, protein supplementation, and treatment with an antibacterial drug clinically effective against *C. difficile* colitis.

Ruptures of the shoulder, hand, and Achilles tendons that required surgical repair or resulted in prolonged disability have been reported with norfloxacin. Norfloxacin should be discontinued if the patient experiences pain, inflammation, or rupture of a tendon. Patients should rest and refrain from exercise until the diagnosis of tendinitis or tendon rupture has been confidently excluded. Tendon rupture can occur at any time during or after therapy with norfloxacin.

Norfloxacin has not been shown to be effective in the treatment of syphilis. Antimicrobial agents used in high doses for short periods of time to treat gonorrhea may mask or delay the symptoms of incubating syphilis. All patients with gonorrhea should have a serologic test for syphilis at the time of diagnosis. Patients treated with norfloxacin should have a follow-up serologic test for syphilis after 3 months.

PRECAUTIONS

GENERAL

Needle-shaped crystals were found in the urine of some volunteers who received either placebo, 800 mg norfloxacin, or 1600 mg norfloxacin (at or twice the recommended daily dose, respectively) while participating in a double-blind, crossover study comparing single doses of norfloxacin with placebo. While crystalluria is not expected to occur under usual conditions with a dosage regimen of 400 mg bid, as a precaution, the daily recommended dosage should not be exceeded and the patient should drink sufficient fluids to ensure a proper state of hydration and adequate urinary output.

Alteration in dosage regimen is necessary for patients with impaired renal function (see DOSAGE AND ADMINISTRATION).

Moderate to severe phototoxicity reactions have been observed in patients who are exposed to excessive sunlight while receiving some members of this drug class. Excessive sunlight should be avoided. Therapy should be discontinued if phototoxicity occurs.

Rarely, hemolytic reactions have been reported in patients with latent or actual defects in glucose-6-phosphate dehydrogenase activity who take quinolone antibacterial agents, including norfloxacin. (See ADVERSE REACTIONS.)

Quinolones, including norfloxacin, may exacerbate the signs of myasthenia gravis and lead to life threatening weakness of the respiratory muscles. Caution should be exercised when using quinolones, including norfloxacin, in patients with myasthenia gravis (see ADVERSE REACTIONS).

INFORMATION FOR THE PATIENT

Patients should be advised:

- To drink fluids liberally.
- That norfloxacin should be taken at least 1 hour before or at least 2 hours after a meal or ingestion of milk and/or other dairy products.
- That multivitamins or other products containing iron or zinc, antacids or didanosine chewable/buffered tablets or the pediatric powder for oral solution, should not be taken within the 2 hour period before or within the 2 hour period after taking norfloxacin. (See DRUG INTERACTIONS.)

- That norfloxacin can cause dizziness and lightheadedness and, therefore, patients should know how they react to norfloxacin before they operate an automobile or machinery or engage in activities requiring mental alertness and coordination.
- To discontinue treatment and inform their physician if they experience pain, inflammation, or rupture of a tendon, and to rest and refrain from exercise until the diagnosis of tendinitis or tendon rupture has been confidently excluded.
- That norfloxacin may be associated with hypersensitivity reactions, even following the first dose, and to discontinue the drug at the first sign of a skin rash or other allergic reaction.
- To avoid undue exposure to excessive sunlight while receiving norfloxacin and to discontinue therapy if phototoxicity occurs.
- That some quinolones may increase the effects of theophylline and/or caffeine. (See DRUG INTERACTIONS.)
- That convulsions have been reported in patients taking quinolones, including norfloxacin, and to notify their physician before taking this drug if there is a history of this condition.

LABORATORY TESTS

As with any potent antibacterial agent, periodic assessment of organ system functions, including renal, hepatic, and hematopoietic, is advisable during prolonged therapy.

CARCINOGENESIS, MUTAGENESIS, AND IMPAIRMENT OF FERTILITY

No increase in neoplastic changes was observed with norfloxacin as compared to controls in a study in rats, lasting up to 96 weeks at doses 8-9 times, based on a patient weight of 50 kg, the usual human dose (on a mg/kg basis).

Norfloxacin was tested for mutagenic activity in a number of *in vivo* and *in vitro* tests. Norfloxacin had no mutagenic effect in the dominant lethal test in mice and did not cause chromosomal aberrations in hamsters or rats at doses 30-60 times, based on a patient weight of 50 kg, the usual human dose (on a mg/kg basis). Norfloxacin had no mutagenic activity *in vitro* in the Ames microbial mutagen test, Chinese hamster fibroblasts and V-79 mammalian cell assay. Although norfloxacin was weakly positive in the Rec-assay for DNA repair, all other mutagenic assays were negative including a more sensitive test (V-79).

Norfloxacin did not adversely affect the fertility of male and female mice at oral doses up to 30 times, based on a patient weight of 50 kg, the usual human dose (on a mg/kg basis).

PREGNANCY, TERATOGENIC EFFECTS, PREGNANCY CATEGORY C

Norfloxacin has been shown to produce embryonic loss in monkeys when given in doses 10 times, based on a patient weight of 50 kg, the maximum daily total human dose (on a mg/kg basis). At this dose, peak plasma levels obtained in monkeys were approximately 2 times those obtained in humans. There has been no evidence of a teratogenic effect in any of the animal species tested (rat, rabbit, mouse, monkey) at 6-50 times, based on a patient weight of 50 kg, the maximum daily human dose (on a mg/kg basis). There are, however, no adequate and well controlled studies in pregnant women. Norfloxacin should be used during pregnancy only if the potential benefit justifies the potential risk to the fetus.

NURSING MOTHERS

It is not known whether norfloxacin is excreted in human milk.

When a 200 mg dose of norfloxacin was administered to nursing mothers, norfloxacin was not detected in human milk. However, because the dose studied was low, because other drugs in this class are secreted in human milk, and because of the potential for serious adverse reactions from norfloxacin in nursing infants, a decision should be made to discontinue nursing or to discontinue the drug, taking into account the importance of the drug to the mother.

PEDIATRIC USE

The safety and effectiveness of oral norfloxacin in pediatric patients and adolescents below the age of 18 years have not been established. Norfloxacin causes arthropathy in juvenile animals of several animal species. (See WARNINGS and ANIMAL PHARMACOLOGY.)

DRUG INTERACTIONS

Elevated plasma levels of theophylline have been reported with concomitant quinolone use. There have been reports of theophylline-related side effects in patients on concomitant therapy with norfloxacin and theophylline. Therefore, monitoring of theophylline plasma levels should be considered and dosage of theophylline adjusted as required.

Elevated serum levels of cyclosporine have been reported with concomitant use of cyclosporine with norfloxacin. Therefore cyclosporine serum levels should be monitored and appropriate cyclosporine dosage adjustments made when these drugs are used concomitantly.

Quinolones, including norfloxacin, may enhance the effects of the oral anticoagulant warfarin or its derivatives. When these products are administered concomitantly, prothrombin time or other suitable coagulation tests should be closely monitored.

Diminished urinary excretion of norfloxacin has been reported during the concomitant administration of probenecid and norfloxacin.

The concomitant use of nitrofurantoin is not recommended since nitrofurantoin may antagonize the antibacterial effect of norfloxacin in the urinary tract.

Multivitamins, or other products containing iron or zinc, antacids or sucralfate should not be administered concomitantly with, or within 2 hours of, the administration of norfloxacin, because they may interfere with absorption resulting in lower serum and urine levels of norfloxacin.

Didanosine chewable/buffered tablets or the pediatric powder for oral solution should not be administered concomitantly with, or within 2 hours of, the administration of norfloxacin, because these products may interfere with absorption resulting in lower serum and urine levels of norfloxacin.

Some quinolones have also been shown to interfere with the metabolism of caffeine. This may lead to reduced clearance of caffeine and a prolongation of its plasma half-life.

ADVERSE REACTIONS

SINGLE-DOSE STUDIES

In clinical trials involving 82 healthy subjects and 228 patients with gonorrhea, treated with a single dose of norfloxacin, 6.5% reported drug-related adverse experiences. However, the following incidence figures were calculated without reference to drug relationship.

The most common adverse experiences (>1.0%) were: Dizziness (2.6%), nausea (2.6%), headache (2.0%), and abdominal cramping (1.6%).

Additional reactions (0.3%-1.0%) were: Anorexia, diarrhea, hyperhidrosis, asthenia, anal/rectal pain, constipation, dyspepsia, flatulence, tingling of the fingers, and vomiting.

Laboratory adverse changes considered drug-related were reported in 4.5% of patients/subjects. *These laboratory changes were:* Increased AST (SGOT) (1.6%), decreased WBC (1.3%), decreased platelet count (1.0%), increased urine protein (1.0%), decreased hematocrit and hemoglobin (0.6%), and increased eosinophils (0.6%).

MULTIPLE-DOSE STUDIES

In clinical trials involving 52 healthy subjects and 1980 patients with urinary tract infections or prostatitis, treated with multiple doses of norfloxacin, 3.6% reported drug-related adverse experiences. However, the incidence figures below were calculated without reference to drug relationship.

The most common adverse experiences (>1.0%) were: Nausea (4.2%), headache (2.8%), dizziness (1.7%), and asthenia (1.3%).

Additional reactions (0.3%-1.0%) were: Abdominal pain, back pain, constipation, diarrhea, dry mouth, dyspepsia/heartburn, fever, flatulence, hyperhidrosis, loose stools, pruritus, rash, somnolence, and vomiting.

Less frequent reactions (0.1%-0.2%) included: Abdominal swelling, allergies, anorexia, anxiety, bitter taste, blurred vision, bursitis, chest pain, chills, depression, dysmenorrhea, edema, erythema, foot or hand swelling, insomnia, mouth ulcer, myocardial infarction, palpitation, pruritus ani, renal colic, sleep disturbances, and urticaria.

Abnormal laboratory values observed in these patients/subjects were: Eosinophilia (1.5%), elevation of ALT (SGPT) (1.4%), decreased WBC and/or neutrophil count (1.4%), elevation of AST (SGOT) (1.4%), and increased alkaline phosphatase (1.1%). Those occurring less frequently included increased BUN, increased LDH, increased serum creatinine, decreased hematocrit, and glycosuria.

POST MARKETING

The most frequently reported adverse reaction in post-marketing experience is rash.

CNS effects characterized as generalized seizures, myoclonus and tremors have been reported with norfloxacin (see WARNINGS). Visual disturbances have been reported with drugs in this class.

The following additional adverse reactions have been reported since the drug was marketed:

Hypersensitivity Reactions: Hypersensitivity reactions have been reported including anaphylactoid reactions, angioedema, dyspnea, vasculitis, urticaria, arthritis, arthralgia and myalgia (see WARNINGS).

Skin: Toxic epidermal necrolysis, Stevens-Johnson syndrome and erythema multiforme, exfoliative dermatitis, photosensitivity.

Gastrointestinal: Pseudomembranous colitis, hepatitis, jaundice including cholestatic jaundice and elevated liver function tests, pancreatitis (rare), stomatitis. The onset of pseudomembranous colitis symptoms may occur during or after antibacterial treatment. (See WARNINGS.)

Renal: Interstitial nephritis, renal failure.

Nervous System/Psychiatric: Peripheral neuropathy, Guillain-Barre syndrome, ataxia, paresthesia; psychic disturbances including psychotic reactions and confusion.

Musculoskeletal: Tendinitis, tendon rupture; exacerbation of myasthenia gravis (see PRECAUTIONS).

Hematologic: Neutropenia, leukopenia, hemolytic anemia, sometimes associated with glucose-6-phosphate dehydrogenase deficiency; thrombocytopenia.

Special Senses: Transient hearing loss (rare), tinnitus, diplopia, dysgeusia.

Other adverse events reported with quinolones include: Agranulocytosis, albuminuria, candiduria, crystalluria, cylindruria, dysphagia, elevation of blood glucose, elevation of serum cholesterol, elevation of serum potassium, elevation of serum triglycerides, hematuria, hepatic necrosis, symptomatic hypoglycemia, nystagmus, postural hypotension, prolongation of prothrombin time, and vaginal candidiasis.

DOSAGE AND ADMINISTRATION

Norfloxacin tablets should be taken at least 1 hour before or at least 2 hours after a meal or ingestion of milk and/or other dairy products. Multivitamins, other products containing iron or zinc, antacids containing magnesium and aluminum, sucralfate, or didanosine chewable/buffered tablets or the pediatric powder for oral solution, should not be taken within 2 hours of administration of norfloxacin. Norfloxacin tablets should be taken with a glass of water. Patients receiving norfloxacin should be well hydrated (see PRECAUTIONS).

NORMAL RENAL FUNCTION

The recommended daily dose of norfloxacin is as described in TABLE 6.

RENAL IMPAIRMENT

Norfloxacin may be used for the treatment of urinary tract infections in patients with renal insufficiency. In patients with a creatinine clearance rate of 30 ml/min/1.73 m^2 or less, the recommended dosage is one 400 mg tablet once daily for the duration given above. At this dosage, the urinary concentration exceeds the MICs for most urinary pathogens susceptible to norfloxacin, even when the creatinine clearance is less than 10 ml/min/1.73 m^2.

When only the serum creatinine level is available, the following formula (based on sex, weight, and age of the patient) may be used to convert this value into creatinine clearance. The serum creatinine should represent a steady state of renal function.

Males: [(weight in kg) × (140 - age)] ÷ [(72) × serum creatinine (mg/100 ml)]

Females: (0.85) × (above value)

TABLE 6

Infection Description	Unit Dose	Frequency	Duration
Urinary Tract			
Uncomplicated UTI's (cystitis) due to *E. coli, K. pneumoniae*, or *P. mirabilis*	400 mg	q12h	3 days
Uncomplicated UTI's due to other indicated organisms	400 mg	q12h	7-10 days
Complicated UTI's	400 mg	q12h	10-21 days
Sexually Transmitted Diseases			
Uncomplicated gonorrhea	800 mg	single dose	1 day
Prostatitis			
Acute or chronic	400 mg	q12h	28 days

ELDERLY

Elderly patients being treated for urinary tract infections who have a creatinine clearance of greater than 30 ml/min/1.73 m^2 should receive the dosages recommended under Normal Renal Function.

Elderly patients being treated for urinary tract infections who have a creatinine clearance of 30 ml/min/1.73 m^2 or less should receive 400 mg once daily as recommended under Renal Impairment.

ANIMAL PHARMACOLOGY

Norfloxacin and related drugs have been shown to cause arthropathy in immature animals of most species tested (see WARNINGS).

Crystalluria has occurred in laboratory animals tested with norfloxacin. In dogs, needle-shaped drug crystals were seen in the urine at doses of 50 mg/kg/day. In rats, crystals were reported following doses of 200 mg/kg/day.

Embryo lethality and slight maternotoxicity (vomiting and anorexia) were observed in cynomolgus monkeys at doses of 150 mg/kg/day or higher.

Ocular toxicity, seen with some related drugs, was not observed in any norfloxacin-treated animals.

HOW SUPPLIED

Noroxin tablets 400 mg are dark pink, oval shaped, film-coated tablets, coded "MSD 705" on one side and "NOROXIN" on the other.

Storage: Store at 25°C (77°F); excursions permitted to 15-30°C (59-86°F). Keep container tightly closed.

PRODUCT LISTING - EQUIVALENTS NOT AVAILABLE

Solution - Ophthalmic - 0.3%

5 ml	$22.54	CHIBROXIN, Merck & Company Inc	00006-3526-03

Tablet - Oral - 400 mg

4's	$12.48	NOROXIN, Southwood Pharmaceuticals Inc	58016-0658-04
14's	$54.09	NOROXIN, Allscripts Pharmaceutical Company	54569-0191-02
15's	$63.00	NOROXIN, Physicians Total Care	54868-0889-05
20's	$58.00	NOROXIN, Southwood Pharmaceuticals Inc	58016-0658-20
20's	$81.05	NOROXIN, Merck & Company Inc	00006-0705-20
20's	$83.61	NOROXIN, Physicians Total Care	54868-0889-01
40's	$166.04	NOROXIN, Physicians Total Care	54868-0889-03
100's	$339.91	NOROXIN, Roberts Pharmaceutical Corporation	54092-0097-52
100's	$399.35	NOROXIN, Merck & Company Inc	00006-0705-68

Norgestrel *(001902)*

Categories: Contraception; Pregnancy Category X; FDA Approved 1973 Oct
Drug Classes: Contraceptives; Hormones/hormone modifiers; Progestins
Brand Names: Ovrette
Foreign Brand Availability: Neogest (England)
Cost of Therapy: $35.95 (Contraception; Ovrette; 0.75 mg; 1 tablet/day; 28 day supply)

DESCRIPTION

Each Ovrette tablet contains 0.075 mg of norgestrel (*dl*-13-beta- ethyl-17-alpha-ethinyl-17-beta-hydroxygon-4-en-3-one). The inactive ingredients present are cellulose, FD&C Yellow 5, lactose, magnesium stearate, and polacrilin potassium.

Each Ovrette tablet contains 0.075 mg of a single active steroid ingredient, norgestrel, a totally synthetic progestogen. The available data suggest that the d(-)enantiomeric form of norgestrel is the biologically active portion. This form amounts to 0.0375 mg per Ovrette tablet.

For prescribing information refer to Ethinyl Estradiol; Norgestrel.

HOW SUPPLIED

Ovrette tablets (norgestrel tablets) are available in containers of 28 yellow, round tablets marked "Wyeth" and "62".

PRODUCT LISTING - EQUIVALENTS NOT AVAILABLE

Tablet - Oral - 0.075 mg

28 x 6	$215.70	OVRETTE, Wyeth-Ayerst Laboratories	00008-0062-01

Nortriptyline Hydrochloride *(001903)*

For related information, see the comparative table section in Appendix A.

Categories: Depression; FDA Approved 1964 Nov; Pregnancy Category D
Drug Classes: Antidepressants, tricyclic
Brand Names: Pamelor
Foreign Brand Availability: Allegron (Australia; Belgium; England); Ateben (Argentina); Aventyl (Canada; England; Ireland; Malaysia; South-Africa); Kareon (Argentina); Martimil (Spain); Noritren (Denmark; Finland; Italy; Japan; Norway; Sweden); Norline (Thailand); Norpress (New-Zealand); Nortrilen (Austria; Bahrain; Belgium; Benin; Bulgaria; Burkina-Faso; Cyprus; Egypt; Ethiopia; Gambia; Germany; Ghana; Greece; Guinea; Hong-Kong; Iran; Iraq; Israel; Ivory-Coast; Jordan; Kenya; Kuwait; Lebanon; Liberia; Libya; Malawi; Mali; Mauritania; Mauritius; Morocco; Netherlands; Niger; Nigeria; Oman; Qatar; Republic-of-Yemen; Saudi-Arabia; Senegal; Seychelles; Sierra-Leone; South-Africa; Sudan; Switzerland; Syria; Tanzania; Thailand; Tunia; Uganda; United-Arab-Emirates; Zambia; Zimbabwe); Nortrix (Portugal); Nortyline (Thailand); Norventyl (Canada); Ortrip (Thailand); Paxtibi (Spain); Sensaval (Sweden); Sensival (India; Japan); Vividyl (Italy)
Cost of Therapy: $306.58 (Depression; Pamelor; 25 mg; 3 capsules/day; 30 day supply)
$6.26 (Depression; Generic Capsule; 25 mg; 3 capsules/day; 30 day supply)

DESCRIPTION

Nortriptyline hydrochloride is 1-propanamine, 3-(10,11-dihydro-5*H*-dibenzo[a,d]cyclo-hepten-5-ylidene)-N-methyl-, hydrochloride.

PAMELOR CAPSULES

10, 25, 50, and 75 mg Capsules

Active ingredient: Nortriptyline hydrochloride..

10, 25, and 75 mg Capsules

Inactive ingredients: D&C yellow no. 10, FD&C yellow no. 6, gelatin, silicone fluid, sodium lauryl sulfate, starch, and titanium dioxide.

May also include: Benzyl alcohol, butylparaben, edetate calcium disodium, methylparaben, propylparaben, silicon dioxide, and sodium propionate.

50 mg Capsules

Inactive indredients: Gelatin, silicone fluid, sodium lauryl sulfate, starch, and titanium dioxide.

May also include: Benzyl alcohol, butylparaben, edetate calcium disodium, methylparaben, propylparaben, silicon dioxide, sodium bisulfite (capsule shell only), and sodium propionate.

PAMELOR SOLUTION

Active ingredient: Nortriptyline hydrochloride.

Inactive ingredients: Alcohol, benzoic acid, flavoring, purified water, and sorbitol.

CLINICAL PHARMACOLOGY

The mechanism of mood elevation by tricyclic antidepressants is at present unknown. Nortriptyline HCl is not a monoamine oxidase inhibitor. It inhibits the activity of such diverse agents as histamine, 5-hydroxytryptamine, and acetylcholine. It increases the pressor effect of norepinephrine but blocks the pressor response of phenethylamine. Studies suggest that nortriptyline HCl interferes with the transport, release, and storage of catecholamines. Operant conditioning techniques in rats and pigeons suggest that nortriptyline HCl has a combination of stimulant and depressant properties.

INDICATIONS AND USAGE

Nortriptyline HCl is indicated for the relief of symptoms of depression. Endogenous depressions are more likely to be alleviated than are other depressive states.

NON-FDA APPROVED INDICATIONS

Nortriptyline has also been used in the treatment of neuropathic pain, chronic pain, and panic disorder although these uses are not explicitly approved by the FDA. Additionally, some investigators have suggested a role for nortriptyline in the treatment of chronic tinnitus and the depression often associated with chronic tinnitus.

CONTRAINDICATIONS

The use of nortriptyline HCl or other tricyclic antidepressants concurrently with a monoamine oxidase (MAO) inhibitor is contraindicated. Hyperpyretic crises, severe convulsions, and fatalities have occurred when similar tricyclic antidepressants were used in such combinations. It is advisable to have discontinued the MAO inhibitor for at least 2 weeks before treatment with nortriptyline HCl is started. Patients hypersensitive to nortriptyline HCl should not be given the drug.

Cross-sensitivity between nortriptyline HCl and other dibenzazepines is a possibility.

Nortriptyline HCl is contraindicated during the acute recovery period after myocardial infarction.

WARNINGS

Patients with cardiovascular disease should be given nortriptyline HCl only under close supervision because of the tendency of the drug to produce sinus tachycardia and to prolong the conduction time. Myocardial infarction, arrhythmia, and strokes have occurred. The antihypertensive action of guanethidine and similar agents may be blocked. Because of its anticholinergic activity, nortriptyline HCl should be used with great caution in patients who have glaucoma or a history of urinary retention. Patients with a history of seizures should be followed closely when nortriptyline HCl is administered, in as much as this drug is known to lower the convulsive threshold. Great care is required if nortriptyline HCl is given to hyperthyroid patients or to those receiving thyroid medication, since cardiac arrhythmias may develop.

Nortriptyline HCl may impair the mental and/or physical abilities required for the performance of hazardous tasks, such as operating machinery or driving a car; therefore, the patient should be warned accordingly.

Excessive consumption of alcohol in combination with nortriptyline therapy may have a potentiating effect, which may lead to the danger of increased suicidal attempts or overdosage, especially in patients with histories of emotional disturbances or suicidal ideation.

The concomitant administration of quinidine and nortriptyline may result in a significantly longer plasma half-life, higher AUC, and lower clearance of nortriptyline.

USE IN PREGNANCY

Safe use of nortriptyline HCl during pregnancy and lactation has not been established; therefore, when the drug is administered to pregnant patients, nursing mothers, or women of childbearing potential, the potential benefits must be weighed against the possible hazards. Animal reproduction studies have yielded inconclusive results.

PEDIATRIC USE

This drug is not recommended for use in children, since safety and effectiveness in the pediatric age group have not been established.

PRECAUTIONS

The use of nortriptyline HCl in schizophrenic patients may result in an exacerbation of the psychosis or may activate latent schizophrenic symptoms. If the drug is given to overactive or agitated patients, increased anxiety and agitation may occur. In manic-depressive patients, nortriptyline HCl may cause symptoms of the manic phase to emerge.

Troublesome patient hostility may be aroused by the use of nortriptyline HCl. Epileptiform seizures may accompany its administration, as is true of other drugs of its class.

When it is essential, the drug may be administered with electroconvulsive therapy, although the hazards may be increased. Discontinue the drug for several days, if possible, prior to elective surgery.

The possibility of a suicidal attempt by a depressed patient remains after the initiation of treatment; in this regard, it is important that the least possible quantity of drug be dispensed at any given time.

Both elevation and lowering of blood sugar levels have been reported.

GERIATRIC USE

Glinical studies of nortriptyline HCl did not include sufficient numbers of subjects aged 65 and over to determine whether they respond differently from younger subjects. Other reported clinical experience indicates that, as with other tricyclic antidepressants, hepatic adverse events (characterized mainly by jaundice and elevated liver enzymes) are observed very rarely in geriatric patients and deaths associated with cholestatic liver damage have been reported in isolated instances. Cardiovascular function, particularly arrhythmias and fluctuations in blood pressure, should be monitored. There have also been reports of confusional states following trycyclic antidepressant administration in the elderly. Higher plasma concentrations of the active nortriptyline metabolite, 10-hydroxynortriptyline, have also been reported in elderly patients. As with other trycyclic antidepressants, dose selection for an elderly patient should usually be limited to the smallest effective total daily dose (see DOSAGE AND ADMINISTRATION).

DRUG INTERACTIONS

Administration of reserpine during therapy with a tricyclic antidepressant has been shown to produce a "stimulating" effect in some depressed patients.

Close supervision and careful adjustment of the dosage are required when nortriptyline HCl is used with other anticholinergic drugs and sympathomimetic drugs.

Concurrent administration of cimetidine and tricyclic antidepressants can produce clinically significant increases in the plasma concentrations of the tricyclic antidepressant. The patient should be informed that the response to alcohol may be exaggerated.

A case of significant hypoglycemia has been reported in a Type II diabetic patient maintained on chlorpropamide (250 mg/day), after the addition of nortriptyline (125 mg/day).

DRUGS METABOLIZED BY P450 2D6

The biochemical activity of the drug metabolizing isozyme cytochrome P450 2D6 (debrisoquin hydroxylase) is reduced in a subset of the Caucasian population (about 7-10% of Caucasians are so called "poor metabolizers"); reliable estimates of the prevalence of reduced P450 2D6 isozyme activity among Asian, African and other populations are not yet available. Poor metabolizers have higher than expected plasma concentrations of tricyclic antidepressants (TCAs) when given usual doses. Depending on the fraction of drug metabolized by P450 2D6, the increase in plasma concentration may be small, or quite large (8-fold increase in plasma AUC of the TCA).

In addition, certain drugs inhibit the activity of this isozyme and make normal metabolizers resemble poor metabolizers. An individual who is stable on a given dose of TCA may become abruptly toxic when given one of these inhibiting drugs as concomitant therapy. The drugs that inhibit cytochrome P450 2D6 include some that are not metabolized by the enzyme (quinidine; cimetidine) and many that are substrates of P450 2D6 (many other antidepressants, phenothiazines, and the Type 1C antiarrhythmic propafenone and flecainide). While all the selective serotonin reuptake inhibitors (SSRIs), *e.g.*, fluoxetine, sertraline, and paroxetine, inhibit P450 2D6, they may vary in the extent of inhibition. The extent to which SSRI TCA interactions may pose clinical problems will depend on the degree of inhibition and the pharmacokinetics of the SSRI involved. Nevertheless, caution is indicated in the co-administration of TCAs with any of the SSRIs and also in switching from one class to the other. Of particular importance, sufficient time must elapse before initiating TCA treatment in a patient being withdrawn from fluoxetine, given the long half-life of the parent and active metabolite (at least 5 weeks may be necessary).

Concomitant use of tricyclic antidepressants with drugs that can inhibit cytochrome P450 2D6 may require lower doses than usually prescribed for either the tricyclic antidepressant or the other drug. Furthermore, whenever one of these other drugs is withdrawn from co-therapy, an increased dose of tricyclic antidepressant may be required. It is desirable to monitor TCA plasma levels whenever a TCA is going to be co-administered with another drug known to be an inhibitor of P450 2D6.

ADVERSE REACTIONS

Note: Included in the following list are a few adverse reactions that have not been reported with this specific drug. However, the pharmacologic similarities among the tricyclic antidepressant drugs require that each of the reactions be considered when nortriptyline is administered.

Cardiovascular: Hypotension, hypertension, tachycardia, palpitation, myocardial infarction, arrhythmias, heart block, stroke.

Psychiatric: Confusional states (especially in the elderly) with hallucinations, disorientation, delusions; anxiety, restlessness, agitation; insomnia, panic, nightmares; hypomania; exacerbation of psychosis.

Neurologic: Numbness, tingling, paresthesias of extremities; incoordination, ataxia, tremors; peripheral neuropathy; extrapyramidal symptoms; seizures, alteration in EEG patterns; tinnitus.

Anticholinergic: Dry mouth and, rarely, associated sublingual adenitis; blurred vision, disturbance of accommodation, mydriasis; constipation, paralytic ileus; urinary retention, delayed micturition, dilation of the urinary tract.

Allergic: Skin rash, petechiae, urticaria, itching, photosensitization (avoid excessive exposure to sunlight); edema (general or of face and tongue), drug fever, cross-sensitivity with other tricyclic drugs.

Hematologic: Bone marrow depression, including agranulocytosis; eosinophilia; purpura; thrombocytopenia.

Gastrointestinal: Nausea and vomiting, anorexia, epigastric distress, diarrhea, peculiar taste, stomatitis, abdominal cramps, black tongue.

Endocrine: Gynecomastia in the male, breast enlargement and galactorrhea in the female; increased or decreased libido, impotence; testicular swelling; elevation or depression of blood sugar levels; syndrome of inappropriate ADH (antidiuretic hormone) secretion.

Other: Jaundice (simulating obstructive), altered liver function; weight gain or loss; perspiration; flushing; urinary frequency, nocturia; drowsiness, dizziness, weakness, fatigue; headache; parotid swelling; alopecia.

WITHDRAWAL SYMPTOMS

Though these are not indicative of addiction, abrupt cessation of treatment after prolonged therapy may produce nausea, headache, and malaise.

DOSAGE AND ADMINISTRATION

Nortriptyline HCl is not recommended for children.

Nortriptyline HCl is administered orally in the form of capsules or liquid. Lower than usual dosages are recommended for elderly patients and adolescents. Lower dosages are also recommended for outpatients than for hospitalized patients who will be under close supervision. The physician should initiate dosage at a low level and increase it gradually, noting carefully the clinical response and any evidence of intolerance. Following remission, maintenance medication may be required for a longer period of time at the lowest dose that will maintain remission.

If a patient develops minor side effects, the dosage should be reduced. The drug should be discontinued promptly if adverse effects of a serious nature or allergic manifestations occur.

Usual Adult Dose: 25 mg three or four times daily; dosage should begin at a low level and be increased as required. As an alternate regimen, the total daily dosage may be given once a day. When doses above 100 mg daily are administered, plasma levels of nortriptyline should be monitored and maintained in the optimum range of 50-150 ng/ml. Doses above 150 mg/day are not recommended.

Elderly and Adolescent Patients: 30-50 mg/day, in divided doses, or the total daily dosage may be given once a day.

HOW SUPPLIED

PAMELOR CAPSULES

Pamelor (nortirptyline HCl) capsules equivalent to 10, 25, 50 or 75 mg of base are available.

10 mg: Branded "SANDOZ" on one half, "PAMELOR 10 mg" other half.
25 mg: Branded "SANDOZ" on one half, "PAMELOR 25 mg" other half.
50 mg: Branded "SANDOZ" on one half, "PAMELOR 50 mg" other half.
75 mg: Branded "SANDOZ" on one half, "PAMELOR 75 mg" other half.

Storage: Below 30°C (86°F); tight container.

PAMELOR SOLUTION

Pamelor (nortriptyline HCl) solution, equivalent to 10 mg base per 5 ml, is supplied in 16 fluid ounce bottles. Alcohol content 4%.

Storage: Store at 25°C (77°F); excursions permitted to 15-30°C (59-86°F); tight, light-resistant container.

PRODUCT LISTING - RATED THERAPEUTICALLY EQUIVALENT

Capsule - Oral - 10 mg

30 x 25	$290.78	GENERIC, Sky Pharmaceuticals Packaging, Inc	63739-0189-03
30's	$10.53	GENERIC, Heartland Healthcare Services	61392-0361-30
30's	$10.53	GENERIC, Heartland Healthcare Services	61392-0361-39
30's	$14.30	GENERIC, St. Mary'S Mpp	60760-0508-30
30's	$21.34	PAMELOR, Allscripts Pharmaceutical Company	54569-0225-00
31 x 10	$125.92	GENERIC, Vangard Labs	00615-1306-53
31's	$10.88	GENERIC, Heartland Healthcare Services	61392-0361-31
32 x 10	$125.92	GENERIC, Vangard Labs	00615-1306-63
32's	$11.23	GENERIC, Heartland Healthcare Services	61392-0361-32
45's	$15.80	GENERIC, Heartland Healthcare Services	61392-0361-45
60's	$21.06	GENERIC, Heartland Healthcare Services	61392-0361-60
90's	$31.59	GENERIC, Heartland Healthcare Services	61392-0361-90
100's	$10.19	FEDERAL UPPER LIMIT, H.C.F.A. F F P	99999-1903-09
100's	$38.15	GENERIC, Major Pharmaceuticals Inc	00904-7787-60
100's	$38.15	GENERIC, Major Pharmaceuticals Inc	00904-7795-60

N

100's $38.15 GENERIC, Major Pharmaceuticals Inc 00904-7939-60
100's $38.20 GENERIC, Mutual/United Research Laboratories 00677-1555-01
100's $38.65 GENERIC, Teva Pharmaceuticals Usa 00093-0810-01
100's $38.80 GENERIC, Watson/Schein Pharmaceuticals Inc 00364-2508-90
100's $39.00 GENERIC, Creighton Products Corporation 50752-0250-05
100's $39.19 GENERIC, Watson/Schein Pharmaceuticals Inc 00364-2508-01
100's $39.60 GENERIC, Dixon-Shane Inc 17236-0003-01
100's $40.50 GENERIC, Watson/Schein Pharmaceuticals Inc 00591-5786-01
100's $40.65 GENERIC, Creighton Products Corporation 50752-0250-06
100's $41.10 GENERIC, Geneva Pharmaceuticals 00781-2630-01
100's $41.15 GENERIC, Ivax Corporation 00182-1190-01
100's $41.25 GENERIC, Mylan Pharmaceuticals Inc 00378-1410-01
100's $44.60 GENERIC, Udl Laboratories Inc 51079-0803-20
100's $44.94 GENERIC, Geneva Pharmaceuticals 00781-2630-13
100's $70.16 PAMELOR, Novartis Pharmaceuticals 00078-0086-05
100's $77.45 PAMELOR, Novartis Pharmaceuticals 00078-0086-06
200 x 5 $406.19 GENERIC, Vangard Labs 00615-1306-43

Capsule - Oral - 25 mg
15's $12.21 GENERIC, Allscripts Pharmaceutical Company 54569-3849-01
25's $22.17 GENERIC, Udl Laboratories Inc 51079-0804-19
30 x 25 $589.13 GENERIC, Sky Pharmaceuticals Packaging, Inc 63739-0190-03
30's $20.08 GENERIC, Heartland Healthcare Services 61392-0364-30
30's $20.08 GENERIC, Heartland Healthcare Services 61392-0364-39
30's $23.55 GENERIC, Allscripts Pharmaceutical Company 54569-3849-00
30's $23.55 GENERIC, Allscripts Pharmaceutical Company 54569-3894-00
30's $38.60 PAMELOR, Pharma Pac 52959-0163-30
31 x 10 $240.13 GENERIC, Vangard Labs 00615-1307-53
31's $20.75 GENERIC, Heartland Healthcare Services 61392-0364-31
32 x 10 $240.13 GENERIC, Vangard Labs 00615-1307-63
32's $21.42 GENERIC, Heartland Healthcare Services 61392-0364-32
45's $30.12 GENERIC, Heartland Healthcare Services 61392-0364-45
50's $10.13 GENERIC, Pd-Rx Pharmaceuticals 55289-0099-50
50's $11.50 GENERIC, Dhs Inc 55887-0745-50
60's $40.17 GENERIC, Heartland Healthcare Services 61392-0364-60
90's $60.25 GENERIC, Heartland Healthcare Services 61392-0364-90
100's $6.95 GENERIC, Creighton Products Corporation 50752-0251-05
100's $14.06 FEDERAL UPPER LIMIT, H.C.F.A. F F P 99999-1903-11
100's $74.38 GENERIC, Creighton Products Corporation 50752-0251-06
100's $76.35 GENERIC, Major Pharmaceuticals Inc 00904-7788-60
100's $76.35 GENERIC, Major Pharmaceuticals Inc 00904-7940-60
100's $77.00 GENERIC, Mutual/United Research Laboratories 00677-1556-01
100's $77.20 GENERIC, Teva Pharmaceuticals Usa 00093-0811-01
100's $79.42 GENERIC, Dixon-Shane Inc 17236-0005-01
100's $80.31 GENERIC, Watson/Schein Pharmaceuticals Inc 00364-2509-01
100's $80.31 GENERIC, Watson/Schein Pharmaceuticals Inc 00591-5787-01
100's $81.90 GENERIC, Geneva Pharmaceuticals 00781-2631-01
100's $81.99 GENERIC, Ivax Corporation 00182-1191-01
100's $82.00 GENERIC, Mylan Pharmaceuticals Inc 00378-2325-01
100's $88.68 GENERIC, Udl Laboratories Inc 51079-0804-20
100's $128.72 PAMELOR, Novartis Pharmaceuticals 00078-0087-06
100's $189.58 PAMELOR, Novartis Pharmaceuticals 00078-0087-05
100's $340.64 PAMELOR, Mallinckrodt Medical Inc 00406-9911-01
200 x 5 $774.61 GENERIC, Vangard Labs 00615-1307-43

Capsule - Oral - 50 mg
15's $24.92 GENERIC, Pharma Pac 52959-0519-15
30's $37.17 GENERIC, Heartland Healthcare Services 61392-0367-30
30's $37.17 GENERIC, Heartland Healthcare Services 61392-0367-39
30's $50.33 GENERIC, Pharma Pac 52959-0519-30
31 x 10 $450.00 GENERIC, Vangard Labs 00615-1315-53
31's $38.41 GENERIC, Heartland Healthcare Services 61392-0367-31
32's $39.64 GENERIC, Heartland Healthcare Services 61392-0367-32
45's $55.75 GENERIC, Heartland Healthcare Services 61392-0367-45
60's $74.34 GENERIC, Heartland Healthcare Services 61392-0367-60
60's $101.40 GENERIC, Pharma Pac 52959-0519-60
90's $111.50 GENERIC, Heartland Healthcare Services 61392-0367-90
100's $17.22 FEDERAL UPPER LIMIT, H.C.F.A. F F P 99999-1903-13
100's $137.66 GENERIC, Creighton Products Corporation 50752-0252-06
100's $145.55 GENERIC, Teva Pharmaceuticals Usa 00093-0812-01
100's $149.50 GENERIC, Mutual/United Research Laboratories 00677-1557-01
100's $149.95 GENERIC, Major Pharmaceuticals Inc 00904-7941-60
100's $151.37 GENERIC, Dixon-Shane Inc 17236-0006-01
100's $151.80 GENERIC, Watson/Schein Pharmaceuticals Inc 00364-2510-01
100's $151.80 GENERIC, Watson/Schein Pharmaceuticals Inc 00591-5788-01
100's $151.95 GENERIC, Creighton Products Corporation 50752-0252-05
100's $154.55 GENERIC, Ivax Corporation 00182-1192-01
100's $154.55 GENERIC, Mylan Pharmaceuticals Inc 00378-3250-01
100's $154.55 GENERIC, Geneva Pharmaceuticals 00781-2632-01
100's $167.17 GENERIC, Udl Laboratories Inc 51079-0805-20
100's $263.81 PAMELOR, Novartis Pharmaceuticals 00078-0078-05
100's $270.54 PAMELOR, Novartis Pharmaceuticals 00078-0078-06
100's $641.95 PAMELOR, Mallinckrodt Medical Inc 00406-9912-01

Capsule - Oral - 75 mg
30's $64.53 GENERIC, Heartland Healthcare Services 61392-0370-30
30's $64.53 GENERIC, Heartland Healthcare Services 61392-0370-39
30's $1434.00 GENERIC, Medirex Inc 57480-0826-06
31's $66.68 GENERIC, Heartland Healthcare Services 61392-0370-31
32's $68.83 GENERIC, Heartland Healthcare Services 61392-0370-32
45's $96.80 GENERIC, Heartland Healthcare Services 61392-0370-45
60's $129.06 GENERIC, Heartland Healthcare Services 61392-0370-60
90's $193.59 GENERIC, Heartland Healthcare Services 61392-0370-90
100's $22.03 FEDERAL UPPER LIMIT, H.C.F.A. F F P 99999-1903-14
100's $206.48 GENERIC, Watson/Schein Pharmaceuticals Inc 00364-2511-90
100's $209.90 GENERIC, Creighton Products Corporation 50752-0253-06
100's $212.50 GENERIC, Major Pharmaceuticals Inc 00904-7742-60
100's $212.50 GENERIC, Major Pharmaceuticals Inc 00904-7790-60
100's $212.50 GENERIC, Major Pharmaceuticals Inc 00904-7798-60
100's $212.50 GENERIC, Major Pharmaceuticals Inc 00904-7942-60
100's $221.00 GENERIC, Creighton Products Corporation 50752-0253-05
100's $221.36 GENERIC, Watson/Schein Pharmaceuticals Inc 00364-2511-01
100's $221.36 GENERIC, Watson/Schein Pharmaceuticals Inc 00591-5789-01
100's $221.78 GENERIC, Dixon-Shane Inc 17236-0007-01
100's $221.95 GENERIC, Teva Pharmaceuticals Usa 00093-0813-01
100's $235.50 GENERIC, Ivax Corporation 00182-1193-01
100's $235.50 GENERIC, Mylan Pharmaceuticals Inc 00378-4175-01
100's $235.50 GENERIC, Geneva Pharmaceuticals 00781-2633-01
100's $978.49 PAMELOR, Novartis Pharmaceuticals 00078-0079-05

Solution - Oral - 10 mg/5 ml
12.50 ml x 40 $104.00 GENERIC, Pharmaceutical Assoc Inc Div Beach Products 00121-0678-12
473 ml $41.60 GENERIC, Pharmaceutical Assoc Inc Div Beach Products 00121-0678-16
473 ml $48.50 GENERIC, Ranbaxy Laboratories 63304-0202-01
473 ml $55.52 AVENTYL HCL, Lilly, Eli and Company 00002-2468-05
480 ml $195.85 PAMELOR, Novartis Pharmaceuticals 00078-0016-33

PRODUCT LISTING - RATED NOT THERAPEUTICALLY EQUIVALENT

Capsule - Oral - 10 mg
100's $50.59 AVENTYL HCL, Lilly, Eli and Company 00002-0817-02

Capsule - Oral - 25 mg
100's $100.99 AVENTYL HCL, Lilly, Eli and Company 00002-0819-02

PRODUCT LISTING - EQUIVALENTS NOT AVAILABLE

Capsule - Oral - 10 mg
12's $5.40 GENERIC, Southwood Pharmaceuticals Inc 58016-0519-12
12's $5.40 GENERIC, Southwood Pharmaceuticals Inc 58016-0934-12
15's $6.75 GENERIC, Southwood Pharmaceuticals Inc 58016-0519-15
15's $6.75 GENERIC, Southwood Pharmaceuticals Inc 58016-0934-15
20's $9.00 GENERIC, Southwood Pharmaceuticals Inc 58016-0519-20
20's $9.00 GENERIC, Southwood Pharmaceuticals Inc 58016-0934-20
30's $4.25 GENERIC, Physicians Total Care 54868-2835-02
30's $12.27 GENERIC, Allscripts Pharmaceutical Company 54569-4146-01
30's $13.50 GENERIC, Southwood Pharmaceuticals Inc 58016-0519-30
30's $13.50 GENERIC, Southwood Pharmaceuticals Inc 58016-0934-30
30's $14.12 GENERIC, Pharma Pac 52959-0358-30
60's $6.88 GENERIC, Physicians Total Care 54868-2835-01
60's $24.53 GENERIC, Allscripts Pharmaceutical Company 54569-4146-00
60's $24.58 GENERIC, Pharma Pac 52959-0358-60
60's $27.32 GENERIC, Southwood Pharmaceuticals Inc 58016-0519-60
100's $10.25 GENERIC, Physicians Total Care 54868-2835-03
100's $45.54 GENERIC, Southwood Pharmaceuticals Inc 58016-0519-00
100's $45.54 GENERIC, Southwood Pharmaceuticals Inc 58016-0934-00
100's $170.73 PAMELOR, Mallinckrodt Medical Inc 00406-9910-01

Capsule - Oral - 25 mg
15's $17.40 GENERIC, Southwood Pharmaceuticals Inc 58016-0491-15
15's $17.40 GENERIC, Southwood Pharmaceuticals Inc 58016-0693-15
20's $23.20 GENERIC, Southwood Pharmaceuticals Inc 58016-0491-20
20's $23.20 GENERIC, Southwood Pharmaceuticals Inc 58016-0693-20
25's $4.03 GENERIC, Physicians Total Care 54868-2480-04
30's $4.57 GENERIC, Physicians Total Care 54868-2480-02
30's $29.22 GENERIC, Pharma Pac 52959-0359-30
30's $34.80 GENERIC, Southwood Pharmaceuticals Inc 58016-0491-30
30's $34.80 GENERIC, Southwood Pharmaceuticals Inc 58016-0693-30
60's $7.27 GENERIC, Physicians Total Care 54868-2480-01
60's $49.70 GENERIC, Pharma Pac 52959-0359-60
60's $69.60 GENERIC, Southwood Pharmaceuticals Inc 58016-0491-60
90's $104.40 GENERIC, Southwood Pharmaceuticals Inc 58016-0491-90
100's $11.22 GENERIC, Physicians Total Care 54868-2480-00
100's $116.00 GENERIC, Southwood Pharmaceuticals Inc 58016-0491-00
100's $116.00 GENERIC, Southwood Pharmaceuticals Inc 58016-0693-00

Capsule - Oral - 50 mg
15's $25.72 GENERIC, Southwood Pharmaceuticals Inc 58016-0508-15
15's $25.72 GENERIC, Southwood Pharmaceuticals Inc 58016-0944-15
30's $51.30 GENERIC, Southwood Pharmaceuticals Inc 58016-0508-30
30's $51.30 GENERIC, Southwood Pharmaceuticals Inc 58016-0944-30
60's $102.89 GENERIC, Southwood Pharmaceuticals Inc 58016-0508-60
100's $14.71 GENERIC, Physicians Total Care 54868-2481-01
100's $171.48 GENERIC, Southwood Pharmaceuticals Inc 58016-0508-00
100's $171.48 GENERIC, Southwood Pharmaceuticals Inc 58016-0944-00

Capsule - Oral - 75 mg
12's $31.32 GENERIC, Southwood Pharmaceuticals Inc 58016-0875-12
12's $31.32 GENERIC, Southwood Pharmaceuticals Inc 58016-0945-12
15's $39.15 GENERIC, Southwood Pharmaceuticals Inc 58016-0875-15
15's $39.15 GENERIC, Southwood Pharmaceuticals Inc 58016-0945-15
20's $52.20 GENERIC, Southwood Pharmaceuticals Inc 58016-0875-20

20's	$52.20	GENERIC, Southwood Pharmaceuticals Inc	58016-0945-20
30's	$46.64	GENERIC, Prescript Pharmaceuticals	00247-0370-30
30's	$78.30	GENERIC, Southwood Pharmaceuticals Inc	58016-0875-30
30's	$78.30	GENERIC, Southwood Pharmaceuticals Inc	58016-0945-30
100's	$261.42	GENERIC, Southwood Pharmaceuticals Inc	58016-0875-00
100's	$261.42	GENERIC, Southwood Pharmaceuticals Inc	58016-0945-00
100's	$978.49	PAMELOR, Mallinckrodt Medical Inc	00406-9913-01

Nystatin (001908)

Categories: Candidiasis; Pregnancy Category C; FDA Approved 1964 Jul; WHO Formulary
Drug Classes: Antifungals; Antifungals, topical; Dermatologics
Brand Names: Barstatin; Bio-Statin; Candex; Korostatin; **Mycostatin**; Mykinac; Nilstat; Nysert; Nystex; Nystop; O-V Statin; Pedi-Dry; Vagistat
Foreign Brand Availability: Acronistina (Ecuador); Biofanal (Germany); Biofanal Mundgel (Germany); Candida-Lokalicid (Germany); Candio-Hermal (Austria; Germany); Canstat (South-Africa); Fungistat (India); Kandistatin (Indonesia); Lystin (Hong-Kong; Malaysia; Thailand); Micostatin (Argentina; Colombia; Ecuador; Mexico; Peru); Moronal (Germany); Mycostatin (Japan); Mycocide (Taiwan); Mycosantin (China); Mycostatine (Korea); Mykoderm (Germany); Nadostine (Taiwan); Nyaderm (Canada); Nystacid (Finland); Nystan (England); Nystatin (Israel); Oranyst (Israel); Scanytin (Taiwan)

DESCRIPTION

CREAM, TOPICAL POWDER, AND OINTMENT

Nystatin cream, topical powder, and ointment are for dermatological use.

Nystatin cream contains the antifungal antibiotic nystatin at a concentration of 100,000 units per gram in an aqueous, perfumed vanishing cream base containing aluminum hydroxide concentrated wet gel, titanium dioxide, propylene glycol, cetearyl alcohol (and) ceteareth-20, white petrolatum, sorbitol solution, glyceryl monostearate, polyethylene glycol monostearate, sorbic acid, and simethicone.

Nystatin topical powder provides, in each gram, 100,000 units nystatin dispersed in talc.

Nystatin ointment provides 100,000 units nystatin per gram in Plastibase (plasticized hydrocarbon gel), a polyethylene and mineral oil gel base.

ORAL SUSPENSION (FOR EXTEMPORANEOUS PREPARATION OF)

This antifungal antibiotic is obtained from *Streptomyces noursei.* It is known to be a mixture, but the composition has not been completely elucidated. Nystatin A is closely related to amphotericin B. Each is a macrocyclic lactone containing a ketal ring, an all-*trans* polyene system, and a mycosamine (3-amino-3-deoxy-rhamose) moiety.

It has a molecular formula of $C_{47}H_{75}NO_{17}$ and a molecular weight of 926.11.

Nystatin is a ready-to-use, nonsterile powder, which contains no excipients or preservatives, for oral administration. It is available in containers of 50, 150, and 500 million units, and 2 and 5 billion units. Each milligram contains a minimum of 5000 units.

ORAL SUSPENSION AND ORAL TABLETS

Nystatin is an antifungal antibiotic which is both fungistatic and fungicidal *in vitro* against a wide variety of yeasts and yeast-like fungi. It is a polyene antibiotic of undetermined structural formula that is obtained from *Streptomyces noursei.*

Nystatin oral suspension is provided for oral administration containing 100,000 units nystatin per milliliter. *Inactive ingredients:* Alcohol (not >1% v/v), carboxymethylcellulose sodium, flavors, glycerin, methylparaben, propylparaben, saccharin sodium, sodium phosphate, sucrose (50% w/v), and purified water.

Nystatin oral tablets are provided for oral administration as coated tablets containing 500,000 units nystatin. *Inactive ingredients:* Cellulose, colorants (FD&C blue no. 2 and yellow no. 6), corn starch, flavor, lactose, magnesium stearate, povidone, stearic acid, and other ingredients.

VAGINAL TABLETS

Nystatin is an antimycotic polyene antibiotic obtained from *Streptomyces noursei.*

Nystatin vaginal tablets are available as oval-shaped, compressed tablets for intravaginal administration, each containing 100,000 units nystatin.

PASTILLES

Nystatin is a polyene antifungal antibiotic obtained from *Streptomyces noursei.*

Nystatin pastilles are round, light-to-dark gold-colored troches designed to dissolve slowly in the mouth. Each pastille provides 200,000 units nystatin. *Inactive ingredients:* Anise oil, cinnamon oil, gelatin, sucrose, and other ingredients.

CLINICAL PHARMACOLOGY

CREAM, TOPICAL POWDER, AND OINTMENT

Nystatin is an antifungal antibiotic which is both fungistatic and fungicidal *in vitro* against a wide variety of yeasts and yeast-like fungi. It probably acts by binding to sterols in the cell membrane of the fungus with a resultant change in membrane permeability allowing leakage of intracellular components. Nystatin is a polyene antibiotic of undetermined structural formula that is obtained from *Streptomyces noursei,* and is the first well tolerated antifungal antibiotic of dependable efficacy for the treatment of cutaneous, oral, and intestinal infections caused by *Candida (Monilia) albicans* and other Candida species. It exhibits no appreciable activity against bacteria.

Nystatin provides specific therapy for all localized forms of candidiasis. Symptomatic relief is rapid, often occurring within 24-72 hours after the initiation of treatment. Cure is effected both clinically and mycologically in most cases of localized candidiasis.

ORAL SUSPENSION (FOR EXTEMPORANEOUS PREPARATION OF), ORAL SUSPENSION, AND ORAL TABLETS

Nystatin probably acts by binding to sterols in the cell membrane of the fungus with a resultant change in membrane permeability allowing leakage of intracellular components. It exhibits no appreciable activity against bacteria or trichomonads.

Following oral administration, nystatin is sparingly absorbed with no detectable blood levels when given in the recommended doses. Most of the orally administered nystatin is passed unchanged in the stool.

VAGINAL TABLETS

Nystatin is both fungistatic and fungicidal *in vitro* against a wide variety of yeasts and yeast-like fungi. Nystatin acts by binding to sterols in the cell membrane of sensitive fungi with a resultant change in membrane permeability allowing leakage of intracellular components. Nystatin exhibits no appreciable activity against bacteria, protozoa, trichomonads, or viruses.

Nystatin is not absorbed from intact skin or mucous membranes.

PASTILLES

Nystatin is both fungistatic and fungicidal *in vitro* against a wide variety of yeasts and yeast-like fungi. *Candida albicans* demonstrates no significant resistance to nystatin *in vitro* on repeated subculture in increasing levels of nystatin; other *Candida* species become quite resistant. Generally, resistance does not develop *in vivo.* Nystatin acts by binding to sterols in the cell membrane of susceptible fungi with a resultant change in membrane permeability allowing leakage of intracellular components. Nystatin exhibits no activity against bacteria, protozoa, trichomonads, or viruses.

PHARMACOKINETICS

Gastrointestinal absorption of nystatin is insignificant. Most orally administered nystatin is passed unchanged in the stool. Significant concentrations of nystatin may appear occasionally in the plasma of patients with renal insufficiency during oral therapy with conventional dosage forms.

Mean nystatin concentrations in excess of those required *in vitro* to inhibit growth of clinically significant *Candida* persisted in saliva for approximately 2 hours after the start of oral dissolution of 2 nystatin pastilles (400,000 units nystatin) administered simultaneously to 12 healthy volunteers.

INDICATIONS AND USAGE

CREAM, TOPICAL POWDER, AND OINTMENT

Nystatin topical preparations are indicated in the treatment of cutaneous or mucocutaneous mycotic infections caused by *Candida (Monilia) albicans* and other *Candida* species.

ORAL SUSPENSION (FOR EXTEMPORANEOUS PREPARATION OF)

For the treatment of intestinal and oral cavity infections caused by *Candida (Monilia) albicans.*

ORAL SUSPENSION AND PASTILLES

Nystatin oral suspension and pastilles are indicated for the treatment of candidiasis in the oral cavity.

ORAL TABLETS

Nystatin oral tablets are intended for the treatment of intestinal candidiasis.

VAGINAL TABLETS

Nystatin vaginal tablets are effective for the local treatment of vulvovaginal candidiasis (moniliasis). The diagnosis should be confirmed, prior to therapy, by KOH smears and/or cultures. Other pathogens commonly associated with vulvovaginitis (Trichomonas and *Haemophilus vaginalis*) do not respond to nystatin and should be ruled out by appropriate laboratory methods.

CONTRAINDICATIONS

Nystatin is contraindicated in patients with a history of hypersensitivity to any of their components.

PRECAUTIONS

GENERAL

Cream, Topical Powder, and Ointment

Should a reaction of hypersensitivity occur the drug should be immediately withdrawn and appropriate measures taken.

These preparations are not for ophthalmic use.

Oral Suspension and Oral Tablets

Usage in Pregnancy: No adverse effects or complications have been attributed to nystatin in infants born to women treated with nystatin.

Vaginal Tablets

Discontinue treatment if sensitization or irritation is reported during use.

Pastilles

This medication is not to be used for the treatment of systemic mycoses. In order to achieve maximum effect from the medication, pastilles must be allowed to dissolve slowly in the mouth; therefore, patients for whom the pastille is prescribed, including children and the elderly, must be competent to utilize the dosage form as intended.

If irritation or hypersensitivity develops with nystatin pastilles, treatment should be discontinued and appropriate therapy instituted.

INFORMATION FOR THE PATIENT

Vaginal Tablets

The patient should be informed of symptoms of sensitization or irritation and told to report them promptly.

The patient should be warned against interruption or discontinuation of medication even during menstruation and even though symptomatic relief may occur within a few days.

N

The patient should be advised that adjunctive measures such as therapeutic douches are unnecessary and sometimes inadvisable, but cleansing douches may be used by nonpregnant women, if desired, for esthetic purposes.

Pastilles

Patients taking this medication should receive the following information and instructions:

Use as directed; the medication is not for any disorder other than for which it was prescribed.

Allow the pastille to dissolve slowly in the mouth; **do not chew or swallow the pastille.**

The patient should be advised regarding replacement of any missed doses.

There should be no interruption or discontinuation of medication until the prescribed course of treatment is completed even though symptomatic relief may occur within a few days.

If symptoms of local irritation develop, the physician should be notified promptly.

Good oral hygiene, including proper care of dentures, is particularly important for denture wearers.

LABORATORY TESTS

Vaginal Tablets

If there is a lack of response to nystatin vaginal tablets, appropriate microbiological studies should be repeated to confirm the diagnosis and rule out other pathogens before instituting another course of antimycotic therapy (see INDICATIONS AND USAGE).

Pastilles

If there is a lack of therapeutic response, appropriate microbiological studies (*e.g.*, KOH smears and/or cultures) should be repeated to confirm the diagnosis of candidiasis and rule out other pathogens before instituting another course of therapy.

CARCINOGENESIS, MUTAGENESIS, AND IMPAIRMENT OF FERTILITY

Vaginal Tablets

Long-term studies in animals have not been performed to evaluate carcinogenic potential, mutagenesis, or whether this medication affects fertility in females.

There have been no reports that use of nystatin vaginal tablets by pregnant women increases the risk of fetal abnormalities or affects later growth, development and functional maturation of the child. Nevertheless, because the possibility of harm cannot be ruled out, nystatin vaginal tablets should be used during pregnancy only if the physician considers it essential to the welfare of the patient.

Animal reproduction studies have not been conducted with nystatin vaginal tablets.

Pastilles

Studies have not been performed to evaluate carcinogenic or mutagenic potential, or possible impairment of fertility in males or females.

Animal reproduction studies have not been conducted with nystatin pastilles. It is also not known whether nystatin pastilles can cause fetal harm when administered to a pregnant woman or can affect reproduction capacity. Nystatin pastilles should be dispensed to a pregnant woman only if clearly needed.

PEDIATRIC USE

Vaginal Tablets

Safety and effectiveness in children have not been established.

Pastilles

See General.

ADVERSE REACTIONS

CREAM, TOPICAL POWDER, OINTMENT, AND ORAL TABLETS

Nystatin is virtually nontoxic and nonsensitizing and is well tolerated by all age groups including debilitated infants, even on prolonged administration.

If irritation on topical application should occur, discontinue medication.

Large oral doses have occasionally produced diarrhea, gastrointestinal distress, nausea, and vomiting.

ORAL SUSPENSION (FOR EXTEMPORANEOUS PREPARATION OF), AND ORAL SUSPENSION

Nystatin is generally well tolerated by all age groups including debilitated infants, even on prolonged administration. Large oral doses have occasionally produced diarrhea, gastrointestinal distress, and possible irritation of the stomach that may result in nausea and vomiting. Rash, including urticaria has been reported rarely. Stevens-Johnson syndrome has been reported very rarely.

VAGINAL TABLETS

Nystatin is virtually nontoxic and nonsensitizing and is well tolerated by all age groups, even on prolonged administration. Rarely, irritation or sensitization may occur (see PRECAUTIONS).

PASTILLES

Nystatin is generally well tolerated by all age groups, even during prolonged use. Rarely, oral irritation or sensitization may occur. Nausea has been reported occasionally during therapy.

Large oral doses of nystatin have occasionally produced diarrhea, gastrointestinal distress, nausea, and vomiting. Rash, including urticaria has been reported rarely. Stevens-Johnson syndrome has been reported very rarely.

DOSAGE AND ADMINISTRATION

CREAM, TOPICAL POWDER, AND OINTMENT

The cream and the ointment should be applied liberally to affected areas twice daily or as indicated until healing is complete. The powder should be applied to candidal lesions 2 or 3 times daily until lesions have healed. For fungal infection of the feet caused by *Candida* species, the powder should be dusted freely on the feet as well as in shoes and socks. Nystatin topical powder does not stain skin or mucous membranes and provides a simple, convenient means of treatment. The cream is usually preferred to the ointment in candidiasis involving intertriginous areas; very moist lesions, however, are best treated with the topical dusting powder.

The preparations do not stain skin or mucous membranes and they provide a simple, convenient means of treatment.

ORAL SUSPENSION (FOR EXTEMPORANEOUS PREPARATION OF)

Infections of the Oral Cavity Caused by Candida (Monilia) albicans

Infants: 200,000 units 4 times daily.

Children and Adults: 400,000-600,000 units 4 times daily (1/2 dose in each side of mouth).

Note: Limited clinical studies in premature and low birth weight infants indicate that 100,000 units 4 times daily is effective.

Local treatment should be continued at least 48 hours after perioral symptoms have disappeared and cultures returned to normal.

It is recommended that the drug be retained in the mouth as long as possible before swallowing.

Intestinal Candidiasis (Moniliasis)

Usual Dosage: 500,000-1 million units (approximately 1/8-1/4 teaspoonful) 3 times daily. Treatment should generally be continued for at least 48 hours after clinical cure to prevent relapse.

Note: The potency of this product cannot be assured for longer than 90 days after the container is first opened.

ORAL SUSPENSION

Infants: 2 ml (200,000 units nystatin) 4 times daily (1 ml in each side of the mouth).

Children and Adults: 4-6 ml (400,000-600,000 units nystatin) 4 times daily (1/2 of dose in each side of mouth). The preparation should be retained in the mouth as long as possible before swallowing.

Note: Limited clinical studies in premature and low birth weight infants indicate that 1 ml 4 times daily is effective.

Continue treatment for at least 48 hours after perioral symptoms have disappeared and cultures returned to normal.

ORAL TABLETS

The usual therapeutic dosage is 1-2 tablets (500,000-1 million units nystatin) 3 times daily. Treatment should generally be continued for at least 48 hours after clinical cure to prevent relapse.

VAGINAL TABLETS

The usual dosage is 1 tablet (100,000 units nystatin) daily for 2 weeks. The tablets should be deposited high in the vagina by means of the applicator. Instructions for the Patient are enclosed in each package.

PASTILLES

Children and Adults: The recommended dose is 1 or 2 pastilles (200,000 or 400,000 units nystatin) 4 or 5 times daily for as long as 14 days if necessary. The dosage regimen should be continued for at least 48 hours after disappearance of oral symptoms.

Dosage should be discontinued if symptoms persist after the initial 14 day period of treatment (see PRECAUTIONS, Laboratory Tests).

Administration: Pastilles must be allowed to dissolve slowly in the mouth, and should not be chewed or swallowed whole.

HOW SUPPLIED

Nilstat Nystatin (for extemporaneous preparation of oral suspension) is available in 150 million, 1 billion, and 2 billion units.

Mycostatin pastilles are available in 200,000 units.

STORAGE

Pastilles and Oral Suspension (for extemporaneous preparation of): Refrigerate 2-8°C (36-46°F), protect from light, and dispense in a tight, light-resistant container.

Oral Suspension: Store at room temperature; avoid freezing.

Topical Powder and Vaginal Tablets: Store at controlled room temperature 15-30°C (59-86°F).

Oral Tablets: Store at room temperature; avoid excessive heat.

PRODUCT LISTING - RATED THERAPEUTICALLY EQUIVALENT

Size	Price	Source	NDC
Cream - Topical - 100,000 us/gm			
30 gm	$2.27	FEDERAL UPPER LIMIT, H.C.F.A. F F P	99999-1908-15
Cream - Topical - 100000 U/Gm			
15 gm	$1.80	GENERIC, Thames Pharmacal Company Inc	49158-0149-20
15 gm	$1.88	GENERIC, Alpharma Uspd Makers Of Barre and Nmc	00472-1600-15
15 gm	$2.08	GENERIC, Clay-Park Laboratories Inc	45802-0059-35
15 gm	$2.15	GENERIC, Moore, H.L. Drug Exchange Inc	00839-7702-47
15 gm	$2.20	GENERIC, Major Pharmaceuticals Inc	00904-2706-36
15 gm	$2.30	GENERIC, Ivax Corporation	00182-0982-51

15 gm	$2.30	GENERIC, Moore, H.L. Drug Exchange Inc	00839-6130-47
15 gm	$2.71	GENERIC, Taro Pharmaceuticals U.S.A. Inc	51672-1289-01
15 gm	$2.75	GENERIC, Alpharma Uspd Makers Of Barre and Nmc	00472-0163-15
15 gm	$2.80	GENERIC, Fougera	00168-0054-15
15 gm	$8.57	GENERIC, Savage Laboratories	00281-3208-44
28 gm	$5.37	GENERIC, Udl Laboratories Inc	51079-0270-65
30 gm	$2.80	GENERIC, Thames Pharmacal Company Inc	49158-0149-08
30 gm	$3.05	GENERIC, Alpharma Uspd Makers Of Barre and Nmc	00472-1600-30
30 gm	$3.19	GENERIC, Clay-Park Laboratories Inc	45802-0059-11
30 gm	$3.70	GENERIC, Ivax Corporation	00182-0982-56
30 gm	$3.75	GENERIC, Major Pharmaceuticals Inc	00904-2706-31
30 gm	$4.25	GENERIC, Moore, H.L. Drug Exchange Inc	00839-6130-49
30 gm	$5.96	GENERIC, Taro Pharmaceuticals U.S.A. Inc	51672-1289-02
30 gm	$6.00	GENERIC, Alpharma Uspd Makers Of Barre and Nmc	00472-0163-30
30 gm	$6.77	GENERIC, Fougera	00168-0054-30
30 gm	$12.85	GENERIC, Savage Laboratories	00281-3208-45
30 gm	$29.71	MYCOSTATIN TOPICAL, Westwood Squibb Pharmaceutical Corporation	00003-0579-31

Ointment - Topical - 100,000 us/gm

15 gm	$1.53	FEDERAL UPPER LIMIT, H.C.F.A. F F P	99999-1908-16

Ointment - Topical - 100000 U/Gm

15 gm	$1.92	GENERIC, Alpharma Uspd Makers Of Barre and Nmc	00472-1650-15
15 gm	$2.08	GENERIC, Clay-Park Laboratories Inc	45802-0048-35
15 gm	$2.20	GENERIC, Qualitest Products Inc	00603-7821-74
15 gm	$2.23	GENERIC, Moore, H.L. Drug Exchange Inc	00839-7128-47
15 gm	$2.39	GENERIC, Ivax Corporation	00182-1678-51
15 gm	$2.43	GENERIC, Watson/Schein Pharmaceuticals Inc	00364-7379-72
15 gm	$2.46	GENERIC, Major Pharmaceuticals Inc	00904-2305-36
15 gm	$2.75	GENERIC, Alpharma Uspd Makers Of Barre and Nmc	00472-0166-15
15 gm	$2.80	GENERIC, Fougera	00168-0007-15
15 gm	$8.91	GENERIC, Savage Laboratories	00281-3212-44
30 gm	$3.19	GENERIC, Clay-Park Laboratories Inc	45802-0048-11
30 gm	$3.28	GENERIC, Alpharma Uspd Makers Of Barre and Nmc	00472-1650-30
30 gm	$3.44	GENERIC, Moore, H.L. Drug Exchange Inc	00839-7128-49
30 gm	$3.60	GENERIC, Major Pharmaceuticals Inc	00904-2305-31
30 gm	$3.70	GENERIC, Ivax Corporation	00182-1678-56
30 gm	$3.99	GENERIC, Watson/Rugby Laboratories Inc	00536-4781-28
30 gm	$6.00	GENERIC, Alpharma Uspd Makers Of Barre and Nmc	00472-0166-30
30 gm	$6.77	GENERIC, Fougera	00168-0007-30

Powder - Topical - 100000 U/Gm

15 gm	$27.46	GENERIC, Paddock Laboratories Inc	00574-2008-15
30 gm	$53.83	GENERIC, Paddock Laboratories Inc	00574-2008-30

Suspension - Oral - 100,000 us/ml

60 ml	$5.10	FEDERAL UPPER LIMIT, H.C.F.A. F F P	99999-1908-12

Suspension - Oral - 100000 U/ml

1 ml x 50	$52.00	GENERIC, Xactdose Inc	50962-0252-01
2 ml x 50	$55.00	GENERIC, Xactdose Inc	50962-0252-02
5 ml x 40	$46.80	GENERIC, Roxane Laboratories Inc	00054-8607-16
5 ml x 50	$64.00	GENERIC, Xactdose Inc	50962-0252-05
5 ml x 100	$68.00	GENERIC, Raway Pharmacal Inc	00686-0307-10
5 ml x 100	$120.00	GENERIC, Fougera	00168-0037-03
5 ml x 100	$120.00	GENERIC, Alpharma Uspd Makers Of Barre and Nmc	50962-0251-61
10 ml x 50	$66.10	GENERIC, Udl Laboratories Inc	51079-0732-10
10 ml x 50	$120.00	GENERIC, Alpharma Uspd Makers Of Barre and Nmc	50962-0250-60
60 ml	$4.75	GENERIC, Raway Pharmacal Inc	00686-0960-67
60 ml	$7.36	GENERIC, Moore, H.L. Drug Exchange Inc	00839-7703-64
60 ml	$8.00	GENERIC, Roxane Laboratories Inc	00054-3607-46
60 ml	$8.64	GENERIC, Aligen Independent Laboratories Inc	00405-3450-56
60 ml	$8.84	GENERIC, Moore, H.L. Drug Exchange Inc	00839-6698-64
60 ml	$9.46	GENERIC, Geneva Pharmaceuticals	00781-6105-61
60 ml	$14.80	GENERIC, Fougera	00168-0037-60
60 ml	$15.73	GENERIC, Lederle Laboratories	00005-5429-18
60 ml	$16.10	GENERIC, Major Pharmaceuticals Inc	00904-2761-03
60 ml	$16.35	GENERIC, Mutual/United Research Laboratories	00677-0836-25
60 ml	$16.40	GENERIC, Alpharma Uspd Makers Of Barre and Nmc	00472-1320-02
60 ml	$16.40	GENERIC, Bausch and Lomb	24208-0413-21
60 ml	$16.40	GENERIC, Morton Grove Pharmaceuticals Inc	60432-0537-60
60 ml	$16.49	GENERIC, Qualitest Products Inc	00603-1480-49
60 ml	$16.81	GENERIC, Savage Laboratories	00281-0037-60
60 ml	$21.63	GENERIC, Cardinal Pharmaceuticals	63874-0727-60
60 ml	$32.29	MYCOSTATIN, Bristol-Myers Squibb	00003-0588-60
480 ml	$51.50	GENERIC, Moore, H.L. Drug Exchange Inc	00839-6698-69
480 ml	$52.51	GENERIC, Aligen Independent Laboratories Inc	00405-3450-16
480 ml	$63.88	GENERIC, Watson/Schein Pharmaceuticals Inc	00364-2075-16
480 ml	$64.35	GENERIC, Major Pharmaceuticals Inc	00904-2761-16
480 ml	$77.11	GENERIC, Geneva Pharmaceuticals	00781-6105-16
480 ml	$81.54	GENERIC, Mutual/United Research Laboratories	00677-0836-33
480 ml	$87.18	GENERIC, Ivax Corporation	00182-1546-40
480 ml	$87.79	GENERIC, Bausch and Lomb	24208-0413-29
480 ml	$87.79	GENERIC, Bausch and Lomb	24208-0960-94
480 ml	$97.45	GENERIC, Alpharma Uspd Makers Of Barre and Nmc	00472-1320-16
480 ml	$97.45	GENERIC, Qualitest Products Inc	00603-1480-58
480 ml	$97.54	GENERIC, Morton Grove Pharmaceuticals Inc	60432-0537-16
480 ml	$104.61	GENERIC, Lederle Laboratories	00005-5429-65
480 ml	$134.93	MYCOSTATIN, Bristol-Myers Squibb	00003-0588-10

Tablet - Oral - 500000 U

100's	$18.90	GENERIC, Interstate Drug Exchange Inc	00814-5495-14
100's	$24.92	GENERIC, Auro Pharmaceutical	55829-0396-10
100's	$25.45	GENERIC, Ivax Corporation	00182-1369-01
100's	$25.95	GENERIC, Geneva Pharmaceuticals	00781-1305-01
100's	$25.95	GENERIC, Martec Pharmaceuticals Inc	52555-0119-01
100's	$26.12	GENERIC, Moore, H.L. Drug Exchange Inc	00839-6282-06
100's	$28.27	GENERIC, Aligen Independent Laboratories Inc	00405-4714-01
100's	$31.95	GENERIC, Eon Labs Manufacturing Inc	00185-0750-01
100's	$32.00	GENERIC, Par Pharmaceutical Inc	49884-0119-01
100's	$56.35	GENERIC, Major Pharmaceuticals Inc	00904-0672-60
100's	$58.08	GENERIC, Qualitest Products Inc	00603-4830-21
100's	$63.68	GENERIC, Mutual Pharmaceutical Co Inc	53489-0400-01
100's	$68.08	GENERIC, Teva Pharmaceuticals Usa	00093-0983-01
100's	$68.08	GENERIC, Mutual/United Research Laboratories	00677-0613-01
100's	$71.55	MYCOSTATIN, Bristol-Myers Squibb	00003-0580-53

Tablet - Vaginal - 100000 U

15's	$10.63	GENERIC, Aligen Independent Laboratories Inc	00405-4719-15
15's	$12.89	GENERIC, Moore, H.L. Drug Exchange Inc	00839-6125-11
15's	$29.95	GENERIC, Qualitest Products Inc	00603-4831-13
15's	$32.31	GENERIC, Major Pharmaceuticals Inc	00904-2707-48
15's	$36.71	GENERIC, Odyssey Pharmaceutical	65473-0705-09
30's	$8.10	GENERIC, Interstate Drug Exchange Inc	00814-5501-04
30's	$19.63	GENERIC, Aligen Independent Laboratories Inc	00405-4719-30
30's	$23.02	GENERIC, Moore, H.L. Drug Exchange Inc	00839-6125-19
30's	$39.95	GENERIC, Qualitest Products Inc	00603-4831-16
30's	$44.01	GENERIC, Major Pharmaceuticals Inc	00904-2707-46

PRODUCT LISTING - EQUIVALENTS NOT AVAILABLE

Capsule - Oral - 500000 U

100's	$55.20	GENERIC, Bio-Tech Pharmacal Inc	53191-0009-01

Capsule - Oral - 1000000 U

100's	$78.00	GENERIC, Bio-Tech Pharmacal Inc	53191-0192-01

Cream - Topical - 100000 U/Gm

15 gm	$2.25	GENERIC, Consolidated Midland Corporation	00223-4378-15
15 gm	$2.88	GENERIC, Physicians Total Care	54868-0242-01
15 gm	$4.19	GENERIC, Prescript Pharmaceuticals	00247-0108-15
15 gm	$5.60	GENERIC, Southwood Pharmaceuticals Inc	58016-3056-01
15 gm	$5.82	GENERIC, Cardinal Pharmaceuticals	63874-0805-15
15 gm	$7.73	GENERIC, Pharma Pac	52959-0557-03
15 gm	$12.74	GENERIC, Allscripts Pharmaceutical Company	54569-1125-00
30 gm	$3.00	GENERIC, Consolidated Midland Corporation	00223-4378-30
30 gm	$3.88	GENERIC, Physicians Total Care	54868-0242-00
30 gm	$5.04	GENERIC, Prescript Pharmaceuticals	00247-0108-30
30 gm	$6.83	GENERIC, Southwood Pharmaceuticals Inc	58016-3057-01
30 gm	$7.10	GENERIC, Cardinal Pharmaceuticals	63874-0805-30
30 gm	$9.33	GENERIC, Pharma Pac	52959-0557-01
30 gm	$25.47	GENERIC, Allscripts Pharmaceutical Company	54569-1155-00

Lozenge - Oral - 200000 U

30's	$31.40	MYCOSTATIN PASTILLES, Bristol-Myers Squibb	00003-0543-20

Ointment - Topical - 100000 U/Gm

15 gm	$1.98	GENERIC, Cardinal Pharmaceuticals	63874-0840-15
15 gm	$2.25	GENERIC, Consolidated Midland Corporation	00223-4379-15
15 gm	$2.99	GENERIC, Physicians Total Care	54868-1425-00
15 gm	$4.04	GENERIC, Allscripts Pharmaceutical Company	54569-1104-00
15 gm	$4.97	GENERIC, Southwood Pharmaceuticals Inc	58016-3058-01
30 gm	$3.00	GENERIC, Consolidated Midland Corporation	00223-4379-30
30 gm	$3.41	GENERIC, Cardinal Pharmaceuticals	63874-0840-30

N

Powder - Topical - 100000 U/Gm

Size	Price	Product	NDC
15 gm	$26.58	MYCOSTATIN TOPICAL, Southwood Pharmaceuticals Inc	58016-3155-01
15 gm	$30.51	MYCOSTATIN TOPICAL, Westwood Squibb Pharmaceutical Corporation	00003-0593-20
60 gm	$25.50	PEDI-DRI, Pedinol Pharmacal Inc	00884-0394-02
60 gm	$65.00	PEDI-DRI, Pedinol Pharmacal Inc	00884-0396-02

Suspension - Oral - 100000 U/ml

Size	Price	Product	NDC
5 ml x 50	$70.00	GENERIC, Alpharma Uspd Makers Of Barre and Nmc	50962-0251-60
60 ml	$5.86	GENERIC, Physicians Total Care	54868-0243-01
60 ml	$7.33	GENERIC, Prescript Pharmaceuticals	00247-0024-60
60 ml	$8.95	GENERIC, Consolidated Midland Corporation	00223-6572-60
60 ml	$9.65	GENERIC, Southwood Pharmaceuticals Inc	58016-1022-01
60 ml	$11.78	GENERIC, Allscripts Pharmaceutical Company	54569-1018-00
480 ml	$52.25	GENERIC, Allscripts Pharmaceutical Company	54569-4042-00

Tablet - Oral - 500000 U

Size	Price	Product	NDC
20's	$12.88	GENERIC, Allscripts Pharmaceutical Company	54569-0270-05
40's	$9.38	GENERIC, Pd-Rx Pharmaceuticals	55289-0130-40
100's	$17.36	GENERIC, Physicians Total Care	54868-3492-00
100's	$55.31	GENERIC, Southwood Pharmaceuticals Inc	58016-0143-00

Tablet - Vaginal - 100000 U

Size	Price	Product	NDC
15's	$5.50	GENERIC, Consolidated Midland Corporation	00223-1378-01
15's	$7.59	GENERIC, Southwood Pharmaceuticals Inc	58016-9005-01
15's	$31.90	GENERIC, Allscripts Pharmaceutical Company	54569-1247-00
15's	$34.72	GENERIC, Prescript Pharmaceuticals	00247-0181-15
15's	$43.31	GENERIC, Physicians Total Care	54868-1459-01
30's	$7.50	GENERIC, Consolidated Midland Corporation	00223-1378-02
30's	$66.09	GENERIC, Prescript Pharmaceuticals	00247-0181-30

Nystatin; Triamcinolone Acetonide *(001909)*

For complete prescribing information, refer to the CD-ROM included with the book.

Categories: Candidiasis; Pregnancy Category C; FDA Approved 1985 May
Drug Classes: Antifungals, topical; Corticosteroids, topical; Dermatologics
Brand Names: Myco-Triacet II; Mycogen II; **Mycolog II**; Mytrex; NGT

N

DESCRIPTION

Nystatin/triamcinolone acetonide for dermatologic use contains the antifungal agent nystatin and the synthetic corticosteroid triamcinolone acetonide.

Nystatin is a polyene antimycotic obtained from *Streptomyces noursei*. It is a yellow to light tan powder with a cereal-like odor, very slightly soluble in water, and slightly to sparingly soluble in alcohol.

Triamcinolone acetonide is designated chemically is 9-fluoro-11β,16α,17,21-tetrahydroxypregna-1,4-diene-3,20-dione cyclic 16,17-acetal with acetone. The white to cream crystalline powder has a slight odor, is practically insoluble in water, and very soluble in alcohol.

Nystatin and Triamcinolone Acetonide Cream is a soft, smooth, cream having a light yellow to buff color. Each gram provides 100,000 units nystatin and 1.0 mg triamcinolone acetonide in an aqueous perfumed vanishing cream base with aluminum hydroxide concentrated wet get, titanium dioxide, glyceryl monostearate, polyethylene glycol monostearate, simethicone, sorbic acid, propylene glycol, white petrolatum, cetearyl alcohol (and) ceteareth-20, and sorbitol solution.

Nystatin and Triamcinolone Acetonide Ointment provides, in each gram 100,000 units nystatin and triamcinolone acetonide in a protective ointment base, plasticized hydrocarbon gel, a polyethylene and mineral oil gel base.

Storage: Store at room temperature; avoid freezing.

INDICATIONS AND USAGE

Nystatin/triamcinolone acetonide is indicated for the treatment of cutaneous candidiasis; it has been demonstrated that the nystatin-steroid combination provides greater benefit than the nystatin component alone during the first few days of treatment.

CONTRAINDICATIONS

This preparation is contraindicated in those patients with a history of hypersensitivity to any of its components.

DOSAGE AND ADMINISTRATION

Nystatin/triamcinolone acetonide is usually applied to the affected areas twice daily in the morning and evening by gently and thoroughly massaging the preparation into the skin. The cream/ointment should be discontinued if symptoms persist after 25 days of therapy.

Nystatin/triamcinolone acetonide should *not* be used with occlusive dressings.

PRODUCT LISTING - RATED THERAPEUTICALLY EQUIVALENT

Cream - Topical - 100,000 us/gm;0.1%

Size	Price	Product	NDC
30 gm	$2.93	FEDERAL UPPER LIMIT, H.C.F.A. F F P	99999-1909-08

Cream - Topical - 100000 U/Gm;0.1%

Size	Price	Product	NDC
2 gm x 12	$12.43	GENERIC, Savage Laboratories	00281-0081-08
15 gm	$1.90	GENERIC, Thames Pharmacal Company Inc	49158-0214-20
15 gm	$2.05	GENERIC, Clay-Park Laboratories Inc	45802-0026-35
15 gm	$2.70	GENERIC, Moore, H.L. Drug Exchange Inc	00839-7137-47
15 gm	$2.70	GENERIC, Moore, H.L. Drug Exchange Inc	00839-7701-47
15 gm	$3.25	GENERIC, Major Pharmaceuticals Inc	00904-2574-36
15 gm	$3.29	GENERIC, Watson/Rugby Laboratories Inc	00536-4910-20
15 gm	$4.25	GENERIC, Alpharma Uspd Makers Of Barre and Nmc	00472-0150-15
15 gm	$4.30	GENERIC, Fougera	00168-0081-15
15 gm	$4.31	GENERIC, Taro Pharmaceuticals U.S.A. Inc	51672-1263-01
15 gm	$5.95	GENERIC, Marlop Pharmaceuticals Inc	12939-0403-15
15 gm	$19.50	MYCOLOG-II, Southwood Pharmaceuticals Inc	58016-9411-01
15 gm	$19.99	MYCOLOG-II, Allscripts Pharmaceutical Company	54569-0775-00
15 gm	$20.82	MYCOLOG-II, Bristol-Myers Squibb	00003-0566-30
15 gm	$24.61	GENERIC, Savage Laboratories	00281-0081-15
30 gm	$3.54	GENERIC, Physicians Total Care	54868-4083-00
30 gm	$3.60	GENERIC, Thames Pharmacal Company Inc	49158-0214-68
30 gm	$3.93	GENERIC, Clay-Park Laboratories Inc	45802-0026-11
30 gm	$4.45	GENERIC, Geneva Pharmaceuticals	00781-7600-03
30 gm	$4.71	GENERIC, Moore, H.L. Drug Exchange Inc	00839-7137-49
30 gm	$4.71	GENERIC, Moore, H.L. Drug Exchange Inc	00839-7701-49
30 gm	$4.80	GENERIC, Watson/Rugby Laboratories Inc	00536-4910-28
30 gm	$4.95	GENERIC, Major Pharmaceuticals Inc	00904-2574-31
30 gm	$5.30	GENERIC, Ivax Corporation	00182-1799-56
30 gm	$6.60	GENERIC, Alpharma Uspd Makers Of Barre and Nmc	00472-0150-30
30 gm	$6.63	GENERIC, Fougera	00168-0081-30
30 gm	$6.64	GENERIC, Taro Pharmaceuticals U.S.A. Inc	51672-1263-02
30 gm	$30.40	GENERIC, Savage Laboratories	00281-0081-30
30 gm	$35.20	MYCOLOG-II, Bristol-Myers Squibb	00003-0566-60
60 gm	$5.90	GENERIC, Thames Pharmacal Company Inc	49158-0214-24
60 gm	$6.20	GENERIC, Clay-Park Laboratories Inc	45802-0026-37
60 gm	$7.90	GENERIC, Moore, H.L. Drug Exchange Inc	00839-7137-50
60 gm	$7.90	GENERIC, Moore, H.L. Drug Exchange Inc	00839-7701-50
60 gm	$7.95	GENERIC, Geneva Pharmaceuticals	00781-7600-35
60 gm	$8.20	GENERIC, Major Pharmaceuticals Inc	00904-2574-02
60 gm	$8.75	GENERIC, Watson/Rugby Laboratories Inc	00536-4910-25
60 gm	$11.25	GENERIC, Alpharma Uspd Makers Of Barre and Nmc	00472-0150-60
60 gm	$11.28	GENERIC, Fougera	00168-0081-60
60 gm	$11.29	GENERIC, Taro Pharmaceuticals U.S.A. Inc	51672-1263-03
60 gm	$16.35	GENERIC, Marlop Pharmaceuticals Inc	12939-0403-60
60 gm	$35.38	GENERIC, Savage Laboratories	00281-0081-60
60 gm	$60.23	MYCOLOG-II, Bristol-Myers Squibb	00003-0566-65
120 gm	$12.94	GENERIC, Clay-Park Laboratories Inc	45802-0026-52
120 gm	$14.40	GENERIC, Major Pharmaceuticals Inc	00904-2574-22
120 gm	$15.90	GENERIC, Ivax Corporation	00182-1799-57
454 gm	$45.99	GENERIC, Thames Pharmacal Company Inc	49158-0214-16
454 gm	$47.03	GENERIC, Clay-Park Laboratories Inc	45802-0026-05

Ointment - Topical - 100,000 us/gm;0.1%

Size	Price	Product	NDC
30 gm	$2.93	FEDERAL UPPER LIMIT, H.C.F.A. F F P	99999-1909-11

Ointment - Topical - 100000 U/Gm;0.1%

Size	Price	Product	NDC
15 gm	$2.77	GENERIC, Moore, H.L. Drug Exchange Inc	00839-7153-47
15 gm	$3.00	GENERIC, Qualitest Products Inc	00603-7811-74
15 gm	$3.15	GENERIC, Ivax Corporation	00182-1800-51
15 gm	$3.25	GENERIC, Major Pharmaceuticals Inc	00904-2699-36
15 gm	$4.25	GENERIC, Alpharma Uspd Makers Of Barre and Nmc	00472-0155-15
15 gm	$4.30	GENERIC, Fougera	00168-0089-15
15 gm	$4.31	GENERIC, Taro Pharmaceuticals U.S.A. Inc	51672-1272-01
15 gm	$11.95	GENERIC, Savage Laboratories	00281-0089-15
15 gm	$20.82	MYCOLOG-II, Bristol-Myers Squibb	00003-0466-30
30 gm	$4.71	GENERIC, Moore, H.L. Drug Exchange Inc	00839-7153-49
30 gm	$5.10	GENERIC, Qualitest Products Inc	00603-7811-78
30 gm	$5.30	GENERIC, Ivax Corporation	00182-1800-56
30 gm	$5.95	GENERIC, Major Pharmaceuticals Inc	00904-2699-31
30 gm	$6.60	GENERIC, Alpharma Uspd Makers Of Barre and Nmc	00472-0155-30
30 gm	$6.63	GENERIC, Fougera	00168-0089-30
30 gm	$6.64	GENERIC, Taro Pharmaceuticals U.S.A. Inc	51672-1272-02
30 gm	$21.14	GENERIC, Savage Laboratories	00281-0089-30
30 gm	$35.20	MYCOLOG-II, Bristol-Myers Squibb	00003-0466-60
60 gm	$8.85	GENERIC, Ivax Corporation	00182-1800-52
60 gm	$8.96	GENERIC, Qualitest Products Inc	00603-7811-88
60 gm	$9.00	GENERIC, Clay-Park Laboratories Inc	45802-0027-37
60 gm	$10.50	GENERIC, Major Pharmaceuticals Inc	00904-2699-02

60 gm	$11.00	GENERIC, Moore, H.L. Drug Exchange Inc	00839-7153-50
60 gm	$11.25	GENERIC, Alpharma Uspd Makers Of Barre and Nmc	00472-0155-60
60 gm	$11.28	GENERIC, Fougera	00168-0089-60
60 gm	$11.29	GENERIC, Taro Pharmaceuticals U.S.A. Inc	51672-1272-03
60 gm	$60.23	MYCOLOG-II, Bristol-Myers Squibb	00003-0466-65
120 gm	$13.90	GENERIC, Alpharma Uspd Makers Of Barre and Nmc	23317-0155-04

PRODUCT LISTING - EQUIVALENTS NOT AVAILABLE

Cream - Topical - 100000 U/Gm;0.1%

15 gm	$2.99	GENERIC, Physicians Total Care	54868-0295-01
15 gm	$3.23	GENERIC, Allscripts Pharmaceutical Company	54569-5060-00
15 gm	$3.23	GENERIC, Allscripts Pharmaceutical Company	54569-7095-00
15 gm	$3.25	GENERIC, Consolidated Midland Corporation	00223-4221-15
15 gm	$3.57	GENERIC, Cardinal Pharmaceuticals	63874-0813-15
15 gm	$4.73	GENERIC, Prescript Pharmaceuticals	00247-0216-15
15 gm	$7.15	GENERIC, Allscripts Pharmaceutical Company	54569-0774-00
15 gm	$14.48	GENERIC, Southwood Pharmaceuticals Inc	58016-3053-01
15 gm	$15.77	GENERIC, Pharma Pac	52959-0558-03
30 gm	$5.50	GENERIC, Consolidated Midland Corporation	00223-4221-30
30 gm	$6.08	GENERIC, Cardinal Pharmaceuticals	63874-0813-30
30 gm	$6.11	GENERIC, Prescript Pharmaceuticals	00247-0216-30
30 gm	$7.32	GENERIC, Physicians Total Care	54868-0295-02
30 gm	$8.94	GENERIC, Marlop Pharmaceuticals Inc	12939-0403-30
30 gm	$11.39	GENERIC, Allscripts Pharmaceutical Company	54569-2148-00
30 gm	$23.70	GENERIC, Southwood Pharmaceuticals Inc	58016-3054-01
30 gm	$24.36	GENERIC, Pharma Pac	52959-0558-01
60 gm	$2.99	GENERIC, Physicians Total Care	54868-0295-03
60 gm	$10.06	GENERIC, Cardinal Pharmaceuticals	63874-0813-60
60 gm	$12.50	GENERIC, Consolidated Midland Corporation	00223-4221-60
120 gm	$18.00	GENERIC, Consolidated Midland Corporation	00223-4221-12
454 gm	$57.50	GENERIC, Consolidated Midland Corporation	00223-4221-16

Ointment - Topical - 100000 U/Gm;0.1%

15 gm	$3.25	GENERIC, Consolidated Midland Corporation	00223-4224-15
15 gm	$5.25	GENERIC, Southwood Pharmaceuticals Inc	58016-3055-01
15 gm	$6.98	GENERIC, Pharma Pac	52959-0559-03
15 gm	$8.22	GENERIC, Allscripts Pharmaceutical Company	52959-1120-00
15 gm	$8.22	GENERIC, Allscripts Pharmaceutical Company	54569-1120-00
30 gm	$5.50	GENERIC, Consolidated Midland Corporation	00223-4224-30
30 gm	$11.25	GENERIC, Pharma Pac	52959-0559-07
30 gm	$13.83	GENERIC, Allscripts Pharmaceutical Company	52959-1143-00
30 gm	$13.83	GENERIC, Allscripts Pharmaceutical Company	54569-1143-00
60 gm	$12.50	GENERIC, Consolidated Midland Corporation	00223-4224-60
120 gm	$19.50	GENERIC, Consolidated Midland Corporation	00223-4224-12
454 gm	$57.50	GENERIC, Consolidated Midland Corporation	00223-4224-16

Octreotide Acetate *(001912)*

Categories: Acromegaly; Carcinoid tumor, adjunct; Diarrhea, carcinoid tumor; Diarrhea, vasoactive intestinal peptide tumor; Vasoactive intestinal peptide tumor, adjunct; Pregnancy Category B; FDA Approved 1988 Oct; Orphan Drugs
Drug Classes: Antidiarrheals; Gastrointestinals; Hormones/hormone modifiers
Brand Names: Sandostatin
Foreign Brand Availability: Sandostatin LAR (Australia; Canada; Korea; New-Zealand; Singapore; Taiwan); Sandostatina (Italy; Mexico; Portugal); Sandostatina LAR (Colombia); Sandostatine (Belgium; France; Netherlands)

DESCRIPTION

Note: The trade names have been used throughout this monograph for clarity.

SANDOSTATIN

Sandostatin (octreotide acetate) injection, a cyclic octapeptide prepared as a clear sterile solution of octreotide, acetate salt, in a buffered lactic acid solution for administration by deep subcutaneous (intrafat) or intravenous injection. Octreotide acetate, known chemically as L-Cysteinamide, D-phenylalanyl-L-cysteinyl-L-phenylalanyl-D-tryptophyl-L-lysyl-L-threonyl-N-[2-hydroxy-1-(hydroxymethyl)propyl]-, cyclic (2→7)-disulfide; [R-(R*, R*)] acetate salt, is a long-acting octapeptide with pharmacologic actions mimicking those of the natural hormone somatostatin.

Sandostatin Injection is available as: Sterile 1 ml ampuls in 3 strengths, containing 50, 100, or 500 µg octreotide (as acetate), and sterile 5 ml multi-dose vials in 2 strengths, containing 200 and 1000 µg/ml of octreotide (as acetate).

Each ampul also contains: Lactic acid, 3.4 mg; mannitol, 45 mg; sodium bicarbonate, qs to pH 4.2 ± 0.3; water for injection, qs to 1 ml.

Each ml of the multi-dose vials also contains: Lactic acid, 3.4 mg mannitol, 45 mg; phenol, 5.0 mg; sodium bicarbonate, qs to pH 4.2 ± 0.3; water for injection, qs to 1 ml.

Lactic acid and sodium bicarbonate are added to provide a buffered solution, pH to 4.2 ± 0.3.

The molecular weight of octreotide acetate is 1019.3 (free peptide, $C_{49}H_{66}N_{10}O_{10}S_2$).

SANDOSTATIN LAR DEPOT

Octreotide is the acetate salt of a cyclic octapeptide. It is a long-acting octapeptide with pharmacologic properties mimicking those of the natural hormone somatostatin. Octreotide is known chemically as L-Cysteinamide, D-phenylalanyl-L-cysteinyl-L-phenylalanyl-Dtryptophyl-L-lysyl-L-threonyl-N-[2-hydroxy-1-(hydroxy-methyl) propyl]-, cyclic (2→7)-disulfide; [R-(R*,R*)].

Sandostatin LAR Depot (octreotide acetate for injectable suspension) is available in a vial containing the sterile drug product, which when mixed with diluent, becomes a suspension that is given as a monthly intragluteal injection. The octreotide is uniformly distributed within the microspheres which are made of a biodegradeable glucose star polymer, D,L-lactic and glycolic acids copolymer. Sterile mannitol is added to the microspheres to improve suspendability.

Sandostatin LAR Depot is available as: sterile 5 ml vials in 3 strengths delivering 10, 20 or 30 mg octreotide free peptide. See TABLE 1 for the amount each vial of Sandostatin LAR Depot delivers.

TABLE 1

Name of Ingredient	10 mg	20 mg	30 mg
Octreotide acetate	11.2 mg*	22.4 mg*	33.6 mg*
D, L-lactic and glycolic acids copolymer	188.8 mg	377.6 mg	566.4 mg
Mannitol	41.0 mg	81.9 mg	122.9 mg

* Equivalent to 10/20/30 mg octreotide base.

Each vial of diluent contains: Carboxymethylcellulose sodium, 10.0 mg; mannitol, 12.0 mg; water for injection, 2.0 ml.

The molecular weight of octreotide is 1019.3 (free peptide, $C_{49}H_{66}N_{10}O_{10}S_2$).

CLINICAL PHARMACOLOGY

SANDOSTATIN

Sandostatin exerts pharmacologic actions similar to the natural hormone, somatostatin. It is an even more potent inhibitor of growth hormone, glucagon, and insulin than somatostatin. Like somatostatin, it also suppresses LH response to GnRH, decreases splanchnic blood flow, and inhibits release of serotonin, gastrin, vasoactive intestinal peptide, secretin, motilin, and pancreatic polypeptide.

By virtue of these pharmacological actions, Sandostatin has been used to treat the symptoms associated with metastatic carcinoid tumors (flushing and diarrhea), and Vasoactive Intestinal Peptide (VIP) secreting adenomas (watery diarrhea).

Sandostatin substantially reduces growth hormone and/or IGF-I (somatomedin C) levels in patients with acromegaly.

Single doses of Sandostatin have been shown to inhibit gallbladder contractility and to decrease bile secretion in normal volunteers. In controlled clinical trials the incidence of gallstone or biliary sludge formation was markedly increased (see WARNINGS, Sandostatin).

Sandostatin suppresses secretion of thyroid stimulating hormone (TSH).

Pharmacokinetics

After subcutaneous injection, octreotide is absorbed rapidly and completely from the injection site. Peak concentrations of 5.2 ng/ml (100 µg dose) were reached 0.4 hours after dosing. Using a specific radioimmunoassay, intravenous and subcutaneous doses were found to be bioequivalent. Peak concentrations and area under the curve values were dose proportional both after subcutaneous or intravenous single doses up to 400 µg and with multiple doses of 200 µg tid (600 µg/day). Clearance was reduced by about 66% suggesting non-linear kinetics of the drug at daily doses of 600 µg/day as compared to 150 µg/day. The relative decrease in clearance with doses above 600 µg/day is not defined.

In healthy volunteers the distribution of octreotide from plasma was rapid ($T\alpha_{1/2}$ = 0.2 h), the volume of distribution (Vdss) was estimated to be 13.6 L, and the total body clearance was 10 L/h.

In blood, the distribution into the erythrocytes was found to be negligible and about 65% was bound in the plasma in a concentration-independent manner. Binding was mainly to lipoprotein and, to a lesser extent, to albumin.

The elimination of octreotide from plasma had an apparent half-life of 1.7 hours compared with 1-3 minutes with the natural hormone. The duration of action of Sandostatin is variable but extends up to 12 hours depending upon the type of tumor. About 32% of the dose is excreted unchanged into the urine. In an elderly population, dose adjustments may be necessary due to a significant increase in the half-life (46%) and a significant decrease in the clearance (26%) of the drug.

In patients with acromegaly, the pharmacokinetics differ somewhat from those in healthy volunteers. A mean peak concentration of 2.8 ng/ml (100 µg dose) was reached in 0.7 hours after subcutaneous dosing. The volume of distribution (Vdss) was estimated to be 21.6 ± 8.5 L and the total body clearance was increased to 18 L/h. The mean percent of the drug bound was 41.2%. The disposition and elimination half-lives were similar to normals.

In patients with severe renal failure requiring dialysis, clearance was reduced to about half that found in normal subjects (from approximately 10 L/h to 4.5 L/h). The effect of hepatic diseases on the disposition of octreotide is unknown.

SANDOSTATIN LAR DEPOT

Sandostatin LAR Depot is a long-acting dosage form consisting of microspheres of the biodegradable glucose star polymer, D,L-lactic and glycolic acids copolymer, containing octreotide. It maintains all of the clinical and pharmacological characteristics of the immediate-release dosage form Sandostatin Injection with the added feature of slow release of octreotide from the site of injection, reducing the need for frequent administration. This slow release occurs as the polymer biodegrades, primarily through hydrolysis. Sandostatin LAR Depot is designed to be injected intramuscularly (intragluteally) once every 4 weeks.

Octreotide exerts pharmacologic actions similar to the natural hormone, somatostatin. It is an even more potent inhibitor of growth hormone, glucagon, and insulin than somatostatin. Like somatostatin, it also suppresses LH response to GnRH, decreases splanchnic blood flow, and inhibits release of serotonin, gastrin, vasoactive intestinal peptide, secretin, motilin, and pancreatic polypeptide.

By virtue of these pharmacological actions, octreotide has been used to treat the symptoms associated with metastatic carcinoid tumors (flushing and diarrhea), and Vasoactive Intestinal Peptide (VIP) secreting adenomas (watery diarrhea).

Octreotide substantially reduces and in many cases can normalize growth hormone and/or IGF-1 (somatomedin C) levels in patients with acromegaly.

Single doses of Sandostatin Injection given subcutaneously have been shown to inhibit gallbladder contractility and to decrease bile secretion in normal volunteers. In controlled clinical trials the incidence of gallstone or biliary sludge formation was markedly increased (see WARNINGS, Sandostatin LAR Depot).

Octreotide may cause clinically significant suppression of thyroid stimulating hormone (TSH).

Pharmacokinetics

The magnitude and duration of octreotide serum concentrations after an intramuscular injection of the long-acting depot formulation Sandostatin LAR Depot reflect the release of drug from the microsphere polymer matrix. Drug release is governed by the slow biodegradation of the microspheres in the muscle, but once present in the systemic circulation, octreotide distributes and is eliminated according to its known pharmacokinetic properties which are as follows:

Pharmacokinetics of Octreotide Acetate

According to data obtained with the immediate-release formulation, Sandostatin Injection solution, after subcutaneous injection, octreotide is absorbed rapidly and completely from the injection site. Peak concentrations of 5.2 ng/ml (100 μg dose) were reached 0.4 hours after dosing. Using a specific radioimmunoassay, intravenous and subcutaneous doses were found to be bioequivalent. Peak concentrations and area-under-the-curve values were dose proportional both after subcutaneous or intravenous single doses up to 400 μg and with multiple doses of 200 μg tid (600 μg/day). Clearance was reduced by about 66% suggesting non-linear kinetics of the drug at daily doses of 600 μg/day as compared to 150 μg/day. The relative decrease in clearance with doses above 600 μg/day is not defined.

In healthy volunteers the distribution of octreotide from plasma was rapid ($T\alpha_{1/2}$ = 0.2 h), the volume of distribution (Vdss) was estimated to be 13.6 L and the total body clearance was 10 L/h.

In blood, the distribution of octreotide into the erythrocytes was found to be negligible and about 65% was bound in the plasma in a concentration-independent manner. Binding was mainly to lipoprotein and, to a lesser extent, to albumin.

The elimination of octreotide from plasma had an apparent half-life of 1.7 hours, compared with the 1-3 minutes with the natural hormone, somatostatin. The duration of action of subcutaneously administered Sandostatin Injection solution is variable but extends up to 12 hours depending upon the type of tumor, necessitating multiple daily dosing with this immediate-release dosage form. About 32% of the dose is excreted unchanged into the urine. In an elderly population, dose adjustments may be necessary due to a significant increase in the half-life (46%) and a significant decrease in the clearance (26%) of the drug.

In patients with acromegaly, the pharmacokinetics differ somewhat from those in healthy volunteers. A mean peak concentration of 2.8 ng/ml (100 μg dose) was reached in 0.7 hours after subcutaneous dosing. The volume of distribution (Vdss) was estimated to be 21.6 ± 8.5 L and the total body clearance was increased to 18 L/h. The mean percent of the drug bound was 41.2%. The disposition and elimination half-lives were similar to normals.

In patients with severe renal failure requiring dialysis, clearance was reduced to about half that found in healthy subjects (from approximately 10 L/h to 4.5 L/h).

The effect of hepatic diseases on the disposition of octreotide is unknown.

Pharmacokinetics of Sandostatin LAR Depot

After a single IM injection of the long-acting depot dosage form Sandostatin LAR Depot in healthy volunteer subjects, the serum octreotide concentration reached a transient initial peak of about 0.03 ng/ml/mg within 1 hour after administration progressively declining over the following 3-5 days to a nadir of <0.01 ng/ml/mg, then slowly increasing and reaching a plateau about 2-3 weeks post injection. Plateau concentrations were maintained over a period of nearly 2-3 weeks, showing dose proportional peak concentrations of about 0.07 ng/ml/mg. After about 6 weeks post injection, octreotide concentration slowly decreased, to <0.01 ng/ml/mg by weeks 12-13, concomitant with the terminal degradation phase of the polymer matrix of the dosage form. The relative bioavailability of the long-acting release Sandostatin LAR Depot compared to immediate-release Sandostatin Injection solution given subcutaneously was 60-63%.

In patients with acromegaly, the octreotide concentrations after single doses of 10, 20, and 30 mg Sandostatin LAR Depot were dose proportional. The transient day 1 peak, amounting to 0.3 ng/ml, 0.8 ng/ml, and 1.3 ng/ml, respectively, was followed by plateau concentrations of 0.5 ng/ml, 1.3 ng/ml, and 2.0 ng/ml, respectively, achieved about 3 weeks post injection. These plateau concentrations were maintained for nearly 2 weeks.

Following multiple doses of Sandostatin LAR Depot given every 4 weeks, steady-state octreotide serum concentrations were achieved after the third injection. Concentrations were dose proportional and higher by a factor of approximately 1.6-2.0 compared to the concentrations after a single dose. The steady-state octreotide concentrations were 1.2 ng/ml and 2.1 ng/ml, respectively, at trough and 1.6 ng/ml and 2.6 ng/ml, respectively, at peak with 20 and 30 mg Sandostatin LAR Depot given every 4 weeks. No accumulation of octreotide beyond that expected from the overlapping release profiles occurred over a duration of up to 28 monthly injections of Sandostatin LAR Depot. With the long-acting depot formulation Sandostatin LAR Depot administered IM every 4 weeks the peak-to-trough variation in octreotide concentrations ranged from 44-68%, compared to the 163-209% variation encountered with the daily subcutaneous tid regimen of Sandostatin Injection solution.

In patients with carcinoid tumors, the mean octreotide concentrations after 6 doses of 10 mg, 20 mg, and 30 mg Sandostatin LAR Depot administered by IM injection every 4 weeks were 1.2 ng/ml, 2.5 ng/ml, and 4.2 ng/ml, respectively. Concentrations were dose proportional and steady-state concentrations were reached after two injections of 20 and 30 mg and after three injections of 10 mg.

Sandostatin LAR Depot has not been studied in patients with renal impairment.

Sandostatin LAR Depot has not been studied in patients with hepatic impairment.

INDICATIONS AND USAGE

SANDOSTATIN

Acromegaly

Sandostatin is indicated to reduce blood levels of growth hormone and IGF-I (somatomedin C) in acromegaly patients who have had inadequate response to or cannot be treated with surgical resection, pituitary irradiation, and bromocriptine mesylate at maximally tolerated doses. The goal is to achieve normalization of growth hormone and IGF-I (somatomedin C) levels (see DOSAGE AND ADMINISTRATION, Sandostatin). In patients with acromegaly, Sandostatin reduces growth hormone to within normal ranges in 50% of patients and reduces IGF-I (somatomedin C) to within normal ranges in 50-60% of patients. Since the effects of pituitary irradiation may not become maximal for several years, adjunctive therapy with Sandostatin to reduce blood levels of growth hormone and IGF-I (somatomedin C) offers potential benefit before the effects of irradiation are manifested.

Improvement in clinical signs and symptoms or reduction in tumor size or rate of growth were not shown in clinical trials performed with Sandostatin; these trials were not optimally designed to detect such effects.

Carcinoid Tumors

Sandostatin is indicated for the symptomatic treatment of patients with metastatic carcinoid tumors where it suppresses or inhibits the severe diarrhea and flushing episodes associated with the disease.

Sandostatin studies were not designed to show an effect on the size, rate of growth or development of metastases.

Vasoactive Intestinal Peptide Tumors (VIPomas)

Sandostatin is indicated for the treatment of the profuse watery diarrhea associated with VIP-secreting tumors. Sandostatin studies were not designed to show an effect on the size, rate of growth or development of metastases.

SANDOSTATIN LAR DEPOT

Acromegaly

Sandostatin LAR Depot is indicated for long-term maintenance therapy in acromegalic patients for whom medical treatment is appropriate and who have been shown to respond to and can tolerate Sandostatin Injection. The goal of treatment in acromegaly is to reduce GH and IGF-1 levels to normal. Sandostatin LAR Depot can be used in patients who have had an inadequate response to surgery or in those for whom surgical resection is not an option. It may also be used in patients who have received radiation and have had an inadequate therapeutic response (see DOSAGE AND ADMINISTRATION, Sandostatin LAR Depot).

Carcinoid Tumors

Sandostatin LAR Depot is indicated for long-term treatment of the severe diarrhea and flushing episodes associated with metastatic carcinoid tumors in patients in whom initial treatment with Sandostatin Injection has been shown to be effective and tolerated.

Vasoactive Intestinal Peptide Tumors (VIPomas)

Sandostatin LAR Depot is indicated for long-term treatment of the profuse watery diarrhea associated with VIP-secreting tumors in patients in whom initial treatment with Sandostatin Injection has been shown to be effective and tolerated.

In patients with acromegaly, carcinoid syndrome and VIPomas, the effect of Sandostatin Injection and Sandostatin LAR Depot on tumor size, rate of growth and development of metastases, has not been determined.

NON-FDA APPROVED INDICATIONS

Data have suggested that octreotide may be useful in the treatment of idiopathic pseudoobstruction, severe diarrhea in AIDS, diabetes mellitus, carcinoid syndrome, dumping syndrome following gastric surgery, insulinoma, glucagonoma, gastrinoma, thyrotropin-secreting tumors, small bowel or pancreatic fistulae, esophageal varices, peptic ulcer hemorrhage, metastatic liver endocrine tumors and primary hepacelluar carcinoma. However, these uses have not been approved by the FDA and further clinical trials are needed.

CONTRAINDICATIONS

SANDOSTATIN

Sensitivity to this drug or any of its components.

SANDOSTATIN LAR DEPOT

Sensitivity to this drug or any of its components.

WARNINGS

SANDOSTATIN

Single doses of Sandostatin have been shown to inhibit gallbladder contractility and decrease bile secretion in normal volunteers. In clinical trials (primarily patients with acromegaly or psoriasis), the incidence of biliary tract abnormalities was 63% (27% gallstones, 24% sludge without stones, 12% biliary duct dilatation). The incidence of stones or sludge in patients who received Sandostatin for 12 months or longer was 52%. Less than 2% of patients treated with Sandostatin for 1 month or less developed gallstones. The incidence of gallstones did not appear related to age, sex or dose. Like patients without gallbladder abnormalities, the majority of patients developing gallbladder abnormalities on ultrasound had gastrointestinal symptoms. The symptoms were not specific for gallbladder disease. A few patients developed acute cholecystitis, ascending cholangitis, biliary obstruction, cholestatic hepatitis, or pancreatitis during Sandostatin therapy or following its withdrawal. One patient developed ascending cholangitis during Sandostatin therapy and died.

SANDOSTATIN LAR DEPOT

Adverse events that have been reported in patients receiving Sandostatin Injection can also be expected in patients receiving Sandostatin LAR Depot. Incidence figures in the WARNINGS, Sandostatin LAR Depot and ADVERSE REACTIONS, Sandostatin LAR Depot, are those obtained in clinical trials of Sandostatin Injection and Sandostatin LAR Depot.

Gallbladder and Related Events

Single doses of Sandostatin Injection have been shown to inhibit gallbladder contractility and decrease bile secretion in normal volunteers. In clinical trials with Sandostatin Injection (primarily patients with acromegaly or psoriasis) in patients who had not previously received octreotide, the incidence of biliary tract abnormalities was 63% (27% gallstones, 24% sludge without stones, 12% biliary duct dilatation). The incidence of stones or sludge in patients who received Sandostatin Injection for 12 months or longer was 52%. The incidence of gallbladder abnormalities did not appear to be related to age, sex or dose but was related to duration of exposure.

In clinical trials 52% of acromegalic patients, most of whom received Sandostatin LAR Depot for 12 months or longer, developed new biliary abnormalities including gallstones, microlithiasis, sediment, sludge and dilatation. The incidence of new cholelithiasis was 22%, of which 7% were microstones.

In clinical trials 62% of malignant carcinoid patients who received Sandostatin LAR Depot for up to 18 months developed new biliary abnormalities including gallstones, sludge and dilatation. New gallstones occurred in a total of 24% of patients.

Across all trials, a few patients developed acute cholecystitis, ascending cholangitis, biliary obstruction, cholestatic hepatitis, or pancreatitis during octreotide therapy or following its withdrawal. One patient developed ascending cholangitis during Sandostatin Injection therapy and died. Despite the high incidence of new gallstones in patients receiving octreotide, 1% of patients developed acute symptoms requiring cholecystectomy.

PRECAUTIONS

SANDOSTATIN

General

Sandostatin alters the balance between the counter-regulatory hormones, insulin, glucagon and growth hormone, which may result in hypoglycemia or hyperglycemia. Sandostatin also suppresses secretion of thyroid stimulating hormone, which may result in hypothyroidism. Cardiac conduction abnormalities have also occurred during treatment with Sandostatin. However, the incidence of these adverse events during long-term therapy was determined vigorously only in acromegaly patients who, due to their underlying disease and/or the subsequent treatment they receive, are at an increased risk for the development of diabetes mellitus, hypothyroidism, and cardiovascular disease. Although the degree to which these abnormalities are related to Sandostatin therapy is not clear, new abnormalities of glycemic control, thyroid function and ECG developed during Sandostatin therapy as described below.

The hypoglycemia or hyperglycemia which occurs during Sandostatin therapy is usually mild, but may result in overt diabetes mellitus or necessitate dose changes in insulin or other hypoglycemic agents. Hypoglycemia and hyperglycemia occurred on Sandostatin in 3% and 16% of acromegalic patients, respectively. Severe hyperglycemia, subsequent pneumonia, and death following initiation of Sandostatin therapy was reported in one patient with no history of hyperglycemia.

In acromegalic patients, 12% developed biochemical hypothyroidism only, 8% developed goiter, and 4% required initiation of thyroid replacement therapy while receiving Sandostatin. Baseline and periodic assessment of thyroid function (TSH, total and/or free T_4) is recommended during chronic therapy.

In acromegalics, bradycardia (<50 bpm) developed in 25%; conduction abnormalities occurred in 10% and arrhythmias occurred in 9% of patients during Sandostatin therapy. Other EKG changes observed included QT prolongation, axis shifts, early repolarization, low voltage, R/S transition, and early R wave progression. These ECG changes are not uncommon in acromegalic patients. Dose adjustments in drugs such as beta-blockers that have bradycardia effects may be necessary. In one acromegalic patient with severe congestive heart failure, initiation of Sandostatin therapy resulted in worsening of CHF with improvement when drug was discontinued. Confirmation of a drug effect was obtained with a positive rechallenge.

Several cases of pancreatitis have been reported in patients receiving Sandostatin therapy. Sandostatin may alter absorption of dietary fats in some patients.

In patients with severe renal failure requiring dialysis, the half-life of Sandostatin may be increased, necessitating adjustment of the maintenance dosage.

Depressed vitamin B_{12} levels and abnormal Schilling's tests have been observed in some patients receiving Sandostatin therapy, and monitoring of vitamin B_{12} levels is recommended during chronic Sandostatin therapy.

Information for the Patient

Careful instruction in sterile subcutaneous injection technique should be given to the patients and to other persons who may administer Sandostatin Injection.

Laboratory Tests

Laboratory tests that may be helpful as biochemical markers in determining and following patient response depend on the specific tumor. Based on diagnosis, measurement of the following substances may be useful in monitoring the progress of therapy:

Acromegaly: Growth Hormone, IGF-I (somatomedin C).

Responsiveness to Sandostatin may be evaluated by determining growth hormone levels at 1-4 hour intervals for 8-12 hours post dose. Alternatively, a single measurement of IGF-I (somatomedin C) level may be made 2 weeks after drug initiation or dosage change.

Carcinoid: 5-HIAA (urinary 5-hydroxyindole acetic acid), plasma serotonin, plasma Substance P.

VIPoma: VIP (plasma vasoactive intestinal peptide).

Baseline and periodic total and/or free T_4 measurements should be performed during chronic therapy (see PRECAUTIONS, Sandostatin, General).

Drug/Laboratory Test Interactions

No known interference exists with clinical laboratory tests, including amine or peptide determinations.

Carcinogenesis, Mutagenesis, and Impairment of Fertility

Studies in laboratory animals have demonstrated no mutagenic potential of Sandostatin.

No carcinogenic potential was demonstrated in mice treated subcutaneously for 85-99 weeks at doses up to 2000 μg/kg/day (8× the human exposure based on body surface area). In a 116 week subcutaneous study in rats, a 27% and 12% incidence of injection site sarcomas or squamous cell carcinomas was observed in males and females, respectively, at the highest dose level of 1250 μg/kg/day (10× the human exposure based on body surface area) compared to an incidence of 8-10% in the vehicle control groups. The increased incidence of injection site tumors was most probably caused by irritation and the high sensitivity of the rat to repeated subcutaneous injections at the same site. Rotating injection sites would prevent chronic irritation in humans. There have been no reports of injection site tumors in patients treated with Sandostatin for up to 5 years. There was also a 15% incidence of uterine adenocarcinomas in the 1250 μg/kg/day females compared to 7% in the saline control females and 0% in the vehicle control females. The presence of endometritis coupled with the absence of corpora lutea, the reduction in mammary fibroadenomas, and the presence of uterine dilatation suggest that the uterine tumors were associated with estrogen dominance in the aged female rats which does not occur in humans.

Sandostatin did not impair fertility in rats at doses up to 1000 μg/kg/day, which represents 7× the human exposure based on body surface area.

Pregnancy Category B

Reproduction studies have been performed in rats and rabbits at doses up to 16 times the highest human dose based on body surface area and have revealed no evidence of impaired fertility or harm to the fetus due to Sandostatin. There are, however, no adequate and well-controlled studies in pregnant women. Because animal reproduction studies are not always predictive of human response, this drug should be used during pregnancy only if clearly needed.

Nursing Mothers

It is not known whether this drug is excreted in human milk. Because many drugs are excreted in milk, caution should be exercised when Sandostatin is administered to a nursing woman.

Pediatric Use

Experience with Sandostatin in the pediatric population is limited. The youngest patient to receive the drug was 1 month old. Doses of 1-10 μg/kg body weight were well tolerated in the young patients. A single case of an infant (nesidioblastosis) was complicated by a seizure thought to be independent of Sandostatin therapy.

SANDOSTATIN LAR DEPOT

See ADVERSE REACTIONS, Sandostatin LAR Depot.

General

Growth hormone secreting tumors may sometimes expand and cause serious complications (*e.g.*, visual field defects). Therefore, all patients with these tumors should be carefully monitored.

Octreotide alters the balance between the counter-regulatory hormones, insulin, glucagon and growth hormone, which may result in hypoglycemia or hyperglycemia. Octreotide also suppresses secretion of thyroid stimulating hormone, which may result in hypothyroidism. Cardiac conduction abnormalities have also occurred during treatment with octreotide.

Glucose Metabolism

The hypoglycemia or hyperglycemia which occurs during octreotide therapy is usually mild, but may result in overt diabetes mellitus or necessitate dose changes in insulin or other hypoglycemic agents. Severe hyperglycemia, subsequent pneumonia, and death following initiation of Sandostatin Injection therapy was reported in one patient with no history of hyperglycemia (see ADVERSE REACTIONS, Sandostatin LAR Depot).

Thyroid Function

Hypothyroidism has been reported in acromegaly and carcinoid patients receiving octreotide therapy. Baseline and periodic assessment of thyroid function (TSH, total and/or free T_4) is recommended during chronic octreotide therapy (see ADVERSE REACTIONS, Sandostatin LAR Depot).

Cardiac Function

In both acromegalic and carcinoid syndrome patients, bradycardia, arrhythmias and conduction abnormalities have been reported during octreotide therapy. Other EKG changes were observed such as QT prolongation, axis shifts, early repolarization, low voltage, R/S transition, early R wave progression, and non-specific ST-T wave changes. The relationship of these events to octreotide acetate is not established because many of these patients have underlying cardiac disease (see PRECAUTIONS, Sandostatin LAR Depot). Dose adjustments in drugs such as beta-blockers that have bradycardia effects may be necessary. In one acromegalic patient with severe congestive heart failure, initiation of Sandostatin Injection therapy resulted in worsening of CHF with improvement when drug was discontinued. Con-

O

firmation of a drug effect was obtained with a positive rechallenge (see ADVERSE REACTIONS, Sandostatin LAR Depot).

Nutrition

Octreotide may alter absorption of dietary fats in some patients.

Depressed vitamin B_{12} levels and abnormal Schilling's tests have been observed in some patients receiving octreotide therapy, and monitoring of vitamin B_{12} levels is recommended during therapy with Sandostatin LAR Depot.

Octreotide has been investigated for the reduction of excessive fluid loss from the GI tract in patients with conditions producing such a loss. If such patients are receiving total parenteral nutrition (TPN), serum zinc may rise excessively when the fluid loss is reversed. Patients on TPN and octreotide should have periodic monitoring of zinc levels.

Information for the Patient

Patients with carcinoid tumors and VIPomas should be advised to adhere closely to their scheduled return visits for reinjection in order to minimize exacerbation of symptoms.

Patients with acromegaly should also be urged to adhere to their return visit schedule to help assure steady control of GH and IGF-1 levels.

Laboratory Tests

Laboratory tests that may be helpful as biochemical markers in determining and following patient response depend on the specific tumor. Based on diagnosis, measurement of the following substances may be useful in monitoring the progress of therapy:

Acromegaly: Growth Hormone, IGF-1 (somatomedin C).

Responsiveness to octreotide may be evaluated by determining growth hormone levels at 1-4 hour intervals for 8-12 hours after subcutaneous injection of Sandostatin Injection (not Sandostatin LAR Depot). Alternatively, a single measurement of IGF-1 (somatomedin C) level may be made 2 weeks after initiation of Sandostatin Injection or dosage change. After patients are switched from Sandostatin Injection to Sandostatin LAR Depot, GH and IGF-1 determinations may be made after 3 monthly injections of Sandostatin LAR Depot. (Steady-state serum levels of octreotide are reached only after a period of 3 months of monthly injections.) Growth hormone can be determined using the mean of 4 assays taken at 1 hour intervals. Somatomedin C can be determined with a single assay. All GH and IGF-1 determinations should be made 4 weeks after the previous Sandostatin LAR Depot.

Carcinoid: 5-HIAA (urinary 5-hydroxyindole acetic acid), plasma serotonin, plasma Substance P.

VIPoma: VIP (plasma vasoactive intestinal peptide).

Baseline and periodic total and/or free T_4 measurements should be performed during chronic therapy (see PRECAUTIONS, Sandostatin LAR Depot, General).

Drug/Laboratory Test Interactions

No known interference exists with clinical laboratory tests, including amine or peptide determinations.

Carcinogenesis, Mutagenesis, and Impairment of Fertility

Studies in laboratory animals have demonstrated no mutagenic potential of Sandostatin. No mutagenic potential of the polymeric carrier in Sandostatin LAR Depot, D,L-lactic and glycolic acids copolymer, was observed in the Ames mutagenicity test.

No carcinogenic potential was demonstrated in mice treated subcutaneously with octreotide for 85-99 weeks at doses up to 2000 μg/kg/day (8× the human exposure based on body surface area). In a 116 week subcutaneous study in rats administered octreotide, a 27% and 12% incidence of injection site sarcomas or squamous cell carcinomas was observed in males and females, respectively, at the highest dose level of 1250 μg/kg/day (10× the human exposure based on body surface area) compared to an incidence of 8-10% in the vehicle control groups. The increased incidence of injection site tumors was most probably caused by irritation and the high sensitivity of the rat to repeated subcutaneous injections at the same site. Rotating injection sites would prevent chronic irritation in humans. There have been no reports of injection site tumors in patients treated with Sandostatin Injection for at least 5 years. There was also a 15% incidence of uterine adenocarcinomas in the 1250 μg/kg/day females compared to 7% in the saline control females and 0% in the vehicle control females. The presence of endometritis coupled with the absence of corpora lutea, the reduction in mammary fibroadenomas, and the presence of uterine dilatation suggest that the uterine tumors were associated with estrogen dominance in the aged female rats which does not occur in humans.

Octreotide did not impair fertility in rats at doses up to 1000 μg/kg/day, which represents 7× the human exposure based on body surface area.

Pregnancy Category B

Reproduction studies have been performed in rats and rabbits at doses up to 16 times the highest human dose based on body surface area and have revealed no evidence of impaired fertility or harm to the fetus due to octreotide. There are, however, no adequate and well-controlled studies in pregnant women. Because animal reproduction studies are not always predictive of human response, this drug should be used during pregnancy only if clearly needed.

Nursing Mothers

It is not known whether this drug is excreted in human milk. Because many drugs are excreted in milk, caution should be exercised when Sandostatin LAR Depot is administered to a nursing woman.

Pediatric Use

Sandostatin LAR Depot has not been studied in pediatric patients.

Experience with Sandostatin Injection in the pediatric population is limited. Its use has been primarily in patients with congenital hyperinsulinism (also called nesidioblastosis). The youngest patient to receive the drug was 1 month old. At doses of 1-40 μg/kg body weight/day, the majority of side effects observed were gastrointestinal- steatorrhea, diarrhea, vomiting and abdominal distension. Poor growth has been reported in several patients treated with Sandostatin Injection for more than 1 year; catch-up growth occurred after Sandostatin Injection was discontinued. A 16-month-old male with enterocutaneous fistula developed sudden abdominal pain and increased nasogastric drainage and died 8 hours after receiving a single 100 μg subcutaneous dose of Sandostatin Injection.

DRUG INTERACTIONS

SANDOSTATIN

Sandostatin has been associated with alterations in nutrient absorption, so it may have an effect on absorption of orally administered drugs. Concomitant administration of Sandostatin with cyclosporine may decrease blood levels of cyclosporine and result in transplant rejection.

Patients receiving insulin, oral hypoglycemic agents, beta blockers, calcium channel blockers, or agents to control fluid and electrolyte balance, may require dose adjustments of these therapeutic agents.

SANDOSTATIN LAR DEPOT

Octreotide has been associated with alterations in nutrient absorption, so it may have an effect on absorption of orally administered drugs. Concomitant administration of octreotide injection with cyclosporine may decrease blood levels of cyclosporine and result in transplant rejection.

Patients receiving insulin, oral hypoglycemic agents, beta-blockers, calcium channel blockers, or agents to control fluid and electrolyte balance, may require dose adjustments of these therapeutic agents.

ADVERSE REACTIONS

SANDOSTATIN

Gallbladder Abnormalities

Gallbladder abnormalities, especially stones and/or biliary sludge, frequently develop in patients on chronic Sandostatin therapy (see WARNINGS, Sandostatin).

Cardiac

In acromegalics, sinus bradycardia (<50 bpm) developed in 25%; conduction abnormalities occurred in 10% and arrhythmias developed in 9% of patients during Sandostatin therapy (see PRECAUTIONS, Sandostatin, General).

Gastrointestinal

Diarrhea, loose stools, nausea and abdominal discomfort were each seen in 34-61% of acromegalic patients in US studies although only 2.6% of the patients discontinued therapy due to these symptoms. These symptoms were seen in 5-10% of patients with other disorders.

The frequency of these symptoms was not dose-related, but diarrhea and abdominal discomfort generally resolved more quickly in patients treated with 300 μg/day than in those treated with 750 μg/day. Vomiting, flatulence, abnormal stools, abdominal distention, and constipation were each seen in less than 10% of patients.

Hypo/Hyperglycemia

Hypoglycemia and hyperglycemia occurred in 3% and 16% of acromegalic patients, respectively, but only in about 1.5% of other patients. Symptoms of hypoglycemia were noted in approximately 2% of patients.

Hypothyroidism

In acromegalics, biochemical hypothyroidism alone occurred in 12% while goiter occurred in 6% during Sandostatin therapy (see PRECAUTIONS, Sandostatin, General). In patients without acromegaly, hypothyroidism has only been reported in several isolated patients and goiter has not been reported.

Other Adverse Events

Pain on injection was reported in 7.7%, headache in 6% and dizziness in 5%. Pancreatitis was also observed (see WARNINGS, Sandostatin and PRECAUTIONS, Sandostatin).

Other Adverse Events 1-4%

Other events (relationship to drug not established), each observed in 1-4% of patients, included fatigue, weakness, pruritus, joint pain, backache, urinary tract infection, cold symptoms, flu symptoms, injection site hematoma, bruise, edema, flushing, blurred vision, pollakiuria, fat malabsorption, hair loss, visual disturbance and depression.

Other Adverse Events <1%

Events reported in less than 1% of patients and for which relationship to drug is not established are listed:

Gastrointestinal: Hepatitis, jaundice, increase in liver enzymes, GI bleeding, hemorrhoids, appendicitis, gastric/peptic ulcer, gallbladder polyp.

Integumentary: Rash, cellulitis, petechiae, urticaria, basal cell carcinoma.

Musculoskeletal: Arthritis, joint effusion, muscle pain, Raynaud's phenomenon.

Cardiovascular: Chest pain, shortness of breath, thrombophlebitis, ischemia, congestive heart failure, hypertension, hypertensive reaction, palpitations, orthostatic BP decrease, tachycardia.

CNS: Anxiety, libido decrease, syncope, tremor, seizure, vertigo, Bell's Palsy, paranoia, pituitary apoplexy, increased intraocular pressure, amnesia, hearing loss, neuritis.

Respiratory: Pneumonia, pulmonary nodule, status asthmaticus.

Endocrine: Galactorrhea, hypoadrenalism, diabetes insipidus, gynecomastia, amenorrhea, polymenorrhea, oligomenorrhea, vaginitis.

Urogenital: Nephrolithiasis, hematuria.

Hematologic: Anemia, iron deficiency, epistaxis.

Miscellaneous: Otitis, allergic reaction, increased CK, weight loss.

Evaluation of 20 patients treated for at least 6 months has failed to demonstrate titers of antibodies exceeding background levels. However, antibody titers to Sandostatin were subsequently reported in 3 patients and resulted in prolonged duration of drug action in 2 pa-

O

tients. Anaphylactoid reactions, including anaphylactic shock, have been reported in several patients receiving Sandostatin.

SANDOSTATIN LAR DEPOT

See WARNINGS, Sandostatin LAR Depot and PRECAUTIONS, Sandostatin LAR Depot.

Gallbladder abnormalities, especially stones and/or biliary sludge, frequently develop in patients on chronic octreotide therapy (see WARNINGS, Sandostatin LAR Depot). Few patients, however, develop acute symptoms requiring cholecystectomy.

Cardiac

In acromegalics, sinus bradycardia (<50 bpm) developed in 25%; conduction abnormalities occurred in 10% and arrhythmias developed in 9% of patients during Sandostatin Injection therapy. Electrocardiograms were performed only in carcinoid patients receiving Sandostatin LAR Depot. In carcinoid syndrome patients sinus bradycardia developed in 19%; conduction abnormalities occurred in 9%, and arrhythmias developed in 3%. The relationship of these events to octreotide acetate is not established because many of these patients have underlying cardiac disease (see PRECAUTIONS, Sandostatin LAR Depot).

Gastrointestinal

The most common symptoms are gastrointestinal. The overall incidence of the most frequent of these symptoms in clinical trials of acromegalic patients treated for approximately 1 to 4 years is shown in TABLE 5.

TABLE 5 *Number (%) of Acromegalic Patients With Common GI Adverse Events*

Adverse Event	Sandostatin Injection SC tid n=114	Sandostatin LAR Depot q 28 Days n=261
Diarrhea	66 (57.9%)	95 (36.4%)
Abdominal pain or discomfort	50 (43.9%)	76 (29.1%)
Flatulence	15 (13.2%)	67 (25.7%)
Constipation	10 (8.8%)	49 (18.8%)
Nausea	34 (29.8%)	27 (10.3%)
Vomiting	5 (4.4%)	17 (6.5%)

Only 2.6% of the patients on Sandostatin Injection in US clinical trials discontinued therapy due to these symptoms. No acromegalic patient receiving Sandostatin LAR Depot discontinued therapy for a GI event.

In patients receiving Sandostatin LAR Depot the incidence of diarrhea was dose-related. Diarrhea, abdominal pain, and nausea developed primarily during the first month of treatment with Sandostatin LAR Depot. Thereafter, new cases of these events were uncommon. The vast majority of these events were mild-to-moderate in severity.

In rare instances gastrointestinal adverse effects may resemble acute intestinal obstruction, with progressive abdominal distention, severe epigastric pain, abdominal tenderness, and guarding.

Dyspepsia, steatorrhea, discoloration of feces, and tenesmus were reported in 4-6% of patients.

In a clinical trial of carcinoid syndrome, nausea, abdominal pain, and flatulence were reported in 27-38% and constipation or vomiting in 15-21% of patients treated with Sandostatin LAR Depot. Diarrhea was reported as an adverse event in 14% of patients but since most of the patients had diarrhea as a symptom of carcinoid syndrome, it is difficult to assess the actual incidence of drug-related diarrhea.

Hypo/Hyperglycemia

In acromegaly patients treated with either Sandostatin Injection or Sandostatin LAR Depot, hypoglycemia occurred in approximately 2% and hyperglycemia in approximately 15% of patients. In carcinoid patients, hypoglycemia occurred in 4% and hyperglycemia in 27% of patients treated with Sandostatin LAR Depot (see PRECAUTIONS, Sandostatin LAR Depot).

Hypothyroidism

In acromegaly patients receiving Sandostatin Injection, 12% developed biochemical hypothyroidism, 8% developed goiter, and 4% required initiation of thyroid replacement therapy while receiving Sandostatin Injection. In acromegalics treated with Sandostatin LAR Depot hypothyroidism was reported as an adverse event in 2% and goiter in 2%. Two patients receiving Sandostatin LAR Depot, required initiation of thyroid hormone replacement therapy. In carcinoid patients, hypothyroidism has only been reported in isolated patients and goiter has not been reported (see PRECAUTIONS, Sandostatin LAR Depot).

Pain at the Injection Site

Pain on injection, which is generally mild-to-moderate, and short-lived (usually about 1 hour) is dose-related, being reported by 2%, 9%, and 11% of acromegalics receiving doses of 10 mg, 20 mg, and 30 mg, respectively, of Sandostatin LAR Depot. In carcinoid patients, where a diary was kept, pain at the injection site was reported by about 20-25% at a 10 mg dose and about 30-50% at the 20 and 30 mg dose.

Other Adverse Events 16-20%

Other adverse events (relationship to drug not established) in acromegalic and/or carcinoid syndrome patients receiving Sandostatin LAR Depot were upper respiratory infection, flu-like symptoms, fatigue, dizziness, headache, malaise, fever, dyspnea, back pain, chest pain, arthropathy.

Other Adverse Events 5-15%

Other adverse events (relationship to drug not established) occurring in an incidence of 5-15% in patients receiving Sandostatin LAR Depot were:

Body as a Whole: Asthenia, rigors, allergy.
Cardiovascular: Hypertension, peripheral edema.
Central and Peripheral Nervous System: Paresthesia, hypoesthesia.
Gastrointestinal: Dyspepsia, anorexia, hemorrhoids.
Hearing and Vestibular: Earache.
Heart Rate and Rhythm: Palpitations.
Hematologic: Anemia.
Metabolic and Nutritional: Dehydration, weight decrease.
Musculoskeletal System: Myalgia, leg cramps, arthralgia.
Psychiatric: Depression, anxiety, confusion, insomnia.
Resistance Mechanism: Viral infection, otitis media.
Respiratory System: Coughing, pharyngitis, rhinitis, sinusitis.
Skin and Appendages: Rash, pruritus, increased sweating.
Urinary System: Urinary tract infection, renal calculus.

Other Adverse Events 1-4%

Other events (relationship to drug not established), each occurring in an incidence of 1-4% in patients receiving Sandostatin LAR Depot and reported by at least 2 patients were:

Application Site: Injection site inflammation.
Body as a Whole: Syncope, ascites, hot flushes.
Cardiovascular: Cardiac failure, angina pectoris, hypertension aggravated.
Central and Peripheral Nervous System: Vertigo, abnormal gait, neuropathy, neuralgia, tremor, dysphonia, hyperkinesia, hypertonia.
Gastrointestinal: Rectal bleeding, melena, gastritis, gastroenteritis, colitis, gingivitis, taste perversion, stomatitis, glossitis, dry mouth, dysphagia, steatorrhea, diverticulitis.
Hearing and Vestibular: Tinnitus.
Heart Rate and Rhythm: Tachycardia.
Liver and Biliary: Jaundice.
Metabolic and Nutritional: Hypokalemia, cachexia, gout, hypoproteinemia.
Platelet, Bleeding, Clotting: Pulmonary embolism, epistaxis.
Psychiatric: Amnesia, somnolence, nervousness, hallucinations.
Reproductive, Female: Menstrual irregularities, breast pain.
Reproductive, Male: Impotence.
Resistance Mechanism: Cellulitis, renal abcess, moniliasis, bacterial infection.
Respiratory System: Bronchitis, pneumonia, pleural effusion.
Skin and Appendages: Alopecia, urticaria, acne.
Urinary System: Incontinence, albuminuria.
Vascular: Cerebral vascular disorder, phlebitis, hematoma.
Vision: Abnormal vision.

Rare Adverse Events

Other events (relationship to drug not established) of potential clinical significance occurring rarely (<1%) in clinical trials of octreotide either as Sandostatin Injection or Sandostatin LAR Depot, or reported post-marketing in patients with acromegaly, carcinoid syndrome, or other disorders include:

Body as a Whole: Anaphylactoid reactions, including anaphylactic shock, facial edema, generalized edema, abdomen enlarged, malignant hyperpyrexia.
Cardiovascular: Aneurysm, myocardial infarction, angina pectoris, aggravated, pulmonary hypertension, cardiac arrest, orthostatic hypotension.
Central and Peripheral Nervous System: Hemiparesis, paresis, convulsions, paranoia, pituitary apoplexy, visual field defect, migraine, aphasia, scotoma, Bell's palsy.
Endocrine Disorders: Hypoadrenalism, diabetes insipidus, gynecomastia, galactorrhea.
Gastrointestinal: GI hemorrhage, intestinal obstruction, hepatitis, increase in liver enzymes, fatty liver, peptic/gastric ulcer, gallbladder polyp, appendicitis, pancreatitis.
Hearing and Vestibular: Deafness.
Heart Rate and Rhythm: Atrial fibrillation.
Hematologic: Pancytopenia, thrombocytopenia.
Metabolic and Nutritional: Renal insufficiency, creatinine increased, CK increased, diabetes mellitus.
Musculoskeletal: Raynaud's syndrome, arthritis, joint effusion.
Neoplasms: Breast carcinoma, basal cell carcinoma.
Platelet, Bleeding, and Clotting: Arterial thrombosis of the arm.
Psychiatric: Suicide attempt, libido decrease.
Reproductive, Female: Lactation, nonpuerperal.
Respiratory: Pulmonary nodule, status asthmaticus, pneumothorax.
Skin and Appendages: Cellulitis, petechiae, urticaria.
Urinary System: Renal failure, hematuria.
Vascular: Intracranial hemorrhage, retinal vein thrombosis.
Vision: Glaucoma.

Antibodies to Octreotide

Studies to date have shown that antibodies to octreotide develop in up to 25% of patients treated with octreotide acetate. These antibodies do not influence the degree of efficacy response to octreotide; however, in two acromegalic patients who received Sandostatin Injection, the duration of GH suppression following each injection was about twice as long as in patients without antibodies. It has not been determined whether octreotide antibodies will also prolong the duration of GH suppression in patients being treated with Sandostatin LAR Depot.

DOSAGE AND ADMINISTRATION

SANDOSTATIN

Sandostatin may be administered subcutaneously or intravenously. Subcutaneous injection is the usual route of administration of Sandostatin for control of symptoms. Pain with subcutaneous administration may be reduced by using the smallest volume that will deliver the desired dose. Multiple subcutaneous injections at the same site within short periods of time should be avoided. Sites should be rotated in a systematic manner.

Parenteral drug products should be inspected visually for particulate matter and discoloration prior to administration. **Do not use if particulates and/or discoloration are observed.** Proper sterile technique should be used in the preparation of parenteral admixtures to minimize the possibility of microbial contamination. **Sandostatin is not compatible in Total Parenteral Nutrition (TPN) solutions because of the formation of a glycosyl octreotide conjugate which may decrease the efficacy of the product.**

Sandostatin is stable in sterile isotonic saline solutions or sterile solutions of dextrose 5% in water for 24 hours. It may be diluted in volumes of 50-200 ml and infused intravenously over 15-30 minutes or administered by IV push over 3 minutes. In emergency situations (*e.g.,* carcinoid crisis) it may be given by rapid bolus.

The initial dosage is usually 50 µg administered twice or three times daily. Upward dose titration is frequently required. Dosage information for patients with specific tumors follows.

Acromegaly

Dosage may be initiated at 50 µg tid. Beginning with this low dose may permit adaptation to adverse gastrointestinal effects for patients who will require higher doses. IGF-I (somatomedin C) levels every 2 weeks can be used to guide titration. Alternatively, multiple growth hormone levels at 0-8 hours after Sandostatin administration permit more rapid titration of dose. The goal is to achieve growth hormone levels less than 5 ng/ml or IGF-I (somatomedin C) levels less than 1.9 U/ml in males and less than 2.2 U/ml in females. The dose most commonly found to be effective is 100 µg tid, but some patients require up to 500 µg tid for maximum effectiveness. Doses greater than 300 µg/day seldom result in additional biochemical benefit, and if an increase in dose fails to provide additional benefit, the dose should be reduced. IGF-I (somatomedin C) or growth hormone levels should be reevaluated at 6 month intervals.

Sandostatin should be withdrawn yearly for approximately 4 weeks from patients who have received irradiation to assess disease activity. If growth hormone or IGF-I (somatomedin C) levels increase and signs and symptoms recur, Sandostatin therapy may be resumed.

Carcinoid Tumors

The suggested daily dosage of Sandostatin during the first 2 weeks of therapy ranges from 100-600 µg/day in 2-4 divided doses (mean daily dosage is 300 µg). In the clinical studies, the median daily maintenance dosage was approximately 450 µg, but clinical and biochemical benefits were obtained in some patients with as little as 50 µg, while others required doses up to 1500 µg/day. However, experience with doses above 750 µg/day is limited.

VIPomas

Daily dosages of 200-300 µg in 2-4 divided doses are recommended during the initial 2 weeks of therapy (range 150-750 µg) to control symptoms of the disease. On an individual basis, dosage may be adjusted to achieve a therapeutic response, but usually doses above 450 µg/day are not required.

SANDOSTATIN LAR DEPOT

Sandostatin LAR Depot must be administered under the supervision of a physician. It is important to closely follow the mixing instructions included in the packaging. Sandostatin LAR Depot must be administered immediately after mixing. Sandostatin LAR Depot should be administered intragluteally at 4 week intervals. Administration of Sandostatin LAR Depot at intervals greater than 4 weeks is not recommended because there is no adequate information on whether such patients could be satisfactorily controlled. Deltoid injections are to be avoided because of significant discomfort at the injection site when given in that area. **Sandostatin LAR Depot should never be administered by the IV or SC routes.** The following dosage regimens are recommended.

Acromegaly

Patients Not Currently Receiving Octreotide Acetate

Patients not currently receiving octreotide acetate should begin therapy with Sandostatin Injection given subcutaneously in an initial dose of 50 µg tid. Beginning with this low dose may permit adaptation to adverse gastrointestinal effects for patients who require higher doses. Multiple growth hormone (GH) determinations at 0-8 hours after a subcutaneous Sandostatin Injection will guide dosage titration. The goal is to attempt to normalize GH and IGF-1 (somatomedin C) levels. Most patients require doses of 100-200 µg tid for maximum effect but some patients require up to 500 µg tid. Injection sites should be rotated in a systematic manner to avoid irritation.

Although responsiveness of GH to octreotide acetate can be ascertained quickly, patients should be maintained on Sandostatin Injection SC for at least 2 weeks to determine tolerance to octreotide.

The most common adverse events are gastrointestinal, which usually begin within the first few days of administration and usually subside within 2-8 weeks. In clinical trials, <3% of patients discontinued Sandostatin Injection because of GI symptoms.

Patients who are considered to be "responders" to the drug, based on GH and IGF-1 levels, and who tolerate the drug, can then be switched to Sandostatin LAR Depot in the dosage scheme described under Patients Currently Receiving Sandostatin Injection.

Patients Currently Receiving Sandostatin Injection

Patients currently receiving Sandostatin Injection can be switched directly to Sandostatin LAR Depot in a dose of 20 mg given IM intragluteally at 4 week intervals for 3 months. **(Deltoid injections are to be avoided because of significant discomfort at the injection site when given in that area.)** Gluteal injection sites should be alternated to avoid irritation.

At the end of 3 months Sandostatin LAR Depot dosage may be continued at the same level or increased or decreased based on the following regimen:

GH ≤2.5 ng/ml, IGF-1 normal and clinical symptoms controlled: maintain Sandostatin LAR Depot dosage at 20 mg every 4 weeks.

GH >2.5 ng/ml, IGF-1 elevated, and/or clinical symptoms uncontrolled, increase Sandostatin LAR Depot dosage to 30 mg every 4 weeks.

GH ≤1 ng/ml, IGF-1 normal and clinical symptoms controlled, reduce Sandostatin LAR Depot dosage to 10 mg every 4 weeks.

Patients whose GH, IGF-1, and symptoms are not adequately controlled at a dose of 30 mg may have the dose increased to 40 mg every 4 weeks. Doses higher than 40 mg are not recommended.

Administration of Sandostatin LAR Depot at intervals greater than 4 weeks is not recommended because there is no adequate information on whether such patients could be satisfactorily controlled.

In patients who have received pituitary irradiation, Sandostatin LAR Depot Depot should be withdrawn yearly for approximately 8 weeks to assess disease activity. If GH or IGF-1 levels increase and signs and symptoms recur, Sandostatin LAR Depot Depot therapy may be resumed.

Special Populations: Renal Failure

In patients with renal failure requiring dialysis, the half-life of octreotide may be increased, necessitating adjustment of the maintenance dosage (see CLINICAL PHARMACOLOGY, Sandostatin LAR Depot and CLINICAL PHARMACOLOGY, Sandostatin LAR Depot, Pharmacokinetics of Octreotide).

Carcinoid Tumors and VIPomas

Patients Not Currently Receiving Octreotide Acetate

Patients not currently receiving octreotide acetate should begin therapy with Sandostatin Injection given subcutaneously. The suggested daily dosage for carcinoid tumors during the first 2 weeks of therapy ranges from 100-600 µg/day in 2-4 divided doses (mean daily dosage is 300 µg). Some patients may require doses up to 1500 µg/day. The suggested daily dosage for VIPomas is 200-300 µg in 2-4 divided doses (range 150-750 µg); dosage may be adjusted on an individual basis to control symptoms but usually doses above 450 µg/day are not required.

Sandostatin Injection should be continued for at least 2 weeks. Thereafter, patients who are considered "responders" to octreotide acetate and who tolerate the drug may be switched to Sandostatin LAR Depot in the dosage regimen described Patients Currently Receiving Sandostatin Injection.

Patients Currently Receiving Sandostatin Injection

Patients currently receiving Sandostatin Injection can be switched to Sandostatin LAR Depot in a dosage of 20 mg given IM intragluteally at 4 week intervals for 2 months. **Deltoid injections are to be avoided because of significant discomfort at the injection site when given in that area.** Gluteal injection sites should be alternated to avoid irritation. Because of the need for serum octreotide to reach therapeutically effective levels following initial injection of Sandostatin LAR Depot, carcinoid tumor and VIPoma patients should continue to receive Sandostatin Injection SC for at least 2 weeks in the same dosage they were taking before the switch. Failure to continue subcutaneous injections for this period may result in exacerbation of symptoms. (Some patients may require 3 or 4 weeks of such therapy.)

After 2 months of a 20 mg dosage of Sandostatin LAR Depot, dosage may be increased to 30 mg every 4 weeks if symptoms are not adequately controlled. Patients who achieve good control on a 20 mg dose may have their dose lowered to 10 mg for a trial period. If symptoms recur, dosage should then be increased to 20 mg every 4 weeks. Many patients can, however, be satisfactorily maintained at a 10 mg dosage every 4 weeks. A dose of 10 mg is not recommended as a starting dose, however, because therapeutically effective levels of octreotide are reached more rapidly with a 20 mg dose.

Dosages higher than 30 mg are not recommended because there is no information on their usefulness.

Despite good overall control of symptoms, patients with carcinoid tumors and VIPomas often experience periodic exacerbation of symptoms (regardless of whether they are being maintained on Sandostatin Injection or Sandostatin LAR Depot). During these periods they may be given Sandostatin Injection SC for a few days at the dosage they were receiving prior to switch to Sandostatin LAR Depot. When symptoms are again controlled, the Sandostatin Injection SC can be discontinued.

Administration of Sandostatin LAR Depot at intervals greater than 4 weeks is not recommended because there is no adequate information on whether such patients could be adequately controlled.

Special Populations: Renal Failure

In patients with renal failure requiring dialysis, the half-life of octreotide may be increased, necessitating adjustment of the maintenance dosage (see CLINICAL PHARMACOLOGY, Sandostatin LAR Depot and CLINICAL PHARMACOLOGY, Sandostatin LAR Depot, Pharmacokinetics of Octreotide).

HOW SUPPLIED

SANDOSTATIN

Sandostatin Injection is available in 1 ml ampuls containing 50, 100, and 500 µg/ml octreotide (as acetate) and 5 ml multi-dose vials containing 200 and 1000 µg/ml octreotide (as acetate).

Storage

For prolonged storage, Sandostatin ampuls and multi-dose vials should be stored at refrigerated temperatures 2-8°C (36-46°F) and protected from light. At room temperature, (20-30°C or 70-86°F), Sandostatin is stable for 14 days if protected from light. The solution can be allowed to come to room temperature prior to administration. Do not warm artificially. After initial use, multiple dose vials should be discarded within 14 days. Ampuls should be opened just prior to administration and the unused portion discarded.

SANDOSTATIN LAR DEPOT

Sandostatin LAR Depot is available in single use kits containing a 5 ml vial of 10, 20 or 30 mg strength, a 2 ml vial of diluent, a 5 ml sterile plastic syringe, two sterile 1½" 20 gauge needles, and three alcohol wipes. An instruction booklet for the preparation of drug suspension for injection is also included with each kit.

Storage

For prolonged storage, Sandostatin LAR Depot should be stored at refrigerated temperatures 2-8°C (36-46°F) and protected from light until the time of use. Sandostatin LAR Depot drug product kit should remain at room temperature for 30-60 minutes prior to preparation of the drug suspension. However, after preparation the drug suspension must be administered immediately.

PRODUCT LISTING - EQUIVALENTS NOT AVAILABLE

Powder For Injection - Intramuscular - 10 mg
1's $1535.23 SANDOSTATIN LAR DEPOT, Novartis Consumer Health 00078-0340-84

Powder For Injection - Intramuscular - 20 mg
1's $1867.20 SANDOSTATIN LAR DEPOT, Novartis Consumer Health 00078-0341-84

Powder For Injection - Intramuscular - 30 mg
1's $2509.11 SANDOSTATIN LAR DEPOT, Novartis Consumer Health 00078-0342-84

Solution - Injectable - 50 mcg/ml
1 ml x 20 $199.60 SANDOSTATIN, Novartis Pharmaceuticals 00078-0180-03

Solution - Injectable - 100 mcg/ml
1 ml x 20 $387.00 SANDOSTATIN, Novartis Pharmaceuticals 00078-0181-03

Solution - Injectable - 200 mcg/ml
5 ml $199.43 SANDOSTATIN, Novartis Pharmaceuticals 00078-0183-25

Solution - Injectable - 500 mcg/ml
1 ml x 20 $1866.00 SANDOSTATIN, Novartis Pharmaceuticals 00078-0182-03

Solution - Injectable - 1000 mcg/ml
5 ml $981.31 SANDOSTATIN, Novartis Pharmaceuticals 00078-0184-25

Ofloxacin *(003016)*

For related information, see the comparative table section in Appendix A.

Categories: Bronchitis, chronic, acute exacerbation; Conjunctivitis, infectious; Gonorrhea; Infection, cervix; Infection, ear, external; Infection, ear, middle; Infection, lower respiratory tract; Infection, skin and skin structures; Infection, urinary tract; Pneumonia, community-acquired; Prostatitis; Ulcer, corneal; Urethritis; Pregnancy Category C; FDA Approved 1990 Dec; Orphan Drugs

Drug Classes: Antibiotics, quinolones; Anti-infectives, ophthalmic; Ophthalmics

Brand Names: **Floxin**; Ocuflox

Foreign Brand Availability: Akilen (Indonesia); Baccidal (Korea); Bactocin (Mexico); Danoflox (Indonesia); Effexin (Korea); Exocin (Ireland); Exocine (France); Flobacin (Italy); Floxal (Germany); Floxil (Mexico); Floxstat (Colombia; Costa-Rica; Dominican-Republic; Ecuador; El-Salvador; Guatemala; Honduras; Mexico; Nicaragua; Panama); Fugacin (Korea); Inoflox (Malaysia; Philippines); Kinflocin (Taiwan); Kinoxacin (Korea); Loxinter (Indonesia); Marfloxacin (Hong-Kong); Novecin (Bahrain; Cyprus; Egypt; Iran; Iraq; Jordan; Kuwait; Lebanon; Libya; Oman; Qatar; Republic-of-Yemen; Saudi-Arabia; Syria; United-Arab-Emirates); Nufafloqo (Indonesia); Obide (Korea); Occidal (Thailand); Ofcin (Singapore; Taiwan); Oflin (India); Oflocee (Thailand); Oflocet (France); Oflocin (Italy); Oflodal (Taiwan); Oflodex (Israel); O-Flox (Thailand); Oflox (Colombia; Israel; Peru); Ofloxin (Thailand); Operan (Korea); Orocin (Korea); Pharflox (Indonesia); Qinolon (Philippines); Qipro (Indonesia); Quinolon (Thailand); Rilox (Indonesia); Sinflo (Taiwan); Tabrin (Greece); Taravid (Bahrain; Cyprus; Egypt; Iran; Iraq; Israel; Jordan; Kuwait; Lebanon; Libya; Oman; Qatar; Republic-of-Yemen; Saudi-Arabia; Syria; United-Arab-Emirates); Tariflox (Indonesia); Tarivid (Austria; Belgium; Benin; Bulgaria; Burkina-Faso; China; Czech-Republic; Denmark; England; Ethiopia; Finland; Gambia; Germany; Ghana; Guinea; Hungary; India; Indonesia; Ireland; Israel; Ivory-Coast; Japan; Kenya; Korea; Liberia; Malawi; Malaysia; Mali; Mauritania; Mauritius; Morocco; Netherlands; Niger; Nigeria; Norway; Portugal; Senegal; Seychelles; Sierra-Leone; Singapore; South-Africa; Spain; Sudan; Sweden; Switzerland; Tanzania; Thailand; Tunia; Uganda; Zambia; Zimbabwe); Tarivid Eye Ear (Hong-Kong); Tructum (Peru); Uro Tarivid (Bahrain; Cyprus; Egypt; Iran; Iraq; Jordan; Kuwait; Lebanon; Libya; Oman; Qatar; Republic-of-Yemen; Saudi-Arabia; Syria; United-Arab-Emirates); Viotisone (Thailand); Zanocin (India)

Cost of Therapy: $120.85 (Infection; Floxin; 400 mg; 2 tablets/day; 10 day supply)

DESCRIPTION

TABLETS AND INTRAVENOUS INFUSION

Floxin Tablets and IV are synthetic broad-spectrum antimicrobial agents for oral or intravenous administration. Chemically, ofloxacin, a fluorinated carboxyquinolone, is the racemate, (±)-9-fluoro-2,3-dihydro-3-methyl-10-(4-methyl-1-piperazinyl)-7-oxo-7H-pyrido[1,2,3-de]-1,4-benzoxazine-6-carboxylic acid. Its empirical formula is $C_{18}H_{20}FN_3O_4$, and its molecular weight is 361.4. Ofloxacin is an off-white to pale yellow crystalline powder. The molecule exists as a zwitterion at the pH conditions in the small intestine. The relative solubility characteristics of ofloxacin at room temperature, as defined by USP nomenclature, indicate that ofloxacin is considered to be *soluble* in aqueous solutions with pH between 2 and 5. It is *sparingly* to *slightly soluble* in aqueous solutions with pH 7 (solubility falls to 4 mg/ml) and *freely soluble* in aqueous solutions with pH above 9. Ofloxacin has the potential to form stable coordination compounds with many metal ions. This *in vitro* chelation potential has the following formation order: $Fe^{+3}>Al^{+3}>Cu^{+2}>Ni^{+2}>Pb^{+2}>Zn^{+2}>Mg^{+2}>Ca^{+2}>Ba^{+2}$.

Tablets

Floxin tablets contain the following inactive ingredients: anhydrous lactose, corn starch, hydroxypropyl cellulose, hydroxypropyl methylcellulose, magnesium stearate, polyethylene glycol, polysorbate 80, sodium starch glycolate, titanium dioxide and may also contain synthetic yellow iron oxide.

Intravenous Infusion

Floxin IV in single-use vials is a sterile, preservative-free aqueous solution of ofloxacin with pH ranging from 3.5-5.5. Floxin IV in pre-mixed bottles and in pre-mixed flexible containers are sterile, preservative-free aqueous solutions of ofloxacin with pH ranging from 3.8-5.8. The color of Floxin IV may range from light yellow to amber. This does not adversely affect product potency. Floxin IV in single-use vials contains ofloxacin in water for injection. Floxin IV in pre-mixed bottles and in pre-mixed flexible containers are dilute, non-pyrogenic, nearly isotonic pre-mixed solutions that contain ofloxacin in 5% dextrose (D_5W). Hydrochloric acid and sodium hydroxide may have been added to adjust the pH.

The flexible container is fabricated from a specially formulated non-plasticized, thermoplastic copolyester (CR3). The amount of water that can permeate from the container into the overwrap is insufficient to affect the solution significantly. Solutions in contact with the flexible container can leach out certain of the container's chemical components in very small amounts within the expiration period. The suitability of the container material has been confirmed by tests in animals according to USP biological tests for plastic containers.

OPHTHALMIC SOLUTION AND OTIC SOLUTION

Ocuflox 0.3% is a sterile ophthalmic solution. It is a fluorinated carboxyquinolone anti-infective for topical ophthalmic use. Ofloxacin otic solution 0.3% is a sterile aqueous anti-infective (anti-bacterial) solution for otic use.

Chemically, ofloxacin has three condensed 6-membered rings made up of a fluorinated carboxyquinolone with a benzoxazine ring. The chemical name is: (±)-9-fluoro-2, 3-dihydro-3-methyl-10-(4-methyl-1-piperazinyl)-7-oxo-7H-pyrido[1, 2, 3-de]-1, 4 benzoxazine-6-carboxylic acid.

Ocuflox 0.3% contains: *Active:* Ofloxacin 0.3% (3 mg/ml); *Preservative:* Benzalkonium chloride (0.005%); *Inactives:* Sodium chloride and purified water. May also contain hydrochloric acid and/or sodium hydroxide to adjust pH.

Floxin Otic contains 0.3% (3mg/ml) ofloxacin with benzalkonium chloride (0.0025%), sodium chloride (0.9%), and water for injection. Hydrochloric acid and sodium hydroxide are added to adjust the pH to 6.5 ± 0.5.

Ofloxacin ophthalmic solution is unbuffered and formulated with a pH of 6.4 (range: 6.0-6.8). It has an osmolality of 300 mOsm/kg. Ofloxacin is a fluorinated 4-quinolone which differs from other fluorinated 4-quinolones in that there is a six member (pyridobenzoxazine) ring from positions 1-8 of the basic ring structure.

CLINICAL PHARMACOLOGY

PHARMACOKINETICS

Tablets and Intravenous Infusion

In vitro, approximately 32% of the drug in plasma is protein bound.

The single dose and steady-state plasma profiles of ofloxacin injection were comparable in extent of exposure (AUC) to those of ofloxacin tablets when the injectable and tablet formulations of ofloxacin were administered in equal doses (mg/mg) to the same group of subjects. The mean steady-state AUC(0-12) attained after the intravenous administration of 400 mg over 60 min was 43.5 μg·h/ml; the mean steady-state AUC(0-12) attained after the oral administration of 400 mg was 41.2 μg·h/ml (two one-sided t-test, 90% confidence interval was 103-109).

Between 0 and 6 hours following the administration of a single 200 mg oral dose of ofloxacin to 12 healthy volunteers, the average urine ofloxacin concentration was approximately 220 μg/ml. Between 12 and 24 hours after administration, the average urine ofloxacin level was approximately 34 μg/ml.

Following oral administration of recommended therapeutic doses, ofloxacin has been detected in blister fluid, cervix, lung tissue, ovary, prostatic fluid, prostatic tissue, skin, and sputum. The mean concentration of ofloxacin in each of these various body fluids and tissues after 1 or more doses was 0.8-1.5 times the concurrent plasma level. Inadequate data are presently available on the distribution or levels of ofloxacin in the cerebrospinal fluid or brain tissue.

Following the administration of oral doses of ofloxacin to healthy elderly volunteers (64-74 years of age) with normal renal function, the apparent half-life of ofloxacin was 7-8 hours, as compared to approximately 6 hours in younger adults. Drug absorption, however, appears to be unaffected by age.

Clearance of ofloxacin is reduced in patients with impaired renal function (creatinine clearance rate ≤50 ml/min), and dosage adjustment is necessary. (See PRECAUTIONS, General and DOSAGE AND ADMINISTRATION.)

Tablets

Ofloxacin has a pyridobenzoxazine ring that appears to decrease the extent of parent compound metabolism. Between 65 and 80% of an administered oral dose of ofloxacin is excreted unchanged via the kidneys within 48 hours of dosing. Studies indicate that less than 5% of an administered dose is recovered in the urine as the desmethyl or N-oxide metabolites. Four (4%) to 8% of an ofloxacin dose is excreted in the feces. This indicates a small degree of biliary excretion of ofloxacin. The administration of ofloxacin with food does not affect the C_{max} and AUC (∞) of the drug, but T_{max} is prolonged.

Following oral administration, the bioavailability of ofloxacin in the tablet formulation is approximately 98%. Maximum serum concentrations are achieved 1-2 hours after an oral dose. Absorption of ofloxacin after single or multiple doses of 200-400 mg is predictable, and the amount of drug absorbed increases proportionately with the dose.

Ofloxacin has biphasic elimination. Following multiple oral doses at steady-state administration, the half-lives are approximately 4-5 hours and 20-25 hours. However, the longer half-life represents less than 5% of the total AUC. Accumulation at steady-state can be estimated using a half-life of 9 hours. The total clearance and volume of distribution are approximately similar after single or multiple doses. Elimination is mainly by renal excretion. TABLE 1 shows mean peak serum concentrations in healthy 70-80 kg male volunteers after single oral doses of 200, 300, or 400 mg of ofloxacin or after multiple oral doses of 400 mg.

TABLE 1

Oral Dose	Serum Concentration 2 hours after admin.	Area Under the Curve [AUC(0-∞)]
200 mg single dose	1.5 μg/ml	14.1 μg·h/ml
300 mg single dose	2.4 μg/ml	21.2 μg·h/ml
400 mg single dose	2.9 μg/ml	31.4 μg·h/ml
400 mg steady state	4.6 μg/ml	61.0 μg·h/ml

Steady-state concentrations were attained after 4 oral doses and the area under the curve (AUC) was approximately 40% higher than the AUC after single doses. Therefore, after multiple-dose administration of 200 mg and 300 mg doses, peak serum levels of 2.2 μg/ml and 3.6 μg/ml, respectively, are predicted at steady-state.

Intravenous Infusion

Following a single 60-minute intravenous infusion of 200 mg or 400 mg of ofloxacin to normal volunteers, the mean maximum plasma concentrations attained were 2.7 and 4.0 μg/ml, respectively; the concentrations at 12 hours after dosing were 0.3 and 0.7 μg/ml, respectively.

Steady-state concentrations were attained after 4 doses, and the area under the curve (AUC) was approximately 40% higher than the AUC after a single dose. The mean peak and trough plasma steady-state levels attained following intravenous administration of 200 mg of ofloxacin q12h for 7 days were 2.9 and 0.5 μg/ml, respectively. Following intravenous doses of 400 mg of ofloxacin q12h, the mean peak and trough plasma steady-state levels ranged, in two different studies, from 5.5-7.2 μg/ml and 1.2-1.9 μg/ml, respectively.

Following 7 days of intravenous administration, the elimination half-life of ofloxacin was 6 hours (range 5-10 hours). The total clearance and the volume of distribution were approximately 15 L/h and 120 L, respectively.

Elimination of ofloxacin is primarily by renal excretion. Approximately 65% of a dose is excreted renally within 48 hours. Studies indicate that <5% of an administered dose is recovered in the urine as the desmethyl or N-oxide metabolites. Four (4%) to 8% of an ofloxacin dose is excreted in the feces. This indicates a small degree of biliary excretion of ofloxacin.

Ophthalmic Solution

Serum, urine and tear concentrations of ofloxacin were measured in 30 healthy women at various time points during a 10 day course of treatment with ofloxacin ophthalmic solution. The mean serum ofloxacin concentration ranged from 0.4-1.9 ng/ml. Maximum ofloxacin concentration increased from 1.1 ng/ml on day 1-1.9 ng/ml on day 11 after 4 times daily dosing for 10½ days. Maximum serum ofloxacin concentrations after 10 days of topical ophthalmic dosing were more than 1000 times lower than those reported after standard oral doses of ofloxacin.

Tear ofloxacin concentrations ranged from 5.7 to 31 μg/g during the 40 minute period following the last dose on day 11. Mean tear concentration measured 4 hours after topical ophthalmic dosing was 9.2 μg/g.

Corneal tissue concentrations of 4.4 μg/ml were observed 4 hours after beginning topical ocular application of 2 drops of ofloxacin ophthalmic solution every 30 minutes. Ofloxacin was excreted in the urine primarily unmodified.

Otic Solution

Drug concentrations in serum (in subjects with tympanostomy tubes and perforated tympanic membranes), in otorrhea, and in mucosa of the middle ear (in subjects with perforated tympanic membranes) were determined following otic administration of ofloxacin solution. In two single-dose studies, mean ofloxacin serum concentrations were low in adult patients with tympanostomy tubes, with and without otorrhea, after otic administration of a 0.3% solution [4.1 ng/ml (n=3) and 5.4 ng/ml (n=5), respectively]. In adults with perforated tympanic membranes, the maximum serum drug level of ofloxacin detected was 10 ng/ml after administration of a 0.3% solution. Ofloxacin was detectable in the middle ear mucosa of some adult subjects with perforated tympanic membranes (11 of 16 subjects). The variability of ofloxacin concentration in middle ear mucosa was high. The concentrations ranged from 1.2 to 602 μg/g after otic administration of a 0.3% solution. Ofloxacin was present in high concentrations in otorrhea (389-2850 μg/g, n=13) 30 minutes after otic administration of a 0.3% solution in subjects with chronic suppurative otitis media and perforated tympanic membranes. However, the measurement of ofloxacin in the otorrhea does not necessarily reflect the exposure of the middle ear to ofloxacin.

MICROBIOLOGY

Tablet and Intravenous Infusion

Ofloxacin has *in vitro* activity against a broad spectrum of gram-positive and gram-negative aerobic and anaerobic bacteria. Ofloxacin is often bactericidal at concentrations equal to or slightly greater than inhibitory concentrations. Ofloxacin is thought to exert a bactericidal effect on susceptible microorganisms by inhibiting DNA gyrase, an essential enzyme that is a critical catalyst in the duplication, transcription, and repair of bacterial DNA.

Ofloxacin has been shown to be active against most strains of the following microorganisms both *in vitro* and in specific clinical infections; (see INDICATIONS AND USAGE).

Gram-Positive Aerobes: *Staphylococcus aureus, Streptococcus pneumoniae, Streptococcus pyogenes.*

Gram-Negative Aerobes: *Citrobacter diversus, Enterobacter aerogenes, Escherichia coli, Haemophilus influenzae, Klebsiella pneumoniae, Neisseria gonorrhoeae, Proteus mirabilis, Pseudomonas aeruginosa.*

Other: *Chlamydia trachomatis.*

The following *in vitro* data are available, but their clinical significance is unknown.

Ofloxacin exhibits *in vitro* minimum inhibitory concentrations (MICs) of 2 μg/ml or less against most (≥90%) strains of the following microorganisms; however, the safety and effectiveness of ofloxacin in treating clinical infections due to these microorganisms have not been established in adequate and well-controlled clinical trials:

Gram-Positive Aerobes: *Staphylococcus epidermidis* (excluding methicillin-resistant strains), *Staphylococcus haemolyticus, Staphylococcus saprophyticus.*

Gram-Negative Aerobes: *Acinetobacter calcoaceticus, Aeromonas caviae, Aeromonas hydrophila, Bordetella parapertussis, Bordetella pertussis, Citrobacter freundii, Enterobacter cloacae, Haemophilus ducreyi, Klebsiella oxytoca, Moraxella catarrhalis, Morganella morganii, Proteus vulgaris, Providencia rettgeri, Providencia stuartii, Serratia marcescens, Vibrio parahaemolyticus.*

Anaerobes: *Clostridium perfringens, Gardnerella vaginalis.*

Other Organisms: *Chlamydia pneumoniae, Legionella pneumophila, Mycobacterium tuberculosis* (including multiple drug-resistant strains), *Mycoplasma hominis, Mycoplasma pneumoniae, Ureaplasma urealyticum.*

Ofloxacin has not been shown to be active against *Treponema pallidum*. (See WARNINGS.)

Many strains of other streptococcal species, *Enterococcus* species, and anaerobes are resistant to ofloxacin.

Resistance to ofloxacin due to spontaneous mutation *in vitro* is a rare occurrence (range: 10^{-9} to 10^{-11}). To date, emergence of resistance has been relatively uncommon in clinical practice. With the exception of *Pseudomonas aeruginosa* (10%), less than a 4% rate of resistance emergence has been reported for most other species. Although cross-resistance has been observed between ofloxacin and other fluoroquinolones, some organisms resistant to other quinolones may be susceptible to ofloxacin.

Otic Solution

Ofloxacin has *in vitro* activity against a wide range of gram-negative and gram-positive microorganisms. Ofloxacin exerts its antibacterial activity by inhibiting DNA gyrase, a bacterial topoisomerase. DNA gyrase is an essential enzyme which controls DNA topology and assists in DNA replication, repair, deactivation, and transcription. Cross-resistance has been observed between ofloxacin and other fluoroquinolones. There is generally no cross-resistance between ofloxacin and other classes of antibacterial agents such as beta-lactams or aminoglycosides.

Ofloxacin has been shown to be active against most strains of the following microorganisms, both *in vitro* and clinically in otic infections as described in the INDICATIONS AND USAGE.

Aerobes, Gram-Positive: *Staphylococcus aureus, Streptococcus pneumoniae.*

Aerobes, Gram-Negative: *Haemophilus influenzae, Moraxella catarrhalis, Proteus mirabilis, Pseudomonas aeruginosa.*

SUSCEPTIBILITY TESTING

Dilution Techniques

Quantitative methods are used to determine antimicrobial minimal inhibitory concentrations (MICs). These MICs provide estimates of the susceptibility of bacteria to antimicrobial compounds. The MICs should be determined using a standardized procedure. Standardized procedures are based on a dilution method[1] (broth or agar) or equivalent with standardized inoculum concentrations and standardized concentrations of ofloxacin powder. The MIC values should be interpreted according to the criteria in TABLE 2.

TABLE 2

MIC (μg/ml)	Interpretation
≤ 2	Susceptible (S)
4	Intermediate (I)
≥ 8	Resistant (R)

A report of "Susceptible" indicates that the pathogen is likely to be inhibited if the antimicrobial compound in the blood reaches the concentrations usually achievable. A report of "Intermediate" indicates that the result should be considered equivocal, and, if the microorganism is not fully susceptible to alternative, clinically feasible drugs, the test should be repeated. This category implies possible clinical applicability in body sites where the drug is physiologically concentrated or in situations where high dosage of drug can be used. This category also provides a buffer zone which prevents small uncontrolled technical factors from causing major discrepancies in interpretation. A report of "Resistant" indicates that the pathogen is not likely to be inhibited if the antimicrobial compound in the blood reaches the concentrations usually achievable; other therapy should be selected.

Standardized susceptibility test procedures require the use of laboratory control microorganisms to control the technical aspects of the laboratory procedures. Standard ofloxacin powder should provide MIC values in TABLE 3.

TABLE 3

Microorganism		MIC (μg/ml)
Escherichia coli	ATCC 25922	0.015-0.12
Staphylococcus aureus	ATCC 29213	0.12-1.0
Pseudomonas aeruginosa	ATCC 27853	1.0-8.0
Haemophilus influenzae	ATCC 49247	0.016-0.06
Neisseria gonorrhoeae	ATCC 49226	0.004-0.016

Diffusion Techniques

Quantitative methods that require measurement of zone diameters also provide reproducible estimates of the susceptibility of bacteria to antimicrobial compounds. One such standardized procedure[2] requires the use of standardized inoculum concentrations. This procedure uses paper disks impregnated with 5 μg ofloxacin to test the susceptibility of microorganisms to ofloxacin.

Reports from the laboratory providing results of the standard single-disk susceptibility test with a 5 μg ofloxacin disk should be interpreted according to TABLE 4.

TABLE 4

Zone Diameter (mm)	Interpretation
≥16	Susceptible (S)
13-15	Intermediate (I)
≤12	Resistant (R)

Interpretation should be as stated above for results using dilution techniques. Interpretation involves correlation of the diameter obtained in the disk test with the MIC for ofloxacin.

As with standardized dilution techniques, diffusion methods require the use of laboratory control microorganisms that are used to control the technical aspects of the laboratory procedures. For the diffusion technique, the 5 μg ofloxacin disk should provide the following zone diameters in these laboratory test quality control strains (see TABLE 5).

TABLE 5

Microorganism		Zone Diameter (mm)
Escherichia coli	ATCC 25922	29-33
Pseudomonas aeruginosa	ATCC 27853	17-21
Haemophilus influenzae	ATCC 49247	31-40
Neisseria gonorrhoeae	ATCC 49226	43-51
Staphylococcus aureus	ATCC 25923	24-28

INDICATIONS AND USAGE

TABLETS AND INTRAVENOUS INFUSION

Ofloxacin tablets and IV are indicated for the treatment of adults with mild to moderate infections (unless otherwise indicated) caused by susceptible strains of the designated microorganisms in the infections listed- (*For Intravenous Infusion:* when intravenous administration offers a route of administration advantageous to the patient, [*e.g.,* patient cannot tolerate an oral dosage form]). See DOSAGE AND ADMINISTRATION for specific recommendations.

The safety and effectiveness of the intravenous formulation in treating patients with severe infections have not been established.

NOTE: IN THE ABSENCE OF VOMITING OR OTHER FACTORS INTERFERING WITH THE ABSORPTION OF ORALLY ADMINISTERED DRUG, PATIENTS RECEIVE ESSENTIALLY THE SAME SYSTEMIC ANTIMICROBIAL THERAPY AFTER EQUIVALENT DOSES OF OFLOXACIN ADMINISTERED BY EITHER THE ORAL OR THE INTRAVENOUS ROUTE. THEREFORE, THE INTRAVENOUS FORMULATION DOES NOT PROVIDE A HIGHER DEGREE OF EFFICACY OR MORE POTENT ANTIMICROBIAL ACTIVITY THAN AN EQUIVALENT DOSE OF THE ORAL FORMULATION OF OFLOXACIN.

- ***Acute Bacterial Exacerbation of Chronic Bronchitis:*** Due to *Haemophilus influenzae* or *Streptococcus pneumoniae.*
- ***Community-Acquired Pneumonia:*** Due to *Haemophilus influenzae* or *Streptococcus pneumoniae.*
- ***Uncomplicated Skin and Skin Structure Infections:*** Due to *Staphylococcus aureus, Streptococcus pyogenes,* or *Proteus mirabilis**.
- ***Acute, Uncomplicated Urethral and Cervical Gonorrhea:*** Due to *Neisseria gonorrhoeae.* (See WARNINGS.)
- ***Nongonococcal Urethritis and Cervicitis:*** Due to *Chlamydia trachomatis.* (See WARNINGS.)
- ***Mixed Infections of the Urethra and Cervix:*** Due to *Chlamydia trachomatis* and *Neisseria gonorrhoeae.* (See WARNINGS.)
- ***Acute Pelvic Inflammatory Disease:*** (including severe infection) Due to *Chlamydia trachomatis* and/or *Neisseria gonorrhoeae.* (See WARNINGS.) *NOTE:* if anaerobic microorganisms are suspected of contributing to the infection, appropriate therapy for anaerobic pathogens should be administered.
- ***Uncomplicated Cystitis:*** Due to *Citrobacter diversus, Enterobacter aerogenes, Escherichia coli, Klebsiella pneumoniae, Proteus mirabilis, or Pseudomonas aeruginosa**.
- ***Complicated Urinary Tract Infections:*** Due to *Escherichia coli, Klebsiella pneumoniae, Proteus mirabilis, Citrobacter diversus**, or *Pseudomonas aeruginosa**.
- ***Prostatitis:*** Due to *Escherichia coli.*
- *Although treatment of infections due to this organism in this organ system demonstrated a clinically significant outcome, efficacy was studies in fewer than 10 patients.

Appropriate culture and susceptibility tests should be performed before treatment in order to isolate and identify organisms causing the infection and to determine their susceptibility to ofloxacin. Therapy with ofloxacin may be initiated before results of these tests are known; once results become available, appropriate therapy should be continued.

As with other drugs in this class, some strains of *Pseudomonas aeruginosa* may develop resistance fairly rapidly during treatment with ofloxacin. Culture and susceptibility testing performed periodically during therapy will provide information not only on the therapeutic effect of the antimicrobial agent but also on the possible emergence of bacterial resistance.

OPHTHALMIC SOLUTION

Ofloxacin ophthalmic solution is indicated for the treatment of infections caused by susceptible strains of the following bacteria in the conditions listed below:

Conjunctivitis

Gram-Positive Bacteria: *Staphylococcus aureus, Staphylococcus epidermidis, Streptococcus pneumoniae.*

Gram-Negative Bacteria: *Enterobacter cloacae, Haemophilus influenzae, Proteus mirabilis, Pseudomonas aeruginosa.*

Corneal Ulcers

Gram-Positive Bacteria: *Staphylococcus aureus, Staphylococcus epidermidis, Streptococcus pneumoniae.*

Gram-Negative Bacteria: *Pseudomonas aeruginosa, Serratia marcescens**.

Anaerobic Species: *Propionibacterium acnes.*

*Efficacy for this organism was studied in fewer than 10 infections.

OTIC SOLUTION

Ofloxacin otic solution 0.3% is indicated for the treatment of infections caused by susceptible strains of the designated microorganisms in the specific conditions listed below:

Otitis Externa: in adults and pediatric patients, 1 year and older, due to *Staphylococcus aureus* and *Pseudomonas aeruginosa.*

Chronic Suppurative Otitis Media: in patients 12 years and older with perforated tympanic membranes due to *Staphylococcus aureus, Proteus mirabilis, and Pseudomonas aeruginosa.*

Acute Otitis Media: in pediatric patients 1 year and older with tympanostomy tubes due to *Staphylococcus aureus, Streptococcus pneumoniae, Haemophilus influenzae, Moraxella catarrhalis,* and *Pseudomonas aeruginosa.*

NON-FDA APPROVED INDICATIONS

Ofloxacin is being used with increasing frequency in the treatment of multiple-drug-resistant tuberculosis; however, the optimal use for this condition has not yet been clearly established. Additionally, ofloxacin has been used to treat gastrointestinal, bone and joint infections. Currently, none of these uses have been approved by the FDA.

CONTRAINDICATIONS

Ofloxacin is contraindicated in persons with a history of hypersensitivity to ofloxacin, to other quinolones, or to any of the components in this medication.

WARNINGS

TABLETS AND INTRAVENOUS INFUSION

THE SAFETY AND EFFICACY OF OFLOXACIN IN CHILDREN, ADOLESCENTS (UNDER THE AGE OF 18 YEARS), PREGNANT WOMEN, AND LACTATING WOMEN HAVE NOT BEEN ESTABLISHED. (SEE PRECAUTIONS: Pediatric Use; Pregnancy, Teratogenic Effects, Pregnancy Category C; andNursing Mothers.)

In the immature rat, the oral administration of ofloxacin at 5-16 times the recommended maximum human dose based on mg/kg or 1-3 times based on mg/m^2 increased the incidence and severity of osteochondrosis. The lesions did not regress after 13 weeks of drug withdrawal. Other quinolones also produce similar erosions in the weight-bearing joints and other signs of arthropathy in immature animals of various species. (See ANIMAL PHARMACOLOGY.)

Serious and occasionally fatal hypersensitivity (anaphylactic/anaphylactöid) reactions have been reported in patients receiving therapy with quinolones, including ofloxacin. These reactions often occur following the first dose. Some reactions were accompanied by cardiovascular collapse, hypotension/shock, seizure, loss of consciousness, tingling, angioedema (including tongue, laryngeal, throat or facial edema/swelling), airway obstruction (including bronchospasm, shortness of breath and acute respiratory distress), dyspnea, urticaria/hives, itching, and other serious skin reactions. A few patients had a history of hypersensitivity reactions. The drug should be discontinued immediately at the first appearance of a skin rash or any other sign of hypersensitivity. Serious acute hypersensitivity reactions may require treatment with epinephrine and other resuscitative measures, including oxygen, intravenous fluids, antihistamines, corticosteroids, pressor amines, and airway management, as clinically indicated. (See PRECAUTIONS and ADVERSE REACTIONS.)

Convulsions, increased intracranial pressure, and toxic psychosis have been reported in patients receiving quinolones, including ofloxacin. Quinolones, including ofloxacin, may also cause central nervous system stimulation which may lead to: tremors, restlessness/agitation, nervousness/anxiety, lightheadedness, confusion, hallucinations, paranoia and depression, nightmares, insomnia, and rarely suicidal thoughts or acts. These reactions may occur following the first dose. If these reactions occur in patients receiving ofloxacin, the drug should be discontinued and appropriate measures instituted. As with all quinolones, ofloxacin should be used with caution in patients with a known or suspected CNS disorder that may predispose to seizures or lower the seizure threshold (*e.g.,* severe cerebral arteriosclerosis, epilepsy, etc.) or in the presence of other risk factors that may predispose to seizures or lower the seizure threshold (*e.g.,* certain drug therapy, renal dysfunction, etc.). See PRECAUTIONS, General; PRECAUTIONS, Information for the Patient; DRUG INTERACTIONS and ADVERSE REACTIONS.

Serious and sometimes fatal events, some due to hypersensitivity, and some due to uncertain etiology, have been reported in patients receiving therapy with quinolones including ofloxacin. These events may be severe and generally occur following the administration of multiple doses. Clinical manifestations may include one or more of the following: fever, rash or severe dermatologic reactions (*e.g.,* toxic epidermal necrolysis, Stevens-Johnson Syndrome); vasculitis, arthralgia, myalgia, serum sickness; allergic pneumonitis; interstitial nephritis, acute renal insufficiency/failure; hepatitis, jaundice, acute hepatic necrosis/failure; anemia including hemolytic and aplastic, thrombocytopenia, including thrombotic thrombocytopenic purpura, leukopenia, agranulocytosis, pancytopenia, and/or other hematologic abnormalities. The drug should be discontinued immediately at the first appearance of a skin rash or any other sign of hypersensitivity and supportive measures instituted. (See PRECAUTIONS and ADVERSE REACTIONS.)

Pseudomembranous colitis has been reported with nearly all antibacterial agents, including ofloxacin, and may range in severity from mild to life-threatening. Therefore, it is important to consider this diagnosis in patients who present with diarrhea subsequent to the administration of any antibacterial agents.

Treatment with antibacterial agents alters the normal flora of the colon and may permit overgrowth of clostridia. Studies indicate a toxin produced by *Clostridium difficile* is one primary cause of "antibiotic-associated colitis".

After the diagnosis of pseudomembranous colitis has been established, therapeutic measures should be initiated. Mild cases of pseudomembranous colitis usually respond to drug discontinuation alone. In moderate to severe cases, consideration should be given to management with fluids and electrolytes, protein supplementation, and treatment with an antibacterial drug clinically effective against *C. difficile* colitis. (See ADVERSE REACTIONS.)

Ruptures of the shoulder, hand, and Achilles tendons that required surgical repair or resulted in prolonged disability have been reported with ofloxacin and other quinolones. Ofloxacin should be discontinued if the patient experiences pain, inflammation, or rupture of a tendon. Patients should rest and refrain from exercise until the diagnosis of tendinitis or tendon rupture has been confidently excluded. Tendon rupture can occur at any time during or after therapy with ofloxacin.

Ofloxacin has not been shown to be effective in the treatment of syphilis. Antimicrobial agents used in high doses for short periods of time to treat gonorrhea may mask or delay the symptoms of incubating syphilis. All patients with gonorrhea should have a serologic test for syphilis at the time of diagnosis. Patients treated with ofloxacin for gonorrhea should have a follow-up serologic test for syphilis after 3 months and, if positive, treatment with an appropriate antimicrobial should be instituted.

OPHTHALMIC SOLUTION

NOT FOR INJECTION.

Ofloxacin ophthalmic solution should not be injected subconjunctivally, nor should it be introduced directly into the anterior chamber of the eye.

Serious and occasionally fatal hypersensitivity (anaphylactic) reactions, some following the first dose, have been reported in patients receiving systemic quinolones, including ofloxacin. Some reactions were accompanied by cardiovascular collapse, loss of consciousness, angioedema (including laryngeal, pharyngeal or facial edema), airway obstruction, dyspnea, urticaria, and itching. A rare occurrence of Stevens-Johnson syndrome, which progressed to toxic epidermal necrolysis, has been reported in a patient who was receiving topical ophthalmic ofloxacin. If an allergic reaction to ofloxacin occurs, discontinue the drug. Serious acute hypersensitivity reactions may require immediate emergency treatment. Oxygen and airway management, including intubation should be administered as clinically indicated.

OTIC SOLUTION

NOT FOR OPHTHALMIC USE.

NOT FOR INJECTION.

Serious and occasionally fatal hypersensitivity (anaphylactic) reactions, some following the first dose, have been reported in patients receiving systemic quinolones, including ofloxacin. Some reactions were accompanied by cardiovascular collapse, loss of consciousness, angioedema (including laryngeal, pharyngeal or facial edema), airway obstruction, dyspnea, urticaria, and itching. If an allergic reaction to ofloxacin is suspected, stop the drug. Serious acute hypersensitivity reactions may require immediate emergency treatment. Oxygen and airway management, including intubation, should be administered as clinically indicated.

PRECAUTIONS

GENERAL

Intravenous Infusion

Because a rapid or bolus intravenous injection may result in hypotension, **OFLOXACIN INJECTION SHOULD ONLY BE ADMINISTERED BY SLOW INTRAVENOUS INFUSION OVER A PERIOD OF 60 MINUTES. (SEE DOSAGE AND ADMINISTRATION.)**

Tablets and Intravenous Infusion

Adequate hydration of patients receiving ofloxacin should be maintained to prevent the formation of a highly concentrated urine.

Administer ofloxacin with caution in the presence of renal or hepatic insufficiency/impairment. In patients with known or suspected renal or hepatic insufficiency/impairment, careful clinical observation and appropriate laboratory studies should be performed prior to and during therapy since elimination of ofloxacin may be reduced. In patients with impaired renal function (creatinine clearance ≤50 mg/ml), alteration of the dosage regimen is necessary. (See CLINICAL PHARMACOLOGY and DOSAGE AND ADMINISTRATION.)

Moderate to severe phototoxicity reactions have been observed in patients exposed to direct sunlight while receiving some drugs in this class, including ofloxacin. Excessive sunlight should be avoided. Therapy should be discontinued if phototoxicity (*e.g.,* a skin eruption) occurs.

As with other quinolones, ofloxacin should be used with caution in any patient with a known or suspected CNS disorder that may predispose to seizures or lower the seizure threshold (*e.g.,* severe cerebral arteriosclerosis, epilepsy) or in the presence of other risk factors that may predispose to seizures or lower the seizure threshold (*e.g.,* certain drug therapy, renal dysfunction). (See WARNINGS and DRUG INTERACTIONS.)

A possible interaction between oral hypoglycemic drugs (*e.g.,* glyburide/glibenclamide) or with insulin and fluoroquinolone antimicrobial agents have been reported resulting in a potentiation of the hypoglycemic action of these drugs. The mechanism for this interaction is not known. If a hypoglycemic reaction occurs in a patient being treated with ofloxacin, discontinue ofloxacin immediately and consult a physician. (See DRUG INTERACTIONS and ADVERSE REACTIONS.)

As with any potent drug, periodic assessment of organ system functions, including renal, hepatic, and hematopoietic, is advisable during prolonged therapy. (See WARNINGS and ADVERSE REACTIONS.)

Intravenous Infusion

Because a rapid or bolus intravenous injection may result in hypotension, **OFLOXACIN INJECTION SHOULD ONLY BE ADMINISTERED BY SLOW INTRAVENOUS INFUSION OVER A PERIOD OF 60 MINUTES.** (See DOSAGE AND ADMINISTRATION.)

Ophthalmic Solution

As with other anti-infectives, prolonged use may result in overgrowth of nonsusceptible organisms, including fungi. If superinfection occurs discontinue use and institute alternative therapy. Whenever clinical judgment dictates, the patient should be examined with the aid of magnification, such as slit lamp biomicroscopy and, where appropriate, fluorescein staining. Ofloxacin should be discontinued at the first appearance of a skin rash or any other sign of hypersensitivity reaction.

The systemic administration of quinolones, including ofloxacin, has led to lesions or erosions of the cartilage in weight-bearing joints and other signs of arthropathy in immature animals of various species. Ofloxacin, administered systemically at 10 mg/kg/day in young dogs (equivalent to 110 times the maximum recommended daily *adult ophthalmic* dose) has been associated with these types of effects.

Otic Solution

As with other anti-infective preparations, prolonged use may result in over-growth of non-susceptible organisms, including fungi. If the infection is not improved after 1 week, cultures should be obtained to guide further treatment. If otorrhea persists after a full course of therapy, or if two or more episodes of otorrhea occur within 6 months, further evaluation is recommended to exclude an underlying condition such as cholesteatoma, foreign body, or a tumor.

The systemic administration of quinolones, including ofloxacin at doses much higher than given or absorbed by the otic route, has led to lesions or erosions of the cartilage in weight-bearing joints and other signs of arthropathy in immature animals of various species.

Young growing guinea pigs dosed in the middle ear with 0.3% ofloxacin otic solution showed no systemic effects, lesions or erosions of the cartilage in weight-bearing joints, or other signs of arthropathy. No drug-related structural or functional changes of the cochlea and no lesions in the ossicles were noted in the guinea pig following otic administration of 0.3% ofloxacin for 1 month.

No signs of local irritation were found when 0.3% ofloxacin was applied topically in the rabbit eye. Ofloxacin was also shown to lack dermal sensitizing potential in the guinea pig maximization study.

INFORMATION FOR THE PATIENT

Tablets and Intravenous Infusion

Patients should be advised:

- To drink fluids liberally if able to take fluids by the oral route.
- ***Tablets:*** That oxfloxacin can be taken without regard to meals.
- That ofloxacin may cause neurologic adverse effects (*e.g.,* dizziness, lightheadedness) and that patients should know how they react to ofloxacin before they operate an automobile or machinery or engage in activities requiring mental alertness and coordination. (See WARNINGS and ADVERSE REACTIONS.)
- That ofloxacin may be associated with hypersensitivity reactions, even following the first dose, to discontinue the drug at the first sign of a skin rash, hives or other skin reactions, a rapid heartbeat, difficulty in swallowing or breathing, any swelling suggesting angioedema (*e.g.,* swelling of the lips, tongue, face; tightness of the throat, hoarseness), or any other symptom of an allergic reaction. (See WARNINGS and ADVERSE REACTIONS.)
- To avoid excessive sunlight or artificial ultraviolet light while receiving ofloxacin and to discontinue therapy if phototoxicity (*e.g.,* skin eruption) occurs.
- To discontinue treatment and inform their physician if they experience pain, inflammation, or rupture of a tendon, and to rest and refrain from exercise until the diagnosis of tendinitis or tendon rupture has been confidently excluded.
- That if they are diabetic and are being treated with insulin or an oral hypoglycemic drug, to discontinue ofloxacin immediately if a hypoglycemic reaction occurs and consult a physician. (See General and DRUG INTERACTIONS.)
- That convulsions have been reported in patients taking quinolones, including ofloxacin, and to notify their physician before taking this drug if there is a history of this condition.
- ***Tablets:*** That mineral supplements, vitamins with iron or minerals, calcium-, aluminum- or magnesium-based antacids or sucralfate should not be taken within the 2 hour period before or within the 2 hour period after taking ofloxacin. (See DRUG INTERACTIONS.)

Ophthalmic Solution

Avoid contaminating the applicator tip with material from the eye, fingers or other source.

Systemic quinolones, including ofloxacin, have been associated with hypersensitivity reactions, even following a single dose. Discontinue use immediately and contact your physician at the first sign of a rash or allergic reaction.

Otic Solution

Avoid contaminating the applicator tip with material from the fingers or other sources. This precaution is necessary if the sterility of the drops is to be preserved. Systemic quinolones, including ofloxacin, have been associated with hypersensitivity reactions, even following a single dose. Discontinue use immediately and contact your physician at the first sign of a rash or allergic reaction.

Otitis Externa

Prior to administration of ofloxacin otic in patients with otitis externa, the solution should be warmed by holding the bottle in the hand for 1 or 2 minutes to avoid dizziness which may result from the instillation of a cold solution. The patient should lie with the affected ear upward, and then the drops should be instilled. This position should be maintained for 5 minutes to facilitate penetration of the drops into the ear canal. Repeat, if necessary, for the opposite ear (see DOSAGE AND ADMINISTRATION).

Acute Otitis Media and Chronic Suppurative Otitis Media

In pediatric patients (from 1-12 years old) with acute otitis media with tympanostomy tubes and in patients with chronic suppurative otitis media with perforated tympanic membranes, prior to administration, the solution should be warmed by holding the bottle in the hand for 1 or 2 minutes to avoid dizziness which may result from the instillation of a cold solution. The patient should lie with the affected ear upward, and then the drops should be instilled. The tragus should then be pumped 4 times by pushing inward to facilitate penetration of the drops into the middle ear. This position should be maintained for 5 minutes. Repeat, if necessary, for the opposite ear (see DOSAGE AND ADMINISTRATION).

CARCINOGENESIS, MUTAGENESIS, AND IMPAIRMENT OF FERTILITY

Long-term studies to determine the carcinogenic potential of ofloxacin have not been conducted.

Ofloxacin was not mutagenic in the Ames bacterial test, *in vitro* and *in vivo* cytogenetic assay, sister chromatid exchange (Chinese Hamster and human cell lines), unscheduled DNA repair (UDS) using human fibroblasts, dominant lethal assay, or mouse micronucleus assay. Ofloxacin was positive in the UDS test using rat hepatocyte, and Mouse Lymphoma Assay.

Otic Solution

Long-term studies to determine the carcinogenic potential of ofloxacin have not been conducted. Ofloxacin was not mutagenic in the Ames test, the sister chromatid exchange assay (Chinese hamster and human cell lines), the unscheduled DNA synthesis (UDS) assay using human fibroblasts, the dominant lethal assay, or the mouse micronucleus assay. Ofloxacin was positive in the rat hepatocyte UDS assay, and in the mouse lymphoma assay. In rats, ofloxacin did not affect male or female reproductive performance at oral doses up to 360 mg/kg/day. This would be over 1000 times the maximum recommended clinical dose, based upon body surface area, assuming total absorption of ofloxacin from the ear of a patient treated with ofloxacin otic twice per day.

PREGNANCY, TERATOGENIC EFFECTS, PREGNANCY CATEGORY C

Ofloxacin had not been shown to have any teratogenic effects at oral doses as high as 810 mg/kg/day (11 times the recommended maximum human dose based on mg/m^2 or 50 times based on mg/kg) and 160 mg/kg/day (4 times the reommended maximum human dose based on mg/m^2 or 10 times based on mg/kg) when administered to pregnant rats and rabbits, respectively. Additional studies in rats with oral doses up to 360 mg/kg/day (5 times the recommended maximum human dose based on mg/m^2 or 23 times based on mg/kg) demonstrated no adverse effect on late fetal development, labor, delivery, lactation, neonatal viability, or growth of the newborn. Doses equivalent to 50 and 10 were fetotoxic (*i.e.*, decreased fetal body weight and increased fetal mortality) in rats and rabbits, respectively. Minor skeletal variations were reported in rats receiving doses of 810 mg/kg/day, which is more than 10 times higher than the recommended maximum human dose based on mg/m^2.

There are, however, no adequate and well-controlled studies in pregnant women. Ofloxacin should be used during pregnancy only if the potential benefit justifies the potential risk to the fetus. (See WARNINGS.)

Otic Solution

Ofloxacin has been shown to have an embryocidal effect in rats at a dose of 810 mg/kg/day and in rabbits at 160 mg/kg/day.

These dosages resulted in decreased fetal body weights and increased fetal mortality in rats and rabbits, respectively. Minor fetal skeletal variations were reported in rats receiving doses of 810 mg/kg/day. Ofloxacin has not been shown to be teratogenic at doses as high as 810 mg/kg/day and 160 mg/kg/day when administered to pregnant rats and rabbits, respectively.

Ofloxacin has not been shown to have any adverse effects on the developing embryo or fetus at doses relevant to the amount of ofloxacin that will be delivered ototopically at the recommended clinical doses.

NONTERATOGENIC EFFECTS

Otic Solution

Additional studies in the rat demonstrated that doses up to 360 mg/kg/day during late gestation had no adverse effects on late fetal develoopment, labor, delivery, lactation, neonatal viability, or growth of the newborn. There are, however, no adequate and well-controlled studies in pregnant women. Ofloxacin otic should be used during pregnancy only if the potential benefit justifies the potential risk to the fetus.

NURSING MOTHERS

In lactating females, a single 200 mg oral dose of ofloxacin resulted in concentrations of ofloxacin in milk that were similar to those found in plasma. It is not known whether ofloxacin is excreted in human milk following topical ophthalmic and otic administration. Because of the potential for serious adverse reactions from ofloxacin in nursing infants, a decision should be made whether to discontinue nursing or to discontinue the drug, taking into account the importance of the drug to the mother. (See WARNINGS and ADVERSE REACTIONS).

PEDIATRIC USE

Safety and effectiveness in children and adolescents below the age of 18 years have not been established. Ofloxacin causes arthropathy (arthrosis) and osteochondrosis in juvenile animals of several species. (See WARNINGS.)

Otic Solution

No changes in hearing function occurred in 30 pediatric subjects treated with ofloxacin otic and tested for audiometric parameters. Although safety and efficacy have been demonstrated in pediatric patients 1 year and older, safety and effectiveness in infants below the age of 1 year have not been established. Although quinolones, including ofloxacin, have been shown to cause arthropathy in immature animals after systemic administration, young growing guinea pigs dosed in the middle ear with 0.3% ofloxacin otic solution for 1 month showed no systemic effects, quinolone-induced lesions, erosions of the cartilage in weight-bearing joints, or other signs of arthropathy.

DRUG INTERACTIONS

TABLETS AND INTRAVENOUS INFUSION

Antacids, Sucralfate, Metal Cations, Multivitamins: *Tablets:* Quinolones form chelates with alkaline earth and transition metal cations. Administration of quinolones with antacids containing calcium, magnesium, or aluminum, with sucralfate, with divalent or trivalent cations such as iron, or with multivitamins containing zinc may substantially interfere with the absorption of quinolones resulting in systemic levels considerably lower than desired. These agents should not be taken within the 2 hour period before or within the 2 hour period after ofloxacin administration. (See DOSAGE AND ADMINISTRATION.) *Intravenous Infusion:* There are no data concerning an interaction of **intravenous** quinolones with **oral** antacids, sucralfate, multivitamins, or metal cations. However, no quinolone should be co-administered with any solution containing multivalent cations, (*e.g.,* magnesium,) through the same intravenous line. (See DOSAGE AND ADMINISTRATION.)

Caffeine: Interactions between ofloxacin and caffeine have not been detected.

Cimetidine: Cimetidine has demonstrated interference with the elimination of some quinolones. This interference has resulted in significant increases in half-life and AUC of some quinolones. The potential for interaction between ofloxacin and cimetidine has not been studied.

Cyclosporine: Elevated serum levels of cyclosporine have been reported with concomitant use of cyclosporine with some other quinolones. The potential for interaction between ofloxacin and cyclosporine has not been studied.

Drugs Metabolized By Cytochrome P450 Enzymes: Most quinolone antimicrobial drugs inhibit cytochrome P450 enzyme activity. This may result in a prolonged half-life for some drugs that are also metabolized by this system (*e.g.,* cyclosporine, theophylline/methylxanthines, warfarin) when co-administered with quinolones. The extent of this inhibition varies among different quinolones. (See DRUG INTERACTIONS.)

Non-Steroidal Anti-Inflammatory Drugs: The concomitant administration of a non-steroidal anti-inflammatory drug, with a quinolone, including ofloxacin, may increase the risk of CNS stimulation and convulsive seizures. (See WARNINGS and PRECAUTIONS, General.)

Probenecid: The concomitant use of probenecid with certain other quinolones has been reported to affect renal tubular secretion. The effect of probenecid on the elimination of ofloxacin has not been studied.

Theophylline: Steady-state theophylline levels may increase when ofloxacin and theophylline are administered concurrently. As with other quinolones, concomitant administration of ofloxacin may prolong the half-life of theophylline, elevate serum theoplylline levels, and increase the risk of theophylline-related adverse reactions. Theophylline levels should be closely monitored and theophylline dosage adjustments made, if appropriate, when ofloxacin is co-administered. Adverse reactions (including seizures) may occur with or without an elevation in the serum theophylline level. (See WARNINGS and PRECAUTIONS, General.)

Warfarin: Some quinolones have been reported to enhance the effects of the oral anticoagulant warfarin or its derivatives. Therefore, if a quinolone antimicrobial is administered concomitantly with warfarin or its derivatives, the prothrombin time or other suitable coagulation test should be closely monitored.

Antidiabetic Agents (e.g., insulin, glyburide/glibenclamide): Since disturbances of blood glucose, including hyperglycemia and hypoglycemia, have been reported in patients treated concurrently with quinolones and an antidiabetic agent, careful monitoring of blood glucose is recommended when these agents are used concomitantly. (See PRECAUTIONS, General and PRECAUTIONS, Information for the Patient.)

OPHTHALMIC SOLUTION

Specific drug interaction studies have not been conducted with oflaxacin ophthalmic solution. However, the systemic administration of some quinolones has been shown to elevate plasma concentrations of theophylline, interfere with the metabolism of caffeine, and enhance the effects of the oral anticoagulant warfarin and its derivatives, and has been associated with transient elevations in serum creatinine in patients receiving cyclosporine concomitantly.

OTIC SOLUTION

Specific drug interaction studies have not been conducted with ofloxacin otic.

ADVERSE REACTIONS

TABLETS AND INTRAVENOUS INFUSION

The following is a compilation of the data for ofloxacin based on clinical experience with both the oral and intravenous formulations. The incidence of drug-related adverse reactions in patients during Phase 2 and 3 clinical trials was 11%. Among patients receiving multiple-dose therapy, 4% discontinued ofloxacin due to adverse experiences.

In clinical trials, the following events were considered likely to be drug-related in patients receiving multiple doses of ofloxacin: Nausea 3%, insomnia 3%, headache 1%, dizziness 1%, diarrhea 1%, vomiting 1%, rash 1%, pruritus 1%, external genital pruritus in women 1%, vaginitis 1%, dysgeusia 1%.

In clinical trials, the most frequently reported adverse events, regardless of relationship to drug, were: Nausea 10%, headache 9%, insomnia 7%, external genital pruritus in women 6%, dizziness 5%, vaginitis 5%, diarrhea 4%, vomiting 4%.

In clinical trials, the following events, regardless of relationship to drug, occurred in 1-3% of patients: Abdominal pain and cramps, chest pain, decreased appetite, dry mouth, dysgeusia, fatigue, flatulence, gastrointestinal distress, nervousness, pharyngitis, pruritus, fever, rash, sleep disorders, somnolence, trunk pain, vaginal discharge, visual disturbances, and constipation.

Additional events, occurring in clinical trials at a rate of less than 1%, regardless of relationship to drug, were:

Body as a Whole: Asthenia, chills, malaise, extremity pain, pain, epistaxis.

Cardiovascular System: Cardiac arrest, edema, hypertension, hypotension, palpitations, vasodilation.

Gastrointestinal System: Dyspepsia.

Genital/Reproductive System: Burning, irritation, pain and rash of the female genitalia, dysmenorrhea, menorrhagia, metrorrhagia.

Musculoskeletal System: Arthralgia, myalgia.

Nervous System: Seizures, anxiety, cognitive change, depression, dream abnormality, euphoria, hallucinations, paresthesia, syncope, vertigo, tremor, confusion.

Nutritional/Metabolic: Thirst, weight loss.

Respiratory System: Respiratory arrest, cough, rhinorrhea.

Skin/Hypersensitivity: Angiodema, diaphoresis, urticaria, vasculitis.

Special Senses: Decreased hearing acuity, tinnitus, photophobia.

Urinary System: Dysuria, urinary frequency, urinary retention.

The following laboratory abnormalities appeared in $\geq$1.0% of patients receiving multiple doses of ofloxacin. It is not known whether these abnormalities were caused by the drug or the underlying conditions being treated.

Hematopoietic: Anemia, leukopenia, leukocytosis, neutropenia, neutrophilia, increased band forms, lymphocytopenia, eosinophilia, lymphocytosis, thrombocytopenia, thrombocytosis, elevated ESR.

Hepatic: Elevated: alkaline phosphatase, AST (SGOT), ALT (SGPT).

Serum Chemistry: Hyperglycemia, hypoglycemia, elevated creatinine, elevated BUN.

Urinary: Glucosuria, proteinuria, alkalinuria, hyposthenuria, hematuria, pyuria.

O

Post-Marketing Adverse Events

Additional adverse events, regardless of relationship to drug, reported from worldwide marketing experience with quinolones, including ofloxacin:

Clinical

Cardiovascular System: Cerebral thrombosis, pulmonary edema, tachycardia, hypotension/shock, syncope.

Endocrine/Metabolic: Hyper- or hypoglycemia, especially in diabetic patients on insulin or oral hypoglycemic agents (see PRECAUTIONS, General and DRUG INTERACTIONS).

Gastrointestinal System: Hepatic dysfunction including: hepatic necrosis, jaundice (cholestatic or hepatocellular), hepatitis; instestinal perforation; pseudomembranous colitis (the onset of pseudomembranous colitis symptoms may occur during or after antimicrobial treatment), GI hemorrhage; hiccough, painful oral mucosa, pyrosis (see WARNINGS).

Genital/Reproductive System: Vaginal candidiasis.

Hematopoietic: Anemia, including hemolytic and aplastic; hemorrhage, pancytopenia, agranulocytosis, leukopenia, reversible bone marrow depression, thrombocytopenia, thrombotic thrombocytopenic purpura, petechiae, ecchymosis/burning (see WARNINGS).

Musculoskeletal: Tendinitis/rupture: weakness; rhabdomyolysis.

Nervous System: Nightmares; suicidal thoughts or acts, disorientation, psychotic reactions, paranoia; phobia, agitation, restlessness, agressiveness/hostility, manic reaction, emotional lability; peripheral neuropathy, ataxia, incoordination; possible exacerbation of: myasthenia gravis and extrapyramidal disorders; dysphasia, lightheadedness (See WARNINGS and PRECAUTIONS.)

Respiratory System: Dyspnea, bronchospasm, allergic pneumonitis, stridor (see WARNINGS).

Skin/Hypersensitivity: Anaphylactic (-toid) reactions/shock; purpura, serum sickness, erythema multiforme/Stevens-Johnson Syndrome, erythema nodosum, exfoliative dermatitis, hyperpigmentation, toxic epidermal necrolysis, conjunctivitis, photosensitivity, vesiculobullous eruption (see WARNINGS and PRECAUTIONS).

Special Senses: Diplopia, nystagmus, blurred vision, disturbances of: taste, smell, hearing and equilibrium, usually reversible following discontinuation.

Urinary System: Anuria, polyuria, renal calculi, renal failure, interstitial nephritis, hematuria (see WARNINGS and PRECAUTIONS).

Laboratory

Hematopoietic: Prolongation of prothrombin time.

Serum Chemistry: Acidosis, elevation of: serum triglycerides, serum cholesterol, serum potassium, liver function tests including: GGTP, LDH, bilirubin.

Urinary: Albuminuria, candiduria.

In clinical trials using multiple-dose therapy, ophthalmologic abnormalities, including cataracts and multiple punctate lenticular opacities, have been noted in patients undergoing treatment with other quinolones. The relationship of the drugs to these events is not presently established.

CRYSTALLURIA and CYLINDRURIA HAVE BEEN REPORTED with other quinolones.

Intravenous Infusion

Local injection site reactions (phlebitis, swelling, erythema) were reported in approximately 2% of patients treated with the 3.63 mg/ml final infusion concentration of intravenous ofloxacin used in the clinical safety trials. The final infusion concentration of intravenous ofloxacin in the commercially available intravenous preparations is 4.0 mg/ml. To date, individuals administered the 4.0 mg/ml concentration of the intravenous ofloxacin have demonstrated clinically acceptable rates of local injection site reactions. Due to the small difference in concentration, significant differences in local site reactions are unexpected with the 4.0 mg/ml concentration.

OPHTHALMIC SOLUTION

The most frequently reported drug-related adverse reaction was transient ocular burning or discomfort. Other reported reactions include stinging, redness, itching, chemical conjunctivitis/keratitis, periocular/facial edema, foreign body sensation, photophobia, blurred vision, tearing, dryness, and eye pain. Rare reports of dizziness have been received.

OTIC SOLUTION

In the Phase III registration trials, a total of 885 subjects were treated with ofloxacin otic solution. This included 229 subjects with otitis externa (with intact tympanic membranes) and 656 subjects with acute otitis media with tympanostomy tubes or chronic suppurative otitis media with perforated tympanic membranes. The reported treatment-related adverse events are listed in TABLE 6.

Subjects With Otitis Externa

The treatment-related adverse events listed in TABLE 6 occurred in 1% or more of the subjects with intact tympanic membranes.

TABLE 6

Adverse Event	Frequency (n=229)
Pruritus	4%
Application site reaction	3%
Dizziness	1%
Earache	1%
Vertigo	1%

The following treatment-related adverse events were each reported in a single subject: dermatitis, eczema, erythematous rash, follicular rash, rash, hypoaesthesia, tinnitus, dyspepsia, hot flushes, flushing, and otorrhagia.

Subjects With Acute Otitis Media With Tympanostomy Tubes and Subjects With Chronic Suppurative Otitis Media With Perforated Tympanic Membranes

The treatment-related adverse events listed in occurred in 1% or more of the subjects with non-intact tympanic membranes.

TABLE 7

Adverse Event	Frequency (n=656)
Taste perversion	7%
Earache	1%
Pruritus	1%
Paraesthesia	1%
Rash	1%
Dizziness	1%

Other treatment-related adverse reactions reported in subjects with non-intact tympanic membranes included: diarrhea (0.6%), nausea (0.3%), vomiting (0.3%), dry mouth (0.5%), headache (0.3%), vertigo (0.5%), otorrhagia (0.6%), tinnitus (0.3%), fever (0.3%). The following treatment-related adverse events were each reported in a single subject: application site reaction, otitis externa, urticaria, abdominal pain, dysaesthesia, hyperkinesia, halitosis, inflammation, pain, insomnia, coughing, pharyngitis, rhinitis, sinusitis, and tachycardia.

DOSAGE AND ADMINISTRATION

TABLETS AND INTRAVENOUS INFUSION

TABLE 8 *Patients With Normal Renal Function*

Infection	Unit Daily Dose	Frequency	Duration	Dose
Exacerbation of chronic bronchitis	400 mg	q12h	10 days	800 mg
Comm. acq. pneumonia	400 mg	q12h	10 days	800 mg
Uncomplicated skin and skin structure infections	400 mg	q12h	10 days	800 mg
Acute, uncomplicated urethral and cervical gonorrhea	400 mg	Single dose	1 day	400 mg
Nongonococcal cervicitis/ urethritis due to *C. trachomatis*	300 mg	q12h	7 days	600 mg
Mixed infection of the urethra and cervix due to *C. trachomatis* and *N. gonorrhoeae*	300 mg	q12h	7 days	600 mg
Acute pelvic inflammatory disease	400 mg	q12h	10-14 days	800 mg
Uncomplicated cystitis due to *E. coli* or *K. pneumoniae*	200 mg	q12h	3 days	400 mg
Uncomplicated cystitis due to other approved pathogens	200 mg	q12h	7 days	400 mg
Complicated UTI's	200 mg	q12h	10 days	400 mg
Prostatitis due to *E. coli*	300 mg	q12h	6 wks†	600 mg

* Due to the designated pathogens. (See INDICATIONS AND USAGE.)

† Because there are no safety data presently available to support the use of the intravenous formulation of ofloxacin for more than 10 days, therapy after 10 days should be switched to the oral tablet formulation or other appropriate therapy.

Patients With Impaired Renal Function

Dosage should be adjusted for patients with a creatinine clearance ≤50 ml/min.

After a normal initial dose, dosage should be adjusted as follows (see TABLE 9).

TABLE 9

Creatinine Clearance	Maintenance Dose	Frequency
20-50 ml/min	the usual recommended unit dose	q24h
<20 ml/min	½ the usual recommended unit dose	q24h

When only the serum creatinine is known, the formula may be used to estimate creatinine clearance.

Men: [Weight (kg) × (140-age)] ÷ [72 × serum creatinine (mg/dl)]

Women: 0.85 × the value calculated for men.

The serum creatinine should represent a steady-state of renal function.

Patients With Cirrhosis

The excretion of ofloxacin may be reduced in patients with severe liver function disorders (*e.g.,* cirrhosis with or without ascites). A maximum dose of 400 mg of ofloxacin per day should therefore not be exceeded.

Tablets

The usual dose of ofloxacin tablets are 200-400 mg orally every 12 hours as described in the dosing chart (TABLE 8). These recommendations apply to patients with normal renal function (*i.e.,* creatinine clearance >50 ml/min). For patients with altered renal function (*i.e.,* creatinine clearance ≤50 ml/min), see Patients With Impaired Renal Function.

Antacids containing calcium, magnesium, or aluminum; sucralfate; divalent or trivalent cations such as iron; or multivitamins containing zinc should not be taken within the 2 hour period before, or within the 2 hour period after ofloxacin administrations. (See PRECAUTIONS.)

Intravenous Infusion

Ofloxacin IV should only be administered by **intravenous** infusion. It is not for intramuscular, intrathecal, intraperitoneal, or subcutaneous administration.

CAUTION: RAPID OR BOLUS INTRAVENOUS INFUSION MUST BE AVOIDED.

Ofloxacin injection should be infused intravenously slowly over a period of not less than 60 minutes. (See PRECAUTIONS.)

Single-use vials require dilution prior to administration. (See Preparation of Ofloxacin Injection for Administration.)

The usual dose of ofloxacin injection IV is 200-400 mg administered by slow infusion over 60 minutes every 12 hours as described in the dosing chart (TABLE 8). These recommendations apply to patients with mild to moderate infection and normal renal function (*i.e.*, creatinine clearance >50 ml/min). For patients with altered renal function (*i.e.*, creatinine clearance ≤50 ml/min), see Patients With Impaired Renal Function.

OPHTHALMIC SOLUTION

The recommended dosage regimen for the treatment of **bacterial conjunctivitis** is:

Days 1 and 2: Instill 1-2 drops every 2-4 hours in the affected eye(s).

Days 3 through 7: Instill 1-2 drops 4 times daily.

The recommended dosage regimen for the treatment of **bacterial corneal ulcer** is:

Days 1 and 2: Instill 1-2 drops into the affected eye every 30 minutes, while awake. Awaken at approximately 4 and 6 hours after retiring and instill 1-2 drops.

Days 3 through 7-9: Instill 1-2 drops hourly, while awake.

Days 7-9 through treatment completion: Instill 1-2 drops, 4 times daily.

OTIC SOLUTION

Otitis Externa

The recommended dosage regimen for the treatment of otitis externa is: *For pediatric patients (from 1-12 years old):* Five (5) drops (0.25 ml, 0.75 mg ofloxacin) instilled into the affected ear twice daily for 10 days. *For patients 12 years and older:* Ten (10) drops (0.5 ml, 1.5 mg ofloxacin) instilled into the affected ear twice daily for 10 days.

The solution should be warmed by holding the bottle in the hand for 1 or 2 minutes to avoid dizziness which may result from the instillation of a cold solution. The patient should lie with the affected ear upward, and then the drops should be instilled. This position should be maintained for 5 minutes to facilitate penetration of the drops into the ear canal. Repeat, if necessary, for the opposite ear.

Acute Otitis Media in Pediatric Patients With Tympanostomy Tubes

The recommended dosage regimen for the treatment of acute otitis media in pediatric patients (from 1-12 years old) with tympanostomy tubes is:

Five (5) drops (0.25 ml, 0.75 mg ofloxacin) instilled into the affected ear twice daily for 10 days. The solution should be warmed by holding the bottle in the hand for 1 or 2 minutes to avoid dizziness which may result from the instillation of a cold solution. The patient should lie with the affected ear upward, and then the drops should be instilled. The tragus should then be pumped 4 times by pushing inward to facilitate penetration of the drops into the middle ear. This position should be maintained for 5 minutes. Repeat, if necessary, for the opposite ear.

Chronic Suppurative Otitis Media With Perforated Tympanic Membranes

The recommended dosage regimen for the treatment of chronic suppurative otitis media with perforated tympanic membranes in patients 12 years and older is:

Ten (10) drops (0.5 ml, 1.5 mg ofloxacin) instilled into the affected ear twice daily for 14 days. The solution should be warmed by holding the bottle in the hand for 1 or 2 minutes to avoid dizziness which may result from the instillation of a cold solution. The patient should lie with the affected ear upward, before instilling the drops. The tragus should then be pumped 4 times by pushing inward to facilitate penetration into the middle ear. This position should be maintained for 5 minutes. Repeat, if necessary, for the opposite ear.

INTRAVENOUS INFUSION

Preparation of Ofloxacin Injection for Administration

Ofloxacin Intravenous Infusion in Single-Use Vials

Ofloxacin IV is supplied in single-use vials containing a concentrated ofloxacin solution with the equivalent of 400 mg of ofloxacin in Water for Injection. The 10 ml vials contain 40 mg of ofloxacin/ml. **THESE OFLOXACIN IV SINGLE-USE VIALS MUST BE FURTHER DILUTED WITH AN APPROPRIATE SOLUTION PRIOR TO INTRAVENOUS ADMINISTRATION**. (See Compatible Intravenous Solutions.) The concentration of the resulting diluted solution should be 4 mg/ml prior to administration.

This parenteral drug product should be inspected visually for discoloration and particulate matter prior to administration.

Since no preservative or bacteriostatic agent is present in this product, aseptic technique must be used in preparation of the final parenteral solution. **Since the vials are for single-use only, any unused portion should be discarded.**

Since only limited data are available on the compatibility of ofloxacin intravenous injection with other intravenous substances, **additives or other medications should not be added to ofloxacin IV in single-use vials or infused simultaneously through the same intravenous line.** If the same intravenous line is used for sequential infusion of several different drugs, the line should be flushed before and after infusion of ofloxacin IV with an infusion solution compatible with ofloxacin IV and with any other drug(s) administrated via this common line.

Prepare the desired dosage of ofloxacin according to TABLE 10.

TABLE 10

Desired Dosage Strength	From 10 ml Vial, Withdraw Volume	Volume of Diluent	Infusion Time
200 mg	5 ml	qs 50 ml	60 min
300 mg	7.5 ml	qs 75 ml	60 min
400 mg	10 ml	qs 100 ml	60 min

For example, to prepare a 200 mg dose using the 10 ml vial (40 mg/ml), withdraw 5 ml and dilute with a compatible intravenous solution to a total volume of 50 ml.

Compatible Intravenous Solutions

Any of the intravenous solutions listed in TABLE 11 may be used to prepare a 4 mg/ml ofloxacin solution with the appropriate pH values.

TABLE 11

Intravenous Fluids	pH of 4 mg/ml Floxin IV Solution
0.9% Sodium chloride injection	4.69
5% Dextrose injection	4.57
5% Dextrose/0.9% NaCl injection	4.56
5% Dextrose in lactated Ringer's	4.94
5% Sodium bicarbonate injection	7.95
Plasma-Lyte 56/5% dextrose injection	5.02
5% Dextrose, 0.45% sodium chloride, and 0.15% potassium chloride injection	4.64
Sodium lactate injection (M/6)	5.64
Water for injection	4.66

Ofloxacin Intravenous Infusion Pre-Mixed in Single-Use Flexible Containers

Ofloxacin IV is also supplied in 50 ml and 100 ml flexible containers containing a premixed, ready-to-use ofloxacin solution in D_5W for single-use. **NO FURTHER DILUTION OF THIS PREPARATION IS NECESSARY. Each 50 ml pre-mixed flexible container already contains a dilute solution with the equivalent of 200 mg of ofloxacin (4 mg/ml) in 5% Detrose (D_5W). Each 100 ml pre-mixed bottle already contains a dilute solution with the equivalent of 400 mg of ofloxacin (4 mg/ml) in 5% dextrose (D_5W).**

This parenteral drug product should be inspected visually for discoloration and particulate matter prior to administration.

Since no preservative or bacteriostatic agent is present in this product, aseptic technique must be used in preparation of the final parenteral solution. **Since the pre-mixed flexible containers are for single-use only, any unused portion should be discarded.**

Since only limited data are available on the compatibility of ofloxacin intravenous injection with other intravenous substances, **additives or other medications should not be added to ofloxacin IV in flexible containers or infused simultaneously through the same intravenous line.** If the same intravenous line is used for sequential infusion of several different drugs, the line should be flushed before and after infusion of ofloxacin IV with an infusion solution compatible with ofloxacin IV and with any other drug(s) administrated via this common line.

Stability of Ofloxacin Intravenous Infusion as Supplied

When stored under recommended conditions, ofloxacin IV, as supplied in 10 ml vials, and 50 ml and 100 ml flexible containers, is stable through the expiration date printed on the label.

Stability of Ofloxacin Intravenous Infusion Following Dilution

Ofloxacin IV, when diluted in a compatible intravenous fluid to a concentration between 0.4 mg/ml and 4 mg/ml, is stable for 72 hours when stored at or below 75°F or 24°C and for 14 days when stored under refrigeration at 41°F or 5°C in glass bottles or plastic intravenous containers. Solutions that are diluted in a compatible intravenous solution and frozen in glass bottles or plastic intravenous containers are stable for 6 months when stored at -4°F or-20°C. Once thawed, the solution is stable for up to 14 days, if refrigerated at 2-8°C (36-46°F). **THAW FROZEN SOLUTIONS AT ROOM TEMPERATURE (77°F OR 25°C) OR IN A REFRIGERATOR (46°F OR 8°C). DO NOT FORCE THAW BY MICROWAVE IRRADIATION OR WATER BATH IMMERSION. DO NOT REFREEZE AFTER INITIAL THAWING.**

OPHTHALMIC SOLUTION

The recommended dosage regimen for the treatment of **bacterial conjunctivitis** is:

Days 1 and 2: Instill 1-2 drops every 2-4 hours in the affected eye(s).

Days 3 through 7: Instill 1-2 drops 4 times daily.

The recommended dosage regimen for the treatment of **bacterial corneal ulcer** is:

Days 1 and 2: Instill 1-2 drops into the affected eye every 30 minutes, while awake. Awaken at approximately 4 and 6 hours after retiring and instill 1-2 drops.

Days 3 through 7-9: Instill 1-2 drops hourly, while awake.

Days 7-9 through treatment completion: Instill 1-2 drops, 4 times daily.

ANIMAL PHARMACOLOGY

TABLETS AND INTRAVENOUS INFUSION

Ofloxacin, as well as other drugs of the quinolone class, has been shown to cause arthropathies (arthrosis) in immature dogs and rats. In addition, these drugs are associated with an increased incidence of osteochondrosis in rats as compared to the incidence observed in vehicle-treated rats. (See WARNINGS.) There is no evidence of arthropathies in fully mature dogs at intravenous doses up to 3 times the recommended maximum human dose (on a mg/m^2 basis or 5 times based on a mg/kg basis), for a 1 week exposure period.

Long-term, high-dose systemic use of other quinolones in experimental animals has caused lenticular opacities; however, this finding was not observed in any animal studies with ofloxacin.

Reduced serum globulin and protein levels were observed in animals treated with other quinolones. In one ofloxacin study, minor decreases in serum globulin and protein levels were noted in female cynomolgus monkeys dosed orally with 40 mg/kg ofloxacin daily for 1 year. These changes, however, were considered to be within normal limits for monkeys.

Crystalluria and ocular toxicity were not observed in any animals treated with ofloxacin.

HOW SUPPLIED

TABLETS

Floxin tablets are supplied as 200 mg light yellow, 300 mg white, and 400 mg pale gold flim-coated tablets. Each tablet is distinguished by "Floxin" and the appropriate strength.

Storage: Floxin tablets should be stored in well-closed containers. Store below 30°C (86°F).

IV SINGLE-USE VIALS

Floxin IV is supplied in single-use vials. Each vial contains a concentrated solution with the equivalent of 400 mg of ofloxacin.

Storage: Floxin IV in single-use vials should be stored at controlled room temperature 15-30°C (59-86°F) and protected from light.

IV PRE-MIXED IN FLEXIBLE CONTAINERS

Floxin IV pre-mixed in flexible containers is supplied as a single-use, pre-mixed solution in 50 and 100 ml flexible containers. Each contains a dilute solution with the equivalent of 200 mg or 400 mg of ofloxacin, respectively, in 5% dextrose (D_5W).

Storage: Floxin IV pre-mixed in flexible containers should be stored at or below 25°C or 77°F; however, brief exposure up to 40°C or 104°F does not adversely affect the product. Avoid excessive heat and protect from freezing and light.

OPHTHALMIC SOLUTION

Ocuflox 0.3% is supplied sterile in plastic dropper bottles in 1, 5, and 10 ml sizes.

Storage: Store at 15-25° C (59-77° F).

OTIC SOLUTION

Floxin Otic 0.3% is supplied in plastic dropper bottles containing 5 ml.

Storage: Store at 15-25°C (59-77°F).

PRODUCT LISTING - EQUIVALENTS NOT AVAILABLE

Size	Price	Product	NDC
Solution - Ophthalmic - 0.3%			
5 ml	$32.60	OCUFLOX, Allscripts Pharmaceutical Company	54569-4160-00
5 ml	$34.55	OCUFLOX, Southwood Pharmaceuticals Inc	58016-6498-01
5 ml	$35.31	OCUFLOX, Physicians Total Care	54868-3900-00
5 ml	$36.75	OCUFLOX, Pharma Pac	52959-0607-05
5 ml	$39.55	OCUFLOX, Allergan Inc	11980-0779-05
10 ml	$69.08	OCUFLOX, Southwood Pharmaceuticals Inc	58016-8711-01
10 ml	$79.05	OCUFLOX, Allergan Inc	11980-0779-10
Solution - Otic - 0.3%			
5 ml	$40.71	FLOXIN OTIC, Daiichi Pharmaceuticals	63395-0101-05
10 ml	$65.40	FLOXIN OTIC, Daiichi Pharmaceuticals	63395-0101-10
Tablet - Oral - 200 mg			
6's	$24.98	FLOXIN, Allscripts Pharmaceutical Company	54569-3268-00
6's	$74.55	FLOXIN, Pd-Rx Pharmaceuticals	55289-0030-06
50's	$248.63	FLOXIN, Janssen Pharmaceuticals	00062-1540-02
Tablet - Oral - 300 mg			
6's	$40.11	FLOXIN, Pd-Rx Pharmaceuticals	55289-0263-06
14's	$69.33	FLOXIN, Allscripts Pharmaceutical Company	54569-3872-00
14's	$93.92	FLOXIN, Pd-Rx Pharmaceuticals	55289-0263-14
50's	$295.88	FLOXIN, Ortho Mcneil Pharmaceutical	00062-1541-02
Tablet - Oral - 400 mg			
1's	$4.98	FLOXIN, Allscripts Pharmaceutical Company	54569-3293-02
1's	$8.42	FLOXIN, Pd-Rx Pharmaceuticals	55289-0059-79
1's	$9.36	FLOXIN, Prescript Pharmaceuticals	00247-0260-01
2's	$15.38	FLOXIN, Prescript Pharmaceuticals	00247-0260-02
3's	$21.38	FLOXIN, Prescript Pharmaceuticals	00247-0260-03
4's	$27.39	FLOXIN, Prescript Pharmaceuticals	00247-0260-04
6's	$39.41	FLOXIN, Prescript Pharmaceuticals	00247-0260-06
10's	$55.76	FLOXIN, Pharma Pac	52959-0216-10
10's	$63.45	FLOXIN, Prescript Pharmaceuticals	00247-0260-10
14's	$73.12	FLOXIN, Allscripts Pharmaceutical Company	54569-3293-00
14's	$73.86	FLOXIN, Pharma Pac	52959-0216-14
14's	$87.47	FLOXIN, Prescript Pharmaceuticals	00247-0260-14
20's	$99.58	FLOXIN, Allscripts Pharmaceutical Company	54569-3293-01
20's	$101.90	FLOXIN, Pharma Pac	52959-0216-20
20's	$123.53	FLOXIN, Prescript Pharmaceuticals	00247-0260-20
21's	$129.54	FLOXIN, Prescript Pharmaceuticals	00247-0260-21
28's	$235.62	FLOXIN, Pd-Rx Pharmaceuticals	55289-0059-28
50's	$303.80	FLOXIN, Prescript Pharmaceuticals	00247-0260-50
60's	$363.88	FLOXIN, Prescript Pharmaceuticals	00247-0260-60
100's	$604.24	FLOXIN, Prescript Pharmaceuticals	00247-0260-00
100's	$624.06	FLOXIN, Ortho Mcneil Pharmaceutical	00062-1542-01
118's	$712.40	FLOXIN, Prescript Pharmaceuticals	00247-0260-52

Olanzapine *(003301)*

Categories: Schizophrenia; Bipolar affective disorder; Mania; Pregnancy Category C; FDA Approved 1996 Sep
Drug Classes: Antipsychotics
Brand Names: Zyprexa
Foreign Brand Availability: Dozic (Colombia); Olansek (Austria; Belgium; Bulgaria; Czech-Republic; Denmark; England; Finland; France; Germany; Greece; Hungary; Ireland; Italy; Netherlands; Norway; Poland; Portugal; Slovenia; Spain; Sweden; Switzerland; Turkey); Oleanz (India); Zelta (Colombia); Zyprexa Velotab (Austria; Belgium; Bulgaria; Czech-Republic; Denmark; England; Finland; France; Germany; Greece; Hungary; Ireland; Italy; Netherlands; Norway; Poland; Portugal; Slovenia; Spain; Sweden; Switzerland; Turkey); Zyprexa Zydis (New-Zealand)
Cost of Therapy: $289.14 (Schizophrenia; Zyprexa; 10 mg; 1 tablets/day; 30 day supply)
$324.42 (Schizophrenia; Zyprexa Zydis; 10 mg; 1 tablets/day; 30 day supply)

DESCRIPTION

Olanzapine is a psychotropic agent that belongs to the thienobenzodiazepine class. The chemical designation is 2-methyl-4-(4-methyl-1-piperazinyl)-10*H*-thieno[2,3-*b*] [1,5]benzodiazepine. The molecular formula is $C_{17}H_{20}N_4S$, which corresponds to a molecular weight of 312.44. Olanzapine is a yellow crystalline solid, which is practically insoluble in water.

TABLETS

Zyprexa (olanzapine) tablets are intended for oral administration only.

Each Zyprexa tablet contains olanzapine equivalent to 2.5 mg (8 μmol), 5 mg (16 μmol), 7.5 mg (24 μmol), 10 mg (32 μmol), or 15 mg (48 μmol), or 20 mg (64 μmol). Inactive ingredients are carnauba wax, crospovidone, hydroxypropyl cellulose, hydroxypropyl methylcellulose, lactose, magnesium stearate, microcrystalline cellulose, and other inactive ingredients. The color coating contains titanium dioxide (all strengths) and FD&C blue no. 2 aluminum lake (15 mg), or synthetic red iron oxide (20 mg). The 2.5, 5.0, 7.5, and 10 mg tablets are imprinted with edible ink which contains FD&C blue no. 2 aluminum lake.

ORALLY DISINTEGRATING TABLETS

Zyprexa Zydis (olanzapine) orally disintegrating tablets is intended for oral administration only.

Each orally disintegrating tablet contains olanzapine equivalent to 5 mg (16 μmol) or 10 mg (32 μmol). It begins disintegrating in the mouth within seconds, allowing its contents to be subsequently swallowed with or without liquid. Zyprexa Zydis orally disintegrating tablets also contain the following inactive ingredients: gelatin, mannitol, aspartame, sodium methyl paraben, and sodium propyl paraben.

CLINICAL PHARMACOLOGY

PHARMACODYNAMICS

Olanzapine is a selective monoaminergic antagonist with high affinity binding to the following receptors: serotonin $5HT_{2A/2C}$ (Ki=4 and 11 nM, respectively), dopamine D_{1-4} (Ki=11-31 nM), muscarinic M_{1-5} (Ki=1.9-25 nM), histamine H_1 (Ki=7 nM), and adrenergic α_1 receptors (Ki=19 nM). Olanzapine binds weakly to $GABA_A$, BZD, and β adrenergic receptors (Ki >10 μM).

The mechanism of action of olanzapine, as with other drugs having efficacy in schizophrenia, is unknown. However, it has been proposed that this drug's efficacy in schizophrenia is mediated through a combination of dopamine and serotonin type 2 ($5HT_2$) antagonism. The mechanism of action of olanzapine in the treatment of acute manic episodes associated with Bipolar I Disorder is unknown.

Antagonism at receptors other than dopamine and $5HT_2$ with similar receptor affinities may explain some of the other therapeutic and side effects of olanzapine. Olanzapine's antagonism of muscarinic M_{1-5} receptors may explain its anticholinergic effects. Olanzapine's antagonism of histamine H_1 receptors may explain the somnolence observed with this drug. Olanzapine's antagonism of adrenergic α_1 receptors may explain the orthostatic hypotension observed with this drug.

PHARMACOKINETICS

Olanzapine is well absorbed and reaches peak concentrations in approximately 6 hours following an oral dose. It is eliminated extensively by first pass metabolism, with approximately 40% of the dose metabolized before reaching the systemic circulation. Food does not affect the rate or extent of olanzapine absorption. Pharmacokinetic studies showed that olanzapine tablets and orally disintegrating tablets dosage forms are bioequivalent.

Olanzapine displays linear kinetics over the clinical dosing range. Its half-life ranges from 21-54 hours (5th to 95th percentile; mean of 30 hours), and apparent plasma clearance ranges from 12-47 L/h (5th to 95th percentile; mean of 25 L/h).

Administration of olanzapine once daily leads to steady state concentrations in about 1 week that are approximately twice the concentrations after single doses. Plasma concentrations, half-life, and clearance of olanzapine may vary between individuals on the basis of smoking status, gender, and age (see Special Populations).

Olanzapine is extensively distributed throughout the body, with a volume of distribution of approximately 1000 L. It is 93% bound to plasma proteins over the concentration range of 7-1100 ng/ml, binding primarily to albumin and α_1-acid glycoprotein.

METABOLISM AND ELIMINATION

Following a single oral dose of ^{14}C labeled olanzapine, 7% of the dose of olanzapine was recovered in the urine as unchanged drug, indicating that olanzapine is highly metabolized. Approximately 57% and 30% of the dose was recovered in the urine and feces, respectively. In the plasma, olanzapine accounted for only 12% of the AUC for total radioactivity, indicating significant exposure to metabolites. After multiple dosing, the major circulating metabolites were the 10-N-glucuronide, present at steady state at 44% of the concentration of olanzapine, and 4'-N-desmethyl olanzapine, present at steady state at 31% of the concentration of olanzapine. Both metabolites lack pharmacological activity at the concentrations observed.

Direct glucuronidation and cytochrome P450 (CYP) mediated oxidation are the primary metabolic pathways for olanzapine. *In vitro* studies suggest that CYPs 1A2 and 2D6, and the flavin-containing mono-oxygenase system are involved in olanzapine oxidation. CYP2D6 mediated oxidation appears to be a minor metabolic pathway *in vivo*, because the clearance of olanzapine is not reduced in subjects who are deficient in this enzyme.

SPECIAL POPULATIONS

Renal Impairment

Because olanzapine is highly metabolized before excretion and only 7% of the drug is excreted unchanged, renal dysfunction alone is unlikely to have a major impact on the pharmacokinetics of olanzapine. The pharmacokinetic characteristics of olanzapine were similar in patients with severe renal impairment and normal subjects, indicating that dosage adjustment based upon the degree of renal impairment is not required. In addition, olanzapine is not removed by dialysis. The effect of renal impairment on metabolite elimination has not been studied.

Hepatic Impairment

Although the presence of hepatic impairment may be expected to reduce the clearance of olanzapine, a study of the effect of impaired liver function in subjects (n=6) with clinically significant (Childs Pugh Classification A and B) cirrhosis revealed little effect on the pharmacokinetics of olanzapine.

Age

In a study involving 24 healthy subjects, the mean elimination half-life of olanzapine was about 1.5 times greater in elderly (>65 years) than in nonelderly subjects (≤65 years). Caution should be used in dosing the elderly, especially if there are other factors that might additively influence drug metabolism and/or pharmacodynamic sensitivity (see DOSAGE AND ADMINISTRATION).

Gender

Clearance of olanzapine is approximately 30% lower in women than in men. There were, however, no apparent differences between men and women in effectiveness or adverse effects. Dosage modifications based on gender should not be needed.

Smoking Status

Olanzapine clearance is about 40% higher in smokers than in nonsmokers, although dosage modifications are not routinely recommended.

Race

No specific pharmacokinetic study was conducted to investigate the effects of race. A cross-study comparison between data obtained in Japan and data obtained in the US suggests that exposure to olanzapine may be about 2-fold greater in the Japanese when equivalent doses are administered. Clinical trial safety and efficacy data, however, did not suggest clinically significant differences among Caucasian patients, patients of African descent, and a third pooled category including Asian and Hispanic patients. Dosage modifications for race are, therefore, not recommended.

Combined Effects

The combined effects of age, smoking, and gender could lead to substantial pharmacokinetic differences in populations. The clearance in young smoking males, for example, may be 3 times higher than that in elderly nonsmoking females. Dosing modification may be necessary in patients who exhibit a combination of factors that may result in slower metabolism of olanzapine (see DOSAGE AND ADMINISTRATION).

INDICATIONS AND USAGE

SCHIZOPHRENIA

Olanzapine is indicated for the treatment of schizophrenia.

The efficacy of olanzapine was established in short-term (6 week) controlled trials of schizophrenic inpatients.

The effectiveness of oral olanzapine at maintaining a treatment response in schizophrenic patients who had been stable on olanzapine for approximately 8 weeks and were then followed for a period of up to 8 months has been demonstrated in a placebo-controlled trial. Nevertheless, the physician who elects to use olanzapine for extended periods should periodically re-evaluate the long-term usefulness of the drug for the individual patient (see DOSAGE AND ADMINISTRATION).

BIPOLAR MANIA

Olanzapine is indicated for the short-term treatment of acute manic episodes associated with Bipolar I Disorder.

The efficacy of olanzapine was established in 2 placebo-controlled trials (one 3-week and one 4-week) with patients meeting DSM-IV criteria for Bipolar I Disorder who currently displayed an acute manic or mixed episode with or without psychotic features.

The effectiveness of olanzapine for longer-term use, that is, for more than 4 weeks treatment of an acute episode, and for prophylactic use in mania, has not been systematically evaluated in controlled clinical trials. Therefore, physicians who elect to use olanzapine for extended periods should periodically re-evaluate the long-term risks and benefits of the drug for the individual patient (see DOSAGE AND ADMINISTRATION).

CONTRAINDICATIONS

Olanzapine is contraindicated in patients with a known hypersensitivity to the product.

WARNINGS

NEUROLEPTIC MALIGNANT SYNDROME (NMS)

A potentially fatal symptom complex sometimes referred to as Neuroleptic Malignant Syndrome (NMS) has been reported in association with administration of antipsychotic drugs, including olanzapine. Clinical manifestations of NMS are hyperpyrexia, muscle rigidity, altered mental status and evidence of autonomic instability (irregular pulse or blood pressure, tachycardia, diaphoresis and cardiac dysrhythmia). Additional signs may include elevated creatinine phosphokinase, myoglobinuria (rhabdomyolysis), and acute renal failure.

The diagnostic evaluation of patients with this syndrome is complicated. In arriving at a diagnosis, it is important to exclude cases where the clinical presentation includes both serious medical illness (*e.g.*, pneumonia, systemic infection, etc.) and untreated or inadequately treated extrapyramidal signs and symptoms (EPS). Other important considerations in the differential diagnosis include central anticholinergic toxicity, heat stroke, drug fever, and primary central nervous system pathology.

The management of NMS should include: (1) immediate discontinuation of antipsychotic drugs and other drugs not essential to concurrent therapy; (2) intensive symptomatic treatment and medical monitoring; and (3) treatment of any concomitant serious medical problems for which specific treatments are available. There is no general agreement about specific pharmacological treatment regimens for NMS.

If a patient requires antipsychotic drug treatment after recovery from NMS, the potential reintroduction of drug therapy should be carefully considered. The patient should be carefully monitored, since recurrences of NMS have been reported.

TARDIVE DYSKINESIA

A syndrome of potentially irreversible, involuntary, dyskinetic movements may develop in patients treated with antipsychotic drugs. Although the prevalence of the syndrome appears to be highest among the elderly, especially elderly women, it is impossible to rely upon prevalence estimates to predict, at the inception of antipsychotic treatment, which patients are likely to develop the syndrome. Whether antipsychotic drug products differ in their potential to cause tardive dyskinesia is unknown.

The risk of developing tardive dyskinesia and the likelihood that it will become irreversible are believed to increase as the duration of treatment and the total cumulative dose of antipsychotic drugs administered to the patient increase. However, the syndrome can develop, although much less commonly, after relatively brief treatment periods at low doses.

There is no known treatment for established cases of tardive dyskinesia, although the syndrome may remit, partially or completely, if antipsychotic treatment is withdrawn. Antipsychotic treatment, itself, however, may suppress (or partially suppress) the signs and symptoms of the syndrome and thereby may possibly mask the underlying process. The effect that symptomatic suppression has upon the long-term course of the syndrome is unknown.

Given these considerations, olanzapine should be prescribed in a manner that is most likely to minimize the occurrence of tardive dyskinesia. Chronic antipsychotic treatment should generally be reserved for patients (1) who suffer from a chronic illness that is known to respond to antipsychotic drugs; and (2) for whom alternative, equally effective, but potentially less harmful treatments are not available or appropriate. In patients who do require chronic treatment, the smallest dose and the shortest duration of treatment producing a satisfactory clinical response should be sought. The need for continued treatment should be reassessed periodically.

If signs and symptoms of tardive dyskinesia appear in a patient on olanzapine, drug discontinuation should be considered. However, some patients may require treatment with olanzapine despite the presence of the syndrome.

PRECAUTIONS

GENERAL

Orthostatic Hypotension

Olanzapine may induce orthostatic hypotension associated with dizziness, tachycardia, and in some patients, syncope, especially during the initial dose-titration period, probably reflecting its α_1-adrenergic antagonistic properties. Syncope was reported in 0.6% (15/2500) of olanzapine-treated patients in Phase 2 and 3 studies. The risk of orthostatic hypotension and syncope may be minimized by initiating therapy with 5 mg qd (see DOSAGE AND ADMINISTRATION). A more gradual titration to the target dose should be considered if hypotension occurs. Olanzapine should be used with particular caution in patients with known cardiovascular disease (history of myocardial infarction or ischemia, heart failure, or conduction abnormalities), cerebrovascular disease, and conditions which would predispose patients to hypotension (dehydration, hypovolemia, and treatment with antihypertensive medications).

Seizures

During premarketing testing, seizures occurred in 0.9% (22/2500) of olanzapine-treated patients. There were confounding factors that may have contributed to the occurrence of seizures in many of these cases. Olanzapine should be used cautiously in patients with a history of seizures or with conditions that potentially lower the seizure threshold, *e.g.*, Alzheimer's dementia. Conditions that lower the seizure threshold may be more prevalent in a population of 65 years or older.

Hyperprolactinemia

As with other drugs that antagonize dopamine D_2 receptors, olanzapine elevates prolactin levels, and a modest elevation persists during chronic administration. Tissue culture experiments indicate that approximately one-third of human breast cancers are prolactin dependent *in vitro*, a factor of potential importance if the prescription of these drugs is contemplated in a patient with previously detected breast cancer of this type. Although disturbances such as galactorrhea, amenorrhea, gynecomastia, and impotence have been reported with prolactin-elevating compounds, the clinical significance of elevated serum prolactin levels is unknown for most patients. As is common with compounds which increase prolactin release, an increase in mammary gland neoplasia was observed in the olanzapine carcinogenicity studies conducted in mice and rats (see Carcinogenesis). However, neither clinical studies nor epidemiologic studies have shown an association between chronic administration of this class of drugs and tumorigenesis in humans; the available evidence is considered too limited to be conclusive.

Transaminase Elevations

In placebo-controlled studies, clinically significant ALT (SGPT) elevations (≥3 times the upper limit of the normal range) were observed in 2% (6/243) of patients exposed to olan-

O

zapine compared to none (0/115) of the placebo patients. None of these patients experienced jaundice. In 2 of these patients, liver enzymes decreased toward normal despite continued treatment and in 2 others, enzymes decreased upon discontinuation of olanzapine. In the remaining 2 patients, one, seropositive for hepatitis C, had persistent enzyme elevation for 4 months after discontinuation, and the other had insufficient follow-up to determine if enzymes normalized.

Within the larger premarketing database of about 2400 patients with baseline SGPT ≤90 IU/L, the incidence of SGPT elevation to >200 IU/L was 2% (50/2381). Again, none of these patients experienced jaundice or other symptoms attributable to liver impairment and most had transient changes that tended to normalize while olanzapine treatment was continued.

Among all 2500 patients in clinical trials, about 1% (23/2500) discontinued treatment due to transaminase increases.

Caution should be exercised in patients with signs and symptoms of hepatic impairment, in patients with pre-existing conditions associated with limited hepatic functional reserve, and in patients who are being treated with potentially hepatotoxic drugs. Periodic assessment of transaminases is recommended in patients with significant hepatic disease (see Laboratory Tests).

Potential for Cognitive and Motor Impairment

Somnolence was a commonly reported adverse event associated with olanzapine treatment, occurring at an incidence of 26% in olanzapine patients compared to 15% in placebo patients. This adverse event was also dose related. Somnolence led to discontinuation in 0.4% (9/2500) of patients in the premarketing database.

Since olanzapine has the potential to impair judgment, thinking, or motor skills, patients should be cautioned about operating hazardous machinery, including automobiles, until they are reasonably certain that olanzapine therapy does not affect them adversely.

Body Temperature Regulation

Disruption of the body's ability to reduce core body temperature has been attributed to antipsychotic agents. Appropriate care is advised when prescribing olanzapine for patients who will be experiencing conditions which may contribute to an elevation in core body temperature, *e.g.*, exercising strenuously, exposure to extreme heat, receiving concomitant medication with anticholinergic activity, or being subject to dehydration.

Dysphagia

Esophageal dysmotility and aspiration have been associated with antipsychotic drug use. Two olanzapine-treated patients (2/407) in two studies in patients with Alzheimer's disease died from aspiration pneumonia during or within 30 days of the termination of the double-blind portion of their respective studies; there were no deaths in the placebo-treated patients. One of these patients had experienced dysphagia prior to the development of aspiration pneumonia. Aspiration pneumonia is a common cause of morbidity and mortality in patients with advanced Alzheimer's disease. Olanzapine and other antipsychotic drugs should be used cautiously in patients at risk for aspiration pneumonia.

Suicide

The possibility of a suicide attempt is inherent in schizophrenia and in bipolar disorder, and close supervision of high-risk patients should accompany drug therapy. Prescriptions for olanzapine should be written for the smallest quantity of tablets consistent with good patient management, in order to reduce the risk of overdose.

O

Use in Patients With Concomitant Illness

Clinical experience with olanzapine in patients with certain concomitant systemic illnesses (see CLINICAL PHARMACOLOGY, Special Populations, Renal Impairment and Hepatic Impairment) is limited.

Olanzapine exhibits *in vitro* muscarinic receptor affinity. In premarketing clinical trials with olanzapine, olanzapine was associated with constipation, dry mouth, and tachycardia, all adverse events possibly related to cholinergic antagonism. Such adverse events were not often the basis for discontinuations from olanzapine, but olanzapine should be used with caution in patients with clinically significant prostatic hypertrophy, narrow angle glaucoma, or a history of paralytic ileus.

In a fixed-dose study of olanzapine (olanzapine at doses of 5, 10, and 15 mg/day) and placebo in nursing home patients (mean age: 83 years, range: 61-97; median Mini-Mental State Examination (MMSE): 5, range: 0-22) having various psychiatric symptoms in association with Alzheimer's disease, the following treatment-emergent adverse events were reported in all (each and every) olanzapine-treated groups at an incidence of either (1) 2-fold or more in excess of the placebo-treated group, where at least 1 placebo-treated patient was reported to have experienced the event; or (2) at least 2 cases if no placebo-treated patient was reported to have experienced the event: somnolence, abnormal gait, fever, dehydration, and back pain. The rate of discontinuation in this study for olanzapine was 12% vs 4% with placebo. Discontinuations due to abnormal gait (1% for olanzapine vs 0% for placebo), accidental injury (1% for olanzapine vs 0% for placebo), and somnolence (3% for olanzapine vs 0% for placebo) were considered to be drug-related. As with other CNS-active drugs, olanzapine should be used with caution in elderly patients with dementia (see PRECAUTIONS).

Olanzapine has not been evaluated or used to any appreciable extent in patients with a recent history of myocardial infarction or unstable heart disease. Patients with these diagnoses were excluded from premarketing clinical studies. Because of the risk of orthostatic hypotension with olanzapine, caution should be observed in cardiac patients (see Orthostatic Hypotension).

INFORMATION FOR THE PATIENT

Physicians are advised to discuss the following issues with patients for whom they prescribe olanzapine.

Orthostatic Hypotension: Patients should be advised of the risk of orthostatic hypotension, especially during the period of initial dose titration and in association with the use of concomitant drugs that may potentiate the orthostatic effect of olanzapine, *e.g.*, diazepam or alcohol (see DRUG INTERACTIONS).

Interference With Cognitive and Motor Performance: Because olanzapine has the potential to impair judgment, thinking, or motor skills, patients should be cautioned about operating hazardous machinery, including automobiles, until they are reasonably certain that olanzapine therapy does not affect them adversely.

Pregnancy: Patients should be advised to notify their physician if they become pregnant or intend to become pregnant during therapy with olanzapine.

Nursing: Patients should be advised not to breastfeed an infant if they are taking olanzapine.

Concomitant Medication: Patients should be advised to inform their physicians if they are taking, or plan to take, any prescription or over-the-counter drugs, since there is a potential for interactions.

Alcohol: Patients should be advised to avoid alcohol while taking olanzapine.

Heat Exposure and Dehydration: Patients should be advised regarding appropriate care in avoiding overheating and dehydration.

Phenylketonurics (Orally Disintegrating Tablets Only): Olanzapine orally disintegrating tablets contain phenylalanine (0.34 and 0.45 mg per 5 and 10 mg tablet, respectively).

LABORATORY TESTS

Periodic assessment of transaminases is recommended in patients with significant hepatic disease (see Transaminase Elevations).

CARCINOGENESIS, MUTAGENESIS, AND IMPAIRMENT OF FERTILITY

Carcinogenesis

Oral carcinogenicity studies were conducted in mice and rats. Olanzapine was administered to mice in two 78-week studies at doses of 3, 10, 30/20 mg/kg/day (equivalent to 0.8-5 times the maximum recommended human daily dose [MRHD] on a mg/m^2 basis) and 0.25, 2, 8 mg/kg/day (equivalent to 0.06-2 times the MRHD on a mg/m^2 basis). Rats were dosed for 2 years at doses of 0.25, 1, 2.5, 4 mg/kg/day (males) and 0.25, 1, 4, 8 mg/kg/day (females) (equivalent to 0.13-2 and 0.13-4 times the MRHD on a mg/m^2 basis, respectively). The incidence of liver hemangiomas and hemangiosarcomas was significantly increased in one mouse study in female mice dosed at 8 mg/kg/day (2 times the MRHD on a mg/m^2 basis). These tumors were not increased in another mouse study in females dosed at 10 or 30/20 mg/kg/day (2-5 times the MRHD on a mg/m^2 basis); in this study, there was a high incidence of early mortalities in males of the 30/20 mg/kg/day group. The incidence of mammary gland adenomas and adenocarcinomas was significantly increased in female mice dosed at ≥2 mg/kg/day and in female rats dosed at ≥4 mg/kg/day (0.5 and 2 times the MRHD on a mg/m^2 basis, respectively). Antipsychotic drugs have been shown to chronically elevate prolactin levels in rodents. Serum prolactin levels were not measured during the olanzapine carcinogenicity studies; however, measurements during subchronic toxicity studies showed that olanzapine elevated serum prolactin levels up to 4-fold in rats at the same doses used in the carcinogenicity study. An increase in mammary gland neoplasms has been found in rodents after chronic administration of other antipsychotic drugs and is considered to be prolactin mediated. The relevance for human risk of the finding of prolactin-mediated endocrine tumors in rodents is unknown (see General, Hyperprolactinemia).

Mutagenesis

No evidence of mutagenic potential for olanzapine was found in the Ames reverse mutation test, *in vivo* micronucleus test in mice, the chromosomal aberration test in Chinese hamster ovary cells, unscheduled DNA synthesis test in rat hepatocytes, induction of forward mutation test in mouse lymphoma cells, or *in vivo* sister chromatid exchange test in bone marrow of Chinese hamsters.

Impairment of Fertility

In a fertility and reproductive performance study in rats, male mating performance, but not fertility, was impaired at a dose of 22.4 mg/kg/day and female fertility was decreased at a dose of 3 mg/kg/day (11 and 1.5 times the MRHD on a mg/m^2 basis, respectively). Discontinuance of olanzapine treatment reversed the effects on male mating performance. In female rats, the precoital period was increased and the mating index reduced at 5 mg/kg/day (2.5 times the MRHD on a mg/m^2 basis). Diestrous was prolonged and estrous delayed at 1.1 mg/kg/day (0.6 times the MRHD on a mg/m^2 basis); therefore olanzapine may produce a delay in ovulation.

PREGNANCY CATEGORY C

In reproduction studies in rats at doses of up to 18 mg/kg/day and in rabbits at doses of up to 30 mg/kg/day (9 and 30 times the MRHD on a mg/m^2 basis, respectively) no evidence of teratogenicity was observed. In a rat teratology study, early resorptions and increased numbers of nonviable fetuses were observed at a dose of 18 mg/kg/day (9 times the MRHD on a mg/m^2 basis). Gestation was prolonged at 10 mg/kg/day (5 times the MRHD on a mg/m^2 basis). In a rabbit teratology study, fetal toxicity (manifested as increased resorptions and decreased fetal weight) occurred at a maternally toxic dose of 30 mg/kg/day (30 times the MRHD on a mg/m^2 basis).

Placental transfer of olanzapine occurs in rat pups.

There are no adequate and well-controlled trials with olanzapine in pregnant females. Seven pregnancies were observed during clinical trials with olanzapine, including 2 resulting in normal births, one resulting in neonatal death due to a cardiovascular defect, three therapeutic abortions, and one spontaneous abortion. Because animal reproduction studies are not always predictive of human response, this drug should be used during pregnancy only if the potential benefit justifies the potential risk to the fetus.

LABOR AND DELIVERY

Parturition in rats was not affected by olanzapine. The effect of olanzapine on labor and delivery in humans is unknown.

NURSING MOTHERS

Olanzapine was excreted in milk of treated rats during lactation. It is not known if olanzapine is excreted in human milk. It is recommended that women receiving olanzapine should not breastfeed.

PEDIATRIC USE

Safety and effectiveness in pediatric patients have not been established.

GERIATRIC USE

Of the 2500 patients in premarketing clinical studies with olanzapine, 11% (263) were 65 years of age or over. In patients with schizophrenia, there was no indication of any different tolerability of olanzapine in the elderly compared to younger patients. Studies in patients with various psychiatric symptoms in association with Alzheimer's disease have suggested that there may be a different tolerability profile in this population compared to younger patients with schizophrenia. As with other CNS-active drugs, olanzapine should be used with caution in elderly patients with dementia. Also, the presence of factors that might decrease pharmacokinetic clearance or increase the pharmacodynamic response to olanzapine should lead to consideration of a lower starting dose for any geriatric patient (see PRECAUTIONS and DOSAGE AND ADMINISTRATION).

DRUG INTERACTIONS

The risks of using olanzapine in combination with other drugs have not been extensively evaluated in systematic studies. Given the primary CNS effects of olanzapine, caution should be used when olanzapine is taken in combination with other centrally acting drugs and alcohol.

Because of its potential for inducing hypotension, olanzapine may enhance the effects of certain antihypertensive agents.

Olanzapine may antagonize the effects of levodopa and dopamine agonists.

THE EFFECT OF OTHER DRUGS ON OLANZAPINE

Agents that induce CYP1A2 or glucuronyl transferase enzymes, such as omeprazole and rifampin, may cause an increase in olanzapine clearance. Inhibitors of CYP1A2 (*e.g.,* fluvoxamine) could potentially inhibit olanzapine elimination. Because olanzapine is metabolized by multiple enzyme systems, inhibition of a single enzyme may not appreciably decrease olanzapine clearance.

CHARCOAL

The administration of activated charcoal (1 g) reduced the C_{max} and AUC of olanzapine by about 60%. As peak olanzapine levels are not typically obtained until about 6 hours after dosing, charcoal may be a useful treatment for olanzapine overdose.

CIMETIDINE AND ANTACIDS

Single doses of cimetidine (800 mg) or aluminum- and magnesium-containing antacids did not affect the oral bioavailability of olanzapine.

CARBAMAZEPINE

Carbamazepine therapy (200 mg bid) causes an approximately 50% increase in the clearance of olanzapine. This increase is likely due to the fact that carbamazepine is a potent inducer of CYP1A2 activity. Higher daily doses of carbamazepine may cause an even greater increase in olanzapine clearance.

ETHANOL

Ethanol (45 mg/70 kg single dose) did not have an effect on olanzapine pharmacokinetics.

FLUOXETINE

Fluoxetine (60 mg single dose or 60 mg daily for 8 days) causes a small (mean 16%) increase in the maximum concentration of olanzapine and a small (mean 16%) decrease in olanzapine clearance. The magnitude of the impact of this factor is small in comparison to the overall variability between individuals, and therefore dose modification is not routinely recommended.

VALPROATE

Studies *in vitro* using human liver microsomes determined that olanzapine has little potential to inhibit the major metabolic pathway, glucuronidation, of valproate. Further, valproate has little effect on the metabolism of olanzapine *in vitro.* Thus, a clinically significant pharmacokinetic interaction between olanzapine and valproate is unlikely.

WARFARIN

Warfarin (20 mg single dose) did not affect olanzapine pharmacokinetics.

EFFECT OF OLANZAPINE ON OTHER DRUGS

In vitro studies utilizing human liver microsomes suggest that olanzapine has little potential to inhibit CYP1A2, CYP2C9, CYP2C19, CYP2D6, and CYP3A. Thus, olanzapine is unlikely to cause clinically important drug interactions mediated by these enzymes.

Single doses of olanzapine did not affect the pharmacokinetics of imipramine or its active metabolite desipramine, and warfarin. Multiple doses of olanzapine did not influence the kinetics of diazepam and its active metabolite N-desmethyldiazepam, lithium, ethanol, or biperiden. However, the coadministration of either diazepam or ethanol with olanzapine potentiated the orthostatic hypotension observed with olanzapine. Multiple doses of olanzapine did not affect the pharmacokinetics of theophylline or its metabolites.

ADVERSE REACTIONS

The information below is derived from a clinical trial database for olanzapine consisting of 4189 patients with approximately 2665 patient-years of exposure. This database includes: (1) 2500 patients who participated in multiple-dose premarketing trials in schizophrenia and Alzheimer's disease representing approximately 1122 patient-years of exposure as of February 14, 1995; (2) 182 patients who participated in premarketing bipolar mania trials representing approximately 66 patient-years of exposure; (3) 191 patients who participated in a trial of patients having various psychiatric symptoms in association with Alzheimer's disease representing approximately 29 patient-years of exposure; and (4) 1316 patients from 43 additional clinical trials as of May 1, 1997.

The conditions and duration of treatment with olanzapine varied greatly and included (in overlapping categories) open-label and double-blind phases of studies, inpatients and outpatients, fixed-dose and dose-titration studies, and short-term or longer-term exposure. Adverse reactions were assessed by collecting adverse events, results of physical examinations, vital signs, weights, laboratory analytes, ECGs, chest x-rays, and results of ophthalmologic examinations.

Certain portions of the discussion below relating to objective or numeric safety parameters, namely, dose-dependent adverse events, vital sign changes, weight gain, laboratory changes, and ECG changes are derived from studies in patients with schizophrenia and have not been duplicated for bipolar mania. However, this information is also generally applicable to bipolar mania.

Adverse events during exposure were obtained by spontaneous report and recorded by clinical investigators using terminology of their own choosing. Consequently, it is not possible to provide a meaningful estimate of the proportion of individuals experiencing adverse events without first grouping similar types of events into a smaller number of standardized event categories. In the tables and tabulations that follow, standard COSTART dictionary terminology has been used initially to classify reported adverse events.

The stated frequencies of adverse events represent the proportion of individuals who experienced, at least once, a treatment-emergent adverse event of the type listed. An event was considered treatment-emergent if it occurred for the first time or worsened while receiving therapy following baseline evaluation. The reported events do not include those event terms which were so general as to be uninformative. Events listed elsewhere in labeling may not be repeated below. It is important to emphasize that, although the events occurred during treatment with olanzapine, they were not necessarily caused by it. The entire label should be read to gain a complete understanding of the safety profile of olanzapine.

The prescriber should be aware that the figures in the tables and tabulations cannot be used to predict the incidence of side effects in the course of usual medical practice where patient characteristics and other factors differ from those that prevailed in the clinical trials. Similarly, the cited frequencies cannot be compared with figures obtained from other clinical investigations involving different treatments, uses, and investigators. The cited figures, however, do provide the prescribing physician with some basis for estimating the relative contribution of drug and nondrug factors to the adverse event incidence in the population studied.

INCIDENCE OF ADVERSE EVENTS IN SHORT-TERM, PLACEBO-CONTROLLED TRIALS

The following findings are based on the short-term, placebo-controlled premarketing trials for schizophrenia and bipolar mania and a subsequent trial of patients having various psychiatric symptoms in association with Alzheimer's disease.

Adverse events associated with discontinuation of treatment in short-term, placebo-controlled trials

Schizophrenia: Overall, there was no difference in the incidence of discontinuation due to adverse events (5% for olanzapine vs 6% for placebo). However, discontinuations due to increases in SGPT were considered to be drug-related (2% for olanzapine vs 0% for placebo) (see PRECAUTIONS).

Bipolar Mania: Overall, there was no difference in the incidence of discontinuation due to adverse events (2% for olanzapine vs 2% for placebo).

Commonly observed adverse events in short-term, placebo-controlled trials

The most commonly observed adverse events associated with the use of olanzapine (incidence of 5% or greater) and not observed at an equivalent incidence among placebo-treated patients (olanzapine incidence at least twice that for placebo) are shown in TABLE 1 and TABLE 2.

TABLE 1 *Common Treatment-Emergent Adverse Events Associated With the Use of Olanzapine in 6 Week Trials*

Schizophrenia

	Percentage of Patients Reporting Event	
	Olanzapine	Placebo
Adverse Event	(n=248)	(n=118)
Postural hypotension	5%	2%
Constipation	9%	3%
Weight gain	6%	1%
Dizziness	11%	4%
Personality disorder*	8%	4%
Akathisia	5%	1%

* Personality disorder is the COSTART term for designating nonaggressive objectionable behavior.

TABLE 2 *Common Treatment-Emergent Adverse Events Associated With the Use of Olanzapine in 3 and 4 Week Trials*

Bipolar Mania

	Percentage of Patients Reporting Event	
	Olanzapine	Placebo
Adverse Event	(n=125)	(n=129)
Asthenia	15%	6%
Dry mouth	22%	7%
Constipation	11%	5%
Dyspepsia	11%	5%
Increased appetite	6%	3%
Somnolence	35%	13%
Dizziness	18%	6%
Tremor	6%	3%

Adverse events occurring at an incidence of 2% or more among olanzapine-treated patients in short-term, placebo-controlled trials

TABLE 3 enumerates the incidence, rounded to the nearest percent, of treatment-emergent adverse events that occurred in 2% or more of patients treated with olanzapine (doses ≥2.5 mg/day) and with incidence greater than placebo who participated in the acute phase of placebo-controlled trials.

TABLE 3 *Treatment-Emergent Adverse Events Incidence in Short-Term, Placebo-Controlled Clinical Trials**

	Percentage of Patients Reporting Event	
	Olanzapine	Placebo
Body System/Adverse Event	**(n=532)**	**(n=294)**
Body as a Whole		
Accidental injury	12%	8%
Asthenia	10%	9%
Fever	6%	2%
Back pain	5%	2%
Chest pain	3%	1%
Cardiovascular System		
Postural hypotension	3%	1%
Tachycardia	3%	1%
Hypertension	2%	1%
Digestive System		
Dry mouth	9%	5%
Constipation	9%	4%
Dyspepsia	7%	5%
Vomiting	4%	3%
Increased appetite	3%	2%
Hemic and Lymphatic System		
Ecchymosis	5%	3%
Metabolic and Nutritional Disorders		
Weight gain	5%	3%
Peripheral edema	3%	1%
Musculoskeletal System		
Extremity pain (other than joint)	5%	3%
Joint pain	5%	3%
Nervous System		
Somnolence	29%	13%
Insomnia	12%	11%
Dizziness	11%	4%
Abnormal gait	6%	1%
Tremor	4%	3%
Akathisia	3%	2%
Hypertonia	3%	2%
Articulation impairment	2%	1%
Respiratory System		
Rhinitis	7%	6%
Cough increased	6%	3%
Pharyngitis	4%	3%
Special Senses		
Amblyopia	3%	2%
Urogenital System		
Urinary incontinence	2%	1%
Urinary tract infection	2%	1%

* Events reported by at least 2% of patients treated with olanzapine, except the following events which had an incidence equal to or less than placebo: abdominal pain, agitation, anorexia, anxiety, apathy, confusion, depression, diarrhea, dysmenorrhea.†Hhallucinations, headache, hostility, hyperkinesia, myalgia, nausea, nervousness, paranoid reaction, personality disorder.‡, rash, thinking abnormal, weight loss.

† Denominator used was for females only (olanzapine, n=201; placebo, n=114).

‡ Personality disorder is the COSTART term for designating nonaggressive objectionable behavior.

ADDITIONAL FINDINGS OBSERVED IN CLINICAL TRIALS

The following findings are based on clinical trials.

Dose dependency of adverse events in short-term, placebo-controlled trials

Extrapyramidal Symptoms

TABLE 4 enumerates the percentage of patients with treatment-emergent extrapyramidal symptoms as assessed by categorical analyses of formal rating scales during acute therapy in a controlled clinical trial comparing olanzapine at 3 fixed doses with placebo in the treatment of schizophrenia.

TABLE 4 *Treatment-Emergent Extrapyramidal Symptoms Assessed by Rating Scales Incidence in a Fixed Dosage Range, Placebo-Controlled Clinical Trial Acute Phase**

	Percentage of Patients			
		Olanzapine		
	Placebo	**5 ± 2.5 mg/day**	**10 ± 2.5 mg/day**	**15 ± 2.5 mg/day**
Parkinsonism†	15%	14%	12%	14%
Akathisia‡	23%	16%	19%	27%

* No statistically significant differences.

† Percentage of patients with a Simpson-Angus Scale total score >3.

‡ Percentage of patients with a Barnes Akathisia Scale global score ≥2.

TABLE 5 enumerates the percentage of patients with treatment-emergent extrapyramidal symptoms as assessed by spontaneously reported adverse events during acute therapy in the same controlled clinical trial comparing olanzapine at 3 fixed doses with placebo in the treatment of schizophrenia.

TABLE 5 *Treatment-Emergent Extrapyramidal Symptoms Assessed by Adverse Events Incidence in a Fixed Dosage Range, Placebo-Controlled Clinical Trial Acute Phase*

	Percentage of Patients Reporting Event			
		Olanzapine		
	Placebo (n=68)	**5 ± 2.5 mg/day (n=65)**	**10 ± 2.5 mg/day (n=64)**	**15 ± 2.5 mg/day (n=69)**
Dystonic events†	1%	3%	2%	3%
Parkinsonism events‡	10%	8%	14%	20%
Akathisia events§	1%	5%	11%*	10%*
Dyskinetic events¤	4%	0%	2%	1%
Residual events¶	1%	2%	5%	1%
Any extrapyramidal event	16%	15%	25%	32%*

* Statistically significantly different from placebo.

† Patients with the following COSTART terms were counted in this category: dystonia, generalized spasm, neck rigidity, oculoyric crisis, opisthontonos, torticollis.

‡ Patients with the following COSTART terms were counted in this category: akinesia, cogwheel rigidity, extrapyramidal syndrome, hypertonia, hypokinesia, masked facies, tremor.

§ Patients with the following COSTART terms were counted in this category: akathisia, hyperkinesia.

¤ Patients with the following COSTART terms were counted in this category: buccoglossal syndrome, choreoathetosis, dyskinesia, tardive dyskinesia.

¶ Patients with the following COSTART terms were counted in this category: movement disorder, myoclonus, twitching.

Other Adverse Events

TABLE 6 addresses dose relatedness for other adverse events using data from a schizophrenia trial involving fixed dosage ranges. It enumerates the percentage of patients with treatment-emergent adverse events for the three fixed-dose range groups and placebo. The data were analyzed using the Cochran-Armitage test, excluding the placebo group, and TABLE 6 includes only those adverse events for which there was a statistically significant trend.

TABLE 6

	Percentage of Patients Reporting Event			
		Olanzapine		
Adverse Event	**Placebo (n=68)**	**5 ± 2.5 mg/day (n=65)**	**10 ± 2.5 mg/day (n=64)**	**15 ± 2.5 mg/day (n=69)**
Asthenia	15%	8%	9%	20%
Dry mouth	4%	3%	5%	13%
Nausea	9%	0%	2%	9%
Somnolence	16%	20%	30%	39%
Tremor	3%	0%	5%	7%

Vital Sign Changes

Olanzapine is associated with orthostatic hypotension and tachycardia (see PRECAUTIONS).

Weight Gain

In placebo-controlled, 6-week studies, weight gain was reported in 5.6% of olanzapine patients compared to 0.8% of placebo patients. Olanzapine patients gained an average of 2.8 kg, compared to an average 0.4 kg weight loss in placebo patients; 29% of olanzapine patients gained greater than 7% of their baseline weight, compared to 3% of placebo patients. A categorization of patients at baseline on the basis of body mass index (BMI) revealed a significantly greater effect in patients with low BMI compared to normal or overweight patients; nevertheless, weight gain was greater in all three olanzapine groups compared to the placebo group. During long-term continuation therapy with olanzapine (238 median days of exposure), 56% of olanzapine patients met the criterion for having gained greater than 7% of their baseline weight. Average weight gain during long-term therapy was 5.4 kg.

Laboratory Changes

An assessment of the premarketing experience for olanzapine revealed an association with asymptomatic increases in SGPT, SGOT, and GGT (see PRECAUTIONS). Olanzapine administration was also associated with increases in serum prolactin (see PRECAUTIONS), with an asymptomatic elevation of the eosinophil count in 0.3% of patients, and with an increase in CPK.

Given the concern about neutropenia associated with other psychotropic compounds and the finding of leukopenia associated with the administration of olanzapine in several animal models (see ANIMAL PHARMACOLOGY), careful attention was given to examination of hematologic parameters in premarketing studies with olanzapine. There was no indication of a risk of clinically significant neutropenia associated with olanzapine treatment in the premarketing database for this drug.

ECG Changes

Between-group comparisons for pooled placebo-controlled trials revealed no statistically significant olanzapine/placebo differences in the proportions of patients experiencing potentially important changes in ECG parameters, including QT, QTc, and PR intervals. Olanzapine use was associated with a mean increase in heart rate of 2.4 beats per minute compared to no change among placebo patients. This slight tendency to tachycardia may be related to olanzapine's potential for inducing orthostatic changes (see PRECAUTIONS).

OTHER ADVERSE EVENTS OBSERVED DURING THE PREMARKETING EVALUATION OF OLANZAPINE

Following is a list of terms that reflect treatment-emergent adverse events reported by patients treated with olanzapine (at multiple doses ≥1 mg/day) in clinical trials (4189 patients, 2665 patient-years of exposure). This listing does not include those events already listed in previous tables or elsewhere in labeling, those events for which a drug cause was remote, those event terms which were so general as to be uninformative, and those events reported only once which did not have a substantial probability of being acutely life-threatening.

Events are further categorized by body system and listed in order of decreasing frequency according to the following definitions: *Frequent adverse events* are those occurring in at least 1/100 patients (only those not already listed in the tabulated results from placebo-controlled trials appear in this listing); *infrequent adverse events* are those occurring in 1/100 to 1/1000 patients; *rare events* are those occurring in fewer than 1/1000 patients:

Body as a Whole: *Frequent:* Dental pain, flu syndrome, intentional injury, and suicide attempt; *Infrequent:* Abdomen enlarged, chills, chills and fever, face edema, malaise, moniliasis, neck pain, neck rigidity, pelvic pain, and photosensitivity reaction; *Rare:* Hangover effect and sudden death.

Cardiovascular System: *Frequent:* Hypotension; *Infrequent:* Bradycardia, cerebrovascular accident, congestive heart failure, heart arrest, hemorrhage, migraine, pallor, palpitation, vasodilatation, and ventricular extrasystoles; *Rare:* Arteritis, atrial fibrillation, heart failure, and pulmonary embolus.

Digestive System: *Frequent:* Increased salivation and thirst; *Infrequent:* Dysphagia, eructation, fecal impaction, fecal incontinence, flatulence, gastritis, gastroenteritis, gingivitis, hepatitis, melena, mouth ulceration, nausea and vomiting, oral moniliasis, periodontal abscess, rectal hemorrhage, stomatitis, tongue edema, and tooth caries; *Rare:* Aphthous stomatitis, enteritis, esophageal ulcer, esophagitis, glossitis, ileus, intestinal obstruction, liver fatty deposit, and tongue discoloration.

Endocrine System: *Infrequent:* Diabetes mellitus; *Rare:* Diabetic acidosis and goiter.

Hemic and Lymphatic System: *Frequent:* Leukopenia; *Infrequent:* Anemia, cyanosis, leukocytosis, lymphadenopathy, thrombocythemia, and thrombocytopenia; *Rare:* Normocytic anemia.

Metabolic and Nutritional Disorders: *Infrequent:* Acidosis, alkaline phosphatase increased, bilirubinemia, dehydration, hypercholesteremia, hyperglycemia, hyperlipemia, hyperuricemia, hypoglycemia, hypokalemia, hyponatremia, lower extremity edema, upper extremity edema, and water intoxication; *Rare:* Gout, hyperkalemia, hypernatremia, hypoproteinemia, and ketosis.

Musculoskeletal System: *Frequent:* Joint stiffness and twitching; *Infrequent:* Arthritis, arthrosis, bursitis, leg cramps, and myasthenia; *Rare:* Bone pain, myopathy, osteoporosis, and rheumatoid arthritis.

Nervous System: *Frequent:* Abnormal dreams, emotional lability, euphoria, libido decreased, paresthesia, and schizophrenic reaction; *Infrequent:* Alcohol misuse, amnesia, antisocial reaction, ataxia, CNS stimulation, cogwheel rigidity, coma, delirium, depersonalization, dysarthria, facial paralysis, hypesthesia, hypokinesia, hypotonia, incoordination, libido increased, obsessive-compulsive symptoms, phobias, somatization, stimulant misuse, stupor, stuttering, tardive dyskinesia, tobacco misuse, vertigo, and withdrawal syndrome; *Rare:* Akinesia, circumoral paresthesia, encephalopathy, neuralgia, neuropathy, nystagmus, paralysis, and subarachnoid hemorrhage.

Respiratory System: *Frequent:* Dyspnea; *Infrequent:* Apnea, aspiration pneumonia, asthma, atelectasis, epistaxis, hemoptysis, hyperventilation, laryngitis, pneumonia, and voice alteration; *Rare:* Hiccup, hypoventilation, hypoxia, lung edema, and stridor.

Skin and Appendages: *Frequent:* Sweating; *Infrequent:* Alopecia, contact dermatitis, dry skin, eczema, maculopapular rash, pruritus, seborrhea, skin ulcer, and vesiculobullous rash; *Rare:* Hirsutism, pustular rash, skin discoloration, and urticaria.

Special Senses: *Frequent:* Conjunctivitis; *Infrequent:* Abnormality of accommodation, blepharitis, cataract, corneal lesion, deafness, diplopia, dry eyes, ear pain, eye hemorrhage, eye inflammation, eye pain, ocular muscle abnormality, taste perversion, and tinnitus; *Rare:* Glaucoma, keratoconjunctivitis, macular hypopigmentation, miosis, mydriasis, and pigment deposits lens.

Urogenital System: *Frequent:* Amenorrhea*, hematuria, metrorrhagia*, and vaginitis*; *Infrequent:* Abnormal ejaculation*, breast pain, cystitis, decreased menstruation*, dysuria, female lactation, glycosuria, impotence*, increased menstruation*, menorrhagia*, polyuria, premenstrual syndrome*, pyuria, urinary frequency, urinary retention, urination impaired, uterine fibroids enlarged*, and vaginal hemorrhage*; *Rare:* Albuminuria, gynecomastia, mastitis, oliguria, and urinary urgency.

*Adjusted for gender.

POSTINTRODUCTION REPORTS

Adverse events reported since market introduction which were temporally (but not necessarily causally) related to olanzapine therapy include the following: diabetic coma and priapism.

DOSAGE AND ADMINISTRATION

SCHIZOPHRENIA

Usual Dose

Olanzapine should be administered on a once-a-day schedule without regard to meals, generally beginning with 5-10 mg initially, with a target dose of 10 mg/day within several days. Further dosage adjustments, if indicated, should generally occur at intervals of not less than 1 week, since steady state for olanzapine would not be achieved for approximately 1 week in the typical patient. When dosage adjustments are necessary, dose increments/decrements of 5 mg qd are recommended.

Efficacy in schizophrenia was demonstrated in a dose range of 10-15 mg/day in clinical trials. However, doses above 10 mg/day were not demonstrated to be more efficacious than the 10 mg/day dose. An increase to a dose greater than the target dose of 10 mg/day (*i.e.*, to a dose of 15 mg/day or greater) is recommended only after clinical assessment. The safety of doses above 20 mg/day has not been evaluated in clinical trials.

Dosing in Special Populations

The recommended starting dose is 5 mg in patients who are debilitated, who have a predisposition to hypotensive reactions, who otherwise exhibit a combination of factors that may result in slower metabolism of olanzapine (*e.g.*, nonsmoking female patients ≥65 years of age), or who may be more pharmacodynamically sensitive to olanzapine (see CLINICAL PHARMACOLOGY; DRUG INTERACTIONS; and PRECAUTIONS, Use in Patients With Concomitant Illness). When indicated, dose escalation should be performed with caution in these patients.

Maintenance Treatment

While there is no body of evidence available to answer the question of how long the patient treated with olanzapine should remain on it, the effectiveness of oral olanzapine, 10-20 mg/day, in maintaining treatment response in schizophrenic patients who had been stable on olanzapine for approximately 8 weeks and were then followed for a period of up to 8 months has been demonstrated in a placebo-controlled trial. Patients should be periodically reassessed to determine the need for maintenance treatment with appropriate dose.

BIPOLAR MANIA

Usual Dose

Olanzapine should be administered on a once-a-day schedule without regard to meals, generally beginning with 10 or 15 mg. Dosage adjustments, if indicated, should generally occur at intervals of not less than 24 hours, reflecting the procedures in the placebo-controlled trials. When dosage adjustments are necessary, dose increments/decrements of 5 mg qd are recommended.

Short-term (3-4 weeks) antimanic efficacy was demonstrated in a dose range of 5-20 mg/day in clinical trials. The safety of doses above 20 mg/day has not been evaluated in clinical trials.

Dosing in Special Populations

See Schizophrenia, Dosing in Special Populations.

Maintenance Treatment

There is no body of evidence available from controlled trials to guide a clinician in the longer-term management of a patient who improves during treatment of an acute manic episode with olanzapine. While it is generally agreed that pharmacological treatment beyond an acute response in mania is desirable, both for maintenance of the initial response and for prevention of new manic episodes, there are no systematically obtained data to support the use of olanzapine in such longer-term treatment (*i.e.*, beyond 3-4 weeks).

ADMINISTRATION OF OLANZAPINE ORALLY DISINTEGRATING TABLETS

After opening sachet, peel back foil on blister. Do not push tablet through foil. Immediately upon opening the blister, using dry hands, remove tablet and place entire olanzapine orally disintegrating tablet in the mouth. Tablet disintegration occurs rapidly in saliva so it can be easily swallowed with or without liquid.

ANIMAL PHARMACOLOGY

In animal studies with olanzapine, the principal hematologic findings were reversible peripheral cytopenias in individual dogs dosed at 10 mg/kg (17 times the MRHD on a mg/m^2 basis), dose-related decreases in lymphocytes and neutrophils in mice, and lymphopenia in rats. A few dogs treated with 10 mg/kg developed reversible neutropenia and/or reversible hemolytic anemia between 1 and 10 months of treatment. Dose-related decreases in lymphocytes and neutrophils were seen in mice given doses of 10 mg/kg (equal to 2 times the MRHD on a mg/m^2 basis) in studies of 3 months' duration. Nonspecific lymphopenia, consistent with decreased body weight gain, occurred in rats receiving 22.5 mg/kg (11 times the MRHD on a mg/m^2 basis) for 3 months or 16 mg/kg (8 times the MRHD on a mg/m^2 basis) for 6 or 12 months. No evidence of bone marrow cytotoxicity was found in any of the species examined. Bone marrows were normocellular or hypercellular, indicating that the reductions in circulating blood cells were probably due to peripheral (nonmarrow) factors.

HOW SUPPLIED

ZYPREXA TABLETS

Zyprexa 2.5, 5, 7.5, and 10 mg tablets are white, round, and imprinted in blue ink with "LILLY" and the tablet number. The tablet numbers are *2.5 mg:* Tablet no. "4112"; *5 mg:* Tablet no. "4115"*7.5 mg:* Tablet no. "4116"; *10 mg:* Tablet no. "4117".

The 15 mg tablets are elliptical, blue, and debossed with "LILLY" and tablet number "4415".

The 20 mg tablets are elliptical, pink, and debossed with "LILLY" and tablet number "4420".

ZYPREXA ZYDIS ORALLY DISINTEGRATING TABLETS

Zyprexa Zydis orally disintegrating tablets are yellow, round, and debossed with the tablet strength. The tablets are available as 5 and 10 mg tablets. *5 mg:* Debossed with "5" and tablet no. "4453"; *10 mg:* Debossed with "10" and tablet no. "4454".

STORAGE

Store at controlled room temperature, 20-25°C (68-77°F). Protect from light and moisture.

PRODUCT LISTING - EQUIVALENTS NOT AVAILABLE

Tablet - Oral - 2.5 mg

60's	$322.10	ZYPREXA, Lilly, Eli and Company	00002-4112-60
100's	$536.84	ZYPREXA, Lilly, Eli and Company	00002-4112-33

Tablet - Oral - 5 mg

60's	$380.44	ZYPREXA, Lilly, Eli and Company	00002-4115-60

100's	$634.07	ZYPREXA, Lilly, Eli and Company	00002-4115-33
Tablet - Oral - 7.5 mg			
60's	$435.72	ZYPREXA, Lilly, Eli and Company	00002-4116-60
100's	$726.19	ZYPREXA, Lilly, Eli and Company	00002-4116-33
Tablet - Oral - 10 mg			
60's	$578.28	ZYPREXA, Lilly, Eli and Company	00002-4117-60
100's	$963.79	ZYPREXA, Lilly, Eli and Company	00002-4117-33
Tablet - Oral - 15 mg			
60's	$867.41	ZYPREXA, Lilly, Eli and Company	00002-4415-60
100's	$1445.69	ZYPREXA, Lilly, Eli and Company	00002-4415-33
Tablet - Oral - 20 mg			
60's	$1154.88	ZYPREXA, Lilly, Eli and Company	00002-4420-60
100's	$1924.79	ZYPREXA, Lilly, Eli and Company	00002-4420-33
Tablet, Disintegrating - Oral - 5 mg			
30's	$225.49	ZYPREXA ZYDIS, Lilly, Eli and Company	00002-4453-85
Tablet, Disintegrating - Oral - 10 mg			
30's	$324.42	ZYPREXA ZYDIS, Lilly, Eli and Company	00002-4454-85
Tablet, Disintegrating - Oral - 15 mg			
100's	$468.98	ZYPREXA ZYDIS, Lilly, Eli and Company	00002-4455-85
Tablet, Disintegrating - Oral - 20 mg			
30's	$612.72	ZYPREXA ZYDIS, Lilly, Eli and Company	00002-4456-85

Olmesartan Medoxomil *(003555)*

For related information, see the comparative table section in Appendix A.

Categories: Hypertension, essential; FDA Approved 2002 Apr; Pregnancy Category C, 1st Trimester; Pregnancy Category D, 2nd & 3rd Trimesters
Drug Classes: Angiotensin II receptor antagonists
Brand Names: **Benicar**
Cost of Therapy: $39.38 (Hypertension; Benicar; 20 mg; 1 tablet/day; 30 day supply)

WARNING

USE IN PREGNANCY

When used in pregnancy during the second and third trimesters, drugs that act directly on the renin-angiotensin system can cause injury and even death to the developing fetus. When pregnancy is detected, olmesartan medoxomil should be discontinued as soon as possible. See WARNINGS, Fetal/Neonatal Morbidity and Mortality.

DESCRIPTION

Benicar (olmesartan medoxomil), a prodrug, is hydrolyzed to olmesartan during absorption from the gastrointestinal tract. Olmesartan is a selective AT_1 subtype angiotensin II receptor antagonist.

Olmesartan medoxomil is described chemically as 2,3-dihydroxy-2-butenyl 4-(1-hydroxy-1-methylethyl)-2-propyl-1-[*p*-(*o*-1H-tetrazol-5-ylphenyl)benzyl]imidazole-5-carboxylate, cyclic 2,3-carbonate.

Its empirical formula is $C_{29}H_{30}N_6O_6$.

Olmesartan medoxomil is a white to light yellowish-white powder or crystalline powder with a molecular weight of 558.59. It is practically insoluble in water and sparingly soluble in methanol. Olmesartan medoxomil is available for oral use as film-coated tablets containing 5, 20, or 40 mg of olmesartan medoxomil and the following inactive ingredients: hydroxypropylcellulose, lactose, lowsubstituted hydroxypropylcellulose, magnesium stearate, microcrystalline cellulose, talc, titanium dioxide, and (5 mg only) yellow iron oxide.

CLINICAL PHARMACOLOGY

MECHANISM OF ACTION

Angiotensin II is formed from angiotensin I in a reaction catalyzed by angiotensin converting enzyme (ACE, kininase II). Angiotensin II is the principal pressor agent of the renin-angiotensin system, with effects that include vasoconstriction, stimulation of synthesis and release of aldosterone, cardiac stimulation and renal reabsorption of sodium. Olmesartan blocks the vasoconstrictor effects of angiotensin II by selectively blocking the binding of angiotensin II to the AT_1 receptor in vascular smooth muscle. Its action is, therefore, independent of the pathways for angiotensin II synthesis.

An AT_2 receptor is found also in many tissues, but this receptor is not known to be associated with cardiovascular homeostasis. Olmesartan has more than a 12,500-fold greater affinity for the AT_1 receptor than for the AT_2 receptor.

Blockade of the renin-angiotensin system with ACE inhibitors, which inhibit the biosynthesis of angiotensin II from angiotensin I, is a mechanism of many drugs used to treat hypertension. ACE inhibitors also inhibit the degradation of bradykinin, a reaction also catalyzed by ACE. Because olmesartan medoxomil does not inhibit ACE (kininase II), it does not affect the response to bradykinin. Whether this difference has clinical relevance is not yet known.

Blockade of the angiotensin II receptor inhibits the negative regulatory feedback of angiotensin II on renin secretion, but the resulting increased plasma renin activity and circulating angiotensin II levels do not overcome the effect of olmesartan on blood pressure.

PHARMACOKINETICS

General

Olmesartan medoxomil is rapidly and completely bioactivated by ester hydrolysis to olmesartan during absorption from the gastrointestinal tract. Olmesartan appears to be eliminated in a biphasic manner with a terminal elimination half-life of approximately 13 hours. Olmesartan shows linear pharmacokinetics following single oral doses of up to 320 mg and multiple oral doses of up to 80 mg. Steady-state levels of olmesartan are achieved within 3-5 days and no accumulation in plasma occurs with once-daily dosing.

The absolute bioavailability of olmesartan is approximately 26%. After oral administration, the peak plasma concentration (C_{max}) of olmesartan is reached after 1-2 hours. Food does not affect the bioavailability of olmesartan.

Metabolism and Excretion

Following the rapid and complete conversion of olmesartan medoxomil to olmesartan during absorption, there is virtually no further metabolism of olmesartan. Total plasma clearance of olmesartan is 1.3 L/h, with a renal clearance of 0.6 L/h. Approximately 35% to 50% of the absorbed dose is recovered in urine while the remainder is eliminated in feces via the bile.

Distribution

The volume of distribution of olmesartan is approximately 17 L. Olmesartan is highly bound to plasma proteins (99%) and does not penetrate red blood cells. The protein binding is constant at plasma olmesartan concentrations well above the range achieved with recommended doses.

In rats, olmesartan crossed the blood-brain barrier poorly, if at all. Olmesartan passed across the placental barrier in rats and was distributed to the fetus. Olmesartan was distributed to milk at low levels in rats.

SPECIAL POPULATIONS

Pediatric

The pharmacokinetics of olmesartan have not been investigated in patients <18 years of age.

Geriatrics

The pharmacokinetics of olmesartan were studied in the elderly (≥65 years). Overall, maximum plasma concentrations of olmesartan were similar in young adults and the elderly. Modest accumulation of olmesartan was observed in the elderly with repeated dosing; AUC(ss,τ) was 33% higher in elderly patients, corresponding to an approximate 30% reduction in CLR.

Gender

Minor differences were observed in the pharmacokinetics of olmesartan in women compared to men. AUC and C_{max} were 10-15% higher in women than in men.

Renal Insufficiency

In patients with renal insufficiency, serum concentrations of olmesartan were elevated compared to subjects with normal renal function. After repeated dosing, the AUC was approximately tripled in patients with severe renal impairment (creatinine clearance <20 ml/min). The pharmacokinetics of olmesartan in patients undergoing hemodialysis has not been studied.

Hepatic Insufficiency

Increases in AUC(0-∞) and C_{max} were observed in patients with moderate hepatic impairment compared to those in matched controls, with an increase in AUC of about 60%.

DRUG INTERACTIONS

See DRUG INTERACTIONS.

PHARMACODYNAMICS

Olmesartan medoxomil doses of 2.5 to 40 mg inhibit the pressor effects of angiotensin I infusion. The duration of the inhibitory effect was related to dose, with doses of olmesartan medoxomil >40 mg giving >90% inhibition at 24 hours.

Plasma concentrations of angiotensin I and angiotensin II and plasma renin activity (PRA) increase after single and repeated administration of olmesartan medoxomil to healthy subjects and hypertensive patients. Repeated administration of up to 80 mg olmesartan medoxomil had minimal influence on aldosterone levels and no effect on serum potassium.

INDICATIONS AND USAGE

Olmesartan medoxomil is indicated for the treatment of hypertension. It may be used alone or in combination with other antihypertensive agents.

CONTRAINDICATIONS

Olmesartan medoxomil is contraindicated in patients who are hypersensitive to any component of this product.

WARNINGS

FETAL/NEONATAL MORBIDITY AND MORTALITY

Drugs that act directly on the renin-angiotensin system can cause fetal and neonatal morbidity and death when administered to pregnant women. Several dozen cases have been reported in the world literature of patients who were taking angiotensin converting enzyme inhibitors. When pregnancy is detected, olmesartan medoxomil should be discontinued as soon as possible.

The use of drugs that act directly on the renin-angiotensin system during the second and third trimesters of pregnancy has been associated with fetal and neonatal injury, including hypotension, neonatal skull hypoplasia, anuria, reversible or irreversible renal failure and death. Oligohydramnios has also been reported, presumably resulting from decreased fetal function; oligohydramnios in this setting has been associated with fetal limb contractures, craniofacial deformation and hypoplastic lung development. Prematurity, intrauterine growth retardation and patent ductus arteriosus have also been reported, although it is not clear whether these occurrences were due to exposure to the drug.

These adverse effects do not appear to have resulted from intrauterine drug exposure that has been limited to the first trimester. Mothers whose embryos and fetuses are exposed to an angiotensin II receptor antagonist only during the first trimester should be so informed. Nonetheless, when patients become pregnant, physicians should have the patient discontinue the use of olmesartan medoxomil as soon as possible.

Rarely (probably less often than once in every thousand pregnancies), no alternative to a drug acting on the renin-angiotensin system will be found. In these rare cases, the mothers should be apprised of the potential hazards to their fetuses and serial ultrasound examinations should be performed to assess the intra-amniotic environment.

If oligohydramnios is observed, olmesartan medoxomil should be discontinued unless it is considered life-saving for the mother. Contraction stress testing (CST), a nonstress test (NST) or biophysical profiling (BPP) may be appropriate, depending upon the week of pregnancy. Patients and physicians should be aware, however, that oligohydramnios may not appear until after the fetus has sustained irreversible injury.

Infants with histories of *in utero* exposure to an angiotensin II receptor antagonist should be closely observed for hypotension, oliguria and hyperkalemia. If oliguria occurs, attention should be directed toward support of blood pressure and renal perfusion. Exchange transfusion or dialysis may be required as means of reversing hypotension and/or substituting for disordered renal function.

There is no clinical experience with the use of olmesartan medoxomil in pregnant women. No teratogenic effects were observed when olmesartan medoxomil was administered to pregnant rats at oral doses up to 1000 mg/kg/day (240 times the maximum recommended human dose [MRHD] of olmesartan medoxomil on a mg/m^2 basis) or pregnant rabbits at oral doses up to 1 mg/kg/day (half the MRHD on a mg/m^2 basis; higher doses could not be evaluated for effects on fetal development as they were lethal to the does). In rats, significant decreases in pup birth weight and weight gain were observed at doses ≥1.6 mg/kg/day, and delays in developmental milestones and dose-dependent increases in the incidence of dilation of the renal pelvis were observed at doses ≥8 mg/kg/day. The no observed effect dose for developmental toxicity in rats is 0.3 mg/kg/day, about one-tenth the MRHD of 40 mg/day.

HYPOTENSION IN VOLUME- OR SALT-DEPLETED PATIENTS

In patients with an activated renin-angiotensin system, such as volume- and/or salt-depleted patients (*e.g.,* those being treated with high doses of diuretics), symptomatic hypotension may occur after initiation of treatment with olmesartan medoxomil. Treatment should start under close medical supervision. If hypotension does occur, the patient should be placed in the supine position and, if necessary, given an intravenous infusion of normal saline (see DOSAGE AND ADMINISTRATION). A transient hypotensive response is not a contraindication to further treatment, which usually can be continued without difficulty once the blood pressure has stabilized.

PRECAUTIONS

GENERAL

Impaired Renal Function

As a consequence of inhibiting the renin-angiotensin-aldosterone system, changes in renal function may be anticipated in susceptible individuals treated with olmesartan medoxomil. In patients whose renal function may depend upon the activity of the renin-angiotensin-aldosterone system (*e.g.,* patients with severe congestive heart failure), treatment with angiotensin converting enzyme inhibitors and angiotensin receptor antagonists has been associated with oliguria and/or progressive azotemia and (rarely) with acute renal failure and/or death. Similar results may be anticipated in patients treated with olmesartan medoxomil. (See CLINICAL PHARMACOLOGY, Special Populations.)

In studies of ACE inhibitors in patients with unilateral or bilateral renal artery stenosis, increases in serum creatinine or blood urea nitrogen (BUN) have been reported. There has been no long-term use of olmesartan medoxomil in patients with unilateral or bilateral renal artery stenosis, but similar results may be expected.

INFORMATION FOR THE PATIENT

Pregnancy

Female patients of childbearing age should be told about the consequences of second and third trimester exposure to drugs that act on the renin-angiotensin system and they should be told also that these consequences do not appear to have resulted from intrauterine drug exposure that has been limited to the first trimester. These patients should be asked to report pregnancies to their physicians as soon as possible.

CARCINOGENESIS, MUTAGENESIS, AND IMPAIRMENT OF FERTILITY

Olmesartan medoxomil was not carcinogenic when administered by dietary administration to rats for up to 2 years. The highest dose tested (2000 mg/kg/day) was, on a mg/m^2 basis, about 480 times the maximum recommended human dose (MRHD) of 40 mg/day. Two carcinogenicity studies conducted in mice, a 6 month gavage study in the p53 knockout mouse and a 6 month dietary administration study in the Hras2 transgenic mouse, at doses of up to 1000 mg/kg/day (about 120 times the MRHD), revealed no evidence of a carcinogenic effect of olmesartan medoxomil.

Both olmesartan medoxomil and olmesartan tested negative in the *in vitro* Syrian hamster embryo cell transformation assay and showed no evidence of genetic toxicity in the Ames (bacterial mutagenicity) test. However, both were shown to induce chromosomal aberrations in cultured cells *in vitro* (Chinese hamster lung). Olmesartan medoxomil also tested positive for thymidine kinase mutations in the *in vitro* mouse lymphoma assay (olmesartan not tested). Olmesartan medoxomil tested negative *in vivo* for mutations in the MutaMouse intestine and kidney, for DNA damage in the rat kidney (comet assay) and for clastogenicity in mouse bone marrow (micronucleus test) at oral doses of up to 2000 mg/kg (olmesartan not tested).

Fertility of rats was unaffected by administration of olmesartan medoxomil at dose levels as high as 1000 mg/kg/day (240 times the MRHD) in a study in which dosing was begun 2 (female) or 9 (male) weeks prior to mating.

PREGNANCY CATEGORIES C (FIRST TRIMESTER) AND D (SECOND AND THIRD TRIMESTERS)

See WARNINGS, Fetal/Neonatal Morbidity and Mortality.

NURSING MOTHERS

It is not known whether olmesartan is excreted in human milk, but olmesartan is secreted at low concentration in the milk of lactating rats. Because of the potential for adverse effects on the nursing infant, a decision should be made whether to discontinue nursing or discontinue the drug, taking into account the importance of the drug to the mother.

PEDIATRIC USE

Safety and effectiveness in pediatric patients have not been established.

GERIATRIC USE

Of the total number of hypertensive patients receiving olmesartan medoxomil in clinical studies, more than 20% were 65 years of age and over, while more than 5% were 75 years of age and older. No overall differences in effectiveness or safety were observed between elderly patients and younger patients. Other reported clinical experience has not identified differences in responses between the elderly and younger patients, but greater sensitivity of some older individuals cannot be ruled out.

DRUG INTERACTIONS

No significant drug interactions were reported in studies in which olmesartan medoxomil was co-administered with digoxin or warfarin in healthy volunteers. The bioavailability of olmesartan was not significantly altered by the co-administration of antacids [$Al(OH)_3$/$Mg(OH)_2$]. Olmesartan medoxomil is not metabolized by the cytochrome P450 system and has no effects on P450 enzymes; thus, interactions with drugs that inhibit, induce or are metabolized by those enzymes are not expected.

ADVERSE REACTIONS

Olmesartan medoxomil has been evaluated for safety in more than 3825 patients/subjects, including more than 3275 patients treated for hypertension in controlled trials. This experience included about 900 patients treated for at least 6 months and more than 525 for at least 1 year. Treatment with olmesartan medoxomil was well tolerated, with an incidence of adverse events similar to placebo. Events generally were mild, transient and had no relationship to the dose of olmesartan medoxomil.

The overall frequency of adverse events was not dose-related. Analysis of gender, age and race groups demonstrated no differences between olmesartan medoxomil and placebo-treated patients. The rate of withdrawals due to adverse events in all trials of hypertensive patients was 2.4% (*i.e.,* 79/3278) of patients treated with olmesartan medoxomil and 2.7% (*i.e.,* 32/1179) of control patients. In placebo-controlled trials, the only adverse event that occurred in more than 1% of patients treated with olmesartan medoxomil and at a higher incidence versus placebo was dizziness (3% vs 1%).

The following adverse events occurred in placebo-controlled clinical trials at an incidence of more than 1% of patients treated with olmesartan medoxomil, but also occurred at about the same or greater incidence in patients receiving placebo: back pain, bronchitis, creatine phosphokinase increased, diarrhea, headache, hematuria, hyperglycemia, hypertriglyceridemia, inflicted injury, influenza-like symptoms, pharyngitis, rhinitis, sinusitis and upper respiratory tract infection.

The incidence of cough was similar in placebo (0.7%) and olmesartan medoxomil (0.9%) patients.

Other (potentially important) adverse events that have been reported with an incidence of greater than 0.5%, whether or not attributed to treatment, in the more than 3100 hypertensive patients treated with olmesartan medoxomil monotherapy in controlled or open-label trials are listed below.

Body as a Whole: Chest pain, fatigue, pain, peripheral edema.
Central and Peripheral Nervous System: Vertigo.
Gastrointestinal: Abdominal pain, dyspepsia, gastroenteritis, nausea.
Heart Rate and Rhythm Disorders: Tachycardia.
Metabolic and Nutritional Disorders: Hypercholesterolemia, hyperlipemia, hyperuricemia.
Musculoskeletal: Arthralgia, arthritis, myalgia, skeletal pain.
Psychiatric Disorders: Insomnia.
Skin and Appendages: Rash.
Urinary System: Urinary tract infection.

Facial edema was reported in 5 patients receiving olmesartan medoxomil. Angioedema has been reported with other angiotensin II antagonists.

LABORATORY TEST FINDINGS

In controlled clinical trials, clinically important changes in standard laboratory parameters were rarely associated with administration of olmesartan medoxomil.

Hemoglobin and Hematocrit: Small decreases in hemoglobin and hematocrit (mean decreases of approximately 0.3 g/dl and 0.3 volume percent, respectively) were observed.

Liver Function Tests: Elevations of liver enzymes and/or serum bilirubin were observed infrequently. Five patients (0.1%) assigned to olmesartan medoxomil and one patient (0.2%) assigned to placebo in clinical trials were withdrawn because of abnormal liver chemistries (transaminases or total bilirubin). Of the 5 olmesartan medoxomil patients, 3 had elevated transaminases, which were attributed to alcohol use, and 1 had a single elevated bilirubin value, which normalized while treatment continued.

DOSAGE AND ADMINISTRATION

Dosage must be individualized. The usual recommended starting dose of olmesartan medoxomil is 20 mg once daily when used as monotherapy in patients who are not volume-contracted. For patients requiring further reduction in blood pressure after 2 weeks of therapy, the dose of olmesartan medoxomil may be increased to 40 mg. Doses above 40 mg do not appear to have greater effect. Twice-daily dosing offers no advantage over the same total dose given once daily.

No initial dosage adjustment is recommended for elderly patients, for patients with moderate to marked renal impairment (creatinine clearance <40 ml/min) or with moderate to marked hepatic dysfunction (see CLINICAL PHARMACOLOGY, Special Populations).

For patients with possible depletion of intravascular volume (*e.g.,* patients treated with diuretics, particularly those with impaired renal function), olmesartan medoxomil should be initiated under close medical supervision and consideration should be given to use of a lower starting dose (see WARNINGS, Hypotension in Volume- and Salt-Depleted Patients).

Olmesartan medoxomil may be administered with or without food.

If blood pressure is not controlled by olmesartan medoxomil alone, a diuretic may be added. Olmesartan medoxomil may be administered with other antihypertensive agents.

HOW SUPPLIED

Benicar is supplied in:

5 mg: Yellow, round, film-coated tablets containing 5 mg of olmesartan medoxomil, debossed with "Sankyo" on one side and "C12" on the other side.

20 mg: White, round, film-coated tablets containing 20 mg of olmesartan medoxomil, debossed with "Sankyo" on one side and "C14" on the other side.

40 mg: White, oval-shaped, film-coated tablets containing 40 mg of olmesartan medoxomil, debossed with "Sankyo" on one side and "C15" on the other side.

Storage: Store at 20-25°C (68-77°F).

PRODUCT LISTING - EQUIVALENTS NOT AVAILABLE

Tablet - Oral - 5 mg			
30's	$39.38	BENICAR, Sankyo Parke Davis	65597-0101-30
Tablet - Oral - 20 mg			
10 x 10	$131.25	BENICAR, Sankyo Parke Davis	65597-0103-10
30's	$39.38	BENICAR, Sankyo Parke Davis	65597-0103-30
90's	$118.13	BENICAR, Sankyo Parke Davis	65597-0103-90
Tablet - Oral - 40 mg			
10 x 10	$131.25	BENICAR, Sankyo Parke Davis	65597-0104-10
30's	$39.38	BENICAR, Sankyo Parke Davis	65597-0104-30
90's	$118.13	BENICAR, Sankyo Parke Davis	65597-0104-90

Olopatadine Hydrochloride *(003317)*

Categories: Conjunctivitis, allergic; Pregnancy Category C; FDA Approved 1996 Dec
Drug Classes: Antihistamines, H1; Ophthalmics
Brand Names: Patanol
Cost of Therapy: $60.38 (Allergic Conjunctivitis; Patanol Solution; 0.1%; 5 ml; 6 drops/day; variable day supply)

DESCRIPTION

Olopatadine HCl ophthalmic solution 0.1% is a sterile ophthalmic solution containing olopatadine, a relatively selective H_1-receptor antagonist and inhibitor of histamine release from the mast cell for topical administration to the eyes. Olopatadine HCl is a white, crystalline, water-soluble powder with a molecular weight of 373.88. The chemical name is 11-[(Z)-3-(dimethylamino)propylidene]-6-11-dihydrodibenz[b,e] oxepin-2-acetic acid hydrochloride.

Each ml of patanol 0.1% contains: *Active:* 1.11 olopatadine hydrochloride equivalent to 1 mg olopatadine. *Preservative:* Benzalkonium chloride 0.01%. *Inactives:* Dibasic sodium phosphate; sodium chloride; hydrochloric acid/sodium hydroxide (adjust pH); and purified water. It has a pH of approximately 7 and an osmolality of approximately 300 mOsmol/kg.

CLINICAL PHARMACOLOGY

Olopatadine is an inhibitor of the release of histamine from the mast cell and a relatively selective histamine H_1-antagonist that inhibits the *in vivo* and *in vitro* type 1 immediate hypersensitivity reaction. Olopatadine is devoid of effects on alpha-adrenergic, dopamine, muscarinic type 1 and 2, and seratonin receptors. Following topical ocular administration in man, olopatadine was shown to have low systemic exposure. Two studies in normal volunteers (totaling 24 subjects) dosed bilaterally with olopatadine 0.15% ophthalmic solution once every 12 hours for 2 weeks demonstrated plasma concentrations to be generally below the quantitation limit of the assay (<0.5 ng/ml). Samples in which olopatadine was quantifiable were typically found within 2 hours of dosing and ranged from 0.5-1.3 ng/ml. The half-life in plasma was approximately 3 hours, and ellimination was predominantly through renal excretion. Approximately 60-70% of the dose was recovered in the urine as parent drug. Two metabolites, the mono-desmethyl and the N-oxide, were detected at low concentrations in the urine. Results from conjunctival antigen challenge studies demonstrated that olopatadine HCl ophthalmic solution 0.1%, when subjects were challenged with antigen both initially and up to 8 hours after dosing, was significantly more effective than its vehicle in preventing ocular itching associated with allergic conjunctivitis.

INDICATIONS AND USAGE

Olopatadine HCl ophthalmic solution 0.1% is indicated for the temporary prevention of itching of the eye due to allergic conjunctivitis.

CONTRAINDICATIONS

Olopatadine HCl ophthalmic solution 0.1% is contraindicated in persons with a known hypersensitivity to olopatadine HCl or any components of this product.

WARNINGS

Olopatadine HCl ophthalmic solution 0.1% is for topical use only and not for injection or oral use.

PRECAUTIONS

INFORMATION FOR THE PATIENT

To prevent contaminating the dropper tip and solution, care should be taken not to touch the eyelids or surrounding areas with the dropper tip of the bottle. Keep bottle tightly closed when not in use.

Patients should be advised not to wear contact lenses if their eye is red. Olopatadine HCl ophthalmic solution 0.1% should not be used to treat contact lens irritation. The preservative in patanol, benzalkonium chloride, may be absorbed by soft contact lenses. Patients who wear soft contact lenses and whose eyes are not red, should be instructed to wait at least ten minutes after instilling olopatadine HCl ophthalmic solution 0.1% before they insert their contact lenses.

CARCINOGENESIS, MUTAGENESIS, AND IMPAIRMENT OF FERTILITY

Olopatadine administered orally was not carcinogenic in mice and rats in doses up to 500 mg/kg/day and 200 mg/kg/day, respectively. Based on a 40 µl drop size, these doses were 78,125 and 31,250 times higher than the maximum recommended ocular human dose (MROHD). No mutagenic potential was observed when olopatadine was tested in an *in vitro* bacterial reverse mutation (Ames) test, an *in vitro* mammalian chromosome aberration assay or an *in vivo* mouse micronucleus test. Olopatadine administered to male and female rats at oral doses of 62,500 times MROHD level resulted in a slight decrease in the fertility index and reduced implantation rate; no effects on reproductive function were observed at doses of 7800 times the maximum recommended ocular human use level.

PREGNANCY CATEGORY C

Olopatadine was found not to be teratogenic in rats and rabbits. However, rats treated at 600 mg/kg/day, or 93,750 times the MROHD and rabbits treated at 400 mg/kg/day, or 62,500 times the MROHD, during organogenesis showed a decrease in live fetuses. There are, however no adequated and well controlled studies in pregnant women. Because animal studies are not always predictive of human responses, this drug should be used in pregnant women only if the potential benefit to the mother justifies the potential risk to the embryo or fetus.

NURSING MOTHERS

Olopatadine has been identified in the milk of nursing rats following oral administration. It is not known whether topical ocular administration could result in sufficient systemic absorption to produce detectable quantities in the human breast milk. Nevertheless, caution should be exercised when olopatadine HCl ophthalmic solution 0.1% is administered to a nursing mother.

PEDIATRIC USE

Safety and effectiveness in pediatric patients below the age of 3 years have not been established.

ADVERSE REACTIONS

Headaches were reported at an incidence of 7%. The following adverse experiences were reported in less than 5% of patients: Asthenia, burning or stinging, cold syndrome, dry eye, foreign body sensation, hyperemia, keratitis, lid edema, pharyngitis, pruritus, rhinitis, sinusitis, and taste perversion. Some of these events were similar to the underlying disease being studied.

DOSAGE AND ADMINISTRATION

The recommended dose is 1-2 drops in each affected eye 2 times per day at an interval of 6-8 hours.

HOW SUPPLIED

Patanol (olopatadine HCl ophthalmic solution 0.1%) is supplied in 5 ml plastic DROP-TAINER dispensers.

Storage: Store at 4-30°C (39-86°F).

PRODUCT LISTING - EQUIVALENTS NOT AVAILABLE

Solution - Ophthalmic - 0.1%			
5 ml	$60.38	PATANOL, Allscripts Pharmaceutical Company	54569-4470-00
5 ml	$70.25	PATANOL, Alcon Laboratories Inc	00065-0271-05

Olsalazine Sodium *(003017)*

Categories: Colitis, ulcerative; Pregnancy Category C; FDA Approved 1990 Jul
Drug Classes: Gastrointestinals; Salicylates
Brand Names: Dipentum
Cost of Therapy: $171.00 (Ulcerative Colitis; Dipentum; 250 mg; 4 capsules/day; 30 day supply)

DESCRIPTION

The active ingredient in Dipentum capsules (olsalazine sodium) is the sodium salt of a salicylate, disodium 3,3'-azobis (6-hydroxybenzoate) a compound that is effectively bioconverted to 5-aminosalicylic acid (5-ASA), which has anti-inflammatory activity in ulcerative colitis. Its empirical formula is $C_{14}H_8N_2Na_2O_6$ with a molecular weight of 346.21.

Olsalazine sodium is a yellow crystalline powder which melts with decomposition at 240°C. It is the sodium salt of a weak acid, soluble in water and DMSO, and practically insoluble in ethanol, chloroform, and ether. Olsalazine sodium has acceptable stability under acidic or basic conditions.

Dipentum is supplied in hard gelatin capsules for oral administration. The inert ingredient in each 250 mg capsule of olsalazine sodium is magnesium stearate. *The capsule shell has the following inactive ingredients:* Black iron oxide, caramel, gelatin, and titanium dioxide.

CLINICAL PHARMACOLOGY

After oral administration, olsalazine has limited systemic bioavailability. Based on oral and intravenous dosing studies, approximately 2.4% of a single 1.0 g oral dose is absorbed. Less than 1% of olsalazine is recovered in the urine. The remaining 98-99% of an oral dose will reach the colon where each molecule is rapidly converted into 2 molecules of 5-aminosalicylic acid (5-ASA) by colonic bacteria and the low prevailing redox potential found in this environment. The liberated 5-ASA is absorbed slowly resulting in very high local concentrations in the colon.

The conversion of olsalazine to mesalamine (5-ASA) in the colon is similar to that of sulfasalazine, which is converted into sulfapyridine and mesalamine. It is thought that the mesalamine component is therapeutically active in ulcerative colitis.[1] The usual dose of sulfasalazine for maintenance of remission in patients with ulcerative colitis is 2 g daily, which would provide approximately 0.8 g of mesalamine to the colon. More than 0.9 g of mesalamine would usually be made available in the colon from 1 g of olsalazine.

The mechanism of action of mesalamine (and sulfasalazine) is unknown, but appears to be topical rather than systemic. Mucosal production of arachidonic acid (AA) metabolites, both through the cyclooxygenase pathways, *i.e.,* prostanoids, and through the lipoxygenase pathways, *i.e.,* leukotrienes (LTs) and hydroxyeicosatetraenoic acids (HETEs) is increased in patients with chronic inflammatory bowel disease, and it is possible that mesalamine diminishes inflammation by blocking cyclooxygenase and inhibiting prostaglandin (PG) production in the colon.

PHARMACOKINETICS

The pharmacokinetics of olsalazine are similar in both healthy volunteers and in patients with ulcerative colitis. Maximum serum concentrations of olsalazine appear after approximately 1 hour, and, even after a 1.0 g single dose are low, *e.g.,* 1.6-6.2 μmol/L. Olsalazine, has a very short serum half-life, approximately 0.9 hours. Olsalazine is more than 99% bound to plasma proteins. It does not interfere with protein binding of warfarin. The urinary recovery of olsalazine is below 1%. Total recovery of oral ^{14}C-labeled olsalazine in animals and humans ranges from 90-97%.

Approximately 0.1% of an oral dose of olsalazine is metabolized in the liver to olsalazine-O-sulfate (olsalazine-S). Olsalazine-S, in contrast to olsalazine has a half-life of 7 days. Olsalazine-S accumulates to steady state within 2-3 weeks.

Patients on daily doses of 1.0 g olsalazine for 2-4 years show a stable plasma concentration of olsalazine-S (3.3-12.4 μmol/L). Olsalazine-S, is more than 99% bound to plasma proteins. Its long half-life is mainly due to slow dissociation from the protein binding site. Less than 1% of both olsalazine and olsalazine-S appears undissociated in plasma.

5-Aminosalicylic Acid (5-ASA)

Serum concentration of 5-ASA are detected after 4-8 hours. The peak levels of 5-ASA after an oral dose of 1.0 g olsalazine are low, *i.e.,* 0 to 4.3 μmol/L. Of the total 5-ASA found in the urine, more than 90% is in the form of N-acetyl-5-ASA (Ac-5-ASA). Only small amounts of 5-ASA are detected.

N-acetyl-5-ASA (Ac-5-ASA), the major metabolite of 5-ASA found in plasma and urine, is acetylated (deactivated) in at least 2 sites, the colonic epithelium and the liver. Ac-5-ASA is found in the serum, with peak values of 1.7-8.7 μmol/L after a single 1.0 g dose. Approximately 20% of the total 5-ASA is recovered in the urine, where it is found almost exclusively as Ac-5-ASA. The remaining 5-ASA is partially acetylated and is excreted in the feces. From fecal dialysis, the concentration of 5-ASA in the colon following olsalazine has been calculated to be 18-49 mmol/L. No accumulation of 5-ASA or Ac-5-ASA in plasma has been detected. 5-ASA and Ac-5-ASA are 74 and 81%, respectively, bound to plasma proteins.

INDICATIONS AND USAGE

Olsalazine is indicated for the maintenance of remission of ulcerative colitis in patients who are intolerant of sulfasalazine.

CONTRAINDICATIONS

Hypersensitivity to salicylates.

PRECAUTIONS

GENERAL

Overall, approximately 17% of subjects receiving olsalazine in clinical studies reported diarrhea sometime during therapy. This diarrhea resulted in withdrawal of treatment in 6% of patients. This diarrhea appears to be dose related, although it may be difficult to distinguish from the underlying symptoms of the disease.

Exacerbation of the symptoms of colitis thought to have been caused by mesalamine or sulfasalazine has been noted.

Although renal abnormalities were not reported in clinical trials with olsalazine, there have been rare reports from post-marketing experience (see ADVERSE REACTIONS). Therefore, the possibility of renal tubular damage due to absorbed mesalamine or its n-acetylated metabolite, as noted in ANIMAL PHARMACOLOGY must be kept in mind, particularly for patients with pre-existing renal disease. In these patients, monitoring with urinalysis, BUN and creatinine determinations is advised.

INFORMATION FOR THE PATIENT

Patients should be instructed to take olsalazine with food. The drug should be taken in evenly divided doses. Patients should be informed that about 17% of subjects receiving olsalazine during clinical studies reported diarrhea sometime during therapy. If diarrhea occurs, patients should contact their physician.

DRUG/LABORATORY TEST INTERACTIONS

None known.

CARCINOGENESIS, MUTAGENESIS, AND IMPAIRMENT OF FERTILITY

In a 2 year oral rat carcinogenicity study, olsalazine was tested in male and female Wistar rats at daily doses of 200, 400, and 800 mg/kg/day (approximately 10-40 times the human maintenance dose, based on a patient weight of 50 kg and a human dose of 1 g). Urinary bladder transitional cell carcinomas were found in 3 male rats (6%, p=0.022, exact trend test) receiving 40 times the human dose and were not found in untreated male controls. In the same study, urinary bladder transitional cell carcinoma and papilloma occurred in 2 untreated control female rats (2%). No such tumors were found in any of the female rats treated at doses up to 40 times the human dose.

In an 18 month oral mouse carcinogenicity study, olsalazine was tested in male and female CD-1 mice at daily doses of 500, 1000, and 2000 mg/kg/day (approximately 25-100 times the human maintenance dose). Liver hemangiosarcomata were found in 2 male mice (4%) receiving olsalazine at 100 times the human dose, while no such tumor occurred in the other treated male mice groups or any of the treated female mice. The observed incidence of this tumor is within the 4% incidence in historical controls.

Olsalazine was not mutagenic in *in vitro* Ames tests, mouse lymphoma cell mutation assays, human lymphocyte chromosomal aberration tests and the *in vivo* rat bone marrow cell chromosomal aberration test.

Olsalazine in a dose range of 100-400 mg/kg/day (approximately 5-20 times the human maintenance dose) did not influence the fertility of male or female rats. The oligospermia and infertility in men associated with sulfasalazine have not been reported with olsalazine.

PREGNANCY, TERATOGENIC EFFECTS, PREGNANCY CATEGORY C

Olsalazine has been shown to produce fetal developmental toxicity as indicated by reduced fetal weights, retarded ossifications and immaturity of the fetal visceral organs when given during organogenesis to pregnant rats in doses 5-20 times the human dose (100-400 mg/kg). There are no adequate and well-controlled studies in pregnant women. Olsalazine should be used during pregnancy only if the potential benefit justifies the potential risk to the fetus.

NURSING MOTHERS

Oral administration of olsalazine to lactating rats in doses 5-20 times the human dose produced growth retardation in their pups. It is not known whether this drug is excreted in human milk. Because many drugs are excreted in human milk, caution should be exercised when olsalazine is administered to a nursing woman.

PEDIATRIC USE

Safety and effectiveness in a pediatric population have not been established.

GERIATRIC USE

Clinical studies of olsalazine sodium did not include sufficient numbers of subjects aged 65 and over to determine whether they respond differently from younger subjects. Other reported clinical experience has not identified differences in responses between the elderly and younger patients. In general, elderly patients should be treated with caution due to the greater frequency of decreased hepatic, renal, or cardiac function, co-existence of other disease, as well as concomitant drug therapy.

DRUG INTERACTIONS

Increased prothrombin time in patients taking concomitant warfarin has been reported.

ADVERSE REACTIONS

Olsalazine has been evaluated in ulcerative colitis patients in remission as well as those with acute disease. Both sulfasalazine-tolerant and intolerant patients have been studied in controlled clinical trials. Overall, 10.4% of patients discontinued olsalazine because of an adverse experience compared with 6.7% of placebo patients. The most commonly reported adverse reactions leading to treatment withdrawal were diarrhea or loose stools (olsalazine 5.9%; placebo 4.8%), abdominal pain and rash or itching (slightly more than 1% of patients receiving olsalazine). Other adverse reactions to olsalazine leading to withdrawal occurred in fewer than 1% of patients (see TABLE 1).

TABLE 1 *Adverse Reactions Resulting in Withdrawal From Controlled Studies*

	Total	
	Olsalazine (n=441)	Placebo (n=208)
Diarrhea/loose stools	26 (5.9%)	10 (4.8%)
Nausea	3	2
Abdominal pain	5 (1.1%)	0
Rash/itching	5 (1.1%)	0
Headache	3	0
Heartburn	2	0
Rectal bleeding	1	0
Insomnia	1	0
Dizziness	1	0
Anorexia	1	0
Light headedness	1	0
Depression	1	0
Miscellaneous	4 (0.9%)	3 (1.4%)
Total number of patients withdrawn	46 (10.4%)	14 (6.7%)

For those controlled studies, the comparative incidences of adverse reactions reported in 1% or more patients treated with olsalazine or placebo are provided in TABLE 2.

Over 2500 patients have been treated with olsalazine in various controlled and uncontrolled clinical studies. In these as well as in the post-marketing experience, olsalazine was administered mainly to patients intolerant to sulfasalazine. There have been rare reports of the following adverse effects in patients receiving olsalazine. These were often difficult to distinguish from possible symptoms of the underlying disease or from the effects of prior and/or concomitant therapy. A causal relationship to the drug has not been demonstrated for some of these reactions.

Digestive: Pancreatitis, diarrhea with dehydration, increased blood in stool, rectal bleeding, flare in symptoms, rectal discomfort, epigastric discomfort, flatulence.

In a double-blind, placebo-controlled study, increased frequency and severity of diarrhea were reported in patients randomized to olsalazine 500 mg bid with concomitant pelvic radiation.

Rare cases of granulomatous hepatitis and nonspecific, reactive hepatitis have been reported in patients receiving olsalazine. Additionally, a patient developed mild cholestatic hepatitis during treatment with sulfasalazine and experienced the same

TABLE 2 *Comparative Incidence (%) of Adverse Effects Reported By 1% or More of Ulcerative Colitis Patients Treated With Olsalazine or Placebo in Double Blind Controlled Studies*

Adverse Event	Olsalazine (n=441)	Placebo (n=208)
Digestive System		
Diarrhea	11.1%	6.7%
Abdominal pain/cramps	10.1%	7.2%
Nausea	5.0%	3.9%
Dyspepsia	4.0%	4.3%
Bloating	1.5%	1.4%
Anorexia	1.3%	1.9%
Vomiting	1.0%	—
Stomatitis	1.0%	—
Increased blood in stool	—	3.4%
CNS/Psychiatric		
Headache	5.0%	4.8%
Fatigue/drowsiness/lethargy	1.8%	2.9%
Depression	1.5%	—
Vertigo/dizziness	1.0%	—
Insomnia	—	2.4%
Skin		
Rash	2.3%	1.4%
Itching	1.3%	—
Musculoskeletal		
Arthralgia/joint pain	4.0%	2.9%
Miscellaneous		
Upper respiratory infection	1.5%	—

symptoms 2 weeks later after the treatment was changed to olsalazine. Withdrawal of olsalazine led to complete recovery in these cases.

Neurologic: Paresthesia, tremors, insomnia, mood swings, irritability, fever, chills, rigors.

Dermatologic: Erythema nodosum, photosensitivity, erythema, hot flashes, alopecia.

Musculoskeletal: Muscle cramps.

Cardiovascular/Pulmonary: Pericarditis, second degree heart block, interstitial pulmonary disease, hypertension, orthostatic hypotension, peripheral edema, chest pains, tachycardia, palpitations, bronchospasm, shortness of breath.

A patient who developed thyroid disease 9 days after starting olsalazine sodium was given propranolol and radioactive iodine and subsequently developed shortness of breath and nausea. The patient died 5 days later with signs and symptoms of acute diffuse myocarditis.

Genitourinary: Frequency, dysuria, hematuria, proteinuria, nephrotic syndrome, interstitial nephritis, impotence, menorrhagia.

Hematologic: Leukopenia, neutropenia, lymphopenia, eosinophilia, thrombocytopenia, anemia, hemolytic anemia, reticulocytosis.

Laboratory: ALT (SGPT) or AST (SGOT) elevated beyond the normal range.

Special Senses: Tinnitus, dry mouth, dry eyes, watery eyes, blurred vision.

O

POSTMARKETING REPORTS

The following events have been identified during post-approval use of products which contain (or are metabolized to) mesalamine in clinical practice. Because they are reported voluntarily from a population of unknown size, estimates of frequency cannot be made. These events have been chosen for inclusion due to a combination of seriousness, frequency of reporting, or potential causal connection to mesalamine:

Gastrointestinal: Reports of hepatotoxicity, including elevated liver function tests (SGOT/AST, SGPT/ALT, GGT, LDH, alkaline phosphatase, bilirubin), jaundice, cholestatic jaundice, cirrhosis, and possible hepatocellular damage including liver necrosis and liver failure. Some of these cases were fatal. One case of Kawasaki-like syndrome, which included hepatic function changes, was also reported.

DOSAGE AND ADMINISTRATION

The usual dosage in adults for maintenance of remission is 1.0 g/day in 2 divided doses.

ANIMAL PHARMACOLOGY

Preclinical subacute and chronic toxicity studies in rats have shown the kidney to be the major target organ of olsalazine toxicity. At an oral daily dose of 400 mg/kg or higher, olsalazine treatment produced nephritis and tubular necrosis in a 4 week study; interstitial nephritis and tubular calcinosis in a 6 month study, and renal fibrosis, mineralization, and transitional cell hyperplasia in a 1 year study.

HOW SUPPLIED

DIPENTUM CAPSULES

Beige colored capsules, containing 250 mg olsalazine sodium imprinted with "DIPENTUM 250 mg" on the capsule shell.

Storage: Store at 25°C (77°F). Excursions permitted to 15-30°C (59-86°F).

PRODUCT LISTING - EQUIVALENTS NOT AVAILABLE

Capsule - Oral - 250 mg

100's $142.50 DIPENTUM, Pharmacia and Upjohn 00013-0105-01

Omalizumab (003602)

Categories: Asthma; Pregnancy Category B; FDA Approved 2003 Jun
Drug Classes: Monoclonal antibodies
Brand Names: Xolair

DESCRIPTION

For Subcutaneous Use

Xolair is a recombinant DNA-derived humanized IgG1κ monoclonal antibody that selectively binds to human immunoglobulin E (IgE). The antibody has a molecular weight of approximately 149 kilodaltons. Xolair is produced by a Chinese hamster ovary cell suspension culture in a nutrient medium containing the antibiotic gentamicin. Gentamicin is not detectable in the final product.

Xolair is a sterile, white, preservative-free, lyophilized powder contained in a single-use vial that is reconstituted with sterile water for injection (SWFI), and administered as a subcutaneous (SC) injection. A Xolair vial contains 202.5 mg of omalizumab, 145.5 mg sucrose, 2.8 mg L-histidine hydrochloride monohydrate, 1.8 mg L-histidine, and 0.5 mg polysorbate 20, and is designed to deliver 150 mg of omalizumab in 1.2 ml after reconstitution with 1.4 ml SWFI.

CLINICAL PHARMACOLOGY

MECHANISM OF ACTION

Omalizumab inhibits the binding of IgE to the high-affinity IgE receptor (FcεRI) on the surface of mast cells and basophils. Reduction in surface-bound IgE on FcεRI-bearing cells limits the degree of release of mediators of the allergic response. Treatment with omalizumab also reduces the number of FcεRI receptors on basophils in atopic patients.

PHARMACOKINETICS

After SC administration, omalizumab is absorbed with an average absolute bioavailability of 62%. Following a single SC dose in adult and adolescent patients with asthma, omalizumab was absorbed slowly, reaching peak serum concentrations after an average of 7-8 days. The pharmacokinetics of omalizumab are linear at doses greater than 0.5 mg/kg. Following multiple doses of omalizumab, areas under the serum concentration-time curve from Day 0 to Day 14 at steady-state were up to 6-fold of those after the first dose.

In vitro, omalizumab forms complexes of limited size with IgE. Precipitating complexes and complexes larger than 1 million daltons in molecular weight are not observed *in vitro* or *in vivo*. Tissue distribution studies in cynomolgus monkeys showed no specific uptake of ^{125}I-omalizumab by any organ or tissue. The apparent volume of distribution in patients following SC administration was 78 ± 32 ml/kg.

Clearance of omalizumab involves IgG clearance processes as well as clearance via specific binding and complex formation with its target ligand, IgE. Liver elimination of IgG includes degradation in the liver reticuloendothelial system (RES) and endothelial cells. Intact IgG is also excreted in bile. In studies with mice and monkeys, omalizumab:IgE complexes were eliminated by interactions with Fcγ receptors within the RES at rates that were generally faster than IgG clearance. In asthma patients omalizumab serum elimination half-life averaged 26 days, with apparent clearance averaging 2.4 ± 1.1 ml/kg/day. In addition, doubling body weight approximately doubled apparent clearance.

PHARMACODYNAMICS

In clinical studies, serum free IgE levels were reduced in a dose dependent manner within 1 hour following the first dose and maintained between doses. Mean serum free IgE decrease was greater than 96% using recommended doses. Serum total IgE levels (*i.e.*, bound and unbound) increased after the first dose due to the formation of omalizumab:IgE complexes, which have a slower elimination rate compared with free IgE. At 16 weeks after the first dose, average serum total IgE levels were 5-fold higher compared with pre-treatment when using standard assays. After discontinuation of omalizumab dosing, the omalizumab-induced increase in total IgE and decrease in free IgE were reversible, with no observed rebound in IgE levels after drug washout. Total IgE levels did not return to pre-treatment levels for up to 1 year after discontinuation of omalizumab.

SPECIAL POPULATIONS

The population pharmacokinetics of omalizumab were analyzed to evaluate the effects of demographic characteristics. Analyses of these limited data suggest that no dose adjustments are necessary for age (12-76 years), race, ethnicity, or gender.

INDICATIONS AND USAGE

Omalizumab is indicated for adults and adolescents (12 years of age and above) with moderate to severe persistent asthma who have a positive skin test or *in vitro* reactivity to a perennial aeroallergen and whose symptoms are inadequately controlled with inhaled corticosteroids. Omalizumab has been shown to decrease the incidence of asthma exacerbations in these patients. Safety and efficacy have not been established in other allergic conditions.

CONTRAINDICATIONS

Omalizumab should not be administered to patients who have experienced a severe hypersensitivity reaction to omalizumab (see WARNINGS, Anaphylaxis).

WARNINGS

MALIGNANCY

Malignant neoplasms were observed in 20 of 4127 (0.5%) omalizumab-treated patients compared with 5 of 2236 (0.2%) control patients in clinical studies of asthma and other allergic disorders. The observed malignancies in omalizumab-treated patients were a variety of types, with breast, non-melanoma skin, prostate, melanoma, and parotid occurring more than once, and five other types occurring once each. The majority of patients were observed for less than 1 year. The impact of longer exposure to omalizumab or use in patients at higher risk for malignancy (*e.g.*, elderly, current smokers) is not known (see ADVERSE REACTIONS).

ANAPHYLAXIS

Anaphylaxis has occurred within 2 hours of the first or subsequent administration of omalizumab in 3 (<0.1%) patients without other identifiable allergic triggers. These events included urticaria and throat and/or tongue edema (see ADVERSE REACTIONS). Patients should be observed after injection of omalizumab, and medications for the treatment of severe hypersensitivity reactions including anaphylaxis should be available. If a severe hypersensitivity reaction to omalizumab occurs, therapy should be discontinued (see CONTRAINDICATIONS).

PRECAUTIONS

GENERAL

Omalizumab has not been shown to alleviate asthma exacerbations acutely and should not be used for the treatment of acute bronchospasm or status asthmaticus.

CORTICOSTEROID REDUCTION

Systemic or inhaled corticosteroids should not be abruptly discontinued upon initiation of omalizumab therapy. Decreases in corticosteroids should be performed under the direct supervision of a physician and may need to be performed gradually.

INFORMATION FOR THE PATIENT

Patients receiving omalizumab should be told not to decrease the dose of, or stop taking any other asthma medications unless otherwise instructed by their physician. Patients should be told that they may not see immediate improvement in their asthma after beginning omalizumab therapy.

LABORATORY TESTS

Serum total IgE levels increase following administration of omalizumab due to formation of omalizumab:IgE complexes (see CLINICAL PHARMACOLOGY and DOSAGE AND ADMINISTRATION). Elevated serum total IgE levels may persist for up to 1 year following discontinuation of omalizumab. Serum total IgE levels obtained less than 1 year following discontinuation may not reflect steady-state free IgE levels and should not be used to reassess the dosing regimen.

CARCINOGENESIS, MUTAGENESIS, AND IMPAIRMENT OF FERTILITY

No long-term studies have been performed in animals to evaluate the carcinogenic potential of omalizumab.

No evidence of mutagenic activity was observed in Ames tests using six different strains of bacteria with and without metabolic activation at omalizumab concentrations up to 5000 μg/ml.

The effects of omalizumab on male and female fertility have been assessed in cynomolgus monkey studies. Administration of omalizumab at doses up to and including 75 mg/kg/week did not elicit reproductive toxicity in male cynomolgus monkeys and did not inhibit reproductive capability, including implantation, in female cynomolgus monkeys. These doses provide a 2- to 16-fold safety factor based on total dose and 2- to 5-fold safety factor based on AUC over the range of adult clinical doses.

PREGNANCY CATEGORY B

Reproduction studies in cynomolgus monkeys have been conducted with omalizumab. Subcutaneous doses up to 75 mg/kg (12-fold the maximum clinical dose) of omalizumab did not elicit maternal toxicity, embryotoxicity, or teratogenicity when administered throughout organogenesis and did not elicit adverse effects on fetal or neonatal growth when administered throughout late gestation, delivery, and nursing.

IgG molecules are known to cross the placental barrier. There are no adequate and well-controlled studies of omalizumab in pregnant women. Because animal reproduction studies are not always predictive of human response, omalizumab should be used during pregnancy only if clearly needed.

NURSING MOTHERS

The excretion of omalizumab in milk was evaluated in female cynomolgus monkeys receiving SC doses of 75 mg/kg/week. Neonatal plasma levels of omalizumab after *in utero* exposure and 28 days of nursing were between 11% and 94% of the maternal plasma level. Milk levels of omalizumab were 1.5% of maternal blood concentration. While omalizumab presence in human milk has not been studied, IgG is excreted in human milk and therefore it is expected that omalizumab will be present in human milk. The potential for omalizumab absorption or harm to the infant are unknown; caution should be exercised when administering omalizumab to a nursing woman.

PEDIATRIC USE

Safety and effectiveness in pediatric patients below the age of 12 have not been established.

GERIATRIC USE

In clinical trials 134 patients 65 years of age or older were treated with omalizumab. Although there were no apparent age-related differences observed in these studies, the number of patients aged 65 and over is not sufficient to determine whether they respond differently from younger patients.

DRUG INTERACTIONS

No formal drug interaction studies have been performed with omalizumab. The concomitant use of omalizumab and allergen immunotherapy has not been evaluated.

ADVERSE REACTIONS

The most serious adverse reactions occurring in clinical studies with omalizumab are malignancies and anaphylaxis (see WARNINGS). The observed incidence of malignancy among omalizumab-treated patients (0.5%) was numerically higher than among patients in control groups (0.2%). Anaphylactic reactions were rare but temporally associated with omalizumab administration.

The adverse reactions most commonly observed among patients treated with omalizumab included injection site reaction (45%), viral infections (23%), upper respiratory tract infection (20%), sinusitis (16%), headache (15%), and pharyngitis (11%). These events were observed at similar rates in omalizumab-treated patients and control patients. These were also the most frequently reported adverse reactions resulting in clinical intervention (*e.g.*, discontinuation of omalizumab, or the need for concomitant medication to treat an adverse reaction).

Because clinical trials are conducted under widely varying conditions, adverse reaction rates observed in the clinical trials of one drug cannot be directly compared with rates in the clinical trials of another drug and may not reflect the rates observed in medical practice.

The data described above reflect omalizumab exposure for 2076 adult and adolescent patients ages 12 and older, including 1687 patients exposed for 6 months and 555 exposed for 1 year or more, in either placebo-controlled or other controlled asthma studies. The mean age of patients receiving omalizumab was 42 years, with 134 patients 65 years of age or older; 60% were women, and 85% Caucasian. Patients received omalizumab 150-375 mg every 2 or 4 weeks or, for patients assigned to control groups, standard therapy with or without a placebo.

TABLE 4 shows adverse events that occurred ≥1% more frequently in patients receiving omalizumab than in those receiving placebo in the placebo-controlled asthma studies. Adverse events were classified using preferred terms from the International Medical Nomenclature (IMN) dictionary. Injection site reactions were recorded separately from the reporting of other adverse events and are described following TABLE 4.

TABLE 4 *Adverse Events ≥1% More Frequent in Omalizumab-Treated Patients*

Adverse Event	Omalizumab n=738	Placebo n=717
Body as a Whole		
Pain	7%	5%
Fatigue	3%	2%
Musculoskeletal System		
Arthralgia	8%	6%
Fracture	2%	1%
Leg pain	4%	2%
Arm pain	2%	1%
Nervous System		
Dizziness	3%	2%
Skin and Appendages		
Pruritus	2%	1%
Dermaitits	2%	1%
Special Senses		
Earache	2%	1%

Age (among patients under age 65), race, and gender did not appear to affect the between group differences in the rates of adverse events.

INJECTION SITE REACTIONS

Injection site reactions of any severity occurred at a rate of 45% in omalizumab-treated patients compared with 43% in placebo-treated patients. The types of injection site reactions included: bruising, redness, warmth, burning, stinging, itching, hive formation, pain, indurations, mass, and inflammation.

Severe injection-site reactions occurred more frequently in omalizumab-treated patients compared with patients in the placebo group (12% vs 9%).

The majority of injection site reactions occurred within 1 hour-post injection, lasted less than 8 days, and generally decreased in frequency at subsequent dosing visits.

IMMUNOGENICITY

Low titers of antibodies to omalizumab were detected in approximately 1/1723 (<0.1%) of patients treated with omalizumab. The data reflect the percentage of patients whose test results were considered positive for antibodies to omalizumab in an ELISA assay and are highly dependent on the sensitivity and specificity of the assay. Additionally, the observed incidence of antibody positivity in the assay may be influenced by several factors including sample handling, timing of sample collection, concomitant medications, and underlying disease. Therefore, comparison of the incidence of antibodies to omalizumab with the incidence of antibodies to other products may be misleading.

Allergic symptoms, including urticaria, dermatitis, and pruritus were observed in patients treated with omalizumab. There were also 3 cases of anaphylaxis observed within 2 hours of omalizumab administration in which there were no other identifiable allergic triggers (see WARNINGS, Anaphylaxis).

DOSAGE AND ADMINISTRATION

Omalizumab 150-375 mg is administered SC every 2 or 4 weeks. Because the solution is slightly viscous, the injection may take 5-10 seconds to administer. Doses (mg) and dosing frequency are determined by serum total IgE level (IU/ml), measured before the start of treatment, and body weight (kg). See the dose determination charts below (TABLE 5 and TABLE 6) for appropriate dose assignment. Doses of more than 150 mg are divided among more than 1 injection site to limit injections to not more than 150 mg per site.

DOSE ADJUSTMENT

Total IgE levels are elevated during treatment and remain elevated for up to 1 year after the discontinuation of treatment. Therefore, re-testing of IgE levels during omalizumab treatment cannot be used as a guide for dose determination. Dose determination after treatment interruptions lasting less than 1 year should be based on serum IgE levels obtained at the initial dose determination. Total serum IgE levels may be re-tested for dose determination if treatment with omalizumab has been interrupted for 1 year or more.

Doses should be adjusted for significant changes in body weight. (See TABLE 5 and TABLE 6.)

TABLE 5 *ADMINISTRATION EVERY 4 WEEKS: Omalizumab Doses (mg) Administered by SC Injection Every 4 Weeks for Adults and Adolescents (12 Years of Age and Older) With Asthma*

Pre-Treatment Serum IgE (IU/ml)	Body Weight (kg) 30 to 60	>60 to 70	>70 to 90	>90 to 150
≥30-100	150	150	150	300
>100-200	300	300	300	*
>200-300	300	*	*	*
>300-400	*	*	*	*
>400-500	*	*	*	*
>500-600	*	*	*	*

* See TABLE 6.

TABLE 6 *ADMINISTRATION EVERY 2 WEEKS: Omalizumab Doses (mg) Administered by Subcutaneous Injection Every 2 Weeks for Adults and Adolescents (12 Years of Age and Older) With Asthma*

Pre-Treatement Serum IgE (IU/ml)	Body Weight (kg) 30 to 60	>60 to 70	>70 to 90	>90 to 150
≥30-100	*	*	*	*
>100-200	*	*	*	225
>200-300	*	225	225	300
>300-400	225	225	300	†
>400-500	300	300	375	†
>500-600	300	375	†	†
>600-700	375	†	†	†

* See TABLE 5.
† **DO NOT USE.**

STABILITY AND STORAGE

Omalizumab should be shipped at controlled ambient temperature [≤30°C (≤86°F)]. Omalizumab should be stored under refrigerated conditions 2-8°C (36-46°F). Do not use beyond the expiration date stamped on carton.

Omalizumab is for single-use only and contains no preservatives. The solution may be used for SC administration within 8 hours following reconstitution when stored in the vial at 2-8°C (36-46°F), or within 4 hours of reconstitution when stored at room temperature.

Reconstituted omalizumab vials should be protected from direct sunlight.

HOW SUPPLIED

Xolair is supplied as a lyophilized, sterile powder in a single-use, 5 cc vial that is designed to deliver 150 mg of omalizumab upon reconstitution with 1.4 ml SWFI.

Omeprazole *(001916)*

For related information, see the comparative table section in Appendix A.

Categories: Adenoma, multiple endocrine; Esophagitis, erosive; Mastocytosis, systemic; Gastroesophageal Reflux Disease; Ulcer, duodenal; Ulcer, gastric; Zollinger-Ellison syndrome; Pregnancy Category C; FDA Approved 1989 Sep

Drug Classes: Gastrointestinals; Proton pump inhibitors

Brand Names: Losec; **Prilosec**

Foreign Brand Availability: Acidex (Ecuador); Aleprozil (Mexico); Antra (Germany; Italy; Switzerland); Audazol (Spain); Azoran (Mexico); Baromezole (Korea); Desec (Thailand); Domer (Mexico); Dudencer (Indonesia); Duogas (Thailand); Epirazole (Bahrain; Cyprus; Egypt; Iran; Iraq; Jordan; Kuwait; Lebanon; Libya; Oman; Qatar; Republic-of-Yemen; Saudi-Arabia; Syria; United-Arab-Emirates); Gasec (Bahamas; Barbados; Belize; Bermuda; Curacao; Guyana; Jamaica; Netherland-Antilles; Puerto-Rico; Surinam; Trinidad); Gastop (Peru); Gastroloc (Germany); H-Etom (Colombia); Hyposec (Bahrain; Cyprus; Egypt; Iran; Iraq; Jordan; Kuwait; Lebanon; Libya; Oman; Qatar; Republic-of-Yemen; Saudi-Arabia; Syria; United-Arab-Emirates); Inhibitron (Mexico); Inhipump (Indonesia); Logastric (Belgium); Lomac (India); Lopraz (Bahrain; Cyprus; Egypt; Iran; Iraq; Jordan; Kuwait; Lebanon; Libya; Oman; Qatar; Republic-of-Yemen; Saudi-Arabia; Syria; United-Arab-Emirates); Losec MUPS (Philippines); Madiprazole (Thailand); Maxor (Australia); Medoprazole (Benin; Burkina-Faso; Ethiopia; Gambia; Ghana; Guinea; Ivory-Coast; Kenya; Liberia; Malawi; Mali; Mauritania; Mauritius; Morocco; Niger; Nigeria; Senegal; Seychelles; Sierra-Leone; Sudan; Tanzania; Tunia; Uganda; Zambia; Zimbabwe); Medral (Mexico); Meiceral (Thailand); Mepzol (Korea); Miracid (Thailand); Mopral (France; Mexico); Nocid (Thailand); Ocid (India; Singapore); Olexin (Mexico); Omed (Benin; Burkina-Faso; Ethiopia; Gambia; Ghana; Guinea; India; Ivory-Coast; Kenya; Liberia; Malawi; Mali; Mauritania; Mauritius; Morocco; Niger; Nigeria; Senegal; Seychelles; Sierra-Leone; Sudan; Tanzania; Tunia; Uganda; Zambia; Zimbabwe); Omedar (Bahrain; Cyprus; Egypt; Iran; Iraq; Jordan; Kuwait; Lebanon; Libya; Oman; Qatar; Republic-of-Yemen; Saudi-Arabia; Syria; United-Arab-Emirates); Omelon (Taiwan); OMEP (Germany); Omepril (Ecuador); Omepral (Japan); Omeprazon (Japan); Omeq (Korea); Omesec (Singapore); Omez (Thailand); Omezin (Korea); Omezol (Bahrain; Cyprus; Egypt; India; Iran; Iraq; Jordan; Kuwait; Lebanon; Libya; Oman; Qatar; Republic-of-Yemen; Saudi-Arabia; Syria; United-Arab-Emirates); Omezole (Singapore); Omezzol (Ecuador); Omizac (Bahrain; India; Republic-Of-Yemen); Omisec (Bahrain; Cyprus; Egypt; Iran; Iraq; Jordan; Kuwait; Lebanon; Libya; Oman; Qatar; Republic-of-Yemen; Saudi-Arabia; Syria; United-Arab-Emirates); OMP (China; Korea); OMZ (Indonesia); Opal (Peru); Oprax (Peru); Ozoken (Mexico); Parizac (Spain); Penrazole (Singapore); Peptidin (Colombia); Peptilcer (India); Peptizole (Thailand); Pra-Sec (Korea); Prazidec (Mexico); Prazole (Korea); Proceptin (Singapore); Prohibit (Indonesia); Ramezol (Korea); Result (Korea); Roweprazol (Costa-Rica; Dominican-Republic; El-Salvador; Guatemala; Honduras; Nicaragua; Panama); Severon (Thailand); Stomacer (Indonesia); Stomec (Thailand); Stozole (India); Suifac (Mexico); Ulcozol (Colombia; Peru); Ulnor (Germany); Ulsen (Mexico); Vulcasid (Mexico); Xoprin (Peru); Zefxon (Thailand); Zimor (Singapore); Zoltum (France)

Cost of Therapy: $415.27 (GERD; Prilosec; 20 mg; 1 capsule/day; 30 day supply)
$248.03 (GERD; Prilosec; 10 mg; 2 capsules/day; 30 day supply)
$178.20 (Gastric Ulcer; Prilosec; 40 mg; 1 capsule/day; 30 day supply)

DESCRIPTION

The active ingredient in Prilosec (omeprazole) delayed-release capsules is a substituted benzimidazole, 5-methoxy-2-[[(4-methoxy-3,5-dimethyl-2-pyridinyl)methyl]sulfinyl]-1*H*-benzimidazole, a compound that inhibits gastric acid secretion. Its empirical formula is $C_{17}H_{19}N_3O_3S$, with a molecular weight of 345.42.

Omeprazole is a white to off-white crystalline powder which melts with decomposition at about 155°C. It is a weak base, freely soluble in ethanol and methanol, and slightly soluble in acetone and isopropanol and very slightly soluble in water. The stability of omeprazole is a function of pH; it is rapidly degraded in acid media, but has acceptable stability under alkaline conditions.

Prilosec is supplied as delayed-release capsules for oral administration. Each delayed-release capsule contains either 10, 20, or 40 mg of omeprazole in the form of enteric-coated granules with the following inactive ingredients: cellulose, disodium hydrogen phosphate, hydroxypropyl cellulose, hydroxypropyl methylcellulose, lactose, mannitol, sodium lauryl sulfate and other ingredients. The capsule shells have the following inactive ingredients: gelatin, FD&C blue no. 1, FD&C red no. 40, D&C red no. 28, titanium dioxide, synthetic black iron oxide, isopropanol, butyl alcohol, FD&C blue no. 2, D&C red no. 7 calcium lake, and, in addition, the 10 and 40 mg capsule shells also contain D&C yellow no. 10.

CLINICAL PHARMACOLOGY

PHARMACOKINETICS AND METABOLISM

Omeprazole

Omeprazole delayed-release capsules contain an enteric-coated granule formulation of omeprazole (because omeprazole is acid-labile), so that absorption of omeprazole begins only after the granules leave the stomach. Absorption is rapid, with peak plasma levels of omeprazole occurring within 0.5-3.5 hours. Peak plasma concentrations of omeprazole and AUC are approximately proportional to doses up to 40 mg, but because of a saturable first-pass effect, a greater than linear response in peak plasma concentration and AUC occurs with doses greater than 40 mg. Absolute bioavailability (compared to intravenous administration) is about 30-40% at doses of 20-40 mg, due in large part to presystemic metabolism. In healthy subjects the plasma half-life is 0.5 to 1 hour, and the total body clearance is 500-600 ml/min. Protein binding is approximately 95%.

The bioavailability of omeprazole increases slightly upon repeated administration of omeprazole delayed-release capsules.

Following single dose oral administration of a buffered solution of omeprazole, little if any unchanged drug was excreted in urine. The majority of the dose (about 77%) was eliminated in urine as at least 6 metabolites. Two were identified as hydroxyomeprazole and the corresponding carboxylic acid. The remainder of the dose was recoverable in feces. This implies a significant biliary excretion of the metabolites of omeprazole. Three metabolites have been identified in plasma — the sulfide and sulfone derivatives of omeprazole, and hydroxyomeprazole. These metabolites have very little or no antisecretory activity.

In patients with chronic hepatic disease, the bioavailability increased to approximately 100% compared to an IV dose, reflecting decreased first-pass effect, and the plasma half-life of the drug increased to nearly 3 hours compared to the half-life in normals of 0.5 to 1 hour. Plasma clearance averaged 70 ml/min, compared to a value of 500-600 ml/min in normal subjects.

In patients with chronic renal impairment, whose creatinine clearance ranged between 10 and 62 ml/min/1.73 m^2, the disposition of omeprazole was very similar to that in healthy volunteers, although there was a slight increase in bioavailability. Because urinary excretion is a primary route of excretion of omeprazole metabolites, their elimination slowed in proportion to the decreased creatinine clearance.

The elimination rate of omeprazole was somewhat decreased in the elderly, and bioavailability was increased. Omeprazole was 76% bioavailable when a single 40 mg oral dose of omeprazole (buffered solution) was administered to healthy elderly volunteers, versus 58% in young volunteers given the same dose. Nearly 70% of the dose was recovered in urine as metabolites of omeprazole and no unchanged drug was detected. The plasma clearance of omeprazole was 250 ml/min (about half that of young volunteers) and its plasma half-life averaged 1 hour, about twice that of young healthy volunteers.

In pharmacokinetic studies of single 20 mg omeprazole doses, an increase in AUC of approximately 4-fold was noted in Asian subjects compared to Caucasians.

Dose adjustment, particularly where maintenance of healing of erosive esophagitis is indicated, for the hepatically impaired and Asian subjects should be considered.

Omeprazole delayed-release capsule 40 mg was bioequivalent when administered with and without applesauce. However, omeprazole delayed-release capsule 20 mg was not bioequivalent when administered with and without applesauce. When administered with applesauce, a mean 25% reduction in C_{max} was observed without a significant change in AUC for omeprazole delayed-release capsule 20 mg. The clinical relevance of this finding is unknown.

The pharmacokinetics of omeprazole have been investigated in pediatric patients of different ages.

TABLE 1 *Pharmacokinetic Parameters of Omeprazole Following Single and Repeated Oral Administration in Pediatric Populations Compared to Adults*

Single or Repeated Oral Dosing/ Parameter	Children† <20 kg 2-5 years 10 mg	>20 kg 6-16 years 20 mg	Adults‡ (mean 76 kg) 23-29 years (n=12)
Single Dosing			
C_{max}* (ng/ml)	288 (n=10)	495 (n=49)	668
AUC* (ng h/ml)	511 (n=7)	1140 (n=32)	1220
Repeated Dosing			
C_{max}* (ng/ml)	539 (n=4)	851 (n=32)	1458
AUC* (ng h/ml)	1179 (n=2)	2276 (n=23)	3352

* Plasma concentration adjusted to an oral dose of 1 mg/kg.
† Data from single and repeated dose studies.
‡ Data from a single and repeated dose study.
Note: Doses of 10, 20 and 40 mg omeprazole as enteric-coated granules.

Following comparable mg/kg doses of omeprazole, younger children (2-5 years) have lower AUCs than children 6-16 years or adults; AUCs of the latter 2 groups did not differ. (See DOSAGE AND ADMINISTRATION, Pediatric Patients.)

PHARMACOKINETICS

Combination Therapy With Antimicrobials

Omeprazole 40 mg daily was given in combination with clarithromycin 500 mg every 8 hours to healthy adult male subjects. The steady state plasma concentrations of omeprazole were increased (C_{max}, AUC(0-24), and $T_{1/2}$ increases of 30%, 89%, and 34% respectively) by the concomitant administration of clarithromycin. The observed increases in omeprazole plasma concentration were associated with the following pharmacological effects. The mean 24 hour gastric pH value was 5.2 when omeprazole was administered alone and 5.7 when co-administered with clarithromycin.

The plasma levels of clarithromycin and 14-hydroxy-clarithromycin were increased by the concomitant administration of omeprazole. For clarithromycin, the mean C_{max} was 10% greater, the mean C_{min} was 27% greater, and the mean AUC(0-8) was 15% greater when clarithromycin was administered with omeprazole than when clarithromycin was administered alone. Similar results were seen for 14-hydroxy-clarithromycin, the mean C_{max} was 45% greater, the mean C_{min} was 57% greater, and the mean AUC(0-8) was 45% greater. Clarithromycin concentrations in the gastric tissue and mucus were also increased by concomitant administration of omeprazole.

TABLE 2 *Clarithromycin Tissue Concentrations 2 Hours After Dose**

Tissue	Clarithromycin	Clarithromycin + Omeprazole
Antrum	10.48 ± 2.01 (n=5)	19.96 ± 4.71 (n=5)
Fundus	20.81 ± 7.64 (n=5)	24.25 ± 6.37 (n=5)
Mucus	4.15 ± 7.74 (n=4)	39.29 ± 32.79 (n=4)

* Mean ±SD (μg/g).

For information on clarithromycin pharmacokinetics and microbiology, consult the clarithromycin package insert, CLINICAL PHARMACOLOGY section.

The pharmacokinetics of omeprazole, clarithromycin, and amoxicillin have not been adequately studied when all 3 drugs are administered concomitantly.

For information on amoxicillin pharmacokinetics and microbiology, see the amoxicillin package insert, ACTIONS, PHARMACOLOGY and MICROBIOLOGY sections.

PHARMACODYNAMICS

Mechanism of Action

Omeprazole belongs to a new class of antisecretory compounds, the substituted benzimidazoles, that do not exhibit anticholinergic or H_2 histamine antagonistic properties, but that suppress gastric acid secretion by specific inhibition of the H^+/K^+ ATPase enzyme system at the secretory surface of the gastric parietal cell. Because this enzyme system is regarded as the acid (proton) pump within the gastric mucosa, omeprazole has been characterized as a gastric acid-pump inhibitor, in that it blocks the final step of acid production. This effect is dose-related and leads to inhibition of both basal and stimulated acid secretion irrespective of the stimulus. Animal studies indicate that after rapid disappearance from plasma, omeprazole can be found within the gastric mucosa for a day or more.

Antisecretory Activity

After oral administration, the onset of the antisecretory effect of omeprazole occurs within 1 hour, with the maximum effect occurring within 2 hours. Inhibition of secretion is about 50% of maximum at 24 hours and the duration of inhibition lasts up to 72 hours. The antisecretory effect thus lasts far longer than would be expected from the very short (less than 1 hour) plasma half-life, apparently due to prolonged binding to the parietal H^+/K^+ ATPase enzyme. When the drug is discontinued, secretory activity returns gradually, over 3-5 days. The inhibitory effect of omeprazole on acid secretion increases with repeated once-daily dosing, reaching a plateau after 4 days.

Results from numerous studies of the antisecretory effect of multiple doses of 20 and 40 mg of omeprazole in normal volunteers and patients are shown in TABLE 3. The "max" value represents determinations at a time of maximum effect (2-6 hours after dosing), while "min" values are those 24 hours after the last dose of omeprazole.

TABLE 3 *Range of Mean Values From Multiple Studies of the Mean Antisecretory Effects of Omeprazole After Multiple Daily Dosing*

Parameter	Omeprazole 20 mg		Omeprazole 40 mg	
% Decrease In	Max	Min	Max	Min
Basal acid output	78*	58-80	94*	80-93
Peak acid output	79*	50-59	88*	62-68
24 h Intragastric acidity		80-97		92-94

* Single studies.

Single daily oral doses of omeprazole ranging from a dose of 10-40 mg have produced 100% inhibition of 24 hour intragastric acidity in some patients.

Enterochromaffin-Like (ECL) Cell Effects

In 24 month carcinogenicity studies in rats, a dose-related significant increase in gastric carcinoid tumors and ECL cell hyperplasia was observed in both male and female animals (see PRECAUTIONS, Carcinogenesis, Mutagenesis, and Impairment of Fertility). Carcinoid tumors have also been observed in rats subjected to fundectomy or long-term treatment with other proton pump inhibitors or high doses of H_2-receptor antagonists.

Human gastric biopsy specimens have been obtained from more than 3000 patients treated with omeprazole in long-term clinical trials. The incidence of ECL cell hyperplasia in these studies increased with time; however, no case of ECL cell carcinoids, dysplasia, or neoplasia has been found in these patients. However, these studies are of insufficient duration and size to rule out the possible influence of long-term administration of omeprazole on the development of any premalignant or malignant conditions.

Serum Gastrin Effects

In studies involving more than 200 patients, serum gastrin levels increased during the first 1-2 weeks of once-daily administration of therapeutic doses of omeprazole in parallel with inhibition of acid secretion. No further increase in serum gastrin occurred with continued treatment. In comparison with histamine H_2-receptor antagonists, the median increases produced by 20 mg doses of omeprazole were higher (1.3- to 3.6-fold vs 1.1- to 1.8-fold increase). Gastrin values returned to pretreatment levels, usually within 1-2 weeks after discontinuation of therapy.

Other Effects

Systemic effects of omeprazole in the CNS, cardiovascular, and respiratory systems have not been found to date. Omeprazole, given in oral doses of 30 or 40 mg for 2-4 weeks, had no effect on thyroid function, carbohydrate metabolism, or circulating levels of parathyroid hormone, cortisol, estradiol, testosterone, prolactin, cholecystokinin, or secretin.

No effect on gastric emptying of the solid and liquid components of a test meal was demonstrated after a single dose of omeprazole 90 mg. In healthy subjects, a single IV dose of omeprazole (0.35 mg/kg) had no effect on intrinsic factor secretion. No systematic dose-dependent effect has been observed on basal or stimulated pepsin output in humans.

However, when intragastric pH is maintained at 4.0 or above, basal pepsin output is low, and pepsin activity is decreased.

As do other agents that elevate intragastric pH, omeprazole administered for 14 days in healthy subjects produced a significant increase in the intragastric concentrations of viable bacteria. The pattern of the bacterial species was unchanged from that commonly found in saliva. All changes resolved within 3 days of stopping treatment.

The course of Barrett's esophagus in 106 patients was evaluated in a US. double-blind controlled study of omeprazole 40 mg bid for 12 months followed by 20 mg bid for 12 months or ranitidine 300 mg bid for 24 months. No clinically significant impact on Barrett's mucosa by antisecretory therapy was observed. Although neosquamous epithelium developed during antisecretory therapy, complete elimination of Barrett's mucosa was not achieved. No significant difference was observed between treatment groups in development of dysplasia in Barrett's mucosa and no patient developed esophageal carcinoma during treatment. No significant differences between treatment groups were observed in development of ECL cell hyperplasia, corpus atrophic gastritis, corpus intestinal metaplasia, or colon polyps exceeding 3 mm in diameter (see also CLINICAL PHARMACOLOGY, Enterochromaffin-like (ECL) Cell Effects).

MICROBIOLOGY

Omeprazole and clarithromycin dual therapy and omeprazole, clarithromycin, and amoxicillin triple therapy have been shown to be active against most strains of *Helicobacter pylori in vitro* and in clinical infections as described in INDICATIONS AND USAGE.

Helicobacter — Helicobacter pylori

Pretreatment Resistance

Clarithromycin pretreatment resistance rates were 3.5% (4/113) in the omeprazole/clarithromycin dual therapy studies (M93-067, M93-100) and 9.3% (41/439) in omeprazole/clarithromycin/amoxicillin triple therapy studies (126, 127, M96-446).

Amoxicillin pretreatment susceptible isolates (≤0.25 μg/ml) were found in 99.3% (436/439) of the patients in the omeprazole/clarithromycin/amoxicillin triple therapy studies (126, 127, M96-446). Amoxicillin pretreatment minimum inhibitory concentrations (MICs) >0.25 μg/ml occurred in 0.7% (3/439) of the patients, all of whom were in the clarithromycin and amoxicillin study arm. One patient had an unconfirmed pretreatment amoxicillin minimum inhibitory concentration (MIC) of >256 μg/ml by Etest.

Clarithromycin Susceptibility Test Results and Clinical/Bacteriological Outcomes

TABLE 4 *Clarithromycin Susceptibility Test Results and Clinical/Bacteriological Outcomes**

		Clarithromycin Post-Treatment Results				
			H. pylori Positive — Not Eradicated			
			Post-Treatment Susceptibility Results			
Clarithromycin Pretreatment Results		*H. pylori* Negative — Eradicated	S†	I†	R†	No MIC
Dual Therapy — (omeprazole 40 mg qd/clarithromycin 500 mg tid for 14 days followed by omeprazole 20 mg qd for another 14 days) (Studies M93-067, M93-100)						
Susceptible†	108	72	1		26	9
Intermediate†	1				1	
Resistant†	4				4	
Triple Therapy — (omeprazole 20 mg bid/clarithromycin 500 mg bid/amoxicillin 1 g bid for 10 days — Studies 126, 127, M96-446; followed by omeprazole 20 mg qd for another 18 days — Studies 126, 127)						
Susceptible†	171	153	7		3	8
Intermediate†						
Resistant†	14	4	1		6	3

* Includes only patients with pretreatment clarithromycin susceptibility test results.
† Susceptible (S) MIC ≤0.25 μg/ml, Intermediate (I) MIC 0.5-1.0 μg/ml, Resistant (R) MIC ≥2 μg/ml.

Patients not eradicated of *H. pylori* following omeprazole/clarithromycin/amoxicillin triple therapy or omeprazole/clarithromycin dual therapy will likely have clarithromycin resistant *H. pylori* isolates. Therefore, clarithromycin susceptibility testing should be done, if possible. *Patients with clarithromycin resistant H. pylori should not be treated with any of the following: Omeprazole/clarithromycin dual therapy, omeprazole/clarithromycin/*

amoxicillin triple therapy, or other regimens which include clarithromycin as the sole antimicrobial agent.

Amoxicillin Susceptibility Test Results and Clinical/Bacteriological Outcomes

In the triple therapy clinical trials, 84.9% (157/185) of the patients in the omeprazole/clarithromycin/amoxicillin treatment group who had pretreatment amoxicillin susceptible MICs (≤0.25 μg/ml) were eradicated of *H. pylori* and 15.1% (28/185) failed therapy. Of the 28 patients who failed triple therapy, 11 had no post-treatment susceptibility test results and 17 had post-treatment *H. pylori* isolates with amoxicillin susceptible MICs. Eleven of the patients who failed triple therapy also had post-treatment *H. pylori* isolates with clarithromycin resistant MICs.

Susceptibility Test for Helicobacter pylori

The reference methodology for susceptibility testing of *H. pylori* is agar dilution MICs.[1] One (1) to 3 μl of an inoculum equivalent to a No. 2 McFarland standard (1×10^7 - 1×10^8 CFU/ml for *H. pylori*) are inoculated directly onto freshly prepared antimicrobial containing Mueller-Hinton agar plates with 5% aged defibrinated sheep blood (≥2 weeks old). The agar dilution plates are incubated at 35°C in a microaerobic environment produced by a gas generating system suitable for campylobacters. After 3 days of incubation, the MICs are recorded as the lowest concentration of antimicrobial agent required to inhibit growth of the organism. The clarithromycin and amoxicillin MIC values should be interpreted according to the criteria in TABLE 5.

TABLE 5

Clarithromycin MIC*	Interpretation
≤0.25 μg/ml	Susceptible (S)
0.5 μg/ml	Intermediate (I)
≥1.0 μg/ml	Resistant (R)
Amoxicillin MIC*†	**Interpretation**
≤0.25 μg/ml	Susceptible (S)

* These are tentative breakpoints for the agar dilution methodology and they should not be used to interpret results obtained using alternative methods.
† There were not enough organisms with MICs >0.25 μg/ml to determine a resistance breakpoint.

Standardized susceptibility test procedures require the use of laboratory control microorganisms to control the technical aspects of the laboratory procedures. Standard clarithromycin and amoxicillin powders should provide the MIC values shown in TABLE 6.

TABLE 6

Microorganism	Antimicrobial Agent	MIC*
H. pylori ATCC 43504	Clarithromycin	0.016-0.12 μg/ml
H. pylori ATCC 43504	Amoxicillin	0.016-0.12 μg/ml

* These are quality control ranges for the agar dilution methodology and they should not be used to control test results obtained using alternative methods.

INDICATIONS AND USAGE

DUODENAL ULCER

Omeprazole delayed-release capsules are indicated for short-term treatment of active duodenal ulcer. Most patients heal within 4 weeks. Some patients may require an additional 4 weeks of therapy.

Omeprazole delayed-release capsules, in combination with clarithromycin and amoxicillin, are indicated for treatment of patients with *H. pylori* infection and duodenal ulcer disease (active or up to 1 year history) to eradicate *H. pylori.*

Omeprazole delayed-release capsules, in combination with clarithromycin, are indicated for treatment of patients with *H. pylori* infection and duodenal ulcer disease to eradicate *H. pylori.*

Eradication of *H. pylori* has been shown to reduce the risk of duodenal ulcer recurrence (see DOSAGE AND ADMINISTRATION).

Among patients who fail therapy, omeprazole with clarithromycin is more likely to be associated with the development of clarithromycin resistance as compared with triple therapy. In patients who fail therapy, susceptibility testing should be done. If resistance to clarithromycin is demonstrated or susceptibility testing is not possible, alternative antimicrobial therapy should be instituted. (See CLINICAL PHARMACOLOGY, Microbiology, and the clarithromycin package insert, MICROBIOLOGY section.)

GASTRIC ULCER

Omeprazole delayed-release capsules are indicated for short-term treatment (4-8 weeks) of active benign gastric ulcer.

TREATMENT OF GASTROESOPHAGEAL REFLUX DISEASE (GERD)

Symptomatic GERD

Omeprazole delayed-release capsules are indicated for the treatment of heartburn and other symptoms associated with GERD.

Erosive Esophagitis

Omeprazole delayed-release capsules are indicated for the short-term treatment (4-8 weeks) of erosive esophagitis which has been diagnosed by endoscopy.

The efficacy of omeprazole used for longer than 8 weeks in these patients has not been established. In the rare instance of a patient not responding to 8 weeks of treatment, it may be helpful to give up to an additional 4 weeks of treatment. If there is recurrence of erosive esophagitis or GERD symptoms (*e.g.*, heartburn), additional 4-8 week courses of omeprazole may be considered.

MAINTENANCE OF HEALING OF EROSIVE ESOPHAGITIS

Omeprazole delayed-release capsules are indicated to maintain healing of erosive esophagitis.

Controlled studies do not extend beyond 12 months.

PATHOLOGICAL HYPERSECRETORY CONDITIONS

Omeprazole delayed-release capsules are indicated for the long-term treatment of pathological hypersecretory conditions (*e.g.*, Zollinger-Ellison syndrome, multiple endocrine adenomas and systemic mastocytosis).

NON-FDA APPROVED INDICATIONS

Omeprazole is also used for duodenal ulcer maintenance, although not FDA-approved.

CONTRAINDICATIONS

OMEPRAZOLE

Omeprazole delayed-release capsules are contraindicated in patients with known hypersensitivity to any component of the formulation.

CLARITHROMYCIN

Clarithromycin is contraindicated in patients with a known hypersensitivity to any macrolide antibiotic.

Concomitant administration of clarithromycin with cisapride, pimozide, or terfenadine is contraindicated. There have been post-marketing reports of drug interactions when clarithromycin and/or erythromycin are co-administered with cisapride, pimozide, or terfenadine resulting in cardiac arrhythmias (QT prolongation, ventricular tachycardia, ventricular fibrillation, and torsades de pointes) most likely due to inhibition of hepatic metabolism of these drugs by erythromycin and clarithromycin. Fatalities have been reported. (Please refer to full prescribing information for clarithromycin before prescribing.)

AMOXICILLIN

Amoxicillin is contraindicated in patients with a history of allergic reaction to any of the penicillins. (Please refer to full prescribing information for amoxicillin before prescribing.)

WARNINGS

CLARITHROMYCIN

CLARITHROMYCIN SHOULD NOT BE USED IN PREGNANT WOMEN EXCEPT IN CLINICAL CIRCUMSTANCES WHERE NO ALTERNATIVE THERAPY IS APPROPRIATE. IF PREGNANCY OCCURS WHILE TAKING CLARITHROMYCIN, THE PATIENT SHOULD BE APPRISED OF THE POTENTIAL HAZARD TO THE FETUS. (See WARNINGS in prescribing information for clarithromycin.)

AMOXICILLIN

SERIOUS AND OCCASIONALLY FATAL HYPERSENSITIVITY (ANAPHYLACTIC) REACTIONS HAVE BEEN REPORTED IN PATIENTS ON PENICILLIN THERAPY. THESE REACTIONS ARE MORE LIKELY TO OCCUR IN INDIVIDUALS WITH A HISTORY OF PENICILLIN HYPERSENSITIVITY AND/OR A HISTORY OF SENSITIVITY TO MULTIPLE ALLERGENS. BEFORE INITIATING THERAPY WITH AMOXICILLIN, CAREFUL INQUIRY SHOULD BE MADE CONCERNING PREVIOUS HYPERSENSITIVITY REACTIONS TO PENICILLINS, CEPHALOSPORINS OR OTHER ALLERGENS. IF AN ALLERGIC REACTION OCCURS, AMOXICILLIN SHOULD BE DISCONTINUED AND APPROPRIATE THERAPY INSTITUTED. **SERIOUS ANAPHYLACTIC REACTIONS REQUIRE IMMEDIATE EMERGENCY TREATMENT WITH EPINEPHRINE. OXYGEN, INTRAVENOUS STEROIDS AND AIRWAY MANAGEMENT, INCLUDING INTUBATION, SHOULD ALSO BE ADMINISTERED AS INDICATED.** (See WARNINGS in prescribing information for amoxicillin.)

ANTIMICROBIALS

Pseudomembranous colitis has been reported with nearly all antibacterial agents and may range in severity from mild to life-threatening. Therefore, it is important to consider this diagnosis in patients who present with diarrhea subsequent to the administration of antibacterial agents. (See WARNINGS in prescribing information for clarithromycin and amoxicillin.)

Treatment with antibacterial agents alters the normal flora of the colon and may permit overgrowth of clostridia. Studies indicate that a toxin produced by *Clostridium difficile* is a primary cause of "antibiotic-associated colitis."

After the diagnosis of pseudomembranous colitis has been established, therapeutic measures should be initiated. Mild cases of pseudomembranous colitis usually respond to discontinuation of the drug alone. In moderate to severe cases, consideration should be given to management with fluids and electrolytes, protein supplementation, and treatment with an antibacterial drug clinically effective against *Clostridium difficile* colitis.

PRECAUTIONS

GENERAL

Symptomatic response to therapy with omeprazole does not preclude the presence of gastric malignancy.

Atrophic gastritis has been noted occasionally in gastric corpus biopsies from patients treated long-term with omeprazole.

INFORMATION FOR THE PATIENT

Omeprazole delayed-release capsules should be taken before eating. Patients should be cautioned that the omeprazole delayed-release capsule should not be opened, chewed or crushed, and should be swallowed whole.

For patients who have difficulty swallowing capsules, the contents of a omeprazole delayed-release capsule can be added to applesauce. One tablespoon of applesauce should be added to an empty bowl and the capsule should be opened. All of the pellets inside the capsule should be carefully emptied on the applesauce. The pellets should be mixed with the applesauce and then swallowed immediately with a glass of cool water to ensure complete swallowing of the pellets. The applesauce used should not be hot and should be soft enough to be swallowed without chewing. The pellets should not be chewed or crushed. The pellets/applesauce mixture should not be stored for future use.

CARCINOGENESIS, MUTAGENESIS, AND IMPAIRMENT OF FERTILITY

In two 24 month carcinogenicity studies in rats, omeprazole at daily doses of 1.7, 3.4, 13.8, 44.0, and 140.8 mg/kg/day (approximately 4-352 times the human dose, based on a patient weight of 50 kg and a human dose of 20 mg) produced gastric ECL cell carcinoids in a dose-related manner in both male and female rats; the incidence of this effect was markedly higher in female rats, which had higher blood levels of omeprazole. Gastric carcinoids seldom occur in the untreated rat. In addition, ECL cell hyperplasia was present in all treated groups of both sexes. In 1 of these studies, female rats were treated with 13.8 mg omeprazole/kg/day (approximately 35 times the human dose) for 1 year, then followed for an additional year without the drug. No carcinoids were seen in these rats. An increased incidence of treatment-related ECL cell hyperplasia was observed at the end of 1 year (94% treated versus 10% controls). By the second year the difference between treated and control rats was much smaller (46% vs 26%) but still showed more hyperplasia in the treated group. An unusual primary malignant tumor in the stomach was seen in 1 rat (2%). No similar tumor was seen in male or female rats treated for 2 years. For this strain of rat no similar tumor has been noted historically, but a finding involving only 1 tumor is difficult to interpret. A 78 week mouse carcinogenicity study of omeprazole did not show increased tumor occurrence, but the study was not conclusive. A 26 week p53± transgenic mouse carcinogenicity study was not positive.

Omeprazole was not mutagenic in an *in vitro* Ames *Salmonella typhimurium* assay, an *in vitro* mouse lymphoma cell assay and an *in vivo* rat liver DNA damage assay. A mouse micronucleus test at 625 and 6250 times the human dose gave a borderline result, as did an *in vivo* bone marrow chromosome aberration test. A second mouse micronucleus study at 2000 times the human dose, but with different (suboptimal) sampling times, was negative.

In a rat fertility and general reproductive performance test, omeprazole in a dose range of 13.8-138.0 mg/kg/day (approximately 35-345 times the human dose) was not toxic or deleterious to the reproductive performance of parental animals.

PREGNANCY CATEGORY C

Omeprazole

Teratology studies conducted in pregnant rats at doses up to 138 mg/kg/day (approximately 345 times the human dose) and in pregnant rabbits at doses up to 69 mg/kg/day (approximately 172 times the human dose) did not disclose any evidence for a teratogenic potential of omeprazole.

In rabbits, omeprazole in a dose range of 6.9-69.1 mg/kg/day (approximately 17-172 times the human dose) produced dose-related increases in embryo-lethality, fetal resorptions and pregnancy disruptions. In rats, dose-related embryo/fetal toxicity and postnatal developmental toxicity were observed in offspring resulting from parents treated with omeprazole 13.8-138.0 mg/kg/day (approximately 35-345 times the human dose). There are no adequate or well-controlled studies in pregnant women. Sporadic reports have been received of congenital abnormalities occurring in infants born to women who have received omeprazole during pregnancy. Omeprazole should be used during pregnancy only if the potential benefit justifies the potential risk to the fetus.

Clarithromycin

See WARNINGS and full prescribing information for clarithromycin before using in pregnant women.

NURSING MOTHERS

It is not known whether omeprazole is excreted in human milk. In rats, omeprazole administration during late gestation and lactation at doses of 13.8 to 138 mg/kg/day (35-345 times the human dose) resulted in decreased weight gain in pups. Because many drugs are excreted in human milk, because of the potential for serious adverse reactions in nursing infants from omeprazole, and because of the potential for tumorigenicity shown for omeprazole in rat carcinogenicity studies, a decision should be made whether to discontinue nursing or to discontinue the drug, taking into account the importance of the drug to the mother.

PEDIATRIC USE

The safety and effectiveness of omeprazole have been established in the age group 2-16 years for the treatment of acid-related gastrointestinal diseases, including the treatment of symptomatic GERD, treatment of erosive esophagitis, and the maintenance of healing of erosive esophagitis. The safety and effectiveness of omeprazole have not been established for pediatric patients less than 2 years of age. Use of omeprazole in the age group 2-16 years is supported by evidence from adequate and well-controlled studies of omeprazole in adults with additional clinical, pharmacokinetic, and safety studies performed in pediatric patients (see CLINICAL PHARMACOLOGY, Pharmacokinetics and Metabolism, Omeprazole).

Treatment of Gastroesophageal Reflux Disease (GERD)

Symptomatic GERD

In an uncontrolled, open-label study of patients aged 2-16 years with a history of symptoms suggestive of nonerosive GERD, 113 patients were assigned to receive a single daily dose of omeprazole (10 or 20 mg, based on body weight) either as an intact capsule or as an open capsule in applesauce. Results showed success rates of 60% (10 mg omeprazole) and 59% (20 mg omeprazole) in reducing the number and intensity of either pain-related symptoms or vomiting/regurgitation episodes.

Erosive Esophagitis

In an uncontrolled, open-label dose-titration study, healing of erosive esophagitis in pediatric patients aged 1-16 years required doses that ranged from 0.7-3.5 mg/kg/day (80 mg/day). Doses were initiated at 0.7 mg/kg/day. Doses were increased in increments of 0.7 mg/kg/day (if intraesophageal pH showed a pH of <4 for less than 6% of a 24 hour study). After titration, patients remained on treatment for 3 months. Forty-four percent (44%) of the patients were healed on a dose of 0.7 mg/kg body weight; most of the remaining patients were healed with 1.4 mg/kg after an additional 3 months' treatment. Erosive esophagitis was healed in 51 of 57 (90%) children who completed the first course of treatment in the healing phase of the study. In addition, after 3 months of treatment, 33% of the children had no overall symptoms, 57% had mild reflux symptoms, and 40% had less frequent regurgitation/vomiting.

Maintenance of Healing of Erosive Esophagitis

In an uncontrolled, open-label study of maintenance of healing of erosive esophagitis in 46 pediatric patients, 54% of patients required half the healing dose. The remaining patients increased the healing dose (0.7 to a maximum of 2.8 mg/kg/day) either for the entire maintenance period, or returned to half the dose before completion. Of the 46 patients who entered the maintenance phase, 19 (41%) had no relapse. In addition, maintenance therapy in erosive esophagitis patients resulted in 63% of patients having no overall symptoms.

Safety

The safety of omeprazole delayed-release capsules has been assessed in 310 pediatric patients aged 0-16 years and 62 physiologically normal volunteers aged 2-16 years. Of the 310 pediatric patients with acid-related disease, a group of 46 who had documented healing of erosive esophagitis after 3 months of treatment continued on maintenance therapy for up to 749 days.

Omeprazole delayed-release capsules administered to pediatric patients was generally well tolerated with an adverse event profile resembling that in adults. Unique to the pediatric population, however, adverse events of the respiratory system were most frequently reported in both the 0-2 year and 2-16 year age groups (46.2% and 18.5%, respectively). Similarly, otitis media was frequently reported in the 0-2 year age group (22.6%), and accidental injuries were reported frequently in the 2-16 year age group (3.8%).

GERIATRIC USE

Omeprazole was administered to over 2000 elderly individuals (≥65 years of age) in clinical trials in the US and Europe. There were no differences in safety and effectiveness between the elderly and younger subjects. Other reported clinical experience has not identified differences in response between the elderly and younger subjects, but greater sensitivity of some older individuals cannot be ruled out.

Pharmacokinetic studies have shown the elimination rate was somewhat decreased in the elderly and bioavailability was increased. The plasma clearance of omeprazole was 250 ml/min (about half that of young volunteers) and its plasma half-life averaged 1 hour, about twice that of young healthy volunteers. However, no dosage adjustment is necessary in the elderly. (See CLINICAL PHARMACOLOGY.)

DRUG INTERACTIONS

OTHER

Omeprazole can prolong the elimination of diazepam, warfarin, and phenytoin, drugs that are metabolized by oxidation in the liver. Although in normal subjects no interaction with theophylline or propranolol was found, there have been clinical reports of interaction with other drugs metabolized via the cytochrome P450 system (*e.g.,* cyclosporine, disulfiram, benzodiazepines). Patients should be monitored to determine if it is necessary to adjust the dosage of these drugs when taken concomitantly with omeprazole.

Because of its profound and long lasting inhibition of gastric acid secretion, it is theoretically possible that omeprazole may interfere with absorption of drugs where gastric pH is an important determinant of their bioavailability (*e.g.,* ketoconazole, ampicillin esters, and iron salts). In the clinical trials, antacids were used concomitantly with the administration of omeprazole.

COMBINATION THERAPY WITH CLARITHROMYCIN

Coadministration of omeprazole and clarithromycin have resulted in increases in plasma levels of omeprazole, clarithromycin, and 14-hydroxy-clarithromycin. (See also CLINICAL PHARMACOLOGY, Pharmacokinetics, Combination Therapy With Antimicrobials.)

Concomitant administration of clarithromycin with cisapride, pimozide, or terfenadine is contraindicated.

There have been reports of an interaction between erythromycin and astemizole resulting in QT prolongation and torsades de pointes. Concomitant administration of erythromycin and astemizole is contraindicated. Because clarithromycin is also metabolized by cytochrome P450, concomitant administration of clarithromycin with astemizole is not recommended. (See also CONTRAINDICATIONS, Clarithromycin. Please refer to full prescribing information for clarithromycin before prescribing.)

ADVERSE REACTIONS

Omeprazole delayed-release capsules were generally well tolerated during domestic and international clinical trials in 3096 patients.

In the US clinical trial population of 465 patients (including duodenal ulcer, Zollinger-Ellison syndrome and resistant ulcer patients), the following adverse experiences were reported to occur in 1% or more of patients on therapy with omeprazole. Numbers in parentheses indicate percentages of the adverse experiences considered by investigators as possibly, probably, or definitely related to the drug (TABLE 19).

The following adverse reactions which occurred in 1% or more of omeprazole-treated patients have been reported in international double-blind, and open-label, clinical trials in which 2631 patients and subjects received omeprazole (TABLE 20).

Additional adverse experiences occurring in <1% of patients or subjects in domestic and/or international trials, or occurring since the drug was marketed, are shown below within each body system. In many instances, the relationship to omeprazole was unclear.

Body as a Whole: Allergic reactions, including, rarely, anaphylaxis (see also Skin), fever, pain, fatigue, malaise, abdominal swelling.

Cardiovascular: Chest pain or angina, tachycardia, bradycardia, palpitation, elevated blood pressure, peripheral edema.

Gastrointestinal: Pancreatitis (some fatal), anorexia, irritable colon, flatulence, fecal discoloration, esophageal candidiasis, mucosal atrophy of the tongue, dry mouth.

TABLE 19

	Omeprazole (n=465)	Placebo (n=64)	Ranitidine (n=195)
Headache	6.9 (2.4%)	6.3	7.7 (2.6%)
Diarrhea	3.0 (1.9%)	3.1 (1.6%)	2.1 (0.5%)
Abdominal pain	2.4 (0.4%)	3.1	2.1
Nausea	2.2 (0.9%)	3.1	4.1 (0.5%)
URI	1.9	1.6	2.6
Dizziness	1.5 (0.6%)	0.0	2.6 (1.0%)
Vomiting	1.5 (0.4%)	4.7	1.5 (0.5%)
Rash	1.5 (1.1%)	0.0	0.0
Constipation	1.1 (0.9%)	0.0	0.0
Cough	1.1	0.0	1.5
Asthenia	1.1 (0.2%)	1.6 (1.6%)	1.5 (1.0%)
Back pain	1.1	0.0	0.5

TABLE 20 *Incidence of Adverse Experiences ≥1% — Causal Relationship Not Assessed*

	Omeprazole (n=2631)	Placebo (n=120)
Body as a Whole, Site Unspecified		
Abdominal pain	5.2%	3.3%
Asthenia	1.3%	0.8%
Digestive System		
Constipation	1.5%	0.8%
Diarrhea	3.7%	2.5%
Flatulence	2.7%	5.8%
Nausea	4.0%	6.7%
Vomiting	3.2%	10.0%
Acid regurgitation	1.9%	3.3%
Nervous System/Psychiatric		
Headache	2.9%	2.5%

During treatment with omeprazole, gastric fundic gland polyps have been noted rarely. These polyps are benign and appear to be reversible when treatment is discontinued.

Gastro-duodenal carcinoids have been reported in patients with ZE syndrome on long-term treatment with omeprazole. This finding is believed to be a manifestation of the underlying condition, which is known to be associated with such tumors.

Hepatic: Mild and, rarely, marked elevations of liver function tests [ALT (SGPT), AST (SGOT), γ-glutamyl transpeptidase, alkaline phosphatase, and bilirubin (jaundice)]. In rare instances, overt liver disease has occurred, including hepatocellular, cholestatic, or mixed hepatitis, liver necrosis (some fatal), hepatic failure (some fatal), and hepatic encephalopathy.

Metabolic/Nutritional: Hyponatremia, hypoglycemia, weight gain.

Musculoskeletal: Muscle cramps, myalgia, muscle weakness, joint pain, leg pain.

Nervous System/Psychiatric: Psychic disturbances including depression, aggression, hallucinations, confusion, insomnia, nervousness, tremors, apathy, somnolence, anxiety, dream abnormalities; vertigo; paresthesia; hemifacial dysesthesia.

Respiratory: Epistaxis, pharyngeal pain.

Skin: Rash and, rarely, cases of severe generalized skin reactions including toxic epidermal necrolysis (TEN; some fatal), Stevens-Johnson syndrome, and erythema multiforme (some severe); purpura and/or petechiae (some with rechallenge); skin inflammation, urticaria, angioedema, pruritus, alopecia, dry skin, hyperhidrosis.

Special Senses: Tinnitus, taste perversion.

Urogenital: Interstitial nephritis (some with positive rechallenge), urinary tract infection, microscopic pyuria, urinary frequency, elevated serum creatinine, proteinuria, hematuria, glycosuria, testicular pain, gynecomastia.

Hematologic: Rare instances of pancytopenia, agranulocytosis (some fatal), thrombocytopenia, neutropenia, anemia, leucocytosis, and hemolytic anemia have been reported.

The incidence of clinical adverse experiences in patients greater than 65 years of age was similar to that in patients 65 years of age or less.

COMBINATION THERAPY FOR H. PYLORI ERADICATION

In clinical trials using either dual therapy with omeprazole and clarithromycin, or triple therapy with omeprazole, clarithromycin, and amoxicillin, no adverse experiences peculiar to these drug combinations have been observed. Adverse experiences that have occurred have been limited to those that have been previously reported with omeprazole, clarithromycin, or amoxicillin.

Triple Therapy (omeprazole/clarithromycin/amoxicillin)

The most frequent adverse experiences observed in clinical trials using combination therapy with omeprazole, clarithromycin, and amoxicillin (n=274) were diarrhea (14%), taste perversion (10%), and headache (7%). None of these occurred at a higher frequency than that reported by patients taking the antimicrobial drugs alone.

For more information on clarithromycin or amoxicillin, refer to the respective package inserts, ADVERSE REACTIONS sections.

Dual Therapy (omeprazole/clarithromycin)

Adverse experiences observed in controlled clinical trials using combination therapy with omeprazole and clarithromycin (n=346) which differed from those previously described for omeprazole alone were: taste perversion (15%), tongue discoloration (2%), rhinitis (2%), pharyngitis (1%), and flu syndrome (1%).

For more information on clarithromycin, refer to the clarithromycin package insert, ADVERSE REACTIONS section.

DOSAGE AND ADMINISTRATION

SHORT-TERM TREATMENT OF ACTIVE DUODENAL ULCER

The recommended adult oral dose of omeprazole is 20 mg once daily. Most patients heal within 4 weeks. Some patients may require an additional 4 weeks of therapy. (See INDICATIONS AND USAGE.)

H. PYLORI ERADICATION FOR THE REDUCTION OF THE RISK OF DUODENAL ULCER RECURRENCE

Triple Therapy (omeprazole/clarithromycin/amoxicillin)

The recommended adult oral regimen is omeprazole 20 mg plus clarithromycin 500 mg plus amoxicillin 1000 mg each given twice daily for 10 days. In patients with an ulcer present at the time of initiation of therapy, an additional 18 days of omeprazole 20 mg once daily is recommended for ulcer healing and symptom relief.

Dual Therapy (omeprazole/clarithromycin)

The recommended adult oral regimen is omeprazole 40 mg once daily plus clarithromycin 500 mg tid for 14 days. In patients with an ulcer present at the time of initiation of therapy, an additional 14 days of omeprazole 20 mg once daily is recommended for ulcer healing and symptom relief.

Please refer to clarithromycin full prescribing information for CONTRAINDICATIONS and WARNINGS, and for information regarding dosing in elderly and renally impaired patients (PRECAUTIONS: General and Geriatric Use; and DRUG INTERACTIONS).

Please refer to amoxicillin full prescribing information for CONTRAINDICATIONS and WARNINGS.

GASTRIC ULCER

The recommended adult oral dose is 40 mg once a day for 4-8 weeks. (See INDICATIONS AND USAGE, Gastric Ulcer.)

GASTROESOPHAGEAL REFLUX DISEASE (GERD)

The recommended adult oral dose for the treatment of patients with symptomatic GERD and no esophageal lesions is 20 mg daily for up to 4 weeks. The recommended adult oral dose for the treatment of patients with erosive esophagitis and accompanying symptoms due to GERD is 20 mg daily for 4-8 weeks. (See INDICATIONS AND USAGE.)

MAINTENANCE OF HEALING OF EROSIVE ESOPHAGITIS

The recommended adult oral dose is 20 mg daily.

PATHOLOGICAL HYPERSECRETORY CONDITIONS

The dosage of omeprazole in patients with pathological hypersecretory conditions varies with the individual patient. The recommended adult oral starting dose is 60 mg once a day. Doses should be adjusted to individual patient needs and should continue for as long as clinically indicated. Doses up to 120 mg tid have been administered. Daily dosages of greater than 80 mg should be administered in divided doses. Some patients with Zollinger-Ellison syndrome have been treated continuously with omeprazole for more than 5 years.

Pediatric Patients

For the treatment of GERD or other acid-related disorders, the recommended dose for pediatric patients 2 years of age and older is shown in TABLE 21.

TABLE 21

Patient Weight	Omeprazole Dose
<20 kg	10 mg
≥20 kg	20 mg

On a per kg basis, the doses of omeprazole required to heal erosive esophagitis are greater than those for adults.

For pediatric patients unable to swallow an intact capsule, see Alternative Administration Options below.

Alternative Administration Options

For patients who have difficulty swallowing capsules, the contents of a omeprazole delayed-release capsule can be added to applesauce. One tablespoon of applesauce should be added to an empty bowl and the capsule should be opened. All of the pellets inside the capsule should be carefully emptied on the applesauce. The pellets should be mixed with the applesauce and then swallowed immediately with a glass of cool water to ensure complete swallowing of the pellets. The applesauce used should not be hot and should be soft enough to be swallowed without chewing. The pellets should not be chewed or crushed. The pellets/applesauce mixture should not be stored for future use.

No dosage adjustment is necessary for patients with renal impairment or for the elderly.

Omeprazole delayed-release capsules should be taken before eating. In the clinical trials, antacids were used concomitantly with omeprazole.

Patients should be cautioned that the omeprazole delayed-release capsule should not be opened, chewed or crushed, and should be swallowed whole.

HOW SUPPLIED

Prilosec delayed-release capsules are available as follows:

10 mg: Opaque, hard gelatin, apricot and amethyst colored capsules, coded "606" on cap and "PRILOSEC 10" on the body.

20 mg: Opaque, hard gelatin, amethyst colored capsules, coded "742" on cap and "PRILOSEC 20" on body.

40 mg: Opaque, hard gelatin, apricot and amethyst colored capsules, coded "743" on cap and "PRILOSEC 40" on the body.

Storage: Store Prilosec delayed-release capsules in a tight container protected from light and moisture. Store between 15 and 30°C (59 and 86°F).

PRODUCT LISTING - EQUIVALENTS NOT AVAILABLE

Capsule, Enteric Coated - Oral - 10 mg

Qty	Price	Product	NDC
30's	$107.12	PRILOSEC, Allscripts Pharmaceutical Company	54569-4828-00
30's	$124.02	PRILOSEC, Astra-Zeneca Pharmaceuticals	00186-0606-31
100's	$413.39	PRILOSEC, Astra-Zeneca Pharmaceuticals	00186-0606-28
100's	$413.39	PRILOSEC, Astra-Zeneca Pharmaceuticals	00186-0606-68

Capsule, Enteric Coated - Oral - 20 mg

Qty	Price	Product	NDC
2's	$8.28	PRILOSEC, Allscripts Pharmaceutical Company	54569-3267-02
6's	$32.07	PRILOSEC, Quality Care Pharmaceuticals Inc	62682-4001-06
10's	$49.75	PRILOSEC, Pharma Pac	52959-0536-10
14's	$65.00	PRILOSEC, Pharma Pac	52959-0536-14
28's	$176.84	PRILOSEC, Pd-Rx Pharmaceuticals	55289-0394-28
30's	$121.60	PRILOSEC, Physicians Total Care	54868-2169-01
30's	$124.18	PRILOSEC, Allscripts Pharmaceutical Company	54569-3267-00
30's	$124.58	GENERIC, Kremers Urban	62175-0118-32
30's	$125.24	PRILOSEC, Cheshire Drugs	55175-2819-03
30's	$127.61	PRILOSEC, Pharma Pac	52959-0536-30
30's	$138.44	PRILOSEC, Astra-Zeneca Pharmaceuticals	00186-0742-31
30's	$138.44	PRILOSEC, Southwood Pharmaceuticals Inc	58016-0327-30
60's	$267.88	PRILOSEC, Southwood Pharmaceuticals Inc	58016-0327-60
90's	$340.32	PRILOSEC, Allscripts Pharmaceutical Company	54569-8550-00
100's	$376.81	PRILOSEC, Astra-Zeneca Pharmaceuticals	61113-0742-28
100's	$403.95	PRILOSEC, Physicians Total Care	54868-2169-00
100's	$415.27	GENERIC, Kremers Urban	62175-0118-37
100's	$461.44	PRILOSEC, Astra-Zeneca Pharmaceuticals	00186-0742-28
100's	$461.47	PRILOSEC, Southwood Pharmaceuticals Inc	58016-0327-00

Capsule, Enteric Coated - Oral - 40 mg

Qty	Price	Product	NDC
30's	$190.70	PRILOSEC, Astra-Zeneca Pharmaceuticals	61113-0743-31
30's	$198.65	PRILOSEC, Astra-Zeneca Pharmaceuticals	00186-0743-31
100's	$594.00	PRILOSEC, Astra-Zeneca Pharmaceuticals	00186-0743-28
100's	$594.00	PRILOSEC, Astra-Zeneca Pharmaceuticals	61113-0743-28
100's	$594.00	PRILOSEC, Astra-Zeneca Pharmaceuticals	61113-0743-68
100's	$662.18	PRILOSEC, Astra-Zeneca Pharmaceuticals	00186-0743-68

Ondansetron Hydrochloride *(003031)*

Categories: Nausea, postoperative; Nausea, secondary to cancer chemotherapy; Nausea, secondary to radiation therapy; Vomiting, postoperative; Vomiting, secondary to cancer chemotherapy; Vomiting, secondary to radiation therapy; Pregnancy Category B; FDA Approved 1991 Jan; Patent Expiration 2005 Jun

Drug Classes: Antiemetics/antivertigo; Serotonin receptor antagonists

Brand Names: **Zofran**

Foreign Brand Availability: Bryterol (Colombia); Cedantron (Indonesia); Emeset (China; India; Korea); Modifical (Colombia); Narfoz (Indonesia); Onsia (Thailand); Sakisozin (Japan); Vomceran (Indonesia); Zetron (Thailand); Zofran Zydis (Korea); Zofron (Greece); Zophren (France)

Cost of Therapy: \$133.45 (Nausea; Zofran; 8 mg; 2 tablets/day; 2 day supply)
\$125.89 (Nausea; Zofran ODT; 8 mg; 2 tablets/day; 2 day supply)

HCFA JCODE(S): J2405 1 mg IV

IM-IV

DESCRIPTION

The active ingredient in Zofran injection and Zofran injection premixed is ondansetron hydrochloride (HCl), the racemic form of ondansetron and a selective blocking agent of the serotonin 5-HT_3 receptor type. Chemically it is (±)1,2,3, 9-tetrahydro-9-methyl-3-[(2-methyl-1H-imidazol-1-yl)methyl]-4H-carbazol-4-one, monohydrochloride, dihydrate.

The empirical formula is $C_{18}H_{19}N_3O{\cdot}HCl{\cdot}2H_2O$, representing a molecular weight of 365.9.

Ondansetron HCl is a white to off-white powder that is soluble in water and normal saline.

STERILE INJECTION FOR INTRAVENOUS (IV) OR INTRAMUSCULAR (IM) ADMINISTRATION

Each 1 ml of aqueous solution in the 2 ml single-dose vial contains 2 mg of ondansetron as the hydrochloride dihydrate; 9.0 mg of sodium chloride, and 0.5 mg of citric acid monohydrate and 0.25 mg of sodium citrate dihydrate, as buffers in water for injection.

Each 1 ml of aqueous solution in the 20 ml multidose vial contains 2 mg of ondansetron as the hydrochloride dihydrate; 8.3 mg of sodium chloride, 0.5 mg of citric acid monohydrate, and 0.25 mg of sodium citrate dihydrate, as buffers; and 1.2 mg of methylparaben, and 0.15 mg of propylparaben, as preservatives in water for injection.

Zofran injection is a clear, colorless, nonpyrogenic, sterile solution. The pH of the injection solution is 3.3-4.0.

STERILE, PREMIXED SOLUTION FOR IV ADMINISTRATION IN SINGLE-DOSE, FLEXIBLE PLASTIC CONTAINERS

Each 50 ml contains ondansetron 32 mg (as the hydrochloride dihydrate); dextrose 2500 mg; and citric acid 26 mg and sodium citrate 11.5 mg as buffers in water for injection. It contains no preservatives. The osmolarity of this solution is 270 mOsm/L (approx.), and the pH is 3.0-4.0.

The flexible plastic container is fabricated from a specially formulated, nonplasticized, thermoplastic co-polyester (CR3). Water can permeate from inside the container into the overwrap but not in amounts sufficient to affect the solution significantly. Solutions inside the plastic container also can leach out certain of the chemical components in very small amounts before the expiration period is attained. However, the safety of the plastic has been confirmed by tests in animals according to USP biological standards for plastic containers.

CLINICAL PHARMACOLOGY

PHARMACODYNAMICS

Ondansetron is a selective 5-HT_3 receptor antagonist. While ondansetron's mechanism of action has not been fully characterized, it is not a dopamine-receptor antagonist. Serotonin receptors of the 5-HT_3 type are present both peripherally on vagal nerve terminals and centrally in the chemoreceptor trigger zone of the area postrema. It is not certain whether ondansetron's antiemetic action in chemotherapy-induced emesis is mediated centrally, peripherally, or in both sites. However, cytotoxic chemotherapy appears to be associated with release of serotonin from the enterochromaffin cells of the small intestine. In humans, urinary 5-HIAA (5-hydroxyindoleacetic acid) excretion increases after cisplatin administration in parallel with the onset of emesis. The released serotonin may stimulate the vagal afferents through the 5-HT_3 receptors and initiate the vomiting reflex.

In animals, the emetic response to cisplatin can be prevented by pretreatment with an inhibitor of serotonin synthesis, bilateral abdominal vagotomy and greater splanchnic nerve section, or pretreatment with a serotonin 5-HT_3 receptor antagonist.

In normal volunteers, single IV doses of 0.15 mg/kg of ondansetron had no effect on esophageal motility, gastric motility, lower esophageal sphincter pressure, or small intestinal transit time. In another study in 6 normal male volunteers, a 16 mg dose infused over 5 minutes showed no effect of the drug on cardiac output, heart rate, stroke volume, blood pressure, or electrocardiogram (ECG). Multiday administration of ondansetron has been shown to slow colonic transit in normal volunteers. Ondansetron has no effect on plasma prolactin concentrations.

In a gender-balanced pharmacodynamic study (n=56), ondansetron 4 mg administered intravenously or intramuscularly was dynamically similar in the prevention of emesis and nausea using the ipecacuanha model of emesis. Both treatments were well tolerated.

Ondansetron does not alter the respiratory depressant effects produced by alfentanil or the degree of neuromuscular blockade produced by atracurium. Interactions with general or local anesthetics have not been studied.

PHARMACOKINETICS

Ondansetron is extensively metabolized in humans, with approximately 5% of a radiolabeled dose recovered as the parent compound from the urine. The primary metabolic pathway is hydroxylation on the indole ring followed by glucuronide or sulfate conjugation.

Although some nonconjugated metabolites have pharmacologic activity, these are not found in plasma at concentrations likely to significantly contribute to the biological activity of ondansetron.

In vitro metabolism studies have shown that ondansetron is a substrate for human hepatic cytochrome P-450 enzymes, including CYP1A2, CYP2D6, and CYP3A4. In terms of overall ondansetron turnover, CYP3A4 played the predominant role. Because of the multiplicity of metabolic enzymes capable of metabolizing ondansetron, it is likely that inhibition or loss of one enzyme (*e.g.,* CYP2D6 genetic deficiency) will be compensated by others and may result in little change in overall rates of ondansetron elimination. Ondansetron elimination may be affected by cytochrome P-450 inducers. In a pharmacokinetic study of 16 epileptic patients maintained chronically on carbamazepine or phenytoin, reduction in AUC, C_{max} and $T_{1/2}$ of ondansetron was observed. This resulted in a significant increase in clearance. However, on the basis of available data, no dosage adjustment is recommended (see DRUG INTERACTIONS).

In normal volunteers, the following mean pharmacokinetic data have been determined following a single 0.15 mg/kg IV dose.

TABLE 1 *Pharmacokinetics in Normal Volunteers*

	Age-Group		
	19-40	61-74	≥75
	n=11	n=12	n=11
Peak plasma concentration (ng/ml)	102	106	170
Mean elimination half-life (h)	3.5	4.7	5.5
Plasma clearance (L/h/kg)	0.381	0.319	0.262

A reduction in clearance and increase in elimination half-life are seen in patients over 75 years of age. In clinical trials with cancer patients, safety and efficacy were similar in patients over 65 years of age and those under 65 years of age; there was an insufficient number of patients over 75 years of age to permit conclusions in that age-group. No dosage adjustment is recommended in the elderly.

In patients with mild-to-moderate hepatic impairment, clearance is reduced 2-fold and mean half-life is increased to 11.6 hours compared to 5.7 hours in normals. In patients with severe hepatic impairment (Child-Pugh score[1] of 10 or greater), clearance is reduced 2- to 3-fold and apparent volume of distribution is increased with a resultant increase in half-life to 20 hours. In patients with severe hepatic impairment, a total daily dose of 8 mg should not be exceeded.

Due to the very small contribution (5%) of renal clearance to the overall clearance, renal impairment was not expected to significantly influence the total clearance of ondansetron. However, ondansetron mean plasma clearance was reduced by about 41% in patients with severe renal impairment (creatinine clearance <30 ml/min). This reduction in clearance is variable and was not consistent with an increase in half-life. No reduction in dose or dosing frequency in these patients is warranted.

In adult cancer patients, the mean elimination half-life was 4.0 hours, and there was no difference in the multidose pharmacokinetics over a 4 day period. In a study of 21 pediatric cancer patients (aged 4-18 years) who received 3 IV doses of 0.15 mg/kg of ondansetron at 4 hour intervals, patients older than 15 years of age exhibited ondansetron pharmacokinetic parameters similar to those of adults. Patients aged 4-12 years generally showed higher clearance and somewhat larger volume of distribution than adults. Most pediatric patients younger than 15 years of age with cancer had a shorter (2.4 hours) ondansetron plasma half-life than patients older than 15 years of age. It is not known whether these differences in ondansetron plasma half-life may result in differences in efficacy between adults and some young pediatric patients.

In a study of 21 pediatric patients (aged 3-12 years) who were undergoing surgery requiring anesthesia for a duration of 45 minutes to 2 hours, a single IV dose of ondansetron, 2 mg (3-7 years) or 4 mg (8-12 years), was administered immediately prior to anesthesia induction. Mean weight-normalized clearance and volume of distribution values in these pediatric surgical patients were similar to those previously reported for young adults. Mean terminal half-life was slightly reduced in pediatric patients (range, 2.5 to 3 hours) in comparison with adults (range, 3 to 3.5 hours).

In normal volunteers (19-39 years old, n=23), the peak plasma concentration was 264 ng/ml following a single 32 mg dose administered as a 15 minute IV infusion. The mean elimination half-life was 4.1 hours. Systemic exposure to 32 mg of ondansetron was not proportional to dose as measured by comparing dose-normalized AUC values to an 8 mg dose. This is consistent with a small decrease in systemic clearance with increasing plasma concentrations.

A study was performed in normal volunteers (n=56) to evaluate the pharmacokinetics of a single 4 mg dose administered as a 5 minute infusion compared to a single IM injection. Systemic exposure as measured by mean AUC was equivalent, with values of 156 [95% CI 136, 180] and 161 [95% CI 137, 190] ng·h/ml for IV and IM groups, respectively. Mean peak plasma concentrations were 42.9 [95% CI 33.8, 54.4] ng/ml at 10 minutes after IV infusion and 31.9 [95% CI 26.3, 38.6] ng/ml at 41 minutes after IM injection. The mean elimination half-life was not affected by route of administration.

Plasma protein binding of ondansetron as measured *in vitro* was 70-76%, with binding constant over the pharmacologic concentration range (10-500 ng/ml). Circulating drug also distributes into erythrocytes.

A positive lymphoblast transformation test to ondansetron has been reported, which suggests immunologic sensitivity to ondansetron.

INDICATIONS AND USAGE

Prevention of nausea and vomiting associated with initial and repeat courses of emetogenic cancer chemotherapy, including high-dose cisplatin. Efficacy of the 32 mg single dose beyond 24 hours in these patients has not been established.

Prevention of postoperative nausea and/or vomiting. As with other antiemetics, routine prophylaxis is not recommended for patients in whom there is little expectation that nausea and/or vomiting will occur postoperatively. In patients where nausea and/or vomiting must be avoided postoperatively, ondansetron HCl injection is recommended even where the incidence of postoperative nausea and/or vomiting is low. For patients who do not receive prophylactic ondansetron HCl injection and experience nausea and/or vomiting postoperatively, ondansetron HCl injection may be given to prevent further episodes.

CONTRAINDICATIONS

Ondansetron HCl injection and ondansetron HCl injection premixed are contraindicated for patients known to have hypersensitivity to the drug.

WARNINGS

Hypersensitivity reactions have been reported in patients who have exhibited hypersensitivity to other selective 5-HT_3 receptor antagonists.

PRECAUTIONS

Ondansetron is not a drug that stimulates gastric or intestinal peristalsis. It should not be used instead of nasogastric suction. The use of ondansetron in patients following abdominal surgery or in patients with chemotherapy-induced nausea and vomiting may mask a progressive ileus and/or gastric distention.

CARCINOGENESIS, MUTAGENESIS, AND IMPAIRMENT OF FERTILITY

Carcinogenic effects were not seen in 2 year studies in rats and mice with oral ondansetron doses up to 10 and 30 mg/kg/day, respectively. Ondansetron was not mutagenic in standard tests for mutagenicity. Oral administration of ondansetron up to 15 mg/kg/day did not affect fertility or general reproductive performance of male and female rats.

PREGNANCY, TERATOGENIC EFFECTS, PREGNANCY CATEGORY B

Reproduction studies have been performed in pregnant rats and rabbits at IV doses up to 4 mg/kg/day and have revealed no evidence of impaired fertility or harm to the fetus due to ondansetron. There are, however, no adequate and well-controlled studies in pregnant women. Because animal reproduction studies are not always predictive of human response, this drug should be used during pregnancy only if clearly needed.

NURSING MOTHERS

Ondansetron is excreted in the breast milk of rats. It is not known whether ondansetron is excreted in human milk. Because many drugs are excreted in human milk, caution should be exercised when ondansetron is administered to a nursing woman.

PEDIATRIC USE

Little information is available about dosage in pediatric patients under 2 years of age (see DOSAGE AND ADMINISTRATION for use in pediatric patients 4-18 years of age receiving cancer chemotherapy or for use in pediatric patients 2-12 years of age receiving general anesthesia).

GERIATRIC USE

Of the total number of subjects enrolled in cancer chemotherapy-induced and postoperative nausea and vomiting in US- and foreign-controlled clinical trials, 862 were 65 years of age and over. No overall differences in safety or effectiveness were observed between these subjects and younger subjects, and other reported clinical experience has not identified differences in responses between the elderly and younger patients, but greater sensitivity of some older individuals cannot be ruled out. Dosage adjustment is not needed in patients over the age of 65 (see CLINICAL PHARMACOLOGY).

DRUG INTERACTIONS

Ondansetron does not itself appear to induce or inhibit the cytochrome P-450 drug-metabolizing enzyme system of the liver. Because ondansetron is metabolized by hepatic cytochrome P-450 drug-metabolizing enzymes, inducers or inhibitors of these enzymes may change the clearance and, hence, the half-life of ondansetron. On the basis of limited available data, no dosage adjustment is recommended for patients on these drugs. Tumor response to chemotherapy in the P 388 mouse leukemia model is not affected by ondansetron. In humans, carmustine, etoposide, and cisplatin do not affect the pharmacokinetics of ondansetron.

In a crossover study in 76 pediatric patients, IV ondansetron did not increase blood levels of high-dose methotrexate.

ADVERSE REACTIONS

CHEMOTHERAPY-INDUCED NAUSEA AND VOMITING

The adverse events in TABLE 10 have been reported in individuals receiving ondansetron at a dosage of three 0.15 mg/kg doses or as a single 32 mg dose in clinical trials. These patients were receiving concomitant chemotherapy, primarily cisplatin, and IV fluids. Most were receiving a diuretic.

TABLE 10 *Principal Adverse Events in Comparative Trials*

	Ondansetron Injection			
	0.15 mg/kg × 3	32 mg × 1	Metoclopramide	Placebo
	n=419	n=220	n=156	n=34
Diarrhea	16%	8%	44%	18%
Headache	17%	25%	7%	15%
Fever	8%	7%	5%	3%
Akathisia	0%	0%	6%	0%
Acute dystonic reactions*	0%	0%	5%	0%

* See Neurological.

The following have been reported during controlled clinical trials:

Cardiovascular: Rare cases of angina (chest pain), electrocardiographic alterations, hypotension, and tachycardia have been reported. In many cases, the relationship to ondansetron HCl injection was unclear.

Gastrointestinal: Constipation has been reported in 11% of chemotherapy patients receiving multiday ondansetron.

Hepatic: In comparative trials in cisplatin chemotherapy patients with normal baseline values of aspartate transaminase (AST) and alanine transaminase (ALT), these enzymes have been reported to exceed twice the upper limit of normal in approximately 5% of patients. The increases were transient and did not appear to be related to dose or duration of therapy. On repeat exposure, similar transient elevations in transaminase values occurred in some courses, but symptomatic hepatic disease did not occur.

Integumentary: Rash has occurred in approximately 1% of patients receiving ondansetron.

Neurological: There have been rare reports consistent with, but not diagnostic of, extrapyramidal reactions in patients receiving ondansetron HCl injection, and rare cases of grand mal seizure. The relationship to ondansetron HCl was unclear.

Other: Rare cases of hypokalemia have been reported. The relationship to ondansetron HCl injection was unclear.

POSTOPERATIVE NAUSEA AND VOMITING

The adverse events in TABLE 11 have been reported in ≥2% of adults receiving ondansetron at a dosage of 4 mg IV over 2-5 minutes in clinical trials. Rates of these events were not significantly different in the ondansetron and placebo groups. These patients were receiving multiple concomitant perioperative and postoperative medications.

TABLE 11 *Adverse Events in ≥2% of Adults Receiving Ondansetron at a Dosage of 4 mg IV Over 2-5 Minutes in Clinical Trials*

	Ondansetron Inj. 4 mg IV	Placebo
	n=547	n=547
Headache	92 (17%)	77 (14%)
Dizziness	67 (12%)	88 (16%)
Musculoskeletal pain	57 (10%)	59 (11%)
Drowsiness/sedation	44 (8%)	37 (7%)
Shivers	38 (7%)	39 (7%)
Malaise/fatigue	25 (5%)	30 (5%)
Injection site reaction	21 (4%)	18 (3%)
Urinary retention	17 (3%)	15 (3%)
Postoperative CO_2-related pain*	12 (2%)	16 (3%)
Chest pain (unspecified)	12 (2%)	15 (3%)
Anxiety/agitation	11 (2%)	16 (3%)
Dysuria	11 (2%)	9 (2%)
Hypotension	10 (2%)	12 (2%)
Fever	10 (2%)	6 (1%)
Cold sensation	9 (2%)	8 (1%)
Pruritus	9 (2%)	3 (<1%)
Paresthesia	9 (2%)	2 (<1%)

* Sites of pain included abdomen, stomach, joints, rib cage, shoulder.

Pediatric Use

The adverse events in TABLE 12 were the most commonly reported adverse events in pediatric patients receiving ondansetron (a single 0.1 mg/kg dose for pediatric patients weighing 40 kg or less, or 4 mg for pediatric patients weighing more than 40 kg) administered intravenously over at least 30 seconds. Rates of these events were not significantly different in the ondansetron and placebo groups. These patients were receiving multiple concomitant perioperative and postoperative medications.

TABLE 12 *Frequency of Adverse Events From Controlled Studies in Pediatric Patients*

Adverse Event	Ondansetron n=755	Placebo n=731
Wound problem	80 (11%)	86 (12%)
Anxiety/agitation	49 (6%)	47 (6%)
Headache	44 (6%)	43 (6%)
Drowsiness/sedation	41 (5%)	56 (8%)
Pyrexia	32 (4%)	41 (6%)

OBSERVED DURING CLINICAL PRACTICE

In addition to adverse events reported from clinical trials, the following events have been identified during post-approval use of IV formulations of ondansetron HCl. Because they are reported voluntarily from a population of unknown size, estimates of frequency cannot be made. The events have been chosen for inclusion due to a combination of their seriousness, frequency of reporting, or potential causal connection to ondansetron HCl.

Cardiovascular: Arrhythmias (including ventricular and supraventricular tachycardia, premature ventricular contractions, and atrial fibrillation), bradycardia, electrocardiographic alterations (including second-degree heart block and ST segment depression), palpitations, and syncope.

General: Flushing. Rare cases of hypersensitivity reactions, sometimes severe (*e.g.*, anaphylaxis/anaphylactoid reactions, angioedema, bronchospasm, cardiopulmonary arrest, hypotension, laryngeal edema, laryngospasm, shock, shortness of breath, stridor) have also been reported.

Hepatobiliary: Liver enzyme abnormalities have been reported. Liver failure and death have been reported in patients with cancer receiving concurrent medications including potentially hepatotoxic cytotoxic chemotherapy and antibiotics. The etiology of the liver failure is unclear.

Local Reactions: Pain, redness, and burning at site of injection.

Lower Respiratory: Hiccups.

Neurological: Oculogyric crisis, appearing alone, as well as with other dystonic reactions.

Skin: Urticaria.

Special Senses: Transient blurred vision, in some cases associated with abnormalities of accommodation, and transient dizziness during or shortly after IV infusion.

DOSAGE AND ADMINISTRATION

PREVENTION OF CHEMOTHERAPY-INDUCED NAUSEA AND VOMITING

The recommended IV dosage of ondansetron HCl is a single 32 mg dose or three 0.15 mg/kg doses. A single 32 mg dose is infused over 15 minutes beginning 30 minutes before the start of emetogenic chemotherapy. The recommended infusion rate should not be exceeded. With the 3 dose (0.15 mg/kg) regimen, the first dose is infused over 15 minutes beginning 30 minutes before the start of emetogenic chemotherapy. Subsequent doses (0.15 mg/kg) are administered 4 and 8 hours after the first dose of ondansetron HCl.

Ondansetron HCl injection should not be mixed with solutions for which physical and chemical compatibility have not been established. In particular, this applies to alkaline solutions as a precipitate may form.

Vial

DILUTE BEFORE USE. Ondansetron HCl injection should be diluted in 50 ml of 5% dextrose injection or 0.9% sodium chloride injection before administration.

Flexible Plastic Container

Ondansetron HCl injection premixed, 32 mg in 5% dextrose, 50 ml, **REQUIRES NO DILUTION.**

Pediatric Use

On the basis of the limited available information (see CLINICAL PHARMACOLOGY, Pharmacokinetics), the dosage in pediatric patients 4-18 years of age should be three 0.15 mg/kg doses. Little information is available about dosage in pediatric patients 3 years of age and younger.

Geriatric Use

The dosage recommendation is the same as for the general population.

PREVENTION OF POSTOPERATIVE NAUSEA AND VOMITING

The recommended IV dosage of ondansetron HCl for adults is 4 mg **undiluted** administered intravenously in not less than 30 seconds, preferably over 2-5 minutes, immediately before induction of anesthesia, or postoperatively if the patient experiences nausea and/or vomiting occurring shortly after surgery. Alternatively, 4 mg **undiluted** may be administered intramuscularly as a single injection for adults. While recommended as a fixed dose for patients weighing more than 40 kg, few patients above 80 kg have been studied. In patients who do not achieve adequate control of postoperative nausea and vomiting following a single, prophylactic, preinduction, IV dose of ondansetron 4 mg, administration of a second IV dose of 4 mg ondansetron postoperatively does not provide additional control of nausea and vomiting.

Vial

Ondansetron HCl injection **REQUIRES NO DILUTION FOR ADMINISTRATION FOR POSTOPERATIVE NAUSEA AND VOMITING.**

Pediatric Use

The recommended IV dosage of ondansetron HCl for pediatric patients (2-12 years of age) is a single 0.1 mg/kg dose for pediatric patients weighing 40 kg or less, or a single 4 mg dose for pediatric patients weighing more than 40 kg. The rate of administration should not be less than 30 seconds, preferably over 2-5 minutes. Little information is available about dosage in pediatric patients younger than 2 years of age.

Geriatric Use

The dosage recommendation is the same as for the general population.

DOSAGE ADJUSTMENT FOR PATIENTS WITH IMPAIRED RENAL FUNCTION

The dosage recommendation is the same as for the general population. There is no experience beyond first day administration of ondansetron.

DOSAGE ADJUSTMENT FOR PATIENTS WITH IMPAIRED HEPATIC FUNCTION

In patients with severe hepatic impairment (Child-Pugh[1] score of 10 or greater), a single maximal daily dose of 8 mg to be infused over 15 minutes beginning 30 minutes before the start of the emetogenic chemotherapy is recommended. There is no experience beyond first day administration of ondansetron.

STABILITY

Ondansetron HCl injection is stable at room temperature under normal lighting conditions for 48 hours after dilution with the following IV fluids: 0.9% sodium chloride injection, 5% dextrose injection, 5% dextrose and 0.9% sodium chloride injection, 5% dextrose and 0.45% sodium chloride injection, and 3% sodium chloride injection.

Although ondansetron HCl injection is chemically and physically stable when diluted as recommended, sterile precautions should be observed because diluents generally do not contain preservative. After dilution, do not use beyond 24 hours.

Note: Parenteral drug products should be inspected visually for particulate matter and discoloration before administration whenever solution and container permit.

Precaution: Occasionally, ondansetron precipitates at the stopper/vial interface in vials stored upright. Potency and safety are not affected. If a precipitate is observed, resolubilize by shaking the vial vigorously.

HOW SUPPLIED

ZOFRAN INJECTION

Zofran injection, 2 mg/ml, is supplied in 2 ml single-dose vials and 20 ml multidose vials.
Storage: Store between 2 and 30°C (36 and 86°F). Protect from light.

ZOFRAN INJECTION PREMIXED

Zofran injection premixed, 32 mg/50 ml, in 5% dextrose, contains no preservatives and is supplied as a sterile, premixed solution for IV administration in single-dose, flexible plastic containers.

Storage: Store between 2 and 30°C (36 and 86°F). Protect from light. Avoid excessive heat. Protect from freezing.

ORAL

DESCRIPTION

The active ingredient in Zofran tablets and Zofran oral solution is ondansetron hydrochloride (HCl) as the dihydrate, the racemic form of ondansetron and a selective blocking agent of the serotonin 5-HT_3 receptor type. Chemically it is (±)1,2,3,9-tetrahydro-9-methyl-3-[(2-methyl-1H-imidazol-1-yl)methyl]-4H-carbazol-4-one, monohydrochloride, dihydrate.

The empirical formula is $C_{18}H_{19}N_3O{\cdot}HCl{\cdot}2H_2O$, representing a molecular weight of 365.9.

Ondansetron HCl dihydrate is a white to off-white powder that is soluble in water and normal saline.

The active ingredient in Zofran ODT orally disintegrating tablets is ondansetron base, the racemic form of ondansetron, and a selective blocking agent of the serotonin 5-HT_3 receptor type. Chemically it is (±)1,2,3,9-tetrahydro-9-methyl-3-[(2-methyl-1H-imidazol-1-yl)methyl]-4H-carbazol-4-one.

The empirical formula is $C_{18}H_{19}N_3O$ representing a molecular weight of 293.4.

Each 4 mg Zofran tablet for oral administration contains ondansetron HCl dihydrate equivalent to 4 mg of ondansetron. Each 8 mg Zofran tablet for oral administration contains ondansetron HCl dihydrate equivalent to 8 mg of ondansetron. Each 24 mg Zofran tablet for oral administration contains ondansetron HCl dihydrate equivalent to 24 mg of ondansetron. Each tablet also contains the inactive ingredients lactose, microcrystalline cellulose, pregelatinized starch, hydroxypropyl methylcellulose, magnesium stearate, titanium dioxide, triacetin, iron oxide yellow (8 mg tablet only), and iron oxide red (24 mg tablet only).

Each 4 mg Zofran ODT orally disintegrating tablet for oral administration contains 4 mg ondansetron base. Each 8 mg Zofran ODT orally disintegrating tablet for oral administration contains 8 mg ondansetron base. Each Zofran ODT tablet also contains the inactive ingredients aspartame, gelatin, mannitol, methylparaben sodium, propylparaben sodium, and strawberry flavor. Zofran ODT tablets are a freeze-dried, orally administered formulation of ondansetron which rapidly disintegrates on the tongue and does not require water to aid dissolution or swallowing.

Each 5 ml of Zofran oral solution contains 5 mg of ondansetron HCl dihydrate equivalent to 4 mg of ondansetron. Zofran oral solution contains the inactive ingredients citric acid anhydrous, purified water, sodium benzoate, sodium citrate, sorbitol, and strawberry flavor.

CLINICAL PHARMACOLOGY

PHARMACODYNAMICS

Ondansetron is a selective 5-HT_3 receptor antagonist. While its mechanism of action has not been fully characterized, ondansetron is not a dopamine-receptor antagonist. Serotonin receptors of the 5-HT_3 type are present both peripherally on vagal nerve terminals and centrally in the chemoreceptor trigger zone of the area postrema. It is not certain whether ondansetron's antiemetic action is mediated centrally, peripherally, or in both sites. However, cytotoxic chemotherapy appears to be associated with release of serotonin from the enterochromaffin cells of the small intestine. In humans, urinary 5-HIAA (5-hydroxyindoleacetic acid) excretion increases after cisplatin administration in parallel with the onset of emesis. The released serotonin may stimulate the vagal afferents through the 5-HT_3 receptors and initiate the vomiting reflex.

In animals, the emetic response to cisplatin can be prevented by pretreatment with an inhibitor of serotonin synthesis, bilateral abdominal vagotomy and greater splanchnic nerve section, or pretreatment with a serotonin 5-HT_3 receptor antagonist.

In normal volunteers, single intravenous (IV) doses of 0.15 mg/kg of ondansetron had no effect on esophageal motility, gastric motility, lower esophageal sphincter pressure, or small intestinal transit time. Multiday administration of ondansetron has been shown to slow colonic transit in normal volunteers. Ondansetron has no effect on plasma prolactin concentrations.

Ondansetron does not alter the respiratory depressant effects produced by alfentanil or the degree of neuromuscular blockade produced by atracurium. Interactions with general or local anesthetics have not been studied.

PHARMACOKINETICS

Ondansetron is extensively metabolized in humans, with approximately 5% of a radiolabeled dose recovered from the urine as the parent compound. The primary metabolic pathway is hydroxylation on the indole ring followed by subsequent glucuronide or sulfate conjugation. Although some nonconjugated metabolites have pharmacologic activity, these are not found in plasma at concentrations likely to significantly contribute to the biological activity of ondansetron.

In vitro metabolism studies have shown that ondansetron is a substrate for human hepatic cytochrome P-450 enzymes, including CYP1A2, CYP2D6, and CYP3A4. In terms of overall ondansetron turnover, CYP3A4 played the predominant role. Because of the multiplicity of metabolic enzymes capable of metabolizing ondansetron, it is likely that inhibition or loss of 1 enzyme (*e.g.*, CYP2D6 genetic deficiency) will be compensated by others and may result in little change in overall rates of ondansetron elimination. Ondansetron elimination may be affected by cytochrome P-450 inducers. In a pharmacokinetic study of 16 epileptic patients maintained chronically on carbamazepine or phenytoin, reduction in AUC, C_{max} and $T_{½}$ of ondansetron was observed. This resulted in a significant increase in clearance. However, on the basis of available data, no dosage adjustment is recommended (see DRUG INTERACTIONS).

Ondansetron is well absorbed from the gastrointestinal tract and undergoes some first-pass metabolism. Mean bioavailability in healthy subjects, following administration of a single 8 mg tablet, is approximately 56%.

Ondansetron systemic exposure does not increase proportionately to dose. AUC from a 16 mg tablet was 24% greater than predicted from an 8 mg tablet dose. This may reflect some reduction of first-pass metabolism at higher oral doses. Bioavailability is also slightly enhanced by the presence of food but unaffected by antacids.

Gender differences were shown in the disposition of ondansetron given as a single dose. The extent and rate of ondansetron's absorption is greater in women than men. Slower clearance in women, a smaller apparent volume of distribution (adjusted for weight), and higher absolute bioavailability resulted in higher plasma ondansetron levels. These higher plasma levels may in part be explained by differences in body weight between men and women. It is not known whether these gender-related differences were clinically important. More detailed pharmacokinetic information is contained in TABLE 13 and TABLE 14 taken from two studies.

TABLE 13 *Pharmacokinetics in Normal Volunteers: Single 8 mg Ondansetron HCl Tablet Dose*

	Age-Group (Years)					
	18-40		61-74		≥75	
	M	F	M	F	M	F
Mean weight (kg)	69.0	62.7	77.5	60.2	78.0	67.6
n=	6	5	6	6	5	6
Peak plasma concentration (ng/ml)	26.2	42.7	24.1	52.4	37.0	46.1
Time of peak plasma concentration (h)	2.0	1.7	2.1	1.9	2.2	2.1
Mean elimination half-life (h)	3.1	3.5	4.1	4.9	4.5	6.2
Systemic plasma clearance L/h/kg	0.403	0.354	0.384	0.255	0.277	0.249
Absolute bioavailability	0.483	0.663	0.585	0.643	0.619	0.747

TABLE 14 *Pharmacokinetics in Normal Volunteers: Single 24 mg Ondansetron HCl Tablet Dose*

	Age-Group (Years)	
	18-43	
	M	F
Mean weight (kg)	84.1	71.8
n=	8	8
Peak plasma concentration (ng/ml)	125.8	194.4
Time of peak plasma concentration (h)	1.9	1.6
Mean elimination half-life (h)	4.7	5.8

A reduction in clearance and increase in elimination half-life are seen in patients over 75 years of age. In clinical trials with cancer patients, safety and efficacy was similar in patients over 65 years of age and those under 65 years of age; there was an insufficient number of patients over 75 years of age to permit conclusions in that age-group. No dosage adjustment is recommended in the elderly.

In patients with mild-to-moderate hepatic impairment, clearance is reduced 2-fold and mean half-life is increased to 11.6 hours compared to 5.7 hours in normals. In patients with severe hepatic impairment (Child-Pugh score[1] of 10 or greater), clearance is reduced 2- to 3-fold and apparent volume of distribution is increased with a resultant increase in half-life to 20 hours. In patients with severe hepatic impairment, a total daily dose of 8 mg should not be exceeded.

Due to the very small contribution (5%) of renal clearance to the overall clearance, renal impairment was not expected to significantly influence the total clearance of ondansetron. However, ondansetron oral mean plasma clearance was reduced by about 50% in patients with severe renal impairment (creatinine clearance <30 ml/min). This reduction in clearance is variable and was not consistent with an increase in half-life. No reduction in dose or dosing frequency in these patients is warranted.

Plasma protein binding of ondansetron as measured *in vitro* was 70-76% over the concentration range of 10-500 ng/ml. Circulating drug also distributes into erythrocytes.

Four (4) and 8 mg doses of either ondansetron HCl oral solution or ondansetron HCl orally disintegrating tablets are bioequivalent to corresponding doses of ondansetron HCl tablets and may be used interchangeably. One 24 mg ondansetron HCl tablet is bioequivalent to and interchangeable with three 8 mg ondansetron HCl tablets.

INDICATIONS AND USAGE

1. Prevention of nausea and vomiting associated with highly emetogenic cancer chemotherapy, including cisplatin ≥50 mg/m².
2. Prevention of nausea and vomiting associated with initial and repeat courses of moderately emetogenic cancer chemotherapy.
3. Prevention of nausea and vomiting associated with radiotherapy in patients receiving either total body irradiation, single high-dose fraction to the abdomen, or daily fractions to the abdomen.
4. Prevention of postoperative nausea and/or vomiting. As with other antiemetics, routine prophylaxis is not recommended for patients in whom there is little expectation that nausea and/or vomiting will occur postoperatively. In patients where nausea and/or vomiting must be avoided postoperatively, ondansetron HCl tablets, ondansetron HCl orally disintegrating tablets, and ondansetron HCl oral solution are recommended even where the incidence of postoperative nausea and/or vomiting is low.

CONTRAINDICATIONS

Ondansetron HCl tablets, orally disintegrating tablets, and oral solution are contraindicated for patients known to have hypersensitivity to the drug.

WARNINGS

Hypersensitivity reactions have been reported in patients who have exhibited hypersensitivity to other selective 5-HT_3 receptor antagonists.

PRECAUTIONS

Ondansetron is not a drug that stimulates gastric or intestinal peristalsis. It should not be used instead of nasogastric suction. The use of ondansetron in patients following abdominal surgery or in patients with chemotherapy-induced nausea and vomiting may mask a progressive ileus and/or gastric distension.

INFORMATION FOR THE PATIENT

Phenylketonurics: Phenylketonuric patients should be informed that ondansetron HCl orally disintegrating tablets contain phenylalanine (a component of aspartame). Each 4 and 8 mg orally disintegrating tablet contains <0.03 mg phenylalanine.

Patients should be instructed not to remove ondansetron HCl ODT tablets from the blister until just prior to dosing. The tablet should not be pushed through the foil. With dry hands, the blister backing should be peeled completely off the blister. The tablet should be gently removed and immediately placed on the tongue to dissolve and be swallowed with the saliva. Peelable illustrated stickers are affixed to the product carton that can be provided with the prescription to ensure proper use and handling of the product.

USE IN SURGICAL PATIENTS

The coadministration of ondansetron had no effect on the pharmacokinetics and pharmacodynamics of temazepam.

CARCINOGENESIS, MUTAGENESIS, AND IMPAIRMENT OF FERTILITY

Carcinogenic effects were not seen in 2 year studies in rats and mice with oral ondansetron doses up to 10 and 30 mg/kg/day, respectively. Ondansetron was not mutagenic in standard tests for mutagenicity. Oral administration of ondansetron up to 15 mg/kg/day did not affect fertility or general reproductive performance of male and female rats.

PREGNANCY, TERATOGENIC EFFECTS, PREGNANCY CATEGORY B

Reproduction studies have been performed in pregnant rats and rabbits at daily oral doses up to 15 and 30 mg/kg/day, respectively, and have revealed no evidence of impaired fertility or harm to the fetus due to ondansetron. There are, however, no adequate and well-controlled studies in pregnant women. Because animal reproduction studies are not always predictive of human response, this drug should be used during pregnancy only if clearly needed.

NURSING MOTHERS

Ondansetron is excreted in the breast milk of rats. It is not known whether ondansetron is excreted in human milk. Because many drugs are excreted in human milk, caution should be exercised when ondansetron is administered to a nursing woman.

PEDIATRIC USE

Little information is available about dosage in pediatric patients 4 years of age or younger (see CLINICAL PHARMACOLOGY and DOSAGE AND ADMINISTRATION for use in pediatric patients 4-18 years of age).

GERIATRIC USE

Of the total number of subjects enrolled in cancer chemotherapy-induced and postoperative nausea and vomiting in US and foreign -controlled clinical trials, for which there were subgroup analyses, 938 were 65 years of age and over. No overall differences in safety or effectiveness were observed between these subjects and younger subjects, and other reported clinical experience has not identified differences in responses between the elderly and younger patients, but greater sensitivity of some older individuals cannot be ruled out. Dosage adjustment is not needed in patients over the age of 65 (see CLINICAL PHARMACOLOGY).

DRUG INTERACTIONS

Ondansetron does not itself appear to induce or inhibit the cytochrome P-450 drug-metabolizing enzyme system of the liver. Because ondansetron is metabolized by hepatic cytochrome P-450 drug-metabolizing enzymes, inducers or inhibitors of these enzymes may change the clearance and, hence, the half-life of ondansetron. On the basis of available data, no dosage adjustment is recommended for patients on these drugs. Tumor response to chemotherapy in the P 388 mouse leukemia model is not affected by ondansetron. In humans, carmustine, etoposide, and cisplatin do not affect the pharmacokinetics of ondansetron.

In a crossover study in 76 pediatric patients, IV ondansetron did not increase blood levels of high-dose methotrexate.

ADVERSE REACTIONS

The following have been reported as adverse events in clinical trials of patients treated with ondansetron, the active ingredient of ondansetron HCl. A causal relationship to therapy with ondansetron HCl has been unclear in many cases.

CHEMOTHERAPY-INDUCED NAUSEA AND VOMITING

The adverse events in TABLE 17 have been reported in ≥5% of adult patients receiving a single 24 mg ondansetron HCl tablet in two trials. These patients were receiving concurrent highly emetogenic cisplatin-based chemotherapy regimens (cisplatin dose ≥50 mg/m^2).

TABLE 17 *Principal Adverse Events in US Trials: Single Day Therapy With 24 mg Ondansetron HCl Tablets — Highly Emetogenic Chemotherapy*

	Ondansetron		
	24 mg qd	8 mg bid	32 mg qd
Event	n=300	n=124	n=117
Headache	33 (11%)	16 (13%)	17 (15%)
Diarrhea	13 (4%)	9 (7%)	3 (3%)

The adverse events in TABLE 18 have been reported in ≥5% of adults receiving either 8 mg of ondansetron HCl tablets 2 or 3 times a day for 3 days or placebo in four trials. These patients were receiving concurrent moderately emetogenic chemotherapy, primarily cyclophosphamide-based regimens.

TABLE 18 *Principal Adverse Events in US Trials: 3 Days of Therapy With 8 mg Ondansetron HCl Tablets — Moderately Emetogenic Chemotherapy*

	Ondansetron		
	8 mg bid	8 mg tid	Placebo
Event	n=242	n=415	n=262
Headache	58 (24%)	113 (27%)	34 (13%)
Malaise/fatigue	32 (13%)	37 (9%)	6 (2%)
Constipation	22 (9%)	26 (6%)	1 (<1%)
Diarrhea	15 (6%)	16 (4%)	10 (4%)
Dizziness	13 (5%)	18 (4%)	12 (5%)

Central Nervous System: There have been rare reports consistent with, but not diagnostic of, extrapyramidal reactions in patients receiving ondansetron.

Hepatic: In 723 patients receiving cyclophosphamide-based chemotherapy in US clinical trials, AST and/or ALT values have been reported to exceed twice the upper limit of normal in approximately 1-2% of patients receiving ondansetron HCl tablets. The increases were transient and did not appear to be related to dose or duration of therapy. On repeat exposure, similar transient elevations in transaminase values occurred in some courses, but symptomatic hepatic disease did not occur. The role of cancer chemotherapy in these biochemical changes cannot be clearly determined. There have been reports of liver failure and death in patients with cancer receiving concurrent medications including potentially hepatotoxic cytotoxic chemotherapy and antibiotics. The etiology of the liver failure is unclear.

Integumentary: Rash has occurred in approximately 1% of patients receiving ondansetron.

Other: Rare cases of anaphylaxis, bronchospasm, tachycardia, angina (chest pain), hypokalemia, electrocardiographic alterations, vascular occlusive events, and grand mal seizures have been reported. Except for bronchospasm and anaphylaxis, the relationship to ondansetron HCl was unclear.

RADIATION-INDUCED NAUSEA AND VOMITING

The adverse events reported in patients receiving ondansetron HCl tablets and concurrent radiotherapy were similar to those reported in patients receiving ondansetron HCl tablets and concurrent chemotherapy. The most frequently reported adverse events were headache, constipation, and diarrhea.

POSTOPERATIVE NAUSEA AND VOMITING

The adverse events in TABLE 19 have been reported in ≥5% of patients receiving ondansetron HCl tablets at a dosage of 16 mg orally in clinical trials. With the exception of headache, rates of these events were not significantly different in the ondansetron and placebo groups. These patients were receiving multiple concomitant perioperative and postoperative medications.

TABLE 19 *Frequency of Adverse Events From Controlled Studies With Ondansetron HCl Tablets — Postoperative Nausea and Vomiting*

Adverse Event	Ondansetron 16 mg (n=550)	Placebo (n=531)
Wound problem	152 (28%)	162 (31%)
Drowsiness/sedation	112 (20%)	122 (23%)
Headache	49 (9%)	27 (5%)
Hypoxia	49 (9%)	35 (7%)
Pyrexia	45 (8%)	34 (6%)
Dizziness	36 (7%)	34 (6%)
Gynecological disorder	36 (7%)	33 (6%)
Anxiety/agitation	33 (6%)	29 (5%)
Bradycardia	32 (6%)	30 (6%)
Shiver(s)	28 (5%)	30 (6%)
Urinary retention	28 (5%)	18 (3%)
Hypotension	27 (5%)	32 (6%)
Pruritus	27 (5%)	20 (4%)

Preliminary observations in a small number of subjects suggest a higher incidence of headache when ondansetron HCl orally disintegrating tablets are taken with water, when compared to without water.

OBSERVED DURING CLINICAL PRACTICE

In addition to adverse events reported from clinical trials, the following events have been identified during post-approval use of oral formulations of ondansetron HCl. Because they are reported voluntarily from a population of unknown size, estimates of frequency cannot be made. The events have been chosen for inclusion due to a combination of their seriousness, frequency of reporting, or potential causal connection to ondansetron HCl.

General: Flushing. Rare cases of hypersensitivity reactions, sometimes severe (*e.g.*, anaphylaxis/anaphylactoid reactions, angioedema, bronchospasm, shortness of breath, hypotension, laryngeal edema, stridor) have also been reported. Laryngospasm, shock, and cardiopulmonary arrest have occurred during allergic reactions in patients receiving injectable ondansetron.

Hepatobiliary: Liver enzyme abnormalities.

Lower Respiratory: Hiccups.

Neurology: Oculogyric crisis, appearing alone, as well as with other dystonic reactions.

Skin: Urticaria.

DOSAGE AND ADMINISTRATION

PREVENTION OF NAUSEA AND VOMITING ASSOCIATED WITH HIGHLY EMETOGENIC CANCER CHEMOTHERAPY

The recommended adult oral dosage of ondansetron HCl is a single 24 mg tablet administered 30 minutes before the start of single day highly emetogenic chemotherapy, including cisplatin ≥50 mg/m^2. Multiday, single-dose administration of ondansetron HCl 24 mg tablets has not been studied.

Pediatric Use

There is no experience with the use of 24 mg ondansetron HCl tablets in pediatric patients.

Geriatric Use

The dosage recommendation is the same as for the general population.

PREVENTION OF NAUSEA AND VOMITING ASSOCIATED WITH MODERATELY EMETOGENIC CANCER CHEMOTHERAPY

The recommended adult oral dosage is one 8 mg ondansetron HCl tablet or one 8 mg ondansetron HCl ODT tablet or 10 ml (2 teaspoonfuls equivalent to 8 mg of ondansetron) of ondansetron HCl oral solution given twice a day. The first dose should be administered 30 minutes before the start of emetogenic chemotherapy, with a subsequent dose 8 hours after the first dose. One 8 mg ondansetron HCl tablet or one 8 mg ondansetron HCl ODT tablet or 10 ml (2 teaspoonfuls equivalent to 8 mg of ondansetron) of ondansetron HCl oral solution should be administered twice a day (every 12 hours) for 1-2 days after completion of chemotherapy.

Pediatric Use

For pediatric patients 12 years of age and older, the dosage is the same as for adults. For pediatric patients 4-11 years of age, the dosage is one 4 mg ondansetron HCl tablet or one 4 mg ondansetron HCl ODT tablet or 5 ml (1 teaspoonful equivalent to 4 mg of ondansetron) of ondansetron HCl oral solution given 3 times a day. The first dose should be administered 30 minutes before the start of emetogenic chemotherapy, with subsequent doses 4 and 8 hours after the first dose. One 4 mg ondansetron HCl tablet or one 4 mg ondansetron HCl ODT tablet or 5 ml (1 teaspoonful equivalent to 4 mg of ondansetron) of ondansetron HCl oral solution should be administered 3 times a day (every 8 hours) for 1-2 days after completion of chemotherapy.

Geriatric Use

The dosage is the same as for the general population.

PREVENTION OF NAUSEA AND VOMITING ASSOCIATED WITH RADIOTHERAPY, EITHER TOTAL BODY IRRADIATION, OR SINGLE HIGH-DOSE FRACTION OR DAILY FRACTIONS TO THE ABDOMEN

The recommended oral dosage is one 8 mg ondansetron HCl tablet or one 8 mg ondansetron HCl ODT tablet or 10 ml (2 teaspoonfuls equivalent to 8 mg of ondansetron) of ondansetron HCl oral solution given 3 times a day.

For total body irradiation, one 8 mg ondansetron HCl tablet or one 8 mg ondansetron HCl ODT tablet or 10 ml (2 teaspoonfuls equivalent to 8 mg of ondansetron) of ondansetron HCl oral solution should be administered 1-2 hours before each fraction of radiotherapy administered each day.

For single high-dose fraction radiotherapy to the abdomen, one 8 mg ondansetron HCl tablet or one 8 mg ondansetron HCl ODT tablet or 10 ml (2 teaspoonfuls equivalent to 8 mg of ondansetron) of ondansetron HCl oral solution should be administered 1-2 hours before radiotherapy, with subsequent doses every 8 hours after the first dose for 1-2 days after completion of radiotherapy.

For daily fractionated radiotherapy to the abdomen, one 8 mg ondansetron HCl tablet or one 8 mg ondansetron HCl ODT tablet or 10 ml (2 teaspoonfuls equivalent to 8 mg of ondansetron) of ondansetron HCl oral solution should be administered 1-2 hours before radiotherapy, with subsequent doses every 8 hours after the first dose for each day radiotherapy is given.

Pediatric Use

There is no experience with the use of ondansetron HCl tablets, ondansetron HCl ODT tablets, or ondansetron HCl oral solution in the prevention of radiation-induced nausea and vomiting in pediatric patients.

Geriatric Use

The dosage recommendation is the same as for the general population.

POSTOPERATIVE NAUSEA AND VOMITING

The recommended dosage is 16 mg given as two 8 mg ondansetron HCl tablets or two 8 mg ondansetron HCl ODT tablets or 20 ml (4 teaspoonfuls equivalent to 16 mg of ondansetron) of ondansetron HCl oral solution 1 hour before induction of anesthesia.

Pediatric Use

There is no experience with the use of ondansetron HCl tablets, ondansetron HCl ODT tablets, or ondansetron HCl oral solution in the prevention of postoperative nausea and vomiting in pediatric patients.

Geriatric Use

The dosage is the same as for the general population.

DOSAGE ADJUSTMENT FOR PATIENTS WITH IMPAIRED RENAL FUNCTION

The dosage recommendation is the same as for the general population. There is no experience beyond first day administration of ondansetron.

DOSAGE ADJUSTMENT FOR PATIENTS WITH IMPAIRED HEPATIC FUNCTION

In patients with severe hepatic impairment (Child-Pugh[1] score of 10 or greater), clearance is reduced and apparent volume of distribution is increased with a resultant increase in plasma half-life. In such patients, a total daily dose of 8 mg should not be exceeded.

HOW SUPPLIED

ZOFRAN TABLETS

4 and 8 mg Tablets

4 mg: Zofran tablets, 4 mg (ondansetron HCl dihydrate equivalent to 4 mg of ondansetron), are white, oval, film-coated tablets engraved with "Zofran" on one side and "4" on the other.
8 mg: Zofran tablets, 8 mg (ondansetron HCl dihydrate equivalent to 8 mg of ondansetron), are yellow, oval, film-coated tablets engraved with "Zofran" on one side and "8" on the other.
Storage: Store between 2 and 30°C (36 and 86°F). Protect from light.

24 mg Tablets

Zofran tablets, 24 mg (ondansetron HCl dihydrate equivalent to 24 mg of ondansetron), are pink, oval, film-coated tablets engraved with "GX CF7" on one side and "24" on the other.
Storage: Store between 2 and 30°C (36 and 86°F).

ZOFRAN ODT ORALLY DISINTEGRATING TABLETS

Zofran ODT orally disintegrating tablets, 4 mg (as 4 mg ondansetron base) are white, round and plano-convex tablets debossed with a "Z4" on one side.

Zofran ODT orally disintegrating tablets, 8 mg (as 8 mg ondansetron base) are white, round and plano-convex tablets debossed with a "Z8" on one side.
Storage: Store between 2 and 30°C (36 and 86°F).

ZOFRAN ORAL SOLUTION

Zofran oral solution, a clear, colorless to light yellow liquid with a characteristic strawberry odor, contains 5 mg of ondansetron HCl dihydrate equivalent to 4 mg of ondansetron per 5 ml in amber glass bottles of 50 ml with child-resistant closures.
Storage: Store upright between 15 and 30°C (59 and 86°F). Protect from light.

PRODUCT LISTING - EQUIVALENTS NOT AVAILABLE

Solution - Injectable - 2 mg/ml

2 ml x 5	$128.24	ZOFRAN, Allscripts Pharmaceutical Company	54569-4198-00
2 ml x 5	$133.55	ZOFRAN, Glaxosmithkline	00173-0442-02
20 ml	$267.09	ZOFRAN, Glaxosmithkline	00173-0442-00

Solution - Intravenous - 32 mg/50 ml

50 ml	$1290.06	ZOFRAN, Glaxosmithkline	00173-0461-00

Solution - Oral - 4 mg/5 ml

50 ml	$203.28	ZOFRAN, Glaxosmithkline	00173-0489-00

Tablet - Oral - 4 mg

3's	$52.27	ZOFRAN, Physicians Total Care	54868-3508-00
3's	$60.10	ZOFRAN, Glaxosmithkline	00173-0446-04
30's	$479.20	ZOFRAN, Physicians Total Care	54868-3508-01
30's	$600.88	ZOFRAN, Glaxosmithkline	00173-0446-00
100's	$2002.56	ZOFRAN, Glaxosmithkline	00173-0446-02

Tablet - Oral - 8 mg

3's	$94.01	ZOFRAN, Physicians Total Care	54868-3509-00
3's	$100.06	ZOFRAN, Glaxosmithkline	00173-0447-04
9's	$238.26	ZOFRAN, Allscripts Pharmaceutical Company	54569-4872-00
30's	$1000.85	ZOFRAN, Glaxosmithkline	00173-0447-00
100's	$3336.06	ZOFRAN, Glaxosmithkline	00173-0447-02

Tablet - Oral - 24 mg

1's	$79.42	ZOFRAN, Glaxosmithkline	00173-0680-00

Tablet, Disintegrating - Oral - 4 mg

10 x 3	$566.84	ZOFRAN ODT, Glaxosmithkline	00173-0569-00

Tablet, Disintegrating - Oral - 8 mg

10 x 3	$944.16	ZOFRAN ODT, Glaxosmithkline	00173-0570-00
10's	$314.71	ZOFRAN ODT, Glaxosmithkline	00173-0570-04

Oprelvekin *(003367)*

Categories: Thrombocytopenia; Thrombocytopenia, secondary to cancer chemotherapy; FDA Approved 1997 Dec; Pregnancy Category C; Orphan Drugs
Drug Classes: Hematopoietic agents
Brand Names: **Neumega**
HCFA JCODE(S): J2355 5 mg SC

DESCRIPTION

Interleukin eleven (IL-11) is a thrombopoietic growth factor that directly stimulates the proliferation of hematopoietic stem cells and megakaryocyte progenitor cells and induces megakaryocyte maturation resulting in increased platelet production. IL-11 is a member of a family of human growth factors which includes human growth hormone, granulocyte colony-stimulating factor (G-CSF), and other growth factors.

Oprelvekin, the active ingredient in Neumega, is produced in *Escherichia coli (E. coli)* by recombinant DNA methods. The protein has a molecular mass of approximately 19,000 daltons, and is non-glycosylated. The polypeptide is 177 amino acids in length and differs from the 178 amino acid length of native IL-11 only in lacking the amino-terminal proline residue. This alteration has not resulted in measurable differences in bioactivity either *in vitro* or *in vivo*.

Neumega is available for subcutaneous administration in single-use vials containing 5 mg of Oprelvekin (specific activity approximately 8×10^6 units/mg) as a sterile, lyophilized powder with 23 mg glycine, 1.6 mg dibasic sodium phosphate heptahydrate, and 0.55 mg monobasic sodium phosphate monohydrate. When reconstituted with 1 ml of sterile water for injection, the resulting solution has a pH of 7.0 and a concentration of 5 mg/ml.

CLINICAL PHARMACOLOGY

The primary hematopoietic activity of oprelvekin is stimulation of megakaryocytopoiesis and thrombopoiesis. Oprelvekin has shown potent thrombopoietic activity in animal models of compromised hematopoiesis, including moderately to severely myelosuppressed mice and nonhuman primates. In these models, oprelvekin improved platelet nadirs and accelerated platelet recoveries compared to controls.

Preclinical studies have shown that mature megakaryocytes which develop during *in vivo* treatment with oprelvekin are ultrastructurally normal. Platelets produced in response to oprelvekin were morphologically and functionally normal and possessed a normal life-span.

IL-11 has also been shown to have non-hematopoietic activities in animals including: the regulation of intestinal epithelium growth (enhanced healing of gastrointestinal lesions), the inhibition of adipogenesis, the induction of acute phase protein synthesis, inhibition of proinflammatory cytokine production by macrophages, and the stimulation of osteoclastogenesis and neurogenesis.

IL-11 is produced by bone marrow stromal cells and is part of the cytokine family that shares the gp130 signal transducer. Primary osteoblasts and mature osteoclasts express mRNAs for both IL-11 receptor (IL-11R alpha) and gp130. Both bone-forming and bone-resorbing cells are potential targets of IL-11.[1]

PHARMACOKINETICS

The pharmacokinetics of oprelvekin have been evaluated in studies in healthy, adult subjects and oncology patients receiving chemotherapy. In a study in which a single 50 µg/kg subcutaneous dose was administered to 18 men, the peak serum concentration (C_{max}) of 17.4 ± 5.4 ng/ml (mean ±SD) was reached at 3.2 ± 2.4 hours (T_{max}) following dosing. The terminal half life was 6.9 ± 1.7 hours. In a second study in which single 75 µg/kg subcutaneous and intravenous doses were administered to 24 healthy subjects, the pharmacokinetic profiles were similar between men and women. The absolute bioavailability of oprelvekin was >80%. In a study in which multiple, subcutaneous doses of both 25 and 50 µg/kg were administered to cancer patients receiving chemotherapy, oprelvekin did not accumulate and clearance of oprelvekin was not impaired following multiple doses.

Oprelvekin was also administered to 28 infants, children, and adolescents receiving ICE (ifosfamide, carboplatin, etoposide) chemotherapy. Analysis of data from 23 pediatric patients showed that C_{max} and T_{max} were comparable to the adult population. The mean ±SD area under the concentration-time curve (AUC) for pediatric patients (8 months to 17 years), receiving 50 or 100 µg/kg was 137 ± 56 ng·h/ml or 237 ± 20 ng·h/ml, respectively, compared with 189 ± 41 ng·h/ml in adults receiving 50 µg/kg. Available data suggest that clearance of IL-11 decreases with patient age, and that clearance in infants and children (8 months to 11 years) is approximately 1.2- to 1.6-fold higher than adults and adolescents (ages 12 and over).

In preclinical studies in rats, radiolabeled oprelvekin was rapidly cleared from the serum and distributed to highly perfused organs. The kidney was the primary route of elimination. The amount of intact oprelvekin in urine was low, indicating that the molecule was metabolized before excretion.

PHARMACODYNAMICS

In a study in which oprelvekin was administered to non-myelosuppressed cancer patients, daily subcutaneous dosing for 14 days with oprelvekin increased the platelet count in a dose-dependent manner. Platelet counts began to increase relative to baseline between 5 and 9 days after the start of dosing with oprelvekin. After cessation of treatment, platelet counts continued to increase for up to 7 days then returned toward baseline within 14 days. No change in platelet reactivity as measured by platelet activation in response to ADP, and platelet aggregation in response to ADP, epinephrine, collagen, ristocetin and arachidonic acid has been observed in association with oprelvekin treatment.

In a randomized, double-blind, placebo-controlled study in normal volunteers, subjects receiving oprelvekin had a mean increase in plasma volume of >20%, and all subjects receiving oprelvekin had at least a 10% increase in plasma volume. Red blood cell volume decreased similarly (due to repeated phlebotomy) in the oprelvekin and placebo groups. As a result, whole blood volume increased approximately 10% and hemoglobin concentration decreased approximately 10% in subjects receiving oprelvekin compared with subjects receiving placebo. Mean 24 hour sodium excretion decreased, and potassium excretion did not increase, in subjects receiving oprelvekin compared with subjects receiving placebo.

INDICATIONS AND USAGE

Oprelvekin is indicated for the prevention of severe thrombocytopenia and the reduction of the need for platelet transfusions following myelosuppressive chemotherapy in patients with nonmyeloid malignancies who are at high risk of severe thrombocytopenia. Efficacy was demonstrated in patients who had experienced severe thrombocytopenia following the previous chemotherapy cycle. Oprelvekin is not indicated following myeloablative chemotherapy.

CONTRAINDICATIONS

Oprelvekin is contraindicated in patients with a history of hypersensitivity to oprelvekin or any component of the product.

WARNINGS

Oprelvekin is known to cause fluid retention (see CLINICAL PHARMACOLOGY, Pharmacodynamics), and it should be used with caution in patients with clinically evident congestive heart failure, patients who may be susceptible to developing congestive heart failure, and patients with a history of heart failure who are well-compensated and receiving appropriate medical therapy (see PRECAUTIONS, Fluid Retention).

Close monitoring of fluid and electrolyte status should be performed in patients receiving chronic diuretic therapy. Sudden deaths have occurred in Oprelvekin-treated patients receiving chronic diuretic therapy and ifosfamide who developed severe hypokalemia (see ADVERSE REACTIONS).

PRECAUTIONS

GENERAL

Dosing with oprelvekin should begin 6-24 hours following the completion of chemotherapy dosing. The safety and efficacy of oprelvekin given immediately prior to or concurrently with cytotoxic chemotherapy have not been established (see DOSAGE AND ADMINISTRATION).

Oprelvekin has not been evaluated in patients receiving chemotherapy regimens of greater than 5 days duration or regimens associated with delayed myelosuppression (*e.g.*, nitrosoureas, mitomycin-C).

The parenteral administration of oprelvekin should be attended by appropriate precautions in case allergic reactions occur (see CONTRAINDICATIONS).

FLUID RETENTION

Patients receiving oprelvekin have commonly experienced mild to moderate fluid retention as indicated by peripheral edema or dyspnea on exertion. Weight gain has been uncommon. The fluid retention is reversible within several days following discontinuation of oprelvekin. In some patients, preexisting pleural effusions have increased during administration of oprelvekin. Preexisting fluid collections, including pericardial effusions or ascites, should be monitored. Drainage should be considered if medically indicated. Capillary leak syndrome has not been observed following treatment with oprelvekin.

Moderate decreases in hemoglobin concentration, hematocrit, and red blood cell count (~10-15%) without a decrease in red blood cell mass have been observed. These changes are predominantly due to an increase in plasma volume (dilutional anemia) that is primarily related to renal sodium and water retention. The decrease in hemoglobin concentration typically begins within 3-5 days of the initiation of oprelvekin, and is reversible over approximately a week following discontinuation of oprelvekin.

During dosing with oprelvekin, fluid balance should be monitored and appropriate medical management is advised. If a diuretic is used, fluid and electrolyte balance should be carefully monitored. Oprelvekin should be used with caution in patients who may develop fluid retention as a result of associated medical conditions or whose medical condition may be exacerbated by fluid retention.

CARDIOVASCULAR EVENTS

Oprelvekin should be used with caution in patients with a history of atrial arrhythmia, and only after consideration of the potential risks in relation to anticipated benefit. Transient atrial arrhythmias (atrial fibrillation or atrial flutter) have occurred in approximately 10% of patients following treatment with oprelvekin. In some patients this may be due to increased plasma volume associated with fluid retention (See PRECAUTIONS, Fluid Retention); oprelvekin has been shown not to be directly arrhythmogenic. Arrhythmias have usually been brief in duration and without clinical sequelae; some were asymptomatic. Conversion to sinus rhythm typically occurred spontaneously or after rate-control drug therapy. Most patients have continued to receive oprelvekin without recurrence of atrial arrhythmia. A retrospective analysis of data from clinical studies of oprelvekin suggests that advancing age and other conditions associated with an increased risk of atrial arrhythmias such as use of cardiac medications and a history of doxorubicin exposure are risk factors for the development of atrial fibrillation or atrial flutter in patients receiving oprelvekin. Ventricular arrhythmias have not been attributed to the use of oprelvekin.

OPHTHALMOLOGIC EVENTS

Transient, mild visual blurring has occasionally been reported by patients treated with oprelvekin. Papilledema has been reported in approximately 1.5% of patients treated with oprelvekin following repeated cycles of exposure. Nonhuman primates treated with oprelvekin at a dose of 1000 μg/kg SC once daily for 4-13 weeks developed papilledema which was not associated with inflammation or any other histologic abnormality and was reversible after dosing was discontinued. Oprelvekin should be used with caution in patients with preexisting papilledema, or with tumors involving the central nervous system since it is possible that papilledema could worsen or develop during treatment.

ANTIBODY FORMATION/ALLERGIC REACTIONS

A small proportion (1%) of patients receiving oprelvekin in clinical studies developed antibodies to oprelvekin and transient rashes were occasionally observed at the injection site following oprelvekin administration. The presence of these antibodies or injection site reactions have not been correlated with clinical symptoms such as anaphylactoid reactions or a loss of clinical response to oprelvekin. No anaphylactoid or other severe adverse allergic reactions were reported in clinical studies following single or repeated doses of oprelvekin.

INFORMATION FOR THE PATIENT

In situations when the physician determines that oprelvekin may be used outside of the hospital or office setting, persons who will be administering oprelvekin should be instructed as to the proper dose, and the method for reconstituting and administering oprelvekin (see DOSAGE AND ADMINISTRATION). If home use is prescribed, patients should be instructed in the importance of proper disposal and cautioned against the reuse of needles, syringes, drug product, and diluent. A puncture resistant container should be used by the patient for the disposal of used needles.

Patients should be informed of the most common adverse reactions associated with oprelvekin administration, including those symptoms related to fluid retention (see ADVERSE REACTIONS and PRECAUTIONS). Mild to moderate peripheral edema and shortness of breath on exertion can occur within the first week of treatment and may continue for the duration of administration of oprelvekin. Patients who have preexisting pleural or other effusions or a history of congestive heart failure should be advised to contact their physician for worsening of dyspnea. Most patients who receive oprelvekin develop some anemia. Patients who are older or who have other risk factors for the development of atrial arrhythmias should be cautioned to contact their physician if symptoms attributable to atrial arrhythmia develop and are not transient. Female patients of childbearing potential should be advised of the possible risks to the fetus of oprelvekin (see PRECAUTIONS, Pregnancy Category C).

LABORATORY TESTS

A complete blood count should be obtained prior to chemotherapy and at regular intervals during oprelvekin therapy (see DOSAGE AND ADMINISTRATION). Platelet counts should be monitored during the time of the expected nadir and until adequate recovery has occurred (post-nadir counts ≥50,000).

CARCINOGENESIS, MUTAGENESIS, AND IMPAIRMENT OF FERTILITY

No studies have been performed to assess the carcinogenic potential of oprelvekin. *In vitro*, oprelvekin did not stimulate the growth of tumor colony-forming cells harvested from patients with a variety of human malignancies. Oprelvekin has been shown to be non-genotoxic in *in vitro* studies. These data suggest that oprelvekin is not mutagenic. Although prolonged estrus cycles have been noted at 2-20 times the human dose, no effects on fertility have been observed in rats treated with oprelvekin at doses up to 1000 μg/kg/day.

PREGNANCY CATEGORY C

Oprelvekin has been shown to have embryocidal effects in pregnant rats and rabbits when given in doses of 0.2 to 20 times the human dose. There are no adequate and well-controlled studies of oprelvekin in pregnant women. Oprelvekin should be used during pregnancy only if the potential benefit justifies the potential risk to the fetus.

Oprelvekin has been tested in studies of fertility and early embryonic development in rats and in studies of organogenesis (teratogenicity) in rats and rabbits. Parental toxicity has been observed when oprelvekin is given at doses of 2 to 20 times the human dose (≥100 μg/kg/day) in the rat and when given in doses of 0.02 to 2.0 times the human dose (≥1 μg/kg/day) in the rabbit. Findings in the rat consisted of transient hypoactivity and dyspnea after administration, as well as prolonged estrus cycle, increased early embryonic deaths and decreased numbers of live fetuses. In addition, low fetal body weights and a reduced number of ossified sacral and caudal vertebrae (*i.e.*, retarded fetal development) occurred in rats at 20 times the human dose, but no long-term behavioral or developmental abnormalities were evident. Findings in the rabbits consisted of decreased (fecal/urine) eliminations (the only toxicity noted at 1 μg/kg/day) as well as decreased food consumption, body weight loss, abortion, increased embryonic and fetal deaths, and decreased numbers of live fetuses. There have been no teratogenic effects of oprelvekin observed in rabbits.

NURSING MOTHERS

It is not known if oprelvekin is excreted in human milk. Because many drugs are excreted in human milk and because of the potential for serious adverse reactions in nursing infants from oprelvekin, a decision should be made whether to discontinue nursing or to discontinue the drug, taking into account the importance of the drug to the mother.

PEDIATRIC USE

Efficacy trials have not been conducted in a pediatric population. Preliminary data are available from an ongoing pharmacokinetic study in 28 patients ages 8 months to 17 years who have been treated with oprelvekin at doses of 25-100 μg/kg following ICE (ifosfamide, etoposide, carboplatin) chemotherapy. Oprelvekin treatment was given once daily for a maximum of 28 days in up to eight cycles. Based upon this study, a dose of 75-100 μg/kg in the pediatric population will produce plasma levels consistent with those obtained in adults given 50 μg/kg (see CLINICAL PHARMACOLOGY, Pharmacokinetics).

Adverse events in this pediatric open-label, non-comparative study were generally similar to those observed using oprelvekin at a dose of 50 μg/kg in the randomized chemotherapy studies in adults. Most adverse events that were associated with oprelvekin in adults occurred either with similar or lower frequency in the pediatric study compared with adults. The incidences of tachycardia (46% [13/28]) and conjunctival injection (50% [14/28]) in the pediatric study were higher than in adults (see ADVERSE REACTIONS). There was no evidence of a dose-response relationship for any of the oprelvekin-associated adverse events among the pediatric patients.

No studies have been performed to assess the long-term effects of oprelvekin on growth and development. In growing rodents treated with 100, 300, or 1000 μg/kg/day for a minimum of 28 days, thickening of femoral and tibial growth plates was noted, which did not completely resolve after a 28 day non-treatment period. In a nonhuman primate toxicology study of oprelvekin, animals treated for 2-13 weeks at doses of 10-1000 μg/kg showed partially reversible joint capsule and tendon fibrosis and periosteal hyperostosis. The clinical significance of these findings is not known. An asymptomatic, laminated periosteal reaction in the diaphyses of the femur, tibia and fibula has been observed in 1 patient during pediatric trials involving multiple courses of oprelvekin treatment. The relationship of these findings to treatment with oprelvekin is unclear.

DRUG INTERACTIONS

Most patients in trials evaluating oprelvekin were treated concomitantly with Filgrastim (granulocyte colony-stimulating factor [G-CSF]) with no adverse effect of oprelvekin on the activity of G-CSF. No information is available on the clinical use of Sargramostim (granulocyte-macrophage colony-stimulating factor [GM-CSF]) with oprelvekin. However, in a study in nonhuman primates in which oprelvekin and GM-CSF were coadministered, there were no adverse interactions between oprelvekin and GM-CSF and no apparent difference in the pharmacokinetic profile of oprelvekin.

Drug interactions between oprelvekin and other drugs have not been fully evaluated. Based on *in vitro* and nonclinical *in vivo* evaluations of oprelvekin, drug-drug interactions with known substrates of P450 enzymes would not be predicted.

ADVERSE REACTIONS

Three hundred eight (308) subjects, with ages ranging from 8 months to 75 years, have been exposed to oprelvekin treatment. Subjects have received up to 6 (8 in pediatric patients) sequential courses of oprelvekin treatment, with each course lasting from 1-28 days. Apart from the sequelae of the underlying malignancy or cytotoxic chemotherapy, most adverse events were mild or moderate in severity and reversible after discontinuation of oprelvekin dosing.

In general, the incidence and type of adverse events were similar between oprelvekin 50 μg/kg and placebo groups. The following adverse events, occurring in ≥10% of patients, were observed at equal or greater frequency in placebo-treated patients: asthenia, pain, chills, abdominal pain, infection, anorexia, constipation, dyspepsia, ecchymosis, myalgia, bone pain, nervousness, and alopecia. Selected adverse events that occurred in oprelvekin-treated patients are listed in TABLE 3.

TABLE 3 *Selected Adverse Events*

Body System / Adverse Event	Placebo n=67	50 μg/kg n=69
Body as a Whole		
Edema*	10 (15%)	41 (59%)
Neutropenic fever	28 (42%)	33 (48%)
Headache	24 (36%)	28 (41%)
Fever	19 (28%)	25 (36%)
Cardiovascular System		
Tachycardia*	2 (3%)	14 (20%)
Vasodilatation	6 (9%)	13 (19%)
Palpitations*	2 (3%)	10 (14%)
Syncope	4 (6%)	9 (13%)
Atrial fibrillation/flutter*	1 (1%)	8 (12%)
Digestive System		
Nausea/vomiting	47 (70%)	53 (77%)
Mucositis	25 (37%)	30 (43%)
Diarrhea	22 (33%)	30 (43%)
Oral moniliasis*	1 (1%)	10 (14%)
Nervous System		
Dizziness	19 (28%)	26 (38%)
Insomnia	18 (27%)	23 (33%)
Respiratory System		
Dyspnea*	15 (22%)	33 (48%)
Rhinitis	21 (31%)	29 (42%)
Cough increased	15 (22%)	20 (29%)
Pharyngitis	11 (16%)	17 (25%)
Pleural effusions*	0 (0%)	7 (10%)
Skin and Appendages		
Rash	11 (16%)	17 (25%)
Special Senses		
Conjunctival injection*	2 (3%)	13 (19%)

* Occurred in significantly more oprelvekin-treated patients than in placebo-treated patients.

The following adverse events also occurred more frequently in cancer patients receiving oprelvekin than in those receiving placebo: amblyopia, paresthesia, dehydration, skin discoloration, exfoliative dermatitis, and eye hemorrhage; a statistically significant association of oprelvekin to these events has not been established. Other than a higher incidence of severe asthenia in oprelvekin treated patients (10 [14%] in oprelvekin patients versus 2 [3%] in placebo patients), the incidence of severe or life-threatening adverse events was comparable in the oprelvekin and placebo treatment groups.

The incidence of fever, neutropenic fever, flu-like symptoms, thrombocytosis, thrombotic events, the average number of units of red blood cells transfused per patient, and the duration of neutropenia <500 cells/μl were similar in the oprelvekin 50 μg/kg and placebo groups.

Two patients with cancer treated with oprelvekin experienced sudden death which the investigator considered possibly or probably related to oprelvekin. Both deaths occurred in patients with severe hypokalemia (<3.0 mEq/L) who had received high doses of ifosfamide and were receiving daily doses of a diuretic. The relationship of these deaths to oprelvekin remains unclear.

ABNORMAL LABORATORY VALUES

The most common laboratory abnormality reported in patients in clinical trials was a decrease in hemoglobin concentration predominantly as a result of expansion of the plasma volume (see PRECAUTIONS, Fluid Retention). The increase in plasma volume is also associated with a decrease in the serum concentration of albumin and several other proteins (*e.g.*, transferrin and gamma globulins). A parallel decrease in calcium without clinical effects has been documented.

After daily SC injections, treatment with oprelvekin resulted in a 2-fold increase in plasma fibrinogen. Other acute-phase proteins also increased. These protein levels returned to normal after dosing with oprelvekin was discontinued. Von Willebrand factor (vWF) concentrations increased with a normal multimer pattern in healthy subjects receiving oprelvekin.

DOSAGE AND ADMINISTRATION

The Neumega vial contains a powder which must be reconstituted prior to injection in 1 ml of sterile water for injection provided with oprelvekin. Powdered oprelvekin and sterile water for injection should be stored in a refrigerator at 2-8°C (36-46°F). DO NOT FREEZE.

A new vial of Neumega and sterile water for injection should be used to prepare each dose. Do not use Neumega or sterile water for injection beyond the expiration date printed on the vial. Any unused portion of reconstituted Neumega medication or sterile water for injection remaining in the vial should be discarded. Because neither oprelvekin powder for injection nor its accompanying sterile water for injection contain a preservative, the single-use vials should not be reentered or reused.

Oprelvekin should be used as soon as possible following reconstitution and must be used within 3 hours of reconstitution. The reconstituted oprelvekin solution can be stored in the vial for up to 3 hours either at room temperature up to 25°C (77°F), or in the refrigerator at 2-8°C (36-46°F). THE RECONSTITUTED SOLUTION SHOULD NOT BE STORED IN A SYRINGE.

NOTE: Follow aseptic technique in reconstitution and administration as demonstrated by the health care professional.

The recommended dose of oprelvekin in adults is 50 μg/kg given once daily. Oprelvekin should be administered subcutaneously as a single injection in either the abdomen, thigh, or hip (or upper arm if not self-injecting). Based upon a pharmacokinetic study, a dose of 75-100 μg/kg in the pediatric population will produce plasma levels consistent with those obtained in adults given 50 μg/kg (see CLINICAL PHARMACOLOGY, Pharmacokinetics).

Dosing should be initiated 6-24 hours after the completion of chemotherapy. Platelet counts should be monitored periodically to assess the optimal duration of therapy. Dosing should be continued until the post-nadir platelet count is ≥50,000 cells/μl. In controlled clinical studies, doses were administered in courses of 10-21 days. Dosing beyond 21 days per treatment course is not recommended.

Treatment with oprelvekin should be discontinued at least 2 days before starting the next planned cycle of chemotherapy.

HOW SUPPLIED

Neumega is supplied as a sterile, white, preservative-free, lyophilize powder in vials containing 5 mg oprelvekin. Neumega is available in boxes containing one single-dose oprelvekin vial and one 5 ml vial of diluent for oprelvekin (sterile water for injection); and boxes containing seven single-dose oprelvekin vials and seven 5 ml vials of diluent for oprelvekin (sterile water for injection).

Storage: Lyophilized oprelvekin and diluent should be stored in a refrigerator at 2-8°C (36-46°F). DO NOT FREEZE. Reconstituted oprelvekin must be used within 3 hours of reconstitution and can be stored in the vial either at 2-8°C (36-46°F) or at room temperature up to 25°C (77°F).

PRODUCT LISTING - EQUIVALENTS NOT AVAILABLE

Solution - Subcutaneous - 5 mg

1's	$282.00	NEUMEGA, Genetics Institute	58394-0004-01
7's	$1973.75	NEUMEGA, Genetics Institute	58394-0004-02

Orlistat (003436)

Categories: Obesity, management; FDA Approved 1999 April; Pregnancy Category B

Drug Classes: Gastrointestinals; Lipase inhibitors

Brand Names: **Xenical**

Cost of Therapy: $118.80 (Weight Loss; Xenical; 120 mg; 3 capsules/day; 30 day supply)

DESCRIPTION

Orlistat is a lipase inhibitor for obesity management that acts by inhibiting the absorption of dietary fats.

Orlistat is (S)-2-formylamino-4-methyl-pentanoic acid (S)-1-[[(2S,3S)-3-hexyl-4-oxo-2-oxetanyl]methyl]-dodecyl ester. Its empirical formula is $C_{29}H_{53}NO_5$, and its molecular weight is 495.7. It is a single diastereomeric molecule that contains four chiral centers, with a negative optical rotation in ethanol at 529 nm.

Orlistat is a white to off-white crystalline powder. Orlistat is practically insoluble in water, freely soluble in chloroform, and very soluble in methanol and ethanol. Orlistat has no pKa within the physiological pH range.

Xenical is available for oral administration in dark-blue, hard-gelatin capsules, with light-blue imprinting. Each capsule contains 120 mg of the active ingredient, orlistat. The capsules also contain the inactive ingredients microcrystalline cellulose, sodium starch glycolate, sodium lauryl sulfate, povidone, and talc. Each capsule shell contains gelatin, titanium dioxide, and FD&C blue no. 1, with printing of pharmaceutical glaze, titanium dioxide, and FD&C blue no. 1 aluminum lake.

CLINICAL PHARMACOLOGY

MECHANISM OF ACTION

Orlistat is a reversible inhibitor of lipases. It exerts its therapeutic activity in the lumen of the stomach and small intestine by forming a covalent bond with the active serine residue site of gastric and pancreatic lipases. The inactivated enzymes are thus unavailable to hydrolyze dietary fat in the form of triglycerides into absorbable free fatty acids and monoglycerides. As undigested triglycerides are not absorbed, the resulting caloric deficit may have a positive effect on weight control. Systemic absorption of the drug is therefore not needed for activity. At the recommended therapeutic dose of 120 mg three times a day, orlistat inhibits dietary fat absorption by approximately 30%.

PHARMACOKINETICS

Absorption

Systemic exposure to orlistat is minimal. Following oral dosing with 360 mg ^{14}C-orlistat, plasma radioactivity peaked at approximately 8 hours; plasma concentrations of intact orlistat were near the limits of detection (<5 ng/ml). In therapeutic studies involving monitoring of plasma samples, detection of intact orlistat in plasma was sporadic and concentrations were low (<10 ng/ml or 0.02 μM), without evidence of accumulation, and consistent with minimal absorption.

The average absolute bioavailability of intact orlistat was assessed in studies with male rats at oral doses of 150 and 1000 mg/kg/day and in male dogs at oral doses of 100 and 1000 mg/kg/day and found to be 0.12%, 0.59% in rats and 0.7%, 1.9% in dogs, respectively.

Distribution

In vitro orlistat was >99% bound to plasma proteins (lipoproteins and albumin were major binding proteins). Orlistat minimally partitioned into erythrocytes.

Metabolism

Based on animal data, it is likely that the metabolism of orlistat occurs mainly within the gastrointestinal wall. Based on an oral ^{14}C-orlistat mass balance study in obese patients, two metabolites, M1 (4-member lactone ring hydrolyzed) and M3 (M1 with N-formyl leucine moiety cleaved), accounted for approximately 42% of total radioactivity in plasma. M1 and M3 have an open beta-lactone ring and extremely weak lipase inhibitory activity (1000- and 2500-fold less than orlistat, respectively). In view of this low inhibitory activity and the low plasma levels at the therapeutic dose (average of 26 ng/ml and 108 ng/ml for M1 and M3, respectively, 2-4 hours after a dose), these metabolites are considered pharmacologically inconsequential. The primary metabolite M1 had a short half-life (approximately 3 hours) whereas the secondary metabolite M3 disappeared at a slower rate (half-life approximately 13.5 hours). In obese patients, steady-state plasma levels of M1, but not M3, increased in proportion to orlistat doses.

Elimination

Following a single oral dose of 360 mg ^{14}C-orlistat in both normal weight and obese subjects, fecal excretion of the unabsorbed drug was found to be the major route of elimination. Orlistat and its M1 and M3 metabolites were also subject to biliary excretion. Approximately 97% of the administered radioactivity was excreted in feces; 83% of that was found to be unchanged orlistat. The cumulative renal excretion of total radioactivity was <2% of the given dose of 360 mg ^{14}C-orlistat. The time to reach complete excretion (fecal plus urinary) was 3-5 days. The disposition of orlistat appeared to be similar between normal weight and obese subjects. Based on limited data, the half-life of the absorbed orlistat is in the range of 1-2 hours.

Special Populations

Because the drug is minimally absorbed, studies in special populations (geriatric, pediatric, different races, patients with renal and hepatic insufficiency) were not conducted.

Drug-Drug Interactions

Drug-drug interaction studies indicate that orlistat had no effect on pharmacokinetics and/or pharmacodynamics of alcohol, digoxin, glyburide, nifedipine (extended-release tablets), oral contraceptives, phenytoin, pravastatin, or warfarin. Alcohol did not affect the pharmacodynamics of orlistat.

OTHER SHORT-TERM STUDIES

In several studies of up to 6 weeks duration, the effects of therapeutic doses of orlistat on gastrointestinal and systemic physiological processes were assessed in normal-weight and obese subjects. Postprandial cholecystokinin plasma concentrations were lowered after multiple doses of orlistat in two studies but not significantly different from placebo in two other experiments. There were no clinically significant changes observed in gallbladder motility, bile composition or lithogenicity, or colonic cell proliferation rate, and no clinically significant reduction of gastric emptying time or gastric acidity. In addition, no effects on plasma triglyceride levels or systemic lipases were observed with the administration of orlistat in these studies. In a 3 week study of 28 healthy male volunteers, orlistat (120 mg three times a day) did not significantly affect the balance of calcium, magnesium, phosphorus, zinc, copper, and iron.

DOSE-RESPONSE RELATIONSHIP

A simple maximum effect (E_{max}) model was used to define the dose-response curve of the relationship between orlistat daily dose and fecal fat excretion as representative of gastrointestinal lipase inhibition. The dose-response curve demonstrated a steep portion for doses up to approximately 400 mg daily, followed by a plateau for higher doses. At doses greater than 120 mg three times a day, the percentage increase in effect was minimal.

INDICATIONS AND USAGE

Orlistat is indicated for obesity management including weight loss and weight maintenance when used in conjunction with a reduced-calorie diet. Orlistat is also indicated to reduce the risk for weight regain after prior weight loss. Orlistat is indicated for obese patients with an initial body mass index (BMI) ≥ 30 kg/m^2 or ≥ 27 kg/m^2 in the presence of other risk factors (*e.g.,* hypertension, diabetes, dyslipidemia).

TABLE 5A, TABLE 5B, and TABLE 5C illustrate body mass index (BMI) according to a variety of weights and heights. The BMI is calculated by dividing weight in kilograms by height in meters squared. For example, a person who weighs 180 lb and is 5'5″ would have a BMI of 30.

TABLE 5A *Body Mass Index (BMI), kg/m²**

Height	Weight (lb) 120	130	140	150	160	170	180
4'10″	25	27	29	31	34	36	38
4'11″	24	26	28	30	32	34	36
5'0″	23	25	27	29	31	33	35
5'1″	23	25	27	28	30	32	34
5'2″	22	24	26	27	29	31	33
5'3″	21	23	25	27	28	30	32
5'4″	21	22	24	26	28	29	31
5'5″	20	22	23	25	27	28	30
5'6″	19	21	23	24	26	27	29
5'7″	19	20	22	24	25	27	28
5'8″	18	20	21	23	24	26	27
5'9″	18	19	21	22	24	25	27
5'10″	17	19	20	22	23	24	26
5'11″	17	18	20	21	22	24	25
6'0″	16	18	19	20	22	23	24
6'1″	16	17	19	20	21	22	24
6'2″	15	17	18	19	21	22	23

* **Conversion Factors:** Weight in lb ÷ 2.2 = weight in kilograms (kg); height in inches × 0.0254 = height in meters (m); 1 foot = 12 inches.

TABLE 5B *Body Mass Index (BMI), kg/m²**

Height	Weight (lb) 190	200	210	220	230	240	250
4'10″	40	42	44	46	48	50	52
4'11″	38	40	43	45	47	49	51
5'0″	37	39	41	43	45	47	49
5'1″	36	38	40	42	44	45	47
5'2″	35	37	38	40	42	44	46
5'3″	34	36	37	39	41	43	44
5'4″	33	34	36	38	40	41	43
5'5″	32	33	35	37	38	40	42
5'6″	31	32	34	36	37	39	40
5'7″	30	31	33	35	36	38	39
5'8″	29	30	32	34	35	37	38
5'9″	28	30	31	33	34	36	37
5'10″	27	29	30	32	33	35	36
5'11″	27	28	29	31	32	34	35
6'0″	26	27	29	30	31	33	34
6'1″	25	26	28	29	30	32	33
6'2″	24	26	27	28	30	31	32

* **Conversion Factors:** Weight in lb ÷ 2.2 = weight in kilograms (kg); height in inches × 0.0254 = height in meters (m); 1 foot = 12 inches.

TABLE 5C *Body Mass Index (BMI), kg/m²**

Height	Weight (lb) 260	270	280	290	300	310	320
4'10″	54	57	59	61	63	65	67
4'11″	53	55	57	59	61	63	65
5'0″	51	53	55	57	59	61	63
5'1″	49	51	53	55	57	59	61
5'2″	48	49	51	53	55	57	59
5'3″	46	48	50	51	53	55	57
5'4″	45	46	48	50	52	53	55
5'5″	43	45	47	48	50	52	53
5'6″	42	44	45	47	49	50	52
5'7″	41	42	44	46	47	49	50
5'8″	40	41	43	44	46	47	49
5'9″	38	40	41	43	44	46	47
5'10″	37	39	40	42	43	45	46
5'11″	36	38	39	41	42	43	45
6'0″	35	37	38	39	41	42	43
6'1″	34	36	37	38	40	41	42
6'2″	33	35	36	37	39	40	41

* **Conversion Factors:** Weight in lb ÷ 2.2 = weight in kilograms (kg); height in inches × 0.0254 = height in meters (m); 1 foot = 12 inches.

CONTRAINDICATIONS

Orlistat is contraindicated in patients with chronic malabsorption syndrome or cholestasis, and in patients with known hypersensitivity to orlistat or to any component of this product.

O

WARNINGS

MISCELLANEOUS

Organic causes of obesity (*e.g.*, hypothyroidism) should be excluded before prescribing orlistat.

Preliminary data from an orlistat and cyclosporine drug interaction study indicate a reduction in cyclosporine plasma levels when orlistat was coadministered with cyclosporine. Therefore, orlistat and cyclosporine should not be coadministered. To reduce the chance of a drug-drug interaction, cyclosporine should be taken at least 2 hours before or after orlistat in patients taking both drugs. In addition, in those patients whose cyclosporine levels are being measured, more frequent monitoring should be considered.

PRECAUTIONS

GENERAL

Patients should be advised to adhere to dietary guidelines (see DOSAGE AND ADMINISTRATION). Gastrointestinal events (see ADVERSE REACTIONS) may increase when orlistat is taken with a diet high in fat (>30% total daily calories from fat). The daily intake of fat should be distributed over 3 main meals. If orlistat is taken with any 1 meal very high in fat, the possibility of gastrointestinal effects increases.

Patients should be counseled to take a multivitamin supplement that contains fat-soluble vitamins to ensure adequate nutrition because orlistat has been shown to reduce the absorption of some fat-soluble vitamins and beta-carotene. In addition, the levels of vitamin D and beta-carotene may be low in obese patients compared with non-obese subjects. The supplement should be taken once a day at least 2 hours before or after the administration of orlistat, such as at bedtime.

TABLE 6 illustrates the percentage of patients on orlistat and placebo who developed a low vitamin level on two or more consecutive visits during 1 and 2 years of therapy in studies in which patients were not previously receiving vitamin supplementation.

TABLE 6 *Incidence of Low Vitamin Values on Two or More Consecutive Visits*

Nonsupplemented patients with normal baseline values — first and second year

	Placebo*	Orlistat*
Vitamin A	1.0%	2.2%
Vitamin D	6.6%	12.0%
Vitamin E	1.0%	5.8%
Beta-carotene	1.7%	6.1%

* Treatment designates placebo plus diet or orlistat plus diet.

Some patients may develop increased levels of urinary oxalate following treatment with orlistat. Caution should be exercised when prescribing orlistat to patients with a history of hyperoxaluria or calcium oxalate nephrolithiasis.

Weight-loss induction by orlistat may be accompanied by improved metabolic control in diabetics, which might require a reduction in dose of oral hypoglycemic medication (*e.g.*, sulfonylureas, metformin) or insulin.

MISUSE POTENTIAL

As with any weight-loss agent, the potential exists for misuse of orlistat in inappropriate patient populations (*e.g.*, patients with anorexia nervosa or bulimia). See INDICATIONS AND USAGE for recommended prescribing guidelines.

INFORMATION FOR THE PATIENT

Patients should read the Patient Information accompanying their prescription before starting treatment with orlistat and each time their prescription is renewed.

CARCINOGENESIS, MUTAGENESIS, AND IMPAIRMENT OF FERTILITY

Carcinogenicity studies in rats and mice did not show a carcinogenic potential for orlistat at doses up to 1000 mg/kg/day and 1500 mg/kg/day, respectively. For mice and rats, these doses are 38 and 46 times the daily human dose calculated on an area under concentration versus time curve basis of total drug-related material.

Orlistat had no detectable mutagenic or genotoxic activity as determined by the Ames test, a mammalian forward mutation assay (V79/HPRT), an *in vitro* clastogenesis assay in peripheral human lymphocytes, an unscheduled DNA synthesis assay (UDS) in rat hepatocytes in culture, and an *in vivo* mouse micronucleus test.

When given to rats at a dose of 400 mg/kg/day in a fertility and reproduction study, orlistat had no observable adverse effects. This dose is 12 times the daily human dose calculated on a body surface area (mg/m^2) basis.

PREGNANCY, TERATOGENIC EFFECTS, PREGNANCY CATEGORY B

Teratogenicity studies were conducted in rats and rabbits at doses up to 800 mg/kg/day. Neither study showed embryotoxicity or teratogenicity. This dose is 23 and 47 times the daily human dose calculated on a body surface area (mg/m^2) basis for rats and rabbits, respectively.

The incidence of dilated cerebral ventricles was increased in the mid- and high-dose groups of the rat teratology study. These doses were 6 and 23 times the daily human dose calculated on a body surface area (mg/m^2) basis for the mid- and high-dose levels, respectively. This finding was not reproduced in two additional rat teratology studies at similar doses.

There are no adequate and well-controlled studies of orlistat in pregnant women. Because animal reproductive studies are not always predictive of human response, orlistat is not recommended for use during pregnancy.

NURSING MOTHERS

It is not known if orlistat is secreted in human milk. Therefore, orlistat should not be taken by nursing women.

PEDIATRIC USE

The safety and efficacy of orlistat in pediatric patients have not been established.

GERIATRIC USE

Clinical studies of orlistat did not include sufficient numbers of patients aged 65 years and older to determine whether they respond differently from younger patients.

DRUG INTERACTIONS

ALCOHOL

In a multiple-dose study in 30 normal-weight subjects, coadministration of orlistat and 40 g of alcohol (*e.g.*, approximately 3 glasses of wine) did not result in alteration of alcohol pharmacokinetics, orlistat pharmacodynamics (fecal fat excretion), or systemic exposure to orlistat.

CYCLOSPORINE

Preliminary data from an orlistat and cyclosporine drug interaction study indicate a reduction in cyclosporine plasma levels when orlistat was coadministered with cyclosporine (see WARNINGS).

DIGOXIN

In 12 normal-weight subjects receiving orlistat 120 mg three times a day for 6 days, orlistat did not alter the pharmacokinetics of a single dose of digoxin.

FAT-SOLUBLE VITAMIN SUPPLEMENTS AND ANALOGUES

A pharmacokinetic interaction study showed a 30% reduction in beta-carotene supplement absorption when concomitantly administered with orlistat. Orlistat inhibited absorption of a vitamin E acetate supplement by approximately 60%. The effect of orlistat on the absorption of supplemental vitamin D, vitamin A, and nutritionally-derived vitamin K is not known at this time.

GLYBURIDE

In 12 normal-weight subjects receiving orlistat 80 mg three times a day for 5 days, orlistat did not alter the pharmacokinetics or pharmacodynamics (blood glucose-lowering) of glyburide.

NIFEDIPINE (EXTENDED-RELEASE TABLETS)

In 17 normal-weight subjects receiving orlistat 120 mg three times a day for 6 days, orlistat did not alter the bioavailability of nifedipine (extended-release tablets).

ORAL CONTRACEPTIVES

In 20 normal-weight female subjects, the treatment of orlistat 120 mg three times a day for 23 days resulted in no changes in the ovulation-suppressing action of oral contraceptives.

PHENYTOIN

In 12 normal-weight subjects receiving orlistat 120 mg three times a day for 7 days, orlistat did not alter the pharmacokinetics of a single 300 mg dose of phenytoin.

PRAVASTATIN

In a 2-way crossover study of 24 normal-weight, mildly hypercholesterolemic patients receiving orlistat 120 mg three times a day for 6 days, orlistat did not affect the pharmacokinetics of pravastatin.

WARFARIN

In 12 normal-weight subjects, administration of orlistat 120 mg three times a day for 16 days did not result in any change in either warfarin pharmacokinetics (both R- and S-enantiomers) or pharmacodynamics (prothrombin time and serum Factor VII). Although undercarboxylated osteocalcin, a marker of vitamin K nutritional status, was unaltered with orlistat administration, vitamin K levels tended to decline in subjects taking orlistat. Therefore, as vitamin K absorption may be decreased with orlistat, patients on chronic stable doses of warfarin who are prescribed orlistat should be monitored closely for changes in coagulation parameters.

ADVERSE REACTIONS

COMMONLY OBSERVED

Based on first and second year data — orlistat 120 mg three times a day versus placebo.

Gastrointestinal (GI) symptoms were the most commonly observed treatment-emergent adverse events associated with the use of orlistat in double-blind, placebo-controlled clinical trials and are primarily a manifestation of the mechanism of action. (Commonly observed is defined as an incidence of ≥5% and an incidence in the orlistat 120 mg group that is at least twice that of placebo.)

TABLE 7 *Commonly Observed Adverse Events*

	Year 1		Year 2	
	Orlistat*	Placebo*	Orlistat*	Placebo*
Adverse Event	(n=1913)	(n=1466)	(n=613)	(n=524)
Oily spotting	26.6%	1.3%	4.4%	0.2%
Flatus with discharge	23.9%	1.4%	2.1%	0.2%
Fecal urgency	22.1%	6.7%	2.8%	1.7%
Fatty/oily stool	20.0%	2.9%	5.5%	0.6%
Oily evacuation	11.9%	0.8%	2.3%	0.2%
Increased defecation	10.8%	4.1%	2.6%	0.8%
Fecal incontinence	7.7%	0.9%	1.8%	0.2%

* Treatment designates orlistat 3 times a day plus diet or placebo plus diet.

These and other commonly observed adverse reactions were generally mild and transient, and they decreased during the second year of treatment. In general, the first occurrence of these events was within 3 months of starting therapy. Overall, approximately 50% of all episodes of GI adverse events associated with orlistat treatment lasted for less than 1 week, and a majority lasted for no more than 4 weeks. However, GI adverse events may occur in some individuals over a period of 6 months or longer.

DISCONTINUATION OF TREATMENT

In controlled clinical trials, 8.8% of patients treated with orlistat discontinued treatment due to adverse events, compared with 5.0% of placebo-treated patients. For orlistat, the most common adverse events resulting in discontinuation of treatment were gastrointestinal.

INCIDENCE IN CONTROLLED CLINICAL TRIALS

TABLE 8 lists other treatment-emergent adverse events from seven multicenter, double-blind, placebo-controlled clinical trials that occurred at a frequency of ≥2% among patients treated with orlistat 120 mg three times a day and with an incidence that was greater than placebo during year 1 and year 2, regardless of relationship to study medication.

TABLE 8 *Other Treatment-Emergent Adverse Events From Seven Placebo-Controlled Clinical Trials*

	Year 1		Year 2	
Body System/Adverse Event	Orlistat* (n=1913)	Placebo* (n=1466)	Orlistat* (n=613)	Placebo* (n=524)
Gastrointestinal System				
Abdominal pain/discomfort	25.5%	21.4%	—	—
Nausea	8.1%	7.3%	3.6%	2.7%
Infectious diarrhea	5.3%	4.4%	—	—
Rectal pain/discomfort	5.2%	4.0%	3.3%	1.9%
Tooth disorder	4.3%	3.1%	2.9%	2.3%
Gingival disorder	4.1%	2.9%	2.0%	1.5%
Vomiting	3.8%	3.5%	—	—
Respiratory System				
Influenza	39.7%	36.2%	—	—
Upper respiratory infection	38.1%	32.8%	26.1%	25.8%
Lower respiratory infection	7.8%	6.6%	—	—
Ear, nose & throat symptoms	2.0%	1.6%	—	—
Musculoskeletal System				
Back pain	13.9%	12.1%	—	—
Pain lower extremities	—	—	10.8%	10.3%
Arthritis	5.4%	4.8%	—	—
Myalgia	4.2%	3.3%	—	—
Joint disorder	2.3%	2.2%	—	—
Tendonitis	—	—	2.0%	1.9%
Central Nervous System				
Headache	30.6%	27.6%	—	—
Dizziness	5.2%	5.0%	—	—
Body as a Whole				
Fatigue	7.2%	6.4%	3.1%	1.7%
Sleep disorder	3.9%	3.3%	—	—
Skin & Appenedages				
Rash	4.3%	4.0%	—	—
Dry skin	2.1%	1.4%	—	—
Reproductive, Female				
Menstrual irregularity	9.8%	7.5%	—	—
Vaginitis	3.8%	3.6%	2.6%	1.9%
Urinary System				
Urinary tract infection	7.5%	7.3%	5.9%	4.8%
Psychiatric Disorder				
Psychiatric anxiety	4.7%	2.9%	2.8%	2.1%
Depression	—	—	3.4%	2.5%
Hearing & Vestibular Disorders				
Otitis	4.3%	3.4%	2.9%	2.5%
Cardiovascular Disorders				
Pedal edema	—	—	2.8%	1.9%

* Treatment designates orlistat 120 mg three times a day plus diet or placebo plus diet.
— None reported at a frequency ≥2% and greater than placebo.

OTHER CLINICAL STUDIES OR POSTMARKETING SURVEILLANCE

Rare cases of hypersensitivity have been reported with the use of orlistat. Signs and symptoms have included pruritus, rash, urticaria, angioedema, and anaphylaxis. Preliminary data from an orlistat and cyclosporine drug interaction study indicate a reduction in cyclosporine plasma levels when orlistat was coadministered with cyclosporine (see WARNINGS).

DOSAGE AND ADMINISTRATION

The recommended dose of orlistat is one 120 mg capsule three times a day with each main meal containing fat (during or up to 1 hour after the meal).

The patient should be on a nutritionally balanced, reduced-calorie diet that contains approximately 30% of calories from fat. The daily intake of fat, carbohydrate, and protein should be distributed over 3 main meals. If a meal is occasionally missed or contains no fat, the dose of orlistat can be omitted.

Because orlistat has been shown to reduce the absorption of some fat-soluble vitamins and beta-carotene, patients should be counseled to take a multivitamin containing fat-soluble vitamins to ensure adequate nutrition. The supplement should be taken at least 2 hours before or after the administration of orlistat, such as at bedtime.

Doses above 120 mg three times a day have not been shown to provide additional benefit.

Based on fecal fat measurements, the effect of orlistat is seen as soon as 24-48 hours after dosing. Upon discontinuation of therapy, fecal fat content usually returns to pretreatment levels within 48-72 hours.

The safety and effectiveness of orlistat beyond 2 years have not been determined at this time.

HOW SUPPLIED

Xenical is a dark-blue, 2-piece, no. 1 opaque hard-gelatin capsule imprinted with "Roche" and "XENICAL 120" in light-blue ink containing pellets of powder.

STORAGE

Store at 25°C (77°F); excursions permitted to 15-30°C (59-86°F) [controlled room temperature]. Keep bottle tightly closed.

Xenical should not be used after the given expiration date.

PRODUCT LISTING - EQUIVALENTS NOT AVAILABLE

Capsule - Oral - 120 mg

14's	$18.48	XENICAL, Allscripts Pharmaceutical Company	54569-4742-03
21's	$27.72	XENICAL, Allscripts Pharmaceutical Company	54569-4742-04
28's	$36.96	XENICAL, Allscripts Pharmaceutical Company	54569-4742-05
30's	$39.60	XENICAL, Allscripts Pharmaceutical Company	54569-4742-02
42's	$55.44	XENICAL, Allscripts Pharmaceutical Company	54569-4742-06
60's	$79.20	XENICAL, Allscripts Pharmaceutical Company	54569-4742-01
90's	$118.80	XENICAL, Allscripts Pharmaceutical Company	54569-4742-00
90's	$123.75	XENICAL, Roche Laboratories	00004-0256-52

Orphenadrine Citrate (001920)

Categories: Pain, musculoskeletal; Pregnancy Category C; FDA Approved 1959 Nov
Drug Classes: Musculoskeletal agents; Relaxants, skeletal muscle
Brand Names: Banflex; Flexoject; Flexon; Flexor; Marflex; Mio-Rel; Myolin; Myophen; Myotrol; Neocyten; Noradex; **Norflex**; O'Flex; Orflagen; Orfro; Orphenate; Qualaflex; Tega-Flex
Foreign Brand Availability: Biorfen (England); Biorphen (England); Distalene (Argentina); Disipal (Canada; Denmark; Norway; Sweden); Erilax (Korea); Neekxin (Korea); Neexin (Korea); Orpherin (Korea); Opheryl (Korea); Prolongatum (Sweden); Slaxin (Korea)
Cost of Therapy: $46.20 (Musculoskeletal Pain; Norflex; 100 mg; 2 tablets/day; 10 day supply)
$33.01 (Musculoskeletal Pain; Generic Tablets; 100 mg; 2 tablets/day; 10 day supply)
HCFA JCODE(S): J2360 up to 60 mg IV, IM

DESCRIPTION

Orphenadrine citrate is the citrate salt of orphenadrine (2-dimethylaminoethyl 2-methylbenzhydryl ether citrate). It occurs as a white, crystalline powder having a bitter taste. It is practically odorless; sparingly soluble in water, slightly soluble in alcohol.

Each orphenadrine citrate extended release tablet contains 100 mg orphenadrine citrate. Orphenadrine citrate extended release tablets also contain: calcium stearate, ethylcellulose, and lactose. Orphenadrine citrate injection contains 60 mg of orphenadrine citrate in aqueous solution in each ampul. Orphenadrine citrate injection also contains: sodium bisulfite, 2.0 mg; sodium chloride, 5.8 mg; sodium hydroxide, to adjust pH; and water for injection, qs to 2 ml.

CLINICAL PHARMACOLOGY

The mode of therapeutic action has not been clearly identified, but may be related to its analgesic properties. Orphenadrine citrate also possesses anti-cholinergic actions.

INDICATIONS AND USAGE

Orphenadrine citrate is indicated as an adjunct to rest, physical therapy, and other measures for the relief of discomfort associated with acute painful musculoskeletal conditions. The mode of action of the drug has not been clearly identified, but may be related to its analgesic properties. Orphenadrine citrate does not directly relax tense skeletal muscles in man.

CONTRAINDICATIONS

Contraindicated in patients with glaucoma, pyloric or duodenal obstruction, stenosing peptic ulcers, prostatic hypertrophy or obstruction of the bladder neck, cardio-spasm (megaesophagus) and myasthenia gravis.

Contraindicated in patients who have demonstrated a previous hypersensitivity to the drug.

WARNINGS

Some patients may experience transient episodes of light-headedness, dizziness or syncope. Orphenadrine citrate may impair the ability of the patient to engage in potentially hazardous activities such as operating machinery or driving a motor vehicle; ambulatory patients should therefore be cautioned accordingly.

Orphenadrine citrate injection contains sodium bisulfite, a sulfite that may cause allergic-type reactions including anaphylactic symptoms and life-threatening or less severe asthmatic episodes in certain susceptible people. The overall prevalence of sulfite sensitivity in the general population is unknown and probably low. Sulfite sensitivity is seen more frequently in asthmatic than nonasthmatic people.

PREGNANCY CATEGORY C

Animal reproduction studies have not been conducted with orphenadrine citrate. It is also not known whether orphenadrine citrate can cause fetal harm when administered to a pregnant woman or can affect reproduction capacity. Orphenadrine citrate should be given to a pregnant woman only if clearly needed.

O

USE IN CHILDREN

Safety and effectiveness in children have not been established.

PRECAUTIONS

Confusion, anxiety and tremors have been reported in few patients receiving propoxyphene and orphenadrine concomitantly. As these symptoms may be simply due to an additive effect, reduction to dosage and/or discontinuation of one or both agents is recommended in such cases.

Orphenadrine citrate should be used with caution in patients with tachycardia, cardiac decompensation, coronary insufficiency, cardiac arrhythmias.

Safety of continuous long-term therapy with orphenadrine has not been established. Therefore, if orphenadrine is prescribed for prolonged use, periodic monitoring of blood, urine and liver function values is recommended.

ADVERSE REACTIONS

Adverse reactions of orphenadrine are mainly due to the mild anti-cholinergic action of orphenadrine, and are usually associated with higher dosage. Dryness of the mouth is usually the first adverse effect to appear. When the daily dose is increased, possible adverse effects include: tachycardia, palpitation, urinary hesitancy or retention, blurred vision, dilation of pupils, increased ocular tension, weakness, nausea, vomiting, headache, dizziness, constipation, drowsiness, hypersensitivity reactions, pruritus, hallucinations, agitation, tremor, gastric irritation, and rarely urticaria and other dermatoses. Infrequently, an elderly patient may experience some degree of mental confusion. These adverse reactions can usually be eliminated by reduction in dosage. Very rare cases of aplastic anemia associated with the use of orphenadrine tablets have been reported. No causal relationship has been established.

Rare instances of anaphylactic reaction have been reported associated with the intramuscular injection of orphenadrine citrate injection.

DOSAGE AND ADMINISTRATION

Tablets: *Adults:* Two tablets per day; 1 in the morning and 1 in the evening.

Injection: *Adults:* One 2 ml ampul (60 mg) intravenously or intramuscularly; may be repeated every 12 hours. Relief may be maintained by 1 orphenadrine citrate tablet twice daily.

HOW SUPPLIED

Norflex tablets are round, white tablets imprinted with "3M" on one side and "221" on the other.

Norflex injection is available in 2 ml ampules containing 60 mg of orphenadrine citrate in aqueous solution.

Storage: Store at controlled room temperature, 15-30°C (59-86°F).

PRODUCT LISTING - RATED THERAPEUTICALLY EQUIVALENT

Solution - Injectable - 30 mg/ml

Size	Price	Product	NDC
2 ml x 6	$97.38	NORFLEX INJECTABLE, Allscripts Pharmaceutical Company	54569-1894-01
2 ml x 6	$135.00	NORFLEX INJECTABLE, 3M Pharmaceuticals	00089-0540-06
10 ml	$6.25	GENERIC, Major Pharmaceuticals Inc	00904-0858-10
10 ml	$6.95	GENERIC, Keene Pharmaceuticals Inc	00588-5901-70
10 ml	$7.50	GENERIC, C.O. Truxton Inc	00463-1092-10
10 ml	$8.00	GENERIC, Cmc-Consolidated Midland Corporation	00223-8200-10
10 ml	$9.25	GENERIC, Roberts/Hauck Pharmaceutical Corporation	43797-0115-12
10 ml	$12.00	GENERIC, Forest Pharmaceuticals	00456-1092-10
10 ml	$12.34	GENERIC, Hyrex Pharmaceuticals	00314-0549-10
10 ml	$22.65	GENERIC, Merz Pharmaceuticals	00259-0322-10
10 ml	$29.90	GENERIC, International Ethical Laboratories Inc	11584-1016-05
50 ml	$142.50	GENERIC, International Ethical Laboratories Inc	11584-1016-02

Tablet, Extended Release - Oral - 100 mg

Size	Price	Product	NDC
2's	$8.45	NORFLEX, Prescript Pharmaceuticals	00247-0324-02
8's	$23.74	NORFLEX, Prescript Pharmaceuticals	00247-0324-08
10's	$19.75	NORFLEX, Southwood Pharmaceuticals Inc	58016-0498-10
10's	$23.10	NORFLEX, Allscripts Pharmaceutical Company	54569-0839-03
10's	$26.66	NORFLEX, Pharma Pac	52959-0178-10
10's	$28.84	NORFLEX, Prescript Pharmaceuticals	00247-0324-10
14's	$32.34	NORFLEX, Allscripts Pharmaceutical Company	54569-0839-00
14's	$36.39	NORFLEX, Pharma Pac	52959-0178-14
14's	$39.02	NORFLEX, Prescript Pharmaceuticals	00247-0324-14
14's	$51.84	NORFLEX, Pd-Rx Pharmaceuticals	55289-0646-14
15's	$38.89	NORFLEX, Pharma Pac	52959-0178-15
15's	$41.94	NORFLEX, Physicians Total Care	54868-1056-03
15's	$55.07	NORFLEX, Pd-Rx Pharmaceuticals	55289-0646-15
20's	$46.20	NORFLEX, Allscripts Pharmaceutical Company	54569-0839-02
20's	$54.31	NORFLEX, Prescript Pharmaceuticals	00247-0324-20
20's	$55.09	NORFLEX, Pharma Pac	52959-0178-20
20's	$55.53	NORFLEX, Physicians Total Care	54868-1056-01
20's	$68.33	NORFLEX, Pd-Rx Pharmaceuticals	55289-0646-20
21's	$56.86	NORFLEX, Prescript Pharmaceuticals	00247-0324-21
28's	$74.69	NORFLEX, Prescript Pharmaceuticals	00247-0324-28
30's	$69.30	NORFLEX, Allscripts Pharmaceutical Company	54569-0839-01
30's	$75.75	NORFLEX, Pharma Pac	52959-0178-30
30's	$78.18	NORFLEX, Physicians Total Care	54868-1056-04
30's	$79.79	NORFLEX, Prescript Pharmaceuticals	00247-0324-30
50's	$129.51	NORFLEX, Physicians Total Care	54868-1056-05
100's	$182.25	FEDERAL UPPER LIMIT, H.C.F.A. F F P	99999-1920-01
100's	$207.67	GENERIC, Geneva Pharmaceuticals	00781-1649-01
100's	$217.29	GENERIC, Global Pharmaceutical Corporation	00115-2011-01
100's	$217.45	GENERIC, Watson/Schein Pharmaceuticals Inc	00591-2830-01
100's	$217.50	GENERIC, Mylan Pharmaceuticals Inc	00378-3358-01
100's	$218.42	GENERIC, Eon Labs Manufacturing Inc	00185-0022-01
100's	$231.00	NORFLEX, 3M Pharmaceuticals	00089-0221-10
100's	$257.25	NORFLEX, Physicians Total Care	54868-1056-00
250's	$441.05	GENERIC, Watson/Schein Pharmaceuticals Inc	00364-2830-04

PRODUCT LISTING - EQUIVALENTS NOT AVAILABLE

Solution - Injectable - 30 mg/ml

Size	Price	Product	NDC
10 ml	$19.75	ANTIFLEX, Clint Pharmaceutical Inc	55553-0129-10

Tablet, Extended Release - Oral - 100 mg

Size	Price	Product	NDC
2's	$3.91	GENERIC, Prescript Pharmaceuticals	00247-0368-02
7's	$11.57	GENERIC, Southwood Pharmaceuticals Inc	58016-0248-07
10's	$6.14	GENERIC, Prescript Pharmaceuticals	00247-0368-10
10's	$16.50	GENERIC, Southwood Pharmaceuticals Inc	58016-0248-10
10's	$21.75	GENERIC, Allscripts Pharmaceutical Company	54569-0838-03
10's	$23.68	GENERIC, Pharma Pac	52959-0527-10
12's	$19.80	GENERIC, Southwood Pharmaceuticals Inc	58016-0248-12
14's	$7.26	GENERIC, Prescript Pharmaceuticals	00247-0368-14
14's	$23.10	GENERIC, Southwood Pharmaceuticals Inc	58016-0248-14
14's	$30.45	GENERIC, Allscripts Pharmaceutical Company	54569-0838-02
14's	$32.75	GENERIC, Pharma Pac	52959-0527-14
15's	$26.60	GENERIC, Physicians Total Care	54868-4102-00
15's	$34.58	GENERIC, Southwood Pharmaceuticals Inc	58016-0248-15
15's	$34.95	GENERIC, Pharma Pac	52959-0527-15
20's	$8.94	GENERIC, Prescript Pharmaceuticals	00247-0368-20
20's	$33.00	GENERIC, Southwood Pharmaceuticals Inc	58016-0248-20
20's	$45.97	GENERIC, Pharma Pac	52959-0527-20
21's	$34.65	GENERIC, Southwood Pharmaceuticals Inc	58016-0248-21
28's	$46.21	GENERIC, Southwood Pharmaceuticals Inc	58016-0248-28
30's	$11.73	GENERIC, Prescript Pharmaceuticals	00247-0368-30
30's	$49.51	GENERIC, Southwood Pharmaceuticals Inc	58016-0248-30
30's	$65.25	GENERIC, Allscripts Pharmaceutical Company	54569-0838-01
30's	$68.49	GENERIC, Pharma Pac	52959-0527-30
40's	$66.01	GENERIC, Southwood Pharmaceuticals Inc	58016-0248-40
50's	$115.25	GENERIC, Southwood Pharmaceuticals Inc	58016-0248-50
60's	$99.02	GENERIC, Southwood Pharmaceuticals Inc	58016-0248-60
90's	$148.53	GENERIC, Southwood Pharmaceuticals Inc	58016-0248-90
100's	$9.50	GENERIC, Cmc-Consolidated Midland Corporation	00223-1170-01
100's	$165.03	GENERIC, Southwood Pharmaceuticals Inc	58016-0248-00
100's	$217.45	GENERIC, Watson/Schein Pharmaceuticals Inc	00364-2830-01

Oseltamivir Phosphate *(003452)*

Categories: Influenza virus infection; FDA Approved 1999 Oct; Pregnancy Category C

Drug Classes: Antivirals

Foreign Brand Availability: Tamiflu (Australia; Canada; England; France; Hong-Kong; Ireland; Israel; Korea; New-Zealand; Philippines; Singapore)

Cost of Therapy: $59.54 (Influenza; Tamiflu; 75 mg; 2 capsules/day; 5 day supply)

DESCRIPTION

Tamiflu (oseltamivir phosphate) is available as a capsule containing 75 mg oseltamivir for oral use, in the form of oseltamivir phosphate, and as a powder for oral suspension, which when constituted with water as directed contains 12 mg/ml oseltamivir base. In addition to the active ingredient, each capsule contains pregelatinized starch, talc, povidone K 30, croscarmellose sodium, and sodium stearyl fumarate. The capsule shell contains gelatin, titanium dioxide, yellow iron oxide, black iron oxide, and red iron oxide. Each capsule is printed with blue ink, which includes FD&C blue no. 2 as the colorant. In addition to the active ingredient, the powder for oral suspension contains xanthan gum, monosodium citrate, sodium benzoate, sorbitol, saccharin sodium, titanium dioxide, and tutti-frutti flavoring.

Oseltamivir phosphate is a white crystalline solid with the chemical name (3R,4R,5S)-4-acetylamino-5-amino-3(1-ethylpropoxy)-1-cyclohexene-1-carboxylic acid, ethyl ester, phosphate (1:1). The chemical formula is $C_{16}H_{28}N_2O_4$ (free base). The molecular weight is 312.4 for oseltamivir free base and 410.4 for oseltamivir phosphate salt.

CLINICAL PHARMACOLOGY

MICROBIOLOGY

Mechanism of Action

Oseltamivir is an ethyl ester prodrug requiring ester hydrolysis for conversion to the active form, oseltamivir carboxylate. The proposed mechanism of action of oseltamivir is via inhibition of influenza virus neuraminidase with the possibility of alteration of virus particle aggregation and release.

Antiviral Activity In Vitro

The antiviral activity of oseltamivir carboxylate against laboratory strains and clinical isolates of influenza virus was determined in cell culture assays. The concentrations of oseltamivir carboxylate required for inhibition of influenza virus were highly variable depending on the assay method used and the virus tested. The 50% and 90% inhibitory concentrations (IC50 and IC90) were in the range of 0.0008 μM to >35 μM and 0.004 μM to >100 μM, respectively (1 μM = 0.284 μg/ml). The relationship between the *in vitro* antiviral activity in cell culture and the inhibition of influenza virus replication in humans has not been established.

Drug Resistance

Influenza A virus isolates with reduced susceptibility to oseltamivir carboxylate have been recovered *in vitro* by passage of virus in the presence of increasing concentrations of oseltamivir carboxylate. Genetic analysis of these isolates showed that reduced susceptibility to oseltamivir carboxylate is associated with mutations that result in amino acid changes in the viral neuraminidase or viral hemagglutinin or both.

In clinical studies of postexposure and seasonal prophylaxis, determination of resistance was limited by the low overall incidence rate of influenza infection and prophylactic effect of oseltamivir phosphate.

In clinical studies in the treatment of naturally acquired infection with influenza virus, 1.3% (4/301) of posttreatment isolates in adult patients and adolescents, and 8.6% (9/105) in pediatric patients aged 1-12 years showed emergence of influenza variants with decreased neuraminidase susceptibility to oseltamivir carboxylate.

Genotypic analysis of these variants showed a specific mutation in the active site of neuraminidase compared to pretreatment isolates. The contribution of resistance due to alterations in the viral hemagglutinin has not been fully evaluated.

Cross-Resistance

Cross-resistance between zanamivir-resistant influenza mutants and oseltamivir-resistant influenza mutants has been observed *in vitro.*

Due to limitations in the assays available to detect drug-induced shifts in virus susceptibility, an estimate of the incidence of oseltamivir resistance and possible cross-resistance to zanamivir in clinical isolates cannot be made. However, 1 of the 3 oseltamivir-induced mutations in the viral neuraminidase from clinical isolates is the same as 1 of the 3 mutations observed in zanamivir-resistant virus.

Insufficient information is available to fully characterize the risk of emergence of oseltamivir phosphate resistance in clinical use.

Immune Response

No influenza vaccine interaction study has been conducted. In studies of naturally acquired and experimental influenza, treatment with oseltamivir phosphate did not impair normal humoral antibody response to infection.

PHARMACOKINETICS

Absorption and Bioavailability

Oseltamivir is readily absorbed from the gastrointestinal tract after oral administration of oseltamivir phosphate and is extensively converted predominantly by hepatic esterases to oseltamivir carboxylate. At least 75% of an oral dose reaches the systemic circulation as oseltamivir carboxylate. Exposure to oseltamivir is less than 5% of the total exposure after oral dosing (see TABLE 1).

TABLE 1 *Mean (% CV) Pharmacokinetic Parameters of Oseltamivir and Oseltamivir Carboxylate After a Multiple 75 mg Capsule Twice Daily Oral Dose (n=20)*

Parameter	Oseltamivir	Oseltamivir Carboxylate
C_{max} (ng/ml)	65.2 (26)	348 (18)
AUC(0-12h) (ng·h/ml)	112 (25)	2719 (20)

Plasma concentrations of oseltamivir carboxylate are proportional to doses up to 500 mg given twice daily (see DOSAGE AND ADMINISTRATION).

Coadministration with food has no significant effect on the peak plasma concentration (551 ng/ml under fasted conditions and 441 ng/ml under fed conditions) and the area under the plasma concentration time curve (6218 ng·h/ml under fasted conditions and 6069 ng·h/ml under fed conditions) of oseltamivir carboxylate.

Distribution

The volume of distribution (Vss) of oseltamivir carboxylate, following intravenous administration in 24 subjects, ranged between 23 and 26 liters.

The binding of oseltamivir carboxylate to human plasma protein is low (3%). The binding of oseltamivir to human plasma protein is 42%, which is insufficient to cause significant displacement-based drug interactions.

Metabolism

Oseltamivir is extensively converted to oseltamivir carboxylate by esterases located predominantly in the liver. Neither oseltamivir nor oseltamivir carboxylate is a substrate for, or inhibitor of, cytochrome P450 isoforms.

Elimination

Absorbed oseltamivir is primarily (>90%) eliminated by conversion to oseltamivir carboxylate. Plasma concentrations of oseltamivir declined with a half-life of 1-3 hours in most subjects after oral administration. Oseltamivir carboxylate is not further metabolized and is eliminated in the urine. Plasma concentrations of oseltamivir carboxylate declined with a half-life of 6-10 hours in most subjects after oral administration. Oseltamivir carboxylate is eliminated entirely (>99%) by renal excretion. Renal clearance (18.8 L/h) exceeds glomerular filtration rate (7.5 L/h) indicating that tubular secretion occurs, in addition to glomerular filtration. Less than 20% of an oral radiolabeled dose is eliminated in feces.

SPECIAL POPULATIONS

Renal Impairment

Administration of 100 mg of oseltamivir phosphate twice daily for 5 days to patients with various degrees of renal impairment showed that exposure to oseltamivir carboxylate is inversely proportional to declining renal function. Oseltamivir carboxylate exposures in patients with normal and abnormal renal function administered various dose regimens of oseltamivir are described in TABLE 2.

TABLE 2 *Oseltamivir Carboxylate Exposures in Patients With Normal and Reduced Serum Creatinine Clearance*

	C_{max}	C_{min}	AUC(48)
Normal Renal Function			
75 mg qd	259*	39*	7,476*
75 mg bid	348*	138*	10,876*
150 mg bid	705*	288*	21,864*
Impaired Renal Function			
Creatinine Clearance <10 ml/min			
CAPD†	766	62	17,381
Hemodialysis‡	850	48	12,429
Creatinine Clearance >10 and <30 ml/min			
75 mg daily	1638	864	62,636
75 mg alternate days	1175	209	21,999
30 mg daily	655	346	25,054

* Observed values. All other values are predicted.
† 30 mg weekly.
‡ 30 mg alternate HD cycle.
AUC normalized to 48 hours.

Pediatric Patients

The pharmacokinetics of oseltamivir and oseltamivir carboxylate have been evaluated in a single dose pharmacokinetic study in pediatric patients aged 5-16 years (n=18) and in a small number of pediatric patients aged 3-12 years (n=5) enrolled in a clinical trial. Younger pediatric patients cleared both the prodrug and the active metabolite faster than adult patients resulting in a lower exposure for a given mg/kg dose. For oseltamivir carboxylate, apparent total clearance decreases linearly with increasing age (up to 12 years). The pharmacokinetics of oseltamivir in pediatric patients over 12 years of age are similar to those in adult patients.

Geriatric Patients

Exposure to oseltamivir carboxylate at steady-state was 25-35% higher in geriatric patients (age range 65-78 years) compared to young adults given comparable doses of oseltamivir. Half-lives observed in the geriatric patients were similar to those seen in young adults. Based on drug exposure and tolerability, dose adjustments are not required for geriatric patients for either treatment or prophylaxis (see DOSAGE AND ADMINISTRATION, Special Dosage Instructions).

INDICATIONS AND USAGE

TREATMENT OF INFLUENZA

Oseltamivir phosphate is indicated for the treatment of uncomplicated acute illness due to influenza infection in patients 1 year of age and older who have been symptomatic for no more than 2 days.

PROPHYLAXIS OF INFLUENZA

Oseltamivir phosphate is indicated for the prophylaxis of influenza in adult patients and adolescents 13 years and older.

Oseltamivir phosphate is not a substitute for early vaccination on an annual basis as recommended by the Centers for Disease Control's Immunization Practices Advisory Committee.

CONTRAINDICATIONS

Oseltamivir phosphate is contraindicated in patients with known hypersensitivity to any of the components of the product.

PRECAUTIONS

GENERAL

There is no evidence for efficacy of oseltamivir phosphate in any illness caused by agents other than influenza viruses Types A and B.

Use of oseltamivir phosphate should not affect the evaluation of individuals for annual influenza vaccination in accordance with guidelines of the Center for Disease Control and Prevention Advisory Committee on Immunization Practices.

Efficacy of oseltamivir phosphate in patients who begin treatment after 40 hours of symptoms has not been established.

Efficacy of oseltamivir phosphate in the treatment of subjects with chronic cardiac disease and/or respiratory disease has not been established. No difference in the incidence of complications was observed between the treatment and placebo groups in this population. No information is available regarding treatment of influenza in patients with any medical condition sufficiently severe or unstable to be considered at imminent risk of requiring hospitalization.

Safety and efficacy of repeated treatment or prophylaxis courses have not been studied.

Efficacy of oseltamivir phosphate for treatment or prophylaxis has not been established in immunocompromised patients.

Serious bacterial infections may begin with influenza-like symptoms or may coexist with or occur as complications during the course of influenza. Oseltamivir phosphate has not been shown to prevent such complications.

Hepatic Impairment: The safety and pharmacokinetics in patients with hepatic impairment have not been evaluated.

Renal Impairment: Dose adjustment is recommended for patients with a serum creatinine clearance <30 ml/min (see DOSAGE AND ADMINISTRATION).

INFORMATION FOR THE PATIENT

Patients should be instructed to begin treatment with oseltamivir phosphate as soon as possible from the first appearance of flu symptoms. Similarly, prevention should begin as soon as possible after exposure, at the recommendation of a physician.

Patients should be instructed to take any missed doses as soon as they remember, except if it is near the next scheduled dose (within 2 hours), and then continue to take oseltamivir phosphate at the usual times.

Oseltamivir phosphate is not a substitute for a flu vaccination. Patients should continue receiving an annual flu vaccination according to guidelines on immunization practices.

CARCINOGENESIS, MUTAGENESIS, AND IMPAIRMENT OF FERTILITY

Long-term carcinogenicity tests with oseltamivir are underway but have not been completed. However, a 26 week dermal carcinogenicity study of oseltamivir carboxylate in FVB/Tg.AC transgenic mice was negative. The animals were dosed at 40, 140, 400 or 780 mg/kg/day in two divided doses. The highest dose represents the maximum feasible dose based on the solubility of the compound in the control vehicle. A positive control, tetradecanoyl phorbol-13-acetate administered at 2.5 μg per dose 3 times per week gave a positive response.

Oseltamivir was found to be non-mutagenic in the Ames test and the human lymphocyte chromosome assay with and without enzymatic activation and negative in the mouse micronucleus test. It was found to be positive in a Syrian Hamster Embryo (SHE) cell transformation test. Oseltamivir carboxylate was non-mutagenic in the Ames test and the L5178Y mouse lymphoma assay with and without enzymatic activation and negative in the SHE cell transformation test.

In a fertility and early embryonic development study in rats, doses of oseltamivir at 50, 250, and 1500 mg/kg/day were administered to females for 2 weeks before mating, during mating, and until day 6 of pregnancy. Males were dosed for 4 weeks before mating, during, and for 2 weeks after mating. There were no effects on fertility, mating performance or early embryonic development at any dose level. The highest dose was approximately 100 times the human systemic exposure [AUC(0-24h)] of oseltamivir carboxylate.

PREGNANCY CATEGORY C

There are insufficient human data upon which to base an evaluation of risk of oseltamivir phosphate to the pregnant woman or developing fetus. Studies for effects on embryo-fetal development were conducted in rats (50, 250, and 1500 mg/kg/day) and rabbits (50, 150, and 500 mg/kg/day) by the oral route. Relative exposures at these doses were, respectively, 2, 13, and 100 times human exposure in the rat and 4, 8, and 50 times human exposure in the rabbit. Pharmacokinetic studies indicated that fetal exposure was seen in both species. In the rat study, minimal maternal toxicity was reported in the 1500 mg/kg/day group. In the rabbit study, slight and marked maternal toxicities were observed, respectively, in the 150 and 500 mg/kg/day groups. There was a dose-dependent increase in the incidence rates of a variety of minor skeletal abnormalities and variants in the exposed offspring in these studies. However, the individual incidence rate of each skeletal abnormality or variant remained within the background rates of occurrence in the species studied.

Because animal reproductive studies may not be predictive of human response and there are no adequate and well-controlled studies in pregnant women, oseltamivir phosphate should be used during pregnancy only if the potential benefit justifies the potential risk to the fetus.

O

NURSING MOTHERS

In lactating rats, oseltamivir and oseltamivir carboxylate are excreted in the milk. It is not known whether oseltamivir or oseltamivir carboxylate is excreted in human milk. Oseltamivir phosphate should, therefore, be used only if the potential benefit for the lactating mother justifies the potential risk to the breast-fed infant.

PEDIATRIC USE

The safety and efficacy of oseltamivir phosphate in pediatric patients younger than 1 year of age have not been established.

GERIATRIC USE

The safety of oseltamivir phosphate has been established in clinical studies which enrolled 741 subjects (374 received placebo and 362 received oseltamivir phosphate). Some seasonal variability was noted in the clinical efficacy outcomes.

Safety and efficacy have been demonstrated in elderly residents of nursing homes who took oseltamivir phosphate for up to 42 days for the prevention of influenza. Many of these individuals had cardiac and/or respiratory disease, and most had received vaccine that season.

DRUG INTERACTIONS

Information derived from pharmacology and pharmacokinetic studies of oseltamivir suggests that clinically significant drug interactions are unlikely.

Oseltamivir is extensively converted to oseltamivir carboxylate by esterases, located predominantly in the liver. Drug interactions involving competition for esterases have not been extensively reported in literature. Low protein binding of oseltamivir and oseltamivir carboxylate suggests that the probability of drug displacement interactions is low.

In vitro studies demonstrate that neither oseltamivir nor oseltamivir carboxylate is a good substrate for P450 mixed-function oxidases or for glucuronyl transferases.

Cimetidine, a non-specific inhibitor of cytochrome P450 isoforms and competitor for renal tubular secretion of basic or cationic drugs, has no effect on plasma levels of oseltamivir or oseltamivir carboxylate.

Clinically important drug interactions involving competition for renal tubular secretion are unlikely due to the known safety margin for most of these drugs, the elimination characteristics of oseltamivir carboxylate (glomerular filtration and anionic tubular secretion) and the excretion capacity of these pathways. Coadministration of probenecid results in an approximate 2-fold increase in exposure to oseltamivir carboxylate due to a decrease in active anionic tubular secretion in the kidney. However, due to the safety margin of oseltamivir carboxylate, no dose adjustments are required when coadministering with probenecid.

Coadministration with amoxicillin does not alter plasma levels of either compound, indicating that competition for the anionic secretion pathway is weak.

In 6 subjects, multiple doses of oseltamivir did not affect the single-dose pharmacokinetics of acetaminophen.

ADVERSE REACTIONS

TREATMENT STUDIES IN ADULT PATIENTS

A total of 1171 patients who participated in adult Phase 3 controlled clinical trials for the treatment of influenza were treated with oseltamivir phosphate. The most frequently reported adverse events in these studies were nausea and vomiting. These events were generally of mild to moderate degree and usually occurred on the first 2 days of administration. Less than 1% of subjects discontinued prematurely from clinical trials due to nausea and vomiting.

Adverse events that occurred with an incidence of ≥1% in 1440 patients taking placebo or oseltamivir phosphate 75 mg twice daily in adult Phase 3 treatment studies are shown in TABLE 3. This summary includes 945 healthy young adults and 495 "at risk" patients (elderly patients and patients with chronic cardiac or respiratory disease). Those events reported numerically more frequently in patients taking oseltamivir phosphate compared with placebo were nausea, vomiting, bronchitis, insomnia, and vertigo.

TABLE 3 *Most Frequent Adverse Events in Studies in Naturally Acquired Influenza*

	Treatment		Prophylaxis	
Adverse Event	**Placebo (n=716)**	**Oseltamivir 75 mg bid (n=724)**	**Placebo (n=1434)**	**Oseltamivir 75 mg qd (n=1480)**
Nausea (without vomiting)	40 (5.6%)	72 (9.9%)	56 (3.9%)	104 (7.0%)
Vomiting	21 (2.9%)	68 (9.4%)	15 (1.0%)	31 (2.1%)
Diarrhea	70 (9.8%)	48 (6.6%)	38 (2.6%)	48 (3.2%)
Bronchitis	15 (2.1%)	17 (2.3%)	17 (1.2%)	11 (0.7%)
Abdominal pain	16 (2.2%)	16 (2.2%)	23 (1.6%)	30 (2.0%)
Dizziness	25 (3.5%)	15 (2.1%)	21 (1.5%)	24 (1.6%)
Headache	14 (2.0%)	13 (1.8%)	251 (17.5%)	298 (20.1%)
Cough	12 (1.7%)	9 (1.2%)	86 (6.0%)	83 (5.6%)
Insomnia	6 (0.8%)	8 (1.1%)	14 (1.2%)	18 (1.2%)
Vertigo	4 (0.6%)	7 (1.0%)	3 (0.2%)	4 (0.3%)
Fatigue	7 (1.0%)	7 (1.0%)	107 (7.5%)	117 (7.9%)

Adverse events included are: all events reported in the treatment studies with frequency ≥1% in the oseltamivir 75 mg bid group.

Additional adverse events occurring in <1% of patients receiving oseltamivir phosphate for treatment included unstable angina, anemia, pseudomembranous colitis, humerus fracture, pneumonia, pyrexia, and peritonsillar abscess.

PROPHYLAXIS STUDIES

A total of 3434 subjects (adolescents, healthy adults, and elderly) participated in Phase 3 prophylaxis studies, of whom 1480 received the recommended dose of 75 mg once daily for up to 6 weeks. Adverse events were qualitatively very similar to those seen in the treatment studies, despite a longer duration of dosing (see TABLE 3). Events reported more frequently in subjects receiving oseltamivir phosphate compared to subjects receiving placebo in prophylaxis studies, and more commonly than in treatment studies, were aches and pains, rhinorrhea, dyspepsia, and upper respiratory tract infections. However, the difference in incidence between oseltamivir phosphate and placebo for these events was less than 1%. There were no clinically relevant differences in the safety profile of the 942 elderly subjects who received oseltamivir phosphate or placebo, compared with the younger population.

TREATMENT STUDIES IN PEDIATRIC PATIENTS

A total of 1032 pediatric patients aged 1-12 years (including 698 otherwise healthy pediatric patients aged 1-12 years and 334 asthmatic pediatric patients aged 6-12 years) participated in Phase 3 studies of oseltamivir phosphate given for the treatment of influenza. A total of 515 pediatric patients received treatment with oseltamivir phosphate oral suspension.

Adverse events occurring in >1% of pediatric patients receiving oseltamivir phosphate treatment are listed in TABLE 4. The most frequently reported adverse event was vomiting. Other events reported more frequently by pediatric patients treated with oseltamivir phosphate included abdominal pain, epistaxis, ear disorder, and conjunctivitis. These events generally occurred once and resolved despite continued dosing. They did not cause discontinuation of drug in the vast majority of cases.

The adverse event profile in adolescents is similar to that described for adult patients and pediatric patients aged 1-12 years.

OBSERVED DURING CLINICAL PRACTICE FOR TREATMENT

The following adverse reactions have been identified during postmarketing use of oseltamivir phosphate. Because these reactions are reported voluntarily from a population of uncertain size, it is not possible to reliably estimate their frequency or establish a causal relationship to oseltamivir phosphate exposure.

General: Rash, swelling of the face or tongue, toxic epidermal necrolysis.

Digestive: Hepatitis, liver function tests abnormal.

Cardiac: Arrhythmia.

Neurologic: Seizure, confusion.

Metabolic: Aggravation of diabetes.

TABLE 4 *Adverse Events Occurring on Treatment in >1% of Pediatric Patients Enrolled in Phase 3 Trials of Oseltamivir Phosphate Treatment of Naturally Acquired Influenza*

Adverse Event	Placebo (n=517)	Oseltamivir 2 mg/kg twice daily (n=515)
Vomiting	48 (9.3%)	77 (15.0%)
Diarrhea	55 (10.6%)	49 (9.5%)
Otitis media	58 (11.2%)	45 (8.7%)
Abdominal pain	20 (3.9%)	24 (4.7%)
Asthma (including aggravated)	19 (3.7%)	18 (3.5%)
Nausea	22 (4.3%)	17 (3.3%)
Epistaxis	13 (2.5%)	16 (3.1%)
Pneumonia	17 (3.3%)	10 (1.9%)
Ear disorder	6 (1.2%)	9 (1.7%)
Sinusitis	13 (2.5%)	9 (1.7%)
Bronchitis	11 (2.1%)	8 (1.6%)
Conjunctivitis	2 (0.4%)	5 (1.0%)
Dermatitis	10 (1.9%)	5 (1.0%)
Lymphadenopathy	8 (1.5%)	5 (1.0%)
Tympanic membrane disorder	6 (1.2%)	5 (1.0%)

DOSAGE AND ADMINISTRATION

Oseltamivir phosphate may be taken with or without food (see CLINICAL PHARMACOLOGY, Pharmacokinetics). However, when taken with food, tolerability may be enhanced in some patients.

STANDARD DOSAGE

Treatment of Influenza

Adults and Adolescents

The recommended oral dose of oseltamivir phosphate for treatment of influenza in adults and adolescents 13 years and older is 75 mg twice daily for 5 days. Treatment should begin within 2 days of onset of symptoms of influenza.

Pediatric Patients

The recommended oral dose of oseltamivir phosphate oral suspension for pediatric patients 1 year and older or adult patients who cannot swallow a capsule is shown in TABLE 5.

TABLE 5

Body Weight		Recommended Dose for 5 Days
≤15 kg	≤33 lb	30 mg twice daily
>15 to 23 kg	>33 to 51 lb	45 mg twice daily
>23 to 40 kg	>51 to 88 lb	60 mg twice daily
>40 kg	>88 lb	75 mg twice daily

An oral dosing dispenser with 30, 45, and 60 mg graduations is provided with the oral suspension; the 75 mg dose can be measured using a combination of 30 and 45 mg. It is recommended that patients use this dispenser. In the event that the dispenser provided is lost or damaged, another dosing syringe or other device may be used to deliver the following volumes: 2.5 ml (½ tsp) for children ≤15 kg; 3.8 ml (¾ tsp) for >15 to 23 kg; 5.0 ml (1 tsp) for >23 to 40 kg; and 6.2 ml (1¼ tsp) for >40 kg.

Prophylaxis of Influenza

The recommended oral dose of oseltamivir phosphate for prophylaxis of influenza in adults and adolescents 13 years and older following close contact with an infected individual is 75 mg once daily for at least 7 days. Therapy should begin within 2 days of exposure. The recommended dose for prophylaxis during a community outbreak of influenza is 75 mg once daily. Safety and efficacy have been demonstrated for up to 6 weeks. The duration of protection lasts for as long as dosing is continued.

SPECIAL DOSAGE INSTRUCTIONS

Hepatic Impairment

The safety and pharmacokinetics in patients with hepatic impairment have not been evaluated.

Renal Impairment

For plasma concentrations of oseltamivir carboxylate predicted to occur following various dosing schedules in patients with renal impairment, see CLINICAL PHARMACOLOGY, Special Populations.

Treatment of Influenza: Dose adjustment is recommended for patients with creatinine clearance between 10 and 30 ml/min receiving oseltamivir phosphate for the treatment of influenza. In these patients it is recommended that the dose be reduced to 75 mg of oseltamivir phosphate once daily for 5 days. No recommended dosing regimens are available for patients undergoing routine hemodialysis and continuous peritoneal dialysis treatment with end-stage renal disease.

Prophylaxis of Influenza: For the prophylaxis of influenza, dose adjustment is recommended for patients with creatinine clearance between 10 and 30 ml/min receiving oseltamivir phosphate. In these patients it is recommended that the dose be reduced to 75 mg of oseltamivir phosphate every other day or 30 mg oseltamivir phosphate oral suspension every day. No recommended dosing regimens are available for patients undergoing routine hemodialysis and continuous peritoneal dialysis treatment with end-stage renal disease.

Pediatric Patients

The safety and efficacy of oseltamivir phosphate for prophylaxis in pediatric patients younger than 13 years of age have not been established. The safety and efficacy of oseltamivir phosphate for treatment in pediatric patients younger than 1 year of age have not been established.

Geriatric Patients

No dose adjustment is required for geriatric patients (see CLINICAL PHARMACOLOGY, Special Populations and PRECAUTIONS).

HOW SUPPLIED

CAPSULES

Tamiflu capsules are supplied as 75 mg (75 mg free base equivalent of the phosphate salt) grey/light yellow hard gelatin capsules. "ROCHE" is printed in blue ink on the grey body and "75 mg" is printed in blue ink on the light yellow cap.

Storage

Store at 25°C (77°F); excursions permitted to 15-30°C (59-86°F).

ORAL SUSPENSION

Tamiflu oral suspension is supplied as a white powder blend for constitution to a white tutti-frutti-flavored suspension.

Storage

Dry Powder: Store at 25°C (77°F); excursions permitted to 15-30°C (59-86°F).

Constituted Suspension: Store under refrigeration at 2-8°C (36-46°F). Do not freeze.

PRODUCT LISTING - RATED THERAPEUTICALLY EQUIVALENT

Powder For Reconstitution - Oral - 12 mg/ml

25 ml	$34.85	TAMIFLU, Roche Laboratories	00004-0810-95

PRODUCT LISTING - EQUIVALENTS NOT AVAILABLE

Capsule - Oral - 75 mg

10's	$59.54	TAMIFLU, Allscripts Pharmaceutical Company	54569-4888-00
10's	$69.70	TAMIFLU, Roche Laboratories	00004-0800-85

Powder For Reconstitution - Oral - 12 mg/ml

75 ml	$63.12	TAMIFLU, Roche Laboratories	00004-0810-09

Oxacillin Sodium *(001923)*

Categories: Infection, staphylococcal, penicillinase-producing; Pregnancy Category B; FDA Approved 1973 Jul
Drug Classes: Antibiotics, penicillins
Brand Names: Bactocill; Dicloxal OX; Prostaphlin; Staphaloxin; Wydox
Foreign Brand Availability: Bristopen (France); Prostafilina (Colombia); Stapenor (Germany)
Cost of Therapy: $80.76 (Infection; Bactocill Injection; 1 g; 2 g/day; 10 day supply)
$67.00 (Infection; Generic Injection; 1 g; 2 g/day; 10 day supply)
HCFA JCODE(S): J2700 up to 250 mg IM, IV

DESCRIPTION

Oxacillin sodium is an antibacterial agent of the isoxazolyl penicillin series, chemicall it is 4-thia-1-azabicyclo(3.2.0)heptane-2-carboxylic acid, 3,3 dimethyl-6-(((5-methyl-3-phenyl-4-isoxazolyl)carbonyl) amino)-7-oxo-monosodium salt, monohydrate, (2S-(2α,5α,6β)).

The molecular formula is $C_{19}H_{18}N_3NaO_5S{\cdot}H_2O$, the molecular weight is 441.43.

CAPSULES AND ORAL SOLUTION

Oxacillin sodium is an antibacterial agent of the isoxazolyl penicillin series. It is a penicillinase-resistant, acid resistant, semi-synthetic penicillin suitable for oral administration. Oxacillin sodium is available for administration as an oral solution and capsules.

Inactive ingredient in oxacillin sodium capsules: Lactose, magnesium stearate and FD&C yellow no. 6.

Inactive ingredients in oxacillin sodium oral solution are: FD&C red no. 40, natural & artificial flavorings, potassium alginate, sodium benzoate, sodium citrate, sodium saccharin, and sucrose.

INJECTION

Oxacillin sodium for injection is a semisynthetic antibiotic substance derived from 6-amino-penicillanic acid. It is the sodium salt in a parenteral dosage form. Each gram of oxacillin sodium contains approximately 2.5 mEq of sodium and is buffered with 20 mg dibasic sodium phosphate.

Storage: Store sterile powder at controlled room temperature 15-30°C (59-86° F).

CLINICAL PHARMACOLOGY

MICROBIOLOGY

Penicillinase-resistant penicillins exert a bactericidal action against penicillin-susceptible microorganisms during the state of active multiplication. All penicillins inhibit the biosynthesis of the bacterial cell wall.

The drugs in this class are highly resistant to inactivation by staphylococcal penicillinase and are active against penicillinase producing and non-penicillinase producing strains of *Staphylococcus aureus.*

The penicillinase-resistant penicillins are active *in vitro* against a variety of other bacteria.

Susceptibility Testing

Quantitative methods of susceptibility testing that require measurement of zone diameters or minimal inhibitory concentrations (MICs) give the most precise estimates of antibiotic susceptibility. One such procedure has been recommended for use with discs to test susceptibility to this class of drugs. Interpretations correlate diameters on the disc test with MIC values. A penicillinase-resistant class disk may be used to determine microbial susceptibility to cloxacillin, dicloxacillin, methicillin, nafcillin, and oxacillin. With this procedure, employing a 5 microgram methicillin sodium disc, a report from the laboratory of "susceptible" (zone of at least 14 mm) indicates that the infecting organism is likely to respond to therapy. A report of "resistant" (zone of less than 10 mm) indicates that the infecting organism is not likely to respond to therapy. A report of "intermediate susceptibility" (zone of 10 to 13 mm) suggests that the organism might be susceptible if high doses of the antibiotic are used, or if the infection is confined to tissues and fluids (*e.g.*, urine), in which high antibiotic levels are attained.

In general, all staphylococci should be tested against the penicillin G disc and against the methicillin disc. Routine methods of antibiotic susceptibility testing may fail to detect strains of organisms resistant to the penicillinase-resistant penicillins. For this reason, the use of large inocula and the 48 hour incubation periods may be necessary to obtain accurate susceptibility studies with these antibiotics. Bacterial strains which are resistant to one of the penicillinase-resistant penicillins should be considered resistant to all of the drugs in the class.

PHARMACOKINETICS

Capsules and Oral Solution

Oxacillin sodium is resistant to destruction by acid. Absorption of oxacillin sodium after oral administration is rapid but incomplete. A single 250 mg oral dose gives a 1-hour peak serum level of 1.65 μg/ml. A-500 mg dose peaks at about 2.6 μg/ml. Peak serum levels with the oral solution occur somewhat earlier, about one-half hour after dosing. A single dose of 250 mg oral solution gives a peak serum level of 1.9 μg/ml; of 500 mg 4.8 μg/ml.

Once absorbed, oxacillin sodium binds to serum protein, mainly albumin. The degree of protein binding reported varies with the method of study and the investigator, but generally has been found to be 94.2 ± 2.1%. Oral absorption of oxacillin is delayed when the drug is administered after meals.

Oxacillin sodium, with normal doses, has insignificant concentrations in the cerebrospinal and ascitic fluids. It is found in therapeutic concentrations in the pleural, bile, and amniotic fluids. Oxacillin is rapidly excreted as unchanged drug in the urine by glomerular filtration and active tubular secretion.

Injection

Oxacillin sodium, with normal doses, has significant concentrations in the cerebrospinal and ascitic fluids. It is found in therapeutic concentrations in the pleural, bile, and amniotic fluids. Oxacillin is rapidly excreted as unchanged drug in the urine by glomerular filtration and active tubular secretion.

Oxacillin sodium binds to serum protein, mainly albumin. The degree of protein binding reported varies with the method of study and the investigator, but generally has been found to be 94.2 ± 2.1%.

Intramuscular injections give peak serum levels 30 minutes after injection. A 250 mg dose gives a level of 5.3 μg/ml while a 500 mg dose peaks at 10.9 μg/ml. Intravenous injection gives a peak about 5 minutes after the injection is completed. Slow IV dosing with 500 mg gives a 5 minute peak of 43 μg/ml with a half-life of 20-30 minutes.

INDICATIONS AND USAGE

The penicillinase-resistant penicillins are indicated in the treatment of infections caused by penicillinase-producing staphylococci which have demonstrated susceptibility to the drugs. Culture and susceptibility tests should be performed initially to determine the causative organisms and their sensitivity to the drug (see CLINICAL PHARMACOLOGY, Microbiology, Susceptibility Testing).

The penicillinase-resistant penicillins may be used to initiate therapy in suspected cases of resistant staphylococcal infections prior to the availability of laboratory test results. The penicillinase-resistant penicillins should not be used in infections caused by organisms susceptible to penicillin G. If the susceptibility tests indicate that the infection is due to an organism other than a resistant staphylococcus, therapy should not be continued with a penicillinase-resistant penicillin.

CONTRAINDICATIONS

A history of hypersensitivity (anaphylactic) reaction to any penicillin is a contraindication.

WARNINGS

Serious and occasionally fatal hypersensitivity (anaphylactic shock with collapse) reactions have occurred in patients receiving penicillin. The incidence of anaphylactic shock in all penicillin-treated patients is between 0.015 and 0.04%. Anaphylactic shock resulting in death has occurred in approximately 0.002% of the patients treated. Although anaphylaxis is more frequent following a parenteral administration, it has occurred in patients receiving oral penicillins.

When penicillin therapy is indicated, it should be initiated only after a comprehensive patient drug and allergy history has been obtained. If an allergic reaction occurs, the drug should be discontinued and the patient should receive supportive treatment, e.g., artificial maintenance of ventilation, pressor amines, antihistamines, and corticosteroids. Individuals with a history of penicillin hypersensitivity may also experience allergic reactions when treated with a cephalosporin.

PRECAUTIONS

GENERAL

Penicillinase-resistant penicillins should generally not be administered to patients with a history of sensitivity to any penicillin.

Penicillin should be used with caution in individuals with histories of significant allergies and/or asthma. Whenever allergic reactions occur, penicillin should be withdrawn unless, in the opinion of the physician, the condition being treated is life-threatening and amenable only to penicillin therapy.

The oral route of administration should not be relied upon in patients with severe illness, or with nausea, vomiting, gastric dilation, cardiospasm, or intestinal hypermotility. Occasionally patients will not absorb therapeutic amounts of orally administered penicillin.

The use of antibiotics may result in overgrowth of nonsusceptible organisms. If new infections due to bacteria or fungi occur, the drug should be discontinued and appropriate measures taken.

INFORMATION FOR THE PATIENT

Capsules and Oral Solution

Patients receiving penicillins should be given the following information and instructions by the physician:

Patients should be told that penicillin is an antibacterial agent which will work with the body's natural defenses to control certain types of infections. They should be told that the drug should not be taken if they have had an allergic reaction to any form of penicillin previously, and to inform the physician of any allergies or previous allergic reactions to any drugs they may have had (see WARNINGS).

Patients who have previously experienced an anaphylactic to penicillin should be instructed to wear a medical identification tag or bracelet.

Because most antibacterial agents taken by mouth are best absorbed on an empty stomach, patients should be directed, unless circumstances warrant otherwise, to take penicillin 1 hour before meals or 2 hours after eating (see CLINICAL PHARMACOLOGY, Pharmacokinetics, Injection).

Patients should be told to take the entire course of therapy prescribed, even if fever and other symptoms have stopped (see PRECAUTIONS, General).

If any of the following reactions occur, stop taking your prescription and notify the physician: shortness of breath, wheezing, skin rash, mouth irritation, black tongue, sore throat, nausea, vomiting, diarrhea, fever, swollen joints, or any unusual bleeding or bruising (see ADVERSE REACTIONS).

Do not take any additional medications without physician approval, including nonprescription drugs such as antacids, laxatives, or vitamins.

Discard any liquid forms of penicillin after 7 days if stored at room temperature or after 14 days if refrigerated.

LABORATORY TESTS

Bacteriologic studies to determine the causative organisms and their susceptibility to the penicillinase-resistant penicillins should be performed (see CLINICAL PHARMACOLOGY, Microbiology). In the treatment of suspected staphylococcal infections, therapy should be changed to another active agent if culture tests fail to demonstrate the presence of staphylococci.

Periodic assessment of organ system function including renal, hepatic, and hematopoietic should be made during prolonged therapy with the penicillinase-resistant penicillins.

Blood cultures, white blood cell, and differential cell counts should be obtained prior to initiation of therapy and at least weekly during therapy with penicillinase-resistant penicillins.

Periodic urinalysis, blood urea in nitrogen; and creatinine determinations should be performed during therapy with the penicillinase-resistant penicillins and dosage alterations should be considered if these values become elevated. If any impairment of renal function is suspected or known to exist, a reduction in the total dosage should be considered and blood levels monitored to avoid possible neurotoxic reactions. (See DOSAGE AND ADMINISTRATION.)

SGOT and SGPT values should be obtained periodically during therapy to monitor for possible liver function abnormalities.

CARCINOGENESIS, MUTAGENESIS, AND IMPAIRMENT OF FERTILITY

No long-term animal studies have been conducted with these drugs.

Studies on reproduction (nafcillin) in rats and rabbits reveal no fetal or maternal abnormalities before conception and continuously through weaning (one generation).

PREGNANCY CATEGORY B

Reproduction studies performed in the mouse, rat, and rabbit have revealed no evidence of impaired fertility or harm to the fetus due to the penicillinase-resistant penicillins. Human experience with the penicillins during pregnancy has not shown any positive evidence of adverse effects on the fetus. There are, however, no adequate or well-controlled studies in pregnant women showing conclusively that harmful effects of these drugs on the fetus can be excluded. Because animal reproduction studies are not always predictive of human response, this drug should be used during pregnancy only if clearly needed.

NURSING MOTHERS

Penicillins are excreted in breast milk. Caution should be exercised when penicillins are administered to a nursing woman.

PEDIATRIC USE

Because of incompletely developed renal function in newborns, penicillinase-resistant penicillins (especially methicillin) may not be completely excreted, with abnormally high blood levels resulting. Frequent blood levels are advisable in this group with dosage adjustments when necessary. All newborns treated with penicillins should be monitored closely for clinical and laboratory evidence of toxic or adverse effects (see DOSAGE AND ADMINISTRATION).

DRUG INTERACTIONS

Tetracycline, a bacteriostatic antibiotic, may antagonize the bactericidal effect of penicillin and concurrent use of these drugs should be avoided.

ADVERSE REACTIONS

BODY AS A WHOLE

The reported incidence of allergic reactions to penicillins ranges from 0.7-10% (see WARNINGS). Sensitization is usually the result of treatment but some individuals have had immediate reactions to penicillin when first treated. In such cases, it is thought that the patients may have had prior exposure to the drug via trace amounts present in milk and vaccines.

Two types of allergic reactions to penicillin are noted clinically: immediate and delayed.

Immediate reactions usually occur within 20 minutes of administration and range in severity from urticaria and pruritus to angioneurotic edema, laryngospasm, bronchospasm, hypotension, vascular collapse, and death. Such immediate anaphylactic reactions are very rare (see WARNINGS) and usually occur after parenteral therapy but have occurred in patients receiving oral therapy. Another type of immediate reaction, an accelerated reaction, may occur between 20 minutes and 48 hours after administration and may include urticaria, pruritus, and fever. Although laryngeal edema, laryngospasm, and hypotension occasionally occur, fatality is uncommon.

Delayed allergic reactions to penicillin therapy usually occur after 48 hours and sometimes as late as 2-4 weeks after initiation of therapy. Manifestations of this type of reaction include serum sickness-like symptoms (*i.e.*, fever, malaise, urticaria, myalgia, arthralgia, abdominal pain) and various skin rashes. Nausea, vomiting, diarrhea, stomatitis, black or "hairy" tongue, and other symptoms of gastrointestinal irritation may occur, especially during oral penicillin therapy.

NERVOUS SYSTEM REACTIONS

Neurotoxic reactions similar to those observed with penicillin G may occur with large intravenous doses of the penicillinase-resistant penicillins especially in patients with renal insufficiency.

UROGENITAL REACTIONS

Renal tubular damage and interstitial nephritis have been associated with the administration of methicillin sodium and infrequently with the administration of nafcillin and oxacillin. Manifestations of this reaction may include rash, fever, eosinophilia, hematuria, proteinuria, and renal insufficiency. Methicillin-induced nephropathy does not appear to be dose-related and is generally reversible upon prompt discontinuation of therapy.

GASTROINTESTINAL REACTIONS

Pseudomembranous colitis has been reported with the use of oxacillin sodium (and other broad spectrum antibiotics); therefore, it is important to consider its diagnosis in patients who develop diarrhea in association with antibiotic use.

Treatment with broad spectrum antibiotic alters normal flora of the colon and may permit overgrowth of clostridia. Studies indicate a toxin produced by *Clostridium difficile* is one primary cause of antibiotic-associated colitis. Cholestyramine and colestipol resins have been shown to bind the toxin *in vitro.*

Mild cases of colitis may respond to drug discontinuance alone.

Moderate to severe cases should be managed with fluid, electrolyte and protein supplementation as indicated.

When the colitis is not relieved by drug discontinuance or when it is severe, oral vancomycin is the treatment of choice for antibiotic-associated pseudomembranous colitis produced by *C. difficile.* Other causes of colitis should also be considered.

METABOLIC REACTIONS

Agranulocytosis, neutropenia, and bone marrow depression have been associated with the use of methicillin sodium, nafcillin, oxacillin, and cloxacillin. Hepatotoxicity, characterized by fever, nausea, and vomiting associated with abnormal liver function tests, mainly elevated SGOT levels, has been associated with the use of oxacillin and cloxacillin.

DOSAGE AND ADMINISTRATION

The penicillinase-resistant penicillins are available for oral administration and for intramuscular and intravenous injection. The sodium salts of methicillin, oxacillin, and nafcillin may be administered parenterally and the sodium salts of cloxacillin, dicloxacillin, oxacillin, and nafcillin are available for oral use.

Bacteriologic studies to determine the causative organisms and their sensitivity to the penicillinase-resistant penicillins should always be performed. Duration of therapy varies with the type and severity of infection as well as the overall condition of the patient; therefore, it should be determined by the clinical and bacteriological response of the patient. In severe staphylococcal infections, therapy with penicillinase-resistant penicillins should be continued for at least 14 days. Therapy should be continued for at least 48 hours after the patient has become afebrile, asymptomatic, and cultures are negative. The treatment of endocarditis and osteomyelitis may require a longer term of therapy.

Concurrent administration of the penicillinase-resistant penicillins and probenecid increases and prolongs serum penicillin levels. Probenecid decreases the apparent volume of distribution and slows the rate of excretion by competitively inhibiting renal tubular secretion of penicillin. Penicillin-probenecid therapy is generally limited to those infections where very high serum levels of penicillin are necessary.

Oral preparations of the penicillinase-resistant penicillins should not be used as initial therapy in serious, life-threatening infections. Oral therapy with the penicillinase-resistant penicillins may be used to follow-up the previous use of a parenteral agent as soon as the clinical condition warrants. For intramuscular gluteal injections, care should be taken to avoid sciatic nerve injury. With intravenous administration, particularly in elderly patients, care should be taken because of the possibility of thrombophlebitis. (See TABLE 1.)

DIRECTIONS FOR DISPENSING ORAL SOLUTION

Prepare these formulations at the time of dispensing. For ease in preparation, add water to the bottle in two portions and shake well after each addition. Add the total amount of water as directed on the package being dispensed. The reconstituted formulation is stable or 3 days at room temperature or 14 days under refrigeration.

STABILITY

Stability studies on oxacillin sodium at concentrations of 0.5 mg/ml and 2 mg/ml in various intravenous solutions listed below indicate the drug will lose less than 10% activity at room temperature (70°F) during a 6 hour period.

IV Solution

5% Dextrose in normal saline
10% D-fructose in water
10% D-fructose in normal saline
Lactated potassic saline injection

TABLE 1 *Recommended Dosage for Oxacillin Sodium for Injection*

Adults	Infants and Children 40 kg (88 lb)	Other Recommendations
250-500 mg IM or IV every 4-6 hours (mild to moderate infections)	50 mg/kg/day IM or IV in equally divided doses every 6 hours (mild to moderate infections)	
1 g IM or IV every 4-6 hours severe infections)	100 mg/kg/day IM or IV in equally divided doses every 4-6 hours (severe infections)	Premature and neonates 25 mg/kg/day IM or IV

TABLE 2A *Stability Periods for Oxacillin Sodium for Injection*

Concentration	Sterile Water for Injection	Isotonic Sodium Chloride	M/6 Molar Sodium Lactate Solution	%5 Dextrose in Water
Room Temperature (25°C)				
10-100 mg/ml	4 days	4 days		
10-30 mg/ml			24 hours	
0.5-2 mg/ml				6 hours
Refrigeration (4°C)				
10-100 mg/ml	7 days	7 days		
10-30 mg/ml			4 days	4 days
Frozen (-15°C)				
50-100 mg/ml	30 days			
250 mg/1.5 ml	30 days			
100 mg/ml		30 days		
10-100 mg/ml			30 days	30 days

TABLE 2B *Stability Periods for Oxacillin Sodium for Injection*

Concentration	5% Dextrose in 0.45% NaCl	10% Invert Sugar	Lactated Ringer's Solution
Room Temperature (25°C)			
10-30 mg/ml	24 hours		
0.5-2 mg/ml		6 hours	6 hours
Refrigeration (4°C)			
10-30 mg/ml	4 days	4 days	4 days
Frozen (-15°C)			
10-100 mg/ml	30 days	30 days	30 days

10% Invert sugar in normal saline
10% Invert sugar plus 0.3% potassium chloride in water
Travert 10% electrolyte #1
Travert 10% electrolyte #2
Travert 10% electrolyte #3

Only those solutions listed above should be used for the intravenous infusion of oxacillin sodium. The concentration of the antibiotic should fall within the range specified. The drug concentration and the rate and volume of the infusion should be adjusted so that the total dose of oxacillin is administered before the drug loses its stability in the solution in use.

If another agent is used in conjunction with oxacillin therapy, it should not be physically mixed with oxacillin but should be administered separately.

O

PRODUCT LISTING - RATED THERAPEUTICALLY EQUIVALENT

Capsule - Oral - 250 mg			
40's	$12.10	GENERIC, Allscripts Pharmaceutical Company	54569-1880-00
100's	$20.95	GENERIC, Raway Pharmacal Inc	00686-3115-09
100's	$28.71	GENERIC, Qualitest Products Inc	00603-4927-21
100's	$28.75	GENERIC, Major Pharmaceuticals Inc	00904-2709-60
100's	$29.42	GENERIC, Geneva Pharmaceuticals	00781-2004-01
100's	$29.90	GENERIC, Aligen Independent Laboratories Inc	00405-4726-01
100's	$29.99	GENERIC, Ivax Corporation	00182-1340-01
100's	$30.50	BACTOCILL, Glaxosmithkline	00029-6010-30
100's	$37.43	GENERIC, Interstate Drug Exchange Inc	00814-5587-14
Capsule - Oral - 500 mg			
20's	$11.00	GENERIC, Allscripts Pharmaceutical Company	54569-2708-01
100's	$33.15	GENERIC, Raway Pharmacal Inc	00686-3117-09
100's	$53.20	GENERIC, Major Pharmaceuticals Inc	00904-2710-60
100's	$53.45	GENERIC, Moore, H.L. Drug Exchange Inc	00839-6413-06
100's	$54.45	GENERIC, Qualitest Products Inc	00603-4928-21
100's	$54.68	GENERIC, Geneva Pharmaceuticals	00781-2006-01
100's	$55.29	GENERIC, Aligen Independent Laboratories Inc	00405-4727-01
100's	$56.45	GENERIC, Ivax Corporation	00182-1341-01
100's	$56.85	BACTOCILL, Glaxosmithkline	00029-6015-30
Powder For Injection - Injectable - 1 Gm			
10's	$33.50	GENERIC, Bristol-Myers Squibb	00015-7981-99
10's	$34.60	GENERIC, Bristol-Myers Squibb	00015-7981-89
10's	$36.00	GENERIC, Bristol-Myers Squibb	00015-7981-95
10's	$40.38	BACTOCILL, Glaxosmithkline	00029-6025-07
10's	$61.80	GENERIC, Bristol-Myers Squibb	00003-2712-10
10's	$83.21	GENERIC, Geneva Pharmaceuticals	00781-3762-46
10's	$83.30	GENERIC, Bristol-Myers Squibb	00003-2712-20
Powder For Injection - Injectable - 2 Gm			
1's	$5.22	GENERIC, Bristol-Myers Squibb	00015-7970-18
1's	$51.40	GENERIC, Bristol-Myers Squibb	00015-7970-20
10's	$52.20	GENERIC, Bristol-Myers Squibb	00015-7970-89

10's	$53.00	BACTOCILL, Glaxosmithkline	00029-6028-40
10's	$60.60	GENERIC, Bristol-Myers Squibb	00015-7970-96
10's	$62.94	BACTOCILL, Glaxosmithkline	00029-6028-07
10's	$64.20	GENERIC, Bristol-Myers Squibb	00015-7970-99
10's	$213.80	GENERIC, Bristol-Myers Squibb	00015-7970-22
10's	$252.80	GENERIC, Bristol-Myers Squibb	00015-7970-21

Powder For Injection - Injectable - 4 Gm

10's	$117.84	BACTOCILL, Glaxosmithkline	00029-6030-26

Powder For Injection - Injectable - 10 Gm

10's	$299.28	BACTOCILL, Glaxosmithkline	00029-6032-21
10's	$412.60	GENERIC, Bristol-Myers Squibb	00015-7103-98
10's	$594.60	GENERIC, Bristol-Myers Squibb	00003-2715-25

Powder For Injection - Injectable - 500 mg

10's	$13.68	GENERIC, Bristol-Myers Squibb	00015-7979-99
10's	$31.70	GENERIC, Bristol-Myers Squibb	00003-2711-10

Powder For Reconstitution - Oral - 250 mg/5 ml

100 ml	$5.80	GENERIC, Ivax Corporation	00182-7069-70
100 ml	$5.95	GENERIC, Qualitest Products Inc	00603-6584-64
100 ml	$14.58	GENERIC, Bristol-Myers Squibb	00015-7985-40

Solution - Intravenous - 1 Gm/50 ml

50 ml x 24	$533.04	GENERIC, Baxter I.V. Systems Division	00338-1013-41

PRODUCT LISTING - EQUIVALENTS NOT AVAILABLE

Capsule - Oral - 250 mg

20's	$7.59	GENERIC, Prescript Pharmaceuticals	00247-0182-20
40's	$11.82	GENERIC, Prescript Pharmaceuticals	00247-0182-40

Powder For Injection - Injectable - 1 Gm

1's	$3.60	GENERIC, Bristol-Myers Squibb	00015-7981-28
1's	$26.80	GENERIC, Bristol-Myers Squibb	00015-7981-20
1's	$27.60	GENERIC, Bristol-Myers Squibb	00015-7981-18
10's	$111.10	GENERIC, Bristol-Myers Squibb	00015-7981-22

Powder For Injection - Injectable - 10 Gm

1's	$33.01	GENERIC, Bristol-Myers Squibb	00015-7103-28

Powder For Injection - Injectable - 500 mg

1's	$13.70	GENERIC, Bristol-Myers Squibb	00015-7979-20

Powder For Reconstitution - Oral - 250 mg/5 ml

100 ml	$3.75	GENERIC, Raway Pharmacal Inc	00686-4157-32

Solution - Intravenous - 2 Gm/50 ml

1500 ml x 24	$767.28	GENERIC, Baxter I.V. Systems Division	00338-1015-41

Oxaliplatin *(003567)*

Categories: Carcinoma, colorectal; Pregnancy Category D; FDA Approved 2002 Aug
Drug Classes: Antineoplastics, platinum agents
Brand Names: Eloxatin
Foreign Brand Availability: Heloxatin (Peru); Oplat (Colombia)

WARNING

Oxaliplatin for injection should be administered under the supervision of a qualified physician experienced in the use of cancer chemotherapeutic agents. Appropriate management of therapy and complications is possible only when adequate diagnostic and treatment facilities are readily available.

Anaphylactic-like reactions to oxaliplatin have been reported, and may occur within minutes of oxaliplatin administration. Epinephrine, corticosteroids, and antihistamines have been employed to alleviate symptoms. (See WARNINGS and ADVERSE REACTIONS.)

DESCRIPTION

Oxaliplatin is an antineoplastic agent with the molecular formula $C_8H_{14}N_2O_4Pt$ and the chemical name of *cis*-[(1*R*,2*R*)-1,2-cyclohexanediamine-*N*,*N'*] [oxalato(2-)-*O*,*O'*] platinum. Oxaliplatin is an organoplatinum complex in which the platinum atom is complexed with 1,2-diaminocyclohexane (DACH) and with an oxalate ligand as a leaving group.

The molecular weight is 397.3. Oxaliplatin is slightly soluble in water at 6 mg/ml, very slightly soluble in methanol, and practically insoluble in ethanol and acetone.

Eloxatin is supplied in vials containing 50 or 100 mg of oxaliplatin as a sterile, preservative-free lyophilized powder for reconstitution. Lactose monohydrate is present as an inactive ingredient at 450 and 900 mg in the 50 and 100 mg dosage strengths, respectively.

CLINICAL PHARMACOLOGY

MECHANISM OF ACTION

Oxaliplatin undergoes nonenzymatic conversion in physiologic solutions to active derivatives via displacement of the labile oxalate ligand. Several transient reactive species are formed, including monoaquo and diaquo DACH platinum, which covalently bind with macromolecules. Both inter- and intra-strand Pt-DNA cross-links are formed. Crosslinks are formed between the *N7* positions of two adjacent guanines (GG), adjacent adenine-guanines (AG), and guanines separated by an intervening nucleotide (GNG). These crosslinks inhibit DNA replication and transcription. Cytotoxicity is cell-cycle nonspecific.

PHARMACOLOGY

In vivo studies have shown antitumor activity of oxaliplatin against colon carcinoma. In combination with 5-fluorouracil (5-FU), oxaliplatin exhibits *in vitro* and *in vivo* antiproliferative activity greater than either compound alone in several tumor models [HT29 (colon), GR (mammary), and L1210 (leukemia)].

HUMAN PHARMACOKINETICS

The reactive oxaliplatin derivatives are present as a fraction of the unbound platinum in plasma ultrafiltrate. The decline of ultrafilterable platinum levels following oxaliplatin administration is triphasic, characterized by two relatively short distribution phases ($T_{1/2}\alpha$; 0.43 hours and $T_{1/2}\beta$; 16.8 hours) and a long terminal elimination phase ($T_{1/2}\gamma$; 391 hours). Pharmacokinetic parameters obtained after a single 2 hour IV infusion of oxaliplatin at a dose of 85 mg/m^2 expressed as ultrafilterable platinum were C_{max} of 0.814 µg/ml and volume of distribution of 440 L.

Interpatient and intrapatient variability in ultrafilterable platinum exposure [AUC(0-48)] assessed over 3 cycles was moderate to low (23% and 6%, respectively). A pharmacodynamic relationship between platinum ultrafiltrate levels and clinical safety and effectiveness has not been established.

DISTRIBUTION

At the end of a 2 hour infusion of oxaliplatin, approximately 15% of the administered platinum is present in the systemic circulation. The remaining 85% is rapidly distributed into tissues or eliminated in the urine. In patients, plasma protein binding of platinum is irreversible and is greater than 90%. The main binding proteins are albumin and gamma-globulins. Platinum also binds irreversibly and accumulates (approximately 2-fold) in erythrocytes, where it appears to have no relevant activity. No platinum accumulation was observed in plasma ultrafiltrate following 85 mg/m^2 every 2 weeks.

METABOLISM

Oxaliplatin undergoes rapid and extensive nonenzymatic biotransformation. There is no evidence of cytochrome P450-mediated metabolism *in vitro*.

Up to 17 platinum-containing derivatives have been observed in plasma ultrafiltrate samples from patients, including several cytotoxic species (monochloro DACH platinum, dichloro DACH platinum, and monoaquo and diaquo DACH platinum) and a number of noncytotoxic, conjugated species.

ELIMINATION

The major route of platinum elimination is renal excretion. At 5 days after a single 2 hour infusion of oxaliplatin, urinary elimination accounted for about 54% of the platinum eliminated, with fecal excretion accounting for only about 2%. Platinum was cleared from plasma at a rate (10-17 L/h) that was similar to or exceeded the average human glomerular filtration rate (GFR; 7.5 L/h). There was no significant effect of gender on the clearance of ultrafilterable platinum. The renal clearance of ultrafilterable platinum is significantly correlated with GFR. (See ADVERSE REACTIONS.)

PHARMACOKINETICS IN SPECIAL POPULATIONS

Renal Impairment

The AUC(0-48h) of platinum in the plasma ultrafiltrate increases as renal function decreases. The AUC(0-48h) of platinum in patients with mild (creatinine clearance, CLCR 50-80 ml/min), moderate (CLCR 30 to <50 ml/min) and severe renal (CLCR <30 ml/min) impairment is increased by about 60, 140 and 190%, respectively, compared to patients with normal renal function (CLCR >80 ml/min). (See PRECAUTIONS and ADVERSE REACTIONS.)

Drug-Drug Interactions

No pharmacokinetic interaction between 85 mg/m^2 of oxaliplatin and infusional 5-FU has been observed in patients treated every 2 weeks, but increases of 5-FU plasma concentrations by approximately 20% have been observed with doses of 130 mg/m^2 of oxaliplatin administered every 3 weeks. *In vitro,* platinum was not displaced from plasma proteins by the following medications: erythromycin, salicylate, sodium valproate, granisetron, and paclitaxel. *In vitro,* oxaliplatin is not metabolized by, nor does it inhibit, human cytochrome P450 isoenzymes. No P450-mediated drug-drug interactions are therefore anticipated in patients.

Since platinum containing species are eliminated primarily through the kidney, clearance of these products may be decreased by co-administration of potentially nephrotoxic compounds, although this has not been specifically studied.

INDICATIONS AND USAGE

Oxaliplatin, used in combination with infusional 5-FU/LV, is indicated for the treatment of patients with metastatic carcinoma of the colon or rectum whose disease has recurred or progressed during or within 6 months of completion of first line therapy with the combination of bolus 5-FU/LV and irinotecan.

The approval of oxaliplatin is based on response rate and an interim analysis showing improved time to radiographic progression. No results are available at this time that demonstrate a clinical benefit, such as improvement of disease-related symptoms or increased survival.

CONTRAINDICATIONS

Oxaliplatin should not be administered to patients with a history of known allergy to oxaliplatin or other platinum compounds.

WARNINGS

As in the case for other platinum compounds, hypersensitivity and anaphylactic/anaphylactoid reactions to oxaliplatin have been reported (see ADVERSE REACTIONS). These allergic reactions were similar in nature and severity to those reported with other platinum-containing compounds, *i.e.*, rash, urticaria, erythema, pruritus, and, rarely, bronchospasm and hypotension. These reactions occur within minutes of administration and should be managed with appropriate supportive therapy. Drug-related deaths associated with platinum compounds from this reaction have been reported.

PREGNANCY CATEGORY D

Oxaliplatin may cause fetal harm when administered to a pregnant woman. Pregnant rats were administered 1 mg/kg/day oxaliplatin (less than one-tenth the recommended human dose based on body surface area) during gestation days 1-5 (pre-implantation), 6-10, or 11-16 (during organogenesis). Oxaliplatin caused developmental mortality (increased early resorptions) when administered on days 6-10 and 11-16 and adversely affected fetal growth (decreased fetal weight, delayed ossification) when administered on days 6-10. If this drug is used during pregnancy or if the patient becomes pregnant while taking this drug, the patient should be apprised of the potential hazard to the fetus. Women of childbearing potential should be advised to avoid becoming pregnant while receiving treatment with oxaliplatin.

PRECAUTIONS

GENERAL

Oxaliplatin should be administered under the supervision of a qualified physician experienced in the use of cancer chemotherapeutic agents. Appropriate management of therapy and complications is possible only when adequate diagnostic and treatment facilities are readily available.

NEUROPATHY

Neuropathy was graded using a study-specific neurotoxicity scale, which was different than the National Cancer Institute Common Toxicity Criteria, Version 2.0 (NCI CTC) (see Neurotoxicity Scale). Oxaliplatin is associated with 2 types of neuropathy:

An acute, reversible primarily peripheral sensory neuropathy that is of early onset, occurring within hours or 1-2 days of dosing, that resolves within 14 days, and that frequently recurs with further dosing. The symptoms may be precipitated or exacerbated by exposure to cold temperature or cold objects and they usually present as transient paresthesia, dysesthesia and hypoesthesia in the hands, feet, perioral area, or throat. Jaw spasm, abnormal tongue sensation, dysarthria, eye pain, and a feeling of chest pressure have also been observed. The acute, reversible pattern of sensory neuropathy was observed in about 56% of study patients who received oxaliplatin with infusional 5-FU/LV. In any individual cycle acute neurotoxicity was observed in approximately 30% of patients. Ice (mucositis prophylaxis) should be avoided during the infusion of oxaliplatin because cold temperature can exacerbate acute neurological symptoms. (See DOSAGE AND ADMINISTRATION, Dose Modification Recommendations.)

An acute syndrome of pharyngolaryngeal dysesthesia seen in 1-2% of patients is characterized by subjective sensations of dysphagia or dyspnea, without any laryngospasm or bronchospasm (no stridor or wheezing).

A persistent (>14 days), primarily peripheral, sensory neuropathy that is usually characterized by paresthesias, dysethesias, hypoesthesias, but may also include deficits in proprioception that can interfere with daily activities (*e.g.*, writing, buttoning, swallowing, and difficulty walking from impaired proprioception). These forms of neuropathy occurred in 48% of the study patients receiving oxaliplatin with infusional 5-FU/LV. Persistent neuropathy can occur without any prior acute neuropathy event. The majority of the patients (80%) who developed Grade 3 persistent neuropathy progressed from prior Grade 1 or 2 events. These symptoms may improve in some patients upon discontinuation of oxaliplatin.

Neurotoxicity Scale:

The grading scale for paresthesias/dysesthesias was: Grade 1, resolved and did not interfere with functioning; Grade 2, interfered with function but not daily activities; Grade 3, pain or functional impairment that interfered with daily activities; Grade 4, persistent impairment that is disabling or life-threatening.

PULMONARY TOXICITY

Oxaliplatin has been associated with pulmonary fibrosis (0.7% of study patients), which may be fatal. In case of unexplained respiratory symptoms such as non-productive cough, dyspnea, crackles, or radiological pulmonary infiltrates, oxaliplatin should be discontinued until further pulmonary investigation excludes interstitial lung disease or pulmonary fibrosis.

INFORMATION FOR THE PATIENT

Patients and patients' caregivers should be informed of the expected side effects of oxaliplatin, particularly its neurologic effects, both the acute, reversible effects, and the persistent neurosensory toxicity. Patients should be informed that the acute neurosensory toxicity may be precipitated or exacerbated by exposure to cold or cold objects. Patients should be instructed to avoid cold drinks, use of ice, and should cover exposed skin prior to exposure to cold temperature or cold objects.

Patients must be adequately informed of the risk of low blood cell counts and instructed to contact their physician immediately should fever, particularly if associated with persistent diarrhea, or evidence of infection develop.

Patients should be instructed to contact their physician if persistent vomiting, diarrhea, signs of dehydration, cough or breathing difficulties occur, or signs of allergic reaction appear.

LABORATORY TESTS

Standard monitoring of the white blood cell count with differential, hemoglobin, platelet count, and blood chemistries (including ALT, AST, bilirubin and creatinine) is recommended before each oxaliplatin cycle (see DOSAGE AND ADMINISTRATION).

LABORATORY TEST INTERACTIONS

None known.

CARCINOGENESIS, MUTAGENESIS, AND IMPAIRMENT OF FERTILITY

Long-term animal studies have not been performed to evaluate the carcinogenic potential of oxaliplatin. Oxaliplatin was not mutagenic to bacteria (Ames test) but was mutagenic to mammalian cells *in vitro* (L5178Y mouse lymphoma assay). Oxaliplatin was clastogenic both *in vitro* (chromosome aberration in human lymphocytes) and *in vivo* (mouse bone marrow micronucleus assay).

In a fertility study, male rats were given oxaliplatin at 0, 0.5, 1, or 2 mg/kg/day for 5 days every 21 days for a total of 3 cycles prior to mating with females that received two cycles of oxaliplatin on the same schedule. A dose of 2 mg/kg/day (less than one-seventh the recommended human dose on a body surface area basis) did not affect pregnancy rate, but caused developmental mortality (increased early resorptions, decreased live fetuses, decreased live births) and delayed growth (decreased fetal weight). Testicular damage, characterized by degeneration, hypoplasia, and atrophy, was observed in dogs administered oxaliplatin at 0.75 mg/kg/day × 5 days every 28 days for 3 cycles. A no effect level was not identified. This daily dose is approximately one-sixth of the recommended human dose on a body surface area basis.

PREGNANCY CATEGORY D

See WARNINGS.

NURSING MOTHERS

It is not known whether oxaliplatin or its derivatives are excreted in human milk. Because many drugs are excreted in human milk and because of the potential for serious adverse reactions in nursing infants from oxaliplatin, a decision should be made whether to discontinue nursing or delay the use of the drug, taking into account the importance of the drug to the mother.

PEDIATRIC USE

The safety and effectiveness of oxaliplatin in pediatric patients have not been established.

PATIENTS WITH RENAL IMPAIRMENT

The safety and effectiveness of the combination of oxaliplatin and infusional 5-FU/LV in patients with renal impairment has not been evaluated. The combination of oxaliplatin and infusional 5-FU/LV should be used with caution in patients with preexisting renal impairment since the primary route of platinum elimination is renal. Clearance of ultrafilterable platinum is decreased in patients with mild, moderate, and severe renal impairment. A pharmacodynamic relationship between platinum ultrafiltrate levels and clinical safety and effectiveness has not been established. (See CLINICAL PHARMACOLOGY and ADVERSE REACTIONS.)

GERIATRIC USE

No significant effect of age on the clearance of ultrafilterable platinum has been observed. In the randomized clinical trial of oxaliplatin, 95 patients treated with oxaliplatin and infusional 5-FU/LV were <65 years and 55 patients were ≥65 years. The rates of overall adverse events, including Grade 3 and 4 events, were similar across and within arms in the different age groups. The incidence of diarrhea, dehydration, hypokalemia, and fatigue were higher in patients ≥65 years old.

DRUG INTERACTIONS

No specific cytochrome P-450-based drug interaction studies have been conducted. No pharmacokinetic interaction between 85 mg/m^2 oxaliplatin and infusional 5-FU has been observed in patients treated every 2 weeks. Increases of 5-FU plasma concentrations by approximately 20% have been observed with doses of 130 mg/m^2 oxaliplatin dosed every 3 weeks. Since platinum containing species are eliminated primarily through the kidney, clearance of these products may be decreased by coadministration of potentially nephrotoxic compounds; although, this has not been specifically studied. (See CLINICAL PHARMACOLOGY.)

ADVERSE REACTIONS

More than 1500 patients with advanced colorectal cancer have been treated in clinical studies with oxaliplatin either as a single agent or in combination with other medications. The most common adverse reactions were peripheral sensory neuropathies, neutropenia, nausea, emesis, and diarrhea (see PRECAUTIONS). Four-hundred and fifty (450) patients (about 150 receiving the combination of oxaliplatin and 5-FU/LV) were studied in a randomized trial in patients with refractory and relapsed colorectal cancer. The adverse event profile in this study was similar to that seen in other studies and the adverse reactions in this trial are shown in TABLES 5-8.

Thirteen percent (13%) of patients in the oxaliplatin and infusional 5-FU/LV-combination arm and 18% in the infusional 5-FU/LV arm had to discontinue treatment because of adverse effects related to gastrointestinal or hematologic adverse events, or neuropathies. Both 5-FU and oxaliplatin are associated with gastrointestinal and hematologic adverse events. When oxaliplatin is administered in combination with infusional 5-FU, the incidence of these events is increased.

The incidence of death within 30 days of treatment, regardless of causality, was 5% with the oxaliplatin and infusional 5-FU/LV combination, 8% with oxaliplatin alone, and 7% with infusional 5-FU/LV. Of the 7 deaths that occurred on the oxaliplatin and infusional 5-FU/LV combination arm within 30 days of stopping treatment, 3 may have been treatment-related, associated with gastrointestinal bleeding or dehydration.

TABLE 5A and TABLE 5B provide adverse events reported in the study in decreasing order of frequency in the oxaliplatin and infusional 5-FU/LV combination arm for events with overall incidences ≥5% and for Grade 3/4 events with incidences ≥1%. TABLE 5A and TABLE 5B do not include hematologic and blood chemistry abnormalities; these are shown separately in TABLE 7.

TABLE 6 provides adverse events reported in the study in decreasing order of frequency in the oxaliplatin and infusional 5-FU/LV combination arm for events with overall incidences ≥5% but with incidences <1% NCI Grade 3/4 events.

Adverse events were similar in men and women and in patients <65 and ≥65 years, but older patients may have been more susceptible to dehydration, diarrhea, hypokalemia and fatigue. The following additional adverse events, at least possibly related to treatment and potentially important, were reported in ≥2% and <5% of the patients in the oxaliplatin and infusional 5-FU/LV combination arm (listed in decreasing order of frequency): anxiety, myalgia, erythematous rash, increased sweating, conjunctivitis, weight decrease, dry mouth, rectal hemorrhage, depression, ataxia, ascites, hemorrhoids, muscle weakness, nervousness, tachycardia, abnormal micturition frequency, dry skin, pruritus, hemoptysis, purpura, vaginal hemorrhage, melena, somnolence, pneumonia, proctitis, involuntary muscle contractions, intestinal obstruction, gingivitis, tenesmus, hot flashes, enlarged abdomen, urinary incontinence.

O

TABLE 5A *Adverse Experience Reported in Colorectal Cancer Clinical Trial**

Adverse Event (WHO/Preferred)	5-FU/LV (n=142) All Grades	5-FU/LV (n=142) Grade 3/4	Oxaliplatin (n=153) All Grades	Oxaliplatin (n=153) Grade 3/4
Any event	98%	41%	100%	46%
Fatigue	52%	6%	61%	9%
Diarrhea	44%	3%	46%	4%
Nausea	59%	4%	64%	4%
Neuropathy	17%	0%	76%	7%
Acute	10%	0%	65%	5%
Persistent	9%	0%	43%	3%
Vomiting	27%	4%	37%	4%
Stomatitis	32%	3%	14%	0%
Abdominal pain	31%	5%	31%	7%
Fever	23%	1%	25%	1%
Anorexia	20%	1%	20%	2%
Dyspnea	11%	2%	13%	7%
Back pain	16%	4%	11%	0%
Coughing	9%	0%	11%	0%
Edema	13%	1%	10%	1%
Pain	9%	3%	14%	3%
Injection site reaction	5%	1%	9%	0%
Thromboembolism	4%	2%	2%	1%
Hypokalemia	3%	1%	3%	2%
Dehydration	6%	4%	5%	3%
Chest pain	4%	1%	5%	1%
Febrile neutropenia	1%	1%	0%	0%
Gastroesophageal reflux	3%	0%	1%	0%

* ≥5% of all patients and with ≥1% NCI Grade 3/4 events.

TABLE 5B *Adverse Experience Reported In Colorectal Cancer Clinical Trial**

Adverse Event (WHO/Preferred)	Oxaliplatin + 5-FU/LV (n=150) All Grades	Oxaliplatin + 5-FU/LV (n=150) Grade 3/4
Any event	99%	73%
Fatigue	68%	7%
Diarrhea	67%	11%
Nausea	65%	11%
Neuropathy	73%	7%
Acute	56%	2%
Persistent	48%	6%
Vomiting	40%	9%
Stomatitis	37%	3%
Abdominal pain	33%	4%
Fever	29%	1%
Anorexia	29%	3%
Dyspnea	20%	4%
Back pain	19%	3%
Coughing	19%	1%
Edema	15%	1%
Pain	15%	2%
Injection site reaction	10%	3%
Thromboembolism	9%	8%
Hypokalemia	9%	4%
Dehydration	8%	3%
Chest pain	8%	1%
Febrile neutropenia	6%	6%
Gastroesophageal reflux	5%	2%

* ≥5% of all patients and with ≥1% NCI Grade 3/4 events.

TABLE 6 *Adverse Experience Reported in Colorectal Cancer Clinical Trial**

Adverse Event (WHO/Preferred)	5-FU/LV (n=142) All Grades	Oxaliplatin (n=153) All Grades	Oxaliplatin + 5-FU/LV (n=150) All Grades
Constipation	23%	31%	32%
Headache	8%	13%	17%
Rhinitis	4%	6%	15%
Dyspepsia	10%	7%	14%
Taste perversion	1%	5%	13%
Dizziness	8%	7%	13%
Hand-foot syndrome	13%	1%	11%
Flushing	2%	3%	10%
Peripheral edema	11%	5%	10%
Allergic reaction	1%	3%	10%
Arthralgia	10%	7%	10%
Upper respiratory tract infection	4%	7%	10%
Pharyngitis	10%	2%	9%
Rash	5%	5%	9%
Insomnia	4%	11%	9%
Epistaxis	1%	2%	9%
Mucositis	10%	2%	7%
Alopecia	3%	3%	7%
Abnormal lacrimation	6%	1%	7%
Rigors	6%	9%	7%
Hematuria	4%	0%	6%
Dysuria	1%	1%	6%
Hiccup	0%	2%	5%
Flatulence	6%	3%	5%

* ≥5% of all patients but with <1% NCI Grade 3/4 events.

HEMATOLOGIC

TABLE 7 lists the hematologic changes occurring in ≥5% of patients, based on laboratory values and NCI Grade.

TABLE 7 *Adverse Hematologic Experiences (≥5% of patients)*

Hematology Parameter	5-FU/LV (n=142) All Grades	5-FU/LV (n=142) Grade 3/4	Oxaliplatin (n=153) All Grades	Oxaliplatin (n=153) Grade 3/4	Oxaliplatin + 5-FU/LV (n=150) All Grades	Oxaliplatin + 5-FU/LV (n=150) Grade 3/4
Anemia	68%	2%	64%	1%	81%	2%
Leukopenia	34%	1%	13%	0%	76%	19%
Neutropenia	25%	5%	7%	0%	73%	44%
Thrombocytopenia	20%	0%	30%	3%	64%	4%

Thrombocytopenia

Thrombocytopenia was frequently reported with the combination of oxaliplatin and infusional 5-FU/LV. The incidence of Grade 3/4 thrombocytopenia was 4%. Grade 3/4 hemorrhagic events were reported at low frequency and the incidence of these events was similar for the combination of oxaliplatin and infusional 5-FU/LV and the infusional 5-FU/LV control group. The incidence of all hemorrhagic events, however, was higher on the oxaliplatin combination arm compared to the 5-FU/LV arm. These events included gastrointestinal bleeding, hematuria and epistaxis.

Neutropenia

Neutropenia was frequently observed with the combination of oxaliplatin and infusional 5-FU/LV, with Grade 3 and 4 events reported in 27% and 17% of previously treated patients, respectively. The incidence of febrile neutropenia was 1% in the infusional 5-FU/LV arm and 6% (less than 1% of cycles) in the oxaliplatin and infusional 5-FU/LV combination arm.

GASTROINTESTINAL

In patients receiving the combination of oxaliplatin and infusional 5-FU/LV, the incidence of Grade 3 and 4 nausea, vomiting, diarrhea, and mucositis/stomatitis increased compared to infusional 5-FU/LV controls (see TABLE 5A and TABLE 5B).

The incidence of gastrointestinal adverse events appears to be similar across cycles. Premedication with antiemetics, including 5-HT$_3$ blockers, is recommended. Diarrhea and mucositis may be exacerbated by the addition of oxaliplatin to infusional 5-FU/LV, and should be managed with appropriate supportive care. Since cold temperature can exacerbate acute neurological symptoms, ice (mucositis prophylaxis) should be avoided during the infusion of oxaliplatin.

DERMATOLOGIC

Oxaliplatin did not increase the incidence of alopecia compared to infusional 5-FU/LV alone. No complete alopecia was reported. The incidence of hand-foot syndrome was 13% in the infusional 5-FU/LV arm and 11% in the oxaliplatin and infusional 5-FU/LV combination arm.

Care of Intravenous Site

Extravasation may result in local pain and inflammation that may be severe and lead to complications, including necrosis. Injection site reaction, including redness, swelling, and pain have been reported.

NEUROLOGIC

Oxaliplatin is consistently associated with 2 types of peripheral neuropathy (see PRECAUTIONS, Neuropathy). Seventy-four percent (74%) of patients experienced neuropathy. The incidence of overall and Grade 3/4 persistent peripheral neuropathy was 48% and 6%, respectively, in the study. These events can occur without any prior acute event. The majority of the patients (80%) that developed Grade 3 persistent neuropathy progressed from prior Grade 1 or 2 events. The median number of cycles administered on the oxaliplatin with infusional 5-FU/LV combination arm was 6 cycles. In clinical trials that have studied similar administration schedules of this combination regimen, (median cycles ranged 10-12), a higher incidence (17%) of Grade 3/4 persistent neurotoxicity was observed.

ALLERGIC REACTIONS

Hypersensitivity to oxaliplatin has been observed (<1% Grade 3/4) in clinical studies. These allergic reactions, which can be fatal, were similar in nature and severity to those reported with other platinum-containing compounds — *i.e.*, rash, urticaria, erythema, pruritus, and, rarely, bronchospasm and hypotension. These reactions are usually managed with standard epinephrine, corticosteroid, and antihistamine therapy, (see WARNINGS for anaphylactic/anaphylactoid reactions).

RENAL

About 10% of patients in all groups had some degree of elevation of serum creatinine. The incidence of Grade 3/4 elevations in serum creatinine in the oxaliplatin and infusional 5-FU/LV combination arm was 1%.

HEPATIC

TABLE 8 lists the clinical chemistry changes associated with hepatic toxicity occurring in ≥5% of patients, based on laboratory values and NCI CTC Grade.

THROMBOEMBOLISM

The incidence of thromboembolic events was 4% in the infusional 5-FU/LV arm, and 9% in the oxaliplatin and infusional 5-FU/LV combination arm.

TABLE 8 *Adverse Hepatic — Clinical Chemistry Experience (≥5% of patients)*

Clinical Chemistry	5-FU/LV (n=142) All Grades	Grade 3/4	Oxaliplatin (n=153) All Grades	Grade 3/4	Oxaliplatin + 5-FU/LV (n=150) All Grades	Grade 3/4
ALT (SGPT-ALAT)	28%	3%	36%	1%	31%	0%
AST (SGOT-ASAT)	39%	2%	54%	4%	47%	0%
Total bilirubin	22%	6%	13%	5%	13%	1%

POSTMARKETING EXPERIENCE

The following events have been reported from worldwide postmarketing experience:

Body as a whole: Angioedema, anaphylactic shock.

Central and peripheral nervous system disorders: Loss of deep tendon reflexes, dysarthria, Lhermittes' sign, cranial nerve palsies, fasciculations.

Gastrointestinal system disorders: Severe diarrhea/vomiting resulting in hypokalemia, metabolic acidosis; ileus; intestinal obstruction, pancreatitis.

Hearing and vestibular system disorders: Deafness.

Platelet, bleeding, and clotting disorders: Immuno-allergic thrombocytopenia.

Red blood cell disorders: Hemolytic uremic syndrome.

Respiratory system disorders: Pulmonary fibrosis, and other interstitial lung diseases.

Vision disorders: Decrease of visual acuity, visual field disturbance, optic neuritis.

DOSAGE AND ADMINISTRATION

The recommended dose schedule given every 2 weeks is as follows:

Day 1: Oxaliplatin 85 mg/m^2 IV infusion in 250-500 ml D5W and leucovorin 200 mg/m^2 IV infusion in D5W both given over 120 minutes at the same time in separate bags using a Y-line, followed by 5-FU 400 mg/m^2 IV bolus given over 2-4 minutes, followed by 5-FU 600 mg/m^2 IV infusion in 500 ml D5W (recommended) as a 22 hour continuous infusion.

Day 2: Leucovorin 200 mg/m^2 IV infusion over 120 minutes, followed by 5-FU 400 mg/m^2 IV bolus given over 2-4 minutes, followed by 5-FU 600 mg/m^2 IV infusion in 500 ml D5W (recommended) as a 22 hour continuous infusion.

Repeat cycle every 2 weeks.

The administration of oxaliplatin does not require prehydration.

Premedication with antiemetics, including 5-HT$_3$ blockers with or without dexamethasone, is recommended.

For information on 5-fluorouracil and leucovorin, see the respective package inserts.

DOSE MODIFICATION RECOMMENDATIONS

Prior to subsequent therapy cycles, patients should be evaluated for clinical toxicities and laboratory tests (see PRECAUTIONS, Laboratory Tests). Neuropathy was graded using a study-specific neurotoxicity scale (see PRECAUTIONS, Neuropathy). Other toxicities were graded by the NCI CTC, Version 2.0.

Prolongation of infusion time for oxaliplatin from 2 hours to 6 hours decreases the C_{max} by an estimated 32% and may mitigate acute toxicities. The infusion time for infusional 5-FU and leucovorin do not need to be changed.

For patients who experience persistent Grade 2 neurosensory events that do not resolve, a dose reduction of oxaliplatin to 65 mg/m^2 should be considered. For patients with persistent Grade 3 neurosensory events, discontinuing therapy should be considered. The infusional 5-FU/LV regimen need not be altered.

A dose reduction of oxaliplatin to 65 mg/m^2 and infusional 5-FU by 20% (300 mg/m^2 bolus and 500 mg/m^2 22 hour infusion) is recommended for patients after recovery from Grade 3/4 gastrointestinal (despite prophylactic treatment) or Grade 3/4 hematologic toxicity (neutrophils $<1.5 \times 10^9$/L, platelets $<100 \times 10^9$/L).

PREPARATION OF INFUSION SOLUTION

RECONSTITUTION OR FINAL DILUTION MUST NEVER BE PERFORMED WITH A SODIUM CHLORIDE SOLUTION OR OTHER CHLORIDE-CONTAINING SOLUTIONS.

The lyophilized powder is reconstituted by adding 10 ml (for the 50 mg vial) or 20 ml (for the 100 mg vial) of water for injection or 5% dextrose injection. **Do not administer the reconstituted solution without further dilution.** The reconstituted solution must be further diluted in an infusion solution of 250-500 ml of 5% dextrose injection.

After reconstitution in the original vial, the solution may be stored up to 24 hours under refrigeration [2-8°C (36-46°F)]. After final dilution with 250-500 ml of 5% dextrose injection, the shelf life is **6 hours at room temperature [20-25°C (68-77°F)] or up to 24 hours under refrigeration [2-8°C (36-46°F)].** Oxaliplatin is not light sensitive.

Oxaliplatin is incompatible in solution with alkaline medications or media (such as basic solutions of 5-FU) and must not be mixed with these or administered simultaneously through the same infusion line. **The infusion line should be flushed with D5W prior to administration of any concomitant medication.**

Parenteral drug products should be inspected visually for particulate matter and discoloration prior to administration and discarded if present.

Needles or intravenous administration sets containing aluminum parts that may come in contact with oxaliplatin should not be used for the preparation or mixing of the drug. Aluminum has been reported to cause degradation of platinum compounds.

HANDLING AND DISPOSAL

As with other potentially toxic anticancer agents, care should be exercised in the handling and preparation of infusion solutions prepared from oxaliplatin. The use of gloves is recommended. If a solution of oxaliplatin contacts the skin, wash the skin immediately and thoroughly with soap and water. If oxaliplatin contacts the mucous membranes, flush thoroughly with water.

Procedures for the handling and disposal of anticancer drugs should be considered. Several guidelines on the subject have been published.[1-8] There is no general agreement that all of the procedures recommended in the guidelines are necessary or appropriate.

HOW SUPPLIED

Eloxatin is supplied in clear, glass, single-use vials with gray elastomeric stoppers and aluminum flip-off seals containing 50 or 100 mg of oxaliplatin as a sterile, preservative-free lyophilized powder for reconstitution. Lactose monohydrate is also present as an inactive ingredient.

50 mg: Single-use vial with green flip-off seal.

100 mg: Single-use vial with dark blue flip-off seal.

Storage: Store under normal lighting conditions at 25°C (77°F); excursions permitted to 15-30°C (59-86°F).

PRODUCT LISTING - EQUIVALENTS NOT AVAILABLE

Powder For Injection - Intravenous - 50 mg

1's $994.26 ELOXATIN, Sanofi Winthrop Pharmaceuticals 00024-0596-02

Powder For Injection - Intravenous - 100 mg

1's $1988.53 ELOXATIN, Sanofi Winthrop Pharmaceuticals 00024-0597-04

Oxaprozin *(003140)*

For related information, see the comparative table section in Appendix A.

Categories: Arthritis, osteoarthritis; Arthritis, rheumatoid; FDA Approved 1992 Oct; Pregnancy Category C
Drug Classes: Analgesics, non-narcotic; Nonsteroidal anti-inflammatory drugs
Brand Names: **Daypro**
Foreign Brand Availability: Deflam (South-Africa); Duraprox (Portugal)
Cost of Therapy: $122.60 (Osteoarthritis; Daypro; 600 mg; 2 tablets/day; 30 day supply)
$88.87 (Osteoarthritis; Generic Tablets; 600 mg; 2 tablets/day; 30 day supply)

DESCRIPTION

Daypro (oxaprozin) is a nonsteroidal anti-inflammatory drug (NSAID), chemically designated as 4,5-diphenyl-2-oxazole-propionic acid.

The empirical formula for oxaprozin is $C_{18}H_{15}NO_3$, and the molecular weight is 293. Oxaprozin is a white to off-white powder with a slight odor and a melting point of 162-163°C. It is slightly soluble in alcohol and insoluble in water, with an octanol/water partition coefficient of 4.8 and physiologic pH (7.4). The pK_a in water is 4.3.

Daypro oral caplets contain 600 mg of oxaprozin.

Inactive ingredients in Daypro oral caplets are microcrystalline cellulose, hydroxypropyl methylcellulose, methylcellulose, magnesium stearate, polacrilin potassium, starch, polyethylene glycol, and titanium dioxide.

CLINICAL PHARMACOLOGY

PHARMACODYNAMICS

Oxaprozin is a nonsteroidal anti-inflammatory drug (NSAID) that exhibits anti-inflammatory, analgesic, and antipyretic properties in animal models. The mechanism of action of oxaprozin, like that of other NSAIDs, is not completely understood but may be related to prostaglandin synthetase inhibition.

PHARMACOKINETICS

See TABLE 1.

Absorption

Oxaprozin is 95% absorbed after oral administration. Food may reduce the rate of absorption of oxaprozin, but the extent of absorption is unchanged. Antacids do not significantly affect the extent and rate of oxaprozin absorption.

TABLE 1 *Oxaproxin Pharmacokinetics Parameters [Mean (% CV)] (1200 mg)*

Healthy Adults (19-78 Years)	Total Drug Single n=35	Total Drug Multiple n=12	Unbound Drug Single n=35	Unbound Drug Multiple n=12
T_{max} (h)	3.09 (39)	2.44 (40)	3.03 (48)	2.33 (35)
Oral clearance (L/h/70 kg)	0.150 (24)	0.301 (29)	136 (24)	102 (45)
Apparent volume of distribution at steady-state (Vd/F; L/70 kg)	11.7 (13)	16.7 (14)	6230 (28)	2420 (38)
Elimination half-life (h)	54.9 (49)	41.4 (27)	27.8 (34)	19.5 (15)

Distribution

In dose proportionality studies utilizing 600, 1200 and 1800 mg doses, the pharmacokinetics of oxaprozin in healthy subjects demonstrated nonlinear kinetics of both the total and unbound drug in opposite directions, *i.e.,* dose exposure related increase in the clearance of total drug and decrease in the clearance of the unbound drug. Decreased clearance of the unbound drug was related predominantly to a decrease in the volume of distribution and not an increase in the half-life. This phenomenon is considered to have minimal impact on drug accumulation upon multiple dosing.

The apparent volume of distribution (Vd/F) of total oxaprozin is approximately 11-17 L/70 kg. Oxaprozin is 99% bound to plasma proteins, primarily to albumin. At therapeutic drug concentrations, the plasma protein binding of oxaprozin is saturable, resulting in a higher proportion of the free drug as the total drug concentration is increased. With increases in single doses or following repetitive once-daily dosing, the apparent volume of distribution and clearance of total drug increased, while that of unbound drug decreased due to the effects of nonlinear protein binding. Oxaprozin penetrates into synovial tissues of rheumatoid arthritis patients with oxaprozin concentrations 2- and 3-fold greater than in plasma and synovial fluid, respectively. Oxaprozin is expected to be excreted in human milk based on its physical-chemical properties, however, the amount of oxaprozin excreted in breast milk has not been evaluated.

Metabolism

Several oxaprozin metabolites have been identified in human urine or feces.

Oxaprozin is primarily metabolized by the liver, by both microsomal oxidation (65%) and glucuronic acid conjugation (35%). Ester and ether glucuronide are the major conjugated metabolites of oxaprozin. On chronic dosing, metabolites do not accumulate in the plasma of patients with normal renal function. Concentrations of the metabolites in plasma are very low.

Oxaprozin's metabolites do not have significant pharmacologic activity. The major ester and ether glucuronide conjugated metabolites have been evaluated along with oxaprozin in receptor binding studies and *in vivo* animal models and have demonstrated no activity. A small amount (<5%) of active phenolic metabolites are produced, but the contribution to overall activity is limited.

Excretion

Approximately 5% of the oxaprozin dose is excreted unchanged in the urine. Sixty-five percent (65%) of the dose is excreted in the urine and 35% in the feces as metabolite. Biliary excretion of unchanged oxaprozin is a minor pathway, and enterohepatic recycling of oxaprozin is insignificant. Upon chronic dosing the accumulation half-life is approximately 22 hours. The elimination half-life is approximately twice the accumulation half-life due to increased binding and decreased clearance at lower concentrations.

SPECIAL POPULATIONS

Pediatric Patients

A population pharmacokinetic study indicated no clinically important age dependent changes in the apparent clearance of unbound oxaprozin between adult rheumatoid arthritis patients (n=40) and juvenile rheumatoid arthritis (JRA) patients (≥6 years, n=44) when adjustments were made for differences in body weight between these patient groups. The extent of protein binding of oxaprozin at various therapeutic total plasma concentrations was also similar between the adult and pediatric patient groups. Pharmacokinetic model-based estimates of daily exposure [AUC(0-24)] to unbound oxaprozin in JRA patients relative to adult rheumatoid arthritis patients suggest dose to body weight range relationships as shown in TABLE 2. No pharmacokinetic data are available for pediatric patients under 6 years of age (see PRECAUTIONS, Pediatric Use).

***TABLE 2** Dose to Body Weight Range to Achieve Similar Steady-State Exposure [AUC (0-24h)] to Unbound Oxaprozin in JRA Patients Relative to 70 kg Adult Rheumatoid Arthritis Patients Administered Oxaprozin 1200 mg qd**

Dose	Body Weight Range
600 mg	22-31 kg
900 mg	32-54 kg
1200 mg	≥55 kg

* Model-based nomogram derived from unbound oxaprozin steady-state drug plasma concentrations of JRA patients weighing 22.1-42.7 kg or ≥45.0 kg administered oxaprozin 600 or 1200 mg qd for 14 days, respectively.

Geriatric

As with any NSAID, caution should be exercised in treating the elderly (65 years and older). No dosage adjustment is necessary in the elderly for pharmacokinetics reasons, although many elderly may need a reduced dose due to low body weight or disorders associated with aging.

A multiple dose study comparing the pharmacokinetics of oxaprozin (1200 mg qd) in 20 young (21-44 years) adults and 20 elderly (64-83 years) adults, did not show any statistically significant differences between age groups.

Race

Pharmacokinetics differences due to race have not been identified.

Hepatic Insufficiency

Approximately 95% of oxaprozin is metabolized by the liver. However, patients with well compensated cirrhosis do not require reduced doses of oxaprozin as compared to patients with normal hepatic function. Nevertheless, caution should be observed in patients with severe hepatic dysfunction.

Cardiac Failure

Well-compensated cardiac failure does not affect the plasma protein binding or the pharmacokinetics of oxaprozin.

Renal Insufficiency

The pharmacokinetics of oxaprozin have been investigated in patients with renal insufficiency. Oxaprozin's renal clearance decreased proportionally with creatinine clearance (CRCL), but since only about 5% of oxaprozin dose is excreted unchanged in the urine, the decrease in total body clearance becomes clinically important only in those subjects with highly decreased CRCL. Oxaprozin is not significantly removed from the blood in patients undergoing hemodialysis or CAPD due to its high protein binding. Oxaprozin plasma protein binding may decrease in patients with severe renal deficiency. Dosage adjustment may be necessary in patients with renal insufficiency (see PRECAUTIONS, General, Renal Effects).

INDICATIONS AND USAGE

Oxaprozin is indicated for relief of the signs and symptoms of osteoarthritis, adult rheumatoid arthritis and juvenile rheumatoid arthritis.

CONTRAINDICATIONS

Oxaprozin is contraindicated in patients with known hypersensitivity to oxaprozin. Oxaprozin should not be given to patients who have experienced asthma, urticaria, or allergic-type reactions after taking aspirin or other NSAIDs. Severe, rarely fatal, anaphylactic-like reactions to NSAIDs have been reported in such patients (see WARNINGS, Anaphylactic Reactions and PRECAUTIONS, General, Preexisting Asthma).

WARNINGS

GASTROINTESTINAL (GI) EFFECTS — RISK OF GI ULCERATION, BLEEDING, AND PERFORATION

Serious gastrointestinal toxicity, such as inflammation, bleeding, ulceration, and perforation of the stomach, small intestine, or large intestine, can occur at any time, with or without warning symptoms, in patients treated with nonsteroidal anti-inflammatory drugs (NSAIDs). Minor upper gastrointestinal problems, such as dyspepsia, are common and may also occur at any time during NSAID therapy. Therefore, physicians and patients should remain alert for ulceration and bleeding, even in the absence of previous GI tract symptoms. Patients should be informed about the signs and/or symptoms of serious GI toxicity and the steps to take if they occur.

The utility of periodic laboratory monitoring has not been demonstrated, nor has it been adequately assessed. Only 1 in 5 patients, who develop a serious upper GI adverse event on NSAID therapy, is symptomatic. It has been demonstrated that upper GI ulcers, gross bleeding or perforation, caused by NSAIDs, appear to occur in approximately 1% of patients treated for 3-6 months, and in about 2-4% of patients treated for 1 year. These trends continue thus, increasing the likelihood of developing a serious GI event at some time during the course of therapy. However, even short term therapy is not without risk.

NSAIDs should be prescribed with extreme caution in those with a prior history of ulcer disease or gastrointestinal bleeding. Most spontaneous reports of fatal GI events are in elderly or debilitated patients and therefore special care should be taken in treating this population. **To minimize the potential risk for an adverse GI event, the lowest effective dose should be used for the shortest possible duration.** For high risk patients, alternate therapies that do not involve NSAIDs should be considered.

Studies have shown that patients with a prior history of peptic ulcer disease and/or gastrointestinal bleeding and who use NSAIDs, have a greater than 10-fold risk for developing a GI bleed than patients with neither of these risk factors. In addition to a past history of ulcer disease, pharmacoepidemiological studies have identified several other co-therapies or co-morbid conditions that may increase the risk for GI bleeding such as: treatment with oral corticosteroids, treatment with anticoagulants, longer duration of NSAID therapy, smoking, alcoholism, older age and poor general health status.

ANAPHYLACTIC REACTIONS

As with other NSAIDs, anaphylactoid reactions may occur in patients without known prior exposure to oxaprozin. Oxaprozin should not be given to patients with the aspirin triad. This symptom complex typically occurs in asthmatic patients who experience rhinitis with or without nasal polyps, or who exhibit severe, potentially fatal bronchospasm after taking aspirin or other NSAIDs (see CONTRAINDICATIONS and PRECAUTIONS, General, Preexisting Asthma). Emergency help should be sought in cases where an anaphylactoid reaction occurs.

ADVANCED RENAL DISEASE

In cases with advanced kidney disease, treatment with oxaprozin is not recommended. If oxaprozin therapy must be initiated, close monitoring of the patient's kidney function is advisable (see PRECAUTIONS, General, Renal Effects).

PREGNANCY

In late pregnancy, as with other NSAIDs, oxaprozin should be avoided because it may cause premature closure of the ductus arteriosus.

PRECAUTIONS

GENERAL

Oxaprozin cannot be expected to substitute for corticosteroids or to treat corticosteroid insufficiency. Abrupt discontinuation of corticosteroids may lead to disease exacerbation. Patients on prolonged corticosteroid therapy should have their therapy tapered slowly if a decision is made to discontinue corticosteroids.

The pharmacological activity of oxaprozin in reducing fever and inflammation may diminish the utility of these diagnostic signs in detecting complications of presumed noninfectious, painful conditions.

Hepatic Effects

Borderline elevations of 1 or more liver tests may occur in up to 15% of patients taking NSAIDs including oxaprozin. These laboratory abnormalities may progress, remain unchanged, or may be transient with continued therapy. Notable elevations of ALT or AST (approximately 3 or more times the upper limit of normal) have been reported in approximately 1% of patients in clinical trials with NSAIDs. In addition, rare cases of severe hepatic reactions, including jaundice and fatal fulminate hepatitis, liver necrosis and hepatic failure, some of them with fatal outcomes have been reported.

A patient with symptoms and/or signs suggesting liver dysfunction, or in whom an abnormal liver test has occurred, should be evaluated for evidence of the development of a more severe hepatic reaction while on therapy with oxaprozin. If clinical signs and symptoms consistent with liver disease develop, or if systemic manifestations occur (*e.g.*, eosinophilia, rash, etc.), oxaprozin should be discontinued.

Renal Effects

Caution should be used when initiating treatment with oxaprozin in patients with considerable dehydration. It is advisable to rehydrate patients first and then start therapy with oxaprozin. Caution is also recommended in patients with preexisting kidney disease (see WARNINGS, Advanced Renal Disease).

As with other NSAIDs, long-term administration of oxaprozin has resulted in renal papillary necrosis and other renal medullary changes. Renal toxicity has also been seen in patients in which renal prostaglandins have a compensatory role in the maintenance of renal perfusion. In these patients, administration of a nonsteroidal anti-inflammatory drug may cause a dose-dependent reduction in prostaglandin formation and, secondarily, in renal blood flow, which may precipitate overt renal decompensation. Patients at greatest risk of this reaction are those with impaired renal function, heart failure, liver dysfunction, those taking diuretics and ACE inhibitors, and the elderly. Discontinuation of nonsteroidal anti-inflammatory drug therapy is usually followed by recovery to the pretreatment state.

Oxaprozin metabolites are eliminated primarily by the kidneys. The extent to which the metabolites may accumulate in patients with renal failure has not been studied. As with other NSAIDs, metabolites of which are excreted by the kidney, patients with significantly impaired renal function should be more closely monitored.

Photosensitivity

Oxaprozin has been associated with rash and/or mild photosensitivity in dermatologic testing. An increased incidence of rash on sun-exposed skin was seen in some patients in the clinical trials.

Hematological Effects

Anemia is sometimes seen in patients receiving NSAIDs, including oxaprozin. This may be due to fluid retention, gastrointestinal blood loss, or an incompletely described effect upon erythrogenesis. Patients on long-term treatment with oxaprozin should have their hemoglobin or hematocrit values determined if they exhibit any signs or symptoms of anemia.

All drugs which inhibit the biosynthesis of prostaglandins may interfere to some extent with platelet function and vascular responses to bleeding.

NSAIDs inhibit platelet aggregation and have been shown to prolong bleeding time in some patients. Unlike aspirin, their effect on platelet function is quantitatively less, of shorter duration, and reversible. Oxaprozin does not generally affect platelet counts, prothrombin time (PT), or partial thromboplastin time (PTT). Patients receiving oxaprozin who may be adversely affected by alterations in platelet function, such as those with coagulation disorders or patients receiving anticoagulants, should be carefully monitored.

Fluid Retention and Edema

Fluid retention and edema have been observed in some patients taking NSAIDs. Therefore, as with other NSAIDs, oxaprozin should be used with caution in patients with fluid retention, hypertension, or heart failure.

Preexisting Asthma

Patients with asthma may have aspirin-sensitive asthma. The use of aspirin in patients with aspirin-sensitive asthma has been associated with the severe bronchospasm which can be fatal. Since cross reactivity, including bronchospasm, between aspirin and other nonsteroidal anti-inflammatory drugs has been reported in such aspirin-sensitive patients, oxaprozin should not be administered to patients with this form of aspirin sensitivity and should be used with caution in patients with preexisting asthma.

INFORMATION FOR THE PATIENT

Oxaprozin, like other drugs of its class, can cause discomfort and, rarely, more serious side effects, such as gastrointestinal bleeding, which may result in hospitalization and even fatal outcomes. Although serious gastrointestinal tract ulcerations and bleeding can occur without warning symptoms, patients should be alert for the signs and symptoms of ulcerations and bleeding, and should ask for medical advice when observing any indicative sign or symptoms. Patients should be apprised of the importance of this follow-up (see WARNINGS, Risk of GI Ulceration, Bleeding, and Perforation).

Patients should report to their physicians the signs or symptoms of gastrointestinal ulceration or bleeding, skin rash, weight gain, or edema.

Patients should be informed of the warning signs and symptoms of hepatotoxicity (*e.g.*, nausea, fatigue, lethargy, pruritus, jaundice, right upper quadrant tenderness, and "flu-like" symptoms). If these occur, patients should be instructed to stop therapy and seek immediate medical therapy.

Patients should also be instructed to seek immediate emergency help in the case of an anaphylactoid reaction (see WARNINGS).

In late pregnancy, as with other NSAIDs, oxaprozin should be avoided because it will cause premature closure of the ductus arteriosus.

LABORATORY TESTS

Patients on long-term treatment with NSAIDs should have their CBC and a chemistry profile checked periodically. If clinical signs and symptoms consistent with liver or renal disease develop, systemic manifestations occur (*e.g.* eosinophilia, rash, *etc.*) or if abnormal liver tests persist or worsen, oxaprozin should be discontinued.

LABORATORY TEST INTERACTIONS

False-positive urine immunoassay screening tests for benzodiazepines have been reported in patients taking oxaprozin. This is due to lack of specificity of the screening tests. False-positive test results may be expected for several days following discontinuation of oxaprozin therapy. Confirmatory tests, such as gas chromatography/mass spectrometry, will distinguish oxaprozin from benzodiazepines.

CARCINOGENESIS, MUTAGENESIS, AND IMPAIRMENT OF FERTILITY

In oncogenicity studies, oxaprozin administration for 2 years was associated with the exacerbation of liver neoplasms (hepatic adenomas and carcinomas) in male CD mice, but not in female CD mice or rats. The significance of this species-specific finding to man is unknown.

Oxaprozin did not display mutagenic potential. Results from the Ames test, forward mutation in yeast and Chinese hamster ovary (CHO) cells, DNA repair testing in CHO cells, micronucleus testing in mouse bone marrow, chromosomal aberration testing in human lymphocytes, and cell transformation testing in mouse fibroblast all showed no evidence of genetic toxicity or cell-transforming ability.

Oxaprozin administration was not associated with impairment of fertility in male and female rats at oral doses up to 200 mg/kg/day (1180 mg/m^2); the usual human dose is 17 mg/kg/day (629 mg/m^2). However, testicular degeneration was observed in beagle dogs treated with 37.5 to 150 mg/kg/day (750-3000 mg/m^2) of oxaprozin for 6 months, or 37.5 mg/kg/day for 42 days, a finding not confirmed in other species. The clinical relevance of this finding is not known.

PREGNANCY CATEGORY C

Teratogenic Effects

Teratology studies with oxaprozin were performed in mice, rats, and rabbits. In mice and rats, no drug-related developmental abnormalities were observed at 50-200 mg/kg/day of oxaprozin (225-900 mg/m^2). However, in rabbits, infrequent malformed fetuses were observed in dams treated with 7.5 to 30 mg/kg/day of oxaprozin (the usual human dosage range). Animal reproductive studies are not always predictive of human response. There are no adequate or well-controlled studies in pregnant women. Oxaprozin should be used during pregnancy only if the potential benefits justify the potential risks to the fetus.

Nonteratogenic Effects

Because of the known effects of nonsteroidal anti-inflammatory drugs on the fetal cardiovascular system (closure of ductus arteriosus), use during pregnancy (particularly late pregnancy) should be avoided.

LABOR AND DELIVERY

In rat studies with NSAIDs, as with other drugs known to inhibit prostaglandin synthesis, an increased incidence of dystocia, delayed parturition, and decreased pup survival occurred. The effects of oxaprozin on labor and delivery in pregnant women are unknown.

NURSING MOTHERS

It is not known whether this drug is excreted in human milk. Because many drugs are excreted in human milk and because of the potential for serious adverse reactions in nursing infants from oxaprozin, a decision should be made whether to discontinue nursing or to discontinue the drug, taking into account the importance of the drug to the mother.

PEDIATRIC USE

Safety and effectiveness of oxaprozin in pediatric patients less than 6 years of age have not been established. The effectiveness of oxaprozin for the treatment of the signs and symptoms of juvenile rheumatoid arthritis (JRA) in pediatric patients aged 6-16 years is supported by evidence from adequate and well controlled studies in adult rheumatoid arthritis patients, and is based on an extrapolation of the demonstrated efficacy of oxaprozin in adults with rheumatoid arthritis and the similarity in the course of the disease and the drug's mechanism of effect between these 2 patient populations. Use of oxaprozin in JRA patients 6-16 years of age is also supported by the following pediatric studies.

The pharmacokinetic profile and tolerability of oxaprozin were assessed in JRA patients relative to adult rheumatoid arthritis patients in a 14 day multiple dose pharmacokinetic study. Apparent clearance of unbound oxaprozin in JRA patients was reduced compared to adult rheumatoid arthritis patients, but this reduction could be accounted for by differences in body weight (see CLINICAL PHARMACOLOGY, Special Populations, Pediatric Patients). No pharmacokinetic data are available for pediatric patients under 6 years. Adverse events were reported by approximately 45% of JRA patients versus an approximate 30% incidence of adverse events in the adult rheumatoid arthritis patient cohort. Most of the adverse events were related to the gastrointestinal tract and were mild to moderate.

In a 3 month open label study, 10-20 mg/kg/day of oxaprozin were administered to 59 JRA patients. Adverse events were reported by 58% of JRA patients. Most of those reported were generally mild to moderate, tolerated by the patients, and did not interfere with continuing treatment. Gastrointestinal symptoms were the most frequently reported adverse effects and occurred at a higher incidence than those historically seen in controlled studies in adults. Fifty two (52) patients completed 3 months of treatment with a mean daily dose of 20 mg/kg. Of 30 patients who continued treatment (19-48 week range total treatment duration), 9 (30%) experienced rash on sun-exposed areas of the skin and 5 of those discontinued treatment. Controlled clinical trials with oxaprozin in pediatric patients have not been conducted.

GERIATRIC USE

No adjustment of the dose of oxaprozin is necessary in the elderly for *pharmacokinetic* reasons, although many elderly may need to receive a reduced dose because of low body weight or disorders associated with aging. No significant differences in the pharmacokinetic profile for oxaprozin were seen in studies in the healthy elderly (see CLINICAL PHARMACOLOGY, Special Populations, Geriatric).

Of the total number of subjects evaluated in four placebo controlled clinical studies of oxaprozin, 39% were 65 and over, and 11% were 75 and over. No overall differences in safety or effectiveness were observed between these subjects and younger subjects, and other reported clinical experience has not identified differences in responses between the elderly and younger patients, but greater sensitivity of some older individuals cannot be ruled out.

Although selected elderly patients in controlled clinical trials tolerated oxaprozin as well as younger patients, caution should be exercised in treating the elderly, and extra care should be taken when choosing a dose. As with any NSAID, the elderly are likely to tolerate adverse reactions less well than younger patients.

Oxaprozin is substantially excreted by the kidney, and the risk of toxic reactions to oxaprozin may be greater in patients with impaired renal function. Because elderly patients are more likely to have decreased renal function, care should be taken in dose selection, and it may be useful to monitor renal function (see PRECAUTIONS, General, Renal Effects).

DRUG INTERACTIONS

Aspirin: Concomitant administration of oxaprozin and aspirin is not recommended because oxaprozin displaces salicylates from plasma protein binding sites. Coadministration would be expected to increase the risk of salicylate toxicity.

Methotrexate: Coadministration of oxaprozin with methotrexate results in approximately a 36% reduction in apparent oral clearance of methotrexate. A reduction in methotrexate dosage may be considered due to the potential for increased methotrexate toxicity associated with the increased exposure.

ACE-Inhibitors: Reports suggest that NSAIDs may diminish the antihypertensive effect of ACE-inhibitors. Oxaprozin has been shown to alter the pharmacokinetics of enalapril [significant decrease in dose-adjusted AUC(0-24) and C_{max}] and its active metabolite enalaprilat [significant increase in dose-adjusted AUC(0-24)]. This interaction should be given consideration in patients taking NSAIDs concomitantly with ACE-inhibitors.

Furosemide: Clinical studies, as well as post marketing observations, have shown that oxaprozin can reduce the natriuretic effect of furosemide and thiazides in some patients. This response has been attributed to inhibition of renal prostaglandin synthesis. During concomitant therapy with NSAIDs, the patient should be observed closely for signs of renal failure (see PRECAUTIONS, General, Renal Effects), as well as to assure diuretic efficacy.

Lithium: Coadministration of oxaprozin with lithium carbonate can cause an increase in serum lithium levels. Whenever oxaprozin is added to or removed from patients on lithium therapy, therapeutic drug monitoring of lithium levels should be performed.

Glyburide: While oxaprozin does alter the pharmacokinetics of glyburide, coadministration of oxaprozin to Type II non-insulin dependent diabetic patients did not affect the area under the glucose concentration curve nor the magnitude or duration of control.

Warfarin: The effects of warfarin and NSAIDs on gastrointestinal (GI) bleeding are synergistic, such that users of both drugs together have a risk of serious GI bleeding higher than that of users of either drug alone.

H_2-Receptor Antagonists: The total body clearance of oxaprozin was reduced by 20% in subjects who concurrently received therapeutic doses of cimetidine or ranitidine; no other pharmacokinetic parameter was affected. A change of clearance of this magnitude lies within the range of normal variation and is unlikely to produce a clinically detectable difference in the outcome of therapy.

Beta-Blockers: Subjects receiving 1200 mg oxaprozin qd with 100 mg metoprolol bid exhibited statistically significant but transient increases in sitting and standing blood pressures after 14 days. Therefore, as with all NSAIDs, routine blood pressure monitoring should be considered in these patients when starting oxaprozin therapy.

Other Drugs: The coadministration of oxaprozin and antacids, acetaminophen, or conjugated estrogens resulted in no statistically significant changes in pharmacokinetic parameters in single- and/or multiple-dose studies. The interaction of oxaprozin with cardiac glycosides has not been studied.

ADVERSE REACTIONS

Adverse reaction data were derived from patients who received oxaprozin in multidose, controlled, and open-label clinical trials, and from worldwide marketing experience. Rates for events occurring in more than 1% of patients, and for most of the less common events, are based on 2253 patients who took 1200-1800 mg oxaprozin per day in clinical trials. Of these, 1721 were treated for at least 1 month, 971 for at least 3 months, and 366 for more than 1 year. Rates for the rarer events and for events reported from worldwide marketing experience are difficult to estimate accurately and are only listed as less than 1%.

INCIDENCE GREATER THAN 1%

In clinical trials or in patients taking other NSAIDs (indicated by double asterisks**), the following adverse reactions occurred at an incidence greater than 1%. Reactions occurring in 3-9% of patients treated with oxaprozin are indicated by an asterisk (*); those reactions occurring in less than 3% of patients are unmarked.

Cardiovascular System: Edema**.

Digestive System: Abdominal pain/distress, anorexia, constipation*, diarrhea*, dyspepsia*, flatulence, gastrointestinal ulcers** (gastric/duodenal), gross bleeding/perforation**, heartburn**, liver enzyme elevations**, nausea*, vomiting.

Hematologic System: Anemia**, increased bleeding time**.

Nervous System: CNS inhibition (depression, sedation, somnolence, or confusion), disturbance of sleep, dizziness**, headache**.

Skin and Appendages: Pruritus**, rash*.

Special Senses: Tinnitus.

Urogenital System: Abnormal renal function**, dysuria or frequency.

INCIDENCE LESS THAN 1%

The following adverse reactions were reported in clinical trials, from worldwide marketing experience (*in italics*) or in patients taking other NSAIDs (double asterisks**).

Body as a Whole: Drug hypersensitivity reactions including anaphylaxis, fever**, infection**, sepsis**, *serum sickness.*

Cardiovascular System: Edema, blood pressure changes, congestive heart failure**, hypertension**, palpitations, tachycardia**, syncope**.

Digestive System: Alteration in taste, dry mouth**, esophagitis**, gastritis**, glossitis**, hematemesis**, jaundice**, peptic ulceration and/or GI bleeding (see WARNINGS), liver function abnormalities including *hepatitis* (see PRECAUTIONS), stomatitis, hemorrhoidal or rectal bleeding, *pancreatitis.*

Hematologic System: *Agranulocytosis,* anemia, ecchymoses, eosinophilia**, melena**, *pancytopenia, purpura***, thrombocytopenia, leukopenia.

Metabolic System: Weight changes.

Nervous System: Anxiety**, asthenia**, confusion**, depression**, dream abnormalities**, drowsiness**, insomnia**, malaise, nervousness**, paresthesia**, somnolence**, tremors**, vertigo**, weakness.

Respiratory System: Asthma**, dyspnea**, pulmonary infections, pneumonia**, sinusitis, symptoms of upper respiratory tract infection, respiratory depression**.

Skin: Alopecia, angioedema**, pruritus, urticaria, photosensitivity, *pseudoporphyria, exfoliative dermatitis, erythema multiforme, Stevens-Johnson syndrome,* sweat**, *toxic epidermal necrolysis (Lyell's syndrome).*

Special Senses: Blurred vision, conjunctivitis, hearing decrease.

Urogenital: *Acute interstitial nephritis,* cystitis**, dysuria**, hematuria, increase in menstrual flow, *nephrotic syndrome,* oliguria/ polyuria**, proteinuria**, renal insufficiency, *acute renal failure,* decreased menstrual flow.

DOSAGE AND ADMINISTRATION

RHEUMATOID ARTHRITIS

For relief of the signs and symptoms of rheumatoid arthritis, the usual recommended dose is 1200 mg (two 600-mg caplets) given orally once a day (see Individualization Of Dosage).

OSTEOARTHRITIS

For relief of the signs and symptoms of osteoarthritis, the usual recommended dose is 1200 mg (two 600-mg caplets) given orally once a day (see Individualization Of Dosage).

JUVENILE RHEUMATOID ARTHRITIS:

For the relief of the signs and symptoms of JRA in patients 6-16 years of age, the recommended dose given orally once per day should be based on body weight of the patient as given in TABLE 3 (see also DOSAGE AND ADMINISTRATION, Individualization Of Dosage).

TABLE 3

Body Weight Range	Dose
22-31 kg	600 mg
32-54 kg	900 mg
≥55 kg	1200 mg

See CLINICAL PHARMACOLOGY,Special Populations, and Pediatric Patients.

INDIVIDUALIZATION OF DOSAGE

As with other NSAIDs, the lowest dose should be sought for each patient. Therefore, after observing the response to initial therapy with oxaprozin, the dose and frequency should be adjusted to suit an individual patient's needs. In osteoarthritis and rheumatoid arthritis and juvenile rheumatoid arthritis, the dosage should be individualized to the lowest effective dose of oxaprozin to minimize adverse effects. The maximum recommended total daily dose of oxaprozin in adults is 1800 mg (26 mg/kg, whichever is *lower*) in divided doses. In children, doses greater than 1200 mg have not been studied.

Patients of low body weight should initiate therapy with 600 mg once daily. Patients with severe renal impairment or on dialysis should also initiate therapy with 600 mg once daily. If there is insufficient relief of symptoms in such patients, the dose may be cautiously increased to 1200 mg, but only with close monitoring (see CLINICAL PHARMACOLOGY, Special Populations).

In adults, in cases where a quick onset of action is important, the pharmacokinetics of oxaprozin allow therapy to be started with a one-time loading dose of 1200-1800 mg (not to exceed 26 mg/kg). Doses larger than 1200 mg/day on a chronic basis should be reserved for patients who weigh more than 50 kg, have normal renal and hepatic function, are at low risk of peptic ulcer, and whose severity of disease justifies maximal therapy. Physicians should ensure that patients are tolerating doses in the 600-1200 mg/day range without gastroenterologic, renal, hepatic, or dermatologic adverse effects before advancing to the larger doses. Most patients will tolerate once-a-day dosing with oxaprozin, although divided doses may be tried in patients unable to tolerate single doses.

SAFETY AND HANDLING

Oxaprozin is supplied as a solid dosage form in closed containers, is not known to produce contact dermatitis, and poses no known risk to healthcare workers. It may be disposed of in accordance with applicable local regulations governing the disposal of pharmaceuticals.

HOW SUPPLIED

Daypro 600 mg Caplets: White, capsule-shaped, scored, film-coated, with "DAYPRO" debossed on 1 side and "1381" on the other side.

Storage: Keep bottles tightly closed. Store at 25°C (77°F); excursions permitted to 15-30°C (59-86°F. Dispense in a tight, light-resistant container with a child resistant closure. Protect the unit dose from light.

PRODUCT LISTING - RATED THERAPEUTICALLY EQUIVALENT

Tablet - Oral - 600 mg

2's	$3.16	DAYPRO, Allscripts Pharmaceutical Company	54569-3702-05
10's	$21.07	DAYPRO, Dhs Inc	55887-0894-10
14's	$29.50	DAYPRO, Dhs Inc	55887-0894-14
14's	$39.38	DAYPRO, Pharma Pac	52959-0252-14
15's	$23.67	DAYPRO, Allscripts Pharmaceutical Company	54569-3702-01
15's	$35.63	DAYPRO, Pd-Rx Pharmaceuticals	55289-0453-15
15's	$40.85	DAYPRO, Pharma Pac	52959-0252-15
20's	$40.81	DAYPRO, St. Mary'S Mpp	60760-0381-20
20's	$54.50	DAYPRO, Pharma Pac	52959-0252-20
21's	$57.23	DAYPRO, Pharma Pac	52959-0252-21
24's	$65.42	DAYPRO, Pharma Pac	52959-0252-24

28's	$58.99	DAYPRO, Dhs Inc	55887-0894-28
28's	$76.23	DAYPRO, Pharma Pac	52959-0252-28
30's	$52.02	DAYPRO, Allscripts Pharmaceutical Company	54569-3702-00
30's	$53.73	DAYPRO, St. Mary'S Mpp	60760-0381-30
30's	$63.21	DAYPRO, Dhs Inc	55887-0894-30
30's	$68.25	DAYPRO, Pd-Rx Pharmaceuticals	55289-0453-30
30's	$81.64	DAYPRO, Pharma Pac	52959-0252-30
40's	$90.00	DAYPRO, Pd-Rx Pharmaceuticals	55289-0453-40
42's	$66.26	DAYPRO, Allscripts Pharmaceutical Company	54569-3702-02
42's	$94.35	DAYPRO, Pd-Rx Pharmaceuticals	55289-0453-42
42's	$113.72	DAYPRO, Pharma Pac	52959-0252-42
45's	$121.01	DAYPRO, Pharma Pac	52959-0252-45
60's	$94.66	DAYPRO, Allscripts Pharmaceutical Company	54569-3702-04
60's	$104.94	DAYPRO, St. Mary'S Mpp	60760-0381-60
60's	$133.50	DAYPRO, Pd-Rx Pharmaceuticals	55289-0453-60
60's	$160.18	DAYPRO, Pharma Pac	52959-0252-60
63's	$99.40	DAYPRO, Allscripts Pharmaceutical Company	54569-3702-03
100's	$148.11	GENERIC, Warrick Pharmaceuticals Corporation	59930-1508-01
100's	$151.25	GENERIC, Dr. Reddy'S Laboratories, Inc	55111-0170-01
100's	$151.48	GENERIC, Eon Labs Manufacturing Inc	00815-0141-01
100's	$151.49	GENERIC, Par Pharmaceutical Inc	49884-0723-01
100's	$163.40	GENERIC, Eon Labs Manufacturing Inc	00185-0141-01
100's	$163.40	GENERIC, Purepac Pharmaceutical Company	00228-2614-11
100's	$204.33	DAYPRO, Pharmacia Corporation	00025-1381-31
100's	$210.49	DAYPRO, Pharmacia Corporation	00025-1381-34
100's	$263.24	DAYPRO, Pharma Pac	52959-0252-01
180's	$218.11	DAYPRO, Allscripts Pharmaceutical Company	54569-8615-00

PRODUCT LISTING - EQUIVALENTS NOT AVAILABLE

Tablet - Oral - 600 mg

10's	$18.15	GENERIC, Southwood Pharmaceuticals Inc	58016-0574-10
12's	$21.78	GENERIC, Southwood Pharmaceuticals Inc	58016-0574-12
14's	$25.42	GENERIC, Southwood Pharmaceuticals Inc	58016-0574-14
15's	$27.23	GENERIC, Southwood Pharmaceuticals Inc	58016-0574-15
20's	$36.31	GENERIC, Southwood Pharmaceuticals Inc	58016-0574-20
28's	$50.83	GENERIC, Southwood Pharmaceuticals Inc	58016-0574-28
30's	$46.80	GENERIC, Pharma Pac	52959-0800-30
30's	$54.46	GENERIC, Southwood Pharmaceuticals Inc	58016-0574-30
40's	$72.62	GENERIC, Southwood Pharmaceuticals Inc	58016-0574-40
60's	$108.92	GENERIC, Southwood Pharmaceuticals Inc	58016-0574-60
100's	$149.80	GENERIC, Greenstone Limited	59762-5002-01
100's	$181.54	GENERIC, Southwood Pharmaceuticals Inc	58016-0574-00

Oxazepam *(001926)*

Categories: Anxiety disorder, generalized; DEA Class CIV; FDA Approved 1966 Sep; Pregnancy Category D
Drug Classes: Anxiolytics; Benzodiazepines
Brand Names: **Serax**; Wakezepam
Foreign Brand Availability: Adumbran (Argentina; Austria; Germany; Greece; Portugal; Spain); Alepam (Australia; Taiwan); Alopam (Denmark; Finland; Norway; Sweden); Anxiolit (Austria; Greece; Switzerland); Anxiolit Retard (Switzerland); Apo-Oxazepam (Canada); Azutranquil (Germany); Benzotran (New-Zealand); Durazepam (Germany); Enidrel (Argentina); Hilong (Japan); Medopam (South-Africa); Murelax (Australia; New-Zealand); Nesontil (Argentina); Noctazepam (Germany); Noripam (South-Africa); Opamox (Finland); Oxahexal (Germany); Oxaline (South-Africa); Oxepam (Finland); Ox-Pam (New-Zealand); Praxiten (Argentina; Austria; Greece); Primizum (Japan); Propax (Japan); Psiquiwas (Spain; Taiwan); Purata (South-Africa); Quilibrex (Italy); Serepax (Australia; Denmark; Greece; India; South-Africa); Seresta (Belgium; France; Netherlands; Switzerland); Sobile (Spain); Sobril (Norway; Sweden); Vaben (Israel); Wakazepam (Japan)
Cost of Therapy: $92.41 (Anxiety; Serax; 10 mg; 3 capsules/day; 30 day supply)
$16.56 (Anxiety; Generic Capsules; 10 mg; 3 capsules/day; 30 day supply)

DESCRIPTION

Oxazepam is the first of a chemically series of compounds known as the 3-hydroxybenzodiazepinones. A therapeutic agent providing versatility and flexibility in control of common emotional disturbances, this product exerts prompt action in a wide variety of disorders associated with anxiety, tension, agitation, and irritability, and anxiety associated with depression. In tolerance and toxicity studies on several animal species, this product reveals significantly greater safety factors than related compounds (chlordiazepoxide and diazepam) and manifests a wide separation of effective doses and doses inducing side effects.

Serax capsules contain 10, 15, or 30 mg oxazepam. The inactive ingredients present are FD&C red 40, gelatin, lactose, titanium dioxide, and other ingredients. Each dosage strength also contains the following: *10 mg:* D&C red 22, D&C red 28, and FD&C blue 1; *15 mg:* FD&C yellow 6; *30 mg:* D&C red 28 and FD&C blue 1.

Serax tablets contain 15 mg oxazepam. The inactive ingredients present are FD&C yellow 5, lactose, magnesium stearate, methylcellulose, and polacrilin potassium.

Oxazepam is 7 chloro-1,3-dihydro-3-hydroxy-5-phenyl-2N-1,4-benzodiazepin-2-one. A white crystalline powder with a molecular weight of 286.7.

CLINICAL PHARMACOLOGY

Pharmacokinetic testing in 12 volunteers demonstrated that when given as a single 30 mg dose, the capsule, tablet, and suspension were equivalent in extent of absorption. For the capsule and tablet, peak plasma levels averaged 450 ng/ml and were observed to occur about 3 hours after dosing. The mean elimination half-life for oxazepam was approximately 8.2 hours (range 5.7-10.9 hours).

This product has a single, major inactive metabolite in man, a glucuronide excreted in the urine.

Age (<80 years old) does not appear to have a clinically significant effect on oxazepam kinetics. A statistically significant increase in elimination half-life in the very elderly (>80 years of age) as compared to younger subjects has been reported, due to a 30% increase in volume of distribution, as well as a 50% reduction in unbound clearance of oxazepam in the very elderly. (See PRECAUTIONS, General.)

INDICATIONS AND USAGE

Oxazepam is indicated for the management of anxiety disorders or for the short-term relief of the symptoms of anxiety. Anxiety or tension associated with the stress of everyday life usually does not require treatment with an anxiolytic.

Anxiety associated with depression is also responsive to oxazepam therapy.

This product has been found particularly useful in the management of anxiety, tension, agitation, and irritability in older patients.

Alcoholics with acute tremulousness, inebriation, or with anxiety associated with alcohol withdrawal are responsive to therapy.

The effectiveness of oxazepam in long-term use, that is, more than 4 months, has not been assessed by systematic clinical studies. The physician should periodically reassess the usefulness of the drug for the individual patient.

CONTRAINDICATIONS

History of previous hypersensitivity reaction to oxazepam. Oxazepam is not indicated in psychoses.

WARNINGS

As with other CNS-acting drugs, patients should be cautioned against driving automobiles or operating dangerous machinery until it is known that they do not become drowsy or dizzy on oxazepam therapy.

Patients should be warned that the effects of alcohol or other CNS depressant drugs may be additive to those of oxazepam, possibly requiring adjustment of dosage or elimination of such agents.

PHYSICAL AND PSYCHOLOGICAL DEPENDENCE

Withdrawal symptoms, similar in character to those noted with barbiturates and alcohol (convulsions, tremor, abdominal and muscle cramps, vomiting, and sweating), have occurred following abrupt discontinuance of oxazepam. The more severe withdrawal symptoms have usually been limited to those patients who received excessive doses over an extended period of time. Generally milder withdrawal symptoms (*e.g.*, dysphoria and insomnia) have been reported following abrupt discontinuance of benzodiazepines taken continuously at therapeutic levels for several months. Consequently, after extended therapy, abrupt discontinuation should generally be avoided and a gradual dosage-tapering schedule followed. Addiction-prone individuals (such as drug addicts or alcoholics) should be under careful surveillance when receiving oxazepam or other psychotropic agents because of the predisposition of such patients to habituation and dependence.

USE IN PREGNANCY

An increased risk of congenital malformations associated with the use of minor tranquilizers (chlordiazepoxide, diazepam, and meprobamate) during the first trimester of pregnancy has been suggested in several studies. Oxazepam, a benzodiazepine derivative, has not been studied adequately to determine whether it, too, may be associated with an increased risk of fetal abnormality. Because use of these drugs is rarely a matter of urgency, their use during this period should almost always be avoided. The possibility that a woman of childbearing potential may be pregnant at the time of institution of therapy should be considered. Patients should be advised that if they become pregnant during therapy or intend to become pregnant they should communicate with their physician about the desirability of discontinuing the drug.

PRECAUTIONS

GENERAL

Although hypotension has occurred only rarely, oxazepam should be administered with caution to patients in whom a drop in blood pressure might lead to cardiac complications. This is particularly true in the elderly patient.

Oxazepam 15 mg tablets, *but none of the other* available dosage forms *of this product,* contain FD&C yellow 5 (tartrazine) which may cause allergic-type reactions (including bronchial asthma) in certain susceptible individuals. Although the overall incidence of FD&C yellow 5 (tartrazine) sensitivity in the general population is low, it is frequently seen in patients who also have aspirin hypersensitivity.

INFORMATION FOR THE PATIENT

To assure the safe and effective use of oxazepam, patients should be informed that, since benzodiazepines may produce psychological and physical dependence, it is advisable that they consult with their physician before either increasing the dose or abruptly discontinuing this drug.

PEDIATRIC USE

Safety and effectiveness in pediatric patients under 6 years of age have not been established. Absolute dosage for pediatric patients 6-12 years of age is not established.

GERIATRIC USE

Clinical studies of oxazepam were not adequate to determine whether subjects aged 65 and over respond differently than younger subjects. Age (<80 years old) does not appear to have a clinically significant effect on oxazepam kinetics (see CLINICAL PHARMACOLOGY).

Clinical circumstances, some of which may be more common in the elderly, such as hepatic or renal impairment, should be considered. Greater sensitivity of some older individuals to the effects of oxazepam (*e.g.*, sedation, hypotension, paradoxical excitation) cannot be ruled out (see PRECAUTIONS, General and ADVERSE REACTIONS). In general, dose

O

selection for oxazepam for elderly patients should be cautious, usually starting at the lower end of the dosing range (see DOSAGE AND ADMINISTRATION).

ADVERSE REACTIONS

The necessity for discontinuation of therapy due to undesirable effects has been rare. Transient, mild drowsiness is commonly seen in the first few days of therapy. If it persists, the dosage should be reduced. In few instances, dizziness, vertigo, headache, and rarely syncope have occurred either alone or together with drowsiness. Mild paradoxical reactions, *i.e.*, excitement, stimulation of affect, have been reported in psychiatric patients; these reactions may be secondary to relief of anxiety and usually appear in the first 2 weeks of therapy.

Other side effects occurring during oxazepam therapy include rare instances of nausea, lethargy, edema, slurred speech, tremor, altered libido, and minor diffuse skin rashes — morbilliform, urticarial, and maculopapular. Such side effects have been infrequent and are generally controlled with reduction of dosage. A case of an extensive fixed drug eruption also has been reported.

Although rare, leukopenia and hepatic dysfunction including jaundice have been reported during therapy. Periodic blood counts and liver-function tests are advisable.

Ataxia with oxazepam has been reported in rare instances and does not appear to be specifically related to dose or age.

Although the following side reactions have not as yet been reported with oxazepam, they have occurred with related compounds (chlordiazepoxide and diazepam): paradoxical excitation with severe rage reactions, hallucinations, menstrual irregularities, change in EEG pattern, blood dyscrasias including agranulocytosis, blurred vision, diplopia, incontinence, stupor, disorientation, fever, and euphoria.

Transient amnesia or memory impairment has been reported in association with the use of benzodiazepines.

DOSAGE AND ADMINISTRATION

Because of the flexibility of this product and the range of emotional disturbances responsive to it, dosage should be individualized for maximum beneficial effects (see TABLE 1).

TABLE 1

Usual Dose	
Mild-to-moderate anxiety, with associated tension, irritability, agitation, or related symptoms of functional origin or secondary to organic disease.	10-15 mg, 3 or 4 times daily
Severe anxiety syndromes, agitation, or anxiety associated with depression.	15-30 mg, 3 or 4 times daily
Older patients with anxiety, tension, irritability, and agitation.	Initial dosage: 10 mg, 3 times daily. If necessary, increase cautiously to 15 mg, 3 or 4 times daily.
Alcoholics with acute inebriation, tremulousness, or anxiety on withdrawal.	15-30 mg, 3 or 4 times daily.

This product is not indicated in pediatric patients under 6 years of age. Absolute dosage for pediatric patients 6-12 years of age is not established.

ANIMAL PHARMACOLOGY

In mice, oxazepam exerts an anticonvulsant (anti-Metrazol) activity at 50% effective doses of about 0.6 mg/kg orally. (Such anticonvulsant activity of benzodiazepines correlates with their tranquilizing properties.) To produce ataxia (rotabar test) and sedation (abolition of spontaneous motor activity), the 50% effective doses of this product are greater than 5 mg/kg orally. Thus, about 10 times the therapeutic (anticonvulsant) dose must be given before ataxia ensues, indicating a wide separation of effective doses and doses inducing side effects.

In evaluation of antianxiety activity of compounds, conflict behavioral tests in rats differentiate continuous response for food in the presence of anxiety-provoking stress (shock) from drug-induced motor incoordination. This product shows significant separation of doses required to relieve anxiety and doses producing sedation or ataxia. Ataxia-producing doses exceed those of related CNS-acting drugs.

Acute oral LD_{50} in mice is greater than 5000 mg/kg, compared to 800 mg/kg for a related compound (chlordiazepoxide).

Subacute toxicity studies in dogs for 4 weeks at 480 mg/kg daily showed no specific changes; at 960 mg/kg, 2 out of 8 died with evidence of circulatory collapse. This wide margin of safety is significant compared to chlordiazepoxide HCl, which showed nonspecific changes in 6 dogs at 80 mg/kg. On chlordiazepoxide, 2 out of 6 died with evidence of circulatory collapse at 127 mg/kg, and 6 out of 6 died at 200 mg/kg daily. Chronic toxicity studies of oxazepam in dogs at 120 mg/kg/day for 52 weeks produced no toxic manifestation.

Fatty metamorphosis of the liver has been noted in 6 week toxicity studies in rats given this product at 0.5% of the diet. Such accumulations of fat are considered reversible, as there is no liver necrosis or fibrosis. Breeding studies in rats through two successive litters did not produce fetal abnormality. Oxazepam has not been adequately evaluated for mutagenic activity.

In a carcinogenicity study, oxazepam was administered with diet to rats for 2 years. Male rats receiving 30 times the maximum human dose showed a statistical increase, when compared to controls, in benign thyroid follicular cell tumors, testicular interstitial cell adenomas, and prostatic adenomas. An earlier published study reported that mice fed dietary dosages of 35 or 100 times the human daily dose of oxazepam for 9 months developed a dose-related increase in liver adenomas.[1] In an independent analysis of some of the microscopic slides from this mouse study, several of these tumors were classified as liver carcinomas. At this time, there is no evidence that clinical use of oxazepam is associated with tumors.

HOW SUPPLIED

Serax capsules and tablets are available in the following dosage strengths:

10 mg capsules: White and pink capsule marked "SERAX", "10", and "327".

15 mg capsules: White and red capsule marked "SERAX", "15", and "328".

30 mg capsules: White and maroon capsule marked "SERAX", "30", and "329".

15 mg tablets: Yellow, five-sided, flat-faced, beveled edge tablet with a raised "S" on one side and "SERAX" and "15" on the other side.

Storage: Store at room temperature, approximately 25°C (77°F). Keep tightly closed. Dispense in tight container.

PRODUCT LISTING - RATED THERAPEUTICALLY EQUIVALENT

Capsule - Oral - 10 mg

Qty	Price	Product	NDC
30's	$8.99	GENERIC, Heartland Healthcare Services	61392-0373-30
30's	$8.99	GENERIC, Heartland Healthcare Services	61392-0373-39
31's	$9.29	GENERIC, Heartland Healthcare Services	61392-0373-31
32's	$9.59	GENERIC, Heartland Healthcare Services	61392-0373-32
45's	$13.49	GENERIC, Heartland Healthcare Services	61392-0373-45
60's	$17.98	GENERIC, Heartland Healthcare Services	61392-0373-60
90's	$26.97	GENERIC, Heartland Healthcare Services	61392-0373-90
100's	$18.40	GENERIC, Esi Lederle Generics	00641-4508-86
100's	$23.34	GENERIC, Moore, H.L. Drug Exchange Inc	00839-7501-06
100's	$24.92	GENERIC, Caremark Inc	00339-4023-12
100's	$25.94	GENERIC, Aligen Independent Laboratories Inc	00405-0132-01
100's	$28.00	GENERIC, Martec Pharmaceuticals Inc	52555-0233-01
100's	$28.37	GENERIC, Auro Pharmaceutical	55829-0867-10
100's	$53.63	FEDERAL UPPER LIMIT, H.C.F.A. F F P	99999-1926-02
100's	$57.75	GENERIC, Major Pharmaceuticals Inc	00904-1890-60
100's	$74.50	GENERIC, Esi Lederle Generics	59911-5876-01
100's	$86.21	GENERIC, Purepac Pharmaceutical Company	00228-2067-10
100's	$86.99	GENERIC, Ivax Corporation	00172-4804-60
100's	$87.08	GENERIC, Geneva Pharmaceuticals	00781-2809-01
100's	$102.68	SERAX, Faulding Pharmaceutical Company	63857-0327-10

Capsule - Oral - 15 mg

Qty	Price	Product	NDC
30's	$8.99	GENERIC, Heartland Healthcare Services	61392-0376-30
30's	$9.90	GENERIC, Heartland Healthcare Services	61392-0376-39
31's	$10.23	GENERIC, Heartland Healthcare Services	61392-0376-31
32's	$10.56	GENERIC, Heartland Healthcare Services	61392-0376-32
45's	$13.49	GENERIC, Heartland Healthcare Services	61392-0376-45
60's	$17.98	GENERIC, Heartland Healthcare Services	61392-0376-60
90's	$26.97	GENERIC, Heartland Healthcare Services	61392-0376-90
100's	$23.80	GENERIC, Esi Lederle Generics	00641-4509-86
100's	$32.18	GENERIC, Caremark Inc	00339-4025-12
100's	$32.70	GENERIC, Aligen Independent Laboratories Inc	00405-0133-01
100's	$33.30	GENERIC, Auro Pharmaceutical	55829-0868-10
100's	$34.16	GENERIC, Moore, H.L. Drug Exchange Inc	00839-7502-06
100's	$36.30	GENERIC, Martec Pharmaceuticals Inc	52555-0234-01
100's	$69.63	GENERIC, Major Pharmaceuticals Inc	00904-1891-60
100's	$75.92	GENERIC, Udl Laboratories Inc	51079-0478-20
100's	$76.24	FEDERAL UPPER LIMIT, H.C.F.A. F F P	99999-1926-05
100's	$93.00	GENERIC, Esi Lederle Generics	59911-5877-01
100's	$108.85	GENERIC, Purepac Pharmaceutical Company	00228-2069-10
100's	$108.99	GENERIC, Ivax Corporation	00172-4805-60
100's	$109.95	GENERIC, Geneva Pharmaceuticals	00781-2810-01
100's	$129.64	SERAX, Faulding Pharmaceutical Company	63857-0328-10

Capsule - Oral - 30 mg

Qty	Price	Product	NDC
30's	$13.38	GENERIC, Heartland Healthcare Services	61392-0379-30
30's	$13.38	GENERIC, Heartland Healthcare Services	61392-0379-39
31's	$13.82	GENERIC, Heartland Healthcare Services	61392-0379-31
32's	$14.27	GENERIC, Heartland Healthcare Services	61392-0379-32
45's	$20.07	GENERIC, Heartland Healthcare Services	61392-0379-45
60's	$26.76	GENERIC, Heartland Healthcare Services	61392-0379-60
90's	$40.14	GENERIC, Heartland Healthcare Services	61392-0379-90
100's	$33.80	GENERIC, Esi Lederle Generics	00641-4510-86
100's	$42.14	GENERIC, Caremark Inc	00339-4027-12
100's	$42.78	GENERIC, Moore, H.L. Drug Exchange Inc	00839-7503-06
100's	$43.42	GENERIC, Aligen Independent Laboratories Inc	00405-0134-01
100's	$49.00	GENERIC, Martec Pharmaceuticals Inc	52555-0235-01
100's	$49.01	GENERIC, Watson/Schein Pharmaceuticals Inc	00364-2153-01
100's	$49.55	GENERIC, Auro Pharmaceutical	55829-0869-10
100's	$104.25	GENERIC, Major Pharmaceuticals Inc	00904-1892-60
100's	$111.96	FEDERAL UPPER LIMIT, H.C.F.A. F F P	99999-1926-08
100's	$136.00	GENERIC, Esi Lederle Generics	59911-5878-01
100's	$157.43	GENERIC, Purepac Pharmaceutical Company	00228-2073-10
100's	$159.02	GENERIC, Geneva Pharmaceuticals	00781-2811-01
100's	$163.02	GENERIC, Udl Laboratories Inc	51079-0479-20
100's	$163.99	GENERIC, Ivax Corporation	00172-4806-60
100's	$176.89	SERAX, Faulding Pharmaceutical Company	00008-0052-02
100's	$187.50	GENERIC, Faulding Pharmaceutical Company	63857-0329-10

Tablet - Oral - 15 mg

Qty	Price	Product	NDC
100's	$129.64	SERAX, Faulding Pharmaceutical Company	00008-0317-01

PRODUCT LISTING - EQUIVALENTS NOT AVAILABLE

Capsule - Oral - 15 mg

30's	$15.86	GENERIC, Physicians Total Care	54868-2182-01
30's	$28.12	GENERIC, Pharmaceutical Corporation Of America	51655-0854-24
90's	$82.36	GENERIC, Pharmaceutical Corporation Of America	51655-0854-26
100's	$47.04	GENERIC, Physicians Total Care	54868-2182-02

Capsule - Oral - 30 mg

30's	$42.40	GENERIC, Pharmaceutical Corporation Of America	51655-0855-24

Tablet - Oral - 15 mg

100's	$129.64	SERAX, Faulding Pharmaceutical Company	63857-0332-10

Oxcarbazepine *(003468)*

Categories: Seizures, partial; FDA Approved 2000 Jan; Pregnancy Category C
Drug Classes: Anticonvulsants
Foreign Brand Availability: Oxrate (India); Timox (Germany); Trileptal (Australia; Austria; Bahrain; Bulgaria; China; Colombia; Cyprus; Denmark; Egypt; England; Finland; France; Greece; Hong-Kong; Indonesia; Iran; Iraq; Ireland; Jordan; Korea; Kuwait; Lebanon; Libya; Malaysia; Mexico; Netherlands; New-Zealand; Oman; Peru; Philippines; Qatar; Republic-of-Yemen; Saudi-Arabia; Switzerland; Syria; United-Arab-Emirates); Trileptin (Israel)
Cost of Therapy: $213.74 (Epilepsy; Trileptal; 600 mg; 2 tablets/day; 30 day supply)

DESCRIPTION

Trileptal is an antiepileptic drug available as 150, 300, and 600 mg film-coated tablets for oral administration. Trileptal is also available as a 300 mg/5 ml (60 mg/ml) oral suspension. Oxcarbazepine is 10,11-Dihydro-10-oxo-5*H*-dibenz[b,*f*]azepine-5-carboxamide.

Oxcarbazepine is a white to faintly orange crystalline powder. It is slightly soluble in chloroform, dichloromethane, acetone, and methanol and practically insoluble in ethanol, ether, and water. Its molecular weight is 252.27.

TABLETS

Trileptal film-coated tablets contain the following inactive ingredients: Colloidal silicon dioxide, crospovidone, hydroxypropyl methylcellulose, magnesium stearate, microcrystalline cellulose, polyethylene glycol, talc and titanium dioxide, yellow iron oxide.

ORAL SUSPENSION

Trileptal oral suspension contains the following inactive ingredients: Ascorbic acid; dispersible cellulose; ethanol; macrogol stearate; methyl parahydroxybenzoate; propylene glycol; propyl parahydroxybenzoate; purified water; sodium saccharin; sorbic acid; sorbitol; yellow-plum-lemon aroma.

CLINICAL PHARMACOLOGY

MECHANISM OF ACTION

The pharmacological activity of oxcarbazepine is primarily exerted through the 10-monohydroxy metabolite (MHD) of oxcarbazepine (see Metabolism and Excretion). The precise mechanism by which oxcarbazepine and MHD exert their antiseizure effect is unknown; however, *in vitro* electrophysiological studies indicate that they produce blockade of voltage-sensitive sodium channels, resulting in stabilization of hyperexcited neural membranes, inhibition of repetitive neuronal firing, and diminution of propagation of synaptic impulses. These actions are thought to be important in the prevention of seizure spread in the intact brain. In addition, increased potassium conductance and modulation of high-voltage activated calcium channels may contribute to the anticonvulsant effects of the drug. No significant interactions of oxcarbazepine or MHD with brain neurotransmitter or modulator receptor sites have been demonstrated.

PHARMACODYNAMICS

Oxcarbazepine and its active metabolite (MHD) exhibit anticonvulsant properties in animal seizure models. They protected rodents against electrically induced tonic extension seizures and, to a lesser degree, chemically induced clonic seizures, and abolished or reduced the frequency of chronically recurring focal seizures in Rhesus monkeys with aluminum implants. No development of tolerance (*i.e.*, attenuation of anticonvulsive activity) was observed in the maximal electroshock test when mice and rats were treated daily for 5 days and 4 weeks, respectively, with oxcarbazepine or MHD.

PHARMACOKINETICS

Following oral administration of oxcarbazepine tablets, oxcarbazepine is completely absorbed and extensively metabolized to its pharmacologically active 10-monohydroxy metabolite (MHD). The half-life of the parent is about 2 hours, while the half-life of MHD is about 9 hours, so that MHD is responsible for most antiepileptic activity.

Based on MHD concentrations, oxcarbazepine tablets and suspension were shown to have similar bioavailability.

After single dose administration of oxcarbazepine tablets to healthy male volunteers under fasted conditions, the median T_{max} was 4.5 (range 3-13) hours. After single dose administration of oxcarbazepine oral suspension to healthy male volunteers under fasted conditions, the median T_{max} was 6 hours.

In a mass balance study in people, only 2% of total radioactivity in plasma was due to unchanged oxcarbazepine, with approximately 70% present as MHD, and the remainder attributable to minor metabolites.

Effect of Food: Food has no effect on the rate and extent of absorption of oxcarbazepine from oxcarbazepine tablets. Although not directly studied, the oral bioavailability of the oxcarbazepine suspension is unlikely to be affected under fed conditions. Therefore, oxcarbazepine tablets and suspension can be taken with or without food.

Steady-state plasma concentrations of MHD are reached within 2-3 days in patients when oxcarbazepine is given twice a day. At steady-state the pharmacokinetics of MHD are linear and show dose proportionality over the dose range of 300-2400 mg/day.

Distribution

The apparent volume of distribution of MHD is 49 liters.

Approximately 40% of MHD is bound to serum proteins, predominantly to albumin. Binding is independent of the serum concentration within the therapeutically relevant range. Oxcarbazepine and MHD do not bind to alpha-1-acid glycoprotein.

Metabolism and Excretion

Oxcarbazepine is rapidly reduced by cytosolic enzymes in the liver to its 10-monohydroxy metabolite, MHD, which is primarily responsible for the pharmacological effect of oxcarbazepine. MHD is metabolized further by conjugation with glucuronic acid. Minor amounts (4% of the dose) are oxidized to the pharmacologically inactive 10,11-dihydroxy metabolite (DHD).

Oxcarbazepine is cleared from the body mostly in the form of metabolites which are predominantly excreted by the kidneys. More than 95% of the dose appears in the urine, with less than 1% as unchanged oxcarbazepine. Fecal excretion accounts for less than 4% of the administered dose. Approximately 80% of the dose is excreted in the urine either as glucuronides of MHD (49%) or as unchanged MHD (27%); the inactive DHD accounts for approximately 3% and conjugates of MHD and oxcarbazepine account for 13% of the dose.

Special Populations

Hepatic Impairment

The pharmacokinetics and metabolism of oxcarbazepine and MHD were evaluated in healthy volunteers and hepatically-impaired subjects after a single 900 mg oral dose. Mild-to-moderate hepatic impairment did not affect the pharmacokinetics of oxcarbazepine and MHD. No dose adjustment for oxcarbazepine is recommended in patients with mild-to-moderate hepatic impairment. The pharmacokinetics of oxcarbazepine and MHD have not been evaluated in severe hepatic impairment.

Renal Impairment

There is a linear correlation between creatinine clearance and the renal clearance of MHD. When oxcarbazepine is administered as a single 300 mg dose in renally impaired patients (creatinine clearance <30 ml/min), the elimination half-life of MHD is prolonged to 19 hours, with a 2-fold increase in AUC. Dose adjustment for oxcarbazepine is recommended in these patients (see PRECAUTIONS and DOSAGE AND ADMINISTRATION).

Pediatric Use

After a single-dose administration of 5 or 15 mg/kg of oxcarbazepine, the dose-adjusted AUC values of MHD were 30-40% lower in children below the age of 8 years than in children above 8 years of age. The clearance in children greater than 8 years old approaches that of adults.

Geriatric Use

Following administration of single (300 mg) and multiple (600 mg/day) doses of oxcarbazepine to elderly volunteers (60-82 years of age), the maximum plasma concentrations and AUC values of MHD were 30-60% higher than in younger volunteers (18-32 years of age). Comparisons of creatinine clearance in young and elderly volunteers indicate that the difference was due to age-related reductions in creatinine clearance.

Gender

No gender related pharmacokinetic differences have been observed in children, adults, or the elderly.

Race

No specific studies have been conducted to assess what effect, if any, race may have on the disposition of oxcarbazepine.

INDICATIONS AND USAGE

Oxcarbazepine is indicated for use as monotherapy or adjunctive therapy in the treatment of partial seizures in adults with epilepsy and as adjunctive therapy in the treatment of partial seizures in children ages 4-16 with epilepsy.

CONTRAINDICATIONS

Oxcarbazepine tablets should not be used in patients with a known hypersensitivity to oxcarbazepine or to any of its components.

WARNINGS

HYPONATREMIA

Clinically significant hyponatremia (sodium <125 mmol/L) can develop during oxcarbazepine use. In the 14 controlled epilepsy studies 2.5% of oxcarbazepine treated patients (38/1524) had a sodium of less than 125 mmol/L at some point during treatment, compared to no such patients assigned placebo or active control (carbamazepine and phenobarbital for adjunctive and monotherapy substitution studies, and phenytoin and valproate for the monotherapy initiation studies). Clinically significant hyponatremia generally occurred during the first 3 months of treatment with oxcarbazepine, although there were patients who first developed a serum sodium <125 mmol/L more than 1 year after initiation of therapy. Most patients who developed hyponatremia were asymptomatic but patients in the clinical trials were frequently monitored and some had their oxcarbazepine dose reduced, discontinued, or had their fluid intake restricted for hyponatremia. Whether or not these maneuvers prevented the occurrence of more severe events is unknown. Cases of symptomatic hyponatremia have been reported during post-marketing use. In clinical trials, patients whose treatment with oxcarbazepine was discontinued due to hyponatremia generally experienced normalization of serum sodium within a few days without additional treatment.

Measurement of serum sodium levels should be considered for patients during maintenance treatment with oxcarbazepine, particularly if the patient is receiving other medications known to decrease serum sodium levels (for example, drugs associated with inappropriate ADH secretion) or if symptoms possibly indicating hyponatremia develop (*e.g.*, nausea, malaise, headache, lethargy, confusion, or obtundation, or increase in seizure frequency or severity).

PATIENTS WITH A PAST HISTORY OF HYPERSENSITIVITY REACTION TO CARBAMAZEPINE

Patients who have had hypersensitivity reactions to carbamazepine should be informed that approximately 25-30% of them will experience hypersensitivity reactions with oxcarbazepine. For this reason patients should be specifically questioned about any prior experience with carbamazepine, and patients with a history of hypersensitivity reactions to carbamazepine should ordinarily be treated with oxcarbazepine only if the potential benefit justifies the potential risk. If signs or symptoms of hypersensitivity develop, oxcarbazepine should be discontinued immediately.

WITHDRAWAL OF AEDS

As with all antiepileptic drugs, oxcarbazepine should be withdrawn gradually to minimize the potential of increased seizure frequency.

PRECAUTIONS

COGNITIVE/NEUROPSYCHIATRIC ADVERSE EVENTS

Use of oxcarbazepine has been associated with central nervous system related adverse events. The most significant of these can be classified into three general categories: (1) cognitive symptoms including psychomotor slowing, difficulty with concentration, and speech or language problems; (2) somnolence or fatigue; and (3) coordination abnormalities, including ataxia and gait disturbances.

In one large, fixed dose study, oxcarbazepine was added to existing AED therapy (up to three concomitant AEDs). By protocol, the dosage of the concomitant AEDs could not be reduced as oxcarbazepine was added, reduction in oxcarbazepine dosage was not allowed if intolerance developed, and patients were discontinued if unable to tolerate their highest target maintenance doses. In this trial, 65% of patients were discontinued because they could not tolerate the 2400 mg/day dose of oxcarbazepine on top of existing AEDs. The adverse events seen in this study were primarily CNS related and the risk for discontinuation was dose related.

In this trial, 7.1% of oxcarbazepine-treated patients and 4% of placebo-treated patients experienced a cognitive adverse event. The risk of discontinuation for these events was about 6.5 times greater on oxcarbazepine than on placebo. In addition, 26% of oxcarbazepine-treated patients and 12% of placebo-treated patients experienced somnolence. The risk of discontinuation for somnolence was about 10 times greater on oxcarbazepine than on placebo. Finally 28.7% of oxcarcarbazepine treated patients and 6.4% of placebo treated patients experienced ataxia or gait disturbances. The risk of discontinuation for these events was about 7 times greater on oxcarbazepine than on placebo.

In a single placebo-controlled monotherapy trial evaluating 2400 mg/day of oxcarbazepine, no patients in either treatment group discontinued double-blind treatment because of cognitive adverse events, somnolence, ataxia, or gait disturbance.

In the two dose-controlled conversion to monotherapy trials comparing 2400 mg/day and 300 mg/day oxcarbazepine, 1.1% of patients in the 2400 mg/day group discontinued double-blind treatment because of somnolence or cognitive adverse events compared to 0% in the 300 mg/day group. In these trials, no patients discontinued because of ataxia or gait disturbances in either treatment group.

INFORMATION FOR THE PATIENT

Patients who have exhibited hypersensitivity reactions to carbamazepine should be informed that approximately 25-30% of these patients may experience hypersensitivity reactions with oxcarbazepine. (See WARNINGS.)

Female patients of childbearing age should be warned that the concurrent use of oxcarbazepine with hormonal contraceptives may render this method of contraception less effective. (See DRUG INTERACTIONS.) Additional non-hormonal forms of contraception are recommended when using oxcarbazepine.

Caution should be exercised if alcohol is taken in combination with oxcarbazepine therapy, due to a possible additive sedative effect.

Patients should be advised that oxcarbazepine may cause dizziness and somnolence. Accordingly, patients should be advised not to drive or operate machinery until they have gained sufficient experience on oxcarbazepine to gauge whether it adversely affects their ability to drive or operate machinery.

LABORATORY TESTS

Serum sodium levels below 125 mmol/L have been observed in patients treated with oxcarbazepine (see WARNINGS). Experience from clinical trials indicates that serum sodium levels return toward normal when the oxcarbazepine dosage is reduced or discontinued, or when the patient was treated conservatively (*e.g.*, fluid restriction).

Laboratory data from clinical trials suggest that oxcarbazepine use was associated with decreases in T_4, without changes in T_3 or TSH.

DRUG/LABORATORY TEST INTERACTIONS

There are no known interactions of oxcarbazepine with commonly used laboratory tests.

CARCINOGENESIS, MUTAGENESIS, AND IMPAIRMENT OF FERTILITY

In 2 year carcinogenicity studies, oxcarbazepine was administered in the diet at doses of up to 100 mg/kg/day to mice and by gavage at doses of up to 250 mg/kg to rats, and the pharmacologically active 10-hydroxy metabolite (MHD) was administered orally at doses of up to 600 mg/kg/day to rats. In mice, a dose-related increase in the incidence of hepatocellular adenomas was observed at oxcarbazepine doses ≥70 mg/kg/day or approximately 0.1 times the maximum recommended human dose [MRHD] on a mg/m² basis. In rats, the incidence of hepatocellular carcinomas was increased in females treated with oxcarbazepine at doses ≥25 mg/kg/day (0.1 times the MRHD on a mg/m² basis), and incidences of hepatocellular adenomas and/or carcinomas were increased in males and females treated with MHD at doses of 600 mg/kg/day (2.4 times the MRHD on a mg/m² basis) and ≥250 mg/kg/day (equivalent to the MRHD on a mg/m² basis), respectively. There was an increase in the incidence of benign testicular interstitial cell tumors in rats at 250 mg oxcarbazepine/kg/day and at ≥250 mg MHD/kg/day, and an increase in the incidence of granular cell tumors in the cervix and vagina in rats at 600 mg MHD/kg/day.

Oxcarbazepine increased mutation frequencies in the Ames test *in vitro* in the absence of metabolic activation in 1 of 5 bacterial strains. Both oxcarbazepine and MHD produced increases in chromosomal aberrations and polyploidy in the Chinese hamster ovary assay *in vitro* in the absence of metabolic activation. MHD was negative in the Ames test, and no mutagenic or clastogenic activity was found with either oxcarbazepine or MHD in V79 Chinese hamster cells *in vitro*. Oxcarbazepine and MHD were both negative for clastogenic or aneugenic effects (micronucleus formation) in an *in vivo* rat bone marrow assay.

In a fertility study in which rats were administered MHD (50, 150, or 450 mg/kg) orally prior to and during mating and early gestation, estrous cyclicity was disrupted and numbers of corpora lutea, implantations, and live embryos were reduced in females receiving the highest dose (approximately 2 times the MRHD on a mg/m² basis).

PREGNANCY CATEGORY C

Increased incidences of fetal structural abnormalities and other manifestations of developmental toxicity (embryolethality, growth retardation) were observed in the offspring of animals treated with either oxcarbazepine or its active 10-hydroxy metabolite (MHD) during pregnancy at doses similar to the maximum recommended human dose.

When pregnant rats were given oxcarbazepine (30, 300, or 1000 mg/kg) orally throughout the period of organogenesis, increased incidences of fetal malformations (craniofacial, cardiovascular, and skeletal) and variations were observed at the intermediate and high doses (approximately 1.2 and 4 times, respectively, the maximum recommended human dose [MRHD] on a mg/m² basis). Increased embryofetal death and decreased fetal body weights were seen at the high dose. Doses ≥300 mg/kg were also maternally toxic (decreased body weight gain, clinical signs), but there is no evidence to suggest that teratogenicity was secondary to the maternal effects.

In a study in which pregnant rabbits were orally administered MHD (20, 100, or 200 mg/kg) during organogenesis, embryofetal mortality was increased at the highest dose (1.5 times the MRHD on a mg/m² basis). This dose produced only minimal maternal toxicity.

In a study in which female rats were dosed orally with oxcarbazepine (25, 50, or 150 mg/kg) during the latter part of gestation and throughout the lactation period, a persistent reduction in body weights and altered behavior (decreased activity) were observed in offspring exposed to the highest dose (0.6 times the MRHD on a mg/m² basis). Oral administration of MHD (25, 75, or 250 mg/kg) to rats during gestation and lactation resulted in a persistent reduction in offspring weights at the highest dose (equivalent to the MRHD on a mg/m² basis).

There are no adequate and well-controlled clinical studies of oxcarbazepine in pregnant women; however, oxcarbazepine is closely related structurally to carbamazepine, which is considered to be teratogenic in humans. Given this fact, and the results of the animal studies described, it is likely that oxcarbazepine is a human teratogen. Oxcarbazepine should be used during pregnancy only if the potential benefit justifies the potential risk to the fetus.

LABOR AND DELIVERY

The effect of oxcarbazepine on labor and delivery in humans has not been evaluated.

NURSING MOTHERS

Oxcarbazepine and its active metabolite (MHD) are excreted in human breast milk. A milk-to-plasma concentration ratio of 0.5 was found for both. Because of the potential for serious adverse reactions to oxcarbazepine in nursing infants, a decision should be made about whether to discontinue nursing or to discontinue the drug in nursing women, taking into account the importance of the drug to the mother.

PATIENTS WITH RENAL IMPAIRMENT

In renally-impaired patients (creatinine clearance <30 ml/min), the elimination half-life of MHD is prolonged with a corresponding 2-fold increase in AUC (see CLINICAL PHARMACOLOGY, Pharmacokinetics). Oxcarbazepine therapy should be initiated at one-half the usual starting dose and increased, if necessary, at a slower than usual rate until the desired clinical response is achieved.

PEDIATRIC USE

Oxcarbazepine has been shown to be effective as adjunctive therapy for partial seizures in patients aged 4-16 years old. Oxcarbazepine has been given to about 623 patients between the ages of 3-17 in controlled clinical trials (185 treated as monotherapy) and about 615 patients between the ages of 3-17 in other trials. (See ADVERSE REACTIONS for a description of the adverse events associated with oxcarbazepine use in this population.)

GERIATRIC USE

There were 52 patients over age 65 in controlled clinical trials and 565 patients over the age of 65 in other trials. Following administration of single (300 mg) and multiple (600 mg/day) doses of oxcarbazepine in elderly volunteers (60-82 years of age), the maximum plasma concentrations and AUC values of MHD were 30-60% higher than in younger volunteers (18-32 years of age). Comparisons of creatinine clearance in young and elderly volunteers indicate that the difference was due to age-related reductions in creatinine clearance.

DRUG INTERACTIONS

Oxcarbazepine can inhibit CYP2C19 and induce CYP3A4/5 with potentially important effects on plasma concentrations of other drugs. In addition, several AEDs that are cythochrome P450 inducers can decrease plasma concentrations of oxcarbazepine and MHD.

Oxcarbazepine was evaluated in human liver microsomes to determine its capacity to inhibit the major cytochrome P450 enzymes responsible for the metabolism of other drugs. Results demonstrate that oxcarbazepine and its pharmacologically active 10-monohydroxy metabolite (MHD) have little or no capacity to function as inhibitors for most of the human cytochrome P450 enzymes evaluated (CYP1A2, CYP2A6, CYP2C9, CYP2D6, CYP2E1, CYP4A9, and CYP4A11) with the exception of CYP2C19 and CYP3A4/5. Although inhibition of CYP3A4/5 by oxcarbazepine and MHD did occur at high concentrations, it is not likely to be of clinical significance. The inhibition of CYP2C19 by oxcarbazepine and MHD, however, is clinically relevant (see TABLE 2).

In vitro, the UDP-glucuronyl transferase level was increased, indicating induction of this enzyme. Increases of 22% with MHD and 47% with oxcarbazepine were observed. As MHD, the predominant plasma substrate, is only a weak inducer of UDP-glucuronyl transferase, it is unlikely to have an effect on drugs that are mainly eliminated by conjugation through UDP-glucuronyl transferase (*e.g.*, valproic acid, lamotrigine).

In addition, oxcarbazepine and MHD induce a subgroup of the cytochrome P450 3A family (CYP3A4 and CYP3A5) responsible for the metabolism of dihydropyridine calcium antagonists and oral contraceptives, resulting in a lower plasma concentration of these drugs.

As binding of MHD to plasma proteins is low (40%), clinically significant interactions with other drugs through competition for protein binding sites are unlikely.

ANTIEPILEPTIC DRUGS

Potential interactions between oxcarbazepine and other AEDs were assessed in clinical studies. The effect of these interactions on mean AUCs and C_{min} are summarized in TABLE 2.

TABLE 2 *Summary of AED Interactions With Oxcarbazepine*

AED Co-administered	Dose of AED (mg/day)	Oxcarbazepine Dose (mg/day)	Influence of Oxcarbazepine on AED Concentration (mean change, 90% CI)	Influence of AED on MHD Concentration (mean change, 90% CI)
Carbamazepine	400-2000	900	nc*	40% decrease [CI: 17% decrease, 57% decrease]
Phenobarbital	100-150	600-1800	14% increase [CI: 2% increase, 24% increase]	25% decrease [CI: 12% decrease, 51% decrease]
Phenytoin	250-500	600-1800 >1200-2400	nc*† up to 40% increase‡ [CI: 12% increase, 60% increase]	30% decrease [CI: 3% decrease, 48% decrease]
Valproic acid	400-2800	600-1800	nc*	18% decrease [CI: 13% decrease, 40% decrease]

* nc denotes a mean change of less than 10%.
† Pediatrics.
‡ Mean increase in adults at high oxcarbazepine doses.

In vivo, the plasma levels of phenytoin increased by up to 40%, when oxcarbazepine was given at doses above 1200 mg/day. Therefore, when using doses of oxcarbazepine greater than 1200 mg/day during adjunctive therapy, a decrease in the dose of phenytoin may be required. The increase of phenobarbital level, however, is small (15%) when given with oxcarbazepine.

Strong inducers of cytochrome P450 enzymes (*i.e.*, carbamazepine, phenytoin, and phenobarbital) have been shown to decrease the plasma levels of MHD (29-40%).

No autoinduction has been observed with oxcarbazepine.

HORMONAL CONTRACEPTIVES

Co-administration of oxcarbazepine with an oral contraceptive has been shown to influence the plasma concentrations of the two hormonal components, ethinylestradiol (EE) and levonorgestrel (LNG). The mean AUC values of EE were decreased by 48% [90% CI: 22-65] in one study and 52% [90% CI: 38-52] in another study [1,2]. The mean AUC values of LNG were decreased by 32% [90% CI: 20-45] in one study and 52% [90% CI: 42-52] in another study. Therefore, concurrent use of oxcarbazepine with hormonal contraceptives may render these contraceptives less effective (see DRUG INTERACTIONS). Studies with other oral or implant contraceptives have not been conducted.

CALCIUM ANTAGONISTS

After repeated co-administration of oxcarbazepine, the AUC of felodipine was lowered by 28% [90% CI: 20-33].

Verapamil produced a decrease of 20% [90% CI: 18-27] of the plasma levels of MHD.

OTHER DRUG INTERACTIONS

Cimetidine, erythromycin, and dextropropoxyphene had no effect on the pharmacokinetics of MHD. Results with warfarin show no evidence of interaction with either single or repeated doses of oxcarbazepine.

ADVERSE REACTIONS

MOST COMMON ADVERSE EVENTS IN ALL CLINICAL STUDIES

Adjunctive Therapy/Monotherapy in Adults Previously Treated With Other AEDs

The most commonly observed (≥5%) adverse experiences seen in association with oxcarbazepine and substantially more frequent than in placebo treated patients were: dizziness, somnolence, diplopia, fatigue, nausea, vomiting, ataxia, abnormal vision, abdominal pain, tremor, dyspepsia, and abnormal gait.

Approximately 23% of these 1537 adult patients discontinued treatment because of an adverse experience. The adverse experiences most commonly associated with discontinuation were: dizziness (6.4%), diplopia (5.9%), ataxia (5.2%), vomiting (5.1%), nausea (4.9%), somnolence (3.8%), headache (2.9%), fatigue (2.1%), abnormal vision (2.1%), tremor (1.8%), abnormal gait (1.7%), rash (1.4%), and hyponatremia (1.0%).

Monotherapy in Adults Not Previously Treated With Other AEDs

The most commonly observed (≥5%) adverse experiences seen in association with oxcarbazepine in these patients were similar to those in previously treated patients.

Approximately 9% of these 295 adult patients discontinued treatment because of an adverse experience. The adverse experiences most commonly associated with discontinuation were: dizziness (1.7%), nausea (1.7%), rash (1.7%), headache (1.4%).

Adjunctive Therapy/Monotherapy in Pediatric Patients Previously Treated With Other AEDs

The most commonly observed (≥5%) adverse experiences seen in association with oxcarbazepine in these patients were similar to those seen in adults.

Approximately 11% of these 456 pediatric patients discontinued treatment because of an adverse experience. The adverse experiences most commonly associated with discontinuation were: somnolence (2.4%), vomiting (2.0%), ataxia (1.8%), diplopia (1.3%), dizziness (1.3%), fatigue (1.1%), and nystagmus (1.1%).

Incidence in Controlled Clinical Studies

The prescriber should be aware that the figures in TABLE 3, TABLE 4, TABLE 5, and TABLE 6 cannot be used to predict the frequency of adverse experiences in the course of usual medical practice where patient characteristics and other factors may differ from those prevailing during clinical studies. Similarly, the cited frequencies cannot be directly compared with figures obtained from other clinical investigations involving different treatments, uses, or investigators. An inspection of these frequencies, however, does provide the prescriber with one basis to estimate the relative contribution of drug and nondrug factors to the adverse event incidences in the population studied.

Controlled Clinical Studies of Adjunctive Therapy/Monotherapy in Adults Previously Treated With Other AEDs

TABLE 3 lists treatment-emergent signs and symptoms that occurred in at least 2% of adult patients with epilepsy treated with oxcarbazepine or placebo as adjunctive treatment and were numerically more common in the patients treated with any dose of oxcarbazepine. TABLE 4 lists treatment-emergent signs and symptoms in patients converted from other AEDs to either high dose oxcarbazepine or low dose (300 mg) oxcarbazepine. Note that in some of these monotherapy studies patients who dropped out during a preliminary tolerability phase are not included in the tables.

TABLE 3 *Treatment-Emergent Adverse Event Incidence in a Controlled Clinical Study of Adjunctive Therapy in Adults**

Body System	Oxcarbazepine Dosage (mg/day)			
	600	1200	2400	Placebo
Adverse Event	n=163	n=171	n=126	n=166
Body as a Whole				
Fatigue	15%	12%	15%	7%
Asthenia	6%	3%	6%	5%
Edema legs	2%	1%	2%	1%
Weight increase	1%	2%	2%	1%
Feeling abnormal	0%	1%	2%	0%
Cardiovascular System				
Hypotension	0%	1%	2%	0%
Digestive System				
Nausea	15%	25%	29%	10%
Vomiting	13%	25%	36%	5%
Pain abdominal	10%	13%	11%	5%
Diarrhea	5%	6%	7%	6%
Dyspepsia	5%	5%	6%	2%
Constipation	2%	2%	6%	4%
Gastritis	2%	1%	2%	1%
Metabolic and Nutritional Disorders				
Hyponatremia	3%	1%	2%	1%
Musculoskeletal System				
Muscle weakness	1%	2%	2%	0%
Sprains and strains	0%	2%	2%	1%
Nervous System				
Headache	32%	28%	26%	23%
Dizziness	26%	32%	49%	13%
Somnolence	20%	28%	36%	12%
Ataxia	9%	17%	31%	5%
Nystagmus	7%	20%	26%	5%
Gait abnormal	5%	10%	17%	1%
Insomnia	4%	2%	3%	1%
Tremor	3%	8%	16%	5%
Nervousness	2%	4%	2%	1%
Agitation	1%	1%	2%	1%
Coordination abnormal	1%	3%	2%	1%
EEG abnormal	0%	0%	2%	0%
Speech disorder	1%	1%	3%	0%
Confusion	1%	1%	2%	1%
Cranial injury NOS	1%	0%	2%	1%
Dysmetria	1%	2%	3%	0%
Thinking abnormal	0%	2%	4%	0%
Respiratory System				
Rhinitis	2%	4%	5%	4%
Skin and Appendages				
Acne	1%	2%	2%	0%
Special Senses				
Diplopia	14%	30%	40%	5%
Vertigo	6%	12%	15%	2%
Vision abnormal	6%	14%	13%	4%
Accommodation abnormal	0%	0%	2%	0%

* Events in at least 2% of patients treated with 2400 mg/day of oxcarbazepine and numerically more frequent than in the placebo group.

TABLE 4 *Treatment-Emergent Adverse Event Incidence in Controlled Clinical Studies of Monotherapy in Adults Previously Treated With Other AEDs**

Body System	Oxcarbazepine Dosage (mg/day) 2400	300
Adverse Event	n=86	n=86
Body as a Whole — General Disorder		
Fatigue	21%	5%
Fever	3%	0%
Allergy	2%	0%
Edema generalized	2%	1%
Pain chest	2%	0%
Digestive System		
Nausea	22%	7%
Vomiting	15%	5%
Diarrhea	7%	5%
Dyspepsia	6%	1%
Anorexia	5%	3%
Pain abdominal	5%	3%
Mouth dry	3%	0%
Hemorrhage rectum	2%	0%
Toothache	2%	1%
Hemic and Lymphatic System		
Lymphadenopathy	2%	0%
Infections and Infestations		
Infection viral	7%	5%
Infection	2%	0%
Metabolic and Nutritional Disorders		
Hyponatremia	5%	0%
Thirst	2%	0%
Nervous System		
Headache	31%	15%
Dizziness	28%	8%
Somnolence	19%	5%
Anxiety	7%	5%
Ataxia	7%	1%
Confusion	7%	0%
Nervousness	7%	0%
Insomnia	6%	3%
Tremor	6%	3%
Amnesia	5%	1%
Convulsions aggravated	5%	2%
Emotional lability	3%	2%
Hypoesthesia	3%	1%
Coordination abnormal	2%	1%
Nystagmus	2%	0%
Speech disorder	2%	0%
Respiratory System		
Upper respiratory tract infection	10%	5%
Coughing	5%	0%
Bronchitis	3%	0%
Pharyngitis	3%	0%
Skin and Appendages		
Hot flushes	2%	1%
Purpura	2%	0%
Special Senses		
Vision abnormal	14%	2%
Diplopia	12%	1%
Taste perversion	5%	0%
Vertigo	3%	0%
Ear ache	2%	1%
Ear infection NOS	2%	0%
Urogenital and Reproductive System		
Urinary tract infection	5%	1%
Micturition frequency	2%	1%
Vaginitis	2%	0%

* Events in at least 2% of patients treated with 2400 mg/day of oxcarbazepine and numerically more frequent than in the low dose control group.

TABLE 5 *Treatment-Emergent Adverse Event Incidence in a Controlled Clinical Study of Monotherapy in Adults Not Previously Treated With Other AEDs**

Body System	Oxcarbazepine	Placebo
Adverse Event	n=55	n=49
Body as a Whole		
Falling down NOS	4%	0%
Digestive System		
Nausea	16%	12%
Diarrhea	7%	2%
Vomiting	7%	6%
Constipation	5%	0%
Dyspepsia	5%	4%
Musculoskeltal System		
Pain back	4%	2%
Nervous System		
Dizziness	22%	6%
Headache	13%	10%
Ataxia	5%	0%
Nervousness	5%	2%
Amnesia	4%	2%
Coordination abnormal	4%	2%
Tremor	4%	0%
Respiratory System		
Upper respiratory tract infection	7%	0%
Epistaxis	4%	0%
Infection chest	4%	0%
Sinusitis	4%	2%
Skin and Appendages		
Rash	4%	2%
Special Senses		
Vision abnormal	4%	0%

* Events in at least 2% of patients treated with oxcarbazepine and numerically more frequent than in the placebo group.

TABLE 6 *Treatment-Emergent Adverse Event Incidence in Controlled Clinical Studies of Adjunctive Therapy/Monotherapy in Pediatric Patients Previously Treated With Other AEDs**

Body System	Oxcarbazepine	Placebo
Adverse Event	n=171	n=139
Body as a Whole		
Fatigue	13%	9%
Allergy	2%	0%
Asthenia	2%	1%
Digestive System		
Vomiting	33%	14%
Nausea	19%	5%
Constipation	4%	1%
Dyspepsia	2%	0%
Nervous System		
Headache	31%	19%
Somnolence	31%	13%
Dizziness	28%	8%
Ataxia	13%	4%
Nystagmus	9%	1%
Emotional lability	8%	4%
Gait abnormal	8%	3%
Tremor	6%	4%
Speech disorder	3%	1%
Concentration impaired	2%	1%
Convulsions	2%	1%
Muscle contractions involuntary	2%	1%
Respiratory System		
Rhinitis	10%	9%
Pneumonia	2%	1%
Skin and Appendages		
Bruising	4%	2%
Sweating increased	3%	0%
Special Senses		
Diplopia	17%	1%
Vision abnormal	13%	1%
Vertigo	2%	0%

* Events in at least 2% of patients treated with oxcarbazepine and numerically more frequent than in the placebo group.

Controlled Clinical Study of Monotherapy in Adults Not Previously Treated With Other AEDs

TABLE 5 lists treatment-emergent signs and symptoms in a controlled clinical study of monotherapy in adults not previously treated with other AEDs that occurred in at least 2% of adult patients with epilepsy treated with oxcarbazepine or placebo and were numerically more common in the patients treated with oxcarbazepine.

Controlled Clinical Studies of Adjunctive Therapy/Monotherapy in Pediatric Patients Previously Treated With Other AEDs

TABLE 6 lists treatment-emergent signs and symptoms that occurred in at least 2% of pediatric patients with epilepsy treated with oxcarbazepine or placebo as adjunctive treatment and were numerically more common in the patients treated with oxcarbazepine.

OTHER EVENTS OBSERVED IN ASSOCIATION WITH THE ADMINISTRATION OF OXCARBAZEPINE

In the paragraphs that follow, the adverse events other than those in TABLE 3, TABLE 4, TABLE 5, and TABLE 6 or text, that occurred in a total of 565 children and 1574 adults exposed to oxcarbazepine and that are reasonably likely to be related to drug use are presented. Events common in the population, events reflecting chronic illness and events likely to reflect concomitant illness are omitted particularly if minor. They are listed in order of decreasing frequency. Because the reports cite events observed in open label and uncontrolled trials, the role of oxcarbazepine in their causation cannot be reliably determined.

Body as a Whole: Fever, malaise, pain chest precordial, rigors, weight decrease.

Cardiovascular System: Bradycardia, cardiac failure, cerebral hemorrhage, hypertension, hypotension postural, palpitation, syncope, tachycardia.

Digestive System: Appetite increased, blood in stool, cholelithiasis, colitis, duodenal ulcer, dysphagia, enteritis, eructation, esophagitis, flatulence, gastric ulcer, gingival bleeding, gum hyperplasia, hematemesis, hemorrhage rectum, hemorrhoids, hiccup, mouth dry, pain biliary, pain right hypochondrium, retching, sialoadenitis, stomatitis, stomatitis ulcerative.

Hemic and Lymphatic System: Leukopenia, thrombocytopenia.

Laboratory Abnormality: Gamma-GT increased, hyperglycemia, hypocalcemia, hypoglycemia, hypokalemia, liver enzymes elevated, serum transaminase increased.

Musculoskeletal System: Hypertonia muscle.

Nervous System: Aggressive reaction, amnesia, anguish, anxiety, apathy, aphasia, aura, convulsions aggravated, delirium, delusion, depressed level of consciousness, dysphonia, dystonia, emotional lability, euphoria, extrapyramidal disorder, feeling drunk, hemiplegia, hyperkinesia, hyperreflexia, hypoesthesia, hypokinesia, hyporeflexia, hypotonia, hysteria, libido decreased, libido increased, manic reaction, migraine, muscle contractions involuntary, nervousness, neuralgia, oculogyric crisis, panic disorder, paralysis, paroniria, personality disorder, psychosis, ptosis, stupor, tetany.

Respiratory System: Asthma, dyspnea, epistaxis, laryngismus, pleurisy.

Skin and Appendages: Acne, alopecia, angioedema, bruising, dermatitis contact, eczema, facial rash, flushing, folliculitis, heat rash, hot flushes, photosensitivity reaction, pruritus genital, psoriasis, purpura, rash erythematous, rash maculopapular, vitiligo, urticaria.

Special Senses: Accommodation abnormal, cataract, conjunctival hemorrhage, edema eye, hemianopia, mydriasis, otitis externa, photophobia, scotoma, taste perversion, tinnitus, xerophthalmia.

Surgical and Medical Procedures: Procedure dental oral, procedure female reproductive, procedure musculoskeletal, procedure skin.

Urogenital and Reproductive System: Dysuria, hematuria, intermenstrual bleeding, leukorrhea, menorrhagia, micturition frequency, pain renal, pain urinary tract, polyuria, priapism, renal calculus.

Other: Systemic lupus erythematosus.

POST-MARKETING AND OTHER EXPERIENCE

The following adverse events not seen in controlled clinical trials have been observed in named patient programs or post-marketing experience:

Body as a Whole: Multiorgan hypersensitivity disorders characterized by features such as rash, fever, lymphadenopathy, abnormal liver function tests, eosinophilia and arthralgia.

Skin and Appendages: Erythema multiforme, Stevens-Johnson syndrome, toxic epidermal necrolysis.

DOSAGE AND ADMINISTRATION

Oxcarbazepine is recommended as adjunctive treatment and monotherapy in the treatment of partial seizures in adults and as adjunctive treatment for partial seizures in children ages 4-16. All dosing should be given in a twice a day (bid) regimen. Oxcarbazepine oral suspension and film-coated tablets may be interchanged at equal doses.

Oxcarbazepine should be kept out of the reach and sight of children.

Before using oxcarbazepine oral suspension, shake the bottle well and prepare the dose immediately afterwards. The prescribed amount of oral suspension should be withdrawn from the bottle using the oral dosing syringe supplied. Oxcarbazepine oral suspension can be mixed in a small glass of water just prior to administration or, alternatively, may be swallowed directly from the syringe. After each use, close the bottle and rinse the syringe with warm water and allow it to dry thoroughly.

Oxcarbazepine can be taken with or without food (see CLINICAL PHARMACOLOGY, Pharmacokinetics).

ADULTS

Adjunctive Therapy

Treatment with oxcarbazepine should be initiated with a dose of 600 mg/day, given in a bid regimen. If clinically indicated, the dose may be increased by a maximum of 600 mg/day at approximately weekly intervals; the recommended daily dose is 1200 mg/day. Daily doses above 1200 mg/day show somewhat greater effectiveness in controlled trials, but most patients were not able to tolerate the 2400 mg/day dose, primarily because of CNS effects. It is recommended that the patient be observed closely and plasma levels of the concomitant AEDs be monitored during the period of oxcarbazepine titration, as these plasma levels may be altered, especially at oxcarbazepine doses greater than 1200 mg/day (see DRUG INTERACTIONS).

Conversion to Monotherapy

Patients receiving concomitant AEDs may be converted to monotherapy by initiating treatment with oxcarbazepine at 600 mg/day (given in a bid regimen) while simultaneously initiating the reduction of the dose of the concomitant AEDs. The concomitant AEDs should be completely withdrawn over 3-6 weeks, while the maximum dose of oxcarbazepine should be reached in about 2-4 weeks. Oxcarbazepine may be increased as clinically indicated by a maximum increment of 600 mg/day at approximately weekly intervals to achieve the recommended daily dose of 2400 mg/day. A daily dose of 1200 mg/day has been shown in one study to be effective in patients in whom monotherapy has been initiated with oxcarbazepine. Patients should be observed closely during this transition phase.

Initiation of Monotherapy

Patients not currently being treated with AEDs may have monotherapy initiated with oxcarbazepine. In these patients, oxcarbazepine should be initiated at a dose of 600 mg/day (given in a bid regimen); the dose should be increased by 300 mg/day every third day to a dose of 1200 mg/day. Controlled trials in these patients examined the effectiveness of a 1200 mg/day dose; a dose of 2400 mg/day has been shown to be effective in patients converted from other AEDs to oxcarbazepine monotherapy (see Conversion to Monotherapy).

PEDIATRIC PATIENTS AGE 4-16

Adjunctive Therapy

Treatment should be initiated at a daily dose of 8-10 mg/kg generally not to exceed 600 mg/day, given in a bid regimen. The target maintenance dose of oxcarbazepine should be achieved over 2 weeks, and is dependent upon patient weight, according to TABLE 7.

TABLE 7

Weight	Dose
20-29 kg	900 mg/day
29.1-39 kg	1200 mg/day
>39 kg	1800 mg/day

In the clinical trial, in which the intention was to reach these target doses, the median daily dose was 31 mg/kg with a range of 6-51 mg/kg.

The pharmacokinetics of oxcarbazepine are similar in older children (age >8 years) and adults. However, younger children (age <8 years) have an increased clearance (by about 30-40%) compared with older children and adults. In the controlled trial, pediatric patients 8 years old and below received the highest maintenance doses.

Children below 2 years of age have not been studied in controlled clinical trials.

PATIENTS WITH HEPATIC IMPAIRMENT

In general, dose adjustments are not required in patients with mild-to-moderate hepatic impairment (see CLINICAL PHARMACOLOGY, Pharmacokinetics, Special Populations).

PATIENTS WITH RENAL IMPAIRMENT

In patients with impaired renal function (creatine clearance <30 ml/min) oxcarbazepine therapy should be initiated at one-half the usual starting dose (300 mg/day) and increased slowly to achieve the desired clinical response (see CLINICAL PHARMACOLOGY, Pharmacokinetics, Special Populations).

HOW SUPPLIED

TRILEPTAL FILM-COATED TABLETS

150 mg: Yellow, ovaloid, slightly biconvex, scored on both sides. Imprinted with "T/D" on one side and "C/G" on the other side.

300 mg: Yellow, ovaloid, slightly biconvex, scored on both sides. Imprinted with "TE/TE" on one side and "CG/CG" on the other side.

600 mg: Yellow, ovaloid, slightly biconvex, scored on both sides. Imprinted with "TF/TF" on one side and "CG/CG" on the other side.

Storage

Store at 25°C (77°F); excursions permitted to 15-30°C (59-86°F). Dispense in tight container.

TRILEPTAL ORAL SUSPENSION

300 mg/5 ml (60 mg/ml): Off-white to slightly brown or slightly red oral suspension. Available in amber glass bottles containing 250 ml of oral suspension. Supplied with a 10 ml dosing syringe and press-in bottle adapter.

Storage

Store Trileptal oral suspension in the original container. Shake well before using.

Use within 7 weeks of first opening the bottle.

Store at 25°C (77°F); excursions permitted to 15-30°C (59-86°F).

PRODUCT LISTING - EQUIVALENTS NOT AVAILABLE

Suspension - Oral - 300 mg/5 ml

250 ml	$98.11	TRILEPTAL, Novartis Pharmaceuticals	00078-0357-52

Tablet - Oral - 150 mg

100's	$106.14	TRILEPTAL, Novartis Pharmaceuticals	00078-0336-05
100's	$111.44	TRILEPTAL, Novartis Pharmaceuticals	00078-0336-06

Tablet - Oral - 300 mg

100's	$193.81	TRILEPTAL, Novartis Pharmaceuticals	00078-0337-05
100's	$203.50	TRILEPTAL, Novartis Pharmaceuticals	00078-0337-06

Tablet - Oral - 600 mg

100's	$356.24	TRILEPTAL, Novartis Pharmaceuticals	00078-0338-05
100's	$374.05	TRILEPTAL, Novartis Pharmaceuticals	00078-0338-06

Oxiconazole Nitrate *(001927)*

Categories: Pityriasis; Tinea corporis; Tinea cruris; Tinea pedis; Tinea versicolor; Pregnancy Category B; FDA Approved 1988 Dec
Drug Classes: Antifungals, topical; Dermatologics
Brand Names: Oxistat
Foreign Brand Availability: Derimine (Japan); Myfungar (Germany; Mexico; Switzerland); Oceral (Austria; Portugal; Switzerland); Oceral GB (Germany); Okinazole (Japan); Oxizole (Canada); Sylos Vaginal Tab (Korea)
Cost of Therapy: $17.08 (Fungal Infection; Oxistat Cream; 1%; 15 g; 2 applications/day; variable day supply)

DESCRIPTION

For Topical Dermatologic Use Only — Not for Ophthalmic or Intravaginal Use.

Oxistat cream and lotion formulations contain the antifungal active compound oxiconazole nitrate. Both formulations are for topical dermatological use only.

Chemically, oxiconazole nitrate is 2′,4′-dichloro-2-imidazol-1-ylacetophenone (*Z*)-[*O*-(2,4-dichlorobenzyl)oxime], mononitrate.

The compound has the empirical formula $C_{18}H_{13}ON_3Cl_4 \cdot HNO_3$, and a molecular weight of 492.15.

Oxiconazole nitrate is a nearly white crystalline powder, soluble in methanol; sparingly soluble in ethanol, chloroform, and acetone; and very slightly soluble in water.

Oxistat Cream contains 10 mg of oxiconazole per gram of cream in a white to off-white, opaque cream base of purified water, white petrolatum, stearyl alcohol, propylene glycol, polysorbate 60, cetyl alcohol, and benzoic acid 0.2% as a preservative.

Oxistat Lotion contains 10 mg of oxiconazole per gram of lotion in a white to off-white, opaque lotion base of purified water, white petrolatum, stearyl alcohol, propylene glycol, polysorbate 60, cetyl alcohol, and benzoic acid 0.2% as a preservative.

CLINICAL PHARMACOLOGY

PHARMACOKINETICS

The penetration of oxiconazole nitrate into different layers of the skin was assessed using an *in vitro* permeation technique with human skin. Five (5) hours after application of 2.5 mg/cm^2 of oxiconazole nitrate cream onto human skin, the concentration of oxiconazole nitrate was demonstrated to be 16.2 μmol in the epidermis, 3.64 μmol in the upper corium, and 1.29 μmol in the deeper corium. Systemic absorption of oxiconazole nitrate is low. Using radiolabeled drug, less than 0.3% of the applied dose of oxiconazole nitrate was recovered in the urine of volunteer subjects up to 5 days after application of the cream formulation.

Neither *in vitro* nor *in vivo* studies have been conducted to establish relative activity between the lotion and cream formulations.

MICROBIOLOGY
Oxiconazole nitrate is an imidazole derivative whose antifungal activity is derived primarily from the inhibition of ergosterol biosynthesis, which is critical for cellular membrane integrity. It has *in vitro* activity against a wide range of pathogenic fungi.

Oxiconazole has been shown to be active against most strains of the following organisms both *in vitro* and in clinical infections at indicated body sites (see INDICATIONS AND USAGE):

Epidermophyton floccosum.
Trichophyton mentagrophytes.
Trichophyton rubrum.
Malassezia furfur.

The following *in vitro* data are available; **however, their clinical significance is unknown.** Oxiconazole exhibits satisfactory *in vitro* minimum inhibitory concentrations (MICs) against most strains of the following organisms; however, the safety and efficacy of oxiconazole in treating clinical infections due to these organisms have not been established in adequate and well-controlled clinical trials:

Candida albicans.
Microsporum audouini.
Microsporum canis.
Microsporum gypseum.
Trichophyton tonsurans.
Trichophyton violaceum.

INDICATIONS AND USAGE

Oxiconazole nitrate cream and lotion are indicated for the topical treatment of the following dermal infections: tinea pedis, tinea cruris, and tinea corporis due to *Trichophyton rubrum, Trichophyton mentagrophytes,* or *Epidermophyton floccosum.* Oxiconazole nitrate cream is indicated for the topical treatment of tinea (pityriasis) versicolor due to *Malassezia furfur* (see DOSAGE AND ADMINISTRATION).

Oxiconazole nitrate cream may be used in pediatric patients for tinea corporis, tinea cruris, tinea pedis, and tinea (pityriasis) versicolor; however, these indications for which oxiconazole nitrate cream has been shown to be effective rarely occur in children below the age of 12.

CONTRAINDICATIONS

Oxiconazole cream and lotion are contraindicated in individuals who have shown hypersensitivity to any of their components.

WARNINGS

Oxiconazole cream and lotion is not for ophthalmic or intravaginal use.

PRECAUTIONS

GENERAL
Oxiconazole nitrate cream and lotion are for external dermal use only. Avoid introduction of oxiconazole nitrate cream or lotion into the eyes or vagina. If a reaction suggesting sensitivity or chemical irritation should occur with the use of oxiconazole nitrate cream or lotion, treatment should be discontinued and appropriate therapy instituted. If signs of epidermal irritation should occur, the drug should be discontinued.

O

INFORMATION FOR THE PATIENT
The patient should be instructed to:

1. Use oxiconazole nitrate as directed by the physician. The hands should be washed after applying the medication to the affected area(s). Avoid contact with the eyes, nose, mouth, and other mucous membranes. Oxiconazole nitrate is for external use only.
2. Use the medication for the **full** treatment time recommended by the physician, even though symptoms may have improved. Notify the physician if there is no improvement after 2-4 weeks, or sooner if the condition worsens (see below).
3. Inform the physician if the area of application shows signs of increased irritation, itching, burning, blistering, swelling, or oozing.
4. Avoid the use of occlusive dressings unless otherwise directed by the physician.
5. Do not use this medication for any disorder other than that for which it was prescribed.

CARCINOGENESIS, MUTAGENESIS, AND IMPAIRMENT OF FERTILITY
Although no long-term studies in animals have been performed to evaluate carcinogenic potential, no evidence of mutagenic effect was found in 2 mutation assays (Ames test and Chinese hamster V79 *in vitro* cell mutation assay) or in 2 cytogenetic assays (human peripheral blood lymphocyte *in vitro* chromosome aberration assay and *in vivo* micronucleus assay in mice).

Reproductive studies revealed no impairment of fertility in rats at oral doses of 3 mg/kg/day in females (one time the human dose based on mg/m^2) and 15 mg/kg/day in males (4 times the human dose based on mg/m^2). However, at doses above this level, the following effects were observed: a reduction in the fertility parameters of males and females, a reduction in the number of sperm in vaginal smears, extended estrous cycle, and a decrease in mating frequency.

PREGNANCY, TERATOGENIC EFFECTS, PREGNANCY CATEGORY B
Reproduction studies have been performed in rabbits, rats, and mice at oral doses up to 100, 150, and 200 mg/kg/day (57, 40, and 27 times the human dose based on mg/m^2), respectively, and revealed no evidence of harm to the fetus due to oxiconazole nitrate. There are, however, no adequate and well-controlled studies in pregnant women. Because animal reproduction studies are not always predictive of human response, this drug should be used during pregnancy only if clearly needed.

NURSING MOTHERS
Because oxiconazole is excreted in human milk, caution should be exercised when the drug is administered to a nursing woman.

PEDIATRIC USE
Oxiconazole nitrate cream may be used in pediatric patients for tinea corporis, tinea cruris, tinea pedis, and tinea (pityriasis) versicolor; however, these indications for which oxiconazole nitrate cream has been shown to be effective rarely occur in children below the age of 12.

GERIATRIC USE
A limited number of patients at or above 65 years of age (n=508) have been treated with oxiconazole nitrate cream in US and non-US clinical trials, and a limited number (n=43) have been treated with oxiconazole nitrate lotion in US clinical trials. The number of patients is too small to permit separate analysis of efficacy and safety. No adverse events were reported with oxiconazole nitrate lotion in geriatric patients, and the adverse reactions reported with oxiconazole nitrate cream in this population were similar to those reported by younger patients. Based on available data, no adjustment of dosage of oxiconazole nitrate cream and lotion in geriatric patients is warranted.

DRUG INTERACTIONS

Potential drug interactions between oxiconazole nitrate and other drugs have not been systematically evaluated.

ADVERSE REACTIONS

During clinical trials, of 955 patients treated with oxiconazole nitrate cream, 1%, 41 (4.3%) reported adverse reactions thought to be related to drug therapy. These reactions included pruritus (1.6%); burning (1.4%); irritation and allergic contact dermatitis (0.4% each); folliculitis (0.3%); erythema (0.2%); and papules, fissure, maceration, rash, stinging, and nodules (0.1% each).

In a controlled, multicenter clinical trial of 269 patients treated with oxiconazole nitrate lotion, 1%, 7 (2.6%) reported adverse reactions thought to be related to drug therapy. These reactions included burning and stinging (0.7% each) and pruritus, scaling, tingling, pain, and dyshidrotic eczema (0.4% each).

DOSAGE AND ADMINISTRATION

Oxiconazole nitrate cream or lotion should be applied to affected and immediately surrounding areas once to twice daily in patients with tinea pedis, tinea corporis, or tinea cruris. Oxiconazole nitrate cream should be applied once daily in the treatment of tinea (pityriasis) versicolor. Tinea corporis, tinea cruris, and tinea (pityriasis) versicolor should be treated for 2 weeks and tinea pedis for 1 month to reduce the possibility of recurrence. If a patient shows no clinical improvement after the treatment period, the diagnosis should be reviewed.
Note: Tinea (pityriasis) versicolor may give rise to hyperpigmented or hypopigmented patches on the trunk that may extend to the neck, arms, and upper thighs. Treatment of the infection may not immediately result in restoration of pigment to the affected sites. Normalization of pigment following successful therapy is variable and may take months, depending on individual skin type and incidental sun exposure. Although tinea (pityriasis) versicolor is not contagious, it may recur because the organism that causes the disease is part of the normal skin flora.
Geriatric Use: In studies where geriatric patients (65 years of age or older, see PRECAUTIONS) have been treated with oxiconazole nitrate cream or lotion, safety did not differ from that in younger patients; therefore, no dosage adjustment is recommended.

HOW SUPPLIED

OXISTAT CREAM
Oxistat Cream, 1% is supplied in 15, 30, and 60 g tubes.
Storage: Store between 15 and 30°C (59 and 86°F).

OXISTAT LOTION
Oxistat Lotion, 1% is supplied in a 30 ml bottle.
Storage: Store between 15 and 30°C (59 and 86°F). Shake well before using.

PRODUCT LISTING - EQUIVALENTS NOT AVAILABLE

Cream - Topical - 1%			
15 gm	$17.08	OXISTAT, Dura Pharmaceuticals	51479-0423-00
30 gm	$32.33	OXISTAT, Dura Pharmaceuticals	51479-0423-01
60 gm	$43.55	OXISTAT, Dura Pharmaceuticals	51479-0423-04
Lotion - Topical - 1%			
30 ml	$28.73	OXISTAT, Dura Pharmaceuticals	51479-0448-01

Oxybutynin *(001930)*

Categories: Bladder, neurogenic; Bladder, overactive; Dysuria; Incontinence, urinary, urge; Urinary frequency; Urinary urgency; Pregnancy Category B; FDA Approved 1975 Jul
Drug Classes: Anticholinergics; Relaxants, urinary tract
Brand Names: **Ditropan**; Ditropan XL; Oxytrol
Foreign Brand Availability: Cystonorm (Germany); Cystrin (England; Ireland); Delifon (Colombia); Diutropin (Thailand); Dridase (Germany; Netherlands); Driptane (Philippines); Iliaden (Peru); Lenditro (South-Africa); Mutum CR (Colombia); Nefryl (Mexico); Novitropan (Israel); Oxyb (Germany); Oxyban (Taiwan); Oyrobin (Korea); Tavor (Mexico); Tropan (India); Uricont (Israel); Zatur Ge (France)
Cost of Therapy: $38.59 (Urinary Incontinence; Ditropan; 5 mg; 2 tablets/day; 30 day supply)
$9.17 (Urinary Incontinence; Generic Tablets; 5 mg; 2 tablets/day; 30 day supply)
$87.95 (Urinary Incontinence; Ditropan XL; 5 mg; 1 tablet/day; 30 day supply)

ORAL

DESCRIPTION

Oxybutynin chloride is an antispasmodic, anticholinergic agent. Chemically, oxybutynin chloride is d,l(racemic)4-diethylamino-2-butynyl phenylcyclohexylglycolate hydrochloride. The empirical formula of oxybutynin chloride is $C_{22}H_{31}NO_3 \cdot HCl$.

Oxybutynin chloride is a white crystalline solid with a molecular weight of 393.9. It is readily soluble in water and acids, but relatively insoluble in alkalis.

Oxybutynin chloride tablets, extended-release tablets and syrup are for oral administration.

TABLETS

Each scored biconvex, engraved blue tablet contains 5 mg of oxybutynin chloride.
Oxybutynin chloride tablets also contain: Calcium stearate, FD&C blue no. 1 lake, lactose, and microcrystalline cellulose.

EXTENDED-RELEASE TABLETS

Each oxybutynin chloride extended-release tablet contains 5, 10, or 15 mg of oxybutynin chloride, formulated as a once-a-day controlled-release tablet for oral administration. Oxybutynin chloride is administered as a racemate of R- and S-enantiomers.
Oxybutynin chloride extended-release tablets also contains the following inert ingredients: Cellulose acetate, hydroxypropyl methylcellulose, lactose, magnesium stearate, polyethylene glycol, polyethylene oxide, synthetic iron oxides, titanium dioxide, polysorbate 80, sodium chloride, and butylated hydroxytoluene.

System Components and Performance

Oxybutynin chloride extended-release tablets use osmotic pressure to deliver oxybutynin chloride at a controlled rate over approximately 24 hours. The system, which resembles a conventional tablet in appearance, comprises an osmotically active bilayer core surrounded by a semipermeable membrane. The bilayer core is composed of a drug layer containing the drug and excipients, and a push layer containing osmotically active components. There is a precision-laser drilled orifice in the semipermeable membrane on the drug-layer side of the tablet. In an aqueous environment, such as the gastrointestinal tract, water permeates through the membrane into the tablet core, causing the drug to go into suspension and the push layer to expand. This expansion pushes the suspended drug out through the orifice. The semipermeable membrane controls the rate at which water permeates into the tablet core, which in turn controls the rate of drug delivery. The controlled rate of drug delivery into the gastrointestinal lumen is thus independent of pH or gastrointestinal motility. The function of oxybutynin chloride extended-release tablets depends on the existence of an osmotic gradient between the contents of the bilayer core and the fluid in the gastrointestinal tract. Since the osmotic gradient remains constant, drug delivery remains essentially constant. The biologically inert components of the tablet remain intact during gastrointestinal transit and are eliminated in the feces as an insoluble shell.

SYRUP

Each 5 ml of syrup contains 5 mg of oxybutynin chloride.
Oxybutynin chloride syrup also contains: Citric acid, FD&C green no. 3, glycerin, methylparaben, flavor, sodium citrate, sorbitol, sucrose, and water.

CLINICAL PHARMACOLOGY

Oxybutynin chloride exerts a direct antispasmodic effect on smooth muscle and inhibits the muscarinic action of acetylcholine on smooth muscle. Oxybutynin chloride exhibits only one-fifth of the anticholinergic activity of atropine on the rabbit detrusor muscle, but 4-10 times the antispasmodic activity. No blocking effects occur at skeletal neuromuscular junctions or autonomic ganglia (antinicotinic effects).

Oxybutynin chloride relaxes bladder smooth muscle. In patients with conditions characterized by involuntary bladder contractions, cystometric studies have demonstrated that oxybutynin chloride increases bladder (vesical) capacity, diminishes the frequency of uninhibited contractions of the detrusor muscle, and delays the initial desire to void. Oxybutynin chloride thus decreases urgency and the frequency of both incontinent episodes and voluntary urination.

Antimuscarinic activity resides predominantly in the R-isomer. A metabolite, desethyloxybutynin, has pharmacological activity similar to that of oxybutynin in *in vitro* studies.

TABLETS AND SYRUP

Pharmacokinetics

Absorption

Following oral administration of oxybutynin, oxybutynin is rapidly absorbed achieving C_{max} within an hour, following which plasma concentration decreases with an effective half-life of approximately 2-3 hours. The absolute bioavailability of oxybutynin is reported to be about 6% (range 1.6-10.9%) for both the tablet and syrup. Wide interindividual variation in pharmacokinetic parameters is evident following oral administration of oxybutynin.

The mean pharmacokinetic parameters for R- and S-oxybutynin are summarized in TABLE 1. The plasma concentration-time profiles for R- and S-oxybutynin are similar in shape.

TABLE 1 *Mean (SD) R- and S-Oxybutynin Pharmacokinetic Parameters Following 3 Doses of Oxybutynin Chloride 5 mg Administered Every 8 Hours (n=23)*

Parameters (units)	R-Oxybutyin	S-Oxybutynin
C_{max} (ng/ml)	3.6 (2.2)	7.8 (4.1)
T_{max} (h)	0.89 (0.34)	0.65 (0.32)
AUC(t) (ng·h/ml)	22.6 (11.3)	35.0 (17.3)
AUC(∞) (ng·h/ml)	24.3 (12.3)	37.3 (18.7)

Oxybutynin chloride steady-state pharmacokinetics was also studied in 23 pediatric patients with detrusor overactivity associated with a neurological condition (*e.g.,* spina bifida). These pediatric patients were on oxybutynin chloride tablets (n=11) with total daily dose ranging from 7.5 to 15 mg (0.22-0.53 mg/kg) or oxybutynin chloride syrup (n=12) with total daily dose ranging from 5 to 22.5 mg (0.26-0.75 mg/kg). Overall, most patients (86.9%) were taking a total daily oxybutynin chloride dose between 10 and 15 mg. Sparse sampling technique was used to obtain serum samples. When all available data are normalized to an equivalent of 5 mg twice daily oxybutynin chloride, the mean pharmacokinetic parameters derived for R- and S-oxybutynin and R- and S-desethyloxybutynin are summarized in TABLE 2A (for tablet) and TABLE 2B (for syrup). The plasma-time concentration profile for R- and S-oxybutynin are similar in shape.

TABLE 2A *Mean ± SD R- and S-Oxybutynin and R- and S-Desethyloxybutynin Pharmacokinetic Parameters in Children Aged 5-15 Following Administration of 7.5 to 15 mg Total Daily Dose of Oxybutynin Chloride Tablets (n=11)**

	R-Oxybutyin	S-Oxybutynin	R-Desethyl-oxybutynin	S-Desethyl-oxybutynin
C_{max}† (ng/ml)	6.1 ± 3.2	10.1 ± 7.5	55.4 ± 17.9	28.2 ± 10.0
T_{max} (h)	1.0	1.0	2.0	2.0
AUC‡ (ng·h/ml)	19.8 ± 7.4	28.4 ± 12.7	238.8 ± 77.6	119.5 ± 50.7

* **All available data normalized to an equivalent of oxybutynin chloride tablets 5 mg bid or tid at steady-state.**
† Reflects C_{max} for pooled data.
‡ AUC(0-end of dosing interval).

TABLE 2B *Mean ± SD R- and S-Oxybutynin and R- and S-Desethyloxybutynin Pharmacokinetic Parameters in Children Aged 5-15 Following Administration of 5 to 22.5 mg Total Daily Dose of Oxybutynin Chloride Syrup (n=12)**

	R-Oxybutyin	S-Oxybutynin	R-Desethyl-oxybutynin	S-Desethyl-oxybutynin
C_{max}† (ng/ml)	5.7 ± 6.2	7.3 ± 7.3	54.2 ± 34.0	27.8 ± 20.7
T_{max} (h)	1.0	1.0	1.0	1.0
AUC‡ (ng·h/ml)	16.3 ± 17.1	20.2 ± 20.8	209.1 ± 174.2	99.1 ± 87.5

* **All available data normalized to an equivalent of oxybutynin chloride syrup 5 mg bid or tid at steady-state.**
† Reflects C_{max} for pooled data.
‡ AUC(0-end of dosing interval).

Food Effects

Data in the literature suggests that oxybutynin solution coadministered with food resulted in a slight delay in absorption and an increase in its bioavailability by 25% (n=18).[1]

Distribution

Plasma concentrations of oxybutynin decline biexponentially following IV or oral administration. The volume of distribution is 193 L after IV administration of 5 mg oxybutynin chloride.

Metabolism

Oxybutynin is metabolized primarily by the cytochrome P450 enzyme systems, particularly CYP3A4 found mostly in the liver and gut wall. Its metabolic products include phenylcyclohexylglycolic acid, which is pharmacologically inactive, and desethyloxybutynin, which is pharmacologically active.

Excretion

Oxybutynin is extensively metabolized by the liver, with less than 0.1% of the administered dose excreted unchanged in the urine. Also, less than 0.1% of the administered dose is excreted as the metabolite desethyloxybutynin.

EXTENDED-RELEASE TABLETS

Pharmacokinetics

Absorption

Following the first dose of oxybutynin chloride extended-release tablets, oxybutynin plasma concentrations rise for 4-6 hours; thereafter steady concentrations are maintained for up to 24 hours, minimizing fluctuations between peak and trough concentrations associated with oxybutynin.

The relative bioavailabilities of R- and S-oxybutynin from oxybutynin chloride extended-release tablets are 156% and 187%, respectively, compared with oxybutynin. The mean pharmacokinetic parameters for R- and S-oxybutynin are summarized in TABLE 3. The plasma concentration-time profiles for R- and S-oxybutynin are similar in shape.

TABLE 3 *Mean (SD) R- and S-Oxybutynin Pharmacokinetic Parameters Following a Single Dose of Oxybutynin Chloride Extended-Release Tablets 10 mg (n=43)*

Parameters (units)	R-Oxybutynin	S-Oxybutynin
C_{max} (ng/ml)	1.0 (0.6)	1.8 (1.0)
T_{max} (h)	12.7 (5.4)	11.8 (5.3)
T½ (h)	13.2 (6.2)	12.4 (6.1)
AUC(0-48) (ng·h/ml)	18.4 (10.3)	34.2 (16.9)
AUC(∞) (ng·h/ml)	21.3 (12.2)	39.5 (21.2)

Steady-state oxybutynin plasma concentrations are achieved by Day 3 of repeated oxybutynin chloride extended-release tablets dosing, with no observed drug accumulation or change in oxybutynin and desethyloxybutynin pharmacokinetic parameters.

Oxybutynin chloride extended-release tablets steady-state pharmacokinetics was studied in 19 children aged 5-15 years with detrusor overactivity associated with a neurological condition (*e.g.,* spina bifida). The children were on oxybutynin chloride extended-release tablets total daily dose ranging from 5-20 mg (0.10-0.77 mg/kg). Sparse sampling technique was used to obtain serum samples. When all available data are normalized to an equivalent of 5 mg/day oxybutynin chloride extended-release tablets, the mean pharmacokinetic parameters derived for R- and S-oxybutynin and R- and S-desethyloxybutynin are summarized in TABLE 4. The plasma-time concentration profiles for R- and S-oxybutynin are similar in shape.

TABLE 4 *Mean ± SD R- and S-Oxybutynin and R- and S-Desethyloxybutynin Pharmacokinetic Parameters in Children Aged 5-15 Following Administration of 5-20 mg Oxybutynin Chloride Extended-Release Tablets Once Daily (n=19)**

	R-Oxybutynin	S-Oxybutynin	R-Desethyl-oxybutynin	S-Desethyl-oxybutynin
C_{max} (ng/ml)	0.7 ± 0.4	1.3 ± 0.8	7.8 ± 3.7	4.2 ± 2.3
T_{max} (h)	5.0	5.0	5.0	5.0
AUC (ng·h/ml)	12.8 ± 7.0	23.7 ± 14.4	125.1 ± 66.7	73.6 ± 47.7

*** All available data normalized to an equivalent of oxybutynin chloride extended-release tablets 5 mg once daily.**

Food Effects
The rate and extent of absorption and metabolism of oxybutynin are similar under fed and fasted conditions.

Distribution
Plasma concentrations of oxybutynin decline biexponentially following IV or oral administration. The volume of distribution is 193 L after IV administration of 5 mg oxybutynin chloride.

Metabolism
Oxybutynin is metabolized primarily by the cytochrome P450 enzyme systems, particularly CYP3A4 found mostly in the liver and gut wall. Its metabolic products include phenylcyclohexylglycolic acid, which is pharmacologically inactive, and desethyloxybutynin, which is pharmacologically active. Following oxybutynin chloride extended-release tablets administration, plasma concentrations of R- and S-desethyloxybutynin are 73% and 92%, respectively, of concentrations observed with oxybutynin.

Excretion
Oxybutynin is extensively metabolized by the liver, with less than 0.1% of the administered dose excreted unchanged in the urine. Also, less than 0.1% of the administered dose is excreted as the metabolite desethyloxybutynin.

Dose Proportionality
Pharmacokinetic parameters of oxybutynin and desethyloxybutynin (C_{max} and AUC) following administration of 5-20 mg of oxybutynin chloride extended-release tablets are dose proportional.

Special Populations
Geriatric: The pharmacokinetics of oxybutynin chloride extended-release tablets were similar in all patients studied (up to 78 years of age).

Pediatric: The pharmacokinetics of oxybutynin chloride extended-release tablets were evaluated in 19 children aged 5-15 years with detrusor overactivity associated with a neurological condition (*e.g.,* spina bifida). The pharmacokinetics of oxybutynin chloride extended-release tablets in these pediatric patients were consistent with those reported for adults (see TABLE 3 and TABLE 4).

Gender: There are no significant differences in the pharmacokinetics of oxybutynin in healthy male and female volunteers following administration of oxybutynin chloride extended-release tablets.

Race: Available data suggest that there are no significant differences in the pharmacokinetics of oxybutynin based on race in healthy volunteers following administration of oxybutynin chloride extended-release tablets.

Renal Insufficiency: There is no experience with the use of oxybutynin chloride extended-release tablets in patients with renal insufficiency.

Hepatic Insufficiency: There is no experience with the use of oxybutynin chloride extended-release tablets in patients with hepatic insufficiency.

Drug-Drug Interactions: See DRUG INTERACTIONS.

INDICATIONS AND USAGE

TABLETS AND SYRUP

Oxybutynin chloride is indicated for the relief of symptoms of bladder instability associated with voiding in patients with uninhibited neurogenic or reflex neurogenic bladder (*i.e.,* urgency, frequency, urinary leakage, urge incontinence, dysuria).

EXTENDED-RELEASE TABLETS

Oxybutynin chloride extended-release tablets are a once-daily controlled-release tablet indicated for the treatment of overactive bladder with symptoms of urge urinary incontinence, urgency, and frequency.

Oxybutynin chloride extended-release tablets is also indicated in the treatment of pediatric patients aged 6 years and older with symptoms of detrusor overactivity associated with a neurological condition (*e.g.,* spina bifida).

NON-FDA APPROVED INDICATIONS

Although not FDA approved, oxybutynin has been used as an antispasmodic in the symptomatic treatment of various GI disorders, following transurethral surgery, and in conjunction with intermittent self-catheterization and chronic indwelling catheterization.

CONTRAINDICATIONS

Oxybutynin chloride is contraindicated in patients with urinary retention, gastric retention and other severe decreased gastrointestinal motility conditions, uncontrolled narrow-angle glaucoma and in patients who are at risk for these conditions.

Oxybutynin chloride is also contraindicated in patients who have demonstrated hypersensitivity to the drug substance or other components of the product.

PRECAUTIONS

GENERAL

Oxybutynin chloride should be used with caution in the frail elderly, in patients with hepatic or renal impairment and in patients with myasthenia gravis.

Oxybutynin chloride may aggravate the symptoms of hyperthyroidism, coronary heart disease, congestive heart failure, cardiac arrhythmias, hiatal hernia, tachycardia, hypertension, myasthenia gravis, and prostatic hypertrophy.

Urinary Retention

Oxybutynin chloride should be administered with caution to patients with clinically significant bladder outflow obstruction because of the risk of urinary retention (see CONTRAINDICATIONS).

Gastrointestinal Disorders

Oxybutynin chloride should be administered with caution to patients with gastrointestinal obstructive disorders because of the risk of gastric retention (see CONTRAINDICATIONS).

Administration of oxybutynin chloride tablets to patients with ulcerative colitis may suppress intestinal motility to the point of producing a paralytic ileus and precipitate or aggravate toxic megacolon, a serious complication of the disease.

Oxybutynin chloride, like other anticholinergic drugs, may decrease gastrointestinal motility and should be used with caution in patients with conditions such as ulcerative colitis, and intestinal atony.

Oxybutynin chloride should be used with caution in patients who have gastroesophageal reflux and/or who are concurrently taking drugs (such as bisphosphonates) that can cause or exacerbate esophagitis.

As with any other nondeformable material, caution should be used when administering oxybutynin chloride extended-release tablets to patients with preexisting severe gastrointestinal narrowing (pathologic or iatrogenic). There have been rare reports of obstructive symptoms in patients with known strictures in association with the ingestion of other drugs in nondeformable controlled-release formulations.

INFORMATION FOR THE PATIENT

Patients should be informed that heat prostration (fever and heat stroke due to decreased sweating) can occur when anticholinergics such as oxybutynin chloride are administered in the presence of high environmental temperature.

Because anticholinergic agents such as oxybutynin may produce drowsiness (somnolence) or blurred vision, patients should be advised to exercise caution.

Patients should be informed that alcohol may enhance the drowsiness caused by anticholinergic agents such as oxybutynin.

Patients should be informed that oxybutynin chloride extended-release tablets should be swallowed whole with the aid of liquids. Patients should not chew, divide, or crush tablets. The medication is contained within a nonabsorbable shell designed to release the drug at a controlled rate. The tablet shell is eliminated from the body; patients should not be concerned if they occasionally notice in their stool something that looks like a tablet.

CARCINOGENESIS, MUTAGENESIS, AND IMPAIRMENT OF FERTILITY

A 24 month study in rats at dosages of oxybutynin chloride of 20, 80 and 160 mg/kg/day showed no evidence of carcinogenicity. These doses are approximately 6, 25 and 50 times the maximum human exposure, based on surface area.

Oxybutynin chloride showed no increase of mutagenic activity when tested in *Schizosaccharomyces pompholiciformis, Saccharomyces cerevisiae* and *Salmonella typhimurium* test systems.

Reproduction studies using oxybutynin chloride in the hamster, rabbit, rat, and mouse have shown no definite evidence of impaired fertility.

PREGNANCY CATEGORY B

Reproduction studies using oxybutynin chloride in the hamster, rabbit, rat, and mouse have shown no definite evidence of impaired fertility or harm to the animal fetus. The safety of oxybutynin chloride administered to women who are or who may become pregnant has not been established. Therefore, oxybutynin chloride should not be given to pregnant women unless, in the judgment of the physician, the probable clinical benefits outweigh the possible hazards.

NURSING MOTHERS

It is not known whether this drug is excreted in human milk. Because many drugs are excreted in human milk, caution should be exercised when oxybutynin chloride is administered to a nursing woman.

PEDIATRIC USE

Tablets and Syrup

The safety and efficacy of oxybutynin chloride administration have been demonstrated for pediatric patients 5 years of age and older (see DOSAGE AND ADMINISTRATION: Tablets and Syrup).

The safety and efficacy of oxybutynin chloride tablets and syrup were studied in 30 and in 26 children, respectively, in a 24 week, open-label trial. Patients were aged 5-15 years, all had symptoms of detrusor overactivity in association with a neurological condition (*e.g.,* spina bifida), all used clean intermittent catheterization, and all were current users of oxybutynin chloride. Study results demonstrated that the administration of oxybutynin chloride was associated with improvement in clinical and urodynamic parameters.

At total daily doses ranging from 5-15 mg, treatment with oxybutynin chloride tablets was associated with an increase from baseline in mean urine volume per catheterization from 122-145 ml, an increase from baseline in mean urine volume after morning awakening from 148-168 ml, and an increase from baseline in the mean percentage of catheterizations without a leaking episode from 43-61%. Urodynamic results in these patients were consistent with the clinical results. Treatment with oxybutynin chloride tablets was associated with an increase from baseline in maximum cystometric capacity from 230-279 ml, a decrease from baseline in mean detrusor pressure at maximum cystometric capacity from 36 to 33 cm

H_2O, and a reduction in the percentage of patients demonstrating uninhibited detrusor contractions (of at least 15 cm H_2O) from 39% to 20%.

At total daily doses ranging from 5-30 mg, treatment with oxybutynin chloride syrup was associated with an increase from baseline in mean urine volume per catheterization from 113-133 ml, an increase from baseline in mean urine volume after morning awakening from 143-165 ml, and an increase from baseline in the mean percentage of catheterizations without a leaking episode from 34-63%. Urodynamic results were consistent with these clinical results. Treatment with oxybutynin chloride syrup was associated with an increase from baseline in maximum cystometric capacity from 192-294 ml, a decrease from baseline in mean detrusor pressure at maximum cystometric capacity from 46 to 37 cm H_2O, and a reduction in the percentage of patients demonstrating uninhibited detrusor contractions (of at least 15 cm H_2O) from 67% to 28%.

As there is insufficient clinical data for pediatric populations under age 5, oxybutynin chloride is not recommended for this age group.

Extended-Release Tablets

The safety and efficacy of oxybutynin chloride extended-release tablets were studied in 60 children in a 24 week, open-label trial. Patients were aged 6-15 years, all had symptoms of detrusor overactivity in association with a neurological condition (*e.g.,* spina bifida), all used clean intermittent catheterization, and all were current users of oxybutynin chloride. Study results demonstrated that administration of oxybutynin chloride extended-release tablets 5-20 mg/day was associated with an increase from baseline in mean urine volume per catheterization from 108-136 ml, an increase from baseline in mean urine volume after morning awakening from 148-189 ml, and an increase from baseline in the mean percentage of catheterizations without a leaking episode from 34-51%.

Urodynamic results were consistent with clinical results. Administration of oxybutynin chloride extended-release tablets resulted in an increase from baseline in mean maximum cystometric capacity from 185-254 ml, a decrease from baseline in mean detrusor pressure at maximum cystometric capacity from 44 to 33 cm H_2O, and a reduction in the percentage of patients demonstrating uninhibited detrusor contractions (of at least 15 cm H_2O) from 60% to 28%.

Oxybutynin chloride extended-release tablets is not recommended in pediatric patients who can not swallow the tablet whole without chewing, dividing, or crushing, or in children under the age of 6 (see DOSAGE AND ADMINISTRATION, Extended-Release Tablets).

GERIATRIC USE

Tablets and Syrup

Clinical studies of oxybutynin chloride did not include sufficient numbers of subjects age 65 and over to determine whether they respond differently from younger patients. Other reported clinical experience has not identified differences in responses between healthy elderly and younger patients; however, a lower initial starting dose of 2.5 mg given 2 or 3 times a day has been recommended for the frail elderly due to a prolongation of the elimination half-life from 2-3 hours to 5 hours.[2,3,4] In general, dose selection for an elderly patient should be cautious, usually starting at the low end of the dosing range, reflecting the greater frequency of decreased hepatic, renal or cardiac function, and of concomitant disease or other drug therapy.

Extended-Release Tablets

The rate and severity of anticholinergic effects reported by patients less than 65 years old and those 65 years and older were similar (see CLINICAL PHARMACOLOGY, Extended-Release Tablets, Pharmacokinetics, Special Populations, Gender).

DRUG INTERACTIONS

The concomitant use of oxybutynin with other anticholinergic drugs or with other agents which produce dry mouth, constipation, somnolence (drowsiness), and/or other anticholinergic-like effects may increase the frequency and/or severity of such effects.

Anticholinergic agents may potentially alter the absorption of some concomitantly administered drugs due to anticholinergic effects on gastrointestinal motility. This may be of concern for drugs with a narrow therapeutic index.

Mean oxybutynin chloride plasma concentrations were approximately 3- to 4-fold higher when oxybutynin chloride tablets were administered with ketoconazole, and 2-fold higher when oxybutynin chloride extended-release tablets were administered with ketoconazole, a potent CYP3A4 inhibitor.

Other inhibitors of the cytochrome P450 3A4 enzyme system, such as antimycotic agents (*e.g.,* itraconazole and miconazole) or macrolide antibiotics (*e.g.,* erythromycin and clarithromycin), may alter oxybutynin mean pharmacokinetic parameters (*i.e.,* C_{max} and AUC). The clinical relevance of such potential interactions is not known. Caution should be used when such drugs are coadministered.

ADVERSE REACTIONS

TABLETS AND SYRUP

The safety and efficacy of oxybutynin chloride was evaluated in a total of 199 patients in three clinical trials comparing oxybutynin chloride with oxybutynin chloride extended-release tablets (see TABLE 6). These participants were treated with oxybutynin chloride 5-20 mg/day for up to 6 weeks. TABLE 6 shows the incidence of adverse events judged by investigator to be at least possibly related to treatment and reported by at least 5% of patients.

The most common adverse events reported by patients receiving oxybutynin chloride 5-20 mg/day were the expected side effects of anticholinergic agents. The incidence of dry mouth was dose-related.

In addition, the following adverse events were reported by 2 to <5% of patients using oxybutynin chloride (5-20 mg/day) in all studies:

General: Asthenia, dry nasal and sinus mucous membranes.
Cardiovascular: Palpitation.
Metabolic and Nutritional System: Peripheral edema.
Nervous System: Insomnia, nervousness, confusion.
Skin: Dry skin.
Special Senses: Dry eyes, taste perversion.

TABLE 6 *Incidence (%) of Adverse Events Reported by >5% of Patients Using Oxybutynin Chloride (5-20 mg/day)*

Body System / Adverse Event	Oxybutynin Chloride (5-20 mg/day) (n=199)
General	
Abdominal pain	6.5%
Headache	6.0%
Digestive	
Dry mouth	71.4%
Constipation	12.6%
Nausea	10.1%
Dyspepsia	7.0%
Diarrhea	5.0%
Nervous	
Dizziness	15.6%
Somnolence	12.6%
Special Senses	
Blurred vision	9.0%
Urogenital	
Urination impaired	10.6%
Post void residuals increase	5.0%
Urinary tract infection	5.0%

Other adverse events that have been reported include: Tachycardia, hallucinations, cycloplegia, mydriasis, impotence, suppression of lactation, vasodilatation, rash, decreased gastrointestinal motility, flatulence, urinary retention, convulsions and decreased sweating.

EXTENDED-RELEASE TABLETS

The safety and efficacy of oxybutynin chloride extended-release tablets was evaluated in a total of 580 participants who received oxybutynin chloride extended-release tablets in clinical trials (429 patients, 151 healthy volunteers). These participants were treated with 5-30 mg/day for up to 4.5 months. Safety information is provided for 429 patients from three controlled clinical studies and one open label study (TABLE 7). The adverse events are reported regardless of causality.

TABLE 7 *Incidence (%) of Adverse Events Reported by ≥5% of Patients Using Oxybutynin Chloride Extended-Release Tablets (5-30 mg/day)*

Body System / Adverse Event	Oxybutynin Chloride Extended-Release Tablets (5-30 mg/day) (n=429)
General	
Headache	9.8%
Asthenia	6.8%
Pain	6.8%
Digestive	
Dry mouth	60.8%
Constipation	13.1%
Diarrhea	9.1%
Nausea	8.9%
Dyspepsia	6.8%
Nervous	
Somnolence	11.9%
Dizziness	6.3%
Respiratory	
Rhinitis	5.6%
Special Senses	
Blurred vision	7.7%
Dry eyes	6.1%
Urogenital	
Urinary tract infection	5.1%

The most common adverse events reported by patients receiving 5-30 mg/day oxybutynin chloride extended-release tablets were the expected side effects of anticholinergic agents. The incidence of dry mouth was dose-related.

The discontinuation rate for all adverse events was 6.8%. The most frequent adverse event causing early discontinuation of study medication was nausea (1.9%), while discontinuation due to dry mouth was 1.2%.

In addition, the following adverse events were reported by 2 to <5% of patients using oxybutynin chloride extended-release tablets (5-30 mg/day) in all studies:

General: Abdominal pain, dry nasal and sinus mucous membranes, accidental injury, back pain, flu syndrome.
Cardiovascular: Hypertension, palpitation, vasodilation.
Digestive: Flatulence, gastroesophageal reflux.
Musculoskeletal: Arthritis.
Nervous: Insomnia, nervousness, confusion.
Respiratory: Upper respiratory tract infection, cough, sinusitis, bronchitis, pharyngitis.
Skin: Dry skin, rash.
Urogenital: Impaired urination (hesitancy), increased post void residual volume, urinary retention, cystitis.

Additional rare adverse events reported from worldwide post-marketing experience with oxybutynin chloride extended-release tablets include: Peripheral edema, cardiac arrhythmia, tachycardia, hallucinations, convulsions, and impotence.

Additional adverse events reported with some other oxybutynin chloride formulations include: Cycloplegia, mydriasis, and suppression of lactation.

O

DOSAGE AND ADMINISTRATION

TABLETS

Adults: The usual dose is one 5 mg tablet 2-3 times a day. The maximum recommended dose is one 5 mg tablet 4 times a day. A lower starting dose of 2.5 mg two or three times a day is recommended for the frail elderly.

Pediatric patients over 5 years of age: The usual dose is one 5 mg tablet 2 times a day. The maximum recommended dose is one 5 mg tablet 3 times a day.

SYRUP

Adults: The usual dose is 1 teaspoon (5 mg/5 ml) syrup 2-3 times a day. The maximum recommended dose is 1 teaspoon (5 mg/5 ml) syrup 4 times a day. A lower starting dose of 2.5 mg two or three times a day is recommended for the frail elderly.

Pediatric patients over 5 years of age: The usual dose is 1 teaspoon (5 mg/5 ml) 2 times a day. The maximum recommended dose is 1 teaspoon (5 mg/5 ml) 3 times a day.

EXTENDED-RELEASE TABLETS

Oxybutynin chloride extended-release tablets must be swallowed whole with the aid of liquids, and must not be chewed, divided, or crushed.

Oxybutynin chloride extended-release tablets may be administered with or without food.

Adults: The recommended starting dose of oxybutynin chloride extended-release tablets is 5 mg once daily. Dosage may be adjusted in 5 mg increments to achieve a balance of efficacy and tolerability (up to a maximum of 30 mg/day). In general, dosage adjustment may proceed at approximately weekly intervals.

Pediatric patients aged 6 years of age and older: The recommended starting dose of oxybutynin chloride extended-release tablets is 5 mg once daily. Dosage may be adjusted in 5 mg increments to achieve a balance of efficacy and tolerability (up to a maximum of 20 mg/day).

HOW SUPPLIED

TABLETS

Ditropan tablets are supplied as blue scored tablets (5 mg) engraved with "DITROPAN" on one side with "92" and "00", separated by a horizontal score, on the other side.
Storage: Store at controlled room temperature (59-86°F).
Dispense in tight, light-resistant container.

SYRUP

Ditropan syrup (5 mg/5 ml) is supplied in bottles of 16 fl oz (473 ml).
Storage: Store at controlled room temperature (59-86°F).
Dispense in tight, light-resistant container.

EXTENDED-RELEASE TABLETS

Ditropan XL tablets are available in 3 dosage strengths, 5 mg (pale yellow), 10 mg (pink) and 15 mg (gray) and are imprinted with "5 XL", "10 XL" or "15 XL".
Storage: Store at 25°C (77°F); excursions permitted to 15-30°C (59-86°F). Protect from moisture and humidity.

TRANSDERMAL

O

DESCRIPTION

Oxytrol, oxybutynin transdermal system, is designed to deliver oxybutynin continuously and consistently over a 3-4 day interval after application to intact skin. Oxytrol is available as a 39 cm^2 system containing 36 mg of oxybutynin. Oxytrol has a nominal *in vivo* delivery rate of 3.9 mg oxybutynin per day through skin of average permeability (interindividual variation in skin permeability is approximately 20%).

Oxybutynin is an antispasmodic, anticholinergic agent. Oxybutynin is administered as a racemate of R- and S-isomers. Chemically, oxybutynin is d,l(racemic)4-diethylamino-2-butynyl phenylcyclohexylglycolate. The empirical formula of oxybutynin is $C_{22}H_{31}NO_3$.

Oxybutynin is a white powder with a molecular weight of 357. It is soluble in alcohol, but relatively insoluble in water.

TRANSDERMAL SYSTEM COMPONENTS

Oxytrol is a matrix-type transdermal system composed of 3 layers. Layer 1 (backing film) is a thin flexible polyester/ethylene-vinyl acetate film that provides the matrix system with occlusivity and physical integrity and protects the adhesive/drug layer. Layer 2 (adhesive/drug layer) is a cast film of acrylic adhesive containing oxybutynin and triacetin. Layer 3 (release liner) is two overlapped siliconized polyester strips that are peeled off and discarded by the patient prior to applying the matrix system.

CLINICAL PHARMACOLOGY

The free base form of oxybutynin is pharmacologically equivalent to oxybutynin hydrochloride. Oxybutynin acts as a competitive antagonist of acetylcholine at postganglionic muscarinic receptors, resulting in relaxation of bladder smooth muscle. In patients with conditions characterized by involuntary detrusor contractions, cystometric studies have demonstrated that oxybutynin increases maximum urinary bladder capacity and increases the volume to first detrusor contraction. Oxybutynin thus decreases urinary urgency and the frequency of both incontinence episodes and voluntary urination.

Oxybutynin is a racemic (50:50) mixture of R- and S-isomers. Antimuscarinic activity resides predominantly in the R-isomer. The active metabolite, N-desethyloxybutynin, has pharmacological activity on the human detrusor muscle that is similar to that of oxybutynin in *in vitro* studies.

PHARMACOKINETICS

Absorption

Oxybutynin is transported across intact skin and into the systemic circulation by passive diffusion across the stratum corneum. The average daily dose of oxybutynin absorbed from the 39 cm^2 oxybutynin transdermal system is 3.9 mg. The average (SD) nominal dose, 0.10 (0.02) mg oxybutynin per cm^2 surface area, was obtained from analysis of residual oxybutynin content of systems worn over a continuous 4 day period during 303 separate occasions in 76 healthy volunteers. Following application of the first oxybutynin transdermal 3.9 mg/day system, oxybutynin plasma concentration increases for approximately 24-48 hours, reaching average maximum concentrations of 3-4 ng/ml. Thereafter, steady concentrations are maintained for up to 96 hours. Absorption of oxybutynin is bioequivalent when oxybutynin transdermal is applied to the abdomen, buttocks, or hip.

Steady-state conditions are reached during the second oxybutynin transdermal application. Average steady-state plasma concentrations were 3.1 ng/ml for oxybutynin and 3.8 ng/ml for N-desethyloxybutynin. TABLE 8 provides a summary of pharmacokinetic parameters of oxybutynin in healthy volunteers after single and multiple applications of oxybutynin transdermal.

TABLE 8 *Mean (SD) Oxybutynin Pharmacokinetic Parameters From Single and Multiple Dose Studies in Healthy Men and Women Volunteers After Application of Oxybutynin Transdermal on Abdomen*

	Oxybutynin Single Dose		Oxybutynin Multiple Dose	
C_{max} (SD) (ng/ml)	3.0 (0.8)	3.4 (1.1)	6.6 (2.4)	4.2 (1.0)
T_{max}* (h)	48	36	10	28
C_{avg} (SD) (ng/ml)	—	—	4.2 (1.1)	3.1 (0.7)
AUC (SD) (ng/ml×h)	245 (59)†	279 (99)†	408 (108)‡	259 (57)§

* T_{max} given as median.
† AUC(∞).
‡ AUC(0-96).
§ AUC(0-84).

Distribution

Oxybutynin is widely distributed in body tissues following systemic absorption. The volume of distribution was estimated to be 193 L after IV administration of 5 mg oxybutynin chloride.

Metabolism

Oxybutynin is metabolized primarily by the cytochrome P450 enzyme systems, particularly CYP3A4, found mostly in the liver and gut wall. Metabolites include phenylcyclohexylglycolic acid, which is pharmacologically inactive, and N-desethyloxybutynin, which is pharmacologically active.

After oral administration of oxybutynin, pre-systemic first-pass metabolism results in an oral bioavailability of approximately 6% and higher plasma concentration of the N-desethyl metabolite compared to oxybutynin. The plasma concentration AUC ratio of N-desethyl metabolite to parent compound following a single 5 mg oral dose of oxybutynin chloride was 11.9:1.

Transdermal administration of oxybutynin bypasses the first-pass gastrointestinal and hepatic metabolism, reducing the formation of the N-desethyl metabolite. Only small amounts of CYP3A4 are found in skin, limiting pre-systemic metabolism during transdermal absorption. The resulting plasma concentration AUC ratio of N-desethyl metabolite to parent compound following multiple oxybutynin transdermal applications was 1.3:1.

Following IV administration, the elimination half-life of oxybutynin is approximately 2 hours. Following removal of oxybutynin transdermal, plasma concentrations of oxybutynin and N-desethyloxybutynin decline with an apparent half-life of approximately 7-8 hours.

Excretion

Oxybutynin is extensively metabolized by the liver, with less than 0.1% of the administered dose excreted unchanged in the urine. Also, less than 0.1% of the administered dose is excreted as the metabolite N-desethyloxybutynin.

Special Populations

Geriatric: The pharmacokinetics of oxybutynin and N-desethyloxybutynin were similar in all patients studied.

Pediatric: The pharmacokinetics of oxybutynin and N-desethyloxybutynin were not evaluated in individuals younger than 18 years of age. See PRECAUTIONS, Pediatric Use.

Gender: There were no significant differences in the pharmacokinetics of oxybutynin in healthy male and female volunteers following application of oxybutynin transdermal.

Race: Available data suggest that there are no significant differences in the pharmacokinetics of oxybutynin based on race in healthy volunteers following administration of oxybutynin transdermal. Japanese volunteers demonstrated a somewhat lower metabolism of oxybutynin to N-desethyloxybutynin compared to Caucasian volunteers.

Renal Insufficiency: There is no experience with the use of oxybutynin transdermal in patients with renal insufficiency.

Hepatic Insufficiency: There is no experience with the use of oxybutynin transdermal in patients with hepatic insufficiency.

Drug-Drug Interactions: See DRUG INTERACTIONS.

ADHESION

Adhesion was periodically evaluated during the Phase 3 studies. Of the 4746 oxybutynin transdermal evaluations in the Phase 3 trials, 20 (0.4%) were observed at clinic visits to have become completely detached and 35 (0.7%) became partially detached during routine clinic use. Similar to the pharmacokinetic studies, >98% of the systems evaluated in the Phase 3 studies were assessed as being ≥75% attached and thus would be expected to perform as anticipated.

INDICATIONS AND USAGE

Oxybutynin transdermal is indicated for the treatment of overactive bladder with symptoms of urge urinary incontinence, urgency, and frequency.

CONTRAINDICATIONS

Oxybutynin transdermal is contraindicated in patients with urinary retention, gastric retention, or uncontrolled narrow-angle glaucoma and in patients who are at risk for these conditions. Oxybutynin transdermal is also contraindicated in patients who have demonstrated hypersensitivity to oxybutynin or other components of the product.

PRECAUTIONS

GENERAL

Oxybutynin transdermal should be used with caution in patients with hepatic or renal impairment.

Urinary Retention

Oxybutynin transdermal should be administered with caution to patients with clinically significant bladder outflow obstruction because of the risk of urinary retention (see CONTRAINDICATIONS).

Gastrointestinal Disorders

Oxybutynin transdermal should be administered with caution to patients with gastrointestinal obstructive disorders because of the risk of gastric retention (see CONTRAINDICATIONS).

Oxybutynin transdermal, like other anticholinergic drugs, may decrease gastrointestinal motility and should be used with caution in patients with conditions such as ulcerative colitis, intestinal atony, and myasthenia gravis. Oxybutynin transdermal should be used with caution in patients who have gastroesophageal reflux and/or who are concurrently taking drugs (such as bisphosphonates) that can cause or exacerbate esophagitis.

INFORMATION FOR THE PATIENT

Patients should be informed that heat prostration (fever and heat stroke due to decreased sweating) can occur when anticholinergics such as oxybutynin are used in a hot environment. Because anticholinergic agents such as oxybutynin may produce drowsiness (somnolence) or blurred vision, patients should be advised to exercise caution. Patients should be informed that alcohol may enhance the drowsiness caused by anticholinergic agents such as oxybutynin.

Oxybutynin transdermal should be applied to dry, intact skin on the abdomen, hip, or buttock. A new application site should be selected with each new system to avoid re-application to the same site within 7 days. Details on use of the system are explained in the patient information leaflet that should be dispensed with the product.

CARCINOGENESIS, MUTAGENESIS, AND IMPAIRMENT OF FERTILITY

A 24 month study in rats at dosages of oxybutynin chloride of 20, 80 and 160 mg/kg showed no evidence of carcinogenicity. These doses are approximately 6, 25 and 50 times the maximum exposure in humans taking an oral dose based on body surface area.

Oxybutynin chloride showed no increase of mutagenic activity when tested in *Schizosaccharomyces pompholiciformis, Saccharomyces cerevisiae*, and *Salmonella typhimurium* test systems. Reproduction studies with oxybutynin chloride in the mouse, rat, hamster, and rabbit showed no definite evidence of impaired fertility.

PREGNANCY, TERATOGENIC EFFECTS, PREGNANCY CATEGORY B

Reproduction studies with oxybutynin chloride in the mouse, rat, hamster, and rabbit showed no definite evidence of impaired fertility or harm to the animal fetus. Subcutaneous administration to rats at doses up to 25 mg/kg (approximately 50 times the human exposure based on surface area) and to rabbits at doses up to 0.4 mg/kg (approximately 1 times the human exposure) revealed no evidence of harm to the fetus due to oxybutynin chloride. The safety of oxybutynin transdermal administration to women who are or who may become pregnant has not been established. Therefore, oxybutynin transdermal should not be given to pregnant women unless, in the judgment of the physician, the probable clinical benefits outweigh the possible hazards.

NURSING MOTHERS

It is not known whether oxybutynin is excreted in human milk. Because many drugs are excreted in human milk, caution should be exercised when oxybutynin transdermal is administered to a nursing woman.

PEDIATRIC USE

The safety and efficacy of oxybutynin transdermal in pediatric patients have not been established.

GERIATRIC USE

Of the total number of patients in the clinical studies of oxybutynin transdermal, 49% were 65 and over. No overall differences in safety or effectiveness were observed between these subjects and younger subjects, and other reported clinical experience has not identified differences in response between elderly and younger patients, but greater sensitivity of some older individuals cannot be ruled out (see CLINICAL PHARMACOLOGY, Pharmacokinetics, Special Populations, Geriatric).

DRUG INTERACTIONS

The concomitant use of oxybutynin with other anticholinergic drugs or with other agents that produce dry mouth, constipation, somnolence, and/or other anticholinergic-like effects may increase the frequency and/or severity of such effects.

Anticholinergic agents may potentially alter the absorption of some concomitantly administered drugs due to anticholinergic effects on gastrointestinal motility.

Pharmacokinetic studies have not been performed with patients concomitantly receiving cytochrome P450 enzyme inhibitors, such as antimycotic agents (*e.g.*, ketoconazole, itraconazole, and miconazole) or macrolide antibiotics (*e.g.*, erythromycin and clarithromycin). No specific drug-drug interaction studies have been performed with oxybutynin transdermal.

ADVERSE REACTIONS

The safety of oxybutynin transdermal was evaluated in a total of 417 patients who participated in two Phase 3 clinical efficacy and safety studies and an open-label extension. Additional safety information was collected in Phase 1 and Phase 2 trials. In the two pivotal studies, a total of 246 patients received oxybutynin transdermal during the 12 week treatment periods. A total of 411 patients entered the open-label extension and of those, 65 patients and 52 patients received oxybutynin transdermal for at least 24 weeks and at least 36 weeks, respectively.

No deaths were reported during treatment. No serious adverse events related to treatment were reported.

Adverse events reported in the pivotal trials are summarized in TABLE 11 and TABLE 12.

TABLE 11 *Number (%) of Adverse Events Occurring in ≥2% of Oxybutynin Transdermal-Treated Patients and Greater in Oxybutynin Transdermal Group Than in Placebo Group (Study 1)*

Adverse Event*	Placebo (n=132)	Oxybutynin Transdermal (3.9 mg/day) (n=125)
Application site pruritus	8 (6.1%)	21 (16.8%)
Dry mouth	11 (8.3%)	12 (9.6%)
Application site erythema	3 (2.3%)	7 (5.6%)
Application site vesicles	0 (0.0%)	4 (3.2%)
Diarrhea	3 (2.3%)	4 (3.2%)
Dysuria	0 (0.0%)	3 (2.4%)

* Includes adverse events judged by the investigator as possibly, probably or definitely treatment-related.

TABLE 12 *Number (%) of Adverse Events Occurring in ≥2% of Oxybutynin Transdermal-Treated Patients and Greater in Oxybutynin Transdermal Group Than in Placebo Group (Study 2)*

Adverse Event*	Placebo (n=117)	Oxybutynin Transdermal (3.9 mg/day) (n=121)
Application site pruritus	5 (4.3%)	17 (14.0%)
Application site erythema	2 (1.7%)	10 (8.3%)
Dry mouth	2 (1.7%)	5 (4.1%)
Constipation	0 (0.0%)	4 (3.3%)
Application site rash	1 (0.9%)	4 (3.3%)
Application site macules	0 (0.0%)	3 (2.5%)
Abnormal vision	0 (0.0%)	3 (2.5%)

* Includes adverse events judged by the investigator as possibly, probably or definitely treatment-related.

Other adverse events reported by >1% of oxybutynin transdermal-treated patients, and judged by the investigator to be possibly, probably or definitely related to treatment include: abdominal pain, nausea, flatulence, fatigue, somnolence, headache, flushing, rash, application site burning and back pain.

Most treatment-related adverse events were described as mild or moderate in intensity. Severe application site reactions were reported by 6.4% of oxybutynin transdermal-treated patients in Study 1 and by 5.0% of oxybutynin transdermal-treated patients in Study 2.

Treatment-related adverse events that resulted in discontinuation were reported by 11.2% of oxybutynin transdermal-treated patients in Study 1 and 10.7% of oxybutynin transdermal-treated patients in Study 2. Most of these were secondary to application site reaction. In the two pivotal studies, no patient discontinued oxybutynin transdermal treatment due to dry mouth.

In the open-label extension, the most common treatment-related adverse events were: application site pruritus, application site erythema and dry mouth.

DOSAGE AND ADMINISTRATION

Oxybutynin transdermal should be applied to dry, intact skin on the abdomen, hip, or buttock. A new application site should be selected with each new system to avoid re-application to the same site within 7 days.

The dose of oxybutynin transdermal is one 3.9 mg/day system applied twice weekly (every 3-4 days).

HOW SUPPLIED

Oxytrol 3.9 mg/day (oxybutynin transdermal system). Each 39 cm^2 system imprinted with Oxytrol 3.9 mg/day contains 36 mg oxybutynin for nominal delivery of 3.9 mg oxybutynin per day when dosed in a twice weekly regimen.

Storage: Store at 25°C (77°F); excursions permitted to 15-30°C (59-86°F). Protect from moisture and humidity. Do not store outside the sealed pouch. Apply immediately after removal from the protective pouch. Discard used Oxytrol in household trash in a manner that prevents accidental application or ingestion by children, pets, or others.

PRODUCT LISTING - RATED THERAPEUTICALLY EQUIVALENT

Syrup - Oral - 5 mg/5 ml

5 ml	$78.00	GENERIC, Pharmaceutical Assoc Inc Div Beach Products	00121-0671-05
473 ml	$33.80	GENERIC, Pharmaceutical Assoc Inc Div Beach Products	00121-0671-16
473 ml	$39.99	GENERIC, Boca Pharmacal Inc	64376-0402-16

473 ml	$51.95	GENERIC, Morton Grove Pharmaceuticals Inc	60432-0092-16
473 ml	$52.49	GENERIC, Cypress Pharmaceutical Inc	60258-0071-16
473 ml	$105.25	DITROPAN, Alza	17314-9201-04
480 ml	$38.95	GENERIC, Qualitest Products Inc	00603-1490-58
480 ml	$39.98	GENERIC, Silarx Pharmaceuticals Inc	54838-0510-80
480 ml	$66.32	GENERIC, Apotex Usa Inc	60505-6008-09
Tablet - Oral - 5 mg			
25's	$11.15	GENERIC, Udl Laboratories Inc	51079-0628-19
30 x 25	$331.65	GENERIC, Sky Pharmaceuticals Packaging, Inc	63739-0195-01
30 x 25	$331.65	GENERIC, Sky Pharmaceuticals Packaging, Inc	63739-0195-03
30's	$13.36	GENERIC, Heartland Healthcare Services	61392-0138-30
30's	$13.36	GENERIC, Heartland Healthcare Services	61392-0138-39
30's	$16.31	GENERIC, Qualitest Products Inc	00603-4975-16
31 x 10	$141.79	GENERIC, Vangard Labs	00615-3512-53
31 x 10	$141.79	GENERIC, Vangard Labs	00615-3512-63
31's	$13.81	GENERIC, Heartland Healthcare Services	61392-0138-31
32's	$14.25	GENERIC, Heartland Healthcare Services	61392-0138-32
45's	$20.04	GENERIC, Heartland Healthcare Services	61392-0138-45
60's	$26.73	GENERIC, Heartland Healthcare Services	61392-0138-60
60's	$32.62	GENERIC, Qualitest Products Inc	00603-4975-20
90's	$40.09	GENERIC, Heartland Healthcare Services	61392-0138-90
90's	$48.94	GENERIC, Qualitest Products Inc	00603-4975-02
100's	$12.60	FEDERAL UPPER LIMIT, H.C.F.A. F F P	99999-1930-01
100's	$19.31	GENERIC, Us Trading Corporation	56126-0404-11
100's	$25.00	GENERIC, Raway Pharmacal Inc	00686-0628-20
100's	$26.61	GENERIC, Auro Pharmaceutical	55829-0397-10
100's	$31.50	GENERIC, Alza	00575-1900-01
100's	$31.96	GENERIC, Dixon-Shane Inc	17236-0850-11
100's	$36.50	GENERIC, Parmed Pharmaceuticals Inc	00349-8827-01
100's	$37.53	GENERIC, Moore, H.L. Drug Exchange Inc	00839-7504-06
100's	$38.20	GENERIC, Major Pharmaceuticals Inc	00904-2821-60
100's	$38.59	GENERIC, Ivax Corporation	00182-1289-01
100's	$38.60	GENERIC, Geneva Pharmaceuticals	00781-1629-01
100's	$38.60	GENERIC, Martec Pharmaceuticals Inc	52555-0105-01
100's	$38.60	GENERIC, Martec Pharmaceuticals Inc	52555-0685-01
100's	$38.68	GENERIC, Aligen Independent Laboratories Inc	00405-4735-01
100's	$39.99	GENERIC, Geneva Pharmaceuticals	00781-1629-13
100's	$40.45	GENERIC, Mutual/United Research Laboratories	00677-1759-01
100's	$40.45	GENERIC, Dixon-Shane Inc	17236-0850-01
100's	$44.36	GENERIC, Ivax Corporation	00182-1289-89
100's	$44.59	GENERIC, Udl Laboratories Inc	51079-0628-20
100's	$47.86	GENERIC, Watson Laboratories Inc	52544-0779-01
100's	$54.38	GENERIC, Vintage Pharmaceuticals Inc	00254-4853-28
100's	$54.38	GENERIC, Qualitest Products Inc	00603-4975-21
100's	$54.38	GENERIC, Sidmak Laboratories Inc	50111-0456-01
100's	$56.32	GENERIC, Rosemont Pharmaceutical Corporation	00832-0038-00
100's	$61.96	GENERIC, Major Pharmaceuticals Inc	00904-2821-61
100's	$64.32	DITROPAN, Aventis Pharmaceuticals	00088-1375-47
100's	$70.20	DITROPAN, Aventis Pharmaceuticals	00088-1375-49
100's	$85.08	DITROPAN, Alza	17314-9200-03
100's	$97.14	DITROPAN, Alza	17314-9200-01
120's	$61.99	GENERIC, Qualitest Products Inc	00603-4975-22
180's	$92.98	GENERIC, Qualitest Products Inc	00603-4975-04
270's	$139.48	GENERIC, Qualitest Products Inc	00603-4975-03

PRODUCT LISTING - EQUIVALENTS NOT AVAILABLE

Tablet - Oral - 5 mg			
30's	$5.52	GENERIC, Physicians Total Care	54868-2157-01
30's	$9.71	GENERIC, Southwood Pharmaceuticals Inc	58016-0908-30
30's	$11.58	GENERIC, Allscripts Pharmaceutical Company	54569-1990-00
90's	$35.56	GENERIC, Pharmaceutical Corporation Of America	51655-0665-26
100's	$15.28	GENERIC, Physicians Total Care	54868-2157-02
100's	$38.60	GENERIC, Watson/Rugby Laboratories Inc	00536-5672-01
Tablet, Extended Release - Oral - 5 mg			
100's	$293.18	DITROPAN XL, Alza	17314-8500-01
Tablet, Extended Release - Oral - 10 mg			
100's	$304.70	DITROPAN XL, Alza	17314-8501-01
Tablet, Extended Release - Oral - 15 mg			
100's	$337.48	DITROPAN XL, Alza	17314-8502-01

Oxycodone Hydrochloride *(001932)*

For related information, see the comparative table section in Appendix A.

Categories: Pain, moderate to moderately severe; DEA Class CII; FDA Pre 1938 Drugs; FDA Approved 1995 Dec
Drug Classes: Analgesics, narcotic
Brand Names: Oxycontin; Roxicodone
Foreign Brand Availability: Codix 5 (Colombia); Endone (Australia); Oxicontin (Colombia); Oxycod (Israel); Oxycontin CR (Korea); Oxycontin LP (France); OxyContin (Israel); Oxygesic (Germany); Oxy IR (Canada); Supeudol (Canada)
Cost of Therapy: $8.69 (Pain; Roxicodone; 5 mg; 4 tablets/day; 7 day supply)
$18.81 (Pain; Oxycontin, Extended Release; 10 mg; 2 tablets/day; 7 day supply)

WARNING

Note: The trade name has been used throughout this monograph for clarity.

OxyContin is an opioid agonist and a Schedule II controlled substance with an abuse liability similar to morphine.Oxycodone can be abused in a manner similar to other opioid agonists, legal or illicit. This should be considered when prescribing or dispensing OxyContin in situations where the physician or pharmacist is concerned about an increased risk of misuse, abuse, or diversion.

OxyContin tablets are a controlled-release oral formulation of oxycodone hydrochloride indicated for the management of moderate to severe pain when a continuous, around-the-clock analgesic is needed for an extended period of time.

OxyContin tablets are NOT intended for use as a prn analgesic.

OxyContin 80 mg and 160 mg tablets ARE FOR USE IN OPIOID-TOLERANT PATIENTS ONLY. These tablet strengths may cause fatal respiratory depression when administered to patients not previously exposed to opioids.

OxyContin TABLETS ARE TO BE SWALLOWED WHOLE AND ARE NOT TO BE BROKEN, CHEWED, OR CRUSHED. TAKING BROKEN, CHEWED, OR CRUSHED OxyContin TABLETS LEADS TO RAPID RELEASE AND ABSORPTION OF A POTENTIALLY FATAL DOSE OF OXYCODONE.

DESCRIPTION

OxyContin (oxycodone hydrochloride controlled-release) tablets are an opioid analgesic supplied in 10, 20, 40, 80, and 160 mg tablet strengths for oral administration. The tablet strengths describe the amount of oxycodone per tablet as the hydrochloride salt.

The molecular formula for oxycodone hydrochloride is: $C_{18}H_{21}NO_4$·HCl, the molecular weight is: 351.83. The chemical formula is: 4,5-epoxy-14-hydroxy-3-methoxy-17-methylmorphinan-6-one hydrochloride.

Oxycodone is a white, odorless crystalline powder derived from the opium alkaloid, thebaine. Oxycodone hydrochloride dissolves in water (1 g in 6-7 ml). It is slightly soluble in alcohol (octanol water partition coefficient 0.7). The tablets contain the following inactive ingredients: ammonio methacrylate copolymer, hydroxypropyl methylcellulose, lactose, magnesium stearate, povidone, red iron oxide (20 mg strength tablet only), stearyl alcohol, talc, titanium dioxide, triacetin, yellow iron oxide (40 mg strength tablet only), yellow iron oxide with FD&C blue no. 2 (80 mg strength tablet only), FD&C blue no. 2 (160 mg strength tablet only) and other ingredients.

CLINICAL PHARMACOLOGY

Oxycodone is a pure agonist opioid whose principal therapeutic action is analgesia. Other members of the class known as opioid agonists include substances such as morphine, hydromorphone, fentanyl, codeine, and hydrocodone. Pharmacological effects of opioid agonists include anxiolysis, euphoria, feelings of relaxation, respiratory depression, constipation, miosis, and cough suppression, as well as analgesia. Like all pure opioid agonist analgesics, with increasing doses there is increasing analgesia, unlike with mixed agonist/antagonists or non-opioid analgesics, where there is a limit to the analgesic effect with increasing doses. With pure opioid agonist analgesics, there is no defined maximum dose; the ceiling to analgesic effectiveness is imposed only by side effects, the more serious of which may include somnolence and respiratory depression.

CENTRAL NERVOUS SYSTEM

The precise mechanism of the analgesic action is unknown. However, specific CNS opioid receptors for endogenous compounds with opioid-like activity have been identified throughout the brain and spinal cord and play a role in the analgesic effects of this drug.

Oxycodone produces respiratory depression by direct action on brain stem respiratory centers. The respiratory depression involves both a reduction in the responsiveness of the brain stem respiratory centers to increases in carbon dioxide tension and to electrical stimulation.

Oxycodone depresses the cough reflex by direct effect on the cough center in the medulla. Antitussive effects may occur with doses lower than those usually required for analgesia.

Oxycodone causes miosis, even in total darkness. Pinpoint pupils are a sign of opioid overdose but are not pathognomonic (*e.g.*, pontine lesions of hemorrhagic or ischemic origin may produce similar findings). Marked mydriasis rather than miosis may be seen with hypoxia in the setting of OxyContin overdose.

GASTROINTESTINAL TRACT AND OTHER SMOOTH MUSCLE

Oxycodone causes a reduction in motility associated with an increase in smooth muscle tone in the antrum of the stomach and duodenum. Digestion of food in the small intestine is delayed and propulsive contractions are decreased. Propulsive peristaltic waves in the colon are decreased, while tone may be increased to the point of spasm resulting in constipation. Other opioid-induced effects may include a reduction in gastric, biliary and pancreatic secretions, spasm of sphincter of Oddi, and transient elevations in serum amylase.

CARDIOVASCULAR SYSTEM

Oxycodone may produce release of histamine with or without associated peripheral vasodilation. Manifestations of histamine release and/or peripheral vasodilation may include pruritus, flushing, red eyes, sweating, and/or orthostatic hypotension.

CONCENTRATION - EFFICACY RELATIONSHIPS

Studies in normal volunteers and patients reveal predictable relationships between oxycodone dosage and plasma oxycodone concentrations, as well as between concentration and certain expected opioid effects, such as pupillary constriction, sedation, overall "drug effect", analgesia and feelings of "relaxation".

As with all opioids, the minimum effective plasma concentration for analgesia will vary widely among patients, especially among patients who have been previously treated with potent agonist opioids. As a result, patients must be treated with individualized titration of dosage to the desired effect. The minimum effective analgesic concentration of oxycodone for any individual patient may increase over time due to an increase in pain, the development of a new pain syndrome and/or the development of analgesic tolerance.

CONCENTRATION - ADVERSE EXPERIENCE RELATIONSHIPS

OxyContin tablets are associated with typical opioid-related adverse experiences. There is a general relationship between increasing oxycodone plasma concentration and increasing frequency of dose-related opioid adverse experiences such as nausea, vomiting, CNS effects, and respiratory depression. In opioid-tolerant patients, the situation is altered by the development of tolerance to opioid-related side effects, and the relationship is not clinically relevant.

As with all opioids, the dose must be individualized (see DOSAGE AND ADMINISTRATION), because the effective analgesic dose for some patients will be too high to be tolerated by other patients.

PHARMACOKINETICS AND METABOLISM

The activity of OxyContin tablets is primarily due to the parent drug oxycodone. OxyContin tablets are designed to provide controlled delivery of oxycodone over 12 hours.

Breaking, chewing or crushing OxyContin tablets eliminates the controlled delivery mechanism and results in the rapid release and absorption of a potentially fatal dose of oxycodone.

Oxycodone release from OxyContin tablets is pH independent. Oxycodone is well absorbed from OxyContin tablets with an oral bioavailability of 60-87%. The relative oral bioavailability of OxyContin to immediate-release oral dosage forms is 100%. Upon repeated dosing in normal volunteers in pharmacokinetic studies, steady-state levels were achieved within 24-36 hours. Dose proportionality and/or bioavailability has been established for the 10, 20, 40, 80, and 160 mg tablet strengths for both peak plasma levels (C_{max}) and extent of absorption (AUC). Oxycodone is extensively metabolized and eliminated primarily in the urine as both conjugated and unconjugated metabolites. The apparent elimination half-life of oxycodone following the administration of OxyContin was 4.5 hours compared to 3.2 hours for immediate-release oxycodone.

Absorption

About 60-87% of an oral dose of oxycodone reaches the central compartment in comparison to a parenteral dose. This high oral bioavailability is due to low pre-systemic and/or first-pass metabolism. In normal volunteers, the $T_{1/2}$ of absorption is 0.4 hours for immediate-release oral oxycodone. In contrast, OxyContin tablets exhibit a biphasic absorption pattern with two apparent absorption half-times of 0.6 and 6.9 hours, which describes the initial release of oxycodone from the tablet followed by a prolonged release.

Plasma Oxycodone by Time

Dose proportionality has been established for the 10, 20, 40, and 80 mg tablet strengths for both peak plasma concentrations (C_{max}) and extent of absorption (AUC) (see TABLE 1). Another study established that the 160 mg tablet is bioequivalent to 2 × 80 mg tablets as well as to 4 × 40 mg for both peak plasma concentrations (C_{max}) and extent of absorption (AUC) (see TABLE 2). Given the short half-life of elimination of oxycodone from OxyContin, steady-state plasma concentrations of oxycodone are achieved within 24-36 hours of initiation of dosing with OxyContin tablets. In a study comparing 10 mg of OxyContin every 12 hours to 5 mg of immediate-release oxycodone every 6 hours, the two treatments were found to be equivalent for AUC and C_{max}, and similar for C_{min} (trough) concentrations. There was less fluctuation in plasma concentrations for the OxyContin tablets than for the immediate-release formulation.

TABLE 1

Regimen / Dosage Form	AUC (ng·h/ml)*	C_{max} (ng/ml)	T_{max} (hours)	Trough Conc. (ng/ml)
	Mean [% coefficient variation]			
Single Dose				
10 mg†	100.7 [26.6]	10.6 [20.1]	2.7 [44.1]	n.a.
20 mg†	207.5 [35.9]	21.4 [36.6]	3.2 [57.9]	n.a.
40 mg†	423.1 [33.3]	39.3 [34.0]	3.1 [77.4]	n.a.
80 mg†‡	1085.5 [32.3]	98.5 [32.1]	2.1 [52.3]	n.a.
Multiple Dose				
10 mg† q12h	103.6 [38.6]	15.1 [31.0]	3.2 [69.5]	7.2 [48.1]
5 mg immediate release q6h	99.0 [36.2]	15.5 [28.8]	1.6 [49.7]	7.4 [50.9]

* For single-dose AUC=AUC(0-∞); for multiple-dose AUC=AUC(0-T).
† Oxycodone hydrochloride controlled-release tablets.
‡ Data obtained while volunteers received naltrexone which can enhance absorption.

OxyContin is NOT INDICATED FOR RECTAL ADMINISTRATION. Data from a study involving 21 normal volunteers show that OxyContin tablets administered per rectum resulted in an AUC 39% greater and a C_{max} 9% higher than tablets administered by mouth. Therefore, there is an increased risk of adverse events with rectal administration.

TABLE 2

Regimen / Dosage Form	AUC(∞) (ng·h/ml)*	C_{max} (ng/ml)	T_{max} (hours)	Trough Conc. (ng/ml)
	Mean [% coefficient variation]			
Single Dose†				
4 × 40 mg‡	1935.3 [34.7]	152.0 [28.9]	2.56 [42.3]	n.a.
2 × 80 mg‡	1859.3 [30.1]	153.4 [25.1]	2.78 [69.3]	n.a.
1 × 160 mg‡	1856.4 [30.5]	156.4 [24.8]	2.54 [36.4]	n.a.

* For single-dose AUC=AUC(0-∞).
† Data obtained while volunteers received naltrexone which can enhance absorption.
‡ Oxycodone hydrochloride controlled-release tablets.

Food Effects

Food has no significant effect on the extent of absorption of oxycodone from OxyContin. However, the peak plasma concentration of oxycodone increased by 25% when a OxyContin 160 mg tablet was administered with a high-fat meal.

Distribution

Following intravenous administration, the volume of distribution (Vss) for oxycodone was 2.6 L/kg. Oxycodone binding to plasma protein at 37°C and a pH of 7.4 was about 45%. Once absorbed, oxycodone is distributed to skeletal muscle, liver, intestinal tract, lungs, spleen, and brain. Oxycodone has been found in breast milk (see PRECAUTIONS).

Metabolism

Oxycodone hydrochloride is extensively metabolized to noroxycodone, oxymorphone, and their glucuronides. The major circulating metabolite is noroxycodone with an AUC ratio of 0.6 relative to that of oxycodone. Noroxycodone is reported to be a considerably weaker analgesic than oxycodone. Oxymorphone, although possessing analgesic activity, is present in the plasma only in low concentrations. The correlation between oxymorphone concentrations and opioid effects was much less than that seen with oxycodone plasma concentrations. The analgesic activity profile of other metabolites is not known.

The formation of oxymorphone, but not noroxycodone, is mediated by cytochrome P450 2D6 and, as such, its formation can, in theory, be affected by other drugs (see Drug-Drug Interactions).

Excretion

Oxycodone and its metabolites are excreted primarily via the kidney. The amounts measured in the urine have been reported as follows: free oxycodone up to 19%; conjugated oxycodone up to 50%; free oxymorphone 0%; conjugated oxymorphone ≤14%; both free and conjugated noroxycodone have been found in the urine but not quantified. The total plasma clearance was 0.8 L/min for adults.

Special Populations

Elderly

The plasma concentrations of oxycodone are only nominally affected by age, being 15% greater in elderly as compared to young subjects.

Gender

Female subjects have, on average, plasma oxycodone concentrations up to 25% higher than males on a body weight adjusted basis. The reason for this difference is unknown.

Renal Impairment

Data from a pharmacokinetic study involving 13 patients with mild to severe renal dysfunction (creatinine clearance <60 ml/min) show peak plasma oxycodone and noroxycodone concentrations 50% and 20% higher, respectively, and AUC values for oxycodone, noroxycodone, and oxymorphone 60%, 50%, and 40% higher than normal subjects, respectively. This is accompanied by an increase in sedation but not by differences in respiratory rate, pupillary constriction, or several other measures of drug effect. There was an increase in $T_{1/2}$ of elimination for oxycodone of only 1 hour (see PRECAUTIONS).

Hepatic Impairment

Data from a study involving 24 patients with mild to moderate hepatic dysfunction show peak plasma oxycodone and noroxycodone concentrations 50% and 20% higher, respectively, than normal subjects. AUC values are 95% and 65% higher, respectively. Oxymorphone peak plasma concentrations and AUC values are lower by 30% and 40%. These differences are accompanied by increases in some, but not other, drug effects. The $T_{1/2}$ elimination for oxycodone increased by 2.3 hours (see PRECAUTIONS).

Drug-Drug Interactions

See DRUG INTERACTIONS.

Oxycodone is metabolized in part by cytochrome P450 2D6 to oxymorphone which represents less than 15% of the total administered dose. This route of elimination may be blocked by a variety of drugs (*e.g.,* certain cardiovascular drugs including amiodarone and quinidine as well as polycyclic anti-depressants). However, in a study involving 10 subjects using quinidine, a known inhibitor of cytochrome P450 2D6, the pharmacodynamic effects of oxycodone were unchanged.

Pharmacodynamics

A single-dose, double-blind, placebo- and dose-controlled study was conducted using OxyContin (10, 20, and 30 mg) in an analgesic pain model involving 182 patients with moderate to severe pain. Twenty (20) and 30 mg of OxyContin were superior in reducing pain compared with placebo, and this difference was statistically significant. The onset of analgesic action with OxyContin occurred within 1 hour in most patients following oral administration.

INDICATIONS AND USAGE

OxyContin tablets are a controlled-release oral formulation of oxycodone hydrochloride indicated for the management of moderate to severe pain when a continuous, around-the-clock analgesic is needed for an extended period of time.

OxyContin is **NOT** intended for use as a prn analgesic.

Physicians should individualize treatment in every case, initiating therapy at the appropriate point along a progression from non-opioid analgesics, such as non-steroidal anti-inflammatory drugs and acetaminophen to opioids in a plan of pain management such as outlined by the World Health Organization, the Agency for Healthcare Research and Quality (formerly known as the Agency for Health Care Policy and Research), the Federation of State Medical Boards Model Guidelines, or the American Pain Society.

OxyContin is not indicated for pain in the immediate postoperative period (the first 12-24 hours following surgery), or if the pain is mild, or not expected to persist for an extended period of time. OxyContin is only indicated for postoperative use if the patient is already receiving the drug prior to surgery or if the postoperative pain is expected to be moderate to severe and persist for an extended period of time. Physicians should individualize treatment, moving from parenteral to oral analgesics as appropriate. (See American Pain Society guidelines.)

CONTRAINDICATIONS

OxyContin is contraindicated in patients with known hypersensitivity to oxycodone, or in any situation where opioids are contraindicated. This includes patients with significant respiratory depression (in unmonitored settings or the absence of resuscitative equipment), and patients with acute or severe bronchial asthma or hypercarbia. OxyContin is contraindicated in any patient who has or is suspected of having paralytic ileus.

WARNINGS

OXYCONTIN TABLETS ARE TO BE SWALLOWED WHOLE, AND ARE NOT TO BE BROKEN, CHEWED OR CRUSHED. TAKING BROKEN, CHEWED OR CRUSHED OXYCONTIN TABLETS LEADS TO RAPID RELEASE AND ABSORPTION OF A POTENTIALLY FATAL DOSE OF OXYCODONE.

OxyContin 80 and 160 mg tablets ARE FOR USE IN OPIOID-TOLERANT PATIENTS ONLY. These tablet strengths may cause fatal respiratory depression when administered to patients not previously exposed to opioids.

OxyContin 80 and 160 mg tablets are for use only in opioid-tolerant patients requiring daily oxycodone equivalent dosages of 160 mg or more for the 80 mg tablet and 320 mg or more for the 160 mg tablet. Care should be taken in the prescribing of these tablet strengths. Patients should be instructed against use by individuals other than the patient for whom it was prescribed, as such inappropriate use may have severe medical consequences, including death.

MISUSE, ABUSE AND DIVERSION OF OPIOIDS

Oxycodone is an opioid agonist of the morphine-type. Such drugs are sought by drug abusers and people with addiction disorders and are subject to criminal diversion.

Oxycodone can be abused in a manner similar to other opioid agonists, legal or illicit. This should be considered when prescribing or dispensing OxyContin in situations where the physician or pharmacist is concerned about an increased risk of misuse, abuse, or diversion.

OxyContin has been reported as being abused by crushing, chewing, snorting, or injecting the dissolved product. These practices will result in the uncontrolled delivery of the opioid and pose a significant risk to the abuser that could result in overdose and death (see WARNINGS).

Concerns about abuse, addiction, and diversion should not prevent the proper management of pain. The development of addiction to opioid analgesics in properly managed patients with pain has been reported to be rare. However, data are not available to establish the true incidence of addiction in chronic pain patients.

Healthcare professionals should contact their State Professional Licensing Board, or State Controlled Substances Authority for information on how to prevent and detect abuse or diversion of this product.

INTERACTIONS WITH ALCOHOL AND DRUGS OF ABUSE

Oxycodone may be expected to have additive effects when used in conjunction with alcohol, other opioids, or illicit drugs that cause central nervous system depression.

RESPIRATORY DEPRESSION

Respiratory depression is the chief hazard from oxycodone, the active ingredient in OxyContin, as with all opioid agonists. Respiratory depression is a particular problem in elderly or debilitated patients, usually following large initial doses in non-tolerant patients, or when opioids are given in conjunction with other agents that depress respiration.

Oxycodone should be used with extreme caution in patients with significant chronic obstructive pulmonary disease or cor pulmonale, and in patients having a substantially decreased respiratory reserve, hypoxia, hypercapnia, or pre-existing respiratory depression. In such patients, even usual therapeutic doses of oxycodone may decrease respiratory drive to the point of apnea. In these patients alternative non-opioid analgesics should be considered, and opioids should be employed only under careful medical supervision at the lowest effective dose.

HEAD INJURY

The respiratory depressant effects of opioids include carbon dioxide retention and secondary elevation of cerebrospinal fluid pressure, and may be markedly exaggerated in the presence of head injury, intracranial lesions, or other sources of pre-existing increased intracranial pressure. Oxycodone produces effects on pupillary response and consciousness which may obscure neurologic signs of further increases in intracranial pressure in patients with head injuries.

HYPOTENSIVE EFFECT

OxyContin may cause severe hypotension. There is an added risk to individuals whose ability to maintain blood pressure has been compromised by a depleted blood volume, or after concurrent administration with drugs such as phenothiazines or other agents which compromise vasomotor tone. Oxycodone may produce orthostatic hypotension in ambulatory patients. Oxycodone, like all opioid analgesics of the morphinetype, should be administered with caution to patients in circulatory shock, since vasodilation produced by the drug may further reduce cardiac output and blood pressure.

PRECAUTIONS

GENERAL

Opioid analgesics have a narrow therapeutic index in certain patient populations, especially when combined with CNS depressant drugs, and should be reserved for cases where the benefits of opioid analgesia outweigh the known risks of respiratory depression, altered mental state, and postural hypotension.

Use of OxyContin is associated with increased potential risks and should be used only with caution in the following conditions: acute alcoholism; adrenocortical insufficiency (*e.g.*, Addison's disease); CNS depression or coma; delirium tremens; debilitated patients; kyphoscoliosis associated with respiratory depression; myxedema or hypothyroidism; prostatic hypertrophy or urethral stricture; severe impairment of hepatic, pulmonary or renal function; and toxic psychosis.

The administration of oxycodone may obscure the diagnosis or clinical course in patients with acute abdominal conditions. Oxycodone may aggravate convulsions in patients with convulsive disorders, and all opioids may induce or aggravate seizures in some clinical settings.

INTERACTIONS WITH OTHER CNS DEPRESSANTS

OxyContin should be used with caution and started in a reduced dosage (1/3 to 1/2 of the usual dosage) in patients who are concurrently receiving other central nervous system depressants including sedatives or hypnotics, general anesthetics, phenothiazines, other tranquilizers, and alcohol. Interactive effects resulting in respiratory depression, hypotension, profound sedation, or coma may result if these drugs are taken in combination with the usual doses of OxyContin.

INTERACTIONS WITH MIXED AGONIST/ANTAGONIST OPIOID ANALGESICS

Agonist/antagonist analgesics (*i.e.*, pentazocine, nalbuphine, and butorphanol) should be administered with caution to a patient who has received or is receiving a course of therapy with a pure opioid agonist analgesic such as oxycodone. In this situation, mixed agonist/antagonist analgesics may reduce the analgesic effect of oxycodone and/or may precipitate withdrawal symptoms in these patients.

AMBULATORY SURGERY AND POSTOPERATIVE USE

OxyContin is not indicated for pre-emptive analgesia (administration pre-operatively for the management of postoperative pain).

OxyContin is not indicated for pain in the immediate postoperative period (the first 12-24 hours following surgery) for patients not previously taking the drug, because its safety in this setting has not been established.

OxyContin is not indicated for pain in the postoperative period if the pain is mild or not expected to persist for an extended period of time.

OxyContin is only indicated for postoperative use if the patient is already receiving the drug prior to surgery or if the postoperative pain is expected to be moderate to severe and persist for an extended period of time. Physicians should individualize treatment, moving from parenteral to oral analgesics as appropriate (See American Pain Society guidelines).

Patients who are already receiving OxyContin tablets as part of ongoing analgesic therapy may be safely continued on the drug if appropriate dosage adjustments are made considering the procedure, other drugs given, and the temporary changes in physiology caused by the surgical intervention (see DOSAGE AND ADMINISTRATION).

OxyContin and other morphine-like opioids have been shown to decrease bowel motility. Ileus is a common postoperative complication, especially after intra-abdominal surgery with opioid analgesia. Caution should be taken to monitor for decreased bowel motility in postoperative patients receiving opioids. Standard supportive therapy should be implemented.

USE IN PANCREATIC/BILIARY TRACT DISEASE

Oxycodone may cause spasm of the sphincter of Oddi and should be used with caution in patients with biliary tract disease, including acute pancreatitis. Opioids like oxycodone may cause increases in the serum amylase level.

TOLERANCE AND PHYSICAL DEPENDENCE

Tolerance is the need for increasing doses of opioids to maintain a defined effect such as analgesia (in the absence of disease progression or other external factors). Physical dependence is manifested by withdrawal symptoms after abrupt discontinuation of a drug or upon administration of an antagonist. Physical dependence and tolerance are not unusual during chronic opioid therapy.

The opioid abstinence or withdrawal syndrome is characterized by some or all of the following: restlessness, lacrimation, rhinorrhea, yawning, perspiration, chills, myalgia, and mydriasis. Other symptoms also may develop, including: irritability, anxiety, backache, joint pain, weakness, abdominal cramps, insomnia, nausea, anorexia, vomiting, diarrhea, or increased blood pressure, respiratory rate, or heart rate.

In general, opioids should not be abruptly discontinued (see DOSAGE AND ADMINISTRATION, Cessation of Therapy).

INFORMATION FOR PATIENTS/CAREGIVERS

If clinically advisable, patients receiving OxyContin tablets or their caregivers should be given the following information by the physician, nurse, pharmacist, or caregiver:

1. Patients should be aware that OxyContin tablets contain oxycodone, which is a morphine-like substance.

2. Patients should be advised that OxyContin tablets were designed to work properly only if swallowed whole. OxyContin tablets will release all their contents at once if broken, chewed, or crushed, resulting in a risk of fatal overdose.
3. Patients should be advised to report episodes of breakthrough pain and adverse experiences occurring during therapy. Individualization of dosage is essential to make optimal use of this medication.
4. Patients should be advised not to adjust the dose of OxyContin without consulting the prescribing professional.
5. Patients should be advised that OxyContin may impair mental and/or physical ability required for the performance of potentially hazardous tasks (*e.g.*, driving, operating heavy machinery).
6. Patients should not combine OxyContin with alcohol or other central nervous system depressants (sleep aids, tranquilizers) except by the orders of the prescribing physician, because dangerous additive effects may occur, resulting in serious injury or death.
7. Women of childbearing potential who become, or are planning to become, pregnant should be advised to consult their physician regarding the effects of analgesics and other drug use during pregnancy on themselves and their unborn child.
8. Patients should be advised that OxyContin is a potential drug of abuse. They should protect it from theft, and it should never be given to anyone other than the individual for whom it was prescribed.
9. Patients should be advised that they may pass empty matrix "ghosts" (tablets) via colostomy or in the stool, and that this is of no concern since the active medication has already been absorbed.
10. Patients should be advised that if they have been receiving treatment with OxyContin for more than a few weeks and cessation of therapy is indicated, it may be appropriate to taper the OxyContin dose, rather than abruptly discontinue it, due to the risk of precipitating withdrawal symptoms. Their physician can provide a dose schedule to accomplish a gradual discontinuation of the medication.
11. Patients should be instructed to keep OxyContin in a secure place out of the reach of children. When OxyContin is no longer needed, the unused tablets should be destroyed by flushing down the toilet.

USE IN DRUG AND ALCOHOL ADDICTION

OxyContin is an opioid with no approved use in the management of addictive disorders. Its proper usage in individuals with drug or alcohol dependence, either active or in remission, is for the management of pain requiring opioid analgesia.

CARCINOGENESIS, MUTAGENESIS, AND IMPAIRMENT OF FERTILITY

Studies of oxycodone to evaluate its carcinogenic potential have not been conducted.

Oxycodone was not mutagenic in the following assays: Ames *Salmonella* and *E. coli* test with and without metabolic activation at doses of up to 5000 µg, chromosomal aberration test in human lymphocytes in the absence of metabolic activation at doses of up to 1500 µg/ml and with activation 48 hours after exposure at doses of up to 5000 µg/ml, and in the *in vivo* bone marrow micronucleus test in mice (at plasma levels of up to 48 µg/ml). Oxycodone was clastogenic in the human lymphocyte chromosomal assay in the presence of metabolic activation in the human chromosomal aberration test (at greater than or equal to 1250 µg/ml) at 24 but not 48 hours of exposure and in the mouse lymphoma assay at doses of 50 µg/ml or greater with metabolic activation and at 400 µg/ml or greater without metabolic activation.

PREGNANCY, TERATOGENIC EFFECTS, PREGNANCY CATEGORY C

Reproduction studies have been performed in rats and rabbits by oral administration at doses up to 8 mg/kg and 125 mg/kg, respectively. These doses are 3 and 46 times a human dose of 160 mg/day, based on mg/kg basis. The results did not reveal evidence of harm to the fetus due to oxycodone. There are, however, no adequate and well-controlled studies in pregnant women. Because animal reproduction studies are not always predictive of human response, this drug should be used during pregnancy only if clearly needed.

LABOR AND DELIVERY

OxyContin is not recommended for use in women during and immediately prior to labor and delivery because oral opioids may cause respiratory depression in the newborn. Neonates whose mothers have been taking oxycodone chronically may exhibit respiratory depression and/or withdrawal symptoms, either at birth and/or in the nursery.

NURSING MOTHERS

Low concentrations of oxycodone have been detected in breast milk. Withdrawal symptoms can occur in breast-feeding infants when maternal administration of an opioid analgesic is stopped. Ordinarily, nursing should not be undertaken while a patient is receiving OxyContin because of the possibility of sedation and/or respiratory depression in the infant.

PEDIATRIC USE

Safety and effectiveness of OxyContin have not been established in pediatric patients below the age of 18. **It must be remembered that OxyContin tablets cannot be crushed or divided for administration.**

GERIATRIC USE

In controlled pharmacokinetic studies in elderly subjects (greater than 65 years) the clearance of oxycodone appeared to be slightly reduced. Compared to young adults, the plasma concentrations of oxycodone were increased approximately 15% (see CLINICAL PHARMACOLOGY, Pharmacokinetics and Metabolism). Of the total number of subjects (445) in clinical studies of OxyContin, 148 (33.3%) were age 65 and older (including those age 75 and older) while 40 (9.0%) were age 75 and older. In clinical trials with appropriate initiation of therapy and dose titration, no untoward or unexpected side effects were seen in the elderly patients who received OxyContin. Thus, the usual doses and dosing intervals are appropriate for these patients. As with all opioids, the starting dose should be reduced to 1/3 to 1/2 of the usual dosage in debilitated, non-tolerant patients. Respiratory depression is the chief hazard in elderly or debilitated patients, usually following large initial doses in non-tolerant patients, or when opioids are given in conjunction with other agents that depress respiration.

LABORATORY MONITORING

Due to the broad range of plasma concentrations seen in clinical populations, the varying degrees of pain, and the development of tolerance, plasma oxycodone measurements are usually not helpful in clinical management. Plasma concentrations of the active drug substance may be of value in selected, unusual or complex cases.

HEPATIC IMPAIRMENT

A study of OxyContin in patients with hepatic impairment indicates greater plasma concentrations than those with normal function. The initiation of therapy at 1/3 to 1/2 the usual doses and careful dose titration is warranted.

RENAL IMPAIRMENT

In patients with renal impairment, as evidenced by decreased creatinine clearance (<60 ml/min), the concentrations of oxycodone in the plasma are approximately 50% higher than in subjects with normal renal function. Dose initiation should follow a conservative approach. Dosages should be adjusted according to the clinical situation.

GENDER DIFFERENCES

In pharmacokinetic studies, opioid-naive females demonstrate up to 25% higher average plasma concentrations and greater frequency of typical opioid adverse events than males, even after adjustment for body weight. The clinical relevance of a difference of this magnitude is low for a drug intended for chronic usage at individualized dosages, and there was no male/female difference detected for efficacy or adverse events in clinical trials.

DRUG INTERACTIONS

Opioid analgesics, including OxyContin, may enhance the neuromuscular blocking action of skeletal muscle relaxants and produce an increased degree of respiratory depression.

Oxycodone is metabolized in part to oxymorphone via cytochrome P450 2D6. While this pathway may be blocked by a variety of drugs (*e.g.*, certain cardiovascular drugs including amiodarone and quinidine as well as polycyclic antidepressants), such blockade has not yet been shown to be of clinical significance with this agent. Clinicians should be aware of this possible interaction, however.

USE WITH CNS DEPRESSANTS

OxyContin, like all opioid analgesics, should be started at 1/3 to 1/2 of the usual dosage in patients who are concurrently receiving other central nervous system depressants including sedatives or hypnotics, general anesthetics, phenothiazines, centrally acting anti-emetics, tranquilizers, and alcohol because respiratory depression, hypotension, and profound sedation or coma may result. No specific interaction between oxycodone and monoamine oxidase inhibitors has been observed, but caution in the use of any opioid in patients taking this class of drugs is appropriate.

ADVERSE REACTIONS

The safety of OxyContin was evaluated in double-blind clinical trials involving 713 patients with moderate to severe pain of various etiologies. In open-label studies of cancer pain, 187 patients received OxyContin in total daily doses ranging from 20-640 mg/day. The average total daily dose was approximately 105 mg/day.

Serious adverse reactions which may be associated with OxyContin tablet therapy in clinical use are those observed with other opioid analgesics, including respiratory depression, apnea, respiratory arrest, and (to an even lesser degree) circulatory depression, hypotension, or shock.

The non-serious adverse events seen on initiation of therapy with OxyContin are typical opioid side effects. These events are dose-dependent, and their frequency depends upon the dose, the clinical setting, the patient's level of opioid tolerance, and host factors specific to the individual. They should be expected and managed as a part of opioid analgesia. The most frequent (>5%) include: constipation, nausea, somnolence, dizziness, vomiting, pruritus, headache, dry mouth, sweating, and asthenia.

In many cases the frequency of these events during initiation of therapy may be minimized by careful individualization of starting dosage, slow titration, and the avoidance of large swings in the plasma concentrations of the opioid. Many of these adverse events will cease or decrease in intensity as OxyContin therapy is continued and some degree of tolerance is developed.

Clinical trials comparing OxyContin with immediate-release oxycodone and placebo revealed a similar adverse event profile between OxyContin and immediate-release oxycodone. The most common adverse events (>5%) reported by patients at least once during therapy were as shown in TABLE 3.

TABLE 3

	Number of Patients		
	Controlled-Release (n=227)	Immediate-Release (n=225)	Placebo (n=45)
Constipation	23%	26%	7%
Nausea	23%	27%	11%
Somnolence	23%	24%	4%
Dizziness	13%	16%	9%
Pruritus	13%	12%	2%
Vomiting	12%	14%	7%
Headache	7%	8%	7%
Dry mouth	6%	7%	2%
Asthenia	6%	7%	—
Sweating	5%	6%	2%

The following adverse experiences were reported in OxyContin-treated patients with an incidence between 1 and 5%. In descending order of frequency they were anorexia, ner-

O

vousness, insomnia, fever, confusion, diarrhea, abdominal pain, dyspepsia, rash, anxiety, euphoria, dyspnea, postural hypotension, chills, twitching, gastritis, abnormal dreams, thought abnormalities, and hiccups.

The following adverse reactions occurred in less than 1% of patients involved in clinical trials or were reported in postmarketing experience.

General: Accidental injury, chest pain, facial edema, malaise, neck pain, pain.

Cardiovascular: Migraine, syncope, vasodilation, ST depression.

Digestive: Dysphagia, eructation, flatulence, gastrointestinal disorder, increased appetite, nausea and vomiting, stomatitis, ileus.

Hemic and Lymphatic: Lymphadenopathy.

Metabolic and Nutritional: Dehydration, edema, hyponatremia, peripheral edema, syndrome of inappropriate antidiuretic hormone secretion, thirst.

Nervous: Abnormal gait, agitation, amnesia, depersonalization, depression, emotional lability, hallucination, hyperkinesia, hypesthesia, hypotonia, malaise, paresthesia, seizures, speech disorder, stupor, tinnitus, tremor, vertigo, withdrawal syndrome with or without seizures.

Respiratory: Cough increased, pharyngitis, voice alteration.

Skin: Dry skin, exfoliative dermatitis, urticaria.

Special Senses: Abnormal vision, taste perversion.

Urogenital: Amenorrhea, decreased libido, dysuria, hematuria, impotence, polyuria, urinary retention, urination impaired.

DOSAGE AND ADMINISTRATION

GENERAL PRINCIPLES

OXYCONTIN IS AN OPIOID AGONIST AND A SCHEDULE II CONTROLLED SUBSTANCE WITH AN ABUSE LIABILITY SIMILAR TO MORPHINE. OXYCODONE, LIKE MORPHINE AND OTHER OPIOIDS USED IN ANALGESIA, CAN BE ABUSED AND IS SUBJECT TO CRIMINAL DIVERSION.

OXYCONTIN TABLETS ARE TO BE SWALLOWED WHOLE, AND ARE NOT TO BE BROKEN, CHEWED OR CRUSHED. TAKING BROKEN, CHEWED OR CRUSHED OXYCONTIN TABLETS LEADS TO RAPID RELEASE AND ABSORPTION OF A POTENTIALLY FATAL DOSE OF OXYCODONE.

One OxyContin 160 mg tablet is comparable to two 80 mg tablets when taken on an empty stomach. With a high-fat meal, however, there is a 25% greater peak plasma concentration following one 160 mg tablet. Dietary caution should be taken when patients are initially titrated to 160 mg tablets (see DOSAGE AND ADMINISTRATION).

In treating pain it is vital to assess the patient regularly and systematically. Therapy should also be regularly reviewed and adjusted based upon the patient's own reports of pain and side effects and the health professional's clinical judgment.

OxyContin tablets are a controlled-release oral formulation of oxycodone hydrochloride indicated for the management of moderate to severe pain when a continuous, around-the-clock analgesic is needed for an extended period of time. The controlled-release nature of the formulation allows OxyContin to be effectively administered every 12 hours (see CLINICAL PHARMACOLOGY, Pharmacokinetics and Metabolism). While symmetric (same dose AM and PM), around-the-clock, q12h dosing is appropriate for the majority of patients, some patients may benefit from asymmetric (different dose given in AM than in PM) dosing, tailored to their pain pattern. It is usually appropriate to treat a patient with only one opioid for around-the-clock therapy.

Physicians should individualize treatment using a progressive plan of pain management such as outlined by the World Health Organization, the American Pain Society and the Federation of State Medical Boards Model Guidelines. Health care professionals should follow appropriate pain management principles of careful assessment and ongoing monitoring (see BOXED WARNING).

INITIATION OF THERAPY

It is critical to initiate the dosing regimen for each patient individually, taking into account the patient's prior opioid and non-opioid analgesic treatment. Attention should be given to:

1. The general condition and medical status of the patient;
2. The daily dose, potency, and kind of the analgesic(s) the patient has been taking;
3. The reliability of the conversion estimate used to calculate the dose of oxycodone;
4. The patient's opioid exposure and opioid tolerance (if any);
5. Special safety issues associated with conversion to OxyContin doses at or exceeding 160 mg q12h (see Special Instructions for OxyContin 80 and 160 mg Tablets); and
6. The balance between pain control and adverse experiences.

Care should be taken to use low initial doses of OxyContin in patients who are not already opioid-tolerant, especially those who are receiving concurrent treatment with muscle relaxants, sedatives, or other CNS active medications (see DRUG INTERACTIONS).

For initiation of OxyContin therapy for patients previously taking opioids, the conversion ratios from Foley, KM. [NEJM, 1985; 313:84-95], found below, are a reasonable starting point, although not verified in well-controlled, multiple-dose trials.

Experience indicates a reasonable starting dose of OxyContin for patients who are taking non-opioid analgesics and require continuous around-the-clock therapy for an extended period of time is 10 mg q12h. If a non-opioid analgesic is being provided, it may be continued. OxyContin should be individually titrated to a dose that provides adequate analgesia and minimizes side effects.

1. Using standard conversion ratio estimates (see TABLE 4), multiply the mg/day of the previous opioids by the appropriate multiplication factors to obtain the equivalent total daily dose of oral oxycodone.
2. When converting from oxycodone, divide the 24 hour oxycodone dose in half to obtain the twice a day (q12h) dose of OxyContin.
3. Round down to a dose which is appropriate for the tablet strengths available (10, 20, 40, 80, and 160 mg tablets).
4. Discontinue all other around-the-clock opioid drugs when OxyContin therapy is initiated.
5. No fixed conversion ratio is likely to be satisfactory in all patients, especially patients receiving large opioid doses. The recommended doses shown in TABLE 4 are only a starting point, and close observation and frequent titration are indicated until patients are stable on the new therapy.

***TABLE 4** Multiplication Factors for Converting the Daily Dose of Prior Opioids to the Daily Dose of Oral Oxycodone**

(mg/day Prior Opioid × Factor = mg/day Oral Oxycodone)

	Oral Prior Opioid	Parenteral Prior Opioid
Oxycodone	1	—
Codeine	0.15	—
Hydrocodone	0.9	—
Hydromorphone	4	20
Levorphanol	7.5	15
Meperidine	0.1	0.4
Methadone	1.5	3
Morphine	0.5	3

* **To be used only for conversion to oral oxycodone.** For patients receiving high-dose parenteral opioids, a more conservative conversion is warranted. For example, for high-dose parenteral morphine, use 1.5 instead of 3 as a multiplication factor.

In all cases, supplemental analgesia (see Supplemental Analgesia) should be made available in the form of a suitable short-acting analgesic.

OxyContin can be safely used concomitantly with usual doses of non-opioid analgesics and analgesic adjuvants, provided care is taken to select a proper initial dose (see PRECAUTIONS).

CONVERSION FROM TRANSDERMAL FENTANYL TO OXYCONTIN

Eighteen (18) hours following the removal of the transdermal fentanyl patch, OxyContin treatment can be initiated. Although there has been no systematic assessment of such conversion, a conservative oxycodone dose, approximately 10 mg q12h of OxyContin, should be initially substituted for each 25 µg/h fentanyl transdermal patch. The patient.should be followed closely for early titration, as there is very limited clinical experience with this conversion.

MANAGING EXPECTED OPIOID ADVERSE EXPERIENCES

Most patients receiving opioids, especially those who are opioid-naive, will experience side effects. Frequently the side effects from OxyContin are transient, but may require evaluation and management. Adverse events such as constipation should be anticipated and treated aggressively and prophylactically with a stimulant laxative and/or stool softener. Patients do not usually become tolerant to the constipating effects of opioids.

Other opioid-related side effects such as sedation and nausea are usually self-limited and often do not persist beyond the first few days. If nausea persists and is unacceptable to the patient, treatment with antiemetics or other modalites may relieve these symptoms and should be considered.

Patients receiving OxyContin may pass an intact matrix "ghost" in the stool or via colostomy. These ghosts contain little or no residual oxycodone and are of no clinical consequence.

INDIVIDUALIZATION OF DOSAGE

Once therapy is initiated, pain relief and other opioid effects should be frequently assessed. Patients should be titrated to adequate effect (generally mild or no pain with the regular use of no more than 2 doses of supplemental analgesia per 24 hours). Patients who experience breakthrough pain may require dosage adjustment or rescue medication. Because steady-state plasma concentrations are approximated within 24-36 hours, dosage adjustment may be carried out every 1-2 days. It is most appropriate to increase the q12h dose, not the dosing frequency. There is no clinical information on dosing intervals shorter than q12h. As a guideline, except for the increase from 10-20 mg q12h, the total daily oxycodone dose usually can be increased by 25-50% of the current dose at each increase.

If signs of excessive opioid-related adverse experiences are observed, the next dose may be reduced. If this adjustment leads to inadequate analgesia, a supplemental dose of immediate-release oxycodone may be given. Alternatively, non-opioid analgesic adjuvants may be employed. Dose adjustments should be made to obtain an appropriate balance between pain relief and opioid-related adverse experiences.

If significant adverse events occur before the therapeutic goal of mild or no pain is achieved, the events should be treated aggressively. Once adverse events are under control, upward titration should continue to an acceptable level of pain control.

During periods of changing analgesic requirements, including initial titration, frequent contact is recommended between physician, other members of the healthcare team, the patient and the caregiver/family.

SPECIAL INSTRUCTIONS FOR OXYCONTIN 80 AND 160 MG TABLETS

(For use in opioid-tolerant patients only.)

OxyContin 80 and 160 mg tablets are for use only in opioid-tolerant patients requiring daily oxycodone equivalent dosages of 160 mg or more for the 80 mg tablet and 320 mg or more for the 160 mg tablet. Care should be taken in the prescribing of these tablet strengths. Patients should be instructed against use by individuals other than the patient for whom it was prescribed, as such inappropriate use may have severe medical consequences, including death.

One OxyContin 160 mg tablet is comparable to two 80 mg tablets when taken on an empty stomach. With a high-fat meal, however, there is a 25% greater peak plasma concentration following one 160 mg tablet. Dietary caution should be taken when patients are initially titrated to 160 mg tablets.

SUPPLEMENTAL ANALGESIA

Most patients given around-the-clock therapy with controlled-release opioids may need to have immediate-release medication available for exacerbations of pain or to prevent pain that occurs predictably during certain patient activities (incident pain).

MAINTENANCE OF THERAPY

The intent of the titration period is to establish a patient-specific q12h dose that will maintain adequate analgesia with acceptable side effects for as long as pain relief is necessary. Should pain recur then the dose can be incrementally increased to re-establish pain control. The method of therapy adjustment outlined above should be employed to re-establish pain control.

During chronic therapy, especially for non-cancer pain syndromes, the continued need for around-the-clock opioid therapy should be reassessed periodically (*e.g.*, every 6-12 months) as appropriate.

CESSATION OF THERAPY

When the patient no longer requires therapy with OxyContin tablets, doses should be tapered gradually to prevent signs and symptoms of withdrawal in the physically dependent patient.

CONVERSION FROM OXYCONTIN TO PARENTERAL OPIOIDS

To avoid overdose, conservative dose conversion ratios should be followed.

SAFETY AND HANDLING

OxyContin tablets are solid dosage forms that contain oxycodone which is a controlled substance. Like morphine, oxycodone is controlled under Schedule II of the Controlled Substances Act.

OxyContin has been targeted for theft and diversion by criminals. Healthcare professionals should contact their State Professional Licensing Board or State Controlled Substances Authority for information on how to prevent and detect abuse or diversion of this product.

HOW SUPPLIED

OXYCONTIN (OXYCODONE HYDROCHLORIDE CONTROLLED-RELEASE) TABLETS ARE SUPPLIED IN:

10 mg: Round, unscored, white-colored, convex tablets bearing the symbol "OC" on one side and "10" on the other.

20 mg: Round, unscored, pink-colored, convex tablets bearing the symbol "OC" on one side and "20" on the other.

40 mg: Round, unscored, yellow-colored, convex tablets bearing the symbol "OC" on one side and "40" on the other.

80 mg: Round, unscored, green-colored, convex tablets bearing the symbol "OC" on one side and "80" on the other.

160 mg: Modified caplet-shaped, unscored, blue-colored, convex tablets bearing the symbol "OC" on one side and "160" on the other.

STORAGE

Store at 25°C (77°F); excursions permitted between 15-30°C (59-86°F).

Dispense in tight, light-resistant container.

PRODUCT LISTING - EQUIVALENTS NOT AVAILABLE

Package	Price	Product	NDC
Capsule - Oral - 5 mg			
10 x 10	$35.39	GENERIC, Ethex Corporation	58177-0041-11
100's	$29.30	GENERIC, Ethex Corporation	58177-0041-04
100's	$30.60	GENERIC, Mallinckrodt Medical Inc	00406-0554-01
100's	$33.21	GENERIC, Amide Pharmaceutical Inc	52152-0187-02
100's	$39.37	OXYIR, Purdue Frederick Company	59011-0201-10
Concentrate - Oral - 20 mg/ml			
30 ml	$34.42	GENERIC, Ethex Corporation	58177-0914-01
30 ml	$35.00	GENERIC, Mallinckrodt Medical Inc	00406-8558-30
30 ml	$40.56	ROXICODONE, Roxane Laboratories Inc	00054-3683-44
30 ml	$43.43	OXYFAST, Purdue Frederick Company	59011-0225-20
Solution - Oral - 5 mg/5 ml			
5 ml x 40	$56.00	ROXICODONE, Roxane Laboratories Inc	00054-8782-16
500 ml	$37.00	GENERIC, Mallinckrodt Medical Inc	00406-8555-50
500 ml	$41.65	ROXICODONE, Roxane Laboratories Inc	00054-3682-63
Tablet - Oral - 5 mg			
25 x 4	$68.75	PERCOLONE, Endo Laboratories Llc	63481-0132-75
100's	$31.04	ROXICODONE, Roxane Laboratories Inc	00054-4657-25
100's	$32.99	GENERIC, Amide Pharmaceutical Inc	52152-0165-11
100's	$35.09	GENERIC, Mallinckrodt Medical Inc	00406-0552-01
100's	$35.75	GENERIC, Ethex Corporation	58177-0315-04
100's	$35.99	GENERIC, Amide Pharmaceutical Inc	52152-0165-02
100's	$41.05	GENERIC, Mallinckrodt Medical Inc	00406-0552-62
100's	$41.05	GENERIC, Ethex Corporation	58177-0315-11
100's	$42.49	ROXICODONE, Roxane Laboratories Inc	00054-8657-24
100's	$61.53	GENERIC, Endo Laboratories Llc	60951-0657-70
100's	$68.75	PERCOLONE, Endo Laboratories Llc	63481-0132-70
Tablet - Oral - 15 mg			
100's	$74.94	ROXICODONE, Elan Pharmaceuticals	00054-4658-25
Tablet - Oral - 30 mg			
25 x 4	$183.13	ROXICODONE, Roxane Laboratories Inc	00054-8665-24
100's	$144.43	ROXICODONE, Elan Pharmaceuticals	00054-4665-25
Tablet, Extended Release - Oral - 10 mg			
25's	$36.53	OXYCONTIN, Purdue Frederick Company	59011-0100-25
100's	$134.39	OXYCONTIN, Purdue Frederick Company	59011-0100-10
Tablet, Extended Release - Oral - 20 mg			
25's	$69.91	OXYCONTIN, Purdue Frederick Company	59011-0103-25
100's	$257.16	OXYCONTIN, Purdue Frederick Company	59011-0103-10
Tablet, Extended Release - Oral - 40 mg			
25's	$123.96	OXYCONTIN, Purdue Frederick Company	59011-0105-25
100's	$456.30	OXYCONTIN, Purdue Frederick Company	59011-0105-10
Tablet, Extended Release - Oral - 80 mg			
25's	$233.25	OXYCONTIN, Purdue Frederick Company	59011-0107-25
100's	$858.08	OXYCONTIN, Purdue Frederick Company	59011-0107-10
Tablet, Extended Release - Oral - 160 mg			
25's	$413.75	OXYCONTIN, Purdue Frederick Company	59011-0109-25
100's	$1617.94	OXYCONTIN, Purdue Frederick Company	59011-0109-10

Oxymorphone Hydrochloride *(001935)*

For related information, see the comparative table section in Appendix A.

Categories: Anesthesia, adjunct; Anxiety, secondary to dyspnea; Pain, moderate to severe; Pain, obstetrical; DEA Class CII; Pregnancy Category C; FDA Approved 1959 Apr
Drug Classes: Analgesics, narcotic
Brand Names: **Numorphan**
HCFA JCODE(S): J2410 up to 1 mg IV, SC, IM

DESCRIPTION

Oxymorphone hydrochloride is a semi-synthetic narcotic substitute for morphine, is a potent analgesic.

Oxymorphone hydrochloride occurs as a white or slightly off-white, odorless powder, sparingly soluble in alcohol and ether, but freely soluble in water.

Numorphan injection is available in two concentrations, 1 and 1.5 mg of oxymorphone hydrochloride per ml. Both strengths contain sodium chloride 0.8%; with methylparaben 0.18%, propylparaben 0.02% and sodium dithionite 0.1%, as preservatives. pH is adjusted with sodium hydroxide.

CLINICAL PHARMACOLOGY

Oxymorphone HCl is a potent narcotic analgesic. Administered parenterally, 1 mg of oxymorphone HCl is approximately equivalent in analgesic activity to 10 mg of morphine sulfate.

The onset of action is rapid; initial effects are usually perceived within 5-10 minutes. Its duration of action is approximately 3-6 hours.

Oxymorphone HCl produces mild sedation and causes little depression of the cough reflex. These properties make it particularly useful in postoperative patients.

INDICATIONS AND USAGE

Oxymorphone HCl is indicated for the relief of moderate to severe pain. This drug is also indicated parenterally for preoperative medication, for support of anesthesia, for obstetrical analgesia, and for relief of anxiety in patients with dyspnea associated with acute left ventricular failure and pulmonary edema.

CONTRAINDICATIONS

Oxymorphone HCl in children under 12 years of age has not been established. This drug should not be used in patients known to be hypersensitive to morphine analogs.

WARNINGS

May be habit forming: As with other narcotic drugs, tolerance and addiction may develop. The addicting potential of the drug appears to be about the same as for morphine.

Like other narcotic-containing medications, oxymorphone HCl is subject to the Federal Controlled Substances Act.

Sulfites Sensitivity: Oxymorphone HCl contains sodium dithionite, a sulfite that may cause allergic-type reactions including anaphylactic symptoms and life-threatening or less severe asthmatic episodes in certain susceptible people. The overall prevalence of sulfite sensitivity in the general population is unknown and probably low. Sulfite sensitivity is seen more frequently in asthmatic than in nonasthmatic people.

PRECAUTIONS

The same care and caution should be taken when administering oxymorphone HCl as when other potent analgesics are used. It should be borne in mind that some respiratory depression may occur as with all potent narcotics especially when other analgesic and/or anesthetic drugs with depressant action have been given shortly before administration of oxymorphone HCl.

The respiratory depressant effects of narcotics and their capacity to elevate cerebrospinal fluid pressure may be markedly exaggerated in the presence of head injury, other intracranial lesions or a pre-existing increase in intracranial pressure.

Furthermore, narcotics produce adverse reactions which may obscure the clinical course of patients with head injuries.

As with other analgesics, caution must also be exercised in elderly and debilitated patients and in patients who are known to be sensitive to central nervous system depressants, such as those with cardiovascular, pulmonary, or hepatic disease, in hypothyroidism (myxedema), acute alcoholism, delirium tremens, convulsive disorders, bronchial asthma and kyphoscoliosis. Debilitated and elderly patients and those with severe liver diseases should receive smaller doses of oxymorphone HCl.

DRUG INTERACTIONS

Interactions with other central nervous system depressants: Patients receiving other narcotic analgesics, general anesthetics, phenothiazines, other tranquilizers, sedatives, hypnotics or other CNS depressants (including alcohol) concomitantly with oxymorphone HCl may exhibit an additive CNS depression. When such combined therapy is contemplated, the dose of one or both agents should be reduced.

Safe use in pregnancy has not been established (relative to possible adverse effects on fetal development). As with other analgesics, the use of oxymorphone HCl in pregnancy, in nursing mothers, or in women of child-bearing potential requires that the possible benefits of the drug be weighted against the possible hazards to the mother and child.

ADVERSE REACTIONS

As with all potent narcotic analgesics, possible side effects include drowsiness, nausea, vomiting, miosis, itching, dysphoria, light-headedness, and headache. Respiratory depression may occur with oxymorphone as with other narcotics.

DOSAGE AND ADMINISTRATION

USUAL ADULT DOSAGE OF OXYMORPHONE HCl INJECTION

Subcutaneous or Intramuscular administration: Initially 1 mg to 1.5 mg, repeated every 4-6 hours as needed.

Intravenous: 0.5 mg initially.

In nondebilitated patients the dose can be cautiously increased until satisfactory pain relief is obtained. For analgesia during labor 0.5 to 1 mg intramuscularly is recommended.

PRODUCT LISTING - EQUIVALENTS NOT AVAILABLE

Solution - Injectable - 1 mg/ml			
1 ml x 10	$29.50	NUMORPHAN HCL, Endo Laboratories Llc	63481-0444-10
1 ml x 10	$38.75	NUMORPHAN HCL, Dupont Pharmaceuticals	00590-0370-10
Solution - Injectable - 1.5 mg/ml			
1 ml x 10	$36.25	NUMORPHAN HCL, Endo Laboratories Llc	63481-0445-01
1 ml x 10	$50.69	NUMORPHAN HCL, Dupont Pharmaceuticals	00590-0373-10
10 ml	$49.00	NUMORPHAN HCL, Dupont Pharmaceuticals	00590-0374-01
Suppository - Rectal - 5 mg			
6's	$27.50	NUMORPHAN HCL, Dupont Pharmaceuticals	00590-0761-06
6's	$29.19	NUMORPHAN HCL, Endo Laboratories Llc	63481-0761-06

Oxytocin (001945)

Categories: Hemorrhage, postpartum; Labor, induction; Lactation, postpartum; Pregnancy Category X; FDA Approved 1980 Nov; WHO Formulary

Drug Classes: Hormones/hormone modifiers; Oxytocics; Stimulants, uterine

Brand Names: **Pitocin**; Syntocinon

Foreign Brand Availability: Fetusin (Philippines); NeOxyn (Philippines); Orasthin (Germany); Oxytocin S INJ (Indonesia); Oxiton INJ (Korea); Oxitone (Bahrain; Cyprus; Egypt; Iran; Iraq; Israel; Jordan; Kuwait; Lebanon; Libya; Oman; Peru; Qatar; Republic-of-Yemen; Saudi-Arabia; Syria; United-Arab-Emirates); Partocon INJ (Finland; Sweden); Pitocin INJ (India); Piton S (Indonesia); Piton S INJ (Bahrain; Cyprus; Egypt; Iran; Iraq; Jordan; Kuwait; Lebanon; Libya; Netherlands; Oman; Qatar; Republic-of-Yemen; Saudi-Arabia; Syria; Taiwan; United-Arab-Emirates); Synthetic Oxytocin INJ (India); Syntocinon INJ (Australia; Austria; Belgium; Benin; Bulgaria; Burkina-Faso; Denmark; England; Ethiopia; Finland; France; Gambia; Ghana; Guinea; Hong-Kong; Indonesia; Ireland; Italy; Ivory-Coast; Kenya; Liberia; Malawi; Malaysia; Mali; Mauritania; Mauritius; Morocco; Netherlands; New-Zealand; Niger; Nigeria; Philippines; Senegal; Seychelles; Sierra-Leone; South-Africa; Spain; Sudan; Sweden; Switzerland; Taiwan; Tanzania; Tunia; Uganda; Zambia; Zimbabwe); Syntocinon Spray (Austria; Denmark; Norway; South-Africa; Sweden; Switzerland); Utron INJ (Israel); Xitocin (Mexico)

HCFA JCODE(S): J2590 up to 10 units IV, IM

DESCRIPTION

INJECTION

Pitocin (oxytocin injection) is a sterile, clear, colorless solution of synthetic oxytocin, for intravenous infusion or intramuscular injection. Pitocin is a nonapeptide found in pituitary extracts from mammals. It is standardized to contain 10 units of oxytocic hormone/ml and contains 0.5% Chloretone (chlorobutanol, a chloroform derivative) as a preservative, with the pH adjusted with acetic acid. The hormone is prepared synthetically to avoid possible concentration with vasopressin (ADH) and other small polypeptides with biologic activity. Pitocin has the empirical formula $C_{43}H_{66}N_{12}O_{12}S_2$ (molecular weight 1007.19).

Storage: Store between 15 and 25°C (59° and 77°F).

NASAL SPRAY

Each ml contains 40 Units (International Units) oxytocin and the following: chlorobutanol, max, 0.05%; citric acid; dried sodium phosphate, glycerin; methylparaben; propylparaben; purified water; sodium chloride; sorbitol solution.

Oxytocin is one of the polypeptide hormones of the pituitary gland. The pharmacologic and clinical properties of oxytocin nasal solution (nasal spray) are identical with the oxytocic and galactokinetic principle of the natural hormone.

Synthetic oxytocin has the formula $C_{43}H_{66}N_{12}O_{12}S_2$, with a molecular weight of 1007.19

Since oxytocin, a polypeptide, is subject to inactivation by the proteolytic enzymes of the alimentary tract, it is **not absorbed from the gastrointestinal tract.**

Storage: Store below 77°F; DO NOT FREEZE.

CLINICAL PHARMACOLOGY

INJECTION

Uterine motility depends on the formation of the contractile protein actomyosin under the influence of the Ca^{2+}-dependent phosphorylating enzyme myosin light-chain kinase. Oxytocin promotes contractions by increasing the intracellular Ca^{2+}. Oxytocin has specific receptors in the myometrium and the receptor concentration increases greatly during pregnancy, reaching a maximum in early labor at term. The response to a given dose of oxytocin is very individualized and depends on the sensitivity of the uterus, which is determined by the oxytocin receptor concentration. However, the physician should be aware of the fact that oxytocin even in its pure form has inherent pressor and antidiuretic properties which may become manifest when large doses are administered. These properties are though to be due to the fact that oxytocin and vasopressin differ in regard to only two of the eight amino acids (see PRECAUTIONS).

Oxytocin is distributed throughout the extracellular fluid. Small amounts of the drug probably reach the fetal circulation. Oxytocin has a plasma half-life of about 1-6 minutes which is decreased in late pregnancy and during lactation. Following intravenous administration of oxytocin, uterine response occurs almost immediately and subsides within 1 hour. Following intramuscular injection of the drug, uterine response occurs within 3-5 minutes and persists for 2-3 hours. Its rapid removal from plasma is accomplished largely by the kidney and the liver. Only small amounts are excreted in urine unchanged.

NASAL SPRAY

Oxytocin nasal spray acts specifically on the myoepithelial elements surrounding the alveoli of the breast, and making up the walls of the lactiferous ducts, causing their smooth muscle fibers to contract and thus force milk into the large ducts of the sinuses where it is more readily available to the baby. Oxytocin does not possess galactopoietic properties and its use is intended only for the purpose of milk ejection.

Pharmacokinetics

Oxytocin nasal solution (nasal spray) is promptly absorbed by the nasal mucosa to enter the systemic circulation. Intranasal application of the spray preparation, however, is a practical and effective method of administration. Half-life is extremely short - less than 10 minutes - and oxytocin is then rapidly removed from the plasma by the kidney, liver, and lactating mammary gland. The enzyme oxytocinase is believed to be elaborated by placental and uterine tissues. This enzyme inactivates the hormone by cleavage of the cysteine- tyrosine peptide bond. Excretion is mainly urinary following inactivation of metabolites.[2]

INDICATIONS AND USAGE

INJECTION

IMPORTANT NOTICE

Elective induction of labor is defined as the initiation of labor in a pregnant individual who has no medical indications for induction. Since the available data are inadequate to evaluate the benefits-to-risks considerations. Oxytocin is not indicated for elective induction of labor.

Antepartum

Oxytocin is indicated for the initiation or improvement of uterine contractions, where this is desirable and considered suitable for reasons of fetal or maternal concern, in order to achieve vaginal delivery. It is indicated for (1) induction of labor in patients with a medical indication for initiation of labor, such as Rh problems, maternal diabetes, preeclampsia at or near term, when delivery is in the best interest of mother and fetus or when membranes are prematurely ruptured and delivery is indicated; (2) stimulation or reinforcement of labor, as in selected cases of uterine inertia; (3) as adjunctive therapy in the management of incomplete or inevitable abortion. In the first trimester, curettage is generally considered primary therapy. In second trimester abortion, oxytocin infusion will often be successful in emptying the uterus. Other means of therapy, however, may be required in such cases.

Postpartum

Oxytocin is indicated to produce uterine contractions during the third stage of labor and to control postpartum bleeding or hemorrhage.

NASAL SPRAY

Oxytocin nasal solution (nasal spray) is indicated to assist the initial postpartum milk ejection from the breasts once milk formulation has commenced.

CONTRAINDICATIONS

INJECTION

Antepartum use of oxytocin is contraindicated in any of the following circumstances:

- Where there is significant cephalopelvic disproportion;
- In unfavorable fetal positions or presentations, such as transverse lies, which are undeliverable without conversion prior to delivery;
- In obstetrical emergencies where the benefit-to-risk ratio for either the fetus or the mother favors surgical intervention;
- In fetal distress where delivery is not imminent;
- Where adequate uterine activity fails to achieve satisfactory progress;
- Where the uterus is already hyperactive or hypertonic;
- In cases where vaginal delivery is contraindicated, such as invasive cervical carcinoma, active herpes genitalis, total placenta previa, vase previa, and cord presentation or prolapse of the cord;
- In patients with hypersensitivity to the drug.

NASAL SPRAY

Pregnancy and hypersensitivity are the only known contraindications.

WARNINGS

INJECTION

Oxytocin, when given for induction of labor on augmentation of uterine activity, should be administered only by the intravenous route and with adequate medical supervision in a hospital.

PRECAUTIONS

GENERAL

Injection

All patients receiving intravenous oxytocin must be under continuous observation by trained personnel who have a thorough knowledge of the drug and qualified to identify complications. A physician qualified to manage any complications should be immediately available. Electric fetal monitoring provides the best means for early detection of overdosage. However, it must be born in mind that only intrauterine pressure recording can accurately measure the intrauterine pressure during contractions. A fetal scalp electrode provides a more dependable recording of the fetal heart rate than any external monitoring system.

When properly administered, oxytocin should stimulate uterine contractions similar to those seen in normal labor. Overstimulation of the uterus by improper administration can be hazardous to both mother and fetus. Even with proper administration and adequate supervision, hypertonic contractions can occur in patients whose uteri are hypersensitive to oxytocin. This fact must be considered by the physician in exercising his judgement regarding patient selection.

Except in unusual circumstances, oxytocin should not be administered in the following conditions: fetal distress, partial placenta previa, prematurity, borderline cephalopelvic disproportion, and major surgery on the cervix or uterus including cesarean section, overdistention of the uterus, grand multiparity, or past history of uterine sepsis or of traumatic delivery. Because of the variability of the combinations of factors which may be present in the conditions listed above, the definition of "unusual circumstances" must be left to the judgment of the physician. The decision can only be made by carefully weighing the potential benefits which oxytocin can provide in a given case against rare but definite potential for the drug to produce hypertonicity or tetanic spasm.

Maternal deaths due to hypertensive episodes, subarachnoid hemorrhage, rupture of the uterus, fetal deaths due to various cases have been reported associated with the use of parenteral oxytocic drugs for induction of labor or the augmentation in the first and second stages of labor

Oxytocin has been shown to have an intrinsic antidiuretic effect, acting to increase water reabsorption from the glomerular filtrate. Consideration should, therefore, be given to the possibility of water intoxication, particularly when oxytocin is administered continuously by infusion and the patient is receiving fluids by mouth.

When oxytocin is used for induction or reinforcement of already existent labor, patients should be carefully selected. Pelvic adequacy must be considered and maternal and fetal conditions evaluated before the drug is administered.

CARCINOGENESIS, MUTAGENESIS, AND IMPAIRMENT OF FERTILITY

There are no animal or human studies on the carcinogenicity and mutagenicity of this drug, nor is there any information on its effect on fertility.

PREGNANCY

Injection

Pregnancy, Teratogenic Effects

Animal reproduction studies have not been conducted with oxytocin. There are no known indications for use in the first trimester of pregnancy other than in relation to spontaneous or induced abortion. Based on the wide experience with this drug and its chemical structure and pharmacological properties, it would not be expected to present a risk of fetal abnormalities when used as indicated.

Nonteratogenic Effects

See ADVERSE REACTIONS in the fetus or infant.

Nasal Spray

Pregnancy Category X

See CONTRAINDICATIONS.

Oxytocin nasal solution, (nasal spray) is contraindicated during pregnancy since it may provoke a uterotonic effect to precipitate contractions and abortions. Its proper use is during the first week postpartum, as needed.

LABOR AND DELIVERY

See INDICATIONS AND USAGE.

Nasal Spray

No particular information regarding any special care to be exercised by the practitioner for safe and effective use of the drug is known at this time.

INFORMATION FOR THE PATIENT

Nasal Spray

The squeeze bottle should be held in an upright position when administering the drug to the nose and the patient should be in an sitting position rather than lying down. If preferred, the solution can be instilled in drop form by inverting the squeeze bottle and exerting very gentle pressure on its walls.

NURSING MOTHERS

Nasal Spray

While harmful effects on the newborn have not been reported, it should be noted that Oxytocin nasal solution, (nasal spray) is intended to be used only for **initial** milk propulsion and ejection during the first week postpartum, and not for continued use. Caution shall be exercised when oxytocin nasal solution, (nasal spray) is administered to a nursing mother since oxytocin is known to be excreted in human milk.

DRUG INTERACTIONS

INJECTION

Severe hypertension has been reported when oxytocin was given 3-4 hours following prophylactic administration of a vasoconstrictor in conjunction with caudal block anesthesia. Cyclopropane anesthesia may modify oxytocin's cardiovascular effects, so as to produce unexpected results such as hypotension. Maternal sinus bradycardia with abnormal atrioventricular rhythms has also been noted when oxytocin was used concomitantly with cyclopropane anesthesia.

ADVERSE REACTIONS

INJECTION

The following adverse reactions have been reported in the mother: Anaphylactic reaction, nausea, postpartum hemorrhage, vomiting, cardiac arrhythmia, premature ventricular contractions, fatal afibrinogenemia, pelvic hematoma.

Excessive dosage or hypersensitivity to the drug may result in uterine hypertonicity, spasm, tetanic contraction, or rupture of the uterus.

The possibility of increased blood loss and afibrinogenemia should be kept in mind when administering the drug.

Severe water intoxication with convulsions and coma has occurred, associated with a slow oxytocin infusion over a 24 hour period. Maternal death due to oxytocin-induced water intoxication has been reported.

The following adverse reactions have been reported in the fetus or infant: *Due to induced uterine motility:* Bradycardia, premature ventricular contractions and other arrhythmias, permanent CNS or brain damage, fetal death. *Due to use of oxytocin in the mother:* Low Apgar scores at 5 minutes, neonatal jaundice, neonatal retinal hemorrhage.

NASAL SPRAY

Lack of efficacy has been the most frequent adverse effect (7 cases), followed by nasal irritation and/or rhinorrhea, uterine bleeding, excessive uterine contractions, and lacrimation.

One case each of seizure and "psychotic state" are the most severe reactions reported. No other reactions have been described.[3]

DOSAGE AND ADMINISTRATION

INJECTION

Parenteral drug products should be inspected visually for particulate matter and discoloration prior to administration whenever solution and container permit.

The dosage of oxytocin is determined by uterine response. The following dosage information is based upon the various regimens and indications in general use.

Induction or Stimulation of Labor

Intravenous infusion (drip method) is the only acceptable method of parenteral administration of oxytocin for the induction or stimulation of labor. Accurate control of the rate of infusion flow is essential and is best accomplished by an infusion pump. It is convenient to piggyback the oxytocin infusion on a physiologic electrolyte solution, permitting the oxytocin infusion to be stopped abruptly without interrupting the electrolyte infusion. This is done in the following way.

Administration

The initial dose should be 0.5-1 mU/min (equal to 3-6 ml of the dilute oxytocin solution per hour). At 30-60 minute intervals the dose should be gradually increased in the increments desired frequency of contractions has been reached and labor has progressed to 5-6 cm dilation, the dose may be reduced by similar increments.

Studies of the concentrations of oxytocin in the maternal plasma during oxytocin infusion have shown that infusion rates up to 6 mU/min give the same oxytocin levels that are found in spontaneous labor. At term, higher infusion rates should be given with great care, and rates exceeding 9-10 mU/min are rarely required. Before term, when the sensitivity of the uterus is lower because of a lower concentration of oxytocin receptors, a higher infusion rate may be required.

Monitoring

Electronically monitor the uterine activity and the fetal heart rate throughout the infusion of oxytocin. Attention should be given to tonus, amplitude and frequency of contractions and to the fetal heart rate in relation to uterine contractions. If uterine contractions become too powerful, the infusion can be abruptly stopped and oxytocic stimulation of the uterine musculature will soon wane. (See PRECAUTIONS.)

Discontinue the infusion of oxytocin immediately in the event of uterine and hyperactivity and/or fetal distress. Administer oxygen to the mother, who preferably should be put in a lateral position. The condition of mother and fetus should immediately be evaluated by the responsible physician and appropriate steps taken.

Control of Postpartum Uterine Bleeding

Intravenous infusion (drip method): If the patient has an intravenous infusion running, 10-40 units of oxytocin may be added to the bottle, depending on the amount of electrolyte or dextrose solution remaining (maximum 40 units to 1000 ml). Adjust the infusion rate to sustain uterine concentration and control uterine atony.

Intramuscular Administration: Ten (10) units (1 ml) of oxytocin can be given after the delivery of the placenta.

Treatment of Incomplete, Inevitable or Elective Abortion

Intravenous infusion of 10 units of oxytocin added to 500 ml of a physiologic saline solution or 5% dextrose in-water solution may help the uterus contract after a suction or sharp curettage for an incomplete, inevitable or elective abortion.

Subsequent to intra-amniotic injection of hypertonic saline, professionals, urea, etc., for midtrimester elective abortion, the injection-to-abortion time may be shortened by infusion of oxytocin at the rate of 10-20 milliunits (20-40 drops) per minute. The total dose should not exceed 30 units in a 12 hour period due to the risk of water intoxication.

NASAL SPRAY

One spray into one or both nostrils 2-3 minutes before nursing or pumping of breasts.

PRODUCT LISTING - RATED THERAPEUTICALLY EQUIVALENT

Solution - Injectable - 10 IU/ml

Size	Price	Product	NDC
1 ml x 10	$12.47	PITOCIN, Allscripts Pharmaceutical Company	54569-3056-00
1 ml x 10	$26.00	PITOCIN, Monarch Pharmaceuticals Inc	61570-0416-03
1 ml x 25	$33.75	PITOCIN, Monarch Pharmaceuticals Inc	61570-0416-05
1 ml x 25	$41.80	GENERIC, King Pharmaceuticals Inc	60793-0416-05
1 ml x 25	$75.00	GENERIC, American Pharmaceutical Partners	63323-0012-01
10 ml	$8.05	PITOCIN, Monarch Pharmaceuticals Inc	61570-0416-06
10 ml x 25	$453.25	GENERIC, American Pharmaceutical Partners	63323-0012-10
25 ml	$31.17	PITOCIN, Allscripts Pharmaceutical Company	54569-3914-00

Paclitaxel (003073)

Categories: Carcinoma, breast; Carcinoma, ovarian; Carcinoma, lung; Sarcoma, Kaposi's; FDA Approved 1992 Dec; Pregnancy Category D; Patent Expiration 1999 May; Orphan Drugs
Drug Classes: Antineoplastics, antimitotics
Brand Names: Taxol
Foreign Brand Availability: Anzatax (Australia; Hong-Kong; Philippines; Taiwan; Thailand); Biotax (Israel); Bristaxol (Mexico); Ifaxol (Mexico); Intaxel (India; Thailand); Medixel (Israel); Parexel (Colombia); Paxene (Austria; Belgium; Bulgaria; Czech-Republic; Denmark; England; Finland; France; Germany; Greece; Hungary; Ireland; Italy; Netherlands; Norway; Poland; Portugal; Slovenia; Spain; Sweden; Switzerland; Turkey); Praxel (Mexico)
HCFA JCODE(S): J9265 30 mg IV

WARNING

Paclitaxel injection should be administered under the supervision of a physician experienced in the use of cancer chemotherapeutic agents. Appropriate management of complications is possible only when adequate diagnostic and treatment facilities are readily available.

Anaphylaxis and severe hypersensitivity reactions characterized by dyspnea and hypotension requiring treatment, angioedema, and generalized urticaria have occurred in 2-4% of patients receiving paclitaxel in clinical trials. Fatal reactions have occurred in patients despite premedication. All patients should be pretreated with corticosteroids, diphenhydramine, and H_2 antagonists. (See DOSAGE AND ADMINISTRATION.) Patients who experience severe hypersensitivity reactions to paclitaxel should not be rechallenged with the drug.

Paclitaxel therapy should not be given to patients with solid tumors who have baseline neutrophil counts of less than 1500 cells/mm^3 and should not be given to patients with AIDS-related Kaposi's sarcoma if the baseline neutrophil count is less than 1000 cells/mm^3. In order to monitor the occurrence of bone marrow suppression, primarily neutropenia, which may be severe and result in infection, it is recommended that frequent peripheral blood cell counts be performed on all patients receiving paclitaxel.

DESCRIPTION

Taxol injection is a clear colorless to slightly yellow viscous solution. It is supplied as a nonaqueous solution intended for dilution with a suitable parenteral fluid prior to intravenous infusion. Taxol is available in 30 mg (5 ml), 100 mg (16.7 ml), and 300 mg (50 ml) multidose vials. Each ml of sterile nonpyrogenic solution contains 6 mg paclitaxel, 527 mg of purified Cremophor EL (polyoxyethylated castor oil) and 49.7% (v/v) dehydrated alcohol.

Paclitaxel is a natural product with antitumor activity. Taxol is obtained via a semi-synthetic process from *Taxus baccata*. The chemical name for paclitaxel is 5β,20-Epoxy-1,2α,4,7β,10β,13α-hexahydroxytax-11-en-9-one 4,10-diacetate 2-benzoate 13-ester with (2*R*,3*S*)-*N*-benzoyl-3-phenylisoserine.

Paclitaxel is a white to off-white crystalline powder with the empirical formula $C_{47}H_{51}NO_{14}$ and a molecular weight of 853.9. It is highly lipophilic, insoluble in water, and melts at around 216-217°C.

CLINICAL PHARMACOLOGY

Paclitaxel is a novel antimicrotubule agent that promotes the assembly of microtubules from tubulin dimers and stabilizes microtubules by preventing depolymerization. This stability results in the inhibition of the normal dynamic reorganization of the microtubule network that is essential for vital interphase and mitotic cellular functions. In addition, paclitaxel induces abnormal arrays or "bundles" of microtubules throughout the cell cycle and multiple asters of microtubules during mitosis.

Following intravenous administration of paclitaxel, paclitaxel plasma concentrations declined in a biphasic manner. The initial rapid decline represents distribution to the peripheral compartment and elimination of the drug. The later phase is due, in part, to a relatively slow efflux of paclitaxel from the peripheral compartment.

Pharmacokinetic parameters of paclitaxel following 3 and 24 hour infusions of paclitaxel at dose levels of 135 and 175 mg/m^2 were determined in a Phase 3 randomized study in ovarian cancer patients and are summarized in TABLE 1.

TABLE 1 *Summary of Pharmacokinetic Parameters — Mean Values*

	24 Hour Infusion		3 Hour Infusion	
	Dose (mg/m^2)			
	135 (n=2)	175 (n=4)	135 (n=7)	175 (n=5)
C_{max} (ng/ml)	195	365	2170	3650
AUC(0-∞) (ng·h/ml)	6300	7993	7952	15007
T-HALF (h)	52.7	15.7	13.1	20.2
CL_T (L/h/m^2)	21.7	23.8	17.7	12.2

C_{max} = Maximum plasma concentration.
AUC(0-∞) = Area under the plasma concentration-time curve from time 0 to infinity.
CL_T = Total body clearance.

It appeared that with the 24 hour infusion of paclitaxel, a 30% increase in dose (135 vs 175 mg/m^2) increased the C_{max} by 87%, whereas the AUC(0-∞) remained proportional. However, with a 3 hour infusion, for a 30% increase in dose, the C_{max} and AUC(0-∞) were increased by 68% and 89%, respectively. The mean apparent volume of distribution at steady state, with the 24 hour infusion of paclitaxel, ranged from 227-688 L/m^2, indicating extensive extravascular distribution and/or tissue binding of paclitaxel.

The pharmacokinetics of paclitaxel were also evaluated in adult cancer patients who received single doses of 15-135 mg/m^2 given by 1 hour infusions (n=15), 30-275 mg/m^2 given by 6 hour infusions (n=36), and 200-275 mg/m^2 given by 24 hour infusions (n=54) in Phase 1 & 2 studies. Values for CLT and volume of distribution were consistent with the findings in the Phase 3 study. The pharmacokinetics of paclitaxel in patients with AIDS-related Kaposi's sarcoma have not been studied.

In vitro studies of binding to human serum proteins, using paclitaxel concentrations ranging from 0.1 to 50 μg/ml, indicate that between 89-98% of drug is bound; the presence of cimetidine, ranitidine, dexamethasone, or diphenhydramine did not affect protein binding of paclitaxel.

After intravenous administration of 15-275 mg/m^2 doses of paclitaxel injection as 1, 6, or 24 hour infusions, mean values for cumulative urinary recovery of unchanged drug ranged from 1.3-12.6% of the dose, indicating extensive non-renal clearance. In 5 patients administered a 225 or 250 mg/m^2 dose of radiolabeled paclitaxel as a 3 hour infusion, a mean of 71% of the radioactivity was excreted in the feces in 120 hours, and 14% was recovered in the urine. Total recovery of radioactivity ranged from 56-101% of the dose. Paclitaxel represented a mean of 5% of the administered radioactivity recovered in the feces, while metabolites, primarily 6α-hydroxypaclitaxel, accounted for the balance. *In vitro* studies with human liver microsomes and tissue slices showed that paclitaxel was metabolized primarily to 6α-hydroxypaclitaxel by the cytochrome P450 isozyme CYP2C8; and to two minor metabolites, 3′-*p*-hydroxypaclitaxel and 6α, 3′-*p*-dihydroxypaclitaxel, by CYP3A4. *In vitro*, the metabolism of paclitaxel to 6α-hydroxypaclitaxel was inhibited by a number of agents (ketoconazole, verapamil, diazepam, quinidine, dexamethasone, cyclosporin, teniposide, etoposide, and vincristine), but the concentrations used exceeded those found *in vivo* following normal therapeutic doses. Testosterone, 17α -ethinyl estradiol, retinoic acid, and quercetin, a specific inhibitor of CYP2C8, also inhibited the formation of 6α-hydroxypaclitaxel *in vitro*. The pharmacokinetics of paclitaxel may also be altered *in vivo* as a result of interactions with compounds that are substrates, inducers, or inhibitors of CYP2C8 and/or CYP3A4. (See DRUG INTERACTIONS.) The effect of renal or hepatic dysfunction on the disposition of paclitaxel has not been investigated.

Possible interactions of paclitaxel with concomitantly administered medications have not been formally investigated.

INDICATIONS AND USAGE

Paclitaxel is indicated as first-line and subsequent therapy for the treatment of advanced carcinoma of the ovary. As first-line therapy, paclitaxel is indicated in combination with cisplatin.

Paclitaxel is indicated for the adjuvant treatment of node-positive breast cancer administered sequentially to standard doxorubicin-containing combination chemotherapy. In the clinical trial, there was an overall favorable effect on disease-free and overall survival in the total population of patients with receptor-positive and receptor-negative tumors, but the benefit has been specifically demonstrated by available data (median follow-up 30 months) only in the patients with estrogen and progesterone receptor-negative tumors.

Paclitaxel is indicated for the treatment of breast cancer after failure of combination chemotherapy for metastatic disease or relapse within 6 months of adjuvant chemotherapy. Prior therapy should have included an anthracycline unless clinically contraindicated.

Paclitaxel, in combination with cisplatin, is indicated for the first-line treatment of non-small cell lung cancer in patients who are not candidates for potentially curative surgery and/or radiation therapy.

Paclitaxel is indicated for the second-line treatment of AIDS-related Kaposi's sarcoma.

CONTRAINDICATIONS

Paclitaxel is contraindicated in patients who have a history of hypersensitivity reactions to paclitaxel or other drugs formulated in Cremophor EL (polyoxyethylated castor oil).

Paclitaxel should not be used in patients with solid tumors who have baseline neutrophil counts of <1500 cells/mm^3 or in patients with AIDS-related Kaposi's sarcoma with baseline neutrophil counts of <1000 cells/mm^3.

WARNINGS

Anaphylaxis and severe hypersensitivity reactions characterized by dyspnea and hypotension requiring treatment, angioedema, and generalized urticaria have occurred in 2-4% of patients receiving paclitaxel in clinical trials. Fatal reactions have occurred in patients despite premedication. All patients should be pretreated with corticosteroids, diphenhydramine, and H_2 antagonists. (See DOSAGE AND ADMINISTRATION.) Patients who experience severe hypersensitivity reactions to paclitaxel should not be rechallenged with the drug.

Bone marrow suppression (primarily neutropenia) is dose-dependent and is the dose-limiting toxicity. Neutrophil nadirs occurred at a median of 11 days. Paclitaxel should not be administered to patients with baseline neutrophil counts of less than 1500 cells/mm^3 (<1000 cells/mm^3 for patients with KS). Frequent monitoring of blood counts should be instituted during paclitaxel treatment. Patients should not be re-treated with subsequent cycles of paclitaxel until neutrophils recover to a level >1500 cells/mm^3 (>1000 cells/mm^3 for patients with KS) and platelets recover to a level >100,000 cells/mm^3.

Severe conduction abnormalities have been documented in <1% of patients during paclitaxel therapy and in some cases requiring pacemaker placement. If patients develop significant conduction abnormalities during paclitaxel infusion, appropriate therapy should be administered and continuous cardiac monitoring should be performed during subsequent therapy with paclitaxel.

PREGNANCY

Paclitaxel can cause fetal harm when administered to a pregnant woman. Administration of paclitaxel during the period of organogenesis to rabbits at doses of 3.0 mg/kg/day (about 0.2 the daily maximum recommended human dose on a mg/m^2 basis) caused embryo- and fetotoxicity, as indicated by intrauterine mortality, increased resorptions, and increased fetal deaths. Maternal toxicity was also observed at this dose. No teratogenic effects were observed at 1.0 mg/kg/day (about 1/15 the daily maximum recommended human dose on a mg/m^2 basis); teratogenic potential could not be assessed at higher doses due to extensive fetal mortality.

There are no adequate and well-controlled studies in pregnant women. If paclitaxel is used during pregnancy, or if the patient becomes pregnant while receiving this drug, the patient should be apprised of the potential hazard to the fetus. Women of childbearing potential should be advised to avoid becoming pregnant.

PRECAUTIONS

Contact of the undiluted concentrate with plasticized polyvinyl chloride (PVC) equipment or devices used to prepare solutions for infusion is not recommended. In order to minimize patient exposure to the plasticizer DEHP [di-(2-ethylhexyl)phthalate], which may be leached from PVC infusion bags or sets, diluted paclitaxel injection solutions should preferably be stored in bottles (glass, polypropylene) or plastic bags (polypropylene, polyolefin) and administered through polyethylene-lined administration sets.

Paclitaxel should be administered through an in-line filter with a microporous membrane not greater than 0.22 microns. Use of filter devices such as IVEX-2 filters which incorporate short inlet and outlet PVC-coated tubing has not resulted in significant leaching of DEHP.

HEMATOLOGY

Paclitaxel therapy should not be administered to patients with baseline neutrophil counts of less than 1500 cells/mm^3. In order to monitor the occurrence of myelotoxicity, it is recommended that frequent peripheral blood cell counts be performed on all patients receiving paclitaxel. Patients should not be re-treated with subsequent cycles of paclitaxel until neutrophils recover to a level >1500 cells/mm^3 and platelets recover to a level >100,000 cells/mm^3. In the case of severe neutropenia (<500 cells/mm^3 for 7 days or more) during a course of paclitaxel therapy, a 20% reduction in dose for subsequent courses of therapy is recommended.

For patients with advanced HIV disease and poor-risk AIDS-related Kaposi's sarcoma, paclitaxel, at the recommended dose for this disease, can be initiated and repeated if the neutrophil count is at least 1000 cells/mm^3.

HYPERSENSITIVITY REACTIONS

Patients with a history of severe hypersensitivity reactions to products containing Cremophor EL (*e.g.*, cyclosporin for injection concentrate and teniposide for injection concentrate) should not be treated with paclitaxel. In order to avoid the occurrence of severe hypersensitivity reactions, all patients treated with paclitaxel should be premedicated with corticosteroids (such as dexamethasone), diphenhydramine and H_2 antagonists (such as cimetidine or ranitidine). Minor symptoms such as flushing, skin reactions, dyspnea, hypotension, or tachycardia do not require interruption of therapy. However, severe reactions, such as hypotension requiring treatment, dyspnea requiring bronchodilators, angioedema, or generalized urticaria require immediate discontinuation of paclitaxel and aggressive symptomatic therapy. Patients who have developed severe hypersensitivity reactions should not be rechallenged with paclitaxel.

CARDIOVASCULAR

Hypotension, bradycardia, and hypertension have been observed during administration of paclitaxel, but generally do not require treatment. Occasionally paclitaxel infusions must be interrupted or discontinued because of initial or recurrent hypertension. Frequent vital sign monitoring, particularly during the first hour of paclitaxel infusion, is recommended. Continuous cardiac monitoring is not required except for patients with serious conduction abnormalities. (See WARNINGS.)

NERVOUS SYSTEM

Although the occurrence of peripheral neuropathy is frequent, the development of severe symptomatology is unusual and requires a dose reduction of 20% for all subsequent courses of paclitaxel.

Paclitaxel contains dehydrated alcohol, 396 mg/ml; consideration should be given to possible CNS and other effects of alcohol. (See Pediatric Use.)

HEPATIC

There is evidence that the toxicity of paclitaxel is enhanced in patients with elevated liver enzymes. Caution should be exercised when administering paclitaxel to patients with moderate to severe hepatic impairment and dose adjustments should be considered.

INJECTION SITE REACTION

Injection site reactions, including reactions secondary to extravasation, were usually mild and consisted of erythema, tenderness, skin discoloration, or swelling at the injection site. These reactions have been observed more frequently with the 24 hour infusion than with the 3 hour infusion. Recurrence of skin reactions at a site of previous extravasation following administration of paclitaxel at a different site, *i.e.*, "recall", has been reported rarely.

Rare reports of more severe events such as phlebitis, cellulitis, induration, skin exfoliation, necrosis, and fibrosis have been received as part of the continuing surveillance of paclitaxel safety. In some cases the onset of the injection site reaction either occurred during a prolonged infusion or was delayed by a week to ten days.

A specific treatment for extravasation reactions is unknown at this time. Given the possibility of extravasation, it is advisable to closely monitor the infusion site for possible infiltration during drug administration.

CARCINOGENESIS, MUTAGENESIS, AND IMPAIRMENT OF FERTILITY

The carcinogenic potential of paclitaxel has not been studied.

Paclitaxel has been shown to be clastogenic *in vitro* (chromosome aberrations in human lymphocytes) and *in vivo* (micronucleus test in mice). Paclitaxel was not mutagenic in the Ames test or the CHO/HGPRT gene mutation assay.

Administration of paclitaxel prior to and during mating produced impairment of fertility in male and female rats at doses equal to or greater than 1 mg/kg/day (about 0.04 the daily maximum recommended human dose on a mg/m^2 basis). At this dose, paclitaxel caused reduced fertility and reproductive indices, and increased embryo- and fetotoxicity. (See WARNINGS.)

PREGNANCY CATEGORY D

See WARNINGS.

NURSING MOTHERS

It is not known whether the drug is excreted in human milk. Following intravenous administration of carbon-14 labeled paclitaxel to rats on days 9-10 postpartum, concentrations of radioactivity in milk were higher than in plasma and declined in parallel with the plasma concentrations. Because many drugs are excreted in human milk and because of the potential for serious adverse reactions in nursing infants, it is recommended that nursing be discontinued when receiving paclitaxel therapy.

PEDIATRIC USE

The safety and effectiveness of paclitaxel in pediatric patients have not been established.

There have been reports of central nervous system (CNS) toxicity (rarely associated with death) in a clinical trial in pediatric patients in which paclitaxel was infused intravenously over 3 hours at doses ranging from 350-420 mg/m^2. The toxicity is most likely attributable to the high dose of the ethanol component of the paclitaxel injection vehicle given over a short infusion time. The use of concomitant antihistamines may intensify this effect. Although a direct effect of the paclitaxel itself cannot be discounted, the high doses used in this study (over twice the recommended adult dosage) must be considered in assessing the safety of paclitaxel for use in this population.

INFORMATION FOR THE PATIENT

See the Patient Information Leaflet that is distributed with the prescription.

DRUG INTERACTIONS

In a Phase 1 trial using escalating doses of paclitaxel (110-200 mg/m^2) and cisplatin (50 or 75 mg/m^2) given as sequential infusions, myelosuppression was more profound when paclitaxel was given after cisplatin than with the alternate sequence (*i.e.*, paclitaxel before cisplatin). Pharmacokinetic data from these patients demonstrated a decrease in paclitaxel clearance of approximately 33% when paclitaxel was administered following cisplatin.

The metabolism of paclitaxel is catalyzed by cytochrome P450 isoenzymes CYP2C8 and CYP3A4. In the absence of formal clinical drug interaction studies, caution should be exercised when administering paclitaxel concomitantly with known substrates or inhibitors of the cytochrome P450 isoenzymes CYP2C8 and CYP3A4. (See CLINICAL PHARMACOLOGY.)

Potential interactions between paclitaxel, a substrate of CYP3A4, and protease inhibitors (ritonavir, saquinavir, indinavir, and nelfinavir), which are substrates and/or inhibitors of CYP3A4, have not been evaluated in clinical trials.

Reports in the literature suggest that plasma levels of doxorubicin (and its active metabolite doxorubicinol) may be increased when paclitaxel and doxorubicin are used in combination.

ADVERSE REACTIONS

POOLED ANALYSIS OF ADVERSE EVENT EXPERIENCES FROM SINGLE-AGENT STUDIES

Data in TABLE 9 are based on the experience of 812 patients (493 with ovarian carcinoma and 319 with breast carcinoma) enrolled in 10 studies who received single-agent paclitaxel. Two hundred and seventy-five (275) patients were treated in eight Phase 2 studies with paclitaxel doses ranging from 135-300 mg/m^2 administered over 24 hours (in four of these studies, G-CSF was administered as hematopoietic support). Three hundred and one (301) patients were treated in the randomized Phase 3 ovarian carcinoma study which compared two doses (135 or 175 mg/m^2) and two schedules (3 or 24 hours) of paclitaxel. Two hundred and thirty-six (236) patients with breast carcinoma received paclitaxel (135 or 175 mg/m^2) administered over 3 hours in a controlled study.

None of the observed toxicities were clearly influenced by age.

DISEASE-SPECIFIC ADVERSE EVENT EXPERIENCES FIRST-LINE OVARY IN COMBINATION

For the 1084 patients who were evaluable for safety in the Phase 3 first-line ovary combination therapy studies, TABLE 10 shows the incidence of important adverse events. For both studies, the analysis of safety was based on all courses of therapy (six courses for the GOG-111 study and up to nine courses for the Intergroup study).

Second-Line Ovary

For the 403 patients who received single-agent paclitaxel injection in the Phase 3 second-line ovarian carcinoma study, TABLE 11 shows the incidence of important adverse events.

Myelosuppression was dose and schedule related, with the schedule effect being more prominent. The development of severe hypersensitivity reactions (HSRs) was rare; 1% of the patients and 0.2% of the courses overall. There was no apparent dose or schedule effect seen for the HSRs. Peripheral neuropathy was clearly dose-related, but schedule did not appear to affect the incidence.

Adjuvant Breast

For the Phase 3 adjuvant breast carcinoma study, TABLE 12 shows the incidence of important severe adverse events for the 3121 patients (total population) who were evaluable for safety as well as for a group of 325 patients (early population) who, per the study protocol, were monitored more intensively than other patients.

The incidence of an adverse event for the total population likely represents an underestimation of the actual incidence given that safety data were collected differently based on enrollment cohort. However, since safety data were collected consistently across regimens, the safety of the sequential addition of paclitaxel injection following AC therapy may be compared with AC therapy alone. Compared to patients who received AC alone, patients who received AC followed by paclitaxel experienced more Grade III/IV neurosensory toxicity, more Grade III/IV myalgia/arthralgia, more Grade III/IV neurologic pain (5% vs 1%), more Grade III/IV flu-like symptoms (5% vs 3%), and more Grade III/IV hyperglycemia (3% vs 1%). During the additional four courses of treatment with paclitaxel, two deaths (0.1%) were attributed to treatment. During paclitaxel treatment, Grade IV neutropenia was reported for 15% of patients, Grade II/III neurosensory toxicity for 15%, Grade II/III myalgias for 23%, and alopecia for 46%.

P

TABLE 9 *Summary* of Adverse Events in Patients With Solid Tumors Receiving Single-Agent Paclitaxel*

	Percent of Patients (n=812)
Bone Marrow	
Neutropenia	
$<2000/mm^3$	90%
$<500/mm^3$	52%
Leukopenia	
$<4000/mm^3$	90%
$<1000/mm^3$	17%
Thrombocytopenia	
$<100,000/mm^3$	20%
$<50,000/mm^3$	7%
Anemia	
<11 g/dl	78%
<8 g/dl	16%
Infections	30%
Bleeding	14%
Red cell transfusions	25%
Platelet transfusions	2%
Hypersensitivity Reactions†	
All	41%
Severe‡	2%
Cardiovascular	
Vital sign changes§	
Bradycardia (n=537)	3%
Hypotension (n=532)	12%
Significant cardiovascular events	1%
Abnormal ECG	
All patients	23%
Patients with normal baseline (n=559)	14%
Peripheral Neuropathy	
Any symptoms	60%
Severe symptoms‡	3%
Myalgia/Arthralgia	
Any symptoms	60%
Severe symptoms‡	8%
Gastrointestinal	
Nausea and vomiting	52%
Diarrhea	38%
Mucositis	31%
Alopeica	87%
Hepatic (patients with normal baseline and on study data)	
Bilibruin elevations (n=765)	7%
Alkaline phosphatase elevations (n=575)	22%
AST (SGOT) elevations (n=591)	19%
Injection Site Reactions	13%

* Based on worst course analysis.
† All patients received premedication.
‡ Severe events are defined as at least Grade III toxicity.
§ During the first 3 hours of infusion.

The incidences of severe hematologic toxicities, infections, mucositis, and cardiovascular events increased with higher doses of doxorubicin.

Breast Cancer After Failure of Initial Chemotherapy

For the 458 patients who received single-agent paclitaxel in the Phase 3 breast carcinoma study, TABLE 13 shows the incidence of important adverse events by treatment arm (each arm was administered by a 3 hour infusion).

Myelosuppression and peripheral neuropathy were dose related. There was one severe hypersensitivity reaction (HSR) observed at the dose of 135 mg/m^2.

First-Line NSCLC in Combination

In the study conducted by the Eastern Cooperative Oncology Group (ECOG), patients were randomized to either paclitaxel (P) 135 mg/m^2 as a 24 hour infusion in combination with cisplatin (c) 75 mg/m^2, paclitaxel (P) 250 mg/m^2 as a 24 hour infusion in combination with cisplatin (c) 75 mg/m^2 with G-CSF support, or cisplatin (c) 75 mg/m^2 on day 1, followed by etoposide (VP) 100 mg/m^2 on days 1, 2 and 3 (control).

TABLE 14 shows the incidence of important adverse events.

Toxicity was generally more severe in the high-dose paclitaxel injection treatment arm (P250/c75) than in the low-dose paclitaxel arm (T135/c75). Compared to the cisplatin/etoposide arm, patients in the low-dose paclitaxel arm experienced more arthralgia/myalgia of any grade and more severe neutropenia. The incidence of febrile neutropenia was not reported in this study.

Kaposi's Sarcoma

TABLE 15 shows the frequency of important adverse events in the 85 patients with KS treated with two different single-agent paclitaxel regimens.

As demonstrated in TABLE 15, toxicity was more pronounced in the study utilizing paclitaxel at a dose of 135 mg/m^2 every 3 weeks than in the study utilizing paclitaxel at a dose of 100 mg/m^2 every 2 weeks. Notably, severe neutropenia (76% vs 35%), febrile neutropenia (55% vs 9%), and opportunistic infections (76% vs 54%) were more common with the former dose and schedule. The differences between the two studies with respect to dose escalation and use of hematopoietic growth factors, as described above, should be taken into account. Note also that only 26% of the 85 patients in these studies received concomitant treatment with protease inhibitors, whose effect on paclitaxel metabolism has not yet been studied.

ADVERSE EVENT EXPERIENCES BY BODY SYSTEM

Unless otherwise noted, the following discussion refers to the overall safety database of 812 patients with solid tumors treated with single-agent paclitaxel in clinical studies. Toxicities that occurred with greater severity or frequency in previously untreated patients with ova-

TABLE 10 *Frequency* of Important Adverse Events in the Phase 3 First-Line Ovarian Carcinoma Studies*

	Intergroup		GOG-111	
	P175/3† c75‡ (n=339)	C750‡ c75‡ (n=336)	P135/24† c75‡ (n=196)	C750‡ c75‡ (n=213)
Bone Marrow				
Neutropenia				
$<2000/mm^3$	91%§	95%§	96%	92%
$<500/mm^3$	33%§	43%§	81%§	58%§
Thrombocytopenia				
$<100,000/mm^3$¤	21%§	33%§	26%	30%
$<50,000/mm^3$	3%§	7%§	10%	9%
Anemia				
<11 g/dl¶	96%	97%	88%	86%
<8 g/dl	3%§	8%§	13%	9%
Infections	25%	27%	21%	15%
Febrile neutropenia	4%	7%	15%§	4%§
Hypersensitivity Reaction				
All	11%§	6%§	8%§**	1%§**
Severe††	1%	1%	3%§**	—§**
Neurotoxicity‡‡				
Any symptoms	87%§	52%§	25%	20%
Severe symptoms††	21%§	2%§	3%§	—§
Nausea and Vomiting				
Any symptoms	88%	93%	65%	69%
Severe symptoms††	18%	24%	10%	11%
Myalgia/Arthralgia				
Any symptoms	60%§	27%§	9%§	2%§
Severe symptoms††	6%§	1%§	1%	—
Diarrhea				
Any symptoms	37%§	29%§	16%§	8%§
Severe symptoms††	2%	3%	4%	1%
Asthenia				
Any symptoms	NC	NC	17%§	10%§
Severe symptoms††	NC	NC	1%	1%
Alopecia				
Any symptoms	96%§	89%§	55%§	37%§
Severe symptoms††	51%§	21%§	6%	8%

* Based on worst course analysis.
† Paclitaxel (P) dose in mg/m^2/infusion duration in hours.
† Cyclophosphamide (C) or cisplatin (c) dose in mg/m^2.
§ $p < 0.05$ by Fisher exact test.
¤ $<130,000/mm^3$ in the Intergroup study.
¶ <12 g/dl in the Intergroup study.
** All patients received premedication.
†† Severe events are defined as at least Grade III toxicity.
‡‡ In the GOG-111 study, neurotoxicity was collected as peripheral neuropathy and in the Intergroup study, neurotoxicity was collected as either neuromotor or neurosensory symptoms.
NC Not Collected.

TABLE 11 *Frequency* of Important Adverse Events in the Phase 3 Second-Line Ovarian Carcinoma Study*

	175/3† (n=95)	175/24† (n=105)	135/3† (n=98)	135/24† (n=105)
Bone Marrow				
Neutropenia				
$<2000/mm^3$	78%	98%	78%	98%
$<500/mm^3$	27%	75%	14%	67%
Thrombocytopenia				
$<100,000/mm^3$	4%	18%	8%	6%
$<50,000/mm^3$	1%	7%	2%	1%
Anemia				
<11 g/dl	84%	90%	68%	88%
<8 g/dl	11%	12%	6%	10%
Infections	26%	29%	20%	18%
Hypersensitivity Reaction‡				
All	41%	45%	38%	45%
Severe§	2%	0%	2%	1%
Peripheral Neuropathy				
Any symptoms	63%	60%	55%	42%
Severe symptoms§	1%	2%	0%	0%
Mucositis				
Any symptoms	17%	35%	21%	25%
Severe symptoms§	0%	3%	0%	2%

* Based on worst course analysis.
† Paclitaxel dose in mg/m^2/infusion duration in hours.
‡ All patients received premedication.
§ Severe events are defined as at least Grade III toxicity.

rian carcinoma or NSCLC who received paclitaxel in combination with cisplatin or in patients with breast cancer who received paclitaxel after doxorubicin/cyclophosphamide in the adjuvant setting and that occurred with a difference that was clinically significant in these populations are also described. The frequency and severity of important adverse events for the Phase 3 ovarian carcinoma, breast carcinoma, NSCLC, and the Phase 2 Kaposi's sarcoma studies are presented above in tabular form by treatment arm. In addition, rare events have been reported from postmarketing experience or from other clinical studies. The frequency and severity of adverse events have been generally similar for patients receiving paclitaxel for the treatment of ovarian, breast, or lung carcinoma or Kaposi's sarcoma, but patients with AIDS-related Kaposi's sarcoma may have more frequent and severe hematologic toxicity, infections, and febrile neutropenia. These patients require a lower dose intensity and supportive care. Toxicities that were observed only in or were noted to have

TABLE 12 *Frequency* of Important Severe† Adverse Events in the Phase 3 Adjuvant Breast Carcinoma Study*

	Early Population		Total Population	
	AC	AC followed by P	AC	AC followed by P
	(n=166)	(n=159)	(n=1551)	(n=1570)
Bone Marrow‡				
Neutropenia				
$<500/mm^3$	79%	76%	48%	50%
Thrombocytopenia				
$<50,000/mm^3$	27%	25%	11%	11%
Anemia				
<8 g/dl	17%	21%	8%	8%
Infections	6%	14%	5%	6%
Fever without infection	—	3%	<1%	1%
Hypersensitivity Reaction§	1%	4%	1%	2%
Cardiovascular Events	1%	2%	1%	2%
Neuromotor Toxicity	1%	1%	<1%	1%
Neurosensory Toxicity	—	3%	<1%	3%
Myalgia/Arthralgia	—	2%	<1%	2%
Nausea/Vomiting	13%	18%	8%	9%
Mucositis	13%	4%	6%	5%

* Based on worst course analysis.
† Severe events are defined as at least Grade III toxicity.
‡ The incidence of febrile neutropenia was not reported in this study.
§ All patients were to receive premedication.
AC Patients received 600 mg/m^2 cyclophosphamide and doxorubicin (AC) at doses of either 60 mg/m^2, 75 mg/m^2, or 90 mg/m^2 (with prophylactic G-CSF support and ciprofloxacin), every 3 weeks for four courses.
P Paclitaxel (P) following four courses of AC at a dose of 175 mg/m^2/3 hours every 3 weeks for four courses.

TABLE 13 *Frequency* of Important Adverse Events in the Phase 3 Study of Breast Cancer After Failure of Initial Chemotherapy or Within 6 Months of Adjuvant Chemotherapy*

	175/3†	135/3†
	(n=229)	(n=229)
Bone Marrow		
Neutropenia		
$<2000/mm^3$	90%	81%
$<500/mm^3$	28%	19%
Thrombocytopenia		
$<100,000/mm^3$	11%	7%
$<50,000/mm^3$	3%	2%
Anemia		
<11 g/dl	55%	47%
<8 g/dl	4%	2%
Infections	23%	15%
Febrile neutropenia	2%	2%
Hypersensitivity Reaction‡		
All	36%	31%
Severe§	0%	<1%
Peripheral Neuropathy		
Any symptoms	70%	46%
Severe symptoms§	7%	3%
Mucositis		
Any symptoms	23%	17%
Severe symptoms§	3%	<1%

* Based on worst course analysis.
† Paclitaxel dose in mg/m^2/infusion duration in hours.
‡ All patients received premedication.
§ Severe events are defined as at least Grade III toxicity.

occurred with greater severity in the population with Kaposi's sarcoma and that occurred with a difference that was clinically significant in this population are described.

Hematologic

Bone marrow suppression was the major dose-limiting toxicity of paclitaxel. Neutropenia, the most important hematologic toxicity, was dose and schedule dependent and was generally rapidly reversible. Among patients treated in the Phase 3 second-line ovarian study with a 3 hour infusion, neutrophil counts declined below 500 cells/mm^3 in 14% of the patients treated with a dose of 135 mg/m^2 compared to 27% at a dose of 175 mg/m^2 (p=0.05). In the same study, severe neutropenia (<500 cells/mm^3) was more frequent with the 24 hour than with the 3 hour infusion; infusion duration had a greater impact on myelosuppression than dose. Neutropenia did not appear to increase with cumulative exposure and did not appear to be more frequent nor more severe for patients previously treated with radiation therapy.

In the study where paclitaxel was administered to patients with ovarian carcinoma at a dose of 135 mg/m^2/24 hours in combination with cisplatin versus the control arm of cyclosphosphamide plus cisplatin, the incidences of grade IV neutropenia and of febrile neutropenia were significantly greater in the paclitaxel plus cisplatin arm than in the control arm. Grade IV neutropenia occurred in 81% on the paclitaxel injection plus cisplatin arm versus 58% on the cyclophosphamide plus cisplatin arm, and febrile neutropenia occurred in 15% and 4% respectively. On the paclitaxel/cisplatin arm, there were 35/1074 (3%) courses with fever in which Grade IV neutropenia was reported at some time during the course. When paclitaxel followed by cisplatin was administered to patients with advanced NSCLC in the ECOG study, the incidences of Grade IV neutropenia were 74% (paclitaxel 135 mg/m^2/24 hours followed by cisplatin) and 65% (paclitaxel 250 mg/m^2/24 hours fol-

TABLE 14 *Frequency* of Important Adverse Events in the Phase 3 Study for First-Line NSCLC*

	P135/24†	P250/24‡	VP100§
	c75	c75	c75
	(n=195)	(n=197)	(n=196)
Bone Marrow			
Neutropenia			
$<2000/mm^3$	89%	86%	84%
$<500/mm^3$	74%¤	65%	55%
Thrombocytopenia			
<normal	48%	68%	62%
$<50,000/mm^3$	6%	12%	16%
Anemia			
<normal	94%	96%	95%
<8 g/dl	22%	19%	28%
Infections	38%	31%	35%
Hypersensitivity Reaction¶			
All	16%	27%	13%
Severe**	1%	4%¤	1%
Arthralgia/Myalgia			
Any symptoms	21%¤	42%¤	9%
Severe symptoms**	3%	11%	1%
Nausea/Vomiting			
Any symptoms	85%	87%	81%
Severe symptoms**	27%	29%	22%
Mucositis			
Any symptoms	18%	28%	16%
Severe symptoms**	1%	4%	2%
Neuromotor Toxicity			
Any symptoms	37%	47%	44%
Severe symptoms**	6%	12%	7%
Neurosensory Toxicity			
Any symptoms	48%	61%	25%
Severe symptoms**	13%	28%¤	8%
Cardiovascular Events			
Any symptoms	33%	39%	24%
Severe symptoms**	13%	12%	8%

* Based on worst course analysis.
† Paclitaxel (P) dose in mg/m^2/infusion duration in hours; cisplatin (c) dose in mg/m^2.
‡ Paclitaxel dose in mg/m^2/infusion duration in hours with G-CSF support; cisplatin dose in mg/m^2.
§ Etoposide (VP) dose in mg/m^2 was administered IV on days 1, 2 and 3; cisplatin dose in mg/m^2.
¤ $p < 0.05$.
¶ All patients received premedication.
** Severe events are defined as at least Grade III toxicity.

TABLE 15 *Frequency* of Important Adverse Events in the AIDS-Related Kaposi's Sarcoma Studies*

	Study CA139-174	Study CA139-281
	Paclitaxel 135/3† q3wk	Paclitaxel 100/3† q2wk
	(n=29)	(n=56)
Bone Marrow		
Neutropenia		
$<2000/mm^3$	100%	95%
$<500/mm^3$	76%	35%
Thrombocytopenia		
$<100,000/mm^3$	52%	27%
$<50,000/mm^3$	17%	5%
Anemia		
<11 g/dl	86%	73%
<8 g/dl	34%	25%
Febrile neutropenia	55%	9%
Opportunistic Infection		
Any	76%	54%
Cytomegalovirus	45%	27%
Herpes simplex	38%	11%
Pneumocystis carinii	14%	21%
M. avium-intracellulare	24%	4%
Candidiasis, esophageal	7%	9%
Cryptosporidiosis	7%	7%
Cryptococcal meningitis	3%	2%
Leukoencephalopathy	—	2%
Hypersensitivity Reaction‡		
All	14%	9%
Cardiovascular		
Hypotension	17%	9%
Bradycardia	3%	—
Peripheral Neuropathy		
Any	79%	46%
Severe§	10%	2%
Myalgia/Arthralgia		
Any	93%	48%
Severe§	14%	16%
Gastrointestinal		
Nausea or vomiting	69%	70%
Diarrhea	90%	73%
Mucositis	45%	20%
Renal (creatinine elevation)		
Any	34%	18%
Severe§	7%	5%
Discontinuation for Drug Toxicity	7%	16%

* Based on worst course analysis.
† Paclitaxel dose in mg/m^2/infusion duration in hours.
‡ All patients received premedication.
§ Severe events are defined as at least Grade III toxicity.

P

lowed by cisplatin and G-CSF) compared with 55% in patients who received cisplatin/etoposide.

Fever was frequent (12% of all treatment courses). Infectious episodes occurred in 30% of all patients and 9% of all courses; these episodes were fatal in 1% of all patients, and included sepsis, pneumonia and peritonitis. In the Phase 3 second-line ovarian study, infectious episodes were reported in 20% and 26% of the patients treated with a dose of 135 mg/m^2 or 175 mg/m^2 given as 3 hour infusions, respectively. Urinary tract infections and upper respiratory tract infections were the most frequently reported infectious complications. In the immunosuppressed patient population with advanced HIV disease and poor-risk AIDS-related Kaposi's sarcoma, 61% of the patients reported at least one opportunistic infection. The use of supportive therapy, including G-CSF, is recommended for patients who have experienced severe neutropenia. (See DOSAGE AND ADMINISTRATION.)

Thrombocytopenia was uncommon, and almost never severe (<50,000 cells/mm^3). Twenty percent (20%) of the patients experienced a drop in their platelet count below 100,000 cells/mm^3 at least once while on treatment; 7% had a platelet count <50,000 cells/mm^3 at the time of their worst nadir. Bleeding episodes were reported in 4% of all courses and by 14% of all patients but most of the hemorrhagic episodes were localized and the frequency of these events was unrelated to the paclitaxel dose and schedule. In the Phase 3 second-line ovarian study, bleeding episodes were reported in 10% of the patients; no patients treated with the 3 hour infusion received platelet transfusions. In the adjuvant breast carcinoma trial, the incidence of severe thrombocytopenia and platelet transfusions increased with higher doses of doxorubicin.

Anemia (Hb <11 g/dl) was observed in 78% of all patients and was severe (Hb <8 g/dl) in 16% of the cases. No consistent relationship between dose or schedule and the frequency of anemia was observed. Among all patients with normal baseline hemoglobin, 69% became anemic on study but only 7% had severe anemia. Red cell transfusions were required in 25% of all patients and in 12% of those with normal baseline hemoglobin levels.

Hypersensitivity Reactions (HSRs)

All patients received premedication prior to paclitaxel (see WARNINGS and PRECAUTIONS, Hypersensitivity Reactions). The frequency and severity of HSRs were not affected by the dose or schedule of paclitaxel administration. In the Phase 3 second-line ovarian study, the 3 hour infusion was not associated with a greater increase in HSRs when compared to the 24 hour infusion. Hypersensitivity reactions were observed in 20% of all courses and in 41% of all patients. These reactions were severe in less than 2% of the patients and 1% of the courses. No severe reactions were observed after course 3 and severe symptoms occurred generally within the first hour of paclitaxel infusion. The most frequent symptoms observed during these severe reactions were dyspnea, flushing, chest pain, and tachycardia.

The minor hypersensitivity reactions consisted mostly of flushing (28%), rash (12%), hypotension (4%), dyspnea (2%), tachycardia (2%), and hypertension (1%). The frequency of hypersensitivity reactions remained relatively stable during the entire treatment period.

Rare reports of chills and reports of back pain in association with hypersensitivity reactions have been received as part of the continuing surveillance of paclitaxel safety.

Cardiovascular

Hypotension, during the first 3 hours of infusion, occurred in 12% of all patients and 3% of all courses administered. Bradycardia, during the first 3 hours of infusion, occurred in 3% of all patients and 1% of all courses. In the Phase 3 second-line ovarian study, neither dose nor schedule had an effect on the frequency of hypotension and bradycardia. These vital sign changes most often caused no symptoms and required neither specific therapy nor treatment discontinuation. The frequency of hypotension and bradycardia were not influenced by prior anthracycline therapy.

Significant cardiovascular events possibly related to single-agent paclitaxel occurred in approximately 1% of all patients. These events included syncope, rhythm abnormalities, hypertension and venous thrombosis. One of the patients with syncope treated with paclitaxel at 175 mg/m^2 over 24 hours had progressive hypotension and died. The arrhythmias included asymptomatic ventricular tachycardia, bigeminy and complete AV block requiring pacemaker placement. Among patients with NSCLC treated with paclitaxel in combination with cisplatin in the Phase 3 study, significant cardiovascular events occurred in 12-13%. This apparent increase in cardiovascular events is possibly due to an increase in cardiovascular risk factors in patients with lung cancer.

Electrocardiogram (ECG) abnormalities were common among patients at baseline. ECG abnormalities on study did not usually result in symptoms, were not dose-limiting, and required no intervention. ECG abnormalities were noted in 23% of all patients. Among patients with a normal ECG prior to study entry, 14% of all patients developed an abnormal tracing while on study. The most frequently reported ECG modifications were non-specific repolarization abnormalities, sinus bradycardia, sinus tachycardia, and premature beats. Among patients with normal ECGs at baseline, prior therapy with anthracyclines did not influence the frequency of ECG abnormalities.

Cases of myocardial infarction have been reported rarely. Congestive heart failure has been reported typically in patients who have received other chemotherapy, notably anthracyclines. (See DRUG INTERACTIONS.)

Rare reports of atrial fibrillation and supraventricular tachycardia have been received as part of the continuing surveillance of paclitaxel safety.

Respiratory

Rare reports of interstitial pneumonia, lung fibrosis, and pulmonary embolism have been received as part of the continuing surveillance of paclitaxel safety. Rare reports of radiation pneumonitis have been received in patients receiving concurrent radiotherapy.

Neurologic

The assessment of neurologic toxicity was conducted differently among the studies as evident from the data reported in each individual study (see TABLES 9-15). Moreover, the frequency and severity of neurologic manifestations were influenced by prior and/or concomitant therapy with neurotoxic agents.

In general, the frequency and severity of neurologic manifestations were dose-dependent in patients receiving single-agent paclitaxel injection. Peripheral neuropathy was observed in 60% of all patients (3% severe) and in 52% (2% severe) of the patients without pre-existing neuropathy. The frequency of peripheral neuropathy increased with cumulative dose. Neurologic symptoms were observed in 27% of the patients after the first course of treatment and in 34-51% from course 2 to 10. Peripheral neuropathy was the cause of paclitaxel discontinuation in 1% of all patients. Sensory symptoms have usually improved or resolved within several months of paclitaxel discontinuation. Pre-existing neuropathies resulting from prior therapies are not a contraindication for paclitaxel therapy.

In the Intergroup first-line ovarian carcinoma study (see TABLE 10), neurotoxicity included reports of neuromotor and neurosensory events. The regimen with paclitaxel 175 mg/m^2 given by 3 hour infusion plus cisplatin 75 mg/m^2 resulted in a greater incidence and severity of neurotoxicity than the regimen containing cyclophosphamide and cisplatin, 87% (21% severe) versus 52% (2% severe), respectively. The duration of grade III or IV neurotoxicity cannot be determined with precision for the Intergroup study since the resolution dates of adverse events were not collected in the case report forms for this trial and complete follow-up documentation was available only in a minority of these patients. In the GOG first-line ovarian carcinoma study, neurotoxicity was reported as peripheral neuropathy. The regimen with paclitaxel 135 mg/m^2 given by 24 hour infusion plus cisplatin 75 mg/m^2 resulted in an incidence of neurotoxicity that was similar to the regimen containing cyclophosphamide plus cisplatin, 25% (3% severe) versus 20% (0% severe), respectively. Cross-study comparison of neurotoxicity in the Intergroup and GOG trials suggests that when paclitaxel is given in combination with cisplatin 75 mg/m^2, the incidence of severe neurotoxicity is more common at a paclitaxel dose of 175 mg/m^2 given by 3 hour infusion (21%) than at a dose of 135 mg/m^2 given by 24 hour infusion (3%).

In patients with NSCLC, administration of paclitaxel followed by cisplatin resulted in a greater incidence of severe neurotoxicity compared to the incidence in patients with ovarian or breast cancer treated with single-agent paclitaxel. Severe neurosensory symptoms were noted in 13% of NSCLC patients receiving paclitaxel 135 mg/m^2 by 24 hour infusion followed by cisplatin 75 mg/m^2 and 8% of NSCLC patients receiving cisplatin/etoposide (see TABLE 14).

Other than peripheral neuropathy, serious neurologic events following paclitaxel administration have been rare (<1%) and have included grand mal seizures, syncope, ataxia, and neuroencephalopathy.

Rare reports of autonomic neuropathy resulting in paralytic ileus have been received as part of the continuing surveillance of paclitaxel safety. Optic nerve and/or visual disturbances (scintillating scotomata) have also been reported, particularly in patients who have received higher doses than those recommended. These effects generally have been reversible. However, rare reports in the literature of abnormal visual evoked potentials in patients have suggested persistent optic nerve damage. Postmarketing reports of ototoxicity (hearing loss and tinnitus) have also been received.

Arthralgia/Myalgia

There was no consistent relationship between dose or schedule of paclitaxel and the frequency or severity of arthralgia/myalgia. Sixty percent (60%) of all patients treated experienced arthralgia/myalgia; 8% experienced severe symptoms. The symptoms were usually transient, occurred 2 or 3 days after paclitaxel administration, and resolved within a few days. The frequency and severity of musculoskeletal symptoms remained unchanged throughout the treatment period.

Hepatic

No relationship was observed between liver function abnormalities and either dose or schedule of paclitaxel administration. Among patients with normal baseline liver function 7%, 22%, and 19% had elevations in bilirubin, alkaline phosphatase, and AST (SGOT), respectively. Prolonged exposure to paclitaxel was not associated with cumulative hepatic toxicity.

Rare reports of hepatic necrosis and hepatic encephalopathy leading to death have been received as part of the continuing surveillance of paclitaxel safety.

Renal

Among the patients treated for Kaposi's sarcoma with paclitaxel, 5 patients had renal toxicity of grade III or IV severity. One patient with suspected HIV nephropathy of grade IV severity had to discontinue therapy. The other 4 patients had renal insufficiency with reversible elevations of serum creatinine.

Gastrointestinal (GI)

Nausea/vomiting, diarrhea, and mucositis were reported by 52%, 38%, and 31% of all patients, respectively. These manifestations were usually mild to moderate. Mucositis was schedule dependent and occurred more frequently with the 24 hour than with the 3 hour infusion.

In patients with poor-risk AIDS-related Kaposi's sarcoma, nausea/vomiting, diarrhea, and mucositis were reported by 69%, 79%, and 28% of patients, respectively. One-third of patients with Kaposi's sarcoma complained of diarrhea prior to study start.

In the first-line Phase 3 ovarian carcinoma studies, the incidence of nausea and vomiting when paclitaxel was administered in combination with cisplatin appeared to be greater compared with the database for single-agent paclitaxel in ovarian and breast carcinoma. In addition, diarrhea of any grade was reported more frequently compared to the control arm, but there was no difference for severe diarrhea in these studies.

Rare reports of intestinal obstruction, intestinal perforation, pancreatitis, ischemic colitis, and dehydration have been received as part of the continuing surveillance of paclitaxel safety. Rare reports of neutropenic enterocolitis (typhlitis), despite the coadministration of G-CSF, were observed in patients treated with paclitaxel alone and in combination with other chemotherapeutic agents.

Injection Site Reaction

Injection site reactions, including reactions secondary to extravasation, were usually mild and consisted of erythema, tenderness, skin discoloration, or swelling at the injection site. These reactions have been observed more frequently with the 24 hour infusion than with the 3 hour infusion. Recurrence of skin reactions at a site of previous extravasation following administration of paclitaxel at a different site, *i.e.*, "recall", has been reported rarely.

Rare reports of more severe events such as phlebitis, cellulitis, induration, skin exfoliation, necrosis, and fibrosis have been received as part of the continuing surveillance of paclitaxel safety. In some cases the onset of the injection site reaction either occurred during a prolonged infusion or was delayed by a week to ten days.

A specific treatment for extravasation reactions is unknown at this time. Given the possibility of extravasation, it is advisable to closely monitor the infusion site for possible infiltration during drug administration.

OTHER CLINICAL EVENTS

Alopecia was observed in almost all (87%) of the patients. Transient skin changes due to paclitaxel injection-related hypersensitivity reactions have been observed, but no other skin toxicities were significantly associated with paclitaxel administration. Nail changes (changes in pigmentation or discoloration of nail bed) were uncommon (2%). Edema was reported in 21% of all patients (17% of those without baseline edema); only 1% had severe edema and none of these patients required treatment discontinuation. Edema was most commonly focal and disease-related. Edema was observed in 5% of all courses for patients with normal baseline and did not increase with time on study.

Rare reports of skin abnormalities related to radiation recall as well as reports of maculopapular rash, pruritus, Stevens-Johnson syndrome, and toxic epidermal necrolysis have been received as part of the continuing surveillance of paclitaxel safety.

Reports of asthenia and malaise have been received as part of the continuing surveillance of paclitaxel safety. In the Phase 3 trial of paclitaxel 135 mg/m^2 over 24 hours in combination with cisplatin as first-line therapy of ovarian cancer, asthenia was reported in 17% of the patients, significantly greater than the 10% incidence observed in the control arm of cyclophosphamide/ cisplatin.

ACCIDENTAL EXPOSURE

Upon inhalation, dyspnea, chest pain, burning eyes, sore throat, and nausea have been reported. Following topical exposure, events have included tingling, burning, and redness.

DOSAGE AND ADMINISTRATION

Note: Contact of the undiluted concentrate with plasticized PVC equipment or devices used to prepare solutions for infusion is not recommended. In order to minimize patient exposure to the plasticizer DEHP [di-(2-ethylhexyl)phthalate], which may be leached from PVC infusion bags or sets, diluted paclitaxel solutions should be stored in bottles (glass, polypropylene) or plastic bags (polypropylene, polyolefin) and administered through polyethylene-lined administration sets.

All patients should be premedicated prior to paclitaxel administration in order to prevent severe hypersensitivity reactions. Such premedication may consist of dexamethasone 20 mg PO administered approximately 12 and 6 hours before paclitaxel, diphenhydramine (or its equivalent) 50 mg IV 30-60 minutes prior to paclitaxel, and cimetidine (300 mg) or ranitidine (50 mg) IV 30-60 minutes before paclitaxel.

For patients with **carcinoma of the ovary,** the following regimens are recommended:

1. For previously untreated patients with carcinoma of the ovary, one of the following recommended regimens may be given every 3 weeks. In selecting the appropriate regimen, differences in toxicities should be considered (see TABLE 10).
   a. Paclitaxel administered intravenously over 3 hours at a dose of 175 mg/m^2 followed by cisplatin at a dose of 75 mg/m^2; or
   b. Paclitaxel administered intravenously over 24 hours at a dose of 135 mg/m^2 followed by cisplatin at a dose of 75 mg/m^2.
2. In patients previously treated with chemotherapy for carcinoma of the ovary, paclitaxel has been used at several doses and schedules; however, the optimal regimen is not yet clear. The recommended regimen is paclitaxel 135 mg/m^2 or 175 mg/m^2 administered intravenously over 3 hours every 3 weeks.

For patients with **carcinoma of the breast,** the following regimens are recommended:

1. For the adjuvant treatment of node-positive breast cancer, the recommended regimen is paclitaxel, at a dose of 175 mg/m^2 intravenously over 3 hours every 3 weeks for four courses administered sequentially to doxorubicin-containing combination chemotherapy. The clinical trial used four courses of doxorubicin and cyclophosphamide.
2. After failure of initial chemotherapy for metastatic disease or relapse within 6 months of adjuvant chemotherapy, paclitaxel at a dose of 175 mg/m^2 administered intravenously over 3 hours every 3 weeks has been shown to be effective.

For patients with **non-small cell lung carcinoma,** the recommended regimen, given every 3 weeks, is paclitaxel administered intravenously over 24 hours at a dose of 135 mg/m^2 followed by cisplatin, 75 mg/m^2.

For patients with **AIDS-related Kaposi's sarcoma,** paclitaxel administered at a dose of 135 mg/m^2 given intravenously over 3 hours every 3 weeks or at a dose of 100 mg/m^2 given intravenously over 3 hours every 2 weeks is recommended (dose intensity 45-50 mg/m^2/week). In the two clinical trials evaluating these schedules, the former schedule (135 mg/m^2 every 3 weeks) was more toxic than the latter. In addition, all patients with low performance status were treated with the latter schedule (100 mg/m^2 every 2 weeks).

Based upon the immunosuppression in patients with advanced HIV disease, the following modifications are recommended in these patients:

1. Reduce the dose of dexamethasone as one of the three premedication drugs to 10 mg PO (instead of 20 mg PO);
2. Initiate or repeat treatment with paclitaxel only if the neutrophil count is at least 1000 cells/mm^3;
3. Reduce the dose of subsequent courses of paclitaxel by 20% for patients who experience severe neutropenia (neutrophil $<$500 cells/mm^3 for a week or longer); and
4. Initiate concomitant hematopoietic growth factor (G-CSF) as clinically indicated.

For the therapy of patients with solid tumors (ovary, breast, and NSCLC), courses of paclitaxel should not be repeated until the neutrophil count is at least 1500 cells/mm^3 and the platelet count is at least 100,000 cells/mm^3. Paclitaxel should not be given to patients with AIDS-related Kaposi's sarcoma if the baseline or subsequent neutrophil count is less than 1000 cells/mm^3. Patients who experience severe neutropenia (neutrophil $<$500 cells/mm^3 for a week or longer) or severe peripheral neuropathy during paclitaxel injection therapy should have dosage reduced by 20% for subsequent courses of paclitaxel. The incidence of neurotoxicity and the severity of neutropenia increase with dose.

PREPARATION AND ADMINISTRATION PRECAUTIONS

Paclitaxel is a cytotoxic anticancer drug and, as with other potentially toxic compounds, caution should be exercised in handling paclitaxel. The use of gloves is recommended. If paclitaxel solution contacts the skin, wash the skin immediately and thoroughly with soap and water. Following topical exposure, events have included tingling, burning, and redness. If paclitaxel contacts mucous membranes, the membranes should be flushed thoroughly with water. Upon inhalation, dyspnea, chest pain, burning eyes, sore throat, and nausea have been reported.

Given the possibility of extravasation, it is advisable to closely monitor the infusion site for possible infiltration during drug administration. (See PRECAUTIONS, Injection Site Reaction.)

PREPARATION FOR INTRAVENOUS ADMINISTRATION

Paclitaxel must be diluted prior to infusion. Paclitaxel should be diluted in 0.9% sodium chloride injection, 5% dextrose injection, 5% dextrose and 0.9% sodium chloride injection, or 5% dextrose in Ringer's injection to a final concentration of 0.3-1.2 mg/ml. The solutions are physically and chemically stable for up to 27 hours at ambient temperature (approximately 25°C) and room lighting conditions. Parenteral drug products should be inspected visually for particulate matter and discoloration prior to administration whenever solution and container permit.

Upon preparation, solutions may show haziness, which is attributed to the formulation vehicle. No significant losses in potency have been noted following simulated delivery of the solution through IV tubing containing an in-line (0.22 micron) filter.

Data collected for the presence of the extractable plasticizer DEHP [di-(2-ethylhexyl)phthalate] show that levels increase with time and concentration when dilutions are prepared in PVC containers. Consequently, the use of plasticized PVC containers and administration sets is not recommended. Paclitaxel solutions should be prepared and stored in glass, polypropylene, or polyolefin containers. Non-PVC containing administration sets, such as those which are polyethylene-lined, should be used.

Paclitaxel should be administered through an in-line filter with a microporous membrane not greater than 0.22 microns. Use of filter devices such as IVEX-2 filters which incorporate short inlet and outlet PVC-coated tubing has not resulted in significant leaching of DEHP.

The Chemo Dispensing Pin device or similar devices with spikes should not be used with vials of paclitaxel since they can cause the stopper to collapse resulting in loss of sterile integrity of the paclitaxel solution.

STABILITY

Unopened vials of paclitaxel injection are stable until the date indicated on the package when stored between 20-25°C (68-77°F), in the original package. Neither freezing nor refrigeration adversely affects the stability of the product. Upon refrigeration components in the paclitaxel vial may precipitate, but will redissolve upon reaching room temperature with little or no agitation. There is no impact on product quality under these circumstances. If the solution remains cloudy or if an insoluble precipitate is noted, the vial should be discarded. Solutions for infusion prepared as recommended are stable at ambient temperature (approximately 25°C) and lighting conditions for up to 27 hours.

HOW SUPPLIED

Taxol injection is available in 30 mg/5 ml, 100 mg/16.7 ml, and 300 mg/50 ml multidose vials.

Storage: Store the vials in original cartons between 20-25°C (68-77°F). Retain in the original package to protect from light.

HANDLING AND DISPOSAL

Procedures for proper handling and disposal of anticancer drugs should be considered. Several guidelines on this subject have been published.[1-7] There is no general agreement that all of the procedures recommended in the guidelines are necessary or appropriate.

PRODUCT LISTING - RATED THERAPEUTICALLY EQUIVALENT

Solution - Intravenous - 30 mg/5 ml

Size	Price	Product	NDC
5 ml	$140.25	GENERIC, Abbott Pharmaceutical	00074-4335-01
5 ml	$170.70	GENERIC, Udl Laboratories Inc	51079-0961-01
5 ml	$175.35	TAXOL, Bristol-Myers Squibb	00015-3475-30
5 ml	$182.63	GENERIC, Bedford Laboratories	55390-0114-05
16.70 ml	$467.50	GENERIC, Abbott Pharmaceutical	00074-4335-02
16.70 ml	$571.60	GENERIC, Udl Laboratories Inc	51079-0962-01
16.70 ml	$608.76	GENERIC, Bedford Laboratories	55390-0114-20
25 ml	$863.60	GENERIC, Ivax Corporation	00172-3756-75
30 ml	$172.72	GENERIC, Ivax Corporation	00172-3754-73
50 ml	$1400.00	GENERIC, Abbott Pharmaceutical	00074-4335-04
50 ml	$1725.10	GENERIC, Udl Laboratories Inc	51079-0963-01
50 ml	$1727.19	GENERIC, Ivax Corporation	00172-3753-77
50 ml	$1826.25	GENERIC, Bedford Laboratories	55390-0114-50

PRODUCT LISTING - EQUIVALENTS NOT AVAILABLE

Solution - Intravenous - 30 mg/5 ml

Size	Price	Product	NDC
5 ml	$175.32	TAXOL, Bristol-Myers Squibb	00015-3475-20
5 ml	$175.32	TAXOL, Bristol-Myers Squibb	00015-3475-27
5 ml	$175.32	TAXOL, Bristol-Myers Squibb	00015-3475-29
5 ml	$182.63	TAXOL, Bristol-Myers Squibb	00015-3456-20
16.70 ml	$584.51	TAXOL, Bristol-Myers Squibb	00015-3476-30
16.70 ml	$608.76	TAXOL, Bristol-Myers Squibb	00015-3476-20
50 ml	$1753.49	TAXOL, Bristol-Myers Squibb	00015-3479-11
50 ml	$1826.25	TAXOL, Bristol-Myers Squibb	00015-3456-99

Palivizumab

(003423)

Categories: Infection, upper respiratory tract, prevention; FDA Approved 1998 Jun; Pregnancy Category C
Drug Classes: Antivirals; Monoclonal antibodies
Brand Names: Synagis
Foreign Brand Availability: Abbosynagis (Israel)

DESCRIPTION

Synagis is a humanized monoclonal antibody (IgG1κ) produced by recombinant DNA technology, directed to an epitope in the A antigenic site of the F protein of respiratory syncytial virus (RSV). Palivizumab is a composite of human (95%) and murine (5%) antibody sequences. The human heavy chain sequence was derived from the constant domains of human IgG1 and the variable framework regions of the V_H genes Cor[1] and Cess.[2] The human light chain sequence was derived from the constant domain of Cκ and the variable framework regions of the V_L gene K104 with Jκ-4.[3] The murine sequences were derived from a murine monoclonal antibody, Mab 1129,[4] in a process which involved the grafting of the murine complementarity determining regions into the human antibody frameworks. Palivizumab is composed of two heavy chains and two light chains and has a molecular weight of approximately 148,000 Daltons.

Palivizumab is supplied as a sterile lyophilized product for reconstitution with sterile water for injection. Reconstituted palivizumab is to be administered by intramuscular injection only. Upon reconstitution, palivizumab contains the following excipients: 47 mM histidine, 3.0 mM glycine and 5.6% mannitol and the active ingredient, palivizumab, at a concentration of 100 milligrams per vial. The reconstituted solution should appear clear or slightly opalescent.

Storage: Upon receipt and until reconstitution for use, Synagis should be stored at 2-8°C (35.6-46.4°F) in its original container. Do not freeze. Do not use beyond the expiration date.

CLINICAL PHARMACOLOGY

MECHANISM OF ACTION

Palivizumab exhibits neutralizing and fusion-inhibitory activity against RSV. These activities inhibit RSV replication in laboratory experiments. Although resistant RSV strains may be isolated in laboratory studies, a panel of 57 clinical RSV isolates were all neutralized by palivizumab.[5] Palivizumab serum concentrations of ≥40 μg/ml have been shown to reduce pulmonary RSV replication in the cotton rat model of RSV infection by 100-fold.[5] The *in vivo* neutralizing activity of the active ingredient in palivizumab was assessed in a randomized, placebo-controlled study of 35 pediatric patients tracheally intubated because of RSV disease. In these patients, palivizumab significantly reduced the quantity of RSV in the lower respiratory tract compared to control patients.[6]

PHARMACOKINETICS

In studies in adult volunteers palivizumab had a pharmacokinetic profile similar to a human IgG1 antibody in regard to the volume of distribution and the half-life (mean 18 days). In pediatric patients less than 24 months of age, the mean half-life of palivizumab was 20 days and monthly intramuscular doses of 15 mg/kg achieved mean ±SD 30 day trough serum drug concentrations of 37 ± 21 μg/ml after the first injection, 57 ± 41 μg/ml after the second injection, 68 ± 51 μg/ml after the third injection and 72 ± 50 μg/ml after the fourth injection.[7] In pediatric patients given palivizumab for a second season, the mean ±SD serum concentrations following the first and fourth injections were 61 ± 17 μg/ml and 86 ± 31 μg/ml, respectively.

INDICATIONS AND USAGE

Palivizumab is indicated for the prevention of serious lower respiratory tract disease caused by respiratory syncytial virus (RSV) in pediatric patients at high risk of RSV disease. Safety and efficacy were established in infants with bronchopulmonary dysplasia (BPD) and infants with a history of prematurity (≤35 weeks gestational age).

CONTRAINDICATIONS

Palivizumab should not be used in pediatric patients with a history of a severe prior reaction to palivizumab or other components of this product.

WARNINGS

Anaphylactoid reactions following the administration of palivizumab have not been observed but can occur following the administration of proteins. **If anaphylaxis or severe allergic reaction occurs, administer epinephrine (1:1000) and provide supportive care as required.**

PRECAUTIONS

GENERAL

Palivizumab is for intramuscular use only. As with any intramuscular injection, palivizumab should be given with caution to patients with thrombocytopenia or any coagulation disorder.

The safety and efficacy of palivizumab have not been demonstrated for treatment of established RSV disease.

The single-use vial of palivizumab does not contain a preservative. Injections should be given within 6 hours after reconstitution.

IMMUNOGENICITY

In the IMpact-RSV trial, the incidence of anti-humanized antibody following the fourth injection was 1.1% in the placebo group and 0.7% in the palivizumab group. In pediatric patients receiving palivizumab for a second season, 1 of 56 patients had transient, low titer reactivity. This reactivity was not associated with adverse events or alteration in palivizumab serum concentrations.

CARCINOGENESIS, MUTAGENESIS, AND IMPAIRMENT OF FERTILITY

Carcinogenesis, mutagenesis and reproductive toxicity studies have not performed.

PREGNANCY CATEGORY C

Palivizumab is not indicated for adult usage and animal reproduction studies have not been conducted. It is also not known whether palivizumab can cause fetal harm when administered to a pregnant woman or could affect reproductive capacity.

DRUG INTERACTIONS

No formal drug-drug interaction studies were conducted. In the IMpact-RSV trial, the proportions of patients in the placebo and palivizumab groups who received routine childhood vaccines, influenza vaccine, bronchodilators or corticosteroids were similar and no incremental increase in adverse reactions was observed among patients receiving these agents.

ADVERSE REACTIONS

In the combined pediatric prophylaxis studies of pediatric patients with BPD or prematurity involving 520 subjects receiving placebo and 1168 subjects receiving palivizumab, the proportions of subjects in the placebo and palivizumab groups who experienced any adverse event or any serious adverse event were similar.

Most of the safety information was derived from the IMpact-RSV trial. In this study, palivizumab was discontinued in 5 patients: 2 because of vomiting and diarrhea, 1 because of erythema and moderate induration at the site of the fourth injection, and 2 because of pre-existing medical conditions which required management (1 with congenital anemia and 1 with pulmonary venous stenosis requiring cardiac surgery). Deaths in study patients occurred in 5 of 500 placebo recipients and 4 of 1002 palivizumab recipients. Sudden infant death syndrome was responsible for 2 of these deaths in the placebo group and 1 death in the palivizumab group. Adverse events which occurred in more than 1% of patients receiving palivizumab in the IMpact-RSV study for which the incidence in the palivizumab group was 1% greater than in the placebo group are shown in TABLE 1.

TABLE 1 *Adverse Events Occurring in IMpact-RSV Study at Greater Frequency in the Palivizumab Group*

% of Patients With:	Placebo n=500	Palivizumab n=1002
Upper respiratory infection	49.0%	52.6%
Otitis media	40.0%	41.9%
Rhinitis	23.4%	28.7%
Rash	22.4%	25.6%
Pain	6.8%	8.5%
Hernia	5.0%	6.3%
SGOT increased	3.8%	4.9%
Pharyngitis	1.4%	2.6%

Other adverse events reported in more than 1% of the palivizumab group included: cough, wheeze, bronchiolitis, pneumonia, bronchitis, asthma, croup, dyspnea, sinusitis, apnea, failure to thrive, nervousness, diarrhea, vomiting, and gastroenteritis, SGPT increase, liver function abnormality, study drug injections site reaction, conjunctivitis, viral infection, oral monilia, fungal dermatitis, eczema, seborrhea, anemia and flu syndrome. The incidence of these adverse events was similar between the palivizumab and placebo groups.

DOSAGE AND ADMINISTRATION

The recommended dose of palivizumab is 15 mg/kg of body weight. Patients, including those who develop an RSV infection, should receive monthly doses throughout the RSV season. The first dose should be administered prior to commencement of the RSV season. In the northern hemisphere, the RSV season typically commences in November and lasts through April, but it may begin earlier or persist later in certain communities.

Palivizumab should be administered in a dose of 15 mg/kg intramuscularly using aseptic technique, preferably in the anterolateral aspect of the thigh. The gluteal muscle should not be used routinely as an injection site because of the risk of damage to the sciatic nerve. The dose per month = [)patient weight (kg) × 15 mg/kg) ÷ (100 mg/ml of palivizumab)]. Injection volumes over 1 ml should be given as a divided dose.

Preparation for Administration

To reconstitute, remove the tab portion of the vial cap and clean the rubber stopper with 70% ethanol or equivalent.

Slowly add 1.0 ml of sterile water for injection to a 100 mg vial. The vial should be gently swirled for 30 seconds to avoid foaming. DO NOT SHAKE VIAL.

Reconstituted palivizumab should stand at room temperature for a minimum of 20 minutes until the solution clarifies.

Reconstituted palivizumab does not contain a preservative and should be administered within 6 hours of reconstitution.

To prevent the transmission of hepatitis viruses or other infectious agents from one person to another, sterile disposable syringes and needles should be used. Do not reuse syringes and needles.

PRODUCT LISTING - EQUIVALENTS NOT AVAILABLE

Injection - Intramuscular - 50 mg

1's	$694.59	SYNAGIS, Medimmune	60574-4112-01

Injection - Intramuscular - 100 mg

1's	$1311.56	SYNAGIS, Medimmune	60574-4111-01

Pamidronate Disodium (003067)

Categories: Hypercalcemia, secondary to neoplasia; Osteolysis, secondary to breast cancer; Osteolysis, secondary to multiple myeloma; Paget's disease; Pregnancy Category C; FDA Approved 1991 Oct
Drug Classes: Bisphosphonates
Brand Names: Aredia
Foreign Brand Availability: Aredronet (India); Pamisol (Singapore); Panolin (Korea); Panorin (Korea)
HCFA JCODE(S): J2430 per 30 mg IV

DESCRIPTION

Aredia, pamidronate disodium (APD), is a bone-resorption inhibitor available in 30 or 90 mg vials for intravenous (IV) administration. Each 30 mg and 90 mg vial contains, respectively, 30 mg and 90 mg of sterile, lyophilized pamidronate disodium and 470 mg and 375 mg of mannitol. The pH of a 1% solution of pamidronate disodium in distilled water is approximately 8.3. Pamidronate disodium, a member of the group of chemical compounds known as bisphosphonates, is an analog of pyrophosphate. Pamidronate disodium is designated chemically as phosphonic acid (3-amino-1-hydroxypropylidene) bis-, disodium salt, pentahydrate, (APD).

Pamidronate disodium is a white-to-practically-white powder. It is soluble in water and in 2 N sodium hydroxide, sparingly soluble in 0.1 N hydrochloric acid and in 0.1 N acetic acid, and practically insoluble in organic solvents. Its molecular formula is $C_3H_9NO_7P_2Na_2{\cdot}5H_2O$ and its molecular weight is 369.1.

Inactive Ingredients: Mannitol and phosphoric acid (for adjustment to pH 6.5 prior to lyophilization).

CLINICAL PHARMACOLOGY

The principal pharmacologic action of pamidronate disodium is inhibition of bone resorption. Although the mechanism of antiresorptive action is not completely understood, several factors are thought to contribute to this action. Pamidronate disodium adsorbs to calcium phosphate (hydroxyapatite) crystals in bone and may directly block dissolution of this mineral component of bone. *In vitro* studies also suggest that inhibition of osteoclast activity contributes to inhibition of bone resorption. In animal studies, at doses recommended for the treatment of hypercalcemia, pamidronate disodium inhibits bone resorption apparently without inhibiting bone formation and mineralization. Of relevance to the treatment of hypercalcemia of malignancy is the finding that pamidronate disodium inhibits the accelerated bone resorption that results from osteoclast hyperactivity induced by various tumors in animal studies.

PHARMACOKINETICS

Cancer patients (n=24) who had minimal or no bony involvement were given an IV infusion of 30, 60, or 90 mg of pamidronate disodium over 4 hours and 90 mg of pamidronate disodium over 24 hours (see TABLE 1).

TABLE 1 *Mean (SD, CV%) Pamidronate Pharmacokinetic Parameters in Cancer Patients (n=6 for each group)*

Dose (infusion rate)	Max. Concentration (µg/ml)	% of Dose Excreted in Urine	Total Clearance (ml/min)	Renal Clearance (ml/min)
30 mg (4 h)	0.73 (0.14, 19.1%)	43.9 (14.0, 31.9%)	136 (44, 32.4%)	58 (27, 46.5%)
60 mg (4 h)	1.44 (0.57, 39.6%)	47.4 (47.4%, 54.4%)	88 (56, 63.6%)	42 (28, 66.7%)
90 mg (4 h)	2.61 (0.74, 28.3%)	45.3 (25.8, 56.9%)	103 (37, 35.9%)	44 (16, 36.4%)
90 mg (24 h)	1.38 (1.97, 142.7%)	47.5 (10.2, 21.5%	101 (58, 57.4%)	52 (42, 80.8%)

Distribution

The mean ±SD body retention of pamidronate was calculated to be 54 ± 16% of the dose over 120 hours.

Metabolism

Pamidronate is not metabolized and is exclusively eliminated by renal excretion.

Excretion

After administration of 30, 60, and 90 mg of pamidronate disodium over 4 hours, and 90 mg of pamidronate disodium over 24 hours, an overall mean ±SD of 46 ± 16% of the drug was excreted unchanged in the urine within 120 hours. Cumulative urinary excretion was linearly related to dose. The mean ±SD elimination half-life is 28 ± 7 hours. Mean ±SD total and renal clearances of pamidronate were 107 ± 50 ml/min and 49 ± 28 ml/min, respectively. The rate of elimination from bone has not been determined.

Special Populations

There are no data available on the effects of age, gender, or race on the pharmacokinetics of pamidronate.

Pediatric

Pamidronate is not labeled for use in the pediatric population.

Renal Insufficiency

The pharmacokinetics of pamidronate were studied in cancer patients (n=19) with normal and varying degrees of renal impairment. Each patient received a single 90 mg dose of pamidronate disodium infused over 4 hours. The renal clearance of pamidronate in patients was found to closely correlate with creatinine clearance. A trend toward a lower percentage of drug excreted unchanged in urine was observed in renally impaired patients. Adverse experiences noted were not found to be related to changes in renal clearance of pamidronate. Given the recommended dose, 90 mg infused over 4 hours, excessive accumulation of pamidronate in renally impaired patients is not anticipated if pamidronate is administered on a monthly basis.

Hepatic Insufficiency

There are no human pharmacokinetic data for pamidronate disodium in patients who have hepatic insufficiency.

Drug-Drug Interactions

There are no human pharmacokinetic data for drug interactions with pamidronate disodium.

After IV administration of radiolabeled pamidronate in rats, approximately 50-60% of the compound was rapidly absorbed by bone and slowly eliminated from the body by the kidneys. In rats given 10 mg/kg bolus injections of radiolabeled pamidronate disodium, approximately 30% of the compound was found in the liver shortly after administration and was then redistributed to bone or eliminated by the kidneys over 24-48 hours. Studies in rats injected with radiolabeled pamidronate disodium showed that the compound was rapidly cleared from the circulation and taken up mainly by bones, liver, spleen, teeth, and tracheal cartilage. Radioactivity was eliminated from most soft tissues within 1-4 days; was detectable in liver and spleen for 1 and 3 months, respectively; and remained high in bones, trachea, and teeth for 6 months after dosing. Bone uptake occurred preferentially in areas of high bone turnover. The terminal phase of elimination half-life in bone was estimated to be approximately 300 days.

PHARMACODYNAMICS

Serum phosphate levels have been noted to decrease after administration of pamidronate disodium, presumably because of decreased release of phosphate from bone and increased renal excretion as parathyroid hormone levels, which are usually suppressed in hypercalcemia associated with malignancy, return toward normal. Phosphate therapy was administered in 30% of the patients in response to a decrease in serum phosphate levels. Phosphate levels usually returned toward normal within 7-10 days.

Urinary calcium/creatinine and urinary hydroxyproline/creatinine ratios decrease and usually return to within or below normal after treatment with pamidronate disodium. These changes occur within the first week after treatment, as do decreases in serum calcium levels, and are consistent with an antiresorptive pharmacologic action.

HYPERCALCEMIA OF MALIGNANCY

Osteoclastic hyperactivity resulting in excessive bone resorption is the underlying pathophysiologic derangement in metastatic bone disease and hypercalcemia of malignancy. Excessive release of calcium into the blood as bone is resorbed results in polyuria and gastrointestinal disturbances, with progressive dehydration and decreasing glomerular filtration rate. This, in turn, results in increased renal resorption of calcium, setting up a cycle of worsening systemic hypercalcemia. Correction of excessive bone resorption and adequate fluid administration to correct volume deficits are therefore essential to the management of hypercalcemia.

Most cases of hypercalcemia associated with malignancy occur in patients who have breast cancer; squamous-cell tumors of the lung or head and neck; renal-cell carcinoma; and certain hematologic malignancies, such as multiple myeloma and some types of lymphomas. A few less-common malignancies, including vasoactive intestinal-peptide-producing tumors and cholangiocarcinoma, have a high incidence of hypercalcemia as a metabolic complication. Patients who have hypercalcemia of malignancy can generally be divided into 2 groups, according to the pathophysiologic mechanism involved.

In humoral hypercalcemia, osteoclasts are activated and bone resorption is stimulated by factors such as parathyroid-hormone-related protein, which are elaborated by the tumor and circulate systemically. Humoral hypercalcemia usually occurs in squamous-cell malignancies of the lung or head and neck or in genitourinary tumors such as renal-cell carcinoma or ovarian cancer. Skeletal metastases may be absent or minimal in these patients.

Extensive invasion of bone by tumor cells can also result in hypercalcemia due to local tumor products that stimulate bone resorption by osteoclasts. Tumors commonly associated with locally mediated hypercalcemia include breast cancer and multiple myeloma.

Total serum calcium levels in patients who have hypercalcemia of malignancy may not reflect the severity of hypercalcemia, since concomitant hypoalbuminemia is commonly present. Ideally, ionized calcium levels should be used to diagnose and follow hypercalcemic conditions; however, these are not commonly or rapidly available in many clinical situations. Therefore, adjustment of the total serum calcium value for differences in albumin levels is often used in place of measurement of ionized calcium; several nomograms are in use for this type of calculation (see DOSAGE AND ADMINISTRATION).

INDICATIONS AND USAGE

HYPERCALCEMIA OF MALIGNANCY

Pamidronate disodium, in conjunction with adequate hydration, is indicated for the treatment of moderate or severe hypercalcemia associated with malignancy, with or without bone metastases. Patients who have either epidermoid or non-epidermoid tumors respond to treatment with pamidronate disodium. Vigorous saline hydration, an integral part of hypercalcemia therapy, should be initiated promptly and an attempt should be made to restore the urine output to about 2 L/day throughout treatment. Mild or asymptomatic hypercalcemia may be treated with conservative measures (*i.e.*, saline hydration, with or without loop diuretics). Patients should be hydrated adequately throughout the treatment, but overhydration, especially in those patients who have cardiac failure, must be avoided. Diuretic therapy should not be employed prior to correction of hypovolemia. The safety and efficacy of pamidronate disodium in the treatment of hypercalcemia associated with hyperparathyroidism or with other non-tumor-related conditions has not been established.

PAGET'S DISEASE

Pamidronate disodium is indicated for the treatment of patients with moderate to severe Paget's disease of bone. The effectiveness of pamidronate disodium was demonstrated pri-

P

marily in patients with serum alkaline phosphatase ≥3 times the upper limit of normal. Pamidronate disodium therapy in patients with Paget's disease has been effective in reducing serum alkaline phosphatase and urinary hydroxyproline levels by ≥50% in at least 50% of patients, and by ≥30% in at least 80% of patients. Pamidronate disodium therapy has also been effective in reducing these biochemical markers in patients with Paget's disease who failed to respond, or no longer responded to other treatments.

OSTEOLYTIC BONE METASTASES OF BREAST CANCER AND OSTEOLYTIC LESIONS OF MULTIPLE MYELOMA

Pamidronate disodium is indicated, in conjunction with standard antineoplastic therapy, for the treatment of osteolytic bone metastases of breast cancer and osteolytic lesions of multiple myeloma. The pamidronate disodium treatment effect appeared to be smaller in the study of breast cancer patients receiving hormonal therapy than in the study of those receiving chemotherapy, however, overall evidence of clinical benefit has been demonstrated.

CONTRAINDICATIONS

Pamidronate disodium is contraindicated in patients with clinically significant hypersensitivity to pamidronate disodium or other bisphosphonates.

WARNINGS

DUE TO THE RISK OF CLINICALLY SIGNIFICANT DETERIORATION IN RENAL FUNCTION, WHICH MAY PROGRESS TO RENAL FAILURE, SINGLE DOSES OF PAMIDRONATE DISODIUM SHOULD NOT EXCEED 90 MG (see DOSAGE AND ADMINISTRATION for appropriate infusion durations).

Bisphosphonates, including pamidronate disodium, have been associated with renal toxicity manifested as deterioration of renal function and potential renal failure.

Patients who receive pamidronate disodium should have serum creatinine assessed prior to each treatment. Patients treated with pamidronate disodium for bone metastases should have the dose withheld if renal function has deteriorated. (See DOSAGE AND ADMINISTRATION.)

In both rats and dogs, nephropathy has been associated with IV (bolus and infusion) administration of pamidronate disodium.

Two 7 day IV infusion studies were conducted in the dog wherein pamidronate disodium was given for 1, 4, or 24 hours at doses of 1-20 mg/kg for up to 7 days. In the first study, the compound was well tolerated at 3 mg/kg (1.7 × highest recommended human dose [HRHD] for a single IV infusion) when administered for 4 or 24 hours, but renal findings such as elevated BUN and creatinine levels and renal tubular necrosis occurred when 3 mg/kg was infused for 1 hour and at doses of ≥10 mg/kg. In the second study, slight renal tubular necrosis was observed in 1 male at 1 mg/kg when infused for 4 hours. Additional findings included elevated BUN levels in several treated animals and renal tubular dilation and/or inflammation at ≥1 mg/kg after each infusion time.

Pamidronate disodium was given to rats at doses of 2, 6, and 20 mg/kg and to dogs at doses of 2, 4, 6, and 20 mg/kg as a 1 hour infusion, once a week, for 3 months followed by a 1 month recovery period. In rats, nephrotoxicity was observed at ≥6 mg/kg and included increased BUN and creatinine levels and tubular degeneration and necrosis. These findings were still present at 20 mg/kg at the end of the recovery period. In dogs, moribundity/death and renal toxicity occurred at 20 mg/kg as did kidney findings of elevated BUN and creatinine levels at ≥6 mg/kg and renal tubular degeneration at ≥4 mg/kg. The kidney changes were partially reversible at 6 mg/kg. In both studies, the dose level that produced no adverse renal effects was considered to be 2 mg/kg (1.1 × HRHD for a single IV infusion).

P

PREGNANCY: PAMIDRONATE DISODIUM SHOULD NOT BE USED DURING PREGNANCY

Pamidronate disodium may cause fetal harm when administered to a pregnant woman. (See PRECAUTIONS, Pregnancy Category D.)

There are no studies in pregnant women using pamidronate disodium. If the patient becomes pregnant while taking this drug, the patient should be apprised of the potential harm to the fetus. Women of childbearing potential should be advised to avoid becoming pregnant.

Studies conducted in young rats have reported the disruption of dental dentine formation following single- and multi-dose administration of bisphosphonates. The clinical significance of these findings is unknown.

PRECAUTIONS

GENERAL

Standard hypercalcemia-related metabolic parameters, such as serum levels of calcium, phosphate, magnesium, and potassium, should be carefully monitored following initiation of therapy with pamidronate disodium. Cases of asymptomatic hypophosphatemia (12%), hypokalemia (7%), hypomagnesemia (11%), and hypocalcemia (5-12%), were reported in pamidronate disodium-treated patients. Rare cases of symptomatic hypocalcemia (including tetany) have been reported in association with pamidronate disodium therapy. If hypocalcemia occurs, short-term calcium therapy may be necessary. In Paget's disease of bone, 17% of patients treated with 90 mg of pamidronate disodium showed serum calcium levels below 8 mg/dl.

RENAL INSUFFICIENCY

Pamidronate disodium is excreted intact primarily via the kidney, and the risk of renal adverse reactions may be greater in patients with impaired renal function. Patients who receive pamidronate disodium should have serum creatinine assessed prior to each treatment. In patients receiving pamidronate disodium for bone metastases, who show evidence of deterioration in renal function, pamidronate disodium treatment should be withheld until renal function returns to baseline (see WARNINGS and DOSAGE AND ADMINISTRATION).

Pamidronate disodium has not been tested in patients who have class Dc renal impairment (creatinine >5.0 mg/dl), and has been tested in few multiple myeloma patients with serum creatinine ≥3.0 mg/dl (see CLINICAL PHARMACOLOGY, Pharmacokinetics). For the treatment of bone metastases, the use of pamidronate disodium in patients with severe renal impairment is not recommended. In other indications, clinical judgment should determine whether the potential benefit outweighs the potential risk in such patients.

LABORATORY TESTS

Patients who receive pamidronate disodium should have serum creatinine assessed prior to each treatment. Serum calcium, electrolytes, phosphate, magnesium, and CBC, differential, and hematocrit/hemoglobin must be closely monitored in patients treated with pamidronate disodium. Patients who have preexisting anemia, leukopenia, or thrombocytopenia should be monitored carefully in the first 2 weeks following treatment.

CARCINOGENESIS, MUTAGENESIS, AND IMPAIRMENT OF FERTILITY

In a 104 week carcinogenicity study (daily oral administration) in rats, there was a positive dose response relationship for benign adrenal pheochromocytoma in males (P <0.00001). Although this condition was also observed in females, the incidence was not statistically significant. When the dose calculations were adjusted to account for the limited oral bioavailability of pamidronate disodium in rats, the lowest daily dose associated with adrenal pheochromocytoma was similar to the intended clinical dose. Adrenal pheochromocytoma was also observed in low numbers in the control animals and is considered a relatively common spontaneous neoplasm in the rat. Pamidronate disodium (daily oral administration) was not carcinogenic in an 80 week study in mice.

Pamidronate disodium was nonmutagenic in 6 mutagenicity assays: Ames test, *Salmonella* and *Escherichia*/liver-microsome test, nucleus-anomaly test, sister-chromatid-exchange study, point-mutation test, and micronucleus test in the rat.

In rats, decreased fertility occurred in first-generation offspring of parents who had received 150 mg/kg of pamidronate disodium orally; however, this occurred only when animals were mated with members of the same dose group. Pamidronate disodium has not been administered intravenously in such a study.

PREGNANCY CATEGORY D

See WARNINGS.

There are no adequate and well-controlled studies in pregnant women.

Bolus IV studies conducted in rats and rabbits determined that pamidronate disodium produces maternal toxicity and embryo/fetal effects when given during organogenesis at doses of 0.6-8.3 times the highest recommended human dose for a single IV infusion. As it has been shown that pamidronate disodium can cross the placenta in rats and has produced marked maternal and nonteratogenic embryo/fetal effects in rats and rabbits, it should not be given to women during pregnancy.

NURSING MOTHERS

It is not known whether pamidronate disodium is excreted in human milk. Because many drugs are excreted in human milk, caution should be exercised when pamidronate disodium is administered to a nursing woman.

PEDIATRIC USE

Safety and effectiveness of pamidronate disodium in pediatric patients have not been established.

DRUG INTERACTIONS

Concomitant administration of a loop diuretic had no effect on the calcium-lowering action of pamidronate disodium.

Caution is indicated when pamidronate disodium is used with other potentially nephrotoxic drugs.

ADVERSE REACTIONS

CLINICAL STUDIES

Hypercalcemia of Malignancy

Transient mild elevation of temperature by at least 1°C was noted 24-48 hours after administration of pamidronate disodium in 34% of patients in clinical trials. In the saline trial, 18% of patients had a temperature elevation of at least 1°C 24-48 hours after treatment.

Drug-related local soft-tissue symptoms (redness, swelling or induration and pain on palpation) at the site of catheter insertion were most common in patients treated with 90 mg of pamidronate disodium. Symptomatic treatment resulted in rapid resolution in all patients.

Rare cases of uveitis, iritis, scleritis, and episcleritis have been reported, including 1 case of scleritis, and 1 case of uveitis upon separate rechallenges.

Five of 231 patients (2%) who received pamidronate disodium during the 4 US controlled hypercalcemia clinical studies were reported to have had seizures, 2 of whom had preexisting seizure disorders. None of the seizures were considered to be drug-related by the investigators. However, a possible relationship between the drug and the occurrence of seizures cannot be ruled out. It should be noted that in the saline arm 1 patient (4%) had a seizure.

There are no controlled clinical trials comparing the efficacy and safety of 90 mg pamidronate disodium over 24 hours to 2 hours in patients with hypercalcemia of malignancy. However, a comparison of data from separate clinical trials suggests that the overall safety profile in patients who received 90 mg pamidronate disodium over 24 hours is similar to those who received 90 mg pamidronate disodium over 2 hours. The only notable differences observed were an increase in the proportion of patients in the pamidronate disodium 24 hour group who experienced fluid overload and electrolyte/mineral abnormalities.

At least 15% of patients treated with pamidronate disodium for hypercalcemia of malignancy also experienced the following adverse events during a clinical trial:

General: Fluid overload, generalized pain.
Cardiovascular: Hypertension.
Gastrointestinal: Abdominal pain, anorexia, constipation, nausea, vomiting.
Genitourinary: Urinary tract infection.
Musculoskeletal: Bone pain.
Laboratory Abnormality: Anemia, hypokalemia, hypomagnesemia, hypophosphatemia.

Many of these adverse experiences may have been related to the underlying disease state. TABLE 6 lists the adverse experiences considered to be treatment-related during comparative, controlled US trials.

***TABLE 6** Treatment-Related Adverse Experiences Reported in Three US Controlled Clinical Trials*

	Pamidronate Disodium			Didronel	
	60 mg*	60 mg†	90 mg†	7.5‡	Saline
	n=23	n=73	n=17	n=35	n=23
General					
Edema	0%	1%	0%	0%	0%
Fatigue	0%	0%	12%	0%	0%
Fever	26%	19%	18%	9%	0%
Fluid overload	0%	0%	0%	6%	0%
Infusion-site reaction	0%	4%	18%	0%	0%
Moniliasis	0%	0%	6%	0%	0%
Rigors	0%	0%	0%	0%	4%
Gastrointestinal					
Abdominal pain	0%	1%	0%	0%	0%
Anorexia	4%	1%	12%	0%	0%
Constipation	4%	0%	6%	3%	0%
Diarrhea	0%	1%	0%	0%	0%
Dyspepsia	4%	0%	0%	0%	0%
Gastrointestinal hemorrhage	0%	0%	6%	0%	0%
Nausea	4%	0%	18%	6%	0%
Stomatitis	0%	1%	0%	3%	0%
Vomiting	4%	0%	0%	0%	0%
Respiratory					
Dyspnea	0%	0%	0%	3%	0%
Rales	0%	0%	6%	0%	0%
Rhinitis	0%	0%	6%	0%	0%
Upper respiratory infection	0%	3%	0%	0%	0%
CNS					
Anxiety	0%	0%	0%	0%	4%
Convulsions	0%	0%	0%	3%	0%
Insomnia	0%	1%	0%	0%	0%
Nervousness	0%	0%	0%	0%	4%
Psychosis	4%	0%	0%	0%	0%
Somnolence	0%	1%	6%	0%	0%
Taste perversion	0%	0%	0%	3%	0%
Cardiovascular					
Atrial fibrillation	0%	0%	6%	0%	4%
Atrial flutter	0%	1%	0%	0%	0%
Cardiac failure	0%	1%	0%	0%	0%
Hypertension	0%	0%	6%	0%	4%
Syncope	0%	0%	6%	0%	0%
Tachycardia	0%	0%	6%	0%	4%
Endocrine					
Hypothyroidism	0%	0%	6%	0%	0%
Hemic and Lymphatic					
Anemia	0%	0%	6%	0%	0%
Leukopenia	4%	0%	0%	0%	0%
Neutropenia	0%	1%	0%	0%	0%
Thrombocytopenia	0%	1%	0%	0%	0%
Musculoskeletal					
Myalgia	0%	1%	0%	0%	0%
Urogenital					
Uremia	4%	0%	0%	0%	0%
Laboratory Abnormalities					
Hypocalcemia	0%	1%	12%	0%	0%
Hypokalemia	4%	4%	18%	0%	0%
Hypomagnesemia	4%	10%	12%	3%	4%
Hypophosphatemia	0%	9%	18%	3%	0%
Abnormal liver function	0%	0%	0%	3%	0%

* Over 4 h.
† Over 24 h.
‡ Mg/kg × 3 days.

Paget's Disease

Transient mild elevation of temperature >1°C above pretreatment baseline was noted within 48 hours after completion of treatment in 21% of the patients treated with 90 mg of pamidronate disodium in clinical trials.

Drug-related musculoskeletal pain and nervous system symptoms (dizziness, headache, paresthesia, increased sweating) were more common in patients with Paget's disease treated with 90 mg of pamidronate disodium than in patients with hypercalcemia of malignancy treated with the same dose.

Adverse experiences considered to be related to trial drug, which occurred in at least 5% of patients with Paget's disease treated with 90 mg of pamidronate disodium in 2 US clinical trials, were fever, nausea, back pain, and bone pain.

At least 10% of all pamidronate disodium-treated patients with Paget's disease also experienced the following adverse experiences during clinical trials:

Cardiovascular: Hypertension.

Musculoskeletal: Arthrosis, bone pain.

Nervous System: Headache.

Most of these adverse experiences may have been related to the underlying disease state.

Osteolytic Bone Metastases of Breast Cancer and Osteolytic Lesions of Multiple Myeloma

The most commonly reported (>15%) adverse experiences occurred with similar frequencies in the pamidronate disodium and placebo treatment groups, and most of these adverse experiences may have been related to the underlying disease state or cancer therapy (see TABLE 7).

***TABLE 7** Commonly Reported Adverse Experiences in Three US Controlled Clinical Trials*

	APD over 4 h	PLA	APD over 2 h	PLA	All APD	PLA
	n=205	n=187	n=367	n=386	n=572	n=573
General						
Asthenia	16.1%	17.1%	25.6%	19.2%	22.2%	18.5%
Fatigue	31.7%	28.3%	40.3%	28.8%	37.2%	29.0%
Fever	38.5%	38.0%	38.1%	32.1%	38.5%	34.0%
Metastases	1.0%	3.0%	31.3%	24.4%	20.5%	17.5%
Pain	13.2%	11.8%	15.0%	18.1%	14.3%	16.1%
Digestive System						
Anorexia	17.1%	17.1%	31.1%	24.9%	26.0%	22.3%
Constipation	28.3%	31.7%	36.0%	38.6%	33.2%	35.1%
Diarrhea	26.8%	26.8%	29.4%	30.6%	28.5%	29.7%
Dyspepsia	17.6%	13.4%	18.3%	15.0%	22.6%	17.5%
Nausea	35.6%	37.4%	63.5%	59.1%	53.5%	51.8%
Pain, abdominal	19.5%	16.0%	24.3%	18.1%	22.6%	17.5%
Vomiting	16.6%	19.8%	46.3%	39.1%	35.7%	32.8%
Hemic and Lymphatic						
Anemia	47.8%	41.7%	39.5%	36.8%	42.5%	38.4%
Granulocytopenia	20.5%	15.5%	19.3%	20.5%	19.8%	18.8%
Thrombocytopenia	16.6%	17.1%	12.5%	14.0%	14.0%	15.0%
Musculoskeletal System						
Arthralgias	10.7%	7.0%	15.3%	12.7%	13.6%	10.8%
Myalgia	25.4%	15.0%	26.4%	22.5%	26.0%	20.1%
Skeletal pain	61.0%	71.7%	70.0%	75.4%	66.8%	74.0%
CNS						
Anxiety	7.8%	9.1%	18.0%	16.8%	14.3%	14.3%
Headache	24.4%	19.8%	27.2%	23.6%	26.2%	22.3%
Insomnia	17.1%	17.2%	25.1%	19.4%	22.2%	19.0%
Respiratory System						
Coughing	26.3%	22.5%	25.3%	19.7%	25.7%	20.6%
Dyspnea	22.0%	21.4%	35.1%	24.4%	30.4%	23.4%
Pleural effusion	2.9%	4.3%	15.0%	9.1%	10.7%	7.5%
Sinusitis	14.6%	16.6%	16.1%	10.4%	15.6%	12.0%
Upper resp. tract infection	32.2%	28.3%	19.6%	20.2%	24.1%	22.9%
Urogenital System						
Urinary tract infection	15.6%	9.1%	20.2%	17.6%	18.5%	15.6%

APD Pamidronate disodium 90 mg.
PLA Placebo.

Of the toxicities commonly associated with chemotherapy, the frequency of vomiting, anorexia, and anemia were slightly more common in the pamidronate disodium patients whereas stomatitis and alopecia occurred at a frequency similar to that in placebo patients. In the breast cancer trials, mild elevations of serum creatinine occurred in 18.5% of pamidronate disodium patients and 12.3% of placebo patients. Mineral and electrolyte disturbances, including hypocalcemia, were reported rarely and in similar percentages of pamidronate disodium-treated patients compared with those in the placebo group. The reported frequencies of hypocalcemia, hypokalemia, hypophosphatemia, and hypomagnesemia for pamidronate disodium-treated patients were 3.3%, 10.5%, 1.7% and 4.4%, respectively, and for placebo-treated patients were 1.2%, 12%, 1.7% and 4.5%, respectively. In previous hypercalcemia of malignancy trials, patients treated with pamidronate disodium (60 or 90 mg over 24 hours) developed electrolyte abnormalities more frequently (see Hypercalcemia of Malignancy).

Arthralgias and myalgias were reported slightly more frequently in the pamidronate disodium group than in the placebo group (13.6% and 26% vs 10.8% and 20.1%, respectively).

In multiple myeloma patients, there were 5 pamidronate disodium-related serious and unexpected adverse experiences. Four of these were reported during the 12 month extension of the multiple myeloma trial. Three of the reports were of worsening renal function developing in patients with progressive multiple myeloma or multiple myeloma-associated amyloidosis. The fourth report was the adult respiratory distress syndrome developing in a patient recovering from pneumonia and acute gangrenous cholecystitis. One pamidronate disodium-treated patient experienced an allergic reaction characterized by swollen and itchy eyes, runny nose, and scratchy throat within 24 hours after the sixth infusion.

In the breast cancer trials, there were 4 pamidronate disodium-related adverse experiences, all moderate in severity, that caused a patient to discontinue participation in the trial. One was due to interstitial pneumonitis, another to malaise and dyspnea. One pamidronate disodium patient discontinued the trial due to a symptomatic hypocalcemia. Another pamidronate disodium patient discontinued therapy due to severe bone pain after each infusion, which the investigator felt was trial-drug-related.

RENAL TOXICITY

In a study of the safety and efficacy of pamidronate disodium 90 mg (2 hour infusion) versus zoledronic acid 4 mg (15 minute infusion) in bone metastases patients with multiple myeloma or breast cancer, renal deterioration was defined as an increase in serum creatinine of 0.5 mg/dl for patients with normal baseline creatinine (<1.4 mg/dl) or an increase of 1.0 mg/dl for patients with an abnormal baseline creatinine (≥1.4 mg/dl). The following are data on the incidence of renal deterioration in patients in this trial. (See TABLE 8.)

P

TABLE 8 *Incidence of Renal Function Deterioration in Multiple Myeloma and Breast Cancer Patients With Normal and Abnormal Serum Creatinine at Baseline**

Patient Population/ Baseline Creatinine	Pamidronate Disodium 90 mg/2 h		Zoledronic Acid 4 mg/15 min	
Normal	20/246 n/N	(8.1%)	23/246 n/N	(9.3%)
Abnormal	2/22 n/N	(9.1%)	1/26 n/N	(3.8%)
Total	22/268 n/N	(8.2%)	24/272 n/N	(8.8%)

* Patients were randomized following the 15 minute infusion amendment for the zoledronic acid arm.

POST-MARKETING EXPERIENCE

Rare instances of allergic manifestations have been reported, including hypotension, dyspnea, or angioedema, and, very rarely, anaphylactic shock. Pamidronate disodium is contraindicated in patients with clinically significant hypersensitivity to pamidronate disodium or other bisphosphonates (see CONTRAINDICATIONS).

DOSAGE AND ADMINISTRATION

HYPERCALCEMIA OF MALIGNANCY

Consideration should be given to the severity of as well as the symptoms of hypercalcemia. Vigorous saline hydration alone may be sufficient for treating mild, asymptomatic hypercalcemia. Overhydration should be avoided in patients who have potential for cardiac failure. In hypercalcemia associated with hematologic malignancies, the use of glucocorticoid therapy may be helpful.

Moderate Hypercalcemia

The recommended dose of pamidronate disodium in moderate hypercalcemia (corrected serum calcium* of approximately 12-13.5 mg/dl) is 60-90 mg given as a SINGLE-DOSE, IV infusion over 2-24 hours. Longer infusions (*i.e.*, >2 hours) may reduce the risk for renal toxicity, particularly in patients with pre-existing renal insufficiency.

Severe Hypercalcemia

The recommended dose of pamidronate disodium in severe hypercalcemia (corrected serum calcium* >13.5 mg/dl) is 90 mg given as a SINGLE-DOSE, IV infusion over 2-24 hours. Longer infusions (*i.e.*, >2 hours) may reduce the risk for renal toxicity, particularly in patients with pre-existing renal insufficiency.

*Albumin-corrected serum calcium (CCa, mg/dl) = serum calcium, mg/dl + 0.8 (4.0 serum albumin, g/dl).

Retreatment

A limited number of patients have received more than 1 treatment with pamidronate disodium for hypercalcemia. Retreatment with pamidronate disodium, in patients who show complete or partial response initially, may be carried out if serum calcium does not return to normal or remain normal after initial treatment. **It is recommended that a minimum of 7 days elapse before retreatment, to allow for full response to the initial dose.** The dose and manner of retreatment is identical to that of the initial therapy.

PAGET'S DISEASE

The recommended dose of pamidronate disodium in patients with moderate to severe Paget's disease of bone is 30 mg daily, administered as a 4 hour infusion on 3 consecutive days for a total dose of 90 mg.

Retreatment

A limited number of patients with Paget's disease have received more than 1 treatment of pamidronate disodium in clinical trials. When clinically indicated, patients should be retreated at the dose of initial therapy.

Osteolytic Bone Lesions of Multiple Myeloma

The recommended dose of pamidronate disodium in patients with osteolytic bone lesions of multiple myeloma is 90 mg administered as a 4 hour infusion given on a monthly basis.

Patients with marked Bence-Jones proteinuria and dehydration should receive adequate hydration prior to pamidronate disodium infusion.

Limited information is available on the use of pamidronate disodium in multiple myeloma patients with a serum creatinine ≥3.0 mg/dl.

Patients who receive pamidronate disodium should have serum creatinine assessed prior to each treatment. Treatment should be withheld for renal deterioration. In a clinical study, renal deterioration was defined as follows:

- For patients with normal baseline creatinine, increase of 0.5 mg/dl.
- For patients with abnormal baseline creatinine, increase of 1.0 mg/dl.

In this clinical study, pamidronate disodium treatment was resumed only when the creatinine returned to within 10% of the baseline value.

The optimal duration of therapy is not yet known, however, in a study of patients with myeloma, final analysis after 21 months demonstrated overall benefits.

Osteolytic Bone Metastases of Breast Cancer

The recommended dose of pamidronate disodium in patients with osteolytic bone metastases is 90 mg administered over a 2 hour infusion given every 3-4 weeks.

Pamidronate disodium has been frequently used with doxorubicin, fluorouracil, cyclophosphamide, methotrexate, mitoxantrone, vinblastine, dexamethasone, prednisone, melphalan, vincristine, megesterol, and tamoxifen. It has been given less frequently with etoposide, cisplatin, cytarabine, paclitaxel, and aminoglutethimide.

Patients who receive pamidronate disodium should have serum creatinine assessed prior to each treatment. Treatment should be withheld for renal deterioration. In a clinical study, renal deterioration was defined as follows:

- For patients with normal baseline creatinine, increase of 0.5 mg/dl.
- For patients with abnormal baseline creatinine, increase of 1.0 mg/dl.

In this clinical study, pamidronate disodium treatment was resumed only when the creatinine returned to within 10% of the baseline value.

The optimal duration of therapy is not known, however, in 2 breast cancer studies, final analyses performed after 24 months of therapy demonstrated overall benefit.

PREPARATION OF SOLUTION

Reconstitution

Pamidronate disodium is reconstituted by adding 10 ml of sterile water for injection to each vial, resulting in a solution of 30 mg/10 ml or 90 mg/10 ml. The pH of the reconstituted solution is 6.0-7.4. The drug should be completely dissolved before the solution is withdrawn.

Method of Administration

DUE TO THE RISK OF CLINICALLY SIGNIFICANT DETERIORATION IN RENAL FUNCTION, WHICH MAY PROGRESS TO RENAL FAILURE, SINGLE DOSES OF PAMIDRONATE DISODIUM SHOULD NOT EXCEED 90 MG. (SEE WARNINGS.)

There must be strict adherence to the intravenous administration recommendations for pamidronate disodium in order to decrease the risk of deterioration in renal function.

Hypercalcemia of Malignancy

The daily dose must be administered as an IV infusion over at least 2-24 hours for the 60 and 90 mg doses. The recommended dose should be diluted in 1000 ml of sterile 0.45% or 0.9% sodium chloride, or 5% dextrose injection. This infusion solution is stable for up to 24 hours at room temperature.

Paget's Disease

The recommended dose of 30 mg should be diluted in 500 ml of sterile 0.45% or 0.9% sodium chloride or 5% dextrose injection and administered over a 4 hour period for 3 consecutive days.

Osteolytic Bone Metastases of Breast Cancer

The recommended dose of 90 mg should be diluted in 250 ml of sterile 0.45% or 0.9% sodium chloride or 5% dextrose injection and administered over a 2 hour period every 3-4 weeks.

Osteolytic Bone Lesions of Multiple Myeloma

The recommended dose of 90 mg should be diluted in 500 ml of sterile 0.45% or 0.9% sodium chloride or 5% dextrose injection and administered over a 4 hour period on a monthly basis.

Pamidronate disodium must not be mixed with calcium-containing infusion solutions, such as Ringer's solution and should be given in a single IV solution and line separate from all other drugs.

***Note:* Parenteral drug products should be inspected visually for particulate matter and discoloration prior to administration, whenever solution and container permit.**

HOW SUPPLIED

Aredia Is Available in:

30 mg: Each vial contains 30 mg of sterile, lyophilized pamidronate disodium and 470 mg of mannitol.

90 mg: Each vial contains 90 mg of sterile, lyophilized pamidronate disodium and 375 mg of mannitol.

STORAGE

Pamidronate disodium reconstituted with sterile water for injection may be stored under refrigeration at 2-8°C (36-46°F) for up to 24 hours.

Do not store above 30°C (86°F).

PRODUCT LISTING - RATED THERAPEUTICALLY EQUIVALENT

Powder For Injection - Intravenous - 30 mg

1's	$290.00	GENERIC, American Pharmaceutical Partners	63323-0734-10
1's	$291.53	PAMIDRONATE DISODIUM, Bedford Laboratories	55390-0127-01
1's	$291.53	PAMIDRONATE DISODIUM, Bedford Laboratories	55390-0204-01

Powder For Injection - Intravenous - 90 mg

1's	$872.00	GENERIC, American Pharmaceutical Partners	63323-0735-10
1's	$874.59	PAMIDRONATE DISODIUM, Bedford Laboratories	55390-0129-01

PRODUCT LISTING - EQUIVALENTS NOT AVAILABLE

Powder For Injection - Intravenous - 30 mg

1's	$1119.44	PAMIDRONATE DISODIUM, Gensia Sicor Pharmaceuticals Inc	00703-4075-19
4's	$1119.44	AREDIA, Novartis Pharmaceuticals	00083-2601-04

Powder For Injection - Intravenous - 60 mg

1's	$428.97	AREDIA, Novartis Pharmaceuticals	00083-2606-01
1's	$559.72	GENERIC, Faulding Pharmaceutical Company	61703-0325-18

Powder For Injection - Intravenous - 90 mg

1's	$839.60	AREDIA, Novartis Pharmaceuticals	00083-2609-01

1's	$839.60	PAMIDRONATE DISODIUM, Gensia Sicor Pharmaceuticals Inc	00703-4085-11
1's	$839.60	PAMIDRONATE DISODIUM, Bedford Laboratories	55390-0206-01

Pancrelipase (001949)

Categories: Bypass, gastrointestinal, adjunct; Cystic fibrosis, adjunct; Obstruction, pancreatic duct, secondary to neoplasm; Pancreatectomy, adjunct; Pancreatitis, chronic; FDA Pre 1938 Drugs; Pregnancy Category C
Drug Classes: Enzymes, gastrointestinal; Gastrointestinals
Brand Names: Amylase; Amylase Lipase Protease; **Cotazym-S**; Creon; Creon 5; Encron 10; Encron-10; Entolase; Enzymase 16; Festalan; Ilozyme; Ku-Zyme Hp; Lipase; Panase; Pancote; Pancrease; Pancreatic Enzyme; Pancreatin 10; Pancrelipase 10000; Pancrelipase Mt 16; Pancrelipase Mt-16; Pancron 10; Panokase; Promylin; Protease; Protilase; Protilase Mt 16; Ultrase; Ultrase Mt; Vio-Moore; Zymase
Foreign Brand Availability: Combizym (New-Zealand); Combizym Compositum (New-Zealand); Cotazym (Canada); Cotazym-65 B (Canada); Cotazym ECS (New-Zealand); Cotazym-S Forte (Australia); Krebsilasi (Italy); Pancrease HL (England); Pancrease MT 4 (Canada); Pancrease MT 10 (Canada); Pancrease MT 16 (Canada); Pancrex (Italy); Pankrease (South-Africa); Panzytrat (New-Zealand); Prolipase (Austria; Switzerland); Vitazyme (Malaysia)

DESCRIPTION

Pancrelipase capsules are a pancreatic enzyme supplement for oral administration. Pancrelipase, the active ingredient in Pancrease and Pancrease MT capsules, is a natural product harvested by extraction from the pancreas of the hog. Pancrelipase powder is a slightly brown amorphous powder with a faint characteristic odor. It is partly soluble in water and practically insoluble in alcohol or ether.

MICROSPHERES

Pancrease capsules contain enteric-coated microspheres of porcine pancreatic enzyme concentrate in the following theoretical quantities:

Lipase: 4500 units
Amylase: 20,000 units
Protease: 25,000 units

Inactive ingredients are povidone, sodium starch glycolate, sugar (sucrose) spheres, cellulose acetate phthalate, diethyl phthalate, talc, corn starch, titanium dioxide, gelatin, and other trace ingredients.

MICROTABLETS

Pancrease MT capsules contain enteric-coated microtablets of porcine pancreatic enzyme concentrate in the following theoretical quantities:

Each Pancrease MT 4 capsule contains:
Lipase: 4000 units
Amylase: 12,000 units
Protease: 12,000 units

Each Pancrease MT 10 capsule contains:
Lipase: 10,000 units
Amylase: 30,000 units
Protease: 30,000 units

Each Pancrease MT 16 capsule contains:
Lipase: 16,000 units
Amylase: 48,000 units
Protease: 48,000 units

Each Pancrease MT 25 capsule contains:
Lipase: 25,000 units
Amylase: 75,000 units
Protease: 75,000 units

Inactive ingredients are cellulose, crospovidone, magnesium stearate, colloidal silicon dioxide, methacrylic acid copolymer, triethyl citrate, talc, polydimethylsiloxane, wax, gelatin, iron oxide, polysorbate 80, sodium lauryl sulfate, titanium dioxide, and other trace ingredients.

CLINICAL PHARMACOLOGY

The enteric-coated microspheres and microtablets contained in pancrelipase and pancrelipate MT resist gastric inactivation and deliver enzymes into the duodenum. The enzymes in pancrelipase act locally in the gastrointestinal tract. The enzymes are present in the form of pH-sensitive enteric-coated microspheres or microtablets of less than 3 mm in diameter which are filled into gelatin capsules. The microspheres and microtablets, which are released from the capsule into the stomach, are enteric coated to resist inactivation at low pH. Once released the microspheres and microtablets are distributed into the stomach and pass into the duodenum where, when the pH reaches approximately 5.5, the enteric coating begins to dissolve and the release of the enzymes is initiated. The enzymes catalyze the hydrolysis of fats into glycerol and fatty acids, protein into proteoses and derived substances, and starch into dextrins and sugars. Duodenal availability studies in adults indicate that following oral administration of pancrelipase microspheres and microtablets to adults, measurable levels of enzymes are present in the duodenum. Once they have accomplished their digestive function the enzymes may be digested in the intestine. The constituents may be partially absorbed and subsequently excreted in the urine. Any undigested enzymes are excreted in the feces.

PRECLINICAL

Studies in a small number of rats administered indomethacin or ibuprofen and pancrelipase enzymes concomitantly revealed intestinal and liver lesions. The clinical significance of these findings is not known.

INDICATIONS AND USAGE

Pancrelipase microspheres and microtablets are indicated for the treatment of steatorrhea secondary to pancreatic insufficiency such as cystic fibrosis or chronic alcoholic pancreatitis.

CONTRAINDICATIONS

Pancrelipase microspheres and microtablets are contraindicated in patients known to be hypersensitive to pork protein or any other component of this product.

WARNINGS

Cases of fibrotic strictures in the colon have been reported primarily in cystic fibrosis patients with the use of enzyme supplements, generally at dosages above the recommended range. Some cases required surgery including resection of the bowel. If symptoms suggestive of gastrointestinal obstruction occur, the possibility of bowel strictures should be considered.

Any change in pancreatic enzyme replacement therapy (*e.g.*, dose or brand of medication) should be made cautiously and only under medical supervision. It is recommended that therapy be initiated at a low dose, followed by titration to an effective dose. The titration schedule should be guided by measured changes in 3 day fecal fat excretion. (See DOSAGE AND ADMINISTRATION.)

PRECAUTIONS

GENERAL

TO PROTECT THE ENTERIC COATING, MICROSPHERES AND MICROTABLETS SHOULD NOT BE CRUSHED OR CHEWED. Intact capsules should be swallowed with liquids at mealtime. If an intact capsule can not be swallowed, it may be opened and the contents taken with small amounts of food that do not require chewing. (See DOSAGE AND ADMINISTRATION.)

INFORMATION FOR THE PATIENT

Patients should be advised that:

- Pancrelipase microspheres and microtablets must not be crushed or chewed;
- Intact capsules should be swallowed with liquid at mealtimes;
- The microspheres and microtablets from opened capsules should be swallowed immediately and not be retained in the mouth;
- Doses should only be taken with meals or snacks;
- Fluids should be consumed liberally while dosing with pancrelipase microspheres and microtablets;
- Any change in pancreatic enzyme replacement therapy (*e.g.*, dose or brand of medication) should be made only under medical supervision.

PREGNANCY, TERATOGENIC EFFECTS, PREGNANCY CATEGORY B

Reproduction studies have been conducted in rats and rabbits at doses 0.44 times and 0.35 times the maximum daily human dose, respectively, and have revealed no evidence of impaired fertility or harm to the fetus due to pancrelipase microspheres or microtablets. No fertility or peri-/postnatal studies have been performed in animals. There are, however, no adequate and well-controlled studies in pregnant women. Because animal reproduction studies are not always predictive of human response, this drug should be used during pregnancy only if clearly needed.

NURSING MOTHERS

Pancreatic enzymes act locally in the gastrointestinal tract and are not likely to be systemically absorbed. Some of the constituent amino and nucleic acids are likely to be absorbed along with dietary proteins. The possibility of the protein constituents appearing in the breast milk can not be excluded.

PEDIATRIC USE

Colonic strictures, particularly in children with cystic fibrosis, have been associated with doses generally above the recommended dosing range. (See WARNINGS.) Patients currently receiving doses >2500 lipase units/kg/meal or 4000 lipase units/g fat/day should be re-evaluated and the dosage either immediately decreased or titrated downward to the lowest effective clinical dose as assessed by 3 day fecal fat excretion.

GERIATRIC USE

Studies on the relationship of age to the effects of pancrelipase have not been conducted. However, geriatric-specific problems that would limit the usefulness of this medication in the elderly are not expected.

ADVERSE REACTIONS

Clinical evidence indicates that pancrelipase microspheres and microtablets are well-tolerated.

MICROSPHERES

The most frequently reported adverse events resulting from the post-marketing experience with pancrelipase microspheres were gastrointestinal and include diarrhea, abdominal pain, intestinal obstruction, vomiting, flatulence, nausea, constipation, melena, and perianal irritation. Frequently reported adverse events in other body systems included weight decrease and pain. Hyperuricemia and hyperuricosuria have been reported with the use of pancrelipase products, primarily with non-enteric coated formulations. Cases of fibrosing colonopathy have been reported primarily in cystic fibrosis patients. (See WARNINGS.)

MICROTABLETS

The most frequently reported adverse events resulting from the post-marketing experience with pancrelipase microtablets were gastrointestinal in nature and include diarrhea, abdominal pain, intestinal obstruction, vomiting, intestinal stenosis, and constipation. Frequently reported adverse events in other body systems include dermatitis. Hyperuricemia and hyperuricosuria have been reported with the use of pancrelipase products, primarily with non-enteric coated formulations. Cases of fibrosing colonopathy have been reported primarily in cystic fibrosis patients. (See WARNINGS.)

DOSAGE AND ADMINISTRATION

GENERAL

Patients with pancreatic insufficiency should consume a high-calorie diet with unrestricted fat which is appropriate for age and clinical status. A nutritional assessment should be performed regularly as a component of routine care and additionally, when dosing of pancreatic enzyme replacement is altered.

Dosage should be individualized and determined by the degree of steatorrhea and the fat content of the diet. Therapy should be initiated at the lowest possible dose and gradually increased until the desired control of steatorrhea is obtained. Dosage should be adjusted based on 3 day fecal fat studies.

Pancrelipase microspheres and microtablets should only be taken with meals or snacks.

It is important to ensure that patients ingest a liberal amount of liquids to maintain adequate hydration while dosing with pancrelipase microspheres and microtablets.

Whenever possible, pancrelipase microspheres and microtablets should be swallowed intact with generous amounts of liquid. However, if swallowing of capsules is difficult, they may be opened and the microspheres or microtablets sprinkled onto a small quantity of soft food on a teaspoon or tablespoon and ingested immediately. Foods which do not require chewing and have a pH lower than 7.3 are recommended. Examples of such foods are apricot, banana and sweet potato baby foods, applesauce, instant pudding and gelatin snacks. Contact of the microspheres with foods having a pH greater than 7.3 (*e.g.*, milk, custard, ice cream, and many other dairy products) can dissolve the protective enteric coating and destroy enzyme activity.

To avoid irritation of the mouth, lips, and tongue, opened pancrelipase microspheres and microtablets should be swallowed immediately before regular feedings or meals to minimize the likelihood that the microspheres are retained in the mouth. Proteolytic enzymes present in pancrelipase, when retained in the mouth, may begin to digest the mucous membranes and cause ulcerations.

There is considerable variation among individuals in response to enzymes with respect to control of steatorrhea; therefore, a range of doses is suggested.

Infants (up to 12 months)

Fat-Consumption Scheme

2000-4000 lipase units per 120 ml of formula or per breast feeding. This provides approximately 450-900 lipase units/g of fat ingested (based on 4.5 g of fat per 120 ml standard cow's milk-based infant formula).

Higher doses are used in infants because on average, infants ingest 5 g of fat/kg of body weight per day, whereas adults tend to ingest about 2 g of fat/kg/day.

Children and Older

Weight-Based Scheme

<4 years: Begin with 1000 lipase units/kg/meal to a maximum of 2500 lipase units/kg/meal.

>4 Years

Begin with 400 lipase units/kg/meal to a maximum of 2500 lipase units/kg/meal.

Enzyme doses, expressed as lipase units/kg/meal, should be decreased in older patients since they weigh more but tend to ingest less fat/kg. Usually, half the mealtime dose is given with a snack. The total daily dose reflects approximately 3 meals and 2-3 snacks per day.

If doses greater than 2500 lipase units/kg/meal (4000 lipase units/g fat/day) are required to control malabsorption, further investigation is warranted to rule out other causes of malabsorption. Doses greater than 2500 lipase units/kg/meal should be used with caution and only if they are documented to be effective by 3 day fecal fat measures. It is unknown whether doses above 2500 lipase units/kg/meal are safe.

Colonic strictures, particularly in children with cystic fibrosis, have been associated with doses generally above the recommended dosing range. (See WARNINGS.) Patients currently receiving doses >2500 lipase units/kg/meal or 4000 lipase units/g fat/day should be re-evaluated and the dosage either immediately decreased or titrated downward to the lowest effective clinical dose as assessed by 3 day fecal fat excretion.

HOW SUPPLIED

PANCREASE CAPSULES

Microspheres

Pancrease capsules are supplied as white body, clear cap, dye-free capsules.

Pancrease capsules are imprinted with "McNEIL" and "Pancrease".

Storage: Pancrease capsules should be stored in a dry place below 25°C (77°F) in well-closed containers. Do not refrigerate.

Microtablets

Pancrease MT capsules are supplied as follows:

MT 4: Yellow opaque body, clear cap capsules imprinted with "McNEIL" and "PANCREASE MT 4".

MT 10: Pink opaque body, clear cap capsules imprinted with "McNEIL" and "PANCREASE MT 10".

MT 16: Salmon opaque body, clear cap capsules imprinted with "McNEIL" and "PANCREASE MT 16".

MT 20: White opaque body, cap with yellow band capsules imprinted with "McNEIL" and "PANCREASE MT 20".

Storage: Pancrease MT capsules should be stored in a dry place below 25°C (77°F) in well-closed containers. Do not refrigerate.

PRODUCT LISTING - EQUIVALENTS NOT AVAILABLE

Capsule - Oral - 15000 U;12000 U;15000 U

100's	$61.88	KU-ZYME, Schwarz Pharma	00091-4122-01

Capsule - Oral - 30000 U;8000 U;30000 U

100's	$22.36	COTAZYM, Organon	00052-0382-91
100's	$25.95	GENERIC, Breckenridge Inc	51991-0655-01
100's	$26.67	COTAZYM, Organon	00052-0381-91
100's	$61.88	KU-ZYME HP, Schwarz Pharma	00091-3525-01

Capsule - Oral - 30000 U;24000 U;30000 U

100's	$74.71	KUTRASE, Schwarz Pharma	00091-4175-01

Capsule, Extended Release - Oral - 12000 U;4000 U;12000 U

100's	$42.08	PANCREASE MT 4, Janssen Pharmaceuticals	00045-0341-60

Capsule, Extended Release - Oral - 16600 U;5000 U;18750 U

100's	$42.28	GENERIC, Global Pharmaceutical Corporation	00115-7057-01
100's	$49.70	CREON 5, Solvay Pharmaceuticals Inc	00032-1205-01
250's	$97.18	CREON 5, Solvay Pharmaceuticals Inc	00032-1205-07
250's	$103.57	GENERIC, Global Pharmaceutical Corporation	00115-7057-05

Capsule, Extended Release - Oral - 20000 U;4000 U;25000 U

100's	$25.30	GENERIC, Qualitest Products Inc	00603-5021-21
100's	$28.24	GENERIC, Watson/Rugby Laboratories Inc	00536-4929-01
100's	$29.50	GENERIC, Ivax Corporation	00182-1554-01
250's	$61.40	GENERIC, Qualitest Products Inc	00603-5021-24

Capsule, Extended Release - Oral - 20000 U;4500 U;25000 U

100's	$32.50	GENERIC, Major Pharmaceuticals Inc	00904-5413-60
100's	$36.99	LIPRAM, Global Pharmaceutical Corporation	00115-7004-01
100's	$37.70	GENERIC, Ethex Corporation	58177-0031-04
100's	$38.99	GENERIC, Mutual Pharmaceutical Co Inc	00677-1653-01
100's	$38.99	GENERIC, Mutual/United Research Laboratories	53489-0320-01
100's	$40.81	LIPRAM, Global Pharmaceutical Corporation	00115-7035-01
100's	$47.93	ULTRASE, Scandipharm Inc	58914-0045-10
100's	$48.62	PANCREASE, Physicians Total Care	54868-1557-01
100's	$50.43	PANCREASE, Janssen Pharmaceuticals	00045-0095-60
250's	$59.98	GENERIC, Major Pharmaceuticals Inc	00904-5413-70
250's	$87.87	LIPRAM, Global Pharmaceutical Corporation	00115-7004-05
250's	$94.29	GENERIC, Ethex Corporation	58177-0031-06
250's	$96.96	LIPRAM, Global Pharmaceutical Corporation	00115-7035-05
250's	$127.20	PANCREASE, Janssen Pharmaceuticals	00045-0095-69

Capsule, Extended Release - Oral - 20000 U;5000 U;20000 U

100's	$30.25	COTAZYM-S, Organon	00052-0389-91
100's	$36.06	COTAZYM-S, Organon	00052-0388-91

Capsule, Extended Release - Oral - 24000 U;12000 U;24000 U

100's	$66.39	ZYMASE, Organon	00052-0394-91
100's	$68.39	ZYMASE, Organon	00052-0393-91

Capsule, Extended Release - Oral - 25000 U;4000U;25000U

100's	$61.85	GENERIC, Digestive Care Inc	59767-0002-01

Capsule, Extended Release - Oral - 30000 U;10000 U;30000 U

100's	$72.95	PANGESTYME CN 10, Ethex Corporation	58177-0029-04
100's	$77.06	GENERIC, Global Pharmaceutical Corporation	00115-7040-01
100's	$105.16	PANCREASE MT 10, Janssen Pharmaceuticals	00045-0342-60

Capsule, Extended Release - Oral - 33200 U;10000 U;37500 U

100's	$61.50	LIPRAM-CR, Global Pharmaceutical Corporation	00115-7003-01
100's	$67.93	LIPRAM-CR, Global Pharmaceutical Corporation	00115-7036-01
100's	$73.95	GENERIC, Mutual/United Research Laboratories	00677-1654-01
100's	$97.76	CREON 10, Solvay Pharmaceuticals Inc	00032-1210-01
250's	$147.57	LIPRAM-CR, Global Pharmaceutical Corporation	00115-7003-05
250's	$163.01	LIPRAM-CR, Global Pharmaceutical Corporation	00115-7036-05
250's	$176.89	GENERIC, Mutual/United Research Laboratories	00677-1654-03
250's	$176.89	GENERIC, Mutual/United Research Laboratories	53489-0321-03
250's	$239.64	CREON 10, Solvay Pharmaceuticals Inc	00032-1210-07

Capsule, Extended Release - Oral - 39000 U;12000 U;39000 U

100's	$74.55	GENERIC, Ethex Corporation	58177-0048-04
100's	$80.48	GENERIC, Global Pharmaceutical Corporation	00115-7042-01
100's	$98.78	ULTRASE MT 12, Scandipharm Inc	58914-0002-10

Capsule, Extended Release - Oral - 40000 U;8000 U;45000 U

100's	$112.15	PANCRECARB MS-8, Digestive Care Inc	59767-0001-01
250's	$253.67	PANCRECARB MS-8, Digestive Care Inc	59767-0001-02

Capsule, Extended Release - Oral - 48000 U;16000 U;48000 U

100's	$99.50	GENERIC, Pecos Pharmaceutical	59879-0122-01
100's	$118.23	GENERIC, Mutual/United Research Laboratories	00677-1655-01
100's	$119.20	PANGESTYME MT 16, Ethex Corporation	58177-0028-04
100's	$123.73	GENERIC, Global Pharmaceutical Corporation	00115-7023-01
100's	$168.85	PANCREASE MT 16, Janssen Pharmaceuticals	00045-0343-60

Capsule, Extended Release - Oral - 56000 U;20000 U;44000 U

100's	$154.11	GENERIC, Global Pharmaceutical Corporation	00115-7055-01
100's	$210.29	PANCREASE MT 20, Janssen Pharmaceuticals	00045-0346-60

Capsule, Extended Release - Oral - 59000 U;18000 U;59000 U

100's	$116.87	PANGESTYME NL 18, Ethex Corporation	58177-0049-04

100's	$126.16	LIPRAM-UL 18, Global Pharmaceutical Corporation	00115-7041-01
100's	$154.86	ULTRASE MT 18, Scandipharm Inc	58914-0018-10
Capsule, Extended Release - Oral - 65000 U;20000 U;65000 U			
100's	$129.17	PANGESTYME NL 18, Ethex Corporation	58177-0050-04
100's	$139.42	GENERIC, Global Pharmaceutical Corporation	00115-7043-01
100's	$141.00	GENERIC, Mutual/United Research Laboratories	00677-1776-01
100's	$141.46	GENERIC, Ethex Corporation	58177-0030-04
100's	$171.14	ULTRASE MT 20, Scandipharm Inc	58914-0004-10
Capsule, Extended Release - Oral - 66400 U;20000 U;75000 U			
100's	$146.97	GENERIC, Global Pharmaceutical Corporation	00115-7024-01
100's	$189.56	CREON 20, Solvay Pharmaceuticals Inc	00032-1220-01
250's	$356.71	GENERIC, Global Pharmaceutical Corporation	00115-7024-05
250's	$460.39	CREON 20, Solvay Pharmaceuticals Inc	00032-1220-07
Powder For Reconstitution - Oral - 70000 U;16800 U;70000 U/0.7 Gm			
240 gm	$144.86	VIOKASE, Paddock Laboratories Inc	00574-9115-25
240 gm	$159.35	VIOKASE, Scandipharm Inc	58914-0115-08
Tablet - Oral - 30000 U;8000 U;30000 U			
100's	$12.81	GENERIC, Moore, H.L. Drug Exchange Inc	00839-7618-06
100's	$17.22	GENERIC, Econolab	55053-0320-01
100's	$29.48	GENERIC, Global Pharmaceutical Corporation	00115-7029-01
100's	$29.95	GENERIC, Ethex Corporation	58177-0416-04
100's	$31.65	GENERIC, Ivax Corporation	00182-1741-01
100's	$37.43	GENERIC, Major Pharmaceuticals Inc	00904-3472-60
100's	$40.71	VIOKASE 8, Scandipharm Inc	58914-0111-10
Tablet - Oral - 30000 U;11000 U;30000 U			
250's	$139.23	ILOZYME, Savage Laboratories	00281-2001-19
Tablet - Oral - 60000 U;16000 U;60000 U			
100's	$67.20	VIOKASE 16, Paddock Laboratories Inc	00574-9116-63
100's	$73.92	VIOKASE 16, Scandipharm Inc	58914-0116-10

Pantoprazole Sodium *(003467)*

For related information, see the comparative table section in Appendix A.

Categories: Esophagitis, erosive; Gastroesophageal Reflux Disease; FDA Approved 2000 Feb; Pregnancy Category B
Drug Classes: Gastrointestinals; Proton pump inhibitors
Brand Names: **Protonix**
Foreign Brand Availability: Controloc (Egypt; Iran; Israel; Jordan; Singapore; Thailand); Eupantol (France); Inipomp (France); Pantodac (India); Pantodar (Bahrain; Cyprus; Egypt; Iran; Iraq; Jordan; Kuwait; Lebanon; Libya; Oman; Qatar; Republic-of-Yemen; Saudi-Arabia; Syria; United-Arab-Emirates); Pantoloc (Austria; Canada; China; Denmark; Hong-Kong; Korea; Philippines; Taiwan); Pantozol (Bahrain; Cyprus; Egypt; Germany; India; Indonesia; Iran; Iraq; Jordan; Kuwait; Lebanon; Libya; Mexico; Netherlands; Oman; Qatar; Republic-of-Yemen; Saudi-Arabia; Syria; United-Arab-Emirates); Rifun 40 (Germany); Somac (Australia; New-Zealand); Ulcepraz (Philippines); Zoltum (Peru); Zurcal (Austria; Colombia; Mexico; Peru); Zurcazol (Greece)
Cost of Therapy: $108.75 (GERD; Protonix; 40 mg; 1 tablet/day; 30 day supply)

INTRAVENOUS

DESCRIPTION

Note: The trade names have been used throughout this monograph for clarity.

The active ingredient in Protonix IV (pantoprazole sodium) for injection is a substituted benzimidazole, sodium 5-(difluoromethoxy)-2-[[(3,4-dimethoxy-2-pyridinyl)methyl] sulfinyl]-1H-benzimidazole, a compound that inhibits gastric acid secretion. Its empirical formula is $C_{16}H_{14}F_2N_3NaO_4S$, with a molecular weight of 405.4.

Pantoprazole sodium is a white to off-white crystalline powder and is racemic. Pantoprazole has weakly basic and acidic properties. Pantoprazole sodium is freely soluble in water, very slightly soluble in phosphate buffer at pH 7.4, and practically insoluble in n-hexane. The stability of the compound in aqueous solution is pH-dependent. The rate of degradation increases with decreasing pH. The reconstituted solution of Protonix IV for injection is in the pH range 9.0-10.0.

Protonix IV for injection is supplied as a freeze-dried powder in a clear glass vial fitted with a rubber stopper and crimp seal containing pantoprazole sodium, equivalent to 40 mg of pantoprazole.

CLINICAL PHARMACOLOGY

PHARMACOKINETICS

Pantoprazole peak serum concentration (C_{max}) and area under the serum concentration-time curve (AUC) increase in a manner proportional to intravenous (IV) doses from 10-80 mg. Pantoprazole does not accumulate and its pharmacokinetics are unaltered with multiple daily dosing. Following the administration of Protonix IV for injection, the serum concentration of pantoprazole declines biexponentially with a terminal elimination half-life of approximately 1 hour. In extensive metabolizers (see Metabolism) with normal liver function receiving a 40 mg dose of Protonix IV for injection by constant rate over 15 minutes, the peak concentration (C_{max}) is 5.52 µg/ml and the total area under the plasma concentration versus time curve (AUC) is 5.4 µg·h/ml. The total clearance is 7.6-14.0 L/h and the apparent volume of distribution is 11.0-23.6 L.

Distribution

The apparent volume of distribution of pantoprazole is approximately 11.0-23.6 L, distributing mainly in extracellular fluid. The serum protein binding of pantoprazole is about 98%, primarily to albumin.

Metabolism

Pantoprazole is extensively metabolized in the liver through the cytochrome P450 (CYP) system. Pantoprazole metabolism is independent of the route of administration (IV or oral). The main metabolic pathway is demethylation, by CYP2C19, with subsequent sulfation; other metabolic pathways include oxidation by CYP3A4. There is no evidence that any of the pantoprazole metabolites have significant pharmacologic activity. CYP2C19 displays a known genetic polymorphism due to its deficiency in some sub-populations (*e.g.,* 3% of Caucasians and African-Americans and 17-23% of Asians). Although these sub-populations of slow pantoprazole metabolizers have elimination half-life values from 3.5-10.0 hours, they still have minimal accumulation (≤23%) with once daily dosing.

Elimination

After administration of a single IV dose of ^{14}C-labeled pantoprazole to healthy, normal metabolizer subjects, approximately 71% of the dose was excreted in the urine with 18% excreted in the feces through biliary excretion. There was no renal excretion of unchanged pantoprazole.

Special Populations

Geriatric

After repeated IV administration in elderly subjects (65-76 years of age), pantoprazole AUC and elimination half-life values were similar to those observed in younger subjects. No dosage adjustment is recommended based on age.

Pediatric

The pharmacokinetics of pantoprazole have not been investigated in patients <18 years of age.

Gender

After oral administration there is a modest increase in pantoprazole AUC and C_{max} in women compared to men. However, weight-normalized clearance values are similar in women and men. No dosage adjustment is warranted based on gender (also see PRECAUTIONS, Use in Women).

Renal Impairment

In patients with severe renal impairment, pharmacokinetic parameters for pantoprazole were similar to those of healthy subjects. No dosage adjustment is necessary in patients with renal impairment or in patients undergoing hemodialysis.

Hepatic Impairment

Oral administration studies (absolute bioavailability is approximately 70%) were performed in patients with mild to severe hepatic impairment. Maximum pantoprazole concentrations increased only slightly (1.5-fold) relative to healthy subjects. Although serum elimination half-life values increased to 7-9 hours and AUC values increased by 5- to 7-fold in hepatic-impaired patients, these increases were no greater than those observed in slow CYP2C19 metabolizers, where no dosage adjustment is warranted. These pharmacokinetic changes in hepatic-impaired patients result in minimal drug accumulation following once daily multiple-dose administration equal to or less than 21%. No dosage adjustment is needed in patients with mild to severe hepatic impairment.

DRUG-DRUG INTERACTIONS

Pantoprazole is metabolized mainly by CYP2C19 and to minor extents by CYPs 3A4, 2D6 and 2C9. In *in vivo* drug-drug interaction studies with CYP2C19 substrates (diazepam [also a CYP3A4 substrate] and phenytoin [also a CYP3A4 inducer]), nifedipine, midazolam, and clarithromycin (CYP3A4 substrates), metoprolol (a CYP2D6 substrate), diclofenac (a CYP2C9 substrate) and theophylline (a CYP1A2 substrate) in healthy subjects, the pharmacokinetics of pantoprazole were not significantly altered. It is, therefore, expected that other drugs metabolized by CYPs 2C19, 3A4, 2D6, 2C9 and 1A2 would not significantly affect the pharmacokinetics of pantoprazole. *In vivo* studies also suggest that pantoprazole does not significantly affect the kinetics of other drugs (cisapride, theophylline, diazepam [and its active metabolite, desmethyldiazepam], phenytoin, warfarin, metoprolol, nifedipine, carbamazepine, midazolam, clarithromycin, and oral contraceptives) metabolized by CYPs 2C19, 3A4, 2D6, 2C9 and 1A2. Therefore, it is expected that pantoprazole would not significantly affect the pharmacokinetics of other drugs metabolized by these isozymes. Dosage adjustment of such drugs is not necessary when they are coadministered with pantoprazole. In other *in vivo* studies, digoxin, ethanol, glyburide, antipyrine, caffeine, metronidazole, and amoxicillin had no clinically relevant interactions with pantoprazole. Although no significant drug-drug interactions have been observed in clinical studies, the potential for significant drug-drug interactions with more than once daily dosing with high doses of pantoprazole has not been studied in poor metabolizers or individuals who are hepatically impaired.

Because of profound and long lasting inhibition of gastric acid secretion, pantoprazole may interfere with absorption of drugs where gastric pH is an important determinant of their bioavailability (*e.g.,* ketoconazole, ampicillin esters, and iron salts).

PHARMACODYNAMICS

Mechanism of Action

Pantoprazole is a proton pump inhibitor (PPI) that suppresses the final step in gastric acid production by covalently binding to the (H^+, K^+)-ATPase enzyme system at the secretory surface of the gastric parietal cell. This effect leads to inhibition of both basal and stimulated gastric acid secretion irrespective of the stimulus. The binding to the (H^+, K^+)-ATPase results in a duration of antisecretory effect that persists longer than 24 hours for all doses tested.

Antisecretory Activity

The magnitude and time course for inhibition of pentagastrin-stimulated acid output (PSAO) by single doses (20-120 mg) of Protonix IV for injection were assessed in a single-dose, open-label, placebo-controlled, dose-response study. The results of this study are shown in TABLE 1. Healthy subjects received a continuous infusion for 25 hours of penta-

P

gastrin (PG) at 1 μg/kg/h, a dose known to produce submaximal gastric acid secretion. The placebo group showed a sustained, continuous acid output for 25 hours, validating the reliability of the testing model. Protonix IV for injection had an onset of antisecretory activity within 15-30 minutes of administration. Doses of 20-80 mg of Protonix IV for injection substantially reduced the 24 hour cumulative PSAO in a dose-dependent manner, despite a short plasma elimination half-life. Complete suppression of PSAO was achieved with 80 mg within approximately 2 hours and no further significant suppression was seen with 120 mg. The duration of action of Protonix IV for injection was 24 hours.

TABLE 1 *Gastric Acid Output (mEq/h, Mean ± SD) and % Inhibition* (Mean ± SD) of Pentagastrin-Stimulated Acid Output Over 24 Hours Following a Single Dose of Protonix IV for Injection† in Healthy Subjects*

	Placebo (n=4)	20 mg (n=4-6)	40 mg (n=8)	80 mg (n=8)
2 Hours				
Acid output	39 ± 21	13 ± 18	5 ± 5	0.1 ± 0.2
% Inhibition	NA	47 ± 27	82 ± 11	96 ± 6
4 Hours				
Acid output	26 ± 14	6 ± 8	4 ± 4	0.3 ± 0.4
% Inhibition	NA	83 ± 21	90 ± 11	99 ± 1
12 Hours				
Acid output	32 ± 20	20 ± 20	11 ± 10	2 ± 2
% Inhibition	NA	54 ± 44	81 ± 13	90 ± 7
24 Hours				
Acid output	38 ± 24	30 ± 23	16 ± 12	7 ± 4
% Inhibition	NA	45 ± 43	52 ± 36	63 ± 18

* Compared to individual subject baseline prior to treatment with Protonix IV for injection. NA = not applicable.

† Inhibition of gastric acid output and the percent inhibition of stimulated acid output in response to Protonix IV for injection may be higher after repeated doses.

In one study of gastric pH in healthy subjects, pantoprazole was administered orally (40 mg enteric coated tablets) or intravenously (40 mg) once daily for 5 days and pH was measured for 24 hours following the fifth dose. The outcome measure was median % of time that pH was ≥4 and the results were similar for IV and oral medications; however, the clinical significance of this parameter is unknown.

Serum Gastrin Effects

Serum gastrin concentrations were assessed in a placebo-controlled 5 day study of IV pantoprazole with 40 and 60 mg doses. Following the last dose on Day 5, the median 24 hour serum gastrin concentrations were elevated by 3- to 4-fold compared to placebo in both 40 and 60 mg dose groups. However, by 24 hours following the last dose median serum gastrin concentrations for both groups returned to normal levels.

During 6 days of repeated administration of Protonix IV for injection in patients with Zollinger-Ellison Syndrome, consistent changes of serum gastrin concentrations from baseline were not observed.

Enterochromaffin-Like (ECL) Cell Effects

There are no data available on the effects of IV pantoprazole on ECL cells.

In a nonclinical study in Sprague-Dawley rats, lifetime exposure (24 months) to pantoprazole at doses of 0.5-200 mg/kg/day resulted in dose-related increases in gastric ECL-cell proliferation and gastric neuroendocrine (NE)-cell tumors. Gastric NE-cell tumors in rats may result from chronic elevation of serum gastrin concentrations. The high density of ECL cells in the rat stomach makes this species highly susceptible to the proliferative effects of elevated gastrin concentrations produced by proton pump inhibitors. However, there were no observed elevations in serum gastrin following the administration of pantoprazole at a dose of 0.5 mg/kg/day. In a separate study, a gastric NE-cell tumor without concomitant ECL-cell proliferative changes was observed in 1 female rat following 12 months of dosing with pantoprazole at 5 mg/kg/day and a 9 month off-dose recovery (see PRECAUTIONS, Carcinogenesis, Mutagenesis, and Impairment of Fertility).

Other Effects

No clinically relevant effects of pantoprazole on cardiovascular, respiratory, ophthalmic, or central nervous system function have been detected. In a clinical pharmacology study, pantoprazole 40 mg given orally once daily for 2 weeks had no effect on the levels of the following hormones: cortisol, testosterone, triiodothyronine (T3), thyroxine (T4), thyroid-stimulating hormone, thyronine-binding protein, parathyroid hormone, insulin, glucagon, renin, aldosterone, follicle-stimulating hormone, luteinizing hormone, prolactin and growth hormone.

INDICATIONS AND USAGE

TREATMENT OF GASTROESOPHAGEAL REFLUX DISEASE ASSOCIATED WITH A HISTORY OF EROSIVE ESOPHAGITIS

Protonix IV for injection is indicated for short-term treatment (7-10 days) of patients having gastroesophageal reflux disease (GERD) with a history of erosive esophagitis, **as an alternative to oral therapy in patients who are unable to continue taking Protonix delayed-release tablets.** Safety and efficacy of Protonix IV for injection as an initial treatment of patients having GERD with a history of erosive esophagitis have not been demonstrated.

PATHOLOGICAL HYPERSECRETION ASSOCIATED WITH ZOLLINGER-ELLISON SYNDROME

Protonix IV for injection is indicated for the treatment of pathological hypersecretory conditions associated with Zollinger-Ellison Syndrome or other neoplastic conditions.

CONTRAINDICATIONS

Protonix IV for injection is contraindicated in patients with known hypersensitivity to the formulation.

PRECAUTIONS

GENERAL

Immediate Hypersensitivity Reactions: Anaphylaxis has been reported with use of IV pantoprazole. This may require emergency medical treatment.

Injection Site Reactions: Thrombophlebitis was associated with the administration of IV pantoprazole.

Hepatic Effects: Mild, transient transaminase elevations have been observed in clinical studies. The clinical significance of this finding in a large population of subjects administered IV pantoprazole is unknown. (See ADVERSE REACTIONS.)

Symptomatic response to therapy with pantoprazole does not preclude the presence of gastric malignancy.

Treatment with Protonix IV for injection should be discontinued as soon as the patient is able to resume treatment with Protonix delayed-release tablets.

CARCINOGENESIS, MUTAGENESIS, AND IMPAIRMENT OF FERTILITY

In a 24 month carcinogenicity study, Sprague-Dawley rats were treated orally with doses of 0.5-200 mg/kg/day, about 0.1-40 times the exposure on a body surface area basis, of a 50 kg person dosed at 40 mg/day. In the gastric fundus, treatment at 0.5-200 mg/kg/day produced enterochromaffin-like (ECL) cell hyperplasia and benign and malignant neuroendocrine cell tumors in a dose-related manner. In the forestomach, treatment at 50 and 200 mg/kg/day (about 10 and 40 times the recommended human dose on a body surface area basis) produced benign squamous cell papillomas and malignant squamous cell carcinomas. Rare gastrointestinal tumors associated with pantoprazole treatment included an adenocarcinoma of the duodenum at 50 mg/kg/day, and benign polyps and adenocarcinomas of the gastric fundus at 200 mg/kg/day. In the liver, treatment at 0.5-200 mg/kg/day produced dose-related increases in the incidences of hepatocellular adenomas and carcinomas. In the thyroid gland, treatment at 200 mg/kg/day produced increased incidences of follicular cell adenomas and carcinomas for both male and female rats.

Sporadic occurrences of hepatocellular adenomas and a hepatocellular carcinoma were observed in Sprague-Dawley rats exposed to pantoprazole in 6 and 12 month oral toxicity studies.

In a 24 month carcinogenicity study, Fischer 344 rats were treated orally with doses of 5-50 mg/kg/day, approximately 1-10 times the recommended human dose based on body surface area. In the gastric fundus, treatment at 5-50 mg/kg/day produced enterochromaffin-like (ECL) cell hyperplasia and benign and malignant neuroendocrine cell tumors. Dose selection for this study may not have been adequate to comprehensively evaluate the carcinogenic potential of pantoprazole.

In a 24 month carcinogenicity study, B6C3F1 mice were treated orally with doses of 5-150 mg/kg/day, 0.5-15 times the recommended human dose based on body surface area. In the liver, treatment at 150 mg/kg/day produced increased incidences of hepatocellular adenomas and carcinomas in female mice. Treatment at 5-150 mg/kg/day also produced gastric fundic ECL cell hyperplasia.

Pantoprazole was positive in the *in vitro* human lymphocyte chromosomal aberration assays, in one of two mouse micronucleus tests for clastogenic effects, and in the *in vitro* Chinese hamster ovarian cell/HGPRT forward mutation assay for mutagenic effects. Equivocal results were observed in the *in vivo* rat liver DNA covalent binding assay. Pantoprazole was negative in the *in vitro* Ames mutation assay, the *in vitro* unscheduled DNA synthesis (UDS) assay with rat hepatocytes, the *in vitro* AS52/GPT mammalian cell-forward gene mutation assay, the *in vitro* thymidine kinase mutation test with mouse lymphoma L5178Y cells, and the *in vivo* rat bone marrow cell chromosomal aberration assay. A 26 week p53 ± transgenic mouse carcinogenicity study was not positive.

Pantoprazole at oral doses up to 500 mg/kg/day in male rats (98 times the recommended human dose based on body surface area) and 450 mg/kg/day in female rats (88 times the recommended human dose based on body surface area) was found to have no effect on fertility and reproductive performance.

PREGNANCY, TERATOGENIC EFFECTS, PREGNANCY CATEGORY B

Teratology studies have been performed in rats at IV doses up to 20 mg/kg/day (4 times the recommended human dose based on body surface area) and rabbits at IV doses up to 15 mg/kg/day (6 times the recommended human dose based on body surface area) and have revealed no evidence of impaired fertility or harm to the fetus due to pantoprazole. There are, however, no adequate and well-controlled studies in pregnant women. Because animal reproduction studies are not always predictive of human response, this drug should be used during pregnancy only if clearly needed.

NURSING MOTHERS

Pantoprazole and its metabolites are excreted in the milk of rats. It is not known whether pantoprazole is excreted in human milk. Many drugs which are excreted in human milk have a potential for serious adverse reactions in nursing infants. Based on the potential for tumorigenicity shown for pantoprazole in rodent carcinogenicity studies, a decision should be made whether to discontinue nursing or to discontinue the drug, taking into account the benefit of the drug to the mother.

PEDIATRIC USE

Safety and effectiveness in pediatric patients have not been established.

USE IN WOMEN

No gender-related differences in the safety profile of IV pantoprazole were seen in international trials involving 166 men and 120 women with erosive esophagitis associated with GERD. Erosive esophagitis healing rates in the 221 women treated with oral pantoprazole in US clinical trials were similar to those found in men. The incidence rates of adverse events were also similar between men and women.

GERIATRIC USE

No age-related differences in the safety profile of IV pantoprazole were seen in international trials involving 86 elderly (≥65 years old) and 200 younger (<65 years old) patients with erosive esophagitis associated with GERD. Erosive esophagitis healing rates in the 107 elderly patients (≥65 years old) treated with oral pantoprazole in US clinical trials were

P

similar to those found in patients under the age of 65. The incidence rates of adverse events and laboratory abnormalities in patients aged 65 years and older were similar to those associated with patients younger than 65 years of age.

LABORATORY TESTS

There have been reports of false-positive urine screening for tetrahydrocannabinol (THC) in patients receiving pantoprazole.

DRUG INTERACTIONS

See CLINICAL PHARMACOLOGY, Drug-Drug Interactions.

ADVERSE REACTIONS

SAFETY EXPERIENCE WITH IV PANTOPRAZOLE

Intravenous pantoprazole has been studied in clinical trials in several populations including patients having GERD with a history of erosive esophagitis, patients with Zollinger-Ellison Syndrome and healthy subjects. Adverse experiences occurring in >1% of patients treated with IV pantoprazole (n=714) in domestic or international clinical trials are shown below by body system. In most instances, the relationship to pantoprazole was unclear.

Body as a Whole: Abdominal pain, headache, injection site reaction (including thrombophlebitis and abscess).
Digestive System: Constipation, dyspepsia, nausea, diarrhea.
Nervous System: Insomnia.
Respiratory System: Rhinitis.

Head-to-head comparative studies between Protonix IV for injection and oral Protonix, other proton pump inhibitors (oral or IV), or H2 receptor antagonists (oral or IV) have been limited. The available information does not provide sufficient evidence to distinguish the safety profile of these regimens.

SAFETY EXPERIENCE WITH ORAL PANTOPRAZOLE

In short-term clinical trials in patients with erosive esophagitis associated with GERD treated with oral pantoprazole, the following adverse events, regardless of causality, occurred at a rate of ≥1%.

Body as a Whole: Headache, asthenia, back pain, chest pain, neck pain, flu syndrome, infection, pain.
Cardiovascular System: Migraine.
Digestive System: Diarrhea, flatulence, abdominal pain, eructation, constipation, dyspepsia, gastroenteritis, gastrointestinal disorder, nausea, rectal disorder, vomiting.
Hepato-Biliary System: Liver function tests abnormal, SGPT increased.
Metabolic and Nutritional: Hyperglycemia, hyperlipemia.
Musculoskeletal System: Arthralgia.
Nervous System: Insomnia, anxiety, dizziness, hypertonia.
Respiratory System: Bronchitis, cough increased, dyspnea, pharyngitis, rhinitis, sinusitis, upper respiratory tract infection.
Skin and Appendages: Rash.
Urogenital System: Urinary frequency, and urinary tract infection.

Additional adverse experiences occurring in <1% of patients with erosive esophagitis associated with GERD receiving oral pantoprazole based on pooled results from either short-term domestic or international trials are shown below within each body system. In most instances, the relationship to pantoprazole was unclear.

Body as a Whole: Abscess, allergic reaction, chills, cyst, face edema, fever, generalized edema, heat stroke, hernia, laboratory test abnormal, malaise, moniliasis, neoplasm, non-specified drug reaction.
Cardiovascular System: Abnormal electrocardiogram, angina pectoris, arrhythmia, cardiovascular disorder, chest pain substernal, congestive heart failure, hemorrhage, hypertension, hypotension, myocardial ischemia, palpitation, retinal vascular disorder, syncope, tachycardia, thrombophlebitis, thrombosis, vasodilatation.
Digestive System: Anorexia, aphthous stomatitis, cardiospasm, colitis, dry mouth, duodenitis, dysphagia, enteritis, esophageal hemorrhage, esophagitis, gastrointestinal carcinoma, gastrointestinal hemorrhage, gastrointestinal moniliasis, gingivitis, glossitis, halitosis, hematemesis, increased appetite, melena, mouth ulceration, oral moniliasis, periodontal abscess, periodontitis, rectal hemorrhage, stomach ulcer, stomatitis, stools abnormal, tongue discoloration, ulcerative colitis.
Endocrine System: Diabetes mellitus, glycosuria, goiter.
Hepato-Biliary System: Biliary pain, hyperbilirubinemia, cholecystitis, cholelithiasis, cholestatic jaundice, hepatitis, alkaline phosphatase increased, gamma glutamyl transpeptidase increased, SGOT increased.
Hemic and Lymphatic System: Anemia, ecchymosis, eosinophilia, hypochromic anemia, iron deficiency anemia, leukocytosis, leukopenia, thrombocytopenia.
Metabolic And Nutritional: Dehydration, edema, gout, peripheral edema, thirst, weight gain, weight loss.
Musculoskeletal System: Arthritis, arthrosis, bone disorder, bone pain, bursitis, joint disorder, leg cramps, neck rigidity, myalgia, tenosynovitis.
Nervous System: Abnormal dreams, confusion, convulsion, depression, dry mouth, dysarthria, emotional lability, hallucinations, hyperkinesia, hypesthesia, libido decreased, nervousness, neuralgia, neuritis, paresthesia, reflexes decreased, sleep disorder, somnolence, thinking abnormal, tremor, vertigo.
Respiratory System: Asthma, epistaxis, hiccup, laryngitis, lung disorder, pneumonia, voice alteration.
Skin and Appendages: Acne, alopecia, contact dermatitis, dry skin, eczema, fungal dermatitis, hemorrhage, herpes simplex, herpes zoster, lichenoid dermatitis, maculopapular rash, pain, pruritus, skin disorder, skin ulcer, sweating, urticaria.
Special Senses: Abnormal vision, amblyopia, cataract specified, deafness, diplopia, ear pain, extraocular palsy, glaucoma, otitis externa, taste perversion, tinnitus.
Urogenital System: Albuminuria, balanitis, breast pain, cystitis, dysmenorrhea, dysuria, epididymitis, hematuria, impotence, kidney calculus, kidney pain, nocturia, prostatic disorder, pyelonephritis, scrotal edema, urethral pain, urethritis, urinary tract disorder, urination impaired, vaginitis.

POSTMARKETING REPORTS

The postmarketing safety profile of IV pantoprazole (from an estimate of over 700,000 patients) is not substantially different from that of oral pantoprazole (described below).

There have been spontaneous reports of adverse events with postmarketing use of IV or oral pantoprazole. These reports include anaphylaxis (including anaphylactic shock); angioedema (Quincke's edema); anterior ischemic optic neuropathy; severe dermatologic reactions, including erythema multiforme, Stevens-Johnson syndrome, and toxic epidermal necrolysis (TEN, some fatal); hepatocellular damage leading to jaundice and hepatic failure; pancreatitis; pancytopenia; and rhabdomyolysis. In addition, also observed have been confusion, hypokinesia, speech disorder, increased salivation, vertigo, nausea, tinnitus, and blurred vision.

LABORATORY VALUES

In US clinical trials of patients having GERD with a history of erosive esophagitis and international clinical trials of patients with erosive esophagitis associated with GERD, the overall percentages of transaminase elevations did not increase during treatment with IV pantoprazole. For other laboratory parameters, there were no clinically important changes identified.

In two US controlled trials of oral pantoprazole in patients with erosive esophagitis associated with GERD, 0.4% of the patients on 40 mg oral pantoprazole experienced SGPT elevations of greater than 3 times the upper limit of normal at the final treatment visit. Except in those patients where there was a clear alternative explanation for a laboratory value change, such as intercurrent illness, the elevations tended to be mild and sporadic. The following changes in laboratory parameters were reported as adverse events: creatinine increased, hypercholesterolemia, and hyperuricemia.

DOSAGE AND ADMINISTRATION

Protonix IV for injection admixtures should be administered intravenously through a dedicated line, using the in-line filter provided. **The filter must be used** to remove the precipitate that may form when the reconstituted drug product is mixed with IV solutions. Studies have shown that filtration does not alter the amount of drug that is available for administration. If administration through a Y-site is desirable, the in-line filter must be positioned below the Y-site that is closest to the patient. The IV line should be flushed before and after administration of Protonix IV for injection with either 5% dextrose injection, 0.9% sodium chloride injection, or lactated Ringer's injection. Protonix IV for injection should not be simultaneously administered through the same line with other IV solutions.

Treatment with Protonix IV for injection should be discontinued as soon as the patient is able to resume treatment with Protonix delayed-release tablets. Also, data on the safe and effective dosing for conditions other than those described in INDICATIONS AND USAGE, such as life-threatening upper gastrointestinal bleeds, are not available. Protonix IV 40 mg once daily does not raise gastric pH to levels sufficient to contribute to the treatment of such life-threatening conditions.

Parenteral routes of administration other than IV are not recommended.

No dosage adjustment is necessary in patients with renal impairment, hepatic impairment, or for elderly patients. No dosage adjustment is necessary in patients undergoing hemodialysis.

TREATMENT OF GASTROESOPHAGEAL REFLUX DISEASE ASSOCIATED WITH A HISTORY OF EROSIVE ESOPHAGITIS

The recommended adult dose, **as an alternative to continued oral therapy,** is 40 mg pantoprazole given once daily by IV infusion for 7-10 days. Safety and efficacy of Protonix IV for injection as a treatment of patients having GERD with a history of erosive esophagitis for more than 10 days have not been demonstrated (see INDICATIONS AND USAGE).

Protonix IV for injection should be reconstituted with 10 ml of 0.9% sodium chloride injection, and further diluted (admixed) with 100 ml of 5% dextrose injection, 0.9% sodium chloride injection, or lactated Ringer's injection, to a final concentration of approximately 0.4 mg/ml. The reconstituted solution may be stored for up to 2 hours at room temperature prior to further dilution; the admixed solution may be stored for up to 12 hours at room temperature prior to IV infusion. Neither the reconstituted solution nor the admixed solution need to be protected from light.

Protonix IV for injection admixtures should be administered intravenously over a period of approximately 15 minutes at a rate not greater than 3 mg/min (7 ml/min).

PATHOLOGICAL HYPERSECRETION ASSOCIATED WITH ZOLLINGER-ELLISON SYNDROME

The dosage of Protonix IV for injection in patients with pathological hypersecretory conditions associated with Zollinger-Ellison Syndrome or other neoplastic conditions varies with individual patients. The recommended adult dosage is 80 mg q12h. The frequency of dosing can be adjusted to individual patient needs based on acid output measurements. In those patients who need a higher dosage, 80 mg q8h is expected to maintain acid output below 10 mEq/h. Daily doses higher than 240 mg or administered for more than 6 days have not been studied. Transition from oral to IV and from IV to oral formulations of gastric acid inhibitors should be performed in such a manner to ensure continuity of effect of suppression of acid secretion. Patients with Zollinger-Ellison Syndrome may be vulnerable to serious clinical complications of increased acid production even after a short period of loss of effective inhibition.

Each vial of Protonix IV for injection should be reconstituted with 10 ml of 0.9% sodium chloride injection. The contents of the 2 vials should be combined and further diluted (admixed) with 80 ml of 5% dextrose injection, 0.9% sodium chloride injection, or lactated Ringer's injection, to a total volume of 100 ml with a final concentration of approximately 0.8 mg/ml. The reconstituted solution may be stored for up to 2 hours at room temperature prior to further dilution; the admixed solution may be stored for up to 12 hours at room temperature prior to IV infusion. Neither the reconstituted solution nor the admixed solution need to be protected from light.

Protonix IV for injection should be administered intravenously over a period of approximately 15 minutes at a rate not greater than 6 mg/min (7 ml/min).

HOW SUPPLIED

Protonix IV for injection is supplied as a freeze-dried powder containing 40 mg of pantoprazole per vial.

STORAGE

Store Protonix IV for injection vials at 2-8°C (36-46°F) and protect from light.
Caution: The reconstituted product should not be frozen.
Store the provided in-line filters at room temperature.

ORAL

DESCRIPTION

Note: The trade names have been used throughout this monograph for clarity.
The active ingredient in Protonix (pantoprazole sodium) delayed-release tablets is a substituted benzimidazole, sodium 5-(difluoromethoxy)-2-[[(3,4-dimethoxy-2-pyridinyl)methyl] sulfinyl]-1*H*-benzimidazole sesquihydrate, a compound that inhibits gastric acid secretion. Its empirical formula is $C_{16}H_{14}F_2N_3NaO_4S \times 1.5\ H_2O$, with a molecular weight of 432.4.

Pantoprazole sodium sesquihydrate is a white to off-white crystalline powder and is racemic. Pantoprazole has weakly basic and acidic properties. Pantoprazole sodium sesquihydrate is freely soluble in water, very slightly soluble in phosphate buffer at pH 7.4, and practically insoluble in n-hexane.

The stability of the compound in aqueous solution is pH-dependent. The rate of degradation increases with decreasing pH. At ambient temperature, the degradation half-life is approximately 2.8 hours at pH 5.0 and approximately 220 hours at pH 7.8.

Protonix is supplied as a delayed-release tablet for oral administration, available in 2 strengths. Each delayed-release tablet contains 45.1 mg or 22.6 mg of pantoprazole sodium sesquihydrate (equivalent to 40 mg or 20 mg pantoprazole, respectively) with the following inactive ingredients: calcium stearate, crospovidone, hydromellose, iron oxide, mannitol, methacrylic acid copolymer, polysorbate 80, povidone, propylene glycol, sodium carbonate, sodium lauryl sulfate, titanium dioxide, and triethyl citrate.

CLINICAL PHARMACOLOGY

PHARMACOKINETICS

Protonix is prepared as an enteric-coated tablet so that absorption of pantoprazole begins only after the tablet leaves the stomach. Peak serum concentration (C_{max}) and area under the serum concentration time curve (AUC) increase in a manner proportional to oral and IV doses from 10-80 mg. Pantoprazole does not accumulate and its pharmacokinetics are unaltered with multiple daily dosing. Following oral or IV administration, the serum concentration of pantoprazole declines biexponentially with a terminal elimination half-life of approximately 1 hour. In extensive metabolizers (see Metabolism) with normal liver function receiving an oral dose of the enteric-coated 40 mg pantoprazole tablet, the peak concentration (C_{max}) is 2.5 μg/ml, the time to reach the peak concentration (T_{max}) is 2.5 hours and the total area under the plasma concentration versus time curve (AUC) is 4.8 μg·h/ml. When pantoprazole is given with food, its T_{max} is highly variable and may increase significantly. Following IV administration of pantoprazole to extensive metabolizers, its total clearance is 7.6-14.0 L/h and its apparent volume of distribution is 11.0-23.6 L.

Absorption

P

The absorption of pantoprazole is rapid, with a C_{max} of 2.5 μg/ml that occurs approximately 2.5 hours after single or multiple oral 40 mg doses. Pantoprazole is well absorbed; it undergoes little first-pass metabolism resulting in an absolute bioavailability of approximately 77%. Pantoprazole absorption is not affected by concomitant administration of antacids. Administration of pantoprazole with food may delay its absorption up to 2 hours or longer; however, the C_{max} and the extent of pantoprazole absorption (AUC) are not altered. Thus, pantoprazole may be taken without regard to timing of meals.

Distribution

The apparent volume of distribution of pantoprazole is approximately 11.0-23.6 L, distributing mainly in extracellular fluid. The serum protein binding of pantoprazole is about 98%, primarily to albumin.

Metabolism

Pantoprazole is extensively metabolized in the liver through the cytochrome P450 (CYP) system. Pantoprazole metabolism is independent of the route of administration (IV or oral). The main metabolic pathway is demethylation, by CYP2C19, with subsequent sulfation; other metabolic pathways include oxidation by CYP3A4. There is no evidence that any of the pantoprazole metabolites have significant pharmacologic activity. CYP2C19 displays a known genetic polymorphism due to its deficiency in some sub-populations (*e.g.*, 3% of Caucasians and African-Americans and 17-23% of Asians). Although these sub-populations of slow pantoprazole metabolizers have elimination half-life values of 3.5-10.0 hours, they still have minimal accumulation (≤23%) with once daily dosing.

Elimination

After a single oral or IV dose of ^{14}C-labeled pantoprazole to healthy, normal metabolizer volunteers, approximately 71% of the dose was excreted in the urine with 18% excreted in the feces through biliary excretion. There was no renal excretion of unchanged pantoprazole.

Special Populations

Geriatric

Only slight to moderate increases in pantoprazole AUC (43%) and C_{max} (26%) were found in elderly volunteers (64-76 years of age) after repeated oral administration, compared with younger subjects. No dosage adjustment is recommended based on age.

Pediatric

The pharmacokinetics of pantoprazole have not been investigated in patients <18 years of age.

Gender

There is a modest increase in pantoprazole AUC and C_{max} in women compared to men. However, weight-normalized clearance values are similar in women and men. No dosage adjustment is needed based on gender (also see PRECAUTIONS, Use in Women).

Renal Impairment

In patients with severe renal impairment, pharmacokinetic parameters for pantoprazole were similar to those of healthy subjects. No dosage adjustment is necessary in patients with renal impairment or in patients undergoing hemodialysis.

Hepatic Impairment

In patients with mild to severe hepatic impairment, maximum pantoprazole concentrations increased only slightly (1.5-fold) relative to healthy subjects. Although serum half-life values increased to 7-9 hours and AUC values increased by 5- to 7-fold in hepatic-impaired patients, these increases were no greater than those observed in slow CYP2C19 metabolizers, where no dosage frequency adjustment is warranted. These pharmacokinetic changes in hepatic-impaired patients result in minimal drug accumulation following once daily multiple-dose administration. No dosage adjustment is needed in patients with mild to severe hepatic impairment.

DRUG-DRUG INTERACTIONS

Pantoprazole is metabolized mainly by CYP2C19 and to minor extents by CYPs 3A4, 2D6 and 2C9. In *in vivo* drug-drug interaction studies with CYP2C19 substrates (diazepam [also a CYP3A4 substrate] and phenytoin [also a CYP3A4 inducer]), nifedipine, midazolam, and clarithromycin (CYP3A4 substrates), metoprolol (a CYP2D6 substrate), diclofenac (a CYP2C9 substrate) and theophylline (a CYP1A2 substrate) in healthy subjects, the pharmacokinetics of pantoprazole were not significantly altered. It is, therefore, expected that other drugs metabolized by CYPs 2C19, 3A4, 2D6, 2C9 and 1A2 would not significantly affect the pharmacokinetics of pantoprazole. *In vivo* studies also suggest that pantoprazole does not significantly affect the kinetics of other drugs (cisapride, theophylline, diazepam [and its active metabolite, desmethyldiazepam], phenytoin, warfarin, metoprolol, nifedipine, carbamazepine, midazolam, clarithromycin, and oral contraceptives) metabolized by CYPs 2C19, 3A4, 2C9, 2D6 and 1A2. Therefore, it is expected that pantoprazole would not significantly affect the pharmacokinetics of other drugs metabolized by these isozymes. Dosage adjustment of such drugs is not necessary when they are coadministered with pantoprazole. In other *in vivo* studies, digoxin, ethanol, glyburide, antipyrine, caffeine, metronidazole, and amoxicillin had no clinically relevant interactions with pantoprazole. Although no significant drug-drug interactions have been observed in clinical studies, the potential for significant drug-drug interactions with more than once daily dosing with high doses of pantoprazole has not been studied in poor metabolizers or individuals who are hepatically impaired.

PHARMACODYNAMICS

Mechanism of Action

Pantoprazole is a proton pump inhibitor (PPI) that suppresses the final step in gastric acid production by covalently binding to the (H^+,K^+)-ATPase enzyme system at the secretory surface of the gastric parietal cell. This effect leads to inhibition of both basal and stimulated gastric acid secretion irrespective of the stimulus. The binding to the (H^+,K^+)-ATPase results in a duration of antisecretory effect that persists longer than 24 hours for all doses tested.

Antisecretory Activity

Under maximal acid stimulatory conditions using pentagastrin, a dose-dependent decrease in gastric acid output occurs after a single dose of oral (20-80 mg) or a single dose of IV (20-120 mg) pantoprazole in healthy volunteers. Pantoprazole given once daily results in increasing inhibition of gastric acid secretion. Following the initial oral dose of 40 mg pantoprazole, a 51% mean inhibition was achieved by 2.5 hours. With once a day dosing for 7 days the mean inhibition was increased to 85%. Pantoprazole suppressed acid secretion in excess of 95% in half of the subjects. Acid secretion had returned to normal within a week after the last dose of pantoprazole; there was no evidence of rebound hypersecretion.

In a series of dose-response studies pantoprazole, at oral doses ranging from 20-120 mg, caused dose-related increases in median basal gastric pH and in the percent of time gastric pH was >3 and >4. Treatment with 40 mg of pantoprazole produced optimal increases in gastric pH which were significantly greater than the 20 mg dose. Doses higher than 40 mg (60, 80, 120 mg) did not result in further significant increases in median gastric pH. The effects of pantoprazole on median pH from one double-blind crossover study are shown in TABLE 3.

TABLE 3 *Effect of Single Daily Doses of Oral Pantoprazole on Intragastric pH*

		Median pH on Day 7		
Time	Placebo	20 mg	40 mg	80 mg
8 AM - 8 AM (24 hours)	1.3	2.9*	3.8*†	3.9*†
8 AM - 10 PM (daytime)	1.6	3.2*	4.4*†	4.8*†
10 PM - 8 AM (nighttime)	1.2	2.1*	3.0*	2.6*

* Significantly different from placebo.
† Significantly different from 20 mg.

Serum Gastrin Effects

Fasting serum gastrin levels were assessed in two double-blind studies of the acute healing of erosive esophagitis (EE) in which 682 patients with gastroesophageal reflux disease (GERD) received 10, 20, or 40 mg of Protonix for up to 8 weeks. At 4 weeks of treatment there was an increase in mean gastrin levels of 7, 35, and 72% over pretreatment values in the 10, 20, and 40 mg treatment groups, respectively. A similar increase in serum gastrin levels was noted at the 8 week visit with mean increases of 3, 26, and 84% for the three pantoprazole dose groups. Median serum gastrin levels remained within normal limits during maintenance therapy with Protonix delayed-release tablets.

In long-term international studies involving over 800 patients, a 2- to 3-fold mean increase from the pretreatment fasting serum gastrin level was observed in the initial months of treatment with pantoprazole at doses of 40 mg/day during GERD maintenance studies and 40 mg or higher per day in patients with refractory GERD. Fasting serum gastrin levels generally remained at approximately 2-3 times baseline for up to 4 years of periodic follow-up in clinical trials.

Following healing of gastric or duodenal ulcers with pantoprazole treatment, elevated gastrin levels return to normal by at least 3 months.

Enterochromaffin-Like (ECL) Cell Effects

In 39 patients treated with oral pantoprazole 40-240 mg daily (majority receiving 40-80 mg) for up to 5 years, there was a moderate increase in ECL-cell density starting after the first year of use which appeared to plateau after 4 years.

In a nonclinical study in Sprague-Dawley rats, lifetime exposure (24 months) to pantoprazole at doses of 0.5-200 mg/kg/day resulted in dose-related increases in gastric ECL-cell proliferation and gastric neuroendocrine (NE)-cell tumors. Gastric NE-cell tumors in rats may result from chronic elevation of serum gastrin concentrations. The high density of ECL cells in the rat stomach makes this species highly susceptible to the proliferative effects of elevated gastrin concentrations produced by proton pump inhibitors. However, there were no observed elevations in serum gastrin following the administration of pantoprazole at a dose of 0.5 mg/kg/day. In a separate study, a gastric NE-cell tumor without concomitant ECL-cell proliferative changes was observed in 1 female rat following 12 months of dosing with pantoprazole at 5 mg/kg/day and a 9 month off-dose recovery. (See PRECAUTIONS, Carcinogenesis, Mutagenesis, and Impairment of Fertility.)

Other Effects

No clinically relevant effects of pantoprazole on cardiovascular, respiratory, ophthalmic, or central nervous system function have been detected. In a clinical pharmacology study, pantoprazole 40 mg given once daily for 2 weeks had no effect on the levels of the following hormones: cortisol, testosterone, triiodothyronine (T3), thyroxine (T4), thyroid-stimulating hormone (TSH), thyronine-binding protein, parathyroid hormone, insulin, glucagon, renin, aldosterone, follicle-stimulating hormone, luteinizing hormone, prolactin and growth hormone.

In two 1 year studies of GERD patients treated with pantoprazole 40 or 20 mg, there were changes from baseline in overall levels of T3, T4, and TSH.

INDICATIONS AND USAGE

SHORT-TERM TREATMENT OF EROSIVE ESOPHAGITIS ASSOCIATED WITH GASTROESOPHAGEAL REFLUX DISEASE (GERD)

Protonix delayed-release tablets are indicated for the short-term treatment (up to 8 weeks) in the healing and symptomatic relief of erosive esophagitis. For those patients who have not healed after 8 weeks of treatment, an additional 8 week course of Protonix may be considered.

MAINTENANCE OF HEALING OF EROSIVE ESOPHAGITIS

Protonix delayed-release tablets are indicated for maintenance of healing of erosive esophagitis and reduction in relapse rates of daytime and nighttime heartburn symptoms in patients with GERD. Controlled studies did not extend beyond 12 months.

PATHOLOGICAL HYPERSECRETORY CONDITIONS INCLUDING ZOLLINGER-ELLISON SYNDROME

Protonix delayed-release tablets are indicated for the long-term treatment of pathological hypersecretory conditions, including Zollinger-Ellison syndrome.

CONTRAINDICATIONS

Protonix delayed-release tablets are contraindicated in patients with known hypersensitivity to any component of the formulation.

PRECAUTIONS

GENERAL

Symptomatic response to therapy with pantoprazole does not preclude the presence of gastric malignancy.

Owing to the chronic nature of erosive esophagitis, there may be a potential for prolonged administration of pantoprazole. In long-term rodent studies, pantoprazole was carcinogenic and caused rare types of gastrointestinal tumors. The relevance of these findings to tumor development in humans is unknown.

INFORMATION FOR THE PATIENT

Patients should be cautioned that Protonix delayed-release tablets should not be split, crushed or chewed. The tablets should be swallowed whole, with or without food in the stomach. Concomitant administration of antacids does not affect the absorption of pantoprazole.

CARCINOGENESIS, MUTAGENESIS, AND IMPAIRMENT OF FERTILITY

In a 24 month carcinogenicity study, Sprague-Dawley rats were treated orally with doses of 0.5-200 mg/kg/day, about 0.1-40 times the exposure on a body surface area basis, of a 50 kg person dosed at 40 mg/day. In the gastric fundus, treatment at 0.5-200 mg/kg/day produced enterochromaffin-like (ECL) cell hyperplasia and benign and malignant neuroendocrine cell tumors in a dose-related manner. In the forestomach, treatment at 50 and 200 mg/kg/day (about 10 and 40 times the recommended human dose on a body surface area basis) produced benign squamous cell papillomas and malignant squamous cell carcinomas. Rare gastrointestinal tumors associated with pantoprazole treatment included an adenocarcinoma of the duodenum at 50 mg/kg/day, and benign polyps and adenocarcinomas of the gastric fundus at 200 mg/kg/day. In the liver, treatment at 0.5-200 mg/kg/day produced dose-related increases in the incidences of hepatocellular adenomas and carcinomas. In the thyroid gland, treatment at 200 mg/kg/day produced increased incidences of follicular cell adenomas and carcinomas for both male and female rats.

Sporadic occurrences of hepatocellular adenomas and a hepatocellular carcinoma were observed in Sprague-Dawley rats exposed to pantoprazole in 6 and 12 month toxicity studies.

In a 24 month carcinogenicity study, Fischer 344 rats were treated orally with doses of 5-50 mg/kg/day, approximately 1-10 times the recommended human dose based on body surface area. In the gastric fundus, treatment at 5-50 mg/kg/day produced enterochromaffin-like (ECL) cell hyperplasia and benign and malignant neuroendocrine cell tumors. Dose selection for this study may not have been adequate to comprehensively evaluate the carcinogenic potential of pantoprazole.

In a 24 month carcinogenicity study, B6C3F1 mice were treated orally with doses of 5-150 mg/kg/day, 0.5 to 15 times the recommended human dose based on body surface area. In the liver, treatment at 150 mg/kg/day produced increased incidences of hepatocellular adenomas and carcinomas in female mice. Treatment at 5-150 mg/kg/day also produced gastric fundic ECL cell hyperplasia.

A 26 week p53 ± transgenic mouse carcinogenicity study was not positive.

Pantoprazole was positive in the *in vitro* human lymphocyte chromosomal aberration assays, in one of two mouse micronucleus tests for clastogenic effects, and in the *in vitro* Chinese hamster ovarian cell/HGPRT forward mutation assay for mutagenic effects. Equivocal results were observed in the *in vivo* rat liver DNA covalent binding assay. Pantoprazole was negative in the *in vitro* Ames mutation assay, the *in vitro* unscheduled DNA synthesis (UDS) assay with rat hepatocytes, the *in vitro* AS52/GPT mammalian cell-forward gene mutation assay, the *in vitro* thymidine kinase mutation test with mouse lymphoma L5178Y cells, and the *in vivo* rat bone marrow cell chromosomal aberration assay.

Pantoprazole at oral doses up to 500 mg/kg/day in male rats (98 times the recommended human dose based on body surface area) and 450 mg/kg/day in female rats (88 times the recommended human dose based on body surface area) was found to have no effect on fertility and reproductive performance.

PREGNANCY, TERATOGENIC EFFECTS, PREGNANCY CATEGORY B

Teratology studies have been performed in rats at oral doses up to 450 mg/kg/day (88 times the recommended human dose based on body surface area) and rabbits at oral doses up to 40 mg/kg/day (16 times the recommended human dose based on body surface area) and have revealed no evidence of impaired fertility or harm to the fetus due to pantoprazole. There are, however, no adequate and well-controlled studies in pregnant women. Because animal reproduction studies are not always predictive of human response, this drug should be used during pregnancy only if clearly needed.

NURSING MOTHERS

Pantoprazole and its metabolites are excreted in the milk of rats. It is not known whether pantoprazole is excreted in human milk. Many drugs which are excreted in human milk have a potential for serious adverse reactions in nursing infants. Based on the potential for tumorigenicity shown for pantoprazole in rodent carcinogenicity studies, a decision should be made whether to discontinue nursing or to discontinue the drug, taking into account the benefit of the drug to the mother.

PEDIATRIC USE

Safety and effectiveness in pediatric patients have not been established.

USE IN WOMEN

Erosive esophagitis healing rates in the 221 women treated with Protonix delayed-release tablets in US clinical trials were similar to those found in men. In the 122 women treated long-term with Protonix 40 or 20 mg, healing was maintained at a rate similar to that in men. The incidence rates of adverse events were also similar for men and women.

LABORATORY TESTS

There have been reports of false-positive urine screening tests for tetrahydrocannabinol (THC) in patients receiving pantoprazole.

GERIATRIC USE

In short-term US clinical trials, erosive esophagitis healing rates in the 107 elderly patients (≥65 years old) treated with Protonix were similar to those found in patients under the age of 65. The incidence rates of adverse events and laboratory abnormalities in patients aged 65 years and older were similar to those associated with patients younger than 65 years of age.

DRUG INTERACTIONS

Pantoprazole is metabolized through the cytochrome P450 system, primarily the CYP2C19 and CYP3A4 isozymes, and subsequently undergoes Phase II conjugation. Based on studies evaluating possible interactions of pantoprazole with other drugs, no dosage adjustment is needed with concomitant use of the following: theophylline, cisapride, antipyrine, caffeine, carbamazepine, diazepam, diclofenac, digoxin, ethanol, glyburide, an oral contraceptive (levonorgestrel/ethinyl estradiol), metoprolol, nifedipine, phenytoin, warfarin, midazolam, clarithromycin, metronidazole, or amoxicillin. Clinically relevant interactions of pantoprazole with other drugs with the same metabolic pathways are not expected. Therefore, when coadministered with pantoprazole, adjustment of the dosage of pantoprazole or of such drugs may not be necessary. There was also no interaction with concomitantly administered antacids.

Because of profound and long lasting inhibition of gastric acid secretion, pantoprazole may interfere with absorption of drugs where gastric pH is an important determinant of their bioavailability (*e.g.*, ketoconazole, ampicillin esters, and iron salts).

ADVERSE REACTIONS

Worldwide, more than 11,100 patients have been treated with pantoprazole in clinical trials involving various dosages and duration of treatment. In general, pantoprazole has been well tolerated in both short-term and long-term trials.

In two US controlled clinical trials involving Protonix 10, 20, or 40 mg doses for up to 8 weeks, there were no dose-related effects on the incidence of adverse events. The following adverse events considered by investigators to be possibly, probably or definitely related to drug occurred in 1% or more in the individual studies of GERD patients on therapy with Protonix (see TABLE 8).

TABLE 8 *Most Frequent Adverse Events Reported as Drug Related in Short-Term Domestic Trials*

	Study 300 — US		Study 301 — US	
	Protonix	Placebo	Protonix	Nizatidine
Study Event	(n=521)	(n=82)	(n=161)	(n=82)
Headache	6%	6%	9%	13%
Diarrhea	4%	1%	6%	6%
Flatulence	2%	2%	4%	0%
Abdominal pain	1%	2%	4%	4%
Rash	<1%	0%	2%	0%
Eructation	1%	1%	0%	0%
Insomnia	<1%	2%	1%	1%
Hyperglycemia	1%	0%	<1%	0%

Note: Only adverse events with an incidence greater than or equal to the comparators are shown.

In international short-term double-blind or open-label, clinical trials involving 20-80 mg/day, the following adverse events were reported to occur in 1% or more of 2805 GERD patients receiving pantoprazole for up to 8 weeks. (See TABLE 9.)

TABLE 9 *Adverse Events in GERD Patients in Short-Term International Trials*

	Pantoprazole	Ranitidine	Omeprazole	Famotidine
	Total	300 mg	20 mg	40 mg
Study Event	(n=2805)	(n=594)	(n=474)	(n=239)
Headache	2%	3%	2%	1%
Diarrhea	2%	2%	2%	<1%
Abdominal pain	1%	1%	<1%	<1%

In two US controlled clinical trials involving Protonix 10, 20, or 40 mg doses for up to 12 months, the following adverse events considered by investigators to be possibly, probably or definitely related to drug occurred in 1% or more of GERD patients on long-term therapy. (See TABLE 10.)

TABLE 10 *Most Frequent Adverse Events Reported as Drug Related in Long-Term Domestic Trials*

	Protonix	Ranitidine
Study Event	(n=536)	(n=185)
Headache	5%	2%
Abdominal pain	3%	1%
Liver function tests abnormal	2%	<1%
Nausea	2%	2%
Vomiting	2%	2%

Note: Only adverse events with an incidence greater than or equal to the comparators are shown.

In addition, in these short- and long-term domestic and international trials, the following treatment-emergent events, regardless of causality, occurred at a rate of ≥1% in pantoprazole-treated patients: anxiety, arthralgia, asthenia, back pain, bronchitis, chest pain, constipation, cough increased, dizziness, dyspepsia, dyspnea, flu syndrome, gastroenteritis, gastrointestinal disorder, hyperlipemia, hypertonia, infection, liver function tests abnormal, migraine, nausea, neck pain, pain, pharyngitis, rectal disorder, rhinitis, SGPT increased, sinusitis, upper respiratory tract infection, urinary frequency, urinary tract infection, and vomiting.

Additional treatment-emergent adverse experiences occurring in <1% of pantoprazole-treated patients from these trials are listed below by body system. In most instances the relationship to pantoprazole was unclear.

Body as a Whole: Abscess, allergic reaction, chills, cyst, face edema, fever, generalized edema, heat stroke, hernia, laboratory test abnormal, malaise, moniliasis, neoplasm, non-specified drug reaction, photosensitivity reaction.

Cardiovascular System: Abnormal electrocardiogram, angina pectoris, arrhythmia, atrial fibrillation/flutter, cardiovascular disorder, chest pain substernal, congestive heart failure, hemorrhage, hypertension, hypotension, myocardial infarction, myocardial ischemia, palpitation, retinal vascular disorder, syncope, tachycardia, thrombophlebitis, thrombosis, vasodilatation.

Digestive System: Anorexia, aphthous stomatitis, cardiospasm, colitis, dry mouth, duodenitis, dysphagia, enteritis, esophageal hemorrhage, esophagitis, gastrointestinal carcinoma, gastrointestinal hemorrhage, gastrointestinal moniliasis, gingivitis, glossitis, halitosis, hematemesis, increased appetite, melena, mouth ulceration, oral moniliasis, periodontal abscess, periodontitis, rectal hemorrhage, stomach ulcer, stomatitis, stools abnormal, tongue discoloration, ulcerative colitis.

Endocrine System: Diabetes mellitus, glycosuria, goiter.

Hepato-Biliary System: Biliary pain, hyperbilirubinemia, cholecystitis, cholelithiasis, cholestatic jaundice, hepatitis, alkaline phosphatase increased, gamma glutamyl transpeptidase increased, SGOT increased.

Hemic and Lymphatic System: Anemia, ecchymosis, eosinophilia, hypochromic anemia, iron deficiency anemia, leukocytosis, leukopenia, thrombocytopenia.

Metabolic and Nutritional: Dehydration, edema, gout, peripheral edema, thirst, weight gain, weight loss.

Musculoskeletal System: Arthritis, arthrosis, bone disorder, bone pain, bursitis, joint disorder, leg cramps, neck rigidity, myalgia, tenosynovitis.

Nervous System: Abnormal dreams, confusion, convulsion, depression, dry mouth, dysarthria, emotional lability, hallucinations, hyperkinesia, hypesthesia, libido decreased, nervousness, neuralgia, neuritis, neuropathy, paresthesia, reflexes decreased, sleep disorder, somnolence, thinking abnormal, tremor, vertigo.

Respiratory System: Asthma, epistaxis, hiccup, laryngitis, lung disorder, pneumonia, voice alteration.

Skin and Appendages: Acne, alopecia, contact dermatitis, dry skin, eczema, fungal dermatitis, hemorrhage, herpes simplex, herpes zoster, lichenoid dermatitis, maculopapular rash , pruritus, skin disorder, skin ulcer, sweating, urticaria.

Special Senses: Abnormal vision, amblyopia, cataract specified, deafness, diplopia, ear pain, extraocular palsy, glaucoma, otitis externa, taste perversion, tinnitus.

Urogenital System: Albuminuria, balanitis, breast pain, cystitis, dysmenorrhea, dysuria, epididymitis, hematuria, impotence, kidney calculus, kidney pain, nocturia, prostatic disorder, pyelonephritis, scrotal edema, urethral pain, urethritis, urinary tract disorder, urination impaired, vaginitis.

In an open-label US clinical trial conducted in 35 patients with pathological hypersecretory conditions treated with Protonix for up to 27 months, the adverse events reported were consistent with the safety profile of the drug in other populations.

POSTMARKETING REPORTS

There have been spontaneous reports of adverse events with the postmarketing use of pantoprazole. These reports include anaphylaxis (including anaphylactic shock); angioedema (Quincke's edema); anterior ischemic optic neuropathy; severe dermatological reactions, including erythema multiforme, Stevens-Johnson syndrome, and toxic epidermal necrolysis (TEN, some fatal); hepatocellular damage leading to jaundice and hepatic failure; pancreatitis; pancytopenia; and rhabdomyolysis. In addition, also observed have been confusion, hypokinesia, speech disorder, increased salivation, vertigo, nausea, tinnitus, and blurred vision.

LABORATORY VALUES

In two US controlled, short-term trials in patients with erosive esophagitis associated with GERD, 0.4 % of the patients on Protonix 40 mg experienced SGPT elevations of greater than 3 times the upper limit of normal at the final treatment visit. In two US controlled, long-term trials in patients with erosive esophagitis associated with GERD, none of 178 patients (0%) on Protonix 40 mg and 2 of 181 patients (1.1%) on Protonix 20 mg, experienced significant transaminase elevations at 12 months (or earlier if a patient discontinued prematurely). Significant elevations of SGOT or SGPT were defined as values at least 3 times the upper limit of normal that were non-sporadic and had no clear alternative explanation. The following changes in laboratory parameters were reported as adverse events: creatinine increased, hypercholesterolemia, and hyperuricemia.

DOSAGE AND ADMINISTRATION

TREATMENT OF EROSIVE ESOPHAGITIS

The recommended adult oral dose is 40 mg given once daily for up to 8 weeks. For those patients who have not healed after 8 weeks of treatment, an additional 8 week course of Protonix may be considered. (See INDICATIONS AND USAGE.)

MAINTENANCE OF HEALING OF EROSIVE ESOPHAGITIS

The recommended adult oral dose is one Protonix 40 mg delayed-release tablet, taken daily.

PATHOLOGICAL HYPERSECRETORY CONDITIONS INCLUDING ZOLLINGER-ELLISON SYNDROME

The dosage of Protonix in patients with pathological hypersecretory conditions varies with the individual patient. The recommended adult starting dose is 40 mg twice daily. Dosage regimens should be adjusted to individual patient needs and should continue for as long as clinically indicated. Doses up to 240 mg daily have been administered. Some patients have been treated continuously with Protonix for more than 2 years.

No dosage adjustment is necessary in patients with renal impairment, hepatic impairment or for elderly patients. No dosage adjustment is necessary in patients undergoing hemodialysis.

Protonix delayed-release tablets should be swallowed whole, with or without food in the stomach. If patients are unable to swallow a 40 mg tablet, two 20 mg tablets may be taken. Concomitant administration of antacids does not affect the absorption of Protonix.

Patients should be cautioned that Protonix delayed-release tablets should not be split, chewed or crushed.

HOW SUPPLIED

Protonix delayed-release tablets are supplied as 40 mg yellow oval biconvex delayed-release tablets imprinted with "PROTONIX" (brown ink) on one side.

Protonix is supplied as 20 mg yellow oval biconvex delayed-release tablets imprinted with "P20" (brown ink) on one side.

Storage: Store Protonix delayed-release tablets at 20-25°C (68-77°F); excursions permitted to 15-30°C (59-86°F).

PRODUCT LISTING - EQUIVALENTS NOT AVAILABLE

Powder For Injection - Intravenous - 40 mg

25's $687.50 PROTONIX IV, Wyeth-Ayerst Laboratories 00008-0923-03

Tablet, Enteric Coated - Oral - 20 mg
90's $326.25 PROTONIX, Wyeth-Ayerst Laboratories 00008-0843-81
Tablet, Enteric Coated - Oral - 40 mg
90's $326.25 PROTONIX, Wyeth-Ayerst Laboratories 00008-0841-81
100's $362.50 PROTONIX, Wyeth-Ayerst Laboratories 00008-0841-99

Paricalcitol (003390)

Categories: Hyperparathyroidism, secondary to renal failure; FDA Approved 1998 Apr; Pregnancy Category C
Drug Classes: Vitamins/minerals
Brand Names: Zemplar

DESCRIPTION

Zemplar is a synthetically manufactured vitamin D analog. It is available as a sterile, clear, colorless, aqueous solution for intravenous injection. Each ml contains paricalcitol, 5 μg; propylene glycol, 30% (v/v); and alcohol, 20% (v/v).

Paricalcitol is a white powder chemically designated as 19-nor-1α,3β,25-trihydroxy-9,10-secoergosta-5(Z),7(E),22(E)-triene.

The molecular formula is $C_{27}H_{44}O_3$ and the molecular weight is 416.65.

CLINICAL PHARMACOLOGY

MECHANISM OF ACTION

Paricalcitol is a synthetic vitamin D analog. Vitamin D and paricalcitol have been shown to reduce parathyroid hormone (PTH) levels.

PHARMACOKINETICS

Distribution

The pharmacokinetics of paricalcitol have been studied in patients with chronic renal failure (CRF) requiring hemodialysis. Paricalcitol is administered as an intravenous bolus injection. Within 2 hours after administering doses ranging from 0.04-0.24 μg/kg, concentrations of paricalcitol decreased rapidly; thereafter, concentrations of paricalcitol declined log-linearly with a mean half-life of about 15 hours. No accumulation of paricalcitol was observed with multiple dosing.

Elimination

In healthy subjects, plasma radioactivity after a single 0.16 μg/kg intravenous bolus dose of ^{3}H-paricalcitol (n=4) was attributed to parent drug. Paricalcitol was eliminated primarily by hepatobiliary excretion, as 74% of the radioactive dose was recovered in feces and only 16% was found in urine.

Metabolism

Several unknown metabolites were detected in both the urine and feces, with no detectable paricalcitol in the urine. These metabolites have not been characterized and have not been identified. Together, these metabolites contributed 51% of the urinary radioactivity and 59% of the fecal radioactivity. *In vitro* plasma protein binding of paricalcitol was extensive (>99.9%) and nonsaturable over the concentration range of 1-100 ng/ml.

TABLE 1 *Paricalcitol Pharmacokinetic Characteristics in CRF Patients (0.24 μg/kg dose)*

Parameter		Values (Mean ±SD)
C_{max} (5 min. after bolus)	n=6	1850 ± 664 (pg/ml)
AUC(0-∞)	n=5	27382 ± 8230 (pg·h/ml)
CL	n=5	0.72 ± 0.24 (L/h)
Vss	n=5	6 ± 2 (L)

Laboratory Tests

In placebo-controlled studies, paricalcitol reduced serum total alkaline phosphatase levels.

SPECIAL POPULATIONS

Paricalcitol pharmacokinetics have not been investigated in special populations (geriatric, pediatric, hepatic insufficiency) or for drug-drug interactions. Pharmacokinetics were not gender-dependent.

INDICATIONS AND USAGE

Paricalcitol is indicated for the prevention and treatment of secondary hyperparathyroidism associated with chronic renal failure. Studies in patients with chronic renal failure show that paricalcitol suppresses PTH levels with no significant difference in the incidence of hypercalcemia or hyperphosphatemia when compared to placebo. However, the serum phosphorus, calcium and calcium × phosphorus product (Ca × P) may increase when paricalcitol is administered.

CONTRAINDICATIONS

Paricalcitol should not be given to patients with evidence of vitamin D toxicity, hypercalcemia, or hypersensitivity to any ingredient in this product (see PRECAUTIONS, General).

WARNINGS

Acute overdose of paricalcitol may cause hypercalcemia, and require emergency attention. During dose adjustment, serum calcium and phosphorus levels should be monitored closely (*e.g.*, twice weekly). If clinically significant hypercalcemia develops, the dose should be reduced or interrupted. Chronic administration of paricalcitol may place patients at risk of hypercalcemia, elevated Ca × P product, and metastatic calcification.

Signs and symptoms of vitamin D intoxication associated with hypercalcemia include:

Early: Weakness, headache, somnolence, nausea, vomiting, dry mouth, constipation, muscle pain, bone pain, and metallic taste.

Late: Anorexia, weight loss, conjunctivitis (calcific), pancreatitis, photophobia, rhinorrhea, pruritus, hyperthermia, decreased libido, elevated BUN, hypercholesterolemia, elevated AST and ALT, ectopic calcification, hypertension, cardiac arrhythmias, somnolence, death, and, rarely, overt psychosis.

Treatment of patients with clinically significant hypercalcemia consists of immediate dose reduction interruption of paricalcitol therapy and includes a low calcium diet, withdrawal of calcium supplements, patient mobilization, attention to fluid and electrolyte imbalances, assessment of electrocardiographic abnormalities (critical in patient receiving digitalis), and hemodialysis or peritoneal dialysis against a calcium-free dialysate, as warranted. Serum calcium levels should be monitored frequently until normocalcemia ensues.

Phosphate or vitamin D-related compounds should not be taken concomitantly with paricalcitol.

PRECAUTIONS

GENERAL

Digitalis toxicity is potentiated by hypercalcemia of any cause, so caution should be applied when digitalis compounds are prescribed concomitantly with paricalcitol. Adynamic bone lesions may develop if PTH levels are suppressed to abnormal levels.

INFORMATION FOR THE PATIENT

The patient should be instructed that, to ensure effectiveness of paricalcitol therapy, it is important to adhere to a dietary regimen of calcium supplementation and phosphorus restriction. Appropriate types of phosphate-binding compounds may be needed to control serum phosphorus levels in patients with chronic renal failure (CRF), but excessive use of aluminum containing compounds should be avoided. Patients should also be carefully informed about the symptoms of elevated calcium.

ESSENTIAL LABORATORY TESTS

During the initial phase of medication, serum calcium and phosphorus should be determined frequently (*e.g.*, twice weekly). Once dosage has been established, serum calcium and phosphorus should be measured at least monthly. Measurements of serum or plasma PTH are recommended every 3 months. An intact PTH (iPTH) assay is recommended for reliable detection of biologically active PTH in patients with CRF. During dose adjustment of paricalcitol, laboratory tests may be required more frequently.

CARCINOGENESIS, MUTAGENESIS, AND IMPAIRMENT OF FERTILITY

Longterm studies in animals to evaluate the carcinogenic potential of paricalcitol have not been completed. Paricalcitol did not exhibit genetic toxicity *in vitro* with or without metabolic activation in the microbial mutagenesis assay (Ames Assay), mouse lymphoma mutagenesis assay (L5178Y), or a human lymphocyte cell chromosomal aberration assay. There was also no evidence of genetic toxicity in an *in vivo* mouse micronucleus assay. Paricalcitol had no effect on fertility (male or female) in rats at intravenous doses up to 20 μg/kg/dose [equivalent to 13 times the highest recommended human dose (0.24 μg/kg) based on surface area, mg/m^2].

PREGNANCY CATEGORY C

Paricalcitol has been shown to cause minimal decreases in fetal viability (5%) when administered daily to rabbits at a dose 0.5 times the 0.24 μg/kg human dose (based on surface area, mg/m^2) and when administered to rats at a dose 2 times the 0.24 μg/kg human dose (based on plasma levels of exposure). At the highest dose tested (20 μg/kg 3 times per week in rats, 13 times the 0.24 μg/kg human dose based on surface area), there was a significant increase of the mortality of newborn rats at doses that were maternally toxic (hypercalcemia). No other effects on offspring development were observed. Paricalcitol was not teratogenic at the doses tested.

There are no adequate and well-controlled studies in pregnant women. Paricalcitol should be used during pregnancy only if the potential benefit justifies the potential risk to the fetus.

NURSING MOTHERS

It is not known whether paricalcitol is excreted in human milk. Because many drugs are excreted in human milk, caution should be exercised when paricalcitol is administered to a nursing woman.

PEDIATRIC USE

Safety and efficacy of paricalcitol in pediatric patients have not been established.

GERIATRIC USE

Of the 40 patients receiving paricalcitol in the three Phase 3 placebo-controlled CRF studies, 10 patients were 65 years or over. In these studies, no overall differences in efficacy or safety were observed between patients 65 years or older and younger patients.

DRUG INTERACTIONS

Specific interaction studies were not performed. Digitalis toxicity is potentiated by hypercalcemia of any cause, so caution should be applied when digitalis compounds are prescribed concomitantly with paricalcitol.

ADVERSE REACTIONS

Paricalcitol has been evaluated for safety in clinical studies in 454 CRF patients.

In four, placebo-controlled, double-blind, multicenter studies, discontinuation of therapy due to any adverse event occurred in 6.5% of 62 patients treated with paricalcitol and 2.0% of 51 patients treated with placebo for 1-3 months. Adverse events occurring with greater frequency in the paricalcitol group at a frequency of 2% or greater, regardless of causality, are presented in TABLE 3.

A patient who reported the same medical term more than once was counted only once for that medical term.

Safety parameters (changes in mean Ca, P, Ca × P) in an open-label safety study up to 13 months in duration support the long-term safety of paricalcitol in this patient population.

P

TABLE 3 *Adverse Event Incidence Rates for All Treated Patients in All Placebo-Controlled Studies*

Adverse Event	Paricalcitol (n=62)	Placebo (n=51)
Overall	71%	78%
Body as a Whole		
Chills	5%	0%
Feeling unwell	3%	0%
Fever	5%	2%
Flu	5%	4%
Sepsis	5%	2%
Cardiovascular System		
Palpitation	3%	0%
Digestive System		
Dry mouth	3%	2%
Gastrointestinal bleeding	5%	2%
Nausea	13%	8%
Vomiting	8%	4%
Metabolic and Nutritional Disorders		
Edema	7%	0%
Nervous System		
Light-headedness	5%	2%
Respiratory System		
Pneumonia	5%	0%

DOSAGE AND ADMINISTRATION

The currently accepted target range for iPTH levels in CRF patients is no more than 1.5 to 3 times the non-uremic upper limit of normal.

The recommended initial dose of paricalcitol is 0.04 μg/kg to 0.1 μg/kg (2.8-7 μg) administered as a bolus dose no more frequently than every other day at any time during dialysis. Doses as high as 0.24 μg/kg (16.8 μg) have been safely administered.

If a satisfactory response is not observed, the dose may be increased by 2-4 μg at 2-4 week intervals. During any dose adjustment period, serum calcium and phosphorus levels should be monitored more frequently, and if an elevated calcium level or a Ca × P product greater than 75 is noted, the drug dosage should be immediately reduced or interrupted until these parameters are normalized. Then, paricalcitol should be reinitiated at a lower dose. Doses may need to be decreased as the PTH levels decrease in response to therapy. Thus, incremental dosing must be individualized.

TABLE 4 is a suggested approach in dose titration.

TABLE 4 *Suggested Dosing Guidelines*

PTH Level	Paricalcitol Dose
The same or increasing	Increase
Decreasing by <30%	Increase
Decreasing by >30%, <60%	Maintain
Decreasing by >60%	Decrease
1½ to 3 to three times upper limit of normal	Maintain

Parenteral drug products should be inspected visually for particulate matter and discoloration prior to administration whenever solution and container permit.

Discard unused portion.

HOW SUPPLIED

Zemplar 5 μg/ml is supplied as 1 and 2 ml single-dose Fliptop vials.

Storage: Store at 25°C (77°F). Excursions permitted to 15-30°C (59-86°F).

PRODUCT LISTING - RATED THERAPEUTICALLY EQUIVALENT

Solution - Intravenous - 5 mcg/ml

1 ml x 100	$721.00	ZEMPLAR, Abbott Pharmaceutical	00074-1658-01
2 ml x 100	$5282.76	ZEMPLAR, Abbott Pharmaceutical	00074-1658-02

PRODUCT LISTING - EQUIVALENTS NOT AVAILABLE

Solution - Intravenous - 2 mcg/ml

1 ml x 100	$1056.88	ZEMPLAR, Abbott Pharmaceutical	00074-4637-01

Paroxetine Hydrochloride *(003130)*

For related information, see the comparative table section in Appendix A.

Categories: Anxiety disorder, generalized; Anxiety disorder, social; Depression; Obsessive compulsive disorder; Panic disorder; Posttraumatic stress disorder; Pregnancy Category C; FDA Approved 1992 Dec

Drug Classes: Antidepressants, serotonin specific reuptake inhibitors

Brand Names: Paxil; Seroxat

Foreign Brand Availability: Aropax 20 (Australia; Mexico; New-Zealand; South-Africa); Deroxat (France); Paroxet (Peru); Paxan (Colombia); Paxtine (Australia); Paxxet (Israel); Tagonis (Germany); XET (India)

Cost of Therapy: $81.45 (Depression; Paxil; 20 mg; 1 tablet/day; 30 day supply)
$79.40 (Obsessive-Compulsive Disorder; Paxil; 40 mg; 1 tablet/day; 30 day supply)

DESCRIPTION

Note: The trade names have been used throughout this monograph for clarity.

PAXIL

Paxil (paroxetine hydrochloride) is an orally administered psychotropic drug. It is the hydrochloride salt of a phenylpiperidine compound identified chemically as (-)-*trans-4R*-(4′-fluorophenyl)-3*S*-[(3′,4′-methylenedioxyphenoxy)methyl] piperidine hydrochloride hemihydrate and has the empirical formula of $C_{19}H_{20}FNO_3 \cdot HCl \cdot ½H_2O$. The molecular weight is 374.8 (329.4 as free base).

Paroxetine hydrochloride is an odorless, off-white powder, having a melting point range of 120-138°C and a solubility of 5.4 mg/ml in water.

Tablets

Each film-coated tablet contains paroxetine hydrochloride equivalent to paroxetine as follows: *10 mg:* Yellow (scored); *20 mg:* Pink (scored); *30 mg:* Blue; *40 mg:* Green. Inactive ingredients consist of dibasic calcium phosphate dihydrate, hypromellulose, magnesium stearate, polyethylene glycols, polysorbate 80, sodium starch glycolate, titanium dioxide and one or more of the following: D&C red no. 30, D&C yellow no. 10, FD&C blue no. 2, FD&C yellow no. 6.

Suspension for Oral Administration

Each 5 ml of orange-colored, orange-flavored liquid contains paroxetine hydrochloride equivalent to paroxetine, 10 mg. Inactive ingredients consist of polacrilin potassium, microcrystalline cellulose, propylene glycol, glycerin, sorbitol, methyl paraben, propyl paraben, sodium citrate dihydrate, citric acid anhydrate, sodium saccharin, flavorings, FD&C yellow no. 6 and simethicone emulsion.

PAXIL CR

Paxil CR is an orally administered psychotropic drug with a chemical structure unrelated to other selective serotonin reuptake inhibitors or to tricyclic, tetracyclic or other available antidepressant or antipanic agents. It is the hydrochloride salt of a phenylpiperidine compound identified chemically as (-)-trans-4R-(4′-fluorophenyl)-3S-[(3′,4′-methylenedioxyphenoxy)methyl]piperidine hydrochloride hemihydrate and has the empirical formula of $C_{19}H_{20}FNO_3 \cdot HCl \cdot ½H_2O$. The molecular weight is 374.8 (329.4 as free base).

Paroxetine HCl is an odorless, off-white powder, having a melting point range of 120-138°C and a solubility of 5.4 mg/ml in water.

Each enteric, film-coated, controlled-release tablet contains paroxetine hydrochloride equivalent to paroxetine as follows: *12.5 mg:* Yellow; *25 mg:* Pink; *37.5 mg:* Blue. One layer of the tablet consists of a degradable barrier layer and the other contains the active material in a hydrophilic matrix.

Inactive ingredients consist of hydroxypropyl methylcellulose, polyvinylpyrrolidone, lactose monohydrate, magnesium stearate, colloidal silicon dioxide, glyceryl behenate, methacrylic acid copolymer type C, sodium lauryl sulfate, polysorbate 80, talc, triethyl citrate, and one or more of the following colorants: yellow ferric oxide, red ferric oxide, D&C red no. 30, D&C yellow no. 6, D&C yellow no. 10, FD&C blue no. 2.

CLINICAL PHARMACOLOGY

PAXIL

Pharmacodynamics

The efficacy of paroxetine in the treatment of major depressive disorder, social anxiety disorder, obsessive compulsive disorder (OCD), panic disorder (PD), generalized anxiety disorder (GAD) and posttraumatic stress disorder (PTSD) is presumed to be linked to potentiation of serotonergic activity in the central nervous system resulting from inhibition of neuronal reuptake of serotonin (5-hydroxy-tryptamine, 5-HT). Studies at clinically relevant doses in humans have demonstrated that paroxetine blocks the uptake of serotonin into human platelets. *In vitro* studies in animals also suggest that paroxetine is a potent and highly selective inhibitor of neuronal serotonin reuptake and has only very weak effects on norepinephrine and dopamine neuronal reuptake. *In vitro* radioligand binding studies indicate that paroxetine has little affinity for muscarinic, alpha$_1$-, alpha$_2$-, beta-adrenergic-, dopamine (D_2)-, 5-HT_1-, 5-HT_2- and histamine (H_1)-receptors; antagonism of muscarinic, histaminergic and alpha$_1$-adrenergic receptors has been associated with various anticholinergic, sedative and cardiovascular effects for other psychotropic drugs.

Because the relative potencies of paroxetine's major metabolites are at most 1/50 of the parent compound, they are essentially inactive.

Pharmacokinetics

Paroxetine is equally bioavailable from oral suspension and tablet.

Paroxetine hydrochloride is completely absorbed after oral dosing of a solution of the hydrochloride salt. In a study in which normal male subjects (n=15) received 30 mg tablets daily for 30 days, steady-state paroxetine concentrations were achieved by approximately 10 days for most subjects, although it may take substantially longer in an occasional patient. At steady-state, mean values of C_{max}, T_{max}, C_{min} and $T_{½}$ were 61.7 ng/ml (CV 45%), 5.2 hours (CV 10%), 30.7 ng/ml (CV 67%) and 21.0 hours (CV 32%), respectively. The steady-state C_{max} and C_{min} values were about 6 and 14 times what would be predicted from single-dose studies. Steady-state drug exposure based on AUC(0-24) was about 8 times greater than would have been predicted from single-dose data in these subjects. The excess accumulation is a consequence of the fact that one of the enzymes that metabolizes paroxetine is readily saturable.

In steady-state dose proportionality studies involving elderly and nonelderly patients, at doses of 20-40 mg daily for the elderly and 20-50 mg daily for the nonelderly, some nonlinearity was observed in both populations, again reflecting a saturable metabolic pathway. In comparison to C_{min} values after 20 mg daily, values after 40 mg daily were only about 2-3 times greater than doubled.

The effects of food on the bioavailability of paroxetine were studied in subjects administered a single-dose with and without food. AUC was only slightly increased (6%) when drug was administered with food but the C_{max} was 29% greater, while the time to reach peak plasma concentration decreased from 6.4 hours post-dosing to 4.9 hours.

Paroxetine is extensively metabolized after oral administration. The principal metabolites are polar and conjugated products of oxidation and methylation, which are readily cleared. Conjugates with glucuronic acid and sulfate predominate, and major metabolites have been isolated and identified. Data indicate that the metabolites have no more than 1/50 the potency of the parent compound at inhibiting serotonin uptake. The metabolism of paroxetine is accomplished in part by cytochrome P450 2D6. Saturation of this enzyme at clinical doses appears to account for the nonlinearity of paroxetine kinetics with increasing dose and increasing duration of treatment. The role of this enzyme in paroxetine metabolism also suggests potential drug-drug interactions (see PRECAUTIONS, Paxil).

Approximately 64% of a 30 mg oral solution dose of paroxetine was excreted in the urine with 2% as the parent compound and 62% as metabolites over a 10 day post-dosing period. About 36% was excreted in the feces (probably via the bile), mostly as metabolites and less than 1% as the parent compound over the 10 day post-dosing period.

Distribution

Paroxetine distributes throughout the body, including the CNS, with only 1% remaining in the plasma.

Protein Binding

Approximately 95% and 93% of paroxetine is bound to plasma protein at 100 ng/ml and 400 ng/ml, respectively. Under clinical conditions, paroxetine concentrations would normally be less than 400 ng/ml. Paroxetine does not alter the *in vitro* protein binding of phenytoin or warfarin.

Renal and Liver Disease

Increased plasma concentrations of paroxetine occur in subjects with renal and hepatic impairment. The mean plasma concentrations in patients with creatinine clearance below 30 ml/min was approximately 4 times greater than seen in normal volunteers. Patients with creatinine clearance of 30-60 ml/min and patients with hepatic functional impairment had about a 2-fold increase in plasma concentrations (AUC, C_{max}).

The initial dosage should therefore be reduced in patients with severe renal or hepatic impairment, and upward titration, if necessary, should be at increased intervals (see DOSAGE AND ADMINISTRATION, Paxil).

Elderly Patients

In a multiple-dose study in the elderly at daily paroxetine doses of 20, 30 and 40 mg, C_{min} concentrations were about 70-80% greater than the respective C_{min} concentrations in nonelderly subjects. Therefore the initial dosage in the elderly should be reduced (see DOSAGE AND ADMINISTRATION, Paxil).

PAXIL CR

Pharmacodynamics

The efficacy of paroxetine in the treatment of major depressive disorder and panic disorder is presumed to be linked to potentiation of serotonergic activity in the central nervous system resulting from inhibition of neuronal reuptake of serotonin (5-hydroxy-tryptamine, 5-HT). Studies at clinically relevant doses in humans have demonstrated that paroxetine blocks the uptake of serotonin into human platelets. *In vitro* studies in animals also suggest that paroxetine is a potent and highly selective inhibitor of neuronal serotonin reuptake and has only very weak effects on norepinephrine and dopamine neuronal reuptake. *In vitro* radioligand binding studies indicate that paroxetine has little affinity for muscarinic, alpha$_1$-, alpha$_2$-, beta-adrenergic-, dopamine (D_2)-, 5-HT$_1$-, 5-HT$_2$- and histamine (H_1)-receptors; antagonism of muscarinic, histaminergic and alpha$_1$-adrenergic receptors has been associated with various anticholinergic, sedative and cardiovascular effects for other psychotropic drugs.

Because the relative potencies of paroxetine's major metabolites are at most 1/50 of the parent compound, they are essentially inactive.

Pharmacokinetics

Paxil CR tablets contain a degradable polymeric matrix designed to control the dissolution rate of paroxetine over a period of approximately 4-5 hours. In addition to controlling the rate of drug release *in vivo,* an enteric coat delays the start of drug release until Paxil CR tablets have left the stomach.

Paroxetine HCl is completely absorbed after oral dosing of a solution of the hydrochloride salt. In a study in which normal male and female subjects (n=23) received single oral doses of Paxil CR at four dosage strengths (12.5 mg, 25 mg, 37.5 mg and 50 mg), paroxetine C_{max} and AUC(0-∞) increased disproportionately with dose (as seen also with immediate-release formulations). Mean C_{max} and AUC(0-∞) values at these doses were 2.0, 5.5, 9.0, and 12.5 ng/ml, and 121, 261, 338, and 540 ng·h/ml, respectively. T_{max} was observed typically between 6 and 10 hours post-dose, reflecting a reduction in absorption rate compared with immediate-release formulations. The mean elimination half-life of paroxetine was 15-20 hours throughout this range of single Paxil CR doses. The bioavailability of 25 mg Paxil CR is not affected by food.

During repeated administration of Paxil CR (25 mg once daily), steady-state was reached within 2 weeks (*i.e.,* comparable to immediate-release formulations). In a repeat-dose study in which normal male and female subjects (n=23) received Paxil CR (25 mg daily), mean steady-state C_{max}, C_{min} and AUC(0-24) values were 30 ng/ml, 20 ng/ml and 550 ng·h/ml, respectively.

Based on studies using immediate-release formulations, steady-state drug exposure based on AUC(0-24) was several-fold greater than would have been predicted from single-dose data. The excess accumulation is a consequence of the fact that one of the enzymes that metabolizes paroxetine is readily saturable.

In steady-state dose proportionality studies involving elderly and nonelderly patients, at doses of the immediate-release formulation of 20-40 mg daily for the elderly and 20-50 mg daily for the nonelderly, some nonlinearity was observed in both populations, again reflecting a saturable metabolic pathway. In comparison to C_{min} values after 20 mg daily, values after 40 mg daily were only about 2-3 times greater than doubled.

Paroxetine is extensively metabolized after oral administration. The principal metabolites are polar and conjugated products of oxidation and methylation, which are readily cleared. Conjugates with glucuronic acid and sulfate predominate, and major metabolites have been isolated and identified. Data indicate that the metabolites have no more than 1/50 the potency of the parent compound at inhibiting serotonin uptake. The metabolism of paroxetine is accomplished in part by cytochrome P450 2D6. Saturation of this enzyme at clinical doses appears to account for the nonlinearity of paroxetine kinetics with increasing dose and increasing duration of treatment. The role of this enzyme in paroxetine metabolism also suggests potential drug-drug interactions (see PRECAUTIONS, Paxil CR).

Approximately 64% of a 30 mg oral solution dose of paroxetine was excreted in the urine with 2% as the parent compound and 62% as metabolites over a 10 day post-dosing period. About 36% was excreted in the feces (probably via the bile), mostly as metabolites and less than 1% as the parent compound over the 10 day post-dosing period.

Distribution

Paroxetine distributes throughout the body, including the CNS, with only 1% remaining in the plasma.

Protein Binding

Approximately 95% and 93% of paroxetine is bound to plasma protein at 100 ng/ml and 400 ng/ml, respectively. Under clinical conditions, paroxetine concentrations would normally be less than 400 ng/ml. Paroxetine does not alter the *in vitro* protein binding of phenytoin or warfarin.

Renal and Liver Disease

Increased plasma concentrations of paroxetine occur in subjects with renal and hepatic impairment. The mean plasma concentrations in patients with creatinine clearance below 30 ml/min was approximately 4 times greater than seen in normal volunteers. Patients with creatinine clearance of 30-60 ml/min and patients with hepatic functional impairment had about a 2-fold increase in plasma concentrations (AUC, C_{max}).

The initial dosage should therefore be reduced in patients with severe renal or hepatic impairment, and upward titration, if necessary, should be at increased intervals (see DOSAGE AND ADMINISTRATION, Paxil CR).

Elderly Patients

In a multiple-dose study in the elderly at daily doses of 20, 30 and 40 mg of the immediate-release formulation, C_{min} concentrations were about 70-80% greater than the respective C_{min} concentrations in nonelderly subjects. Therefore the initial dosage in the elderly should be reduced (see DOSAGE AND ADMINISTRATION, Paxil CR).

INDICATIONS AND USAGE

PAXIL

Major Depressive Disorder

Paxil is indicated for the treatment of major depressive disorder.

The efficacy of Paxil in the treatment of a major depressive episode was established in 6 week controlled trials of outpatients whose diagnoses corresponded most closely to the DSM-III category of major depressive disorder. A major depressive episode implies a prominent and relatively persistent depressed or dysphoric mood that usually interferes with daily functioning (nearly every day for at least 2 weeks); it should include at least 4 of the following 8 symptoms: change in appetite, change in sleep, psychomotor agitation or retardation, loss of interest in usual activities or decrease in sexual drive, increased fatigue, feelings of guilt or worthlessness, slowed thinking or impaired concentration, and a suicide attempt or suicidal ideation.

The effects of Paxil in hospitalized depressed patients has not been adequately studied.

The efficacy of Paxil in maintaining a response in major depressive disorder for up to 1 year was demonstrated in a placebo-controlled trial. Nevertheless, the physician who elects to use Paxil for extended periods should periodically re-evaluate the long-term usefulness of the drug for the individual patient.

Obsessive Compulsive Disorder

Paxil is indicated for the treatment of obsessions and compulsions in patients with obsessive compulsive disorder (OCD) as defined in the DSM-IV. The obsessions or compulsions cause marked distress, are time-consuming, or significantly interfere with social or occupational functioning.

The efficacy of Paxil was established in two 12 week trials with obsessive compulsive outpatients whose diagnoses corresponded most closely to the DSM-IIIR category of obsessive compulsive disorder.

Obsessive compulsive disorder is characterized by recurrent and persistent ideas, thoughts, impulses or images (obsessions) that are ego-dystonic and/or repetitive, purposeful and intentional behaviors (compulsions) that are recognized by the person as excessive or unreasonable.

Long-term maintenance of efficacy was demonstrated in a 6 month relapse prevention trial. In this trial, patients assigned to paroxetine showed a lower relapse rate compared to patients on placebo. Nevertheless, the physician who elects to use Paxil for extended periods should perisodically re-evaluate the long-term usefulness of the drug for the individual patient (see DOSAGE AND ADMINISTRATION, Paxil).

Panic Disorder

Paxil is indicated for the treatment of panic disorder, with or without agoraphobia, as defined in DSM-IV. Panic disorder is characterized by the occurrence of unexpected panic attacks and associated concern about having additional attacks, worry about the implications or consequences of the attacks, and/or a significant change in behavior related to the attacks.

The efficacy of Paxil was established in three 10-12 week trials in panic disorder patients whose diagnoses corresponded to the DSM-IIIR category of panic disorder.

Panic disorder (DSM-IV) is characterized by recurrent unexpected panic attacks, *i.e.,* a discrete period of intense fear or discomfort in which four (or more) of the following symptoms develop abruptly and reach a peak within 10 minutes: (1) palpitations, pounding heart, or accelerated heart rate; (2) sweating; (3) trembling or shaking; (4) sensations of shortness of breath or smothering; (5) feeling of choking; (6) chest pain or discomfort; (7) nausea or abdominal distress; (8) feeling dizzy, unsteady, lightheaded, or faint; (9) derealization (feelings of unreality) or depersonalization (being detached from oneself); (10) fear of losing control; (11) fear of dying; (12) paresthesias (numbness or tingling sensations); (13) chills or hot flushes.

P

Long-term maintenance of efficacy was demonstrated in a 3 month relapse prevention trial. In this trial, patients with panic disorder assigned to paroxetine demonstrated a lower relapse rate compared to patients on placebo. Nevertheless, the physician who prescribes Paxil for extended periods should periodically re-evaluate the long-term usefulness of the drug for the individual patient.

Social Anxiety Disorder

Paxil is indicated for the treatment of social anxiety disorder, also known as social phobia, as defined in DSM-IV (300.23). Social anxiety disorder is characterized by a marked and persistent fear of one or more social or performance situations in which the person is exposed to unfamiliar people or to possible scrutiny by others. Exposure to the feared situation almost invariably provokes anxiety, which may approach the intensity of a panic attack. The feared situations are avoided or endured with intense anxiety or distress. The avoidance, anxious anticipation, or distress in the feared situation(s) interferes significantly with the person's normal routine, occupational or academic functioning, or social activities or relationships, or there is marked distress about having the phobias. Lesser degrees of performance anxiety or shyness generally do not require psychopharmacological treatment.

The efficacy of Paxil was established in three 12 week trials in adult patients with social anxiety disorder (DSM-IV). Paxil has not been studied in children or adolescents with social phobia.

The effectiveness of Paxil in long-term treatment of social anxiety disorder, *i.e.,* for more than 12 weeks, has not been systematically evaluated in adequate and well-controlled trials. Therefore, the physician who elects to prescribe Paxil for extended periods should periodically re-evaluate the long-term usefulness of the drug for the individual patient (see DOSAGE AND ADMINISTRATION, Paxil).

Generalized Anxiety Disorder

Paxil is indicated for the treatment of Generalized Anxiety Disorder (GAD), as defined in DSM-IV. Anxiety or tension associated with the stress of everyday life usually does not require treatment with an anxiolytic.

The efficacy of Paxil in the treatment of GAD was established in two 8 week placebo-controlled trials in adults with GAD. Paxil has not been studied in children or adolescents with Generalized Anxiety Disorder.

Generalized Anxiety Disorder (DSM-IV) is characterized by excessive anxiety and worry (apprehensive expectation) that is persistent for at least 6 months and which the person finds difficult to control. It must be associated with at least 3 of the following 6 symptoms: restlessness or feeling keyed up or on edge, being easily fatigued, difficulty concentrating or mind going blank, irritability, muscle tension, sleep disturbance.

The efficacy of Paxil in maintaining a response in patients with Generalized Anxiety Disorder, who responded during an 8 week acute treatment phase while taking Paxil and were then observed for relapse during a period of up to 24 weeks, was demonstrated in a placebo-controlled trail (see CLINICAL STUDIES). Nevertheless, the physician who elects to prescribe Paxil for extended periods should periodically re-evaluate the long-term usefulness of the drug for the individual patient (see DOSAGE AND ADMINISTRATION, Paxil).

Posttraumatic Stress Disorder

Paxil is indicated for the treatment of Posttraumatic Stress Disorder (PTSD).

The efficacy of Paxil in the treatment of PTSD was established in two 12 week placebo-controlled trials in adults with PTSD (DSM-IV).

PTSD, as defined by DSM-IV, requires exposure to a traumatic event that involved actual or threatened death or serious injury, or threat to the physical integrity of self or others, and a response which involves intense fear, helplessness, or horror. Symptoms that occur as a result of exposure to the traumatic event include reexperiencing of the event in the form of intrusive thoughts, flashbacks or dreams, and intense psychological distress and physiological reactivity on exposure to cues to the event; avoidance of situations reminiscent of the traumatic event, inability to recall details of the event, and/or numbing of general responsiveness manifested as diminished interest in significant activities, estrangement from others, restricted range of affect, or sense of foreshortened future; and symptoms of autonomic arousal including hypervigilance, exaggerated startle response, sleep disturbance, impaired concentration, and irritability or outbursts of anger. A PTSD diagnosis requires that the symptoms are present for at least a month and that they cause clinically significant distress or impairment in social, occupational, or other important areas of functioning.

The efficacy of Paxil in maintaining a response in patients with Generalized Anxiety Disorder, who responded during an 8 week acute treatment phase while taking Paxil and were then observed for relapse during a period of up to 24 weeks, was demonstrated in a placebo-controlled trial. Nevertheless, the efficacy of Paxil in longer-term treatment of PTSD, *i.e.,* for more than 12 weeks, has not been systematically evaluated in placebo-controlled trials. Therefore, the physician who elects to prescribe Paxil for extended periods should periodically re-evaluate the long-term usefulness of the drug for the individual patient (see DOSAGE AND ADMINISTRATION, Paxil).

PAXIL CR

Major Depressive Disorder

Paxil CR is indicated for the treatment of major depressive disorder.

The efficacy of Paxil CR in the treatment of a major depressive episode was established in two 12 week controlled trials of outpatients whose diagnoses corresponded to the DSM-IV category of major depressive disorder (see CLINICAL PHARMACOLOGY, Paxil CR).

A major depressive episode (DSM-IV) implies a prominent and relatively persistent (nearly every day for at least 2 weeks) depressed mood or loss of interest or pleasure in nearly all activities, representing a change from previous functioning, and includes the presence of at least 5 of the following 9 symptoms during the same 2 week period: depressed mood, markedly diminished interest or pleasure in usual activities, significant change in weight and/or appetite, insomnia or hypersomnia, psychomotor agitation or retardation, increased fatigue, feelings of guilt or worthlessness, slowed thinking or impaired concentration, a suicide attempt or suicidal ideation.

The antidepressant action of paroxetine in hospitalized depressed patients has not been adequately studied.

Paxil CR has not been systematically evaluated beyond 12 weeks in controlled clinical trials; however, the effectiveness of immediate-release paroxetine HCl in maintaining a response in major depressive disorder for up to 1 year has been demonstrated in a placebo-controlled trial (see CLINICAL PHARMACOLOGY, Paxil CR). The physician who elects to use Paxil CR for extended periods should periodically re-evaluate the long-term usefulness of the drug for the individual patient.

Panic Disorder

Paxil CR is indicated for the treatment of panic disorder, with or without agoraphobia, as defined in DSM-IV. Panic disorder is characterized by the occurrence of unexpected panic attacks and associated concern about having additional attacks, worry about the implications or consequences of the attacks, and/or a significant change in behavior related to the attacks.

The efficacy of Paxil CR was established in two 10 week trials in panic disorder patients whose diagnoses corresponded to the DSM-IV category of panic disorder.

Panic disorder (DSM-IV) is characterized by recurrent unexpected panic attacks, *i.e.,* a discrete period of intense fear or discomfort in which four (or more) of the following symptoms develop abruptly and reach a peak within 10 minutes: (1) palpitations, pounding heart, or accelerated heart rate; (2) sweating; (3) trembling or shaking; (4) sensations of shortness of breath or smothering; (5) feeling of choking; (6) chest pain or discomfort; (7) nausea or abdominal distress; (8) feeling dizzy, unsteady, lightheaded, or faint; (9) derealization (feelings of unreality) or depersonalization (being detached from oneself); (10) fear of losing control; (11) fear of dying; (12) paresthesias (numbness or tingling sensations); (13) chills or hot flushes.

Long-term maintenance of efficacy with the immediate-release formulation of paroxetine was demonstrated in a 3 month relapse prevention trial. In this trial, patients with panic disorder assigned to immediate-release paroxetine demonstrated a lower relapse rate compared to patients on placebo (see CLINICAL PHARMACOLOGY, Paxil CR). Nevertheless, the physician who prescribes Paxil CR for extended periods should periodically re-evaluate the long-term usefulness of the drug for the individual patient.

NON-FDA APPROVED INDICATIONS

Paroxetine may also have clinical utility in a number of other disorders including eating disorders, substance abuse, headaches, premenstrual dysphoric disorder, premature ejaculation, migraine prophylaxis, chronic pain, primary insomnia, and episodic rages in Tourette's disorder patients. The drug has shown efficacy when used in the prevention of depression induced by high-dose interferon alfa. Preliminary results also report paroxetine to be effective in improving the negative symptoms of schizophrenia. However, further studies on the use of paroxetine for these indications are needed and none of these uses are approved by the FDA.

CONTRAINDICATIONS

PAXIL

Concomitant use in patients taking either monoamine oxidase inhibitors (MAOIs) or thioridazine is contraindicated (see WARNINGS, Paxil and PRECAUTIONS, Paxil).

Paxil is contraindicated in patients with a hypersensitivity to paroxetine or any of the inactive ingredients in Paxil.

PAXIL CR

Concomitant use in patients taking either monoamine oxidase inhibitors (MAOIs) or thioridazine is contraindicated (see WARNINGS, Paxil CR and PRECAUTIONS, Paxil CR).

Paxil CR is contraindicated in patients with a hypersensitivity to paroxetine or to any of the inactive ingredients in Paxil CR.

WARNINGS

PAXIL

Potential for Interaction With Monoamine Oxidase Inhibitors

In patients receiving another serotonin reuptake inhibitor drug in combination with a monoamine oxidase inhibitor (MAOI), there have been reports of serious, sometimes fatal, reactions including hyperthermia, rigidity, myoclonus, autonomic instability with possible rapid fluctuations of vital signs, and mental status changes that include extreme agitation progressing to delirium and coma. These reactions have also been reported in patients who have recently discontinued that drug and have been started on a MAOI. Some cases presented with features resembling neuroleptic malignant syndrome. While there are no human data showing such an interaction with Paxil, limited animal data on the effects of combined use of paroxetine and MAOIs suggest that these drugs may act synergistically to elevate blood pressure and evoke behavioral excitation. Therefore, it is recommended that Paxil not be used in combination with an MAOI, or within 14 days of discontinuing treatment with an MAOI. At least 2 weeks should be allowed after stopping Paxil before starting a MAOI.

Potential Interaction With Thioridazine

Thioridazine administration alone produces prolongation of the QTc interval, which is associated with serious ventricular arrhythmias, such as torsade de pointes-type arrhythmias, and sudden death. This effect appears to be dose related.

An *in vivo* study suggests that drugs which inhibit P450 2D6, such as paroxetine, will elevate plasma levels of thioridazine. Therefore, it is recommended that paroxetine not be used in combination with thioridazine (see CONTRAINDICATIONS, Paxil and PRECAUTIONS, Paxil).

PAXIL CR

Potential for Interaction With Monoamine Oxidase Inhibitors

In patients receiving another serotonin reuptake inhibitor drug in combination with a monoamine oxidase inhibitor (MAOI), there have been reports of serious, sometimes fatal, reactions including hyperthermia, rigidity, myoclonus, autonomic instability with possible rapid fluctuations of vital signs, and mental status changes that include extreme agitation progressing to delirium and coma. These reactions have also been

P

reported in patients who have recently discontinued that drug and have been started on a MAOI. Some cases presented with features resembling neuroleptic malignant syndrome. While there are no human data showing such an interaction with paroxetine HCl, limited animal data on the effects of combined use of paroxetine and MAOIs suggest that these drugs may act synergistically to elevate blood pressure and evoke behavioral excitation. Therefore, it is recommended that Paxil CR not be used in combination with an MAOI, or within 14 days of discontinuing treatment with a MAOI. At least 2 weeks should be allowed after stopping Paxil CR before starting a MAOI.

Potential Interaction With Thioridazine

Thioridazine administration alone produces prolongation of the QTc interval, which is associated with serious ventricular arrhythmias, such as torsade de pointes-type arrhythmias, and sudden death. This effect appears to be dose related.

An *in vivo* study suggests that drugs which inhibit P450 2D6, such as paroxetine, will elevate plasma levels of thioridazine. Therefore, it is recommended that paroxetine not be used in combination with thioridazine (see CONTRAINDICATIONS, Paxil CR and PRECAUTIONS, Paxil CR).

PRECAUTIONS

PAXIL

General

Activation of Mania/Hypomania

During premarketing testing, hypomania or mania occurred in approximately 1.0% of Paxil-treated unipolar patients compared to 1.1% of active-control and 0.3% of placebo-treated unipolar patients. In a subset of patients classified as bipolar, the rate of manic episodes was 2.2% for Paxil and 11.6% for the combined active-control groups. As with all drugs effective in the treatment of major depressive disorder, Paxil should be used cautiously in patients with a history of mania.

Seizures

During premarketing testing, seizures occurred in 0.1% of Paxil-treated patients, a rate similar to that associated with other drugs effective in the treatment of major depressive disorder. Paxil should be used cautiously in patients with a history of seizures. It should be discontinued in any patient who develops seizures.

Suicide

The possibility of a suicide attempt is inherent in major depressive disorder and may persist until significant remission occurs. Close supervision of high-risk patients should accompany initial drug therapy. Prescriptions for Paxil should be written for the smallest quantity of tablets consistent with good patient management, in order to reduce the risk of overdose.

Because of well-established comorbidity between major depressive disorder and other psychiatric disorders, the same precautions observed when treating patients with major depressive disorder should be observed when treating patients with other psychiatric disorders.

Discontinuation of Treatment With Paxil

Recent clinical trials supporting the various approved indications for Paxil employed a taper phase regimen, rather than an abrupt discontinuation of treatment. The taper phase regimen used in GAD and PTSD clinical trials involved an incremental decrease in the daily dose by 10 mg/day at weekly intervals. When a daily dose of 20 mg/day was reached, patients were continued on this dose for 1 week before treatment was stopped.

With this regimen in those studies, the following adverse events were reported at an incidence of 2% or greater for Paxil and were at least twice that reported for placebo: abnormal dreams (2.3% vs 0.5%), paresthesia (2.0% vs 0.4%), and dizziness (7.1% vs 1.5%). In the majority of patients, these events were mild to moderate and were self-limiting and did not require medical intervention. During Paxil marketing, there have been spontaneous reports of similar adverse events, which may have no causal relationship to the drug, upon the discontinuation of Paxil (particularly when abrupt), including the following: dizziness, sensory disturbances (*e.g.,* paresthesias such as electric shock sensations), agitation, anxiety, nausea, and sweating. These events are generally self-limiting. Similar events have been reported for other selective serotonin reuptake inhibitors.

Patients should be monitored for these symptoms when discontinuing treatment, regardless of the indication for which Paxil is being prescribed. A gradual reduction in the dose rather than abrupt cessation is recommended whenever possible. If intolerable symptoms occur following a decrease in the dose or upon discontinuation of treatment, then resuming the previously prescribed dose may be considered. Subsequently, the physician may continue decreasing the dose but at a more gradual rate (see DOSAGE AND ADMINISTRATION, Paxil).

Hyponatremia

Several cases of hyponatremia have been reported. The hyponatremia appeared to be reversible when Paxil was discontinued. The majority of these occurrences have been in elderly individuals, some in patients taking diuretics or who were otherwise volume depleted.

Abnormal Bleeding

There have been several reports of abnormal bleeding (mostly ecchymosis and purpura) associated with paroxetine treatment, including a report of impaired platelet aggregation. While a causal relationship to paroxetine is unclear, impaired platelet aggregation may result from platelet serotonin depletion and contribute to such occurrences.

Use in Patients With Concomitant Illness

Clinical experience with Paxil in patients with certain concomitant systemic illness is limited. Caution is advisable in using Paxil in patients with diseases or conditions that could affect metabolism or hemodynamic responses.

As with other SSRIs, mydriasis has been infrequently reported in premarketing studies with Paxil. A few cases of acute angle closure glaucoma associated with paroxetine therapy have been reported in the literature. As mydriasis can cause acute angle closure in patients with narrow angle glaucoma, caution should be used when Paxil is prescribed for patients with narrow angle glaucoma.

Paxil has not been evaluated or used to any appreciable extent in patients with a recent history of myocardial infarction or unstable heart disease. Patients with these diagnoses were excluded from clinical studies during the product's premarket testing. Evaluation of electrocardiograms of 682 patients who received Paxil in double-blind, placebo-controlled trials, however, did not indicate that Paxil is associated with the development of significant ECG abnormalities. Similarly, Paxil does not cause any clinically important changes in heart rate or blood pressure.

Increased plasma concentrations of paroxetine occur in patients with severe renal impairment (creatinine clearance <30 ml/min) or severe hepatic impairment. A lower starting dose should be used in such patients (see DOSAGE AND ADMINISTRATION, Paxil).

Information for the Patient

Physicians are advised to discuss the following issues with patients for whom they prescribe Paxil:

Interference with cognitive and motor performance: Any psychoactive drug may impair judgment, thinking or motor skills. Although in controlled studies Paxil has not been shown to impair psychomotor performance, patients should be cautioned about operating hazardous machinery, including automobiles, until they are reasonably certain that Paxil therapy does not affect their ability to engage in such activities.

Completing course of therapy: While patients may notice improvement with Paxil therapy in 1-4 weeks, they should be advised to continue therapy as directed.

Concomitant medication: Patients should be advised to inform their physician if they are taking, or plan to take, any prescription or over-the-counter drugs, since there is a potential for interactions.

Alcohol: Although Paxil has not been shown to increase the impairment of mental and motor skills caused by alcohol, patients should be advised to avoid alcohol while taking Paxil.

Pregnancy: Patients should be advised to notify their physician if they become pregnant or intend to become pregnant during therapy.

Nursing: Patients should be advised to notify their physician if they are breast-feeding an infant (see Nursing Mothers).

Laboratory Tests

There are no specific laboratory tests recommended.

Carcinogenesis, Mutagenesis, and Impairment of Fertility

Carcinogenesis

Two year carcinogenicity studies were conducted in rodents given paroxetine in the diet at 1, 5, and 25 mg/kg/day (mice) and 1, 5, and 20 mg/kg/day (rats). These doses are up to 2.4 (mouse) and 3.9 (rat) times the maximum recommended human dose (MRHD) for major depressive disorder, social anxiety disorder, GAD and PTSD on a mg/m^2 basis. Because the MRHD for major depressive disorder is slightly less than that for OCD (50 mg vs 60 mg), the doses used in these carcinogenicity studies were only 2.0 (mouse) and 3.2 (rat) times the MRHD for OCD. There was a significantly greater number of male rats in the high-dose group with reticulum cell sarcomas (1/100, 0/50, 0/50 and 4/50 for control, low-, middle- and high-dose groups, respectively) and a significantly increased linear trend across dose groups for the occurrence of lymphoreticular tumors in male rats. Female rats were not affected. Although there was a dose-related increase in the number of tumors in mice, there was no drug-related increase in the number of mice with tumors. The relevance of these findings to humans is unknown.

Mutagenesis

Paroxetine produced no genotoxic effects in a battery of 5 *in vitro* and 2 *in vivo* assays that included the following: bacterial mutation assay, mouse lymphoma mutation assay, unscheduled DNA synthesis assay, and tests for cytogenetic aberrations *in vivo* in mouse bone marrow and *in vitro* in human lymphocytes and in a dominant lethal test in rats.

Impairment of Fertility

A reduced pregnancy rate was found in reproduction studies in rats at a dose of paroxetine of 15 mg/kg/day which is 2.9 times the MRHD for major depressive disorder, social anxiety disorder, GAD and PTSD or 2.4 times the MRHD for OCD on a mg/m^2 basis.

Irreversible lesions occurred in the reproductive tract of male rats after dosing in toxicity studies for 2-52 weeks. These lesions consisted of vacuolation of epididymal tubular epithelium at 50 mg/kg/day and atrophic changes in the seminiferous tubules of the testes with arrested spermatogenesis at 25 mg/kg/day (9.8 and 4.9 times the MRHD for major depressive disorder, social anxiety disorder and GAD; 8.2 and 4.1 times the MRHD for OCD and PD on a mg/m^2 basis).

Pregnancy, Teratogenic Effects, Pregnancy Category C

Reproduction studies were performed at doses up to 50 mg/kg/day in rats and 6 mg/kg/day in rabbits administered during organogenesis. These doses are equivalent to 9.7 (rat) and 2.2 (rabbit) times the maximum recommended human dose (MRHD) for major depressive disorder, social anxiety disorder, GAD and PTSD (50 mg) and 8.1 (rat) and 1.9 (rabbit) times the MRHD for OCD, on a mg/m^2 basis. These studies have revealed no evidence of teratogenic effects. However, in rats, there was an increase in pup deaths during the first 4 days of lactation when dosing occurred during the last trimester of gestation and continued throughout lactation. This effect occurred at a dose of 1 mg/kg/day or 0.19 times (mg/m^2) the MRHD for major depressive disorder, social anxiety disorder, GAD and PTSD, and at 0.16 times (mg/m^2) the MRHD for OCD. The no-effect dose for rat pup mortality was not determined. The cause of these deaths is not known. There are no adequate and well-controlled studies in pregnant women. Because animal reproduction studies are not always predictive of human response, this drug should be used during pregnancy only if the potential benefit justifies the potential risk to the fetus.

Labor and Delivery

The effect of paroxetine on labor and delivery in humans is unknown.

P

Nursing Mothers
Like many other drugs, paroxetine is secreted in human milk, and caution should be exercised when Paxil is administered to a nursing woman.

Pediatric Use
Safety and effectiveness in the pediatric population have not been established.

Geriatric Use
In worldwide premarketing Paxil clinical trials, 17% of Paxil-treated patients (approximately 700) were 65 years of age or older. Pharmacokinetic studies revealed a decreased clearance in the elderly, and a lower starting dose is recommended; there were, however, no overall differences in the adverse event profile between elderly and younger patients, and effectiveness was similar in younger and older patients (see CLINICAL PHARMACOLOGY, Paxil and DOSAGE AND ADMINISTRATION, Paxil).

PAXIL CR
General
Activation of Mania/Hypomania
During premarketing testing of immediate-release paroxetine HCl, hypomania or mania occurred in approximately 1.0% of paroxetine-treated unipolar patients compared to 1.1% of active-control and 0.3% of placebo-treated unipolar patients. In a subset of patients classified as bipolar, the rate of manic episodes was 2.2% for immediate-release paroxetine and 11.6% for the combined active-control groups.

Among 760 patients with major depressive disorder or panic disorder treated with Paxil CR in controlled clinical studies, there were no reports of mania or hypomania. As with all drugs effective in the treatment of major depressive disorder, Paxil CR should be used cautiously in patients with a history of mania.

Seizures
During premarketing testing of immediate-release paroxetine HCl, seizures occurred in 0.1% of paroxetine-treated patients, a rate similar to that associated with other drugs effective in the treatment of major depressive disorder.

Among 760 patients who received Paxil CR in controlled clinical trials in major depressive disorder or panic disorder, one patient (0.1%) experienced a seizure. Paxil CR should be used cautiously in patients with a history of seizures. It should be discontinued in any patient who develops seizures.

Suicide
The possibility of a suicide attempt is inherent in major depressive disorder and may persist until significant remission occurs. Close supervision of high-risk patients should accompany initial drug therapy. Prescriptions for Paxil CR should be written for the smallest quantity of tablets consistent with good patient management, in order to reduce the risk of overdose.

Because of well-established comorbidity between major depressive disorder and other psychiatric disorders, the same precautions observed when treating patients with major depressive disorder should be observed when treating patients with other psychiatric disorders.

Discontinuation of Treatment With Paxil CR
Adverse events while discontinuing therapy with Paxil CR were not systematically evaluated in the clinical trials. However, recent clinical trials supporting the various approved indications for immediate-release paroxetine HCl employed a taper phase regimen, rather than an abrupt discontinuation of treatment. The taper phase regimen used in generalized anxiety disorder and posttraumatic stress disorder immediate-release paroxetine HCl clinical trials involved an incremental decrease in the daily dose by 10 mg/day at weekly intervals. When a daily dose of 20 mg/day was reached, patients were continued on this dose for 1 week before treatment was stopped.

With this regimen in those studies, the following adverse events were reported at an incidence of 2% or greater for immediate-release paroxetine HCl and were at least twice that reported for placebo: abnormal dreams (2.3% vs 0.5%), paresthesia (2.0% vs 0.4%), and dizziness (7.1% vs 1.5%). In the majority of patients, these events were mild to moderate and were self-limiting and did not require medical intervention.

During marketing of immediate-release paroxetine HCl, there have been spontaneous reports of similar adverse events, which may have no causal relationship to the drug, upon discontinuation of immediate-release paroxetine HCl (particularly when abrupt), including the following: dizziness, sensory disturbances (*e.g.*, paresthesias such as electric shock sensations), agitation, anxiety, nausea, and sweating.

These events are generally self-limiting. Similar events have been reported for other selective serotonin reuptake inhibitors.

Patients should be monitored for these symptoms when discontinuing treatment, regardless of the indication for which Paxil CR is being prescribed. A gradual reduction in the dose rather than abrupt cessation is recommended whenever possible. If intolerable symptoms occur following a decrease in dose or upon discontinuation of treatment, then resuming the previously prescribed dose may be considered. Subsequently, the physician may continue decreasing the dose but at a more gradual rate (see DOSAGE AND ADMINISTRATION, Paxil CR).

Hyponatremia
Several cases of hyponatremia have been reported with immediate-release paroxetine HCl.

The hyponatremia appeared to be reversible when paroxetine was discontinued. The majority of these occurrences have been in elderly individuals, some in patients taking diuretics or who were otherwise volume depleted.

Abnormal Bleeding
There have been several reports of abnormal bleeding (mostly ecchymosis and purpura) associated with immediate-release paroxetine HCl treatment, including a report of impaired platelet aggregation. While a causal relationship to paroxetine is unclear, impaired platelet aggregation may result from platelet serotonin depletion and contribute to such occurrences.

Use in Patients With Concomitant Illness
Clinical experience with immediate-release paroxetine HCl in patients with certain concomitant systemic illness is limited. Caution is advisable in using Paxil CR in patients with diseases or conditions that could affect metabolism or hemodynamic responses.

As with other SSRIs, mydriasis has been infrequently reported in premarketing studies with paroxetine HCl. A few cases of acute angle closure glaucoma associated with therapy with immediate-release paroxetine have been reported in the literature. As mydriasis can cause acute angle closure in patients with narrow angle glaucoma, caution should be used when Paxil CR is prescribed for patients with narrow angle glaucoma.

Paxil CR or the immediate-release formulation has not been evaluated or used to any appreciable extent in patients with a recent history of myocardial infarction or unstable heart disease. Patients with these diagnoses were excluded from clinical studies during premarket testing. Evaluation of electrocardiograms of 682 patients who received immediate-release paroxetine HCl in double-blind, placebo-controlled trials, however, did not indicate that paroxetine is associated with the development of significant ECG abnormalities. Similarly, paroxetine HCl does not cause any clinically important changes in heart rate or blood pressure.

Increased plasma concentrations of paroxetine occur in patients with severe renal impairment (creatinine clearance <30 ml/min) or severe hepatic impairment. A lower starting dose should be used in such patients (see DOSAGE AND ADMINISTRATION, Paxil CR).

Information for the Patient
Physicians are advised to discuss the following issues with patients for whom they prescribe Paxil CR:

Paxil CR tablets should not be chewed or crushed, and should be swallowed whole.

Interference with cognitive and motor performance: Any psychoactive drug may impair judgment, thinking or motor skills. Although in controlled studies immediate-release paroxetine HCl has not been shown to impair psychomotor performance, patients should be cautioned about operating hazardous machinery, including automobiles, until they are reasonably certain that Paxil CR therapy does not affect their ability to engage in such activities.

Completing course of therapy: While patients may notice improvement with Paxil CR therapy in 1-4 weeks, they should be advised to continue therapy as directed.

Concomitant medication: Patients should be advised to inform their physician if they are taking, or plan to take, any prescription or over-the-counter drugs, since there is a potential for interactions.

Alcohol: Although immediate-release paroxetine HCl has not been shown to increase the impairment of mental and motor skills caused by alcohol, patients should be advised to avoid alcohol while taking Paxil CR.

Pregnancy: Patients should be advised to notify their physician if they become pregnant or intend to become pregnant during therapy.

Nursing: Patients should be advised to notify their physician if they are breast-feeding an infant (see Nursing Mothers).

Laboratory Tests
There are no specific laboratory tests recommended.

Carcinogenesis, Mutagenesis, and Impairment of Fertility
Carcinogenesis
Two year carcinogenicity studies were conducted in rodents given paroxetine in the diet at 1, 5, and 25 mg/kg/day (mice) and 1, 5, and 20 mg/kg/day (rats). These doses are up to approximately 2 (mouse) and 3 (rat) times the maximum recommended human dose (MRHD) on a mg/m^2 basis. There was a significantly greater number of male rats in the high-dose group with reticulum cell sarcomas (1/100, 0/50, 0/50 and 4/50 for control, low-, middle- and high-dose groups, respectively) and a significantly increased linear trend across dose groups for the occurrence of lymphoreticular tumors in male rats. Female rats were not affected. Although there was a dose-related increase in the number of tumors in mice, there was no drug-related increase in the number of mice with tumors. The relevance of these findings to humans is unknown.

Mutagenesis
Paroxetine produced no genotoxic effects in a battery of 5 *in vitro* and 2 *in vivo* assays that included the following: bacterial mutation assay, mouse lymphoma mutation assay, unscheduled DNA synthesis assay, and tests for cytogenetic aberrations *in vivo* in mouse bone marrow and *in vitro* in human lymphocytes and in a dominant lethal test in rats.

Impairment of Fertility
A reduced pregnancy rate was found in reproduction studies in rats at a dose of paroxetine of 15 mg/kg/day which is approximately twice the MRHD on a mg/m^2 basis. Irreversible lesions occurred in the reproductive tract of male rats after dosing in toxicity studies for 2-52 weeks. These lesions consisted of vacuolation of epididymal tubular epithelium at 50 mg/kg/day and atrophic changes in the seminiferous tubules of the testes with arrested spermatogenesis at 25 mg/kg/day (approximately 8 and 4 times the MRHD on a mg/m^2 basis).

Pregnancy Category C
Reproduction studies were performed at doses up to 50 mg/kg/day in rats and 6 mg/kg/day in rabbits administered during organogenesis. These doses are approximately 8 (rat) and 2 (rabbit) times the maximum recommended human dose (MRHD) on a mg/m^2 basis. These studies have revealed no evidence of teratogenic effects. However, in rats, there was an increase in pup deaths during the first 4 days of lactation when dosing occurred during the last trimester of gestation and continued throughout lactation. This effect occurred at a dose of 1 mg/kg/day or approximately one-sixth of the MRHD on a mg/m^2 basis. The no-effect dose for rat pup mortality was not determined. The cause of these deaths is not known. There are no adequate and well-controlled studies in pregnant women. This drug should be used during pregnancy only if the potential benefit justifies the potential risk to the fetus.

Labor and Delivery
The effect of paroxetine on labor and delivery in humans is unknown.

Nursing Mothers

Like many other drugs, paroxetine is secreted in human milk, and caution should be exercised when Paxil CR is administered to a nursing woman.

Pediatric Use

Safety and effectiveness in the pediatric population have not been established.

Geriatric Use

In worldwide premarketing clinical trials with immediate-release paroxetine HCl, 17% of paroxetine-treated patients (approximately 700) were 65 years of age or older. Pharmacokinetic studies revealed a decreased clearance in the elderly, and a lower starting dose is recommended; there were, however, no overall differences in the adverse event profile between elderly and younger patients, and effectiveness was similar in younger and older patients (see CLINICAL PHARMACOLOGY, Paxil CR and DOSAGE AND ADMINISTRATION, Paxil CR).

In a controlled study focusing specifically on elderly patients with major depressive disorder, Paxil CR was demonstrated to be safe and effective in the treatment of elderly patients (>60 years of age) with major depressive disorder. (See TABLE 12.)

DRUG INTERACTIONS

PAXIL

Tryptophan

As with other serotonin reuptake inhibitors, an interaction between paroxetine and tryptophan may occur when they are coadministered. Adverse experiences, consisting primarily of headache, nausea, sweating and dizziness, have been reported when tryptophan was administered to patients taking Paxil. Consequently, concomitant use of Paxil with tryptophan is not recommended.

Monoamine Oxidase Inhibitors

See CONTRAINDICATIONS, Paxil and WARNINGS, Paxil.

Thioridazine

See CONTRAINDICATIONS, Paxil and WARNINGS, Paxil.

Warfarin

Preliminary data suggest that there may be a pharmacodynamic interaction (that causes an increased bleeding diathesis in the face of unaltered prothrombin time) between paroxetine and warfarin. Since there is little clinical experience, the concomitant administration of Paxil and warfarin should be undertaken with caution.

Sumatriptan

There have been rare postmarketing reports describing patients with weakness, hyperreflexia, and incoordination following the use of a selective serotonin reuptake inhibitor (SSRI) and sumatriptan. If concomitant treatment with sumatriptan and an SSRI (*e.g.*, fluoxetine, fluvoxamine, paroxetine, sertraline) is clinically warranted, appropriate observation of the patient is advised.

Drugs Affecting Hepatic Metabolism

The metabolism and pharmacokinetics of paroxetine may be affected by the induction or inhibition of drug-metabolizing enzymes.

Cimetidine

Cimetidine inhibits many cytochrome P450 (oxidative) enzymes. In a study where Paxil (30 mg qd) was dosed orally for 4 weeks, steady-state plasma concentrations of paroxetine were increased by approximately 50% during coadministration with oral cimetidine (300 mg tid) for the final week. Therefore, when these drugs are administered concurrently, dosage adjustment of Paxil after the 20 mg starting dose should be guided by clinical effect. The effect of paroxetine on cimetidine's pharmacokinetics was not studied.

Phenobarbital

Phenobarbital induces many cytochrome P450 (oxidative) enzymes. When a single oral 30 mg dose of Paxil was administered at phenobarbital steady-state (100 mg qd for 14 days), paroxetine AUC and $T_{1/2}$ were reduced (by an average of 25% and 38%, respectively) compared to paroxetine administered alone. The effect of paroxetine on phenobarbital pharmacokinetics was not studied. Since Paxil exhibits nonlinear pharmacokinetics, the results of this study may not address the case where the two drugs are both being chronically dosed. No initial Paxil dosage adjustment is considered necessary when coadministered with phenobarbital; any subsequent adjustment should be guided by clinical effect.

Phenytoin

When a single oral 30 mg dose of Paxil was administered at phenytoin steady-state (300 mg qd for 14 days), paroxetine AUC and $T_{1/2}$ were reduced (by an average of 50% and 35%, respectively) compared to Paxil administered alone. In a separate study, when a single oral 300 mg dose of phenytoin was administered at paroxetine steady-state (30 mg qd for 14 days), phenytoin AUC was slightly reduced (12% on average) compared to phenytoin administered alone. Since both drugs exhibit nonlinear pharmacokinetics, the above studies may not address the case where the two drugs are both being chronically dosed. No initial dosage adjustments are considered necessary when these drugs are coadministered; any subsequent adjustments should be guided by clinical effect (see ADVERSE REACTIONS, Paxil, Postmarketing Reports).

Drugs Metabolized by Cytochrome P450 2D6

Many drugs, including most drugs effective in the treatment of major depressive disorder (paroxetine, other SSRIs and many tricyclics), are metabolized by the cytochrome P450 isozyme P450 2D6. Like other agents that are metabolized by P450 2D6, paroxetine may significantly inhibit the activity of this isozyme. In most patients (>90%), this P450 2D6 isozyme is saturated early during Paxil dosing. In one study, daily dosing of Paxil (20 mg qd) under steady-state conditions increased single-dose desipramine (100 mg) C_{max}, AUC and $T_{1/2}$ by an average of approximately 2-, 5- and 3-fold, respectively. Concomitant use of Paxil with other drugs metabolized by cytochrome P450 2D6 has not been formally studied but may require lower doses than usually prescribed for either Paxil or the other drug.

Therefore, coadministration of Paxil with other drugs that are metabolized by this isozyme, including certain drugs effective in the treatment of major depressive disorder (*e.g.*, nortriptyline, amitriptyline, imipramine, desipramine and fluoxetine), phenothiazines and Type 1C antiarrhythmics (*e.g.*, propafenone, flecainide and encainide), or that inhibit this enzyme (*e.g.*, quinidine), should be approached with caution.

However, due to the risk of serious ventricular arrhythmias and sudden death potentially associated with elevated plasma levels of thioridazine, paroxetine and thioridazine should not be coadministered (see CONTRAINDICATIONS, Paxil and WARNINGS, Paxil).

At steady-state, when the P450 2D6 pathway is essentially saturated, paroxetine clearance is governed by alternative P450 isozymes which, unlike P450 2D6, show no evidence of saturation (see Tricyclic Antidepressants).

Drugs Metabolized by Cytochrome P450 3A4

An *in vivo* interaction study involving the coadministration under steady-state conditions of paroxetine and terfenadine, a substrate for cytochrome P450 3A4, revealed no effect of paroxetine on terfenadine pharmacokinetics. In addition, *in vitro* studies have shown ketoconazole, a potent inhibitor of P450 3A4 activity, to be at least 100 times more potent than paroxetine as an inhibitor of the metabolism of several substrates for this enzyme, including terfenadine, astemizole, cisapride, triazolam, and cyclosporin. Based on the assumption that the relationship between paroxetine's *in vitro* Ki and its lack of effect on terfenadine's *in vivo* clearance predicts its effect on other 3A4 substrates, paroxetine's extent of inhibition of 3A4 activity is not likely to be of clinical significance.

Tricyclic Antidepressants (TCAs)

Caution is indicated in the coadministration of tricyclic antidepressants (TCAs) with Paxil, because paroxetine may inhibit TCA metabolism. Plasma TCA concentrations may need to be monitored, and the dose of TCA may need to be reduced, if a TCA is coadministered with Paxil (see Drugs Metabolized by Cytochrome P450 2D6).

Drugs Highly Bound to Plasma Protein

Because paroxetine is highly bound to plasma protein, administration of Paxil to a patient taking another drug that is highly protein bound may cause increased free concentrations of the other drug, potentially resulting in adverse events. Conversely, adverse effects could result from displacement of paroxetine by other highly bound drugs.

Alcohol

Although Paxil does not increase the impairment of mental and motor skills caused by alcohol, patients should be advised to avoid alcohol while taking Paxil.

Lithium

A multiple-dose study has shown that there is no pharmacokinetic interaction between Paxil and lithium carbonate. However, since there is little clinical experience, the concurrent administration of paroxetine and lithium should be undertaken with caution.

Digoxin

The steady-state pharmacokinetics of paroxetine was not altered when administered with digoxin at steady-state. Mean digoxin AUC at steady-state decreased by 15% in the presence of paroxetine. Since there is little clinical experience, the concurrent administration of paroxetine and digoxin should be undertaken with caution.

Diazepam

Under steady-state conditions, diazepam does not appear to affect paroxetine kinetics. The effects of paroxetine on diazepam were not evaluated.

Procyclidine

Daily oral dosing of Paxil (30 mg qd) increased steady-state AUC(0-24), C_{max} and C_{min} values of procyclidine (5 mg oral qd) by 35%, 37% and 67%, respectively, compared to procyclidine alone at steady-state. If anticholinergic effects are seen, the dose of procyclidine should be reduced.

Beta-Blockers

In a study where propranolol (80 mg bid) was dosed orally for 18 days, the established steady-state plasma concentrations of propranolol were unaltered during coadministration with Paxil (30 mg qd) for the final 10 days. The effects of propranolol on paroxetine have not been evaluated (see ADVERSE REACTIONS, Paxil, Postmarketing Reports).

Theophylline

Reports of elevated theophylline levels associated with Paxil treatment have been reported. While this interaction has not been formally studied, it is recommended that theophylline levels be monitored when these drugs are concurrently administered.

Electroconvulsive Therapy (ECT)

There are no clinical studies of the combined use of ECT and Paxil.

PAXIL CR

Tryptophan

As with other serotonin reuptake inhibitors, an interaction between paroxetine and tryptophan may occur when they are coadministered. Adverse experiences, consisting primarily of headache, nausea, sweating and dizziness, have been reported when tryptophan was administered to patients taking immediate-release paroxetine. Consequently, concomitant use of Paxil CR with tryptophan is not recommended.

Monoamine Oxidase Inhibitors

See CONTRAINDICATIONS, Paxil CR and WARNINGS, Paxil CR.

P

Thioridazine
See CONTRAINDICATIONS, Paxil CR and WARNINGS, Paxil CR.

Warfarin
Preliminary data suggest that there may be a pharmacodynamic interaction (that causes an increased bleeding diathesis in the face of unaltered prothrombin time) between paroxetine and warfarin. Since there is little clinical experience, the concomitant administration of Paxil CR and warfarin should be undertaken with caution.

Sumatriptan
There have been rare postmarketing reports describing patients with weakness, hyperreflexia, and incoordination following the use of a selective serotonin reuptake inhibitor (SSRI) and sumatriptan. If concomitant treatment with sumatriptan and an SSRI (*e.g.*, fluoxetine, fluvoxamine, paroxetine, sertraline) is clinically warranted, appropriate observation of the patient is advised.

Drugs Affecting Hepatic Metabolism
The metabolism and pharmacokinetics of paroxetine may be affected by the induction or inhibition of drug-metabolizing enzymes.

Cimetidine
Cimetidine inhibits many cytochrome P450 (oxidative) enzymes. In a study where immediate-release paroxetine (30 mg qd) was dosed orally for 4 weeks, steady-state plasma concentrations of paroxetine were increased by approximately 50% during coadministration with oral cimetidine (300 mg tid) for the final week. Therefore, when these drugs are administered concurrently, dosage adjustment of Paxil CR after the 25 mg starting dose should be guided by clinical effect. The effect of paroxetine on cimetidine's pharmacokinetics was not studied.

Phenobarbital
Phenobarbital induces many cytochrome P450 (oxidative) enzymes. When a single oral 30 mg dose of immediate-release paroxetine was administered at phenobarbital steady-state (100 mg qd for 14 days), paroxetine AUC and T½ were reduced (by an average of 25% and 38%, respectively) compared to paroxetine administered alone. The effect of paroxetine on phenobarbital pharmacokinetics was not studied. Since paroxetine exhibits nonlinear pharmacokinetics, the results of this study may not address the case where the two drugs are both being chronically dosed. No initial Paxil CR dosage adjustment is considered necessary when coadministered with phenobarbital; any subsequent adjustment should be guided by clinical effect.

Phenytoin
When a single oral 30 mg dose of immediate-release paroxetine was administered at phenytoin steady-state (300 mg qd for 14 days), paroxetine AUC and T½ were reduced (by an average of 50% and 35%, respectively) compared to immediate-release paroxetine administered alone. In a separate study, when a single oral 300 mg dose of phenytoin was administered at paroxetine steady-state (30 mg qd for 14 days), phenytoin AUC was slightly reduced (12% on average) compared to phenytoin administered alone. Since both drugs exhibit nonlinear pharmacokinetics, the above studies may not address the case where the two drugs are both being chronically dosed. No initial dosage adjustments are considered necessary when Paxil CR is coadministered with phenytoin; any subsequent adjustments should be guided by clinical effect (see ADVERSE REACTIONS, Paxil CR, Postmarketing Reports).

Drugs Metabolized by Cytochrome P450 2D6
Many drugs, including most drugs effective in the treatment of major depressive disorder (paroxetine, other SSRIs, and many tricyclics), are metabolized by the cytochrome P450 isozyme P450 2D6. Like other agents that are metabolized by P450 2D6, paroxetine may significantly inhibit the activity of this isozyme. In most patients (>90%), this P450 2D6 isozyme is saturated early during paroxetine dosing. In one study, daily dosing of immediate-release paroxetine (20 mg qd) under steady-state conditions increased single-dose desipramine (100 mg) C_{max}, AUC, and T½ by an average of approximately 2-, 5-, and 3-fold respectively. Concomitant use of Paxil CR with other drugs metabolized by cytochrome P450 2D6 has not been formally studied but may require lower doses than usually prescribed for either Paxil CR or the other drug.

Therefore, coadministration of Paxil CR with other drugs that are metabolized by this isozyme, including certain drugs effective in the treatment of major depressive disorder (*e.g.*, nortriptyline, amitriptyline, imipramine, desipramine and fluoxetine), phenothiazines and Type 1C antiarrhythmics (*e.g.*, propafenone, flecainide and encainide), or that inhibit this enzyme (*e.g.*, quinidine), should be approached with caution.

However, due to the risk of serious ventricular arrhythmias and sudden death potentially associated with elevated plasma levels of thioridazine, paroxetine and thioridazine should not be coadministered (see CONTRAINDICATIONS, Paxil CR and WARNINGS, Paxil CR).

At steady-state, when the P450 2D6 pathway is essentially saturated, paroxetine clearance is governed by alternative P450 isozymes which, unlike P450 2D6, show no evidence of saturation (see Tricyclic Antidepressants).

Drugs Metabolized by Cytochrome P450 3A4
An *in vivo* interaction study involving the coadministration under steady-state conditions of paroxetine and terfenadine, a substrate for P450 3A4, revealed no effect of paroxetine on terfenadine pharmacokinetics. In addition, *in vitro* studies have shown ketoconazole, a potent inhibitor of P450 3A4 activity, to be at least 100 times more potent than paroxetine as an inhibitor of the metabolism of several substrates for this enzyme, including terfenadine, astemizole, cisapride, triazolam, and cyclosporin. Based on the assumption that the relationship between paroxetine's *in vitro* Ki and its lack of effect on terfenadine's *in vivo* clearance predicts its effect on other 3A4 substrates, paroxetine's extent of inhibition of 3A4 activity is not likely to be of clinial significance.

Tricyclic Antidepressants (TCA)
Caution is indicated in the coadministration of tricyclic antidepressants (TCAs) with Paxil CR, because paroxetine may inhibit TCA metabolism. Plasma TCA concentrations may need to be monitored, and the dose of TCA may need to be reduced, if a TCA is coadministered with Paxil CR (see Drugs Metabolized by Cytochrome P450 2D6).

Drugs Highly Bound to Plasma Protein
Because paroxetine is highly bound to plasma protein, administration of Paxil CR to a patient taking another drug that is highly protein bound may cause increased free concentrations of the other drug, potentially resulting in adverse events. Conversely, adverse effects could result from displacement of paroxetine by other highly bound drugs.

Alcohol
Although paroxetine does not increase the impairment of mental and motor skills caused by alcohol, patients should be advised to avoid alcohol while taking Paxil CR.

Lithium
A multiple-dose study with immediate-release paroxetine HCl has shown that there is no pharmacokinetic interaction between paroxetine and lithium carbonate. However, since there is little clinical experience, the concurrent administration of Paxil CR and lithium should be undertaken with caution.

Digoxin
The steady-state pharmacokinetics of paroxetine was not altered when administered with digoxin at steady-state. Mean digoxin AUC at steady-state decreased by 15% in the presence of paroxetine. Since there is little clinical experience, the concurrent administration of Paxil CR and digoxin should be undertaken with caution.

Diazepam
Under steady-state conditions, diazepam does not appear to affect paroxetine kinetics. The effects of paroxetine on diazepam were not evaluated.

Procyclidine
Daily oral dosing of immediate-release paroxetine (30 mg qd) increased steady-state AUC(0-24), C_{max} and C_{min} values of procyclidine (5 mg oral qd) by 35%, 37% and 67%, respectively, compared to procyclidine alone at steady-state. If anticholinergic effects are seen, the dose of procyclidine should be reduced.

Beta-Blockers
In a study where propranolol (80 mg bid) was dosed orally for 18 days, the established steady-state plasma concentrations of propranolol were unaltered during coadministration with immediate-release paroxetine (30 mg qd) for the final 10 days. The effects of propranolol on paroxetine have not been evaluated (see ADVERSE REACTIONS, Paxil CR, Postmarketing Reports).

Theophylline
Reports of elevated theophylline levels associated with immediate-release paroxetine treatment have been reported. While this interaction has not been formally studied, it is recommended that theophylline levels be monitored when these drugs are concurrently administered.

Electroconvulsive Therapy (ECT)
There are no clinical studies of the combined use of ECT and Paxil CR.

ADVERSE REACTIONS

PAXIL

Associated With Discontinuation of Treatment
Twenty percent (20%) (1199/6145) of Paxil patients in worldwide clinical trials in major depressive disorder and 16.1% (84/522), 11.8% (64/542), 9.4% (44/469), 10.7% (79/735) and 11.7% (79/676) of Paxil patients in worldwide trials in social anxiety disorder, OCD, panic disorder, GAD and PTSD, respectively, discontinued treatment due to an adverse event. The most common events (≥1%) associated with discontinuation and considered to be drug related (*i.e.*, those events associated with dropout at a rate approximately twice or greater for Paxil compared to placebo) are listed in TABLE 2A and TABLE 2B.

Commonly Observed Adverse Events

Major Depressive Disorder
The most commonly observed adverse events associated with the use of paroxetine (incidence of 5% or greater and incidence for Paxil at least twice that for placebo, derived from TABLE 3) were: asthenia, sweating, nausea, decreased appetite, somnolence, dizziness, insomnia, tremor, nervousness, ejaculatory disturbance and other male genital disorders.

Obsessive Compulsive Disorder
The most commonly observed adverse events associated with the use of paroxetine (incidence of 5% or greater and incidence for Paxil at least twice that of placebo, derived from TABLE 4A and TABLE 4B) were: nausea, dry mouth, decreased appetite, constipation, dizziness, somnolence, tremor, sweating, impotence and abnormal ejaculation.

Panic Disorder
The most commonly observed adverse events associated with the use of paroxetine (incidence of 5% or greater and incidence for Paxil at least twice that for placebo, derived from TABLE 4A and TABLE 4B) were: asthenia, sweating, decreased appetite, libido decreased, tremor, abnormal ejaculation, female genital disorders and impotence.

Social Anxiety Disorder
The most commonly observed adverse events associated with the use of paroxetine (incidence of 5% or greater and incidence for Paxil at least twice that for placebo, derived from

TABLE 2A

	Major Depressive Disorder		OCD		Panic Disorder	
	Paxil	Placebo	Paxil	Placebo	Paxil	Placebo
CNS						
Somnolence	2.3%	0.7%	—		1.9%	0.3%
Insomnia	—	—	1.7%	0%	1.3%	0.3%
Agitation	1.1%	0.5%	—			
Tremor	1.1%	0.3%	—			
Anxiety	—	—	—			
Dizziness	—	—	1.5%	0%		
Gastrointestinal						
Constipation	—		1.1%	0%		
Nausea	3.2%	1.1%	1.9%	0%	3.2%	1.2%
Diarrhea	1.0%	0.3%	—			
Dry mouth	1.0%	0.3%	—			
Vomiting	1.0%	0.3%	—			
Other						
Asthenia	1.6%	0.4%	1.9%	0.4%		
Abnormal ejaculation*	1.6%	0%	2.1%	0%		
Sweating	1.0%	0.3%	—			
Impotence*	—		1.5%	0%		

Where numbers are not provided the incidence of the adverse events in Paxil patients was not >1% or was not greater than or equal to 2 times the incidence of placebo.
* Incidence corrected for gender.

TABLE 2B

	Social Anxiety Disorder		Generalized Anxiety Disorder		PTSD	
	Paxil	Placebo	Paxil	Placebo	Paxil	Placebo
CNS						
Somnolence	3.4%	0.3%	2.0%	0.2%	2.8%	0.6%
Insomnia	3.1%	0%			—	—
Agitation					—	—
Tremor	1.7%	0%			1.0%	0.2%
Anxiety	1.1%	0%			—	—
Dizziness	1.9%	0%	1.0%	0.2%	—	—
Gastrointestinal						
Constipation					—	—
Nausea	4.0%	0.3%	2.0%	0.2%	2.2%	0.6%
Diarrhea						
Dry mouth					—	—
Vomiting	1.0%	0%			—	—
Flatulence	1.0%	0.3%			—	—
Other						
Asthenia	2.5%	0.6%	1.8%	0.2%	1.6%	0.2%
Abnormal ejaculation*	4.9%	0.6%	2.5%	0.5%	—	—
Sweating	1.1%	0%	1.1%	0.2%	—	—
Impotence*					—	—
Libido decreased	1.0%	0%			—	—

Where numbers are not provided the incidence of the adverse events in Paxil patients was not >1% or was not greater than or equal to 2 times the incidence of placebo.
* Incidence corrected for gender.

TABLE 3 *Treatment-Emergent Adverse Experience Incidence in Placebo-Controlled Clinical Trials for Major Depressive Disorder**

Body System / Preferred Term	Paxil (n=421)	Placebo (n=421)
Body as a Whole		
Headache	18%	17%
Asthenia	15%	6%
Cardiovascular		
Palpitation	3%	1%
Vasodilation	3%	1%
Dermatologic		
Sweating	11%	2%
Rash	2%	1%
Gastrointestinal		
Nausea	26%	9%
Dry mouth	18%	12%
Constipation	14%	9%
Diarrhea	12%	8%
Decreased appetite	6%	2%
Flatulence	4%	2%
Oropharynx disorder†	2%	0%
Dyspepsia	2%	1%
Musculoskeletal		
Myopathy	2%	1%
Myalgia	2%	1%
Myasthenia	1%	0%
Nervous System		
Somnolence	23%	9%
Dizziness	13%	6%
Insomnia	13%	6%
Tremor	8%	2%
Nervousness	5%	3%
Anxiety	5%	3%
Paresthesia	4%	2%
Libido decreased	3%	0%
Drugged feeling	2%	1%
Confusion	1%	0%
Respiration		
Yawn	4%	0%
Special Senses		
Blurred vision	4%	1%
Taste perversion	2%	0%
Urogenital System		
Ejaculatory disturbance‡§	13%	0%
Other male genital disorders‡¤	10%	0%
Urinary frequency	3%	1%
Urination disorder¶	3%	0%
Female genital disorders‡**	2%	0%

* Events reported by at least 1% of patients treated with Paxil are included, except the following events which had an incidence on placebo ≥ Paxil: abdominal pain, agitation, back pain, chest pain, CNS stimulation, fever, increased appetite, myoclonus, pharyngitis, postural hypotension, respiratory disorder (includes mostly "cold symptoms" or "URI"), trauma and vomiting.
† Includes mostly "lump in throat" and "tightness in throat".
‡ Percentage corrected for gender.
§ Mostly "ejaculatory delay."
¤ Includes "anorgasmia", "erectile difficulties", "delayed ejaculation/orgasm", and "sexual dysfunction", and "impotence."
¶ Includes mostly "difficulty with micturition" and "urinary hesitancy."
** Includes mostly "anorgasmia" and "difficulty reaching climax/orgasm."

TABLE 4A and TABLE 4B) were: sweating, nausea, dry mouth, constipation, decreased appetite, somnolence, tremor, libido decreased, yawn, abnormal ejaculation, female genital disorders and impotence.

Generalized Anxiety Disorder

The most commonly observed adverse events associated with the use of paroxetine (incidence of 5% or greater and incidence for Paxil at least twice that for placebo, derived from TABLE 5) were: asthenia, infection, constipation, decreased appetite, dry mouth, nausea, libido decreased, somnolence, tremor, sweating, and abnormal ejaculation.

Posttraumatic Stress Disorder

The most commonly observed adverse events associated with the use of paroxetine (incidence of 5% or greater and incidence for Paxil at least twice that for placebo, derived from TABLE 5 below) were: asthenia, sweating, nausea, dry mouth, diarrhea, decreased appetite, somnolence, libido decreased, abnormal ejaculation, female genital disorders, and impotence.

Incidence in Controlled Clinical Trials

The prescriber should be aware that the figures in the tables following cannot be used to predict the incidence of side effects in the course of usual medical practice where patient characteristics and other factors differ from those which prevailed in the clinical trials. Similarly, the cited frequencies cannot be compared with figures obtained from other clinical investigations involving different treatments, uses and investigators. The cited figures, however, do provide the prescribing physician with some basis for estimating the relative contribution of drug and nondrug factors to the side effect incidence rate in the populations studied.

Major Depressive Disorder

TABLE 3 enumerates adverse events that occurred at an incidence of 1% or more among paroxetine-treated patients who participated in short-term (6 week) placebo-controlled trials in which patients were dosed in a range of 20-50 mg/day. Reported adverse events were classified using a standard COSTART-based Dictionary terminology.

Obsessive Compulsive Disorder, Panic Disorder and Social Anxiety Disorder

TABLE 4A and TABLE 4B enumerates adverse events that occurred at a frequency of 2% or more among OCD patients on Paxil who participated in placebo-controlled trials of 12 weeks duration in which patients were dosed in a range of 20-60 mg/day or among patients with panic disorder on Paxil who participated in placebo-controlled trials of 10-12 weeks duration in which patients were dosed in a range of 10-60 mg/day or among patients with social anxiety disorder on Paxil who participated in placebo-controlled trials of 12 weeks duration in which patients were dosed in a range of 20-50 mg/day.

Generalized Anxiety Disorder and Posttraumatic Stress Disorder

TABLE 5 enumerates adverse events that occurred at a frequency of 2% or more among GAD patients on Paxil who participated in placebo-controlled trials of 8 weeks duration in which patients were dosed in a range of 10-50 mg/day or among PTSD patients on Paxil who participated in placebo-controlled trials of 12 weeks duration in which patients were dosed in a range of 20-50 mg/day.

Dose Dependency of Adverse Events

A comparison of adverse event rates in a fixed-dose study comparing Paxil 10, 20, 30 and 40 mg/day with placebo in the treatment of major depressive disorder revealed a clear dose dependency for some of the more common adverse events associated with Paxil use, as shown in TABLE 6.

In a fixed-dose study comparing placebo and Paxil 20, 40 and 60 mg in the treatment of OCD, there was no clear relationship between adverse events and the dose of Paxil to which patients were assigned. No new adverse events were observed in the Paxil 60 mg dose group compared to any of the other treatment groups.

In a fixed-dose study comparing placebo and Paxil 10, 20 and 40 mg in the treatment of panic disorder, there was no clear relationship between adverse events and the dose of Paxil to which patients were assigned, except for asthenia, dry mouth, anxiety, libido decreased, tremor and abnormal ejaculation. In flexible-dose studies, no new adverse events were observed in patients receiving Paxil 60 mg compared to any of the other treatment groups.

In a fixed-dose study comparing placebo and Paxil 20, 40 and 60 mg in the treatment of social anxiety disorder, for most of the adverse events, there was no clear relationship between adverse events and the dose of Paxil to which patients were assigned.

TABLE 4A *Treatment-Emergent Adverse Experience Incidence in Placebo-Controlled Clinical Trials for Obsessive Compulsive Disorder**

Body System / Preferred Term	Paxil (n=542)	Placebo (n=265)
Body as a Whole		
Asthenia	22%	14%
Chest pain	3%	2%
Chills	2%	1%
Cardiovascular		
Vasodilation	4%	1%
Palpitation	2%	0%
Dermatologic		
Sweating	9%	3%
Rash	3%	2%
Gastrointestinal		
Nausea	23%	10%
Dry mouth	18%	9%
Constipation	16%	6%
Diarrhea	10%	10%
Decreased appetite	9%	3%
Increased appetite	4%	3%
Nervous System		
Insomnia	24%	13%
Somnolence	24%	7%
Dizziness	12%	6%
Tremor	11%	1%
Nervousness	9%	8%
Libido decreased	7%	4%
Abnormal dreams	4%	1%
Concentration impaired	3%	2%
Depersonalization	3%	0%
Myoclonus	3%	0%
Amnesia	2%	1%
Special Senses		
Abnormal vision	4%	2%
Taste perversion	2%	0%
Urogenital System		
Abnormal ejaculation†	23%	1%
Female genital disorder†	3%	0%
Impotence†	8%	1%
Urinary frequency	3%	1%
Urination impaired	3%	0%
Urinary tract infection	2%	1%

* Events reported by at least 2% of OCD Paxil-treated patients are included, except the following events which had an incidence on placebo ≥ Paxil: abdominal pain, agitation, anxiety, back pain, cough increased, depression, headache, hyperkinesia, infection, paresthesia, pharyngitis, respiratory disorder, rhinitis and sinusitis.
† Percentage corrected for gender.

In a fixed-dose study comparing placebo and Paxil 20 and 40 mg in the treatment of generalized anxiety disorder, for most of the adverse events, there was no clear relationship between adverse events and the dose of Paxil to which patients were assigned, except for the following adverse events: asthenia, constipation, and abnormal ejaculation.

In a fixed-dose study comparing placebo and Paxil 20 and 40 mg in the treatment of posttraumatic stress disorder, for most of the adverse events, there was no clear relationship between adverse events and the dose of Paxil to which patients were assigned, except for impotence and abnormal ejaculation.

P

Adaptation to Certain Adverse Events

Over a 4-6 week period, there was evidence of adaptation to some adverse events with continued therapy (*e.g.,* nausea and dizziness), but less to other effects (*e.g.,* dry mouth, somnolence and asthenia).

Male and Female Sexual Dysfunction With SSRIs

Although changes in sexual desire, sexual performance and sexual satisfaction often occur as manifestations of a psychiatric disorder, they may also be a consequence of pharmacologic treatment. In particular, some evidence suggests that selective serotonin reuptake inhibitors (SSRIs) can cause such untoward sexual experiences.

Reliable estimates of the incidence and severity of untoward experiences involving sexual desire, performance and satisfaction are difficult to obtain, however, in part because patients and physicians may be reluctant to discuss them. Accordingly, estimates of the incidence of untoward sexual experience and performance cited in product labeling, are likely to underestimate their actual incidence.

In placebo-controlled clinical trials involving more than 3200 patients, the ranges for the reported incidence of sexual side effects in males and females with major depressive disorder, OCD, panic disorder, social anxiety disorder, GAD and PTSD are displayed in TABLE 7.

There are no adequate and well-controlled studies examining sexual dysfunction with paroxetine treatment.

Paroxetine treatment has been associated with several cases of priapism. In those cases with a known outcome, patients recovered without sequelae.

While it is difficult to know the precise risk of sexual dysfunction associated with the use of SSRIs, physicians should routinely inquire about such possible side effects.

Weight and Vital Sign Changes

Significant weight loss may be an undesirable result of treatment with Paxil for some patients but, on average, patients in controlled trials had minimal (about 1 lb) weight loss versus smaller changes on placebo and active control. No significant changes in vital signs (systolic and diastolic blood pressure, pulse and temperature) were observed in patients treated with Paxil in controlled clinical trials.

TABLE 4B *Treatment-Emergent Adverse Experience Incidence in Placebo-Controlled Clinical Trials for Panic Disorder and Social Anxiety Disorder**

	Panic Disorder		Social Anxiety Disorder	
Body System	**Paxil**	**Placebo**	**Paxil**	**Placebo**
Preferred Term	**(n=469)**	**(n=324)**	**(n=425)**	**(n=339)**
Body as a Whole				
Asthenia	14%	5%	22%	14%
Abdominal pain	4%	3%	—	—
Back pain	3%	2%	—	—
Chills	2%	1%	—	—
Trauma	—	—	3%	1%
Dermatologic				
Sweating	14%	6%	9%	2%
Gastrointestinal				
Nausea	23%	17%	25%	7%
Dry mouth	18%	11%	9%	3%
Constipation	8%	5%	5%	2%
Diarrhea	12%	7%	9%	6%
Decreased appetite	7%	3%	8%	2%
Dyspepsia	—	—	4%	2%
Flatulence	—	—	4%	2%
Increased appetite	2%	1%	—	—
Vomiting	—	—	2%	1%
Musculoskeletal				
Myalgia	—	—	4%	3%
Nervous System				
Insomnia	18%	10%	21%	16%
Somnolence	19%	11%	22%	5%
Dizziness	14%	10%	11%	7%
Tremor	9%	1%	9%	1%
Nervousness	—	—	8%	7%
Libido decreased	9%	1%	12%	1%
Agitation	5%	4%	3%	1%
Anxiety	5%	4%	5%	4%
Concentration impaired	—	—	4%	1%
Myoclonus	3%	2%	2%	1%
Respiratory System				
Rhinitis	3%	0%	—	—
Pharyngitis	—	—	4%	2%
Yawn	—	—	5%	1%
Special Senses				
Abnormal vision	—	—	4%	1%
Urogenital System				
Abnormal ejaculation†	21%	1%	28%	1%
Dysmenorrhea	—	—	5%	4%
Female genial disorder†	9%	1%	9%	1%
Impotence†	5%	0%	5%	1%
Urinary frequency	2%	0%	—	—
Urinary tract infection	2%	1%	—	—

* Events reported by at least 2% of panic disorder and social anxiety disorder Paxil-treated patients are included, except the following events which had an incidence on placebo ≥ Paxil: *Panic disorder* : Abnormal dreams, abnormal vision, chest pain, cough increased, depersonalization, depression, dysmenorrhea, dyspepsia, flu syndrome, headache, infection, myalgia, nervousness, palpitation, paresthesia, pharyngitis, rash, respiratory disorder, sinusitis, taste perversion, trauma, urination impaired and vasodilation. *Social anxiety disorder* : Abdominal pain, depression, headache, infection, respiratory disorder, and sinusitis.
† Percentage corrected for gender.

ECG Changes

In an analysis of ECGs obtained in 682 patients treated with Paxil and 415 patients treated with placebo in controlled clinical trials, no clinically significant changes were seen in the ECGs of either group.

Liver Function Tests

In placebo-controlled clinical trials, patients treated with Paxil exhibited abnormal values on liver function tests at no greater rate than that seen in placebo-treated patients. In particular, the Paxil-vs-placebo comparisons for alkaline phosphatase, SGOT, SGPT and bilirubin revealed no differences in the percentage of patients with marked abnormalities.

Other Events Observed During the Premarketing Evaluation of Paxil

During its premarketing assessment in major depressive disorder, multiple doses of Paxil were administered to 6145 patients in Phase 2 and 3 studies. The conditions and duration of exposure to Paxil varied greatly and included (in overlapping categories) open and double-blind studies, uncontrolled and controlled studies, inpatient and outpatient studies, and fixed-dose and titration studies. During premarketing clinical trials in OCD, panic disorder, social anxiety disorder, generalized anxiety disorder and posttraumatic stress disorder, 542, 469, 522, 735 and 676 patients, respectively, received multiple doses of Paxil. Untoward events associated with this exposure were recorded by clinical investigators using terminology of their own choosing. Consequently, it is not possible to provide a meaningful estimate of the proportion of individuals experiencing adverse events without first grouping similar types of untoward events into a smaller number of standardized event categories.

In the tabulations that follow, reported adverse events were classified using a standard COSTART-based Dictionary terminology. The frequencies presented, therefore, represent the proportion of the 9089 patients exposed to multiple doses of Paxil who experienced an event of the type cited on at least one occasion while receiving Paxil. All reported events are included except those already listed in TABLES 3-5, those reported in terms so general as to be uninformative and those events where a drug cause was remote. It is important to emphasize that although the events reported occurred during treatment with paroxetine, they were not necessarily caused by it.

Events are further categorized by body system and listed in order of decreasing frequency according to the following definitions: *frequent* adverse events are those occurring on one or more occasions in at least 1/100 patients (only those not already listed in the tabulated results from placebo-controlled trials appear in this listing); *infrequent* adverse events are

TABLE 5 *Treatment-Emergent Adverse Experience Incidence in Placebo-Controlled Clinical Trials for Generalized Anxiety Disorder and Posttraumatic Stress Disorder**

	Generalized Anxiety Disorder		Posttraumatic Stress Disorder	
Body System	**Paxil**	**Placebo**	**Paxil**	**Placebo**
Preferred Term	**(n=735)**	**(n=529)**	**(n=676)**	**(n=504)**
Body as a Whole				
Asthenia	14%	6%	12%	4%
Headache	17%	14%	—	—
Infection	6%	3%	5%	4%
Abdominal pain			4%	3%
Trauma			6%	5%
Cardiovascular				
Vasodilation	3%	1%	2%	1%
Dermatologic				
Sweating	6%	2%	5%	1%
Gastrointestinal				
Nausea	20%	5%	19%	8%
Dry mouth	11%	5%	10%	5%
Constipation	10%	2%	5%	3%
Diarrhea	9%	7%	11%	5%
Decreased appetite	5%	1%	6%	3%
Vomiting	3%	2%	3%	2%
Dyspepsia	—	—	5%	3%
Nervous System				
Insomnia	11%	8%	12%	11%
Somnolence	15%	5%	16%	5%
Dizziness	6%	5%	6%	5%
Tremor	5%	1%	4%	1%
Nervousness	4%	3%	—	—
Libido decreased	9%	2%	5%	2%
Abnormal dreams			3%	2%
Respiratory System				
Respiratory disorder	7%	5%	—	—
Sinusitis	4%	3%	—	—
Yawn	4%	—	2%	<1%
Special Senses				
Abnormal vision	2%	1%	3%	1%
Urogenital System				
Abnormal ejaculation†	25%	2%	13%	2%
Female genital disorder†	4%	1%	5%	1%
Impotence	4%	3%	9%	1%

* Events reported by at least 2% of GAD and PTSD Paxil-treated patients are included, except the following events which had an incidence on placebo ≥Paxil: *GAD* : Abdominal pain, back pain, trauma, dyspepsia, myalgia, and pharyngitis. *PTSD* : Back pain, headache, anxiety, depression, nervousness, respiratory disorder, pharyngitis and sinusitis.

† Percentage corrected for gender.

TABLE 6 *Treatment-Emergent Adverse Experience Incidence in a Dose-Comparison Trial in the Treatment of Major Depressive Disorder**

Body System	**Placebo**	**Paxil 10 mg**	**Paxil 20 mg**	**Paxil 30 mg**	**Paxil 40 mg**
Preferred Term	**n=51**	**n=102**	**n=104**	**n=101**	**n=102**
Body as a Whole					
Asthenia	0.0%	2.9%	10.6%	13.9%	12.7%
Dermatology					
Sweating	2.0%	1.0%	6.7%	8.9%	11.8%
Gastrointestinal					
Constipation	5.9%	4.9%	7.7%	9.9%	12.7%
Decreased appetite	2.0%	2.0%	5.8%	4.0%	4.9%
Diarrhea	7.8%	9.8%	19.2%	7.9%	14.7%
Dry mouth	2.0%	10.8%	18.3%	15.8%	20.6%
Nausea	13.7%	14.7%	26.9%	34.7%	36.3%
Nervous System					
Anxiety	0.0%	2.0%	5.8%	5.9%	5.9%
Dizziness	3.9%	6.9%	6.7%	8.9%	12.7%
Nervousness	0.0%	5.9%	5.8%	4.0%	2.9%
Paresthesia	0.0%	2.9%	1.0%	5.0%	5.9%
Somnolence	7.8%	12.7%	18.3%	20.8%	21.6%
Tremor	0.0%	0.0%	7.7%	7.9%	14.7%
Special Senses					
Blurred vision	2.0%	2.9%	2.9%	2.0%	7.8%
Urogenital System					
Abnormal ejaculation	0.0%	5.8%	6.5%	10.6%	13.0%
Impotence	0.0%	1.9%	4.3%	6.4%	1.9%
Male genital disorders	0.0%	3.8%	8.7%	6.4%	3.7%

* Rule for including adverse events in table: incidence at least 5% for one of paroxetine groups and ≥ twice the placebo incidence for at least one paroxetine group.

those occurring in 1/100 to 1/1000 patients; *rare* events are those occurring in fewer than 1/1000 patients. Events of major clinical importance are also described in PRECAUTIONS, Paxil.

Body as a Whole: *Infrequent:* Allergic reaction, chills, face edema, malaise, neck pain; *Rare:* Adrenergic syndrome, cellulitis, moniliasis, neck rigidity, pelvic pain, peritonitis, sepsis, ulcer.

Cardiovascular System: *Frequent:* Hypertension, tachycardia; *Infrequent:* Bradycardia, hematoma, hypotension, migraine, syncope; *Rare:* Angina pectoris, arrhythmia nodal, atrial fibrillation, bundle branch block, cerebral ischemia, cerebrovascular accident, congestive heart failure, heart block, low cardiac output, myocardial infarct, myocardial ischemia, pallor, phlebitis, pulmonary embolus, supraventricular extrasystoles, thrombophlebitis, thrombosis, varicose vein, vascular headache, ventricular extrasystoles.

TABLE 7 *Incidence of Sexual Adverse Events in Controlled Clinical Trials*

	Paxil	**Placebo**
n (males)	**1446**	**1042**
Decreased libido	6-15%	0-5%
Ejaculatory disturbance	13-28%	0-2%
Impotence	2-9%	0-3%
n (females)	**1822**	**1340**
Decreased libido	0-9%	0-2%
Orgasmic disturbance	2-9%	0-1%

Digestive System: *Infrequent:* Bruxism, colitis, dysphagia, eructation, gastritis, gastroenteritis, gingivitis, glossitis, increased salivation, liver function tests abnormal, rectal hemorrhage, ulcerative stomatitis; *Rare:* Aphthous stomatitis, bloody diarrhea, bulimia, cardiospasm, cholelithiasis, duodenitis, enteritis, esophagitis, fecal impactions, fecal incontinence, gum hemorrhage, hematemesis, hepatitis, ileitis, ileus, intestinal obstruction, jaundice, melena, mouth ulceration, peptic ulcer, salivary gland enlargement, sialadenitis, stomach ulcer, stomatitis, tongue discoloration, tongue edema, tooth caries.

Endocrine System: *Rare:* Diabetes mellitus, goiter, hyperthyroidism, hypothyroidism, thyroiditis.

Hemic and Lymphatic Systems: *Infrequent:* Anemia, leukopenia, lymphadenopathy, purpura; *Rare:* Abnormal erythrocytes, basophilia, bleeding time increased, eosinophilia, hypochromic anemia, iron deficiency anemia, leukocytosis, lymphedema, abnormal lymphocytes, lymphocytosis, microcytic anemia, monocytosis, normocytic anemia, thrombocythemia, thrombocytopenia.

Metabolic and Nutritional: *Frequent:* Weight gain; *Infrequent:* Edema, peripheral edema, SGOT increased, SGPT increased, thirst, weight loss; *Rare:* Alkaline phosphatase increased, bilirubinemia, BUN increased, creatinine phosphokinase increased, dehydration, gamma globulins increased, gout, hypercalcemia, hypercholesteremia, hyperglycemia, hyperkalemia, hyperphosphatemia, hypocalcemia, hypoglycemia, hypokalemia, hyponatremia, ketosis, lactic dehydrogenase increased, non-protein nitrogen (NPN) increased.

Musculoskeletal System: *Frequent:* Arthralgia; *Infrequent:* Arthritis, arthrosis; *Rare:* Bursitis, myositis, osteoporosis, generalized spasm, tenosynovitis, tetany.

Nervous System: *Frequent:* Emotional lability, vertigo; *Infrequent:* Abnormal thinking, alcohol abuse, ataxia, dystonia, dyskinesia, euphoria, hallucinations, hostility, hypertonia, hypesthesia, hypokinesia, incoordination, lack of emotion, libido increased, manic reaction, neurosis, paralysis, paranoid reaction; *Rare:* Abnormal gait, akinesia, antisocial reaction, aphasia, choreoathetosis, circumoral paresthesias, convulsion, delirium, delusions, diplopia, drug dependence, dysarthria, extrapyramidal syndrome, fasciculations, grand mal convulsion, hyperalgesia, hysteria, manic-depressive reaction, meningitis, myelitis, neuralgia, neuropathy, nystagmus, peripheral neuritis, psychotic depression, reflexes decreased, reflexes increased, stupor, torticollis, trismus, withdrawal syndrome.

Respiratory System: *Infrequent:* Asthma, bronchitis, dyspnea, epistaxis, hyperventilation, pneumonia, respiratory flu; *Rare:* Emphysema, hemoptysis, hiccups, lung fibrosis, pulmonary edema, sputum increased, stridor, voice alteration.

Skin and Appendages: *Frequent:* Pruritus; *Infrequent:* Acne, alopecia, contact dermatitis, dry skin, ecchymosis, eczema, herpes simplex, photosensitivity, urticaria; *Rare:* Angioedema, erythema nodosum, erythema multiforme, exfoliative dermatitis, fungal dermatitis, furunculosis, herpes zoster, hirsutism, maculopapular rash, seborrhea, skin discoloration, skin hypertrophy, skin ulcer, sweating decreased, vesiculobullous rash.

Special Senses: *Frequent:* Tinnitus; *Infrequent:* Abnormality of accommodation, conjunctivitis, ear pain, eye pain, keratoconjunctivitis, mydriasis, otitis media; *Rare:* Amblyopia, anisocoria, blepharitis, cataract, conjunctival edema, corneal ulcer, deafness, exophthalmos, eye hemorrhage, glaucoma, hyperacusis, night blindness, otitis externa, parosmia, photophobia, ptosis, retinal hemorrhage, taste loss, visual field defect.

Urogenital System: *Infrequent:* Amenorrhea, breast pain, cystitis, dysuria, hematuria, menorrhagia, nocturia, polyuria, urinary incontinence, urinary retention, urinary urgency, vaginitis; *Rare:* Abortion, breast atrophy, breast enlargement, endometrial disorder, epididymitis, female lactation, fibrocystic breast, kidney calculus, kidney pain, leukorrhea, mastitis, metrorrhagia, nephritis, oliguria, salpingitis, urethritis, urinary casts, uterine spasm, urolith, vaginal hemorrhage, vaginal moniliasis.

Postmarketing Reports

Voluntary reports of adverse events in patients taking Paxil that have been received since market introduction and not listed above that may have no causal relationship with the drug include acute pancreatitis, elevated liver function tests (the most severe cases were deaths due to liver necrosis, and grossly elevated transaminases associated with severe liver dysfunction), Guillain-Barré syndrome, toxic epidermal necrolysis, priapism, syndrome of inappropriate ADH secretion, symptoms suggestive of prolactinemia and galactorrhea, neuroleptic malignant syndrome-like events; extrapyramidal symptoms which have included akathisia, bradykinesia, cogwheel rigidity, dystonia, hypertonia, oculogyric crisis which has been associated with concomitant use of pimozide, tremor and trismus; serotonin syndrome, associated in some cases with concomitant use of serotonergic drugs and with drugs which may have impaired Paxil metabolism (symptoms have included agitation, confusion, diaphoresis, hallucinations, hyperreflexia, myoclonus, shivering, tachycardia and tremor), status epilepticus, acute renal failure, pulmonary hypertension, allergic alveolitis, anaphylaxis, eclampsia, laryngismus, optic neuritis, porphyria, ventricular fibrillation, ventricular tachycardia (including torsade de pointes), thrombocytopenia, hemolytic anemia, and events related to impaired hematopoiesis (including aplastic anemia, pancytopenia, bone marrow aplasia, and agranulocytosis), and vasculitic snydromes (such as Henoch-Schönlein purpura. There has been a case report of an elevated phenytoin level after 4 weeks of Paxil and phenytoin coadministration. There has been a case report of severe hypotension when Paxil was added to chronic metoprolol treatment.

PAXIL CR

The information included in "Adverse Findings Observed in Short-Term, Placebo-Controlled Trials With Paxil CR" is based on data from six placebo-controlled clinical trials. Three of these studies were conducted in patients with major depressive disorder and three studies were done in patients with panic disorder. Two of the studies in major depressive disorder, which enrolled patients in the age range 18-65 years, are pooled. Information from a third study of major depressive disorder, which focused on elderly patients (ages 60-88), is presented separately as is the information from the panic disorder studies. Information on additional adverse events associated with Paxil CR and the immediate-release formulation of paroxetine HCl is included in a separate subsection (see Other Events Observed During the Clinical Development of Paxil CR).

Adverse Findings Observed in Short-Term, Placebo-Controlled Trials With Paxil CR

Adverse Events Associated With Discontinuation of Treatment

Major Depressive Disorder

Ten percent (21/212) of Paxil CR patients discontinued treatment due to an adverse event in a pool of two studies of patients with major depressive disorder. The most common events (≥1%) associated with discontinuation and considered to be drug related (*i.e.,* those events associated with dropout at a rate approximately twice or greater for Paxil CR compared to placebo) included the following (see TABLE 8).

TABLE 8

	Paxil CR (n=212)	Placebo (n=211)
Nausea	3.7%	0.5%
Asthenia	1.9%	0.5%
Dizziness	1.4%	0.0%
Somnolence	1.4%	0.0%

In a placebo-controlled study of elderly patients with major depressive disorder, 13% (13/104) of Paxil CR patients discontinued due to an adverse event. Events meeting the above criteria included the following (see TABLE 9).

TABLE 9

	Paxil CR (n=104)	Placebo (n=109)
Nausea	2.9%	0.0%
Headache	1.9%	0.9%
Depression	1.9%	0.0%
LFTs abnormal	1.9%	0.0%

Panic Disorder

Eleven percent (50/444) of Paxil CR patients in panic disorder studies discontinued treatment due to an adverse event. Events meeting the above criteria included the following (see TABLE 10).

TABLE 10

	Paxil CR (n=444)	Placebo (n=445)
Nausea	2.9%	0.4%
Insomnia	1.8%	0.0%
Headache	1.4%	0.2%
Asthenia	1.1%	0.0%

Commonly Observed Adverse Events

Major Depressive Disorder

The most commonly observed adverse events associated with the use of Paxil CR in a pool of two trials (incidence of 5.0% or greater and incidence for Paxil CR at least twice that for placebo, derived from TABLE 11) were: abnormal ejaculation, abnormal vision, constipation, decreased libido, diarrhea, dizziness, female genital disorders, nausea, somnolence, sweating, trauma, tremor, and yawning.

Using the same criteria, the adverse events associated with the use of Paxil CR in a study of elderly patients with major depressive disorder were: abnormal ejaculation, constipation, decreased appetite, dry mouth, impotence, infection, libido decreased, sweating, and tremor.

Panic Disorder

In the pool of panic disorder studies, the adverse events meeting these criteria were: abnormal ejaculation, somnolence, impotence, libido decreased, tremor, sweating, and female genital disorders (generally anorgasmia or difficulty achieving orgasm).

Incidence in Controlled Clinical Trials

TABLE 11 enumerates adverse events that occurred at an incidence of 1% or more among Paxil CR-treated patients, aged 18-65, who participated in two short-term (12 week) placebo-controlled trials in major depressive disorder in which patients were dosed in a range of 25 to 62.5 mg/day.

TABLE 12 enumerates adverse events reported at an incidence of 5% or greater among elderly Paxil CR-treated patients (ages 60-88) who participated in a short-term (12 week) placebo-controlled trial in major depressive disorder in which patients were dosed in a range of 12.5 to 50 mg/day.

TABLE 13 enumerates adverse events reported at an incidence of 1% or greater among Paxil CR-treated patients (ages 19-72) who participated in short-term (10 week) placebo-controlled trials in panic disorder in which patients were dosed in a range of 12.5 to 75 mg/day.

Reported adverse events were classified using a standard COSTART-based Dictionary terminology.

The prescriber should be aware that these figures cannot be used to predict the incidence of side effects in the course of usual medical practice where patient characteristics and other factors differ from those which prevailed in the clinical trials. Similarly, the cited frequencies cannot be compared with figures obtained from other clinical investigations involving different treatments, uses and investigators. The cited figures, however, do provide the prescribing physician with some basis for estimating the relative contribution of drug and non-drug factors to the side effect incidence rate in the population studied.

TABLE 11 *Treatment Emergent Adverse Events Occurring in ≥1% of Paxil CR Patients in a Pool of Two Studies in Major Depressive Disorder*†*

Body System / Adverse Event	Paxil CR (n=212)	Placebo (n=211)
Body as a Whole		
Headache	27%	20%
Asthenia	14%	9%
Infection‡	8%	5%
Abdominal pain	7%	4%
Back pain	5%	3%
Trauma§	5%	1%
Pain¤	3%	1%
Allergic reaction¶	2%	1%
Cardiovascular System		
Tachycardia	1%	0%
Vasodilation**	2%	0%
Digestive System		
Nausea	22%	10%
Diarrhea	18%	7%
Dry mouth	15%	8%
Constipation	10%	4%
Flatulence	6%	4%
Decreased appetite	4%	2%
Vomiting	2%	1%
Nervous System		
Somnolence	22%	8%
Insomnia	17%	9%
Dizziness	14%	4%
Libido decreased	7%	3%
Tremor	7%	1%
Hypertonia	3%	1%
Paresthesia	3%	1%
Agitation	2%	1%
Confusion	1%	0%
Respiratory System		
Yawn	5%	0%
Rhinitis	4%	1%
Cough increased	2%	1%
Bronchitis	1%	0%
Skin and Appendages		
Sweating	6%	2%
Photosensitivity	2%	0%
Special Senses		
Abnormal vision††	5%	1%
Taste perversion	2%	0%
Urogential System		
Abnormal ejaculation‡‡ §§	26%	1%
Female genital disorder‡‡ ¤¤	10%	<1%
Impotence‡‡	5%	3%
Urinary tract infection	3%	1%
Menstrual disorder‡‡	2%	<1%
Vaginitis‡‡	2%	0%

* Adverse events for which the Paxil CR reporting incidence was less than or equal to the placebo incidence are not included. These events are: abnormal dreams, anxiety, arthralgia, depersonalization, dysmenorrhea, dyspepsia, hyperkinesia, increased appetite, myalgia, nervousness, pharyngitis, purpura, rash, respiratory disorder, sinusitis, urinary frequency, and weight gain.
† <1% means greater than zero and less than 1%.
‡ Mostly flu.
§ A wide variety of injuries with no obvious pattern.
¤ Pain in a variety of locations with no obvious pattern.
¶ Most frequently seasonal allergic symptoms.
** Usually flushing.
†† Mostly blurred vision.
‡‡ Based on the number of males or females.
§§ Mostly anorgasmia or delayed ejaculation.
¤¤ Mostly anorgasmia or delayed orgasm.

Dose Dependency of Adverse Events

A comparison of adverse event rates in a fixed-dose study comparing immediate-release paroxetine with placebo in the treatment of major depressive disorder revealed a clear dose dependency for some of the more common adverse events associated with the use of immediate-release paroxetine.

Male and Female Sexual Dysfunction With SSRIs

Although changes in sexual desire, sexual performance and sexual satisfaction often occur as manifestations of a psychiatric disorder, they may also be a consequence of pharmacologic treatment. In particular, some evidence suggests that selective serotonin reuptake inhibitors (SSRIs) can cause such untoward sexual experiences.

Reliable estimates of the incidence and severity of untoward experiences involving sexual desire, performance and satisfaction are difficult to obtain, however, in part because patients and physicians may be reluctant to discuss them. Accordingly, estimates of the incidence of

TABLE 12 *Treatment Emergent Adverse Events Occurring in ≥5% of Paxil CR Patients in a Study of Elderly Patients With Major Depressive Disorder*†*

Body System / Adverse Event	Paxil CR (n=104)	Placebo (n=109)
Body as a Whole		
Headache	17%	13%
Asthenia	15%	14%
Trauma	8%	5%
Infection	6%	2%
Digestive System		
Dry mouth	18%	7%
Diarrhea	15%	9%
Constipation	13%	5%
Dyspepsia	13%	10%
Decreased appetite	12%	5%
Flatulence	8%	7%
Nervous System		
Somnolence	21%	12%
Insomnia	10%	8%
Dizziness	9%	5%
Libido decreased	8%	<1%
Tremor	7%	0%
Skin and Appendages		
Sweating	10%	<1%
Urogenital System		
Abnormal ejaculation‡§	17%	3%
Impotence‡	9%	3%

* Adverse events for which the Paxil CR reporting incidence was less than or equal to the placebo incidence are not included. These events are nausea and respiratory disorder.
† <1% means greater than zero and less than 1%.
‡ Based on the number of males.
§ Mostly anorgasmia or delayed ejaculation.

TABLE 13 *Treatment-Emergent Adverse Events Occuring in ≥1% of Paxil CR Patients in a Pool of Three Panic Disorder Studies*†*

Body System / Adverse Event	Paxil CR (n=444)	Placebo (n=445)
Body as a Whole		
Asthenia	15%	10%
Abdominal pain	6%	4%
Trauma‡	5%	4%
Cardiovascular System		
Vasodilatation§	3%	2%
Digestive System		
Nausea	23%	17%
Dry mouth	13%	9%
Diarrhea	12%	9%
Constipation	9%	6%
Decreased appetite	8%	6%
Metabolic/Nutritional Disorders		
Weight loss	1%	0%
Musculoskeletal System		
Myalgia	5%	3%
Nervous System		
Insomnia	20%	11%
Somnolence	20%	9%
Libido decreased	9%	4%
Nervousness	8%	7%
Tremor	8%	2%
Anxiety	5%	4%
Agitation	3%	2%
Hypertonia¤	2%	<1%
Myoclonus	2%	<1%
Respiratory System		
Sinusitis	8%	5%
Yawning	3%	0%
Skin and Appendages		
Sweating	7%	2%
Special Senses		
Abnormal vision¶	3%	<1%
Urogenital System		
Abnormal ejaculation**,††	27%	3%
Impotence**	10%	1%
Female genital disorders‡‡,§§	7%	1%
Urinary frequency	2%	<1%
Urination impaired	2%	<1%
Vaginitis‡‡	1%	<1%

* Adverse events for which the Paxil CR reporting rate was less than or equal to the placebo rate are not included. These events are: abnormal dreams, allergic reaction, back pain, bronchitis, chest pain, concentration impaired, confusion, cough increased, depression, dizziness, dysmenorrhea, dyspepsia, fever, flatulence, headache, increased appetite, infection, menstrual disorder, migraine, pain, paresthesia, pharyngitis, respiratory disorder, rhinitis, tachycardia, taste perversion, thinking abnormal, urinary tract infection, and vomiting.
† <1% means greater than zero and less than 1%.
‡ Various physical injuries.
§ Mostly flushing.
¤ Mostly muscle tightness or stiffness.
¶ Mostly blurred vision.
** Based on the number of male patients.
† Mostly anorgasmia or delayed ejaculation.
‡‡ Based on the number of female patients.
§§ Mostly anorgasmia or difficulty achieving orgasm.

untoward sexual experience and performance cited in product labeling, are likely to underestimate their actual incidence.

The percentage of patients reporting symptoms of sexual dysfunction in the pool of two placebo-controlled trials in non-elderly patients with major depressive disorder and in the pool of three placebo-controlled trials in patients with panic disorder are as follows (see TABLE 14).

TABLE 14

	Major Depressive Disorder		Panic Disorder	
	Paxil CR	Placebo	Paxil CR	Placebo
n (males)	78	78	162	194
Decreased libido	10%	5%	9%	6%
Ejaculatory disturbance	26%	1%	27%	3%
Impotence	5%	3%	10%	1%
n (females)	134	133	282	251
Decreased libido	4%	2%	8%	2%
Orgasmic disturbance	10%	<1%	7%	1%

There are no adequate, controlled studies examining sexual dysfunction with paroxetine treatment.

Paroxetine treatment has been associated with several cases of priapism. In those cases with a known outcome, patients recovered without sequelae.

While it is difficult to know the precise risk of sexual dysfunction associated with the use of SSRIs, physicians should routinely inquire about such possible side effects.

Weight and Vital Sign Changes

Significant weight loss may be an undesirable result of treatment with paroxetine for some patients but, on average, patients in controlled trials with Paxil CR, or the immediate-release formulation, had minimal weight loss (about 1 pound). No significant changes in vital signs (systolic and diastolic blood pressure, pulse and temperature) were observed in patients treated with Paxil CR, or immediate-release paroxetine HCl, in controlled clinical trials.

ECG Changes

In an analysis of ECGs obtained in 682 patients treated with immediate-release paroxetine and 415 patients treated with placebo in controlled clinical trials, no clinically significant changes were seen in the ECGs of either group.

Liver Function Tests

In a pool of two placebo-controlled clinical trials, patients treated with Paxil CR or placebo exhibited abnormal values on liver function tests at comparable rates. In particular, the controlled-release paroxetine-vs-placebo comparisons for alkaline phosphatase, SGOT, SGPT and bilirubin revealed no differences in the percentage of patients with marked abnormalities.

In a study of elderly patients with major depressive disorder, 3 of 104 Paxil CR patients and none of 109 placebo patients experienced liver transaminase elevations of potential clinical concern. Two (2) of the Paxil CR patients dropped out of the study due to abnormal liver function tests; the third patient experienced normalization of transaminase levels with continued treatment. Also, in the pool of three studies of patients with panic disorder, 4 of 444 Paxil CR patients and none of 445 placebo patients experienced liver transaminase elevations of potential clinical concern. Elevations in all 4 patients decreased substantially after discontinuation of Paxil CR. The clinical significance of these findings is unknown.

In placebo-controlled clincial trials with the immediate release formulation of paroxetine, patients exhibited abnormal values on liver function tests at no greater rate than that seen in placebo-treated patients.

Other Events Observed During the Clinical Development of Paxil CR

The following adverse events were reported during the clinical development of Paxil CR tablets and/or the clinical development of the immediate-release formulation of paroxetine.

Adverse events for which frequencies are provided below occurred in clinical trials with the controlled-release formulation of paroxetine. During its premarketing assessment in major depressive disorder and panic disorder, multiple doses of Paxil CR were administered to 760 patients in Phase 3 double-blind, controlled, outpatient studies. Untoward events associated with this exposure were recorded by clinical investigators using terminology of their own choosing. Consequently, it is not possible to provide a meaningful estimate of the proportion of individuals experiencing adverse events without first grouping similar types of untoward events into a smaller number of standardized event categories.

In the tabulations that follow, reported adverse events were classified using a COSTART-based dictionary. The frequencies presented, therefore, represent the proportion of the 760 patients exposed to Paxil CR controlled-release who experienced an event of the type cited on at least one occasion while receiving Paxil CR. All reported events are included except those already listed in TABLE 11, TABLE 12, or TABLE 13 and those events where a drug cause was remote. If the COSTART term for an event was so general as to be uninformative, it was deleted or, when possible, replaced with a more informative term. It is important to emphasize that although the events reported occurred during treatment with paroxetine, they were not necessarily caused by it.

Events are further categorized by body system and listed in order of decreasing frequency according to the following definitions: *frequent* adverse events are those occurring on one or more occasions in at least 1/100 patients (only those not already listed in the tabulated results from placebo-controlled trials appear in this listing); *infrequent* adverse events are those occurring in 1/100 to 1/1000 patients.

Adverse events for which frequencies are not provided occurred during the premarketing assessment of immediate-release paroxetine in Phase 2 and 3 studies of major depressive disorder, obsessive compulsive disorder, panic disorder, social anxiety disorder, generalized anxiety disorder, and posttraumatic stress disorder. The conditions and duration of exposure to immediate-release paroxetine varied greatly and included (in overlapping categories) open and double-blind studies, uncontrolled and controlled studies, inpatient and outpatient studies, and fixed-dose and titration studies. Only those events not previously listed for controlled-release paroxetine are included. The extent to which these events may be associated with Paxil CR is unknown.

P

Events are listed alphabetically within the respective body system. Events of major clinical importance are also described in PRECAUTIONS, Paxil CR.

Body as a Whole: *Infrequent:* Anaphylactoid reaction, chills, flu syndrome, malaise; also observed were adrenergic syndrome, face edema, neck rigidity, sepsis.

Cardiovascular System: *Frequent:* Hypertension, hypotension; *Infrequent:* Angina pectoris, bradycardia, bundle branch block, palpitation, postural hypotension, syncope; also observed were arrhythmia nodal, atrial fibrillation, cerebrovascular accident, congestive heart failure, hematoma, low cardiac output, myocardial infarct, myocardial ischemia, pallor, phlebitis, pulmonary embolus, supraventricular extrasystoles, thrombophlebitis, thrombosis, vascular headache, ventricular extrasystoles.

Digestive System: *Infrequent:* Bruxism, dysphagia, eructation, gastroenteritis, gastroesophageal reflux, gingivitis, glossitis, gum hyperplasia, hemorrhoids, hepatosplenomegaly, increased salivation, intestinal obstruction, melena, pancreatitis, peptic ulcer, rectal hemorrhage, stomach ulcer, toothache, ulcerative stomatitis; also observed were aphthous stomatitis, bloody diarrhea, bulimia, cardiospasm, cholelithiasis, colitis, duodenitis, enteritis, esophagitis, fecal impactions, fecal incontinence, gastritis, gum hemorrhage, hematemesis, hepatitis, ileitis, ileus, jaundice, mouth ulceration, salivary gland enlargement, sialadenitis, stomatitis, throat tightness, tongue discoloration, tongue edema.

Endocrine System: *Infrequent:* Hyperthyroidism, ovarian cyst, testes pain; also observed were diabetes mellitus, goiter, hypothyroidism, thyroiditis.

Hemic and Lymphatic System: *Infrequent:* Anemia, eosinophilia, leukocytosis, leukopenia, lymphadenopathy, thrombocytopenia; also observed were anisocytosis, basophilia, bleeding time increased, hypochromic anemia, lymphedema, lymphocytosis, lymphopenia, microcytic anemia, monocytosis, normocytic anemia, thrombocythemia.

Metabolic and Nutritional Disorders: *Infrequent:* Bilirubinemia, dehydration, generalized edema, hyperglycemia, hyperkalemia, hypokalemia, peripheral edema, SGOT increased, SGPT increased, thirst; also observed were alkaline phosphatase increased, BUN increased, creatinine phosphokinase increased, gamma globulins increased, gout, hypercalcemia, hypercholesteremia, hyperphosphatemia, hypocalcemia, hypoglycemia, hyponatremia, ketosis, lactic dehydrogenase increased, non-protein nitrogen (NPN) increased.

Musculoskeletal System: *Infrequent:* Arthritis, bursitis, myasthenia, myopathy, myositis, tendonitis; also observed were generalized spasm, osteoporosis, tenosynovitis, tetany.

Nervous System: *Infrequent:* Amnesia, ataxia, convulsion, diplopia, dystonia, emotional lability, hallucinations, hypesthesia, hypokinesia, incoordination, neuralgia, neuropathy, nystagmus, paralysis, paranoid reaction, vertigo, withdrawal syndrome; also observed were abnormal gait, akathisia, akinesia, aphasia, choreoathetosis, circumoral paresthesia, delirium, delusions, dysarthria, dyskinesia, euphoria, extrapyramidal syndrome, fasciculations, grand mal convulsion, hostility, hyperalgesia, irritability, libido increased, manic reaction, manic-depressive reaction, meningitis, myelitis, peripheral neuritis, psychosis, psychotic depression, reflexes decreased, reflexes increased, stupor, torticollis, trismus.

Respiratory System: *Infrequent:* Asthma, dyspnea, epistaxis, laryngitis, pneumonia, stridor; also observed were dysphonia, emphysema, hemoptysis, hiccups, hyperventilation, lung fibrosis, pulmonary edema, respiratory flu, sputum increased.

Skin and Appendages: *Infrequent:* Acne, alopecia, dry skin, eczema, exfoliative dermatitis, furunculosis, pruritus, seborrhea, urticaria; also observed were angioedema, ecchymosis, erythema multiforme, erythema nodosum, hirsutism, maculopapular rash, skin discoloration, skin hypertrophy, skin ulcer, sweating decreased, vesiculobullous rash.

Special Senses: *Infrequent:* Abnormality of accommodation, conjunctivitis, earache, keratoconjunctivitis, mydriasis, photophobia, retinal hemorrhage, tinnitus, visual field defect; also observed were amblyopia, anisocoria, blepharitis, blurred vision, cataract, conjunctival edema, corneal ulcer, deafness, exophthalmos, glaucoma, hyperacusis, night blindness, parosmia, ptosis, taste loss.

Urogenital System: *Infrequent:* Albuminuria, amenorrhea*, breast enlargement*, breast pain*, cystitis, dysuria, hematuria, kidney calculus, menorrhagia*, nocturia, prostatitis*, urinary incontinence, urinary retention; also observed were breast atrophy, ejaculatory disturbance, endometrial disorder, epididymitis, female lactation, fibrocystic breast, leukorrhea, mastitis, metrorrhagia, nephritis, oliguria, polyuria, pyuria, salpingitis, urinary casts, urethritis, urinary urgency, urolith, uterine spasm, vaginal hemorrhage.

*Based on the number of men and women as appropriate.

Postmarketing Reports

Voluntary reports of adverse events in patients taking immediate-release paroxetine HCl that have been received since market introduction and not listed above that may have no causal relationship with the drug include acute pancreatitis, elevated liver function tests (the most severe cases were deaths due to liver necrosis, and grossly elevated transaminases associated with severe liver dysfunction), Guillain-Barré syndrome, toxic epidermal necrolysis, priapism, syndrome of inappropriate ADH secretion, symptoms suggestive of prolactinemia and galactorrhea, neuroleptic malignant syndrome-like events; extrapyramidal symptoms which have included akathisia, bradykinesia, cogwheel rigidity, dystonia, hypertonia, oculogyric crisis which has been associated with concomitant use of pimozide, tremor and trismus; serotonin syndrome, associated in some cases with concomitant use of serotonergic drugs and with drugs which may have impaired paroxetine metabolism (symptoms have included agitation, confusion, diaphoresis, hallucinations, hyperreflexia, myoclonus, shivering, tachycardia and tremor); status epilepticus, acute renal failure, pulmonary hypertension, allergic alveolitis, anaphylaxis, eclampsia, laryngismus, optic neuritis, porphyria, ventricular fibrillation, ventricular tachycardia (including torsade de pointes), thrombocytopenia, hemolytic anemia, events related to impaired hematopoiesis (including aplastic anemia, pancytopenia, bone marrow aplasia, and agranulocytosis), and vasculitic syndromes (such as Henoch-Schönlein purpura). There has been a case report of an elevated phenytoin level after 4 weeks of immediate-release paroxetine and phenytoin coadministration. There has been a case report of severe hypotension when immediate-release paroxetine was added to chronic metoprolol treatment.

DOSAGE AND ADMINISTRATION

PAXIL

Major Depressive Disorder

Usual Initial Dosage

Paxil should be administered as a single daily dose with or without food, usually in the morning. The recommended initial dose is 20 mg/day. Patients were dosed in a range of 20-50 mg/day in the clinical trials demonstrating the effectiveness of Paxil in the treatment of major depressive disorder. As with all drugs effective in the treatment of major depressive disorder, the full effect may be delayed. Some patients not responding to a 20 mg dose may benefit from dose increases, in 10 mg/day increments, up to a maximum of 50 mg/day. Dose changes should occur at intervals of at least 1 week.

Maintenance Therapy

There is no body of evidence available to answer the question of how long the patient treated with Paxil should remain on it. It is generally agreed that acute episodes of major depressive disorder require several months or longer of sustained pharmacologic therapy. Whether the dose needed to induce remission is identical to the dose needed to maintain and/or sustain euthymia is unknown.

Systematic evaluation of the efficacy of Paxil has shown that efficacy is maintained for periods of up to 1 year with doses that averaged about 30 mg.

Obsessive Compulsive Disorder

Usual Initial Dosage

Paxil should be administered as a single daily dose with or without food, usually in the morning. The recommended dose of Paxil in the treatment of OCD is 40 mg daily. Patients should be started on 20 mg/day and the dose can be increased in 10 mg/day increments. Dose changes should occur at intervals of at least 1 week. Patients were dosed in a range of 20-60 mg/day in the clinical trials demonstrating the effectiveness of Paxil in the treatment of OCD. The maximum dosage should not exceed 60 mg/day.

Maintenance Therapy

Long-term maintenance of efficacy was demonstrated in a 6 month relapse prevention trial. In this trial, patients with OCD assigned to paroxetine demonstrated a lower relapse rate compared to patients on placebo. OCD is a chronic condition, and it is reasonable to consider continuation for a responding patient. Dosage adjustments should be made to maintain the patient on the lowest effective dosage, and patients should be periodically reassessed to determine the need for continued treatment.

Panic Disorder

Usual Initial Dosage

Paxil should be administered as a single daily dose with or without food, usually in the morning. The target dose of Paxil in the treatment of panic disorder is 40 mg/day. Patients should be started on 10 mg/day. Dose changes should occur in 10 mg/day increments and at intervals of at least 1 week. Patients were dosed in a range of 10-60 mg/day in the clinical trials demonstrating the effectiveness of Paxil. The maximum dosage should not exceed 60 mg/day.

Maintenance Therapy

Long-term maintenance of efficacy was demonstrated in a 3 month relapse prevention trial. In this trial, patients with panic disorder assigned to paroxetine demonstrated a lower relapse rate compared to patients on placebo. Panic disorder is a chronic condition, and it is reasonable to consider continuation for a responding patient. Dosage adjustments should be made to maintain the patient on the lowest effective dosage, and patients should be periodically reassessed to determine the need for continued treatment.

Social Anxiety Disorder

Usual Initial Dosage

Paxil should be administered as a single daily dose with or without food, usually in the morning. The recommended and initial dosage is 20 mg/day. In clinical trials the effectiveness of Paxil was demonstrated in patients dosed in a range of 20-60 mg/day. While the safety of Paxil has been evaluated in patients with social anxiety disorder at doses up to 60 mg/day, available information does not suggest any additional benefit for doses above 20 mg/day.

Maintenance Therapy

There is no body of evidence available to answer the question of how long the patient treated with Paxil should remain on it. Although the efficacy of Paxil beyond 12 weeks of dosing has not been demonstrated in controlled clinical trials, social anxiety disorder is recognized as a chronic condition, and it is reasonable to consider continuation of treatment for a responding patient. Dosage adjustments should be made to maintain the patient on the lowest effective dosage, and patients should be periodically reassessed to determine the need for continued treatment.

Generalized Anxiety Disorder

Usual Initial Dosage

Paxil should be administered as a single daily dose with or without food, usually in the morning. In clinical trials the effectiveness of Paxil was demonstrated in patients dosed in a range of 20-50 mg/day. The recommended starting dosage and the established effective dosage is 20 mg/day. There is not sufficient evidence to suggest a greater benefit to doses higher than 20 mg/day. Dose changes should occur in 10 mg/day increments and at intervals of at least 1 week.

Maintenance Therapy
Systematic evaluation of continuing Paxil for periods of up to 24 weeks in patients with Generalized Anxiety Disorder who had responded while taking Paxil during an 8 week acute treatment phase has demonstrated a benefit of such maintenance. Nevertheless, patients should be periodically reassessed to determine the need for maintenance treatment.

Posttraumatic Stress Disorder
Usual Initial Dosage
Paxil should be administered as a single daily dose with or without food, usually in the morning. The recommended starting dosage and the established effective dosage is 20 mg/day. In one clinical trial, the effectiveness of Paxil was demonstrated in patients dosed in a range of 20-50 mg/day. However, in a fixed-dose study, there was not sufficient evidence to suggest a greater benefit for a dose of 40 mg/day compared to 20 mg/day. Dose changes, if indicated, should occur in 10 mg/day increments and at intervals of at least 1 week.

Maintenance Therapy
There is no body of evidence available to answer the question of how long the patient treated with Paxil should remain on it. Although the efficacy of Paxil beyond 12 weeks of dosing has not been demonstrated in controlled clinical trials, PTSD is recognized as a chronic condition, and it is reasonable to consider continuation of treatment for a responding patient. Dosage adjustments should be made to maintain the patient on the lowest effective dosage, and patients should be periodically reassessed to determine the need for continued treatment.

Dosage for Elderly or Debilitated, and Patients With Severe Renal or Hepatic Impairment
The recommended initial dose is 10 mg/day for elderly patients, debilitated patients, and/or patients with severe renal or hepatic impairment. Increases may be made if indicated. Dosage should not exceed 40 mg/day.

Switching Patients To or From a Monoamine Oxidase Inhibitor
At least 14 days should elapse between discontinuation of a MAOI and initiation of Paxil therapy. Similarly, at least 14 days should be allowed after stopping Paxil before starting a MAOI.

Discontinuation of Treatment With Paxil
Symptoms associated with discontinuation of Paxil have been reported (see PRECAUTIONS, Paxil). Patients should be monitored for these symptoms when discontinuing treatment, regardless of the indication for which Paxil is being prescribed. A gradual reduction in the dose rather than abrupt cessation is recommended whenever possible. If intolerable symptoms occur following a decrease in the dose or upon discontinuation of treatment, then resuming the previously prescribed dose may be considered. Subsequently, the physician may continue decreasing the dose but at a more gradual rate.
NOTE: SHAKE SUSPENSION WELL BEFORE USING.

PAXIL CR
Major Depressive Disorder
Usual Initial Dosage
Paxil CR should be administered as a single daily dose, usually in the morning, with or without food. The recommended initial dose is 25 mg/day. Patients were dosed in a range of 25 to 62.5 mg/day in the clinical trials demonstrating the effectiveness of Paxil CR in the treatment of major depressive disorder. As with all drugs effective in the treatment of major depressive disorder, the full effect may be delayed. Some patients not responding to a 25 mg dose may benefit from dose increases, in 12.5 mg/day increments, up to a maximum of 62.5 mg/day. Dose changes should occur at intervals of at least 1 week.

Patients should be cautioned that the Paxil CR tablet should not be chewed or crushed, and should be swallowed whole.

Maintenance Therapy
There is no body of evidence available to answer the question of how long the patient treated with Paxil CR should remain on it. It is generally agreed that acute episodes of major depressive disorder require several months or longer of sustained pharmacologic therapy. Whether the dose of an antidepressant needed to induce remission is identical to the dose needed to maintain and/or sustain euthymia is unknown.

Systematic evaluation of the efficacy of immediate-release paroxetine HCl has shown that efficacy is maintained for periods of up to 1 year with doses that averaged about 30 mg, which corresponds to a 37.5 mg dose of Paxil CR, based on relative bioavailability considerations (see CLINICAL PHARMACOLOGY, Paxil CR, Pharmacokinetics).

Panic Disorder
Usual Initial Dosage
Paxil CR should be administered as a single daily dose, usually in the morning. Patients should be started on 12.5 mg/day. Dose changes should occur in 12.5 mg/day increments and at intervals of at least 1 week. Patients were dosed in a range of 12.5 to 75 mg/day in the clinical trials demonstrating the effectiveness of Paxil CR. The maximum dosage should not exceed 75 mg/day.

Patients should be cautioned that the Paxil CR tablet should not be chewed or crushed, and should be swallowed whole.

Maintenance Therapy
Long-term maintenance of efficacy with the immediate-release formulation of paroxetine was demonstrated in a 3 month relapse prevention trial. In this trial, patients with panic disorder assigned to immediate-release paroxetine demonstrated a lower relapse rate compared to patients on placebo. Panic disorder is a chronic condition, and it is reasonable to consider continuation for a responding patient. Dosage adjustments should be made to maintain the patient on the lowest effective dosage, and patients should be periodically reassessed to determine the need for continued treatment.

Dosage for Elderly or Debilitated, and Patients With Severe Renal or Hepatic Impairment
The recommended initial dose of Paxil CR is 12.5 mg/day for elderly patients, debilitated patients, and/or patients with severe renal or hepatic impairment. Increases may be made if indicated. Dosage should not exceed 50 mg/day.

Switching Patients To or From a Monoamine Oxidase Inhibitor
At least 14 days should elapse between discontinuation of a MAOI and initiation of Paxil CR therapy. Similarly, at least 14 days should be allowed after stopping Paxil CR before starting a MAOI.

Discontinuation of Treatment With Paxil CR
Symptoms associated with discontinuation of immediate-release paroxetine HCl have been reported (see PRECAUTIONS, Paxil CR). Patients should be monitored for these symptoms when discontinuing treatment, regardless of the indication for which Paxil CR is being prescribed. A gradual reduction in the dose rather than abrupt cessation is recommended whenever possible. If intolerable symptoms occur following a decrease in the dose or upon discontinuation of treatment, then resuming the previously prescribed dose may be considered. Subsequently, the physician may continue decreasing the dose but at a more gradual rate.

HOW SUPPLIED

PAXIL TABLETS

Paxil is supplied as film-coated, modified-oval tablets as follows:

10 mg: Yellow, scored tablets engraved on the front with "PAXIL" and on the back with "10".

20 mg: Pink, scored tablets engraved on the front with "PAXIL" and on the back with "20".

30 mg: Blue tablets engraved on the front with "PAXIL" and on the back with "30".

40 mg: Green tablets engraved on the front with "PAXIL" and on the back with "40".

Storage: Store tablets between 15 and 30°C (59 and 86°F).

PAXIL ORAL SUSPENSION
Orange-colored, orange-flavored, 10 mg/5 ml, in 250 ml white bottles.
Storage: Store suspension at or below 25°C (77°F).

PAXIL CR

Paxil CR is supplied as an enteric film-coated, controlled-release, round tablet, as follows:

12.5 mg: Yellow tablets, engraved with "Paxil CR" and "12.5".

25 mg: Pink tablets, engraved with "Paxil CR" and "25".

37.5 mg: Blue tablets, engraved with "Paxil CR" and "37.5".

Storage: Store at or below 25°C (77°F).

PRODUCT LISTING - EQUIVALENTS NOT AVAILABLE

Suspension - Oral - 10 mg/5 ml			
250 ml	$140.49	PAXIL, Glaxosmithkline	00029-3215-48
Tablet - Oral - 10 mg			
30's	$69.95	PAXIL, Allscripts Pharmaceutical Company	54569-4787-00
30's	$73.49	PAXIL, Physicians Total Care	54868-4065-00
30's	$80.50	PAXIL, Pharma Pac	52959-0639-30
30's	$81.19	PAXIL, Southwood Pharmaceuticals Inc	58016-0661-30
30's	$84.44	PAXIL, Glaxosmithkline	00029-3210-13
60's	$162.38	PAXIL, Southwood Pharmaceuticals Inc	58016-0661-60
90's	$243.57	PAXIL, Southwood Pharmaceuticals Inc	58016-0661-90
100's	$270.63	PAXIL, Southwood Pharmaceuticals Inc	58016-0661-00
Tablet - Oral - 20 mg			
10's	$24.33	PAXIL, Southwood Pharmaceuticals Inc	58016-0372-10
10's	$24.33	PAXIL, Southwood Pharmaceuticals Inc	58016-0485-10
14's	$30.63	PAXIL, Allscripts Pharmaceutical Company	54569-3810-01
15's	$50.25	PAXIL, Pharma Pac	52959-0360-15
20's	$48.60	PAXIL, Southwood Pharmaceuticals Inc	58016-0372-20
20's	$48.60	PAXIL, Southwood Pharmaceuticals Inc	58016-0485-20
20's	$66.40	PAXIL, Pharma Pac	52959-0360-20
30's	$57.00	PAXIL, Cheshire Drugs	55175-2715-03
30's	$57.85	PAXIL, Compumed Pharmaceuticals	00403-4753-30
30's	$65.64	PAXIL, Allscripts Pharmaceutical Company	54569-3810-00
30's	$74.02	PAXIL, Physicians Total Care	54868-2976-02
30's	$80.51	PAXIL, Quality Care Pharmaceuticals Inc	60346-0993-30
30's	$81.45	PAXIL, Southwood Pharmaceuticals Inc	58016-0485-30
30's	$87.61	PAXIL, Pd-Rx Pharmaceuticals	55289-0216-30
30's	$88.10	PAXIL, Glaxosmithkline	00029-3211-13
30's	$99.30	PAXIL, Pharma Pac	52959-0360-30
40's	$97.20	PAXIL, Southwood Pharmaceuticals Inc	58016-0372-40
40's	$97.20	PAXIL, Southwood Pharmaceuticals Inc	58016-0485-40
60's	$162.90	PAXIL, Southwood Pharmaceuticals Inc	58016-0485-60
60's	$192.00	PAXIL, Pharma Pac	52959-0360-60
90's	$170.91	PAXIL, Allscripts Pharmaceutical Company	54569-8609-00
90's	$218.70	PAXIL, Southwood Pharmaceuticals Inc	58016-0372-90
90's	$218.70	PAXIL, Southwood Pharmaceuticals Inc	58016-0485-90
100's	$220.05	PAXIL, Physicians Total Care	54868-2976-00
100's	$271.50	PAXIL, Southwood Pharmaceuticals Inc	58016-0485-00
100's	$293.74	PAXIL, Glaxosmithkline	00029-3211-20
100's	$299.73	PAXIL, Glaxosmithkline	00029-3211-21
Tablet - Oral - 30 mg			
30's	$72.37	PAXIL, Physicians Total Care	54868-3526-00
30's	$90.76	PAXIL, Glaxosmithkline	00029-3212-13
Tablet - Oral - 40 mg			
15's	$39.70	PAXIL, Allscripts Pharmaceutical Company	54569-4901-01
30's	$79.40	PAXIL, Allscripts Pharmaceutical Company	54569-4901-00
30's	$95.88	PAXIL, Glaxosmithkline	00029-3213-13
Tablet, Extended Release - Oral - 12.5 mg			
30's	$84.44	PAXIL CR, Glaxosmithkline	00029-3206-13

P

Tablet, Extended Release - Oral - 25 mg
30's $88.10 PAXIL CR, Glaxosmithkline 00029-3207-13
Tablet, Extended Release - Oral - 37.5 mg
30's $90.76 PAXIL CR, Glaxosmithkline 00029-3208-13

Pegaspargase *(003199)*

Categories: Leukemia, acute lymphoblastic; FDA Approved 1994 Feb; Pregnancy Category C; Orphan Drugs
Drug Classes: Antineoplastics, enzymes
Brand Names: Oncaspar; L-Asparaginase
HCFA JCODE(S): J9266 per single dose vial IM, IV

DESCRIPTION

Oncaspar, the ENZON trademark for pegaspargase, is a modified version of the enzyme L-asparaginase. It is an oncolytic agent used in combination chemotherapy for the treatment of patients with acute lymphoblastic leukemia who are hypersensitive to native forms of L-asparaginase (as described in CLINICAL PHARMACOLOGY).

The generic name for Oncaspar is pegaspargase. The chemical name is monomethoxypolyethylene glycol succinimidyl L-asparaginase. L- asparaginase is modified by covalently conjugating units of monomethoxypolyethylene glycol (PEG), molecular weight of 5000, to the enzyme, forming the active ingredient PEG-L-asparaginase. The L- asparaginase (L-asparagine amidohydrolase, type EC-2, EC 3.5.1.1) used in the manufacture of Oncaspar is derived from *Escherichia coli.* ENZON purchases the enzyme L-asparaginase in bulk from Merck, Sharp and Dohme, Division of Merck & Co., Inc., West Point, PA 19486, US License Number 2. Merck & Co., Inc. supplies bulk L-asparaginase as a licensed intermediate for further manufacture by ENZON into PEG-L-asparaginase. Merck & Co., Inc. can only assume responsibility for the bulk intermediate supplied to ENZON.

Oncaspar is supplied as an isotonic sterile solution in phosphate buffered saline, pH 7.3, for intramuscular or intravenous administration only. The solution is clear, colorless and contains no preservatives. It is supplied in 5 ml single-dose vials.

Oncaspar activity is expressed in International Units (IU) according to the recommendation of the International Union of Biochemistry. One IU of L-asparaginase is defined as that amount of enzyme required to generate 1 μmol of ammonia per minute at pH 7.3 and 37°C.

Each milliliter of Oncaspar contains:
PEG-L-asparaginase: 750 IU ± 20%
Monobasic sodium phosphate: 1.20 mg ± 5%
Dibasic sodium phosphate: 5.58 mg ± 5%
Sodium chloride: 8.50 mg ± 5%
Water for injection: qs to 1.0 ml

The specific activity of Oncaspar is at least 85 IU per milligram protein.

CLINICAL PHARMACOLOGY

Leukemic cells are unable to synthesize asparagine due to a lack of asparagine synthetase and are dependent on an exogenous source of asparagine for survival. Rapid depletion of asparagine which results from treatment with the enzyme L-asparaginase, kills the leukemic cells. Normal cells, however, are less affected by the rapid depletion due to their ability to synthesize asparagine. This is an approach to therapy based on a specific metabolic defect in some leukemic cells which do not produce asparagine synthetase.[1]

In a study in predominately L-asparaginase naive adult patients with leukemia and lymphoma, initial plasma levels of L-asparaginase following intravenous administration were determined. Plasma half-life did not appear to be influenced by dose levels, and it could not be correlated with age, sex, surface area, renal or hepatic function, diagnosis or extent of disease. Apparent volume of distribution was equal to estimated plasma volume. L-asparaginase was measurable for at least 15 days following the initial treatment with pegaspargase. The enzyme could not be detected in the urine.[2]

In a study of newly diagnosed pediatric patients with acute lymphoblastic leukemia (ALL) who received either a single intramuscular injection of pegaspargase (2500 IU/m^2), *E. coli* L-asparaginase (25,000 IU/m^2), or *Erwinia* L-asparaginase (25,000 IU/m^2) the plasma half-lives for the 3 forms of L-asparaginase were as seen in TABLE 1.[3]

TABLE 1 *Plasma Half-Lives of 3 Forms of L-Asparaginase*

Treatment Group		Mean (Days)	Standard Deviation
Oncaspar	n=10	5.73	3.24
E. coli L-asparaginase	n=17	1.24	0.17
Erwinia L-asparaginase	n=10	0.65	0.13

In this same study of newly diagnosed pediatric ALL patients, the *in vivo* early leukemic cell kill after a single intramuscular injection of native *E. coli* L-asparaginase (25,000 IU/m^2), *Erwinia* L-asparaginase (25,000 IU/m^2), and pegaspargase (25,000 IU/m^2) during a 5 day "investigational window" was studied.[4] Bone marrow aspirates were taken before and 5 days after a single dose of 1 of the 3 different forms of L- asparaginase. Rhodamine-124 (RH-123), a selectively incorporated fluorescent mitochondrial dye, was used in an *in vitro* assay on the bone marrow aspirates to ascertain cell viability. The percent reduction of viable lymphoblasts at day 5 for each group is presented in TABLE 2.[4]

In three pharmacokinetic studies, 37 relapsed ALL patients received pegaspargase at 2500 IU/m^2 every 2 weeks. The plasma half-life of pegaspargase was 3.24 ± 1.83 days in 9 patients who were previously hypersensitive to native L-asparaginase and 5.69 ± 3.25 days in 28 non-hypersensitive patients. The area under the curve was 9.50 ± 3.95 IU/ml/day in the previously hypersensitive patients, and 9.83 ± 5.94 IU/ml/day in the non-hypersensitive patients.

TABLE 2

Rhodamine-123 (*In Vivo* Cell Kill)

Treatment Group		% Reduction of Viable Lymphoblasts at Day 5 Mean ±SD
Oncaspar	n=21	55.7 ± 10.2
E. coli L-asparaginase	n=28	57.8 ± 10.1
Erwinia L-asparaginase	n=19	57.9 ± 13.8

HYPERSENSITIVITY REACTIONS

Hypersensitivity reactions to *E. coli*L-asparaginase have been reported in the literature in 3-73% of patients.[1] Patients in pegaspargase clinical studies were considered to be previously hypersensitive if they experienced a systemic rash, urticaria, bronchospasm, laryngeal edema, or hypotension following administration of any form of native L- asparaginase. Patients were also considered to be previously hypersensitive if they experienced local erythema, urticaria, or swelling, greater than 2 centimeters, for at least 10 minutes following administration of any form of native L-asparaginase. The National Cancer Institute Common Toxicity Criteria (CTC) were used to classify the severity of the hypersensitivity reactions. These are: *Grade 1:* Transient rash (mild); *Grade 2:* Mild bronchospasm (moderate); *Grade 3:* Moderate bronchospasm and/or serum sickness (severe); *Grade 4:* Hypotension and/or anaphylaxis (life-threatening). Additionally, most transient local urticaria were considered Grade 2 hypersensitivity reactions, while most sustained urticaria distant from the injection site were considered Grade 3 hypersensitivity reactions. In general, the moderate to life-threatening hypersensitivity reactions were considered dose-limiting; that is, they required L-asparaginase treatment to be discontinued.

In separate studies, pegaspargase was administered intravenously to 48 patients and intramuscularly to 126 patients. The incidence of hypersensitivity reactions when pegaspargase was administered intramuscularly was 30% in patients who were previously hypersensitive to native L-asparaginase and 11% in non-hypersensitive patients (p-value of 0.007). The incidence of hypersensitivity reactions when pegaspargase was administered intravenously was 60% in patients who were previously hypersensitive to native L-asparaginase and 12% in non-hypersensitive patients. Since only 5 previously hypersensitive patients received pegaspargase intravenously, no meaningful analysis of the incidence of hypersensitivity reactions was possible between either the previously hypersensitive and non-hypersensitive patients, or between the intravenous and intramuscular routes of administration.

The overall incidence of hypersensitivity reactions in 174 patients who received pegaspargase in five clinical studies is shown in TABLE 3.

TABLE 3 *Incidence of Oncaspar Hypersensitivity Reactions*

Patient Status	n	CTC Grade of Hypersensitivity Reaction 1	2	3	4	Total
Previously hypersensitive patients	62	7	8	4	1	20 (32%)
Non-hypersensitive patients	112	5	4	1	1	11 (10%)
Total patients	174	12	12	5	2	31 (18%)

The probability of a previously hypersensitive or non-hypersensitive patient completing 8 doses of pegaspargase therapy without developing a dose-limiting hypersensitivity reaction was 77% and 95%, respectively.

All of the 62 hypersensitive patients treated with pegaspargase in five clinical studies had previously hypersensitivity reactions to 1 or more of the native forms of L-asparaginase. Of the 35 patients who had previous hypersensitivity reactions to *E. coli* L-asparaginase only, 5 (14%) had pegaspargase dose-limiting hypersensitivity reactions. Of the 27 patients who had hypersensitivity reactions to both *E. coli* and *Erwinia* L-asparaginase, 7 (26%) had pegaspargase dose- limiting hypersensitivity reactions. The overall incidence of dose- limiting hypersensitivity reactions in 174 patients treated with pegaspargase was 9% (19% in 62 hypersensitive and 3% in 112 non-hypersensitive patients). Of the total of 9% dose-limiting hypersensitivity reactions, 1% were anaphylactic (CTC Grade 4) and the other 8% were ≤ CTC Grade 3.

CLINICAL ACTIVITY

Pegaspargase was evaluated as part of combination therapy in four open label studies comprising 42 multiply-relapsed, previously hypersensitive acute leukemia patients [39 (93%) with ALL] at a dose of 2,000 or 2500 IU/m^2 administered intramuscularly or intravenously every 14 days during induction combination chemotherapy. The reinduction response rate was 50% (36% complete remissions and 14% partial remissions), with a 95% confidence interval of 35%-65%. This response rate is comparable to that reported in the literature for relapsed patients treated with native L-asparaginase as part of combination chemotherapy.[1]

Pegaspargase was also shown to have some activity as a single agent in multiply-relapsed hypersensitive ALL patients, the majority of whom were pediatric. Treatment with pegaspargase resulted in 3 responses (1 complete remission and 2 partial remissions) in 9 previously hypersensitive patients who would not have been able to receive any further L-asparaginase treatment.

Pegaspargase was also studied in non-hypersensitive, relapsed ALL patients who were randomized to receive 2 doses of pegaspargase at 2500 IU/m^2 every 14 days or twelve doses of *E. coli* L- asparaginase at 10,000 IU/m^{2}3 times a week during a 28 induction combination chemotherapy regimen (which included vincristine and prednisone). Although the enrollment in this study was too small to be conclusive, the data showed that for 20 patients there was no significant difference between the overall response rates of 60% and 50%, respectively, or the complete remission rates of 50% and 50%, respectively.

Pegaspargase was administered during maintenance therapy regimens to 33 previously hypersensitive patients. The average number of doses received during maintenance therapy was 5.8 (range of 1-24) and the average duration of maintenance therapy was 126 (range of 1-513) days for this patient population.

INDICATIONS AND USAGE

Pegaspargase is indicated for patients with acute lymphoblastic leukemia who require L-asparaginase in their treatment regimen, but have developed hypersensitivity to the native forms of L-asparaginase (see CLINICAL PHARMACOLOGY). Pegaspargase, like native L-asparaginase, is generally used in combination with other chemotherapeutic agents, such as vincristine, methotrexate, cytarabine, daunorubicin, and doxorubicin.[1,5] Use of pegaspargase as a single agent should only be undertaken when multi-agent chemotherapy is judged to be inappropriate for the patient.

CONTRAINDICATIONS

Pegaspargase is contraindicated in patients with pancreatitis or a history of pancreatitis. Pegaspargase is contraindicated in patients who have had significant hemorrhagic events associated with prior L-asparaginase therapy. Pegaspargase is also contraindicated in patients who have had previous serious allergic reactions, such as generalized urticaria, bronchospasm, laryngeal edema, hypotension, or other unacceptable adverse reactions to pegaspargase.

WARNINGS

It is recommended that pegaspargase be given under the supervision of an individual who is qualified by training and experience to administer cancer chemotherapeutic agents.

Especially in patients with known hypersensitivity to the other forms of L-asparaginase, hypersensitivity reactions to pegaspargase, including life-threatening anaphylaxis, may occur during therapy. As a routine precaution, patients should be kept under observation for 1 hour with resuscitation equipment and other agents necessary to treat anaphylaxis (epinephrine, oxygen, intravenous steroids, etc.) available.

PRECAUTIONS

GENERAL

This drug may be a contact irritant, and the solution must be handled and administered with care. Gloves are recommended. Inhalation of vapors and contact with skin or mucous membranes, especially those of the eyes, must be avoided. In case of contact, wash with copious amounts of water for at least 15 minutes. Anaphylactic reactions require the immediate use of epinephrine, oxygen, intravenous steroids, and antihistamines. Patients taking pegaspargase are at higher than usual risk for bleeding problems, especially with simultaneous use of other drugs that have anticoagulant properties, such as aspirin, and non-steroidal anti-inflammatories (see DRUG INTERACTIONS). Pegaspargase may have immunosuppressive activity. Therefore, it is possible that use of the drug in patients may predispose the patient to infection. Severe hepatic and central nervous system toxicity following multi-agent chemotherapy that includes pegaspargase may occur. Caution appears warranted when treating patients with pegaspargase given in combination with hepatotoxic agents, particularly when liver dysfunction is present.

Patients undergoing pegaspargase therapy must be carefully monitored and the therapeutic regimen adjusted according to response and toxicity. Physicians using a given treatment regimen incorporating pegaspargase should be thoroughly familiar with its benefits and risks.

INFORMATION FOR THE PATIENT

Patients should be informed of the possibility of hypersensitivity reactions, including immediate anaphylaxis, to pegaspargase. Patients taking pegaspargase are at higher than usual risk for bleeding problems. Patients should be instructed that the simultaneous use of pegaspargase with other drugs that may increase the risk of bleeding should be avoided (see DRUG INTERACTIONS). Pegaspargase may affect the ability of the liver to function normally in some patients. Therapy with pegaspargase may increase the toxicity of other medications (see DRUG INTERACTIONS). Pegaspargase may have immunosuppressive activity. Therefore, it is possible that use of the drug in patients may predispose the patient to infection. Patients should notify their physicians of any adverse reactions that occur.

LABORATORY TESTS

A fall in circulating lymphoblasts is often noted after initiating therapy. This may be accompanied by a marked rise in serum uric acid. As a guide to the effects of therapy, the patient's peripheral blood count and bone marrow should be monitored.

Frequent serum amylase determinations should be obtained to detect early evidence of pancreatitis (see CONTRAINDICATIONS). Blood sugar should be monitored during therapy with pegaspargase because hyperglycemia may occur. When using pegaspargase in conjunction with hepatotoxic chemotherapy, patients should be monitored for liver dysfunction. Pegaspargase may affect a number of plasma proteins; therefore, monitoring of fibrinogen, PT, and PTT may be indicated.

CARCINOGENESIS, MUTAGENESIS, AND IMPAIRMENT OF FERTILITY

Long-term carcinogenic studies in animals have not been performed with pegaspargase nor have studies been performed on impairment of fertility. Pegaspargase did no exhibit a mutagenic effect when tested against *Salmonella typhimurium* strains in the Ames assay.

PREGNANCY CATEGORY C

Animal reproduction studies have not been conducted with pegaspargase. It is also not known whether pegaspargase can cause fetal harm when administered to a pregnant woman or can affect reproduction capacity. Pegaspargase should be given to a pregnant woman only if clearly needed.

NURSING MOTHERS

It is not known whether pegaspargase is excreted in human milk. Because many drugs are excreted in human milk and because of the potential for serious adverse reactions due to pegaspargase in nursing infants, a decision should be made to discontinue nursing or discontinue the drug, taking into account the importance of the drug to the mother.

DRUG INTERACTIONS

Unfavorable interactions of L-asparaginase with some antitumor agents have been demonstrated.[1] It is recommended, therefore, that pegaspargase be used in combination regimens only by physicians familiar with the benefits and risks of a given regimen. Depletion of serum proteins by pegaspargase may increase the toxicity of other drugs which are protein bound. Additionally, during the period of its inhibition of protein synthesis and cell replication, pegaspargase may interfere with the action of drugs such as methotrexate, which require cell replication for their lethal effects. Pegaspargase may interfere with the enzymatic detoxification of other drugs, particularly in the liver. Physicians using a given treatment regimen should be thoroughly familiar with its benefits and risks.

Imbalances in coagulation factors have been noted with the use of pegaspargase predisposing to bleeding and/or thrombosis. Caution should be used when administering any concurrent anticoagulant therapy, such as coumadin, heparin, dipyridamole, aspirin, or nonsteroidal anti- inflammatories.

ADVERSE REACTIONS

Adverse reactions have been reported in adults and pediatric patients. Overall, the adult patients treated with pegaspargase had a somewhat higher incidence of known L-asparaginase toxicities, except for hypersensitivity reactions, than the pediatric patients treated with pegaspargase.

Excluding hypersensitivity reactions, the most frequently occurring known L-asparaginase related toxicities and adverse experiences reported for the 174 patients in clinical studies were chemical hepatotoxicities and coagulopathies, the majority of which did not result in any significant clinical events. The incidence of significant clinical events included clinical pancreatitis (1%), hyperglycemia requiring insulin therapy (3%), and thrombosis (4%).

The following adverse reactions related to pegaspargase were reported for 174 patients in five clinical studies.

The adverse reactions reported most frequently (greater than 5%) were allergic reactions (which may have included rash, erythema, edema, pain, fever, chills, urticaria, dyspnea, or bronchospasm), SGPT increase, nausea and/or vomiting, fever, and malaise.

The adverse reactions reported occasionally (greater than 1% but less than 5%) were anaphylactic reactions, dyspnea, injection site hypersensitivity, lip edema, rash, urticaria, abdominal pain, chills, pain in the extremities, hypotension, tachycardia, thrombosis, anorexia, diarrhea, jaundice, abnormal liver function test, decreased anticoagulant effect, disseminated intravascular coagulation, decreased fibrinogen, hemolytic anemia, leukopenia, pancytopenia, thrombocytopenia, increased thromboplastin, injection site pain, injection site reaction, bilirubinemia, hyperglycemia, hyperuricemia, hypoglycemia, hypoproteinemia, peripheral edema, increased SGOT, arthralgia, myalgia, convulsion, headache, night sweats, and paresthesia.

The adverse reactions reported rarely (less than 1%) were bronchospasm, petechial rash, face edema, lesional edema, sepsis, septic shock, chest pain, endocarditis, hypertension, constipation, flatulence, gastrointestinal pain, hepatomegaly, increased appetite, liver fatty deposits, coagulation disorder, increased coagulation time, decreased platelet count, purpura, increased amylase, edema, excessive thirst, hyperammonemia, hyponatremia, weight loss, bone pain, joint disorder, confusion, dizziness, emotional lability, somnolence, increased cough, epistaxis, upper respiratory infection, erythema simplex, pruritus, hematuria, increased urinary frequency, and abnormal kidney function.

The following pegaspargase related adverse reactions have been observed in patients with hematologic malignancies, primarily acute lymphoblastic leukemia (approximately 75%), non-Hodgkins lymphoma (approximately 13%), acute myelogenous leukemia (approximately 3%), and a variety of solid tumors (approximately 9%):

HYPERSENSITIVITY REACTIONS

A variety of hypersensitivity reactions have occurred. These reactions may be acute or delayed, and include acute anaphylaxis, bronchospasm, dyspnea, urticaria, arthralgia, erythema, induration, edema, pain, tenderness, hives, swelling, lip edema, chills, fever, and skin rashes (see WARNINGS and CONTRAINDICATIONS).

PANCREATIC FUNCTION

Pancreatitis, sometimes fulminant and fatal, has occurred. Increased serum amylase and lipase have also occurred.

LIVER FUNCTION

A variety of liver function abnormalities have been observed, including elevations of SGOT, SGPT, and bilirubin (direct and indirect). Jaundice, ascites, and hypoalbuminemia, which may be associated with peripheral edema, have been observed. These abnormalities usually are reversible on discontinuance of therapy, and some reversal may occur during the course of therapy. Fatty changes in the liver and liver failure have occurred.

HEMATOLOGIC

Hypofibrinogenemia, prolonged prothrombin times, prolonged partial thromboplastin times, and decreased antithrombin III have been observed. Superficial and deep venous thrombosis, sagittal sinus thrombosis, venous catheter thrombosis, and atrial thrombosis have occurred. Leukopenia, agranulocytosis, pancytopenia, thrombocytopenia, disseminated intravascular coagulation, severe hemolytic anemia, and anemia have been observed. Clinical hemorrhage, which may be fatal; easy bruisability, and ecchymosis have also been observed.

METABOLIC

Mild to severe hyperglycemia has been observed in low incidence, and usually responds to discontinuation of pegaspargase and the judicious use of intravenous fluid and insulin. Hypoglycemia, increased thirst and hyponatremia, uric acid nephropathy, hyperuricemia, hypoproteinemia, and peripheral edema have also been observed. Hypoalbuminemia, proteinuria, weight loss, and metabolic acidosis have occurred. Therapy with pegaspargase is associated with an increase in blood ammonia during the conversion of L-asparagine to aspartic acid by the enzyme.

NEUROLOGIC

Status epilepticus and temporal lobe seizures, somnolence, coma, malaise, mental status changes, dizziness, emotional lability, headache, lip numbness, finger paresthesia, mood changes, night sweats, and a Parkinson-like syndrome have occurred. Mild to severe confusion, disorientation, and paresthesia have also occurred. These side effects usually have reversed spontaneously after treatment was stopped.

RENAL

Increased BUN, increased creatinine, increased urinary frequency, hematuria due to thrombopenia, severe hemorrhagic cystitis, renal dysfunction, and renal failure have been observed.

CARDIOVASCULAR

Chest pain, subacute bacterial endocarditis, hypertension, severe hypotension, and tachycardia have occurred.

DIGESTIVE

Anorexia, constipation, decreased appetite, diarrhea, indigestion, flatulence, gas, gastrointestinal pain, mucositis, hepatomegaly, elevated gamma-glutamyltranspeptidase, increased appetite, mouth tenderness, severe colitis, and nausea and/or vomiting have been observed.

MUSCULOSKELETAL

Diffuse and local musculoskeletal pain, arthralgia, joint stiffness, and cramps have occurred.

RESPIRATORY

Cough, epistaxis, severe bronchospasm, and upper respiratory infection have been observed.

SKIN/APPENDAGES

Itching, alopecia, fever blister, purpura, hand whiteness and fungal changes, nail whiteness and ridging, erythema simplex, jaundice, and petechial rash have occurred.

GENERAL

Localized edema, injection site reactions (including pain, swelling, or redness), malaise, infection, sepsis, fatigue, and septic shock may occur.

DOSAGE AND ADMINISTRATION

As a component of selected multiple agent regimens, the recommended dose of pegaspargase is 2500 IU/m^2 every 14 days by either the intramuscular or intravenous route of administration.

The preferred route of administration, however, is the intramuscular route because of the lower incidence of hepatotoxicity, coagulopathy, and gastrointestinal and renal disorders compared to the intravenous route of administration.

The safety and effectiveness of pegaspargase have been established in patients with known previous hypersensitivity to L-aparaginase whose ages ranged from 1-21 years old. The recommended dose of pegaspargase for children with a body surface area $\geq$0.6 m^2 is 2500 IU/m^2 administered every 14 days. The recommended dose of pegaspargase for children with a body surface area for children with a body surface area $<$ 0.6 m^{2}is $<$0.6 m^2 is 82.5 IU/kg administered every 14 days.

Do not administer pegaspargase if there is any indication that the drug has been frozen. Although there may not be an apparent change in the appearance of the drug, pegaspargase's activity is destroyed after freezing.

When administering pegaspargase intramuscularly, the volume at a single injection site should be limited to 2 ml. If the volume to be administered is greater than 2 ml, multiple injection sites should be used.

When administered intravenously, pegaspargase should be given over a period of 1-2 hours in 100 ml of sodium chloride or dextrose injection 5%, through an infusion that is already running.

Anaphylactic reactions require the immediate use of antihistamines, epinephrine, oxygen, and intravenous steroids.

Use pegaspargase as the sole induction agent should be undertaken only in an unusual situation when a combined regimen, which uses other chemotherapeutic agents such as vincristine, methotrexate, cytarabine, daunorubicin, or doxorubicin is inappropriate because of toxicity or other specific patient-related factors, or in patients refractory to other therapy. When pegaspargase is to be used as the sole induction agent, the recommended dosage regimen is also 2500 IU/m^2 every 14 days.

When a remission is obtained, appropriate maintenance therapy may be instituted. pegaspargase may be used as part of a maintenance regimen.

Parenteral drug products should be inspected visually for particulate matter, cloudiness or discoloration prior to administration, whenever solution and container permit.

HOW SUPPLIED

ONCASPAR

Use only one dose per vial; do not re-enter the vial. Discard unused portions. Do not save unused drug for later administration.

Sterile solution for injection in ready to use single-use vials. Preservative free.

5 ml per vial containing 750 IU/ml Oncaspar in a clear, colorless, phosphate buffered saline solution, pH 7.3. Each vial contains 3.750 IU of Oncaspar.

HANDLING AND STORAGE

Avoid excessive agitation. DO NOT SHAKE.

Keep refrigerated at 2-8°C (36-46°F).

Do not use if cloudy or if precipitate is present.

Do not use if stored at room temperature for more than 48 hours.

DO NOT FREEZE. Do not use product if it is known to have been frozen. Freezing destroys activity, which cannot be detected visually.

PRODUCT LISTING - RATED THERAPEUTICALLY EQUIVALENT

Solution - Injectable - 750 IU/ml

5 ml $1391.21 ONCASPAR, Aventis Pharmaceuticals 00075-0640-05

Pegfilgrastim *(003548)*

Categories: Neutropenia; FDA Approved 2002 Jan; Pregnancy Category C
Drug Classes: Hematopoietic agents
Brand Names: Neulasta

DESCRIPTION

Note: The trade names have been used throughout this monograph for clarity.

Neulasta (pegfilgrastim) is a covalent conjugate of recombinant methionyl human G-CSF (Filgrastim) and monomethoxypolyethylene glycol. Filgrastim is a water-soluble 175 amino acid protein with a molecular weight of approximately 19 kilodaltons (kD). Filgrastim is obtained from the bacterial fermentation of a strain of *Escherichia coli* transformed with a genetically engineered plasmid containing the human G-CSF gene. To produce pegfilgrastim, a 20 kD monomethoxypolyethylene glycol molecule is covalently bound to the N-terminal methionyl residue of Filgrastim. The average molecular weight of pegfilgrastim is approximately 39 kD.

Neulasta is supplied in 0.6 ml prefilled syringes for subcutaneous (SC) injection. Each syringe contains 6 mg pegfilgrastim (based on protein weight), in a sterile, clear, colorless, preservative-free solution (pH 4.0) containing acetate (0.35 mg), sorbitol (30.0 mg), polysorbate 20 (0.02 mg), and sodium (0.02 mg) in water for injection.

CLINICAL PHARMACOLOGY

Both Filgrastim and pegfilgrastim are Colony Stimulating Factors that act on hematopoietic cells by binding to specific cell surface receptors thereby stimulating proliferation, differentiation, commitment, and end cell functional activation.[1,2] Studies on cellular proliferation, receptor binding, and neutrophil function demonstrate that Filgrastim and pegfilgrastim have the same mechanism of action. Pegfilgrastim has reduced renal clearance and prolonged persistence *in vivo* as compared to Filgrastim.

PHARMACOKINETICS

The pharmacokinetics and pharmacodynamics of Neulasta were studied in 379 patients with cancer. The pharmacokinetics of Neulasta were nonlinear in cancer patients and clearance decreased with increases in dose. Neutrophil receptor binding is an important component of the clearance of Neulasta, and serum clearance is directly related to the number of neutrophils. For example, the concentration of Neulasta declined rapidly at the onset of neutrophil recovery that followed myelosuppressive chemotherapy. In addition to numbers of neutrophils, body weight appeared to be a factor. Patients with higher body weights experienced higher systemic exposure to Neulasta after receiving a dose normalized for body weight. A large variability in the pharmacokinetics of Neulasta was observed in cancer patients. The half-life of Neulasta ranged from 15-80 hours after SC injection.

SPECIAL POPULATIONS

No gender-related differences were observed in the pharmacokinetics of Neulasta, and no differences were observed in the pharmacokinetics of geriatric patients ($\geq$65 years of age) compared to younger patients ($<$65 years of age) (see PRECAUTIONS, Geriatric Use). The pharmacokinetic profile in pediatric populations or in patients with hepatic or renal insufficiency has not been assessed.

INDICATIONS AND USAGE

Neulasta is indicated to decrease the incidence of infection, as manifested by febrile neutropenia, in patients with non-myeloid malignancies receiving myelosuppressive anti-cancer drugs associated with a clinically significant incidence of febrile neutropenia.

CONTRAINDICATIONS

Neulasta is contraindicated in patients with known hypersensitivity to *E. coli*-derived proteins, pegfilgrastim, Filgrastim, or any other component of the product.

WARNINGS

SPLENIC RUPTURE

RARE CASES OF SPLENIC RUPTURE HAVE BEEN REPORTED FOLLOWING THE ADMINISTRATION OF THE PARENT COMPOUND OF NEULASTA, FILGRASTIM, FOR PBPC MOBILIZATION IN BOTH HEALTHY DONORS AND PATIENTS WITH CANCER. SOME OF THESE CASES WERE FATAL. NEULASTA HAS NOT BEEN EVALUATED IN THIS SETTING, THEREFORE, NEULASTA SHOULD NOT BE USED FOR PBPC MOBILIZATION. PATIENTS RECEIVING NEULASTA WHO REPORT LEFT UPPER ABDOMINAL OR SHOULDER TIP PAIN SHOULD BE EVALUATED FOR AN ENLARGED SPLEEN OR SPLENIC RUPTURE.

ADULT RESPIRATORY DISTRESS SYNDROME (ARDS)

Adult respiratory distress syndrome (ARDS) has been reported in neutropenic patients with sepsis receiving Filgrastim, the parent compound of Neulasta, and is postulated to be secondary to an influx of neutrophils to sites of inflammation in the lungs. Neutropenic patients receiving Neulasta who develop fever, lung infiltrates, or respiratory distress should be evaluated for the possibility of ARDS. In the event that ARDS occurs, Neulasta should be discontinued and/or withheld until resolution of ARDS and patients should receive appropriate medical management for this condition.

ALLERGIC REACTIONS

Allergic-type reactions, including anaphylaxis, skin rash and urticaria, occurring on initial or subsequent treatment have been reported with the parent compound of Neulasta,

Filgrastim. In some cases, symptoms have recurred with rechallenge, suggesting a causal relationship. Allergic-type reactions to Neulasta have not been observed in clinical trials. If a serious allergic reaction or an anaphylactic reaction occurs, appropriate therapy should be administered and further use of Neulasta should be discontinued.

SICKLE CELL DISEASE

Severe sickle cell crises have been reported in patients with sickle cell disease (specifically homozygous sickle cell anemia, sickle/hemoglobin C disease, and sickle/β+ thalassemia) who received Filgrastim, the parent compound of pegfilgrastim, for PBPC mobilization or following chemotherapy. One of these cases was fatal. Pegfilgrastim should be used with caution in patients with sickle cell disease, and only after careful consideration of the potential risks and benefits. Patients with sickle cell disease who receive Neulasta should be kept well hydrated and monitored for the occurrence of sickle cell crises. In the event of severe sickle cell crisis supportive care should be administered, and interventions to ameliorate the underlying event, such as therapeutic red blood cell exchange transfusion, should be considered.

PRECAUTIONS

GENERAL

Use With Chemotherapy and/or Radiation Therapy

Neulasta should not be administered in the period between 14 days before and 24 hours after administration of cytotoxic chemotherapy (see DOSAGE AND ADMINISTRATION) because of the potential for an increase in sensitivity of rapidly dividing myeloid cells to cytotoxic chemotherapy.

The use of Neulasta has not been studied in patients receiving chemotherapy associated with delayed myelosuppression (*e.g.,* nitrosoureas, mitomycin C).

The administration of Neulasta concomitantly with 5-fluorouracil or other antimetabolites has not been evaluated in patients. Administration of pegfilgrastim at 0, 1 and 3 days before 5-fluorouracil resulted in increased mortality in mice; administration of pegfilgrastim 24 hours after 5-fluorouracil did not adversely affect survival.

The use of Neulasta has not been studied in patients receiving radiation therapy.

POTENTIAL EFFECT ON MALIGNANT CELLS

Pegfilgrastim is a growth factor that primarily stimulates neutrophils and neutrophil precursors; however, the G-CSF receptor through which pegfilgrastim and Filgrastim act has been found on tumor cell lines, including some myeloid, T-lymphoid, lung, head and neck, and bladder tumor cell lines. The possibility that pegfilgrastim can act as a growth factor for any tumor type cannot be excluded. Use of Neulasta in myeloid malignancies and myelodysplasia (MDS) has not been studied. In a randomized study comparing the effects of the parent compound of Neulasta, Filgrastim, to placebo in patients undergoing remission induction and consolidation chemotherapy for acute myeloid leukemia, important differences in remission rate between the two arms were excluded. Disease-free survival and overall survival were comparable; however, the study was not designed to detect important differences in these endpoints.[3]

INFORMATION FOR THE PATIENT

Patients should be informed of the possible side effects of Neulasta, and be instructed to report them to the prescribing physician. Patients should be informed of the signs and symptoms of allergic drug reactions and be advised of appropriate actions. Patients should be counseled on the importance of compliance with their Neulasta treatment, including regular monitoring of blood counts.

If it is determined that a patient or caregiver can safely and effectively administer Neulasta at home, appropriate instruction on the proper use of Neulasta should be provided for patients and their caregivers, including careful review of the "Information for Patients and Caregivers" insert. Patients and caregivers should be cautioned against the reuse of needles, syringes, or drug product, and be thoroughly instructed in their proper disposal. A puncture-resistant container for the disposal of used syringes and needles should be available.

LABORATORY MONITORING

To assess a patient's hematologic status and ability to tolerate myelosuppressive chemotherapy, a complete blood count and platelet count should be obtained before chemotherapy is administered. Regular monitoring of hematocrit value and platelet count is recommended.

CARCINOGENESIS, MUTAGENESIS, AND IMPAIRMENT OF FERTILITY

No mutagenesis studies were conducted with pegfilgrastim. The carcinogenic potential of pegfilgrastim has not been evaluated in long-term animal studies. In a toxicity study of 6 months duration in rats given once weekly SC injections of up to 1000 μg/kg of pegfilgrastim (approximately 23-fold higher than the recommended human dose), no precancerous or cancerous lesions were noted.

When administered once weekly via SC injections to male and female rats at doses up to 1000 μg/kg prior to, and during mating, reproductive performance, fertility and sperm assessment parameters were not affected.

PREGNANCY CATEGORY C

Pegfilgrastim has been shown to have adverse effects in pregnant rabbits when administered SC every other day during gestation at doses as low as 50 μg/kg/dose (approximately 4-fold higher than the recommended human dose). Decreased maternal food consumption, accompanied by a decreased maternal body weight gain and decreased fetal body weights were observed at 50-1000 μg/kg/dose. Pegfilgrastim doses of 200 and 250 μg/kg/dose resulted in an increased incidence of abortions. Increased post-implantation loss due to early resorptions, was observed at doses of 200-1000 μg/kg/dose and decreased numbers of live rabbit fetuses were observed at pegfilgrastim doses of 200-1000 μg/kg/dose, given every other day.

Subcutaneous injections of pegfilgrastim of up to 1000 μg/kg/dose every other day during the period of organogenesis in rats were not associated with an embryotoxic or fetotoxic outcome. However, an increased incidence (compared to historical controls) of wavy ribs was observed in rat fetuses at 1000 μg/kg/dose every other day. Very low levels (<0.5%) of pegfilgrastim crossed the placenta when administered subcutaneously to pregnant rats every other day during gestation.

Once weekly SC injections of pegfilgrastim to female rats from day 6 of gestation through day 18 of lactation at doses up to 1000 μg/kg/dose did not result in any adverse maternal effects. There were no deleterious effects on the growth and development of the offspring and no adverse effects were found upon assessment of fertility indices.

There are no adequate and well-controlled studies in pregnant women. Neulasta should be used during pregnancy only if the potential benefit to the mother justifies the potential risk to the fetus.

NURSING MOTHERS

It is not known whether pegfilgrastim is excreted in human milk. Because many drugs are excreted in human milk, caution should be exercised when Neulasta is administered to a nursing woman.

PEDIATRIC USE

The safety and effectiveness of Neulasta in pediatric patients have not been established. The 6 mg fixed dose single-use syringe formulation should not be used in infants, children and smaller adolescents weighing less than 45 kg.

GERIATRIC USE

Of the 465 subjects with cancer who received Neulasta in clinical studies, 85 (18%) were age 65 and over, and 14 (3%) were age 75 and over. No overall differences in safety or effectiveness were observed between these patients and younger patients; however, due to the small number of elderly subjects, small but clinically relevant differences cannot be excluded.

DRUG INTERACTIONS

No formal drug interaction studies between Neulasta and other drugs have been performed. Drugs such as lithium may potentiate the release of neutrophils; patients receiving lithium and Neulasta should have more frequent monitoring of neutrophil counts.

ADVERSE REACTIONS

See WARNINGS: Splenic Rupture, ARDS, Allergic Reactions, and Sickle Cell Disease.

Safety data are based upon 465 subjects with lymphoma and solid tumors (breast, lung, and thoracic tumors) enrolled in six randomized clinical studies. Subjects received Neulasta after nonmyeloablative cytotoxic chemotherapy. Most adverse experiences were attributed by the investigators to the underlying malignancy or cytotoxic chemotherapy and occurred at similar rates in subjects who received Neulasta (n=465) or Filgrastim (n=331). These adverse experiences occurred at rates between 72% and 15% and included: nausea, fatigue, alopecia, diarrhea, vomiting, constipation, fever, anorexia, skeletal pain, headache, taste perversion, dyspepsia, myalgia, insomnia, abdominal pain, arthralgia, generalized weakness, peripheral edema, dizziness, granulocytopenia, stomatitis, mucositis, and neutropenic fever.

The most common adverse event attributed to Neulasta in clinical trials was medullary bone pain, reported in 26% of subjects, which was comparable to the incidence in Filgrastim-treated patients. This bone pain was generally reported to be of mild-to-moderate severity. Approximately 12% of all subjects utilized non-narcotic analgesics and less than 6% utilized narcotic analgesics in association with bone pain. No patient withdrew from study due to bone pain.

In clinical studies, leukocytosis (WBC counts $>100 \times 10^9$/L) was observed in less than 1% of 465 subjects with non-myeloid malignancies receiving Neulasta. Leukocytosis was not associated with any adverse effects.

In subjects receiving Neulasta in clinical trials, the only serious event that was not deemed attributable to underlying or concurrent disease, or to concurrent therapy was a case of hypoxia.

Reversible elevations in LDH, alkaline phosphatase, and uric acid, which did not require treatment intervention, were observed. The incidences of these changes, presented for Neulasta relative to Filgrastim, were: LDH (19% vs 29%), alkaline phosphatase (9% vs 16%), and uric acid (8% vs 9% [1% of reported cases for both treatment groups were classified as severe]).

IMMUNOGENICITY

As with all therapeutic proteins, there is a potential for immunogenicity. The incidence of antibody development in patients receiving Neulasta has not been adequately determined. While available data suggest that a small proportion of patients developed binding antibodies to Filgrastim or pegfilgrastim, the nature and specificity of these antibodies has not been adequately studied. No neutralizing antibodies have been detected using a cell-based bioassay in 46 patients who apparently developed binding antibodies. The detection of antibody formation is highly dependent on the sensitivity and specificity of the assay, and the observed incidence of antibody positivity in an assay may be influenced by several factors including sample handling, concomitant medications, and underlying disease. Therefore, comparison of the incidence of antibodies to Neulasta with the incidence of antibodies to other products may be misleading.

Cytopenias resulting from an antibody response to exogenous growth factors have been reported on rare occasions in patients treated with other recombinant growth factors. There is a theoretical possibility that an antibody directed against pegfilgrastim may cross-react with endogenous G-CSF, resulting in immune-mediated neutropenia, but this has not been observed in clinical studies.

DOSAGE AND ADMINISTRATION

The recommended dosage of Neulasta is a single SC injection of 6 mg administered once per chemotherapy cycle. Neulasta should not be administered in the period between 14 days before and 24 hours after administration of cytotoxic chemotherapy (see PRECAUTIONS).

The 6 mg fixed dose formulation should not be used in infants, children and smaller adolescents weighing less than 45 kg.

Neulasta should be visually inspected for discoloration and particulate matter before administration. Neulasta should not be administered if discoloration or particulates are observed.

Neulasta is supplied in prefilled syringes with UltraSafe Needle Guards. Following administration of Neulasta from the prefilled syringe, the UltraSafe Needle Guard should be activated to prevent accidental needle sticks. To activate the UltraSafe Needle Guard, place your hands behind the needle, grasp the guard with one hand, and slide the guard forward until the needle is completely covered and the guard clicks into place. NOTE: If an audible click is not heard, the needle guard may not be completely activated. The prefilled syringe should be disposed of by placing the entire prefilled syringe with guard activated into an approved puncture-proof container.

HOW SUPPLIED

Neulasta is supplied as a preservative-free solution containing 6 mg (0.6 ml) of pegfilgrastim (10 mg/ml) in a single-dose syringe with a 27 gauge, ½ inch needle with an UltraSafe Needle Guard.

STORAGE

Neulasta should be stored refrigerated at 2-8°C (36-46°F); syringes should be kept in their carton to protect from light until time of use. Shaking should be avoided. Before injection, Neulasta may be allowed to reach room temperature for a maximum of 48 hours but should be protected from light. Neulasta left at room temperature for more than 48 hours should be discarded. Freezing should be avoided; however, if accidentally frozen, Neulasta should be allowed to thaw in the refrigerator before administration. If frozen a second time, Neulasta should be discarded.

PRODUCT LISTING - EQUIVALENTS NOT AVAILABLE

Injection - Subcutaneous - 6 mg/0.6 ml

1 each $2950.00 NEULASTA, Amgen 55513-0190-01

Peginterferon alfa-2a (003580)

Categories: Hepatitis C; Pregnancy Category X; FDA Approved 2002 Dec
Drug Classes: Antivirals; Immunomodulators
Brand Names: Pegasys

WARNING

Alpha interferons, including peginterferon alfa-2a (peginterferon alfa-2a), may cause or aggravate fatal or life-threatening neuropsychiatric, autoimmune, ischemic, and infectious disorders. Patients should be monitored closely with periodic clinical and laboratory evaluations. Therapy should be withdrawn in patients with persistently severe or worsening signs or symptoms of these conditions. In many, but not all cases, these disorders resolve after stopping peginterferon alfa-2a therapy (see WARNINGS and ADVERSE REACTIONS).

Use With Ribavirin

Ribavirin, including Copegus, may cause birth defects and/or death of the fetus. Extreme care must be taken to avoid pregnancy in female patients and in female partners of male patients. Ribavirin causes hemolytic anemia. The anemia associated with ribavirin therapy may result in a worsening of cardiac disease. Ribavirin is genotoxic and mutagenic and should be considered a potential carcinogen (see ribavirin package insert for additional information and other warnings).

DESCRIPTION

Peginterferon alfa-2a, is a covalent conjugate of recombinant alfa-2a interferon (approximate molecular weight [MW] 20,000 daltons) with a single branched bis-monomethoxy polyethylene glycol (PEG) chain (approximate MW 40,000 daltons). The PEG moiety is linked at a single site to the interferon alfa moiety via a stable amide bond to lysine. Peginterferon alfa-2a has an approximate molecular weight of 60,000 daltons. Interferon alfa-2a is produced using recombinant DNA technology in which a cloned human leukocyte interferon gene is inserted into and expressed in *Escherichia coli.*

Each vial contains approximately 1.2 ml of solution to deliver 1.0 ml of drug product. Subcutaneous (SC) administration of 1.0 ml delivers 180 µg of drug product (expressed as the amount of interferon alfa-2a), 8.0 mg sodium chloride, 0.05 mg polysorbate 80, 10.0 mg benzyl alcohol, 2.62 mg sodium acetate trihydrate, and 0.05 mg acetic acid. The solution is colorless to light yellow and the pH is 6.0 ± 0.01.

CLINICAL PHARMACOLOGY

PHARMACODYNAMICS

Interferons bind to specific receptors on the cell surface initiating intracellular signaling via a complex cascade of protein-protein interactions leading to rapid activation of gene transcription. Interferon-stimulated genes modulate many biological effects including the inhibition of viral replication in infected cells, inhibition of cell proliferation, and immunomodulation. The clinical relevance of these in vitro activities is not known.

Peginterferon alfa-2a stimulates the production of effector proteins such as serum neopterin and 2′, 5′-oligoadenylate synthetase.

PHARMACOKINETICS

Maximal serum concentrations (C_{max}) occur between 72-96 hours post dose. The C_{max} and AUC measurements of peginterferon alfa-2a increase in a dose-related manner. Week 48 mean trough concentrations (16 ng/ml; range 4-28) at 168 hours post dose are approximately 2-fold higher than week 1 mean trough concentrations (8 ng/ml; range 0-15). Steady-state serum levels are reached within 5-8 weeks of once weekly dosing. The peak to trough ratio at week 48 is approximately 2.0.

The mean systemic clearance in healthy subjects given peginterferon alfa-2a was 94 ml/h, which is 48 approximately 100- fold lower than that for interferon alfa-2a (interferon alfa-2b). The mean terminal half- life after SC dosing in patients with chronic hepatitis C was 80 hours (range 50-140 hours) compared to 5.1 hours (range 3.7-8.5 hours) for interferon alfa-2b.

SPECIAL POPULATIONS

Gender and Age

Peginterferon alfa-2a administration yielded similar pharmacokinetics in male and female healthy subjects. The AUC was increased from 1295-1663 ng·h/ml in subjects older than 62 years taking 180 µg peginterferon alfa-2a, but peak concentrations were similar (9 vs 10 ng/ml) in those older and younger than 62 years.

Pediatric Patients

The pharmacokinetics of peginterferon alfa-2a have not been adequately studied in pediatric patients.

Renal Dysfunction

In patients with end stage renal disease undergoing hemodialysis, there is a 25-45% reduction in peginterferon alfa-2a clearance (see PRECAUTIONS, Renal Impairment).

The pharmacokinetics of ribavirin following administration of ribavirin have not been studied in patients with renal impairment and there are limited data from clinical trials on administration of ribavirin in patients with creatinine clearance <50 ml/min. Therefore, patients with creatinine clearance <50 ml/min should not be treated with ribavirin (see WARNINGS and DOSAGE AND ADMINISTRATION).

Effect of Food on Absorption of Ribavirin

Bioavailability of a single oral dose of ribavirin was increased by co-administration with a high-fat meal. The absorption was slowed (T_{max} was doubled) and the AUC(0-192h) and C_{max} increased by 42% and 66%, respectively, when ribavirin was taken with a high-fat meal compared with fasting conditions (see DOSAGE AND ADMINISTRATION).

DRUG INTERACTIONS

Nucleoside Analogues

Ribavirin has been shown in vitro to inhibit phosphorylation of zidovudine and stavudine which could lead to decreased anti-retroviral activity. Exposure to didanosine or its active metabolite (dideoxyadenosine 5′-triphosphate) is increased when didanosine is co-administered with ribavirin (see DRUG INTERACTIONS).

INDICATIONS AND USAGE

Peginterferon alfa-2a, alone or in combination with ribavirin, is indicated for the treatment of adults with chronic hepatitis C virus infection who have compensated liver disease and have not been previously treated with interferon alpha.

CONTRAINDICATIONS

Peginterferon alfa-2a is contraindicated in patients with:

- Hypersensitivity to peginterferon alfa-2a or any of its components.
- Autoimmune hepatitis.
- Hepatic decompensation (Child-Pugh class B and C) before or during treatment.

Peginterferon alfa-2a is contraindicated in neonates and infants because it contains benzyl alcohol. Benzyl alcohol is associated with an increased incidence of neurologic and other complications in neonates and infants, which are sometimes fatal.

Peginterferon alfa-2a and ribavirin combination therapy is additionally contraindicated in:

- Patients with known hypersensitivity to ribavirin or to any component of the tablet.
- Women who are pregnant.
- Men whose female partners are pregnant.
- Patients with hemoglobinopathies (*e.g.*, thalassemia major, sickle-cell anemia).

WARNINGS

GENERAL

Patients should be monitored for the following serious conditions, some of which may become life threatening. Patients with persistently severe or worsening signs or symptoms should have their therapy withdrawn (see BOXED WARNING).

NEUROPSYCHIATRIC

Life-threatening or fatal neuropsychiatric reactions may manifest in patients receiving therapy with peginterferon alfa-2a and include suicide, suicidal ideation, depression, relapse of drug addiction and drug overdose. These reactions may occur in patients with and without previous psychiatric illness.

Peginterferon alfa-2a should be used with extreme caution in patients who report a history of depression. Neuropsychiatric adverse events observed with alpha interferon treatment include aggressive behavior, psychoses, hallucinations, bipolar disorders and mania. Physicians should monitor all patients for evidence of depression and other psychiatric symptoms. Patients should be advised to report any sign or symptom of depression or suicidal ideation to their prescribing physicians. In severe cases, therapy should be stopped immediately and psychiatric intervention instituted (see ADVERSE REACTIONS and DOSAGE AND ADMINISTRATION).

INFECTIONS

Serious and severe bacterial infections, some fatal, have been observed in patients treated with alpha interferons including peginterferon alfa-2a. Some of the infections have been associated with neutropenia. Peginterferon alfa-2a should be discontinued in patients who develop severe infections and appropriate antibiotic therapy instituted.

BONE MARROW TOXICITY

Peginterferon alfa-2a suppresses bone marrow function and may result in severe cytopenias. Ribavirin may potentiate the neutropenia and lymphopenia induced by alpha interferons including peginterferon alfa-2a. Very rarely alpha interferons may be associated with aplas-

P

tic anemia. It is advised that complete blood counts (CBC) be obtained pre-treatment and monitored routinely during therapy (see PRECAUTIONS, Laboratory Tests).

Peginterferon alfa-2a and ribavirin should be used with caution in patients with baseline neutrophil counts <1500 cells/mm^3, with baseline platelet counts <90,000 cells/mm^3 or baseline hemoglobin <10 g/dl. Peginterferon alfa-2a therapy should be discontinued, at least temporarily, in patients who develop severe decreases in neutrophil and/or platelet counts (see DOSAGE AND ADMINISTRATION, Dose Modification).

CARDIOVASCULAR DISORDERS

Hypertension, supraventricular arrhythmias, chest pain, and myocardial infarction have been observed in patients treated with peginterferon alfa-2a.

Peginterferon alfa-2a should be administered with caution to patients with preexisting cardiac disease. Because cardiac disease may be worsened by ribavirin- induced anemia, patients with a history of significant or unstable cardiac disease should not use ribavirin (see WARNINGS, Anemia and the ribavirin package insert).

HYPERSENSITIVITY

Severe acute hypersensitivity reactions (*e.g.,* urticaria, angioedema, bronchoconstriction, anaphylaxis) have been rarely observed during alpha interferon and ribavirin therapy. If such reaction occurs, therapy with peginterferon alfa-2a and ribavirin should be discontinued and appropriate medical therapy immediately instituted.

ENDOCRINE DISORDERS

Peginterferon alfa-2a causes or aggravates hypothyroidism and hyperthyroidism. Hyperglycemia, hypoglycemia, and diabetes mellitus have been observed to develop in patients treated with peginterferon alfa-2a. Patients with these conditions at baseline who cannot be effectively treated by medication should not begin peginterferon alfa-2a therapy. Patients who develop these conditions during treatment and cannot be controlled with medication may require discontinuation of peginterferon alfa-2a therapy.

AUTOIMMUNE DISORDERS

Development or exacerbation of autoimmune disorders including myositis, hepatitis, ITP, psoriasis, rheumatoid arthritis, interstitial nephritis, thyroiditis, and systemic lupus erythematosus have been reported in patients receiving alpha interferon. Peginterferon alfa-2a should be used with caution in patients with autoimmune disorders.

PULMONARY DISORDERS

Dyspnea, pulmonary infiltrates, pneumonia, bronchiolitis obliterans, interstitial pneumonitis and sarcoidosis, some resulting in respiratory failure and/or patient deaths, may be induced or aggravated by peginterferon alfa-2a or alpha interferon therapy. Patients who develop persistent or unexplained pulmonary infiltrates or pulmonary function impairment should discontinue treatment with peginterferon alfa-2a.

COLITIS

Ulcerative, and hemorrhagic/ischemic colitis, sometimes fatal, have been observed within 12 weeks of starting alpha interferon treatment. Abdominal pain, bloody diarrhea, and fever are the typical manifestations of colitis. Peginterferon alfa-2a should be discontinued immediately if these symptoms develop. The colitis usually resolves within 1-3 weeks of discontinuation of alpha interferon.

PANCREATITIS

Pancreatitis, sometimes fatal, has occurred during alpha interferon and ribavirin treatment. Peginterferon alfa-2a and ribavirin should be suspended if symptoms or signs suggestive of pancreatitis are observed. Peginterferon alfa-2a and ribavirin should be discontinued in patients diagnosed with pancreatitis.

OPHTHALMOLOGIC DISORDERS

Decrease or loss of vision, retinopathy including macular edema, retinal artery or vein thrombosis, retinal hemorrhages and cotton wool spots, optic neuritis, and papilledema are induced or aggravated by treatment with peginterferon alfa-2a or other alpha interferons. All patients should receive an eye examination at baseline. Patients with preexisting ophthalmologic disorders (*e.g.,* diabetic or hypertensive retinopathy) should receive periodic ophthalmologic exams during interferon alpha treatment. Any patient who develops ocular symptoms should receive a prompt and complete eye examination. Peginterferon alfa-2a treatment should be discontinued in patients who develop new or worsening ophthalmologic disorders.

USE WITH RIBAVIRIN

Also, see ribavirin package insert.

Ribavirin may cause birth defects and/or death of the exposed fetus. Extreme care must be taken to avoid pregnancy in female patients and in female partners of male patients taking peginterferon alfa-2a and ribavirin combination therapy. RIBAVIRIN THERAPY SHOULD NOT BE STARTED UNLESS A REPORT OF A NEGATIVE PREGNANCY TEST HAS BEEN OBTAINED IMMEDIATELY PRIOR TO INITIATION OF THERAPY. Women of childbearing potential and men must use 2 forms of effective contraception during treatment and for at least 6 months after treatment has concluded. Routine monthly pregnancy tests must be performed during this time (see BOXED WARNING, CONTRAINDICATIONS, PRECAUTIONS, Information for the Patient, and the ribavirin package insert).

ANEMIA

The primary toxicity of ribavirin is hemolytic anemia. Hemoglobin <10 g/dl was observed in approximately 13% of ribavirin and peginterferon alfa-2a treated patients in clinical trials (see PRECAUTIONS, Laboratory Tests). The anemia associated with ribavirin occurs within 1-2 weeks of initiation of therapy with maximum drop in hemoglobin observed during the first 8 weeks. BECAUSE THE INITIAL DROP IN HEMOGLOBIN MAY BE SIGNIFICANT, IT IS ADVISED THAT HEMOGLOBIN OR HEMATOCRIT BE OBTAINED PRETREATMENT AND AT WEEK 2 AND WEEK 4 OF THERAPY OR MORE FREQUENTLY IF CLINICALLY INDICATED. Patients should then be followed as clinically appropriate.

Fatal and nonfatal myocardial infarctions have been reported in patients with anemia caused by ribavirin. Patients should be assessed for underlying cardiac disease before initiation of ribavirin therapy. Patients with pre-existing cardiac disease should have electrocardiograms administered before treatment, and should be appropriately monitored during therapy. If there is any deterioration of cardiovascular status, therapy should be suspended or discontinued (see DOSAGE AND ADMINISTRATION, Dose Modification, Ribavirin). Because cardiac disease may be worsened by drug-induced anemia, patients with a history of significant or unstable cardiac disease should not use ribavirin (see ribavirin package insert).

RENAL

It is recommended that renal function be evaluated in all patients started on ribavirin. Ribavirin should not be administered to patients with creatinine clearance <50 ml/min (see CLINICAL PHARMACOLOGY, Special Populations).

PRECAUTIONS

GENERAL

The safety and efficacy of peginterferon alfa-2a alone or in combination with ribavirin for the treatment of hepatitis C have not been established in:

- Patients who have failed other alpha interferon treatments.
- Liver or other organ transplant recipients.
- Patients co-infected with human immunodeficiency virus (HIV) or hepatitis B virus (HBV).

RENAL IMPAIRMENT

A 25-45% higher exposure to peginterferon alfa-2a is seen in subjects undergoing hemodialysis. In patients with impaired renal function, signs and symptoms of interferon toxicity should be closely monitored. Doses of peginterferon alfa-2a should be adjusted accordingly. Peginterferon alfa-2a should be used with caution in patients with creatinine clearance <50 ml/min (see DOSAGE AND ADMINISTRATION, Dose Modification).

INFORMATION FOR THE PATIENT

Patients receiving peginterferon alfa-2a alone or in combination with ribavirin should be directed in its appropriate use, informed of the benefits and risks associated with treatment, and referred to the peginterferon alfa-2a and, if applicable, ribavirin medication guides.

Peginterferon alfa-2a and ribavirin combination therapy must not be used by women who are pregnant or by men whose female partners are pregnant. Ribavirin therapy should not be initiated until a report of a negative pregnancy test has been obtained immediately before starting therapy. Female patients of childbearing potential and male patients with female partners of childbearing potential must be advised of the teratogenic/embryocidal risks and must be instructed to practice effective contraception during ribavirin therapy and for 6 months posttherapy. Patients should be advised to notify the physician immediately in the event of a pregnancy (see CONTRAINDICATIONS and WARNINGS).

Women of childbearing potential and men must use 2 forms of effective contraception during treatment and during the 6 months after treatment has concluded; routine monthly pregnancy tests must be performed during this time (see CONTRAINDICATIONS and ribavirin package insert).

If pregnancy does occur during treatment or during 6 months post-therapy, the patient must be advised of the significant teratogenic risk of ribavirin therapy to the fetus. To monitor maternal-fetal outcomes of pregnant women exposed to ribavirin, the Copegus Pregnancy Registry has been established. Physicians and patients are strongly encouraged to register by calling 1-800-526-6367.

Patients should be advised that laboratory evaluations are required before starting therapy and periodically thereafter (see Laboratory Tests). Patients should be instructed to remain well hydrated, especially during the initial stages of treatment. Patients should be advised to take ribavirin with food.

Patients should be informed that it is not known if therapy with peginterferon alfa-2a alone or in combination with ribavirin will prevent transmission of HCV infection to others or prevent cirrhosis, liver failure or liver cancer that might result from HCV infection. Patients who develop dizziness, confusion, somnolence, and fatigue should be cautioned to avoid driving or operating machinery.

If home use is prescribed, a puncture-resistant container for the disposal of used needles and syringes should be supplied to the patients. Patients should be thoroughly instructed in the importance of proper disposal and cautioned against any reuse of any needles and syringes. The full container should be disposed of according to the directions provided by the physician (see medication guide that comes with the prescription).

LABORATORY TESTS

Before beginning peginterferon alfa-2a or peginterferon alfa-2a and ribavirin combination therapy, standard hematological and biochemical laboratory tests are recommended for all patients. Pregnancy screening for women of childbearing potential must be performed.

After initiation of therapy, hematological tests should be performed at 2 weeks and 4 weeks and biochemical tests should be performed at 4 weeks. Additional testing should be performed periodically during therapy. In the clinical studies, the CBC (including hemoglobin level and white blood cell and platelet counts) and chemistries (including liver function tests and uric acid) were measured at 1, 2, 4, 6, and 8, and then every 4 weeks or more frequently if abnormalities were found. Thyroid stimulating hormone (TSH) was measured every 12 weeks. Monthly pregnancy testing should be performed during combination therapy and for 6 months after discontinuing therapy.

The entrance criteria used for the clinical studies of peginterferon alfa-2a may be considered as a guideline to acceptable baseline values for initiation of treatment:

- Platelet count ≥90,000 cells/mm^3 (as low as 75,000 cells/mm^3 in patients with cirrhosis).
- Caution should be exercised in initiating treatment in any patient with baseline risk of severe anemia (*e.g.,* spherocytosis, history of GI bleeding).
- Absolute neutrophil count (ANC) ≥1500 cells/mm^3.

P

- Serum creatinine concentration <1.5 × upper limit of normal.
- TSH and T4 within normal limits or adequately controlled thyroid function.

Peginterferon alfa-2a treatment was associated with decreases in WBC, ANC, lymphocytes and platelet counts often starting within the first 2 weeks of treatment (see ADVERSE REACTIONS). Dose reduction is recommended in patients with hematologic abnormalities (see DOSAGE AND ADMINISTRATION, Dose Modification).

While fever is commonly caused by peginterferon alfa-2a therapy, other causes of persistent fever must be ruled out, particularly in patients with neutropenia (see WARNINGS, Infections).

Transient elevations in ALT (2- to 5-fold above baseline) were observed in some patients receiving peginterferon alfa-2a, and were not associated with deterioration of other liver function tests. When the increase in ALT levels is progressive despite dose reduction or is accompanied by increased bilirubin, peginterferon alfa-2a therapy should be discontinued (see DOSAGE AND ADMINISTRATION, Dose Modification).

CARCINOGENESIS, MUTAGENESIS, AND IMPAIRMENT OF FERTILITY

Carcinogenesis

Peginterferon alfa-2a has not been tested for its carcinogenic potential.

Mutagenesis

Peginterferon alfa-2a did not cause DNA damage when tested in the Ames bacterial mutagenicity assay and in the *in vitro* chromosomal aberration assay in human lymphocytes, either in the presence or absence of metabolic activation.

Use With Ribavirin

Ribavirin is genotoxic and mutagenic. The carcinogenic potential of ribavirin has not been fully determined. In a p53 (+/-) mouse carcinogenicity study at doses up to the maximum tolerated dose of 100 mg/kg/day ribavirin was not oncogenic. However, on a body surface area basis, this dose was 0.5 times maximum recommended human 24 hour dose of ribavirin. A study in rats to assess the carcinogenic potential of ribavirin is ongoing.

Mutagenesis

See ribavirin package insert.

Impairment of Fertility

Peginterferon alfa-2a may impair fertility in women. Prolonged menstrual cycles and/or 437 amenorrhea were observed in female cynomolgus monkeys given SC injections of 600 μg/kg/dose (7200 μg/m^2/dose) of peginterferon alfa-2a every other day for 1 month, at approximately 180 times the recommended weekly human dose for a 60 kg person (based on body surface area). Menstrual cycle irregularities were accompanied by both a decrease and delay in the peak 17β-estradiol and progesterone levels following administration of peginterferon alfa-2a to female monkeys. A return to normal menstrual rhythm followed cessation of treatment. Every other day dosing with 100 μg/kg (1200 μg/m^2) peginterferon alfa-2a (equivalent to approximately 30 times the recommended human dose) had no effects on cycle duration or reproductive hormone status.

The effects of peginterferon alfa-2a on male fertility have not been studied. However, no adverse effects on fertility were observed in male Rhesus monkeys treated with non-pegylated interferon alfa-2a for 5 months at doses up to 25 × 10^6 IU/kg/day (see ribavirin package insert).

PREGNANCY CATEGORY C

Peginterferon alfa-2a has not been studied for its teratogenic effect. Non-pegylated interferon alfa-2a treatment of pregnant Rhesus monkeys at approximately 20-500 times the human weekly dose resulted in a statistically significant increase in abortions. No teratogenic effects were seen in the offspring delivered at term. Peginterferon alfa-2a should be assumed to have abortifacient potential. There are no adequate and well-controlled studies of peginterferon alfa-2a in pregnant women. Peginterferon alfa-2a is to be used during pregnancy only if the potential benefit justifies the potential risk to the fetus. Peginterferon alfa-2a is recommended for use in women of childbearing potential only when they are using effective contraception during therapy.

PREGNANCY CATEGORY X: USE WITH RIBAVIRIN

Significant teratogenic and/or embryocidal effects have been demonstrated in all animal species exposed to ribavirin. Ribavirin therapy is contraindicated in women who are pregnant and in the male partners of women who are pregnant (see CONTRAINDICATIONS, WARNINGS, and the ribavirin package insert).

If pregnancy occurs in a patient or partner of a patient during treatment or during the 6 months after treatment cessation, such cases should be reported to the Copegus Pregnancy Registry at 1-800-526-6367.

NURSING MOTHERS

It is not known whether peginterferon or ribavirin or its components are excreted in human milk. The effect of orally ingested peginterferon or ribavirin from breast milk on the nursing infant has not been evaluated. Because of the potential for adverse reactions from the drugs in nursing infants, a decision must be made whether to discontinue nursing or discontinue peginterferon alfa-2a and ribavirin treatment.

PEDIATRIC USE

The safety and effectiveness of peginterferon alfa-2a, alone or in combination with ribavirin in patients below the age of 18 years have not been established.

Peginterferon alfa-2a contains benzyl alcohol. Benzyl alcohol has been reported to be associated with an increased incidence of neurological and other complications in neonates and infants, which are sometimes fatal (see CONTRAINDICATIONS).

GERIATRIC USE

Younger patients have higher virologic response rates than older patients. Clinical studies of peginterferon alfa-2a alone or in combination with ribavirin did not include sufficient numbers of subjects aged 65 or over to determine whether they respond differently from younger subjects. Adverse reactions related to alpha interferons, such as CNS, cardiac, and systemic (*e.g.*, flu- like) effects may be more severe in the elderly and caution should be exercised in the use of peginterferon alfa-2a in this population. Peginterferon alfa-2a and ribavirin are excreted by the kidney, and the risk of toxic reactions to this therapy may be greater in patients with impaired renal function. Because elderly patients are more likely to have decreased renal func tion, care should be taken in dose selection and it may be useful to monitor renal function. Peginterferon alfa-2a should be used with caution in patients with creatinine clearance <50 ml/min and ribavirin should not be administered to patients with creatinine clearance <50 ml/min.

DRUG INTERACTIONS

Treatment with peginterferon alfa-2a once weekly for 4 weeks in healthy subjects was associated with an inhibition of P450 1A2 and a 25% increase in theophylline AUC. Theophylline serum levels should be monitored and appropriate dose adjustments considered for patients given both theophylline and peginterferon alfa-2a (see PRECAUTIONS). There was no effect on the pharmacokinetics of representative drugs metabolized by CYP 2C9, CYP 2C19, CYP 2D6 or CYP 3A4. In patients with chronic hepatitis C treated with peginterferon alfa-2a in combination with ribavirin, peginterferon alfa-2a treatment did not affect ribavirin distribution or clearance.

NUCLEOSIDE ANALOGUES

Didanosine

Co-administration of ribavirin and didanosine is not recommended. Reports of fatal hepatic failure, as well as peripheral neuropathy, pancreatitis, and symptomatic hyperlactatemia/lactic acidosis have been reported in clinical trials (see CLINICAL PHARMACOLOGY, Drug Interactions).

Stavudine and Zidovudine

Ribavirin can antagonize the in vitro antiviral activity of stavudine and zidovudine against HIV. Therefore, concomitant use of ribavirin with either of these drugs should be avoided.

ADVERSE REACTIONS

Peginterferon alfa-2a alone or in combination with ribavirin causes a broad variety of serious adverse reactions (see BOXED WARNING and WARNINGS). In all studies, one or more serious adverse reactions occurred in 10% of patients receiving peginterferon alfa-2a alone or in combination with ribavirin.

The most common life-threatening or fatal events induced or aggravated by peginterferon alfa-2a and ribavirin were depression, suicide, relapse of drug abuse/overdose, and bacterial infections; each occurred at a frequency of <1%.

Nearly all patients in clinical trials experienced one or more adverse events. The most commonly reported adverse reactions were psychiatric reactions, including depression, irritability, anxiety, and flu-like symptoms such as fatigue, pyrexia, myalgia, headache and rigors.

Overall 11% of patients receiving 48 weeks of therapy with peginterferon alfa-2a either alone (7%) or in combination with ribavirin (10%) discontinued therapy. The most common reasons for discontinuation of therapy were psychiatric, flu-like syndrome (*e.g.*, lethargy, fatigue, headache), dermatologic and gastrointestinal disorders.

The most common reason for dose modification in patients receiving combination therapy was for laboratory abnormalities; neutropenia (20%) and thrombocytopenia (4%) for peginterferon alfa-2a and anemia (22%) for ribavirin. Peginterferon alfa-2a dose was reduced in 12% of patients receiving 1000-1200 mg ribavirin for 48 weeks and in 7% of patients receiving 800 mg ribavirin for 24 weeks. ribavirin dose was reduced in 21% of patients receiving 1000-1200 mg ribavirin for 48 weeks and 12% in patients receiving 800 mg ribavirin for 24 weeks.

Because clinical trials are conducted under widely varying and controlled conditions, adverse reaction rates observed in clinical trials of a drug cannot be directly compared to rates in the clinical trials of another drug. Also, the adverse event rates listed here may not predict the rates observed in a broader patient population in clinical practice.

Patients treated for 24 weeks with peginterferon alfa-2a and 800 mg ribavirin were observed to have lower incidence of serious adverse events (3% vs 10%), Hgb <10g/dl (3% vs 15%), dose modification of peginterferon alfa-2a (30% vs 36%) and ribavirin (19% vs 38%) and of withdrawal from treatment (5% vs 15%) compared to patients treated for 48 weeks with peginterferon alfa-2a and 1000 or 1200 mg ribavirin. On the other hand the overall incidence of adverse events appeared to be similar in the 2 treatment groups.

The most common serious adverse event (3%) was bacterial infection (*e.g.*, sepsis, osteomyelitis, endocarditis, pyelonephritis, pneumonia). Other SAEs occurred at a frequency of <1% and included: suicide, suicidal ideation, psychosis, aggression, anxiety, drug abuse and drug overdose, angina, hepatic dysfunction, fatty liver, cholangitis, arrhythmia, diabetes mellitus, autoimmune phenomena (*e.g.*, hyperthyroidism, hypothyroidism, sarcoidosis, systemic lupus erythematosis, rheumatoid arthritis) peripheral neuropathy, aplastic anemia, peptic ulcer, gastrointestinal bleeding, pancreatitis, colitis, corneal ulcer, pulmo nary embolism, coma, myositis, and cerebral hemorrhage.

LABORATORY TEST VALUES

Hemoglobin

The hemoglobin concentration decreased below 12g/dl in 17% (median Hgb drop = 2.2 g/dl) of monotherapy and 52% (median Hgb drop = 3.7 g/dl) of combination therapy patients. Severe anemia (Hgb <10 g/dl) was encountered in 13% of patients receiving combination therapy and 2% of monotherapy recipients. Dose modification for anemia was required in 22% of ribavirin recipients treated for 48 weeks. Hemoglobin decreases in peginterferon alfa-2a monotherapy were generally mild and did not require dose modification (see DOSAGE AND ADMINISTRATION, Dose Modification).

Neutrophils

Decreases in neutrophil count below normal were observed in 95% of patients treated with peginterferon alfa-2a either alone or in combination with ribavirin. Severe potentially life-threatening neutropenia (ANC <0.5 × 10^9/L) occurred in approximately 5% of patients

TABLE 4 *Adverse Reactions Occurring in ≥5% of Patients in Hepatitis C Clinical Trials (Pooled Studies 1, 2, 3, and Study 4)*

	Peginterferon alfa-2a 180 µg 48 wk† n=559	Roferon-A*† n=554	Peginterferon alfa-2a 180 µg + 1000 mg or 1200 mg Copegus 48 wk‡ n=451	Intron A + 1000 mg or 1200 mg Rebetol 48 wk‡ n=443
Application Site Disorders				
Injection site reaction	22%	18%	23%	16%
Endocrine Disorders				
Hypothyroidism	3%	2%	4%	5%
Flu-Like Symptoms and Signs				
Fatigue/asthenia	56%	57%	65%	68%
Pyrexia	37%	41%	41%	55%
Rigors	35%	44%	25%	37%
Pain	11%	12%	10%	9%
Gastrointestinal				
Nausea/ vomiting	24%	33%	25%	29%
Diarrhea	16%	16%	11%	10%
Abdominal pain	15%	15%	8%	9%
Dry mouth	6%	3%	4%	7%
Dyspepsia	<1%	1%	6%	5%
Hematologic§				
Lymphopenia	3%	5%	14%	12%
Anemia	2%	1%	11%	11%
Neutropenia	21%	8%	27%	8%
Thrombocytopenia	5%	2%	5%	<1%
Metobolic and Nutritional				
Anorexia	17%	17%	24%	26%
Weight decrease	4%	3%	10%	10%
Musculoskeletal, Connective Tissue and Bone				
Myalgia	37%	38%	40%	49%
Arthralgia	28%	29%	22%	23%
Back pain	9%	10%	5%	5%
Neurological				
Headache	54%	58%	43%	49%
Dizziness (excluding vertigo)	16%	12%	14%	14%
Memory impairment	5%	4%	6%	5%
Psychiatric				
Irritability/ anxiety/ nervousness	19%	22%	33%	38%
Insomnia	19%	23%	30%	37%
Depression	18%	19%	20%	28%
Concentration impairment	8%	10%	10%	13%
Mood alteration	3%	2%	5%	6%
Resistance Mechanism Disorders				
Overall	10%	6%	12%	10%
Respiratory, Thoracic and Mediastinal				
Dyspnea	4%	2%	13%	14%
Cough	4%	3%	10%	7%
Dyspnea exertional	<1%	<1%	4%	7%
Skin and Subcutaneous Tissue				
Alopecia	23%	30%	28%	33%
Pruritus	12%	8%	19%	18%
Dermatitis	8%	3%	16%	13%
Dry skin	4%	3%	10%	13%
Rash	5%	4%	8%	5%
Sweating increased	6%	7%	6%	5%
Eczema	1%	1%	5%	4%
Visual Disorders				
Vision blurred	4%	2%	5%	2%

* Pooled studies 1, 2, and 3.
† Either 3 MIU or 6/3 MIU of interferon alfa-2b.
‡ Study 4.
§ Severe hematologic abnormalities.

receiving peginterferon alfa-2a either alone or in combination with ribavirin. Seventeen percent (17%) of patients receiving peginterferon alfa-2a monotherapy and 20-24% of patients receiving peginterferon alfa-2a/ribavirin combination therapy required modification of interferon dosage for neutropenia. Two percent of patients required permanent reductions of peginterferon alfa-2a dosage and <1% required permanent discontinuation. Median neutrophil counts return to pre-treatment levels 4 weeks after cessation of therapy (see DOSAGE AND ADMINISTRATION, Dose Modification).

Lymphocytes

Decreases in lymphocyte count are induced by interferon alpha therapy. Lymphopenia was observed during both monotherapy (86%) and combination therapy with peginterferon alfa-2a and ribavirin (94%). Severe lymphopenia (<0.5 x 10^9/L) occurred in approximately 5% of monotherapy patients and 14% of combination peginterferon alfa-2a and ribavirin therapy recipients. Dose adjustments were not required by protocol. Median lymphocyte counts return to pre-treatment levels after 4-12 weeks of the cessation of therapy. The clinical significance of the lymphopenia is not known.

Platelets

Platelet counts decreased in 52% of patients treated with peginterferon alfa-2a alone (median drop 45% from baseline), 33% of patients receiving combination with ribavirin (median drop 30% from baseline). Median platelet counts return to pretreatment levels 4 weeks after the cessation of therapy.

Triglycerides

Triglyceride levels are elevated in patients receiving alfa interferon therapy and were elevated in the majority of patients participating in clinical studies receiving either peginterferon alfa-2a alone or in combination with ribavirin. Random levels higher ≥400 mg/dl were observed in about 20% of patients.

ALT Elevations

Less than 1% of patients experienced marked elevations (5- to 10-fold above baseline) in ALT levels during treatment. These transaminase elevations were on occasion associated with hyperbilirubinemia and were managed by dose reduc tion or discontinuation of study treatment. Liver function test abnormalities were generally transient. One case was attributed to autoimmune hepatitis, which persisted beyond study medication discontinuation (see DOSAGE AND ADMINISTRATION, Dose Modification).

Thyroid Function

Peginterferon alfa-2a alone or in combination with ribavirin was associated with the development of abnormalities in thyroid laboratory values, some with associated clinical manifestations. Hypothyroidism or hyperthyroidism requiring treatment, dose modification or discontinuation occurred in 4% and 1% of peginterferon alfa-2a treated patients and 4% and 2% of peginterferon alfa-2a and ribavirin treated patients, respectively. Approximately half of the patients, who developed thyroid abnormalities during peginterferon alfa-2a treatment, still had abnormalities during the follow-up period (see PRECAUTIONS, Laboratory Tests).

Immunogenicity

Nine percent (71/834) of patients treated with peginterferon alfa-2a with or without ribavirin developed binding antibodies to interferon alfa-2a, as assessed by an ELISA assay. Three percent of patients (25/835) receiving peginterferon alfa-2a with or without ribavirin, developed low-titer neutralizing antibodies (using an assay of a sensitivity of 100 INU/ml).

The clinical and pathological significance of the appearance of serum neutralizing antibodies is unknown. No apparent correlation of antibody development to clinical response or adverse events was observed. The percentage of patients whose test results were considered positive for antibodies is highly dependent on the sensitivity and specificity of the assays.

Additionally the observed incidence of antibody positivity in these assays may be influenced by several factors including sample timing and handling, concomitant medications, and underlying disease. For these reasons, comparison of the incidence of antibodies to peginterferon alfa-2a with the incidence of antibodies to these products may be misleading.

DOSAGE AND ADMINISTRATION

There are no safety and efficacy data on treatment for longer than 48 weeks. Consideration should be given to discontinuing therapy after 12-24 weeks of therapy if the patient has failed to demonstrate an early virologic response.

PEGINTERFERON ALFA-2A

The recommended dose of peginterferon alfa-2a monotherapy is 180 µg (1.0 ml) once weekly for 48 weeks by subcutaneous administration in the abdomen or thigh.

PEGINTERFERON ALFA-2A AND RIBAVIRIN COMBINATION

The recommended dose of peginterferon alfa-2a when used in combination with ribavirin is 180 µg (1.0 ml) once weekly. The recommended dose of ribavirin and duration for peginterferon alfa-2a/ribavirin therapy is based on viral genotype (see TABLE 5).

The daily dose of ribavirin is 800-1200 mg administered orally in 2 divided doses. The dose should be individualized to the patient depending on baseline disease characteristics (*e.g.*, genotype), response to therapy, and tolerability of the regimen.

Since ribavirin absorption increases when administered with a meal, patients are advised to take ribavirin with food.

TABLE 5 *Peginterferon alfa-2a and Ribavirin Dosing Recommendations*

Genotype	Peginterferon alfa-2a Dose	Copegus Dose	Duration
Genotype 1, 4	180 µg	<75 kg = 1000 mg ≥75 kg = 1200 mg	48 weeks 48 weeks
Genotype 2, 3	180 µg	800 mg	24 weeks

Genotypes showed no increased response to treatment beyond 24 weeks.
Data on genotypes 5 and 6 are insufficient for dosing recommendations.

A patient should self-inject peginterferon alfa-2a only if the physician determines that it is appropriate and the patient agrees to medical follow-up as necessary and training in proper injection technique has been provided to him/her (see illustrated Peginterferon alfa-2a Medication Guide included with the prescription for directions on injection site preparation and injection instructions).

Peginterferon alfa-2a should be inspected visually for particulate matter and discoloration before administration, and not used if particulate matter is visible or product is discolored. Vials with particulate matter or discoloration should be returned to the pharmacist.

DOSE MODIFICATION

If severe adverse reactions or laboratory abnormalities develop during combination ribavirin/peginterferon alfa-2a therapy, the dose should be modified or discontinued, if appropriate, until the adverse reactions abate. If intolerance persists after dose adjustment, ribavirin/peginterferon alfa-2a therapy should be discontinued.

Peginterferon alfa-2a

General

When dose modification is required for moderate to severe adverse reactions (clinical and/or laboratory), initial dose reduction to 135 µg (0.75 ml) is generally adequate. However, in some cases, dose reduction to 90 µg (0.5 ml) may be needed. Following improvement of the adverse reaction, re-escalation of the dose may be considered (see WARNINGS, PRECAUTIONS, and ADVERSE REACTIONS).

Hematological

TABLE 6 *Peginterferon alfa-2a Hematological Dose Modification Guidelines*

Laboratory Values	Peginterferon alfa-2a Dose Reduction	Discontinue Peginterferon alfa-2a if:
ANC <750/mm^3	135 µg	ANC <500/mm^3, treatment should be suspended until ANC values return to more than 1000/mm^3. Reinstitute at 90 µg and monitor ANC
Platelet <50,000/mm^3	90 µg	Platelet count <25,000/mm^3

Psychiatric: Depression

TABLE 7 *Guidelines for Modification or Discontinuation of Peginterferon alfa-2a and for Scheduling Visits for Patients With Depression*

	Depression Severity		
	Mild	Moderate	Severe
Initial Management (4-8 Weeks)			
Dose modification	No change	Decrease peginterferon alfa-2a dose to 135 µg (in some cases dose reduction to 90 µg may be needed)	Discontinue peginterferon alfa-2a permanently
Visit schedule	Evaluate once weekly by visit and/or phone	Evaluate once weekly (office visit at least every other week)	Obtain immediate psychiatric consultation
Depression			
Remains stable	Continue weekly visit schedule	Consider psychiatric consultation. Continue reduced dosing	Psychiatric therapy necessary
Improves	Resume normal visit schedule	If symptoms improve and are stable for 4 weeks, may resume normal visit schedule. Continue reduced dosing or return to normal dose	Psychiatric therapy necessary
Worsens	(See moderate or severe depression)	(See severe depression)	Psychiatric therapy necessary

Renal Function

In patients with end-stage renal disease requiring hemodialysis, dose reduction to 135 µg peginterferon alfa-2a is recommended. Signs and symptoms of interferon toxicity should be closely monitored.

Liver Function

In patients with progressive ALT increases above baseline values, the dose of peginterferon alfa-2a should be reduced to 135 µg. If ALT increases are progressive despite dose reduction or accompanied by increased bilirubin or evidence of hepatic decompensation, therapy should be immediately discontinued.

Ribavirin

TABLE 8 *Ribavirin Dosage Modification Guidelines*

Laboratory Values	Reduce Only Copegus Dose to 600 mg/day* if:	Discontinue Copegus if:
Hemoglobin in patients with no cardiac disease	<10 g/dl	<8.5 g/dl
Hemoglobin in patients with history of stable cardiac disease	≥2 g/dl decrease in hemoglobin during any 4 week period treatment	<12 g/dl despite 4 weeks at reduced dose

* One 200 mg tablet in the morning and two 200 mg tablets in the evening.

Once ribavirin has been withheld due to a laboratory abnormality or clinical manifestation, an attempt may be made to restart ribavirin at 600 mg daily and further increase the dose to 800 mg daily depending upon the physician's judgment. However, it is not recommended that ribavirin be increased to the original dose (1000 mg or 1200 mg).

Renal Impairment

Ribavirin should not be used in patients with creatinine clearance <50 ml/min (see WARNINGS and the ribavirin package insert).

HOW SUPPLIED

SINGLE DOSE VIAL

Each Pegasys 180 µg single use, clear glass vial provides 1.0 ml containing 180 µg peginterferon alfa-2a for SC injection.

MONTHLY CONVENIENCE PACK

Four vials of Pegasys, 180 µg single use, in a box with 4 syringes and 8 alcohol swabs. Each syringe is a 1 ml (1 cc) 695 volume syringe supplied with a 27 gauge, ½ inch needle with needle-stick protection device.

STORAGE

Store in the refrigerator at 36-46°F (2-8°C). Do not freeze or shake. Protect from light. Vials are for single use only. Discard any unused portion.

PRODUCT LISTING - EQUIVALENTS NOT AVAILABLE

Solution - Subcutaneous - 180 mcg/ml

1 ml	$363.75	PEGASYS, Roche Laboratories	00004-0350-09
2 ml x 4	$1455.00	PEGASYS, Roche Laboratories	00004-0350-39

Pegvisomant (003588)

Categories: Acromegaly; Pregnancy Category B; FDA Approved 2003 Mar
Drug Classes: Hormones/hormone modifiers
Brand Names: Somavert
Cost of Therapy: $2,812.50 (Acromegaly; Somavert; 10 mg/vial; 10 mg/day; 30 day supply)

DESCRIPTION

Somavert contains pegvisomant for injection, an analog of human growth hormone (GH) that has been structurally altered to act as a GH receptor antagonist.

Pegvisomant is a protein of recombinant DNA origin containing 191 amino acid residues to which several polyethylene glycol (PEG) polymers are covalently bound (predominantly 4-6 PEG/protein molecule). The molecular weight of the protein of pegvisomant is 21,998 Daltons. The molecular weight of the PEG portion of pegvisomant is approximately 5,000 Daltons. The predominant molecular weights of pegvisomant are thus approximately 42,000, 47,000, and 52,000 Daltons. Pegvisomant is synthesized by a specific strain of *Escherichia coli* bacteria that has been genetically modified by the addition of a plasmid that carries a gene for GH receptor antagonist. Biological potency is determined using a cell proliferation bioassay.

Somavert is supplied as a sterile, white lyophilized powder intended for subcutaneous (SC) injection after reconstitution with 1 ml of sterile water for injection. Somavert is available in single-dose sterile vials containing 10, 15, or 20 mg of pegvisomant protein (approximately 10, 15, and 20 U activity, respectively). Vials containing 10, 15, and 20 mg of pegvisomant protein correspond to approximately 21, 32, and 43 mg pegvisomant, respectively. Each vial also contains 1.36 mg of glycine, 36.0 mg of mannitol, 1.04 mg of sodium phosphate dibasic anhydrous, and 0.36 mg of sodium phosphate monobasic monohydrate.

Somavert is supplied in packages that include a plastic vial containing diluent. Sterile water for injection, is a sterile, nonpyrogenic preparation of water for injection that contains no bacteriostat, antimicrobial agent, or added buffer, and is supplied in single-dose containers to be used as a diluent.

CLINICAL PHARMACOLOGY

MECHANISM OF ACTION

Pegvisomant selectively binds to growth hormone (GH) receptors on cell surfaces, where it blocks the binding of endogenous GH, and thus interferes with GH signal transduction. Inhibition of GH action results in decreased serum concentrations of insulin-like growth factor-I (IGF-I), as well as other GH-responsive serum proteins, including IGF binding protein-3 (IGFBP-3), and the acid-labile subunit (ALS).

PHARMACOKINETICS

Absorption

Following SC administration, peak serum pegvisomant concentrations are not generally attained until 33-77 hours after administration. The mean extent of absorption of a 20 mg SC dose was 57%, relative to a 10 mg intravenous dose.

Distribution

The mean apparent volume of distribution of pegvisomant is 7 L (12% coefficient of variation), suggesting that pegvisomant does not distribute extensively into tissues. After a single SC administration, exposure (C_{max}, AUC) to pegvisomant increases disproportionately with increasing dose. Mean ± SEM serum pegvisomant concentrations after 12 weeks of therapy with daily doses of 10, 15, and 20 mg were 6,600 ± 1,330; 16,000 ± 2,200; and 27,000 ± 3,100 ng/ml, respectively.

Metabolism and Elimination

The pegvisomant molecule contains covalently bound polyethylene glycol polymers in order to reduce the clearance rate. Clearance of pegvisomant following multiple doses is lower than seen following a single dose. The mean total body systemic clearance of pegvisomant following multiple doses is estimated to range between 36 to 28 ml/h for SC doses ranging from 10-20 mg/day, respectively. Clearance of pegvisomant was found to increase with body weight. Pegvisomant is eliminated from serum with a mean half-life of approximately 6 days following either single or multiple doses. Less than 1% of administered drug is recovered in the urine over 96 hours. The elimination route of pegvisomant has not been studied in humans.

DRUG-DRUG INTERACTIONS

In clinical studies, patients on opioids often needed higher serum pegvisomant concentrations to achieve appropriate IGF-I suppression compared with patients not receiving opioids. The mechanism of this interaction is not known (see DRUG INTERACTIONS).

SPECIAL POPULATIONS

Renal: No pharmacokinetic studies have been conducted in patients with renal insufficiency.

Hepatic: No pharmacokinetic studies have been conducted in patients with hepatic insufficiency.

Geriatric: No pharmacokinetic studies have been conducted in elderly subjects.

Pediatric: No pharmacokinetic studies have been conducted in pediatric subjects.

Gender: No gender effect on the pharmacokinetics of pegvisomant was found in a population pharmacokinetic analysis.

Race: The effect of race on the pharmacokinetics of pegvisomant has not been studied.

INDICATIONS AND USAGE

Pegvisomant is indicated for the treatment of acromegaly in patients who have had an inadequate response to surgery and/or radiation therapy and/or other medical therapies, or for whom these therapies are not appropriate. The goal of treatment is to normalize serum IGF-I levels.

CONTRAINDICATIONS

Pegvisomant is contraindicated in patients with a history of hypersensitivity to any of its components. The stopper on the vial of pegvisomant contains latex.

PRECAUTIONS

GENERAL

Tumor Growth

Tumors that secrete growth hormone (GH) may expand and cause serious complications. Therefore, all patients with these tumors, including those who are receiving pegvisomant, should be carefully monitored with periodic imaging scans of the sella turcica. During clinical studies of pegvisomant, 2 patients manifested progressive tumor growth. Both patients had, at baseline, large globular tumors impinging on the optic chiasm, which had been relatively resistant to previous anti-acromegalic therapies. Overall, mean tumor size was unchanged during the course of treatment with pegvisomant in the clinical studies.

Glucose Metabolism

GH opposes the effects of insulin on carbohydrate metabolism by decreasing insulin sensitivity; thus, glucose tolerance may increase in some patients treated with pegvisomant. Although none of the acromegalic patients with diabetes mellitus who were treated with pegvisomant during the clinical studies had clinically relevant hypoglycemia, these patients should be carefully monitored and doses of anti-diabetic drugs reduced as necessary.

GH Deficiency

A state of functional GH deficiency may result from administration of pegvisomant, despite the presence of elevated serum GH levels. Therefore, during treatment with pegvisomant, patients should be carefully observed for the clinical signs and symptoms of a GH-deficient state, and serum IGF-I concentrations should be monitored and maintained within the age-adjusted normal range (by adjustment of the dose of pegvisomant).

LIVER TESTS (LTS)

Elevations of serum concentrations of alanine aminotransferase (ALT) and aspartate aminotransferase (AST) greater than 10 times the upper limit of normal (ULN) were reported in 2 patients (0.8%) exposed to pegvisomant during pre-marketing clinical studies. One patient was rechallenged with pegvisomant, and the recurrence of elevated transaminase levels suggested a probable causal relationship between administration of the drug and the elevation in liver enzymes. A liver biopsy performed on the second patient was consistent with chronic hepatitis of unknown etiology. In both patients, the transaminase elevations normalized after discontinuation of the drug.

During the pre-marketing clinical studies, the incidence of elevations in ALT greater than 3 times but less than or equal to 10 times the ULN in patients treated with pegvisomant and placebo were 1.2% and 2.1%, respectively.

Elevations in ALT and AST levels were not associated with increased levels of serum total bilirubin (TBIL) and alkaline phosphatase (ALP), with the exception of 2 patients with minimal associated increases in ALP levels (*i.e.,* less than 3 times ULN). The transaminase elevations did not appear to be related to the dose of pegvisomant administered, generally occurred within 4-12 weeks of initiation of therapy, and were not associated with any identifiable biochemical, phenotypic, or genetic predictors.

Baseline serum ALT, AST, TBIL, and ALP levels should be obtained prior to initiating therapy with pegvisomant. TABLE 3 lists recommendations regarding initiation of treatment with pegvisomant, based on the results of these liver tests (LTs).

TABLE 3 *Initiation of Treatment With Pegvisomant Based on Results of Liver Tests*

Baseline LT Levels/Recommendations
Normal
May treat with pegvisomant. Monitor LTs at monthly intervals during the first 6 months of treatment, quarterly for the next 6 months, and then biannually for the next year.
Elevated, but less than or equal to 3 times ULN
May treat with pegvisomant; however, monitor LTs monthly for at least 1 year after initiation of therapy and then biannually for the next year.
Greater than 3 times ULN
Do not treat with pegvisomant until a comprehensive workup establishes the cause of the patient's liver dysfunction. Determine if cholelithiasis or choledocholithiasis is present, particularly in patients with a history of prior therapy with somatostatin analogs. Based on the workup, consider initiation of therapy with pegvisomant. If the decision is to treat, LTs and clinical symptoms should be monitored very closely.

If a patient develops LT elevations, or any other signs or symptoms of liver dysfunction while receiving pegvisomant, the following patient management is recommended (TABLE 4).

TABLE 4 *Continuation of Treatment With Pegvisomant Based on Results of Liver Tests*

LT Levels and Clinical Signs/Symptoms	Recommendations
Greater than or equal to 3 but less than 5 times ULN (without signs/symptoms of hepatitis or other liver injury, or increase in serum TBIL).	May continue therapy with pegvisomant. However, monitor LTs weekly to determine if further increases occur (see below). In addition, perform a comprehensive hepatic workup to discern if an alternative cause of liver dysfunction is present.
At least 5 times ULN, or transaminase elevations at least 3 times ULN associated with any increase in serum TBIL (with or without signs/symptoms of hepatitis or other liver injury).	Discontinue pegvisomant immediately. Perform a comprehensive hepatic workup, including serial LTs, to determine if and when serum levels return to normal. If LTs normalize (regardless of whether an alternative cause of the liver dysfunction is discovered), consider cautious reinitiation of therapy with pegvisomant, with frequent LT monitoring.
Signs or symptoms suggestive of hepatitis or other liver injury (*e.g.,* jaundice, bilirubinuria, fatigue, nausea, vomiting, right upper quadrant pain, ascites, unexplained edema, easy bruisability).	Immediately perform a comprehensive hepatic workup. If liver injury is confirmed, the drug should be discontinued.

INFORMATION FOR THE PATIENT

Patients and any other persons who may administer pegvisomant should be carefully instructed by a health care professional on how to properly reconstitute and inject the product (see instructions that are distributed with the prescription).

Patients should be informed about the need for serial monitoring of LTs, and told to immediately discontinue therapy and contact their physician if they become jaundiced. In addition, patients should be made aware that serial IGF-I levels will need to be obtained to allow their physician to properly adjust the dose of pegvisomant.

LABORATORY TESTS

Liver Tests

Recommendations for monitoring LTs are stated above [see Liver Tests (LTs)].

IGF-I Levels

Treatment with pegvisomant should be evaluated by monitoring serum IGF-I concentrations 4-6 weeks after therapy is initiated or any dose adjustments are made and at least every 6 months after IGF-I levels have normalized. The goals of treatment should be to maintain a patient's serum IGF-I concentration within the age-adjusted normal range and to control the signs and symptoms of acromegaly.

GH Levels

Pegvisomant interferes with the measurement of serum GH concentrations by commercially available GH assays (see Drug/Laboratory Test Interactions). Furthermore, even when accurately determined, GH levels usually increase during therapy with pegvisomant. Therefore, treatment with pegvisomant should not be adjusted based on serum GH concentrations.

DRUG/LABORATORY TEST INTERACTIONS

Pegvisomant has significant structural similarity to GH, which causes it to cross-react in commercially available GH assays. Because serum concentrations of pegvisomant at therapeutically effective doses are generally 100-1000 times higher than endogenous serum GH levels seen in patients with acromegaly, commercially available GH assays will overestimate true GH levels. Treatment with pegvisomant should therefore not be monitored or adjusted based on serum GH concentrations reported from these assays. Instead, monitoring and dose adjustments should only be based on serum IGF-I levels.

CARCINOGENESIS, MUTAGENESIS, AND IMPAIRMENT OF FERTILITY

Standard 2 year rodent bioassays have not been performed with pegvisomant. Pegvisomant was not mutagenic in the Ames assay or clastogenic in the *in vitro* chromosomal aberration test in human lymphocytes. Pegvisomant was found to have no effect on fertility and reproductive performance of female rabbits at SC doses up to 10 mg/kg/day (10 times the maximum human therapeutic exposure based on body surface area, mg/m^2).

PREGNANCY CATEGORY B

Early embryonic development and teratology studies were conducted in pregnant rabbits with pegvisomant at SC doses of 1, 3, and 10 mg/kg/day. There was no evidence of teratogenic effects associated with pegvisomant treatment during organogenesis. At the 10 mg/kg/day dose (10 times the maximum human therapeutic dose based on body surface area), a reproducible, slight increase in post-implantation loss was observed in both studies. There are no adequate and well-controlled studies in pregnant women. Because animal reproduction studies are not always predictive of human responses, pegvisomant should be used during pregnancy only if clearly needed.

NURSING MOTHERS

It is not known whether pegvisomant is excreted in human milk. Because many drugs are excreted in milk, caution should be exercised when pegvisomant is administered to a nursing woman.

PEDIATRIC USE

The safety and effectiveness of pegvisomant in pediatric patients have not been established.

GERIATRIC USE

Clinical studies of pegvisomant did not include sufficient numbers of subjects aged 65 and over to determine whether they respond differently from younger subjects. In general, dose selection for an elderly patient should be cautious, usually starting at the low end of the dosing range, reflecting the greater frequency of decreased hepatic, renal, or cardiac function, and of concomitant disease or other drug therapy.

DRUG INTERACTIONS

Acromegalic patients with diabetes mellitus being treated with insulin and/or oral hypoglycemic agents may require dose reductions of these therapeutic agents after the initiation of therapy with pegvisomant.

In clinical studies, patients on opioids often needed higher serum pegvisomant concentrations to achieve appropriate IGF-I suppression compared with patients not receiving opioids. The mechanism of this interaction is not known.

ADVERSE REACTIONS

LABORATORY CHANGES

Elevations of serum concentrations of ALT and AST greater than 10 times the ULN were reported in 2 subjects (0.8%) exposed to pegvisomant in pre-approval clinical studies [see PRECAUTIONS, Liver Tests (LTs)].

GENERAL

Nine acromegalic patients (9.6%) withdrew from pre-marketing clinical studies because of adverse events, including 2 patients with marked transaminase elevations [see PRECAUTIONS, Liver Tests (LTs)], 1 patient with lipohypertrophy at the injection sites, and 1 patient with substantial weight gain. The majority of reported adverse events were of mild to moderate intensity and limited duration. Most adverse events did not appear to be dose dependent. TABLE 5 shows the incidence of treatment-emergent adverse events that were reported in at least 2 patients treated with pegvisomant and at frequencies greater than placebo during the 12 week, placebo-controlled study.

TABLE 5 *Number of Patients (%) With Acromegaly Reporting Adverse Events in a 12 Week Placebo-Controlled Study With Pegvisomant**

	Pegvisomant			
	10 mg/day	15 mg/day	20 mg/day	Placebo
Event	n=26	n=26	n=28	n=32
Body as a Whole				
Infection†	6 (23%)	0	0	2 (6%)
Pain	2 (8%)	1 (4%)	4 (14%)	2 (6%)
Injection site reaction	2 (8%)	1 (4%)	3 (11%)	0
Accidental injury	2 (8%)	1 (4%)	0	1 (3%)
Back pain	2 (8%)	0	1 (4%)	1 (3%)
Flu syndrome	1 (4%)	3 (12%)	2 (7%)	0
Chest pain	1 (4%)	2 (8%)	0	0
Digestive				
Abnormal liver function tests	3 (12%)	1 (4%)	1 (4%)	1 (3%)
Diarrhea	1 (4%)	0	4 (14%)	1 (3%)
Nausea	0	2 (8%)	4 (14%)	1 (3%)
Nervous				
Dizziness	2 (8%)	1 (4%)	1 (4%)	2 (6%)
Paresthesia	0	0	2 (7%)	2 (6%)
Metabolic and Nutritional Disorders				
Peripheral edema	2 (8%)	0	1 (4%)	0
Cardiovascular				
Hypertension	0	2 (8%)	0	0
Respiratory				
Sinusitis	2 (8%)	0	1 (4%)	1 (3%)

* Table includes only those events that were reported in at least 2 patients and at a higher incidence in patients treated with pegvisomant than in patients treated with placebo.

† The 6 events coded as "infection" in the group treated with pegvisomant 10 mg were reported as cold symptoms (3), upper respiratory infection (1), blister (1), and ear infection (1). The 2 events in the placebo group were reported as cold symptoms (1) and chest infection (1).

IMMUNOGENICITY

In pre-marketing clinical studies, approximately 17% of the patients developed low titer, non-neutralizing anti-GH antibodies. Although the presence of these antibodies did not appear to impact the efficacy of pegvisomant, the long-term clinical significance of these antibodies is not known. No assay for anti-pegvisomant antibodies is commercially available for patients receiving pegvisomant.

DOSAGE AND ADMINISTRATION

A loading dose of 40 mg of pegvisomant should be administered subcutaneously under physician supervision. The patient should then be instructed to begin daily SC injections of 10 mg of pegvisomant. Serum IGF-I concentrations should be measured every 4-6 weeks, at which time the dosage of pegvisomant should be adjusted in 5 mg increments if IGF-I levels are still elevated (or 5 mg decrements if IGF-I levels have decreased below the normal range). While the goals of therapy are to achieve (and then maintain) serum IGF-I concentrations within the age-adjusted normal range and to alleviate the signs and symptoms of acromegaly, titration of dosing should be based on IGF-I levels. It is unknown whether patients who remain symptomatic while achieving normalized IGF-I levels would benefit from increased dosing with pegvisomant.

The maximum daily maintenance dose should not exceed 30 mg.

Pegvisomant is supplied as a lyophilized powder. Each vial of pegvisomant should be reconstituted with 1 ml of the diluent provided in the package (sterile water for injection). Instructions regarding reconstitution and administration are included in the package of pegvisomant and should be closely followed. To prepare the solution, withdraw 1 ml of sterile water for injection and inject it into the vial of pegvisomant, aiming the stream of liquid against the glass wall. Hold the vial between the palms of both hands and gently roll it to dissolve the powder. **DO NOT SHAKE THE VIAL,** as this may cause denaturation of pegvisomant. Discard the diluent vial containing the remaining water for injection. After reconstitution, each vial of pegvisomant contains 10, 15, or 20 mg of pegvisomant protein in 1 ml of solution. Parenteral drug products should be inspected visually for particulate matter and discoloration prior to administration. The solution should be clear after reconstitution. If the solution is cloudy, do not inject it. Only 1 dose should be administered from each vial. Pegvisomant should be administered within 6 hours after reconstitution.

HOW SUPPLIED

Somavert is available in single-dose, sterile glass vials in 10, 15, and 20 mg (as protein) strengths.

Each package of Somavert also includes a single-dose LifeShield plastic fliptop vial containing 10 ml of sterile water for injection.

The stopper on the vial of Somavert contains latex.

Storage: Prior to reconstitution, Somavert should be stored in a refrigerator at 2-8°C (36-46°F). Protect from freezing.

After reconstitution, Somavert should be administered within 6 hours. Only 1 dose should be administered from each vial.

Pemirolast Potassium *(003491)*

Categories: Conjunctivitis, allergic; FDA Approved 1999 Sep; Pregnancy Category C
Drug Classes: Mast cell stabilizers; Ophthalmics
Brand Names: Alamast
Foreign Brand Availability: Alegysal (Korea; Philippines)
Cost of Therapy: $56.70 (Allergic Conjunctivitis; Alamast; 0.1%; 10 mg; 8 drops/day; variable day supply)

DESCRIPTION

Alamast (pemirolast potassium ophthalmic solution) is a sterile, aqueous ophthalmic solution with a pH of approximately 8.0 containing 0.1% of the mast cell stabilizer, pemirolast potassium, for topical administration to the eyes. Pemirolast potassium is a slightly yellow, water-soluble powder with a molecular weight of 266.3.

The chemical formula is $C_{10}H_7KN_6O$.

The chemical name is 9-methyl-3-(1H-tetrazol-5-yl)-4H-pyrido[1,2-α] pyrimidin-4-one potassium.

Each ml contains: *Active:* Pemirolast potassium 1 mg (0.1%); *Preservative:* Lauralkonium chloride 0.005%; *Inactives:* Glycerin, dibasic sodium phosphate, monobasic sodium phosphate, phosphoric acid and/or sodium hydroxide to adjust pH, and purified water. The osmolality of Alamast ophthalmic solution is approximately 240 mOsmol/kg.

CLINICAL PHARMACOLOGY

MECHANISM OF ACTION

Pemirolast potassium is a mast cell stabilizer that inhibits the *in vivo* Type I immediate hypersensitivity reaction.

In vitro and *in vivo* studies have demonstrated that pemirolast potassium inhibits the antigen-induced release of inflammatory mediators (*e.g.*, histamine, leukotriene C_4, D_4, E_4) from human mast cells.

In addition, pemirolast potassium inhibits the chemotaxis of eosinophils into ocular tissue and blocks the release of mediators from human eosinophils.

Although the precise mechanism of action is unknown, the drug has been reported to prevent calcium influx into mast cells upon antigen stimulation.

PHARMACOKINETICS

Topical ocular administration of 1-2 drops of pemirolast potassium ophthalmic solution in each eye 4 times daily in 16 healthy volunteers for 2 weeks resulted in detectable concentrations in the plasma. The mean (±SE) peak plasma level of 4.7 ± 0.8 ng/ml occurred at 0.42 ± 0.05 hours and the mean $t_{1/2}$ was 4.5 ± 0.2 hours. When a single 10 mg pemirolast potassium dose was taken orally, a peak plasma concentration of 0.723 μg/ml was reached.

Following topical administration, about 10-15% of the dose was excreted unchanged in the urine.

INDICATIONS AND USAGE

Pemirolast potassium ophthalmic solution is indicated for the prevention of itching of the eye due to allergic conjunctivitis. Symptomatic response to therapy (decreased itching) may be evident within a few days, but frequently requires longer treatment (up to 4 weeks).

CONTRAINDICATIONS

Pemirolast potassium ophthalmic solution is contraindicated in patients with previously demonstrated hypersensitivity to any of the ingredients of this product.

WARNINGS

For topical ophthalmic use only. Not for injection or oral use.

PRECAUTIONS

INFORMATION FOR THE PATIENT

To prevent contaminating the dropper tip and solution, do not touch the eyelids or surrounding areas with the dropper tip. Keep the bottle tightly closed when not in use.

Patients should be advised not to wear contact lenses if their eyes are red. Pemirolast potassium ophthalmic solution should not be used to treat contact lens related irritation. The preservative in Alamast, lauralkonium chloride, may be absorbed by soft contact lenses. Patients who wear soft contact lenses and whose eyes are not red should be instructed to wait at least 10 minutes after instilling pemirolast potassium ophthalmic solution before they insert their contact lenses.

CARCINOGENESIS, MUTAGENESIS, AND IMPAIRMENT OF FERTILITY

Pemirolast potassium was not mutagenic or clastogenic when tested in a series of bacterial and mammalian tests for gene mutation and chromosomal injury *in vitro* nor was it clastogenic when tested *in vivo* in rats.

Pemirolast potassium had no effect on mating and fertility in rats at oral doses up to 250 mg/kg (approximately 20,000-fold the human dose at 2 drops/eye, 40 μl/drop, qid for a 50 kg adult). A reduced fertility and pregnancy index occurred in the F_1 generation when F_0 dams were treated with 400 mg/kg pemirolast potassium during late pregnancy and lactation period (approximately 30,000-fold the human dose).

PREGNANCY

Teratogenic Effects, Pregnancy Category C

Pemirolast potassium caused an increased incidence of thymic remnant in the neck, interventricular septal defect, fetuses with wavy rib, splitting of thoracic vertebral body, and reduced numbers of ossified sternebrae, sacral and caudal vertebrae, and metatarsi when rats were given oral doses ≥250 mg/kg (approximately 20,000-fold the human dose at 2 drops/eye, 40 µl/drop, qid for a 50 kg adult) during organogenesis. Increased incidence of dilation of renal pelvis/ureter in the fetuses and neonates was also noted when rats were given an oral dose of 400 mg/kg pemirolast potassium (approximately 30,000-fold the human dose). Pemirolast potassium was not teratogenic in rabbits given oral doses up to 150 mg/kg (approximately 12,000-fold the human dose) during the same time period. There are no adequate and well-controlled studies in pregnant women. Because animal reproductive studies are not always predictive of human response, pemirolast potassium ophthalmic solution should be used during pregnancy only if the benefit outweighs the risk.

Nonteratogenic Effects

Pemirolast potassium produced increased pre- and post-implantation losses, reduced embryo/fetal and neonatal survival, decreased neonatal body weight, and delayed neonatal development in rats receiving an oral dose at 400 mg/kg (approximately 30,000-fold the human dose). Pemirolast potassium also caused a reduction in the number of corpus lutea, the number of implantations, and number of live fetuses in the F_1 generation in rats when F_0 dams were given oral dosages ≥250 mg/kg (approximately 20,000-fold the human dose) during late gestation and the lactation period.

NURSING MOTHERS

Pemirolast potassium is excreted in the milk of lactating rats at concentrations higher than those in plasma. It is not known whether pemirolast potassium is excreted in human milk. Because many drugs are excreted in human milk, caution should be exercised when pemirolast potassium ophthalmic solution is administered to a nursing woman.

PEDIATRIC USE

Safety and effectiveness in pediatric patients below the age of 3 years have not been established.

ADVERSE REACTIONS

In clinical studies lasting up to 17 weeks with pemirolast potassium ophthalmic solution, headache, rhinitis, and cold/flu symptoms were reported at an incidence of 10-25%. The occurrence of these side effects was generally mild. Some of these events were similar to the underlying ocular disease being studied.

The following ocular and non-ocular adverse reactions were reported at an incidence of less than 5%:

Ocular: Burning, dry eye, foreign body sensation, and ocular discomfort. *Non-Ocular:* Allergy, back pain, bronchitis, cough, dysmenorrhea, fever, sinusitis, and sneezing/nasal congestion.

DOSAGE AND ADMINISTRATION

The recommended dose is 1-2 drops in each affected eye 4 times daily.

Symptomatic response to therapy (decreased itching) may be evident within a few days, but frequently requires longer treatment (up to 4 weeks).

HOW SUPPLIED

Alamast (pemirolast potassium ophthalmic solution), 0.1% is supplied as follows: 10 ml in a white, low density polyethylene bottle with a controlled dropper tip, and a white polypropylene screw cap.

Storage: Store at 15-25°C (59-77°F).

PRODUCT LISTING - EQUIVALENTS NOT AVAILABLE

Solution - Ophthalmic - 0.1%

10 ml $56.70 ALAMAST, Santen Inc 65086-0711-10

Pemoline *(001963)*

Categories: Attention deficit hyperactivity disorder; Pregnancy Category B; DEA Class CIV; FDA Approved 1975 Jan
Drug Classes: Stimulants, central nervous system
Brand Names: Cylert
Foreign Brand Availability: Betanamin (Japan); Hyperilex (Germany); Tradon (Germany)
Cost of Therapy: $78.36 (Attention Deficit Hyperactivity Disorder; Generic Tablets; 18.75 mg; 3 tablets/day; 30 day supply)

WARNING

PEMOLINE SHOULD NOT BE USED BY PATIENTS UNTIL THERE HAS BEEN A COMPLETE DISCUSSION OF THE RISKS AND BENEFITS OF PEMOLINE THERAPY AND WRITTEN INFORMED CONSENT HAS BEEN OBTAINED. A SUPPLY OF PATIENT INFORMATION/CONSENT FORMS ARE AVAILABLE, FREE OF CHARGE, BY CALLING 847-937-7302. PERMISSION TO USE THE PATIENT INFORMATION/CONSENT FORM BY PHOTOCOPY REPRODUCTION IS HEREBY GRANTED BY ABBOTT LABORATORIES.

Because of its association with life threatening hepatic failure, pemoline should not ordinarily be considered as first line drug therapy for ADHD (see INDICATIONS AND USAGE). Because pemoline provides an observable symptomatic benefit, patients who fail to show substantial clinical benefit within 3 weeks of completing dose titration, should be withdrawn from pemoline therapy.

WARNING — Cont'd

Since pemoline's marketing in 1975, 15 cases of acute hepatic failure have been reported to the FDA. While the absolute number of reported cases is not large, the rate of reporting ranges from 4-17 times the rate expected in the general population. This estimate may be conservative because of under reporting and because the long latency between initiation of pemoline treatment and the occurrence of hepatic failure may limit recognition of the association. If only a portion of actual cases were recognized and reported, the risk could be substantially higher.

Of the 15 cases reported as of December 1998, 12 resulted in death or liver transplantation, usually within 4 weeks of the onset of signs and symptoms of liver failure. The earliest onset of hepatic abnormalities occurred 6 months after initiation of pemoline. Although some reports described dark urine and nonspecific prodromal symptoms (*e.g.*, anorexia, malaise, and gastrointestinal symptoms), in other reports it was not clear if any prodromal symptoms preceded the onset of jaundice.

Treatment with pemoline should be initiated only in individuals without liver disease and with normal baseline liver function tests. It is not clear if baseline and periodic liver function testing are predictive of these instances of acute liver failure; however it is generally believed that early detection of drug-induced hepatic injury along with immediate withdrawal of the suspect drug enhances the likelihood for recovery. Accordingly, the following liver monitoring program is recommended: Serum ALT (SGPT) levels should be determined at baseline, and every 2 weeks thereafter. If pemoline therapy is discontinued and then restarted, liver function test monitoring should be done at baseline and reinitiated at the frequency above.

Pemoline should be discontinued if serum ALT (SGPT) is increased to a clinically significant level, or any increase ≥2 times the upper limit of normal, or if clinical signs and symptoms suggest liver failure (see PRECAUTIONS).

The physician who elects to use pemoline should obtain written informed consent from the patient prior to initiation of pemoline therapy.

DESCRIPTION

Pemoline is a central nervous system stimulant. Pemoline is structurally dissimilar to the amphetamines and methylphenidate.

It is an oxazolidine compound and is chemically identified as 2-amino-5-phenyl-2-oxazolin-4-one.

Pemoline is a white, tasteless, odorless powder, relatively insoluble (less than 1 mg/ml) in water, chloroform, ether, acetone, and benzene; its solubility in 95% ethyl alcohol is 2.2 mg/ml.

Cylert is supplied as tablets containing 18.75, 37.5 or 75 mg of pemoline for oral administration. Cylert is also available as chewable tablets containing 37.5 mg of pemoline.

Cylert Inactive Ingredients

18.75 mg Tablet: Corn starch, gelatin, lactose, magnesium hydroxide, polyethylene glycol, and talc.

37.5 mg Tablet: Corn starch, FD&C yellow no. 6, gelatin, lactose, magnesium hydroxide, polyethylene glycol, and talc.

37.5 mg Chewable Tablet: Corn starch, FD&C yellow no. 6, magnesium hydroxide, magnesium stearate, mannitol, polyethylene glycol, povidone, talc, and artificial flavor.

75 mg Tablet: Corn starch, gelatin, iron oxide, lactose, magnesium hydroxide, polyethylene glycol, and talc.

CLINICAL PHARMACOLOGY

METABOLISM

Pemoline has a pharmacological activity similar to that of other known central nervous system stimulants; however, it has minimal sympathomimetic effects. Although studies indicate that pemoline may act in animals through dopaminergic mechanisms, the exact mechanism and site of action of the drug in humans is not known.

There is neither specific evidence which clearly establishes the mechanism whereby pemoline produces its mental and behavioral effects in children, nor conclusive evidence regarding how these effects relate to the condition of the central nervous system.

Pemoline has a gradual onset of action. Using the recommended schedule of dosage titration, significant clinical benefit may not be evident until the third or fourth week of drug administration.

ABSORPTION

Pemoline is rapidly absorbed from the gastrointestinal tract. Approximately 50% is bound to plasma proteins. The serum half-life of pemoline is approximately 12 hours. Peak serum levels of the drug occur within 2-4 hours after ingestion of a single dose. Multiple dose studies in adults at several dose levels indicate that steady state is reached in approximately 2-3 days. In animals given radiolabeled pemoline, the drug was widely and uniformly distributed throughout the tissues, including the brain.

METABOLISM

Pemoline is metabolized by the liver. Metabolites of pemoline include pemoline conjugate, pemoline dione, mandelic acid, and unidentified polar compounds. Pemoline is excreted primarily by the kidneys with approximately 50% excreted unchanged and only minor fractions present as metabolites.

INDICATIONS AND USAGE

Pemoline is indicated in Attention Deficit Hyperactivity Disorder (ADHD). Because of its association with life threatening hepatic failure, pemoline should not ordinarily be considered as first line therapy for ADHD (see BOXED WARNING).

Pemoline therapy should be part of a total treatment program which typically includes other remedial measures (psychological, educational, social) for a stabilizing effect in children with a behavioral syndrome characterized by the following group of developmentally inappropriate symptoms: moderate to severe distractibility, short attention span, hyperactivity, emotional lability, and impulsivity. The diagnosis of this syndrome should not be made with finality when these symptoms are only of comparatively recent origin. Nonlocalizing (soft) neurological signs, learning disability, and abnormal EEG may or may not be present, and a diagnosis of central nervous system dysfunction may or may not be warranted.

CONTRAINDICATIONS

Pemoline is contraindicated in patients with known hypersensitivity or idiosyncrasy to the drug. Pemoline should not be administered to patients with impaired hepatic function (see BOXED WARNING and ADVERSE REACTIONS).

WARNINGS

Decrements in the predicted growth (*i.e.,* weight gain and/or height) rate have been reported with the long-term use of stimulants in children. Therefore, patients requiring long-term therapy should be carefully monitored.

PRECAUTIONS

GENERAL

Clinical experience suggests that in psychotic children, administration of pemoline may exacerbate symptoms of behavior disturbance and thought disorder.

Pemoline should be administered with caution to patients with significantly impaired renal function.

INFORMATION FOR THE PATIENT

Patients should be informed that pemoline therapy has been associated with liver abnormalities ranging from reversible liver function test increases that do not cause any symptoms to liver failure, which may result in death. Patients should be informed that the risk of liver failure in the general population is relatively rare; however patients taking pemoline are at a greater risk of developing liver failure than that expected in the general population. At present, there is no way to predict who is likely to develop liver failure; however only patients without liver disease and with normal baseline liver function tests should initiate pemoline therapy. Patients should be advised to follow their doctor's directives for liver function tests prior to and during pemoline therapy. Patients should be advised to be alert for signs of liver dysfunction (jaundice, anorexia, gastrointestinal complaints, malaise, etc.) and to report them to their doctor immediately if they should occur.

The physician who elects to use pemoline should obtain written informed consent from patients prior to initiation of pemoline therapy.

LABORATORY TESTS

Since pemoline's market introduction, there have been reports of elevated liver enzymes associated with its use. Many of these patients had this increase detected several months after starting pemoline. Most patients were asymptomatic, with the increase in liver enzymes returning to normal after pemoline was discontinued.

Treatment with pemoline should be initiated only in individuals without liver disease and with normal baseline liver function tests. It is not clear if baseline and periodic liver function testing are predictive of these instances of acute liver failure; however it is generally believed that early detection of drug-induced hepatic injury along with immediate withdrawal of the suspect drug enhances the likelihood for recovery. Accordingly, the following liver monitoring program is recommended.

Serum ALT (SGPT) levels should be determined at baseline, and every 2 weeks thereafter. If pemoline therapy is discontinued and then restarted, liver function test monitoring should be done at baseline and reinitiated at the frequency above. Pemoline should be discontinued if serum ALT (SGPT) is increased to a clinically significant level, or any increase ≥2 times the upper limit of normal, or if clinical signs and symptoms suggest liver failure (see BOXED WARNING).

CARCINOGENESIS, MUTAGENESIS, AND IMPAIRMENT OF FERTILITY

Carcinogenesis

Long-term studies have been conducted in rats with doses as high as 150 mg/kg/day for 18 months. There was no significant difference in the incidence of any neoplasm between treated and control animals.

Mutagenesis

Data are not available concerning long-term effects on mutagenicity in animals or humans.

Impairment of Fertility

The results of studies in which rats were given 18.75 and 37.5 mg/kg/day indicated that pemoline did not affect fertility in males or females at those doses.

PREGNANCY, TERATOGENIC EFFECTS, PREGNANCY CATEGORY B

Reproduction studies have been performed in rats and rabbits at doses of 18.75 and 37.5 mg/kg/day and have revealed no evidence of impaired fertility or harm to the fetus. There are, however, no adequate and well-controlled studies in pregnant women. Because animal reproduction studies are not always predictive of human response, this drug should be used during pregnancy only if clearly needed.

NONTERATOGENIC EFFECTS

Studies in rats have shown an increased incidence of stillbirths and cannibalization when pemoline was administered at a dose of 37.5 mg/kg/day. Postnatal survival of offspring was reduced at doses of 18.75 and 37.5 mg/kg/day.

NURSING MOTHERS

It is not known whether this drug is excreted in human milk. Because many drugs are excreted in human milk, caution should be exercised when pemoline is administered to a nursing woman.

PEDIATRIC USE

Safety and effectiveness in children below the age of 6 years have not been established.

Long-term effects of pemoline in children have not been established (see WARNINGS).

CNS stimulants, including pemoline, have been reported to precipitate motor and phonic tics and Tourette's syndrome. Therefore, clinical evaluation for tics and Tourette's syndrome in children and their families should precede use of stimulant medications.

Drug treatment is not indicated in all cases of ADHD and should be considered only in light of complete history and evaluation of the child. The decision to prescribe pemoline should depend on the physician's assessment of the chronicity and severity of the child's symptoms and their appropriateness for his/her age. Prescription should not depend solely on the presence of one or more of the behavioral characteristics.

DRUG INTERACTIONS

The interaction of pemoline with other drugs has not been studied in humans. Patients who are receiving pemoline concurrently with other drugs, especially drugs with CNS activity, should be monitored carefully.

Decreased seizure threshold has been reported in patients receiving pemoline concomitantly with *antiepileptic medications.*

ADVERSE REACTIONS

The following are adverse reactions in decreasing order of severity within each category associated with pemoline.

Hepatic: There have been reports of hepatic dysfunction, ranging from asymptomatic reversible increases in liver enzymes to hepatitis, jaundice, and fatal hepatic failure, in patients taking pemoline (see BOXED WARNING and PRECAUTIONS).

Hematopoietic: There have been isolated reports of aplastic anemia.

Central Nervous System: The following CNS effects have been reported with the use of pemoline: convulsive seizures; literature reports indicate that pemoline may precipitate attacks of Gilles de la Tourette syndrome; hallucinations; dyskinetic movements of the tongue, lips, face, and extremities; abnormal oculomotor function including nystagmus and oculogyric crisis; mild depression; dizziness; increased irritability; headache; and drowsiness.

Insomnia is the most frequently reported side effect of pemoline; it usually occurs early in therapy prior to an optimum therapeutic response. In the majority of cases it is transient in nature or responds to a reduction in dosage.

Gastrointestinal: Anorexia and weight loss may occur during the first weeks of therapy. In the majority of cases it is transient in nature; weight gain usually resumes within 3-6 months.

Nausea and stomachache have also been reported.

Genitourinary: A case of elevated acid phosphatase in association with prostatic enlargement has been reported in a 63 year old male who was treated with pemoline for sleepiness. The acid phosphatase normalized with discontinuation of pemoline and was again elevated.

Miscellaneous: Suppression of growth has been reported with the long-term use of stimulants in children. (See WARNINGS.) Skin rash has been reported with pemoline.

If adverse reactions are of a significant or protracted nature, dosage should be reduced or the drug discontinued.

DOSAGE AND ADMINISTRATION

Pemoline is administered as a single oral dose each morning. The recommended starting dose is 37.5 mg/day. This daily dose should be gradually increased by 18.75 mg at 1 week intervals until the desired clinical response is obtained. The effective daily dose for most patients will range from 56.25 to 75 mg. The maximum recommended daily dose of pemoline is 112.5 mg.

Clinical improvement with pemoline is gradual. Using the recommended schedule of dosage titration, significant benefit may not be evident until the third or fourth week of drug administration. Because pemoline provides an observable symptomatic benefit, patients who fail to show substantial clinical benefit within 3 weeks of completing dose titration, should be withdrawn from pemoline therapy.

Where possible, drug administration should be interrupted occasionally to determine if there is a recurrence of behavioral symptoms sufficient to require continued therapy.

HOW SUPPLIED

Cylert is supplied as monogrammed, grooved tablets in three dosage strengths: 18.75 mg (white), 37.5 mg (orange-colored), and 75 mg (tan-colored).

Cylert chewable: Supplied as 37.5 mg monogrammed, grooved tablets (orange-colored).

Recommended storage: Store below 30°C (86°F).

PRODUCT LISTING - RATED THERAPEUTICALLY EQUIVALENT

Tablet - Oral - 18.75 mg			
100's	$87.07	GENERIC, Geneva Pharmaceuticals	00781-1731-01
100's	$87.08	GENERIC, Qualitest Products Inc	00603-5055-21
100's	$88.73	GENERIC, Apothecon Inc	62269-0391-24
100's	$90.53	GENERIC, Mallinckrodt Medical Inc	00406-1552-01
100's	$90.59	GENERIC, Teva Pharmaceuticals Usa	00093-9541-01
100's	$99.70	GENERIC, Amide Pharmaceutical Inc	52152-0197-02
100's	$117.80	CYLERT, Abbott Pharmaceutical	00074-6025-13
Tablet - Oral - 37.5 mg			
100's	$136.88	GENERIC, Qualitest Products Inc	00603-5056-21
100's	$136.88	GENERIC, Teva Pharmaceuticals Usa	00781-1741-01
100's	$136.88	GENERIC, Bristol-Myers Squibb	62269-0392-24
100's	$151.38	GENERIC, Teva Pharmaceuticals Usa	00093-9524-01
100's	$157.22	GENERIC, Amide Pharmaceutical Inc	52152-0161-02
100's	$185.15	CYLERT, Abbott Pharmaceutical	00074-6057-13
Tablet - Oral - 75 mg			
100's	$236.28	GENERIC, Mallinckrodt Medical Inc	00406-1558-01
100's	$236.34	GENERIC, Geneva Pharmaceuticals	00781-1751-01
100's	$236.34	GENERIC, Bristol-Myers Squibb	62269-0393-24

100's	$236.35	GENERIC, Qualitest Products Inc	00603-5057-21
100's	$261.38	GENERIC, Teva Pharmaceuticals Usa	00093-9472-01
100's	$271.48	GENERIC, Amide Pharmaceutical Inc	52152-0162-02
100's	$319.73	CYLERT, Abbott Pharmaceutical	00074-6073-13

Tablet, Chewable - Oral - 37.5 mg

100's	$136.81	GENERIC, Mallinckrodt Medical Inc	00406-1554-01
100's	$155.19	GENERIC, Mallinckrodt Medical Inc	00406-8854-01
100's	$155.22	GENERIC, Teva Pharmaceuticals Usa	00093-9577-01
100's	$155.22	GENERIC, Teva Pharmaceuticals Usa	38245-0577-01
100's	$171.38	GENERIC, Amide Pharmaceutical Inc	52152-0186-02
100's	$201.84	CYLERT, Abbott Pharmaceutical	00074-6088-13

Penbutolol Sulfate *(001964)*

For complete prescribing information, refer to the CD-ROM included with the book.

For related information, see the comparative table section in Appendix A.

Categories: Hypertension, essential; Pregnancy Category C; FDA Approved 1989 Jan
Drug Classes: Antiadrenergics, beta blocking
Brand Names: Levatol
Foreign Brand Availability: Betapresin (Mexico); Betapressin (Austria; Germany; Japan; Korea; Netherlands)
Cost of Therapy: $49.92 (Hypertension; Levatol; 20 mg; 1 tablet/day; 30 day supply)

DESCRIPTION

Penbutolol sulfate is a synthetic β-receptor antagonist for oral administration. The chemical name of penbutolol sulfate is (S)-1-tert-butylamino-3-(o-cyclopentylphenoxy)-2-propanol sulfate. It is provided as the levorotatory isomer.

The empirical formula for penbutolol sulfate is: $C_{36}H_{60}N_2O_8S$.

Its molecular weight is 680.94. A dose of 20 mg is equivalent to 29.4 μmol.

Penbutolol is a white, odorless, crystalline powder.

Levatol is available as tablets for oral administration. Each tablet contains 20 mg of penbutolol sulfate. It also contains corn starch, D&C yellow no. 10, lactose, magnesium stearate, povidone, silicon dioxide, talc, titanium dioxide, and other inactive ingredients.

INDICATIONS AND USAGE

Penbutolol sulfate is indicated in the treatment of mild to moderate arterial hypertension. It may be used alone or in combination with other antihypertensive agents, especially thiazide-type diuretics.

NON-FDA APPROVED INDICATIONS

Penbutolol has been used without FDA approval for the treatment of angina pectoris.

CONTRAINDICATIONS

Penbutolol sulfate is contraindicated in patients with cardiogenic shock, sinus bradycardia, second and third degree atrioventricular conduction block, bronchial asthma, and those with known hypersensitivity to this product (see WARNINGS).

WARNINGS

CARDIAC FAILURE

Sympathetic stimulation may be essential for supporting circulatory function in patients with heart failure, and its inhibition by β-adrenergic receptor blockade may precipitate more severe failure. Although β-blockers should be avoided in overt congestive heart failure, penbutolol sulfate can, if necessary, by used with caution in patients with a history of cardiac failure who are well compensated, on treatment with vasodilators, digitalis and/or diuretics. Both digitalis and penbutolol slow AV conduction. Beta-adrenergic receptor antagonists do not inhibit the inotropic action of digitalis on heart muscle. If cardiac failure persists, treatment with penbutolol sulfate should be discontinued.

PATIENTS WITHOUT HISTORY OF CARDIAC FAILURE

Continued depression of the myocardium with β-blocking agents over a period of time can, in some cases, lead to cardiac failure. At the first evidence of heart failure, patients receiving penbutolol sulfate should be given appropriate treatment, and the response should be closely observed. If cardiac failure continues despite adequate intervention with appropriate drugs, penbutolol sulfate should be withdrawn (gradually, if possible).

EXACERBATION OF ISCHEMIC HEART DISEASE FOLLOWING ABRUPT WITHDRAWAL

Hypersensitivity to catecholamines has been observed in patients who were withdrawn from therapy with β-blocking agents; exacerbation of angina and, in some cases, myocardial infarction have occurred after abrupt discontinuation of such therapy. When discontinuing penbutolol sulfate, particularly in patients with ischemic heart disease the dosage should be reduced gradually over a period of 1-2 weeks and the patient should be monitored carefully. If angina becomes more pronounced or acute coronary insufficiency develops, administration of penbutolol sulfate should be reinstated promptly, at least on a temporary basis, and appropriate measures should be taken for the management of unstable angina. Patients should be warned against interruption or discontinuation of therapy without the physician's advice. Because coronary artery disease is common and may not be recognized, it may not be prudent to discontinue penbutolol sulfate abruptly, even in patients who are being treated only for hypertension.

NONALLERGIC BRONCHOSPASM (E.G., CHRONIC BRONCHITIS, EMPHYSEMA)

Penbutolol sulfate is contraindicated in bronchial asthma. In general, patients with bronchospastic diseases should not receive β-blockers. Penbutolol sulfate should be administered with caution because it may block bronchodilation produced by endogenous catecholamine stimulation of β-2 receptors.

ANESTHESIA AND MAJOR SURGERY

The necessity, or desirability, of withdrawal of a β-blocking therapy prior to major surgery is controversial. Beta-adrenergic receptor blockade impairs the ability of the heart to respond to β-adrenergically mediated reflex stimuli. Although this might be of benefit in preventing arrhythmic response, the risk of excessive myocardial depression during general anesthesia may be enhanced and difficulty in restarting and maintaining the heart beat has been reported with β-blockers. If treatment is continued, particular care should be taken when using anesthetic agents that depress the myocardium, such as ether, cyclopropane, and trichloroethylene, and it is prudent to use the lowest possible dose of penbutolol sulfate. Penbutolol sulfate like other β-blockers, is a competitive inhibitor of β-receptor agonists, and its effect on the heart can be reversed by cautious administration of such agents (*e.g.,* dobutamine or isoproterenol. Manifestations of excessive vagal tone (*e.g.,* profound bradycardia, hypotension) may be corrected with atropine 1-3 mg IV in divided doses.

DIABETES MELLITUS AND HYPOGLYCEMIA

Beta-adrenergic receptor blockade may prevent the appearance of signs and symptoms of acute hypoglycemia, such as tachycardia and blood pressure changes. This is especially important in patients with labile diabetes. Beta-blockade also reduces the release of insulin in response to hyperglycemia; therefore, it may be necessary to adjust the dose of hypoglycemic drugs. Beta-adrenergic blockade may also impair the homeostatic response to hypoglycemia; in that event, the spontaneous recovery from hypoglycemia may be delayed during treatment with β-adrenergic receptor antagonists.

THYROTOXICOSIS

Beta-adrenergic blockade may mask certain clinical signs (*e.g.,* tachycardia) of hyperthyroidism. Patients suspected of developing thyrotoxicosis should be managed carefully to avoid abrupt withdrawal of β-adrenergic receptor blockers that might precipitate a thyroid storm.

DOSAGE AND ADMINISTRATION

The usual starting and maintenance dose of penbutolol sulfate, used alone in combination with other antihypertensive agents, such as thiazide-type diuretics, is 20 mg given once daily.

Doses of 40 and 80 mg have been well tolerated but have not been shown to give a greater antihypertensive effect. The full effect of a 20 or 40 mg dose is seen by the end of 2 weeks. A dose of 10 mg also lowers blood pressure, but the full effect is not seen for 4-6 weeks.

PRODUCT LISTING - EQUIVALENTS NOT AVAILABLE

Tablet - Oral - 20 mg

100's	$166.40	LEVATOL, Schwarz Pharma	00091-4500-15

Penciclovir *(003304)*

Categories: Herpes labialis; Infection, herpes simplex virus; Pregnancy Category B; FDA Approved 1996 Sep
Drug Classes: Antivirals
Brand Names: Denavir
Foreign Brand Availability: Vectavir (Bahamas; Barbados; Belize; Benin; Bermuda; Burkina-Faso; Costa-Rica; Curacao; Dominican-Republic; El-Salvador; Ethiopia; Gambia; Germany; Ghana; Guatemala; Guinea; Guyana; Honduras; Israel; Ivory-Coast; Jamaica; Kenya; Liberia; Malawi; Mali; Mauritania; Mauritius; Morocco; Netherland-Antilles; Nicaragua; Niger; Nigeria; Panama; Puerto-Rico; Senegal; Seychelles; Sierra-Leone; Sudan; Surinam; Tanzania; Trinidad; Tunia; Uganda; Zambia; Zimbabwe)
Cost of Therapy: $22.90 (Herpes Labialis; Denavir Cream; 10 mg/g; 1.5 g; 8 applications/day; variable day supply)

DESCRIPTION

For Dermatologic Use Only.

Penciclovir is an antiviral agent active against herpes viruses. Denavir is available for topical administration as a 1% white cream. Each gram of Denavir contains 10 mg of penciclovir and the following inactive ingredients: cetomacrogol 1000 BP, cetostearyl alcohol, mineral oil, propylene glycol, purified water and white petrolatum.

Chemically, penciclovir is known as 9-[4-hydroxy-3-(hydroxymethyl) butyl]guanine. Its molecular formula is $C_{10}H_{15}N_5O_3$; its molecular weight is 253.26. It is a synthetic acyclic guanine derivative.

Penciclovir is a white to pale yellow solid. At 20°C it has a solubility of 0.2 mg/ml in methanol, 1.3 mg/ml in propylene glycol, and 1.7 mg/ml in water. In aqueous buffer (pH 2) the solubility is 10.0 mg/ml. Penciclovir is not hygropscopic. Its partition coefficient in n-octanol/water at pH 7.5 is 0.024 (logP = -1.62).

CLINICAL PHARMACOLOGY

MICROBIOLOGY

Mechanism of Antiviral Activity

The antiviral compound penciclovir has *in vitro* inhibitory activity against herpes simplex virus types 1 (HSV-1) and 2 (HSV-2). In cells infected with HSV-1 or HSV-2, viral thymidine kinase phosphorylates penciclovir to a monophosphate form which, in turn, is converted to penciclovir triphosphate by cellular kinases. *In vitro* studies demonstrate that penciclovir triphosphate inhibits HSV polymerase competitively with deoxyguanosine triphosphate. Consequently, herpes viral DNA synthesis and, therefore, replication are selectively inhibited.

Antiviral Activity In Vitro and In Vivo

In cell culture studies, penciclovir has antiviral activity against HSV-1 and HSV-2. Sensitivity test results, expressed as the concentration of the drug required to inhibit growth of the virus by 50% (IC_{50}) or 99% (IC_{99}) in cell culture, vary depending upon a number of factors, including the assay protocols. See TABLE 1.

P

TABLE 1

Method of Assay / Virus Type	Cell Type	IC_{50} (µg/ml)	IC_{99} (µg/ml)
Plaque Reduction			
HSV-1 (c.i.)	MRC-5	0.2-0.6	
HSV-1 (c.i.)	WISH	0.04-0.5	
HSV-2 (c.i.)	MRC-5	0.9-2.1	
HSV-2 (c.i.)	WISH	0.1-0.8	
Virus Yield Reduction			
HSV-1 (c.i.)	MRC-5		0.4-0.5
HSV-2 (c.i.)	MRC-5		0.6-0.7
DNA Synthesis Inhibition			
HSV-1 (SC16)	MRC-5	0.04	
HSV-2 (MS)	MRC-5	0.05	

(c.i.) Clinical isolates. The latent state of any herpes virus not known to respond to any antiviral therapy.

Drug Resistance

Penciclovir-resistant mutants of HSV can result from qualitative changes in viral thymidine kinase or DNA polymerase. The most commonly encountered acyclovir-resistant mutants that are deficient in viral thymidine kinase are also resistant to penciclovir.

PHARMACOKINETICS

Measurable penciclovir concentration were not detected in plasma or urine of healthy male volunteers (n=12) following single or repeat application of the 1% cream at a dose of 180 mg penciclovir daily (approximately 67 times the estimated usual clinical dose).

Pediatric Patients

The systemic absorption of penciclovir following topical administration has not been evaluated in patients <18 years of age. However, a multicenter open label study was initiated and 1% penciclovir cream was well tolerated in children 12-17 years old with recurrent herpes labialis.

INDICATIONS AND USAGE

Penciclovir cream is indicated for the treatment of recurrent herpes labialis (cold sores) in adults and children 12 years and over.

CONTRAINDICATIONS

Penciclovir is contraindicated in patients with known hypersensitivity to the product or any of its components.

PRECAUTIONS

GENERAL

Penciclovir should only be used on herpes labialis on the lips and face. Because no data are available, application to human mucous membranes is not recommended. Particular care should be taken to avoid application in or near the eyes since it may cause irritation. The effect of penciclovir has not been established in immunocompromised patients.

CARCINOGENESIS, MUTAGENESIS, AND IMPAIRMENT OF FERTILITY

In clinical trials, systemic drug exposure following the topical administration of penciclovir cream was negligible, as the penciclovir content of all plasma and urine samples was below the limit of assay detection (0.1 µg/ml and 10 µg/ml, respectively). However, for the purpose of inter-species dose comparisons presented in the following sections, an assumption of 100% absorption of penciclovir from the topically applied product has been used. Based on use of the maximal recommended topical dose of penciclovir of 0.05 mg/kg/day and an assumption of 100% absorption, the maximum theoretical plasma AUC(0-24h) for penciclovir is approximately 0.129 µg·h/ml.

Carcinogenesis

Two year carcinogenicity studies were conducted with famciclovir (the oral prodrug of penciclovir) in rats and mice. An increase in the incidence of mammary adenocarcinoma (a common tumor in female rats of the strain used) was seen in female rats receiving 600 mg/kg/day (approximately 395× the maximum theoretical human exposure to penciclovir following application of the topical product, based on area under the plasma concentration curve comparison [24 hr AUC]). No increases in tumor incidence were seen among male rats treated at doses up to 240 mg/kg/day (approximately 190× the maximum theoretical human AUC for penciclovir), or in male and female mice at doses up to 600 mg/kg/day (approximately 100× the maximum theoretical human AUC for penciclovir).

Mutagenesis

When tested *in vitro*, penciclovir did not cause an increase in gene mutation in the Ames assay using multiple strains of *S. typhimurium* or *E. coli* (at up to 20,000 µg/plate), nor did it cause an increase in unscheduled DNA repair in mammalian HeLa S3 cells (at up to 5000 µg/ml). However, an increase in clastogenic responses was seen with penciclovir in the L5178Y mouse lymphoma cell assay (at doses ≥1000 µg/ml) and, in human lymphocytes incubated *in vitro* at doses ≥250 µg/ml. When tested *in vivo*, penciclovir caused an increase in micronuclei in mouse bone marrow following the intravenous (IV) administration of doses ≥500 mg/kg (≥810 times the maximum human dose, based on body surface area conversion.)

Impairment of Fertility

Testicular toxicity was observed in multiple animal species (rats and dogs) following repeated IV administration of penciclovir (160 mg/kg/day and 100 mg/kg/day, respectively, approximately 1155 and 3255× the maximum theoretical human AUC). Testicular changes seen in both species included atrophy of the seminiferous tubules and reductions in epididymal sperm counts and/or an increased incidence of sperm with abnormal morphology or reduced motility. Adverse testicular effects were related to an increasing dose or duration of exposure to penciclovir. No adverse testicular or reproductive effects (fertility and reproductive function) were observed in rats after 10-13 weeks dosing at 80 mg/kg/day, or testicular effects in dogs after 13 weeks dosing at 30 mg/kg/day (575 and 845× the maximum theoretical human AUC, respectively). Intravenously administered penciclovir had no effect on fertility or reproductive performance in female rats at doses of up to 80 mg/kg/day [260× the maximum human dose (BSA)].

There was no evidence of any clinically significant effects on sperm count, motility or morphology in 2 placebo-controlled clinical trails of famciclovir (the oral prodrug of penciclovir, 250 mg bid daily; n=66) in immunocompetent men with recurrent genital herpes, when dosing and follow-up were maintained for 18 and 8 weeks, respectively (approximately 2 and 1 spermatogenic cycles in the human).

PREGNANCY, TERATOGENIC EFFECTS, PREGNANCY CATEGORY B

No adverse effects on the course and outcome of pregnancy or on fetal development were noted in rats and rabbits following the IV administration of penciclovir at doses of 80 and 60 mg/kg/day, respectively (estimated human equivalent doses of 13 and 18 mg/kg/day for the rat and rabbit, respectively, based on body surface area conversion; the body surface area doses being 260 and 355× the maximum recommended dose following topical application of the penciclovir cream). There are, however, no adequate and well-controlled studies in pregnant women. Because animal reproduction studies are not always predictive of human response, penciclovir should be used during pregnancy only if clearly needed.

NURSING MOTHERS

There is no information on whether penciclovir is excreted in human milk after topical administration. However, following oral administration of famciclovir (the oral prodrug of penciclovir) to lactating rats, penciclovir was excreted in breast milk at concentrations higher than those seen in the plasma. Therefore, a decision should be made whether to discontinue the drug, taking into account the importance of the drug to the mother. There are no data on the safety of penciclovir in newborns.

PEDIATRIC USE

In 102 patients, ages 12-17, the overall incidence of adverse events was lower and the incidence of treatment related adverse events was similar to that in adult patients in clinical trials.

GERIATRIC USE

In 74 patients ≥65 years of age, the adverse events profile was comparable to that observed in younger patients.

ADVERSE REACTIONS

In two double-blind, placebo-controlled trials, 1516 patients were treated with penciclovir cream and 1541 with placebo. The most frequently reported adverse event was headache, which occurred in 5.3% of the patients treated with penciclovir and 5.8% of the placebo-treated patients. The rates of reported local adverse reactions are shown in TABLE 2. One or more local adverse reactions were reported by 2.7% of the patients treated with penciclovir and 3.9% of the placebo-treated patients.

TABLE 2 *Local Adverse Reactions Reported in Phase 3 Trials*

	Penciclovir n=1516	Placebo n=1541
Application site reaction	1.3%	1.8%
Hypesthesia/local anesthesia	0.9%	1.4%
Taste perversion	0.2%	0.3%
Pruritus	0.0%	0.3%
Pain	0.0%	0.1%
Rash (erythematous)	0.1%	0.1%
Allergic reaction	0.0%	0.1%

Two studies, enrolling 108 healthy subjects, were conducted to evaluate the dermal tolerance of 5% penciclovir cream (a 5-fold higher concentration than the commercial formulation) compared to vehicle using repeated occluded patch testing methodology. The 5% penciclovir cream induced mild erythema in approximately one-half of the subjects exposed, an irritancy profile similar to the vehicle control in terms of severity and proportion of subjects with a response. No evidence of sensitization was observed.

POST-MARKETING EXPERIENCE

In worldwide post-marketing experience with penciclovir in the treatment of recurrent herpes labialis in adults the following adverse events have been reported: application site reaction, decreased therapeutic response, aggravated condition, urticaria, local edema, oral/pharyngeal edema, pain, pruritus, paresthesia, skin discoloration, erythematous rash, parosmia, and headache.

DOSAGE AND ADMINISTRATION

Penciclovir should be applied every 2 hours during waking hours for a period of 4 days. Treatment should be started as early as possible (*i.e.,* during the prodrome or when lesions appear).

HOW SUPPLIED

Denavir is supplied in a 1.5 g tube containing 10 mg of penciclovir per gram.
Storage: Store at controlled room temperature, 20-25°C (68-77°F).

PRODUCT LISTING - EQUIVALENTS NOT AVAILABLE

Cream - Topical - 1%

1.50 gm	$22.90	DENAVIR, Allscripts Pharmaceutical Company	54569-4947-00
1.50 gm	$24.05	DENAVIR, Glaxosmithkline Healthcare	00135-0315-52
1.50 gm	$26.45	DENAVIR, Novartis Consumer Health	00078-0369-64

Penicillamine *(001965)*

Categories: Arthritis, rheumatoid; Cystinuria; Wilson's disease; FDA Approved 1978 Nov; Pregnancy Category D; WHO Formulary
Drug Classes: Chelators; Cystine depleting agents; Disease modifying antirheumatic drugs
Brand Names: **Cuprimine**; Depen; Mercaptyl
Foreign Brand Availability: Adaleen (Mexico); Artamin (Austria; Korea); Atamir (Denmark); Cupripen (Spain); D-Penil (Peru); Distamine (England; Netherlands; Switzerland); D-Penamine (Australia; New-Zealand); Kelatin (Belgium; Netherlands); Kelatine (Portugal); Metalcaptase (Japan); Penicillamine (South-Africa); Pendramine (England); Sufortanon (Spain)
Cost of Therapy: $104.34 (Wilson's Disease; Cuprimine; 250 mg; 3 capsules/day; 30 day supply)
$69.56 (Rheumatoid Arthritis; Cuprimine; 250 mg; 2 capsules/day; 30 day supply)

WARNING

Physicians planning to use penicillamine should thoroughly familiarize themselves with its toxicity, special dosage considerations, and therapeutic benefits. Penicillamine should never be used casually. Each patient should remain constantly under the close supervision of the physician. Patients should be warned to report promptly any symptoms suggesting toxicity.

DESCRIPTION

Penicillamine is a chelating agent used in the treatment of Wilson's disease. It is also used to reduce cystine excretion in cystinuria and to treat patients with severe, active rheumatoid arthritis unresponsive to conventional therapy (see INDICATIONS AND USAGE). It is 3-mercapto-D-valine. It is a white or practically white, crystalline powder, freely soluble in water, slightly soluble in alcohol, and insoluble in ether, acetone, benzene, and carbon tetrachloride.

The empirical formula is $C_5H_{11}NO_2S$, giving it a molecular weight of 149.21.

It reacts readily with formaldehyde or acetone to form a thiazolidine-carboxylic acid.

Cuprimine capsules for oral administration contain either 125 or 250 mg of penicillamine. Each capsule contains the following inactive ingredients: D&C yellow 10, gelatin, lactose, magnesium stearate, and titanium dioxide. The 125 mg capsule also contains iron oxide.

CLINICAL PHARMACOLOGY

Penicillamine is a chelating agent recommended for the removal of excess copper in patients with Wilson's disease. From *in vitro* studies which indicate that one atom of copper combines with two molecules of penicillamine, it would appear that 1 g of penicillamine should be followed by the excretion of about 200 mg of copper; however, the actual amount excreted is about 1% of this.

Penicillamine also reduces excess cystine excretion in cystinuria. This is done, at least in part, by disulfide interchange between penicillamine and cystine, resulting in formation of penicillamine-cysteine disulfide, a substance that is much more soluble than cystine and is excreted readily.

Penicillamine interferes with the formation of cross-links between tropocollagen molecules and cleaves them when newly formed.

The mechanism of action of penicillamine in rheumatoid arthritis is unknown although it appears to suppress disease activity. Unlike cytotoxic immunosuppressants, penicillamine markedly lowers lgM rheumatoid factor but produces no significant depression in absolute levels of serum immunoglobulins. Also unlike cytotoxic immunosuppressants which act on both, penicillamine *in vitro* depresses T-cell activity but not B-cell activity.

In vitro, penicillamine dissociates macroglobulins (rheumatoid factor) although the relationship of the activity to its effect in rheumatoid arthritis is not known.

In rheumatoid arthritis, the onset of therapeutic response to penicillamine may not be seen for 2 or 3 months. In those patients who respond, however, the first evidence of suppression of symptoms such as pain, tenderness, and swelling is generally apparent within 3 months. The optimum duration of therapy has not been determined. If remissions occur, they may last from months to years, but usually require continued treatment (see DOSAGE AND ADMINISTRATION).

In all patients receiving penicillamine, it is important that penicillamine be given on an empty stomach, at least 1 hour before meals or 2 hours after meals, and at least 1 hour apart from any other drug, food, or milk. This permits maximum absorption and reduces the likelihood of inactivation by metal binding in the gastrointestinal tract.

Methodology for determining the bioavailability of penicillamine is not available; however, penicillamine is known to be a very soluble substance.

INDICATIONS AND USAGE

Penicillamine is indicated in the treatment of Wilson's disease, cystinuria, and in patients with severe, active rheumatoid arthritis who have failed to respond to an adequate trial of conventional therapy. Available evidence suggests that penicillamine is not of value in ankylosing spondylitis.

WILSON'S DISEASE

Wilson's disease (hepatolenticular degeneration) results from the interaction of an inherited defect and an abnormality in copper metabolism. The metabolic defect, which is the consequence of the autosomal inheritance of one abnormal gene from each parent, manifests itself in a greater positive copper balance than normal. As a result, copper is deposited in several organs and appears eventually to produce pathologic effects most prominently seen in the brain, where degeneration is widespread; in the liver, where fatty infiltration, inflammation, and hepatocellular damage progress to postnecrotic cirrhosis; in the kidney, where tubular and glomerular dysfunction results; and in the eye, where characteristic corneal copper deposits are known as Kayser-Fleischer rings.

Two types of patients require treatment for Wilson's disease: (1) the symptomatic, and (2) the asymptomatic in whom it can be assumed the disease will develop in the future if the patient is not treated.

Diagnosis, suspected on the basis of family or individual history, physical examination, or a low serum concentration of ceruloplasmin*, is confirmed by the demonstration of Kayser-Fleischer rings or, particularly in the asymptomatic patient, by the quantitative demonstration in a liver biopsy specimen of a concentration of copper in excess of 250 μg/g dry weight.

Treatment has two objectives:

To minimize dietary intake and absorption of copper.

To promote excretion of copper deposited in tissues.

The first objective is attained by a daily diet that contains no more than 1 or 2 mg of copper. Such a diet should exclude, most importantly, chocolate, nuts, shellfish, mushrooms, liver, molasses, broccoli, and cereals enriched with copper, and be composed to as great an extent as possible of foods with a low copper content. Distilled or demineralized water should be used if the patient's drinking water contains more than 0.1 mg of copper per liter.

For the second objective, a copper chelating agent is used.

In symptomatic patients this treatment usually produces marked neurologic improvement, fading of Kayser-Fleischer rings, and gradual amelioration of hepatic dysfunction and psychic disturbances.

Clinical experience to date suggests that life is prolonged with the above regimen.

Noticeable improvement may not occur for 1-3 months. Occasionally, neurologic symptoms become worse during initiation of therapy with penicillamine. Despite this, the drug should not be discontinued permanently, although temporary interruption may result in clinical improvement of the neurological symptoms but it carries an increased risk of developing a sensitivity reaction upon resumption of therapy (see WARNINGS).

Treatment of asymptomatic patients has been carried out for over 10 years. Symptoms and signs of the disease appear to be prevented indefinitely if daily treatment with penicillamine can be continued.

CYSTINURIA

Cystinuria is characterized by excessive urinary excretion of the dibasic amino acids, arginine, lysine, ornithine, and cystine, and the mixed disulfide of cysteine and homocysteine. The metabolic defect that leads to cystinuria is inherited as an autosomal, recessive trait. Metabolism of the affected amino acids is influenced by at least two abnormal factors: (1) defective gastrointestinal absorption and (2) renal tubular dysfunction.

Arginine, lysine, ornithine, and cysteine are soluble substances, readily excreted. There is no apparent pathology connected with their excretion in excessive quantities.

Cystine, however, is so slightly soluble at the usual range of urinary pH that it is not excreted readily, and so crystallizes and forms stones in the urinary tract. Stone formation is the only known pathology in cystinuria.

Normal daily output of cystine is 40-80 mg. In cystinuria, output is greatly increased and may exceed 1 g/day. At 500-600 mg/day, stone formation is almost certain. When it is more than 300 mg/day, treatment is indicated.

Conventional treatment is directed at keeping urinary cystine diluted enough to prevent stone formation, keeping the urine alkaline enough to dissolve as much cystine as possible, and minimizing cystine production by a diet low in methionine (the major dietary precursor of cystine). Patients must drink enough fluid to keep urine specific gravity below 1.010, take enough alkali to keep urinary pH at 7.5 to 8, and maintain a diet low in methionine. This diet is not recommended in growing children and probably is contraindicated in pregnancy because of its low protein content (see PRECAUTIONS).

When these measures are inadequate to control recurrent stone formation, penicillamine may be used as additional therapy. When patients refuse to adhere to conventional treatment, penicillamine may be a useful substitute. It is capable of keeping cystine excretion to near normal values, thereby hindering stone formation and the serious consequences of pyelonephritis and impaired renal function that develop in some patients.

RHEUMATOID ARTHRITIS

Because penicillamine can cause severe adverse reactions, its use in rheumatoid arthritis should be restricted to patients who have severe, active disease and who have failed to respond to an adequate trial of conventional therapy. Even then, benefit-to-risk ratio should be carefully considered. Other measures, such as rest, physiotherapy, salicylates, and corticosteroids should be used, when indicated, in conjunction with penicillamine (see PRECAUTIONS).

*For quantitative test for serum ceruloplasmin see: Morell, A.G.; Windsor, J.; Sternlieb, I.; Scheinberg, I.H.: Measurement of the concentration of ceruloplasmin in serum by determination of its oxidase activity, in "Laboratory Diagnosis of Liver Disease", F.W. Sunderman; F.W. Sunderman, Jr. (eds.), St. Louis, Warren H. Green, Inc., 1968, pp. 193-195.

CONTRAINDICATIONS

Except for the treatment of Wilson's disease or certain cases of cystinuria, use of penicillamine during pregnancy is contraindicated (see WARNINGS).

Although breast milk studies have not been reported in animals or humans, mothers on therapy with penicillamine should not nurse their infants.

Patients with a history of penicillamine-related aplastic anemia or agranulocytosis should not be restarted on penicillamine (see WARNINGS and ADVERSE REACTIONS).

Because of its potential for causing renal damage, penicillamine should not be administered to rheumatoid arthritis patients with a history or other evidence of renal insufficiency.

WARNINGS

The use of penicillamine has been associated with fatalities due to certain diseases such as aplastic anemia, agranulocytosis, thrombocytopenia, Good-pasture's syndrome, and myasthenia gravis.

Because of the potential for serious hematological and renal adverse reactions to occur at any time, routine urinalysis, white and differential blood cell count, hemoglobin determination, and direct platelet count must be done every 2 weeks for at least the first 6 months

P

of penicillamine therapy and monthly thereafter. Patients should be instructed to report promptly the development of signs and symptoms of granulocytopenia and/or thrombocytopenia such as fever, sore throat, chills, bruising or bleeding. The above laboratory studies should then be promptly repeated.

Leukopenia and thrombocytopenia have been reported to occur in up to 5% of patients during penicillamine therapy. Leukopenia is of the granulocytic series and may or may not be associated with an increase in eosinophils. A confirmed reduction in, WBC below 3500/mm^3 mandates discontinuance of penicillamine therapy. Thrombocytopenia may be on an idiosyncratic basis, with decreased or absent megakaryocytes in the marrow, when it is part of an aplastic anemia. In other cases the thrombocytopenia is presumably on an immune basis since the number of megakaryocytes in the marrow has been reported to be normal or sometimes increased. The development of a platelet count below 100,000/mm^3, even in the absence of clinical bleeding, requires at least temporary cessation of penicillamine therapy. A progressive fall in either platelet count or WBC in three successive determinations, even though values are still within the normal range, likewise requires at least temporary cessation.

Proteinuria and/or hematuria may develop during therapy and may be warning signs of membranous glomerulopathy which can progress to a nephrotic syndrome. Close observation of these patients is essential. In some patients the proteinuria disappears with continued therapy; in others, penicillamine must be discontinued. When a patient develops proteinuria or hematuria the physician must ascertain whether it is a sign of drug-induced glomerulopathy or is unrelated to penicillamine.

Rheumatoid arthritis patients who develop moderate degrees of proteinuria may be continued cautiously on penicillamine therapy, provided that quantitative 24 hour urinary protein determinations are obtained at intervals of 1-2 weeks. Penicillamine dosage should not be increased under these circumstances. Proteinuria which exceeds 1 g/24 hours, or proteinuria which progressively increasing, requires either discontinuance of the drug or a reduction in the dosage. In some patients, proteinuria has been reported to clear following reduction in dosage.

In rheumatoid arthritis patients penicillamine should be discontinued if unexplained gross hematuria or persistent microscopic hematuria develops.

In patients with Wilson's disease or cystinuria the risks of continued penicillamine therapy in patients manifesting potentially serious urinary abnormalities must be weighed against the expected therapeutic benefits.

When penicillamine is used in cystinuria, an annual x-ray for renal stones is advised. Cystine stones form rapidly, sometimes in 6 months.

Up to 1 year or more may be required for any urinary abnormalities to disappear after penicillamine has been discontinued.

Because of rare reports of intrahepatic cholestasis and toxic hepatitis, liver function tests are recommended every 6 months for the duration of therapy.

Goodpasture's syndrome has occurred rarely. The development of abnormal urinary findings associated with hemoptysis and pulmonary infiltrates on x-ray requires immediate cessation of penicillamine.

Obliterative bronchiolitis has been reported rarely. The patient should be cautioned to report immediately pulmonary symptoms such as exertion, dyspnea, unexplained cough or wheezing. Pulmonary function studies should be considered at that time.

Myasthenic syndrome sometimes progressing to myasthenia gravis has been reported. Ptosis and diplopia, with weakness of the extraocular muscles are often early signs of myasthenia. In the majority of cases, symptoms of myasthenia have receded after withdrawal of penicillamine.

Most of the various forms of pemphigus have occurred during treatment with penicillamine. Pemphigus vulgaris and pemphigus foliaceus are reported most frequently, usually as a late complication of therapy. The seborrhea-like characteristics of pemphigus foliaceus may obscure an early diagnosis. When pemphigus is suspected, penicillamine should be discontinued. Treatment has consisted of high doses of corticosteroids alone or, in some cases, concomitantly with an immunosuppressant. Treatment may be required for only a few weeks or months, but may need to be continued for more than a year.

Once instituted for Wilson's disease or cystinuria, treatment with penicillamine should, as a rule, be continued on a daily basis. Interruptions for even a few days have been followed by sensitivity reactions after reinstitution of therapy.

USE IN PREGNANCY

Penicillamine has been shown to be teratogenic in rats when given in doses 6 times higher than the highest dose recommended for human use. Skeletal defects, cleft palates and fetal toxicity (resorptions) has been reported.

There are no controlled studies on the use of penicillamine in pregnant women. Although normal outcomes have been reported, characteristic congenital cutis laxa and associated birth defects have been reported in infants born of mothers who received therapy with penicillamine during pregnancy. Penicillamine should be used in women of childbearing potential only when the expected benefits outweigh the possible hazards. Women on therapy with penicillamine who are of childbearing potential should be apprised of this risk advised to report promptly any missed menstrual periods or other indications of possible pregnancy, and followed closely for early recognition of pregnancy.

WILSON'S DISEASE

Reported experience shows that continued treatment with penicillamine throughout pregnancy protects the mother against relapse of the Wilson's disease, and that discontinuation of penicillamine has deleterious effects on the mother.

If penicillamine is administered during pregnancy to patients with Wilson disease, it is recommended that the daily dosage be limited to 1 g. If cesarean section is planned, the daily dosage should be limited to 250 mg during the last 6 weeks of pregnancy and postoperatively until wound healing is complete.

CYSTINURIA

If possible, penicillamine should not be given during pregnancy to women with cystinuria (see CONTRAINDICATIONS). There are reports of women with cystinuria on therapy with penicillamine who gave birth to infants with generalized connective tissue defects who died following abdominal surgery. If stones continue to form in these patients, the benefits of therapy to the mother must be evaluated against the risk to the fetus.

RHEUMATOID ARTHRITIS

Penicillamine should not be administered to rheumatoid arthritis patients who are pregnant (see CONTRAINDICATIONS) and should be discontinued promptly in patients in whom pregnancy is suspected or diagnosed.

There is a report that a woman with rheumatoid arthritis treated with less than 1 g a day of penicillamine during pregnancy gave birth (cesarean delivery) to an infant with growth retardation, flattened face with broad nasal bridge, low set ears, short neck with loose skin folds, and unusually lax body skin.

PRECAUTIONS

Some patients may experience drug fever, a marked febrile response tp penicillamine, usually in the second to third week following initiation of therapy. Drug fever may sometimes be accompanied by a macular cutaneous eruption.

In the case of drug fever in patients with Wilson's disease or cystinuria penicillamine should be temporarily discontinued until the reaction subsides. Then penicillamine should be reinstituted with a small dose that is gradually increased until the desired dosage is attained. Systemic steroid therapy may be necessary, and is usually helpful, in such patients in whom toxic reactions develop a second or third time.

In the case of drug fever in rheumatoid arthritis patients, because other treatments are available, penicillamine should be discontinued and another therapeutic alternative tried since experience indicates that the febrile reaction will recur in a very high percentage of patients upon readministration of penicillamine.

The skin and mucous membranes should be observed for allergic reactions. Early and late rashes have occurred. Early rash occurs during the first few months of treatment and is more common. It is usually a generalized pruritic, erythematous, maculopapular or morbilliform rash and resembles the allergic rash seen with other drugs. Early rash usually disappears within days after stopping penicillamine and seldom recurs when the drug is restarted at a lower dosage. Pruritus and early rash may often be controlled by the concomitant administration of antihistamines. Less commonly, a late rash may be seen, usually after 6 months or more of treatment, and requires discontinuation of penicillamine. It is usually on the trunk, is accompanied by intense pruritus, and is usually unresponsive to topical corticosteroid therapy. Late rash may take weeks to disappear after penicillamine is stopped and usually recurs if the drug is restarted.

The appearance of a drug eruption accompanied by fever, arthralgia, lymphadenopathy or other allergic manifestations usually requires discontinuation of penicillamine.

Certain patients will develop a positive antinuclear antibody (ANA) test and some of these may show a lupus erythematosus-like syndrome similar to drug-induced lupus associated with other drugs. The lupus erythematosus-like syndrome is not associated with hypocomplementemia and may be present without nephropathy. The development of a positive ANA test does not mandate discontinuance of the drug; however, the physician should be alerted to the possibility that a lupus erythematosus-like syndrome may develop in the future.

Some patients may develop oral ulcerations which in some cases have the appearance of aphthous stomatitis. The stomatitis usually recurs on rechallenge but often clears on a lower dosage. Although rare, cheilosis, glossitis and gingivostomatitis have also been reported. These oral lesions are frequently dose-related and may preclude further increase in penicillamine dosage or require discontinuation of the drug.

Hypogeusia (a blunting or diminution in taste perception) has occurred in some patients. This may last 2-3 months or more and may develop into a total loss of taste; however, it is usually self-limited despite continued penicillamine treatment. Such taste impairment is rare in patients with Wilson's disease.

Penicillamine should not be used in patients who are receiving concurrently gold therapy, antimalarial or cytotoxic drugs, oxyphenbutazone or phenylbutazone because these drugs are also associated with similar serious hematologic and renal adverse reactions. Patients who have had gold salt therapy discontinued due to a major toxic reaction may be at greater risk of serious adverse reactions with penicillamine but not necessarily of the same type.

Patients who are allergic to penicillin may theoretically have cross-sensitivity to penicillamine. The possibility of reactions from contamination of penicillamine by trace amounts of penicillin has been eliminated now that penicillamine is being produced synthetically rather than as a degradation product of penicillin.

Because of their dietary restrictions, patients with Wilson's disease and cystinuria should be given 25 mg/day of pyridoxine during therapy, since penicillamine increases the requirement for this vitamin. Patients also may receive benefit from a multivitamin preparation, although there is no evidence that deficiency of any vitamin other than pyridoxine is associated with penicillamine. In Wilson's disease, multivitamin preparations must be copper-free.

Rheumatoid arthritis patients whose nutrition is impaired should also be given a daily supplement of pyridoxine. Mineral supplements should not be given, since they may block the response to penicillamine.

Iron deficiency may develop, especially in children and in menstruating women. In Wilson's disease, this may be a result of adding the effects of the low copper diet, which is probably also low in iron, and the penicillamine to the effects of blood loss or growth. In cystinuria, a low methionine diet may contribute to iron deficiency, since it is necessarily low in protein. If necessary, iron may be given in short courses, but a period of 2 hours should elapse between administration of penicillamine and iron, since orally administered iron has been shown to reduce the effects of penicillamine.

Penicillamine causes an increase in the amount of soluble collagen. In the rat this results in inhibition of normal healing and also a decrease in tensile strength of intact skin. In man this may be the cause of increased skin friability at sites especially subject to pressure or trauma, such as shoulders, elbows, knees, toes, and buttocks. Extravasations of blood may occur and may appear as pupuric areas, with external bleeding if the skin is broken, or as vesicles containing dark blood. Neither type is progressive. There is no apparent association with bleeding elsewhere in the body and no associated coagulation defect has been found. Therapy with penicillamine may be continued in the presence of these lesions. They may not recur if dosage is reduced. Other reported effects probably due to the action of penicillamine on collagen are excessive wrinkling of the skin and development of small, white papules at venipuncture and surgical sites.

The effects of penicillamine on collagen and elastin make it advisable to consider a reduction in dosage to 250 mg/day, when surgery is contemplated. Reinstitution of full therapy should be delayed until wound healing is complete.

CARCINOGENESIS

Long-term animal carcinogenicity studies have not been done with penicillamine. There is a report that 5 of 10 autoimmune disease-prone NZB hybrid mice developed lymphocytic leukemia after 6 months' intraperitoneal treatment with a dose of 400 mg/kg penicillamine 5 days per week.

NURSING MOTHERS

See CONTRAINDICATIONS.

USAGE IN CHILDREN

The efficacy of penicillamine in juvenile rheumatoid arthritis has not been established.

*Scheinberg, I.H.; Sternlieb, I.: N. Engl. J. Med. *293:*1300-1302, Dec. 18, 1975

ADVERSE REACTIONS

Penicillamine is a drug with a high incidence of untoward reactions, some of which are potentially fatal. Therefore, it is mandatory that patients receiving penicillamine therapy remain under close medical supervision throughout the period of drug administration (see WARNINGS) and PRECAUTIONS.

Reported incidences (%) for the most commonly occurring adverse reactions in rheumatoid arthritis patients are noted, based on 17 representative clinical trials reported in the literature (1270 patients).

ALLERGIC

Generalized pruritus, early and late rashes (5%), pemphigus (see WARNINGS), and drug eruptions which may be accompanied by fever, arthralgia, or lymphadenopathy have occurred (see WARNINGS and PRECAUTIONS). Some patients may show a lupus erythematosus-like syndrome similar to drug-induced lupus produced by other pharmacological agents (see PRECAUTIONS).

Urticaria and exfoliative dermatitis have occurred.

Thyroiditis has been reported; hypoglycemia in association with anti-insulin antibodies has been reported. These reactions are extremely rare.

Some patients may develop a migratory polyarthralgia, often with objective synovitis (see DOSAGE AND ADMINISTRATION).

GASTROINTESTINAL

Anorexia, epigastric pain, nausea, vomiting, or occasional diarrhea may occur (17%).

Isolated cases of reactivated peptic ulcer have occurred, as have hepatic dysfunction and pancreatitis. Intrahepatic cholestasis and toxic hepatitis have been reported rarely. There have been a few reports of increased serum alkaline phosphatase, lactic dehydrogenase, and positive cephalin flocculation and thymol turbidity tests.

Some patients may report a blunting, diminution, or total loss of taste perception (12%); or may develop oral ulcerations. Although rare, cheilosis, glossitis, and gingivostomatitis have been reported (see PRECAUTIONS).

Gastrointestinal side effects are usually reversible following cessation of therapy.

HEMATOLOGICAL

Penicillamine can cause bone marrow depression (see WARNINGS). Leukopenia (2%) and thrombocytopenia (4%) have occurred. Fatalities have been reported as a result of thrombocytopenia, agranulocytosis, aplastic anemia, and sideroblastic anemia.

Thrombotic thrombocytopenic purpura, hemolytic anemia, red cell aplasia, monocytosis, leukocytosis, eosinophilia, and thrombocytosis have also been reported.

RENAL

Patients on penicillamine therapy may develop proteinuria (6%) and/or hematuria which, in some, may progress to the development of the nephrotic syndrome as a result of an immune complex membranous glomerulopathy (see WARNINGS).

CENTRAL NERVOUS SYSTEM

Tinnitus, optic neuritis and peripheral sensory and motor neuropathies (including polyradiculoneuropathy, *i.e.,* Guillain-Barré syndrome) have been reported. Muscular weakness may or may not occur with the peripheral neuropathies. Visual and psychic disturbances have been reported.

NEUROMUSCULAR

Myasthenia gravis (see WARNINGS).

OTHER

Adverse reactions that have been reported rarely include thrombophlebitis; hyperpyrexia (see PRECAUTIONS); falling hair or alopecia; lichen planus; polymyositis; dermatomyositis; mammary hyperplasia; elastosis perforans serpiginosa; toxic epidermal necrolysis; anetoderma (cutaneous macular atrophy); and Goodpasture's syndrome, a severe and ultimately fatal glomerulonephritis associated with intra-alveolar hemorrhage (see WARNINGS). Fatal renal vasculitis has also been reported. Allergic alveolitis, obliterative bronchiolitis, interstitial pneumonitis and pulmonary fibrosis have been reported in patients with severe rheumatoid arthritis, some of whom were receiving penicillamine. Bronchial asthma also has been reported.

Increased skin friability, excessive wrinkling of skin, and development of small white papules at venipuncture and surgical sites have been reported (see PRECAUTIONS).

The chelating action of the drug may cause increased excretion of other heavy metals such as zinc, mercury and lead.

There have been reports associating penicillamine with leukemia. However, circumstances involved in these reports are such that a cause and effect relationship to the drug has not been established.

DOSAGE AND ADMINISTRATION

In all patients receiving penicillamine, it is important that penicillamine be given on an empty stomach, at least 1 hour before meals or 2 hours after meals, and at least 1 hour apart from any other drug, food, or milk. Because penicillamine increases the requirement for pyridoxine, patients may require a daily supplement of pyridoxine (see PRECAUTIONS).

WILSON'S DISEASE

Optimal dosage can be determined by measurement of urinary copper excretion and the determination of free copper in the serum. The urine must be collected in copper-free glassware, and should be quantitatively analyzed for copper before and soon after initiation of therapy with penicillamine.

Determination of 24 hour urinary copper excretion is of greatest value in the first week of therapy with penicillamine. In the absence of any drug reaction, a dose between 0.75 and 1.5 g that results in an initial 24 hour cupriuresis of over 2 mg should be continued for about 3 months, by which time the most reliable method of monitoring maintenance treatment is the determination of free copper in the serum. This equals the difference between quantitatively determined total copper and ceruloplasmin-copper. Adequately treated patients will usually have less than 10 µg free copper/dl of serum. It is seldom necessary to exceed a dosage of 2 g/day. If the patient is intolerant to therapy with penicillamine, alternative treatment is trientine hydrochloride.

In patients who cannot tolerate as much as 1 g/day initially, initiating dosage with 250 mg/day, and increasing gradually to the requisite amount, gives closer control of the effects of the drug and may help to reduce the incidence of adverse reactions.

CYSTINURIA

It is recommended that penicillamine be used along with conventional therapy. By reducing urinary cystine, it decreases crystalluria and stone formation. In some instances, it has been reported to decrease the size of, and even to dissolve, stones already formed.

The usual dosage of penicillamine in the treatment of cystinuria is 2 g/day for adults, with a range of 1-4 g/day. For children, dosage can be based on 30 mg/kg/day. The total daily amount should be divided into four doses. If four equal doses are not feasible, give the larger portion at bedtime. If adverse reactions necessitate a reduction in dosage, it is important to retain the bedtime dose.

Initiating dosage with 250 mg/day, and increasing gradually to the requisite amount, gives closer control of the effects of the drug and may help to reduce the incidence of adverse reactions.

In addition to taking penicillamine, patients should drink copiously. It is especially important to drink about a pint of fluid at bedtime and another pint once during the night when urine is more concentrated and more acid than during the day. The greater the fluid intake, the lower the required dosage of penicillamine.

Dosage must be individualized to an amount that limits cystine excretion to 100-200 mg/day in those with no history of stones, and below 100 mg/day in those who have had stone formation and/or pain. Thus, in determining dosage, the inherent tubular defect, the patient's size, age, and rate of growth, and his diet and water intake all must be taken into consideration.

The standard nitroprusside cyanide test has been reported useful as a qualitative measure of the effective dose*: Add 2 ml of freshly prepared 5% sodium cyanide to 5 ml of a 24 hour aliquot of protein-free urine and let stand 10 minutes. Add 5 drops of freshly prepared 5% sodium nitroprusside and mix. Cystine will turn the mixture magenta. If the result is negative, it can be assumed that cystine excretion is less than 100 mg/g creatinine.

Although penicillamine is rarely excreted unchanged, it also will turn the mixture magenta. If there is any question as to which substance is causing the reaction, a ferric chloride test can be done to eliminate doubt: Add 3% ferric chloride dropwise to the urine. Penicillamine will turn the urine an immediate and quickly fading blue. Cystine will not produce any change in appearance.

RHEUMATOID ARTHRITIS

The principal rule of treatment with penicillamine in rheumatoid arthritis is patience. The onset of therapeutic response is typically delayed. Two (2) or 3 months may be required before the first evidence of a clinical response is noted (see CLINICAL PHARMACOLOGY).

When treatment with penicillamine has been interrupted because of adverse reactions or other reasons, the drug should be reintroduced cautiously by starting with a lower dosage and increasing slowly.

Initial Therapy

The currently recommended dosage regimen in rheumatoid arthritis begins with a single daily dose of 125 or 250 mg which is thereafter increased at 1-3 month intervals, by 125 or 250 mg/day, as patient response and tolerance indicate. If a satisfactory remission of symptoms is achieved, the dose associated with the remission should be continued (see Maintenance Therapy). If there is no improvement and there are no signs of potentially serious toxicity after 2-3 months of treatment with doses of 500-750 mg/day, increases of 250 mg/day at 2-3 month intervals may be continued until a satisfactory remission occurs (see Maintenance Therapy) or signs of toxicity develop (see WARNINGS and PRECAUTIONS). If there is no discernible improvement after 3-4 months of treatment with 1000-1500 mg of penicillamine/day, it may be assumed the patient will not respond and penicillamine should be discontinued.

Maintenance Therapy

The maintenance dosage of penicillamine must be individualized, and may require adjustment during the course of treatment. Many patients respond satisfactorily to a dosage within the 500-750 mg/day range. Some need less.

Changes in maintenance dosage levels may not be reflected clinically or in the erythrocyte sedimentation rate for 2-3 months after each dosage adjustment.

P

Some patients will subsequently require an increase in the maintenance dosage to achieve maximal disease suppression. In those patients who do respond, but who evidence incomplete suppression of their disease after the first 6-9 months of treatment, the daily dosage of penicillamine may be increased by 125 or 250 mg/day at 3 month intervals. It is unusual in current practice to employ a dosage in excess of 1 g/day, but up to 1.5 g/day has sometimes been required.

Management of Exacerbations

During the course of treatment some patients may experience an exacerbation of disease activity following an initial good response. These may be self-limited and can subside within twelve weeks. They are usually controlled by the addition of non-steroidal anti-inflammatory drugs, and only if the patient has demonstrated a true "escape" phenomenon (as evidenced by failure of the flare to subside within this time period) should an increase in the maintenance dose ordinarily be considered.

In the rheumatoid patient, migratory polyarthralgia due to penicillamine is extremely difficult to differentiate from an exacerbation of the rheumatoid arthritis. Discontinuance or a substantial reduction in dosage of penicillamine for up to several weeks will usually determine which of these processes is responsible for the arthralgia.

Duration of Therapy

The optimum duration of therapy with penicillamine in rheumatoid arthritis has not been determined. If the patient has been in remission for 6 months or more, a gradual, stepwise dosage reduction in decrements of 125 or 250 mg/day at approximately 3 month intervals may be attempted.

Concomitant Drug Therapy

Penicillamine should not be used in patients who are receiving gold therapy, antimalarial or cytotoxic drugs, oxyphenbutazone, or phenylbutazone (see PRECAUTIONS). Other measures, such as salicylates, other non-steroidal anti-inflammatory drugs, or systemic corticosteroids, may be continued when penicillamine is initiated. After improvement commences, analgesic and anti-inflammatory drugs may be slowly discontinued as symptoms permit. Steroid withdrawal must be done gradually, and many months of treatment with penicillamine may be required before steroids can be completely eliminated.

Dosage Frequency

Based on clinical experience dosages up to 500 mg/day can be given as a single daily dose. Dosages in excess of 500 mg/day should be administered in divided doses.

PRODUCT LISTING - EQUIVALENTS NOT AVAILABLE

Capsule - Oral - 125 mg			
100's	$81.19	CUPRIMINE, Merck & Company Inc	00006-0672-68
Capsule - Oral - 250 mg			
100's	$115.93	CUPRIMINE, Merck & Company Inc	00006-0602-68
Tablet - Oral - 250 mg			
100's	$294.83	DEPEN, Wallace Laboratories	00037-4401-01

Penicillin G Benzathine (001966)

For related information, see the comparative table section in Appendix A.

Categories: Bejel; Infection, upper respiratory tract; Pinta; Rheumatic fever; Syphilis; Yaws; Pregnancy Category B; FDA Approved 1952 Jun; WHO Formulary

Drug Classes: Antibiotics, penicillins

Brand Names: Benzathine Benzylpenicillin; **Bicillin L-A**; Permapen

Foreign Brand Availability: Benzacillin (Korea); Benzanil Simple (Mexico); Benzetacil (Ecuador; Spain); Benzetacil A.P. (Mexico); Benzetacil L.A. (Colombia; Ecuador); Benzilfan (Mexico); Bicillin LA 1.2 (South-Africa); Bicillin LA 2.4 (South-Africa); Cepacilina (Spain); Diaminocillina (Italy); Durabiotic (Israel); Extencilline (France); Lentopenil (Mexico); Lutecilina (Colombia); Penadur (Switzerland); Penadur L.A. (Belgium; Greece; Switzerland); Penadur L-A (Thailand); Penadur LA (Bahrain; Benin; Burkina-Faso; Cyprus; Egypt; Ethiopia; Gambia; Ghana; Guinea; Hong-Kong; Indonesia; Iran; Iraq; Ivory-Coast; Jordan; Kenya; Kuwait; Lebanon; Liberia; Libya; Malawi; Malaysia; Mali; Mauritania; Mauritius; Morocco; Niger; Nigeria; Oman; Philippines; Qatar; Republic-of-Yemen; Saudi-Arabia; Senegal; Seychelles; Sierra-Leone; Sudan; Syria; Tanzania; Tunia; Uganda; United-Arab-Emirates; Zambia; Zimbabwe); Pencom (India); Penadur - LA (Bahamas; Barbados; Belize; Bermuda; Curacao; Guyana; Jamaica; Netherland-Antilles; Surinam; Trinidad); Pen-Di-Ben (Dominican-Republic; El-Salvador; Guatemala; Honduras; Nicaragua; Panama); Penidural (Netherlands); Penidure LA 6 (India); Penidure LA 12 (India); Penidure LA 24 (India); Penilente (Benin; Burkina-Faso; Ethiopia; Gambia; Ghana; Guinea; Ivory-Coast; Kenya; Liberia; Malawi; Mali; Mauritania; Mauritius; Morocco; Niger; Nigeria; Senegal; Seychelles; Sierra-Leone; Sudan; Tanzania; Tunia; Uganda; Zambia; Zimbabwe); Penilente - LA (South-Africa); Retarpen (Austria; Bahrain; Costa-Rica; Cyprus; Dominican-Republic; Ecuador; Egypt; El-Salvador; Guatemala; Honduras; Iran; Iraq; Jordan; Kuwait; Lebanon; Libya; Nicaragua; Oman; Panama; Qatar; Republic-of-Yemen; Saudi-Arabia; Singapore; Syria; United-Arab-Emirates); Tardocillin 1200 (Germany); Wycillina A P (Italy)

HCFA JCODE(S): J0530 up to 600,000 units IM; J0550 up to 2,400,000 units IM; J0560 up to 600,000 units IM; J0570 up to 1,200,000 units IM; J0580 up to 2,400,000 units IM

DESCRIPTION

Sterile penicillin G benzathine suspension, is prepared by the reaction of dibenzylethylene diamine with two molecules of penicillin G. It is chemically designated as 3,3-dimethyl-7-oxo-6-(2-phenylacetamido)-4-thia-1-azabicyclo(3.2.0)heptane-2-carboxylic acid compound with *N,N'*-dibenzylethylenediamine (2:1), tetrahydrate.

It is available for deep intramuscular injection. It contains sterile penicillin G benzathine in aqueous suspension with sodium citrate buffer and, as w/v, approximately 0.5% lecithin, 0.6% carboxymethylcellulose, 0.6% povidone, 0.1% methylparaben, and 0.01% propylparaben. It occurs as a white, crystalline powder and is very slightly soluble in water and sparingly soluble in alcohol.

Sterile penicillin G benzathine suspension in the multiple-dose vial formulation is viscous and opaque. It contains the equivalent of 300,000 units per ml of penicillin G as the benzathine salt. Read CONTRAINDICATIONS, WARNINGS, PRECAUTIONS, and DOSAGE AND ADMINISTRATION prior to use.

CLINICAL PHARMACOLOGY

GENERAL

Penicillin G benzathine has an extremely low solubility and, thus, the drug is slowly released from intramuscular injection sites. The drug is hydrolyzed to penicillin G. This combination of hydrolysis and slow absorption results in blood serum levels much lower but much more prolonged than other parenteral penicillins.

Intramuscular administration of 300,000 units of penicillin G benzathine in adults results in blood levels of 0.03-0.05 units per ml, which are maintained for 4-5 days. Similar blood levels may persist for 10 days following administration of 600,000 units and for 14 days following administration of 1,200,000 units. Blood concentrations of 0.003 units per ml may still be detectable 4 weeks following administration of 1,200,000 units.

Approximately 60% of penicillin G is bound to serum protein. The drug is distributed throughout the body tissues in widely varying amounts. Highest levels are found in the kidneys with lesser amounts in the liver, skin, and intestines. Penicillin G penetrates into all other tissues and the spinal fluid to a lesser degree. With normal kidney function, the drug is excreted rapidly by tubular excretion. In neonates and young infants and in individuals with impaired kidney function, excretion is considerably delayed.

MICROBIOLOGY

Penicillin G exerts a bactericidal action against penicillin-susceptible microorganisms during the stage of active multiplication. It acts through the inhibition of biosynthesis of cell-wall mucopeptide. It is not active against the penicillinase-producing bacteria, which include many strains of staphylococci.

The following *in vitro* data are available, but their clinical significance is unknown. Penicillin G exerts high *in vitro* activity against staphylococci (except penicillinase-producing strains), streptococci (Groups A, C, G, H, L, and M), and pneumococci. Other organisms susceptible to penicillin G are *Neisseria gonorrhoeae, Corynebacterium diphtheriae, Bacillus anthracis,* Clostridia species, *Actinomyces bovis, Streptobacillus moniliformis, Listeria monocytogenes,* and *Leptospira* species. *Treponema pallidum* is extremely susceptible to the bactericidal action of penicillin G.

Susceptibility Test

If the Kirby-Bauer method of disc susceptibility is used, a 20 unit penicillin disc should give a zone greater than 28 mm when tested against a penicillin-susceptible bacterial strain.

INDICATIONS AND USAGE

Intramuscular penicillin G benzathine is indicated in the treatment of infections due to penicillin-G-sensitive microorganisms that are susceptible to the low and very prolonged serum levels common to this particular dosage form. Therapy should be guided by bacteriological studies (including sensitivity tests) and by clinical response.

The following infections will usually respond to adequate dosage of intramuscular penicillin G benzathine:

Mild-to-moderate infections of the upper-respiratory tract due to susceptible streptococci.

Venereal Infections: Syphilis, yaws, bejel, and pinta.

Medical conditions in which penicillin G benzathine therapy is indicated as prophylaxis:

Rheumatic Fever and/or Chorea: Prophylaxis with penicillin G benzathine has proven effective in preventing recurrence of these conditions. It has also been used as follow-up prophylactic therapy for rheumatic heart disease and acute glomerulonephritis.

CONTRAINDICATIONS

A history of a previous hypersensitivity reaction to any of the penicillins is a contraindication.

Do not inject into or near an artery or nerve.

WARNINGS

Penicillin G benzathine should only be prescribed for the indications listed in this insert.

Serious and occasionally fatal hypersensitivity (anaphylactoid) reactions have been reported in patients receiving penicillin. Although anaphylaxis is more frequent following parenteral administration, it has occurred in patients on oral penicillins. These reactions are more apt to occur in individuals with a history of sensitivity to multiple allergens.

There are reports of patients with a history of penicillin hypersensitivity reactions who experienced severe hypersensitivity reactions when treated with a cephalosporin. Before therapy with a penicillin, careful inquiry should be made about previous hypersensitivity reactions to penicillins, cephalosporins, and other allergens. If an allergic reaction occurs, the drug should be discontinued and appropriate therapy should be instituted. Serious anaphylactoid reactions require immediate emergency treatment with epinephrine. Oxygen, intravenous steroids, airway management, including intubation, should also be administered as indicated.

Inadvertent intravascular administration, including inadvertent direct intraarterial injection or injection immediately adjacent to arteries, of sterile penicillin G benzathine suspension and other penicillin preparations has resulted in severe neurovascular damage, including transverse myelitis with permanent paralysis, gangrene requiring amputation of digits and more proximal portions of extremities, and necrosis and sloughing at and surrounding the injection site. Such severe effects have been reported following injections into the buttock, thigh, and deltoid areas. Other serious complications of suspected intravascular administration which have been reported include immediate pallor, mottling, or cyanosis of the extremity both distal and proximal to the injection site, followed by bleb formation; severe edema requiring anterior and/or posterior compartment fasciotomy in the lower extremity. The above-described severe effects and complications have most often occurred in infants and small children. Prompt consultation with an appropriate specialist is indicated if any evidence of compromise of the blood supply occurs at, proximal to, or distal to the site of injection.[1-9] See CONTRAINDICATIONS, PRECAUTIONS and DOSAGE AND ADMINISTRATION.

Quadriceps femoris fibrosis and atrophy have been reported following repeated intramuscular injections of penicillin preparations into the anterolateral thigh.

Injection into or near a nerve may result in permanent neurological damage.

PRECAUTIONS

GENERAL

Penicillin should be used with caution in individuals with histories of significant allergies and/or asthma.

Care should be taken to avoid intravenous or intraarterial administration, or injection into or near major peripheral nerves or blood vessels, since such injection may produce neurovascular damage. See CONTRAINDICATIONS, WARNINGS and DOSAGE AND ADMINISTRATION.

Prolonged use of antibiotics may promote the overgrowth of nonsusceptible organisms, including fungi. Should superinfection occur, appropriate measures should be taken.

LABORATORY TESTS

In streptococcal infections, therapy must be sufficient to eliminate the organism; otherwise, the sequelae of streptococcal disease may occur. Cultures should be taken following completion of treatment to determine whether streptococci have been eradicated.

PREGNANCY CATEGORY B

Reproduction studies performed in the mouse, rat, and rabbit have revealed no evidence of impaired fertility or harm to the fetus due to penicillin G. Human experience with the penicillins during pregnancy has not shown any positive evidence of adverse effects on the fetus. There are, however, no adequate and well-controlled studies in pregnant women showing conclusively that harmful effects of these drugs on the fetus can be excluded. Because animal reproduction studies are not always predictive of human response, this drug should be used during pregnancy only if clearly needed.

NURSING MOTHERS

Soluble penicillin G is excreted in breast milk. Caution should be exercised when penicillin G benzathine is administered to a nursing woman.

CARCINOGENESIS, MUTAGENESIS, AND IMPAIRMENT OF FERTILITY

No long-term animal studies have been conducted with this drug.

PEDIATRIC USE

See INDICATIONS AND USAGE and DOSAGE AND ADMINISTRATION.

DRUG INTERACTIONS

Tetracycline, a bacteriostatic antibiotic, may antagonize the bactericidal effect of penicillin, and concurrent use of these drugs should be avoided.

Concurrent administration of penicillin and probenecid increases and prolongs serum penicillin levels by decreasing the apparent volume of distribution and slowing the rate of excretion by competitively inhibiting renal tubular secretion of penicillin.

ADVERSE REACTIONS

As with other penicillins, untoward reactions of the sensitivity phenomena are likely to occur, particularly in individuals who have previously demonstrated hypersensitivity to penicillins or in those with a history of allergy, asthma, hay fever, or urticaria.

As with other treatments for syphilis, the Jarisch-Herxheimer reaction has been reported. The following have been reported with parenteral penicillin G:

General: Hypersensitivity reactions including the following: skin eruptions (maculopapular to exfoliative dermatitis), urticaria, laryngeal edema, fever, eosinophilia; other serum-sicknesslike reactions (including chills, fever, edema, arthralgia, and prostration); anaphylaxis. Note: Urticaria, other skin rashes, and serum-sicknesslike reactions may be controlled with antihistamines and, if necessary, systemic corticosteroids.

Whenever such reactions occur, penicillin G should be discontinued unless, in the opinion of the physician, the condition being treated is life-threatening and amenable only to therapy with penicillin G. Serious anaphylactic reactions require the immediate use of epinephrine, oxygen, and intravenous steroids.

Hematologic: Hemolytic anemia, leukopenia, thrombocytopenia.

Neurologic: Neuropathy.

Urogenital: Nephropathy.

DOSAGE AND ADMINISTRATION

Streptococcal (Group A) Upper Respiratory Infections (for example, pharyngitis):

Adults: A single injection of 1,200,000 units.

Older children: A single injection of 900,000 units.

Infants and children (under 60 lb): 300,000 to 600,000 units.

Syphilis:

Primary, Secondary, and Latent: 2,400,000 units (1 dose).

Late (tertiary and neurosyphilis): 2,400,000 units at 7 day intervals for three doses.

Congenital: *Under 2 years of age:* 50,000 units/kg/body weight; *Ages 2-12 years:* Adjust dosage based on adult dosage schedule.

Yaws, Bejel, and Pinta:

1,200,000 units (1 injection).

PROPHYLAXIS — FOR RHEUMATIC FEVER AND GLOMERULONEPHRITIS

Following an acute attack, penicillin G benzathine (parenteral) may be given in doses of 1,200,000 units once a month or 600,000 units every 2 weeks.

Administer by DEEP INTRAMUSCULAR INJECTION in the upper, outer quadrant of the buttock. In infants and small children, the midlateral aspect of the thigh may be preferable. When doses are repeated, vary the injection site.

After selection of the proper site and insertion of the needle into the selected muscle, aspirate by pulling back on the plunger. While maintaining negative pressure for 2-3 seconds, carefully observe the barrel of the syringe immediately proximal to the needle hub for appearance of blood or any discoloration. Blood or "typical blood color" may *not* be seen if a blood vessel has been entered — only a mixture of blood and sterile penicillin G benzathine suspension. The appearance of any discoloration is reason to withdraw the needle and discard the syringe. If it is elected to inject at another site, a new syringe and needle should be used. If no blood or discoloration appears, inject the contents of the syringe slowly. Discontinue delivery of the dose if the subject complains of severe immediate pain at the injection site or if in infants and young children symptoms or signs occur suggesting onset of severe pain.

Because of the high concentration of suspended material in this product, the needle may be blocked if the injection is not made at a slow, steady rate.

Parenteral drug products should be inspected visually for particulate matter and discoloration prior to administration whenever solution and container permit.

PRODUCT LISTING - RATED NOT THERAPEUTICALLY EQUIVALENT

Suspension - Intramuscular - G Benzathine 600000 U/ml

Size	Price	Product	NDC
1 ml x 10	$102.54	BICILLIN L-A, Allscripts Pharmaceutical Company	54569-1917-01
1 ml x 10	$131.69	BICILLIN L-A, Wyeth-Ayerst Laboratories	00008-0021-37
1 ml x 10	$178.40	BICILLIN L-A, Monarch Pharmaceuticals Inc	61570-0146-10
2 ml	$15.61	BICILLIN L-A, Allscripts Pharmaceutical Company	54569-1409-01
2 ml	$20.64	BICILLIN L-A, Physicians Total Care	54868-0753-00
2 ml x 10	$59.50	ISOJECT PERMAPEN, Pfizer U.S. Pharmaceuticals	00049-0210-35
2 ml x 10	$190.01	BICILLIN L-A, Physicians Total Care	54868-0753-01
2 ml x 10	$228.06	BICILLIN L-A, Wyeth-Ayerst Laboratories	00008-0021-35
2 ml x 10	$309.00	BICILLIN L-A, Monarch Pharmaceuticals Inc	61570-0147-10
4 ml x 10	$389.44	BICILLIN L-A, Allscripts Pharmaceutical Company	54569-2200-00
4 ml x 10	$467.33	BICILLIN L-A, Wyeth-Ayerst Laboratories	00008-0021-12
4 ml x 10	$633.10	BICILLIN L-A, Monarch Pharmaceuticals Inc	61570-0148-10
20 ml	$156.08	BICILLIN L-A, Allscripts Pharmaceutical Company	54569-1409-00

PRODUCT LISTING - EQUIVALENTS NOT AVAILABLE

Suspension - Intramuscular - G Benzathine 300000 U/ml

Size	Price	Product	NDC
10 ml	$30.55	BICILLIN L-A, Physicians Total Care	54868-3349-00

Penicillin G Potassium *(001968)*

For related information, see the comparative table section in Appendix A.

Categories: Actinomycosis; Anthrax; Arthritis, gonorrheal; Arthritis, infectious; Bacteremia; Bacteremia, secondary to tooth extraction, prevention; Chorea, prevention; Diphtheria; Empyema; Endocarditis, gonorrheal; Endocarditis, prevention; Erysipelas; Gonorrhea; Infection, lower respiratory tract; Infection, skin and skin structures; Infection, upper respiratory tract; Meningitis; Pericarditis; Pneumonia; Rat bite fever; Rheumatic fever, prophylaxis; Scarlet fever; Syphilis; Syphilis, congenital; Tetanus; Vincent's gingivitis; Vincent's pharyngitis; Pregnancy Category B; FDA Approved 1966 Feb; WHO Formulary

Drug Classes: Antibiotics, penicillins

Brand Names: Pfizerpen

Foreign Brand Availability: Cristapen (Argentina); K-Cillin (Taiwan); Megacillin (Canada); Novopen-G (Canada); Pentids (India)

HCFA JCODE(S): J2540 up to 600,000 units IM, IV

DESCRIPTION

TABLETS

Active ingredients: Penicillin G potassium.

Inactive ingredients: Calcium carbonate, povidone, magnesium stearate, sodium starch glycolate, sodium lauryl sulfate, and other trace inactive ingredients (NO sulfiting agents).

Penicillin G potassium is provided is oral dosage form as white compressed tablets buffered with calcium carbonate.

Storage

Store at 15-30°C (59-86°F).

Dispense in a tight, child-resistant container.

INJECTION

Buffered penicillin G potassium for Injection is a sterile, pyrogen-free powder for reconstitution. Buffered penicillin G potassium for injection is an antibacterial agent for IM, continuous drip, intrapleural or other local infusion, and intrathecal administration.

Each million units contains approximately 6.8 mg of sodium (0.3 mEq) and 65.6 mg of potassium (1.68 mEq).

Chemically, this drug is monopotassium 3,3-dimethyl-7-oxo-6-(2-phenylacetamido)-4-thia-l'azabicyclo(3.2.0) heptane-2-carboxylate. It has a molecular weight of 372.48.

Penicillin G potassium is a colorless or white crystal, or a white crystalline powder which is odorless, or practically so, and moderately hygroscopic. Penicillin G potassium is very soluble in water. The pH of the reconstituted product is between 6.0-8.5.

CLINICAL PHARMACOLOGY

Penicillin G exerts a bactericidal action against penicillin-sensitive micro-organisms during the stage of active multiplication. It acts through the inhibition of biosynthesis of cell wall mucopeptide. It is not active against the penicillinase producing bacteria, which include many strains of staphylococci. Penicillin G exerts high *in vitro* activity against the non-

P

penicillinase producing bacteria, which include many strains of staphylococci. Penicillin G exerts high *in vitro* activity against staphylococci (except penicillinase-producing strains), streptococci (groups A, C, G, H, L, and M) and pneumococci. Other organisms, sensitive to penicillin G are *Neisseria gonorrhoeae, Corynebacterium diphtheriae, Bacillus anthracis,* Clostridia, *Actinomycesbovis, Streptobacillus moniliformis, Listeria monocytogenes,* and Leptospira. *Treponema palladium* is extremely sensitive to the bactericidal action of penicillin G. Some species of gram-negative bacilli are sensitive to moderate to high concentrations of the drug obtained with intravenous administration. These include most strains of *Escherichia coli,* all strains of *Proteus mirabilis,* Salmonella and Shigella and some strains of *Aerobacter aerogenes* and *Alcaligenes faecalis.*

TABLETS

Oral preparations of penicillin G are only slightly affected by normal gastric acidity (pH of 2-3.5); however a pH below 2.0 may partially or totally inactivate penicillin G. Oral penicillin G is absorbed in the upper small intestine, chiefly the duodenum; however, based on serum level and urinary excretion data only approximately 30% of the dose is absorbed. For this reason 4-5 times the dose of oral penicillin G must be given to obtain a blood level comparable to that obtained with parenteral penicillin G. Since gastric acidity, stomach emptying time and other factors affecting may vary considerably, serum levels may be appreciably reduced to non-therapeutic levels in certain individuals.

Approximately 60% of penicillin G is bound to serum protein. The drug is distributed throughout the body tissues in widely varying amounts. Highest levels are found in the kidneys with lesser amounts in the liver, skin and intestines. Penicillin G penetrates into all other tissues to a lesser degree with very limited amounts found in the cerebrospinal fluid. With normal kidney function the drug is excreted rapidly by tubular excretion. In neonates and young infants and in individuals with impaired kidney function, excretion is considerably delayed. Approximately 20% of a dose of oral penicillin G is excreted in the urine under normal circumstances.

INJECTION

Aqueous penicillin G is rapidly absorbed following both intramuscular and subcutaneous injection. Initial blood levels following parenteral administration are high but not transient. Penicillins bind to serum proteins, mainly albumin. Therapeutic levels of the penicillins are easily achieved under normal circumstances in extracellular fluid and most other body tissues. Penicillins are distributed in varying degrees into pleural, pericardial, peritoneal, ascitic, synovial, and interstitial fluids. Penicillins are excreted in breast milk. Penetration into the cerebrospinal fluid, eyes, and prostate is poor. Penicillins are rapidly excreted in the urine by glomerular filtration and active tubular secretion, primarily as unchanged drug. Approximately 60% of the total dose of 300,000 units is excreted in the urine within this 5 hour period. For this reason high and frequent doses are required to maintain the elevated serum levels desirable in treating certain severe infections in individuals with normal kidney function. In neonates and young infants, and in individuals with impaired kidney function, excretion is considerably delayed.

Penicillin acts synergistically with gentamicin or tobramycin against many strains of enterococci.

Susceptibility Testing

Penicillin G Susceptibility Powder or 10 units penicillin G Susceptibility Discs may be used to determine microbial susceptibility to penicillin G using one of the following standard methods recommended by the National Committee for Laboratory Standards:

M2-M3, "Performance Standards for Antimicrobial Disk Susceptibility Tests"
M7-A, "Methods for Dilution Antimicrobial Susceptibility Tests for Bacteria that Grow Aerobically"
M11-A, "Reference Agar Dilution Procedure for Antimicrobial Susceptibility Testing of Anaerobic Bacteria"
M17-P, "Alternative Methods for Antimicrobial Susceptibility Testing of Anaerobic Bacteria"

Tests should be interpreted by the criteria in TABLE 1 and TABLE 2.

TABLE 1 *Zone Diameter, Nearest Whole mm*

	Susceptible	Moderately Susceptible	Resistant
Staphylococci	≥29	—	≤28
N. gonorrhoeae	≥20	—	≤19
Enterococci	—	≥15	≤14
Non-enterococcal streptococci and *L. monocytogenes*	≥28	20-27	≤19

TABLE 2 *Approximate MIC Correlates*

	Susceptible	Resistant
Staphylococci	≤0.1 μg/ml	β-lactamase
N. gonorrhoeae	≤0.1 μg/ml	β-lactamase
Enterococci	—	≥16 μg/ml
Non-enterococcal streptococci and *L. monocytogenes*	≤0.12 μg/ml	≥ 4 μg/ml

Interpretations of susceptible, intermediate, and resistant correlate zone size diameters with MIC values. A laboratory report of "susceptible" indicates that the suspected causative microorganism most likely will respond to therapy with penicillin G. A laboratory test of "resistant" indicates that the infecting microorganism most likely will not respond to therapy. A laboratory report of "moderately susceptible" indicates that the microorganism is most likely susceptible if a high dose of penicillin G is used, or if the infection is such that high levels of penicillin G may be attained, as in urine. A report of "intermediate" using the disk diffusion method may be considered an equivocal result, and dilution tests may be indicated.

Control organisms are recommended for susceptibility testing. Each time the test is performed the following organisms should be included. The range for zones of inhibition is shown below:

Control Organism: (ATCC 25923)
Zone of Inhibition Range: 27-35

INDICATIONS AND USAGE

TABLETS

Oral penicillin G is indicated in the treatment of mild to moderately severe infections due to penicillin G sensitive micro-organisms that are sensitive to the low serum levels common to this particular dosage form. Therapy should be guided by bacteriological studies (including sensitivity tests) and by clinical response.

NOTE: Severe pneumonia, empyema, bacteremia, pericarditis, meningitis, and arthritis should not be treated with oral penicillin during the acute stage.

Indicated surgical procedures should be performed.

The following infections will usually respond to adequate dosage of oral penicillin G.

Streptococcal Infections: (Group A) (without bacteremia). Mild to moderate infections of the upper respiratory tract, skin and soft tissue infections, scarlet fever, and mild very erysipelas.

Note: Streptococci in groups A, C, H, G, L and M are very sensitive to penicillin G. Other groups, including group D (enterococcus) are resistant.

Pneumococcal Infections: Mild to moderately severe infections of the respiratory tract.

Staphylococcal Infections: Penicillin G sensitive. Mild infections of the skin and soft tissues.

Note: Reports indicate an increasing number of strains of staphylococci resistant to penicillin G, emphasizing the need for culture and sensitivity studies in treating suspected staphylococcal infections.

Fusospirochetosis: (Vincent's gingivitis and pharyngitis) - Mild to moderately severe infection of the oropharynx usually respond with oral penicillin G.

Note: Necessary dental care should be accomplished in infections involving the gum tissue.

Medical conditions in which oral penicillin G therapy is indicated as prophylaxis:

For the prevention of recurrence following rheumatic fever and/or chorea. Prophylaxis with oral penicillin G on a continuing basis has proven effective in preventing recurrence of these conditions.

Prevention of bacteremia following tooth extraction.

Note: Oral penicillin G should not be used as adjunctive prophylaxis for genito-urinary instrumentation or surgery, lower intestinal tract surgery, sigmoidoscopy and childbirth.

Oral penicillin G is not recommended for short-term prevention of bacterial endocarditis in patients with valvular heart disease undergoing dental or surgical procedures.

INJECTION

Aqueous penicillin G (parenteral) is indicated in the therapy of severe infections caused by penicillin G susceptible microorganisms when rapid and high penicillin levels are required in the conditions listed below. Therapy should be guided by bacteriological studies (including susceptibility tests) and by clinical response.

The following infections will usually respond to adequate dosage of aqueous penicillin G (parenteral):

Note: Streptococci in groups A, C, H, G, L, and M are very sensitive to penicillin G. Some group D organisms are sensitive to the high serum levels obtained with aqueous penicillin G.

Aqueous penicillin G (parenteral) is the penicillin dosage form of choice for bacteremia, empyema, severe pneumonia, pericarditis, endocarditis, meningitis, and other severe infections caused by sensitive trains of the gram-positive species listed above.

Pneumococcal Infections: *Staphylococcal infections* penicillin G sensitive.

Other Infections: Anthrax, Actinomycosis, Clostridial infections (including tetanus), Diphtheria (to prevent carrier state), Erysipeloid (*Erysipelothrix insidiosa*) endocarditis.

Fusospirochetal Infections: Severe infections of the oropharynx (Vincent's), lower respiratory tract and genital area due to *Fusobacterium fusiformisans* spirochetes.

Gram-Negative Bacillary Infections (Bacteremias): (*E. coli, A. aerogenes, A. faecalis,* Salmonella, Shigella and *P. mirabilis*), Listeria infections (*Listeria monocytogenes*), Meningitis and endocarditis, Pasteurella infections (*Pasteurella multocida*), Bacteremia and meningitis, Rat-bite fever (*Spirillum minus* or *Streptobacillus moniliformis*), Gonorrheal endocarditis and arthritis (*N. gonorrhoeae*), Syphilis (*T. pallidum*) including congenital syphilis, Meningococcic meningitis.

Although no controlled clinical efficacy studies have been conducted, aqueous crystalline penicillin G for injection and penicillin G procaine suspension have been suggested by the American Heart Association and the American Dental Association for use as part of a combined parenteral-oral regimen for prophylaxis against bacterial endocarditis in patients with congenital heart disease or rheumatic, or other acquired valvular heart disease when they undergo dental procedures and surgical procedures of the upper respiratory tract.[1] Since it may happen that *alpha* hemolytic streptococci relatively resistant to penicillin may be found when patients are receiving continuous oral penicillin for secondary prevention of rheumatic fever, prophylactic agents other than penicillin may be chosen for these patients and prescribed in addition to their continuous rheumatic fever prophylactic regimen.

Note: When selecting antibiotics for the prevention of bacterial endocarditis the physician or dentist should read the full joint statement of the American Heart Association and the American Dental Association.[1]

CONTRAINDICATIONS

A previous hypersensitivity reaction to any penicillin is a contraindication.

WARNINGS

Serious and occasionally fatal hypersensitivity (anaphylactoid) reactions have been reported in patients on penicillin therapy. Although anaphylaxis is more frequent following parenteral therapy, it has occurred in patients on oral penicillins. These reactions are more apt to occur in individuals with history of sensitivity to multiple allergens.

There have been well documented reports of individuals with a history of penicillin hypersensitivity reactions who have experienced severe hypersensitivity reactions when treated with a cephalosporin. Before therapy with a penicillin, careful inquiry should be made concerning previous hypersensitivity reactions to penicillin, cephalosporins, and other allergens.

TABLETS

If an allergic reaction occurs, the drug should be discontinued and the patient treated with the usual agents *e.g.*, pressor amines, antihistamines and corticosteroids.

INJECTION

If an allergic reaction occurs, the drug should be discontinued and the appropriate therapy instituted. Serious anaphylactoid reactions require immediate emergency treatment with epinephrine. Oxygen, intravenous steroids, and airway management including intubation, should also be administered as indicated.

PRECAUTIONS

Penicillin should be used with caution in individuals with histories of significant allergies and/or asthma.

The oral route of administration should not be relied upon in patients with severe illness, or with nausea, vomiting gastric dilatation, cardiospasm or intestinal hypermotility.

Occasional patients will not absorb therapeutic amounts of orally administered penicillin.

In streptococcal infections, therapy must be sufficient to eliminate that organism (10 days minimum); otherwise the sequelae or streptococcal disease may occur. Culture should be taken following completion of treatment to determine whether streptococci have been eradicated.

TABLETS

Prolonged use of antibiotics may promote the overgrowth of nonsusceptible organisms, including fungi. Should superinfection occur, appropriate measures should be taken.

INJECTION

Intramuscular Therapy

Care should be taken to avoid intravenous or accidental intraarterial administration, or injection into or near major peripheral nerves or blood vessels, since such injections may produce neurovascular damage. Particular care should be taken with IV administration because of the possibility of thrombophlebitis.

The use of antibiotics may result in overgrowth of nonsusceptible organisms. Constant observation of the patient is essential. If new infections due to bacteria or fungi appear during therapy, the drug should be discontinued and appropriate measures taken. Whenever allergic reactions occur, penicillin should be withdrawn unless, in the opinion of the physician, the condition being treated is life threatening and amenable only to penicillin therapy.

Aqueous penicillin G by the intravenous route in high doses (above 10 million units), should be administered slowly because of the adverse effects of electrolyte imbalance from either the potassium or sodium content of the penicillin. Potassium penicillin G contains 1.7 mEg potassium and 0.3 mEq sodium per million units. The patient's renal, cardiac, and vascular status should be evaluated and if impairment of function is suspected or known to exist a reduction in the total dosage should be evaluated and if impairment of function is suspected or known to exist a reduction in the total dosage should be considered. Frequent evaluation of electrolyte balance, renal and hematopoietic function is recommended during therapy when high doses of intravenous aqueous penicillin G are used.

Laboratory Tests

In prolonged therapy with penicillin, periodic evaluation of the renal, hepatic, and hematopoietic systems is recommended foe organ system dysfunction. This is particularly important in prematures, neonates and other infants, and when high doses are used.

Positive Coomb's tests have been reported after large intravenous doses.

Monitor serum potassium and implement corrective measures when necessary.

When treating gonococcal infections in which primary and secondary syphilis are suspected, proper diagnostic procedures, including dark field examinations, should be done before receiving penicillin and monthly serological tests made for at least 4 months. All cases of penicillin treated syphilis should receive clinical and serological examinations every 6 months for 2-3 years.

In suspected staphylococcal infections, proper laboratory studies, including susceptibility tests, should be performed.

In streptococcal infections, cultures should be taken following completion of treatment to determine whether streptococci have been eradicated. Therapy must be sufficient to eliminate the organism (a minimum of 10 days); otherwise the sequelae of streptococcal disease (*e.g.*, endocarditis, rheumatic fever) may occur.

Carcinogenesis, Mutagenesis, and Impairment of Fertility

No information on long-term studies are available on the carcinogenesis, mutagenesis, ot the impairment of fertility with the use of penicillins.

Pregnancy, Teratogenic Effects, Pregnancy Category B

Reproduction studies performed in the mouse, rat, and rabbit have revealed no evidence of impaired fertility or harm to the fetus due to penicillin G. Human experience with the penicillins during pregnancy has not shown any positive evidence of adverse effects on the fetus. There are, however, no adequate and well controlled studies in pregnant women showing conclusively that harmful effects of these drugs on the fetus can be excluded. Because animal reproduction studies are not always predictive of human response, this drug should be used during pregnancy only if clearly needed.

Nursing Mothers

Penicillins are excreted in human milk. Caution should be exercised wen penicillin G is administered to a nursing woman.

Pediatric Use

Penicillins are excreted largely unchanged by the kidney. Because of incompletely developed renal function in infants, the rate of elimination will be slow. Use caution in administering to newborns and evaluate organ system function frequently.

DRUG INTERACTIONS

Concurrent administration of bacteriostatic antibiotics (*e.g.*, erythromycin, tetracycline) may diminish the bactericidal effects of penicillins by slowing the rate of bacterial growth. Bactericidal agents work most effective against the immature cell wall of rapidly proliferating microorganisms. This has been demonstrated *in vitro;* however, the clinical significance of this interaction is not well documented. There are few clinical situations in which the concurrent use of "static" and "cidal" antibiotics are indicated. However, in selected circumstances in which such therapy is appropriate, using adequate doses of antibacterial agents and beginning penicillin therapy first, should minimize the potential for interaction.

Penicillin blood levels may be prolonged by concurrent administration of probenecid which blocks the renal tubular secretion of penicillins.

Displacement of penicillin from plasma protein binding sites will elevate the level of free penicillin in the serum.

ADVERSE REACTIONS

TABLETS

Although the incidence of reactions to oral penicillin has been reported with much less frequency than following parenteral therapy, it should be remembered that all degrees of hypersensitivity including fatal anaphylaxis, have been reported with oral penicillin.

The most common reactions to oral penicillin are nausea, vomiting, epigastric distress, diarrhea, and black hairy tongue. The hypersensitivity reactions reported are skin eruptions (maculo-papular to exfoliative dermatitis), urticaria and other serum sickness reactions, laryngeal edema and anaphylaxis. Fever and eosinophilia may frequently be the only reaction observed. Hemolytic anemia, leukopenia, thrombocytopenia, neuropathy, and nephropathy are infrequent reactions and usually associated with high doses of parenteral penicillin.

INJECTION

Penicillin is a substance of low toxicity but does have a significant index of sensitization. The following hypersensitivity reactions have been reported: skin rashes ranging from maculopapular eruptions to exfoliative dermatitis; urticaria; and reactions resembling serum sickness, including chills, fever, edema, arthralgia and prostration. Severe and occasionally fatal anaphylaxis has occurred (see WARNINGS).

Hemolytic anemia, leucopenia, thrombocytopenia, nephropathy, and neuropathy are rarely observed adverse reactions and are usually associated with high intravenous dosage. Patients given continuous intravenous therapy with penicillin G potassium in high dosage (10 million to 100 million units daily) may suffer severe or even fatal potassium poisoning, particularly if renal insufficiency is present. Hyperreflexia, convulsions, and coma may be indicative of this syndrome.

Cardiac arrhythmias and cardiac arrest may also occur. (High dosage of penicillin G sodium may result in congestive heart failure due to high sodium intake.)

The Jarisch-Herxheimer reaction has been reported in patients treated for syphilis.

DOSAGE AND ADMINISTRATION

TABLETS

The dosage of penicillin G (oral) should be determined according to the sensitivity of the causative micro-organism and the severity of infection, and adjusted to the clinical response of the patient.

Oral penicillin G should be given at least 1 hour before or 2 hours after meals. The usual dosage recommendation for adults and children 12 years and over is as follows:

Streptococcal Infections

Mild to moderately severe-of the upper respiratory tract and including scarlet fever and mild erysipelas.

200,000-250,000 units q6-8h for 10 days for mild infections.

400,000-5000,000 units q8h for 10 days for moderately severe infections.

800,000 units may be given q12h.

Pneumococcal Infections

Mild to moderately severe-of the respiratory tract, including otitis media.

400,000-5000,000 units q6h until the patient has been afebrile for at least 2 days.

Staphylococcal Infections

Mild infections of skin and soft tissue (culture and sensitivity tests should be performed).

200,000-5000,000 units q6-8h until infection is cured.

Fusospirochetosis (Vincent's Infection) of the Oropharynx

Mild to moderately severe infections.

400,000-500,000 units q6-8h.

For the prevention of recurrence following rheumatic fever and/or chorea:

200,000-250,000 units twice daily on a continuing basis.

Note: Therapy for children 12 years of age is calculated on the basis of body weight. For infants and small children the suggested dose is 25,000 to 90,000 units per kg per day in 3-6 divided doses.

INJECTION

Severe infections due to susceptible strains of streptococci, pneumococci and staphylococci: Bacteremia, pneumonia, endocarditis, pericarditis, empyema, meningitis, and other severe infections — a minimum of 5 million units daily.

P

Syphilis: Aqueous Penicillin G may be used in the treatment of acquired and congenital syphilis, but because of necessity of frequent dosage, hospitalization is recommended. Dosage and duration of therapy will be determined by age of patient and stage of the disease.

Gonorrheal endocarditis: A minimum of 5 million units daily.

Meningococcic meningitis: 1-2 million units by the IM route every 2 hours, or continuous IV drip of 20-30 million units daily.

Actinomycosis: 1-6 million units/day for cervicofacial cases; 10- 20 million units daily for thoracic and abdominal disease.

Clostridial infections: 20 million units/day; penicillin is adjunctive therapy to antitoxin.

Fusospirochetal infections: Severe infections of oropharynx, lower respiratory tract, and genital area — 5-10 million units/day.

Rat-bite fever (spirillum minus or streptobacillus moniliformis): 12-15 million units/day for 3-4 weeks.

Listeria Infections (Listeria Monocytogenes):

Neonates: 500,000 to 1 million units/day.

Adults with Meningitis: 15-20 million units/day for 2 weeks.

Adults with Endocarditis: 15-20 million units/day for 4 weeks.

Pasteurella Infections (Pasteurella multocida):

Bacteremia and meningitis—4-6 million units/day for 2 weeks.

Erysipeloid (Erysipelothrix insidiosa):

Endocarditis: 20-20 million units/day for 4-6 weeks.

Gram-Negative Bacillary Infections (*E. Coli, Enterobacter Aerogens, A Faecalis* Salmonella, Shigella and *Proteus mirabilis*).):

Bacteremia: 20-80 units day.

Diphtheria: (carrier state); 300,000-400,000 units of penicillin/day in divided doses for 10-12 days.

Anthrax: A minimum of 5 million units of penicillin/day in divided doses until cure is effected.

For prophylaxis against bacterial endocarditis (American Heart Association, 1977. Prevention of bacterial endocarditis. Circulation. **56** :139A-143A) in patients with congenital heart disease or rheumatic or other acquired valvular heart disease, when undergoing dental procedures or surgical procedures of the upper respiratory tract, use a combined parenteral-oral regimen. One million units of aqueous crystalline-penicillin G (30,000 units/kg in children) intramuscularly, mixed with 600,000 units of procaine penicillin G (600,000 units for children) should be given one-half to one hour before the procedure. Oral penicillin V (phenoxymethyl penicillin), 500 mg for adults or 250 mg for children less than 60 lb, should be given every 6 hours for 8 doses. Doses for children should not exceed recommendations for adults for a single dose or for a 24 hour period.

Reconstitution

Buffered penicillin G potassium for Injection is highly water soluble. It may be dissolved in small amounts of water for injection, or sterile isotonic sodium chloride solution for parenteral use. All solutions should be stored in a refrigerator. When refrigerated, penicillin solutions may be stored for 7 days without significant loss of potency.

Penicillin G potassium for Injection may be given intramuscularly or by continuous drip for dosages of 500,000; 1,000,000; or 5,000,000 units. It is also suitable for intrapleural, intraarticulare, and other local instillations.

THE 20,000,000 UNIT DOSAGE MAY BE ADMINISTERED BY INTRAVENOUS INFUSION ONLY.

Intramuscular Injection: Keep total volume of injection small. The IM route is the preferred route of administration. Solutions containing up to 100,000 units of penicillin per ml of diluent may be used with a minimum of discomfort. Greater concentrations of penicillin G per ml is physically possible and may be employed where therapy demands. When larger doses are required, it may be advisable to administer aqueous solutions of penicillin by means of continuous IV drip.

Continuous Intravenous Drip: Determine the volume of fluid and rate of its administration required by the patient in a 24 hour period in the usual manner of fluid therapy, and add the appropriate daily dosage of penicillin to this fluid. For example, if an adult patient requires 2 L of fluid in 24 hours and a daily dosage of 10 million units of penicillin, add 5 million units to 1 L and adjust the rate of flow so the liter will be infused in 12 hours.

Intrapleural or Other Local Infusions: If fluid is aspirated, give infusion in a volume equal to ¼ or ½ the amount of fluid aspirated, otherwise, prepare as for intramuscular injection.

Intrathecal Use: The intrathecal use of penicillin in meningitis must be highly individualized. It should be employed only with full consideration of the possible irritating effects of penicillin when used by this route. The preferred route of therapy in bacterial meningitides is intravenous, supplemented by intravenous injection.

Parenteral drug products should be inspected visually for particulate matter and discoloration prior to administration, whenever solution and container permit.

Sterile solution may be left in the refrigerator for 1 week without significant loss of potency.

PRODUCT LISTING - RATED THERAPEUTICALLY EQUIVALENT

Powder For Injection - Injectable - G Potassium 1000000 U

10's	$9.25	GENERIC, Bristol-Myers Squibb	00003-0634-41

Powder For Injection - Injectable - G Potassium 5000000 U

10's	$34.44	PFIZERPEN, Pfizer U.S. Pharmaceuticals	00049-0520-83

Powder For Injection - Injectable - G Potassium 20000000 U

1's	$10.09	PFIZERPEN, Pfizer U.S. Pharmaceuticals	00049-0530-28

Solution - Intravenous - G Potassium 1000000 U/50 ml

1500 ml x 24	$316.80	GENERIC, Baxter I.V. Systems Division	00338-1021-41

PRODUCT LISTING - EQUIVALENTS NOT AVAILABLE

Powder For Injection - Injectable - G Potassium 5000000 U

10's	$309.96	GENERIC, Geneva Pharmaceuticals	00781-6135-95
10's	$314.40	GENERIC, Physicians Total Care	54868-3480-00
10's	$344.40	GENERIC, Watson/Schein Pharmaceuticals Inc	00364-2906-38
50's	$2108.75	GENERIC, Geneva Pharmaceuticals	00781-6153-97

Powder For Injection - Injectable - G Potassium 20000000 U

10's	$162.50	GENERIC, Watson/Schein Pharmaceuticals Inc	00364-2908-61

Solution - Intravenous - G Potassium 2000000 U/50 ml

1500 ml	$329.70	GENERIC, Baxter I.V. Systems Division	00338-1023-41

Solution - Intravenous - G Potassium 3000000 U/50 ml

1500 ml x 24	$342.30	GENERIC, Baxter I.V. Systems Division	00338-1025-41

Penicillin G Procaine *(001969)*

For related information, see the comparative table section in Appendix A.

Categories: Anthrax; Bacteremia; Bejel; Endocarditis, prevention; Erysipelas; Gonorrhea; Infection, ear, middle; Infection, skin and skin structures; Infection, upper respiratory tract; Pinta; Rat bite fever; Scarlet fever; Syphilis; Vincent's gingivitis; Vincent's pharyngitis; Yaws; Pregnancy Category B; FDA Approved 1948 Nov; WHO Formulary
Drug Classes: Antibiotics, penicillins
Brand Names: Crysticillin AS; Duracillin AS; **Pfizerpen AS**; Provaine Pencillin; Wycillin
Foreign Brand Availability: Aquilina (Spain); Farmaproina (Spain); Fradicilina 600 (Spain); Kemopen (Indonesia); Novocillin (South-Africa); Penicil (Mexico); Procapen (Finland); Procillin (South-Africa)
HCFA JCODE(S): J2510 up to 600,000 units IM, IV

DESCRIPTION

Penicillin G procaine is a highly potent antibacterial agent effective against a wide variety of pathogenic organisms. It is an equimolecular compound of procaine and penicillin G in aqueous suspension for intramuscular administration.

Penicillin G procaine is supplied in 10 ml vials (3,000,000 units).

Chemically, Penicillin G procaine is: 3,3-Dimethyl-7-oxo-6-(2-phenylacetamido)-4-thia-1-azabicyclo (3.2.0) heptane-2-carboxylic acid compound with 2-(diethylamino) ethyl-*p*-aminobenzoate (1:1) monohydrate.

It has a molecular weight of 588.72.

Penicillin G procaine is a white, fine crystal, or a white, very fine microcrystalline powder. Penicillin G procaine is odorless or practically so and 1 gram is soluble in 250 ml water. The pH of the aqueous suspension is between 5.0-7.5.

Storage: The product should be stored between 2-8°C (36-46°F).

CLINICAL PHARMACOLOGY

Penicillin G procaine is an equimolecular compound of procaine and penicillin G administered intramuscularly as a suspension. It dissolves slowly at the site of injection, giving a plateau type of blood level at about 4 hours, which falls slowly over a period of the next 15-20 hours.

Approximately 60% of penicillin G is bound to serum protein. The drug is distributed throughout the body tissues in widely varying amounts. Highest levels are found in the kidneys with lesser amounts in the liver, skin, and intestines. Penicillin G penetrates into all other tissues to a lesser degree with a very small level found in the cerebrospinal fluid. With normal kidney function the drug is excreted rapidly by tubular excretion. In neonates and young infants, and in individuals with impaired kidney function, excretion is considerably delayed. Approximately 60-90% of a dose of parenteral penicillin G is excreted in the urine within 24-36 hours. Penicillin G crosses the placental barrier and is found in the amniotic fluid and cord serum.

MICROBIOLOGY

Penicillin G exerts a bactericidal action against penicillin-susceptible microorganisms during the stage of active multiplication. It acts through the inhibition of biosynthesis of cell wall mucopeptide. It is not active against the penicillinase-producing bacteria, which include many strains of staphylococci. While *in vitro* studies have demonstrated the susceptibility of most strains of the following organisms, clinical efficacy for infections other than those included in INDICATIONS AND USAGE has not been documented. Penicillin G exerts high *in vitro* activity against staphylococci (except penicillinase-producing strains), streptococci (groups A, C, G, H, L, and M), and pneumococci. Other organisms sensitive to penicillin G are *N. gonorrhoeae, Corynebacterium diphtheriae, Bacillus anthracis,* Clostridia, *Actinomyces bovis, Streptobacillus moniliformis, Listeria monocytogenes,* and Leptospira. *Treponema pallidum* is extremely sensitive to the bactericidal action of penicillin G.

Penicillin acts synergistically with gentamicin or tobramycin against many strains of enterococci.

Susceptibility Testing

Penicillin G Susceptibility Powder or 10 units Penicillin G Susceptibility Discs may be used to determine microbial susceptibility to penicillin G using one of the following standard methods recommended by the National Committee for Laboratory Standards:

M2-A3, "Performance Standards for Antimicrobial Disk Susceptibility Tests"

M7-A, "Methods for Dilution Antimicrobial Susceptibility Tests for Bacteria that Grow Aerobically"

M11-A, "Reference Agar Dilution Procedure for Antimicrobial Susceptibility Testing of Anaerobic Bacteria"

M17-P, "Alternative Methods for Antimicrobial susceptibility Testing of Anaerobic Bacteria"

Tests should be interpreted by the following criteria (TABLE 1A and TABLE 1B):

P

TABLE 1A

	Zone Diameter, Nearest Whole mm		
	Susceptible	Moderately Susceptible	Resistant
Staphylococci	≥29	—	≤28
N. gonorrhoeae	≥20	—	≤19
Enterococci	—	≥15	≤14
Non-enterococcal streptococci and *L. monocytogenes*	≥28	20-27	≤19

TABLE 1B

	Approximate MIC Correlates	
	Susceptible	Resistant
Staphylococci	≤0.1 mcg/ml	β-lactamase
N. gonorrhoeae	≤0.1 mcg/ml	β-lactamase
Enterococci	—	≥16 mcg/ml
Non-enterococcal streptococci and *L. monocytogenes*	≤0.12 mcg/ml	≥4 mcg/ml

Interpretations of susceptible, intermediate, and resistant correlate zone size diameters with MIC values. A laboratory report of "susceptible" indicates that the suspected causative microorganism most likely will respond to therapy with penicillin G. A laboratory report of "resistant" indicates that the infecting microorganism most likely will not respond to therapy. A laboratory report of "moderately susceptible" indicates that the microorganism is most likely susceptible if a high dosage of penicillin G is used, or if the infection is such that high levels of penicillin G may be attained as in urine. A report of "intermediate" using the disk diffusion method may be considered an equivocal result, and dilution tests may be indicated.

Control organisms are recommended for susceptibility testing. Each time the test is performed the following organisms should be included. The range for zones of inhibition is shown below (TABLE 2):

TABLE 2

Control Organism	Zone of Inhibition Range
Staphylococcus aureus (ATCC 25923)	27-35

INDICATIONS AND USAGE

Penicillin G procaine is indicated in the treatment of moderately severe infections in both adults and children due to penicillin G-susceptible microorganisms that are susceptible to the low and persistent serum levels common to this particular dosage form in the indications listed below. Therapy should be guided by bacteriological studies (including susceptibility tests) and by clinical response.

NOTE: When high sustained serum levels are required, aqueous penicillin G either IM or IV should be used.

The following infections will usually respond to adequate dosages of intramuscular penicillin G procaine.

Streptococcal Infections Group A (Without Bacteremia): Moderately severe to severe to severe infections of the upper respiratory tract (including middle ear infections - otitis media), skin and soft tissue infections, scarlet fever, and erysipelas.

NOTE: Streptococci in groups A, C, H, G, L, and M are very sensitive to penicillin G. Other groups, including group D (enterococcus) are resistant. Aqueous penicillin is recommended for streptococcal infections with bacteremia.

Pneumococcal Infections: Moderately severe infections of the respiratory tract (including middle ear infections-otitis media).

NOTE: Severe pneumonia, empyema, bacteremia, pericarditis, meningitis, peritonitis, and purulent or septic arthritis of pneumococcal etiology are better treated with aqueous penicillin G during the acute stage.

Staphylococcal Infections: Penicillin G-sensitive. Moderately severe infections of the skin and soft tissues.

NOTE: Reports indicate an increasing number of strains of staphylococci resistant to penicillin G emphasizing the need for culture and sensitivity studies in treating suspected staphylococcal infections.

Indicated surgical procedures should be performed.

***Fusospirochetosis* (Vincent's Gingivitis And Pharyngitis):** Moderately severe infections of the oropharynx respond to therapy with penicillin G procaine.

NOTE: Necessary dental care should be accomplished in infections involving the gum tissue.

***Treponema pallidum*:** (Syphilis); all stages.

***N. gonorrhoeae*:** Acute and chronic (without bacteremia).

Yaws, Bejel, Pinta: *C. diphtheriae*-penicillin G procaine as an adjunct to antitoxin for prevention of the carrier stage.

Anthrax: *Streptobacillus moniliformis* and *Spirillum minus* infections (rat bite fever).

Erysipeloid: Subacute bacterial endocarditis (group A streptococcus) only in extremely sensitive infections.

PROPHYLAXIS AGAINST BACTERIAL ENDOCARDITIS

Although no controlled clinical efficacy studies have been conducted, aqueous crystalline penicillin G for injection and penicillin G procaine suspension have been suggested by the American Heart Association and the American Dental Association for use as part of a combined parenteral-oral regimen for prophylaxis against bacterial endocarditis in patients with congenital heart disease or rheumatic, or other acquired valvular heart disease when they undergo dental procedures and surgical procedures of the upper respiratory tract.[1] Since it may happen that *alpha* hemolytic streptococci relatively resistant to penicillin may be found when patients are receiving continuous oral penicillin for secondary prevention of rheumatic fever, prophylactic agents other than penicillin may be chosen for these patients and prescribed in addition to their continuous rheumatic fever prophylactic regimen.

NOTE: When selecting antibiotics for the prevention of bacterial endocarditis the physician or dentist should read the full joint statement of the American Heart Association and the American Dental Association.[1]

CONTRAINDICATIONS

A previous hypersensitivity reaction to any penicillin or procaine is a contraindication.

WARNINGS

Serious and occasionally fatal hypersensitivity (anaphylactoid) reactions have been reported in patients on penicillin therapy. These reactions are more likely to occur in individuals with a history of penicillin hypersensitivity and/or a history of sensitivity to multiple allergens. There have been reports of individuals with a history of penicillin hypersensitivity who have experienced severe reactions when treated with cephalosporins. Before initiating therapy with any penicillin, careful inquiry should be made concerning previous hypersensitivity reactions to penicillin, cephalosporins, or other allergens. If an allergic reaction occurs, the drug should be discontinued and the appropriate therapy instituted. Serious anaphylactoid reactions require immediate emergency treatment with epinephrine. Oxygen, intravenous steroids, and airway management-including intubation, should be administered as indicated.

Immediate toxic reactions to procaine may occur in some individuals, particularly when a large single dose is administered in the treatment of gonorrhea (4.8 million units). These reactions may be manifested by mental disturbances including anxiety, confusion, agitation, depression, weakness, seizures, hallucinations, combativeness, and expressed "fear of impending death." The reactions noted in carefully controlled studies occurred in approximately 1 in 500 patients treated for gonorrhea. Reactions are transient, lasting from 15-30 minutes.

PRECAUTIONS

GENERAL

Penicillin should be used with caution in individuals with histories of significant allergies and/or asthma.

INTRAMUSCULAR THERAPY

Care should be taken to avoid intravenous or accidental intraarterial administration, or injection into or near major peripheral nerves or blood vessels, since such injections may produce neurovascular damage.

As with all intramuscular preparations, Penicillin G procaine should be injected well within the body of a relatively large muscle. *Adults:* The preferred site is the upper outer quadrant of the buttock (*i.e.,* gluteus maximus), or the mid-lateral thigh. *Children:* It is recommended that intramuscular injections be given preferably in the mid-lateral muscles of the thigh. In infants and small children the periphery of the upper outer quadrant of the gluteal region should only be used when necessary, such as in burn patients, in order to minimize the possibility of damage to the sciatic nerve.

The deltoid area should be used only if well developed, such as in certain adults and older children, and then only with caution to avoid radial nerve injury. Intramuscular injections should not be made into the lower and mid-third of the upper arm. As with all intramuscular injections, aspiration is necessary to help avoid inadvertent injection into a blood vessel.

In streptococcal infections, therapy must be sufficient to eliminate the organism (10 days minimum), otherwise the sequelae of streptococcal disease may occur. Cultures should be taken following completion of treatment to determine whether streptococci have been eradicated.

The use of antibiotics may result in overgrowth of nonsusceptible organisms. Constant observation of the patient is essential. If new infections due to bacteria or fungi appear during therapy, the drug should be discontinued and appropriate measures taken. whenever allergic reactions occur, penicillin should be withdrawn unless, in the opinion of the physician, the condition being treated is life threatening and amenable only to penicillin therapy.

A small percentage of patients are sensitive to procaine. If there is a history of sensitivity make the usual test: Inject intradermally 0.1 ml of a 1-2 percent solution. Development of an erythema, wheal, flare, or eruption indicates procaine sensitivity. Sensitivity should be treated by the usual methods, including barbiturates, and penicillin G procaine preparations should not be used. Antihistamines appear beneficial in treatment of procaine reactions.

LABORATORY TESTS

In prolonged therapy with penicillin, periodic evaluation of the renal, hepatic, and hematopoietic systems is recommended. This is particularly important in prematures, neonates and other infants, and when high doses are used.

When treating gonococcal infections in which primary or secondary syphilis may be suspected, proper diagnostic procedures, including dark field examinations, should be done. In all cases in which concomitant syphilis is suspected, monthly serological tests should be made for at least 4 months. All cases of penicillin treated syphilis should receive clinical and serological examinations every 6 months for 2-3 years.

In suspected staphylococcal infections, proper laboratory studies, including susceptibility tests, should be performed.

In streptococcal infections, cultures should be taken following completion of treatment to determine whether streptococci have been eradicated.

CARCINOGENESIS, MUTAGENESIS, AND IMPAIRMENT OF FERTILITY

No information or long-term studies are available on the carcinogenesis, mutagenesis, or the impairment of fertility with the use of penicillin.

PREGNANCY, TERATOGENIC EFFECTS, PREGNANCY CATEGORY B

Reproduction studies performed in the mouse, rat, and rabbit have revealed no evidence of impaired fertility or harm to the fetus due to penicillin G. Human experience with the peni-

P

cillins during pregnancy has not shown any positive evidence of adverse effects on the fetus. There are, however, no adequate and well controlled studies in pregnant women showing conclusively that harmful effects of these drugs on the fetus can be excluded. Because animal reproduction studies are not always predictive of human response, this drug should be used during pregnancy only if clearly needed.

NURSING MOTHERS

Penicillin G procaine has been reported in milk. Caution should be exercised when penicillin G is administered to a nursing woman.

PEDIATRIC USE

Penicillins are excreted largely unchanged by the kidney. Because of incompletely developed renal function in infants, the rate of elimination will be slow. Use caution in administering to newborns and evaluate organ system function frequently.

DRUG INTERACTIONS

Concurrent administration of bacteriostatic antibiotics (*e.g.,* erythromycin, tetracycline) may diminish the bactericidal effects of penicillins by slowing the rate of bacterial growth. Bactericidal agents work most effectively against the immature cell wall of rapidly proliferating microorganisms. This has been demonstrated *in vitro;* however, the clinical significance of this interaction is not well documented. There are few clinical situations in which the concurrent use of "static" and "cidal" antibiotics are indicated. However, in selected circumstances in which such therapy is appropriate, using adequate doses of antibacterial agents and beginning penicillin therapy first, should minimize the potential for interaction.

Penicillin blood levels may be prolonged by concurrent administration of probenecid which blocks the renal tubular secretion of penicillins.

Displacement of penicillins from plasma protein binding sites will elevate the level of free penicillin in the serum.

ADVERSE REACTIONS

Penicillin is a substance of low toxicity, but does possess a significant index of sensitization. The following hypersensitivity reactions associated with use of penicillin have been reported: skin rashes, ranging from maculopapular eruptions to exfoliative dermatitis; urticaria; serum sickness-like reactions, including chills, fever, edema, arthralgia, and prostration. Severe and often fatal anaphylaxis has been reported (see WARNINGS). As with other treatments for syphilis, the Jarisch-Herxheimer reaction has been reported.

Procaine toxicity manifestations have been reported (see WARNINGS). Procaine hypersensitivity reactions have not been reported with this drug.

DOSAGE AND ADMINISTRATION

PEDIATRIC DOSAGE SCHEDULE

In children under 3 months of age, the absorption of aqueous penicillin G produces such high and sustained levels that penicillin G procaine dosage forms offer no advantages and are usually unnecessary.

In children under 12 years of age, dosage should be adjusted in accordance with the age and weight of the child, and the severity of the infection.

Under 2 years of age, the dose may be divided between the two buttocks if necessary.

Penicillin G procaine (aqueous) is for intramuscular injection only.

RECOMMENDED DOSAGE FOR PENICILLIN G PROCAINE AQUEOUS

Pneumonia: *Pneumococcal*, moderately severe (uncomplicated): 600,000-1,000,000 units daily.

Streptococcal Infections: Group A, moderately severe to severe tonsillitis, erysipelas, scarlet fever, upper respiratory tract, skin and soft tissue: 600,000-1,000,000 units daily for a minimum of 10 days.

Staphylococcal Infections: Moderately severe to severe: 600,000-1,000,000 units daily.

Bacterial Endocarditis: Group A streptococci, only in extremely sensitive infections: 600,000-1,000,000 units daily. For prophylaxis against bacterial endocarditis[1] in patients with congenital heart disease or rheumatic or other acquired valvular heart disease, when undergoing dental procedures or surgical procedures of the upper respiratory tract, use a combined parenteral-oral regimen. One million units of aqueous crystalline penicillin G (30,000 units/kg in children) intramuscularly, mixed with 600,000 units penicillin G (600,000 units for children) should be given ½-1 hour before the procedure. Oral penicillin V (phenoxymethyl penicillin), 500 mg for adults or 250 mg for children less than 60 lb, should be given every 6 hours for 8 doses. Doses for children should not exceed recommendations for adults for a single dose or for a 24 hour period.

Syphilis: Primary, secondary and latent with a negative spinal fluid in adults and children over 12 years of age: 600,000 units daily for 8 days, total 4,800,000 units.

Late (tertiary neurosyphilis and latent syphilis): With positive spinal fluid examination or no spinal fluid examination): 600,000 units daily for 10-15 days, total 6-9 million units.

Congenital Syphilis (early and late): 50,000 units/kg per day for a minimum of 10 days.

Yaws, Bejel, and Pinta: Treatment as syphilis in corresponding stage of disease.

Gonorrheal Infections (uncomplicated): Men or women-4.8 million units intramuscularly divided into at least 2 doses and injected at different sites at one visit, together with 1 gram of oral probenecid, preferably given at least 30 minutes prior to the injection. *NOTE:* Gonorrheal endocarditis should be treated intensively with aqueous penicillin G.

Diphtheria Adjunctive Therapy With Antitoxin: 300,000-600,000 units daily.

Diphtheria Carrier State: 300,000 units daily for 10 days.

Anthrax Cutaneous: 600,000-1,000,000 units/day.

Vincent's Infection (Fusospirochetosis): 600,000-1,000,000 units/day.

Erysipeloid: 600,000-1,000,000 units/day.

Streptobacillus moniliformis and Spirillum minus (rat bite fever): 600,000-1,000,000 units/day.

Parenteral drug products should be inspected visually for particulate matter and discoloration prior to administration, whenever solution and container permit.

CDC GUIDELINES FOR TREATMENT OF SEXUALLY TRANSMITTED DISEASES

Neurosyphilis[2] (as an alternative to the recommended regimen of penicillin G aqueous): 2 to 4 million units/day plus probenecid 500 mg orally 4 times daily, both for 10-14 days; many recommend benzathine penicillin G 2.4 million units weekly for 3 doses following the completion of this regimen.

Congenital Syphilis:[2] *Symptomatic and asymptomatic infants:* 50,000 units/kg/day (administered once IM) for 10-14 days.

PRODUCT LISTING - EQUIVALENTS NOT AVAILABLE

Suspension - Intramuscular - G Benzathine;Procaine 150000 U;150000 U/ml			
10 ml	$21.85	BICILLIN C-R, Allscripts Pharmaceutical Company	54569-2316-00
Suspension - Intramuscular - G Benzathine;Procaine 300000 U;300000 U/ml			
2 ml x 10	$125.50	BICILLIN C-R, Monarch Pharmaceuticals Inc	61570-0139-10
2 ml x 10	$141.58	BICILLIN C-R, Wyeth-Ayerst Laboratories	00008-0026-36
2 ml x 10	$151.51	BICILLIN C-R, Allscripts Pharmaceutical Company	54569-1545-00
2 ml x 10	$246.30	BICILLIN C-R, Monarch Pharmaceuticals Inc	61570-0140-10
4 ml x 10	$303.23	BICILLIN C-R, Allscripts Pharmaceutical Company	54569-1850-01
Suspension - Intramuscular - G Benzathine;Procaine 900000 U;300000 U/2 ml			
2 ml x 10	$157.69	BICILLIN C-R, Allscripts Pharmaceutical Company	54569-1859-00
2 ml x 10	$157.69	BICILLIN C-R, Allscripts Pharmaceutical Company	54596-1859-00
2 ml x 10	$228.90	BICILLIN C-R, Monarch Pharmaceuticals Inc	61570-0144-10
2 ml x 10	$256.40	BICILLIN C-R, Monarch Pharmaceuticals Inc	61570-0143-10
Suspension - Intramuscular - G Procaine 600000 U/ml			
1 ml x 10	$70.88	WYCILLIN, Allscripts Pharmaceutical Company	54569-2380-00
1 ml x 10	$95.30	WYCILLIN, Esi Lederle Generics	00008-0018-34
1 ml x 10	$101.00	GENERIC, Monarch Pharmaceuticals Inc	61570-0085-10
1 ml x 10	$101.00	WYCILLIN, Monarch Pharmaceuticals Inc	61570-0149-10
2 ml x 10	$158.60	WYCILLIN, Esi Lederle Generics	00008-0018-35
2 ml x 10	$168.10	GENERIC, Monarch Pharmaceuticals Inc	61570-0086-10
2 ml x 10	$168.10	WYCILLIN, Monarch Pharmaceuticals Inc	61570-0150-10

Penicillin V Potassium *(001971)*

For related information, see the comparative table section in Appendix A.

Categories: Chorea, prevention; Endocarditis, prevention; Erysipelas; Infection, skin and skin structures; Infection, upper respiratory tract; Rheumatic fever, prophylaxis; Scarlet fever; Vincent's gingivitis; Vincent's pharyngitis; Pregnancy Category B; FDA Approved 1957 Sep; WHO Formulary

Drug Classes: Antibiotics, penicillins

Brand Names: Beepen-VK; Pen Vee K; Penicillin VK; Veetids

Foreign Brand Availability: Abbocillin VK (Australia); Anapenil (Mexico); Apo-Pen-VK (Canada); Arcasin (Germany); Beapen (Malaysia); Cilacil (Argentina); Cilicaine VK (Australia; New-Zealand); Cliacil (Argentina); Crystapen V (India); Distaquaine V-K (England); DuraPenicillin (Germany); Fenocin (Indonesia); Fenoxcillin (Denmark); Fenoxypen (Norway; Sweden); Isocillin (Germany); Kavipen (Mexico); L.P.V. (Australia); Len V.K. (South-Africa); Megacilina Oral (Peru); Megacillin Oral (Germany); Milcopen (Finland); Nadopen-V (Canada); Newcillin (Japan); Novo-VK (South-Africa); Novopen-VK (Canada); Oracillin VK (South-Africa); Orvek (Bahrain; Cyprus; Egypt; Iran; Iraq; Jordan; Kuwait; Lebanon; Libya; Oman; Qatar; Republic-of-Yemen; Saudi-Arabia; Syria; United-Arab-Emirates); Ospen (France; Malaysia); Ospen 250 (Austria); Pen V (Hong-Kong); Penbeta (Germany); Penoral (Argentina); Pentacillin (Philippines); Pentid (Argentina); Pentranex (Philippines); Pen-Vi-K (Mexico); Primcillin (Denmark); Rafapen V-K (Israel); Robicillin VK (Bahrain; Cyprus; Egypt; Iran; Iraq; Jordan; Kuwait; Lebanon; Libya; Oman; Qatar; Republic-of-Yemen; Saudi-Arabia; Syria; United-Arab-Emirates); Rocilin (Denmark); Servipen-V (Thailand); Trepopen VK (Philippines); V-Cil-K (Bahamas; Barbados; Belize; Benin; Bermuda; Burkina-Faso; Curacao; Ethiopia; Gambia; Ghana; Guinea; Guyana; Ireland; Ivory-Coast; Jamaica; Kenya; Liberia; Malawi; Mali; Mauritania; Mauritius; Morocco; Netherland-Antilles; Niger; Nigeria; Senegal; Seychelles; Sierra-Leone; Sudan; Surinam; Tanzania; Trinidad; Tunia; Uganda; Zambia; Zimbabwe); V-Cillin K (Benin; Burkina-Faso; Ethiopia; Gambia; Ghana; Guinea; Ivory-Coast; Kenya; Liberia; Malawi; Mali; Mauritania; Mauritius; Morocco; Niger; Nigeria; Senegal; Seychelles; Sierra-Leone; South-Africa; Sudan; Tanzania; Tunia; Uganda; Zambia; Zimbabwe); V-Kal-K (Japan); V-Pen (Israel); V-Penicillin Kalium (Japan); Vepicombin (Denmark)

Cost of Therapy: $2.20 (Infection; Generic Tablets; 250 mg; 4 tablets/day; 10 day supply)

DESCRIPTION

Penicillin V potassium is the potassium salt of penicillin V. This chemically improved form combines acid stability with immediate solubility and rapid absorption. It is designated 4-thia-1-azabicyclo[3.2.0]-heptane-2-carboxylic acid, 3,3 -dimethyl-7-oxo-6-[(phenoxyacetyl)amino]-, monopotassium salt, [2S-(2α,5α,6β)]-. The empirical formula is $C_{16}H_{17}KN_2O_5S$, and the molecular weight is 388.48.

Each tablet contains penicillin V potassium equivalent to 250 mg (400,000 units) or 500 mg (800,000 units) penicillin V. The tablets also contain lactose, magnesium stearate, povidone, starch, stearic acid, and other inactive ingredients.

After being mixed as directed, each 5 ml of the oral solution will contain penicillin V potassium equivalent to 250 mg (400,000 units) penicillin V. The suspension also contains citric acid, FD&C red no. 40, flavors, saccharin, sodium citrate, and sucrose.

The potassium content of the tablets and oral solution is listed in TABLE 1.

Storage: Tablets should be stored at controlled room temperature, 59-86°F (15-30°C).

CLINICAL PHARMACOLOGY

Penicillin V potassium is bactericidal against penicillin-susceptible microorganisms during the stage of active multiplication. It produces its effect by inhibiting biosynthesis of cell-

TABLE 1

Size	Potassium (mEq)	Potassium (mg)
Tablets		
250 mg (400,000 units)	0.72	28.06
500 mg (800,000 units)	1.44	56.12
Oral Solution		
250 mg (400,000 units) 5 ml	0.72	28.06

wall mucopeptide. It is not active against the penicillinase-producing bacteria, which include many strains of staphylococci. The drug exerts high *in vitro* activity against staphylococci (except penicillinase-producing strains), streptococci (groups A, C, G, H, L, and M), and pneumococci. Other organisms susceptible *in vitro* to penicillin V are *Corynebacterium diphtheriae, Bacillus anthracis,* clostridia, *Actinomyces bovis, Streptobacillus moniliformis, Listeria monocytogenes, Leptospira,* and *Neisseria gonorrhoeae. Treponema pallidium* is extremely susceptible.

Penicillin V potassium has the distinct advantage over penicillin G in being resistant to inactivation by gastric acid. It may be given with meals; however, blood levels are slightly higher when the drug is given on an empty stomach. Average blood levels are 2-5 times higher than those following the same dose of oral penicillin G and also show much less individual variation.

Once absorbed, about 80% of penicillin V potassium is bound to serum protein. Tissue levels are highest in the kidneys, and lesser amounts appear in the liver, skin, and intestines. Small concentrations are found in all other body tissues and the cerebrospinal fluid. The drug is excreted as rapidly as it is absorbed in individuals with normal kidney function; however, recovery of the drug from the urine indicates that only about 25% of the dose given is absorbed. In neonates, young infants, and individuals with impaired kidney function, excretion is considerably delayed.

INDICATIONS AND USAGE

Penicillin V potassium is indicated in the treatment of mild to moderately severe infections due to microorganisms whose susceptibility to penicillin G is within the range of serum levels common to this particular dosage form. Therapy should be guided by bacteriologic studies (including susceptibility tests) and by clinical response.

NOTE: Severe pneumonia, empyema, bacteremia, pericarditis, meningitis, and arthritis should not be treated with penicillin V during the acute stage.

Indicated surgical procedures should be performed.

The following infections will usually respond to adequate dosage of penicillin V:

Streptococcal Infections (without bacteremia): Mild to moderate infections of the upper respiratory tract, scarlet fever, and mild erysipelas. *NOTE:* Streptococci groups A, C, G, H, L, and M are very susceptible to penicillin. Other groups, including group D (enterococcus), are resistant.

Pneumococcal Infections: Mild to moderately severe infections of the respiratory tract.

Staphylococcal Infections Susceptible to Penicillin G: Mild infections of the skin and soft tissues. *NOTE:* Reports indicate an increasing number of strains of staphylococci resistant to penicillin G, which emphasizes the need for culture and susceptibility studies in treating suspected staphylococcal infections.

Fusospirochetosis (Vincent's gingivitis and pharyngitis): Mild to moderately severe infections of the oropharynx usually respond to therapy with oral penicillin. *NOTE:* Necessary dental care should be accomplished in infections involving the gum tissue.

Medical conditions in which oral penicillin therapy is indicated as prophylaxis: To prevent recurrence following rheumatic fever and/or chorea. Prophylaxis with oral penicillin on a continuing basis has proved effective in preventing recurrence of these conditions.

Although no controlled clinical efficacy studies have been conducted, penicillin V has been suggested by the American Heart Association and the American Dental Association for use as an oral regimen for prophylaxis against bacterial endocarditis in patients with congenital heart disease or rheumatic or other acquired valvular heart disease when they undergo dental procedures and surgical procedures of the respiratory tract.[1]

Since α-hemolytic streptococci relatively resistant to penicillin may be found when patients are receiving continuous oral penicillin for secondary prevention of rheumatic fever, prophylactic agents other than penicillin may be chosen for these patients and prescribed in addition to their continuous prophylactic regimen for rheumatic fever.

Oral penicillin should not be used as adjunctive prophylaxis for genitourinary instrumentation or surgery, lower intestinal tract surgery, sigmoidoscopy, and childbirth.

NOTE: When selecting antibiotics for the prevention of bacterial endocarditis, the physician or dentist should read the full joint statement of the American Heart Association and the American Dental Association.[1]

CONTRAINDICATIONS

A previous hypersensitivity reaction to any penicillin is a contraindication.

WARNINGS

SERIOUS AND OCCASIONALLY FATAL HYPERSENSITIVITY (ANAPHYLACTIC) REACTIONS HAVE BEEN REPORTED IN PATIENTS RECEIVING PENICILLIN THERAPY. THESE REACTIONS ARE MORE LIKELY TO OCCUR IN INDIVIDUALS WITH A HISTORY OF PENICILLIN HYPERSENSITIVITY AND/OR A HISTORY OF SENSITIVITY TO MULTIPLE ALLERGENS. THERE HAVE BEEN REPORTS OF INDIVIDUALS WITH A HISTORY OF PENICILLIN HYPERSENSITIVITY WHO HAVE EXPERIENCED SEVERE REACTIONS WHEN TREATED WITH CEPHALOSPORINS. BEFORE INITIATING THERAPY WITH PENICILLIN V POTASSIUM, CAREFUL INQUIRY SHOULD BE MADE CONCERNING PREVIOUS HYPERSENSITIVITY REACTIONS TO PENICILLINS, CEPHALOSPORINS, OR OTHER ALLERGENS. IF AN ALLERGIC REACTION OCCURS, PENICILLIN V POTASSIUM SHOULD BE DISCONTINUED AND APPROPRIATE THERAPY INSTITUTED. **SERIOUS ANAPHYLACTIC REACTIONS REQUIRE IMMEDIATE EMERGENCY TREATMENT WITH EPINEPHRINE. OXYGEN, INTRAVENOUS STEROIDS, AND AIRWAY MANAGEMENT, INCLUDING INTUBATION, SHOULD ALSO BE ADMINISTRATED AS INDICATED.**

Pseudomembranous colitis has been reported with nearly all antibacterial agents including penicillins, and may range in severity from mild to life-threatening. Therefore, it is important to consider this diagnosis in patients who present with diarrhea subsequent to the administration of antibacterial agents.

Treatment with antibacterial agents alters the normal flora of the colon and may permit overgrowth of clostridia. Studies indicate that a toxin produced by *Clostridium difficile* is one primary cause of "antibiotic-associated colitis."

After the diagnosis of pseudomembranous colitis has been established, therapeutic measures should be initiated. Mild cases of pseudomembranous colitis usually respond to drug discontinuation alone. In moderate to severe cases, consideration should be given to management with fluids and electrolytes, protein supplementation, and treatment with an antibacterial drug clinically effective against *C. difficile* colitis.

PRECAUTIONS

Penicillin should be used with caution in individuals with histories of significant allergies and/or asthma.

The oral route of administration should not be relied upon in patients with severe illness or with nausea, vomiting, gastric dilatation, cardiospasm, or intestinal hypermotility.

Occasional patients will not absorb therapeutic amounts of orally administered penicillin.

In streptococcal infections, therapy must be sufficient to eliminate the organism (a minimum of 10 days); otherwise, the sequelae of streptococcal disease may occur. Cultures should be taken following completion of treatment to determine whether streptococci have been eradicated.

Prolonged use of antibiotics may promote the overgrowth of nonsusceptible organisms, including fungi. If superinfection occurs, appropriate measures should be taken.

ADVERSE REACTIONS

Although reactions have been reported much less frequently after oral than after parenteral penicillin therapy, it should be remembered that all degrees of hypersensitivity, including fatal anaphylaxis, have been observed with oral penicillin.

The most common reactions to oral penicillin are nausea, vomiting, epigastric distress, diarrhea, and black, hairy tongue. The hypersensitivity reactions noted are skin eruptions (ranging from maculopapular to exfoliative dermatitis); urticaria; reactions resembling serum sickness, including chills, fever, edema, arthralgia, and prostration; laryngeal edema; and anaphylaxis. Fever and eosinophilia may frequently be the only reactions observed. Hemolytic anemia, leukopenia, thrombocytopenia, neuropathy, and nephropathy are infrequent reactions and are usually associated with high doses of parenteral penicillin.

DOSAGE AND ADMINISTRATION

The dosage of penicillin V potassium should be determined according to the susceptibility of the causative microorganism and the severity of infection and should be adjusted to the clinical response of the patient.

The usual dosage recommendations for adults and children 12 years and over are as follows:

Streptococcal Infections: Mild to moderately severe infections of the upper respiratory tract, including scarlet fever and mild erysipelas: 200,000-500,000 units every 6-8 hours for 10 days.

Pneumococcal Infections: Mild to moderately severe infections of the respiratory tract, including otitis media: 400,000-500,000 units every 6 hours until the patient has been afebrile for at least 2 days.

Staphylococcal Infections: Mild infections of skin and soft tissue (culture and susceptibility tests should be performed): 400,000-500,000 units every 6-8 hours.

Fusospirochetosis (Vincent's Infection) of the Oropharynx: Mild to moderately severe infections: 400,000-500,000 units every 6-8 hours.

Prophylaxis in the Following Conditions: To prevent recurrence following rheumatic fever and/or chorea: 200,000-250,000 units twice daily on a continuing basis.

For prophylaxis against bacterial endocarditis[1] in patients with congenital heart disease or rheumatic or other acquired valvular heart disease when undergoing dental procedures or surgical procedures of the upper respiratory tract, 1 of 2 regimens may be selected:

(1) For the oral regimen, the usual adult dosage is 2 g of penicillin V (1 g for children less than 30 kg) 1 hour before the procedure and then 1 g (500 mg for children less than 30 kg) 6 hours later.

(2) For patients unable to take oral antibiotics, 2,000,000 units of aqueous penicillin G (50,000 units/kg for children) IV or IM may be substituted 30-60 minutes before the procedure and 1,000,000 units (25,000 units/kg for children) 6 hours later.

For patients with prosthetic valves and for those at highest risk for endocarditis, ampicillin, 1-2 g (50 mg/kg for children), plus gentamicin, 1.5 mg/kg (2 mg/kg for children), IM or IV, may be given one- half hour prior to the procedure, followed by 1 g of oral penicillin V 6 hours later. Alternatively, the parenteral regimen should be repeated once every 8 hours later.

Children's antibiotic dosages should not exceed the maximum adult doses.

NOTE: Therapy for children under 12 years of age is calculated on the basis of body weight. For infants and small children, the suggested daily dose is 25,000-90,000 units (15-50 mg)/kg in 3-6 divided doses.

After being mixed, the solution should be stored in a refrigerator. It may be kept for 14 days without significant loss of potency. Shake well before using. Keep tightly closed.

PRODUCT LISTING - RATED THERAPEUTICALLY EQUIVALENT

Powder For Reconstitution - Oral - V Potassium 125 mg/5 ml

Size	Price	Manufacturer	NDC
100 ml	$1.74	GENERIC, Moore, H.L. Drug Exchange Inc	00839-5189-73
100 ml	$2.16	GENERIC, Ivax Corporation	00182-0276-70
100 ml	$2.16	GENERIC, Major Pharmaceuticals Inc	00904-4001-04
100 ml	$2.25	GENERIC, Interstate Drug Exchange Inc	00814-5875-54

P

Size	Price	Supplier	NDC
100 ml	$2.28	GENERIC, Qualitest Products Inc	00603-6605-64
100 ml	$2.48	GENERIC, Bristol-Myers Squibb	00003-0681-44
100 ml	$2.48	GENERIC, Teva Pharmaceuticals Usa	00093-5198-73
100 ml	$2.51	GENERIC, Aligen Independent Laboratories Inc	00405-3500-60
100 ml	$6.25	GENERIC, Pharma Pac	52959-0560-00
200 ml	$3.34	GENERIC, Teva Pharmaceuticals Usa	00093-4125-74
200 ml	$3.34	GENERIC, Ivax Corporation	00182-0276-73
200 ml	$3.34	GENERIC, Qualitest Products Inc	00603-6605-68
200 ml	$3.34	GENERIC, Major Pharmaceuticals Inc	00904-4001-08
200 ml	$3.64	GENERIC, Bristol-Myers Squibb	00003-0681-54
200 ml	$3.64	GENERIC, Teva Pharmaceuticals Usa	00093-5198-74
200 ml	$3.92	GENERIC, Aligen Independent Laboratories Inc	00405-3500-70

Powder For Reconstitution - Oral - V Potassium 250 mg/5 ml

Size	Price	Supplier	NDC
100 ml	$2.21	GENERIC, Moore, H.L. Drug Exchange Inc	00839-5190-73
100 ml	$2.60	GENERIC, Glaxosmithkline	00029-6170-23
100 ml	$2.78	GENERIC, Bristol-Myers Squibb	00003-0682-44
100 ml	$2.78	GENERIC, Teva Pharmaceuticals Usa	00093-5199-73
100 ml	$2.93	GENERIC, Interstate Drug Exchange Inc	00814-5878-54
100 ml	$2.95	GENERIC, Teva Pharmaceuticals Usa	00093-4127-73
100 ml	$2.95	GENERIC, Ivax Corporation	00182-0308-70
100 ml	$2.95	GENERIC, Major Pharmaceuticals Inc	00904-4004-04
100 ml	$3.03	GENERIC, Aligen Independent Laboratories Inc	00405-3525-60
100 ml	$3.08	GENERIC, Qualitest Products Inc	00603-6606-64
200 ml	$3.42	GENERIC, Moore, H.L. Drug Exchange Inc	00839-5190-78
200 ml	$4.02	GENERIC, Bristol-Myers Squibb	00003-0682-54
200 ml	$4.02	GENERIC, Teva Pharmaceuticals Usa	00093-5199-74
200 ml	$4.66	GENERIC, Interstate Drug Exchange Inc	00814-5878-60
200 ml	$5.07	GENERIC, Ivax Corporation	00182-0308-73
200 ml	$5.08	GENERIC, Qualitest Products Inc	00603-6606-68
200 ml	$5.08	GENERIC, Major Pharmaceuticals Inc	00904-4004-08
200 ml	$5.42	GENERIC, Aligen Independent Laboratories Inc	00405-3525-70

Powder For Reconstitution - Oral - 250 mg/5 ml

Size	Price	Supplier	NDC
200 ml	$3.30	FEDERAL UPPER LIMIT, H.C.F.A. F F P	99999-1971-18

Tablet - Oral - V Potassium 250 mg

Size	Price	Supplier	NDC
10's	$3.84	GENERIC, Pd-Rx Pharmaceuticals	55289-0206-10
20's	$4.70	GENERIC, Pd-Rx Pharmaceuticals	55289-0206-20
20's	$4.95	GENERIC, Dhs Inc	55887-0830-20
25's	$10.62	GENERIC, Pd-Rx Pharmaceuticals	55289-0206-97
28's	$5.00	GENERIC, Pd-Rx Pharmaceuticals	55289-0206-28
28's	$6.87	GENERIC, Dhs Inc	55887-0830-28
30's	$5.10	GENERIC, Pd-Rx Pharmaceuticals	55289-0206-30
30's	$7.38	GENERIC, Dhs Inc	55887-0830-30
40's	$3.26	GENERIC, Pd-Rx Pharmaceuticals	58864-0379-40
40's	$3.71	GENERIC, Golden State Medical	60429-0147-40
40's	$5.50	GENERIC, Pd-Rx Pharmaceuticals	55289-0206-40
40's	$9.88	GENERIC, Dhs Inc	55887-0830-40
40's	$14.50	GENERIC, Med-Pro Inc	53978-5042-06
100's	$5.50	GENERIC, Major Pharmaceuticals Inc	00904-2449-60
100's	$5.50	GENERIC, Major Pharmaceuticals Inc	00904-2450-60
100's	$7.20	GENERIC, Aligen Independent Laboratories Inc	00405-4762-01
100's	$7.20	GENERIC, Aligen Independent Laboratories Inc	00405-4768-01
100's	$7.36	GENERIC, Moore, H.L. Drug Exchange Inc	00839-5187-06
100's	$7.36	GENERIC, Moore, H.L. Drug Exchange Inc	00839-5188-06
100's	$8.15	GENERIC, Ivax Corporation	00182-0869-01
100's	$8.15	GENERIC, Mylan Pharmaceuticals Inc	00378-0195-01
100's	$9.25	GENERIC, Mylan Pharmaceuticals Inc	00378-0111-01
100's	$12.60	GENERIC, Udl Laboratories Inc	51079-0615-20
100's	$23.46	GENERIC, Bristol-Myers Squibb	00003-0115-50
100's	$23.46	GENERIC, Teva Pharmaceuticals Usa	00093-5194-01
100's	$23.46	GENERIC, Geneva Pharmaceuticals	00781-1205-01

Tablet - Oral - V Potassium 500 mg

Size	Price	Supplier	NDC
15's	$4.60	GENERIC, Pd-Rx Pharmaceuticals	55289-0207-15
20's	$3.55	GENERIC, Circle Pharmaceuticals Inc	00659-0130-20
20's	$4.90	GENERIC, Pd-Rx Pharmaceuticals	55289-0207-20
28's	$5.30	GENERIC, Pd-Rx Pharmaceuticals	55289-0207-28
30's	$5.42	GENERIC, Pd-Rx Pharmaceuticals	55289-0207-30
40's	$2.99	GENERIC, Circle Pharmaceuticals Inc	00659-0130-40
40's	$6.53	GENERIC, Golden State Medical	60429-0148-40
40's	$7.00	GENERIC, Pd-Rx Pharmaceuticals	55289-0207-40
40's	$22.80	GENERIC, Med-Pro Inc	53978-5055-06
100's	$9.24	GENERIC, Teva Pharmaceuticals Usa	00093-1173-01
100's	$9.24	GENERIC, Teva Pharmaceuticals Usa	00093-1174-01
100's	$9.90	GENERIC, Major Pharmaceuticals Inc	00904-2451-60
100's	$9.90	GENERIC, Major Pharmaceuticals Inc	00904-2452-60
100's	$10.43	GENERIC, Interstate Drug Exchange Inc	00814-5870-14
100's	$10.43	GENERIC, Interstate Drug Exchange Inc	00814-5871-14
100's	$11.68	GENERIC, Moore, H.L. Drug Exchange Inc	00839-1766-06
100's	$11.68	GENERIC, Moore, H.L. Drug Exchange Inc	00839-6393-06
100's	$12.25	GENERIC, Aligen Independent Laboratories Inc	00405-4763-01
100's	$12.25	GENERIC, Aligen Independent Laboratories Inc	00405-4769-01
100's	$15.33	GENERIC, Qualitest Products Inc	00603-5068-21
100's	$15.35	GENERIC, Ivax Corporation	00182-0115-01
100's	$15.35	GENERIC, Ivax Corporation	00182-1537-01
100's	$15.35	GENERIC, Mylan Pharmaceuticals Inc	00378-0112-01
100's	$15.35	GENERIC, Mylan Pharmaceuticals Inc	00378-0198-01
100's	$24.60	GENERIC, Udl Laboratories Inc	51079-0616-20
100's	$39.88	GENERIC, Bristol-Myers Squibb	00003-0116-50
100's	$39.88	GENERIC, Teva Pharmaceuticals Usa	00093-5195-01
100's	$39.88	GENERIC, Geneva Pharmaceuticals	00781-1655-01

PRODUCT LISTING - EQUIVALENTS NOT AVAILABLE

Powder For Reconstitution - Oral - V Potassium 125 mg/5 ml

Size	Price	Supplier	NDC
100 ml	$2.53	GENERIC, Physicians Total Care	54868-4125-01
100 ml	$4.62	GENERIC, Prescript Pharmaceuticals	00247-0106-00
100 ml	$4.70	GENERIC, Southwood Pharmaceuticals Inc	58016-1026-01
200 ml	$3.37	GENERIC, Physicians Total Care	54868-4125-02
200 ml	$5.89	GENERIC, Prescript Pharmaceuticals	00247-0106-79
200 ml	$6.22	GENERIC, Southwood Pharmaceuticals Inc	58016-1027-01
200 ml	$6.22	GENERIC, Southwood Pharmaceuticals Inc	58016-1027-06

Powder For Reconstitution - Oral - V Potassium 250 mg/5 ml

Size	Price	Supplier	NDC
100 ml	$2.35	GENERIC, Circle Pharmaceuticals Inc	00659-6124-80
100 ml	$2.88	GENERIC, Physicians Total Care	54868-1780-01
100 ml	$2.95	GENERIC, Allscripts Pharmaceutical Company	54569-2933-00
100 ml	$4.79	GENERIC, Prescript Pharmaceuticals	00247-0014-00
100 ml	$5.25	GENERIC, Southwood Pharmaceuticals Inc	58016-1028-01
150 ml	$5.96	GENERIC, Pharma Pac	52959-1172-01
200 ml	$4.05	GENERIC, Physicians Total Care	54868-1780-02
200 ml	$6.21	GENERIC, Prescript Pharmaceuticals	00247-0014-79
200 ml	$7.10	GENERIC, Pharma Pac	52959-1172-02
200 ml	$7.70	GENERIC, Southwood Pharmaceuticals Inc	58016-1029-01
200 ml x 12	$5.07	GENERIC, Allscripts Pharmaceutical Company	54569-8004-00

Tablet - Oral - V Potassium 250 mg

Size	Price	Supplier	NDC
2's	$3.41	GENERIC, Prescript Pharmaceuticals	00247-0069-02
3's	$3.44	GENERIC, Prescript Pharmaceuticals	00247-0069-03
4's	$3.46	GENERIC, Prescript Pharmaceuticals	00247-0069-04
5's	$3.48	GENERIC, Prescript Pharmaceuticals	00247-0069-05
6's	$3.52	GENERIC, Prescript Pharmaceuticals	00247-0069-06
8's	$3.56	GENERIC, Prescript Pharmaceuticals	00247-0069-08
9's	$3.59	GENERIC, Prescript Pharmaceuticals	00247-0069-09
10's	$1.22	GENERIC, Southwood Pharmaceuticals Inc	58016-0146-10
10's	$3.62	GENERIC, Prescript Pharmaceuticals	00247-0069-10
12's	$0.98	GENERIC, Allscripts Pharmaceutical Company	54569-2702-06
12's	$1.47	GENERIC, Southwood Pharmaceuticals Inc	58016-0146-12
12's	$3.67	GENERIC, Prescript Pharmaceuticals	00247-0069-12
15's	$3.75	GENERIC, Prescript Pharmaceuticals	00247-0069-15
16's	$1.95	GENERIC, Southwood Pharmaceuticals Inc	58016-0146-16
16's	$3.78	GENERIC, Prescript Pharmaceuticals	00247-0069-16
20's	$1.32	GENERIC, Allscripts Pharmaceutical Company	54569-2702-00
20's	$2.10	GENERIC, Circle Pharmaceuticals Inc	00659-0125-20
20's	$2.45	GENERIC, Pharmaceutical Corporation Of America	51655-0009-52
20's	$2.45	GENERIC, Southwood Pharmaceuticals Inc	58016-0146-20
20's	$3.88	GENERIC, Prescript Pharmaceuticals	00247-0069-20
20's	$13.87	GENERIC, Pharma Pac	52959-0333-20
21's	$2.57	GENERIC, Southwood Pharmaceuticals Inc	58016-0146-21
21's	$3.91	GENERIC, Prescript Pharmaceuticals	00247-0069-21
24's	$2.94	GENERIC, Southwood Pharmaceuticals Inc	58016-0146-24
24's	$3.99	GENERIC, Prescript Pharmaceuticals	00247-0069-24
24's	$16.09	GENERIC, Pharma Pac	52959-0333-24
28's	$2.10	GENERIC, Circle Pharmaceuticals Inc	00659-0125-28
28's	$2.28	GENERIC, Allscripts Pharmaceutical Company	54569-2702-02
28's	$3.03	GENERIC, Pharmaceutical Corporation Of America	51655-0009-29
28's	$3.43	GENERIC, Southwood Pharmaceuticals Inc	58016-0146-28
28's	$18.57	GENERIC, Pharma Pac	52959-0333-28
30's	$2.44	GENERIC, Allscripts Pharmaceutical Company	54569-2702-03
30's	$2.80	GENERIC, Physicians Total Care	54868-1171-03
30's	$3.67	GENERIC, Southwood Pharmaceuticals Inc	58016-0146-30
30's	$4.15	GENERIC, Prescript Pharmaceuticals	00247-0069-30
30's	$19.27	GENERIC, Pharma Pac	52959-0333-30
32's	$4.20	GENERIC, Prescript Pharmaceuticals	00247-0069-32
40's	$2.31	GENERIC, Pharmaceutical Corporation Of America	51655-0009-51
40's	$2.89	GENERIC, Circle Pharmaceuticals Inc	00659-0125-40
40's	$3.25	GENERIC, Allscripts Pharmaceutical Company	54569-2702-04
40's	$3.29	GENERIC, Physicians Total Care	54868-1171-01
40's	$4.41	GENERIC, Prescript Pharmaceuticals	00247-0069-40
40's	$4.90	GENERIC, Southwood Pharmaceuticals Inc	58016-0146-40
40's	$22.66	GENERIC, Pharma Pac	52959-0333-40
44's	$4.52	GENERIC, Prescript Pharmaceuticals	00247-0069-44
100's	$5.93	GENERIC, Interstate Drug Exchange Inc	00814-5863-14
100's	$5.93	GENERIC, Interstate Drug Exchange Inc	00814-5866-14
100's	$6.00	GENERIC, Prescript Pharmaceuticals	00247-0069-00
100's	$12.24	GENERIC, Southwood Pharmaceuticals Inc	58016-0146-00

Tablet - Oral - V Potassium 500 mg

Size	Price	Supplier	NDC
1's	$3.42	GENERIC, Prescript Pharmaceuticals	00247-0068-01
2's	$3.48	GENERIC, Prescript Pharmaceuticals	00247-0068-02
3's	$3.55	GENERIC, Prescript Pharmaceuticals	00247-0068-03
4's	$0.57	GENERIC, Allscripts Pharmaceutical Company	54569-3503-01
4's	$3.62	GENERIC, Prescript Pharmaceuticals	00247-0068-04
6's	$1.38	GENERIC, Southwood Pharmaceuticals Inc	58016-0147-06
6's	$3.75	GENERIC, Prescript Pharmaceuticals	00247-0068-06

P

8's	$3.88	GENERIC, Prescript Pharmaceuticals	00247-0068-08
10's	$2.30	GENERIC, Southwood Pharmaceuticals Inc	58016-0147-10
10's	$4.01	GENERIC, Prescript Pharmaceuticals	00247-0068-10
12's	$1.70	GENERIC, Allscripts Pharmaceutical Company	54569-2710-01
12's	$2.76	GENERIC, Southwood Pharmaceuticals Inc	58016-0147-12
12's	$4.15	GENERIC, Prescript Pharmaceuticals	00247-0068-12
14's	$4.28	GENERIC, Prescript Pharmaceuticals	00247-0068-14
15's	$3.45	GENERIC, Southwood Pharmaceuticals Inc	58016-0147-15
15's	$4.34	GENERIC, Prescript Pharmaceuticals	00247-0068-15
16's	$3.68	GENERIC, Southwood Pharmaceuticals Inc	58016-0147-16
16's	$4.41	GENERIC, Prescript Pharmaceuticals	00247-0068-16
20's	$2.83	GENERIC, Allscripts Pharmaceutical Company	54569-2710-02
20's	$3.01	GENERIC, Physicians Total Care	54868-1173-05
20's	$4.60	GENERIC, Southwood Pharmaceuticals Inc	58016-0147-20
20's	$4.68	GENERIC, Prescript Pharmaceuticals	00247-0068-20
20's	$43.43	GENERIC, Pharma Pac	52959-0213-20
21's	$4.74	GENERIC, Prescript Pharmaceuticals	00247-0068-21
21's	$4.83	GENERIC, Southwood Pharmaceuticals Inc	58016-0147-21
24's	$4.94	GENERIC, Prescript Pharmaceuticals	00247-0068-24
24's	$5.52	GENERIC, Southwood Pharmaceuticals Inc	58016-0147-24
24's	$51.94	GENERIC, Pharma Pac	52959-0213-24
25's	$5.01	GENERIC, Prescript Pharmaceuticals	00247-0068-25
28's	$3.96	GENERIC, Allscripts Pharmaceutical Company	54569-2710-04
28's	$5.21	GENERIC, Prescript Pharmaceuticals	00247-0068-28
28's	$6.44	GENERIC, Southwood Pharmaceuticals Inc	58016-0147-28
28's	$60.32	GENERIC, Pharma Pac	52959-0213-28
30's	$3.72	GENERIC, Physicians Total Care	54868-1173-01
30's	$4.24	GENERIC, Allscripts Pharmaceutical Company	54569-2710-05
30's	$5.34	GENERIC, Prescript Pharmaceuticals	00247-0068-30
30's	$6.90	GENERIC, Southwood Pharmaceuticals Inc	58016-0147-30
30's	$64.34	GENERIC, Pharma Pac	52959-0213-30
32's	$5.47	GENERIC, Prescript Pharmaceuticals	00247-0068-32
40's	$4.69	GENERIC, Physicians Total Care	54868-1173-02
40's	$5.65	GENERIC, Allscripts Pharmaceutical Company	54569-2710-06
40's	$6.00	GENERIC, Prescript Pharmaceuticals	00247-0068-40
40's	$7.98	GENERIC, Pharmaceutical Corporation Of America	51655-0010-51
40's	$9.20	GENERIC, Southwood Pharmaceuticals Inc	58016-0147-40
40's	$72.33	GENERIC, Pharma Pac	52959-0213-40
50's	$11.50	GENERIC, Southwood Pharmaceuticals Inc	58016-0147-50
60's	$13.80	GENERIC, Southwood Pharmaceuticals Inc	58016-0147-60
100's	$9.05	GENERIC, Physicians Total Care	54868-1173-00
100's	$23.01	GENERIC, Southwood Pharmaceuticals Inc	58016-0147-00

Pentamidine Isethionate *(001975)*

Categories: Pneumonia, pneumocystis carinii; Pregnancy Category C; FDA Approved 1984 Oct; WHO Formulary; Orphan Drugs
Drug Classes: Antiprotozoals
Brand Names: Nebupent; **Pentam 300**
Foreign Brand Availability: Benambex (Japan); Pentacarinat (Austria; Bahamas; Barbados; Belgium; Belize; Bermuda; Canada; Curacao; Denmark; England; Finland; France; Germany; Greece; Guyana; Israel; Italy; Jamaica; Netherland-Antilles; Netherlands; New-Zealand; Norway; Peru; Portugal; South-Africa; Spain; Surinam; Sweden; Switzerland; Thailand; Trinidad)
HCFA JCODE(S): J2545 per 300 mg INH

DESCRIPTION

INHALATION SOLUTION

NebuPent (pentamidine isethionate), an anti-protozoal agent, is a sterile and nonpyrogenic lyophilized product. After reconstitution with sterile water for injection, NebuPent is administered by inhalation via the Respirgard II nebulizer [Marquest, Englewood, CO]. (See DOSAGE AND ADMINISTRATION.)

INJECTION

Pentam 300 (sterile pentamidine isethionate),

an anti-protozoal agent, is a nonpyrogenic lyophilized product. After reconstitution, it should be administered by intramuscular or intravenous (IM or IV) routes. (See DOSAGE AND ADMINISTRATION.)

Pentamidine isethionate is a white crystalline powder soluble in water and glycerin and insoluble in ether, acetone, and chloroform. It is chemically designated as 4,4'-diamidino-diphenoxypentane di-(β-hydroxyethanesulfonate) with the following empirical formula: $C_{23}H_{36}N_4O_{10}S_2$ with a molecular weight of 592.68.

Each Vial Contains: Pentamidine isethionate - 300 mg

Storage: Store the dry product at controlled room temperature 15-30°C (59-86°F). Protect the dry product and reconstituted solution from light.

Discard unused portions.

CLINICAL PHARMACOLOGY

MICROBIOLOGY

Inhalation Solution and Injection

Pentamidine isethionate, an aromatic diamidine, is known to have activity against *Pneumocystis carinii*. The mode of action is not fully understood. *In vitro* studies with mammalian tissues and the protozoan *Crithidia oncopelti* indicate that the drug interferes with nuclear metabolism producing inhibition of the synthesis of DNA, RNA, phospholipids and proteins.

PHARMACOKINETICS

Inhalation Solution

In 5 AIDS patients with suspected *Pneumocystis carinii* pneumonia (PCP), the mean concentrations of pentamidine determined 18-24 hours after inhalation therapy were 23.2 ng/ml (range 5.1 to 43.0 ng/ml) in bronchoalveolar lavage fluid and 705 ng/ml (range, 140-1336 ng/ml) in sediment after administration of a 300 mg single dose via the Respirgard II nebulizer. In 3 AIDS patients with suspected PCP, the mean concentrations of pentamidine determined 18-24 hours after a 4 mg/kg intravenous dose were 2.6 ng/ml (range 1.5-4.0 ng/ml) in bronchoalveolar lavage fluid and 9.3 ng/ml (range, 6.9-12.8 ng/ml) in sediment. In the patients who received aerosolized pentamidine, the peak plasma levels of pentamidine were at or below the lower limit of detection of the assay (2.3 ng/ml).

Following a single 2 hour intravenous infusion of 4 mg/kg of pentamidine isethionate to 6 AIDS patients, the mean plasma Cmax, T 1/2 and clearance were 612 ± 371 ng/ml, 6.4 ± 1.3 hr and 248 ± 91 l/hr respectively. In another study of aerosolized pentamidine in 13 AIDS patients with acute PCP who received 4 mg/kg/day administered via the Ultra Vent jet nebulizer, peak plasma levels of pentamidine averaged 18.8 ± 11.9 ng/ml after the first dose. During the next 14 days of repeated dosing, the highest observed Cmax averaged 20.5 ± 21.2 ng/ml. In a third study, following daily administration of 600 mg of inhaled pentamidine isethionate with the Respirgard II nebulizer for 21 days in 11 patients with acute PCP, mean plasma levels measured shortly after the 21st dose averaged 11.8 ± 10.0 ng/ml. Plasma concentrations after aerosol administration are substantially lower than those observed after a comparable intravenous dose. The extent of pentamidine accumulation and distribution following chronic inhalation therapy are not known.

In rats, intravenous administration of a 5 mg/kg dose resulted in concentrations of pentamidine in the liver and kidney that were 87.5 and 62.3-fold higher, respectively, than levels in those organs following 5 mg/kg administered as an aerosol.

No pharmacokinetic data are available following aerosol administration of pentamidine in humans with impaired hepatic or renal function.

Injection

Little is known about the drug's pharmacokinetics. Preliminary studies have shown that in 7 patients treated with daily IM doses of pentamidine at 4 mg/kg for 10-12 days, plasma concentrations were between 0.3 and 0.5 μg/ml. The levels did not appreciably change with time after injection or from day to day. Higher plasma levels were encountered in patients with an elevated BUN. The patients continued to excrete decreasing amounts of pentamidine in urine up to 6-8 weeks after cessation of the treatment.

Tissue distribution has been studied in mice given a single intraperitoneal injection of pentamidine at 10 mg/kg. The concentration in the kidneys was the highest followed by that in the liver. In mice, pentamidine was excreted unchanged, primarily via the kidneys with some elimination in the feces. The ratio of amounts excreted in the urine and feces (4:1) was constant over the period of study.

INDICATIONS AND USAGE

INHALATION SOLUTION

Pentamidine isethionate is indicated for the prevention of *Pneumocystis carinii* pneumonia (PCP) in high-risk, HIV-infected patients defined by one or both of the following criteria:

- A history of one or more episodes of PCP.
- A peripheral CD4+ (T4 helper/inducer) lymphocyte count less than or equal to 200/mm^3.

These indications are based on the results of an 18 month randomized, dose-response trial in high risk HIV-infected patients and on existing epidemiological data from natural history studies.

The patient population of the controlled trial consisted of 408 patients, 237 of whom had a history of one or more episodes of PCP. The remaining patients without a history of PCP included 55 patients with Kaposi's sarcoma and 116 patients with other AIDS diagnoses, ARC or asymptomatic HIV infection. Patients were randomly assigned to receive pentamidine isethionate via the Respirgard II nebulizer at 1 of the following 3 doses: 30 mg every 2 weeks (n=135), 150 mg every 2 weeks (n=134) or 300 mg every 4 weeks (n=139). The results of the trial demonstrated a significant protective effect ($p<0.01$) against PCP with the 300 mg every 4 week dosage regimen compared to the 30 mg every 2 week dosage regimen. The 300 mg dose regimen reduced the risk of developing PCP by 50-70% compared to the 30 mg regimen. A total of 293 patients (72% of all patients) also received zidovudine at sometime during the trial.

The analysis of the data demonstrated the efficacy of the 300 mg dose even after adjusting for the effect of zidovudine.

The results of the trial further demonstrate that the dose and frequency of dosing are important to the efficacy of pentamidine isethionate prophylaxis in that multiple analyses consistently demonstrated a trend toward greater efficacy with 300 mg every 4 weeks as compared to 150 mg every 2 weeks.

No dose-response was observed for reduction in overall mortality; however, mortality from PCP was low in all 3 dosage groups.

INJECTION

Pentam 300 (sterile pentamidine isethionate) is indicated for the treatment of pneumonia due to *Pneumocystis carinii*.

NON-FDA APPROVED INDICATIONS

Pentamidine is also used as a second-line agent in the treatment of leishmaniasis and some forms of African trypanosomiasis (rare diseases in the United States).

CONTRAINDICATIONS

INHALATION SOLUTION

Pentamidine isethionate is contraindicated in patients with a history of an anaphylactic reaction to inhaled or parenteral pentamidine isethionate.

INJECTION

Once the diagnosis of *Pneumocystis carinii* pneumonia has been firmly established, there are no absolute contraindications to the use of pentamidine isethionate.

WARNINGS

INHALATION SOLUTION

The potential for development of acute PCP still exists in patients receiving pentamidine isethionate prophylaxis. Therefore, any patient with symptoms suggestive of the presence of a pulmonary infection, including but not limited to dyspnea, fever or cough, should receive a thorough medical evaluation and appropriate diagnostic tests for possible acute PCP as well as for other opportunistic and non-opportunistic pathogens. The use of pentamidine isethionate may alter the clinical and radiographic features of PCP and could result in an atypical presentation, including but not limited to mild disease or focal infection.

Prior to initiating pentamidine isethionate prophylaxis, symptomatic patients should be evaluated appropriately to exclude the presence of PCP. The recommended dose of pentamidine isethionate for the prevention of PCP is insufficient to treat acute PCP.

INJECTION

Fatalities due to severe hypotension, hypoglycemia, acute pancreatitis and cardiac arrhythmias have been reported in patients treated with pentamidine isethionate, both by the IM and IV routes. Severe hypotension may result after a single dose (see PRECAUTIONS.) The administration of the drug should, therefore, be limited to the patients in whom*Pneumocystis carinii* has been demonstrated. Patients should be closely monitored for the development of serious adverse reactions (see PRECAUTIONS and ADVERSE REACTIONS).

PRECAUTIONS

INHALATION SOLUTION

IMPORTANT: DO NOT MIX THE NEBUPENT SOLUTION WITH ANY OTHER DRUGS. DO NOT USE THE RESPIRGARD II NEBULIZER TO ADMINISTER A BRONCHODILATOR. (See DOSAGE AND ADMINISTRATION.)

PULMONARY

Inhalation of pentamidine isethionate may induce bronchospasm or cough. This has been noted particularly in some patients who have a history of smoking or asthma. In clinical trials, cough and bronchospasm were the most frequently reported adverse experiences associated with pentamidine isethionate administration (38% and 15%, respectively of patients receiving the 300 mg dose); however less than 1% of the doses were interrupted or terminated due to these effects. For the majority of patients, cough and bronchospasm were controlled by administration of an aerosolized bronchodilator (only 1% of patients withdrew from the study due to treatment-associated cough or bronchospasm). In patients who experience bronchospasm or cough, administration of an inhaled bronchodilator prior to giving each pentamidine isethionate dose may minimize recurrence of the symptoms.

GENERAL

Inhalation Solution

The extent and consequence of pentamidine accumulation following chronic inhalation therapy are not known. As a result, patients receiving pentamidine isethionate should be closely monitored for the development of serious adverse reactions that have occurred in patients receiving parenteral pentamidine, including hypotension, hypoglycemia, hyperglycemia, hypocalcemia, anemia, thrombocytopenia, leukopenia, hepatic or renal dysfunction, ventricular tachycardia, pancreatitis and Stevens-Johnson syndrome.

Extrapulmonary infection with *P. carinii* has been reported infrequently. Most, but not all, of the cases have been reported in patients who have a history of PCP. The presence of extrapulmonary pneumocystosis should be considered when evaluating patients with unexplained signs and symptoms.

Cases of acute pancreatitis have been reported in patients receiving aerosolized pentamidine. Pentamidine isethionate should be discontinued if signs or symptoms of acute pancreatitis develop.

Injection

Pentamidine isethionate should be used with caution in patients with hypertension, hypotension, hypoglycemia, hyperglycemia, hypocalcemia, leukopenia, thrombocytopenia, anemia, and hepatic or renal dysfunction.

Patients may develop sudden, severe hypotension after a single dose of pentamidine isethionate, whether given IV or IM. Therefore, patients receiving the drug should be lying down and the blood pressure should be monitored closely during administration of the drug and several times thereafter until the blood pressure is stable. Equipment for emergency resuscitation should be readily available. If pentamidine isethionate is administered IV, it should be infused over a period of 60 minutes.

Pentamidine isethionate-induced hypoglycemia has been associated with pancreatic islet cell necrosis and inappropriately high plasma insulin concentrations. Hyperglycemia and diabetes mellitus, with or without preceding hypoglycemia, have also occurred, sometimes several months after therapy with pentamidine isethionate. Therefore, blood glucose levels should be monitored daily during therapy with pentamidine isethionate, and several times thereafter.

LABORATORY TESTS

The following tests should be carried out before, during and after therapy:

a) Daily blood urea nitrogen and serum creatinine determinations.
b) Daily blood glucose determinations.
c) Complete blood count and platelet count.
d) Liver function test, including bilirubin, alkaline phosphatase, AST (SGOT), and ALT (SGPT).
e) Serum calcium determinations.
f) Electrocardiograms at regular intervals.

CARCINOGENESIS, MUTAGENESIS, AND IMPAIRMENT OF FERTILITY

No studies have been conducted to evaluate the potential of pentamidine isethionate as a carcinogen, mutagen, or cause of impaired fertility.

PREGNANCY CATEGORY C

Animal reproduction studies have not been conducted with pentamidine isethionate. It is also not known whether pentamidine isethionate can cause fetal harm when administered to a pregnant woman or can affect reproduction capacity. Pentamidine isethionate should be given to a pregnant woman only if clearly needed. Pentamidine isethionate should not be given to a pregnant woman unless the potential benefits are judged to outweigh the unknown risk.

NURSING MOTHERS

Inhalation Solution

It is not known whether pentamidine isethionate is excreted in human milk. Because of the potential for serious adverse reactions in nursing infants from pentamidine isethionate, a decision should be made whether to discontinue nursing or to discontinue the drug, taking into account the importance of the drug to the mother. Because many drugs are excreted in human milk, pentamidine isethionate should not be given to a nursing mother unless the potential benefits are judged to outweigh the unknown risk.

PEDIATRIC USE

Inhalation Solution: The safety and effectiveness of pentamidine isethionate in children have not been established.

DRUG INTERACTIONS

INHALATION SOLUTION

While specific studies on drug interactions with pentamidine isethionate have not been conducted, the majority of patients in clinical trials received concomitant medications, including zidovudine, with no reported interactions.

ADVERSE REACTIONS

INHALATION SOLUTION

The most frequent adverse effects attributable to pentamidine isethionate administration are cough and bronchospasm (reported by 38% and 15%, respectively, of patients receiving 300 mg every 4 weeks).

The most frequently reported adverse experiences in the controlled clinical trials in which 607 patients were treated with pentamidine isethionate (139 patients at 300 mg every 4 weeks, 232 at 150 mg every 2 weeks, 101 at 100 mg every 2 weeks and 135 at 30 mg every 2 weeks) using the Respirgard II nebulizer were as follows:

53-72%: fatigue, bad (metallic) taste, shortness of breath and decreased appetite; 31-47%: dizziness and rash; 10-23%: nausea, pharyngitis, chest pain or congestion, night sweats, chills and vomiting.

In nearly all cases neither the relationship to treatment or underlying disease nor the severity of adverse experiences was recorded.

Other less frequently occurring adverse experiences (reported by greater than 1% and up to 5% of patients in two clinical trials) were pneumothorax, diarrhea, headache, anemia (generally associated with zidovudine use), myalgia, abdominal pain and edema.

From a total experience with 1130 patients adverse events reported with a frequency of 1% or less were as follows. No causal relationship to treatment has been established for these adverse events.

General: Allergic reaction and extrapulmonary pneumocystosis.

Cardiovascular: Tachycardia, hypotension, hypertension, palpitations, syncope, cerebrovascular accident, vasodilation and vasculitis.

Metabolic: Hypoglycemia, hyperglycemia, and hypocalcemia.

Gastrointestinal: Gingivitis, dyspepsia, oral ulcer/abscess, gastritis, gastric ulcer, hypersalivation, dry mouth, splenomegaly, melena, hematochezia, esophagitis, colitis, and pancreatitis.

Hematological: Pancytopenia, neutropenia, eosinophilia and thrombocytopenia.

Hepatorenal: Hepatitis, hepatomegaly, hepatic dysfunction, renal failure, flank pain and nephritis.

Musculoskeletal: Arthralgia.

Neurological: Tremors, confusion, anxiety, memory loss, seizure, neuropathy, paresthesia, insomnia, hypesthesia, drowsiness, emotional lability, vertigo, paranoia, neuralgia, hallucination, depression and unsteady gait.

Respiratory: Rhinitis, laryngitis, laryngospasm, hyperventilation, hemoptysis, gagging, eosinophilic or interstitial pneumonitis, pleuritis, cyanosis, tachypnea, and rales.

Skin: Pruritus, erythema, dry skin, desquamation and urticaria.

Special Senses: Eye discomfort, conjunctivitis, blurred vision, blepharitis and loss of taste and smell.

Urogenital: Incontinence.

Reproductive: Miscarriage.

INJECTION

CAUTION: Fatalities due to severe hypotension, hypoglycemia, acute pancreatitis and cardiac arrhythmias have been reported in patients treated with pentamidine isethionate, both by the IM and IV routes. The administration of the drug should, therefore, be limited to the patients in whom *Pneumocystis carinii* has been demonstrated.

Of 424 patients treated with pentamidine isethionate, 244 (57.5%) developed some adverse reaction. Most of the patients had the acquired immunodeficiency syndrome (AIDS). In the following (TABLE 1), "Severe" refers to life-threatening reactions or reactions that required immediate corrective measures and led to discontinuation of pentamidine isethionate.

DOSAGE AND ADMINISTRATION

INHALATION SOLUTION

IMPORTANT: PENTAMIDINE ISETHIONATE MUST BE DISSOLVED ONLY IN STERILE WATER FOR INJECTION. DO NOT USE SALINE SOLUTION FOR RECONSTITUTION BECAUSE THE DRUG WILL PRECIPITATE. DO NOT MIX THE PENTAMIDINE ISETHIONATE SOLUTION WITH ANY OTHER DRUGS. DO NOT USE THE RESPIRGARD II NEBULIZER TO ADMINISTER A BRONCHODILATOR.

TABLE 1

Adverse Reactions	Number	%
Severe		
Leukopenia (<1000/mm^3)	12	2.8
Hypoglycemia (<25 mg/dl)	10	2.4
Thrombocytopenia (<20,000/mm^3)	7	1.7
Hypotension (<60 mm Hg systolic)	4	0.9
Acute renal failure (serum creatinine >6 mg/dl)	2	0.5
Hypocalcemia	1	0.2
Stevens-Johnson syndrome	1	0.2
Ventricular tachycardia	1	0.2
Total number of patients with severe effects*	37	8.7
Moderate		
Elevated serum creatinine (2.4-6.0 mg/dl)	98	23.1
Sterile abscess, pain, or induration at the site of IM injection	47	11.1
Elevated liver function tests	37	8.7
Leukopenia	32	7.5
Nausea, anorexia	25	5.9
Hypotension	17	4.0
Fever	15	3.5
Hypoglycemia	15	3.5
Rash	14	3.3
Bad taste in mouth	7	1.7
Confusion/hallucinations	7	1.7
Anemia	5	1.2
Neuralgia	4	0.9
Thrombocytopenia	4	0.9
Hyperkalemia	3	0.7
Phlebitis	3	0.7
Dizziness (without hypotension)	2	0.5
Other moderate adverse reactions†	5	1.2
Total number of patients with moderate adverse reactions*	207	48.8

* Patients total may not equal sum of reactions, since some patients had more than one reaction.
† Each of the following moderate adverse reactions was reported in 1 patient: Hypocalcemia, abnormal ST segment of electrocardiogram, bronchospasm, diarrhea, and hyperglycemia.

RECONSTITUTION

The contents of 1 vial (300 mg) must be dissolved in 6 mL sterile water for injection. Place the entire reconstituted contents of the vial into the Respirgard II nebulizer reservoir for administration.

DOSAGE

The recommended adult dosage of pentamidine isethionate for the prevention of *Pneumocystis carinii* pneumonia is 300 mg once every 4 weeks administered via the Respirgard II nebulizer.

The dose should be delivered until the nebulizer chamber is empty (approximately 30-45 minutes). The flow rate should be 5-7 liters per minute from a 40-50 pounds per square inch (PSI) air or oxygen source. Alternatively, a 40-50 PSI air compressor can be used with flow limited by setting the flowmeter at 5-7 liters per minute or by setting the pressure at 22-25 PSI. Low pressure (less than 20 PSI) compressors should not be used.

STABILITY

Freshly prepared solutions for aerosol use are recommended. After reconstitution with sterile water, the pentamidine isethionate solution is stable for 48 hours in the original vial at room temperature if protected from light.

Store the dry product at controlled room temperature 15-30°C (59-86°F).

Protect the dry product and the reconstituted solution from light.

INJECTION

Pentamidine isethionate should be administered IM or IV only. The recommended regimen for adults and children is 4 mg/kg once a day for 14 days. The benefits and risks of therapy with pentamidine isethionate for more than 14 days are not well defined.

INTRAMUSCULAR INJECTION

The contents of 1 vial (300 mg) should be dissolved in 3 ml of sterile water for injection. The calculated daily dose should then be withdrawn and administered by deep IM injection.

INTRAVENOUS INJECTION

The contents of 1 vial should first be dissolved in 3-5 ml of sterile water for injection, or 5% dextrose injection. The calculated dose of pentamidine isethionate should then be withdrawn and diluted further in 50-250 ml of 5% dextrose injection. **The diluted IV solutions containing pentamidine isethionate should be infused over a period of 60 minutes.**

Aseptic technique should be employed in preparation of all solutions. Parenteral drug products should be inspected visually for particulate matter and discoloration prior to administration.

Stability: Intravenous infusion solutions of pentamidine isethionate at 1 mg and 2.5 mg/ml prepared in 5% dextrose injection are stable at room temperature for up to 24 hours.

PRODUCT LISTING - RATED THERAPEUTICALLY EQUIVALENT

Powder For Injection - Injectable - 300 mg

1's	$47.20	GENERIC, Abbott Pharmaceutical	00074-4548-01
1's	$94.50	GENERIC, Vha Supply	00074-4548-49

PRODUCT LISTING - EQUIVALENTS NOT AVAILABLE

Powder For Injection - Injectable - 300 mg

1's	$540.00	GENERIC, Pasadena Research Laboratories Inc	00418-3001-03
3's	$61.25	GENERIC, Taylor Pharmaceuticals	00418-0512-99
10's	$987.50	GENERIC, American Pharmaceutical Partners	63323-0113-10

Powder For Reconstitution - Inhalation - 300 mg

1's	$98.75	NEBUPENT, American Pharmaceutical Partners	63323-0877-15

Pentazocine Lactate (001977)

For related information, see the comparative table section in Appendix A.

Categories: Anesthesia, adjunct; Pain, moderate to severe; DEA Class CIV; Pregnancy Category C; FDA Approved 1967 Jul
Drug Classes: Analgesics, narcotic agonist-antagonist
Brand Names: **Talwin**
Foreign Brand Availability: Fortral (Australia; France; Germany; Netherlands; New-Zealand); Fortwin (Benin; Burkina-Faso; Ethiopia; Gambia; Ghana; Guinea; India; Ivory-Coast; Kenya; Liberia; Malawi; Mali; Mauritania; Mauritius; Morocco; Niger; Nigeria; Senegal; Seychelles; Sierra-Leone; Sudan; Tanzania; Thailand; Tunia; Uganda; Zambia; Zimbabwe); Liticon (Italy); Ospronim (South-Africa); Pentafen (Italy); Pentawin (India); Sosegon (Bahrain; Benin; Burkina-Faso; Cyprus; Ecuador; Egypt; Ethiopia; Gambia; Ghana; Guinea; Iran; Iraq; Ivory-Coast; Jordan; Kenya; Kuwait; Lebanon; Liberia; Libya; Malawi; Mali; Mauritania; Mauritius; Morocco; Niger; Nigeria; Oman; Portugal; Qatar; Republic-of-Yemen; Saudi-Arabia; Senegal; Seychelles; Sierra-Leone; Sudan; Syria; Tanzania; Tunia; Uganda; United-Arab-Emirates; Zambia; Zimbabwe); Susevin (India)

DESCRIPTION

Pentazocine lactate injection is a member of the benzozocine series (also known as the benzomorphan series). Chemically, pentazocine lactate is 1,2,3,4,5,6-hexahydro-6,11-dimethyl-3-(3-methyl-2-butenyl)-2,6-methano-3-benzazocin-8-ol lactate, a white, crystalline substance soluble in acidic aqueous solutions.

Multiple-Dose Vial: Each ml contains pentazocine lactate equivalent to 30 mg base and 2 mg acetone sodium bisulfite, 1.5 mg sodium chloride, and 1 mg methylparaben as perservative, in water for injection.

Carpuject Cartridge Unit: Each ml contains pentazocine lactate equivalent to 30 mg base, 1 mg acetone sodium bisulfite, and 2.2 mg sodium chloride, in water for injection.

Ampul: Each ml contains pentazocine lactate equivalent to 30 mg base and 2.8 mg sodium chloride, in water for injection.

The pH of Talwin solutions is adjusted between 4 and 5 with lactic acid or sodium hydroxide. The air in the ampuls, vials, and cartridge units has been displaced by nitrogen gas.

CLINICAL PHARMACOLOGY

Pentazocine lactate is a potent analgesic and 30 mg is usually as effective an analgesic as morphine 10 mg or meperidine 75-100 mg; however, a few studies suggest the pentazocine lactate to morphine ratio may range from 20-40 mg pentazocine lactate to 10 mg morphine. The duration of analgesia may sometimes be less than that of morphine. Analgesia usually occurs within 15-20 minutes after intramuscular or subcutaneous injection and within 2-3 minutes after intravenous injection. Pentazocine lactate weakly antagonizes the analgesic effects of morphine, meperidine, and phenazocine; in addition, it produces incomplete reversal of cardiovascular, respiratory, and behavioral depression induced by morphine and meperidine. Pentazocine lactate has about 1/50 the antagonistic activity of nalorphine. It also has sedative activity.

Clinical data indicate that differences in various pharmacokinetic parameters may be observed with increasing age. In one study, elderly patients exhibited a longer mean elimination half-life, a lower mean total plasma clearance, and a larger mean area under the concentration-time curve than younger patients.

INDICATIONS AND USAGE

For the relief of moderate to severe pain. Pentazocine lactate may also be used for preoperative or preanesthetic medication and as a supplement to surgical anesthesia.

CONTRAINDICATIONS

Pentazocine lactate should not be administered to patients who are hypersensitive to it.

WARNINGS

DRUG DEPENDENCE

Special care should be exercised in prescribing pentazocine for emotionally unstable patients and for those with a history of drug misuse. Such patients should be closely supervised when greater than 4 or 5 days of therapy is contemplated. There have been instances of psychological and physical dependence on pentazocine lactate in patients with such a history and, rarely, in patients without such a history. Extended use of parenteral pentazocine lactate may lead to physical or psychological dependence in some patients. When pentazocine lactate is abruptly discontinued, withdrawal symptoms such as abdominal cramps, elevated temperature, rhinorrhea, restlessness, anxiety, and lacrimation may occur. However, even when these have occurred, discontinuance has been accomplished with minimal difficulty. In the rare patient in whom more than minor difficulty has been encountered, reinstitution of parenteral pentazocine lactate with gradual withdrawal has ameliorated the patient's symptoms. Substituting methadone or other narcotics for pentazocine lactate in the treatment of the pentazocine abstinence syndrome should be avoided. There have been rare reports of possible abstinence syndromes in newborns after prolonged use of pentazocine lactate during pregnancy.

In prescribing parenteral pentazocine lactate for chronic use, particularly if the drug is to be self-administered, the physician should take precautions to avoid increases in dose and frequency of injection by the patient.

Just as with all medication, the oral form of pentazocine lactate is preferable for chronic administration.

TISSUE DAMAGE AT INJECTION SITES

Severe sclerosis of the skin, subcutaneous tissues, and underlying muscle have occurred at the injection sites of patients who have received multiple doses of pentazocine lactate. Constant rotation of injection sites is, therefore, essential. In addition, animal studies have demonstrated that pentazocine lactate is tolerated less well subcutaneously than intramuscularly. (See DOSAGE AND ADMINISTRATION.)

HEAD INJURY AND INCREASED INTRACRANIAL PRESSURE

As in the case of other potent analgesics, the potential of pentazocine lactate injection for elevating cerebrospinal fluid pressure may be attributed to CO_2 retention due to the respiratory depressant effects of the drug. These effects may be markedly exaggerated in the presence of head injury, other intracranial lesions, or a preexisting increase in intracranial pressure. Furthermore, pentazocine lactate can produce effects which may obscure the clinical course of patients with head injuries. In such patients, pentazocine lactate must be used with extreme caution and only if its use is deemed essential.

USE IN PREGNANCY

Safe use of pentazocine lactate during pregnancy (other than labor) has not been established. Animal reproduction studies have not demonstrated teratogenic or embryotoxic effects. However, pentazocine lactate should be administered to pregnant patients (other than labor) only when, in the judgment of the physician, the potential benefits outweigh the possible hazards. Patients receiving pentazocine lactate during labor have experienced no adverse effects other than those that occur with commonly used analgesics. Pentazocine lactate should be used with caution in women delivering premature infants.

ACUTE CNS MANIFESTATIONS

Patients receiving therapeutic doses of pentazocine have experienced hallucinations (usually visual), disorientation, and confusion which have cleared spontaneously within a period of hours. The mechanism of this reaction is not known. Such patients should be closely observed and vital signs checked. If the drug is reinstituted, it should be done with caution since these acute CNS manifestations may recur.

Due to the potential for increased CNS depressant effects, alcohol should be used with caution in patients who are currently receiving pentazocine.

PEDIATRIC USE

The safety and efficacy of pentazocine lactate as preoperative or preanesthetic medication have been established in pediatric patients 1-16 years of age. Use of pentazocine lactate in these age groups is supported by evidence from adequate and controlled studies in adults with additional data from published controlled trials in pediatric patients. The safety and efficacy of pentazocine lactate as a premedication for sedation have not been established in pediatric patients less than one year old. Information on the safety profile of pentazocine lactate as a postoperative analgesic in children less than 16 years is limited.

GERIATRIC USE

Elderly patients may be more sensitive to the analgesic effects of pentazocine lactate than younger patients. See DOSAGE AND ADMINISTRATION.

Clinical data indicate that differences in various pharmacokinetic parameters of pentazocine lactate may exist between elderly and younger patients. See CLINICAL PHARMACOLOGY.

Sedating drugs may cause confusion and oversedation in the elderly; elderly patients generally should be started on low doses of pentazocine lactate and observed closely.

This drug is known to be substantially excreted by the kidney, and the risk of toxic reactions to this drug may be greater in patients with impaired renal function. Because elderly patients are more likely to have decreased renal function, care should be taken in dose selection, and it may be useful to monitor renal function.

AMBULATORY PATIENTS

Since sedation, dizziness, and occasional euphoria have been noted, ambulatory patients should be warned not to operate machinery, drive cars, or unnecessarily expose themselves to hazards.

MYOCARDIAL INFARCTION

Caution should be exercised in the intravenous use of pentazocine for patients with acute myocardial infarction accompanied by hypertension or left ventricular failure. Data suggest that intravenous administration of pentazocine increases systemic and pulmonary arterial pressure and systemic vascular resistance in patients with acute myocardial infarction.

NOTE: Acetone sodium bisulfite, a sulfite that may cause allergic-type reactions including anaphylactic symptoms and life-threatening or less severe asthmatic episodes in certain susceptible people, is contained in both Carpuject Sterile Cartridge Units and multiple-dose vials. The overall prevalence of sulfite sensitivity in the general population in unknown and probably low. Sulfite sensitivity is seen more frequently in asthmatic than in nonasthmatic people.

The ampuls in the Uni-Amp Pak and the Uni-Nest Pak do not contain acetone sodium bisulfite.

PRECAUTIONS

CERTAIN RESPIRATORY CONDITIONS

The possibility that pentazocine lactate may cause respiratory depression should be considered in treatment of patients with bronchial asthma. Pentazocine lactate should be administered only with caution and in low dosage to patients with respiratory depression (*e.g.*, from other medication, uremia, or severe infection), severely limited respiratory reserve, obstructive respiratory conditions, or cyanosis.

IMPAIRED RENAL OR HEPATIC FUNCTION

Although laboratory tests have not indicated that pentazocine lactate causes or increases renal or hepatic impairment, the drug should be administered with caution to patients with such impairment. Extensive liver disease appears to predispose to greater side effects (*e.g.*, marked apprehension, anxiety, dizziness, sleepiness) from the usual clinical dose, and may be the result of decreased metabolism of the drug by the liver.

BILIARY SURGERY

Narcotic drug products are generally considered to elevate biliary tract pressure for varying periods following their administration. Some evidence suggests that pentazocine may differ from other marketed narcotics in this respect (*i.e.*, it causes little or no elevation in biliary tract pressures). The clinical significance of these findings, however, is not yet known.

PATIENTS RECEIVING NARCOTICS

Pentazocine lactate is a mild narcotic antagonist. Some patients previously given narcotics, including methadone for the daily treatment of narcotic dependence, have experienced withdrawal symptoms after receiving pentazocine lactate.

CNS EFFECT

Caution should be used when pentazocine lactate is administered to patients prone to seizures; seizures have occurred in a few such patients in association with the use of pentazocine lactate although no cause and effect relationship has been established.

USE IN ANESTHESIA

Concomitant use of CNS depressants with parenteral pentazocine lactate may produce additive CNS depression. Adequate equipment and facilities should be available to identify and treat systemic emergencies should they occur.

ADVERSE REACTIONS

The Most Commonly Occurring Reactions Are: Nausea, dizziness or lightheadedness, vomiting, euphoria.

DERMATOLOGIC REACTIONS

Soft tissue induration, nodules, and cutaneous depression can occur at injection sites. Ulceration (sloughing) and severe sclerosis of the skin and subcutaneous tissues (and, rarely underlying muscle) have been reported after multiple doses. Other reported dermatologic reactions include diaphoresis, sting on injection, flushed skin including plethora, dermatitis including pruritus.

Infrequently Occurring Reactions Are:

Respiratory: Respiratory depression, dyspnea, transient apnea in a small number of newborn infants whose mothers received pentazocine lactate during labor.

Cardiovascular: Circulatory depression, shock, hypertension.

CNS Effects: Dizziness, lightheadedness, hallucinations, sedation, euphoria, headache, confusion, disorientation; *infrequently* weakness, disturbed dreams, insomnia, syncope, visual blurring and focusing difficulty, depression; and *rarely* tremor, irritability, excitement, tinnitus.

Gastrointestinal: Constipation, dry mouth.

Other: Urinary retention, headache, paresthesia, alterations in rate or strength of uterine contractions during labor.

Rarely Reported Reactions Include:

Neuromuscular and Psychiatric: Muscle tremor, insomnia, disorientation, hallucinations.

Gastrointestinal: Taste alteration, diarrhea and cramps.

Ophthalmic: Blurred vision, nystagmus, diplopia, miosis.

Hematologic: Depression of white bloods cells (especially granulocytes), which is usually reversible, moderate transient eosinophilia.

Other: Tachycardia, weakness or faintness, chills; allergic reactions including edema of the face, toxic epidermal necrolysis.

See WARNINGS: Acute CNS Manifestations and Drug Dependence.

DOSAGE AND ADMINISTRATION

Caution: Pentazocine lactate should not be mixed in the same syringe with soluble barbiturates because precipitation will occur.

ADULTS, EXCLUDING PATIENTS IN LABOR

The recommended single parenteral dose is 30 mg by intramuscular, subcutaneous, or intravenous route. This may be repeated every 3-4 hours. Doses in excess of 30 mg intravenously or 60 mg intramuscularly or subcutaneously are not recommended. Total daily dosage should not exceed 360 mg. Elderly patients may be more sensitive to the analgesic effects of pentazocine lactate than younger patients. Elderly patients generally should be started on low doses of pentazocine lactate and observed closely.

The subcutaneous route of administration should be used only when necessary because of possible severe tissue damage at injection sites (see WARNINGS). When frequent injections are needed, the drug should be administered intramuscularly. In addition, constant rotation of injection sites (*e.g.*, the upper outer quadrants of the buttocks, mid-lateral aspects of the thighs, and the deltoid areas) is essential.

ADULTS, PATIENTS IN LABOR

A single, intramuscular 30 mg dose has been most commonly administered. An intravenous 20 mg dose has given adequate pain relief to some patients in labor when contractions become regular, and this dose may be given 2 or 3 times at 2-3 hour intervals, as needed.

PEDIATRIC PATIENTS EXCLUDING PATIENTS LESS THAN 1 YEAR OLD

The recommended single parenteral dose as premedication for sedation is 0.5 mg/kg by intramuscular route.

HOW SUPPLIED

Talwin injection is supplied in the following dosage forms and strengths:

Multiple-Dose Vial: 30 mg/ml in 10 ml volume.

Carpuject Cartridge Unit: 30 mg/ml in 1 and 2 ml volumes.

Ampul: 30 mg/ml in 1 ml volume.

Storage: Store at controlled room temperature 15-30°C (59-86°F).

PRODUCT LISTING - EQUIVALENTS NOT AVAILABLE

Solution - Injectable - 30 mg/ml

1 ml x 10	$24.94	TALWIN LACTATE, Abbott Pharmaceutical	00074-1937-01
1 ml x 25	$126.50	TALWIN LACTATE, Abbott Pharmaceutical	00074-1941-11
1 ml x 25	$137.45	TALWIN LACTATE, Abbott Pharmaceutical	00074-1941-01
2 ml x 10	$29.93	TALWIN LACTATE, Abbott Pharmaceutical	00074-1938-02
2 ml x 25	$147.55	TALWIN LACTATE, Sanofi Winthrop Pharmaceuticals	00024-1926-04
10 ml	$33.41	TALWIN LACTATE, Sanofi Winthrop Pharmaceuticals	00024-1916-01
10 ml	$33.41	TALWIN LACTATE, Allscripts Pharmaceutical Company	54569-1903-01
10 ml	$35.57	TALWIN LACTATE, Physicians Total Care	54868-2530-00
10 ml	$43.79	TALWIN LACTATE, Abbott Pharmaceutical	00074-1920-10

Pentobarbital Sodium *(001978)*

Categories: Preanesthesia; Insomnia; Sedation; Status epilepticus; Pregnancy Category D; DEA Class CII; DEA Class CIII; FDA Approved 1973 Sep
Drug Classes: Anticonvulsants; Barbiturates; Preanesthetics; Sedatives/hypnotics
Brand Names: Carbrital; Nembutal; Sodium Pentobarbital
Foreign Brand Availability: Embutal (Argentina); Medinox Mono (Germany); Mintal (Japan); Sombutol (Finland)
Cost of Therapy: $5.79 (Insomnia; Nembutal; 100 mg; 1 capsule/day; 10 day supply)
HCFA JCODE(S): J2515 per 50 mg IM, IV, OTH

DESCRIPTION

WARNING-MAY BE HABIT FORMING. The barbiturates are nonselective central nervous system depressants which are primarily used as sedative hypnotics. The barbiturates and their sodium salts are subject to control under the Federal Controlled Substances Act.

Barbiturates and substituted pyrimidine derivatives in which the basic structure common to these drugs is barbituric acid, a substance which has no central nervous system (CNS) activity. CNS activity is obtained by substituting alkenyl, or aryl groups on the pyrimidine ring. Pentobarbital sodium) is chemically represented by sodium 5-ethyl-5-(1-methylbutyl) barbiturate.

CAPSULES, SUPPOSITORIES, AND INJECTION

The sodium salt of pentobarbital occurs as a white, slightly bitter powder which is freely soluble in water and alcohol but practically insoluble in benzene and ether.

CAPSULES

Pentobarbital sodium capsules for oral administration contain either 50 or 100 mg of pentobarbital sodium.
Storage: Store below 30°C (86°F).

ELIXIR

Pentobarbital elixir for oral use contains 18.2 mg pentobarbital (equivalent to 20 mg pentobarbital sodium) per 5 ml.
Storage: Store below 30°C (86°F). Avoid freezing.
Dispense in a tight, light-resistant, glass container.

SUPPOSITORIES

Each rectal suppository contains either 30, 60, 120, or 200 mg of pentobarbital sodium.
Storage: Store in a refrigerator (36-46°F).

SOLUTION

Pentobarbital sodium injection is a sterile solution for intravenous or intramuscular injection. Each ml contains pentobarbital sodium 50 mg, in a vehicle of propylene glycol, 40%, alcohol, 10% and water for injection, to volume. The pH is adjusted to approximately 9.5 with hydrochloric acid and/or sodium hydroxide.
Storage: Exposure of pharmaceutical products to heat should be minimized. Avoid excessive heat. Protect from freezing. It is recommended that the product be stored at room temperature 30°C (86°F); however, brief exposure up to 40°C (104°F) does not adversely affect the product.

CLINICAL PHARMACOLOGY

Barbiturates are capable of producing all levels of CNS mood alteration from excitation to mild sedation, to hypnosis, and deep coma. Overdosage can produce death. In high enough therapeutic doses, barbiturates induce anesthesia.

Barbiturates depress the sensory cortex, decrease motor activity, alter cerebellar function, and produce drowsiness, sedation, and hypnosis.

Barbiturate-induced sleep differs from physiological sleep. Sleep laboratory studies have demonstrated that barbiturates reduce the amount of time spent in the rapid eye movement (REM) phase of sleep or dreaming stage. Also, Stages III and IV sleep are decreased. Following abrupt cessation of barbiturates used regularly, patients may experience markedly increased dreaming, nightmares, and/or insomnia. Therefore, withdrawal of a single therapeutic dose over 5 or 6 days has been recommended to lessen the REM rebound and disturbed sleep which contribute to drug withdrawal syndrome (for example, decrease the dose from 3 to 2 doses a day for 1 week).

In studies, secobarbital sodium and pentobarbital sodium have been found to lose most of their effectiveness for both inducing and maintaining sleep by the end of 2 weeks of continued drug administration at fixed doses. The short-, intermediate-, and, to a lesser degree, long-acting barbiturates have been widely prescribed for treating insomnia. Although the clinical literature abounds with claims that the short-acting barbiturates are superior for producing sleep while the intermediate-acting compounds are more effective in maintaining sleep, controlled studies have failed to demonstrate these differential effects. Therefore, as sleep medications, the barbiturates are of limited value beyond short-term use.

Barbiturates have little analgesic action at subanesthetic doses. Rather, in subanesthetic doses these drugs may increase the reaction to painful stimuli. All barbiturates exhibit anticonvulsant activity in anesthetic doses. However, of the drugs in this class, only phenobarbital, mephobarbital, and metharbital have been clinically demonstrated to be effective as oral anticonvulsants in subhypnotic doses.

Barbiturates are respiratory depressants. The degree of respiratory depression is dependent upon dose. With hypnotic doses, respiratory depression produced by barbiturates is similar to that which occurs during physiologic sleep with slight decrease in blood pressure and heart rate.

Studies in laboratory animals have shown that barbiturates cause reduction in the tone and contractility of the uterus, ureters, and urinary bladder. However, concentrations of the drugs required to produce this effect in humans are not reached with sedative-hypnotic doses.

Barbiturates do not impair normal hepatic function, but have been shown to induce liver microsomal enzymes, thus increasing and/or altering the metabolism of barbiturates and other drugs. (See DRUG INTERACTIONS.)

PHARMACOKINETICS

Barbiturates are absorbed in varying degrees following oral, rectal, or parenteral administration. The salts are more rapidly absorbed than are the acids. The rate of absorption is increased if the sodium salt is ingested as a dilute solution or taken on an empty stomach.

The onset of action for oral or rectal administration varies from 20-60 minutes. For IM administration, the onset of action is slightly faster. Following IV administration, the onset of action ranges from almost immediately for pentobarbital sodium to 5 minutes for phenobarbital sodium. Maximal CNS depression may not occur until 15 minutes or more after IV administration for phenobarbital sodium.

Duration of action, which is related to the rate at which the barbiturates are redistributed throughout the body, varies among persons and in the same person from time to time.

No studies have demonstrated that the different routes of administration are equivalent with respect to bioavailability.

Barbiturates are weak acids that are absorbed and rapidly distributed to all tissues and fluids with high concentrations in the brain, liver, and kidneys. Lipid solubility of the barbiturates is the dominant factor in their distribution within the body. The more lipid soluble the barbiturate, the more rapidly it penetrates all tissues of the body. Barbiturates are bound to plasma and tissue proteins to a varying degree of binding increasing directly as function of lipid solubility.

Phenobarbital has the lowest lipid solubility, lowest plasma binding, lowest brain protein binding, the longest delay in onset of activity, and the longest duration of action. At the opposite extreme is secobarbital which has the highest lipid solubility, plasma protein binding, brain protein binding, the shortest delay in onset of activity, and the shortest duration of action. Butabarbital is classified as an intermediate barbiturate.

The plasma half-life for pentobarbital in adults is 15-50 hours and appears to be dose dependent.

Barbiturates are metabolized primarily by the hepatic microsomal enzyme system, and the metabolic products are excreted in the urine, and less commonly, in the feces. Approximately 25-50% of a dose of aprobarbital or phenobarbital is eliminated unchanged in the urine, whereas the amount of other barbiturates excreted unchanged in the urine is negligible. The excretion of unmetabolized barbiturate is one feature that distinguishes the long-acting category from those belonging to other categories which are almost entirely metabolized. The inactive metabolites of the barbiturates are excreted as conjugates of glucuronic acid.

CAPSULES AND ELIXIR

In TABLE 1, the barbiturates are classified according to their duration of action. This classification should not be used to predict the exact duration of effect, but the grouping of drugs should be used as a guide in the selection of barbiturates.

TABLE 1 *Classification, Onset, and Duration of Action of Commonly used Barbiturates Taken Orally*

Classification	Onset of action	Duration of action
Long-acting Phenobarbital.	1 hour or longer	10-12 hours
Intermediate Amobarbital Butabarbital.	3/4-1 hour	6-8 hours
Short-acting Pentobarbital Secobarbital.	10-15 minutes	3-4 hours

INDICATIONS AND USAGE

CAPSULES, ELIXIR, AND INJECTION

Oral

a. Sedatives.
b. Hypnotics, for the short-term treatment of insomnia, since they appear to lose their effectiveness for sleep induction and sleep maintenance after 2 weeks. (See CLINICAL PHARMACOLOGY.)
c. Preanesthetics.

SUPPOSITORIES

Barbiturates administered rectally are absorbed from the colon and are used when oral or parenteral administration may be undesirable.

Rectal

a. Sedative.

b. Hypnotic, for the short-term treatment of insomnia, since they appear to lose their effectiveness for sleep induction and sleep maintenance after 2 weeks (see CLINICAL PHARMACOLOGY).

INJECTION

Parenteral

a. Sedatives.

b. Hypnotics, for the short-term treatment of insomnia, since they appear to lose their effectiveness for sleep induction and sleep maintenance after 2 weeks (see CLINICAL PHARMACOLOGY).

c. Preanesthetics.

d. Anticonvulsant, in anesthetic doses, in the emergency control of certain acute convulsive episodes, *e.g.,* those associated with status epilepticus, cholera, eclampsia, meningitis, tetanus, and toxic reactions to strychnine or local anesthetics.

NON-FDA APPROVED INDICATIONS

Pentobarbital has also been used to induce coma in the setting of intracranial hypertension and for the treatment of withdrawal from other barbiturates and hypnotics although these uses are not FDA approved.

CONTRAINDICATIONS

Barbiturates are contraindicated in patients with known barbiturate sensitivity. Barbiturates are also contraindicated in patients with a history of manifest or latent porphyria.

WARNINGS

1. ***Habit Forming:*** Barbiturates may be habit forming. Tolerance, psychological and physical dependence may occur with continued use. (See Pharmacokinetics). Patients who have psychological dependence on barbiturates may increase the dosage or decrease the dosage interval without consulting a physician and may subsequently develop a physical dependence on barbiturates. To minimize the possibility of overdosage or the development of dependence, the prescribing and dispensing of sedative-hypnotic barbiturates should be limited to the amount required for the interval until the next appointment. Abrupt cessation after prolonged use in the dependent person may result in withdrawal symptoms, including delirium, convulsions, and possibly death. Barbiturates should be withdrawn gradually from any patient known to be taking excessive dosage over long periods of time.
2. ***Acute or Chronic Pain:*** Caution should be exercised when barbiturates are administered to patients with acute or chronic pain, because paradoxical excitement could be induced or important symptoms could be masked. However, the use of barbiturates as sedatives in the postoperative surgical period and as adjuncts to cancer chemotherapy is well established.
3. ***Use in Pregnancy:*** Barbiturates can cause fetal damage when administered to a pregnant women. Retrospective, case-controlled studies have suggested a connection of barbiturates and a higher than expected incidence of fetal abnormalities. Following oral or parenteral administration, barbiturates readily cross the placental barrier and are distributed throughout fetal tissues with highest concentrations found in the placenta, fetal liver, and brain. It is presumed that this effect will also be seen following rectal administration.
4. ***Synergistic Effects:*** The concomitant use of alcohol or other CNS depressants may produce additive CNS depressant effects.

Withdrawal symptoms occur in infants born to mothers who receive barbiturates throughout the last trimester of pregnancy. If this drug is used during pregnancy, or if the patient becomes pregnant while taking this drug, the patient should be apprised of the potential hazard to the fetus.

P

INJECTION

IV Administration: Too rapid administration may cause respiratory depression, apnea, laryngospasm or vasodilation with fall in blood pressure.

Fetal blood levels approach maternal blood levels following parenteral administration.

PRECAUTIONS

GENERAL

Barbiturates may be habit forming. Tolerance and psychological and physical dependence may occur with continuing use. Barbiturates should be administered with caution, if at all, to patients who are mentally depressed, have suicidal tendencies, or a history of drug abuse.

Elderly or debilitated patients may react to barbiturates with marked excitement, depression, and confusion. In some persons, barbiturates repeatedly produce excitement rather than depression.

In patients with hepatic damage, barbiturates should be administered with caution and initially in reduced doses. Barbiturates should not be administered to patients showing the premonitory signs of hepatic coma.

The 100 mg dosage strength of pentobarbital sodium capsules contains FD&C yellow no. 5 (tartrazine) which may cause allergic-type reactions (including bronchial asthma) in certain susceptible individuals. Although the overall incidence of FD&C yellow no. 5 (tartrazine) sensitivity in the general population is low, it is frequently seen in patients who also have aspirin hypersensitivity.

Parenteral solutions of barbiturates are highly alkaline. Therefore, extreme care should be taken to avoid perivascular extravasation or intra-arterial injection. Extravascular injection may cause local tissue damage with subsequent necrosis; consequences of intra-arterial injection may vary from transient pain to gangrene of the limb. Any complaint of pain in the limb warrants stopping the injection.

Capsules

The 100 mg dosage strength of pentobarbital sodium capsules contains FD&C yellow no. 5 (tartrazine) which may cause allergic-type reactions (including bronchial asthma) in certain susceptible individuals. Although the overall incidence of FD&C yellow no. 5 (tartrazine) sensitivity in the general population is low, it is frequently seen in patients who also have aspirin hypersensitivity.

INFORMATION FOR THE PATIENT

Practitioners should give the following information and instructions to patients receiving barbiturates.

1. The use of barbiturates carries with it an associated risk of psychological and/or physical dependence. The patients should be warned against increasing the dose of the drug without consulting a physician.
2. Barbiturates may impair mental and/or physical abilities required for the performance of potentially hazardous tasks (*e.g.,* driving, operating machinery, etc.).
3. Alcohol should not be consumed while taking barbiturates with other CNS depressants (*e.g.,* alcohol, narcotics, tranquilizers, and antihistamines) may result in additional CNS depressant effects.

LABORATORY TESTS

Prolonged therapy with barbiturates should be accompanied by periodic laboratory evaluation of organ systems, including hematopoietic, renal, and hepatic systems. (See PRECAUTIONS, General and ADVERSE REACTIONS.)

CARCINOGENESIS

1. ***Animal Data:*** Phenobarbital sodium is carcinogenic in mice and rats after lifetime administration. In mice, it produced benign and malignant liver cell tumors. In rats, benign liver cell tumors were observed very late in life.
2. ***Human Data:*** In a 29 year epidemiological study of 9136 patients who were treated on an anticonvulsant protocol that included phenobarbital, results indicated a higher than normal incidence of hepatic carcinoma. Previously some of these patients were treated with thorotrast, a drug that is known to produce hepatic carcinomas. Thus, this study did not provide sufficient evidence that phenobarbital sodium is carcinogenic in humans.

Data from one retrospective study of 235 children in which the types of barbiturates are not identified suggested an association between exposure to barbiturates prenatally and an increased incidence of brain tumor. (Gold, E., *et al.,* "Increased Risk of Brain Tumors in Children Exposed to Barbiturates," Journal of National Cancer Institute, 61: 1031-1034, 1978).

PREGNANCY

1. ***Pregnancy, Teratogenic Effects, Pregnancy Category D:*** See WARNINGS, Use in Pregnancy.
2. ***Nonteratogenic Effects:*** Reports of infants suffering from long-term barbiturate exposure in utero included the acute withdrawal syndrome of seizures and hyperirritability from birth to a delayed onset of up to 14 days.

LABOR AND DELIVERY

Hypnotic doses of these barbiturates do not appear to significantly impair uterine a activity during labor. Full anesthetic doses of barbiturates decrease the force and frequency of uterine contractions. Administration of sedative-hypnotic barbiturates to the mother during labor may result in respiratory depression in the newborn. Premature infants are particularly susceptible to the depressant effects of barbiturates. If barbiturates are used during labor and delivery, resuscitation equipment should be available.

Data are currently not available to evaluate the effect of these barbiturates when forceps delivery or other intervention is necessary. Also, data are not available to determine the effect of these barbiturates on the later growth, development, and functional maturation of the child.

NURSING MOTHERS

Caution should be exercised when a barbiturate is administered to a nursing woman since small amounts of barbiturates are excreted in the milk.

DRUG INTERACTIONS

Most reports of clinically significant drug interactions occurring with the barbiturates have involved phenobarbital. However, the application of these data to other barbiturates appears valid and warrants serial blood level determinations of the relevant drugs when there are multiple therapies.

1. ***Anticoagulants:*** Phenobarbital lowers the plasma levels of dicumarol (name previously used: bishydroxycoumarin) and causes a decrease in anticoagulant activity as measured by the prothrombin time. Barbiturates can induce hepatic microsomal enzymes resulting in increased metabolism and decreased anticoagulant response of oral anticoagulants (*e.g.,* warfarin, acenocoumarol, dicumarol and phenprocoumon). Patients stabilized on anticoagulant therapy may require dosage adjustments if barbiturates are added to or withdrawn from their dosage regimen.
2. ***Corticosteroids:*** Barbiturates appear to enhance the metabolism of exogenous corticosteroids probably through the induction of hepatic microsomal enzymes. Patients stabilized on corticosteroid therapy may require dosage adjustments if barbiturates are added to or withdrawn from their dosage regimen.
3. ***Griseofulvin:*** Phenobarbital appears to interfere with the absorption of orally administered griseofulvin, thus decreasing its blood level. The effect of the resultant decreased blood levels of griseofulvin on therapeutic response has not been established. However, it would be preferable to avoid concomitant administration of these drugs.
4. ***Doxycycline:*** Phenobarbital has been shown to shorten the half-life of doxycycline for as long as 2 weeks after barbiturate therapy is discontinued.

This mechanism is probably through the induction of hepatic microsomal enzymes that metabolize the antibiotic. If phenobarbital and doxycycline are administered concurrently, the clinical response to doxycycline should be monitored closely.

5. ***Phenytoin, Sodium Valproate, Valproic Acid:*** The effect of barbiturates on the metabolism of phenytoin appears to be variable. Some investigators report an accelerating effect, while others report no effect. Because the effect of barbiturates on the metabolism of phenytoin is not predictable, phenytoin and barbiturate blood levels should be monitored more frequently if these drugs are given concurrently. Sodium valproate and valproic acid appear to decrease barbiturate metabolism; therefore, barbiturate blood levels should be monitored and appropriate dosage adjustments made as indicated.
6. ***Central Nervous System Depressants:*** The concomitant use of other central nervous system depressants, including other sedatives or hypnotics, antihistamines, tranquilizers, or alcohol, may produce additive depressant effects.
7. ***Monoamine Oxidase Inhibitors (MAOI):*** MAOI prolong the effects of barbiturates probably because metabolism of the barbiturate is inhibited.
8. ***Estradiol, Estrone, Progesterone and Other Steroidal Hormones:*** Pretreatment with or concurrent administration of phenobarbital may decrease the effect of estradiol by increasing its metabolism. There have been reports of patients treated with antiepileptic drugs (*e.g.*, phenobarbital) who became pregnant while taking oral contraceptives. An alternate contraceptive method might be suggested to women taking phenobarbital.

ADVERSE REACTIONS

The following adverse reactions and their incidence were compiled from surveillance of thousands of hospitalized patients. Because such patients may be less aware of certain of the milder adverse effects of barbiturates, the incidence of these reactions may be somewhat higher in fully ambulatory patients.

More Than 1 in 100 Patients: The most common adverse reaction estimated to occur at a rate of 1-3 patients per 100 is: *Nervous System:* Somnolence.

Less Than 1 in 100 Patients: Adverse reactions estimated to occur at a rate of less than 1 in 100 patients listed below, grouped by organ system, and by decreasing order of occurrence are:

Nervous System: Agitation, confusion, hyperkinesia, ataxia, CNS depression, nightmares, nervousness, psychiatric disturbance, hallucinations, insomnia, anxiety, dizziness, thinking abnormality.

Respiratory System: Hypoventilation, apnea.

Cardiovascular System: Bradycardia, hypotension, syncope.

Digestive System: Nausea, vomiting, constipation.

Other Reported Reactions: Headache, injection site reactions, hypersensitivity reactions (angioedema, skin rashes, exfoliative dermatitis), fever, liver damage, megaloblastic anemia following chronic phenobarbital use.

DOSAGE AND ADMINISTRATION

CAPSULES

Adults

The usual hypnotic dose consists of 100 mg at bedtime.

Children

The preoperative dose is 2-6 mg/kg/24 hours (maximum 100 mg), depending on age, weight, and the desired degree of sedation.

The proper hypnotic dose for children must be judged on the basis of individual age and weight.

Dosages of barbiturates must be individualized with full knowledge of their particular characteristics and recommended rate of administration. Factors of consideration are the patient's age, weight, and condition.

Special Patient Population

Dosage should be reduced in the elderly or debilitated because these patients may be more sensitive to barbiturates. Dosage should be reduced for patients with impaired renal function or hepatic disease.

ELIXIR

Adults

Daytime sedation can ordinarily be provided by one 5 ml teaspoonful of the elixir taken 3 or 4 times per day.

The usual hypnotic dose consists of the equivalent to 100 mg pentobarbital sodium provided by 5 teaspoonfuls pentobarbital elixir.

Children

Daytime sedation can be provided by 2-6 mg/kg/24 hours, depending on age, weight, and the desired degree of sedation.

The proper hypnotic dose for children must be judged on the basis of individual age and weight.

Dosages of barbiturates must be individualized with full knowledge of their particular characteristics and recommended rate of administration. Factors of consideration are the patient's age, weight and condition.

Special Patient Population

Dosage should be reduced in the elderly or debilitated because these patients may be more sensitive to barbiturates. Dosage should be reduced for patients with impaired renal function or hepatic disease.

SUPPOSITORIES

Typical hypnotic doses for adults and children are given below. These are intended only as a guide, and administration should be adjusted to the individual needs of each patient. For sedation, in children 5-14 years and in adults, reduce dose appropriately.

Adults (average to above average weight): One 120 mg or one 200 mg suppository.

Children: *12-14 years (80-110 lbs.):* One 60 mg or one 120 mg suppository; *5-12 years (40-80 lbs.):* One 60 mg suppository; *1-4 years (20-40 lbs.):* One 30 mg or one 60 mg suppository; *2 months-1 year (10-20 lbs.):* One 30 mg suppository.

Suppositories should not be divided.

Dosages of barbiturates must be individualized with full knowledge of their particular characteristics and recommended rate of administration. Factors of consideration are the patient's age, weight, and condition.

Special Patient Population: Dosage should be reduced in the elderly or debilitated because these patients more sensitive to barbiturates. Dosage should be reduced for patients with impaired renal function or hepatic disease.

INJECTION

Dosages of barbiturates must be individualized with full knowledge of their particular characteristics and recommended rate of administration. Factors of consideration are the patient's age, weight, and condition. Parenteral routes should be used only when oral administration is impossible or impractical.

Intramuscular Administration

IM injection of the sodium salts of barbiturates should be made deeply into a large muscle, and a volume of 5 ml should not be exceeded at any one site because of possible tissue irritation. After IM injection of a hypnotic dose, the patient's vital signs should be monitored. The usual adult dosage of pentobarbital sodium solution is 150-200 mg as a single IM injection; the recommended pediatric dosage ranges from 2-6 mg/kg as a single IM injection not to exceed 100 mg.

Intravenous Administration

Pentobarbital sodium solution should not be admixed with any other medication or solution. IV injection is restricted to conditions in which other routes are not feasible, either because the patient is unconscious (as in cerebral hemorrhage, eclampsia, or status epilepticus), or because the patient resists (as in delirium), or because prompt action is imperative. Slow IV injection is essential, and patients should be carefully observed during administration. This requires that blood pressure, respiration, and cardiac function be maintained, vital signs be recorded, and equipment for resuscitation and artificial ventilation be available. The rate of IV injection should not exceed 50 mg/min for pentobarbital sodium.

There is no average intravenous dose of pentobarbital sodium solution that can be relied on to produce similar effects in different patients. The possibility of overdose and respiratory depression is remote when the drug is injected slowly in fractional doses.

A commonly used initial dose for the 70 kg adult is 100 mg. Proportional reduction in dosage should be made for pediatric or debilitated patients. At least one minute is necessary to determine the full effect of intravenous pentobarbital. If necessary, additional small increments of the drug may be given up to a total of from 200-500 mg for normal adults.

Anticonvulsant Use

In convulsive states, dosage of pentobarbital sodium solution should be kept to a minimum to avoid compounding the depression which may follow convulsions. The injection must be made slowly with due regard to the time required for the drug to penetrate the blood-brain barrier.

Special Patient Population: Dosage should be reduced in the elderly or debilitated because these patients may be more sensitive to barbiturates. Dosage should be reduced for patients with impaired renal function or hepatic disease.

Inspection: Parenteral drug products should be inspected visually for particulate matter and discoloration prior to administration, whenever solution containers permit. Solutions for injection showing evidence of precipitation should not be used.

PRODUCT LISTING - RATED THERAPEUTICALLY EQUIVALENT

Capsule - Oral - 50 mg

100's	$42.82	NEMBUTAL SODIUM, Abbott Pharmaceutical	00074-3150-11

Capsule - Oral - 100 mg

100's	$67.08	NEMBUTAL SODIUM, Abbott Pharmaceutical	00074-3114-01

Solution - Injectable - 50 mg/ml

2 ml x 25	$66.16	NEMBUTAL SODIUM, Abbott Pharmaceutical	00074-6899-04
20 ml	$37.30	NEMBUTAL SODIUM, Abbott Pharmaceutical	00074-3778-04
50 ml	$69.59	NEMBUTAL SODIUM, Abbott Pharmaceutical	00074-3778-05

Pentostatin *(003065)*

Categories: Leukemia, hairy cell; Pregnancy Category D; FDA Approved 1991 Oct; Orphan Drugs
Drug Classes: Antineoplastics, antimetabolites
Brand Names: **Nipent**
Foreign Brand Availability: Coforin (Japan)
HCFA JCODE(S): J9268 per 10 mg IV

WARNING

Pentostatin for Injection should be administered under the supervision of a physician qualified and experienced in the use of cancer chemotherapeutic agents. The use of higher doses than those specified (see DOSAGE AND ADMINISTRATION) is not recommended. Dose-limiting severe renal, liver, pulmonary, and CNS toxicities occurred in Phase 1 studies that used pentostatin at higher doses (20-50 mg/m² in divided doses over 5 days) than recommended.

In a clinical investigation in patients with refractory chronic lymphocytic leukemia using pentostatin at the recommended dose in combination with fludarabine phosphate, 4 of 6 patients entered in the study had severe or fatal pulmonary toxicity. The use of pentostatin in combination with fludarabine phosphate is not recommended.

DESCRIPTION

Nipent (pentostatin for injection) is supplied as a sterile, apyrogenic, lyophilized powder in single-dose vials for intravenous administration. Each vial contains 10 mg of pentostatin and 50 mg of mannitol. The pH of the final product is maintained between 7.0 and 8.5 by addition of sodium hydroxide or hydrochloric acid.

Pentostatin, also known as 2′-deoxycoformycin (DCF), is a potent inhibitor of the enzyme adenosine deaminase and is isolated from fermentation cultures of *Streptomyces antibioticus*. Pentostatin is known chemically as (R)-3-(2-deoxy-β-D-*erythro*-pentofuranosyl)-3,6,7,8-tetrahydroimidazo(4,5-d)(1,3)diazepin-8-ol with a molecular formula of $C_{11}H_{16}N_4O_4$ and a molecular weight of 268.27.

Pentostatin is a white to off-white solid, freely soluble in distilled water.

CLINICAL PHARMACOLOGY

MECHANISM OF ACTION

Pentostatin is a potent transition state inhibitor of the enzyme adenosine deaminase (ADA). The greatest activity of ADA is found in cells of the lymphoid system with T-cells having higher activity than B-cells and T-cell malignancies higher ADA activity than B-cell malignancies. Pentostatin inhibition of ADA, particularly in the presence of adenosine or deoxyadenosine, leads to cytotoxicity, and this is believed to be due to elevated intracellular levels of dATP which can block DNA synthesis through inhibition of ribonucleotide reductase. Pentostatin can also inhibit RNA synthesis as well as cause increased DNA damage. In addition to elevated dATP, these mechanisms may contribute to the overall cytotoxic effect of pentostatin. The precise mechanism of pentostatin's antitumor effect, however, in hairy cell leukemia is not known.

PHARMACOKINETICS/DRUG METABOLISM

A tissue distribution and whole-body autoradiography study in the rat revealed that radioactivity concentrations were highest in the kidneys with very little central nervous system penetration.

In man, following a single dose of 4 mg/m² of pentostatin infused over 5 minutes, the distribution half-life was 11 minutes, the mean terminal half-life was 5.7 hours, the mean plasma clearance was 68 ml/min/m², and approximately 90% of the dose was excreted in the urine as unchanged pentostatin and/or metabolites as measured by adenosine deaminase inhibitory activity. The plasma protein binding of pentostatin is low, approximately 4%.

A positive correlation was observed between pentostatin clearance and creatinine clearance (CRCL) in patients with creatinine clearance values ranging from 60-130 ml/min.[1] Pentostatin half-life in patients with renal impairment (CRCL <50 ml/min, n=2) was 18 hours, which was much longer than that observed in patients with normal renal function (CRCL >60 ml/min, n=14), about 6 hours.

INDICATIONS AND USAGE

Pentostatin is indicated as single agent treatment for adult patients with alpha-interferon-refractory hairy cell leukemia (HCL). Alpha-interferon-refractory disease is defined as progressive disease after a minimum of 3 months of alpha-interferon treatment or no response after a minimum of 6 months of alpha-interferon treatment.

NON-FDA APPROVED INDICATIONS

The drug has also shown activity against chronic lymphocytic leukemia (refractory to conventional chemotherapy) and previously treated prolymphocytic leukemia. Modest activity has also been shown in the treatment of adult T-cell leukemia/lymphoma, acute lymphoblastic leukemia and non-Hodgkin's lymphoma. Use of pentostatin for the treatment of these conditions has not been approved by the FDA.

CONTRAINDICATIONS

Pentostatin is contraindicated in patients who have demonstrated hypersensitivity to pentostatin.

WARNINGS

See BOXED WARNING.

Patients with hairy cell leukemia may experience myelosuppression primarily during the first few courses of treatment. Patients with infections prior to pentostatin treatment have in some cases developed worsening of their condition leading to death, whereas others have achieved complete response. Patients with infection should be treated only when the potential benefit of treatment justifies the potential risk to the patient. Efforts should be made to control the infection before treatment is initiated or resumed.

In patients with progressive hairy cell leukemia, the initial courses of pentostatin treatment were associated with worsening of neutropenia. Therefore, frequent monitoring of complete blood counts during this time is necessary. If severe neutropenia continues beyond the initial cycles, patients should be evaluated for disease status, including a bone marrow examination.

Elevations in liver function tests occurred during treatment with pentostatin and were generally reversible.

Renal toxicity was observed at higher doses in early studies; however, in patients treated at the recommended dose, elevations in serum creatinine were usually minor and reversible. There were some patients who began treatment with normal renal function who had evidence of mild to moderate toxicity at a final assessment. (See DOSAGE AND ADMINISTRATION.)

Rashes, occasionally severe, were commonly reported and may worsen with continued treatment. Withholding of treatment may be required. (See DOSAGE AND ADMINISTRATION.)

PREGNANCY CATEGORY D

Pentostatin can cause fetal harm when administered to a pregnant woman. Pentostatin was administered intravenously at doses of 0, 0.01, 0.1, or 0.75 mg/kg/day (0, 0.06, 0.6, and 4.5 mg/m²) to pregnant rats on days 6 through 15 of gestation. Drug-related maternal toxicity occurred at doses of 0.1 and 0.75 mg/kg/day (0.6 and 4.5 mg/m²). Teratogenic effects were observed at 0.75 mg/kg/day (4.5 mg/m²) manifested by increased incidence of various skeletal malformations. In a dose range-finding study, pentostatin was administered intravenously to rats at doses of 0, 0.05, 0.1, 0.5, 0.75, or 1 mg/kg/day (0, 0.3, 0.6, 3, 4.5, 6 mg/m²) on days 6 through 15 of gestation. Fetal malformations that were observed were an omphalocele at 0.05 mg/kg (0.3 mg/m²), gastroschisis at 0.75 mg/kg and 1 mg/kg (4.5 and 6 mg/m²), and a flexure defect of the hindlimbs at 0.75 mg/kg (4.5 mg/m²). Pentostatin was also shown to be teratogenic in mice when administered as a single 2 mg/kg (6 mg/m²) intraperitoneal injection on day 7 of gestation. Pentostatin was not teratogenic in rabbits when administered intravenously on days 6 through 18 of gestation at doses of 0, 0.005, 0.01, or 0.02 mg/kg/day (0, 0.015, 0.03, or 0.06 mg/m²); however maternal toxicity, abortions, early deliveries, and deaths occurred in all drug-treated groups. There are no adequate and well-controlled studies in pregnant women. If pentostatin is used during pregnancy, or if the patient becomes pregnant while taking (receiving) this drug, the patient should be apprised of the potential hazard to the fetus. Women of childbearing potential receiving pentostatin should be advised to avoid becoming pregnant.

PRECAUTIONS

GENERAL

Therapy with pentostatin requires regular patient observation and monitoring of hematologic parameters and blood chemistry values. If severe adverse reactions occur, the drug should be withheld (see DOSAGE AND ADMINISTRATION), and appropriate corrective measures should be taken according to the clinical judgment of the physician.

Pentostatin treatment should be withheld or discontinued in patients showing evidence of nervous system toxicity.

INFORMATION FOR THE PATIENT

Patients should be advised of the signs and symptoms of adverse events associated with pentostatin therapy. (See ADVERSE REACTIONS.)

LABORATORY TESTS

Prior to initiating therapy with pentostatin, renal function should be assessed with a serum creatinine and/or a creatinine clearance assay. (See CLINICAL PHARMACOLOGY and DOSAGE AND ADMINISTRATION.) Complete blood counts and serum creatinine should be performed before each dose of pentostatin and at other appropriate periods during therapy (see DOSAGE AND ADMINISTRATION.) Severe neutropenia has been observed following the early courses of treatment with pentostatin and therefore frequent monitoring of complete blood counts is recommended during this time. If hematologic parameters do not improve with subsequent courses, patients should be evaluated for disease status, including a bone marrow examination. Periodic monitoring of the peripheral blood for hairy cells should be performed to assess the response to treatment.

In addition, bone marrow aspirates and biopsies may be required at 2-3 month intervals to assess the response to treatment.

CARCINOGENESIS, MUTAGENESIS, AND IMPAIRMENT OF FERTILITY

Carcinogenesis

No animal carcinogenicity studies have been conducted with pentostatin.

Mutagenesis

Pentostatin was nonmutagenic when tested in *Salmonella typhimurium* strains TA-98, TA-1535, TA-1537, and TA-1538. When tested with strain TA-100, a repeatable statistically significant response trend was observed with and without metabolic activation. The response was 2.1- to 2.2-fold higher than the background at 10 mg/plate, the maximum possible drug concentration. Formulated pentostatin was clastogenic in the in vivo mouse bone marrow micronucleus assay at 20, 120, and 240 mg/kg. Pentostatin was not mutagenic to V79 Chinese hamster lung cells at the HGPRT locus exposed 3 hours to concentrations of 1 to 3 mg/ml, with or without metabolic activation. Pentostatin did not significantly increase chromosomal aberrations in V79 Chinese hamster lung cells exposed 3 hours to 1-3 mg/ml in the presence or absence of metabolic activation.

Impairment of Fertility

No fertility studies have been conducted in animals; however, in a 5 day intravenous toxicity study in dogs, mild seminiferous tubular degeneration was observed with doses of 1 and 4 mg/kg. The possible adverse effects on fertility in humans have not been determined.

PREGNANCY CATEGORY D:

See WARNINGS.

NURSING MOTHERS

It is not known whether pentostatin is excreted in human milk. Because many drugs are excreted in human milk, and because of the potential for serious adverse reactions in nursing infants from pentostatin, a decision should be made whether to discontinue nursing or discontinue the drug, taking into account the importance of pentostatin to the mother.

PEDIATRIC USE

Safety and effectiveness in children or adolescents have not been established.

DRUG INTERACTIONS

Allopurinol and pentostatin are both associated with skin rashes. Based on clinical studies in 25 refractory patients who received both pentostatin and allopurinol, the combined use of pentostatin and allopurinol did not appear to produce a higher incidence of skin rashes than observed with pentostatin alone. There has been a report of one patient who received both drugs and experienced a hypersensitivity vasculitis that resulted in death. It was unclear whether this adverse event and subsequent death resulted from the drug combination.

Biochemical studies have demonstrated that pentostatin enhances the effects of vidarabine, a purine nucleoside with antiviral activity. The combined use of vidarabine and pentostatin may result in an increase in adverse reactions associated with each drug. The therapeutic benefit of the drug combination has not been established.

The combined use of pentostatin and fludarabine phosphate is not recommended because it may be associated with an increased risk of fatal pulmonary toxicity (see WARNINGS.)

ADVERSE REACTIONS

The following adverse events were reported during clinical studies with pentostatin in patients with hairy cell leukemia who were refractory to alpha-interferon therapy. Most patients experienced an adverse event. The drug association of these adverse events in particular cases is uncertain as they may be associated with the disease itself (*e.g.*, fever, infection, anemia), but other events, such as the gastrointestinal symptoms, hematologic suppression, rashes, and abnormal liver function tests, can in many cases be attributed to the drug. Most adverse events that were assessed for severity were either mild (52% of reports) or moderate (26% of reports) and diminished in frequency with continued therapy. Eleven percent of patients withdrew from treatment due to an adverse event.

TABLE 1 lists adverse events that occurred in at least 21 (11%) of 197 alpha-interferon-refractory patients with hairy cell leukemia.

TABLE 1

Adverse Event*	(n=197)
Leukopenia	118 (60%)
Nausea and Vomiting	104 (53%)
Fever	83 (42%)
Infection	70 (36%)
Anemia	68 (35%)
Thrombocytopenia	64 (32%)
Fatigue	57 (29%)
Rash	52 (26%)
Nausea	43 (22%)
Pain	40 (20%)
Hepatic Disorder/Elevated Liver Function Tests	38 (19%)
Skin Disorder	34 (17%)
Increased Cough	33 (17%)
Upper Respiratory Infection	31 (16%)
Anorexia	32 (16%)
Genitourinary Disorder	30 (15%)
Diarrhea	29 (15%)
Headache	25 (13%)
Lung Disorder	24 (12%)
Allergic Reaction	22 (11%)
Chills	22 (11%)
Myalgia	22 (11%)
Neurologic Disorder, CNS	21 (11%)

* Occurring in at least 11% of patients

Adverse events that occurred in 3% to 10% of alpha-interferon-refractory patients are as follows. The drug relatedness of many of these adverse events is uncertain.

Body as a Whole: Death, sepsis, chest pain, abdominal pain, back pain, flu syndrome, asthenia, malaise, and neoplasm

Cardiovascular System: Arrhythmia, abnormal electrocardiogram, thrombophlebitis, and hemorrhage

Digestive System: Constipation, flatulence, and stomatitis

Hemic and Lymphatic System: Ecchymosis, lymphadenopathy, and petechia

Metabolic and Nutritional System: Weight loss, peripheral edema, increased lactate dehydrogenase (LDH)

Musculoskeletal System: Arthralgia

Nervous System: Anxiety, confusion, depression, dizziness, insomnia, nervousness, paresthesia, somnolence, and abnormal thinking

Respiratory System: Bronchitis, dyspnea, epistaxis, lung edema, pneumonia, pharyngitis, rhinitis, and sinusitis

Skin and Appendages: Eczema, dry skin, herpes simplex, herpes zoster, maculopapular rash, pruritus, seborrhea, skin discoloration, sweating, and vesiculobullous rash

Special Senses: Abnormal vision, conjunctivitis, ear pain, and eye pain

Urogenital System: Hematuria and dysuria, increased BUN, and increased creatinine

The remaining adverse events occurred in less than 3% of patients; their relationship to pentostatin is uncertain: *Body as a Whole:* abscess, enlarged abdomen, ascites, cellulitis, cyst, face edema, fibrosis, granuloma, hernia, injection-site hemorrhage, injection-site inflammation, moniliasis, neck rigidity, pelvic pain, photosensitivity reaction, anaphylactoid reaction, immune system disorder, mucous membrane disorder, neck pain; *Cardiovascular System:* aortic stenosis, arterial anomaly, cardiomegaly, congestive heart failure, flushing, cardiac arrest, hypertension, myocardial infarct, palpitation, shock, and varicose vein; *Digestive System:* colitis, dysphagia, eructation, gastritis, gastrointestinal hemorrhage, gum hemorrhage, hepatitis, hepatomegaly, intestinal obstruction, jaundice, leukoplakia, melena, periodontal abscess, proctitis, abnormal stools, dyspepsia, esophagitis, gingivitis, hepatic failure, mouth disorder; *Hemic and Lymphatic System:* abnormal erythrocytes, leucocytosis, pancytopenia, purpura, splenomegaly, eosinophilia, hematologic disorder, hemolysis, lymphoma-like reaction, thrombocythemia; *Metabolic and Nutritional System:* acidosis, increased creatine phosphokinase, dehydration, diabetes mellitus, increased gamma globulins, gout, abnormal healing, hypocholesterolemia, weight gain, hyponatremia; *Musculoskeletal System:* arthritis, bone pain, osteomyelitis, pathological fracture;*Nervous System:* agitation, amnesia, apathy, ataxia, central nervous system depression, coma, convulsion, abnormal dreams, depersonalization, emotional lability, facial paralysis, abnormal gait, hyperesthesia, hypesthesia, hypertonia, incoordination, decreased libido, neuropathy, postural dizziness, decreased reflexes, stupor, tremor, vertigo; *Respiratory System:* asthma, atelectasis, hemoptysis, hyperventilation, hypoventilation, laryngitis, larynx edema, lung fibrosis, pleural effusion, pneumothorax, pulmonary embolus, increased sputum; *Skin and Appendages:* acne, alopecia, contact dermatitis, exfoliative dermatitis, fungal dermatitis, psoriasis, benign skin neoplasm, subcutaneous nodule, skin hypertrophy, urticaria; *Special Senses:* blepharitis, cataract, deafness, diplopia, exophthalmos, lacrimation disorder, optic neuritis, otitis media, parosmia, retinal detachment, taste perversion, tinnitus; *Urogenital System:* albuminuria, fibrocystic breast, glycosuria, gynecomastia, hydronephrosis, kidney failure, oliguria, polyuria, pyuria, toxic nephropathy, urinary frequency, urinary retention, urinary tract infection, urinary urgency, impaired urination, urolithiasis, and vaginitis.

One patient with hairy cell leukemia treated with pentostatin during another clinical study developed unilateral uveitis with vision loss.

DOSAGE AND ADMINISTRATION

It is recommended that patients receive hydration with 500-1000 ml of 5% dextrose in 0.5 normal saline or equivalent before pentostatin administration. An additional 500 ml of 5% dextrose or equivalent should be administered after pentostatin is given.

The recommended dosage of pentostatin for the treatment of alpha-interferon-refractory hairy cell leukemia is 4 mg/m^2 every other week. Pentostatin may be administered intravenously by bolus injection or diluted in a larger volume and given over 20-30 minutes. See Preparation of Intravenous Solution.

Higher doses are not recommended.

No extravasation injuries were reported in clinical studies.

The optimal duration of treatment has not been determined. In the absence of major toxicity and with observed continuing improvement, the patient should be treated until a complete response has been achieved. Although not established as required, the administration of two additional doses has been recommended following the achievement of a complete response.

All patients receiving pentostatin at 6 months should be assessed for response to treatment. If the patient has not achieved a complete or partial response, treatment with pentostatin should be discontinued.

If the patient has achieved a partial response, pentostatin treatment should be continued in an effort to achieve a complete response. At any time thereafter that a complete response is achieved, two additional doses of pentostatin are recommended. Pentostatin treatment should then be stopped. If the best response to treatment at the end of 12 months is a partial response, it is recommended that treatment with pentostatin be stopped.

Withholding or discontinuation of individual doses may be needed when severe adverse reactions occur. Drug treatment should be withheld in patients with severe rash, and withheld or discontinued in patients showing evidence of nervous system toxicity.

Pentostatin treatment should be withheld in patients with active infection occurring during the treatment but may be resumed when the infection is controlled.

Patients who have elevated serum creatinine should have their dose withheld and a creatinine clearance determined. There are insufficient data to recommend a starting or a subsequent dose for patients with impaired renal function (creatinine clearance <60 ml/min).

Patients with impaired renal function should be treated only when the potential benefit justifies the potential risk. Two patients with impaired renal function (creatinine clearances 50-60 ml/min) achieved complete response without unusual adverse events when treated with 2 mg/m^2.

No dosage reduction is recommended at the start of therapy with pentostatin in patients with anemia, neutropenia, or thrombocytopenia. In addition, dosage reductions are not recommended during treatment in patients with anemia and thrombocytopenia if patients can be otherwise supported hematologically. Pentostatin should be temporarily withheld if the absolute neutrophil count falls during treatment below 200 cells/mm^3 in a patient who had an initial neutrophil count greater than 500 cells/mm^3 and may be resumed when the count returns to predose levels.

PREPARATION OF INTRAVENOUS SOLUTION

1. Procedures for proper handling and disposal of anticancer drugs should be followed. Several guidelines on this subject have been published.[2-7] There is no general agreement that all of the procedures recommended in the guidelines are necessary or appropriate. Spills and wastes should be treated with a 5% sodium hypochlorite solution prior to disposal.
2. Protective clothing including polyethylene gloves must be worn.
3. Transfer 5 ml of sterile water for injection to the vial containing pentostatin and mix thoroughly to obtain complete dissolution of a solution yielding 2 mg/ml. Parenteral drug products should be inspected visually for particulate matter and discoloration prior to administration.
4. Pentostatin may be given intravenously by bolus injection or diluted in a larger volume (25-50 ml) with 5% dextrose injection or 0.9% sodium chloride injection. Dilution of the entire contents of a reconstituted vial with 25 ml or 50 ml provides a pentostatin concentration of 0.33 mg/ml or 0.18 mg/ml respectively for the diluted solutions.
5. Pentostatin solution when diluted for infusion with 5% dextrose injection or 0.9% sodium chloride injection does not interact with PVC infusion containers or administration sets at concentrations of 0.18-0.33 mg/ml.

STABILITY

Pentostatin vials are stable at refrigerated storage temperature 2-8°C (36-46°F) for the period stated on the package. Vials reconstituted or reconstituted and further diluted as directed may be stored at room temperature and ambient light but should be used within 8 hours because Nipent contains no preservatives.

Storage: Store pentostatin vials under refrigerated storage conditions 2-8°C (36-46°F).

PRODUCT LISTING - EQUIVALENTS NOT AVAILABLE

Powder For Injection - Intravenous - 10 mg

1's	$1440.00	NIPENT, Parke-Davis	67201-0800-01
1's	$1934.44	NIPENT, Supergen Inc	62701-0800-01

P

Pentoxifylline (001980)

Categories: Claudication, intermittent; Pregnancy Category C; FDA Approved 1984 Aug
Drug Classes: Hemorrheologic agents; Xanthine derivatives
Brand Names: Trental
Foreign Brand Availability: Agapurin (Singapore; Thailand); Artal (Finland); Azupentat (Germany); Carpental S.R. (Korea); Ceretal (Taiwan); C-Vex (Philippines); Elorgan (Spain); Erytral (Indonesia); Fixoten (Mexico); Flexital (Philippines); Harine (Korea); Hemovas (Spain); Ipentol (Taiwan); Kentadin (Mexico); Oxopurin 400 SR (Israel); Penphylline (Taiwan); Pentox (Philippines); Pentoxi (Switzerland); Pentoxifilin (Colombia); Pentoxine (Bahrain; Cyprus; Egypt; Iran; Iraq; Jordan; Kuwait; Lebanon; Libya; Oman; Qatar; Republic-of-Yemen; Saudi-Arabia; Syria; United-Arab-Emirates); Perencal (Korea); Peridane (Mexico); Pexal (Bahamas; Barbados; Belize; Bermuda; Curacao; Guyana; Jamaica; Netherland-Antilles; Surinam; Trinidad); Pexol (Peru); Platof (Indonesia); Tarontal (Greece; Indonesia); Torental (Belgium; France); Trenfyl (Indonesia); Trenlin SR (Singapore)
Cost of Therapy: \$59.29 (Intermittent Claudication; Trental; 400 mg; 3 tablets/day; 30 day supply)
\$40.95 (Intermittent Claudication; Generic Tablets; 400 mg; 3 tablets/day; 30 day supply)

DESCRIPTION

Trental (pentoxifylline) tablets for oral administration contain 400 mg of the active drug and the following inactive ingredients: D&C red no. 27 aluminum lake or FD&C red no. 3, hydroxypropyl methylcellulose, magnesium stearate, polyethylene glycol, povidone, talc, titanium dioxide, and other ingredients in a controlled-release formulation. Trental is a tri-substituted xanthine derivative designated chemically as 1-(5-oxohexyl)-3, 7-dimethylxanthine that, unlike theophylline, is a hemorrheologic agent, (*i.e.*, an agent that affects blood viscosity). Pentoxifylline is soluble in water and ethanol, and sparingly soluble in toluene.

CLINICAL PHARMACOLOGY

MODE OF ACTION

Pentoxifylline and its metabolites improve the flow properties of blood by decreasing its viscosity. In patients with chronic peripheral arterial disease, this increases blood flow to the affected microcirculation and enhances tissue oxygenation. The precise mode of action of pentoxifylline and the sequence of events leading to clinical improvement are still to be defined. Pentoxifylline administration has been shown to produce dose related hemorrheologic effects, lowering blood viscosity, and improving erythrocyte flexibility. Leukocyte properties of hemorrheologic importance have been modified in animal and *in vitro* human studies. Pentoxifylline has been shown to increase leukocyte deformability and to inhibit neutrophil adhesion and activation. Tissue oxygen levels have been shown to be significantly increased by therapeutic doses of pentoxifylline in patients with peripheral arterial disease.

PHARMACOKINETICS AND METABOLISM

After oral administration in aqueous solution pentoxifylline is almost completely absorbed. It undergoes a first-pass effect and the various metabolites appear in plasma very soon after dosing. Peak plasma levels of the parent compound and its metabolites are reached within 1 hour. The major metabolites are Metabolite I (1-[5-hydroxyhexyl]-3,7-dimethylxanthine) and Metabolite V (1-[3-carboxypropyl]-3, 7-dimethylxanthine), and plasma levels of these metabolites are 5 and 8 times greater, respectively, than pentoxifylline.

Following oral administration of aqueous solutions containing 100-400 mg of pentoxifylline, the pharmacokinetics of the parent compound and Metabolite I are dose-related and not proportional (non-linear), with half-life and area under the blood-level time curve (AUC) increasing with dose. The elimination kinetics of Metabolite V are not dose-dependent. The apparent plasma half-life of pentoxifylline varies from 0.4-0.8 hours and the apparent plasma half-lives of its metabolites vary from 1 to 1.6 hours. There is no evidence of accumulation or enzyme induction (Cytochrome P450) following multiple oral doses.

P

Excretion is almost totally urinary; the main biotransformation product is Metabolite V. Essentially no parent drug is found in the urine. Despite large variations in plasma levels of parent compound and its metabolites, the urinary recovery of Metabolite V is consistent and shows dose proportionality. Less than 4% of the administered dose is recovered in feces. Food intake shortly before dosing delays absorption of an immediate-release dosage form but does not affect total absorption. The pharmacokinetics and metabolism of pentoxifylline have not been studied in patients with renal and/or hepatic dysfunction, but AUC was increased and elimination rate decreased in an older population (60-68 years) compared to younger individuals (22-30 years).

After administration of the 400 mg controlled-release pentoxifylline tablet, plasma levels of the parent compound and its metabolites reach their maximum within 2-4 hours and remain constant over an extended period of time. Coadministration of pentoxifylline tablets with meals resulted in an increase in mean C_{max} and AUC by about 28% and 13% for pentoxifylline, respectively. C_{max} for metabolite I also increased by about 20%. The controlled release of pentoxifylline from the tablet eliminates peaks and troughs in plasma levels for improved gastrointestinal tolerance.

INDICATIONS AND USAGE

Pentoxifylline is indicated for the treatment of patients with intermittent claudication on the basis of chronic occlusive arterial disease of the limbs. Pentoxifylline can improve function and symptoms but is not intended to replace more definitive therapy, such as surgical bypass, or removal of arterial obstructions when treating peripheral vascular disease.

NON-FDA APPROVED INDICATIONS

Pentoxifylline has also been studied in the treatment of vascular complications of diabetes, cerebrovascular disease, and other circulatory disorders, however firm guidelines for use in these conditions are not yet available. Preliminary data also suggests that pentoxifylline may offer a protective effect against cyclosporine-induced nephrotoxicity in transplant patients.

CONTRAINDICATIONS

Pentoxifylline should not be used in patients with recent cerebral and/or retinal hemorrhage or in patients who have previously exhibited intolerance to this product or methylxanthines such as caffeine, theophylline, and theobromine.

PRECAUTIONS

GENERAL

Patients with chronic occlusive arterial disease of the limbs frequently show other manifestations of arteriosclerotic disease. Pentoxifylline has been used safely for treatment of peripheral arterial disease in patients with concurrent coronary artery and cerebrovascular diseases, but there have been occasional reports of angina, hypotension, and arrhythmia. Controlled trials do not show that pentoxifylline causes such adverse effects more often than placebo, but, as it is a methylxanthine derivative, it is possible some individuals will experience such responses. Patients on warfarin should have more frequent monitoring of prothrombin times, while patients with other risk factors complicated by hemorrhage (*e.g.*, recent surgery, peptic ulceration, cerebral and/or retinal bleeding) should have periodic examinations for bleeding including hematocrit and/or hemoglobin.

CARCINOGENESIS, MUTAGENESIS, AND IMPAIRMENT OF FERTILITY

Long-term studies of the carcinogenic potential of pentoxifylline were conducted in mice and rats by dietary administration of the drug at doses up to 450 mg/kg (approximately 19 times the maximum recommended human daily dose (MRHD) in both species when based on body weight; 1.5 times the MRHD in the mouse and 3.3 times the MRHD in the rat when based on body surface area). In mice, the drug was administered for 18 months, whereas in rats, the drug was administered for 18 months followed by an additional 6 months without drug exposure. In the rat study, there was a statistically significant increase in benign mammary fibroadenomas in females of the 450 mg/kg group. The relevance of this finding to human use is uncertain. Pentoxifylline was devoid of mutagenic activity in various strains of *Salmonella* (Ames test) and in cultured mammalian cells (unscheduled DNA synthesis test) when tested in the presence and absence of metabolic activation. It was also negative in the *in vivo* mouse micronucleus test.

PREGNANCY CATEGORY C

Teratogenicity studies have been performed in rats and rabbits using oral doses up to 576 and 264 mg/kg, respectively. On a weight basis, these doses are 24 and 11 times the maximum recommended human daily dose (MRHD); on a body surface area basis, they are 4.2 and 3.5 times the MRHD. No evidence of fetal malformation was observed. Increased resorption was seen in rats of the 576 mg/kg group. There are no adequate and well controlled studies in pregnant women. Pentoxifylline should be used during pregnancy only if the potential benefit justifies the potential risk to the fetus.

NURSING MOTHERS

Pentoxifylline and its metabolites are excreted in human milk. Because of the potential for tumorigenicity shown for pentoxifylline in rats, a decision should be made whether to discontinue nursing or discontinue the drug, taking into account the importance of the drug to the mother.

PEDIATRIC USE

Safety and effectiveness in pediatric patients have not been established.

DRUG INTERACTIONS

Although a causal relationship has not been established, there have been reports of bleeding and/or prolonged prothrombin time in patients treated with pentoxifyline with and without anticoagulants or platelet aggregation inhibitors. Patients on warfarin should have more frequent monitoring of prothrombin times, while patients with other risk factors complicated by hemorrhage (*e.g.*, recent surgery, peptic ulceration) should have periodic examinations for bleeding including hematocrit and/or hemoglobin. Concomitant administration of pentoxifyline and theophylline-containing drugs leads to increased theophylline levels and theophylline toxicity in some individuals. Such patients should be closely monitored for signs of toxicity and have their theophylline dosage adjusted as necessary. Pentoxifyline has been used concurrently with antihypertensive drugs, beta blockers, digitalis, diuretics, antidiabetic agents, and antiarrhythmics, without observed problems. Small decreases in blood pressure have been observed in some patients treated with pentoxifyline; periodic systemic blood pressure monitoring is recommended for patients receiving concomitant antihypertensive therapy. If indicated, dosage of the antihypertensive agents should be reduced.

ADVERSE REACTIONS

Clinical trials were conducted using either controlled-release pentoxifylline tablets for up to 60 weeks or immediate-release pentoxifyline capsules for up to 24 weeks. Dosage ranges in the tablet studies were 400 mg bid to tid and in the capsule studies, 200-400 mg tid. TABLE 1 summarizes the incidence (in percent) of adverse reactions considered drug related, as well as the numbers of patients who received controlled-release pentoxifyline tablets, immediate-release pentoxifyline capsules, or the corresponding placebos. The incidence of adverse reactions was higher in the capsule studies (where dose related increases were seen in digestive and nervous system side effects) than in the tablet studies. Studies with the capsule include domestic experience, whereas studies with the controlled-release tablets were conducted outside the U.S.

TABLE 1 indicates that in the tablet studies few patients discontinued because of adverse effects.

Pentoxifyline has been marketed in Europe and elsewhere since 1972. In addition to the above symptoms, the following have been reported spontaneously since marketing or occurred in other clinical trials with an incidence of less than 1%; the causal relationship was uncertain:

Cardiovascular: Dyspnea, edema, hypotension.
Digestive: Anorexia, cholecystitis, constipation, dry mouth/thirst.
Nervous: Anxiety, confusion, depression, seizures.
Respiratory: Epistaxis, flu-like symptoms, laryngitis, nasal congestion.
Skin and Appendages: Brittle fingernails, pruritus, rash, urticaria, angioedema.
Special Senses: Blurred vision, conjunctivitis, earache, scotoma.
Miscellaneous: Bad taste, excessive salivation, leukopenia, malaise, sore throat/swollen neck glands, weight change.

A few rare events have been reported spontaneously worldwide since marketing in 1972. Although they occurred under circumstances in which a causal relationship with pentoxi-

TABLE 1 *Incidence (%) of Side effects*

	Controlled-Release Tablets		Immediate-Release Capsules	
	Commercially Available		Used only for Controlled Clinical Trials	
	Pentoxifylline	Placebo	Pentoxifylline	Placebo
(Numbers of patients at risk)	(321)	(128)	(177)	(138)
Discontinued for side effect	3.1%	0%	9.6%	7.2%
Cardiovascular System				
Angina/chest pain	0.3%	—	1.1%	2.2%
Arrhythmia/ palpitation	—	—	1.7%	0.7%
Flushing	—	—	2.3%	0.7%
Digestive System				
Abdominal discomfort	—	—	4.0%	1.4%
Belching/flatus/ bloating	0.6%	—	9.0%	3.6%
Diarrhea	—	—	3.4%	2.9%
Dyspepsia	2.8%	4.7%	9.6%	2.9%
Nausea	2.2%	0.8%	28.8%	8.7%
Vomiting	1.2%	—	4.5%	0.7%
Nervous System				
Agitation/ nervousness	—	—	1.7%	0.7%
Dizziness	1.9%	3.1%	11.9%	4.3%
Drowsiness	—	—	1.1%	5.8%
Headache	1.2%	1.6%	6.2%	5.8%
Insomnia	—	—	2.3%	2.2%
Tremor	0.3%	0.8%	—	—
Blurred vision	—	—	2.3%	1.4%

fylline could not be established, they are listed to serve as information for physicians. *Cardiovascular:* Angina, arrhythmia, tachycardia, anaphylactoid reactions. *Digestive:* Hepatitis, jaundice, increased liver enzymes; and *Hemic and Lymphatic:* Decreased serum fibrinogen, pancytopenia, aplastic anemia, leukemia, purpura, thrombocytopenia.

DOSAGE AND ADMINISTRATION

The usual dosage of pentoxifyline in controlled-release tablet form is 1 tablet (400 mg) three times a day with meals.

While the effect of pentoxifyline may be seen within 2-4 weeks, it is recommended that treatment be continued for at least 8 weeks. Efficacy has been demonstrated in double-blind clinical studies of 6 months duration.

Digestive and central nervous system side effects are dose related. If patients develop these side effects it is recommended that the dosage be lowered to 1 tablet twice a day (800 mg/day). If side effects persist at this lower dosage, the administration of pentoxifyline should be discontinued.

HOW SUPPLIED

Trental is available for oral administration as 400 mg pink film-coated oblong tablets imprinted "Trental".

STORAGE

Store between 15-30°C (59-86°F).

Dispense in well-closed, light-resistant containers.

Protect blisters from light.

PRODUCT LISTING - RATED THERAPEUTICALLY EQUIVALENT

Tablet, Extended Release - Oral - 400 mg

10 x 10	$66.56	GENERIC, Major Pharmaceuticals Inc	00904-5448-61
25 x 30	$453.38	GENERIC, Sky Pharmaceuticals Packaging, Inc	63739-0260-03
25's	$14.45	GENERIC, Udl Laboratories Inc	51079-0889-19
30's	$27.01	TRENTAL, Physicians Total Care	54868-0374-03
31 x 10	$171.81	GENERIC, Vangard Labs	00615-4523-53
31 x 10	$171.81	GENERIC, Vangard Labs	00615-4523-63
60's	$44.71	TRENTAL, Allscripts Pharmaceutical Company	54569-0668-01
90's	$64.47	GENERIC, Zoetica Pharmaceutical	64909-0001-90
100's	$31.47	FEDERAL UPPER LIMIT, H.C.F.A. F F P	99999-1980-01
100's	$45.50	GENERIC, Sidmak Laboratories Inc	50111-0609-01
100's	$55.45	GENERIC, Dixon-Shane Inc	17236-0862-01
100's	$59.40	GENERIC, Upsher-Smith Laboratories Inc	00245-0027-11
100's	$59.48	GENERIC, Global Pharmaceutical Corporation	00115-7044-01
100's	$59.50	GENERIC, Teva Pharmaceuticals Usa	00093-5116-01
100's	$59.51	GENERIC, Apotex Usa Inc	60505-0033-06
100's	$59.51	GENERIC, Andrx Pharmaceuticals	62037-0951-01
100's	$59.90	GENERIC, Major Pharmaceuticals Inc	00904-5448-60
100's	$60.75	GENERIC, Mylan Pharmaceuticals Inc	00378-0357-01
100's	$61.99	GENERIC, Upsher-Smith Laboratories Inc	00245-0027-01
100's	$64.05	GENERIC, Purepac Pharmaceutical Company	00228-2611-11
100's	$64.05	GENERIC, Purepac Pharmaceutical Company	00228-2747-11
100's	$65.71	GENERIC, Udl Laboratories Inc	51079-0889-20
100's	$65.88	TRENTAL, Southwood Pharmaceuticals Inc	58016-0568-00
100's	$74.52	TRENTAL, Allscripts Pharmaceutical Company	54569-0668-00
100's	$81.20	TRENTAL, Aventis Pharmaceuticals	00039-0078-10
100's	$84.75	TRENTAL, Aventis Pharmaceuticals	00039-0078-11
100's	$86.63	TRENTAL, Physicians Total Care	54868-0374-01
270's	$152.69	TRENTAL, Allscripts Pharmaceutical Company	54569-8544-00

PRODUCT LISTING - EQUIVALENTS NOT AVAILABLE

Tablet, Extended Release - Oral - 400 mg

90's	$54.89	GENERIC, Golden State Medical	60429-0703-90

Pergolide Mesylate *(001986)*

Categories: Parkinson's disease; Pregnancy Category B; FDA Approved 1988 Dec
Drug Classes: Antiparkinson agents; Dermatologics; Ergot alkaloids and derivatives
Brand Names: **Permax**
Foreign Brand Availability: Celance (China; Costa-Rica; Dominican-Republic; El-Salvador; England; France; Guatemala; Guyana; Hong-Kong; Ireland; Japan; Korea; Nicaragua; Panama; Peru; Philippines; Taiwan; Thailand); Parkotil (Germany); Pergolide (Israel)
Cost of Therapy: $33.64 (Parkinsonism; Permax; 0.05 mg; 3 tablets/day; 30 day supply)

DESCRIPTION

Permax (pergolide mesylate) is an ergot derivative dopamine receptor agonist at both D_1 and D_2 receptor sites. Pergolide mesylate is chemically designated as 8β-[(Methylthio)methyl]-6-propylergoline monomethanesulfonate.

The empirical formula is $C_{19}H_{26}N_2S{\cdot}CH_4O_3S$, representing a molecular weight of 410.60.

Pergolide mesylate is provided for oral administration in tablets containing 0.05 mg (0.159 μmol), 0.25 mg (0.795 μmol), or 1 mg (3.18 μmol) pergolide as the base. The tablets also contain croscarmellose sodium, iron oxide, lactose, magnesium stearate, and povidone. The 0.05 mg tablet also contains L-methionine, and the 0.25 mg tablet also contains FD&C blue no. 2.

CLINICAL PHARMACOLOGY

PHARMACODYNAMICS

Pergolide mesylate is a potent dopamine receptor agonist. Pergolide is 10-1000 times more potent than bromocriptine on a milligram per milligram basis in various *in vitro* and *in vivo* test systems. Pergolide mesylate inhibits the secretion of prolactin in humans; it causes a transient rise in serum concentrations of growth hormone and a decrease in serum concentrations of luteinizing hormone. In Parkinson's disease, pergolide mesylate is believed to exert its therapeutic effect by directly stimulating postsynaptic dopamine receptors in the nigrostriatal system.

PHARMACOKINETICS (ABSORPTION, DISTRIBUTION, METABOLISM, AND ELIMINATION)

Information on oral systemic bioavailability of pergolide mesylate is unavailable because of the lack of a sufficiently sensitive assay to detect the drug after the administration of a single dose. However, following oral administration of ^{14}C radiolabeled pergolide mesylate, approximately 55% of the administered radioactivity can be recovered from the urine and 5% from expired CO_2, suggesting that a significant fraction is absorbed. Nothing can be concluded about the extent of presystemic clearance, if any.

Data on postabsorption distribution of pergolide are unavailable.

At least 10 metabolites have been detected, including N-despropylpergolide, pergolide sulfoxide, and pergolide sulfone. Pergolide sulfoxide and pergolide sulfone are dopamine agonists in animals. The other detected metabolites have not been identified and it is not known whether any other metabolites are active pharmacologically.

The major route of excretion is the kidney.

Pergolide is approximately 90% bound to plasma proteins. This extent of protein binding may be important to consider when pergolide mesylate is coadministered with other drugs known to affect protein binding.

INDICATIONS AND USAGE

Pergolide mesylate is indicated as adjunctive treatment to levodopa/carbidopa in the management of the signs and symptoms of Parkinson's disease.

Evidence to support the efficacy of pergolide mesylate as an antiparkinsonian adjunct was obtained in a multicenter study enrolling 376 patients with mild to moderate Parkinson's disease who were intolerant to *l*-dopa/carbidopa as manifested by moderate to severe dyskinesia and/or on-off phenomena. On average, the patients evaluated had been on *l*-dopa/carbidopa for 3.9 years (range, 2 days to 16.8 years). The administration of pergolide mesylate permitted a 5-30% reduction in the daily dose of *l*-dopa. On average, these patients treated with pergolide mesylate maintained an equivalent or better clinical status than they exhibited at baseline.

NON-FDA APPROVED INDICATIONS

Pergolide has also been reported to be effective in the treatment of hyperprolactinemia, restless legs syndrome, and nocturnal myoclonus syndrome. However, none of these uses has been approved by the FDA and further clinical trials are needed.

CONTRAINDICATIONS

Pergolide mesylate is contraindicated in patients who are hypersensitive to this drug or other ergot derivatives.

WARNINGS

SYMPTOMATIC HYPOTENSION

In clinical trials, approximately 10% of patients taking pergolide mesylate with *l*-dopa versus 7% taking placebo with *l*-dopa experienced symptomatic orthostatic and/or sustained hypotension, especially during initial treatment. With gradual dosage titration, tolerance to the hypotension usually develops. It is therefore important to warn patients of the risk, to

P

begin therapy with low doses, and to increase the dosage in carefully adjusted increments over a period of 3-4 weeks (see DOSAGE AND ADMINISTRATION).

HALLUCINOSIS

In controlled trials, pergolide mesylate with *l*-dopa caused hallucinosis in about 14% of patients as opposed to 3% taking placebo with *l*-dopa. This was of sufficient severity to cause discontinuation of treatment in about 3% of those enrolled; tolerance to this untoward effect was not observed.

FATALITIES

In the placebo-controlled trial, 2 of 187 patients treated with placebo died as compared with 1 of 189 patients treated with pergolide mesylate. Of the 2299 patients treated with pergolide mesylate in premarketing studies evaluated as of October 1988, 143 died while on the drug or shortly after discontinuing it. Because the patient population under evaluation was elderly, ill, and at high risk for death, it seems unlikely that pergolide mesylate played any role in these deaths, but the possibility that pergolide shortens survival of patients cannot be excluded with absolute certainty.

In particular, a case-by-case review of the clinical course of the patients who died failed to disclose any unique set of signs, symptoms, or laboratory results that would suggest that treatment with pergolide caused their deaths. Sixty-eight percent (68%) of the patients who died were 65 years of age or older. No death (other than a suicide) occurred within the first month of treatment; most of the patients who died had been on pergolide for years. A relative frequency of the causes of death by organ system are: pulmonary failure/pneumonia, 35%; cardiovascular, 30%; cancer, 11%; unknown, 8.4%; infection, 3.5%; extrapyramidal syndrome, 3.5%; stroke, 2.1%; dysphagia, 2.1%; injury, 1.4%; suicide, 1.4%; dehydration, 0.7%; glomerulonephritis, 0.7%.

SERIOUS INFLAMMATION AND FIBROSIS

There have been rare reports of pleuritis, pleural effusion, pleural fibrosis, pericarditis, pericardial effusion, cardiac valvulopathy involving 1 or more valves, or retroperitoneal fibrosis in patients taking pergolide. In some cases, symptoms or manifestations of cardiac valvulopathy improved after discontinuation of pergolide. Pergolide should be used with caution in patients with a history of these conditions, particularly those patients who experienced the events while taking ergot derivatives. Patients with a history of such events should be carefully monitored clinically and with appropriate radiographic and laboratory studies while taking pergolide.

PRECAUTIONS

GENERAL

Caution should be exercised when administering pergolide mesylate to patients prone to cardiac dysrhythmias.

In a study comparing pergolide mesylate and placebo, patients taking pergolide mesylate were found to have significantly more episodes of atrial premature contractions (APCs) and sinus tachycardia.

The use of pergolide mesylate in patients on *l*-dopa may cause and/or exacerbate preexisting states of confusion and hallucinations (see WARNINGS) and preexisting dyskinesia. Also, the abrupt discontinuation of pergolide mesylate in patients receiving it chronically as an adjunct to *l*-dopa may precipitate the onset of hallucinations and confusion; these may occur within a span of several days. Discontinuation of pergolide should be undertaken gradually whenever possible, even if the patient is to remain on *l*-dopa.

A symptom complex resembling the neuroleptic malignant syndrome (NMS) (characterized by elevated temperature, muscular rigidity, altered consciousness, and autonomic instability), with no other obvious etiology, has been reported in association with rapid dose reduction, withdrawal of, or changes in antiparkinsonian therapy, including pergolide.

INFORMATION FOR THE PATIENT

Because pergolide mesylate may cause somnolence, patients should be cautioned about operating hazardous machinery, including automobiles, until they are reasonably certain that pergolide mesylate therapy does not affect them adversely. Due to the possible additive sedative effects, caution should also be used when patients are taking other CNS depressants in combination with pergolide mesylate.

Patients and their families should be informed of the common adverse consequences of the use of pergolide mesylate (see ADVERSE REACTIONS) and the risk of hypotension (see WARNINGS).

Patients should be advised to notify their physician if they become pregnant or intend to become pregnant during therapy.

Patients should be advised to notify their physician if they are breast feeding an infant.

LABORATORY TESTS

No specific laboratory tests are deemed essential for the management of patients on pergolide mesylate. Periodic routine evaluation of all patients, however, is appropriate.

CARCINOGENESIS, MUTAGENESIS, AND IMPAIRMENT OF FERTILITY

A 2 year carcinogenicity study was conducted in mice using dietary levels of pergolide mesylate equivalent to oral doses of 0.6, 3.7, and 36.4 mg/kg/day in males and 0.6, 4.4, and 40.8 mg/kg/day in females. A 2 year study in rats was conducted using dietary levels equivalent to oral doses of 0.04, 0.18, and 0.88 mg/kg/day in males and 0.05, 0.28, and 1.42 mg/kg/day in females. The highest doses tested in the mice and rats were approximately 340 and 12 times the maximum human oral dose administered in controlled clinical trials (6 mg/day equivalent to 0.12 mg/kg/day).

A low incidence of uterine neoplasms occurred in both rats and mice. Endometrial adenomas and carcinomas were observed in rats. Endometrial sarcomas were observed in mice. The occurrence of these neoplasms is probably attributable to the high estrogen/progesterone ratio that would occur in rodents as a result of the prolactin-inhibiting action of pergolide mesylate. The endocrine mechanisms believed to be involved in the rodents are not present in humans. However, even though there is no known correlation between uterine malignancies occurring in pergolide-treated rodents and human risk, there are no human data to substantiate this conclusion.

Pergolide mesylate was evaluated for mutagenic potential in a battery of tests that included an Ames bacterial mutation assay, a DNA repair assay in cultured rat hepatocytes, an *in vitro* mammalian cell gene mutation assay in cultured L5178Y cells, and a determination of chromosome alteration in bone marrow cells of Chinese hamsters. A weak mutagenic response was noted in the mammalian cell gene mutation assay only after metabolic activation with rat liver microsomes. No mutagenic effects were obtained in the 2 other *in vitro* assays and in the *in vivo* assay. The relevance of these findings in humans is unknown.

A fertility study in male and female mice showed that fertility was maintained at 0.6 and 1.7 mg/kg/day but decreased at 5.6 mg/kg/day. Prolactin has been reported to be involved in stimulating and maintaining progesterone levels required for implantation in mice and, therefore, the impaired fertility at the high dose may have occurred because of depressed prolactin levels.

PREGNANCY CATEGORY B

Reproduction studies were conducted in mice at doses of 5, 16, and 45 mg/kg/day and in rabbits at doses of 2, 6, and 16 mg/kg/day. The highest doses tested in mice and rabbits were 375 and 133 times the 6 mg/day maximum human dose administered in controlled clinical trials. In these studies, there was no evidence of harm to the fetus due to pergolide mesylate.

There are, however, no adequate and well-controlled studies in pregnant women. Among women who received pergolide mesylate for endocrine disorders in premarketing studies, there were 33 pregnancies that resulted in healthy babies and 6 pregnancies that resulted in congenital abnormalities (3 major, 3 minor); a causal relationship has not been established. Because human data are limited and because animal reproduction studies are not always predictive of human response, this drug should be used during pregnancy only if clearly needed.

NURSING MOTHERS

It is not known whether this drug is excreted in human milk. The pharmacologic action of pergolide mesylate suggests that it may interfere with lactation. Because many drugs are excreted in human milk and because of the potential for serious adverse reactions to pergolide mesylate in nursing infants, a decision should be made whether to discontinue nursing or to discontinue the drug, taking into account the importance of the drug to the mother.

PEDIATRIC USE

Safety and effectiveness in pediatric patients have not been established.

GERIATRIC USE

Of the total number of subjects in clinical studies of pergolide mesylate, 78 were 65 and over. There were no apparent differences in efficacy between these subjects and younger subjects. There was an increased incidence of confusion, somnolence, and peripheral edema in patients 65 and over. Other reported clinical experience has not identified differences in responses between the elderly and younger patients, but greater sensitivity of some older individuals cannot be ruled out. This drug is known to be substantially excreted by the kidney, and the risk of toxic reactions to this drug may be greater in patients with impaired renal function. Because elderly patients are more likely to have decreased renal function, care should be taken in dose selection, and it may be useful to monitor renal function.

DRUG INTERACTIONS

Dopamine antagonists, such as the neuroleptics (phenothiazines, butyrophenones, thioxanthenes) or metoclopramide, ordinarily should not be administered concurrently with pergolide mesylate (a dopamine agonist); these agents may diminish the effectiveness of pergolide mesylate.

Because pergolide mesylate is approximately 90% bound to plasma proteins, caution should be exercised if pergolide mesylate is coadministered with other drugs known to affect protein binding.

ADVERSE REACTIONS

COMMONLY OBSERVED

In premarketing clinical trials, the most commonly observed adverse events associated with use of pergolide mesylate which were not seen at an equivalent incidence among placebo-treated patients were: nervous system complaints, including dyskinesia, hallucinations, somnolence, and insomnia; digestive complaints, including nausea, constipation, diarrhea, and dyspepsia; and respiratory system complaints, including rhinitis.

ASSOCIATED WITH DISCONTINUATION OF TREATMENT

Twenty-seven percent (27%) of approximately 1200 patients receiving pergolide mesylate for treatment of Parkinson's disease in premarketing clinical trials in the US and Canada discontinued treatment due to adverse events. The events most commonly causing discontinuation were related to the nervous system (15.5%), primarily hallucinations (7.8%), and confusion (1.8%).

FATALITIES

See WARNINGS.

INCIDENCE IN CONTROLLED CLINICAL TRIALS

TABLE 1 enumerates adverse events that occurred at a frequency of 1% or more among patients taking pergolide mesylate who participated in the premarketing controlled clinical trials comparing pergolide mesylate with placebo. In a double-blind, controlled study of 6 months' duration, patients with Parkinson's disease were continued on *l*-dopa/carbidopa and were randomly assigned to receive either pergolide mesylate or placebo as additional therapy.

The prescriber should be aware that these figures cannot be used to predict the incidence of side effects in the course of usual medical practice where patient characteristics and other factors differ from those which prevailed in the clinical trials. Similarly, the cited frequencies cannot be compared with figures obtained from other clinical investigations involving different treatments, uses, and investigators. The cited figures, however, do provide the prescribing physician with some basis for estimating the relative contribution of drug and nondrug factors to the side-effect incidence rate in the population studied.

TABLE 1 *Incidence of Treatment-Emergent Adverse Experiences in the Placebo-Controlled Clinical Trial*

Body System/ Adverse Event*	Percentage of Patients Reporting Events	
	Pergolide Mesylate (n=189)	Placebo (n=187)
Body as a Whole		
Pain	7.0%	2.1%
Abdominal pain	5.8%	2.1%
Injury, accident	5.8%	7.0%
Headache	5.3%	6.4%
Asthenia	4.2%	4.8%
Chest pain	3.7%	2.1%
Flu syndrome	3.2%	2.1%
Neck pain	2.7%	1.6%
Back pain	1.6%	2.1%
Surgical procedure	1.6%	<1%
Chills	1.1%	0%
Face edema	1.1%	0%
Infection	1.1%	0%
Cardiovascular		
Postural hypotension	9.0%	7.0%
Vasodilatation	3.2%	<1%
Palpitation	2.1%	<1%
Hypotension	2.1%	<1%
Syncope	2.1%	1.1%
Hypertension	1.6%	1.1%
Arrhythmia	1.1%	<1%
Myocardial infarction	1.1%	<1%
Digestive		
Nausea	24.3%	12.8%
Constipation	10.6%	5.9%
Diarrhea	6.4%	2.7%
Dyspepsia	6.4%	2.1%
Anorexia	4.8%	2.7%
Dry mouth	3.7%	<1%
Vomiting	2.7%	1.6%
Hemic and Lymphatic		
Anemia	1.1%	<1%
Metabolic and Nutritional		
Peripheral edema	7.4%	4.3%
Edema	1.6%	0%
Weight gain	1.6%	0%
Musculoskeletal		
Arthralgia	1.6%	2.1%
Bursitis	1.6%	<1%
Myalgia	1.1%	<1%
Twitching	1.1%	0%
Nervous System		
Dyskinesia	62.4%	24.6%
Dizziness	19.1%	13.9%
Hallucinations	13.8%	3.2%
Dystonia	11.6%	8.0%
Confusion	11.1%	9.6%
Somnolence	10.1%	3.7%
Insomnia	7.9%	3.2%
Anxiety	6.4%	4.3%
Tremor	4.2%	7.5%
Depression	3.2%	5.4%
Abnormal dreams	2.7%	4.3%
Personality disorder	2.1%	<1%
Psychosis	2.1%	0%
Abnormal gait	1.6%	1.6%
Akathisia	1.6%	0%
Extrapyramidal syndrome	1.6%	1.1%
Incoordination	1.6%	<1%
Paresthesia	1.6%	3.2%
Akinesia	1.1%	1.1%
Hypertonia	1.1%	0%
Neuralgia	1.1%	<1%
Speech disorder	1.1%	1.6%
Respiratory System		
Rhinitis	12.2%	5.4%
Dyspnea	4.8%	1.1%
Epistaxis	1.6%	<1%
Hiccup	1.1%	0%
Skin and Appendages		
Rash	3.2%	2.1%
Sweating	2.1%	2.7%
Special Senses		
Abnormal vision	5.8%	5.4%
Diplopia	2.1%	0%
Taste perversion	1.6%	0%
Eye disorder	1.1%	0%
Urogenital System		
Urinary frequency	2.7%	6.4%
Urinary tract infection	2.7%	3.7%
Hematuria	1.1%	<1%

* Events reported by at least 1% of patients receiving pergolide mesylate are included.

EVENTS OBSERVED DURING THE PREMARKETING EVALUATION OF PERGOLIDE MESYLATE

This section reports event frequencies evaluated as of October 1988 for adverse events occurring in a group of approximately 1800 patients who took multiple doses of pergolide mesylate. The conditions and duration of exposure to pergolide mesylate varied greatly, involving well-controlled studies as well as experience in open and uncontrolled clinical settings. In the absence of appropriate controls in some of the studies, a casual relationship between these events and treatment with pergolide mesylate cannot be determined.

The following enumeration by organ system describes events in terms of their relative frequency of reporting in the data base. Events of major clinical importance are also described in WARNINGS and PRECAUTIONS.

The following definitions of frequency are used: *frequent* adverse events are defined as those occurring in at least 1/100 patients; *infrequent* adverse events are those occurring in 1/100 to 1/1000 patients; *rare* events are those occurring in fewer than 1/1000 patients.

Body as a Whole: *Frequent:* Headache, asthenia, accidental injury, pain, abdominal pain, chest pain, back pain, flu syndrome, neck pain, fever. *Infrequent:* Facial edema, chills, enlarged abdomen, malaise, neoplasm, hernia, pelvic pain, sepsis, cellulitis, moniliasis, abscess, jaw pain, hypothermia. *Rare:* Acute abdominal syndrome, LE syndrome.

Cardiovascular System: *Frequent:* Postural hypotension, syncope, hypertension, palpitations, vasodilatations, congestive heart failure. *Infrequent:* Myocardial infarction, tachycardia, heart arrest, abnormal electrocardiogram, angina pectoris, thrombophlebitis, bradycardia, ventricular extrasystoles, cerebrovascular accident, ventricular tachycardia, cerebral ischemia, atrial fibrillation, varicose vein, pulmonary embolus, AV block, shock. *Rare:* Vasculitis, pulmonary hypertension, pericarditis, migraine, heart block, cerebral hemorrhage.

Digestive System: *Frequent:* Nausea, vomiting, dyspepsia, diarrhea, constipation, dry mouth, dysphagia. *Infrequent:* Flatulence, abnormal liver function tests, increased appetite, salivary gland enlargement, thirst, gastroenteritis, gastritis, periodontal abscess, intestinal obstruction, nausea and vomiting, gingivitis, esophagitis, cholelithiasis, tooth caries, hepatitis, stomach ulcer, melena, hepatomegaly, hematemesis, eructation. *Rare:* Sialadenitis, peptic ulcer, pancreatitis, jaundice, glossitis, fecal incontinence, duodenitis, colitis, cholecystitis, aphthous stomatitis, esophageal ulcer.

Endocrine System: *Infrequent:* Hypothyroidism, adenoma, diabetes mellitus, ADH inappropriate. *Rare:* Endocrine disorder, thyroid adenoma.

Hemic and Lymphatic System: *Frequent:* Anemia. *Infrequent:* Leukopenia, lymphadenopathy, leukocytosis, thrombocytopenia, petechia, megaloblastic anemia, cyanosis. *Rare:* Purpura, lymphocytosis, eosinophilia, thrombocythemia, acute lymphoblastic leukemia, polycythemia, splenomegaly.

Metabolic and Nutritional System: *Frequent:* Peripheral edema, weight loss, weight gain. *Infrequent:* Dehydration, hypokalemia, hypoglycemia, iron deficiency anemia, hyperglycemia, gout, hypercholesteremia. *Rare:* Electrolyte imbalance, cachexia, acidosis, hyperuricemia.

Musculoskeletal System: *Frequent:* Twitching, myalgia, arthralgia. *Infrequent:* Bone pain, tenosynovitis, myositis, bone sarcoma, arthritis. *Rare:* Osteoporosis, muscle atrophy, osteomyelitis.

Nervous System: *Frequent:* Dyskinesia, dizziness, hallucinations, confusion, somnolence, insomnia, dystonia, paresthesia, depression, anxiety, tremor, akinesia, extrapyramidal syndrome, abnormal gait, abnormal dreams, incoordination, psychosis, personality disorder, nervousness, choreoathetosis, amnesia, paranoid reaction, abnormal thinking. *Infrequent:* Akathisia, neuropathy, neuralgia, hypertonia, delusions, convulsion, libido increased, euphoria, emotional lability, libido decreased, vertigo, myoclonus, coma, apathy, paralysis, neurosis, hyperkinesia, ataxia, acute brain syndrome, torticollis, meningitis, manic reaction, hypokinesia, hostility, agitation, hypotonia. *Rare:* Stupor, neuritis, intracranial hypertension, hemiplegia, facial paralysis, brain edema, myelitis, hallucinations and confusion after abrupt discontinuation.

Respiratory System: *Frequent:* Rhinitis, dyspnea, pneumonia, pharyngitis, cough increased. *Infrequent:* Epistaxis, hiccup, sinusitis, bronchitis, voice alteration, hemoptysis, asthma, lung edema, pleural effusion, laryngitis, emphysema, apnea, hyperventilation. *Rare:* Pneumothorax, lung fibrosis, larynx edema, hypoxia, hypoventilation, hemothorax, carcinoma of lung.

Skin and Appendages System: *Frequent:* Sweating, rash. *Infrequent:* Skin discoloration, pruritus, acne, skin ulcer, alopecia, dry skin, skin carcinoma, seborrhea, hirsutism, herpes simplex, eczema, fungal dermatitis, herpes zoster. *Rare:* Vesiculobullous rash, subcutaneous nodule, skin nodule, skin benign neoplasm, lichenoid dermatitis.

Special Senses System: *Frequent:* Abnormal vision, diplopia. *Infrequent:* Otitis media, conjunctivitis, tinnitus, deafness, taste perversion, ear pain, eye pain, glaucoma, eye hemorrhage, photophobia, visual field defect. *Rare:* Blindness, cataract, retinal detachment, retinal vascular disorder.

Urogenital System: *Frequent:* Urinary tract infection, urinary frequency, urinary incontinence, hematuria, dysmenorrhea. *Infrequent:* Dysuria, breast pain, menorrhagia, impotence, cystitis, urinary retention, abortion, vaginal hemorrhage, vaginitis, priapism, kidney calculus, fibrocystic breast, lactation, uterine hemorrhage, urolithiasis, salpingitis, pyuria, metrorrhagia, menopause, kidney failure, breast carcinoma, cervical carcinoma. *Rare:* Amenorrhea, bladder carcinoma, breast engorgement, epididymitis, hypogonadism, leukorrhea, nephrosis, pyelonephritis, urethral pain, uricaciduria, withdrawal bleeding.

POSTINTRODUCTION REPORTS

Voluntary reports of adverse events temporally associated with pergolide that have been received since market introduction and which may have no causal relationship with the drug, include the following: neuroleptic malignant syndrome.

DOSAGE AND ADMINISTRATION

Administration of pergolide mesylate should be initiated with a daily dosage of 0.05 mg for the first 2 days. The dosage should then be gradually increased by 0.1 or 0.15 mg/day every third day over the next 12 days of therapy. The dosage may then be increased by 0.25 mg/day every third day until an optimal therapeutic dosage is achieved.

Pergolide mesylate is usually administered in divided doses 3 times/day. During dosage titration, the dosage of concurrent *l*-dopa/carbidopa may be cautiously decreased.

In clinical studies, the mean therapeutic daily dosage of pergolide mesylate was 3 mg/day. The average concurrent daily dosage of *l*-dopa/carbidopa (expressed as *l*-dopa) was ap-

P

proximately 650 mg/day. The efficacy of pergolide mesylate at doses above 5 mg/day has not been systematically evaluated.

HOW SUPPLIED

PERMAX TABLETS (MODIFIED RECTANGLE SHAPE, SCORED)

0.05 mg: Ivory, debossed with A 024.
0.25 mg: Green, debossed with A 025.
1 mg: Pink, debossed with A 026.

Storage: Store at 25°C (77°F); excursions permitted to 15-30°C (59-86°F).

PRODUCT LISTING - EQUIVALENTS NOT AVAILABLE

Tablet - Oral - 0.05 mg

30's	$37.44	PERMAX, Elan Pharmaceuticals	59075-0615-30
100's	$37.38	PERMAX, Amarin Pharmaceuticals	65234-0024-30
100's	$112.32	GENERIC, Teva Pharmaceuticals Usa	00093-7160-01

Tablet - Oral - 0.25 mg

100's	$186.29	GENERIC, Teva Pharmaceuticals Usa	00093-7159-01
100's	$206.99	PERMAX, Elan Pharmaceuticals	59075-0625-10
100's	$207.00	PERMAX, Amarin Pharmaceuticals	65234-0025-10

Tablet - Oral - 1 mg

100's	$381.34	PERMAX, Elan Pharmaceuticals	59075-0630-10
100's	$401.66	GENERIC, Teva Pharmaceuticals Usa	00093-7161-01
100's	$446.29	PERMAX, Amarin Pharmaceuticals	65234-0026-10

Perindopril Erbumine *(003453)*

For related information, see the comparative table section in Appendix A.

Categories: Hypertension, essential; FDA Approved 1999 Jul; Pregnancy Category C, 1st Trimester; Pregnancy Category D, 2nd & 3rd Trimesters
Drug Classes: Angiotensin converting enzyme inhibitors
Brand Names: **Aceon**
Cost of Therapy: $36.30 (Hypertension; Aceon; 4 mg; 1 tablet/day; 30 day supply)

WARNING

USE IN PREGNANCY:

When used in pregnancy during the second and third trimesters, ACE inhibitors can cause injury and even death to the developing fetus. When pregnancy is detected, perindopril erbumine should be discontinued as soon as possible. (See WARNINGS, Fetal/Neonatal Morbidity and Mortality.)

DESCRIPTION

Perindopril erbumine is the tert-butylamine salt of perindopril, the ethyl ester of a non-sulfhydryl angiotensin converting enzyme (ACE) inhibitor. Perindopril erbumine is chemically described as (2S,3αS,7αS)-1-[(S)-N-[(S)-1-Carboxy-butyl]alanyl]hexahydro-2-indolinecarboxylic acid, 1-ethyl ester, compound with tert-butylamine (1:1). Its molecular formula is $C_{19}H_{32}N_2O_5C_4H_{11}N$.

Perindopril erbumine is a white, crystalline powder with a molecular weight of 368.47 (free acid) or 441.61 (salt form). It is freely soluble in water (60% w/w), alcohol and chloroform.

Perindopril is the free acid form of perindopril erbumine, is a pro-drug and metabolized *in vivo* by hydrolysis of the ester group to form perindoprilat, the biologically active metabolite.

Aceon tablets are available in 2, 4, and 8 mg strengths for oral administration. In addition to perindopril erbumine, each tablet contains the following inactive ingredients: colloidal silica (hydrophobic), lactose, magnesium stearate and microcrystalline cellulose. The 4 mgand 8 mg tablets also contain iron oxide.

CLINICAL PHARMACOLOGY

MECHANISM OF ACTION

Perindopril erbumine is a pro-drug for perindoprilat, which inhibits ACE in human subjects and animals. The mechanism through which perindoprilat lowers blood pressure is believed to be primarily inhibition of ACE activity. ACE is a peptidyl dipeptidase that catalyzes conversion of the inactive decapeptide, angiotensin I, to the vasoconstrictor, angiotensin II. Angiotensin II is a potent peripheral vasoconstrictor, which stimulates aldosterone secretion by the adrenal cortex, and provides negative feedback on renin secretion. Inhibition of ACE results in decreased plasma angiotensin II, leading to decreased vasoconstriction, increased plasma renin activity and decreased aldosterone secretion. The latter results in diuresis and natriuresis and may be associated with a small increase of serum potassium.

ACE is identical to kininase II, an enzyme that degrades bradykinin. Whether increased levels of bradykinin, a potent vasodepressor peptide, play a role in the therapeutic effects of perindopril erbumine remains to be elucidated.

While the principal mechanism of perindopril in blood pressure reduction is believed to be through the renin-angiotensin-aldosterone system, ACE inhibitors have some effect even in apparent low-renin hypertension. Perindopril has been studied in relatively few black patients, usually a low-renin population, and the average response of diastolic blood pressure to perindopril was about half the response seen in nonblacks, a finding consistent with previous experience of other ACE inhibitors.

After administration of perindopril, ACE is inhibited in a dose- and blood concentration-related fashion, with the maximal inhibition of 80-90% attained by 8 mg persisting for 10-12 hours. Twenty-four (24) hour ACE inhibition is about 60% after these doses. The degree of ACE inhibition achieved by a given dose appears to diminish over time (the ID_{50} increases). The pressor response to an angiotensin I infusion is reduced by perindopril, but this effect is not as persistent as the effect on ACE; there is about 35% inhibition at 24 hours after a 12 mg dose.

PHARMACOKINETICS

Oral administration of perindopril erbumine results in its rapid absorption with peak plasma concentrations occurring at approximately 1 hour. The absolute oral bioavailability of perindopril is about 75%. Following absorption, approximately 30-50% of systemically available perindopril is hydrolyzed to its active metabolite, perindoprilat, which has a mean bioavailability of about 25%. Peak plasma concentrations of perindoprilat are attained 3-7 hours after perindopril administration. The presence of food in the gastrointestinal tract does not affect the rate or extent of absorption of perindopril but reduces bioavailability of perindoprilat by about 35%. (See DRUG INTERACTIONS, Food Interaction.)

With 4, 8, and 16 mg doses of perindopril erbumine, C_{max} and AUC of perindopril and perindoprilat increase in a linear and dose-proportional manner following both single oral dosing and at steady state during a once-a-day multiple dosing regimen.

Perindopril exhibits multiexponential pharmacokinetics following oral administration. The mean half-life of perindopril associated with most of its elimination is approximately 0.8-1.0 hours. At very low plasma concentrations of perindopril (<3 ng/ml), there is a prolonged terminal elimination half-life, similar to that seen with other ACE inhibitors, that results from slow dissociation of perindopril from plasma/tissue ACE binding sites. Perindopril does not accumulate with a once-a-day multiple dosing regimen. Mean total body clearance of perindopril is 219-362 ml/min and its mean renal clearance is 23.3- 28.6 ml/min.

Perindopril is extensively metabolized following oral administration, with only 4-12% of the dose recovered unchanged in the urine. Six metabolites resulting from hydrolysis, glucuronidation and cyclization via dehydration have been identified. These include the active ACE inhibitor, perindoprilat (hydrolyzed perindopril), perindopril and perindoprilat glucuronides, dehydrated perindopril and the diastereoisomers of dehydrated perindoprilat. In humans, hepatic esterase appears to be responsible for the hydrolysis of perindopril.

The active metabolite, perindoprilat, also exhibits multiexponential pharmacokinetics following the oral administration of perindopril erbumine. Formation of perindoprilat is gradual with peak plasma concentrations occurring between 3 and 7 hours. The subsequent decline in plasma concentration shows an apparent mean half-life of 3-10 hours for the majority of the elimination, with a prolonged terminal elimination half-life of 30-120 hours resulting from slow dissociation of perindoprilat from plasma/tissue ACE binding sites. During repeated oral once-daily dosing with perindopril, perindoprilat accumulates about 1.5- to 2.0-fold and attains steady state plasma levels in 3-6 days. The clearance of perindoprilat and its metabolites is almost exclusively renal.

Approximately 60% of circulating perindopril is bound to plasma proteins, and only 10-20% of perindoprilat is bound. Therefore, drug interactions mediated through effects on protein binding are not anticipated.

At usual antihypertensive dosages, little radioactivity (<5% of the dose) was distributed to the brain after administration of ^{14}C-perindopril to rats.

Radioactivity was detectable in fetuses and in milk after administration of ^{14}C-perindopril to pregnant and lactating rats.

ELDERLY PATIENTS

Plasma concentrations of both perindopril and perindoprilat in elderly patients (>70 years) are approximately twice those observed in younger patients, reflecting both increased conversion of perindopril to perindoprilat and decreased renal excretion of perindoprilat. (See PRECAUTIONS, Geriatric Use.)

HEART FAILURE PATIENTS

Perindoprilat clearance is reduced in congestive heart failure patients, resulting in a 40% higher dose interval AUC. (See DOSAGE AND ADMINISTRATION.)

PATIENTS WITH RENAL INSUFFICIENCY

With perindopril erbumine doses of 2-4 mg, perindoprilat AUC increases with decreasing renal function. At creatinine clearances of 30-80 ml/min, AUC is about double that of 100 ml/min. When creatinine clearance drops below 30 ml/min, AUC increases more markedly.

In a limited number of patients studied, perindopril dialysis clearance ranged from 41.7-76.7 ml/min (mean 52.0 ml/min). Perindoprilat dialysis clearance ranged from 37.4-91.0 ml/min (mean 67.2 ml/min). (See DOSAGE AND ADMINISTRATION.)

PATIENTS WITH HEPATIC INSUFFICIENCY

The bioavailability of perindoprilat is increased in patients with impaired hepatic function. Plasma concentrations of perindoprilat in patients with impaired liver function were about 50% higher than those observed in healthy subjects or hypertensive patients with normal liver function.

PHARMACODYNAMICS

In placebo-controlled studies of perindopril monotherapy (2-16 mg qd) in patients with a mean blood pressure of about 150/100 mm Hg, 2 mg had little effect, but doses of 4-16 mg lowered blood pressure. The 8 and 16 mg doses were indistinguishable, and both had a greater effect than the 4 mg dose. The magnitude of the blood pressure effect was similar in the standing and supine positions, generally about 1 mm Hg greater on standing. In these studies, doses of 8 and 16 mg/day gave supine, trough blood pressure reductions of 9-15/5 to 6 mm Hg. When once-daily and twice-daily dosing were compared, the bid regimen was generally slightly superior, but by not more than about 0.5-1 mm Hg. After 2-16 mg doses of perindopril, the trough mean systolic and diastolic blood pressure effects were approximately equal to the peak effects (measured 3-7 hours after dosing). Trough effects were about 75-100% of peak effects. When perindopril was given to patients receiving 25 mg hydrochlorothiazide, it had an added effect similar in magnitude to its effect as monotherapy, but 2-8 mg doses were approximately equal in effectiveness. In general, the effect of perindopril occurred promptly, with effects increasing slightly over several weeks.

In hemodynamic studies carried out in animal models of hypertension, blood pressure reduction after perindopril administration was accompanied by a reduction in peripheral arterial resistance and improved arterial wall compliance. In studies carried out in patients with essential hypertension, the reduction in blood pressure was accompanied by a reduction in peripheral resistance with no significant changes in heart rate or glomerular filtration rate. An increase in the compliance of large arteries was also observed, suggesting a direct effect on arterial smooth muscle, consistent with the results of animal studies.

Formal interaction studies of perindopril erbumine have not been carried out with antihypertensive agents other than thiazides. Limited experience in controlled and uncontrolled trials coadministering perindopril erbumine with a calcium channel blocker, a loop diuretic or triple therapy (beta-blocker, vasodilator and a diuretic) do not suggest any unexpected interactions. In general, ACE inhibitors have less than additive effects when given with beta-adrenergic blockers, presumably because both work in part through the renin angiotension system. A controlled pharmacokinetic study has shown no effect on plasma digoxin concentrations when coadministered with perindopril erbumine. (See DRUG INTERACTIONS.)

In uncontrolled studies in patients with insulin-dependent diabetes, perindopril did not appear to affect glycemic control. In long-term use, no effect on urinary protein excretion was seen in these patients.

The effectiveness of perindopril erbumine was not influenced by sex and it was less effective in blacks than in nonblacks. In elderly patients (≥60 years), the mean blood pressure effect was somewhat smaller than in younger patients, although the difference was not significant.

INDICATIONS AND USAGE

Perindopril erbumine is indicated for the treatment of patients with essential hypertension. Perindopril erbumine may be used alone or given with other classes of antihypertensives, especially thiazide diuretics.

When using perindopril erbumine, consideration should be given to the fact that another angiotensin converting enzyme inhibitor (captopril) has caused agranulocytosis, particularly in patients with renal impairment or collagen vascular disease. Available data are insufficient to determine whether perindopril erbumine has a similar potential. (See WARNINGS.)

In considering use of perindopril erbumine, it should be noted that in controlled trials ACE inhibitors have an effect on blood pressure that is less in black patients than in nonblacks. In addition, it should be noted that black patients receiving ACE inhibitor monotherapy have been reported to have a higher incidence of angioedema compared to nonblacks. (See WARNINGS, Angioedema.)

NON-FDA APPROVED INDICATIONS

ACE inhibitors are also used for the treatment of heart failure, left ventricular dysfunction following myocardial infarction (MI), and diabetic nephropathy (greater than 500 mg/day proteinuria). Data have shown that the use of some ACE inhibitors improves survival and exercise tolerance and reduces the incidence of overt heart failure and subsequent hospitalizations in patients with recent MI. Data have also shown that the use of ACE inhibitors reduces the 3 year incidence of heart failure and related hospitalization in patients with asymptomatic left ventricular dysfunction.

CONTRAINDICATIONS

Perindopril erbumine is contraindicated in patients known to be hypersensitive to this product or to any other ACE inhibitor. Perindopril erbumine is also contraindicated in patients with a history of angioedema related to previous treatment with an ACE inhibitor.

WARNINGS

ANAPHYLACTOID AND POSSIBLY RELATED REACTIONS

Presumably because angiotensin-converting enzyme inhibitors affect the metabolism of eicosanoids and polypeptides, including endogenous bradykinin, patients receiving ACE inhibitors (including perindopril erbumine) may be subject to a variety of adverse reactions, some of them serious.

Angioedema

Angioedema involving the face, extremities, lips, tongue, glottis and/or larynx has been reported in patients treated with ACE inhibitors, including perindopril erbumine (0.1% of patients treated with perindopril erbumine in US clinical trials). In such cases, perindopril erbumine should be promptly discontinued and the patient carefully observed until the swelling disappears. In instances where swelling has been confined to the face and lips, the condition has generally resolved without treatment, although antihistamines have been useful in relieving symptoms. Angioedema associated with involvement of the tongue, glottis or larynx may be fatal due to airway obstruction. Appropriate therapy, such as subcutaneous epinephrine solution 1:1000 (0.3-0.5 ml), should be promptly administered. Patients with a history of angioedema unrelated to ACE inhibitor therapy may be at increased risk of angioedema while receiving an ACE inhibitor.

Anaphylactoid Reactions During Desensitization

Two patients undergoing desensitizing treatment with hymenoptera venom while receiving ACE inhibitors sustained life-threatening anaphylactoid reactions. In the same patients, these reactions were avoided when ACE inhibitors were temporarily withheld, but they reappeared upon inadvertent rechallenge.

Anaphylactoid Reactions During Membrane Exposure

Anaphylactoid reactions have been reported in patients dialyzed with high-flux membranes and treated concomitantly with an ACE inhibitor. Anaphylactoid reactions have also been reported in patients undergoing low-density lipoprotein apheresis with dextran sulfate absorption.

HYPOTENSION

Like other ACE inhibitors, perindopril erbumine can cause symptomatic hypotension. Perindopril erbumine has been associated with hypotension in 0.3% of uncomplicated hypertensive patients in US placebo-controlled trials. Symptoms related to orthostatic hypotension were reported in another 0.8% of patients.

Symptomatic hypotension associated with the use of ACE inhibitors is more likely to occur in patients who have been volume and/or salt-depleted, as a result of prolonged diuretic therapy, dietary salt restriction, dialysis, diarrhea or vomiting. Volume and/or salt depletion should be corrected before initiating therapy with perindopril erbumine. (See DOSAGE AND ADMINISTRATION.)

In patients with congestive heart failure, with or without associated renal insufficiency, ACE inhibitors may cause excessive hypotension, and may be associated with oliguria or azotemia, and rarely with acute renal failure and death. In patients with ischemic heart disease or cerebrovascular disease such an excessive fall in blood pressure could result in a myocardial infarction or a cerebrovascular accident.

In patients at risk of excessive hypotension, perindopril erbumine therapy should be started under very close medical supervision. Patients should be followed closely for the first 2 weeks of treatment and whenever the dose of perindopril erbumine and/or diuretic is increased.

If excessive hypotension occurs, the patient should be placed immediately in a supine position and, if necessary, treated with an intravenous infusion of physiological saline. Perindopril erbumine treatment can usually be continued following restoration of volume and blood pressure.

NEUTROPENIA/ANGRANULOCYTOSIS

Another ACE inhibitor, captopril, has been shown to cause agranulocytosis and bone marrow depression, rarely in uncomplicated patients but more frequently in patients with renal impairment, especially patients with a collagen vascular disease such as systemic lupus erythematosis or scleroderma. Available data from clinical trials of perindopril erbumine are insufficient to show whether perindopril erbumine causes agranulocytosis at similar rates.

FETAL/NEONATAL MORBIDITY AND MORTALITY

ACE inhibitors can cause fetal and neonatal morbidity and death when administered to pregnant women. Several dozen cases have been reported in the world literature. When pregnancy is detected, ACE inhibitors should be discontinued as soon as possible.

The use of ACE inhibitors during the second and third trimesters of pregnancy has been associated with fetal and neonatal injury, including hypotension, neonatal skull hypoplasia, anuria, reversible or irreversible renal failure and death. Oligohydramnios has also been reported, presumably resulting from decreased fetal renal function; oligohydramnios in this setting has been associated with fetal limb contractures, craniofacial deformation and hypoplastic lung development. Prematurity, intrauterine growth retardation and patent ductus arteriosus have also been reported, although it is not clear whether these occurrences were due to the ACE-inhibitor exposure.

These adverse effects do not appear to have resulted from intrauterine ACE-inhibitor exposure that has been limited to the first trimester. Mothers whose embryos and fetuses are exposed to ACE inhibitors only during the first trimester should be so informed. Nonetheless, when patients become pregnant, physicians should make every effort to discontinue the use of perindopril erbumine as soon as possible.

Rarely (probably less often than once in every thousand pregnancies), no alternative to ACE inhibitors will be found. In these rare cases, the mothers should be apprised of the potential hazards to their fetuses, and serial ultrasound examinations should be performed to assess the intra-amniotic environment.

If oligohydramnios is observed, perindopril erbumine should be discontinued unless it is considered life-saving for the mother. Contraction stress testing (CST), a non-stress test (NST) or biophysical profiling (BPP) may be appropriate, depending upon the week of pregnancy. Patients and physicians should be aware, however, that oligohydramnios may not appear until after the fetus has sustained irreversible injury.

Infants with histories of *in utero* exposure to ACE inhibitors should be closely observed for hypotension, oliguria and hyperkalemia. If oliguria occurs, attention should be directed toward support of blood pressure and renal perfusion. Exchange transfusion or dialysis may be required as means of reversing hypotension and/or substituting for disordered renal function. Perindopril, which crosses the placenta, can theoretically be removed from the neonatal circulation by these means, but limited experience has not shown that such removal is central to the treatment of these infants.

No teratogenic effects of perindopril were seen in studies of pregnant rats, mice, rabbits and cynomologous monkeys. On a mg/m basis, the doses used in these studies were 6 times (in mice), 670 times (in rats), 50 times (in rabbits) and 17 times (in monkeys) the maximum recommended human dose (assuming a 50 kg adult). On a mg/kg basis, these multiples are 60 times (in mice), 3.750 times (in rats), 150 times (in rabbits) and 50 times (in monkeys) the maximum recommended human dose.

HEPATIC FAILURE

Rarely, ACE inhibitors have been associated with a syndrome that starts with cholestatic jaundice and progresses to fulminant hepatic necrosis and (sometimes) death. The mechanism of this syndrome is not understood. Patients receiving ACE inhibitors who develop jaundice or marked elevations of hepatic enzymes should discontinue the ACE inhibitor and receive appropriate medical follow-up.

PRECAUTIONS

GENERAL

Impaired Renal Function

As a consequence of inhibiting the renin-angiotensin-aldosterone system, changes in renal function may be anticipated in susceptible individuals.

Hypertensive Patients With Congestive Heart Failure

In patients with severe congestive heart failure, where renal function may depend on the activity of the renin-angiotensin-aldosterone system, treatment with ACE inhibitors, including perindopril erbumine, may be associated with oliguria and/or progressive azotemia, and rarely with acute renal failure and/or death.

P

Hypertensive Patients With Renal Artery Stenosis

In hypertensive patients with unilateral or bilateral renal artery stenosis, increases in blood urea nitrogen and serum creatinine may occur. Experience with ACE inhibitors suggests that these increases are usually reversible upon discontinuation of the drug. In such patients, renal function should be monitored during the first few weeks of therapy.

Some hypertensive patients without apparent pre-existing renal vascular disease have developed increases in blood urea nitrogen and serum creatinine, usually minor and transient. These increases are more likely to occur in patients treated concomitantly with a diuretic and in patients with pre-existing renal impairment. Reduction of dosages of perindopril erbumine, the diuretic or both may be required. In some cases, discontinuation of either or both drugs may be necessary.

Evaluation of hypertensive patients should always include an assessment of renal function. (See DOSAGE AND ADMINISTRATION.)

Hyperkalemia

Elevations of serum potassium have been observed in some patients treated with ACE inhibitors, including perindopril erbumine. In US controlled clinical trials, 1.4% of the patients receiving perindopril erbumine and 2.3% of patients receiving placebo showed increased serum potassium levels to greater than 5.7 mEq/L. Most cases were isolated single values that did not appear clinically relevant and were rarely a cause for withdrawal. Risk factors for the development of hyperkalemia include renal insufficiency, diabetes mellitus and the concomitant use of agents such as potassium-sparing diuretics, potassium supplements and/or potassium-containing salt substitutes. Drugs associated with increases in serum potassium should be used cautiously, if at all, with perindopril erbumine. (See DRUG INTERACTIONS.)

Cough

Presumably due to the inhibition of the degradation of endogenous bradykinin, persistent nonproductive cough has been reported with all ACE inhibitors, always resolving after discontinuation of therapy. ACE inhibitor-induced cough should be considered in the differential diagnosis of cough. In controlled trials with perindopril, cough was present in 12% of perindopril patients and 4.5% of patients given placebo.

Surgery/Anesthesia

In patients undergoing surgery or during anesthesia with agents that produce hypotension, perindopril erbumine may block angiotensin II formation that would otherwise occur secondary to compensatory renin release. Hypotension attributable to this mechanism can be corrected by volume expansion.

INFORMATION FOR THE PATIENT

Angioedema

Angioedema, including laryngeal edema, can occur with ACE inhibitor therapy, especially following the first dose. Patients should be told to report immediately signs or symptoms suggesting angioedema (swelling of face, extremities, eyes, lips, tongue, hoarseness or difficulty in swallowing or breathing) and to take no more drug before consulting a physician.

Symptomatic Hypotension

As with any antihypertensive therapy, patients should be cautioned that lightheadedness can occur, especially during the first few days of therapy and that it should be reported promptly. Patients should be told that if fainting occurs, perindopril erbumine should be discontinued and a physician consulted.

All patients should be cautioned that inadequate fluid intake or excessive perspiration, diarrhea or vomiting can lead to an excessive fall in blood pressure in association with ACE inhibitor therapy.

Hyperkalemia

Patients should be advised not to use potassium supplements or salt substitutes containing potassium without a physician's advice.

Neutropenia

Patients should be told to report promptly any indication of infection (*e.g.*, sore throat, fever) which could be a sign of neutropenia.

Pregnancy

Female patients of childbearing age should be told about the consequences of second and third trimester exposure to ACE inhibitors, and they should also be told that these consequences do not appear to have resulted from intrauterine ACE-inhibitor exposure that has been limited to the first trimester. These patients should be asked to report pregnancies to their physicians as soon as possible.

CARCINOGENESIS, MUTAGENESIS, AND IMPAIRMENT OF FERTILITY

Carcinogenesis

No evidence of carcinogenic effect was observed in studies in rats and mice when perindopril was administered at dosages up to 20 times (mg/kg) or 2-4 times (mg/m^2) the maximum proposed clinical doses (16 mg/day) for 104 weeks.

Mutagenesis

No genotoxic potential was detected for perindopril erbumine, perindoprilat and other metabolites in various *in vitro* and *in vivo* investigations, including the Ames test, the *Saccharomyces cerevisiae* D4 test, cultured human lymphocytes, TK ± mouse lymphoma assay, mouse and rat micronucleus tests and Chinese hamster bone marrow assay.

Impairment of Fertility

There was no meaningful effect on reproductive performance or fertility in the rat given up to 30 times (mg/kg) or 6 times (mg/m^2) the proposed maximum clinical dosage of perindopril erbumine during the period of spermatogenesis in males or oogenesis and gestation in females.

PREGNANCY CATEGORY C (FRIST TRIMESTER) AND PREGNANCY CATEGORY D (SECOND AND THIRD TRIMESTERS)

See WARNINGS, Fetal/Neonatal Morbidity and Mortality.

NURSING MOTHERS

Milk of lactating rats contained radioactivity following administration ^{14}C-perindopril. It is not known whether perindopril is secreted in human milk. Because many drugs are secreted in human milk, caution should be exercised when perindopril erbumine is given to nursing mothers.

PEDIATRIC USE

Safety and effectiveness of perindopril erbumine in pediatric patients have not been established.

GERIATRIC USE

The mean blood pressure effect of perindopril was somewhat smaller in patients over 60 than in younger patients, although the difference was not significant. Plasma concentrations of both perindopril and perindoprilat were increased in elderly patients compared to concentrations in younger patients. No adverse effects were clearly increased in older patients with the exception of dizziness and possibly rash. Experience with perindopril erbumine in elderly patients at daily doses exceeding 8 mg is limited.

DRUG INTERACTIONS

DIURETICS

Patients on diuretics, and especially those started recently, may occasionally experience an excessive reduction of blood pressure after initiation of perindopril erbumine therapy. The possibility of hypotensive effects can be minimized by either discontinuing the diuretic or increasing the salt intake prior to initiation of treatment with perindopril. If diuretics cannot be interrupted, close medical supervision should be provided with the first dose of perindopril erbumine, for at least 2 hours and until blood pressure has stabilized for another hour. (See WARNINGS and DOSAGE AND ADMINISTRATION.)

The rate and extent of perindopril absorption and elimination are not affected by concomitant diuretics. The bioavailability of perindoprilat was reduced by diuretics, however, and this was associated with a decrease in plasma ACE inhibition.

POTASSIUM SUPPLEMENTS AND POTASSIUM-SPARING DIURETICS

Perindopril erbumine may increase serum potassium because of its potential to decrease aldosterone production. Use of potassium-sparing diuretics (spironolactone, amiloride, triamterene and others), potassium supplements or other drugs capable of increasing serum potassium (indomethacin, heparin, cyclosporine and others) can increase the risk of hyperkalemia. Therefore, if concomitant use of such agents is indicated, they should be given with caution and the patient's serum potassium should be monitored frequently.

LITHIUM

Increased serum lithium and symptoms of lithium toxicity have been reported in patients receiving concomitant lithium and ACE inhibitor therapy. These drugs should be coadministered with caution and frequent monitoring of serum lithium concentration is recommended. Use of a diuretic may further increase the risk of lithium toxicity.

DIGOXIN

A controlled pharmacokinetic study has shown no effect on plasma digoxin concentrations when coadministered with perindopril erbumine, but an effect of digoxin on the plasma concentration of perindopril/perindoprilat has not been excluded.

GENTAMICIN

Animal data have suggested the possibility of interaction between perindopril and gentamicin. However, this has not been investigated in human studies. Coadministration of both drugs should proceed with caution.

FOOD INTERACTION

Oral administration of perindopril erbumine with food does not significantly lower the rate or extent of perindopril absorption relative to the fasted state. However, the extent of biotransformation of perindopril to the active metabolite, perindoprilat, is reduced approximately 43%, resulting in a reduction in the plasma ACE inhibition curve of approximately 20%, probably clinically insignificant. In clinical trials, perindopril was generally administered in a non-fasting state.

ADVERSE REACTIONS

Perindopril erbumine has been evaluated for safety in approximately 3400 patients with hypertension in US and foreign clinical trials. Perindopril erbumine was in general well-tolerated in the patient populations studied, the side effects were usually mild and transient. Although dizziness was reported more frequently in placebo patients (8.5%) than in perindopril patients (8.2%), the incidence appeared to increase with an increase in perindopril dose.

The data presented here are based on results from the 1417 perindopril erbumine-treated patients who participated in the US clinical trials. Over 220 of these patients were treated with perindopril erbumine for at least 1 year.

In placebo-controlled US clinical trials, the incidence of premature discontinuation of therapy due to adverse events was 6.5% in patients treated with perindopril erbumine and 6.7% in patients treated with placebo. The most common causes were cough, headache, asthenia and dizziness.

Among 1012 patients in placebo-controlled US trials, the overall frequency of reported adverse events was similar in patients treated with perindopril erbumine and in those treated with placebo (approximately 75% in each group). Adverse events that occurred in 1% or greater of the patients and that were more common for perindopril than placebo by at least 1% (regardless of whether they were felt to be related to study drug) are shown in the first

TABLE 1 *Frequency of Adverse Events (%)*

	All Adverse Events		Possibly-or-Probably Related Adverse Events	
	Perindopril n=789	Placebo n=223	Perindopril n=789	Placebo n=223
Cough	12.0%	4.5%	6.0%	1.6%
Back pain	5.8%	3.1%	0.0%	0.0%
Sinusitis	5.2%	3.6%	0.6%	0.0%
Viral infection	3.4%	1.6%	0.3%	0.0%
Upper extremity pain	2.8%	1.4%	0.2%	0.0%
Hypertonia	2.7%	1.4%	0.2%	0.0%
Dyspepsia	1.9%	0.9%	0.3%	0.0%
Fever	1.5%	0.5%	0.3%	0.0%
Proteinuria	1.5%	0.5%	1.0%	0.5%
Ear infection	1.3%	0.0%	0.0%	0.0%
Palpitation	1.1%	0.0%	0.9%	0.0%

two columns below. Of these adverse events, those considered possibly or probably related to study drug are shown in the last two columns.

Of these, cough was the reason for withdrawal in 1.3% of perindopril and 0.4% of placebo patients. While dizziness was not reported more frequently in the perindopril group (8.2%) than in the placebo group (8.5%), it was clearly increased with dose, suggesting a causal relationship with perindopril. Other commonly reported complaints (1% or greater), regardless of causality, include headache (23.8%), upper respiratory infection (8.6%), asthenia (7.9%), rhinitis (4.8%), low extremity pain (4.7%), diarrhea (4.3%), edema (3.9%), pharyngitis (3.3%), urinary tract infection (2.8%), abdominal pain (2.7%), sleep disorder (2.5%), chest pain (2.4%), injury, paresthesia, nausea, rash (each 2.3%), seasonal allergy, depression (each 2.0%), abnormal ECG (1.8%), ALT increase (1.7%), tinnitus, vomiting (each 1.5%), neck pain, male sexual dysfunction (each 1.4%), triglyceride increase, somnolence (each 1.3%), joint pain, nervousness, myalgia, menstrual disorder (each 1.1%), flatulence and arthritis (each 1.0%), but none of those was more frequent by at least 1% on perindopril than on placebo. Depending on the specific adverse event, approximately 30-70% of the common complaints were considered possibly or probably related to treatment.

Below is a list (by body system) of adverse experiences reported in 0.3-1% of patients in US placebo-controlled studies without regard to attribution to therapy. Less frequent but medically important adverse events are also included, the incidence of these events is given in parentheses.

Body as a Whole: Malaise, pain, cold/hot sensation, chills, fluid retention, orthostatic symptoms, anaphylactic reaction, facial edema, angioedema (0.1%).

Gastrointestinal: Constipation, dry mouth, dry mucous membrane, appetite increased, gastroenteritis.

Respiratory: Posterior nasal drip, bronchitis, rhinorrhea, throat disorder, dyspnea, sneezing, epistaxis, hoarseness, pulmonary fibrosis (<0.1%).

Urogenital: Vaginitis, kidney stone, flank pain, urinary frequency, urinary retention.

Cardiovascular: Hypotension, ventricular extrasystole, myocardial infarction, vasodilation, syncope, abnormal conduction, heart murmur, orthostatic hypotension.

Endocrine: Gout.

Hematology: Hematoma, ecchymosis.

Musculoskeletal: Arthralgia, myalgia.

CNS: Migraine, amnesia, vertigo, cerebral vascular accident (0.2%).

Psychiatric: Anxiety, psychosexual disorder.

Dermatology: Sweating, skin infection, tinea, pruritus, dry skin, erythema, fever blisters, purpura (0.1%).

Special Senses: Conjunctivitis, earache.

Laboratory: Potassium decrease, uric acid increase, alkaline phosphatase increase, cholesterol increase, AST increase, creatinine increase, hematuria, glucose increase.

When perindopril erbumine was given concomitantly with thiazide diuretics, adverse events were generally reported at the same rate as those for perindopril erbumine alone, except for a higher incidence of abnormal laboratory findings known to be related to treatment with thiazide diuretics alone (*e.g.,* increases in serum uric acid, triglycerides and cholesterol and decreases in serum potassium).

POTENTIAL ADVERSE EFFECTS REPORTED WITH ACE INHIBITORS

Other medically important adverse effects reported with other available ACE inhibitors include: cardiac arrest, eosinophilic pneumonitis, neutropenia/agranulocytosis, pancytopenia, anemia (including hemolytic and aplastic), thrombocytopenia, acute renal failure, nephritis, hepatic failure, jaundice (hepatocellular or cholestatic), symptomatic hyponatremia, bullous pemphigus, exfoliative dermatitis and a syndrome which may include: arthralgia/arthritis, vasculitis, serositis, myalgia, fever, rash or other dermatologic manifestations, a positive ANA, leukocytosis, eosinophilia or an elevated ESR. Many of these adverse effects have also been reported for perindopril.

FETAL/NEONATAL MORBIDITY AND MORTALITY

See WARNINGS, Fetal/Neonatal Morbidity and Mortality.

CLINICAL LABORATORY TEST FINDINGS

Hematology, clinical chemistry and urinalysis parameters have been evaluated in US placebo-controlled trials. In general, there were no clinically significant trends in laboratory test findings.

Hyperkalemia: In clinical trials, 1.4% of the patients receiving perindopril erbumine and 2.3% of the patients receiving placebo showed serum potassium levels greater than 5.7 mEq/L. (See PRECAUTIONS.)

BUN/Serum Creatinine Elevations: Elevations, usually transient and minor, of BUN and serum creatinine have been observed. In placebo-controlled clinical trials, the proportion of patients experiencing increases in serum creatinine were similar in the perindopril erbumine and placebo treatment groups. Rapid reduction of long-standing or markedly elevated blood pressure by any antihypertensive therapy can result in decreases in the glomerular filtration rate and, in turn, lead to increases in BUN or serum creatinine. (See PRECAUTIONS.)

Hematology: Small decreases in hemoglobin and hematocrit occur frequently in hypertensive patients treated with perindopril erbumine, but are rarely of clinical importance. In controlled clinical trials, no patient was discontinued from therapy due to the development of anemia. Leukopenia (including neutropenia) was observed in 0.1% of patients in US clinical trials (see WARNINGS).

Liver Function Tests: Elevations in ALT (1.6% perindopril erbumine vs 0.9% placebo) and AST (0.5% perindopril erbumine vs 0.4% placebo) have been observed in US placebo-controlled clinical trials. The elevations were generally mild and transient and resolved after discontinuation of therapy.

DOSAGE AND ADMINISTRATION

USE IN UNCOMPLICATED HYPERTENSIVE PATIENTS

In patients with essential hypertension, the recommended initial dose is 4 mg once a day. The dosage may be titrated upward until blood pressure, when measured just before the next dose, is controlled or to a maximum of 16 mg/day. The usual maintenance dose range is 4-8 mg administered as a single daily dose. Perindopril erbumine may also be administered in two divided doses. When once-daily dosing was compared to twice-daily dosing in clinical studies, the bid regimen was generally slightly superior, but not by more than about 0.5-1.0 mm Hg.

USE IN THE ELDERLY PATIENTS

As in younger patients, the recommended initial dosages of perindopril erbumine for the elderly (>65 years) is 4 mg daily in one or in two divided doses. The daily dosage may be titrated upward until blood pressure, when measured just before the next dose, is controlled, but experience with perindopril erbumine is limited in the elderly at doses exceeding 8 mg. Dosages above 8 mg should be administered with caution and under close medical supervision. (See PRECAUTIONS, Geriatric Use.)

USE IN CONCOMITANT DIURETICS

If blood pressure is not adequately controlled with perindopril alone, a diuretic may be added. In patients currently being treated with a diuretic, symptomatic hypotension occasionally can occur following the initial dose of perindopril. To reduce likelihood of such reaction, the diuretic should, if possible, be discontinued 2-3 days prior to beginning of perindopril erbumine therapy. (See WARNINGS.) Then, if blood pressure is not controlled with perindopril erbumine alone, the diuretic should be resumed.

If the diuretic cannot be discontinued, an initial dose of 2-4 mg daily in one or in two divided doses should be used with careful medical supervision for several hours and until blood pressure has stabilized. The dosage should then be titrated as described above. (See WARNINGS and DRUG INTERACTIONS.)

USE IN PATIENTS WITH IMPAIRED RENAL FUNCTION

Kinetic data indicate that perindopril elimination is decreased in renally impaired patients, with a marked increase in accumulation when creatinine clearance drops below 30 ml/min. In such patients (creatinine clearance <30 ml/min), safety and efficacy of perindopril erbumine have not been established. For patients with lesser degrees of impairment (creatinine clearance above 30 ml/min), the initial dosage should be 2 mg/day and dosage should not exceed 8 mg/day due to limited clinical experience. During dialysis, perindopril is removed with the same clearance as in patients with normal renal function.

HOW SUPPLIED

Aceon tablets are available in:

2 mg: Scored one side, white, oblong (debossed "ACEON 2" on one side and debossed with "SLV" on both sides of score on the other side).

4 mg: Scored one side, pink, oblong (debossed "ACEON 4" on one side and debossed with "SLV" on both sides of score on the other side).

8 mg: Scored one side, salmon-colored, oblong (debossed "ACEON 8" on one side and debossed with "SLV" on both sides of score on the other side).

Storage: Store at controlled room temperature 20-25°C (68-77°F). Protect from moisture.

PRODUCT LISTING - EQUIVALENTS NOT AVAILABLE

Tablet - Oral - 2 mg
100's $120.99 ACEON, Solvay Pharmaceuticals Inc 00032-1101-01
Tablet - Oral - 4 mg
100's $120.99 ACEON, Solvay Pharmaceuticals Inc 00032-1102-01
Tablet - Oral - 8 mg
100's $185.55 ACEON, Solvay Pharmaceuticals Inc 00032-1103-01

P

Perphenazine (001988)

Categories: Nausea; Schizophrenia; Vomiting; FDA Approved 1957 Feb; Pregnancy Category C
Drug Classes: Antiemetics/antivertigo; Antipsychotics; Phenothiazines
Brand Names: Trilifon; **Trilafon**
Foreign Brand Availability: APO-Perphenazine (Canada; Malaysia); Decentan (Austria; Germany; Spain); Fentazin (England; Ireland); F-Mon (Japan); Leptopsique (Mexico); Peratsin (Finland); Pernamed (Thailand); Perphenan (Israel); Pernazine (Thailand); Perzine-P (Thailand); Porazine (Thailand); Trilifan Retard (France); Trimin (Bahrain; Cyprus; Egypt; Iran; Iraq; Israel; Jordan; Korea; Kuwait; Lebanon; Libya; Oman; Qatar; Republic-of-Yemen; Saudi-Arabia; Syria; United-Arab-Emirates); Triomin (Taiwan)
Cost of Therapy: $105.94 (Psychotic Disorders; Trilafon; 4 mg; 3 tablets/day; 30 day supply)
$49.37 (Psychotic Disorders; Generic Tablets; 4 mg; 3 tablets/day; 30 day supply)
HCFA JCODE(S): J3310 up to 5 mg IM, IV

DESCRIPTION

Trilafon products contain perphenazine (4-[3-(2-chlorophenothiazin-10-yl)propyl]-1-piperazineethanol), a piperazinyl phenothiazine having the chemical formula, $C_{21}H_{26}ClN_3OS$. They are available as **tablets,** 2, 4, 8, and 16 mg; and **injection,** perphenazine 5 mg/1 ml.

The inactive ingredients for Trilafon Tablets, 2, 4, 8, and 16 mg, include: Acacia, black iron oxide, butylparaben, calcium phosphate, calcium sulfate, carnauba wax, corn starch, lactose, magnesium stearate, sugar, titanium dioxide, and white wax.

The inactive ingredients for Trilafon Injection include: Citric acid, sodium bisulfite, sodium hydroxide, and water.

CLINICAL PHARMACOLOGY

MECHANISM OF ACTION

Perphenazine has actions at all levels of the central nervous system, particularly the hypothalamus. However, the site and mechanism of action of therapeutic effect are not known.

PHARMACOKINETICS

Following oral administration of perphenazine tablets, mean peak plasma perphenazine concentrations were observed between 1-3 hours. The plasma elimination half-life of perphenazine was independent of dose and ranged between 9 and 12 hours. In a study in which normal volunteers (n=12) received perphenazine 4 mg q8h for 5 days, steady-state concentrations of perphenazine were reached within 72 hours. Mean (%CV) C_{max} and C_{min} values for perphenazine and 7-hydroxyperphenazine at steady-state are listed in TABLE 1.

TABLE 1

Parameter	Perphenazine	7-Hydroxyperphenazine
C_{max} (pg/ml)	984 (43)	509 (25)
C_{min} (pg/ml)	442 (76)	350 (56)

Peak 7-hydroxyperphenazine concentrations were observed between 2-4 hours with a terminal phase half-life ranging between 9.9-18.8 hours. Perphenazine is extensively metabolized in the liver to a number of metabolites by sulfoxidation, hydroxylation, dealkylation, and glucuronidation. The pharmacokinetics of perphenazine covary with the hydroxylation of debrisoquine which is mediated by cytochrome P450 2D6 (CYP 2D6) and thus is subject to genetic polymorphism — *i.e.,* 7-10% of Caucasians and a low percentage of Asians have little or no activity and are called "poor metabolizers". Poor metabolizers of CYP 2D6 will metabolize perphenazine more slowly and will experience higher concentrations compared with normal or "extensive" metabolizers.

P

INDICATIONS AND USAGE

Perphenazine is indicated for use in the treatment of schizophrenia; and for the control of severe nausea and vomiting in adults.

Perphenazine has not been shown effective for the management of behavioral complications in patients with mental retardation.

CONTRAINDICATIONS

Perphenazine products are contraindicated in comatose or greatly obtunded patients and in patients receiving large doses of central nervous system depressants (barbiturates, alcohol, narcotics, analgesics, or antihistamines); in the presence of existing blood dyscrasias, bone marrow depression, or liver damage; and in patients who have shown hypersensitivity to perphenazine products, their components, or related compounds.

Perphenazine products are also contraindicated in patients with suspected or established subcortical brain damage, with or without hypothalamic damage, since a hyperthermic reaction with temperatures in excess of 104°F may occur in such patients, sometimes not until 14-16 hours after drug administration. Total body ice-packing is recommended for such a reaction; antipyretics may also be useful.

WARNINGS

Tardive dyskinesia, a syndrome consisting of potentially irreversible, involuntary, dyskinetic movements, may develop in patients treated with antipsychotic drugs. Older patients are at increased risk for development of tardive dyskinesia. Although the prevalence of the syndrome appears to be highest among the elderly, especially elderly women, it is impossible to rely upon prevalence estimates to predict, at the inception of antipsychotic treatment, which patients are likely to develop the syndrome. Whether antipsychotic drug products differ in their potential to cause tardive dyskinesia is unknown.

Both the risk of developing the syndrome and the likelihood that it will become irreversible are believed to increase as the duration of treatment and the total cumulative dose of antipsychotic drugs administered to the patient increase. However, the syndrome can develop, although much less commonly, after relatively brief treatment periods at low doses.

There is no known treatment for established cases of tardive dyskinesia, although the syndrome may remit, partially or completely, if antipsychotic treatment is withdrawn. Antipsychotic treatment itself, however, may suppress (or partially suppress) the signs and symptoms of the syndrome, and thereby may possibly mask the underlying disease process. The effect that symptomatic suppression has upon the long-term course of the syndrome is unknown.

Given these considerations, especially in the elderly, antipsychotics should be prescribed in a manner that is most likely to minimize the occurrence of tardive dyskinesia. Chronic antipsychotic treatment should generally be reserved for patients who suffer from a chronic illness that (1) is known to respond to antipsychotic drugs, and (2) for whom alternative, equally effective, but potentially less harmful treatments are not available or appropriate. In patients who do require chronic treatment, the smallest dose and the shortest duration of treatment producing a satisfactory clinical response should be sought. The need for continued treatment should be reassessed periodically.

If signs and symptoms of tardive dyskinesia appear in a patient on antipsychotics, drug discontinuation should be considered. However, some patients may require treatment despite the presence of the syndrome.

(For further information about the description of tardive dyskinesia and its clinical detection, please refer to PRECAUTIONS, Information for the Patient and ADVERSE REACTIONS.)

Perphenazine **injection** contains sodium bisulfite, a sulfite that may cause allergic-type reactions including anaphylactic symptoms and life-threatening or less severe asthmatic episodes in certain susceptible people. The overall prevalence of sulfite sensitivity is seen more frequently in asthmatic than in nonasthmatic people.

NEUROLEPTIC MALIGNANT SYNDROME (NMS)

A potentially fatal symptom complex, sometimes referred to as Neuroleptic Malignant Syndrome (NMS), has been reported in association with antipsychotic drugs. Clinical manifestations of NMS are hyperpyrexia, muscle rigidity, altered mental status and evidence of autonomic instability (irregular pulse or blood pressure, tachycardia, diaphoresis, and cardiac dysrhythmias).

The diagnostic evaluation of patients with this syndrome is complicated. In arriving at a diagnosis, it is important to identify cases where the clinical presentation includes both serious medical illness (*e.g.,* pneumonia, systemic infection, etc.) and untreated or inadequately treated extrapyramidal signs and symptoms (EPS). Other important considerations in the differential diagnosis include central anticholinergic toxicity, heat stroke, drug fever, and primary central nervous system (CNS) pathology.

The management of NMS should include (1) immediate discontinuation of antipsychotic drugs and other drugs not essential to concurrent therapy, (2) intensive symptomatic treatment and medical monitoring, and (3) treatment of any concomitant serious medical problems for which specific treatments are available. There is no general agreement about specific pharmacological treatment regimens for uncomplicated NMS.

If a patient requires antipsychotic drug treatment after recovery from NMS, the reintroduction of drug therapy should be carefully considered. The patient should be carefully monitored, since recurrences of NMS have been reported.

If hypotension develops, epinephrine should not be administered since its action is blocked and partially reversed by perphenazine. If a vasopressor is needed, norepinephrine may be used. Severe, acute hypotension has occurred with the use of phenothiazines and is particularly likely to occur in patients with mitral insufficiency or pheochromocytoma. Rebound hypertension may occur in pheochromocytoma patients.

Perphenazine products can lower the convulsive threshold in susceptible individuals; they should be used with caution in alcohol withdrawal and in patients with convulsive disorders. If the patient is being treated with an anticonvulsant agent, increased dosage of that agent may be required when perphenazine products are used concomitantly.

Perphenazine products should be used with caution in patients with psychic depression.

Perphenazine may impair the mental and/or physical abilities required for the performance of hazardous tasks such as driving a car or operating machinery; therefore, the patient should be warned accordingly.

Perphenazine products are not recommended for pediatric patients under 12 years of age.

USE IN PREGNANCY

Safe use of perphenazine during pregnancy and lactation has not been established; therefore, in administering the drug to pregnant patients, nursing mothers, or women who may become pregnant, the possible benefits must be weighed against the possible hazards to mother and child.

PRECAUTIONS

The possibility of suicide in depressed patients remains during treatment and until significant remission occurs. This type of patient should not have access to large quantities of this drug.

As with all phenothiazine compounds, perphenazine should not be used indiscriminately. Caution should be observed in giving it to patients who have previously exhibited severe adverse reactions to other phenothiazines. Some of the untoward actions of perphenazine tend to appear more frequently when high doses are used. However, as with other phenothiazine compounds, patients receiving perphenazine products in any dosage should be kept under close supervision.

Antipsychotic drugs elevate prolactin levels; the elevation persists during chronic administration. Tissue culture experiments indicate that approximately one-third of human breast cancers are prolactin dependent *in vitro,* a factor of potential importance if the prescription of these drugs is contemplated in a patient with a previously detected breast cancer. Although disturbances such as galactorrhea, amenorrhea, gynecomastia, and impotence have been reported, the clinical significance of elevated serum prolactin levels is unknown for most patients. An increase in mammary neoplasms has been found in rodents after chronic administration of antipsychotic drugs. Neither clinical studies nor epidemiologic studies conducted to date, however, have shown an association between chronic administration of these drugs and mammary tumorigenesis; the available evidence is considered too limited to be conclusive at this time.

The antiemetic effect of perphenazine may obscure signs of toxicity due to overdosage of other drugs, or render more difficult the diagnosis of disorders such as brain tumors or intestinal obstruction.

A significant, not otherwise explained, rise in body temperature may suggest individual intolerance to perphenazine, in which case it should be discontinued.

Patients on large doses of a phenothiazine drug who are undergoing surgery should be watched carefully for possible hypotensive phenomena. Moreover, reduced amounts of anesthetics or central nervous system depressants may be necessary.

Since phenothiazines and central nervous system depressants (opiates, analgesics, antihistamines, barbiturates) can potentiate each other, less than the usual dosage of the added drug is recommended and caution is advised when they are administered concomitantly.

Use with caution in patients who are receiving atropine or related drugs because of additive anticholinergic effects and also in patients who will be exposed to extreme heat or phosphorus insecticides.

The use of alcohol should be avoided, since additive effects and hypotension may occur. Patients should be cautioned that their response to alcohol may be increased while they are being treated with perphenazine products. The risk of suicide and the danger of overdose may be increased in patients who use alcohol excessively due to its potentiation of the drug's effect.

Blood counts and hepatic and renal functions should be checked periodically. The appearance of signs of blood dyscrasias requires the discontinuance of the drug and institution of appropriate therapy. If abnormalities in hepatic tests occur, phenothiazine treatment should be discontinued. Renal function in patients on long-term therapy should be monitored; if blood urea nitrogen (BUN) becomes abnormal, treatment with the drug should be discontinued.

The use of phenothiazine derivatives in patients with diminished renal function should be undertaken with caution.

Use with caution in patients suffering from respiratory impairment due to acute pulmonary infections, or in chronic respiratory disorders such as severe asthma or emphysema.

In general, phenothiazines, including perphenazine, do not produce psychic dependence. Gastritis, nausea and vomiting, dizziness, and tremulousness have been reported following abrupt cessation of high-dose therapy. Reports suggest that these symptoms can be reduced by continuing concomitant antiparkinson agents for several weeks after the phenothiazine is withdrawn.

The possibility of liver damage, corneal and lenticular deposits, and irreversible dyskinesias should be kept in mind when patients are on long-term therapy.

Because photosensitivity has been reported, undue exposure to the sun should be avoided during phenothiazine treatment.

INFORMATION FOR THE PATIENT

This information is intended to aid in the safe and effective use of this medication. It is not a disclosure of all possible adverse or intended effects.

Given the likelihood that a substantial proportion of patients exposed chronically to antipsychotics will develop tardive dyskinesia, it is advised that all patients in whom chronic use is contemplated be given, if possible, full information about this risk. The decision to inform patients and/or their guardians must obviously take into account the clinical circumstances and the competency of the patient to understand the information provided.

GERIATRIC USE

Clinical studies of perphenazine products did not include sufficient numbers of subjects aged 65 and over to determine whether elderly subjects respond differently from younger subjects. Other reported clinical experience has not identified differences in responses between the elderly and younger patients. In general, dose selection for an elderly patient should be cautious, usually starting at the low end of the dosing range, reflecting the greater frequency of decreased hepatic function, concomitant disease or other drug therapy.

Geriatric patients are particularly sensitive to the side effects of antipsychotics, including perphenazine. These side effects include extrapyramidal symptoms (tardive dyskinesia, antipsychotic-induced parkinsonism, akathisia), anticholinergic effects, sedation and orthostatic hypotension (see WARNINGS). Elderly patients taking psychotropic drugs may be at increased risk for falling and consequent hip fractures. Elderly patients should be started on lower doses and observed closely.

DRUG INTERACTIONS

Metabolism of a number of medications, including antipsychotics, antidepressants, β-blockers, and antiarrhythmics, occurs through the cytochrome P450 2D6 isoenzyme (debrisoquine hydroxylase). Approximately 10% of the Caucasian population has reduced activity of this enzyme, so-called "poor" metabolizers. Among other populations the prevalence is not known. Poor metabolizers demonstrate higher plasma concentrations of antipsychotic drugs at usual doses, which may correlate with emergence of side effects. In one study of 45 elderly patients suffering from dementia treated with perphenazine, the 5 patients who were prospectively identified as poor P450 2D6 metabolizers had reported significantly greater side effects during the first 10 days of treatment than the 40 extensive metabolizers, following which the groups tended to converge. Prospective phenotyping of elderly patients prior to antipsychotic treatment may identify those at risk for adverse events.

The concomitant administration of other drugs that inhibit the activity of P450 2D6 may acutely increase plasma concentrations of antipsychotics. Among these are tricyclic antidepressants and selective serotonin reuptake inhibitors, *e.g.,* fluoxetine, sertraline and paroxetine. When prescribing these drugs to patients already receiving antipsychotic therapy, close monitoring is essential and dose reduction may become necessary to avoid toxicity. Lower doses than usually prescribed for either the antipsychotic or the other drug may be required.

ADVERSE REACTIONS

Not all of the following adverse reactions have been reported with this specific drug; however, pharmacological similarities among various phenothiazine derivatives require that each be considered. With the piperazine group (of which perphenazine is an example), the extrapyramidal symptoms are more common, and others (*e.g.,* sedative effects, jaundice, and blood dyscrasias) are less frequently seen.

CNS Effects:

Extrapyramidal Reactions: Opisthotonus, trismus, torticollis, retrocollis, aching and numbness of the limbs, motor restlessness, oculogyric crisis, hyperreflexia, dystonia, including protrusion, discoloration, aching and rounding of the tongue, tonic spasm of the masticatory muscles, tight feeling in the throat, slurred speech, dysphagia, akathisia, dyskinesia, parkinsonism, and ataxia. Their incidence and severity usually increase with an increase in dosage, but there is considerable individual variation in the tendency to develop such symptoms. Extrapyramidal symptoms can usually be controlled by the concomitant use of effective antiparkinsonian drugs, such as benztropine mesylate, and/or by reduction in dosage. In some instances, however, these extrapyramidal reactions may persist after discontinuation of treatment with perphenazine.

Persistent Tardive Dyskinesia: As with all antipsychotic agents, tardive dyskinesia may appear in some patients on long-term therapy or may appear after drug therapy has been discontinued. Although the risk appears to be greater in elderly patients on high-dose therapy, especially females, it may occur in either sex and in children. The symptoms are persistent and in some patients appear to be irreversible. The syndrome is characterized by rhythmical, involuntary movements of the tongue, face, mouth, or jaw (*e.g.,* protrusion of tongue, puffing of cheeks, puckering of mouth, chewing movements). Sometimes these may be accompanied by involuntary movements of the extremities. There is no known effective treatment for tardive dyskinesia; antiparkinsonism agents usually do not alleviate the symptoms of this syndrome. It is suggested that all antipsychotic agents be discontinued if these symptoms appear. Should it be necessary to reinstitute treatment, or increase the dosage of the agent, or switch to a different antipsychotic agent, the syndrome may be masked. It has been reported that fine, vermicular movements of the tongue may be an early sign of the syndrome, and if the medication is stopped at that time the syndrome may not develop.

Other CNS Effects: Include cerebral edema; abnormality of cerebrospinal fluid proteins; convulsive seizures, particularly in patients with EEG abnormalities or a history of such disorders; and headaches.

Neuroleptic malignant syndrome has been reported in patients treated with antipsychotic drugs (see WARNINGS for further information).

Drowsiness may occur, particularly during the first or second week, after which it generally disappears. If troublesome, lower the dosage. Hypnotic effects appear to be minimal, especially in patients who are permitted to remain active.

Adverse behavioral effects include paradoxical exacerbation of psychotic symptoms, catatonic-like states, paranoid reactions, lethargy, paradoxical excitement, restlessness, hyperactivity, nocturnal confusion, bizarre dreams, and insomnia.

Hyperreflexia has been reported in the newborn when a phenothiazine was used during pregnancy.

Autonomic Effects:

Dry mouth or salivation, nausea, vomiting, diarrhea, anorexia, constipation, obstipation, fecal impaction, urinary retention, frequency or incontinence, bladder paralysis, polyuria, nasal congestion, pallor, myosis, mydriasis, blurred vision, glaucoma, perspiration, hypertension, hypotension, and change in pulse rate occasionally may occur. Significant autonomic effects have been infrequent in patients receiving less than 24 mg perphenazine daily.

Adynamic ileus occasionally occurs with phenothiazine therapy and if severe can result in complications and death. It is of particular concern in psychiatric patients, who may fail to seek treatment of the condition.

Allergic Effects:

Urticaria, erythema, eczema, exfoliative dermatitis, pruritus, photosensitivity, asthma, fever, anaphylactoid reactions, laryngeal edema, and angioneurotic edema; contact dermatitis in nursing personnel administering the drug; and in extremely rare instances, individual idiosyncrasy or hypersensitivity to phenothiazines has resulted in cerebral edema, circulatory collapse, and death.

Endocrine Effects:

Lactation, galactorrhea, moderate breast enlargement in females and gynecomastia in males on large doses, disturbances in the menstrual cycle, amenorrhea, changes in libido, inhibition of ejaculation, syndrome of inappropriate ADH (antidiuretic hormone) secretion, false positive pregnancy tests, hyperglycemia, hypoglycemia, glycosuria.

Cardiovascular Effects:

Postural hypotension, tachycardia (especially with sudden marked increase in dosage), bradycardia, cardiac arrest, faintness, and dizziness. Occasionally the hypotensive effect may produce a shock-like condition. ECG changes, nonspecific (quinidinelike effect) usually reversible, have been observed in some patients receiving phenothiazine antipsychotics.

Sudden death has occasionally been reported in patients who have received phenothiazines. In some cases the death was apparently due to cardiac arrest; in others, the cause appeared to be asphyxia due to failure of the cough reflex. In some patients, the cause could not be determined nor could it be established that the death was due to the phenothiazine.

Hematological Effects:

Agranulocytosis, eosinophilia, leukopenia, hemolytic anemia, thrombocytopenic purpura, and pancytopenia. Most cases of agranulocytosis have occurred between the fourth and tenth weeks of therapy. Patients should be watched closely, especially during that period, for the sudden appearance of sore throat or signs of infection. If white blood cell and differential cell counts show significant cellular depression, discontinue the drug and start appropriate therapy. However, a slightly lowered white count is not in itself an indication to discontinue the drug.

Other Effects:

Special considerations in long-term therapy include pigmentation of the skin, occurring chiefly in the exposed areas; ocular changes consisting of deposition of fine particulate matter in the cornea and lens, progressing in more severe cases to star-shaped lenticular opacities; epithelial keratopathies; and pigmentary retinopathy. *Also Noted:* Peripheral edema, reversed epinephrine effect, increase in PBI not attributable to an increase in thyroxine, parotid swelling (rare), hyperpyrexia, systemic lupus erythematosuslike syndrome, increases in appetite and weight, polyphagia, photophobia, and muscle weakness.

Liver damage (biliary stasis) may occur. Jaundice may occur, usually between the second and fourth weeks of treatment, and is regarded as a hypersensitivity reaction. Incidence is low. The clinical picture resembles infectious hepatitis but with laboratory features of obstructive jaundice. It is usually reversible; however, chronic jaundice has been reported.

Side effects with intramuscular perphenazine **injection** have been infrequent and transient. Dizziness or significant hypotension after treatment with perphenazine **injection** is a rare occurrence.

DOSAGE AND ADMINISTRATION

Dosage must be individualized and adjusted according to the severity of the condition and the response obtained. As with all potent drugs, the best dose is the lowest dose that will produce the desired clinical effect. Since extrapyramidal symptoms increase in frequency and severity with increased dosage, it is important to employ the lowest effective dose. These symptoms have disappeared upon reduction of dosage, withdrawal of the drug, or administration of an antiparkinsonian agent.

Prolonged administration of doses exceeding 24 mg daily should be reserved for hospitalized patients or patients under continued observation for early detection and management of adverse reactions. An antiparkinsonian agent, such as trihexyphenidyl hydrochloride or benztropine mesylate, is valuable in controlling drug-induced extrapyramidal symptoms.

PERPHENAZINE TABLETS

Suggested dosages for tablets for various conditions follow:

Moderately disturbed nonhospitalized patients with schizophrenia: Tablets 4-8 mg tid initially; reduce as soon as possible to minimum effective dosage.

Hospitalized patients with schizophrenia: Tablets 8-16 mg bid to qid; avoid dosages in excess of 64 mg daily.

Severe nausea and vomiting in adults: Tablets 8-16 mg daily in divided doses; 24 mg occasionally may be necessary; early dosage reduction is desirable.

PERPHENAZINE INJECTION

Intramuscular Administration

The injection is used when rapid effect and prompt control of acute or intractable conditions is required or when oral administration is not feasible. Perphenazine injection, administered by deep intramuscular injection, is well tolerated. The injection should be given with the patient seated or recumbent, and the patient should be observed for a short period after administration.

Therapeutic effect is usually evidenced in 10 minutes and is maximal in 1-2 hours. The average duration of effective action is 6 hours, occasionally 12-24 hours.

Pediatric dosage has not yet been established. Pediatric patients over 12 years may receive the lowest limit of adult dosage.

The usual initial dose is 5 mg (1 ml). This may be repeated every 6 hours. Ordinarily, the total daily dosage should not exceed 15 mg in ambulatory patients or 30 mg in hospitalized patients. When required for satisfactory control of symptoms in severe conditions, an initial 10 mg intramuscular dose may be given. Patients should be placed on oral therapy as soon as practicable. Generally, this may be achieved within 24 hours. In some instances, however, patients have been maintained on injectable therapy for several months. It has been established that perphenazine **injection** is more potent than perphenazine **tablets.** Therefore, equal or higher dosage should be used when the patient is transferred to oral therapy after receiving the injection.

Schizophrenia: While 5 mg of the **injection** has a definite tranquilizing effect, it may be necessary to use 10 mg doses to initiate therapy in severely agitated schizophrenic states. Most patients will be controlled and amenable to oral therapy within a maximum of 24-48 hours. Acute schizophrenic conditions (hysteria, panic reaction) often respond well to a single dose, whereas in chronic conditions, several injections may be required. When transferring patients to oral therapy, it is suggested that increased dosage be employed to maintain adequate clinical control. This should be followed by gradual reduction to the minimal maintenance dose which is effective.

Severe nausea and vomiting in adults: To obtain rapid control of vomiting, administer 5 mg (1 ml); in rare instances it may be necessary to increase the dose to 10 mg; in general, higher doses should be given only to hospitalized patients.

Intravenous Administration

The intravenous administration of perphenazine **injection** is seldom required. This route of administration should be used with particular caution and care, and only when absolutely necessary to control severe vomiting, intractable hiccoughs, or acute conditions, such as violent retching during surgery. Its use should be limited to recumbent hospitalized adults in doses not exceeding 5 mg. When employed in this manner, intravenous injection ordinarily should be given as a diluted solution by either fractional injection or a slow drip infusion. In the surgical patient, slow infusion of not more than 5 mg is preferred. When administered in divided doses, perphenazine **injection** should be diluted to 0.5 mg/ml (1 ml mixed with 9 ml of physiologic saline solution), and not more than 1 mg/injection given at not less than 1-2 minute intervals. Intravenous injection should be discontinued as soon as symptoms are controlled and should not exceed 5 mg. The possibility of hypotensive and extrapyramidal side effects should be considered and appropriate means for management kept available. Blood pressure and pulse should be monitored continuously during intravenous administration. Pharmacologic and clinical studies indicate that intravenous administration of norepinephrine should be useful in alleviating the hypotensive effect.

ELDERLY PATIENTS

With increasing age, plasma concentrations of perphenazine/daily ingested dose increase. Geriatric dosages of perphenazine preparations have not been established, but initiation of lower dosages is recommended. Optimal clinical effect or benefit may require lower doses for a longer duration. Dosing of perphenazine may occur before bedtime, if required.

HOW SUPPLIED

TRILAFON TABLETS

2 mg: Gray, sugar-coated tablets branded in black with the Schering trademark and the numbers, "1229".

4 mg: Gray, sugar-coated tablets branded in green with the Schering trademark and the numbers, "1232".

8 mg: Gray, sugar-coated tablets branded in blue with the Schering trademark and the numbers, "1251".

16 mg: Gray, sugar-coated tablets branded in red with the Schering trademark and the numbers, "1237".

Storage: Store between 2 and 25°C (36 and 77°F).

TRILAFON INJECTION

Trilafon injection is available in a 5 mg/ml, 1 ml ampule for intramuscular or intravenous use.

Storage: Store between 2 and 30°C (36 and 86°F). Keep package closed to protect from light. Exposure may cause discoloration. Slight yellowish discoloration will not alter potency or therapeutic efficacy; if markedly discolored, ampule should be discarded. **Protect from light. Store in carton until completely used.**

PRODUCT LISTING - RATED THERAPEUTICALLY EQUIVALENT

Tablet - Oral - 2 mg			
7's	$5.58	GENERIC, Prescript Pharmaceuticals	00247-0796-07
14's	$7.80	GENERIC, Prescript Pharmaceuticals	00247-0796-14
30's	$12.88	GENERIC, Prescript Pharmaceuticals	00247-0796-30
30's	$15.12	GENERIC, Heartland Healthcare Services	61392-0082-30
30's	$15.12	GENERIC, Heartland Healthcare Services	61392-0082-39
31 x 10	$166.94	GENERIC, Vangard Labs	00615-3584-53
31's	$15.62	GENERIC, Heartland Healthcare Services	61392-0082-31
32's	$16.13	GENERIC, Heartland Healthcare Services	61392-0082-32
45's	$22.68	GENERIC, Heartland Healthcare Services	61392-0082-45
60's	$30.24	GENERIC, Heartland Healthcare Services	61392-0082-60
90's	$45.36	GENERIC, Heartland Healthcare Services	61392-0082-90
100's	$10.03	GENERIC, Richmond Pharmaceuticals	54738-0550-01
100's	$28.01	FEDERAL UPPER LIMIT, H.C.F.A. F F P	99999-1988-01
100's	$40.90	GENERIC, Major Pharmaceuticals Inc	00904-1872-60
100's	$42.86	GENERIC, Moore, H.L. Drug Exchange Inc	00839-7423-06
100's	$45.50	GENERIC, Martec Pharmaceuticals Inc	52555-0380-01
100's	$45.95	GENERIC, Martec Pharmaceuticals Inc	52555-0569-01
100's	$45.99	GENERIC, Vintage Pharmaceuticals Inc	00254-4940-28
100's	$45.99	GENERIC, Qualitest Products Inc	00603-5090-21
100's	$46.00	GENERIC, Ivax Corporation	00172-3667-60
100's	$46.00	GENERIC, Warrick Pharmaceuticals Corporation	59930-1600-01
100's	$46.93	GENERIC, Major Pharmaceuticals Inc	00904-1872-61
100's	$53.89	GENERIC, Medirex Inc	57480-0442-01
100's	$68.82	GENERIC, Geneva Pharmaceuticals	00781-1046-01
100's	$77.42	GENERIC, Geneva Pharmaceuticals	00781-1046-13
100's	$86.03	TRILAFON, Schering Corporation	00085-0705-04
Tablet - Oral - 4 mg			
7's	$6.32	GENERIC, Prescript Pharmaceuticals	00247-0797-07
14's	$9.28	GENERIC, Prescript Pharmaceuticals	00247-0797-14
30's	$16.06	GENERIC, Prescript Pharmaceuticals	00247-0797-30
30's	$17.99	GENERIC, Heartland Healthcare Services	61392-0081-30
30's	$17.99	GENERIC, Heartland Healthcare Services	61392-0081-39
31 x 10	$231.26	GENERIC, Vangard Labs	00615-3585-53
31's	$18.59	GENERIC, Heartland Healthcare Services	61392-0081-31
32's	$19.19	GENERIC, Heartland Healthcare Services	61392-0081-32
45's	$26.99	GENERIC, Heartland Healthcare Services	61392-0081-45
50's	$24.53	GENERIC, Prescript Pharmaceuticals	00247-0797-50
60's	$35.98	GENERIC, Heartland Healthcare Services	61392-0081-60
90's	$53.97	GENERIC, Heartland Healthcare Services	61392-0081-90
100's	$13.74	GENERIC, Richmond Pharmaceuticals	54738-0551-01
100's	$34.48	FEDERAL UPPER LIMIT, H.C.F.A. F F P	99999-1988-03
100's	$54.85	GENERIC, Major Pharmaceuticals Inc	00904-1873-60
100's	$55.22	GENERIC, Aligen Independent Laboratories Inc	00405-4780-01
100's	$58.25	GENERIC, Moore, H.L. Drug Exchange Inc	00839-7424-06
100's	$60.28	GENERIC, Major Pharmaceuticals Inc	00904-1873-61
100's	$64.15	GENERIC, Medirex Inc	57480-0443-01
100's	$64.90	GENERIC, Martec Pharmaceuticals Inc	52555-0381-01
100's	$64.90	GENERIC, Martec Pharmaceuticals Inc	52555-0570-01
100's	$64.99	GENERIC, Vintage Pharmaceuticals Inc	00254-4941-28
100's	$64.99	GENERIC, Qualitest Products Inc	00603-5091-21
100's	$65.00	GENERIC, Ivax Corporation	00172-3668-60
100's	$65.00	GENERIC, Warrick Pharmaceuticals Corporation	59930-1603-01
100's	$94.17	GENERIC, Geneva Pharmaceuticals	00781-1047-01
100's	$105.93	GENERIC, Geneva Pharmaceuticals	00781-1047-13
100's	$117.71	TRILAFON, Schering Corporation	00085-0940-05
Tablet - Oral - 8 mg			
7's	$6.96	GENERIC, Prescript Pharmaceuticals	00247-0798-07
14's	$10.58	GENERIC, Prescript Pharmaceuticals	00247-0798-14
30's	$18.84	GENERIC, Prescript Pharmaceuticals	00247-0798-30
30's	$29.40	GENERIC, Heartland Healthcare Services	61392-0142-30
30's	$29.40	GENERIC, Heartland Healthcare Services	61392-0142-39
31 x 10	$306.13	GENERIC, Vangard Labs	00615-4511-53
31's	$30.38	GENERIC, Heartland Healthcare Services	61392-0142-31
32's	$31.36	GENERIC, Heartland Healthcare Services	61392-0142-32
45's	$44.10	GENERIC, Heartland Healthcare Services	61392-0142-45
60's	$58.80	GENERIC, Heartland Healthcare Services	61392-0142-60
90's	$88.20	GENERIC, Heartland Healthcare Services	61392-0142-90
100's	$12.23	GENERIC, Richmond Pharmaceuticals	54738-0552-01

P

100's	$65.60	GENERIC, Major Pharmaceuticals Inc	00904-1874-60
100's	$67.30	GENERIC, Aligen Independent Laboratories Inc	00405-4781-01
100's	$70.19	GENERIC, Moore, H.L. Drug Exchange Inc	00839-7425-06
100's	$71.38	GENERIC, Major Pharmaceuticals Inc	00904-1874-61
100's	$77.85	GENERIC, Martec Pharmaceuticals Inc	52555-0382-01
100's	$77.95	GENERIC, Martec Pharmaceuticals Inc	52555-0571-01
100's	$77.99	GENERIC, Vintage Pharmaceuticals Inc	00254-4942-28
100's	$77.99	GENERIC, Qualitest Products Inc	00603-5092-21
100's	$78.00	GENERIC, Ivax Corporation	00172-3669-60
100's	$78.00	GENERIC, Warrick Pharmaceuticals Corporation	59930-1605-01
100's	$98.00	GENERIC, Medirex Inc	57480-0444-01
100's	$114.25	GENERIC, Geneva Pharmaceuticals	00781-1048-01
100's	$128.52	GENERIC, Geneva Pharmaceuticals	00781-1048-13
100's	$142.81	TRILAFON, Schering Corporation	00085-0313-05
Tablet - Oral - 16 mg			
7's	$7.99	GENERIC, Prescript Pharmaceuticals	00247-0799-07
14's	$12.62	GENERIC, Prescript Pharmaceuticals	00247-0799-14
30's	$23.21	GENERIC, Prescript Pharmaceuticals	00247-0799-30
31 x 10	$353.46	GENERIC, Vangard Labs	00615-4512-53
100's	$27.71	GENERIC, Richmond Pharmaceuticals	54738-0553-01
100's	$63.77	FEDERAL UPPER LIMIT, H.C.F.A. F F P	99999-1988-08
100's	$71.52	GENERIC, Major Pharmaceuticals Inc	00904-1875-61
100's	$89.25	GENERIC, Major Pharmaceuticals Inc	00904-1875-60
100's	$90.82	GENERIC, Aligen Independent Laboratories Inc	00405-4782-01
100's	$95.18	GENERIC, Moore, H.L. Drug Exchange Inc	00839-7426-06
100's	$107.55	GENERIC, Martec Pharmaceuticals Inc	52555-0383-01
100's	$107.55	GENERIC, Martec Pharmaceuticals Inc	52555-0572-01
100's	$107.99	GENERIC, Vintage Pharmaceuticals Inc	00254-4943-28
100's	$107.99	GENERIC, Qualitest Products Inc	00603-5093-21
100's	$108.00	GENERIC, Ivax Corporation	00172-3670-60
100's	$108.00	GENERIC, Warrick Pharmaceuticals Corporation	59930-1610-01
100's	$114.10	GENERIC, Geneva Pharmaceuticals	00781-1049-13
100's	$153.70	GENERIC, Geneva Pharmaceuticals	00781-1049-01
100's	$192.13	TRILAFON, Schering Corporation	00085-0077-05

PRODUCT LISTING - EQUIVALENTS NOT AVAILABLE

Concentrate - Oral - 16 mg/5 ml			
118 ml	$39.73	GENERIC, Pharmaceutical Assoc Inc Div Beach Products	00121-0673-04
118 ml	$44.64	TRILAFON, Schering Corporation	00085-0363-02
Solution - Injectable - 5 mg/ml			
1 ml x 100	$782.50	TRILAFON, Schering Corporation	00085-0012-04
Tablet - Oral - 4 mg			
30's	$10.24	GENERIC, Physicians Total Care	54868-2686-00
Tablet - Oral - 8 mg			
100's	$27.69	GENERIC, Physicians Total Care	54868-2687-01

Phenelzine Sulfate *(001999)*

For related information, see the comparative table section in Appendix A.

Categories: Depression; FDA Approved 1961 Jun; Pregnancy Category C
Drug Classes: Antidepressants, monoamine oxidase inhibitors
Brand Names: Nardil
Foreign Brand Availability: Nardelzine (Belgium; Spain)
Cost of Therapy: $48.74 (Depression; Nardil; 15 mg; 3 tablets/day; 30 day supply)

DESCRIPTION

Phenelzine sulfate is a potent inhibitor of monoamine oxidase (MAO). Chemically, it is a hydrazine derivative.

Each tablet contains phenelzine sulfate equivalent to 15 mg of phenelzine base. Also contains: acacia; calcium carbonate; carnauba wax; corn starch; FD&C yellow no. 6; gelatin; kaolin; magnesium stearate; mannitol; pharmaceutical glaze; povidone; sucrose; talc; white wax; white wheat flour.

CLINICAL PHARMACOLOGY

Monoamine oxidase is a complex enzyme system, widely distributed throughout the body. Drugs that inhibit monoamine oxidase in the laboratory are associated with a number of clinical effects. Thus, it is unknown whether MAO inhibition *per se*, other pharmacologic actions, or an interaction of both, is responsible for the clinical effects observed. Therefore, the physician should become familiar with all the effects produced by drugs of this class.

INDICATIONS AND USAGE

Phenelzine sulfate has been found to be effective in depressed patients clinically characterized as "atypical," "nonendogenous," or "neurotic." These patients often have mixed anxiety and depression and phobic or hypochondriacal features. There is less conclusive evidence of its usefulness with severely depressed patients with endogenous features.

Phenelzine sulfate should rarely be the first antidepressant drug used. Rather, it is more suitable for use with patients who have failed to respond to the drugs more commonly used for these conditions.

CONTRAINDICATIONS

Phenelzine sulfate is contraindicated in patients with known sensitivity to the drug, pheochromocytoma, congestive heart failure, a history of liver disease, or abnormal liver function tests.

The potentiation of sympathomimetic substances and related compounds by MAO inhibitors may result in hypertensive crises (see WARNINGS). Therefore, patients being treated with phenelzine sulfate should not take **sympathomimetic drugs** (including amphetamines, cocaine, methylphenidate, dopamine, epinephrine and norepinephrine) or related compounds (including methyldopa, L-dopa, L-tryptophan, L-tyrosine, and phenylalanine). Hypertensive crises during phenelzine sulfate therapy may also be caused by the ingestion of foods with a high concentration of tyramine or dopamine. Therefore, patients being treated with phenelzine sulfate should avoid high protein food that has undergone protein breakdown by aging, fermentation, pickling, smoking, or bacterial contamination; patients should also avoid cheeses (especially aged varieties), pickled herring, beer, wine, liver, yeast extract (including brewer's yeast in large quantities), dry sausage (including Genoa salami, hard salami, pepperoni, and Lebanon bologna), pods of broad beans (fava beans), and yogurt. Excessive amounts of caffeine and chocolate may also cause hypertensive reactions.

WARNINGS

Important

The most serious reactions to phenelzine sulfate involve changes in blood pressure.Hypertensive Crises: The most important reaction associated with phenelzine sulfate administration is the occurrence of hypertensive crises, which have sometimes been fatal.These crises are characterized by some or all of the following symptoms: Occipital headache which may radiate frontally, palpitation, neck stiffness or soreness, nausea, vomiting, sweating (sometimes with fever and sometimes with cold, clammy skin), dilated pupils, and photophobia. Either tachycardia or bradycardia may be present and can be associated with constricting chest pain.Note: Intracranial bleeding has been reported in association with the increase in blood pressure.

Blood pressure should be observed frequently to detect evidence of any pressor response in all patients receiving phenelzine sulfate. Therapy should be discontinued immediately upon the occurrence of palpitation or frequent headaches during therapy.

RECOMMENDED TREATMENT IN HYPERTENSIVE CRISIS

If a hypertensive crisis occurs, phenelzine sulfate should be discontinued immediately and therapy to lower blood pressure should be instituted immediately. On the basis of present evidence, phentolamine is recommended. (The dosage reported for phentolamine is 5 mg intravenously.) Care should be taken to administer this drug slowly in order to avoid producing an excessive hypotensive effect. Fever should be managed by means of external cooling.

WARNING TO THE PATIENT

All patients should be warned that the following foods, beverages and medications must be avoided while taking phenelzine sulfate, and for 2 weeks after discontinuing use.

Foods and Beverages to Avoid

Meat and Fish: Pickled herring, liver, dry sausage (including Genoa salami, hard salami, pepperoni, and Lebanon bologna).
Vegetables: Broad bean pods (fava bean pods).
Dairy Products: Cheese (cottage cheese and cream cheese are allowed), yogurt.
Beverages: Beer and wine, alcohol-free and reduced-alcohol beer and wine products.
Miscellaneous: Yeast extract (including brewer's yeast in large quantities), excessive amounts of chocolate and caffeine.

Also, any spoiled or improperly refrigerated, handled or stored protein-rich foods such as meats, fish, and dairy products, including foods that may have undergone protein changes by aging, pickling, fermentation, or smoking to improve flavor should be avoided.

OTC Medications to Avoid

Cold and cough preparations (including those containing dextromethorphan)
Nasal decongestants (tablets, drops or spray)
Hay-fever medications
Sinus medications
Asthma inhalant medications
Antiappetite medicines
Weight-reducing preparations
"Pep" pills
L-tryptophan containing preparations

Also, certain prescription drugs should be avoided. Therefore, patients under the care of another physician or dentist should inform him/her that they are taking phenelzine sulfate.

Patients should be warned that the use of the above foods, beverages or medications may cause a reaction characterized by headache and other serious symptoms due to a rise in blood pressure, with the exception of dextromethorphan which may cause reactions similar to those seen with meperidine.

Patients should be instructed to report promptly the occurrence of headache or other unusual symptoms.

USE IN PREGNANCY

The safe use of phenelzine sulfate during pregnancy or lactation has not been established. The potential benefit of this drug, if used during pregnancy, lactation or in women of childbearing age, should be weighed against the possible hazard to the mother or fetus.

Doses of phenelzine sulfate in pregnant mice well exceeding the maximum recommended human dose have caused a significant decrease in the number of viable offspring per mouse. In addition, the growth of young dogs and rats has been retarded by doses exceeding the maximum human dose.

USE IN CHILDREN

Phenelzine sulfate is not recommended for patients under 16 years of age, since there are no controlled studies of safety in this age group.

Phenelzine sulfate, as with other hydrazine derivatives, has been reported to induce pulmonary and vascular tumors in an uncontrolled lifetime study in mice.

PRECAUTIONS

In depressed patients, the possibility of suicide should always be considered and adequate precautions taken. It is recommended that careful observations of patients undergoing phenelzine sulfate treatment be maintained until control of depression is achieved. If necessary, additional measures (ECT, hospitalization, etc) should be instituted.

All patients undergoing treatment with phenelzine sulfate should be closely followed for symptoms of postural hypotension. Hypotensive side effects have occurred in hypertensive as well as normal and hypotensive patients. Blood pressure usually returns to pretreatment levels rapidly when the drug is discontinued or the dosage is reduced.

Because the effect of phenelzine sulfate on the convulsive threshold may be variable, adequate precautions should be taken when treating epileptic patients.

Of the more severe side effects that have been reported with any consistency, hypomania has been the most common. This reaction has been largely limited to patients in whom disorders characterized by hyperkinetic symptoms coexist with, but are obscured by, depressive affect; hypomania usually appeared as depression improved. If agitation is present, it may be increased with phenelzine sulfate. Hypomania and agitation have also been reported at higher than recommended doses or following long-term therapy.

Phenelzine sulfate may cause excessive stimulation in schizophrenic patients; in manic-depressive states it may result in a swing from a depressive to a manic phase.

MAO inhibitors, including phenelzine sulfate, potentiate hexobarbital hypnosis in animals. Therefore, barbiturates should be given at a reduced dose with phenelzine sulfate.

MAO inhibitors inhibit the destruction of serotonin and norepinephrine, which are believed to be released from tissue stores by rauwolfia alkaloids. Accordingly, caution should be exercised when rauwolfia is used concomitantly with an MAO inhibitor, including phenelzine sulfate.

There is conflicting evidence as to whether or not MAO inhibitors affect glucose metabolism or potentiate hypoglycemic agents. This should be kept in mind if phenelzine sulfate is administered to diabetics.

DRUG INTERACTIONS

Phenelzine sulfate should not be used in combination with dextromethorphan or with CNS depressants such as alcohol and certain narcotics. Excitation, seizures, delirium, hyperpyrexia, circulatory collapse, coma, and death have been reported in patients receiving MAOI therapy who have been given a single dose of meperidine. Phenelzine sulfate should not be administered together with or in rapid succession to other MAO inhibitors because HYPERTENSIVE CRISES and convulsive seizures, fever, marked sweating, excitation, delirium, tremor, coma, and circulatory collapse may occur (TABLE 1).

TABLE 1 *List of MAO Inhibitors*

Generic Name	Trademark
Pargyline hydrochloride	Eutonyl (Abbott Laboratories)
Pargyline hydrochloride and methyclothiazide	Eutron (Abbott Laboratories)
Furazolidone	Furoxone (Eaton Laboratories)
Isocarboxazid	Marplan (Roche)
Procarbazine	Matulane (Roche)
Tranylcypromine	Parnate (Smith Kline & French Laboratories)

Phenelzine sulfate should also not be used in combination with buspirone HCl, since several cases of elevated blood pressure have been reported in patients taking MAO inhibitors who were then given buspirone HCl. At least 10 days should elapse between the discontinuation of phenelzine sulfate and the institution of another antidepressant or buspirone HCl, or the discontinuation of another MAO inhibitor and the institution of phenelzine sulfate.

There have been reports of serious reactions (including hyperthermia, rigidity, myoclonic movements and death) when fluoxetine has been combined with an MAO inhibitor. Therefore, phenelzine sulfate should not be used in combination with fluoxetine. Allow at least 5 weeks between discontinuation of fluoxetine and initiation of phenelzine sulfate and at least 10 days between discontinuation of phenelzine sulfate and initiation of fluoxetine.

Patients taking phenelzine sulfate should not undergo elective surgery requiring general anesthesia. Also they should not be given cocaine or local anesthesia containing sympathomimetic vasoconstrictors. The possible combined hypotensive effects of phenelzine sulfate and spinal anesthesia should be kept in mind. Phenelzine sulfate should be discontinued at least 10 days prior to elective surgery.

CONCOMITANT USE WITH DIBENZAZEPINE DERIVATIVE DRUGS

If the decision is made to administer phenelzine sulfate concurrently with other antidepressant drugs, or within less than 10 days after discontinuation of antidepressant therapy, the patient should be cautioned by the physician regarding the possibility of adverse drug interaction (TABLE 2).

Phenelzine sulfate should be used with caution in combination with antihypertensive drugs, including thiazide diuretics and β-blockers, since exaggerated hypotensive effects may result. MAO inhibitors including phenelzine sulfate, are contraindicated in patients receiving guanethidine.

ADVERSE REACTIONS

Phenelzine sulfate is a potent inhibitor of monoamine oxidase. Because this enzyme is widely distributed throughout the body, diverse pharmacologic effects can be expected to occur. When they occur, such effects tend to be mild or moderate in severity (see below), often subside as treatment continues, and can be minimized by adjusting dosage; rarely is it necessary to institute counteracting measures or to discontinue phenelzine sulfate.

TABLE 2 *Phenelzine Sulfate, Drug Interactions*

Generic Name	Trademark
Nortriptyline hydrochloride	Aventyl (Eli Lilly & Co)
Amitriptyline hydrochloride	Elavil (Merck Sharp & Dohme)
Amitriptyline hydrochloride	Endep (Roche)
Perphenazine and amitriptyline Hydrochloride	Etrafon (Schering Corporation)
Perphenazine and amitriptyline Hydrochloride	Triavil (Merck Sharp & Dohme)
Clomipramine hydrochloride	Anafranil (CIBA-Geigy)
Desipramine hydrochloride	Norpramin (Merrell-National)
Desipramine hydrochloride	Pertofrane (USV)
Imipramine hydrochloride	Tofranil (Geigy)
Doxepin	Adapin (Pennwalt)
Doxepin	Sinequan (Pfizer)
Carbamazepine	Tegretol (Geigy)
Cyclobenzaprine HCl	Flexeril (Merck Sharp & Dohme)
Amoxapine	Asendin (Lederle)
Maprotiline HCl	Ludiomil (CIBA)
Trimipramine maleate	Surmontil (Wyeth)
Protriptyline HCl	Vivactil (Merck Sharp & Dohme)

Common Side Effects Include:

Nervous System: Dizziness, headache, drowsiness, sleep disturbances (including insomnia and hypersomnia), fatigue, weakness, tremors, twitching, myoclonic movements, hyperreflexia.

Gastrointestinal: Constipation, dry mouth, gastrointestinal disturbances, elevated serum transaminases (without accompanying signs and symptoms).

Metabolic: Weight gain.

Cardiovascular: Postural hypotension, edema.

Genitourinary: Sexual disturbances, *i.e.*, anorgasmia and ejaculatory disturbances.

Less common mild to moderate side effects (some of which have been reported in a single patient or by a single physician) include:

Nervous System: Jitteriness, palilalia, euphoria, nystagmus, paresthesias.

Genitourinary: Urinary retention.

Metabolic: Hypernatremia.

Dermatologic: Skin rash, sweating.

Special Senses: Blurred vision, glaucoma.

Although reported less frequently, and sometimes only once, additional severe side effects include:

Nervous System: Ataxia, shock-like coma, toxic delirium, manic reaction, convulsions, acute anxiety reaction, precipitation of schizophrenia, transient respiratory and cardiovascular depression following ECT.

Gastrointestinal: To date, fatal progressive necrotizing hepatocellular damage has been reported in very few patients. Reversible jaundice.

Hematologic: Leukopenia.

Metabolic: Hypermetabolic syndrome (which may include, but is not limited to, hyperpyrexia, tachycardia, tachypnea, muscular rigidity, elevated CK levels, metabolic acidosis, hypoxia, coma and may resemble an overdose).

Respiratory: Edema of the glottis.

Withdrawal may be associated with nausea, vomiting and malaise.

An uncommon withdrawal syndrome following abrupt withdrawal of phenelzine sulfate has been infrequently reported. Signs and symptoms of this syndrome generally commence 24-72 hours after drug discontinuation and may range from vivid nightmares with agitation to frank psychosis and convulsions. This syndrome generally responds to reinstitution of low- dose phenelzine sulfate therapy followed by cautious downward titration and discontinuation.

DOSAGE AND ADMINISTRATION

Initial Dose: The usual starting dose of phenelzine sulfate is 1 tablet (15 mg) 3 times a day.

Early Phase Treatment: Dosage should be increased to at least 60 mg/day at a fairly rapid pace consistent with patient tolerance. It may be necessary to increase dosage up to 90 mg/day to obtain sufficient MAO inhibition. Many patients do not show a clinical response until treatment at 60 mg has been continued for at least 4 weeks.

Maintenance Dose: After maximum benefit from phenelzine sulfate is achieved, dosage should be reduced slowly over several weeks. Maintenance dose may be as low as 1 tablet, 15 mg, a day or every other day, and should be continued for as long as is required.

HOW SUPPLIED

Each orange-coated Nardil tablet bears the P-D 270 monogram and contains phenelzine sulfate equivalent to 15 mg of phenelzine base.

Storage: Store between 15-30°C (59-86°F).

PRODUCT LISTING - EQUIVALENTS NOT AVAILABLE

Tablet - Oral - 15 mg

100's	$54.15	NARDIL, Parke-Davis	00071-0270-24

Phenobarbital (002005)

Categories: Insomnia; Preanesthesia; Sedation; Seizures, generalized tonic-clonic; Seizures, partial; Status epilepticus; Pregnancy Category D; DEA Class CIV; FDA Pre 1938 Drugs; WHO Formulary
Drug Classes: Anticonvulsants; Barbiturates; Preanesthetics; Sedatives/hypnotics
Brand Names: Luminal; Solfoton
Foreign Brand Availability: Andral (Philippines); Atrofen (Dominican-Republic); Barbilettae (Finland); Barbiphenyl (Finland); Fenemal (Denmark; Norway); Fenemal NM Pharma (Sweden); Fenobarbital (Ecuador); Gardenal (Belgium; France; Greece; India; South-Africa; Spain); Gardenale (Italy); Lethyl (South-Africa); Linasen (Japan); Luminal (Argentina; Belgium; Germany; India; Philippines; Spain); Luminale (Italy); Luminaletas (Argentina; Spain); Luminaletten (Germany); Luminalettes (Belgium); Menobarb (Thailand); Phenobal (Japan); Phenobarbitone (Australia; New-Zealand); Phenotal (Thailand)
Cost of Therapy: $0.06 (Insomnia; Generic Tablets; 30 mg; 1 tablet/day; 10 day supply)
$0.80 (Epilepsy; Generic Tablets; 60 mg; 1 tablet/day; 30 day supply)
HCFA JCODE(S): J2560 up to 120 mg IM, IV

DESCRIPTION

The barbiturates are nonselective central nervous system (CNS) depressants which are primarily used as sedative hypnotics and are also anticonvulsants in subhypnotic doses. The barbiturates and their sodium salts are subject to control under the Federal Controlled Substances Act.

Barbiturates are substituted pyrimidine derivatives in which the basic structure common to these drugs is barbituric acid, a substance which has no CNS activity. CNS activity is obtained by substituting alkyl, alkenyl, or aryl groups on the pyrimidine ring. Phenobarbital is 5- ethyl-t-phenylbarbituric acid and has the empirical formula $C_{12}H_{12}N_2O_3$. Its molecular weight is 232.24.

TABLETS

The tablets contain 15 mg (0.064 mmol), 30 mg (0.129 mmol), 60 mg (0.258 mmol), or 100 mg (0.431 mmol) phenobarbital. The tablets also contain cornstarch, lactose, magnesium, stearate, and talc.

Phenobarbital occurs as white, odorless, glistening, small crystals or as white, crystalline powder. It is very slightly soluble in water and is soluble in alcohol.

Storage: Keep tightly closed. Store at controlled room temperature, 15-30°C (59-86°F).

INJECTABLE

Do not use if solution is discolored or contains a precipitate.

The sodium salt of phenobarbital is available as a sterile parenteral solution. It occurs as a white, slightly bitter powder or crystals; it is very soluble in alcohol, and practically insoluble in ether or chloroform.

In the TUBEX and TUBEX BLUE POINTE (Wyeth) Sterile Cartridge Units each milliliter contains 30, 60, or 130 mg phenobarbital sodium in a special vehicle containing 10% alcohol and approximately 75% propylene glycol; when required during manufacture, the pH is adjusted with hydrochloric acid.

Storage: Store at room temperature, approximately 25°C (77°F).

Phenobarbital is designated chemically as 5-ethyl-5-phenylbarbiturate.

CLINICAL PHARMACOLOGY

Barbiturates are capable of producing all levels of CNS mood alteration from excitation to mild sedation, to hypnosis, and deep coma. Overdosage can produce death. In high enough therapeutic doses, barbiturates induce anesthesia.

Barbiturates depress the sensory cortex, decrease motor activity, alter cerebellar function, and produce drowsiness, sedation, and hypnosis.

Barbiturate-induced sleep differs from physiological sleep. Sleep laboratory studies have demonstrated that barbiturates reduce the amount of time spent in the rapid-eye-movement (REM) phase of sleep or dreaming stage. Also, Stages III and IV sleep are decreased. Following abrupt cessation of barbiturates used regularly, patients may experience markedly increased dreaming, nightmares, and/or insomnia. Therefore, withdrawal of a single therapeutic dose over 5 or 6 days has been recommended to lessen the REM rebound and disturbed sleep which contribute to drug-withdrawal syndrome (for example, decrease the dose from 3-2 doses a day for 1 week).

The short, intermediate and, to a lesser degree, long-acting barbiturates have been widely prescribed for treating insomnia. Although the clinical literature abounds with claims that the short-acting barbiturates are superior for producing sleep while the intermediate- acting compounds are more effective in maintaining sleep, controlled studies have failed to demonstrate these differential effects. Therefore, as sleep medications, the barbiturates are of limited value beyond short-term use.

Barbiturates have little analgesic action at subanesthetic doses. Rather, in subanesthetic doses these drugs may increase the reaction to painful stimuli. All barbiturates exhibit anticonvulsant activity in anesthetic doses. However, of the drugs in this class, only phenobarbital, mephobarbital, and metharbital are effective as oral anticonvulsants in subhypnotic doses.

Barbiturates are respiratory depressants. The degree of respiratory depression is dependent upon dose. With hypnotic doses, respiratory depression produced by barbiturates is similar to that which occurs during physiologic sleep with slight decrease in blood pressure and heart rate.

Studies in laboratory animals have shown that barbiturates cause reduction in the tone and contractility of the uterus, ureters, and urinary bladder. However, concentrations of the drugs required to produce this effect in humans are not reached with sedative-hypnotic doses.

Barbiturates do not impair normal hepatic function, but have been shown to induce liver microsomal enzymes, thus increasing and/or altering the metabolism of barbiturates and other drugs. (See DRUG INTERACTIONS.)

PHARMACOKINETICS

Barbiturates are absorbed in varying degrees following oral, rectal, or parenteral administration. The salts are more rapidly absorbed than are the acids. The rate of absorption is increased if the sodium salt is ingested as a dilute solution or taken on an empty stomach.

Duration of action, which is related to the rate at which the barbiturates are redistributed throughout the body, varies among persons and in the same person from time to time.

Phenobarbital is classified as a long-acting barbiturate when taken orally. Its onset of action is 1 hour or longer, and its duration of action ranges from 10-12 hours.

No studies have demonstrated that the different routes of administration are equivalent with respect to bioavailability.

Barbiturates are weak acids that are absorbed and rapidly distributed to all tissues and fluids with high concentrations in the brain, liver, and kidneys. Lipid solubility of the barbiturates is the dominant factor in their distribution within the body. The more lipid soluble the barbiturate, the more rapidly it penetrates all tissues of the body. Barbiturates are bound to plasma and tissue proteins to a varying degree, with the degree of binding increasing directly as a function of lipid solubility.

Phenobarbital has the lowest lipid solubility, lowest plasma binding, lowest brain-protein binding, the longest delay in onset of activity, and the longest duration of action.

Phenobarbital plasma half-life values in adults range from 53-118 hours (mean 79 hours) and 60-180 hours (mean 110 hours) in children and newborns (age 48 hours or less).

Barbiturates are metabolized primarily by the hepatic microsomal enzyme system, and the metabolic products are excreted in the urine, and less commonly, in the feces. Approximately 25-50 percent of a dose of phenobarbital is eliminated unchanged in the urine, whereas the amount of other barbiturates excreted unchanged in the urine is negligible. The excretion of unmetabolized barbiturate is one feature that distinguishes the long-acting category from those belonging to other categories which are almost entirely metabolized. The inactive metabolites of the barbiturates are excreted as conjugates of glucuronic acid.

ADDITIONAL INFORMATION FOR INJECTION

Following IV administration, the onset of action is 5 minutes for phenobarbital sodium. Maximal CNS depression may not occur until 15 minutes or more after IV administration. The onset of action of IM administration of barbiturates is slightly faster than the oral route. The onset of action of the oral route varies between 20 and 60 minutes.

INDICATIONS AND USAGE

- Sedative
- Hypnotic, for the short-term treatment of insomnia, since barbiturates appear to lose their effectiveness for sleep induction and sleep maintenance after 2 weeks (see CLINICAL PHARMACOLOGY).
- Preanesthetic
- ***Tablets:*** *Anticonvulsant:* For the treatment of generalized and partial seizures.
- ***Injection:*** For the treatment of generalized tonic-clonic and cortical focal seizures. And, in the emergency control of certain acute convulsive episodes, *e.g.*, those associated with status epilepticus, cholera, eclampsia, meningitis, tetanus, and toxic reactions to strychnine or local anesthetics. Phenobarbital sodium may be administered IM or IV as an anticonvulsant for emergency use. When administered IV, it may require 15 or more minutes before reaching peak concentrations in the brain. Therefore, injecting phenobarbital sodium until the convulsions stop may cause the brain level to exceed that required to control the convulsions and lead to severe barbiturate- induced depression.

NON-FDA APPROVED INDICATIONS

Phenobarbital has also been used for the treatment of hyperbilirubinemia and for the treatment of withdrawal from other barbiturates and hypnotics although these uses are not FDA approved.

CONTRAINDICATIONS

Barbiturates are contraindicated in patients with known barbiturate sensitivity. Barbiturates are also contraindicated in patients with a history of manifest or latent porphyria or marked impairment of liver function, or with severe respiratory disease where dyspnea or obstruction is evident. Large doses are contraindicated in nephritic subjects. Barbiturates should not be administered to persons with known previous addiction to the sedative/hypnotic group, since ordinary doses may be ineffectual and may contribute to further addiction.

Intra-arterial administration is contraindicated. Its consequences vary from transient pain to gangrene. Subcutaneous administration produces tissue irritation, ranging from tenderness and redness to necrosis, and it not recommended. (See DOSAGE AND ADMINISTRATION, Treatment of Adverse Effects Due to Inadvertent Error in Administration.)

WARNINGS

HABIT-FORMING

Barbiturates may be habit-forming. Tolerance, psychological and physical dependence may occur with continued use. (See CLINICAL PHARMACOLOGY, Pharmacokinetics. Patients who have psychological dependence on barbiturates may increase the dosage or decrease the dosage interval without consulting a physician and may subsequently develop a physical dependence on barbiturates. To minimize the possibility of overdosage or the development of dependence, the prescribing and dispensing of sedative-hypnotic barbiturates should be limited to the amount required for the interval until the next appointment. Abrupt cessation after prolonged use in the dependent person may result in withdrawal symptoms, including delirium, convulsions, and possibly death. Barbiturates should be withdrawn gradually from any patient known to be taking excessive dosage over long periods of time.

IV ADMINISTRATION

Too-rapid administration may cause respiratory depression, apnea, laryngospasm, or vasodilation with fall in blood pressure.

ACUTE OR CHRONIC PAIN

Caution should be exercised when barbiturates are administered to patients with acute or chronic pain, because paradoxical excitement could be induced or important symptoms could be masked. However, the use of barbiturates as sedatives in the postoperative surgical period and as adjuncts to cancer chemotherapy is well established.

P

USE IN PREGNANCY

Barbiturates can cause fetal damage when administered to a pregnant woman. Retrospective, case-controlled studies have suggested a connection between the maternal consumption of barbiturates and a higher than expected incidence of fetal abnormalities. Following oral or parenteral administration, barbiturates readily cross the placental barrier and are distributed throughout fetal tissues, with highest concentration found in the placenta, fetal liver, and brain. Fetal blood levels approach maternal blood levels following parenteral administration.

Withdrawal symptoms occur in infants born to mothers who receive barbiturates throughout the last trimester of pregnancy. If phenobarbital is used during pregnancy, or if the patient becomes pregnant while taking this drug, the patient should be apprised of the potential hazard to the fetus.

SYNERGISTIC EFFECTS

The concomitant use of alcohol or other CNS depressants may produce additive CNS depressant effects.

PRECAUTIONS

GENERAL

Barbiturates may be habit-forming. Tolerance and psychological and physical dependence may occur with continuing use. Barbiturates should be administered with caution, if at all, to patients who are mentally depressed, have suicidal tendencies, or a history of drug abuse.

Elderly or debilitated patients may react to barbiturates with marked excitement, depression, and confusion. In some persons, barbiturates repeatedly produce excitement rather than depression.

In patients with hepatic damage, barbiturates should be administered with caution and initially in reduced doses. Barbiturates should not be administered to patients showing the premonitory signs of hepatic coma.

Untoward reactions may occur in the presence of fever, hyperthyroidism, diabetes mellitus, and severe anemia.

Intramuscular injection should be confined to a total volume of 5 ml and made in a large muscle in order to avoid possible tissue irritation.

Parenteral solutions of barbiturates are highly alkaline. Therefore, extreme care should be taken to avoid perivascular extravasation or intra-arterial injection.

Extravascular injection may cause local tissue damage with subsequent necrosis; consequences of intra-arterial injection may vary from transient pain to gangrene of the limb. Any complaint of pain in the limb warrants stopping the injection.

INFORMATION FOR THE PATIENT

Practitioners should give the following information and instructions to patients receiving barbiturates:

The use of barbiturates carries with it an associated risk of psychological and/or physical dependence. The patient should be warned against increasing the dose of the drug without consulting a physician.

Barbiturates may impair mental and/or physical abilities required for the performance of potentially hazardous tasks (*e.g.*, driving, operating machinery, etc.).

Alcohol should not be consumed while taking barbiturates. Concurrent use of the barbiturates with other CNS depressants (*e.g.*, alcohol, narcotics, tranquilizers, and antihistamines) may result in additional CNS depressant effects.

LABORATORY TESTS

Prolonged therapy with barbiturates should be accompanied by periodic laboratory evaluation of organ systems, including hematopoietic, renal, and hepatic systems. (See PRECAUTIONS, General and ADVERSE REACTIONS).

CARCINOGENESIS, MUTAGENESIS, AND IMPAIRMENT OF FERTILITY

Animal Data

Phenobarbital sodium is carcinogenic in mice and rats after lifetime administration. In mice, it produced benign and malignant liver-cell tumors. In rats, benign liver-cell tumors were observed very late in life.

Human Data

In a 29 year epidemiological study of 9136 patients who were treated on an anticonvulsant protocol which included phenobarbital, results indicated a higher than normal incidence of hepatic carcinoma. Previously, some of these patients were treated with thorotrast, a drug which is known to produce hepatic carcinomas. Thus, this study did not provide sufficient evidence that phenobarbital sodium is carcinogenic in humans.

A retrospective study of 84 children with brain tumors matched to 73 normal controls and 78 cancer controls (malignant disease other than brain tumors) suggested an association between exposure to barbiturates prenatally and an increased incidence of brain tumors.

PREGNANCY CATEGORY D

Teratogenic Effects

See WARNINGS, Use in Pregnancy.

Nonteratogenic Effects

Reports of infants suffering from long- term barbiturate exposure *in utero* included the acute withdrawal syndrome of seizures and hyperirritability from birth to a delayed onset of up to 14 days.

LABOR AND DELIVERY

Hypnotic doses of these barbiturates do not appear to significantly impair uterine activity during labor. Full anesthetic doses of barbiturates decrease the force and frequency of uterine contractions. Administration of sedative-hypnotic barbiturates to the mother during labor may result in respiratory depression in the newborn. Premature infants are particularly susceptible to the depressant effects of barbiturates. If barbiturates are used during labor and delivery, resuscitation equipment should be available.

Data are currently not available to evaluate the effect of these barbiturates when forceps delivery or other intervention is necessary. Also, data are not available to determine the effect of these barbiturates on the later growth, development, and functional maturation of the child.

NURSING MOTHERS

Caution should be exercised when a barbiturate is administered to a nursing woman, since small amounts of barbiturates are excreted in the milk.

DRUG INTERACTIONS

ANTICOAGULANTS

Phenobarbital lowers the plasma levels of dicumarol (name previously used: bishydroxycoumarin) and causes a decrease in anticoagulant activity as measured by the prothrombin time. Barbiturates can induce hepatic microsomal enzymes, resulting in increased metabolism and decreased anticoagulant response of oral anticoagulants (*e.g.*, warfarin, acenocoumarol, dicumarol, and phenprocoumon). Patients stabilized on anticoagulant therapy may require dosage adjustments if barbiturates are added to or withdrawn from their dosage regimen.

CORTICOSTEROIDS

Barbiturates appear to enhance the metabolism of exogenous corticosteroids, probably through the induction of hepatic microsomal enzymes. Patients stabilized on corticosteroid therapy may require dosage adjustments if barbiturates are added to or withdrawn from their dosage regimen.

GRISEOFULVIN

Phenobarbital appears to interfere with the absorption of orally administered griseofulvin, thus decreasing its blood level. The effect of the resultant decreased blood levels of griseofulvin on therapeutic response has not been established. However, it would be preferable to avoid concomitant administration of these drugs.

DOXYCYCLINE

Phenobarbital has been shown to shorten the half- life of doxycycline for as long as 2 weeks after barbiturate therapy is discontinued.

This mechanism is probably through the induction of hepatic microsomal enzymes that metabolize the antibiotic. If phenobarbital and doxycycline are administered concurrently, the clinical response to doxycycline should be monitored closely.

PHENYTOIN, SODIUM VALPROATE, VALPROIC ACID

The effect of barbiturates on the metabolism of phenytoin appears to be variable. Some investigators report an accelerating effect, while others report no effect. Because the effect of barbiturates on the metabolism of phenytoin is not predictable, phenytoin and barbiturate blood levels should be monitored more frequently if these drugs are given concurrently. Sodium valproate and valproic acid appear to decrease barbiturate metabolism; therefore, barbiturate blood levels should be monitored and appropriate dosage adjustments made as indicated.

CENTRAL NERVOUS SYSTEM DEPRESSANTS

The concomitant use of other central nervous system depressants, including other sedatives or hypnotics, antihistamines, tranquilizers, or alcohol, may produce additive depressant effects.

MONOAMINE OXIDASE INHIBITORS (MAOI)

MAOI prolong the effects of barbiturates, probably because metabolism of the barbiturate is inhibited.

ESTRADIOL, ESTRONE, PROGESTERONE, AND OTHER STEROIDAL HORMONES

Pretreatment with or concurrent administration of phenobarbital may decrease the effect of estradiol by increasing its metabolism. There have been reports of patients treated with antiepileptic drugs (*e.g.*, phenobarbital) who became pregnant while taking oral contraceptives. An alternate contraceptive method might be suggested to women taking phenobarbital.

ADVERSE REACTIONS

The following adverse reactions and their incidence were compiled from surveillance of thousands of hospitalized patients. Because such patients may be less aware of certain of the milder adverse effects of barbiturates, the incidence of these reactions may be somewhat higher in fully ambulatory patients.

MORE THAN 1 IN 100 PATIENTS

The most common adverse reaction estimated to occur at a rate of 1-3 patients per 100 is:

Nervous System: Somnolence.

LESS THAN 1 IN 100 PATIENTS

Adverse reactions estimated to occur at a rate of less than 1 in 100 patients listed below, grouped by organ system, and by decreasing order of occurrence are:

Nervous System: Agitation, confusion, hyperkinesia, ataxia, CNS depression, nightmares, nervousness, psychiatric disturbance, hallucinations, insomnia, anxiety, dizziness, thinking abnormality.

Respiratory System: Hypoventilation, apnea.

Cardiovascular System: Bradycardia, hypotension, syncope.

Digestive System: Nausea, vomiting, constipation.

Other Reported Reactions: Headache, injection-site reactions, hypersensitivity reactions (angioedema, skin rashes, exfoliative dermatitis), fever, liver damage, megaloblastic anemia following chronic phenobarbital use.

DOSAGE AND ADMINISTRATION

Dosages of barbiturates must be individualized with full knowledge of their particular characteristics and recommended rate of administration. Factors of consideration are the patient's age, weight, and condition.

TABLETS

Sedation

For sedation, the drug may be administered in single doses of 30-120 mg repeated at intervals; frequency will be determined by the patient's response. It is generally considered that no more than 400 mg of phenobarbital should be administered during a 24 hour period.

Adults

Daytime Sedation: 30-120 mg daily in 2-3 divided doses.

Oral Hypnotic: 100-200 mg.

Anticonvulsant Use

Clinical laboratory reference values should be used to determine the therapeutic anticonvulsant level of phenobarbital in the serum. To achieve the blood levels considered therapeutic in children, higher per-kilogram dosages are generally necessary for phenobarbital and most other anticonvulsants. In children and infants, phenobarbital at a loading dose of 15-20 mg/kg produces blood levels of about 20 μg/ml shortly after administration

Phenobarbital has been used in the treatment and prophylaxis of febrile seizures. However, it has not been established that prevention of febrile seizures influences the subsequent development of epilepsy.

Adults: 60-200 mg/day.

Children: 3-6 mg/kg/day.

Special Patient Populations

Dosage should be reduced in the elderly or debilitated because these patients may be more sensitive to barbiturates. Dosage should be reduced for patients with impaired renal function or hepatic disease.

INJECTION

Suggested doses of phenobarbital sodium for specific indications:

Pediatric dosage recommended by the American Academy of Pediatrics (intended as a guide):

Preoperative Sedation: 1-3 mg/kg IM or IV

Anticonvulsion: 4-6 mg/kg/day for 7-10 days to blood level of 10-15 μg/ml or 10-15 mg/kg/day IM or IV

Status Epilepticus: 15-20 mg/kg over 10-15 minutes IV

Adult Dosage (intended as a guide):

Daytime Sedation: 30-120 mg daily in 2-3 divided doses IM or IV

Bedtime Hypnosis: 100-320 mg IM or IV

Preoperative Sedation: IM only; 100-200 mg 60-90 minutes before surgery

Acute Convulsions: 200-320 mg IM or IV, repeated in 6 hours as necessary.

Parenteral routes should be used only when oral administration is impossible or impractical.

The TUBEX BLUE POINTE Sterile Cartridge Unit (Wyeth) is suitable for substances to be administered intravenously only. It is intended for use with injection sets specifically manufactured as "needle-less" injection systems. TUBEX BLUE POINTE (Wyeth) is compatible with Abbott's Life- Shield pre-pierced reseal injection site, Baxter's InterLink Injection Site, and B. Braun Medical's SafSite Reflux Valve. Consult manufacturer's recommendations regarding "Directions for Use" of the "needle-less" system. It is also intended for admixture with, and convenient administration of, various medicaments when using Drug Vial Adapters for "needle-less" injection systems.

The TUBEX Sterile Cartridge-Needle Unit (Wyeth) is suitable for substances to be administered intravenously or intramuscularly.

IM injection of the sodium salts of barbiturates should be made deeply into a large muscle, and a volume of 5 ml should not be exceeded at any one site because of possible tissue irritation. After IM injection of a hypnotic dose, the patient's vital signs should be monitored.

IV injection is restricted to conditions in which other routes are not feasible, either because the patient is unconscious (as in cerebral hemorrhage, eclampsia, or status epilepticus), or because the patient resists (as in delirium), or because prompt action is imperative. Slow IV injection is essential, and patients should be carefully observed during administration. This requires that blood pressure, respiration, and cardiac function be maintained, vital signs be recorded, and equipment for resuscitation and ventilation be available. The rate of IV injection for adults should not exceed 60 mg/mn for phenobarbital sodium.

Any vein may be used, but preference should be given to a larger vein (to minimize the risk of irritation with the possibility of resultant thrombosis). Avoid administration into varicose veins, because circulation there is retarded. Inadvertent injection into or adjacent to an artery has resulted in gangrene requiring amputation of an extremity or a portion thereof. Careful technique, including aspiration, is necessary to avoid inadvertent intra-arterial injection.

Treatment of Adverse Effects Due To Inadvertent Error in Administration

Extravasation into subcutaneous tissues causes tissue irritation. This may vary from slight tenderness and redness to necrosis. Recommended treatment includes the application of moist heat and the injection of 0.05% procaine solution into the affected area.

Intra-arterial injection of any barbiturate must be avoided. The accidental intra-arterial injection of a small amount of the solution may cause spasm and severe pain along the course of the artery. The injection should be terminated if the patient complains of pain or if other indications of accidental intra-arterial injection occur, such as a white hand with cyanosed skin or patches of discolored skin and delayed onset of hypnosis.

The consequences of intra-arterial injection of phenobarbital can vary from transient pain to gangrene. It is not possible to formulate strict rules for management of such accidents. The following procedures have been suggested: 1) release of the tourniquet or restrictive garments to permit dilution of injected drug, 2) relief of arterial spasm by injecting 10 ml of a 1% procaine solution into the artery and, if considered necessary, brachial plexus block, 3) prevention of thrombosis by early anticoagulant therapy, and 4) supportive treatment.

Anticonvulsant Use

A therapeutic anticonvulsant level of phenobarbital in the serum is 10-25 μg/ml. To achieve the blood levels considered therapeutic in children, higher per-kilogram dosages are generally necessary for phenobarbital and higher per-kilogram dosages are generally necessary for phenobarbital and most other anticonvulsants. In children and infants, phenobarbital at loading doses of 15-20 mg/kg produces blood levels of about 20 μg/ml shortly after administration.

In status epilepticus, it is imperative to achieve therapeutic blood levels of a barbiturate (or other anticonvulsants) as rapidly as possible. When administered intravenously, phenobarbital sodium may require 15 minutes or more to attain peak concentrations in the brain. If phenobarbital sodium is injected continuously until the convulsions stop, the brain concentration would continue to rise and could eventually exceed that required to control the seizures. A barbiturate-induced depression may occur along with a postictal depression once the seizures are controlled, therefore, it is important to use the minimal amount required, and to wait for the anticonvulsant effect to develop before administering a second dose.

Phenobarbital has been used in the treatment and prophylaxis of febrile seizures. However, it has not been established that prevention of febrile seizures influences the subsequent development of epilepsy.

Special Patient Population

Dosage should be reduced in the elderly or debilitated because these patients may be more sensitive to barbiturates. Dosage should be reduced for patients with impaired renal function or hepatic disease.

Inspection

Parenteral drug products should be inspected visually for particulate matter and discoloration prior to administration, whenever solution and container permit. Solutions for injection showing evidence of precipitation should not be used.

PRODUCT LISTING - RATED THERAPEUTICALLY EQUIVALENT

Elixir - Oral - 20 mg/5 ml			
480 ml	$5.28	GENERIC, Cenci, H.R. Labs Inc	00556-0112-16
3840 ml	$31.10	GENERIC, Cenci, H.R. Labs Inc	00556-0112-28
Tablet - Oral - 15 mg			
30's	$1.95	GENERIC, Heartland Healthcare Services	61392-0382-30
30's	$1.95	GENERIC, Heartland Healthcare Services	61392-0382-39
31's	$2.01	GENERIC, Heartland Healthcare Services	61392-0382-31
60's	$3.90	GENERIC, Heartland Healthcare Services	61392-0382-60
90's	$5.85	GENERIC, Heartland Healthcare Services	61392-0382-90
100's	$4.32	GENERIC, Auro Pharmaceutical	55829-0857-10
Tablet - Oral - 30 mg			
30's	$2.08	GENERIC, Heartland Healthcare Services	61392-0391-30
30's	$2.08	GENERIC, Heartland Healthcare Services	61392-0391-39
31's	$2.15	GENERIC, Heartland Healthcare Services	61392-0391-31
32's	$2.22	GENERIC, Heartland Healthcare Services	61392-0391-32
60's	$4.16	GENERIC, Heartland Healthcare Services	61392-0391-60
60's	$6.24	GENERIC, Heartland Healthcare Services	61392-0391-65
90's	$6.24	GENERIC, Heartland Healthcare Services	61392-0391-90
100's	$5.67	GENERIC, Auro Pharmaceutical	55829-0858-10
Tablet - Oral - 60 mg			
100's	$4.81	GENERIC, Auro Pharmaceutical	55829-0859-10
Tablet - Oral - 64.8 mg			
30's	$2.30	GENERIC, Heartland Healthcare Services	61392-0392-30
30's	$2.30	GENERIC, Heartland Healthcare Services	61392-0392-39
31's	$2.38	GENERIC, Heartland Healthcare Services	61392-0392-31
60's	$4.60	GENERIC, Heartland Healthcare Services	61392-0392-60

PRODUCT LISTING - EQUIVALENTS NOT AVAILABLE

Elixir - Oral - 15 mg/5 ml			
5 ml x 100	$33.20	GENERIC, Pharmaceutical Assoc Inc Div Beach Products	00121-0518-05
10 ml x 100	$34.30	GENERIC, Pharmaceutical Assoc Inc Div Beach Products	00121-0518-10
20 ml x 100	$38.20	GENERIC, Pharmaceutical Assoc Inc Div Beach Products	00121-0518-20
Elixir - Oral - 20 mg/5 ml			
4 ml x 100	$23.76	GENERIC, Pharmaceutical Assoc Inc Div Beach Products	00121-0531-03
5 ml x 100	$25.25	GENERIC, Pharmaceutical Assoc Inc Div Beach Products	00121-0531-05
5 ml x 100	$46.00	GENERIC, Roxane Laboratories Inc	00054-8704-04
7.50 ml x 100	$29.15	GENERIC, Pharmaceutical Assoc Inc Div Beach Products	00121-0531-07
7.50 ml x 100	$48.00	GENERIC, Roxane Laboratories Inc	00054-8701-04
15 ml x 100	$30.55	GENERIC, Pharmaceutical Assoc Inc Div Beach Products	00121-0531-15
480 ml	$3.65	GENERIC, Bio Pharm Inc	59741-0136-16
480 ml	$4.51	GENERIC, Liquipharm Inc	54198-0130-16
480 ml	$5.31	GENERIC, Vintage Pharmaceuticals Inc	00254-9355-58
480 ml	$5.31	GENERIC, Qualitest Products Inc	00603-1508-58
480 ml	$5.76	GENERIC, Aligen Independent Laboratories Inc	00405-0155-16
480 ml	$5.95	GENERIC, Pharmaceutical Assoc Inc Div Beach Products	00121-0531-16
480 ml	$5.95	GENERIC, Century Pharmaceuticals Inc	00436-0585-16
480 ml	$5.95	GENERIC, Allscripts Pharmaceutical Company	54569-2031-00
480 ml	$6.10	GENERIC, Moore, H.L. Drug Exchange Inc	00839-5398-69

480 ml	$7.73	GENERIC, Major Pharmaceuticals Inc	00904-1015-16
480 ml	$8.45	GENERIC, Ivax Corporation	00182-0314-40
480 ml	$8.45	GENERIC, Alpharma Uspd Makers Of Barre and Nmc	00472-1015-16
960 ml	$7.78	GENERIC, Century Pharmaceuticals Inc	00436-0585-32
3840 ml	$22.27	GENERIC, Liquipharm Inc	54198-0130-28
3840 ml	$29.18	GENERIC, Morton Grove Pharmaceuticals Inc	60432-0026-28
3840 ml	$30.00	GENERIC, C.O. Truxton Inc	00463-9018-28
3840 ml	$31.49	GENERIC, Halsey Drug Company Inc	00879-0049-28
3840 ml	$34.94	GENERIC, Major Pharmaceuticals Inc	00904-1015-28
3840 ml	$35.71	GENERIC, Ivax Corporation	00182-0314-41
3840 ml	$38.02	GENERIC, Century Pharmaceuticals Inc	00436-0585-28
3840 ml	$44.31	GENERIC, Alpharma Uspd Makers Of Barre and Nmc	00472-1015-28
Solution - Injectable - 30 mg/ml			
1 ml x 10	$22.36	GENERIC, Esi Lederle Generics	00008-0499-50
1 ml x 10	$29.90	GENERIC, Esi Lederle Generics	00008-0499-01
Solution - Injectable - 60 mg/ml			
1 ml x 10	$25.54	GENERIC, Allscripts Pharmaceutical Company	54569-3282-00
1 ml x 10	$32.00	LUMINAL, Abbott Pharmaceutical	00074-2343-01
1 ml x 10	$32.54	LUMINAL, Abbott Pharmaceutical	00074-2343-31
Solution - Injectable - 65 mg/ml			
1 ml x 25	$42.50	GENERIC, Esi Lederle Generics	00641-0476-25
Solution - Injectable - 130 mg/ml			
1 ml x 10	$36.60	GENERIC, Esi Lederle Generics	00008-0304-01
1 ml x 10	$41.10	LUMINAL, Abbott Pharmaceutical	00074-2349-01
1 ml x 10	$43.10	LUMINAL, Abbott Pharmaceutical	00074-2349-31
1 ml x 25	$50.50	GENERIC, Esi Lederle Generics	00641-0477-25
1 ml x 100	$475.00	LUMINAL, Abbott Pharmaceutical	00074-1540-01
Tablet - Oral - 15 mg			
100's	$0.54	GENERIC, Global Pharmaceutical Corporation	00115-4211-01
100's	$0.54	GENERIC, Global Pharmaceutical Corporation	00115-4212-01
100's	$0.54	GENERIC, Global Pharmaceutical Corporation	00115-4214-01
100's	$2.50	GENERIC, Cmc-Consolidated Midland Corporation	00223-1430-01
100's	$3.35	GENERIC, Lilly, Eli and Company	00002-1031-02
100's	$4.41	GENERIC, Ranbaxy Laboratories	63304-0741-01
100's	$4.86	GENERIC, Major Pharmaceuticals Inc	00904-3815-61
100's	$5.92	GENERIC, Roxane Laboratories Inc	00054-8703-25
Tablet - Oral - 16.2 mg			
100's	$2.90	GENERIC, Jones Pharma Inc	52604-6712-01
100's	$3.90	GENERIC, Qualitest Products Inc	00603-5165-21
150's	$11.50	GENERIC, Sky Pharmaceuticals Packaging, Inc	63739-0200-15
Tablet - Oral - 30 mg			
6's	$2.44	GENERIC, Southwood Pharmaceuticals Inc	58016-0826-06
9's	$0.11	GENERIC, Allscripts Pharmaceutical Company	54569-0938-02
30's	$0.36	GENERIC, Allscripts Pharmaceutical Company	54569-0938-01
50's	$6.20	GENERIC, Southwood Pharmaceuticals Inc	58016-0826-50
100's	$0.64	GENERIC, Global Pharmaceutical Corporation	00115-4229-01
100's	$0.64	GENERIC, Global Pharmaceutical Corporation	00115-4231-01
100's	$1.20	GENERIC, Allscripts Pharmaceutical Company	54569-0938-00
100's	$2.75	GENERIC, Cmc-Consolidated Midland Corporation	00223-1431-01
100's	$3.43	GENERIC, Lilly, Eli and Company	00002-1032-02
100's	$3.60	GENERIC, Qualitest Products Inc	00603-5166-21
100's	$3.89	GENERIC, Ohm Laboratories Inc	51660-0785-01
100's	$4.18	GENERIC, Ranbaxy Laboratories	63304-0742-01
100's	$5.31	GENERIC, Vintage Pharmaceuticals Inc	00254-5012-28
100's	$6.95	GENERIC, Roxane Laboratories Inc	00054-8705-25
Tablet - Oral - 32.4 mg			
90's	$3.15	GENERIC, Qualitest Products Inc	00603-5166-02
100's	$2.68	GENERIC, Jones Pharma Inc	52604-6722-01
150's	$11.78	GENERIC, Sky Pharmaceuticals Packaging, Inc	63739-0201-15
Tablet - Oral - 60 mg			
100's	$2.66	GENERIC, Vintage Pharmaceuticals Inc	00254-5013-28
100's	$3.25	GENERIC, Cmc-Consolidated Midland Corporation	00223-1432-01
100's	$5.07	GENERIC, Lilly, Eli and Company	00002-1037-02
100's	$5.75	GENERIC, Qualitest Products Inc	00603-5167-21
100's	$5.87	GENERIC, Vangard Labs	00615-0418-47
100's	$6.20	GENERIC, Ranbaxy Laboratories	63304-0743-01
100's	$7.27	GENERIC, Roxane Laboratories Inc	00054-8708-25
Tablet - Oral - 64.8 mg			
100's	$4.40	GENERIC, Jones Pharma Inc	52604-6731-01
Tablet - Oral - 97.2 mg			
100's	$5.63	GENERIC, Jones Pharma Inc	52604-6740-01
Tablet - Oral - 100 mg			
30's	$7.15	GENERIC, West Ward Pharmaceutical Corporation	00143-1458-01
100's	$3.31	GENERIC, Vintage Pharmaceuticals Inc	00254-5014-28
100's	$3.75	GENERIC, Cmc-Consolidated Midland Corporation	00223-1433-01
100's	$6.42	GENERIC, Lilly, Eli and Company	00002-1033-02
100's	$6.65	GENERIC, Vangard Labs	00615-0423-47
100's	$6.95	GENERIC, Qualitest Products Inc	00603-5168-21
100's	$7.30	GENERIC, Ranbaxy Laboratories	51660-0787-01
100's	$7.45	GENERIC, Roxane Laboratories Inc	00054-8707-25
100's	$7.85	GENERIC, Ranbaxy Laboratories	63304-0744-01

P

Phentermine Hydrochloride *(002016)*

Categories: Obesity, exogenous; DEA Class CIV; Pregnancy Category B; FDA Approved 1973 Aug
Drug Classes: Anorexiants; Stimulants, central nervous system
Brand Names: Adipex-P; Dapex-37.5; **Fastin**; Obe-Nix; Oby-Cap; Oby-Trim; Ona-Mast; Panbesyl; Phentercot; Phentride; T-Diet; Teramin; Tora; Umi-Pex 30; Zantryl
Foreign Brand Availability: Minobese-Forte (South-Africa); Panbesy (Hong-Kong; Malaysia; Thailand); Panbesyl Nyscaps (Belgium); Redusa (Hong-Kong); Umine (New-Zealand)
Cost of Therapy: $1.73 (Weight Loss; Generic Tablets; 30 mg; 1 capsule/day; 30 day supply)

DESCRIPTION

Each Fastin capsule contains phentermine hydrochloride, 30 mg (equivalent to 24 mg phentermine).

Phentermine hydrochloride is a white crystalline powder, very soluble in water and alcohol. Chemically, the product is phenyl-tertiary-butylamine hydrochloride. *Fastin Inactive Ingredients:* FD&C blue no. 1, invert sugar, methylcellulose, polyethylene glycol, starch, sucrose and titanium dioxide. The branding ink used on the gelatin capsules contains: aluminum lake, ethyl alcohol, FD&C blue no. 1 , isopropyl alcohol, n-butyl alcohol, pharmaceutical shellac (modified) or refined shellac (food grade) and propylene glycol.

CLINICAL PHARMACOLOGY

Phentermine HCl is a sympathomimetic amine with pharmacologic activity similar to the prototype drugs of this class used in obesity, the amphetamines. Actions include central nervous system stimulation and elevation of blood pressure. Tachyphylaxis and tolerance have been demonstrated with all drugs of this class in which these phenomena have been looked for.

Drugs of this class used in obesity are commonly known as "anorectics" or "anorexigenics." It has not been established that the action of such drugs in treating obesity is primarily one of appetite suppression. Other central nervous system actions, or metabolic effects, may be involved, for example.

Adult obese subjects instructed in dietary management and treated with "anorectic" drugs lose more weight on the average than those treated with placebo and diet, as determined in relatively short-term clinical trials.

The magnitude of increased weight loss of drug-treated patients over placebo-treated patients is only a fraction of a pound a week. The rate of weight loss is greatest in the first weeks of therapy for both drug and placebo subjects and tends to decrease in succeeding weeks. The possible origins of the increased weight loss due to the various drug effects are not established. The amount of weight loss associated with the use of an "anorectic" drug varies from trial to trial, and the increased weight loss appears to be related in part to variables other than the drugs prescribed, such as the physician-investigator, the population treated, and the diet prescribed. Studies do not permit conclusions as to the relative importance of the drug and non-drug factors on weight loss.

The natural history of obesity is measured in years, whereas the studies cited are restricted to a few weeks' duration; thus, the total impact of drug-induced weight loss over that of diet alone must be considered clinically limited.

INDICATIONS AND USAGE

Phentermine HCl is indicated as a short-term (a few weeks) adjunct in a regimen of weight reduction based on exercise, behavioral modification and caloric restriction in the management of exogenous obesity for patients with an initial body mass index ≥ 30 kg/m^2, or ≥ 27 kg/m^2 in the presence of other risk factors (*e.g.*, hypertension, diabetes, hyperlipidemia).

The limited usefulness of agents of this class (see CLINICAL PHARMACOLOGY) should be measured against possible risk factors inherent in their use as described in WARNINGS.

CONTRAINDICATIONS

Advanced arteriosclerosis, cardiovascular disease, moderate to severe hypertension, hyperthyroidism, known hypersensitivity or idiosyncrasy to the sympathomimetic amines, glaucoma.

Agitated states.

Patients with a history of drug abuse.

During or within 14 days following the administration of monoamine oxidase inhibitors (hypertensive crises may result).

WARNINGS

Phentermine HCl capsules are indicated only as short-term monotherapy for the management of exogenous obesity. The safety and efficacy of combination therapy with phentermine and any other drug products for weight loss, including selective serotonin reuptake inhibitors (*e.g.*, fluoxetine, sertraline, fluvoxamine, paroxetine), have not been established. Therefore, coadministration of these drug products for weight loss is not recommended.

Primary Pulmonary Hypertension (PPH) — a rare, frequently fatal disease of the lungs — has been reported to occur in patients receiving a combination of phentermine with fenfluramine or dexfenfluramine. The possibility of an association between PPH and the use of phentermine alone cannot be ruled out; there have been rare cases of PPH in patients who reportedly have taken phentermine alone. The initial symptom of PPH is usually dyspnea. Other initial symptoms include: angina pectoris, syncope or lower extremity edema. Patients should be advised to report immediately any deterioration in exercise tolerance. Treatment should be discontinued in patients who develop new, unexplained symptoms of dyspnea, angina pectoris, syncope or lower extremity edema.

VALVULAR HEART DISEASE

Serious, regurgitant cardiac valvular disease, primarily affecting the mitral, aortic and/or tricuspid valves, has been reported in otherwise healthy persons who had taken a combination of phentermine with fenfluramine or dexfenfluramine for weight loss. The etiology of these valvulopathies has not been established and their course in individuals after the drugs are stopped is not known. The possibility of an association between valvular heart disease and the use of phentermine alone cannot be ruled out; there have been rare cases of valvular heart disease in patients who reportedly have taken phentermine alone.

Tolerance to the anorectic effect usually develops within a few weeks. When this occurs, the recommended dose should not be exceeded in an attempt to increase the effect; rather, the drug should be discontinued.

Phentermine HCl may impair the ability of the patient to engage in potentially hazardous activities such as operating machinery or driving a motor vehicle; the patient should therefore be cautioned accordingly.

Usage With Alcohol: Concomitant use of alcohol with phentermine HCl may result in an adverse drug interaction.

PRECAUTIONS

GENERAL

Caution is to be exercised in prescribing phentermine HCl for patients with even mild hypertension.

Insulin requirements in diabetes mellitus may be altered in association with the use of phentermine HCl and the concomitant dietary regimen.

Phentermine HCl may decrease the hypotensive effect of guanethidine.

The least amount feasible should be prescribed or dispensed at one time in order to minimize the possibility of overdosage.

CARCINOGENESIS, MUTAGENESIS, AND IMPAIRMENT OF FERTILITY

Studies have not been performed with phentermine HCl to determine the potential for carcinogenesis, mutagenesis, or impairment of fertility.

PREGNANCY, TERATOGENIC EFFECTS, PREGNANCY CATEGORY C

Animal reproduction studies have not been conducted with phentermine HCl. It is also not known whether phentermine HCl can cause fetal harm when administered to a pregnant woman or can affect reproductive capacity. Phentermine HCl should be given to a pregnant woman only if clearly needed.

NURSING MOTHERS

Because of the potential for serious adverse reactions in nursing infants, a decision should be made whether to discontinue nursing or to discontinue the drug, taking into account the importance of the drug to the mother.

PEDIATRIC USE

Safety and effectiveness in pediatric patients have not been established.

DRUG INTERACTIONS

Concomitant use of alcohol with phentermine HCl may result in an adverse drug interaction.

ADVERSE REACTIONS

Cardiovascular: Primary pulmonary hypertension and/or regurgitant cardiac valvular disease (see WARNINGS), palpitation, tachycardia, elevation of blood pressure.

Central Nervous System: Overstimulation, restlessness, dizziness, insomnia, euphoria, dysphoria, tremor, headache; rarely psychotic episodes at recommended doses.

Gastrointestinal: Dryness of the mouth, unpleasant taste, diarrhea, constipation, other gastrointestinal disturbances.

Allergic: Urticaria.

Endocrine: Impotence, changes in libido.

DOSAGE AND ADMINISTRATION

Exogenous Obesity: One capsule at approximately 2 hours after breakfast for appetite control. Late evening medication should be avoided because of the possibility of resulting insomnia.

Administration of 1 capsule (30 mg) daily has been found to be adequate in depression of the appetite for 12-14 hours.

Phentermine HCl is not recommended for use in patients 16 years of age and under.

HOW SUPPLIED

Blue and clear capsules with blue and white beads containing 30 mg phentermine HCl (equivalent to 24 mg phentermine) imprinted with "BEECHAM" on cap and product name "FASTIN" on body.

Storage: Store at room temperature.

PRODUCT LISTING - RATED THERAPEUTICALLY EQUIVALENT

Capsule, Extended Release - Oral - 15 mg

100's	$125.37	GENERIC, Eon Labs Manufacturing Inc	00185-0644-01

Capsule, Extended Release - Oral - 30 mg

100's	$5.78	GENERIC, Interstate Drug Exchange Inc	00814-6077-14
100's	$5.93	GENERIC, Interstate Drug Exchange Inc	00814-6078-14
100's	$7.35	GENERIC, Rexar Pharmacal	00478-5469-01
100's	$10.05	GENERIC, Aligen Independent Laboratories Inc	00405-4796-01
100's	$11.96	GENERIC, Mutual/United Research Laboratories	00677-0460-01
100's	$18.00	GENERIC, Watson/Rugby Laboratories Inc	00536-4236-01
100's	$25.02	GENERIC, King Pharmaceuticals Inc	60793-0009-01
100's	$31.95	GENERIC, Camall Company	00147-0198-10
100's	$31.95	GENERIC, Camall Company	00147-0201-10
100's	$31.95	GENERIC, Camall Company	00147-0202-10
100's	$73.50	T-DIET, Jones Pharma Inc	52604-0010-01
100's	$93.00	ZANTRYL, Ion Laboratories Inc	11808-0555-01
100's	$96.64	GENERIC, Major Pharmaceuticals Inc	00904-3921-60
100's	$101.00	GENERIC, Able Laboratories Inc	53265-0259-10
100's	$103.35	GENERIC, Eon Labs Manufacturing Inc	00185-0647-01
100's	$103.35	GENERIC, Mutual/United Research Laboratories	00677-1823-01
100's	$130.65	GENERIC, Major Pharmaceuticals Inc	00904-0614-60
100's	$131.98	GENERIC, Eon Labs Manufacturing Inc	00185-5000-01

Capsule, Extended Release - Oral - 37.5 mg

100's	$38.95	GENERIC, Camall Company	00147-0234-10
100's	$38.95	GENERIC, Camall Company	00147-0235-10
100's	$38.95	GENERIC, Camall Company	00147-0251-10
100's	$38.95	GENERIC, Camall Company	00147-0253-10
100's	$38.95	GENERIC, Camall Company	00147-0254-10
100's	$70.95	GENERIC, Camall Company	00147-0231-10
100's	$85.91	GENERIC, Abana Pharmaceuticals	12463-0217-01
100's	$157.00	GENERIC, Amide Pharmaceutical Inc	52152-0167-02
100's	$174.76	ADIPEX-P, Gate Pharmaceuticals	57844-0019-01

Tablet - Oral - 8 mg

100's	$15.65	GENERIC, Camall Company	00147-0136-10

Tablet, Extended Release - Oral - 37.5 mg

100's	$23.00	GENERIC, Ivax Corporation	00182-0205-01
100's	$35.81	GENERIC, Pan American Laboratories	00525-0509-01
100's	$39.80	GENERIC, Camall Company	00147-0232-10
100's	$70.95	GENERIC, Camall Company	00147-0248-10
100's	$150.00	GENERIC, Able Laboratories Inc	53265-0257-10
100's	$152.25	GENERIC, Purepac Pharmaceutical Company	00228-3016-11
100's	$152.25	GENERIC, Mutual/United Research Laboratories	00677-1824-01
100's	$154.25	GENERIC, Amide Pharmaceutical Inc	52152-0159-02
100's	$171.68	ADIPEX-P, Gate Pharmaceuticals	57844-0009-01

PRODUCT LISTING - EQUIVALENTS NOT AVAILABLE

Capsule, Extended Release - Oral - Resin 15 mg

100's	$106.25	IONAMIN, Celltech Pharmacueticals Inc	00585-0903-71
100's	$232.80	IONAMIN, Celltech Pharmacueticals Inc	53014-0903-71

Capsule, Extended Release - Oral - Resin 30 mg

100's	$266.68	IONAMIN, Celltech Pharmacueticals Inc	53014-0904-71

Capsule, Extended Release - Oral - 15 mg

6's	$17.10	GENERIC, Pharma Pac	52959-0426-06
7's	$19.51	GENERIC, Pharma Pac	52959-0426-07
14's	$24.91	GENERIC, Pharma Pac	52959-0426-14
15's	$26.11	GENERIC, Pharma Pac	52959-0426-15
24's	$30.31	GENERIC, Pharma Pac	52959-0426-24
28's	$35.35	GENERIC, Pharma Pac	52959-0426-28
30's	$38.11	GENERIC, Pharma Pac	52959-0426-30

Capsule, Extended Release - Oral - 18.75 mg

7's	$3.35	GENERIC, Allscripts Pharmaceutical Company	54569-2669-00
15's	$7.18	GENERIC, Allscripts Pharmaceutical Company	54569-2669-01
21's	$10.05	GENERIC, Allscripts Pharmaceutical Company	54569-2669-03
30's	$14.35	GENERIC, Allscripts Pharmaceutical Company	54569-2669-02
100's	$30.95	GENERIC, Camall Company	00147-0249-10
100's	$66.84	GENERIC, Mcr/American Pharmaceuticals Inc	58605-0508-01

Capsule, Extended Release - Oral - 30 mg

7's	$8.47	GENERIC, Pharma Pac	52959-0440-07
14's	$4.45	GENERIC, Southwood Pharmaceuticals Inc	58016-0861-14
15's	$18.15	GENERIC, Pharma Pac	52959-0440-15
30's	$5.81	GENERIC, Southwood Pharmaceuticals Inc	58016-0861-30
30's	$36.30	GENERIC, Pharma Pac	52959-0440-30
60's	$10.28	GENERIC, Southwood Pharmaceuticals Inc	58016-0861-60

Capsule, Extended Release - Oral - 37.5 mg

100's	$52.89	GENERIC, Mcr/American Pharmaceuticals Inc	58605-0503-01

Tablet - Oral - 8 mg

100's	$54.07	GENERIC, Mcr/American Pharmaceuticals Inc	58605-0504-01

Tablet, Extended Release - Oral - 37.5 mg

100's	$152.25	GENERIC, Qualitest Products Inc	00603-5192-21

Phentolamine Mesylate *(002017)*

Categories: Diagnosis, pheochromocytoma; Hypertension, secondary to pheochromocytoma; Pheochromocytoma; Pregnancy Category C; FDA Approved 1953 Mar

Drug Classes: Antiadrenergics, alpha blocking

Brand Names: **Regitine**

Foreign Brand Availability: Regitin (Czech-Republic; Denmark; Germany; Hungary; Switzerland); Regitina (Peru); Rogitine (England; Ireland); Z-Max (Mexico; Peru)

HCFA JCODE(S): J2760 up to 5 mg IM, IV

DESCRIPTION

Phentolamine mesylate, is an antihypertensive, available in vials for intravenous and intramuscular administration. Each vial contains phentolamine mesylate USP, 5 mg, and mannitol USP, 25 mg, in sterile, lyophilized form.

P

Phentolamine mesylate is 4,5-dihydro-2-(N-(*m*-hydroxyphenyl)-N-(*p*-methylphenyl)amin omethyl)-1*H*-imidazole 1:1 methanesulfonate.

Phentolamine mesylate is a white or off-white, odorless crystalline powder with a molecular weight of 377.46. Its solutions are acid to litmus. It is freely soluble in water and in alcohol, and slightly soluble in chloroform. It melts at about 178°C.

Storage: Store between 59 and 86°F.

CLINICAL PHARMACOLOGY

Phentolamine mesylate produces an alpha-adrenergic block of relatively short duration. It also has direct, but less marked, positive inotropic and chronotropic effects on cardiac muscle and vasodilator effects on vascular smooth muscle.

Phentolamine mesylate has a half-life in the blood of 19 minutes following intravenous administration. Approximately 13% of a single intravenous dose appears in the urine as unchanged drug.

INDICATIONS AND USAGE

Phentolamine mesylate is indicated for the prevention or control of hypertensive episodes that may occur in a patient with pheochromocytoma as a result of stress or manipulation during preoperative preparation and surgical excision.

Phentolamine mesylate is indicated for the prevention of treatment of dermal necrosis and sloughing following intravenous administration or extravasation of norepinephrine.

Phentolamine mesylate is also indicated for the diagnosis of pheochromocytoma by the phentolamine mesylate blocking test.

NON-FDA APPROVED INDICATIONS

Phentolamine has been used without FDA approval for the prevention of dermal necrosis following extravasation of dopamine or accidental injection of epinephrine and for the treatment (with papaverine) of male impotence.

CONTRAINDICATIONS

Myocardial infarction, history of myocardial infarction, coronary insufficiency, angina, or other evidence suggestive of coronary artery disease; hypersensitivity to phentolamine or related compounds.

WARNINGS

Myocardial infarction, cerebrovascular spasm, and cerebrovascular occlusion have been reported to occur following the administration of phentolamine mesylate, usually in association with marked hypotensive episodes.

For screening tests in patients with hypertension, the generally available urinary assay of catecholamines or other biochemical assays have largely replaced the phentolamine mesylate and other pharmacological tests for reasons of accuracy and safety. None of the chemical or pharmacological tests is infallible in the diagnosis of pheochromocytoma. The phentolamine mesylate blocking test is not the procedure of choice and should be reserved for cases in which additional confirmatory evidence is necessary and the relative risks involved in conducting the test have been considered.

PRECAUTIONS

GENERAL

Tachycardia and cardiac arrhythmias may occur with the use of phentolamine mesylate or other alpha-adrenergic blocking agents. When possible, administration of cardiac glycosides should be deferred until cardiac rhythm returns to normal.

P

CARCINOGENESIS, MUTAGENESIS, AND IMPAIRMENT OF FERTILITY

Long-term carcinogenicity studies, mutagenicity studies, and fertility studies have not been conducted with phentolamine mesylate.

PREGNANCY CATEGORY C

Administration of phentolamine mesylate to pregnant rats and mice at oral doses 24-30 times the usual daily human dose (based on a 60 kg human) resulted in slightly decreased growth and slight skeletal immaturity of the fetuses. Immaturity was manifested by increased incidence of incomplete or unossified calcanei and phalangeal nuclei of the hind limb and of incompletely ossified sternebrae. At oral doses 60 times the usual daily human dose (based on a 60 kg human), a slightly lower rate of implantation was found in the rat. Phentolamine mesylate did not affect embryonic or fetal development in the rabbit at oral doses 20 times the usual daily human dose (based on a 60 kg human). No teratogenic or embryotoxic effects were observed in the rat, mouse, or rabbit studies.

There are no adequate and well-controlled studies in pregnant women. Phentolamine mesylate should be used during pregnancy only if the potential benefit justifies the potential risk to the fetus.

NURSING MOTHERS

It is not known whether this drug is excreted in human milk. Because many drugs are excreted in human milk and because of the potential for serious adverse reactions in nursing infants from phentolamine mesylate, a decision should be made whether to discontinue nursing or to discontinue the drug, taking into account the importance of the drug to the mother.

PEDIATRIC USE

See DOSAGE AND ADMINISTRATION.

DRUG INTERACTIONS

See DOSAGE AND ADMINISTRATION, Preparation.

ADVERSE REACTIONS

Acute and prolonged hypotensive episodes, tachycardia, and cardiac arrhythmias have been reported. In addition, weakness, dizziness, flushing, orthostatic hypotension, nasal stuffiness, nausea, vomiting, and diarrhea may occur.

DOSAGE AND ADMINISTRATION

The reconstituted solution should be used upon preparation and should not be stored.

Note: Parenteral drug products should be inspected visually for particulate matter and discoloration prior to administration, whenever solution and container permit.

PREVENTION OR CONTROL OF HYPERTENSIVE EPISODES IN THE PATIENT WITH PHEOCHROMOCYTOMA

For preoperative reduction of elevated blood pressure, 5 mg of phentolamine mesylate (1 mg for children) is injected intravenously or intramuscularly 1 or 2 hours before surgery, and repeated if necessary.

During surgery, phentolamine mesylate (5 mg for adults, 1 mg for children) is administered intravenously as indicated, to help prevent or control paroxysms of hypertension, tachycardia, respiratory depression, convulsions, or other effects of epinephrine intoxication. (Postoperatively norepinephrine may be given to control the hypotension that commonly follows complete removal of a pheochromocytoma.)

PREVENTION OR TREATMENT OF DERMAL NECROSIS AND SLOUGHING FOLLOWING INTRAVENOUS ADMINISTRATION OR EXTRAVASATION OF NOREPINEPHRINE.

For Prevention: 10 mg of phentolamine mesylate is added to each liter of solution containing norepinephrine. The pressor effect of norepinephrine is not affected.

For Treatment: 5-10 mg of phentolamine mesylate in 10 ml of saline is injected into the area of extravasation within 12 hours.

DIAGNOSIS OF PHEOCHROMOCYTOMA - PHENTOLAMINE MESYLATE BLOCKING TEST

The test is most reliable in detecting pheochromocytoma in patients with sustained hypertension and least reliable in those with paroxysmal hypertension. False-positive tests may occur in patients with hypertension without pheochromocytoma.

Intravenous

Preparation

CONTRAINDICATIONS and WARNINGS, and PRECAUTIONS should be reviewed. Sedatives, analgesics, and all other medications except those that might be deemed essential (such as digitalis and insulin) are withheld for at least 24 hours, and preferably 48-72 hours, prior to the test. Antihypertensive drugs are withheld until blood pressure returns to the untreated, hypertensive level. This test is not performed on a patient who is normotensive.

Procedure

The patient is kept at rest in the supine position throughout the test, preferably in a quiet, darkened room. Injection of phentolamine mesylate is delayed until blood pressure is stabilized, as evidenced by blood pressure readings taken every 10 minutes for at least 30 minutes.

Five milligrams of phentolamine mesylate is dissolved in 1 ml of Sterile Water for Injection. The dose for adults is 5 mg; for children, 1 mg.

The syringe needle is inserted into the vein, and injection is delayed until pressor response to venipuncture has subsided.

Phentolamine mesylate is injected rapidly. Blood pressure is recorded immediately after injection, at 30 second intervals for the first 3 minutes, and at 60 second intervals for the next 7 minutes.

Interpretation

A positive response, suggestive of pheochromocytoma, is indicated when the blood pressure is reduced more than 35 mm Hg systolic and 25 mm Hg diastolic. A typical positive response is a reduction in pressure of 60 mm Hg systolic and 25 mm Hg diastolic. Usually, maximal effect is evident within 2 minutes after injection. A return to preinjection pressure commonly occurs within 15-30 minutes but may occur more rapidly.

If blood pressure decreases to a dangerous level, the patient should be treated as outlined under OVERDOSAGE.

A positive response should always be confirmed by other diagnostic procedures, preferably by measurement of urinary catecholamines or their metabolites.

A negative response is indicated when the blood pressure is elevated, unchanged, or reduced less than 35 mm Hg systolic and 25 mm Hg diastolic after injection of phentolamine mesylate. A negative response to this test does not exclude the diagnosis of pheochromocytoma especially in patients with paroxysmal hypertension in whom the incidence of false-negative responses is high.

Intramuscular

If the intramuscular test for pheochromocytoma is preferred, preparation is the same as for the intravenous test. Five milligrams of phentolamine mesylate is then dissolved in 1 ml of Sterile Water of Injection. The dose for adults is 5 mg intramuscularly; for children 3 mg. Blood pressure is recorded every 5 minutes for 30-45 minutes following injection. A positive response is indicated when the blood pressure is reduced 35 mm Hg systolic and 25 mm Hg diastolic, or more, within 20 minutes following injection.

PRODUCT LISTING - RATED THERAPEUTICALLY EQUIVALENT

Powder For Injection - Injectable - 5 mg

1's	$35.00	GENERIC, Bedford Laboratories	55390-0113-01

PRODUCT LISTING - EQUIVALENTS NOT AVAILABLE

Powder For Injection - Injectable - 5 mg

1's	$35.00	GENERIC, Allscripts Pharmaceutical Company	54569-4702-00

Phenylephrine Hydrochloride *(002020)*

Categories: Anesthesia, adjunct; Cycloplegia; Funduscopy, adjunct; Hypotension; Mydriasis; Surgery, ophthalmic, adjunct; Tachycardia, paroxysmal supraventricular; Uveitis; Pregnancy Category C; FDA Pre 1938 Drugs
Drug Classes: Adrenergic agonists; Decongestants, ophthalmic; Ophthalmics
Brand Names: Ah-Chew D; Ak-Dilate; Dilatair; I-Phrine; Murocoll-2; Mydfrin; **Neo-Synephrine**; Neofrin; Ocu-Phrin; Phenylephrine Hcl; Ricobid-D; Spectro-Dilate; Spectro-Nephrine; Storz-Fen
Foreign Brand Availability: Af-Taf (Israel); Albalon Relief (New-Zealand); Drosin (India); Efrin-10 (Israel); Efrisel (Indonesia); Isopto Frin (Australia; Belgium; Czech-Republic; Ecuador; Malaysia; New-Zealand); Metaoxedrin (Denmark; Norway; Sweden); Minims Phenylephrine Hydrochloride (England); Minims Phenylephrine HCL 10% (South-Africa); Nefrin-Ofteno (Costa-Rica; Dominican-Republic; El-Salvador; Guatemala; Honduras; Nicaragua; Panama); Neosynephrine (Belgium; Sweden); Neo-Synephrine Ophthalmic Viscous 10% (Australia); Neosynephrine 10% Chibret (France); Neosynephrine Faure 10% (France); Neosynephrin-POS (Korea); Oftan-Metaoksedrin (Finland); Optistin (Italy); Phenylephrine (Netherlands); Prefrin (Austria; Bahrain; Cyprus; Ecuador; Egypt; Greece; Hong-Kong; Indonesia; Iran; Iraq; Israel; Jordan; Kuwait; Lebanon; Libya; New-Zealand; Oman; Qatar; Republic-of-Yemen; Saudi-Arabia; South-Africa; Syria; Thailand; United-Arab-Emirates); Pupiletto Forte (India); Vistafrin (Spain); Vistosan (Germany)
HCFA JCODE(S): J2370 up to 1 ml SC, IM, IV

WARNING

PHYSICIANS SHOULD THOROUGHLY FAMILIARIZE THEMSELVES WITH THE COMPLETE CONTENTS OF THIS INSERT BEFORE PRESCRIBING PHENYLEPHRINE HYDROCHLORIDE.

DESCRIPTION

(Note: This monograph contains information on the 2.5% ophthalmic solution, the 10% ophthalmic solution, and the 1% injection). Phenylephrine HCl is a sterile topical ophthalmic solution.
Established Name: Phenylephrine Hydrochloride
Chemical Name (2.5%, 10%, and Injection): Benzenemethanol, 3-hydroxy-α-((methylamino)methyl)-,hydrochloride (*S*)-.
Each ml Contains: *Active:* Phenylephrine HCl 2.5%. *Preservative:* Benzalkonium Chloride 0.01%. *Inactive:* Boric Acid, Sodium Bisulfite, Edetate Disodium, Sodium Hydroxide and/or Hydrochloric Acid (to adjust pH), Purified Water.

CLINICAL PHARMACOLOGY

2.5%/10% Solution: Phenylephrine HCl 2.5% is an alpha receptor sympathetic agonist used in local ocular disorders because of its vasoconstrictor and mydriatic action. It exhibits rapid and moderately prolonged action, and it produces little rebound vasodilatation. Systemic side effects are uncommon.
The action of different concentrations of ophthalmic solutions of phenylephrine HCl 2.5% is shown in TABLE 1.

***TABLE 1** Phenylephrine HCl, Clinical Pharmacology*

	Mydriasis		
Strength of Solution	Maximal	Recovery Time	Paralysis of Accommodation
2.5	15-60 min	3 hours	trace
10	10-60 min	6 hours	slight

1% Injection: Phenylephrine HCl provides vasoconstriction that lasts longer than that of epinephrine and ephedrine. Responses are more sustained than those to epinephrine, lasting 20 minutes after intravenous and as long as 50 minutes after subcutaneous injection. It's action on the heart contrasts sharply with that of epinephrine and ephedrine, in that it slows the heart rate and increases the stroke output, producing no disturbance in the rhythm of the pulse.
Phenylephrine is a powerful postsynaptic alpha-receptor stimulant with little effect on the beta receptors of the heart. In therapeutic doses it produces little if any stimulation of either spinal cord or cerebrum. a singular advantage of this drug is the fact that repeated injections produce comparable effects.

The predominant actions of phenylephrine are on the cardiovascular system. Parenteral administration causes a rise in systolic and diastolic pressures in man and other species. Accompanying the pressure response to phenylephrine is a marked reflex bradycardia that can be blocked by atropine; after atropine, large doses of the drug increase the heart rate only slightly. In man, cardiac output is slightly decreased and peripheral resistance is considerably increased. Circulation time is slightly prolonged, and venous pressure is slightly increased; venous constriction is not marked. Most vascular beds are constricted; renal splanchnic, cutaneous, and limb blood flows are reduced but coronary blood blow is increased. Pulmonary vessels are constricted, and pulmonary arterial pressure is raised.

The drug is a powerful vasoconstrictor, with properties very similar to those of norepinephrine but almost completely lacking the chronotropic and inotropic actions on the heart. Cardiac irregularities are seen only very rarely even with large doses.

INDICATIONS AND USAGE

2.5%/10% Solution: Phenylephrine HCl is recommended as a vasoconstrictor, decongestant, and mydriatic in a variety of ophthalmic conditions and procedures. Some of its uses are for pupillary dilatation in uveitis (to prevent or aid in the disruption of posterior synechia formation), for many ophthalmic surgical procedures and for refraction without cycloplegia. Phenylephrine HCl 2.5% may also be used for funduscopy, and other diagnostic procedures.
1% Injection: Phenylephrine HCl 1% injection is intended for the maintenance of an adequate level of blood pressure during spinal and inhalation anesthesia and for the treatment of vascular failure in shock, shocklike states, and drug-induced hypotension, or hypersensitivity. It is also employed to overcome paroxysmal superventricular tachycardia, to prolong spinal anesthesia, and as a vasoconstrictor in regional analgesia.

CONTRAINDICATIONS

Ophthalmic solutions, (both strengths), of phenylephrine HCl are contraindicated in patients with anatomically narrow angles or narrow angle glaucoma. Phenylephrine HCl may be contraindicated in some low birth weight infants and some elderly adults with severe arteriosclerotic cardiovascular or cerebrovascular disease. Phenylephrine HCl may be contraindicated during intraocular operative procedures when the corneal epithelial barrier has been disturbed. This preparation is also contraindicated in persons with a known sensitivity to phenylephrine HCl or any of its components.
Additional Information for the 10% Solution: Contraindicated in infants and in patients with aneurysms.
1% Injection: Phenylephrine HCl injection should not be used with patients with severe hypertension, ventricular tachycardia, or in patients who are hypersensitive to it.

WARNINGS

10% Solution: There have been reports associating the use of phenylephrine HCl 10% ophthalmic solutions with the development of serious cardiovascular reactions, including ventricular arrhythmias and myocardial infarctions. These episodes, some ending fatally, have usually occurred in elderly patients with preexisting cardiovascular diseases.
1% Injection: If used in conjunction with oxytocic drugs, the pressure effect of sympathomimetic pressor amines is potentiated. The obstetrician should be warned that some oxytocic drugs may cause severe persistent hypertension and that even a rupture of a cerebral blood vessel may occur during the postpartum period.
Contains sodium metabisulfite, a sulfite that may cause allergic-type reactions including anaphylactic symptoms and life-threatening or less severe asthmatic episodes in certain susceptible people. The overall prevalence of sulfite sensitivity in the general population is unknown and probably low. Sulfite sensitivity is seen more frequently in asthmatic than in nonasthmatic people.

PRECAUTIONS

Both Solution Strengths: Ordinarily, any mydriatic, including phenylephrine HCl, is contraindicated in patients with glaucoma, since it may occasionally raise intraocular pressure. However, when temporary dilatation of the pupil may free adhesions, this advantage may temporarily outweigh the danger from coincident dilatation of the pupil. Rebound miosis has been reported in older persons one day after receiving phenylephrine HCl ophthalmic solutions, and reinstillation of the drug may produce less mydriasis than previously. This may be of clinical importance in dilating the pupils of older subjects prior to retinal detachment or cataract surgery. The lacrimal sac should be compressed by digital pressure for one minute after instillation to avoid excessive systemic absorption.
Due to a strong action of the drug on the dilator muscle, older individuals may also develop transient pigment floaters in the aqueous humor 40 to 45 minutes following the administration of phenylephrine HCl ophthalmic solution. The appearance may be similar to anterior uveitis or to a microscopic hyphema. To prevent pain, a drop of suitable topical anesthetic may be applied before using. Prolonged exposure to air or strong light may cause oxidation and discoloration. Do not use if solution is brown or contains a precipitate.
Additional Information for the 10% Solution: A significant elevation in blood pressure is rare but has been reported following conjunctival instillation of recommended doses of phenylephrine HCl 10%. Caution, therefore, should be exercised in administering the 10% solutions to children of low body weight, the elderly, and patients with insulin-dependent diabetes, hypertension, hyperthyroidism, generalized arteriosclerosis, or cardiovascular disease. The posttreatment blood pressure of these patients, and any patients who develop symptoms, should be carefully monitored.
To prevent pain, a drop of suitable topical anesthetic may be applied before using the 10 percent ophthalmic solution.

It has ben reported that the concomitant use of phenylephrine HCl 10% ophthalmic solutions and systemic beta blockers has caused acute hypertension and, in one case, the rupture of a congenital cerebral aneurysm. This drug may potentiate the cardiovascular depressant effects of potent inhalation anesthetic agents.
1% Injection: Should be employed only with extreme caution in elderly patients or in patients with hyperthyroidism, bradycardia, partial heart block, myocardial disease, or severe arteriosclerosis.
Vasopressors, particularly metaraminol, may cause serious cardiac arrhythmias during halothane anesthesia and therefore should be used only with great caution or not at all.

The pressor effect of sympathomimetic pressor amines is markedly potentiated in patients receiving MAO inhibitors. Therefore, when initiating pressor therapy in these patients, the initial dose should be small and used with due caution. The pressor response of adrenergic agents may also be potentiated by tricyclic antidepressants.
Carcinogenesis, Mutagenesis, and Impairment of Fertility: No long-term animal studies have been done to evaluate the potential of phenylephrine HCl injection in these areas.
Pregnancy Category C: Animal reproduction studies have not been conducted with this drug. It is also not known whether phenylephrine HCl injection can cause fetal harm when administered to a pregnant woman or can affect reproduction capacity. This drug should be given to a pregnant women only if clearly needed.
Labor and Delivery: If vasopressor drugs are either used to correct hypotension or added to the local anesthetic solution, the obstetrician should be cautioned that some oxytocic drugs may cause severe persistent hypertension and that a rupture of a cerebral blood vessel may occur during the postpartum period (see WARNINGS.)
Nursing Mothers: It is not known whether this drug is excreted in human milk. Because many are excreted in human milk, caution should be exercised when phenylephrine HCl injection is administered to a nursing woman.
Pediatric Use: To combat hypotension during special anesthesia in children, a dose of 0.5 mg to 1 mg per 25 pounds body weight, administered subcutaneously or IM, is recommended.

DRUG INTERACTIONS

2.5% Solution: Not for intraocular use. As with other adrenergic drugs, when it is administered simultaneously with, or up to 21-days after, administration of monoamine oxidase

P

(MAO) inhibitors, careful supervision and adjustment of dosages are required since exaggerated adrenergic effects may result. The pressor response of adrenergic agents may also be potentiated by tricyclic antidepressants. Systemic side effects are more common in patients taking beta adrenergic blocking agents such as propranolol.

ADVERSE REACTIONS

(Pertains only to the injection)
Headache, reflex bradycardia, excitability, restlessness, and rarely arrhythmias.

DOSAGE AND ADMINISTRATION

2.5% SOLUTION

Vasoconstriction and Pupil Dilatation: Phenylephrine HCl 2.5% is especially useful when rapid and powerful dilatation of the pupil without cycloplegia and reduction of congestion in the capillary bed are desired. A drop of a suitable topical anesthetic may be applied, followed in a few minutes by 1 drop of the on the upper limbus. The anesthetic prevents stinging and consequent dilution of the solution by lacrimation. It may occasionally be necessary to repeat the instillation after one hour, again preceded by the use of the topical anesthetic.

Uveitis

Posterior Synechia: Phenylephrine HCl 2.5% may be used in patients with uveitis when synechiae are present or may develop. The formation of synechia may be prevented by the use of this ophthalmic solution and atropine or other cycloplegics to produce wide dilatation of the pupil. For recently formed posterior synechiae one drop of may be applied to the upper surface of the cornea and be repeated as necessary, not to exceed three times. Treatment may be continued the following day, if necessary. Atropine sulfate and the application of hot compresses should also be used if indicated.

MYDRIATICS/CYCLOPLEGICS

Glaucoma: Phenylephrine HCl 2.5% may be used with miotics in patients with open angle glaucoma. It reduces the difficulties experienced by the patient because of the small field produced by miosis, and still it permits and often supports the effect of the miotic in lowering the intraocular pressure in open angle glaucoma. Hence, there may be marked improvement in visual acuity after using phenylephrine HCl 2.5% in conjunction with miotic drugs.

Surgery: When a short-acting mydriatic is needed for wide dilatation of the pupil before intraocular surgery, phenylephrine HCl 2.5% (or the 10%) may be applied topically from 30 to 60 minutes before the operation.

Refraction: Phenylephrine HCl 2.5% may be used effectively to increase mydriasis with homatropine hydrobromide, cyclopentolate hydrochloride, tropicamide hydrochloride and atropine sulfate.

For Adults: One drop of the preferred cycloplegic is placed in each eye, followed in 5 minutes by one drop of phenylephrine HCl 2.5%.

Since adequate cycloplegia is achieved at different time intervals after the instillation of the necessary number of drops, different cycloplegics will require different waiting periods to achieve adequate cycloplegia.

For Children: For a "one application method," phenylephrine HCl 2.5% may be combined with one of the preferred rapid acting cycloplegics to produce adequate cycloplegia.

Ophthalmoscopic Examination: One drop of phenylephrine HCl 2.5% is placed in each eye. Sufficient mydriasis to permit examination is produced in 15 to 30 minutes. Dilatation lasts from one to three hours.

P

Diagnostic Procedures: Provocative Test for Angle Closure Glaucoma: phenylephrine HCl 2.5% may be used cautiously as a provocative test when interval narrow angle closure glaucoma is suspected. Intraocular tension and gonioscopy are performed prior to and after dilatation of the pupil with phenylephrine HCl. A "significant" intraocular pressure (IOP) rise combined with gonioscopic evidence of angle closure indicates an anterior segment anatomy capable of angle closure. A negative test does not rule this out. This pharmacologically induced angle closure glaucoma may not simulate real life conditions and other causes for transient elevations of IOP should be excluded.

Retinoscopy (Shadow Test): When dilatation of the pupil without cycloplegic action is desired for retinoscopy, may be used.

NOTE: Heavily pigmented irides may require larger doses in all of the above procedures.

Blanching Test: One or two drops of phenylephrine HCl 2.5% should be applied to the injected eye. After five minutes, examine for perilimbal blanching. If blanching occurs, the congestion is superficial and probably does not indicate iridocyclitis.

10% SOLUTION

Vasoconstriction and Pupil Dilatation: (same as 2.5%, please see above)

Uveitis

Posterior Synechiae: (also see 2.5%, above). Phenylephrine HCl 10% ophthalmic solution may be used in patients with uveitis when synechiae are present or may develop. The formation of synechiae may be prevented by the use of the 10% solution and atropine to produce wide dilation of the pupil. It should be emphasized, however, that the vasoconstrictor effect of this drug may be antagonistic to the increase of local blood flow in uveal infection. To free recently formed posterior synechiae, 1 drop of the 10 percent ophthalmic solution may be applied to the upper surface of the cornea. On the following day, treatment may be continued if necessary. In the interim, hot compresses should be applied for five or ten minutes three times a day, with 1 drop of a 1 or 2 percent solution of atropine sulfate before and after each series of compresses.

Glaucoma: In certain patients with glaucoma, temporary reduction of intraocular tension may be attained by producing vasoconstriction of the intraocular vessels; this may be accompanied by placing 1 drop of the 10 % solution on the upper surface of the cornea. This treatment may be repeated as often as necessary.

1% INJECTION

Generally injected subcutaneously, intramuscularly, slowly intravenously, or in dilute solution as a continuous IV infusion. In patients with paroxysmal superventricular tachycardia and, if indicated, in case of emergency, phenylephrine HCl is administered directly intravenously. The dose should be adjusted according to the pressure response. Dosage calculations are shown in TABLE 2.

TABLE 2 *Dosage Calculations*

Dose Required	Use Phenylephrine HCl 1%
10 mg	1 ml
5 mg	0.5 ml
1 mg	0.1 ml

For convenience in intermittent IV administration, dilute 1 ml phenylephrine HCl 1% with 9 ml Sterile Water for Injection, USP, to yield 0.1% phenylephrine HCl (TABLE 3).

TABLE 3 *Phenylephrine HCl, DOSAGE AND ADMINISTRATION*

Dose Required	Use Diluted Phenylephrine HCl (0.1%)
0.1 mg	0.1 ml
0.2 mg	0.2 ml
0.5 mg	0.5 ml

Mild or Moderate Hypotension: *Subcutaneously or Intramuscularly:* Usual dose, from 1 mg to 10 mg. Initial dose should not exceed 5 mg. *Intravenously:* Usual dose, 0.2 mg. Range, from 0.1 mg to 0.5 mg. Initial dose should not exceed 0.5 mg.

Injections should not be repeated more often than every 10 to 15 minutes. A 5 mg IM dose should raise blood pressure for one to two hours. A 0.5 mg IV dose should elevate the pressure for about 15 minutes.

SEVERE HYPOTENSION AND SHOCK - INCLUDING DRUG-RELATED HYPOTENSION

Blood volume depletion should always be corrected as fully as possible before any vasopressor is administered. When, as an emergency measure, intra-aortic pressures must be maintained to prevent cerebral or coronary artery ischemia, phenylephrine HCl can be administered before and concurrently with blood volume replacement.

Hypotension and occasionally severe shock may result from overdosage or idiosyncracy following the administration of certain drugs, especially adrenergic and ganglionic blocking agents, rauwolfia and veratrum alkaloids, and phenothiazine tranquilizers. patients who receive a phenothiazine derivative as preoperative medication are especially susceptible to these reactions. As an adjunct in the management of such episodes, phenylephrine HCl 1% is a suitable agent for restoring blood pressure.

Higher initial and maintenance doses of phenylephrine HCl are required in patients with persistent or untreated severe hypotension or shock. Hypotension produced by powerful peripheral adrenergic blocking agents, chlorpromazine, or pheochromocytometoctomy may also require more intensive therapy.

Continuous Infusion: Add 10 mg of the drug (1 ml of 1 percent solution) to 500 ml of Dextrose Injection, USP, or Sodium Chloride Injection, USP (providing a 1:50,000 solution). To raise the blood pressure rapidly, start to infusion at about 100 µg to 180 µg per minute (based on 20 drops per ml this would be 100 to 180 drops per minute). When the blood pressure is stabilized (at a low normal level for the individual), a maintenance rate of 40 µg to 60 µg per minute usually suffices (based on 20 drops per ml this would be 40 µg to 60 µg per minute). If the drop size of the infusion system varies from the 20 drops per ml, the dose must be adjusted accordingly.

If a prompt initial pressor response is not obtained, additional increments of phenylephrine HCl (10 mg or more) are added to the infusion bottle. The rate of flow is then adjusted until the desired blood pressure level is obtained. (In some cases, a more potent vasopressor such as norepinephrine biurate, may be required). Hypertension should be avoided. The blood pressure should be checked frequently. Headache and/or bradycardia may indicate hypertension. Arrhythmias are rare.

SPINAL ANESTHESIA-HYPOTENSION

Routine parenteral use of phenylephrine HCl has been recommended for the prophylaxis and treatment of hypotension during spinal anesthesia. It is best administered subcutaneously or intramuscularly three to four minutes before injection of the spinal anesthetic. The total requirement for high anesthetic levels is usually 3 mg, and for the lower levels, 2 mg. For hypotensive emergencies during spinal anesthesia, this drug may be given IV, using an initial dose of 0.2 mg. Any subsequent dose should not exceed the previous dose by more than 0.1 mg to 0.2 mg and no more than 0.5 mg should be administered in a single dose. To combat hypotension during spinal anesthesia in children, a dose of 0.5 mg to 1 mg per 25 pounds body weight, administered subcutaneously or IM, is recommended.

PROLONGATION OF SPINAL ANESTHESIA

The addition of 2 mg to 5 mg of phenylephrine HCl to the anesthetic solution increases the duration of motor block by as much as approximately 50% without any increase in the incidence of complications such as nausea, vomiting, or blood pressure disturbances.

VASOCONSTRICTOR FOR REGIONAL ANALGESIA

Concentrations about 10 times those employed when epinephrine is used as a vasoconstrictor are recommended. The optimum strength is 1:20,000 (made by adding 1 mg of phenylephrine HCl to every 20 ml of local anesthetic solution). Some pressor responses can be expected when 2 mg or more are injected.

PAROXYSMAL SUPERVENTRICULAR TACHYCARDIA

Rapid IV Injection (within 20 to 30 seconds) is recommended; the initial dose should not exceed 0.5 mg, and subsequent doses, which are determined by the initial blood pressure response, should not exceed the preceding dose by more than 0.1 mg to 0.2 mg and should never exceed 1 mg.

Protect from light if removed from carton or dispensing bin.

Storage: *(2.5 and 10% Solutions):* Store at 36° to 80°F. Protect from light and excessive heat.

PRODUCT LISTING - RATED THERAPEUTICALLY EQUIVALENT

Solution - Injectable - 10 mg/ml

Size	Price	Manufacturer	NDC
1 ml x 25	$33.75	GENERIC, Gensia Sicor Pharmaceuticals Inc	00703-1631-04

PRODUCT LISTING - EQUIVALENTS NOT AVAILABLE

Size	Price	Manufacturer	NDC
Liquid - Oral - 5 mg/5 ml			
120 ml	$10.98	DESPEC-SF, International Ethical Laboratories Inc	11584-0453-04
Solution - Injectable - 10 mg/ml			
1 ml x 25	$18.75	GENERIC, Baxter Pharmaceutical Products, Inc	10019-0163-12
1 ml x 25	$33.25	GENERIC, International Medication Systems, Limited	00548-8301-25
1 ml x 25	$78.25	GENERIC, American Regent Laboratories Inc	00517-0299-25
5 ml	$390.75	GENERIC, American Regent Laboratories Inc	00517-0405-25
5 ml x 25	$143.50	GENERIC, Baxter Pharmaceutical Products, Inc	10019-0163-01
10 ml	$1.33	GENERIC, International Medication Systems, Limited	00548-8301-00
Solution - Ophthalmic - 2.5%			
2 ml	$3.73	GENERIC, Bausch and Lomb	24208-0740-59
2 ml	$3.94	GENERIC, Prescript Pharmaceuticals	00247-0048-02
2 ml	$4.10	GENERIC, Akorn Inc	17478-0200-20
3 ml	$4.10	GENERIC, Falcon Pharmaceuticals, Ltd.	61314-0342-01
3 ml	$134.28	MYDFRIN, Alcon Laboratories Inc	00065-0342-03
5 ml	$2.63	OCU-PHRIN, Ocumed Inc	51944-4470-05
5 ml	$3.50	GENERIC, Cmc-Consolidated Midland Corporation	00223-6695-05
5 ml	$4.14	GENERIC, Bausch and Lomb	24208-0740-02
5 ml	$4.15	GENERIC, Falcon Pharmaceuticals, Ltd.	61314-0342-02
5 ml	$4.81	GENERIC, Prescript Pharmaceuticals	00247-0048-05
5 ml	$6.43	GENERIC, Physicians Total Care	54868-2812-01
5 ml	$19.50	MYDFRIN, Alcon Laboratories Inc	00998-0342-05
15 ml	$3.00	OCU-PHRIN, Ocumed Inc	51944-4470-02
15 ml	$3.90	GENERIC, Cmc-Consolidated Midland Corporation	00223-6695-15
15 ml	$4.00	GENERIC, Miza Pharmaceutcials Dba Optopics Laboratories Corporation	55238-0718-15
15 ml	$4.90	GENERIC, Bausch and Lomb	24208-0740-06
15 ml	$6.19	GENERIC, Ocusoft	54799-0530-15
15 ml	$6.70	GENERIC, Akorn Inc	17478-0200-12
15 ml	$7.72	GENERIC, Prescript Pharmaceuticals	00247-0048-15
15 ml	$11.60	GENERIC, Southwood Pharmaceuticals Inc	58016-6097-01
15 ml	$24.37	NEO-SYNEPHRINE OPHTHALMIC, Allscripts Pharmaceutical Company	54569-2304-00
15 ml	$30.23	NEO-SYNEPHRINE OPHTHALMIC, Sanofi Winthrop Pharmaceuticals	00024-1358-01
Solution - Ophthalmic - 10%			
1 ml x 12	$30.63	GENERIC, Ciba Vision Ophthalmics	00058-0780-12
2 ml	$4.76	GENERIC, Akorn Inc	17478-0205-20
5 ml	$3.00	OCU-PHRIN, Ocumed Inc	51944-4475-35
5 ml	$4.00	GENERIC, Cmc-Consolidated Midland Corporation	00223-6696-05
5 ml	$6.70	GENERIC, Akorn Inc	17478-0205-10
5 ml	$7.20	GENERIC, Allscripts Pharmaceutical Company	54569-1442-00
5 ml	$28.03	NEO-SYNEPHRINE OPHTHALMIC, Sanofi Winthrop Pharmaceuticals	00024-1362-01
5 ml	$28.89	NEO-SYNEPHRINE OPHTHALMIC, Sanofi Winthrop Pharmaceuticals	00024-1359-01
15 ml	$3.68	OCU-PHRIN, Ocumed Inc	51944-4475-02
15 ml	$4.95	GENERIC, Cmc-Consolidated Midland Corporation	00223-6696-15
Suppository - Rectal - 0.25%			
12's	$5.50	RECTASOL, Bio Pharm Inc	59741-0302-12

Phenytoin Sodium *(002030)*

Categories: Seizures, complex partial; Seizures, generalized tonic-clonic; Seizures, secondary to neurosurgery; FDA Approval Pre 1982; Pregnancy Category D

Drug Classes: Anticonvulsants; Hydantoins

Brand Names: **Dilantin**; Dilantin Kapseals; Diphen; Diphentoin; Diphenylan Sodium; Dyatoin; Phenytex; Prompt Phenytoin Sodium

Foreign Brand Availability: Aleviatin (Japan); Antisacer (Portugal); Cumatil (Colombia); Difhydan (Denmark); Dintoina (Italy); Diphantoine (Belgium); Diphantoine-Z (Netherlands); Ditoin (Hong-Kong; Malaysia; Thailand); Ditomed (Thailand); Epamin (Argentina; Canada; CIS; Colombia; Ecuador; Mexico; Peru); Epanutin (Austria; Bahrain; Belgium; Benin; Burkina-Faso; Cyprus; Egypt; England; Ethiopia; Finland; Gambia; Germany; Ghana; Greece; Guinea; Hungary; Iran; Iraq; Ireland; Israel; Ivory-Coast; Jordan; Kenya; Kuwait; Lebanon; Liberia; Libya; Malawi; Mali; Mauritania; Mauritius; Morocco; Netherlands; Niger; Nigeria; Oman; Qatar; Republic-of-Yemen; Saudi-Arabia; Senegal; Seychelles; Sierra-Leone; South-Africa; Spain; Sudan; Sweden; Switzerland; Syria; Tanzania; Tunia; Turkey; Uganda; United-Arab-Emirates; Zambia; Zimbabwe); Epilan-D (Austria); Epilantin (Philippines; Switzerland); Epileptin (Taiwan); Eptoin (India); Felantin (Peru); Fenatoin NM (Sweden); Fenidantoin S 100 (Mexico); Fenitron (Mexico); Fenytoin (Denmark; Germany); Hidanil (Colombia); Hydantin (Finland); Hydantol (Japan); Lehydan (Sweden); Nuctane (Mexico); Phenhydan (Austria; Germany; Switzerland); Phenilep (Indonesia); Phenytoin KP (Thailand); Pyoredol (Argentina); Vasilcon (Philippines)

Cost of Therapy: $27.82 (Epilepsy; Dilantin Kapseals; 100 mg; 3 capsules/day; 30 day supply)
$40.41 (Epilepsy; Generic Capsules; 100 mg; 3 capsules/day; 30 day supply)

HCFA JCODE(S): J1165 per 50 mg IM, IV

DESCRIPTION

Phenytoin sodium is an antiepileptic drug. Phenytoin sodium is related to the barbiturates in chemical structure, but has a five-membered ring. The chemical name is sodium 5,5-diphenyl-2, 4-imidazolidinedione.

Each Dilantin (extended phenytoin sodium) capsule contains 30 or 100 mg phenytoin sodium. Also contains lactose, confectioner's sugar, talc, and magnesium stearate. The capsule shell and band contain colloidal silicon dioxide, FD&C red no. 3, gelatin, glyceryl monooleate, sodium lauryl sulfate. The dilantin 30 mg capsule shell and band also contain citric acid, FD&C blue no. 1, sodium benzoate, titanium dioxide. The dilantin 100 mg capsule shell and band also contain FD&C yellow no. 6, purified water, and polyethylene glycol 200. Product *in vivo* performance is characterized by a slow and extended rate of absorption with peak blood concentrations expected in 4-12 hours as contrasted to *Prompt Phenytoin Sodium Capsules,* with a rapid rate of absorption with peak blood concentration expected in 1.5-3 hours.

CLINICAL PHARMACOLOGY

Phenytoin is an antiepileptic drug which can be useful in the treatment of epilepsy. The primary site of action appears to be the *motor cortex* where spread of seizure activity is inhibited. Possibly by promoting sodium efflux from neurons, phenytoin tends to *stabilize* the threshold against hyperexcitability caused by excessive stimulation or environmental changes capable of reducing membrane sodium gradient. This includes the reduction of posttetanic potentiation at synapses. Loss of posttetanic potentiation prevents cortical seizure foci from detonating adjacent cortical areas. Phenytoin reduces the maximal activity of brain stem centers responsible for the tonic phase of tonic-clonic (grand mal) seizures.

The plasma half-life in man after oral administration of phenytoin averages 22 hours, with a range of 7-42 hours. Steady-state therapeutic levels are achieved at least 7-10 days (5-7 half-lives) after initiation of therapy with recommended doses of 300 mg/day.

When serum level determinations are necessary, they should be obtained at least 5-7 half-lives after treatment initiation, dosage change, or addition or subtraction of another drug to the regimen so that equilibrium or steady-state will have been achieved. Trough levels provide information about clinically effective serum level range and confirm patient compliance and are obtained just prior to the patient's next scheduled dose. Peak levels indicate an individual's threshold for emergence of dose-related side effects and are obtained at the time of expected peak concentration. For phenytoin sodium capsules kapseals peak serum levels occur 4-12 hours after administration.

Optimum control without clinical signs of toxicity occurs more often with serum levels between 10 and 20 μg/ml, although some mild cases of tonic-clonic (grand mal) epilepsy may be controlled with lower serum levels of phenytoin.

In most patients maintained at a steady dosage, stable phenytoin serum levels are achieved. There may be wide interpatient variability in phenytoin serum levels with equivalent dosages. Patients with unusually low levels may be noncompliant or hypermetabolizers of phenytoin. Unusually high levels result from liver disease, congenital enzyme deficiency or drug interactions which result in metabolic interference. The patient with large variations in phenytoin plasma levels, despite standard doses, presents a difficult clinical problem. Serum level determinations in such patients may be particularly helpful. As phenytoin is highly protein bound, free phenytoin levels may be altered in patients whose protein binding characteristics differ from normal.

Most of the drug is excreted in the bile as inactive metabolites which are then reabsorbed from the intestinal tract and excreted in the urine. Urinary excretion of phenytoin and its metabolites occurs partly with glomerular filtration but, more importantly, by tubular secretion. Because phenytoin is hydroxylated in the liver by an enzyme system which is saturable at high plasma levels, small incremental doses may increase the half-life and produce very substantial increases in serum levels, when these are in the upper range. The steady-state level may be disproportionately increased, with resultant intoxication, from an increase in dosage of 10% or more.

INDICATIONS AND USAGE

Phenytoin sodium capsules is indicated for the control of generalized tonic-clonic (grand mal) and complex partial (psychomotor, temporal lobe) seizures and prevention and treatment of seizures occurring during or following neurosurgery.

Phenytoin serum level determinations may be necessary for optimal dosage adjustments (see DOSAGE AND ADMINISTRATION and CLINICAL PHARMACOLOGY).

NON-FDA APPROVED INDICATIONS

Phenytoin has also been used for the treatment of trigeminal neuralgia (and other neuralgias) and migraine. Additionally, phenytoin possesses antiarrhythmic activity and has been used in the treatment of ventricular tachycardia, paroxysmal supraventricular tachycardia and arrhythmias associated with digitalis glycoside toxicity. (Currently, phenytoin is rarely used as an antiarrhythmic agent, but may occasionally play a role in the treatment of arrhythmias associated with digitalis excess.) Phenytoin has been reported to be effective in the treatment of rheumatoid arthritis and discoid lupus erythematosus. Phenytoin has also been used topically to speed the healing of chronic skin ulcers. Low doses of phenytoin have been reported to be effectively increase HDL-C levels in men with low levels of HDL-C. However, none of these uses is approved by the FDA and standard dosage recommendations for these indications are not available.

CONTRAINDICATIONS

Phenytoin is contraindicated in those patients who are hypersensitive to phenytoin or other hydantoins.

WARNINGS

Abrupt withdrawal of phenytoin in epileptic patients may precipitate status epilepticus. When, in the judgment of the clinician, the need for dosage reduction, discontinuation, or substitution of alternative antiepileptic medication arises, this should be done gradually. However, in the event of an allergic or hypersensitivity reaction, rapid substitution of alternative therapy may be necessary. In this case, alternative therapy should be an antiepileptic drug not belonging to the hydantoin chemical class.

There have been a number of reports suggesting a relationship between phenytoin and the development of lymphadenopathy (local or generalized) including benign lymph node hyperplasia, pseudolymphoma, lymphoma, and Hodgkin's disease. Although a cause and effect relationship has not been established, the occurrence of lymphadenopathy indicates the need to differentiate such a condition from other types of lymph node pathology. Lymph node involvement may occur with or without symptoms and signs resembling serum sickness, *e.g.*, fever, rash, and liver involvement.

In all cases of lymphadenopathy, follow-up observation for an extended period is indicated and every effort should be made to achieve seizure control using alternative antiepileptic drugs.

Acute alcoholic intake may increase phenytoin serum levels, while chronic alcohol use may decrease serum levels.

In view of isolated reports associating phenytoin with exacerbation of porphyria, caution should be exercised in using this medication in patients suffering from this disease.

USE IN PREGNANCY

A number of reports suggests an association between the use of antiepileptic drugs by women with epilepsy and a higher incidence of birth defects in children born to these women. Data are more extensive with respect to phenytoin and phenobarbital, but these are also the most commonly prescribed antiepileptic drugs; less systematic or anecdotal reports suggest a possible similar association with the use of all known antiepileptic drugs.

The reports suggesting a higher incidence of birth defects in children of drug-treated epileptic women cannot be regarded as adequate to prove a definite cause and effect relationship. There are intrinsic methodologic problems in obtaining adequate data on drug teratogenicity in humans; genetic factors or the epileptic condition itself may be more important than drug therapy in leading to birth defects. The great majority of mothers on antiepileptic medication deliver normal infants. It is important to note that antiepileptic drugs should not be discontinued in patients in whom the drug is administered to prevent major seizures, because of the strong possibility of precipitating status epilepticus with attendant hypoxia and threat to life. In individual cases where the severity and frequency of the seizure disorder are such that the removal of medication does not pose a serious threat to the patient, discontinuation of the drug may be considered prior to and during pregnancy, although it cannot be said with any confidence that even minor seizures do not pose some hazard to the developing embryo or fetus. The prescribing physician will wish to weigh these considerations in treating or counseling epileptic women of childbearing potential.

In addition to the reports of increased incidence of congenital malformation, such as cleft lip/palate and heart malformations, in children of women receiving phenytoin and other antiepileptic drugs, there have more recently been reports of a fetal hydantoin syndrome. This consists of prenatal growth deficiency, microcephaly and mental deficiency in children born to mothers who have received phenytoin, barbiturates, alcohol, or trimethadione. However, these features are all inter-related and are frequently associated with intrauterine growth retardation from other causes.

There have been isolated reports of malignancies, including neuroblastoma, in children whose mothers received phenytoin during pregnancy.

An increase in seizure frequency during pregnancy occurs in a high proportion of patients, because of altered phenytoin absorption or metabolism. Periodic measurement of serum phenytoin levels is particularly valuable in the management of a pregnant epileptic patient as a guide to an appropriate adjustment of dosage. However, postpartum restoration of the original dosage will probably be indicated.

Neonatal coagulation defects have been reported within the first 24 hours in babies born to epileptic mothers receiving phenobarbital and/or phenytoin. Vitamin K has been shown to prevent or correct this defect and has been recommended to be given to the mother before delivery and to the neonate after birth.

PRECAUTIONS

GENERAL

The liver is the chief site of biotransformation of phenytoin; patients with impaired liver function, elderly patients, or those who are gravely ill may show early signs of toxicity.

A small percentage of individuals who have been treated with phenytoin has been shown to metabolize the drug slowly. Slow metabolism may be due to limited enzyme availability and lack of induction; it appears to be genetically determined.

Phenytoin should be discontinued if a skin rash appears (see WARNINGS regarding drug discontinuation). If the rash is exfoliative, purpuric, or bullous or if lupus erythematosus, Stevens-Johnson syndrome, or toxic epidermal necrolysis is suspected, use of this drug should not be resumed and alternative therapy should be considered. (See ADVERSE REACTIONS.) If the rash is of a milder type (measles-like or scarlatiniform), therapy may be resumed after the rash has completely disappeared. If the rash recurs upon reinstitution of therapy, further phenytoin medication is contraindicated.

Phenytoin and other hydantoins are contraindicated in patients who have experienced phenytoin hypersensitivity. Additionally, caution should be exercised if using structurally similar compounds (*e.g.*, barbiturates, succinimides, oxazolidinediones and other related compounds) in these same patients.

Hyperglycemia, resulting from the drug's inhibitory effects on insulin release, has been reported. Phenytoin may also raise the serum glucose level in diabetic patients.

Osteomalacia has been associated with phenytoin therapy and is considered to be due to phenytoin's interference with vitamin D metabolism.

Phenytoin is not indicated for seizures due to hypoglycemic or other metabolic causes. Appropriate diagnostic procedures should be performed as indicated.

Phenytoin is not effective for absence (petit mal) seizures. If tonic-clonic (grand mal) and absence (petit mal) seizures are present, combined drug therapy is needed.

Serum levels of phenytoin sustained above the optimal range may produce confusional states referred to as "delirium," "psychosis," or "encephalopathy," or rarely irreversible cerebellar dysfunction. Accordingly, at the first sign of acute toxicity, plasma levels are recommended. Dose reduction of phenytoin therapy is indicated if plasma levels are excessive; if symptoms persist, termination is recommended. (See WARNINGS.)

INFORMATION FOR THE PATIENT

Patients taking phenytoin should be advised of the importance of adhering strictly to the prescribed dosage regimen, and of informing the physician of any clinical condition in which it is not possible to take the drug orally as prescribed, *e.g.*, surgery, etc.

Patients should also be cautioned on the use of other drugs or alcoholic beverages without first seeking the physician's advice.

Patients should be instructed to call their physician if skin rash develops.

The importance of good dental hygiene should be stressed in order to minimize the development of gingival hyperplasia and its complications.

Do not use capsules which are discolored.

LABORATORY TESTS

Phenytoin serum level determinations may be necessary to achieve optimal dosage adjustments.

DRUG/LABORATORY TEST INTERACTIONS

Phenytoin may cause decreased serum levels of protein-bound iodine (PBI). It may also produce lower than normal values for dexamethasone or metyrapone tests. Phenytoin may cause increased serum levels of glucose, alkaline phosphatase, and gamma glutamyl transpeptidase (GGT).

CARCINOGENESIS

See WARNINGS for information on carcinogenesis.

PREGNANCY

See WARNINGS.

NURSING MOTHERS

Infant breast-feeding is not recommended for women taking this drug because phenytoin appears to be secreted in low concentrations in human milk.

DRUG INTERACTIONS

There are many drugs which may increase or decrease phenytoin levels or which phenytoin may affect. Serum level determinations for phenytoin are especially helpful when possible drug interactions are suspected. The most commonly occurring drug interactions are listed.

1. Drugs which may increase phenytoin serum levels include: acute alcohol intake, amiodarone, chloramphenicol, chlordiazepoxide, diazepam, dicumarol, disulfiram, estrogens, H_2-antagonists, halothane, isoniazid, methylphenidate, phenothiazines, phenylbutazone, salicylates, succinimides, sulfonamides, tolbutamide, trazodone.
2. Drugs which may decrease phenytoin levels include: carbamazepine, chronic alcohol abuse, reserpine, and sucralfate. Moban brand of molindone hydrochloride contains calcium ions which interfere with the absorption of phenytoin. Ingestion times of phenytoin and antacid preparations containing calcium should be staggered in patients with low serum phenytoin levels to prevent absorption problems.
3. Drugs which may either increase or decrease phenytoin serum levels include: phenobarbital, sodium valproate, and valproic acid. Similarly, the effect of phenytoin on phenobarbital, valproic acid and sodium valproate serum levels is unpredictable.
4. Although not a true drug interaction, tricyclic antidepressants may precipitate seizures in susceptible patients and phenytoin dosage may need to be adjusted.
5. Drugs whose efficacy is impaired by phenytoin include: corticosteroids, coumarin anticoagulants, digitoxin, doxycycline, estrogens, furosemide, oral contraceptives, quinidine, rifampin, theophylline, vitamin D.

ADVERSE REACTIONS

CENTRAL NERVOUS SYSTEM

The most common manifestations encountered with phenytoin therapy are referable to this system and are usually dose-related. These include nystagmus, ataxia, slurred speech, decreased coordination and mental confusion. Dizziness, insomnia, transient nervousness, motor twitchings, and headaches have also been observed. There have also been rare reports of phenytoin induced dyskinesias, including chorea, dystonia, tremor and asterixis, similar to those induced by phenothiazine and other neuroleptic drugs.

A predominantly sensory peripheral polyneuropathy has been observed in patients receiving long-term phenytoin therapy.

GASTROINTESTINAL SYSTEM

Nausea, vomiting, constipation, toxic hepatitis and liver damage.

INTEGUMENTARY SYSTEM

Dermatological manifestations sometimes accompanied by fever have included scarlatiniform or morbilliform rashes. A morbilliform rash (measles-like) is the most common; other types of dermatitis are seen more rarely. Other more serious forms which may be fatal have included bullous, exfoliative or purpuric dermatitis, lupus erythematosus, Stevens-Johnson syndrome, and toxic epidermal necrolysis (see PRECAUTIONS).

HEMOPOIETIC SYSTEM

Hemopoietic complications, some fatal, have occasionally been reported in association with administration of phenytoin. These have included thrombocytopenia, leukopenia, granulocytopenia, agranulocytosis, and pancytopenia with or without bone marrow suppression. While macrocytosis and megaloblastic anemia have occurred, these conditions usually respond to folic acid therapy. Lymphadenopathy including benign lymph node hyperplasia, pseudolymphoma, lymphoma, and Hodgkin's disease have been reported (see WARNINGS).

CONNECTIVE TISSUE SYSTEM

Coarsening of the facial features, enlargement of the lips, gingival hyperplasia, hypertrichosis and Peyronie's disease.

CARDIOVASCULAR

Periarteritis nodosa.

IMMUNOLOGIC

Hypersensitivity syndrome (which may include, but is not limited to, symptoms such as arthralgias, eosinophilia, fever, liver dysfunction, lymphadenopathy or rash), systemic lupus erythematosus, and immunoglobulin abnormalities.

DOSAGE AND ADMINISTRATION

Serum concentrations should be monitored in changing from extended phenytoin sodium capsules to prompt phenytoin sodium capsules, and from the sodium salt to the free acid form.

Extended phenytoin sodium capsules, extended phenytoin sodium parenteral, and extended phenytoin sodium capsules with phenobarbital are formulated with the sodium salt of phenytoin. The free acid form of phenytoin is used in phenytoin sodium capsules-30 pediatric and phenytoin sodium capsules-125 suspensions and phenytoin sodium capsules infatabs. Because there is approximately an 8% increase in drug content with the free acid form over that of the sodium salt, dosage adjustments and serum level monitoring may be necessary when switching from a product formulated with the free acid to a product formulated with the sodium salt and vice versa.

GENERAL

Dosage should be individualized to provide maximum benefit. In some cases, serum blood level determinations may be necessary for optimal dosage adjustments—the clinically effective serum level is usually 10-20 μg/ml. With recommended dosage, a period of 7-10 days may be required to achieve steady-state blood levels with phenytoin and changes in dosage (increase or decrease) should not be carried out at intervals shorter than 7-10 days.

ADULT DOSAGE

Divided Daily Dosage

Patients who have received no previous treatment may be started on one 100 mg extended phenytoin sodium capsule 3times daily and the dosage then adjusted to suit individual requirements. For most adults, the satisfactory maintenance dosage will be 1 capsule 3-4 times a day. An increase up to 2 capsules 3 times a day may be made, if necessary.

Once-a-Day Dosage

In adults, if seizure control is established with divided doses of three 100 mg phenytoin sodium capsules capsules daily, once-a-day dosage with 300 mg of extended phenytoin sodium capsules may be considered. Studies comparing divided doses of 300 mg with a single daily dose of this quantity indicated absorption, peak plasma levels, biologic half-life, difference between peak and minimum values, and urinary recovery were equivalent. Once-a-day dosage offers a convenience to the individual patient or to nursing personnel for institutionalized patients and is intended to be used only for patients requiring this amount of drug daily. A major problem in motivating noncompliant patients may also be lessened when the patient can take this drug once a day. However, patients should be cautioned not to miss a dose, inadvertently.

Only extended phenytoin sodium capsules are recommended for once-a-day dosing. Inherent differences in dissolution characteristics and resultant absorption rates of phenytoin due to different manufacturing procedures and/or dosage forms preclude such recommendation for other phenytoin products. When a change in the dosage form or brand is prescribed, careful monitoring of phenytoin serum levels should be carried out.

Loading Dose

Some authorities have advocated use of an oral loading dose of phenytoin in adults who require rapid steady-state serum levels and where intravenous administration is not desirable. This dosing regimen should be reserved for patients in a clinic or hospital setting where phenytoin serum levels can be closely monitored. Patients with a history of renal or liver disease should not receive the oral loading regimen.

Initially, one gram of phenytoin capsules is divided into 3 doses (400 mg, 300 mg, 300 mg) and administered at two-hourly intervals. Normal maintenance dosage is then instituted 24 hours after the loading dose, with frequent serum level determinations.

PEDIATRIC DOSAGE

Initially, 5 mg/kg/day in two or three equally divided doses, with subsequent dosage individualized to a maximum of 300 mg daily. A recommended daily maintenance dosage is usually 4-8 mg/kg. Children over 6 years old may require the minimum adult dose (300 mg/day).

HOW SUPPLIED

FOR ORAL USE

Dilantin 100 mg: Kapseal 362, transparent no. 3 capsule with an orange band.
Dilantin 30 mg: Kapseal 365, transparent no. 4 capsule with a pink band.
Dilantin-125 Suspension: 125 mg phenytion/5 ml with a maximum alcohol content not greater than 0.6%.
Dilantin Infatabs: Each contain 50 mg phenytoin.
Storage: Store below 30°C (86°F). Protect from light and moisture.

FOR PARENTERAL USE

Steri-Dose 4488: Dilantin ready-mixed solution containing 50 mg phenytoin sodium per milliliter.
Dilantin Ready-Mixed Solution: Solution contains 50 mg phenytoin sodium per milliliter.
Storage: Store below 30°C (86°F).

PRODUCT LISTING - RATED THERAPEUTICALLY EQUIVALENT

Package	Price	Product, Manufacturer	NDC
Capsule, Extended Release - Oral - 100 mg			
5's	$1.35	DILANTIN KAPSEALS, Allscripts Pharmaceutical Company	54569-0161-06
6's	$1.62	DILANTIN KAPSEALS, Allscripts Pharmaceutical Company	54569-0161-08
9's	$2.43	DILANTIN KAPSEALS, Allscripts Pharmaceutical Company	54569-0161-07
10's	$6.06	DILANTIN KAPSEALS, Pd-Rx Pharmaceuticals	55289-0152-10
25's	$7.70	GENERIC, Udl Laboratories Inc	51079-0905-19
25's	$11.79	DILANTIN KAPSEALS, Pd-Rx Pharmaceuticals	55289-0152-97
30's	$8.09	DILANTIN KAPSEALS, Allscripts Pharmaceutical Company	54569-0161-02
30's	$14.64	GENERIC, Physicians Total Care	54868-0040-02
60's	$27.61	GENERIC, Physicians Total Care	54868-0040-01
100's	$26.80	GENERIC, Mylan Pharmaceuticals Inc	00378-1560-01
100's	$26.97	DILANTIN KAPSEALS, Allscripts Pharmaceutical Company	54569-0161-00
100's	$27.65	GENERIC, Udl Laboratories Inc	51079-0905-20
100's	$30.91	DILANTIN KAPSEALS, Parke-Davis	00071-0362-24
100's	$34.11	DILANTIN KAPSEALS, Parke-Davis	00071-0362-40
100's	$44.90	GENERIC, Physicians Total Care	54868-0040-00
270's	$58.64	DILANTIN KAPSEALS, Allscripts Pharmaceutical Company	54569-8567-00
Solution - Injectable - 50 mg/ml			
2 ml x 10	$15.10	GENERIC, Abbott Pharmaceutical	00074-1844-02
2 ml x 10	$23.75	GENERIC, Abbott Pharmaceutical	00074-1844-32
2 ml x 25	$98.75	GENERIC, Esi Lederle Generics	00641-0493-25
5 ml x 10	$26.30	GENERIC, Abbott Pharmaceutical	00074-1844-05
5 ml x 25	$53.75	GENERIC, Abbott Pharmaceutical	00074-1844-15
5 ml x 25	$117.25	GENERIC, Esi Lederle Generics	00641-2555-45

PRODUCT LISTING - RATED NOT THERAPEUTICALLY EQUIVALENT

Package	Price	Product, Manufacturer	NDC
Capsule - Oral - 100 mg			
100's	$7.13	GENERIC, Interstate Drug Exchange Inc	00814-2580-14
100's	$24.50	GENERIC, Ivax Corporation	00172-2057-60
Solution - Injectable - 50 mg/ml			
2 ml x 25	$43.64	GENERIC, Abbott Pharmaceutical	00074-1317-01
5 ml x 25	$51.25	GENERIC, Abbott Pharmaceutical	00074-1317-02

PRODUCT LISTING - EQUIVALENTS NOT AVAILABLE

Package	Price	Product, Manufacturer	NDC
Capsule - Oral - 100 mg			
10's	$2.17	DILANTIN, Southwood Pharmaceuticals Inc	58016-0907-10
12's	$2.61	DILANTIN, Southwood Pharmaceuticals Inc	58016-0907-12
15's	$3.26	DILANTIN, Southwood Pharmaceuticals Inc	58016-0907-15
30's	$6.52	DILANTIN, Southwood Pharmaceuticals Inc	58016-0907-30
100's	$21.72	DILANTIN, Southwood Pharmaceuticals Inc	58016-0907-00
Capsule, Extended Release - Oral - 30 mg			
100's	$26.66	DILANTIN KAPSEALS, Parke-Davis	00071-0365-24
Solution - Injectable - 50 mg/ml			
2 ml x 25	$15.50	GENERIC, Raway Pharmacal Inc	00686-0034-02
10 ml x 25	$23.00	GENERIC, Raway Pharmacal Inc	00686-0034-05

P

Phytonadione (002035)

Categories: Deficiency, vitamin K; Hemorrhagic disease of the newborn; Hypoprothrombinemia; Toxicity, coumarin; Pregnancy Category C; FDA Approved 1956 Sep; WHO Formulary
Drug Classes: Hemostatics; Vitamins/minerals
Brand Names: Aquamephyton; **Konakion**; Mephyton; Phytomenadione; Vitamin K1 Roche
Foreign Brand Availability: Haemokion (Bahrain; Cyprus; Egypt; Iran; Iraq; Jordan; Kuwait; Lebanon; Libya; Oman; Qatar; Republic-of-Yemen; Saudi-Arabia; Syria; United-Arab-Emirates); Kaywan (Indonesia; Korea); Kenadion (India); Konakion 10 mg (Austria; Finland; Hungary); Konakion (10 mg) (Bahrain; Costa-Rica; Cyprus; Dominican-Republic; Egypt; El-Salvador; England; Germany; Ghana; Guatemala; Honduras; Iran; Iraq; Ireland; Italy; Jordan; Kenya; Kuwait; Lebanon; Libya; Mexico; Netherlands; Nicaragua; Oman; Panama; Qatar; Republic-of-Yemen; Saudi-Arabia; South-Africa; Sweden; Switzerland; Syria; Tanzania; Uganda; United-Arab-Emirates; Zambia); Konakion MM Paediatric (Bahamas; Barbados; Belize; Bermuda; Curacao; Guyana; Jamaica; Netherland-Antilles; Puerto-Rico; Surinam; Trinidad); Konakion MM Pediatric (Australia; Colombia; Mexico); Microka (Mexico); Vitak (Japan); Vitamin K (Hong-Kong)
HCFA JCODE(S): J3430 per 1 mg IM, SC, IV

IM-IV-SC

WARNING

INTRAVENOUS AND INTRAMUSCULAR USE

Severe reactions, including fatalities, have occurred during and immediately after INTRAVENOUS injection of phytonadione, even when precautions have been taken to dilute the phytonadione and to avoid rapid infusion. Severe reactions, including fatalities, have also been reported following INTRAMUSCULAR administration. Typically these severe reactions have resembled hypersensitivity or anaphylaxis, including shock and cardiac and/or respiratory arrest. Some patients have exhibited these severe reactions on receiving phytonadione for the first time. Therefore the INTRAVENOUS and INTRAMUSCULAR routes should be restricted to those situations where the subcutaneous route is not feasible and the serious risk involved is considered justified.

DESCRIPTION

Phytonadione is a vitamin, which is a clear, yellow to amber, viscous, odorless or nearly odorless liquid. It is insoluble in water, soluble in chloroform and slightly soluble in ethanol. It has a molecular weight of 450.70.

Phytonadione is 2-methyl-3-phytyl-1,4-naphthoquinone. Its empirical formula is $C_{31}H_{46}O_2$.

AquaMephyton injection is a yellow, sterile, aqueous colloidal solution of vitamin K_1, with a pH of 5.0-7.0, available for injection by the intravenous(IV), intramuscular (IM), and subcutaneous (SC) routes. Each milliliter contains:

Active Ingredient: Phytonadione: 2 or 10 mg.
Inactive Ingredients: Polyoxyethylated fatty acid derivative: 70 mg; *Dextrose:* 37.5 mg; *Water for injection, qs:* 1 ml; *Added as preservative:* Benzyl alcohol 0.9%.

CLINICAL PHARMACOLOGY

Phytonadione aqueous colloidal solution of vitamin K_1 for parenteral injection, possesses the same type and degree of activity as does naturally-occurring vitamin K, which is necessary for the production via the liver of active prothrombin (factor II), proconvertin (factor VII), plasma thromboplastin component (factor IX), and Stuart factor (factor X). The prothrombin test is sensitive to the levels of three of these four factors — II, VII, and X. Vitamin K is an essential cofactor for a microsomal enzyme that catalyzes the post-translational carboxylation of multiple, specific, peptide-bound glutamic acid residues in inactive hepatic precursors of factors II, VII, IX, and X. The resulting gamma-carboxyglutamic acid residues convert the precursors into active coagulation factors that are subsequently secreted by liver cells into the blood.

Phytonadione is readily absorbed following IM administration. After absorption, phytonadione is initially concentrated in the liver, but the concentration declines rapidly. Very little vitamin K accumulates in tissues. Little is known about the metabolic fate of vitamin K. Almost no free unmetabolized vitamin K appears in bile or urine.

In normal animals and humans, phytonadione is virtually devoid of pharmacodynamic activity. However, in animals and humans deficient in vitamin K, the pharmacological action of vitamin K is related to its normal physiological function, that is, to promote the hepatic biosynthesis of vitamin K dependent clotting factors.

The action of the aqueous colloidal solution, when administered intravenously, is generally detectable within an hour or 2 and hemorrhage is usually controlled within 3-6 hours. A normal prothrombin level may often be obtained in 12-14 hours.

In the prophylaxis and treatment of hemorrhagic disease of the newborn, phytonadione has demonstrated a greater margin of safety than that of the water-soluble vitamin K analogues.

INDICATIONS AND USAGE

Phytonadione is indicated in the following coagulation disorders which are due to faulty formation of factors II, VII, IX and X when caused by vitamin K deficiency or interference with vitamin K activity.

Phytonadione injection is indicated in:

- Anticoagulant-induced prothrombin deficiency caused by coumarin or indanedione derivatives.
- Prophylaxis and therapy of hemorrhagic disease of the newborn.
- Hypoprothrombinemia due to antibacterial therapy.
- Hypoprothrombinemia secondary to factors limiting absorption or synthesis of vitamin K, *e.g.*, obstructive jaundice, biliary fistula, sprue, ulcerative colitis, celiac disease, intestinal resection, cystic fibrosis of the pancreas, and regional enteritis.
- Other drug-induced hypoprothrombinemia where it is definitely shown that the result is due to interference with vitamin K metabolism, *e.g.*, salicylates.

CONTRAINDICATIONS

Hypersensitivity to any component of this medication.

WARNINGS

Benzyl alcohol as a preservative in bacteriostatic sodium chloride injection has been associated with toxicity in newborns. Data are unavailable on the toxicity of other preservatives in this age group. There is no evidence to suggest that the small amount of benzyl alcohol contained in phytonadione, when used as recommended, is associated with toxicity.

An immediate coagulant effect should not be expected after administration of phytonadione. It takes a minimum of 1-2 hours for measurable improvement in the prothrombin time. Whole blood or component therapy may also be necessary if bleeding is severe.

Phytonadione will not counteract the anticoagulant action of heparin.

When vitamin K_1 is used to correct excessive anticoagulant-induced hypoprothrombinemia, anticoagulant therapy still being indicated, the patient is again faced with the clotting hazards existing prior to starting the anticoagulant therapy. Phytonadione is not a clotting agent, but overzealous therapy with vitamin K_1 may restore conditions which originally permitted thromboembolic phenomena. Dosage should be kept as low as possible, and prothrombin time should be checked regularly as clinical conditions indicate.

Repeated large doses of vitamin K are not warranted in liver disease if the response to initial use of the vitamin is unsatisfactory. Failure to respond to vitamin K may indicate that the condition being treated is inherently unresponsive to vitamin K.

PRECAUTIONS

GENERAL

Vitamin K_1 is fairly rapidly degraded by light; therefore, always protect phytonadione from light. Store phytonadione in closed original carton until contents have been used. (See also HOW SUPPLIED, Storage.)

LABORATORY TESTS

Prothrombin time should be checked regularly as clinical conditions indicate.

CARCINOGENESIS, MUTAGENESIS, AND IMPAIRMENT OF FERTILITY

Studies of carcinogenicity, mutagenesis or impairment of fertility have not been conducted with phytonadione.

PREGNANCY CATEGORY C

Animal reproduction studies have not been conducted with phytonadione. It is also not known whether phytonadione can cause fetal harm when administered to a pregnant woman or can affect reproduction capacity. Phytonadione should be given to a pregnant woman only if clearly needed.

NURSING MOTHERS

It is not known whether this drug is excreted in human milk. Because many drugs are excreted in human milk, caution should be exercised when phytonadione is administered to a nursing woman.

PEDIATRIC USE

Hemolysis, jaundice, and hyperbilirubinemia in newborns, particularly in premature infants, may be related to the dose of phytonadione. Therefore, the recommended dose should not be exceeded (see ADVERSE REACTIONS and DOSAGE AND ADMINISTRATION).

DRUG INTERACTIONS

Temporary resistance to prothrombin-depressing anticoagulants may result, especially when larger doses of phytonadione are used. If relatively large doses have been employed, it may be necessary when reinstituting anticoagulant therapy to use somewhat larger doses of the prothrombin-depressing anticoagulant, or to use one which acts on a different principle, such as heparin sodium.

ADVERSE REACTIONS

Deaths have occurred after IV and IM administration. (See BOXED WARNING.)

Transient "flushing sensations" and "peculiar" sensations of taste have been observed, as well as rare instances of dizziness, rapid and weak pulse, profuse sweating, brief hypotension, dyspnea, and cyanosis.

Pain, swelling, and tenderness at the injection site may occur.

The possibility of allergic sensitivity, including an anaphylactoid reaction, should be kept in mind.

Infrequently, usually after repeated injection, erythematous, indurated, pruritic plaques have occurred; rarely, these have progressed to scleroderma-like lesions that have persisted for long periods. In other cases, these lesions have resembled erythema perstans.

Hyperbilirubinemia has been observed in the newborn following administration of phytonadione. This has occurred rarely and primarily with doses above those recommended. (See PRECAUTIONS, Pediatric Use.)

DOSAGE AND ADMINISTRATION

Whenever possible, phytonadione should be given by the SC route (see BOXED WARNING). When IV administration is considered unavoidable, the drug should be injected very slowly, not exceeding 1 mg/min.

Protect from light at all times.

Parenteral drug products should be inspected visually for particulate matter and discoloration prior to administration, whenever solution and container permit.

DIRECTIONS FOR DILUTION

Phytonadione may be diluted with 0.9% sodium chloride injection, 5% dextrose injection, or 5% dextrose and sodium chloride injection. Benzyl alcohol as a preservative has been associated with toxicity in newborns. *Therefore, all of the above diluents should be preservative-free* (see WARNINGS). *Other diluents should not be used.* When dilutions are indicated, administration should be started immediately after mixture with the diluent, and unused portions of the dilution should be discarded, as well as unused contents of the ampul.

PROPHYLAXIS OF HEMORRHAGIC DISEASE OF THE NEWBORN

The American Academy of Pediatrics recommends that vitamin K_1 be given to the newborn. A single IM dose of phytonadione 0.5 to 1 mg within 1 hour of birth is recommended.

TREATMENT OF HEMORRHAGIC DISEASE OF THE NEWBORN

Empiric administration of vitamin K_1 should not replace proper laboratory evaluation of the coagulation mechanism. A prompt response (shortening of the prothrombin time in 2-4 hours) following administration of vitamin K_1 is usually diagnostic of hemorrhagic disease of the newborn, and failure to respond indicates another diagnosis or coagulation disorder.

Phytonadione 1 mg should be given either subcutaneously or intramuscularly. Higher doses may be necessary if the mother has been receiving oral anticoagulants.

Whole blood or component therapy may be indicated if bleeding is excessive. This therapy, however, does not correct the underlying disorder and phytonadione should be given concurrently.

ANTICOAGULANT-INDUCED PROTHROMBIN DEFICIENCY IN ADULTS

To correct excessively prolonged prothrombin time caused by oral anticoagulant therapy — 2.5 to 10 mg or up to 25 mg initially is recommended. In rare instances 50 mg may be required. Frequency and amount of subsequent doses should be determined by prothrombin time response or clinical condition (see WARNINGS). If in 6-8 hours after parenteral administration the prothrombin time has not been shortened satisfactorily, the dose should be repeated.

TABLE 1 *Summary of Dosage Guidelines (See Circular Text for Details)*

Newborns	Dosage
Hemorrhagic Disease of the Newborn	
Prophylaxis	0.5-1 mg IM within 1 hour of birth
Treatment	1 mg SC or IM (higher doses may be necessary if the mother has been receiving oral anticoagulants)
Adults	**Initial Dosage**
Anticoagulant-Induced Prothrombin Deficiency (caused by coumarin or indanedione derivatives)	2.5-10 mg or up to 25 mg (rarely 50 mg)
Hypoprothrombinemia due to other causes (antibiotics; salicylates or other drugs; factors limiting absorption or synthesis)	2.5-25 mg or more (rarely up to 50 mg)

In the event of shock or excessive blood loss, the use of whole blood or component therapy is indicated.

HYPOPROTHROMBINEMIA DUE TO OTHER CAUSES IN ADULTS

A dosage of 2.5 to 25 mg or more (rarely up to 50 mg) is recommended, the amount and route of administration depending upon the severity of the condition and response obtained.

If possible, discontinuation or reduction of the dosage of drugs interfering with coagulation mechanisms (such as salicylates, antibiotics) is suggested as an alternative to administering concurrent phytonadione. The severity of the coagulation disorder should determine whether the immediate administration of phytonadione is required in addition to discontinuation or reduction of interfering drugs.

HOW SUPPLIED

AquaMephyton injection is a yellow, sterile, aqueous colloidal solution and is supplied in 10 mg of vitamin K_1 per ml and 1 mg of vitamin K_1 per 0.5 ml.

Storage: Store container in original carton. Always protect AquaMephyton from light. Store container in closed original carton until contents have been used. (See PRECAUTIONS, General.)

ORAL

DESCRIPTION

Phytonadione is a vitamin which is a clear, yellow to amber, viscous, and nearly odorless liquid. It is insoluble in water, soluble in chloroform and slightly soluble in ethanol. It has a molecular weight of 450.70.

Phytonadione is 2-methyl-3-phytyl-1,4-naphthoquinone. Its empirical formula is $C_{31}H_{46}O_2$.

Mephyton tablets containing 5 mg of phytonadione are yellow, compressed tablets, scored on one side. Inactive ingredients are acacia, calcium phosphate, colloidal silicon dioxide, lactose, magnesium stearate, starch, and talc.

CLINICAL PHARMACOLOGY

Phytonadione tablets possess the same type and degree of activity as does naturally-occurring vitamin K, which is necessary for the production via the liver of active prothrombin (factor II), proconvertin (factor VII), plasma thromboplastin component (factor IX), and Stuart factor (factor X). The prothrombin test is sensitive to the levels of three of these four factors — II, VII, and X. Vitamin K is an essential cofactor for a microsomal enzyme that catalyzes the post-translational carboxylation of multiple, specific, peptide-bound glutamic acid residues in inactive hepatic precursors of factors II, VII, IX, and X. The resulting gamma-carboxyglutamic acid residues convert the precursors into active coagulation factors that are subsequently secreted by liver cells into the blood.

Oral phytonadione is adequately absorbed from the gastrointestinal tract only if bile salts are present. After absorption, phytonadione is initially concentrated in the liver, but the concentration declines rapidly. Very little vitamin K accumulates in tissues. Little is known about the metabolic fate of vitamin K. Almost no free unmetabolized vitamin K appears in bile or urine.

In normal animals and humans, phytonadione is virtually devoid of pharmacodynamic activity. However, in animals and humans deficient in vitamin K, the pharmacological action of vitamin K is related to its normal physiological function; that is, to promote the hepatic biosynthesis of vitamin K-dependent clotting factors.

Phytonadione tablets generally exert their effect within 6-10 hours.

INDICATIONS AND USAGE

Phytonadione is indicated in the following coagulation disorders which are due to faulty formation of factors II, VII, IX and X when caused by vitamin K deficiency or interference with vitamin K activity.

Phytonadione tablets are indicated in:

- Anticoagulant-induced prothrombin deficiency caused by coumarin or indanedione derivatives.
- Hypoprothrombinemia secondary to antibacterial therapy.
- Hypoprothrombinemia secondary to administration of salicylates.
- Hypoprothrombinemia secondary to obstructive jaundice or biliary fistulas but only if bile salts are administered concurrently, since otherwise the oral vitamin K will not be absorbed.

CONTRAINDICATIONS

Hypersensitivity to any component of this medication.

WARNINGS

An immediate coagulant effect should not be expected after administration of phytonadione.

Phytonadione will not counteract the anticoagulant action of heparin.

When vitamin K_1 is used to correct excessive anticoagulant-induced hypoprothrombinemia, anticoagulant therapy still being indicated, the patient is again faced with the clotting hazards existing prior to starting the anticoagulant therapy. Phytonadione is not a clotting agent, but overzealous therapy with vitamin K_1 may restore conditions which originally permitted thromboembolic phenomena. Dosage should be kept as low as possible, and prothrombin time should be checked regularly as clinical conditions indicate.

Repeated large doses of vitamin K are not warranted in liver disease if the response to initial use of the vitamin is unsatisfactory. Failure to respond to vitamin K may indicate a congenital coagulation defect or that the condition being treated is unresponsive to vitamin K.

PRECAUTIONS

GENERAL

Vitamin K_1 is fairly rapidly degraded by light; therefore, always protect phytonadione from light. Store phytonadione in closed original carton until contents have been used. (See also HOW SUPPLIED, Storage.)

LABORATORY TESTS

Prothrombin time should be checked regularly as clinical conditions indicate.

CARCINOGENESIS, MUTAGENESIS, AND IMPAIRMENT OF FERTILITY

Studies of carcinogenicity or impairment of fertility have not been performed with phytonadione. Phytonadione at concentrations up to 2000 μg/plate with or without metabolic activation, was negative in the Ames microbial mutagen test.

PREGNANCY CATEGORY C

Animal reproduction studies have not been conducted with phytonadione. It is also not known whether phytonadione can cause fetal harm when administered to a pregnant woman or can affect reproduction capacity. Phytonadione should be given to a pregnant woman only if clearly needed.

PEDIATRIC USE

Safety and effectiveness in pediatric patients have not been established with phytonadione. Hemolysis, jaundice, and hyperbilirubinemia in newborns, particularly in premature infants, have been reported with vitamin K.

NURSING MOTHERS

It is not known whether this drug is excreted in human milk. Because many drugs are excreted in human milk, caution should be exercised when phytonadione is administered to a nursing woman.

DRUG INTERACTIONS

Temporary resistance to prothrombin-depressing anticoagulants may result, especially when larger doses of phytonadione are used. If relatively large doses have been employed, it may be necessary when reinstituting anticoagulant therapy to use somewhat larger doses of the prothrombin-depressing anticoagulant, or to use one which acts on a different principle, such as heparin sodium.

ADVERSE REACTIONS

Transient "flushing sensations" and "peculiar" sensations of taste have been observed with parenteral phytonadione, as well as rare instances of dizziness, rapid and weak pulse, profuse sweating, brief hypotension, dyspnea, and cyanosis.

Hyperbilirubinemia has been observed in the newborn following administration of parenteral phytonadione. This has occurred rarely and primarily with doses above those recommended.

DOSAGE AND ADMINISTRATION

ANTICOAGULANT-INDUCED PROTHROMBIN DEFICIENCY IN ADULTS

To correct excessively prolonged prothrombin times caused by oral anticoagulant therapy — 2.5 to 10 mg or up to 25 mg initially is recommended. In rare instances 50 mg may be required. Frequency and amount of subsequent doses should be determined by prothrombin time response or clinical condition. (See WARNINGS.) If, in 12-48 hours after oral admin-

TABLE 2 *Summary of Dosage Guidelines (See Circular Text for Details)*

Adults	Initial Dosage
Anticoagulant-Induced Prothrombin Deficiency (caused by coumarin or indanedione derivatives)	2.5-10 mg or up to 25 mg (rarely 50 mg)
Hypoprothrombinemia due to other causes (antibiotics; salicylates or other drugs; factors limiting absorption or synthesis)	2.5-25 mg or more (rarely up to 50 mg)

istration, the prothrombin time has not been shortened satisfactorily, the dose should be repeated.

HYPOPROTHROMBINEMIA DUE TO OTHER CAUSES IN ADULTS

If possible, discontinuation or reduction of the dosage of drugs interfering with coagulation mechanisms (such as salicylates, antibiotics) is suggested as an alternative to administering concurrent phytonadione. The severity of the coagulation disorder should determine whether the immediate administration of phytonadione is required in addition to discontinuation or reduction of interfering drugs.

A dosage of 2.5 to 25 mg or more (rarely up to 50 mg) is recommended, the amount and route of administration depending upon the severity of the condition and response obtained.

The oral route should be avoided when the clinical disorder would prevent proper absorption. Bile salts must be given with the tablets when the endogenous supply of bile to the gastrointestinal tract is deficient.

HOW SUPPLIED

Mephyton Tablets

5 mg vitamin K_1: Yellow, round, scored, compressed tablets, coded "MSD 43" on one side and "MEPHYTON" on the other.

Storage: Store in a tightly closed container at 25°C (77°F); excursions permitted to 15-30°C (59-86°F). Always protect Mephyton from light. Store in tightly closed original container and carton until contents have been used. (See PRECAUTIONS, General.)

PRODUCT LISTING - RATED NOT THERAPEUTICALLY EQUIVALENT

Solution - Injectable - 1 mg/0.5 ml

Size	Price	Product	NDC
0.50 ml x 25	$64.50	AQUAMEPHYTON, Merck & Company Inc	00006-7784-33
1 ml x 25	$67.75	GENERIC, Abbott Pharmaceutical	00074-9157-01
1 ml x 25	$125.00	GENERIC, Celltech Pharmacueticals Inc	00548-1140-00

Solution - Injectable - 10 mg/ml

Size	Price	Product	NDC
1 ml x 6	$35.46	AQUAMEPHYTON, Merck & Company Inc	00006-7780-64
1 ml x 25	$125.50	AQUAMEPHYTON, Merck & Company Inc	00006-7780-66
1 ml x 25	$129.50	GENERIC, Abbott Pharmaceutical	00074-9158-01
5 ml	$24.35	AQUAMEPHYTON, Physicians Total Care	54868-3806-00

PRODUCT LISTING - EQUIVALENTS NOT AVAILABLE

Tablet - Oral - 5 mg

Size	Price	Product	NDC
10's	$6.95	MEPHYTON, Pharma Pac	52959-0424-10
10's	$9.53	MEPHYTON, Pd-Rx Pharmaceuticals	55289-0793-10
12's	$11.78	GENERIC, Prescript Pharmaceuticals	00247-0082-12
14's	$12.15	MEPHYTON, Pd-Rx Pharmaceuticals	55289-0793-14
14's	$13.18	GENERIC, Prescript Pharmaceuticals	00247-0082-14
16's	$14.58	GENERIC, Prescript Pharmaceuticals	00247-0082-16
20's	$16.13	MEPHYTON, Pd-Rx Pharmaceuticals	55289-0793-20
20's	$17.39	GENERIC, Prescript Pharmaceuticals	00247-0082-20
30's	$18.68	MEPHYTON, Allscripts Pharmaceutical Company	54569-1476-03
100's	$65.33	MEPHYTON, Merck & Company Inc	00006-0043-68
100's	$73.51	GENERIC, Prescript Pharmaceuticals	00247-0082-00

P

Pilocarpine *(002036)*

Categories: Glaucoma, angle-closure; Glaucoma, open-angle; Hypertension, ocular; Xerostomia; Sjogren's syndrome; FDA Approved 1984 Oct; Pregnancy Category C; Orphan Drugs; WHO Formulary

Drug Classes: Cholinergics; Miotics; Ophthalmics

Brand Names: Adsorbocarpine; Akarpine; I-Pilopine; Isopto Carpine; Ocu-Carpine; Pilokair; Pilopine HS; Pilosol; Pilostat; Salagen; Spectro-Pilo; Storzine

Foreign Brand Availability: Asthenopin (Philippines); Cendo Carpine (Indonesia); Glaucocarpine (Israel); Isopto Carpina (Argentina; Ecuador; Peru); Isopto Pilocarpine (France); Liocarpina (Italy); Miocarpine (Canada); O.P.D. (Taiwan); Ocucarpine (Korea); Ocusert P-20 (Japan); Ocusert P-40 (Japan); Ocusert Pilo-20 (Australia; England); Ocusert Pilo-40 (Australia; England); Ocusert Pilocarpine (England); Oftan-Pilocarpin (Finland); P.V. Carpine Liquifilm Ophthalimic Solution (Australia; New-Zealand); Pil Ofteno (Mexico); Pilo Grin (Mexico); Pilocarpin (Korea); Pilocarpol (Germany); Pilogel (Germany; Italy; South-Africa; Taiwan); Pilogel HS (Hong-Kong; Philippines); Pilokarpin Isopto (Denmark); Pilomann (Philippines); Pilomin (India); Pilopt Eye Drops (Australia; New-Zealand); Pilotonina (Italy); Sanpilo (Taiwan); Sno Pilo (England); Spersacarpine (Hong-Kong; Malaysia; Philippines; Sweden; Switzerland; Taiwan); Vistacarpin (Germany); Ximex Opticar (Indonesia)

Cost of Therapy: $154.31 (Sjögren's Syndrome; Salagen; 5 mg; 4 tablets/day; 30 day supply)
$20.37 (Glaucoma; Isopto Carpine Ophth. Solution; 1%; 15 ml; 2 drops/day; variable day supply)
$2.65 (Glaucoma; Generic Ophth. Solution; 1%; 15 ml; 6 drops/day; variable day supply)

OPHTHALMIC

DESCRIPTION

Note: The trade names have been used throughout this monograph for clarity.

ISOPTO CARPINE

Isopto Carpine (pilocarpine hydrochloride) is a cholinergic prepared as a sterile topical ophthalmic solution.

Chemical Name: 2(3*H*)-furanone, 3-ethyldihydro-4-[(1-methyl-1*H*-imidazol-5-yl)-methyl]-, monohydrochloride, (3*S-cis*)-.

Each ml contains:

Active: Pilocarpine hydrochloride 1, 2, 4, 6, or 8%.

Preservative: Benzalkonium chloride 0.01%.

Vehicle: 0.5% Hydroxypropyl methylcellulose 2910.

Inactive: Boric acid, sodium citrate, sodium chloride (present in 1% only); hydrochloric acid and/or sodium hydroxide (to adjust pH); purified water.

OCUSERT

Ocusert pilocarpine system is an elliptically shaped unit designed for continuous release of pilocarpine following placement in the cul-de-sac of the eye. Clinical evaluation in appropriate patients has demonstrated therapeutic efficacy of the system in the eye for 1 week. Two strengths are available, Pilo-20 and Pilo-40.

Ocusert systems contain a core reservoir consisting of pilocarpine and alginic acid. Pilocarpine is designated chemically as 2(3H)-Furanone,3-ethyldihydro-4[(1-methyl-1H-imidazol-5-yl)methyl]-,(3S-cis)-.

The core is surrounded by a hydrophobic ethylene/vinyl acetate (EVA) copolymer membrane which controls the diffusion of pilocarpins, which increases the rate of diffusion of pilocarpine across the EVA membrane. Of the total content of pilocarpine in the Pilo-20 or Pilo-40 system (5 µg or 11 µg, respectively), a portion serves as the thermodynamic diffusional energy source to release the drug and remains in the unit at the end of the week's use. The alginic acid component of the core is not released from the system. The readily visible white margin around the system contains titanium dioxide. The Pilo-20 system is 5.7 × 13.4 mm on its axes and 0.3 mm thick; the Pilo-40 system is 5.5 × 13 mm on its axes and 0.5 mm thick.

Release Rate Concept

With the Ocusert system form of therapy, the particular strength is described by the rated release, the mean release rate of drug from the system over 7 days, in µg/h. To cover the range of drug therapy needed to control the increased intraocular pressure associated with the glaucomas, 2 rated releases of pilocarpine from the Ocusert system are available, 20 and 40 µg/h, for 1 week.

During the first few hours of the 7 day time course, the release rate is higher than that prevailing over the remainder of the 1 week period. The system releases drug at 3 times the rated value in the first hours and drops to the rated value in approximately 6 hours. A total of 0.3-0.7 µg pilocarpine (Pilo-20 or Pilo-40, respectively) is released during this initial 6 hour period (1 drop of 2% pilocarpine ophthalmic solution contains 1 µg pilocarpine). During the remainder of the 7 day period the release rate is within ±20% of the rated value.

PILOPINE HS

Pilopine HS (pilocarpine hydrochloride ophthalmic gel) 4% is a sterile topical ophthalmic aqueous gel which contains more than 90% water and employs Carbopol 940, a synthetic high molecular weight cross-linked polymer of acrylic acid, to impart a high viscosity. The active ingredient, pilocarpine hydrochloride, is a cholinergic.

Chemical Name: 2(3*H*)-furanone, 3-ethyldihydro-4-[(1-methyl-1*H*-imidazol-5-yl)-methyl]-, monohydrochloride,(3S-cis)-.

Pilopine HS Gel — Each gram contains:

Active: Pilocarpine hydrochloride 4% (40 µg).

Preservative: Benzalkonium chloride 0.008%.

Inactive: Carbopol 940, edetate disodium, hydrochloric acid and/or sodium hydroxide (to adjust pH) and purified water.

CLINICAL PHARMACOLOGY

ISOPTO CARPINE

Pilocarpine is a direct acting cholinergic parasympathomimetic agent which acts through direct stimulation of muscarinic neuro receptors and smooth muscle such as the iris and secretory glands. Pilocarpine produces miosis through contraction of the iris sphincter, causing increased tension on the scleral spur and opening of the trabecular mesh work spaces to facilitate outflow of aqueous humor. Outflow resistance is thereby reduced, lowering intraocular pressure.

OCUSERT

Pilocarpine is released from the Ocusert system as soon as it is placed in contact with the conjunctival surfaces. Pilocarpine is a direct acting parasympathomimetic drug which produces pupillary constriction, stimulates the ciliary muscle, and increases aqueous humor outflow facility. Because of its action on ciliary muscle, pilocarpine induces transient myopia, generally more pronounced in younger patients. In association with the increase in outflow facility, there is a decrease in intraocular pressure.

Preclinical Results

The levels of ^{14}C-pilocarpine in the ocular tissues of rabbits following Ocusert system and eyedrop administration have been determined. The Ocusert system produces constant low pilocarpine levels in the ciliary body and iris. Following ^{14}C-pilocarpine eyedrop treatment, the initial levels of pilocarpine in the cornea, aqueous humor, ciliary body and iris are 3-5 times higher than the corresponding levels with the Ocusert system, declining over the next 6 hours to approximately the tissue concentrations maintained by the Ocusert system. In contrast, in the conjunctiva, lens, and vitreous the ^{14}C-pilocarpine concentrations remain consistently high from eyedrops and do not return to the constant low levels maintained by the Ocusert system. Pilocarpine does not accumulate in ocular tissues during Ocusert system use. These studies in rabbits have not been done in humans.

PILOPINE HS

Pilocarpine is a direct acting cholinergic parasympathomimetic agent which acts through direct stimulation of muscarinic neuro receptors and smooth muscle such as the iris and secretory glands. Pilocarpine produces miosis through contraction of the iris sphincter, causing increased tension on the scleral spur and opening of the trabecular meshwork spaces to facilitate outflow of aqueous humor. Outflow resistance is thereby reduced, lowering intraocular pressure.

INDICATIONS AND USAGE

ISOPTO CARPINE

Pilocarpine HCl is a miotic (parasympathomimetic) used to control intraocular pressure. It may be used in combination with other miotics, beta blockers, carbonic anhydrase inhibitors, sympathomimetics, or hyperosmotic agents.

OCUSERT

Ocusert pilocarpine system is indicated for control of elevated intraocular pressure in pilocarpine responsive patients. Clinical studies have demonstrated Ocusert system efficacy in certain glaucomatous patients.

The patient should be instructed on the use of the Ocusert system and should read the package insert instructions for use. The patient should demonstrate to the ophthalmologist his ability to place, adjust and remove the units.

Concurrent Therapy

Ocusert systems have been used concomitantly with various ophthalmic medications. The release rate of pilocarpine from the Ocusert system is not influenced by carbonic anhydrase inhibitors, epinephrine or timolol ophthalmic solutions, fluorescein, or anesthetic, antibiotic, or anti-inflammatory steroid ophthalmic solutions. Systemic reactions consistent with an increased rate of absorption from the eye of an autonomic drug, such as epinephrine, have been observed. The occurrence of mild bulbar conjunctival edema, which is frequently present with epinephrine ophthalmic solutions, is not influenced by the Ocusert pilocarpine system.

PILOPINE HS

Pilocarpine HCl is a miotic (parasympathomimetic) used to control intraocular pressure. It may be used in combination with other miotics, beta blockers, carbonic anhydrase inhibitors, sympathomimetics or hyperosmotic agents.

NON-FDA APPROVED INDICATIONS

Dilute pilocarpine solutions are used in the diagnosis of Adie tonic pupil; however this use is not approved by the FDA.

CONTRAINDICATIONS

ISOPTO CARPINE

Miotics are contraindicated where constriction is undesirable such as in acute iritis, in those persons showing hypersensitivity to any of their components, and in pupillary block glaucoma.

OCUSERT

Ocusert pilocarpine system is contraindicated where pupillary constriction is undesirable, such as for glaucomas associated with acute inflammatory disease of the anterior segment of the eye, and glaucomas occurring or persisting after extracapsular cataract extraction where posterior synechiae may occur.

PILOPINE HS

Miotics are contraindicated where constriction is undesirable, such as in acute iritis, and in those persons showing hypersensitivity to any of their components.

WARNINGS

ISOPTO CARPINE

For topical use only. NOT FOR INJECTION.

OCUSERT

Patients with acute infectious conjunctivitis or keratitis should be given special consideration and evaluation prior to the use of the Ocusert pilocarpine system.

Damaged or deformed systems should not be placed or retained in the eye. Systems believed to be associated with an unexpected increase in drug action should be removed and replaced with a new system.

PILOPINE HS

For topical use only.

PRECAUTIONS

ISOPTO CARPINE

General

The miosis usually causes difficulty in dark adaptation. Patient should be advised to exercise caution in night driving and other hazardous occupations in poor illumination.

Carcinogenesis, Mutagenesis, and Impairment of Fertility

There have been no long-term studies done using pilocarpine in animals to evaluate carcinogenic potential.

Pregnancy Category C

Animal reproduction studies have not been conducted with pilocarpine. It is also not known whether pilocarpine can cause fetal harm when administered to a pregnant woman or can affect reproduction capacity. Pilocarpine should be given to a pregnant woman only if clearly needed.

Nursing Mothers

It is not known whether this drug is excreted in human milk. Because many drugs are excreted in human milk, caution should be exercised when pilocarpine is administered to a nursing woman.

Information for the Patient

Do not touch dropper tip to any surface, as this may contaminate the solution.

OCUSERT

General

Ocusert pilocarpine system safety in retinal detachment patients and in patients with filtration blebs has not been established. The conjunctival erythema and edema associated with epinephrine ophthalmic solutions are not substantially altered by concomitant Ocusert pilocarpine system therapy. The use of pilocarpine drops should be considered when intense miosis is desired in certain ocular conditions.

Carcinogenesis, Mutagenesis, and Impairment of Fertility

No long-term carcinogenicity and reproduction studies in animals have been conducted with the Ocusert system.

Pregnancy Category C

Although the use of the Ocusert pilocarpine system has not been reported to have adverse effect on pregnancy, the safety of its use in pregnant women has not been absolutely established. While systemic absorption of pilocarpine from the Ocusert system is highly unlikely, pregnant women should use it only if clearly needed.

Nursing Mothers

It is not known whether pilocarpine is excreted in human milk. Because many drugs are excreted in human milk, caution should be exercised when the Ocusert system is used by a nursing woman.

Pediatric Use

Safety and effectiveness in children have not been established.

PILOPINE HS

General

The miosis usually causes difficulty in dark adaptation. Patient should be advised to exercise caution in night driving and other hazardous occupations in poor illumination.

Information for the Patient

Do not touch tube tip to any surface, as this may contaminate the gel.

Carcinogenesis, Mutagenesis, and Impairment of Fertility

There have been no long-term studies done using pilocarpine HCl in animals to evaluate carcinogenic potential.

Pregnancy Category C

Animal reproduction studies have not been conducted with pilocarpine HCl. It is also not known whether pilocarpine HCl can cause fetal harm when administered to a pregnant woman or can affect reproduction capacity. Pilopine HS gel should be given to a pregnant woman only if clearly needed.

Nursing Mothers

It is not known whether this drug is excreted in human milk. Because many drugs are excreted in human milk, caution should be exercised when pilocarpine HCl is administered to a nursing woman.

Pediatric Use

Safety and effectiveness in pediatric patients have not been established.

DRUG INTERACTIONS

OCUSERT

Although ophthalmic solutions have been used effectively in conjunction with the Ocusert system, systemic reactions consistent with an increased rate of absorption from the eye of an autonomic drug, such as epinephrine, have been observed. In rare instances, reactions of this type can be severe.

ADVERSE REACTIONS

ISOPTO CARPINE

Transient symptoms of stinging and burning may occur. Ciliary spasm, conjunctival vascular congestion, temporal or supraorbital headache, and induced myopia may occur. This is especially true in younger individuals who have recently started administration. Reduced visual acuity in poor illumination is frequently experienced by older individuals and individuals with lens opacity. As with all miotics, rare cases of retinal detachment have been reported when used in certain susceptible individuals. Lens opacity may occur with prolonged use of pilocarpine.

OCUSERT

Ciliary spasm is encountered with pilocarpine usage but is not a contraindication to continued therapy unless the induced myopia is debilitating to the patient. Irritation from pilocarpine has been infrequently encountered and may require cessation of therapy depending on the judgement of the physician. True allergic reactions are uncommon but require discontinuation of therapy should they occur. Corneal abrasion and visual impairment have been reported with use of the Ocusert System.

Although withdrawal of the peripheral iris from the anterior chamber angle by miosis may reduce the tendency for narrow angle closure, miotics can occasionally precipitate angle closure by increasing the resistance to aqueous flow from posterior to anterior chamber.

Miotic agents may also cause retinal detachment; thus, care should be exercised with all miotic therapy especially in young myopic patients.

Some patients may notice signs of conjunctival irritation, including mild erythema with or without a slight increase in mucous secretion when they first use Ocusert pilocarpine systems. These symptoms tend to lessen or disappear after the first week of therapy. In rare instances a sudden increase in pilocarpine effects has been reported during system use.

PILOPINE HS

The following adverse experiences associated with pilocarpine therapy have been reported: lacrimation, burning or discomfort, temporal or periorbital headache, ciliary spasm, conjunctival vascular congestion, superficial keratitis and induced myopia. Systemic reactions following topical administration are extremely rare, but occasional patients are peculiarly sensitive to develop sweating and gastrointestinal overactivity following suggested dosage and administration. Ocular reactions usually occur during initiation of therapy and often will not persist with continued therapy. Reduced visual acuity in poor illumination is frequently experienced in older individuals and in those with lens opacity. A subtle corneal granularity was observed in about 10% of patients treated with Pilopine HS gel. Cases of retinal detachment have been reported during treatment with miotic agents; especially in young myopic patients. Lens opacity may occur with prolonged use of pilocarpine.

DOSAGE AND ADMINISTRATION

ISOPTO CARPINE

Two drops topically in the eye(s) up to 3 or 4 times daily as directed by a physician. Under selected conditions, more frequent instillations may be indicated. Individuals with heavily pigmented irides may require higher strengths.

OCUSERT

Initiation of Therapy

A patient whose intraocular pressure has been controlled by 1 or 2% pilocarpine eyedrop solution has a higher probability of pressure control with the Pilo-20 system than a patient who has used a higher strength pilocarpine solution and might require Pilo-40 therapy. However, there is no direct correlation between the Ocusert system (Pilo-20 or Pilo-40) and the strength of pilocarpine eyedrop solutions required to achieve a given level of pressure lowering. The Ocusert system reduces the amount of drug necessary to achieve adequate medical control; therefore, therapy may be started with the Ocusert Pilo-20 system irrespective of the strength of pilocarpine solution the patient previously required. Because of the patient's age, family history, and disease status or progression, however, the ophthalmologist may elect to begin therapy with the Pilo-40. The patient should then return during the first week of therapy for evaluation of his intraocular pressure, and as often thereafter as the ophthalmologist deems necessary.

If the pressure is satisfactorily reduced with the Ocusert Pilo-20 system the patient should continue its use, replacing each unit every 7 days. If the physician desires intraocular pressure reduction greater than that achieved by the Pilo-20 system, the patient should be transferred to the Pilo-40 system. If necessary, an epinephrine ophthalmic solution or a carbonic anhydrase inhibitor may be used concurrently with Ocusert system.

After a satisfactory therapeutic regimen has been established with the Ocusert pilocarpine system, the frequency of follow-up should be determined by the ophthalmologist according to the status of the patient's disease process.

Placement and Removal of the Ocusert System

The Ocusert system is readily placed in the eye by the patient, according to patient instructions provided in the package. The instructions also describe procedures for removal of the system. It is strongly recommended that the patient's ability to manage the placement and removal of the system be reviewed at the first patient visit after initiation of therapy.

Since the pilocarpine-induced myopia from the Ocusert systems may occur during the first several hours of therapy (average of 1.4 diopters in a group of young subjects), the patient should be advised to place the system into the conjunctial cul-de-sac at bedtime. By morning the induced myopia is at a stable level (about 0.5 diopters or less in young subjects).

Sanitary Handling

Patients should be instructed to wash their hands thoroughly with soap and water before touching or manipulating the Ocusert system. In the event a displaced unit contacts unclean surfaces, rinsing with cool tap water before replacing is advisable. Obviously bacteriologically contaminated units should be discarded and replaced with a fresh unit.

Ocusert System Retention in the Eye

During the initial adaptation period, the Ocusert unit may slip out of the conjunctival cul-de-sac onto the cheek. The patient is usually aware of such movement and can replace the unit without difficulty.

In those patients in whom retention of the Ocusert unit is a problem, superior cul-de-sac placement is often more desirable. The Ocusert unit can be manipulated from the lower to the upper conjunctival cul-de-sac by a gentle digital massage through the lid, a technique readily learned by the patient. If possible the unit should be moved before sleep to the upper conjunctival cul-de-sac for best retention. Should the unit slip out of the conjunctival cul-de-sac during sleep, its ocular hypotensive effect following loss continues for a period of time comparable to that following instillation of eyedrops. The patient should be instructed to check for the presence of the Ocusert unit before retiring at night and upon arising.

PILOPINE HS

Apply a one-half inch ribbon in the lower conjunctival sac of the affected eye(s) once a day at bedtime.

HOW SUPPLIED

ISOPTO CARPINE

Isopto Carpine is available in:

1%: 15 and 30 ml plastic Drop-Tainer dispensers.
2%: 15 and 30 ml plastic Drop-Tainer dispensers.
4%: 15 and 30 ml plastic Drop-Tainer dispensers.
6%: 15 ml plastic Drop-Tainer dispensers.
8%: 15 ml plastic Drop-Tainer dispensers.

Storage: Store at 8-27°C (46-80°F).

OCUSERT

Ocusert Pilo-20 or Pilo-40 systems are available in packages containing 8 individual sterile systems.

Storage and Handling: Store under refrigeration (36-46°F).

PILOPINE HS

Pilopine HS gel is supplied as a 4% sterile aqueous gel in 4 g tubes with ophthalmic tip.

Storage: Store at room temperature 2-27°C (36-80°F). Avoid excessive heat. Do not freeze.

ORAL

DESCRIPTION

Note: The trade names have been used throughout this monograph for clarity.

Salagen tablets contain pilocarpine hydrochloride, a cholinergic agonist for oral use. Pilocarpine hydrochloride is a hygroscopic, odorless, bitter tasting white crystal or powder, which is soluble in water and alcohol and virtually insoluble in most non-polar solvents. Pilocarpine hydrochloride, with a chemical name of (3*S*-*cis*)-2(3*H*)-furanone, 3-ethyldihydro-4-[(1-methyl-1*H*-imidazol-5-yl)methyl] monohydrochloride, has a molecular weight of 244.72.

Each Salagen tablet for oral administration contains 5 µg of pilocarpine hydrochloride. Inactive ingredients in the tablet, the tablet's film coating, polishing, and branding are: carnauba wax, hydroxypropyl methylcellulose, iron oxide, microcrystalline cellulose, stearic acid, titanium dioxide and other ingredients.

CLINICAL PHARMACOLOGY

PHARMACODYNAMICS

Pilocarpine is a cholinergic parasympathomimetic agent exerting a broad spectrum of pharmacologic effects with predominant muscarinic action. Pilocarpine, in appropriate dosage, can increase secretion by the exocrine glands. The sweat, salivary, lacrimal, gastric, pancreatic, and intestinal glands and the mucous cells of the respiratory tract may be stimulated. When applied topically to the eye as a single dose it causes miosis, spasm of accommodation, and may cause a transitory rise in intraocular pressure followed by a more persistent fall. Dose-related smooth muscle stimulation of the intestinal tract may cause increased tone, increased motility, spasm, and tenesmus. Bronchial smooth muscle tone may increase. The tone and motility of urinary tract, gallbladder, and biliary duct smooth muscle may be enhanced. Pilocarpine may have paradoxical effects on the cardiovascular system. The expected effect of a muscarinic agonist is vasodepression, but administration of pilocarpine may produce hypertension after a brief episode of hypotension. Bradycardia and tachycardia have both been reported with use of pilocarpine.

In a study of 12 healthy male volunteers there was a dose-related increase in unstimulated salivary flow following single 5 and 10 µg oral doses of Salagen tablets. This effect of pilocarpine on salivary flow was time-related with an onset at 20 minutes and a peak effect at 1 hour with a duration of 3-5 hours (see Pharmacokinetics).

Head and Neck Cancer Patients

In a 12 week randomized, double-blind, placebo-controlled study in 207 patients (placebo, n=65; 5 µg, n=73; 10 µg, n=69), increases from baseline (means 0.072 and 0.112 ml/min, ranges -0.690 to 0.728 and -0.380 to 1.689) of whole saliva flow for the 5 µg (63%) and 10 µg (90%) tablet, respectively, were seen 1 hour after the first dose of Salagen tablets. Increases in unstimulated parotid flow were seen following the first dose (means 0.025 and 0.046 ml/min, ranges 0 to 0.414 and -0.070 to 1.002 ml/min for the 5 µg and 10 µg dose, respectively). In this study, no correlation existed between the amount of increase in salivary flow and the degree of symptomatic relief.

Sjögren's Syndrome Patients

In two 12 week randomized, double-blind, placebo-controlled studies in 629 patients (placebo, n=253; 2.5 µg, n=121; 5 µg, n=255; 5 to 7.5 µg, n=114), the ability of Salagen tablets to stimulate saliva production was assessed. In these trials using varying doses of Salagen tablets (2.5-7.5 µg), the rate of saliva production was plotted against time. An area under the curve (AUC) representing the total amount of saliva produced during the observation interval was calculated. Relative to placebo, an increase in the amount of saliva being produced was observed following the first dose of Salagen tablets and was maintained throughout the duration (12 weeks) of the trials in an approximate dose response fashion.

PHARMACOKINETICS

In a multiple-dose pharmacokinetic study in male volunteers following 2 days of 5 or 10 µg of oral pilocarpine HCl tablets given at 8 AM, noontime, and 6 PM, the mean elimination half-life was 0.76 hours for the 5 µg dose and 1.35 hours for the 10 µg dose. T_{max} values were 1.25 hours and 0.85 hours. C_{max} values were 15 and 41 ng/ml. The AUC trapezoidal values were 33 h(ng/ml) and 108 h(ng/ml), respectively, for the 5 µg and 10 µg doses following the last 6 hour dose.

Pharmacokinetics in elderly male volunteers (n=11) were comparable to those in younger men. In 5 healthy elderly female volunteers, the mean C_{max} and AUC were approximately twice that of elderly males and young normal male volunteers.

When taken with a high fat meal by 12 healthy male volunteers, there was a decrease in the rate of absorption of pilocarpine from Salagen tablets. Mean T_{max}s were 1.47 and 0.87 hours, and mean C_{max}s were 51.8 and 59.2 ng/ml for fed and fasted, respectively.

Limited information is available about the metabolism and elimination of pilocarpine in humans. Inactivation of pilocarpine is thought to occur at neuronal synapses and probably in plasma. Pilocarpine and its minimally active or inactive degradation products, including pilocarpic acid, are excreted in the urine. Pilocarpine does not bind to human or rat plasma proteins over a concentration range of 5-25,000 ng/ml. The effect of pilocarpine on plasma protein binding of other drugs has not been evaluated.

In patients with mild to moderate hepatic impairment (n=12), administration of a single 5 μg dose resulted in a 30% decrease in total plasma clearance and a doubling of exposure (as measured by AUC). Peak plasma levels were also increased by about 30% and half-life was increased to 2.1 hours.

There were no significant differences in the pharmacokinetics of oral pilocarpine in volunteer subjects (n=8) with renal insufficiency (mean creatinine clearances 25.4 ml/min; range 9.8-40.8 ml/min) compared to the pharmacokinetics previously observed in normal volunteers.

INDICATIONS AND USAGE

Salagen tablets are indicated for (1) the treatment of symptoms of dry mouth from salivary gland hypofunction caused by radiotherapy for cancer of the head and neck; and (2) the treatment of symptoms of dry mouth in patients with Sjögren's syndrome.

CONTRAINDICATIONS

Salagen tablets are contraindicated in patients with uncontrolled asthma, known hypersensitivity to pilocarpine, and when miosis is undesirable, *e.g.*, in acute iritis and in narrow-angle (angle closure) glaucoma.

WARNINGS

CARDIOVASCULAR DISEASE

Patients with significant cardiovascular disease may be unable to compensate for transient changes in hemodynamics or rhythm induced by pilocarpine. Pulmonary edema has been reported as a complication of pilocarpine toxicity from high ocular doses given for acute angle-closure glaucoma. Pilocarpine should be administered with caution in and under close medical supervision of patients with significant cardiovascular disease.

OCULAR

Ocular formulations of pilocarpine have been reported to cause visual blurring which may result in decreased visual acuity, especially at night and in patients with central lens changes, and to cause impairment of depth perception. Caution should be advised while driving at night or performing hazardous activities in reduced lighting.

PULMONARY DISEASE

Pilocarpine has been reported to increase airway resistance, bronchial smooth muscle tone, and bronchial secretions. Pilocarpine HCl should be administered with caution to and under close medical supervision in patients with controlled asthma, chronic bronchitis, or chronic obstructive pulmonary disease requiring pharmacotherapy.

PRECAUTIONS

GENERAL

Pilocarpine toxicity is characterized by an exaggeration of its parasympathomimetic effects. These may include: headache, visual disturbance, lacrimation, sweating, respiratory distress, gastrointestinal spasm, nausea, vomiting, diarrhea, atrioventricular block, tachycardia, bradycardia, hypotension, hypertension, shock, mental confusion, cardiac arrhythmia, and tremors.

The dose-related cardiovascular pharmacologic effects of pilocarpine include hypotension, hypertension, bradycardia, and tachycardia.

Pilocarpine should be administered with caution to patients with known or suspected cholelithiasis or biliary tract disease. Contractions of the gallbladder or biliary smooth muscle could precipitate complications including cholecystitis, cholangitis, and biliary obstruction.

Pilocarpine may increase ureteral smooth muscle tone and could theoretically precipitate renal colic (or "ureteral reflux"), particularly in patients with nephrolithiasis.

Cholinergic agonists may have dose-related central nervous system (CNS) effects. This should be considered when treating patients with underlying cognitive or psychiatric disturbances.

HEPATIC INSUFFICIENCY

Based on decreased plasma clearance observed in patients with moderate hepatic impairment, the starting dose in these patients should be 5 μg twice daily, followed by adjustment based on therapeutic response and tolerability. Patients with mild hepatic insufficiency (Child-Pugh score of 5-6) do not require dosage reductions. To date, pharmacokinetic studies in subjects with severe hepatic impairment (Child-Pugh score of 10-15) have not been carried out. The use of pilocarpine in these patients is not recommended.

TABLE 1 *Child-Pugh Scoring System for Hepatic Impairment*

Clinical and Biochemical Measurements	Points Scored for Increasing Abnormality 1	2	3
Encephalopathy (Grade)*	None	1 and 2	3 and 4
Ascites	Absent	Slight	Moderate
Bilirubin (μg/100 ml)	1-2	2-3	>3
Albumin (g/100 ml)	3-5	2.8-3.5	<2.8
Prothrombin time (second prolonged)	1-4	4-6	>6
For Primary Biliary Cirrhosis			
Bilirubin (μg/100 ml)	1-4	4-10	>10

* According to grading of Trey, Burns, and Saunders (1966).

INFORMATION FOR THE PATIENT

Patients should be informed that pilocarpine may cause visual disturbances, especially at night, that could impair their ability to drive safely.

If a patient sweats excessively while taking pilocarpine HCl and cannot drink enough liquid, the patient should consult a physician. Dehydration may develop.

CARCINOGENESIS, MUTAGENESIS, AND IMPAIRMENT OF FERTILITY

Lifetime oral carcinogenicity studies were conducted in CD-1 mice and Sprague-Dawley rats. Pilocarpine did not induce tumors in mice at any dosage studied (up to 30 μg/kg/day, which yielded a systemic exposure approximately 50 times larger than the maximum systemic exposure observed clinically). In rats, a dosage of 18 μg/kg/day, which yielded a systemic exposure approximately 100 times larger than the maximum systemic exposure observed clinically, resulted in a statistically significant increase in the incidence of benign pheochromocytomas in both males and females, and a statistically significant increase in the incidence of hepatocellular adenomas in female rats. The tumorigenicity observed in rats was observed only at a large multiple of the maximum labeled clinical dose, and may not be relevant to clinical use.

No evidence that pilocarpine has the potential to cause genetic toxicity was obtained in a series of studies that included: (1) bacterial assays (*Salmonella* and *E. coli*) for reverse gene mutations; (2) an *in vitro* chromosome aberration assay in a Chinese hamster ovary cell line; (3) an *in vivo* chromosome aberration assay (micronucleus test) in mice; and (4) a primary DNA damage assay (unscheduled DNA synthesis) in rat hepatocyte primary cultures.

Oral administration of pilocarpine to male and female rats at a dosage of 18 μg/kg/day, which yielded a systemic exposure approximately 100 times larger than the maximum systemic exposure observed clinically, resulted in impaired reproductive function, including reduced fertility, decreased sperm motility, and morphologic evidence of abnormal sperm. It is unclear whether the reduction in fertility was due to effects on male animals, female animals, or both males and females. In dogs, exposure to pilocarpine at a dosage of 3 μg/kg/day [approximately 3 times the maximum recommended human dose when compared on the basis of body surface area (μg/m^2) estimates] for 6 months resulted in evidence of impaired spermatogenesis. The data obtained in these studies suggest that pilocarpine may impair the fertility of male and female humans. Pilocarpine HCl tablets should be administered to individuals who are attempting to conceive a child only if the potential benefit justifies potential impairment of fertility.

PREGNANCY, TERATOGENIC EFFECTS, PREGNANCY CATEGORY C

Pilocarpine was associated with a reduction in the mean fetal body weight and an increase in the incidence of skeletal variations when given to pregnant rats at a dosage of 90 μg/kg/day [approximately 26 times the maximum recommended dose for a 50 kg human when compared on the basis of body surface area (μg/m^2) estimates]. These effects may have been secondary to maternal toxicity. In another study, oral administration of pilocarpine to female rats during gestation and lactation at a dosage of 36 μg/kg/day [approximately 10 times the maximum recommended dose for a 50 kg human when compared on the basis of body surface area (μg/m^2) estimates] resulted in an increased incidence of stillbirths; decreased neonatal survival and reduced mean body weight of pups were observed at dosages of 18 μg/kg/day [approximately 5 times the maximum recommended dose for a 50 kg human when compared on the basis of body surface area (μg/m^2) estimates] and above. There are no adequate and well-controlled studies in pregnant women. Salagen tablets should be used during pregnancy only if the potential benefit justifies the potential risk to the fetus.

NURSING MOTHERS

It is not known whether this drug is excreted in human milk. Because many drugs are excreted in human milk and because of the potential for serious adverse reactions in nursing infants from Salagen tablets, a decision should be made whether to discontinue nursing or to discontinue the drug, taking into account the importance of the drug to the mother.

P

PEDIATRIC USE

Safety and effectiveness in pediatric patients have not been established.

GERIATRIC USE

Head and Neck Cancer Patients

In the placebo-controlled clinical trials the mean age of patients was approximately 58 years (range 19-80). Of these patients, 97/369 (61/217 receiving pilocarpine) were over the age of 65 years. In the healthy volunteer studies, 15/150 subjects were over the age of 65 years. In both study populations, the adverse events reported by those over 65 years and those 65 years and younger were comparable. Of the 15 elderly volunteers (5 women, 10 men), the 5 women had higher C_{max}s and AUCs than the men. (See CLINICAL PHARMACOLOGY, Pharmacokinetics.)

Sjögren's Syndrome Patients

In the placebo-controlled clinical trials, the mean age of patients was approximately 55 years (range 21-85). The adverse events reported by those over 65 years and those 65 years and younger were comparable except for notable trends for urinary frequency, diarrhea, and dizziness (see ADVERSE REACTIONS).

DRUG INTERACTIONS

Pilocarpine should be administered with caution to patients taking beta-adrenergic antagonists because of the possibility of conduction disturbances. Drugs with parasympathomimetic effects administered concurrently with pilocarpine would be expected to result in additive pharmacologic effects.

Pilocarpine might antagonize the anticholinergic effects of drugs used concomitantly. These effects should be considered when anticholinergic properties may be contributing to the therapeutic effect of concomitant medication (*e.g.*, atropine, inhaled ipratropium).

While no formal drug interaction studies have been performed, the following concomitant drugs were used in at least 10% of patients in either or both Sjögren's efficacy studies: acetylsalicylic acid, artificial tears, calcium, conjugated estrogens, hydroxychloroquine sulfate, ibuprofen, levothyroxine sodium, medroxyprogesterone acetate, methotrexate, multivitamins, naproxen, omeprazole, paracetamol, and prednisone.

ADVERSE REACTIONS

HEAD AND NECK CANCER PATIENTS

In controlled studies, 217 patients received pilocarpine, of whom 68% were men and 32% were women. Race distribution was 91% Caucasian, 8% Black, and 1% of other origin. Mean age was approximately 58 years. The majority of patients were between 50 and 64 years (51%), 33% were 65 years and older and 16% were younger than 50 years of age.

The most frequent adverse experiences associated with Salagen tablets were a consequence of the expected pharmacologic effects of pilocarpine.

TABLE 2

Adverse Event	10 μg tid (30 μg/day) n=121	5 μg tid (15 μg/day) n=141	Placebo (tid) n=152
Sweating	68%	29%	9%
Nausea	15%	6%	4%
Rhinitis	14%	5%	7%
Diarrhea	7%	4%	5%
Chills	15%	3%	<1%
Flushing	13%	8%	3%
Urinary frequency	12%	9%	7%
Dizziness	12%	5%	4%
Asthenia	12%	6%	3%

In addition, the following adverse events (≥3% incidence) were reported at dosages of 15-30 μg/day in the controlled clinical trials (see TABLE 3).

TABLE 3

Adverse Event	Pilocarpine HCl 5-10 μg tid (15-30 μg/day) n=212	Placebo (tid) n=152
Headache	11%	8%
Dyspepsia	7%	5%
Lacrimation	6%	8%
Edema	5%	4%
Abdominal pain	4%	4%
Amblyopia	4%	2%
Vomiting	4%	1%
Pharyngitis	3%	8%
Hypertension	3%	1%

The following events were reported with treated head and neck cancer patients at incidences of 1-2% at dosages of 7.5 to 30 μg/day:

Abnormal vision, conjunctivitis, dysphagia, epistaxis, myalgias, pruritus, rash, sinusitis, tachycardia, taste perversion, tremor, voice alteration.

The following events were reported rarely in treated head and neck cancer patients (<1%) — Causal Relation is Unknown:

Body as a Whole: Body odor, hypothermia, mucous membrane abnormality.
Cardiovascular: Bradycardia, ECG abnormality, palpitations, syncope.
Digestive: Anorexia, increased appetite, esophagitis, gastrointestinal disorder, tongue disorder.
Hematologic: Leukopenia, lymphadenopathy.
Nervous: Anxiety, confusion, depression, abnormal dreams, hyperkinesia, hypesthesia, nervousness, paresthesias, speech disorder, twitching.
Respiratory: Increased sputum, stridor, yawning.
Skin: Seborrhea.
Special Senses: Deafness, eye pain, glaucoma.
Urogenital: Dysuria, metrorrhagia, urinary impairment.

In long-term treatment were 2 patients with underlying cardiovascular disease of whom one experienced a myocardial infarct and another an episode of syncope. The association with drug is uncertain.

SJÖGREN'S SYNDROME PATIENTS

In controlled studies, 376 patients received pilocarpine, of whom 5% were men and 95% were women. Race distribution was 84% Caucasian, 9% Oriental, 3% Black, and 4% of other origin. Mean age was 55 years. The majority of patients were between 40 and 69 years (70%), 16% were 70 years and older and 14% were younger than 40 years of age. Of these patients, 161/629 (89/376 receiving pilocarpine) were over the age of 65 years. The adverse events reported by those over 65 years and those 65 years and younger were comparable except for notable trends for urinary frequency, diarrhea, and dizziness. The incidences of urinary frequency and diarrhea in the elderly were about double those in the non-elderly. The incidence of dizziness was about 3 times as high in the elderly as in the non-elderly. These adverse experiences were not considered to be serious. In the 2 placebo-controlled studies, the most common adverse events related to drug use were sweating, urinary frequency, chills, and vasodilatation (flushing). The most commonly reported reason for patient discontinuation of treatment was sweating. Expected pharmacologic effects of pilocarpine include the following adverse experiences associated with Salagen tablets (see TABLE 4).

In addition, the following adverse events (≥3% incidence) were reported at dosing of 20 μg/day in the controlled clinical trials (see TABLE 5).

The following events were reported in Sjögren's patients at incidences of 1-2% at dosing of 20 μg/day:

Accidental injury, allergic reaction, back pain, blurred vision, constipation, increased cough, edema, epistaxis, face edema, fever, flatulence, glossitis, lab test abnormalities, including chemistry, hematology, and urinalysis, myalgia, palpitation, pruritus, somnolence, stomatitis, tachycardia, tinnitus, urinary incontinence, urinary tract infection, vaginitis.

TABLE 4

Adverse Event	Pilocarpine HCl 5 μg qid (20 μg/day) n=255	Placebo (qid) n=253
Sweating	40%	7%
Urinary frequency	10%	4%
Nausea	9%	9%
Flushing	9%	2%
Rhinitis	7%	8%
Diarrhea	6%	7%
Chills	4%	2%
Increased salivation	3%	0%
Asthenia	2%	2%

TABLE 5

Adverse Event	Pilocarpine HCl 5 μg qid (20 μg/day) n=255	Placebo (qid) n=253
Headache	13%	19%
Flu syndrome	9%	9%
Dyspepsia	7%	7%
Dizziness	6%	7%
Pain	4%	2%
Sinusitis	4%	5%
Abdominal pain	3%	4%
Vomiting	3%	1%
Pharyngitis	2%	5%
Rash	2%	3%
Infection	2%	6%

The following events were reported rarely in treated Sjögren's patients (<1%) at dosing of 10-30 μg/day — Causal Relation is Unknown:

Body as a Whole: Chest pain, cyst, death, moniliasis, neck pain, neck rigidity, photosensitivity reaction.
Cardiovascular: Angina pectoris, arrhythmia, ECG abnormality, hypotension, hypertension, intracranial hemorrhage, migraine, myocardial infarction.
Digestive: Anorexia, bilirubinemia, cholelithiasis, colitis, dry mouth, eructation, gastritis, gastroenteritis, gastrointestinal disorder, gingivitis, hepatitis, abnormal liver function tests, melena, nausea and vomiting, pancreatitis, parotid gland enlargement, salivary gland enlargement, sputum increased, taste loss, tongue disorder, tooth disorder.
Hematologic: Hematuria, lymphadenopathy, abnormal platelets, thrombocythemia, thrombocytopenia, thrombosis, abnormal WBC.
Metabolic and Nutritional: Peripheral edema, hypoglycemia.
Musculoskeletal: Arthralgia, arthritis, bone disorder, spontaneous bone fracture, pathological fracture, myasthenia, tendon disorder, tenosynovitis.
Nervous: Aphasia, confusion, depression, abnormal dreams, emotional lability, hyperkinesia, hypesthesia, insomnia, leg cramps, nervousness, paresthesias, abnormal thinking, tremor.
Respiratory: Bronchitis, dyspnea, hiccup, laryngismus, laryngitis, pneumonia, viral infection, voice alteration.
Skin: Alopecia, contact dermatitis, dry skin, eczema, erythema nodosum, exfoliative dermatitis, herpes simplex, skin ulcer, vesiculobullous rash.
Special Senses: Cataract, conjunctivitis, dry eyes, ear disorder, ear pain, eye disorder, eye hemorrhage, glaucoma, lacrimation disorder, retinal disorder, taste perversion, abnormal vision.
Urogenital: Breast pain, dysuria, mastitis, menorrhagia, metrorrhagia, ovarian disorder, pyuria, salpingitis, urethral pain, urinary urgency, vaginal hemorrhage, vaginal moniliasis.

The following adverse experiences have been reported rarely with ocular pilocarpine: A-V block, agitation, ciliary congestion, confusion, delusion, depression, dermatitis, middle ear disturbance, eyelid twitching, malignant glaucoma, iris cysts, macular hole, shock, and visual hallucination.

DOSAGE AND ADMINISTRATION

Regardless of the indication, the starting dose in patients with moderate hepatic impairment should be 5 μg twice daily, followed by adjustment based on therapeutic response and tolerability. Patients with mild hepatic insufficiency do not require dosage reductions. The use of pilocarpine in patients with severe hepatic insufficiency is not recommended. If needed, refer to PRECAUTIONS, Hepatic Insufficiency for definitions of mild, moderate and severe hepatic impairment.

HEAD AND NECK CANCER PATIENTS

The recommended initial dose of Salagen tablets is 1 tablet (5 μg) taken 3 times a day. Dosage should be adjusted according to therapeutic response and tolerance. The usual dosage range is 3-6 tablets or 15-30 μg/day. (Not to exceed 2 tablets per dose.) Although early improvement may be realized, at least 12 weeks of uninterrupted therapy with Salagen tablets may be necessary to assess whether a beneficial response will be achieved. The incidence of the most common adverse events increases with dose. The lowest dose that is tolerated and effective should be used for maintenance.

SJöGREN'S SYNDROME PATIENTS

The recommended dose of Salagen tablets is 1 tablet (5 μg) taken 4 times/day. Efficacy was established by 6 weeks of use.

HOW SUPPLIED

Salagen tablets, 5 μg, are white, film coated, round tablets, coded "MGI 705". Each tablet contains 5 μg pilocarpine HCl.

Storage: Store at controlled room temperature 15-30°C (59-86°F).

PRODUCT LISTING - RATED THERAPEUTICALLY EQUIVALENT

Solution - Ophthalmic - 3%

15 ml	$8.13	GENERIC, Aligen Independent Laboratories Inc	00405-6122-15

Solution - Ophthalmic - 6%

15 ml	$12.46	GENERIC, Aligen Independent Laboratories Inc	00405-6124-15

PRODUCT LISTING - EQUIVALENTS NOT AVAILABLE

Crystal - Compounding - 100%

1 gm	$19.50	GENERIC, A-A Spectrum Quality Products	49452-5400-01
1 gm	$23.70	GENERIC, Gallipot Inc	51552-0477-01
5 gm	$46.80	GENERIC, A-A Spectrum Quality Products	49452-5400-02
25 gm	$210.40	GENERIC, A-A Spectrum Quality Products	49452-5400-03

Gel - Ophthalmic - 4%

3.50 gm	$35.75	PILOPINE-HS, Allscripts Pharmaceutical Company	54569-3655-00
4 gm	$42.44	PILOPINE-HS, Alcon Laboratories Inc	00065-0215-35
15 ml	$7.05	GENERIC, Interstate Drug Exchange Inc	00814-6125-42
15 ml	$8.15	GENERIC, Hi-Tech Pharmacal Company Inc	50383-0008-15

Insert - Ophthalmic - 20 mcg/Hr

8's	$51.55	GENERIC, Physicians Total Care	54868-2799-00

Insert - Ophthalmic - 40 mcg/Hr

8's	$45.13	GENERIC, Akorn Inc	17478-0229-05
8's	$51.55	GENERIC, Physicians Total Care	54868-2800-00

Solution - Ophthalmic - Nitrate 1%

15 ml	$11.59	PILAGAN WITH C CAP, Allergan Inc	11980-0879-45

Solution - Ophthalmic - Nitrate 2%

15 ml	$12.04	PILAGAN WITH C CAP, Allergan Inc	11980-0878-45

Solution - Ophthalmic - Nitrate 4%

15 ml	$12.49	PILAGAN WITH C CAP, Allergan Inc	11980-0877-45

Solution - Ophthalmic - 0.25%

15 ml	$17.25	ISOPTO CARPINE, Physicians Total Care	54868-3401-00

Solution - Ophthalmic - 0.5%

15 ml	$1.68	OCU-CARPINE, Ocumed Inc	51944-4535-02
15 ml	$1.68	OCU-CARPINE, Ocumed Inc	51944-4535-42
15 ml	$3.07	GENERIC, Physicians Total Care	54868-2110-00
15 ml	$4.19	GENERIC, Moore, H.L. Drug Exchange Inc	00839-6076-31
15 ml	$4.28	GENERIC, Caremark Inc	00339-5963-52
15 ml	$4.80	GENERIC, Martec Pharmaceuticals Inc	52555-0995-01
15 ml	$4.82	GENERIC, Steris Laboratories Inc	00402-0860-15
15 ml	$4.98	GENERIC, Miza Pharmaceutcials Dba Optopics Laboratories Corporation	52238-0750-15
15 ml	$6.62	PILOSTAT, Bausch and Lomb	24208-0806-15
15 ml	$11.62	PILOCAR, Ciba Vision Ophthalmics	00058-2514-15
15 ml	$12.21	PILOCAR, Ciba Vision Ophthalmics	58768-0514-15
15 ml x 2	$5.01	GENERIC, Aligen Independent Laboratories Inc	00405-6119-15

Solution - Ophthalmic - 1%

1 ml x 12	$27.69	PILOCAR, Ciba Vision Ophthalmics	00058-0781-12
1 ml x 12	$29.40	PILOCAR, Ciba Vision Ophthalmics	58768-0781-12
1 ml x 12	$35.28	PILOCAR, Ciba Vision Ophthalmics	58768-0515-12
2 ml x 12	$57.75	GENERIC, Alcon Laboratories Inc	00065-0728-12
15 ml	$1.95	OCU-CARPINE, Ocumed Inc	51944-4410-02
15 ml	$1.95	OCU-CARPINE, Ocumed Inc	51944-4410-42
15 ml	$2.65	GENERIC, Paco Pharmaceutical Services, Inc	52967-0550-45
15 ml	$3.03	GENERIC, Physicians Total Care	54868-1200-00
15 ml	$3.39	GENERIC, Logen	00820-0101-25
15 ml	$4.13	GENERIC, Interstate Drug Exchange Inc	00814-6094-42
15 ml	$4.49	GENERIC, Miza Pharmaceutcials Dba Optopics Laboratories Corporation	52238-0751-15
15 ml	$4.85	GENERIC, Hi-Tech Pharmacal Company Inc	50383-0007-15
15 ml	$4.93	GENERIC, Moore, H.L. Drug Exchange Inc	00839-5517-31
15 ml	$5.11	GENERIC, Qualitest Products Inc	00603-7247-41
15 ml	$5.26	GENERIC, Caremark Inc	00339-5965-52
15 ml	$5.30	GENERIC, Mutual/United Research Laboratories	00677-0910-30
15 ml	$5.50	GENERIC, Cmc-Consolidated Midland Corporation	00223-6700-15
15 ml	$5.60	GENERIC, Aligen Independent Laboratories Inc	00405-6120-15
15 ml	$5.67	GENERIC, Allscripts Pharmaceutical Company	54569-1196-00
15 ml	$5.83	GENERIC, Ivax Corporation	00182-0301-64
15 ml	$6.50	GENERIC, Martec Pharmaceuticals Inc	52555-0996-01
15 ml	$6.56	GENERIC, Akorn Inc	17478-0223-12
15 ml	$7.50	GENERIC, Major Pharmaceuticals Inc	00904-2714-35
15 ml	$7.95	GENERIC, Watson/Schein Pharmaceuticals Inc	00364-7131-72
15 ml	$7.95	GENERIC, Steris Laboratories Inc	00402-0863-15
15 ml	$7.95	GENERIC, Allscripts Pharmaceutical Company	54569-4356-00
15 ml	$8.00	GENERIC, Geneva Pharmaceuticals	00781-7040-85
15 ml	$8.30	GENERIC, Ivax Corporation	00182-0301-66
15 ml	$9.20	GENERIC, Falcon Pharmaceuticals, Ltd.	61314-0203-15
15 ml	$9.21	PILOSTAT, Bausch and Lomb	24208-0676-15
15 ml	$10.24	GENERIC, Southwood Pharmaceuticals Inc	58016-6403-01
15 ml	$12.54	PILOCAR, Ciba Vision Ophthalmics	58768-0515-15
15 ml	$17.06	GENERIC, Southwood Pharmaceuticals Inc	58016-6103-01
15 ml	$23.00	ISOPTO CARPINE, Alcon Laboratories Inc	00998-0203-15
15 ml x 2	$9.22	GENERIC, Aligen Independent Laboratories Inc	00405-6120-22
15 ml x 2	$9.90	GENERIC, Major Pharmaceuticals Inc	00904-2714-30
15 ml x 2	$26.95	PILOCAR, Ciba Vision Ophthalmics	00058-2515-34
15 ml x 2	$28.84	PILOCAR, Ciba Vision Ophthalmics	58768-0515-34
30 ml	$12.08	GENERIC, Qualitest Products Inc	00603-7249-42

Solution - Ophthalmic - 2%

1 ml x 12	$29.06	PILOCAR, Ciba Vision Ophthalmics	00058-0782-12
1 ml x 12	$29.40	PILOCAR, Ciba Vision Ophthalmics	58768-0782-12
1 ml x 12	$35.28	PILOCAR, Ciba Vision Ophthalmics	58768-0516-12
2 ml x 12	$57.72	GENERIC, Alcon Laboratories Inc	00065-0752-12
15 ml	$2.02	OCU-CARPINE, Ocumed Inc	51944-4415-02
15 ml	$2.02	OCU-CARPINE, Ocumed Inc	51944-4415-42
15 ml	$3.60	GENERIC, Physicians Total Care	54868-1167-01
15 ml	$3.75	GENERIC, Paco Pharmaceutical Services, Inc	52967-0551-45
15 ml	$4.40	GENERIC, Logen	00820-0102-25
15 ml	$5.70	GENERIC, Interstate Drug Exchange Inc	00814-6096-42
15 ml	$6.14	GENERIC, Aligen Independent Laboratories Inc	00405-6121-15
15 ml	$6.14	GENERIC, Miza Pharmaceutcials Dba Optopics Laboratories Corporation	52238-0752-15
15 ml	$6.50	GENERIC, Qualitest Products Inc	00603-7249-41
15 ml	$6.76	GENERIC, Caremark Inc	00339-5967-52
15 ml	$6.93	GENERIC, Allscripts Pharmaceutical Company	54569-1191-00
15 ml	$6.95	GENERIC, Moore, H.L. Drug Exchange Inc	00839-5518-31
15 ml	$6.95	GENERIC, Major Pharmaceuticals Inc	00904-2715-35
15 ml	$6.95	GENERIC, Hi-Tech Pharmacal Company Inc	50383-0009-15
15 ml	$7.20	GENERIC, Ivax Corporation	00182-0303-64
15 ml	$7.50	GENERIC, Cmc-Consolidated Midland Corporation	00223-6701-15
15 ml	$7.70	GENERIC, Martec Pharmaceuticals Inc	52555-0997-01
15 ml	$10.03	GENERIC, Steris Laboratories Inc	00402-0864-15
15 ml	$10.03	GENERIC, Allscripts Pharmaceutical Company	54569-4357-00
15 ml	$10.10	GENERIC, Geneva Pharmaceuticals	00781-7042-85
15 ml	$10.24	GENERIC, Southwood Pharmaceuticals Inc	58016-6088-01
15 ml	$11.79	PILOSTAT, Bausch and Lomb	24208-0681-15
15 ml	$11.80	GENERIC, Falcon Pharmaceuticals, Ltd.	61314-0204-15
15 ml	$12.54	PILOCAR, Ciba Vision Ophthalmics	58768-0516-15
15 ml	$23.50	ISOPTO CARPINE, Alcon Laboratories Inc	00998-0204-15
15 ml x 2	$6.56	GENERIC, Akorn Inc	17478-0224-12
15 ml x 2	$11.65	GENERIC, Ivax Corporation	00182-0303-66
15 ml x 2	$11.90	GENERIC, Major Pharmaceuticals Inc	00904-2715-30
15 ml x 2	$13.43	GENERIC, Aligen Independent Laboratories Inc	00405-6121-22
15 ml x 2	$29.06	PILOCAR, Ciba Vision Ophthalmics	58768-0516-34
30 ml	$33.00	ADSORBOCARPINE, Alcon Laboratories Inc	00998-0204-30

Solution - Ophthalmic - 3%

15 ml	$2.17	OCU-CARPINE, Ocumed Inc	51944-4540-02
15 ml	$2.17	OCU-CARPINE, Ocumed Inc	51944-4540-42
15 ml	$6.20	GENERIC, Moore, H.L. Drug Exchange Inc	00839-5519-31
15 ml	$6.74	GENERIC, Qualitest Products Inc	00603-7251-41
15 ml	$6.75	GENERIC, Major Pharmaceuticals Inc	00904-2716-35
15 ml	$6.84	GENERIC, Miza Pharmaceutcials Dba Optopics Laboratories Corporation	52238-0753-15
15 ml	$7.40	GENERIC, Caremark Inc	00339-5969-52
15 ml	$7.50	GENERIC, Ivax Corporation	00182-0304-64
15 ml	$7.90	GENERIC, Watson/Schein Pharmaceuticals Inc	00364-7133-72
15 ml	$7.90	GENERIC, Martec Pharmaceuticals Inc	52555-0998-01
15 ml	$8.00	GENERIC, Sidmak Laboratories Inc	50111-0813-20
15 ml	$10.68	PILOSTAT, Bausch and Lomb	24208-0811-15
15 ml	$12.75	PILOCAR, Ciba Vision Ophthalmics	00058-2517-15
15 ml x 2	$30.05	PILOCAR, Ciba Vision Ophthalmics	00058-2517-34

Solution - Ophthalmic - 4%

1 ml x 12	$27.69	PILOCAR, Ciba Vision Ophthalmics	00058-0783-12
1 ml x 12	$29.40	PILOCAR, Ciba Vision Ophthalmics	58768-0783-12
1 ml x 12	$35.28	PILOCAR, Ciba Vision Ophthalmics	58768-0518-12
2 ml x 12	$55.20	GENERIC, Alcon Laboratories Inc	00065-0756-12
15 ml	$2.35	OCU-CARPINE, Ocumed Inc	51944-4420-02
15 ml	$2.35	OCU-CARPINE, Ocumed Inc	51944-4420-42
15 ml	$4.50	GENERIC, Paco Pharmaceutical Services, Inc	52967-0552-45
15 ml	$4.79	GENERIC, Physicians Total Care	54868-1168-01
15 ml	$7.04	GENERIC, Qualitest Products Inc	00603-7253-41
15 ml	$7.09	GENERIC, Miza Pharmaceutcials Dba Optopics Laboratories Corporation	52238-0754-15
15 ml	$7.49	GENERIC, Moore, H.L. Drug Exchange Inc	00839-5520-31
15 ml	$7.51	GENERIC, Caremark Inc	00339-5971-52

P

Size	Price	Description	NDC
15 ml	$7.88	GENERIC, Aligen Independent Laboratories Inc	00405-6123-15
15 ml	$7.96	GENERIC, Allscripts Pharmaceutical Company	54569-1222-00
15 ml	$8.10	GENERIC, Ivax Corporation	00182-0305-64
15 ml	$8.16	GENERIC, Akorn Inc	17478-0226-12
15 ml	$8.20	GENERIC, Martec Pharmaceuticals Inc	52555-0999-01
15 ml	$8.50	GENERIC, Cmc-Consolidated Midland Corporation	00223-6702-15
15 ml	$9.50	GENERIC, Major Pharmaceuticals Inc	00904-2717-35
15 ml	$9.51	GENERIC, Allscripts Pharmaceutical Company	54569-4358-00
15 ml	$11.15	GENERIC, Geneva Pharmaceuticals	00781-7044-85
15 ml	$11.15	PILOSTAT, Bausch and Lomb	24208-0686-15
15 ml	$11.15	GENERIC, Falcon Pharmaceuticals, Ltd.	61314-0206-15
15 ml	$13.45	PILOCAR, Ciba Vision Ophthalmics	58768-0518-15
15 ml	$15.00	PILOCAR, Ciba Vision Ophthalmics	00058-2518-15
15 ml	$24.75	ISOPTO CARPINE, Alcon Laboratories Inc	00998-0206-15
15 ml x 2	$11.04	GENERIC, Southwood Pharmaceuticals Inc	58016-6037-01
15 ml x 2	$12.50	GENERIC, Ivax Corporation	00182-0305-66
15 ml x 2	$14.21	GENERIC, Aligen Independent Laboratories Inc	00405-6123-22
15 ml x 2	$14.30	GENERIC, Major Pharmaceuticals Inc	00904-2717-30
15 ml x 2	$24.37	PILOCAR, Ciba Vision Ophthalmics	00058-2518-34
15 ml x 2	$32.59	PILOCAR, Ciba Vision Ophthalmics	58768-0518-34
30 ml	$35.00	ISOPTO CARPINE, Alcon Laboratories Inc	00998-0206-30
Solution - Ophthalmic - 5%			
15 ml	$2.60	OCU-CARPINE, Ocumed Inc	51944-4545-02
15 ml	$2.60	OCU-CARPINE, Ocumed Inc	51944-4545-42
15 ml	$10.00	GENERIC, Sidmak Laboratories Inc	50111-0815-20
15 ml	$11.88	ISOPTO CARPINE, Alcon Laboratories Inc	00998-0207-15
Solution - Ophthalmic - 6%			
15 ml	$2.95	OCU-CARPINE, Ocumed Inc	51944-4550-02
15 ml	$2.95	OCU-CARPINE, Ocumed Inc	51944-4550-42
15 ml	$5.50	GENERIC, Paco Pharmaceutical Services, Inc	52967-0553-45
15 ml	$8.91	GENERIC, Apotex Usa Inc	60505-7491-05
15 ml	$9.46	GENERIC, Physicians Total Care	54868-1203-00
15 ml	$10.15	GENERIC, Moore, H.L. Drug Exchange Inc	00839-5521-31
15 ml	$10.80	GENERIC, Miza Pharmaceutcials Dba Optopics Laboratories Corporation	52238-0756-15
15 ml	$11.63	GENERIC, Caremark Inc	00339-5973-52
15 ml	$12.15	GENERIC, Hi-Tech Pharmacal Company Inc	50383-0012-15
15 ml	$13.05	GENERIC, Qualitest Products Inc	00603-7257-41
15 ml	$13.05	PILOSTAT, Bausch and Lomb	24208-0821-15
15 ml	$13.20	GENERIC, Falcon Pharmaceuticals, Ltd.	61314-0208-15
15 ml	$14.64	PILOCAR, Ciba Vision Ophthalmics	58768-0519-15
15 ml	$21.35	GENERIC, Southwood Pharmaceuticals Inc	58016-6327-01
15 ml	$25.56	ISOPTO CARPINE, Alcon Laboratories Inc	00998-0208-15
15 ml x 2	$28.20	PILOCAR, Ciba Vision Ophthalmics	58768-0519-34
15 ml x 2	$30.88	PILOCAR, Ciba Vision Ophthalmics	00058-2519-34
Solution - Ophthalmic - 8%			
2 ml	$55.20	GENERIC, Alcon Laboratories Inc	00065-0758-12
15 ml	$28.92	ISOPTO CARPINE, Alcon Laboratories Inc	00998-0209-15
Tablet - Oral - 5 mg			
100's	$128.59	SALAGEN, Physicians Total Care	54868-3447-01
100's	$153.60	SALAGEN, Mgi Pharma Inc	58063-0705-10

P

Pimecrolimus *(003542)*

Categories: Dermatitis, atopic; FDA Approved 2001 Dec; Pregnancy Category C
Drug Classes: Dermatologics; Immunosuppressives
Brand Names: Elidel

DESCRIPTION

FOR DERMATOLOGIC USE ONLY

NOT FOR OPHTHALMIC USE

Elidel cream 1% contains the compound pimecrolimus, the 33-epi-chloro-derivative of the macrolactam ascomycin.

Chemically, pimecrolimus is (1R,9S,12S,13R,14S,17R,18E,21S,23S,24R,25S,27R)-12-[(1E)-2-{(1R,3R,4S)-4-chloro-3-methoxycyclohexyl}-1-methylvinyl]-17-ethyl-1,14-dihydroxy-23,25-dimethoxy-13,19,21,27-tetramethyl-11,28-dioxa-4-aza-tricyclo[22.3.1.$0^{4,9}$]octacos-18-ene-2,3,10,16-tetraone.

The compound has the empirical formula $C_{43}H_{68}ClNO_{11}$ and the molecular weight of 810.47.

Pimecrolimus is a white to off-white fine crystalline powder. It is soluble in methanol and ethanol and insoluble in water.

Each gram of Elidel cream 1% contains 10 mg of pimecrolimus in a whitish cream base of benzyl alcohol, cetyl alcohol, citric acid, mono- and di-glycerides, oleyl alcohol, propylene glycol, sodium cetostearyl sulphate, sodium hydroxide, stearyl alcohol, triglycerides, and water.

CLINICAL PHARMACOLOGY

MECHANISM OF ACTION/PHARMACODYNAMICS

The mechanism of action of pimecrolimus in atopic dermatitis is not known. While the following have been observed, the clinical significance of these observations in atopic dermatitis is not known. It has been demonstrated that pimecrolimus binds with high affinity to macrophilin-12 (FKBP-12) and inhibits the calcium-dependent phosphatase, calcineurin. As a consequence, it inhibits T cell activation by blocking the transcription of early cytokines. In particular, pimecrolimus inhibits at nanomolar concentrations Interleukin-2 and interferon gamma (Th1-type) and Interleukin-4 and Interleukin-10 (Th2-type) cytokine synthesis in human T cells. In addition, pimecrolimus prevents the release of inflammatory cytokines and mediators from mast cells *in vitro* after stimulation by antigen/IgE.

PHARMACOKINETICS

Absorption

In adult patients being treated for atopic dermatitis [13-62% Body Surface Area (BSA) involvement] for periods up to a year, blood concentrations of pimecrolimus are routinely either at or below the limit of quantification of the assay (<0.5 ng/ml). In those subjects with detectable blood levels they are routinely <2 ng/ml and show no sign of drug accumulation with time. Because of the low systemic absorption of pimecrolimus following topical application the calculation of standard pharmacokinetic measures such as AUC, C_{max}, $T_{1/2}$, etc. cannot be reliably done.

Distribution

In vitro studies of the protein binding of pimecrolimus indicate that it is 74-87% bound to plasma proteins.

Metabolism

Following the administration of a single oral radiolabeled dose of pimecrolimus numerous circulating O-demethylation metabolites were seen. Studies with human liver microsomes indicate that pimecrolimus is metabolized *in vitro* by the CYP3A sub-family of metabolizing enzymes. No evidence of skin mediated drug metabolism was identified *in vivo* using the minipig or *in vitro* using stripped human skin.

Elimination

Based on the results of the aforementioned radiolabeled study, following a single oral dose of pimecrolimus ~81% of the administered radioactivity was recovered, primarily in the feces (78.4%) as metabolites. Less than 1% of the radioactivity found in the feces was due to unchanged pimecrolimus.

SPECIAL POPULATIONS

Pediatrics

The systemic exposure to pimecrolimus from pimecrolimus cream 1% was investigated in 26 pediatric patients with atopic dermatitis (20-69% BSA involvement) between the ages of 2-14 years. Following twice daily application for 3 weeks, blood concentrations of pimecrolimus were consistently low (<3 ng/ml), with the majority of the blood samples being below the limit of quantification (0.5 ng/ml). However, the children (20 children out of the total 23 children investigated) had at least one detectable blood level as compared to the adults (13 adults out of the total 25 adults investigated) over a 3 week treatment period. Due to the low and erratic nature of the blood levels observed, no correlation could be made between amount of cream, degree of BSA involvement, and blood concentrations. In general, the blood concentrations measured in adult atopic dermatitis patients were comparable to those seen in the pediatric population.

In a second group of 22 pediatric patients aged 3-23 months with 10-92% BSA involvement, a higher proportion of detectable blood levels was seen ranging from 0.1 to 2.6 ng/ml (limit of quantification 0.1 ng/ml). This increase in the absolute number of positive blood levels may be due to the larger surface area to body mass ratio seen in these younger subjects. In addition, a higher incidence of upper respiratory symptoms/infections was also seen relative to the older age group in the PK studies. At this time a causal relationship between these findings and pimecrolimus use cannot be ruled out. Use of pimecrolimus in this population is not recommended (see PRECAUTIONS, Pediatric Use).

Renal Insufficiency

The effect of renal insufficiency on the pharmacokinetics of topically administered pimecrolimus has not been evaluated. Given the very low systemic exposure of pimecrolimus via the topical route, no change in dosing is required.

Hepatic Insufficiency

The effect of hepatic insufficiency on the pharmacokinetics of topically administered pimecrolimus has not been evaluated. Given the very low systemic exposure of pimecrolimus via the topical route, no change in dosing is required.

INDICATIONS AND USAGE

Pimecrolimus cream 1% is indicated for short-term and intermittent long-term therapy in the treatment of *mild to moderate* atopic dermatitis in non-immunocompromised patients 2 years of age and older, in whom the use of alternative, conventional therapies is deemed inadvisable because of potential risks, or in the treatment of patients who are not adequately responsive to or intolerant of alternative, conventional therapies (see DOSAGE AND ADMINISTRATION).

CONTRAINDICATIONS

Pimecrolimus cream 1% is contraindicated in individuals with a history of hypersensitivity to pimecrolimus or any of the components of the cream.

PRECAUTIONS

GENERAL

Pimecrolimus cream 1% should not be applied to areas of active cutaneous viral infections.

Studies have not evaluated the safety and efficacy of pimecrolimus cream in the treatment of clinically infected atopic dermatitis. Before commencing treatment with pimecrolimus cream, clinical infections at treatment sites should be cleared.

While patients with atopic dermatitis are predisposed to superficial skin infections including eczema herpeticum (Kaposi's varicelliform eruption), treatment with pimecrolimus cream may be associated with an increased risk of varicella zoster virus infection (chicken pox or shingles), herpes simplex virus infection, or eczema herpeticum. In the presence of these skin infections, the balance of risks and benefits associated with pimecrolimus cream use should be evaluated.

In clinical studies, 14 cases of lymphadenopathy (0.9%) were reported while using pimecrolimus cream. These cases of lymphadenopathy were usually related to infections and noted to resolve upon appropriate antibiotic therapy. Of these 14 cases, the majority had either a clear etiology or were known to resolve. Patients who receive pimecrolimus cream and who develop lymphadenopathy should have the etiology of their lymphadenopathy investigated. In the absence of a clear etiology for the lymphadenopathy, or in the presence of acute infectious mononucleosis, discontinuation of pimecrolimus cream should be considered. Patients who develop lymphadenopathy should be monitored to ensure that the lymphadenopathy resolves.

In clinical studies, 15 cases of skin papilloma or warts (1%) were observed in patients using pimecrolimus cream. The youngest patient was age 2 and the oldest was age 12. In cases where there is worsening of skin papillomas or they do not respond to conventional therapy, discontinuation of pimecrolimus cream should be considered until complete resolution of the warts is achieved.

The enhancement of ultraviolet carcinogenicity is not necessarily dependent on phototoxic mechanisms. Despite the absence of observed phototoxicity in humans (see ADVERSE REACTIONS), pimecrolimus cream shortened the time to skin tumor formation in an animal photo-carcinogenicity study (see Carcinogenesis, Mutagenesis, and Impairment of Fertility). Therefore, it is prudent for patients to minimize or avoid natural or artificial sunlight exposure.

The use of pimecrolimus cream in patients with Netherton's Syndrome is not recommended due to the potential for increased systemic absorption of pimecrolimus.

There are no data to support use of pimecrolimus in immunocompromised patients.

The use of pimecrolimus cream may cause local symptoms such as skin burning. Localized symptoms are most common during the first few days of pimecrolimus cream application and typically improve as the lesions of atopic dermatitis resolve. Most application site reactions lasted no more than 5 days, were mild to moderate in severity, and started within 1-5 days of treatment. (See ADVERSE REACTIONS.)

INFORMATION FOR THE PATIENT

Patients using pimecrolimus should receive the following information and instructions:

Patients should use pimecrolimus cream as directed by the physician. Pimecrolimus cream is for external use on the skin only. As with any topical medication, patients or caregivers should wash hands after application if hands are not an area for treatment.

Patients should minimize or avoid exposure to natural or artificial sunlight (tanning beds or UVA/B treatment) while using pimecrolimus cream.

Patients should not use this medication for any disorder other than that for which it was prescribed.

Patients should report any signs or symptoms of adverse reactions to their physician.

Therapy should be discontinued after signs and symptoms of atopic dermatitis have resolved. Treatment with pimecrolimus should be resumed at the first signs or symptoms of recurrence.

Use of pimecrolimus may cause reactions at the site of application such as a mild to moderate feeling of warmth and/or sensation of burning. Patients should see a physician if an application site reaction is severe or persists for more than 1 week.

The patient should contact the physician if no improvement in the atopic dermatitis is seen following 6 weeks of treatment, or if at any time the condition worsens.

CARCINOGENESIS, MUTAGENESIS, AND IMPAIRMENT OF FERTILITY

In a 2 year rat dermal carcinogenicity study using pimecrolimus cream, a statistically significant increase in the incidence of follicular cell adenoma of the thyroid was noted in low, mid and high dose male animals compared to vehicle and saline control male animals. Follicular cell adenoma of the thyroid was noted in the dermal rat carcinogenicity study at the lowest dose of 2 mg/kg/day [0.2% pimecrolimus cream; 1.5× the Maximum Recommended Human Dose (MRHD) based on AUC comparisons]. No increase in the incidence of follicular cell adenoma of the thyroid was noted in the oral carcinogenicity study in male rats up to 10 mg/kg/day (66× MRHD based on AUC comparisons). However, oral studies may not reflect continuous exposure or the same metabolic profile as by the dermal route. In a mouse dermal carcinogenicity study using pimecrolimus in an ethanolic solution, no increase in incidence of neoplasms was observed in the skin or other organs up to the highest dose of 4 mg/kg/day (0.32% pimecrolimus in ethanol) 27× MRHD based on AUC comparisons. However, lymphoproliferative changes (including lymphoma) were noted in a 13 week repeat dose dermal toxicity study conducted in mice using pimecrolimus in an ethanolic solution at a dose of 25 mg/kg/day (47× MRHD based on AUC comparisons). No lymphoproliferative changes were noted in this study at a dose of 10 mg/kg/day (17× MRHD based on AUC comparison). However, the latency time to lymphoma formation was shortened to 8 weeks after dermal administration of pimecrolimus dissolved in ethanol at a dose of 100 mg/kg/day (179-217× MRHD based on AUC comparisons).

In a mouse oral (gavage) carcinogenicity study, a statistically significant increase in the incidence of lymphoma was noted in high dose male and female animals compared to vehicle control male and female animals. Lymphomas were noted in the oral mouse carcinogenicity study at a dose of 45 mg/kg/day (258-340× MRHD based on AUC comparisons). No drug-related tumors were noted in the mouse oral carcinogenicity study at a dose of 15 mg/kg/day (60-133× MRHD based on AUC comparisons). In an oral (gavage) rat carcinogenicity study, a statistically significant increase in the incidence of benign thymoma was noted in 10 mg/kg/day pimecrolimus treated male and female animals compared to vehicle control treated male and female animals. In addition, a significant increase in the incidence of benign thymoma was noted in another oral (gavage) rat carcinogenicity study in 5 mg/kg/day pimecrolimus treated male animals compared to vehicle control treated male animals. No drug-related tumors were noted in the rat oral carcinogenicity study at a dose of 1 mg/kg/day male animals (1.1× MRHD based on AUC comparisons) and at a dose of 5 mg/kg/day for female animals (21× MRHD based on AUC comparisons).

In a 52 week dermal photo-carcinogenicity study, the median time to onset of skin tumor formation was decreased in hairless mice following chronic topical dosing with concurrent exposure to UV radiation (40 weeks of treatment followed by 12 weeks of observation) with the pimecrolimus cream vehicle alone. No additional effect on tumor development beyond the vehicle effect was noted with the addition of the active ingredient, pimecrolimus, to the vehicle cream.

A battery of *in vitro* genotoxicity tests, including Ames assay, mouse lymphoma L5178Y assay, and chromosome aberration test in V79 Chinese hamster cells and an *in vivo* mouse micronucleus test revealed no evidence for a mutagenic or clastogenic potential for the drug.

An oral fertility and embryofetal developmental study in rats revealed estrus cycle disturbances, post-implantation loss and reduction in litter size at the 45 mg/kg/day dose (38× MRHD based on AUC comparisons). No effect on fertility in female rats was noted at 10 mg/kg/day (12× MRHD based on AUC comparisons). No effect on fertility in male rats was noted at 45 mg/kg/day (23× MRHD based on AUC comparisons), which was the highest dose tested in this study.

PREGNANCY, TERATOGENIC EFFECTS, PREGNANCY CATEGORY C

There are no adequate and well-controlled studies of topically administered pimecrolimus in pregnant women. The experience with pimecrolimus cream when used by pregnant women is too limited to permit assessment of the safety of its use during pregnancy.

In dermal embryofetal developmental studies, no maternal or fetal toxicity was observed up to the highest practicable doses tested, 10 mg/kg/day (1% pimecrolimus cream) in rats (0.14× MRHD based on body surface area) and 10 mg/kg/day (1% pimecrolimus cream) in rabbits (0.65× MRHD based on AUC comparisons). The 1% pimecrolimus cream was administered topically for 6 hours/day during the period of organogenesis in rats and rabbits (gestational days 6-21 in rats and gestational days 6-20 in rabbits).

A combined oral fertility and embryofetal developmental study was conducted in rats and an oral embryofetal developmental study was conducted in rabbits. Pimecrolimus was administered during the period of organogenesis (2 weeks prior to mating until gestational day 16 in rats, gestational days 6-18 in rabbits) up to dose levels of 45 mg/kg/day in rats and 20 mg/kg/day in rabbits. In the absence of maternal toxicity, indicators of embryofetal toxicity (post-implantation loss and reduction in litter size) were noted at 45 mg/kg/day (38× MRHD based on AUC comparisons) in the oral fertility and embryofetal developmental study conducted in rats. No malformations in the fetuses were noted at 45 mg/kg/day (38× MRHD based on AUC comparisons) in this study. No maternal toxicity, embryotoxicity or teratogenicity were noted in the oral rabbit embryofetal developmental toxicity study at 20 mg/kg/day (3.9× MRHD based on AUC comparisons), which was the highest dose tested in this study.

An oral peri- and post-natal developmental study was conducted in rats. Pimecrolimus was administered from gestational day 6 through lactational day 21 up to a dose level of 40 mg/kg/day. Only 2 of 22 females delivered live pups at the highest dose of 40 mg/kg/day. Postnatal survival, development of the F1 generation, their subsequent maturation and fertility were not affected at 10 mg/kg/day (12× MRHD based on AUC comparisons), the highest dose evaluated in this study.

Pimecrolimus was transferred across the placenta in oral rat and rabbit embryofetal developmental studies.

There are, however, no adequate and well-controlled studies in pregnant women. Because animal reproduction studies are not always predictive of human response, this drug should be used only if clearly needed during pregnancy.

NURSING MOTHERS

It is not known whether this drug is excreted in human milk. Because of the potential for serious adverse reactions in nursing infants from pimecrolimus, a decision should be made whether to discontinue nursing or to discontinue the drug, taking into account the importance of the drug to the mother.

PEDIATRIC USE

Pimecrolimus cream may be used in pediatric patients 2 years of age and older. Three Phase 3 pediatric studies were conducted involving 1114 patients 2-17 years of age. Two studies were 6 week randomized vehicle-controlled studies with a 20 week open-label phase and one was a vehicle-controlled long-term (up to 1 year) safety study with the option for sequential topical corticosteroid use. Of these patients 542 (49%) were 2-6 years of age. In the short-term studies, 11% of pimecrolimus patients did not complete these studies and 1.5% of pimecrolimus patients discontinued due to adverse events. In the 1 year study, 32% of pimecrolimus patients did not complete this study and 3% of pimecrolimus patients discontinued due to adverse events. Most discontinuations were due to unsatisfactory therapeutic effect.

The most common local adverse event in the short-term studies of pimecrolimus cream in pediatric patients ages 2-17 was application site burning (10% vs 13% vehicle); the incidence in the long-term study was 9% pimecrolimus vs 7% vehicle (see ADVERSE REACTIONS). Adverse events that were more frequent (>5%) in patients treated with pimecrolimus cream compared to vehicle were headache (14% vs 9%) in the short-term trial. Nasopharyngitis (26% vs 21%), influenza (13% vs 4%), pharyngitis (8% vs 3%), viral infection (7% vs 1%), pyrexia (13% vs 5%), cough (16% vs 11%), and headache (25% vs 16%) were increased over vehicle in the 1 year safety study (see ADVERSE REACTIONS). In 843 patients ages 2-17 years treated with pimecrolimus cream, 9 (0.8%) developed eczema herpeticum (5 on pimecrolimus cream alone and 4 on pimecrolimus cream used in sequence with cortico-steroids). In 211 patients on vehicle alone, there were no cases of eczema herpeticum. The majority of adverse events were mild to moderate in severity.

Pimecrolimus cream is not recommended for use in pediatric patients below the age of 2 years. Two Phase 3 studies were conducted involving 436 infants age 3-23 months. One 6 week randomized vehicle-controlled study with a 20 week open-label phase and one long term safety study were conducted. In the 6 week study, 11% of pimecrolimus and 48% of vehicle patients did not complete this study; no patient in either group discontinued due to adverse events. Infants on pimecrolimus cream had an increased incidence of some adverse events compared to vehicle. In the 6 week vehicle-controlled study these adverse events included pyrexia (32% vs 13% vehicle), URI (24% vs 14%), nasopharyngitis (15% vs 8%), gastroenteritis (7% vs 3%), otitis media (4% vs 0%), and diarrhea (8% vs 0%). In the open-label phase of the study, for infants who switched to pimecrolimus cream from vehicle, the incidence of the above-cited adverse events approached or equaled the incidence of those

TABLE 2A *Treatment Emergent Adverse Events (≥1%) in Pimecrolimus Treatment Groups*

	Pediatric Patients* Vehicle-Controlled (6 weeks)		Pediatric Patients* Open-Label (20 weeks)
	Pimecrolimus (n=267)	Vehicle (n=136)	Pimecrolimus (n=355)
At least 1 AE	182 (68.2%)	97 (71.3%)	240 (72.0%)
Infections and Infestations			
Upper respiratory tract infection NOS	38 (14.2%)	18 (13.2%)	65 (19.4%)
Nasopharyngitis	27 (10.1%)	10 (7.4%)	32 (19.6%)
Skin infection NOS	8 (3.0%)	9 (5.1%)	18 (5.4%)
Influenza	8 (3.0%)	1 (0.7%)	22 (6.6%)
Ear infection NOS	6 (2.2%)	2 (1.5%)	19 (5.7%)
Otitis media	6 (2.2%)	1 (0.7%)	10 (3.0%)
Impetigo	5 (1.9%)	3 (2.2%)	12 (3.6%)
Bacterial infection	4 (1.5%)	3 (2.2%)	4 (1.2%)
Folliculitis	3 (1.1%)	1 (0.7%)	3 (0.9%)
Sinusitis	3 (1.1%)	1 (0.7%)	11 (3.3%)
Pneumonia NOS	3 (1.1%)	1 (0.7%)	5 (1.5%)
Pharyngitis NOS	2 (0.7%)	2 (1.5%)	3 (0.9%)
Pharyngitis streptococcal	2 (0.7%)	2 (1.5%)	10 (3.0%)
Molluscum contagiosum	2 (0.7%)	0	4 (1.2%)
Staphylococcal infection	1 (0.4%)	5 (3.7%)	7 (2.1%)
Bronchitis NOS	1 (0.4%)	3 (2.2%)	4 (1.2%)
Herpes simplex	1 (0.4%)	0	4 (1.2%)
Tonsillitis NOS	1 (0.4%)	0	3 (0.9%)
Viral infection NOS	2 (0.7%)	1 (0.7%)	1 (0.3%)
Gastroenteritis NOS	0	3 (2.2%)	2 (0.6%)
Chickenpox	2 (0.7%)	0	3 (0.9%)
Skin papilloma	1 (0.4%)	0	2 (0.6%)
Tonsillitis acute NOS	0	0	0
Upper respiratory tract infection viral NOS	1 (0.4%)	0	3 (0.9%)
Herpes simplex dermatitis	0	0	1 (0.3%)
Bronchitis acute NOS	0	0	0
Eye infection NOS	0	0	0
General Disorders and Administration Site Conditions			
Application site burning	28 (10.4%)	17 (12.5%)	5 (1.5%)
Pyrexia	20 (7.5%)	12 (8.8%)	41 (12.2%)
Application site reaction NOS	8 (3.0%)	7 (5.1%)	7 (2.1%)
Application site irritation	8 (3.0%)	8 (5.9%)	3 (0.9%)
Influenza like illness	1 (0.4%)	0	2 (0.6%)
Application site erythema	1 (0.4%)	0	0
Application site pruritus	3 (1.1%)	2 (1.5%)	2 (0.6%)
Respiratory, Thoracic and Mediastinal Disorders			
Cough	31 (11.6%)	11 (8.1%)	31 (9.3%)
Nasal congestion	7 (2.6%)	2 (1.5%)	6 (1.8%)
Rhinorrhea	5 (1.9%)	1 (0.7%)	3 (0.9%)
Asthma aggravated	4 (1.5%)	3 (2.2%)	13 (3.9%)
Sinus congestion	3 (1.1%)	1 (0.7%)	2 (0.6%)
Rhinitis	1 (0.4%)	0	5 (1.5%)
Wheezing	1 (0.4%)	1 (0.7%)	4 (1.2%)
Asthma NOS	2 (0.7%)	1 (0.7%)	11 (3.3%)
Epistaxis	0	1 (0.7%)	0
Dyspnea NOS	0	0	0
Gastrointestinal Disorders			
Abdominal pain upper	11 (4.1%)	6 (4.4%)	10 (3.0%)
Sore throat	9 (3.4%)	5 (3.7%)	15 (5.4%)
Vomiting NOS	8 (3.0%)	6 (4.4%)	14 (4.2%)
Diarrhea NOS	3 (1.1%)	1 (0.7%)	2 (0.6%)
Nausea	1 (0.4%)	3 (2.2%)	4 (1.2%)
Abdominal pain NOS	1 (0.4%)	1 (0.7%)	5 (1.5%)
Toothache	1 (0.4%)	1 (0.7%)	2 (0.6%)
Constipation	1 (0.4%)	0	2 (0.6%)
Loose stools	0	1 (0.7%)	4 (1.2%)
Reproductive System and Breast Disorders			
Dysmenorrhea	3 (1.1%)	0	5 (1.5%)
Eye Disorders			
Conjuctivitis NEC	2 (0.7%)	1 (0.7%)	7 (2.1%)
Skin & Subcutaneous Tissue Disorders			
Urticaria	3 (1.1%)	0	1 (0.3%)
Acne NOS	0	1 (0.7%)	1 (0.3%)
Immune System Disorders			
Hypersensitivity NOS	11 (4.1%)	6 (4.4%)	16 (4.8%)
Injury and Poisoning			
Accident NOS	3 (1.1%)	1 (0.7%)	1 (0.3%)
Laceration	2 (0.7%)	1 (0.7%)	5 (1.5%)
Musculoskeletal, Connective Tissue and Bone Disorders			
Back pain	1 (0.4%)	2 (1.5%)	1 (0.3%)
Arthralgias	0	0	1 (0.3%)
Ear and Labyrinth Disorders			
Earache	2 (0.7%)	1 (0.7%)	0
Nervous System Disorders			
Headache	37 (13.9%)	12 (8.8%)	38 (11.3%)

* Ages 2-17 years.

patients who remained on pimecrolimus cream. In the 6 month safety data, 16% of pimecrolimus and 35% of vehicle patients discontinued early and 1.5% of pimecrolimus and 0% of vehicle patients discontinued due to adverse events. Infants on pimecrolimus cream had a greater incidence of some adverse events as compared to vehicle. These included pyrexia (30% vs 20%), URI (21% vs 17%), cough (15% vs 9%), hypersensitivity (8% vs 2%), teething (27% vs 22%), vomiting (9% vs 4%), rhinitis (13% vs 9%), viral rash (4% vs 0%), rhinorrhea (4% vs 0%), and wheezing (4% vs 0%).

The effects of pimecrolimus cream on the developing immune system in infants are unknown.

TABLE 2B *Treatment Emergent Adverse Events (≥1%) in Pimecrolimus Treatment Groups*

	Pediatric Patients* Vehicle-Controlled (1 year)		Adult Active Comparator (1 year)
	Pimecrolimus (n=272)	Vehicle (n=75)	Pimecrolimus (n=328)
At least 1 AE	230 (84.6%)	56 (74.7%)	256 (78.0%)
Infections and Infestations			
Upper respiratory tract infection NOS	13 (4.8%)	6 (8.0%)	14 (4.3%)
Nasopharyngitis	72 (26.5%)	16 (21.3%)	25 (7.6%)
Skin infection NOS	6 (2.2%)	3 (4.0%)	21 (6.4%)
Influenza	36 (13.2%)	3 (4.0%)	32 (9.8%)
Ear infection NOS	9 (3.3%)	1 (1.3%)	2 (0.6%)
Otitis media	8 (2.9%)	4 (5.3%)	2 (0.6%)
Impetigo	11 (4.0%)	4 (5.3%)	8 (2.4%)
Bacterial infection	3 (1.1%)	0	6 (1.8%)
Folliculitis	6 (2.2%)	3 (4.0%)	20 (6.1%)
Sinusitis	6 (2.2%)	1 (1.3%)	2 (0.6%)
Pneumonia NOS	0	1 (1.3%)	1 (0.3%)
Pharyngitis NOS	22 (8.1%)	2 (2.7%)	3 (0.9%)
Pharyngitis streptococcal	0	<1%	0
Molluscum contagiosum	5 (1.8%)	0	0
Staphylococcal infection	0	<1%	3 (0.9%)
Bronchitis NOS	29 (10.7%)	6 (8.0%)	8 (2.4%)
Herpes simplex	9 (3.3%)	2 (2.7%)	13 (4.0%)
Tonsillitis NOS	17 (6.3%)	0	2 (0.6%)
Viral infection NOS	18 (6.6%)	1 (1.3%)	0
Gastroenteritis NOS	20 (7.4%)	2 (2.7%)	6 (1.8%)
Chickenpox	8 (2.9%)	3 (4.0%)	1 (0.3%)
Skin papilloma	9 (3.3%)	<1%	0
Tonsillitis acute NOS	7 (2.6%)	0	0
Upper respiratory tract infection viral NOS	4 (1.5%)	0	1 (0.3%)
Herpes simplex dermatitis	4 (1.5%)	0	2 (0.6%)
Bronchitis acute NOS	4 (1.5%)	0	0
Eye infection NOS	3 (1.1%)	<1%	1 (0.3%)
General Disorders and Administration Site Conditions			
Application site burning	23 (8.5%)	5 (6.7%)	85 (25.9%)
Pyrexia	34 (12.5%)	4 (5.3%)	4 (1.2%)
Application site reaction NOS	9 (3.3%)	2 (2.7%)	48 (14.6%)
Application site irritation	1 (0.4%)	3 (4.0%)	21 (6.4%)
Influenza like illness	5 (1.8%)	2 (2.7%)	6 (1.8%)
Application site erythema	6 (2.2%)	0	7 (2.1%)
Application site pruritus	5 (1.8%)	0	18 (5.5%)
Respiratory, Thoracic and Mediastinal Disorders			
Cough	43 (15.8%)	8 (10.7%)	8 (2.4%)
Nasal congestion	4 (1.5%)	1 (1.3%)	2 (0.6%)
Rhinorrhea	1 (0.4%)	1 (1.3%)	0
Asthma aggravated	3 (1.1%)	1 (1.3%)	0
Sinus congestion	<1%	<1%	3 (0.9%)
Rhinitis	12 (4.4%)	5 (6.7%)	7 (2.1%)
Wheezing	2 (0.7%)	<1%	0
Asthma NOS	10 (3.7%)	2 (2.7%)	8 (2.4%)
Epistaxis	9 (3.3%)	1 (1.3%)	1 (0.3%)
Dyspnea NOS	5 (1.8%)	1 (1.3%)	2 (0.6%)
Gastrointestinal Disorders			
Abdominal pain upper	15 (5.5%)	5 (6.7%)	1 (0.3%)
Sore throat	22 (8.1%)	4 (5.3%)	12 (3.7%)
Vomiting NOS	18 (6.6%)	6 (8.0%)	2 (0.6%)
Diarrhea NOS	21 (7.7%)	4 (5.3%)	7 (2.1%)
Nausea	11 (4.0%)	5 (6.7%)	6 (1.8%)
Abdominal pain NOS	12 (4.4%)	3 (4.0%)	1 (0.3%)
Toothache	7 (2.6%)	1 (1.3%)	2 (0.6%)
Constipation	10 (3.7%)	<1%	0
Loose stools	<1%	<1%	0
Reproductive System and Breast Disorders			
Dysmenorrhea	3 (1.1%)	1 (1.3%)	4 (1.2%)
Eye Disorders			
Conjuctivitis NEC	6 (2.2%)	3 (4.0%)	10 (3.0%)
Skin & Subcutaneous Tissue Disorders			
Urticaria	1 (0.4%)	<1%	3 (0.9%)
Acne NOS	4 (1.5%)	<1%	6 (1.8%)
Immune System Disorders			
Hypersensitivity NOS	14 (5.1%)	1 (1.3%)	11 (3.4%)
Injury and Poisoning			
Accident NOS	<1%	1 (1.3%)	0
Laceration	<1%	<1%	0
Musculoskeletal, Connective Tissue and Bone Disorders			
Back pain	<1%	0	6 (1.8%)
Arthralgias	3 (1.1%)	1 (1.3%)	5 (1.5%)
Ear and Labyrinth Disorders			
Earache	8 (2.9%)	2 (2.7%)	0
Nervous System Disorders			
Headache	69 (25.4%)	12 (16.0%)	23 (7.0%)

* Ages 2-17 years.

GERIATRIC USE

Nine (9) patients ≥65 years old received pimecrolimus cream in Phase 3 studies. Clinical studies of pimecrolimus did not include sufficient numbers of patients aged 65 and over to assess efficacy and safety.

DRUG INTERACTIONS

Potential interactions between pimecrolimus and other drugs, including immunizations, have not been systematically evaluated. Due to the very low blood levels of pimecrolimus detected in some patients after topical application, systemic drug interactions are not expected, but cannot be ruled out. The concomitant administration of known CYP3A family of inhibitors in patients with widespread and/or erythrodermic disease should be done with caution. Some examples of such drugs are erythromycin, itraconazole, ketoconazole, fluconazole, calcium channel blockers and cimetidine.

ADVERSE REACTIONS

In human dermal safety studies, pimecrolimus cream 1% did not induce contact sensitization, phototoxicity, or photoallergy, nor did it show any cumulative irritation.

In a 1 year safety study in pediatric patients age 2-17 years old involving sequential use of pimecrolimus cream and a topical corticosteroid, 43% of pimecrolimus patients and 68% of vehicle patients used corticosteroids during the study. Corticosteroids were used for more than 7 days by 34% of pimecrolimus patients and 54% of vehicle patients. An increased incidence of impetigo, skin infection, superinfection (infected atopic dermatitis), rhinitis, and urticaria were found in the patients that had used pimecrolimus cream and topical corticosteroid sequentially as compared to pimecrolimus cream alone.

In 3 randomized, double-blind vehicle-controlled pediatric studies and one active-controlled adult study, 843 and 328 patients respectively, were treated with pimecrolimus cream. In these clinical trials, 48 (4%) of the 1171 pimecrolimus patients and 13 (3%) of 408 vehicle-treated patients discontinued therapy due to adverse events. Discontinuations for AEs were primarily due to application site reactions, and cutaneous infections. The most common application site reaction was application site burning, which occurred in 8-26% of patients treated with pimecrolimus cream.

TABLE 2A and TABLE 2B depict the incidence of adverse events pooled across the 2 identically designed 6 week studies with their open label extensions and the 1 year safety study for pediatric patients ages 2-17. Data from the adult active-controlled study is also included in this table. Adverse events are listed regardless of relationship to study drug.

DOSAGE AND ADMINISTRATION

Apply a thin layer of pimecrolimus cream 1% to the affected skin twice daily and rub in gently and completely. Pimecrolimus may be used on all skin surfaces, including the head, neck, and intertriginous areas.

Pimecrolimus should be used twice daily for as long as signs and symptoms persist. Treatment should be discontinued if resolution of disease occurs. If symptoms persist beyond 6 weeks, the patient should be re-evaluated.

The safety of pimecrolimus cream under occlusion, which may promote systemic exposure, has not been evaluated. **Pimecrolimus cream should not be used with occlusive dressings.**

HOW SUPPLIED

Elidel cream 1% is available in tubes of 15, 30, and 100 g.

Storage: Store at 25°C (77°F); excursions permitted to 15-30°C (59-86°F). Do not freeze.

PRODUCT LISTING - EQUIVALENTS NOT AVAILABLE

Cream - Topical - 1%

15 gm	$27.36	ELIDEL, Novartis Pharmaceuticals	00078-0375-40
30 gm	$53.95	ELIDEL, Novartis Pharmaceuticals	00078-0375-46
100 gm	$170.31	ELIDEL, Novartis Pharmaceuticals	00078-0375-63

Pimozide *(002038)*

Categories: Tourette's syndrome; Pregnancy Category C; FDA Approved 1984 Jul
Drug Classes: Antipsychotics
Brand Names: **Orap**; Pimodac
Foreign Brand Availability: Orap (1 mg) (Bahrain; Benin; Burkina-Faso; Cyprus; Egypt; Ethiopia; Gambia; Ghana; Guinea; Hong-Kong; Indonesia; Iran; Iraq; Ivory-Coast; Jordan; Kenya; Kuwait; Lebanon; Liberia; Libya; Malawi; Mali; Mauritania; Mauritius; Morocco; Niger; Nigeria; Oman; Qatar; Republic-of-Yemen; Saudi-Arabia; Senegal; Seychelles; Sierra-Leone; South-Africa; Sudan; Syria; Tanzania; Thailand; Tunia; Uganda; United-Arab-Emirates; Zambia; Zimbabwe); Orap (4 mg) (Bahrain; Cyprus; Egypt; Iran; Iraq; Israel; Jordan; Kuwait; Lebanon; Libya; Oman; Qatar; Republic-of-Yemen; Saudi-Arabia; Syria; United-Arab-Emirates); Orap Forte (4 mg) (Bahrain; Benin; Burkina-Faso; Cyprus; Egypt; Ethiopia; Gambia; Ghana; Guinea; Hong-Kong; Indonesia; Iran; Iraq; Israel; Ivory-Coast; Jordan; Kenya; Kuwait; Lebanon; Liberia; Libya; Malawi; Mali; Mauritania; Mauritius; Morocco; Niger; Nigeria; Oman; Peru; Qatar; Republic-of-Yemen; Saudi-Arabia; Senegal; Seychelles; Sierra-Leone; Sudan; Syria; Tanzania; Thailand; Tunia; Uganda; United-Arab-Emirates; Zambia; Zimbabwe); Pizide (Thailand)
Cost of Therapy: $50.27 (Tourette's Syndrome; Orap; 1 mg; 2 tablets/day; 30 day supply)

DESCRIPTION

Pimozide is an orally active antipsychotic agent of the diphenylbutylpiperidine series. The structural formula of pimozide, 1-[1- [4,4-bis(4-fluorophenyl)-butyl]-4-piperidinyl]-1,3-dihydro-2*H*-benzimidazol-2-one.

The solubility of pimozide in water is less than 0.01 mg/ml; it is slightly soluble in most organic solvents.

Each white pimozide tablet contains 2 mg of pimozide and the following inactive ingredients: calcium stearate, cellulose, lactose and corn starch.

CLINICAL PHARMACOLOGY

PHARMACODYNAMIC ACTIONS

Pimozide is an orally active antipsychotic drug product which shares with other antipsychotics the ability to blockade dopaminergic receptors on neurons in the central nervous system. Although its exact mode of action has not been established, the ability of pimozide to suppress motor and phonic tics in Tourette's Disorder is thought to be a function of its dopaminergic blocking activity. However, receptor blockade is often accompanied by a series of secondary alterations in central dopamine metabolism and function which may contribute to both pimozide's therapeutic and untoward effects. In addition, pimozide, in common with other antipsychotic drugs, has various effects on other central nervous system receptor systems which are not fully characterized.

METABOLISM AND PHARMACOKINETICS

More than 50% of a dose of pimozide is absorbed after oral administration. Based on the pharmacokinetic and metabolic profile, pimozide appears to undergo significant first pass metabolism. Peak serum levels occur generally six to eight hours (range 4-12 hours) after dosing. Pimozide is extensively metabolized, primarily by N-dealkylation in the liver. Two major metabolites have been identified, 1-(4-piperidyl)-2-benzimidazolinone and 4,4-bis(4-fluorophenyl) butyric acid. The antipsychotic activity of these metabolites is undetermined. The major route of elimination of pimozide and its metabolites is through the kidney.

The mean serum elimination half-life of pimozide in schizophrenic patients was approximately 55 hours. There was a 13-fold interindividual difference in the area under the serum pimozide level-time curve and an equivalent degree of variation in peak serum levels among patients studied. The significance of this is unclear since there are few correlations between plasma levels and clinical findings.

Effects of food, disease or concomitant medication upon the absorption, distribution, metabolism and elimination of pimozide are not known.

INDICATIONS AND USAGE

Pimozide is indicated for the suppression of motor and phonic tics in patients with Tourette's Disorder who have failed to respond satisfactorily to standard treatment. Pimozide is not intended as a treatment of first choice nor is it intended for the treatment for tics that are merely annoying or cosmetically troublesome. Pimozide should be reserved for use in Tourette's Disorder patients whose development and/or daily life function is severely compromised by the presence of motor and phonic tics.

Evidence supporting approval of Pimozide for use in Tourette's Disorder was obtained in two controlled clinical investigations which enrolled patients between the ages of 8 and 53 years. Most subjects in the two trials were 12 or older.

CONTRAINDICATIONS

Pimozide is contraindicated in the treatment of simple tics or tics other than those associated with Tourette's Disorder.

Pimozide should not be used in patients taking drugs that may, themselves, cause motor and phonic tics (*e.g.*, pemoline, methylphenidate and amphetamines) until such patients have been withdrawn from these drugs to determine whether or not the drugs, rather than Tourette's Disorder, are responsible for the tics.

Because pimozide prolongs the QT interval of the electrocardiogram it is contraindicated in patients with congenital long QT syndrome, patients with a history of cardiac arrhythmias, or patients taking other drugs which prolong the QT interval of the electrocardiogram (see DRUG INTERACTIONS.)

Pimozide is contraindicated in patients with severe toxic central nervous system depression or comatose states from any cause.

Pimozide is contraindicated in patients with hypersensitivity to it. As it is not known whether cross-sensitivity exists among the antipsychotics, pimozide should be used with appropriate caution in patients who have demonstrated hypersensitivity to other antipsychotic drugs.

WARNINGS

The use of pimozide in the treatment of Tourette's Disorder involves different risk/benefit considerations than when antipsychotic drugs are used to treat other conditions. Consequently, a decision to use pimozide should take into consideration the following (see also PRECAUTIONS, Information for the Patient).

TARDIVE DYSKINESIA

A syndrome consisting of potentially irreversible, involuntary, dyskinetic movements may develop in patients treated with antipsychotic drugs. Although the prevalence of the syndrome appears to be highest among the elderly, especially elderly women, it is impossible to rely upon prevalence estimates to predict, at the inception of antipsychotic treatment, which patients are likely to develop the syndrome. Whether antipsychotic drug products differ in their potential to cause tardive dyskinesia is unknown.

Both the risk of developing tardive dyskinesia and the likelihood that it will become irreversible are believed to increase as the duration of treatment and the total cumulative dose of antipsychotic drugs administered to the patient increase. However, the syndrome can develop, although much less commonly, after relatively brief treatment periods at low doses.

There is no known treatment for established cases of tardive dyskinesia, although the syndrome may remit, partially or completely, if antipsychotic treatment is withdrawn. Antipsychotic treatment, itself, however, may suppress (or partially suppress) the signs and symptoms of the syndrome and thereby possibly mask the underlying process. The effect that symptomatic suppression has upon the long-term course of the syndrome is unknown.

Given these considerations, antipsychotic drugs should be prescribed is a manner that is most likely to minimize the occurrence of tardive dyskinesia. Chronic antipsychotic treatment should generally be reserved for patients who suffer from a chronic illness that, 1) is known to respond to antipsychotic drugs, and, 2) for whom alternative, equally effective, but potentially less harmful treatments are not available or appropriate. In patients who do require chronic treatment, the smallest dose and the shortest duration of treatment producing a satisfactory clinical response should be sought. The need for continued treatment should be reassessed periodically.

If signs and symptoms of tardive dyskinesia appear in a patient on antipsychotics, drug discontinuation should be considered. However, some patients may require treatment despite the presence of the syndrome.

(For further information about the description of tardive dyskinesia and its clinical detection, please refer to ADVERSE REACTIONS and PRECAUTIONS- Information for Patients.)

NEUROLEPTIC MALIGNANT SYNDROME (NMS)

A potentially fatal syndrome complex sometimes referred to as Neuroleptic Malignant Syndrome (NMS) has been reported in association with antipsychotic drugs. Clinical manifestations of NMS are hyperpyrexia, muscle rigidity, altered mental status (including catatonic signs) and evidence of autonomic instability (irregular pulse or blood pressure, tachycardia,

P

diaphoresis, and cardiac dysrhythmias). Additional signs may include elevated creatinine phosphokinase, myoglobinuria (rhabdomyolysis) and acute renal failure.

The diagnostic evaluation of patients with this syndrome is complicated. In arriving at a diagnosis, it is important to identify cases where the clinical presentation includes both serious medical illness (*e.g.*, pneumonia, systemic infection, etc.) and untreated or inadequately treated extrapyramidal signs and symptoms (EPS). Other important considerations in the differential diagnosis include central anticholinergic toxicity, heat stroke, drug fever and primary central nervous system (CNS) pathology.

The management of NMS should include (1) immediate discontinuation of antipsychotic drugs and other drugs not essential to concurrent therapy, (2) intensive symptomatic treatment and medical monitoring, and (3) treatment of any concomitant serious medical problems for which specific treatments are available. There is no general agreement about specific pharmacological treatment regimens for uncomplicated NMS.

If a patient requires antipsychotic drug treatment after recovery from NMS, the potential reintroduction of drug therapy should be carefully considered. The patient should be carefully monitored, since recurrences of NMS have been reported.

Hyperpyrexia, not associated with the above symptom complex, has been reported with other antipsychotic drugs.

OTHER

Sudden, unexpected deaths have occurred in experimental studies of conditions other than Tourette's Disorder. These deaths occurred while patients were receiving dosages in the range of 1 mg per kg. One possible mechanisms for such deaths is prolongations of the QT interval predisposing patients to ventricular arrhythmia. An electrocardiogram should be performed before pimozide treatment is initiated and periodically thereafter, especially during the period of dose adjustment.

Pimozide may have a tumorigenic potential. Based on studies conducted in mice, it is known that pimozide can produce a dose related increase in pituitary tumors. The full significance of this finding is not known, but should be taken into consideration in the physician's and patient's decisions to use this drug product. This finding should be given special consideration when the patient is young and chronic use of pimozide is anticipated. (See PRECAUTIONS, Carcinogenesis, Mutagenesis, and Impairment of Fertility.)

PRECAUTIONS

GENERAL

Pimozide may impair the mental and/or physical abilities required for the performance of potentially hazardous tasks, such as driving a car or operating machinery, especially during the first few days of therapy.

Pimozide produces anticholinergic side effects and should be used with caution in individuals whose conditions may be aggravated by anticholinergic activity.

Pimozide should be administered cautiously to patients with impairment of liver or kidney function, because it is metabolized by the liver and excreted by the kidneys.

Antipsychotics should be administered with caution to patients receiving anticonvulsant medication, with a history of seizures, or with EEG abnormalities, because they may lower the convulsive threshold. If indicated, adequate anticonvulsant therapy should be maintained concomitantly.

INFORMATION FOR THE PATIENT

Treatment with pimozide exposes the patient to serious risks. A decision to use pimozide chronically in Tourette's Disorder is one that deserves full consideration by the patient (or patient's family) as well as by the treating physician. Because the goal of treatment is symptomatic improvement, the patient's view of the need for treatment and assessment of response are critical in evaluating the impact of therapy and weighing its benefits against the risks. Since the physician is the primary source of information about the use of a drug in any disease it is recommended that the following information be discussed with patients and/or their families.

Pimozide is intended only for use in patients with Tourette's Disorder whose symptoms are severe and who cannot tolerate, or who do not respond to Haldol (haloperidol).

Given the likelihood that a proportion of patients exposed chronically to antipsychotics will develop tardive dyskinesia, it is advised that all patients in whom chronic use is contemplated be given, if possible, full information about this risk. The decision to inform patients and/or their guardians must obviously take into account the clinical circumstances and the competency of the patient to understand the information provided.

There is limited information available on the use of pimozide in children under 12 years of age.

The information available on pimozide from foreign marketing experience and from U.S. clinical trials indicate that pimozide has a side effect profile similar to that of other antipsychotic drugs. Patients should be informed that all types of side effects associated with the use of antipsychotics may be associated with the use of pimozide.

In addition, sudden unexpected deaths have occurred in patients taking high doses of pimozide for conditions other than Tourette's Disorder. These deaths may have been the result of an effect of pimozide upon the heart. Therefore, patients should be instructed not to exceed the prescribed dose of pimozide and they should realize the need for the initial ECG and for follow-up ECGs during treatment.

Also, pimozide, at a dose about 15 times that given humans, caused an increase in the number of benign tumors of the pituitary gland in female mice. It is not possible to say how important this is. Similar tumors were not seen in rats given pimozide, nor at lower doses in mice, which is reassuring. However, any such finding must be considered to suggest a possible risk of long term use of the drug.

LABORATORY TESTS

An ECG should be done at baseline and periodically thereafter throughout the period of dose adjustment. Any indication of prolongation of the QT_c interval beyond an absolute limit of 0.47 seconds (children) or 0.52 seconds (adults), or more than 25% above the patient's original baseline should be considered a basis for stopping further dose increase (see CONTRAINDICATIONS) and considering a lower dose.

Since hypokalemia has been associated with ventricular arrhythmias, potassium insufficiency, secondary to diuretics, diarrhea, or other cause, should be corrected before pimozide therapy is initiated and normal potassium maintained during therapy.

CARCINOGENESIS, MUTAGENESIS, AND IMPAIRMENT OF FERTILITY

Carcinogenicity studies were conducted in mice and rats. In mice, pimozide causes a dose-related increase in pituitary and mammary tumors.

When mice were treated for up to 18 months with pimozide, pituitary gland changes developed in females only. These changes were characterized as hyperplasia at doses approximating the human dose and adenoma at doses about fifteen times the maximum recommended human dose on a mg per kg basis. The mechanism for the induction of pituitary tumors in mice is not known.

Mammary gland tumors in female mice were also increased, but these tumors are expected in rodents treated with antipsychotic drugs which elevate prolactin levels. Chronic administration of an antipsychotic also causes elevated prolactin levels in humans. Tissue culture experiments indicate that approximately one-third of human breast cancers are prolactin-dependent *in vitro*, a factor of potential importance if the prescription of these drugs is contemplated in a patient with a previously detected breast cancer. Although disturbances such as galactorrhea, amenorrhea, gynecomastia, and impotence have been reported with antipsychotic drugs, the clinical significance of elevated serum prolactin levels is unknown for most patients. Neither clinical studies nor epidemiologic studies conducted to date have shown an association between chronic administration of these drugs and mammary tumorigenesis. The available evidence, however, is considered too limited to be conclusive at this time.

In a 24 month carcinogenicity study in rats, animals received up to 50 times the maximum recommended human dose. No increased incidence of overall tumors or tumors at any site was observed in either sex. Because of the limited number of animals surviving this study, the meaning of these results is unclear.

Pimozide did not have mutagenic activity in the Ames test with four bacterial test strains, in the mouse dominant lethal test or in the micronucleus test in rats.

Reproduction studies in animals were not adequate to assess all aspects of fertility. Nevertheless, female rats administered pimozide had prolonged estrus cycles, an effect also produced by other antipsychotic drugs.

PREGNANCY CATEGORY C

Reproduction studies performed in rats and rabbits at oral doses up to 8 times the maximum human dose did not reveal evidence of teratogenicity. In the rat, however, this multiple of the human dose resulted in decreased pregnancies and in the retarded development of fetuses. These effects are thought to be due to an inhibition or delay in implantation which is also observed in rodents administered other antipsychotic drugs. In the rabbit, maternal toxicity, mortality, decreased weight gain, and embryotoxicity including increased resorptions were dose related. Because animal reproduction studies are not always predictive of human response, pimozide should be given to a pregnant woman only if the potential benefits to treatment clearly outweigh the potential risks.

LABOR AND DELIVERY

This drug has no recognized use in labor or delivery.

NURSING MOTHERS

It is not known whether pimozide is excreted in human milk. Because many drugs are excreted in human milk and because of the potential for tumorigenicity and unknown cardiovascular effects in the infant, a decision should be made whether to discontinue nursing or to discontinue the drug, taking into account the importance of the drug to the mother.

PEDIATRIC USE

Although Tourette's Disorder most often has its onset between the ages of 2 and 15 years, information on the use and efficacy of pimozide in patients less than 12 years of age is limited.

A 24 week open label study in 36 children between the age of 2 and 12 demonstrated that pimozide has a similiar safety profile in this age group as in older patients and there were no safety findings that would preclude its use in this age group.

Because its use and safety have not been evaluated in other childhood disorders, pimozide is not recommended for use in any condition other than Tourette's Disorder.

DRUG INTERACTIONS

Because pimozide prolongs the QT interval of the electrocardiogram, an additive effect on QT interval would be anticipated if administered with other drugs such as phenothiazines, tricyclic antidepressants or antiarrhythmic agents, which prolong the QT interval. Such concomitant administration should not be undertaken (see CONTRAINDICATIONS.)

Pimozide may be capable of potentiating CNS depressants, including analgesics, sedatives, anxiolytics, and alcohol.

ADVERSE REACTIONS

GENERAL

Extrapyramidal Reactions

Neuromuscular (extrapyramidal) reactions during the administration of pimozide have been reported frequently, often during the first few days of treatment. In most patients, these reactions involved Parkinson-like symptoms which, when first observed, were usually mild to moderately severe and usually reversible.

Other types of neuromuscular reactions (motor restlessness, dystonia, akathisia, hyperreflexia, opisthotonos, oculogyric crises) have been reported far less frequently. Severe extrapyramidal reactions have been reported to occur at relatively low doses. Generally the occurrence and severity of most extrapyramidal symptoms are dose related since they occur at relatively high doses and have been shown to disappear or become less severe when the dose is reduced. Administration of antiparkinson drugs such as benztropine mesylate or trihexyphenidyl hydrochloride may be required for control of such reactions. It should be noted that persistent extrapyramidal reactions have been reported and that the drug may have to be discontinued in such cases.

Withdrawal Emergent Neurological Signs

Generally, patients receiving short term therapy experience no problems with abrupt discontinuation of antipsychotic drugs. However, some patients on maintenance treatment experience transient dyskinetic signs after abrupt withdrawal. In certain of these cases the dyskinetic movements are indistinguishable from the syndrome described below under "Tardive Dyskinesia" except for duration. It is not known whether gradual withdrawal of antipsychotic drugs will reduce the rate of occurrence of withdrawal emergent neurological signs but until further evidence becomes available, it seems reasonable to gradually withdraw use of pimozide.

Tardive Dyskinesia

Pimozide may be associated with persistent dyskinesias. Tardive dyskinesias. Tardive dyskinesia, a syndrome consisting of potentially irreversible, involuntary, dyskinetic movements, may appear in some patients on long-term therapy or may occur after drug therapy has been discontinued. The risk appears to be greater in elderly patients on long-term therapy or may occur after drug therapy has been discontinued. The risk appears to be greater in elderly patients on high-dose therapy, especially females. The symptoms are persistent and in some patients appear irreversible. The syndrome is characterized by rhythmical involuntary movements of tongue, face, mouth or jaw (*e.g.,* protrusion of tongue, puffing of cheeks, puckering of mouth, chewing movements). Sometimes these may be accompanied by involuntary movements of extremities and the trunk.

There is no known effective treatment for tardive dyskinesia; antiparkinson agents usually do not alleviate the symptoms of this syndrome. It is suggested that all antipsychotic agents be discontinued if these symptoms appear. Should it be necessary to reinstitute treatment, or increase the dosage of the agent, or switch to a different antipsychotic agent, this syndrome may be masked.

It has been reported that fine vermicular movement of the tongue may be an early sign of tardive dyskinesia and if the medication is stopped at that time the full syndrome may not develop.

Electrocardiographic Changes

Electrocardiographic changes have been observed in clinical trials of pimozide in Tourette's Disorder and schizophrenia. These have included prolongation of the QT interval, flattening, notching and inversion of the T wave and the appearance of U waves. Sudden, unexpected deaths and grand mal seizure have occurred at doses above 20 mg/day.

Neuroleptic Malignant Syndrome

Neuroleptic malignant syndrome (NMS) has been reported with pimozide. (See WARNINGS for further information concerning NMS.)

Hyperpyrexia

Hyperpyrexia has been reported with other antipsychotic drugs.

CLINICAL TRIALS

The following adverse reaction tabulation (TABLE 1) was derived from 20 patients in a 6 week long placebo controlled clinical trial of pimozide in Tourette's Disorder.

The following adverse event tabulation was derived from 36 children (age 2-12) in a 24 week open trial of pimozide in Tourette's Disorder. (See TABLE 2)

Because clinical investigational experience with pimozide in Tourette's Disorder is limited, uncommon adverse reactions may not have been detected. The physician should consider that other adverse reactions associated with antipsychotics may occur.

TABLE 1

Body System/ Adverse Reaction	Pimozide (n=20)	Placebo (n=20)
Body as a Whole		
Headache	1	2
Gastrointestinal		
Dry Mouth	5	1
Diarrhea	1	0
Nausea	0	2
Vomiting	0	1
Constipation	4	2
Eructations	0	1
Thirsty	1	0
Appetite increase	1	0
Endocrine		
Menstrual disorder	0	1
Breast secretions	0	1
Musculoskeletal		
Muscle cramps	0	1
Muscle tightness	3	0
Stooped posture	2	0
CNS		
Drowsiness	7	3
Sedation	14	5
Insomnia	2	2
Dizziness	0	1
Akathisia	8	0
Rigidity	2	0
Speech disorder	2	0
Handwriting change	1	0
Akinesia	8	0
Psychiatric		
Depression	2	3
Excitement	0	1
Nervous	1	0
Adverse behavior effect	5	0
Special Senses		
Visual disturbance	4	0
Taste change	1	0
Sensitivity of eyes to light	1	0
Decreased accommodation	4	1
Spots before eyes	0	1
Urogenital		
Impotence	3	0

TABLE 2 *Pimozide, Adverse Reactions*

Body System/ Adverse Reaction	All Events (n=36)	Drug-Related Events (n=36)
Body as a Whole		
Asthenia	9 (25.0%)	5 (13.8%)
Headache	8 (22.2%)	1 (2.7%)
Gastrointestinal		
Dysphagia	1 (2.7%)	1 (2.7%)
Increased Salivation	5 (13.8%)	2 (5.5%)
Musculoskeletal		
Myalgia	1 (2.7%)	1 (2.7%)
Central Nervous System		
Dreaming Abnormal	1 (2.7%)	1 (2.7%)
Hyperkinesia	2 (5.5%)	1 (2.7%)
Somnolence	10 (27.7%)	9 (25.0%)
Torticollis	1 (2.7%)	1 (2.7%)
Tremor, Limbs	1 (2.7%)	1 (2.7%)
Psychiatric		
Adverse Behavior Effect	10 (27.7%)	8 (22.2%)
Nervous	3 (8.3%)	2 (5.5%)
Skin		
Rash	3 (8.3%)	1 (2.7%)
Special Senses		
Visual Disturbances	2 (5.5%)	1 (2.7%)
Cardiovascular		
ECG Abnormal	1 (2.7%)	1 (2.7%)

OTHER ADVERSE REACTIONS

In addition to the adverse reactions listed above, those listed below have been reported in US clinical trials of pimozide in conditions other than Tourette's Disorder.

Body as a Whole: Asthenia, chest pain, periorbital edema

Cardiovascular/Respiratory: Postural hypotension, hypotension, hypertension, tachycardia, palpitations

Gastrointestinal: Increased salivation, nausea, vomiting anorexia, GI distress

Endocrine: Loss of libido

Metabolic/Nutritional: Weight gain, weight loss

Central Nervous System: Dizziness, tremor, parkinsonism, fainting, dyskinesia

Psychiatric: Excitement

Skin: Rash, sweating, skin irritation

Special Senses: Blurred vision, cataracts

Urogenital: Nocturia, urinary frequency

POSTMARKETING REPORTS

The following experiences were described in spontaneous postmarketing reports. These reports do not provide sufficient information to establish a clear causal relationship with the use of pimozide.

Hematologic: Hemolytic anemia.

Other: Seizure has been reported in one patient.

DOSAGE AND ADMINISTRATION

GENERAL

The suppression of tics by pimozide requires a slow and gradual introduction of the drug. The patient's dose should be carefully adjusted to a point where the suppression of tics and the relief afforded is balanced against the untoward side effects of the drug.

An ECG should be done at baseline and periodically thereafter, especially during the period of dose adjustment (see WARNINGS and PRECAUTIONS, Laboratory Tests).

Periodic attempts should be made to reduce the dosage of pimozide to see whether or not tics persist at the level and extent first identified. In attempts to reduce the dosage of pimozide, consideration should be given to the possibility that increases of tic intensity and frequency may represent a transient, withdrawal related phenomenon rather than a return of disease symptoms. Specifically, one to two weeks should be allowed to elapse before one concludes that an increase in tic manifestations is a function of the underlying disease syndrome rather than a response to drug withdrawal. A gradual withdrawal recommended in any case.

CHILDREN

Reliable dose response data for the effects of pimozide on tic manifestations in Tourette's Disorder patients below the age of twelve are not available. Treatment should be initiated at a dose of 0.05 mg/kg preferably taken once at bedtime. The dose may be increased every third day to a maximum of 0.2 mg/kg not to exceed 10 mg/day.

ADULTS

In general, treatment with pimozide should be initiated with a dose of 1-2 mg a day in divided doses. The dose may be increased thereafter every other day. Most patients are maintained at less than 0.2 mg/kg/day, or 10 mg/day, whichever is less. Doses greater than 0.2 mg/kg/day or 10 mg/day are not recommended.

ANIMAL PHARMACOLOGY

A chronic study in dogs indicated that pimozide caused gingival hyperplasia when administered for several months at about 5 times the maximum recommended human dose. This condition was reversible after withdrawal. This condition has not been observed following chronic administration of pimozide to man.

P

HOW SUPPLIED

Pimozide 2 mg tablets, white, scored, debossed "LEMMON" and "ORAP 2".

Dispense in a tight, light-resistant container as defined in the official compendium.

Pharmacist: Dispense in child resistant container.

PRODUCT LISTING - EQUIVALENTS NOT AVAILABLE

Tablet - Oral - 1 mg

100's	$83.78	ORAP, Gate Pharmaceuticals	57844-0151-01

Tablet - Oral - 2 mg

100's	$111.70	ORAP, Gate Pharmaceuticals	57844-0187-01

Pindolol *(002039)*

For complete prescribing information, refer to the CD-ROM included with the book.

For related information, see the comparative table section in Appendix A.

Categories: Hypertension, essential; Pregnancy Category B; FDA Approved 1982 Sep
Drug Classes: Antiadrenergics, beta blocking
Brand Names: Bedrenal; Betadren; **Visken**
Foreign Brand Availability: Apo-Pindol (Malaysia); Apo-Pindolol (New-Zealand); Barbloc (Australia; Taiwan); Betapindol (Switzerland); Blocklin (Taiwan); Carvisken (Japan); Decreten (Denmark; Norway); Dranolis (Greece); Durapindol (Germany); Hexapindol (Denmark; Norway; Sweden); Nonspi (Germany); Novo-Pindol (Canada); Pidol (Taiwan); Pinbetol (Germany); Pinden (Israel); Pindol (New-Zealand); Pindomex (Finland); Pindoreal (Germany); Pinloc (Finland); Pyndale (Philippines); Pinsken (Thailand); Treparasen (Greece); Viskeen (Netherlands); Viskeen Retard (Netherlands); Viskene (Portugal); Vypen (New-Zealand)
Cost of Therapy: $10.48 (Hypertension; Generic Tablets; 5 mg; 2 tablets/day; 30 day supply)

DESCRIPTION

Pindolol, a synthetic beta-adrenergic receptor blocking agent with intrinsic sympathomimetic activity is 1-(Indol-4-yloxy)-3-(isopropylamino)-2-propanol.

Pindolol is a white to off-white odorless powder soluble in organic solvents and aqueous acids. Pindolol is intended for oral administration.

5 MG AND 10 MG TABLETS

Active Ingredient: Pindolol
Inactive Ingredients: Colloidal silicon dioxide, magnesium stearate, microcrystalline cellulose, and pregelatinized starch.
Storage: Store at controlled room temperature, 15-30°C (59-86°F). Dispense in a tight, light-resistant container.

INDICATIONS AND USAGE

Pindolol is indicated in the management of hypertension. It may be used alone or concomitantly with other antihypertensive agents, particularly with a thiazide-type diuretic.

NON-FDA APPROVED INDICATIONS

It has been used without FDA approval for the treatment of angina pectoris and vasovagal syncope.

P

CONTRAINDICATIONS

Pindolol is contraindicated in:

1. Bronchial asthma.
2. Overt cardiac failure.
3. Cardiogenic shock.
4. Second and third degree heart block.
5. Severe bradycardia (see WARNINGS).

WARNINGS

CARDIAC FAILURE

Sympathetic stimulation may be a vital component supporting circulatory function in patients with congestive heart failure, and its inhibition by beta-blockade may precipitate more severe failure. Although beta-blockers should be avoided in overt congestive heart failure, if necessary, pindolol can be used with caution in patients with a history of failure who are well-compensated, usually with digitalis and diuretics. Beta-adrenergic blocking agents do not abolish the inotropic action of digitalis on heart muscle.

IN PATIENTS WITHOUT A HISTORY OF CARDIAC FAILURE

In patients with latent cardiac insufficiency, continued depression of the myocardium with beta-blocking agents over a period of time can in some cases lead to cardiac failure. At the first sign or symptom of impending cardiac failure, patients should be fully digitalized and/or be given a diuretic, and the response observed closely. If cardiac failure continues, despite adequate digitalization and diuretic, pindolol therapy should be withdrawn (gradually if possible).

EXACERBATION OF ISCHEMIC HEART DISEASE FOLLOWING ABRUPT WITHDRAWAL

Hypersensitivity to catecholamines has been observed in patients withdrawn from beta-blockers therapy; exacerbation of angina and, in some cases, myocardial infarction have occurred after *abrupt* discontinuation of such therapy. When discontinuing chronically administered pindolol, particularly in patients with ischemic heart disease, the dosage should be gradually reduced over a period of 1 to 2 weeks and the patient should be carefully monitored. If angina markedly worsens or acute coronary insufficiency develops, pindolol administration should be reinstituted promptly, at least temporarily, and other measures appropriate for the management of unstable angina should be taken. Patients should be warned against interruption or discontinuation of therapy without the physician's advice. Because coronary artery disease is common and may be unrecognized, it may be prudent not to discontinue pindolol therapy abruptly even in patients treated only for hypertension.

NONALLERGIC BRONCHOSPASM (E.G., CHRONIC BRONCHITIS, EMPHYSEMA)

Patients with bronchospastic disease should in general not receive beta-blockers. Pindolol should be administered with caution since it may block bronchodilation produced by endogenous or exogenous catecholamine stimulation of $beta_2$ receptors.

MAJOR SURGERY

Because beta blockade impairs the ability of the heart to respond to reflex stimuli and may increase the risks of general anesthesia and surgical procedures, resulting in protracted hypotension or low cardiac output, it has generally been suggested that such therapy should be withdrawn several days prior to surgery. Recognition of the increased sensitivity to catecholamines of patients of patients recently withdrawn from beta-blocker therapy, however, has made this recommendation controversial. If possible, beta-blockers should be withdrawn well before surgery takes place. In the event of emergency surgery, the anesthesiologist should be informed that the patient is on beta-blocker therapy.

The effects of pindolol can be reversed by administration of beta-receptor agonists such as isoproterenol, dopamine, dobutamine, or norepinephrine. Difficulty in restarting and maintaining the heart beat has also been reported with beta-adrenergic receptor blocking agents.

DIABETES AND HYPOGLYCEMIA

Beta-adrenergic blockade may prevent the appearance of premonitory signs and symptoms (*e.g.*, tachycardia and blood pressure changes) of acute hypoglycemia. This is especially important with labile diabetics. Beta-blockade also reduces the release of insulin in response to hyperglycemia; therefore, it may be necessary to adjust the dose of antidiabetic drugs.

THYROTOXICOSIS

Beta-adrenergic blockade may mask certain clinical signs (*e.g.*, tachycardia) of hyperthyroidism. Patients suspected of developing thyrotoxicosis should be managed carefully to avoid abrupt withdrawal of beta-blockade, which might precipitate a thyroid crisis.

DOSAGE AND ADMINISTRATION

The dose of pindolol should be individualized. The recommended initial dose of pindolol is 5 mg bid alone or in combination with other antihypertensive agents. An antihypertensive response usually occurs within the first week of treatment. Maximal response, however, may take as long as or occasionally longer than two weeks. If a satisfactory reduction in blood pressure does not occur within 3-4 weeks, the dose may be adjusted in increments of 10 mg per day at these intervals up to a maximum of 60 mg/day.

PRODUCT LISTING - RATED THERAPEUTICALLY EQUIVALENT

Tablet - Oral - 5 mg

30's	$16.73	GENERIC, Heartland Healthcare Services	61392-0395-30
30's	$16.73	GENERIC, Heartland Healthcare Services	61392-0395-39
31's	$17.29	GENERIC, Heartland Healthcare Services	61392-0395-31
32's	$17.84	GENERIC, Heartland Healthcare Services	61392-0395-32
45's	$25.09	GENERIC, Heartland Healthcare Services	61392-0395-45
60's	$33.45	GENERIC, Heartland Healthcare Services	61392-0395-60
90's	$50.18	GENERIC, Heartland Healthcare Services	61392-0395-90
100's	$15.37	FEDERAL UPPER LIMIT, H.C.F.A. F F P	99999-2039-02
100's	$40.16	GENERIC, Vangard Labs	00615-3547-13
100's	$58.00	GENERIC, Par Pharmaceutical Inc	49884-0442-01
100's	$59.98	GENERIC, Qualitest Products Inc	00603-5220-21
100's	$61.05	GENERIC, Aligen Independent Laboratories Inc	00405-4804-01
100's	$61.16	GENERIC, Purepac Pharmaceutical Company	00228-2534-10
100's	$65.25	GENERIC, Major Pharmaceuticals Inc	00904-7893-60
100's	$66.95	GENERIC, Moore, H.L. Drug Exchange Inc	00839-7761-06
100's	$67.11	GENERIC, Mutual Pharmaceutical Co Inc	53489-0430-01
100's	$67.40	GENERIC, Martec Pharmaceuticals Inc	52555-0545-01
100's	$67.95	GENERIC, Geneva Pharmaceuticals	00781-1168-01
100's	$69.00	GENERIC, Bristol-Myers Squibb	59772-8804-10
100's	$69.30	GENERIC, Ivax Corporation	00172-4217-60
100's	$69.30	GENERIC, Mylan Pharmaceuticals Inc	00378-0052-01
100's	$69.30	GENERIC, Mutual/United Research Laboratories	00677-1457-01
100's	$69.30	GENERIC, Martec Pharmaceuticals Inc	52555-0454-01

Tablet - Oral - 10 mg

30's	$36.29	GENERIC, Heartland Healthcare Services	61392-0018-30
30's	$36.29	GENERIC, Heartland Healthcare Services	61392-0018-39
31's	$37.50	GENERIC, Heartland Healthcare Services	61392-0018-31
32's	$38.71	GENERIC, Heartland Healthcare Services	61392-0018-32
45's	$54.44	GENERIC, Heartland Healthcare Services	61392-0018-45
60's	$72.59	GENERIC, Heartland Healthcare Services	61392-0018-60
90's	$108.88	GENERIC, Heartland Healthcare Services	61392-0018-90
100's	$17.46	GENERIC, Bristol-Myers Squibb	59772-8805-10
100's	$19.73	FEDERAL UPPER LIMIT, H.C.F.A. F F P	99999-2039-05
100's	$62.02	GENERIC, Vangard Labs	00615-3506-13
100's	$79.51	GENERIC, Qualitest Products Inc	00603-5221-21
100's	$79.90	GENERIC, Par Pharmaceutical Inc	49884-0443-01
100's	$81.24	GENERIC, Purepac Pharmaceutical Company	00228-2535-10
100's	$84.11	GENERIC, Aligen Independent Laboratories Inc	00405-4805-01
100's	$86.50	GENERIC, Major Pharmaceuticals Inc	00904-7894-60
100's	$88.20	GENERIC, Mutual Pharmaceutical Co Inc	53489-0431-01
100's	$89.63	GENERIC, Moore, H.L. Drug Exchange Inc	00839-7762-06
100's	$93.50	GENERIC, Geneva Pharmaceuticals	00781-1169-01

100's	$93.50	GENERIC, Martec Pharmaceuticals Inc	52555-0546-01
100's	$93.52	GENERIC, Mutual/United Research Laboratories	00677-1458-01
100's	$94.50	GENERIC, Mylan Pharmaceuticals Inc	00378-0127-01
100's	$94.50	GENERIC, Martec Pharmaceuticals Inc	52555-0455-01
100's	$96.20	GENERIC, Ivax Corporation	00172-4218-60

Pioglitazone Hydrochloride *(003441)*

For related information, see the comparative table section in Appendix A.

Categories: Diabetes mellitus; FDA Approved 1999 Jul; Pregnancy Category C
Drug Classes: Antidiabetic agents; Thiazolidinediones
Foreign Brand Availability: Actos (Australia; Austria; Belgium; Bulgaria; Colombia; Czech-Republic; Denmark; England; Finland; France; Germany; Greece; Hong-Kong; Hungary; Indonesia; Ireland; Italy; Netherlands; New-Zealand; Norway; Philippines; Poland; Portugal; Slovenia; South-Africa; Spain; Sweden; Switzerland; Thailand; Turkey); Glitase (India); Glustin (Austria; Belgium; Bulgaria; Czech-Republic; Denmark; England; Finland; France; Germany; Greece; Hungary; Ireland; Italy; Netherlands; Norway; Poland; Portugal; Slovenia; Spain; Sweden; Switzerland; Turkey); Pioglit (India); Zactos (Mexico)
Cost of Therapy: $99.89 (Diabetes mellitus; Actos; 15 mg; 1 tablet/day; 30 day supply)

DESCRIPTION

Pioglitazone hydrochloride is an oral antidiabetic agent that acts primarily by decreasing insulin resistance. Pioglitazone hydrochloride is used in the management of Type 2 diabetes mellitus (also known as non-insulin-dependent diabetes mellitus [NIDDM] or adult-onset diabetes). Pharmacological studies indicate that pioglitazone hydrochloride improves sensitivity to insulin in muscle and adipose tissue and inhibits hepatic gluconeogenesis. Pioglitazone hydrochloride improves glycemic control while reducing circulating insulin levels.

Pioglitazone [(±)-5-[[4-[2-(5-ethyl-2-pyridinyl)ethoxy]phenyl]methyl]-2,4-] thiazolidinedione monohydrochloride belongs to a different chemical class and has a different pharmacological action than the sulfonylureas, metformin, or the α-glucosidase inhibitors. The molecule contains one asymmetric carbon, and the compound is synthesized and used as the racemic mixture. The two enantiomers of pioglitazone inter-convert *in vivo*. No differences were found in the pharmacologic activity between the two enantiomers.

Pioglitazone hydrochloride is an odorless white crystalline powder that has a molecular formula of $C_{19}H_{20}N_2O_3S{\cdot}HCl$ and a molecular weight of 392.90 daltons. It is soluble in N,N-dimethylformamide, slightly soluble in anhydrous ethanol, very slightly soluble in acetone and acetonitrile, practically insoluble in water, and insoluble in ether.

Actos is available as a tablet for oral administration containing 15, 30, or 45 mg of pioglitazone (as the base) formulated with the following excipients: lactose monohydrate, hydroxypropylcellulose, carboxymethylcellulose calcium, and magnesium stearate.

CLINICAL PHARMACOLOGY

MECHANISM OF ACTION

Pioglitazone HCl is a thiazolidinedione antidiabetic agent that depends on the presence of insulin for its mechanism of action. Pioglitazone HCl decreases insulin resistance in the periphery and in the liver resulting in increased insulin-dependent glucose disposal and decreased hepatic glucose output. Unlike sulfonylureas, pioglitazone is not an insulin secretagogue. Pioglitazone is a potent and highly selective agonist for peroxisome proliferator-activated receptor-gamma (PPARγ). PPAR receptors are found in tissues important for insulin action such as adipose tissue, skeletal muscle, and liver. Activation of PPARγ nuclear receptors modulates the transcription of a number of insulin responsive genes involved in the control of glucose and lipid metabolism.

In animal models of diabetes, pioglitazone reduces the hyperglycemia, hyperinsulinemia, and hypertriglyceridemia characteristic of insulin-resistant states such as Type 2 diabetes. The metabolic changes produced by pioglitazone result in increased responsiveness of insulin-dependent tissues and are observed in numerous animal models of insulin resistance.

Since pioglitazone enhances the effects of circulating insulin (by decreasing insulin resistance), it does not lower blood glucose in animal models that lack endogenous insulin.

PHARMACOKINETICS AND DRUG METABOLISM

Serum concentrations of total pioglitazone (pioglitazone plus active metabolites) remain elevated 24 hours after once daily dosing. Steady-state serum concentrations of both pioglitazone and total pioglitazone are achieved within 7 days. At steady-state, two of the pharmacologically active metabolites of pioglitazone, Metabolites III (M-III) and IV (M-IV), reach serum concentrations equal to or greater than pioglitazone. In both healthy volunteers and in patients with Type 2 diabetes, pioglitazone comprises approximately 30-50% of the peak total pioglitazone serum concentrations and 20-25% of the total area under the serum concentration-time curve (AUC).

Maximum serum concentration (C_{max}), AUC, and trough serum concentrations (C_{min}) for both pioglitazone and total pioglitazone increase proportionally at doses of 15 and 30 mg/day. There is a slightly less than proportional increase for pioglitazone and total pioglitazone at a dose of 60 mg/day.

Absorption

Following oral administration, in the fasting state, pioglitazone is first measurable in serum within 30 minutes, with peak concentrations observed within 2 hours. Food slightly delays the time to peak serum concentration to 3-4 hours, but does not alter the extent of absorption.

Distribution

The mean apparent volume of distribution (Vd/F) of pioglitazone following single-dose administration is 0.63 ± 0.41 (mean ±SD) L/kg of body weight. Pioglitazone is extensively protein bound (>99%) in human serum, principally to serum albumin. Pioglitazone also binds to other serum proteins, but with lower affinity. Metabolites M-III and M-IV also are extensively bound (>98%) to serum albumin.

Metabolism

Pioglitazone is extensively metabolized by hydroxylation and oxidation; the metabolites also partly convert to glucuronide or sulfate conjugates. Metabolites M-II and M-IV (hydroxy derivatives of pioglitazone) and M-III (keto derivative of pioglitazone) are pharmacologically active in animal models of Type 2 diabetes. In addition to pioglitazone, M-III and M-IV are the principal drug-related species found in human serum following multiple dosing. At steady-state, in both healthy volunteers and in patients with Type 2 diabetes, pioglitazone comprises approximately 30-50% of the total peak serum concentrations and 20-25% of the total AUC.

Pioglitazone incubated with expressed human P450 or human liver microsomes results in the formation of M-IV and to a much lesser degree, M-II. The major cytochrome P450 isoforms involved in the hepatic metabolism of pioglitazone are CYP2C8 and CYP3A4 with contributions from a variety of other isoforms including the mainly extrahepatic CYP1A1. Ketoconazole inhibited up to 85% of hepatic pioglitazone metabolism *in vitro* at a concentration equal molar to pioglitazone. Pioglitazone did not inhibit P450 activity when incubated with human P450 liver microsomes. *In vivo* human studies have not been performed to investigate any induction of CYP3A4 by pioglitazone.

Excretion and Elimination

Following oral administration, approximately 15-30% of the pioglitazone dose is recovered in the urine. Renal elimination of pioglitazone is negligible, and the drug is excreted primarily as metabolites and their conjugates. It is presumed that most of the oral dose is excreted into the bile either unchanged or as metabolites and eliminated in the feces.

The mean serum half-life of pioglitazone and total pioglitazone ranges from 3-7 hours and 16-24 hours, respectively. Pioglitazone has an apparent clearance, CL/F, calculated to be 5-7 L/h.

SPECIAL POPULATIONS

Renal Insufficiency

The serum elimination half-life of pioglitazone, M-III, and M-IV remains unchanged in patients with moderate (creatinine clearance 30-60 ml/min) to severe (creatinine clearance <30 ml/min) renal impairment when compared to normal subjects. No dose adjustment in patients with renal dysfunction is recommended (see DOSAGE AND ADMINISTRATION).

Hepatic Insufficiency

Compared with normal controls, subjects with impaired hepatic function (Child-Pugh Grade B/C) have an approximate 45% reduction in pioglitazone and total pioglitazone mean peak concentrations but no change in the mean AUC values.

Pioglitazone HCl therapy should not be initiated if the patient exhibits clinical evidence of active liver disease or serum transaminase levels (ALT) exceed 2.5 times the upper limit of normal (see PRECAUTIONS, General, Hepatic Effects).

Elderly

In healthy elderly subjects, peak serum concentrations of pioglitazone and total pioglitazone are not significantly different, but AUC values are slightly higher and the terminal half-life values slightly longer than for younger subjects. These changes were not of a magnitude that would be considered clinically relevant.

Pediatrics

Pharmacokinetic data in the pediatric population are not available.

Gender

The mean C_{max} and AUC values were increased 20-60% in females. As monotherapy and in combination with sulfonylurea, metformin, or insulin, pioglitazone HCl improved glycemic control in both males and females. In controlled clinical trials, hemoglobin A_{1c} (HbA_{1c}) decreases from baseline were generally greater for females than for males (average mean difference in HbA_{1c} 0.5%). Since therapy should be individualized for each patient to achieve glycemic control, no dose adjustment is recommended based on gender alone.

Ethnicity

Pharmacokinetic data among various ethnic groups are not available.

DRUG-DRUG INTERACTIONS

The following drugs were studied in healthy volunteers with a co-administration of pioglitazone HCl 45 mg once daily. Listed below are the results:

Fexofenadine HCl: Co-administration of pioglitazone HCl for 7 days with 60 mg fexofenadine administered orally twice daily resulted in no significant effect on pioglitazone pharmacokinetics. Pioglitazone HCl had no significant effect on fexofenadine pharmacokinetics.

Glipizide: Co-administration of pioglitazone HCl and 5 mg glipizide administered orally once daily for 7 days did not alter the steady-state pharmacokinetics of glipizide.

Digoxin: Co-administration of pioglitazone HCl with 0.25 mg digoxin administered orally once daily for 7 days did not alter the steady-state pharmacokinetics of digoxin.

Warfarin: Co-administration of pioglitazone HCl for 7 days with warfarin did not alter the steady-state pharmacokinetics of warfarin. Pioglitazone HCl has no clinically significant effect on prothrombin time when administered to patients receiving chronic warfarin therapy.

Metformin: Co-administration of a single dose of metformin (1000 mg) and pioglitazone HCl after 7 days of pioglitazone HCl did not alter the pharmacokinetics of the single dose of metformin.

Midazolam: Administration of pioglitazone HCl for 15 days followed by a single 7.5 mg dose of midazolam syrup resulted in a 26% reduction in midazolam C_{max} and AUC.

Ranitidine HCl: Co-administration of pioglitazone HCl for 7 days with ranitidine administered orally twice daily for either 4 or 7 days resulted in no significant effect on

P

pioglitazone pharmacokinetics. Pioglitazone HCl showed no significant effect on ranitidine pharmacokinetics.

Nifedipine ER: Co-administration of pioglitazone HCl for 7 days with 30 mg nifedipine ER administered orally once daily for 4 days to male and female volunteers resulted in a $\log_e$ transformed AUC ratio of 0.88 (CI 0.81-0.95). In view of the high variability of nifedipine pharmacokinetics, the clinical significance of this finding is unknown.

Oral Contraceptives: See PRECAUTIONS.

Cytochrome P450: See PRECAUTIONS.

PHARMACODYNAMICS AND CLINICAL EFFECTS

Clinical studies demonstrate that pioglitazone HCl improves insulin sensitivity in insulin-resistant patients. Pioglitazone HCl enhances cellular responsiveness to insulin, increases insulin-dependent glucose disposal, improves hepatic sensitivity to insulin, and improves dysfunctional glucose homeostasis. In patients with Type 2 diabetes, the decreased insulin resistance produced by pioglitazone HCl results in lower blood glucose concentrations, lower plasma insulin levels, and lower HbA_{1c} values. Based on results from an open-label extension study, the glucose lowering effects of pioglitazone HCl appear to persist for at least 1 year. In controlled clinical trials, pioglitazone HCl in combination with sulfonylurea, metformin, or insulin had an additive effect on glycemic control.

Patients with lipid abnormalities were included in clinical trials with pioglitazone HCl. Overall, patients treated with pioglitazone HCl had mean decreases in triglycerides, mean increases in HDL cholesterol, and no consistent mean changes in LDL and total cholesterol.

In a 26 week, placebo-controlled, dose-ranging study, mean triglyceride levels decreased in the 15, 30, and 45 mg pioglitazone HCl dose groups compared to a mean increase in the placebo group. Mean HDL levels increased to a greater extent in patients treated with pioglitazone HCl than in the placebo-treated patients. There were no consistent differences for LDL and total cholesterol in patients treated with pioglitazone HCl compared to placebo (see TABLE 1).

TABLE 1 *Lipids in a 26 Week Placebo-Controlled Dose-Ranging Study*

		Pioglitazone HCl Once Daily		
	Placebo	**15 mg**	**30 mg**	**45 mg**
Triglycerides (mg/dl)	n=79	n=79	n=84	n=77
Baseline (mean)	262.8	283.8	261.1	259.7
Percent change from baseline (mean)	4.8%	-9.0%	-9.6%	-9.3%
HDL Cholesterol (mg/dl)	n=79	n=79	n=83	n=77
Baseline (mean)	41.7	40.4	40.8	40.7
Percent change from baseline (mean)	8.1%	14.1%	12.2%	19.1%
LDL Cholesterol (mg/dl)	n=65	n=63	n=74	n=62
Baseline (mean)	138.8	131.9	135.6	126.8
Percent change from baseline (mean)	4.8%	7.2%	5.2%	6.0%
Total Cholesterol (mg/dl)	n=79	n=79	n=84	n=77
Baseline (mean)	224.6	220.0	222.7	213.7
Percent change from baseline (mean)	4.4%	4.6%	3.3%	6.4%

In the two other monotherapy studies (24 and 16 weeks) and in combination therapy studies with sulfonylurea (16 weeks) and metformin (16 weeks), the results were generally consistent with the data above. For patients treated with pioglitazone HCl, the placebo-corrected mean changes from baseline decreased 5-26% for triglycerides and increased 6-13% for HDL cholesterol.

In the combination therapy study with insulin (16 weeks), the placebo-corrected mean percent change from baseline in triglyceride values for patients treated with pioglitazone HCl was also decreased. A placebo-corrected mean change from baseline in LDL cholesterol of 7% was observed for the 15 mg dose group. Similar results to those noted above for HDL and total cholesterol were observed.

INDICATIONS AND USAGE

Pioglitazone HCl is indicated as an adjunct to diet and exercise to improve glycemic control in patients with Type 2 diabetes (non-insulin-dependent diabetes mellitus, NIDDM). Pioglitazone HCl is indicated for monotherapy. Pioglitazone HCl is also indicated for use in combination with a sulfonylurea, metformin, or insulin when diet and exercise plus the single agent does not result in adequate glycemic control.

Management of Type 2 diabetes should also include nutritional counseling, weight reduction as needed, and exercise. These efforts are important not only in the primary treatment of Type 2 diabetes, but also to maintain the efficacy of drug therapy.

CONTRAINDICATIONS

Pioglitazone HCl is contraindicated in patients with known hypersensitivity to this product or any of its components.

WARNINGS

CARDIAC FAILURE AND OTHER CARDIAC EFFECTS

Pioglitazone HCl, like other thiazolidinediones, can cause fluid retention when used alone or in combination with other antidiabetic agents, including insulin. Fluid retention may lead to or exacerbate heart failure. Patients should be observed for signs and symptoms of heart failure (see PRECAUTIONS, Information for the Patient). Pioglitazone HCl should be discontinued if any deterioration in cardiac status occurs. Patients with New York Heart Association (NYHA) Class III and IV cardiac status were not studied during clinical trials; therefore, pioglitazone HCl is not recommended in these patients (see PRECAUTIONS, General, Cardiovascular).

In one 16 week US double-blind, placebo-controlled clinical trial involving 566 patients with Type 2 diabetes, pioglitazone HCl at doses of 15 and 30 mg in combination with insulin were compared to insulin therapy alone. This trial included patients with long-standing diabetes and a high prevalence of pre-existing medical conditions as follows: arterial hypertension (57.2%), peripheral neuropathy (22.6%), coronary heart disease (19.6%), retinopathy (13.1%), myocardial infarction (8.8%), vascular disease (6.4%), angina pectoris (4.4%), stroke and/or transient ischemic attack (4.1%), and congestive heart failure (2.3%).

In this study 2 of the 191 patients receiving 15 mg pioglitazone HCl plus insulin (1.1%) and 2 of the 188 patients receiving 30 mg pioglitazone HCl plus insulin (1.1%) developed congestive heart failure compared with none of the 187 patients on insulin therapy alone. All 4 of these patients had previous histories of cardiovascular conditions including coronary artery disease, previous CABG procedures, and myocardial infarction.

Analysis of data from this study did not identify specific factors that predict increased risk of congestive heart failure on combination therapy with insulin.

PRECAUTIONS

GENERAL

Pioglitazone HCl exerts its antihyperglycemic effect only in the presence of insulin. Therefore, pioglitazone HCl should not be used in patients with Type 1 diabetes or for the treatment of diabetic ketoacidosis.

Hypoglycemia

Patients receiving pioglitazone HCl in combination with insulin or oral hypoglycemic agents may be at risk for hypoglycemia, and a reduction in the dose of the concomitant agent may be necessary.

Cardiovascular

In US placebo-controlled clinical trials that excluded patients with New York Heart Association (NYHA) Class III and IV cardiac status, the incidence of serious cardiac adverse events related to volume expansion was not increased in patients treated with pioglitazone HCl as monotherapy or in combination with sulfonylureas or metformin versus placebo-treated patients. In insulin combination studies, a small number of patients with a history of previously existing cardiac disease developed congestive heart failure when treated with pioglitazone HCl in combination with insulin (see WARNINGS). Patients with NYHA Class III and IV cardiac status were not studied in pioglitazone HCl clinical trials. Pioglitazone HCl is not indicated in patients with NYHA Class III or IV cardiac status.

In postmarketing experience with pioglitazone HCl, cases of congestive heart failure have been reported in patients both with and without previously known heart disease.

Edema

Pioglitazone HCl should be used with caution in patients with edema. In all US clinical trials, edema was reported more frequently in patients treated with pioglitazone HCl than in placebo-treated patients (see ADVERSE REACTIONS). In postmarketing experience, reports of initiation or worsening of edema have been received.

Weight Gain

Dose related weight gain was seen with pioglitazone HCl alone and in combination with other hypoglycemic agents (TABLE 6). The mechanism of weight gain is unclear but probably involves a combination of fluid retention and fat accumulation.

TABLE 6 *Weight Changes (kg) From Baseline During Double-Blind Clinical Trials With Pioglitazone HCl: Median (25th/75th Percentile)*

	Control Group	Pioglitazone HCl		
	(Placebo)	**15 mg**	**30 mg**	**45 mg**
Monotherapy	-1.4 (-2.7/0.0) n=256	0.9 (-0.5/3.4) n=79	1.0 (-0.9/3.4) n=188	2.6 (0.2/5.4) n=79
Combination Therapy				
Sulfonylurea	-0.5 (-1.8/0.7) n=187	2.0 (0.2/3.2) n=183	2.7 (1.1/4.5) n=186	N/A
Metformin	-1.4 (-3.2/0.3) n=160	N/A	1.4 (-0.9/3.0) n=167	N/A
Insulin	0.2 (-1.4/1.4) n=182	2.3 (0.5/4.3) n=190	3.6 (1.4/5.9) n=188	N/A

Ovulation

Therapy with pioglitazone HCl, like other thiazolidinediones, may result in ovulation in some premenopausal anovulatory women. As a result, these patients may be at an increased risk for pregnancy while taking pioglitazone HCl. Thus, adequate contraception in premenopausal women should be recommended. This possible effect has not been investigated in clinical studies so the frequency of this occurence is not known.

Hematologic

Pioglitazone HCl may cause decreases in hemoglobin and hematocrit. Across all clinical studies, mean hemoglobin values declined by 2-4% in patients treated with pioglitazone HCl. These changes primarily occurred within the first 4-12 weeks of therapy and remained relatively constant thereafter. These changes may be related to increased plasma volume and have not been associated with any significant hematologic clinical effects (see ADVERSE REACTIONS, Laboratory Abnormalities).

Hepatic Effects

Another drug of the thiazolidinedione class, troglitazone, has been associated with idiosyncratic hepatotoxicity, and very rare cases of liver failure, liver transplants, and death have been reported during postmarketing clinical use. In pre-approval controlled clinical trials in patients with Type 2 diabetes, troglitazone was more frequently associated with clinically significant elevations of hepatic enzymes (ALT >3 times the upper limit of normal) compared to placebo, and very rare cases of reversible jaundice were reported.

In pre-approval clinical studies worldwide, over 4500 subjects have been treated with pioglitazone HCl. In US clinical studies, over 2500 patients with Type 2 diabetes received pioglitazone HCl. There was no evidence of drug-induced hepatotoxicity or elevation of ALT levels in the clinical studies.

During pre-approval placebo-controlled clinical trials in the US, a total of 4 of 1526 (0.26%) patients treated with pioglitazone HCl and 2 of 793 (0.25%) placebo-treated patients had ALT values ≥3 times the upper limit of normal. The ALT elevations in patients treated with pioglitazone HCl were reversible and were not clearly related to therapy with pioglitazone HCl.

In postmarketing experience with pioglitazone HCl, reports of hepatitis and of hepatic enzyme elevations to 3 or more times the upper limit of normal have been received. Very rarely, these reports have involved hepatic failure with and without fatal outcome, although causality has not been established.

Pioglitazone is structurally related to troglitazone, a thiazolidinedione no longer marketed in the US, which was associated with idiosyncratic hepatotoxicity and rare cases of liver failure, liver transplants and death during postmarketing clinical use.

Pending the availability of the results of additional large, long-term controlled clinical trials and additional postmarketing safety data, it is recommended that patients treated with pioglitazone HCl undergo periodic monitoring of liver enzymes.

Serum ALT (alanine aminotranferase) levels should be evaluated prior to the initiation of therapy with pioglitazone HCl in all patients, every 2 months for the first year of therapy, and periodically thereafter. Liver function tests should also be obtained for patients if symptoms suggestive of hepatic dysfunction occur, *e.g.*, nausea, vomiting, abdominal pain, fatigue, anorexia, dark urine. The decision whether to continue the patient on therapy with pioglitazone HCl should be guided by clinical judgement pending laboratory evaluations. If jaundice is observed, drug therapy should be discontinued.

Therapy with pioglitazone HCl should not be initiated if the patient exhibits clinical evidence of active liver disease or the ALT levels exceed 2.5 times the upper limit of normal. Patients with mildly elevated liver enzymes (ALT levels at 1 to 2.5 times the upper limit of normal) at baseline or any time during therapy with pioglitazone HCl should be evaluated to determine the cause of the liver enzyme elevation. Initiation or continuation of therapy with pioglitazone HCl in patients with mildly elevated liver enzymes should proceed with caution and include the appropriate clinical follow-up which may include more frequent liver enzyme monitoring. If serum transaminase levels are increased (ALT >2.5 times the upper limit of normal), liver function tests should be evaluated more frequently until the levels return to normal or pretreatment values. If ALT levels exceed 3 times the upper limit of normal, the test should be repeated as soon as possible. If ALT levels remain >3 times the upper limit of normal or if the patient is jaundiced, pioglitazone HCl therapy should be discontinued.

There are no data available to evaluate the safety of pioglitazone HCl in patients who experienced liver abnormalities, hepatic dysfunction, or jaundice while on troglitazone. Pioglitazone HCl should not be used in patients who experienced jaundice while taking troglitazone.

LABORATORY TESTS

FBG and HbA_{1c} measurements should be performed periodically to monitor glycemic control and the therapeutic response to pioglitazone HCl.

Liver enzyme monitoring is recommended prior to initiation of therapy with pioglitazone HCl in all patients and periodically therafter (see General, Hepatic Effects and ADVERSE REACTIONS, Laboratory Abnormalities, Serum Transaminase Levels).

INFORMATION FOR THE PATIENT

It is important to instruct patients to adhere to dietary instructions and to have blood glucose and glycosylated hemoglobin tested regularly. During periods of stress such as fever, trauma, infection, or surgery, medication requirements may change and patients should be reminded to seek medical advice promptly.

Patients who experience an unusually rapid increase in weight or edema or who develop shortness of breath or other symptoms of heart failure while on pioglitazone HCl should immediately report these symptoms to their physician.

Patients should be told that blood tests for liver function will be performed prior to the start of therapy, every 2 months for the first year, and periodically thereafter. Patients should be told to seek immediate medical advice for unexplained nausea, vomiting, abdominal pain, fatigue, anorexia, or dark urine.

Patients should be told to take pioglitazone HCl once daily. Pioglitazone HCl can be taken with or without meals. If a dose is missed on 1 day, the dose should not be doubled the following day.

When using combination therapy with insulin or oral hypoglycemic agents, the risks of hypoglycemia, its symptoms and treatment, and conditions that predispose to its development should be explained to patients and their family members.

Therapy with pioglitazone HCl, like other thiazolidinediones, may result in ovulation in some premenopausal anovulatory women. As a result, these patients may be at an increased risk for pregnancy while taking pioglitazone HCl. Thus, adequate contraception in premenopausal women should be recommended. This possible effect has not been investigated in clinical studies so the frequency of this occurrence is not known.

CARCINOGENESIS, MUTAGENESIS, AND IMPAIRMENT OF FERTILITY

A 2 year carcinogenicity study was conducted in male and female rats at oral doses up to 63 mg/kg (approximately 14 times the maximum recommended human oral dose of 45 mg based on mg/m^2). Drug-induced tumors were not observed in any organ except for the urinary bladder. Benign and/or malignant transitional cell neoplasms were observed in male rats at 4 mg/kg/day and above (approximately equal to the maximum recommended human oral dose based on mg/m^2). The relationship of these findings in male rats to humans is unclear. A 2 year carcinogenicity study was conducted in male and female mice at oral doses up to 100 mg/kg/day (approximately 11 times the maximum recommended human oral dose based on mg/m^2). No drug-induced tumors were observed in any organ.

During prospective evaluation of urinary cytology involving more than 1800 patients receiving pioglitazone HCl in clinical trials up to 1 year in duration, no new cases of bladder tumors were identified. Occasionally, abnormal urinary cytology results indicating possible malignancy were observed in both patients treated with pioglitazone HCl (0.72%) and patients treated with placebo (0.88%).

Pioglitazone HCl was not mutagenic in a battery of genetic toxicology studies, including the Ames bacterial assay, a mammalian cell forward gene mutation assay (CHO/HPRT and AS52/XPRT), an *in vitro* cytogenetics assay using CHL cells, an unscheduled DNA synthesis assay, and an *in vivo* micronucleus assay.

No adverse effects upon fertility were observed in male and female rats at oral doses up to 40 mg/kg pioglitazone HCl daily prior to and throughout mating and gestation (approximately 9 times the maximum recommended human oral dose based on mg/m^2).

PREGNANCY CATEGORY C

Pioglitazone was not teratogenic in rats at oral doses up to 80 mg/kg or in rabbits given up to 160 mg/kg during organogenesis (approximately 17 and 40 times the maximum recommended human oral dose based on mg/m^2, respectively). Delayed parturition and embryotoxicity (as evidenced by increased postimplantation losses, delayed development and reduced fetal weights) were observed in rats at oral doses of 40 mg/kg/day and above (approximately 10 times the maximum recommended human oral dose based on mg/m^2). No functional or behavioral toxicity was observed in offspring of rats. In rabbits, embryotoxicity was observed at an oral dose of 160 mg/kg (approximately 40 times the maximum recommended human oral dose based on mg/m^2). Delayed postnatal development, attributed to decreased body weight, was observed in offspring of rats at oral doses of 10 mg/kg and above during late gestation and lactation periods (approximately 2 times the maximum recommended human oral dose based on mg/m^2).

There are no adequate and well-controlled studies in pregnant women. Pioglitazone HCl should be used during pregnancy only if the potential benefit justifies the potential risk to the fetus.

Because current information strongly suggests that abnormal blood glucose levels during pregnancy are associated with a higher incidence of congenital anomalies, as well as increased neonatal morbidity and mortality, most experts recommend that insulin be used during pregnancy to maintain blood glucose levels as close to normal as possible.

NURSING MOTHERS

Pioglitazone is secreted in the milk of lactating rats. It is not known whether pioglitazone HCl is secreted in human milk. Because many drugs are excreted in human milk, pioglitazone HCl should not be administered to a breast-feeding woman.

PEDIATRIC USE

Safety and effectiveness of pioglitazone HCl in pediatric patients have not been established.

ELDERLY USE

Approximately 500 patients in placebo-controlled clinical trials of pioglitazone HCl were 65 and over. No significant differences in effectiveness and safety were observed between these patients and younger patients.

DRUG INTERACTIONS

Oral Contraceptives: Administration of another thiazolidinedione with an oral contraceptive containing ethinyl estradiol and norethindrone reduced the plasma concentrations of both hormones by approximately 30%, which could result in loss of contraception. The pharmacokinetics of coadministration of pioglitazone HCl and oral contraceptives have not been evaluated in patients receiving pioglitazone HCl and an oral contraceptive. Therefore, additional caution regarding contraception should be exercised in patients receiving pioglitazone HCl and an oral contraceptive.

The cytochrome P450 isoform CYP3A4 is partially responsible for the metabolism of pioglitazone. Specific formal pharmacokinetic interaction studies have not been conducted with pioglitazone HCl and other drugs metabolized by this enzyme such as: erythromycin, astemizole, cisapride, corticosteroids, cyclosporine, HMG-CoA reductase inhibitors, tacrolimus, trizolam, and trimetrexate, as well as inhibitory drugs such as ketoconazole and itraconazole. *In vitro,* ketoconazole appears to significantly inhibit the metabolism of pioglitazone (see CLINICAL PHARMACOLOGY, Pharmacokinetics and Drug Metabolism, Metabolism). Pending the availability of additional data, patients receiving ketoconazole concomitantly with pioglitazone HCl should be evaluated more frequently with respect to glycemic control.

ADVERSE REACTIONS

In worldwide clinical trials, over 3700 patients with Type 2 diabetes have been treated with pioglitazone HCl. In US clinical trials, over 2500 patients have received pioglitazone HCl, over 1100 patients have been treated for 6 months or longer, and over 450 patients for 1 year or longer.

The overall incidence and types of adverse events reported in placebo-controlled clinical trials of pioglitazone HCl monotherapy at doses of 7.5, 15, 30, or 45 mg once daily are shown in TABLE 7.

TABLE 7 *Placebo-Controlled Clinical Studies of Pioglitazone HCl Monotherapy**

	Placebo n=259	Pioglitazone HCl n=606
Upper respiratory tract infection	8.5%	13.2%
Headache	6.9%	9.1%
Sinusitis	4.6%	6.3%
Myalgia	2.7%	5.4%
Tooth disorder	2.3%	5.3%
Diabetes mellitus aggravated	8.1%	5.1%
Pharyngitis	0.8%	5.1%

* Adverse events reported at a frequency ≥5% of patients treated with pioglitazone HCl.

For most clinical adverse events the incidence was similar for groups treated with pioglitazone HCl monotherapy and those treated in combination with sulfonylureas, metformin, and insulin. There was an increase in the occurrence of edema in the patients treated with pioglitazone HCl and insulin compared to insulin alone.

In the pioglitazone HCl plus insulin trial (n=379), 10 patients treated with pioglitazone HCl plus insulin developed dyspnea and also, at some point during the therapy developed either weight change or edema. Seven (7) of these 10 patients received diuretics to treat these symptoms. This was not reported in the insulin plus placebo group.

The incidence of withdrawals from clinical trials due to an adverse event other than hyperglycemia was similar for patients treated with placebo (2.8%) or pioglitazone HCl (3.3%).

Mild to moderate hypoglycemia was reported during combination therapy with sulfonylurea or insulin. Hypoglycemia was reported for 1% of placebo-treated patients and 2% of patients when pioglitazone HCl was used in combination with a sulfonylurea. In combination with insulin, hypoglycemia was reported for 5% of placebo-treated patients, 8% for patients treated with 15 mg of pioglitazone HCl, and 15% for patients treated with 30 mg of pioglitazone HCl (see PRECAUTIONS, General, Hypoglycemia).

In US double-blind studies, anemia was reported for 1.0% of patients treated with pioglitazone HCl and 0.0% of placebo-treated patients in monotherapy studies. Anemia was reported for 1.6% of patients treated with pioglitazone HCl and 1.6% of placebo-treated patients in combination with insulin. Anemia was reported for 0.3% of patients treated with pioglitazone HCl and 1.6% of placebo-treated patients in combination with sulfonylurea. Anemia was reported for 1.2% of patients treated with pioglitazone HCl and 0.0% of placebo-treated patients in combination with metformin.

In monotherapy studies, edema was reported for 4.8% of patients treated with pioglitazone HCl versus 1.2% of placebo-treated patients. In combination therapy studies, edema was reported for 7.2% of patients treated with pioglitazone HCl and sulfonylureas compared to 2.1% of patients on sulfonylureas alone. In combination therapy studies with metformin, edema was reported in 6.0% of patients on combination therapy compared to 2.5% of patients on metformin alone. In combination therapy studies with insulin, edema was reported in 15.3% of patients on combination therapy compared to 7.0% of patients on insulin alone. Most of these events were considered mild or moderate in intensity (see PRECAUTIONS, General, Edema).

In one 16 week clinical trial of insulin plus pioglitazone HCl combination therapy, more patients developed congestive heart failure on combination therapy (1.1%) compared to none on insulin alone (see WARNINGS, Cardiac Failure and Other Cardiac Effects).

LABORATORY ABNORMALITIES

Hematologic

Pioglitazone HCl may cause decreases in hemoglobin and hematocrit. Across all clinical studies, mean hemoglobin values declined by 2-4% in patients treated with pioglitazone HCl. These changes generally occurred within the first 4-12 weeks of therapy and remained relatively stable thereafter. These changes may be related to increased plasma volume associated with pioglitazone HCl therapy and have not been associated with any significant hematologic clinical effects.

Serum Transaminase Levels

During placebo-controlled clinical trials in the US, a total of 4 of 1526 (0.26%) patients treated with pioglitazone HCl and 2 of 793 (0.25%) placebo-treated patients had ALT values ≥3 times the upper limit of normal. During all clinical studies in the US, 11 of 2561 (0.43%) patients treated with pioglitazone HCl had ALT values ≥3 times the upper limit of normal. All patients with follow-up values had reversible elevations in ALT. In the population of patients treated with pioglitazone HCl, mean values for bilirubin, AST, ALT, alkaline phosphatase, and GGT were decreased at the final visit compared with baseline. Fewer than 0.12% of patients treated with pioglitazone HCl were withdrawn from clinical trials in the US due to abnormal liver function tests.

P

In pre-approval clinical trials, there were no cases of idiosyncratic drug reactions leading to hepatic failure (see PRECAUTIONS, General, Hepatic Effects).

CPK Levels

During required laboratory testing in clinical trials, sporadic, transient elevations in creatine phosphokinase levels (CPK) were observed. A single, isolated elevation to greater than 10 times the upper limit of normal (values of 2150-8610) was noted in 7 patients. Five of these patients continued to receive pioglitazone HCl and the other 2 patients had completed receiving study medication at the time of the elevated value. These elevations resolved without any apparent clinical sequelae. The relationship of these events to pioglitazone HCl therapy is unknown.

DOSAGE AND ADMINISTRATION

Pioglitazone HCl should be taken once daily without regard to meals.

The management of antidiabetic therapy should be individualized. Ideally, the response to therapy should be evaluated using HbA_{1c} which is a better indicator of long-term glycemic control than FBG alone. HbA_{1c} reflects glycemia over the past 2-3 months. In clinical use, it is recommended that patients be treated with pioglitazone HCl for a period of time adequate to evaluate change in HbA_{1c} (3 months) unless glycemic control deteriorates.

MONOTHERAPY

Pioglitazone HCl monotherapy in patients not adequately controlled with diet and exercise may be initiated at 15 or 30 mg once daily. For patients who respond inadequately to the initial dose of pioglitazone HCl, the dose can be increased in increments up to 45 mg once daily. For patients not responding adequately to monotherapy, combination therapy should be considered.

COMBINATION THERAPY

Sulfonylureas: Pioglitazone HCl in combination with a sulfonylurea may be initiated at 15 or 30 mg once daily. The current sulfonylurea dose can be continued upon initiation of pioglitazone HCl therapy. If patients report hypoglycemia, the dose of the sulfonylurea should be decreased.

Metformin: Pioglitazone HCl in combination with metformin may be initiated at 15 or 30 mg once daily. The current metformin dose can be continued upon initiation of pioglitazone HCl therapy. It is unlikely that the dose of metformin will require adjustment due to hypoglycemia during combination therapy with pioglitazone HCl.

Insulin: Pioglitazone HCl in combination with insulin may be initiated at 15 or 30 mg once daily. The current insulin dose can be continued upon initiation of pioglitazone HCl therapy. In patients receiving pioglitazone HCl and insulin, the insulin dose can be decreased by 10-25% if the patient reports hypoglycemia or if plasma glucose concentrations decrease to less than 100 mg/dl. Further adjustments should be individualized based on glucose-lowering response.

MAXIMUM RECOMMENDED DOSE

The dose of pioglitazone HCl should not exceed 45 mg once daily since doses higher than 45 mg once daily have not been studied in placebo-controlled clinical studies. No placebo-controlled clinical studies of more than 30 mg once daily have been conducted in combination therapy.

Dose adjustment in patients with renal insufficiency is not recommended (see CLINICAL PHARMACOLOGY, Pharmacokinetics and Drug Metabolism).

Therapy with pioglitazone HCl should not be initiated if the patient exhibits clinical evidence of active liver disease or increased serum transaminase levels (ALT greater than 2.5 times the upper limit of normal) at start of therapy (see PRECAUTIONS, General, Hepatic Effects and CLINICAL PHARMACOLOGY, Special Populations, Hepatic Insufficiency). Liver enzyme monitoring is recommended in all patients prior to initiation of therapy with pioglitazone HCl and periodically thereafter (see PRECAUTIONS, General, Hepatic Effects).

There are no data on the use of pioglitazone HCl in patients under 18 years of age; therefore, use of pioglitazone HCl in pediatric patients is not recommended.

No data are available on the use of pioglitazone HCl in combination with another thiazolidinedione.

ANIMAL PHARMACOLOGY

Heart enlargement has been observed in mice (100 mg/kg), rats (4 mg/kg and above) and dogs (3 mg/kg) treated orally with pioglitazone HCl (approximately 11, 1, and 2 times the maximum recommended human oral dose for mice, rats, and dogs, respectively, based on mg/m^2). In a 1 year rat study, drug-related early death due to apparent heart dysfunction occurred at an oral dose of 160 mg/kg/day (approximately 35 times the maximum recommended human oral dose based on mg/m^2). Heart enlargement was seen in a 13 week study in monkeys at oral doses of 8.9 mg/kg and above (approximately 4 times the maximum recommended human oral dose based on mg/m^2), but not in a 52 week study at oral doses up to 32 mg/kg (approximately 13 times the maximum recommended human oral dose based on mg/m^2).

HOW SUPPLIED

Actos is available in 15, 30, and 45 mg tablets as follows:

15 mg: White to off-white, round, convex, non-scored tablet with "ACTOS" on one side, and "15" on the other.

30 mg: White to off-white, round, flat, non-scored tablet with "ACTOS" on one side, and "30" on the other.

45 mg: White to off-white, round, flat, non-scored tablet with "ACTOS" on one side, and "45" on the other.

Storage: Store at 25°C (77°F); excursions permitted to 15-30°C (59-86°F). Keep container tightly closed, and protect from moisture and humidity.

PRODUCT LISTING - EQUIVALENTS NOT AVAILABLE

Tablet - Oral - 15 mg			
30's	$85.50	ACTOS, Allscripts Pharmaceutical Company	54569-4880-00
30's	$99.90	ACTOS, Takeda Pharmaceuticals America	64764-0151-04
90's	$299.68	ACTOS, Takeda Pharmaceuticals America	64764-0151-05
Tablet - Oral - 30 mg			
30's	$136.90	ACTOS, Allscripts Pharmaceutical Company	54569-4881-00
30's	$159.94	ACTOS, Takeda Pharmaceuticals America	64764-0301-14
90's	$479.84	ACTOS, Takeda Pharmaceuticals America	64764-0301-15
Tablet - Oral - 45 mg			
30's	$148.50	ACTOS, Allscripts Pharmaceutical Company	54569-4882-00
30's	$173.50	ACTOS, Takeda Pharmaceuticals America	64764-0451-24
90's	$520.50	ACTOS, Takeda Pharmaceuticals America	64764-0451-25

Piperacillin Sodium *(002042)*

For related information, see the comparative table section in Appendix A.

Categories: Bacteremia; Cellulitis, pelvic; Endometritis; Gonorrhea; Infection, bone; Infection, gynecologic; Infection, intra-abdominal; Infection, joint; Infection, lower respiratory tract; Infection, skin and skin structures; Infection, urinary tract; Pelvic inflammatory disease; Prophylaxis, perioperative; Septicemia; Pregnancy Category B; FDA Approved 1981 Dec

Drug Classes: Antibiotics, penicillins

Brand Names: Pipracil

Foreign Brand Availability: Acopex (Korea); Avocin (Italy); Cypercil (Philippines); Ivacin (Denmark; Sweden); Pentcillin (Japan); Picillin (Israel; Italy); Picillina (Taiwan); Pipcil (Belgium; Netherlands); Piperacin (Korea); Piperilline (France); Pipracin (Israel); Pipraks (Bahrain; Cyprus; Egypt; Iran; Iraq; Jordan; Kuwait; Lebanon; Libya; Oman; Qatar; Republic-of-Yemen; Saudi-Arabia; Syria; United-Arab-Emirates); Pipril (Australia; Austria; Bahrain; Cyprus; Egypt; Finland; Greece; Hungary; Iran; Iraq; Israel; Jordan; Kuwait; Lebanon; Libya; New-Zealand; Oman; Qatar; Republic-of-Yemen; Saudi-Arabia; South-Africa; Spain; Switzerland; Syria; Taiwan; United-Arab-Emirates); Piprilin (Portugal); Pitamycin (Taiwan)

Cost of Therapy: $884.76 (Infection; Pipracil Injection; 3 g; 12 g/day; 10 day supply)

DESCRIPTION

Piperacillin sodium is a semisynthetic broad-spectrum penicillin for parenteral use derived from D(-)-α-aminobenzylpenicillin. The chemical name of piperacillin sodium is (2S-(2α,5α,6β(S*)))-6-(((((4-ethyl-2,3-dioxo-1-

piperazinyl)carbonyl)amino)phenylacetyl)amino)-3,3-dimethyl-7-oxo-4-thia-1-azabicyclo(3.2.0)heptane-2-carboxylic acid, monosodium salt.

Piperacillin sodium is a white to off-white hygroscopic cryodesiccated crystalline powder which is readily soluble in water and gives a colorless to pale-yellow solution. The pH of the aqueous solution is 5.5-7.5 One (1) g contains 1.85mEq (42.5mg) of sodium (Na+).

Storage: This product should be stored at controlled room temperature 15-30°C (59-86°F).

CLINICAL PHARMACOLOGY

INTRAVENOUS ADMINISTRATION

In healthy adult volunteers, mean serum levels immediately after a 2-3 minute intravenous injection of 2, 4 or 6 g were 305, 412, and 775 µg/ml. Serum levels lack dose proportionally (TABLE 1A and TABLE 1B and TABLE 2A and TABLE 2B).

TABLE 1A *Piperacillin Serum Levels in Adults (µg/ml) After a 2-3 Minute IV Injection*

DOSE	0	10 min	20 min	30 min	1 h	1.5 h
2	305 (159-615)	202 (164-225)	156 (52-165)	67 (41-88)	40 (25-57)	24 (18-31)
4	412 (389-484)	344 (315-379)	295 (269-330)	117 (98-138)	93 (78-110)	60 (50-67)
6	775 (695-849)	609 (530-670)	563 (492-630)	325 (292-363)	208 (180-239)	138 (115-175)

TABLE 1B *Piperacillin Serum Levels in Adults (µg/ml) After a 2-3 Minute IV Injection*

DOSE	2 h	3 h	4 h	6 h	8 h
2	20 (14-24)	8 (3-11)	3 (2-4)	2 (<0.6-3)	—
4	36 (26-51)	20 (17-24)	8 (7-11)	4 (3.7-4.1)	0.9 (0.7-1)
6	90 (71-113)	38 (29-53)	33 (25-44)	8 (3-19)	3.2 (<2-6)

TABLE 2A *Piperacillin Serum Levels in Adults (µg/ml) After a 30 Minute IV Infusion*

DOSE	0	5 min	10 min	15 min	30 min
4	244 (155-298)	215 (169-247)	186 (140-209)	177 (142-213)	141 (122-156)
6	353 (324-371)	298 (242-339)	298 (232-331)	272 (219-314)	229 (185-249)

TABLE 2B *Piperacillin Serum Levels in Adults (µg/ml) After a 30 Minute IV Infusion*

DOSE	45 min	1h	1.5 h	2h	4 h	6 h	7.5 h
4	146 (110-265)	105 (85-133)	72 (53-105)	53 (36-69)	15 (6-24)	4 (1-9)	2 (0.5-3)
6	180 (144-209)	149 (117-171)	104 (89-113)	73 (66-94)	22 (12-39)	1 (5-49)	— —

A 30 minute infusion of 6 g every 6 h gave, on the fourth day, a mean peak serum concentration of 420 µg/ml.

INTRAMUSCULAR ADMINISTRATION

Piperacillin sodium is rapidly absorbed after intramuscular injection. In healthy volunteers, the mean peak serum concentration occurs approximately 30 minutes after a single dose of 2 g and is about 36 µg/ml. The oral administration of 1 g probenecid before injection produces an increase in piperacillin peak serum level of about 30%. The area under the curve (AUC) is increased by approximately 60%.

GENERAL

Piperacillin sodium is not absolved when given orally. Peak serum concentrations ate attained approximately 30 minutes after intramuscular injections and immediately after completion of intravenous injection or infusion. The serum half-life in healthy volunteers ranges from 36 minutes to 1 hour and 12 minutes. The mean elimination half-life of piperacillin sodium in healthy adult volunteers is 54 minutes following administration of 2 g and 63 minutes following 6 g. As with other penicillins, piperacillin sodium is eliminated primarily by glomerular filtration and tubular secretion; it is excreted rapidly as unchanged drug in high concentration in the urine. Approximately 60-80% of the administered dose is excreted in the urine in the first 24 hours. Piperacillin urine concentrations, determined by microbioassay, were as high as 14,100 µg/ml following a 6 g intravenous dose and 8500 µg/ml following a 4 g intravenous dose. These urine drug concentrations remained well above 1000 µg/ml throughout the dosing interval. The elimination half-life is increased 2-fold in mild to moderate renal impairment and 5-fold to 6-fold in severe impairment. Piperacillin sodium binding to human serum proteins is 16%. The drug is widely distributed in human tissues and body fluids, including bone, prostate, and heart and reaches high concentrations in bile. After a 4 gram bolus, maximum biliary concentrations averaged 3205 µg/ml. It penetrates into the cerebrospinal fluid in the presence of inflamed meninges. Because piperacillin sodium is excreted by the biliary route as well as by the renal route, it can be used safely in appropriate dosage (see DOSAGE AND ADMINISTRATION) in patients with severely restricted kidney function, and can be used effectively in treatment of hepatobiliary infections.

MICROBIOLOGY

Piperacillin sodium is an antibiotic which exerts its bactericidal activity by inhibiting both septum and cell wall synthesis. It is active against a variety of gram-positive and gram-negative aerobic and anaerobic bacteria. *In vitro*, piperacillin is active against most strains of clinical isolates of the following microorganisms (TABLE 3).

TABLE 3

Aerobic and Facultatively Anaerobic Organisms

Gram-negative bacteria	
Escherichia coli	*Salmonella* species*
Proteus mirabilis	*Shigella* species*
Proteus vulgaris	*Pseudomonas aeruginosa*
Morganella morganii	*Pseudomonas* species
(formerly *Proteus morganii*)	including *P cepacia*,*
Providencia rettgeri	*P maltophilia,* P fluorescens*
(formerly *Proteus rettgeri*)	*Acinetobacter* species
Serratia species including	(formerly *Mima-herellea*)
S marcescens and *S liquefaciens*	*Haemophilus influenzae* (non-β-lactamase-producing strains)
Klebsiella pneumoniae	*Neisseria gonorrhoeae*
Klebsiella species	*Neisseria meningitidis**
Enterobacter species including	*Moraxella* species*
E aerogenes and *E cloacae*	*Yersinia* species*
Citrobacter species including	(formerly *pasteurella*)
C freundii and *C diversus*	*Streptococcus pneumoniae*
Gram-positive bacteria	*Streptococcus viridans*
Group D streptococci including	*Staphylococcus aureus*
Enterococci (Streptococcus faecalis,	(non-penicillinase-producing)*
S faucium)	*Staphylococcus epidermidis*
Non-enterococci*	(non-penicillinase-producing)*
β-hemolytic streptococci including	*Clostridium* species including
Group A *Streptococcus (S pyogenes)*	*C perfringens* and *C difficile**
Group B *Streptococcus (S agalactiae)*	*Eubacterium* species
Anaerobic bacteria	*Fusobacterium* species
Actinomyces species*	*F nucleatum* and *F necrophorum*
Bacteroides species including	*Peptococcus* species
B fragilis group (*B fragilis*,	*Peptostreptococcus* species
including *B vulgatus)*	*Veillonella* species
Non-*B fragilis* group	
(*B melaninogenicus*)	
*B asaccharolyticus**	

* Piperacillin has been shown to be active *in vitro* against these organisms; however, clinical efficacy has not yet been established.

In vitro, piperacillin sodium is inactivated by staphylococcal β-lactamase and β-lactamase produced by gram-negative bacteria. However, it is active against β-lactamase-producing gonococci. Many strains of gram-negative organisms resistant to certain antibiotics have been found to be susceptible to piperacillin sodium.

Piperacillin sodium has excellent activity against gram-positive organisms, including enterococci (*S faecalis*). It is active against obligate anaerobes such as *Bacteroides* species and also against *C difficile* (which has been associated with pseudomembranous colitis).

Piperacillin is active against many gram-negative bacteria including *Enterobacteriaceae, klebsiella, Serratia, Pseudomonas, E coli, Proteus,* and *Citrobacter*, and, in addition, it is active against anaerobes and enterococci.

In vitro tests show piperacillin to act synergistically with aminoglycoside antibiotics against most isolates of *P aeruginosa*.

SUSCEPTIBILITY TESTING

The use of a 100 µg piperacillin antibiotic disk with susceptibility test methods which measure zone diameter gives an accurate estimation of susceptibility of organisms to piperacillin sodium. The following standard procedure† has been recommended for use with disks for testing antimicrobials. †NCCLS Approved Standard; M2-A2 (Formerly ASM-2) Performance Standards for Antimicrobic Disk Susceptibility Tests, Second Edition, available from the National Committee of Clinical Laboratory Standards.

With this type of procedure, a report of "susceptible" from the laboratory indicates that the infecting organism is likely to respond to therapy. A report of "intermediate susceptibility" suggests that the organism would be susceptible if high dosage is used or if the infection is confined to tissues and fluids (*e.g.,* urine) in which high antibiotic levels are obtained. A report of "resistant" indicates that the infecting organism is not likely to respond to therapy. With the piperacillin disk, a zone of 18 mm or greater indicates susceptibility, zone sizes of 14 mm or less indicate resistance, and zone sizes of 15-17 mm indicate intermediate susceptibility.

Haemophilus and *Neisseria* species which give zones of $\geq$29 mm are susceptible; resistant strains give zones of $\leq$28 mm. The above interpretive criteria are based on the use of the standardized procedure. Antibiotic susceptibility testing requires carefully prescribed procedures. Susceptibility tests are biased to a considerable degree when different methods are used.

The standardized procedure requires the use of control organisms. The 100 µg piperacillin disk should give zone diameters between 24 and 30 mm for *E. coli* ATCC No. 25922 and between 25 and 33 mm for *pseudomonas aeruginosa* ATCC No. 27853.

Dilution methods such as those described in the International Collaborative study‡ have been used to determine susceptibility of organisms to piperacillin sodium.

‡*Acta Pathol Microbial Scand* (B) 1971; suppl 217.

Enterobacteriaceae, Pseudomonas species and *Acinetobacter* sp. are considered susceptible if the minimal inhibitory concentration (MIC) of piperacillin is no greater than 64 µg/ml and are considered resistant if the MIC is greater than 128 µg/ml.

Haemophilus and *Neisseria* species are considered susceptible if the MIC of piperacillin is $\leq$ to 1 µg/ml.

When anaerobic organisms are isolated from infection sites, it is recommended that other tests such as the modified Broth-Disk Method (Wilkins TD and Thiel T: *Antimicrob Agents*

P

Chemother 1973; 3:350-356) be used to determine the antibiotic susceptibility of these slowly growing organisms.

INDICATIONS AND USAGE

Therapeutic: Piperacillin sodium is indicated for the treatment of serious infections caused by susceptible strains of the designated organisms in the conditions as listed below.

Intra-Abdominal Infections: Including hepatobiliary and surgical infections caused by *E. coli, P. aeruginosa*, enterococci, *Clostridium* sp., anaerobic cocci, and *Bacteroides* sp., including *B. fragilis.*

Urinary Tract infections: Caused by *E. coli, Klebsiella* sp., *P. aeruginosa, Proteus* sp., including *P. mirabilis*, and enterococci.

Gynecologic Infections: Including endometritis, pelvic inflammatory disease, pelvic cellulitis caused by *Bacteroides* sp. including *B. fragilis*, anaerobic cocci, *Neisseria gonorrhoeae*, and enterococci (*S. faecalis*). *Septicemia*, including bacteremia caused by *E. coli, Klebsiella* sp., *Enterobacter* sp., *Serratia* sp., *P. mirabilis, S. pneumoniae*, enterococci, *P. aeruginosa, Bacteroides* sp. and anaerobic cocci.

Lower Respiratory Tract Infections: Caused by *E. coli, Klebsiella* sp., *Enterobacter* sp., *Pseudomonas aeruginosa, Serratia* sp., *H. influenzae, Bacteroides* sp., and anaerobic cocci. Although improvement has been noted in patients with cystic fibrosis, lasting bacterial eradication may not necessarily be achieved.

Skin and Skin Structure Infections: Caused by *E. coli, Klebsiella* sp., *Serratia* sp., *Acinetobacter* sp., *Enterobacter* sp., *Pseudomonas aeruginosa*, indole-positive *Proteus* sp., *proteus mirabilis, Bacteroides* sp., including *B. fragilis*, anaerobic cocci, and enterococci.

Bone and Joint Infections: Caused by *P. aeruginosa*, enterococci, *Bacteroides* sp., and anaerobic cocci.

Gonococcal Infections: Piperacillin sodium has been effective in the treatment of uncomplicated gonococcal urethritis.

Piperacillin sodium has also been shown to be clinically effective for the treatment of infections at various sites caused by *Streptococcus* species including Group A β-hemolytic *Streptococcus* and *S. pneumoniae*; however, infections caused by these organisms are ordinarily treated with more narrow spectrum penicillins. Because of its broad spectrum of bactericidal activity against gram-positive and gram-negative aerobic and anaerobic bacteria, piperacillin sodium is particularly useful for the treatment of mixed infections and presumptive therapy prior to the identification of the causative organisms.

Also piperacillin sodium may be administered as single drug therapy in some situations where normally 2 antibiotics might be employed.

Piperacillin has been successfully used with aminoglycosides, especially in patients with impaired host defenses. Both drugs should be used in full therapeutic doses.

Appropriate cultures should be made for susceptibility testing before initiating therapy and therapy adjusted, if appropriate, once the results are known.

PROPHYLAXIS

Piperacillin sodium is indicated for prophylactic use in surgery including intra-abdominal (gastrointestinal and biliary) procedures, vaginal hysterectomy, abdominal hysterectomy, and cesarean section. Effective prophylactic use depends on the time of administration and piperacillin sodium should be given ½-1 hour before the operation so that effective levels can be achieved in the site prior to the procedure.

The prophylactic use of piperacillin should be stopped within 24 hours, since continuing administration of any antibiotic increased the possibility of adverse reactions, but in the majority of surgical procedures, does not reduce the incidence of subsequent infections. If there are signs of infection, specimens for culture should be obtained for identification of the causative organism so that appropriate therapy can be instituted.

P

CONTRAINDICATIONS

A history of allergic reactions to any of the penicillins and/or cephalosporins.

WARNINGS

Serious and occasionally fatal hypersensitivity (anaphylactic) reactions have been reported in patients receiving therapy with penicillins. These reactions are more apt to occur in persons with a history of sensitivity to multiple allergens.

There have been reports of patients with a history of penicillin hypersensitivity who have experienced severe hypersensitivity reactions when treated with a cephalosporin. Before initiating therapy with piperacillin sodium, careful inquiry should be made concerning previous hypersensitivity reactions to penicillins, cephalosporins, and other allergens. If an allergic reaction occurs during therapy with piperacillin sodium, the antibiotic should be discontinued. The usual agents (antihistamines, pressor amines, and corticosteroids) should be readily available. SERIOUS ANAPHYLACTOID REACTIONS REQUIRE IMMEDIATE EMERGENCY TREATMENT WITH EPINEPHRINE. OXYGEN AND INTERVENOUS CORTICOSTEROIDS AND AIRWAY MANAGEMENT INCLUDING INTUBATION SHOULD ALSO BE ADMINISTERED AS NECESSARY.

PRECAUTIONS

GENERAL

While piperacillin possesses the characteristic low toxicity of the penicillin group of antibiotics, periodic assessment of organ system functions including renal, hepatic, and hematopoietic during prolonged therapy is advisable.

Bleeding manifestations have occurred in some patients receiving β-lactam antibiotics, including piperacillin. These reactions have sometimes been associated with abnormalities of coagulation tests such as clotting time, platelet aggregation and prothrombin time and are more likely to occur in patients with renal failure.

If bleeding manifestations occur, the antibiotic should be discontinued and appropriate therapy instituted.

The possibility of the emergence of resistant organisms which might cause superinfections should be kept in mind, particularly during prolonged treatment. If this occurs, appropriate measures should be taken.

As with other penicillins, patients may experience neuromuscular excitability or convulsions if higher than recommended doses are given intravenously.

Piperacillin sodium is a monosodium salt containing 1.85 mEq of Na + per g. This should be considered when treating patients requiring restricted salt intake. Periodic electrolyte determinations should be made in patients with low potassium reserves, and the possibility of hypokalemia should be kept in mind with patients who have potentially low potassium reserves and who are receiving cytotoxic therapy or diuretics.

Antimicrobials used in high doses for short periods to treat gonorrhea may mask or delay the symptoms of incubating syphilis. Therefore, prior to treatment, patients with gonorrhea should also be evaluated for syphilis. Specimens for darkfield examination should be obtained from patients with any suspected primary lesion, and serologic tests should be performed. In all cases where concomitant syphilis is suspected, monthly serological tests should be made for a minimum of 4 months.

As with other semisynthetic penicillins, piperacillin sodium therapy has been associated with an increased incidence of fever and rash in cystic fibrosis patients.

PREGNANCY CATEGORY B

Although reproduction studies in mice and rats performed at doses up to 4 times the human dose have shown no evidence of impaired fertility or harm to the fetus, safety of piperacillin sodium use in pregnant women has not been determined by adequate and well-controlled studies. Because animal reproduction studies are not always predictive of human response, this drug should be used during pregnancy only if clearly needed. It has been found to cross the placenta in rats.

NURSING MOTHERS

Caution should be exercised when piperacillin sodium is administered to nursing mothers. It is excreted in low concentrations in milk.

PEDIATRIC USE

Dosages for children under age of 12 have not been established. The safety of piperacillin sodium in neonates is not known. In dog neonates dilated renal tubules and peritubular hyalinization occurred following administer of piperacillin sodium.

DRUG INTERACTIONS

The mixing of piperacillin with an aminoglycoside *in vitro* can result in substantial inactivation of the aminoglycosides.

ADVERSE REACTIONS

Piperacillin sodium is generally well tolerated. The most common adverse reactions have been local in nature, following intravenous or intramuscular injection.

The following adverse reactions may occur:

Local Reactions: In clinical trials thrombophlebitis was noted in 4% of patients. Pain, erythema, and/or induration at the injection site occurred in 2% of patients. Less frequent reactions including ecchymosis, deep vein thrombosis and hematomas have also occurred.

Gastrointestinal: Diarrhea and loose stools were noted in 2% of patients. Other less frequent reactions included vomiting, nausea, increases in liver enzymes, (LDH, SGOT, SGPT), hyperbilirubinemia, cholestatic hepatitis, bloody diarrhea and, rarely, pseudomembranous colitis.

Hypersensitivity Reactions: Anaphylactoid reactions, see WARNINGS. Rash was noted in 1% patients. Other less frequent findings included pruritus, vesicular eruptions, positive Coombs tests. Other dermatologic manifestations, such as erythema multiforme and Stevens-Johnson syndrome have been reported rarely.

Renal: Elevations of creatinine or BUN, and rarely, interstitial nephritis.

Central Nervous System: Headache, dizziness, fatigue.

Hemic and Lymphatic: Reversible leukopenia, leukopenia, thrombocytopenia and/or eosinophilia have been reported. As with other β-lactam antibiotics, reversible leukopenia (neutropenia) is more apt to occur in patients prolonged therapy at high dosages or in association with drugs known to cause this reaction.

Serum Electrolytes: Individuals with liver disease or individuals receiving cytotoxic therapy or diuretics were reported rarely to demonstrate a decrease in serum potassium concentrations with high of piperacillin.

Skeletal: Rarely, prolonged muscle relaxation.

Other: Superinfection, including candidiasis. Hemorrhagic manifestations.

DOSAGE AND ADMINISTRATION

Piperacillin sodium may be administered by the intramuscular route (see NOTE) or intravenously or given in a 3-5 minute intravenous injection. The usual dosage of piperacillin sodium for serious infections is 3-4 g given every 4-6 hours as a 20-30 minute infusion. For serious infections, the intravenous route should be used.

Piperacillin sodium should not be mixed with an aminoglycoside in a syringe or infusion bottle since this can result in inactivation of the aminoglycoside.

The maximum daily dose for adults is usually 24 g/day, although higher doses have been used. Intramuscular injections (see NOTE) should be limited to 2 g per injection site. This route of administration has been used primarily in the treatment of patients with uncomplicated gonorrhea and urinary tract infections.[1]

NOTE: THE ADD-VANTAGE VAIL IS *NOT* FOR IM USE (TABLE 4).

The average duration of piperacillin sodium treatment is from 7-10 days, except in the treatment of gynecologic infections, in which it is from 3-10 days; the duration should be guided by the patient's clinical and bacteriological progress. For most acute infections, treatment should be continued for at least 48-72 hours after the patient becomes asymptomatic. Antibiotic therapy for group A β-hemolytic streptococcal infections should be maintained for at least 10 days to reduce the risk of rheumatic fever or glomerulonephritis.

When piperacillin sodium is given concurrently with aminoglycosides, both drugs should be used in full therapeutic doses.

Renal Impairment: See TABLE 5.

TABLE 4 *Dosage Recommendations*

Type of Infection	Used Total Daily Dose
Serious infections such as septicemia, nosocomial pneumonia, intraabdominal infections, aerobic and anaerobic gynecologic infections, and skin and soft tissue infections	12-18 g/d IV (200-300 mg/kg/d) in divided doses every 4-6 h
Completed urinary tract infections	8-16 g/d IV (125-200 mg/kg/d) in divided doses every 6-8 h
Uncomplicated urinary tract infections and most community-acquired pneumonia	6-8 g/d IM or IV (100-125 mg/kg/d) in divided doses every 6-12 h
Uncomplicated gonorrhea infections	2 g IM* as a one-time dose

* One (1) g of probenecid given orally ½ hour prior to injection.

TABLE 5 *Dosage in Renal Impairment*

Creatinine Clearance ml/min	Urinary Tract Infection (uncomplicated)	Urinary Tract Infection (complicated)	Serious Systemic Infection
>40	No dosage adjustment necessary		
20-40	No dosage adjustment necessary	9 g/day 3 g every 8 h	12 g/day 4 g every 8 h
<20	6 g/day 3 g every 12 h	6 g/day 3 g every 12 h	8 g/day 4 g every 12 h

For patients on hemodialysis the maximum daily dose is 6 g/day (2 g every 8 h). In addition, because hemodialysis removes 30-50% of piperacillin in 4 hours, 1 g additional dose should be administered following each dialysis period.

For patients with renal failure and hepatic insufficiency, measurement of serum level of piperacillin sodium will provide additional guidance for adjusting dosage.

PROPHYLAXIS

When possible, piperacillin sodium should be administered as a 20-30 minute infusion just prior to anesthesia. Administration while the patient is awake will facilitate identification of possible adverse reactions during drug infusion (see TABLE 6).

TABLE 6

Indication	1st Dose	2nd Dose	3rd Dose
Intra-abdominal Surgery	2g IV just prior to surgery	2g during surgery	2g every 6 h Post-Op for no more than 24 h
Vaginal Hysterectomy	2g IV just prior to surgery	2g 6 h after 1st dose	2g 12 h after 1st dose
Cesarean Section	2g IV after cord is clamped	2g 4 h after 1st dose	2g 8 h after 1st dose
Abdominal Hysterectomy	2g IV just prior to surgery	2g on return to recovery room	2g after 6 h

Infants and Children: Dosage in infants and children under 12 years of age have not been established.

PRODUCT RECONSTITUTION/DOSAGE PREPARATION

Conventional Vials: See TABLE 7.

TABLE 7 *Diluents for Reconstitution*

Sterile water for injection	Sodium chloride injection
Bacteriostatic water for injection	Bacteriostatic sodium
Chloride	
Either parabens or benzyl alcohol	Injection
	Dextrose 5% in water
	Dextrose 5% and 0.9% sodium chloride
	*Lidocaine HCl 0.5-1% (without epinephrine)

* For Intramuscular Use Only. Lidocaine is contraindicated in patients with a known history of hypersensitivity to local anesthetics of the amide type.

Conventional Vials: See TABLE 8.

TABLE 8

Intravenous Solutions	Intravenous Admixtures
Dextrose 5% in water	Normal saline (+ KCI 40 mEq)
0.9% sodium chloride	5% dextrose in water (+ KCI 40mEq)
Dextrose 5% and 0.9% sodium chloride	5% dextrose/normal saline (+ KCI 40 mEq)
Lactated Ringer's injection	Ringer's injection (+ KCI 40mEq)
Dextran 6% in 9% sodium chloride	Lactated Ringer's injection (+ KCI 40 mEq)

ADD-VANTAGEVIALS

ADD-Vantage System Admixtures: Dextrose 5% in water (50 or 100 ml); 0.9% sodium chloride (50 or 100 ml)

INTRAVENOUS ADMINISTRATION

Reconstitution Directions for Conventional Vials

Reconstitute each gram of piperacillin sodium with at least 5 ml of a suitable diluent (except lidocaine HCl 0.5%-1% without epinephrine) listed above. Shake well until dissolved. Reconstituted solution may be further diluted to the desired volume (*e.g.,* 50 or 100 ml) in the above listed intravenous solutions and admixtures.

Reconstitution Directions for ADD-Vantage Vials

See Instruction Sheet provided in box.

Reconstitution Directions for Pharmacy Bulk Vial

Reconstitute the 40 g vial with 172 ml of a suitable diluent (except Lidocaine HCL 0.5%-1% without epinephrine) listed above to achieve a concentration of 1 g per 5 ml.

DIRECTION OF ADMINISTRATION

Intermittent IV Infusion

Infuse diluted solution over period of about 30 minutes. During infusion it is desirable to discontinue the primary intravenous solution.

Intravenous Injection (bolus)

Reconstituted solution should be injected slowly over a 3-5 minute period to help avoid vein irritation.

Intramuscular Administration (conventional vials only)

Reconstitution Direction

Reconstitute each gram of piperacillin sodium with 2 ml of a suitable diluent listed above to achieve a concentration of 1 g per 2.5 ml. Shake well until dissolved.

Direction for Administration

When indicated by clinical and bacteriological findings, intramuscular administration of 6-8 g daily of piperacillin sodium, in divided doses, may be utilized for initiation of therapy. In addition, intramuscular administration of the drug may be considered for maintenance therapy after clinical and bacteriologic improvement has been obtained with intravenous piperacillin sodium treatment. Intramuscular administration should not exceed 2 g per injection at any 1 site.

The preferred site is the upper outer quadrant of the buttock (*i.e.,* gluteus maximus).

The deltoid area should be used only if well-developed, and then caution to avoid radial nerve injury. Intramuscular injections should not be made into the lower or mid-third of the upper arm.

STABILITY OF PIPERACILLIN SODIUM FOLLOWING RECONSTITUTION

Piperacillin sodium is stable in both glass and plastic when reconstituted with recommended diluents when diluted with the intravenous solutions and intravenous admixtures indicated above.

Extensive stability studies have demonstrated chemical stability (potency, pH, and clarity) through 24 hours at room temperature, up to 1 week refrigerated, and up to 1 month frozen (-10-20°). (Note: The 40 g Pharmacy Bulk vial should not be frozen after reconstitution.) Appropriate consideration of aseptic technique and individual hospital policy, however, may recommend discarding unused portions after storage for 48 hours under refrigeration and discarding after 24 hours storage at room temperature.

ADD-VANTAGE SYSTEM

Stability studies with the ad-mixed ADD-Vantage system have demonstrated chemical stability (potency, pH and clarity) through 24 hours at room temperature. (Note: The ad-mixed ADD-Vantage should not be refrigerated or frozen after reconstitution.)

Additional stability data available upon request.

PRODUCT LISTING - EQUIVALENTS NOT AVAILABLE

Powder For Injection - Injectable - 2 Gm

10's	$147.48	PIPRACIL, Wyeth-Ayerst Laboratories	00206-3879-16

Powder For Injection - Injectable - 3 Gm

10's	$221.19	PIPRACIL, Wyeth-Ayerst Laboratories	00206-3882-55
10's	$227.18	PIPRACIL, Wyeth-Ayerst Laboratories	00206-3882-28

Powder For Injection - Injectable - 4 Gm

10's	$294.89	PIPRACIL, Wyeth-Ayerst Laboratories	00206-3880-25
10's	$302.88	PIPRACIL, Wyeth-Ayerst Laboratories	00206-3880-29

Piperacillin Sodium; Tazobactam Sodium *(003186)*

For related information, see the comparative table section in Appendix A.

Categories: Abscess, cutaneous; Appendicitis; Bacteremia; Cellulitis; Cellulitis, pelvic; Endometritis; Gonorrhea; Infection, bone; Infection, gynecologic; Infection, intra-abdominal; Infection, joint; Infection, lower respiratory tract; Infection, skin and skin structures; Infection, urinary tract; Pelvic inflammatory disease; Peritonitis; Pneumonia, community-acquired; Prophylaxis, perioperative; Septicemia; FDA Approved 1993 Oct; Pregnancy Category B

Drug Classes: Antibiotics, penicillins

Brand Names: Tazosyn; **Zosyn**

Foreign Brand Availability: Tazobac (Germany; Switzerland); Tazocel (Spain); Tazocilline (France); Tazocin (Australia; Bahrain; Canada; China; Colombia; Costa-Rica; Cyprus; Dominican-Republic; Egypt; El-Salvador; England; Guatemala; Honduras; Hong-Kong; Indonesia; Iran; Iraq; Ireland; Israel; Jordan; Korea; Kuwait; Lebanon; Libya; Mexico; Netherlands; New-Zealand; Nicaragua; Oman; Panama; Qatar; Republic-of-Yemen; Saudi-Arabia; Singapore; South-Africa; Syria; Taiwan; Thailand; United-Arab-Emirates); Tazopril (Ecuador)

Cost of Therapy: $648.40 (Infection; Zosyn Injection; 3 g; 0.375 g; 12 g/day; 10 day supply)

DESCRIPTION

Note: The trade name has been used throughout this monograph for clarity.

Piperacillin sodium is an injectable antibacterial combination product consisting of the semisynthetic antibiotic piperacillin sodium and the beta-lactamase inhibitor tazobactam sodium for intravenous administration.

Piperacillin sodium is derived from D(-)-α-aminobenzylpenicillin. The chemical name of piperacillin sodium is sodium (2*S*,5*R*,6*R*)-6-[(*R*)-2-(4-ethyl-2,3-dioxo-1-piperazine-carboxyamido)-2-phenylacetamido]-3,3-dimethyl-7-oxo-4-thia-1-azabicyclo[3.2.0]-heptane-2-carboxylate. The chemical formula is $C_{23}H_{26}N_5NaO_7S$ and the molecular weight is 539.5.

Tazobactam sodium, a derivative of the penicillin nucleus, is a penicillinic acid sulfone. Its chemical name is sodium (2*S*,3*S*,5*R*)-3-methyl-7-oxo-3-(1*H*-1,2,3-triazol-1-ylmethyl)-4-thia-1-azabicyclo-[3.2.0]heptane-2-carboxylate-4,4-dioxide. The chemical formula is $C_{10}H_{11}N_4NaO_5S$ and the molecular weight is 322.3.

Zosyn parenteral combination is a white to off-white sterile, cryodesiccated powder consisting of piperacillin and tazobactam as their sodium salts packaged in glass vials. The product does not contain excipients or preservatives.

Each Zosyn 2.25 g single dose vial contains an amount of drug sufficient for withdrawal of piperacillin sodium equivalent to 2 g of piperacillin and tazobactam sodium equivalent to 0.25 g of tazobactam.

Each Zosyn 3.375 g single dose vial contains an amount of drug sufficient for withdrawal of piperacillin sodium equivalent to 3 g of piperacillin and tazobactam sodium equivalent to 0.375 g of tazobactam.

Each Zosyn 4.5 single dose vial contains an amount of drug sufficient for withdrawal of piperacillin sodium equivalent to 4 g of piperacillin and tazobactam sodium equivalent to 0.5 g of tazobactam.

Zosyn is a monosodium salt of piperacillin and a monosodium salt of tazobactam containing a total of 2.35 mEq (54 mg) of Na^+ per gram of piperacillin in the combination product.

Storage: Zosyn vials should be stored at controlled room temperature 15-30°C (59-86°F) prior to reconstitution.

CLINICAL PHARMACOLOGY

Peak plasma concentrations of piperacillin and tazobactam are attained immediately after completion of an intravenous infusion of Zosyn. Piperacillin plasma concentrations, following a 30 minute infusion of Zosyn, were similar to those attained when equivalent doses of piperacillin were administered alone, with mean peak plasma concentrations of approximately 134, 142, and 298 μg/ml for the 2.25 g, 3.375 g, and 4.5 g Zosyn doses, respectively. The corresponding mean peak plasma concentrations of tazobactam were 15 μg/ml, 24 μg/ml, and 34 μg/ml, respectively.

Following a 30 minute IV infusion of 3.375 g Piperacillin STS every 6 hours, steady-state plasma concentrations of piperacillin and tazobactam were similar to those attained after the first dose. In like manner, steady-state plasma concentrations were not different from those attained after the first dose when 2.25 or 4.5 g doses of Piperacillin STS were administered via 30 minute infusion every 6 hours.

Steady-state plasma concentrations after 30 minute infusions every 6 hours are provided in TABLE 1A and TABLE 1B.

Following single or multiple piperacillin STS doses to healthy subjects, the plasma half-life of piperacillin and of tazobactam ranged from 0.7-1.2 hours and were unaffected by dose or duration of infusion.

Piperacillin is metabolized to a minor microbiologically active desethyl metabolite. Tazobactam is metabolized to a single metabolite that lacks pharmacological and antibacterial activities. Both piperacillin and tazobactam are eliminated via the kidney by glomerular filtration and tubular secretion. Piperacillin is excreted rapidly as unchanged drug with 68% of the administered dose excreted in the urine. Tazobactam and its metabolite are eliminated primarily by renal excretion with 80% of the administered dose excreted as unchanged drug and the remainder as the single metabolite. Piperacillin, tazobactam, and desethyl piperacillin are also secreted into the bile.

Both piperacillin and tazobactam are approximately 30% bound to plasma proteins. The protein binding of either piperacillin or tazobactam is unaffected by the presence of the other compound. Protein binding of the tazobactam metabolite is negligible.

Piperacillin and tazobactam are widely distributed into tissues and body fluids including intestinal mucosa, gallbladder, lung, female reproductive tissues (uterus, ovary, and fallopian tube), interstitial fluid, and bile. Mean tissue concentrations are generally 50-100% of those in plasma. Distribution of piperacillin and tazobactam into cerebrospinal fluid is low in subjects with non-inflamed meninges, as with other penicillins.

After the administration of single doses of piperacillin/tazobactam to subjects with renal impairment, the half-life of piperacillin and of tazobactam increases with decreasing creatinine clearance. At creatinine clearance below 20 ml/min, the increase in half-life is 2-fold for piperacillin and 4-fold for tazobactam compared to subjects with normal renal function. Dosage adjustments for Piperacillin STS are recommended when creatinine clearance is below 40 ml/min in patients receiving the usual recommended daily dose of Piperacillin STS. (See DOSAGE AND ADMINISTRATION for specific recommendations for the treatment of patients with renal insufficiency.)

Hemodialysis removes 30-40% of a piperacillin/tazobactam dose with an additional 5% of the tazobactam dose removed as the tazobactam metabolite. Peritoneal dialysis removes approximately 6% and 21% of the piperacillin and tazobactam doses, respectively, with up to 16% of the tazobactam dose removed as the tazobactam metabolite. For dosage recommendation for patients undergoing hemodialysis, see DOSAGE AND ADMINISTRATION.

The half-life of piperacillin and of tazobactam increases by approximately 25% and 18%, respectively, in patients with hepatic cirrhosis compared to healthy subjects. However, this difference does not warrant dosage adjustment of Piperacillin STS due to hepatic cirrhosis.

METABOLISM

Piperacillin sodium exerts bactericidal activity by inhibiting septum formation and cell wall synthesis. *In vitro*, piperacillin is active against a variety of gram-positive and gram-negative aerobic and anaerobic bacteria. Tazobactam sodium, which has very little intrinsic microbiologic activity due to its very low level of binding to penicillin-binding proteins, is a β-lactamase inhibitor of the Richmond-Sykes class III (Bush class 2b & 2b′) penicillinases and cephalosporinases. It varies in its ability to inhibit class II and IV (2a & 4) penicillinases. Tazobactam does not induce chromosomally-mediated β-lactamases at tazobactam levels achieved with the recommended dosing regimen.

TABLE 1A *Steady State Mean Plasma Concentrations In Adults After 30 Minute Intravenous Infusion of Piperacillin/Tazobactam Every 6 Hours*

Piperacillin

	Piperacillin/Tazobactam* Dose		
	2.25 g **n=8**	**3.375 g** **n=6**	**4.5 g** **n=8**
Plasma Concentrations (μg/ml)			
30 minutes	134 (14)	242 (12)	298 (14)
1 hour	57 (14)	106 (8)	141 (19)
2 hours	17.1 (23)	34.6 (20)	46.6 (28)
3 hours	5.2 (32)	11.5 (19)	16.4 (29)
4 hours	2.5 (35)	5.1 (22)	6.9 (29)
6 hours	0.9 (14)†	1.0 (10)	1.4 (30)
AUC(0-6) (μg·h/ml)	131 (14)	242 (10)	322 (16)

* Piperacillin and tazobactam were given in combination.
† n=4
Note: Numbers in parentheses are coefficients of variation (%CV).

TABLE 1B *Steady State Mean Plasma Concentrations In Adults After 30 Minute Intravenous Infusion of Piperacillin/Tazobactam Every 6 Hours*

Tazobactam

	Piperacillin/Tazobactam* Dose		
	2.25 g **n=8**	**3.375 g** **n=6**	**4.5 g** **n=8**
Plasma Concentrations (μg/ml)			
30 minutes	14.8 (14)	24.2 (14)	33.8 (15)
1 hour	7.2 (22)	10.7 (7)	17.3 (16)
2 hours	2.6 (30)	4.0 (18)	6.8 (24)
3 hours	1.1 (35)	1.4 (21)	2.8 (25)
4 hours	0.7 (6)†	1.4 (16)‡	1.3 (30)
6 hours	<0.5	<0.5	<0.5
AUC(0-6) (μg·h/ml)	16.0 (21)	25.0 (8)	39.8 (15)

* Piperacillin and tazobactam were given in combination.
† n=3
‡ n=4
Note: Numbers in parentheses are coefficients of variation (%CV).

Piperacillin/tazobactam has been shown to be active against most strains of the following piperacillin resistant β-lactamase producing microorganisms both *in vitro* and in clinical infections as described in INDICATIONS AND USAGE.

Gram-Positive Aerobes:

Staphylococcus aureus (NOT methicillin-resistant strains)

Gram-Negative Aerobes:

Escherichia coli
Haemophilus influenzae (NOT ampicillin-resistant β-lactamase negative strains)

Gram-Negative Anaerobes:

Bacteroides fragilis group (*B. fragilis, B. ovatus, B. thetaiotaomicron*, or *B. vulgatus*)

The following *in vitro* data are available; **but their clinical significance is unknown.**

Piperacillin/tazobactam exhibits *in vitro* minimal inhibitory concentrations (MICs) of 16 μg/ml or less against most (≥90%) strains of the following microorganisms (or MICs of 1 μg/ml or less against *Haemophilus* species or *Neisseria* species or MICs of 8 μg/ml or less against *Staphylococcus* species); however, the safety and effectiveness of piperacillin/tazobactam in treating clinical infections due to these microorganisms have not been established in adequate and well-controlled clinical trials.

Gram-Positive Aerobes:

*Enterococcus faecalis**
Staphylococcus epidermis (NOT methicillin/oxacillin-resistant strains)
*Streptococcus agalactiae**
*Streptococcus pneumoniae**
*Streptococcus pyogenes**
Viridans group *streptococci**

* These are not beta-lactamase producing strains and, therefore, are susceptible to piperacillin alone.

Gram-Negative Anaerobes:

Klebsiella oxytoca
Klebsiella pneumoniae
Klebsiella catarrhalis
Morganella morganii
Neisseria gonorrhoeae
Neisseria meningitidis
Proteus mirabilis
Proteus vulgaris
Serratia marcescens

Gram-Positive Anaerobes:

Bacteroides distasonis
Fusobacterium nucleatum
Prevotella melaninogenica (formerly *Bacteroides melaninogenicus*)

SUSCEPTIBILITY TESTING

Dilution Techniques

Quantitative methods that are used to determine minimum inhibitory concentrations provide reproducible estimates of the susceptibility of bacteria to antimicrobial compounds. One such standardized procedure uses a dilution method[1] (broth, agar, or microdilution) or equivalent with piperacillin and tazobactam standard powders. MIC values should be determined using serial dilutions of piperacillin combined with a fixed concentration of 4 μg/ml tazobactam. The MIC values obtained should be interpreted according to the criteria found in TABLE 2.

TABLE 2

MIC (μg/ml)	Interpretation
For *Enterobacteriaceae:*	
≤16	Susceptible (S)
32-64	Intermediate (I)
≤128	Resistant (R)
For *Haemophilus* species:	
≤1	Susceptible (S)
≥2	Resistant (R)
For *Staphylococcus* species:	
≤8	Susceptible (S)
≥16	Resistant (R)

A report of "Susceptible" indicates that the pathogen is likely to be inhibited by usually achievable concentrations of the antimicrobial compound in the blood. A report of "Intermediate" indicates that the result should be considered equivocal, and, if the microorganism is not fully susceptible to alternative, clinically feasible drugs, the test should be repeated. This category implies clinical applicability in body sites where the drug is physiologically concentrated or in situations where high dosage of drug can be used. This category also provides a buffer zone that prevents small uncontrolled technical factors from causing major discrepancies in interpretation. A report of "Resistant" indicates that usually achievable concentrations of the antimicrobial compound in the blood are unlikely to be inhibitory and other therapy should be selected.

Measurement of MIC or MBC and achieved compound concentrations may be appropriate to guide therapy in some infections. (See CLINICAL PHARMACOLOGY for further information on drug concentrations achieved in infected body sites and other pharmacokinetic properties of this antimicrobial product.)(See TABLE 3.)

TABLE 3

Microorganism	Zone Diameter
Escherichia coli ATCC 25922	1-4 mm
Escherichia coli ATCC 35218	0.5-2 mm
Haemophilus influenzae ATCC 49247	0.06-0.5 mm
Staphylococcus aureus ATCC 29213	0.25-2 mm

Anaerobic Techniques

For anaerobic bacteria, the susceptibility to piperacillin/tazobactam can be determined by the reference agar dilution method or by alternate standardized test methods.[2]

For *Bacteroides* species, the dilution and zone diameters should be interpreted as seen in TABLE 4.

TABLE 4

MIC (μg/ml)	Interpretation
≤16	Susceptible (S)
≥32	Resistant (R)

Serial dilutions of piperacillin combined with a fixed concentration of 4 μg/ml tazobactam should provide the MIC values found in TABLE 5.

TABLE 5

Microorganism	MIC (μg/ml)
Bacteroides fragilis ATCC 25285	0.12-0.5
Bacteroides thetaiotaomicron ATCC 29741	4-16

Diffusion Techniques

Quantitative methods that require measurement of zone diameters provide reproducible estimates of the susceptibility of bacteria to antimicrobial compounds. One such standardized procedure[3] that has been recommended for use with disks to test the susceptibility of microorganisms to piperacillin/tazobactam uses the 100 μg/10 μg piperacillin/tazobactam disk. Interpretation involves correlation of the diameter obtained in the disk test with the MIC for piperacillin/tazobactam.

Reports from the laboratory giving results of the standard single-disk susceptibility test 100 μg/10 μg piperacillin/tazobactam disk should be interpreted according to the criteria found in TABLE 6.

Interpretation is as stated above for results using dilution techniques.

As with standardized dilution techniques, diffusion susceptibility test procedures require the use of laboratory control microorganisms. The 100 μg/10 μg piperacillin/tazobactam disk should give the following zone diameters in these laboratory test quality control strains (TABLE 7).

TABLE 6

Zone Diameter (mm)	Interpretation
For *Enterobacteriaceae:*	
≥21	Susceptible (S)
18-20	Intermediate (I)
≤17	Resistant (R)
For *Staphylococcus* species:	
≥20	Susceptible (S)
≤19	Resistant (R)

TABLE 7

Microorganism	Zone Diameter
Escherichia coli ATCC 25922	24-30 mm
Escherichia coli ATCC 35218	24-30 mm
Staphylococcus aureus ATCC 25923	27-36 mm

INDICATIONS AND USAGE

Piperacillin STS is indicated for the treatment of patients with moderate to severe infections caused by piperacillin resistant, piperacillin/tazobactam susceptible, β-lactamase producing strains of the designated microorganisms in the specified conditions listed below:

Appendicitis (complicated by rupture or abscess) and peritonitis caused by piperacillin resistant, β-lactamase producing strains of *Escherichia coli* or the following members of the *Bacteroides fragilis* group: *B. fragilis, B. ovatus, B. thetaiotaomicron,* or *B. vulgatus.* The individual members of this group were studied in less than 10 cases.

Uncomplicated and complicated skin and skin structure infections, including cellulitis, cutaneous abscesses, and ischemic/diabetic foot infections caused by piperacillin resistant, β-lactamase producing strains of *Staphylococcus aureus.*

Postpartum endometritis or pelvic inflammatory disease caused by piperacillin resistant, β-lactamase producing strains of *Escherichia coli.*

Community-acquired pneumonia (moderate severity only) caused by piperacillin resistant, β-lactamase producing strains of *Haemophilus influenzae.*

Clinical trial data for the treatment of complicated urinary tract infections demonstrated inadequate efficacy at the dosage regimen of Piperacillin STS studied (*i.e.,* 3.375 g every 8 hours). There are no other adequate and well controlled trial data to support the use of this product in the treatment of complicated urinary tract infections.

A study for the treatment of nosocomial lower respiratory tract infections was initiated with Piperacillin STS as monotherapy at 3.375 g every 6 hours. This study was terminated because of an unacceptable level of efficacy at this dosage.

As a combination product, Piperacillin STS is indicated only for the specified conditions listed above. Infections caused by piperacillin susceptible organisms for which piperacillin has been shown to be effective are also amenable to Piperacillin STS treatment due to its piperacillin content. The tazobactam component of this combination product does not decrease the activity of the piperacillin component against piperacillin susceptible organisms. Therefore, the treatment of mixed infections caused by piperacillin susceptible organisms and piperacillin resistant, β-lactamase producing organisms susceptible to Piperacillin STS should not require the addition of another antibiotic.

Piperacillin STS is useful as presumptive therapy in the indicated conditions prior to the identification of causative organisms because of its broad spectrum of bactericidal activity against gram-positive and gram-negative anaerobic organisms.

Appropriate cultures should usually be performed before initiating antimicrobial treatment in order to isolate and identify the organisms causing infection and to determine their susceptibility to Piperacillin STS. Antimicrobial therapy should be adjusted, if appropriate, once the results of culture(s) and antimicrobial susceptibility testing are known.

CONTRAINDICATIONS

Piperacillin STS is contraindicated in patients with a history of allergic reactions to any of the penicillins, cephalosporins, or β-lactamase inhibitors.

WARNINGS

SERIOUS AND OCCASIONALLY FATAL HYPERSENSITIVITY (ANAPHYLACTIC) REACTIONS HAVE BEEN REPORTED IN PATIENTS IN PENICILLIN THERAPY. THESE REACTIONS ARE MORE LIKELY TO OCCUR IN INDIVIDUALS WITH A HISTORY OF PENICILLIN HYPERSENSITIVITY OR A HISTORY OF SENSITIVITY TO MULTIPLE ALLERGENS. THERE HAVE BEEN REPORTS OF INDIVIDUALS WITH A HISTORY OF PENICILLIN HYPERSENSITIVITY WHO HAVE EXPERIENCED SEVERE REACTIONS WHEN TREATED WITH CEPHALOSPORINS. BEFORE INITIATING THERAPY WITH PIPERACILLIN STS, CAREFUL INQUIRY SHOULD BE MADE CONCERNING PREVIOUS HYPERSENSITIVITY REACTIONS TO PENICILLINS, CEPHALOSPORINS, OR OTHER ALLERGENS. IF AN ALLERGIC REACTION OCCURS, PIPERACILLIN STS SHOULD BE DISCONTINUED AND APPROPRIATE THERAPY INSTITUTED. **SERIOUS ANAPHYLACTIC REACTIONS REQUIRE IMMEDIATE EMERGENCY TREATMENT WITH EPINEPHRINE. OXYGEN, INTRAVENOUS STEROIDS, AND AIRWAY MANAGEMENT, INCLUDING INTUBATION, SHOULD ALSO BE ADMINISTERED AS INDICATED.**

Pseudomembranous colitis has been reported with nearly all antibacterial agents, including piperacillin/tazobactam, and may range in severity from mild to life-threatening. Therefore, it is important to consider this diagnosis in patients who present with diarrhea subsequent to the administration of antibacterial agents.

Treatment with antibacterial agents alters the normal flora of the colon and may permit overgrowth of clostridia. Studies indicate that a toxin produced by *Clostridium difficile* is one primary cause of "antibiotic-associated colitis."

After the diagnosis of pseudomembranous colitis has been established, therapeutic measures should be initiated. Mild cases of pseudomembranous colitis usually respond to drug discontinuation alone. In moderate to severe cases, consideration should be given to management with fluids and electrolytes, protein supplementation, and treatment with an antibacterial drug clinically effective against *Clostridium difficile* colitis.

PRECAUTIONS

GENERAL

Bleeding manifestations have occurred in some patients receiving β-lactam antibiotics, including piperacillin. These reactions have sometimes been associated with abnormalities of coagulation tests such as clotting time, platelet aggregation, and prothrombin time and are more likely to occur in patients with renal failure. If bleeding manifestations occur, Piperacillin STS should be discontinued and appropriate therapy instituted.

The possibility of the emergence of resistant organisms that might cause superinfections should be kept in mind. If this occurs, appropriate measures should be taken.

As with other penicillins, patients may experience neuromuscular excitability or convulsions if higher than recommended doses are given intravenously (particularly in the presence of renal failure).

Piperacillin STS is a monosodium salt of piperacillin and a monosodium salt of tazobactam and contains a total of 2.35 mEq (54 mg) of Na^+ per gram of piperacillin in the combination product. This should be considered when treating patients requiring restricted salt intake. Periodic electrolyte determinations should be performed in patients with low potassium reserves, and the possibility of hypokalemia should be kept in mind with patients who have potentially low potassium reserves and who are receiving cytotoxic therapy for diuretics.

As with other semisynthetic penicillins, piperacillin therapy has been associated with an increased incidence of fever and rash in cystic fibrosis patients.

LABORATORY TESTS

Periodic assessment of hematopoietic function should be performed, especially with prolonged therapy, (*i.e.*, ≥21 days). (See ADVERSE REACTIONS, Adverse Laboratory Events.)

DRUG/LABORATORY TEST INTERACTIONS

As with other penicillins, the administration of Piperacillin STS may result in a false-positive reaction for glucose in the urine using a copper-reduction method (Clinitest). It is recommended that glucose tests based on enzymatic glucose oxidase reactions (such as Diastix or Tes-Tape) be used.

CARCINOGENESIS, MUTAGENESIS, AND IMPAIRMENT OF FERTILITY

Long term carcinogenicity studies in animals have not been conducted with piperacillin/tazobactam, piperacillin, or tazobactam.

Piperacillin/Tazobactam

Piperacillin/tazobactam was negative in microbial mutagenicity assays at concentrations up to 14.84/1.86 μg/plate. Piperacillin/tazobactam was negative in the unscheduled DNA synthesis (UDS) test at concentrations up to 5689/711 μg/ml. Piperacillin/tazobactam was negative in a mammalian point mutation (Chinese hamster ovary cell HPRT) assay at concentrations up to 8000/1000 μg/ml. Piperacillin/tazobactam was negative in a mammalian cell (BALB/c-3T3) transformation assay at concentrations up to 8/1 μg/ml.*In vivo,* piperacillin/tazobactam did not induce chromosomal aberrations in rats dosed IV with 1500/187.5 mg/kg; this dose is similar to the maximum recommended human daily dose on a body-surface-area basis (mg/m^2).

Piperacillin

Piperacillin was negative in microbial mutagenicity assays at concentrations up to 50 μg/plate. There was no DNA damage in bacteria (Rec assay) exposed to piperacillin at concentrations up to 200 μg/disk. Piperacillin was negative in the UDS test at concentrations up to 10,000 μg/ml. In a mammalian point mutation (mouse lymphoma cells) assay, piperacillin was positive at concentrations ≥2500 μg/ml. Piperacillin was negative in a cell (BALB/c-3T3) transformation assay at concentrations up to 3000 μg/ml. *In vivo,* piperacillin did not induce chromosomal aberrations in mice at IV doses up to 1500 mg/kg/day. These doses are half (mice) or similar (rats) to the maximum recommended human daily dose based on body-surface area (mg/m^2). In another *in vivo* test, there was no dominant lethal effect when piperacillin was administered to rats at IV doses up to 2000 mg/kg/day, which is similar to the maximum recommended human daily dose based on body-surface area (mg/m^2). When mice were administered piperacillin at IV doses up to 2000 mg/kg/day, which is half the maximum recommended human daily dose based on body-surface area (mg/m^2), urine from these animals was not mutagenic when tested in a microbial mutagenicity assay. Bacteria injected into the peritoneal cavity of mice administered piperacillin at IV doses up to 2000 mg/kg/day did not show increased mutation frequencies.

Tazobactam

Tazobactam was negative in microbial mutagenicity assays at concentrations up to 330 μg/plate. Tazobactam was negative in the UDS test at concentrations up to 2000 μg/ml. Tazobactam was negative in a mammalian point mutation (Chinese hamster ovary cell HPRT) assay at concentrations up to 5000 μg/ml. In another mammalian point mutation (mouse lymphoma cells) assay, tazobactam was positive at concentrations ≥3000 μg/ml. Tazobactam was negative in a cell (BALB/c-3T3) transformation assay at concentrations up to 900 μg/ml. In an *in vitro* cytogenetics (Chinese hamster lung cells) assay, tazobactam was negative at concentrations up to 3000 μg/ml. *In vivo,* tazobactam did not induce chromosomal aberrations in rats at IV doses up to 5000 mg/kg, which is 23 times the maximum recommended human daily dose based on body-surface area (mg/m^2).

PREGNANCY CATEGORY B

Piperacillin/Tazobactam

Reproduction studies have performed in rats and have revealed no evidence of impaired fertility due to piperacillin/tazobactam administered up to a dose which is similar to the maximum recommended human daily dose based on body-surface area (mg/m^2).

Teratology studies have been performed in mice and rats and have revealed no evidence of harm to the fetus due to piperacillin/tazobactam administered up to a dose which is 1-2 times and 2-3 times the human dose of piperacillin and tazobactam, respectively, based on body-surface area (mg/m^2).

Piperacillin

Reproduction and teratology studies have been performed in mice and rats and have revealed no evidence of impaired fertility or harm to the fetus due to piperacillin administered up to a dose which is half (mice) or similar (rats) to the maximum recommended human daily dose based on body-surface area (mg/m^2).

Tazobactam

Reproduction studies have been performed in rats and have revealed no evidence of harm to the fetus due to tazobactam administered at doses up to 3 times the maximum recommended human daily dose based on body-surface area (mg/m^2).

Teratology studies have been performed in mice and rats and have revealed no evidence of harm to the fetus due to tazobactam administered at doses up to 6 and 14 times, respectively, the human dose based on body-surface area (mg/m^2). In rats, tazobactam crosses the placenta. Concentrations in the fetus are less than or equal to 10% of that found in maternal plasma.

There are, however, no adequate and well-controlled studies with the piperacillin/tazobactam combination or with piperacillin or tazobactam alone in pregnant women. Because animal reproduction studies are not always predictive of the human response, this drug should be used during pregnancy only if clearly needed.

NURSING MOTHERS

Piperacillin is excreted in low concentrations in human milk; tazobactam concentrations in human milk have not been studied. Caution should be exercised when Piperacillin STS is administered to a nursing woman.

PEDIATRIC USE

Safety and efficacy in children below the age of 12 years have not been established.

GERIATRIC USE

Patients over 65 years are **not** at an increased risk of developing adverse effects solely because of age. However, dosage should be adjusted in the presence of renal insufficiency. (See DOSAGE AND ADMINISTRATION.)

DRUG INTERACTIONS

AMINOGLYCOSIDES

The mixing of Piperacillin STS with an aminoglycoside *in vitro* can result in substantial inactivation of the aminoglycoside. (See DOSAGE AND ADMINISTRATION, Compatible Intravenous Diluents.)

When Piperacillin STS is co-administered with tobramycin, the area under the curve, renal clearance, and urinary recovery of tobramycin were decreased by 11%, 32%, and 38%, respectively. The alterations in the pharmacokinetics of tobramycin when administered in combination with piperacillin/tazobactam may be due to *in vivo* and *in vitro* inactivation of tobramycin in the presence of piperacillin/tazobactam. The inactivation of aminoglycosides in the presence of penicillin class drugs has been recognized. It has been postulated that penicillin-aminoglycoside complexes form; these complexes are microbiologically inactive and of unknown toxicity. In patients with severe renal dysfunction (*i.e.*, chronic hemodialysis patients), the pharmacokinetics of tobramycin are significantly altered when tobramycin is administered in combination with piperacillin.[4] The alteration of tobramycin pharmacokinetics and the potential toxicity of the penicillin-aminoglycoside complexes in patients with mild to moderate renal dysfunction who are administered an aminoglycoside in combination with piperacillin/tazobactam is unknown.

PROBENECID

Probenecid administered concomitantly with Piperacillin STS prolongs the half-life of piperacillin by 21% and of tazobactam by 71%.

VANCOMYCIN

No pharmacokinetic interactions have been noted between Piperacillin STS and vancomycin.

HEPARIN

Coagulation parameters should be tested more frequently and monitored regularly during simultaneous administration of high doses of heparin, oral anticoagulants, or other drugs that may affect the blood coagulation system or the thrombocyte function.

VECURONIUM

Piperacillin when used concomitantly with vecuronium has been implicated in the prolongation of the neuromuscular blockade of vecuronium. Piperacillin STS (piperacillin/tazobactam) could produce the same phenomenon if given along with vecuronium. Due to their similar mechanism of action, it is expected that the neuromuscular blockade produced by any of the non-depolarizing muscle relaxants could be prolonged in the presence of piperacillin (See monograph for vecuronium bromide).

ADVERSE REACTIONS

During the clinical investigations, 2621 patients worldwide were treated with Piperacillin STS in phase 3 trials. In the key North American clinical trials (n=830 patients), 90% of the adverse events reported were mild to moderate in severity and transient in nature. However, in 3.2% of the patients treated worldwide, Piperacillin STS was discontinued because of adverse events primarily involving the skin (1.3%), including rash and pruritus; the gastrointestinal system (0.9%), including diarrhea, nausea, and vomiting; and allergic reactions (0.5%).

Adverse local reactions that were reported, irrespective of relationship to therapy with Piperacillin STS, were phlebitis (1.3%), injection site reaction (0.5%), pain (0.2%), inflammation (0.2%), thrombophlebitis (0.2%), and edema (0.1%).

ADVERSE CLINICAL EVENTS

Based on patients from the North American trials (n=1063), the events with the highest incidence in patients, irrespective of relationship to Piperacillin STS therapy, were diarrhea (11.3%); headache (7.7%); constipation (7.7%); nausea (6.9%); insomnia (6.6%); rash (4.2%), including maculopapular, bullous, urticarial, and eczematoid; vomiting (3.3%); dyspepsia (3.3%); pruritus (3.1%); stool changes (2.4%); fever (2.4%); agitation (2.1%); pain (1.7%); moniliasis (1.6%); hypertension (1.6%); dizziness (1.4%); abdominal pain (1.3%); chest pain (1.3%); edema (1.2%); anxiety (1.2%); rhinitis (1.2%); and dyspnea (1.1%).

Additional adverse systemic clinical events reported in 1.0% or less of the patients are listed below within each body system:

Autonomic Nervous System: Hypotension, ileus, syncope.
Body as a Whole: Rigors, back pain, malaise.
Cardiovascular: Tachycardia, including supraventricular and ventricular; bradycardia; arrhythmia, including atrial fibrillation, ventricular fibrillation, cardiac arrest, cardiac failure, circulatory failure, myocardial infarction.
Central Nervous System: Tremor, convulsions, vertigo.
Gastrointestinal: Melena, flatulence, hemorrhage, gastritis, hiccough, ulcerative stomatitis.
Pseudomembranous colitis was reported in 1 patient during the clinical trials. The onset of pseudomembranous colitis symptoms may occur during or after antibacterial treatment. (See WARNINGS.)
Hearing: Tinnitus.
Hypersensitivity: Anaphylaxis.
Metabolic and Nutritional: Symptomatic hypoglycemia, thirst.
Musculoskeletal: Myalgia, arthralgia.
Platelet, Bleeding, Clotting: Mesenteric embolism, purpura, epistaxis, pulmonary embolism (see PRECAUTIONS, General).
Psychiatric: Confusion, hallucination, depression.
Reproductive, Female: Leukorrhea, vaginitis.
Respiratory: Pharyngitis, pulmonary edema, bronchospasm, coughing.
Skin and Appendages: Genital pruritus, diaphoresis.
Special Senses: Taste perversion.
Urinary: Retention, dysuria, oliguria, hematuria, incontinence.
Vision: Photophobia.
Vascular (Extracardiac): Flushing.

ADVERSE LABORATORY EVENTS

Changes in laboratory parameters, without regard to drug relationship, include:

Hematologic: Decreases in hemoglobin and hematocrit, thrombocytopenia, increases in platelet count, eosinophilia, leukopenia, neutropenia. The leukopenia/neutropenia associated with Piperacillin STS administration appears to be reversible and most frequently associated with prolonged administration, (*i.e.,* ≥21 days of therapy). These patients were withdrawn from therapy; some had accompanying systemic symptoms (*e.g.,* fever, rigors, chills).
Coagulation: Positive direct Coombs' test, prolonged prothrombin time, prolonged partial thromboplastin time.
Hepatic: Transient elevations of AST (SGOT), ALT (SGPT), alkaline phosphatase, bilirubin.
Renal: Increases in serum creatinine, blood urea nitrogen.
Urinalysis: Proteinuria, hematuria, pyuria.

Additional laboratory events include abnormalities in electrolytes (*i.e.,* increases and decreases in sodium, potassium, and calcium), hyperglycemia, decreases in total protein or albumin.

The following adverse reactions have also been reported for sterile piperacillin sodium:

Skin and Appendages: Erythema multiforme and Stevens-Johnson syndrome, rarely reported.
Gastrointestinal: Cholestatic hepatitis.
Renal: Rarely, interstitial hepatitis.
Skeletal: Prolonged muscle relaxation (see DRUG INTERACTIONS).

DOSAGE AND ADMINISTRATION

Piperacillin STS should be administered by intravenous administration over 30 minutes.

The usual total daily dose of Piperacillin STS for adults is 12 g/1.5 g, given as 3.375 g every 6 hours.

RENAL INSUFFICIENCY

In patients with renal insufficiency, the intravenous dose should be adjusted to the degree of actual renal function impairment. The recommended daily doses are as in TABLE 8.

TABLE 8

Creatinine Clearance	Recommended Dosage Regimen
>40 ml/min	12 g/1.5 g/day in divided doses of 3.375 g q6h
20-40 ml/min	8 g/1.0 g/day in divided doses of 2.25 g q6h
<20 ml/min	6 g/0.75 g/day in divided doses of 2.25 g q8h

For patients on hemodialysis, the maximum dose is 2.25 g Piperacillin STS q 8 hours. In addition, because hemodialysis removes 30-40% of a Piperacillin STS dose in 4 hours, one additional dose of 0.75 g Piperacillin STS should be administered following each dialysis period. For patients with renal failure, measurement of serum levels of piperacillin and tazobactam will provide additional guidance for adjusting dosage.

DURATION OF THERAPY

The usual duration of Piperacillin STS treatment is from 7 to 10 days. The duration should be guided by the severity of the infection and the patient's clinical and bacteriological progress.

INTRAVENOUS ADMINISTRATION

Reconstitute Piperacillin STS per gram of piperacillin with 5 ml of a compatible reconstitution diluent from the list provided below. Shake well until dissolved. Single dose vials should be used immediately after reconstitution. Discard any unused portion after 24 hours if stored at room temperature, or after 48 hours if stored at refrigerated temperature [2-8°C (36-46°F)].

COMPATIBLE INTRAVENOUS DILUENTS

0.9% sodium chloride for injection; sterile water for injection; dextrose 5%; bacteriostatic saline/parabens; bacteriostatic water/parabens; bacteriostatic saline/benzyl alcohol; and bacteriostatic water/benzyl alcohol.

Reconstituted Piperacillin STS solution should be further diluted (recommended volume per dose of 50-150 ml) in a compatible intravenous diluent solution listed below. Administer by infusion over a period of at least 30 minutes. During the infusion it is desirable to discontinue the primary infusion solution.

COMPATIBLE INTRAVENOUS DILUENT SOLUTIONS

0.9% sodium chloride for injection; sterile water for injection; dextrose 5%; and dextran 6% in saline.

Maximum recommended volume per dose of sterile water for injection is 50 ml.

LACTATED RINGERS SOLUTION IS NOT COMPATIBLE WITH PIPERACILLIN STS

When concomitant therapy with aminoglycosides is indicated, Piperacillin STS and the aminoglycoside should be reconstituted and administered separately, due to the *in vitro* inactivation of aminoglycoside by the penicillin. (See DRUG INTERACTIONS.)

Piperacillin STS can be used in ambulatory intravenous infusion pumps.

STABILITY OF PIPERACILLIN STS FOLLOWING RECONSTITUTION

Piperacillin STS is stable in glass and plastic containers (plastic syringes, IV bags, and tubing) when reconstituted with acceptable diluents.

Stability studies in the IV bags have demonstrated chemical stability [potency, pH of reconstituted solution, and clarity of solution] for up to 24 hours at room temperature and up to 1 week at refrigerated temperature. Piperacillin STS contains no preservatives. Appropriate consideration of aseptic technique should not be used.

Stability of Piperacillin STS in an ambulatory intravenous infusion pump has been demonstrated for a period of 12 hours at room temperature. Each dose was reconstituted and diluted to a volume of 37.5 ml or 25 ml. One day supplies of dosing solution were aseptically transferred into the medication reservoir (IV bags or cartridge). The reservoir was fitted to a preprogrammed ambulatory intravenous infusion pump per the manufacturer's instructions. Stability of Piperacillin STS is not affected when administered using an ambulatory intravenous infusion pump.

Parenteral drug products should be inspected visually for particulate matter and discoloration prior to administration, whenever solution and container permit.

PRODUCT LISTING - EQUIVALENTS NOT AVAILABLE

Powder For Injection - Intravenous - 2 Gm;0.25 Gm

10's	$108.08	ZOSYN, Wyeth-Ayerst Laboratories	00206-8452-16
10's	$111.25	ZOSYN, Wyeth-Ayerst Laboratories	00206-8452-17

Powder For Injection - Intravenous - 3 Gm;0.375 Gm

10's	$162.10	ZOSYN, Wyeth-Ayerst Laboratories	00206-8454-55
10's	$165.29	ZOSYN, Wyeth-Ayerst Laboratories	00206-8454-17

Powder For Injection - Intravenous - 4 Gm;0.5 Gm

10's	$205.33	ZOSYN, Wyeth-Ayerst Laboratories	00206-8455-25
10's	$208.35	ZOSYN, Wyeth-Ayerst Laboratories	00206-8455-17

Powder For Injection - Intravenous - 36 Gm;4.5 Gm

1's	$194.55	ZOSYN, Wyeth-Ayerst Laboratories	00206-8620-11

Solution - Intravenous - 2 Gm;0.25 Gm/50 ml

24's	$293.81	ZOSYN, Wyeth-Ayerst Laboratories	00206-8820-02

Solution - Intravenous - 3 Gm;0.375 Gm/50 ml

24's	$440.70	ZOSYN, Wyeth-Ayerst Laboratories	00206-8821-02

Solution - Intravenous - 4 Gm;0.5 Gm/100 ml

12's	$279.13	ZOSYN, Wyeth-Ayerst Laboratories	00206-8822-02

Pirbuterol Acetate *(002046)*

For related information, see the comparative table section in Appendix A.

Categories: Asthma; Pregnancy Category C; FDA Approved 1986 Dec
Drug Classes: Adrenergic agonists; Bronchodilators
Brand Names: **Maxair**
Foreign Brand Availability: Exirel (Austria; Zimbabwe); Spirolair (Belgium)
Cost of Therapy: $40.21 (Asthma; Maxair Autohaler; 0.2 mg/inh; 14 g; 8 inhalations/day; 37 day supply)

DESCRIPTION

The active component of Maxair inhaler is (R,S)α^6-{[(1,1-dimethylethyl)amino]methy}-3-hydroxy-2,6-pyridine-dimethanol monoacetate salt, and is a beta-2 adrenergic bronchodilator.

Pirbuterol acetate is a white, crystalline racemic mixture of two optically active isomers. It is a powder, freely soluble in water, with a molecular weight of 300.3 and empirical formula of $C_{12}H_{20}N_2O_3{\cdot}C_2H_4O_2$.

Maxair inhaler is a metered dose aerosol unit for oral inhalation. It provides a fine-particle suspension of pirbuterol acetate in the propellant mixture of trichloromonofluoromethane and dichlorodifluoromethane, with sorbitan trioleate. Each actuation delivers from the mouthpiece pirbuterol acetate equivalent to 0.2 mg of pirbuterol with the majority of particles less than 5 microns in diameter. Each canister provides at least 300 inhalations.

P

CLINICAL PHARMACOLOGY

In vitro studies and *in vivo* pharmacologic studies have demonstrated that pirbuterol acetate has preferential effect on beta-2 adrenergic receptors compared with isoproterenol. While it is recognized that beta-2 adrenergic receptors are the predominant receptors in bronchial smooth muscle, recent data indicate that there is a population of beta-2 receptors in the human heart, existing in a concentration between 10-50%. The precise function of these, however, is not yet established (see WARNINGS).

The pharmacologic effects of beta adrenergic agonist drugs, including pirbuterol acetate, are at least in part attributable to stimulation through beta adrenergic receptors of intracellular adenyl cyclase, the enzyme which catalyzes the conversion of adenosine triphosphate (ATP) to cyclic-3'5'-adenosine monophosphate (c-AMP). Increased c-AMP levels are associated with relaxation of bronchial smooth muscle and inhibition of release of mediators of immediate hypersensitivity from cells, especially from mast cells.

Bronchodilator activity of pirbuterol acetate was manifested clinically by an improvement in various pulmonary function parameters (FEV_1, MMF, PEFR, airway resistance [RAW] and conductance [GA/V_{tg}]).

In controlled double-blind single dose clinical trials, the onset of improvement in pulmonary function occurred within 5 minutes in most patients as determined by forced expiratory volume in one second (FEV_1). FEV_1 and MMF measurements also showed that maximum improvement in pulmonary function generally occurred 30-60 minutes following 1 or 2 inhalations of pirbuterol (0.2-0.4 mg).

The duration of action of pirbuterol acetate is maintained for 5 hours (the time at which the last observations were made) in a substantial number of patients, based on a 15% or greater increase in FEV_1. In controlled repetitive dose studies of 12 weeks' duration, 74% of 156 patients on pirbuterol and 62% of 141 patients on metaproterenol showed a clinically significant improvement based on a 15% or greater increase in FEV_1 on at least half of the days. Onset and duration were equivalent to that seen in single dose studies. Continued effectiveness was demonstrated over the 12 week period in the majority (94%) of responding patients; however, chronic dosing was associated with the development of tachyphylaxis (tolerance) to the bronchodilator effect in some patients in both treatment groups.

A placebo-controlled double-blind single dose study (24 patients per treatment group), utilizing continuous Holter monitoring for 5 hours after drug administration, showed no significant difference in ectopic activity between the placebo control group and pirbuterol acetate at the recommended dose (0.2-0.4 mg), and twice the recommended dose (0.8 mg). As with other inhaled beta adrenergic agonists, supraventricular and ventricular ectopic beats have been seen with pirbuterol acetate (see WARNINGS).

Recent studies in laboratory animals (minipigs, rodents, and dogs) recorded the occurrence of cardiac arrhythmias and sudden death (with histologic evidence of myocardial necrosis) when beta agonists and methylxanthines were administered concurrently. The significance of these findings when applied to humans is currently unknown.

PHARMACOKINETICS

As expected by extrapolation from oral data, systemic blood levels of pirbuterol are below the limit of assay sensitivity (2-5 ng/ml) following inhalation of doses up to 0.8 mg (twice the maximum recommended dose). A mean of 51% of the dose is recovered in urine as pirbuterol plus its sulfate conjugate following administration by aerosol. Pirbuterol is not metabolized by catechol-O-methyltransferase. The percent of administered dose recovered as pirbuterol plus its sulfate conjugate does not change significantly over the dose range of 0.4- 0.8 mg and is not significantly different from that after oral administration of pirbuterol. the plasma half-life measured after oral administration is about 2 hours.

INDICATIONS AND USAGE

Pirbuterol acetate inhaler is indicated for the prevention and reversal of bronchospasm in patients with reversible bronchospasm including asthma. It may be used with or without concurrent theophylline and/or steroid therapy.

CONTRAINDICATIONS

Pirbuterol acetate is contraindicated in patients with a history of hypersensitivity to any of its ingredients.

WARNINGS

As with other beta adrenergic aerosols, pirbuterol acetate should not be used in excess. Controlled clinical studies and other clinical experience have shown that pirbuterol acetate, like other inhaled beta adrenergic agonists, can produce a significant cardiovascular effect in some patients, as measured by pulse rate, blood pressure, symptoms, and/or ECG changes. As with other beta adrenergic aerosols, the potential for paradoxical bronchospasm (which can be life threatening) should be kept in mind. If it occurs, the preparation should be discontinued immediately and alternative therapy instituted.

Fatalities have been reported in association with excessive use of inhaled sympathomimetic drugs.

The contents of pirbuterol acetate inhaler are under pressure. Do not puncture. Do not use or store near heat or open flame. Exposure to temperature above 120°F may cause bursting. Never throw container into fire or incinerator. Keep out of reach of children.

PRECAUTIONS

GENERAL

Since pirbuterol is a sympathomimetic amine, it should be used with caution in patients with cardiovascular disorders, including ischemic heart disease, hypertension, or cardiac arrhythmias, in patients with hyperthyroidism or diabetes mellitus, and in patients who are unusually responsive to sympathomimetic amines or who have convulsive disorders. Significant changes in systolic and diastolic blood pressure could be expected to occur in some patients after use of any beta adrenergic aerosol bronchodilator.

INFORMATION FOR THE PATIENT

Pirbuterol acetate effects may last up to 5 hours or longer. It should not be used more often than recommended and the patient should not increase the number of inhalations or frequency of use without first asking the physician. If symptoms of asthma get worse, adverse reactions occur, or the patient does not respond to the usual dose, the patient should be instructed to contact the physician immediately. The patient should be advised to read the Patient Instructions that are distributed with the prescription.

CARCINOGENESIS, MUTAGENESIS, AND IMPAIRMENT OF FERTILITY

Pirbuterol HCl administered in the diet to rats for 24 months and to mice for 18 months was free of carcinogenic activity at doses corresponding to 200 times the maximum human inhalation dose. In addition, the intragastric intubation of the drug at doses corresponding to 6250 times the maximum recommended human daily inhalation dose resulted in no increase in tumors in a 12 month rat study. Studies with pirbuterol revealed no evidence of mutagenesis. Reproduction studies in rats revealed no evidence of impaired fertility.

PREGNANCY, TERATOGENIC EFFECTS, PREGNANCY CATEGORY C

Reproductions studies have been performed in rats and rabbits by the inhalation route at doses up to 12 times (rat) and 16 times (rabbit) the maximum human inhalation dose and have revealed no significant findings. Animal reproduction studies in rats at *oral doses* up to 300 mg/kg and in rabbits at oral doses up to 100 mg/kg have shown no adverse effect on reproductive behavior, fertility, litter size, peri- and postnatal viability or fetal development. In rabbits at the highest dose level given, 300 mg/kg, abortions and fetal mortality were observed. There are no adequate and well controlled studies in pregnant women and pirbuterol acetate should be used during pregnancy only if the potential benefit justifies the potential risk to the fetus.

NURSING MOTHERS

It is not known whether pirbuterol acetate is excreted in human milk. Therefore, pirbuterol acetate should be used during nursing only if the potential benefit justifies the possible risk to the newborn.

PEDIATRIC USE

Pirbuterol acetate inhaler is not recommended for patients under the age of 12 years because of insufficient clinical data to establish safety and effectiveness.

DRUG INTERACTIONS

Other beta adrenergic aerosol bronchodilators should not be used concomitantly with pirbuterol acetate because they may have additive effects. Beta adrenergic agonists should be administered with caution to patients being treated with monoamine oxidase inhibitors or tricyclic antidepressants, since the action of beta adrenergic agonists on the vascular system may be potentiated.

ADVERSE REACTIONS

The following rates of adverse reactions to pirbuterol are based on single and multiple dose clinical trials involving 761 patients, 400 of whom received multiple doses (mean duration of treatment was 2.5 months and maximum was 19 months).

The following were the adverse reactions reported more frequently than 1 in 100 patients:

CNS: Nervousness (6.9%), tremor (6.0%), headache (2.0%), dizziness (1.2%).
Cardiovascular: Palpitations (1.7%), tachycardia (1.2%).
Respiratory: Cough (1.2%).
Gastrointestinal: Nausea (1.7%).

The following adverse reactions occurred less frequently than 1 in 100 patients and there may be a causal relationship with pirbuterol.

CNS: Depression, anxiety, confusion, insomnia, weakness, hyperkinesia, syncope.
Cardiovascular: Hypotension, skipped beats, chest pain.
Gastrointestinal: Dry mouth, glossitis, abdominal pain/cramps, anorexia, diarrhea, stomatitis, nausea, and vomiting.
Ear, Nose and Throat: Smell/taste changes, sore throat.
Dermatologic: Rash, pruritus.
Other: Numbness in extremities, alopecia, bruising, fatigue, edema, weight gain, flushing.

Other adverse reactions were reported with a frequency of less than 1 in 100 patients but a causal relationship between pirbuterol and the reaction could not be determined: migraine, productive cough, wheezing, and dermatitis.

The following rates of adverse reactions during 3 month controlled clinical trials involving 310 patients are noted. TABLE 1 does not include mild reactions.

DOSAGE AND ADMINISTRATION

The usual dose for adults and children 12 years and older is 2 inhalations (0.4 mg) repeated every 4-6 hours. One inhalation (0.2 mg) repeated every 4-6 hours may be sufficient for some patients.

A total daily dose of 12 inhalations should not be exceeded.

If a previously effective dosage regimen fails to provide the usual relief, medical advice should be sought immediately as this is often a sign of seriously worsening asthma which would require reassessment of therapy.

HOW SUPPLIED

Each actuation of Maxair delivers pirbuterol acetate equivalent to 0.2 mg of pirbuterol from the mouthpiece.

Note: The statement below is required by the Federal government's Clean Air Act for all products containing or manufactured with chlorofluorocarbons (CFC's).

WARNING: Contains trichloromonofluoromethane and dichlorodifluoromethane, substances which harm public health and environment by destroying ozone in the upper atmosphere.

Store between 15-30°C (59-86°F).

TABLE 1 *Percent of Patients with Moderate to Severe Adverse Reactions*

Adverse Reaction	Pirbuterol (N=157)	Metaproterenol (N=153)
Central Nervous System		
Tremors	1.3%	3.3%
Nervousness	4.5%	2.6%
Headache	1.3%	2.0%
Weakness	0%	1.3%
Drowsiness	0%	0.7%
Dizziness	0.6%	0%
Cardiovascular		
Palpitations	1.3%	1.3%
Tachycardia	1.3%	2.0%
Respiratory		
Chest Pain/tightness	1.3%	0%
Cough	0%	0.7%
Gastrointestinal		
Nausea	1.3%	2.0%
Diarrhea	1.3%	0.7%
Dry mouth	1.3%	1.3%
Vomiting	0%	0.7%
Dermatological		
Skin reaction	0%	0.7%
Rash	0%	1.3%
Other		
Bruising	0.6%	0%
Smell/taste change	0.6%	0%
Backache	0%	0.7%
Fatigue	0%	0.7%
Hoarseness	0%	0.7%
Nasal congestion	0%	0.7%

PRODUCT LISTING - EQUIVALENTS NOT AVAILABLE

Aerosol with Adapter - Inhalation - 0.2 mg/Inh

14 gm	$40.75	MAXAIR AUTOHALER, Physicians Total Care	54868-2821-01
14 gm	$56.76	MAXAIR, Allscripts Pharmaceutical Company	54569-4615-00
14 gm	$79.69	MAXAIR AUTOHALER, 3M Pharmaceuticals	00089-0815-21
25.60 gm	$26.64	MAXAIR, Allscripts Pharmaceutical Company	54569-2253-00

Piroxicam *(002047)*

For related information, see the comparative table section in Appendix A.

Categories: Arthritis, osteoarthritis; Arthritis, rheumatoid; FDA Approved 1982 Apr; Pregnancy Category B; Pregnancy Category D, 3rd Trimester

Drug Classes: Analgesics, non-narcotic; Nonsteroidal anti-inflammatory drugs

Brand Names: **Feldene**

Foreign Brand Availability: Antiflog (Italy); Apo-Piroxicam (Canada; New-Zealand); Arpyrox (Indonesia); Artrilase (Dominican-Republic); Atidem (Peru); Baxo (Japan); Benoxicam (Indonesia); Brexic (India); Brexicam (Costa-Rica; Dominican-Republic; El-Salvador; Guatemala; Honduras; Nicaragua; Panama); Brexin (Bahrain; Cyprus; Egypt; Iran; Iraq; Jordan; Kuwait; Lebanon; Libya; Oman; Qatar; Republic-of-Yemen; Saudi-Arabia; Syria; Taiwan; United-Arab-Emirates); Brexodin (Mexico); Camrox (Korea); Candyl-D (Australia); Capxidin (Singapore); Citoken T (Mexico); Dacam (Finland); Desinflam (Peru); Dixonal (Mexico); Doblexan (Spain); Dolonex (India); Exipan (Israel); Facicam (Mexico); Felcicam (Korea); Felden (Austria; Denmark; Finland; Germany; Norway; Sweden; Switzerland); Feldene Gel (Benin; Burkina-Faso; Ethiopia; Gambia; Ghana; Guinea; Ivory-Coast; Kenya; Liberia; Malawi; Mali; Mauritania; Mauritius; Morocco; Niger; Nigeria; Senegal; Seychelles; Sierra-Leone; Sudan; Tanzania; Thailand; Tunia; Uganda; Zambia; Zimbabwe); Felxicam (Hong-Kong; Malaysia); Felrox (Thailand); Flamic Gel (Thailand); Flaxine (Philippines); Flexirox (France); Flogosan (Mexico); Floglugen (Taiwan); Focus (Taiwan); Fulden (Korea); Hotemin (Hong-Kong; Malaysia); Indene (Indonesia); Infeld (Indonesia); Inflamene (Brazil; Indonesia); Konshien (Taiwan); Kydoflam (Colombia); Larapam (England); Macroxam (Philippines); Mobilis (Australia); Movon-20 (India); Movon Gel (India); Moxicam (Thailand); Novopirocam (Canada); Nu-Pirox (Canada); Osteral (Mexico); Parixam (Philippines); Piraldene (Peru); Piram (Thailand); Piram-D (New-Zealand); Pirax (Thailand); Pirkam (Denmark); Pirocutan (Germany); Pirocutan Gel (Germany); Pirohexal-D (Australia); Pirom (Denmark); Priorheum (Germany); Pirox (India); Piroxan (Mexico); Piroxedol (Colombia); Piroxicam (Colombia); Piroxim (Bahrain; Benin; Burkina-Faso; Colombia; Cyprus; Egypt; Ethiopia; Gambia; Ghana; Guinea; Iran; Iraq; Ivory-Coast; Jordan; Kenya; Kuwait; Lebanon; Liberia; Libya; Malawi; Mali; Mauritania; Mauritius; Morocco; Niger; Nigeria; Oman; Qatar; Republic-of-Yemen; Saudi-Arabia; Senegal; Seychelles; Sierra-Leone; Sudan; Syria; Tanzania; Tunia; Uganda; United-Arab-Emirates; Zambia; Zimbabwe); Piroxton (Korea); Pixicam (South-Africa); Posidene (Thailand); Proxalyoc (France); Pyrocaps (South-Africa); Pyroxy (Thailand); Raxicam (Philippines); Rexicam (Indonesia); Rheugesic (South-Africa); Rosic (Indonesia); Rosiden (Korea); Rosiden Gel (Korea); Rosig (Australia); Rosig-D (Australia); Roxicam (Bahrain; Cyprus; Egypt; Iran; Iraq; Jordan; Kuwait; Lebanon; Libya; Oman; Qatar; Republic-of-Yemen; Saudi-Arabia; South-Africa; Syria; United-Arab-Emirates); Roxium (Thailand); Ruvamed (Greece); Scandene (Indonesia); Sefdene (Hong-Kong); Sinalgico (Argentina); Sofden (Indonesia); Sotilen (Bahrain; Benin; Burkina-Faso; Cyprus; Egypt; Ethiopia; Gambia; Ghana; Guinea; Hong-Kong; Iran; Iraq; Ivory-Coast; Jordan; Kenya; Kuwait; Lebanon; Liberia; Libya; Malawi; Mali; Mauritania; Mauritius; Morocco; Niger; Nigeria; Oman; Qatar; Republic-of-Yemen; Saudi-Arabia; Senegal; Seychelles; Sierra-Leone; Sudan; Syria; Taiwan; Tanzania; Thailand; Tunia; Uganda; United-Arab-Emirates; Zambia; Zimbabwe); Stopen (Colombia); Tropidene (Indonesia); Unicam (Bahrain; Cyprus; Egypt; Iran; Iraq; Jordan; Kuwait; Lebanon; Libya; Oman; Qatar; Republic-of-Yemen; Saudi-Arabia; Syria; United-Arab-Emirates); Vidapirocam (Hong-Kong); Xicalom (Indonesia); Xicam (Thailand); Xycam (South-Africa); Zitumex (Greece); Zunden (Italy)

Cost of Therapy: $77.99 (Osteoarthritis; Feldene; 20 mg; 1 capsule/day; 30 day supply)
$3.27 (Osteoarthritis; Generic Capsules; 20 mg; 1 capsule/day; 30 day supply)

DESCRIPTION

Piroxicam is 4-Hydroxy-2-methyl-*N*-2-pyridinyl-2*H*-1,2-benzothiazine-3-carboxamide 1,1-dioxide, an oxicam. Members of the oxicam family are not carboxylic acids, but they are acidic by virtue of the enolic 4-hydroxy substituent. Piroxicam occurs as a white crystalline solid, sparingly soluble in water, dilute acid and most organic solvents. It is slightly soluble in alcohols and in aqueous alkaline solution. It exhibits a weakly acidic 4-hydroxy proton (pKa 5.1) and a weakly basic pyridyl nitrogen (pKa 1.8).

Molecular Formula: $C_{15}H_{13}N_3O_4S$

Molecular Weight: 331.35

Inert Ingredients in the Formulations Are: Hard gelatin capsules (which may contain blue 1, red 3, and other inert ingredients); lactose; magnesium stearate; sodium lauryl sulfate; starch.

Storage: STORE AT CONTROLLED ROOM TEMPERATURE 15-30°C (59-86°F). PROTECT FROM LIGHT. Dispense in a tight, light-resistant container using a child-resistant closure.

CLINICAL PHARMACOLOGY

Piroxicam has shown anti-inflammatory, analgesic, and antipyretic properties in animals. Edema, erythema, tissue proliferation, fever, and pain can all be inhibited in laboratory animals by the administration of piroxicam. It is effective regardless of the etiology of the inflammation. The mode of action of piroxicam is not fully established at this time. However, a common mechanism for the above effects may exist in the ability of piroxicam to inhibit the biosynthesis of prostaglandins, known mediators of inflammation.

It is established that piroxicam does not act by stimulating the pituitary-adrenal axis.

Piroxicam is well absorbed following oral administration. Drug plasma concentrations are proportional for 10 and 20 mg doses, generally peak within 3-5 hours after medication, and subsequently decline with a mean half-life of 50 hours (range of 30-86 hours, although values outside of this range have been encountered).

This prolonged half-life results in the maintenance of relatively stable plasma concentrations throughout the day on once daily doses and to significant drug accumulation upon multiple dosing. A single 20 mg dose generally produces peak piroxicam plasma levels of 1.5 to 2 μg/ml, while maximum drug plasma concentrations, after repeated daily ingestion of 20 mg piroxicam, usually stabilize at 3-8 μg/ml. Most patients approximate steady state plasma levels within 7-12 days. Higher levels, which approximate steady state at 2-3 weeks, have been observed in patients in whom longer plasma half-lives of piroxicam occurred.

Piroxicam and its biotransformation products are excreted in urine and feces, with about twice as much appearing in the urine as the feces with about twice as much appearing in the urine as the feces. Metabolism occurs by hydroxylation at the 5 position of the pyridyl side chain and conjugation of this product; by cyclodehydration; and by a sequence of reactions involving hydrolysis of the amide linkage, decarboxylation, ring contraction, and N-demethylation. Less than 5% of the daily dose is excreted unchanged.

Concurrent administration of aspirin (3900 mg/day) and piroxicam (20 mg/day), resulted in a reduction of plasma levels of piroxicam to about 80% of their normal values. The use of piroxicam in conjunction with aspirin is not recommended because data are inadequate to demonstrate that the combination produces greater improvement than that achieved with aspirin alone and the potential for adverse reactions is increased. The effects of impaired renal function or hepatic disease on plasma levels have not been established.

Piroxicam, like salicylates and other nonsteroidal anti-inflammatory agents, is associated with symptoms of gastrointestinal tract irritation (see ADVERSE REACTIONS). However, in a study utilizing ^{51}Cr-tagged red blood cells, 20 mg of piroxicam administered as a single dose for 4 days did not result in a significant increase in fecal blood loss and did not detectably affect the gastric mucosa. In the same study a total daily dose of 3900 mg of aspirin, *i.e.*, 972 mg qid, caused a significant increase in fecal blood loss and mucosal lesions as demonstrated by gastroscopy.

In controlled clinical trials, the effectiveness of piroxicam has been established for both acute exacerbations and long-term management of rheumatoid arthritis and osteoarthritis.

The therapeutic effects of piroxicam are evident early in the treatment of both diseases with a progressive increase in response over several (8-12) weeks. Efficacy is seen in terms of pain relief and, when present, subsidence of inflammation.

Doses of 20 mg/day piroxicam display a therapeutic effect comparable to therapeutic doses of aspirin, with a lower incidence of minor gastrointestinal effects and tinnitus.

Piroxicam has been administered concomitantly with fixed doses of gold and corticosteroids. The existence of a "steroid-sparing" effect has not been adequately studied to date.

INDICATIONS AND USAGE

Piroxicam is indicated for acute or long-term use in the relief of signs and symptoms of the following:

1. Osteoarthritis.
2. Rheumatoid arthritis.

Dosage recommendations for use in children have not been established.

NON-FDA APPROVED INDICATIONS

While not FDA approved indications, piroxicam is also effective in the management of ankylosing spondylitis and acute gout.

CONTRAINDICATIONS

Piroxicam should not be used in patients who have previously exhibited hypersensitivity to it, or in individuals with the syndrome comprised of bronchospasm, nasal polyps, and angioedema precipitated by aspirin or other nonsteroidal anti-inflammatory drugs.

WARNINGS

RISK OF GI ULCERATION, BLEEDING, AND PERFORATION WITH NSAID THERAPY

Serious gastrointestinal toxicity such as bleeding, ulceration, and perforation can occur at any time, with or without warning symptoms, in patients treated chronically with NSAID therapy. Although minor upper gastrointestinal problems, such as dyspepsia, are common, usually developing early in therapy, physicians should remain alert for ulceration and bleeding in patients treated chronically with NSAIDs even in the absence of previous GI tract symptoms. In patients observed in clinical trials of several months to 2 years of duration, symptomatic upper GI ulcers, gross bleeding or perforation appear to occur in approximately 1% of patients treated for 3-6 months, and in about 2-4% of patients treated for 1 year. Physicians should inform patients about the signs and/or symptoms of serious GI toxicity and what steps to take if they occur.

Studies to date have not identified any subset of patients not at risk of developing peptic ulceration and bleeding. Except for a prior history of serious GI events and other risk factors known to be associated with peptic ulcer disease, such as alcoholism, smoking, etc., no risk

P

factors (*e.g.*, age, sex) have been associated with increased risk. Elderly or debilitated patients seem to tolerate ulceration or bleeding less well than other individuals and most spontaneous reports of fatal GI events are in this population. Studies to date are inconclusive concerning the relative risk of various NSAIDs in causing such reactions. High doses of any NSAID probably carry a greater risk of these reactions, although controlled clinical trials showing this do not exist in most cases. In considering the use of relatively large doses (within the recommended dosage range), sufficient benefit should be anticipated to offset the potential increased risk of GI toxicity.

PRECAUTIONS

RENAL EFFECTS

As with other nonsteroidal anti-inflammatory drugs, long-term administration of piroxicam to animals has resulted in renal papillary necrosis and other abnormal renal pathology. In humans there have been reports of acute interstitial nephritis with hematuria, proteinuria, and occasionally, nephrotic syndrome.

A second form of renal toxicity has been seen in patients with prerenal conditions leading to a reduction in renal blood flow or blood volume, where the renal prostaglandins have a supportive role in the maintenance of renal perfusion. In these patients administration of an NSAID may cause a dose-dependent reduction in prostaglandin formation and may precipitate overt renal decompensation. Patients at greatest risk of this reaction are those with impaired renal function, heart failure, liver dysfunction, those taking diuretics, and the elderly. Discontinuation of NSAID therapy is typically followed by recovery to the pretreatment state.

Because of extensive renal excretion of piroxicam and its biotransformation products (less than 5% of the daily dose excreted unchanged, see CLINICAL PHARMACOLOGY, lower doses of piroxicam should be anticipated in patients with impaired renal function, and they should be carefully monitored.

Although other nonsteroidal anti-inflammatory drugs do not have the same direct effects on platelets that aspirin does, all drugs inhibiting prostaglandin biosynthesis do interfere with platelet function to some degree; therefore, patients who may be adversely affected by such an action should be carefully observed when piroxicam is administered.

Because of reports of adverse eye findings with nonsteroidal anti-inflammatory agents, it is recommended that patients who develop visual complaints during treatment with piroxicam have ophthalmic evaluation.

As with other nonsteroidal anti-inflammatory drugs, borderline elevations of one or more liver tests may occur in up to 15% of patients. These abnormalities may progress, may remain essentially unchanged, or may be transient with continued therapy. The SGPT (ALT) test is probably the most sensitive indicator of liver dysfunction. Meaningful (3 times the upper limit of normal) elevations of SGPT or SGOT (AST) occurred in controlled clinical trials in less than 1% of patients. A patient with symptoms and/or signs suggesting liver dysfunction, or in whom an abnormal liver test has occurred, should be evaluated for evidence of the development of more severe hepatic reaction while on therapy with piroxicam. Severe hepatic reactions, including jaundice and cases of fatal hepatitis, have been reported with piroxicam. Although such reactions are rare, if abnormal liver tests persist or worsen, if clinical signs and symptoms consistent with liver disease develop, or if systemic manifestations occur (*e.g.*, eosinophilia, rash, etc.), piroxicam should be discontinued. (See also ADVERSE REACTIONS.)

Although at the recommended dose of 20 mg/day of piroxicam increased fecal blood loss due to gastrointestinal irritation did not occur (see CLINICAL PHARMACOLOGY), in about 4% of the patients treated with piroxicam alone or concomitantly with aspirin, reductions in hemoglobin and hematocrit values were observed. Therefore, these values should be determined if signs or symptoms of anemia occur.

Peripheral edema has been observed in approximately 2% of the patients treated with piroxicam. Therefore, as with other nonsteroidal anti-inflammatory drugs, piroxicam should be used with caution in patients with heart failure, hypertension or other conditions predisposing to fluid retention, since its usage may be associated with a worsening of these conditions.

A combination of dermatological and/or allergic signs and symptoms suggestive of serum sickness have occasionally occurred in conjunction with the use of piroxicam. These include arthralgias, pruritus, fever, fatigue, and rash including vesiculo bullous reactions and exfoliative dermatitis.

INFORMATION FOR THE PATIENT

Piroxicam, like other drugs of its class, is not free of side effects. The side effects of these drugs can cause discomfort and, rarely, there are more serious side effects, such as gastrointestinal bleeding, which may result in hospitalization and even fatal outcomes.

NSAIDs (Nonsteroidal Anti-Inflammatory Drugs) are often essential agents in the management of arthritis, but they also may be commonly employed for conditions which are less serious.

Physicians may wish to discuss with their patients the potential risks (see WARNINGS, PRECAUTIONS, and ADVERSE REACTIONS) and likely benefits of NSAID treatment, particularly when the drugs are used for less serious conditions where treatment without NSAIDs may represent an acceptable alternative to both the patient and physician.

LABORATORY TESTS

Because serious GI tract ulceration and bleeding can occur without warning symptoms, physicians should follow chronically treated patients for the signs and symptoms of ulceration and bleeding and should inform them of the importance of this follow-up (see WARNINGS, Risk of GI Ulceration, Bleeding and Perforation With NSAID Therapy).

CARCINOGENESIS, MUTAGENESIS, AND IMPAIRMENT OF FERTILITY

Subacute and chronic toxicity studies have been carried out in rats, mice, dogs, and monkeys.

The pathology most often seen was that characteristically associated with the animal toxicology of anti-inflammatory agents: renal papillary necrosis (see PRECAUTIONS) and gastrointestinal lesions.

In classical studies in laboratory animals piroxicam did not show any teratogenic potential.

Reproductive studies revealed no impairment of fertility in animals.

PREGNANCY AND NURSING MOTHERS

Like other drugs which inhibit the synthesis and release of prostaglandins, piroxicam increased the incidence of dystocia and delayed parturition in pregnant animals when piroxicam administration was continued late into pregnancy. Gastrointestinal tract toxicity was increased in pregnant females in the last trimester of pregnancy compared to non-pregnant females or females in earlier trimesters of pregnancy.

Piroxicam is not recommended for use in nursing mothers or in pregnant women because of the animal findings and since safety for such use has not been established in humans.

PEDIATRIC USE

Dosage recommendations and indications for use in children have not been established.

DRUG INTERACTIONS

Piroxicam is highly protein bound, and, therefore, might be expected to displace other protein-bound drugs. Although this has not occurred in *in vitro* studies with coumarin-type anticoagulants, interactions with coumarin-type anticoagulants have been reported with piroxicam since marketing, therefore, physicians should closely monitor patients for a change in dosage requirements when administering piroxicam to patients on coumarin-type anticoagulants and other highly protein-bound drugs.

Plasma levels of piroxicam are depressed to approximately 80% of their normal values when piroxicam is administered in conjunction with aspirin (3900 mg/day) (see CLINICAL PHARMACOLOGY).

Nonsteroidal anti-inflammatory agents, including piroxicam, have been reported to increase steady state plasma lithium levels. It is recommended that plasma lithium levels be monitored when initiating, adjusting, and discontinuing piroxicam.

ADVERSE REACTIONS

The incidence of adverse reactions to piroxicam is based on clinical trials involving approximately 2300 patients, about 400 of whom were treated for more than 1 year and 170 for more than 2 years. About 30% of all patients receiving daily doses of 20 mg of piroxicam experienced side effects. Gastrointestinal symptoms were the most prominent side effects—occurring in approximately 20% of the patients, which in most instances did not interfere with the course of therapy. Of the patients experiencing gastrointestinal side effects, approximately 5% discontinued therapy with an overall incidence of peptic ulceration of about 1%.

Other than the gastrointestinal symptoms, edema, dizziness, headache, changes in hematological parameters, and rash have been reported in a small percentage of patients. Routine ophthalmoscopy and slit-lamp examinations have revealed no evidence of ocular changes in 205 patients followed from 3-24 months while on therapy.

INCIDENCE GREATER THAN 1%

The following adverse reactions occurred more frequently than 1 in 100:

Gastrointestinal: Stomatitis, anorexia, epigastric distress,* nausea,* constipation, abdominal discomfort, flatulence, diarrhea, abdominal pain, indigestion.

Hematologic: Decreases in hemoglobin* and hematocrit* (see PRECAUTIONS), anemia, leukopenia, eosinophilia.

Dermatologic: Pruritus, rash.

Central Nervous System: Dizziness, somnolence, vertigo.

Urogenital: BUN and creatinine elevations (see PRECAUTIONS).

Body as a Whole: Headache, malaise.

Special Senses: Tinnitus.

Cardiovascular/Respiratory: Edema (see PRECAUTIONS).

*Reactions occurring in 3-9% of patients treated with piroxicam. Reactions occurring in 1-3% of patients are unmarked.

INCIDENCE LESS THAN 1% (CAUSAL RELATIONSHIP PROBABLE)

The following adverse reactions occurred less frequently than 1 in 100. The probability exists that there is a causal relationship between piroxicam and these reactions.

Gastrointestinal: Liver function abnormalities, jaundice, hepatitis (see PRECAUTIONS), vomiting, hematemesis, melena, gastrointestinal bleeding, perforation and ulceration (see WARNINGS), dry mouth.

Hematologic: Thrombocytopenia, petechial rash, ecchymosis, bone marrow depression including aplastic anemia, epistaxis.

Dermatologic: Sweating, erythema, bruising, desquamation, exfoliative dermatitis, erythema multiforme, toxic epidermal necrolysis, Stevens-Johnson syndrome, vesiculo bullous reaction, photoallergic skin reactions.

Central Nervous System: Depression, insomnia, nervousness.

Urogenital: Hematuria, proteinuria, interstitial nephritis, renal failure, hyperkalemia, glomerulitis, papillary necrosis, nephrotic syndrome (see PRECAUTIONS).

Body as a Whole: Pain (colic), fever, flu-like syndrome (see PRECAUTIONS).

Special Senses: Swollen eyes, blurred vision, eye irritations.

Cardiovascular/Respiratory: Hypertension, worsening of congestive heart failure (see PRECAUTIONS), exacerbation of angina.

Metabolic: Hypoglycemia, hyperglycemia, weight increase, weight decrease.

Hypersensitivity: Anaphylaxis, bronchospasm, urticaria/angioedema, vasculitis, "serum sickness" (see PRECAUTIONS).

INCIDENCE LESS THAN 1% (CAUSAL RELATIONSHIP UNKNOWN):

Other adverse reactions were reported with a frequency of less than 1 in 100, but a causal relationship between piroxicam and the reaction could not be determined.

Gastrointestinal: Pancreatitis.

Dermatologic: Onycholysis, loss of hair.

Central Nervous System: Akathisia, hallucinations, mood alterations, dream abnormalities, mental confusion, paresthesias.

Urogenital System: Dysuria.
Body as a Whole: Weakness.
Cardiovascular/Respiratory: Palpitations, dyspnea.
Hypersensitivity: Positive ANA.
Special Senses: Transient hearing loss.
Hematologic: Hemolytic anemia.

DOSAGE AND ADMINISTRATION

RHEUMATOID ARTHRITIS, OSTEOARTHRITIS

It is recommended that piroxicam therapy be initiated and maintained at a single daily dose of 20 mg. If desired the daily dose may be divided. Because of the long half-life of piroxicam, steady-state blood levels are not reached for 7-12 days. Therefore although the therapeutic effects of piroxicam are evident early in treatment, there is a progressive increase in response over several weeks and the effect of therapy should not be assessed for two weeks.

Dosage recommendations and indications for use in children have not been established.

PRODUCT LISTING - RATED THERAPEUTICALLY EQUIVALENT

Capsule - Oral - 10 mg

10's	$9.06	GENERIC, Pd-Rx Pharmaceuticals	55289-0515-10
30's	$36.29	GENERIC, Heartland Healthcare Services	61392-0398-30
30's	$36.29	GENERIC, Heartland Healthcare Services	61392-0398-39
31's	$37.50	GENERIC, Heartland Healthcare Services	61392-0398-31
32's	$38.71	GENERIC, Heartland Healthcare Services	61392-0398-32
45's	$54.44	GENERIC, Heartland Healthcare Services	61392-0398-45
60's	$72.59	GENERIC, Heartland Healthcare Services	61392-0398-60
90's	$108.88	GENERIC, Heartland Healthcare Services	61392-0398-90
100's	$8.91	FEDERAL UPPER LIMIT, H.C.F.A. F F P	99999-2047-01
100's	$41.63	GENERIC, Roxane Laboratories Inc	00054-8660-25
100's	$86.39	GENERIC, Roxane Laboratories Inc	00054-2660-25
100's	$117.60	GENERIC, Geneva Pharmaceuticals	00781-2507-01
100's	$118.77	GENERIC, Qualitest Products Inc	00603-5222-21
100's	$119.36	GENERIC, West Point Pharma	59591-0617-68
100's	$120.15	GENERIC, Moore, H.L. Drug Exchange Inc	00839-7734-06
100's	$120.94	GENERIC, Watson Laboratories Inc	52544-0712-01
100's	$121.50	GENERIC, Rexall Group	60814-0701-01
100's	$125.75	GENERIC, Aligen Independent Laboratories Inc	00405-4807-01
100's	$125.75	GENERIC, Par Pharmaceutical Inc	49884-0440-01
100's	$127.00	GENERIC, Major Pharmaceuticals Inc	00904-7697-60
100's	$127.00	GENERIC, Major Pharmaceuticals Inc	00904-7845-60
100's	$131.10	GENERIC, Martec Pharmaceuticals Inc	52555-0972-01
100's	$131.19	GENERIC, Mutual/United Research Laboratories	00677-1713-01
100's	$131.20	GENERIC, Ivax Corporation	00182-1933-01
100's	$132.03	GENERIC, Moore, H.L. Drug Exchange Inc	00839-7773-06
100's	$134.10	GENERIC, Mylan Pharmaceuticals Inc	00378-1010-01
100's	$140.80	GENERIC, Teva Pharmaceuticals Usa	00093-0756-01
100's	$140.80	GENERIC, Ranbaxy Laboratories	63304-0690-01
100's	$145.02	GENERIC, Udl Laboratories Inc	51079-0742-20

Capsule - Oral - 20 mg

7's	$12.48	GENERIC, Pd-Rx Pharmaceuticals	55289-0052-07
7's	$27.40	FELDENE, Pharma Pac	52959-0066-07
7's	$33.23	FELDENE, Pd-Rx Pharmaceuticals	55289-0471-07
10's	$13.29	GENERIC, Pd-Rx Pharmaceuticals	55289-0052-10
10's	$33.02	FELDENE, Prescript Pharmaceuticals	00247-0057-10
10's	$39.80	FELDENE, Pharma Pac	52959-0066-10
10's	$43.43	FELDENE, Pd-Rx Pharmaceuticals	55289-0471-10
14's	$14.40	GENERIC, Pd-Rx Pharmaceuticals	55289-0052-14
14's	$41.71	FELDENE, Allscripts Pharmaceutical Company	54569-0272-07
14's	$69.65	FELDENE, Pd-Rx Pharmaceuticals	55289-0471-14
15's	$47.86	FELDENE, Prescript Pharmaceuticals	00247-0057-15
18's	$59.15	FELDENE, Pharma Pac	52959-0066-18
20's	$16.05	GENERIC, Pd-Rx Pharmaceuticals	55289-0052-20
20's	$56.73	GENERIC, St. Mary'S Mpp	60760-0020-20
20's	$59.59	FELDENE, Allscripts Pharmaceutical Company	54569-0272-05
20's	$62.71	FELDENE, Prescript Pharmaceuticals	00247-0057-20
20's	$64.30	FELDENE, Pharma Pac	52959-0066-20
21's	$16.80	GENERIC, Pd-Rx Pharmaceuticals	55289-0052-21
30's	$24.00	GENERIC, Pd-Rx Pharmaceuticals	55289-0052-30
30's	$57.75	GENERIC, Heartland Healthcare Services	61392-0401-30
30's	$57.75	GENERIC, Heartland Healthcare Services	61392-0401-39
30's	$82.59	GENERIC, St. Mary'S Mpp	60760-0020-30
30's	$85.93	FELDENE, Pharma Pac	52959-0066-30
30's	$89.38	FELDENE, Allscripts Pharmaceutical Company	54569-0272-01
30's	$92.38	FELDENE, Prescript Pharmaceuticals	00247-0057-30
30's	$149.27	FELDENE, Pd-Rx Pharmaceuticals	55289-0471-30
31's	$59.68	GENERIC, Heartland Healthcare Services	61392-0401-31
32's	$61.60	GENERIC, Heartland Healthcare Services	61392-0401-32
45's	$86.63	GENERIC, Heartland Healthcare Services	61392-0401-45
60's	$115.50	GENERIC, Heartland Healthcare Services	61392-0401-60
60's	$181.40	FELDENE, Prescript Pharmaceuticals	00247-0057-60
90's	$173.25	GENERIC, Heartland Healthcare Services	61392-0401-90
90's	$270.41	FELDENE, Prescript Pharmaceuticals	00247-0057-90
100's	$11.31	FEDERAL UPPER LIMIT, H.C.F.A. F F P	99999-2047-03
100's	$59.63	GENERIC, Roxane Laboratories Inc	00054-8661-25
100's	$78.17	GENERIC, Vangard Labs	00615-0389-13
100's	$140.43	GENERIC, Roxane Laboratories Inc	00054-2661-25
100's	$201.25	GENERIC, Geneva Pharmaceuticals	00781-2508-01
100's	$203.90	GENERIC, Mova Pharmaceutical Corporation	55370-0170-07
100's	$203.90	GENERIC, Mova Pharmaceutical Corporation	55370-0841-07
100's	$203.92	GENERIC, Qualitest Products Inc	00603-5223-21
100's	$204.21	GENERIC, West Point Pharma	59591-0640-68
100's	$207.00	GENERIC, Dupont Pharmaceuticals	00056-0260-70
100's	$208.00	GENERIC, Rexall Group	60814-0700-01
100's	$212.99	GENERIC, Teva Pharmaceuticals Usa	62584-0826-01
100's	$215.19	GENERIC, Aligen Independent Laboratories Inc	00405-4808-01
100's	$215.19	GENERIC, Par Pharmaceutical Inc	49884-0441-01
100's	$217.50	GENERIC, Major Pharmaceuticals Inc	00904-5063-60
100's	$217.50	GENERIC, Major Pharmaceuticals Inc	00904-7698-60
100's	$217.50	GENERIC, Major Pharmaceuticals Inc	00904-7812-60
100's	$225.57	GENERIC, Moore, H.L. Drug Exchange Inc	00839-7774-06
100's	$231.35	GENERIC, Ivax Corporation	00182-1934-01
100's	$231.35	GENERIC, Watson Laboratories Inc	52544-0713-01
100's	$241.37	GENERIC, Moore, H.L. Drug Exchange Inc	00839-7735-06
100's	$251.35	GENERIC, Mylan Pharmaceuticals Inc	00378-2020-01
100's	$251.35	GENERIC, Martec Pharmaceuticals Inc	52555-0973-01
100's	$259.95	FELDENE, Pharma Pac	52959-0066-00
100's	$263.90	GENERIC, Teva Pharmaceuticals Usa	00093-0757-01
100's	$263.90	GENERIC, Ranbaxy Laboratories	63304-0691-01
100's	$271.82	GENERIC, Udl Laboratories Inc	51079-0743-20
100's	$300.09	FELDENE, Prescript Pharmaceuticals	00247-0057-00
100's	$328.09	FELDENE, Pfizer U.S. Pharmaceuticals	00069-3230-66

PRODUCT LISTING - EQUIVALENTS NOT AVAILABLE

Capsule - Oral - 10 mg

7's	$10.67	GENERIC, Southwood Pharmaceuticals Inc	58016-0705-07
10's	$15.20	GENERIC, Pharma Pac	52959-0398-10
10's	$15.25	GENERIC, Southwood Pharmaceuticals Inc	58016-0705-10
14's	$21.35	GENERIC, Southwood Pharmaceuticals Inc	58016-0705-14
15's	$22.87	GENERIC, Southwood Pharmaceuticals Inc	58016-0705-15
20's	$30.40	GENERIC, Pharma Pac	52959-0398-20
20's	$30.49	GENERIC, Southwood Pharmaceuticals Inc	58016-0705-20
21's	$29.57	GENERIC, Allscripts Pharmaceutical Company	54569-3974-00
21's	$31.90	GENERIC, Pharma Pac	52959-0398-21
21's	$32.02	GENERIC, Southwood Pharmaceuticals Inc	58016-0705-21
28's	$42.69	GENERIC, Southwood Pharmaceuticals Inc	58016-0705-28
30's	$44.69	GENERIC, Pharma Pac	52959-0398-30
30's	$45.74	GENERIC, Southwood Pharmaceuticals Inc	58016-0705-30
40's	$60.99	GENERIC, Southwood Pharmaceuticals Inc	58016-0705-40
50's	$76.23	GENERIC, Southwood Pharmaceuticals Inc	58016-0705-50
60's	$91.48	GENERIC, Southwood Pharmaceuticals Inc	58016-0705-60
90's	$137.22	GENERIC, Southwood Pharmaceuticals Inc	58016-0705-90
100's	$127.90	GENERIC, Pharma Pac	52959-0398-00
100's	$152.47	GENERIC, Southwood Pharmaceuticals Inc	58016-0705-00
100's	$179.66	FELDENE, Pfizer U.S. Pharmaceuticals	00069-3220-66
126's	$192.11	GENERIC, Southwood Pharmaceuticals Inc	58016-0705-97

Capsule - Oral - 20 mg

5's	$3.62	GENERIC, Prescript Pharmaceuticals	00247-0092-05
7's	$3.73	GENERIC, Prescript Pharmaceuticals	00247-0092-07
7's	$18.47	GENERIC, Allscripts Pharmaceutical Company	54569-3693-02
7's	$19.65	GENERIC, Southwood Pharmaceuticals Inc	58016-0666-07
7's	$20.80	GENERIC, Alpharma Uspd Makers Of Barre and Nmc	63874-0362-07
7's	$23.63	GENERIC, Pharma Pac	52959-0232-07
9's	$26.41	GENERIC, Pharma Pac	52959-0232-09
10's	$2.22	GENERIC, Physicians Total Care	54868-2199-04
10's	$3.88	GENERIC, Prescript Pharmaceuticals	00247-0092-10
10's	$24.96	GENERIC, Alpharma Uspd Makers Of Barre and Nmc	63874-0362-10
10's	$26.39	GENERIC, Allscripts Pharmaceutical Company	54569-3693-01
10's	$28.07	GENERIC, Southwood Pharmaceuticals Inc	58016-0666-10
10's	$33.39	GENERIC, Pharma Pac	52959-0232-10
14's	$4.09	GENERIC, Prescript Pharmaceuticals	00247-0092-14
14's	$16.09	GENERIC, Pharmaceutical Corporation Of America	51655-0567-84
14's	$35.19	GENERIC, Allscripts Pharmaceutical Company	54569-3693-00
14's	$39.30	GENERIC, Southwood Pharmaceuticals Inc	58016-0666-14
14's	$44.10	GENERIC, Pharma Pac	52959-0232-14
15's	$4.15	GENERIC, Prescript Pharmaceuticals	00247-0092-15
15's	$39.52	GENERIC, Alpharma Uspd Makers Of Barre and Nmc	63874-0362-15
15's	$39.59	GENERIC, Allscripts Pharmaceutical Company	54569-3693-05
15's	$42.11	GENERIC, Southwood Pharmaceuticals Inc	58016-0666-15
15's	$47.25	GENERIC, Pharma Pac	52959-0232-15
18's	$56.70	GENERIC, Pharma Pac	52959-0232-18
20's	$4.41	GENERIC, Prescript Pharmaceuticals	00247-0092-20
20's	$52.00	GENERIC, Alpharma Uspd Makers Of Barre and Nmc	63874-0362-20
20's	$52.78	GENERIC, Allscripts Pharmaceutical Company	54569-3693-03
20's	$63.00	GENERIC, Pharma Pac	52959-0232-20
21's	$58.95	GENERIC, Southwood Pharmaceuticals Inc	58016-0666-21
21's	$66.15	GENERIC, Pharma Pac	52959-0232-21
28's	$78.60	GENERIC, Southwood Pharmaceuticals Inc	58016-0666-28
30's	$4.40	GENERIC, Physicians Total Care	54868-2199-01
30's	$4.94	GENERIC, Prescript Pharmaceuticals	00247-0092-30

P

30's	$71.76	GENERIC, Alpharma Uspd Makers Of Barre and Nmc	63874-0362-30
30's	$79.17	GENERIC, Allscripts Pharmaceutical Company	54569-3693-04
30's	$84.21	GENERIC, Southwood Pharmaceuticals Inc	58016-0666-30
30's	$94.50	GENERIC, Pharma Pac	52959-0232-30
40's	$112.28	GENERIC, Southwood Pharmaceuticals Inc	58016-0666-40
50's	$140.35	GENERIC, Southwood Pharmaceuticals Inc	58016-0666-50
60's	$168.42	GENERIC, Southwood Pharmaceuticals Inc	58016-0666-60
90's	$191.62	GENERIC, Allscripts Pharmaceutical Company	54569-8521-00
90's	$267.30	GENERIC, Southwood Pharmaceuticals Inc	58016-0666-90
100's	$10.90	GENERIC, Physicians Total Care	54868-2199-05
100's	$257.92	GENERIC, Alpharma Uspd Makers Of Barre and Nmc	63874-0362-01
100's	$280.70	GENERIC, Southwood Pharmaceuticals Inc	58016-0666-00
126's	$374.85	GENERIC, Southwood Pharmaceuticals Inc	58016-0666-97

Plicamycin *(002053)*

For complete prescribing information, refer to the CD-ROM included with the book.

Categories: Carcinoma, testicular; Hypercalcemia, secondary to neoplasia; Hypercalciuria, secondary to neoplasia; Pregnancy Category X; FDA Approved 1970 May
Drug Classes: Antineoplastics, antibiotics
Brand Names: ***Mithracin***; Mithramycin
HCFA JCODE(S): J9270 2,500 mcg IV

WARNING

FOR INTRAVENOUS USE

IT IS RECOMMENDED THAT PLICAMYCIN BE ADMINISTERED ONLY TO HOSPITALIZED PATIENTS BY OR UNDER THE SUPERVISION OF A QUALIFIED PHYSICIAN WHO IS EXPERIENCED IN THE USE OF CANCER CHEMOTHERAPEUTIC AGENTS, BECAUSE OF THE POSSIBILITY OF SEVERE REACTIONS. FACILITIES FOR THE DETERMINATION OF NECESSARY LABORATORY STUDIES MUST BE MADE AVAILABLE.

SEVERE THROMBOCYTOPENIA, A HEMORRHAGIC TENDENCY AND EVEN DEATH MAY RESULT FROM THE USE OF MITHRACIN. ALTHOUGH SEVERE TOXICITY IS MORE APT TO OCCUR IN PATIENTS WHO HAVE FAR-ADVANCED DISEASE OR ARE OTHERWISE CONSIDERED POOR RISKS FOR THERAPY, SERIOUS TOXICITY MAY ALSO OCCASIONALLY OCCUR EVEN IN PATIENTS WHO ARE IN RELATIVELY GOOD CONDITION.

IN THE TREATMENT OF EACH PATIENT, THE PHYSICIAN MUST WEIGH CAREFULLY THE POSSIBILITY OF ACHIEVING THERAPEUTIC BENEFIT VERSUS THE RISK OF TOXICITY WHICH MAY OCCUR WITH MITHRACIN THERAPY. THE FOLLOWING DATA CONCERNING THE USE OF MITHRACIN IN THE TREATMENT OF TESTICULAR TUMORS, HYPERCALCEMIC AND/OR HYPERCALCIURIC CONDITIONS ASSOCIATED WITH VARIOUS ADVANCED MALIGNANCIES SHOULD BE THOROUGHLY REVIEWED BEFORE ADMINISTERING THIS COMPOUND.

DESCRIPTION

Plicamycin is a yellow crystalline compound which is produced by a microorganism, *Streptomyces plicatus.* Plicamycin is available as a freeze-dried, sterile preparation for IV administration. Each vial contains 2500 µg of plicamycin with 100 mg of mannitol and disodium phosphate to adjust pH 7. After reconstitution with sterile water for injection, the solution has a pH of 7. The drug is unstable in acid solutions with a pH below 4.

Plicamycin is an antineoplastic agent. It has an empirical formula of $C_{52}H_{76}O_{24}$.

INDICATIONS AND USAGE

Plicamycin is a potent antineoplastic agent which has been shown to be useful in the treatment of carefully selected hospitalized patients with malignant tumors of the testis in whom successful treatment by surgery and/or radiation is impossible. Also, on the basis of limited clinical experience to date, it may be considered in the treatment of certain symptomatic patients with hypercalcemia and hypercalciuria with a variety of advanced neoplasms.

The use of plicamycin in other types of neoplastic disease is not recommended at the present time.

NON-FDA APPROVED INDICATIONS

The drug has been reported to have efficacy in the treatment of Paget's disease. However, use in the treatment of Paget's disease has not been approved by the FDA and further studies are needed.

CONTRAINDICATIONS

Plicamycin is contraindicated in patients with thrombocytopenia, thrombocytopathy, coagulation disorder or an increased susceptibility to bleeding due to other causes. Plicamycin should not be administered to any patient with impairment of blood marrow function.

Plicamycin may cause fetal harm when administered to pregnant women. Plicamycin is contraindicated in women who are or may become pregnant. If this drug is used during pregnancy, or if the patient becomes pregnant while taking the drug, the patient should be apprised of the potential hazard to the fetus.

WARNINGS

See BOXED WARNING.

DOSAGE AND ADMINISTRATION

The daily dose of plicamycin is based on the patient's body weight. If a patient has abnormal fluid retention such as edema, hydrothorax or ascites, if the patient's ideal weight rather than actual body weight should calculate the dose.

TREATMENT OF TESTICULAR TUMORS

In the treatment of patients with testicular tumors the recommended daily dose of plicamycin is 25-30 µg/kg of body weight. Therapy should be continued for a period of 8-10 days unless significant side effects or toxicity occur during therapy. A course of therapy consisting of more than 10 daily doses is not recommended. Individuals daily doses should not exceed 30 µg/kg of body weight.

In those patients with responsive tumors, some degree of regression is usually evident within 3 or 4 weeks following the initial course of therapy. If tumors masses remain unchanged following an initial course of therapy, additional courses of therapy at monthly intervals are warranted.

When a significant tumor regression is obtained, it is suggested that additional courses of therapy be given at monthly intervals until a complete regression of tumor masses is achieved or until definite tumor progression of new tumor masses occur in spite of continued therapy.

TREATMENT OF HYPERCALCEMIA AND HYPERCALCIURIA

Reversal of hypercalcemia and hypercalciuria associated with advanced malignancy the recommended course of treatment with plicamycin is 25 µg/kg of body weight per day for 3 or 4 days.

If the desired degree of reversal of hypercalcemia or hypercalciuria is not achieved with the initial course of therapy, additional courses of therapy may be administrated at intervals of one week or more to achieve the desired result or to maintain serum calcium and urinary calcium excretion at normal levels. It may be possible to maintain normal calcium balance with single, weekly doses or with a schedule of 2 or 3 doses per week.

NOTE: BECAUSE OF THE DRUG'S TOXICITY AND THE LIMITED CLINICAL EXPERIENCE TO DATE IN THESE INDICATIONS, THE FOLLOWING RECOMMENDATIONS SHOULD BE KEPT IN MIND BY THE PHYSICIAN.

1. CONSIDER CASES OF HYPERCALCEMIA AND HYPERCALCIURIA NOT RESPONSIVE TO CONVENTIONAL TREATMENT.

2. APPLY THE SAME CONTRAINDICATIONS AND PRECAUTIONARY MEASURES AS IN ANTITUMOR TREATMENT.

3. RENAL FUNCTION SHOULD BE CAREFULLY MONITORED BEFORE, DURING, AND AFTER TREATMENT.

4. BENEFITS OF USE DURING PREGNANCY OR IN WOMEN OF CHILDBEARING AGE SHOULD BE WEIGHED AGAINST THE POTENTIAL TOXICITY TO EMBRYO OR FETUS.

ADMINISTRATION

By IV administration only. The appropriate daily dose of plicamycin should be diluted in one liter of 5% Dextrose Injection, USP or Sodium Chloride Injection, USP and administered by slow IV infusion over a period of 4-6 hours. Rapid direct IV injection of Mithracin should be avoided as it may be associated with a higher incidence and greater severity of gastrointestinal side effects. Extravasation of solutions of Mithracin may cause local irritation and cellulitis at injection sites. Should thrombophlebitis or perivascular cellulitis occur, the infusion should be terminated and reinstituted at another site. The application of moderate heat to the site of extravasation may help to disperse the compound and minimize discomfort and local tissue irritation. The use of antiemetic compounds prior to and during treatment with Mithracin may be helpful in relieving nausea and vomiting.

Procedures for proper handling and disposal of anti-cancer drugs should be considered.[2] Several guidelines on this subject have been published.[3-8] There is no general agreement that all procedures recommended in the guidelines are necessary or appropriate.

PRODUCT LISTING - EQUIVALENTS NOT AVAILABLE

Powder For Injection - Intravenous - 2.5 mg

10's	$987.36	MITHRACIN, Bayer	00026-8161-15

Pneumococcal Vaccine *(002055)*

For complete prescribing information, refer to the CD-ROM included with the book.

Categories: Immunization, pneumococcal; Pregnancy Category C; FDA Approval Pre 1982
Drug Classes: Vaccines
Brand Names: Pneumovax 23; ***Pnu-Imune 23***
Foreign Brand Availability: Moniarix (Benin; Burkina-Faso; Ethiopia; Gambia; Ghana; Guinea; Ivory-Coast; Kenya; Liberia; Malawi; Mali; Mauritania; Mauritius; Morocco; Niger; Nigeria; Senegal; Seychelles; Sierra-Leone; Sudan; Tanzania; Tunia; Uganda; Zambia; Zimbabwe); Pneumo 23 (Canada; Colombia; France; Hong-Kong; Italy; Malaysia; New-Zealand; Philippines; Taiwan; Thailand); Pneumo 23 Imovax (Israel); Pneumovax (Japan); Pneumovax II (England; Ireland); Prevenar (Australia); Prevnar (Austria; Belgium; Bulgaria; Czech-Republic; Denmark; England; Finland; France; Germany; Greece; Hungary; Ireland; Italy; Netherlands; Norway; Poland; Portugal; Slovenia; Spain; Sweden; Switzerland; Turkey)

DESCRIPTION

Pneumococcal vaccine polyvalent, is a sterile, liquid vaccine for intramuscular or subcutaneous injection. It consists of a mixture of highly purified capsular polysaccharides from the 23 most prevalent or invasive pneumococcal types accounting for at least 90% of pneumococcal blood isolates and at least 85% of all pneumococcal isolates from sites which are generally sterile as determined by ongoing surveillance of US data.[1]

Pneumococcal vaccine polyvalent is manufactured according to methods developed by the Merck Sharp & Dohme Research Laboratories. Each 0.5 ml dose of vaccine contains 25 µg of each polysaccharide type dissolved in isotonic saline solution containing 0.25% phenol as preservative.

Type 6B pneumococcal polysaccharide exhibits somewhat greater stability in purified form than does Type 6A.[1] A high degree of cross-reactivity between the two types has been demonstrated in adult volunteers.[2,3] Therefore, Type 6B has replaced Type 6A, which had been used in the 14-valent vaccine. Although contained in the 14-valent vaccine, Type 25 is not included in pneumococcal vaccine polyvalent because it has recently become a rare isolate in many parts of the world including the United States, Canada and Europe.[2] (see TABLE 1.)

TABLE 1 *Pneumococcal Vaccine Polyvalent, Description 23 Pneumococcal Capsular Types Included in PNEUMOVAX 23*

Nomenclature	Pneumococcal Types
Danish	1 2 3 4 5 6B 7F 8 9N 9V 10A 11A 12F 14 15B 17F 18C 19F 19A 20 22F 23F 33F
US	1 2 3 4 5 26 51 8 9 68 34 43 12 14 54 17 56 19 57 20 22 23 70

Storage: Store unopened and opened vials at 2-8°C (36-46°F). The vaccine is used directly as supplied. No dilution or reconstitution is necessary. Phenol 0.25% added as preservative. All vaccine must be discarded after the expiration date.

INDICATIONS AND USAGE

Pneumococcal vaccine polyvalent is indicated for immunization against pneumococcal disease caused by those pneumococcal types included in the vaccine. Effectiveness of the vaccine in the prevention of pneumococcal pneumonia and pneumococcal bacteremia has been demonstrated in controlled trials.

Pneumococcal vaccine polyvalent *will not immunize against capsular types of pneumococcus other than those contained in the vaccine.*

Use in selected individuals over 2 years of age as follows: (1) patients who have anatomical asplenia or who have splenic dysfunction due to sickle cell disease or other causes; (2) persons with chronic illnesses in which there is an increased risk of pneumococcal disease, such as functional impairment of cardiorespiratory, hepatic and renal systems; (3) persons 50 years of age or older; (4) patients with other chronic illnesses who may be at greater risk of developing pneumococcal infection or experiencing more severe pneumococcal illness as a result of alcohol abuse or coexisting diseases including diabetes mellitus, chronic cerebrospinal fluid leakage, or conditions associated with immunosuppression;[22] (5) patients with Hodgkin's disease if immunization can be given at least 10 days prior to treatment. For maximal antibody response immunization should be given at least 14 days prior to the start of treatment with radiation or chemotherapy. Immunization of patients less than 10 days prior to or during treatment is not recommended.[23] (See CONTRAINDICATIONS.)

Use in communities. Persons over 2 years of age as follows: (1) closed groups such as those in residential schools, nursing homes and other institutions. (To decrease the likelihood of acute outbreaks of pneumococcal disease in closed institutional populations where there is increased risk that the disease may be severe, vaccination of the entire closed population should be considered where there are no other contraindications.[22]); (2) groups epidemiologically at risk in the community when there is a generalized outbreak in the population due to a single pneumococcal type included in the vaccine; (3) patients at high risk of influenza complications, particularly pneumonia.[7]

Pneumococcal vaccine polyvalent may not be effective in preventing infection resulting from basilar skull fracture or from external communication with cerebrospinal fluid.

Simultaneous administration of pneumococcal polysaccharide vaccine and whole-virus influenza vaccine give satisfactory antibody response with out increasing the occurrence of adverse reactions.[24] Simultaneous administration of the pneumococcal vaccine and split-virus influenza vaccine may also be expected to yield satisfactory results.[25]

REVACCINATION

Routine revaccination of adults previously vaccinated with PNEUMOVAX 23 is not recommended because an increased incidence and severity of adverse reactions have been reported among healthy adults revaccinated with pneumococcal vaccines at intervals under 3 years.[2,15] This was probably due to sustained high antibody levels.[26]

Based on a clinical study, revaccination with PNEUMOVAX 23 is recommended for adults at highest risk of fatal pneumococcal infection who were initially vaccinated with PNEUMOVAX (pneumococcal vaccine polyvalent, MSD) (14-valent) without serious or severe reaction 4 or more years previously.[30]*

Children at highest risk for pneumococcal infection (*e.g.,* children with asplenia, sickle cell disease or nephrotic syndrome) may have lower peak antibody levels and/or more rapid antibody decline than do healthy adults.[27,31] There is evidence that some of these high-risk children, (*e.g.,* asplenic children) benefit from revaccination with vaccine containing antigen types 7F, 8, 19F.[33,34] The Immunization Practices Advisory Committee (ACIP) recommends that revaccination after 3-5 years should be considered for children at highest risk for pneumococcal infection (*e.g.,* children with asplenia, sickle cell disease or nephrotic syndrome) who would be 10 years old or younger at revaccination.[35]

***NOTE:** The Immunization Practices Advisory Committee (ACIP) has stated that, without more information: persons who received the 14-valent pneumococcal vaccine should not be routinely revaccinated with the 23-valent vaccine, as increased coverage is modest and duration of protection is not well defined. However, revaccination with the 23-valent vaccine should be strongly considered for persons who received the 14-valent vaccine if they are at highest risk of fatal pneumococcal infection (*e.g.,* asplenic patients). Revaccination should also be considered for adults at highest risk who received the 23-valent vaccine ≥ 6 years before and for those shown to have rapid decline in pneumococcal antibody levels (*e.g.,* patients with nephrotic syndrome, renal failure, or transplant recipients).[35]

CONTRAINDICATIONS

Hypersensitivity to any component of the vaccine. Epinephrine injection (1:1000) must be immediately available should an acute anaphylactoid reaction occur due to any component of the vaccine.

Revaccination of adults with pneumococcal vaccine polyvalent is contraindicated except as described under **INDICATIONS AND USAGE**.

Patients with Hodgkin's disease immunized less than 7-10 days prior to immunosuppressive therapy have in some instances been found to have post-immunization antibody levels below their pre-immunization levels.[23] Because of these results, immunization less than 10 days prior to or during treatment is contraindicated.

Patients with Hodgkin's disease who have received extensive chemotherapy and/or nodal irradiation have been shown to have an impaired antibody response to a 12-valent pneumococcal vaccine.[28] Because, in some intensively treated patients, administration of that vaccine depressed pre-existing levels of antibody to some pneumococcal types, pneumococcal vaccine polyvalent is not recommended at this time for patients who have received these forms of therapy for Hodgkin's disease.

WARNINGS

If the vaccine is used in persons receiving immunosuppressive therapy, the expected serum antibody response may not be obtained.

Intradermal administration may cause severe local reactions.

DOSAGE AND ADMINISTRATION

Do not inject intravenously. Intradermal administration should be avoided.

Parenteral drug products should be inspected visually for particulate matter and discoloration prior to administration, whenever solution and container permit. Pneumococcal vaccine polyvalent is a clear, colorless solution.

Administer a single 0.5 ml dose of pneumococcal vaccine polyvalent subcutaneously or intramuscularly (preferably in the deltoid muscle or lateral mid-thigh), with appropriate precautions to avoid intravascular administration.

SINGLE-DOSE AND 5-DOSE VIALS

For Syringe Use Only

Withdraw 0.5 ml from the vial using a sterile needle and syringe free of preservatives, antiseptics and detergents.

It is important to use a separate sterile syringe and needle for each individual patient to prevent transmission of hepatitis B and other infectious agents from 1 person to another.

PRODUCT LISTING - EQUIVALENTS NOT AVAILABLE

Solution - Injectable - Strength n/a

0.50 ml	$65.31	PNEUMOVAX 23, Allscripts Pharmaceutical Company	54569-1412-00
0.50 ml x 5	$61.81	PNEUMOVAX 23, Merck & Company Inc	00006-4741-00
0.50 ml x 5	$93.01	PNU-IMUNE 23, Lederle Laboratories	00005-2309-33
0.50 ml x 5	$107.30	PNEUMOVAX 23, Merck & Company Inc	00006-4894-00
0.50 ml x 10	$183.30	PNEUMOVAX 23, Merck & Company Inc	00006-4943-00
2.50 ml	$71.07	PNEUMOVAX 23, Physicians Total Care	54868-3339-01
2.50 ml	$81.65	PNEUMOVAX 23, Merck & Company Inc	00006-4739-00
2.50 ml	$82.93	PNU-IMUNE 23, Lederle Laboratories	00005-2309-31
2.50 ml	$97.61	PNU-IMUNE 23, Physicians Total Care	54868-0707-00

Suspension - Intramuscular - Pediatric

0.50 ml x 5	$362.50	PREVNAR, Wyeth-Ayerst Laboratories	00005-1970-67

Polio Vaccine, Inactivated (002060)

For complete prescribing information, refer to the CD-ROM included with the book.

Categories: Immunization, poliomyelitis; Pregnancy Category C; FDA Approval Pre 1982
Drug Classes: Vaccines
Brand Names: Ipol; Poliovax
Foreign Brand Availability: Imovax Polio (Finland; Hong-Kong; Israel); Polio Salk "Sero" (Austria)

DESCRIPTION

Poliovirus vaccine, inactivated, produced by Pasteur Merieux Serums & Vaccins S.A., is a sterile suspension of three types of poliovirus: Type 1 (Mahoney), Type 2 (MEF-1), and Type 3 (Saukett). The viruses are grown in cultures of VERO cells, a continuous line of monkey kidney cells, by the microcarrier technique. The viruses are concentrated, purified, and made noninfectious by inactivation with formaldehyde. Each sterile immunizing dose (0.5 ml) of trivalent vaccine is formulated to contain 40 D antigen units of Type 1, 8 D antigen units of Type 2, and 32 D antigen units of Type 3 poliovirus, determined by comparison to a reference preparation. The poliovirus vaccine is dissolved in phosphate buffered saline. Also present are 0.5% of 2-phenoxyethanol and a maximum of 0.02% of formaldehyde per dose as preservatives. Neomycin, streptomycin and polymyxin B are used in vaccine production, and although purification procedures eliminate measurable amounts, less than 5 ng neomycin, 200 ng streptomycin and 25 ng polymyxin B per dose may still be present. The vaccine is clear and colorless and should be administered subcutaneously.

Storage: The vaccine is stable if stored in the refrigerator between 2°C and 8°C (35-46°F). *The vaccine must not be frozen.*

INDICATIONS AND USAGE

Poliovirus vaccine, inactivated is indicated for active immunization of infants, children and adults for the prevention of poliomyelitis. Recommendations on the use of live and inactivated poliovirus vaccines are described in the ACIP Recommendations[18,19] and the 1988 American Academy of Pediatrics Red Book.[20]

INFANTS, CHILDREN, AND ADOLESCENTS

General Recommendations

It is recommended that all infants, unimmunized children and adolescents not previously immunized be vaccinated routinely against paralytic poliomyelitis.[18] Poliovirus vaccine, inactivated should be offered to individuals who have refused Poliovirus Vaccine Live Oral Trivalent (OPV) or in whom OPV is contraindicated. Parents should be adequately informed of the risks and benefits of both inactivated and oral polio vaccines so that they can make an informed choice (Report of An Evaluation of Poliomyelitis Vaccine Policy Options, Institute of Medicine, National Academy of Sciences, Washington, D.C., 1988).

OPV should not be used in households with immunodeficient individuals because OPV is excreted in the stool by healthy vaccinees and can infect an immunocompromised household member, which may result in paralytic disease. In a household with an immunocompromised member, only poliovirus vaccine, inactivated should be used for all those requiring poliovirus immunization.[20]

Children Incompletely Immunized

Children of all ages should have their immunization status reviewed and be considered for supplemental immunization as follows for adults. Time intervals between doses longer than those recommended for routine primary immunization do not necessitate additional doses as long as a final total of 4 doses is reached (See DOSAGE AND ADMINISTRATION.)

Previous clinical poliomyelitis (usually due to only a single poliovirus type) or incomplete immunization with OPV are not contraindications to completing the primary series of immunization with poliovirus vaccine, inactivated.

ADULTS

General Recommendations

Routine primary poliovirus vaccination of adults (generally those 18 years of age or older) residing in the US is not recommended. Adults who have increased risk of exposure to either vaccine or wild poliovirus and have not been adequately immunized should receive polio vaccination in accordance with the schedule given in the DOSAGE AND ADMINISTRATION section.[16]

The following categories of adults run an increased risk of exposure to wild polioviruses:[19]

- Travelers to regions or countries where poliomyelitis is endemic or epidemic.
- Health care workers in close contact with patients who may be excreting polioviruses.
- Laboratory workers handling specimens that may contain polioviruses.
- Members of communities or specific population groups with disease caused by wild polioviruses.
- Incompletely vaccinated or unvaccinated adults in a household (or other close contacts) with children given OPV provided that the immunization of the child can be assured and not unduly delayed. The adult should be informed of the small OPV related risk to the contact.

IMMUNODEFICIENCY AND ALTERED IMMUNE STATUS

Patients with recognized immunodeficiency are at greater risk of developing paralysis when exposed to live poliovirus than persons with a normal immune system. Under no circumstances should oral live poliovirus vaccine be used in such patients or introduced into a household where such a patient resides.[18]

Poliovirus vaccine, inactivated should be used in all patients with immunodeficiency diseases and members of such patients' households when vaccination of such persons is indicated. This includes patients with asymptomatic HIV infection, AIDS or AIDS Related Complex, severe combined immunodeficiency, hypogammaglobulinemia, or agammaglobulinemia; altered immune states due to diseases such as leukemia, lymphoma, or generalized malignancy; or an immune system compromised by treatment with corticosteroids, alkylating drugs, antimetabolites or radiation. Patients with an altered immune state may or may not develop a protective response against paralytic poliomyelitis after administration of poliovirus vaccine, inactivated.[21]

CONTRAINDICATIONS

Poliovirus vaccine, inactivated is contraindicated in persons with a history of hypersensitivity to any component of the vaccine, including neomycin, streptomycin and polymyxin B.

If anaphylaxis or anaphylactic shock occurs within 24 hours of administration of a dose of vaccine, no further doses should be given.

Vaccination of persons with any acute, febrile illness should be deferred until after recovery; however, minor illnesses such as mild upper respiratory infections are not in themselves reasons for postponing vaccine administration.

WARNINGS

Neomycin, streptomycin, and polymyxin B are used in the production of this vaccine. Although purification procedures eliminate measurable amounts of these substances, traces may be present (see DESCRIPTION) and allergic reactions may occur in persons sensitive to these substances.

DOSAGE AND ADMINISTRATION

Parenteral drug products should be inspected visually for particulate matter and/or discoloration prior to administration. If these conditions exist, vaccine should not be administered.

After preparation of the injection site, immediately administer the vaccine subcutaneously. In infants and small children, the mid-lateral aspect of the thigh is the preferred site. In adults the vaccine should be administered in the deltoid area.

Care should be taken to avoid administering the injection into or near blood vessels and nerves. After aspiration, if blood or any suspicious discoloration appears in the syringe, do not inject but discard contents and repeat procedures using a new dose of vaccine administered at a different site. DO NOT ADMINISTER VACCINE INTRAVENOUSLY.

CHILDREN

Primary Immunization

A primary series of poliovirus vaccine, inactivated consists of three 0.5 ml doses administered subcutaneously. The interval between the first 2 doses should be at least 4 weeks, but preferably 8 weeks. The first 2 doses are usually administered with DTP immunization and are given at 2 and 4 months of age. The third dose should follow at least 6 months but preferably 12 months after the second dose. It may be desirable to administer this dose with MMR and other vaccines, but at a different site, in children 15-18 months of age. All children who received a primary series of poliovirus vaccine, inactivated, or a combination of IPV and OPV, should be given a booster dose of OPV or IPV before entering school, unless the final (third dose) of the primary series was administered on or after the fourth birthday.[18]

The need to routinely administer additional doses is unknown at this time.[18]

A final total of 4 doses is necessary to complete a series of primary and booster doses. Children and adolescents with a previously incomplete series of IPV should receive sufficient additional doses to reach this number.

ADULTS

Unvaccinated Adults

For unvaccinated adults at increased risk of exposure to poliovirus, a primary series of poliovirus vaccine, inactivated is recommended. While the responses of adults to primary series have not been studied, the recommended schedule for adults is 2 doses given at a 1 to 2 month interval and a third dose given 6 to 12 months later. If less than 3 months but more than 2 months are available before protection is needed, 3 doses of poliovirus vaccine, inactivated should be given at least 1 month apart. Likewise, if only 1 or 2 months are available, 2 doses of poliovirus vaccine, inactivated should be given at least 1 month apart. If less than 1 month is available, a single dose of either OPV or IPV is recommended.

Incompletely Vaccinated Adults

Adults who are at an increased risk of exposure to poliovirus and who have had at least 1 dose of OPV, fewer than 3 doses of conventional IPV or a combination of conventional IPV or OPV totalling fewer than 3 doses should receive at least 1 dose of OPV or poliovirus vaccine, inactivated. Additional doses needed to complete a primary series should be given if time permits.

Completely Vaccinated Adults

Adults who are at an increased risk of exposure to poliovirus and who have previously completed a primary series with one or a combination of polio vaccines can be given a dose of either OPV or IPV.[19]

PRODUCT LISTING - EQUIVALENTS NOT AVAILABLE

Suspension - Subcutaneous - Strength n/a

0.50 ml	$19.50	IPOL, Allscripts Pharmaceutical Company	54569-3246-00
0.50 ml	$20.60	IPOL, Compumed Pharmaceuticals	00403-4961-18
0.50 ml	$29.79	IPOL, Aventis Pharmaceuticals	49281-0860-51
0.50 ml	$31.68	IPOL, Physicians Total Care	54868-4105-00
0.50 ml x 10	$314.90	IPOL, Aventis Pharmaceuticals	49281-0860-52
5 ml	$206.40	IPOL, Allscripts Pharmaceutical Company	54569-4812-00
5 ml	$270.58	IPOL, Aventis Pharmaceuticals	49281-0860-10

Polio Vaccine, Oral Live (002061)

For complete prescribing information, refer to the CD-ROM included with the book.

Categories: Immunization, poliomyelitis; Pregnancy Category C; FDA Approval Pre 1982; WHO Formulary

Drug Classes: Vaccines

Brand Names: **Orimune**

Foreign Brand Availability: Buccopol Berna (Hong-Kong; Malaysia; Peru); Imovax Polio (Korea); Imovax Polio Sabin (Taiwan); OPV-Merieux (South-Africa); Oral Polio Vaccine (Benin; Burkina-Faso; Ethiopia; Gambia; Ghana; Guinea; Israel; Ivory-Coast; Kenya; Liberia; Malawi; Mali; Mauritania; Mauritius; Morocco; Niger; Nigeria; Senegal; Seychelles; Sierra-Leone; Sudan; Tanzania; Tunia; Uganda; Zambia; Zimbabwe); Oral Poliomyelitis Vaccine-Sabine (Australia); Oral Virelon (Germany; New-Zealand); Polio Sabin (Ecuador; Israel; Mexico; Philippines; Taiwan; Thailand); Polio Sabin Oral (Austria); Polio "Sabin" Oral Vaccine (Czech-Republic); Polio Sabin OS (Italy); Polio Sabin-S (Germany); Polio-Kovax (Korea); Polioral (Israel; Korea; Malaysia; Mexico; Philippines; South-Africa; Taiwan; Thailand); Polioral Trivalent (Bahrain; Cyprus; Egypt; Iran; Iraq; Jordan; Kuwait; Lebanon; Libya; Oman; Qatar; Republic-of-Yemen; Saudi-Arabia; Syria; United-Arab-Emirates); Tri-Polio (Korea)

DESCRIPTION

Poliovirus vaccine, oral live trivalent is a mixture of three types of attenuated polioviruses that have been propagated in monkey kidney cell culture. The cells are grown in the presence of Eagle's basal medium consisting of Earle's balanced salt solution containing amino acids, antibiotics, and calf serum. After cell growth, the medium is removed and replaced with fresh medium containing the inoculating virus but no calf serum. The final vaccine is diluted with a modified cell-culture maintenance medium containing sorbitol. Each dose (0.5 ml) contains less than 25 μg of each of the antibiotics, streptomycin and neomycin.

Potency of the vaccine is expressed in terms of the amount of virus (log10) contained in the recommended dose as tissue culture infective doses (TCID50). The human dose of vaccine containing all three virus types shall be constituted to have infectivity titers in the final container material of (10 to power 5.4) to (10 to power 6.4) for Type 1, (10 to power 4.5) to (10 to power 5.5) for Type 2, and (10 to power 5.2) to (10 to power 6.2) for Type 3, when the primary monkey kidney tube titration method is used. If the more sensitive Hep-2 microtitration procedure is employed to determine the infectivity titers in each human dose, then equivalent vaccine is achieved with numerical infectivity titers of (10 to power 6.0) to (10 to power 7.0) for Type 1, (10 to power 5.1) to (10 to power 6.1) for Type 2, and (10 to power 5.8) to (10 to power 6.8) for Type 3.

STORAGE

To maintain potency of poliovirus vaccine live oral trivalent, it is necessary to store this vaccine at a temperature which will maintain ice continuously in a solid state (below 0°C, or 32°F). However, since the vaccine contains sorbitol it may remain fluid at temperature above -14°C (+7°F). Ice cubes that remain frozen continuously when stored in the same freezer compartment will confirm that the temperature is appropriate for storage of poliovirus vaccine live oral trivalent. If frozen, the vaccine must be completely thawed prior to use. A container of vaccine that has been frozen and then is thawed may be carried through a maximum of 10 freeze-thaw cycles, provided the temperature does not exceed 8°C (46°F) during the periods of thaw, and provided the total cumulative duration of thaw does not exceed 24 hours. If the 24 hour period is exceeded, the vaccine must be used within 30 days, during which time it must be stored at a temperature between 2-8°C (36-46°F). Ideally, a poliovirus vaccine live oral trivalent dispette should be removed from the freezer and thawed immediately prior to use.

INDICATIONS AND USAGE

THIS VACCINE IS INDICATED FOR USE IN THE PREVENTION OF POLIOMYELITIS CAUSED BY POLIOVIRUS TYPES 1, 2, and 3.

INFANTS FROM 6-12 WEEKS OF AGE, ALL UNIMMUNIZED CHILDREN, AND ADOLESCENTS up to age 18 are the usual candidates for routine prophylaxis.

The Immunization Practices Advisory Committee (ACIP) of the Public Health Service states that trivalent oral poliovirus vaccine (OPV) and inactivated poliovirus vaccine (IPV) are both effective in preventing poliomyelitis.

The choice of OPV as the preferred poliovirus vaccine for primary administration to children in the United States has been made by the ACIP, the Committee on Infectious Diseases of the American Academy of Pediatrics, and a special expert committee of the Institute of Medicine, National Academy of Science. OPV is preferred because it induces intestinal immunity, is simple to administer, is well accepted by patients, results in immunization of some contacts of vaccinated persons, and has a record of having essentially eliminated disease associated with wild poliovirus in this country. OPV is also recommended for control of epidemic poliomyelitis.

IPV is specifically indicated for use in immunodeficient individuals, their household contacts, or in certain adults (See CONTRAINDICATIONS and Use In Adults for details).

Prior to immunization, the parent, guardian, or adult patient should be informed of the two types of poliovirus vaccines available, the risks and benefits of each to the individual and to the community, and the reasons why recommendations are made for giving specific vaccines under certain circumstances.

Past history of clinical poliomyelitis or prior vaccination with IPV in otherwise healthy individuals does not preclude the administration of OPV when otherwise indicated.

The simultaneous administration of OPV, diphtheria and tetanus toxoids and pertussis vaccine (DTP), and/or measles-mumps-rubella vaccine (MMR), has resulted in seroconversion rates and rates of side effects similar to those observed when the vaccines are administered separately.

Administration of Immune Globulin (IG), if necessary, within 7 days prior to immunization with OPV does not reduce the antibody response to OPV based on a study conducted in Peace Corps volunteers.

USE IN ADULTS

Routine primary poliovirus immunization of adults (generally those 18 years of age or older), residing in the United States, is not recommended by the Immunization Practices Advisory Committee (ACIP). Immunization is recommended by the ACIP for certain adults who are at greater risk of exposure to wild polioviruses than the general population, including travelers to areas where poliomyelitis is endemic or epidemic, members of communities or specific population groups with disease caused by wild polioviruses, laboratory workers handling specimens that may contain polioviruses, and health care workers in close contact with patients who might be excreting polioviruses as follows: UNIMMUNIZED ADULTS-primary immunization with enhanced-potency IPV is recommended. However, if less than 1 month is available before protection is needed, a single dose of either OPV or enhanced-potency IPV is recommended, with the remaining doses given later if the person remains at increased risk. INCOMPLETELY IMMUNIZED ADULTS who have had 1) at least one dose OPV, 2) fewer than three doses of conventional IPV, or 3) a combination of conventional IPV and OPV totaling fewer than three doses, should receive at least one dose of OPV or enhanced-potency IPV. Additional doses needed to complete a primary series should be given prior to exposure, if time permits. ADULTS WHO HAVE COMPLETED A PRIMARY SERIES with any one or a combination of polio vaccines may be given a dose of OPV or enhanced-potency IPV. Immunization with IPV may be undertaken in unimmunized or inadequately immunized adults in households in which children are to be given OPV.

EPIDEMIC CONTROL

Poliovirus vaccine, oral live trivalent has been recommended for epidermic control. Within an epidemic are, OPV should be provided for all persons over 6 weeks of age who have not been completely immunized or whose immunization status is unknown, with the exceptions noted under immunodeficiency. (See CONTRAINDICATIONS.)

In certain tropical endemic areas, where poliomyelitis has been increasing in recent years, the physician may wish to administer OPV to the infant at birth. Because successful immunization is less likely in new born infants, a complete series of OPV should follow the neonatal dose beginning when the infants are 2 months old. If the physician elects to immunize the infant at birth, it may be prudent to wait until the child is 3 days old, and to recommend abstention from breast-feeding for 2-3 hours before and after oral immunization to minimize exposure of the vaccine viruses to colostrum and to permit the establishment of the vaccine viruses in the gut.

CONTRAINDICATIONS

UNDER NO CIRCUMSTANCES SHOULD THIS VACCINE BE ADMINISTERED PARENTERALLY.

Poliovirus vaccine liver oral trivalent must not be administered to patients with immune deficiency diseases such as combined immunodeficiency, hypogammaglobulinemia and agammaglobulinemia. Further, poliovirus vaccine live oral trivalent must not be administered to patients with altered immune states, such as those occurring in human immunodeficiency virus (HIV) infection, thymic abnormalities, leukemia, lymphoma, generalized malignancy or advanced debilitating conditions, or by lowered resistance from therapy with corticosteroids, alkylating drugs, antimetabolites, or radiation. Because vaccine viruses are excreted by the vaccinee, and may spread to contacts, poliovirus vaccine live oral trivalent should not be used in families with immunodeficient members.

Recipients of the vaccine should avoid close household-type contact with all persons with altered immune status for at least 6-8 weeks.

Because of the possibility of immunodeficiency in other children born to a family in which there has been one such case, opv should not be given to a member of a household in which there is a family history of immunodeficiency until the immune status of the intended recipient and other children in the family is determined to be normal.

Immunization of all persons in the above described circumstances should be with ipv.

WARNINGS

UNDER NO CIRCUMSTANCES SHOULD THIS VACCINE BE ADMINISTERED PARENTERALLY.

Immunization should be deferred during the course of any febrile illness or acute infection. In addition, immunization should be deferred in the presence of persistent vomiting or diarrhea, or suspected gastroenteritis infection. Other viruses (including poliovirus and other enteroviruses) may compromise the desired response to this vaccine, since their presence in the intestinal tract may interfere with the replication of the attenuated strains of poliovirus.

DOSAGE AND ADMINISTRATION

Poliovirus vaccine, oral live trivalent is to be administered ORALLY, UNDER THE SUPERVISION OF A PHYSICIAN. UNDER NO CIRCUMSTANCES SHOULD THIS VACCINE BE ADMINISTERED PARENTERALLY. For convenience, the vaccine is supplied in a disposable pipette containing a single dose of 0.5 ml which should be administered directly into the mouth of the vaccinee. Breast feeding does not interfere with successful immunization when OPV is administered according to the following schedule.

PRIMARY SERIES

The primary series consists of three doses.

Infants

The ACIP and AAP recommend that the first dose of OPV be administered when the infant is approximately 2 months (6-12 weeks) of age. The second dose should be given not less than 6 and preferably 8 weeks later, commonly at 4 months of age. A third dose of OPV should be given when the child is approximately 15-18 months of age to complete the primary series, but may be given at any time between 12 and 24 months of age. In endemic areas an additional dose administered 2 months after the second dose is desirable.

Older Children and Adolescents (up to 18 years of age)

Unimmunized children and adolescents should receive two doses given not less than 6 and preferably 8 weeks apart, followed by a third dose 6-12 months after the second dose. If there is substantial risk of exposure to polio, the third dose should be given 6-8 weeks after the second dose.

Children at any age who are unimmunized or partially immunized should receive the number of doses necessary to complete the required series of three doses. If the schedule has been interrupted, the series does not need to be reinitiated.

Adults

See INDICATIONS AND USAGE. Where OPV is given to unimmunized adults the dosage regimen is ad indicated for older children and adolescents.

Supplemental Doses/School Entry

On entering elementary school, all children who have completed the primary series should be given a single follow-up dose of OPV (all others should complete the primary series). The fourth supplemental dose is not required in those who received the third primary dose on or after their fourth birthday. The ACIP and AAP do not recommend routine booster doses of vaccine beyond that given at the time of entering school. It has been shown that over 95% of children studied 5 years after full immunization with oral polio vaccine had protective antibodies to all three types of poliovirus.

INCREASED RISK: If an individual who has completed a primary series is subjected to a substantially increased risk because of personal contact, travel, or occupation, a single dose of OPV may be given.

SIMULTANEOUS ADMINISTRATION WITH OTHER VACCINE

The simultaneous administration of OPV, diphtheria and tetanus toxoids and pertussis vaccine (DTP) and/or measles-mumps-rubella vaccine (MMR), has resulted in seroconversion rates and rates of side effects similar to those observed when the vaccines are administered separately. The AAP states that OPV, DTP, MMR and/or Haemophilus b conjugate vaccines may be given concomitantly.

COLOR CHANGE

This vaccine contains phenol red as a pH indicator. The usual color of the vaccine is pink, although some containers of vaccine, shipped or stored in dry ice, may exhibit a yellow coloration due to the very low temperature or possible absorption of carbon dioxide. The color of the vaccine prior to use (red- pink-yellow) has no effect on the virus or efficacy of the vaccine.

P

Polymyxin B Sulfate; Trimethoprim Sulfate (002067)

Categories: Blepharoconjunctivitis; Conjunctivitis, infectious; Pregnancy Category C; FDA Approved 1988 Oct
Drug Classes: Antibiotics, folate antagonists; Antibiotics, polymyxins; Antibiotics, sulfonamides; Anti-infectives, ophthalmic; Ophthalmics
Brand Names: Polytrim
Foreign Brand Availability: Destrim (Colombia)
Cost of Therapy: $21.88 (Bacterial Conjunctivitis; Polytrim Ophthalmic Solution; 10000u; 1 mg/ml; 6 drops/day; 7 day supply)
$17.23 (Bacterial Conjunctivitis; Generic Ophthalmic Solution; 10000u; 1 mg/ml; 6 drops/day; 7 day supply)

DESCRIPTION

Polytrim ophthalmic solution (trimethoprim sulfate and polymyxin B sulfate) is a sterile antimicrobial solution for topical ophthalmic use. Each ml contains trimethoprim sulfate equivalent to 1 mg trimethoprim and polymyxin B sulfate 10,000 units. The vehicle contains benzalkonium chloride 0.004% (added as a preservative) and the inactive ingredients sodium chloride, sodium hydroxide or sulfuric acid (added to adjust pH), and water for injection.

Trimethoprim sulfate, 2,4-diamino-5-(3,4,5-trimethoxybenzyl)pyrimidine sulfate (2:1), is a white, odorless, crystalline powder with a molecular weight of 678.72.

Polymyxin B sulfate is the sulfate salt of polymyxin B_1 and B_2, which are produced by the growth of *Bacillus polymyxa* (Prazmowski) Migula (Fam. Bacillaceae). It has a potency of not less than 6,000 Polymyxin B units per mg, calculated on an anhydrous basis.

CLINICAL PHARMACOLOGY

Trimethoprim is a synthetic antibacterial drug active against a wide variety of aerobic gram-positive and gram-negative ophthalmic pathogens. Trimethoprim blocks the production of tetrahydrofolic acid from dihydrofolic acid by binding to and reversibly inhibiting the enzyme dihydrofolate reductase. This binding is very much stronger for the bacterial enzyme than for the corresponding mammalian enzyme. For that reason, trimethoprim selectively interferes with bacterial biosynthesis of nucleic acids and proteins.

Polymyxin B, a cyclic lipopeptide antibiotic, is rapidly bactericidal for a variety of gram-negative organisms, especially *Pseudomonas aeruginosa*. It increases the permeability of the bacterial cell membrane by interacting with the phospholipid components of the membrane.

When used topically, trimethoprim and polymyxin B absorption through intact skin and mucous membranes is insignificant.

Blood samples were obtained from 11 human volunteers at 20 minutes, 1 hour and 3 hours following instillation in the eye of 2 drops of ophthalmic solution containing 1 mg trimethoprim and 10,000 units polymyxin B per ml. Peak serum concentrations were approximately 0.03 μg/ml trimethoprim and 1 unit/ml polymyxin B.

MICROBIOLOGY

In vitro studies have demonstrated that the anti-infective components of Polymyxin B-S-T-S are active against the following bacterial pathogens that are capable of causing external infections of the eye:

Trimethoprim: *Staphylococcus aureus* and *Staphylococcus epidermidis, Streptococcus pyogenes, Streptococcus faecalis, Streptococcus pneumoniae, Haemophilus influenzae, Haemophilus aegyptius, Escherichia coli, Klebsiella pneumoniae, Proteus mirabilis* (indole-negative), *Proteus vulgaris* (indole-positive), *Enterobacter aerogenes,* and *Serratia marcescens.*

Polymyxin B: *Pseudomonas aeruginosa, Escherichia coli, Klebsiella pneumoniae, Enterobacter aerogenes* and *Haemophilus influenzae.*

P

INDICATIONS AND USAGE

Polymyxin B; trimethoprim ophthalmic solution is indicated in the treatment of surface ocular bacterial infections, including acute bacterial conjunctivitis, and blepharoconjunctivitis, caused by susceptible strains of the following microorganisms: *Staphylococcus aureus, Staphylococcus epidermidis, Streptococcus pneumoniae, Streptococcus viridans, Haemophilus influenzae* and *Pseudomonas aeruginosa.**

* Efficacy for this organism in this organ system was studied in fewer than 10 infections.

CONTRAINDICATIONS

Polymyxin B; trimethoprim ophthalmic solution is contraindicated in patients with known hypersensitivity to any of its components.

WARNINGS

NOT FOR INJECTION INTO THE EYE. If a sensitivity reaction to Polymyxin B/Trimethoprim occurs, discontinue use. Polymyxin B; trimethoprim ophthalmic solution is not indicated for the prophylaxis or treatment of ophthalmia neonatorum.

PRECAUTIONS

GENERAL

As with other antimicrobial preparations, prolonged use may result in overgrowth of nonsusceptible organisms, including fungi. If superinfection occurs, appropriate therapy should be initiated.

INFORMATION FOR THE PATIENT

Avoid contaminating the applicator tip with material from the eye, fingers, or other source. This precaution is necessary if the sterility of the drops is to be maintained.

If redness, irritation, swelling or pain persists or increases, discontinue use immediately and contact your physician.

CARCINOGENESIS, MUTAGENESIS, AND IMPAIRMENT OF FERTILITY

Carcinogenesis

Long-term studies in animals to evaluate carcinogenic potential have not been conducted with polymyxin B sulfate or trimethoprim.

Mutagenesis

Trimethoprim was demonstrated to be non-mutagenic in the Ames assay. In studies at two laboratories no chromosomal damage was detected in cultured Chinese hamster ovary cells at concentrations approximately 500 times human plasma levels after oral administration; at concentrations approximately 1000 times human plasma levels after oral administration in these same cells a low level of chromosomal damage was induced at one of the laboratories. Studies to evaluate mutagenic potential have not been conducted with polymyxin B sulfate.

Impairment of Fertility

Polymyxin B sulfate has been reported to impair the motility of equine sperm, but its effects on male or female fertility are unknown.

No adverse effects on fertility or general reproductive performance were observed in rats given trimethoprim in oral dosages as high as 70 mg/kg/day for males and 14 mg/kg/day for females.

PREGNANCY, TERATOGENIC EFFECTS, PREGNANCY CATEGORY C

Animal reproduction studies have not been conducted with polymyxin B sulfate. It is not known whether polymyxin B sulfate can cause fetal harm when administered to a pregnant woman or can affect reproduction capacity.

Trimethoprim has been shown to be teratogenic in the rat when given in oral doses 40 times the human dose. In some rabbit studies, the overall increase in fetal loss (dead and resorbed and malformed conceptuses) was associated with oral doses 6 times the human therapeutic dose.

While there are no large well-controlled studies on the use of trimethoprim in pregnant women, Brumfitt and Pursell, in a retrospective study, reported the outcome of 186 pregnancies during which the mother received either placebo or oral trimethoprim in combination with sulfamethoxazole. The incidence of congenital abnormalities was 4.5% (3 of 66) in those who received placebo and 3.3% (4 of 120) in those receiving trimethoprim and sulfamethoxazole. There were no abnormalities in the 10 children whose mothers received the drug during the first trimester. In a separate survey, Brumfitt and Pursell also found no congenital abnormalities in 35 children whose mothers had received oral trimethoprim and sulfamethoxazole at the time of conception or shortly thereafter.

Because trimethoprim may interfere with folic acid metabolism, trimethoprim should be used during pregnancy only if the potential benefit justifies the potential risk to the fetus.

Nonteratogenic Effects

The oral administration of trimethoprim to rats at a dose of 70 mg/kg/day commencing with the last third of gestation and continuing through parturition and lactation caused no deleterious effects on gestation or pup growth and survival.

NURSING MOTHERS

It is not known whether this drug is excreted in human milk. Because many drugs are excreted in human milk, caution should be exercised when Polymyxin B/Trimethoprim Opthalmic Solution is administered to a nursing woman.

PEDIATRIC USE

Safety and effectiveness in children below the age of 2 months have not been established (see WARNINGS.)

ADVERSE REACTIONS

The most frequent adverse reaction to polymyxin B; trimethoprim ophthalmic solution is local irritation consisting of increased redness, burning, stinging, and/or itching. This may occur on instillation, within 48 hours, or at any time with extended use. There are also multiple reports of hypersensitivity reactions consisting of lid edema, itching, increased redness, tearing, and/or circumocular rash.

Photosensitivity has been reported in patients taking oral trimethoprim.

DOSAGE AND ADMINISTRATION

ADULTS

In mild to moderate infections, instill one drop in the affected eye(s) every three hours (maximum of 6 doses per day) for a period of 7 to 10 days.

PEDIATRIC USE

Clinical studies have shown Polymyxin B/Trimethoprim to be safe and effective for use in children over two months of age. The dosage regimen is the same as for adults.

HOW SUPPLIED

A sterile ophthalmic solution, each ml contains trimethoprim sulfate equivalent to 1 mg trimethoprim and polymyxin B sulfate 10,000 units in a plastic dropper bottle of 10 ml.
Storage: Store at 15-25°C (59-77°F) and protect from light.

PRODUCT LISTING - RATED THERAPEUTICALLY EQUIVALENT

Solution - Ophthalmic - 10000 U;1 mg/ml

Size	Price	Product	NDC
10 ml	$17.23	GENERIC, Pacific Pharma	60758-0908-10
10 ml	$17.42	GENERIC, Bausch and Lomb	24208-0315-10
10 ml	$17.42	GENERIC, Falcon Pharmaceuticals, Ltd.	61314-0628-10
10 ml	$17.50	GENERIC, Akorn Inc	17478-0703-11
10 ml	$19.50	GENERIC, Cheshire Drugs	55175-2746-01
10 ml	$21.88	POLYTRIM, Southwood Pharmaceuticals Inc	58016-6336-01
10 ml	$30.19	POLYTRIM, Allscripts Pharmaceutical Company	54569-2867-00
10 ml	$34.55	POLYTRIM, Allergan Inc	00023-7824-10

10 ml $34.68 POLYTRIM, Physicians Total Care 54868-1148-00
Solution - Opthalmic - 10,000 us/ml;EQ 1 mg/ml
10 ml $12.36 FEDERAL UPPER LIMIT, H.C.F.A. F F P 99999-2067-01

PRODUCT LISTING - EQUIVALENTS NOT AVAILABLE

Solution - Ophthalmic - 10000 U;1 mg/ml
10 ml $27.75 GENERIC, Southwood Pharmaceuticals Inc 58016-5561-01
10 ml $28.64 GENERIC, Pharma Pac 52959-0609-10

Polythiazide *(002068)*

Categories: Edema; Hypertension, essential; FDA Approved 1961 Sep; Pregnancy Category D
Drug Classes: Diuretics, thiazide and derivatives
Brand Names: **Renese**
Foreign Brand Availability: Drenusil (Germany); Nephril (Ireland)
Cost of Therapy: $19.35 (Hypertension; Renese; 2 mg; 1 tablet/day; 30 day supply)

DESCRIPTION

Polythiazide is designated generically as polythiazide, and chemically as 2*H*-1,2,4-Benzothiadiazine-7-sulfonamide, 6-chloro-3,4-dihydro-2- methyl-3-(((2,2,2-trifluoroethyl) thio)methyl)-,1,1-dioxide. It is a white crystalline substance, insoluble in water but readily soluble in alkaline solution.

Inert Ingredients: dibasic calcium phosphate; lactose; magnesium stearate; polyethylene glycol; sodium laurel sulfate; starch; vanillin. The 2 mg tablets also contain: Yellow 6; Yellow 10.

CLINICAL PHARMACOLOGY

The mechanism of action results in an interference with the renal tubular mechanism of electrolyte reabsorption. At maximal therapeutic dosage all thiazides are approximately equal in their diuretic potency. The mechanism whereby thiazides function in the control of hypertension is unknown.

INDICATIONS AND USAGE

Polythiazide is indicated as adjunctive therapy in edema associated with congestive heart failure, hepatic cirrhosis, and corticosteroid and estrogen therapy.

Polythiazide has also been found useful in edema due to various forms of renal dysfunction as: Nephrotic syndrome; Acute glomerulonephritis; and Chronic renal failure.

Polythiazide is indicated in the management of hypertension either as the sole therapeutic agent or to enhance the effectiveness of other antihypertensive drugs in the more severe forms of hypertension.

USAGE IN PREGNANCY

The routine use of diuretics in an otherwise healthy woman is inappropriate and exposes mother and fetus to unnecessary hazard. Diuretics do not prevent development of toxemia of pregnancy, and there is no satisfactory evidence that they are useful in the treatment of developed toxemia.

Edema during pregnancy may arise from pathological causes or from the physiologic and mechanical consequences of pregnancy. Thiazides are indicated in pregnancy when edema is due to pathologic causes, just as they are in the absence of pregnancy (however, see WARNINGS, below). Dependent edema in pregnancy, resulting from restriction of venous return by the expanded uterus, is properly treated through elevation of the lower extremities and use of support hose; use of diuretics to lower intravascular volume in this case is illogical and unnecessary. There is hypervolemia during normal pregnancy which is harmful to neither the fetus nor the mother (in the absence of cardiovascular disease), but which is associated with edema, including generalized edema, in the majority of pregnant women. If this edema produces discomfort, increased recumbency will often provide relief. In rare instances, this edema may cause extreme discomfort which is not relieved by rest. In these cases, a short course of diuretics may provide relief and may be appropriate.

CONTRAINDICATIONS

Anuria. Hypersensitivity to this or other sulfonamide derived drugs.

WARNINGS

Thiazides should be used with caution in severe renal disease. In patients with renal disease, thiazides may precipitate azotemia. Cumulative effects of the drug may develop in patients with impaired renal function.

Thiazides should be used with caution in patients with impaired hepatic function or progressive liver disease, since minor alterations of fluid and electrolyte balance may precipitate hepatic coma.

Thiazides may add to or potentiate the action of other antihypertensive drugs. Potentiation occurs with ganglionic or peripheral adrenergic blocking drugs.

Sensitivity reactions may occur in patients with a history of allergy or bronchial asthma.

The possibility of exacerbation or activation of systemic lupus erythematosus has been reported.

USE IN PREGNANCY

Thiazides cross the placental barrier and appear in cord blood. The use of thiazides in pregnant women requires that the anticipated benefit be weighed against possible hazards to the fetus. These hazards include fetal or neonatal jaundice, thrombocytopenia, and possibly other adverse reactions which have occurred in the adult.

NURSING MOTHERS

Thiazides appear in breast milk. If use of the drug is deemed essential, the patient should stop nursing.

PRECAUTIONS

Periodic determination of serum electrolytes to detect possible electrolyte imbalance should be performed at appropriate intervals.

All patients receiving thiazide therapy should be observed for clinical signs of fluid or electrolyte imbalance; namely, hyponatremia, hypochloremic alkalosis, and hypokalemia. Serum and urine electrolyte determinations are particularly important when the patient is vomiting excessively or receiving parenteral fluids. Medication such as digitalis may also influence serum electrolytes. Warning signs, irrespective of cause, are: dryness of mouth, thirst, weakness, lethargy, drowsiness, restlessness, muscle pains or cramps, muscular fatigue, hypotension, oliguria, tachycardia, and gastrointestinal disturbances such as nausea and vomiting.

Hypokalemia may develop with thiazides as with any other potent diuretic, especially with brisk diuresis, when severe cirrhosis is present, or during concomitant use of corticosteroids or ACTH.

Interference with adequate oral electrolyte intake will also contribute to hypokalemia. Digitalis therapy may exaggerate metabolic effects of hypokalemia especially with reference to myocardial activity.

Any chloride deficit is generally mild and usually does not require specific treatment except under extraordinary circumstances (as in liver disease or renal disease). Dilutional hyponatremia may occur in edematous patients in hot weather; appropriate therapy is water restriction, rather than administration of salt except in rare instances when the hyponatremia is life threatening. In actual salt depletion, appropriate replacement is the therapy of choice.

Hyperuricemia may occur or frank gout may be precipitated in certain patients receiving thiazide therapy.

Insulin requirements in diabetic patients may be increased, decreased, or unchanged. Latent diabetes mellitus may become manifest during thiazide administration.

Thiazide drugs may increase the responsiveness to tubocurarine.

The antihypertensive effects of the drug may be enhanced in the postsympathectomy patient.

Thiazides may decrease arterial responsiveness to norepinephrine. This diminution is not sufficient to preclude effectiveness of the pressor agent for therapeutic use.

If progressive renal impairment becomes evident, as indicated by a rising nonprotein nitrogen or blood urea nitrogen, a careful reappraisal of therapy is necessary with consideration given to withholding or discontinuing diuretic therapy.

Thiazides may decrease serum PBI levels without signs of thyroid disturbance.

ADVERSE REACTIONS

Gastrointestinal System Reactions: Anorexia, gastric irritation, nausea, vomiting, cramping, diarrhea, constipation, jaundice (intrahepatic cholestatic jaundice), pancreatitis

Central Nervous System Reactions: Dizziness, vertigo, paresthesias, headache, xanthopsia

Hematologic Reactions: Leukopenia, agranulocytosis, thrombocytopenia, aplastic anemia

Dermatologic/Hypersensitivity Reactions: Purpura, photosensitivity, rash, urticaria, necrotizing angiitis, (vasculitis), (cutaneous vasculitis)

Cardiovascular Reaction: Orthostatic hypotension may occur and may be aggravated by alcohol, barbiturates or narcotics.

Other: Hyperglycemia, glycosuria, hyperuricemia, muscle spasm, weakness, restlessness

Whenever adverse reactions are moderate or severe, thiazide dosage should be reduced or therapy withdrawn.

DOSAGE AND ADMINISTRATION

Therapy should be individualized according to patient response. This therapy should be titrated to gain maximal therapeutic response as well as the minimal dose possible to maintain that therapeutic response. The usual dosage of Polythiazide tablets for diuretic therapy is 1-4 mg daily, and for antihypertensive therapy is 2-4 mg daily.

HOW SUPPLIED

Polythiazide (polythiazide) tablets are available as:

1 mg: White, scored tablets.
2 mg: Yellow, scored tablets.
4 mg: White, scored tablets.

PRODUCT LISTING - EQUIVALENTS NOT AVAILABLE

Tablet - Oral - 1 mg
100's $49.29 RENESE, Pfizer U.S. Pharmaceuticals 00069-3750-66
Tablet - Oral - 2 mg
100's $64.50 RENESE, Pfizer U.S. Pharmaceuticals 00069-3760-66

Polythiazide; Prazosin Hydrochloride *(002069)*

Categories: Hypertension, essential; Pregnancy Category C; FDA Approval Pre 1982
Drug Classes: Antiadrenergics, alpha blocking; Antiadrenergics, peripheral; Diuretics, thiazide and derivatives
Brand Names: **Minizide**
Cost of Therapy: $118.71 (Hypertension; Minizide; 0.5 mg; 5 mg; 3 capsules/day; 30 day supply)

WARNING

This fixed combination drug is not indicated for initial therapy of hypertension. Hypertension requires therapy titrated to the individual patient. If the fixed combination represents the dose so determined,

P

> **WARNING — Cont'd**
> **its use may be more convenient in patient management. The treatment of hypertension is not static, but must be re-evaluated as conditions in each patient warrant.**

DESCRIPTION

FOR COMPLETE PRESCRIBING INFORMATION REFER TO THE INDIVIDUAL DRUG MONOGRAPHS (POLYTHIAZIDE; PRAZOSIN HYDROCHLORIDE).

DOSAGE AND ADMINISTRATION

POLYTHIAZIDE; PRAZOSIN HCl

Dosage: as determined by individual titration of prazosin HCl and polythiazide. (See BOXED WARNING.)

Usual polythiazide; prazosin HCl dosage is 1 capsule two or three times daily, the strength depending upon individual requirement following titration.

The following is a general guide to the administration of the individual components of polythiazide; prazosin HCl:

Prazosin HCl

Initial Dose: 1 mg two or three times a day.

Maintenance Dose: Dosage may be slowly increased to a total daily dose of 20 mg given in divided doses. The therapeutic dosages most commonly employed have ranged from 6 mg to 15 mg daily given in divided doses. Doses higher than 20 mg usually do not increase efficacy, however a few patients may benefit from further increases up to a daily dose of 40 mg given in divided doses. After initial titration some patients can be maintained adequately on a twice daily dosage regimen.

Use With Other Drugs: When adding a diuretic or other antihypertensive agent, the dose of prazosin HCl should be reduced to 1 mg or 2 mg three times a day and retitration then carried out.

Polythiazide

The usual dose of polythiazide for antihypertensive therapy is 2 to 4 mg daily.

HOW SUPPLIED

TABLE 1

Strength	Components	Color	Capsule Code	Pkg. Size
Minizide 1	1 mg prazosin + 0.5 mg polythiazide	Blue-Green	430	100's
Minizide 2	2 mg prazosin + 0.5 mg polythiazide	Blue-Green/ Pink	432	100's
Minizide 5	5 mg prazosin + 0.5 mg polythiazide	Blue-Green/ Blue	436	100's

PRODUCT LISTING - EQUIVALENTS NOT AVAILABLE

Capsule - Oral - 0.5 mg;1 mg
100's $78.40 MINIZIDE, Pfizer U.S. Pharmaceuticals 00069-4300-66

Capsule - Oral - 0.5 mg;2 mg
100's $86.96 MINIZIDE, Pfizer U.S. Pharmaceuticals 00069-4320-66

Capsule - Oral - 0.5 mg;5 mg
100's $131.90 MINIZIDE, Pfizer U.S. Pharmaceuticals 00069-4360-66

Porfimer Sodium *(003228)*

For complete prescribing information, refer to the CD-ROM included with the book.

Categories: Carcinoma, esophageal; Carcinoma, lung; Pregnancy Category C; FDA Approved 1995 Dec; Orphan Drugs
Drug Classes: Antineoplastics, miscellaneous
Brand Names: Photofrin
HCFA JCODE(S): J9600 75 mg IV

DESCRIPTION

Photofrin (porfimer sodium) for injection is a photosensitizing agent used in the photodynamic therapy (PDT) of tumors. Following reconstitution of the freeze-dried product with 5% dextrose injection or 0.9% sodium chloride injection, it is injected intravenously. This is followed 40-50 hours later by illumination of the tumor with laser light (630 nm wavelength). Photofrin is not a single chemical entity; it is a mixture of oligomers formed by ether and ester linkages of up to 8 porphyrin units. It is a dark red to reddish brown cake or powder. Each vial of Photofrin contains 75 mg of porfimer sodium as a sterile freeze-dried cake or powder. Hydrochloric acid and/or sodium hydroxide may be added during manufacture to adjust pH. There are no preservatives or other additives.

INDICATIONS AND USAGE

Photodynamic therapy with porfimer sodium is indicated for:

- Palliation of patients with completely obstructing esophageal cancer, or of patients with partially obstructing esophageal cancer who, in the opinion of their physician, cannot be satisfactorily treated with Nd:YAG laser therapy.
- Reduction of obstruction and palliation of symptoms in patients with completely or partially obstructing endobronchial nonsmall cell lung cancer (NSCLC).
- Treatment of microinvasive endobronchial NSCLC in patients for whom surgery and radiotherapy are not indicated.

CONTRAINDICATIONS

Porfimer sodium is contraindicated in patients with porphyria or in patients with known allergies to porphyrins.

PDT is contraindicated in patients with an existing tracheoesophageal or bronchoesophageal fistula.

PDT is contraindicated in patients with tumors eroding into a major blood vessel.

WARNINGS

Following injection with porfimer sodium precautions must be taken to avoid exposure of skin and eyes to direct sunlight or bright indoor light.

ESOPHAGEAL CANCER

If the esophageal tumor is eroding into the trachea or bronchial tree, the likelihood of tracheoesophageal or bronchoesophageal fistula resulting from treatment is sufficiently high that PDT is not recommended.

Patients with esophageal varices should be treated with extreme caution. Light should not be given directly to the variceal area because of the high risk of bleeding.

ENDOBRONCHIAL CANCER

Patients should be assessed for the possibility that a tumor may be eroding into a pulmonary blood vessel (see CONTRAINDICATIONS). Patients at high risk for fatal hemoptysis include those with large, centrally located tumors, those with cavitating tumors or those with extensive tumor extrinsic to the bronchus.

If the endobronchial tumor invades deeply into the bronchial wall, the possibility exists for fistula formation upon resolution of tumor.

PDT should be used with extreme caution for endobronchial tumors in locations where treatment-induced inflammation could obstruct the main airway, *e.g.,* long or circumferential tumors of the trachea, tumors of the carina that involve both mainstem bronchi circumferentially, or circumferential tumors in the mainstem bronchus in patients with prior pneumonectomy.

DOSAGE AND ADMINISTRATION

Photodynamic therapy with porfimer sodium is a two-stage process requiring administration of both drug and light. The first stage of PDT is the intravenous injection of porfimer sodium at 2 mg/kg. Illumination with laser light 40-50 hours following injection with porfimer sodium constitutes the second stage of therapy. A second laser light application may be given 96-120 hours after injection, preceded by gentle debridement of residual tumor. In clinical studies, debridement via endoscopy was required 2 days after the initial light application. Standard endoscopic techniques are used for light administration and debridement. Practitioners should be fully familiar with the patient's condition and trained in the safe and efficacious treatment of esophageal or endobronchial cancer using photodynamic therapy with porfimer sodium and associated light delivery devices.

Patients may receive a second course of PDT a minimum of 30 days after the initial therapy; up to 3 courses of PDT (each separated by a minimum of 30 days) can be given. Before each course of treatment, patients with esophageal cancer should be evaluated for the presence of a tracheoesophageal or bronchoesophageal fistula (see CONTRAINDICATIONS). In patients with endobronchial lesions who have recently undergone radiotherapy, sufficient time (approximately 4 weeks) should be allowed between the therapies to ensure that the acute inflammation produced by radiotherapy has subsided prior to PDT. All patients should be evaluated for the possibility that the tumor may be eroding into a major blood vessel (see CONTRAINDICATIONS).

PRODUCT LISTING - EQUIVALENTS NOT AVAILABLE

Powder For Injection - Injectable - 75 mg
1's $2740.70 PHOTOFRIN, Scandipharm Inc 58914-0155-75

Potassium Chloride *(002081)*

Categories: Hypokalemia; Pregnancy Category C; FDA Approved 1972 Mar; WHO Formulary
Drug Classes: Electrolyte replacements; Vitamins/minerals
Brand Names: Cena-K; K Tab; K-10; K-Care; K-Dur; K-Lease; K-Lor; K-Lyte Cl; K-Norm; K-Sol; Kaochlor; Kaon Cl; Kaon-Cl; Kay Ciel; Klor-Con; Klorvess; Klotrix; Kolyum; Micro-K; Rum-K; **Slow-K**; Ten-K
Foreign Brand Availability: Acronitol (Greece); Addi-K (Benin; Burkina-Faso; Ethiopia; Gambia; Ghana; Guinea; Ivory-Coast; Kenya; Liberia; Malawi; Malaysia; Mali; Mauritania; Mauritius; Morocco; Niger; Nigeria; Senegal; Seychelles; Sierra-Leone; Sudan; Taiwan; Tanzania; Tunia; Uganda; Zambia; Zimbabwe); Apo-K (Canada; Malaysia); Celeka (Argentina); Chlorvescent (New-Zealand); Clor-K-Zaf (Mexico); Diffu-K (France); Durekal (Finland); Durules-K (Argentina); K-Contin (Benin; Burkina-Faso; Ethiopia; Gambia; Ghana; Guinea; Ivory-Coast; Kenya; Liberia; Malawi; Mali; Mauritania; Mauritius; Morocco; Niger; Nigeria; Senegal; Seychelles; Sierra-Leone; Sudan; Tanzania; Tunia; Uganda; Zambia; Zimbabwe); K-Contin Continus (Korea); K-SR (New-Zealand); K-Tab (Bahamas; Barbados; Belize; Bermuda; Curacao; Guyana; Jamaica; Netherland-Antilles; Surinam; Trinidad); Kaleorid (Denmark; France; Norway; Sweden); Kaliduron (Finland); Kaliglutol (Switzerland); Kalilente (Norway); Kalinor-Retard P (Germany); Kalinorm (Denmark; Finland); Kalinorm Depottab (Norway); Kaliolite (Mexico); Kalipor (Finland; Sweden); Kalipoz (Poland); Kalitabs (Sweden); Kalitrans Retard (Germany); Kalium (Benin; Burkina-Faso; Ethiopia; Gambia; Ghana; Guinea; Ivory-Coast; Kenya; Liberia; Malawi; Mali; Mauritania; Mauritius; Morocco; Netherlands; Niger; Nigeria; Philippines; Senegal; Seychelles; Sierra-Leone; Sudan; Tanzania; Tunia; Uganda; Zambia; Zimbabwe); Kalium-Durettes (Belgium; Netherlands); Kalium Duriles (Germany); Kalium-R (Hungary; Switzerland); Kalium Retard (Norway); Kay-Cee-L (England); KCL Retard (Austria; Bahrain; Cyprus; Czech-Republic; Egypt; Greece; Hungary; Iran; Iraq; Italy; Jordan; Kuwait; Lebanon; Libya; Oman; Qatar; Republic-of-Yemen; Saudi-Arabia; Spain; Syria; United-Arab-Emirates); Keylyte (India); KSR (Australia; Indonesia); Lento-Kalium (Italy); Leo-K (England; Ireland); Micro-K Extentcaps (Bahamas; Barbados; Belize; Bermuda; Curacao; Guyana; Jamaica; Netherland-Antilles; Surinam; Trinidad); Micro-Kalium Retard (Austria); Miopotasio (Spain); Nu-K (England); Plus Kalium Retard (Switzerland); Potasion (Spain); Rekawan (Germany); Rekawan Retard (Austria); Span-K (Australia; Malaysia)
Cost of Therapy: $33.59 (Hypokalemia; K-Dur; 20 mEq; 2 tablets/day; 30 day supply)
$30.30 (Hypokalemia; Genric Tablets; 20 mEq; 2 tablets/day; 30 day supply)
HCFA JCODE(S): J3480 per 2 mEq IV

DESCRIPTION

EXTENDED RELEASE CAPSULES AND TABLETS

Potassium chloride extended release capsules are a solid oral dosage form of potasium chloride containing 10 mEq (750 mg) of potassium chloride [equivalent to 10 mEq (390 mg) of potassium and 10 mEq (360 mg) of chloride] in a microencapsulated capsule. This formulation is intended to slow the release of potassium so that the likelihood of a high localized concentration of potassium chloride within the gastrointestinal tract is reduced.

Potassium chloride extended release capsules are an electrolyte replenisher. The chemical name is potassium chloride, and the structural formula is KCl. Potassium chloride occurs as a white, granular powder or as colorless crystals. It is odorless and has a saline taste. Its solutions are neutral to litmus. It is freely soluble in water and insoluble in alcohol.

Inactive ingredients: Calcium stearate, gelatin, pharmaceutical glaze, povidone, sugar spheres, talc.

Klor-Con extended release tablets are a solid oral dosage form of potassium chloride. Each contains 600 or 750 mg of potassium chloride equivalent to 8mEq or 10mEq of potassium in a wax matrix tablet.

EXTENDED RELEASE FORMULATION FOR LIQUID SUSPENSION

Potassium chloride liquid suspension is an oral dosage form of microencapsulated potassium chloride. Each packet contains 1.5 g of potassium chloride equivalent to 20 mEq of potassium. Potassium chloride liquid suspension is comprised of specially formulated granules. After reconstituting with 2-6 fl oz of water and 1 minute of stirring, the suspension is odorless and tasteless.

Each crystal of potassium chloride (KCl) is microencapsulated with an insoluble polymeric coating which functions as a semipermeable membrane; it allows for the controlled release of potassium and chloride ions over an eight-ten hour period. The controlled release of K+ ions by the microcapsular membrane is intended to reduce the likelihood of a high localized concentration of potassium chloride at any point on the mucosa of the gastrointestinal tract. Fluids pass through the membrane and gradually dissolve the potassium chloride within the microcapsules. The resulting potassium chloride solution slowly diffuses outward through the membrane.

Potassium chloride liquid suspension is an electrolyte replenisher. The chemical name of the active ingredient is potassium chloride and the structural formula is KCI. Potassium chloride occurs as a white, granular powder or as colorless crystals. It is odorless and has a saline taste. Its solutions are neutral to litmus. It is freely soluble in water and insoluble in alcohol.

Inactive Ingredients: Docusate sodium, ethylcellulose, povidone, silicon dioxide, sucrose, and another ingredient.

CLINICAL PHARMACOLOGY

The potassium ion is the principal intracellular cation of most body tissues. Potassium ions participate in a number of essential physiological processes, including the maintenance of intracellular tonicity, the transmission of nerve impulses, the contraction of cardiac, skeletal and smooth muscle and the maintenance of normal renal function.

The intracellular concentration of potassium is approximately 150-160 mEq per liter. The normal adult plasma concentration is 3.5 to 5 mEq per liter. An active ion transport system maintains this gradient across the plasma membrane.

Potassium is a normal dietary constituent and under steady state conditions the amount of potassium absorbed from the gastrointestinal tract is equal to the amount excreted in the urine. The usual dietary intake of potassium is 50-100 mEq per day.

Potassium depletion will occur whenever the rate of potassium loss through renal excretion and/or loss from the gastrointestinal tract exceeds the rate of potassium intake. Such depletion usually develops as a consequence of therapy with diuretics, primary or secondary hyperaldosteronism, diabetic ketoacidosis, or inadequate replacement of potassium in patients on prolonged parenteral nutrition. Depletion can develop rapidly with severe diarrhea, especially if associated with vomiting. Potassium depletion due to these causes is usually accompanied by a concomitant loss of chloride and is manifested by hypokalemia and metabolic alkalosis. Potassium depletion may produce weakness, fatigue, disturbances of cardiac rhythm (primarily ectopic beats), prominent U- waves in the electrocardiogram, and, in advanced cases, flaccid paralysis and/or impaired ability to concentrate urine.

If potassium depletion associated with metabolic alkalosis cannot be managed by correcting the fundamental cause of the deficiency, e.g., where the patient requires long term diuretic therapy, supplemental potassium in the form of high potassium food or potassium chloride may be able to restore normal potassium levels.

In rare circumstances (*e.g.,* patients with renal tubular acidosis) potassium depletion may be associated with metabolic acidosis and hyperchloremia. In such patients potassium replacement should be accomplished with potassium salts other than the chloride, such as potassium bicarbonate, potassium citrate, potassium acetate, or potassium gluconate.

INDICATIONS AND USAGE

EXTENDED RELEASE CAPSULES AND TABLETS

BECAUSE OF REPORTS OF INTESTINAL AND GASTRIC ULCERATION AND BLEEDING WITH EXTENDED RELEASE POTASSIUM CHLORIDE PREPARATIONS, THESE DRUGS SHOULD BE RESERVED FOR THOSE PATIENTS WHO CANNOT TOLERATE OR REFUSE TO TAKE LIQUID OR EFFERVESCENT POTASSIUM PREPARATIONS OR FOR PATIENTS IN WHOM THERE IS A PROBLEM OF COMPLIANCE WITH THESE PREPARATIONS.

1. For the treatment of patients with hypokalemia, with or without metabolic alkalosis; in digitalis intoxication; and in patients with hypokalemic familial periodic paralysis. If hypokalemia is the result of diuretic therapy, consideration should be given to the use of a lower dose of diuretic therapy, which may be sufficient without leading to hypokalemia.
2. For the prevention of hypokalemia in patients who would be at particular risk if hypokalemia were to develop (*e.g.,* digitalized patients or patients with significant cardiac arrhythmias).

The use of potassium salts in patients receiving diuretics for uncomplicated essential hypertension is often unnecessary when such patients have a normal dietary pattern and when low doses of the diuretic are used. Serum potassium levels should be checked periodically, however, and if hypokalemia occurs, dietary supplementation with potassium-containing foods may be adequate to control milder cases. In more severe cases, and if dose adjustment of the diuretic is ineffective or unwarranted, supplementation with potassium salts may be indicated.

EXTENDED RELEASE FORMULATION FOR LIQUID SUSPENSION

BECAUSE OF REPORTS OF INTESTINAL AND GASTRIC ULCERATION AND BLEEDING WITH CONTROLLED RELEASE POTASSIUM CHLORIDE PREPARATIONS, THESE DRUGS SHOULD BE RESERVED FOR THOSE PATIENTS WHO CANNOT TOLERATE OR REFUSE TO TAKE IMMEDIATE RELEASE LIQUIDS/ EFFERVESCENT POTASSIUM PREPARATIONS OR FOR PATIENTS IN WHOM THERE IS A PROBLEM OF COMPLIANCE WITH THESE PREPARATIONS.

1. For the treatment of patients with hypokalemia, with or without metabolic alkalosis; in digitalis intoxication; and in patients with hypokalemic familial periodic paralysis. If hypokalemia is the result of diuretic therapy, consideration should be given to the use of a lower dose of diuretic, which may be sufficient without leading to hypokalemia.
2. For the prevention of hypokalemia in patients who would be at particular risk if hypokalemia were to develop (*e.g.,* digitalized patients or patients with significant cardiac arrhythmias, hepatic cirrhosis with ascites, states of aldosterone excess with normal renal function, potassium losing nephropathy, and certain diarrheal states).

The use of potassium salts in patients receiving diuretics for uncomplicated essential hypertension is often unnecessary when such patients have a normal dietary pattern and when low doses of the diuretic are used. Serum potassium should be checked periodically, however, and if hypokalemia occurs, dietary supplementation with potassium-containing foods may be adequate to control milder cases. In more severe cases, and if dose adjustment of the diuretic is ineffective or unwarranted, supplementation with potassium salts may be indicated.

NON-FDA APPROVED INDICATIONS

The use of potassium chloride as an antihypertensive agent is based on limited data and not approved by the FDA

CONTRAINDICATIONS

Potassium supplements are contraindicated in patients with hyperkalemia, since a further increase in serum potassium concentration in such patients can produce cardiac arrest. Hyperkalemia may complicate any of the following conditions: chronic renal failure, systemic acidosis such as diabetic acidosis, acute dehydration, heat cramps - extended release capsules, extensive tissue breakdown as in severe burns, adrenal insufficiency, or the administration of a potassium-sparing diuretic (*e.g.,* spironolactone, triamterene, amiloride).

Extended and controlled release formulations of potassium chloride have produced esophageal ulceration in certain cardiac patients with esophageal compression due to an enlarged left atrium. Potassium supplementation, when indicated in such patients, should be given as a liquid preparation/an immediate release liquid preparation.

All solid oral dosage forms of potassium chloride are contraindicated in any patient in whom there is structural, pathological (*e.g.,* diabetic gastroparesis) or pharmacologic (use of anticholinergic agents or other agents with anticholinergic properties at sufficient doses to exert anticholinergic effects) cause for arrest or delay in tablet or capsule-passage through the gastrointestinal tract; an oral liquid preparation should be used when indicated in these patients.

WARNINGS

HYPERKALEMIA

In patients with impaired mechanisms for excreting potassium, the administration of potassium salts can produce hyperkalemia and cardiac arrest. This occurs most commonly in patients given potassium by the intravenous route but may also occur in patients given potassium orally. Potentially fatal hyperkalemia can develop rapidly and be asymptomatic. The use of potassium salts in patients with chronic renal disease, or any other condition which impairs potassium excretion, requires particularly careful monitoring of the serum potassium concentration and appropriate dosage adjustment.

INTERACTION WITH POTASSIUM SPARING DIURETICS
Hypokalemia should not be treated by the concomitant administration of potassium salts and a potassium-sparing diuretic (*e.g.*, spironolactone, triamterene or amiloride) since the simultaneous administration of these agents can produce severe hyperkalemia.

INTERACTION WITH ANGIOTENSIN CONVERTING ENZYME INHIBITORS
Angiotensin converting enzyme (ACE) inhibitors (*e.g.*, captopril, enalapril) will produce some potassium retention by inhibiting aldosterone production. Potassium supplements should be given to patients receiving ACE inhibitors only with close monitoring.

GASTROINTESTINAL LESIONS
Solid oral dosage forms of potassium chloride can produce ulcerative and/or stenotic lesions of the gastrointestinal tract and deaths. Based on spontaneous adverse reaction reports, enteric coated preparations of potassium chloride are associated with an increased frequency of small bowel lesions (40-50 per 100,000 patient years) compared to extended and sustained release wax matrix formulations (less than 1 per 100,000 patient years). Because of the lack of extensive marketing experience with microencapsulated products, a comparison between such products and wax matrix or enteric coated products is not available.

EXTENDED RELEASE CAPSULES AND TABLETS
Potassium chloride capsules and tablets are microencapsulated capsules formulated to provide a controlled rate of release of potassium chloride and thus to minimize the possibility of a high local concentration of potassium near the gastrointestinal wall.

EXTENDED RELEASE FORMULATION FOR LIQUID SUSPENSION
Potassium chloride liquid suspension is administered as a liquid suspension of microencapsulated potassium chloride formulated to provide a controlled rate of release of potassium chloride and thus to minimize the possibility of a high local concentration of potassium near the gastrointestinal wall.

DIARRHEA OR DEHYDRATION
Potassium chloride liquid suspension contains, as a dispersing agent, docusate sodium, which also increases stool water and is used as a stool softener. Clinical studies with Potassium chloride liquid suspension indicate that minor changes in stool consistency may be common, although usually are well-tolerated. However, rarely patients may experience diarrhea or cramping abdominal pain. Patients with severe or chronic diarrhea or who are dehydrated ordinarily should not be prescribed potassium chloride liquid suspension.

EXTENDED RELEASE CAPSULES AND TABLETS AND EXTENDED RELEASE FORMULATION FOR LIQUID SUSPENSION
Prospective trials have been conducted in normal human volunteers in which the upper gastrointestinal tract was evaluated by endoscopic inspection before and after 1 week of solid oral potassium chloride therapy. The ability of this model to predict events occurring in usual clinical practice is unknown. Trials which approximated usual clinical practice did not reveal any clear differences between the wax matrix and microencapsulated dosage forms. In contrast, there was a higher incidence of gastric and duodenal lesions in subjects receiving a high dose of a wax matrix extended and controlled release formulation under conditions which did not resemble usual or recommended clinical practice (*i.e.*, 96 mEq per day in divided doses of potassium chloride administered to fasted patients, in the presence of an anticholinergic drug to delay gastric emptying). The upper gastrointestinal lesions observed by endoscopy were asymptomatic and were not accompanied by evidence of bleeding (hemoccult testing). The relevance of these findings to the usual conditions (*i.e.*, non-fasting, no anticholinergic agent, smaller doses) under which extended and controlled release potassium chloride products are used is uncertain; epidemiologic studies have not identified an elevated risk, compared to microencapsulated products, for upper gastrointestinal lesions in patients receiving wax matrix formulations. Potassium chloride extended-release capsules and potassium chloride liquid suspension should be discontinued immediately and the possibility of ulceration, obstruction or perforation considered if severe vomiting, abdominal pain, distention, or gastrointestinal bleeding occurs.

METABOLIC ACIDOSIS
Hypokalemia in patients with metabolic acidosis should be treated with an alkalinizing potassium salt such as potassium bicarbonate, potassium citrate, potassium acetate, or potassium gluconate.

PRECAUTIONS

GENERAL
The diagnosis of potassium depletion is ordinarily made by demonstrating hypokalemia in a patient with a clinical history suggesting some cause for potassium depletion. In interpreting the serum potassium level, the physician should bear in mind that acute alkalosis per se can produce hypokalemia in the absence of a deficit in total body potassium while acute acidosis per se can increase the serum potassium concentration into the normal range even in the presence of a reduced total body potassium.

The treatment of potassium depletion, particularly in the presence of cardiac disease, renal disease, or acidosis requires careful attention to acid-base balance and appropriate monitoring of serum electrolytes, the electrocardiogram, and the clinical status of the patient.
Extended Release Capsules and Tablets: Regular serum potassium determinations are recommended.
Potassium should generally not be given in the immediate postoperative period until urine flow is established.

INFORMATION FOR THE PATIENT
Physicians should consider reminding the patient of the following:
- To take this medicine following the frequency and amount prescribed by the physician. This is especially important if the patient is also taking diuretics and/or digitalis preparations.
- To check with the physician at once if tarry stools or other evidence of gastrointestinal bleeding is noticed.

Extended Release Capsules and Tablets
- To take each dose with meals and with a full glass of water or other liquid.
- To check with the physician if there is trouble swallowing capsules or if the capsules seem to stick in the throat.

Extended Release Formulation for Liquid Suspension
- To take each dose with meals mixed in water or other suitable liquid.
- To inform patients that this product contains as a dispersing agent the stool softener, docusate sodium, which may change stool consistency, or rarely produce diarrhea or cramps.

CARCINOGENESIS, MUTAGENESIS, AND IMPAIRMENT OF FERTILITY
Carcinogenicity, mutagenicity and fertility studies in animals have not been performed. Potassium is a normal dietary constituent.

LABORATORY TESTS
Extended Release Capsules and Tablets
When blood is drawn for analysis of plasma potassium it is important to recognize that artifactual elevations can occur after improper venipuncture technique or as a result of *in vitro* hemolysis of the sample.

PREGNANCY, TERATOGENIC EFFECTS, PREGNANCY CATEGORY C
Animal reproduction studies have not been conducted with potassium chloride capsules and tablets and potassium chloride liquid suspension. It is unlikely that potassium supplementation that does not lead to hyperkalemia would have an adverse effect on the fetus or would affect reproductive capacity.

NURSING MOTHERS
The normal potassium ion content of human milk is about 13 mEq per liter. Since oral potassium becomes part of the (body) potassium pool, so long as body potassium is not excessive, the contribution of potassium chloride supplementation should have little or no effect on the level in human milk.

PEDIATRIC USE
Safety and effectiveness in pediatric patients/children have not been established.

EXTENDED RELEASE FORMULATION FOR LIQUID SUSPENSION
Regular serum potassium determinations are recommended, especially in patients with renal insufficiency or diabetic nephropathy.

When blood is drawn for analysis of plasma potassium, it is important to recognize that artifactual elevations can occur after improper venipuncture technique or as a result of *in vitro* hemolysis of the sample.

DRUG INTERACTIONS

Potassium-sparing diuretic, angiotensin converting enzyme inhibitors: see WARNINGS.

ADVERSE REACTIONS

One of the most severe adverse effects is hyperkalemia (see CONTRAINDICATIONS and WARNINGS).

The most common adverse reactions to the oral potassium salts are nausea, vomiting, flatulence, abdominal pain/discomfort, and diarrhea.

Skin rash has been reported rarely.

EXTENDED RELEASE CAPSULES AND TABLETS
There also have been reports of upper and lower gastrointestinal conditions including obstruction, bleeding, ulceration, and perforation (see CONTRAINDICATIONS and WARNINGS).

These symptoms are due to irritation of the gastrointestinal tract and are best managed by diluting the preparation further, taking the dose with meals, or reducing the amount taken at one time.

EXTENDED RELEASE FORMULATION FOR LIQUID SUSPENSION
Gastrointestinal bleeding and ulceration have been reported in patients treated with microencapsulated KCl (see WARNINGS).

In addition to bleeding and ulceration, perforation and obstruction have been reported in patients treated with solid KCl dosage forms, and may occur with potassium chloride liquid suspension.

These symptoms are due to irritation of the gastrointestinal tract and are best managed by taking the dose with meals, or reducing the amount taken at one time.

In a controlled clinical study, potassium chloride liquid suspension was associated with an increased frequency of gastrointestinal intolerance (*e.g.*, diarrhea, loose stools, abdominal pain, etc.) compared to equal doses (100 mEq/day) of Micro-K Extencaps (see WARNINGS), Diarrhea or Dehydration). This finding was attributed to an inactive ingredient used in the Micro- K LS formulation that is not present in the Micro-K Extencaps formulation.

DOSAGE AND ADMINISTRATION

The usual dietary potassium intake by the average adult is 50-100 mEq per day. Potassium depletion sufficient to cause hypokalemia usually requires the loss of 200 or more mEq of potassium from the total body store.

Dosage must be adjusted to the individual needs of each patient. The dose for the prevention of hypokalemia is typically in the range of 20 mEq per day. Doses of 40-100 mEq per day or more are used for the treatment of potassium depletion. Dosage should be divided if more than 20 mEq per day is given such that no more than 20 mEq is given in a single dose.

EXTENDED RELEASE CAPSULES AND TABLETS
K-Norm Capsules provide 10 mEq of potassium chloride. K-Norm Capsules should be taken with meals and with a glass of water or other liquid. This product should not be taken

on an empty stomach because of its potential for gastric irritation (see WARNINGS). Those patients having difficulty swallowing the capsules may be advised to sprinkle the contents onto a spoonful of soft food to facilitate ingestion.

Each Klor-Con extended release tablet provides 8mEq or 10mEq of potassium chloride. Klor-Con extended release tablets should be taken with meals and with a glass of water or other liquid.

EXTENDED RELEASE FORMULATION FOR LIQUID SUSPENSION

Usual Adult Dose

One (1) potassium chloride liquid suspension 20 mEq packet 1-5 times daily, depending on the requirements of the patient. This product must be suspended in a liquid, preferably water, or sprinkled on food prior to ingestion.

Suspension in Water

Pour contents of packet slowly into approximately 2-6 fluid ounces (1/4 - 3/4 glassful) of water. Stir thoroughly for approximately 1 minute until slightly thickened, then drink. The entire contents of the packet must be used immediately and not stored for future use. Any microcapsule/water mixture should be used immediately and not stored for future use.

Suspension in Liquids Other Than Water

Studies conducted using orange juice, tomato juice, apple juice and milk as the suspending liquid have shown that the quantity of fluid used to suspend 1 potassium chloride liquid suspension packet MUST be limited to **2 fluid ounces (1/4 glassful).** The use of volumes greater than 2 fluid ounces substantially reduces the dose of potassium chloride delivered. If a liquid other than water is used to suspend potassium chloride liquid suspension then the contents of the packet should be slowly poured into **2 fluid ounces (1/4 glassful)** of liquid. Stir thoroughly for approximately 1 minute, then drink. The entire contents of the packet must be used immediately and not stored for future use. Any microcapsule/liquid mixture should be used immediately and not stored for future use.

Sprinkling Contents on Food

Potassium chloride liquid suspension may be given on soft food that may be swallowed easily without chewing, such as applesauce or pudding. After sprinkling the contents of the packet on the food, it should be swallowed immediately without chewing and followed with a glass of cool water, milk, or juice to ensure complete swallowing of all the microcapsules. Do not store microcapsule/food mixture for future use.

HOW SUPPLIED

EXTENDED RELEASE CAPSULES AND TABLETS

K-Norm Capsules are clear/clear hard gelatin capsules, containing 10 mEq (750 mg) of potassium chloride [equivalent to 10 mEq (390 mg) of potassium and 10 mEq (360 mg) of chloride]. Each capsule is imprinted with "K-Norm" on one side and "10" on the other side.

Film coated Klor-Con 8 (blue), imprinted round tablets containing: 600 mg potassium chloride (equivalent to 8 mEq).

Film coated Klor-Con 10 (yellow), imprinted round tablets containing: 750 mg potassium chloride (equivalent to 10 mEq).

Mico-K 8 Extencaps are pale orange capsules monogrammed Mick-K and AHR/5720, each containing 600 mg potassium chloride (equivalent to 8 mEq).

Mico-K 10 Extencaps are pale orange and opaque white capsules monogrammed Mick-K and AHR/5730, each containing 750 mg potassium chloride (equivalent to 10 mEq).

Storage: Store at controlled room temperature 15-30°C (59-86°F). Dispense in container with child-resistant closure.

EXTENDED RELEASE FORMULATION FOR LIQUID SUSPENSION

Micro-K LS containing 1.5 g microencapsulated potassium chloride (equivalent to 20 mEq K) per packet in cartons of 30 and 100 packets.

Storage: Store at controlled room temperature, between 15-30°C (59-86°F).

PRODUCT LISTING - RATED THERAPEUTICALLY EQUIVALENT

Size	Price	Product, Manufacturer	NDC
Capsule, Extended Release - Oral - 8 Meq			
30's	$9.90	MICRO-K, Physicians Total Care	54868-1851-01
100's	$32.49	MICRO-K, Ther-Rx Corporation	64011-0010-04
100's	$34.17	MICRO-K, Ther-Rx Corporation	64011-0010-11
Capsule, Extended Release - Oral - 10 Meq			
30's	$5.10	GENERIC, Heartland Healthcare Services	61392-0402-30
30's	$5.10	GENERIC, Heartland Healthcare Services	61392-0402-39
30's	$8.73	MICRO-K 10, Allscripts Pharmaceutical Company	54569-0660-02
30's	$9.75	MICRO-K 10, Pd-Rx Pharmaceuticals	55289-0899-30
31 x 10	$59.47	GENERIC, Vangard Labs	00615-1318-53
31's	$5.27	GENERIC, Heartland Healthcare Services	61392-0402-31
32 x 10	$59.47	GENERIC, Vangard Labs	00615-1318-63
32's	$5.44	GENERIC, Heartland Healthcare Services	61392-0402-32
60's	$10.20	GENERIC, Heartland Healthcare Services	61392-0402-60
90's	$15.30	GENERIC, Heartland Healthcare Services	61392-0402-90
100's	$14.20	GENERIC, Major Pharmaceuticals Inc	00904-2295-60
100's	$15.75	GENERIC, Interstate Drug Exchange Inc	00814-6200-14
100's	$26.65	MICRO-K 10, Ther-Rx Corporation	64011-0009-11
100's	$29.09	MICRO-K 10, Allscripts Pharmaceutical Company	54569-0660-01
100's	$32.00	GENERIC, Major Pharmaceuticals Inc	00904-2295-61
100's	$32.29	GENERIC, Ethex Corporation	58177-0001-04
100's	$33.91	GENERIC, Ethex Corporation	58177-0001-11
100's	$35.96	MICRO-K 10, Ther-Rx Corporation	64011-0009-04
100's	$35.96	MICRO-K 10, Ther-Rx Corporation	64011-0009-21
Liquid - Oral - 20 Meq/15 ml			
480 ml	$2.21	GENERIC, Cenci, H.R. Labs Inc	00556-0150-16
480 ml	$2.50	GENERIC, Cenci, H.R. Labs Inc	00556-0317-16
480 ml	$2.59	GENERIC, Cenci, H.R. Labs Inc	00556-0434-16
3840 ml	$11.90	GENERIC, Cenci, H.R. Labs Inc	00556-0317-28
3840 ml	$12.00	GENERIC, Cenci, H.R. Labs Inc	00556-0150-28
4000 ml	$11.60	GENERIC, Cenci, H.R. Labs Inc	00556-0434-28
Liquid - Oral - 40 Meq/15 ml			
480 ml	$2.59	GENERIC, Cenci, H.R. Labs Inc	00556-0103-16
480 ml	$2.78	GENERIC, Cenci, H.R. Labs Inc	00556-0442-16
3840 ml	$14.00	GENERIC, Cenci, H.R. Labs Inc	00556-0103-28
3840 ml	$14.59	GENERIC, Cenci, H.R. Labs Inc	00556-0442-28
Powder For Reconstitution - Oral - 20 Meq			
30's	$5.75	GENERIC, Alra	51641-0120-03
100's	$18.50	GENERIC, Alra	51641-0120-01
Solution - Intravenous - 1.5 Meq/ml			
20 ml x 10	$87.88	GENERIC, Abbott Pharmaceutical	00074-4993-19
20 ml x 25	$123.13	GENERIC, Abbott Pharmaceutical	00074-4993-01
Solution - Intravenous - 2 Meq/ml			
5 ml x 25	$14.84	GENERIC, Abbott Pharmaceutical	00074-6635-01
5 ml x 25	$19.75	GENERIC, American Pharmaceutical Partners	63323-0965-05
5 ml x 25	$90.00	GENERIC, Abbott Pharmaceutical	00074-4931-01
5 ml x 25	$141.88	GENERIC, Abbott Pharmaceutical	00074-4991-01
10 ml x 10	$34.00	GENERIC, Abbott Pharmaceutical	00074-4992-18
10 ml x 25	$15.44	GENERIC, Abbott Pharmaceutical	00074-6651-06
10 ml x 25	$31.77	GENERIC, Abbott Pharmaceutical	00074-3907-03
10 ml x 25	$70.94	GENERIC, Abbott Pharmaceutical	00074-4932-01
10 ml x 25	$84.61	GENERIC, Abbott Pharmaceutical	00074-1497-01
10 ml x 25	$191.70	GENERIC, Abbott Pharmaceutical	00074-4992-01
15 ml x 25	$17.22	GENERIC, Abbott Pharmaceutical	00074-6636-01
20 ml x 10	$107.10	GENERIC, Abbott Pharmaceutical	00074-4994-19
20 ml x 25	$20.48	GENERIC, Abbott Pharmaceutical	00074-6653-05
20 ml x 25	$38.00	GENERIC, Abbott Pharmaceutical	00074-3934-02
20 ml x 25	$157.25	GENERIC, Abbott Pharmaceutical	00074-1499-01
20 ml x 25	$222.60	GENERIC, Abbott Pharmaceutical	00074-4994-01
250 ml	$12.00	GENERIC, Baxter I.V. Systems Division	00338-0318-02
250 ml	$35.00	GENERIC, Cmc-Consolidated Midland Corporation	00223-8330-10
250 ml x 12	$74.24	GENERIC, Abbott Pharmaceutical	00074-1513-02
250 ml x 12	$260.28	GENERIC, Baxter I.V. Systems Division	00338-0317-02
250 ml x 12	$523.50	GENERIC, B. Braun/Mcgaw Inc	00264-1940-20
500 ml	$40.00	GENERIC, Cmc-Consolidated Midland Corporation	00223-8331-20
500 ml x 12	$523.20	GENERIC, B. Braun/Mcgaw Inc	00264-1940-10
750 ml	$50.02	GENERIC, Cmc-Consolidated Midland Corporation	00223-8332-30
1000 ml	$120.00	GENERIC, Cmc-Consolidated Midland Corporation	00223-8330-01
Solution - Intravenous - 10 Meq/100 ml			
100 ml x 24	$66.69	GENERIC, Abbott Pharmaceutical	00074-7074-26
Solution - Intravenous - 20 Meq/100 ml			
50 ml x 24	$63.84	GENERIC, Abbott Pharmaceutical	00074-7075-14
50 ml x 80	$1577.20	GENERIC, Abbott Pharmaceutical	00074-7075-36
100 ml x 24	$66.69	GENERIC, Abbott Pharmaceutical	00074-7075-26
Solution - Intravenous - 30 Meq/100 ml			
100 ml x 24	$63.12	GENERIC, Abbott Pharmaceutical	00074-7076-26
Solution - Intravenous - 40 Meq/100 ml			
50 ml x 24	$63.84	GENERIC, Abbott Pharmaceutical	00074-7077-14
100 ml x 24	$63.12	GENERIC, Abbott Pharmaceutical	00074-7077-26
Tablet, Extended Release - Oral - 8 Meq			
10's	$3.90	GENERIC, Pd-Rx Pharmaceuticals	55289-0697-10
30's	$4.65	GENERIC, Heartland Healthcare Services	61392-0403-30
30's	$4.65	GENERIC, Heartland Healthcare Services	61392-0403-39
30's	$5.15	GENERIC, Allscripts Pharmaceutical Company	54569-1899-01
30's	$7.65	GENERIC, Pd-Rx Pharmaceuticals	55289-0697-30
31's	$4.81	GENERIC, Heartland Healthcare Services	61392-0403-31
32's	$4.96	GENERIC, Heartland Healthcare Services	61392-0403-32
45's	$6.98	GENERIC, Heartland Healthcare Services	61392-0403-45
60's	$9.30	GENERIC, Heartland Healthcare Services	61392-0403-60
60's	$10.29	GENERIC, Allscripts Pharmaceutical Company	54569-1899-02
90's	$9.50	GENERIC, Allscripts Pharmaceutical Company	54569-8566-01
90's	$13.95	GENERIC, Heartland Healthcare Services	61392-0403-90
100's	$9.79	GENERIC, Aligen Independent Laboratories Inc	00405-4810-01
100's	$10.25	GENERIC, Moore, H.L. Drug Exchange Inc	00839-7193-06
100's	$10.36	GENERIC, Qualitest Products Inc	00603-5238-21
100's	$10.50	GENERIC, Ivax Corporation	00182-1839-01
100's	$10.85	GENERIC, Major Pharmaceuticals Inc	00904-2300-60
100's	$10.85	GENERIC, Dixon-Shane Inc	17236-0621-01
100's	$10.85	GENERIC, Martec Pharmaceuticals Inc	52555-0481-01
100's	$11.40	GENERIC, Ivax Corporation	00182-1319-01
100's	$12.75	GENERIC, Interstate Drug Exchange Inc	00814-4070-14
100's	$15.50	GENERIC, Ivax Corporation	00182-1839-89
100's	$16.95	GENERIC, Major Pharmaceuticals Inc	00904-3360-60
100's	$17.06	GENERIC, Alra	51641-0175-01
100's	$17.15	GENERIC, Teva Pharmaceuticals Usa	00093-9225-01
100's	$17.15	GENERIC, Copley	38245-0225-10
100's	$17.15	GENERIC, Allscripts Pharmaceutical Company	54569-1899-00
100's	$17.74	GENERIC, Upsher-Smith Laboratories Inc	00245-0040-11
100's	$21.20	GENERIC, Alra	51641-0175-11
100's	$21.84	GENERIC, Upsher-Smith Laboratories Inc	00245-0040-01
100's	$25.00	SLOW-K, Novartis Pharmaceuticals	00078-0320-05
100's	$169.75	GENERIC, Qualitest Products Inc	00603-5237-32
180's	$19.01	GENERIC, Allscripts Pharmaceutical Company	54569-8566-00

Tablet, Extended Release - Oral - 8 meq

Size	Price	Product	NDC
100's	$7.72	FEDERAL UPPER LIMIT, H.C.F.A. F F P	99999-2081-01

Tablet, Extended Release - Oral - 10 Meq

Size	Price	Product	NDC
25's	$11.85	K-DUR 10, Pd-Rx Pharmaceuticals	55289-0190-97
30's	$8.83	K-DUR 10, Allscripts Pharmaceutical Company	54569-3525-00
31 x 10	$59.47	GENERIC, Vangard Labs	00615-4542-53
31 x 10	$59.47	GENERIC, Vangard Labs	00615-4542-63
100's	$15.82	GENERIC, Caremark Inc	00339-5646-12
100's	$24.15	KAON-CL 10, Savage Laboratories	00281-3131-17
100's	$26.83	KAON-CL 10, Savage Laboratories	00281-3131-18
100's	$27.75	GENERIC, Warrick Pharmaceuticals Corporation	59930-1715-01
100's	$27.77	GENERIC, Qualitest Products Inc	00603-5243-21
100's	$28.08	GENERIC, Andrx Pharmaceuticals	62037-0710-01
100's	$29.05	GENERIC, Upsher-Smith Laboratories Inc	00245-0057-11
100's	$33.25	K-DUR 10, Schering Corporation	00085-0263-81
100's	$35.11	K-DUR 10, Schering Corporation	00085-0263-01

Tablet, Extended Release - Oral - 20 Meq

Size	Price	Product	NDC
3's	$1.18	K-DUR 20, Allscripts Pharmaceutical Company	54569-1955-02
6's	$2.35	K-DUR 20, Allscripts Pharmaceutical Company	54569-1955-03
30's	$16.82	K-DUR 20, Allscripts Pharmaceutical Company	54569-1955-01
30's	$19.90	K-DUR 20, Physicians Total Care	54868-0354-01
30's	$20.13	K-DUR 20, Pd-Rx Pharmaceuticals	55289-0079-30
60's	$38.60	K-DUR 20, Physicians Total Care	54868-0354-00
90's	$35.29	K-DUR 20, Allscripts Pharmaceutical Company	54569-8559-00
100's	$41.12	K-DUR 20, Allscripts Pharmaceutical Company	54569-1955-00
100's	$43.23	K-DUR 20, Southwood Pharmaceuticals Inc	58016-0578-00
100's	$50.60	GENERIC, Qualitest Products Inc	00603-5244-21
100's	$52.91	KLOR-CON M20, Upsher-Smith Laboratories Inc	00245-0058-11
100's	$55.99	K-DUR 20, Physicians Total Care	54868-0354-02
100's	$57.35	KLOR-CON M20, Upsher-Smith Laboratories Inc	00245-0058-01
100's	$63.95	K-DUR 20, Schering Corporation	00085-0787-01

PRODUCT LISTING - RATED NOT THERAPEUTICALLY EQUIVALENT

Tablet, Extended Release - Oral - 8 Meq

Size	Price	Product	NDC
100's	$11.96	GENERIC, Abbott Pharmaceutical	00074-7767-13
100's	$17.10	GENERIC, Qualitest Products Inc	00603-5237-21
100's	$21.73	KAON-Cl, Savage Laboratories	00281-0212-17
100's	$24.15	KAON-Cl, Savage Laboratories	00281-0212-18
100's	$36.00	GENERIC, Moore, H.L. Drug Exchange Inc	00839-7736-06

Tablet, Extended Release - Oral - 10 Meq

Size	Price	Product	NDC
30's	$5.68	KLOR-CON 10, Physicians Total Care	54868-1302-01
60's	$7.23	GENERIC, Pd-Rx Pharmaceuticals	55289-0359-60
90's	$21.05	KLOTRIX, Allscripts Pharmaceutical Company	54569-8568-00
100's	$9.92	GENERIC, Moore, H.L. Drug Exchange Inc	00839-7194-06
100's	$10.25	GENERIC, Moore, H.L. Drug Exchange Inc	00839-7737-06
100's	$10.50	GENERIC, Major Pharmaceuticals Inc	00904-2301-60
100's	$11.78	GENERIC, Pd-Rx Pharmaceuticals	55289-0359-01
100's	$17.00	GENERIC, Ivax Corporation	00182-1840-89
100's	$17.85	GENERIC, Alra	51641-0177-11
100's	$20.19	KLOR-CON 10, Physicians Total Care	54868-1302-02
100's	$21.00	GENERIC, Alra	51641-0177-01
100's	$27.75	GENERIC, Apothecon Inc	59772-6910-01
100's	$29.08	GENERIC, Qualitest Products Inc	00603-5241-21
100's	$31.27	KLOR-CON 10, Upsher-Smith Laboratories Inc	00245-0041-11
100's	$35.94	GENERIC, Abbott Pharmaceutical	00074-7763-13
100's	$35.98	KLOTRIX, Bristol-Myers Squibb	00087-0770-41
100's	$36.00	KLOR-CON 10, Upsher-Smith Laboratories Inc	00245-0041-01
100's	$46.78	K-TAB, Physicians Total Care	54868-1304-01
100's	$51.84	K-TAB, Abbott Pharmaceutical	00074-7804-13
100's	$134.00	GENERIC, Mutual/United Research Laboratories	00677-1097-05
100's	$276.26	GENERIC, Qualitest Products Inc	00603-5241-32

PRODUCT LISTING - EQUIVALENTS NOT AVAILABLE

Capsule, Extended Release - Oral - 10 Meq

Size	Price	Product	NDC
12's	$3.79	GENERIC, Physicians Total Care	54868-1317-03
30's	$5.75	GENERIC, Southwood Pharmaceuticals Inc	58016-0989-30
30's	$6.06	GENERIC, Allscripts Pharmaceutical Company	54569-3388-00
30's	$6.30	GENERIC, Pharmaceutical Corporation Of America	51655-0583-24
30's	$7.22	GENERIC, Pd-Rx Pharmaceuticals	55289-0218-30
30's	$7.91	GENERIC, Physicians Total Care	54868-1317-01
60's	$12.12	GENERIC, Allscripts Pharmaceutical Company	54569-3388-01
60's	$14.48	GENERIC, Physicians Total Care	54868-1317-05
80's	$16.16	GENERIC, Allscripts Pharmaceutical Company	54569-3388-05
90's	$14.56	GENERIC, Allscripts Pharmaceutical Company	54569-8548-01
100's	$16.31	K-NORM, Celltech Pharmaceuticals Inc	00585-0010-71
100's	$16.31	K-NORM, Celltech Pharmaceuticals Inc	53014-0010-71
100's	$17.45	GENERIC, Southwood Pharmaceuticals Inc	58016-0989-00
100's	$23.24	GENERIC, Physicians Total Care	54868-1317-02
180's	$29.12	GENERIC, Allscripts Pharmaceutical Company	54569-8548-00

Liquid - Oral - 20 Meq/15 ml

Size	Price	Product	NDC
11 ml x 100	$42.00	GENERIC, Roxane Laboratories Inc	00054-8711-04
15 ml x 100	$22.50	GENERIC, Pharmaceutical Assoc Inc Div Beach Products	00121-0465-15
15 ml x 100	$42.00	GENERIC, Roxane Laboratories Inc	00054-8714-04
22 ml x 100	$37.72	GENERIC, Pharmaceutical Assoc Inc Div Beach Products	00121-0465-22
22 ml x 100	$42.00	GENERIC, Roxane Laboratories Inc	00054-8712-04
30 ml x 100	$23.75	GENERIC, Pharmaceutical Assoc Inc Div Beach Products	00121-0465-30
30 ml x 100	$42.00	GENERIC, Roxane Laboratories Inc	00054-8713-04
120 ml	$11.74	KAY CIEL, Forest Pharmaceuticals	00456-0661-04
473 ml	$3.65	GENERIC, Baker Norton Pharmaceuticals	50732-0625-16
473 ml	$3.79	GENERIC, Baker Norton Pharmaceuticals	50732-0627-16
473 ml	$4.87	GENERIC, Seatrace Pharmaceuticals	00551-0202-01
480 ml	$1.49	GENERIC, Denison Pharmaceuticals Inc	00295-1118-16
480 ml	$1.68	GENERIC, Chemrich Laboratories	10235-1001-06
480 ml	$1.68	GENERIC, Chemrich Laboratories	10235-1033-06
480 ml	$1.75	GENERIC, Veratex Corporation	17022-3147-07
480 ml	$2.11	GENERIC, Major Pharmaceuticals Inc	00904-1006-16
480 ml	$2.26	GENERIC, Century Pharmaceuticals Inc	00436-0522-16
480 ml	$2.50	GENERIC, Cenci, H.R. Labs Inc	00556-0422-16
480 ml	$2.52	KAOCHLOR S-F, Savage Laboratories	00281-3093-51
480 ml	$2.52	GENERIC, Caremark Inc	00339-5959-53
480 ml	$2.74	GENERIC, Cmc-Consolidated Midland Corporation	00223-6589-01
480 ml	$2.78	GENERIC, Geneva Pharmaceuticals	00781-6040-16
480 ml	$3.00	GENERIC, Cmc-Consolidated Midland Corporation	00223-6591-01
480 ml	$3.10	GENERIC, Humco Holding Group	00395-2300-16
480 ml	$3.17	GENERIC, Interstate Drug Exchange Inc	00814-6215-82
480 ml	$3.26	GENERIC, Century Pharmaceuticals Inc	00436-0515-16
480 ml	$3.41	GENERIC, Major Pharmaceuticals Inc	00904-1005-16
480 ml	$3.41	GENERIC, Morton Grove Pharmaceuticals Inc	60432-0006-16
480 ml	$3.53	GENERIC, Ivax Corporation	00182-6120-40
480 ml	$3.80	GENERIC, Ivax Corporation	00182-6099-40
480 ml	$3.90	GENERIC, Vintage Pharmaceuticals Inc	00254-9380-58
480 ml	$3.90	GENERIC, Vintage Pharmaceuticals Inc	00254-9381-58
480 ml	$3.90	GENERIC, Vintage Pharmaceuticals Inc	00254-9383-58
480 ml	$4.03	GENERIC, Purepac Pharmaceutical Company	00228-2318-16
480 ml	$4.03	GENERIC, Moore, H.L. Drug Exchange Inc	00839-5421-69
480 ml	$4.32	GENERIC, Aligen Independent Laboratories Inc	00405-3575-16
480 ml	$4.40	GENERIC, Morton Grove Pharmaceuticals Inc	60432-0492-16
480 ml	$4.61	GENERIC, Emerson Laboratories	00802-3971-16
480 ml	$4.77	GENERIC, Allscripts Pharmaceutical Company	54569-2758-00
480 ml	$4.80	GENERIC, Major Pharmaceuticals Inc	00904-1007-16
480 ml	$4.90	GENERIC, Qualitest Products Inc	00603-1532-58
480 ml	$4.90	GENERIC, Qualitest Products Inc	00603-1534-58
480 ml	$4.90	GENERIC, Qualitest Products Inc	00603-1535-58
480 ml	$5.15	GENERIC, Southwood Pharmaceuticals Inc	58016-5001-01
480 ml	$6.65	GENERIC, Alpharma Uspd Makers Of Barre and Nmc	00472-1000-16
480 ml	$29.11	KAOCHLOR, Savage Laboratories	00281-3103-51
480 ml	$48.00	KAY CIEL, Forest Pharmaceuticals	00456-0661-16
500 ml	$6.83	GENERIC, Roxane Laboratories Inc	00054-3716-63
1000 ml	$11.26	GENERIC, Roxane Laboratories Inc	00054-3716-68
3785 ml	$17.66	GENERIC, Baker Norton Pharmaceuticals	50732-0625-28
3785 ml	$19.58	GENERIC, Baker Norton Pharmaceuticals	50732-0627-28
3840 ml	$10.75	GENERIC, Major Pharmaceuticals Inc	00904-1006-28
3840 ml	$10.75	GENERIC, Chemrich Laboratories	10235-1001-08
3840 ml	$12.29	GENERIC, Century Pharmaceuticals Inc	00436-0515-28
3840 ml	$12.29	GENERIC, Century Pharmaceuticals Inc	00436-0522-28
3840 ml	$12.50	GENERIC, Cmc-Consolidated Midland Corporation	00223-6591-02
3840 ml	$13.44	GENERIC, Moore, H.L. Drug Exchange Inc	00839-5421-70
3840 ml	$13.49	GENERIC, Major Pharmaceuticals Inc	00904-1007-28
3840 ml	$13.82	GENERIC, Cmc-Consolidated Midland Corporation	00223-6589-02
3840 ml	$14.21	GENERIC, Interstate Drug Exchange Inc	00814-6215-86
3840 ml	$17.28	GENERIC, Emerson Laboratories	00802-3971-28
3840 ml	$22.87	GENERIC, Ivax Corporation	00182-6120-41
3840 ml	$23.42	GENERIC, Major Pharmaceuticals Inc	00904-1005-28
3840 ml	$29.95	GENERIC, Vintage Pharmaceuticals Inc	00254-9381-62
3840 ml	$30.22	GENERIC, Qualitest Products Inc	00603-1534-60
3840 ml	$42.55	GENERIC, Alpharma Uspd Makers Of Barre and Nmc	00472-1000-28

Liquid - Oral - 30 Meq/15 ml

Size	Price	Product	NDC
480 ml	$23.60	GENERIC, Fleming and Company	00256-0160-01

Liquid - Oral - 40 Meq/15 ml

Size	Price	Product	NDC
15 ml x 100	$26.60	GENERIC, Pharmaceutical Assoc Inc Div Beach Products	00121-0466-15

P

30 ml x 100	$48.30	GENERIC, Pharmaceutical Assoc Inc Div Beach Products	00121-0466-30
360 ml	$2.56	GENERIC, Chemrich Laboratories	10235-1002-06
473 ml	$3.98	GENERIC, Baker Norton Pharmaceuticals	50732-0626-16
473 ml	$4.92	GENERIC, Seatrace Pharmaceuticals	00551-0203-01
480 ml	$3.02	GENERIC, Cmc-Consolidated Midland Corporation	00223-6592-01
480 ml	$3.41	GENERIC, Aligen Independent Laboratories Inc	00405-3550-16
480 ml	$3.74	GENERIC, Century Pharmaceuticals Inc	00436-0523-16
480 ml	$3.74	GENERIC, Century Pharmaceuticals Inc	00436-0527-16
480 ml	$3.74	GENERIC, Geneva Pharmaceuticals	00781-6790-16
480 ml	$3.98	GENERIC, Interstate Drug Exchange Inc	00814-6216-82
480 ml	$4.03	GENERIC, Moore, H.L. Drug Exchange Inc	00839-5420-69
480 ml	$4.25	GENERIC, Ivax Corporation	00182-6121-40
480 ml	$4.35	GENERIC, Major Pharmaceuticals Inc	00904-1001-16
480 ml	$4.46	GENERIC, Century Pharmaceuticals Inc	00436-0516-16
480 ml	$5.47	GENERIC, Emerson Laboratories	00802-3912-16
480 ml	$5.60	GENERIC, Vintage Pharmaceuticals Inc	00254-9384-58
480 ml	$5.60	GENERIC, Qualitest Products Inc	00603-1536-58
480 ml	$8.91	GENERIC, Alpharma Uspd Makers Of Barre and Nmc	00472-1001-16
480 ml	$26.94	KAON-CL 20%, Savage Laboratories	00281-3113-51
500 ml	$9.23	GENERIC, Roxane Laboratories Inc	00054-3714-63
1000 ml	$15.50	GENERIC, Roxane Laboratories Inc	00054-3714-68
3785 ml	$21.50	GENERIC, Baker Norton Pharmaceuticals	50732-0626-28
3840 ml	$13.44	GENERIC, Century Pharmaceuticals Inc	00436-0516-28
3840 ml	$13.44	GENERIC, Century Pharmaceuticals Inc	00436-0523-28
3840 ml	$13.44	GENERIC, Century Pharmaceuticals Inc	00436-0527-28
3840 ml	$15.36	GENERIC, Cmc-Consolidated Midland Corporation	00223-6592-02
3840 ml	$16.51	GENERIC, Major Pharmaceuticals Inc	00904-1001-28
3840 ml	$19.20	GENERIC, Emerson Laboratories	00802-3912-28

Powder For Reconstitution - Oral - 20 Meq

30's	$3.95	GENERIC, Bajamar Chemical Company Inc	44184-0017-02
30's	$4.92	GENERIC, Major Pharmaceuticals Inc	00904-1899-46
30's	$5.13	GENERIC, Qualitest Products Inc	00603-4173-16
30's	$6.05	GENERIC, Ivax Corporation	00182-1451-17
30's	$6.06	GENERIC, Moore, H.L. Drug Exchange Inc	00839-6715-19
30's	$6.15	GENERIC, Watson/Schein Pharmaceuticals Inc	00364-7378-30
30's	$6.15	GENERIC, Watson Laboratories Inc	00591-7378-30
30's	$6.17	GENERIC, Geneva Pharmaceuticals	00781-8010-30
30's	$6.25	GENERIC, Major Pharmaceuticals Inc	00904-5346-46
30's	$6.26	GENERIC, Upsher-Smith Laboratories Inc	00245-0035-30
30's	$10.00	GENERIC, Physicians Total Care	54868-0356-03
30's	$17.56	GENERIC, Icn Pharmaceuticals Inc	00187-0112-03
30's	$38.99	K-LOR, Abbott Pharmaceutical	00074-7349-30
30's	$47.69	K-LOR, Abbott Pharmaceutical	00074-3611-01
30's	$53.26	KAY CIEL, Forest Pharmaceuticals	00456-0662-70
50's	$15.99	GENERIC, Physicians Total Care	54868-0356-01
100's	$11.95	GENERIC, Major Pharmaceuticals Inc	00904-1899-60
100's	$12.00	GENERIC, Bajamar Chemical Company Inc	44184-0017-04
100's	$18.25	GENERIC, Major Pharmaceuticals Inc	00904-5436-60
100's	$18.78	GENERIC, Upsher-Smith Laboratories Inc	00245-0035-01
100's	$29.47	GENERIC, Physicians Total Care	54868-0356-02
100's	$126.05	K-LOR, Abbott Pharmaceutical	00074-7349-11
100's	$130.80	KAY CIEL, Forest Pharmaceuticals	00456-0662-71
100's	$154.23	K-LOR, Abbott Pharmaceutical	00074-3611-02
120's	$66.56	GENERIC, Icn Pharmaceuticals Inc	00187-0112-12

Powder For Reconstitution - Oral - 25 Meq

30's	$7.41	GENERIC, Upsher-Smith Laboratories Inc	00245-0037-30
100's	$22.23	GENERIC, Upsher-Smith Laboratories Inc	00245-0037-01

Solution - Intravenous - 2 Meq/ml

10 ml	$2.23	GENERIC, Physicians Total Care	54868-0767-00
10 ml x 25	$25.25	GENERIC, American Pharmaceutical Partners	63323-0965-10
10 ml x 100	$99.00	GENERIC, Raway Pharmacal Inc	00686-2110-25
15 ml x 25	$38.90	GENERIC, American Pharmaceutical Partners	63323-0965-15
20 ml x 25	$28.75	GENERIC, American Pharmaceutical Partners	63323-0965-20
20 ml x 100	$99.00	GENERIC, Raway Pharmacal Inc	00686-2210-25
20 ml x 100	$100.00	GENERIC, Raway Pharmacal Inc	00686-2120-25
30 ml	$1.49	GENERIC, Mcguff Company	49072-0571-30
30 ml x 25	$30.50	GENERIC, American Pharmaceutical Partners	63323-0967-30
30 ml x 25	$50.00	GENERIC, Cmc-Consolidated Midland Corporation	00223-8322-30
30 ml x 100	$165.00	GENERIC, Raway Pharmacal Inc	00686-2130-25
50 ml x 24	$351.12	GENERIC, Baxter I.V. Systems Division	00338-0703-41
50 ml x 24	$351.12	GENERIC, Baxter I.V. Systems Division	00338-0705-41

Solution - Intravenous - 10 Meq/100 ml

100 ml x 24	$351.12	GENERIC, Baxter I.V. Systems Division	00338-0709-48

Solution - Intravenous - 20 Meq/100 ml

100 ml x 24	$351.12	GENERIC, Baxter I.V. Systems Division	00338-0705-48

Solution - Intravenous - 30 Meq/100 ml

100 ml x 24	$72.30	GENERIC, Baxter I.V. Systems Division	00338-0707-48

Solution - Intravenous - 40 Meq/100 ml

100 ml x 24	$351.12	GENERIC, Baxter I.V. Systems Division	00338-0703-48

Tablet - Oral - 500 mg

30's	$5.05	GENERIC, Allscripts Pharmaceutical Company	54569-2747-01
100's	$3.53	GENERIC, Camall Company	00147-0238-10
100's	$4.80	GENERIC, Ivax Corporation	00182-1024-01
100's	$6.80	GENERIC, Allscripts Pharmaceutical Company	54569-2747-00

Tablet - Oral - 595 mg

30's	$4.88	GENERIC, Southwood Pharmaceuticals Inc	58016-0982-30

Tablet, Effervescent - Oral - 25 Meq

30's	$19.17	GENERIC, Qualitest Products Inc	00603-3508-16
30's	$39.93	K-LYTE CI, Physicians Total Care	54868-3238-01
30's	$43.07	K-LYTE CI, Bristol-Myers Squibb	00087-0766-41
30's	$43.07	K-LYTE CI, Bristol-Myers Squibb	00087-0767-41
60's	$78.68	K-LYTE CI, Physicians Total Care	54868-3238-02
100's	$127.47	K-LYTE CI, Bristol-Myers Squibb	00087-0766-43
100's	$127.47	K-LYTE CI, Bristol-Myers Squibb	00087-0767-43

Tablet, Effervescent - Oral - 50 Meq

30's	$77.51	K-LYTE CI, Bristol-Myers Squibb	00087-0758-41

Tablet, Extended Release - Oral - 8 Meq

8's	$4.68	GENERIC, Southwood Pharmaceuticals Inc	58016-0564-08
30's	$5.19	GENERIC, Physicians Total Care	54868-0097-02
100's	$13.41	GENERIC, Physicians Total Care	54868-0097-04

Tablet, Extended Release - Oral - 10 Meq

20's	$5.30	GENERIC, Pharma Pac	52959-0651-20
28's	$7.31	GENERIC, Allscripts Pharmaceutical Company	54569-4903-03
30's	$5.81	GENERIC, Southwood Pharmaceuticals Inc	58016-0522-30
30's	$7.83	GENERIC, Allscripts Pharmaceutical Company	54569-4903-01
30's	$12.10	GENERIC, Pharmaceutical Corporation Of America	51655-0511-24
40's	$10.44	GENERIC, Pharma Pac	52959-0651-40
60's	$9.71	GENERIC, Southwood Pharmaceuticals Inc	58016-0522-60
60's	$14.54	GENERIC, Pharmaceutical Corporation Of America	51655-0511-25
60's	$15.66	GENERIC, Allscripts Pharmaceutical Company	54569-4903-02
80's	$20.88	GENERIC, Allscripts Pharmaceutical Company	54569-4903-00
100's	$13.61	GENERIC, Southwood Pharmaceuticals Inc	58016-0522-00
100's	$22.00	GENERIC, Edwards Pharmaceuticals Inc	00485-0064-01
100's	$27.75	GENERIC, Geneva Pharmaceuticals	00781-1526-01
150's	$50.00	GENERIC, Sky Pharmaceuticals Packaging, Inc	63739-0305-15

Tablet, Extended Release - Oral - 20 Meq

10 x 10	$56.45	GENERIC, Ethex Corporation	58177-0202-11
100's	$50.50	GENERIC, Warrick Pharmaceuticals Corporation	59930-1714-01
100's	$52.03	GENERIC, Ethex Corporation	58177-0202-04
100's	$69.31	K-DUR 20, Schering Corporation	00085-0787-81
150's	$92.54	GENERIC, Sky Pharmaceuticals Packaging, Inc	63739-0306-15

Pramipexole Dihydrochloride *(003343)*

Categories: Parkinson's disease; Pregnancy Category C; FDA Approved 1997 Jul
Drug Classes: Antiparkinson agents; Dopaminergics
Brand Names: **Mirapex**
Foreign Brand Availability: Daquiran (Austria; Belgium; Bulgaria; Czech-Republic; Denmark; England; Finland; France; Germany; Greece; Hungary; Ireland; Italy; Netherlands; Norway; Poland; Portugal; Slovenia; Spain; Sweden; Switzerland; Turkey); Mirapexin (Austria; Belgium; Bulgaria; Czech-Republic; Denmark; England; Finland; France; Germany; Greece; Hungary; Ireland; Italy; Netherlands; Norway; Poland; Portugal; Slovenia; Spain; Sweden; Switzerland; Turkey); Pexola (Colombia); Sifrol (Austria; Bahrain; Belgium; Bulgaria; Cyprus; Czech-Republic; Denmark; Egypt; England; Finland; France; Germany; Greece; Hungary; Iran; Iraq; Ireland; Italy; Jordan; Kuwait; Lebanon; Libya; Netherlands; Norway; Oman; Poland; Portugal; Qatar; Republic-of-Yemen; Saudi-Arabia; Slovenia; Spain; Sweden; Switzerland; Syria; Turkey; United-Arab-Emirates)
Cost of Therapy: $200.61 (Parkinsonism; Mirapex; 0.5 mg; 3 tablets/day; 30 day supply)

DESCRIPTION

Mirapex tablets contain pramipexole, a dopamine agonist indicated for the treatment of the signs and symptoms of idiopathic Parkinson's disease. The chemical name of pramipexole dihydrochloride is (*S*)-2-amino-4,5,6,7-tetrahydro-6-(propylamino)benzothiazole dihydrochloride monohydrate. Its empirical formula is $C_{10}H_{17}N_3S{\cdot}2HCl{\cdot}H_2O$, and its molecular weight is 302.27.

Pramipexole dihydrochloride is a white to off-white powder substance. Melting occurs in the range of 296-301°C, with decomposition. Pramipexole dihydrochloride is more than 20% soluble in water, about 8% in methanol, about 0.5% in ethanol, and practically insoluble in dichloromethane.

Mirapex tablets, for oral administration, contain 0.125, 0.25, 0.5, 1.0, or 1.5 mg of pramipexole dihydrochloride monohydrate. *Inactive ingredients:* Mannitol, corn starch, colloidal silicon dioxide, povidone, and magnesium stearate.

CLINICAL PHARMACOLOGY

Pramipexole is a nonergot dopamine agonist with high relative *in vitro* specificity and full intrinsic activity at the D_2 subfamily of dopamine receptors, binding with higher affinity to D_3 than to D_2 or D_4 receptor subtypes. The relevance of D_3 receptor binding in Parkinson's disease is unknown.

The precise mechanism of action of pramipexole as a treatment for Parkinson's disease is unknown, although it is believed to be related to its ability to stimulate dopamine receptors in the striatum. This conclusion is supported by electrophysiologic studies in animals that have demonstrated that pramipexole influences striatal neuronal firing rates via activation of dopamine receptors in the stratum and the substantia nigra, the site of neurons that send projections to the striatum.

PHARMACOKINETICS

Pramipexole is rapidly absorbed, reaching peak concentrations in approximately 2 hours. The absolute bioavailability of pramipexole is greater than 90%, indicating that it is well absorbed and undergoes little presystemic metabolism. Food does not affect the extent of pramipexole absorption, although the time of maximum plasma concentration (T_{max}) is increased by about 1 hour when the drug is taken with a meal.

Pramipexole is extensively distributed, having a volume of distribution of about 500 L (coefficient of variation [CV]=20%). It is about 15% bound to plasma proteins. Pramipexole distributes into red blood cells as indicated by an erythrocyte-to-plasma ratio of approximately 2.

Pramipexole displays linear pharmacokinetics over the clinical dosage range. Its terminal half-life is about 8 hours in young healthy volunteers and about 12 hours in elderly volunteers (see Pharmacokinetics in Special Populations). Steady-state concentrations are achieved within 2 days of dosing.

Metabolism and Elimination

Urinary excretion is the major route of pramipexole elimination, with 90% of a pramipexole dose recovered in urine, almost all as unchanged drug. Non-renal routes may contribute to a small extent to pramipexole elimination, although no metabolites have been identified in plasma or urine. The renal clearance of pramipexole is approximately 400 ml/min (CV=25%), approximately 3 times higher than the glomerular filtration rate. Thus, pramipexole is secreted by the renal tubules, probably by the organic cation transport system.

PHARMACOKINETICS IN SPECIAL POPULATIONS

Because therapy with pramipexole is initiated at a sub-therapeutic dosage and gradually titrated upward according to clinical tolerability to obtain the optimum therapeutic effect, adjustment of the initial dose based on gender, weight, or age is not necessary. However, renal insufficiency, which can cause a large decrease in the ability to eliminate pramipexole, may necessitate dosage adjustment (see Renal Insufficiency).

GENDER

Pramipexole clearance is about 30% lower in women than in men, but most of this difference can be accounted for by differences in body weight. There is no difference in half-life between males and females.

AGE

Pramipexole clearance decreases with age as the half-life and clearance are about 40% longer and 30% lower, respectively, in elderly (aged 65 years or older) compared with young healthy volunteers (aged less than 40 years). This difference is most likely due to the well-known reduction in renal function with age, since pramipexole clearance is correlated with renal function, as measured by creatinine clearance (see Renal Insufficiency).

PARKINSON'S DISEASE PATIENTS

A cross-study comparison of data suggests that the clearance of pramipexole may be reduced by about 30% in Parkinson's disease patients compared with healthy elderly volunteers. The reason for this difference appears to be reduced renal function in Parkinson's disease patients, which may be related to their poorer general health. The pharmacokinetics of pramipexole were comparable between early and advanced Parkinson's disease patients.

PEDIATRIC

The pharmacokinetics of pramipexole in the pediatric population have not been evaluated.

HEPATIC INSUFFICIENCY

The influence of hepatic insufficiency on pramipexole pharmacokinetics has not been evaluated. Because approximately 90% of the recovered dose is excreted in the urine as unchanged drug, hepatic impairment would not be expected to have a significant effect on pramipexole elimination.

RENAL INSUFFICIENCY

The clearance of pramipexole was about 75% lower in patients with severe renal impairment (creatinine clearance approximately 20 ml/min) and about 60% lower in patients with moderate impairment (creatinine clearance approximately 40 ml/min) compared with healthy volunteers. A lower starting and maintenance dose is recommended in these patients (see PRECAUTIONS and DOSAGE AND ADMINISTRATION). In patients with varying degrees of renal impairment, pramipexole clearance correlates well with creatinine clearance. Therefore, creatinine clearance can be used as a predictor of the extent of decrease in pramipexole clearance. Pramipexole clearance is extremely low in dialysis patients, as a negligible amount of pramipexole is removed by dialysis. Caution should be exercised when administering pramipexole to patients with renal disease.

INDICATIONS AND USAGE

Pramipexole dihydrochloride tablets are indicated for the treatment of the signs and symptoms of idiopathic Parkinson's disease.

The effectiveness of pramipexole dihydrochloride was demonstrated in randomized, controlled trials in patients with early Parkinson's disease who were not receiving concomitant levodopa therapy as well as in patients with advanced disease on concomitant levodopa.

NON-FDA APPROVED INDICATIONS

Pramipexole has also been reported to have clinical efficacy in the treatment of restless legs syndrome. However, this use has not been approved by the FDA and further clinical trials regarding this indication are needed.

CONTRAINDICATIONS

Pramipexole dihydrochloride tablets are contraindicated in patients who have demonstrated hypersensitivity to the drug or its ingredients.

WARNINGS

FALLING ASLEEP DURING ACTIVITIES OF DAILY LIVING

Patients treated with pramipexole dihydrochloride have reported falling asleep while engaged in activities of daily living, including the operation of motor vehicles which sometimes resulted in accidents. Although many of these patients reported somnolence while on pramipexole dihydrochloride, some perceived that they had no warning signs such as excessive drowsiness, and believed that they were alert immediately prior to the event. Some of these events have been reported as late as 1 year after the initiation of treatment.

Somnolence is a common occurrence in patients receiving pramipexole dihydrochloride at doses above 1.5 mg/day. Many clinical experts believe that falling asleep while engaged in activities of daily living always occurs in a setting of preexisting somnolence, although patients may not give such a history. For this reason, prescribers should continually reassess patients for drowsiness or sleepiness, especially since some of the events occur well after the start of treatment. Prescribers should also be aware that patients may not acknowledge drowsiness or sleepiness until directly questioned about drowsiness or sleepiness during specific activities.

Before initiating treatment with pramipexole dihydrochloride, patients should be advised of the potential to develop drowsiness and specifically asked about factors that may increase the risk with pramipexole dihydrochloride such as concomitant sedating medications, the presence of sleep disorders, and concomitant medications that increase pramipexole plasma levels (*e.g.,* cimetidine [see DRUG INTERACTIONS]). If a patient develops significant daytime sleepiness or episodes of falling asleep during activities that require active participation (*e.g.,* conversations, eating, etc.), pramipexole dihydrochloride should ordinarily be discontinued. If a decision is made to continue pramipexole dihydrochloride, patients should be advised to not drive and to avoid other potentially dangerous activities. While dose reduction clearly reduces the degree of somnolence, there is insufficient information to establish that dose reduction will eliminate episodes of falling asleep while engaged in activities of daily living.

SYMPTOMATIC HYPOTENSION

Dopamine agonists, in clinical studies and clinical experience, appear to impair the systemic regulation of blood pressure, with resulting orthostatic hypotension, especially during dose escalation. Parkinson's disease patients, in addition, appear to have an impaired capacity to respond to an orthostatic challenge. For these reasons, Parkinson's disease patients being treated with dopaminergic agonists ordinarily require careful monitoring for signs and symptoms of orthostatic hypotension, especially during dose escalation, and should be informed of this risk (see PRECAUTIONS, Information for the Patient).

In clinical trials of pramipexole, however, and despite clear orthostatic effects in normal volunteers, the reported incidence of clinically significant orthostatic hypotension was not greater among those assigned to pramipexole dihydrochloride tablets than among those assigned to placebo. This result is clearly unexpected in light of the previous experience with the risks of dopamine agonist therapy.

While this finding could reflect a unique property of pramipexole, it might also be explained by the conditions of the study and the nature of the population enrolled in the clinical trials. Patients were very carefully titrated, and patients with active cardiovascular disease or significant orthostatic hypotension at baseline were excluded.

HALLUCINATIONS

In the three double-blind, placebo-controlled trials in early Parkinson's disease, hallucinations were observed in 9% (35 of 388) of patients receiving pramipexole dihydrochloride, compared with 2.6% (6 of 235) of patients receiving placebo. In the four double-blind, placebo-controlled trials in advanced Parkinson's disease, where patients received pramipexole dihydrochloride and concomitant levodopa, hallucinations were observed in 16.5% (43 of 260) of patients receiving pramipexole dihydrochloride compared with 3.8% (10 of 264) of patients receiving placebo. Hallucinations were of sufficient severity to cause discontinuation of treatment in 3.1% of the early Parkinson's disease patients and 2.7% of the advanced Parkinson's disease patients compared with about 0.4% of placebo patients in both populations.

Age appears to increase the risk of hallucinations attributable to pramipexole. In the early Parkinson's disease patients, the risk of hallucinations was 1.9 times greater than placebo in patients younger than 65 years and 6.8 times greater than placebo in patients older than 65 years. In the advanced Parkinson's disease patients, the risk of hallucinations was 3.5 times greater than placebo in patients younger than 65 years and 5.2 times greater than placebo in patients older than 65 years.

PRECAUTIONS

GENERAL

Rhabdomyolysis

A single case of rhabdomyolysis occurred in a 49-year-old male with advanced Parkinson's disease treated with pramipexole dihydrochloride tablets. The patient was hospitalized with an elevated CPK (10,631 IU/L). The symptoms resolved with discontinuation of the medication.

Renal

Since pramipexole is eliminated through the kidneys, caution should be exercised when prescribing pramipexole dihydrochloride to patients with renal insufficiency (see DOSAGE AND ADMINISTRATION).

Dyskinesia

Pramipexole dihydrochloride may potentiate the dopaminergic side effects of levodopa and may cause or exacerbate pre-existing dyskinesia. Decreasing the dose of levodopa may ameliorate this side effect.

Retinal Pathology in Albino Rats

Pathologic changes (degeneration and loss of photoreceptor cells) were observed in the retina of albino rats in the 2 year carcinogenicity study. Evaluation of the retinas of albino mice, pigmented rats, monkeys, and minipigs did not reveal similar changes. The potential significance of this effect in humans has not been established, but cannot be disregarded because disruption of a mechanism that is universally present in vertebrates (*i.e.*, disk shedding) may be involved. (See ANIMAL PHARMACOLOGY.)

EVENTS REPORTED WITH DOPAMINERGIC THERAPY

Although the events enumerated below have not been reported in association with the use of pramipexole in its development program, they are associated with the use of other dopaminergic drugs. The expected incidence of these events, however, is so low that even if pramipexole caused these events at rates similar to those attributable to other dopaminergic therapies, it would be unlikely that even a single case would have occurred in a cohort of the size exposed to pramipexole in studies to date.

Withdrawal-Emergent Hyperpyrexia and Confusion

Although not reported with pramipexole in the clinical development program, a symptom complex resembling the neuroleptic malignant syndrome (characterized by elevated temperature, muscular rigidity, altered consciousness, and autonomic instability), with no other obvious etiology, has been reported in association with rapid dose reduction, withdrawal of, or changes in antiparkinsonian therapy.

Fibrotic Complications

Although not reported with pramipexole in the clinical development program, cases of retroperitoneal fibrosis, pulmonary infiltrates, pleural effusion, and pleural thickening have been reported in some patients treated with ergot-derived dopaminergic agents. While these complications may resolve when the drug is discontinued, complete resolution does not always occur.

Although these adverse events are believed to be related to the ergoline structure of these compounds, whether other, nonergot derived dopamine agonists can cause them is unknown.

INFORMATION FOR THE PATIENT

Patients should be instructed to take pramipexole dihydrochloride only as prescribed.

Patients should be alerted to the potential sedating effects associated with pramipexole dihydrochloride, including somnolence and the possibility of falling asleep while engaged in activities of daily living. Since somnolence is a frequent adverse event with potentially serious consequences, patients should neither drive a car nor engage in other potentially dangerous activities until they have gained sufficient experience with pramipexole dihydrochloride to gauge whether or not it affects their mental and/or motor performance adversely. Patients should be advised that if increased somnolence or new episodes of falling asleep during activities of daily living (*e.g.*, watching television, passenger in a car, etc.) are experience at any time during treatment, they should not drive or participate in potentially dangerous activities until they have contacted their physician. Because of possible additive effects, caution should be advised when patients are taking other sedating medications or alcohol in combination with pramipexole dihydrochloride and when taking concomitant medications that increase plasma levels of pramipexole (*e.g.*, cimetidine).

Patients should be informed that hallucinations can occur and that the elderly are at a higher risk than younger patients with Parkinson's disease.

Patients may develop postural (orthostatic) hypotension, with or without symptoms such as dizziness, nausea, fainting or blackouts, and sometimes, sweating. Hypotension may occur more frequently during initial therapy. Accordingly, patients should be cautioned against rising rapidly after sitting or lying down, especially if they have being doing so for prolonged periods and especially at the initiation of treatment with pramipexole dihydrochloride.

Because the teratogenic potential of pramipexole has not been completely established in laboratory animals, and because experience in humans is limited, patients should be advised to notify their physicians if they become pregnant or intend to become pregnant during therapy (see Pregnancy Category C).

Because of the possibility that pramipexole may be excreted in breast milk, patients should be advised to notify their physicians if they intend to breast-feed or are breast-feeding an infant.

If patients develop nausea, they should be advised that taking pramipexole dihydrochloride with food may reduce the occurrence of nausea.

LABORATORY TESTS

During the development of pramipexole dihydrochloride, no systematic abnormalities on routine laboratory testing were noted. Therefore, no specific guidance is offered regarding routine monitoring; the practitioner retains responsibility for determining how best to monitor the patient in his or her care.

DRUG/LABORATORY TEST INTERACTIONS

There are no known interactions between pramipexole dihydrochloride and laboratory tests.

CARCINOGENESIS, MUTAGENESIS, AND IMPAIRMENT OF FERTILITY

Two year carcinogenicity studies with pramipexole have been conducted in mice and rats. Pramipexole was administered in the diet to Chbb:NMRI mice at doses of 0.3, 2, and 10 mg/kg/day (0.3, 2.2, and 11 times the highest recommended clinical dose [1.5 mg tid] on a mg/m^2 basis). Pramipexole was administered in the diet to Wistar rats at 0.3, 2, and 8 mg/kg/day (plasma AUCs equal to 0.3, 2.5, and 12.5 times the AUC in humans receiving 1.5 mg tid). No significant increases in tumors occurred in either species.

Pramipexole was not mutagenic or clastogenic in a battery of assays, including the *in vitro* Ames assay, V79 gene mutation assay for HGPRT mutants, chromosomal aberration assay in Chinese hamster ovary cells, and *in vivo* mouse micronucleus assay.

In rat fertility studies, pramipexole at a dose of 2.5 mg/kg/day (5.4 times the highest clinical dose on a mg/m^2 basis), prolonged estrus cycles and inhibited implantation. These effects were associated with reductions in serum levels of prolactin, a hormone necessary for implantation and maintenance of early pregnancy in rats.

PREGNANCY CATEGORY C

When pramipexole was given to female rats throughout pregnancy, implantation was inhibited at a dose of 2.5 mg/kg/day (5.4 times the highest clinical dose on a mg/m^2 basis). Administration of 1.5 mg/kg/day of pramipexole to pregnant rats during the period of organogenesis (gestation days 7 through 16) resulted in a high incidence of total resorption of embryos. The plasma AUC in rats dosed at this level was 4.3 times the AUC in humans receiving 1.5 mg tid. These findings are thought to be due to the prolactin-lowering effect of pramipexole, since prolactin is necessary for implantation and maintenance of early pregnancy in rats (but not rabbits or humans). Because of pregnancy disruption and early embryonic loss in these studies, the teratogenic potential of pramipexole could not be adequately evaluated. There was no evidence of adverse effects on embryo-fetal development following administration of up to 10 mg/kg/day to pregnant rabbits during organogenesis (plasma AUC was 71 times that in humans receiving 1.5 mg tid). Postnatal growth was inhibited in the offspring of rats treated with 0.5 mg/kg/day (approximately equivalent to the highest clinical dose on a mg/m^2 basis) or greater during the latter part of pregnancy and throughout lactation.

There are no studies of pramipexole in human pregnancy. Because animal reproduction studies are not always predictive of human response, pramipexole should be used during pregnancy only if the potential benefit outweighs the potential risk to the fetus.

NURSING MOTHERS

A single-dose, radio-labeled study showed that drug-related materials were excreted into the breast milk of lactating rats. Concentrations of radioactivity in milk were 3-6 times higher than concentrations in plasma at equivalent time points.

Other studies have shown that pramipexole treatment resulted in an inhibition of prolactin secretion in humans and rats.

It is not known whether this drug is excreted in human milk. Because many drugs are excreted in human milk and because of the potential for serious adverse reactions in nursing infants from pramipexole, a decision should be made as to whether to discontinue nursing or to discontinue the drug, taking into account the importance of the drug to the mother.

PEDIATRIC USE

The safety and efficacy of pramipexole dihydrochloride in pediatric patients has not been established.

GERIATRIC USE

Pramipexole total oral clearance was approximately 30% lower in subjects older than 65 years compared with younger subjects, because of a decline in pramipexole renal clearance due to an age-related reduction in renal function. This resulted in an increase in elimination half-life from approximately 8.5-12 hours. In clinical studies, 38.7% of patients were older than 65 years. There were no apparent differences in efficacy or safety between older and younger patients, except that the relative risk of hallucination associated with the use of pramipexole dihydrochloride was increased in the elderly.

DRUG INTERACTIONS

Carbidopa/Levodopa: Carbidopa/levodopa did not influence the pharmacokinetics of pramipexole in healthy volunteers (n=10). Pramipexole did not alter the extent of absorption (AUC) or the elimination of carbidopa/levodopa, although it caused an increase in levodopa C_{max} by about 40% and a decrease in T_{max} from 2.5 to 0.5 hours.

Selegiline: In healthy volunteers (n=11), selegiline did not influence the pharmacokinetics of pramipexole.

Amantadine: Population pharmacokinetic analysis suggests that amantadine is unlikely to alter the oral clearance of pramipexole (n=54).

Cimetidine: Cimetidine, a known inhibitor of renal tubular secretion of organic bases via the cationic transport system, caused a 50% increase in pramipexole AUC and a 40% increase in half-life (n=12).

Probenecid: Probenecid, a known inhibitor of renal tubular secretion of organic acids via the anionic transporter, did not noticeably influence pramipexole pharmacokinetics (n=12).

Other Drugs Eliminated Via Renal Secretion: Population pharmacokinetic analysis suggests that coadministration of drugs that are secreted by the cationic transport system (*e.g.*, cimetidine, ranitidine, diltiazem, triamterene, verapamil, quinidine, and quinine) decreases the oral clearance of pramipexole by about 20%, while those secreted by the anionic transport system (*e.g.*, cephalosporins, penicillins, indomethacin, hydrochlorothiazide, and chlorpropamide) are likely to have little effect on the oral clearance of pramipexole.

CYP Interactions: Inhibitors of cytochrome P450 enzymes would not be expected to affect pramipexole elimination because pramipexole is not appreciably metabolized by these enzymes *in vivo* or *in vitro*. Pramipexole does not inhibit CYP enzymes CYP1A2, CYP2C9, CYP2C19, CYP2E1, and CYP3A4. Inhibition of CYP2D6 was observed with an apparent Ki of 30 μM, indicating that pramipexole will not inhibit CYP enzymes at plasma concentrations observed following the highest recommended clinical dose (1.5 mg tid).

Dopamine Antagonists: Since pramipexole is a dopamine agonist, it is possible that dopamine antagonists, such as the neuroleptics (phenothiazines, butyrophenones, thioxanthenes) or metoclopramide, may diminish the effectiveness of pramipexole dihydrochloride.

ADVERSE REACTIONS

During the premarketing development of pramipexole, patients with either early or advanced Parkinson's disease were enrolled in clinical trials. Apart from the severity and duration of their disease, the two populations differed in their use of concomitant levodopa therapy. Patients with early disease did not receive concomitant levodopa therapy during treatment with pramipexole; those with advanced Parkinson's disease all received concomitant levodopa treatment. Because these two populations may have differential risks for various adverse events, this section will, in general, present adverse-event data for these two populations separately.

P

Because the controlled trials performed during premarketing development all used a titration design, with a resultant confounding of time and dose, it was impossible to adequately evaluate the effects of dose on the incidence of adverse events.

EARLY PARKINSON'S DISEASE

In the three double-blind, placebo-controlled trials of patients with early Parkinson's disease, the most commonly observed adverse events (>5%) that were numerically more frequent in the group treated with pramipexole dihydrochloride tablets were nausea, dizziness, somnolence, insomnia, constipation, asthenia, and hallucinations.

Approximately 12% of 388 patients with early Parkinson's disease and treated with pramipexole dihydrochloride who participated in the double-blind, placebo-controlled trials discontinued treatment due to adverse events compared with 11% of 235 patients who received placebo. The adverse events most commonly causing discontinuation of treatment were related to the nervous system (see TABLE 1).

TABLE 1

Body System/Adverse Event	Pramipexole Dihydrochloride	Placebo
Nervous System		
Hallucinations	3.1%	0.4%
Dizziness	2.1%	1.0%
Somnolence	1.6%	0.0%
Extrapyramidal syndrome	1.6%	6.4%
Headache	1.3%	0.0%
Confusion	1.0%	0.0%
Gastrointestinal System		
Nausea	2.1%	0.4%

Adverse-Event Incidence in Controlled Clinical Studies in Early Parkinson's Disease

TABLE 2 lists treatment-emergent adverse events that occurred in the double-blind, placebo-controlled studies in early Parkinson's disease that were reported by ≥1% of patients treated with pramipexole dihydrochloride and were numerically more frequent than in the placebo group. In these studies, patients did not receive concomitant levodopa. Adverse events were usually mild or moderate in intensity.

The prescriber should be aware that these figures cannot be used to predict the incidence of adverse events in the course of usual medical practice where patient characteristics and other factors differ from those that prevailed in the clinical studies. Similarly, the cited frequencies cannot be compared with figures obtained from other clinical investigations involving different treatments, uses, and investigators. However, the cited figures do provide the prescribing physician with some basis for estimating the relative contribution of drug and non-drug factors to the adverse-event incidence rate in the population studied.

TABLE 2 *Treatment-Emergent Adverse-Event* Incidence in Double-Blind, Placebo-Controlled Trials in Early Parkinson's Disease*

Events ≥1% of patients treated with pramipexole dihydrochloride and numerically more frequent than in the placebo group

Body System Adverse Event	Pramipexole Dihydrochloride n=388	Placebo n=235
Body as a Whole		
Asthenia	14%	12%
General edema	5%	3%
Malaise	2%	1%
Reaction unevaluable	2%	1%
Fever	1%	0%
Digestive System		
Nausea	28%	18%
Constipation	14%	6%
Anorexia	4%	2%
Dysphagia	2%	0%
Metabolic & Nutritional System		
Peripheral edema	5%	4%
Decreased weight	2%	0%
Nervous System		
Dizziness	25%	24
Somnolence	22%	9%
Insomnia	17%	12%
Hallucinations	9%	3%
Confusion	4%	1%
Amnesia	4%	2%
Hypesthesia	3%	1%
Dystonia	2%	1%
Akathisia	2%	0%
Thinking Abnormalites	2%	0%
Decreased Libido	1%	0%
Myoclonus	1%	0%
Special Senses		
Vision abnormalities	3%	0%
Urogenital System		
Impotence	2%	1%

* Patients may have reported multiple adverse experiences during the study or at discontinuation; thus, patients may be included in more than one category.

Other events reported by 1% or more of patients with early Parkinson's disease and treated with pramipexole dihydrochloride but reported equally or more frequently in the placebo group were: infection, accidental injury, headache, pain, tremor, back pain, syncope, postural hypotension, hypertonia, depression, abdominal pain, anxiety, dyspepsia, flatulence, diarrhea, rash, ataxia, dry mouth, extrapyramidal syndrome, leg cramps, twitching, pharyngitis, sinusitis, sweating, rhinitis, urinary tract infection, vasodilation, flu syndrome, increased saliva, tooth disease, dyspnea, increased cough, gait abnormalities, urinary frequency, vomiting, allergic reaction, hypertension, pruritus, hypokinesia, increased creatine PK, nervousness, dream abnormalities, chest pain, neck pain, paresthesia, tachycardia, vertigo, voice alteration, conjunctivitis, paralysis, accomodation abnormalities, tinnitus, diplopia, and taste perversions.

In a fixed-dose study in early Parkinson's disease, occurrence of the following events increased in frequency as the dose increased over the range from 1.5-6.0 mg/day: postural hypotension, nausea, constipation, somnolence, and amnesia. The frequency of these events was generally 2-fold greater than placebo for pramipexole doses greater than 3 mg/day. The incidence of somnolence with pramipexole at a dose of 1.5 mg/day was comparable to that reported for placebo.

ADVANCED PARKINSON'S DISEASE

In the four double-blind, placebo-controlled trials of patients with advanced Parkinson's disease, the most commonly observed adverse events (>5%) that were numerically more frequent in the group treated with pramipexole dihydrochloride and concomitant levodopa were: postural (orthostatic) hypotension, dyskinesia, extrapyramidal syndrome, insomnia, dizziness, hallucinations, accidental injury, dream abnormalities, confusion, constipation, asthenia, somnolence, dystonia, gait abnormality, hypertonia, dry mouth, amnesia, and urinary frequency.

Approximately 12% of 260 patients with advanced Parkinson's disease who received pramipexole dihydrochloride and concomitant levodopa in the double-blind, placebo-controlled trials discontinued treatment due to adverse events compared with 16% of 264 patients who received placebo and concomitant levodopa. The events most commonly causing discontinuation of treatment were related to the nervous system (see TABLE 3).

TABLE 3

Body System/Adverse Event	Pramipexole Dihydrochloride	Placebo
Nervous System		
Hallucinations	2.7%	0.4%
Dyskinesia	1.9%	0.8%
Extrapyramidal syndrome	1.5%	4.9%
Dizziness	1.2%	1.5%
Confusion	1.2%	2.3%
Cardiovascular System		
Postural (orthostatic) hypotension	2.3%	1.1%

Adverse-Event Incidence in Controlled Clinical Studies in Advanced Parkinson's Disease

TABLE 4 lists treatment-emergent adverse events that occurred in the double-blind, placebo-controlled studies in advanced Parkinson's disease that were reportedly by ≥1% of patients treated with pramipexole dihydrochloride and were numerically more frequent than in the placebo group. In the studies, pramipexole dihydrochloride or placebo was administered to patients who were also receiving concomitant levodopa. Adverse events were usually mild or moderate in intensity.

The prescriber should be aware that these figures cannot be used to predict the incidence of adverse events in the course of usual medical practice where patient characteristics and other factors differ from those that prevailed in the clinical studies. Similarly, the cited frequencies cannot be compared with figures obtained from other clinical investigations involving different treatments, uses, and investigators. However, the cited figures do provide the prescribing physician with some basis for estimating the relative contribution of drug and non-drug factors to the adverse-events incidence rate in the population studied.

Other events reported by 1% or more of patients with advanced Parkinson's disease and treated with pramipexole dihydrochloride but reported equally or more frequently in the placebo group were: nausea, pain, infection, headache, depression, tremor, hypokinesia, anorexia, back pain, dyspepsia, flatulence, ataxia, flu syndrome, sinusitis, diarrhea, myalgia, abdominal pain, anxiety, rash, paresthesia, hypertension, increased saliva, tooth disorder, apathy, hypotension, sweating, vasodilation, vomiting, increased cough, nervousness, pruritus, hypesthesia, neck pain, syncope, arthralgia, dysphagia, palpitations, pharyngitis, vertigo, leg cramps, conjunctivitis, and lacrimation disorders.

ADVERSE EVENTS-RELATIONSHIP TO AGE, GENDER, AND RACE

Among the treatment-emergent adverse events in patients treated with pramipexole dihydrochloride, hallucination appeared to exhibit a positive relationship to age. No gender-related differences were observed. Only a small percentage (4%) of patients enrolled were non-caucasian, therefore, an evaluation of adverse events related to race is not possible.

OTHER ADVERSE EVENTS OBSERVED DURING ALL PHASE 2 AND 3 CLINICAL TRIALS

Pramipexole dihydrochloride has been administered to 1408 individuals during all clinical trials (Parkinson's disease and other patient populations), 648 of whom were in seven double-blind, placebo-controlled Parkinson's disease trials. During these trials, all adverse events were recorded by the clinical investigators using terminology of their own choosing. To provide a meaningful estimate of the proportion of individuals having adverse events, similar types of events were grouped into a smaller number of standardized categories using modified COSTART dictionary terminology. These categories are used in the listing below. The events listed below occurred in less than 1% of the 1408 individuals exposed to pramipexole dihydrochloride and occurred on at least two occasions (on one occasion if the event was serious). All reported events, except those already listed above, are included, without regard to determination of a causal relationship to pramipexole dihydrochloride. Events are listed within body system categories in order of decreasing frequency.

Body as a Whole: Enlarged abdomen, death, fever, suicide attempt.

Cardiovascular System: Peripheral vascular disease, myocardial infarction, angina pectoris, atrial fibrillation, heart failure, arrhythmia, atrial arrhythmia, pulmonary embolism.

Digestive System: Thirst.

Musculoskeletal System: Joint disorder, myasthenia.

TABLE 4 *Treatment-Emergent Adverse-Event* Incidence in Double-Blind, Placebo-Controlled Trials in Advanced Parkinson's Disease*

Events ≥ 1% of patients treated with pramipexole dihydrochloride and numerically more frequent than in the placebo group

Body System / Adverse Event	Pramipexole Dihydrochloride† n=260	Placebo † n=264
Body as a Whole		
Accidental injury	17%	15%
Asthenia	10%	8%
General edema	4%	3%
Chest pain	3%	2%
Malaise	3%	2%
Cardiovascular System		
Postural hypotension	53%	48%
Digestive System		
Constipation	10%	9%
Dry mouth	7%	3%
Metabolic & Nutritional System		
Peripheral edema	2%	1%
Increased creatine PK	1%	0%
Musculoskeletal System		
Arthritis	3%	1%
Twitching	2%	0%
Bursitis	2%	0%
Myasthenia	1%	0%
Nervous System		
Dyskinesia	47%	31%
Extrapyramidal syndrome	28%	26%
Insomnia	27%	22%
Dizziness	26%	25%
Hallucinations	17%	4%
Dream abnormalities	11%	10%
Confusion	10%	7%
Somnolence	9%	6%
Dystonia	8%	7%
Gait abnormalities	7%	5%
Hypertonia	7%	6%
Amnesia	6%	4%
Akathisia	3%	2%
Thinking abnormalities	3%	2%
Paranoid reaction	2%	0%
Delusions	1%	0%
Sleep disorders	1%	0%
Respiratory System		
Dyspnea	4%	3%
Rhinitis	3%	1%
Pneumonia	2%	0%
Skin & Appendages		
Skin disorders	2%	1%
Special Senses		
Accomodation abnormalities	4%	2%
Vision abnormalities	3%	1%
Diplopia	1%	0%
Urogenital System		
Urinary frequency	6%	3%
Urinary tract infection	4%	3%
Urinary incontinence	2%	1%

* Patients may have reported multiple adverse experiences during the study or at discontinuation; thus, patients may be included in more than one category.
† Patients received concomitant levodopa.

Nervous System: Agitation, CNS stimulation, hyperkinesia, psychosis, convulsions.
Respiratory System: Pneumonia.
Special Senses: Cataract, eye disorder, glaucoma.
Urogenital System: Dysuria, abnormal ejaculation, prostate cancer, hematuria, prostate disorder.

FALLING ASLEEP DURING ACTIVITIES OF DAILY LIVING

Patients treated with pramipexole dihydrochloride have reported falling asleep while engaged in activities of daily living, including operation of a motor vehicle which sometimes resulted in accidents (see WARNINGS).

DOSAGE AND ADMINISTRATION

In all clinical studies, dosage was initiated at a subtherapeutic level to avoid intolerable adverse effects and orthostatic hypotension. Pramipexole dihydrochloride should be titrated gradually in all patients. The dosage should be increased to achieve a maximum therapeutic effect, balanced against the principal side effects of dyskinesia, hallucinations, somnolence, and dry mouth.

DOSING IN PATIENTS WITH NORMAL RENAL FUNCTION

Initial Treatment

Dosages should be increased gradually from a starting dose of 0.375 mg/day given in 3 divided doses and should not be increased more frequently than every 5-7 days. A suggested ascending dosage schedule that was used in clinical studies is shown in TABLE 5.

Maintenance Treatment

Pramipexole dihydrochloride tablets were effective and well tolerated over a dosage range of 1.5-4.5 mg/day administered in equally divided doses 3 times per day with or without concomitant levodopa (approximately 800 mg/day).

In a fixed-dose study in early Parkinson's disease patients, doses of 3, 4.5, and 6 mg/day of pramipexole dihydrochloride were not shown to provide any significant benefit beyond that achieved at a daily dose of 1.5 mg/day. However, in the same fixed-dose study, the

TABLE 5 *Ascending Dosage Schedule of Pramipexole Dihydrochloride*

Week	Dosage (mg)	Total Daily Dose (mg)
1	0.125 tid	0.375
2	0.25 tid	0.75
3	0.5 tid	1.50
4	0.75 tid	2.25
5	1.0 tid	3.0
6	1.25 tid	3.75
7	1.5 tid	4.50

following adverse events were dose related: postural hypotension, nausea, constipation, somnolence, and amnesia. The frequency of these events was generally 2-fold greater than placebo for pramipexole doses greater than 3 mg/day. The incidence of somnolence reported with pramipexole at a dose of 1.5 mg/day was comparable to placebo.

When pramipexole dihydrochloride is used in combination with levodopa, a reduction of the levodopa dosage should be considered. In a controlled study in advanced Parkinson's disease, the dosage of levodopa was reduced by an average of 27% from baseline.

DOSING IN PATIENTS WITH RENAL IMPAIRMENT

TABLE 6 *Pramipexole Dosage in the Renally Impaired*

Renal Status	Starting Dose	Maximum Dose
Normal to mild impairment (creatinine Cl >60 ml/min)	0.125 mg tid	1.5 mg tid
Moderate impairment (creatinine Cl = 35-59 ml/min)	0.125 mg bid	1.5 mg bid
Severe impairment (creatinine Cl = 15-34 ml/min)	0.125 mg qd	1.5 mg qd
Very severe impairment (creatine Cl <15 ml/min and hemodialysis patients)	The use of pramipexole dihydrochloride has not been adequately studied in this group of patients.	

DISCONTINUATION OF TREATMENT

It is recommended that pramipexole dihydrochloride be discontinued over a period of 1 week; in some studies, however, abrupt discontinuation was uneventful.

ANIMAL PHARMACOLOGY

RENTINAL PATHOLOGY IN ALBINO RATS

Pathologic changes (degeneration and loss of photoreceptor cells) were observed in the retina of albino rats in the 2 year carcinogenicity study with pramipexole. These findings were first observed during week 76 and were dose dependent in animals receiving 2 or 8 mg/kg/day (plasma AUCs equal to 2.5 and 12.5 times the AUC in humans that received 1.5 mg tid). Similar findings were not present in rats receiving 0.3 mg/kg/day (plasma AUC equal to 0.3 times the AUC in humans that received 1.5 mg tid).

Investigative studies demonstrated that pramipexole reduced the rate of disk shedding from the photoreceptor rod cells of the retina in albino rats, which was associated with enhanced sensitivity to the damaging effects of light. In a comparative study, degeneration and loss of photreceptor cells occurred in albino rats after 13 weeks of treatment with 25 mg/kg/day of pramipexole (54 times the highest clinical dose on a mg/m^2 basis) and constant light (100 lux) but not in pigmented rats exposed to the same dose and higher light intensities (500 lux). Thus, the retina of albino rats is considered to be uniquely sensitive to the damaging effects of pramipexole and light. Similar changes in the retina did not occur in a 2 year carcinogenicity study in albino mice treated with 0.3, 2, or 10 mg/kg/day (0.3, 2.2, and 11 times the highest clinical dose on a mg/m^2 basis). Evaluation of the retinas of monkeys given 0.1, 0.5, or 2.0 mg/kg/day of pramipexole (0.4, 2.2, and 8.6 times the highest clinical dose on a mg/m^2 basis) for 12 months and minipigs given 0.3, 1, or 5 mg/kg/day of pramipexole for 13 weeks also detected no changes.

The potential significance of this effect in humans has not been established, but cannot be disregarded because disruption of a mechanism that is universally present in vetebrates (*i.e.,* disk shedding) may be involved.

FIBRO-OSSEOUS PROLIFERATIVE LESIONS IN MICE

An increased incidence of fibro-osseous proliferative lesions occurred in the femurs of female mice treated for 2 years with 0.3, 2.0, or 10 mg/kg/day (0.3, 2.2, and 11 times the highest clinical dose on a mg/m^2 basis). Lesions occurred at a lower rate in control animals. Similar lesions were not observed in male mice or rats and monkeys of either sex that were treated chronically with pramipexole. The significance of this lesion to humans is unknown.

HOW SUPPLIED

Mirapex tablets are available as follows:

0.125 mg: White, round tablet with "U" on one side and "2" on the reverse side.
0.25 mg: White, oval, scored tablet with "U" twice on one side and "4" twice on the reverse side.
0.5 mg: White, oval, scored tablet with "U" twice on one side and "8" twice on the reverse side.
1.0 mg: White, round, scored tablet with "U" twice on one side and "6" twice on the reverse side.
1.5 mg: White, round, scored tablet with "U" twice on one side and "37" twice on the reverse side.

Storage: Store at 25°C (77°F); excursions permitted to 15-30°C (59-86°F). Protect from light.

PRODUCT LISTING - EQUIVALENTS NOT AVAILABLE

Tablet - Oral - 0.125 mg

63's	$59.39	MIRAPEX, Pharmacia and Upjohn	00009-0002-02

Tablet - Oral - 0.25 mg

90's	$112.60	MIRAPEX, Pharmacia and Upjohn	00009-0004-02

P

100's	$106.24	MIRAPEX, Pharmacia Corporation	00009-0004-06
Tablet - Oral - 0.5 mg			
90's	$200.61	MIRAPEX, Pharmacia and Upjohn	00009-0008-02
100's	$216.55	MIRAPEX, Pharmacia Corporation	00009-0008-03
Tablet - Oral - 1 mg			
90's	$200.61	MIRAPEX, Pharmacia and Upjohn	00009-0006-02
100's	$225.21	MIRAPEX, Pharmacia and Upjohn	00009-0006-06
Tablet - Oral - 1.5 mg			
90's	$200.61	MIRAPEX, Pharmacia and Upjohn	00009-0037-02
100's	$225.21	MIRAPEX, Pharmacia and Upjohn	00009-0037-06

Pravastatin Sodium *(003064)*

For related information, see the comparative table section in Appendix A.

Categories: Atherosclerosis; Coronary heart disease, prevention; Hypercholesterolemia; Hyperlipidemia; Myocardial infarction, prophylaxis; Stroke, prophylaxis; Pregnancy Category X; FDA Approved 1991 Oct
Drug Classes: Antihyperlipidemics; HMG CoA reductase inhibitors
Brand Names: **Pravachol**
Foreign Brand Availability: Astin (Mexico); Bristacol (Spain); Elisor (France); Kenstatin (Mexico); Lipemol (Spain); Lipidal (Israel); Liplat (Spain); Lipostat (England; Ireland; Israel; Philippines); Liprevil (Germany); Mevalotin (China; Germany; Indonesia; Japan; Korea; Taiwan; Thailand); Novales (Indonesia); Prascolend (Mexico); Prastan (Korea); Prava (Slovenia); Pravacol (Portugal); Pravaselect (Italy); Pravasin (Germany); Pravasine (Belgium); Pravastatin Natrium "Mayrho Fer" (Austria); Pravator (India); Pravyl (Colombia); Selectin (Italy); Selektine (Netherlands); Selipran (Switzerland); Vasopran (Korea); Vasten (France); Xipral (Mexico)
Cost of Therapy: $50.64 (Hypercholesterolemia; Pravachol ; 10 mg; 1 tablet/day; 30 day supply)

DESCRIPTION

Pravastatin sodium is one of a new class of lipid-lowering compounds, the HMG-CoA reductase inhibitors, which reduce cholesterol biosynthesis. These agents are competitive inhibitors of 3-hydroxy-3-methylglutaryl-coenzyme A (HMG-CoA) reductase, the enzyme catalyzing the early rate-limiting step in cholesterol biosynthesis, conversion of HMG-CoA to mevalonate.

Pravastatin sodium is designated chemically as 1-naphthalene-heptanoic acid, 1,2,6,7,8,8a-hexahydro-β,δ,6-trihydroxy-2-methyl-8-(2-methyl-1-oxobutoxy)-, monosodium salt, [1S-[1α(βS*,δS*),2α,6α,8β(R*),8aα]]-. The empirical formula is $C_{23}H_{35}NaO_7$, and the molecular weight is 446.52.

Pravastatin sodium is an odorless, white to off-white, fine or crystalline powder. It is a relatively polar hydrophilic compound with a partition coefficient (octanol/water) of 0.59 at a pH of 7.0. It is soluble in methanol and water (>300 mg/ml), slightly soluble in isopropanol, and practically insoluble in acetone, acetonitrile, chloroform, and ether.

Pravachol is available for oral administration as 10, 20, 40 and 80 mg tablets. Inactive ingredients include: croscarmellose sodium, lactose, magnesium oxide, magnesium stearate, microcrystalline cellulose, and povidone. The 10 mg tablet also contains red ferric oxide, the 20 and 80 mg tablets also contain yellow ferric oxide, and the 40 mg tablet also contains green lake blend (mixture of D&C yellow no. 10-aluminum lake and FD&C blue no. 1-aluminum lake).

CLINICAL PHARMACOLOGY

Cholesterol and triglycerides in the bloodstream circulate as part of lipoprotein complexes. These complexes can be separated by density ultracentrifugation into high (HDL), intermediate (IDL), low (LDL), and very low (VLDL) density lipoprotein fractions. Triglycerides (TG) and cholesterol synthesized in the liver are incorporated into very low density lipoproteins (VLDLs) and released into the plasma for delivery to peripheral tissues. In a series of subsequent steps, VLDLs are transformed into intermediate density lipoproteins (IDLs), and cholesterol-rich low density lipoproteins (LDLs). High density lipoproteins (HDLs), containing apolipoprotein A, are hypothesized to participate in the reverse transport of cholesterol from tissues back to the liver.

Pravastatin sodium produces its lipid-lowering effect in 2 ways. First, as a consequence of its reversible inhibition of HMG-CoA reductase activity, it effects modest reductions in intracellular pools of cholesterol. This results in an increase in the number of LDL-receptors on cell surfaces and enhanced receptor-mediated catabolism and clearance of circulating LDL. Second, pravastatin inhibits LDL production by inhibiting hepatic synthesis of VLDL, the LDL precursor.

Clinical and pathologic studies have shown that elevated levels of total cholesterol (Total-C), low density lipoprotein cholesterol (LDL-C), and apolipoprotein B (Apo B — a membrane transport complex for LDL) promote human atherosclerosis. Similarly, decreased levels of HDL-cholesterol (HDL-C) and its transport complex, apolipoprotein A, are associated with the development of atherosclerosis. Epidemiologic investigations have established that cardiovascular morbidity and mortality vary directly with the level of Total-C and LDL-C and inversely with the level of HDL-C. Like LDL, cholesterol-enriched triglyceride-rich lipoproteins, including VLDL, IDL, and remnants, can also promote atherosclerosis. Elevated plasma TG are frequently found in a triad with low HDL-C levels and small LDL particles, as well as in association with non-lipid metabolic risk factors for coronary heart disease. As such, total plasma TG has not consistently been shown to be an independent risk factor for CHD. Furthermore, the independent effect of raising HDL or lowering TG on the risk of coronary and cardiovascular morbidity and mortality has not been determined. In both normal volunteers and patients with hypercholesterolemia, treatment with pravastatin sodium reduced Total-C, LDL-C, and apolipoprotein B. Pravastatin sodium also reduced VLDL-C and TG and produced increases in HDL-C and apolipoprotein A. The effects of pravastatin on Lp (a), fibrinogen, and certain other independent biochemical risk markers for coronary heart disease are unknown. Although pravastatin is relatively more hydrophilic than other HMG-CoA reductase inhibitors, the effect of relative hydrophilicity, if any, on either efficacy or safety has not been established.

In 1 primary (West of Scotland Coronary Prevention Study — WOS)[1] and 2 secondary (Long-Term Intervention With Pravastatin in Ischemic Disease — LIPID[2] and the Cholesterol and Recurrent Events — CARE[3]) prevention studies, pravastatin sodium has been shown to reduce cardiovascular morbidity and mortality across a wide range of cholesterol levels.

PHARMACOKINETICS AND METABOLISM

Pravastatin sodium is administered orally in the active form. In clinical pharmacology studies in man, pravastatin is rapidly absorbed, with peak plasma levels of parent compound attained 1 to 1.5 hours following ingestion. Based on urinary recovery of radiolabeled drug, the average oral absorption of pravastatin is 34% and absolute bioavailability is 17%. While the presence of food in the gastrointestinal tract reduces systemic bioavailability, the lipid-lowering effects of the drug are similar whether taken with, or 1 hour prior, to meals.

Pravastatin undergoes extensive first-pass extraction in the liver (extraction ratio 0.66), which is its primary site of action, and the primary site of cholesterol synthesis and of LDL-C clearance. *In vitro* studies demonstrated that pravastatin is transported into hepatocytes with substantially less uptake into other cells. In view of pravastatin's apparently extensive first-pass hepatic metabolism, plasma levels may not necessarily correlate perfectly with lipid-lowering efficacy. Pravastatin plasma concentrations [including: area under the concentration-time curve (AUC), peak (C_{max}), and steady-state minimum (C_{min})] are directly proportional to administered dose. Systemic bioavailability of pravastatin administered following a bedtime dose was decreased 60% compared to that following an AM dose. Despite this decrease in systemic bioavailability, the efficacy of pravastatin administered once daily in the evening, although not statistically significant, was marginally more effective than that after a morning dose. This finding of lower systemic bioavailability suggests greater hepatic extraction of the drug following the evening dose. Steady-state AUCs, C_{max} and C_{min} plasma concentrations showed no evidence of pravastatin accumulation following once or twice daily administration of pravastatin sodium tablets. Approximately 50% of the circulating drug is bound to plasma proteins. Following single dose administration of ^{14}C-pravastatin, the elimination half-life (T½) for total radioactivity (pravastatin plus metabolites) in humans is 77 hours.

Pravastatin, like other HMG-CoA reductase inhibitors, has variable bioavailability. The coefficient of variation (CV), based on between-subject variability, was 50%-60% for AUC. Pravastatin 20 mg was administered under fasting conditions in adults. The geometric means of C_{max} and AUC ranged from 23.3-26.3 ng/ml and from 54.7-62.2 ng·hr/ml, respectively.

Approximately 20% of a radiolabeled oral dose is excreted in urine and 70% in the feces. After intravenous administration of radiolabeled pravastatin to normal volunteers, approximately 47% of total body clearance was via renal excretion and 53% by non-renal routes (*i.e.*, biliary excretion and biotransformation). Since there are dual routes of elimination, the potential exists both for compensatory excretion by the alternate route as well as for accumulation of drug and/or metabolites in patients with renal or hepatic insufficiency.

In a study comparing the kinetics of pravastatin in patients with biopsy confirmed cirrhosis (n=7) and normal subjects (n=7), the mean AUC varied 18-fold in cirrhotic patients and 5-fold in healthy subjects. Similarly, the peak pravastatin values varied 47-fold for cirrhotic patients compared to 6-fold for healthy subjects.

Biotransformation pathways elucidated for pravastatin include: (a) isomerization to 6-epi pravastatin and the 3α-hydroxyisomer of pravastatin (SQ 31,906), (b) enzymatic ring hydroxylation to SQ 31,945, (c) ω-1 oxidation of the ester side chain, (d) β-oxidation of the carboxy side chain, (e) ring oxidation followed by aromatization, (f) oxidation of a hydroxyl group to a keto group, and (g) conjugation. The major degradation product is the 3α-hydroxy isomeric metabolite, which has one-tenth to one-fortieth the HMG-CoA reductase inhibitory activity of the parent compound.

In a single oral dose study using pravastatin 20 mg, the mean AUC for pravastatin was approximately 27% greater and the mean cumulative urinary excretion (CUE) approximately 19% lower in elderly men (65-75 years old) compared with younger men (19-31 years old). In a similar study conducted in women, the mean AUC for pravastatin was approximately 46% higher and the mean CUE approximately 18% lower in elderly women (65-78 years old) compared with younger women (18-38 years old). In both studies, C_{max}, T_{max} and T½ values were similar in older and younger subjects.

After 2 weeks of once-daily 20 mg oral pravastatin administration, the geometric means of AUC were 80.7 (CV 44%) and 44.8 (CV 89%) ng·hr/ml for children (8-11 years, n=14) and adolescents (12-16 years, n=10), respectively. The corresponding values for C_{max} were 42.4 (CV 54%) and 18.6 ng/ml (CV 100%) for children and adolescents, respectively. No conclusion can be made based on these findings due to the small number of samples and large variability.

INDICATIONS AND USAGE

Therapy with pravastatin sodium should be considered in those individuals at increased risk for atherosclerosis-related clinical events as a function of cholesterol level, the presence or absence of coronary heart disease, and other risk factors.

PRIMARY PREVENTION OF CORONARY EVENTS

In hypercholesterolemic patients without clinically evident coronary heart disease, pravastatin sodium is indicated to:

- Reduce the risk of myocardial infarction.
- Reduce the risk of undergoing myocardial revascularization procedures.
- Reduce the risk of cardiovascular mortality with no increase in death from non-cardiovascular causes.

SECONDARY PREVENTION OF CARDIOVASCULAR EVENTS

In patients with clinically evident coronary heart disease, pravastatin sodium is indicated to:

- Reduce the risk of total mortality by reducing coronary death.
- Reduce the risk of myocardial infarction.
- Reduce the risk of undergoing myocardial revascularization procedures.
- Reduce the risk of stroke and stroke/transient ischemic attack (TIA).
- Slow the progression of coronary atherosclerosis.

HYPERLIPIDEMIA

Pravastatin sodium is indicated as an adjunct to diet to reduce elevated Total-C, LDL-C, Apo B, and TG levels and to increase HDL-C in patients with primary hypercholesterolemia and mixed dyslipidemia (Fredrickson Type IIa and IIb).[8]

Pravastatin sodium is indicated as adjunctive therapy to diet for the treatment of patients with elevated serum triglyceride levels (Fredrickson Type IV).

Pravastatin sodium is indicated for the treatment of patients with primary dysbetalipoproteinemia (Fredrickson Type III) who do not respond adequately to diet.

Pravastatin sodium is indicated as an adjunct to diet and lifestyle modification for treatment of HeFH in children and adolescent patients ages 8 years and older if after an adequate trial of diet the following findings are present:

LDL-C remains ≥190 mg/dl or;

LDL-C remains ≥160 mg/dl and:

- There is a positive family history of premature cardiovascular disease or;
- Two or more other CVD risk factors are present in the patient.

Lipid-altering agents should be used in addition to a diet restricted in saturated fat and cholesterol when the response to diet and other nonpharmacological measures alone have been inadequate.

Prior to initiating therapy with pravastatin, secondary causes for hypercholesterolemia (*e.g.,* poorly controlled diabetes mellitus, hypothyroidism, nephrotic syndrome, dysproteinemias, obstructive liver disease, other drug therapy, alcoholism) should be excluded, and a lipid profile performed to measure Total-C, HDL-C, and TG. For patients with triglycerides (TG) <400 mg/dl (<4.5 mmol/L), LDL-C can be estimated using the following equation:

LDL-C = (Total-C) - (HDL-C) - 1/5 TG

For TG levels >400 mg/dl (>4.5 mmol/L), this equation is less accurate and LDL-C concentrations should be determined by ultracentrifugation. In many hypertriglyceridemic patients, LDL-C may be low or normal despite elevated Total-C. In such cases, HMG-CoA reductase inhibitors are not indicated.

Lipid determinations should be performed at intervals of no less than 4 weeks and dosage adjusted according to the patient's response to therapy.

The National Cholesterol Education Program's Treatment Guidelines are summarized in TABLE 7.

TABLE 7 *NCEP Treatment Guidelines: LDL-C Goals and Cutpoints for Therapeutic Lifestyle Changes and Drug Therapy in Different Risk Categories*

Risk Category	LDL Goal	LDL Level at Which to: Initiate Therapeutic Lifestyle Changes	Consider Drug Therapy
CHD or CHD risk equivalents (10 year risk >20%)	<100 mg/dl	≥100 mg/dl	≥130 mg/dl (100-129: drug optional)*
2+ Risk factors (10 year risk ≤20%)	<130 mg/dl	≥130 mg/dl	10 year risk 10-20%: ≥130 mg/dl 10 year risk <10%: ≥160 mg/dl
0-1 Risk factor†	<160 mg/dl	≥160 mg/dl	≥190 mg/dl (160-189: LDL-lowering drug optional)

CHD Coronary heart disease.
* Some authorities recommend use of LDL-lowering drugs in this category if an LDL-C level of <100 mg/dl cannot be achieved by therapeutic lifestyle changes. Others prefer use of drugs that primarily modify triglycerides and HDL-C, *e.g.,* nicotinic acid or fibrate. Clinical judgment also may call for deferring drug therapy in this subcategory.
† Almost all people with 0-1 risk factor have a 10 year risk <10%; thus, 10 year risk assessment in people with 0-1 risk factor is not necessary.

After the LDL-C goal has been achieved, if the TG is still ≥200 mg/dl, non-HDL-C (total-C minus HDL-C) becomes a secondary target of therapy. Non-HDL-C goals are set 30 mg/dl higher than LDL-C goals for each risk category.

At the time of hospitalization for an acute coronary event, consideration can be given to initiating drug therapy at discharge if the LDL-C is ≥130 mg/dl (see TABLE 7).

Since the goal of treatment is to lower LDL-C, the NCEP recommends that LDL-C levels be used to initiate and assess treatment response. Only if LDL-C levels are not available, should the Total-C be used to monitor therapy.

As with other lipid-lowering therapy, pravastatin sodium is not indicated when hypercholesterolemia is due to hyperalphalipoproteinemia (elevated HDL-C).

The NCEP classification of cholesterol levels in pediatric patients with a familial history of hypercholesterolemia or premature cardiovascular disease is summarized in TABLE 8.

TABLE 8

Category	Total-C	LDL-C
Acceptable	<170 mg/dl	<110 mg/dl
Borderline	170-199 mg/dl	110-129 mg/dl
High	≥200 mg/dl	≥130 mg/dl

NON-FDA APPROVED INDICATIONS

Although not approved by the FDA, pravastatin has been studied in normo-cholesterolemic patients with atherosclerosis to determine if the drug may delay the progression of coronary atherosclerosis.

CONTRAINDICATIONS

Hypersensitivity to any component of this medication.

Active liver disease or unexplained, persistent elevations in liver function tests (see WARNINGS).

PREGNANCY AND LACTATION

Atherosclerosis is a chronic process and discontinuation of lipid-lowering drugs during pregnancy should have little impact on the outcome of long-term therapy of primary hypercholesterolemia. Cholesterol and other products of cholesterol biosynthesis are essential components for fetal development (including synthesis of steroids and cell membranes). Since HMG-CoA reductase inhibitors decrease cholesterol synthesis and possibly the synthesis of other biologically active substances derived from cholesterol, they are contraindicated during pregnancy and in nursing mothers. **Pravastatin should be administered to women of childbearing age only when such patients are highly unlikely to conceive and have been informed of the potential hazards.** If the patient becomes pregnant while taking this class of drug, therapy should be discontinued immediately and the patient apprised of the potential hazard to the fetus (see PRECAUTIONS, Pregnancy Category X).

WARNINGS

LIVER ENZYMES

HMG-CoA reductase inhibitors, like some other lipid-lowering therapies, have been associated with biochemical abnormalities of liver function. In 3 long-term (4.8-5.9 years), placebo-controlled clinical trials (WOS, LIPID, CARE), 19,592 subjects (19,768 randomized), were exposed to pravastatin or placebo. In an analysis of serum transaminase values (ALT, AST), incidences of marked abnormalities were compared between the pravastatin and placebo treatment groups; a marked abnormality was defined as a post-treatment test value greater than 3 times the upper limit of normal for subjects with pretreatment values less than or equal to the upper limit of normal, or 4 times the pretreatment value for subjects with pretreatment values greater than the upper limit of normal but less than 1.5 times the upper limit of normal. Marked abnormalities of ALT or AST occurred with similar low frequency (≤1.2%) in both treatment groups. Overall, clinical trial experience showed that liver function test abnormalities observed during pravastatin therapy were usually asymptomatic, not associated with cholestasis, and did not appear to be related to treatment duration.

It is recommended that liver function tests be performed prior to the initiation of therapy, prior to the elevation of the dose, and when otherwise clinically indicated.

Active liver disease or unexplained persistent transaminase elevations are contraindications to the use of pravastatin (see CONTRAINDICATIONS). Caution should be exercised when pravastatin is administered to patients who have a recent history of liver disease, have signs that may suggest liver disease (*e.g.,* unexplained aminotransferase elevations, jaundice), or are heavy users of alcohol (see CLINICAL PHARMACOLOGY, Pharmacokinetics and Metabolism). Such patients should be closely monitored, started at the lower end of the recommended dosing range, and titrated to the desired therapeutic effect.

Patients who develop increased transaminase levels or signs and symptoms of liver disease should be monitored with a second liver function evaluation to confirm the finding and be followed thereafter with frequent liver function tests until the abnormality(ies) return to normal. Should an increase in AST or ALT of 3 times the upper limit of normal or greater persist, withdrawal of pravastatin therapy is recommended.

SKELETAL MUSCLE

Rare cases of rhabdomyolysis with acute renal failure secondary to myoglobinuria have been reported with pravastatin and other drugs in this class. Uncomplicated myalgia has also been reported in pravastatin-treated patients (see ADVERSE REACTIONS). Myopathy, defined as muscle aching or muscle weakness in conjunction with increases in creatine phosphokinase (CPK) values to greater than 10 times the upper normal limit, was rare (<0.1%) in pravastatin clinical trials. Myopathy should be considered in any patient with diffuse myalgias, muscle tenderness or weakness, and/or marked elevation of CPK. Patients should be advised to report promptly unexplained muscle pain, tenderness or weakness, particularly if accompanied by malaise or fever. **Pravastatin therapy should be discontinued if markedly elevated CPK levels occur or myopathy is diagnosed or suspected. Pravastatin therapy should also be temporarily withheld in any patient experiencing an acute or serious condition predisposing to the development of renal failure secondary to rhabdomyolysis, *e.g.,* sepsis; hypotension; major surgery; trauma; severe metabolic, endocrine, or electrolyte disorders; or uncontrolled epilepsy.**

The risk of myopathy during treatment with another HMG-CoA reductase inhibitor is increased with concurrent therapy with either erythromycin, cyclosporine, niacin, or fibrates. However, neither myopathy nor significant increases in CPK levels have been observed in 3 reports involving a total of 100 post-transplant patients (24 renal and 76 cardiac) treated for up to 2 years concurrently with pravastatin 10-40 mg and cyclosporine. Some of these patients also received other concomitant immunosuppressive therapies. Further, in clinical trials involving small numbers of patients who were treated concurrently with pravastatin and niacin, there were no reports of myopathy. Also, myopathy was not reported in a trial of combination pravastatin (40 mg/day) and gemfibrozil (1200 mg/day), although 4 of 75 patients on the combination showed marked CPK elevations versus 1 of 73 patients receiving placebo. There was a trend toward more frequent CPK elevations and patient withdrawals due to musculoskeletal symptoms in the group receiving combined treatment as compared with the groups receiving placebo, gemfibrozil, or pravastatin monotherapy (see DRUG INTERACTIONS). **The use of fibrates alone may occasionally be associated with myopathy. The combined use of pravastatin and fibrates should be avoided unless the benefit of further alterations in lipid levels is likely to outweigh the increased risk of this drug combination.**

PRECAUTIONS

GENERAL

Pravastatin sodium may elevate creatine phosphokinase and transaminase levels (see ADVERSE REACTIONS). This should be considered in the differential diagnosis of chest pain in a patient on therapy with pravastatin.

HOMOZYGOUS FAMILIAL HYPERCHOLESTEROLEMIA

Pravastatin has not been evaluated in patients with rare homozygous familial hypercholesterolemia. In this group of patients, it has been reported that HMG-CoA reductase inhibitors are less effective because the patients lack functional LDL receptors.

RENAL INSUFFICIENCY

A single 20 mg oral dose of pravastatin was administered to 24 patients with varying degrees of renal impairment (as determined by creatinine clearance). No effect was observed on the pharmacokinetics of pravastatin or its 3α-hydroxy isomeric metabolite (SQ 31,906). A small increase was seen in mean AUC values and half-life ($T_{1/2}$) for the inactive enzymatic ring hydroxylation metabolite (SQ 31,945). Given this small sample size, the dosage administered, and the degree of individual variability, patients with renal impairment who are receiving pravastatin should be closely monitored.

INFORMATION FOR THE PATIENT

Patients should be advised to report promptly unexplained muscle pain, tenderness or weakness, particularly if accompanied by malaise or fever (see WARNINGS, Skeletal Muscle).

ENDOCRINE FUNCTION

HMG-CoA reductase inhibitors interfere with cholesterol synthesis and lower circulating cholesterol levels and, as such, might theoretically blunt adrenal or gonadal steroid hormone production. Results of clinical trials with pravastatin in males and post-menopausal females were inconsistent with regard to possible effects of the drug on basal steroid hormone levels. In a study of 21 males, the mean testosterone response to human chorionic gonadotropin was significantly reduced ($p < 0.004$) after 16 weeks of treatment with 40 mg of pravastatin. However, the percentage of patients showing a ≥50% rise in plasma testosterone after human chorionic gonadotropin stimulation did not change significantly after therapy in these patients. The effects of HMG-CoA reductase inhibitors on spermatogenesis and fertility have not been studied in adequate numbers of patients. The effects, if any, of pravastatin on the pituitary-gonadal axis in pre-menopausal females are unknown. Patients treated with pravastatin who display clinical evidence of endocrine dysfunction should be evaluated appropriately. Caution should also be exercised if an HMG-CoA reductase inhibitor or other agent used to lower cholesterol levels is administered to patients also receiving other drugs (*e.g.,* ketoconazole, spironolactone, cimetidine) they may diminish the levels or activity of steroid hormones.

In a placebo-controlled study of 214 pediatric patients with HeFH, of which 106 were treated with pravastatin (20 mg in the children aged 8-13 years and 40 mg in the adolescents aged 14-18 years) for 2 years, there were no detectable differences seen in any of the endocrine parameters [ACTH, cortisol, DHEAS, FSH, LH, TSH, estradiol (girls) or testosterone (boys)] relative to placebo. There were no detectable differences seen in height and weight changes, testicular volume changes, or Tanner score relative to placebo.

CNS TOXICITY

CNS vascular lesions, characterized by perivascular hemorrhage and edema and mononuclear cell infiltration of perivascular spaces, were seen in dogs treated with pravastatin at a dose of 25 mg/kg/day. These effects in dogs were observed at approximately 59 times the human dose of 80 mg/day, based on AUC. Similar CNS vascular lesions have been observed with several other drugs in this class.

A chemically similar drug in this class produced optic nerve degeneration (Wallerian degeneration of retinogeniculate fibers) in clinically normal dogs in a dose-dependent fashion starting at 60 mg/kg/day, a dose that produced mean plasma drug levels about 30 times higher than the mean drug level in humans taking the highest recommended dose (as measured by total enzyme inhibitory activity). This same drug also produced vestibulocochlear Wallerian-like degeneration and retinal ganglion cell chromatolysis in dogs treated for 14 weeks at 180 mg/kg/day, a dose which resulted in a mean plasma drug level similar to that seen with the 60 mg/kg/day dose.

P

CARCINOGENESIS, MUTAGENESIS, AND IMPAIRMENT OF FERTILITY

In a 2 year study in rats fed pravastatin at doses of 10, 30, or 100 mg/kg body weight, there was an increased incidence of hepatocellular carcinomas in males at the highest dose ($p < 0.01$). These effects in rats were observed at approximately 12 times the human dose (HD) of 80 mg based on body surface area mg/m^2 and at approximately 4 times the human dose, based on AUC.

In a 2 year study in mice fed pravastatin at doses of 250 and 500 mg/kg/day, there was an increased incidence of hepatocellular carcinomas in males and females at both 250 and 500 mg/kg/day ($p < 0.0001$). At these doses, lung adenomas in females were increased ($p=0.013$). These effects in mice were observed at approximately 15 times (250 mg/kg/day) and 23 times (500 mg/kg/day) the human dose of 80 mg, based on AUC. In another 2 year study in mice with doses up to 100 mg/kg/day (producing drug exposures approximately 2 times the human dose of 80 mg, based on AUC), there were no drug-induced tumors.

No evidence of mutagenicity was observed *in vitro,* with or without rat-liver metabolic activation, in the following studies: microbial mutagen tests, using mutant strains of *Salmonella typhimurium* or *Escherichia coli;* a forward mutation assay in L5178Y TK +/- mouse lymphoma cells; a chromosomal aberration test in hamster cells; and a gene conversion assay using *Saccharomyces cerevisiae.* In addition, there was no evidence of mutagenicity in either a dominant lethal test in mice or a micronucleus test in mice.

In a study in rats, with daily doses up to 500 mg/kg, pravastatin did not produce any adverse effects on fertility or general reproductive performance. However, in a study with another HMG-CoA reductase inhibitor, there was decreased fertility in male rats treated for 34 weeks at 25 mg/kg body weight, although this effect was not observed in a subsequent fertility study when this same dose was administered for 11 weeks (the entire cycle of spermatogenesis, including epididymal maturation). In rats treated with this same reductase inhibitor at 180 mg/kg/day, seminiferous tubule degeneration (necrosis and loss of spermatogenic epithelium) was observed. Although not seen with pravastatin, 2 similar drugs in this class caused drug-related testicular atrophy, decreased spermatogenesis, spermatocytic degeneration, and giant cell formation in dogs. The clinical significance of these findings is unclear.

PREGNANCY CATEGORY X

See CONTRAINDICATIONS.

Safety in pregnant women has not been established. Pravastatin was not teratogenic in rats at doses up to 1000 mg/kg daily or in rabbits at doses of up to 50 mg/kg daily. These doses resulted in 10× (rabbit) or 120× (rat) the human exposure based on surface area (mg/m^2).

Rare reports of congenital anomalies have been received following intrauterine exposure to other HMG-CoA reductase inhibitors. In a review[9] of approximately 100 prospectively followed pregnancies in women exposed to simvastatin or lovastatin, the incidences of congenital anomalies, spontaneous abortions and fetal deaths/stillbirths did not exceed what would be expected in the general population. The number of cases is adequate only to exclude a 3- to 4-fold increase in congenital anomalies over the background incidence. In 89% of the prospectively followed pregnancies, drug treatment was initiated prior to pregnancy and was discontinued at some point in the first trimester when pregnancy was identified. As safety in pregnant women has not been established and there is no apparent benefit to therapy with pravastatin sodium during pregnancy (see CONTRAINDICATIONS), treatment should be immediately discontinued as soon as pregnancy is recognized. Pravastatin sodium should be administered to women of child-bearing potential only when such patients are highly unlikely to conceive and have been informed of the potential hazards.

NURSING MOTHERS

A small amount of pravastatin is excreted in human breast milk. Because of the potential for serious adverse reactions in nursing infants, women taking pravastatin sodium should not nurse (see CONTRAINDICATIONS).

PEDIATRIC USE

The safety and effectiveness of pravastatin sodium in children and adolescents from 8-18 years of age have been evaluated in a placebo-controlled study of 2 years duration. Patients treated with pravastatin had an adverse experience profile generally similar to that of patients treated with placebo with influenza and headache commonly reported in both treatment groups. (See ADVERSE REACTIONS, Pediatric Patients.) **Doses greater than 40 mg have not been studied in this population.** For dosing information see DOSAGE AND ADMINISTRATION: Adult Patients and Pediatric Patients.

Double-blind, placebo-controlled pravastatin studies in children less than 8 years of age have not been conducted.

GERIATRIC USE

Two secondary prevention trials with pravastatin (CARE and LIPID) included a total of 6593 subjects treated with pravastatin 40 mg for periods ranging up to 6 years. Across these 2 studies, 36.1% of pravastatin subjects were aged 65 and older and 0.8% were aged 75 and older. The beneficial effect of pravastatin in elderly subjects in reducing cardiovascular events and in modifying lipid profiles was similar to that seen in younger subjects. The adverse event profile in the elderly was similar to that in the overall population. Other reported clinical experience has not identified differences in responses to pravastatin between elderly and younger patients.

Mean pravastatin AUCs are slightly (25-50%) higher in elderly subjects than in healthy young subjects, but mean C_{max}, T_{max} and $T_{1/2}$ values are similar in both age groups and substantial accumulation of pravastatin would not be expected in the elderly (see CLINICAL PHARMACOLOGY, Pharmacokinetics and Metabolism).

DRUG INTERACTIONS

Immunosuppressive drugs, gemfibrozil, niacin (nicotinic acid), erythromycin: See WARNINGS, Skeletal Muscle.

Cytochrome P450 3A4 inhibitors: *In vitro* and *in vivo* data indicate that pravastatin is not metabolized by cytochrome P450 3A4 to a clinically significant extent. This has been shown in studies with known cytochrome P450 3A4 inhibitors (see Diltiazem and Itraconazole). Other examples of cytochrome P450 3A4 inhibitors include ketoconazole, mibefradil, and erythromycin.

Diltiazem: Steady-state levels of diltiazem (a known, weak inhibitor of P450 3A4) had no effect on the pharmacokinetics of pravastatin. In this study, the AUC and C_{max} of another HMG-CoA reductase inhibitor which is known to be metabolized by cytochrome P450 3A4 increased by factors of 3.6 and 4.3, respectively.

Itraconazole: The mean AUC and C_{max} for pravastatin were increased by factors of 1.7 and 2.5, respectively, when given with itraconazole (a potent P450 3A4 inhibitor which also inhibits p-glycoprotein transport) as compared to placebo. The mean $T_{1/2}$ was not affected by itraconazole, suggesting that the relatively small increases in C_{max} and AUC were due solely to increased bioavailability rather than a decrease in clearance, consistent with inhibition of p-glycoprotein transport by itraconazole. This drug transport system is thought to affect bioavailability and excretion of HMG-CoA reductase inhibitors, including pravastatin. The AUC and C_{max} of another HMG-CoA reductase inhibitor which is known to be metabolized by cytochrome P450 3A4 increased by factors of 19 and 17, respectively, when given with itraconazole.

Antipyrine: Since concomitant administration of pravastatin had no effect on the clearance of antipyrine, interactions with other drugs metabolized via the same hepatic cytochrome isozymes are not expected.

Cholestyramine/colestipol: Concomitant administration resulted in an approximately 40-50% decrease in the mean AUC of pravastatin. However, when pravastatin was administered 1 hour before or 4 hours after cholestyramine or 1 hour before colestipol and a standard meal, there was no clinically significant decrease in bioavailability or therapeutic effect. (See DOSAGE AND ADMINISTRATION, Concomitant Therapy.)

Warfarin: Concomitant administration of 40 mg pravastatin had no clinically significant effect on prothrombin time when administered in a study to normal elderly subjects who were stabilized on warfarin.

Cimetidine: The AUC(0-12h) for pravastatin when given with cimetidine was not significantly different from the AUC for pravastatin when given alone. A significant difference was observed between the AUCs for pravastatin when given with cimetidine compared to when administered with antacid.

Digoxin: In a crossover trial involving 18 healthy male subjects given 20 mg pravastatin and 0.2 mg digoxin concurrently for 9 days, the bioavailability parameters of digoxin were not affected. The AUC of pravastatin tended to increase, but the overall bioavailability of pravastatin plus its metabolites SQ 31,906 and SQ 31,945 was not altered.

Cyclosporine: Some investigators have measured cyclosporine levels in patients on pravastatin (up to 20 mg), and to date, these results indicate no clinically meaningful elevations in cyclosporine levels. In one single-dose study, pravastatin levels were found to be increased in cardiac transplant patients receiving cyclosporine.

Gemfibrozil: In a crossover study in 20 healthy male volunteers given concomitant single doses of pravastatin and gemfibrozil, there was a significant decrease in urinary excretion and protein binding of pravastatin. In addition, there was a significant increase in AUC, C_{max}, and T_{max} for the pravastatin metabolite SQ 31,906. Combination therapy with pravastatin and gemfibrozil is generally not recommended. (See WARNINGS, Skeletal Muscle.)

In interaction studies with *aspirin, antacids* (1 hour prior to pravastatin), *cimetidine, nicotinic acid,* or *probucol,* no statistically significant differences in bioavailability were seen when pravastatin sodium was administered.

ADVERSE REACTIONS

Pravastatin is generally well tolerated; adverse reactions have usually been mild and transient. In 4 month long placebo-controlled trials, 1.7% of pravastatin-treated patients and 1.2% of placebo-treated patients were discontinued from treatment because of adverse experiences attributed to study drug therapy; this difference was not statistically significant. (See also PRECAUTIONS, Geriatric Use.)

ADVERSE CLINICAL EVENTS

Short-Term Controlled Trials

All adverse clinical events (regardless of attribution) reported in more than 2% of pravastatin-treated patients in placebo-controlled trials of up to 4 months duration are identified in TABLE 9; also shown are the percentages of patients in whom these medical events were believed to be related or possibly related to the drug.

***TABLE 9** Adverse Events in >2% of Patients Treated With Pravastatin 10-40 mg in Short-Term Placebo-Controlled Trials*

	All Events		Events Attributed to Study Drug	
	Pravastatin	Placebo	Pravastatin	Placebo
Body System/Event	(n=900)	(n=411)	(n=900)	(n=411)
Cardiovascular				
Cardiac chest pain	4.0%	3.4%	0.1%	0.0%
Dermatologic				
Rash	4.0%*	1.1%	1.3%	0.9%
Gastrointestinal				
Nausea/vomiting	7.3%	7.1%	2.9%	3.4%
Diarrhea	6.2%	5.6%	2.0%	1.9%
Abdominal pain	5.4%	6.9%	2.0%	3.9%
Constipation	4.0%	7.1%	2.4%	5.1%
Flatulence	3.3%	3.6%	2.7%	3.4%
Heartburn	2.9%	1.9%	2.0%	0.7%
General				
Fatigue	3.8%	3.4%	1.9%	1.0%
Chest pain	3.7%	1.9%	0.3%	0.2%
Influenza	2.4%*	0.7%	0.0%	0.0%
Musculoskeletal				
Localized pain	10.0%	9.0%	1.4%	1.5%
Myalgia	2.7%	1.0%	0.6%	0.0%
Nervous System				
Headache	6.2%	3.9%	1.7%*	0.2%
Dizziness	3.3%	3.2%	1.0%	0.5%
Renal/Genitourinary				
Urinary abnormality	2.4%	2.9%	0.7%	1.2%
Respiratory				
Common cold	7.0%	6.3%	0.0%	0.0%
Rhinitis	4.0%	4.1%	0.1%	0.0%
Cough	2.6%	1.7%	0.1%	0.0%

* Statistically significantly different from placebo.

The safety and tolerability of pravastatin sodium at a dose of 80 mg in 2 controlled trials with a mean exposure of 8.6 months was similar to that of pravastatin sodium at lower doses except that 4 out of 464 patients taking 80 mg of pravastatin had a single elevation of CK >10 × ULN compared to 0 out of 115 patients taking 40 mg of pravastatin.

LONG-TERM CONTROLLED MORBIDITY AND MORTALITY TRIALS

Adverse event data were pooled from 7 double-blind, placebo-controlled trials (West of Scotland Coronary Prevention study [WOS]; Cholesterol and Recurrent Events study [CARE]; Long-term Intervention with Pravastatin in Ischemic Disease study [LIPID]; Pravastatin Limitation of Atherosclerosis in the Coronary Arteries study [PLAC I]; Pravastatin, Lipids and Atherosclerosis in the Carotids study [PLAC II]; Regression Growth Evaluation Statin Study [REGRESS]; and Kuopio Atherosclerosis Prevention Study [KAPS]) involving a total of 10,764 patients treated with pravastatin 40 mg and 10,719 patients treated with placebo. The safety and tolerability profile in the pravastatin group was comparable to that of the placebo group. Patients were exposed to pravastatin for a mean of 4.0-5.1 years in WOS, CARE, and LIPID and 1.9-2.9 years in PLAC I, PLAC II, KAPS, and REGRESS. In these long-term trials, the most common reasons for discontinuation were mild, non-specific gastrointestinal complaints. Collectively, these 7 trials represent 47,613 patient-years of exposure to pravastatin. Events believed to be of probable, possible, or uncertain relationship to study drug, occurring in at least 1% of patients treated with pravastatin in these studies are identified in TABLE 10.

***TABLE 10** Adverse Events in ≥1% of Patients Treated With Pravastatin 40 mg in Long-Term Placebo-Controlled Trials*

Body System/Event	Pravastatin (n=10,764)	Placebo (n=10,719)
Cardiovascular		
Angina pectoris	3.1%	3.4%
Dermatologic		
Rash	2.1%	2.2%
Gastrointestinal		
Dyspepsia/heartburn	3.5%	3.7%
Abdominal pain	2.4%	2.5%
Nausea/vomiting	1.6%	1.6%
Flatulence	1.2%	1.1%
Constipation	1.2%	1.3%
General		
Fatigue	3.4%	3.3%
Chest pain	2.6%	2.6%
Musculoskeletal		
Musculoskeletal pain (includes arthralgia)	6.0%	5.8%
Muscle cramp	2.0%	1.8%
Myalgia	1.4%	1.4%
Nervous system		
Dizziness	2.2%	2.1%
Headache	1.9%	1.8%
Sleep disturbance	1.0%	0.9%
Depression	1.0%	1.0%
Anxiety/nervousness	1.0%	1.2%
Renal/Genitourinary		
Urinary abnormality (includes dysuria, frequency, nocturia)	1.0%	0.8%
Respiratory		
Dyspnea	1.6%	1.6%
Upper respiratory infection	1.3%	1.3%
Cough	1.0%	1.0%
Special Senses		
Vision disturbance (includes blurred vision, diplopia)	1.6%	1.3%

Events of probable, possible, or uncertain relationship to study drug that occurred in <1.0% of pravastatin-treated patients in the long-term trials included the following; frequencies were similar in placebo-treated patients:

Dermatologic: Pruritus, dermatitis, dryness skin, scalp hair abnormality (including alopecia), urticaria.

Endocrine/Metabolic: Sexual dysfunction, libido change.

Gastrointestinal: Decreased appetite.

General: Fever, flushing.

Immunologic: Allergy, edema head/neck.

Musculoskeletal: Muscle weakness.

Nervous System: Paresthesia, vertigo, insomnia, memory impairment, tremor, neuropathy (including peripheral neuropathy).

Special Senses: Lens opacity, taste disturbance.

POSTMARKETING EXPERIENCE

In addition to the events reported above, as with other drugs in this class, the following events have been reported rarely during postmarketing experience with pravastatin sodium, regardless of causality assessment:

Musculoskeletal: Myopathy, rhabdomyolysis.

Nervous System: Dysfunction of certain cranial nerves (including alteration of taste, impairment of extra-ocular movement, facial paresis), peripheral nerve palsy.

Hypersensitivity: Anaphylaxis, lupus erythematosus-like syndrome, polymyalgia rheumatica, dermatomyositis, vasculitis, purpura, hemolytic anemia, positive ANA, ESR increase, arthritis, arthralgia, asthenia, photosensitivity, chills, malaise, toxic epidermal necrolysis, erythema multiforme, including Stevens-Johnson syndrome.

Gastrointestinal: Pancreatitis, hepatitis, including chronic active hepatitis, cholestatic jaundice, fatty change in liver, cirrhosis, fulminant hepatic necrosis, hepatoma.

Dermatologic: A variety of skin changes (*e.g.,* nodules, discoloration, dryness of mucous membranes, changes to hair/nails).

Reproductive: Gynecomastia.

Laboratory Abnormalities: Elevated alkaline phosphatase and bilirubin; thyroid function abnormalities.

LABORATORY TEST ABNORMALITIES

Increases in serum transaminase (ALT, AST) values and CPK have been observed (see WARNINGS).

Transient, asymptomatic eosinophilia has been reported. Eosinophil counts usually returned to normal despite continued therapy. Anemia, thrombocytopenia, and leukopenia have been reported with HMG-CoA reductase inhibitors.

CONCOMITANT THERAPY

Pravastatin has been administered concurrently with cholestyramine, colestipol, nicotinic acid, probucol and gemfibrozil. Preliminary data suggest that the addition of either probucol or gemfibrozil to therapy with lovastatin or pravastatin is **not** associated with greater reduction in LDL-cholesterol than that achieved with lovastatin or pravastatin alone. No adverse reactions unique to the combination or in addition to those previously reported for each drug alone have been reported. Myopathy and rhabdomyolysis (with or without acute renal failure) have been reported when another HMG-CoA reductase inhibitor was used in combination with immunosuppressive drugs, gemfibrozil, erythromycin, or lipid-lowering doses of nicotinic acid. Concomitant therapy with HMG-CoA reductase inhibitors and these agents is generally not recommended. (See WARNINGS, Skeletal Muscle and DRUG INTERACTIONS.)

PEDIATRIC PATIENTS

In a 2 year double-blind placebo-controlled study involving 100 boys and 114 girls with HeFH, the safety and tolerability profile of pravastatin was generally similar to that of placebo. (See PRECAUTIONS, Pediatric Use.)

DOSAGE AND ADMINISTRATION

The patient should be placed on a standard cholesterol-lowering diet before receiving pravastatin sodium and should continue on this diet during treatment with pravastatin sodium (see TABLE 7).

Pravastatin sodium can be administered orally as a single dose at any time of the day, with or without food. Since the maximal effect of a given dose is seen within 4 weeks, periodic lipid determinations should be performed at this time and dosage adjusted according to the patient's response to therapy and established treatment guidelines.

ADULT PATIENTS

The recommended starting dose is 40 mg once daily. If a daily dose of 40 mg does not achieve desired cholesterol levels, 80 mg once daily is recommended. In patients with a history of significant renal or hepatic dysfunction, a starting dose of 10 mg daily is recommended.

PEDIATRIC PATIENTS

Children (ages 8-13 years, inclusive)

The recommended dose is 20 mg once daily in children 8-13 years of age. Doses greater than 20 mg have not been studied in this patient population.

Adolescents (ages 14-18 years)

The recommended starting dose is 40 mg once daily in adolescents 14-18 years of age. Doses greater than 40 mg have not been studied in this patient population.

Children and adolescents treated with pravastatin should be re-evaluated in adulthood and appropriate changes made to their cholesterol-lowering regimen to achieve adult goals for LDL-C (see TABLE 7).

In patients taking immunosuppressive drugs such as cyclosporine (see WARNINGS, Skeletal Muscle) concomitantly with pravastatin, therapy should begin with 10 mg of pravastatin once-a-day at bedtime and titration to higher doses should be done with caution. Most patients treated with this combination received a maximum pravastatin dose of 20 mg/day.

CONCOMITANT THERAPY

The lipid-lowering effects of pravastatin sodium on total and LDL cholesterol are enhanced when combined with a bile-acid-binding resin. When administering a bile-acid-binding resin (*e.g.*, cholestyramine, colestipol) and pravastatin, pravastatin sodium should be given either 1 hour or more before or at least 4 hours following the resin. (See also ADVERSE REACTIONS, Concomitant Therapy.)

HOW SUPPLIED

Pravachol tablets are supplied as:

10 mg tablets: Pink to peach, rounded, rectangular-shaped, biconvex with a "P" embossed on one side and "PRAVACHOL 10" engraved on the opposite side.

20 mg tablets: Yellow, rounded, rectangular-shaped, biconvex with a "P" embossed on one side and "PRAVACHOL 20" engraved on the opposite side.

40 mg tablets: Green, rounded, rectangular-shaped, biconvex with a "P" embossed on one side and "PRAVACHOL 40" engraved on the opposite side.

80 mg tablets: Yellow, oval-shaped, biconvex with "BMS" embossed on one side and "80" engraved on the opposite side.

Storage: Store at 25°C (77°F); excursions permitted to 15-30°C (59- 86°F). Keep tightly closed (protect from moisture). Protect from light.

PRODUCT LISTING - EQUIVALENTS NOT AVAILABLE

Tablet - Oral - 10 mg			
30's	$68.92	PRAVACHOL, Allscripts Pharmaceutical Company	54569-4346-01
30's	$78.76	PRAVACHOL, Pd-Rx Pharmaceuticals	55289-0104-30
90's	$151.91	PRAVACHOL, Allscripts Pharmaceutical Company	54569-8598-00
90's	$272.83	PRAVACHOL, Bristol-Myers Squibb	00003-5154-05
100's	$168.79	PRAVACHOL, Allscripts Pharmaceutical Company	54569-3840-00
100's	$191.51	PRAVACHOL, Allscripts Pharmaceutical Company	54569-4346-00
Tablet - Oral - 20 mg			
30's	$74.95	PRAVACHOL, Southwood Pharmaceuticals Inc	58016-0425-30
60's	$149.90	PRAVACHOL, Southwood Pharmaceuticals Inc	58016-0425-60
90's	$224.85	PRAVACHOL, Southwood Pharmaceuticals Inc	58016-0425-90
90's	$233.87	PRAVACHOL, Physicians Total Care	54868-2288-00
90's	$277.24	PRAVACHOL, Bristol-Myers Squibb	00003-5178-05
100's	$249.83	PRAVACHOL, Southwood Pharmaceuticals Inc	58016-0425-00
100's	$308.04	PRAVACHOL, Bristol-Myers Squibb	00003-5178-06
Tablet - Oral - 40 mg			
30's	$109.48	PRAVACHOL, Physicians Total Care	54868-3270-00
30's	$118.28	PRAVACHOL, Allscripts Pharmaceutical Company	54569-4610-00
60's	$205.76	PRAVACHOL, Physicians Total Care	54868-3270-01
90's	$406.84	PRAVACHOL, Bristol-Myers Squibb	00003-5194-10
Tablet - Oral - 80 mg			
90's	$406.84	PRAVACHOL, Bristol-Myers Squibb	00003-5195-10

Praziquantel (002099)

Categories: Infection, liver flukes; Schistosomiasis; Pregnancy Category B; FDA Approved 1982 Dec; WHO Formulary
Drug Classes: Antihelmintics
Brand Names: **Biltricide**
Foreign Brand Availability: Cesol (Mexico); Cisticid (Ecuador; Mexico; Peru); Distocide (Bahrain; Cyprus; Egypt; Iran; Iraq; Jordan; Korea; Kuwait; Lebanon; Libya; Oman; Qatar; Republic-of-Yemen; Saudi-Arabia; Syria; United-Arab-Emirates); Ehliten (Mexico); Helmiben (Peru); Kalcide (Taiwan); Mycotricide (Thailand); Opticide (Thailand); Prazite (Thailand); Teniken (Mexico); Z-Queen (Thailand)
Cost of Therapy: $83.31 (Helminth Infection; Biltricide; 600 mg; 7 tablets/day; 1 day supply)

DESCRIPTION

Biltricide (praziquantel) is a trematodicide provided in tablet form for the oral treatment of schistosome infections and infections due to liver fluke.

Praziquantel is 2-(cyclohexylcarbonyl-1,2,3,6,7 11b-hexahydro-4H-pyrazino (2,1-a) isoquinolin-4-one with the molecular formula: $C_{19}H_{24}N_2O_2$.

Praziquantel is a white to nearly white crystalline powder of bitter taste. The compound is stable under normal conditions and melts at 136-140°C with decomposition. The active substance is hygroscopic. Praziquantel is easily soluble in chloroform and dimethylsulfoxide, soluble in ethanol and very slightly soluble in water.

Biltricide tablets contain 600 mg of praziquantel. *Inactive ingrediants:* Corn starch, magnesium stearate, microcrystalline cellulose, povidone, sodium lauryl sulfate, polyethylene glycol, titanium dioxide and HPM cellulose.

CLINICAL PHARMACOLOGY

Praziquantel induces a rapid contraction of schistosomes by a specific effect on the permeability of the cell membrane. The drug further results in vacuolization & disintegration of the schistosome tegument.

After oral administration praziquantel is rapidly absorbed (80%), subjected to a first pass effect, metabolized and eliminated by the kidneys. Maximal serum concentration is achieved 1-3 hours after dosing. The half-life of praziquantel in serum is 0.8-1.5 hours.

INDICATIONS AND USAGE

Praziquantel is indicated for the treatment of infections due to: all species of *Schistosoma* (*e.g., Schistosoma mekongi; Schistosoma japonicum, Schistosoma mansoni* and *Schistosoma hematobium*), and infections due to the liver flukes, *Clonorchis sinensis/Opisthorchis viverrini* (approval of this indication was based on studies in which the two species were not differentiated).

CONTRAINDICATIONS

Praziquantel should not be given to patients who previously have shown hypersensitivity to the drug. Since parasite destruction within the eye may cause irreparable lesions, ocular cysticercosis should not be treated with this compound.

PRECAUTIONS

INFORMATION FOR THE PATIENT

Patients should be warned not to drive a car and not to operate machinery on the day of praziquantel treatment and the following day.

Minimal increases in liver enzymes have been reported in some patients.

When schistosomiasis or fluke infection is found to be associated with cerebral cysticercosis it is advised to hospitalize the patient for the duration of treatment.

MUTAGENESIS, CARCINOGENESIS

Mutagenic effects in Salmonella tests found by one laboratory have not been confirmed in the same tested strain by other laboratories. Long term carcinogenicity studies in rats and golden hamsters did not reveal any carcinogenic effect.

PREGNANCY CATEGORY B

Reproduction studies have been performed in rats and rabbits at doses up to 40 times the human dose and have revealed no evidence of impaired fertility or harm to the fetus due to praziquantel. There are, however, no adequate and well-controlled studies in pregnant women. An increase of the abortion rate was found in rats at 3 times the single human therapeutic dose. While animal reproduction studies are not always predictive of human response, this drug should be used during pregnancy only if clearly needed.

NURSING MOTHERS

Praziquantel appeared in the milk of nursing women at a concentration of about ¼ that of maternal serum. Woman should not nurse on the day of praziquantel treatment and during the subsequent 72 hours.

PEDIATRIC USE

Safety in children under 4 years of age has not been established.

DRUG INTERACTIONS

No data are available regarding interaction of praziquantel with other drugs.

ADVERSE REACTIONS

In general praziquantel is very well tolerated. Side effects are usually mild and transient and do not require treatment. The following side effects were observed generally in order of severity: malaise, headache, dizziness, abdominal discomfort with or without nausea, rise in temperatue and, rarely, urticaria. Such symptoms can, however, also result from the infection itself. Such side effects may be more frequent and/or serious in patients with a heavy worm burden. In patients with liver impairment caused by the infection, no adverse effects of praziquantel have occurred which would necessitate restriction in use.

DOSAGE AND ADMINISTRATION

The dosage recommended for the treatment of schistosomiasis is: 3 × 20 mg/kg bodyweight as a 1 day treatment. **The recommended dose for clonorchiasis and opisthorchiasis is:** 3 × 25 mg/kg as a 1 day treatment. The tablets should be washed down unchewed with some liquid during meals. Keeping the tablets or segments thereof in the mouth can reveal a bitter taste which can promote gagging or vomiting. The interval between the individual doses should not be less than 4 and not more than 6 hours.

HOW SUPPLIED

Biltricide is supplied as a 600 mg white to orange tinged, filmcoated, oblong tablets with 3 scores. The tablet is coded with "BAYER" on one side and "LG" on the reverse side. When broken each of the 4 segments contain 150 mg of active ingrediant so that the dosage can be easily adjusted to the patient's bodyweight.

Segments are broken off by pressing the score (notch) with thumbnails. If ¼ of a tablet is required, this is best achieved by breaking the segment from the outer end.

Storage: Store below 30°C (86°F).

PRODUCT LISTING - EQUIVALENTS NOT AVAILABLE

Tablet - Oral - 600 mg

6's	$71.41	BILTRICIDE, Bayer	00026-2521-06

Prazosin Hydrochloride (002100)

Categories: Hypertension, essential; Pregnancy Category C; FDA Approved 1976 Jun; WHO Formulary
Drug Classes: Antiadrenergics, alpha blocking; Antiadrenergics, peripheral
Brand Names: Minipress
Foreign Brand Availability: Atodel (Malaysia; Philippines); Decliten (Argentina); Duramipress (Germany); Eurex (Germany); Hexapress (Denmark); Hypotens (Israel); Hypovase (England; Ireland); Hyprosin (New-Zealand; Taiwan); Lopress (Thailand); Minipres (Argentina; Costa-Rica; Dominican-Republic; El-Salvador; Guatemala; Honduras; Mexico; Nicaragua; Panama; Spain); Minipres SR (Colombia); Minipress XL (India); Mizosin (Hong-Kong); Patsolin (Finland); Peripress (Denmark; Finland; Norway; Sweden); Polypress (Thailand); Prasig (Australia); Pratisol (Australia; New-Zealand; South-Africa; Taiwan); Pratsiol (Finland); Prazac (Denmark); Prazopress (India); Pressin (Australia)
Cost of Therapy: $65.17 (Hypertension; Minipress; 2 mg; 3 capsules/day; 30 day supply)
$8.39 (Hypertension; Generic Capsules; 2 mg; 3 capsules/day; 30 day supply)

DESCRIPTION

Prazosin hydrochloride, a quinazoline derivative, is the first of a new chemical class of antihypertensives. It is the hydrochloride salt of 1-(4-amino-6,7-dimethoxy-2-quinazolinyl)-4-(2-furoyl)piperazine.

It is a white, crystalline substance, slightly soluble in water and isotonic saline, and has a molecular weight of 419.87. Each 1 mg capsule of Minipress for oral use contains drug equivalent to 1 mg free base.

Inert ingredients in the formulations are: hard gelatin capsules (which may contain blue 1, red 3, red 28, red 40, and other inert ingredients); magnesium stearate; sodium lauryl sulfate; starch; sucrose.

CLINICAL PHARMACOLOGY

The exact mechanism of the hypotensive action of prazosin is unknown. Prazosin causes a decrease in total peripheral resistance and was originally thought to have a direct relaxant action on vascular smooth muscle. Recent animal studies, however, have suggested that the vasodilator effect of prazosin is also related to blockade of postsynaptic *alpha*-adrenoceptors. The results of dog forelimb experiments demonstrate that the peripheral vasodilator effect of prazosin is confined mainly to the level of the resistance vessels (arterioles). Unlike conventional *alpha*-blockers, the antihypertensive action of prazosin is usually not accompanied by a reflex tachycardia. Tolerance has not been observed to develop in long term therapy.

Hemodynamic studies have been carried out in man following acute single dose administration and during the course of long term maintenance therapy. The results confirm that the therapeutic effect is a fall in blood pressure unaccompanied by a clinically significant change in cardiac output, heart rate, renal blood flow and glomerular filtration rate. There is no measurable negative chronotropic effect.

In clinical studies to date, prazosin HCl has not increased plasma renin activity.

In man, blood pressure is lowered in both the supine and standing positions. This effect is most pronounced on the diastolic blood pressure.

Following oral administration, human plasma concentrations reach a peak at about 3 hours with a plasma half-life of 2-3 hours. The drug is highly bound to plasma protein. Bioavailability studies have demonstrated that the total absorption relative to the drug in a 20% alcoholic solution is 90%, resulting in peak levels approximately 65% of that of the drug in solution. Animal studies indicate that prazosin HCl is extensively metabolized, primarily by demethylation and conjugation, and excreted mainly via bile and feces. Less extensive human studies suggest similar metabolism and excretion in man.

In clinical studies in which lipid profiles were followed, there were generally no adverse changes noted between pre- and post-treatment lipid levels.

INDICATIONS AND USAGE

Prazosin HCl is indicated in the treatment of hypertension. It can be used alone or in combination with other antihypertensive drugs such as diuretics or beta-adrenergic blocking agents.

NON-FDA APPROVED INDICATIONS

Prazosin has been used without FDA approval for the treatment of congestive heart failure, Raynaud's vasospasm, and prostatic outflow obstruction. Preliminary studies suggest that it may have beneficial effects on sleep and reducing nightmares in patients with posttraumatic stress disorder. Alone and in combination with terlipressin, prazosin has been studied in the treatment of portal hypertension.

CONTRAINDICATIONS

Prazosin HCl is contraindicated in patients with known sensitivity to quinazolines, prazosin or any of the inert ingredients.

WARNINGS

As with all alpha-blockers, prazosin HCl may cause syncope with sudden loss of consciousness. In most cases this is believed to be due to an excessive postural hypotensive effect, although occasionally the syncopal episode has been preceded by a bout of severe tachycardia with heart rates of 120-160 beats per minute. Syncopal episodes have usually occurred within 30-90 minutes of the initial dose of the drug; occasionally they have been reported in association with rapid dosage increases or the introduction of another antihypertensive drug into the regimen of a patient taking high doses of prazosin HCl. The incidence of syncopal episodes is approximately 1% in patients given an initial dose of 2 mg or greater. Clinical trials conducted during the investigational phase of this drug suggest that syncopal episodes can be minimized by limiting the initial dose of the drug to 1 mg, by subsequently increasing the dosage slowly, and by introducing any additional antihypertensive drugs into the patient's regimen with caution (see DOSAGE AND ADMINISTRATION). Hypotension may develop in patients given prazosin HCl who are also receiving a beta-blocker such as propranolol.

If syncope occurs, the patient should be placed in the recumbent position and treated supportively as necessary. This adverse effect is self-limiting and in most cases does not recur after the initial period of therapy or during subsequent dose titration.

Patients should always be started on the 1 mg capsules of prazosin HCl. The 2 and 5 mg capsules are not indicated for initial therapy.

More common than loss of consciousness are the symptoms often associated with lowering of the blood pressure, namely, dizziness and lightheadedness. The patient should be cautioned about these possible adverse effects and advised what measures to take should they develop. The patient should also be cautioned to avoid situations where injury could result should syncope occur during the initiation of prazosin HCl therapy.

PRECAUTIONS

INFORMATION FOR THE PATIENT

Dizziness or drowsiness may occur after the first dose of this medicine. Avoid driving or performing hazardous tasks for the first 24 hours after taking this medicine or when the dose is increased. Dizziness, lightheadedness or fainting may occur, especially when rising from a lying or sitting position. Getting up slowly may help lessen the problem. These effects may also occur if you drink alcohol, stand for long periods of time, exercise, or if the weather is hot. While taking prazosin HCl, be careful in the amount of alcohol you drink. Also, use extra care during exercise or hot weather, or if standing for long periods. Check with your physician if you have any questions.

DRUG/LABORATORY TEST INTERACTIONS

In a study on 5 patients given from 12-24 mg of prazosin per day for 10-14 days, there was an average increase of 42% in the urinary metabolite of norepinephrine and an average increase in urinary VMA of 17%. Therefore, false positive results may occur in screening tests for pheochromocytoma in patients who are being treated with prazosin. If an elevated VMA is found, prazosin should be discontinued and the patient retested after a month.

LABORATORY TESTS

In clinical studies in which lipid profiles were followed, there were generally no adverse changes noted between pre- and post-treatment lipid levels.

CARCINOGENESIS, MUTAGENESIS, AND IMPAIRMENT OF FERTILITY

No carcinogenic potential was demonstrated in an 18 month study in rats with prazosin HCl at dose levels more than 225 times the usual maximum recommended human dose of 20 mg/day. Prazosin HCl was not mutagenic in *in vivo* genetic toxicology studies. In a fertility and general reproductive performance study in rats, both males and females, treated with 75 mg/kg (225 times the usual maximum recommended human dose), demonstrated decreased fertility while those treated with 25 mg/kg (75 times the usual maximum recommended human dose) did not.

In chronic studies (1 year or more) of prazosin HCl in rats and dogs, testicular changes consisting of atrophy and necrosis occurred at 25 mg/kg/day (75 times the usual maximum recommended human dose). No testicular changes were seen in rats or dogs at 10 mg/kg/day (30 times the usual maximum recommended human dose). In view of the testicular changes observed in animals, 105 patients on long term prazosin HCl therapy were monitored for 17-ketosteroid excretion and no changes indicating a drug effect were observed. In addition, 27 males on prazosin HCl for up to 51 months did not have changes in sperm morphology suggestive of drug effect.

PREGNANCY CATEGORY C

Prazosin HCl has been shown to be associated with decreased litter size at birth, 1, 4, and 21 days of age in rats when given doses more than 225 times the usual maximum recommended human dose. No evidence of drug-related external, visceral, or skeletal fetal abnormalities were observed. No drug-related external, visceral, or skeletal abnormalities were observed in fetuses of pregnant rabbits and pregnant monkeys at doses more than 225 times and 12 times the usual maximum recommended human dose respectively.

The use of prazosin and a beta-blocker for the control of severe hypertension in 44 pregnant women revealed no drug-related fetal abnormalities or adverse effects. Therapy with prazosin was continued for as long as 14 weeks.[1]

Prazosin has also been used alone or in combination with other hypotensive agents in severe hypertension of pregnancy by other investigators. No fetal or neonatal abnormalities have been reported with the use of prazosin.[2]

There are no adequate and well controlled studies which establish the safety of prazosin HCl in pregnant women. Prazosin HCl should be used during pregnancy only if the potential benefit justifies the potential risk to the mother and fetus.

P

NURSING MOTHERS

Prazosin HCl has been shown to be excreted in small amounts in human milk. Caution should be exercised when prazosin HCl is administered to a nursing woman.

USAGE IN CHILDREN

Safety and effectiveness in children have not been established.

DRUG INTERACTIONS

Prazosin HCl has been administered without any adverse drug interaction in limited clinical experience to date with the following:

Cardiac Glycosides: Digitalis and digoxin;
Hypoglycemics: Insulin, chlorpropamide, phenformin, tolazamide, and tolbutamide;
Tranquilizers and Sedatives: Chlordiazepoxide, diazepam, and phenobarbital;
Antigout: Allopurinol, colchicine, and probenecid;
Antiarrhythmics: Procainamide, propranolol (see WARNINGS however), and quinidine; and
Analgesics, Antipyretics and Anti-Inflammatories: Propoxyphene, aspirin, indomethacin, and phenylbutazone.

Addition of a diuretic or other antihypertensive agent to prazosin HCl has been shown to cause an additive hypotensive effect. This effect can be minimized by reducing the prazosin HCl dose to 1-2 mg three times a day, by introducing additional antihypertensive drugs cautiously and then by retitrating prazosin HCl based on clinical response.

ADVERSE REACTIONS

Clinical trials were conducted on more than 900 patients. During these trials and subsequent marketing experience, the most frequent reactions associated with prazosin HCl therapy are: dizziness 10.3%, headache 7.8%, drowsiness 7.6%, lack of energy 6.9%, weakness 6.5%, palpitations 5.3%, and nausea 4.9%. In most instances side effects have disappeared with continued therapy or have been tolerated with no decrease in dose of drug.

Less frequent adverse reactions which are reported to occur in 1-4% of patients are:

Gastrointestinal: Vomiting, diarrhea, constipation.
Cardiovascular: Edema, orthostatic hypotension, dyspnea, syncope.
Central Nervous System: Vertigo, depression, nervousness.
Dermatologic: Rash.
Genitourinary: Urinary frequency.
EENT: Blurred vision, reddened sclera, epistaxis, dry mouth, nasal congestion.

In addition, fewer than 1% of patients have reported the following (in some instances, exact causal relationships have not been established):

Gastrointestinal: Abdominal discomfort and/or pain, liver function abnormalities, pancreatitis.
Cardiovascular: Tachycardia.
Central Nervous System: Paresthesia, hallucinations.
Dermatologic: Pruritus, alopecia, lichen planus.
Genitourinary: Incontinence, impotence, priapism.
EENT: Tinnitus.
Other: Diaphoresis, fever, positive ANA titer, arthralgia.

Single reports of pigmentary mottling and serous retinopathy, and few reports of cataract development or disappearance have been reported. In these instances, the exact causal relationship has not been established because the baseline observations were frequently inadequate.

In more specific slit-lamp and funduscopic studies, which included adequate baseline examinations, no drug-related abnormal ophthalmological findings have been reported.

Literature reports exist associating prazosin HCl therapy with a worsening of pre-existing narcolepsy. A causal relationship is uncertain in these cases.

In post-marketing experience, the following adverse events have been reported:

Autonomic Nervous System: Flushing.
Body as a Whole: Allergic reaction, asthenia, malaise, pain.
Cardiovascular, General: Angina pectoris, hypertension.
Endocrine: Gynecomastia.
Heart Rate/Rhythm: Bradycardia.
Psychiatric: Insomnia.
Skin/Appendages: Urticaria.
Vascular (Extracardiac): Vasculitis.
Vision: Eye pain.

DOSAGE AND ADMINISTRATION

The dose of prazosin HCl should be adjusted according to the patient's individual blood pressure response. The following is a guide to its administration:

INITIAL DOSE

1 mg two or three times a day. (See WARNINGS.)

MAINTENANCE DOSE

Dosage may be slowly increased to a total daily dose of 20 mg given in divided doses. The therapeutic dosages most commonly employed have ranged from 6-15 mg daily given in divided doses. Doses higher than 20 mg usually do not increase efficacy, however a few patients may benefit from further increases up to a daily dose of 40 mg given in divided doses. After initial titration some patients can be maintained adequately on a twice daily dosage regimen.

USE WITH OTHER DRUGS

When adding a diuretic or other antihypertensive agent, the dose of prazosin HCl should be reduced to 1 or 2 mg three times a day and retitration then carried out.

HOW SUPPLIED

Minipress is available in 1, 2, and 5 mg sizes:
1 mg: White capsules coded "431".
2 mg: Pink and white capsules coded "437".
5 mg: Blue and white capsules coded "438".

PRODUCT LISTING - RATED THERAPEUTICALLY EQUIVALENT

Capsule - Oral - 1 mg

20's	$5.43	GENERIC, Allscripts Pharmaceutical Company	54569-2582-03
30's	$8.15	GENERIC, Allscripts Pharmaceutical Company	54569-2582-01
30's	$13.04	GENERIC, Heartland Healthcare Services	61392-0115-30
30's	$13.04	GENERIC, Heartland Healthcare Services	61392-0115-39
30's	$17.43	MINIPRESS, Physicians Total Care	54868-0704-01
31's	$13.47	GENERIC, Heartland Healthcare Services	61392-0115-31
32's	$13.90	GENERIC, Heartland Healthcare Services	61392-0115-32
45's	$19.55	GENERIC, Heartland Healthcare Services	61392-0115-45
60's	$9.65	GENERIC, Pd-Rx Pharmaceuticals	55289-0536-60
60's	$22.40	GENERIC, Major Pharmaceuticals Inc	00904-1040-52
60's	$24.11	GENERIC, Allscripts Pharmaceutical Company	54569-7103-00
60's	$26.07	GENERIC, Heartland Healthcare Services	61392-0115-60
90's	$39.11	GENERIC, Heartland Healthcare Services	61392-0115-90
100's	$8.84	GENERIC, Pd-Rx Pharmaceuticals	55289-0536-01
100's	$10.04	GENERIC, Us Trading Corporation	56126-0463-11
100's	$24.11	GENERIC, Geneva Pharmaceuticals	00781-2211-01
100's	$24.15	GENERIC, Watson/Schein Pharmaceuticals Inc	00364-2389-01
100's	$24.80	GENERIC, Aligen Independent Laboratories Inc	00405-4816-01
100's	$24.89	GENERIC, Allscripts Pharmaceutical Company	54569-7103-01
100's	$26.00	GENERIC, Qualitest Products Inc	00603-5286-21
100's	$26.07	GENERIC, Watson/Schein Pharmaceuticals Inc	00364-2389-90
100's	$26.85	GENERIC, Martec Pharmaceuticals Inc	52555-0279-01
100's	$28.15	GENERIC, Esi Lederle Generics	00005-3473-43
100's	$28.75	GENERIC, Allscripts Pharmaceutical Company	54569-2582-00
100's	$29.36	GENERIC, Udl Laboratories Inc	51079-0630-20
100's	$31.25	GENERIC, Moore, H.L. Drug Exchange Inc	00839-7554-06
100's	$32.00	GENERIC, Mylan Pharmaceuticals Inc	00378-1101-01
100's	$37.60	GENERIC, Auro Pharmaceutical	55829-0677-10
100's	$39.60	GENERIC, Ivax Corporation	00172-4067-60
100's	$48.04	MINIPRESS, Southwood Pharmaceuticals Inc	58016-0549-00
250's	$47.55	GENERIC, Mova Pharmaceutical Corporation	55370-0817-25
250's	$52.92	GENERIC, Moore, H.L. Drug Exchange Inc	00839-7554-09
250's	$57.40	GENERIC, Geneva Pharmaceuticals	00781-2211-25
250's	$59.70	GENERIC, Major Pharmaceuticals Inc	00904-1040-70
250's	$59.70	GENERIC, Major Pharmaceuticals Inc	00904-5095-70
250's	$63.01	GENERIC, Qualitest Products Inc	00603-5286-24
250's	$63.20	GENERIC, Aligen Independent Laboratories Inc	00405-4816-04
250's	$99.00	GENERIC, Ivax Corporation	00172-4067-65
250's	$132.06	MINIPRESS, Pfizer U.S. Pharmaceuticals	00069-4310-71

Capsule - Oral - 2 mg

30's	$15.98	GENERIC, Heartland Healthcare Services	61392-0118-30
30's	$15.98	GENERIC, Heartland Healthcare Services	61392-0118-39
31's	$16.51	GENERIC, Heartland Healthcare Services	61392-0118-31
32's	$17.04	GENERIC, Heartland Healthcare Services	61392-0118-32
45's	$23.96	GENERIC, Heartland Healthcare Services	61392-0118-45
60's	$31.20	GENERIC, Major Pharmaceuticals Inc	00904-1041-52
60's	$31.95	GENERIC, Heartland Healthcare Services	61392-0118-60
90's	$47.93	GENERIC, Heartland Healthcare Services	61392-0118-90
100's	$9.32	GENERIC, Physicians Total Care	54868-1547-01
100's	$12.92	GENERIC, Us Trading Corporation	56126-0464-11
100's	$29.96	GENERIC, Moore, H.L. Drug Exchange Inc	00839-7555-06
100's	$32.80	GENERIC, Aligen Independent Laboratories Inc	00405-4817-01
100's	$33.58	GENERIC, Geneva Pharmaceuticals	00781-2212-01
100's	$34.40	GENERIC, Qualitest Products Inc	00603-5287-21
100's	$34.98	GENERIC, Martec Pharmaceuticals Inc	52555-0280-01
100's	$38.17	GENERIC, Esi Lederle Generics	00005-3474-43
100's	$38.21	GENERIC, Udl Laboratories Inc	51079-0631-20
100's	$40.13	GENERIC, Auro Pharmaceutical	55829-0678-10
100's	$47.25	GENERIC, Mylan Pharmaceuticals Inc	00378-2302-01
100's	$55.15	GENERIC, Ivax Corporation	00172-4068-60
100's	$72.41	MINIPRESS, Physicians Total Care	54868-1290-01
120's	$63.90	GENERIC, Heartland Healthcare Services	61392-0118-34
250's	$49.88	GENERIC, Moore, H.L. Drug Exchange Inc	00839-7555-09
250's	$65.97	GENERIC, Mova Pharmaceutical Corporation	55370-0818-25
250's	$77.96	GENERIC, Esi Lederle Generics	00005-3474-27
250's	$78.03	GENERIC, Aligen Independent Laboratories Inc	00405-4817-04
250's	$83.15	GENERIC, Major Pharmaceuticals Inc	00904-1041-70
250's	$83.15	GENERIC, Major Pharmaceuticals Inc	00904-5096-70
250's	$83.60	GENERIC, Qualitest Products Inc	00603-5287-24

250's	$83.65	GENERIC, Geneva Pharmaceuticals	00781-2212-25
250's	$85.35	GENERIC, Martec Pharmaceuticals Inc	52555-0280-02
250's	$137.85	GENERIC, Ivax Corporation	00172-4068-65
250's	$183.84	MINIPRESS, Pfizer U.S. Pharmaceuticals	00069-4370-71
Capsule - Oral - 5 mg			
30's	$23.84	GENERIC, Heartland Healthcare Services	61392-0112-30
30's	$23.84	GENERIC, Heartland Healthcare Services	61392-0112-39
31's	$24.64	GENERIC, Heartland Healthcare Services	61392-0112-31
32's	$25.43	GENERIC, Heartland Healthcare Services	61392-0112-32
45's	$35.76	GENERIC, Heartland Healthcare Services	61392-0112-45
60's	$40.75	GENERIC, Major Pharmaceuticals Inc	00904-1042-52
60's	$47.68	GENERIC, Heartland Healthcare Services	61392-0112-60
90's	$71.52	GENERIC, Heartland Healthcare Services	61392-0112-90
100's	$17.69	GENERIC, Us Trading Corporation	56126-0465-11
100's	$45.35	GENERIC, Moore, H.L. Drug Exchange Inc	00839-7556-06
100's	$52.19	GENERIC, Aligen Independent Laboratories Inc	00405-4818-01
100's	$57.60	GENERIC, Qualitest Products Inc	00603-5288-21
100's	$57.85	GENERIC, Geneva Pharmaceuticals	00781-2213-01
100's	$60.00	GENERIC, Martec Pharmaceuticals Inc	52555-0281-01
100's	$65.41	GENERIC, Udl Laboratories Inc	51079-0632-20
100's	$78.00	GENERIC, Mylan Pharmaceuticals Inc	00378-3205-01
100's	$87.00	GENERIC, Watson/Schein Pharmaceuticals Inc	00364-2391-90
100's	$93.98	GENERIC, Ivax Corporation	00172-4069-60
250's	$90.45	GENERIC, Moore, H.L. Drug Exchange Inc	00839-7556-09
250's	$124.28	GENERIC, Mova Pharmaceutical Corporation	55370-0819-25
250's	$133.72	GENERIC, Aligen Independent Laboratories Inc	00405-4818-04
250's	$141.60	GENERIC, Geneva Pharmaceuticals	00781-2213-25
250's	$141.70	GENERIC, Qualitest Products Inc	00603-5288-24
250's	$141.70	GENERIC, Major Pharmaceuticals Inc	00904-1042-70
250's	$141.70	GENERIC, Major Pharmaceuticals Inc	00904-5097-70
250's	$195.00	GENERIC, Mylan Pharmaceuticals Inc	00378-3205-25
250's	$234.95	GENERIC, Ivax Corporation	00172-4069-65
250's	$313.39	MINIPRESS, Pfizer U.S. Pharmaceuticals	00069-4380-71

PRODUCT LISTING - EQUIVALENTS NOT AVAILABLE

Capsule - Oral - 1 mg			
30's	$14.40	GENERIC, Southwood Pharmaceuticals Inc	58016-0398-30
60's	$5.48	GENERIC, Physicians Total Care	54868-0705-00
60's	$28.80	GENERIC, Southwood Pharmaceuticals Inc	58016-0398-60
90's	$43.20	GENERIC, Southwood Pharmaceuticals Inc	58016-0398-90
100's	$8.25	GENERIC, Physicians Total Care	54868-0705-01
100's	$48.00	GENERIC, Southwood Pharmaceuticals Inc	58016-0398-00
Capsule - Oral - 2 mg			
30's	$12.32	GENERIC, Allscripts Pharmaceutical Company	54569-2583-01
100's	$49.43	GENERIC, Allscripts Pharmaceutical Company	54569-2583-00
Capsule - Oral - 5 mg			
100's	$15.77	GENERIC, Physicians Total Care	54868-2004-01
100's	$72.16	GENERIC, Allscripts Pharmaceutical Company	54569-2584-00

Prednicarbate (003070)

Categories: Dermatosis, corticosteroid-responsive; FDA Approved 1991 Sep; Pregnancy Category C
Drug Classes: Corticosteroids, topical; Dermatologics
Brand Names: Dermatop
Foreign Brand Availability: Pretop (Korea); Titibe (Korea)

DESCRIPTION

FOR DERMATOLOGIC USE ONLY.
NOT FOR USE IN EYES.

PREDNICARBATE EMOLLIENT CREAM 0.1%

Dermatop E Emollient Cream (prednicarbate emollient cream) 0.1% contains prednicarbate, a synthetic corticosteroid for topical dermatologic use. The chemical name of prednicarbate is 11β,17,21-trihydroxypregna-1,4-diene-3,20-dione17-(ethyl carbonate)21-propionate. Prednicarbate has the empirical formula $C_{27}H_{36}O_8$ and a molecular weight of 488.58. Topical corticosteroids constitute a class of primarily synthetic steroids used topically as anti-inflammatory and antipruritic agents.

Prednicarbate is a practically odorless white to yellow-white powder insoluble to practically insoluble in water and freely soluble in ethanol.

Each gram of Dermatop E Emollient Cream 0.1% contains 1.0 mg of prednicarbate in a base consisting of white petrolatum, purified water, isopropyl myristate, lanolin alcohols, mineral oil, cetostearyl alcohol, aluminum stearate, edetate disodium, lactic acid, and magnesium stearate DAB 9.

PREDNICARBATE EMOLLIENT OINTMENT 0.1%

Dermatop E Emollient Ointment (prednicarbate ointment) 0.1% contains the non-halogenated prednisolone derivative prednicarbate. The topical corticosteroids constitute a class of primarily synthetic steroids used topically as anti-inflammatory and anti-pruritic agents.

Each gram of Dermatop E Emollient Ointment 0.1% contains 0.1 mg of prednicarbate in a base consisting of white petrolatum, octyldodecanol, glycerol mono-, di- and trioleate, glycerin, oleic acid, propylene glycol, butylated hydroxyanisole, and citric acid.

Prednicarbate has the empirical formula $C_{27}H_{36}O_8$ and a molecular weight of 488.58.

CLINICAL PHARMACOLOGY

In common with other topical corticosteroids, prednicarbate has anti-inflammatory, antipruritic, and vasoconstrictive properties. In general, the mechanism of the anti-inflammatory activity of topical steroids is unclear. However, corticosteroids are thought to act by the induction of phospholipase A_2 inhibitory proteins, collectively called lipocortins. It is postulated that these proteins control the biosynthesis of potent mediators of inflammation such as prostaglandins and leukotrienes by inhibiting the release of their common precursor arachidonic acid. Arachidonic acid is released from membrane phospholipids by phospholipase A_2.

PHARMACOKINETICS

The extent of percutaneous absorption of topical corticosteroids is determined by many factors, including the vehicle and the integrity of the epidermal barrier. Use of occlusive dressings with hydrocortisone for up to 24 hours has not been shown to increase penetration; however, occlusion of hydrocortisone for 96 hours does markedly enhance penetration. Topical corticosteroids can be absorbed from normal intact skin. Inflammation and/or other disease processes in the skin increase percutaneous absorption.

Studies performed with prednicarbate emollient cream and ointment 0.1% indicate that the drug product is in the medium range of potency compared with other topical corticosteroids.

INDICATIONS AND USAGE

PREDNICARBATE EMOLLIENT CREAM 0.1%

Prednicarbate emollient cream 0.1% is a medium-potency corticosteroid indicated for the relief of the inflammatory and pruritic manifestations of corticosteroid-responsive dermatoses. Prednicarbate emollient cream 0.1% may be used with caution in pediatric patients 1 year of age or older. The safety and efficacy of drug use for longer than 3 weeks in this population have not been established. Since safety and efficacy of prednicarbate emollient cream 0.1% have not been established in pediatric patients below 1 year of age, its use in this age group is not recommended.

PREDNICARBATE EMOLLIENT OINTMENT 0.1%

Prednicarbate emollient ointment 0.1% is a medium-potency corticosteroid indicated for the relief of the inflammatory and pruritic manifestations of corticosteroid responsive dermatoses.

CONTRAINDICATIONS

Prednicarbate emollient cream and ointment 0.1% are contraindicated in those patients with a history of hypersensitivity to any of the components in the preparations.

PRECAUTIONS

GENERAL

Systemic absorption of topical corticosteroids can produce reversible hypothalamic-pituitary-adrenal (HPA) axis suppression with the potential for glucocorticosteroid insufficiency after withdrawal of treatment. Manifestations of Cushing's syndrome, hyperglycemia, and glucosuria can also be produced in some patients by systemic absorption of topical corticosteroids while on treatment. Patients applying a topical steroid to a large surface area or under occlusion should be evaluated periodically for evidence of HPA-axis suppression. This may be done by using the ACTH stimulation, AM plasma cortisol, and urinary free cortisol tests.

Prednicarbate emollient cream and ointment 0.1% did not produce significant HPA-axis suppression when used at a dose of 30 g/day and 60 g/day, respectively, for a week in patients with extensive psoriasis or atopic dermatitis.

Prednicarbate emollient cream 0.1% did not produce HPA-axis suppression in any of 59 pediatric patients with extensive atopic dermatitis when applied bid for 3 weeks to >20% of the body surface. (See PRECAUTIONS, Pediatric Use.)

If HPA-axis suppression is noted, an attempt should be made to withdraw the drug, to reduce the frequency of application, or to substitute a less potent corticosteroid. Recovery of HPA-axis function is generally prompt and complete upon discontinuation of topical corticosteroids. Infrequently, signs and symptoms of glucocorticosteroid insufficiency may occur requiring supplemental systemic corticosteroids. For information on systemic supplementation, see prescribing information for those products.

Pediatric patients may be more susceptible to systemic toxicity from equivalent doses due to their larger skin surface to body mass ratios. (See PRECAUTIONS, Pediatric Use.)

If irritation develops, prednicarbate emollient cream and ointment 0.1% should be discontinued and appropriate therapy instituted. Allergic contact dermatitis with corticosteroids is usually diagnosed by observing a failure to heal rather than noting a clinical exacerbation, as observed with most topical products not containing corticosteroids. Such an observation should be corroborated with appropriate diagnostic patch testing.

If concomitant skin infections are present or develop, an appropriate antifungal or antibacterial agent should be used.

If a favorable response does not occur promptly, use of prednicarbate emollient cream and ointment 0.1% should be discontinued until the infection has been adequately controlled.

INFORMATION FOR THE PATIENT

Patients using topical corticosteroids should receive the following information and instructions:

- This medication is to be used as directed by the physician. It is for external use only. Avoid contact with the eyes.
- This medication should not be used for any disorder other than that for which it was prescribed.

P

- The treated skin area should not be bandaged, otherwise covered or wrapped so as to be occlusive, unless directed by the physician.
- Patients should report to their physician any signs of local adverse reactions.
- Parents of pediatric patients should be advised not to use this medication in the treatment of diaper dermatitis. This medication should not be applied in the diaper area as diapers or plastic pants may constitute occlusive dressing (see DOSAGE AND ADMINISTRATION).
- This medication should not be used on the face, underarms, or groin areas.

As with other corticosteroids, therapy should be discontinued when control is achieved. If no improvement is seen within 2 weeks, contact the physician.

LABORATORY TESTS

The following tests may be helpful in evaluating patients for HPA-axis suppression:

ACTH stimulation test
AM plasma cortisol test
Urinary free cortisol test

CARCINOGENESIS, MUTAGENESIS, AND IMPAIRMENT OF FERTILITY

In a study of the effect of prednicarbate on fertility, pregnancy, and postnatal development in rats, no effect was noted on the fertility or pregnancy of the parent animals or postnatal development of the offspring after administration of up to 0.80 mg/kg of prednicarbate subcutaneously.

Prednicarbate has been evaluated in the *Salmonella* reversion test (Ames test) over a wide range of concentrations in the presence and absence of an S-9 liver microsomal fraction, and did not demonstrate mutagenic activity. Similarly, prednicarbate did not produce any significant changes in the numbers of micronuclei seen in erythrocytes when mice were given doses ranging from 1-160 mg/kg of the drug.

PREGNANCY, TERATOGENIC EFFECTS, PREGNANCY CATEGORY C

Corticosteroids have been shown to be teratogenic in laboratory animals when administered systemically at relatively low dosage levels. Some corticosteroids have been shown to be teratogenic after dermal application in laboratory animals.

Prednicarbate has been shown to be teratogenic and embryotoxic in Wistar rats and Himalayan rabbits when given subcutaneously during gestation at doses 1900 times and 45 times the recommended topical human dose, assuming a percutaneous absorption of approximately 3%. In the rats, slightly retarded fetal development and an incidence of thickened and wavy ribs higher than the spontaneous rate were noted.

In rabbits, increased liver weights and slight increase in the fetal intrauterine death rate were observed. The fetuses that were delivered exhibited reduced placental weight, increased frequency of cleft palate, ossification disorders in the sternum, omphalocele, and anomalous posture of the forelimbs.

There are no adequate and well-controlled studies in pregnant women on teratogenic effects of prednicarbate. Prednicarbate emollient cream and ointment 0.1% should be used during pregnancy only if the potential benefit justifies the potential risk to the fetus.

NURSING MOTHERS

Systemically administered corticosteroids appear in human milk and could suppress growth, interfere with endogenous corticosteroid production, or cause other untoward effects. It is not known whether topical administration of corticosteroids could result in sufficient systemic absorption to produce detectable quantities in human milk. Because many drugs are excreted in human milk, caution should be exercised when prednicarbate emollient cream or ointment 0.1% is administered to a nursing woman.

P

PEDIATRIC USE

Prednicarbate Emollient Cream 0.1%

Prednicarbate emollient cream 0.1% may be used with caution in pediatric patients 1 year of age or older, although the safety and efficacy of drug use longer than 3 weeks have not been established. The use of prednicarbate emollient cream 0.1% is supported by results of a 3 week, uncontrolled study in 59 pediatric patients between the ages of 4 months and 12 years of age with atopic dermatitis. None of the 59 pediatric patients showed evidence of HPA-axis suppression. Safety and efficacy of prednicarbate emollient cream 0.1% in pediatric patients below 1 year of age have not been established, therefore use in this age group is not recommended. Because of a higher ratio of skin surface area to body mass, pediatric patients are at a greater risk than adults of HPA-axis suppression and Cushing's syndrome when they are treated with topical corticosteroids. They are therefore also at greater risk of adrenal insufficiency during and/or after withdrawal of treatment. In an uncontrolled study in pediatric patients with atopic dermatitis, the incidence of adverse reactions possibly or probably associated with the use of prednicarbate emollient cream 0.1% was limited.

Mild signs of atrophy developed in 5 patients (5/59, 8%) during the clinical trial, with 2 patients exhibiting more than 1 sign. Two patients (2/59, 3%) developed shininess, and 2 patients (2/59, 3%) developed thinness. Three patients (3/59, 5%) were observed with mild telangectasia. It is unknown whether prior use of topical corticosteroids was a contributing factor in the development of telangectasia in 2 of the patients. Adverse effects including striae have also been reported with inappropriate use of topical corticosteroids in infants and children. Pediatric patients applying topical corticosteroids to greater than 20% of body surface are at higher risk for HPA-axis suppression.

HPA-axis suppression, Cushing's syndrome, linear growth retardation, delayed weight gain and intracranial hypertension have been reported in children receiving topical corticosteroids. Manifestations of adrenal suppression in children include low plasma cortisol levels, and absence of response to ACTH stimulation. Manifestations of intracranial hypertension include bulging fontanelles, headaches, and bilateral papilledema.

Prednicarbate emollient cream 0.1% should not be used in the treatment of diaper dermatitis.

Prednicarbate Emollient Ointment 0.1%

Safety and effectiveness of prednicarbate emollient ointment 0.1% in pediatric patients below the age of 10 years have not been established. Because of a higher ratio of skin surface area to body mass, pediatric patients are at a greater risk than adults of HPA-axis suppression when they are treated with topical corticosteroids. They are therefore also at greater risk of glucocorticosteroid insufficiency after withdrawal of treatment and of Cushing's syndrome while on treatment.

Adverse effects including striae have been reported with inappropriate use of topical corticosteroids in pediatric patients. (See PRECAUTIONS.)

HPA-axis suppression, Cushing's syndrome, and intracranial hypertension have been reported in pediatric patients receiving topical corticosteroids. Manifestations of adrenal suppression in pediatric patients include linear growth retardation, delayed weight gain, low plasma cortisol levels, and absence of response to ACTH stimulation. Manifestations of intracranial hypertension include bulging fontanelles, headaches, and bilateral papilledema.

ADVERSE REACTIONS

PREDNICARBATE EMOLLIENT CREAM 0.1%

In controlled adult clinical studies, the incidence of adverse reactions probably or possibly associated with the use of prednicarbate emollient cream 0.1% was approximately 4%. Reported reactions included mild signs of skin atrophy in 1% of treated patients, as well as the following reactions which were reported in less than 1% of patients: pruritus, edema, paresthesia, urticaria, burning, allergic contact dermatitis and rash.

In an uncontrolled study in pediatric patients with atopic dermatitis, the incidence of adverse reactions possibly or probably associated with the use of prednicarbate emollient cream 0.1% was limited. Mild signs of atrophy developed in 5 patients (5/59, 8%) during the clinical trial, with 2 patients exhibiting more than 1 sign. Two patients (2/59, 3%) developed shininess, and 2 patients (2/59, 3%) developed thinness. Three patients (3/59, 5%) were observed with mild telangectasia. It is unknown whether prior use of topical corticosteroids was a contributing factor in the development of telangectasia in 2 of the patients. (See PRECAUTIONS, Pediatric Use.)

The following additional local adverse reactions have been reported infrequently with topical corticosteroids, but may occur more frequently with the use of occlusive dressings. These reactions are listed in an approximate decreasing order of occurrence: folliculitis, acneiform eruptions, hypopigmentation, perioral dermatitis, secondary infection, striae and miliaria.

PREDNICARBATE EMOLLIENT OINTMENT 0.1%

In controlled clinical studies, the incidence of adverse reactions associated with the use of prednicarbate emollient ointment 0.1% was approximately 1.5%. Reported reactions including burning, pruritus, drying, scaling, cracking and pain and irritant dermatitis.

The following additional local adverse reactions are reported infrequently with topical corticosteroids, but may occur more frequently with the use of occlusive dressings and especially with higher potency corticosteroids. These reactions are listed in an approximate decreasing order of occurrence: folliculitis, hypertrichosis, acneiform eruptions, hypopigmentation, perioral dermatitis, allergic contact dermatitis, secondary infection, skin atrophy, striae and miliaria.

DOSAGE AND ADMINISTRATION

Apply a thin film of prednicarbate emollient cream or ointment 0.1% to the affected skin areas twice daily. Rub in gently.

Prednicarbate emollient cream 0.1% may be used in pediatric patients 1 year of age or older. Safety and efficacy of prednicarbate emollient cream 0.1% in pediatric patients for more than 3 weeks of use have not been established. Use in pediatric patients under 1 year of age is not recommended.

As with other corticosteroids, therapy should be discontinued when control is achieved. If no improvement is seen within 2 weeks, reassessment of the diagnosis may be necessary.

Prednicarbate emollient cream or ointment 0.1% should not be used with occlusive dressings unless directed by the physician. Prednicarbate emollient cream or ointment 0.1% should not be applied in the diaper area if the child still requires diapers or plastic pants as these garments may constitute occlusive dressing.

HOW SUPPLIED

DERMATOP E EMOLLIENT CREAM 0.1%

Dermatop E Emollient Cream (prednicarbate emollient cream) 0.1% is supplied in 15 and 60 g tubes.

Storage: Store between 5-25°C (41-77°F).

DERMATOP E EMOLLIENT OINTMENT 0.1%

Dermatop E Emollient Ointment (prednicarbate emollient ointment) 0.1% is supplied in 15 and 60 g tubes.

Storage: Store at controlled room temperature 15-30°C (59-86°F).

PRODUCT LISTING - EQUIVALENTS NOT AVAILABLE

Size	Price	Product, Manufacturer	NDC
Cream - Topical - 0.1%			
15 gm	$14.10	DERMATOP, Aventis Pharmaceuticals	00039-0088-15
15 gm	$21.65	DERMATOP, Janssen Pharmaceuticals	00062-0351-15
15 gm	$21.65	DERMATOP, Aventis Pharmaceuticals	00066-0507-15
60 gm	$34.80	DERMATOP, Aventis Pharmaceuticals	00039-0088-60
60 gm	$53.25	DERMATOP, Janssen Pharmaceuticals	00062-0351-60
60 gm	$53.25	DERMATOP, Aventis Pharmaceuticals	00066-0507-60
Ointment - Topical - 0.1%			
15 gm	$21.65	DERMATOP, Janssen Pharmaceuticals	00062-0352-15
15 gm	$21.65	DERMATOP, Aventis Pharmaceuticals	00066-0508-15
60 gm	$53.25	DERMATOP, Janssen Pharmaceuticals	00062-0352-60
60 gm	$53.25	DERMATOP, Aventis Pharmaceuticals	00066-0508-60

Prednisolone (002102)

For related information, see the comparative table section in Appendix A.

Categories: Adrenocortical insufficiency; Anemia, acquired hemolytic; Anemia, congenital hypoplastic; Ankylosing spondylitis; Arthritis, gouty; Arthritis, osteoarthritis; Arthritis, psoriatic; Arthritis, rheumatoid; Asthma; Berylliosis; Bursitis; Carditis, rheumatic; Chorioretinitis; Choroiditis; Colitis, ulcerative; Conjunctivitis, allergic; Crohn's disease; Dermatitis herpetiformis; Dermatitis, atopic; Dermatitis, contact; Dermatitis, exfoliative; Dermatitis, seborrheic; Dermatomyositis, systemic; Epicondylitis; Erythema multiforme; Erythroblastopenia; Herpes zoster ophthalmicus; Hypercalcemia, secondary to neoplasia; Hyperplasia, congenital adrenal; Hypersensitivity reactions; Iridocyclitis; Iritis; Keratitis, ophthalmic; Leukemia; Loffler's syndrome; Lupus erythematosus, systemic; Lymphoma; Meningitis, tuberculous; Mycosis fungoides; Neuritis, optic; Ophthalmia, sympathetic; Pemphigus; Pneumonitis, aspiration; Polymyositis; Proteinuria; Psoriasis; Purpura, idiopathic thrombocytopenic; Rhinitis, perennial allergic; Rhinitis, seasonal allergic; Sarcoidosis; Serum sickness; Stevens-Johnson syndrome; Synovitis, secondary to osteoarthritis; Tenosynovitis; Thrombocytopenia; Thyroiditis, nonsuppurative; Trichinosis; Tuberculosis, disseminated; Tuberculosis, fulminating; Ulcer, allergic corneal marginal; Uveitis; FDA Approved 1972 Sep; Pregnancy Category B; WHO Formulary
Drug Classes: Corticosteroids
Brand Names: Cortalone; Cotolone; **Delta-Cortef**; Prelone
Foreign Brand Availability: Capsoid (South-Africa); Dermosolon (Germany); Liquipred (France); Lygal Kopftinktur N (Germany); Preconin (Taiwan); Prednecort (Philippines); Prenilone (Thailand); Solupred (France); Ultracortenol (Colombia); Walesolone (Singapore)
Cost of Therapy: $0.80 (Asthma; Generic Tablets; 5 mg; 1 tablet/day; 30 day supply)
HCFA JCODE(S): J7510 5 mg ORAL

DESCRIPTION

Prednisolone syrup contains prednisolone which is a glucocorticoid. Glucocorticoids are adrenocortical steroids, both naturally occurring and synthetic, which are readily absorbed from the gastrointestinal tract. Prednisolone is a white to practically white, odorless crystalline powder. It is very slightly soluble in water, soluble in methanol and in dioxane, sparingly soluble in acetone and in alcohol, slightly soluble in chloroform.

The chemical name for prednisolone is 11β,17,21-trihydroxypregna-1,4-diene-3,20-dione (anhydrous). The molecular weight is 360.45. The molecular formula is $C_{21}H_{28}O_5$.

TABLETS

Each prednisolone tablet contains 5 mg of the anti-inflammatory adrenocortical steroid, prednisolone.

SYRUP

Each 5 ml (teaspoonful) contains 15 mg of prednisolone syrup. In addition, each 5 ml (teaspoonful) contains the following inactive ingredients: benzoic acid 0.1% added as a preservative. It also contains alcohol 5%, citric acid, edetate disodium, FD&C red no. 40, flavor wild cherry, glycerin, propylene glycol, purified water, sodium saccharin and sucrose.

CLINICAL PHARMACOLOGY

Naturally occurring glucocorticoids (hydrocortisone and cortisone), which also have salt-retaining properties, are used as replacement therapy in adrenocortical deficiency states. Their synthetic analogs such as prednisolone are primarily used for their potent anti-inflammatory effects in disorders of many organ systems.

Glucocorticoids cause profound and varied metabolic effects. In addition, they modify the body's immune responses to diverse stimuli.

INDICATIONS AND USAGE

Prednisolone is indicated in the following conditions:

Endocrine Disorders: Primary or secondary adrenocortical insufficiency (hydrocortisone or cortisone is the first choice: synthetic analogs may be used in conjunction with mineralocorticoids where applicable; in infancy mineralocorticoid supplementation is of particular importance): Congenital adrenal hyperplasia, nonsuppurative thyroiditis, hypercalcemia associated with cancer.

Rheumatic Disorders: As adjunctive therapy for short-term administration (to tide the patient over an acute episode or exacerbation) in: Psoriatic arthritis, rheumatoid arthritis—including juvenile rheumatoid arthritis—(selected cases may require low-dose maintenance therapy), ankylosing spondylitis, acute gouty arthritis, acute and subacute bursitis, post-traumatic osteoarthritis, acute nonspecific tenosynovitis, synovitis of osteoarthritis, epicondylitis.

Collagen Diseases: During an exacerbation or as maintenance therapy in selected cases of: Systemic lupus erythematosus, acute rheumatic carditis and systemic dermatomyositis (polymyositis).

Dermatologic Diseases: Pemphigus, exfoliative dermatitis, bullous dermatitis herpetiformis, mycosis fungoides, severe psoriasis, severe erythema multiforme (Stevens-Johnson syndrome), severe seborrheic dermatitis.

Allergic States: Control of severe or incapacitating allergic conditions intractable to adequate trials of conventional treatment: Seasonal or perennial allergic rhinitis, contact dermatitis, atopic dermatitis, serum sickness, drug hypersensitivity reactions, bronchial asthma.

Ophthalmic Diseases: Severe acute and chronic allergic and inflammatory processes involving the eye and its adnexa such as: Allergic conjunctivitis, chorioretinitis, keratitis, anterior segment inflammation, allergic corneal marginal ulcers, diffuse posterior uveitis and choroiditis, herpes zoster ophthalmicus, optic neuritis, iritis and iridocyclitis, sympathetic ophthalmia.

Respiratory Diseases: Symptomatic sarcoidosis, Loeffler's syndrome not manageable by other means, berylliosis, fulminating or disseminated pulmonary tuberculosis when used concurrently with appropriate chemotherapy, aspiration pneumonitis.

Hematologic Disorders: Idiopathic thrombocytopenic purpura in adults, secondary thrombocytopenia in adults, acquired (autoimmune) hemolytic anemia, erythroblastopenia (RBC anemia), congenital (erythroid) hypoplastic anemia.

Neoplastic Diseases: For palliative management of: leukemias and lymphomas in adults, acute leukemia of childhood.

Edematous States: To induce a diuresis or remission of proteinuria in the nephrotic syndrome, without uremia, of the idiopathic type or that due to lupus erythematosus.

Gastrointestinal Diseases: To tide the patient over a critical period of the disease in: ulcerative colitis, regional enteritis.

Miscellaneous: Tuberculous meningitis with subarachnoid block or impending block used concurrently with appropriate antituberculous chemotherapy, trichinosis with neurologic or myocardial involvement.

In addition to the above indications prednisolone syrup is indicated for systemic dermatomyositis (polymyositis).

CONTRAINDICATIONS

Systemic fungal infections.

WARNINGS

In patients on corticosteroid therapy subjected to unusual stress, increased dosage of rapidly acting corticosteroids before, during, and after the stressful situation is indicated.

Corticosteroids may mask some signs of infection and new infections may appear during their use. There may be decreased resistance and inability to localize infection when corticosteroids are used.

Prolonged use of corticosteroids may produce posterior subcapsular cataracts, glaucoma with possible damage to the optic nerves, and may enhance the establishment of secondary ocular infections due to fungi or viruses.

Average and large doses of hydrocortisone or cortisone can cause elevation of blood pressure, salt and water retention, and increased excretion of potassium. These effects are less likely to occur with the synthetic derivatives except when used in large doses. Dietary salt restriction and potassium supplementation may be necessary. All corticosteroids increase calcium excretion.

WHILE ON CORTICOSTEROID THERAPY PATIENTS SHOULD NOT BE VACCINATED AGAINST SMALLPOX. OTHER IMMUNIZATION PROCEDURES SHOULD NOT BE UNDERTAKEN IN PATIENTS WHO ARE ON CORTICOSTEROIDS, ESPECIALLY ON HIGH DOSE, BECAUSE OF POSSIBLE HAZARDS OF NEUROLOGICAL COMPLICATIONS AND A LACK OF ANTIBODY RESPONSE.

Persons who are on drugs which suppress the immune system are more susceptible to infections than healthy individuals. Chickenpox and measles, for example, can have a more serious or even fatal course in nonimmune children or adults on corticosteroids. In such children or adults who have not had these diseases, particular care should be taken to avoid exposure. How the dose, route and duration of corticosteroid administration affects the risk of developing a disseminated infection is not known. The contribution of the underlying disease and/or prior corticosteroid treatment to the risk is also not known. If exposed to chickenpox, prophylaxis with varicella zoster immune globulin (VZIG) may be indicated. If exposed to measles, prophylaxis with pooled intravenous immunoglobulin (IVIG) may be indicated. (See the respective prescribing information for complete VZIG and IVIG prescribing information. If chickenpox develops, treatment with antiviral agents may be considered.

The use of prednisolone in active tuberculosis should be restricted to those cases of fulminating or disseminated tuberculosis in which the corticosteroid is used for the management of the disease in conjunction with an appropriate antituberculous regimen.

If corticosteroids are indicated in patients with latent tuberculosis or tuberculin reactivity, dose observation is necessary as reactivation of the disease may occur. During prolonged corticosteroid therapy, these patients should receive chemoprophylaxis.

P

USE IN PREGNANCY

Since adequate human reproduction studies have not been done with corticosteroids, the use of these drugs in pregnancy, nursing mothers or women of childbearing potential requires that the possible benefits of the drug be weighed against the potential hazards to the mother and embryo or fetus. Infants born of mothers who have received substantial doses of corticosteroids during pregnancy should be carefully observed for signs of hypoadrenalism.

PRECAUTIONS

GENERAL

Drug-induced secondary adrenocortical insufficiency may be minimized by gradual reduction of dosage. This type of relative insufficiency may persist for months after discontinuation of therapy; therefore, in any situation of stress occurring during that period, hormone therapy should be reinstituted. Since mineralocorticoid secretion may be impaired, salt and/or a mineralocorticoid should be administered concurrently.

There is an enhanced effect of corticosteroids on patients with hypothyroidism and in those with cirrhosis.

Corticosteroids should be used cautiously in patients with ocular herpes simplex because of possible corneal perforation.

The lowest possible dose of corticosteroid should be used to control the condition under treatment, and when reduction in dosage is possible, the reduction should be gradual.

Psychic derangements may appear when corticosteroids are used, ranging from euphoria, insomnia, mood swings, personality changes, and severe depression, to frank psychotic manifestations. Also, existing emotional instability or psychotic tendencies may be aggravated by corticosteroids.

Aspirin should be used cautiously in conjunction with corticosteroids in hypoprothrombinemia.

Steroids should be used with caution in nonspecific ulcerative colitis if there is a probability of impending perforation, abscess or other pyogenic infections, diverticulitis, fresh intestinal anastomoses, active or latent peptic ulcer, renal insufficiency, hypertension, osteoporosis, and myasthenia gravis.

Growth and development of infants and children on prolonged corticosteroid therapy should be carefully observed.

INFORMATION FOR THE PATIENT

Patients who are on immunosuppressant doses of corticosteroids should be warned to avoid exposure to chickenpox or measles. Patients should also be advised that if they are exposed, medical advice should be sought without delay.

ADVERSE REACTIONS

Fluid and Electrolyte Disturbances: Sodium retention, fluid retention, congestive heart failure in susceptible patients, potassium loss, hypokalemic alkalosis, hypertension.

Musculoskeletal: Muscle weakness, steroid myopathy, loss of muscle mass, osteoporosis, vertebral compression fractures, aseptic necrosis of femoral and humeral heads, pathological fracture of long bones.

Gastrointestinal: Peptic ulcer with possible perforation and hemorrhage, pancreatitis, abdominal distention, ulcerative esophagitis.

Dermatologic: Impaired wound healing, thin and fragile skin, petechiae and ecchymoses, facial erythema, increased sweating, may supress reactions to skin tests.

Metabolic: Negative nitrogen balance due to protein catabolism.

Neurological: Increased intracranial pressure with papilledema (pseudotumor cerebri) usually after treatment, convulsions, vertigo, headache.

Endocrine: Menstrual irregularities, development of Cushingoid state, secondary adrenocortical and pituitary unresponsiveness (particularly in times of stress, as in trauma, surgery, or illness), suppression of growth in pediatric patients, decreased carbohydrate tolerance, manifestations of latent diabetes mellitus, increased requirements for insulin or oral hypoglycemic agents in diabetics.

Ophthalmic: Posterior subscapular cataracts, increased intraocular pressure, glaucoma, exophthalmos.

DOSAGE AND ADMINISTRATION

Dosage of prednisolone should be individualized according to the severity of the disease and the response of the patient. For pediatric patients, the recommended dosage should be governed by the same considerations rather than strict adherence to the ratio indicated by age or body weight.

Hormone therapy is an adjunct to, and not a replacement for, conventional therapy.

Dosage should be decreased or discontinued gradually when the drug has been administered for more than a few days.

The severity, prognosis, expected duration of the disease, and the reaction of the patient to medication are primary factors in determining dosage.

If a period of spontaneous remission occurs in a chronic condition, treatment should be discontinued.

Blood pressure, body weight, routine laboratory studies, including 2 hour postprandial blood glucose and serum potassium, and a chest Xray should be obtained at regular intervals during prolonged therapy. Upper GI Xrays are desirable in patients with known or suspected peptic ulcer disease.

The initial dosage of prednisolone may vary from 5-60 mg/day depending on the specific disease entity being treated. In situations of less severity, lower doses will generally suffice, while in selected patients higher initial doses may be required. The initial dosage should be maintained or adjusted until a satisfactory response is noted. If after a reasonable period of time there is a lack of satisfactory clinical response, prednisolone should be discontinued and the patient transferred to other appropriate therapy. IT SHOULD BE EMPHASIZED THAT DOSAGE REQUIREMENTS ARE VARIABLE AND MUST BE INDIVIDUALIZED ON THE BASIS OF THE DISEASE UNDER TREATMENT AND THE RESPONSE OF THE PATIENT.

After a favorable response is noted, the proper maintenance dosage should be determined by decreasing the initial drug dosage in small decrements at appropriate time intervals until the lowest dosage which will maintain an adequate clinical response is reached. It should be kept in mind that constant monitoring is needed in regard to drug dosage. Included in the situations which may make dosage adjustments necessary are changes in clinical status secondary to remissions or exacerbations in the disease process, the patient's individual drug responsiveness and the effect of patient exposure to stressful situations not directly related to the disease entity under treatment. In this latter situation it may be necessary to increase the dosage of prednisolone for a period of time consistent with the patient's condition. If after long-term therapy the drug is to be stopped, it is recommended that it be withdrawn gradually rather than abruptly.

ALTERNATE-DAY THERAPY (ADT)

ADT is a corticosteroid dosing regimen in which twice the usual daily dose of corticoid is administered every other morning. The purpose of this mode of therapy is to provide the patient requiring long-term, pharmacologic-dose treatment with the beneficial effects of corticoids while minimizing certain undesirable effects, including pituitary-adrenal suppression, the cushingoid state, corticoid withdrawal symptoms, and growth suppression in children.

The rationale for this treatment schedule is based on two major premises: (1) the anti-inflammatory or therapeutic effect of corticoids persists longer than their physical presence and metabolic effects, and (2) administration of the corticosteroid every other morning allows for reestablishment of more nearly normal hypothalamic-pituitary-adrenal (HPA) activity on the off-steroid day.

A brief review of the HPA physiology may be helpful in understanding this rationale. Acting primarily through the hypothalamus a fall in free cortisol stimulates the pituitary gland to produce increasing amounts of corticotropin (ACTH) while a rise in free cortisol inhibits ACTH secretion. Normally the HPA system is characterized by diurnal (circadian) rhythm. Serum levels of ACTH rise from a low point about 10 PM to a peak level about 6 AM. Increasing levels of ACTH stimulate adrenocortical activity resulting in a rise in plasma cortisol with maximal levels occurring between 2 AM and 8 AM. This rise in cortisol dampens ACTH production and in turn adrenocortical activity. There is a gradual fall in plasma corticoids during the day with lowest levels occurring about midnight.

The diurnal rhythm of the HPA axis is lost in Cushing's disease, a syndrome of adrenocortical hyperfunction characterized by obesity with centripetal fat distribution, thinning of the skin with easy bruisability, muscle wasting with weakness, hypertension, latent diabetes, osteoporosis, electrolyte imbalance, etc. The same clinical findings of hyperadrenocorticism may be noted during long-term, pharmacologic-dose corticoid therapy administered in conventional daily divided doses. It would appear, then, that a disturbance in the diurnal cycle with maintenance of elevated corticoid values during the night may play a significant role in the development of undesirable corticoid effects. Escape from these constantly elevated plasma levels for even short periods of time may be instrumental in protecting against undesirable pharmacologic effects.

During conventional pharmacologic-dose corticosteroid therapy, ACTH production is inhibited with subsequent suppression of cortisol production by the adrenal cortex. Recovery time for normal HPA activity is variable depending upon the dose and duration of treatment. During this time the patient is vulnerable to any stressful situation. Although it has been shown that there is considerably less adrenal suppression following a single morning dose of prednisolone (10 mg) as opposed to a quarter of that dose administered every 6 hours, there is evidence that some suppressive effect on adrenal activity may be carried over into the following day when pharmacologic doses are used. Further, it has been shown that a single dose of certain corticosteroids will produce adrenocortical suppression for 2 or more days. Other corticoids, including methylprednisolone, hydrocortisone, prednisone, and prednisolone are considered to be short-acting (producing adrenocortical suppression for 1 ¼ to 1½ days following a single dose) and thus are recommended for alternate-day therapy.

The following should be kept in mind when considering alternate-day therapy:

1. Basic principles and indications for corticosteroid therapy should apply. The benefits of ADT should not encourage the indiscriminate use of steroids.
2. ADT is a therapeutic technique primarily designed for patients in whom long-term pharmacologic corticoid therapy is anticipated.
3. In less severe disease processes in which corticoid therapy is indicated, it may be possible to initiate treatment with ADT. More severe disease states usually will require daily divided high dose therapy for initial control of the disease process. The initial suppressive dose level should be continued until satisfactory clinical response is obtained, usually 4-10 days in the case of many allergic and collagen diseases. It is important to keep the period of initial suppressive dose as brief as possible particularly when subsequent use of alternate-day therapy is intended.
4. Because of the advantages of ADT, is may be desirable to try patients on this form of therapy who have been on daily corticoids for long periods of time (*e.g.*, patients with rheumatoid arthritis). Since these patients may already have a suppressed HPA axis, establishing them on ADT may be difficult and not always successful; however, it is recommended that regular attempts be made to change them over. It may be helpful to triple or even quadruple the daily maintenance dose and administer this every other day rather than just doubling the daily dose if difficulty is encountered. Once the patient is again controlled, an attempt should be made to reduce this dose to a minimum.
5. As indicated above, certain corticosteroids, because of their prolonged suppressive effect on adrenal activity, are not recommended for alternate-day therapy (*e.g.*, dexamethasone and betamethasone).
6. The maximal activity of the adrenal cortex is between 2 AM and 8 AM and it is minimal between 4 PM and midnight. Exogenous corticosteroids suppress adrenocortical activity the least when given at the time of maximal activity (am).
7. In using ADT it is important, as in all therapeutic situations, to individualize and tailor the therapy to each patient. Complete control of symptoms will not be possible in all patients. An explanation of the benefits of ADT will help the patient to understand and tolerate the possible flare-up in symptoms which may occur in the latter part of the off-steroid day. Other symptomatic therapy may be added or increased at this time if needed.
8. In the event of an acute flare-up of the disease process, it may be necessary to return to a full suppressive daily divided corticoid dose for control. Once control is again established alternate-day therapy may be reinstituted.
9. Although many of the undesirable features of corticosteroid therapy can be minimized by ADT, as in any therapeutic situation, the physician must carefully weigh the benefit-risk ratio for each patient in whom corticoid therapy is being considered.

HOW SUPPLIED

SYRUP

Prednisolone syrup is a cherry flavored red liquid containing 15 mg of prednisolone in each 5 ml (teaspoonful). *Pharmacist:* Dispense with a suitable calibrated measuring device to assure proper measuring of dose.

TABLE 1

Prednisolone (mg)	Teaspoons
15	1
10	2/3
7.5	1/2
5	1/3

Dispense in tight, light resistant and child-resistant containers.

Storage: Store at controlled room temperature 15-30°C (59-86°F). Do not refrigerate.

PRODUCT LISTING - RATED THERAPEUTICALLY EQUIVALENT

Liquid - Oral - 5 mg/5 ml

120 ml	$17.35	GENERIC, Ethex Corporation	58177-0912-03
120 ml	$21.74	PRELONE, Muro Pharmaceuticals Inc	00451-2201-04

Syrup - Oral - 15 mg/5 ml

60 ml	$11.84	PRELONE, Southwood Pharmaceuticals Inc	58016-0673-12
60 ml	$19.24	PRELONE, Allscripts Pharmaceutical Company	54569-4012-01
60 ml	$21.35	PRELONE, Pd-Rx Pharmaceuticals	55289-0952-02
120 ml	$22.44	PRELONE, Southwood Pharmaceuticals Inc	58016-0673-24
120 ml	$23.75	PRELONE, Compumed Pharmaceuticals	00403-2407-84
120 ml	$38.48	PRELONE, Allscripts Pharmaceutical Company	54569-4012-02

Size	Price	Product	NDC
120 ml	$48.69	PRELONE, Pd-Rx Pharmaceuticals	55289-0952-04
120 ml x 2	$76.96	PRELONE, Allscripts Pharmaceutical Company	54569-4012-03
240 ml	$51.65	PRELONE, Compumed Pharmaceuticals	00403-2407-88
240 ml	$74.50	GENERIC, Mylan Pharmaceuticals Inc	00378-3425-24
240 ml	$74.50	GENERIC, Alpharma Uspd Makers Of Barre and Nmc	00472-0212-08
240 ml	$76.96	PRELONE, Allscripts Pharmaceutical Company	54569-4012-04
240 ml	$91.84	PRELONE, Physicians Total Care	54868-3220-00
240 ml	$108.30	PRELONE, Muro Pharmaceuticals Inc	00451-1500-08
480 ml	$99.89	FEDERAL UPPER LIMIT, H.C.F.A. F F P	99999-2102-02
480 ml	$119.20	GENERIC, Mylan Pharmaceuticals Inc	00378-3425-48
480 ml	$119.20	GENERIC, Alpharma Uspd Makers Of Barre and Nmc	00472-0212-16
480 ml	$173.26	PRELONE, Muro Pharmaceuticals Inc	00451-1500-16

PRODUCT LISTING - RATED NOT THERAPEUTICALLY EQUIVALENT

Syrup - Oral - 15 mg/5 ml

Size	Price	Product	NDC
240 ml	$42.44	PRELONE, Southwood Pharmaceuticals Inc	58016-0673-48
240 ml	$82.35	PRELONE, Allscripts Pharmaceutical Company	54569-4012-00

Tablet - Oral - 5 mg

Size	Price	Product	NDC
100's	$2.66	GENERIC, Global Pharmaceutical Corporation	00115-4280-01
100's	$3.23	GENERIC, Interstate Drug Exchange Inc	00814-6250-14
100's	$3.79	GENERIC, Geneva Pharmaceuticals	00781-1540-01
100's	$3.95	GENERIC, Cmc-Consolidated Midland Corporation	00223-1512-01
100's	$4.04	GENERIC, Moore, H.L. Drug Exchange Inc	00839-5076-06
100's	$4.60	GENERIC, Aligen Independent Laboratories Inc	00405-4823-01
100's	$4.95	GENERIC, Major Pharmaceuticals Inc	00904-2155-60
100's	$13.75	GENERIC, Watson/Schein Pharmaceuticals Inc	00364-0217-01
100's	$13.75	GENERIC, Lannett Company Inc	00527-1201-01
100's	$13.75	GENERIC, Watson/Schein Pharmaceuticals Inc	00591-5059-01

PRODUCT LISTING - EQUIVALENTS NOT AVAILABLE

Liquid - Oral - 5 mg/5 ml

Size	Price	Product	NDC
120 ml	$15.45	PRELONE, Allscripts Pharmaceutical Company	54569-4807-00

Syrup - Oral - 15 mg/5 ml

Size	Price	Product	NDC
60 ml x 4	$69.13	GENERIC, Allscripts Pharmaceutical Company	54569-4827-01
120 ml x 2	$71.08	GENERIC, Allscripts Pharmaceutical Company	54569-4827-00
240 ml	$50.88	GENERIC, We Pharmaceuticals Inc	59196-0010-24
240 ml	$70.90	GENERIC, Teva Pharmaceuticals Usa	00093-6118-87
240 ml	$71.08	GENERIC, Allscripts Pharmaceutical Company	54569-4827-02
240 ml	$74.50	GENERIC, Watson/Rugby Laboratories Inc	52544-0520-38
480 ml	$81.60	GENERIC, We Pharmaceuticals Inc	59196-0010-48
480 ml	$113.50	GENERIC, Teva Pharmaceuticals Usa	00093-6118-16
480 ml	$119.20	GENERIC, Watson/Rugby Laboratories Inc	52544-0520-16
480 ml	$119.20	GENERIC, Ethex Corporation	58177-0910-07

Prednisolone Acetate (002103)

For related information, see the comparative table section in Appendix A.

Categories: Blepharitis, nonpurulent; Conjunctivitis, allergic; Conjunctivitis, vernal; Herpes zoster ophthalmicus; Iritis; Keratitis, ophthalmic; Keratoconjunctivitis; Keratoplasty, adjunct; Trauma, corneal; Ulcer, corneal; Pregnancy Category C; FDA Approved 1972 Nov

Drug Classes: Corticosteroids; Corticosteroids, ophthalmic; Ophthalmics

Brand Names: Ak-Tate; Articulose-50; Cotolone; Econopred; Ed-Pred 25; Key-Pred; Medicort 50; Ocu-Pred-A; **Pred Forte**; Pred Mild; Predair-A; Predaject-50; Predalone 50; Predate-50; Predcor-50; Predicort-50; Pri-Cortin; Sholone; Spectro-Tate; Uad Pred

Foreign Brand Availability: Prednigalen (Germany); Predni-Ophtal (Germany)

HCFA JCODE(S): J2650 up to 1 ml IM

DESCRIPTION

Prednisolone Acetate is an adrenocortical steroid prepared as a sterile ophthalmic suspension.

Established name: Prednisolone Acetate

Chemical name: Pregna-1,4-diene-3,20-dione, 21-(acetyloxy)-11,17-dihydroxy-, (11β)-.

Each Pred Forte ml Contains: *Active:* Prednisolone acetate 0.125% or 1.0%. *Preservative:* Benzalkonium chloride 0.01%. *Vehicle:* Hydroxypropyl methylcellulose. *Inactive:* Dried sodium phosphate, polysorbate 80, edetate disodium, glycerin, citric acid and/or sodium hydroxide (to adjust pH), purified water.

CLINICAL PHARMACOLOGY

This drug causes inhibition of the inflammatory response to inciting agents of a mechanical, chemical, or immunological nature. No generally accepted explanation of this steroid property has been advanced.

INDICATIONS AND USAGE

For use in the treatment of inflammatory and allergic conditions: allergic, nonpurulent catarrhal, and vernal conjunctivitis; acute iritis; catarrhal corneal ulcer; corneal injuries; nonpurulent blepharitis; herpes zoster ophthalmicus; nonspecific superficial keratitis; nonpurulent phlyctenular keratoconjunctivitis. 1% may be indicated to suppress graft reaction after keratoplasty.

CONTRAINDICATIONS

Contraindicated in acute superficial herpes simplex keratitis (dendritic keratitis), vaccinia, varicella, and most other viral diseases of the cornea and conjunctiva; tuberculosis; fungal diseases; acute purulent untreated infections which, like other diseases caused by microorganisms, may be masked or enhanced by the presence of the steroid.

WARNINGS

Employment of steroid medication in the treatment of stromal herpes simplex requires great caution; frequent slit lamp microscopy is mandatory. Prolonged use may result in glaucoma, damage to the optic nerve, defects in visual acuity and visual field, posterior subcapsular cataract formation; or may aid in the establishment of secondary ocular infection from pathogens liberated from ocular tissue. In those diseases causing thinning of the cornea, or sclera, perforation has been known to occur with the use of topical steroids.

PRECAUTIONS

During the course of the therapy, if the inflammatory reaction does not respond within a reasonable period, other forms of therapy should be instituted. As fungal infections of the cornea are particularly prone to develop coincidentally with long-term local steroid application, fungus invasion must be considered in any persistent corneal ulceration where a steroid has been used or is in use. Intraocular pressure should be checked frequently. Steroids should be used with caution in glaucoma. This product should not be used without continuing medical supervision.

Usage in Pregnancy: Safety of intensive or protracted use of topical steroids during pregnancy has not been substantiated.

ADVERSE REACTIONS

Glaucoma with optic nerve damage, visual acuity and field defects, posterior subcapsular cataract formation, secondary ocular infections from pathogens including herpes simplex liberated from ocular tissues, perforation of the globe. Viral and fungal infections of the cornea may be exacerbated by the application of steroids.

DOSAGE AND ADMINISTRATION

Two drops topically in the eye(s) four times daily. In cases of bacterial infections, concomitant use of antibiotics or chemotherapeutic agents is mandatory.

PRODUCT LISTING - RATED THERAPEUTICALLY EQUIVALENT

Suspension - Injectable - acetate 50 mg/ml

Size	Price	Product	NDC
10 ml	$18.30	GENERIC, Merz Pharmaceuticals	00259-0310-10
30 ml	$18.55	GENERIC, Ivax Corporation	00182-0939-66

Suspension - Ophthalmic - acetate 1%

Size	Price	Product	NDC
1 ml	$7.96	PRED FORTE, Allergan Inc	11980-0180-01
5 ml	$1.80	OCU-PRED-A, Ocumed Inc	51944-5440-05
5 ml	$12.60	GENERIC, Pacific Pharma	60758-0119-05
5 ml	$12.60	GENERIC, Falcon Pharmaceuticals, Ltd.	61314-0637-05
5 ml	$17.48	PRED FORTE, Southwood Pharmaceuticals Inc	58016-0637-01
5 ml	$21.66	PRED FORTE, Allscripts Pharmaceutical Company	54569-0871-00
5 ml	$23.67	PRED FORTE, Physicians Total Care	54868-0636-01
5 ml	$24.79	PRED FORTE, Allergan Inc	11980-0180-05
5 ml	$31.00	ECONOPRED PLUS, Alcon Laboratories Inc	00998-0637-05
10 ml	$2.25	OCU-PRED-A, Ocumed Inc	51944-5440-00
10 ml	$23.10	GENERIC, Falcon Pharmaceuticals, Ltd.	61314-0637-10
10 ml	$23.15	GENERIC, Pacific Pharma	60758-0119-10
10 ml	$43.29	PRED FORTE, Allscripts Pharmaceutical Company	54569-2868-00
10 ml	$48.69	ECONOPRED PLUS, Alcon Laboratories Inc	00998-0637-10
10 ml	$49.55	PRED FORTE, Allergan Inc	11980-0180-10
15 ml	$34.10	GENERIC, Pacific Pharma	60758-0119-15
15 ml	$34.10	GENERIC, Falcon Pharmaceuticals, Ltd.	61314-0637-15
15 ml	$64.91	PRED FORTE, Allscripts Pharmaceutical Company	54569-1203-00
15 ml	$74.29	PRED FORTE, Allergan Inc	11980-0180-15

Suspension - Ophthalmic - 1%

Size	Price	Product	NDC
10 ml	$16.95	FEDERAL UPPER LIMIT, H.C.F.A. F F P	99999-2103-01

PRODUCT LISTING - RATED NOT THERAPEUTICALLY EQUIVALENT

Suspension - Injectable - acetate 25 mg/ml

Size	Price	Product	NDC
30 ml	$10.91	GENERIC, Moore, H.L. Drug Exchange Inc	00839-5617-36

Suspension - Injectable - acetate 50 mg/ml

Size	Price	Product	NDC
10 ml	$6.25	GENERIC, Roberts/Hauck Pharmaceutical Corporation	43797-0101-12
30 ml	$13.73	GENERIC, Moore, H.L. Drug Exchange Inc	00839-5120-36

PRODUCT LISTING - EQUIVALENTS NOT AVAILABLE

Suspension - Injectable - acetate 25 mg/ml

Size	Price	Product	NDC
10 ml	$5.75	GENERIC, Roberts/Hauck Pharmaceutical Corporation	43797-0027-12

10 ml	$6.00	GENERIC, Cmc-Consolidated Midland Corporation	00223-8345-10
10 ml	$6.90	GENERIC, Hyrex Pharmaceuticals	00314-0695-70
30 ml	$6.45	GENERIC, Veratex Corporation	17022-2638-07
30 ml	$6.50	GENERIC, Cmc-Consolidated Midland Corporation	00223-8345-30
30 ml	$7.75	GENERIC, C.O. Truxton Inc	00463-1019-30
30 ml	$11.63	GENERIC, Interstate Drug Exchange Inc	00814-6255-46
Suspension - Injectable - acetate 40 mg/ml			
10 ml	$14.95	GENERIC, Legere Pharmaceuticals	25332-0121-03
Suspension - Injectable - acetate 50 mg/ml			
10 ml	$4.60	GENERIC, Veratex Corporation	17022-2659-03
10 ml	$5.25	GENERIC, C.O. Truxton Inc	00463-1020-10
10 ml	$5.50	GENERIC, Keene Pharmaceuticals Inc	00588-5352-70
10 ml	$6.25	GENERIC, Med Tek Pharmaceuticals Inc	52349-0108-10
10 ml	$6.50	GENERIC, Cmc-Consolidated Midland Corporation	00223-8346-10
10 ml	$7.50	GENERIC, Cmc-Consolidated Midland Corporation	00223-5346-10
10 ml	$8.00	GENERIC, Dunhall Pharmaceuticals Inc	00217-8404-08
10 ml	$10.00	GENERIC, Forest Pharmaceuticals	00456-0924-10
10 ml	$10.95	GENERIC, Legere Pharmaceuticals	25332-0031-10
10 ml	$12.36	GENERIC, Primedics Laboratories	00684-0115-10
10 ml	$12.75	GENERIC, Clint Pharmaceutical Inc	55553-0249-10
30 ml	$6.95	GENERIC, Veratex Corporation	17022-2659-07
30 ml	$6.98	GENERIC, Hauser, A.F. Inc	52637-0325-10
30 ml	$9.50	GENERIC, Cmc-Consolidated Midland Corporation	00223-8341-30
30 ml	$11.50	GENERIC, Cmc-Consolidated Midland Corporation	00223-8346-30
30 ml	$14.03	GENERIC, Allscripts Pharmaceutical Company	54569-2161-00
30 ml	$14.93	GENERIC, Interstate Drug Exchange Inc	00814-6260-46
Suspension - Injectable - acetate 80 mg/ml			
5 ml	$14.95	GENERIC, Legere Pharmaceuticals	25332-0062-05
Suspension - Ophthalmic - acetate 0.12%			
5 ml	$17.25	PRED MILD, Southwood Pharmaceuticals Inc	58016-6057-01
5 ml	$24.78	PRED MILD, Allergan Inc	11980-0174-05
10 ml	$31.58	PRED MILD, Allscripts Pharmaceutical Company	54569-1858-00
10 ml	$36.14	PRED MILD, Allergan Inc	11980-0174-10
Suspension - Ophthalmic - acetate 0.125%			
5 ml	$4.75	GENERIC, Allscripts Pharmaceutical Company	54569-1226-00
5 ml	$25.69	ECONOPRED, Alcon Laboratories Inc	00998-0635-05
10 ml	$38.50	ECONOPRED, Alcon Laboratories Inc	00998-0635-10
Suspension - Ophthalmic - acetate 1%			
5 ml	$12.60	GENERIC, Southwood Pharmaceuticals Inc	58016-6029-01
5 ml	$13.50	GENERIC, Southwood Pharmaceuticals Inc	58016-6557-05
5 ml	$16.35	GENERIC, Pharma Pac	52959-0265-05

Prednisolone Sodium Phosphate *(002105)*

For related information, see the comparative table section in Appendix A.

Categories: Adrenocortical insufficiency; Anemia, acquired hemolytic; Anemia, congenital hypoplastic; Ankylosing spondylitis; Arthritis, gouty; Arthritis, osteoarthritis; Arthritis, psoriatic; Arthritis, rheumatoid; Asthma; Berylliosis; Bursitis; Carditis, rheumatic; Chorioretinitis; Choroiditis; Colitis, ulcerative; Conjunctivitis, allergic; Crohn's disease; Dermatitis herpetiformis; Dermatitis, atopic; Dermatitis, contact; Dermatitis, exfoliative; Dermatitis, seborrheic; Dermatomyositis, systemic; Epicondylitis; Erythema multiforme; Erythroblastopenia; Herpes zoster ophthalmicus; Hypercalcemia, secondary to neoplasia; Hyperplasia, congenital adrenal; Hypersensitivity reactions; Iridocyclitis; Iritis; Keratitis, ophthalmic; Leukemia; Loffler's syndrome; Lupus erythematosus, systemic; Lymphoma; Meningitis, tuberculous; Mycosis fungoides; Neuritis, optic; Ophthalmia, sympathetic; Pemphigus; Pneumonitis, aspiration; Polymyositis; Proteinuria; Psoriasis; Purpura, idiopathic thrombocytopenic; Rhinitis, perennial allergic; Rhinitis, seasonal allergic; Sarcoidosis; Serum sickness; Stevens-Johnson syndrome; Synovitis, secondary to osteoarthritis; Tenosynovitis; Thrombocytopenia; Thyroiditis, nonsuppurative; Trichinosis; Tuberculosis, disseminated; Tuberculosis, fulminating; Ulcer, allergic corneal marginal; Uveitis; Pregnancy Category C; FDA Approved 1961 Aug

Drug Classes: Corticosteroids; Corticosteroids, ophthalmic; Ophthalmics

Brand Names: Ak-Pred; **Hydeltrasol**; I-Pred; Inflamase; Isolone Forte; Key-Pred Sp; Metreton; Nor-Pred S; Ocu-Pred; Pediapred; Predair; Predair-A; Predate-S; Predicort-Rp; Prednisol; Spectro-Pred

HCFA JCODE(S): J2640 up to 20 mg IV, IM

DESCRIPTION

INJECTION

Prednisolone sodium phosphate, a synthetic adrenocortical steroid, is a white or slightly yellow powder that is slightly hygroscopic and is freely soluble in water. The molecular weight is 484.39. It is designated chemically as 11β, 17-dihydroxy-21-(phosphonooxy) pregna-1,4-diene-3,20-dione disodium salt. The empirical formula is $C_{21}H_{27}Na_2O_8P$.

Hydeltrasol (prednisolone sodium phosphate) injection is a sterile solution (pH 7.0-8.0), sealed under nitrogen, for intravenous, intramuscular, intra-articular, intralesional, and soft tissue administration.

Each milliliter contains prednisolone sodium phosphate equivalent to 20 mg prednisolone phosphate. Inactive ingredients per ml: niacinamide, 25 mg; sodium hydroxide to adjust pH; disodium edetate, 0.5 mg; water for injection, qs 1 ml. Sodium bisulfite, 1 mg, and phenol, 5 mg, added as preservatives.

ORAL LIQUID

Pediapred Oral Liquid is a dye free, colorless to light straw colored, raspberry flavored solution. Each 5 ml (teaspoonful) of Pediapred contains 6.7 mg prednisolone sodium phosphate (5 mg prednisolone base) in a palatable, aqueous vehicle.

Inactive Ingredients: Dibasic sodium phosphate, edetate disodium, methylparaben, purified water, sodium biphosphate, sorbitol, natural and artificial raspberry flavor.

Prednisolone sodium phosphate occurs as white or slightly yellow, friable granules or powder. It is freely soluble in water; soluble in methanol; slightly soluble in alcohol and in chloroform; and very slightly soluble in acetone and in dioxane. The chemical name of prednisolone sodium phosphate is pregna-1,4-diene-3,20-dione, 11, 17-dihydroxy-21-(phosphonooxy)-, disodium salt, (11β)-. The empirical formula is $C_{21}H_{27}Na_2O_8P$; the molecular weight is 484.39.

Pharmacological Category: Glucocorticoid.

OPHTHALMIC SOLUTION

Inflamase Mild and Inflamase Forte (prednisolone sodium phosphate) ophthalmic solutions are sterile solutions for ophthalmic administration having the following compositions:

Inflamase Mild

Prednisolone sodium phosphate: 1.25 mg/ml
(adrenocortical steroid/anti-inflammatory)
(equivalent to Prednisolone Phosphate 1.1 mg/ml)

Inflamase Forte

Prednisolone sodium phosphate: 10 mg/ml
(adrenocortical steroid/anti-inflammatory)
(equivalent to Prednisolone Phosphate 9.1 mg/ml)
in buffered, isotonic solutions containing sodium biphosphate, sodium phosphate anhydrous, sodium chloride, edetate disodium and purified water; preserved with benzalkonium chloride 0.1 mg/ml.

The chemical name for prednisolone sodium phosphate is pregna-1,4-diene-3,20-dione, 11,17-dihydroxy-21-(phosphonooxy)-, disodium salt, (11 β)-. The empirical formula is $C_{21}H_{27}Na_2O_8P$; the molecular weight is 484.39.

CLINICAL PHARMACOLOGY

INJECTION

Hydeltrasol injection has a rapid onset but short duration of action when compared with less soluble preparations. Because of this, it is suitable for the treatment of acute disorders responsive to adrenocortical steroid therapy.

Naturally occurring glucocorticoids (hydrocortisone and cortisone), which also have salt-retaining properties, are used as replacement therapy in adrenocortical deficiency states. Their synthetic analogs, including prednisolone, are primarily used for their potent anti-inflammatory effects in disorders of many organ systems.

Glucocorticoids cause profound and varied metabolic effects. In addition, they modify the body's immune responses to diverse stimuli.

At equipotent anti-inflammatory doses, prednisolone has less tendency to cause salt and water retention than either hydrocortisone or cortisone.

ORAL LIQUID

Prednisolone is a synthetic adrenocortical steroid drug with predominantly glucocorticoid properties. Some of these properties reproduce the physiological actions of endogenous glucocorticosteroids, but others do not necessarily reflect any of the adrenal hormones' normal functions; they are seen only after administration of large therapeutic doses of the drug. The pharmacological effects of prednisolone which are due to its glucocorticoid properties include: promotion of gluconeogenesis; increased deposition of glycogen in the liver; inhibition of the utilization of glucose; anti-insulin activity; increased catabolism of protein; increased lipolysis; stimulation of fat synthesis and storage; increased glomerular filtration rate and resulting increase in urinary excretion of urate (creatinine excretion remains unchanged); and increased calcium excretion.

Decreased production of eosinophils and lymphocytes occurs, but erythropoieses and production of polymorphonuclear leukocytes are stimulated. Anti-inflammatory processes (edema, fibrin deposition, capillary dilatation, migration of leukocytes and phagocytosis) and the later stages of wound healing (capillary proliferation, deposition of collagen, cicatrization) are inhibited. Prednisolone can stimulate secretion of various components of gastric juice. Stimulation of the production of corticotropin may lead to suppression of endogenous corticosteroids. Prednisolone has slight mineralocorticoid activity, whereby entry of sodium into cells and loss of intracellular potassium is stimulated. This is particularly evident in the kidney, where rapid ion exchange leads to sodium retention and hypertension.

Prednisolone is rapidly and well absorbed from the gastrointestinal tract following oral administration. Pediapred oral liquid produces a 20% higher peak plasma level of prednisolone which occurs approximately 15 minutes earlier than the peak seen with tablet formulations. Prednisolone is 70-90% protein-bound in the plasma and it is eliminated from the plasma with a half-life of 2-4 hours. It is metabolized mainly in the liver and excreted in the urine as sulfate and glucuronide conjugates.

OPHTHALMIC SOLUTION

Prednisolone sodium phosphate causes inhibition of the inflammatory response to inciting agents of a mechanical, chemical or immunological nature. No generally accepted explanation of this steroid property has been advanced.

INDICATIONS AND USAGE

INJECTION

By Intravenous or Intramuscular Injection (when oral therapy is not feasible)

Endocrine Disorders: Primary or secondary adrenocortical insufficiency (hydrocortisone or cortisone is the drug of choice; synthetic analogs may be used in conjunction with mineralocorticoids where applicable; in infancy, mineralocorticoid supplementation is of particular importance).

Acute adrenocortical insufficiency (hydrocortisone or cortisone is the drug of choice; mineralocorticoid supplementation may be necessary, particularly when synthetic analogs are used).

Preoperatively, and in the event of serious trauma or illness, in patients with known adrenal insufficiency or when adrenocortical reserve is doubtful.

Congenital adrenal hyperplasia; nonsuppurative thyroiditis; hypercalcemia associated with cancer.

Rheumatic Disorders: As adjunctive therapy for short-term administration (to tide the patient over an acute episode or exacerbation) in: post-traumatic osteoarthritis; synovitis of osteoarthritis; rheumatoid arthritis, including juvenile rheumatoid arthritis (selected cases may require low-dose maintenance therapy).

Acute and subacute bursitis; epicondylitis; acute nonspecific tenosynovitis; acute gouty arthritis; psoriatic arthritis; ankylosing spondylitis.

Collagen Diseases: During an exacerbation or as maintenance therapy in selected cases of: systemic lupus erythematosus; acute rheumatic carditis; systemic dermatomyositis (polymyositis).

Dermatologic Diseases: Pemphigus; severe erythema multiforme (Stevens-Johnson syndrome); exfoliative dermatitis; bullous dermatitis herpetiformis; severe seborrheic dermatitis; severe psoriasis; mycosis fungoides.

Allergic States: Control of severe or incapacitating allergic conditions intractable to adequate trials of conventional treatment in: bronchial asthma; contact dermatitis; atopic dermatitis; serum sickness; seasonal or perennial allergic rhinitis; drug hypersensitivity reactions; urticarial transfusion reactions; acute noninfectious laryngeal edema (epinephrine is the drug of first choice).

Ophthalmic Diseases: Severe acute and chronic allergic and inflammatory processes involving the eye, such as: herpes zoster ophthalmicus; iritis, iridocyclitis; chorioretinitis; diffuse posterior uveitis and choroiditis; optic neuritis; sympathetic ophthalmia; anterior segment inflammation; allergic conjunctivitis; keratitis; allergic corneal marginal ulcers.

Gastrointestinal Diseases: To tide the patient over a critical period of the disease in: ulcerative colitis (systemic therapy); regional enteritis (systemic therapy).

Respiratory Diseases: Symptomatic sarcoidosis; berylliosis; fulminating or disseminated pulmonary tuberculosis when used concurrently with appropriate antituberculous chemotherapy; loeffler's syndrome not manageable by other means; aspiration pneumonitis.

Hematologic Disorders: Acquired (autoimmune) hemolytic anemia.

Idiopathic thrombocytopenic purpura in adults (IV only; IM administration is contraindicated); secondary thrombocytopenia in adults; erythroblastopenia (RBC anemia); congenital (erythroid) hypoplastic anemia.

Neoplastic Diseases: For palliative management of: leukemias and lymphomas in adults; acute leukemia of childhood.

Edematous States: To induce diuresis or remission of proteinuria in the nephrotic syndrome, without uremia, of the idiopathic type, or that due to lupus erythematosus.

Miscellaneous: Tuberculous meningitis with subarachnoid block or impending block when used concurrently with appropriate antituberculous chemotherapy; trichinosis with neurologic or myocardial involvement.

By Intra-Articular or Soft Tissue Injection

As adjunctive therapy for short-term administration (to tide the patient over an acute episode or exacerbation) in: synovitis of osteoarthritis; rheumatoid arthritis; acute and subacute bursitis; acute gouty arthritis; epicondylitis; acute nonspecific tenosynovitis; post-traumatic osteoarthritis.

By Intralesional Injection

Keloids; localized hypertrophic, infiltrated, inflammatory lesions of: lichen planus, psoriatic plaques, granuloma annulare, and lichen simplex chronicus (neurodermatitis); discoid lupus erythematosus; necrobiosis lipoidica diabeticorum; alopecia areata.

May also be useful in cystic tumors of an aponeurosis or tendon (ganglia).

ORAL LIQUID

Pediapred oral liquid is indicated in the following conditions:

Endocrine Disorders: Primary or secondary adrenocortical insufficiency (hydrocortisone or cortisone is the first choice; synthetic analogs may be used in conjunction with mineralocorticoids where applicable; in infancy mineralocorticoid supplementation is of particular importance); congenital adrenal hyperplasia; hypercalcemia associated with cancer; non-suppurative thyroiditis.

Rheumatic Disorders: As adjunctive therapy for short term administration (to tide the patient over an acute episode or exacerbation) in: psoriatic arthritis; rheumatoid arthritis, including juvenile rheumatoid arthritis (selected cases may require low dose maintenance therapy); ankylosing spondylitis; acute and subacute bursitis; acute nonspecific tenosynovitis; acute gouty arthritis; post- traumatic osteoarthritis; synovitis of osteoarthritis; epicondylitis.

Collagen Diseases: During an exacerbation or as maintenance therapy in selected cases of: systemic lupus erythematosus; systemic dermatomyositis (polymyositis); acute rheumatic carditis.

Dermatologic Diseases: Pemphigus; bullous dermatitis herpetiformis; severe erythema multiforme (Stevens-Johnson syndrome); exfoliative dermatitis; mycosis fungoides; severe psoriasis; severe seborrheic dermatitis.

Allergic States: Control of severe or incapacitating allergic conditions intractable to adequate trials of conventional treatment in: seasonal or perennial allergic rhinitis; bronchial asthma; contact dermatitis; atopic dermatitis; serum sickness; drug hypersensitivity reactions.

Ophthalmic Diseases: Severe acute and chronic allergic and inflammatory processes involving the eye and its adnexa such as: allergic conjunctivitis; keratitis; allergic corneal marginal ulcers; herpes zoster ophthalmicus; iritis and iridocyclitis; chorioretinitis; anterior segment inflammation; diffuse posterior uveitis and choroiditis; optic neuritis; sympathetic ophthalmia.

Respiratory Diseases: Symptomatic sarcoidosis; Loeffler's syndrome not manageable by other means; berylliosis; fulminating or disseminated pulmonary tuberculosis when used concurrently with appropriate antituberculous chemotherapy; aspiration pneumonitis.

Hematologic Disorders: Idiopathic thrombocytopenic purpura in adults; secondary thrombocytopenia in adults; acquired (autoimmune) hemolytic anemia; erythroblastopenia (RBC anemia); congenital (erythroid) hypoplastic anemia.

Neoplastic Diseases: For palliative management of: leukemias and lymphomas in adults; acute leukemia of childhood.

Edematous States: To induce a diuresis or remission of proteinuria in the nephrotic syndrome, without uremia, of the idiopathic type or that due to lupus erythematosus.

Gastrointestinal Diseases: To tide the patient over a critical period of the disease in: ulcerative colitis; regional enteritis.

Nervous System: Acute exacerbations of multiple sclerosis.

Miscellaneous: Tuberculous meningitis with subarachnoid block or impending block when used concurrently with appropriate antituberculous chemotherapy; trichinosis with neurologic or myocardial involvement.

OPHTHALMIC SOLUTION

Inflamase Mild and Inflamase Forte ophthalmic solutions are indicated for the treatment of the following conditions: Steroid responsive inflammatory conditions of the palpebral and bulbar conjunctiva, cornea, and anterior segment of the globe, such as allergic conjunctivitis, acne rosacea, superficial punctate keratitis, herpes zoster keratitis, iritis, cyclitis, selected infective conjunctivitis when the inherent hazard of steroid use is accepted to obtain an advisable diminution in edema and inflammation; corneal injury from chemical, radiation, or thermal burns, or penetration of foreign bodies.

Inflamase Forte ophthalmic solution is recommended for moderate to severe inflammations, particularly when unusually rapid control is desired. In stubborn cases of anterior segment eye disease, systemic adrenocortical hormone therapy may be required. When the deeper ocular structures are involved, systemic therapy is necessary.

CONTRAINDICATIONS

Injection: Systemic fungal infections (see WARNINGS) regarding amphotericin B. Hypersensitivity to any component of this product, including sulfites (see WARNINGS).

Oral Liquid: Systemic fungal infections.

Ophthalmic Solution: The use of these preparations is contraindicated in the presence of acute superficial herpes simplex, keratitis, fungal diseases of the ocular structures, acute infectious stages of vaccinia, varicella and most other viral diseases of the cornea and conjunctiva, tuberculosis of the eye and hypersensitivity to a component of this preparation. The use of these preparations is always contraindicated after uncomplicated removal of a superficial corneal foreign body.

WARNINGS

INJECTION

Because rare instances of anaphylactoid reactions have occurred in patients receiving parenteral corticosteroid therapy, appropriate precautionary measures should be taken prior to administration, especially when the patient has a history of allergy to any drug. Anaphylactoid and hypersensitivity reactions have been reported for Injection Hydeltrasol (see ADVERSE REACTIONS).

Injection Hydeltrasol contains sodium bisulfite, a sulfite that may cause allergic-type reactions including anaphylactic symptoms and life-threatening or less severe asthmatic episodes in certain susceptible people. The overall prevalence of sulfite sensitivity in the general population is unknown and probably low. Sulfite sensitivity is seen more frequently in asthmatic than in nonasthmatic people.

Corticosteroids may exacerbate systemic fungal infections and therefore should not be used in the presence of such infections unless they are needed to control drug reactions due to amphotericin B. Moreover, there have been cases reported in which concomitant use of amphotericin B and hydrocortisone was followed by cardiac enlargement and congestive failure.

In patients on corticosteroid therapy subjected to any unusual stress, increased dosage of rapidly acting corticosteroids before, during, and after the stressful situation is indicated.

Drug-induced secondary adrenocortical insufficiency may result from too rapid withdrawal of corticosteroids and may be minimized by gradual reduction of dosage. This type of relative insufficiency may persist for months after discontinuation of therapy; therefore, in any situation of stress occurring during that period, hormone therapy should be reinstituted. If the patient is receiving steroids already, dosage may have to be increased. Since mineralocorticoid secretion may be impaired, salt and/or a mineralocorticoid should be administered concurrently.

Corticosteroids may mask some signs of infection, and new infections may appear during their use. There may be decreased resistance and inability to localize infection when corticosteroids are used. Moreover, corticosteroids may affect the nitroblue-tetrazolium test for bacterial infection and produce false negative results.

In cerebral malaria, a double-blind trial has shown that the use of corticosteroids is associated with prolongation of coma and a higher incidence of pneumonia and gastrointestinal bleeding.

Corticosteroids may activate latent amebiasis. Therefore, it is recommended that latent or active amebiasis be ruled out before initiating corticosteroid therapy in any patient who has spent time in the tropics or any patient with unexplained diarrhea.

Prolonged use of corticosteroids may produce posterior subcapsular cataracts, glaucoma with possible damage to the optic nerves, and may enhance the establishment of secondary ocular infections due to fungi or viruses.

Usage In Pregnancy: Since adequate human reproduction studies have not been done with corticosteroids, use of these drugs in pregnancy or in women of childbearing potential requires that the anticipated benefits be weighed against the possible hazards to the mother and embryo or fetus. Infants born of mothers who have received substantial doses of corticosteroids during pregnancy should be carefully observed for signs of hypoadrenalism.

Corticosteroids appear in breast milk and could suppress growth, interfere with endogenous corticosteroid production, or cause other unwanted effects. Mothers taking pharmacologic doses of corticosteroids should be advised not to nurse.

Average and large doses of cortisone or hydrocortisone can cause elevation of blood pressure, salt and water retention, and increased excretion of potassium. These effects are less likely to occur with the synthetic derivatives except when used in large doses. Dietary salt restriction and potassium supplementation may be necessary. All corticosteroids increase calcium excretion.

Administration of live virus vaccines, including smallpox, is contraindicated in individuals receiving immunosuppressive doses of corticosteroids. If inactivated viral or bacterial vaccines are administered to individuals receiving immunosuppressive doses of corticosteroids, the expected serum antibody response may not be obtained. However, immunization procedures may be undertaken in patients who are receiving corticosteroids as replacement therapy, e.g., for Addison's disease.

Patients who are on drugs which suppress the immune system are more susceptible to infections than healthy individuals. Chickenpox and measles, for example, can have a more serious or even fatal course in non-immune children or adults on corticosteroids. In such children or adults who have not had these diseases, particular care should be taken to avoid exposure. The risk of developing a disseminated infection varies among individuals and can be related to the dose, route and duration of corticosteroid administration as well as to the underlying disease. If exposed to chickenpox, prophylaxis with varicella zoster immune globulin (VZIG) may be indicated. If chickenpox develops, treatment with antiviral agents may be considered. If exposed to measles, prophylaxis with immune globulin (IG) may be indicated. (See the respective package inserts for VZIG and IG for complete prescribing information.)

The use of Hydeltrasol injection in active tuberculosis should be restricted to those cases of fulminating or disseminated tuberculosis in which the corticosteroid is used for the management of the disease in conjunction with appropriate antituberculous regimen.

If corticosteroids are indicated in patients with latent tuberculosis or tuberculin reactivity, close observation is necessary as reactivation of the disease may occur. During prolonged corticosteroid therapy, these patients should receive chemoprophylaxis.

Literature reports suggest an apparent association between use of corticosteroids and left ventricular free wall rupture after a recent myocardial infarction; therefore, therapy with corticosteroids should be used with great caution in these patients.

ORAL LIQUID

In patients on corticosteroid therapy subjected to unusual stress, increased dosage of rapidly acting corticosteroids before, during and after the stressful situation is indicated.

Corticosteroids may mask some signs of infection, and new infections may appear during their use. There may be decreased resistance and inability to localize infection when corticosteroids are used.

Prolonged use of corticosteroids may produce posterior subcapsular cataracts, glaucoma with possible damage to the optic nerves, and may enhance the establishment of secondary ocular infections due to fungi or viruses.

Average and large doses of hydrocortisone or cortisone can cause elevation of blood pressure, salt and water retention, and increased excretion of potassium. These effects are less likely to occur with the synthetic derivatives except when used in large doses. Dietary salt restriction and potassium supplementation may be necessary. All corticosteroids increase calcium excretion. **While on corticosteroid therapy patients should not be vaccinated against smallpox. Other immunization procedures should not be undertaken in patients who are on corticosteroids, especially on high doses, because of possible hazards of neurological complications and a lack of antibody response.**

The use of prednisolone in active tuberculosis should be restricted to those cases of fulminating or disseminated tuberculosis in which the corticosteroid is used for the management of the disease in conjunction with an appropriate antituberculous regimen.

If corticosteroids are indicated in patients with latent tuberculosis or tuberculin reactivity, close observation is necessary as reactivation of the disease may occur. During prolonged corticosteroid therapy these patients should receive chemoprophylaxis.

Persons who are on drugs which suppress the immune system are more susceptible to infections than healthy individuals. Chicken pox and measles, for example, can have a more serious or even fatal course in non-immune children or adults on corticosteroids. In such children or adults who have not had these diseases, particular care should be taken to avoid exposure. How the dose, route and duration of corticosteroid administration affects the risk of developing a disseminated infection is not known. The contribution of the underlying disease and/or prior corticosteroid treatment to the risk is also not known. If exposed to chicken pox, prophylaxis with varicella zoster immune globulin (VZIG) may be indicated. If exposed to measles, prophylaxis with pooled intramuscular immunoglobulin (IG) may be indicated. (See the respective package inserts for complete VZIG and IG prescribing information.) If chicken pox develops, treatment with antiviral agents may be considered.

OPHTHALMIC SOLUTION

NOT FOR INJECTION INTO THE EYE - FOR TOPICAL USE ONLY.

Employment of steroid medication in the treatment of herpes simplex, keratitis involving the stroma requires great caution; frequent slit lamp microscopy is mandatory.

Prolonged use may result in elevated intraocular pressure and/or glaucoma, damage to the optic nerve, defects in visual acuity and fields of vision, posterior subcapsular cataract formation, or may result in secondary ocular infections. Viral, bacterial and fungal infections of the cornea may be exacerbated by the application of steroids. In those diseases causing thinning of the cornea or sclera, perforation has been known to occur with the use of topical steroids. Acute purulent untreated infection of the eye may be masked or activity enhanced by the presence of steroid medication.

These drugs are not effective in mustard gas keratitis and Sjogren's keratoconjunctivitis.

If irritation persists or develops, the patient should be advised to discontinue use and consult prescribing physician.

PRECAUTIONS

INJECTION

This product, like many other steroid formulations, is sensitive to heat. Therefore, it should not be autoclaved when it is desirable to sterilize the exterior of the vial.

Following prolonged therapy, withdrawal of corticosteroids may result in symptoms of the corticosteroid withdrawal syndrome including fever, myalgia, arthralgia, and malaise. This may occur in patients even without evidence of adrenal insufficiency.

There is an enhanced effect of corticosteroids in patients with hypothyroidism and in those with cirrhosis.

Corticosteroids should be used cautiously in patients with ocular herpes simplex for fear of corneal perforation.

The lowest possible dose of corticosteroid should be used to control the condition under treatment, and when reduction in dosage is possible, the reduction must be gradual.

Psychic derangements may appear when corticosteroids are used, ranging from euphoria, insomnia, mood swings, personality changes, and severe depression to frank psychotic manifestations. Also, existing emotional instability or psychotic tendencies may be aggravated by corticosteroids.

Aspirin should be used cautiously in conjunction with corticosteroids in hypoprothrombinemia.

Steroids should be used with caution in nonspecific ulcerative colitis, if there is a probability of impending perforation, abscess, or other pyogenic infection, also in diverticulitis, fresh intestinal anastomoses, active or latent peptic ulcer, renal insufficiency, hypertension, osteoporosis, and myasthenia gravis. Signs of peritoneal irritation following gastrointestinal perforation in patients receiving large doses of corticosteroids may be minimal or absent. Fat embolism has been reported as a possible complication of hypercortisonism.

When large doses are given, some authorities advise that antacids be administered between meals to help to prevent peptic ulcer.

Growth and development of infants and children on prolonged corticosteroid therapy should be carefully followed.

Steroids may increase or decrease motility and number of spermatozoa in some patients.

Phenytoin, phenobarbital, ephedrine, and rifampin may enhance the metabolic clearance of corticosteroids, resulting in decreased blood levels and lessened physiologic activity, thus requiring adjustment in corticosteroid dosage.

The prothrombin time should be checked frequently in patients who are receiving corticosteroids and coumarin anticoagulants at the same time because of reports that corticosteroids have altered the response to these anticoagulants. Studies have shown that the usual effect produced by adding corticosteroids is inhibition of response to coumarins, although there have been some conflicting reports of potentiation not substantiated by studies.

When corticosteroids are administered concomitantly with potassium-depleting diuretics, patients should be observed closely for development of hypokalemia.

Intra-articular injection of a corticosteroid may produce systemic as well as local effects.

Appropriate examination of any joint fluid present is necessary to exclude a septic process.

A marked increase in pain accompanied by local swelling, further restriction of joint motion, fever, and malaise is suggestive of septic arthritis. If this complication occurs and the diagnosis of sepsis is confirmed, appropriate antimicrobial therapy should be instituted.

Injection of a steroid into an infected site is to be avoided.

Corticosteroids should not be injected into unstable joints.

Patients should be impressed strongly with the importance of not overusing joints in which symptomatic benefit has been obtained as long as the inflammatory process remains active.

Frequent intra-articular injection may result in damage to joint tissues.

The slower rate of absorption by intramuscular administration should be recognized.

GENERAL

Oral Liquid

Drug-Induced secondary adrenocortical insufficiency may be minimized by general reduction of dosage. This type of relative insufficiency may persist for months after discontinuation of therapy; therefore, in any situation of stress occurring during that period, hormone therapy should be reinstituted. Since mineralocorticoid secretion may be impaired, salt and/or a mineralocorticoid should be administered concurrently.

There is an enhanced effect of corticosteroids in patients with hypothyroidism and in those with cirrhosis.

Corticosteroids should be used cautiously in patients with ocular herpes simplex because of possible corneal perforation.

The lowest possible dose of corticosteroid should be used to control the condition under treatment, and when reduction in dosage is possible, the reduction should be gradual.

Psychic derangements may appear when corticosteroids are used, ranging from euphoria, insomnia, mood swings, personality changes, and severe depression, to frank psychotic manifestations. Also, existing emotional instability or psychotic tendencies may be aggravated by corticosteroids.

Aspirin should be used cautiously in conjunction with corticosteroids in hypoprothrombinemia.

Steroids should be used with caution in nonspecific ulcerative colitis, if there is a probability of impending perforation, abscess or other pyogenic infection; diverticulitis; fresh intestinal anastomoses; active or latent peptic ulcer; renal insufficiency; hypertension; osteoporosis; and myasthenia gravis.

Growth and development of infants and children on prolonged corticosteroid therapy should be carefully observed.

Although controlled clinical trials have shown corticosteroids to be effective in speeding the resolution of acute exacerbations of multiple sclerosis, they do not show that they affect the ultimate outcome or natural history of the disease. The studies do show that relatively high doses of corticosteroids are necessary to demonstrate a significant effect. (See DOSAGE AND ADMINISTRATION.)

Since complications of treatment with glucocorticoids are dependent on the size of the dose and the duration of treatment, a risk/benefit decision must be made in each individual case as to dose and duration of treatment and as to whether daily or intermittent therapy should be used.

Ophthalmic Solution

As fungal infections of the cornea are particularly prone to develop coincidentally with long-term local steroid applications, fungus invasion must be suspected in any persistent corneal ulceration where a steroid has been used or is in use.

Intraocular pressure should be checked frequently.

INFORMATION FOR THE PATIENT

Injection

Susceptible patients who are on immunosuppressant doses of corticosteroids should be warned to avoid exposure to chickenpox or measles. Patients should also be advised that if they are exposed, medical advice should be sought without delay.

Oral Liquid

Patients should be warned not to discontinue the use of Pediapred abruptly or without medical supervision, to advise any medical attendants that they are taking Pediapred and to seek medical advice at once should they develop fever or other signs of infection.

Persons who are on immunosuppressant doses of corticosteroids should be warned to avoid exposure to chicken pox or measles. Patients should also be advised that if they are exposed, medical advice should be sought without delay.

Ophthalmic Solution

Do not touch dropper tip to any surface as this may contaminate the solution.

PREGNANCY CATEGORY C

Oral Liquid

Prednisolone has been shown to be teratogenic in many species when given in doses equivalent to the human dose. There are no adequate and well controlled studies in pregnant women. Pediapred should be used during pregnancy only if the potential benefit justifies the potential risk to the fetus. Animal studies in which prednisolone has been given to pregnant mice, rats, and rabbits have yielded an increased incidence of cleft palate in the offspring.

Ophthalmic Solution

Animal reproductive studies have not been conducted with prednisolone sodium phosphate. It is also not known whether prednisolone sodium phosphate can cause fetal harm when administered to a pregnant woman or can affect reproductive capacity. Prednisolone sodium phosphate should be given to a pregnant woman only if clearly needed.

The effect of prednisolone sodium phosphate on the later growth, development and functional maturation of the child is unknown.

NURSING MOTHERS

Oral Liquid

Prednisolone is excreted in breast milk, but only to a small (less than 1% of the administered dose) and probably clinically insignificant extent. Caution should be exercised when Pediapred is administered to a nursing woman.

Ophthalmic Solution

It is not known whether this drug is excreted in human milk. Because many drugs are excreted in human milk, caution should be exercised when prednisolone sodium phosphate is administered to a nursing woman.

PEDIATRIC USE

Safety and effectiveness in children have not been established.

DRUG INTERACTIONS

ORAL LIQUID

Drugs such as barbiturates which induce hepatic microsomal drug metabolizing enzyme activity may enhance metabolism of prednisolone and require that the dosage of Pediapred be increased.

ADVERSE REACTIONS

INJECTION

Fluid and Electrolyte Disturbances: Sodium retention; fluid retention; congestive heart failure in susceptible patients; potassium loss; hypokalemic alkalosis; hypertension.
Musculoskeletal: Muscle weakness; steroid myopathy; loss of muscle mass; osteoporosis; vertebral compression fractures; aseptic necrosis of femoral and humeral heads; pathologic fracture of long bones; tendon rupture.
Gastrointestinal: Peptic ulcer with possible subsequent perforation and hemorrhage; perforation of the small and large bowel, particularly in patients with inflammatory bowel disease; pancreatitis; abdominal distention; ulcerative esophagitis.
Dermatologic: Impaired wound healing; thin fragile skin; petechiae and ecchymoses; erythema; increased sweating; may suppress reactions to skin tests; burning or tingling, especially in the perineal area (after IV injection); other cutaneous reactions, such as allergic dermatitis, urticaria, angioneurotic edema.
Neurologic: Convulsions; increased intracranial pressure with papilledema (pseudotumor cerebri) usually after treatment; vertigo; headache; psychic disturbances.
Endocrine: Menstrual irregularities; development of cushingoid state; suppression of growth in children; secondary adrenocortical and pituitary unresponsiveness, particularly in times of stress, as in trauma, surgery, or illness; decreased carbohydrate tolerance; manifestations of latent diabetes mellitus; increased requirements for insulin or oral hypoglycemic agents in diabetics; hirsutism.
Ophthalmic: Posterior subcapsular cataracts; increased intraocular pressure; glaucoma; exophthalmos.
Metabolic: Negative nitrogen balance due to protein catabolism.
Cardiovascular: Myocardial rupture following recent myocardial infarction (see WARNINGS).
Other: Anaphylactoid or hypersensitivity reactions; thromboembolism; weight gain; increased appetite; nausea; malaise.

The following *additional* adverse reactions are related to parenteral corticosteroid therapy:

Rare instances of blindness associated with intralesional therapy around the face and head; hyperpigmentation or hypopigmentation; subcutaneous and cutaneous atrophy; sterile abscess; postinjection flare (following intra-articular use); charcot-like arthropathy.

ORAL LIQUID

Fluid and Electrolyte Disturbances: Sodium retention; fluid retention; congestive heart failure in susceptible patients; potassium loss; hypokalemic alkalosis; hypertension.
Musculoskeletal: Muscle weakness; steroid myopathy; loss of muscle mass; osteoporosis; vertebral compression fractures; aseptic necrosis of femoral and humeral heads; pathologic fracture of long bones.
Gastrointestinal: Peptic ulcer with possible perforation and hemorrhage; pancreatitis; abdominal distention; ulcerative esophagitis.
Dermatologic: Impaired wound healing; thin fragile skin; petechiae and ecchymoses; facial erythema; increased sweating; may suppress reactions to skin tests.
Metabolic: Negative nitrogen balance due to protein catabolism.
Neurological: Convulsions; increased intracranial pressure with papilledema (pseudotumor cerebri) usually after treatment; vertigo; headache.
Endocrine: Menstrual irregularities; development of cushingoid state; secondary adrenocortical and pituitary unresponsiveness, particularly in times of stress, as in trauma, surgery or illness; suppression of growth in children; decreased carbohydrate tolerance; manifestations of latent diabetes mellitus; increased requirements for insulin or oral hypoglycemic agents in diabetes.
Ophthalmic: Posterior subcapsular cataracts; increased intraocular pressure; glaucoma; exophthalmos.

OPHTHALMIC SOLUTION

The following adverse reactions have been reported: glaucoma with optic nerve damage, visual acuity and field defects, posterior subcapsular cataract formation, secondary ocular infections from pathogens including herpes simplex and fungi, and perforation of the globe.

Rarely, filtering blebs have been reported when topical steroids have been used following cataract surgery.

Rarely, stinging or burning may occur.

DOSAGE AND ADMINISTRATION

INJECTION

For intravenous, intramuscular, intra-articular, intralesional, and soft tissue injection. DOSAGE REQUIREMENTS ARE VARIABLE AND MUST BE INDIVIDUALIZED ON THE BASIS OF THE DISEASE AND THE RESPONSE OF THE PATIENT.

Intravenous and Intramuscular Injection

Hydeltrasol injection can be given directly from the vial, or it can be added to sodium chloride injection or dextrose injection and given by intravenous drip.

Benzyl alcohol as a preservative has been associated with toxicity in premature infants. Solutions used for intravenous administration or further dilution of this product should be preservative-free when used in the neonate, especially the premature infant.

When it is mixed with an infusion solution, sterile precautions should be observed. Since infusion solutions generally do not contain preservatives, mixtures should be used within 24 hours.

The initial dosage varies from 4-60 mg a day depending on the disease being treated. In less severe diseases doses lower than 4 mg may suffice, while in severe diseases doses higher than 60 mg may be required. Usually the daily parenteral dose of Hydeltrasol injection is the same as the daily oral dose of prednisolone and the dosage interval is every 4-8 hours.

The initial dosage should be maintained or adjusted until the patient's response is satisfactory. If a satisfactory clinical response does not occur after a reasonable period of time, discontinue Hydeltrasol injection and transfer the patient to other therapy.

After a favorable initial response, the proper maintenance dosage should be determined by decreasing the initial dosage in small amounts to the lowest dosage that maintains an adequate clinical response.

Patients should be observed closely for signs that might require dosage adjustment, including changes in clinical status resulting from remissions or exacerbations of the disease, individual drug responsiveness, and the effect of stress (*e.g.,* surgery, infection, trauma). During stress it may be necessary to increase dosage temporarily.

If the drug is to be stopped after more than a few days of treatment, it usually should be withdrawn gradually.

Intra-articular, Intralesional, and Soft Tissue Injection

Intra-articular, intralesional, and soft tissue injections are generally employed when the affected joints or areas are limited to 1 or 2 sites. Dosage and frequency of injection vary depending on the condition being treated and the site of injection. The usual dose is from 2-30 mg. The frequency usually ranges from once every 3-5 days to once every 2-3 weeks. Frequent intra-articular injection may result in damage to joint tissues. Some of the usual single doses are shown in TABLE 1.

TABLE 1

	Doses	
Site of Injection	**Amount of Injection (ml)**	**Amount of Prednisolone Phosphate (mg)**
Large joints (*e.g.,* knee)	0.5 to 1	10-20
Small joints (*e.g.,* interphalangeal, temporomandibular)	0.2-0.25	4-5
Bursae	0.5-0.75	10-15
Tendon sheaths	0.1-0.25	2-5
Soft tissue infiltration	0.5-1.5	10-30
Ganglia	0.25-0.5	5-10

Hydeltrasol injection is particularly recommended for use in conjunction with one of the less soluble, longer-acting steroids, such as Hydeltra- T.B.A. (prednisolone tebutate) suspension or Hydrocortone Acetate (hydrocortisone acetate) sterile suspension, available for intra-articular and soft tissue injection.

P

ORAL LIQUID

The initial dosage of Pediapred may vary from 5-60 ml (5-60 mg prednisolone base) per day depending on the specific disease entity being treated. In situations of less severity lower doses will generally suffice while in selected patients higher initial doses may be required. The initial dosage should be maintained or adjusted until a satisfactory response is noted. If after a reasonable period of time there is a lack of satisfactory clinical response, Pediapred should be discontinued and the patient transferred to other appropriate therapy. **IT SHOULD BE EMPHASIZED THAT DOSAGE REQUIREMENTS ARE VARIABLE AND MUST BE INDIVIDUALIZED ON THE BASIS OF THE DISEASE UNDER TREATMENT AND THE RESPONSE OF THE PATIENT.** After a favorable response is noted, the proper maintenance dosage should be determined by decreasing the initial drug dosage in small decrements at appropriate time intervals until the lowest dosage which will maintain an adequate clinical response is reached. It should be kept in mind that constant monitoring is needed in regard to drug dosage. Included in the situations which may make dosage adjustments necessary are changes in clinical status secondary to remissions or exacerbations in the disease process, the patient's individual drug responsiveness, and the effect of patient exposure to stressful situations not directly related to the disease entity under treatment; in this latter situation it may be necessary to increase the dosage of Pediapred for a period of time consistent with the patient's condition. If after long term therapy the drug is to be stopped, it is recommended that it be withdrawn gradually rather than abruptly.

In the treatment of acute exacerbations of multiple sclerosis daily doses of 200 mg of prednisolone for a week followed by 80 mg every other day or 4-8 mg dexamethasone every other day for 1 month have been shown to be effective.

For the purpose of comparison, the following is the equivalent milligram dosage of the various glucocorticoids: cortisone, 25; hydrocortisone, 20; prednisolone, 5; prednisone, 5; methylprednisolone, 4; triamcinolone, 4; paramethasone, 2; betamethasone, 0.75; dexamethasone, 0.75. These dose relationships apply only to oral or intravenous administration of these compounds. When these substances or their derivatives are injected intramuscularly or into joint spaces, their relative properties may be greatly altered.

OPHTHALMIC SOLUTION

Depending on the severity of inflammation, instill 1 or 2 drops of solution into the conjunctival sac up to every hour during the day and every 2 hours during the night as necessary as initial therapy.

When a favorable response is observed, reduce dosage to 1 drop every 4 hours.

Later, further reduction in dosage to 1 drop 3-4 times daily may suffice to control symptoms.

The duration of treatment will vary with the type of lesion and may extend from a few days to several weeks, according to therapeutic response. Relapses, more common in chronic active lesions than in self- limiting conditions, usually respond to retreatment.

HOW SUPPLIED

INJECTION

No. 7577X — Injection Hydeltrasol, 20 mg prednisolone phosphate equivalent per ml, is a clear, colorless to slightly yellow solution, and is supplied as follows: 2 ml vials; 5 ml vials; 20 mg/ml 5 ml vial.

Storage: Sensitive to heat. Do not autoclave. Protect from light. Store container in carton until contents have been used.

ORAL LIQUID

Pediapred oral liquid is a colorless to light straw colored solution containing 6.7 mg prednisolone sodium phosphate (5 mg prednisolone base) per 5 ml (teaspoonful).

Store at 4-25°C (39-77°F). May be refrigerated. Keep tightly closed and out of the reach of children.

OPHTHALMIC SOLUTION

STORE AT CONTROLLED ROOM TEMPERATURE, 59-86°F (15-30°C). Protect from light. Keep out of the reach of children.

PRODUCT LISTING - RATED THERAPEUTICALLY EQUIVALENT

Liquid - Oral - Sodium Phosphate 5 mg/5 ml

120 ml	$25.38	GENERIC, Morton Grove Pharmaceuticals Inc	60432-0089-04

Liquid - Oral - Sodium Phosphate 15 mg/5 ml

240 ml	$101.35	GENERIC, Ascent Pediatrics Inc	59439-0455-02

Solution - Injectable - Sodium Phosphate 20 mg/ml

2 ml	$16.25	HYDELTRASOL, Merck & Company Inc	00006-7577-02
5 ml	$35.64	HYDELTRASOL, Merck & Company Inc	00006-7577-03
10 ml	$7.50	GENERIC, Dunhall Pharmaceuticals Inc	00217-8410-08
10 ml	$12.44	GENERIC, Hyrex Pharmaceuticals	00314-0696-70

Solution - Ophthalmic - Sodium Phosphate 0.125%

5 ml	$5.00	GENERIC, Akorn Inc	17478-0218-10
5 ml	$17.68	INFLAMASE MILD, Ciba Vision Ophthalmics	00058-2875-05
5 ml	$18.56	INFLAMASE MILD, Ciba Vision Ophthalmics	58768-0875-05
10 ml	$27.29	INFLAMASE MILD, Ciba Vision Ophthalmics	58768-0875-10

Solution - Ophthalmic - Sodium Phosphate 1%

5 ml	$5.50	GENERIC, Raway Pharmacal Inc	00686-0715-02
5 ml	$7.75	GENERIC, Fougera	00168-0253-03
5 ml	$7.95	GENERIC, Ivax Corporation	00182-7048-62
5 ml	$11.87	GENERIC, Allscripts Pharmaceutical Company	54569-1225-00
5 ml	$13.65	GENERIC, Bausch and Lomb	24208-0715-02
5 ml	$16.18	GENERIC, Akorn Inc	17478-0219-10
5 ml	$18.38	INFLAMASE FORTE, Ciba Vision Ophthalmics	58768-0877-05
5 ml	$18.69	GENERIC, Ocusoft	54799-0550-10
10 ml	$20.09	GENERIC, Bausch and Lomb	24208-0715-10
10 ml	$27.03	INFLAMASE FORTE, Ciba Vision Ophthalmics	58768-0877-10
15 ml	$7.00	GENERIC, Raway Pharmacal Inc	00686-0715-06
15 ml	$9.40	GENERIC, Fougera	00168-0253-15
15 ml	$27.63	GENERIC, Bausch and Lomb	24208-0715-06
15 ml	$32.90	GENERIC, Akorn Inc	17478-0219-12
15 ml	$37.18	INFLAMASE FORTE, Ciba Vision Ophthalmics	58768-0877-15

PRODUCT LISTING - EQUIVALENTS NOT AVAILABLE

Liquid - Oral - Sodium Phosphate 5 mg/5 ml

120 ml	$15.49	PEDIAPRED, Celltech Pharmaceuticals Inc	00585-2250-01
120 ml	$19.79	PEDIAPRED, Southwood Pharmaceuticals Inc	58016-4144-01
120 ml	$21.32	PEDIAPRED, Allscripts Pharmaceutical Company	54569-1335-00
120 ml	$25.68	PEDIAPRED, Physicians Total Care	54868-1720-00
120 ml	$31.37	PEDIAPRED, Celltech Pharmaceuticals Inc	53014-0250-01

Liquid - Oral - Sodium Phosphate 15 mg/5 ml

240 ml	$61.50	GENERIC, We Pharmaceuticals Inc	59196-0012-24

Solution - Ophthalmic - Sodium Phosphate 0.125%

5 ml	$1.73	OCU-PRED, Ocumed Inc	51944-4435-05
5 ml	$11.21	GENERIC, Watson/Schein Pharmaceuticals Inc	58016-6031-01
15 ml	$2.48	OCU-PRED, Ocumed Inc	51944-4435-02

Solution - Ophthalmic - Sodium Phosphate 1%

5 ml	$1.72	GENERIC, Ocumed Inc	51944-4445-05
5 ml	$8.25	GENERIC, Prescript Pharmaceuticals	00247-0046-05
10 ml	$10.61	GENERIC, Steris Laboratories Inc	00402-0857-10
10 ml	$13.15	GENERIC, Prescript Pharmaceuticals	00247-0046-10
15 ml	$2.32	GENERIC, Ocumed Inc	51944-4445-02
15 ml	$18.05	GENERIC, Prescript Pharmaceuticals	00247-0046-15

Prednisone *(002109)*

For related information, see the comparative table section in Appendix A.

Categories: Adrenocortical insufficiency; Anemia, acquired hemolytic; Anemia, congenital hypoplastic; Ankylosing spondylitis; Arthritis, gouty; Arthritis, osteoarthritis; Arthritis, psoriatic; Arthritis, rheumatoid; Asthma; Berylliosis; Bursitis; Carditis, rheumatic; Chorioretinitis; Choroiditis; Colitis, ulcerative; Conjunctivitis, allergic; Crohn's disease; Dermatitis herpetiformis; Dermatitis, atopic; Dermatitis, contact; Dermatitis, exfoliative; Dermatitis, seborrheic; Dermatomyositis, systemic; Epicondylitis; Erythema multiforme; Erythroblastopenia; Herpes zoster ophthalmicus; Hypercalcemia, secondary to neoplasia; Hyperplasia, congenital adrenal; Hypersensitivity reactions; Iridocyclitis; Iritis; Keratitis, ophthalmic; Leukemia; Loffler's syndrome; Lupus erythematosus, systemic; Lymphoma; Meningitis, tuberculous; Mycosis fungoides; Neuritis, optic; Ophthalmia, sympathetic; Pemphigus; Pneumonitis, aspiration; Polymyositis; Proteinuria; Psoriasis; Purpura, idiopathic thrombocytopenic; Rhinitis, perennial allergic; Rhinitis, seasonal allergic; Sarcoidosis; Serum sickness; Stevens-Johnson syndrome; Synovitis, secondary to osteoarthritis; Tenosynovitis; Thrombocytopenia; Thyroiditis, nonsuppurative; Trichinosis; Tuberculosis, disseminated; Tuberculosis, fulminating; Ulcer, allergic corneal marginal; Uveitis; FDA Approved 1955 Sep; Pregnancy Category B

Drug Classes: Corticosteroids

Brand Names: Cordrol; Cortan; Delta-Dome; **Deltasone**; Econosone; Fernisone; Liquid Pred; Meticorten; Orasone; Panasol; Prednicen-M; Prednicot; Sterapred

Foreign Brand Availability: Apo-Prednisone (Canada; New-Zealand); Cortancyl (France); Cutason (Germany); Dacorten (Spain); Decortin (Bulgaria; Germany); Decortisyl (England; Ireland; Philippines); Delcortin (Denmark); Dellacort A (Indonesia); Deltacortene (Italy); Deltacortone (Japan); Deltison (Sweden); Deltisona (Argentina); Di-Adreson (Japan); Drazone (Philippines); Encorton (Poland); Hostacortin (Indonesia); Me-Korti (Finland); Nisona (Peru); Panafcort (Australia; South-Africa); Pehacort (Indonesia); Prednicorm (Germany); Prednicort (Belgium); Prednidib (Mexico); Prednitone (Israel); Pulmison (South-Africa); Sone (Australia); Steerometz (Philippines); Ultracorten (Germany); Winpred (Canada)

Cost of Therapy: $1.13 (Asthma; Deltasone; 5 mg; 1 tablet/day; 30 day supply)
$0.33 (Asthma; Generic Tablets; 5 mg; 1 tablet/day; 30 day supply)

HCFA JCODE(S): J7506 any dose, 100 tabl ORAL

DESCRIPTION

Deltasone tablets contain prednisone which is a glucocorticoid. Glucocorticoids are adrenocortical steroids, both naturally occurring and synthetic, which are readily absorbed from the gastrointestinal tract. Prednisone is a white to practically white, odorless, crystalline powder. It is very slightly soluble in water; slightly soluble in alcohol, in chloroform, in dioxane, and in methanol.

The chemical name for prednisone is pregna-1,4-diene-3,11,20-trione,17,21-dihydroxy- and its molecular weight is 358.43.

Deltasone are available in 5 strengths: 2.5, 5, 10, 20, and 50 mg. *Inactive Ingredients:* **2.5 mg:** Calcium stearate, corn starch, erythrosine sodium, lactose, mineral oil, sorbic acid and sucrose. **5 mg:** Calcium stearate, corn starch, lactose, mineral oil, sorbic acid and sucrose. **10 mg:** Calcium stearate, corn starch, lactose, sorbic acid and sucrose. **20 mg:** Calcium stearate, corn starch, FD&C yellow no. 6, lactose, sorbic acid and sucrose. **50 mg:** Corn starch, lactose, magnesium stearate, sorbic acid, sucrose, and talc.

CLINICAL PHARMACOLOGY

Naturally occurring glucocorticoids (hydrocortisone and cortisone), which also have salt-retaining properties, are used as replacement therapy in adrenocortical deficiency states. Their synthetic analogs are primarily used for their potent anti-inflammatory effects in disorders of many organ systems.

Glucocorticoids cause profound and varied metabolic effects. In addition, they modify the body's immune responses to diverse stimuli.

INDICATIONS AND USAGE

Prednisone tablets are indicated in the following conditions:

1. ***Endocrine Disorders:***
   Primary or secondary adrenocortical insufficiency (hydrocortisone or cortisone is the first choice; synthetic analogs may be used in conjunction with mineralocorticoids where applicable; in infancy mineralocorticoid supplementation is of particular importance).
   Congenital adrenal hyperplasia.
   Hypercalcemia associated with cancer.
   Nonsuppurative thyroiditis.
2. ***Rheumatic Disorders:*** As adjunctive therapy for short-term administration (to tide the patient over an acute episode or exacerbation) in:
   Psoriatic arthritis.
   Rheumatoid arthritis, including juvenile rheumatoid arthritis (selected cases may require low-dose maintenance therapy).
   Ankylosing spondylitis.
   Acute and subacute bursitis.
   Acute nonspecific tenosynovitis.
   Acute gouty arthritis.
   Post-traumatic osteoarthritis.
   Synovitis of osteoarthritis.
   Epicondylitis.
3. ***Collagen Diseases:*** During an exacerbation or as maintenance therapy in selected cases of:
   Systemic lupus erythematosus.
   Systemic dermatomyositis (polymyositis).
   Acute rheumatic carditis.
4. ***Dermatological Diseases:***
   Pemphigus.
   Bullous dermatitis herpetiformis.
   Severe erythema muliforme (Stevens-Johnson syndrome).
   Exfoliative dermatitis.
   Mycosis fungoides.
   Severe psoriasis.
   Severe seborrheic dermatitis.
5. ***Allergic States:*** Control of severe or incapacitating allergic conditions intractable to adequate trials of conventional treatment:
   Seasonal or perennial allergic rhinitis.
   Bronchial asthma.
   Contact dermatitis.
   Atopic dermatitis.
   Serum sickness.
   Drug hypersensitivity reactions.
6. ***Ophthalmic Diseases:*** Severe acute and chronic allergic and inflammatory processes involving the eye and its adnexa such as:
   Allergic corneal marginal ulcers.
   Herpes zoster ophthalmicus.
   Anterior segment inflammation.
   Diffuse posterior uveitis and choroiditis.
   Sympathetic ophthalmia.
   Allergic conjunctivitis.
   Keratitis.
   Chorioretinitis.
   Optic neuritis.
   Iritis and iridocyclitis.
7. ***Respiratory Diseases:***
   Symptomatic sarcoidosis.
   Loeffler's syndrome not manageable by other means.
   Berylliosis.
   Fulminating or disseminated pulmonary tuberculosis when used concurrently with appropriate antituberculous chemotherapy.
   Aspiration pneumonitis.
8. ***Hematologic Disorders:***
   Idiopathic thrombocytopenic purpura in adults.
   Secondary thrombocytopenia in adults.
   Acquired (autoimmune) hemolytic anemia.
   Erythroblastopenia (RBC anemia).
   Congenital (erythroid) hypoplastic anemia.
9. ***Neoplastic Diseases:*** For palliative management of:
   Leukemias and lymphomas in adults.
   Acute leukemia of childhood.
10. ***Edematous States:***
    To induce a diuresis or remission of proteinuria in the nephrotic syndrome, without uremia, of the idiopathic type or that due to lupus erythematosus.
11. ***Gastrointestinal Diseases:*** To tide the patient over a critical period of the disease in:
    Ulcerative colitis.
    Regional enteritis.
12. ***Nervous System:***
    Acute exacerbations of multiple sclerosis.
13. ***Miscellaneous:***
    Tuberculous meningitis with subarachnoid block or impending block when used concurrently with appropriate antituberculous chemotherapy.
    Trichinosis with neurologic or myocardial involvement.

CONTRAINDICATIONS

Systemic fungal infections and known hypersensitivity to components.

WARNINGS

In patients on corticosteroid therapy subjected to unusual stress, increased dosage of rapidly acting corticosteroids before, during, and after the stressful situation is indicated.

Corticosteroids may mask some signs of infection, and new infections may appear during their use. Infections with any pathogen including viral, bacterial, fungal, protozoan or helminthic infections, in any location of the body, may be associated with the use of corticosteroids alone or in combination with other immunosuppressive agents that affect cellular immunity, humoral immunity, or neutrophil function.[1]

These infections may be mild, but can be severe and at times fatal. With increasing doses of corticosteroids, the rate of occurrence of infectious complications increases.[2] There may be decreased resistance and inability to localize infection when corticosteroids are used.

Prolonged use of corticosteroids may produce posterior subcapsular cataracts, glaucoma with possible damage to the optic nerves, and may enhance the establishment of secondary ocular infections due to fungi or viruses.

Use in Pregnancy: Since adequate human reproduction studies have not been done with corticosteroids, the use of these drugs in pregnancy, nursing mothers or women of child-bearing potential requires that the possible benefits of the drug be weighed against the potential hazards to the mother and embryo or fetus. Infants born of mothers who have received substantial doses of corticosteroids during pregnancy should be carefully observed for signs of hypoadrenalism.

Average and large doses of hydrocortisone or cortisone can cause elevation of blood pressure, salt and water retention, and increased excretion of potassium. These effects are less likely to occur with the synthetic derivatives except when used in large doses. Dietary salt restriction and potassium supplementation may be necessary. All corticosteroids increase calcium excretion.

Administration of live or live, attenuated vaccines is contraindicated in patients receiving immunosuppressive doses of corticosteroids. Killed or inactivated vaccines may be administered to patients receiving immunosuppressive doses of corticosteroids; however, the response to such vaccines may be diminished. Indicated immunization procedures may be undertaken in patients receiving nonimmunosuppressive doses of corticosteroids.

The use of prednisone tablets in active tuberculosis should be restricted to those cases of fulminating or disseminated tuberculosis in which the corticosteroid is used for the management of the disease in conjunction with an appropriate anti-tuberculous regimen.

If corticosteroids are indicated in patients with latent tuberculosis or tuberculin reactivity, close observation is necessary as reactivation of the disease may occur. During prolonged corticosteroid therapy, these patients should receive chemoprophylaxis.

Persons who are on drugs which suppress the immune system are more susceptible to infections than healthy individuals. Chicken pox and measles, for example, can have a more serious or even fatal course in non-immune children or adults on corticosteroids. In such children or adults who have not had these diseases, particular care should be taken to avoid exposure. How the dose, route and duration of corticosteroid administration affects the risk of developing a disseminated infection is not known. The contribution of the underlying disease and/or prior corticosteroid treatment to the risk is also not known. If exposed to chicken pox, prophylaxis with varicella zoster immune globulin (VZIG) may be indicated. If exposed to measles, prophylaxis with pooled intramuscular immunoglobulin (IG) may be indicated. (See the respective monographs for complete VZIG and IG prescribing information.) If chicken pox develops, treatment with antiviral agents may be considered. Similarly, corticosteroids should be used with great care in patients with known or suspected Strongyloides (threadworm) infestation. In such patients, corticosteroids-induced immunosuppression may lead to Strongyloides hyperinfection and dissemination with wide-spread larval migration, often accompanied by severe enterocolitis and potentially fatal gram-negative septicemia.

PRECAUTIONS

GENERAL

Drug-induced secondary adrenocortical insufficiency may be minimized by gradual reduction of dosage. This type of relative insufficiency may persist for months after discontinuation of therapy; therefore, in any situation of stress occurring during that period, hormone therapy should be reinstituted. Since mineralocorticoid secretion may be impaired, salt and/or a mineralocorticoid should be administered concurrently.

There is an enhanced effect of corticosteroids on patients with hypothyroidism and in those with cirrhosis.

Corticosteroids should be used cautiously in patients with ocular herpes simplex because of possible corneal perforation.

The lowest possible dose of corticosteroid should be used to control the condition under treatment, and when reduction in dosage is possible, the reduction should be gradual.

Psychic derangements may appear when corticosteroids are used, ranging from euphoria, insomnia, mood swings, personality changes, and severe depression, to frank psychotic manifestations. Also, existing emotional instability or psychotic tendencies may be aggravated by corticosteroids.

Steroids should be used with caution in nonspecific ulcerative colitis, if there is a probability of impending perforation, abscess or other pyogenic infection; diverticulitis; fresh intestinal anastomoses; active or latent peptic ulcer; renal insufficiency; hypertension; osteoporosis; and myasthenia gravis.

Growth and development of infants and children on prolonged corticosteroid therapy should be carefully observed.

Kaposi's sarcoma has been reported to occur in patients receiving corticosteroid therapy. Discontinuation of corticosteroids may result in clinical remission.

Although controlled clinical trials have shown corticosteroids to be effective in speeding the resolution of acute exacerbations of multiple sclerosis, they do not show that corticosteroids affect the ultimate outcome or natural history of the disease. The studies do show that relatively high doses of corticosteroids are necessary to demonstrate a significant effect. (See DOSAGE AND ADMINISTRATION.)

Since complications of treatment with glucocorticoids are dependent on the size of the dose and the duration of treatment, a risk/benefit decision must be made in each individual case as to dose and duration of treatment and as to whether daily or intermittent therapy should be used.

Convulsions have been reported with concurrent use of methylprednisolone and cyclosporin. Since concurrent use of these agents results in a mutual inhibition of metabolism, it is possible that adverse events associated with the individual use of either drug may be more apt to occur.

INFORMATION FOR THE PATIENT

Persons who are on immunosuppressant doses of corticosteroids should be warned to avoid exposure to chicken pox or measles. Patients should also be advised that if they are exposed, medical advice should be sought without delay.

DRUG INTERACTIONS

The pharmacokinetic interactions listed below are potentially clinically important. Drugs that induce hepatic enzymes such as phenobarbital, phenytoin and rifampin may increase the clearance of corticosteroids and may require increases in corticosteroid dose to achieve the desired response. Drugs such as troleandomycin and ketoconazole may inhibit the metabolism of corticosteroids and thus decrease their clearance. Therefore, the dose of corticosteroid should be titrated to avoid steroid toxicity. Corticosteroids may increase the clearance of chronic high dose aspirin. This could lead to decreased salicylate serum levels or increase the risk of salicylate toxicity when corticosteroid is withdrawn. Aspirin should be used cautiously in conjunction with corticosteroids in patients suffering from hypoprothrombinemia. The effect of corticosteroids on oral anticoagulants is variable. There are reports of enhanced as well as diminished effects of anticoagulants when given concurrently with corticosteroids. Therefore, coagulation indices should be monitored to maintain the desired anticoagulant effect.

ADVERSE REACTIONS

Fluid and Electrolyte Disturbances: Sodium retention, fluid retention, congestive heart failure in susceptible patients, potassium loss, hypokalemic alkalosis, and hypertension.

Musculoskeletal: Muscle weakness, steriod myopathy, loss of muscle mass, osteoporosis, tendon rupture, particularly of the Achilles tendon, vertebral compression fractures, aseptic necrosis of femoral and humeral heads, and pathologic fracture of long bones.

Gastrointestinal: Peptic ulcer with possible perforation and hemorrhage; pancreatitis; abdominal distention; ulcerative esophagitis; Increases in alanine transaminase (ALT, SGPT), aspartate transaminase (AST, SGOT) and alkaline phosphatase have been observed following corticosteroid treatment. These changes are usually small, not associated with any clinical syndrome and are reversible upon discontinuation.

Dermatologic: Impaired wound healing, thin fragile skin, petechiae and ecchymoses, facial erythema, increased sweating, and may suppress reactions to skin tests.

Metabolic: Negative nitrogen balance due to protein catabolism.

Neurological: Increased intracranial pressure with papilledema (pseudo-tumor cerebri) usually after treatment, convulsions, vertigo, and headache.

Endocrine: Menstrual irregularities; development of Cushingoid state; secondary adrenocortical and pituitary unresponsiveness, particularly in times of stress, as in trauma, surgery or illness; suppression of growth of children; decreased carbohydrate tolerance; manifestations of latent diabetes mellitus; increased requirements for insulin or oral hypoglycemic agents in diabetics.

Ophthalmic: Posterior subcapsular cataracts, increased intraocular pressure, glaucoma, and exophthalmos.

Additional Reactions: Urticaria and other allergic, anaphylactic or hypersensitivity reactions.

P

DOSAGE AND ADMINISTRATION

The initial dosage of prednisone tablets may vary from 5-60 mg of prednisone per day depending on the specific disease entity being treated. In situations of less severity lower doses will generally suffice while in selected patients higher initial doses may be required. The initial dosage should be maintained or adjusted until a satisfactory response is noted. If after a reasonable period of time there is a lack of satisfactory clinical response, prednisone should be discontinued and the patient transferred to other appropriate therapy. **IT SHOULD BE EMPHASIZED THAT DOSAGE REQUIREMENTS ARE VARIABLE AND MUST BE INDIVIDUALIZED ON THE BASIS OF THE DISEASE UNDER TREATMENT AND THE RESPONSE OF THE PATIENT.** After a favorable response is noted, the proper maintenance dosage should be determined by decreasing the initial drug dosage in small decrements at appropriate time intervals until the lowest dosage which will maintain an adequate clinical response is reached. It should be kept in mind that constant monitoring is needed in regard to drug dosage. Included in the situations which may make dosage adjustments necessary are changes in clinical status secondary to remissions or exacerbations in the disease process, the patient's individual drug responsiveness, and the effect of patient exposure to stressful situations not directly related to the disease entity under treatment; in this latter situation it may be necessary to increase the dosage of prednisone for a period of time consistent with the patient's condition. If after long-term therapy the drug is to be stopped, it is recommended that it be withdrawn gradually rather than abruptly.

MULTIPLE SCLEROSIS

In the treatment of acute exacerbations of multiple sclerosis daily doses of 200 mg of prednisolone for a week followed by 80 mg every other day for 1 month have been shown to be effective. (Dosage range is the same for prednisone and prednisolone.)

ADT (ALTERNATE DAY THERAPY)

ADT is a corticosteroid dosing regimen in which twice the usual daily dose of corticoid is administered every other morning. The purpose of this mode of therapy is to provide the patient requiring long-term pharmacologic dose treatment with the beneficial effects of corticoids while minimizing certain undesirable effects, including pituitary-adrenal suppression, the Cushingoid state, corticoid withdrawal symptoms, and growth suppression in children.

The rationale for this treatment schedule is based on two major premises: (a) the anti-inflammatory or therapeutic effect of corticoids persists longer than their physical presence and metabolic effects and (b) administration of the corticosteroid every other morning allows for re-establishment of more nearly normal hypothalamic-pituitary-adrenal (HPA) activity on the off-steroid day.

A brief review of the HPA physiology may be helpful in understanding this rationale. Acting primarily through the hypothalamus a fall in free cortisol stimulates the pituitary gland to produce increasing amounts of corticotropin (ACTH) while a rise in free cortisol inhibits ACTH secretion. Normally the HPA system is characterized by diurnal (circadian) rhythm. Serum levels of ACTH rise from a low point about 10 pm to a peak level about 6 am. Increasing levels of ACTH stimulate adrenocortical activity resulting in a rise in plasma cortisol with maximal levels occurring between 2 am and 8 am. This rise in cortisol dampens ACTH production and in turn adrenocortical activity. There is a gradual fall in plasma corticoids during the day with lowest levels occurring about midnight.

The diurnal rhythm of the HPA axis is lost in Cushing's disease, a syndrome of adrenocortical hyperfunction characterized by obesity with centripetal fat distribution, thinning of the skin with easy bruisability, muscle wasting with weakness, hypertension, latent diabetes, osteoporosis, electrolyte imbalance, etc. The same clinical findings of hyperadrenocorticism may be noted during long-term pharmacologic dose corticoid therapy administered in conventional daily divided doses. It would appear, then, that a disturbance in the diurnal cycle with maintenance of elevated corticoid values during the night may play a significant role in the development of undesirable corticoid effects. Escape from these constantly elevated plasma levels for even short periods of time may be instrumental in protecting against undesirable pharmacologic effects.

During conventional pharmacologic dose corticosteroid therapy, ACTH production is inhibited with subsequent suppression of cortisol production by the adrenal cortex. Recovery time for normal HPA activity is variable depending upon the dose and duration of treatment. During this time the patient is vulnerable to any stressful situation. Although it has been shown that there is considerably less adrenal suppression following a single morning dose of prednisolone (10 mg) as opposed to a quarter of that dose administered every 6 hours, there is evidence that some suppressive effect on adrenal activity may be carried over into the following day when pharmacologic doses are used. Further, it has been shown that a single dose of certain corticosteroids will produce adrenocortical suppression for 2 or more days. Other corticoids, including methylprednisolone, hydrocortisone, prednisone, and prednisolone, are considered to be short acting (producing adrenocortical suppression for 1¼ to 1½ days following a single dose) and thus are recommended for alternate day therapy.

The following should be kept in mind when considering alternate day therapy:

1. Basic principles and indications for corticosteroid therapy should apply. The benefits of ADT should not encourage the indiscriminate use of steroids.
2. ADT is a therapeutic technique primarily designed for patients in whom long-term pharmacologic corticoid therapy is anticipated.
3. In less severe disease processes in which corticoid therapy is indicated, it may be possible to initiate treatment with ADT. More severe disease states usually will require daily divided high dose therapy for initial control of the disease process. The initial suppressive dose level should be continued until satisfactory clinical response is obtained, usually 4-10 days in the case of many allergic and collagen diseases. It is important to keep the period of initial suppressive dose as brief as possible particularly when subsequent use of alternate day therapy is intended.
4. Once control has been established, two courses are available: (a) change to ADT and then gradually reduce the amount of corticoid given every other day **or** (b) following control of the disease process reduce the daily dose of corticoid to the lowest effective level as rapidly as possible and then change over to an alternate day schedule. Theoretically, course (a) may be preferable.
5. Because of the advantages of ADT, it may be desirable to try patients on this form of therapy who have been on daily corticoids for long periods of time (*e.g.,* patients with rheumatoid arthritis). Since these patients may already have a suppressed HPA axis, establishing them on ADT may be difficult and not always successful. However, it is recommended that regular attempts be made to change them over. It may be helpful to triple or even quadruple the daily maintenance dose and administer this every other day rather than just doubling the daily dose if difficulty is encountered. Once the patient is again controlled, an attempt should be made to reduce this dose to a minimum.
6. As indicated above, certain corticosteroids, because of their prolonged suppressive effect on adrenal activity, are not recommended for alternate day therapy (*e.g.,* dexamethasone and betamethasone).
7. The maximal activity of the adrenal cortex is between 2 am and 8 am, and it is minimal between 4 pm and midnight. Exogenous corticosteroids suppress adrenocortical activity the least, when given at the time of maximal activity (am).
8. In using ADT it is important, as in all therapeutic situations, to individualize and tailor the therapy to each patient. Complete control of symptoms will not be possible in all patients. An explanation of the benefits of ADT will help the patient to understand and tolerate the possible flare-up in symptoms which may occur in the latter part of the off-steroid day. Other symptomatic therapy may be added or increased at this time if needed.
9. In the event of an acute flare-up of the disease process, it may be necessary to return to a full suppressive daily divided corticoid dose for control. Once control is again established alternate day therapy may be re-instituted.
10. Although many of the undesirable features of corticosteroid therapy can be minimized by ADT, as in any therapeutic situation, the physician must carefully weigh the benefit-risk ratio for each patient in whom corticoid therapy is being considered.

HOW SUPPLIED

Deltasone tablets are available as:

2.5 mg: Pink, round, scored, imprinted "Deltasone 2.5"

5 mg: White, round, scored, imprinted "Delatsone 5"

10 mg: White, round, scored, imprinted "Delatsone 10"

20 mg: Peach, round, scored, imprinted "Delatsone 20")
50 mg: White, round, scored, imprinted "Delatsone 50")
Storage: Store at controlled room temperature 20-25°C (68-77°F).

PRODUCT LISTING - RATED THERAPEUTICALLY EQUIVALENT

Solution - Oral - 5 mg/5 ml

5 ml x 40	$36.72	GENERIC, Roxane Laboratories Inc	00054-8722-16
500 ml	$74.97	GENERIC, Roxane Laboratories Inc	00054-3722-63

Tablet - Oral - 1 mg

100's	$3.16	GENERIC, Caremark Inc	00339-5775-12
100's	$17.65	GENERIC, Roxane Laboratories Inc	00054-4741-25
100's	$20.70	METICORTEN, Schering Corporation	00085-0843-03
100's	$21.18	GENERIC, Roxane Laboratories Inc	00054-8739-25

Tablet - Oral - 2.5 mg

100's	$5.02	GENERIC, Roxane Laboratories Inc	00054-4742-25
100's	$5.13	DELTASONE, Pharmacia Corporation	00009-0032-01
100's	$8.19	GENERIC, Roxane Laboratories Inc	00054-8740-25

Tablet - Oral - 5 mg

15's	$1.05	GENERIC, Heartland Healthcare Services	61392-0408-15
21's	$3.05	DELTASONE, Pharmacia and Upjohn	00009-0045-04
21's	$3.90	GENERIC, Major Pharmaceuticals Inc	00904-2157-19
21's	$3.95	GENERIC, Vintage Pharmaceuticals Inc	00254-5094-13
21's	$5.40	GENERIC, Qualitest Products Inc	00603-5332-15
21's	$6.25	GENERIC, Merz Pharmaceuticals	00259-0284-01
21's	$6.95	GENERIC, Merz Pharmaceuticals	00259-0390-21
25's	$1.60	GENERIC, Udl Laboratories Inc	51079-0032-19
30's	$1.95	GENERIC, Major Pharmaceuticals Inc	00904-2157-46
30's	$2.09	GENERIC, Heartland Healthcare Services	61392-0408-30
30's	$2.09	GENERIC, Heartland Healthcare Services	61392-0408-39
30's	$3.23	GENERIC, St. Mary'S Mpp	60760-0138-30
30's	$3.75	GENERIC, Pd-Rx Pharmaceuticals	55289-0373-30
31 x 10	$23.99	GENERIC, Vangard Labs	00615-0536-53
31 x 10	$23.99	GENERIC, Vangard Labs	00615-0536-63
31's	$2.16	GENERIC, Heartland Healthcare Services	61392-0408-31
32's	$2.23	GENERIC, Heartland Healthcare Services	61392-0408-32
36's	$4.13	GENERIC, Pd-Rx Pharmaceuticals	55289-0373-36
42's	$4.47	GENERIC, Pd-Rx Pharmaceuticals	55289-0373-42
45's	$3.14	GENERIC, Heartland Healthcare Services	61392-0408-45
46's	$4.89	GENERIC, Pd-Rx Pharmaceuticals	55289-0373-46
48's	$7.85	GENERIC, Vintage Pharmaceuticals Inc	00254-5094-23
48's	$11.70	GENERIC, Qualitest Products Inc	00603-5332-31
48's	$14.95	GENERIC, Merz Pharmaceuticals	00259-0391-48
55's	$5.42	GENERIC, Pd-Rx Pharmaceuticals	55289-0373-55
60's	$2.55	GENERIC, Major Pharmaceuticals Inc	00904-2157-52
60's	$4.19	GENERIC, Heartland Healthcare Services	61392-0408-60
60's	$5.90	GENERIC, Pd-Rx Pharmaceuticals	55289-0373-60
72's	$7.07	GENERIC, Pd-Rx Pharmaceuticals	55289-0373-72
90's	$6.28	GENERIC, Heartland Healthcare Services	61392-0408-90
100's	$3.03	GENERIC, Caremark Inc	00339-5293-12
100's	$3.30	FEDERAL UPPER LIMIT, H.C.F.A. F F P	99999-2109-06
100's	$3.50	GENERIC, West Ward Pharmaceutical Corporation	00143-1475-01
100's	$3.50	GENERIC, Cmc-Consolidated Midland Corporation	00223-1515-01
100's	$3.50	GENERIC, Major Pharmaceuticals Inc	00904-2157-60
100's	$3.68	GENERIC, Interstate Drug Exchange Inc	00814-6285-14
100's	$3.76	DELTASONE, Pharmacia and Upjohn	00009-0045-05
100's	$4.20	GENERIC, Aligen Independent Laboratories Inc	00405-4828-01
100's	$4.23	GENERIC, Roxane Laboratories Inc	00054-4728-25
100's	$4.59	GENERIC, Moore, H.L. Drug Exchange Inc	00839-5143-06
100's	$4.75	GENERIC, Mutual Pharmaceutical Co Inc	53489-0138-01
100's	$5.08	GENERIC, Geneva Pharmaceuticals	00781-1495-01
100's	$5.46	DELTASONE, Pharmacia and Upjohn	00009-0045-01
100's	$6.00	GENERIC, Raway Pharmacal Inc	00686-0032-20
100's	$6.06	GENERIC, Auro Pharmaceutical	55829-0422-10
100's	$6.37	GENERIC, Udl Laboratories Inc	51079-0032-20
100's	$6.52	GENERIC, Watson/Schein Pharmaceuticals Inc	00364-0218-01
100's	$6.74	GENERIC, Major Pharmaceuticals Inc	00904-2157-61
100's	$7.08	GENERIC, Vangard Labs	00615-0536-13
100's	$7.21	GENERIC, Roxane Laboratories Inc	00054-8724-25
100's	$7.73	GENERIC, Pd-Rx Pharmaceuticals	55289-0373-01
100's	$7.75	GENERIC, Geneva Pharmaceuticals	00781-1495-13
100's	$8.22	GENERIC, Watson/Schein Pharmaceuticals Inc	00591-5052-01
100's	$8.46	GENERIC, Qualitest Products Inc	00603-5332-21
100's	$8.65	GENERIC, Ivax Corporation	00182-0201-89

Tablet - Oral - 10 mg

15's	$1.76	GENERIC, Heartland Healthcare Services	61392-0417-15
20's	$6.08	GENERIC, Pd-Rx Pharmaceuticals	55289-0438-20
21's	$6.17	GENERIC, Pd-Rx Pharmaceuticals	55289-0438-21
21's	$9.45	GENERIC, Vintage Pharmaceuticals Inc	00254-5093-13
21's	$9.45	GENERIC, Qualitest Products Inc	00603-5333-15
21's	$11.95	GENERIC, Allscripts Pharmaceutical Company	54569-3847-00
21's	$13.05	GENERIC, Compumed Pharmaceuticals	00403-1965-18
21's	$15.45	GENERIC, Merz Pharmaceuticals	00259-0364-21
25's	$2.48	GENERIC, Udl Laboratories Inc	51079-0033-19
25's	$5.25	GENERIC, Pd-Rx Pharmaceuticals	55289-0438-97
30's	$3.51	GENERIC, Heartland Healthcare Services	61392-0417-30
30's	$3.51	GENERIC, Heartland Healthcare Services	61392-0417-39
30's	$5.31	GENERIC, Pd-Rx Pharmaceuticals	55289-0438-30
31 x 10	$35.61	GENERIC, Pharmaceutical Corporation Of America	00615-3593-53
31 x 10	$35.61	GENERIC, Pharmaceutical Corporation Of America	00615-3593-63
31's	$3.63	GENERIC, Heartland Healthcare Services	61392-0417-31
32's	$3.74	GENERIC, Heartland Healthcare Services	61392-0417-32
36's	$6.30	GENERIC, Pd-Rx Pharmaceuticals	55289-0438-36
38's	$8.37	GENERIC, Pd-Rx Pharmaceuticals	55289-0438-38
40's	$8.52	GENERIC, Pd-Rx Pharmaceuticals	55289-0438-40
45's	$3.17	GENERIC, Allscripts Pharmaceutical Company	54569-3302-02
45's	$5.27	GENERIC, Heartland Healthcare Services	61392-0417-45
48's	$13.28	GENERIC, Vintage Pharmaceuticals Inc	00254-5093-23
48's	$13.28	GENERIC, Qualitest Products Inc	00603-5333-31
48's	$16.30	GENERIC, Merz Pharmaceuticals	00259-0364-48
48's	$16.80	GENERIC, Merz Pharmaceuticals	00259-0389-48
48's	$16.80	GENERIC, Allscripts Pharmaceutical Company	54569-3798-00
48's	$18.65	GENERIC, Compumed Pharmaceuticals	00403-1967-18
48's	$21.42	GENERIC, Physicians Total Care	54868-3234-00
49's	$18.00	GENERIC, Merz Pharmaceuticals	00259-0389-49
50's	$9.29	GENERIC, Pd-Rx Pharmaceuticals	55289-0438-50
60's	$7.02	GENERIC, Heartland Healthcare Services	61392-0417-60
90's	$10.53	GENERIC, Heartland Healthcare Services	61392-0417-90
100's	$4.83	DELTASONE, Pharmacia and Upjohn	00009-0193-03
100's	$4.95	GENERIC, Caremark Inc	00339-5295-12
100's	$5.25	GENERIC, Major Pharmaceuticals Inc	00904-2141-60
100's	$5.48	FEDERAL UPPER LIMIT, H.C.F.A. F F P	99999-2109-12
100's	$6.09	GENERIC, Roxane Laboratories Inc	00054-4730-25
100's	$6.15	GENERIC, Interstate Drug Exchange Inc	00814-6288-14
100's	$6.62	GENERIC, Moore, H.L. Drug Exchange Inc	00839-1520-06
100's	$7.04	GENERIC, Watson/Schein Pharmaceuticals Inc	00364-0461-01
100's	$7.05	GENERIC, Watson/Rugby Laboratories Inc	00536-4325-01
100's	$7.05	GENERIC, Geneva Pharmaceuticals	00781-1500-01
100's	$7.05	GENERIC, Watson Laboratories Inc	52544-0831-01
100's	$7.24	DELTASONE, Pharmacia and Upjohn	00009-0193-01
100's	$7.76	GENERIC, Aligen Independent Laboratories Inc	00405-4829-01
100's	$7.93	GENERIC, Mutual Pharmaceutical Co Inc	53489-0139-01
100's	$8.40	GENERIC, West Ward Pharmaceutical Corporation	00143-1473-01
100's	$8.85	GENERIC, Roxane Laboratories Inc	00054-8725-25
100's	$8.85	GENERIC, Ivax Corporation	00182-1334-89
100's	$8.87	GENERIC, Watson/Schein Pharmaceuticals Inc	00591-5442-01
100's	$9.50	GENERIC, Cmc-Consolidated Midland Corporation	00223-1516-01
100's	$9.94	GENERIC, Udl Laboratories Inc	51079-0033-20
100's	$9.96	GENERIC, Qualitest Products Inc	00603-5333-21
100's	$9.96	GENERIC, Qualitest Products Inc	00603-5338-21
100's	$11.10	GENERIC, Major Pharmaceuticals Inc	00904-2141-61
100's	$11.50	GENERIC, Allscripts Pharmaceutical Company	54569-0331-07
100's	$11.75	GENERIC, Medirex Inc	57480-0352-01
100's	$12.15	GENERIC, Auro Pharmaceutical	55829-0423-10
100's	$13.71	GENERIC, Pd-Rx Pharmaceuticals	55289-0438-01
200 x 5	$114.87	GENERIC, Pharmaceutical Corporation Of America	00615-3593-43

Tablet - Oral - 20 mg

9's	$0.73	DELTASONE, Allscripts Pharmaceutical Company	54569-4017-00
9's	$2.55	GENERIC, Pd-Rx Pharmaceuticals	55289-0352-09
10's	$3.14	GENERIC, Pd-Rx Pharmaceuticals	55289-0352-10
14's	$3.98	GENERIC, Pd-Rx Pharmaceuticals	55289-0352-14
15's	$4.07	GENERIC, Pd-Rx Pharmaceuticals	55289-0352-15
20's	$4.07	GENERIC, Pd-Rx Pharmaceuticals	55289-0352-20
21's	$4.28	GENERIC, Pd-Rx Pharmaceuticals	55289-0352-21
21's	$4.80	GENERIC, St. Mary'S Mpp	60760-0002-21
25's	$3.81	GENERIC, Udl Laboratories Inc	51079-0022-19
25's	$8.25	GENERIC, Pd-Rx Pharmaceuticals	55289-0352-97
30's	$4.43	GENERIC, Pd-Rx Pharmaceuticals	55289-0352-30
30's	$5.16	GENERIC, Heartland Healthcare Services	61392-0761-30
30's	$5.16	GENERIC, Heartland Healthcare Services	61392-0761-39
31 x 10	$52.66	GENERIC, Vangard Labs	00615-1542-53
31 x 10	$52.66	GENERIC, Vangard Labs	00615-1542-63
31's	$5.33	GENERIC, Heartland Healthcare Services	61392-0761-31
32's	$5.50	GENERIC, Heartland Healthcare Services	61392-0761-32
45's	$7.74	GENERIC, Heartland Healthcare Services	61392-0761-45
60's	$10.32	GENERIC, Heartland Healthcare Services	61392-0761-60
90's	$15.48	GENERIC, Heartland Healthcare Services	61392-0761-90
100's	$6.69	GENERIC, Major Pharmaceuticals Inc	00904-2140-60
100's	$7.58	FEDERAL UPPER LIMIT, H.C.F.A. F F P	99999-2109-15
100's	$8.25	GENERIC, West Ward Pharmaceutical Corporation	00143-1477-01
100's	$8.56	GENERIC, Caremark Inc	00339-5777-12
100's	$10.00	GENERIC, Raway Pharmacal Inc	00686-0022-20
100's	$10.43	GENERIC, Interstate Drug Exchange Inc	00814-6290-14
100's	$10.88	GENERIC, Aligen Independent Laboratories Inc	00405-4830-01
100's	$11.77	GENERIC, Roxane Laboratories Inc	00054-4729-25
100's	$11.79	GENERIC, Mutual Pharmaceutical Co Inc	53489-0140-01
100's	$11.80	GENERIC, Ivax Corporation	00182-1086-89
100's	$11.99	DELTASONE, Pharmacia and Upjohn	00009-0165-01
100's	$12.89	GENERIC, Watson/Rugby Laboratories Inc	00536-4326-01
100's	$12.89	GENERIC, Moore, H.L. Drug Exchange Inc	00839-1517-06
100's	$13.17	GENERIC, Roxane Laboratories Inc	00054-8726-25

P

Qty	Price	Product	NDC
100's	$14.24	GENERIC, Watson/Schein Pharmaceuticals Inc	00364-0442-01
100's	$14.24	GENERIC, Watson Laboratories Inc	52544-0832-01
100's	$15.89	GENERIC, Udl Laboratories Inc	51079-0022-20
100's	$16.37	GENERIC, American Health Packaging	62584-0834-01
100's	$17.61	GENERIC, Auro Pharmaceutical	55829-0424-10
100's	$17.94	GENERIC, Watson/Schein Pharmaceuticals Inc	00591-5443-01
100's	$18.53	GENERIC, Major Pharmaceuticals Inc	00904-2140-61
100's	$19.22	GENERIC, Qualitest Products Inc	00603-5334-21
200 x 5	$169.87	GENERIC, Vangard Labs	00615-1542-43

Tablet - Oral - 50 mg

Qty	Price	Product	NDC
10's	$4.16	GENERIC, Pd-Rx Pharmaceuticals	55289-0330-10
100's	$17.63	GENERIC, Caremark Inc	00339-5296-12
100's	$22.67	GENERIC, Geneva Pharmaceuticals	00781-1450-01
100's	$25.88	GENERIC, Roxane Laboratories Inc	00054-4733-25
100's	$26.95	GENERIC, Watson/Rugby Laboratories Inc	52544-0797-01
100's	$27.33	DELTASONE, Pharmacia and Upjohn	00009-0388-01
100's	$31.06	GENERIC, Roxane Laboratories Inc	00054-8729-25
100's	$32.00	GENERIC, West Ward Pharmaceutical Corporation	00143-1481-25
100's	$34.92	GENERIC, Geneva Pharmaceuticals	00781-1450-13

PRODUCT LISTING - RATED NOT THERAPEUTICALLY EQUIVALENT

Tablet - Oral - 5 mg

Qty	Price	Product	NDC
21's	$7.30	GENERIC, Schwarz Pharma	00131-2228-81
100's	$1.09	GENERIC, Global Pharmaceutical Corporation	00115-4294-01

PRODUCT LISTING - EQUIVALENTS NOT AVAILABLE

Solution - Oral - 5 mg/ml

Qty	Price	Product	NDC
30 ml	$30.84	GENERIC, Roxane Laboratories Inc	00054-3721-44

Solution - Oral - 5 mg/5 ml

Qty	Price	Product	NDC
60 ml	$7.02	GENERIC, Pd-Rx Pharmaceuticals	55289-0859-02
120 ml	$16.57	LIQUID PRED, Muro Pharmaceuticals Inc	00451-1201-04
120 ml	$18.36	GENERIC, Roxane Laboratories Inc	00054-3722-50

Tablet - Oral - 1 mg

Qty	Price	Product	NDC
20's	$4.60	GENERIC, Southwood Pharmaceuticals Inc	58016-0320-20
100's	$6.63	GENERIC, Physicians Total Care	54868-1119-01
120's	$21.18	GENERIC, Allscripts Pharmaceutical Company	54569-1469-01

Tablet - Oral - 5 mg

Qty	Price	Product	NDC
3's	$3.44	GENERIC, Prescript Pharmaceuticals	00247-0072-03
4's	$3.46	GENERIC, Prescript Pharmaceuticals	00247-0072-04
5's	$3.48	GENERIC, Prescript Pharmaceuticals	00247-0072-05
6's	$0.39	GENERIC, Allscripts Pharmaceutical Company	54569-0330-08
8's	$3.56	GENERIC, Prescript Pharmaceuticals	00247-0072-08
10's	$3.62	GENERIC, Prescript Pharmaceuticals	00247-0072-10
12's	$3.67	GENERIC, Prescript Pharmaceuticals	00247-0072-12
12's	$4.06	GENERIC, Pharmaceutical Corporation Of America	51655-0086-27
15's	$0.98	GENERIC, Allscripts Pharmaceutical Company	54569-0330-09
15's	$3.75	GENERIC, Prescript Pharmaceuticals	00247-0072-15
20's	$1.44	GENERIC, Southwood Pharmaceuticals Inc	58016-0218-20
20's	$2.61	GENERIC, Physicians Total Care	54868-0258-04
20's	$3.88	GENERIC, Prescript Pharmaceuticals	00247-0072-20
20's	$5.73	GENERIC, Pharma Pac	52959-0220-20
21's	$1.37	GENERIC, Allscripts Pharmaceutical Company	54569-0330-00
21's	$1.51	GENERIC, Southwood Pharmaceuticals Inc	58016-0218-21
21's	$3.25	GENERIC, First Horizon Pharmaceutical Corporation	60904-0286-20
21's	$3.91	GENERIC, Prescript Pharmaceuticals	00247-0072-21
21's	$5.95	GENERIC, Pharma Pac	52959-0220-21
22's	$3.94	GENERIC, Prescript Pharmaceuticals	00247-0072-22
24's	$0.73	GENERIC, Allscripts Pharmaceutical Company	54569-4026-01
24's	$1.73	GENERIC, Southwood Pharmaceuticals Inc	58016-0218-24
24's	$3.99	GENERIC, Prescript Pharmaceuticals	00247-0072-24
27's	$4.07	GENERIC, Prescript Pharmaceuticals	00247-0072-27
28's	$1.82	GENERIC, Allscripts Pharmaceutical Company	54569-2785-00
28's	$5.40	GENERIC, Allscripts Pharmaceutical Company	54569-3413-00
30's	$1.95	GENERIC, Allscripts Pharmaceutical Company	54569-0330-04
30's	$2.16	GENERIC, Southwood Pharmaceuticals Inc	58016-0218-30
30's	$3.07	GENERIC, Physicians Total Care	54868-0258-01
30's	$4.15	GENERIC, Prescript Pharmaceuticals	00247-0072-30
30's	$4.30	GENERIC, Pharmaceutical Corporation Of America	51655-0086-24
30's	$8.06	GENERIC, Pharma Pac	52959-0220-30
33's	$2.38	GENERIC, Southwood Pharmaceuticals Inc	58016-0218-33
36's	$2.34	GENERIC, Allscripts Pharmaceutical Company	54569-0330-05
36's	$2.59	GENERIC, Southwood Pharmaceuticals Inc	58016-0218-36
36's	$3.37	GENERIC, Physicians Total Care	54868-0258-05
36's	$4.31	GENERIC, Prescript Pharmaceuticals	00247-0072-36
36's	$9.41	GENERIC, Pharma Pac	52959-0220-36
40's	$1.22	GENERIC, Allscripts Pharmaceutical Company	54569-4026-04
40's	$2.88	GENERIC, Southwood Pharmaceuticals Inc	58016-0218-40
40's	$4.41	GENERIC, Prescript Pharmaceuticals	00247-0072-40
40's	$10.35	GENERIC, Pharma Pac	52959-0220-40
42's	$2.73	GENERIC, Allscripts Pharmaceutical Company	54569-4026-00
42's	$4.47	GENERIC, Prescript Pharmaceuticals	00247-0072-42
44's	$4.52	GENERIC, Prescript Pharmaceuticals	00247-0072-44
45's	$4.54	GENERIC, Prescript Pharmaceuticals	00247-0072-45
48's	$4.62	GENERIC, Prescript Pharmaceuticals	00247-0072-48
50's	$3.25	GENERIC, Allscripts Pharmaceutical Company	54569-0330-01
50's	$3.60	GENERIC, Southwood Pharmaceuticals Inc	58016-0218-50
50's	$4.03	GENERIC, Physicians Total Care	54868-0258-03
50's	$4.68	GENERIC, Prescript Pharmaceuticals	00247-0072-50
54's	$4.79	GENERIC, Prescript Pharmaceuticals	00247-0072-54
55's	$1.68	GENERIC, Allscripts Pharmaceutical Company	54569-4026-05
55's	$3.96	GENERIC, Southwood Pharmaceuticals Inc	58016-0218-55
55's	$4.26	GENERIC, Physicians Total Care	54868-0258-06
60's	$3.90	GENERIC, Allscripts Pharmaceutical Company	54569-0330-07
60's	$4.32	GENERIC, Southwood Pharmaceuticals Inc	58016-0218-60
60's	$4.94	GENERIC, Prescript Pharmaceuticals	00247-0072-60
60's	$12.59	GENERIC, Pharma Pac	52959-0220-60
61's	$4.96	GENERIC, Prescript Pharmaceuticals	00247-0072-61
75's	$4.88	GENERIC, Allscripts Pharmaceutical Company	54569-0330-02
75's	$13.11	GENERIC, Pharma Pac	52959-0220-75
80's	$5.47	GENERIC, Prescript Pharmaceuticals	00247-0072-80
100's	$6.00	GENERIC, Prescript Pharmaceuticals	00247-0072-00
100's	$6.38	GENERIC, Physicians Total Care	54868-0258-02
100's	$6.50	GENERIC, Allscripts Pharmaceutical Company	54569-0330-03
100's	$7.20	GENERIC, Southwood Pharmaceuticals Inc	58016-0218-00
100's	$8.46	GENERIC, Qualitest Products Inc	00603-5337-21
100's	$15.52	GENERIC, Pharma Pac	52959-0220-00
118's	$6.48	GENERIC, Prescript Pharmaceuticals	00247-0072-52

Tablet - Oral - 10 mg

Qty	Price	Product	NDC
2's	$3.46	GENERIC, Prescript Pharmaceuticals	00247-0071-02
3's	$3.52	GENERIC, Prescript Pharmaceuticals	00247-0071-03
4's	$0.28	GENERIC, Allscripts Pharmaceutical Company	54569-3302-07
4's	$3.56	GENERIC, Prescript Pharmaceuticals	00247-0071-04
6's	$0.42	GENERIC, Allscripts Pharmaceutical Company	54569-3302-06
6's	$3.67	GENERIC, Prescript Pharmaceuticals	00247-0071-06
8's	$3.78	GENERIC, Prescript Pharmaceuticals	00247-0071-08
10's	$0.71	GENERIC, Allscripts Pharmaceutical Company	54569-0331-00
10's	$3.88	GENERIC, Prescript Pharmaceuticals	00247-0071-10
10's	$4.59	GENERIC, Pharmaceutical Corporation Of America	51655-0020-53
12's	$0.85	GENERIC, Allscripts Pharmaceutical Company	54569-0331-06
12's	$1.56	GENERIC, Southwood Pharmaceuticals Inc	58016-0126-12
12's	$1.56	GENERIC, Southwood Pharmaceuticals Inc	58016-0216-12
12's	$5.43	GENERIC, Pharma Pac	52959-0126-12
14's	$1.82	GENERIC, Southwood Pharmaceuticals Inc	58016-0216-14
14's	$4.09	GENERIC, Prescript Pharmaceuticals	00247-0071-14
15's	$1.06	GENERIC, Allscripts Pharmaceutical Company	54569-0331-01
15's	$1.95	GENERIC, Southwood Pharmaceuticals Inc	58016-0216-15
15's	$2.51	GENERIC, Physicians Total Care	54868-0836-04
15's	$4.15	GENERIC, Prescript Pharmaceuticals	00247-0071-15
15's	$6.54	GENERIC, Pharma Pac	52959-0126-15
18's	$6.78	GENERIC, Pharma Pac	52959-0126-18
20's	$1.41	GENERIC, Allscripts Pharmaceutical Company	54569-3302-01
20's	$2.60	GENERIC, Southwood Pharmaceuticals Inc	58016-0216-20
20's	$2.90	GENERIC, Physicians Total Care	54868-0836-08
20's	$4.41	GENERIC, Prescript Pharmaceuticals	00247-0071-20
20's	$4.83	GENERIC, Pharmaceutical Corporation Of America	51655-0020-52
20's	$7.13	GENERIC, Pharma Pac	52959-0126-20
21's	$1.48	GENERIC, Allscripts Pharmaceutical Company	54569-0331-02
21's	$2.73	GENERIC, Southwood Pharmaceuticals Inc	58016-0216-21
21's	$4.47	GENERIC, Prescript Pharmaceuticals	00247-0071-21
21's	$7.49	GENERIC, Pharma Pac	52959-0126-21
22's	$4.52	GENERIC, Prescript Pharmaceuticals	00247-0071-22
24's	$1.69	GENERIC, Allscripts Pharmaceutical Company	54569-0331-03
24's	$3.12	GENERIC, Southwood Pharmaceuticals Inc	58016-0216-24
24's	$4.62	GENERIC, Prescript Pharmaceuticals	00247-0071-24
25's	$4.68	GENERIC, Prescript Pharmaceuticals	00247-0071-25
25's	$8.57	GENERIC, Pharma Pac	52959-0126-25
27's	$4.79	GENERIC, Prescript Pharmaceuticals	00247-0071-27
28's	$3.64	GENERIC, Southwood Pharmaceuticals Inc	58016-0216-28
28's	$4.84	GENERIC, Prescript Pharmaceuticals	00247-0071-28
30's	$2.12	GENERIC, Allscripts Pharmaceutical Company	54569-0331-05
30's	$3.13	GENERIC, Physicians Total Care	54868-0836-07
30's	$3.90	GENERIC, Southwood Pharmaceuticals Inc	58016-0216-30
30's	$4.43	GENERIC, Pharmaceutical Corporation Of America	51655-0020-24
30's	$4.94	GENERIC, Prescript Pharmaceuticals	00247-0071-30
30's	$9.50	GENERIC, Pharma Pac	52959-0126-30

32's $4.16 GENERIC, Southwood Pharmaceuticals Inc 58016-0216-32
32's $5.05 GENERIC, Prescript Pharmaceuticals 00247-0071-32
35's $5.21 GENERIC, Prescript Pharmaceuticals 00247-0071-35
40's $2.82 GENERIC, Allscripts Pharmaceutical Company 54569-0331-08
40's $4.46 GENERIC, Physicians Total Care 54868-0836-00
40's $5.20 GENERIC, Southwood Pharmaceuticals Inc 58016-0216-40
40's $5.47 GENERIC, Prescript Pharmaceuticals 00247-0071-40
40's $12.47 GENERIC, Pharma Pac 52959-0126-40
42's $2.96 GENERIC, Allscripts Pharmaceutical Company 54569-0331-09
42's $5.58 GENERIC, Prescript Pharmaceuticals 00247-0071-42
42's $13.36 GENERIC, Pharma Pac 52959-0126-42
43's $5.64 GENERIC, Prescript Pharmaceuticals 00247-0071-43
50's $3.53 GENERIC, Allscripts Pharmaceutical Company 54569-0331-04
50's $5.24 GENERIC, Physicians Total Care 54868-0836-03
50's $6.00 GENERIC, Prescript Pharmaceuticals 00247-0071-50
50's $6.50 GENERIC, Southwood Pharmaceuticals Inc 58016-0216-50
50's $15.44 GENERIC, Pharma Pac 52959-0126-50
54's $3.81 GENERIC, Allscripts Pharmaceutical Company 54569-3302-05
60's $6.02 GENERIC, Physicians Total Care 54868-0836-05
60's $6.13 GENERIC, Allscripts Pharmaceutical Company 54569-3302-00
60's $7.80 GENERIC, Southwood Pharmaceuticals Inc 58016-0216-60
60's $17.81 GENERIC, Pharma Pac 52959-0126-60
63's $6.26 GENERIC, Physicians Total Care 54868-0836-09
90's $11.70 GENERIC, Southwood Pharmaceuticals Inc 58016-0216-90
100's $8.48 GENERIC, Physicians Total Care 54868-0836-02
100's $8.65 GENERIC, Prescript Pharmaceuticals 00247-0071-00
100's $13.00 GENERIC, Southwood Pharmaceuticals Inc 58016-0216-00
100's $21.00 GENERIC, Pharma Pac 52959-0126-00

Tablet - Oral - 20 mg

2's $3.54 GENERIC, Prescript Pharmaceuticals 00247-0100-02
3's $0.43 GENERIC, Allscripts Pharmaceutical Company 54569-3043-04
3's $3.64 GENERIC, Prescript Pharmaceuticals 00247-0100-03
4's $3.73 GENERIC, Prescript Pharmaceuticals 00247-0100-04
5's $3.81 GENERIC, Prescript Pharmaceuticals 00247-0100-05
6's $0.85 GENERIC, Allscripts Pharmaceutical Company 54569-3043-02
7's $3.64 GENERIC, Pharma Pac 52959-0127-07
7's $4.00 GENERIC, Prescript Pharmaceuticals 00247-0100-07
8's $1.41 GENERIC, Allscripts Pharmaceutical Company 54569-0332-00
8's $4.09 GENERIC, Prescript Pharmaceuticals 00247-0100-08
9's $1.28 GENERIC, Allscripts Pharmaceutical Company 54569-3043-03
9's $4.19 GENERIC, Prescript Pharmaceuticals 00247-0100-09
10's $1.42 GENERIC, Allscripts Pharmaceutical Company 54569-0332-01
10's $1.65 GENERIC, Southwood Pharmaceuticals Inc 58016-0217-10
10's $3.86 GENERIC, Pharma Pac 52959-0127-10
10's $4.28 GENERIC, Prescript Pharmaceuticals 00247-0100-10
12's $1.71 GENERIC, Allscripts Pharmaceutical Company 54569-3043-01
12's $4.47 GENERIC, Prescript Pharmaceuticals 00247-0100-12
13's $4.55 GENERIC, Prescript Pharmaceuticals 00247-0100-13
14's $1.99 GENERIC, Allscripts Pharmaceutical Company 54569-3043-05
14's $4.65 GENERIC, Prescript Pharmaceuticals 00247-0100-14
15's $2.48 GENERIC, Southwood Pharmaceuticals Inc 58016-0217-15
15's $2.70 GENERIC, Physicians Total Care 54868-1183-01
15's $4.74 GENERIC, Prescript Pharmaceuticals 00247-0100-15
15's $7.07 GENERIC, Pharma Pac 52959-0127-15
16's $2.64 GENERIC, Southwood Pharmaceuticals Inc 58016-0217-16
16's $4.84 GENERIC, Prescript Pharmaceuticals 00247-0100-16
18's $2.56 GENERIC, Allscripts Pharmaceutical Company 54569-0332-09
18's $2.98 GENERIC, Southwood Pharmaceuticals Inc 58016-0217-18
18's $5.02 GENERIC, Prescript Pharmaceuticals 00247-0100-18
20's $3.31 GENERIC, Southwood Pharmaceuticals Inc 58016-0217-20
20's $3.53 GENERIC, Allscripts Pharmaceutical Company 54569-3043-00
20's $3.90 GENERIC, Physicians Total Care 54868-1183-07
20's $5.21 GENERIC, Prescript Pharmaceuticals 00247-0100-20
20's $9.36 GENERIC, Pharma Pac 52959-0127-20
21's $2.99 GENERIC, Allscripts Pharmaceutical Company 54569-0332-02
21's $3.47 GENERIC, Southwood Pharmaceuticals Inc 58016-0217-21
21's $5.29 GENERIC, Prescript Pharmaceuticals 00247-0100-21
21's $9.84 GENERIC, Pharma Pac 52959-0127-21
22's $3.64 GENERIC, Southwood Pharmaceuticals Inc 58016-0217-22
24's $3.97 GENERIC, Southwood Pharmaceuticals Inc 58016-0217-24
25's $11.46 GENERIC, Pharma Pac 52959-0127-25
27's $3.84 GENERIC, Allscripts Pharmaceutical Company 54569-0332-08
27's $5.86 GENERIC, Prescript Pharmaceuticals 00247-0100-27
28's $4.63 GENERIC, Southwood Pharmaceuticals Inc 58016-0217-28
30's $4.07 GENERIC, Physicians Total Care 54868-1183-03
30's $4.27 GENERIC, Allscripts Pharmaceutical Company 54569-0332-03
30's $4.96 GENERIC, Southwood Pharmaceuticals Inc 58016-0217-30
30's $6.13 GENERIC, Prescript Pharmaceuticals 00247-0100-30
30's $12.57 GENERIC, Pharma Pac 52959-0127-30
37's $14.35 GENERIC, Pharma Pac 52959-0127-37
40's $6.61 GENERIC, Southwood Pharmaceuticals Inc 58016-0217-40
40's $7.06 GENERIC, Prescript Pharmaceuticals 00247-0100-40
42's $7.25 GENERIC, Prescript Pharmaceuticals 00247-0100-42
42's $15.80 GENERIC, Pharma Pac 52959-0127-42
50's $7.12 GENERIC, Allscripts Pharmaceutical Company 54569-0332-04
60's $6.81 GENERIC, Physicians Total Care 54868-1183-02
60's $9.92 GENERIC, Southwood Pharmaceuticals Inc 58016-0217-60
90's $11.69 GENERIC, Prescript Pharmaceuticals 00247-0100-90
100's $9.79 GENERIC, Physicians Total Care 54868-1183-00
100's $11.50 GENERIC, Cmc-Consolidated Midland Corporation 00223-1517-01
100's $12.62 GENERIC, Prescript Pharmaceuticals 00247-0100-00
100's $14.24 GENERIC, Allscripts Pharmaceutical Company 54569-0332-05
100's $16.53 GENERIC, Southwood Pharmaceuticals Inc 58016-0217-00
100's $21.84 GENERIC, Pharma Pac 52959-0127-00

Tablet - Oral - 50 mg

5's $1.35 GENERIC, Allscripts Pharmaceutical Company 54569-0333-04
8's $2.16 GENERIC, Allscripts Pharmaceutical Company 54569-0333-00
30's $10.99 GENERIC, Physicians Total Care 54868-0908-00

Prilocaine Hydrochloride *(002112)*

For complete prescribing information, refer to the CD-ROM included with the book.

Categories: Anesthesia, local; Pregnancy Category B; FDA Approved 1965 Nov
Drug Classes: Anesthetics, local
Brand Names: Citanest
Foreign Brand Availability: Xylonest (Germany)

DESCRIPTION

For Local Anesthesia in Dentistry

Prilocaine solutions are sterile nonpyrogenic isotonic solutions that contain a local anesthetic agent with and without epinephrine (as bitartrate) and are administered parenterally by injection. See INDICATIONS AND USAGE for specific uses. The quantitative composition of each available solution is shown in Table 1.

Prilocaine HCl is chemically designated as propanamide, N-2-(2-methyl-phenyl)-2-(propylamino)-, monohydrochloride.

Epinephrine is (-) -3,4-Dihydroxy-α-[(methylamino)methyl]benzyl alcohol. Parenteral drug products should be inspected visually for particulate matter and discoloration prior to administration. The specific quantitative composition of each available solution is shown in TABLE 1.

***TABLE 1** Composition Of Available Injections*

Product I.D.:	Formula (mg/ml) Prilocaine HCl	Epinephrine (as the bitartrate)	Citric Acid	Sodium Metabisulfite	pH
Prilocaine HCl injection	40.0	None	None	None	6.0-7.0
Prilocaine HCl injectionwith epinephrine	40.0	0.005	0.2	0.5	3.3-5.5

Note: Sodium hydroxide and/or hydrochloric acid may be used to adjust the pH of prilocaine Solutions. Filled under nitrogen.

INDICATIONS AND USAGE

Prilocaine HCl 4% and 4% prilocaine HCl with epinephrine injections are indicated for the production of local anesthesia in dentistry by nerve block or infiltration techniques. Only accepted procedures for these techniques as described in standard text books are recommended.

CONTRAINDICATIONS

Prilocaine is contraindicated in patients with a known history of hypersensitivity to local anesthetics of the amide type and in those rare patients with congenital or idiopathic methemoglobinemia.

WARNINGS

DENTAL PRACTITIONERS WHO EMPLOY LOCAL ANESTHETIC AGENTS SHOULD BE WELL VERSED IN DIAGNOSIS AND MANAGEMENT OF EMERGENCIES THAT MAY ARISE FROM THEIR USE. RESUSCITATIVE EQUIPMENT, OXYGEN AND OTHER RESUSCITATIVE DRUGS SHOULD BE AVAILABLE FOR IMMEDIATE USE.

To minimize the likelihood of intravascular injection, aspiration should be performed before the local anesthetic solution is injected. If blood is aspirated, the needle must be repositioned until no return blood can be elicited by aspiration. Note, however, that the absence of blood in the syringe does not assure that intravascular injection will be avoided.

Prilocaine with epinephrine injections contain sodium metabisulfite, a sulfite that may cause allergic-type reactions including anaphylactic symptoms and life-threatening or less severe asthmatic episodes in certain susceptible people. The overall prevalence of sulfite sensitivity in the general population is unknown and probably low. Sulfite sensitivity is seen more frequently in asthmatic than in nonasthmatic people.

DOSAGE AND ADMINISTRATION

The dosage of prilocaine HCl injection and prilocaine HCl with epinephrine injection varies and depends on the physical status of the patient, the area of the oral cavity to be anesthetized, the vascularity of the oral tissues, and the technique of anesthesia. The least volume of solution that results in effective local anesthesia should be administered. For specific techniques and procedures of local anesthesia in the oral cavity, refer to standard textbooks.

Inferior Alveolar Block: There are no practical clinical differences between prilocaine with and without epinephrine when used for inferior alveolar blocks.

Maxillary Infiltration: Prilocaine HCl is recommended for use in maxillary infiltration anesthesia for procedures in which the painful aspects can be completed within 15 minutes after the injection. Prilocaine HCl is therefore especially suited to short procedures in the maxillary anterior teeth. For long procedures, or those involving maxillary posterior teeth where soft tissue numbness is not troublesome to the patient, prilocaine HCl with epinephrine is recommended.

For most routine procedures, initial dosages of 1 to 2 ml of prilocaine HCl injection or prilocaine HCl with epinephrine injection will usually provide adequate infiltration or major nerve block anesthesia. No more than 600 mg (15 ml; 8 cartridges) should ever be administered within a 2 hour period in normal healthy adults.

In children under 10 years of age it is rarely necessary to administer more than one-half cartridge (40 mg) of prilocaine HCl injection or prilocaine HCl with epinephrine injection per procedure to achieve local anesthesia for a procedure involving a single tooth. In maxillary infiltration, this amount will often suffice to the treatment of 2 or even 3 teeth. In the mandibular block, however, satisfactory anesthesia achieved with this amount of drug will allow treatment of the teeth in an entire quadrant.

Aspiration prior to injection is recommended, since it reduces the possibility of intravascular injection, thereby keeping the incidence of side effects and anesthetic failure to a minimum.

NOTE: Parenteral drug products should be inspected visually for particulate matter and discoloration prior to administration whenever the solution and container permit. Solutions that are discolored and/or contain particulate matter should not be used. **Any unused portion of a cartridge of prilocaine HCl or prilocaine HCl with epinephrine injection should be discarded.**

Maximum Recommended Dosages Normal Healthy Adults: No more than 600 mg (8 mg/kg or 4 mg/lb) of prilocaine HCl should be administered as a single injection.

Children: It is difficult to recommend a maximum dose of any drug for children since this varies as a function of age and weight. For children of less than 10 years who have a normal lean body mass and normal body development, the maximum dose may be determined by the application of one of the standard pediatric drug formulas (*e.g.*, Clark's rule). For example, in a child of 5 years weighing 50 lb, the dose of prilocaine hydrochloride should not exceed 150-200 mg (6.6-8.8 mg/kg or 3-4 mg/lb of body weight) when calculated according to Clark's rule.

STERILIZATION, STORAGE AND TECHNICAL PROCEDURES

1. Cartridges of prilocaine HCl injection and prilocaine HCl with epinephrine injection should not be autoclaved, because solutions of epinephrine and the closures employed in cartridges cannot withstand autoclaving temperatures and pressures.
2. If chemical disinfection of anesthetic cartridges is desired, either 91% isopropyl alcohol or 70% ethyl alcohol is recommended. Many commercially available brands of rubbing alcohol, as well as solutions of ethyl alcohol not of U.S.P. grade, contain denaturants that are injurious to rubber and, therefore, are not to be used. It is recommended that chemical disinfection be accomplished by wiping the cartridge cap thoroughly with a pledget of cotton that has been moistened with the recommended alcohol just prior to use. IMMERSION IS NOT RECOMMENDED.
3. Certain metallic ions (mercury, zinc, copper etc.) have been related to swelling and edema after local anesthesia in dentistry. Therefore, chemical disinfectants containing or releasing these ions are not recommended. Antirust tablets usually contain metal ions. Accordingly, aluminum sealed cartridges should not be kept in such solutions.
4. Quaternary ammonium salts, such as benzalkonium chloride, are electrolytically incompatible with aluminum. Cartridges of prilocaine HCl injection and prilocaine HCl with epinephrine injection are sealed with aluminum caps and therefore should not be immersed in any solution containing salts.
5. To avoid leakage of solutions during injection, be sure to penetrate the center of the rubber diaphragm when loading the syringe. An off-center penetration produces an oval shaped puncture that allows leakage around the needle.

Other causes of leakage and breakage include badly worn syringes, aspirating syringes with bent harpoons, the use of syringes not designed to take 1.8 ml cartridges, and inadvertent freezing.

6. Cracking of glass cartridges is most often the result of any attempt to use a cartridge with an extruded plunger. An extruded plunger loses its lubrication and can be forced back into the cartridge only with difficulty. Cartridges with extruded plungers should be discarded.
7. Store at controlled room temperature 25°C (77°F).
8. Solutions containing epinephrine should be protected from light.

P

Primaquine Phosphate (002113)

Categories: Malaria; Malaria, prophylaxis; FDA Approved 1952 Jan; Pregnancy Category C; WHO Formulary
Drug Classes: Antiprotozoals
Brand Names: Primaquine
Foreign Brand Availability: Malaquin (Korea); Malirid (India); Palum (Mexico); PMQ-INGA (India); Primacin (Australia); Vivaquine (Korea)
Cost of Therapy: $13.97 (Malaria; Generic Tablets; 26.3 mg; 1 tablet/day; 14 day supply)

WARNING

PHYSICIANS SHOULD COMPLETELY FAMILIARIZE THEMSELVES WITH THE COMPLETE CONTENTS OF THIS MONOGRAPH BEFORE PRESCRIBING PRIMAQUINE PHOSPHATE.

DESCRIPTION

Primaquine phosphate, USP, is an 8-aminoquinoline synthetic compound for oral administration. Each tablet contains 26.3 mg of primaquine phosphate (equivalent to 15 mg of primaquine base). The dosage is expressed in terms of the base.

Primaquine phosphate is an antimalarial drug.

Chemically, the drug is 8-[(4-Amino-1-methylbutyl)amino]-6- methoxy-quinoline phosphate. *Inactive Ingredients:* Acacia, carnauba wax, gelatin, kaolin, lactose, magnesium stearate, pharmaceutical glaze, precipitated calcium carbonate, starch, sucrose, talc, titanium dioxide, yellow wax.

Storage: Store at room temperature.

CLINICAL PHARMACOLOGY

Primaquine is readily absorbed and rapidly metabolized after ingestion, and only a small proportion of the administered dose is excreted as the parent drug. The plasma concentration reaches a maximum in about 1-2 hours, after a single oral dose (15 mg base) of primaquine. However, the exact mechanism of primaquine is not known.

MICROBIOLOGY

Primaquine is an 8-aminoquinoline compound which eliminates tissue (exo-erythrocytic) infection. Thereby, it prevents the development of the blood (erythrocytic) forms of the parasite which are responsible for relapses in vivax malaria. Primaquine phosphate is also active against gametocytes of Plasmodium falciparum.

INDICATIONS AND USAGE

Primaquine is indicated for the radical cure (prevention or relapse) of vivax malaria.

NON-FDA APPROVED INDICATIONS

While not an FDA approved indication, primaquine is also used in conjunction with clindamycin for the treatment of Pneumocystis carinii pneumonia in patients with severe sulfonamide hypersensitivity.

CONTRAINDICATIONS

Primaquine is contraindicated in acutely ill patients suffering from systemic disease manifested by tendency to granulocytopenia, such as rheumatoid arthritis and lupus erythematosus, and in all patients with known hypersensitivity to it.

Primaquine is also contraindicated in patients receiving concurrently other potentially hemolytic drugs or depressants of myeloid elements of the bone marrow.

Because quinacrine hydrochloride appears to potentiate the toxicity of antimalarial compounds which are structurally related to primaquine, the use of quinacrine in patients receiving primaquine is contraindicated. Similarly, primaquine should not be administered to patients who have received quinacrine recently, as toxicity is increased.

WARNINGS

Primaquine should be discontinued immediately if signs of hemolytic anemia occur (darkening of the urine, marked decrease in hemoglobin or erythrocytic count).

Hemolytic reactions (moderate to severe) may occur in glucose- 6-phosphate dehydrogenase (G-6-PD) deficient Caucasians (particularly in Sardinians, Asians and Mediterranean peoples, and in individuals with a family or personal history of favism). Dark-skinned persons (Negroes, for example) have a great tendency to develop hemolytic anemia (due to congenital deficiency of erythrocytic glucose-6-phosphate dehydrogenase) while receiving primaquine and related drugs.

PRECAUTIONS

GENERAL

If primaquine is prescribed for (1) an individual who has shown a previous idiosyncrasy to primaquine (as manifested by hemolytic anemia, methemoglobinemia, or leukopenia), (2) an individual with a personal or family history of favism, or (3) an individual with erythrocytic glucose-6-phosphate dehydrogenase (G-6-PD) deficiency or nicotinamide adenine dinucleotide (NADH) methemoglobin reductase deficiency, the person should be observed closely for tolerance. The drug should be discontinued immediately if marked darkening of the urine or sudden decrease in hemoglobin concentration or leukocyte count occurs.

Since anemia, methemoglobinemia, and leukopenia have been observed following administration of large doses of primaquine, the adult dosage of 1 tablet (= 15 mg base) daily for fourteen days should not be exceeded.

LABORATORY TESTS

It is advisable to make routine blood examinations (particularly blood cell counts and hemoglobin determinations) during therapy.

NURSING MOTHERS

Caution should be exercised when primaquine is administered to a nursing woman.

PEDIATRIC USE

Safety and effectiveness in children have not been established.

DRUG INTERACTIONS

Potentially hemolytic drugs (*e.g.*, sulfonamides, nitrofurans) or depressants of myeloid elements of the bone marrow (*eg.*, methotrexate, phenylbutazone, chloramphenicol) should not be given concurrently with primaquine. (See CONTRAINDICATIONS.)

Primaquine should not be administered to patients who have recently received quinacrine, as toxicity is increased. (See CONTRAINDICATIONS.)

ADVERSE REACTIONS

Gastrointestinal: Nausea, vomiting, epigastric distress, and abdominal cramps.

Hematologic: Leukopenia, Hemolytic anemia in glucose-6-phosphate dehydrogenase (G-6-PD) deficient individuals, and methemoglobinemia in nicotinamide adenine dinucleotide (NADH) methemoglobin reductase deficient individuals.

DOSAGE AND ADMINISTRATION

Primaquine phosphate is recommended only for the radical cure of vivax malaria, the prevention of relapse in vivax malaria, or following the termination of chloroquine phosphate suppressive therapy in an area where vivax malaria is endemic.

Patients suffering from an attack of vivax malaria or having parasitized red blood cells should receive a course of chloroquine phosphate, which quickly destroys the erythrocytic parasites and terminates the paroxysm. Primaquine should be administered concurrently in order to eradicate the exo-erythrocytic paracytes in a dosage of 1 tablet (equivalent to 15 mg base) daily for 14 days in adults.

PRODUCT LISTING - EQUIVALENTS NOT AVAILABLE

Tablet - Oral - 26.3 mg

100's	$99.80	GENERIC, Sanofi Winthrop Pharmaceuticals	00024-1596-01

Primidone *(002114)*

Categories: Seizures, complex partial; Seizures, generalized tonic-clonic; Seizures, partial; Pregnancy Category B; FDA Approved 1954 Mar

Drug Classes: Anticonvulsants

Brand Names: **Mysoline**

Foreign Brand Availability: Apo-Primidone (Canada); Cyral (Austria); Liskantin (Germany); Mylepsin (Sweden); Mysolin (Bulgaria); Prysoline (Israel)

Cost of Therapy: $89.51 (Epilepsy; Mysoline; 250 mg; 3 tablets/day; 30 day supply)
$7.16 (Epilepsy; Generic Tablets; 250 mg; 3 tablets/day; 30 day supply)

DESCRIPTION

Chemical Name: 5-ethyldihydro-5-phenyl-4,6 (1H, 5H)-pyrimidinedione.

Primadone is a white, crystalline, highly stable substance, M.P. 279-284°C. It is poorly soluble in water (60 mg per 100 ml at 37°C) and in most organic solvents. It possesses no acidic properties, in contrast to its barbiturate analog.

Mysoline 50 mg and 250 mg tablets contain the following inactive ingredients: Microcrystalline cellulose; lactose, methylcellulose, sodium starch glycolate; talc; sodium lauryl sulfate; magnesium stearate; water, purified. Mysoline 250 mg tablets also contain yellow iron oxide.

Mysoline suspension contains these inactive ingredients: Ammonia solution, diluted; citric acid; D&C yellow no. 10; FD&C yellow no. 6; magnesium aluminum silicate; methylparaben; propylparaben; saccharin sodium; sodium alginate; sodium citrate; sodium hypochlorite solution; sorbic acid; sorbitan monolaurate; water, purified; flavors.

CLINICAL PHARMACOLOGY

Primadone raises electro- or chemoshock seizure thresholds or alters seizure patterns in experimental animals. The mechanism(s) of primidone's antiepileptic action is not known.

Primidone *per se* has anticonvulsant activity as do its two metabolites, phenobarbital and phenylethylmalonamide (PEMA). In addition to its anticonvulsant activity, PEMA potentiates the anticonvulsant activity of phenobarbital in experimental animals.

INDICATIONS AND USAGE

Primadone, used alone or concomitantly with other anticonvulsants, is indicated in the control of grand mal, psychomotor, and focal epileptic seizures. It may control grand mal seizures refractory to other anticonvulsant therapy.

NON-FDA APPROVED INDICATIONS

Primidone has been widely used for essential tremor.

CONTRAINDICATIONS

Primidone is contraindicated in:

1. Patients with porphyria.
2. Patients who are hypersensitive to phenobarbital (see CLINICAL PHARMACOLOGY).

WARNINGS

The abrupt withdrawal of antiepileptic medication may precipitate status epilepticus.

The therapeutic efficacy of a dosage regimen takes several weeks before it can be assessed.

USE IN PREGNANCY

The effects of primadone in human pregnancy and nursing infants are unknown. Recent reports suggest an association between the use of anticonvulsant drugs by women with epilepsy and an elevated incidence of birth defects in children born to these women. Data are more extensive with respect to diphenylhydantoin and phenobarbital, but these are also the most commonly prescribed anticonvulsants; less systematic or anecdotal reports suggest a possible similar association with the use of all known anticonvulsant drugs.

The reports suggesting an elevated incidence of birth defects in children of drug-treated epileptic women cannot be regarded as adequate to prove a definite cause-and-effect relationship. There are intrinsic methodologic problems in obtaining adequate data on drug teratogenicity in humans; the possibility also exists that other factors leading to birth defects (*e.g.*, genetic factors or the epileptic condition itself) may be more important than drug therapy. The majority of mothers on anticonvulsant medication deliver normal infants. It is important to note that anticonvulsant drugs should not be discontinued in patients in whom the drug is administered to prevent major seizures because of the strong possibility of precipitating status epilepticus with attendant hypoxia and threat to life. In individual cases where the severity and frequency of the seizure disorders are such that the removal of medication does not pose a serious threat to the patient, discontinuation of the drug may be considered prior to and during pregnancy, although it cannot be said with any confidence that even minor seizures do not pose some hazard to the developing embryo or fetus.

The prescribing physician will wish to weigh these considerations in treating or counseling epileptic women of childbearing potential.

Neonatal hemorrhage, with a coagulation defect resembling vitamin K deficiency, has been described in newborns whose mothers were taking primidone and other anticonvulsants. Pregnant women under anticonvulsant therapy should receive prophylactic vitamin K_1 therapy for 1 month prior to, and during, delivery.

PRECAUTIONS

The total daily dosage should not exceed 2 g. Since primadone therapy generally extends over prolonged periods, a complete blood count and a sequential multiple analysis-12 (SMA-12) test should be made every 6 months.

NURSING MOTHERS

There is evidence that in mothers treated with primidone, the drug appears in the milk in substantial quantities. Since tests for the presence of primidone in biological fluids are too complex to be carried out in the average clinical laboratory, it is suggested that the presence of undue somnolence and drowsiness in nursing newborns of primadone-treated mothers be taken as an indication that nursing should be discontinued.

ADVERSE REACTIONS

The most frequently occurring early side effects are ataxia and vertigo. These tend to disappear with continued therapy, or with reduction of initial dosage. Occasionally, the following have been reported: nausea, anorexia, vomiting, fatigue, hyperirritability, emotional disturbances, sexual impotency, diplopia, nystagmus, drowsiness, and morbilliform skin eruptions. Granulocytopenia, agranulocytosis, and red-cell hypoplasia and aplasia, have been reported rarely. These and, occasionally, other persistent or severe side effects may necessitate withdrawal of the drug. Megaloblastic anemia may occur as a rare idiosyncrasy to primadone and to other anticonvulsants. The anemia responds to folic acid without necessity of discontinuing medication.

DOSAGE AND ADMINISTRATION

ADULT DOSAGE

Patients 8 years of age and older who have received no previous treatment may be started on primadone according to the following regimen using either 50 mg or scored 250 mg primadone tablets:

Days 1-3: 100-125 mg at bedtime.
Days 4-6: 100-125 mg bid.
Days 7-9: 100-125 mg tid.
Day 10 to Maintenance: 250 mg tid.

For most adults and children 8 years of age and over, the usual maintenance dosage is 3-4 250 mg primadone tablets daily in divided doses (250 mg tid or qid). If required, an increase to 5 or 6 250 mg tablets daily may be made, but daily doses should not exceed 500 mg qid (see TABLE 1).

TABLE 1 *Initial: Adults And Children Over 8*

DAY	AM	NOON	PM
1			2 × 50 mg
2			2 × 50 mg
3			2 × 50 mg
4	2 × 50 mg		2 × 50 mg
5	2 × 50 mg		2 × 50 mg
6	2 × 50 mg		2 × 50 mg
7	2 × 50 mg	2 × 50 mg	2 × 50 mg
8	2 × 50 mg	2 × 50 mg	2 × 50 mg
9	2 × 50 mg	2 × 50 mg	2 × 50 mg
10	250 mg	250 mg	250 mg
11	*	*	*
12	*	*	*

* Adjust to maintenance.

Dosage should be individualized to provide maximum benefit. In some cases, serum blood level determinations of primidone may be necessary for optimal dosage adjustment. The clinically effective serum level for primidone is between 5-12 μg/ml.

In Patients Already Receiving Other Anticonvulsants

Primadone should be started at 100-125 mg at bedtime and gradually increased to maintenance level as the other drug is gradually decreased. This regimen should be continued until

P

satisfactory dosage level is achieved for the combination, or the other medication is completely withdrawn. When therapy with primadone alone is the objective, the transition from concomitant therapy should not be completed in less than 2 weeks.

PEDIATRIC DOSAGE

For children under 8 years of age, the following regimen may be used:

Days 1-3: 50 mg at bedtime.
Days 4-6: 50 mg bid.
Days 7-9: 100 mg bid.
Day 10 to Maintenance: 125 mg tid to 250 mg tid.

For children under 8 years of age, the usual maintenance dosage is 125-250 mg 3 times daily or, 10-25 mg/kg/day in divided doses.

HOW SUPPLIED

TABLETS

Each square-shaped, scored, yellow tablet, identified by "MYSOLINE 250" and an embossed M, contains 250 mg of primidone.

Each square-shaped, scored, white tablet, identified by "MYSOLINE 50" and an embossed M, contains 50 mg of primidone.

SUSPENSION

Each 5 ml (teaspoonful) contains 250 mg of primidone.

STORAGE

Store at room temperature, approximately 25°C (77°F).

Dispense in a tight, light-resistant container.

PRODUCT LISTING - RATED THERAPEUTICALLY EQUIVALENT

Tablet - Oral - 50 mg

Qty	Price	Product	NDC
60's	$22.58	MYSOLINE, Physicians Total Care	54868-3689-01
100's	$36.84	MYSOLINE, Physicians Total Care	54868-3689-02
100's	$39.99	GENERIC, Qualitest Products Inc	00603-5369-21
100's	$41.10	GENERIC, Major Pharmaceuticals Inc	00904-5559-60
100's	$43.40	GENERIC, Lannett Company Inc	00527-1301-01
100's	$48.33	MYSOLINE, Elan Pharmaceuticals	59075-0690-10

Tablet - Oral - 250 mg

Qty	Price	Product	NDC
30's	$10.13	GENERIC, Heartland Healthcare Services	61392-0024-30
30's	$10.13	GENERIC, Heartland Healthcare Services	61392-0024-39
31 x 10	$116.21	GENERIC, Vangard Labs	00615-2521-53
31 x 10	$116.21	GENERIC, Vangard Labs	00615-2521-63
31's	$10.46	GENERIC, Heartland Healthcare Services	61392-0024-31
32's	$10.80	GENERIC, Heartland Healthcare Services	61392-0024-32
45's	$15.19	GENERIC, Heartland Healthcare Services	61392-0024-45
60's	$20.25	GENERIC, Heartland Healthcare Services	61392-0024-60
90's	$30.38	GENERIC, Heartland Healthcare Services	61392-0024-90
100's	$7.95	GENERIC, Cmc-Consolidated Midland Corporation	00223-1414-01
100's	$15.00	GENERIC, Us Trading Corporation	56126-0289-11
100's	$34.88	GENERIC, Major Pharmaceuticals Inc	00904-0560-61
100's	$36.03	GENERIC, Moore, H.L. Drug Exchange Inc	00839-1522-06
100's	$36.03	GENERIC, Moore, H.L. Drug Exchange Inc	00839-1552-06
100's	$36.91	GENERIC, Caremark Inc	00339-5659-12
100's	$38.55	GENERIC, Ivax Corporation	00182-0701-01
100's	$41.25	GENERIC, Aligen Independent Laboratories Inc	00405-4836-01
100's	$41.25	GENERIC, Watson/Rugby Laboratories Inc	00536-4373-01
100's	$49.00	GENERIC, Duramed Pharmaceuticals Inc	51285-0939-02
100's	$64.05	FEDERAL UPPER LIMIT, H.C.F.A. F F P	99999-2114-01
100's	$65.00	GENERIC, Mova Pharmaceutical Corporation	55370-0888-07
100's	$77.81	GENERIC, Watson/Schein Pharmaceuticals Inc	00364-0366-01
100's	$77.81	GENERIC, Dixon-Shane Inc	17236-0547-01
100's	$98.60	GENERIC, Major Pharmaceuticals Inc	00904-0560-60
100's	$99.45	MYSOLINE, Allscripts Pharmaceutical Company	54569-0164-02
100's	$99.59	GENERIC, Mutual/United Research Laboratories	00677-0354-01
100's	$99.60	GENERIC, Lannett Company Inc	00527-1231-01
100's	$99.60	GENERIC, Watson Laboratories Inc	00591-5321-01
100's	$99.60	GENERIC, Qualitest Products Inc	00603-5370-21
100's	$161.51	MYSOLINE, Elan Pharmaceuticals	59075-0691-81
100's	$174.44	MYSOLINE, Elan Pharmaceuticals	59075-0691-10
100's	$174.44	MYSOLINE, Xcel Pharmaceuticals Inc	66490-0691-10
100's	$174.44	MYSOLINE, Xcel Pharmaceuticals Inc	66490-0691-81
200 x 5	$374.87	GENERIC, Vangard Labs	00615-2521-43

PRODUCT LISTING - EQUIVALENTS NOT AVAILABLE

Suspension - Oral - 250 mg/5 ml

Qty	Price	Product	NDC
240 ml	$62.95	MYSOLINE, Elan Pharmaceuticals	59075-0692-50

Tablet - Oral - 250 mg

Qty	Price	Product	NDC
30's	$13.70	GENERIC, Physicians Total Care	54868-1691-02
30's	$16.00	GENERIC, Pharmaceutical Corporation Of America	51655-0366-24
100's	$42.54	GENERIC, Physicians Total Care	54868-1691-03
100's	$47.43	GENERIC, Southwood Pharmaceuticals Inc	58016-0877-00

Probenecid *(002115)*

Categories: Arthritis, gouty; FDA Approved 1951 Apr; Pregnancy Category B
Drug Classes: Antigout agents; Uricosurics
Brand Names: **Benemid**; Panuric; Probalan; Solpurin; Urocid
Foreign Brand Availability: Bencid (India; Thailand); Benecid (Japan; Mexico); Benemide (Finland); Benuryl (Canada); Probecid (Finland; Norway; Sweden); Probenemid (Japan); Probenid (Indonesia); Pro-Cid (Australia); Procid (Taiwan)
Cost of Therapy: $5.40 (Gout; Generic Tablets; 500 mg; 2 tablets/day; 30 day supply)

DESCRIPTION

Probenecid is a uricosuric and renal tubular transport blocking agent.

Probenecid is the generic name for 4-((di-propylamino)sulfonyl) benzoic acid (molecular weight 285.36).

Probenecid is a white or nearly white, fine, crystalline powder. Probenecid is soluble in dilute alkali, in alcohol, in chloroform, and in acetone; it is practically insoluble in water and in dilute acids.

Each tablet contains 0.5 g probenecid and the following inactive ingredients: calcium stearate, D&C yellow 10, gelatin, hydroxypropyl methylcellulose, iron oxide, magnesium carbonate, polyethylene glycol, starch, talc, and titanium dioxide.

CLINICAL PHARMACOLOGY

Probenecid is a uricosuric and renal tubular blocking agent. It inhibits the tubular reabsorption of urate, thus increasing the urinary excretion of uric acid and decreasing serum urate levels. Effective uricosuria reduces the miscible urate pool, retards urate deposition, and promotes resorption of urate deposits.

Probenecid inhibits the tubular secretion of penicillin and usually increases penicillin plasma levels by any route the antibiotic is given. A 2-fold to 4-fold elevation has been demonstrated for various penicillins.

Probenecid also has been reported to inhibit the renal transport of many other compounds including aminohippuric acid (PAH), aminosalicylic acid (PAS), indomethacin, sodium iodomethamate and related iodinated organic acids, 17-ketosteroids, pantothenic acid, phenolsulfonphthalein (PSP), sulfonamides, and sulfonylureas. See also DRUG INTERACTIONS.

Probenecid decreases both hepatic and renal excretion of sulfobromophthalein (BSP). The tubular reabsorption of phosphorus is inhibited in hypoparathyroid but not in euparathyroid individuals.

Probenecid does not influence plasma concentrations of salicylates, nor the excretion of streptomycin, chloramphenicol, chlortetracycline, oxytetracycline, or neomycin.

INDICATIONS AND USAGE

For treatment of the hyperuricemia associated with gout and gouty arthritis.

As an adjuvant to therapy with penicillin or with ampicillin, methicillin, oxacillin, cloxacillin, or nafcillin, for elevation and prolongation of plasma levels by whatever route the antibiotic is given.

CONTRAINDICATIONS

Hypersensitivity to this product.

Children under 2 years of age.

Not recommended in persons with known blood dyscrasias or uric acid kidney stones.

Therapy with probenecid should not be started until an acute gouty attack has subsided.

WARNINGS

Exacerbation of gout following therapy with probenecid may occur; in such cases colchicine or other appropriate therapy is advisable.

Probenecid increases plasma concentrations of methotrexate in both animals and humans. In animal studies, increased methotrexate toxicity has been reported. If probenecid is given with methotrexate, the dosage of methotrexate should be reduced and serum levels may need to be monitored.

In patients on probenecid the use of salicylates in either small or large doses is contraindicated because it antagonizes the uricosuric action of probenecid. The biphasic action of salicylates in the renal tubules accounts for the so-called "paradoxical effect" of uricosuric agents. In patients on probenecid who require a mild analgesic agent the use of a acetaminophen rather than small doses of salicylates would be preferred.

Rarely, severe allergic reactions and anaphylaxis have been reported with the use of probenecid. Most of these have been reported to occur within several hours after readministration following prior usage of the drug.

The appearance of hypersensitivity reactions requires cessation of therapy with probenecid.

Use in Pregnancy: Probenecid crosses the placental barrier and appears in cord blood. The use of any drug in women of childbearing potential requires that the anticipated benefit be weighed against possible hazards.

PRECAUTIONS

GENERAL

Hematuria, renal colic, costovertebral pain, and formation of uric acid stones associated with the use of probenecid in gouty patients may be prevented by alkalization of the urine and a liberal fluid intake (*see* DOSAGE AND ADMINISTRATION). In these cases when alkali is administered, the acid-base balance of the patient should be watched.

Use with caution in patients with a history of peptic ulcer.

Probenecid has been used in patients with some renal impairment but dosage requirements may be increased. Probenecid may not be effective in chronic renal insufficiency particularly when the glomerular filtration rate is 30 ml/minute or less. Because of its mechanism of action, probenecid is not recommended in conjunction with a penicillin in the presence of *known* renal impairment.

A reducing substance may appear in the urine of patients receiving probenecid. This disappears with discontinuance of therapy. Suspected glycosuria should be confirmed by using a test specific for glucose.

DRUG INTERACTIONS

When probenecid is used to elevate plasma concentrations of penicillin or other beta-lactams, or when such drugs are given to patients taking probenecid therapeutically, high plasma concentrations of the other drug may increase the incidence of adverse reactions associated with that drug. In the case of penicillin or other beta-lactams, psychic disturbances have been reported.

The use of salicylates antagonizes the uricosuric action of probenecid (see WARNINGS). The uricosuric action of probenecid is also antagonized by pyrazinamide.

Probenecid produces an insignificant increase in free sulfonamide plasma concentrations but a significant increase in total sulfonamide plasma levels. Since probenecid decreases the renal excretion of conjugated sulfonamides, plasma concentrations of the latter should be determined from time to time when a sulfonamide and probenecid are coadministered for prolonged periods. Probenecid may prolong or enhance the action of oral sulfonylureas and thereby increase the risk of hypoglycemia.

It has been reported that patients receiving probenecid require significantly less thiopental for induction of anesthesia. In addition, ketamine and thiopental anesthesia were significantly prolonged in rats receiving probenecid.

The concomitant administration of probenecid increases the mean plasma elimination half-life of a number of drugs which can lead to increased plasma concentrations. These include agents such as indomethacin, acetaminophen, naproxen, ketoprofen, meclofenamate, lorazepam, and rifampin. Although the clinical significance of this observation has not been established, a lower dosage of the drug may be required to produce a therapeutic effect, and increases in dosage of the drug in question should be made cautiously and in small increments when probenecid is being co-administrated. Although specific instances of toxicity due to this potential interaction have not been observed to date, physicians should be alert to this possibility.

Probenecid given concomitantly with sulindac has only a slight effect on plasma sulfide levels, while plasma levels of sulindac and sulfone were increased. Sulindac was shown to produce a modest reduction in the uricosuric action of probenecid, which probably is not significant under most circumstances.

In animals and in humans, probenecid has been reported to increase plasma concentrations of methotrexate (see WARNINGS).

Falsely high readings for theophylline have been reported in an *in vitro* study, using the Schack and Waxler technic, when therapeutic concentrations of theophylline and probenecid were added to human plasma.

ADVERSE REACTIONS

The following adverse reactions have been observed and within each category are listed in order of decreasing severity:

Central Nervous System: headache, dizziness.

Metabolic: precipitation of acute gouty arthritis.

Gastrointestinal: hepatic necrosis, vomiting, nausea, anorexia, sore gums.

Genitourinary: nephrotic syndrome, uric acid stones with or without hematuria, renal colic, costovertebral pain, urinary frequency.

Hypersensitivity: anaphylaxis, fever, urticaria, pruritus.

Hematologic: aplastic anemia, leukopenia, hemolytic anemia which in some patients could be related to genetic deficiency of glucose -6-phosphate dehydrogenase in red blood cells, anemia.

Integumentary: dermatitis, alopecia, flushing.

DOSAGE AND ADMINISTRATION

GOUT

Therapy with probenecid should not be *started* until an acute gouty attack has subsided. However, if and acute attack is precipitated *during* therapy, probenecid may be continued without changing the dosage, and full therapeutic dosage of colchicine or other appropriate therapy should be given to control the acute attack.

The recommended adult dosage is 0.25 g (1/2 tablet of probenecid) twice a day for one week, followed by 0.5 g (1 tablet) twice a day thereafter.

Some degree of renal impairment may be present in patients with gout. A daily dosage of 1 g may be adequate. However, if necessary, the daily dosage may be increased by 0.5 g increments every 4 weeks within tolerance (and usually not above 2 g per day) if symptoms of gouty arthritis are not controlled or the 24 hour uric acid excretion is not above 700 mg. As noted, probenecid may not be effective in chronic renal insufficiency particularly when the glomerular filtration rate is 30 ml/minute or less.

PENICILLIN THERAPY (GONORRHEA)*

1) Uncomplicated gonococcal infection in men and women (urethral, cervical, rectal)

Recommended Regimens**: 4.8 million units of aqueous procaine penicillin G† IM, in at least 2 doses injected at different sites at one visit + 1 g of probenecid orally just before injections *or* 3.5 g of ampicillin† orally + 1 g probenecid orally given simultaneously.

Remarks: *Follow-up:* Obtain urethral and other appropriate cultures from men, and cervical, anal, and other appropriate cultures from women, 7 to 14 days after completion of treatment.

Treatment of Sexual Partners: Persons with known recent exposure to gonorrhea should receive same treatment as those known to have gonorrhea. Examination and treatment of male sex partners of persons with gonorrhea are essential because of high prevalence of non- symptomatic urethral gonococcal infection in such men.

2) Pharyngeal gonococcal infection in men and women

Recommended Regimens**: 4.8 million units of aqueous procaine penicillin G† IM, in at least 2 doses injected at different sites at one visit + 1 g probenecid orally just before injections.

Remarks: Pharyngeal gonococcal infections may be more difficult to treat than anogenital gonorrhea. Post treatment cultures are essential.

3) Uncomplicated gonorrhea in pregnant patients

Recommended Regimens**: 4.8 million units of aqueous procaine penicillin G† IM, in at least 2 doses injected at different sites at one visit *or* 3.5 g of ampicillin† orally + 1 g of probenecid orally given simultaneously

4) Acute gonococcal salpingitis

Recommended Regimens**: *Outpatients:* Aqueous procaine penicillin G† or ampicillin† with probenecid as for gonorrhea in pregnancy, followed by 500 mg of ampicillin 4 times a day for 10 days

Hospitalized Patients: See details in CDC recommendations

Remarks: Follow-up of patients with acute salpingitis is essential. All patients should receive repeat pelvic examinations and cultures for *Neisseria gonorrhoeae* after treatment. Examination and appropriate treatment of male sex partners are essential because of high prevalence of non-symptomatic urethral gonorrhea in such men.

5) Disseminated gonococcal infection (arthritis-dermatitis syndrome)

Recommended Regimens**: 10 million units of aqueous crystalline penicillin G IV a day for 3 days or till significant clinical improvement occurs. May be followed with 500 mg of ampicillin† 4 times a day orally to complete 7 days of treatment *or* 3.5 g of ampicillin† orally with 1 g of probenecid, followed by 500 mg of ampicillin† 4 times a day for at least 7 days

6) Gonococcal infection in children

Recommended Regimens**: For postpubertal children and/or those weighing over 45 kg (100 lb) use the dosage regimens given above for adults. Uncomplicated vulvovaginitis and urethritis: aqueous procaine penicillin G† 75,000 — 100,000 units/kg IM, with probenecid 23 mg/kg orally

Remarks: See CDC recommendations for detailed information about prevention and treatment of neonatal gonococcal infection and gonococcal ophthalmia.

Note: Before treating gonococcal infections in patients with suspected primary or secondary syphilis, perform proper diagnostic procedures including darkfield examinations. If concomitant syphilis is suspected, perform monthly serological tests for at least 4 months.

* Recommended by Venereal Disease Control Advisory Committee, Center for Disease Control, U.S. Department of Health, Education, and Welfare, Public Health Service (Morbidity and Mortality Weekly Report, Vol. *23:* 341, 342, 347, 348, Oct. 11, 1974).

** See CDC recommendations for definition of regimens of choice, alternative regimens, treatment of hypersensitive patients, and other aspects of therapy.

† See prescribing information for detailed information about contraindications, warnings, precautions, and adverse reactions.

Gastric intolerance may be indicative of overdosage, and may be corrected by decreasing the dosage.

As uric acid tends to crystallize out of an acid urine, a liberal fluid intake is recommended, as well as sufficient sodium bicarbonate (3 to 7.5 g daily) or potassium citrate (7.5 g daily) to maintain an alkaline urine (see PRECAUTIONS).

Alkalization of the urine is recommended until the serum urate level returns to normal limits and tophaceous deposits disappear, i.e., during the period when urinary excretion of uric acid is at a high level. Thereafter, alkalization of the urine and the usual restriction of purine-producing foods may be somewhat relaxed.

Probenecid should be continued at the dosage that will maintain normal serum urate levels. When acute attacks have been absent for 6 months or more and serum urate levels remain within normal limits, the daily dosage may be decreased by 0.5 g every 6 months. The maintenance dosage should not be reduced to the point where serum urate levels tend to rise.

PROBENECID AND PENICILLIN THERAPY (GENERAL)

Adults

The recommended dosage is 2 g (4 tablets of probenecid) daily in divided doses. This dosage should be reduced in older patients in whom renal impairment may be present.

Children 2-14 Years of Age

Initial Dose: 25 mg/kg body weight (*or* 0.7 g/square meter body surface).

Maintenance Dose: 40 mg/kg body weight (*or* 1.2 g/square meter body surface) per day, divided into 4 doses.

For children weighing more than 50 kg (110 lb) the adult dosage is recommended.

Probenecid is contraindicated in children under 2 years of age.

The PSP excretion test may be used to determine the effectiveness of probenecid in retarding penicillin excretion and maintaining therapeutic levels. The renal clearance of PSP is reduced to about one-fifth the normal rate when dosage of probenecid is adequate.

PENICILLIN THERAPY (GONORRHEA)

See information above.

(Merck 8/88, 7399021)

PRODUCT LISTING - RATED THERAPEUTICALLY EQUIVALENT

Tablet - Oral - 500 mg

2's	$11.10	GENERIC, Pd-Rx Pharmaceuticals	55289-0715-02
15's	$29.13	GENERIC, Pd-Rx Pharmaceuticals	55289-0715-15
25's	$5.55	GENERIC, Pd-Rx Pharmaceuticals	55289-0715-97
30's	$6.77	GENERIC, Heartland Healthcare Services	61392-0764-30
30's	$6.77	GENERIC, Heartland Healthcare Services	61392-0764-39
31's	$7.00	GENERIC, Heartland Healthcare Services	61392-0764-31
32's	$7.23	GENERIC, Heartland Healthcare Services	61392-0764-32
45's	$10.16	GENERIC, Heartland Healthcare Services	61392-0764-45
60's	$13.55	GENERIC, Heartland Healthcare Services	61392-0764-60
90's	$20.32	GENERIC, Heartland Healthcare Services	61392-0764-90
100's	$13.97	GENERIC, Moore, H.L. Drug Exchange Inc	00839-5081-06

P

100's	$15.85	GENERIC, Aligen Independent Laboratories Inc	00405-4841-01
100's	$15.98	GENERIC, Interstate Drug Exchange Inc	00814-6320-14
100's	$16.20	GENERIC, Pd-Rx Pharmaceuticals	55289-0715-17
100's	$17.00	GENERIC, Martec Pharmaceuticals Inc	52555-0336-01
100's	$17.50	GENERIC, Cmc-Consolidated Midland Corporation	00223-1472-01
100's	$22.58	GENERIC, Us Trading Corporation	56126-0383-11
100's	$70.59	FEDERAL UPPER LIMIT, H.C.F.A. F F P	99999-2115-01
100's	$97.35	GENERIC, Major Pharmaceuticals Inc	00904-2190-60
100's	$98.25	GENERIC, Mylan Pharmaceuticals Inc	00378-0156-01
100's	$98.33	GENERIC, Watson/Schein Pharmaceuticals Inc	00364-0314-01
100's	$98.33	GENERIC, Watson/Schein Pharmaceuticals Inc	00591-5347-01
100's	$219.80	GENERIC, Ivax Corporation	00172-2190-60

PRODUCT LISTING - EQUIVALENTS NOT AVAILABLE

Tablet - Oral - 500 mg

2's	$2.07	GENERIC, Physicians Total Care	54868-0159-01
2's	$3.59	GENERIC, Prescript Pharmaceuticals	00247-0183-02
2's	$4.83	GENERIC, Pharma Pac	52959-0450-02
10's	$4.54	GENERIC, Prescript Pharmaceuticals	00247-0183-10
20's	$5.74	GENERIC, Prescript Pharmaceuticals	00247-0183-20
25's	$6.33	GENERIC, Prescript Pharmaceuticals	00247-0183-25
30's	$6.93	GENERIC, Prescript Pharmaceuticals	00247-0183-30
45's	$8.72	GENERIC, Prescript Pharmaceuticals	00247-0183-45
60's	$13.87	GENERIC, Physicians Total Care	54868-0159-00
100's	$9.00	GENERIC, C.O. Truxton Inc	00463-6318-01
100's	$15.27	GENERIC, Prescript Pharmaceuticals	00247-0183-00
100's	$22.00	GENERIC, Physicians Total Care	54868-0159-02

Procainamide Hydrochloride *(002117)*

Categories: Arrhythmia, ventricular; Tachycardia, ventricular; Pregnancy Category C; FDA Approved 1950 Jun; WHO Formulary
Drug Classes: Antiarrhythmics, class IA
Brand Names: Biocoryl; Procan Sr; Procanbid; Promine; **Pronestyl**; Ritmocamid
Foreign Brand Availability: Amisalin (Taiwan); Cardiorytmin (Finland)
Cost of Therapy: $211.20 (Arrhythmia; Pronestyl; 375 mg; 8 capsules/day; 30 day supply)
$22.32 (Arrhythmia; Generic Tablets; 375 mg; 8 capsules/day; 30 day supply)
$54.00 (Arrhythmia; Generic Extended Release Tablets; 750 mg; 4 capsules/day; 30 day supply)
HCFA JCODE(S): J2690 up to 1 g IM, IV

WARNING

The prolonged administration of procainamide often leads to the development of a positive anti-nuclear antibody (ANA) test, with or without symptoms of a lupus erythematosus-like syndrome. If a positive ANA titer develops, the benefits versus risks of continued procainamide therapy should be assessed.

P

DESCRIPTION

Note: This monograph contains information on procainamide hydrochloride (procainamide HCl) tablets, extended release tablets, capsules, and injection.

Procainamide hydrochloride, a Group 1A cardiac antiarrhythmic drug, is p-amino-N-(2-(diethylamino)ethyl)-benzamide monohydrochloride, molecular weight 271.79.

It differs from procaine which is the p-aminobenzoyl *ester* of 2-(diethylamino)-ethanol. Procainamide as the free base has a pKa of 9.23; the monohydrochloride is very soluble in water. Procainamide hydrochloride is supplied for oral administration as capsules and tablets in potencies of 250, 375, and 500 mg.

INACTIVE INGREDIENTS

Pronestyl Tablets

Calcium silicate, microcrystalline cellulose, colorants (FD&C yellow no. 5 (tartrazine) and yellow no. 6), flavor, povidone, starch, stearic acid, and other ingredients.

Pronestyl Capsules

Colorants (D&C yellow no. 10, except 375 mg; FD&C yellow no. 6), gelatin, lactose (except 500 mg), magnesium stearate, talc, and titanium dioxide.

Pronestyl Extended-Release Tablets

Pronestyl extended-release tablets are available for oral administration as green, film-coated tablets containing 250 mg procainamide hydrochloride, as yellow scored, film-coated tablets containing 500 mg procainamide hydrochloride; as orange, scored, film coated tablets containing 750 mg procainamide hydrochloride; and as red, scored, film-coated tablets containing 1000 mg procainamide hydrochloride.

All strengths of Pronestyl extended release tablets contain candeilla wax; colloidal silicon dioxide; magnesium stearate; titanium dioxide, vanillin; and other ingredients. The individual strengths contain additional ingredients as follows: *250 mg:* D&C yellow no. 10 Al lake; FD&C blue no. 1 Al lake; FD&C yellow no. 6 Al lake; lactose; may also contain methylparaben; or simethicone emulsion and polysorbate 80. *500 mg:* D&C yellow no.10 Al lake; FD &C blue no. 2 Al lake; FD&C yellow no. 6 Al lake; sucrose; may also contain methylparaben; and propylparaben; or simethicone and emulsion and polysorbate 80. *750 mg:* FD&C yellow no. 6 Al lake; may also contain propylene glycol; or simethicone emulsion and polysorbate 80. *1000 mg:* D&C red no. 7 calcium lake; FD&C yellow no. 6 Al lake; propylene glycol.

Pronestyl Injection

Procainamide hydrochloride is available for parenteral use as a sterile, aqueous solution providing 100 mg or 500 mg/ml. The 100 mg/ml concentration in each ml procainamide hydrochloride 100 mg, benzyl alcohol 0.009 ml and sodium metabisulfite 0.9 mg in water for injection. The 500 mg/ml concentration contains in each ml procainamide hydrochloride 500 mg, benzyl alcohol 0.009 ml and sodium metabisulfite 2 mg in water for injection. For both concentrations, pH is 4.0-6.0; sodium hydroxide and/or hydrochloric acid added, if needed, for pH adjustment. Vials are sealed under nitrogen.

STORAGE

Injection

Store at controlled room temperature 15-30°C (59-86°F).

Discard solution if darker than slightly yellow or otherwise discolored.

Oral Forms

Store at room temperature; avoid excessive heat (104° F); protect from moisture.

CLINICAL PHARMACOLOGY

Procainamide (PA) increases the effective refractory period of the atria, and to a lesser extent the bundle of His-Purkinje system and ventricles of the heart. It reduces impulse conduction velocity in the atria, His-Purkinje fibers, and ventricular muscle, but has variable effects on the atrioventricular (A-V) node, a direct slowing action and a weaker vagolytic effect which may speed A-V conduction slightly. Myocardial excitability is reduced in the atria, Purkinje fibers, papillary muscles, and ventricles by an increase in the threshold for excitation, combined with inhibition of ectopic pacemaker activity by retardation of the slow phase of diastolic depolarization, thus decreasing automaticity especially in ectopic sites. Contractility of the undamaged heart is usually not affected by therapeutic concentrations, although slight reduction of cardiac output may occur, and may be significant in the presence of myocardial damage. Therapeutic levels of PA may exert vagolytic effects and produce slight acceleration of heart rate, while high or toxic concentrations may prolong A-V conduction time or induce A-V block, or even cause abnormal automaticity and spontaneous firing, by unknown mechanisms.

The electrocardiogram may reflect these effects by showing slight sinus tachycardia (due to the anticholinergic action) and widened QRS complexes and, less regularly, prolonged Q-T and P-R intervals (due to longer systole and slower conduction), as well as some decrease in QRS and T wave amplitude. These direct effects of PA on electrical activity, conduction, responsiveness, excitability and automaticity are characteristic of a Group 1A antiarrhythmic agent, the prototype for which is quinidine; PA effects are very similar. However, PA has weaker vagal blocking action than does quinidine, does not induce alpha-adrenergic blockade, and is less depressing to cardiac contractility.

Ingested PA is resistant to digestive hydrolysis, and the drug is well absorbed from the entire small intestinal surface, but individual patients vary in their completeness of absorption of PA. Following oral administration of , plasma PA levels reach about 50% of peak in 30 minutes, 90% at an hour, and peak at about 90-120 minutes. About 15-20% of PA is reversibly bound to plasma proteins, and considerable amounts are more slowly and reversibly bound to tissues of the heart, liver, lung, and kidney. The apparent volume of distribution eventually reaches about 2 L/kg body weight with a half-time of approximately 5 minutes. While PA has been shown in the dog to cross the blood-brain barrier, it did not concentrate in the brain at levels higher than in plasma. It is not known if PA crosses the placenta. Plasma esterases are far less active in hydrolysis of PA than of procaine. The half-time for elimination of PA is 3-4 hours in patients with normal renal function, but reduced creatinine clearance and advancing age each prolong the half-time of elimination of PA.

A significant fraction of the circulating PA may be metabolized in hepatocytes to N-acetylprocainamide (NAPA), ranging from 16-21% of an administered dose in "slow acetylators" to 24-33% in "fast-acetylators". Since NAPA also has significant antiarrhythmic activity and somewhat slower renal clearance than PA, both hepatic acetylation rate capability and renal function, as well as age, have significant effects on the effective biologic half-time of therapeutic action of administered PA and the NAPA derivative. Trace amounts may be excreted in the urine as free and conjugated p-aminobenzoic acid, 30-60% as unchanged PA, and 6-52% as the NAPA derivative. Both PA and NAPA are eliminated by active tubular secretion as well as by glomerular filtration. Action of PA on the central nervous system is not prominent, but high plasma concentrations may cause tremors. While therapeutic plasma levels for PA have been reported to be 3-10 µg/ml, certain patients such as those with sustained ventricular tachycardia, may need higher levels for adequate control. This may justify the increased risk of toxicity. Where programmed ventricular stimulation has been used to evaluate efficacy of PA in preventing recurrent ventricular tachyarrhythmias, higher plasma levels (mean, 13.6 µg/ml) of PA were found necessary for adequate control.

ADDITIONAL INFORMATION FOR PROCAINAMIDE HCl INJECTION

Following IM injection, this drug is rapidly absorbed into the blood stream, and, plasma levels peak in about 15-60 minutes, considerably faster than orally administered forms. IV administration of procainamide HCl can produce therapeutic procainamide levels within minutes after the infusion is started.

INDICATIONS AND USAGE

Procainamide HCl is indicated for the treatment of documented ventricular arrhythmias, such as sustained ventricular tachycardia, that, in the judgement of the physician, are life-threatening. Because of the proarrhythmic effects of procainamide HCl, its use with lesser arrythmias is generally not recommended. Treatment of patients with asymptomatic ventricular premature contractions should be avoided.

Initiation of procainamide HCl treatment, as with other antiarrhythmic agents used to treat life-threatening arrythmias, should be carried out in the hospital.

Antiarrhythmic drugs have not been shown to enhance survival in patients with ventricular arrythmias.

Because procainamide has the potential to produce serious hematological disorders (0.5%) particularly leukopenia or agranulocytosis (sometimes fatal), its use should be reserved for patients in whom, in the opinion of the physician, the benefits of treatment clearly outweigh the risks. (See WARNINGS and BOXED WARNING.)

NON-FDA APPROVED INDICATIONS
Procainamide is also used without FDA approval to treat atrial fibrillation.

CONTRAINDICATIONS

COMPLETE HEART BLOCK
Procainamide should not be administered to patients with complete heart block because of its effects in suppressing nodal or ventricular pacemakers and the hazard of asystole. It may be difficult to recognize complete heart block in patients with ventricular tachycardia, but if significant slowing of ventricular rate occurs during PA treatment without evidence of A-V conduction appearing, PA should be stopped. In cases of second degree A-V block or various types of hemiblock, PA should be avoided or discontinued because of the possibility of increased severity of block, unless the ventricular rate is controlled by an electrical pacemaker.

IDIOSYNCRATIC HYPERSENSITIVITY
In patients sensitive to procaine or other ester-type local anesthetics, cross sensitivity to PA is unlikely; however, it should be borne in mind, and PA should not be used if it produces acute allergic dermatitis, asthma, or anaphylactic symptoms.

LUPUS ERYTHEMATOSUS
An established diagnosis of systemic lupus erythematosus is a contraindication to PA therapy, since aggravation of symptoms is highly likely.

TORSADES DE POINTES
In the unusual ventricular arrhythmia called "les torsades de pointes" (Twistings of the points), characterized by alternation of one or more ventricular premature beats in the directions of the QRS complexes on ECG in persons with prolonged Q-T and often enhanced U waves, Group 1A antiarrhythmic drugs are contraindicated. Administration of PA in such cases may aggravate this special type of ventricular extrasystole or tachycardia instead of suppressing it.

WARNINGS

MORTALITY
In the National Heart, Lung and Blood Institute's Cardiac Arrythmia Suppression Trial (CAST), a long-term, multicentered, randomized, double-blind study in patients with asymptomatic non-life-threatening ventricular arrythmias who had had myocardial infarctions more than 6 days but less than 2 years previously, an excessive mortality or non- fatal cardiac arrest rate was seen in patients treated with encainide or flecainide (56/730) compared with that seen in patients assigned to matched placebo-treated groups (22/725). The average duration of treatment with encainide or flecainide in this study was 10 months.

The applicability of these results to other populations (*e.g.*, those without recent myocardial infarctions) or to other antiarrhythmic drugs is uncertain, but at present it is prudent to consider any antiarrhythmic agent to have a significant risk in patients with structural heart disease.

BLOOD DYSCRASIAS: Agranulocytosis, bone marrow depression, neutropenia, hypoplastic anemia and thrombocytopenia in patients receiving procainamide hydrochloride have been reported at a rate of approximately 0.5%. Most of these patients received procainamide within the recommended dosage range. Fatalities have occurred (with approximately 20-25% mortality in reported cases of agranulocytosis). Since most of these events have been noted during the first 12 weeks of therapy, it is recommended that complete blood counts including white cell, differential and platelet counts be performed at weekly intervals for the first 3 months of therapy, and periodically thereafter. Complete blood counts should be performed promptly if the patient develops any signs of infection (such as fever, chills, sore throat or stomatitis), bruising or bleeding. If any of these hematologic disorders are identified, procainamide therapy should be discontinued. Blood counts usually return to normal within 1 month of discontinuation. Caution should be used in patients with pre-existing marrow failure or cytopenia of any type (see ADVERSE REACTIONS).

DIGITALIS INTOXICATION
Caution should be exercised in the use of procainamide in arrhythmias associated with digitalis intoxication. Procainamide can suppress digitalis-induced arrhythmias; however, if there is concomitant marked disturbance of atrioventricular conduction, additional depression of conduction and ventricular asystole or fibrillation may result. Therefore, use of procainamide should be considered only if discontinuation of digitalis, and therapy with potassium, lidocaine, or phenytoin are ineffective.

FIRST DEGREE HEART BLOCK
Caution should be exercised also if the patient exhibits or develops first degree heart block while taking PA, and dosage reduction is advised in such cases. If the block persists despite dosage reduction, continuation of PA administration must be evaluated on the basis of current benefit versus risk of increased heart block.

PREDIGITALIZATION FOR ATRIAL FLUTTER OR FIBRILLATION
Patients with atrial flutter or fibrillation should be cardioverted or digitalized prior to PA administration to avoid enhancement of A-V conduction which may result in ventricular rate acceleration beyond tolerable limits. Adequate digitalization reduces but does not eliminate the possibility of sudden increase in ventricular rate as the atrial rate is slowed by PA in these arrhythmias.

CONGESTIVE HEART FAILURE
For patients in congestive heart failure, and those with acute ischemic heart disease or cardiomyopathy, caution should be used in PA therapy, since even slight depression of myocardial contractility may further reduce cardiac output of the damaged heart.

CONCURRENT OTHER ANTIARRHYTHMIC AGENTS
Concurrent use of PA with other Group 1A antiarrhythmic agents such as quinidine or disopyramide may produce enhanced prolongation of conduction or depression of contractility and hypotension, especially in patients with cardiac decompensation. Such use should be reserved for patients with serious arrhythmias unresponsive to a single drug and employed only if close observation is possible.

RENAL INSUFFICIENCY
Renal insufficiency may lead to accumulation of high plasma levels from conventional oral doses of PA, with effects similar to those of overdosage, unless dosage is adjusted for the individual patient.

MYASTHENIA GRAVIS
Patients with myasthenia gravis may show worsening of symptoms from PA due to its procaine-like effect on diminishing acetylcholine release at skeletal muscle motor nerve endings, so that PA administration may be hazardous without optimal adjustment of anticholinesterase medications and other precautions.

Additional Information for the Injection
This contains sodium metabisulfite, a sulfite that may cause allergic-type reactions including anaphylactic symptoms and life-threatening or less severe asthmatic episodes in certain susceptible people. The overall prevalence of sulfite sensitivity in the general population is unknown and probably low. Sulfite sensitivity is seen more frequently in asthmatic than in non-asthmatic people.

PRECAUTIONS

GENERAL
Immediately after initiation of PA therapy, patients should be closely observed for possible hypersensitivity reactions, especially if procaine or local anesthetic sensitivity is suspected, and for muscular weakness if myasthenia gravis is a possibility.

In conversion of atrial fibrillation to normal sinus rhythm by any means, dislodgement of mural thrombi may lead to embolization, which should be kept in mind.

After a day or so, steady state plasma PA levels are produced following regular oral administration of a given dose of procainamide HCl tablets; procainamide HCl capsules at set intervals, with peak plasma concentrations at about 90-120 minutes after each dose. After achieving and maintaining therapeutic plasma concentrations and satisfactory electrocardiographic and clinical responses, continued frequent periodic monitoring of vital signs and electrocardiograms is advised. If evidence of QRS widening of more than 25% or marked prolongation of the Q-T interval occurs, concern for overdosage is appropriate, and reduction in dosage is advisable if a 50% increase occurs. Elevated serum creatinine or urea nitrogen, reduced creatinine clearance, or history of renal insufficiency, as well as use in older patients (over age 50), provide grounds to anticipate that less than the usual dosage and longer time intervals between doses may suffice, since the urinary elimination of PA and NAPA may be reduced, leading to gradual accumulation beyond normally-predicted amounts. If facilities are available for measurement of plasma PA and NAPA, or acetylation capability, individual dose adjustment for optimal therapeutic levels may be easier, but close observation of clinical effectiveness is the most important criterion.

In the longer term, periodic complete blood counts are useful to detect possible idiosyncratic hematologic effects of PA on neutrophil, platelet or red cell homeostasis; agranulocytosis has been reported to occur occasionally in patients on long-term PA therapy. A rising titer of serum ANA may precede clinical symptoms of the lupoid syndrome (see BOXED WARNING and ADVERSE REACTIONS). If the lupus erythematosus-like syndrome develops in a patient with recurrent life-threatening arrhythmias not controlled by other agents, corticosteroid suppressive therapy may be used concomitantly with PA. Since the PA-induced lupoid syndrome rarely includes the dangerous pathologic renal changes, PA therapy may not necessarily have to be stopped unless the symptoms of serositis and the possibility of further lupoid effects are of greater risk than the benefit of PA in controlling arrhythmias. Patients with rapid acetylation capability are less likely to develop the lupoid syndrome after prolonged PA therapy.

Procainamide HCl tablets contain FD&C yellow no. 5 (tartrazine) which may cause allergic-type reactions (including bronchial asthma) in certain susceptible individuals. Although the overall incidence of FD&C yellow no. 5 (tartrazine) sensitivity in the general population is low, it is frequently seen in patients who also have aspirin hypersensitivity.

Additional Information for the Injection
Blood pressure should be monitored with the patient supine during parenteral, especially intravenous, administration of Procainamide (see DOSAGE AND ADMINISTRATION). There is a possibility that relatively high, although transient, plasma levels of procainamide may be attained and cause hypotension before the procainamide can be disturbed from the plasma volume to its full apparently volume to its full apparent volume of distribution, which is approximately 50 times greater. Therefore, caution should be exercised to avoid overly rapid administration of procainamide. If the blood pressure falls 15 mm Hg or more, procainamide administration should be temporarily discontinued. ECG monitoring is advisable as well, both for observation of the progress and response of the arrhythmia under treatment, and for early detection of any tendency to excessive widening of the QRS complex, prolongation of the P-R interval or any signs of the heat block. Parenteral therapy with procainamide should be limited to use in hospitals in which monitoring and intensive supportive care are available or to emergency situations in which equivalent observation and treatment can be provided.

INFORMATION FOR THE PATIENT
The physician is advised to explain to the patient that close cooperation in adhering to the prescribed dosage schedule is of great importance in controlling the cardiac arrhythmia safely. The patient should understand clearly that more medication is not necessarily better and may be dangerous, that skipping doses or increasing intervals between doses to suit personal convenience may lead to loss of control of the heart problem, and that "making up" missed doses by doubling up later may be hazardous.

The patient should be encouraged to disclose any past history of drug sensitivity, especially to procaine or other local anesthetic agents, or aspirin, and to report any history of kidney disease, congestive heart failure, myasthenia gravis, liver disease, or lupus erythematosus.

The patient should be counseled to report promptly any symptoms of arthralgia, myalgia, fever, chills, skin rash, easy bruising, sore throat or sore mouth, infections, dark urine or icterus, wheezing, muscular weakness, chest or abdominal pain, palpitations, nausea, vomiting, anorexia, diarrhea, hallucinations, dizziness, or depression.

LABORATORY TESTS

Laboratory tests such as complete blood count (CBC), electrocardiogram, and serum creatinine or urea nitrogen may be indicated, depending on the clinical situation, and periodic rechecking of the CBC and ANA may be helpful in early detection of untoward reactions.

DRUG/LABORATORY TEST INTERACTIONS

Suprapharmacologic concentrations of lidocaine and meprobamate may inhibit fluorescence of PA and NAPA, and propranolol shows a native fluorescence close to the PA/NAPA peak wavelengths, so that tests which depend on fluorescence measurement may be affected.

CARCINOGENESIS, MUTAGENESIS, AND IMPAIRMENT OF FERTILITY

Long term studies in animals have not been performed.

PREGNANCY, TERATOGENIC EFFECTS, PREGNANCY CATEGORY C

Animal reproduction studies have not been conducted with PA. It also is not known whether PA can cause fetal harm when administered to a pregnant woman or can affect reproduction capacity. PA should be given to a pregnant woman only if clearly needed.

NURSING MOTHERS

Both PA and NAPA are excreted in human milk, and absorbed by the nursing infant. Because of the potential for serious adverse reactions in nursing infants, a decision to discontinue nursing or the drug should be made, taking into account the importance of the drug to the mother.

PEDIATRIC USE

Safety and effectiveness in children have not been established.

DRUG INTERACTIONS

If other antiarrhythmic drugs are being used, additive effects on the heart may occur with PA administration, and dosage reduction may be necessary (see WARNINGS).

Anticholinergic drugs administered concurrently with PA may produce additive antivagal effects on A-V nodal conduction, although this is not as well documented for PA as for quinidine.

Patients taking PA who require neuromuscular blocking agents such as succinylcholine may require less than usual doses of the latter, due to PA effects on reducing acetylcholine release.

ADVERSE REACTIONS

CARDIOVASCULAR

Hypotension following oral PA administration is rare. Hypotension and serious disturbances of cardiorhythm such as ventricular asystole or fibrillation are more common after intravenous administration (see WARNINGS). Second degree heart block has been reported in 2 of almost 500 patients taking PA orally.

MULTISYSTEM

A lupus erythematosus-like syndrome of arthralgia, pleural or abdominal pain, and sometimes arthritis, pleural effusion, pericarditis, fever, chills, myalgia, and possibly related hematologic or skin lesions is fairly common after prolonged PA administration, perhaps more often in patients who are slow acetylators (see BOXED WARNING and PRECAUTIONS). While some series have reported less than 1 in 500, others have reported the syndrome in up to 30% of patients on long term oral PA therapy. If discontinuation of PA does not reverse the lupoid symptoms, corticosteroid treatment may be effective.

HEMATOLOGIC

Neutropenia, thrombocytopenia, or hemolytic anemia may rarely be encountered. Agranulocytosis has occurred after repeated use of PA, and deaths have been reported. (See BOXED WARNING and WARNINGS.)

SKIN

Angioneurotic edema, urticaria, pruritus, flushing, and maculopapular rash have also occurred occasionally.

GASTROINTESTINAL

Anorexia, nausea, vomiting, abdominal pain, bitter taste, or diarrhea may occur in 3-4% of patients taking oral procainamide. Hepatomegaly with increased serum aminotransferase activity have been reported after a single oral dose.

NERVOUS SYSTEM

Dizziness or giddiness, weakness, mental depression, and psychosis with hallucinations have been reported occasionally.

DOSAGE AND ADMINISTRATION

ORAL FORMS

The oral dose and interval of administration should be adjusted for the individual patient, based on clinical assessment of the degree of underlying myocardial disease, the patient's age, and renal function.

As a general guide, for younger adult patients with normal renal function, an initial total daily oral dose of up to 50 mg/kg of body weight of capsules or tablets may be used, given in divided doses, every 3 hours, to maintain therapeutic blood levels. For older patients, especially those over 50 years of age, or for patients with renal, hepatic, or cardiac insufficiency, lesser amounts or longer intervals may produce adequate blood levels, and decrease the probability of occurrence of dose related adverse reactions.For the tablets and capsules, the total daily dose should be administered in divided doses at 3, 4, or 6 hour intervals and adjusted according to the patient's response (TABLE 1 and TABLE 2).

TABLE 1 *Capsules and Tablets*

*To provide up to 50 mg/kg of body weight/day:**

Patients Weighing		
lb	**kg**	
88-110	40-50	250 mg q3h to 500 mg q6h
132-154	60-70	375 mg q3h to 750 mg q6h
176-198	80-90	500 mg q3h to 1 g q6h
>220	>100	625 mg q3h to 1.25 g q6h

TABLE 2 *Extended Release Tablets*

*To provide up to 50 mg/kg of body weight/day:**

Patients Weighing		
lb	**kg**	
88-110	40-50	500 mg q6h
132-154	60-70	750 mg q6h
176-198	80-90	1 g q6h
>220	>100	1.25 g q6h

* Initial dosage schedule guide only, to be adjusted for each patient individually, based on age, cardiorenal function, blood level (if available), and clinical response.

INJECTION

Procainamide HCl injection is useful for arrhythmias which require immediate suppression and for maintenance of arrhythmia control. IV therapy allows most rapid control of serious arrhythmias, including those following myocardial infarction; it should be carried out in circumstances where close observation and monitoring of the patient are possible, such as hospital or emergency facilities. IM administration is less opt to produce temporary high plasma levels but therapeutic plasma levels are not obtained as rapidly as with IV administration. Oral procainamide dosage forms are preferable for less urgent arrhythmias as well as long-term maintenance after initial parenteral procainamide therapy.

IM administration may be used as an alternative to the oral route for patients with less threatening arrhythmias but who are nauseated or vomiting, who are ordered to receive nothing by mouth preoperatively or who may have malabsorptive problems. An initial dose of 50 mg/kg body weight may be estimated. This amount should be divided into fractional doses of one-eighth to one-quarter to be injected by the IM route every 3-6 hours until oral therapy is possible. If more than three injections are given, the physician may wish to assess the patient factors such as age and renal function , clinical response, and if available, blood levels of procainamide and NAPA in adjusting further doses for that individual. For treatment of arrhythmias associated with anesthesia or surgical operation, the suggested dose is 100-500 mg by IM injection.

IV administration for procainamide HCl injection should be done cautiously to avoid a possible hypotensive response (see PRECAUTIONS). Initial arrhythmia control, under ECG monitoring, may usually be accomplished safely within a half-hour by either of the two methods which follow:

A) Direct injection into a vein or tubing an established infusion line should be done slowly at a rate not to exceed 50 mg per minute. It is advisable to dilute either the 100 mg/ml or the 500 mg/ml concentrations of procainamide HCl injection prior to IV injection to facilitate control of dosage rate. Doses of 100 mg may be administered every 5 minutes at this rate until the arrhythmia is suppressed or until 500 mg has been administered, after which it is advisable to wait 10 minutes or longer to allow for more distribution into tissues before resuming.

B) Alternatively, a loading infusion containing 20 mg of procainamide HCl per ml (1 g diluted to 50 ml with 5% dextrose injection) may be administered at a constant rate of 1 ml/min for 25-30 minutes to deliver 500-600 mg of procainamide. Some effects may be seen after the infusion of the first 100 or 200 mg; it is unusual to require more than 600 mg to achieve satisfactory antiarrhythmic effects.

The maximum advisable dosage to be given either by repeated bolus injections or such loading infusion is 1 g.

To maintain therapeutic levels, a more dilute IV infusion ata concentration of 2 mg/ml is convenient (1 g procainamide HCl in 500 ml of 5% dextrose injection), and may be administered at 1-3 ml/minute. If daily total fluid intake must be limited, a 4 mg/ml concentration (1 g procainamide HCl injection in 250 ml of 5% dextrose injection) administered at 0.5-1.5 ml/minute will deliver an equivalent 2-6 mg per minute. The amount needed in a given patient to maintain therapeutic level should be assessed principally from the clinical response and will depend upon the patient's weight and age, renal elimination, hepatic acetylation rate and cardiac status, but should be adjusted for each patient based upon close observation. A maintenance infusion rate of 50 μg/min/kg body weight to a person with a normal renal procainamide elimination half-time of 3 hours may be expected to produce a plasma level of approximately 6.5 μg/ml (see TABLE 3).

Since the principle route for elimination of procainamide and NAPA is renal excretion, reduced excretion will prolong the half-life of elimination and lower the dose rate needed to maintain therapeutic levels. Advancing age reduces the renal excretion of procainamide and NAPA independently of reductions in creatine clearance; compared to normal young adults, there is approximately 25% reduction at age 50 and 50% at age 75.

IV therapy should be terminated if persistent conduction disturbances or hypotension develop. As soon as the patient's basic cardiac rhythm appears to be stabilized, oral antiarrhythmic maintenance therapy is preferable, if indicated and possible. A period of about 3 to fours (one half-time for renal elimination, ordinarily) should elapse after the last IV dose before administering the first dose of procainamide tablets or capsules.

TABLE 3 *Dilutions and Rates for IV Infusions* Procainamide HCl Injection*

	Final Concentration	Infusion Volume†	Procainamide To Be Added	Infusion Rate
Initial Loading Infusion	20 mg/ml	50 ml	1000 mg	1 ml/min (for up to 25-30 min*)
Maintenance Infusion	2 mg/ml or 4 mg/ml	500 ml 250 ml	1000 mg 1000 mg	1-3 ml/min 0.5-1.5 ml/min

The maintenance infusion rates are calculated to deliver 2-6 mg/min depending on body weight, renal elimination rate and steady-state plasma level needed to maintain control of the arrhythmia*.
The 4 mg/ml maintenance concentration may be preferred if total infusion volume is to be limited.
* Please see text under DOSAGE AND ADMINISTRATION for further details. The flow rate of any IV Procainamide infusion must be monitored closely to avoid transiently high plasma levels and possible hypotension (see PRECAUTIONS).
† All infusions should be made up to final volume with 5% dextrose injection.

Parenteral drug products should be inspected visually for particulate matter and discoloration prior to administration, whenever solution and container permit.

PRODUCT LISTING - RATED THERAPEUTICALLY EQUIVALENT

Capsule - Oral - 250 mg
30's $4.65 GENERIC, Heartland Healthcare Services 61392-0766-30
30's $4.65 GENERIC, Heartland Healthcare Services 61392-0766-39
31's $4.81 GENERIC, Heartland Healthcare Services 61392-0766-31
32's $4.96 GENERIC, Heartland Healthcare Services 61392-0766-32
45's $6.98 GENERIC, Heartland Healthcare Services 61392-0766-45
60's $9.30 GENERIC, Heartland Healthcare Services 61392-0766-60
90's $13.95 GENERIC, Heartland Healthcare Services 61392-0766-90
100's $7.50 GENERIC, Major Pharmaceuticals Inc 00904-2345-60
100's $8.25 GENERIC, Interstate Drug Exchange Inc 00814-6335-14
100's $8.35 GENERIC, Aligen Independent Laboratories Inc 00405-4851-01
100's $8.90 GENERIC, Qualitest Products Inc 00603-5404-21
100's $9.17 GENERIC, Moore, H.L. Drug Exchange Inc 00839-5224-06
100's $9.50 GENERIC, Raway Pharmacal Inc 00686-0101-20
100's $11.72 GENERIC, Major Pharmaceuticals Inc 00904-2345-61
100's $14.50 GENERIC, Cmc-Consolidated Midland Corporation 00223-1456-01
100's $23.18 GENERIC, Ivax Corporation 00172-2345-60
100's $82.94 PRONESTYL, Bristol-Myers Squibb 00003-0758-50
100's $88.21 PRONESTYL, Physicians Total Care 54868-3367-00
250's $17.80 GENERIC, Major Pharmaceuticals Inc 00904-2345-70

Capsule - Oral - 375 mg
30's $5.40 GENERIC, Heartland Healthcare Services 61392-0767-30
30's $5.40 GENERIC, Heartland Healthcare Services 61392-0767-39
31's $5.58 GENERIC, Heartland Healthcare Services 61392-0767-31
32's $5.76 GENERIC, Heartland Healthcare Services 61392-0767-32
45's $8.10 GENERIC, Heartland Healthcare Services 61392-0767-45
60's $10.80 GENERIC, Heartland Healthcare Services 61392-0767-60
90's $16.20 GENERIC, Heartland Healthcare Services 61392-0767-90
100's $9.30 GENERIC, Major Pharmaceuticals Inc 00904-2346-60
100's $9.59 GENERIC, Qualitest Products Inc 00603-5405-21
100's $9.75 GENERIC, Interstate Drug Exchange Inc 00814-6337-14
100's $9.86 GENERIC, Moore, H.L. Drug Exchange Inc 00839-1563-06
100's $11.70 GENERIC, Us Trading Corporation 56126-0291-11
100's $18.00 GENERIC, Ivax Corporation 00172-2346-60
100's $18.00 PRONESTYL, Bristol-Myers Squibb 00003-0756-50
250's $21.40 GENERIC, Major Pharmaceuticals Inc 00904-2346-70

Capsule - Oral - 500 mg
30's $11.60 GENERIC, Heartland Healthcare Services 61392-0768-30
30's $11.60 GENERIC, Heartland Healthcare Services 61392-0768-39
31's $11.98 GENERIC, Heartland Healthcare Services 61392-0768-31
32's $12.37 GENERIC, Heartland Healthcare Services 61392-0768-32
45's $17.40 GENERIC, Heartland Healthcare Services 61392-0768-45
60's $23.19 GENERIC, Heartland Healthcare Services 61392-0768-60
90's $34.79 GENERIC, Heartland Healthcare Services 61392-0768-90
100's $9.20 GENERIC, Major Pharmaceuticals Inc 00904-2347-60
100's $9.72 GENERIC, Qualitest Products Inc 00603-5406-21
100's $11.00 GENERIC, Moore, H.L. Drug Exchange Inc 00839-5050-06
100's $11.25 GENERIC, Interstate Drug Exchange Inc 00814-6340-14
100's $15.50 GENERIC, Raway Pharmacal Inc 00686-0102-20
100's $16.95 GENERIC, Cmc-Consolidated Midland Corporation 00223-1457-01
100's $17.64 GENERIC, Major Pharmaceuticals Inc 00904-2347-61
100's $30.70 GENERIC, Ivax Corporation 00172-2347-60
100's $121.55 PRONESTYL, Bristol-Myers Squibb 00003-0757-50
250's $21.40 GENERIC, Major Pharmaceuticals Inc 00904-2347-70

Solution - Injectable - 100 mg/ml
10 ml $53.40 PRONESTYL, Bristol-Myers Squibb 00003-0759-20
10 ml x 25 $33.84 GENERIC, Abbott Pharmaceutical 00074-1902-01
10 ml x 25 $290.25 GENERIC, Esi Lederle Generics 00641-2587-45

Solution - Injectable - 500 mg/ml
2 ml $40.12 PRONESTYL, Bristol-Myers Squibb 00003-1443-04
2 ml x 10 $56.30 GENERIC, Abbott Pharmaceutical 00074-1826-02
2 ml x 25 $46.02 GENERIC, Abbott Pharmaceutical 00074-1903-01

Tablet - Oral - 375 mg
100's $9.60 GENERIC, Aligen Independent Laboratories Inc 00405-4852-01

Tablet, Extended Release - Oral - 500 mg
30's $11.60 GENERIC, Heartland Healthcare Services 61395-0769-30
30's $11.60 GENERIC, Heartland Healthcare Services 61395-0769-39
31's $11.98 GENERIC, Heartland Healthcare Services 61395-0769-31
32's $12.37 GENERIC, Heartland Healthcare Services 61395-0769-32
45's $17.40 GENERIC, Heartland Healthcare Services 61395-0769-45
60's $23.19 GENERIC, Heartland Healthcare Services 61395-0769-60
90's $34.79 GENERIC, Heartland Healthcare Services 61395-0769-90
100's $25.00 GENERIC, Ivax Corporation 00182-1708-89
100's $29.95 GENERIC, Ivax Corporation 00182-1708-01
100's $80.00 GENERIC, Teva Pharmaceuticals Usa 00093-9188-01

Tablet, Extended Release - Oral - 750 mg
100's $89.74 GENERIC, Teva Pharmaceuticals Usa 00093-9114-01

Tablet, Extended Release - Oral - 1000 mg
100's $150.00 GENERIC, Teva Pharmaceuticals Usa 00093-9117-01

Tablet, Extended Release - Oral - 1000 mg/12 Hours
60's $103.13 PROCANBID, Monarch Pharmaceuticals Inc 61570-0071-60
100's $180.50 PROCANBID, Monarch Pharmaceuticals Inc 61570-0071-70

PRODUCT LISTING - RATED NOT THERAPEUTICALLY EQUIVALENT

Tablet, Extended Release - Oral - 500 mg
100's $86.78 PRONESTYL-SR, Bristol-Myers Squibb 00003-0775-50

PRODUCT LISTING - EQUIVALENTS NOT AVAILABLE

Capsule - Oral - 250 mg
100's $28.65 GENERIC, Physicians Total Care 54868-3468-00

Capsule - Oral - 500 mg
100's $13.63 GENERIC, Physicians Total Care 54868-3469-00

Solution - Injectable - 100 mg/ml
10 ml $4.00 GENERIC, Cmc-Consolidated Midland Corporation 00223-8353-10
10 ml $15.00 GENERIC, Raway Pharmacal Inc 00686-2587-41

Solution - Injectable - 500 mg/ml
2 ml $4.00 GENERIC, C.O. Truxton Inc 00223-8354-02

Tablet - Oral - 250 mg
100's $74.48 PRONESTYL, Bristol-Myers Squibb 00003-0431-50

Tablet - Oral - 375 mg
100's $103.28 PRONESTYL, Bristol-Myers Squibb 00003-0434-50

Tablet - Oral - 500 mg
100's $143.34 PRONESTYL, Bristol-Myers Squibb 00003-0438-50

Tablet, Extended Release - Oral - 250 mg
100's $17.50 GENERIC, Cmc-Consolidated Midland Corporation 00223-1458-01

Tablet, Extended Release - Oral - 500 mg
100's $26.84 GENERIC, Physicians Total Care 54868-0694-01
100's $27.50 GENERIC, Cmc-Consolidated Midland Corporation 00223-1459-01

Tablet, Extended Release - Oral - 500 mg/12 Hours
60's $54.95 PROCANBID, Monarch Pharmaceuticals Inc 61570-0069-60
100's $95.00 PROCANBID, Monarch Pharmaceuticals Inc 61570-0069-01
100's $96.25 PROCANBID, Monarch Pharmaceuticals Inc 61570-0069-70

Tablet, Extended Release - Oral - 750 mg
100's $45.00 GENERIC, Cmc-Consolidated Midland Corporation 00223-1460-01

Tablet, Extended Release - Oral - 1000 mg
100's $47.50 GENERIC, Cmc-Consolidated Midland Corporation 00223-1461-01

Procaine Hydrochloride *(002118)*

Categories: Anesthesia, local; Anesthesia, regional; Anesthesia, spinal; Pregnancy Category C; FDA Approved 1979 Jul
Drug Classes: Anesthetics, local
Brand Names: **Novocain**; Ravocaine-Novocain-Levophed
Foreign Brand Availability: **Novanaest purum 1% (Austria); Novanaest purum 2% (Austria); Procaine Hydrochloride Inj (Australia; New-Zealand); Pasconeural-Injektopas 1% (Germany); Procadolor N (Germany)**

DESCRIPTION

LOCAL ANESTHETIC

Local Anesthetic for Major Infiltration and Peripheral Nerve Block

These Solutions Are Not Intended for Spinal or Epidural Anesthesia or Dental Use

Procaine HCl is a benzoic acid, 4-amino-, 2-(diethylamino) ethyl ester, monohydrochloride, the ester of diethylaminoethanol and para-aminobenzoic acid.

It is a white crystalline, odorless powder that is freely soluble in water, but less soluble in alcohol an has a molecular weight of 272.77

(TABLE 1 shows the composition of solutions).

The solutions are made isotonic with sodium chloride and the pH is adjusted between 3 and 5.5 with sodium hydroxide and/or hydrochloric acid.

Procaine HCl is available as sterile solutions in concentrations of 1% and 2% for injection via local infiltration and peripheral nerve block.

P

TABLE 1 *Composition of Available Solutions*

Each ml contains	1% Ampul	1% Vial	2% Vial
Procaine HCl	10 mg	10 mg	20 mg
Acetone sodium bisulfite	≤1 mg	≤2 mg	≤2 mg
Chlorobutanol	—	≤2.5 mg	≤2.5 mg

Acetone sodium bisulfite is added as an antioxidant in all products, and is added as an antimicrobial preservative in the multiple-dose vial.

SPINAL INJECTION

Procaine hydrochloride, is a benzoic acid, 4-amino-, 2-(diethylamino) ethyl ester, monohydrochloride, the ester of diethylaminoethanol and para-aminobenzoic acid.

It is a white crystalline, odorless powder that is freely soluble in water but less soluble in alcohol. Each ml contains 100 mg procaine HCl and 4 mg acetone sodium bisulfite as antioxidant. DO NOT USE SOLUTIONS IF CRYSTALS, CLOUDINESS, OR DISCOLORATION IS OBSERVED EXAMINE SOLUTIONS CAREFULLY BEFORE USE. REAUTOCLAVING INCREASES LIKELIHOOD OF CRYSTAL FORMATION.

CLINICAL PHARMACOLOGY

LOCAL ANESTHETIC

Local anesthetics block the generation and the conduction of nerve impulses, presumably by increasing the threshold for electrical excitation in the nerve, by slowing the propagation of the nerve impulse, and by reducing the rate of rise of the action potential. In general, the progression of anesthesia is related to the diameter, myelination, and conduction velocity of affected nerve fibers. Clinically, the order of loss of nerve function is as follows: pain, temperature, touch, proprioception, and skeletal muscle tone. Procaine HCl lacks topical anesthetic activity.

Systemic absorption of local anesthetics produces effects on the cardiovascular and the central nervous systems. At blood concentrations achieved with normal therapeutic doses, changes in cardiac conduction, excitability, refractoriness, contractility, and peripheral vascular resistance are minimal. However, toxic blood concentrations depress cardiac conduction and excitability, which may lead to atrioventricular block and ultimately to cardiac arrest. In addition, myocardial contractility is depressed and peripheral vasodilation occurs, leading to decreased cardiac output and arterial blood pressure.

Following systemic absorption, local anesthetics can produce central nervous system stimulation, depression, or both. Apparent central stimulation is manifested as restlessness, tremors and shivering, progressing to convulsions, followed by depression, and coma progressing ultimately to respiratory arrest. However, the local anesthetics have a primary depressant effect on the medulla and on higher centers. The depressed stage may occur without a prior exited stage.

Pharmacokinetics

The rate system absorption of local anesthetics is dependant upon the total dose and concentration of drug administered, the route of administration, the vascularity of the administration site, and the presence or absence of epinephrine in the anesthetic solution. A dilute concentration of epinephrine (1:200,000 or 5 μg/ml) usually reduces the rate of absorption and plasma concentration of procaine HCl. It also will promote local hemostasis and increase the duration of anesthesia.

Onset of anesthesia with procaine HCl is rapid, the time of onset for sensory block ranging from about 2-5 minutes depending upon such factors as the anesthetic technique, the type of block, the concentration of the solution, and the individual patient. The degree of motor blockade produced is dependent on the concentration of the solution.

The duration of anesthesia also varies depending upon the technique and type of block, the concentration, and the individual. Procaine HCl will normally provide anesthesia which is adequate for 1 hour.

The duration of anesthesia also varies depending upon the technique and type of block, the concentration, and the individual. Procaine HCl will normally provide anesthesia which is adequate for 1 hour.

Local anesthetics are bound to plasma proteins in varying degrees. Generally, the lower the plasma concentration of the drug, the higher the percentage of drug bound to plasma.

Local anesthetics appear to cross the placenta by passive diffusion. The rate and degree of diffusion is governed by the degree of plasma protein binding, the degree of ionization, and the degree of lipid solubility. Fetal/maternal ratios of local anesthetics appear to be inversely related to the degree of plasma protein binding, because only the free, unbound drug is available for placental transfer. The extent of placental transfer is also determined by the degree of ionization and lipid solubility of the drug. Lipid, soluble nonionized drugs readily enter the fetal blood from the maternal circulation.

Depending upon the route of administration, local anesthetics are distributed to some extent to all body tissues, with high concentrations found in highly perfused organs such as the liver, lungs, heart, and brain.

Various pharmacokinetics parameters of the local anesthetics can be significantly altered by the presence of hepatic or renal disease, addition of epinephrine, factors affecting urinary pH, renal blood flow, the route of drug administration, and the age of patient. The *in vitro* plasma half-life of procaine HCl in adults is 40 ± 9 seconds and in neonates 84 ± 30 seconds.

Procaine HCl is readily absorbed following parenteral administration and is rapidly hydrolyzed by plasma cholinesterase to para-aminobenzoic acid and diethylaminoethanol.

The para-aminobenzoic acid metabolite inhibits the action of the sulfonamides. (see PRECAUTIONS.)

For procaine HCl, approximately 90% of the para-aminobenzoic acid metabolite and its conjugates and 33% of the diethylaminoethanol metabolite are recovered in the urine, while less than 2% of the administered dose is recovered unchanged in the urine.

SPINAL INJECTION

Procaine HCl stabilizes the neuronal membrane an prevents the initiation and transmission of nerve impulses, thereby effecting local anesthesia. Procaine HCl lacks surface anesthetic activity. The onset of action is rapid (2-5 minutes) and the duration of action is relatively short (average 1-1½ hours), depending upon the anesthetic technique, the type of block, the concentration, and the individual patient.

Procaine HCl is readily absorbed following parenteral administration and is rapidly hydrolyzed by plasma cholinesterase to aminobenzoic acid and diethylaminoethanol.

A vasoconstrictor maybe added to the solution of procaine HCl to promote local hemostasis, delay systemic absorption, and increase duration of anesthesia.

INDICATIONS AND USAGE

LOCAL ANESTHETIC

Procaine HCl is indicated for the production of local or regional analgesia and anesthesia by local infiltration and peripheral nerve block techniques.

The routes of administration and concentrations are: for local infiltration use 0.25 to 0.5% (via dilution) and for peripheral nerve blocks use 0.5% (via dilution), 1% and 2% (see DOSAGE AND ADMINISTRATION for additional information.)

Standard textbooks should be consulted to determine the accepted procedures and techniques for the administration of procaine HCl.

SPINAL INJECTION

Procaine HCl is indicated for spinal anesthesia.

CONTRAINDICATIONS

LOCAL ANESTHETIC

Procaine HCl is contraindicated in patients with a known hypersensitivity to procaine, drugs of a similar chemical configuration, or a para-aminobenzoic acid or its derivatives.

It is also contraindicated in patients with a known hypersensitivity to other components of solutions of procaine HCl.

SPINAL INJECTION

Spinal anesthesia with procaine HCl is contraindicated in patients with generalized septicemia: sepsis at the proposed injection site; certain diseases of the cerebrospinal system, *e.g.*, meningitis, syphilis; and a known hypersensitivity to the drug, drugs of a similar chemical configuration, or aminobenzoic acid or its derivatives.

The decision as to whether or not spinal anesthesia should be used in an individual case should be made by the physician after weighing the advantages with the risks and possible complications.

WARNINGS

LOCAL ANESTHETIC

Contains acetone sodium bisulfite, a sulfite that may cause allergic-type reactions including anaphylactic symptoms and life-threatening or less severe asthmatic episodes in certain susceptible people. The overall prevalence of sulfite sensitivity in the general population is unknown and probably low. Sulfite sensitivity is seen more frequently in asthmatic than in non-asthmatic people.

LOCAL ANESTHETICS SHOULD ONLY BE EMPLOYED BY CLINICIANS WHO ARE WELL VERSED IN DIAGNOSIS AND MANAGEMENT OF DOSE-RELATED TOXICITY AND OTHER ACUTE EMERGENCIES WHICH MIGHT ARISE FROM THE BLOCK TO BE EMPLOYED AND THEN ONLY AFTER INSURING THE IMMEDIATE AVAILABILITY OF OXYGEN, OTHER RESUSCITATIVE DRUGS, CARDIOPULMONARY RESUSCITATIVE EQUIPMENT, AND THE PERSONNEL RESOURCES NEEDED FOR PROPER MANAGEMENT OF TOXIC REACTIONS AND RELATED EMERGENCIES (see also ADVERSE REACTIONS and PRECAUTIONS.) **DELAY IN PROPER MANAGEMENT OF DOSE-RELATED TOXICITY, UNDERVENTILATION FROM ANY CAUSE, AND/OR ALTERED SENSITIVITY MAY LEAD TO THE DEVELOPMENT OF ACIDOSIS, CARDIAC ARREST, AND, POSSIBLY DEATH.**

It is essential that aspiration for blood or cerebrospinal fluid, where applicable, be done prior to injecting any local anesthetic, both the original dose and all subsequent doses, to avoid intravascular or subarachnoid injection.

Reactions resulting in fatality have occurred on rare occasions with the use of local anesthetics, even in the absence of a history of hypersensitivity. Large doses of local anesthetics should not be used in patients with heartblock.

Procaine HCl with epinephrine or other vasopressors should not be used concomitantly with ergot-type oxytocic drugs, because a severe persistent hypertension may occur. Likewise, solutions of procaine HCl containing a vasoconstrictor, such as epinephrine, should be used with extreme caution in patients receiving monoamine oxidase inhibitors (MAOI) or antidepressants of the triptyline or imipramine types, because severe prolonged hypertension or disturbances of cardiac rhythm may occur.

Local anesthetic procedures should be used with caution when there is inflammation and/or sepsis in the region of the proposed injection.

Mixing or the prior or intercurrent use of any local anesthetic with procaine HCl cannot be recommended because of insufficient data on the clinical use of such mixtures.

SPINAL INJECTION

RESUSCITATIVE EQUIPMENT AND DRUGS SHOULD BE IMMEDIATELY AVAILABLE WHENEVER ANY LOCAL ANESTHETIC DRUG IS USED. Spinal anesthesia should not .only be administered by those qualified to do so.

Large doses of local anesthetics should not be used in patients with heartblock.

Reactions resulting in fatality have occurred on rare occasions with the use of local anesthetics, even in the absence of a history of hypersensitivity.

Use in Pregnancy

Safe use of procaine HCl has not been established with respect to adverse effects on fetal development. Careful consideration should be given to this fact before administering this drug to women of childbearing potential particularly during early pregnancy. This does not exclude the use of the drug at term for obstetrical analgesia. Vasopressor agents (administered for the treatment of hypotension or added to the anesthetic solution for vasoconstriction) should be used with extreme caution in the presence of of oxytocic drugs as they may produce severe, persistent hypertension with possible rupture of a cerebral blood vessel.

Solutions which contain a vasoconstrictor should be used with extreme caution in patients receiving drugs known to produce alterations in blood pressure (*i.e.,* monoamine oxidase inhibitors (MAOI), tricyclic antidepressants, phenothiazines, etc), as either severe sustained hypertension or hypotension may occur.

Local anesthetic procedures should be used with caution when there is inflammation and/or sepsis in the region of the proposed injection.

Contains acetone sodium bisulfite, a sulfite that may cause allergic-type reactions including anaphylactic symptoms and life-threatening or less severe asthmatic episodes in certain susceptible people. The overall prevalence of sulfite sensitivity in the general population in unknown and probably low. Sulfite sensitivity is seen more frequently in asthmatic than in non asthmatic people.

PRECAUTIONS

GENERAL

The safety and effectiveness of local and a spinal anesthetic depend on proper dosage, correct technique, adequate precautions, and readiness for emergencies. Resuscitative equipment, oxygen, and other resuscitative drugs should be available for immediate use (see WARNINGS and ADVERSE REACTIONS). During major regional nerve blocks, the patient should have IV fluids running via an indwelling catheter to assure a functioning intravenous pathway. The lowest dosage of local anesthetic that results in effective anesthesia should be used to avoid high plasma levels and serious adverse effects. Injections should be made slowly, with frequent aspirations before and during the injection to avoid intravascular injection. Current opinion favors fractional administration with constant attention to the patient, rather than rapid bolus injection. Syringe aspirations should also be performed before and during each supplemental injection in continuous (intermittent) catheter techniques. An intramuscular injection is still possible even if aspirations for blood are negative.

Injection of repeated doses of local anesthetics may cause significant increases in plasma levels with each repeated dose due to slow accumulation of the drug or its metabolites or to slow metabolic degradation. Tolerance to alleviated blood levels varies with the status of the patient. Debilitated, elderly patients and acutely ill patients should be given reduced doses commensurate with their age and physical status. Local anesthetics should also be used with caution in patients with severe disturbances of cardiac rhythm, shock, heartblock, or hypotension.

Careful and constant monitoring of cardiovascular and respiratory (adequacy of ventilation) vital signs and the patient's state of consciousness should be performed after each local anesthetic injection. It should be kept in mind at such times that restlessness, anxiety, incoherent speech, light-headedness, numbness, and tingling of the mouth and lips, metallic taste, tinnitus, dizziness, blurred vision, tremors, twitching, depression, or drowsiness may be early warning signs of central nervous system toxicity.

Local anesthetic solutions containing a vasoconstrictor should be used cautiously and in carefully circumscribed quantities in the areas of the body supplied by end arteries, or those areas having otherwise compromised blood supply such as digits, nose, external ear, penis. Patients with peripheral vascular disease and hypertensive vascular disease may exhibit an exaggerated vasoconstrictor response. Ischemic injury or necrosis may result.

Procaine HCl should be used with caution in patients with known allergies and sensitivities. A thorough history of the patient's prior experience with procaine HCl or other local anesthetics as well as concomitant or recent drug use should be taken (see CONTRAINDICATIONS and WARNINGS.)

Because ester-type local anesthetics such as procaine HCl are hydrolyzed by plasma cholinesterase produced by the liver and excreted by the kidneys, these drugs, especially repeat doses, should be used cautiously in patients with hepatic disease. Because of their inability to metabolize local anesthetics normally, patients with severe hepatic disease are at a greater risk of developing toxic plasma concentrations. Local anesthetics should also be used with caution in patients with impaired cardiovascular function because they be less able to compensate for functional changes associated with the prolongation of AV conduction produced by these drugs.

Serious dose-related cardiac arrhythmias may occur if preparations containing a vasoconstrictor such as epinephrine are employed in patients during or following the administration of potent inhalation anesthetics. In deciding whether to use these products concurrently in the same patient, the combined action of both agents upon the myocardium, the concentration and volume of vasoconstrictor used, and the time since injection, when applicable, should be taken into account.

Many drugs used during the conduction of anesthesia are considered potential triggering agents for familial malignant hyperthermia. Because it is not known whether ester-type local anesthetics may trigger this reaction and because the need for supplemental general anesthesia cannot be predicted in advance, it is suggested that a standard protocol for management should be available. Early unexplained signs if tachycardia, tachypnea, labile blood pressure, and metabolic acidosis may precede temperature elevation. Successful outcome is dependant on early diagnosis, prompt discontinuance of the suspect triggering agent(s), and institution of treatment, including oxygen therapy, indicated supportive measures, and dantrolene. (Consult dantrolene sodium IV package insert before using).

Uses in Head and Neck Area

Small doses of local anesthetics injected into the head and neck area may produce adverse reactions similar to systemic toxicity seen with unintentional IV injections of larger doses. Confusion, convulsions, respiratory depression and/or respiratory arrest and cardiovascular stimulation or depression have been reported.

These reactions may be due to intra-arterial injection of the local anesthetic with retrograde flow to cerebral circulation. Patients receiving these blocks should have their circulation and respiration monitored and be constantly observed. Resuscitative equipment and personnel for treating adverse reactions should be immediately available. Dosage recommendation should not be exceeded.

INFORMATION FOR THE PATIENT

When appropriate, patients should be informed, in advance, that they may experience temporary loss of sensation and motor activity following proper administration of regional anesthesia. Also, when appropriate, the physician should discuss other information including adverse reactions in the package inserts.

CARCINOGENESIS, MUTAGENESIS, AND IMPAIRMENT OF FERTILITY

Long-term studies in animals of most local anesthetics, including procaine HCl, to evaluate the carcinogenic potentials have not been conducted. Mutagenic potential or the effect on fertility have not been determined. There is no evidence from human data that procaine HCl may be carcinogenic, or mutagenic, or that it impairs fertility.

PREGNANCY CATEGORY C

Animal reproduction studies have not been conducted with procaine HCl. It is not known whether procaine can cause fetal harm when administered to a pregnant woman or can affect reproduction capacity. Procaine HCl should be given to a pregnant women only if clearly needed and the potential benefits outweigh the risk. This does not exclude the use of procaine HCl at term for obstetrical anesthesia or analgesia (see Labor and Delivery.)

LABOR AND DELIVERY

Local anesthetics rapidly cross the placenta, and when used for paracervical or pudendal block anesthesia can cause varying degrees of maternal, fetal, and neonatal toxicity (see CLINICAL PHARMACOLOGY.) The incidence and degree of toxicity depend upon the procedure performed, the type and amount of drug used, and the technique of drug administration. Adverse reactions in the parturient, fetus, and neonate involve alterations of the central nervous system, peripheral vascular tone, and cardiac function.

Maternal hypotension has resulted from regional anesthesia. Local aesthetics produce vasodilation by blocking by blocking sympathetic nerves. Elevating the patient's legs and positioning her on her left side will help prevent decreases in blood pressure. The heart rate also should be monitored continuously and electric fetal monitoring is highly advisable.

Paracervical or pudendal anesthesia may alter the forces of parturition through changes in uterine contractility or maternal expulsive efforts. In one study, paracervical block anesthesia was associated with a decrease in the mean duration of first stage labor and facilitation of cervical dilation. The use of obstetrical anesthesia may increase the need for forceps assistance.

The use of some local anesthetic drug products during labor and delivery may be followed by diminished muscle strength and tone for the first day or 2 of life. The long-term significance of these observations is unknown.

Fetal bradycardia which infrequently follows paracervical block may be indicative of high fetal blood concentrations and procaine with resultant fetal acidosis. Fetal heart rate should be monitored prior to and during paracervical block. Added risk appears to be present in prematurity, toxemia of pregnancy, and fetal distress. The physician should weigh the considering paracervical block in these in these conditions. Careful adherence to recommended dosage is of the utmost importance in paracervical block. Failure to achieve adequate analgesia with these doses should arouse suspicion of intravascular or fetal injection.

Cases compatible with unintended fetal intracranial injection of local anesthetic solution have been reported following intended paracervical or pudendal block or both. Babies so affected present with unexplained neonatal depression at birth, which correlates with high local anesthetic serum levels, and usually manifest seizures within 6 hours. Prompt use of supportive measures combined with forced urinary excretion of the local anesthetic has been used successfully to manage this complication.

Case reports of maternal convulsions and cardiovascular collapse following use of some local anesthetics for paracervical block in early pregnancy (as anesthesia for elective abortion) suggest that systemic absorption under these circumstances may be rapid. The recommended maximum dose of the local anesthetic should not be exceeded. Injection should be made slowly and with frequent aspiration. Allow a 5 minute interval between sides.

It is extremely important to avoid aortocaval compression by the gravid uterus during administration of regional block to parturients. To do this, the patient must be maintained in the left lateral decubitus position or a blanket roll or sandbag may be placed beneath the right hip and the gravid uterus displaced to the left.

NURSING MOTHERS

It is not known whether local anesthetic drugs are excreted in human milk. Because many drugs are excreted in human milk, caution should be exercised when local anesthetics to a nursing woman.

PEDIATRIC USE

See DOSAGE AND ADMINISTRATION.

SPINAL INJECTION

Standard textbooks should be consulted for specific techniques and precautions for various spinal anesthetic procedures. The safety and effectiveness of a spinal anesthetic depend upon proper dosage, correct technique, adequate precautions, and readiness for emergencies. The lowest dosage that results in effective anesthesia should be used to avoid high plasma levels and possible adverse effects. Tolerance varies with the status of the patient. Debilitated, elderly patients, or acutely ill patients should be given reduced doses commensurate with their weight and physical status. Reduced dosages are also indicated for obstetric delivery and patients with increased intra-abdominal pressure.

The decision whether or not to use spinal anesthesia in the following disease states depends on the physician's appraisal of the advantages as opposed to the risk: cardiovascular disease (*i.e.,* shock, hypertension, anemia, etc), pulmonary disease, renal impairment, metabolic or endocrine disorders, gastrointestinal disorders (*i.e.,* intestinal obstruction, peritonitis, etc), or complicated obstetrical deliveries.

PROCAINE HCl SHOULD BE USED WITH CAUTION IN PATIENTS KNOWN WITH DRUG ALLERGIES AND SENSITIVES. A thorough history of patient's prior experience with procaine HCl or local anesthetics as well as concomitant or recent drug use of should be taken (see CONTRAINDICATIONS.) Procaine HCl should not be used in any

P

condition in which a sulfonamide drug is being employed since aminobenzoic acid inhibits the action of sulfonamides.

Solutions containing a vasopressor should be used with caution in the presence of diseases which may adversely affect the cardiovascular system.

Procaine HCl should be used with caution in patients with severe disturbances of cardiac rhythm, shock or heartblock.

DRUG INTERACTIONS

The administration of local anesthetic solutions containing epinephrine or norepinephrine to patients receiving Monoamine oxidase inhibitors tricyclic antidepressants may produce severe, prolonged hypertension. Concurrent use of these agents should generally be avoided. In situations when concurrent therapy is necessary, careful patient monitoring is essential.

Concurrent administration of vasopressor drugs and of ergot-type oxytocic drugs may cause severe, persistent hypertension or cerebrovascular accidents.

Phenothiazines and butyrophenones may reduce or reverse the pressor effect of epinephrine.

The clinical observation has been made that despite adequate sulfonamide therapy local infections have occurred in areas infiltrated with procaine HCl prior to diagnostic punctures and drainage procedures. Therefore, procaine HCl should not be used in any condition in which a sulfonamide drug is being employed since para-aminobenzoic acid inhibits the action of sulfonamide.

ADVERSE REACTIONS

Reactions to procaine are characteristic of those associated with other ester-type local anesthetics. A major cause of adverse reactions to this group of drugs is excessive plasma levels which may be due to overdosage, rapid absorption, inadvertent intravascular injection, or slow metabolic degradation.

A small number of reactions may result from hypersensitivity, idiosyncrasy, or diminished tolerance to normal dosage.

SYSTEMIC

The most commonly encountered acute adverse experiences which demand immediate countermeasures are related to the central nervous system and the cardiovascular system. These adverse experiences are generally dose related and due to high plasma levels, which may result from overdosage, rapid absorption from the injection site, diminished tolerance, or from unintentional intravascular injection of the local anesthetic solution. In addition to systemic dose-related toxicity, unintentional subarachnoid injection or drug during the intended performance of nerve blocks near the vertebral column (especially in the head and neck region), may result in underventilation or apnea ("Total or High Spinal"). Factors influencing plasma protein binding, such as acidosis, systemic diseases which alter protein production, or competition of other drugs for protein binding sites may diminish individual tolerance.

Plasma cholinesterase deficiency may also account for diminished tolerance to ester-type local anesthetics.

CENTRAL NERVOUS SYSTEM REACTIONS

These are characterized by excitation and/or depression. Restlessness, anxiety, dizziness, tinnitus, blurred vision, or tremors may occur, possibly proceeding to convulsions. However, excitement may be transient or absent, with depression being the first manifestation of an adverse reaction. This may quickly be followed by drowsiness merging into unconsciousness and respiratory arrest.

The incidence of convulsions associated with the use of local anesthetics varies with the procedure used and the total dose administered.

CARDIOVASCULAR REACTIONS

High doses or inadvertent intravascular injection may lead to high plasma levels and related depression of the myocardium, decreased cardiac output, heartblock, hypotension (or sometimes hypotension), bradycardia, ventricular arrhythmias, and cardiac arrest. (See WARNINGS and PRECAUTIONS).

ALLERGIC

Allergic-type reactions are rare and may occur as a result of sensitivity to the local anesthetic or to other formulation ingredients, such as the antimicrobial preservative- chlorobutanol contained in multiple-dose vials. These reactions are characterized by signs such urticaria, pruritus, erythema, angioneurotic edema (including laryngeal edema), tachycardia, sneezing, nausea, vomiting, dizziness, syncope, excessive sweating, elevated temperature and, possibly, anaphylactoid-like symptomatology (including severe hypotension). Cross sensitivity among members of the ester-type local anesthetic group has been reported. The usefulness of screening for sensitivity has not been definitely established.

NEUROLOGIC

The incidences of adverse neurologic reactions associated with the use of local anesthetics may be related to the total dose of local anesthetic administered, and are also dependent upon the particular drug used, the route of administration, and the physical status of the patient. Many of these effects may be related to local anesthetic techniques, with or without a contribution from the drug.

TREATMENT OF REACTIONS

Toxic effects of local anesthetics require symptomatic treatment: There is no specific cure. The physician should be prepared to maintain an airway and to support ventilation with oxygen and assisted or controlled respiration as required. Supportive treatment of the cardiovascular system includes intravenous fluids and, when appropriate, vasopressors (preferably those that stimulate the myocardium, such as ephedrine). Convulsions may be controlled with oxygen and by the intravenous administration of diazepam or ultra-short acting barbiturates or a short-acting muscle relaxant (succinylcholine). Intravenous anticonvulsant agents and muscle relaxants should only be administered by those familiar with their use and only when ventilation and oxygenation are assured. In spinal and epidural anesthesia, sympathetic blockade also occurs as a pharmacological reaction, resulting in peripheral vasodilation and often *hypotension*. The extent of the hypotension will usually depend on the number of dermatomes blocked. The blood pressure should therefore be monitored in the early phases of anesthesia. If hypotension occurs, it is readily controlled by vasoconstrictors administered wither by the intramuscular or the intravenous route, the dosage of which would depend on the severity of the hypotension and the response to treatment.

DOSAGE AND ADMINISTRATION

LOCAL ANESTHETIC

The dose of any local anesthetic administered varies with the anesthetic procedure, the area to be anesthetized, the vascularity of the tissue, the number of neuronal segments to be blocked, the depth of anesthesia and degree of muscle relaxation required, the duration of anesthesia desired, individual tolerance, and the physical condition of the patient. The smallest dose and concentration required to produce the desired result should be administered. Dosages of procaine HCl should be reduced for elderly and debilitated patients and patients with cardiac and/or liver disease. The rapid injection of a large volume of local anesthetic solution should be avoided and fractional doses should be used when feasible.

For specific techniques and procedures, refer to standard textbooks.

For infiltration anesthesia, 0.25% or 0.5% solution; 350-600 mg is generally considered to be a single safe total dose. To prepare 60 ml of 0.5% solution (5 mg/ml), dilute 30 ml of the 1% solution with 30 ml sodium chloride injection 0.9%. To prepare 60 ml of a 0.25% solution (2.5 mg/ml), dilute 15 ml of 1% solution with 45 ml sodium chloride injection 0.9%. An anesthetic solution of 0.5 to 1 ml of epinephrine 1:1000 per 100 ml may be added for vasoconstrictive effect (1:200,000 to 1:000,000). (See WARNINGS and PRECAUTIONS).

For peripheral nerve block 0.5% solution (up to 200 ml), 1% solution (up to 100 ml), or 2% solution (up to 50 ml). The use of 2% solution should usually be limited to cases requiring a small volume of anesthetic solution (10-25 ml). An anesthetic solution of 0.5% ml to 1 ml of epinephrine 1:1000 per 100 ml may be added for vasoconstrictive effect (1:200,000 to 1:000,000). (See WARNINGS and PRECAUTIONS).

THE USUAL TOTAL DOSE DURING ONE TREATMENT SHOULD NOT EXCEED 1000 MG.

This product should be inspected visually for particulate matter and discoloration prior to administration whenever solution and container permit. Do not use solutions if crystals, cloudiness, or discoloration is observed. Examine solution carefully before use. Reautoclaving increases likelihood of crystal formation. Solutions which are discarded or which contain particulate matter should be administered.

Unused portions of solutions not containing preservatives should be discarded.

Pediatric Use: In children 15 mg/kg of a 0.5% solution for local infiltration is the maximum recommended dose.

SPINAL INJECTION

As with all local anesthetics, the dose of procaine HCl varies and depends upon the area to be anesthetized, the vascularity of the tissues, the number of neuronal segments to be blocked, individual tolerance, and the technique of anesthesia. The lowest dose needed to provide effective anesthesia should be administered. For specific techniques and procedures, refer to standard textbooks (TABLE 2).

***TABLE 2** Recommended Dosage For Spinal Anesthesia*

	Procaine HCl 10% Solution			
Extent of Anesthesia	**Volume of 10% Solution (ml)**	**Volume of Diluent (ml)**	**Total Dose (mg)**	**Site of Inj. (lumbar interspace)**
Perineum	0.5	0.5	50	4th
Perineum and lower extremities	1	1	100	3rd or 4th
Up to costal margin	2	1	200	2nd, 3rd or 4th

The diluent may be sterile normal saline, sterile distilled water, spinal fluid; and for hyperbaric technique, sterile dextrose solution.

The first rate of injection is 1 ml per 5 seconds. Full anesthesia and fixation usually occurs in 5 minutes.

Sterilization: The drug in intact ampules is sterile. The preferred method of destroying bacteria on the exterior of ampules before opening is heat sterilization (autoclaving). Immersion in antiseptic solution is not recommended.

Autoclave at 15-pound pressure, at 121°C (250°F), for 15 minutes. The diluent dextrose may show some brown discoloration due to carmelization.

Protect solutions from light.

The air in the ampuls has been displaced by nitrogen gas.

PRODUCT LISTING - RATED THERAPEUTICALLY EQUIVALENT

Solution - Injectable - 1%			
2 ml x 25	$85.00	NOVOCAIN, Abbott Pharmaceutical	00074-1808-02
6 ml x 50	$323.50	NOVOCAIN, Abbott Pharmaceutical	00074-1808-06
30 ml x 25	$51.50	GENERIC, Abbott Pharmaceutical	00074-1923-04
Solution - Injectable - 2%			
10 ml	$3.75	GENERIC, C.O. Truxton Inc	00463-1052-01
30 ml	$2.50	GENERIC, Torrance Company	00389-0527-30
30 ml	$4.20	GENERIC, Interstate Drug Exchange Inc	00814-6354-46
30 ml	$4.80	GENERIC, C.O. Truxton Inc	00463-1052-30
30 ml x 25	$59.38	GENERIC, Abbott Pharmaceutical	00074-1953-04
Solution - Injectable - 10%			
2 ml x 25	$54.75	NOVOCAIN, Sanofi Winthrop Pharmaceuticals	00074-1810-02

PRODUCT LISTING - EQUIVALENTS NOT AVAILABLE

Solution - Injectable - 1%

30 ml	$3.50	GENERIC, Cmc-Consolidated Midland Corporation	00223-8350-30

Solution - Injectable - 2%

30 ml	$1.89	GENERIC, Mcguff Company	49072-0587-30
30 ml	$4.00	GENERIC, Cmc-Consolidated Midland Corporation	00223-8362-30

Procarbazine Hydrochloride *(002119)*

Categories: Lymphoma, Hodgkin's; Pregnancy Category D; FDA Approved 1969 Jul; WHO Formulary
Drug Classes: Antineoplastics, miscellaneous
Brand Names: **Matulane**
Foreign Brand Availability: Natulan (Australia; Austria; Bahrain; Belgium; Bulgaria; Cyprus; Czech-Republic; Denmark; Egypt; England; Finland; Germany; Greece; Hungary; Iran; Iraq; Ireland; Israel; Italy; Japan; Jordan; Kuwait; Lebanon; Libya; Malaysia; Netherlands; Norway; Oman; Peru; Poland; Portugal; Qatar; Republic-of-Yemen; Saudi-Arabia; Slovenia; South-Africa; Spain; Sweden; Switzerland; Syria; Turkey; United-Arab-Emirates)
Cost of Therapy: $125.32 (Hodgkin's Disease; Matulane; 50 mg; 6 capsules/day; 30 day supply)

WARNING

It is recommended that procarbazine be given only by or under the supervision of a physician experienced in the use of potent antineoplastic drugs. Adequate clinical and laboratory facilities should be available to patients for proper monitoring of treatment.

DESCRIPTION

Procarbazine hydrochloride, a hydrazine derivative antineoplastic agent, is available as capsules containing the equivalent of 50 mg procarbazine as the hydrochloride. Each capsule also contains corn starch, mannitol and talc. Gelatin capsule shells contain parabens (methyl and propyl), potassium sorbate, titanium dioxide, FD & C yellow no. 6 and D & C yellow no. 10.

Chemically, procarbazine hydrochloride is*N*-isopropyl-α-(2-methylhydrazino)-*p*-toluamide monohydrochloride. It is a white to pale yellow crystalline powder which is soluble but unstable in water or aqueous solutions. The molecular weight of procarbazine hydrochloride is 257.76.

CLINICAL PHARMACOLOGY

The precise mode of cytotoxic action of procarbazine has not been clearly defined. There is evidence that the drug may act by inhibition of protein, RNA and DNA synthesis. Studies have suggested that procarbazine may inhibit transmethylation of methyl groups of methionine into t-RNA. The absence of functional t-RNA could cause the cessation of protein synthesis and consequently DNA and RNA synthesis. In addition, procarbazine may directly damage DNA. Hydrogen peroxide, formed during the auto-oxidation of the drug, may attack protein sulfhydryl groups contained in residual protein which is tightly bound to DNA.

Procarbazine is metabolized primarily in the liver and kidneys. The drug appears to be auto-oxidized to the azo derivative with the release of hydrogen peroxide. The azo derivative isomerizes to the hydrazone, and following hydrolysis splits into a benzylaldehyde derivative and methylhydrazine. The methylhydrazine is further degraded to $CO_2$and CH_4 and possibly hydrazine, whereas the aldehyde is oxidized to *N*-isopropylterephthalamic acid, which is excreted in the urine.

Procarbazine is rapidly and completely absorbed. Following oral administration of 30 mg of ^{14}C-labeled procarbazine, maximum peak plasma radioactive concentrations were reached within 60 minutes.

After intravenous injection, the plasma half-life of procarbazine is approximately 10 minutes. Approximately 70% of the radioactivity is excreted in the urine as *N*-isopropylterephthalamic acid within 24 hours following both oral and intravenous administration of ^{14}C-labeled procarbazine.

Procarbazine crosses the blood-brain barrier and rapidly equilibrates between plasma and cerebrospinal fluid after oral administration.

INDICATIONS AND USAGE

Procarbazine is indicated for use in combination with other anticancer drugs for the treatment of Stage III and IV Hodgkin's disease. Procarbazine HCl is used as part of the MOPP (nitrogen mustard, vincristine, procarbazine, prednisone) regimen.

NON-FDA APPROVED INDICATIONS

Procarbazine has also been used without FDA approval in the treatment of non-Hodgkin's lymphoma, small and large cell carcinomas of the lung, brain tumor, myeloma, melanoma and bronchogenic carcinoma.

CONTRAINDICATIONS

Procarbazine is contraindicated in patients with known hypersensitivity to the drug or inadequate marrow reserve as demonstrated by bone marrow aspiration. Due consideration of this possible state should be given to each patient who has leukopenia, thrombocytopenia or anemia.

WARNINGS

To minimize CNS depression and possible potentiation, barbiturates, antihistamines, narcotics, hypotensive agents or phenothiazines should be used with caution. Ethyl alcohol should not be used since there may be a disulfiram (Antabuse)-like reaction. Because procarbazine HCl exhibits some monoamine oxidase inhibitory activity, sympathomimetic drugs, tricyclic antidepressant drugs (*e.g.*, amitriptyline HCl, imipramine HCl) and other drugs and foods with known high tyramine content, such as wine, yogurt, ripe cheese and bananas, should be avoided. A further phenomenon of toxicity common to many hydrazine derivatives is hemolysis and the appearance of Heinz-Ehrlich inclusion bodies in erythrocytes.

PREGNANCY CATEGORY D

Teratogenic Effects

Procarbazine hydrochloride can cause fetal harm when administered to a pregnant woman. While there are no adequate and well-controlled studies with procarbazine hydrochloride in pregnant women, there are case reports of malformations in the offspring of women who were exposed to procarbazine hydrochloride in combination with other antineoplastic agents during pregnancy. Procarbazine HCl should be used during pregnancy only if the potential benefit justifies the potential risk to the fetus. If this drug is used during pregnancy, or if the patient becomes pregnant while taking this drug, the patient should be apprised of the potential hazard to the fetus. Women of childbearing potential should be advised to avoid becoming pregnant. Procarbazine hydrochloride is teratogenic in the rat when given at doses approximately 4-13 times the maximum recommended human therapeutic dose of 6 mg/kg/day.

Nonteratogenic Effects

Procarbazine hydrochloride has not been adequately studied in animals for its effects on peri- and postnatal development. However, neurogenic tumors were noted in the offspring of rats given intravenous injections of 125 mg/kg of procarbazine hydrochloride on day 22 of gestation. Compounds which inhibit DNA, RNA and protein synthesis might be expected to have adverse effects on peri- and postnatal development.

CARCINOGENESIS, MUTAGENESIS, AND IMPAIRMENT OF FERTILITY

Carcinogenesis

The carcinogenicity of procarbazine hydrochloride in mice, rats and monkeys has been reported in a considerable number of studies. Instances of a second nonlymphoid malignancy, including acute myelocytic leukemia, have been reported in patients with Hodgkin's disease treated with procarbazine in combination with other chemotherapy and/or radiation. The International Agency for Research on Cancer (IARC) considers that there is "sufficient evidence" for the human carcinogenicity of procarbazine hydrochloride when it is given in intensive regimens which include other antineoplastic agents but that there is inadequate evidence of carcinogenicity in humans given procarbazine hydrochloride alone.

Mutagenesis

Procarbazine hydrochloride has been shown to be mutagenic in a variety of bacterial and mammalian test systems.

Impairment of Fertility

Azoospermia and antifertility effects associated with procarbazine hydrochloride administration in combination with other chemotherapeutic agents for treating Hodgkin's disease have been reported in human clinical studies. Since these patients received multicombination therapy, it is difficult to determine to what extent procarbazine hydrochloride alone was involved in the male germ-cell damage. The usual Segment I fertility/reproduction studies in laboratory animals have not been carried out with procarbazine hydrochloride. However, compounds which inhibit DNA, RNA and/or protein synthesis might be expected to have adverse effects on gametogenesis. Unscheduled DNA synthesis in the testis of rabbits and decreased fertility in male mice treated with procarbazine hydrochloride have been reported.

PRECAUTIONS

GENERAL

Undue toxicity may occur if procarbazine HCl is used in patients with impairment of renal and/or hepatic function. When appropriate, hospitalization for the initial course of treatment should be considered.

If radiation or a chemotherapeutic agent known to have marrow-depressant activity has been used, an interval of one month or longer without such therapy is recommended before starting treatment with procarbazine HCl. The length of this interval may also be determined by evidence of bone marrow recovery based on successive bone marrow studies.

Prompt cessation of therapy is recommended if any one of the following occurs:

- ***Central Nervous System:*** Signs or symptoms such as paresthesias, neuropathies or confusion.
- ***Leukopenia:*** White blood count under 4000.
- ***Thrombocytopenia:*** Platelets under 100,000.
- ***Hypersensitivity Reaction***
- ***Stomatitis:*** The first small ulceration or persistent spot soreness around the oral cavity is a signal for cessation of therapy.
- ***Diarrhea:*** Frequent bowel movements or watery stools.
- ***Hemorrhage:*** Bleeding tendencies.

Bone marrow depression often occurs 2-8 weeks after the start of treatment. If leukopenia occurs, hospitalization of the patient may be needed for appropriate treatment to prevent systemic infection.

INFORMATION FOR THE PATIENT

Patients should be warned not to drink alcoholic beverages while on procarbazine HCl therapy since there may be an disulfiram (Antabuse)-like reaction. They should also be cautioned to avoid foods with known high tyramine content such as wine, yogurt, ripe cheese and bananas. Over-the-counter drug preparations which contain antihistamines or sympathomimetic drugs should also be avoided. Patients taking procarbazine HCl should also be warned against the use of prescription drugs without the knowledge and consent of their physician.

LABORATORY TESTS

Baseline laboratory data should be obtained prior to initiation of therapy. The hematologic status as indicated by hemoglobin, hematocrit, white blood count (WBC), differential, reticulocytes and platelets should be monitored closely — at least every 3 or 4 days.

Hepatic and renal evaluation are indicated prior to beginning therapy. Urinalysis, transaminase, alkaline phosphatase and blood urea nitrogen tests should be repeated at least weekly.

CARCINOGENESIS, MUTAGENESIS, AND IMPAIRMENT OF FERTILITY

See WARNINGS.

PREGNANCY CATEGORY D

See WARNINGS.

NURSING MOTHERS

It is not known whether procarbazine HCl is excreted in human milk. Because of the potential for tumorigenicity shown for procarbazine hydrochloride in animal studies, mothers should not nurse while receiving this drug.

DRUG INTERACTIONS

See WARNINGS.

No cross-resistance with other chemotherapeutic agents, radiotherapy or steroids has been demonstrated.

ADVERSE REACTIONS

Leukopenia, anemia and thrombopenia occur frequently. Nausea and vomiting are the most commonly reported side effects.

Other adverse reactions are:

- ***Hematologic:*** Pancytopenia; eosinophilia; hemolytic anemia; bleeding tendencies such as petechiae, purpura, epistaxis and hemoptysis.
- ***Gastrointestinal:*** Hepatic dysfunction, jaundice, stomatitis, hematemesis, melena, diarrhea, dysphagia, anorexia, abdominal pain, constipation, dry mouth.
- ***Neurologic:*** Coma, convulsions, neuropathy, ataxia, paresthesia, nystagmus, diminished reflexes, falling, foot drop, headache, dizziness, unsteadiness.
- ***Cardiovascular:*** Hypotension, tachycardia, syncope.
- ***Ophthalmic:*** Retinal hemorrhage, papilledema, photophobia, diplopia, inability to focus.
- ***Respiratory:*** Pneumonitis, pleural effusion, cough.
- ***Dermatologic:*** Herpes, dermatitis, pruritus, alopecia, hyperpigmentation, rash, urticaria, flushing.
- ***Allergic:*** Generalized allergic reactions.
- ***Genitourinary:*** Hematuria, urinary frequency, nocturia.
- ***Musculoskeletal:*** Pain, including myalgia and arthralgia; tremors.
- ***Psychiatric:*** Hallucinations, depression, apprehension, nervousness, confusion, nightmares.
- ***Endocrine:*** Gynecomastia in prepubertal and early pubertal boys.
- ***Miscellaneous:*** Intercurrent infections, hearing loss, pyrexia, diaphoresis, lethargy, weakness, fatigue, edema, chills, insomnia, slurred speech, hoarseness, drowsiness. Second nonlymphoid malignancies, including acute myelocytic leukemia and malignant myelosclerosis, and azoospermia have been reported in patients with Hodgkin's disease treated with procarbazine in combination with other chemotherapy and/or radiation.

P

DOSAGE AND ADMINISTRATION

The following doses are for administration of the drug as a single agent. When used in combination with other anticancer drugs, the procarbazine HCl dose should be appropriately reduced, e.g., in the MOPP regimen, the procarbazine HCl dose is 100 mg/m^2 daily for 14 days. All dosages are based on the patient's actual weight. However, the estimated lean body mass (dry weight) is used if the patient is obese or if there has been a spurious weight gain due to edema, ascites or other forms of abnormal fluid retention.

ADULTS

To minimize the nausea and vomiting experienced by a high percentage of patients beginning procarbazine HCl therapy, single or divided doses of 2-4 mg/kg/day for the first week are recommended. Daily dosage should then be maintained at 4-6 mg/kg/day until maximum response is obtained or until the white blood count falls below 4000/cmm or the platelets fall below 100,000/cmm. When maximum response is obtained, the dose may be maintained at 1-2 mg/kg/day. Upon evidence of hematologic or other toxicity (see PRECAUTIONS), the drug should be discontinued until there has been satisfactory recovery. After toxic side effects have subsided, therapy may then be resumed at the discretion of the physician, based on clinical evaluation and appropriate laboratory studies, at a dosage of 1-2 mg/kg/day.

CHILDREN

Very close clinical monitoring is mandatory. Undue toxicity, evidenced by tremors, coma and convulsions, has occurred in a few cases. Dosage, therefore, should be individualized. The following dosage schedule is provided as a guideline only.

Fifty (50) mg per square meter of body surface per day is recommended for the first week. Dosage should then be maintained at 100 mg per square meter of body surface per day until maximum response is obtained or until leukopenia or thrombocytopenia occurs. When maximum response is attained, the dose may be maintained at 50 mg per square meter of body surface per day. Upon evidence of hematologic or other toxicity (see PRECAUTIONS), the drug should be discontinued until there has been satisfactory recovery, based on clinical evaluation and appropriate laboratory tests. After toxic side effects have subsided, therapy may then be resumed.

Procedures for proper handling and disposal of anticancer drugs should be considered. Several guidelines on this subject have been published.[1-6] There is no general agreement that all of the procedures recommended in the guidelines are necessary or appropriate.

PRODUCT LISTING - EQUIVALENTS NOT AVAILABLE

Capsule - Oral - 50 mg

100's	$69.62	MATULANE, Sigma-Tau Pharmaceuticals Inc	54482-0053-01

Prochlorperazine (002120)

Categories: Anxiety disorder, generalized; Nausea; Schizophrenia; Vomiting; FDA Approved 1957 Sep; Pregnancy Category C

Drug Classes: Antiemetics/antivertigo; Antipsychotics; Phenothiazines

Brand Names: Compa-Z; **Compazine**; Cotranzine; Prochlorperazine Edisylate; Prochlorperazine Maleate; Ultrazine-10

Foreign Brand Availability: Antinaus (New-Zealand); Dhaperazine (Hong-Kong; Malaysia); Klometil (Finland); Nautisol (Benin; Burkina-Faso; Ethiopia; Gambia; Ghana; Guinea; Ivory-Coast; Kenya; Liberia; Malawi; Mali; Mauritania; Mauritius; Morocco; Niger; Nigeria; Senegal; Seychelles; Sierra-Leone; Sudan; Tanzania; Tunia; Uganda; Zambia; Zimbabwe); Nibromin (Japan); Normalmin (Japan); Novamin (Japan; Taiwan); Pasotomin (Japan); Prochlor (Singapore); Proclozine (Thailand); Stemetil (Australia; Bahamas; Bahrain; Barbados; Belize; Benin; Bermuda; Bulgaria; Burkina-Faso; Canada; Curacao; Cyprus; Denmark; Egypt; England; Ethiopia; Finland; Gambia; Ghana; Guinea; Guyana; India; Indonesia; Iraq; Ireland; Israel; Italy; Ivory-Coast; Jamaica; Kenya; Kuwait; Lebanon; Liberia; Libya; Malawi; Malaysia; Mali; Mauritania; Mauritius; Morocco; Netherland-Antilles; Netherlands; New-Zealand; Niger; Nigeria; Norway; Oman; Peru; Puerto-Rico; Qatar; Republic-of-Yemen; Saudi-Arabia; Senegal; Seychelles; Sierra-Leone; South-Africa; Sudan; Surinam; Sweden; Syria; Tanzania; Thailand; Trinidad; Tunia; Uganda; United-Arab-Emirates; Zambia; Zimbabwe); Stemzine (Australia)

Cost of Therapy: $14.28 (Nausea; Compazine; 5 mg; 3 tablets/day; 7 day supply)
$2.63 (Nausea; Generic Tablets; 5 mg; 3 tablets/day; 7 day supply)
$18.89 (Nausea; Compazine Spansule; 10 mg; 2 capsules/day; 7 day supply)
$92.02 (Psychotic Disorders; Compazine; 10 mg; 3 tablets/day; 30 day supply)
$15.75 (Psychotic Disorders; Generic Tablets; 10 mg; 3 tablets/day; 30 day supply)

HCFA JCODE(S): J0780 up to 10 mg IM, IV

DESCRIPTION

Prochlorperazine is a phenothiazine derivative, present in Compazine tablets and Spansule sustained-release capsules as the maleate. Its chemical name is 2-chloro-10-[3-(4-methyl-1-piperazinyl)propyl]-10H-phenothiazine(Z)-2-butenedioate (1:2).

Compazine vials and syrup contain prochlorperazine as the edisylate salt and Compazine suppositories contain prochlorperazine base. *Empirical formulas (and molecular weights) are:* Prochlorperazine maleate — $C_{20}H_{24}ClN_3S{\cdot}2C_4H_4O_4$ (606.10); prochlorperazine edisylate — $C_{20}H_{24}ClN_3S{\cdot}C_2H_6O_6S_2$ (564.14); and prochlorperazine base — $C_{20}H_{24}ClN_3S$ (373.95).

TABLETS

Each round, yellow-green, coated tablet contains prochlorperazine maleate equivalent to prochloroperazine as follows: 5 mg imprinted "SKF" and "C66"; 10 mg imprinted "SKF" and "C67".

5 and 10 mg Tablets: Inactive ingredients consist of cellulose, lactose, magnesium stearate, polyethylene glycol, sodium croscarmellose, titanium dioxide, D&C yellow no. 10, FD&C blue no. 2, FD&C yellow no. 6, FD&C red no. 40, iron oxide, starch, stearic acid and trace amounts of other inactive ingredients, including aluminum lake dyes.

SPANSULE SUSTAINED-RELEASE CAPSULES

Each Compazine Spansule capsule is so prepared that an initial dose is released promptly and the remaining medication is released gradually over a prolonged period. Food slows absorption of prochloroperazine and decreased C_{max} by 23% and AUC by 13%.

Each capsule, with black cap and natural body, contains prochlorperazine maleate equivalent to prochlorperazine. Inactive ingredients consist of ammonio methacrylate co-polymer, D&C green no. 5, D&C yellow no. 10, FD&C blue no. 1, FD&C blue no. 1 aluminum lake, FD&C red no. 40, FD&C yellow no. 6, gelatin, hydroxypropyl methylcellulose, propylene glycol, silicon dioxide, simethicone emulsion, sodium lauryl sulfate, sorbic acid, sugar spheres, talc, triethyl citrate, and trace amounts of other inactive ingredients.

VIALS

2 ml (5 mg/ml) and 10 ml (5 mg/ml): Each ml contains, in aqueous solution, 5 mg prochlorperazine as the edisylate, 5 mg sodium biphosphate, 12 mg sodium tartrate, 0.9 mg sodium saccharin and 0.75% benzyl alcohol as preservative.

SUPPOSITORIES

Each suppository contains 2½, 5, or 25 mg of prochlorperazine; with glycerin, glyceryl monopalmitate, glyceryl monostearate, hydrogenated cocoanut oil fatty acids and hydrogenated palm kernel oil fatty acids.

SYRUP

Each 5 ml (1 teaspoonful) of clear, yellow-orange, fruit-flavored liquid contains 5 mg of prochlorperazine as the edisylate. Inactive ingredients consist of FD&C yellow no. 6, flavors, polyoxyethylene polyoxypropylene glycol, sodium benzoate, sodium citrate, sucrose, and water.

INDICATIONS AND USAGE

For control of severe nausea and vomiting.

For the treatment of schizophrenia.

Prochlorperazine is effective for the short-term treatment of generalized non-psychotic anxiety. However, prochlorperazine is not the first drug to be used in therapy for most patients with non-psychotic anxiety, because certain risks associated with its use are not shared by common alternative treatments (*e.g.,* benzodiazepines).

When used in the treatment of non-psychotic anxiety, prochlorperazine should not be administered at doses of more than 20 mg/day or for longer than 12 weeks, because the use of prochlorperazine at higher doses or for longer intervals may cause persistent tardive dyskinesia that may prove irreversible (see WARNINGS).

The effectiveness of prochlorperazine as treatment for non-psychotic anxiety was established in 4 week clinical studies of outpatients with generalized anxiety disorder. This evidence does not predict that prochlorperazine will be useful in patients with other nonpsychotic conditions in which anxiety, or signs that mimic anxiety, are found (*e.g.*, physical illness, organic mental conditions, agitated depression, character pathologies, etc.).

Prochlorperazine has not been shown effective in the management of behavioral complications in patients with mental retardation.

NON-FDA APPROVED INDICATIONS

Although not FDA approved, prochlorperazine has been used in the treatment of migraine headaches.

CONTRAINDICATIONS

Do not use in patients with known hypersensitivity to phenothiazines.

Do not use in comatose states or in the presence of large amounts of central nervous system (CNS) depressants (alcohol, barbiturates, narcotics, etc.).

Do not use in pediatric surgery.

Do not use in pediatric patients under 2 years of age or under 20 lb. Do not use in children for conditions for which dosage has not been established.

WARNINGS

The extrapyramidal symptoms which can occur secondary to prochlorperazine may be confused with the CNS signs of an undiagnosed primary disease responsible for the vomiting, *e.g.*, Reye's syndrome or other encephalopathy. The use of prochlorperazine and other potential hepatotoxins should be avoided in children and adolescents whose signs and symptoms suggest Reye's syndrome.

TARDIVE DYSKINESIA

Tardive dyskinesia, a syndrome consisting of potentially irreversible, involuntary, dyskinetic movements, may develop in patients treated with antipsychotic drugs. Although the prevalence of the syndrome appears to be highest among the elderly, especially elderly women, it is impossible to rely upon prevalence estimates to predict, at the inception of antipsychotic drug treatment, which patients are likely to develop the syndrome. Whether antipsychotic drug products differ in their potential to cause tardive dyskinesia is unknown.

Both the risk of developing the syndrome and the likelihood that it will become irreversible are believed to increase as the duration of treatment and the total cumulative dose of antipsychotic drugs administered to the patient increase. However, the syndrome can develop, although much less commonly, after relatively brief treatment periods at low doses.

There is no known treatment for established cases of tardive dyskinesia, although the syndrome may remit, partially or completely, if antipsychotic drug treatment is withdrawn. Antipsychotic drug treatment itself, however, may suppress (or partially suppress) the signs and symptoms of the syndrome and thereby may possibly mask the underlying disease process.

The effect that symptomatic suppression has upon the long-term course of the syndrome is unknown.

Given these considerations, antipsychotic drugs should be prescribed in a manner that is most likely to minimize the occurrence of tardive dyskinesia. Chronic antipsychotic treatment should generally be reserved for patients who suffer from a chronic illness that, (1) is known to respond to antipsychotic drugs, and (2) for whom alternative, equally effective, but potentially less harmful treatments are not available or appropriate. In patients who do require chronic treatment, the smallest dose and the shortest duration of treatment producing a satisfactory clinical response should be sought. The need for continued treatment should be reassessed periodically.

If signs and symptoms of tardive dyskinesia appear in a patient on antipsychotics, drug discontinuation should be considered. However, some patients may require treatment despite the presence of the syndrome.

For further information about the description of tardive dyskinesia and its clinical detection, please refer to the sections on PRECAUTIONS and ADVERSE REACTIONS.

NEUROLEPTIC MALIGNANT SYNDROME (NMS)

A potentially fatal symptom complex sometimes referred to as Neuroleptic Malignant Syndrome (NMS) has been reported in association with antipsychotic drugs. Clinical manifestations of NMS are hyperpyrexia, muscle rigidity, altered mental status and evidence of autonomic instability (irregular pulse or blood pressure, tachycardia, diaphoresis, and cardiac dysrhythmias).

The diagnostic evaluation of patients with this syndrome is complicated. In arriving at a diagnosis, it is important to identify cases where the clinical presentation includes both serious medical illness (*e.g.*, pneumonia, systemic infection, etc.) and untreated or inadequately treated extrapyramidal signs and symptoms (EPS). Other important considerations in the differential diagnosis include central anticholinergic toxicity, heat stroke, drug fever, and primary CNS pathology.

The management of NMS should include (1) immediate discontinuation of antipsychotic drugs and other drugs not essential to concurrent therapy, (2) intensive symptomatic treatment and medical monitoring, and (3) treatment of any concomitant serious medical problems for which specific treatments are available. There is no general agreement about specific pharmacological treatment regimens for uncomplicated NMS.

If a patient requires antipsychotic drug treatment after recovery from NMS, the potential reintroduction of drug therapy should be carefully considered. The patient should be carefully monitored, since recurrences of NMS have been reported.

An encephalopathic syndrome (characterized by weakness, lethargy, fever, tremulousness and confusion, extrapyramidal symptoms, leukocytosis, elevated serum enzymes, BUN and FBS) has occurred in a few patients treated with lithium plus an antipsychotic. In some instances, the syndrome was followed by irreversible brain damage. Because of a possible causal relationship between these events and the concomitant administration of lithium and antipsychotics, patients receiving such combined therapy should be monitored closely for early evidence of neurologic toxicity and treatment discontinued promptly if such signs appear. This encephalopathic syndrome may be similar to or the same as NMS.

Patients with bone marrow depression or who have previously demonstrated a hypersensitivity reaction (*e.g.*, blood dyscrasias, jaundice) with a phenothiazine should not receive any phenothiazine, including prochlorperazine, unless in the judgment of the physician the potential benefits of treatment outweigh the possible hazards.

Prochlorperazine may impair mental and/or physical abilities, especially during the first few days of therapy. Therefore, caution patients about activities requiring alertness (*e.g.*, operating vehicles or machinery).

Phenothiazines may intensify or prolong the action of CNS depressants (*e.g.*, alcohol, anesthetics, narcotics).

USE IN PREGNANCY

Safety for the use of prochlorperazine during pregnancy has not been established. Therefore, prochlorperazine is not recommended for use in pregnant patients except in cases of severe nausea and vomiting that are so serious and intractable that, in the judgment of the physician, drug intervention is required and potential benefits outweigh possible hazards.

There have been reported instances of prolonged jaundice, extrapyramidal signs, hyperreflexia or hyporeflexia in newborn infants whose mothers received phenothiazines.

NURSING MOTHERS

There is evidence that phenothiazines are excreted in the breast milk of nursing mothers. Caution should be exercised when prochlorperazine is administered to a nursing woman.

PRECAUTIONS

The antiemetic action of prochlorperazine may mask the signs and symptoms of overdosage of other drugs and may obscure the diagnosis and treatment of other conditions such as intestinal obstruction, brain tumor and Reye's syndrome (see WARNINGS).

When prochlorperazine is used with cancer chemotherapeutic drugs, vomiting as a sign of the toxicity of these agents may be obscured by the antiemetic effect of prochlorperazine.

Because hypotension may occur, large doses and parenteral administration should be used cautiously in patients with impaired cardiovascular systems. To minimize the occurrence of hypotension after injection, keep patient lying down and observe for at least ½ hour. If hypotension occurs after parenteral or oral dosing, place patient in head-low position with legs raised. If a vasoconstrictor is required, norepinephrine bitatrate and phenylephrine hydrochloride are suitable. Other pressor agents, including epinephrine, should not be used because they may cause a paradoxical further lowering of blood pressure.

Aspiration of vomitus has occurred in a few post-surgical patients who have received prochlorperazine as an antiemetic. Although no causal relationship has been established, this possibility should be borne in mind during surgical aftercare.

Deep sleep, from which patients can be aroused, and coma have been reported, usually with overdosage.

Antipsychotic drugs elevate prolactin levels; the elevation persists during chronic administration. Tissue culture experiments indicate that approximately one-third of human breast cancers are prolactin-dependent *in vitro,* a factor of potential importance if the prescribing of these drugs is contemplated in a patient with a previously detected breast cancer. Although disturbances such as galactorrhea, amenorrhea, gynecomastia and impotence have been reported, the clinical significance of elevated serum prolactin levels is unknown for most patients. An increase in mammary neoplasms has been found in rodents after chronic administration of antipsychotic drugs. Neither clinical nor epidemiologic studies conducted to date, however, have shown an association between chronic administration of these drugs and mammary tumorigenesis; the available evidence is considered too limited to be conclusive at this time.

Chromosomal aberrations in spermatocytes and abnormal sperm have been demonstrated in rodents treated with certain antipsychotics.

As with all drugs which exert an anticholinergic effect, and/or cause mydriasis, prochlorperazine should be used with caution in patients with glaucoma.

Because phenothiazines may interfere with thermoregulatory mechanisms, use with caution in persons who will be exposed to extreme heat.

Phenothiazines can diminish the effect of oral anticoagulants.

Phenothiazines can produce alpha-adrenergic blockade.

Thiazide diuretics may accentuate the orthostatic hypotension that may occur with phenothiazines.

Antihypertensive effects of guanethidine and related compounds may be counteracted when phenothiazines are used concomitantly.

Concomitant administration of propranolol with phenothiazines results in increased plasma levels of both drugs.

Phenothiazines may lower the convulsive threshold; dosage adjustments of anticonvulsants may be necessary. Potentiation of anticonvulsant effects does not occur. However, it has been reported that phenothiazines may interfere with the metabolism of phenytoin and thus precipitate phenytoin toxicity.

The presence of phenothiazines may produce false-positive phenylketonuria (PKU) test results.

LONG-TERM THERAPY

Given the likelihood that some patients exposed chronically to antipsychotics will develop tardive dyskinesia, it is advised that all patients in whom chronic use is contemplated be given, if possible, full information about this risk. The decision to inform patients and/or their guardians must obviously take into account the clinical circumstances and the competency of the patient to understand the information provided.

To lessen the likelihood of adverse reactions related to cumulative drug effect, patients with a history of long-term therapy with prochlorperazine and/or other antipsychotics should be evaluated periodically to decide whether the maintenance dosage could be lowered or drug therapy discontinued.

Children with acute illnesses (*e.g.*, chickenpox, CNS infections, measles, gastroenteritis) or dehydration seem to be much more susceptible to neuromuscular reactions, particularly dystonias, than are adults. In such patients, the drug should be used only under close supervision.

Drugs which lower the seizure threshold, including phenothiazine derivatives, should not be used with metrizamide. As with other phenothiazine derivatives, prochlorperazine should be discontinued at least 48 hours before myelography, should not be resumed for at least 24 hours postprocedure, and should not be used for the control of nausea and vomiting occurring either prior to myelography with metrizamide, or postprocedure.

ADVERSE REACTIONS

Drowsiness, dizziness, amenorrhea, blurred vision, skin reactions, and hypotension may occur. Neuroleptic Malignant Syndrome (NMS) has been reported in association with antipsychotic drugs (see WARNINGS).

Cholestatic jaundice has occurred. If fever with grippe-like symptoms occurs, appropriate liver studies should be conducted. If tests indicate an abnormality, stop treatment. There have been a few observations of fatty changes in the livers of patients who have died while receiving the drug. No causal relationship has been established.

Leukopenia and agranulocytosis have occurred. Warn patients to report the sudden appearance of sore throat or other signs of infection. If white blood cell and differential counts indicate leukocyte depression, stop treatment and start antibiotic and other suitable therapy.

NEUROMUSCULAR (EXTRAPYRAMIDAL) REACTIONS

These symptoms are seen in a significant number of hospitalized mental patients. They may be characterized by motor restlessness, be of the dystonic type, or they may resemble parkinsonism.

Depending on the severity of symptoms, dosage should be reduced or discontinued. If therapy is reinstituted, it should be at a lower dosage. Should these symptoms occur in children or pregnant patients, the drug should be stopped and not reinstituted. In most cases barbiturates by suitable route of administration will suffice. (Or, injectable diphenhydramine may be useful.) In more severe cases, the administration of an anti-parkinsonism agent, except levodopa, usually produces rapid reversal of symptoms. Suitable supportive measures such as maintaining a clear airway and adequate hydration should be employed.

Motor Restlessness

Symptoms May Include: Agitation or jitteriness, and sometimes insomnia. These symptoms often disappear spontaneously. At times these symptoms may be similar to the original neurotic or psychotic symptoms. Dosage should not be increased until these side effects have subsided.

If these symptoms become too troublesome, they can usually be controlled by a reduction of dosage or change of drug. Treatment with anti-parkinsonism agents, benzodiazepines or propranolol may be helpful.

Dystonias

Symptoms May Include: Spasm of the neck muscles, sometimes progressing to torticollis; extensor rigidity of back muscles, sometimes progressing to opisthotonos; carpopedal spasm, trismus, swallowing difficulty, oculogyric crisis and protrusion of the tongue.

These usually subside within a few hours, and almost always within 24-48 hours, after the drug has been discontinued.

In mild cases, reassurance or a barbiturate is often sufficient. *In moderate cases,* barbiturates will usually bring rapid relief. *In more severe adult cases,* the administration of an anti-parkinsonism agent, except levodopa, usually produces rapid reversal of symptoms. *In children,* reassurance and barbiturates will usually control symptoms. (Or, injectable diphenhydramine may be useful. *Note:* See diphenhydramine prescribing information for appropriate children's dosage.) If appropriate treatment with anti-parkinsonism agents or diphenhydramine fails to reverse the signs and symptoms, the diagnosis should be reevaluated.

P

Pseudo-Parkinsonism

Symptoms May Include: Mask-like facies; drooling; tremors; pillrolling motion; cogwheel rigidity; and shuffling gait. Reassurance and sedation are important. In most cases these symptoms are readily controlled when an anti-parkinsonism agent is administered concomitantly. Anti-parkinsonism agents should be used only when required. Generally, therapy of a few weeks to 2 or 3 months will suffice. After this time patients should be evaluated to determine their need for continued treatment. (*Note:* Levodopa has not been found effective in pseudo-parkinsonism.) Occasionally it is necessary to lower the dosage of prochlorperazine or to discontinue the drug.

Tardive Dyskinesia

As with all antipsychotic agents, tardive dyskinesia may appear in some patients on long-term therapy or may appear after drug therapy has been discontinued. The syndrome can also develop, although much less frequently, after relatively brief treatment periods at low doses. This syndrome appears in all age groups. Although its prevalence appears to be highest among elderly patients, especially elderly women, it is impossible to rely upon prevalence estimates to predict at the inception of antipsychotic treatment which patients are likely to develop the syndrome. The symptoms are persistent and in some patients appear to be irreversible. The syndrome is characterized by rhythmical involuntary movements of the tongue, face, mouth or jaw (*e.g.,* protrusion of tongue, puffing of cheeks, puckering of mouth, chewing movements). Sometimes these may be accompanied by involuntary movements of extremities. In rare instances, these involuntary movements of the extremities are the only manifestations of tardive dyskinesia. A variant of tardive dyskinesia, tardive dystonia, has also been described.

There is no known effective treatment for tardive dyskinesia; anti-parkinsonism agents do not alleviate the symptoms of this syndrome. It is suggested that all antipsychotic agents be discontinued if these symptoms appear.

Should it be necessary to reinstitute treatment, or increase the dosage of the agent, or switch to a different antipsychotic agent, the syndrome may be masked.

It has been reported that fine vermicular movements of the tongue may be an early sign of the syndrome and if the medication is stopped at that time the syndrome may not develop.

Contact Dermatitis

Avoid getting the injection solution on hands or clothing because of the possibility of contact dermatitis.

Adverse Reactions Reported With Prochlorperazine or Other Phenothiazine Derivatives

Adverse reactions with different phenothiazines vary in type, frequency and mechanism of occurrence, *i.e.,* some are dose-related, while others involve individual patient sensitivity. Some adverse reactions may be more likely to occur, or occur with greater intensity, in patients with special medical problems, *e.g.,* patients with mitral insufficiency or pheochromocytoma have experienced severe hypotension following recommended doses of certain phenothiazines.

Not all of the following adverse reactions have been observed with every phenothiazine derivative, but they have been reported with 1 or more and should be borne in mind when drugs of this class are administered: extrapyramidal symptoms (opisthotonos, oculogyric crisis, hyperreflexia, dystonia, akathisia, dyskinesia, parkinsonism) some of which have lasted months and even years — particularly in elderly patients with previous brain damage; grand mal and petit mal convulsions, particularly in patients with EEG abnormalities or history of such disorders; altered cerebrospinal fluid proteins; cerebral edema; intensification and prolongation of the action of CNS depressants (opiates, analgesics, antihistamines, barbiturates, alcohol), atropine, heat, organophosphorus insecticides; autonomic reactions (dryness of mouth, nasal congestion, headache, nausea, constipation, obstipation, adynamic ileus, ejaculatory disorders/impotence, priapism, atonic colon, urinary retention, miosis and mydriasis); reactivation of psychotic processes, catatonic-like states; hypotension (sometimes fatal); cardiac arrest; blood dyscrasias (pancytopenia, thrombocytopenic purpura, leukopenia, agranulocytosis, eosinophilia, hemolytic anemia, aplastic anemia); liver damage (jaundice, biliary stasis); endocrine disturbances (hyperglycemia, hypoglycemia, glycosuria, lactation, galactorrhea, gynecomastia, menstrual irregularities, false-positive pregnancy tests); skin disorders (photosensitivity, itching, erythema, urticaria, eczema up to exfoliative dermatitis); other allergic reactions (asthma, laryngeal edema, angioneurotic edema, anaphylactoid reactions); peripheral edema; reversed epinephrine effect; hyperpyrexia; mild fever after large IM doses; increased appetite; increased weight; a systemic lupus erythematosus-like syndrome; pigmentary retinopathy; with prolonged administration of substantial doses, skin pigmentation, epithelial keratopathy, and lenticular and corneal deposits.

EKG changes — particularly nonspecific, usually reversible Q and T wave distortions — have been observed in some patients receiving phenothiazines.

Although phenothiazines cause neither psychic nor physical dependence, sudden discontinuance in long-term psychiatric patients may cause temporary symptoms, *e.g.,* nausea and vomiting, dizziness, tremulousness.

Note: There have been occasional reports of sudden death in patients receiving phenothiazines. In some cases, the cause appeared to be cardiac arrest or asphyxia due to failure of the cough reflex.

DOSAGE AND ADMINISTRATION

NOTES ON INJECTION

Stability: This solution should be protected from light. This is a clear, colorless to pale yellow solution; a slight yellowish discoloration will not alter potency. If markedly discolored, solution should be discarded.

Compatibility: It is recommended that prochlorperazine injection not be mixed with other agents in the syringe.

ADULTS

(For children's dosage and administration, see Children.) Dosage should be increased more gradually in debilitated or emaciated patients.

Elderly Patients

In general, dosages in the lower range are sufficient for most elderly patients. Since they appear to be more susceptible to hypotension and neuromuscular reactions, such patients should be observed closely. Dosage should be tailored to the individual, response carefully monitored and dosage adjusted accordingly. Dosage should be increased more gradually in elderly patients.

To Control Severe Nausea and Vomiting

Adjust dosage to the response of the individual. Begin with the lowest recommended dosage.

Oral Dosage: *Tablets:* Usually one 5 or 10 mg tablet 3 or 4 times daily. Daily dosages above 40 mg should be used only in resistant cases. *Sustained-Release Capsules:* Initially, usually one 15 mg capsule on arising or one 10 mg capsule q12h. Daily doses above 40 mg should be used only in resistant cases.

Rectal Dosage: 25 mg twice daily.

IM Dosage: Initially 5-10 mg (1-2 ml) injected deeply into the upper outer quadrant of the buttock. If necessary, repeat every 3 or 4 hours. Total IM dosage should not exceed 40 mg/day.

IV Dosage: 2.5-10 mg (0.5-2 ml) by slow IV injection or infusion at a rate not to exceed 5 mg/min. Prochlorperazine injection may be administered either undiluted or diluted in isotonic solution. A single dose of the drug should not exceed 10 mg; total IV dosage should not exceed 40 mg/day. When administered IV, do not use bolus injection. Hypotension is a possibility if the drug is given by IV injection or infusion.

Subcutaneous administration is not advisable because of local irritation.

Adult Surgery (for severe nausea and vomiting)

Total parenteral dosage should not exceed 40 mg/day. Hypotension is a possibility if the drug is given by IV injection or infusion.

IM Dosage: 5-10 mg (1-2 ml) 1-2 hours before induction of anesthesia (repeat once in 30 minutes, if necessary), or to control acute symptoms during and after surgery (repeat once if necessary).

IV Dosage: 5-10 mg (1-2 ml) as a slow IV injection or infusion 15-30 minutes before induction of anesthesia, or to control acute symptoms during or after surgery. Repeat once if necessary. Prochlorperazine may be administered either undiluted or diluted in isotonic solution, but a single dose of the drug should not exceed 10 mg. The rate of administration should not exceed 5 mg/min. When administered IV, do not use bolus injection.

In Adult Psychiatric Disorders

Adjust dosage to the response of the individual and according to the severity of the condition. Begin with the lowest recommended dose. Although response ordinarily is seen within a day or 2, longer treatment is usually required before maximal improvement is seen.

Oral Dosage

Non-Psychotic Anxiety: Usual dosage is 5 mg 3 or 4 times daily; by sustained-release capsule, usually one 15 mg capsule on arising or one 10 mg capsule q12h. Do not administer in doses of more than 20 mg/day or for longer than 12 weeks.

Schizophrenia: *In relatively mild conditions,* as seen in private psychiatric practice or in outpatient clinics, dosage is 5 or 10 mg 3-4 times daily. *In moderate to severe conditions,* for hospitalized or adequately supervised patients, usual starting dosage is 10 mg 3 or 4 times daily. Increase dosage gradually until symptoms are controlled or side effects become bothersome. When dosage is increased by small increments every 2 or 3 days, side effects either do not occur or are easily controlled. Some patients respond satisfactorily on 50-75 mg daily. *In more severe disturbances,* optimum dosage is usually 100-150 mg daily.

IM Dosage

For immediate control of adult schizophrenic patients with severe symptomatology, inject an initial dose of 10-20 mg (2-4 ml) deeply into the upper outer quadrant of the buttock. Many patients respond shortly after the first injection. If necessary, however, repeat the initial dose every 2-4 hours (or, in resistant cases, every hour) to gain control of the patient. More than 3 or 4 doses are seldom necessary. After control is achieved, switch patient to an oral form of the drug at the same dosage level or higher. If, in rare cases, parenteral therapy is needed for a prolonged period, give 10-20 mg (2-4 ml) every 4-6 hours. Pain and irritation at the site of injection have seldom occurred.

Subcutaneous administration is not advisable because of local irritation.

CHILDREN

Do not use in pediatric surgery.

Children seem more prone to develop extrapyramidal reactions, even on moderate doses. Therefore, use lowest effective dosage. Tell parents not to exceed prescribed dosage, since the possibility of adverse reactions increases as dosage rises.

Occasionally the patient may react to the drug with signs of restlessness and excitement; if this occurs, do not administer additional doses. Take particular precaution in administering the drug to children with acute illnesses or dehydration [see ADVERSE REACTIONS, Neuromuscular (Extrapyramidal) Reactions, Dystonias].

When writing a prescription for the 2½ mg size suppository, write "2½," not "2.5"; this will help avoid confusion with the 25 mg adult size.

Severe Nausea and Vomiting in Children

Prochlorperazine should not be used in pediatric patients under 20 lb in weight or 2 years of age. It should not be used in conditions for which children's dosages have not been established. Dosage and frequency of administration should be adjusted according to the severity of the symptoms and the response of the patient. The duration of activity following IM administration may last up to 12 hours. Subsequent doses may be given by the same route if necessary.

Oral or Rectal Dosage: More than 1 day's therapy is seldom necessary.

TABLE 1

Weight	Usual Dosage	Not to Exceed
Under 20 lb not recommended		
20-29 lb	2½ mg 1 or 2 times a day	7.5 mg/day
30-39 lb	2½ mg 2 or 3 times a day	10 mg/day
40-85 lb	2½ mg 3 times a day or 5 mg 2 times a day	15 mg/day

IM Dosage: Calculate each dose on the basis of 0.06 mg of the drug per pound of body weight; give by deep IM injection. Control is usually obtained with one dose.

Children With Schizophrenia

Oral or Rectal Dosage: For children 2-12 years, starting dosage is 2½ mg 2-3 times daily. Do not give more than 10 mg the first day. Then increase dosage according to patient's response. FOR AGES 2-5, total daily dosage usually does not exceed 20 mg. FOR AGES 6-12, total daily dosage usually does not exceed 25 mg.

IM Dosage: For ages under 12, calculate each dose on the basis of 0.06 mg of prochlorperazine per pound of body weight; give by deep IM injection. Control is usually obtained with one dose. After control is achieved, switch the patient to an oral form of the drug at the same dosage level or higher.

HOW SUPPLIED

COMPAZINE TABLETS

Each round, yellow-green, coated tablet contains prochlorperazine maleate equivalent to prochlorperazine as follows: 5 mg imprinted "SKF" and "C66"; 10 mg imprinted "SKF" and "C67".

Storage: Store between 15 and 30°C (59 and 86°F). Protect from light.

COMPAZINE SPANSULE CAPSULES

The 10 mg capsule is imprinted "10 mg" and "3344" on the black cap and is imprinted "10 mg" and "SB" on the natural body. The 15 mg capsule is imprinted "15 mg" and "3346" on the black cap and is imprinted "15 mg" and "SB" on the natural body.

Storage: Store between 15 and 30°C (59 and 86°F). Protect from light.

VIALS

Supplied in 2 ml (5 mg/ml) and 10 ml (5 mg/ml) vials. Each ml contains, in aqueous solution, 5 mg prochlorperazine as the edisylate.

Storage: Store prochlorperazine vials below 30°C (86°F). Do not freeze.

SUPPOSITORIES

Each suppository contains 2½, 5, or 25 mg of prochlorperazine.

Storage: Store between 15 and 30°C (59 and 86°F). Protect from light.

SYRUP

Each 5 mg/5 ml (1 teaspoonful) of clear, yellow-orange, fruit-flavored liquid contains 5 mg of prochlorperazine as the edisylate.

Storage: Store between 15 and 30°C (59 and 86°F). Protect from light.

PRODUCT LISTING - RATED THERAPEUTICALLY EQUIVALENT

Package	Price	Product, Manufacturer	NDC
Solution - Injectable - 5 mg/ml			
2 ml	$13.80	COMPAZINE, Glaxosmithkline	00007-3351-01
2 ml x 10	$23.87	GENERIC, Abbott Pharmaceutical	00074-1880-32
2 ml x 25	$65.00	GENERIC, Solo Pak Medical Products Inc	36769-0076-02
2 ml x 25	$102.20	COMPAZINE, Glaxosmithkline	00007-3352-09
2 ml x 25	$129.00	GENERIC, Esi Lederle Generics	00641-0491-25
2 ml x 25	$228.85	COMPAZINE, Glaxosmithkline	00007-3352-16
2 ml x 100	$507.00	COMPAZINE, Glaxosmithkline	00007-3342-76
10 ml	$11.95	PROCHLORPERAZINE EDISYLATE, Prescript Pharmaceuticals	00247-1304-10
10 ml	$12.75	GENERIC, Watson/Rugby Laboratories Inc	00536-2152-70
10 ml	$14.25	GENERIC, Ivax Corporation	00182-3049-63
10 ml	$39.10	COMPAZINE, Allscripts Pharmaceutical Company	54569-1879-01
10 ml	$44.35	COMPAZINE, Glaxosmithkline	00007-3343-01
10 ml	$49.44	COMPAZINE, Prescript Pharmaceuticals	00247-0291-10
10 ml x 25	$309.38	GENERIC, Solo Pak Medical Products Inc	36769-0076-10
Suppository - Rectal - 2.5 mg			
12's	$28.30	GENERIC, Able Laboratories Inc	53265-0243-12
Suppository - Rectal - 5 mg			
12's	$27.70	COMPAZINE, Southwood Pharmaceuticals Inc	58016-3222-01
12's	$31.40	COMPAZINE, Able Laboratories Inc	53265-0244-12
12's	$37.24	COMPAZINE, Glaxosmithkline	00007-3361-03
Suppository - Rectal - 25 mg			
3's	$9.68	COMPAZINE, Allscripts Pharmaceutical Company	54569-0353-02
6's	$19.35	COMPAZINE, Allscripts Pharmaceutical Company	54569-0353-01
6's	$21.56	GENERIC, Pd-Rx Pharmaceuticals	55289-0119-06
6's	$22.98	COMPAZINE, Physicians Total Care	54868-0622-02
12's	$34.00	COMPAZINE, Southwood Pharmaceuticals Inc	58016-3018-03
12's	$36.54	GENERIC, Paddock Laboratories Inc	00574-7226-12
12's	$37.50	GENERIC, G and W Laboratories Inc	00713-0135-12
12's	$37.50	GENERIC, Able Laboratories Inc	53265-0245-12
12's	$38.70	COMPAZINE, Allscripts Pharmaceutical Company	54569-0353-00
12's	$45.37	COMPAZINE, Physicians Total Care	54868-0622-00
12's	$46.09	COMPAZINE, Glaxosmithkline	00007-3362-03
12's	$50.95	COMPAZINE, Pharma Pac	52959-0291-00
Syrup - Oral - 5 mg/5 ml			
118 ml	$24.29	COMPAZINE, Glaxosmithkline	00007-3363-44
Tablet - Oral - 5 mg			
2's	$3.56	GENERIC, Prescript Pharmaceuticals	00247-0825-02
3's	$1.97	COMPAZINE, Allscripts Pharmaceutical Company	54569-0352-02
3's	$3.67	GENERIC, Prescript Pharmaceuticals	00247-0825-03
4's	$3.78	GENERIC, Prescript Pharmaceuticals	00247-0825-04
6's	$3.99	GENERIC, Prescript Pharmaceuticals	00247-0825-06
10's	$4.41	GENERIC, Prescript Pharmaceuticals	00247-0825-10
10's	$7.09	COMPAZINE, Allscripts Pharmaceutical Company	54569-0352-01
12's	$4.62	GENERIC, Prescript Pharmaceuticals	00247-0825-12
12's	$7.87	COMPAZINE, Allscripts Pharmaceutical Company	54569-0352-03
15's	$4.94	GENERIC, Prescript Pharmaceuticals	00247-0825-15
25's	$15.32	GENERIC, Udl Laboratories Inc	51079-0541-19
25's	$24.26	COMPAZINE, Pd-Rx Pharmaceuticals	55289-0113-97
30's	$6.53	GENERIC, Prescript Pharmaceuticals	00247-0825-30
30's	$19.67	COMPAZINE, Allscripts Pharmaceutical Company	54569-0352-00
30's	$23.03	COMPAZINE, Physicians Total Care	54868-1284-02
100's	$39.86	FEDERAL UPPER LIMIT, H.C.F.A. F F P	99999-2120-04
100's	$54.18	GENERIC, Barr Laboratories Inc	00555-0521-02
100's	$54.18	GENERIC, Duramed Pharmaceuticals Inc	51285-0521-02
100's	$56.60	GENERIC, Teva Pharmaceuticals Usa	00093-9643-01
100's	$56.65	GENERIC, Mylan Pharmaceuticals Inc	00378-5105-01
100's	$59.25	GENERIC, Geneva Pharmaceuticals	00781-5020-01
100's	$59.50	GENERIC, Ivax Corporation	00172-3690-60
100's	$59.50	GENERIC, Ivax Corporation	00182-8210-89
100's	$59.50	GENERIC, Lannett Company Inc	00527-1297-01
100's	$59.50	GENERIC, Par Pharmaceutical Inc	49884-0549-01
100's	$59.50	GENERIC, Breckenridge Inc	51991-0196-01
100's	$61.29	GENERIC, Udl Laboratories Inc	51079-0541-20
100's	$68.01	COMPAZINE, Glaxosmithkline	00007-3366-20
100's	$70.88	COMPAZINE, Glaxosmithkline	00007-3366-21
Tablet - Oral - 10 mg			
4's	$15.06	COMPAZINE, Pd-Rx Pharmaceuticals	55289-0033-04

10's	$9.73	COMPAZINE, Allscripts Pharmaceutical Company	54569-0351-01
10's	$13.80	COMPAZINE, Pd-Rx Pharmaceuticals	55289-0033-10
15's	$24.55	COMPAZINE, Pharma Pac	52959-0391-15
20's	$23.06	COMPAZINE, Physicians Total Care	54868-1081-02
25's	$22.38	GENERIC, Udl Laboratories Inc	51079-0542-19
25's	$28.40	GENERIC, Pd-Rx Pharmaceuticals	55289-0224-97
25's	$33.02	COMPAZINE, Pd-Rx Pharmaceuticals	55289-0033-97
30's	$29.18	COMPAZINE, Allscripts Pharmaceutical Company	54569-0351-00
100's	$57.66	FEDERAL UPPER LIMIT, H.C.F.A. F F P	99999-2120-03
100's	$81.40	GENERIC, Apothecon Inc	62269-0276-24
100's	$81.41	GENERIC, Barr Laboratories Inc	00555-0522-02
100's	$81.41	GENERIC, Duramed Pharmaceuticals Inc	51285-0522-02
100's	$85.05	GENERIC, Teva Pharmaceuticals Usa	00093-9652-01
100's	$89.00	GENERIC, Geneva Pharmaceuticals	00781-5021-01
100's	$89.50	GENERIC, Ivax Corporation	00172-3691-60
100's	$89.50	GENERIC, Ivax Corporation	00182-8211-89
100's	$89.50	GENERIC, Mylan Pharmaceuticals Inc	00378-5110-01
100's	$89.50	GENERIC, Lannett Company Inc	00527-1298-01
100's	$89.50	GENERIC, Par Pharmaceutical Inc	49884-0550-01
100's	$89.50	GENERIC, Breckenridge Inc	51991-0197-01
100's	$92.08	GENERIC, Udl Laboratories Inc	51079-0542-20
100's	$102.24	COMPAZINE, Glaxosmithkline	00007-3367-20
100's	$105.20	COMPAZINE, Glaxosmithkline	00007-3367-21

PRODUCT LISTING - EQUIVALENTS NOT AVAILABLE

Capsule, Extended Release - Oral - 10 mg

4's	$9.07	COMPAZINE SPANSULE, Prescript Pharmaceuticals	00247-0218-04
5's	$10.51	COMPAZINE SPANSULE, Prescript Pharmaceuticals	00247-0218-05
6's	$11.93	COMPAZINE SPANSULE, Prescript Pharmaceuticals	00247-0218-06
10's	$17.65	COMPAZINE SPANSULE, Prescript Pharmaceuticals	00247-0218-10
15's	$24.80	COMPAZINE SPANSULE, Prescript Pharmaceuticals	00247-0218-15
20's	$31.94	COMPAZINE SPANSULE, Prescript Pharmaceuticals	00247-0218-20
50's	$67.45	COMPAZINE SPANSULE, Glaxosmithkline	00007-3344-15

Capsule, Extended Release - Oral - 15 mg

50's	$100.25	COMPAZINE SPANSULE, Glaxosmithkline	00007-3346-15

Solution - Injectable - 5 mg/ml

2 ml	$3.64	GENERIC, Allscripts Pharmaceutical Company	54569-3955-01
2 ml x 10	$31.21	GENERIC, Physicians Total Care	54868-4137-00
10 ml	$10.12	GENERIC, Physicians Total Care	54868-0261-00
10 ml	$13.75	GENERIC, C.O. Truxton Inc	00463-1102-10

Suppository - Rectal - 2.5 mg

12's	$33.53	COMPAZINE, Glaxosmithkline	00007-3360-03

Suppository - Rectal - 25 mg

12's	$34.00	GENERIC, Southwood Pharmaceuticals Inc	58016-6506-01
12's	$60.25	GENERIC, Pharma Pac	52959-0355-12

Tablet - Oral - 5 mg

6's	$3.57	GENERIC, Allscripts Pharmaceutical Company	54569-0350-05
10's	$8.80	GENERIC, Pharma Pac	52959-0511-10
12's	$7.14	GENERIC, Allscripts Pharmaceutical Company	54569-0350-03
15's	$13.05	GENERIC, Pharma Pac	52959-0511-15
20's	$11.90	GENERIC, Allscripts Pharmaceutical Company	54569-0350-02
30's	$17.85	GENERIC, Allscripts Pharmaceutical Company	54569-0350-01
100's	$12.50	GENERIC, Cmc-Consolidated Midland Corporation	00223-1524-01
100's	$95.00	GENERIC, Cmc-Consolidated Midland Corporation	00223-1524-02

Tablet - Oral - 10 mg

2's	$4.01	GENERIC, Prescript Pharmaceuticals	00247-0497-02
3's	$4.34	GENERIC, Prescript Pharmaceuticals	00247-0497-03
4's	$3.58	GENERIC, Allscripts Pharmaceutical Company	54569-0355-03
4's	$4.68	GENERIC, Prescript Pharmaceuticals	00247-0497-04
6's	$5.34	GENERIC, Prescript Pharmaceuticals	00247-0497-06
6's	$8.90	GENERIC, Cheshire Drugs	55175-4103-06
9's	$6.33	GENERIC, Prescript Pharmaceuticals	00247-0497-09
10's	$6.66	GENERIC, Prescript Pharmaceuticals	00247-0497-10
10's	$8.95	GENERIC, Allscripts Pharmaceutical Company	54569-0355-02
10's	$9.87	GENERIC, Pharma Pac	52959-0476-10
12's	$7.33	GENERIC, Prescript Pharmaceuticals	00247-0497-12
15's	$8.32	GENERIC, Prescript Pharmaceuticals	00247-0497-15
15's	$10.31	GENERIC, Physicians Total Care	54868-1082-00
15's	$13.43	GENERIC, Allscripts Pharmaceutical Company	54569-0355-01
15's	$13.65	GENERIC, Pharma Pac	52959-0476-15
20's	$9.98	GENERIC, Prescript Pharmaceuticals	00247-0497-20
20's	$19.74	GENERIC, Pharma Pac	52959-0476-20
100's	$17.50	GENERIC, Cmc-Consolidated Midland Corporation	00223-1525-01

Tablet - Oral - 25 mg

100's	$19.50	GENERIC, Cmc-Consolidated Midland Corporation	00223-1526-01

P

Progesterone *(002122)*

Categories: Amenorrhea; Hemorrhage, uterine; Infertility; Pregnancy Category D; FDA Approved 1954 Jun
Drug Classes: Contraceptives; Hormones/hormone modifiers; Progestins
Brand Names: Gesterol 50; Lutolin-S; Progestaject-50; **Progestasert**; Progestrone; Prometrium; Rogest 50
Foreign Brand Availability: Crinone (Canada; Hong-Kong; Korea; Thailand); Cyclogest (Singapore); Endometrin (Israel); Estima Ge (France); Evapause (France); Gepromi (Mexico); Geslutin (Colombia; Mexico); Lutogynestryl Fuerte (Peru); Naturogest (India); Progering (Peru); Progest (India); Progestogel (Hong-Kong); Utrogestan (China; Mexico; South-Africa)
HCFA JCODE(S): J2675 per 50 mg IM

INTRAMUSCULAR

WARNING

THE USE OF PROGESTERONE INJECTION DURING THE FIRST 4 MONTHS OF PREGNANCY IS NOT RECOMMENDED.

Progestational agents have been used beginning with the first trimester of pregnancy in an attempt to prevent habitual abortion. There is no adequate evidence that such use is effective when such drugs are given during the first 4 months of pregnancy. Furthermore, in the vast majority of women, the cause of abortion is a defective ovum, which progestational agents could not be expected to influence. In addition, the use of progestational agents, with their uterine-relaxant properties, in patients with fertilized defective ova may cause a delay in spontaneous abortion. Therefore, the use of such drugs during the first 4 months of pregnancy is not recommended.

Several reports suggest an association between intrauterine exposure to progestational drugs in the first trimester of pregnancy and genital abnormalities in male and female fetuses. The risk of hypospadias, 5-8 per 1000 male births in the general population, may be approximately doubled with exposure to these drugs. There are insufficient data to quantify the risk to exposed female fetuses, but insofar as some of these drugs induce mild virilization of the external genitalia of the female fetus, and because of the increased association of hypospadias in the male fetus, it is prudent to avoid the use of these drugs during the first trimester of pregnancy.

If the patient is exposed to progesterone injection during the first 4 months of pregnancy or if she becomes pregnant while taking this drug, she should be apprised of the potential risks to the fetus.

Intramuscular (IM) Injection: *Important Advice to Physicians:* You are required (in conformance with federal regulations) to give a Patient Package Insert to each premenopausal woman, except those in whom childbearing is impossible, receiving this drug.

DESCRIPTION

Progesterone injection is a sterile solution of progesterone in a suitable vegetable oil available for IM use.

Progesterone occurs as a white or creamy white, crystalline powder. It is odorless and is stable in air. Practically insoluble in water, it is soluble in alcohol, acetone, and dioxane and sparingly soluble in vegetable oils.

Each ml Contains: Progesterone 50 mg, benzyl alcohol 10% as preservative in sesame oil qs.

Storage: Store at controlled room temperature 15-30°C (59-86°F).

CLINICAL PHARMACOLOGY

Transforms proliferative endometrium into secretory endometrium.

Inhibits (at the usual dosage) the secretion of pituitary gonadotropins, which in turn prevents follicular maturation and ovulation.

May also demonstrate some estrogenic, anabolic, or androgenic activity but should not be relied upon.

INDICATIONS AND USAGE

This drug is indicated in amenorrhea and abnormal uterine bleeding due to hormonal imbalance in the absence of organic pathology, such as submucous fibroids or uterine cancer.

CONTRAINDICATIONS

- Thrombophlebitis, thromboembolic disorders, cerebral apoplexy or patients with a past history of these secretions.
- Known or suspected carcinoma of the breast.
- Undiagnosed vaginal bleeding.
- Missed abortion.
- As a diagnostic test for pregnancy (see BOXED WARNING).

WARNINGS

Discontinue medication pending examination if there is a sudden partial or complete loss of vision, or if there is sudden onset of proptosis, diplopia, or migraine. If examination reveals papilledema or retinal vascular lesions, medication should be withdrawn.

Detectable amounts of progestogens have been identified in the milk of mothers receiving them. The effect of this on the nursing infant has not been determined.

Because of the occasional occurrence of thrombophlebitis and pulmonary embolism in patients taking progestogens, the physician should be alert to the earliest manifestation of the disease.

Masculinization of the female fetus has occurred when progestogens have been used in pregnant women.

PRECAUTIONS

GENERAL

The pretreatment physical examination should include special reference to the breast and pelvic organs, as well as Papanicolaou smear.

Because this drug may cause some degree of fluid retention, conditions which might be influenced by this factor, such as epilepsy, migraines, asthma, cardiac, or renal dysfunction, require careful observation.

In cases of breakthrough bleeding, as in all cases of irregular bleeding *per vaginum*, nonfunctional causes should be borne in mind. In cases of undiagnosed vaginal bleeding, adequate diagnostic measures are indicated.

Patients who have a history of psychic depression should be carefully observed and the drug discontinued if the depression recurs to a serious degree.

Any possible influence of prolonged progestin therapy on pituitary, ovarian, adrenal, hepatic, or uterine functions awaits further study.

A decrease in glucose tolerance has been observed in a small percentage of patients on estrogen-progestin combination drugs. The mechanism of this decrease is obscure. For this reason, diabetic patients should be carefully observed while receiving progestin therapy.

The age of the patient constitutes no absolute limiting factor although treatment with progestins may mask the onset of climacteric.

The pathologist should be advised of progestin therapy when relevant specimens are submitted.

Studies of the addition of a progestin product to an estrogen replacement regimen for 7 or more days of a cycle of estrogen administration have reported a lowered incidence of endometrial hyperplasia. Morphological and biochemical studies of endometrium suggest that 10-13 days of a progestin are needed to provide maximal maturation of the endometrium and to eliminate any hyperplastic changes. Whether this will provide protection from endometrial carcinoma has not been clearly established. There are possible additional risks which may be associated with the inclusion of progestin in estrogen replacement regimens. The potential risks include adverse effects on carbohydrate and lipid metabolism. The dosage used may be important in minimizing these adverse effects.

INFORMATION FOR THE PATIENT

See the Patient Instructions that are distributed with the prescription.

LABORATORY TESTS

The following laboratory results may be altered by the concomitant use of an estrogen and a progestogen:

Hepatic Function: Increased sulfobromophthalein retention and other tests.
Coagulation Tests: Increase in prothrombin Factors VII, VIII, IX, and X.
Thyroid Function: Increase in PBI and BEI and a decrease in T_3 uptake values.

CARCINOGENESIS, MUTAGENESIS, AND IMPAIRMENT OF FERTILITY

Metyrapone Test

In dogs, the experimental administration of the progestational agent medroxyprogesterone acetate increased the frequency of mammary nodules. Although nodules occasionally appeared in control animal, they were intermittent in nature, whereas nodules in treated animals were larger, more numerous, persistent, and there were some breast malignancies with metastases. Their significance with respect to humans has not been established.

PREGNANCY CATEGORY D

See WARNINGS and information in the box at the start of this literature.

NURSING MOTHERS

Detectable amounts of progesterone have been identified in the milk of mothers receiving the steroid. Its effect on the nursing infant has not been determined.

Because of the potential for tumorigenicity shown for progesterone in animal studies, a decision should be made whether to discontinue nursing or to discontinue the drug, taking into account the importance of the drug to the mother.

PEDIATRIC USE

Safety and effectiveness in children have not been established.

ADVERSE REACTIONS

The following adverse reactions have been observed in women taking progestogens: Break through bleeding, spotting, change in menstrual flow, amenorrhea, edema, changes in weight (increase or decrease), changes in cervical erosion and cervical secretions, cholestatic jaundice, rash (allergic) with and without pruritus, melasma or chloasma, and mental depression.

A small percentage of patients have local reactions at the site of injection.

The administration of large doses of progesterone (50-100 mg daily) may result in a moderate catabolic effect and a transient increase in sodium and chloride excretion.

The result of a pregnanediol determination may be altered if a patient is being treated with a progestogen.

A statistically significant association has been demonstrated between the use of estrogen-progestin combination drugs and the following serious adverse reactions: Thrombophlebitis; pulmonary embolism and cerebral thrombosis and embolism. For this reason patients on progestin therapy should be carefully observed.

Although available evidence is suggestive of an association, such a relationship has been neither confirmed nor refuted for the following serious, adverse reactions: Beuro-Ocular lesions, *e.g.*, retinal thrombosis and optic neuritis.

The following adverse reactions have been observed in patients receiving estrogen-progestin combination drugs: Rise in blood pressure in susceptible individuals; premenstrual-like syndrome; changes in libido, changes in appetite, cystitis-like syndrome, headache, nervousness, dizziness, fatigue, backache, hirsutism, loss of scalp hair, erythema multiforme, erythema nodosum, hemorrhagic eruption, and itching.

In view of these observations, patients on progestin therapy should be carefully observed for their occurrence.

DOSAGE AND ADMINISTRATION

Progesterone is administered by IM injection. It differs from other commonly used steroids in that it is irritating at the place of injection. This is true whether the preparation is in an oil or an aqueous vehicle. The latter is particularly painful.

AMENORRHEA

Five (5) to 10 mg are given for 6-8 consecutive days. If there has been sufficient ovarian activity to produce a proliferative endometrium, one can expect withdrawal bleeding 48-70 hours after the last injection. This may be followed by spontaneous normal cycles.

FUNCTIONAL UTERINE BLEEDING

Five (5) to 10 mg are given daily for 6 doses. Bleeding may be expected to cease within 6 days. When estrogen is given as well, the administration of progesterone is begun after 2 weeks of estrogen therapy. If menstrual flow begins during the course of injections of progesterone, they are discontinued.

ORAL

DESCRIPTION

Progesterone capsules contain micronized progesterone for oral administration. Progesterone has a molecular weight of 314.47 and an empirical formula of $C_{21}H_{30}O_2$. Progesterone (pregn-4-ene-3,20-dione) is a white or creamy white, odorless, crystalline powder practically insoluble in water, soluble in alcohol, acetone and dioxane and sparingly soluble in vegetable oils, stable in air, melting between 126 and 131°C.

Progesterone is synthesized from a starting material from a plant source and is chemically identical to progesterone of human ovarian origin. Prometrium capsules are available in multiple strengths to afford dosage flexibility for optimum management. Prometrium capsules contain 100 or 200 mg micronized progesterone.

The inactive ingredients for Prometrium capsules 100 mg include: Peanut oil, gelatin, glycerin, lecithin, titanium dioxide, D&C yellow no. 10, and FD&C red no. 40.

The inactive ingredients for Prometrium capsules 200 mg include: Peanut oil, gelatin, glycerin, lecithin, titanium dioxide, D&C yellow no. 10, and FD&C yellow no. 6.

CLINICAL PHARMACOLOGY

Progesterone capsules are an oral dosage form of micronized progesterone which is chemically identical to progesterone of ovarian origin. The oral bioavailability of progesterone is increased through micronization.

PHARMACOKINETICS

Absorption

After oral administration of progesterone as a micronized soft gelatin capsule formulation, maximum serum concentrations were attained within 3 hours. The absolute bioavailability of micronized progesterone is not known. TABLE 1 summarizes the mean pharmacokinetic parameters in postmenopausal women after 5 oral daily doses of progesterone capsules 100 mg as a micronized soft-gelatin capsule formulation.

TABLE 1

Parameter	Progesterone Capsules Dose qd 100 mg	200 mg	300 mg
C_{max}(ng/ml)	17.3 ± 21.9*	38.1 ± 37.8	60.6 ± 72.5
T_{max} (h)	1.5 ± 0.8	2.3 ± 1.4	1.7 ± 0.6
AUC(0-10) (ng·h/ml)	43.3 ± 30.8	101.2 ± 66.0	175.7 ± 170.3

* Mean ±SD.

Serum progesterone concentrations appeared linear and dose proportional following multiple dose administration of progesterone capsules 100 mg over the dose range 100-300 mg/day in postmenopausal women. Although doses greater than 300 mg/day were not studied in females, serum concentrations from a study in male volunteers appeared linear and dose proportional between 100 and 400 mg/day. The pharmacokinetic parameters in male volunteers were generally consistent with those seen in postmenopausal women.

Distribution

Progesterone is approximately 96-99% bound to serum proteins, primarily to serum albumin (50-54%) and transcortin (43-48%).

Metabolism

Progesterone is metabolized primarily by the liver largely to pregnanediols and pregnanolones. Pregnanediols and pregnanolones are conjugated in the liver to glucuronide and sulfate metabolites. Progesterone metabolites which are excreted in the bile may be deconjugated and may be further metabolized in the gut via reduction, dehydroxylation, and epimerization.

Excretion

The glucuronide and sulfate conjugates of pregnanediol and pregnanolone are excreted in the bile and urine. Progesterone metabolites which are excreted in the bile may undergo enterohepatic recycling or may be excreted in the feces.

Special Populations

The pharmacokinetics of progesterone capsules have not been assessed in low body weight or obese patients.

Race

There is insufficient information available from trials conducted with progesterone capsules to compare progesterone pharmacokinetics in different racial groups.

P

Hepatic Insufficiency

No formal studies have evaluated the effect of hepatic disease on the disposition of progesterone. However, since progesterone is metabolized by the liver, use in patients with severe liver dysfunction or disease is contraindicated (see CONTRAINDICATIONS). If treatment with progesterone is indicated in patients with mild to moderate hepatic dysfunction, these patients should be monitored carefully.

Renal Insufficiency

No formal studies have evaluated the effect of renal disease on the disposition of progesterone. Since progesterone metabolites are eliminated mainly by the kidneys, progesterone capsules should be used with caution and only with careful monitoring in patients with renal dysfunction (see PRECAUTIONS).

Food-Drug Interaction

Concomitant food ingestion increased the bioavailability of progesterone capsules relative to a fasting state when administered to postmenopausal women at a dose of 200 mg.

Drug-Drug Interaction

The metabolism of progesterone by human liver microsomes was inhibited by ketoconazole (IC_{50} <0.1 μM). Ketoconazole is a known inhibitor of cytochrome P450 3A4, hence these data suggest that ketoconazole or other known inhibitors of this enzyme may increase the bioavailability of progesterone. The clinical relevance of the *in vitro* findings is unknown.

Coadministration of conjugated estrogens and progesterone capsules to 29 postmenopausal women over a 12 day period resulted in an increase in total estrone concentrations (C_{max} 3.68-4.93 ng/ml) and total equilin concentrations (C_{max} 2.27-3.22 ng/ml) and a decrease in circulating 17β estradiol concentrations (C_{max} 0.037-0.030 ng/ml). The half-life of the conjugated estrogens was similar with coadministration of progesterone capsules. TABLE 2 summarizes the pharmacokinetic parameters.

***TABLE 2** Mean (±SD) Pharmacokinetic Parameters For Estradiol, Estrone and Equilin Following Coadministration of Conjugated Estrogens 0.625 mg and Progesterone Capsules 200 mg For 12 Days to Postmenopausal Women*

	Conjugated Estrogens			Conjugated Estrogens + Progesterone Capsules		
Drug	C_{max} (ng/ml)	T_{max} (h)	AUC(0-24h) (ng·h/ml)	C_{max} (ng/ml)	T_{max} (h)	AUC(0-24h) (ng·h/ml)
Estradiol	0.037 ± 0.048	12.7 ± 9.1	0.676 ± 0.737	0.030 ± 0.032	17.32 ± 1.21	0.561 ± 0.572
Estrone Total*	3.68 ± 1.55	10.6 ± 6.8	61.3 ± 26.36	4.93 ± 2.07	7.5 ± 3.8	85.9 ± 41.2
Equilin Total*	2.27 ± 0.95	6.0 ± 4.0	28.8 ± 13.0	3.22 ± 1.13	5.3 ± 2.6	38.1 ± 20.2

* Total estrogens is the sum of conjugated and unconjugated estrogen.

P

INDICATIONS AND USAGE

Progesterone capsules are indicated for use in the prevention of endometrial hyperplasia in non-hysterectomized postmenopausal women who are receiving conjugated estrogens tablets. They are also indicated for use in secondary amenorrhea.

CONTRAINDICATIONS

- **Known sensitivity to progesterone capsules or its ingredients. Progesterone capsules contain peanut oil and should never be used by patients allergic to peanuts.**
- Known or suspected pregnancy.
- Thrombophlebitis, thromboembolic disorders, cerebral apoplexy, or patients with a past history of these conditions.
- Severe liver dysfunction or disease.
- Known or suspected malignancy of breast or genital organs.
- Undiagnosed vaginal bleeding.
- Missed abortion.
- As a diagnostic test for pregnancy.

WARNINGS

The physician should be alert to the earliest manifestations of thrombotic disorders (thrombophlebitis, cerebrovascular disorders, pulmonary embolism, and retinal thrombosis). Should any of these occur or be suspected, the drug should be discontinued immediately.

Discontinue medication pending examination if there is sudden partial or complete loss of vision, or if there is a sudden onset of proptosis, diplopia or migraine. If examination reveals papilledema or retinal vascular lesions, medication should be withdrawn.

The administration of any drug to nursing mothers should be done only when clearly necessary since many drugs are excreted in human milk. Detectable amounts of progestin have been identified in the milk of mothers receiving progestins. The effect of this on the nursing infant has not been determined.

Retrospective studies of morbidity and mortality in Great Britain and studies of morbidity in the US have shown a statistically significant association between thrombophlebitis, pulmonary embolism, cerebral thrombosis and embolism, and the use of oral contraceptives. The estimate of the relative risk of thromboembolism in the study by Vessey and Doll was about 7-fold, while Sartwell and associates in the US found a relative risk of 4.4, meaning that the users are several times as likely to undergo thromboembolic disease without evident cause as nonusers. The American study also indicated that the risk did not persist after discontinuation of administration, and that it was not enhanced by long-continued administration. The American study was not designed to evaluate a difference between products.

PRECAUTIONS

GENERAL

The pretreatment physical examination should include special reference to breast and pelvic organs, as well as Papanicolaou smear.

Because progesterone may cause some degree of fluid retention, conditions which might be influenced by this factor, such as epilepsy, migraine, asthma, cardiac or renal dysfunction, require careful observation.

In cases of breakthrough bleeding, as in any cases of irregular bleeding per vaginum, nonfunctional causes should be borne in mind. In cases of undiagnosed vaginal bleeding, adequate diagnostic measures are indicated.

Patients who have a history of psychic depression should be carefully observed and the drug discontinued if the depression recurs to a serious degree.

Any possible influence of prolonged progestin therapy on pituitary, ovarian, adrenal, hepatic or uterine functions awaits further study.

Although concomitant use of conjugated estrogens and progesterone capsules did not result in a decrease in glucose tolerance, diabetic patients should be carefully observed while receiving estrogen-progestin therapy.

The pathologist should be advised of progestin therapy when relevant specimens are submitted.

Because of the occurrence of thrombotic disorders (thrombophlebitis, pulmonary embolism, retinal thrombosis, and cerebrovascular disorders) in patients taking estrogen-progestin combinations, the physician should be alert to the earliest manifestation of these disorders.

Transient dizziness may occur in some patients. Use caution when driving a motor vehicle or operating machinery. A small percentage of women may experience extreme dizziness and/or drowsiness during initial therapy. For these women, bedtime dosing is advised.

Rare instances of syncope and hypotension of possible orthostatic origin have been observed in patients taking progesterone capsules.

INFORMATION FOR THE PATIENT

See accompanying Patient Insert which is distributed with the prescription.

General

This product contains peanut oil and should not be used if you are allergic to peanuts.

DRUG/LABORATORY TEST INTERACTIONS

The following laboratory results may be altered by the use of estrogen-progestin combination drugs:

- Increased sulfobromophthalein retention and other hepatic function tests.
- ***Coagulation tests:*** Increase in prothrombin factors VII, VIII, IX and X.
- Metyrapone test.
- Pregnanediol determination.
- ***Thyroid function:*** Increase in PBI, and butanol extractable protein bound iodine and decrease in T3 uptake values.

Fasting and 2 hour plasma insulin and glucose levels following an oral glucose tolerance test (OGTT) and fibrinogen levels were measured in patients receiving progesterone capsules at a dose of 200 mg/day for 12 days per 28 day cycle in combination with conjugated estrogens 0.625 mg/day (n=120). TABLE 6 summarizes this data. Plasma insulin levels 2 hours post-OGTT were decreased from baseline. The fasting plasma glucose and fasting plasma insulin levels were also decreased from baseline. Glucose levels 2 hours post-OGTT were increased slightly. There was no effect on fibrinogen levels.

***TABLE 6** Mean Changes From Baseline in Insulin and Glucose Levels After 36 Months of Treatment*

	Treatment Group Mean (Mean % Change)		
Parameter	Conjugated Estrogens 0.625 mg + Progesterone Capsules 200 mg (cyclical)* n=173-176†	Conjugated Estrogens 0.625 mg (only) n=170-172†	Placebo n=171
OGTT			
Insulin (pmol/L)			
Fasting	-2.2 (-6.2%)	-1.1 (-3.2%)	5.1 (14.2%)
2 hour	-45.2 (-14.5%)	-23.9 (-7.9%)	-29.7 (-9.1%)
Glucose (mg/dl)			
Fasting	-3.0 (-2.9%)	-2.7 (-2.7%)	-1.0 (-0.9%)
2 hour	3.6 (5.2%)	5.0 (7.8%)	2.1 (3.9%)

* There are no significant changes (p <0.05) from conjugated estrogens values.
† Number of subjects (n) varies by parameter.

CARCINOGENESIS, MUTAGENESIS, AND IMPAIRMENT OF FERTILITY

Progesterone has not been tested for carcinogenicity in animals by the oral route of administration. When implanted into female mice, progesterone produced mammary carcinomas, ovarian granulosa cell tumors and endometrial stromal sarcomas.[1] In dogs, long-term intramuscular (IM) injections produced nodular hyperplasia and benign and malignant mammary tumors.[2] Subcutaneous or IM injections of progesterone decreased the latency period and increased the incidence of mammary tumors in rats previously treated with a chemical carcinogen.[3]

Progesterone did not show evidence of genotoxicity in *in vitro* studies for point mutations or for chromosomal damage. *In vivo* studies for chromosome damage have yielded positive results in mice at oral doses of 1000 and 2000 mg/kg.[4] Exogenously administered progesterone has been shown to inhibit ovulation in a number of species and it is expected that high doses given for an extended duration would impair fertility until the cessation of treatment.

PREGNANCY CATEGORY B

Reproductive studies have been performed in mice at doses up to 9 times the human oral dose,[5,6] in rats at doses up to 44 times the human oral dose,[7,8] in rabbits at a dose of 10 µg/day delivered locally within the uterus by an implanted device,[9] in guinea pigs at doses of approximately one-half the human oral dose[10] and in Rhesus monkeys[11] at doses approximately the human dose, all based on body surface area, and have revealed little or no evidence of impaired fertility or harm to the fetus due to progesterone.

Several studies in women exposed to progesterone have not demonstrated any significant increase in fetal malformations.[12] A single case of cleft palate was observed in the child of a woman using progesterone capsules in early pregnancy, although definitive causality has not been established. Rare instances of fetal death have been reported in pregnant women prescribed progesterone capsules for unapproved indications. Because the studies in humans cannot rule out the possibility of harm, progesterone capsules should be used during pregnancy only if indicated (see CONTRAINDICATIONS).

NURSING MOTHERS

The administration of any drug to nursing mothers should be done only when clearly necessary since many drugs are excreted in human milk. Detectable amounts of progestin have been identified in the milk of nursing mothers receiving progestins. The effect of this on the nursing infant has not been determined.

PEDIATRIC USE

The safety and effectiveness of progesterone capsules in pediatric patients have not been established.

ADVERSE REACTIONS

ENDOMETRIAL PROTECTION

TABLE 7 lists adverse experiences which were reported in ≥2% of patients (regardless of relationship to treatment) who received cyclic progesterone capsules, 200 mg daily (12 days/calendar month cycle) with daily 0.625 mg conjugated estrogen, in a multicenter, randomized, double-blind, placebo-controlled clinical trial in 875 postmenopausal women.

TABLE 7 *Adverse Experiences (≥2%) Reported in an 875 Patient Placebo-Controlled Trial in Postmenopausal Women over a 3 Year Period*

	Progesterone Capsules 200 mg With Conjugated Estrogens 0.625 mg (n=178)	Conjugated Estrogens 0.625 mg (only) (n= 175)	Placebo (n=174)
Headache	31%	30%	27%
Breast tenderness	27%	16%	6%
Joint pain	20%	22%	29%
Depression	19%	18%	12%
Dizziness	15%	5%	9%
Abdominal bloating	12%	10%	5%
Hot flashes	11%	14%	35%
Urinary problems	11%	10%	9%
Abdominal pain	10%	13%	10%
Vaginal discharge	10%	10%	3%
Nausea/vomiting	8%	6%	7%
Worry	8%	5%	4%
Chest pain	7%	4%	5%
Diarrhea	7%	7%	4%
Night sweats	7%	5%	17%
Breast pain	6%	6%	2%
Swelling of hands and feet	6%	9%	9%
Vaginal dryness	6%	8%	10%
Constipation	3%	3%	2%
Breast carcinoma	2%	<1%	<1%
Breast excisional biopsy	2%	1%	<1%
Cholecystectomy	2%	<1%	<1%

SECONDARY AMENORRHEA

TABLE 8 lists adverse experiences which were reported in ≥5% of patients receiving progesterone capsules, 400 mg/day, in a multicenter, randomized, double-blind, placebo-controlled clinical trial in estrogen-primed (6 weeks) postmenopausal women receiving conjugated estrogens 0.625 mg/day and cyclic (10 day/calendar month cycle) progesterone capsules at a dose of 400 mg/day, for 3 cycles.

TABLE 8 *Adverse Experiences (≥5%) Reported in Patients Using 400 mg/day in a Placebo-Controlled Trial in Estrogen-Primed Postmenopausal Women*

Adverse Experience	Progesterone Capsules 400 mg n=25	Placebo n=24
Fatigue	8%	4%
Headache	16%	8%
Dizziness	24%	4%
Abdominal distention (bloating)	8%	8%
Abdominal pain (cramping)	20%	13%
Diarrhea	8%	4%
Nausea	8%	0%
Back pain	8%	8%
Musculoskeletal pain	12%	4%
Irritability	8%	4%
Breast pain	16%	8%
Infection viral	12%	0%
Coughing	8%	0%

The most common adverse experiences reported in ≥5% of patients in all progesterone capsules dosage groups studied in this trial (100-400 mg/day) were: Dizziness (16%), breast pain (11%), headache (10%), abdominal pain (10%), fatigue (9%), viral infection (7%), abdominal distention (6%), musculoskeletal pain (6%), emotional lability (6%), irritability (5%), and upper respiratory tract infection (5%).

Other adverse events reported in <5% of patients taking progesterone capsules include:

Autonomic Nervous System Disorders: Dry mouth.

Body as a Whole: Accidental injury, chest pain, fever.

Cardiovascular System Disorders: Hypertension.

Central and Peripheral Nervous System Disorders: Confusion, somnolence, speech disorder.

Gastrointestinal System Disorders: Constipation, dyspepsia, gastroenteritis, hemorrhagic rectum, hiatus hernia, vomiting.

Hearing and Vestibular Disorders: Earache.

Heart Rate and Rhythm Disorders: Palpitation.

Metabolic and Nutritional Disorders: Edema, edema peripheral.

Musculoskeletal System Disorders: Arthritis, leg cramps, hypertonia, muscle disorder, myalgia.

Myo/Endo/Pericardial and Valve Disorders: Angina pectoris.

Psychiatric Disorders: Anxiety, impaired concentration, insomnia, personality disorder.

Reproductive System Disorders: Leukorrhea, uterine fibroid, vaginal dryness, fungal vaginitis, vaginitis.

Resistance Mechanism Disorders: Abscess, herpes simplex.

Respiratory System Disorders: Bronchitis, nasal congestion, pharyngitis, pneumonitis, sinusitis.

Skin and Appendages Disorders: Acne, verruca, wound debridement.

Urinary System Disorders: Urinary tract infection.

Vision Disorders: Abnormal vision.

White Cell and Resistance Disorders: Lymphadenopathy.

The following adverse experiences have been reported with progesterone capsules in other US clinical trials: Increased sweating, asthenia, tooth disorder, anorexia, increased appetite, nervousness, and breast enlargement.

The following spontaneous adverse events have been reported during the marketing of progesterone capsules: Reversible cases of hepatitis and elevated transaminases. These events occurred mainly in patients receiving high doses of up to 1200 mg. Additionally, rare instances of syncope with and without hypotension have been reported.

The following additional adverse experiences have been observed in women taking progestins in general: Breakthrough bleeding, spotting, change in menstrual flow, amenorrhea, changes in weight (increase or decrease), changes in the cervical squamo-columnar junction and cervical secretions, cholestatic jaundice, anaphylactoid reactions and anaphylaxis, rash (allergic) with and without pruritus, melasma or chloasma, pyrexia, and insomnia.

DOSAGE AND ADMINISTRATION

Prevention of Endometrial Hyperplasia: Progesterone capsules should be given as a single daily dose in the evening, 200 mg orally for 12 days sequentially per 28 day cycle, to postmenopausal women with a uterus who are receiving daily conjugated estrogens tablets.

Secondary Amenorrhea: Progesterone capsules may be given as a single daily dose of 400 mg in the evening for 10 days.

HOW SUPPLIED

PROMETRIUM CAPSULES

100 mg: Round, peach-colored capsules branded with black imprint "SV".

200 mg: Oval, pale yellow-colored capsules branded with black imprint "SV2".

Storage

Store at 25°C (77°F). Excursions permitted to 15-30°C (59-86°F).

Dispense in tight, light-resistant container.

Protect from excessive moisture.

VAGINAL

DESCRIPTION

Prochieve (progesterone gel) is a bioadhesive vaginal gel containing micronized progesterone in an emulsion system, which is contained in single use, 1 piece polyethylene vaginal applicators. The carrier vehicle is an oil in water emulsion containing the water swellable, but insoluble polymer, polycarbophil. The progesterone is partially soluble in both the oil and water phase of the vehicle, with the majority of the progesterone existing as a suspension. Physically, Prochieve has the appearance of a soft, white to off-white gel.

The active ingredient, progesterone, is present in either a 4 or an 8% concentration (w/w). The chemical name for progesterone is pregn-4-ene-3,20-dione. It has an empirical formula of $C_{21}H_{30}O_2$ and a molecular weight of 314.5.

Progesterone exists in two polymorphic forms. Form 1, which is the form used in progesterone gel, exists as white orthorhombic prisms with a melting point of 127-131°C.

Each applicator delivers 1.125 g of Prochieve gel containing either 45 mg (4% gel) or 90 mg (8% gel) of progesterone in a base containing glycerin, mineral oil, polycarbophil, carbomer 934P, hydrogenated palm oil glyceride, sorbic acid, sodium hydroxide and purified water.

CLINICAL PHARMACOLOGY

Progesterone is a naturally occurring steroid that is secreted by the ovary, placenta, and adrenal gland. In the presence of adequate estrogen, progesterone transforms a proliferative endometrium into a secretory endometrium. Progesterone is essential for the development of decidual tissue, and the effect of progesterone on the differentiation of glandular epithelia

P

and stroma has been extensively studied. Progesterone is necessary to increase endometrial receptivity for implantation of an embryo. Once an embryo is implanted, progesterone acts to maintain the pregnancy. Normal or near-normal endometrial responses to oral estradiol and intramuscular (IM) progesterone have been noted in functionally agonadal women through the sixth decade of life. Progesterone administration decreases the circulatory levels of gonadotropins.

PHARMACOKINETICS

Absorption

Due to the sustained release properties of progesterone gel, progesterone absorption is prolonged with an absorption half-life of approximately 25-50 hours, and an elimination half-life of 5-20 minutes. Therefore, the pharmacokinetics of progesterone gel are rate-limited by absorption rather than by elimination.

The bioavailability of progesterone in progesterone gel was determined relative to progesterone administered intramuscularly. In a single dose crossover study, 20 healthy, estrogenized postmenopausal women received 45 or 90 mg progesterone vaginally in progesterone gel 4% or progesterone gel 8%, or 45 or 90 mg progesterone intramuscularly. The pharmacokinetic parameters (mean ± standard deviation) are shown in TABLE 9.

TABLE 9 *Single Dose Relative Bioavailability*

	Progesterone Gel 4%	45 mg IM Progesterone	Progesterone Gel 8%	90 mg IM Progesterone
C_{max} (ng/ml)	13.15 ± 6.49	39.06 ± 13.68	14.87 ± 6.32	53.76 ± 14.9
$C_{avg\ 0\text{-}24}$ (ng/ml)	6.94 ± 4.24	22.41 ± 4.92	6.98 ± 3.21	28.98 ± 8.75
AUC(0-96) (ng·h/ml)	288.63 ± 273.72	806.26 ± 102.75	296.78 ± 129.90	1378.91 ± 176.39
T_{max} (h)	5.6 ± 1.84	8.2 ± 6.43	6.8 ± 3.3	9.2 ± 2.7
T½ (h)	55.13 ± 28.04	28.05 ± 16.87	34.8 ± 11.3	19.6 ± 6.0
F (%)	27.6		19.8	

C_{max} = maximum progesterone serum concentration; $C_{avg\ 0\text{-}24}$ = average progesterone serum concentration over 24 hours; AUC(0-96) = area under the drug concentration versus time curve from 0-96 hours post dose; T_{max} = time to maximum progesterone concentration; T½ = elimination half-life; F = relative bioavailability.

The multiple dose pharmacokinetics of progesterone gel 4% and progesterone gel 8% administered every other day and progesterone gel 8% administered daily or twice daily for 12 days were studied in 10 healthy, estrogenized postmenopausal women in two separate studies. Steady state was achieved within the first 24 hours after initiation of treatment. The pharmacokinetic parameters (mean ± standard deviation) after the last administration of progesterone gel 4 or 8% derived from these studies are shown in TABLE 10.

TABLE 10 *Multiple Dose Pharmacokinetics*

	Assisted Reproductive Technology		Secondary Amenorrhea — Every Other Day Dosing	
	Daily Dosing 8%	Twice Daily Dosing 8%	4%	8%
C_{max} (ng/ml)	15.97 ± 5.05	14.57 ± 4.49	13.21 ± 9.46	13.67 ± 3.58
C_{avg} (ng/ml)	8.99 ± 3.53	11.6 ± 3.47	4.05 ± 2.85	6.75 ± 2.83
T_{max} (h)	5.40 ± 0.97	3.55 ± 2.48	6.67 ± 3.16	7.00 ± 2.88
AUC(0-t) (ng·h/ml)	391.98 ± 153.28	138.72 ± 41.58	242.15 ± 167.88	438.36 ± 223.36
T½ (h)	45.00 ± 34.70	25.91 ± 6.15	49.87 ± 31.20	39.08 ± 12.88

Distribution

Progesterone is extensively bound to serum proteins (~96-99%), primarily to serum albumin and corticosteroid binding globulin.

Metabolism

The major urinary metabolite of oral progesterone is 5β-pregnan-3α, 20α-diol glucuronide which is present in plasma in the conjugated form only. Plasma metabolites also include 5β-pregnan-3α-ol-20-one (5β-pregnanolone) and 5a-pregnan-3α-ol-20-one (5α-pregnanolone).

Excretion

Progesterone undergoes both biliary and renal elimination. Following an injection of labeled progesterone, 50-60% of the excretion of progesterone metabolites occurs via the kidney; approximately 10% occurs via the bile and feces, the second major excretory pathway. Overall recovery of labeled material accounts for 70% of an administered dose, with the remainder of the dose not characterized with respect to elimination. Only a small portion of unchanged progesterone is excreted in the bile.

INDICATIONS AND USAGE

ASSISTED REPRODUCTIVE TECHNOLOGY

Progesterone gel 8% is indicated for progesterone supplementation or replacement as part of an Assisted Reproductive Technology ("ART") treatment for infertile women with progesterone deficiency.

SECONDARY AMENORRHEA

Progesterone gel 4% is indicated for the treatment of secondary amenorrhea. Progesterone gel 8% is indicated for use in women who have failed to respond to treatment with progesterone gel 4%.

CONTRAINDICATIONS

Progesterone gel should not be used in individuals with any of the following conditions:

- Known sensitivity to progesterone gel (progesterone or any of the other ingredients).
- Undiagnosed vaginal bleeding.
- Liver dysfunction or disease.
- Known or suspected malignancy of the breast or genital organs.
- Missed abortion.
- Active thrombophlebitis or thromboembolic disorders, or a history of hormone-associated thrombophlebitis or thromboembolic disorders.

WARNINGS

The physician should be alert to the earliest manifestations of thrombotic disorders (thrombophlebitis, cerebrovascular disorders, pulmonary embolism, and retinal thrombosis). Should any of these occur or be suspected, the drug should be discontinued immediately.

Progesterone and progestins have been used to prevent miscarriage in women with a history of recurrent spontaneous pregnancy losses. No adequate evidence is available to show that they are effective for this purpose.

PRECAUTIONS

GENERAL

The pretreatment physical examination should include special reference to breast and pelvic organs, as well as Papanicolaou smear.

In cases of breakthrough bleeding, as in all cases of irregular vaginal bleeding, nonfunctional causes should be considered. In cases of undiagnosed vaginal bleeding, adequate diagnostic measures should be undertaken.

Because progestogens may cause some degree of fluid retention, conditions which might be influenced by this factor (*e.g.*, epilepsy, migraine, asthma, cardiac or renal dysfunction) require careful observation.

The pathologist should be advised of progesterone therapy when relevant specimens are submitted.

Patients who have a history of psychic depression should be carefully observed and the drug discontinued if the depression recurs to a serious degree.

A decrease in glucose tolerance has been observed in a small percentage of patients on estrogen-progestin combination drugs. The mechanism of this decrease is not known. For this reason, diabetic patients should be carefully observed while receiving progestin therapy.

INFORMATION FOR THE PATIENT

The product should not be used concurrently with other local intravaginal therapy. If other local intravaginal therapy is to be used concurrently, there should be at least a 6 hour period before or after progesterone gel administration.

CARCINOGENESIS, MUTAGENESIS, AND IMPAIRMENT OF FERTILITY

Nonclinical toxicity studies to determine the potential of progesterone gel to cause carcinogenicity or mutagenicity have not been performed. The effect of progesterone gel on fertility has not been evaluated in animals.

PREGNANCY

Progesterone gel 8% has been used to support embryo implantation and maintain pregnancies through its use as part of ART treatment regimens in two clinical studies (studies COL1620-007US and COL1620-F01). In the first study (COL1620-007US), 54 progesterone gel-treated women had donor oocyte transfer procedures, and clinical pregnancies occurred in 26 women (48%). The outcomes of these 26 pregnancies were as follows: 1 woman had an elective termination of pregnancy at 19 weeks due to congenital malformations (omphalocele) associated with a chromosomal abnormality; 1 woman pregnant with triplets had an elective termination of her pregnancy; 7 women had spontaneous abortions; and 17 women delivered 25 apparently normal newborns.

In the second study (COL1620-F01), progesterone gel 8% was used in the luteal phase support of women undergoing *in vitro* fertilization ("IVF") procedures. In this multi-center, open-label study, 139 women received progesterone gel 8% once daily beginning within 24 hours of embryo transfer and continuing through Day 30 post-transfer.

Clinical pregnancies assessed at Day 90 post-transfer were seen in 36 (26%) of women. Thirty-two (32) women (23%) delivered newborns and 4 women (3%) had spontaneous abortions. Of the 47 newborns delivered, 1 had a teratoma associated with a cleft palate; 1 had respiratory distress syndrome; 44 were apparently normal and 1 was lost to follow-up.

GERIATRIC USE

The safety and effectiveness in geriatric patients (over age 65) have not been established.

PEDIATRIC USE

Safety and effectiveness in pediatric patients have not been established.

NURSING MOTHERS

Detectable amounts of progestins have been identified in the milk of mothers receiving them. The effect of this on the nursing infant has not been determined.

DRUG INTERACTIONS

No drug interactions have been assessed with progesterone gel.

ADVERSE REACTIONS

ASSISTED REPRODUCTIVE TECHNOLOGY

In a study of 61 women with ovarian failure undergoing a donor oocyte transfer procedure receiving progesterone gel 8% twice daily, treatment-emergent adverse events occurring in 5% or more of the women are shown in TABLE 11.

In a second clinical study of 139 women using progesterone gel 8% once daily for luteal phase support while undergoing an *in vitro* fertilization procedure, treatment-emergent adverse events reported in ≥5% of the women are shown in TABLE 12.

SECONDARY AMENORRHEA

In three studies, 127 women with secondary amenorrhea received estrogen replacement therapy and progesterone gel 4 or 8% every other day for 6 doses. Treatment emergent

TABLE 11 *Treatment-Emergent Adverse Events in ≥5% of Women Receiving Progesterone Gel 8% Twice Daily Study COL1620-007US (n=61)*

Body as a Whole	
Bloating	7%
Cramps NOS	15%
Pain	8%
Central and Peripheral Nervous System	
Dizziness	5%
Headache	13%
Gastrointestinal System	
Nausea	7%
Reproductive, Female	
Breast pain	13%
Moniliasis genital	5%
Vaginal discharge	7%
Skin and Appendages	
Pruritus genital	5%

TABLE 12 *Treatment-Emergent Adverse Events in >5% of Women Receiving Progesterone Gel 8% Once Daily Study COL1620-F01 (n=139)*

Body as a Whole	
Abdominal pain	12%
Perineal pain female	17%
Central and Peripheral Nervous System	
Headache	17%
Gastrointestinal System	
Constipation	27%
Diarrhea	8%
Nausea	22%
Vomiting	5%
Musculoskeletal System	
Arthralgia	8%
Psychiatric	
Depression	11%
Libido decreased	10%
Nervousness	16%
Somnolence	27%
Reproductive, Female	
Breast enlargement	40%
Dyspareunia	6%
Urinary system	
Nocturia	13%

adverse events during estrogen and progesterone gel treatment that occurred in 5% or more of women are shown in TABLE 13.

TABLE 13 *Treatment-Emergent Adverse Events in ≥5% of Women Receiving Estrogen Treatment and Progesterone Gel Every Other Day Studies COL1620-004US, COL1620-005US, COL1620-009US*

	Estrogen + Progesterone Gel 4% n=62	Estrogen + Progesterone Gel 8% n=65
Body as a Whole		
Abdominal pain	3 (5%)	6 (9%)
Appetite increased	3 (5%)	5 (8%)
Bloating	8 (13%)	8 (12%)
Cramps NOS	12 (19%)	17 (26%)
Fatigue	13 (21%)	14 (22%)
Central and Peripheral Nervous System		
Headache	12 (19%)	10 (15%)
Gastrointestinal System		
Nausea	5 (8%)	4 (6%)
Musculoskeletal System		
Back pain	5 (8%)	2 (3%)
Myalgia	5 (8%)	0 (0%)
Psychiatric		
Depression	12 (19%)	10 (15%)
Emotional lability	14 (23%)	14 (22%)
Sleep disorder	11 (18%)	12 (18%)
Reproductive, Female		
Vaginal discharge	7 (11%)	2 (3%)
Resistance Mechanism		
Upper respiratory tract infection	3 (5%)	5 (8%)
Skin and Appendages		
Pruritus genital	1 (2%)	4 (6%)

Additional adverse events reported in women at a frequency <5% in progesterone gel ART and secondary amenorrhea studies and not listed in TABLE 11, TABLE 12 and TABLE 13 include:

Autonomic Nervous System: Mouth dry, sweating increased.
Body as a Whole: Abnormal crying, allergic reaction, allergy, appetite decreased, asthenia, edema, face edema, fever, hot flushes, influenzalike symptoms, water retention, xerophthalmia.
Cardiovascular, General: Syncope.
Central and Peripheral Nervous System: Migraine, tremor.
Gastrointestinal: Dyspepsia, eructation, flatulence, gastritis, toothache.
Metabolic and Nutritional: Thirst.
Musculoskeletal System: Cramps legs, leg pain, skeletal pain.
Neoplasm: Benign cyst.
Platelet, Bleeding & Clotting: Purpura.
Psychiatric: Aggressive reactions, forgetfulness, insomnia.
Red Blood Cell: Anemia.
Reproductive, Female: Dysmenorrhea, premenstrual tension, vaginal dryness.
Resistance Mechanism: Infection, pharyngitis, sinusitis, urinary tract infection.
Respiratory System: Asthma, dyspnea, hyperventilation, rhinitis.
Skin and Appendages: Acne, pruritus, rash, seborrhea, skin discoloration, skin disorder, urticaria.
Urinary System: Cystitis, dysuria, micturition frequency.
Vision Disorders: Conjunctivitis.

DOSAGE AND ADMINISTRATION

ASSISTED REPRODUCTIVE TECHNOLOGY

Progesterone gel 8% is administered vaginally at a dose of 90 mg once daily in women who require progesterone supplementation. Progesterone gel 8% is administered vaginally at a dose of 90 mg twice daily in women with partial or complete ovarian failure who require progesterone replacement. If pregnancy occurs, treatment may be continued until placental autonomy is achieved, up to 10-12 weeks.

SECONDARY AMENORRHEA

Progesterone gel 4% is administered vaginally every other day up to a total of 6 doses. For women who fail to respond, a trial of progesterone gel 8% every other day up to a total of 6 doses may be instituted.

It is important to note that a dosage increase from the 4% gel can only be accomplished by using the 8% gel. Increasing the volume of gel administered does not increase the amount of progesterone absorbed.

SEE PROGESTERONE GEL PATIENT INFORMATION SHEET — HOW TO USE PROGESTERONE GEL WHICH IS DISTRIBUTED WITH THE PRESCRIPTION. **Note:** The PATIENT INFORMATION SHEET contains special instructions for using the applicator at altitudes above 2500 feet in order to avoid a partial release of progesterone gel before vaginal insertion.

HOW SUPPLIED

Prochieve is available in the following strengths:

4% (45 mg) gel: In a single use, 1 piece, disposable, white polyethylene vaginal applicator with a twist-off top. Each applicator contains 1.45 g of gel and delivers 1.125 g of gel.

8% (90 mg) gel: In a single use, 1 piece, disposable, white polyethylene vaginal applicator with a twist-off top. Each applicator contains 1.45 g of gel and delivers 1.125 g of gel.

Each applicator is wrapped and sealed in a foil overwrap.

Storage: Store at 25°C (77°F); excursions permitted to 15-30°C (59-86°F).

PRODUCT LISTING - RATED THERAPEUTICALLY EQUIVALENT

Solution - Intramuscular - 50 mg/ml

10 ml	$8.50	GENERIC, Keene Pharmaceuticals Inc	00588-5056-70
10 ml	$10.95	GENERIC, Roberts/Hauck Pharmaceutical Corporation	43797-0104-12
10 ml	$12.00	GENERIC, Pasadena Research Laboratories Inc	00418-0631-41
10 ml	$12.00	GENERIC, Primedics Laboratories	00684-0113-10
10 ml	$13.00	GENERIC, Cmc-Consolidated Midland Corporation	00223-8381-10
10 ml	$14.41	GENERIC, Hyrex Pharmaceuticals	00314-0060-10
10 ml	$16.36	GENERIC, Moore, H.L. Drug Exchange Inc	00839-5165-30
10 ml	$17.93	GENERIC, Interstate Drug Exchange Inc	00814-6388-40
10 ml	$37.38	GENERIC, American Pharmaceutical Partners	63323-0261-10
10 ml	$38.75	GENERIC, Watson/Schein Pharmaceuticals Inc	00364-6683-54

PRODUCT LISTING - EQUIVALENTS NOT AVAILABLE

Capsule - Oral - 100 mg			
100's	$90.26	PROMETRIUM, Solvay Pharmaceuticals Inc	00032-1708-01
Capsule - Oral - 200 mg			
100's	$171.51	PROMETRIUM, Solvay Pharmaceuticals Inc	00032-1711-01
Gel - Vaginal - 4%			
2.60 gm	$5.00	CRINONE, Wyeth-Ayerst Laboratories	00008-0907-01
2.60 gm x 6	$30.00	CRINONE, Serono Laboratories Inc	44087-0804-06
2.60 gm x 6	$37.50	GENERIC, Columbia Drug Company	55056-0406-01
2.60 gm x 18	$60.48	CRINONE, Wyeth-Ayerst Laboratories	00008-0907-03
Gel - Vaginal - 8%			
2.60 gm	$10.00	CRINONE, Wyeth-Ayerst Laboratories	00008-0908-01
2.60 gm x 6	$60.00	CRINONE, Wyeth-Ayerst Laboratories	00008-0908-02
2.60 gm x 18	$60.00	CRINONE, Serono Laboratories Inc	44087-0808-06
2.60 gm x 18	$180.00	CRINONE, Serono Laboratories Inc	44087-0818-08
2.60 gm x 18	$180.00	GENERIC, Columbia Laboratories Inc	55056-0818-01
Solution - Intramuscular - 50 mg/ml			
10 ml	$10.20	GENERIC, C.O. Truxton Inc	00463-1056-10
10 ml	$16.60	GENERIC, Physicians Total Care	54868-3396-00
10 ml	$29.95	GENERIC, Legere Pharmaceuticals	25332-0081-10
10 ml	$38.75	GENERIC, Watson Laboratories Inc	00591-3128-79

Promethazine Hydrochloride *(002125)*

Categories: Allergic reactions; Anaphylaxis; Conjunctivitis, allergic; Dermographism; Motion sickness; Nausea; Pain, adjunct; Rhinitis, allergic; Rhinitis, vasomotor; Sedation; Urticaria; Vomiting; Pregnancy Category C; DEA Class CV; FDA Approved 1955 Jun; WHO Formulary

Drug Classes: Antiemetics/antivertigo; Antihistamines, H1; Phenothiazines

Brand Names: Anergan; Antiallersin; Avomine; Camergan; Fargan; Metaryl; Pelpica; Pentazine; Phenazine; **Phenergan**; Phenerzine; Phenoject-50; Pilothia; Pipolphene; Pro-50; Promacot; Promergan; Promesan; Prometh; Promethacon; Promethazine Hcl; Promethegan; Prorex; Prozine; Sayomol; Xepagan

Foreign Brand Availability: Allerfen (Italy); Atosil (Germany); Bonnox (Germany); Farganesse (Italy); Fenazine (Bahrain; Cyprus; Egypt; Iran; Iraq; Jordan; Kuwait; Lebanon; Libya; Oman; Qatar; Republic-of-Yemen; Saudi-Arabia; Syria; United-Arab-Emirates); Fenergan (Argentina; Peru); Goodnight (New-Zealand); Hibechin (Japan); Hiberna (Japan); Insomn-Eze (Australia); Lergigan (Sweden); Prome (Indonesia); Proneurin (Germany); Prothiazine (Israel); Pyrethia (Japan)

Cost of Therapy: $70.90 (Nausea; Phenergan; 25 mg; 4 tablets/day; 30 day supply)
$3.06 (Nausea; Generic Tablets; 25 mg; 4 tablets/day; 30 day supply)

HCFA JCODE(S): J2550 up to 50 mg IM, IV

IM-IV

DESCRIPTION

Phenergan (promethazine HCl) injection is a sterile, pyrogen-free solution for deep intramuscular or intravenous administration. Promethazine HCl (10*H*—phenothiazine-10-ethanamine, *N,N*,α-trimethyl-, monohydrochloride, (±)-) is a racemic compound.

Each ml of ampul contains either 25 or 50 mg promethazine HCl with 0.1 mg edetate disodium, 0.04 mg calcium chloride, 0.25 mg sodium metabisulfite, and 5 mg phenol in water for injection. The pH range is 4.0-5.5, buffered with acetic acid-sodium acetate, and it is sealed under nitrogen.

Each ml of the Tubex and Tubex Blunt Pointe Sterile Cartridge Units contains either 25 or 50 mg promethazine HCl with 0.1 mg edetate disodium, 0.04 mg calcium chloride, not more than 5 mg monothioglycerol; and 5 mg phenol in water for injection. The pH range is 4.0-5.5, buffered with sodium acetate-acetic acid, and it is sealed under nitrogen.

Phenergan (promethazine HCl) injection is a clear, colorless solution. The product is light sensitive. It should be inspected before use and discarded if either color or particulate is observed.

CLINICAL PHARMACOLOGY

Promethazine HCl is a phenothiazine derivative which possesses antihistaminic, sedative, antimotion-sickness, antiemetic, and anticholinergic effects. Promethazine is a competitive H_1 receptor antagonist, but does not block the release of histamine. Structural differences from the neuroleptic phenothiazines results in its relative lack (1/10) of dopamine antagonist properties. In therapeutic doses, promethazine HCl produces no significant effects on the cardiovascular system. Clinical effects are generally apparent within 5 minutes of an intravenous injection and within 20 minutes of an intramuscular injection. Duration of action is 4-6 hours, although effects may persist up to 12 hours. Promethazine HCl is metabolized in the liver, with the sulfoxides of promethazine and N-desmethylpromethazine being the predominant metabolites appearing in the urine. Following intravenous administration in healthy volunteers, the plasma half-life for promethazine has been reported to range from 9-16 hours. The mean plasma half-life for promethazine after intramuscular administration in healthy volunteers has been reported to be 9.8 ± 3.4 hours.

INDICATIONS AND USAGE

Promethazine HCl injection is indicated for the following conditions:

- Amelioration of allergic reactions to blood or plasma.
- In anaphylaxis as an adjunct to epinephrine and other standard measures after the acute symptoms have been controlled.
- For other uncomplicated allergic conditions of the immediate type when oral therapy is impossible or contraindicated.
- For sedation and relief of apprehension and to produce light sleep from which the patient can be easily aroused.
- Active treatment of motion sickness.
- Prevention and control of nausea and vomiting associated with certain types of anesthesia and surgery.
- As an adjunct to analgesics for the control of postoperative pain.
- Preoperative, postoperative, and obstetric (during labor) sedation.
- Intravenously in special surgical situations, such as repeated bronchoscopy, ophthalmic surgery, and poor-risk patients, with reduced amounts of meperidine or other narcotic analgesic as an adjunct to anesthesia and analgesia.

NON-FDA APPROVED INDICATIONS

Promethazine has been used for prenatal treatment of erythroblastosis fetalis, although this use is not FDA approved.

CONTRAINDICATIONS

Promethazine HCl injection is contraindicated in comatose states and in patients who have demonstrated an idiosyncrasy or hypersensitivity to promethazine or other phenothiazines.

Under no circumstances should promethazineHCl injection be given by intra-arterial injection due to the likelihood of severe arteriospasm and the possibility of resultant gangrene (see WARNINGS, Inadvertent Intra-Arterial Injection).

Promethazine HCl injection should not be given by the subcutaneous route; evidence of chemical irritation has been noted, and necrotic lesions have resulted on rare occasions following subcutaneous injection. The preferred parenteral route of administration is by deep intramuscular injection.

WARNINGS

SULFITE SENSITIVITY

Promethazine HCl injection (ampuls only) contains sodium metabisulfite, a sulfite that may cause allergic-type reactions, including anaphylactic symptoms and life-threatening or less severe asthma episodes, in certain susceptible people. The overall prevalence of sulfite sensitivity in the general population is unknown and probably low. Sulfite sensitivity is seen more frequently in asthmatic than in nonasthmatic people.

CNS DEPRESSION

Promethazine HCl injection may impair the mental and physical abilities required for the performance of potentially hazardous tasks, such as driving a vehicle or operating machinery. The impairment may be amplified by concomitant use of other central-nervous-system depressants such as alcohol, sedative-hypnotics (including barbiturates), general anesthetics, narcotics, narcotic analgesics, tranquilizers, etc. (see PRECAUTIONS, Information for the Patient).

LOWER SEIZURE THRESHOLD

Promethazine HCl injection may lower seizure threshold and should be used with caution in persons with seizure disorders or in persons who are using concomitant medications, such as narcotics or local anesthetics, which may also affect seizure threshold.

BONE-MARROW DEPRESSION

Promethazine HCl injection should be used with caution in patients with bone-marrow depression. Leukopenia and agranulocytosis have been reported, usually when promethazine HCl has been used in association with other known marrow-toxic agents.

USE IN PEDIATRIC PATIENTS

PROMETHAZINE HCl INJECTION IS NOT RECOMMENDED FOR USE IN PEDIATRIC PATIENTS LESS THAN 2 YEARS OF AGE.

CAUTION SHOULD BE EXERCISED WHEN ADMINISTERING PROMETHAZINE HCl INJECTION TO PEDIATRIC PATIENTS 2 YEARS OF AGE AND OLDER. ANTIEMETICS ARE NOT RECOMMENDED FOR TREATMENT OF UNCOMPLICATED VOMITING IN PEDIATRIC PATIENTS, AND THEIR USE SHOULD BE LIMITED TO PROLONGED VOMITING OF KNOWN ETIOLOGY. THE EXTRAPYRAMIDAL SYMPTOMS WHICH CAN OCCUR SECONDARY TO PROMETHAZINE HCl INJECTION ADMINISTRATION MAY BE CONFUSED WITH THE CNS SIGNS OF UNDIAGNOSED PRIMARY DISEASE, *e.g.*, ENCEPHALOPATHY OR REYE'S SYNDROME. THE USE OF PROMETHAZINE HCl INJECTION SHOULD BE AVOIDED IN PEDIATRIC PATIENTS WHOSE SIGNS AND SYMPTOMS MAY SUGGEST REYE'S SYNDROME OR OTHER HEPATIC DISEASES.

Excessively large dosages of antihistamines, including promethazine HCl injection, in pediatric patients may cause hallucinations, convulsions, and sudden death. In pediatric patients who are acutely ill associated with dehydration, there is an increased susceptibility to dystonias with the use of promethazine HCl injection.

INADVERTENT INTRA-ARTERIAL INJECTION

Due to the close proximity of arteries and veins in the areas most commonly used for intravenous injection, extreme care should be exercised to avoid perivascular extravasation or inadvertent intra-arterial injection. Reports compatible with inadvertent intra-arterial injection of promethazine HCl injection, usually in conjunction with other drugs intended for intravenous use, suggest that pain, severe chemical irritation, severe spasm of distal vessels, and resultant gangrene requiring amputation are likely under such circumstances. Intravenous injection was intended in all the cases reported, but perivascular extravasation or arterial placement of the needle is now suspect. There is no proven successful management of this condition after it occurs, although sympathetic block and heparinization are commonly employed during the acute management because of the results of animal experiments with other known arteriolar irritants. Aspiration of dark blood does not preclude intra-arterial needle placement, because blood is discolored upon contact with promethazine HCl injection. Use of syringes with rigid plungers or of small bore needles might obscure typical arterial backflow if this is relied upon alone.

When used intravenously, promethazine HCl injection should be given in a concentration no greater than 25 mg/ml and at a rate not to exceed 25 mg/min. When administering any irritant drug intravenously, it is usually preferable to inject it through the tubing of an intravenous infusion set that is known to be functioning satisfactorily. In the event that a patient complains of pain during intended intravenous injection of promethazine HCl injection, the injection should be stopped immediately to provide for evaluation of possible arterial placement or perivascular extravasation.

VISUAL INSPECTION

This product is light sensitive and should be inspected before use and discarded if either color or particulate is observed.

OTHER CONSIDERATIONS

Sedative drugs or CNS depressants should be avoided in patients with a history of sleep apnea.

Administration of promethazine has been associated with reported cholestatic jaundice.

PRECAUTIONS

GENERAL

Drugs having anticholingeric properties should be used with caution in patients with narrow-angle glaucoma, prostatic hypertrophy, stenosing peptic ulcer, pyloroduodenal obstruction, and bladder-neck obstruction.

Promethazine HCl injection should be used cautiously in persons with cardiovascular disease or impairment of liver function.

INFORMATION FOR THE PATIENT

Promethazine HCl injection may cause marked drowsiness or impair the mental or physical abilities required for the performance of potentially hazardous tasks, such as driving a vehicle or operating machinery. The use of alcohol, sedative-hypnotics (including barbiturates), general anesthetics, narcotics, narcotic analgesics, tranquilizers, etc., with promethazine HCl injection may enhance impairment. Pediatric patients should be supervised to avoid potential harm in bike riding or in other hazardous activities.

Patients should be advised to report any involuntary muscle movements.

Persistent or worsening pain or burning at the injection site should be reported immediately.

Avoid prolonged exposure to the sun.

LABORATORY TEST INTERACTIONS

The following laboratory tests may be affected in patients who are receiving therapy with promethazine HCl injection:

Pregnancy Tests: Diagnostic pregnancy tests based on immunological reactions between HCG and anti-HCG may result in false-negative or false-positive interpretations.

Glucose Tolerance Test: An increase in glucose tolerance has been reported in patients receiving promethazine HCl injection.

CARCINOGENESIS, MUTAGENESIS, AND IMPAIRMENT OF FERTILITY

Long-term animal studies have not been performed to assess the carcinogenic potential of promethazine HCl injection, nor are there other animal or human data concerning carcinogenicity, mutagenicity, or impairment of fertility. Promethazine HCl injection was nonmutagenic in the Ames *Salmonella* test system.

PREGNANCY CATEGORY C

Teratogenic Effects

Teratogenic effects have not been demonstrated in rat-feeding studies at doses of 6.25 and 12.5 mg/kg (approximately 2.1 and 4.2 times the maximum recommended human daily dose) of promethazine HCl injection. Daily doses of 25 mg/kg intraperitoneally have been found to produce fetal mortality in rats.

There are no adequate and well-controlled studies of promethazine HCl injection in pregnant women. Because animal reproduction studies are not always predictive of human response, promethazine HCl injection should be used during pregnancy only if the potential benefit justifies the potential risk to the fetus.

Adequate studies to determine the action of the drug on parturition, lactation and development of the animal neonate have not been conducted.

Nonteratogenic Effects

Promethazine HCl injection received within 2 weeks of delivery may inhibit platelet aggregation in the newborn.

LABOR AND DELIVERY

Promethazine HCl injection may be used alone or as an adjunct to narcotic analgesics during labor (see DOSAGE AND ADMINISTRATION). Limited data suggest that use of promethazine HCl injection during labor and delivery does not have an appreciable effect on the duration of labor or delivery and does not increase the risk of need for intervention in the newborn. The effect on later growth and development of the newborn is unknown. (See also Nonteratogenic Effects.)

NURSING MOTHERS

It is not known whether promethazine HCl injection is excreted in human milk. Because many drugs are excreted in human milk, caution should be exercised when promethazine HCl injection is administered to a nursing woman.

PEDIATRIC USE

Safety and effectiveness in pediatric patients under 2 years of age have not been established.

Promethazine HCl injection should be used with caution in pediatric patients 2 years of age and older (see WARNINGS, Use in Pediatric Patients).

USE IN GERIATRIC PATIENTS (APPROXIMATELY 60 YEARS OR OLDER)

Since therapeutic requirements for sedative drugs tend to be less in geriatric patients, the dosage should be reduced for these patients.

DRUG INTERACTIONS

CNS DEPRESSANTS

Promethazine HCl injection may increase, prolong, or intensify the sedative action of central-nervous-system depressants, such as alcohol, sedative-hypnotics (including barbiturates), general anesthetics, narcotics, narcotic analgesics, tranquilizers, etc. When given concomitantly with promethazine HCl injection, the dose of barbiturates should be reduced by at least one-half, and the dose of narcotics should be reduced by one-quarter to one-half. Dosage must be individualized. Excessive amounts of promethazine HCl injection relative to a narcotic may lead to restlessness and motor hyperactivity in the patient with pain; these symptoms usually disappear with adequate control of the pain.

EPINEPHRINE

Although reversal of the vasopressor effect of epinephrine has not been reported with promethazine HCl injection, it is recommended that epinephrine NOT be used in the case of promethazine HCl injection overdose.

ANTICHOLINERGICS

Concomitant use of other agents with anticholinergic properties should be undertaken with caution.

MONOAMINE OXIDASE INHIBITORS (MAOI)

Drug interactions, including an increased incidence of extrapyramidal effects, have been reported when some MAOI and phenothiazines are used concomitantly. Although such a reaction has not been reported with promethazine HCl injection, the possibility should be considered.

ADVERSE REACTIONS

CNS EFFECTS

Drowsiness is the most prominent CNS effect of the drug. Extrapyramidal reactions may occur with high doses; this is almost always responsive to a reduction in dosage. Other reported reactions include dizziness, lassitude, tinnitus, incoordination, fatigue, blurred vision, euphoria, diplopia, nervousness, insomnia, tremors, convulsive seizures, oculogyric crises, excitation, catatonic-like states, hysteria, and hallucinations.

CARDIOVASCULAR EFFECTS

Tachycardia, bradycardia, faintness, dizziness, and increases and decreases in blood pressure have been reported following the use of promethazine HCl injection. Venous thrombosis at the injection site has been reported. INTRA-ARTERIAL INJECTION MAY RESULT IN GANGRENE OF THE AFFECTED EXTREMITY (see WARNINGS, Inadvertent Intra-Arterial Injection).

GASTROINTESTINAL EFFECTS

Nausea and vomiting have been reported, usually in association with surgical procedures and combination drug therapy.

ALLERGIC REACTIONS

These include urticaria, dermatitis, asthma, and photosensitivity. Angioneurotic edema has been reported.

OTHER REPORTED REACTIONS

Leukopenia and agranulocytosis, usually when promethazine HCl has been used in association with other known marrow-toxic agents, have been reported. Thrombocytopenic purpura and jaundice of the obstructive type have been associated with the use of promethazine HCl. The jaundice is usually reversible on discontinuation of the drug. Subcutaneous injection has resulted in tissue necrosis. Nasal stuffiness may occur. Dry mouth has been reported.

PARADOXICAL REACTIONS (OVERDOSAGE)

Hyperexcitability and abnormal movements, which have been reported in pediatric patients following a single administration of promethazine HCl injection, may be manifestations of relative overdosage, in which case, consideration should be given to the discontinuation of the promethazine HCl injection and to the use of other drugs. Respiratory depression, nightmares, delirium, and agitated behavior have also been reported in some of these patients.

DOSAGE AND ADMINISTRATION

Parenteral drug products should be inspected visually for particulate matter and discoloration prior to administration, whenever solution and container permit.

Do not use promethazine HCl injection if solution has developed color or contains precipitate.

To avoid the possibility of physical and/or chemical incompatibility, consult specialized literature before diluting with any injectable solution or combining with any other medication. Do not use if there is a precipitate or any sign of incompatibility.

IMPORTANT NOTES ON ADMINISTRATION

The preferred parenteral route of administration for promethazine HCl injection is by deep intramuscular injection. The proper intravenous administration of this product is well-tolerated, but use of this route is not without some hazard. Not for subcutaneous administration.

INADVERTENT INTRA-ARTERIAL INJECTION CAN RESULT IN GANGRENE OF THE AFFECTED EXTREMITY (see WARNINGS, Inadvertent Intra-Arterial Injection). SUBCUTANEOUS INJECTION IS CONTRAINDICATED, AS IT MAY RESULT IN TISSUE NECROSIS (see CONTRAINDICATIONS).

Injection into or near a nerve may result in permanent tissue damage.

When used intravenously, promethazine HCl injection should be given in concentration no greater than 25 mg/ml at a rate not to exceed 25 mg/min; it is preferable to inject through the tubing of an intravenous infusion set that is known to be functioning satisfactorily.

The Tubex Blunt Pointe Sterile Cartridge Unit is suitable for substances to be administered intravenously. It is intended for use with injection sets specifically manufactured as "needle-less" injection systems. Tubex Blunt Pointe is compatible with Abbott's LifeShield Prepierced Reseal injection site, Baxter's Inter-Link injection site, McGaw, Inc's Safe Line injection site, Arrow International, Inc's User-Gard Intermittent Injection Cap, and B. Braun Medical's SafSite reflux valve.

The Tubex Sterile Cartridge Needle Unit is suitable for substances to be administered intravenously or intramuscularly.

ALLERGIC CONDITIONS

The average adult dose is 25 mg. This dose may be repeated within 2 hours if necessary, but continued therapy, if indicated, should be via the oral route as soon as existing circumstances permit. After initiation of treatment, dosage should be adjusted to the smallest amount adequate to relieve symptoms. The average adult dose for amelioration of allergic reactions to blood or plasma is 25 mg.

SEDATION

In hospitalized adult patients, nighttime sedation may be achieved by a dose of 25-50 mg of promethazine HCl injection.

NAUSEA AND VOMITING

For control of nausea and vomiting, the usual adult dose is 12.5-25 mg, not to be repeated more frequently than every 4 hours. When used for control of postoperative nausea and vomiting, the medication may be administered either intramuscularly or intravenously and dosage of analgesics and barbiturates reduced accordingly.

P

PREOPERATIVE AND POSTOPERATIVE USE

As an adjunct to preoperative or postoperative medication, 25-50 mg of promethazine HCl injection in adults may be combined with appropriately reduced doses of analgesics and atropine-like drugs as desired. Dosage of concomitant analgesic or hypnotic medication should be reduced accordingly.

OBSTETRICS

Promethazine HCl injection in doses of 50 mg will provide sedation and relieve apprehension in the early stages of labor. When labor is definitely established, 25-75 mg (average dose, 50 mg) promethazine HCl injection may be given intramuscularly or intravenously with an appropriately reduced dose of any desired narcotic. If necessary, promethazine HCl injection with a reduced dose of analgesic may be repeated once or twice at 4 hour intervals in the course of a normal labor. A maximum total dose of 100 mg of promethazine HCl injection may be administered during a 24 hour period to patients in labor.

PEDIATRIC PATIENTS

Promethazine HCl injection is not recommended for use in pediatric patients less than 2 years of age.

In pediatric patients 2 years of age and older, the dosage should not exceed half that of the suggested adult dose. As an adjunct to premedication, the suggested dose is 0.5 mg/lb of body weight in combination with an appropriately reduced dose of narcotic or barbiturate and the appropriate dose of an atropine-like drug. Antiemetics should not be used in vomiting of unknown etiology in pediatric patients (see WARNINGS, Use in Pediatric Patients).

HOW SUPPLIED

AMPULS

Phenergan (promethazine HCl) injection is available in 1 ml ampuls as follows:

25 mg/ml
50 mg/ml

Storage: Store at controlled room temperature 15-30°C (59-86°F). Protect from light. Keep covered in carton until time of use. Do not use if solution has developed color or contains a precipitate.

ALSO AVAILABLE

Phenergan injection is also available in the following dosage strengths in Tubex Blunt Pointe Sterile Cartridge Units and Sterile Cartridge-Needle Units as follows:

25 mg/ml, 1 ml size Blunt Pointe
25 mg/ml, 1ml size (22 gauge × 1¼ inch needle)
50 mg/ml, 1 ml size (22 gauge × 1¼ inch needle)

ORAL

DESCRIPTION

NOTE: Prescribing information for suppositories is included in this section.

Promethazine hydrochloride is a racemic compound; the empirical formula is $C_{17}H_{20}N_2S{\cdot}HCl$ and its molecular weight is 320.88.

Promethazine HCl, a phenothiazine derivative, is designated chemically as 10*H*—phenothiazine-10-ethanamine, *N,N*,α-trimethyl-, monohydrochloride, (±)-.

Promethazine HCl occurs as a white to faint yellow, practically odorless, crystalline powder which slowly oxidizes and turns blue on prolonged exposure to air. It is soluble in water and freely soluble in alcohol.

SYRUP

Each teaspoon (5 ml) of Phenergan Syrup Plain contains 6.25 mg promethazine hydrochloride in a flavored syrup base with a pH between 4.7 and 5.2. Alcohol 7%. The inactive ingredients present are artificial and natural flavors, citric acid, D&C red 33, D&C yellow 10, FD&C blue 1, FD&C yellow 6, glycerin, saccharin sodium, sodium benzoate, sodium citrate, sodium propionate, water, and other ingredients.

Each teaspoon (5 ml) of Phenergan Syrup Fortis contains 25 mg promethazine hydrochloride in a flavored syrup base with a pH between 5.0 and 5.5. Alcohol 1.5%. The inactive ingredients present are artificial and natural flavors, citric acid, saccharin sodium, sodium benzoate, sodium propionate, water, and other ingredients.

TABLETS AND SUPPOSITORIES

Each tablet of Phenergan contains 12.5, 25, or 50 mg promethazine hydrochloride. The inactive ingredients present are lactose, magnesium stearate, and methylcellulose. Each dosage strength also contains the following: *12.5 mg:* FD&C yellow 6 and saccharin sodium; *25 mg:* Saccharin sodium; *50 mg:* FD&C red 40.

Each rectal suppository of Phenergan contains 12.5, 25, or 50 mg promethazine hydrochloride with ascorbyl palmitate, silicon dioxide, white wax, and cocoa butter. Phenergan suppositories are for rectal administration only.

CLINICAL PHARMACOLOGY

SYRUP

Promethazine is a phenothiazine derivative which differs structurally from the antipsychotic phenothiazines by the presence of a branched side chain and no ring substitution. It is thought that this configuration is responsible for its relative lack (1/10 that of chlorpromazine) of dopaminergic (CNS) action.

Promethazine is an H_1 receptor blocking agent. In addition to its antihistaminic action, it provides clinically useful sedative and antiemetic effects. In therapeutic dosage, promethazine produces no significant effects on the cardiovascular system.

Promethazine is well absorbed from the gastrointestinal tract. Clinical effects are apparent within 20 minutes after oral administration and generally last 4-6 hours, although they may persist as long as 12 hours. Promethazine is metabolized by the liver to a variety of compounds; the sulfoxides of promethazine and N-demethylpromethazine are the predominant metabolites appearing in the urine.

TABLETS AND SUPPOSITORIES

Promethazine is a phenothiazine derivative which differs structurally from the antipsychotic phenothiazines by the presence of a branched side chain and no ring substitution. It is thought that this configuration is responsible for its relative lack (1/10 that of chlorpromazine) of dopamine antagonist properties.

Promethazine is an H_1 receptor blocking agent. In addition to its antihistaminic action, it provides clinically useful sedative and antiemetic effects.

Promethazine is well absorbed from the gastrointestinal tract. Clinical effects are apparent within 20 minutes after oral administration and generally last 4-6 hours, although they may persist as long as 12 hours. Promethazine is metabolized by the liver to a variety of compounds; the sulfoxides of promethazine and N-demethylpromethazine are the predominant metabolites appearing in the urine.

INDICATIONS AND USAGE

SYRUP, TABLETS, AND SUPPOSITORIES

Promethazine HCl is useful for:

- Perennial and seasonal allergic rhinitis.
- Vasomotor rhinitis.
- Allergic conjunctivitis due to inhalant allergens and foods.
- Mild, uncomplicated allergic skin manifestations of urticaria and angioedema.
- Amelioration of allergic reactions to blood or plasma.
- Dermographism.
- Anaphylactic reactions, as adjunctive therapy to epinephrine and other standard measures, after the acute manifestations have been controlled.
- Preoperative, postoperative, or obstetric sedation.
- Prevention and control of nausea and vomiting associated with certain types of anesthesia and surgery.
- Therapy adjunctive to meperidine or other analgesics for control of postoperative pain.
- Sedation in both children and adults, as well as relief of apprehension and production of light sleep from which the patient can be easily aroused.
- Active and prophylactic treatment of motion sickness.
- Antiemetic therapy in postoperative patients.

NON-FDA APPROVED INDICATIONS

Promethazine has been used for prenatal treatment of erythroblastosis fetalis, although this use is not FDA approved.

CONTRAINDICATIONS

SYRUP

Promethazine is contraindicated in individuals known to be hypersensitive or to have had an idiosyncratic reaction to promethazine or to other phenothiazines.

Antihistamines are contraindicated for use in the treatment of lower respiratory tract symptoms including asthma.

TABLETS AND SUPPOSITORIES

Promethazine HCl tablets and suppositories are contraindicated in comatose states, and in individuals known to be hypersensitive or to have had an idiosyncratic reaction to promethazine or to other phenothiazines.

Antihistamines are contraindicated for use in the treatment of lower respiratory tract symptoms including asthma.

WARNINGS

SYRUP

Promethazine may cause marked drowsiness. Ambulatory patients should be cautioned against such activities as driving or operating dangerous machinery until it is known that they do not become drowsy or dizzy from promethazine therapy.

The sedative action of promethazine hydrochloride (HCl) is additive to the sedative effects of central nervous system depressants; therefore, agents such as alcohol, narcotic analgesics, sedatives, hypnotics, and tranquilizers should either be eliminated or given in reduced dosage in the presence of promethazine HCl. When given concomitantly with promethazine HCl, the dose of barbiturates should be reduced by at least one-half, and the dose of analgesic depressants, such as morphine or meperidine, should be reduced by one-quarter to one-half.

Promethazine may lower seizure threshold. This should be taken into consideration when administering to persons with known seizure disorders or when giving in combination with narcotics or local anesthetics which may also affect seizure threshold.

Sedative drugs or CNS depressants should be avoided in patients with a history of sleep apnea.

Antihistamines should be used with caution in patients with narrow-angle glaucoma, stenosing peptic ulcer, pyloroduodenal obstruction, and urinary bladder obstruction due to symptomatic prostatic hypertrophy and narrowing of the bladder neck.

Administration of promethazine has been associated with reported cholestatic jaundice.

TABLETS AND SUPPOSITORIES

CNS Depression

Promethazine HCl tablets and suppositories may impair the mental and/or physical abilities required for the performance of potentially hazardous tasks, such as driving a vehicle or operating machinery. The impairment may be amplified by concomitant use of other central-nervous-system depressants such as alcohol, sedatives/hypnotics (including barbiturates), narcotics, narcotic analgesics general anesthetics, tricyclic antidepressants, and tranquilizers; therefore such agents should either be eliminated or given in reduced dosage in the presence of promethazine HCl (see PRECAUTIONS, Tablets and Suppositories Information for the Patient and DRUG INTERACTIONS, Tablets and Suppositories).

Respiratory Depression

Promethazine HCl tablets and suppositories may lead to potentially fatal respiratory depression.

Use of promethazine HCl tablets and suppositories in patients with compromised respiratory function (*e.g.*, COPD, sleep apnea) should be avoided.

Lower Seizure Threshold
Promethazine HCl tablets and suppositories may lower seizure threshold. It should be used with caution in persons with seizure disorders or in persons who are using concomitant medications, such as narcotics or local anesthetics, which may also affect seizure threshold.

Bone-Marrow Depression
Promethazine HCl tablets and suppositories should be used with caution in patients with bone-marrow depression. Leukopenia and agranulocytosis have been reported, usually when promethazine HCl has been used in association with other known marrow-toxic agents.

Neuroleptic Malignant Syndrome
A potentially fatal symptom complex sometimes referred to as Neuroleptic Malignant Syndrome (NMS) has been reported in association with promethazine HCl alone or in combination with antipsychotic drugs. Clinical manifestations of NMS are hyperpyrexia, muscle rigidity, altered mental status and evidence of autonomic instability (irregular pulse or blood pressure, tachycardia, diaphoresis and cardiac dysrhythmias).

The diagnostic evaluation of patients with this syndrome is complicated. In arriving at a diagnosis, it is important to identify cases where the clinical presentation includes both serious medical illness (*e.g.*, pneumonia, systemic infection, etc.) and untreated or inadequately treated extrapyramidal signs and symptoms (EPS). Other important considerations in the differential diagnosis include central anticholinergic toxicity, heat stroke, drug fever and primary central nervous system (CNS) pathology.

The management of NMS should include (1) immediate discontinuation of promethazine HCl, antipsychotic drugs, if any, and other drugs not essential to concurrent therapy, (2) intensive symptomatic treatment and medical monitoring, and (3) treatment of any concomitant serious medical problems for which specific treatments are available. There is no general agreement about specific pharmacological treatment regimens for uncomplicated NMS.

Since recurrences of NMS have been reported with phenothiazines, the reintroduction of promethazine HCl should be carefully considered.

Use in Pediatric Patients
PROMETHAZINE HCl TABLETS AND SUPPOSITORIES ARE NOT RECOMMENDED FOR USE IN PEDIATRIC PATIENTS LESS THAN 2 YEARS OF AGE.

CAUTION SHOULD BE EXERCISED WHEN ADMINISTERING PROMETHAZINE HCl TABLETS AND SUPPOSITORIES TO PEDIATRIC PATIENTS 2 YEARS OF AGE AND OLDER BECAUSE OF THE POTENTIAL FOR FATAL RESPIRATORY DEPRESSION. ANTIEMETICS ARE NOT RECOMMENDED FOR TREATMENT OF UNCOMPLICATED VOMITING IN PEDIATRIC PATIENTS, AND THEIR USE SHOULD BE LIMITED TO PROLONGED VOMITING OF KNOWN ETIOLOGY. THE EXTRAPYRAMIDAL SYMPTOMS WHICH CAN OCCUR SECONDARY TO PROMETHAZINE HCl TABLETS AND SUPPOSITORIES ADMINISTRATION MAY BE CONFUSED WITH THE CNS SIGNS OF UNDIAGNOSED PRIMARY DISEASE, *e.g.*, ENCEPHALOPATHY OR REYE'S SYNDROME. THE USE OF PROMETHAZINE HCl TABLETS AND SUPPOSITORIES SHOULD BE AVOIDED IN PEDIATRIC PATIENTS WHOSE SIGNS AND SYMPTOMS MAY SUGGEST REYE'S SYNDROME OR OTHER HEPATIC DISEASES.

Excessively large dosages of antihistamines, including promethazine HCl tablets and suppositories, in pediatric patients may cause sudden death. Hallucinations and convulsions have occurred with therapeutic doses and overdoses of promethazine HCl in pediatric patients. In pediatric patients who are acutely ill associated with dehydration, there is an increased susceptibility to dystonias with the use of promethazine HCl.

Other Considerations
Administration of promethazine HCl has been associated with reported cholestatic jaundice.

PRECAUTIONS

SYRUP

General
Promethazine should be used cautiously in persons with cardiovascular disease or with impairment of liver function.

Information for the Patient
Promethazine HCl may cause marked drowsiness or impair the mental and/or physical abilities required for the performance of potentially hazardous tasks, such as driving a vehicle or operating machinery. Ambulatory patients should be told to avoid engaging in such activities until it is known that they do not become drowsy or dizzy from promethazine HCl therapy. Children should be supervised to avoid potential harm in bike riding or in other hazardous activities.

The concomitant use of alcohol or other central nervous system depressants, including narcotic analgesics, sedatives, hypnotics, and tranquilizers, may have an additive effect and should be avoided or their dosage reduced.

Patients should be advised to report any involuntary muscle movements or unusual sensitivity to sunlight.

Drug/Laboratory Test Interactions
The following laboratory tests may be affected in patients who are receiving therapy with promethazine HCl:

Pregnancy Tests: Diagnostic pregnancy tests based on immunological reactions between HCG and anti-HCG may result in false-negative or false-positive interpretations.

Glucose Tolerance Test: An increase in blood glucose has been reported in patients receiving promethazine.

Carcinogenesis, Mutagenesis, and Impairment of Fertility
Long-term animal studies have not been performed to assess the carcinogenic potential of promethazine, nor are there other animal or human data concerning carcinogenicity, mutagenicity, or impairment of fertility with this drug. Promethazine was nonmutagenic in the *Salmonella* test system of Ames.

Pregnancy Category C

Teratogenic Effects
Teratogenic effects have not been demonstrated in rat-feeding studies at doses of 6.25 and 12.5 mg/kg of promethazine HCl. These doses are from approximately 2.1-4.2 times the maximum recommended total daily dose of promethazine for a 50 kg subject, depending upon the indication for which the drug is prescribed. Specific studies to test the action of the drug on parturition, lactation, and development of the animal neonate were not done, but a general preliminary study in rats indicated no effect on these parameters. Although antihistamines, including promethazine, have been found to produce fetal mortality in rodents, the pharmacological effects of histamine in the rodent do not parallel those in man. There are no adequate and well-controlled studies of promethazine in pregnant women. Promethazine HCl should be used during pregnancy only if the potential benefit justifies the potential risk to the fetus.

Nonteratogenic Effects
Promethazine taken within 2 weeks of delivery may inhibit platelet aggregation in the newborn.

Labor and Delivery
Promethazine HCl, in appropriate dosage form, may be used alone or as an adjunct to narcotic analgesics during labor and delivery. (See INDICATIONS AND USAGE, Syrup, Tablets, and Suppositories, and DOSAGE AND ADMINISTRATION, Syrup.)

See also Syrup, Nonteratogenic Effects.

Nursing Mothers
It is not known whether promethazine is excreted in human milk. Caution should be exercised when promethazine is administered to a nursing woman.

Pediatric Use
This product should not be used in children under 2 years of age because safety for such use has not been established.

TABLETS AND SUPPOSITORIES

General
Drugs having anticholingeric properties should be used with caution in patients with narrow-angle glaucoma, prostatic hypertrophy, stenosing peptic ulcer, pyloroduodenal obstruction, and bladder-neck obstruction.

Promethazine HCl tablets and suppositories should be used cautiously in persons with cardiovascular disease or impairment of liver function.

Information for the Patient
Promethazine HCl tablets and suppositories may cause marked drowsiness or impair the mental and/or physical abilities required for the performance of potentially hazardous tasks, such as driving a vehicle or operating machinery. The use of alcohol or other central-nervous-system depressants such as sedatives/hypnotics (including barbiturates), narcotics, narcotic analgesics, general anesthetics, tricyclic antidepressants, and tranquilizers, may enhance impairment (see WARNINGS, Tablets and Suppositories, CNS Depression and DRUG INTERACTIONS, Tablets and Suppositories). Pediatric patients should be supervised to avoid potential harm in bike riding or in other hazardous activities.

Patients should be advised to report any involuntary muscle movements.

Avoid prolonged exposure to the sun.

Drug/Laboratory Test Interactions
The following laboratory tests may be affected in patients who are receiving therapy with promethazine HCl:

Pregnancy Tests: Diagnostic pregnancy tests based on immunological reactions between HCG and anti-HCG may result in false-negative or false-positive interpretations.

Glucose Tolerance Test: An increase in blood glucose has been reported in patients receiving promethazine HCl.

Carcinogenesis, Mutagenesis, and Impairment of Fertility
Long-term animal studies have not been performed to assess the carcinogenic potential of promethazine, nor are there other animal or human data concerning carcinogenicity, mutagenicity, or impairment of fertility with this drug. Promethazine was nonmutagenic in the *Salmonella* test system of Ames.

Pregnancy Category C

Teratogenic Effects
Teratogenic effects have not been demonstrated in rat-feeding studies at doses of 6.25 and 12.5 mg/kg of promethazine HCl. These doses are from approximately 2.1-4.2 times the maximum recommended total daily dose of promethazine for a 50 kg subject, depending upon the indication for which the drug is prescribed. Daily doses of 25 mg/kg intraperitoneally have been found to produce fetal mortality in rats.

Specific studies to test the action of the drug on parturition, lactation, and development of the animal neonate were not done, but a general preliminary study in rats indicated no effect on these parameters. Although antihistamines have been found to produce fetal mortality in rodents, the pharmacological effects of histamine in the rodent do not parallel those in man. There are no adequate and well-controlled studies of promethazine HCL tablets and suppositories in pregnant women.

Promethazine HCl tablets and suppositories should be used during pregnancy only if the potential benefit justifies the potential risk to the fetus.

Nonteratogenic Effects

Promethazine HCl tablets and suppositories administered to a pregnant woman within 2 weeks of delivery may inhibit platelet aggregation in the newborn.

Labor and Delivery

Promethazine HCl may be used alone or as an adjunct to narcotic analgesics during labor (see DOSAGE AND ADMINISTRATION, Tablets and Suppositories). Limited data suggest that use of promethazine HCl during labor and delivery does not have an appreciable effect on the duration of labor or delivery and does not increase the risk of need for intervention in the newborn. The effect on later growth and development of the newborn is unknown. (See also Tablets and Suppositories, Nonteratogenic Effects.)

Nursing Mothers

It is not known whether promethazine HCl is excreted in human milk. Because many drugs are excreted in human milk and because of the potential for serious adverse reactions in nursing infants from promethazine HCl tablets and suppositories, a decision should be made whether to discontinue nursing or to discontinue the drug, taking into account the importance of the drug to the mother.

Pediatric Use

Safety and effectiveness in children under 2 years of age have not been established.

Promethazine HCl tablets and suppositories should be used with caution in pediatric patients 2 years of age and older (see WARNINGS, Tablets and Suppositories, Use in Pediatric Patients).

Use in Geriatric Patients (approximately 60 years or older)

Because therapeutic requirements for sedative drugs tend to be less in elderly patients, the dosage of promethazine HCl tablets and suppositories should be reduced for these patients.

DRUG INTERACTIONS

SYRUP

The sedative action of promethazine is additive to the sedative effects of other central nervous system depressants, including alcohol, narcotic analgesics, sedatives, hypnotics, tricyclic antidepressants, and tranquilizers; therefore, these agents should be avoided or administered in reduced dosage to patients receiving promethazine.

TABLETS AND SUPPOSITORIES

CNS Depressants

Promethazine HCl tablets and suppositories may increase, prolong, or intensify the sedative action of other central-nervous-system depressants, such as alcohol, sedatives/hypnotics (including barbiturates), narcotics, narcotic analgesics, general anesthetics, tricyclic antidepressants, and tranquilizers; therefore, such agents should be avoided or administered in reduced dosage to patients receiving promethazine HCl. When given concomitantly with promethazine HCl tablets and suppositories, the dose of barbiturates should be reduced by at least one-half, and the dose of narcotics should be reduced by one-quarter to one-half. Dosage must be individualized. Excessive amounts of promethazine HCl relative to a narcotic may lead to restlessness and motor hyperactivity in the patient with pain; these symptoms usually disappear with adequate control of pain.

Epinephrine

Because of the potential for promethazine HCl to reverse epinephrine's vasopressor effect, epinephrine should NOT be used to treat hypotension associated with promethazine HCl tablets and suppositories overdose.

Anticholinergics

Concomitant use of other agents with anticholinergic properties should be undertaken with caution.

Monoamine Oxidase Inhibitors (MAOI)

Drug interactions, including an increased incidence of extrapyramidal effects, have been reported when some MAOI and phenothiazines are used concomitantly. This possibility should be considered with promethazine HCl tablets and suppositories.

ADVERSE REACTIONS

SYRUP

Nervous System: Sedation, sleepiness, occasional blurred vision, dryness of mouth, dizziness; rarely confusion, disorientation, and extrapyramidal symptoms such as oculogyric crisis, torticollis, and tongue protrusion (usually in association with parenteral injection or excessive dosage).

Cardiovascular: Increased or decreased blood pressure.

Dermatologic: Rash, rarely photosensitivity.

Hematologic: Rarely leukopenia, thrombocytopenia; agranulocytosis (1 case).

Gastrointestinal: Nausea and vomiting.

TABLETS AND SUPPOSITORIES

Central Nervous System: Drowsiness is the most prominent CNS effect of this drug. Sedation, somnolence, blurred vision, dizziness; confusion, disorientation, and extrapyramidal symptoms such as oculogyric crisis, torticollis, and tongue protrusion; lassitude, tinnitus, incoordination, fatigue, euphoria, nervousness, diplopia, insomnia, tremors, convulsive seizures, excitation, catatonic-like states, hysteria. Hallucinations have also been reported.

Cardiovascular: Increased or decreased blood pressure, tachycardia, bradycardia, faintness.

Dermatologic: Dermatitis, photosensitivity, urticaria.

Hematologic: Leukopenia, thrombocytopenia, thrombocytopenic purpura, agranulocytosis.

Gastrointestinal: Dry mouth, nausea, vomiting, jaundice.

Respiratory: Asthma, nasal stuffiness, respiratory depression (potentially fatal) and apnea (potentially fatal). (See WARNINGS, Tablets and Suppositories, Respiratory Depression.)

Other: Angioneurotic edema. Neuroleptic malignant syndrome (potentially fatal) has also been reported. (See WARNINGS, Tablets and Suppositories, Neuroleptic Malignant Syndrome.)

Paradoxical Reactions

Hyperexcitability and abnormal movements have been reported in patients following a single administration of promethazine HCl. Consideration should be given to the discontinuation of promethazine HCl and to the use of other drugs if these reactions occur. Respiratory depression, nightmares, delirium, and agitated behavior have also been reported in some of these patients.

DOSAGE AND ADMINISTRATION

SYRUP

Allergy

The average oral dose is 25 mg taken before retiring; however, 12.5 mg may be taken before meals and on retiring, if necessary. Children tolerate this product well. Single 25 mg doses at bedtime or 6.25-12.5 mg taken 3 times daily will usually suffice. After initiation of treatment in children or adults, dosage should be adjusted to the smallest amount adequate to relieve symptoms.

Promethazine HCl rectal suppositories may be used if the oral route is not feasible, but oral therapy should be resumed as soon as possible if continued therapy is indicated.

The administration of promethazine HCl in 25 mg doses will control minor transfusion reactions of an allergic nature.

Motion Sickness

The average adult dose is 25 mg taken twice daily. The initial dose should be taken ½ to 1 hour before anticipated travel and be repeated 8-12 hours later, if necessary. On succeeding days of travel, it is recommended that 25 mg be given on arising and again before the evening meal. For children, promethazine HCl tablets, syrup, or rectal suppositories, 12.5-25 mg, twice daily, may be administered.

Nausea and Vomiting

The average effective dose of promethazine HCl for the active therapy of nausea and vomiting in children or adults is 25 mg. When oral medication cannot be tolerated, the dose should be given parenterally (cf. promethazine HCl injection) or by rectal suppository. 12.5-25 mg doses may be repeated, as necessary, at 4-6 hour intervals.

For nausea and vomiting in children, the usual dose is 0.5 mg/lb of body weight, and the dose should be adjusted to the age and weight of the patient and the severity of the condition being treated.

For prophylaxis of nausea and vomiting, as during surgery and the postoperative period, the average dose is 25 mg repeated at 4-6 hour intervals, as necessary.

Sedation

This product relieves apprehension and induces a quiet sleep from which the patient can be easily aroused. Administration of 12.5-25 mg promethazine HCl by the oral route or by rectal suppository at bedtime will provide sedation in children. Adults usually require 25-50 mg for nighttime, presurgical, or obstetrical sedation.

Pre- and Postoperative Use

Promethazine HCl in 12.5-25 mg doses for children and 50 mg doses for adults the night before surgery relieves apprehension and produces a quiet sleep.

For preoperative medication children require doses of 0.5 mg/lb of body weight in combination with an equal dose of meperidine and the appropriate dose of an atropine-like drug.

Usual adult dosage is 50 mg promethazine HCl with an equal amount of meperidine and the required amount of a belladonna alkaloid.

Postoperative sedation and adjunctive use with analgesics may be obtained by the administration of 12.5-25 mg in children and 25-50 mg doses in adults.

Promethazine HCl syrup plain and syrup fortis are not recommended for children under 2 years of age.

TABLETS AND SUPPOSITORIES

Promethazine HCl tablets and rectal suppositories are not recommended for children under 2 years of age (see WARNINGS, Tablets and Suppositories, Use in Pediatric Patients).

Promethazine HCl suppositories are for rectal administration only.

Allergy

The average oral dose is 25 mg taken before retiring; however, 12.5 mg may be taken before meals and on retiring, if necessary. Single 25 mg doses at bedtime or 6.25-12.5 mg taken 3 times daily will usually suffice. After initiation of treatment in children or adults, dosage should be adjusted to the smallest amount adequate to relieve symptoms. The administration of promethazine HCl in 25 mg doses will control minor transfusion reactions of an allergic nature.

Motion Sickness

The average adult dose is 25 mg taken twice daily. The initial dose should be taken ½ to 1 hour before anticipated travel and be repeated 8-12 hours later, if necessary. On succeeding days of travel, it is recommended that 25 mg be given on arising and again before the evening meal. For children, promethazine HCl tablets, syrup, or rectal suppositories, 12.5-25 mg, twice daily, may be administered.

Nausea and Vomiting

Antiemetics should not be used in vomiting of unknown etiology in children and adolescents (see WARNINGS, Tablets and Suppositories, Use in Pediatric Patients).

The average effective dose of promethazine HCl for the active therapy of nausea and vomiting in children or adults is 25 mg. When oral medication cannot be tolerated, the dose should be given parenterally (cf. promethazine HCl injection) or by rectal suppository. 12.5-25 mg doses may be repeated, as necessary, at 4-6 hour intervals.

For nausea and vomiting in children, the usual dose is 0.5 mg/lb of body weight, and the dose should be adjusted to the age and weight of the patient and the severity of the condition being treated.

For prophylaxis of nausea and vomiting, as during surgery and the postoperative period, the average dose is 25 mg repeated at 4-6 hour intervals, as necessary.

Sedation

This product relieves apprehension and induces a quiet sleep from which the patient can be easily aroused. Administration of 12.5-25 mg promethazine HCl by the oral route or by rectal suppository at bedtime will provide sedation in children. Adults usually require 25-50 mg for nighttime, presurgical, or obstetrical sedation.

Pre- and Postoperative Use

Promethazine HCl in 12.5-25 mg doses for children and 50 mg doses for adults the night before surgery relieves apprehension and produces a quiet sleep.

For preoperative medication, children require doses of 0.5 mg/lb of body weight in combination with an appropriately reduced dose of narcotic or barbiturate and the appropriate dose of an atropine-like drug. Usual adult dosage is 50 mg promethazine HCl with an appropriately reduced dose of narcotic or barbiturate and the required amount of a belladonna alkaloid.

Postoperative sedation and adjunctive use with analgesics may be obtained by the administration of 12.5-25 mg in children and 25-50 mg doses in adults.

Promethazine HCl tablets and rectal suppositories are not recommended for children under 2 years of age.

HOW SUPPLIED

SYRUP

Phenergan (promethazine HCl) Syrup Plain is a clear, green solution supplied as follows:

Bottles of 4 fl oz (118 ml).

Bottle of 1 pint (473 ml).

Phenergan Syrup Fortis is a clear, light straw-colored solution supplied as follows:

Bottle of 1 pint (473 mg).

Storage

Keep bottles tightly closed.

Store at room temperature, between 15-25°C (59-77°F).

Protect from light.

Dispense in light-resistant, glass, tight containers.

TABLETS AND SUPPOSITORIES

Phenergan Tablets

Phenergan tablets are available as follows:

12.5 mg: Orange, with "WYETH" on one side and "19" on the scored reverse side.

25 mg: White, with "WYETH" and "27" one side and scored on the reverse side.

50 mg: Pink, with "WYETH" on one side and "227" on the other side.

Storage

Keep tightly closed.

Store at controlled room temperature between 20-25°C (68-77°F).

Protect from light.

Dispense in a light-resistant, tight container.

Use carton to protect contents from light.

Phenergan Suppositories

Phenergan rectal suppositories are available as follows:

12.5 mg: Ivory, torpedo-shaped suppository wrapped in copper-colored foil.

25 mg: Ivory, torpedo-shaped suppository wrapped in light-green foil.

50 mg: Ivory, torpedo-shaped suppository wrapped in blue foil.

Storage

Store refrigerated between 2-8°C (36-46°F).

Dispense in well-closed container.

PRODUCT LISTING - RATED THERAPEUTICALLY EQUIVALENT

Solution - Injectable - 25 mg/ml

1 ml x 10	$11.05	GENERIC, Abbott Pharmaceutical	00074-2312-01
1 ml x 10	$12.00	GENERIC, Abbott Pharmaceutical	00074-2312-11
1 ml x 10	$12.10	GENERIC, Abbott Pharmaceutical	00074-2312-31
1 ml x 10	$45.80	PHENERGAN, Allscripts Pharmaceutical Company	54569-3106-00
1 ml x 25	$59.50	GENERIC, Esi Lederle Generics	00641-1495-35
1 ml x 25	$59.75	GENERIC, Esi Lederle Generics	00641-0928-25
1 ml x 25	$64.70	PHENERGAN, Physicians Total Care	54868-0597-00
1 ml x 25	$73.79	PHENERGAN, Allscripts Pharmaceutical Company	54569-3882-00
1 ml x 25	$77.50	PHENERGAN, Esi Lederle Generics	00008-0063-01
10 ml	$2.25	GENERIC, Vita-Rx Corporation	49727-0746-10
10 ml	$4.00	GENERIC, Cmc-Consolidated Midland Corporation	00223-8393-10
10 ml	$4.45	GENERIC, Roberts/Hauck Pharmaceutical Corporation	43797-0031-12
10 ml	$6.00	GENERIC, Interstate Drug Exchange Inc	00814-6421-40

Solution - Injectable - 50 mg/ml

1 ml x 10	$12.71	GENERIC, Abbott Pharmaceutical	00074-2335-31
1 ml x 10	$13.05	GENERIC, Abbott Pharmaceutical	00074-2335-01
1 ml x 25	$75.00	GENERIC, Esi Lederle Generics	00641-0929-25
1 ml x 25	$75.00	GENERIC, Esi Lederle Generics	00641-1496-35
1 ml x 25	$95.75	PHENERGAN, Esi Lederle Generics	00008-0746-01
10 ml	$2.50	GENERIC, Vita-Rx Corporation	49727-0748-10
10 ml	$4.00	GENERIC, C.O. Truxton Inc	00463-1095-10
10 ml	$4.25	GENERIC, Cmc-Consolidated Midland Corporation	00223-8394-10
10 ml	$4.25	GENERIC, Med Tek Pharmaceuticals Inc	52349-0110-10
10 ml	$5.50	GENERIC, Roberts/Hauck Pharmaceutical Corporation	43797-0032-12
10 ml	$5.77	GENERIC, Forest Pharmaceuticals	00785-8090-10
10 ml	$6.57	GENERIC, General Injectables and Vaccines Inc	52584-0259-10
10 ml	$6.75	GENERIC, Interstate Drug Exchange Inc	00814-6424-40
10 ml	$8.00	GENERIC, Bolan Pharmaceutical Inc	44437-0259-10
10 ml	$8.87	GENERIC, Moore, H.L. Drug Exchange Inc	00839-5158-30
10 ml	$10.25	GENERIC, Forest Pharmaceuticals	00456-1009-10
10 ml	$14.95	GENERIC, Merz Pharmaceuticals	00259-0308-10

Suppository - Rectal - 25 mg

1's	$3.87	PHENERGAN, Allscripts Pharmaceutical Company	54569-0362-03
1's	$8.15	PHENERGAN, Prescript Pharmaceuticals	00247-0205-01
2's	$9.33	PHENERGAN, Physicians Total Care	54868-1933-00
2's	$10.47	PHENERGAN, Pd-Rx Pharmaceuticals	55289-0415-02
2's	$12.95	PHENERGAN, Prescript Pharmaceuticals	00247-0205-02
3's	$17.74	PHENERGAN, Prescript Pharmaceuticals	00247-0205-03
4's	$15.48	PHENERGAN, Allscripts Pharmaceutical Company	54569-0362-00
4's	$20.93	PHENERGAN, Pd-Rx Pharmaceuticals	55289-0415-04
4's	$22.54	PHENERGAN, Prescript Pharmaceuticals	00247-0205-04
6's	$23.22	PHENERGAN, Allscripts Pharmaceutical Company	54569-0362-02
6's	$26.03	PHENERGAN, Pharma Pac	52959-0562-06
6's	$29.57	PHENERGAN, Pd-Rx Pharmaceuticals	55289-0415-06
6's	$32.14	PHENERGAN, Prescript Pharmaceuticals	00247-0205-06
12's	$33.25	PHENERGAN, Southwood Pharmaceuticals Inc	58016-3067-01
12's	$46.45	PHENERGAN, Allscripts Pharmaceutical Company	54569-0362-01
12's	$47.90	PHENERGAN, Pharma Pac	52959-0562-01
12's	$53.04	PHENERGAN, Physicians Total Care	54868-1933-01
12's	$60.18	PHENERGAN, Wyeth-Ayerst Laboratories	00008-0212-01
12's	$60.93	PHENERGAN, Prescript Pharmaceuticals	00247-0205-12

Syrup - Oral - 6.25 mg/5 ml

120 ml	$2.10	GENERIC, Cmc-Consolidated Midland Corporation	00223-6345-01
120 ml	$2.26	GENERIC, Cenci, H.R. Labs Inc	00556-0365-04
120 ml	$2.50	GENERIC, Halsey Drug Company Inc	00879-0539-04
120 ml	$3.06	GENERIC, Major Pharmaceuticals Inc	00904-1508-00
120 ml	$3.17	FEDERAL UPPER LIMIT, H.C.F.A. F F P	99999-2125-01
120 ml	$3.36	GENERIC, Moore, H.L. Drug Exchange Inc	00839-6314-65
120 ml	$3.44	GENERIC, Geneva Pharmaceuticals	00781-6575-04
120 ml	$4.68	GENERIC, Alpharma Uspd Makers Of Barre and Nmc	00472-1504-04
120 ml	$6.79	GENERIC, Pharma Pac	52959-0134-04
120 ml	$7.35	GENERIC, Morton Grove Pharmaceuticals Inc	60432-0608-04
240 ml	$5.83	GENERIC, Alpharma Uspd Makers Of Barre and Nmc	00472-1504-08
240 ml	$13.65	GENERIC, Pharma Pac	52959-0134-08
480 ml	$4.51	GENERIC, Cenci, H.R. Labs Inc	00556-0365-16
480 ml	$4.94	GENERIC, Cmc-Consolidated Midland Corporation	00223-6345-02
480 ml	$5.47	GENERIC, Aligen Independent Laboratories Inc	00405-3600-16
480 ml	$6.19	GENERIC, Moore, H.L. Drug Exchange Inc	00839-6314-69
480 ml	$6.48	GENERIC, Major Pharmaceuticals Inc	00904-1508-16
480 ml	$7.00	GENERIC, Geneva Pharmaceuticals	00781-6575-16
480 ml	$7.28	GENERIC, Esi Lederle Generics	59911-5818-03
480 ml	$7.44	GENERIC, Halsey Drug Company Inc	00879-0539-16
480 ml	$14.04	GENERIC, Alpharma Uspd Makers Of Barre and Nmc	00472-1504-16
480 ml	$22.04	GENERIC, Morton Grove Pharmaceuticals Inc	60432-0608-16
1440 ml	$3.02	GENERIC, Major Pharmaceuticals Inc	00904-1508-20
3840 ml	$27.65	GENERIC, Cmc-Consolidated Midland Corporation	00223-6345-03
3840 ml	$28.80	GENERIC, Cenci, H.R. Labs Inc	00556-0365-28
3840 ml	$31.10	GENERIC, Watson/Rugby Laboratories Inc	00536-1745-90
3840 ml	$33.02	GENERIC, Moore, H.L. Drug Exchange Inc	00839-6314-70
3840 ml	$36.86	GENERIC, Halsey Drug Company Inc	00879-0539-28
3840 ml	$41.86	GENERIC, Ivax Corporation	00182-1737-41
3840 ml	$41.86	GENERIC, Geneva Pharmaceuticals	00781-6575-28
3840 ml	$41.86	GENERIC, Major Pharmaceuticals Inc	00904-1508-28
3840 ml	$84.21	GENERIC, Alpharma Uspd Makers Of Barre and Nmc	00472-1504-28

Syrup - Oral - 25 mg/5 ml

480 ml	$10.99	GENERIC, Cmc-Consolidated Midland Corporation	00223-6344-01

Size	Price	Product	NDC
480 ml	$73.07	PHENERGAN FORTIS, Wyeth-Ayerst Laboratories	00008-0231-01
3840 ml	$77.57	GENERIC, Cmc-Consolidated Midland Corporation	00223-6344-02

Tablet - Oral - 12.5 mg

Size	Price	Product	NDC
100's	$6.50	GENERIC, Esi Lederle Generics	59911-5871-01

Tablet - Oral - 25 mg

Size	Price	Product	NDC
100's	$3.96	GENERIC, Esi Lederle Generics	59911-5872-01

PRODUCT LISTING - RATED NOT THERAPEUTICALLY EQUIVALENT

Suppository - Rectal - 50 mg

Size	Price	Product	NDC
4's	$19.47	GENERIC, Physicians Total Care	54868-1613-01
6's	$33.05	PHENERGAN, Physicians Total Care	54868-1406-01
6's	$35.96	PHENERGAN, Pd-Rx Pharmaceuticals	55289-0639-06
12's	$44.81	PHENERGAN, Southwood Pharmaceuticals Inc	58016-3068-01
12's	$55.07	GENERIC, Physicians Total Care	54868-1613-00
12's	$56.30	GENERIC, Major Pharmaceuticals Inc	00904-1290-12
12's	$59.50	PHENERGAN, Allscripts Pharmaceutical Company	54569-3836-00
12's	$60.41	GENERIC, G and W Laboratories Inc	00713-0132-12
12's	$77.08	PHENERGAN, Wyeth-Ayerst Laboratories	00008-0229-01

Tablet - Oral - 25 mg

Size	Price	Product	NDC
2's	$1.16	GENERIC, Pd-Rx Pharmaceuticals	55289-0464-02
2's	$3.25	GENERIC, Pharma Pac	52959-0534-02
2's	$5.77	PHENERGAN, Pharma Pac	52959-0451-02
10's	$2.87	GENERIC, Pd-Rx Pharmaceuticals	55289-0464-10
10's	$4.60	GENERIC, Pharma Pac	52959-0534-10
12's	$5.66	PHENERGAN, Allscripts Pharmaceutical Company	54569-0358-03
20's	$1.90	GENERIC, Circle Pharmaceuticals Inc	00659-0718-20
20's	$3.48	GENERIC, Pd-Rx Pharmaceuticals	55289-0464-20
20's	$6.75	GENERIC, Pharma Pac	52959-0534-20
25's	$3.87	GENERIC, Pd-Rx Pharmaceuticals	55289-0464-25
25's	$13.28	PHENERGAN, Pd-Rx Pharmaceuticals	55289-0088-25
30's	$4.50	GENERIC, Pd-Rx Pharmaceuticals	55289-0464-30
30's	$9.66	GENERIC, Pharma Pac	52959-0534-30
30's	$16.23	PHENERGAN, Pharma Pac	52959-0451-30
30's	$16.34	PHENERGAN, Physicians Total Care	54868-1285-01
60's	$5.78	GENERIC, Pd-Rx Pharmaceuticals	55289-0464-60
100's	$2.55	GENERIC, Moore, H.L. Drug Exchange Inc	00839-1535-06
100's	$3.15	GENERIC, Major Pharmaceuticals Inc	00904-2329-60
100's	$4.25	GENERIC, Cmc-Consolidated Midland Corporation	00223-1521-01
100's	$5.03	GENERIC, Interstate Drug Exchange Inc	00814-6413-14
100's	$50.64	GENERIC, Geneva Pharmaceuticals	00781-1830-01
100's	$59.08	PHENERGAN, Wyeth-Ayerst Laboratories	00008-0027-02
100's	$59.08	PHENERGAN, Wyeth-Ayerst Laboratories	00008-0027-07

Tablet - Oral - 50 mg

Size	Price	Product	NDC
100's	$4.65	GENERIC, Major Pharmaceuticals Inc	00904-2330-60
100's	$77.62	GENERIC, Geneva Pharmaceuticals	00781-1832-01
100's	$90.54	PHENERGAN, Wyeth-Ayerst Laboratories	00008-0227-01

P

PRODUCT LISTING - EQUIVALENTS NOT AVAILABLE

Solution - Injectable - 25 mg/ml

Size	Price	Product	NDC
1 ml	$4.08	GENERIC, Prescript Pharmaceuticals	00247-0293-01
1 ml x 25	$20.00	GENERIC, Cmc-Consolidated Midland Corporation	00223-8393-01
1 ml x 25	$59.75	GENERIC, Gensia Sicor Pharmaceuticals Inc	00703-2191-04
1 ml x 25	$73.33	GENERIC, Physicians Total Care	54868-4021-00
1 ml x 100	$65.00	GENERIC, Raway Pharmacal Inc	00686-1495-35
10 ml	$10.64	GENERIC, Prescript Pharmaceuticals	00247-0293-10
10 ml	$11.11	GENERIC, Physicians Total Care	54868-2695-00
25 ml	$21.55	GENERIC, Prescript Pharmaceuticals	00247-0293-25

Solution - Injectable - 50 mg/ml

Size	Price	Product	NDC
1 ml x 25	$25.00	GENERIC, Cmc-Consolidated Midland Corporation	00223-8394-01
1 ml x 25	$75.00	GENERIC, Gensia Sicor Pharmaceuticals Inc	00703-2201-04
10 ml	$3.25	PENTAZINE, Century Pharmaceuticals Inc	00436-0280-70
10 ml	$10.95	ANTINAUS 50, Clint Pharmaceutical Inc	55553-0259-10
10 ml	$19.37	GENERIC, Physicians Total Care	54868-0262-00

Suppository - Rectal - 12.5 mg

Size	Price	Product	NDC
1's	$3.38	PHENERGAN, Allscripts Pharmaceutical Company	54569-0361-03
1's	$4.51	PHENERGAN, Physicians Total Care	54868-1932-01
1's	$7.55	PHENERGAN, Prescript Pharmaceuticals	00247-0204-01
2's	$11.74	PHENERGAN, Prescript Pharmaceuticals	00247-0204-02
3's	$15.94	PHENERGAN, Prescript Pharmaceuticals	00247-0204-03
4's	$13.50	PHENERGAN, Allscripts Pharmaceutical Company	54569-0361-00
4's	$19.07	PHENERGAN, Pd-Rx Pharmaceuticals	55289-0414-04
4's	$20.14	PHENERGAN, Prescript Pharmaceuticals	00247-0204-04
6's	$20.25	PHENERGAN, Allscripts Pharmaceutical Company	54569-0361-02
6's	$25.70	PHENERGAN, Pd-Rx Pharmaceuticals	55289-0414-06
6's	$28.53	PHENERGAN, Prescript Pharmaceuticals	00247-0204-06
12's	$30.50	PHENERGAN, Southwood Pharmaceuticals Inc	58016-3066-01
12's	$38.18	PHENERGAN, Pharma Pac	52959-0561-01
12's	$40.51	PHENERGAN, Allscripts Pharmaceutical Company	54569-0361-01
12's	$46.35	PHENERGAN, Physicians Total Care	54868-1932-00
12's	$52.48	PHENERGAN, Wyeth-Ayerst Laboratories	00008-0498-01
12's	$53.71	PHENERGAN, Prescript Pharmaceuticals	00247-0204-12

Suppository - Rectal - 25 mg

Size	Price	Product	NDC
12's	$51.80	GENERIC, Alpharma Uspd Makers Of Barre and Nmc	00472-0096-12
12's	$52.00	PROMETHEGAN, G and W Laboratories Inc	00713-0526-12

Suppository - Rectal - 50 mg

Size	Price	Product	NDC
100's	$45.00	GENERIC, Moore, H.L. Drug Exchange Inc	00839-7492-92

Syrup - Oral - 6.25 mg/5 ml

Size	Price	Product	NDC
118 ml	$4.76	GENERIC, Prescript Pharmaceuticals	00247-0231-52
120 ml	$0.50	PENTAZINE, Century Pharmaceuticals Inc	00436-0580-04
120 ml	$3.25	GENERIC, Cmc-Consolidated Midland Corporation	00223-6347-01
120 ml	$3.97	GENERIC, Allscripts Pharmaceutical Company	54569-1046-00
120 ml	$4.05	GENERIC, Physicians Total Care	54868-1867-00
120 ml	$4.10	GENERIC, Alpharma Uspd Makers Of Barre and Nmc	63874-0712-12
120 ml	$5.66	GENERIC, Southwood Pharmaceuticals Inc	58016-0472-24
120 ml	$6.22	GENERIC, Southwood Pharmaceuticals Inc	58016-4008-01
180 ml	$5.51	GENERIC, Prescript Pharmaceuticals	00247-0231-59
180 ml	$8.48	GENERIC, Southwood Pharmaceuticals Inc	58016-0472-36
480 ml	$1.80	PENTAZINE, Century Pharmaceuticals Inc	00436-0580-16
480 ml	$4.50	GENERIC, Cmc-Consolidated Midland Corporation	00223-6343-01
480 ml	$8.00	GENERIC, Cmc-Consolidated Midland Corporation	00223-6347-02
3840 ml	$11.90	PENTAZINE, Century Pharmaceuticals Inc	00436-0580-28

Tablet - Oral - 12.5 mg

Size	Price	Product	NDC
12's	$4.43	PHENERGAN, Physicians Total Care	54868-0721-00
30's	$8.01	PHENERGAN, Allscripts Pharmaceutical Company	54569-4699-00
100's	$33.44	PHENERGAN, Wyeth-Ayerst Laboratories	00008-0019-01

Tablet - Oral - 25 mg

Size	Price	Product	NDC
2's	$3.78	GENERIC, Prescript Pharmaceuticals	00247-0130-02
4's	$4.20	GENERIC, Prescript Pharmaceuticals	00247-0130-04
5's	$0.36	GENERIC, Allscripts Pharmaceutical Company	54569-4168-00
5's	$4.41	GENERIC, Prescript Pharmaceuticals	00247-0130-05
6's	$4.62	GENERIC, Prescript Pharmaceuticals	00247-0130-06
7's	$4.84	GENERIC, Prescript Pharmaceuticals	00247-0130-07
8's	$5.05	GENERIC, Prescript Pharmaceuticals	00247-0130-08
10's	$0.72	GENERIC, Allscripts Pharmaceutical Company	54569-1754-01
10's	$1.74	GENERIC, Physicians Total Care	54868-1323-01
10's	$2.83	GENERIC, Southwood Pharmaceuticals Inc	58016-0424-10
10's	$5.47	GENERIC, Prescript Pharmaceuticals	00247-0130-10
12's	$0.86	GENERIC, Allscripts Pharmaceutical Company	54569-1754-00
12's	$1.87	GENERIC, Physicians Total Care	54868-1323-02
12's	$3.54	GENERIC, Southwood Pharmaceuticals Inc	58016-0424-12
12's	$4.20	GENERIC, Pharmaceutical Corporation Of America	51655-0084-27
12's	$5.89	GENERIC, Prescript Pharmaceuticals	00247-0130-12
14's	$6.32	GENERIC, Prescript Pharmaceuticals	00247-0130-14
15's	$2.00	GENERIC, Physicians Total Care	54868-1323-04
15's	$4.42	GENERIC, Southwood Pharmaceuticals Inc	58016-0424-15
15's	$6.53	GENERIC, Prescript Pharmaceuticals	00247-0130-15
20's	$2.23	GENERIC, Physicians Total Care	54868-1323-05
20's	$5.90	GENERIC, Southwood Pharmaceuticals Inc	58016-0424-20
20's	$7.59	GENERIC, Prescript Pharmaceuticals	00247-0130-20
24's	$8.44	GENERIC, Prescript Pharmaceuticals	00247-0130-24
30's	$2.15	GENERIC, Allscripts Pharmaceutical Company	54569-1754-09
30's	$2.67	GENERIC, Physicians Total Care	54868-1323-06
30's	$8.85	GENERIC, Southwood Pharmaceuticals Inc	58016-0424-30
30's	$9.71	GENERIC, Prescript Pharmaceuticals	00247-0130-30
40's	$11.82	GENERIC, Prescript Pharmaceuticals	00247-0130-40
50's	$14.75	GENERIC, Southwood Pharmaceuticals Inc	58016-0424-50
100's	$5.14	GENERIC, Physicians Total Care	54868-1323-00
100's	$24.53	GENERIC, Prescript Pharmaceuticals	00247-0130-00
100's	$29.50	GENERIC, Southwood Pharmaceuticals Inc	58016-0424-00
100's	$47.72	GENERIC, Watson Laboratories Inc	00591-5307-01

Tablet - Oral - 50 mg

Size	Price	Product	NDC
60's	$6.31	GENERIC, Physicians Total Care	54868-2844-00
100's	$70.73	GENERIC, Watson Laboratories Inc	00591-5319-01

Propafenone Hydrochloride *(002127)*

Categories: Arrhythmia, paroxysmal atrial fibrillation; Arrhythmia, paroxysmal supraventricular tachycardia; Arrhythmia, ventricular; Tachycardia, ventricular; Pregnancy Category C; FDA Approved 1989 Nov
Drug Classes: Antiarrhythmics, class IC
Brand Names: Arythmol; Norfenon; Normorytmin; Rythmex; **Rythmol**; Rytmonorm
Cost of Therapy: $252.07 (Arrhythmia; Rythmol; 225 mg; 3 tablets/day; 30 day supply)
$209.64 (Arrhythmia; Generic Tablets; 225 mg; 3 tablets/day; 30 day supply)

DESCRIPTION

Rythmol (propafenone hydrochloride) is an antiarrhythmic drug supplied in scored film-coated tablets of 150, 225, and 300 mg for oral administration. Propafenone has some structural similarities to beta-blocking agents.

The molecular formula for propafenone HCl is $C_{21}H_{27}NO_3$·HCl, and is chemically known as 2′-[2-Hydroxy-3-(propylamino)-propoxy]-3-phenylpropiophenone hydrochloride, with a molecular weight of 377.92.

Propafenone HCl occurs as colorless crystals or white crystalline powder with a very bitter taste. It is slightly soluble in water (20°C) chloroform and ethanol. *The following inactive ingredients are contained in Rythmol tablets:* Corn starch, hydroxypropyl methylcellulose, magnesium stearate, polyethylene glycol, polysorbate, povidone, propylene glycol, sodium starch glycolate, and titanium dioxide.

CLINICAL PHARMACOLOGY

MECHANISM OF ACTION

Propafenone HCl is a Class 1C antiarrhythmic drug with local anesthetic effects, and a direct stabilizing action on myocardial membranes. The electrophysiological effect of propafenone HCl manifests itself in a reduction of upstroke velocity (Phase 0) of the monophasic action potential. In Purkinje fibers, and to a lesser extent myocardial fibers, propafenone HCl reduces the fast inward current carried by sodium ions. Diastolic excitability threshold is increased and effective refractory period prolonged. Propafenone reduces spontaneous automaticity and depresses triggered activity.

Studies in anesthetized dogs and isolated organ preparations show that propafenone HCl has beta-sympatholytic activity at about 1/50 the potency of propranolol. Clinical studies employing isoproterenol challenge and exercise testing after single doses of propafenone indicate a beta-adrenergic blocking potency (per mg) about 1/40 that of propranolol in man. In clinical trials, resting heart rate decreases of about 8% were noted at the higher end of the therapeutic plasma concentration range. At very high concentrations *in vitro,* propafenone can inhibit the slow inward current carried by calcium but this calcium antagonist effect probably does not contribute to antiarrhythmic efficacy. Propafenone has local anesthetic activity approximately equal to procaine.

ELECTROPHYSIOLOGY

Electrophysiology studies in patients with ventricular tachycardia have shown that propafenone HCl prolongs atrioventricular conduction while having little or no effect on sinus node function. Both AV nodal conduction time (AH interval) and His-Purkinje conduction time (HV interval) are prolonged. Propafenone has little or no effect on the atrial functional refractory period, but AV nodal functional and effective refractory periods are prolonged. In patients with WPW, propafenone HCl reduces conduction and increases the effective refractory period of the accessory pathway in both directions. Propafenone slows conduction and consequently produces dose related changes in the PR interval and QRS duration. QTc interval does not change.

TABLE 1 *Mean Changes in ECG Intervals**

	Total Daily Dose (mg)							
	337.5 mg		**450 mg**		**675 mg**		**990 mg**	
Interval	**msec**	**%**	**msec**	**%**	**msec**	**%**	**msec**	**%**
RR	-14.5	-1.8	30.6	3.8	31.5	3.9	41.7	5.1
PR	3.6	2.1	19.1	11.6	28.9	17.8	35.6	21.9
QRS	5.6	6.4	5.5	6.1	7.7	8.4	15.6	17.3
QTc	2.7	0.7	-7.5	-1.8	5.0	1.2	14.7	3.7

* Change and percent change based on mean baseline values for each treatment group.

In any individual patient, the above ECG changes cannot be readily used to predict either efficacy or plasma concentration.

Propafenone HCl causes a dose-related and concentration-related decrease in the rate of single and multiple PVCs and can suppress recurrence of ventricular tachycardia. Based on the percent of patients attaining substantial (80-90%) suppression of ventricular ectopic activity, if appears that trough plasma levels of 0.2-1.5 µg/ml can provide good suppression, with higher concentrations giving a greater rate of good response.

When 600 mg/day propafenone was administered to patients with paroxysmal atrial tachyarrhythmias, mean heart rate during arrhythmia decreased 14 beats/min and 37 beats/min for PAF patients and PSVT patients, respectively.

HEMODYNAMICS

Sympathetic stimulation may be a vital component supporting circulatory function in patients with congestive heart failure, and its inhibition by the beta blockade produced by propafenone HCl may in itself aggravate congestive heart failure.

Additionally, like other Class 1C antiarrhythmic drugs, studies in humans have shown that propafenone HCl exerts a negative inotropic effect on the myocardium. Cardiac catheterization studies in patients with moderately impaired ventricular function (mean CI = 2.61 L/min/m^2) utilizing intravenous propafenone infusions (2 mg/kg over 10 min + 2 mg/min for 30 min) that gave mean plasma concentrations of 3.0 µg/ml (well above the therapeutic range of 0.2-1.5 µg/ml) showed significant increases in pulmonary capillary wedge pressure, systemic and pulmonary vascular resistances and depression of cardiac output and cardiac index.

PHARMACOKINETICS AND METABOLISM

Propafenone HCl is nearly completely absorbed after oral administration with peak plasma levels occurring approximately 3.5 hours after administration in most individuals. Propafenone exhibits extensive saturable presystemic biotransformation (first pass effect) resulting in a dose dependent and dosage form dependent absolute bioavailability; *e.g.,* a 150 mg tablet had absolute bioavailability of 3.4%, while a 300 mg tablet had absolute bioavailability of 10.6%. A 300 mg solution which was rapidly absorbed, had absolute bioavailability of 21.4%. At still larger doses, above those recommended, bioavailability increases still further. Decreased liver function also increases bioavailability; bioavailability is inversely related to indocyanine green clearance reaching 60-70% at clearances of 7 ml/min and below. The clearance of propafenone is reduced and the elimination half-life increased in patients with significant hepatic dysfunction (see PRECAUTIONS).

Propafenone HCl follows a nonlinear pharmacokinetic disposition presumably due to saturation of first pass hepatic metabolism as the liver is exposed to higher concentrations of propafenone and shows a very high degree of interindividual variability. For example, for a 3-fold increase in daily dose from 300 to 900 mg/day there is a 10-fold increase in steady-state plasma concentration. The top 25% of patients given 375 mg/day, however, had a mean concentration of propafenone larger than the bottom 25%, and about equal to the second 25%, of patients given a dose of 900 mg. Although food increased peak blood level and bioavailability in a single dose study, during multiple dose administration of propafenone to healthy volunteers food did not change bioavailability significantly.

There are two genetically determined patterns of propafenone metabolism. In over 90% of patients, the drug is rapidly and extensively metabolized with an elimination half-life from 2-10 hours. These patients metabolize propafenone into two active metabolites: 5-hydroxypropafenone and N-depropylpropafenone. *In vitro* preparations have shown these two metabolites to have antiarrhythmic activity comparable to propafenone but in man they both are usually present in concentrations less than 20% of propafenone. Nine (9) additional metabolites have been identified, most in only trace amounts. It is the saturable hydroxylation pathway that is responsible for the nonlinear pharmacokinetic disposition.

In less than 10% of patients (and in any patient also receiving quinidine, see PRECAUTIONS), metabolism of propafenone is slower because the 5-hydroxy metabolite is not formed or is minimally formed. The estimated propafenone elimination half-life ranges from 10-32 hours. Decreased ability to form the 5-hydroxy metabolite of propafenone is associated with a diminished ability to metabolize debrisoquine and a variety of other drugs (encainide, metoprolol, dextromethorphan). In these patients, the N-depropylpropafenone occurs in quantities comparable to the levels occurring in extensive metabolizers. In slow metabolizers propafenone pharmacokinetics are linear.

There are significant differences in plasma concentrations of propafenone in slow and extensive metabolizers, the former achieving concentrations 1.5-2.0 times those of the extensive metabolizers at daily doses of 675-900 mg/day. At low doses the differences are greater, with slow metabolizers attaining concentrations more than five times that of extensive metabolizers. Because the difference decreases at high doses and is mitigated by the lack of the active 5-hydroxy metabolite in the slow metabolizers, and because steady-state conditions are achieved after 4-5 days of dosing in all patients, the recommended dosing regimen is the same for all patients. The greater variability in blood levels require that the drug be titrated carefully in patients with close attention paid to clinical and ECG evidence of toxicity (see DOSAGE AND ADMINISTRATION).

INDICATIONS AND USAGE

In patients without structural heart disease, propafenone HCl is indicated to prolong the time to recurrence of:

- Paroxysmal atrial fibrillation/flutter (PAF) associated with disabling symptoms.
- Paroxysmal supraventricular tachycardia (PSVT) associated with disabling symptoms.

As with other agents, some patients with atrial flutter treated with propafenone have developed 1:1 conduction, producing an increase in ventricular rate. Concomitant treatment with drugs that increase the functional AV refractory period is recommended.

The use of propafenone HCl in patients with chronic atrial fibrillation has not been evaluated. Propafenone HCl should not be used to control ventricular rate during atrial fibrillation.

Propafenone HCl is also indicated for the treatment of:

- Documented ventricular arrhythmias, such as sustained ventricular tachycardia, that, in the judgement of the physician, are life-threatening. Because of the proarrhythmic effects of propafenone HCl, its use with lesser ventricular arrhythmias is not recommended, even if patients are symptomatic, and any use of the drug should be reserved for patients in whom, in the opinion of the physician, the potential benefits outweigh the risks.

Initiation of propafenone HCl treatment, as with other anti-arrhythmics used to treat life-threatening ventricular arrhythmias, should be carried out in the hospital.

Propafenone HCl, like other antiarrhythmic drugs, has not been shown to enhance survival in patients with ventricular or atrial arrhythmias.

P

CONTRAINDICATIONS

Propafenone HCl is contraindicated in the presence of uncontrolled congestive heart failure, cardiogenic shock, sinoatrial, atrioventricular and intraventricular disorders of impulse generation and/or conduction (*e.g.,* sick sinus node syndrome, atrioventricular block) in the absence of an artificial pacemaker, bradycardia, marked hypotension, bronchospastic disorders, manifest electrolyte imbalance, and known hypersensitivity to the drug.

WARNINGS

Mortality:

In the National Heart, Lung and Blood Institute's Cardiac Arrhythmia Suppression Trial (CAST), a long-term, multi-center, randomized, double-blind study in patients with asymptomatic non-life-threatening ventricular arrhythmias who had a myocardial infarction more than 6 days but less than 2 years previously, an increased rate of death or reversed cardiac arrest (7.7%; 56/730) was seen in patients treated with encainide or flecainide (Class 1C antiarrhythmics) compared with that seen in patients assigned to placebo (3.0%; 22/725). The average duration of treatment with encainide or flecainide in this study was 10 months.

The applicability of the CAST results to other populations (*e.g.,* those without recent myocardial infarction) or other antiarrhythmic drugs is uncertain, but at present it is prudent to consider any 1C antiarrhythmic to have a significant risk in patients with structural heart disease. Given the lack of any evidence that these drugs improve survival, antiarrhythmic agents should generally be avoided in patients with non-life-threatening ventricular arrhythmias, even if the patients are experiencing unpleasant, but not life-threatening, symptoms or signs.

PROARRHYTHMIC EFFECTS

Propafenone HCl, like other antiarrhythmic agents, may cause new or worsened arrhythmias. Such proarrhythmic effects range from an increase in frequency of PVCs to the development of more severe ventricular tachycardia, ventricular fibrillation or torsade depointes; *i.e.,* tachycardia that is more sustained or more rapid which may lead to fatal consequences. It is therefore essential that each patient given propafenone HCl be evaluated electrocardiographically and clinically prior to, and during therapy to determine whether the response to propafenone HCl supports continued treatment.

Overall in clinical trials with propafenone, 4.7% of all patients had new or worsened ventricular arrhythmia possibly representing a pro-arrhythmic event (0.7% was an increase in PVCs; 4.0% a worsening, or new appearance, of VT or VF). Of the patients who had worsening of VT (4%), 92% had a history of VT and/or VT/VF, 71% had coronary artery disease, and 68% had a prior myocardial infarction. The incidence of proarrhythmia in patients with less serious or benign arrhythmias, which include patients with an increase in frequency of PVCs, was 1.6%. Although most proarrhythmic events occurred during the first week of therapy, late events also were seen and the CAST study (see Mortality) suggests that an increased risk is present throughout treatment.

In the 474 patient US multicenter trial in patients with symptomatic SVT, 1.9% (9/474) of these patients experienced ventricular tachycardia (VT) or ventricular fibrillation (VF) during the study. However, in 4 of the 9 patients, the ventricular tachycardia was of atrial origin. Six (6) of the 9 patients that developed ventricular arrhythmias did so within 14 days of onset of therapy. About 2.3% (11/474) of all patients had a recurrence of SVT during the study which could have been a change in the patients' arrhythmia behavior or could represent a proarrhythmic event. Case reports in patients treated with propafenone HCl for atrial fibrillation/flutter have included increased PVCs, VT, VF, and death.

NONALLERGIC BRONCHOSPASM (E.G., CHRONIC BRONCHITIS, EMPHYSEMA)

PATIENTS WITH BRONCHOSPASTIC DISEASE SHOULD, IN GENERAL, NOT RECEIVE PROPAFENONE or other agents with beta-adrenergic-blocking activity.

CONGESTIVE HEART FAILURE

During treatment with oral propafenone in patients with depressed baseline function (mean EF = 33.5%), no significant decreases in ejection fraction were seen. In clinical trial experience, new or worsened CHF has been reported in 3.7% of patients with ventricular arrhythmia; of those 0.9% were considered probably or definitely related to propafenone HCl. Of the patients with congestive heart failure probably related to propafenone, 80% had preexisting heart failure and 85% had coronary artery disease. CHF attributable to propafenone HCl developed rarely (<0.2%) in ventricular arrhythmia patients who had no previous history of CHF. CHF occurred in 1.9% of patients studied with PAF or PSVT.

As RYTHMOL exerts both beta blockade and a (dose-related) negative inotropic effect on cardiac muscle, patients with congestive heart failure should be fully compensated before receiving propafenone HCl. If congestive heart failure worsens, propafenone HCl should be discontinued (unless congestive heart failure is due to the cardiac arrhythmia) and, if indicated, restarted at a lower dosage only after adequate cardiac compensation has been established.

CONDUCTION DISTURBANCES

Propafenone HCl slows atrioventricular conduction and also causes first degree AV block. Average PR interval prolongation and increases in QRS duration are closely correlated with dosage increases and concomitant increases in propafenone plasma concentrations. The incidence of first degree, second degree, and third degree AV block observed in 2127 patients was 2.5%, 0.6%, and 0.2%, respectively. Development of second or third degree AV block requires a reduction in dosage or discontinuation of propafenone HCl. Bundle branch block (1.2%) and intraventricular conduction delay (1.1%) have been reported in patients receiving propafenone. Bradycardia has also been reported (1.5%). Experience in patients with sick sinus node syndrome is limited and these patients should not be treated with propafenone.

EFFECTS ON PACEMAKER THRESHOLD

Propafenone HCl may alter both pacing and sensing thresholds of artificial pacemakers. Pacemakers should be monitored and programmed accordingly during therapy.

P

HEMATOLOGIC DISTURBANCES

Agranulocytosis (fever, chills, weakness, and neutropenia) has been reported in patients receiving propafenone. Generally, the agranulocytosis occurred within the first 2 months of propafenone therapy and upon discontinuation of therapy, the white count usually normalized by 14 days. Unexplained fever and/or decrease in white cell count, particularly during the initial 3 months of therapy, warrant consideration of possible agranulocytosis/granulocytopenia. Patients should be instructed to promptly report the development of any signs of infection such as fever, sore throat, or chills.

PRECAUTIONS

HEPATIC DYSFUNCTION

Propafenone is highly metabolized by the liver and should, therefore, be administered cautiously to patients with impaired hepatic function. Severe liver dysfunction increases the bioavailability of propafenone to approximately 70% compared to 3-40% for patients with normal liver function. In 8 patients with moderate to severe liver disease, the mean half-life was approximately 9 hours. As a result, the dose of propafenone given to patients with impaired hepatic function should be approximately 20-30% of the dose given to patients with normal hepatic function (see DOSAGE AND ADMINISTRATION). Careful monitoring for excessive pharmacological effects should be carried out.

RENAL DYSFUNCTION

A considerable percentage of propafenone metabolites (18.5-38% of the dose 48/hours) are excreted in the urine.

Until further data are available, propafenone HCl should be administered cautiously to patients with impaired renal function. These patients should be carefully monitored for signs of overdosage.

ELEVATED ANA TITERS

Positive ANA titers have been reported in patients receiving propafenone. They have been reversible upon cessation of treatment and may disappear even in the face of continued propafenone therapy. These laboratory findings were usually not associated with clinical symptoms, but there is one published case of drug-induced lupus erythematosis (positive rechallenge); it resolved completely upon discontinuation of therapy. Patients who develop an abnormal ANA test should be carefully evaluated and, if persistent or worsening elevation of ANA titers is detected, consideration should be given to discontinuing therapy.

IMPAIRED SPERMATOGENESIS

Reversible disorders of spermatogenesis have been demonstrated in monkeys, dogs and rabbits after high dose intravenous administration. Evaluation of the effects of short-term propafenone administration on spermatogenesis in 11 normal subjects suggests that propafenone produced a reversible, short-term drop (within normal range) in sperm count. Subsequent evaluations in 11 patients receiving propafenone chronically have suggested no effect of propafenone on sperm count.

NEUROMUSCULAR DYSFUNCTION

Exacerbation of myasthenia gravis has been reported during propafenone therapy.

CARCINOGENESIS, MUTAGENESIS, AND IMPAIRMENT OF FERTILITY

Lifetime maximally tolerated oral dose studies in mice (up to 360 mg/kg/day) and rats (up to 270 mg/kg/day) provided no evidence of a carcinogenic potential for propafenone.

Propafenone HCl was not mutagenic when assayed for genotoxicity in (1) mouse Dominant Lethal test, (2) rat bone marrow Chromosome Analysis, (3) Chinese hamster bone marrow and spermatogonia chromosome analysis, (4) Chinese hamster micronucleus test, and (5) Ames bacterial test.

Propafenone administered intravenously to rabbits, dogs, and monkeys has been shown to decrease spermatogenesis. These effects were reversible, were not found following oral dosing of propafenone, were seen only at lethal or sublethal dose levels and were not seen in rats treated either orally or intravenously (see PRECAUTIONS, Impaired Spermatogenesis). Propafenone did not affect fertility rates when administered orally to male and female rats at doses up to 270 mg/kg/day or when administered orally or intravenously to male rabbits at doses of 120 mg/kg/day or 3.5 mg/kg/day, respectively. On a body weight basis, the above noted oral doses in rat and rabbit are 18 times and 8 times, respectively, the maximum recommended daily human dose of 900 mg (based on 60 kg human body weight).

PREGNANCY CATEGORY C

Teratogenic Effects

Propafenone has been shown to be embryotoxic in rabbits and rats when given in doses 10 and 40 times, respectively, the maximum recommended human dose. No teratogenic potential was apparent in either species. There are no adequate and well-controlled studies in pregnant women. Propafenone should be used during pregnancy only if the potential benefit justifies the potential risk to the fetus.

Nonteratogenic Effects

In a perinatal and postnatal study in rats, propafenone, at dose levels of 6 or more times the maximum recommended human dose, produced dose dependent increases in maternal and neonatal mortality, decreased maternal and pup body weight gain and reduced neonatal physiological development.

LABOR AND DELIVERY

It is not known whether the use of propafenone during labor or delivery has immediate or delayed adverse effects on the fetus, or whether it prolongs the duration of labor or increases the need for forceps delivery or other obstetrical intervention.

NURSING MOTHERS

It is not known whether this drug is excreted in human milk. Because many drugs are excreted in human milk and because of the potential for serious adverse reactions in nursing infants from propafenone HCl, a decision should be made whether to discontinue nursing or to discontinue the drug, taking into account the importance of the drug to the mother.

PEDIATRIC USE

The safety and effectiveness of propafenone HCl in pediatric patients have not been established.

GERIATRIC USE

There does not appear to be any age-related differences in adverse reaction rates in the most commonly reported adverse reactions. Because of the possible increased risk of impaired hepatic or renal function in this age group, propafenone HCl should be used with caution. The effective dose may be lower in these patients.

ANIMAL TOXICOLOGY

Renal changes have been observed in the rat following 6 months of oral administration of propafenone at doses of 180 and 360 mg/kg/day (12-24 times the maximum recommended human dose) but not 90 mg/kg/day. Both inflammatory and non-inflammatory changes in the renal tubules with accompanying interstitial nephritis were observed. These lesions were reversible in that they were not found in rats treated at these dosage levels and allowed to recover for 6 weeks. Fatty degenerative changes of the liver were found in rats following chronic administration of propafenone at dose levels 19 times the maximum recommended human dose.

DRUG INTERACTIONS

QUINIDINE

Small doses of quinidine completely inhibit the hydroxylation metabolic pathway, making all patients, in effect, slow metabolizers (see CLINICAL PHARMACOLOGY). There is, as yet, too little information to recommend concomitant use of propafenone and quinidine.

LOCAL ANESTHETICS

Concomitant use of local anesthetics (*i.e.,* during pacemaker implantations, surgery, or dental use) may increase the risks of central nervous system side effects.

DIGITALIS

Propafenone HCl produces dose-related increases in serum digoxin levels ranging from about 35% at 450 mg/day to 85% at 900 mg/day of propafenone without affecting digoxin renal clearance. These elevations of digoxin levels were maintained for up to 16 months during concomitant administration. Plasma digoxin levels of patients on concomitant therapy should be measured, and digoxin dosage should ordinarily be reduced when propafenone is started, especially if a relatively large digoxin dose is used or if plasma concentrations are relatively high.

BETA-ANTAGONISTS

In a study involving healthy subjects, concomitant administration of propafenone and propranolol has resulted in substantial increases in propranolol plasma concentration and elimination half-life with no change in propafenone plasma levels from control values. Similar observations have been reported with metoprolol. Propafenone appears to inhibit the hydroxylation pathway for the two beta-antagonists (just as quinidine inhibits propafenone metabolism). Increased plasma concentrations of metoprolol could overcome its relative cardioselectivity. In propafenone clinical trials, patients who were receiving beta-blockers concurrently did not experience an increased incidence of side effects. While the therapeutic range for beta-blockers is wide, a reduction in dosage may be necessary during concomitant administration with propafenone.

WARFARIN

In a study of 8 healthy subjects receiving propafenone and warfarin concomitantly, mean steady-state warfarin plasma concentrations increased 39% with a corresponding increase in prothrombin times of approximately 25%. It is therefore recommended that prothrombin times be routinely monitored and the dose of warfarin be adjusted if necessary.

CIMETIDINE

Concomitant administration of propafenone and cimetidine in 12 healthy subjects resulted in a 20% increase in steady-state plasma concentrations of propafenone with no detectable changes in electrocardiographic parameters beyond that measured on propafenone alone.

DESIPRAMINE

Concomitant administration of propafenone and desipramine may result in elevated serum desipramine levels. Both desipramine, a tricyclic antidepressant, and propafenone are cleared by oxidative pathways of demthylation and hydroxylation carried out by the hepatic P450 cytochrome.

CYCLOSPORIN

Propafenone therapy may increase levels of cyclosporin.

THEOPHYLLINE

Propafenone may increase theophylline concentration during concomitant therapy with the development of theophylline toxicity.

RIFAMPIN

Rifampin may accelerate the metabolism and decrease the plasma levels and antiarrhythmic efficacy of propafenone.

OTHER

Limited experience with propafenone combined with calcium antagonists and diuretics has been reported without evidence of clinically significant adverse reactions.

ADVERSE REACTIONS

Adverse reactions associated with propafenone HCl occur most frequently in the gastrointestinal, cardiovascular, and central nervous systems. About 20% of patients treated with propafenone HCl have discontinued treatment because of adverse reactions.

Adverse reactions reported for >1.5% of 474 SVT patients who received propafenone in US clinical trials are presented in TABLE 3 by incidence and percent discontinuation, reported to the nearest percent.

TABLE 3 *Adverse Reactions Reported for >1.5% of SVT Patients*

	Incidence (n=480)	% of Patients Who Discontinued
Unusual taste	14%	1.3%
Nausea and/or vomiting	11%	2.9%
Dizziness	9%	1.7%
Constipation	8%	0.2%
Headache	6%	0.8%
Fatigue	6%	1.5%
Blurred vision	3%	0.6%
Weakness	3%	1.3%
Dyspnea	2%	1.0%
Wide complex tachycardia	2%	1.9%
CHF	2%	0.6%
Bradycardia	2%	0.2%
Palpitations	2%	0.2%
Tremor	2%	0.4%
Anorexia	2%	0.2%
Diarrhea	2%	0.4%
Ataxia	2%	0.0%

Results of controlled trials in ventricular arrhythmia patients comparing adverse reaction rates on propafenone and placebo, and on propafenone and quinidine are shown in TABLE 4. Adverse reactions reported in ≥1% of the patients receiving propafenone are shown in TABLE 4, unless they were more frequent on placebo than propafenone. The most common events were unusual taste, dizziness, first degree AV block, intraventricular conduction delay, nausea and/or vomiting, and constipation. Headache was relatively common also, but was not increased compared to placebo.

TABLE 4 *Adverse Reactions Reported for ≥1% of the Ventricular Arrhythmia Patients*

	Propafenone/Placebo Trials		Propafenone/Quinidine Trials	
	Propafenone (n=247)	Placebo (n=111)	Propafenone (n=53)	Quinidine (n=52)
Unusual taste	7%	1%	23%	0%
Dizziness	7%	5%	15%	10%
First degree AV block	5%	1%	2%	0%
Headache(s)	5%	5%	2%	8%
Constipation	4%	0%	6%	2%
Intraventricular conduction delay	4%	0%	—	—
Nausea and/or vomiting	3%	1%	6%	15%
Fatigue	—	—	4%	2%
Palpitations	2%	1%	—	—
Blurred vision	2%	1%	6%	2%
Dry mouth	2%	1%	6%	6%
Dyspnea	2%	3%	4%	0%
Abdominal pain/cramps	—	—	2%	8%
Dyspepsia	—	—	2%	8%
Congestive heart failure	—	—	2%	0%
Fever	—	—	2%	10%
Tinnitus	—	—	2%	2%
Vision, abnormal	—	—	2%	2%
Esophagitis	—	—	2%	0%
Gastroenteritis	—	—	2%	0%
Anxiety	2%	2%	—	—
Anorexia	2%	1%	—	2%
Proarrhythmia	1%	0%	2%	0%
Flatulence	1%	0%	2%	0%
Angina	1%	0%	2%	4%
Second degree AV block	1%	0%	—	—
Bundle branch block	1%	0%	2%	2%
Loss of balance	1%	0%	—	—
Diarrhea	1%	1%	6%	39%

Adverse reactions reported for ≥1% of 2127 ventricular arrhythmia patients who received propafenone in US clinical trials are presented in TABLE 5 by propafenone daily dose. The most common adverse reactions in controlled clinical trials appeared dose related (but note that most patients spent more time at the larger doses), especially dizziness, nausea and/or vomiting, unusual taste, constipation, and blurred vision. Some less common reactions may also have been dose related such as first degree AV block, congestive heart failure, dyspepsia, and weakness. The principal causes of discontinuation were the most common events and are shown in TABLE 5.

In addition, the following adverse reactions were reported less frequently than 1% either in clinical trials or in marketing experience (*adverse events for marketing experience are given in italics*). Causality and relationship to propafenone therapy cannot necessarily be judged from these events.

Cardiovascular System: Atrial flutter, AV dissociation, cardiac arrest, flushing, hot flashes, sick sinus syndrome, sinus pause or arrest, supraventricular tachycardia.

Nervous System: Abnormal dreams, abnormal speech, abnormal vision, *apnea, coma,* confusion, depression, memory loss, numbness, paresthesias, psychosis/mania, seizures (0.3%), tinnitus, unusual smell sensation, vertigo.

Gastrointestinal: A number of patients with liver abnormalities associated with propafenone therapy have been reported in foreign post-marketing experience. Some appeared due to hepatocellular injury, some were cholestatic and some showed a mixed picture. Some of these reports were simply discovered through clinical chemistries, others because of clinical symptoms including fulminant hepatitis and death. One case was rechallenged with a positive outcome. Cholestasis (0.1%), elevated liver enzymes (alkaline phosphatase, serum transaminases) (0.2%), gastroenteritis, hepatitis (0.03%).

Hematologic: Agranulocytosis, anemia, bruising, granulocytopenia, *increased bleeding time,* leukopenia, purpura, thrombocytopenia.

Other: Alopecia, eye irritation, *hyponatremia/inappropriate ADH secretion,* impotence, increased glucose, *kidney failure,* positive ANA (0.7%), *lupus erythematosus,* muscle cramps, muscle weakness, nephrotic syndrome, pain, pruritus.

DOSAGE AND ADMINISTRATION

The dose of propafenone HCl must be individually titrated on the basis of response and tolerance. It is recommended that therapy be initiated with 150 mg propafenone given every 8 hours (450 mg/day). Dosage may be increased at a minimum of 3-4 day intervals to 225 mg every 8 hours (675 mg/day) and, if necessary, to 300 mg every 8 hours (900 mg/day). The usefulness and safety of dosages exceeding 900 mg per day have not been established. In those patients in whom significant widening of the QRS complex or second or third degree AV block occurs, dose reduction should be considered.

As with other antiarrhythmic agents, in the elderly or in patients with marked previous myocardial damage, the dose of propafenone HCl should be increased more gradually during the initial phase of treatment.

HOW SUPPLIED

Rythmol tablets are supplied as scored, round, film-coated tablets containing either 150, 225, or 300 mg of propafenone HCl and embossed with "150", "225", or "300" and an arched triangle on the same side.

Storage: Store at controlled room temperature 15-30°C (59-86°F). Dispense in tight, light-resistant container.

P

TABLE 5 *Adverse Reactions Reported for ≥ 1% of Ventricular Arrhythmia Patients*

n=2127

	Incidence by Total Daily Dose				
	450 mg (n=1430)	600 mg (n=1337)	≥900 mg (n=1333)	Total Incidence (n=2127)	% of Patients Who Discontinued
Dizziness	4%	7%	11%	13%	2.4%
Nausea and/or vomiting	2%	6%	9%	11%	3.4%
Unusual taste	3%	5%	6%	9%	0.7%
Constipation	2%	4%	5%	7%	0.5%
Fatigue	2%	3%	4%	6%	1.0%
Dyspnea	2%	2%	4%	5%	1.6%
Proarrhythmia	2%	2%	3%	5%	4.7%
Angina	2%	2%	3%	5%	0.5%
Headache(s)	2%	3%	3%	5%	1.0%
Blurred vision	1%	2%	3%	4%	0.8%
CHF	1%	2%	3%	4%	1.4%
Ventricular tachycardia	1%	2%	3%	3%	1.2%
Dyspepsia	1%	2%	3%	3%	0.9%
Palpitations	1%	2%	3%	3%	0.5%
Rash	1%	1%	2%	3%	0.8%
AV block, first degree	1%	1%	2%	3%	0.3%
Diarrhea	1%	2%	2%	3%	0.6%
Weakness	1%	2%	2%	2%	0.7%
Dry mouth	1%	1%	1%	2%	0.2%
Syncope/near syncope	1%	1%	1%	2%	0.7%
QRS duration, increased	1%	1%	2%	2%	0.5%
Chest pain	1%	1%	1%	2%	0.2%
Anorexia	1%	1%	2%	2%	0.4%
Abdominal pain, cramps	1%	1%	1%	2%	0.4%
Ataxia	0%	1%	2%	2%	0.2%
Insomnia	0%	1%	1%	2%	0.3%
Premature ventricular contraction(s)	1%	1%	1%	2%	0.1%
Bradycardia	1%	1%	1%	2%	0.5%
Anxiety	1%	1%	1%	2%	0.6%
Edema	1%	0%	1%	1%	0.2%
Tremor(s)	0%	1%	1%	1%	0.3%
Diaphoresis	1%	0	1%	1%	0.3%
Bundle branch block	0%	1%	1%	1%	0.5%
Drowsiness	1%	1%	1%	1%	0.2%
Atrial fibrillation	1%	1%	1%	1%	0.4%
Flatulence	0%	1%	1%	1%	0.1%
Hypotension	0%	1%	1%	1%	0.4%
Intraventricular conduction delay	0%	1%	1%	1%	0.1%
Pain, joints	0%	0%	1%	1%	0.1%

PRODUCT LISTING - RATED THERAPEUTICALLY EQUIVALENT

Tablet - Oral - 150 mg

100's	$142.25	GENERIC, Watson Laboratories Inc	52544-0582-01
100's	$163.58	GENERIC, Mutual/United Research Laboratories	00677-1815-01
100's	$163.58	GENERIC, Mutual Pharmaceutical Co Inc	53489-0551-01
100's	$163.59	GENERIC, Watson Laboratories Inc	00591-0582-01
100's	$163.60	GENERIC, Ethex Corporation	58177-0331-04
100's	$171.87	GENERIC, Ethex Corporation	58177-0331-11
250's	$396.68	GENERIC, Mutual/United Research Laboratories	00677-1815-03

Tablet - Oral - 225 mg

100's	$232.93	GENERIC, Mutual/United Research Laboratories	00677-1816-01
100's	$232.93	GENERIC, Mutual Pharmaceutical Co Inc	53489-0552-01
100's	$232.94	GENERIC, Watson Laboratories Inc	00591-0583-01
100's	$232.94	GENERIC, Watson Laboratories Inc	52544-0583-01
250's	$564.86	GENERIC, Mutual/United Research Laboratories	00677-1816-03
250's	$564.86	GENERIC, Mutual Pharmaceutical Co Inc	53489-0552-03

Tablet - Oral - 300 mg

100's	$296.99	GENERIC, Mutual/United Research Laboratories	00677-1817-01
100's	$296.99	GENERIC, Mutual Pharmaceutical Co Inc	53489-0553-01
250's	$396.68	GENERIC, Mutual Pharmaceutical Co Inc	53489-0551-03
250's	$720.20	GENERIC, Mutual/United Research Laboratories	00677-1817-03
250's	$720.20	GENERIC, Mutual Pharmaceutical Co Inc	53489-0553-03

PRODUCT LISTING - EQUIVALENTS NOT AVAILABLE

Tablet - Oral - 150 mg

100's	$168.40	GENERIC, Udl Laboratories Inc	51079-0996-20
100's	$196.50	RYTHMOL, Knoll Pharmaceutical Company	00044-5022-02
100's	$206.25	RYTHMOL, Knoll Pharmaceutical Company	00044-5022-10

Tablet - Oral - 225 mg

100's	$232.95	GENERIC, Ethex Corporation	58177-0332-04
100's	$280.08	RYTHMOL, Knoll Pharmaceutical Company	00044-5024-02
100's	$280.08	RYTHMOL, Abbott Pharmaceutical	00074-1732-14
100's	$293.98	RYTHMOL, Knoll Pharmaceutical Company	00044-5024-10

Tablet - Oral - 300 mg

100's	$280.36	RYTHMOL, Knoll Pharmaceutical Company	00044-5023-10
100's	$297.00	GENERIC, Ethex Corporation	58177-0333-04
100's	$356.49	RYTHMOL, Knoll Pharmaceutical Company	00044-5023-02

Propofol *(002132)*

Categories: Anesthesia, general; Pregnancy Category B; FDA Approved 1989 Oct
Drug Classes: Anesthetics, general
Brand Names: **Diprivan**
Foreign Brand Availability: Anepol (Korea); Cryotol (Mexico); Diprofol (Israel); Disoprivan (Germany); Fresofol (China; Philippines; Taiwan; Thailand); Pofol (Singapore; Thailand); Propocam (Mexico); Propofol-Lipuro (Colombia); Recofol (Indonesia; Israel; Mexico; Singapore)

DESCRIPTION

Diprivan (propofol) injectable emulsion is a sterile, nonpyrogenic emulsion containing 10 mg/ml of propofol suitable for intravenous administration. Propofol is chemically described as 2,6-diisopropylphenol and has a molecular weight of 178.27.

Propofol is very slightly soluble in water and, thus, is formulated in a white, oil-in-water emulsion. The pKa is 11. The octanol/water partition coefficient for propofol is 6761:1 at a pH of 6-8.5. In addition to the active component, propofol, the formulation also contains soybean oil (100 mg/ml), glycerol (22.5 mg/ml), egg lecithin (12 mg/ml); and disodium edetate (0.005%); with sodium hydroxide to adjust pH. The Diprivan injection emulsion is isotonic and has a pH of 7-8.5.

STRICT ASEPTIC TECHNIQUE MUST ALWAYS BE MAINTAINED DURING HANDLING. PROPOFOL INJECTABLE EMULSION IS A SINGLE-USE PARENTERAL PRODUCT WHICH CONTAINS 0.005% DISODIUM EDETATE TO RETARD THE RATE OF GROWTH OF MICROORGANISMS IN THE EVENT OF ACCIDENTAL EXTRINSIC CONTAMINATION. HOWEVER, PROPOFOL INJECTABLE EMULSION CAN STILL SUPPORT THE GROWTH OF MICROORGANISMS AS IT IS NOT AN ANTIMICROBIALLY PRESERVED PRODUCT UNDER USP STANDARDS. ACCORDINGLY, STRICT ASEPTIC TECHNIQUE MUST STILL BE ADHERED TO. DO NOT USE IF CONTAMINATION IS SUSPECTED. DISCARD UNUSED PORTIONS AS DIRECTED WITHIN THE REQUIRED TIME LIMITS (SEE DOSAGE AND ADMINISTRATION, HANDLING PROCEDURES). THERE HAVE BEEN REPORTS IN WHICH FAILURE TO USE ASEPTIC TECHNIQUE WHEN HANDLING PROPOFOL INJECTABLE EMULSION WAS ASSOCIATED WITH MICROBIAL CONTAMINATION OF THE PRODUCT AND WITH FEVER, INFECTION/SEPSIS, OTHER LIFE-THREATENING ILLNESS, AND/OR DEATH.

CLINICAL PHARMACOLOGY

GENERAL

Propofol injectable emulsion is an intravenous sedative-hypnotic agent for use in the induction and maintenance of anesthesia or sedation. Intravenous injection of a therapeutic dose of propofol produces hypnosis rapidly with minimal excitation, usually within 40 seconds from the start of an injection (the time for one arm-brain circulation). As with other rapidly acting intravenous anesthetic agents, the half-time of the blood-brain equilibration is approximately 1-3 minutes, and this accounts for the rapid induction of anesthesia.

PHARMACODYNAMICS

Pharmacodynamic properties of propofol are dependent upon the therapeutic blood propofol concentrations. Steady state propofol blood concentrations are generally proportional to infusion rates, especially within an individual patient. Undesirable side effects such as cardiorespiratory depression are likely to occur at higher blood concentrations which result from bolus dosing or rapid increase in infusion rate. An adequate interval (3-5 minutes) must be allowed between clinical dosage adjustments in order to assess drug effects.

The hemodynamic effects of propofol injectable emulsion during induction of anesthesia vary. If spontaneous ventilation is maintained, the major cardiovascular effects are arterial hypotension (sometimes greater than a 30% decrease) with little or no change in heart rate and no appreciable decrease in cardiac output. If ventilation is assisted or controlled (positive pressure ventilation), the degree and incidence of decrease in cardiac output are accentuated. Addition of a potent opioid (*e.g.,* fentanyl) when used as a premedicant further decreases cardiac output and respiratory drive.

If anesthesia is continued by infusion of propofol injectable emulsion, the stimulation of endotracheal intubation and surgery may return arterial pressure towards normal. However, cardiac output may remain depressed. Comparative clinical studies have shown that the hemodynamic effects of propofol injectable emulsion during induction of anesthesia are generally more pronounced than with other IV induction agents traditionally used for this purpose.

Clinical and preclinical studies suggest that propofol injectable emulsion is rarely associated with elevation of plasma histamine levels.

Induction of anesthesia with propofol injectable emulsion is frequently associated with apnea in both adult and pediatric patients. In 1573 adult patients who received propofol injectable emulsion (2-2.5 mg/kg), apnea lasted less than 30 seconds in 7% of patients, 30-60 seconds in 24% of patients, and more than 60 seconds in 12% of patients. In 218 pediatric patients from birth through 16 years of age assessable for apnea who received bolus doses of propofol injectable emulsion (1-3.6 mg/kg), apnea lasted less than 30 seconds in 12% of patients, 30-60 seconds in 10% of patients, and more than 60 seconds in 5% of patients.

During maintenance, propofol injectable emulsion causes a decrease in ventilation usually associated with an increase in carbon dioxide tension which may be marked depending upon the rate of administration and other concurrent medications (*e.g.,* opioids, sedatives, etc.).

During monitored anesthesia care (MAC) sedation, attention must be given to the cardiorespiratory effects of propofol injectable emulsion. Hypotension, oxyhemoglobin desaturation, apnea, airway obstruction, and/or oxygen desaturation can occur, especially following a rapid bolus of propofol injectable emulsion. During initiation of MAC sedation, slow infusion or slow injection techniques are preferable over rapid bolus administration, and during maintenance of MAC sedation, a variable rate infusion is preferable over intermittent bolus administration in order to minimize undesirable cardiorespiratory effects. In the elderly, debilitated, or ASA III/IV patients, rapid (single or repeated) bolus dose administration should not be used for MAC sedation. (See WARNINGS.)

Clinical studies in humans and studies in animals show that propofol injectable emulsion does not suppress the adrenal response to ACTH.

Preliminary findings in patients with normal intraocular pressure indicate that propofol injectable emulsion anesthesia produces a decrease in intraocular pressure which may be associated with a concomitant decrease in systemic vascular resistance.

Animal studies and limited experience in susceptible patients have not indicated any propensity of propofol injectable emulsion to induce malignant hyperthermia.

Studies to date indicate that propofol injectable emulsion when used in combination with hypocarbia increases cerebrovascular resistance and decreases cerebral blood flow, cerebral metabolic oxygen consumption, and intracranial pressure. Propofol injectable emulsion does not affect cerebrovascular reactivity to changes in arterial carbon dioxide tension.

Hemosiderin deposits have been observed in the livers of dogs receiving propofol injectable emulsion containing 0.005% disodium edetate over a 4 week period; the clinical significance is unknown.

PHARMACOKINETICS

The proper use of propofol injectable emulsion requires an understanding of the disposition and elimination characteristics of propofol.

The pharmacokinetics of propofol are well described by a three compartment linear model with compartments representing the plasma, rapidly equilibrating tissues, and slowly equilibrating tissues.

Following an IV bolus dose, there is rapid equilibration between the plasma and the highly perfused tissue of the brain, thus accounting for the rapid onset of anesthesia. Plasma levels initially decline rapidly as a result of both rapid distribution and high metabolic clearance. Distribution accounts for about half of this decline following a bolus of propofol.

However, distribution is not constant over time, but decreases as body tissues equilibrate with plasma and become saturated. The rate at which equilibration occurs is a function of the rate and duration of the infusion. When equilibration occurs there is no longer a net transfer of propofol between tissues and plasma.

Discontinuation of the recommended doses of propofol injectable emulsion after the maintenance of anesthesia for approximately 1 hour, or for sedation in the ICU for 1 day, results in a prompt decrease in blood propofol concentrations and rapid awakening. Longer infusions (10 days of ICU sedation) result in accumulation of significant tissue stores of propofol, such that the reduction in circulating propofol is slowed and the time to awakening is increased.

By daily titration of propofol injectable emulsion dosage to achieve only the minimum effective therapeutic concentration, rapid awakening within 10-15 minutes will occur even after long-term administration. If, however, higher than necessary infusion levels have been maintained for a long time, propofol will be redistributed from fat and muscle to the plasma, and this return of propofol from peripheral tissues will slow recovery.

The large contribution of distribution (about 50%) to the fall of propofol plasma levels following brief infusions means that after very long infusions (at steady state), about half the initial rate will maintain the same plasma levels. Failure to reduce the infusion rate in patients receiving propofol injectable emulsion for extended periods may result in excessively high blood concentrations of the drug. Thus, titration to clinical response and daily evaluation of sedation levels are important during use of propofol injectable emulsion infusion for ICU sedation, especially of long duration.

Adults

Propofol clearance ranges from 23-50 ml/kg/min (1.6-3.4 L/min in 70 kg adults). It is chiefly eliminated by hepatic conjugation to inactive metabolites which are excreted by the kidney. A glucuronide conjugate accounts for about 50% of the administered dose. Propofol has a steady state volume of distribution (10 day infusion) approaching 60 L/kg in healthy adults. A difference in pharmacokinetics due to gender has not been observed. The terminal half-life of propofol after a 10 day infusion is 1-3 days.

Geriatrics

With increasing patient age, the dose of propofol needed to achieve a defined anesthetic end point (dose-requirement) decreases. This does not appear to be an age-related change of pharmacodynamics or brain sensitivity, as measured by EEG burst suppression. With increasing patient age pharmacokinetic changes are such that for a given IV bolus dose, higher peak plasma concentrations occur, which can explain the decreased dose requirement. These higher peak plasma concentrations in the elderly can predispose patients to cardiorespiratory effects including hypotension, apnea, airway obstruction, and/or oxygen desaturation. The higher plasma levels reflect an age-related decrease in volume of distribution and reduced intercompartmental clearance. Lower doses are thus recommended for initiation and maintenance of sedation/anesthesia in elderly patients. (See Individualization of Dosage.)

Pediatrics

The pharmacokinetics of propofol were studied in 53 children between the ages of 3 and 12 years who received propofol injectable emulsion for periods of approximately 1-2 hours. The observed distribution and clearance of propofol in these children were similar to adults.

Organ Failure

The pharmacokinetics of propofol do not appear to be different in people with chronic hepatic cirrhosis or chronic renal impairment compared to adults with normal hepatic and renal function. The effects of acute hepatic or renal failure on the pharmacokinetics of propofol have not been studied.

INDIVIDUALIZATION OF DOSAGES

General

STRICT ASEPTIC TECHNIQUE MUST ALWAYS BE MAINTAINED DURING HANDLING. PROPOFOL INJECTABLE EMULSION IS A SINGLE-USE PARENTERAL PRODUCT WHICH CONTAINS 0.005% DISODIUM EDETATE TO RETARD THE RATE OF GROWTH OF MICROORGANISMS IN THE EVENT OF ACCIDENTAL EXTRINSIC CONTAMINATION. HOWEVER, PROPOFOL INJECTABLE EMULSION CAN STILL SUPPORT THE GROWTH OF MICROORGANISMS AS IT IS NOT AN ANTIMICROBIALLY PRESERVED PRODUCT UNDER USP STANDARDS. ACCORDINGLY, STRICT ASEPTIC TECHNIQUE MUST STILL BE ADHERED TO. DO NOT USE IF CONTAMINATION IS SUSPECTED. DISCARD UNUSED PORTIONS AS DIRECTED WITHIN THE REQUIRED TIME LIMITS (SEE DOSAGE AND ADMINISTRATION, HANDLING PROCEDURES). THERE HAVE BEEN REPORTS IN WHICH FAILURE TO USE ASEPTIC TECHNIQUE WHEN HANDLING PROPOFOL INJECTABLE EMULSION WAS ASSOCIATED WITH MICROBIAL CONTAMINATION OF THE PRODUCT AND WITH FEVER, INFECTION/SEPSIS, OTHER LIFE-THREATENING ILLNESS, AND/OR DEATH.

Propofol blood concentrations at steady state are generally proportional to infusion rates, especially in individual patients. Undesirable effects such as cardiorespiratory depression are likely to occur at higher blood concentrations which result from bolus dosing or rapid increases in the infusion rate. An adequate interval (3-5 minutes) must be allowed between clinical dosage adjustments in order to assess drug effects.

When administering propofol injectable emulsion by infusion, syringe pumps, or volumetric pumps are recommended to provide controlled infusion rates. When infusing propofol injectable emulsion to patients undergoing magnetic resonance imaging, metered control devices may be utilized if mechanical pumps are impractical.

Changes in vital signs (increases in pulse rate, blood pressure, sweating, and/or tearing) that indicate a response to surgical stimulation or lightening of anesthesia may be controlled by the administration of propofol injectable emulsion 25 mg (2.5 ml) to 50 mg (5 ml) incremental boluses and/or by increasing the infusion rate.

For minor surgical procedures (*e.g.,* body surface) nitrous oxide (60-70%) can be combined with a variable rate propofol injectable emulsion infusion to provide satisfactory anesthesia. With more stimulating surgical procedures (*e.g.,* intra-abdominal), or if supplementation with nitrous oxide is not provided, administration rate(s) of propofol injectable emulsion and/or opioids should be increased in order to provide adequate anesthesia.

Infusion rates should always be titrated downward in the absence of clinical signs of light anesthesia until a mild response to surgical stimulation is obtained in order to avoid administration of propofol injectable emulsion at rates higher than are clinically necessary. Generally, rates of 50-100 μg/kg/min in adults should be achieved during maintenance in order to optimize recovery times.

Other drugs that cause CNS depression (hypnotics/sedatives, inhalational anesthetics, and opioids) can increase CNS depression induced by propofol. Morphine premedication (0.15 mg/kg) with nitrous oxide 67% in oxygen has been shown to decrease the necessary propofol injection maintenance infusion rate and therapeutic blood concentrations when compared to non-narcotic (lorazepam) premedication.

Induction of General Anesthesia

Adult Patients

Most adult patients under 55 years of age and classified ASA I/II require 2-2.5 mg/kg of propofol injectable emulsion for induction when unpremedicated or when premedicated with oral benzodiazepines or intramuscular opioids. For induction, propofol injectable emulsion should be titrated (approximately 40 mg every 10 seconds) against the response of the patient until the clinical signs show the onset of anesthesia. As with other sedative-hypnotic agents, the amount of intravenous opioid and/or benzodiazepine premedication will influence the response of the patient to an induction dose of propofol injectable emulsion.

Elderly, Debilitated, or ASA III/IV Patients

It is important to be familiar and experienced with the intravenous use of propofol injectable emulsion before treating elderly, debilitated, or ASA III/IV patients. Due to the reduced clearance and higher blood concentrations, most of these patients require approximately 1-1.5 mg/kg (approximately 20 mg every 10 seconds) of propofol injectable emulsion for induction of anesthesia according to their condition and responses. A rapid bolus should not be used, as this will increase the likelihood of undesirable cardiorespiratory depression including hypotension, apnea, airway obstruction, and/or oxygen desaturation. (See DOSAGE AND ADMINISTRATION.)

Pediatric Patients

Most patients aged 3 years through 16 years and classified ASA I or II require 2.5-3.5 mg/kg of propofol injectable emulsion for induction when unpremedicated or when lightly premedicated with oral benzodiazepines or intramuscular opioids. Within this dosage range, younger pediatric patients may require higher induction doses than older pediatric patients. As with other sedative-hypnotic agents, the amount of intravenous opioid and/or benzodiazepine premedication will influence the response of the patient to an induction dose of propofol injectable emulsion. A lower dosage is recommended for pediatric patients classified as ASA III or IV. Attention should be paid to minimize pain on injection when administering propofol injectable emulsion to pediatric patients. Boluses of propofol injectable emulsion may be administered via small veins if pretreated with lidocaine or via antecubital or larger veins (see PRECAUTIONS, General).

Neurosurgical Patients

Slower induction is recommended using boluses of 20 mg every 10 seconds. Slower boluses or infusions of propofol injectable emulsion for induction of anesthesia, titrated to clinical responses, will generally result in reduced induction dosage requirements (1-2 mg/kg). (See PRECAUTIONS and DOSAGE AND ADMINISTRATION.)

Cardiac Anesthesia

Propofol injectable emulsion has been well-studied in patients with coronary artery disease, but experience in patients with hemodynamically significant valvular or congenital heart disease is limited. As with other anesthetic and sedative-hypnotic agents, propofol injectable emulsion in healthy patients causes a decrease in blood pressure that is secondary to decreases in preload (ventricular filling volume at the end of the diastole) and afterload (arterial resistance at the beginning of the systole). The magnitude of these changes is proportional to the blood and effect site concentrations achieved. These concentrations depend upon the dose and speed of the induction and maintenance infusion rates.

In addition, lower heart rates are observed during maintenance with propofol injectable emulsion, possibly due to reduction of the sympathetic activity and/or resetting of the baroreceptor reflexes. Therefore, anticholinergic agents should be administered when increases in vagal tone are anticipated.

As with other anesthetic agents, propofol injectable emulsion reduces myocardial oxygen consumption. Further studies are needed to confirm and delineate the extent of these effects on the myocardium and the coronary vascular system.

Morphine premedication (0.15 mg/kg) with nitrous oxide 67% in oxygen has been shown to decrease the necessary propofol injectable emulsion maintenance infusion rates and therapeutic blood concentrations when compared to non-narcotic (lorazepam) premedication. The rate of propofol injectable emulsion administration should be determined based on the patient's premedication and adjusted according to clinical responses.

A rapid bolus induction should be avoided. A slow rate of approximately 20 mg every 10 seconds until induction onset (0.5-1.5 mg/kg) should be used. In order to assure adequate anesthesia, when propofol injectable emulsion is used as the primary agent, maintenance infusion rates should not be less than 100 μg/kg/min and should be supplemented with analgesic levels of continuous opioid administration. When an opioid is used as the primary agent, propofol injectable emulsion maintenance rates should not be less than 50 μg/kg/min, and care should be taken to ensure amnesia with concomitant benzodiazepines. Higher doses of propofol injectable emulsion will reduce the opioid requirements (see TABLE 1). When propofol injectable emulsion is used as the primary anesthetic, it should not be administered with the high-dose opioid technique, as this may increase the likelihood of hypotension (see PRECAUTIONS, General, Cardiac Anesthesia).

TABLE 1 *Cardiac Anesthesia Techniques*

Primary Agent: Rate	Secondary Agent: Rate*
Propofol Injectable Emulsion *Preinduction anxiolysis:* 25 μg/kg/min *Induction:* 0.5-1.5 mg/kg over 60 seconds *Maintenance (titrated to clinical response):* 100-150 μg/kg/min	Opioid†: 0.05-0.75 μg/kg/min (no bolus)
Opioid‡ *Induction:* 25-50 μg/kg *Maintenance:* 0.2-0.3 μg/kg/min	Propofol injectable emulsion: 50-100 μg/kg/min (no bolus)

* Following induction with primary agent.
† Opioid is defined in terms of fentanyl equivalents, *i.e.*, 1 μg of fentanyl = 5 μg of alfentanil (for bolus) = 10 μg of alfentanil (for maintenance) or = 0.1 μg of sufentanil.
‡ Care should be taken to ensure amnesia with concomitant benzodiazepine therapy.

P

Maintenance of General Anesthesia

Adult Patients

In adults, anesthesia can be maintained by administering propofol injectable emulsion by infusion or intermittent IV bolus injection. The patient's clinical response will determine the infusion rate or the amount and frequency of incremental injections.

Continuous Infusion

Propofol injectable emulsion 100-200 μg/kg/min administered in a variable rate infusion with 60-70% nitrous oxide and oxygen provides anesthesia for patients undergoing general surgery. Maintenance by infusion of propofol injectable emulsion should immediately follow the induction dose in order to provide satisfactory or continuous anesthesia during the induction phase. During this initial period following the induction dose, higher rates of infusion are generally required (150-200 μg/kg/min) for the first 10-15 minutes. Infusion rates should subsequently be decreased 30-50% during the first half-hour of maintenance. Generally, rates of 50-100 μg/kg/min in adults should be achieved during maintenance in order to optimize recovery times.

Other drugs that cause CNS depression (hypnotics/sedatives, inhalational anesthetics, and opioids) can increase the CNS depression induced by propofol.

Intermittent Bolus

Increments of propofol injectable emulsion 25 mg (2.5 ml) to 50 mg (5 ml) may be administered with nitrous oxide in adult patients undergoing general surgery. The incremental boluses should be administered when changes in vital signs indicate a response to surgical stimulation or light anesthesia.

Pediatric Patients

Propofol injectable emulsion administered as a variable rate infusion supplemented with nitrous oxide 60-70% provides satisfactory anesthesia for most children 2 months of age or older, ASA class I or II, undergoing general anesthesia.

In general, for the pediatric population, maintenance by infusion of propofol injectable emulsion at a rate of 200-300 μg/kg/min should immediately follow the induction dose. Following the first half-hour of maintenance, infusion rates of 125-150 μg/kg/min are typically needed. Propofol injectable emulsion SHOULD BE TITRATED TO ACHIEVE THE DESIRED CLINICAL EFFECT. Younger pediatric patients may require higher maintenance infusion rates than older pediatric patients.

Propofol injectable emulsion has been used with a variety of agents commonly used in anesthesia such as atropine, scopolamine, glycopyrrolate, diazepam, depolarizing and non-depolarizing muscle relaxants, and opioid analgesics, as well as with inhalational and regional anesthetic agents.

In the elderly, debilitated, or ASA III/IV patients, rapid bolus doses should not be used, as this will increase cardiorespiratory effects including hypotension, apnea, airway obstruction, and/or oxygen desaturation.

Monitored Anesthesia Care (MAC) Sedation — Adult Patients

When propofol injectable emulsion is administered for MAC sedation, rates of administration should be individualized and titrated to clinical response. In most patients, the rates of propofol injectable emulsion administration will be in the range of 25-75 μg/kg/min.

During initiation of MAC sedation, slow infusion or slow injection techniques are preferable over rapid bolus administration. During maintenance of MAC sedation, a variable rate infusion is preferable over intermittent bolus dose administration. In the elderly, debilitated, or ASA III/IV patients, rapid (single or repeated) bolus dose administration should not be used for MAC sedation. (See WARNINGS.) **A rapid bolus injection can result in undesirable cardiorespiratory depression including hypotension, apnea, airway obstruction, and/or oxygen desaturation.**

Initiation of MAC Sedation

For initiation of MAC sedation, either an infusion or a slow injection method may be utilized while closely monitoring cardiorespiratory function. With the infusion method, sedation may be initiated by infusing propofol injectable emulsion at 100-150 μg/kg/min (6-9 mg/kg/h) for a period of 3-5 minutes and titrating to the desired clinical effect while closely monitoring respiratory function. With the slow injection method for initiation, patients will require approximately 0.5 mg/kg administered over 3-5 minutes and titrated to clinical responses. When propofol injectable emulsion is administered slowly over 3-5 minutes, most patients will be adequately sedated, and the peak drug effect can be achieved while minimizing undesirable cardiorespiratory effects occurring at high plasma levels.

In the elderly, debilitated, or ASA III/IV patients, rapid (single or repeated) bolus dose administration should not be used for MAC sedation. (See WARNINGS.) The rate of administration should be over 3-5 minutes and the dosage of propofol injectable emulsion should be reduced to approximately 80% of the usual adult dosage in these patients according to their condition, responses, and changes in vital signs. (See DOSAGE AND ADMINISTRATION.)

Maintenance of MAC Sedation

For maintenance of sedation, a variable rate infusion method is preferable over an intermittent bolus dose method. With the variable rate infusion method, patients will generally require maintenance rates of 25-75 μg/kg/min (1.5-4.5 mg/kg/h) during the first 10-15 minutes of sedation maintenance. Infusion rates should subsequently be decreased over time to 25-50 μg/kg/min and adjusted to clinical responses. In titrating to clinical effect, allow approximately 2 minutes for onset of peak drug effect.

Infusion rates should always be titrated downward in the absence of clinical signs of light sedation until mild responses to stimulation are obtained in order to avoid sedative administration of propofol injectable emulsion at rates higher than are clinically necessary.

If the intermittent bolus dose method is used, increments of propofol injectable emulsion 10 mg (1 ml) or 20 mg (2 ml) can be administered and titrated to desired clinical effect. With the intermittent bolus method of sedation maintenance, there is the potential for respiratory depression, transient increases in sedation depth, and/or prolongation of recovery.

In the elderly, debilitated, or ASA III/IV patients, rapid (single or repeated) bolus dose administration should not be used for MAC sedation. (See WARNINGS.) The rate of administration and the dosage of propofol injectable emulsion should be reduced to approximately 80% of the usual adult dosage in these patients according to their condition, responses, and changes in vital signs. (See DOSAGE AND ADMINISTRATION.)

Propofol injectable emulsion can be administered as the sole agent for maintenance of MAC sedation during surgical/diagnostic procedures. When propofol injectable emulsion sedation is supplemented with opioid and/or benzodiazepine medications, these agents increase the sedative and respiratory effects of propofol injectable emulsion and may also result in a slower recovery profile. (See DRUG INTERACTIONS.)

ICU Sedation — Adult Patients

See WARNINGS and DOSAGE AND ADMINISTRATION, Handling Procedures.

For intubated, mechanically ventilated adult patients, Intensive Care Unit (ICU) sedation should be initiated slowly with a continuous infusion in order to titrate to desired clinical effect and minimize hypotension. (See DOSAGE AND ADMINISTRATION.)

Across all 6 US/Canadian clinical studies, the mean infusion maintenance rate for all propofol injectable emulsion patients was 27 ± 21 μg/kg/min. The maintenance infusion rates required to maintain adequate sedation ranged from 2.8-130 μg/kg/min. The infusion rate was lower in patients over 55 years of age (approximately 20 μg/kg/min) compared to patients under 55 years of age (approximately 38 μg/kg/min). In these studies, morphine or fentanyl was used as needed for analgesia.

Most adult ICU patients recovering from the effects of general anesthesia or deep sedation will require maintenance rates of 5-50 μg/kg/min (0.3-3 mg/kg/h) individualized and titrated to clinical response. (See DOSAGE AND ADMINISTRATION.) With medical ICU patients or patients who have recovered from the effects of general anesthesia or deep sedation, the rate of administration of 50 μg/kg/min or higher may be required to achieve adequate sedation. These higher rates of administration may increase the likelihood of patients developing hypotension.

Although there are reports of reduced analgesic requirements, most patients received opioids for analgesia during maintenance of ICU sedation. Some patients also received benzodiazepines and/or neuromuscular blocking agents. During long-term maintenance of sedation, some ICU patients were awakened once or twice every 24 hours for assessment of neurologic or respiratory function.

In post-CABG (coronary artery bypass graft) patients, the maintenance rate of propofol administration was usually low (median 11 μg/kg/min) due to the intraoperative administration of high opioid doses. Patients receiving propofol injectable emulsion required 35%

less nitroprusside than midazolam patients; this difference was statistically significant (P <0.05). During initiation of sedation in post-CABG patients, a 15-20% decrease in blood pressure was seen in the first 60 minutes. It was not possible to determine cardiovascular effects in patients with severely compromised ventricular function.

In Medical or Postsurgical ICU studies comparing propofol injectable emulsion to benzodiazepine infusion or bolus, there were no apparent differences in maintenance of adequate sedation, mean arterial pressure, or laboratory findings. Like the comparators, propofol injectable emulsion reduced blood cortisol during sedation while maintaining responsivity to challenges with adrenocorticotropic hormone (ACTH). Case reports from the published literature generally reflect that propofol injectable emulsion has been used safely in patients with a history of porphyria or malignant hyperthermia.

In hemodynamically stable head trauma patients ranging in age from 19-43 years, adequate sedation was maintained with propofol injectable emulsion or morphine (n=7 in each group). There were no apparent differences in adequacy of sedation, intracranial pressure, cerebral perfusion pressure, or neurologic recovery between the treatment groups. In literature reports from Neurosurgical ICU and severely head-injured patients propofol injectable emulsion infusion with or without diuretics and hyperventilation controlled intracranial pressure while maintaining cerebral perfusion pressure. In some patients, bolus doses resulted in decreased blood pressure and compromised cerebral perfusion pressure.

Propofol injectable emulsion was found to be effective in status epilepticus which was refractory to the standard anticonvulsant therapies. For these patients as well as for ARDS/respiratory failure and tetanus patients, sedation maintenance dosages were generally higher than those for other critically ill patient populations.

Abrupt discontinuation of propofol injectable emulsion prior to weaning or for daily evaluation of sedation levels should be avoided. This may result in rapid awakening with associated anxiety, agitation, and resistance to mechanical ventilation. Infusions of propofol injectable emulsion should be adjusted to maintain a light level of sedation through the weaning process or evaluation of sedation level. (See PRECAUTIONS.)

INDICATIONS AND USAGE

Propofol injectable emulsion is an IV sedative-hypnotic agent that can be used for both induction and/or maintenance of anesthesia as part of a balanced anesthetic technique for inpatient and outpatient surgery in adult patients and pediatric patients greater than 3 years of age. Propofol injectable emulsion can also be used for maintenance of anesthesia as part of a balanced anesthetic technique for inpatient and outpatient surgery in adult patients and in pediatric patients greater than 2 months of age. Propofol is not recommended for induction of anesthesia below the age of 3 years or for maintenance of anesthesia below the age of 2 months because its safety and effectiveness have not been established in those populations.

In adult patients, propofol injectable emulsion, when administered intravenously as directed, can be used to initiate and maintain monitored anesthesia care (MAC) sedation during diagnostic procedures. Propofol injectable emulsion may also be used for MAC sedation in conjunction with local/regional anesthesia in patients undergoing surgical procedures. (See PRECAUTIONS.)

Safety, effectiveness and dosing guidelines for propofol injectable emulsion have not been established for MAC sedation/light general anesthesia in the pediatric population undergoing diagnostic or nonsurgical procedures and therefore it is not recommended for this use. (See PRECAUTIONS, Pediatric Use.)

Propofol injectable emulsion should only be administered to intubated, mechanically ventilated adult patients in the Intensive Care Unit (ICU) to provide continuous sedation and control of stress responses. In this setting, propofol injectable emulsion should be administered only by persons skilled in the medical management of critically ill patients and trained in cardiovascular resuscitation and airway management.

Propofol injectable emulsion is not indicated for use in Pediatric ICU sedation since the safety of this regimen has not been established. (See PRECAUTIONS, Pediatric Use.)

Propofol injectable emulsion is not recommended for obstetrics, including cesarean section deliveries. Propofol injectable emulsion crosses the placenta, and as with other general anesthetic agents, the administration of propofol injectable emulsion may be associated with neonatal depression. (See PRECAUTIONS.)

Propofol injectable emulsion is not recommended for use in nursing mothers because propofol injectable emulsion has been reported to be excreted in human milk, and the effects of oral absorption of small amounts of propofol are not known. (See PRECAUTIONS.)

NON-FDA APPROVED INDICATIONS

Propofol has also been used as a sedative in conjunction with regional or local anesthesia for diagnostic procedures, and in other clinical situations such as ophthalmic surgery, cardioversion, laryngeal mask airway insertion, refractory status epilepticus, refractory nausea and vomiting, electroconvulsive therapy, and patient-controlled analgesia; however, these uses are not FDA approved.

CONTRAINDICATIONS

Propofol injectable emulsion is contraindicated in patients with a known hypersensitivity to propofol injectable emulsion or its components, or when general anesthesia or sedation are contraindicated.

WARNINGS

For general anesthesia or monitored anesthesia care (MAC) sedation, propofol injectable emulsion should be administered only by persons trained in the administration of general anesthesia and not involved in the conduct of the surgical/diagnostic procedure. Patients should be continuously monitored, and facilities for maintenance of a patent airway, artificial ventilation, and oxygen enrichment and circulatory resuscitation must be immediately available.

For sedation of intubated, mechanically ventilated adult patients in the Intensive Care Unit (ICU), propofol injectable emulsion should be administered only by persons skilled in the management of critically ill patients and trained in cardiovascular resuscitation and airway management.

In the elderly, debilitated, or ASA III/IV patients, rapid (single or repeated) bolus administration should not be used during general anesthesia or MAC sedation in order to minimize undesirable cardiorespiratory depression, including hypotension, apnea, airway obstruction, and/or oxygen desaturation.

MAC sedation patients should be continuously monitored by persons not involved in the conduct of the surgical or diagnostic procedure; oxygen supplementation should be immediately available and provided where clinically indicated; and oxygen saturation should be monitored in all patients. Patients should be continuously monitored for early signs of hypotension, apnea, airway obstruction, and/or oxygen desaturation. These cardiorespiratory effects are more likely to occur following rapid initiation (loading) boluses or during supplemental maintenance boluses, especially in the elderly, debilitated, or ASA III/IV patients.

Propofol injectable emulsion should not be coadministered through the same IV catheter with blood or plasma because compatibility has not been established. *In vitro* tests have shown that aggregates of the globular component of the emulsion vehicle have occurred with blood/plasma/serum from humans and animals. The clinical significance is not known.

STRICT ASEPTIC TECHNIQUE MUST ALWAYS BE MAINTAINED DURING HANDLING. PROPOFOL INJECTABLE EMULSION IS A SINGLE-USE PARENTERAL PRODUCT WHICH CONTAINS 0.005% DISODIUM EDETATE TO RETARD THE RATE OF GROWTH OF MICROORGANISMS IN THE EVENT OF ACCIDENTAL EXTRINSIC CONTAMINATION. HOWEVER, PROPOFOL INJECTABLE EMULSION CAN STILL SUPPORT THE GROWTH OF MICROORGANISMS AS IT IS NOT AN ANTIMICROBIALLY PRESERVED PRODUCT UNDER USP STANDARDS. ACCORDINGLY, STRICT ASEPTIC TECHNIQUE MUST STILL BE ADHERED TO. DO NOT USE IF CONTAMINATION IS SUSPECTED. DISCARD UNUSED PORTIONS AS DIRECTED WITHIN THE REQUIRED TIME LIMITS (SEE DOSAGE AND ADMINISTRATION, HANDLING PROCEDURES). THERE HAVE BEEN REPORTS IN WHICH FAILURE TO USE ASEPTIC TECHNIQUE WHEN HANDLING PROPOFOL INJECTABLE EMULSION WAS ASSOCIATED WITH MICROBIAL CONTAMINATION OF THE PRODUCT AND WITH FEVER, INFECTION/SEPSIS, OTHER LIFE-THREATENING ILLNESS, AND/OR DEATH.

PRECAUTIONS

GENERAL

Adult and Pediatric Patients

A lower induction dose and a slower maintenance rate of administration should be used in elderly, debilitated, or ASA III/IV patients. (See CLINICAL PHARMACOLOGY, Individualization of Dosages.) Patients should be continuously monitored for early signs of significant hypotension and/or bradycardia. Treatment may include increasing the rate of intravenous fluid, elevation of lower extremities, use of pressor agents, or administration of atropine. Apnea often occurs during induction and may persist for more than 60 seconds. Ventilatory support may be required. Because propofol injectable emulsion is an emulsion, caution should be exercised in patients with disorders of lipid metabolism such as primary hyperlipoproteinemia, diabetic hyperlipemia, and pancreatitis.

Very rarely the use of propofol may be associated with the development of a period of postoperative unconsciousness which may be accompanied by an increase in muscle tone. This may or may not be preceded by a brief period of wakefulness. Recovery is spontaneous. The clinical criteria for discharge from the recovery/day surgery area established for each institution should be satisfied before discharge of the patient from the care of the anesthesiologist.

When propofol injectable emulsion is administered to an epileptic patient, there may be a risk of seizure during the recovery phase.

Attention should be paid to minimize pain on administration of propofol injectable emulsion. Transient local pain can be minimized if the larger veins of the forearm or antecubital fossa are used. Pain during intravenous injection may also be reduced by prior injection of IV lidocaine (1 ml of a 1% solution). Pain on injection occurred frequently in pediatric patients (45%) when a small vein of the hand was utilized without lidocaine pretreatment. With lidocaine pretreatment or when antecubital veins were utilized, pain was minimal (incidence less than 10%) and well-tolerated.

Venous sequelae (phlebitis or thrombosis) have been reported rarely (<1%). In two well-controlled clinical studies using dedicated intravenous catheters, no instances of venous sequelae were observed up to 14 days following induction.

Intra-arterial injection in animals did not induce local tissue effects. Accidental intra-arterial injection has been reported in patients, and, other than pain, there were no major sequelae.

Intentional injection into subcutaneous or perivascular tissues of animals caused minimal tissue reaction. During the post-marketing period, there have been rare reports of local pain, swelling, blisters, and/or tissue necrosis following accidental extravasation of propofol injectable emulsion.

Perioperative myoclonia, rarely including convulsions and opisthotonos, has occurred in temporal relationship in cases in which propofol injectable emulsion has been administered.

Clinical features of anaphylaxis, which may include angioedema, bronchospasm, erythema, and hypotension, occur rarely following propofol injectable emulsion administration, although use of other drugs in most instances makes the relationship to propofol injectable emulsion unclear.

There have been rare reports of pulmonary edema in temporal relationship to the administration of propofol injectable emulsion, although a causal relationship is unknown.

Very rarely, cases of unexplained postoperative pancreatitis (requiring hospital admission) have been reported after anesthesia in which propofol injectable emulsion was one of the induction agents used. Due to a variety of confounding factors in these cases, including concomitant medications, a causal relationship to propofol injectable emulsion is unclear.

Propofol injectable emulsion has no vagolytic activity. Reports of bradycardia, asystole, and rarely, cardiac arrest have been associated with propofol injectable emulsion. Pediatric patients are susceptible to this effect, particularly when fentanyl is given concomitantly. The intravenous administration of anticholinergic agents (*e.g.*, atropine or glycopyrrolate) should be considered to modify potential increases in vagal tone due to concomitant agents (*e.g.*, succinylcholine) or surgical stimuli.

P

Intensive Care Unit Sedation — Adult Patients

See WARNINGS and DOSAGE AND ADMINISTRATION, Handling Procedures.

The administration of propofol injectable emulsion should be initiated as a continuous infusion and changes in the rate of administration made slowly (>5 min) in order to minimize hypotension and avoid acute overdosage. (See CLINICAL PHARMACOLOGY, Individualization of Dosages.)

Patients should be monitored for early signs of significant hypotension and/or cardiovascular depression, which may be profound. These effects are responsive to discontinuation of propofol injectable emulsion, IV fluid administration, and/or vasopressor therapy.

As with other sedative medications, there is wide interpatient variability in propofol injectable emulsion dosage requirements, and these requirements may change with time.

Failure to reduce the infusion rate in patients receiving propofol injectable emulsion for extended periods may result in excessively high blood concentrations of the drug. Thus, titration to clinical response and daily evaluation of sedation levels are important during use of propofol injectable emulsion infusion for ICU sedation, especially of long duration.

Opioids and paralytic agents should be discontinued and respiratory function optimized prior to weaning patients from mechanical ventilation. Infusions of propofol injectable emulsion should be adjusted to maintain a light level of sedation prior to weaning patients from mechanical ventilatory support. Throughout the weaning process, this level of sedation may be maintained in the absence of respiratory depression. Because of the rapid clearance of propofol injectable emulsion, abrupt discontinuation of a patient's infusion may result in rapid awakening of the patient with associated anxiety, agitation, and resistance to mechanical ventilation, making weaning from mechanical ventilation difficult. It is therefore recommended that administration of propofol injectable emulsion be continued in order to maintain a light level of sedation throughout the weaning process until 10-15 minutes prior to extubation, at which time the infusion can be discontinued.

There have been very rare reports of rhdomyolysis associated with the administration of propofol for ICU sedation.

Since propofol injectable emulsion is formulated in an oil-in-water emulsion, elevations in serum triglycerides may occur when propofol injectable emulsion is administered for extended periods of time. Patients at risk of hyperlipidemia should be monitored for increases in serum triglycerides or serum turbidity. Administration of propofol injectable emulsion should be adjusted if fat is being inadequately cleared from the body. A reduction in the quantity of concurrently administered lipids is indicated to compensate for the amount of lipid infused as part of the propofol injectable emulsion formulation; 1 ml of propofol injectable emulsion contains approximately 0.1 g of fat (1.1 kcal).

EDTA is a strong chelator of trace metals — including zinc. Although with propofol injectable emulsion there are no reports of decreased zinc levels or zinc deficiency-related adverse events, propofol injectable emulsion should not be infused for longer than 5 days without providing a drug holiday to safely replace estimated or measured urine zinc losses.

In clinical trials mean urinary zinc loss was approximately 2.5-3.0 mg/day in adult patients and 1.5-2.0 mg/day in pediatric patients.

In patients who are predisposed to zinc deficiency, such as those with burns, diarrhea, and/or major sepsis, the need for supplemental zinc should be considered during prolonged therapy with propofol injectable emulsion.

At high doses (2-3 g/day), EDTA has been reported, on rare occasions, to be toxic to the renal tubules. Studies to-date, in patients with normal or impaired renal function have not shown any alteration in renal function with propofol injectable emulsion containing 0.005% disodium edetate. In patients at risk for renal impairment, urinalysis and urine sediment should be checked before initiation of sedation and then be monitored on alternate days during sedation.

The long-term administration of propofol injectable emulsion to patients with renal failure and/or hepatic insufficiency has not been evaluated.

Neurosurgical Anesthesia

When propofol injectable emulsion is used in patients with increased intracranial pressure or impaired cerebral circulation, significant decreases in mean arterial pressure should be avoided because of the resultant decreases in cerebral perfusion pressure. To avoid significant hypotension and decreases in cerebral perfusion pressure, an infusion or slow bolus of approximately 20 mg every 10 seconds should be utilized instead of rapid, more frequent, and/or larger boluses of propofol injectable emulsion. Slower induction titrated to clinical responses, will generally result in reduced induction dosage requirements (1-2 mg/kg). When increased ICP is suspected, hyperventilation and hypocarbia should accompany the administration of propofol injectable emulsion. (See DOSAGE AND ADMINISTRATION.)

Cardiac Anesthesia

Slower rates of administration should be utilized in premedicated patients, geriatric patients, patients with recent fluid shifts, or patients who are hemodynamically unstable. Any fluid deficits should be corrected prior to administration of propofol injectable emulsion. In those patients where additional fluid therapy may be contraindicated, other measures, *e.g.*, elevation of lower extremities, or use of pressor agents, may be useful to offset the hypotension which is associated with the induction of anesthesia with propofol injectable emulsion.

INFORMATION FOR THE PATIENT

Patients should be advised that performance of activities requiring mental alertness, such as operating a motor vehicle, or hazardous machinery or signing legal documents may be impaired for some time after general anesthesia or sedation.

CARCINOGENESIS, MUTAGENESIS, AND IMPAIRMENT OF FERTILITY

Animal carcinogenicity studies have not been performed with propofol.

In vitro and *in vivo* animal tests failed to show any potential for mutagenicity by propofol. Tests for mutagenicity included the Ames (using *Salmonella* sp) mutation test, gene mutation/gene conversion using *Saccharomyces cerevisiae, in vitro* cytogenetic studies in Chinese hamsters, and a mouse micronucleus test.

Studies in female rats at intravenous doses up to 15 mg/kg/day (approximately equivalent to the recommended human induction dose on a mg/m^2 basis) for 2 weeks before pregnancy to day 7 of gestation did not show impaired fertility. Male fertility in rats was not affected in a dominant lethal study at intravenous doses up to 15 mg/kg/day for 5 days.

PREGNANCY CATEGORY B

Reproduction studies have been performed in rats and rabbits at intravenous doses of 15 mg/kg/day (approximately equivalent to the recommended human induction dose on a mg/m^2 basis) and have revealed no evidence of impaired fertility or harm to the fetus due to propofol. Propofol, however, has been shown to cause maternal deaths in rats and rabbits and decreased pup survival during the lactating period in dams treated with 15 mg/kg/day (approximately equivalent to the recommended human induction dose on a mg/m^2 basis). The pharmacological activity (anesthesia) of the drug on the mother is probably responsible for the adverse effects seen in the offspring. There are, however, no adequate and well-controlled studies in pregnant women. Because animal reproduction studies are not always predictive of human responses, this drug should be used during pregnancy only if clearly needed.

LABOR AND DELIVERY

Propofol injectable emulsion is not recommended for obstetrics, including cesarean section deliveries. Propofol injectable emulsion crosses the placenta, and as with other general anesthetic agents, the administration of propofol injectable emulsion may be associated with neonatal depression.

NURSING MOTHERS

Propofol injectable emulsion is not recommended for use in nursing mothers because propofol injectable emulsion has been reported to be excreted in human milk and the effects of oral absorption of small amounts of propofol are not known.

PEDIATRIC USE

The safety and effectiveness of propofol injectable emulsion have been established for induction of anesthesia in pediatric patients aged 3 years and older and for the maintenance of anesthesia aged 2 months and older.

Propofol injectable emulsion is not recommended for the induction of anesthesia in patients younger than 3 years of age and for the maintenance of anesthesia in patients younger than 2 months of age as safety and effectiveness have not been established.

In pediatric patients, administration of fentanyl concomitantly with propofol injectable emulsion may result in serious brady cardia. (See General.)

Propofol injectable emulsion is not indicated for use in pediatric patients for ICU sedation or for MAC sedation for surgical, nonsurgical or diagnostic procedures as safety and effectiveness have not been established.

There have been anecdotal reports of serious adverse events and death in pediatric patients with upper respiratory tract infections receiving propofol injectable emulsion for ICU sedation.

In one multicenter clinical trial of ICU sedation in critically ill pediatric patients that excluded patients with upper respiratory tract infections, the incidence of mortality observed in patients who received propofol injectable emulsion (n=222) was 9%, while that for patients who received standard sedative agents (n=105) was 4%. While causality has not been established, propofol injectable emulsion is not indicated for sedation in pediatric patients until further studies have been performed to document its safety in that population. (See CLINICAL PHARMACOLOGY, Individualization of Dosages and DOSAGE AND ADMINISTRATION.)

In pediatric patients, abrupt discontinuation following prolonged infusion may result in flushing of the hands and feet, agitation, tremulousness and hyperirritability. Increased incidences of bradycardia (5%), agitation (4%), and jitteriness (9%) have also been observed.

GERIATRIC USE

A lower induction dose and a slower maintenance rate of administration of propofol injectable emulsion should be used in elderly patients. In this group of patients, rapid (single or repeated) bolus administration should not be used in order to minimize undesirable cardiorespiratory depression including hypotension, apnea, airway obstruction and/or oxygen desaturation. All dosing should be titrated according to patient condition and response. (See DOSAGE AND ADMINISTRATION, Summary of Dosage Guidelines and CLINICAL PHARMACOLOGY, Pharmacokinetics, Geriatrics.)

DRUG INTERACTIONS

The induction dose requirements of propofol injectable emulsion may be reduced in patients with intramuscular or intravenous premedication, particularly with narcotics (*e.g.*, morphine, meperidine, and fentanyl, etc.) and combinations of opioids and sedatives (*e.g.*, benzodiazepines, barbiturates, chloral hydrate, droperidol, etc.). These agents may increase the anesthetic or sedative effects of propofol injectable emulsion and may also result in more pronounced decreases in systolic, diastolic, and mean arterial pressures and cardiac output.

During maintenance of anesthesia or sedation, the rate of propofol injectable emulsion administration should be adjusted according to the desired level of anesthesia or sedation and may be reduced in the presence of supplemental analgesic agents (*e.g.*, nitrous oxide or opioids). The concurrent administration of potent inhalational agents (*e.g.*, isoflurane, enflurane, and halothane) during maintenance with propofol injectable emulsion has not been extensively evaluated. These inhalational agents can also be expected to increase the anesthetic or sedative and cardiorespiratory effects of propofol injectable emulsion.

Propofol injectable emulsion does not cause a clinically significant change in onset, intensity or duration of action of the commonly used neuromuscular blocking agents (*e.g.*, succinylcholine and nondepolarizing muscle relaxants).

No significant adverse interactions with commonly used premedications or drugs used during anesthesia or sedation (including a range of muscle relaxants, inhalational agents, analgesic agents, and local anesthetic agents) have been observed in adults. In pediatric patients, administration of fentanyl concomitantly with propofol injectable emulsion may result in serious bradycardia.

ADVERSE REACTIONS

GENERAL

Adverse event information is derived from controlled clinical trials and worldwide marketing experience. In the description below, rates of the more common events represent US/Canadian clinical study results. Less frequent events are also derived from publications and marketing experience in over 8 million patients; there are insufficient data to support an accurate estimate of their incidence rates. These studies were conducted using a variety of premedicants, varying lengths of surgical/diagnostic procedures, and various other anesthetic/sedative agents. Most adverse events were mild and transient.

ANESTHESIA AND MAC SEDATION IN ADULTS

The following estimates of adverse events for propofol injectable emulsion include data from clinical trials in general anesthesia/MAC sedation (n=2889 adult patients). The adverse events listed below as probably causally related are those events in which the actual incidence rate in patients treated with propofol injectable emulsion was greater than the comparator incidence rate in these trials. Therefore, incidence rates for anesthesia and MAC sedation in adults generally represent estimates of the percentage of clinical trial patients which appeared to have probable causal relationship.

The adverse experience profile from reports of 150 patients in the MAC sedation clinical trials is similar to the profile established with propofol injectable emulsion during anesthesia (see below). During MAC sedation clinical trials, significant respiratory events included cough, upper airway obstruction, apnea, hypoventilation, and dyspnea.

ANESTHESIA IN PEDIATRIC PATIENTS

Generally the adverse experience profile from reports of 506 propofol injectable emulsion pediatric patients from 6 days through 16 years of age in the US/Canadian anesthesia clinical trials is similar to the profile established with propofol injectable emulsion during anesthesia in adults (see Pediatric percentages [Peds %] below). Although not reported as an adverse event in clinical trials, apnea is frequently observed in pediatric patients.

ICU SEDATION IN ADULTS

The following estimates of adverse events include data from clinical trials in ICU sedation (n=159 adult patients). Probably related incidence rates for ICU sedation were determined by individual case report form review. Probable causality was based upon an apparent dose response relationship and/or positive responses to rechallenge. In many instances the presence of concomitant disease and concomitant therapy made the causal relationship unknown. Therefore, incidence rates for ICU sedation generally represent estimates of the percentage of clinical trial patients which appeared to have a probable causal relationship.

Incidence Greater Than 1% — Probably Causally Related

Anesthesia/MAC Sedation:

Cardiovascular: Bradycardia; arrhythmia [Peds: 1.2%]; tachycardia nodal [Peds: 1.6%]; hypotension* [Peds: 17%] (see also CLINICAL PHARMACOLOGY) [hypertension Peds: 8%].

Central Nervous System: Movement* [Peds: 17%].

Injection Site: Burning/stinging or pain, 17.6% [Peds: 10%].

Respiratory: Apnea (see also CLINICAL PHARMACOLOGY).

Skin and Appendages: Rash [Peds: 5%]; pruritus [Peds: 2%].

Events without an * or % had an incidence of 1-3%.

* Incidence of events 3-10%.

ICU Sedation:

Cardiovascular: Bradycardia; decreased cardiac output; hypotension 26%.

Metabolic/Nutritional: Hyperlipemia*.

Respiratory: Respiratory acidosis during weaning*.

Events without an * or % had an incidence of 1-3%.

* Incidence of events 3-10%.

Incidence Less Than 1% - Probably Causally Related

Anesthesia/MAC Sedation:

Body as a Whole: Anaphylaxis/anaphylactoid reaction; perinatal disorder; [tachycardia]; [bigeminy]; [bradycardia]; [premature ventricular contractions]; [hemorrhage]; [ECG abnormal]; [arrhythmia atrial]; [fever]; [extremities pain]; [anticholinergic syndrome].

Cardiovascular: Premature atrial contractions; syncope.

Central Nervous System: Hypertonia/dystonia; paresthesia.

Digestive: [Hypersalivation]; [nausea].

Hemic/Lymphatic: [Leykocytosis].

Injection Site: [Phlebitis]; [pruritus].

Metabolic: [Hypomagnesemia].

Musculoskeletal: Myalgia.

Nervous: [Dizziness]; [agitation]; [chills]; [somnolence]; [delirium].

Respiratory: Wheezing; decreased lung function; [cough]; [laryngospasm]; [hypoxia].

Skin and Appendages: Flushing, pruritus.

Special Senses: Amblyopia; [vision abnormal].

Urogenital: Cloudy urine.

ICU Sedation:

Central Nervous System: Agitation.

Urogenital: Green urine.

Incidence Less Than 1% — Causal Relationship Unknown

Anesthesia/MAC Sedation:

Body as a Whole: Asthenia, awareness, chest pain, extremities pain, fever, increased drug effect, neck rigidity/stiffness, trunk pain.

Cardiovascular: Arrhythmia, atrial fibrillation, atrioventricular heart block, bigeminy, bleeding, bundle branch block, cardiac arrest, ECG abnormal, edema, extrasystole, heart block, hypertension, myocardial infarction, myocardial ischemia, premature ventricular contractions, ST segment depression, supraventricular tachycardia, tachycardia, ventricular fibrillation.

Central Nervous System: Abnormal dreams, agitation, amorous behavior, anxiety, bucking/jerking/thrashing, chills/shivering, clonic/myoclonic movement, combativeness, confusion, delirium, depression, dizziness, emotional lability, euphoria, fatigue, hallucinations, headache, hypotonia, hysteria, insomnia, moaning, neuropathy, opisthotonos, rigidity, seizures, somnolence, tremor, twitching.

Digestive: Cramping, diarrhea, dry mouth, enlarged parotid, nausea, swallowing, vomiting.

Hematologic/Lymphatic: Coagulation disorder, leukocytosis.

Injection Site: Hives/itching, phlebitis, redness/discoloration.

Metabolic/Nutritional: Hyperkalemia, hyperlipemia.

Respiratory: Bronchospasm, burning in throat, cough, dyspnea, hiccough, hyperventilation, hypoventilation, hypoxia, laryngospasm, pharyngitis, sneezing, tachypnea, upper airway obstruction.

Skin and Appendages: Conjunctival hyperemia, diaphoresis, urticaria.

Special Senses: Diplopia, ear pain, eye pain, nystagmus, taste perversion, tinnitus.

Urogenital: Oliguria, urine retention.

ICU Sedation:

Body as a Whole: Fever, sepsis, trunk pain whole body weakness.

Cardiovascular: Arrhythmia, atrial fibrillation, bigeminy, cardiac arrest, extrasystole, right heart failure, ventricular tachycardia.

Central Nervous System: Chills/shivering, intracranial hypertension, seizures, somnolence, thinking abnormal.

Digestive: Ileus, liver function abnormal.

Metabolic/Nutritional: BUN increased, creatinine, increased, dehydration, hyperglycemia, metabolic acidosis, osmolality increased.

Respiratory: Hypoxia.

Skin and Appendages: Rash.

Urogenital: Kidney failure.

DOSAGE AND ADMINISTRATION

Dosage and rate of administration should be individualized and titrated to the desired effect, according to clinically relevant factors, including preinduction and concomitant medications, age, ASA physical classification, and level of debilitation of the patient.

The following is abbreviated dosage and administration information which is only intended as a general guide in the use of propofol injectable emulsion. Prior to administering propofol injectable emulsion, it is imperative that the physician review and be completely familiar with the specific dosage and administration information detailed in the CLINICAL PHARMACOLOGY - Individualization of Dosage section.

In the elderly, debilitated, or ASA III/IV patients, rapid bolus doses should not be the method of administration. (See WARNINGS.)

INTENSIVE CARE UNIT SEDATION

STRICT ASEPTIC TECHNIQUE MUST ALWAYS BE MAINTAINED DURING HANDLING. PROPOFOL INJECTABLE EMULSION IS A SINGLE-USE PARENTERAL PRODUCT WHICH CONTAINS 0.005% DISODIUM EDETATE TO RETARD THE RATE OF GROWTH OF MICROORGANISMS IN THE EVENT OF ACCIDENTAL EXTRINSIC CONTAMINATION. HOWEVER, PROPOFOL INJECTABLE EMULSION CAN STILL SUPPORT THE GROWTH OF MICROORGANISMS AS IT IS NOT AN ANTIMICROBIALLY PRESERVED PRODUCT UNDER USP STANDARDS. ACCORDINGLY, STRICT ASEPTIC TECHNIQUE MUST STILL BE ADHERED TO. DO NOT USE IF CONTAMINATION IS SUSPECTED. (See DOSAGE AND ADMINISTRATION, Handling Procedures.)

Propofol injectable emulsion should be individualized according to the patient's condition and response, blood lipid profile, and vital signs. (See PRECAUTIONS, General, Intensive Care Unit Sedation — Adult Patients.) For intubated, mechanically ventilated adult patients, Intensive Care Unit (ICU) sedation should be initiated slowly with a continuous infusion in order to titrate to desired clinical effect and minimize hypotension. When indicated, initiation of sedation should begin at 5 μg/kg/min (0.3 mg/kg/h). The infusion rate should be increased by increments of 5-10 μg/kg/min (0.3-0.6 mg/kg/h) until the desired level of sedation is achieved. A minimum period of 5 minutes between adjustments should be allowed for onset of peak drug effect. Most adult patients require maintenance rates of 5-50 μg/kg/min (0.3-3 mg/kg/h) or higher. Dosages of propofol injectable emulsion should be reduced in patients who have received large dosages of narcotics. Conversely, the propofol injectable emulsion dosage requirement may be reduced by adequate management of pain with analgesic agents. As with other sedative medications, there is interpatient variability in dosage requirements, and these requirements may change with time. (See Summary of Dosage Guidelines.) **EVALUATION OF LEVEL OF SEDATION AND ASSESSMENT OF CNS FUNCTION SHOULD BE CARRIED OUT DAILY THROUGHOUT MAINTENANCE TO DETERMINE THE MINIMUM DOSE OF PROPOFOL INJECTABLE EMULSION REQUIRED FOR SEDATION.** Bolus administration of 10 or 20 mg should only be used to rapidly increase depth of sedation in patients where hypotension is not likely to occur. Patients with compromised myocardial function, intravascular volume depletion, or abnormally low vascular tone (*e.g.,* sepsis) may be more susceptible to hypotension. (See PRECAUTIONS.)

EDTA is a strong chelator of trace metals — including zinc.. Although with propofol injectable emulsion there are no reports of decreased zinc levels or zinc deficiency-related adverse events, propofol injectable emulsion should not be infused for longer than 5 days without providing a drug holiday to safely replace estimated or measured urine zinc losses.

At high doses (2-3 g/day), EDTA has been reported, on rare occasions, to be toxic to the renal tubules. Studies to-date, in patients with normal or impaired renal function have not shown any alteration in renal function with propofol injectable emulsion containing 0.005% disodium edetate. In patients at risk for renal impairment, urinalysis and urine sediment should be checked before initiation of sedation and then be monitored on alternate days during sedation.

SUMMARY OF DOSAGE GUIDELINES

Dosages and rates of administration should be individualized and titrated to clinical response. Safety and dosing requirements for induction of anesthesia in pediatric patients have

P

only been established for children 3 years of age and older. Safety and dosing requirements for the maintenance of anesthesia have only been established for children 2 months of age and older. For complete dosage information, see CLINICAL PHARMACOLOGY, Individualization of Dosages.

Induction of General Anesthesia

Healthy Adults Less Than 55 Years of Age: 40 mg every 10 seconds until induction onset (2-2.5 mg/kg).
Elderly, Debilitated, or ASA III/IV Patients: 20 mg every 10 seconds until induction onset (1-1.5 mg/kg).
Cardiac Anesthesia: 20 mg every 10 seconds until induction onset (0.5-1.5 mg/kg).
Neurosurgical Patients: 20 mg every 10 seconds until induction onset (1-2 mg/kg).
Pediatric Patients - healthy, from 3-16 years of age: 2.5-3.5 mg/kg administered over 20-30 seconds. (See PRECAUTIONS, Pediatric Use and CLINICAL PHARMACOLOGY, Individualization of Dosages).

Maintenance of General Anesthesia

Infusion

Healthy Adults Less Than 55 Years of Age: 100-200 μg/kg/min (6-12 mg/kg/h).
Elderly, Debilitated, ASA III/IV Patients: 50-100 μg/kg/min (3-6 mg/kg/h).
Cardiac Anesthesia, Most Patients Require: *Primary propofol injectable emulsion with secondary opioid:* 100-150 μg/kg/min. *Low-dose propofol injectable emulsion with primary opioid:* 50-100 μg/kg/min.
Neurosurgical Patients: 100-200 μg/kg/min (6-12 mg/kg/h).
Pediatric Patients - healthy, from 2 months to 16 years of age: 125-300 μg/kg/min (7.5-18 mg/kg/h) "Following the first half hour of maintenance, if clinical signs of light anesthesia are not present, the infusion rate should be decreased." (See PRECAUTIONS, Pediatric Use and CLINICAL PHARMACOLOGY, Individualization of Dosagese).

Intermittent Bolus

Healthy Adults Less Than 55 Years of Age: Increments of 20-50 mg as needed.

Initiation of MAC Sedation

Healthy Adults Less Than 55 Years of Age: Slow infusion or slow injection techniques are recommended to avoid apnea or hypotension. Most patients require an infusion of 100-150 μg/kg/min (6-9 mg/kg/h) for 3-5 minutes or a slow injection of 0.5 mg/kg over 3-5 minutes followed immediately by a maintenance infusion.
Elderly, Debilitated, Neurosurgical, or ASA III/IV Patients: Most patients require dosages similar to healthy adults. Rapid boluses are to be avoided (See WARNINGS.)

Maintenance of MAC Sedation

Healthy Adults Less Than 55 Years of Age: A variable rate infusion technique is preferable over an intermittent bolus technique. Most patients require an infusion of 25-75 μg/kg/min (1.5-4.5 mg/kg/h) or incremental bolus doses of 10 or 20 mg.
In Elderly, Debilitated, Neurosurgical, or ASA III/IV Patients: Most patients require 80% of the usual adult dose. A rapid (single or repeated) bolus dose should not be used. (See WARNINGS.)

Initiation and Maintenance of ICU Sedation in Intubated, Mechanically Ventilated

Adult Patients: Because of the residual effects of previous anesthetic or sedative agents, in most patients the initial infusion should be 5 μg/kg/min (0.3 mg/kg/h) for at least 5 minutes. Subsequent increments of 5-10 μg/kg/min (0.3-0.6 mg/kg/h) over 5-10 minutes may be used until desired clinical effect is achieved. Maintenance rates of 5-50 μg/kg/min (0.3-3 mg/kg/h) or higher may be required.
Evaluation of level of sedation and assessment of CNS function should be carried out daily throughout maintenance to determine the minimum dose of propofol injectable emulsion required for sedation.

The tubing and any unused portions of propofol injectable emulsion should be discarded after 12 hours because propofol injectable emulsion contains no preservatives and is capable of supporting rapid growth of microorganisms. (See WARNINGS, and DOSAGE AND ADMINISTRATION.)

COMPATIBILITY AND STABILITY

Propofol injectable emulsion should not be mixed with other therapeutic agents prior to administration.

DILUTION PRIOR TO ADMINISTRATION

Propofol injectable emulsion is provided as a ready to use formulation. However, should dilution be necessary, it should only be diluted with 5% dextrose injection, and it should not be diluted to a concentration less than 2 mg/ml because it is an emulsion. In diluted form it has been shown to be more stable when in contact with glass than with plastic (95% potency after 2 hours of running infusion in plastic).

ADMINISTRATION WITH OTHER FLUIDS

Compatibility of propofol injectable emulsion with the coadministration of blood/serum/plasma has not been established. (See WARNINGS.) When administered using a y-type infusion set, propofol injectable emulsion has been shown to be compatible with the following intravenous fluids.

- 5% Dextrose injection
- Lactated ringers injection
- Lactated ringers and 5% dextrose injection
- 5% Dextrose and 0.45% sodium chloride injection
- 5% Dextrose and 0.2% sodium chloride injection

HANDLING PROCEDURES

General

Parenteral drug products should be inspected visually for particulate matter and discoloration prior to administration whenever solution and container permit.

Clinical experience with the use of in-line filters and propofol injectable emulsion during anesthesia or ICU/MAC sedation is limited. Propofol injectable emulsion should only be administered through a filter with a pore size of 5 μm or greater unless it has been demonstrated that the filter does not restrict the flow of propofol injectable emulsion and/or cause the breakdown of the emulsion. Filters should be used with caution and where clinically appropriate. Continuous monitoring is necessary due to the potential for restrictedflow and/or breakdown of the emulsion.

Do not use if there is evidence of separation of the phases of the emulsion.

Rare cases of self-administration of propofol injectable emulsion by health care professionals have been reported, including some fatalities.

STRICT ASEPTIC TECHNIQUE MUST ALWAYS BE MAINTAINED DURING HANDLING. PROPOFOL INJECTABLE EMULSION IS A SINGLE-USE PARENTERAL PRODUCT; WHICH CONTAINS 0.005% DISODIUM EDETATE TO RETARD THE RATE OF GROWTH OF MICROORGANISMS IN THE EVENT OF ACCIDENTAL EXTRINSIC CONTAMINATION. HOWEVER, PROPOFOL INJECTABLE EMULSION CAN STILL SUPPORT THE GROWTH OF MICROORGANISMS AS IT IS NOT ANTIMICROBIALLY PRESERVED PRODUCT UNDER USP STANDARDS. ACCORDINGLY, STRICT ASEPTIC TECHNIQUES MUST STILL BE ADHERED TO. DO NOT USE IF CONTAMINATION IS SUSPECTED. DISCARD UNUSED PORTIONS AS DIRECTED WITHIN THE REQUIRED TIME LIMITS (SEE DOSAGE AND ADMINISTRATION, HANDLING PROCEDURES). THERE HAVE BEEN REPORTS IN WHICH FAILURE TO USE ASEPTIC TECHNIQUE WHEN HANDLING PROPOFOL INJECTABLE EMULSION WAS ASSOCIATED WITH MICROBIAL CONTAMINATION OF THE PRODUCT AND WITH FEVER, INFECTION/SEPSIS, OTHER LIFE-THREATENING ILLNESS, AND/OR DEATH.

Guidelines for Aseptic Technique for General Anesthesia/MAC Sedation

Propofol injectable emulsion should be prepared for use just prior to initiation of each individual anesthetic/sedative procedure. The ampule neck surface, or vial/pre-filled syringe rubber stopper should be disinfected using 70% isopropyl alcohol. Propofol injectable emulsion should be drawn into sterile syringes immediately after ampules or vials are opened. When withdrawing propofol injectable emulsion from vials, a sterile vent spike should be used. The syringe(s) should be labeled with appropriate information including the date and time the ampule or vial was opened. Administration should commence promptly and be completed within 6 hours after the ampules, vials, or pre-filled syringes have been opened.

Propofol injectable emulsion should be prepared for single-patient use only. Any unused portions of propofol injectable emulsion, reservoirs, dedicated administration tubing and/or solutions containing propofol injectable emulsion must be discarded at the end of the anesthetic procedure or at 6 hours, whichever occurs sooner. The IV line should be flushed every 6 hours and at the end of the anesthetic procedure to remove residual propofol injectable emulsion.

Guidelines for Aseptic Technique for ICU Sedation

Propofol injectable emulsion should be prepared for single-patient use only. When propofol injectable emulsion is administered directly from the vial/pre-filled syringe, strict aseptic techniques must be followed. The vial/pre-filled syringe rubber stopper should be disinfected using 70% isopropyl alcohol. A sterile vent spike and sterile tubing must be used for administration of propofol injectable emulsion. As with other lipid emulsions, the number of IV line manipulations should be minimized. Administration should commence promptly and must be completed within 12 hours after the vial has been spiked. The tubing and any unused portions of propofol injectable emulsion must be discarded after 12 hours.

If propofol injectable emulsion is transferred to a syringe or other container prior to administration, the handling procedures for General Anesthesia/MAC sedation should be followed, and the product should be discarded and administration lines changed after 6 hours.

HOW SUPPLIED

Diprivan injectable emulsion is available in ready to use 20 ml ampoules, 50 ml infusion vials, 100 ml infusion vials, and 50 ml pre-filled syringes containing 10 mg/ml of propofol.

Propofol undergoes oxidative degradation, in the presence of oxygen, and is therefore packaged under nitrogen to eliminate this degradation path.

Storage: Store between 4-22°C (40-72°F). Do not freeze. Shake well before use.

PRODUCT LISTING - RATED THERAPEUTICALLY EQUIVALENT

Emulsion - Intravenous - 10 mg/ml

20 ml x 25	$236.28	GENERIC, Baxter Pharmaceutical Products, Inc	10019-0013-04
20 ml x 25	$332.25	GENERIC, Baxter Pharmaceutical Products, Inc	10019-0013-01
50 ml	$44.28	DIPRIVAN, Astra-Zeneca Pharmaceuticals	00310-0300-54
50 ml x 20	$664.20	GENERIC, Baxter Pharmaceutical Products, Inc	10019-0013-02
100 ml x 10	$664.30	GENERIC, Baxter Pharmaceutical Products, Inc	10019-0013-03

PRODUCT LISTING - EQUIVALENTS NOT AVAILABLE

Emulsion - Intravenous - 10 mg/ml

10 ml x 10	$73.10	GENERIC, Baxter Pharmaceutical Products, Inc	10019-0013-06
20 ml x 20	$374.93	DIPRIVAN, Allscripts Pharmaceutical Company	54569-4340-00
20 ml x 25	$318.90	GENERIC, Baxter Pharmaceutical Products, Inc	10019-0213-01

20 ml x 25	$342.50	DIPRIVAN, Vha Supply	00310-0300-62
20 ml x 25	$421.50	DIPRIVAN, Astra-Zeneca Pharmaceuticals	00310-0300-22
50 ml x 20	$637.68	GENERIC, Baxter Pharmaceutical Products, Inc	10019-0213-02
50 ml x 20	$660.00	GENERIC, Allscripts Pharmaceutical Company	54569-4821-00
50 ml x 20	$749.80	DIPRIVAN, Allscripts Pharmaceutical Company	54569-4073-00
50 ml x 25	$722.40	DIPRIVAN, Vha Supply	00310-0300-65
100 ml x 10	$637.68	GENERIC, Baxter Pharmaceutical Products, Inc	10019-0213-03
100 ml x 10	$694.80	DIPRIVAN, Vha Supply	00310-0300-61

Propoxyphene Hydrochloride *(002133)*

For related information, see the comparative table section in Appendix A.

Categories: Pain, mild to moderate; DEA Class CIV; FDA Approved 1957 Aug; Pregnancy Category C
Drug Classes: Analgesics, narcotic
Brand Names: Darvon; Dolene; Kesso-Gesic; Margesic
Cost of Therapy: $17.25 (Pain; Darvon; 65 mg; 6 capsules/day; 5 day supply)
$2.21 (Pain; Generic Capsules; 65 mg; 6 capsules/day; 5 day supply)

DESCRIPTION

Propoxyphene hydrochloride is an odorless, white crystalline powder with a bitter taste. It is freely soluble in water. Chemically, it is (2*S*,3*R*)-(+)-4-(Dimethylamino)-3-methyl-1,2-diphenyl-2-butanol propionate (ester) hydrochloride.

Each capsule contains 65 mg (172.9 μmol)(No. 65) propoxyphene hydrochloride. It also contains D&C red no. 33, FD&C yellow no. 6, gelatin, magnesium stearate, silicone, starch, titanium dioxide, and other inactive ingredients.

Storage: Store at controlled room temperature, 59-86°F (15-30°C).

CLINICAL PHARMACOLOGY

Propoxyphene is a centrally acting narcotic analgesic agent. Equimolar doses of propoxyphene hydrochloride or napsylate provide similar plasma concentrations. Following administration of 65, 130, or 195 mg of propoxyphene hydrochloride, the bioavailability of propoxyphene is equivalent to that of 100, 200, or 300 mg respectively of propoxyphene napsylate. Peak plasma concentrations of propoxyphene are reached in 2-2½ hours. After a 65 mg oral dose of propoxyphene hydrochloride, peak plasma levels of 0.05 to 0.1 μg/ml are achieved.

Repeated doses of propoxyphene at 6 hour intervals lead to increasing plasma concentrations, with a plateau after the ninth dose at 48 hours.

Propoxyphene is metabolized in the liver to yield norpropoxyphene. Propoxyphene has a half-life of 6-12 hours, whereas that of norpropoxyphene is 30-36 hours.

Norpropoxyphene has substantially less central-nervous-system-depressant effect than propoxyphene but a greater local anesthetic effect, which is similar to that of amitriptyline and antiarrhythmic agents, such as lidocaine and quinidine.

In animal studies in which propoxyphene and norpropoxyphene were continuously infused in large amounts, intracardiac conduction time (P-R and QRS intervals) was prolonged. Any intracardiac conduction delay attributable to high concentrations of norpropoxyphene may be of relatively long duration.

Propoxyphene is a mild narcotic analgesic structurally related to methadone. The potency of propoxyphene hydrochloride is from two-thirds to equal that of codeine.

INDICATIONS AND USAGE

For the relief of mild to moderate pain.

CONTRAINDICATIONS

Hypersensitivity to propoxyphene.

WARNINGS

- **Do not prescribe propoxyphene for patients who are suicidal or addiction-prone.**
- **Prescribe propoxyphene with caution for patients taking tranquilizers or antidepressant drugs and patients who use alcohol in excess.**
- **Tell your patients not to exceed the recommended dose and to limit their intake of alcohol.Propoxyphene products in excessive doses, either along or in combination with other CNS depressants, including alcohol, are a major cause of drug-related deaths. Fatalities within the first hour of overdosage are not uncommon. In a survey of deaths due to overdosage conducted in 1975, in approximately 20% of the fatal cases, death occurred within the first hours (5% occurred within 15 minutes). Propoxyphene should not be taken in doses higher than those recommended by the physician. The judicious prescribing of propoxyphene is essential to the safe use of this drug. With patients who are depressed or suicidal, considerations should be given to the use of non-narcotic analgesics. Patients should be cautioned about the concomitant use of propoxyphene products and alcohol because of potentially serious CNS-additive effects of these agents. Because of its added depressant effects, propoxyphene should be prescribed with caution for those patients whose medical condition requires the concomitant administration of sedatives, tranquilizers, muscle relaxants, antidepressants, or other CNS-depressant drugs. Patients should be advised of the additive depressant effects of these combinations.**

Many of the propoxyphene-related deaths have occurred in patients with previous histories of emotional disturbances or suicidal ideation or attempts as well as histories of misuse of tranquilizers, alcohol, and other CNS-active drugs. Some deaths have occurred as a consequence of the accidental ingestion of excessive quantities of propoxyphene alone or in combination with other drugs. Patients taking propoxyphene should be warned not to exceed the dosage recommended by the physician.

Usage in Ambulatory Patients: Propoxyphene may impair the mental and/or physical abilities required for the performance of potentially hazardous tasks, such as driving a car or operating machinery. The patient should be cautioned accordingly.

PRECAUTIONS

GENERAL

Propoxyphene should be administered with caution to patients with hepatic or renal impairment since higher serum concentrations or delayed elimination may occur.

USAGE IN PREGNANCY

Safe use in pregnancy has not been established relative to possible adverse effects on fetal development. Instances of withdrawal symptoms in the neonate have been reported following usage during pregnancy. Therefore, propoxyphene should not be used in pregnant women unless, in the judgment of the physician, the potential benefits outweigh the possible hazards.

USAGE IN NURSING MOTHERS

Low levels of propoxyphene have been detected in human milk. In postpartum studies involving nursing mothers who were given propoxyphene, no adverse effects were noted in infants receiving mother's milk.

USAGE IN CHILDREN

Propoxyphene is not recommended for use in children, because documented clinical experience has been insufficient to establish safety and a suitable dosage regimen in the pediatric age group.

GERIATRIC USE

The rate of propoxyphene metabolism may be reduced in some patients. Increased dosing interval should be considered.

DRUG INTERACTIONS

The CNS-depressant effect of propoxyphene is additive with that of other CNS depressants, including alcohol.

As is the case with many medicinal agents, propoxyphene may slow the metabolism of a concomitantly administered drug. Should this occur, the higher serum concentrations of that drug may result in increased pharmacologic or adverse effects of that drug. Such occurrences have been reported when propoxyphene was administered to patients on antidepressants, anticonvulsants, or warfarin-like drugs. Sever neurologic signs, including coma, have occurred with concurrent use of carbamazepine.

ADVERSE REACTIONS

In a survey conducted in hospitalized patients, less than 1% of patients taking propoxyphene hydrochloride at recommended doses experienced side effects. The most frequently reported have been dizziness, sedation, nausea, and vomiting. Some of these adverse reactions may be alleviated if the patient lies down.

Other adverse reactions include constipation, abdominal pain, skin rashes, lightheadedness, headache, weakness, euphoria, dysphoria, and minor visual disturbances.

Propoxyphene therapy has been associated with abnormal liver function tests, and, more rarely, with instances of reversible jaundice (including cholestatic jaundice).

Subacute painful myopathy has occurred following chronic propoxyphene overdosage.

DOSAGE AND ADMINISTRATION

Propoxyphene hydrochloride is given orally. The usual dosage is 65 mg propoxyphene hydrochloride every 4 hours as needed for pain. The maximum recommended dose of propoxyphene hydrochloride is 390 mg/day.

Consideration should be given to a reduced total daily dosage in patients with hepatic or renal impairment.

PRODUCT LISTING - RATED THERAPEUTICALLY EQUIVALENT

Capsule - Oral - Hydrochloride 65 mg

100's	$5.80	GENERIC, Alra	51641-0321-01
100's	$7.35	GENERIC, Mutual/United Research Laboratories	00677-0356-01
100's	$7.40	GENERIC, Purepac Pharmaceutical Company	00228-2082-10
100's	$7.48	GENERIC, Aligen Independent Laboratories Inc	00405-0175-01
100's	$8.37	GENERIC, Moore, H.L. Drug Exchange Inc	00839-5098-06
100's	$8.53	GENERIC, Ivax Corporation	00182-0698-01
100's	$8.55	GENERIC, Geneva Pharmaceuticals	00781-2140-01
100's	$8.57	GENERIC, Auro Pharmaceutical	55829-0864-10
100's	$8.63	GENERIC, Interstate Drug Exchange Inc	00814-6457-14
100's	$12.08	GENERIC, Alra	51641-0321-11
100's	$13.52	GENERIC, Ivax Corporation	00172-2186-60
100's	$29.96	GENERIC, Major Pharmaceuticals Inc	00904-7700-61
100's	$30.05	GENERIC, Major Pharmaceuticals Inc	00904-7700-60
100's	$32.50	GENERIC, West Ward Pharmaceutical Corporation	00143-3235-01
100's	$33.30	GENERIC, Teva Pharmaceuticals Usa	00093-0741-01
100's	$33.30	GENERIC, Qualitest Products Inc	00603-5459-21
100's	$57.51	DARVON, Lilly, Eli and Company	00002-0803-02
100's	$64.83	DARVON, Lilly, Eli and Company	00002-0803-33

PRODUCT LISTING - EQUIVALENTS NOT AVAILABLE

Capsule - Oral - Hydrochloride 65 mg

4's	$3.67	GENERIC, Prescript Pharmaceuticals	00247-0154-04
10's	$4.15	GENERIC, Prescript Pharmaceuticals	00247-0154-10
12's	$4.31	GENERIC, Prescript Pharmaceuticals	00247-0154-12
20's	$4.94	GENERIC, Prescript Pharmaceuticals	00247-0154-20
20's	$5.23	GENERIC, Southwood Pharmaceuticals Inc	58016-0214-20
20's	$7.19	GENERIC, Pharma Pac	52959-0334-20
30's	$5.74	GENERIC, Prescript Pharmaceuticals	00247-0154-30
30's	$7.84	GENERIC, Southwood Pharmaceuticals Inc	58016-0214-30

30's	$10.73	GENERIC, Pharma Pac	52959-0334-30
40's	$6.53	GENERIC, Prescript Pharmaceuticals	00247-0154-40
100's	$31.75	GENERIC, Mylan Pharmaceuticals Inc	00378-0129-01
100's	$31.78	GENERIC, Ranbaxy Laboratories	63304-0677-01

Propoxyphene Napsylate (002134)

For related information, see the comparative table section in Appendix A.

Categories: Pain, mild to moderate; DEA Class CIV; FDA Approved 1971 Sep
Drug Classes: Analgesics, narcotic
Brand Names: **Darvon-N**; Doloxene
Cost of Therapy: $25.10 (Pain; Darvon-N; 100 mg; 6 tablets/day; 5 day supply)

DESCRIPTION

Propoxyphene napsylate, USP is an odorless, white crystalline powder with a bitter taste. It is very slightly soluble in water and soluble in methanol, ethanol, chloroform, and acetone. Chemically, it is (αS,1R)-α-[2- (Dimethylamino) -1-methylethyl] -α- phenylphenethyl propionate compound with 2-naphthalenesulfonic acid (1:1) monohydrate. Its molecular weight is 565.72.

Propoxyphene napsylate differs from propoxyphene hydrochloride in that it allows more stable liquid dosage forms and tablet formulations. Because of differences in molecular weight, a dose of 100 mg (176.8 μmol) of propoxyphene napsylate is required to supply an amount of propoxyphene equivalent to that present in 65 mg (172.9 μmol) of propoxyphene hydrochloride.

Each tablet of propoxyphene napsylate contains 100 mg (176.8 μmol) propoxyphene napsylate. The tablet also contains cellulose, cornstarch, iron oxides, lactose, magnesium stearate, silicon dioxide, stearic acid, and titanium dioxide.

CLINICAL PHARMACOLOGY

Propoxyphene is a centrally acting narcotic analgesic agent. Equimolar doses of propoxyphene hydrochloride or napsylate provide similar plasma concentrations. Following administration of 65, 130, or 195 mg of propoxyphene hydrochloride, the bioavailability of propoxyphene is equivalent to that of 100, 200, or 300 mg respectively of propoxyphene napsylate. Peak plasma concentrations of propoxyphene are reached in 2-2½ hours. After a 100 mg oral dose of propoxyphene napsylate, peak plasma levels of 0.05 to 0.1 μg/ml are achieved. The napsylate salt tends to be absorbed more slowly than the hydrochloride. At or near therapeutic doses, this difference is small when compared with that among subjects and among doses.

Because of this several hundredfold difference in solubility, the absorption rate of very large doses of the napsylate salt is significantly lower than that of equimolar doses of the hydrochloride.

Repeated doses of propoxyphene at 6 hour intervals lead to increasing plasma concentrations, with a plateau after the ninth dose at 48 hours.

Propoxyphene is metabolized in the liver to yield norpropoxyphene. Propoxyphene has a half-life of 6-12 hours, whereas that of norpropoxyphene is 30-36 hours.

Norpropoxyphene has substantially less central-nervous-system-depressant effect than propoxyphene but a greater local anesthetic effect, which is similar to that of amitriptyline and antiarrhythmic agents, such as lidocaine and quinidine.

In animal studies in which propoxyphene and norpropoxyphene were continuously infused in large amounts, intracardiac conduction time (PR and QRS intervals) was prolonged. Any intracardiac conduction delay attributable to high concentrations of norpropoxyphene may be of relatively long duration.

Propoxyphene is a mild narcotic analgesic structurally related to methadone. The potency of propoxyphene napsylate is from two-thirds to equal that of codeine.

INDICATIONS AND USAGE

For the relief of mild to moderate pain.

CONTRAINDICATIONS

Hypersensitivity to propoxyphene.

WARNINGS

Do not prescribe propoxyphene for patients who are suicidal or addiction-prone.

Prescribe propoxyphene with caution for patients taking tranquilizers or antidepressant drugs and patients who use alcohol in excess.

Tell your patients not to exceed the recommended dose and to limit their intake of alcohol.

Propoxyphene products in excessive doses, either alone or in combination with other CNS depressants, including alcohol, are a major cause of drug-related deaths. Fatalities within the first hour of overdosage are not uncommon. In a survey of deaths due to overdosage conducted in 1975, in approximately 20% of the fatal cases, death occurred within the first hour (5% occurred within 15 minutes). Propoxyphene should not be taken in doses higher than those recommended by the physician. The judicious prescribing of propoxyphene is essential to the safe use of this drug. With patients who are depressed or suicidal, consideration should be given to the use of non-narcotic analgesics. Patients should be cautioned about the concomitant use of propoxyphene products and alcohol because of potentially serious CNS-additive effects of these agents. Because of its added depressant effects, propoxyphene should be prescribed with caution for those patients whose medical condition requires the concomitant administration of sedatives, tranquilizers, muscle relaxants, antidepressants, or other CNS-depressant drugs. Patients should be advised of the additive depressant effects of these combinations.

Many of the propoxyphene-related deaths have occurred in patients with previous histories of emotional disturbances or suicidal ideation or attempts as well as histories of misuse of tranquilizers, alcohol, and other CNS-active drugs. Some deaths have occurred as a consequence of the accidental ingestion of excessive quantities of propoxyphene alone or in combination with other drugs. Patients taking propoxyphene should be warned not to exceed the dosage recommended by the physician.

DRUG DEPENDENCE

Propoxyphene, when taken in higher-than-recommended doses over long periods of time, can produce drug dependence characterized by psychic dependence and, less frequently, physical dependence and tolerance. Propoxyphene will only partially suppress the withdrawal syndrome in individuals physically dependent on morphine or other narcotics. The abuse liability of propoxyphene is qualitatively similar to that of codeine although quantitatively less, and propoxyphene should be prescribed with the same degree of caution appropriate to the use of codeine.

USAGE IN AMBULATORY PATIENTS

Propoxyphene may impair the mental and/or physical abilities required for the performance of potentially hazardous tasks, such as driving a car or operating machinery. The patient should be cautioned accordingly.

PRECAUTIONS

GENERAL

Propoxyphene should be administered with caution to patients with hepatic or renal impairment since higher serum concentrations or delayed elimination may occur.

USAGE IN PREGNANCY

Safe use in pregnancy has not been established relative to possible adverse effects on fetal development. Instances of withdrawal symptoms in the neonate have been reported following usage during pregnancy. Therefore, propoxyphene should not be used in pregnant women unless, in the judgment of the physician, the potential benefits outweigh the possible hazards.

USAGE IN NURSING MOTHERS

Low levels of propoxyphene have been detected in human milk. In postpartum studies involving nursing mothers who were given propoxyphene, no adverse effects were noted in infants receiving mother's milk.

USAGE IN CHILDREN

Propoxyphene is not recommended for use in children, because documented clinical experience has been insufficient to establish safety and a suitable dosage regimen in the pediatric age group.

GERIATRIC USE

The rate of propoxyphene metabolism may be reduced in some patients. Increased dosing interval should be considered.

A Patient Information Sheet is available for this product.

DRUG INTERACTIONS

The CNS-depressant effect of propoxyphene is additive with that of other CNS depressants, including alcohol.

As is the case with many medicinal agents, propoxyphene may slow the metabolism of a concomitantly administered drug. Should this occur, the higher serum concentrations of that drug may result in increased pharmacologic or adverse effects of that drug. Such occurrences have been reported when propoxyphene was administered to patients on antidepressants, anticonvulsants, or warfarin-like drugs. Severe neurologic signs, including coma, have occurred with concurrent use of carbamazepine.

ADVERSE REACTIONS

In a survey conducted in hospitalized patients, less than 1% of patients taking propoxyphene hydrochloride at recommended doses experienced side effects. The most frequently reported were dizziness, sedation, nausea, and vomiting. Some of these adverse reactions may be alleviated if the patient lies down.

Other adverse reactions include constipation, abdominal pain, skin rashes, lightheadedness, headache, weakness, euphoria, dysphoria, hallucinations, and minor visual disturbances.

Propoxyphene therapy has been associated with abnormal liver function tests and, more rarely, with instances of reversible jaundice (including cholestatic jaundice).

Subacute painful myopathy has occurred following chronic propoxyphene overdosage.

DOSAGE AND ADMINISTRATION

Propoxyphene napsylate is given orally. The usual dosage is 100 mg propoxyphene napsylate every 4 hours as needed for pain. The maximum recommended dose of propoxyphene napsylate is 600 mg per day.

Consideration should be given to a reduced total daily dosage in patients with hepatic or renal impairment.

ANIMAL PHARMACOLOGY

ANIMAL TOXICOLOGY

The acute lethal doses of the hydrochloride and napsylate salts of propoxyphene were determined in 4 species. The results shown in (TABLE 1) indicate that, on a molar basis, the napsylate salt is less toxic than the hydrochloride. This may be due to the relative insolubility and retarded absorption of propoxyphene napsylate.

Some indication of the relative insolubility and retarded absorption of propoxyphene napsylate was obtained by measuring plasma propoxyphene levels in 2 groups of 4 dogs following oral administration of equimolar doses of the 2 salts. The peak plasma concentration observed with propoxyphene hydrochloride was much higher than that obtained after administration of the napsylate salt.

Although none of the animals in this experiment died, 3 of the 4 dogs given propoxyphene hydrochloride exhibited convulsive seizures during the time interval corresponding to the peak plasma levels. The 4 animals receiving the napsylate salt were mildly ataxic but not acutely ill.

TABLE 1 *Acute Oral Toxicity of Propoxyphene*

	LD_{50} (mg/kg) ± SE LD_{50} (mmol/kg)	
Species	**Propoxyphene Hydrochloride**	**Propoxyphene Napsylate**
Mouse	282 ± 39	915 ± 163
	0.75	1.62
Rat	230 ± 44	647 ± 95
	0.61	1.14
Rabbit	ca 82	>183
	0.22	>0.32
Dog	*ca* 100	>183
	0.27	>0.32

HOW SUPPLIED

Darvon: 100 mg, buff (No. 1883)

Storage: Store at controlled room temperature, 59-86°F (15-30°C).

PRODUCT LISTING - EQUIVALENTS NOT AVAILABLE

Tablet - Oral - Napsylate 100 mg

100's	$83.65	DARVON-N, Lilly, Eli and Company	00002-0353-02
100's	$90.99	DARVON-N, Lilly, Eli and Company	00002-0353-33

Propranolol Hydrochloride *(002135)*

For related information, see the comparative table section in Appendix A.

Categories: Angina pectoris; Arrhythmias, atrial fibrillation; Arrhythmias, atrial flutter; Arrhythmias, paroxysmal atrial tachycardia; Arrhythmias, secondary to thyrotoxicosis; Arrhythmias, supraventricular; Extrasystole, atrial; Extrasystole, premature ventricular; Headache, migraine, prophylaxis; Hypertension, essential; Myocardial infarction; Pheochromocytoma, adjunct; Stenosis, hypertrophic subaortic; Tachycardia, digitalis-induced; Tachycardia, sinus; Tachycardia, ventricular; Tremor, essential; Wolff-Parkinson-White syndrome; Pregnancy Category C; FDA Approved 1967 Nov; WHO Formulary

Drug Classes: Antiadrenergics, beta blocking; Antiarrhythmics, class II

Brand Names: **Inderal**; Inderal LA; Inderal Retard; InnoPran XL; Palon

Foreign Brand Availability: Acifol (Mexico); Adrexan (France); Angilol (England; New-Zealand); Angilol LA (New-Zealand); Apo-Propranolol (Canada; New-Zealand); Apsolol (England); Atensin (Benin; Burkina-Faso; Ethiopia; Gambia; Ghana; Guinea; Ivory-Coast; Kenya; Liberia; Malawi; Mali; Mauritania; Mauritius; Morocco; Niger; Nigeria; Senegal; Seychelles; Sierra-Leone; South-Africa; Sudan; Tanzania; Tunia; Uganda; Zambia; Zimbabwe); Avlocardyl (France); Becardin (Hong-Kong); Berkolol (England; Hong-Kong; Ireland); Betabloc (India); Beta-Timelets (Bahrain; Cyprus; Egypt; Germany; Iran; Iraq; Israel; Jordan; Kuwait; Lebanon; Libya; Oman; Qatar; Republic-of-Yemen; Saudi-Arabia; Syria; United-Arab-Emirates); Blocard (Indonesia); Blocaryl (Argentina); Cardinol (New-Zealand); Cardinol LA (New-Zealand); Ciplar (India); Corbeta (India); Deralin (Australia; Israel); Dibudinate (Argentina); Dociton (Germany); Duranol (Philippines); Elbrol (Germany); Emforal (Thailand); Farmadral (Indonesia); Farprolol (Mexico); Frekven (Denmark); Frina (Hungary); Hopranolol (Hong-Kong); Impral (Mexico); Indicardin (Benin; Burkina-Faso; Ethiopia; Gambia; Ghana; Guinea; Ivory-Coast; Kenya; Liberia; Malawi; Mali; Mauritania; Mauritius; Morocco; Niger; Nigeria; Senegal; Seychelles; Sierra-Leone; Sudan; Tanzania; Tunia; Uganda; Zambia; Zimbabwe); Inpanol (Hong-Kong); Noloten (Argentina); Oposim (Argentina); Phanerol (Philippines); Prestoral (Indonesia); Prolol (Hong-Kong; Israel; Thailand); Prolol Plus (Hong-Kong); Propalong (Argentina); Propayerst (Argentina); Propral (Finland); Reducor (Finland); Rexigen (South-Africa); Slow Deralin (Israel); Sumial (Spain); Tenomal (Greece); Tensiflex (Argentina); Waucoton (Greece)

Cost of Therapy: $70.01 (Hypertension; Inderal; 60 mg; 2 tablets/day; 30 day supply)
$2.55 (Hypertension; Generic Tablets; 60 mg; 2 tablets/day; 30 day supply)
$77.70 (Migraine Headache Prophylax; Inderal; 80 mg; 2 tablets/day; 30 day supply)
$2.25 (Migraine Headache Prophylax; Generic Tablets; 80 mg; 2 tablets/day; 30 day supply)
$22.07 (Hypertension; Generic Extended Release Capsules; 80 mg; 1 capsule/day; 30 day supply)
$44.59 (Hypertension; Inderal LA; 80 mg; 1 capsule/day; 30 day supply)
$35.63 (Hypertension; Innopran XL; 80 mg; 1 capsule/day; 30 day supply)

HCFA JCODE(S): J1800 up to 1 mg IV

DESCRIPTION

Note: The trade names have been used throughout this monograph for clarity.

Inderal (propranolol hydrochloride) is a synthetic beta-adrenergic receptor blocking agent chemically described as 1-(Isopropylamino)-3-(1-naphthyloxy)-2-propanol hydrochloride.

Propranolol hydrochloride is a stable, white, crystalline solid which is readily soluble in water and ethanol. Its molecular weight is 295.81.

Propranolol is available as 10, 20, 40, 60, and 80 mg tablets for oral administration and as a 1 mg/ml sterile injectable solution for intravenous administration.

The inactive ingredients contained in Inderal tablets are: Lactose, magnesium stearate, microcrystalline cellulose, and stearic acid. In addition, propranolol 10 mg and 80 mg tablets contain FD&C yellow no. 6 and D&C yellow no. 10; propranolol 20 mg tablets contain FD&C blue no. 1; propranolol 40 mg tablets contain FD&C blue no. 1, FD&C yellow no. 6, and D&C yellow no. 10; propranolol 60 mg tablets contain D&C red no. 30.

LONG-ACTING (LA) CAPSULES

Inderal LA capsules are formulated to provide a sustained release of propranolol hydrochloride. Inderal LA is available as 60, 80, 120, and 160 mg capsules.

Inderal LA capsules contain the following inactive ingredients: Cellulose, ethylcellulose, gelatin capsules, hypromellose, and titanium ddioxide. In addition, Inderal LA 60, 80, and 120 mg capsules contain D&C red no. 28 and FD&C blue no. 1; Inderal LA 160 mg capsules contain FD&C blue no. 1.

EXTENDED-RELEASE CAPSULES

InnoPran XL is a nonselective, beta-adrenergic receptor-blocking agent for oral administration, available as an extended release product. The capsules contain sustained-release beads available as 80 and 120 mg capsules. Each of the beads contains propranolol hydrochloride and is coated with dual membranes. These membranes are designed to retard release of propranolol hydrochloride for several hours after ingestion followed by the sustained release of propranolol.

CLINICAL PHARMACOLOGY

GENERAL

Propranolol is a nonselective beta-adrenergic receptor blocking agent possessing no other autonomic nervous system activity. It specifically competes with beta-adrenergic receptor stimulating agents for available receptor sites. When access to beta-receptor sites is blocked by propranolol HCl, the chronotropic, inotropic, and vasodilator responses to beta-adrenergic stimulation are decreased proportionately.

MECHANISM OF ACTION

The mechanism of the antihypertensive effect of propranolol has not been established. Among the factors that may be involved in contributing to the antihypertensive action are (1) decreased cardiac output, (2) inhibition of renin release by the kidneys, and (3) diminution of tonic sympathetic nerve outflow from vasomotor centers in the brain. Although total peripheral resistance may increase initially, it readjusts to or below the pretreatment level with chronic use. Effects on plasma volume appear to be minor and somewhat variable. Propranolol has been shown to cause a small increase in serum potassium concentration when used in the treatment of hypertensive patients.

In angina pectoris, propranolol generally reduces the oxygen requirement of the heart at any given level of effort by blocking the catecholamine-induced increases in the heart rate, systolic blood pressure, and the velocity and extent of myocardial contraction. Propranolol may increase oxygen requirements by increasing left ventricular fiber length, end diastolic pressure, and systolic ejection period. The net physiologic effect of beta-adrenergic blockade is usually advantageous and is manifested during exercise by delayed onset of pain and increased work capacity. Propranolol exerts its antiarrhythmic effects in concentrations associated with beta-adrenergic blockade, and this appears to be its principal antiarrhythmic mechanism of action. In dosages greater than required for beta blockade, propranolol also exerts a quinidine-like or anesthetic-like membrane action, which affects the cardiac action potential. The significance of the membrane action in the treatment of arrhythmias is uncertain.

The mechanism of the antimigraine effect of propranolol has not been established. Beta-adrenergic receptors have been demonstrated in the pial vessels of the brain.

The specific mechanism of propranolol HCl's antitremor effects has not been established, but beta-2 (noncardiac) receptors may be involved. A central effect is also possible. Clinical studies have demonstrated that propranolol is of benefit in exaggerated physiological and essential (familial) tremor.

Beta-receptor blockade can be useful in conditions in which, because of pathologic or functional changes, sympathetic activity is detrimental to the patient. But there are also situations in which sympathetic stimulation is vital. For example, in patients with severely damaged hearts, adequate ventricular function is maintained by virtue of sympathetic drive, which should be preserved. In the presence of A-V block greater than first degree, beta blockade may prevent the necessary facilitating effect of sympathetic activity on conduction. Beta blockade results in bronchial constriction by interfering with adrenergic bronchodilator activity, which should be preserved in patients subject to bronchospasm.

Absorption

Propranolol is highly lipophilic and is almost completely absorbed after oral administration. However, it undergoes high first-pass metabolism by the liver and on average, only about 25% of propranolol reaches the systemic circulation. Peak effect occurs in 1 to 1.5 hours. The biologic half-life is approximately 4 hours.

There is no simple correlation between dose or plasma level and therapeutic effect, and the dose-sensitivity range as observed in clinical practice is wide. The principal reason for this is that sympathetic tone varies widely between individuals. Since there is no reliable test to estimate sympathetic tone or to determine whether total beta blockade has been achieved, proper dosage requires titration.

LA Capsules

Inderal LA capsules (60, 80, 120, and 160 mg) release propanolol HCl at a controlled and predictable rate. Peak blood levels following dosing with Inderal LA occur at about 6 hours, and the apparent plasma half-life is about 10 hours. When measured at steady-state over a 24 hour period the areas under the propranolol plasma concentration-time curve (AUCs) for the capsules are approximately 60-65% of the AUCs for a comparable divided daily dose of Inderal tablets.The lower AUCs for the capsules are due greater hepatic metabolism of propranolol, resulting from a slower rate of absorption of propranolol. Over a 24 hour period, blood levels are fairly constant for about 12 hours, then decline exponentially.

Inderal LA should not be considered a simple mg-for-mg substitute for conventional propanolol and the blood levels achieved do not match (are lower than) those of 2-4 times daily dosing with the same dose. When changing to Inderal LA from conventional propranolol, a possible need for retitration upwards should be considered, especially to maintain effectiveness at the end of the dosing interval. In most clinical settings, however, such as hypertension or angina where there is little correlation between plasma levels and clinical effect, Inderal LA has been therapeutically equivalent to the same mg dose of conventional Inderal as assessed by 24 hour effects on blood pressure and on 24 hour excercise responses of heart rate, systollic pressure, and rate pressure product. Inderal LA can provide effective beta blockade for a 24 hour period.

InnoPran XL Capsules

A single-dose, food-effect study in 36 healthy subjects showed that a high fat meal administered with propanol HCl extended-release at 10:00 PM, increased the lag time from 3-5 hours and the time to reach the maximum concentration from 11.5-15.4 hours, under fed conditions, with no effect on the AUC. (See DOSAGE AND ADMINISTRATION.)

Following multiple-dose administration of propanol HCl extended-release at 10:00 PM under fasting conditions, the steady-state lag time was between 4-5 hours and propranolol peak plasma concentrations were reached approximately 12-14 hours after dosing. Propranolol trough levels were achieved 24-27 hours after dosing, and persisted for 3-5 hours after the next dose. The elimination half-life of propranolol was approximately 8 hours.

The plasma levels of propranolol showed dose proportional increases after single and multiple administration of 80, 120, and 160 mg of propanol HCl XL.

At steady state, the bioavailability of 160 mg dose of propanol HCl extended-release and propranolol HCl LA capsules did not differ significantly.

Distribution

Approximately 90% of circulating propranolol is bound to plasma proteins (albumin and alpha1 acid glycoprotein). The binding is enantiomer-selective. The S-isomer is preferentially bound to $alpha_1$ glycoprotein and the R-isomer preferentially bound to albumin. The volume of distribution of propranolol is approximately 4 L.

Metabolism and Elimination

Propranolol is extensively metabolized with most metabolites appearing in the urine. Propranolol is metabolized through 3 primary routes: aromatic hydroxylation (mainly 4-hydroxylation), N-dealkylation followed by further side-chain oxidation, and direct glucuronidation. It has been estimated that the percentage contributions of these routes to total metabolism are 42%, 41%, and 17%, respectively, but with considerable variability between individuals. The four major metabolites are propranolol glucuronide, naphthyloxylactic acid, and glucuronic acid and sulfate conjugates of 4-hydroxy propranolol.

In vitro studies have indicated that the aromatic hydroxylation of propranolol is catalyzed mainly by polymorphic CYP2D6. Side-chain oxidation is mediated mainly by CYP1A2 and to some extent by CYP2D6. 4-hydroxy propranolol is a weak inhibitor of CYP2D6.

Propranolol is also a substrate for CYP2C19 and a substrate for the intestinal efflux transporter, p-glycoprotein (p-gp). Studies suggest however that p-gp is not dose-limiting for intestinal absorption of propranolol in the usual therapeutic dose range.

In healthy subjects no difference was observed between CYP2D6 extensive metabolizers (EMs) and poor metabolizers (PMs) with respect to oral clearance or elimination half-life. Partial clearance to 4-hydroxy propranolol was significantly higher and to naphthyloxylactic acid was significantly lower in EMs than PMs.

Enantiomers

Of the two enantiomers of propranolol the S-enantiomer blocks beta-adrenergic receptors. In normal subjects receiving oral doses of racemic propranolol, S-enantiomer concentrations exceeded those of the R-enantiomer by 40-90% as a result of stereoselective hepatic metabolism.

SPECIAL POPULATIONS

Pediatric

The pharmacokinetics of propanol HCl extended-release have not been investigated in patients under 18 years of age.

Geriatric

The pharmacokinetics of propanol HCl extended-release have not been investigated in patients over 65 years of age. In a study of 12 elderly (62-79 years old) and 12 young (25-33 years old) healthy subjects, the clearance of S-enantiomer of propranolol was decreased in the elderly. Additionally, the half-life of both the R- and S-propranolol was prolonged in the elderly compared with the young (11 vs 5 hours).

Gender

In a dose-proportionality study, the pharmacokinetics of propanol HCl extended-release were evaluated in 22 male and 14 female healthy volunteers. Following single doses under fasting conditions, the mean AUC and C_{max} were about 49% and 16% higher for females across the dosage range. The mean elimination half-life was longer in females than in males (11 vs 7.5 hours).

P

Race

A study conducted in 12 Caucasian and 13 African-American male subjects taking propranolol, showed that at steady state, the clearance of R- and S-propranolol were about 76% and 53% higher in African-Americans than in Caucasians, respectively.

Renal Insufficiency

The pharmacokinetics of propanol HCl extended-release have not been evaluated in patients with renal insufficiency. In a study conducted in 5 patients with chronic renal failure, 6 patients on regular dialysis, and 5 healthy subjects, who received a single oral dose of 40 mg of propranolol, the peak plasma concentrations (C_{max}) of propranolol in the chronic renal failure group were 2- to 3-fold higher (161 ± 41 ng/ml) than those observed in the dialysis patients (47 ± 9 ng/ml) and in the healthy subjects (26 ± 1 ng/ml). Propranolol plasma clearance was also reduced in the patients with chronic renal failure.

Chronic renal failure has been associated with a decrease in drug metabolism via down regulation of hepatic cytochrome P450 activity.

Hepatic Insufficiency

The pharmacokinetics of propanol HCl extended-release have not been evaluated in patients with hepatic impairment. However, propranolol is extensively metabolized by the liver. In a study conducted in 7 patients with cirrhosis and 9 healthy subjects receiving 80 mg oral propranolol every 8 hours for 7 doses, the steady-state unbound propranolol concentration in patients with cirrhosis was increased 3-fold in comparison to controls. In cirrhosis, the half-life increased to 11 hours compared to 4 hours (see PRECAUTIONS).

Drug Interactions

Interactions With Substrates, Inhibitors or Inducers of Cytochrome P-450 Enzymes

Because propranolol's metabolism involves multiple pathways in the cytochrome P-450 system (CYP2D6, 1A2, 2C19), administration of propanol HCl extended-release with drugs that are metabolized by, or affect the activity (induction or inhibition) of one or more of these pathways may lead to clinically relevant drug interactions (see DRUG INTERACTIONS).

INDICATIONS AND USAGE

HYPERTENSION

Inderal and Inderal LA are indicated in the management of hypertension. They may be used alone or used in combination with other antihypertensive agents, particularly a thiazide diuretic. Inderal and Inderal LA are not indicated in the management of hypertensive emergencies.

InnoPran XL is indicated in the management of hypertension; it may be used alone or in combination with other antihypertensive agents.

ANGINA PECTORIS DUE TO CORONARY ATHEROSCLEROSISA

Inderal and Inderal LA are indicated for the long-term management of patients with angina pectoris.

CARDIAC ARRHYTHMIAS

Supraventricular Arrhythmias:

Paroxysmal atrial tachycardias, particularly those arrhythmias induced by catecholamines or digitalis or associated with the Wolff-Parkinson-White syndrome. (See WARNINGS, In Patients With Wolff-Parkinson-White Syndrome.)

Persistent sinus tachycardia which is noncompensatory and impairs the well-being of the patient.

Tachycardias and arrhythmias due to thyrotoxicosis when causing distress or increased hazard and when immediate effect is necessary as adjunctive, short-term (2-4 weeks) therapy. May be used with, but not in place of, specific therapy. (See WARNINGS, Thyrotoxicosis.)

Persistent atrial extrasystoles which impair the well-being of the patient and do not respond to conventional measures.

Atrial flutter and fibrillation when ventricular rate cannot be controlled by digitalis alone, or when digitalis is contraindicated.

Ventricular Tachycardias:

Ventricular arrhythmias do not respond to propranolol as predictably as do the supraventricular arrhythmias, but propranolol may be useful for persistent premature ventricular extrasystoles which do not respond to conventional measures and impair the well-being of the patient.

Ventricular tachycardias: With the exception of those induced by catecholamines or digitalis, propranolol is not the drug of first choice. In critical situations when cardioversion techniques or other drugs are not indicated or are not effective, propranolol may be considered. If, after consideration of the risks involved, propranolol is used, it should be given intravenously in low dosage and very slowly. (See DOSAGE AND ADMINISTRATION.) *Care in the administration of propranolol with constant electrocardiographic monitoring is essential as the failing heart requires some sympathetic drive for maintenance of myocardial tone.*

Persistent premature ventricular extrasystoles which do not respond to conventional measures and impair the well-being of the patient.

Tachyarrhythmias of digitalis intoxication: If digitalis-induced tachyarrhythmias persist following discontinuance of digitalis and correction of electrolyte abnormalities, they are usually reversible with *oral* propranolol HCl. Severe bradycardia may occur. Intravenous propranolol hydrochloride is reserved for life-threatening arrhythmias. Temporary maintenance with oral therapy may be indicated. (See DOSAGE AND ADMINISTRATION.)

Resistant tachyarrhythmias due to excessive catecholamine action during anesthesia: Tachyarrhythmias due to excessive catecholamine action during anesthesia may sometimes arise because of release of endogenous catecholamines or administration of catecholamines. When usual measures fail in such arrhythmias, propranolol may be given intravenously to abolish them. All general inhalation anesthetics produce some degree of myocardial depression. Therefore, when propranolol is used to treat arrhythmias during anesthesia, it should be used with extreme caution and constant ECG and central venous pressure monitoring. (See WARNINGS.)

MYOCARDIAL INFARCTION

Inderal is indicated to reduce cardiovascular mortality in patients who have survived the acute phase of myocardial infarction and are clinically stable.

MIGRAINE

Inderal and Inderal LA are indicated for the prophylaxis of common migraine headache. The efficacy of propranolol in the treatment of a migraine attack that has started has not been established, and propranolol is not indicated for such use.

ESSENTIAL TREMOR

Inderal is indicated in the management of familial or hereditary essential tremor. Familial or essential tremor consists of involuntary, rhythmic, oscillatory movements, usually limited to the upper limbs. It is absent at rest but occurs when the limb is held in a fixed posture or position against gravity and during active movement. Propranolol causes a reduction in the tremor amplitude but not in the tremor frequency. Propranolol is not indicated for the treatment of tremor associated with Parkinsonism.

HYPERTROPHIC SUBAORTIC STENOSIS

Inderal and Inderal LA are useful in the management of hypertrophic subaortic stenosis, especially for treatment of exertional or other stress-induced angina, palpitations, and syncope. Inderal and Inderal LA also improves exercise performance. The effectiveness of propranolol hydrochloride in this disease appears to be due to a reduction of the elevated outflow pressure gradient, which is exacerbated by beta-receptor stimulation. Clinical improvement may be temporary.

PHEOCHROMOCYTOMA

After primary treatment with an alpha-adrenergic blocking agent has been instituted, propranolol may be useful as *adjunctive* therapy if the control of tachycardia becomes necessary before of during surgery.

It is hazardous to use propranolol unless alpha-adrenergic blocking drugs are already in use, since this would predispose to serious blood pressure elevation. Blocking only the peripheral dilator (beta) action of epinephrine leaves its constrictor (alpha) action unopposed.

In the event of hemorrhage or shock, there is a disadvantage in having both beta and alpha blockade since the combination prevents the increase in heart rate and peripheral vasoconstriction needed to maintain blood pressure.

With inoperable or metastatic pheochromocytoma, propranolol may be useful as an adjunct to the management of symptoms due to excessive beta-receptor stimulation.

NON-FDA APPROVED INDICATIONS

Propranolol is used without FDA approval for the treatment of symptoms of hyperthyroidism, alcohol withdrawal, anxiety, Parkinsonian tremors, and for the prevention of esophageal variceal hemorrhage in patients with a history of esophageal varices.

CONTRAINDICATIONS

Propranolol is contraindicated in (1) cardiogenic shock, (2) sinus bradycardia and greater than first degree block, (3) bronchial asthma, (4) congestive heart failure (see WARNINGS) unless the failure is secondary to a tachyarrhythmia treatable with propranolol, and (5) in patients with known hypersensitivity to propranolol HCl.

WARNINGS

CARDIAC FAILURE

Sympathetic stimulation may be a vital component supporting circulatory function in patients with congestive heart failure, and its inhibition by beta blockade may precipitate more severe failure. Although beta blockers should be avoided in overt congestive heart failure, if necessary, they can be used with close follow-up in patients with a history of failure who are well compensated and are receiving digitalis and diuretics. Beta-adrenergic blocking agents do not abolish the inotropic action of digitalis on heart muscle.

IN PATIENTS WITHOUT A HISTORY OF HEART FAILURE

Continued use of beta blockers can, in some cases, lead to cardiac failure. Therefore, at the first sign or symptom of heart failure, the patient should be digitalized and/or treated with diuretics, and the response observed closely, or propranolol should be discontinued (gradually, if possible).

In Patients With Angina Pectoris: There have been reports of exacerbation of angina and, in some cases, myocardial infarction, following *abrupt* discontinuance of propranolol therapy. Therefore, when discontinuance of propranolol is planned, the dosage should be gradually reduced over at least a few weeks and the patient should be cautioned against interruption or cessation of therapy without the physician's advice. If propranolol therapy is interrupted and exacerbation of angina occurs, it usually is advisable to reinstitute propranolol therapy and take other measures appropriate for the management of unstable angina pectoris. Since coronary artery disease may be unrecognized, it may be prudent to follow the above advice in patients considered at risk of having occult atherosclerotic heart disease who are given propranolol for other indications.

NONALLERGIC BRONCHOSPASM (E.G., CHRONIC BRONCHITIS, EMPHYSEMA)

PATIENTS WITH BRONCHOSPASTIC DISEASES SHOULD IN GENERAL NOT RECEIVE BETA BLOCKERS. Propranolol should be administered with caution since it may block bronchodilation produced by endogenous and exogenous catecholamine stimulation of beta receptors.

MAJOR SURGERY

The necessity or desirability of withdrawal of beta-blocking therapy prior to major surgery is controversial. It should be noted, however, that the impaired ability of the heart to respond to reflex adrenergic stimuli may augment the risks of general anesthesia and surgical procedures.

Propranolol, like other beta blockers, is a competitive inhibitor of beta-receptor agonists, and its effects can be reversed by administration of such agents, (*e.g.,* dobutamine or isoproterenol). However, such patients may be subject to protracted severe hypotension. Difficulty in starting and maintaining the heartbeat has also been reported with beta blockers.

DIABETES AND HYPOGLYCEMIA

Beta-adrenergic blockage may prevent the appearance of certain premonitory signs and symptoms (pulse rate and pressure changes) of acute hypoglycemica in labile insulin-dependent diabetes. In these patients, it may be more difficult to adjust the dosage of insulin. Hypoglycemic attacks may be accompanied by a precipitous elevation of blood pressure in patients on propranolol.

Propranolol therapy, particularly in infants and children, diabetic or not, has been associated with hypoglycemia especially during fasting as in preparation for surgery. Hypoglycemia also has been found after this type of drug therapy and prolonged physical exertion and has occurred in renal insufficiency, both during dialysis and sporadically, in patients on propranolol.

Acute increases in blood pressure have occurred after insulin-induced hypoglycemia in patients on propranolol.

THYROTOXICOSIS

Beta blockade may mask certain clinical signs of hyperthyroidism. Therefore, abrupt withdrawal of propranolol may be followed by an exacerbation of symptoms of hyperthyroidism, including thyroid storm. Propranolol may change thyroid-function tests, increasing T_4 and reverse T_3 and decreasing T_3.

IN PATIENTS WITH WOLF-PARKINSON-WHITE SYNDROME

Several cases have been reported in which, after propranolol, the tachycardia was replaced by a severe bradycardia requiring a demand pacemaker. In 1 case this resulted after an initial dose of 5 mg propranolol.

PRECAUTIONS

GENERAL

Propranolol should be used with caution in patients with impaired hepatic or renal function. Propranolol HCl is not indicated for the treatment of hypertensive emergencies.

Beta-adrenoreceptor blockade can cause reduction of intraocular pressure. Patients should be told that propranolol may interfere with the glaucoma screening test. Withdrawal may lead to a return of increased intraocular pressure.

CLINICAL LABORATORY TESTS

Elevated blood urea levels in patients with severe heart disease, elevated serum transaminase, alkaline phosphatase, lactate dehydrogenase.

CARCINOGENESIS, MUTAGENESIS, AND IMPAIRMENT OF FERTILITY

In dietary administration studies in which mice and rats were treated with propranolol for up to 18 months at doses of up to 150 mg/kg/day, there was no evidence of drug-related tumorigenesis. In a study in which both male and female rats were exposed to propranolol in their diets at concentrations of up to 0.05%, from 60 days prior to mating and throughout pregnancy and lactation for two generations, there were no effects on fertility. Based on differing results from Ames Tests performed by different laboratories, there is equivocal evidence for a genotoxic effect of propranolol in bacteria (*S. typhimurium* strain TA 1538).

PREGNANCY CATEGORY C

In a series of reproduction and developmental toxicology studies, propranolol was given to rats by gavage or in the diet throughout pregnancy and through lactation. At doses of 150 mg/kg/day (>10 times the maximum recommended human daily dose of propranolol on a body weight basis), but not at doses of 80 mg/kg/day, treatment was associated with embryotoxicity (reduced litter size and increased resorption sites) as well as neonatal toxicity (deaths). Propranolol also was administered (in the feed) to rabbits (throughout pregnancy and lactation) at doses as high as 150 mg/kg/day (>15 times the maximum recommended daily human dose). No evidence of embryo or neonatal toxicity was noted.

There are no adequate and well-controlled studies in pregnant women. Intertwine growth retardation has been reported in neonates whose mothers received propranolol during pregnancy. Neonates whose mothers are receiving propranolol at parturition have exhibited bradycardia, hypoglycemia and respiratory depression. Adequate facilities for monitoring these infants at birth should be available. Propranolol should be used during pregnancy only if the potential benefit justifies the potential risk to the fetus.

NURSING MOTHERS

Propranolol is excreted in human milk. Caution should be exercised when propranolol is administered to a nursing woman.

PEDIATRIC USE

High serum propranolol levels have been noted in patients with Down's syndrome (trisomy 21), suggesting that the bioavailability of propranolol may be increased in patients with this condition.

Evaluation of the effects of propranolol in children, relative to the drug's efficacy and safety, has not been as systematically performed as in adults. Information is available in the medical literature to allow fair estimates, and specific dosing information has been reasonably studied.

Cardiovascular diseases that are common to adults and children are generally as responsive to propranolol intervention in children as they are in adults.

Adverse reactions are also similar, for example, bronchospasm and congestive heart failure related to propranolol therapy have been reported in children and occur through the same mechanisms as previously described in adults.

The normal echocardiogram evolves through a series of changes as the heart matures during growth and development in children. Should echocardiography be used to monitor propranolol therapy in children, the age-related changes in the echocardiogram need to be borne in mind.

GERIATRIC USE

Clinical studies of propranolol did not include sufficient numbers of subjects aged 65 and over to determine whether thay respond differently from younger subjects. Other reported clinical experience has not identified differences in reponses between the elderly and younger patients. In general, dose selection for an elderly patient should be cautious, usually starting at the low end of the dosing range, reflecting the greater frequency of the decreased hepatic, renal or cardiac function, and concomitant disease or other drug therapy.

DRUG INTERACTIONS

CARDIOVASCULAR DRUGS

ACE Inhibitors

When combined with beta-blockers, ACE inhibitors can cause hypotension, particularly in the setting of acute myocardial infarction.

Certain ACE inhibitors have been reported to increase bronchial hyperreactivity when administered with propranolol.

The antihypertensive effects of clonidine may be antagonized by beta-blockers. Propanolol should be administered cautiously to patients withdrawing from clonidine.

Alpha Blockers

Prazosin has been associated with prolongation of first dose hypotension in the presence of beta-blockers.

Postural hypotension has been reported in patients taking both beta-blockers and terazosin or doxazosin.

Antiarrhythmics

Propafenone has negative inotropic and beta-blocking properties that can be additive to those of propranolol.

P

Quinidine increases the concentration of propranolol and produces greater degrees of clinical beta-blockade and may cause postural hypotension.

Disopyramide is a Type 1 antiarrhythmic drug with potent negative inotropic and chronotropic effects and has been associated with severe bradycardia, asystole and heart failure when administered with propranolol.

Amiodarone is an antiarrhythmic agent with negative chronotropic properties that may be additive to those seen with propranolol.

The clearance of lidocaine is reduced with administration of propranolol. Lidocaine toxicity has been reported following coadministration with propranolol.

Caution should be exercised when administering propranolol with drugs that slow A-V nodal conduction, *e.g.,* digitalis, lidocaine and calcium channel blockers.

Calcium Channel Blockers

Caution should be exercised when patients receiving a beta-blocker are administered a calcium-channel-blocking drug with negative inotropic and/or chronotropic effects. Both agents may depress myocardial contractility or atrioventricular conduction.

There have been reports of significant bradycardia, heart failure, and cardiovascular collapse with concurrent use of verapamil and beta-blockers.

Coadministration of propranolol and diltiazem in patients with cardiac disease has been associated with bradycardia, hypotension, high degree heart block, and heart failure.

Inotropic Agents

Patients on long-term therapy with propranolol may experience uncontrolled hypertension if administered epinephrine as a consequence of unopposed alpha-receptor stimulation. Epinephrine is therefore not indicated in the treatment of propranolol overdose.

Isoproterenol and Dobutamine

Propranolol is a competitive inhibitor of beta-receptor agonists, and its effects can be reversed by administration of such agents, *e.g.,* dobutamine or isoproterenol. Also, propranolol may reduce sensitivity to dobutamine stress echocardiography in patients undergoing evaluation for myocardial ischemia.

Reserpine

Patients receiving catecholamine-depleting drugs, such as reserpine and propanol, should be closely observed for excessive reduction of resting sympathetic nervous activity, which may result in hypotension, marked bradycardia, vertigo, syncopal attacks, or orthostatic hypotension. Administration of reserpine with propranolol may also potentiate depression.

NON-CARDIOVASCULAR DRUGS

Anesthetic Agents

Methoxyflurane and trichloroethylene may depress myocardial contractility when administered with propranolol.

Antidepressants

The hypotensive effects of MAO inhibitors or tricyclic antidepressants may be exacerbated when administered with beta-blockers by interfering with the beta-blocking activity of propranolol.

Neuroleptic Drugs

Hypotension and cardiac arrest have been reported with the concomitant use of propranolol and haloperidol.

Non-Steroidal Anti-Inflammatory Drugs

Nonsteroidal anti-inflammatory drugs (NSAIDs) have been reported to blunt the antihypertensive effect of beta-adrenoreceptor blocking agents.

Administration of indomethacin with propranolol may reduce the efficacy of propranolol in reducing blood pressure and heart rate.

Thyroxine

Thyroxine may result in a lower than expected T_3 concentration when used concomitantly with propranolol.

Warfarin

Propranolol when administered with warfarin increases the concentration of warfarin. Prothrombin time, therefore, should be monitored.

Aluminum Hydroxide Gel: Greatly reduces intestinal absorption of propranolol.

Ethanol: Slows the rate of absorption of propranolol.

Phenytoin, Phenobarbitone and Rifampin: Accelerate propranolol clearance.

Chlorpromazine: When used concomitantly with propranolol, results in increased plasma levels of both drugs.

Antipyrine: Has reduced clearance when used concomitantly with propranolol.

Cimetidine: Decreases the hepatic metabolism of propranolol, delaying elimination and increasing blood levels.

Theophylline: Clearance is reduced when used concomitantly with propranolol.

ADVERSE REACTIONS

Most adverse effects have been mild and transient and have rarely required the withdrawal of therapy.

The following adverse events were observed and have been reported with use of formulations of sustained- or immediate-release propranolol:

Cardiovascular: Bradycardia; congestive heart failure; intensification of A-V block; hypotension; paresthesia of hands; thrombocytopenic purpura; arterial insufficiency, usually of the Raynaud type.

Central Nervous System: Light-headedness; mental depression manifested by insomnia, lassitude, weakness, fatigue; reversible mental depression progressing to catatonia; visual disturbances; hallucinations, vivid dreams, an acute reversible syndrome characterized by disorientation for time and place, short term memory loss, emotional lability, slightly clouded sensorium, and decreased performance on neuropsychometrics. Total daily doses above 160 mg (when administered as divided doses of greater than 80 mg each) may be associated with an increased incidence of fatigue, lethargy, and vivid dreams.

Gastrointestinal: Nausea, vomiting, epigastric distress, abdominal cramping, diarrhea, constipation, mesenteric arterial thrombosis, ischemic colitis.

Allergic: Pharyngitis and agranulocytosis, erythematous rash, fever combined with aching and sore throat, laryngospasm, and respiratory distress.

Respiratory: Bronchospasm.

Hematologic: Agranulocytosis, nonthrombocytopenic purpura, thrombocytopenic purpura.

Autoimmune: In extremely rare instances, systemic lupus erythematosus has been reported.

Miscellaneous: Alopecia, LE-like reactions, psoriasiform rashes, dry eyes, male impotence, and Peyronie's disease have been reported rarely. Oculomucocutaneous reactions involving the skin, serous membranes and conjunctivae reported for a beta blocker (practolol) have not been associated with propranolol.

Adverse events occurring at a rate of ≥3%, excluding those reported more commonly in placebo encountered in the propanol HCl extended-release placebo-controlled hypertension trials and are plausibly related to treatment, are shown in TABLE 1.

TABLE 1 *Treatment Emergent Adverse Events Reported In ≥3% of Subjects*

		InnoPran XL	
Body System	Placebo (n=88)	80 mg (n=89)	120 mg (n=85)
Fatigue	3 (3.0%)	4 (5.0%)	6 (7.0%)
Dizziness (except vertigo)	2 (2.0%)	6 (7.0%)	3 (4.0%)
Constipation	0	3 (3.0%)	1 (1.0%)

DOSAGE AND ADMINISTRATION

ORAL

The dosage range for propranolol is different for each indication.

Hypertension

Dosage must be individualized. The usual initial dosage is 40 mg propranolol twice daily, whether used alone or added to a diuretic. Dosage may be increased gradually until adequate blood pressure control is achieved. The usual maintenance dosage is 120-240 mg/day. In some instances a dosage of 640 mg/day may be required. The time needed for full antihypertensive response to a given dosage is variable and may range from a few days to several weeks.

While twice-daily dosing is effective and can maintain a reduction in blood pressure throughout the day, some patients, especially when lower doses are used, may experience a modest rise in blood pressure toward the end of the 12 hour dosing interval. This can be evaluated by measuring blood pressure near the end of the dosing interval to determine whether satisfactory control is being maintained throughout the day. If control is not adequate, a larger dose, or 3 times daily therapy may achieve better control.

Angina Pectoris

Dosage must be individualized. Total daily doses of 80-320 mg, when administered orally, twice a day, 3 times/day, or 4 times/day, have been shown to increase exercise tolerance and to reduce ischemic changes in the ECG. If treatment is to be discontinued, reduce dosage gradually over a period of several weeks. (See WARNINGS.)

Arrhythmias

10-30 mg 3 or 4 times daily, before meals and at bedtime.

Myocardial Infarction

The recommended daily dosage is 180-240 mg/day in divided doses. Although a tid regimen was used in the Beta-Blocker Heart Attack Trial and a qid regimen in the Norwegian Multicenter Trial, there is a reasonable basis for the use of either a tid or bid regimen (see CLINICAL PHARMACOLOGY). The effectiveness and safety of daily dosages greater than 240 mg for prevention of cardiac mortality have not been established. However, higher dosages may be needed to effectively treat coexisting diseases such as angina or hypertension. (See DOSAGE AND ADMINISTRATION.)

Migraine

Dosage must be individualized. The initial oral dose is 80 mg propranolol daily in divided doses. The usual effective dose range is 160-240 mg/day. The dosage may be increased gradually to achieve optimum migraine prophylaxis. If a satisfactory response is not obtained within 4-6 weeks after reaching the maximum dose, propranolol therapy should be discontinued. It may be advisable to withdraw the drug gradually over a period of several weeks.

Essential Tremor

Dosage must be individualized. The initial dosage is 40 mg propranolol twice daily. Optimum reduction of essential tremor is usually achieved with a dose of 120 mg/day. Occasionally, it may be necessary to administer 240-320 mg/day.

Hypertrophic Subaortic Stenosis

20-40 mg 3 or 4 times daily, before meals and at bedtime.

Pheochromocytoma

Preoperatively — 60 mg daily in divided doses for 3 days prior to surgery, concomitantly with an alpha-adrenergic blocking agent.

Management of Inoperable Tumor

30 mg daily in divided doses.

Use in Children

Intravenous administration of propranolol is not recommended in children. Oral dosage for treating hypertension requires individual titration, beginning with a 1.0 mg/kg (body weight)/day dosage regimen (*i.e.,* 0.5 mg/kg bid).

The usual pediatric dosage range is 2-4 mg/kg/day in 2 equally divided doses (*i.e.,* 1.0-2.0 mg/kg bid). Pediatric dosage calculated by weight (recommended) generally produces propranolol plasma levels in a therapeutic range similar to that in adults. On the other hand, pediatric doses calculated on the basis of body surface area (*not* recommended) usually result in plasma levels above the mean adult therapeutic range. Doses above 16 mg/kg/day should not be used in children. If treatment with propranolol is to be discontinued, a gradually decreasing dose titration over a 7-14 day period is necessary.

INTRAVENOUS

Parenteral drug products should be inspected visually for particulate matter and discoloration prior to administration, whenever solution and container permit. Intravenous administration is reserved for life-threatening arrhythmias or those occurring under anesthesia. The usual dose is from 1-3 mg administered under careful monitoring, (*e.g.,* electrocardiographic, central venous pressure). The rate of administration should not exceed 1 mg (1 ml)/ to diminish the possibility of lowering blood pressure and causing cardiac standstill. Sufficient time should be allowed for the drug to reach the site of action even when a slow circulation is present. If necessary, a second dose may be given after 2 minutes. Thereafter, additional drug should not be given in less than 4 hours. Additional propranolol should not be given when the desired alteration in rate and/or rhythm is achieved.

Transference to oral therapy should be made as soon as possible.

The IV administration of propranolol has not been evaluated adequately in the management of hypertensive emergencies.

Inderal LA Capsules

Inderal LA provides propanalol HCl in a sustained-release capsule for administration once daily. If patients are switched from Inderal tablets to Inderal LA capsules, care should be taken to assure that the desired therapeutic effect is maintained. Inderal LA should not be considered a simple mg-for-mg substitute for Inderal. Inderal LA has different kinetics and produces lower blood levels. Retitration may be necessary, especially to maintain effectiveness at the end of the 24 hour dosing interval.

Hypertension

Dosage must be individualized. The usual initial dosage is 80 mg Inderal LA once daily, whether used alone or added to a diuretic. The dosage may be increased to 120 mg once daily or higher until adequate blood pressure control is achieved. The usual maintenance dosage is 120-160 mg once daily. In some instances a dosage of 640 mg may be required. The time needed for full hypertensive response to a given dosage is variable and may range from a few days to several weeks.

Angina Pectoris

Dosage must be individualized. Starting 80 mg Inderal LA once daily, dosage should be gradually increased at 3-7 day intervals until optimal response is obtained. Although individual patients may repond at any dosage level, the average optimal dosage appears to be 160 mg once daily. In angina pectoris, the value and safety of dosage exceeding 320 mg/day have not been established.

If treatment is to be discontinued, reduce dosage gradually over a period of a few weeks (see WARNINGS).

Migrane

Dosage must be individualized. The initial oral dose is 80 mg Inderal LA once daily. The usual effective dose range is 160-240 mg once daily. The dosage may be increased gradually to achieve optimal migrane prophylaxis. If a satisfactory response is not obtained within 4-6 weeks after reaching the maximal dose, Inderal LA therapy should be discontinued. It may be advisable to withdraw the drug gradually over a period of several weeks.

Hypertrophic Subaortic Stenosis

80-160 mg Inderal LA once daily.

Pediatric Dosage

At this time the data on the use of the drug in this age group are too limited to permit adequate directions for use.

InnoPran XL Capsules

InnoPran XL capsules should be administered once daily at bedtime (approximately 10:00 PM) and should be taken consistently either on an empty stomach or with food. The starting dose is 80 mg but dosage should be individualized and titration may be needed to a dose of 120 mg. In the clinical trial, doses of InnoPran XL above 120 mg had no additional effects on blood pressure. The time needed for full antihypertensive response is variable, but is usually achieved within 2-3 weeks.

HOW SUPPLIED

INDERAL TABLETS

Inderal tablets are available containing 10, 20, 40, 60 and 80 mg of propranolol hydrochloride.

10 mg Tablets: Orange, hexagonal-shaped, scored tablets embossed with "I" on one side and imprinted with "INDERAL 10" on the other.

20 mg Tablets: Blue, hexagonal-shaped, scored tablets embossed with "I" on one side and imprinted with "INDERAL 20" on the other.

40 mg Tablets: Green, hexagonal-shaped, scored tablets embossed with "I" on one side and imprinted with "INDERAL 40" on the other.

60 mg Tablets: Pink, hexagonal-shaped, scored tablets embossed with "I" on one side and imprinted with "INDERAL 60" on the other.

80 mg Tablets: Yellow, hexagonal-shaped, scored tablets embossed with "I" on one side and imprinted with "INDERAL 80" on the other.

Storage

Store at controlled room temperature 20-25°C (68-77°F).
Dispense in a well-closed container.

INDERAL INJECTABLE

Each 1 ml ampul contains 1 mg of propranolol HCl in water for injection. The pH is adjusted with citric acid.

Storage

Protect from freezing or excessive heat.

INDERAL LA (LONG-ACTING) CAPSULES

Inderal LA capsules are available containing 60, 80, 120 and 160 mg of propranolol HCl.

60 mg Capsules: White/light-blue capsules identified by 3 narrow bands, 1 wide band and imprinted with "INDERAL LA 60".

80 mg Capsules: Light-blue capsules identified by 3 narrow bands, 1 wide band and imprinted with "INDERAL LA 80".

120 mg Capsules: Light-blue/dark-blue capsules identified by 3 narrow bands, 1 wide band and imprinted with "INDERAL LA 120".

160 mg Capsules: Dark-blue capsules identified by 3 narrow bands, 1 wide band, and imprinted with "INDERAL LA 160".

Storage

Store at controlled room temperature 20-25°C (68-77°F).
Protect from light, moisure, freezing, and excessive heat.
Dispense in a tight, light-resistant container as defined in the USP.

INNOPRAN XL (EXTENDED-RELEASE) CAPSULES

InnoPran XL capsules are available containing 80 mg or 120 mg of propranolol HCl.

80 mg Capsules: Gray/white capsule identified by 2 segmented bands, imprinted with "80", "RD201", and Reliant logo.

120 mg Capsules: Each gray/off-white capsule identified by 3 segmented bands, imprinted with "120", "RD201", and Reliant logo.

Storage

Store at 25°C (77°F); excursions permitted to 15-30°C (59-86°F) in a tightly closed container. The unit dose packaging should be stored in the carton.

PRODUCT LISTING - RATED THERAPEUTICALLY EQUIVALENT

Capsule, Extended Release - Oral - 60 mg			
100's	$62.55	GENERIC, Major Pharmaceuticals Inc	00904-0421-60
100's	$64.00	GENERIC, Qualitest Products Inc	00603-5497-21
100's	$64.92	GENERIC, Moore, H.L. Drug Exchange Inc	00839-7572-06
100's	$65.75	GENERIC, Caremark Inc	00339-5753-12
100's	$67.18	GENERIC, Ivax Corporation	00182-1926-01
100's	$67.36	GENERIC, Aligen Independent Laboratories Inc	00405-4890-01
100's	$68.00	GENERIC, Geneva Pharmaceuticals	00781-2061-01
100's	$68.99	GENERIC, Inwood Laboratories Inc	00258-3609-01
100's	$108.21	GENERIC, Esi Lederle Generics	59911-5470-01
Capsule, Extended Release - Oral - 80 mg			
100's	$73.55	GENERIC, Major Pharmaceuticals Inc	00904-0422-60
100's	$77.28	GENERIC, Qualitest Products Inc	00603-5498-21
100's	$77.34	GENERIC, Moore, H.L. Drug Exchange Inc	00839-7573-06
100's	$78.96	GENERIC, Caremark Inc	00339-5755-12
100's	$79.59	GENERIC, Mutual/United Research Laboratories	00677-1364-01
100's	$81.17	GENERIC, Ivax Corporation	00182-1927-01
100's	$81.36	GENERIC, Aligen Independent Laboratories Inc	00405-4891-01
100's	$99.01	GENERIC, Inwood Laboratories Inc	00258-3610-01
100's	$126.55	GENERIC, Esi Lederle Generics	59911-5471-01
250's	$182.75	GENERIC, Watson/Rugby Laboratories Inc	00536-4912-02
Capsule, Extended Release - Oral - 120 mg			
100's	$90.90	GENERIC, Major Pharmaceuticals Inc	00904-0423-60
100's	$95.75	GENERIC, Caremark Inc	00339-5757-12
100's	$95.90	GENERIC, Qualitest Products Inc	00603-5499-21
100's	$96.24	GENERIC, Moore, H.L. Drug Exchange Inc	00839-7574-06
100's	$96.50	GENERIC, Parmed Pharmaceuticals Inc	00349-8701-01
100's	$97.89	GENERIC, Mutual/United Research Laboratories	00677-1365-01
100's	$101.00	GENERIC, Ivax Corporation	00182-1928-01
100's	$101.00	GENERIC, Inwood Laboratories Inc	00258-3611-01
100's	$132.63	GENERIC, Aligen Independent Laboratories Inc	00405-4892-01
100's	$156.85	GENERIC, Esi Lederle Generics	59911-5473-01
Capsule, Extended Release - Oral - 160 mg			
100's	$118.90	GENERIC, Major Pharmaceuticals Inc	00904-0424-60
100's	$125.00	GENERIC, Qualitest Products Inc	00603-5500-21
100's	$126.02	GENERIC, Moore, H.L. Drug Exchange Inc	00839-7575-06
100's	$128.56	GENERIC, Mutual/United Research Laboratories	00677-1366-01

100's	$129.76	GENERIC, Caremark Inc	00339-5759-12
100's	$132.31	GENERIC, Ivax Corporation	00182-1929-01
100's	$132.31	GENERIC, Inwood Laboratories Inc	00258-3612-01
100's	$137.63	GENERIC, Aligen Independent Laboratories Inc	00405-4893-01
100's	$205.38	GENERIC, Esi Lederle Generics	59911-5479-01
100's	$241.25	INDERAL LA, Wyeth-Ayerst Laboratories	00046-0479-81

Solution - Intravenous - 1 mg/ml

1 ml	$14.27	GENERIC, American Pharmaceutical Partners	63323-0604-01
1 ml x 10	$185.60	INDERAL, Wyeth-Ayerst Laboratories	00046-3265-10
1 ml x 25	$106.30	GENERIC, Bedford Laboratories	55390-0003-10
1 ml x 25	$156.25	GENERIC, Solo Pak Medical Products Inc	39769-0075-02

Solution - Oral - 20 mg/5 ml

5 ml x 40	$56.00	GENERIC, Roxane Laboratories Inc	00054-8764-16
500 ml	$34.65	GENERIC, Roxane Laboratories Inc	00054-3727-63

Solution - Oral - 40 mg/5 ml

5 ml x 40	$79.83	GENERIC, Roxane Laboratories Inc	00054-8765-16
500 ml	$49.51	GENERIC, Roxane Laboratories Inc	00054-3730-63

Tablet - Oral - 10 mg

25's	$4.33	GENERIC, Udl Laboratories Inc	51079-0277-19
30's	$4.67	GENERIC, Heartland Healthcare Services	61392-0420-30
30's	$4.67	GENERIC, Heartland Healthcare Services	61392-0420-39
30's	$103.60	GENERIC, Medirex Inc	57480-0355-06
31 x 10	$56.00	GENERIC, Vangard Labs	00615-2561-53
31 x 10	$56.00	GENERIC, Vangard Labs	00615-2561-63
31's	$4.82	GENERIC, Heartland Healthcare Services	61392-0420-31
32's	$4.98	GENERIC, Heartland Healthcare Services	61392-0420-32
45's	$7.00	GENERIC, Heartland Healthcare Services	61392-0420-45
60's	$4.11	GENERIC, Global Source Management	60429-0227-60
60's	$9.33	GENERIC, Heartland Healthcare Services	61392-0420-60
90's	$6.17	GENERIC, Global Source Management	60429-0227-90
90's	$14.00	GENERIC, Heartland Healthcare Services	61392-0420-90
100's	$2.25	GENERIC, Interstate Drug Exchange Inc	00814-6446-14
100's	$3.53	GENERIC, Us Trading Corporation	56126-0321-11
100's	$4.50	GENERIC, Major Pharmaceuticals Inc	00904-0411-60
100's	$5.00	GENERIC, Raway Pharmacal Inc	00686-0277-20
100's	$5.40	GENERIC, Caremark Inc	00339-5315-12
100's	$5.85	FEDERAL UPPER LIMIT, H.C.F.A. F F P	99999-2135-10
100's	$6.38	GENERIC, Aligen Independent Laboratories Inc	00405-4884-01
100's	$8.94	GENERIC, Purepac Pharmaceutical Company	00228-2327-10
100's	$9.20	GENERIC, Qualitest Products Inc	00603-5489-21
100's	$12.30	GENERIC, Auro Pharmaceutical	55829-0451-10
100's	$18.83	GENERIC, Watson Laboratories Inc	52544-0305-01
100's	$20.29	GENERIC, Udl Laboratories Inc	51079-0277-20
100's	$22.29	GENERIC, Ivax Corporation	00182-1812-89
100's	$24.75	GENERIC, Mylan Pharmaceuticals Inc	00378-0182-01
100's	$24.84	GENERIC, Watson/Schein Pharmaceuticals Inc	00364-0756-01
100's	$27.32	GENERIC, Major Pharmaceuticals Inc	00904-0411-61
100's	$33.53	GENERIC, Watson/Schein Pharmaceuticals Inc	00591-5554-01
100's	$33.55	GENERIC, Sidmak Laboratories Inc	50111-0467-01
100's	$46.31	INDERAL, Wyeth-Ayerst Laboratories	00046-0421-81
120's	$8.20	GENERIC, Golden State Medical	60429-0227-12
120's	$18.66	GENERIC, Heartland Healthcare Services	61392-0420-34
180's	$12.33	GENERIC, Global Source Management	60429-0227-18
200 x 5	$180.65	GENERIC, Vangard Labs	00615-2561-43

Tablet - Oral - 20 mg

10's	$2.78	GENERIC, Pd-Rx Pharmaceuticals	55289-0233-10
25's	$4.37	GENERIC, Pd-Rx Pharmaceuticals	55289-0233-97
25's	$19.73	INDERAL, Pd-Rx Pharmaceuticals	55289-0131-97
30's	$7.07	GENERIC, Heartland Healthcare Services	61392-0423-30
30's	$7.07	GENERIC, Heartland Healthcare Services	61392-0423-39
30's	$157.20	GENERIC, Medirex Inc	57480-0356-06
31 x 10	$86.58	GENERIC, Vangard Labs	00615-2562-53
31 x 10	$86.58	GENERIC, Vangard Labs	00615-2562-63
31's	$7.31	GENERIC, Heartland Healthcare Services	61392-0423-31
32's	$7.55	GENERIC, Heartland Healthcare Services	61392-0423-32
45's	$10.61	GENERIC, Heartland Healthcare Services	61392-0423-45
60's	$5.40	GENERIC, Global Source Management	60429-0164-60
60's	$14.15	GENERIC, Heartland Healthcare Services	61392-0423-60
90's	$4.29	GENERIC, Pd-Rx Pharmaceuticals	55289-0233-90
90's	$8.10	GENERIC, Global Source Management	60429-0164-90
90's	$21.22	GENERIC, Heartland Healthcare Services	61392-0423-90
100's	$2.63	GENERIC, Interstate Drug Exchange Inc	00814-6447-14
100's	$3.74	GENERIC, Us Trading Corporation	56126-0322-11
100's	$4.73	GENERIC, Pd-Rx Pharmaceuticals	55289-0233-01
100's	$5.50	GENERIC, Raway Pharmacal Inc	00686-0278-20
100's	$7.05	FEDERAL UPPER LIMIT, H.C.F.A. F F P	99999-2135-14
100's	$7.84	GENERIC, Caremark Inc	00339-5317-12
100's	$8.97	GENERIC, Aligen Independent Laboratories Inc	00405-4885-01
100's	$12.85	GENERIC, Purepac Pharmaceutical Company	00228-2329-10
100's	$12.85	GENERIC, Richmond Pharmaceuticals	54738-0468-01
100's	$15.25	GENERIC, Geneva Pharmaceuticals	00781-1354-13
100's	$16.21	GENERIC, Auro Pharmaceutical	55829-0452-10
100's	$25.00	GENERIC, Watson Laboratories Inc	52544-0306-01
100's	$26.61	GENERIC, Major Pharmaceuticals Inc	00904-0412-60
100's	$26.75	GENERIC, Mylan Pharmaceuticals Inc	00378-0183-01
100's	$26.88	GENERIC, Watson/Schein Pharmaceuticals Inc	00364-0757-01
100's	$27.09	GENERIC, Udl Laboratories Inc	51079-0278-20
100's	$27.93	GENERIC, Vangard Labs	00615-2562-13
100's	$28.29	GENERIC, Qualitest Products Inc	00603-5490-21
100's	$29.57	GENERIC, Major Pharmaceuticals Inc	00904-0412-61
100's	$32.54	GENERIC, Ivax Corporation	00182-1813-89
100's	$36.29	GENERIC, Watson/Schein Pharmaceuticals Inc	00591-5555-01
100's	$36.30	GENERIC, Sidmak Laboratories Inc	50111-0468-01
100's	$65.00	INDERAL, Wyeth-Ayerst Laboratories	00046-0422-81
120's	$28.30	GENERIC, Heartland Healthcare Services	61392-0423-34
180's	$16.20	GENERIC, Global Source Management	60429-0164-18

Tablet - Oral - 40 mg

30's	$4.80	GENERIC, Pd-Rx Pharmaceuticals	55289-0234-30
30's	$10.65	GENERIC, Heartland Healthcare Services	61392-0430-30
30's	$10.65	GENERIC, Heartland Healthcare Services	61392-0430-39
30's	$237.00	GENERIC, Medirex Inc	57480-0357-06
31 x 10	$130.20	GENERIC, Vangard Labs	00615-2563-53
31 x 10	$130.20	GENERIC, Vangard Labs	00615-2563-63
31's	$11.01	GENERIC, Heartland Healthcare Services	61392-0430-31
32's	$11.36	GENERIC, Heartland Healthcare Services	61392-0430-32
45's	$15.98	GENERIC, Heartland Healthcare Services	61392-0430-45
60's	$5.78	GENERIC, Pd-Rx Pharmaceuticals	55289-0234-60
60's	$21.30	GENERIC, Heartland Healthcare Services	61392-0430-60
90's	$6.11	GENERIC, Pd-Rx Pharmaceuticals	55289-0234-90
90's	$31.95	GENERIC, Heartland Healthcare Services	61392-0430-90
100's	$2.93	GENERIC, Interstate Drug Exchange Inc	00814-6448-14
100's	$3.69	GENERIC, Us Trading Corporation	56126-0323-11
100's	$6.00	GENERIC, Raway Pharmacal Inc	00686-0279-20
100's	$6.50	GENERIC, Pd-Rx Pharmaceuticals	55289-0234-01
100's	$8.48	FEDERAL UPPER LIMIT, H.C.F.A. F F P	99999-2135-18
100's	$11.53	GENERIC, Caremark Inc	00339-5319-12
100's	$12.89	GENERIC, Aligen Independent Laboratories Inc	00405-4886-01
100's	$16.95	GENERIC, Geneva Pharmaceuticals	00781-1364-13
100's	$17.79	GENERIC, Major Pharmaceuticals Inc	00904-0414-60
100's	$18.34	GENERIC, Purepac Pharmaceutical Company	00228-2331-10
100's	$22.23	GENERIC, Auro Pharmaceutical	55829-0453-10
100's	$37.99	GENERIC, Watson Laboratories Inc	52544-0307-01
100's	$40.99	GENERIC, Udl Laboratories Inc	51079-0279-20
100's	$45.27	GENERIC, Ivax Corporation	00182-1814-89
100's	$50.95	GENERIC, Mylan Pharmaceuticals Inc	00378-0184-01
100's	$51.19	GENERIC, Watson/Schein Pharmaceuticals Inc	00364-0758-01
100's	$56.31	GENERIC, Major Pharmaceuticals Inc	00904-0414-61
100's	$69.11	GENERIC, Watson/Schein Pharmaceuticals Inc	00591-5556-01
100's	$69.15	GENERIC, Sidmak Laboratories Inc	50111-0469-01
100's	$84.38	INDERAL, Wyeth-Ayerst Laboratories	00046-0424-81

Tablet - Oral - 60 mg

100's	$5.58	GENERIC, Us Trading Corporation	56126-0392-11
100's	$9.00	GENERIC, Major Pharmaceuticals Inc	00904-0416-60
100's	$13.58	GENERIC, Caremark Inc	00339-5320-12
100's	$28.01	GENERIC, Auro Pharmaceutical	55829-0455-10
100's	$41.45	GENERIC, Qualitest Products Inc	00603-5492-21
100's	$41.47	GENERIC, Sidmak Laboratories Inc	50111-0470-01
100's	$41.47	GENERIC, Watson Laboratories Inc	52544-0352-01
100's	$116.69	INDERAL, Wyeth-Ayerst Laboratories	00046-0426-81

Tablet - Oral - 80 mg

30's	$11.88	GENERIC, Heartland Healthcare Services	61392-0427-30
30's	$11.88	GENERIC, Heartland Healthcare Services	61392-0427-39
31's	$12.28	GENERIC, Heartland Healthcare Services	61392-0427-31
32's	$12.67	GENERIC, Heartland Healthcare Services	61392-0427-32
45's	$17.82	GENERIC, Heartland Healthcare Services	61392-0427-45
60's	$23.76	GENERIC, Heartland Healthcare Services	61392-0427-60
90's	$35.64	GENERIC, Heartland Healthcare Services	61392-0427-90
100's	$4.40	GENERIC, Us Trading Corporation	56126-0324-11
100's	$8.00	GENERIC, Raway Pharmacal Inc	00686-0280-20
100's	$11.40	FEDERAL UPPER LIMIT, H.C.F.A. F F P	99999-2135-25
100's	$17.23	GENERIC, Caremark Inc	00339-5321-12
100's	$21.48	GENERIC, Aligen Independent Laboratories Inc	00405-4888-01
100's	$29.42	GENERIC, Major Pharmaceuticals Inc	00904-0418-60
100's	$31.25	GENERIC, Qualitest Products Inc	00603-5493-21
100's	$34.90	GENERIC, Major Pharmaceuticals Inc	00904-0418-61
100's	$35.72	GENERIC, Auro Pharmaceutical	55829-0454-10
100's	$45.28	GENERIC, Watson Laboratories Inc	52544-0308-01
100's	$48.93	GENERIC, Udl Laboratories Inc	51079-0280-20
100's	$57.62	GENERIC, Ivax Corporation	00182-1815-89
100's	$63.10	GENERIC, Mylan Pharmaceuticals Inc	00378-0185-01
100's	$63.39	GENERIC, Watson/Schein Pharmaceuticals Inc	00364-0760-01
100's	$63.39	GENERIC, Sidmak Laboratories Inc	50111-0471-01
100's	$129.50	INDERAL, Wyeth-Ayerst Laboratories	00046-0428-81

PRODUCT LISTING - EQUIVALENTS NOT AVAILABLE

Capsule, Extended Release - Oral - 60 mg

30's	$65.97	GENERIC, Physicians Total Care	54868-1517-02
100's	$113.86	INDERAL LA, Allscripts Pharmaceutical Company	54569-1634-00
100's	$127.13	INDERAL LA, Wyeth-Ayerst Laboratories	00046-0470-81
100's	$164.74	GENERIC, Physicians Total Care	54868-1517-01

Capsule, Extended Release - Oral - 80 mg

30's	$26.91	GENERIC, Southwood Pharmaceuticals Inc	58016-0136-30
30's	$39.95	INDERAL LA, Allscripts Pharmaceutical Company	54569-0563-00
30's	$46.29	INDERAL LA, Physicians Total Care	54868-0680-00
30's	$58.78	GENERIC, Physicians Total Care	54868-1078-01
60's	$115.90	GENERIC, Physicians Total Care	54868-1078-05
100's	$89.71	GENERIC, Southwood Pharmaceuticals Inc	58016-0136-00

P

100's	$91.16	GENERIC, Southwood Pharmaceuticals Inc	58016-0604-00
100's	$148.63	INDERAL LA, Wyeth-Ayerst Laboratories	00046-0471-81
100's	$181.48	GENERIC, Physicians Total Care	54868-1078-03
Capsule, Extended Release - Oral - 120 mg			
30's	$47.90	INDERAL LA, Physicians Total Care	54868-1442-01
30's	$49.51	INDERAL LA, Allscripts Pharmaceutical Company	54569-0564-00
30's	$94.88	GENERIC, Physicians Total Care	54868-1518-01
100's	$147.67	INDERAL LA, Physicians Total Care	54868-1442-00
100's	$184.25	INDERAL LA, Wyeth-Ayerst Laboratories	00046-0473-81
100's	$239.27	GENERIC, Physicians Total Care	54868-1518-00
Concentrate - Oral - 80 mg/ml			
30 ml	$33.53	GENERIC, Roxane Laboratories Inc	00054-3728-44
Tablet - Oral - 10 mg			
15's	$4.69	GENERIC, Southwood Pharmaceuticals Inc	58016-0528-15
30's	$5.48	GENERIC, Allscripts Pharmaceutical Company	54569-0557-03
30's	$9.38	GENERIC, Southwood Pharmaceuticals Inc	58016-0528-30
40's	$7.30	GENERIC, Allscripts Pharmaceutical Company	54569-0557-00
60's	$18.77	GENERIC, Southwood Pharmaceuticals Inc	58016-0528-60
100's	$2.25	GENERIC, Cmc-Consolidated Midland Corporation	00223-2550-01
100's	$4.74	GENERIC, Physicians Total Care	54868-0052-02
100's	$18.25	GENERIC, Allscripts Pharmaceutical Company	54569-0557-01
100's	$31.28	GENERIC, Southwood Pharmaceuticals Inc	58016-0528-00
Tablet - Oral - 20 mg			
10's	$4.80	GENERIC, Southwood Pharmaceuticals Inc	58016-0529-10
10's	$7.23	GENERIC, Pharma Pac	52959-0212-10
15's	$7.21	GENERIC, Southwood Pharmaceuticals Inc	58016-0529-15
20's	$9.61	GENERIC, Southwood Pharmaceuticals Inc	58016-0529-20
20's	$10.05	GENERIC, Pharma Pac	52959-0212-20
30's	$7.28	GENERIC, Allscripts Pharmaceutical Company	54569-0559-00
30's	$14.41	GENERIC, Southwood Pharmaceuticals Inc	58016-0529-30
50's	$24.02	GENERIC, Southwood Pharmaceuticals Inc	58016-0529-50
60's	$12.94	GENERIC, Pharmaceutical Corporation Of America	51655-0350-24
60's	$14.55	GENERIC, Allscripts Pharmaceutical Company	54569-0559-03
90's	$3.74	GENERIC, Physicians Total Care	54868-0293-00
100's	$2.50	GENERIC, Cmc-Consolidated Midland Corporation	00223-2551-01
100's	$3.97	GENERIC, Physicians Total Care	54868-0293-01
100's	$24.25	GENERIC, Allscripts Pharmaceutical Company	54569-0559-01
100's	$48.04	GENERIC, Southwood Pharmaceuticals Inc	58016-0529-00
120's	$4.44	GENERIC, Physicians Total Care	54868-0293-04
200's	$6.28	GENERIC, Physicians Total Care	54868-0293-03
Tablet - Oral - 40 mg			
15's	$8.55	GENERIC, Southwood Pharmaceuticals Inc	58016-0531-15
30's	$2.47	GENERIC, Physicians Total Care	54868-0053-07
30's	$9.49	GENERIC, Pharmaceutical Corporation Of America	51655-0349-24
30's	$11.06	GENERIC, Allscripts Pharmaceutical Company	54569-0561-03
30's	$17.10	GENERIC, Southwood Pharmaceuticals Inc	58016-0531-30
60's	$22.11	GENERIC, Allscripts Pharmaceutical Company	54569-0561-01
100's	$3.00	GENERIC, Cmc-Consolidated Midland Corporation	00223-2552-01
100's	$4.33	GENERIC, Physicians Total Care	54868-0053-03
100's	$36.85	GENERIC, Allscripts Pharmaceutical Company	54569-0561-02
100's	$56.99	GENERIC, Southwood Pharmaceuticals Inc	58016-0531-00
200's	$7.00	GENERIC, Physicians Total Care	54868-0053-06
Tablet - Oral - 60 mg			
100's	$4.25	GENERIC, Cmc-Consolidated Midland Corporation	00223-2553-01
100's	$40.20	GENERIC, Allscripts Pharmaceutical Company	54569-0442-00
Tablet - Oral - 80 mg			
15's	$13.13	GENERIC, Southwood Pharmaceuticals Inc	58016-0532-15
30's	$2.39	GENERIC, Physicians Total Care	54868-0696-01
30's	$26.25	GENERIC, Southwood Pharmaceuticals Inc	58016-0532-30
100's	$3.75	GENERIC, Cmc-Consolidated Midland Corporation	00223-2554-01
100's	$43.90	GENERIC, Allscripts Pharmaceutical Company	54569-2499-00
100's	$87.50	GENERIC, Southwood Pharmaceuticals Inc	58016-0532-00

Propylthiouracil *(002138)*

Categories: Hyperthyroidism; Pregnancy Category D; FDA Approved 1947 Jul; WHO Formulary
Drug Classes: Antithyroid agents; Hormones/hormone modifiers
Brand Names: Propyl-Thyracil
Foreign Brand Availability: Antiroid (Korea); Propacil (Japan); Propycil (Bulgaria; Czech-Republic; Germany; Portugal); Thyreostat II (Germany); Tiotil (Sweden); Tirostat (Colombia); Uracil (Thailand)
Cost of Therapy: $2.03 (Hyperthyroidism; Generic Tablets; 50 mg; 3 tablets/day; 30 day supply)

DESCRIPTION

Propylthiouracil (6-propyl-2-thiouracil) is one of the thiocarbamide compounds. It is a white, crystalline substance that has a bitter taste and is slightly soluble in water.

Each tablet contains propylthiouracil, 50 mg (293.7 μmol), lactose, sodium lauryl sulfate, starch, stearic acid, and talc.

Propylthiouracil is an antithyroid drug administered orally. The molecular weight is 170.23. The empirical formula is $C_7H_{10}N_2OS$.

CLINICAL PHARMACOLOGY

Propylthiouracil inhibits the synthesis of thyroid hormones and thus is effective in the treatment of hyperthyroidism. The drug does not inactivate existing thyroxine and triiodothyronine that are stored in the thyroid or circulating in the blood nor does it interfere with the effectiveness of thyroid hormones given by mouth or by injection.

Propylthiouracil is readily absorbed from the gastrointestinal tract. It is metabolized rapidly and requires frequent administration. Approximately 35% of the drug is excreted in the urine, intact and in conjugated forms, within 24 hours.

In laboratory animals, various interventions, including propylthiouracil administration, that continuously suppress thyroid function and thereby increase TSH secretion result in thyroid tissue hypertrophy.

INDICATIONS AND USAGE

Propylthiouracil is indicated in the medical treatment of hyperthyroidism. Long-term therapy may lead to remission of the disease. Propylthiouracil may also be used to ameliorate hyperthyroidism in preparation for subtotal thyroidectomy or in radioactive iodine therapy. Propylthiouracil is also used when thyroidectomy is contraindicated or not advisable.

NON-FDA APPROVED INDICATIONS

While not an FDA approved indication, propylthiouracil has been used to treat alcoholic hepatitis. Further evaluation of the safety and efficacy of this use is needed.

CONTRAINDICATIONS

Propylthiouracil is contraindicated in the presence of hypersensitivity to the drug and, in nursing mothers, because the drug is excreted in milk.

WARNINGS

Agranulocytosis is potentially the most serious side effect of propylthiouracil therapy. Patients should be instructed to report any symptoms of agranulocytosis, such as fever or sore throat. Leukopenia, thrombocytopenia, and aplastic anemia (pancytopenia) may also occur. The drug should be discontinued in the presence of agranulocytosis, aplastic anemia (pancytopenia), hepatitis, fever, or exfoliative dermatitis. The patient's bone marrow function should be monitored.

Propylthiouracil can cause fetal harm when administered to a pregnant woman. Because the drug readily crosses placental membranes and can induce goiter and even cretinism in the developing fetus, it is important that a sufficient, but not excessive, dose be given. In many pregnant women, the thyroid dysfunction diminishes as the pregnancy proceeds; consequently, a reduction of dosage may be possible. In some instances, propylthiouracil can be withdrawn 2 or 3 weeks before delivery.

If this drug is used during pregnancy, or if the patient becomes pregnant while taking this drug, the patient should be warned of the potential hazard to the fetus.

Postpartum patients receiving propylthiouracil should not nurse their babies.

Rare reports exist of severe hepatic reactions including encephalopathy fulminant hepatic necrosis, and death in patients receiving propylthiouracil. Symptoms suggestive of hepatic dysfunction (anorexia, pruritus, right upper quadrant pain, etc) should prompt evaluation of liver function. Treatment with propylthiouracil should be discontinued promptly in the event of clinically significant evidence of liver abnormality, including hepatic transaminases in excess of 3 times the upper limit of normal.

PRECAUTIONS

GENERAL

Patients who receive propylthiouracil should be under close surveillance and should be impressed with the necessity of reporting immediately any evidence of illness, particularly sore throat, skin eruptions, fever, headache, or general malaise. In such cases, white-blood-cell and differential counts should be made to determine whether agranulocytosis has developed. Particular care should be exercised with patients who are receiving additional drugs known to cause agranulocytosis.

LABORATORY TESTS

Because propylthiouracil may cause hypoprothrombinemia and bleeding, prothrombin time should be monitored during therapy with the drug, especially before surgical procedures. Thyroid function tests should be monitored periodically during therapy. Once clinical evidence of hyperthyroidism has resolved, the finding of an elevated serum TSH indicates that a lower maintenance dose of propylthiouracil should be employed.

CARCINOGENESIS, MUTAGENESIS, AND IMPAIRMENT OF FERTILITY

Laboratory animals treated with propylthiouracil for >1 year have demonstrated thyroid hyperplasia and carcinoma formation. Such animal findings are seen with continuous sup-

P

pression of thyroid function by sufficient doses of a variety of antithyroid agents, as well as in dietary iodine deficiency, subtotal thyroidectomy, and implantation of autonomous thyrotropic hormone-secreting pituitary tumors. Pituitary adenomas have also been described.

USAGE IN PREGNANCY

Pregnancy Category D: See WARNINGS.

NURSING MOTHERS

The drug appears in human milk and is contraindicated in nursing mothers. See WARNINGS.

PEDIATRIC USE

See DOSAGE AND ADMINISTRATION.

DRUG INTERACTIONS

The activity of anticoagulants may be potentiated by anti-vitamin-K activity attributed to propylthiouracil.

ADVERSE REACTIONS

Major adverse reactions (much less common than the minor adverse reactions) include inhibition of myelopoiesis (agranulocytosis, granulopenia, and thrombocytopenia) aplastic anemia, drug fever, a lupus-like syndrome including splenomegaly, hepatitis, periarteritis, and hypoprothrombinemia and bleeding. Nephritis, interstitial pneumonitis, and erythema nodosum have been reported. Minor adverse reactions include skin rash, urticaria, nausea, vomiting, epigastric distress, arthralgia, paresthesia, loss of taste, abnormal loss of hair, myalgia, headache, pruritus, drowsiness, neuritis, edema, vertigo, skin pigmentation, jaundice, sialadenopathy, and lymphadenopathy. It should be noted that about 10% of patients with untreated hyperthyroidism have leukopenia (white-blood-cell count of less than 4000/cubic mm), often with relative granulopenia.

DOSAGE AND ADMINISTRATION

Propylthiouracil is administered orally. The total daily dosage is usually given in 3 equal doses at approximately 8 hour intervals.

Adult: The initial dosage is 300 mg daily. In patients with severe hyperthyroidism, very large goiters, or both, the beginning dosage usually should be 400 mg daily; an occasional patient will require 600 to 900 mg/day initially. The usual maintenance dosage is 100 to 150 mg daily.

Pediatric: For children 6 to 10 years of age, the initial dosage is 50 to 150 mg daily. For children 10 years and over, the initial dosage is 150 to 300 mg daily. The maintenance dosage is determined by the response of the patient.

Store at controlled room temperature, 15-30°C (59-86°F).

PRODUCT LISTING - RATED NOT THERAPEUTICALLY EQUIVALENT

Tablet - Oral - 50 mg

100's	$2.25	GENERIC, Global Pharmaceutical Corporation	00115-4322-01
100's	$5.25	GENERIC, Interstate Drug Exchange Inc	00814-6465-14
100's	$7.05	GENERIC, Major Pharmaceuticals Inc	00904-2173-60
100's	$8.49	GENERIC, Physicians Total Care	54868-1752-01
100's	$11.81	GENERIC, Esi Lederle Generics	00005-4609-23
100's	$13.50	GENERIC, West Ward Pharmaceutical Corporation	00143-1480-25
100's	$15.67	GENERIC, Purepac Pharmaceutical Company	00228-2348-10
100's	$15.75	GENERIC, West Ward Pharmaceutical Corporation	00143-1480-01

PRODUCT LISTING - EQUIVALENTS NOT AVAILABLE

Tablet - Oral - 50 mg

100's	$8.75	GENERIC, Cmc-Consolidated Midland Corporation	00223-1540-01

P

Protriptyline Hydrochloride (002143)

For related information, see the comparative table section in Appendix A.

Categories: Depression; FDA Approved 1967 Sep; Pregnancy Category C
Drug Classes: Antidepressants, tricyclic
Brand Names: Concordin; Triptil; **Vivactil**
Cost of Therapy: $85.06 (Depression; Vivactil; 5 mg; 3 tablets/day; 30 day supply)
$38.60 (Depression; Generic Tablets; 5 mg; 3 tablets/day; 30 day supply)

DESCRIPTION

Protriptyline HCl is N-methyl-5H-dibenzo [a,d]-cycloheptene-5-propanamine hydrochloride. Its empirical formula is $C_{19}H_{21}N{\cdot}HCl$.

Protriptyline HCl, a dibenzocycloheptene derivative, has a molecular weight of 299.84. It is a white to yellowish powder that is freely soluble in water and soluble in dilute HCl.

Vivactil (protriptyline HCl) is supplied as 5 and 10 mg film coated tablets. Inactive ingredients are calcium phosphate, cellulose, guar gum, hydroxypropyl cellulose, hydroxypropyl methylcellulose, lactose, magnesium stearate, starch, talc, and titanium dioxide. Vivactil 5 mg and 10 mg tablets also contain FD&C yellow 6. Vivactil 10 mg tablets also contain D&C yellow 10.

CLINICAL PHARMACOLOGY

Protriptyline HCl is an antidepressant agent. The mechanism of its antidepressant action in man is not known. It is not a monoamine oxidase inhibitor, and it does not act primarily by stimulation of the central nervous system.

Protriptyline HCl has been found in some studies to have a more rapid onset of action than imipramine or amitriptyline. The initial clinical effect may occur within 1 week. Sedative and tranquilizing properties are lacking. The rate of excretion is slow.

METABOLISM

Metabolic studies indicate that protriptyline is well absorbed from the gastrointestinal tract and is rapidly sequestered in tissues. Relatively low plasma levels are found after administration, and only a small amount of unchanged drug is excreted in the urine of dogs and rabbits. Preliminary studies indicate that demethylation of the secondary amine moiety occurs to a significant extent, and that metabolic transformation probably takes place in the liver. It penetrates the brain rapidly in mice and rats, and moreover that which is present in the brain is almost all unchanged drug.

Studies on the disposition of radioactive protriptyline in human test subjects showed significant plasma levels within 2 hours, peaking at 8-12 hours, then declining gradually.

Urinary excretion studies in the same subjects showed significant amounts of radioactivity in 2 hours. The rate of excretion was slow. Cumulative urinary excretion during 16 days accounted for approximately 50% of the drug. The fecal route of excretion did not seem to be important.

INDICATIONS AND USAGE

Protriptyline HCl is indicated for the treatment of symptoms of mental depression in patients who are under close medical supervision. Its activating properties make it particularly suitable for withdrawn and anergic patients.

NON-FDA APPROVED INDICATIONS

Protriptyline may have a role in the treatment of sleep apnea. However, this use is not approved by the FDA and further clinical testing is required.

CONTRAINDICATIONS

Protriptyline HCl is contraindicated in patients who have shown prior hypersensitivity to it.

It should not be given concomitantly with a monoamine oxidase inhibiting compound. Hyperpyretic crises, severe convulsions, and deaths have occurred in patients receiving tricyclic antidepressant and monoamine oxidase inhibiting drugs simultaneously. When it is desired to substitute protriptyline HCl for a monoamine oxidase inhibitor, a minimum of 14 days should be allowed to elapse after the latter is discontinued. Protriptyline HCl should then be initiated cautiously with gradual increase in dosage until optimum response is achieved.

This drug should not be used during the acute recovery phase following myocardial infarction.

WARNINGS

Protriptyline HCl may block the antihypertensive effect of guanethidine or similarly acting compounds.

Protriptyline HCl should be used with caution in patients with a history of seizures, and, because of its autonomic activity, in patients with a tendency to urinary retention, or increased intraocular tension.

Tachycardia and postural hypotension may occur more frequently with protriptyline HCl than with other antidepressant drugs. Protriptyline HCl should be used with caution in elderly patients and patients with cardiovascular disorders; such patients should be observed closely because of the tendency of the drug to produce tachycardia, hypotension, arrhythmias and prolongation of the conduction time. Myocardial infarction and stroke have occurred with drugs of this class.

On rare occasions, hyperthyroid patients or those receiving thyroid medication may develop arrhythmias when this drug is given.

In patients who may use alcohol excessively, it should be borne in mind that the potentiation may increase the danger inherent in any suicide attempt of overdosage.

USE IN CHILDREN

This drug is not recommended for use in children because safety and effectiveness in the pediatric age group have not been established.

USE IN PREGNANCY

Safe use in pregnancy and lactation has not been established; therefore, use in pregnant women, nursing mothers or women who may become pregnant requires that possible benefits be weighed against possible hazards to mother and child.

In mice, rats, and rabbits, doses about 10 times greater than the recommended human doses had no apparent adverse effects on reproduction.

PRECAUTIONS

GENERAL

When protriptyline HCl is used to treat the depressive component of schizophrenia, psychotic symptoms may be aggravated. Likewise, in manic-depressive psychosis, depressed patients may experience a shift toward the manic phase if they are treated with an antidepressant drug. Paranoid delusions, with or without associated hostility, may be exaggerated. In any of these circumstances, it may be advisable to reduce the dose of protriptyline HCl or to use a major tranquilizing drug concurrently.

Symptoms, such as anxiety or agitation, may be aggravated in overactive or agitated patients.

The possibility of suicide in depressed patients remains during treatment and until significant remission occurs. This type of patient should not have access to large quantities of the drug.

Concurrent administration of protriptyline HCl and electroshock therapy may increase the hazards of therapy. Such treatment should be limited to patients for whom it is essential.

Discontinue the drug several days before elective surgery, if possible.
Both elevation and lowering of blood sugar levels have been reported.

INFORMATION FOR THE PATIENT

While on therapy with protriptyline HCl, patients should be advised as to the possible impairment of mental and/or physical abilities required for performance of hazardous tasks, such as operating machinery or driving a motor vehicle.

DRUG INTERACTIONS

When protriptyline HCl is given with anticholinergic agents or sympathomimetic drugs, including epinephrine combined with local anesthetics, close supervision and careful adjustment of dosages are required.

Hyperpyrexia has been reported when tricyclic antidepressants are administered with anticholinergic agents or with neuroleptic drugs, particularly during hot weather.

Cimetidine is reported to reduce hepatic metabolism of certain tricyclic antidepressants, thereby delaying elimination and increasing steady-state concentrations of these drugs. Clinically significant effects have been reported with the tricyclic antidepressants when used concomitantly with cimetidine. Increases in plasma levels of tricyclic antidepressants, and in the frequency and severity of side effects, particularly anticholinergic, have been reported when cimetidine was added to the drug regimen. Discontinuation of cimetidine in well-controlled patients receiving tricyclic antidepressants and cimetidine may decrease the plasma levels and efficacy of the antidepressants.

It may enhance the response to alcohol and the effects of barbiturates and other ONS depressants.

DRUGS METABOLIZED BY CYTOCHROME P450 2D6

The biochemical activity of the drug-metabolizing isozyme, cytochrome P450 2D6 (debrisoquine hydroxylase), is reduced in a subset of the Caucasian population (about 7-10% of Caucasians are so called "poor metabolizers"); reliable estimates of the prevalence of reduced P450 2D6 isozyme activity among Asian, African, and other populations are not yet available. Poor metabolizers have higher than expected plasma concentrations of tricyclic antidepressants (TCAs) when given usual doses. Depending on the fraction of drug metabolized by P450 2D6, the increase in plasma concentration may be small or quite large (8-fold increase in plasma AUC of the TCA).

In addition, certain drugs inhibit the activity of this isozyme and make normal metabolizers resemble poor metabolizers. An individual who is stable on a given dose of TCA may become abruptly toxic when given 1 of these inhibiting drugs as concomitant therapy. The drugs that inhibit cytochrome P450 2D6 include some that are not metabolized by the enzyme (quinidine; cimetidine) and many that are substrates for P450 2D6 (many other antidepressants, phenothiazines, and the Type 1C antiarrhythmics, propafenone and flecainide). While all the selective serotonin reuptake inhibitors (SSRIs), *e.g.*, fluoxetine, sertraline, and paroxetine inhibit P450 2D6, they may vary in the extent of inhibition. The extent to which SSRI-TCA interactions may pose clinical problems will depend on the degree of inhibition and the pharmacokinetics of the SSRI involved. Nevertheless, caution is indicated in the coadministration of TCAs with any of the SSRIs, and also in switching from 1 class to the other. Of particular importance, sufficient time must elapse before initiating TCA treatment in a patient being withdrawn from fluoxetine, given the long half-life of the parent and active metabolite (at least 5 weeks may be necessary).

Concomitant use of tricyclic antidepressants with drugs that can inhibit cytochrome P450 2D6 may require lower doses than usually prescribed for either the tricyclic antidepressant or the other drug. Furthermore, whenever 1 of these other drugs is withdrawn from co-therapy, an increased dose of tricyclic antidepressant may be required. It is desirable to monitor TCA plasma levels whenever a TCA is going to be coadministered with another drug known to be an inhibitor of P450 2D6.

ADVERSE REACTIONS

Within each category the following adverse reactions are listed in order of decreasing severity. Included in the listing are a few adverse reactions which have not been reported with this specific drug. However, the pharmacological similarities among the tricyclic antidepressant drugs require that each of the reactions be considered when protriptyline is administered. Protriptyline HCl is more likely to aggravate agitation and anxiety and produce cardiovascular reactions such as tachycardia and hypotension.

Cardiovascular: Myocardial infarction; stroke; heart block; arrhythmias; hypolonsion, particularly orthostatic hypotension; hypertension; tachycardia; palpitation.

Psychiatric: Confusional states (especially in the elderly) with hallucinations, disorientation, delusions, anxiety, restlessness, agitation; hypomania; exacerbation of psychosis; insomnia, panic, and nightmares.

Neurological: Seizures; incoordination; ataxia; tremors; peripheral neuropathy; numbness, tingling, and paresthesias of extremities; extrapyramidal symptoms; drowsiness; dizziness; weakness and fatigue; headache; syndrome of inappropriate ADH (antidiuretic hormone) secretion; tinnitus; alteration in EEG patterns.

Anticholinergic: Paralytic ileus; hyperpyrexia; urinary retention, delayed micturition, dilatation of the urinary tract; constipation; blurred vision, disturbance of accommodation, increased intraocular pressure, mydriasis; dry mouth and rarely associated sublingual adenitis.

Allergic: Drug fever; petechiae; skin rash, urticaria, itching, photosensitization (avoid excessive exposure to sunlight); edema (general, or of face and tongue).

Hematologic: Agranulocytosis; bone marrow depression; leukopenia; thrombocytopenia; purpura; eosinophilia.

Gastrointestinal: Nausea and vomiting; anorexia; epigastric distress; diarrhea; peculiar taste; stomatitis; abdominal cramps; black tongue.

Endocrine: Impotence, increased or decreased libido; gynecomastia in the male; breast enlargement and galactorrhea in the female; testicular swelling; elevation or depression of blood sugar levels.

Other: Jaundice (simulating obstructive); altered liver function; parotid swelling; alopecia; flushing; weight gain or loss; urinary frequency, nocturia; perspiration.

Withdrawal Symptoms: Though not indicative of addiction, abrupt cessation of treatment after prolonged therapy may produce nausea, headache, and malaise.

DOSAGE AND ADMINISTRATION

Dosage should be initiated at a low level and increased gradually, noting carefully the clinical response and any evidence of intolerance.

Usual Adult Dosage: Fifteen (15) to 40 mg a day divided into 3 or 4 doses. If necessary, dosage may be increased to 60 mg a day. Dosages above this amount are not recommended. Increases should be made in the morning dose.

Adolescent and Elderly Patients: In general, lower dosages are recommended for these patients. Five (5) mg 3 times a day may be given initially, and increased gradually if necessary. In elderly patients, the cardiovascular system must be monitored closely if the daily dose exceeds 20 mg.

When satisfactory improvement has been reached, dosage should be reduced to the smallest amount that will maintain relief of symptoms.

Minor adverse reactions require reduction in dosage. Major adverse reactions or evidence of hypersensitivity require prompt discontinuation of the drug.

Usage in Children: This drug is not recommended for use in children because safety and effectiveness in the pediatric age group have not been established.

HOW SUPPLIED

Vivactil 5 mg tablets are orange, oval, film coated tablets coded "MSD 26".

Vivactil 10 mg tablets are yellow, oval, film coated tablets coded "MSD 47".

Storage: Store protriptyline HCl in a tightly closed container. Avoid storage at temperatures above 40°C (104°F).

PRODUCT LISTING - RATED THERAPEUTICALLY EQUIVALENT

Tablet - Oral - 5 mg			
100's	$42.89	GENERIC, Ivax Corporation	00182-2643-01
100's	$50.93	GENERIC, Martec Pharmaceuticals Inc	52555-0655-01
100's	$94.51	VIVACTIL, Odyssey Pharmaceutical	65473-0701-01
Tablet - Oral - 10 mg			
100's	$78.80	GENERIC, Martec Pharmaceuticals Inc	52555-0656-01
100's	$136.98	VIVACTIL, Odyssey Pharmaceutical	65473-0702-01

PRODUCT LISTING - EQUIVALENTS NOT AVAILABLE

Tablet - Oral - 10 mg			
100's	$62.17	GENERIC, Ivax Corporation	00182-2644-01

Pyrazinamide *(002150)*

Categories: Tuberculosis; FDA Approved 1971 Jun; Pregnancy Category C; WHO Formulary
Drug Classes: Antimycobacterials
Brand Names: Pirazinamida
Foreign Brand Availability: Braccopiral (Mexico; Philippines); Corsazinmid (Indonesia); Pezetamid (Germany); Piraldina (Bahrain; Cyprus; Egypt; India; Iran; Iraq; Italy; Jordan; Kuwait; Lebanon; Libya; Oman; Qatar; Republic-of-Yemen; Saudi-Arabia; Syria; United-Arab-Emirates); Pirilene (France); Prazina (Indonesia); Pyrafat (Austria; Germany; Hong-Kong); Pyramide (Japan); Pyzamed (Philippines); P-Zide (India); Rozide (South-Africa); Tebrazid (Belgium; Canada; Switzerland); Tisamid (Finland); Zapedia (Philippines); Zinamide (Australia; England; New-Zealand)
Cost of Therapy: $91.29 (Tuberculosis; Generic Tablets; 500 mg; 3 tablets/day; 30 day supply)

P

DESCRIPTION

Pyrazinamide, the pyrazine analogue of nicotinamide, is a white crystalline powder, stable at room temperature, and sparingly soluble in water. Pyrazinamide tablets contain 500 mg of pyrazinamide and the following inactive ingredients: corn starch, magnesium stearate, modified food starch and stearic acid.

Storage: Store at controlled room temperature 15-30°C (59-86°F)

CLINICAL PHARMACOLOGY

Bacteriostatic against *Mycobacterium tuberculosis.*

INDICATIONS AND USAGE

Failure after adequate treatment with primary drugs (that is, isoniazid, streptomycin, aminosalicylic acid) in any form of active tuberculosis. Pyraminazide should only be given with other effective antituberculous agents.

CONTRAINDICATIONS

Severe hepatic damage.

WARNINGS

Pyrazinamide should be used only when close observation of the patient is possible and when laboratory facilities are available for performing frequent reliable liver function tests and blood uric acid determinations.

Pyraminazide should be discontinued and not be resumed if signs of hepatocellular damage or hyperuricemia accompanied by an acute gouty arthritis become manifest.

Use in Children: Safe use of this drug in children has not been established. Because of its potential toxicity, its use in children should be avoided unless crucial to therapy.

PRECAUTIONS

Pretreatment examinations should include *in vitro* susceptability tests of recent cultures of M. tuberculosis from the patient as measured against pyrazinamide and the usual primary drugs; however, there is no reliable *in vitro* test for pyraminazide resistance.

Liver function tests (especially SGPT, SGOT determinations) should be carried out prior to, and every 2-4 weeks during therapy.

This drug should be used with caution in patients with a history of gout or diabetes mellitus, as management may be more difficult.

ADVERSE REACTIONS

The principal untoward effect is a hepatic reaction. This varies from a symptomless abnormality of hepatic cell function, detectable only by laboratory tests, through a mild syndrome of fever, anorexia, malaise, liver tenderness, hepatomegaly and splenomegaly to more serious reactions such as clinical jaundice and rare cases of progressive fulminating acute yellow atrophy and death.

Other reactions are active gout, sideroblastica anemia, and adverse effects on the blood-clotting mechanism or vascular integrity.

DOSAGE AND ADMINISTRATION

Pyraminazide should be administered with at least one other effective antituberculous drug.

Usual adult dose: 20-35 mg/kg/day in 3-4 divided doses; 3.0 grams per day should not be exceeded.

PRODUCT LISTING - RATED THERAPEUTICALLY EQUIVALENT

Tablet - Oral - 500 mg

60's	$68.63	GENERIC, Versapharm Inc	61748-0012-06
90's	$101.35	GENERIC, Versapharm Inc	61748-0012-09
100's	$101.43	GENERIC, Dixon-Shane Inc	17236-0961-01
100's	$109.97	GENERIC, Versapharm Inc	61748-0012-01
100's	$117.66	GENERIC, Versapharm Inc	61748-0012-11
100's	$118.20	GENERIC, American Health Packaging	62584-0848-01
100's	$162.50	GENERIC, Udl Laboratories Inc	51079-0691-20

PRODUCT LISTING - EQUIVALENTS NOT AVAILABLE

Tablet - Oral - 500 mg

100's	$91.75	GENERIC, Esi Lederle Generics	00005-5093-23
120's	$159.31	GENERIC, Physicians Total Care	54868-2487-01

Pyridostigmine Bromide *(002151)*

Categories: Myasthenia gravis; Toxicity, nondepolarizing muscle relaxants; FDA Approved 1959 Jan; WHO Formulary
Drug Classes: Cholinesterase inhibitors; Musculoskeletal agents; Stimulants, muscle
Brand Names: Mestinon
Foreign Brand Availability: Kalymin (Germany)
Cost of Therapy: $199.95 (Myasthenia gravis; Mestinon; 60 mg; 10 tablets/day; 30 day supply)
$179.94 (Myasthenia gravis; Generic Tablets; 60 mg; 10 tablets/day; 30 day supply)
$57.30 (Myasthenia gravis; Mestinon Extended Release; 180 mg; 2 tablets/day; 30 day supply)

INTRAVENOUS

DESCRIPTION

Mestinon (pyridostigmine bromide) is an orally active cholinesterase inhibitor. Chemically, pyridostigmine bromide is 3-hydroxy-1-methylpyridinium bromide dimethylcarbamate.

Each ml contains 5 mg pyridostigmine bromide compounded with 0.296 parabens (methyl and propyl) as preservatives, 0.0296 sodium citrate and pH adjusted to approximately 5.0 with citric acid and, if necessary, sodium hydroxide.

Mestinon injectable is available in 2 ml ampuls.

P

CLINICAL PHARMACOLOGY

ACTIONS

Pyridostigmine bromide facilitates the transmission of impulses across the myoneural junction by inhibiting the destruction of acetylcholine by cholinesterase. Pyridostigmine is an analog of neostigmine but differs from it clinically by having fewer side effects. Currently available data indicate that pyridostigmine may have a significantly lower degree and incidence of bradycardia, salivation and gastrointestinal stimulation. Animal studies using the injectable form of pyridostigmine and human studies using the oral preparation have indicated that pyridostigmine has a longer duration of action than does neostigmine measured under similar circumstances.

INDICATIONS AND USAGE

Pyridostigmine bromide injectable is useful in the treatment of myasthenia gravis and as a reversal agent or antagonist to nondepolarizing muscle relaxants such as curariform drugs and gallamine triethiodide.

NON-FDA APPROVED INDICATIONS

While not approved by the FDA, pyridostigmine has been used as a temporary treatment (if edrophonium is not available) before antivenin is obtained for muscle weakness due to Asian snake envenomation and tetrodotoxin poisoning. It has been used in the past for the treatment of postoperative urinary retention, paralytic ileus, and gastrointestinal motility disorders. Pyridostigmine has also been studied in the treatment of postpolio syndrome; however, it does not appear to have significant beneficial effects.

CONTRAINDICATIONS

Known hypersensitivity to anticholinesterase agents; intestinal and urinary obstructions of mechanical type.

WARNINGS

Pyridostigmine bromide injectable should be used with particular caution in patients with bronchial asthma or cardiac dysrhythmias. Transient bradycardia may occur and be relieved by atropine sulfate. Atropine should also be used with caution in patients with cardiac dysrhythmias. When large doses of pyridostigmine bromide are administered, as during reversal of muscle relaxants, the prior or simultaneous injection of atropine sulfate is advisable. Because of the possibility of hypersensitivity in an occasional patient, atropine and anti-shock medication should always be readily available.

As is true of all cholinergic drugs, overdosage of pyridostigmine bromide may result in cholinergic crisis, a state characterized by increasing muscle weakness which, through involvement of the muscles of respiration, may lead to death.

Myasthenic crisis due to an increase in the severity of the disease is also accompanied by extreme muscle weakness and thus may be difficult to distinguish from cholinergic crisis on a symptomatic basis. Such differentiation is extremely important, since increases in doses of pyridostigmine bromide or other drugs in this class in the presence of cholinergic crisis or of a refractory or "insensitive" state could have grave consequences. Osserman and Genkins[1] indicate that the two types of crisis may be differentiated by the use of edrophonium chloride as well as by clinical judgment. The treatment of the two conditions obviously differs radically. Whereas the presence of *myasthenic* crisis requires more intensive anticholinesterase therapy, *cholinergic crisis,* according to Osserman and Genkins,[1] calls for the prompt withdrawal of all drugs of this type. The immediate use of atropine in cholinergic crisis is also recommended. A syringe containing 1 mg of atropine sulfate should be immediately available to be given in aliquots intravenously to counteract severe cholinergic reactions.

Atropine may also be used to abolish or obtund gastrointestinal side effects or other muscarinic reactions; but such use, by masking signs of overdosage, can lead to inadvertent induction of cholinergic crisis.

For detailed information on the management of patients with myasthenia gravis, the physician is referred to one of the excellent reviews such as those by Osserman and Genkins,[2] Grob[3] or Schwab.[4,5] When used as an antagonist to nondepolarizing muscle relaxants, adequate recovery of voluntary respiration and neuromuscular transmission must be obtained prior to discontinuation of respiratory assistance and there should be continuous patient observation. Satisfactory recovery may be defined by a combination of clinical judgment, respiratory measurements and observation of the effects of peripheral nerve stimulation. If there is any doubt concerning the adequacy of recovery from the effects of the nondepolarizing muscle relaxant, artificial ventilation should be continued until all doubt has been removed.

USE IN PREGNANCY

The safety of pyridostigmine bromide during pregnancy or lactation in humans has not been established. Therefore, use of pyridostigmine bromide in women who may become pregnant requires weighing the drug's potential benefits against its possible hazards to mother and child.

PRECAUTIONS

Pyridostigmine is mainly excreted unchanged by the kidney.[6-8] Therefore, lower doses may be required in patients with renal disease, and treatment should be based on titration of drug dosage to effects.

ADVERSE REACTIONS

The side effects of pyridostigmine bromide are most commonly related to overdosage and generally are of two varieties, muscarinic and nicotinic. Among those in the former group are nausea, vomiting, diarrhea, abdominal cramps, increased peristalsis, increased salivation, increased bronchial secretions, miosis and diaphoresis. Nicotinic side effects are comprised chiefly of muscle cramps, fasciculation and weakness. Muscarinic side effects can usually be counteracted by atropine, but for reasons shown in the preceding section the expedient is not without danger. As with any compound containing the bromide radical, a skin rash may be seen in an occasional patient. Such reactions usually subside promptly upon discontinuance of the medication. Thrombophlebitis has been reported subsequent to intravenous (IV) administration.

DOSAGE AND ADMINISTRATION

FOR MYASTHENIA GRAVIS

To supplement oral dosage, pre- and postoperatively, during labor and postpartum, during myasthenic crisis, or whenever oral therapy is impractical, approximately 1130th of the oral dose of pyridostigmine bromide may be given parenterally, either by intramuscular (IM) or *very slow* IV injection. *The patient must be closely observed for cholinergic reactions, particularly if the IV route is used.*

For details regarding the management of myasthenic patients who are to undergo major surgical procedures, see the article by Foldes.[9]

Neonates of myasthenic mothers may have transient difficulty in swallowing, sucking and breathing. Injectable pyridostigmine bromide may be indicated — by symptomatology and use of the edrophonium chloride test — until pyridostigmine bromide syrup can be taken. To date the world literature consists of less than 100 neonate patients.[10] Of these only 5 were treated with injectable pyridostigmine, with the vast majority of the remaining neonates receiving neostigmine. Dosage requirements of pyridostigmine bromide injectable are minute, ranging from 0.05 mg to 0.15 mg/kg of body weight given intramuscularly. It is important to differentiate between cholinergic and myasthenic crises in neonates. (See WARNINGS.)

Pyridostigmine bromide given parenterally 1 hour before completion of second stage labor enables patients to have adequate strength during labor and provides protection to infants in the immediate postnatal state. For further information on the use of pyridostigmine bromide injectable in neonates of myasthenic mothers, see the article by Namba.[10]

Note: For information on a diagnostic test for myasthenia gravis, and on the evaluation and stabilization of therapy, please see product information on edrophonium chloride.

FOR REVERSAL OF NONDEPOLARIZING MUSCLE RELAXANTS

When pyridostigmine bromide injectable is given intravenously to reverse the action of muscle relaxant drugs, it is recommended that atropine sulfate (0.6-1.2 mg) also be given intravenously immediately prior to the pyridostigmine bromide. Side effects, notably excessive secretions and bradycardia, are thereby minimized. Usually 10 or 20 mg of pyridostigmine bromide will be sufficient for antagonism of the effects of the nondepolarizing muscle relaxants. Although full recovery may occur within 15 minutes in most patients, others may require a half hour or more. Satisfactory reversal can be evident by adequate voluntary respiration, respiratory measurements and use of a peripheral nerve stimulator device. It is recommended that the patient be well ventilated and a patent airway maintained until complete recovery of normal respiration is assured. Once satisfactory reversal has been attained, recurarization has not been reported. For additional information on the use of pyridostigmine bromide for antagonism of nondepolarizing muscle relaxants see the article by Katz[11] and McNall.[12]

Failure of pyridostigmine bromide injectable to provide prompt (within 30 minutes) reversal may occur, *e.g.*, in the presence of extreme debilitation, carcinomatosis, or with concomitant use of certain broad spectrum antibiotics or anesthetic agents, notably ether. Under these circumstances ventilation must be supported by artificial means until the patient has resumed control of his respiration.

ORAL

DESCRIPTION

Pyridostigmine bromide is an orally active cholinesterase inhibitor. Chemically, pyridostigmine bromide is 3-hydroxy-1-methylpyridinium bromide dimethylcarbamate.

Mestinon is available in the following forms:

Syrup containing 60 mg pyridostigmine bromide per teaspoonful in a vehicle containing 5% alcohol, glycerin, lactic acid, sodium benzoate, sorbitol, sucrose, FD&C red no. 40, FD&C blue no. 1, flavors and water.

Tablets containing 60 mg pyridostigmine bromide; each tablet also contains lactose, silicon dioxide and stearic acid.

Timespan tablets containing 180 mg pyridostigmine bromide; each tablet also contains carnauba wax, corn-derived proteins, magnesium stearate, silica gel and tribasic calcium phosphate.

CLINICAL PHARMACOLOGY

ACTIONS

Pyridostigmine bromide inhibits the destruction of acetylcholine by cholinesterase and thereby permits freer transmission of nerve impulses across the neuromuscular junction. Pyridostigmine is an analog of neostigmine, but differs from it in certain clinically significant respects; for example, pyridostigmine is characterized by a longer duration of action and fewer gastrointestinal side effects.

INDICATIONS AND USAGE

Pyridostigmine bromide is useful in the treatment of myasthenia gravis.

NON-FDA APPROVED INDICATIONS

While not approved by the FDA, pyridostigmine has been used as a temporary treatment (if edrophonium is not available) before antivenin is obtained for muscle weakness due to Asian snake envenomation and tetrodotoxin poisoning. It has been used in the past for the treatment of postoperative urinary retention, paralytic ileus, and gastrointestinal motility disorders. Pyridostigmine has also been studied in the treatment of postpolio syndrome; however, it does not appear to have significant beneficial effects.

CONTRAINDICATIONS

Pyridostigmine bromide is contraindicated in mechanical intestinal or urinary obstruction, and particular caution should be used in its administration to patients with bronchial asthma. Care should be observed in the use of atropine for counteracting side effects, as discussed below.

WARNINGS

Although failure of patients to show clinical improvement may reflect underdosage, it can also be indicative of overdosage. As is true of all cholinergic drugs, overdosage of pyridostigmine bromide may result in cholinergic crisis, a state characterized by increasing muscle weakness which, through involvement of the muscles of respiration, may lead to death. Myasthenic crisis due to an increase in the severity of the disease is also accompanied by extreme muscle weakness, and thus may be difficult to distinguish from cholinergic crisis on a symptomatic basis. Such differentiation is extremely important, since increases in doses of pyridostigmine bromide or other drugs of this class in the presence of cholinergic crisis or of a refractory or "insensitive" state could have grave consequences. Osserman and Genkins[1] indicate that the differential diagnosis of the two types of crisis may require the use of edrophonium chloride as well as clinical judgment. The treatment of the two conditions obviously differs radically. Whereas the presence of myasthenic crisis suggests the need for more intensive anticholinesterase therapy, the diagnosis of cholinergic crisis, according to Osserman and Genkins,[1] calls for the prompt *withdrawal* of all drugs of this type. The immediate use of atropine in cholinergic crisis is also recommended.

Atropine may also be used to abolish or obtund gastrointestinal side effects or other muscarinic reactions; but such use, by masking signs of overdosage, can lead to inadvertent induction of cholinergic crisis.

For detailed information on the management of patients with myasthenia gravis, the physician is referred to one of the excellent reviews such as those by Osserman and Genkins,[2] Grob[3] or Schwab.[4,5]

USE IN PREGNANCY

The safety of pyridostigmine bromide during pregnancy or lactation in humans has not been established. Therefore, use of pyridostigmine bromide in women who may become pregnant requires weighing the drug's potential benefits against its possible hazards to mother and child.

PRECAUTIONS

Pyridostigmine is mainly excreted unchanged by the kidney.[6-8] Therefore, lower doses may be required in patients with renal disease, and treatment should be based on titration of drug dosage to effect.[6,7]

ADVERSE REACTIONS

The side effects of pyridostigmine bromide are most commonly related to overdosage and generally are of two varieties, muscarinic and nicotinic. Among those in the former group are nausea, vomiting, diarrhea, abdominal cramps, increased peristalsis, increased salivation, increased bronchial secretions, miosis and diaphoresis. Nicotinic side effects are comprised chiefly of muscle cramps, fasciculation and weakness. Muscarinic side effects can usually be counteracted by atropine, but for reasons shown in the preceding section the expedient is not without danger. As with any compound containing the bromide radical, a skin rash may be seen in an occasional patient. Such reactions usually subside promptly upon discontinuance of the medication.

DOSAGE AND ADMINISTRATION

Pyridostigmine bromide is available in three dosage forms:

Syrup: Raspberry-flavored, containing 60 mg pyridostigmine bromide per teaspoonful (5 ml). This form permits accurate dosage adjustment for children and "brittle" myasthenic patients who require fractions of 60 mg doses. It is more easily swallowed, especially in the morning, by patients with bulbar involvement.

Conventional Tablets: Each containing 60 mg pyridostigmine bromide.

Timespan Tablets: Each containing 180 mg pyridostigmine bromide. This form provides uniformly slow release, hence prolonged duration of drug action; it facilitates control of myasthenic symptoms with fewer individual doses daily. The immediate effect of a 180 mg timespan tablet is about equal to that of a 60 mg conventional tablet; however, its duration of effectiveness, although varying in individual patients, averages 2 1/2 times that of a 60 mg dose.

DOSAGE

The size and frequency of the dosage must be adjusted to the needs of the individual patient.

Syrup and Conventional Tablets: The average dose is ten 60 mg tablets or ten 5 ml teaspoonfuls daily, spaced to provide maximum relief when maximum strength is needed. In severe cases as many as 25 tablets or teaspoonfuls a day may be required, while in mild cases 1-6 tablets or teaspoonfuls a day may suffice.

Timespan Tablets: One to three 180 mg tablets, once or twice daily, will usually be sufficient to control symptoms; however, the needs of certain individuals may vary markedly from this average. The interval between doses should be at least 6 hours. For optimum control, it may be necessary to use the more rapidly acting regular tablets or syrup in conjunction with timespan therapy.

Note: For information on a diagnostic test for myasthenia gravis, and for the evaluation and stabilization of therapy, please see product literature on edrophonium chloride.

HOW SUPPLIED

Mestinon is available as follows:

Syrup: 60 mg pyridostigmine bromide per teaspoonful (5 ml) and 5% alcohol.

Tablets: Scored, 60 mg pyridostigmine bromide each.

Timespan Tablets: Scored, 180 mg pyridostigmine bromide each.

Note: Because of the hygroscopic nature of the timespan tablets, mottling may occur. This does not affect their efficacy.

PRODUCT LISTING - RATED THERAPEUTICALLY EQUIVALENT

Solution - Injectable - 5 mg/ml

2 ml x 10	$50.40	MESTINON, Icn Pharmaceuticals Inc	00187-3011-10

PRODUCT LISTING - EQUIVALENTS NOT AVAILABLE

Syrup - Oral - 60 mg/5 ml			
480 ml	$52.81	MESTINON, Icn Pharmaceuticals Inc	00187-3012-20
Tablet - Oral - 60 mg			
100's	$54.80	MESTINON, Physicians Total Care	54868-3936-00
100's	$59.98	GENERIC, Watson Laboratories Inc	00591-3191-01
100's	$59.98	GENERIC, Geneva Pharmaceuticals	00781-5015-01
100's	$66.65	MESTINON, Icn Pharmaceuticals Inc	00187-3010-30
Tablet, Extended Release - Oral - 180 mg			
30's	$33.70	MESTINON TIMESPAN, Icn Pharmaceuticals Inc	00187-3013-30
100's	$95.50	MESTINON TIMESPAN, Icn Pharmaceuticals Inc	00187-3013-50

Pyridoxine Hydrochloride *(002152)*

Categories: Deficiency, pyridoxine; Pregnancy Category A; FDA Approved 1974 Feb; WHO Formulary
Drug Classes: Vitamins/minerals
Brand Names: Beesix; **Hexa-Betalin**; Rodex; Vitabee 6; Vitamin B-6
Foreign Brand Availability: B(6)-Vicotrat (Germany); Benadon (Bahamas; Barbados; Belize; Bermuda; Curacao; Guyana; Jamaica; Netherland-Antilles; Peru; Puerto-Rico; Surinam; Trinidad); Bexivit (Greece); Bonadon N (Germany); Hexobion 100 (Germany); Pyroxin (Australia)

DESCRIPTION

Pyridoxine hydrochloride, injection, a sterile solution of pyridoxine hydrochloride in water for injection with a pH between 2 and 3.8.

Each vial is preserved with chlorobutanol (chloroform derivative), 0.5%. Sodium hydroxide and/or hydrochloric acid may have been added during manufacture to adjust the pH.

Pyridoxine hydrochloride is a colorless or white crystal or a white crystalline powder. One g dissolves in 5 ml of water. It is stable in air and slowly affected by sunlight. Its chemical name is 2-methyl-3-hydroxy-4,5-bis(hydroxymethyl) pyridine hydrochloride.

CLINICAL PHARMACOLOGY

Natural substances that have vitamin B6 activity are pyridoxine in plants and pyridoxal or pyridoxamine in animals. All 3 are converted to pyridoxal phosphate by the enzyme pyri-

P

doxal kinase. The physiologically active forms of vitamin B6 are pyridoxal phosphate (co-decarboxylase) and pyridoxamine phosphate. Riboflavin is required for the conversion of pyridoxine phosphate to pyridoxal phosphate.

Vitamin B6 acts as a coenzyme in the metabolism of protein, carbohydrate, and fat. In protein metabolism, it participates in the decarboxylation of amino acids, conversion of tryptophan to niacin or to serotonin (5-hydroxytryptamine), deamination, and transamination and transulfuration of amino acids. In carbohydrate metabolism, it is responsible for the breakdown of glycogen to glucose-1-phosphate.

The total adult body pool consists of 16-25 mg of pyridoxine. Its half-life appears to be 15-20 days. Vitamin B6 is degraded to 4-pyridoxic acid in the liver. This metabolite is excreted in the urine.

The need for pyroxidine increases with the amount of protein the diet. The tryptophan load test appears to uncover early vitamin B6 deficiency by detecting xanthinuria. The average adult minimum daily requirement is about 1.25 mg. The "Recommended Dietary Allowance" of the National Academy of Sciences is estimated to be as much as 2 mg for adults and 2.5 mg for pregnant and lactating women. The requirements are more in persons having certain genetic defects or those being treated with isonicotinic acid hydrazide (INH) or oral contraceptives.

INDICATIONS AND USAGE

Pyridoxine hydrochloride injection is effective for the treatment of pyridoxine deficiency as seen in the following:

- Inadequate dietary intake
- Drug-induced deficiency, as from isoniazid (INH) or oral contraceptives
- Inborn errors of metabolism, *e.g.*, vitamin-B6-dependent convulsions or vitamin-B6-responsive anemia.

The parenteral route is indicated when oral administration is not feasible, as in anorexia, nausea and vomiting, and preoperative and postoperative conditions. It is also indicated when gastrointestinal absorption is impaired.

CONTRAINDICATIONS

A history of sensitivity to pyridoxine or to any of the ingredients in pyridoxine is a contraindication.

PRECAUTIONS

GENERAL

Single deficiency, as of pyridoxine alone, is rare. Multiple vitamin deficiency is to be expected in any inadequate diet. Patients treated with levodopa should avoid supplemental vitamins that contain more than 5 mg pyridoxine in the daily dose.

Women taking oral contraceptives may exhibit increased pyridoxine requirements.

PREGNANCY CATEGORY A

The requirement for pyridoxine appears to be increased during pregnancy. Pyridoxine is sometimes of value in the treatment of nausea and vomiting of pregnancy.

NURSING MOTHERS

The need for pyridoxine is increased during lactation.

It is not known whether this drug is excreted in human milk. Because many drugs are excreted in human milk, caution should be exercised when Pyridoxine is administered to a nursing woman.

PEDIATRIC USE

Safety and effectiveness in children have not been established.

DRUG INTERACTIONS

Pyridoxine supplements should not be given to patients receiving levodopa, because the action of the latter drug is antagonized by pyridoxine. However, this vitamin may be used concurrently in patients receiving a preparation containing both carbidopa and levodopa.

ADVERSE REACTIONS

Paresthesia, somnolence, and low serum folic acid levels have been reported.

DOSAGE AND ADMINISTRATION

In cases of dietary deficiency, the dosage is 10-20 mg daily for 3 weeks. Follow-up treatment is recommended daily for several weeks with an oral therapeutic multivitamin preparation containing 2-5 mg pyridoxine. Poor dietary habits should be corrected, an adequate, well-balanced diet should be prescribed.

The vitamin-B6-dependency syndrome may require a therapeutic dosage of as much as 600 mg a day and a daily intake of 30 mg for life.

In deficiencies due to INH, the dosage is 100 mg daily for 3 weeks, followed by a 30-mg maintenance dose daily.

In poisoning caused by ingestion of more than 10 g of INH, an equal amount of pyroxidine should be given—4 g intravenously followed by 1 g intramuscularly every 30 minutes.

This product should be protected from exposure to light.

PRODUCT LISTING - RATED THERAPEUTICALLY EQUIVALENT

Solution - Injectable - 100 mg/ml

Size	Price	Manufacturer	NDC
1 ml x 25	$82.50	GENERIC, American Pharmaceutical Partners	63323-0180-01
10 ml	$3.40	GENERIC, Major Pharmaceuticals Inc	00904-0828-10
10 ml	$4.25	GENERIC, Roberts/Hauck Pharmaceutical Corporation	43797-0030-12
10 ml	$6.45	GENERIC, Ivax Corporation	00182-0500-63

PRODUCT LISTING - EQUIVALENTS NOT AVAILABLE

Solution - Injectable - 100 mg/ml

Size	Price	Manufacturer	NDC
10 ml	$2.95	GENERIC, Keene Pharmaceuticals Inc	00588-5206-70
10 ml	$4.00	GENERIC, Pasadena Research Laboratories Inc	00418-2661-41
10 ml	$4.90	GENERIC, Primedics Laboratories	00684-0147-10
10 ml	$5.50	GENERIC, Cmc-Consolidated Midland Corporation	00223-8403-10
30 ml	$3.19	GENERIC, Mcguff Company	49072-0597-30
30 ml	$5.48	GENERIC, Interstate Drug Exchange Inc	00814-8447-46
30 ml	$7.44	GENERIC, Pasadena Research Laboratories Inc	00418-2661-61
30 ml	$9.00	GENERIC, Cmc-Consolidated Midland Corporation	00223-8404-30

Quazepam (002160)

Categories: Insomnia; Pregnancy Category X; DEA Class CIV; FDA Approved 1985 Dec
Drug Classes: Benzodiazepines; Sedatives/hypnotics
Brand Names: **Doral**; Dormalin; Oniria; Pamerex; Quazium; Quiedorm; Selepam; Temodal
Cost of Therapy: $34.36 (Insomnia; Doral; 15 mg; 1 tablet/day; 10 day supply)

DESCRIPTION

Doral (quazepam) Tablets contain quazepam, a trifluoroethyl benzodiazepine hypnotic agent, having the chemical name 7-chloro-5-(o-fluorophenyl)-1,3-dihydro-1-(2,2,2-trifluoroethyl)-2*H*-1,4-benzo-diazepine-2-thione.

Quazepam has the empirical formula $C_{17}H_{11}ClF_4N_2S$, and a molecular weight of 386.8. It is a white crystalline compound, soluble in ethanol and insoluble in water. Each Doral Tablet contains either 7.5 or 15 mg of quazepam. The inactive ingredients for Doral Tablets 7.5 or 15 mg include cellulose, corn starch, FD&C Yellow No. 6 Al Lake, lactose, magnesium stearate, silicon dioxide, and sodium lauryl sulfate.

CLINICAL PHARMACOLOGY

Central nervous system agents of the 1,4-benzodiazepine class presumably exert their effects by binding to stereo-specific receptors at several sites within the central nervous system (CNS). Their exact mechanism of action is unknown.

In a sleep laboratory study, quazepam significantly decreased sleep latency & total wake time, and significantly increased total sleep time and percent sleep time, for one or more nights. Quazepam 15 mg was effective on the first night of administration. Sleep latency, total wake time and wake time after sleep onset were still decreased and percent sleep time was still increased for several nights after the drug was discontinued. Percent slow wave sleep was decreased, and REM sleep was essentially unchanged. No transient sleep disturbance, such as "rebound insomnia," was observed after withdrawal of the drug in sleep laboratory studies in 12 patients using 15 mg doses.

In outpatient studies, quazepam improved all subjective measures of sleep including sleep induction time, duration of sleep, number of nocturnal awakenings, occurrence of early morning awakening, and sleep quality. Some effects were evident on the first night of administration of quazepam (sleep induction time, number of nocturnal awakenings, and duration of sleep). Residual medication effects ("hangover") were minimal.

Quazepam is rapidly (absorption half-life of about 30 minutes) and well absorbed from the gastrointestinal tract. The peak plasma concentration of quazepam is approximately 20 ng/ml after a 15 mg dose and is obtained at about 2 hours. Quazepam, the active parent compound, is extensively metabolized in the liver; two of the plasma metabolites are 2-oxoquazepam and N-desalkyl-2-oxoquazepam. All three compounds show pharmacological central nervous system activity in animals.

Following administration of ^{14}C-quazepam, approximately 31% of the dose appears in the urine and 23% in the feces over a five-day period; only trace amounts of unchanged drug are present in the urine.

The mean elimination half-life of quazepam and 2-oxoquazepam is 39 hours and that of N-desalkyl-2-oxoquazepam is 73 hours. Steady-state levels of quazepam and 2-oxoquazepam are attained by the seventh daily dose and that of N-desalkyl-2-oxoquazepam by the thirteenth daily dose.

The pharmacokinetics of quazepam and 2-oxoquazepam in geriatric subjects are comparable to those seen in young adults; as with desalkyl metabolites of other benzodiazepines, the elimination half-life of N-desalkyl-2-oxoquazepam in geriatric patients is about twice that of young adults.

The degree of plasma protein binding for quazepam and its two major metabolites is greater than 95%. The absorption, distribution, metabolism, and excretion of benzodiazepines may be altered in various disease states including alcoholism, impaired hepatic function, and impaired renal function.

The type and duration of hypnotic effects and the profile of unwanted effects during administration of benzodiazepine drugs may be influenced by the biologic half-life of administered drug and any active metabolites formed. When half-lives are long, drug or metabolites may accumulate during periods of nightly administration and be associated with impairments of cognitive and/or motor performance during waking hours; the possibility of interaction with other psychoactive drugs or alcohol will be enhanced. In contrast, if half-lives are short, drug and metabolites will be cleared before the next dose is ingested, and carry-over effects related to excessive sedation or CNS depression should be minimal or absent. However, during nightly use for an extended period, pharmacodynamic tolerance or adaptation to some effects of benzodiazepine hypnotics may develop. If the drug has a short half-life of elimination, it is possible that a relative deficiency of the drug or its active metabolites (*i.e.*, in relationship to the receptor site) may occur at some point in the interval between each night's use. This sequence of events may account for two clinical findings reported to occur after several weeks of nightly use of rapidly eliminated benzodiazepine hypnotics, namely, increased wakefulness during the last third of the night, and the appearance of increased signs of daytime anxiety in selected patients.

Quazepam crosses the placental barrier of mice. Quazepam, 2-oxoquazepam and N-desalkyl-2-oxoquazepam are present in breast milk of lactating women, but the total amount found in the milk represents only about 0.1% of the administered dose.

INDICATIONS AND USAGE

Quazepam is indicated for the treatment of insomnia characterized by difficulty in falling asleep, frequent nocturnal awakenings, and/or early morning awakenings. The effectiveness of quazepam has been established in placebo-controlled clinical studies of 5 nights duration in acute and chronic insomnia. The sustained effectiveness of quazepam has been established in chronic insomnia in a sleep lab (polysomnographic) study of 28 nights duration.

Because insomnia is often transient and intermittent, the prolonged administration of quazepam is generally not necessary or recommended. Since insomnia may be a symptom of several other disorders, the possibility that the complaint may be related to a condition for which there is a more specific treatment should be considered.

CONTRAINDICATIONS

Quazepam is contraindicated in patients with known hypersensitivity to this drug or other benzodiazepines, and in patients with established or suspected sleep apnea.

Usage in Pregnancy: Benzodiazepines may cause fetal damage when administered during pregnancy. An increased risk of congenital malformations associated with the use of diazepam and chlordiazepoxide during the first trimester of pregnancy has been suggested in several studies. Transplacental distribution has resulted in neonatal CNS depression following the ingestion of therapeutic doses of a benzodiazepine hypnotic during the last weeks of pregnancy.

Quazepam are contraindicated in pregnancy because the potential risks outweigh the possible advantages of their use during this period. If there is a likelihood of the patient becoming pregnant while receiving quazepam, she should be warned of the potential risk to the fetus. Patients should be instructed to discontinue the drug prior to becoming pregnant. The possibility that a woman of childbearing potential may be pregnant at the time of institution of therapy should be considered. See Pregnancy, Teratogenic Effects.

WARNINGS

Patients receiving benzodiazepines should be cautioned about possible combined effects with alcohol and other CNS depressants. Also, caution patients that an additive effect may occur if alcoholic beverages are consumed during the day following the use of benzodiazepines for nighttime sedation. The potential for this interaction continues for several days following their discontinuance until serum levels of psychoactive metabolites have declined.

Patients should also be cautioned about engaging in hazardous occupations requiring complete mental alertness, such as operating machinery or driving a motor vehicle, after ingesting benzodiazepines, including potential impairment of the performance of such activities which may occur the day following ingestion.

Withdrawal symptoms of the type associated with sedatives/hypnotics (*e.g.*, barbiturates, bromides, etc.) and alcohol have been reported after the discontinuation of benzodiazepines. While these symptoms have been more frequently reported after the discontinuation of excessive benzodiazepine doses, there have also been controlled studies demonstrating the occurrence of such symptoms after discontinuation of therapeutic doses of benzodiazepines, generally following prolonged use (but in some instances after periods as brief as six weeks). It is generally believed that the gradual reduction of dosage will diminish the occurrence of such symptoms.

PRECAUTIONS

GENERAL

Impaired motor and/or cognitive performance attributable to the accumulation of benzodiazepines and their active metabolites following several days of repeated use at their recommended doses is a concern in certain vulnerable patients (*e.g.*, those especially sensitive to the effects of benzodiazepines or those with a reduced capacity to metabolize and eliminate them). Consequently, elderly or debilitated patients and those with impaired renal or hepatic function should be cautioned about the risk and advised to monitor themselves for signs of excessive sedation or impaired coordination.

The possibility of respiratory depression in patients with chronic pulmonary insufficiency should be considered.

When benzodiazepines are administered to depressed patients, there is a risk that the signs and symptoms of depression may be intensified. Consequently, appropriate precautions (*e.g.*, limiting the total prescription size and increased monitoring for suicidal ideation) should be considered.

INFORMATION FOR THE PATIENT

It is suggested that physicians discuss the following information with patients. This information is intended to aid in the safe and effective use of this medication. It is not a disclosure of all possible adverse or intended effects.

1. Inform your physician about any alcohol consumption and medicine you are taking now, including drugs you may buy without a prescription. Alcohol should generally not be used during treatment with hypnotics.
2. Inform your physician if you are planning to become pregnant, if you are pregnant, or if you become pregnant while you are taking this medicine.
3. Inform your physician if you are nursing.
4. Until you experience how this medicine affects you, do not drive a car or operate potentially dangerous machinery, etc.
5. Benzodiazepines may cause daytime sedation, which may persist for several days following drug discontinuation.
6. Patients should be told not to increase the dose on their own and should inform their physician if they believe the drug "does not work anymore".
7. If benzodiazepines are taken on a prolonged and regular basis (even for periods as brief as six weeks), patients should be advised not to stop taking them abruptly or to decrease the dose without consulting their physician, because withdrawal symptoms may occur.

LABORATORY TESTS

Laboratory tests are not ordinarily required in otherwise healthy patients when quazepam is used as recommended.

CARCINOGENESIS, MUTAGENESIS, AND IMPAIRMENT OF FERTILITY

Quazepam showed no evidence of carcinogenicity or other significant pathology in oral oncogenicity studies in mice and hamsters.

Quazepam was tested for mutagenicity using the L5178Y TK +/-Mouse Lymphoma Mutagenesis Assay and Ames Test. The L5178Y TK +/-Assay was equivocal and the Ames Test did not show mutagenic activity.

Reproduction studies in mice conducted with quazepam at doses equal to 60 and 180 times the human dose of 15 mg, and with diazepam at 67 times the human dose, produced slight reductions in the pregnancy rate. Similar reduction in pregnancy rates have been reported in mice dosed with other benzodiazepines, and is believed to be related to the sedative effects of these drugs at high doses.

PREGNANCY CATEGORY X

Teratogenic Effects: (See CONTRAINDICATIONS, Usage in Pregnancy.) Reproduction studies of quazepam in mice at doses up to 400 times the human dose revealed no major drug-related malformations. Minor developmental variations that occurred were delayed ossification of the sternum, vertebrae, distal phalanges and supraoccipital bones, at doses of 66 and 400 times the human dose. Studies with diazepam at 200 times the human dose showed a similar or greater incidence than quazepam. A reproduction study of quazepam in New Zealand rabbits at doses up to 134 times the human dose demonstrated no effect on fetal morphology or development of offspring.

Nonteratogenic Effects: The child born of a mother who is taking benzodiazepines may be at some risk of withdrawal symptoms from the drug during the postnatal period. Neonatal flaccidity has been reported in children born of mothers who had been receiving benzodiazepines.

LABOR AND DELIVERY

Quazepam has no established use in labor or delivery.

NURSING MOTHERS

Quazepam and its metabolites are excreted in the milk of lactating women. Therefore, administration of quazepam to nursing women is not recommended.

PEDIATRIC USE

Safety and effectivenes in children below the age of 18 years have not been established.

DRUG INTERACTIONS

The benzodiazepines, including quazepam, produce additive CNS depressant effects when co-administered with psychotropic medications, anticonvulsants, antihistaminics, ethanol, and other drugs which produce CNS depression.

ADVERSE REACTIONS

Adverse events most frequently encountered in patients treated with quazepam are drowsiness and headache.

Accurate estimates of the incidence of adverse events associated with the use of any drug are difficult to obtain. Estimates are influenced by drug dose, detection technique, setting, physician judgments, etc. Consequently, the table below is presented solely to indicate the relative frequency of adverse events reported in representative controlled clinical studies conducted to evaluate the safety and efficacy of quazepam. The figures cited cannot be used to predict precisely the incidence of such events in the course of usual medical practice. These figures, also, cannot be compared with those obtained from other clinical studies involving related drug products and placebo.

The figures cited below (TABLE 1) are estimates of untoward clinical event incidences of 1% or greater among subjects who participated in the relatively short duration placebo-controlled clinical trials of quazepam.

TABLE 1

	Quazepam 15 mg	Placebo
Number Of Patients	**267**	**268**
	% Of Patients Reporting	
Central Nervous System		
Daytime Drowsiness	12.0	3.3
Headache	4.5	2.2
Fatigue	1.9	0
Dizziness	1.5	<1
Autonomic Nervous System		
Dry Mouth	1.5	<1
Gastrointestinal System		
Dyspepsia	1.1	<1

The following incidences of laboratory abnormalities occurred at a rate of 1% or greater in patients receiving quazepam and the corresponding placebo group. None of these changes were considered to be of physiological significance (TABLE 2).

The following additional events occurred among individuals receiving quazepam at doses equivalent to or greater than those recommended during its clinical testing and development. There is no way to establish whether or not the administration of quazepam caused these events.

Hypokinesia, ataxia, confusion, incoordination, hyperkinesia, speech disorder, and tremor were reported.

Also, depression, nervousness, agitation, amnesia, anorexia, anxiety, apathy, euphoria, impotence, decreased libido, paranoid reaction, nightmares, abnormal thinking, abnormal taste perception, abnormal vision, and cataract were reported.

Q

TABLE 2

	Quazepam		Placebo	
Number Of Patients	234		244	
% of Patients Reporting	**Low**	**High**	**Low**	**High**
Hematology				
Hemoglobin	1.4	0	1.2	0
Hematocrit	1.5	0	1.7	0
Lymphocyte	1.3	1.6	1.2	1.9
Eosinophil	*	1.5	*	1.3
SEG	1.1	*	1.6	*
Monocyte	*	1.1	*	*
Blood Chemistry				
Glucose	*	*	*	1.2
SGOT	*	1.3	*	1.1
Urinalysis				
Specific Gravity	*	*	*	1.1
WBC	0	2.6	0	3.0
RBC	0	*	0	1.1
Epithelial Cells	0	2.5	0	3.2
Crystals	0	*	0	1.0

* These laboratory abnormalities occurred in less than 1% of patients. In addition, abnormalities in the following laboratory tests were observed in less than 1% of the patients evaluated: WBC count, platelet count, total protein, albumin, BUN, creatinine, total bilirubin, alkaline phosphatase, and SGPT.

Also reported were urinary incontinence, palpitations, nausea, constipation, diarrhea, abdominal pain, pruritus, rash, asthenia, and malaise.

The following list provides an overview of adverse experiences that have been reported and are considered to be reasonably related to the administration of benzodiazepines: incontinence, slurred speech, urinary retention, jaundice, dysarthria, dystonia, changes in libido, irritability, and menstrual irregularities.

As with all benzodiazepines, paradoxical reactions such as stimulation, agitation, increased muscle spasticity, sleep disturbances, hallucinations, and other adverse behavioral effects may occur in rare instances and in a random fashion. Should these occur, use of the drug should be discontinued.

There have been reports of withdrawal signs and symptoms of the type associated with withdrawal from CNS depressant drugs following the rapid decrease or the abrupt discontinuation of benzodiazepines.

DOSAGE AND ADMINISTRATION

Adults: Initiate therapy at 15 mg until individual responses are determined. In some patients, the dose may then be reduced to 7.5 mg.

Elderly and debilitated patients: Because the elderly and debilitated may be more sensitive to benzodiazepines, attempts to reduce the nightly dosage after the first one or two nights of therapy are suggested.

Store quazepam tablets between 2 and 30°C (36 and 86°F).

Protect unit doses from excessive moisture.

PRODUCT LISTING - EQUIVALENTS NOT AVAILABLE

Tablet - Oral - 7.5 mg

100's	$314.39	DORAL, Wallace Laboratories	00037-9000-01

Tablet - Oral - 15 mg

100's	$186.66	DORAL, Wallace Laboratories	00037-9002-02
100's	$343.58	DORAL, Wallace Laboratories	00037-9002-01

Q

Quetiapine Fumarate *(003359)*

Categories: Psychosis; Schizophrenia; Pregnancy Category C; FDA Approved 1997 Sep
Drug Classes: Antipsychotics
Brand Names: Seroquel
Cost of Therapy: $261.57 (Schizophrenia; Seroquel; 100 mg; 3 tablets/day; 30 day supply)

DESCRIPTION

Quetiapine fumarate is an antipsychotic drug belonging to a new chemical class, the dibenzothiazepine derivatives. The chemical designation is 2-[2-(4-dibenzo[*b,f*][1,4]thiazepin-11-yl-1-piperazinyl)ethoxy]-ethanol fumarate (2:1)(salt). It is present in tablets as the fumarate salt. All doses and tablet strengths are expressed as milligrams of base, not as fumarate salt. Its molecular formula is $C_{42}H_{50}N_6O_4S_2{\cdot}C_4H_4O_4$ and it has a molecular weight of 883.11 (fumarate salt).

Quetiapine fumarate is a white to off-white crystalline powder which is moderately soluble in water.

Seroquel is supplied for oral administration as 25 mg (peach), 100 mg (yellow) 200 mg (round, white) and 300 mg (capsule-shaped, white) tablets.

Inactive ingredients are povidone, dibasic dicalcium phosphate dihydrate, microcrystalline cellulose, sodium starch glycolate, lactose monohydrate, magnesium stearate, hydroxypropyl methylcellulose, polyethylene glycol, and titanium dioxide.

The 25 mg tablets contain red ferric oxide and yellow ferric oxide and the 100 mg tablets contain only yellow ferric oxide.

CLINICAL PHARMACOLOGY

PHARMACODYNAMICS

Quetiapine fumarate is an antagonist at multiple neurotransmitter receptors in the brain: serotonin $5HT_{1A}$ and $5HT_2$ (IC_{50S} = 717 & 148 nM respectively), dopamine D_1 and D_2 (IC_{50S} = 1268 & 329 nM respectively), histamine H_1 (IC_{50} = 30 nM), and adrenergic α_1 and α_2 receptors (IC_{50S} = 94 & 271 nM, respectively). Quetiapine fumarate has no appreciable affinity at cholinergic muscarinic and benzodiazepine receptors (IC_{50S} >5000 nM).

The mechanism of action of quetiapine fumarate, as with other antipsychotic drugs, is unknown. However, it has been proposed that this drug's therapeutic activity in schizophrenia is mediated through a combination of dopamine type 2 (D_2) and serotonin type 2 ($5HT_2$) antagonism. Antagonism at receptors other than dopamine and $5HT_2$ with similar receptor affinities may explain some of the other effects of quetiapine fumarate.

Quetiapine fumarate's antagonism of histamine H_1 receptors may explain the somnolence observed with this drug.

Quetiapine fumarate's antagonism of adrenergic α_1 receptors may explain the orthostatic hypotension observed with this drug.

PHARMACOKINETICS

Quetiapine fumarate activity is primarily due to the parent drug. The multiple-dose pharmacokinetics of quetiapine are dose-proportional within the proposed clinical dose range, and quetiapine accumulation is predictable upon multiple dosing. Elimination of quetiapine is mainly via hepatic metabolism with a mean terminal half-life of about 6 hours within the proposed clinical dose range. Steady state concentrations are expected to be achieved within 2 days of dosing. Quetiapine is unlikely to interfere with the metabolism of drugs metabolized by cytochrome P450 enzymes.

Absorption

Quetiapine fumarate is rapidly absorbed after oral administration, reaching peak plasma concentrations in 1.5 hours. The tablet formulation is 100% bioavailable relative to solution. The bioavailability of quetiapine is marginally affected by administration with food, with C_{max} and AUC values increased by 25% and 15%, respectively.

Distribution

Quetiapine is widely distributed throughout the body with an apparent volume of distribution of 10 ± 4 L/kg. It is 83% bound to plasma proteins at therapeutic concentrations. *In vitro,* quetiapine did not affect the binding of warfarin or diazepam to human serum albumin. In turn, neither warfarin nor diazepam altered the binding of quetiapine.

Metabolism and Elimination

Following a single oral dose of ^{14}C-quetiapine, less than 1% of the administered dose was excreted as unchanged drug, indicating that quetiapine is highly metabolized. Approximately 73% and 20% of the dose was recovered in the urine and feces, respectively.

Quetiapine is extensively metabolized by the liver. The major metabolic pathways are sulfoxidation to the sulfoxide metabolite and oxidation to the parent acid metabolite; both metabolites are pharmacologically inactive. *In vitro* studies using human liver microsomes revealed that the cytochrome P450 3A4 isoenzyme is involved in the metabolism of quetiapine to its major, but inactive, sulfoxide metabolite.

POPULATION SUBGROUPS

Age

Oral clearance of quetiapine was reduced by 40% in elderly patients (≥65 years, n=9) compared to young patients (n=12), and dosing adjustment may be necessary (see DOSAGE AND ADMINISTRATION).

Gender

There is no gender effect on the pharmacokinetics of quetiapine.

Race

There is no race effect on the pharmacokinetics of quetiapine.

Smoking

Smoking has no effect on the oral clearance of quetiapine.

Renal Insufficiency

Patients with severe renal impairment (CLCR = 10-30 ml/min/1.73 m^2, n=8) had a 25% lower mean oral clearance than normal subjects (CLCR >80 ml/min/1.73 m^2, n=8), but plasma quetiapine concentrations in the subjects with renal insufficiency were within the range of concentrations seen in normal subjects receiving the same dose. Dosage adjustment is therefore not needed in these patients.

Hepatic Insufficiency

Hepatically impaired patients (n=8) had a 30% lower mean oral clearance of quetiapine than normal subjects. In 2 of the 8 hepatically impaired patients, AUC and C_{max} were 3 times higher than those observed typically in healthy subjects. Since quetiapine is extensively metabolized by the liver, higher plasma levels are expected in the hepatically impaired population, and dosage adjustment may be needed (see DOSAGE AND ADMINISTRATION).

Drug-Drug Interactions

In vitro enzyme inhibition data suggest that quetiapine and 9 of its metabolites would have little inhibitory effect on *in vivo* metabolism mediated by cytochromes P450 1A2, 2C9, 2C19, 2D6, and 3A4.

Quetiapine oral clearance is increased by the prototype cytochrome P450 3A4 inducer, phenytoin, and decreased by the prototype cytochrome P450 3A4 inhibitor, ketoconazole. Dose adjustment of quetiapine will be necessary if it is coadministered with phenytoin or ketoconazole (see DRUG INTERACTIONS and DOSAGE AND ADMINISTRATION).

Quetiapine oral clearance is not inhibited by the non-specific enzyme inhibitor, cimetidine.

Quetiapine at doses of 750 mg/day did not affect the single dose pharmacokinetics of antipyrine, lithium, or lorazepam (see DRUG INTERACTIONS).

INDICATIONS AND USAGE

Quetiapine fumarate is indicated for the treatment of schizophrenia.

The efficacy of quetiapine fumarate in schizophrenia was established in short-term (6 week) controlled trials of schizophrenic inpatients (see CLINICAL PHARMACOLOGY).

The effectiveness of quetiapine fumarate in long-term use, that is, for more than 6 weeks, has not been systematically evaluated in controlled trials. Therefore, the physician who elects to use quetiapine fumarate for extended periods should periodically re-evaluate the long-term usefulness of the drug for the individual patient (see DOSAGE AND ADMINISTRATION).

CONTRAINDICATIONS

Quetiapine fumarate is contraindicated in individuals with a known hypersensitivity to this medication or any of its ingredients.

WARNINGS

NEUROLEPTIC MALIGNANT SYNDROME (NMS)

A potentially fatal symptom complex sometimes referred to as Neuroleptic Malignant Syndrome (NMS) has been reported in association with administration of antipsychotic drugs. Two possible cases of NMS [2/2387 (0.1%)] have been reported in clinical trials with quetiapine fumarate. Clinical manifestations of NMS are hyperpyrexia, muscle rigidity, altered mental status, and evidence of autonomic instability (irregular pulse or blood pressure, tachycardia, diaphoresis, and cardiac dysrhythmia). Additional signs may include elevated creatinine phosphokinase, myoglobinuria (rhabdomyolysis), and acute renal failure.

The diagnostic evaluation of patients with this syndrome is complicated. In arriving at a diagnosis, it is important to exclude cases where the clinical presentation includes both serious medical illness (*e.g.*, pneumonia, systemic infection, etc.) and untreated or inadequately treated extrapyramidal signs and symptoms (EPS). Other important considerations in the differential diagnosis include central anticholinergic toxicity, heat stroke, drug fever and primary central nervous system (CNS) pathology.

The management of NMS should include: (1) immediate discontinuation of antipsychotic drugs and other drugs not essential to concurrent therapy; (2) intensive symptomatic treatment and medical monitoring; and (3) treatment of any concomitant serious medical problems for which specific treatments are available. There is no general agreement about specific pharmacological treatment regimens for NMS.

If a patient requires antipsychotic drug treatment after recovery from NMS, the potential reintroduction of drug therapy should be carefully considered. The patient should be carefully monitored since recurrences of NMS have been reported.

TARDIVE DYSKINESIA

A syndrome of potentially irreversible, involuntary, dyskinetic movements may develop in patients treated with antipsychotic drugs. Although the prevalence of the syndrome appears to be highest among the elderly, especially elderly women, it is impossible to rely upon prevalence estimates to predict, at the inception of antipsychotic treatment, which patients are likely to develop the syndrome. Whether antipsychotic drug products differ in their potential to cause tardive dyskinesia is unknown.

The risk of developing tardive dyskinesia and the likelihood that it will become irreversible are believed to increase as the duration of treatment and the total cumulative dose of antipsychotic drugs administered to the patient increase. However, the syndrome can develop, although much less commonly, after relatively brief treatment periods at low doses.

There is no known treatment for established cases of tardive dyskinesia, although the syndrome may remit, partially or completely, if antipsychotic treatment is withdrawn. Antipsychotic treatment, itself, however, may suppress (or partially suppress) the signs and symptoms of the syndrome and thereby may possibly mask the underlying process. The effect that symptomatic suppression has upon the long-term course of the syndrome is unknown.

Given these considerations, quetiapine fumarate should be prescribed in a manner that is most likely to minimize the occurrence of tardive dyskinesia. Chronic antipsychotic treatment should generally be reserved for patients who appear to suffer from a chronic illness that (1) is known to respond to antipsychotic drugs, and (2) for whom alternative, equally effective, but potentially less harmful treatments are not available or appropriate. In patients who do require chronic treatment, the smallest dose and the shortest duration of treatment producing a satisfactory clinical response should be sought. The need for continued treatment should be reassessed periodically.

If signs and symptoms of tardive dyskinesia appear in a patient on quetiapine fumarate, drug discontinuation should be considered. However, some patients may require treatment with quetiapine fumarate despite the presence of the syndrome.

PRECAUTIONS

GENERAL

Orthostatic Hypotension

Quetiapine fumarate may induce orthostatic hypotension associated with dizziness, tachycardia and, in some patients, syncope, especially during the initial dose-titration period, probably reflecting its α_1-adrenergic antagonist properties. Syncope was reported in 1% (22/2162) of the patients treated with quetiapine fumarate, compared with 0% (0/206) on placebo and about 0.5% (2/420) on active control drugs. The risk of orthostatic hypotension and syncope may be minimized by limiting the initial dose to 25 mg bid (see DOSAGE AND ADMINISTRATION). If hypotension occurs during titration to the target dose, a return to the previous dose in the titration schedule is appropriate.

Quetiapine fumarate should be used with particular caution in patients with known cardiovascular disease (history of myocardial infarction or ischemic heard disease, heart failure or conduction abnormalities), cerebrovascular disease or conditions which would predispose patients to hypotension (dehydration, hypovolemia, and treatment with antihypertensive medications).

Cataracts

The development of cataracts was observed in association with quetiapine treatment in chronic dog studies (see ANIMAL PHARMACOLOGY). Lens changes have also been observed in patients during long-term quetiapine fumarate treatment, but a causal relationship to quetiapine fumarate use has not been established. Nevertheless, the possibility of lenticular changes cannot be excluded at this time. Therefore, examination of the lens by methods adequate to detect cataract formation, such as slit lamp exam or other appropriately sensitive methods, is recommended at initiation of treatment or shortly thereafter, and at 6 month intervals during chronic treatment.

Seizures

During clinical trials, seizures occurred in 0.8% (18/2387) of patients treated with quetiapine fumarate compared to 0.5% (1/206) on placebo and 1% (4/420) on active control drugs. As with other antipsychotics quetiapine fumarate should be used cautiously in patients with a history of seizures or with conditions that potentially lower the seizure threshold, *e.g.*, Alzheimer's dementia. Conditions that lower the seizure threshold may be more prevalent in a population of 65 years or older.

Hypothyroidism

Clinical trials with quetiapine fumarate demonstrated a dose-related decrease in total and free thyroxine (T4) of approximately 20% at the higher end of the therapeutic dose range was maximal in the first 2-4 weeks of treatment and maintained without adaptation or progression during more chronic therapy. Generally, these changes were of no clinical significance and TSH was unchanged in most patients, and levels of TBG were unchanged. In nearly all cases, cessation of quetiapine fumarate treatment was associated with a reversal of the effects on total and free T4, irrespective of the duration of treatment. About 0.4% (10/2386) of quetiapine fumarate patients did experience TSH increases. Six (6) of the patients with TSH increases needed replacement thyroid treatment.

Cholesterol and Triglyceride Elevations

In a pool of 3-6 week placebo-controlled trials, quetiapine fumarate-treated patients had increases from baseline in cholesterol and triglyceride of 11% and 17%, respectively, compared to slight decreases for placebo patients. These changes were only weakly related to the increases in weight observed in quetiapine fumarate-treated patients.

Hyperprolactinemia

Although an elevation of prolactin levels was not demonstrated in clinical trials with quetiapine fumarate, increased prolactin levels were observed in rat studies with this compound, and were associated with an increase in mammary gland neoplasia in rats (see Carcinogenesis). Tissue culture experiments indicate that approximately one-third of human breast cancers are prolactin dependent *in vitro,* a factor of potential importance if the prescription of these drugs is contemplated in a patient with previously detected breast cancer. Although disturbances such as galactorrhea, amenorrhea, gynecomastia, and impotence have been reported with prolactin-elevating compounds, the clinical significance of elevated serum prolactin levels is unknown for most patients. Neither clinical studies nor epidemiologic studies conducted to date have shown an association between chronic administration of this class of drugs and tumorigenesis in humans; the available evidence is considered too limited to be conclusive at this time.

Transaminase Elevations

Asymptomatic, transient, and reversible elevations in serum transaminases (primarily ALT) have been reported. The proportions of patients with transaminase elevations of >3 times the upper limits of the normal reference range in a pool of 3-6 week placebo-controlled trials were approximately 6% for quetiapine fumarate compared to 1% for placebo. These hepatic enzyme elevations usually occurred within the first 3 weeks of drug treatment and promptly returned to pre-study levels with ongoing treatment with quetiapine fumarate.

Potential for Cognitive and Motor Impairment

Somnolence was a commonly reported adverse event reported in patients treated with quetiapine fumarate especially during the 3-5 day period of initial dose-titration. In the 3-6 week placebo-controlled trials, somnolence was reported in 18% of patients on quetiapine fumarate compared to 11% of placebo patients. Since quetiapine fumarate has the potential to impair judgment, thinking, or motor skills, patients should be cautioned about performing activities requiring mental alertness, such as operating a motor vehicle (including automobiles) or operating hazardous machinery until they are reasonably certain that quetiapine fumarate therapy does not affect them adversely.

Priapism

One case of priapism in a patient receiving quetiapine fumarate has been reported prior to market introduction. While a causal relationship to use of quetiapine fumarate has not been established, other drugs with alpha-adrenergic blocking effects have been reported to induce priapism, and it is possible that quetiapine fumarate may share this capacity. Severe priapism may require surgical intervention.

Body Temperature Regulation

Although not reported with quetiapine fumarate, disruption of the body's ability to reduce core body temperature has been attributed to antipsychotic agents. Appropriate care is advised when prescribing quetiapine fumarate for patients who will be experiencing conditions which may contribute to an elevation in core body temperature, *e.g.*, exercising strenuously, exposure to extreme heat, receiving concomitant medication with anticholinergic activity, or being subject to dehydration.

Dysphagia

Esophageal dysmotility and aspiration have been associated with antipsychotic drug use. Aspiration pneumonia is a common cause of morbidity and mortality in elderly patients, in particular those with advanced Alzheimer's dementia. Quetiapine fumarate and other antipsychotic drugs should be used cautiously in patients at risk for aspiration pneumonia.

Suicide

The possibility of a suicide attempt is inherent in schizophrenia, and close supervision of high risk patients should accompany drug therapy. Prescriptions for quetiapine fumarate should be written for the smallest quantity of tablets consistent with good patient management in order to reduce the risk of overdose.

Q

Use in Patients With Concomitant Illness
Clinical experience with quetiapine fumarate in patients with certain concomitant systemic illnesses (see CLINICAL PHARMACOLOGY, Population Subgroups: Renal Insufficiency, and Hepatic Insufficiency) is limited.

Quetiapine fumarate has not been evaluated or used to any appreciable extent in patients with a recent history of myocardial infarction or unstable heart disease. Patients with these diagnoses were excluded from premarketing clinical studies. Because of the risk of orthostatic hypotension with quetiapine fumarate, caution should be observed in cardiac patients (see Orthostatic Hypotension).

INFORMATION FOR THE PATIENT

Physicians are advised to discuss the following issues with patients for whom they prescribe quetiapine fumarate.

Orthostatic Hypotension: Patients should be advised of the risk of orthostatic hypotension, especially during the 3-5 day period of initial dose titration, and also at times of re-initiating treatment or increases in dose.

Interference With Cognitive and Motor Performance: Since somnolence was a commonly reported adverse event associated with quetiapine fumarate treatment, patients should be advised of the risk of somnolence, especially during the 3-5 day period of initial dose titration. Patients should be cautioned about performing any activity requiring mental alertness, such as operating a motor vehicle (including automobiles) or operating hazardous machinery, until they are reasonably certain that quetiapine fumarate therapy does not affect them adversely.

Pregnancy: Patients should be advised to notify their physician if they become pregnant or intend to become pregnant during therapy.

Nursing: Patients should be advised not to breast feed if they are taking quetiapine fumarate.

Concomitant Medication: As with other medications, patients should be advised to notify their physicians if they are taking, or plan to take, any prescription or over-the-counter drugs.

Alcohol: Patients should be advised to avoid consuming alcoholic beverages while taking quetiapine fumarate.

Heat Exposure and Dehydration: Patients should be advised regarding appropriate care in avoiding overheating and dehydration.

LABORATORY TESTS

No specific laboratory tests are recommended.

CARCINOGENESIS, MUTAGENESIS, AND IMPAIRMENT OF FERTILITY

Carcinogenesis
Carcinogenicity studies were conducted in C57BL mice and Wistar rats. Quetiapine was administered in the diet to mice at doses of 20, 75, 250, and 750 mg/kg and to rats by gavage at doses of 25, 75, and 250 mg/kg for 2 years. These doses are equivalent to 0.1, 0.5, 1.5, and 4.5 times the maximum human dose (800 mg/day) on a mg/m^2 basis (mice) or 0.3, 0.9, and 3.0 times the maximum human dose on a mg/m^2 basis (rats). There were statistically significant increases in thyroid gland follicular adenomas in male mice at doses of 250 and 750 mg/kg or 1.5 and 4.5 times the maximum human dose on a mg/m^2 basis and in male rats at a dose of 250 mg/kg or 3.0 times the maximum human dose on a mg/m^2 basis. Mammary gland adenocarcinomas were statistically significantly increased in female rats at all doses tested (25, 75, and 250 mg/kg or 0.3, 0.9, and 3.0 times the maximum recommended human dose on a mg/m^2 basis).

Thyroid follicular cell adenomas may have resulted from chronic stimulation of the thyroid gland by thyroid stimulating hormone (TSH) resulting from enhanced metabolism and clearance of thyroxine by rodent liver. Changes in TSH, thyroxine, and thyroxine clearance consistent with this mechanism were observed in subchronic toxicity studies in rat and mouse and in a 1 year toxicity study in rat; however, the results of these studies were not definitive. The relevance of the increases in thyroid follicular cell adenomas to human risk, through whatever mechanism, is unknown.

Antipsychotic drugs have been shown to chronically elevate prolactin levels in rodents. Serum measurements in a 1 year toxicity study showed that quetiapine increased median serum prolactin levels a maximum of 32- and 13-fold in male and female rats, respectively. Increases in mammary neoplasms have been found in rodents after chronic administration of other antipsychotic drugs and are considered to be prolactin-mediated. The relevance of this increased incidence of prolactin-mediated mammary gland tumors in rats to human risk is unknown (see Hyperprolactinemia).

Mutagenesis
The mutagenic potential of quetiapine was tested in six *in vitro* bacterial gene mutation assays and in an *in vitro* mammalian gene mutation assay in Chinese Hamster Ovary cells. However, sufficiently high concentrations of quetiapine may not have been used for all tester strains. Quetiapine did produce a reproducible increase in mutations in one *Salmonella typhimurium* tester strain in the presence of metabolic activation. No evidence of clastogenic potential was obtained in an *in vitro* chromosomal aberration assay in cultured human lymphocytes or in the *in vivo* micronucleus assay in rats.

Impairment of Fertility
Quetiapine decreased mating and fertility in male Sprague-Dawley rats at oral doses of 50 and 150 mg/kg or 0.6 and 1.8 times the maximum human dose on a mg/m^2 basis. Drug-related effects included increases in interval to mate and in the number of matings required for successful impregnation. These effects continued to be observed at 150 mg/kg even after a 2 week period without treatment. The no-effect dose for impaired mating and fertility in male rats was 25 mg/kg, or 0.3 times the maximum human dose on a mg/m^2 basis. Quetiapine adversely affected mating and fertility in female Sprague-Dawley rats at an oral dose of 50 mg/kg, or 0.6 times the maximum human dose on a mg/m^2 basis. Drug-related effects included decreases in matings and in matings resulting in pregnancy, and an increase in the interval to mate. An increase in irregular estrus cycles was observed at doses of 10 and 50 mg/kg, or 0.1 and 0.6 times the maximum human dose on a mg/m^2 basis. The no-effect dose in female rats was 1 mg/kg, or 0.01 times the maximum human dose on a mg/m^2 basis.

PREGNANCY CATEGORY C

The teratogenic potential of quetiapine was studied in Wistar rats and Dutch Belted rabbits dosed during the period of organogenesis. No evidence of a teratogenic effect was detected in rats at doses of 25-200 mg/kg or 0.3-2.4 times the maximum human dose on a mg/m^2 basis or in rabbits at 25-100 mg/kg or 0.6-2.4 times the maximum human dose on a mg/m^2 basis. There was, however, evidence of embryo/fetal toxicity. Delays in skeletal ossification were detected in rat fetuses at doses of 50 and 200 mg/kg (0.6 and 2.4 times the maximum human dose on a mg/m^2 basis) and in rabbits at 50 and 100 mg/kg (1.2 and 2.4 times the maximum human dose on a mg/m^2 basis). Fetal body weight was reduced in rat fetuses at 200 mg/kg and rabbit fetuses at 100 mg/kg (2.4 times the maximum human dose on a mg/m^2 basis for both species). There was an increased incidence of a minor soft tissue anomaly (carpal/tarsal flexure) in rabbit fetuses at a dose of 100 mg/kg (2.4 times the maximum human dose on a mg/m^2 basis). Evidence of maternal toxicity (*i.e.*, decreases in body weight gain and/or death) was observed at the high dose in the rat study and at all doses in the rabbit study. In a peri/postnatal reproductive study in rats, no drug-related effects were observed at doses of 1, 10, and 20 mg/kg or 0.01, 0.12, and 0.24 times the maximum human dose on a mg/m^2 basis. However, in a preliminary peri/postnatal study, there were increases in fetal and pup death, and decreases in mean litter weight at 150 mg/kg, or 3.0 times the maximum human dose on a mg/m^2 basis.

There are no adequate and well-controlled studies in pregnant women and quetiapine should be used during pregnancy only if the potential benefit justifies the potential risk to the fetus.

LABOR AND DELIVERY

The effect of quetiapine fumarate on labor and delivery in humans is unknown.

NURSING MOTHERS

Quetiapine fumarate was excreted in milk of treated animals during lactation. It is not known if quetiapine fumarate is excreted in human milk. It is recommended that women receiving quetiapine fumarate should not breast feed.

PEDIATRIC USE

The safety and effectiveness of quetiapine fumarate in pediatric patients have not been established.

GERIATRIC USE

Of the approximately 2400 patients in clinical studies with quetiapine fumarate, 8% (190) were 65 years of age or over. In general, there was no indication of any different tolerability of quetiapine fumarate in the elderly compared to younger adults. Nevertheless, the presence of factors that might decrease pharmacokinetic clearance, increase the pharmacodynamic response to quetiapine fumarate, or cause poorer tolerance or orthostasis, should lead to consideration of a lower starting dose, slower titration, and careful monitoring during the initial dosing period in the elderly. The mean plasma clearance of quetiapine fumarate was reduced by 30-50% in elderly patients when compared to younger patients (see CLINICAL PHARMACOLOGY, Pharmacokinetics and DOSAGE AND ADMINISTRATION).

DRUG INTERACTIONS

The risks of using quetiapine fumarate in combination with other drugs have not been extensively evaluated in systematic studies. Given the primary CNS effects of quetiapine fumarate, caution should be used when it is taken in combination with other centrally acting drugs. Quetiapine fumarate potentiated the cognitive and motor effects of alcohol in a clinical trial in subjects with selected psychotic disorders, and alcoholic beverages should be avoided while taking quetiapine fumarate.

Because of its potential for inducing hypotension, quetiapine fumarate may enhance the effects of certain antihypertensive agents.

Quetiapine fumarate may antagonize the effects of levodopa and dopamine agonists.

THE EFFECT OF OTHER DRUGS ON QUETIAPINE FUMARATE

Phenytoin: Coadministration of quetiapine (250 mg tid) and phenytoin (100 mg tid) increased the mean oral clearance of quetiapine by 5-fold. Increased doses of quetiapine fumarate may be required to maintain control of symptoms of schizophrenia in patients receiving quetiapine and phenytoin, or other hepatic enzyme inducers (*e.g.*, carbamazepine, barbiturates, rifampin, glucocorticoids). Caution should be taken if phenytoin is withdrawn and replaced with a non-inducer (*e.g.*, valproate) (see DOSAGE AND ADMINISTRATION).

Thioridazine: Thioridazine (200 mg bid) increased the oral clearance of quetiapine (300 mg bid) by 65%.

Cimetidine: Administration of multiple daily doses of cimetidine (400 mg tid for 4 days) resulted in a 20% decrease in the mean oral clearance of quetiapine (150 mg tid). Dosage adjustment for quetiapine is not required when it is given with cimetidine.

P450 3A Inhibitors: Coadministration of ketoconazole (200 mg once daily for 4 days), a potent inhibitor of cytochrome P450 3A, reduced oral clearance of quetiapine by 84%, resulting in a 335% increase in maximum plasma concentration of quetiapine. Caution is indicated when quetiapine fumarate is administered with ketoconazole and other inhibitors of cytochrome P450 3A (*e.g.*, itraconzaole, fluconazole, and erythromycin).

Fluoxetine, Imipramine, Haloperidol, and Risperidone: Coadministration of fluoxetine (60 mg once daily); imipramine (75 mg bid), haloperidol (7.5 mg bid), or risperidone (3 mg bid) with quetiapine (300 mg bid) did not alter the steady-state pharmacokinetics of quetiapine.

EFFECT OF QUETIAPINE ON OTHER DRUGS

Lorazepam: The mean oral clearance of lorazepam (2 mg, single dose) was reduced by 20% in the presence of quetiapine administered as 250 mg tid dosing.

Lithium: Concomitant administration of quetiapine (250 mg tid) with lithium had no effect on any of the steady-state pharmacokinetic parameters of lithium.

Antipyrine: Administration of multiple daily doses up to 750 mg/day (on a tid schedule) of quetiapine to subjects with selected psychotic disorders had no clinically relevant effect on the clearance of antipyrine or urinary recovery of antipyrine metabolites. These results indicate that quetiapine does not significantly induce hepatic enzymes responsible for cytochrome P450 mediated metabolism of antipyrine.

ADVERSE REACTIONS

The premarketing development program for quetiapine fumarate included over 2600 patients and/or normal subjects exposed to 1 or more doses of quetiapine fumarate. Of these 2600 subjects, approximately 2300 were patients who participated in multiple dose effectiveness trials, and their experience corresponded to approximately 865 patient years. The conditions and duration of treatment with quetiapine fumarate varied greatly and included (in overlapping categories) open-label and double-blind phases of studies, inpatients and outpatients, fixed-dose and dose-titration studies, and short-term or longer-term exposure. Adverse reactions were assessed by collecting adverse events, results of physical examinations, vital signs, weights, laboratory analyses, ECGs, and results of ophthalmologic examinations.

Adverse events during exposure were obtained by general inquiry and recorded by clinical investigators using terminology of their own choosing. Consequently, it is not possible to provide a meaningful estimate of the proportion of individuals experiencing adverse events without first grouping similar types of events into a smaller number of standardized event categories. In TABLE 1, TABLE 2, and tabulations that follow, standard COSTART terminology has been used to classify reported adverse events.

The stated frequencies of adverse events represent the proportion of individuals who experienced, at least once, a treatment-emergent adverse event of the type listed. An event was considered treatment emergent if it occurred for the first time or worsened while receiving therapy following baseline evaluation.

ADVERSE FINDINGS OBSERVED IN SHORT-TERM, CONTROLLED TRIALS

Adverse Events Associated With Discontinuation of Treatment in Short-Term, Placebo-Controlled Trials

Overall, there was little difference in the incidence of discontinuation due to adverse events (4% for quetiapine fumarate vs 3% for placebo) in a pool of controlled trials. However, discontinuations due to somnolence and hypotension were considered to be drug related (see PRECAUTIONS).

TABLE 1

Adverse Event	Quetiapine Fumarate	Placebo
Somnolence	0.8%	0%
Hypotension	0.4%	0%

Adverse Events Occurring at an Incidence of 1% or More Among Quetiapine Fumarate Treated Patients in Short-Term, Placebo-Controlled Trials

TABLE 2 enumerates the incidence, rounded to the nearest percent, of treatment-emergent adverse events that occurred during acute therapy (up to 6 weeks) of schizophrenia in 1% or more of patients treated with quetiapine fumarate (doses ranging from 75-750 mg/day) where the incidence in patients treated with quetiapine fumarate was greater than the incidence in placebo-treated patients.

The prescriber should be aware that the figures in TABLE 1, TABLE 2, and the tabulations cannot be used to predict the incidence of side effects in the course of usual medical practice where patient characteristics and other factors differ from those that prevailed in the clinical trials. Similarly, the cited frequencies cannot be compared with figures obtained from other clinical investigations involving different treatments, uses, and investigators. The cited figures, however, do provide the prescribing physician with some basis for estimating the relative contribution of drug and nondrug factors to the side effect incidence in the population studied.

In these studies, the most commonly observed adverse events associated with the use of quetiapine fumarate (incidence of 5% or greater) and observed at a rate on quetiapine fumarate at least twice that of placebo were dizziness (10%), postural hypotension (7%), dry mouth (7%), and dyspepsia (6%).

Explorations for interactions on the basis of gender, age, and race did not reveal any clinically meaningful differences in the adverse event occurrence on the basis of these demographic factors.

DOSE DEPENDENCY OF ADVERSE EVENTS IN SHORT-TERM, PLACEBO-CONTROLLED TRIALS

Dose-Related Adverse Events

Spontaneously elicited adverse event data from a study comparing five fixed doses of quetiapine fumarate (75, 150, 300, 600, and 750 mg/day) to placebo were explored for dose-relatedness of adverse events. Logistic regression analyses revealed a positive dose response ($p < 0.05$) for the following adverse events: dyspepsia, abdominal pain, and weight gain.

Extrapyramidal Symptoms

Data from one 6 week clinical trial comparing five fixed doses of quetiapine fumarate (75, 150, 300, 600, 750 mg/day) provided evidence for the lack of treatment-emergent extrapyramidal symptoms (EPS) and dose-relatedness for EPS associated with quetiapine fumarate treatment. Three methods were used to measure EPS: (1) Simpson-Angus total score (mean change from baseline) which evaluates parkinsonism and akathisia, (2) incidence of spontaneous complaints of EPS (akathisia, akinesia, cogwheel rigidity, extrapyramidal syndrome, hypertonia, hypokinesia, neck rigidity, and tremor), and (3) use of anticholinergic medications to treat emergent EPS.

In three additional placebo-controlled clinical trials using variable doses of quetiapine fumarate, there were no differences between the quetiapine fumarate and placebo treatment groups in the incidence of EPS, as assessed by Simpson-Angus total scores, spontaneous complaints of EPS and the use of concomitant anticholinergic medications to treat EPS.

TABLE 2 *Treatment-Emergent Adverse Experience Incidence in 3-6 Week Placebo-Controlled Clinical Trials**

Body System / Preferred Term	Quetiapine Fumarate (n=510)	Placebo (n=206)
Body as a Whole		
Headache	19%	18%
Asthenia	4%	3%
Abdominal pain	3%	1%
Back pain	2%	1%
Fever	2%	1%
Nervous System		
Somnolence	18%	11%
Dizziness	10%	4%
Digestive System		
Constipation	9%	5%
Dry mouth	7%	3%
Dyspepsia	6%	2%
Cardiovascular System		
Postural hypotension	7%	2%
Tachycardia	7%	5%
Metabolic and Nutritional Disorders		
Weight gain	2%	0%
Skin and Appendages		
Rash	4%	3%
Respiratory System		
Rhinitis	3%	1%
Special Senses		
Ear pain	1%	0%

* Events for which the quatiapine fumarate incidence was equal to or less than placebo are not listed in the table, but included the following: pain, infection, chest pain, hostility, accidental injury, hypertension, hypotension, nausea, vomiting, diarrhea, myalgia, agitation, insomnia, anxiety, nervousness, akathisia, hypertonia, tremor, depression, paresthesia, pharyngitis, dry skin, amblyopia, and urinary tract infection.

TABLE 3

		Quetiapine Fumarate (mg)				
Dose Groups	Placebo	75	150	300	600	750
Parkinsonism	-0.6	-1.0	-1.2	-1.6	-1.8	-1.8
EPS incidence	16%	6%	6%	4%	8%	6%
Anticholinergic medications	14%	11%	10%	8%	12%	11%

Vital Sign Changes

Quetiapine fumarate is associated with orthostatic hypotension (see PRECAUTIONS).

Weight Gain

The proportions of patients meeting a weight gain criterion of ≥7% of body weight were compared in a pool of four 3-6 week placebo-controlled clinical trials, revealing a statistically significantly greater incidence of weight gain for quetiapine fumarate (23%) compared to placebo (6%).

Laboratory Changes

An assessment of the premarketing experience for quetiapine fumarate suggested that it is associated with asymptomatic increases in SGPT and increases in both total cholesterol and triglycerides (see PRECAUTIONS).

An assessment of hematological parameters in short-term, placebo-controlled trials revealed no clinically important differences between quetiapine fumarate and placebo.

ECG Changes

Between group comparisons for pooled placebo-controlled trials revealed to statistically significant quetiapine fumarate/placebo differences in the proportions of patients experiencing potentially important changes in ECG parameters, including QT, QTc, and PR intervals. However, the proportions of patients meeting the criteria for tachycardia were compared in four 3-6 week, placebo-controlled clinical trials revealing a 1% (4/399) incidence for quetiapine fumarate compared to 0.6% (1/156) incidence for placebo. Quetiapine fumarate use was associated with a mean increase in heart rate, assessed by ECG, of 7 beats per minute compared to a mean increase of 1 beat per minute among placebo patients. This slight tendency to tachycardia may be related to quetiapine fumarate's potential for inducing orthostatic changes (see PRECAUTIONS).

OTHER ADVERSE EVENTS OBSERVED DURING THE PRE-MARKETING EVALUATION OF QUETIAPINE FUMARATE

Following is a list of COSTART terms that reflect treatment-emergent adverse events as defined in the introduction to the ADVERSE REACTIONS section reported by patients treated with quetiapine fumarate at multiple doses ≥75 mg/day during any phase of a trial within the premarketing database of approximately 2200 patients. All reported events are included except those already listed in TABLE 2 or elsewhere in labelling, those events for which a drug cause was remote, and those event terms which were so general as to be uninformative. It is important to emphasize that, although the events reported occurred during treatment with quetiapine fumarate, they were not necessarily caused by it.

Events are further categorized by body system and listed in order of decreasing frequency according to the following definitions: *frequent* adverse events are those occurring in at least 1/100 patients (only those not already listed in the tabulated results from placebo-controlled trials appear in this listing); *infrequent* adverse events are those occurring in 1/100 to 1/1000 patients; *rare* events are those occurring in fewer than 1/1000 patients.

Q

Nervous System: *Frequent:* Hypertonia, dysarthria; *Infrequent:* Abnormal dreams, dyskinesia, thinking abnormal, tardive dyskinesia, vertigo, involuntary movements, confusion, amnesia, psychosis, hallucinations, hyperkinesia, libido increased*, urinary retention, incoordination, paranoid reaction, abnormal gait, myoclonus, delusions, manic reaction, apathy, ataxia, depersonalization, stupor, bruxism, catatonic reaction, hemiplegia; *Rare:* Aphasia, buccoglossal syndrome, choreoathetosis, delirium, emotional lability, euphoria, libido decreased*, neuralgia, stuttering, subdural hematoma.

Body as a Whole: *Frequent:* Flu syndrome; *Infrequent:* Neck pain, pelvic pain*, suicide attempt, malaise, photosensitivity reaction, chills, face edema, moniliasis; *Rare:* Abdomen enlarged.

Digestive System: *Frequent:* Anorexia; *Infrequent:* Increased salivation, increased appetite, gamma glutamyl transpeptidase increased, gingivitis, dysphagia, flatulence, gastroenteritis, gastritis, hemorrhoids, stomatitis, thirst, tooth caries, fecal incontinence, gastroesophageal reflux, gum hemorrhage, mouth ulceration, rectal hemorrhage, tongue edema; *Rare:* Glossitis, hematemesis, intestinal obstruction, melena, pancreatitis.

Cardiovascular System: *Frequent:* Palpitation; *Infrequent:* Vasodilatation, QT interval prolonged, migraine, bradycardia, cerebral ischemia, irregular pulse, T wave abnormality, bundle branch block, cerebrovascular accident, deep thrombophlebitis, T wave inversion; *Rare:* Angina pectoris, atrial fibrillation, AV block first degree, congestive heart failure, ST elevated, thrombophlebitis, T wave flattening, ST abnormality, increased QRS duration.

Respiratory System: *Frequent:* Pharyngitis, rhinitis, cough increased, dyspnea; *Infrequent:* Pneumonia, epistaxis, asthma; *Rare:* Hiccup, hyperventilation.

Metabolic and Nutritional System: *Frequent:* Peripheral edema; *Infrequent:* Weight loss, alkaline phosphatase increased, hyperlipemia, alcohol intolerance, dehydration, hyperglycemia, creatinine increased, hypoglycemia; *Rare:* Glycosuria, gout, hand edema, hypokalemia, water intoxication.

Skin and Appendages System: *Frequent:* Sweating; *Infrequent:* Pruritus, acne, eczema, contact dermatitis, maculopapular rash, seborrhea, skin ulcer; *Rare:* Exfolliative dermatitis, psoriasis, skin discoloration.

Urogenital System: *Infrequent:* Dysmenorrhea*, vaginitis*, urinary incontinence, metorrhagia*, impotence*, dysuria, vaginal moniliasis*, abnormal ejaculation*, cystitis, urinary frequency, amenorrhea*, female lactation*, leukorrhea*, vaginal hemorrhage*, vulvovaginitis*, orchitis*; *Rare:* Gynecomastia*, nocturia, polyuria, acute kidney failure.

Special Senses: *Infrequent:* Conjunctivitis, abnormal vision, dry eyes, tinnitus, taste perversion, blepharitis, eye pain; *Rare:* Abnormality of accommodation, deafness, glaucoma.

Musculoskeletal System: *Infrequent:* Pathological fracture, myasthenia, twitching, arthralgia, arthritis, leg cramps, bone pain.

Hemic and Lymphatic System: *Frequent:* Leukopenia; *Infrequent:* Leukocytosis, anemia, ecchymosis, eosinophilia, hypochromic anemia; lymphadenopathy, cyanosis; *Rare:* Hemolysis, thrombocytopenia.

Endocrine System: *Infrequent:* Hypothyroidism, diabetes mellitus; *Rare:* Hyperthyroidism.

*Adjusted for gender.

POST MARKETING EXPERIENCE

Adverse events reported since market introduction which were temporarily related to quetiapine fumarate therapy include the following: rarely leukopenia/neutropenia. If a patient develops a low white cell count consider discontinuation of therapy. Possible risk factors for leukopenia/neutropenia include pre-existing low white cell count and history of drug-induced leukopenia/neutropenia.

DOSAGE AND ADMINISTRATION

USUAL DOSE

Quetiapine fumarate should generally be administered with an initial dose of 25 mg bid, with increases in increments of 25-50 mg bid or tid on the second and third day, as tolerated, to a target dose range of 300-400 mg daily by the fourth day, given bid or tid. Further dosage adjustments, if indicated, should generally occur at intervals of not less than 2 days, as steady state for quetiapine fumarate would not be achieved for approximately 1-2 days in the typical patient. When dosage adjustments are necessary, dose increments/decrements of 25-50 mg bid are recommended. Most efficacy data with quetiapine fumarate were obtained using tid regimens, but in one controlled trial 225 mg bid was also effective.

Efficacy in schizophrenia was demonstrated in a dose range of 150-750 mg/day in the clinical trials supporting the effectiveness of quetiapine fumarate. In a dose response study, doses above 300 mg/day were not demonstrated to be more efficacious than the 300 mg/day dose. In other studies, however, doses in the range of 400-500 mg/day appeared to be needed. The safety of doses above 800 mg/day has not been evaluated in clinical trials.

DOSING IN SPECIAL POPULATIONS

Consideration should be given to a slower rate of dose titration and a lower target dose in the elderly and in patients who are debilitated or who have a predisposition to hypotensive reactions (see CLINICAL PHARMACOLOGY). When indicated, dose escalation should be performed with caution in these patients.

Patients with hepatic impairment should be started on 25 mg/day. The dose should be increased daily in increments of 25-50 mg/day to an effective dose, depending on the clinical response and tolerability of the patient.

The elimination of quetiapine was enhanced in the presence of phenytoin. Higher maintenance doses of quetiapine may be required when it is coadministered with phenytoin and other enzyme inducers such as carbamazepine and phenobarbital (see DRUG INTERACTIONS).

MAINTENANCE TREATMENT

While there is no body of evidence available to answer the question of how long the patient treated with quetiapine fumarate should remain on it, the effectiveness of maintenance treatment is well established for many other drugs used to treat schizophrenia. It is recommended that responding patients be continued on quetiapine fumarate, but at the lowest dose needed to maintain remission. Patients should be periodically reassessed to determine the need for maintenance treatment.

REINITIATION OF TREATMENT IN PATIENTS PREVIOUSLY DISCONTINUED

Although there are no data to specifically address reinitiation of treatment, it is recommended that when restarting patients who have had an interval of less than 1 week off quetiapine fumarate, titration of quetiapine fumarate is not required and the maintenance dose may be reinitiated. When restarting therapy of patients who have been off quetiapine fumarate for more than 1 week, the initial titration schedule should be followed.

SWITCHING FROM OTHER ANTIPSYCHOTICS

There are no systematically collected data to specifically address switching patients with schizophrenia from other antipsychotics to quetiapine fumarate, or concerning concomitant administration with other antipsychotics. While immediate discontinuation of the previous antipsychotic treatment may be acceptable for some patients with schizophrenia, more gradual discontinuation may be most appropriate for others. In all cases, the period of overlapping antipsychotic administration should be minimized. When switching patients with schizophrenia from depot antipsychotics, if medically appropriate, initiate quetiapine fumarate therapy in place of the next scheduled injection. The need for continuing existing EPS medication should be reevaluated periodically.

ANIMAL PHARMACOLOGY

Quetiapine caused a dose-related increase in pigment deposition in thyroid gland in rat toxicity studies which were 4 weeks in duration or longer and in a mouse 2 year carcinogenicity study. Doses were 10-250 mg/kg in rats, 75-750 mg/kg in mice; these doses are 0.1-3.0 and 0.1-4.5 times the maximum recommended human dose (on a mg/m^2 basis), respectively. Pigment deposition was shown to be irreversible in rats. The identity of the pigment could not be determined, but was found to be co-localized with quetiapine in thyroid gland follicular epithelial cells. The functional effects and the relevance of this finding to human risk are unknown.

In dogs receiving quetiapine for 6 or 12 months, but not for 1 month, focal triangular cataracts occurred at the junction of posterior sutures in the outer cortex of the lens at a dose of 100 mg/kg, or 4 times the maximum recommended human dose on a mg/m^2 basis. This finding may be due to inhibition of cholesterol biosynthesis by quetiapine. Quetiapine caused a dose related reduction in plasma cholesterol levels in repeat-dose dog and monkey studies; however, there was no correlation between plasma cholesterol and the presence of cataracts in individual dogs. The appearance of delta-8-cholestanol in plasma is consistent with inhibition of a late stage in cholesterol biosynthesis in these species. There also was a 25% reduction in cholesterol content of the outer cortex of the lens observed in a special study in quetiapine treated female dogs. Drug-related cataracts have not been seen in any other species; however, in a 1 year study in monkeys, a striated appearance of the anterior lens surface was detected in 2/7 females at a dose of 225 mg/kg or 5.5 times the maximum recommended human dose on a mg/m^2 basis.

HOW SUPPLIED

25 mg Tablets: Peach, round, biconvex, film-coated tablets, identified with "SEROQUEL" and "25" on one side and plain on the other side.

100 mg Tablets: Yellow, round, biconvex film-coated tablets, identified with "SEROQUEL" and "100" on one side and plain on the other side.

200 mg Tablets: White, round, biconvex, film-coated tablets, identified with "SEROQUEL" and "200" on one side and plain on the other side.

300 mg Tablets: White, capsule-shaped, biconvex, film-coated tablets, intagliated with "SEROQUEL" on one side and "300" on the other side.

Storage: Store at 25°C (77°F); excursions permitted to 15-30°C (59-86°F).

PRODUCT LISTING - EQUIVALENTS NOT AVAILABLE

Tablet - Oral - 25 mg

100's	$159.69	SEROQUEL, Astra-Zeneca Pharmaceuticals	00310-0275-10
100's	$159.69	SEROQUEL, Astra-Zeneca Pharmaceuticals	00310-0275-39

Tablet - Oral - 100 mg

100's	$290.63	SEROQUEL, Astra-Zeneca Pharmaceuticals	00310-0271-10
100's	$290.63	SEROQUEL, Astra-Zeneca Pharmaceuticals	00310-0271-39

Tablet - Oral - 200 mg

100's	$548.26	SEROQUEL, Astra-Zeneca Pharmaceuticals	00310-0272-10
100's	$548.26	SEROQUEL, Astra-Zeneca Pharmaceuticals	00310-0272-39

Tablet - Oral - 300 mg

60's	$433.14	SEROQUEL, Astra-Zeneca Pharmaceuticals	00310-0274-60
100's	$721.90	SEROQUEL, Astra-Zeneca Pharmaceuticals	00310-0274-39

Quinapril Hydrochloride (003069)

For related information, see the comparative table section in Appendix A.

Categories: Heart failure, congestive; Hypertension, essential; Pregnancy Category D; FDA Approved 1991 Nov
Drug Classes: Angiotensin converting enzyme inhibitors
Brand Names: Accupril
Foreign Brand Availability: Accuprin (Italy); Accupro (Austria; Czech-Republic; Denmark; England; Finland; Germany; Ireland; Sweden; Switzerland); Accupron (Greece); Acequin (Italy); Acuitel (Bahrain; Cyprus; Egypt; France; Iran; Iraq; Jordan; Kuwait; Lebanon; Libya; Mauritius; Oman; Qatar; Republic-of-Yemen; Saudi-Arabia; Syria; United-Arab-Emirates); Acuprel (Spain); Acupril (Mexico; Netherlands); Asig (Australia); Conan (Japan); Korec (France); Quinaten (Colombia); Quinazil (Italy)
Cost of Therapy: $106.84 (Hypertension; Accupril; 20 mg; 1 tablet/day; 30 day supply)

WARNING

Use in Pregnancy

When used in pregnancy during the second and third trimesters, ACE inhibitors can cause injury and even death to the developing fetus. When pregnancy is detected, quinapril HCl should be discontinued as soon as possible. See WARNINGS, Fetal/Neonatal Morbidity and Mortality.

DESCRIPTION

Quinapril hydrochloride is the hydrochloride salt of quinapril, the ethyl ester of a non-sulfhydryl, angiotensin-converting enzyme (ACE) inhibitor, quinaprilat.

Quinapril hydrochloride is chemically described as [3S-[2[R*(R*)],3R*]]-2-[2-[[1-(ethoxycarbonyl)-3-phenylpropyl]amino]-1-oxopropyl]-1,2,3,4-tetrahydro-3-isoquinolinecarboxylic acid, monohydrochloride. Its empirical formula is $C_{25}H_{30}N_2O_5 \cdot HCl$.

Quinapril hydrochloride is a white to off-white amorphous powder that is freely soluble in aqueous solvents.

Accupril tablets contain 5, 10, 20, or 40 mg of quinapril for oral administration. Each tablet also contains candelilla wax, crospovidone, gelatin, lactose, magnesium carbonate, magnesium stearate, synthetic red iron oxide, and titanium dioxide.

CLINICAL PHARMACOLOGY

MECHANISM OF ACTION

Quinapril is deesterified to the principal metabolite, quinaprilat, which is an inhibitor of ACE activity in human subjects and animals. ACE is a peptidyl dipeptidase that catalyzes the conversion of angiotensin I to the vasoconstrictor, angiotensin II. The effect of quinapril in hypertension and in congestive heart failure (CHF) appears to result primarily from the inhibition of circulating and tissue ACE activity, thereby reducing angiotensin II formation. Quinapril inhibits the elevation in blood pressure caused by intravenously administered angiotensin I, but has no effect on the pressor response to angiotensin II, norepinephrine or epinephrine. Angiotensin II also stimulates the secretion of aldosterone from the adrenal cortex, thereby facilitating renal sodium and fluid reabsorption. Reduced aldosterone secretion by quinapril may result in a small increase in serum potassium. In controlled hypertension trials, treatment with quinapril HCl alone resulted in mean increases in potassium of 0.07 mmol/L (see PRECAUTIONS). Removal of angiotensin II negative feedback on renin secretion leads to increased plasma renin activity (PRA).

While the principal mechanism of antihypertensive effect is thought to be through the renin-angiotensin-aldosterone system, quinapril exerts antihypertensive actions even in patients with low renin hypertension. Quinapril HCl was an effective antihypertensive in all races studied, although it was somewhat less effective in blacks (usually a predominantly low renin group) than in non-blacks. ACE is identical to kininase II, an enzyme that degrades bradykinin, a potent peptide vasodilator; whether increased levels of bradykinin play a role in the therapeutic effect of quinapril remains to be elucidated.

PHARMACOKINETICS AND METABOLISM

Following oral administration, peak plasma quinapril concentrations are observed within 1 hour. Based on recovery of quinapril and its metabolites in urine, the extent of absorption is at least 60%. The rate and extent of quinapril absorption are diminished moderately (approximately 25-30%) when quinapril HCl tablets are administered during a high-fat meal. Following absorption, quinapril is deesterified to its major active metabolite, quinaprilat (about 38% of oral dose), and to other minor inactive metabolites. Following multiple oral dosing of quinapril HCl, there is an effective accumulation half-life of quinaprilat of approximately 3 hours, and peak plasma quinaprilat concentrations are observed approximately 2 hours post-dose. Quinaprilat is eliminated primarily by renal excretion, up to 96% of an IV dose, and has an elimination half-life in plasma of approximately 2 hours and a prolonged terminal phase with a half-life of 25 hours. The pharmacokinetics of quinapril and quinaprilat are linear over a single-dose range of 5-80 mg doses and 40-160 mg in multiple daily doses. Approximately 97% of either quinapril or quinaprilat circulating in plasma is bound to proteins.

In patients with renal insufficiency, the elimination half-life of quinaprilat increases as creatinine clearance decreases. There is a linear correlation between plasma quinaprilat clearance and creatinine clearance. In patients with end-stage renal disease, chronic hemodialysis or continuous ambulatory peritoneal dialysis has little effect on the elimination of quinapril and quinaprilat. Elimination of quinaprilat may be reduced in elderly patients (≥65 years) and in those with heart failure; this reduction is attributable to decrease in renal function (see DOSAGE AND ADMINISTRATION). Quinaprilat concentrations are reduced in patients with alcoholic cirrhosis due to impaired deesterification of quinapril. Studies in rats indicate that quinapril and its metabolites do not cross the blood-brain barrier.

PHARMACODYNAMICS AND CLINICAL EFFECTS

Hypertension

Single doses of 20 mg of quinapril HCl provide over 80% inhibition of plasma ACE for 24 hours. Inhibition of the pressor response to angiotensin I is shorter-lived, with a 20 mg dose giving 75% inhibition for about 4 hours, 50% inhibition for about 8 hours, and 20% inhibition at 24 hours. With chronic dosing, however, there is substantial inhibition of angiotensin II levels at 24 hours by doses of 20-80 mg.

Administration of 10-80 mg of quinapril HCl to patients with mild to severe hypertension results in a reduction of sitting and standing blood pressure to about the same extent with minimal effect on heart rate. Symptomatic postural hypotension is infrequent although it can occur in patients who are salt- and/or volume-depleted (see WARNINGS). Antihypertensive activity commences within 1 hour with peak effects usually achieved by 2-4 hours after dosing. During chronic therapy, most of the blood pressure lowering effect of a given dose is obtained in 1-2 weeks. In multiple-dose studies, 10-80 mg/day in single or divided doses lowered systolic and diastolic blood pressure throughout the dosing interval, with a trough effect of about 5-11/3-7 mm Hg. The trough effect represents about 50% of the peak effect. While the dose-response relationship is relatively flat, doses of 40-80 mg were somewhat more effective at trough than 10-20 mg, and twice daily dosing tended to give a somewhat lower trough blood pressure than once daily dosing with the same total dose. The antihypertensive effect of quinapril HCl continues during long-term therapy, with no evidence of loss of effectiveness.

Hemodynamic assessments in patients with hypertension indicate that blood pressure reduction produced by quinapril is accompanied by a reduction in total peripheral resistance and renal vascular resistance with little or no change in heart rate, cardiac index, renal blood flow, glomerular filtration rate, or filtration fraction.

Use of quinapril HCl with a thiazide diuretic gives a blood-pressure lowering effect greater than that seen with either agent alone.

In patients with hypertension, quinapril HCl 10-40 mg was similar in effectiveness to captopril, enalapril, propranolol, and thiazide diuretics.

Therapeutic effects appear to be the same for elderly (≥65 years of age) and younger adult patients given the same daily dosages, with no increase in adverse events in elderly patients.

Heart Failure

In a placebo-controlled trial involving patients with congestive heart failure treated with digitalis and diuretics, parenteral quinaprilat, the active metabolite of quinapril, reduced pulmonary capillary wedge pressure and systemic vascular resistance and increased cardiac output/index. Similar favorable hemodynamic effects were seen with oral quinapril in baseline-controlled trials, and such effects appeared to be maintained during chronic oral quinapril therapy. Quinapril reduced renal hepatic vascular resistance and increased renal and hepatic blood flow with glomerular filtration rate remaining unchanged.

A significant dose response relationship for improvement in maximal exercise tolerance has been observed with quinapril HCl therapy. Beneficial effects on the severity of heart failure as measured by New York Heart Association (NYHA) classification and Quality of Life and on symptoms of dyspnea, fatigue, and edema were evident after 6 months in a double-blind, placebo-controlled study. Favorable effects were maintained for up to 2 years of open label therapy. The effects of quinapril on long-term mortality in heart failure have not been evaluated.

INDICATIONS AND USAGE

HYPERTENSION

Quinapril HCl is indicated for the treatment of hypertension. It may be used alone or in combination with thiazide diuretics.

HEART FAILURE

Quinapril HCl is indicated in the management of heart failure as adjunctive therapy when added to conventional therapy including diuretics and/or digitalis.

In using quinapril HCl, consideration should be given to the fact that another angiotensin-converting enzyme inhibitor, captopril, has caused agranulocytosis, particularly in patients with renal impairment or collagen vascular disease. Available data are insufficient to show that quinapril HCl does not have a similar risk (see WARNINGS).

ANGIOEDEMA IN BLACK PATIENTS

Black patients receiving ACE inhibitor monotherapy have been reported to have a higher incidence of angioedema compared to non-blacks. It should also be noted that in controlled clinical trials ACE inhibitors have an effect on blood pressure that is less in black patients than in non-blacks.

CONTRAINDICATIONS

Quinapril HCl is contraindicated in patients who are hypersensitive to this product and in patients with a history of angioedema related to previous treatment with an ACE inhibitor.

WARNINGS

ANAPHYLACTOID AND POSSIBLY RELATED REACTIONS

Presumably because angiotensin-converting inhibitors affect the metabolism of eicosanoids and polypeptides, including endogenous bradykinin, patients receiving ACE inhibitors (including quinapril HCl) may be subject to a variety of adverse reactions, some of them serious.

Angioedema

Angioedema of the face, extremities, lips, tongue, glottis, and larynx has been reported in patients treated with ACE inhibitors and has been seen in 0.1% of patients receiving quinapril HCl.

In two similarly sized US postmarketing trials that, combined, enrolled over 3,000 black patients and over 19,000 non-blacks, angioedema was reported in 0.30% and 0.55% of blacks (in Study 1 and 2 respectively) and 0.39% and 0.17% of non-blacks.

Angioedema associated with laryngeal edema can be fatal. If laryngeal stridor or angioedema of the face, tongue, or glottis occurs, treatment with quinapril HCl should be

Q

discontinued immediately, the patient treated in accordance with accepted medical care, and carefully observed until the swelling disappears. In instances where swelling is confined to the face and lips, the condition generally resolves without treatment; antihistamines may be useful in relieving symptoms. **Where there is involvement of the tongue, glottis, or larynx likely to cause airway obstruction, emergency therapy including, but not limited to, subcutaneous epinephrine solution 1:1000 (0.3-0.5 ml) should be promptly administered** (see ADVERSE REACTIONS).

Patients With a History of Angioedema: Patients with a history of angioedema unrelated to ACE inhibitor therapy may be at increased risk of angioedema while receiving an ACE inhibitor (see also CONTRAINDICATIONS).

Anaphylactoid Reactions During Desensitization

Two patients undergoing desensitizing treatment with hymenoptera venom while receiving ACE inhibitors sustained life-threatening anaphylactoid reactions. In the same patients, these reactions were avoided when ACE inhibitors were temporarily withheld, but they reappeared upon inadvertent rechallenge.

Anaphylactoid Reactions During Membrane Exposure

Anaphylactoid reactions have been reported in patients dialyzed with high-flux membranes and treated concomitantly with an ACE inhibitor. Anaphylactoid reactions have also been reported in patients undergoing low-density lipoprotein apheresis with dextran sulfate absorption.

HEPATIC FAILURE

Rarely, ACE inhibitors have been associated with a syndrome that starts with cholestatic jaundice and progresses to fulminant hepatic necrosis and (sometimes) death. The mechanism of this syndrome is not understood. Patients receiving ACE inhibitors who develop jaundice or marked elevations of hepatic enzymes should discontinue the ACE inhibitor and receive appropriate medical follow-up.

HYPOTENSION

Excessive hypotension is rare in patients with uncomplicated hypertension treated with quinapril HCl alone. Patients with heart failure given quinapril HCl commonly have some reduction in blood pressure, but discontinuation of therapy because of continuing symptomatic hypotension usually is not necessary when dosing instructions are followed. Caution should be observed when initiating therapy in patients with heart failure (see DOSAGE AND ADMINISTRATION). In controlled studies, syncope was observed in 0.4% of patients (n=3203); this incidence was similar to that observed for captopril (1%) and enalapril (0.8%).

Patients at risk of excessive hypotension, sometimes associated with oliguria and/or progressive azotemia, and rarely with acute renal failure and/or death, include patients with the following conditions or characteristics: heart failure, hyponatremia, high dose diuretic therapy, recent intensive diuresis or increase in diuretic dose, renal dialysis, or severe volume and/or salt depletion of any etiology. It may be advisable to eliminate the diuretic (except in patients with heart failure), reduce the diuretic dose or cautiously increase salt intake (except in patients with heart failure) before initiating therapy with quinapril HCl in patients at risk for excessive hypotension who are able to tolerate such adjustments.

In patients at risk of excessive hypotension, therapy with quinapril HCl should be started under close medical supervision. Such patients should be followed closely for the first 2 weeks of treatment and whenever the dose of quinapril HCl and/or diuretic is increased. Similar considerations may apply to patients with ischemic heart or cerebrovascular disease in whom an excessive fall in blood pressure could result in a myocardial infarction or a cerebrovascular accident.

If excessive hypotension occurs, the patient should be placed in the supine position and, if necessary, receive an IV infusion of normal saline. A transient hypotensive response is not a contraindication to further doses of quinapril HCl, which usually can be given without difficulty once the blood pressure has stabilized. If symptomatic hypotension develops, a dose reduction or discontinuation of quinapril HCl or concomitant diuretic may be necessary.

NEUTROPENIA/AGRANULOCYTOSIS

Another ACE inhibitor, captopril, has been shown to cause agranulocytosis and bone marrow depression rarely in patients with uncomplicated hypertension, but more frequently in patients with renal impairment, especially if they also have a collagen vascular disease, such as systemic lupus erythematosus or scleroderma. Agranulocytosis did occur during quinapril HCl treatment in 1 patient with a history of neutropenia during previous captopril therapy. Available data from clinical trials of quinapril HCl are insufficient to show that, in patients without prior reactions to other ACE inhibitors, quinapril HCl does not cause agranulocytosis at similar rates. As with other ACE inhibitors, periodic monitoring of white blood cell counts in patients with collagen vascular disease and/or renal disease should be considered.

FETAL/NEONATAL MORBIDITY AND MORTALITY

ACE inhibitors can cause fetal and neonatal morbidity and death when administered to pregnant women. Several dozen cases have been reported in the world literature. When pregnancy is detected, ACE inhibitors should be discontinued as soon as possible.

The use of ACE inhibitors during the second and third trimesters of pregnancy has been associated with fetal and neonatal injury, including hypotension, neonatal skull hypoplasia, anuria, reversible or irreversible renal failure, and death. Oligohydramnios has also been reported, presumably resulting from decreased fetal renal function; oligohydramnios in this setting has been associated with fetal limb contractures, craniofacial deformation, and hypoplastic lung development. Prematurity, intrauterine growth retardation, and patent ductus arteriosus have also been reported, although it is not clear whether these occurrences were due to the ACE inhibitor exposure.

These adverse effects do not appear to have resulted from intrauterine ACE inhibitor exposure that has been limited to the first trimester. Mothers whose embryos and fetuses are exposed to ACE inhibitors only during the first trimester should be so informed. Nonetheless, when patients become pregnant, physicians should make every effort to discontinue the use of quinapril HCl as soon as possible.

Rarely (probably less often than once in every 1000 pregnancies), no alternative to ACE inhibitors will be found. In these rare cases, the mothers should be apprised of the potential hazards to their fetuses, and serial ultrasound examinations should be performed to assess the intraamniotic environment.

If oligohydramnios is observed, quinapril HCl should be discontinued unless it is considered life-saving for the mother. Contraction stress testing (CST), a non-stress test (NST), or biophysical profiling (BPP) may be appropriate, depending upon the week of pregnancy. Patients and physicians should be aware, however, that oligohydramnios may not appear until after the fetus has sustained irreversible injury.

Infants with histories of *in utero* exposure to ACE inhibitors should be closely observed for hypotension, oliguria, and hyperkalemia. If oliguria occurs, attention should be directed toward support of blood pressure and renal perfusion. Exchange transfusion or dialysis may be required as a means of reversing hypotension and/or substituting for disordered renal function. Removal of quinapril HCl, which crosses the placenta, from the neonatal circulation is not significantly accelerated by these means.

No teratogenic effects of quinapril HCl were seen in studies of pregnant rats and rabbits. On a mg/kg basis, the doses used were up to 180 times (in rats) and 1 time (in rabbits) the maximum recommended human dose.

PRECAUTIONS

GENERAL

Impaired Renal Function

As a consequence of inhibiting the renin-angiotensin-aldosterone system, changes in renal function may be anticipated in susceptible individuals. In patients with severe heart failure whose renal function may depend on the activity of the renin-angiotensin-aldosterone system, treatment with ACE inhibitors, including quinapril HCl, may be associated with oliguria and/or progressive azotemia and rarely acute renal failure and/or death.

In clinical studies in hypertensive patients with unilateral or bilateral renal artery stenosis, increases in blood urea nitrogen and serum creatinine have been observed in some patients following ACE inhibitor therapy. These increases were almost always reversible upon discontinuation of the ACE inhibitor and/or diuretic therapy. In such patients, renal function should be monitored during the first few weeks of therapy.

Some patients with hypertension or heart failure with no apparent preexisting renal vascular disease have developed increases in blood urea and serum creatinine, usually minor and transient, especially when quinapril HCl has been given concomitantly with a diuretic. This is more likely to occur in patients with preexisting renal impairment. Dosage reduction and/or discontinuation of any diuretic and/or quinapril HCl may be required.

Evaluation of patients with hypertension or heart failure should always include assessment of renal function (see DOSAGE AND ADMINISTRATION).

Hyperkalemia and Potassium-Sparing Diuretics

In clinical trials, hyperkalemia (serum potassium ≥5.8 mmol/L) occurred in approximately 2% of patients receiving quinapril HCl. In most cases, elevated serum potassium levels were isolated values which resolved despite continued therapy. Less than 0.1% of patients discontinued therapy due to hyperkalemia. Risk factors for the development of hyperkalemia include renal insufficiency, diabetes mellitus, and the concomitant use of potassium-sparing diuretics, potassium supplements, and/or potassium-containing salt substitutes, which should be used cautiously, if at all, with quinapril HCl (see DRUG INTERACTIONS).

Cough

Presumably due to the inhibition of the degradation of endogenous bradykinin, persistent non-productive cough has been reported with all ACE inhibitors, always resolving after discontinuation of therapy. ACE inhibitor-induced cough should be considered in the differential diagnosis of cough.

Surgery/Anesthesia

In patients undergoing major surgery or during anesthesia with agents that produce hypotension, quinapril HCl will block angiotensin II formation secondary to compensatory renin release. If hypotension occurs and is considered to be due to this mechanism, it can be corrected by volume expansion.

INFORMATION FOR THE PATIENT

Pregnancy

Female patients of childbearing age should be told about the consequences of second- and third-trimester exposure to ACE inhibitors, and they should also be told that these consequences do not appear to have resulted from intrauterine ACE-inhibitor exposure that has been limited to the first trimester. These patients should be asked to report pregnancies to their physicians as soon as possible.

Angioedema

Angioedema, including laryngeal edema can occur with treatment with ACE inhibitors, especially following the first dose. Patients should be so advised and told to report immediately any signs or symptoms suggesting angioedema (swelling of face, extremities, eyes, lips, tongue, difficulty in swallowing or breathing) and to stop taking the drug until they have consulted with their physician (see WARNINGS).

Symptomatic Hypotension

Patients should be cautioned that lightheadedness can occur, especially during the first few days of quinapril HCl therapy, and that it should be reported to a physician. If actual syncope occurs, patients should be told to not take the drug until they have consulted with their physician (see WARNINGS).

All patients should be cautioned that inadequate fluid intake or excessive perspiration, diarrhea, or vomiting can lead to an excessive fall in blood pressure because of reduction in fluid volume, with the same consequences of lightheadedness and possible syncope.

Patients planning to undergo any surgery and/or anesthesia should be told to inform their physician that they are taking an ACE inhibitor.

Hyperkalemia

Patients should be told not to use potassium supplements or salt substitutes containing potassium without consulting their physician (see PRECAUTIONS).

Neutropenia

Patients should be told to report promptly any indication of infection (*e.g.,* sore throat, fever) which could be a sign of neutropenia.

NOTE: As with many other drugs, certain advice to patients being treated with quinapril HCl is warranted. This information is intended to aid in the safe and effective use of this medication. It is not a disclosure of all possible adverse or intended effects.

CARCINOGENESIS, MUTAGENESIS, AND IMPAIRMENT OF FERTILITY

Quinapril HCl was not carcinogenic in mice or rats when given in doses up to 75 or 100 mg/kg/day (50 to 60 times the maximum human daily dose, respectively, on an mg/kg basis and 3.8 to 10 times the maximum human daily dose when based on an mg/m^2 basis) for 104 weeks. Female rats given the highest dose level had an increased incidence of mesenteric lymph node hemangiomas and skin/subcutaneous lipomas. Neither quinapril nor quinaprilat were mutagenic in the Ames bacterial assay with or without metabolic activation. Quinapril was also negative in the following genetic toxicology studies: *in vitro* mammalian cell point mutation, sister chromatid exchange in cultured mammalian cells, micronucleus test with mice, *in vitro* chromosome aberration with V79 cultured lung cells, and in an *in vivo* cytogenetic study with rat bone marrow. There were no adverse effects on fertility or reproduction in rats at doses up to 100 mg/kg/day (60 and 10 times the maximum daily human dose when based on mg/kg and mg/m^2, respectively).

PREGNANCY CATEGORY C (FIRST TRIMESTER) AND D (SECOND AND THIRD TRIMESTERS)

See WARNINGS, Fetal/Neonatal Morbidity and Mortality.

NURSING MOTHERS

Because quinapril HCl is secreted in human milk, caution should be exercised when this drug is administered to a nursing woman.

PEDIATRIC USE

The safety and effectiveness of quinapril HCl in pediatric patients have not been established.

GERIATRIC USE

Clinical studies of quinapril HCl did not include sufficient numbers of subjects aged 65 and over to determine whether they respond differently from younger subjects. Other reported clinical experience has not identified differences in responses between the elderly and younger patients. In general, dose selection for an elderly patient should be cautious, usually starting at the low end of the dosing range, reflecting the greater frequency of decreased hepatic, renal or cardiac function, and of concomitant disease or other drug therapy.

This drug is known to be substantially excreted by the kidney, and the risk of toxic reactions to this drug may be greater in patients with impaired renal function. Because elderly patients are more likely to have decreased renal function, care should be taken in dose selection, and it may be useful to monitor renal function.

Elderly patients exhibited increased area under the plasma concentration time curve and peak levels for quinaprilat compared to values observed in younger patients; this appeared to relate to decreased renal function rather than to age itself.

DRUG INTERACTIONS

CONCOMITANT DIURETIC THERAPY

As with other ACE inhibitors, patients on diuretics, especially those on recently instituted diuretic therapy, may occasionally experience an excessive reduction of blood pressure after initiation of therapy with quinapril HCl. The possibility of hypotensive effects with quinapril HCl may be minimized by either discontinuing the diuretic or cautiously increasing salt intake prior to initiation of treatment with quinapril HCl. If it is not possible to discontinue the diuretic, the starting dose of quinapril should be reduced (see DOSAGE AND ADMINISTRATION).

AGENTS INCREASING SERUM POTASSIUM

Quinapril can attenuate potassium loss caused by thiazide diuretics and increase serum potassium when used alone. If concomitant therapy of quinapril HCl with potassium-sparing diuretics (*e.g.,* spironolactone, triamterene, or amiloride), potassium supplements, or potassium-containing salt substitutes is indicated, they should be used with caution along with appropriate monitoring of serum potassium (see PRECAUTIONS).

TETRACYCLINE AND OTHER DRUGS THAT INTERACT WITH MAGNESIUM

Simultaneous administration of tetracycline with quinapril HCl reduced the absorption of tetracycline by approximately 28-37%, possibly due to the high magnesium content in quinapril HCl tablets. This interaction should be considered if coprescribing quinapril HCl and tetracycline or other drugs that interact with magnesium.

LITHIUM

Increased serum lithium levels and symptoms of lithium toxicity have been reported in patients receiving concomitant lithium and ACE inhibitor therapy. These drugs should be coadministered with caution and frequent monitoring of serum lithium levels is recommended. If a diuretic is also used, it may increase the risk of lithium toxicity.

OTHER AGENTS

Drug interaction studies of quinapril HCl with other agents showed:

- Multiple dose therapy with propranolol or cimetidine has no effect on the pharmacokinetics of single doses of quinapril HCl.
- The anticoagulant effect of a single dose of warfarin (measured by prothrombin time) was not significantly changed by quinapril co-administration twice-daily.
- Quinapril HCl treatment did not affect the pharmacokinetics of digoxin.
- No pharmacokinetic interaction was observed when single doses of quinapril HCl and hydrochlorothiazide were administered concomitantly.
- Co-administration of multiple 10 mg doses of atorvastatin with 80 mg of quinapril HCl resulted in no significant change in the steady-state pharmacokinetic parmeters of atorvastatin.

ADVERSE REACTIONS

HYPERTENSION

Quinapril HCl has been evaluated for safety in 4960 subjects and patients. Of these, 3203 patients, including 655 elderly patients, participated in controlled clinical trials. Quinapril HCl has been evaluated for long-term safety in over 1400 patients treated for 1 year or more.

Adverse experiences were usually mild and transient.

In placebo-controlled trials, discontinuation of therapy because of adverse events was required in 4.7% of patients with hypertension.

Adverse experiences probably or possibly related to therapy or of unknown relationship to therapy occurring in 1% or more of the 1563 patients in placebo-controlled hypertension trials who were treated with quinapril HCl are shown in TABLE 1.

TABLE 1 *Adverse Events in Placebo-Controlled Trials*

	Incidence (discontinuance)	
	Quinapril HCl	Placebo
(n=1563)	(n=579)	
Headache	5.6 (0.7)	10.9 (0.7)
Dizziness	3.9 (0.8)	2.6 (0.2)
Fatigue	2.6 (0.3)	1.0
Coughing	2.0 (0.5)	0.0
Nausea and/or vomiting	1.4 (0.3)	1.9 (0.2)
Abdominal pain	1.0 (0.2)	0.7

HEART FAILURE

Quinapril HCl has been evaluated for safety in 1222 quinapril HCl treated patients. Of these, 632 patients participated in controlled clinical trials. In placebo-controlled trials, discontinuation of therapy because of adverse events was required in 6.8% of patients with congestive heart failure.

Adverse experiences probably or possibly related or of unknown relationship to therapy occurring in 1% or more of the 585 patients in placebo-controlled congestive heart failure trials who were treated with quinapril HCl are shown in TABLE 2.

TABLE 2

	Incidence (discontinuance)	
	Quinapril HCl	Placebo
(n=585)	(n=295)	
Dizziness	7.7 (0.7)	5.1 (1.0)
Coughing	4.3 (0.3)	1.4
Fatigue	2.6 (0.2)	1.4
Nausea and/or vomiting	2.4 (0.2)	0.7
Chest pain	2.4	1.0
Hypotension	2.9 (0.5)	1.0
Dyspnea	1.9 (0.2)	2.0
Diarrhea	1.7	1.0
Headache	1.7	1.0 (0.3)
Myalgia	1.5	2.0
Rash	1.4 (0.2)	1.0
Back pain	1.2	0.3

See PRECAUTIONS, Cough.

HYPERTENSION AND/OR HEART FAILURE

Clinical adverse experiences probably, possibly, or definitely related, or of uncertain relationship to therapy occurring in 0.5-1.0% (except as noted) of the patients with CHF or hypertension treated with quinapril HCl (with or without concomitant diuretic) in controlled or uncontrolled trials (n=4847) and less frequent, clinically significant events seen in clinical trials or post-marketing experience (the rarer events are in italics) include (listed by body system):

General: Back pain, malaise, viral infections.

Cardiovascular: Palpitation, vasodilation, tachycardia, *heart failure, hyperkalemia, myocardial infarction, cerebrovascular accident, hypertensive crisis, angina pectoris, orthostatic hypotension, cardiac rhythm disturbances, cardiogenic shock.*

Hematology: *Hemolytic anemia.*

Gastrointestinal: Flatulence, dry mouth or throat, constipation, *gastrointestinal hemorrhage, pancreatitis, abnormal liver function tests.*

Nervous/Psychiatric: Somnolence, vertigo, syncope, nervousness, depression, insomnia, paresthesia.

Integumentary: Alopecia, increased sweating, pemphigus, pruritus, *exfoliative dermatitis, photosensitivity reaction, dermatopolymiositis.*

Urogenital: Urinary tract infection, impotence, *acute renal failure, worsening renal failure.*

Respiratory: *Eosinophilic pneumonitis.*

Other: Amblyopia, edema, arthralgia, pharyngitis, *agranulocytosis, hepatitis, thrombocytopenia.*

FETAL/NEONATAL MORBIDITY AND MORTALITY
See WARNINGS, Fetal/Neonatal Morbidity and Mortality.

ANGIOEDEMA
Angioedema has been reported in patients receiving quinapril HCl (0.1%). Angioedema associated with laryngeal edema may be fatal. If angioedema of the face, extremities, lips, tongue, glottis, and/or larynx occurs, treatment with quinapril HCl should be discontinued and appropriate therapy instituted immediately. (See WARNINGS.)

CLINICAL LABORATORY TEST FINDINGS
Hematology: See WARNINGS.
Hyperkalemia: See PRECAUTIONS.
Creatinine and Blood Urea Nitrogen: Increases (>1.25 times the upper limit of normal) in serum creatinine and blood urea nitrogen were observed in 2% and 2%, respectively, of all patients treated with quinapril HCl alone. Increases are more likely to occur in patients receiving concomitant diuretic therapy than in those on quinapril HCl alone. These increases often remit on continued therapy. In controlled studies of heart failure, increases in blood urea nitrogen and serum creatinine were observed in 11% and 8%, respectively, of patients treated with quinapril HCl; most often these patients were receiving diuretics with or without digitalis.

DOSAGE AND ADMINISTRATION

HYPERTENSION
Monotherapy
The recommended initial dosage of quinapril HCl in patients not on diuretics is 10 or 20 mg once daily. Dosage should be adjusted according to blood pressure response measured at peak (2-6 hours after dosing) and trough (predosing). Generally, dosage adjustments should be made at intervals of at least two weeks. Most patients have required dosages of 20, 40, or 80 mg/day, given as a single dose or in two equally divided doses. In some patients treated once daily, the antihypertensive effect may diminish toward the end of the dosing interval. In such patients an increase in dosage or twice daily administration may be warranted. In general, doses of 40-80 mg and divided doses give a somewhat greater effect at the end of the dosing interval.

Concomitant Diuretics
If blood pressure is not adequately controlled with quinapril HCl monotherapy, a diuretic may be added. In patients who are currently being treated with a diuretic, symptomatic hypotension occasionally can occur following the initial dose of quinapril HCl. To reduce the likelihood of hypotension, the diuretic should, if possible, be discontinued 2-3 days prior to beginning therapy with quinapril HCl (see WARNINGS). Then, if blood pressure is not controlled with quinapril HCl alone, diuretic therapy should be resumed.

If the diuretic cannot be discontinued, an initial dose of 5 mg quinapril HCl should be used with careful medical supervision for several hours and until blood pressure has stabilized.

The dosage should subsequently be titrated (as described above) to the optimal response (see WARNINGS, PRECAUTIONS, and DRUG INTERACTIONS).

RENAL IMPAIRMENT
Kinetic data indicate that the apparent elimination half-life of quinaprilat increases as creatinine clearance decreases. Recommended starting doses, based on clinical and pharmacokinetic data from patients with renal impairment, are shown in TABLE 3.

TABLE 3

Creatinine Clearance	Maximum Recommended Initial Dose
>60 ml/min	10 mg
30-60 ml/min	5 mg
10-30 ml/min	2.5 mg
<10 ml/min	Insufficient data for dosage recommendation

Patients should subsequently have their dosage titrated (as described above) to the optimal response.

ELDERLY (≥65 YEARS)
The recommended initial dosage of quinapril HCl in elderly patients is 10 mg given once daily followed by titration (as described above) to the optimal response.

HEART FAILURE
Quinapril HCl is indicated as adjunctive therapy when added to conventional therapy including diuretics and/or digitalis. The recommended starting dose is 5 mg twice daily. This dose may improve symptoms of heart failure, but increases in exercise duration have generally required higher doses. Therefore, if the initial dosage of quinapril HCl is well tolerated, patients should then be titrated at weekly intervals until an effective dose, usually 20-40 mg daily given in 2 equally divided doses, is reached or undesirable hypotension, orthostatis, or azotemia (see WARNINGS) prohibit reaching this dose.

Following the initial dose of quinapril HCl, the patient should be observed under medical supervision for at least 2 hours for the presence of hypotension or orthostatis and, if present, until blood pressure stabilizes. The appearance of hypotension, orthostatis, or azotemia early in dose titration should not preclude further careful dose titration. Consideration should be given to reducing the dose of concomitant diuretics.

DOSE ADJUSTMENTS IN PATIENTS WITH HEART FAILURE AND RENAL IMPAIRMENT OR HYPONATREMIA
Pharmacokinetic data indicate that quinapril elimination is dependent on level of renal function. In patients with heart failure and renal impairment, the recommended initial dose of quinapril HCl is 5 mg in patients with a creatinine clearance above 30 ml/min and 2.5 mg in patients with a creatinine clearance of 10-30 ml/min. There is insufficient data for dosage recommendation in patients with a creatinine clearance less than 10 ml/min. (See Heart Failure, WARNINGS, and DRUG INTERACTIONS.)

If the initial dose is well tolerated, quinapril HCl may be administered the following day as a twice daily regimen. In the absence of excessive hypotension or significant deterioration of renal function, the dose may be increased at weekly intervals based on clinical and hemodynamic response.

HOW SUPPLIED

Accupril tablets are supplied as follows:
5 mg Tablets: Brown, film-coated, elliptical scored tablets, coded "PD 527" on one side and "5" on the other.
10 mg Tablets: Brown, film-coated, triangular tablets, coded "PD 530" on one side and "10" on the other.
20 mg Tablets: Brown, film-coated, round tablets, coded "PD 532" on one side and "20" on the other.
40 mg Tablets: Brown, film-coated, elliptical tablets, coded "PD 535" on one side and "40" on the other.

Dispense in well-closed containers as defined in the USP.
Storage: Store at controlled room temperature 15-30°C (59-86°F). Protect from light.

PRODUCT LISTING - EQUIVALENTS NOT AVAILABLE

Qty	Price	Product	NDC
Tablet - Oral - 5 mg			
30's	$31.43	ACCUPRIL, Physicians Total Care	54868-3307-01
30's	$51.11	ACCUPRIL, Pd-Rx Pharmaceuticals	55289-0552-30
60's	$61.75	ACCUPRIL, Physicians Total Care	54868-3307-00
90's	$106.84	ACCUPRIL, Parke-Davis	00071-0527-23
100's	$118.71	ACCUPRIL, Parke-Davis	00071-0527-40
Tablet - Oral - 10 mg			
7's	$6.36	ACCUPRIL, Allscripts Pharmaceutical Company	54569-3984-01
30's	$27.27	ACCUPRIL, Allscripts Pharmaceutical Company	54569-3984-00
30's	$31.43	ACCUPRIL, Physicians Total Care	54868-2665-01
30's	$51.11	ACCUPRIL, Pd-Rx Pharmaceuticals	55289-0553-30
90's	$106.84	ACCUPRIL, Parke-Davis	00071-0530-23
100's	$118.71	ACCUPRIL, Parke-Davis	00071-0530-40
Tablet - Oral - 20 mg			
30's	$27.27	ACCUPRIL, Allscripts Pharmaceutical Company	54569-3985-00
30's	$31.41	ACCUPRIL, Physicians Total Care	54868-2666-01
30's	$51.11	ACCUPRIL, Pd-Rx Pharmaceuticals	55289-0554-30
50's	$60.97	ACCUPRIL, Physicians Total Care	54868-2666-02
90's	$106.84	ACCUPRIL, Parke-Davis	00071-0532-23
90's	$108.80	ACCUPRIL, Physicians Total Care	54868-2666-03
100's	$118.71	ACCUPRIL, Parke-Davis	00071-0532-40
Tablet - Oral - 40 mg			
30's	$30.50	ACCUPRIL, Allscripts Pharmaceutical Company	54569-4454-00
30's	$30.87	ACCUPRIL, Physicians Total Care	54868-3445-00
30's	$51.11	ACCUPRIL, Pd-Rx Pharmaceuticals	55289-0555-30
90's	$106.84	ACCUPRIL, Parke-Davis	00071-0535-23

Quinidine Gluconate *(002165)*

Categories: Arrhythmia, ventricular; Fibrillation, atrial; Flutter, atrial; Malaria; Tachycardia, ventricular; Pregnancy Category C; FDA Approved 1969 Dec
Drug Classes: Antiarrhythmics, class IA; Antiprotozoals
Brand Names: **Quinaglute Dura-Tabs**
Foreign Brand Availability: Quinaglute Dura-tabs (South-Africa)
Cost of Therapy: $35.10 (Arrhythmia; Quinaglute Dura-Tabs; 324 mg; 2 tablets/day; 30 day supply)
$18.94 (Arrhythmia; Generic Tablets; 324 mg; 2 tablets/day; 30 day supply)

IV-INFUSION

DESCRIPTION

INJECTION
Quinidine is an antimalarial schizonticide and an antiarrhythmic agent with Class Ia activity; it is the d-isomer of quinine and its molecular weight is 324.43. Quinidine gluconate is the gluconate salt of quinidine; its chemical name is cinchonan-9-ol,6′-methoxy-,(9*S*)-,mono-D-gluconate. Its empirical formula is $C_{20}H_{24}N_2O_2 \cdot C_6H_{12}O_7$, and its molecular weight is 520.28, of which 62.3% is quinidine base.

Each vial of quinidine gluconate injection contains 800 mg (1.5 mmol) of quinidine gluconate (500 mg of quinidine in 10 ml of sterile water for injection, 0.005% of edetate disodium, 0.25% phenol, and (as needed) D-gluconic acid δ-lactone to adjust the pH.

CLINICAL PHARMACOLOGY

PHARMACOKINETICS AND METABOLISM
After intramuscular injection of quinidine gluconate, peak serum levels of quinidine are achieved in a little less than 2 hours. This time to peak levels is identical to the time measured when quinidine salts are administered orally.

The volume of distribution of quinidine is typically 2-3 L/kg in healthy young adults, but this may be reduced to as little as 0.5 L/kg in patients with congestive heart failure, or increased to 3-5 L/kg in patients with cirrhosis of the liver. At concentrations of 2-5 mg/L (6.5-16.2 μmol/L), the fraction of quinidine bound to plasma proteins (mainly α_1-acid glycoprotein and to albumin) is 80-88% in adults and older children, but it is lower in pregnant women, and in infants and neonates it may be as low as 50-75%. Because α_1-acid glycoprotein levels are increased in response to stress, serum levels of total quinidine may be greatly increased in settings such as acute myocardial infarction, even though the serum content of unbound (active) drug may remain normal. Protein binding is also increased in chronic renal failure, but binding abruptly descends toward or below normal when heparin is administered for hemodialysis.

Quinidine clearance typically proceeds at 3-5 ml/min/kg in adults, but clearance in pediatric patients may be twice or three times as rapid. The elimination half-life is about 6-8 hours in adults and 3-4 hours in pediatric patients. Quinidine clearance is unaffected by hepatic cirrhosis, so the increased volume of distribution seen in cirrhosis leads to a proportionate increase in the elimination half-life.

Most quinidine is eliminated hepatically via the action of cytochrome P450IIIA4; there are several different hydroxylated metabolites, and some of these have antiarrhythmic activity.

The most important of quinidine's metabolites is 3-hydroxy-quinidine (3HQ), serum levels of which can approach those of quinidine in patients receiving conventional doses of quinidine gluconate. The volume of distribution of 3HQ appears to be larger than that of quinidine, and the elimination half-life of 3HQ is about 12 hours.

As measured by antiarrhythmic effects in animals, by QTc prolongation in human volunteers, or by various *in vitro* techniques, 3HQ has at least half the antiarrhythmic activity of the parent compound, so it may be responsible for a substantial fraction of the effect of quinidine gluconate in chronic use.

When the urine pH is less than 7, about 20% of administered quinidine appears unchanged in the urine, but this fraction drops to as little as 5% when the urine is more alkaline. Renal clearance involves both glomerular filtration and active tubular secretion, moderated by (pH-dependent) tubular reabsorption. The net renal clearance is about 1 ml/min/kg in healthy adults.

When renal function is taken into account, quinidine clearance is apparently independent of patient age.

Assays of serum quinidine levels are widely available, but the results of modern assays may not be consistent with results cited in the older medical literature. The serum levels of quinidine cited in this package insert are those derived from specific assays, using either benzene extraction or (preferably) reverse-phase high-pressure liquid chromatography. In matched samples, older assays might unpredictably have given results that were as much as 2 or 3 times higher. A typical "therapeutic" concentration range is 2-6 mg/L (6.2-18.5 μmol/L).

MECHANISMS OF ACTION

In patients with malaria, quinidine acts primarily as an intraerythrocytic schizonticide, with little effect upon sporozoites or upon pre-erythrocytic parasites. Quinidine is gametocidal to *Plasmodium vivax* and *P. malariae,* but not to *P. falciparum.*

In cardiac muscle and in Purkinje fibers, quinidine depresses the rapid inward depolarizing sodium current, thereby slowing phase-0 depolarization and reducing the amplitude of the action potential without affecting the resting potential. In normal Purkinje fibers, it reduces the slope of phase-4 depolarization, shifting the threshold voltage upward toward zero. The result is slowed conduction and reduced automaticity in all parts of the heart, with increase of the effective refractory period relative to the duration of the action potential in the atria, ventricles, and Purkinje tissues. Quinidine also raises the fibrillation thresholds of the atria and ventricles, and it raises the ventricular *de*fibrillation threshold as well. Quinidine's actions fall into Class Ia in the Vaughan-Williams classification.

By slowing conduction and prolonging the effective refractory period, quinidine can interrupt or prevent reentrant arrhythmias and arrhythmias due to increased automaticity, including atrial flutter, atrial fibrillation, and paroxysmal supraventricular tachycardia.

In patients with the sick sinus syndrome, quinidine can cause marked sinus node depression and bradycardia. In most patients, however, use of quinidine is associated with an increase in sinus rate.

Quinidine prolongs the QT interval in a dose-related fashion. This may lead to increased ventricular automaticity and polymorphic ventricular tachycardias, including *torsades de pointes* (see WARNINGS).

In addition, quinidine has anticholinergic activity, it has negative inotropic activity, and it acts peripherally as an α-adrenergic antagonist (that is, as a vasodilator).

CLINICAL EFFECTS

Malaria

Intravenous quinidine has been associated with clearing of parasitemia and high rates of survival in patients with severe *P. falciparum* malaria and hyperparasitemia. Placebo-controlled trials have not been performed, but clearing of these levels of parasitemia is unprecedented in the absence of effective therapy. Use of quinidine in patients infected with chloroquine-sensitive malaria or in chloroquine-resistant non-falciparum malaria has not been reported.

Maintenance of Sinus Rhythm After Conversion From Atrial Fibrillation

In six clinical trials (published between 1970 and 1984) with a total of 808 patients, quinidine (418 patients) was compared to nontreatment (258 patients) or placebo (132 patients) for the maintenance of sinus rhythm after cardioversion from chronic atrial fibrillation. Quinidine was consistently more efficacious in maintaining sinus rhythm, but a meta-analysis found that mortality in the quinidine-exposed patients (2.9%) was significantly greater than mortality in patients who had not been treated with active drug (0.8%). Supression of atrial fibrillation with quinidine has theoretical patient benefits (*e.g.,* improved exercise tolerance; reduction in hospitalization for cardioversion; lack of arrhythmia-related palpitations, dyspnea, and chest pain; reduced incidence of systemic embolism and/or stroke), but these benefits have never been demonstrated in clinical trials. Some of these benefits (*e.g.,* reduction in stroke incidence) may be achievable by other means (anticoagulation).

By slowing the rate of atrial flutter/fibrillation, quinidine can decrease the degree of atrioventricular block and cause an increase, sometimes marked, in the rate at which supraventricular impulses are successfully conducted by the atrioventricular node, with a resultant paradoxical increase in ventricular rate (see WARNINGS).

Non-Life-Threatening Venricular Arrhythmias

In studies of patients with a variety of ventricular arrhythmias (mainly frequent ventricular premature beats and non-sustained ventricular tachycardia), quinidine (total n=502) has been compared to flecainide (n=141), mexiletine (n=246), propafenone (n=53), and tocainide (n=67). In each of these studies, the mortality in the quinidine group was numerically greater than the mortality in the comparator group. When the studies were combined in a meta-analysis, quinidine was associated with a statistically significant 3-fold relative risk of death.

At therapeutic doses, quinidine's only consistent effect upon the surface electrocardiogram is an increase in the QT interval. This prolongation can be monitored as a guide to safety, and it may provide better guidance than serum drug levels (see WARNINGS).

INDICATIONS AND USAGE

TREATMENT OF MALARIA

Quinidine gluconate injection is indicated for the treatment of life-threatening *Plasmodium falciparum* malaria.

CONVERSION OF ATRIAL FIBRILLATION/FLUTTER

Quinidine gluconate injection is also indicated (when rapid therapeutic effect is required, or when oral therapy is not feasible) as a means of restoring normal sinus rhythm in patients with symptomatic atrial fibrillation/flutter whose symptoms are not adequately controlled by measures that reduce the rate of ventricular response. If this use of quinidine gluconate does not restore sinus rhythm within a reasonable time, then its use should be discontinued.

TREATMENT OF VENTRICULAR ARRHYTHMIAS

Quinidine gluconate injection is also indicated for the treatment of documented ventricular arrhythmias, such as sustained ventricular tachycardia, that in the judgement of the physician are life-threatening. Because of the proarrhythmic effects of quinidine, its use with ventricular arrythmias of lesser severity is generally not recommended, and treatment of patients with asymptomatic ventricular premature contractions should be avoided. Where possible, therapy should be guided by the results of programmed electrical stimulation and/or Holter monitoring with exercise.

Antiarrhythmic drugs (including quinidine) have not been shown to enhance survival in patients with ventricular arrythmias.

CONTRAINDICATIONS

Quinidine is contraindicated in patients who are known to be allergic to it, or who have developed thrombocytopenic purpura during prior therapy with quinidine or quinine.

In the absence of a functioning artificial pacemaker, quinidine is also contraindicated in any patient whose cardiac rhythm is dependent upon a junctional or idioventricular pacemaker, including patients in complete atrioventricular block.

Quinidine is also contraindicated in patients who, like those with myasthenia gravis, might be adversely affected by an anticholinergic agent.

WARNINGS

INAPPROPRIATE INFUSION RATE

Overly rapid infusion of quinidine (see DOSAGE AND ADMINISTRATION) may cause peripheral vascular collapse and severe hypotension.

PROARRHYTHMIC EFFECTS

Like many other drugs (including all other Class Ia antiarrhythmics), quinidine prolongs the QTc interval, and this can lead to *torsades de pointes,* a life-threatening ventricular arrhythmia. The risk of *torsades* is increased by any of bradycardia, hypokalemia, hypomagnesemia, and high serum levels of quinidine, but it may appear in the absence of any of theses risk factors. The best predictor of this arrhythmia appears to be the length of the QTc interval, and quinidine should be used with extreme care in patients who have preexisting long-QT syndromes, who have histories of *torsades de pointes* of any cause, or who have previously responded to quinidine (or other drugs that prolong ventricular repolarization) with marked lengthening of the QTc interval. Estimation of the incidence of *torsades* in patients with therapeutic levels of quinidine is not possible from the available data.

Other ventricular arrhythmias that have been reported with quinidine include frequent extrasystoles, ventricular tachycardia, ventricular flutter, and ventricular fibrillation.

PARADOXICAL INCREASE IN VENTRICULAR RATE IN ATRIAL FLUTTER/FIBRILLATION

When quinidine is administered to patients with atrial flutter/fibrillation, the desired pharmacologic reversion to sinus rhythm may (rarely) be preceded by a slowing of the atrial rate with a consequent increase in the rate of beats conducted to the ventricles. The resulting ventricular rate may be very high (greater than 200 beats/min) and poorly tolerated. This hazard may be decreased if partial atrioventricular block is achieved prior to initiation of quinidine therapy, using conduction-reducing drugs such as **digitalis, verapamil, diltiazem,** or a β-receptor blocking agent.

EXACERBATED BRADYCARDIA IN SICK SINUS SYNDROME

In patients with the sick sinus syndrome, quinidine has been associated with marked sinus node depression and bradycardia.

PHARMACOKINETIC CONSIDERATIONS

Renal or hepatic dysfunction causes the elimination of quinidine to be slowed, while congestive heart failure causes a reduction in quinidine's apparent volume of distribution. Any of these conditions can lead to quinidine toxicity if dosage is not appropriately reduced. In addition, interactions with coadministered drugs can alter the serum concentration and activity of quinidine, leading either to toxicity or to lack of efficacy if the dose of quinidine is not appropriately modified (see DRUG INTERACTIONS).

VAGOLYSIS

Because quinidine opposes the atrial and A-V nodal effects of vagal stimulation, physical or pharmacological vagal maneuvers undertaken to terminate paroxysmal supraventricular tachycardia may be ineffective in patients receiving quinidine.

PRECAUTIONS

HEART BLOCK

In patients without implanted pacemakers who are at high risk of complete atrioventricular block (*e.g.*, those with digitalis intoxication, second-degree atrioventricular block, or severe intraventricular conduction defects), quinidine should be used only with caution.

CARCINOGENESIS, MUTAGENESIS, AND IMPAIRMENT OF FERTILITY

Animal studies to evaluate quinidine's carcinogenic or mutagenic potential have not been performed. Similarly, there are no animal data as to quinidine's potential to impair fertility.

PREGNANCY CATEGORY C

Animal reproductive studies have not been conducted with quinidine. There are no adequate and well-controlled studies in pregnant women. Quinidine should be given to a pregnant woman only if clearly needed.

In one neonate whose mother had received quinidine throughout her pregnancy, the serum level of quinidine was equal to that of the mother, with no apparent ill effect. The level of quinidine in amniotic fluid was about 3 times higher than that found in serum.

LABOR AND DELIVERY

Quinidine is said to be oxytocic in humans, but there are no adequate data as to quinidine's effect (if any) on human labor and delivery.

NURSING MOTHERS

Quinidine is present in human milk at levels slightly lower than those in maternal serum; a human infant ingesting such milk should (scaling directly by weight) be expected to develop serum quinidine levels at least an order of magnitude lower than those of the mother. On the other hand, the pharmacokinetics and pharmacodynamics of quinidine in human infants have not been adequately studied, and neonates' reduced protein binding of quinidine may increase their risk of toxicity at low total serum levels. Administration of quinidine should (if possible) be avoided in lactating women who continue to nurse.

PEDIATRIC USE

In antimalarial trials, quinidine was as safe and effective in pediatric patients as in adults. Notwithstanding the known pharmacokinetic differences between pediatric patients and adults (see CLINICAL PHARMACOLOGY, Pharmacokinetics and Metabolism), pediatric patients in these trials received the same doses (on a mg/kg basis) as adults.

Safety and effectiveness of antiarrhythmic use in pediatric patients have not been established.

GERIATRIC USE

Safety and efficacy of quinidine in elderly patients has not been systematically studied. Clinical studies of quinidine did not include sufficient numbers of subjects aged 65 and over to determine whether they respond differently from younger subjects. The reported clinical experience has not identified differences in responses between the elderly and younger patients. In general, dose selection for an elderly patient should be cautious, usually starting at the low end of the dosing range, reflecting the greater frequency of decreased hepatic, renal or cardiac function and of concomitant disease or other drug therapy.

DRUG INTERACTIONS

ALTERED PHARMACOKINETICS OF QUINIDINE

Drugs that alkalinize the urine (**carbonic-anhydrase inhibitors, sodium bicarbonate, thiazide diuretics**) reduce renal elimination of quinidine.

By pharmacokinetic mechanisms that are not well understood, quinidine levels are increased by coadministration of **amiodarone** or **cimetidine.** Very rarely, and again by mechanisms not understood, quinidine levels are decreased by coadministration of **nifedipine.**

Hepatic elimination of quinidine may be accelerated by coadministration of drugs (**phenobarbital, phenytoin, rifampin**) that induce production of cytochrome P450IIIA4.

Perhaps because of competition for the P450IIIA4 metabolic pathway, quinidine levels rise when **ketaconazole** is administered.

Coadministration of **propranolol** usually does not affect quinidine pharmacokinetics, but in some studies, the β-blocker appeared to cause increases in the peak serum levels of quinidine, decreases in quinidine's volume of distribution and decreases in total quinidine clearance. The effects (if any) of coadministration of **other β-blockers** on quinidine pharmacokinetics have not been adequately studied.

Hepatic clearance of quinidine is significantly reduced during coadministration of **verapamil,** with corresponding increases in serum levels and half-life.

ALTERED PHARMACOKINETICS OF OTHER DRUGS

Quinidine slows the elimination of **digoxin** and simultaneously reduces digoxin's apparent volume of distribution. As a result, serum digoxin levels may be as much as doubled. When quinidine and digoxin are coadministered, digoxin doses usually need to be reduced. Serum levels of **digitoxin** are also raised when quinidine is coadministered, although the effect appears to be smaller.

By a mechanism that is not understood, quinidine potentiates the anticoagulatory action of warfarin, and the anticoagulant dosage may need to be reduced.

Cytochrome P450IID6 is an enzyme critical to the metabolism of many drugs, notably including **mexiletine,** some **phenothiazines,** and most **polycyclic antidepressants.** Constitutional deficiency of cytochrome P450IID6 is found in less than 1% of Orientals, in about 2% of American blacks, and in about 8% of American whites. Testing with debrisoquine is sometimes used to distinguish the P450IID6-deficient "poor metabolizers" from the majority-phenotype "extensive metabolizers".

When drugs whose metabolism is P450IID6-dependent are given to poor metabolizers, the serum levels achieved are higher, sometimes much higher, than the serum levels achieved when identical doses are given to extensive metabolizers. To obtain similar clinical benefit without toxicity, doses given to poor metabolizers may need to be greatly reduced. In the cases of prodrugs whose actions are actually mediated by P450IID6-produced metabolites (for example, **codeine** and **hydrocodone,** whose analgesic and antitussive effects appear to mediated by morphine and hydromorphone, respectively), it may not be possible to achieve the desired clinical benefits in poor metabolizers.

Quinidine is not metabolized by cytochrome P450IID6, but therapeutic serum levels of quinidine inhibit the action of cytochrome P450IID6, effectively converting extensive metabolizers into poor metabolizers. Caution must be exercised whenever quinidine is prescribed together with drugs metabolized by cytochrome P450IID6.

Perhaps by competing for pathways of renal clearance, coadministration of quinidine causes and increase in serum levels of **procainamide.**

Serum levels of **haloperidol** are increased when quinidine is coadministered.

Presumably because both drugs are metabolized by cytochrome P450IIIA4, coadministration of quinidine causes variable slowing of the metabolism of **nifedipine.** Interactions with other dihydropyridine calcium-channel blockers have not been reported, but these agents (including **felodipine, nicardipine,** and **nimodipine**) are all dependent upon P450IIIA4 for metabolism, so similar interactions with quinidine should be anticipated.

ALTERED PHARMACODYNAMICS OF OTHER DRUGS

Quinidine's anticholinergic, vasodilating, and negative inotropic actions may be additive to those of other drugs with these effects, and antagonistic to those of drugs with cholinergic, vasoconstricting, and positive inotropic effects. For example, when quinidine and **verapamil** are coadministered in doses that are each well tolerated as monotherapy, hypotension attributable to additive peripheral α-blockade is sometimes reported.

Quinidine potentiates the actions of depolarizing (succinylcholine, decamethonium) and nondepolarizing (*d*-tubocurarine, pancuronium) neuromuscular blocking agents. These phenomena are not well understood, but they are observed in animal models as well as in humans. In addition, *in vitro* addition of quinidine to the serum of pregnant women reduces the activity of pseudocholinesterase, an enzyme that is essential to the metabolism of succinylcholine.

Diltiazem significantly decreases the clearance and increases the $T_{1/2}$ of quinidine, but quinidine does not alter the kinetics of diltiazem. *Non-interactions of quinidine with other drugs:* Quinidine has no clinically significant effect on the pharmacokinetics of **diltiazem, flecainide, mephenytoin, metoprolol, propafenone, propranolol, quinine, timolol,** or **tocainide.**

Conversely, the pharmacokinetics of quinidine are not significantly affected by **caffeine, ciprofloxacin, digoxin, felodipine, omeprazole,** or **quinine.** Quinidine's pharmacokinetics are also unaffected by cigarette smoking.

ADVERSE REACTIONS

Quinidine preparations have been used for many years, but there are only sparse data from which to estimate the incidence of various adverse reactions. The adverse reactions most frequently reported have consistently been gastro-intestinal, including diarrhea, nausea, vomiting, and heart-burn/esophagitis. In one study of 245 adult outpatients who received quinidine to suppress premature ventricular contractions, the incidence of reported adverse experiences were as shown in TABLE 1. The most serious quinidine-associated adverse reactions are described in WARNINGS.

TABLE 1 *Adverse Experiences in a 245-Patient PVC Trial*

	Incidence (%)
Diarrhea	85 (35%)
"Upper gastrointestinal distress"	55 (22%)
Lightheadedness	37 (15%)
Headache	18 (7%)
Fatigue	17 (7%)
Palpitations	16 (7%)
Angina-like pain	14 (6%)
Weakness	13 (5%)
Rash	11 (5%)
Visual problems	8 (3%)
Change in sleep habits	7 (3%)
Tremor	6 (2%)
Nervousness	5 (2%)
Discoordination	3 (1%)

Intramuscular injections of quinidine gluconate are typically followed by moderate to severe local pain. Some patients will develop tender nodules at the site of injection that persist for several weeks.

Vomiting and diarrhea can occur as isolated reactions to therapeutic levels of quinidine, but they may also be the first signs of **cinchonism,** a syndrome that may also include tinnitus, reversible high-frequency hearing loss, deafness, vertigo, blurred vision, diplopia, photophobia, headache, confusion, and delirium. Cinchonism is most often a sign of chronic quinidine toxicity, but it may appear in sensitive patients after a single moderate dose.

A few cases of **hepatotoxicity,** including granulomatous hepatitis, have been reported in patients receiving quinidine. All of these have appeared during the first few weeks of therapy, and most (not all) have remitted once quinidine was withdrawn.

Autoimmune and inflammatory syndromes associated with quinidine therapy have included fever, urticaria, flushing, exfoliative rash, bronchospasm, pneumonitis, psoriasiform rash, pruritus and lymphadenopathy, hemolytic anemia, vasculitis, thrombocytopenic purpura, uveitis, angioedema, agranulocytosis, the sicca syndrome, arthralgia, myalgia, elevation in serum levels of skeletal-muscle enzymes, and a disorder resembling systemic lupus erythematosus.

Convulsions, apprehension, and ataxia have been reported, but is was not clear that these were not simply the results of hypotension and consequent cerebral hypoperfusion. There are many reports of syncope. Acute psychotic reactions have been reported to follow the first dose of quinidine, but these reactions appear to be extremely rare.

Other adverse reactions occasionally reported include depression, mydriasis, disturbed color perception, night blindness, scotomata, optic neuritis, visual field loss, photosensitivity, and abnormalities of pigmentation.

DOSAGE AND ADMINISTRATION

Because the kinetics of absorption may vary with the patient's peripheral perfusion, intramuscular injection of quinidine gluconate is not recommended.

TREATMENT OF P. FALCIPARUM MALARIA

Two regimens have each been shown to be effective, with or without concomitant exchange transfusion. There are no data indicating that either should be preferred to the other.

In Regimen A, each patient received a **loading dose** of 15 mg/kg of quinidine base (that is, 24 mg/kg of quinidine gluconate) in 250 ml of normal saline infused over 4 hours. Thereafter, each patient received a **maintenance regimen** of 7.5 mg/kg of base (12 mg/kg of quinidine gluconate) infused over 4 hours every 8 hours, starting 8 hours after the beginning of the loading dose. This regimen was continued for 7 days, except that in patients able to swallow, the maintenance infusions were discontinued, and approximately the same daily doses of quinidine were supplied orally, using 300 mg tablets of quinidine sulfate.

In Regimen B, each patient received a **loading dose** of 6.25 mg/kg of quinidine base (that is, 10 mg/kg of quinidine gluconate) in approximately 5 ml/kg of normal saline over 1-2 hours. Thereafter, each patient received a **maintenance infusion** of 12.5 μg/kg/min of base (that is, 20 μg/kg/min of quinidine gluconate). In patients able to swallow, the maintenance infusion was discontinued, and eight-hourly oral quinine sulfate was administered to provide approximately as much daily quinine base as the patient had been receiving quinidine base (for example, each adult patient received 650 mg of quinine sulfate every 8 hours). Quinidine/quinine therapy was continued for 72 hours or until parasitemia had decreased to 1% or less, whichever came first. After completion of quinidine/quinine therapy, adults able to swallow received a single 1500 mg/75 mg dose of sulfadoxine/pyrimethamine or a 7 day course of tetracycline (250 mg four times daily), while those unable to swallow received 7 day courses of intravenous doxycycline hyclate, 100 mg twice daily. Most of the patients described as having been treated with this regimen also underwent exchanged transfusion. Small children have received this regimen without dose adjustment and with apparent good results, notwithstanding the known differences in quinidine pharmacokinetics between pediatric patients and adults (see CLINICAL PHARMACOLOGY).

Even in patients without preexisting cardiac disease, antimalarial use of quinidine has occasionally been associated with hypotension, QTc prolongation, and cinchonism; see WARNINGS.

TREATMENT OF SYMPTOMATIC ATRIAL FIBRILLATION/FLUTTER

A patient receiving an intravenous infusion of quinidine must be carefully monitored, with frequent or continuous electrocardiography and blood-pressure measurement. The infusion should be discontinued as soon as sinus rhythm is restored: the QRS complex widens to 130% of its pre-treatment duration; the QTc interval widens to 130% of its pre-treatment duration, and is then longer than 500 millisecond; P waves disappear; or the patient develops significant tachycardia, symptomatic bradycardia, or hypotension.

To prepare quinidine for infusion, the contents of the supplied vial (80 mg/ml) should be diluted to 50 ml (16 mg/ml) with 5% dextrose. The resulting solution may be stored for up to 24 hours at room temperature or up to 48 hours at 4°C (40°F).

Because quinidine may be absorbed to PVC tubing, tubing length should be minimized. In one study (*Am J Health Syst Pharm.* 1996; 53:655-8), use of 112 inches of tubing resulted in 30% loss of quinidine, but drug loss was less than 3% when only 12 inches of tubing was used.

An infusion of quinidine must be delivered slowly, preferable under control of a volumetric pump, no faster than 0.25 mg/kg/min (that is, no faster than 1 ml/kg/h). During the first few minutes of the infusion, the patient should be monitored especially closely for possible hypersensitive or idiosyncratic reactions.

Most arrhythmias that will respond to intravenous quinidine will respond to a total dose of less than 5 mg/kg, but some patients may require as much as 10 mg/kg. If conversion to sinus rhythm has not been achieved after infusion of 10 mg/kg, then the infusion should be discontinued, and other means of conversion (*e.g.,* direct-current cardioversion) should be considered.

TREATMENT OF LIFE-THREATENING VENTRICULAR ARRHYTHMIAS

Dosing regimens for the use of intravenous quinidine gluconate in controlling life-threatening ventricular arrhythmias have not been adequately studied. Described regimens have generally been similar to the regimen described just above for the treatment of symptomatic atrial fibrillation/flutter.

HOW SUPPLIED

Quinidine gluconate injection is supplied in 80 mg/ml, 10 ml multiple-dose vials.
Storage: Store at 25°C (77°F); excursions permitted to 15-30°C (59-86°F).

ORAL

DESCRIPTION

Quinidine is an antimalarial schizonticide and an antiarrhythmic agent with Class Ia activity; it is the d-isomer of quinine, and its molecular weight is 324.43. Quinidine gluconate is the gluconate salt of quinidine; its chemical name is cinchonan-9-ol,6′-methoxy-,(9*S*)-, mono-D-gluconate.

Its empirical formula is $C_{20}H_{24}N_2O_2 \cdot C_6H_{12}O_7$, and its molecular weight is 520.58, of which 62.3% is quinidine base.

Each Quinaglute Dura-Tabs tablet contains 324 mg of quinidine gluconate (202 mg of quinidine base) in a matrix to provide extended-release; the inactive ingredients include confectioner's sugar, magnesium stearate, corn starch and other ingredients.

CLINICAL PHARMACOLOGY

PHARMACOKINETICS AND METABOLISM

The absolute **bioavailability** of quinidine from quinidine gluconate extended-release tablets is 70-80%. Relative to a solution of quinidine sulfate, the bioavailability of quinidine from quinidine gluconate extended-release tablets is reported to be 1.03. The less-than-complete bioavailability is thought to be due to first-pass elimination by the liver. Peak serum levels generally appear 3-5 hours after dosing; when the drug is taken with food, absorption is increased in both rate (27%) and extent (17%). The rate and extent of absorption of quinidine from quinidine gluconate extended-release tablets are not significantly affected by the coadministration of an aluminum-hydroxide antacid. The rate of absorption of quinidine following the ingestion of grapefruit juice may be decreased.

The **volume of distribution** of quinidine is 2-3 L/kg in healthy young adults, but this may be reduced to as little as 0.5 L/kg in patients with congestive heart failure, or increased to 3-5 L/kg in patients with cirrhosis of the liver. At concentrations of 2-5 mg/L (6.5-16.2 μmol/L), the fraction of quinidine bound to plasma proteins (mainly to α_1-acid glycoprotein and to albumin) is 80-88% in adults and older children, but it is lower in pregnant women, and in infants and neonates it may be as low as 50-70%. Because α_1-acid glycoprotein levels are increased in response to stress, serum levels of total quinidine may be greatly increased in settings such as acute myocardial infarction, even though the serum content of unbound (active) drug may remain normal. Protein binding is also increased in chronic renal failure, but binding abruptly descends toward or below normal when heparin is administered for hemodialysis.

Quinidine **clearance** typically proceeds at 3-5 ml/min/kg in adults, but clearance in children may be twice or three times as rapid. The elimination half-life is 6-8 hours in adults and 3-4 hours in children. Quinidine clearance is unaffected by hepatic cirrhosis, so the increased volume of distribution seen in cirrhosis leads to a proportionate increase in the elimination half-life.

Most quinidine is eliminated hepatically via the action of cytochrome P450IIIA4; there are several different hydroxylated metabolites, and some of these have antiarrhythmic activity.

The most important of quinidine's metabolites is 3-hydroxy-quinidine (3HQ), serum levels of which can approach those of quinidine in patients receiving conventional doses of quinidine gluconate extended-release tablets. The volume of distribution of 3HQ appears to be larger than that of quinidine, and the elimination half-life of 3HQ is about 12 hours.

As measured by antiarrhythmic effects on animals, by QTc prolongation in human volunteers, or by various *in vitro* techniques, 3HQ has at least half the antiarrhythmic activity of the parent compound, so it may be responsible for a substantial fraction of the effect of quinidine gluconate extended-release tablets in chronic use.

When the urine pH is less than 7, about 20% of administered quinidine appears unchanged in the urine, but this fraction drops to as little as 5% when the urine is more alkaline. Renal clearance involves both glomerular filtration and active tubular secretion, moderated by (pH-dependent) tubular reabsorption. The net renal clearance is about 1 ml/min/kg in healthy adults.

When renal function is taken into account, quinidine clearance is apparently independent of patient age.

Assays of serum quinidine levels are widely available, but the results of modern assays may not be consistent with results cited in the older medical literature. The serum levels of quinidine cited in this package insert are those derived from specific assays, using either benzene extraction or (preferably) reverse-phase high-pressure liquid chromatography. In matched samples, older assays might unpredictably have given results that were as much as 2 or 3 times higher. A typical "therapeutic" concentration range is 2-6 mg/L (6.2-18.5 μmol/L).

MECHANISMS OF ACTION

In patients with malaria, quinidine acts primarily as an intra-erythrocytic schizonticide, with little effect upon sporozites or upon pre-erythrocytic parasites. Quinidine is gametocidal to *Plasmodium vivax* and *P. malariae,* but not to *P. falciparum.*

In cardiac muscle and in Purkinje fibers, quinidine depresses the rapid inward depolarizing sodium current, thereby slowing phase-0 depolarization and reducing the amplitude of the action potential without affecting the resting potential. In normal Purkinje fibers, it reduces the slope of phase-4 depolarization, shifting the threshold voltage upward toward zero. The result is slowed conduction and reduced automaticity in all parts of the heart, with increase of the effective refractory period relative to the duration of the action potential in the atria, ventricles, and Purkinje tissues. Quinidine also raises the fibrillation thresholds of the atria and ventricles, and it raises the ventricular *de*fibrillation threshold as well. Quinidine's actions fall into Class Ia in the Vaughn-Williams classification.

By slowing conduction and prolonging the effective refractory period, quinidine can interrupt or prevent reentrant arrhythmias and arrhythmias due to increased automaticity, including atrial flutter, atrial fibrillation, and paroxysmal supraventricular tachycardia.

In patients with the sick sinus syndrome, quinidine can cause marked sinus node depression and bradycardia. In most patients, however, use of quinidine is associated with an increase in the sinus rate.

Like other antiarrhythmic drugs with Class Ia activity, quinidine prolongs the QT interval in a dose-related fashion. This may lead to increased ventricular automaticity and polymorphic ventricular tachycardias, including *torsades de pointes* (see WARNINGS).

In addition, quinidine has anticholinergic activity, it has negative inotropic activity, and it acts peripherally as an α-adrenergic antagonist (that is, as a vasodilator).

CLINICAL EFFECTS

Maintenance of Sinus Rhythm After Conversion From Atrial Fibrillation

In six clinical trials (published between 1970 and 1984) with a total of 808 patients, quinidine (418 patients) was compared to nontreatment (258 patients) or placebo (132 patients) for the maintenance of sinus rhythm after cardioversion from chronic atrial fibrillation. Quinidine was consistently more efficacious in maintaining sinus rhythm, but a meta-analysis found that mortality in the quinidine-exposed patients (2.9%) was significantly greater than mortality in the patients who had not been treated with active drug (0.8%). Suppression of atrial fibrillation with quinidine has theoretical patient benefits (*e.g.,* improved exercise tolerance; reduction in hospitalization for cardioversion; lack of arrhythmia-related palpitations, dyspnea and chest pain; reduced incidence of systemic embolism and/or stroke), but these benefits have never been demonstrated in clinical trials. Some of these benefits (*e.g.*, reduction in stroke incidence) may be achievable by other means (anticoagulation).

By slowing the atrial rate in atrial flutter/fibrillation, quinidine can decrease the degree of atrioventricular block and cause an increase, sometimes marked, in the rate at which supraventricular impulses are successfully conducted by the atrioventricular node, with a resultant paradoxical increase in ventricular rate (see WARNINGS).

Non-Life-Threatening Ventricular Arrhythmias

In studies of patients with a variety of ventricular arrhythmias (mainly frequent ventricular premature beats and non-sustained ventricular tachycardia, quinidine (total n=502) has been compared with flecainide (n=141), mexiletine (n=246), propafenone (n=53), and tocainide (n=67). In each of these studies, the mortality in the quinidine group was numerically greater than the mortality in the comparator group. When the studies were combined in a meta-analysis, quinidine was associated with a statistically significant 3-fold relative risk of death.

At therapeutic doses, quinidine's only consistent effect upon the surface electrocardiogram is an increase in the QT interval. This prolongation can be monitored as a guide to safety, and it may provide better guidance than serum drug levels (see WARNINGS).

INDICATIONS AND USAGE

CONVERSION OF ATRIAL FIBRILLATION/FLUTTER

In patients with symptomatic atrial fibrillation/flutter whose symptoms are not adequately controlled by measures that reduce the rate of ventricular response, quinidine gluconate extended-release tablets is indicated as a means of restoring normal sinus rhythm. If this use of quinidine gluconate extended-release tablets does not restore sinus rhythm within a reasonable time (see DOSAGE AND ADMINISTRATION), then quinidine gluconate extended-release tablets should be discontinued.

REDUCTION OF FREQUENCY OF RELAPSE INTO ATRIAL FIBRILLATION/FLUTTER

Chronic therapy with quinidine gluconate extended-release tablets is indicated for some patients at high risk of symptomatic atrial fibrillation/flutter, generally patients who have had previous episodes of atrial fibrillation/flutter that were so frequent and poorly tolerated as to outweigh, in the judgment of the physician and the patient, the risks of prophylactic therapy with quinidine gluconate extended-release tablets. The increased risk of death should specifically be considered. Quinidine gluconate extended-release tablets should be used only after alternative measures (*e.g.*, use of other drugs to control the ventricular rate) have been found to be inadequate.

In patients with histories of frequent symptomatic episodes of atrial fibrillation/flutter, the goal of therapy should be an increase in the average time between episodes. In most patients, the tachyarrhythmia *will recur* during therapy, and a single recurrence should not be interpreted as therapeutic failure.

SUPPRESSION OF VENTRICULAR ARRHYTHMIAS

Quinidine gluconate extended-release tablets are also indicated for the suppression of recurrent documented ventricular arrhythmias, such as sustained ventricular tachycardia, that in the judgment of the physician are life-threatening. Because of the proarrhythmic effects of quinidine, its use with ventricular arrhythmias of lesser severity is generally not recommended, and treatment of patients with asymptomatic ventricular premature contractions should be avoided. Where possible, therapy should be guided by the results of programmed electrical stimulation and/or Holter monitoring with exercise.

Antiarrhythmic drugs (including quinidine gluconate extended-release tablets) have not been shown to enhance survival in patients with ventricular arrhythmias.

CONTRAINDICATIONS

Quinidine is contraindicated in patients who are known to be allergic to it, or who have developed thrombocytopenic purpura during prior therapy with quinidine or quinine.

In the absence of a functioning artificial pacemaker, quinidine is also contraindicated in any patient whose cardiac rhythm is dependent upon a junctional or idioventricular pacemaker, including patients in complete atrioventricular block.

Quinidine is also contraindicated in patients who, like those with myasthenia gravis, might be adversely affected by an anticholinergic agent.

WARNINGS

MORTALITY

In many trials of antiarrhythmic therapy for non-life-threatening arrhythmias, active antiarrhythmic therapy has resulted in increased mortality; the risk of active therapy is probably greatest in patients with structural heart disease.

In the case of quinidine used to prevent or defer recurrence of atrial flutter/fibrillation, the best available data come from a meta-analysis described in CLINICAL PHARMACOLOGY, Clinical Effects. In the patients studied in the trials there analyzed, the mortality associated with the use of quinidine was more than 3 times as great as the mortality associated with the use of placebo.

Another meta-analysis, also described in CLINICAL PHARMACOLOGY, Clinical Effects, showed that in patients with various non-life-threatening ventricular arrhythmias, the mortality associated with the use of quinidine was consistently greater than that associated with the use of any of a variety of alternative antiarrhythmics.

PROARRHYTHMIC EFFECTS

Like many other drugs (including all other Class Ia antiarrhythmics), quinidine prolongs the QTc interval, and this can lead to *torsades de pointes*, a life-threatening ventricular arrhythmia. The risk of *torsades* is increased by bradycardia, hypokalemia, hypomagnesemia or high serum levels of quinidine, but it may appear in the absence of any of these risk factors. The best predictor of this arrhythmia appears to be the length of QTc interval, and quinidine should be used with extreme care in patients who have preexisting long-QT syndromes, who have histories of *torsades de pointes* of any cause, or who have previously responded to quinidine (or other drugs that prolong ventricular repolarization) with marked lengthening of the QTc interval. Estimation of the incidence of *torsades* in patients with therapeutic levels of quinidine is not possible from the available data.

Other ventricular arrhythmias that have been reported with quinidine include frequent extrasystoles, ventricular tachycardia, ventricular flutter, and ventricular fibrillation.

PARADOXICAL INCREASE IN VENTRICULAR RATE IN ATRIAL FLUTTER/FIBRILLATION

When quinidine is administered to patients with atrial flutter/fibrillation, the desired pharmacologic reversion to sinus rhythm may (rarely) be preceded by a slowing of the atrial rate with a consequent increase in the rate of beats conducted to the ventricles. The resulting ventricular rate may be very high (greater than 200 beats/min) and poorly tolerated. This hazard may be decreased if partial atrioventricular block is achieved prior to initiation of quinidine therapy, using conduction-reducing drugs such as digitalis, verapamil, diltiazem, or a β-receptor blocking agent.

EXACERBATED BRADYCARDIA IN SICK SINUS SYNDROME

In patients with the sick sinus syndrome, quinidine has been associated with marked sinus node depression and bradycardia.

PHARMACOKINETIC CONSIDERATIONS

Renal or hepatic dysfunction causes the elimination of quinidine to be slowed, while congestive heart failure causes a reduction in quinidine's apparent volume of distribution. Any of these conditions can lead to quinidine toxicity if dosage is not appropriately reduced. In addition, interactions with coadministered drugs can alter the serum concentration and activity of quinidine, leading either to toxicity or to lack of efficacy if the dose of quinidine is not appropriately modified. (See DRUG INTERACTIONS.)

VAGOLYSIS

Because quinidine opposes the atrial and A-V nodal effects of vagal stimulation, physical or pharmacological vagal maneuvers undertaken to terminate paroxysmal supraventricular tachycardia may be ineffective in patients receiving quinidine.

PRECAUTIONS

HEART BLOCK

In patients without implanted pacemakers who are at high risk of complete atrioventricular block (*e.g.*, those with digitalis intoxication, second degree atrioventricular block, or severe intraventricular conduction defects), quinidine should be used only with caution.

INFORMATION FOR THE PATIENT

Before prescribing quinidine gluconate extended-release tablets as prophylaxis against recurrence of atrial fibrillation, the physician should inform the patient of the risks and benefits to be expected (see CLINICAL PHARMACOLOGY).

Discussion should include the facts:

- That the goal of therapy will be a reduction (probably not to zero) in the frequency of episodes of atrial fibrillation; and
- That reduced frequency of fibrillatory episodes may be expected, if achieved, to bring symptomatic benefit; but
- That no data are available to show that reduced frequency of fibrillatory episodes will reduce the risks of irreversible harm through stroke or death; and in fact
- That such data as are available suggest that treatment with quinidine gluconate extended-release tablets is likely to increase the patient's risk of death.

CARCINOGENESIS, MUTAGENESIS, AND IMPAIRMENT OF FERTILITY

Animal studies to evaluate quinidine's carcinogenic or mutagenic potential have not been performed. Similarly, there are no animal data as to quinidine's potential to impair fertility.

PREGNANCY CATEGORY C

Animal reproductive studies have not been conducted with quinidine. There are no adequate and well-controlled studies in pregnant women. Quinidine should be given to a pregnant woman only if clearly needed.

In one neonate whose mother had received quinidine throughout her pregnancy, the serum level of quinidine was equal to that of the mother, with no apparent ill effect. The level of quinidine in amniotic fluid was about 3 times higher than that found in serum.

LABOR AND DELIVERY

Quinine is said to be oxytocic in humans, but there are no adequate data as to quinidine's effects (if any) on human labor and delivery.

NURSING MOTHERS

Quinidine is present in human milk at levels slightly lower than those in maternal serum; a human infant ingesting such milk should (scaling directly by weight) be expected to develop serum quinidine levels at least an order of magnitude lower than those of the mother. On the other hand, the pharmacokinetics and pharmacodynamics of quinidine in human infants have not been adequately studied, and neonates' reduced protein binding of quinidine may increase their risk of toxicity at low total serum levels. Administration of quinidine should (if possible) be avoided in lactating women who continue to nurse.

GERIATRIC USE

Safety and efficacy of quinidine in elderly patients have not been systematically studied.

PEDIATRIC USE

In antimalarial trials, quinidine was as safe and effective in pediatric patients as in adults. Notwithstanding the known pharmacokinetic differences between children and adults (see CLINICAL PHARMACOLOGY, Pharmacokinetics and Metabolism), children in these trials received the same doses (on a mg/kg basis) as adults.

Safety and effectiveness of antiarrhythmic use in children have not been established.

DRUG INTERACTIONS

ALTERED PHARMACOKINETICS OF QUINIDINE

Diltiazem significantly decreases the clearance and increases the $T_{½}$ of quinidine, but quinidine does not alter the kinetics of diltiazem.

Drugs that alkalinize the urine (**carbonic-anhydrase inhibitors, sodium bicarbonate, thiazide diuretics**) reduce renal elimination of quinidine.

By pharmacokinetic mechanisms that are not well understood, quinidine levels are increased by coadministration of **amiodarone** or **cimetidine.** Very rarely, and again by mechanisms not understood, quinidine levels are decreased by coadministration of **nifedipine.**

Hepatic elimination of quinidine may be accelerated by coadministration of drugs (**phenobarbital, phenytoin, rifampin**) that induce production of cytochrome P450IIIA4.

Perhaps because of competition for the P450IIIA4 metabolic pathway, quinidine levels rise when **ketaconazole** is coadministered.

Coadministration of **propranolol** usually does not affect quinidine pharmacokinetics, but in some studies the β-blocker appeared to cause increases in the peak serum levels of quinidine, decreases in quinidine's volume of distribution, and decreases in total quinidine clearance. The effects (if any) of coadministration of **other β-blockers** on quinidine pharmacokinetics have not been adequately studied.

Hepatic clearance of quinidine is significantly reduced during coadministration of **verapamil,** with corresponding increases in serum levels and half-life.

Grapefruit Juice: Grapefruit juice inhibits P450 3A4-mediated metabolism of quinidine to 3-hydroxyquinidine. Although the clinical significance of this interaction is unknown, grapefruit juice should be avoided.

Dietary Salt: The rate and extent of quinidine absorption may be affected by changes in dietary salt intake; a decrease in dietary salt intake may lead to an increase in plasma quinidine concentrations.

ALTERED PHARMACOKINETICS OF OTHER DRUGS

Quinidine slows the elimination of **digoxin** and simultaneously reduces digoxin's apparent volume of distribution. As a result, serum digoxin levels may be as much as doubled. When quinidine and digoxin are coadministered, digoxin doses usually need to be reduced. Serum levels of **digitoxin** are also raised when quinidine is coadministered, although the effect appears to be smaller.

By a mechanism that is not understood, quinidine potentiates the anticoagulatory action of **warfarin,** and the anticoagulant dosage may need to be reduced.

Cytochrome P450IID6 is an enzyme critical to the metabolism of many drugs, notably including **mexiletine,** some **phenothiazines,** and most **polycyclic antidepressants.** Constitutional deficiency of cytochrome P450IID6 is found in less than 1% of Orientals, in about 2% of American blacks, and in about 8% of American whites. Testing with debrisoquine is sometimes used to distinguish the P450IID6-deficient "poor metabolizers" from the majority-phenotype "extensive metabolizers".

When drugs whose metabolism is P450IID6-dependent are given to poor metabolizers, the serum levels achieved are higher, sometimes much higher, than the serum levels achieved when identical doses are given to extensive metabolizers. To obtain similar clinical benefit without toxicity, doses given to poor metabolizers may need to be greatly reduced. In the case of prodrugs whose actions are actually mediated by P450IID6-produced metabolites (for example, **codeine** and **hydrocodone,** whose analgesic and antitussive effects appear to be mediated by morphine and hydromorphone, respectively), it may not be possible to achieve the desired clinical benefits in poor metabolizers.

Quinidine is not metabolized by cytochrome P450IID6, but therapeutic serum levels of quinidine inhibit the action of cytochrome P450IID6, effectively converting extensive metabolizers into poor metabolizers. Caution must be exercised whenever quinidine is prescribed together with drugs metabolized by cytochrome P450IID6.

Perhaps by competing for pathways of renal clearance, coadministration of quinidine causes an increase in serum levels of **procainamide.**

Serum levels of **haloperidol** are increased when quinidine is coadministered.

Presumably because both drugs are metabolized by cytochrome P450IIIA4, coadministration of quinidine causes variable slowing of the metabolism of **nifedipine.** Interactions with other dihydropyridine calcium channel blockers have not been reported, but these agents (including **felodipine, nicardipine,** and **nimodipine**) are all dependent upon P450IIIA4 for metabolism, so similar interactions with quinidine should be anticipated.

ALTERED PHARMACODYNAMICS OF OTHER DRUGS

Quinidine's anticholinergic, vasodilating, and negative inotropic actions may be additive to those of other drugs with these effects, and antagonistic to those of drugs with cholinergic, vasoconstricting, and positive inotropic effects. For example, when quinidine and **verapamil** are coadministered in doses that are each well tolerated as monotherapy, hypotension attributable to additive peripheral α-blockade is sometimes reported.

Quinidine potentiates the actions of depolarizing (succinylcholine, decamethonium) and nondepolarizing (*d*-tubocurarine, pancuronium) **neuromuscular blocking agents.** These phenomena are not well understood, but they are observed in animal models as well as in humans. In addition, *in vitro* addition of quinidine to the serum of pregnant women reduces the activity of pseudocholinesterase, an enzyme that is essential to the metabolism of succinylcholine.

Non-Interactions of Quinidine With Other Drugs

Quinidine has no clinically significant effect on the pharmacokinetics of **diltiazem, flecainide, mephenytoin, metoprolol, propafenone, propranolol, quinine, timolol,** or **tocainide.**

Conversely, the pharmacokinetics of quinidine are not significantly affected by **caffeine, ciprofloxacin, digoxin, diltiazem, felodipine, omeprazole,** or **quinine.** Quinidine's pharmacokinetics are also unaffected by cigarette smoking.

ADVERSE REACTIONS

Quinidine preparations have been used for many years, but there are only sparse data from which to estimate the incidence of various adverse reactions. The adverse reactions most frequently reported have consistently been gastrointestinal, including diarrhea, nausea, vomiting, and heartburn/esophagitis.

In the reported study that was closest in character to the predominant approved use of quinidine gluconate extended-release tablets, 86 adult outpatients with atrial fibrillation were followed for 6 months while they received slow-release quinidine bisulfate tablets, 600 mg (approximately 400 mg of quinidine base) twice daily. The incidences of adverse experiences reported more than once were as shown in TABLE 2. The most serious quinidine-associated adverse reactions are described in WARNINGS.

TABLE 2 *Adverse Experiences Reported More Than Once in 86 Patients With Atrial Fibrillation*

	Incidence (%)
Diarrhea	21 (24%)
Fever	5 (6%)
Rash	5 (6%)
Arrhythmia	3 (3%)
Abnormal electrocardiogram	3 (3%)
Nausea/vomitting	3 (3%)
Dizziness	3 (3%)
Headache	3 (3%)
Asthenia	2 (2%)
Cerebral ischemia	2 (2%)

Vomiting and diarrhea can occur as isolated reactions to therapeutic levels of quinidine, but they may also be the first signs of **cinchonism,** a syndrome that may also include tinnitus, reversible high-frequency hearing loss, deafness, vertigo, blurred vision, diplopia, photophobia, headache, confusion, and delirium. Cinchonism is most often a sign of chronic quinidine toxicity, but it may appear in sensitive patients after a single moderate dose.

A few cases of **hepatotoxicity,** including granulomatous hepatitis, have been reported in patients receiving quinidine. All of these have appeared during the first few weeks of therapy, and most (not all) have remitted once quinidine was withdrawn.

Autoimmune and inflammatory syndromes associated with quinidine therapy have included fever, urticaria, flushing, exfoliative rash, bronchospasm, psoriasiform rash, pruritus and lymphadenopathy, hemolytic anemia, vasculitis, thrombocytopenic purpura, uveitis, angioedema, agranulocytosis, the sicca syndrome, arthralgia, myalgia, elevation in serum levels of skeletal-muscle enzymes, a disorder resembling systemic lupus erythematosus, and pneumonitis.

Convulsions, apprehension, and ataxia have been reported, but it is not clear that these were not simply the results of hypotension and consequent cerebral hypoperfusion. There are many reports of syncope. Acute psychotic reactions have been reported to follow the first dose of quinidine, but these reactions appear to be extremely rare.

Other adverse reactions occasionally reported include depression, mydriasis, disturbed color perception, night blindness, scotomata, optic neuritis, visual field loss, photosensitivity, and abnormalities of pigmentation.

DOSAGE AND ADMINISTRATION

The dose of quinidine delivered by quinidine gluconate extended-release tablets may be titrated by breaking a tablet in half. If tablets are crushed or chewed, their extended-release properties will be lost.

The dosage of quinidine varies considerably depending upon the general condition and the cardiovascular state of the patient.

CONVERSION OF ATRIAL FIBRILLATION/FLUTTER TO SINUS RHYTHM

Especially in patients with known structural heart disease or other risk factors for toxicity, initiation or dose-adjustment of treatment with quinidine gluconate extended-release tablets should generally be performed in a setting where facilities and personnel for monitoring and resuscitation are continuously available. Patients with symptomatic atrial fibrillation/flutter should be treated with quinidine gluconate extended-release tablets only after ventricular rate control (*e.g.,* with digitalis or β-blockers) has failed to provide satisfactory control of symptoms.

Adequate trials have not identified an optimal regimen of quinidine gluconate extended-release tablets for conversion of atrial fibrillation/flutter to sinus rhythm. In one reported regimen, the patient first receives 2 tablets (648 mg; 403 mg of quinidine base) of quinidine gluconate extended-release tablets every 8 hours. If this regimen has not resulted in conversion after 3 or 4 doses, then the dose is cautiously increased. If, at any point during administration, the QRS complex widens to 130% of its pre-treatment duration; the QTc interval widens to 130% of its pre-treatment duration and is then longer than 500 milliseconds; P waves disappear; or the patient develops significant tachycardia, symptomatic bradycardia, or hypotension, then quinidine gluconate extended-release tablets are discontinued, and other means of conversion (*e.g.,* direct-current cardioversion) are considered.

In another regimen sometimes used, the patient receives 1 tablet (324 mg; 202 mg of quinidine base) every 8 hours for 2 days; then 2 tablets every 12 hours for 2 days; and finally 2 tablets every 8 hours for up to 4 days. The 4 day stretch may come at one of the lower doses if, in the judgment of the physician, the lower dose is the highest one that will be tolerated. The criteria for discontinuation of treatment with quinidine gluconate extended-release tablets are the same as in the other regimen.

REDUCTION IN THE FREQUENCY OF RELAPSE INTO ATRAIL FIBRILLATION/FLUTTER

In a patient with a history of frequent symptomatic episodes of atrial fibrillation/flutter, the goal of therapy with quinidine gluconate extended-release tablets should be an increase in the average time between episodes. In most patients, the tachyarrhythmia *will recur* during therapy with quinidine gluconate extended-release tablets, and a single recurrence should not be interpreted as therapeutic failure.

Especially in patients with known structural heart disease or other risk factors for toxicity, initiation or dose-adjustment of treatment with quinidine gluconate extended-release tablets should generally be performed in a setting where facilities and personnel for monitoring and

Q

resuscitation are continuously available. Monitoring should be continued for 2 or 3 days after initiation of the regimen on which the patient will be discharged.

Therapy with quinidine gluconate extended-release tablets should be begun with 1 tablet (324 mg; 202 mg of quinidine base) every 8 or 12 hours. If this regimen is well tolerated, if the serum quinidine level is still well within the laboratory's therapeutic range, and if the average time between arrhythmic episodes has not been satisfactorily increased, then the dose may be cautiously raised. The total daily dosage should be reduced if the QRS complex widens to 130% of its pre-treatment duration; the QTc interval widens to 130% of its pre-treatment duration and is then longer than 500 milliseconds; P waves disappear; or the patient develops significant tachycardia, symptomatic bradycardia, or hypotension.

SUPPRESSION OF LIFE-THREATENING VENTRICULAR ARRYTHMIAS

Dosing regimens for the use of quinidine gluconate in suppressing life-threatening ventricular arrhythmias have not been adequately studied. Described regimens have generally been similar to the regimen described just above for the prophylaxis of symptomatic atrial fibrillation/flutter. Where possible, therapy should be guided by the results of programmed electrical stimulation and/or Holter monitoring with exercise.

HOW SUPPLIED

Quinaglute Dura-Tabs tablets are 324 mg white to off-white, round tablets embossed with "C" in a flask design on one side and with a clock-like design on the other.

Storage: Store at 25°C (77°F); excursions permitted to 15-30°C (59-86°F).

PRODUCT LISTING - RATED THERAPEUTICALLY EQUIVALENT

Tablet, Extended Release - Oral - 324 mg

Size	Price	Product	NDC
30's	$14.56	GENERIC, Heartland Healthcare Services	61392-0775-30
30's	$14.56	GENERIC, Heartland Healthcare Services	61392-0775-39
31's	$15.04	GENERIC, Heartland Healthcare Services	61392-0775-31
32's	$15.53	GENERIC, Heartland Healthcare Services	61392-0775-32
45's	$21.84	GENERIC, Heartland Healthcare Services	61392-0775-45
60's	$29.12	GENERIC, Heartland Healthcare Services	61392-0775-60
60's	$70.27	GENERIC, Golden State Medical	60429-0167-60
90's	$43.68	GENERIC, Heartland Healthcare Services	61392-0775-90
90's	$265.90	GENERIC, Golden State Medical	60429-0167-90
100's	$29.00	GENERIC, Raway Pharmacal Inc	00686-0027-20
100's	$31.20	GENERIC, Vita-Rx Corporation	49727-0409-02
100's	$31.56	GENERIC, Aligen Independent Laboratories Inc	00405-4910-01
100's	$31.99	GENERIC, Ivax Corporation	00182-1382-01
100's	$34.63	GENERIC, Moore, H.L. Drug Exchange Inc	00839-6473-06
100's	$41.48	GENERIC, Auro Pharmaceutical	55829-0461-10
100's	$45.00	FEDERAL UPPER LIMIT, H.C.F.A. F F P	99999-2165-04
100's	$45.81	GENERIC, Major Pharmaceuticals Inc	00904-2202-61
100's	$49.93	GENERIC, Watson/Schein Pharmaceuticals Inc	00364-0604-01
100's	$51.04	GENERIC, Caremark Inc	00339-5327-12
100's	$53.63	GENERIC, Major Pharmaceuticals Inc	00904-2202-60
100's	$58.50	QUINAGLUTE DURA-TABS, Berlex Laboratories	50419-0101-10
100's	$58.70	QUINAGLUTE DURA-TABS, Berlex Laboratories	50419-0101-11
100's	$84.03	GENERIC, Mutual Pharmaceutical Co Inc	53489-0141-01
100's	$121.31	GENERIC, Udl Laboratories Inc	51079-0027-20
250's	$48.45	GENERIC, Interstate Drug Exchange Inc	00814-6522-22
250's	$57.95	GENERIC, Aligen Independent Laboratories Inc	00405-4910-04
250's	$65.20	GENERIC, Moore, H.L. Drug Exchange Inc	00839-6473-09
250's	$72.10	GENERIC, Ivax Corporation	00182-1382-02
250's	$121.30	GENERIC, Watson/Schein Pharmaceuticals Inc	00364-0604-04
250's	$122.50	GENERIC, Mutual Pharmaceutical Co Inc	53489-0141-03
250's	$127.94	GENERIC, Major Pharmaceuticals Inc	00904-2202-70
250's	$142.13	QUINAGLUTE DURA-TABS, Berlex Laboratories	50419-0101-25

PRODUCT LISTING - EQUIVALENTS NOT AVAILABLE

Solution - Injectable - 80 mg/ml

Size	Price	Product	NDC
10 ml	$22.46	GENERIC, Lilly, Eli and Company	00002-1407-01

Tablet, Extended Release - Oral - 324 mg

Size	Price	Product	NDC
60's	$30.62	GENERIC, Allscripts Pharmaceutical Company	54569-0496-01
100's	$49.93	GENERIC, Watson/Schein Pharmaceuticals Inc	00591-5538-01
100's	$51.04	GENERIC, Allscripts Pharmaceutical Company	54569-0496-00
100's	$69.04	GENERIC, Physicians Total Care	54868-0698-01
250's	$121.30	GENERIC, Watson/Schein Pharmaceuticals Inc	00591-5538-25

Quinidine Sulfate *(002167)*

Categories: Arrhythmia, ventricular; Fibrillation, atrial; Flutter, atrial; Tachycardia, ventricular; Pregnancy Category C; FDA Approved 1972 Sep; WHO Formulary

Drug Classes: Antiarrhythmics, class IA; Antiprotozoals

Brand Names: Cin-Quin; Quinidex

Foreign Brand Availability: Cardioquinol (Ecuador); Kiditard (Belgium; Netherlands); Kinidin (Bahrain; Cyprus; Denmark; Egypt; Finland; Greece; Iran; Iraq; Ireland; Jordan; Kuwait; Lebanon; Libya; Norway; Oman; Philippines; Qatar; Republic-of-Yemen; Saudi-Arabia; Sweden; Syria; United-Arab-Emirates); Kinidine (Netherlands); Kinidin Durules (Australia; Switzerland); Kinidine Durettes (Belgium); Kinilentin (Denmark); Naticardina (Italy); Quinicardina (Spain); Quinicardine (Peru); Quiniduran (Israel); Quinidurule (Argentina; Mexico); Ritmocor (Italy); Sulfas-Chinidin (Indonesia)

Cost of Therapy: $68.78 (Arrhythmia; Quinidex Extentabs; 300 mg; 2 tablets/day; 30 day supply)
$38.91 (Arrhythmia; Generic Extended Release Tablets; 300 mg; 2 tablets/day; 30 day supply)

DESCRIPTION

Quinidine is an antimalarial schizonticide and an antiarrhythmic agent with Class Ia activity; it is the d-isomer of quinine, and its molecular weight is 324.43. Quinidine sulfate is the sulfate salt of quinidine; its chemical name is cinchonan-9-ol,6′-methoxy-,(9S)-,sulfate(2:1) dihydrate. Its empirical formula is $(C_{20}H_{24}N_2O_2)_2 \cdot H_2SO_4 \cdot 2H_2O$; and its molecular weight is 782.95, of which 82.9% is quinidine base.

Each Quinidex Extentabs tablet contains 300 mg of quinidine sulfate (249 mg of quinidine base) in a formulation to provide extended release; the inactive ingredients are acacia, acetylated monoglycerides, calcium sulfate, carnauba wax, edible ink, FD&C blue 2, gelatin, guar gum, magnesium oxide, magnesium stearate, polysorbates, shellac, sucrose, titanium dioxide, white wax, and other ingredients, one of which is a corn derivative. Tablets may also contain FD&C red 40 and FD&C yellow 6 aluminum lakes.

CLINICAL PHARMACOLOGY

PHARMACOKINETICS

The absolute bioavailability of quinidine from quinidine sulfate is about 70%, but this varies widely (45-100%) between patients. The less-than-complete bioavailability is the result of first-pass metabolism in the liver. Peak serum levels generally appear about 6 hours after dosing.

Although the effect of food upon quinidine sulfate absorption has not been studied, peak serum quinidine levels obtained from immediate-release quinidine sulfate are known to be delayed by nearly an hour (without change in total absorption) when these products are taken with food.

The **volume of distribution** of quinidine is 2-3 L/kg in healthy young adults, but this may be reduced to as little as 0.5 L/kg in patients with congestive heart failure, or increased to 3-5 L/kg in patients with cirrhosis of the liver. At concentrations of 2-5 mg/L (6.5-16.2 μmol/L), the fraction of quinidine bound to plasma proteins (mainly to α_1-acid glycoprotein and to albumin) is 80-88% in adults and older children, but it is lower in pregnant women, and in infants and neonates it may be as low as 50-70%. Because α_1-acid glycoprotein levels are increased in response to stress, serum levels of total quinidine may be greatly increased in settings such as acute myocardial infarction, even though the serum content of unbound (active) drug may remain normal. Protein binding is also increased in chronic renal failure, but binding abruptly descends toward or below normal when heparin is administered for hemodialysis.

Quinidine **clearance** typically proceeds at 3-5 ml/min/kg in adults, but clearance in children may be twice or 3 times as rapid. The elimination half-life is 6-8 hours in adults and 3-4 hours in children. Quinidine clearance is unaffected by hepatic cirrhosis, so the increased volume of distribution seen in cirrhosis leads to a proportionate increase in the elimination half-life.

Most quinidine is eliminated hepatically via the action of cytochrome P450 IIIA4; there are several different hydroxylated metabolites, and some of these have antiarrhythmic activity.

The most important of quinidine's metabolites is 3-hydroxy-quinidine (3HQ), serum levels of which can approach those of quinidine in patients receiving conventional doses of quinidine sulfate. The volume of distribution of 3HQ appears to be larger than that of quinidine, and the elimination half-life of 3HQ is about 12 hours.

As measured by antiarrhythmic effects in animals, by QTc prolongation in human volunteers, or by various *in vitro* techniques, 3HQ has at least half the antiarrhythmic activity of the parent compound, so it may be responsible for a substantial fraction of the effect of quinidine sulfate in chronic use.

When the urine pH is less than 7, about 20% of administered quinidine appears unchanged in the urine, but this fraction drops to as little as 5% when the urine is more alkaline. Renal clearance involves both glomerular filtration and active tubular secretion, moderated by (pH-dependent) tubular reabsorption. The new renal clearance is about 1 ml/min/kg in healthy adults.

When renal function is taken into account, quinidine clearance is apparently independent of patient age.

Assays of serum quinidine levels are widely available, but the results of modern assays may not be consistent with results cited in the older medical literature. The serum levels of quinidine cited in this package insert are those derived from specific assays, using either benzene extraction or (preferably) reverse-phase high-pressure liquid chromatography. In matched samples, older assays might unpredictably have given results that were as much as 2 or 3 times higher. A typical "therapeutic" concentration range is 2-6 mg/L (6.2-18.5 μmol/L).

MECHANISM OF ACTION

In patients with malaria, quinidine acts primarily as an intra-erythrocytic schizonticide, with little effect upon sporozites or upon pre-erythrocytic parasites. Quinidine is gametocidal to *Plasmodium vivax* and *P. malariae*, but not to *P. falciparum.*

In cardiac muscle and in Purkinje fibers, quinidine depresses the rapid inward depolarizing sodium current, thereby slowing phase-0 depolarization and reducing the amplitude of the action potential without affecting the resting potential. In normal Purkinje fibers, it reduces the slope of phase-4 depolarization, shifting the threshold voltage upward toward zero. The result is slowed conduction and reduced automaticity in all parts of the heart, with increase of the effective refractory period relative to the duration of the action potential in the atria, ventricles, and Purkinje tissues. Quinidine also raises the fibrillation thresholds of the atria and ventricles, and it raises the ventricular defibrillation threshold as well. Quinidine's actions fall into Class Ia in the Vaughan-Williams classification.

By slowing conduction and prolonging the effective refractory period, quinidine can interrupt or prevent reentrant arrhythmias and arrhythmias due to increased automaticity, including atrial flutter, atrial fibrillation, and paroxysmal supraventricular tachycardia.

In patients with the sick sinus syndrome, quinidine can cause marked sinus node depression and bradycardia. In most patients, however, use of quinidine is associated with an increase in the sinus rate.

Quinidine prolongs the QT interval in a dose-related fashion. This may lead to increased ventricular automaticity and polymorphic ventricular tachycardias, including *torsades de pointes* (see WARNINGS).

In addition, quinidine has anticholinergic activity, it has negative inotropic activity, and it acts peripherally as an α-adrenergic antagonist (that is, as a vasodilator).

INDICATIONS AND USAGE

CONVERSION OF ATRIAL FIBRILLATION/FLUTTER

In patients with symptomatic atrial fibrillation/flutter whose symptoms are not adequately controlled by measures that reduce the rate of ventricular response, quinidine sulfate is indicated as a means of restoring normal sinus rhythm. If this use of quinidine sulfate does not restore sinus rhythm within a reasonable time (see DOSAGE AND ADMINISTRATION), then quinidine sulfate should be discontinued.

REDUCTION OF FREQUENCY OF RELAPSE INTO ATRIAL FIBRILLATION/FLUTTER

Chronic therapy with quinidine sulfate is indicated for some patients at high risk of symptomatic atrial fibrillation/flutter; generally patients who have had previous episodes of atrial fibrillation/flutter that were so frequent and poorly tolerated as to outweigh, in the judgment of the physician and the patient, the risks of prophylactic therapy with quinidine sulfate. The increased risk of death should specifically be considered. Quinidine sulfate should be used only after alternative measures (*e.g.,* use of other drugs to control ventricular rate) have been found to be inadequate.

In patients with histories of frequent symptomatic episodes of atrial fibrillation/flutter, the goal of therapy should be an increase in the average time between episodes. In most patients, the tachyarrhythmia *will recur* during therapy, and a single recurrence should not be interpreted as therapeutic failure.

SUPPRESSION OF VENTRICULAR ARRHYTHMIAS

Quinidine sulfate is also indicated for the suppression of recurrent documented ventricular arrhythmias, such as sustained ventricular tachycardia, that in the judgment of the physician are life-threatening. Because of the proarrhythmic effects of quinidine, its use with ventricular arrhythmias of lesser severity is generally not recommended, and treatment of patients with asymptomatic ventricular premature contractions should be avoided. Where possible, therapy should be guided by the results of programmed electrical stimulation and/or Holter monitoring with exercise.

Antiarrhythmic drugs (including quinidine sulfate) have not been shown to enhance survival in patients with ventricular arrhythmias.

CONTRAINDICATIONS

Quinidine is contraindicated in patients who are known to be allergic to it, or who have developed thrombocytopenic purpura during prior therapy with quinidine or quinine.

In the absence of a functioning artificial pacemaker, quinidine is also contraindicated in any patient whose cardiac rhythm is dependent upon a junctional or idioventricular pacemaker, including patients in complete atrioventricular block.

Quinidine is also contraindicated in patients who, like those with myasthenia gravis, might be adversely affected by an anticholinergic agent.

WARNINGS

MORTALITY

In many trials of antiarrhythmic therapy for non-life-threatening arrhythmias, active antiarrhythmic therapy has resulted in increased mortality; the risk of active therapy is probably greatest in patients with structural heart disease.

In the case of quinidine used to prevent or defer recurrence of atrial flutter/fibrillation, the best available data come from a meta-analysis. In the patients studied in the trials there analyzed, the mortality associated with the use of quinidine was more than 3 times as great as the mortality associated with the use of placebo.

Another meta-analysis, showed that in patients with various non-life-threatening ventricular arrhythmias, the mortality associated with the use of quinidine was consistently greater than that associated with the use of any of a variety of alternative antiarrhythmics.

PROARRHYTHMIC EFFECTS

Like many other drugs (including all other Class Ia antiarrhythmics), quinidine prolongs the QTc interval, and this can lead to *torsades de pointes,* a life-threatening ventricular arrhythmia. The risk of *torsades* is increased by bradycardia, hypokalemia, hypomagnesemia, or high serum levels of quinidine, but it may appear in the absence of any of these risk factors. The best predictor of this arrhythmia appears to be the length of the QTc interval, and quinidine should be used with extreme care in patients who have preexisting long-QT syndromes, who have histories of *torsades de pointes* of any cause, or who have previously responded to quinidine (or other drugs that prolong ventricular repolarization) with marked lengthening of the QTc interval. Estimation of the incidence of *torsades* in patients with therapeutic levels of quinidine is not possible from the available data.

Other ventricular arrhythmias that have been reported with quinidine include frequent extrasystoles, ventricular tachycardia, ventricular flutter, and ventricular fibrillation.

PARADOXICAL INCREASE IN VENTRICULAR RATE IN ATRIAL FLUTTER/FIBRILLATION

When quinidine is administered to patients with atrial flutter/fibrillation the desired pharmacologic reversion to sinus rhythm may (rarely) be preceded by a showing of the atrial rate with a consequent increase in the rate of beats conducted to the ventricles. The resulting ventricular rate may be very high (greater than 200 beats/minute) and poorly tolerated. This hazard may be decreased if partial atrioventricular block is achieved prior to initiation of quinidine therapy, using conduction-reducing drugs such as digitalis, verapamil, diltiazem, or a β-receptor blocking agent.

EXACERBATED BRADYCARDIA IN SICK SINUS SYNDROME

In patients with the sick sinus syndrome, quinidine has been associated with marked sinus node depression and bradycardia.

PHARMACOKINETIC CONSIDERATIONS

Renal or hepatic dysfunction causes the elimination of quinidine to be slowed, while congestive heart failure causes a reduction in quinidine's apparent volume of distribution. Any of these conditions can lead to quinidine toxicity if dosage is not appropriately reduced. In addition, interactions with coadministered drugs can alter the serum concentration and activity of quinidine, leading either to toxicity or to lack of efficacy if the dose of quinidine is not appropriately modified. (See DRUG INTERACTIONS.)

VAGOLYSIS

Because quinidine opposes the atrial and A-V nodal effects of vagal stimulation, physical or pharmacological vagal maneuvers undertaken to terminate paroxysmal supraventricular tachycardia may be ineffective in patients receiving quinidine.

PRECAUTIONS

GENERAL

All the precautions applying to regular quinidine therapy apply to this product. Hypersensitivity or anaphylactoid reactions to quinidine, although rare, should be considered, especially during the first weeks of therapy. Hospitalization for close clinical observation, electrocardiographic monitoring, and determination of serum quinidine levels are indicated when large doses of quinidine are used or with patients who present an increased risk.

LABORATORY TESTS

Periodic blood counts and liver and kidney function tests should be performed during long-term therapy; the drug should be discontinued if blood dyscrasias or evidence of hepatic or renal dysfunction occurs.

HEART BLOCK

In patients without implanted pacemakers who are at high risk of complete atrioventricular block (*e.g.,* those with digitalis intoxication, second-degree atrioventricular block, or severe intraventricular conduction defects), quinidine should be used only with caution.

INFORMATION FOR THE PATIENT

Before prescribing quinidine sulfate extended-release tablets as prophylaxis against recurrence of atrial fibrillation, the physician should inform the patient of the risks and benefits to be expected (see CLINICAL PHARMACOLOGY).

Discussion should include the facts:

That the goal of therapy will be a reduction (probably not to zero) in the frequency of episodes of atrial fibrillation; and

That reduced frequency of fibrillatory episodes may be expected, if achieved, to bring symptomatic benefit; but

That no data are available to show that reduced frequency of fibrillatory episodes will reduce the risks of irreversible harm through stroke or death; and in fact

That such data as are available suggest that treatment with quinidine sulfate is likely to increase the patient's risk of death.

CARCINOGENESIS, MUTAGENESIS, AND IMPAIRMENT OF FERTILITY

Animal studies to evaluate quinidine's carcinogenic or mutagenic potential have not been performed. Similarly, there are no animal data as to quinidine's potential to impair fertility.

PREGNANCY CATEGORY C

Animal reproductive studies have not been conducted with quinidine. There are no adequate and well-controlled studies in pregnant women. Quinidine should be given to a pregnant woman only if clearly needed.

In 1 neonate whose mother had received quinidine throughout her pregnancy, the serum level of quinidine was equal to that of the mother, with no apparent ill effect. The level of quinidine in amniotic fluid was about 3 times higher than that found in serum.

LABOR AND DELIVERY

Quinine is said to be oxytoxic in humans, but there are no adequate data as to quinidine's effects (if any) on human labor and delivery.

NURSING MOTHERS

Quinidine is present in human milk at levels slightly lower than those in maternal serum; a human infant ingesting such milk should (scaling directly by weight) be expected to develop serum quinidine levels at least an order of magnitude lower than those of the mother. On the other hand, the pharmacokinetics and pharmacodynamics of quinidine in human infants have not been adequately studied, and neonates' reduced protein binding of quinidine may increase their risk of toxicity at low total serum levels. Administration of quinidine should (if possible) be avoided in lactating women who continue to nurse.

PEDIATRIC USE

In antimalarial trials, quinidine was as safe and effective in pediatric patients as in adults. Notwithstanding the known pharmacokinetic differences between the pediatric population and adults (see CLINICAL PHARMACOLOGY, Pharmacokinetics), pediatric patients in these trials received the same doses (on a mg/kg basis) as adults.

Safety and effectiveness of the antiarrhythmic use of quinidine in pediatric patients have not been established in well-controlled clinical trials.

GERIATRIC USE

Clinical studies of quinidine generally were not adequate to determine if significant safety or efficacy differences exist between elderly patients (65 years or older) and younger patients.

Quinidine clearance is apparently independent of age (see CLINICAL PHARMACOLOGY, Pharmacokinetics). However, renal or hepatic dysfunction causes the elimination of quinidine to be slowed (see WARNINGS, Pharmacokinetic Considerations), and since these conditions are more common in the elderly, appropriate dosing reductions should be considered in these individuals.

DRUG INTERACTIONS

ALTERED PHARMACOKINETICS OF QUINIDINE

Drugs that alkalinize the urine **(carbonic-anhydrase inhibitors, sodium bicarbonate, thiazide diuretics)** reduce renal elimination of quinidine.

By pharmacokinetic mechanisms that are not well understood, quinidine levels are increased by coadministration of **amiodarone** or **cimetidine.** Very rarely, and again by mechanisms not understood, quinidine levels are decreased by coadministration of **nifedipine.**

Hepatic elimination of quinidine may be accelerated by coadministration of drugs **(phenobarbital, phenytoin, rifampin)** that induce production of cytochrome P450 IIIA4 (P450 3A4).

Perhaps because of competition for the P450 3A4 metabolic pathway, quinidine levels rise when **ketoconazole** is coadministered.

Coadministration of **propranolol** usually does not affect quinidine pharmacokinetics, but in some studies the β-blocker appeared to cause increases in the peak serum levels of quinidine, decreases in quinidine's volume of distribution, and decreases in total quinidine clearance. The effects (if any) of coadministration of **other β-blockers** on quinidine pharmacokinetics have not been adequately studied.

Diltiazem significantly decreases the clearance and increases the $T_{1/2}$ of quinidine, but quinidine does not alter the kinetics of diltiazem.

Hepatic clearance of quinidine is significantly reduced during coadministration of **verapamil,** with corresponding increases in serum levels and half-life.

Grapefruit juice inhibits P450 3A4-mediated metabolism of quinidine to 3-hydroxyquinidine. Although the clinical significance of this interaction is unknown, grapefruit juice should be avoided.

The rate and extent of quinidine absorption may be affected by changes in **dietary salt** intake; a decrease in dietary salt intake may lead to an increase in plasma quinidine concentrations.

ALTERED PHARMACOKINETICS OF OTHER DRUGS

Quinidine slows the elimination of **digoxin** and simultaneously reduces digoxin's apparent volume of distribution. As a result, serum digoxin levels may be as much as doubled. When quinidine and digoxin are coadministered, digoxin doses usually need to be reduced. Serum levels of **digitoxin** are also raised when quinidine is coadministered, although the effect appears to be smaller.

By a mechanism that is not understood, quinidine potentiates the anticoagulatory action of **warfarin,** and the anticoagulant dosage may need to be reduced.

Cytochrome P450 IID6 (P450 2D6) is an enzyme critical to the metabolism of many drugs, notably including **mexiletine,** some **phenothiazines,** and most **polycyclic antidepressants.** Constitutional deficiency of cytochrome P450 2D6 is found in less than 1% of Orientals, in about 2% of American blacks, and in about 8% of American whites. Testing with debrisoquine is sometimes used to distinguish the P450 2D6-deficient "poor metabolizers" from the majority-phenotype "extensive metabolizers".

When drugs whose metabolism is P450 2D6-dependent are given to poor metabolizers, the serum levels achieved are higher, sometimes much higher, than the serum levels achieved when identical doses are given to extensive metabolizers. To obtain similar clinical benefit without toxicity, doses given to poor metabolizers may need to be greatly reduced. In the cases of prodrugs whose actions are actually mediated by P450 2D6-produced metabolites (for example, **codeine** and **hydrocodone,** whose analgesic and antitussive effects appear to be mediated by morphine and hydromorphone, respectively), it may not be possible to achieve the desired clinical benefits in poor metabolizers.

Quinidine is not metabolized by cytochrome P450 2D6, but therapeutic serum levels of quinidine inhibit the action of cytochrome P450 2D6, effectively converting extensive metabolizers into poor metabolizers. Caution must be exercised whenever quinidine is prescribed together with drugs metabolized by cytochrome P450 2D6.

Perhaps by competing for pathways of renal clearance, coadministration of quinidine causes an increase in serum levels of **procainamide.**

Serum levels of **haloperidol** are increased when quinidine is coadministered.

Presumably because both drugs are metabolized by cytochrome P450 3A4, coadministration of quinidine causes variable slowing of the metabolism of **nifedipine.**

Interactions with other dihydropyridine calcium-channel blockers have not been reported, but these agents (including **felodipine, nicardipine, and nimodipine**) are all dependent upon P450 3A4 for metabolism, so similar interactions with quinidine should be anticipated.

ALTERED PHARMACODYNAMICS OF OTHER DRUGS

Quinidine's anticholinergic, vasodilating, and negative inotropic actions may be additive to those of other drugs with these effects, and antagonistic to those of drugs with cholinergic, vasoconstricting, and positive inotropic effects. For example, when quinidine and **verapamil** are coadministered in doses that are each well tolerated as monotherapy, hypotension attributable to additive peripheral α-blockade is sometimes reported.

Quinidine potentiates the actions of depolarizing (succinylcholine, decamethonium) and nondepolarizing (d-tubocurarine, pancuronium) **neuromuscular blocking agents.** These phenomena are not well understood, but they are observed in animals models as well as in humans. In addition, *in vitro* addition of quinidine to the serum of pregnant women reduces the activity of pseudocholinesterase, an enzyme that is essential to the metabolism of succinylcholine.

NON-INTERACTIONS OF QUINIDINE WITH OTHER DRUGS

Quinidine has no clinically significant effect on the pharmacokinetics of **diltiazem, flecainide, mephenytoin, metoprolol, propafenone, propranolol, quinine, timolol,** or **tocainide.**

Conversely, the pharmacokinetics of quinidine are not significantly affected by **caffeine, ciprofloxacin, digoxin, diltiazem, felodipine, omeprazole,** or **quinine.** Quinidine's pharmacokinetics are also unaffected by cigarette smoking.

ADVERSE REACTIONS

Quinidine preparations have been used for many years, but there are only sparse data from which to estimate the incidence of various adverse reactions. The adverse reactions most frequently reported have consistently been gastrointestinal, including diarrhea, nausea, vomiting, and heartburn/esophagitis. In one study of 245 adult outpatients who received quinidine to suppress premature ventricular contractions, the incidences of reported adverse experiences were as shown in TABLE 1. The most serious quinidine-associated adverse reactions are described above under WARNINGS.

TABLE 1 *Adverse Experiences in a 245-Patient PVC Trial*

Adverse Event	Incidence
Diarrhea	85 (35%)
"Upper gastrointestinal distress"	55 (22%)
Light-headedness	37 (15%)
Headness	18 (7%)
Fatigue	17 (7%)
Palpitations	16 (7%)
Angina-like pain	14 (6%)
Weakness	13 (5%)
Rash	11 (5%)
Visual problems	8 (3%)
Change in sleep habits	7 (3%)
Tremor	6 (2%)
Nervousness	5 (2%)
Discoordination	3 (1%)

Vomiting and diarrhea can occur as isolated reactions to therapeutic levels of quinidine, but they also may be the first signs of **cinchonism,** a syndrome that also may include tinnitus, reversible high-frequency hearing loss, deafness, vertigo, blurred vision, diplopia, photophobia, headache, confusion, and delirium. Cinchonism is most often a sign of chronic quinidine toxicity, but it may appear in sensitive patients after a single moderate dose.

A few cases of **hepatotoxicity,** including granulomatous hepatitis, have been reported in patients receiving quinidine. All of these have appeared during the first few weeks of therapy, and most (not all) have remitted once quinidine was withdrawn.

Autoimmune and inflammatory syndromes associated with quinidine therapy have included pneumonitis, fever, urticaria, flushing, exfoliative rash, bronchospasm, psoriasiform rash, pruritus and lymphadenopathy, hemolytic anemia, vasculitis, thrombocytopenic purpura, uveitis, angioedema, agranulocytosis, the sicca syndrome, arthralgia, myalgia, elevation in serum levels of skeletal-muscle enzymes, and a disorder resembling systemic lupus erythematosus.

Convulsions, apprehension, and ataxia have been reported, but it is not clear that these were not simply the results of hypotension and consequent cerebral hypoperfusion. There are many reports of syncope. Acute psychotic reactions have been reported to follow the first dose of quinidine, but these reactions appear to be extremely rare.

Other adverse reactions occasionally reported include depression, mydriasis, disturbed color perception, night blindness, scotomata, optic neuritis, visual field loss, photosensitivity, and abnormalities of pigmentation.

DOSAGE AND ADMINISTRATION

CONVERSION OF ATRIAL FIBRILLATION/FLUTTER TO SINUS RHYTHM

Especially in patients with known structural heart disease or other risk factors for toxicity, initiation or dose-adjustment of treatment with quinidine sulfate should generally be performed in a setting where facilities and personnel for monitoring and resuscitation are continuously available.

Patients with symptomatic atrial fibrillation/flutter should be treated with quinidine sulfate only after ventricular rate control (*e.g.,* with digitalis or β-blockers) has failed to provide satisfactory control of symptoms. Adequate trials have not identified an optimal regimen of quinidine sulfate for conversion of atrial fibrillation/flutter to sinus rhythm. Therapy with quinidine sulfate should begin with 1 tablet (300 mg; 249 mg of quinidine base) every 8-12 hours. If this regimen is well tolerated, if the serum quinidine level is still well within the laboratory's therapeutic range, and if this regimen has not resulted in conversion, then the dose may be cautiously raised. If, at any point during administration, the QRS complex widens to 130% of its pre-treatment duration; the QTc interval widens to 130% of its pre-treatment duration and is then longer than 500 milliseconds; P waves disappear; or the patient develops significant tachycardia, symptomatic bradycardia, or hypotension, then quinidine sulfate is discontinued, and other means of conversion (*e.g.,* direct-current cardioversion) are considered.

REDUCTION OF FREQUENCY OF RELAPSE INTO ATRIAL FIBRILLATION/FLUTTER

In a patient with a history of frequent symptomatic episodes of atrial fibrillation/flutter, the goal of therapy with quinidine sulfate should be an increase in the average time between episodes. In most patients, the tachyarrhythmia *will recur* during therapy with quinidine sulfate, and a single recurrence should not be interpreted as therapeutic failure.

Especially in patients with known structural heart disease or other risk factors for toxicity, initiation or dose-adjustment of treatment with quinidine sulfate should generally be performed in a setting where facilities and personnel for monitoring and resuscitation are continuously available.

Monitoring should be continued for 2 or 3 days after initiation of the regimen on which the patient will be discharged.

Therapy with quinidine sulfate should begin with 1 tablet (300 mg; 249 mg of quinidine base) every 8-12 hours. If this regimen is well tolerated, if the serum quinidine level is still well within the laboratory's therapeutic range, and if the average time between arrhythmic episodes has not been satisfactorily increased, then the dose may be cautiously raised. The total daily dosage should be reduced if the QRS complex widens to 130% of its pre-treatment duration; the QTc interval widens to 130% of its pre-treatment duration and is then longer than 500 milliseconds; P waves disappear; or the patient develops significant tachycardia, symptomatic bradycardia, or hypotension.

SUPPRESSION OF VENTRICULAR ARRHYTHMIAS

Dosing regimens for the use of quinidine sulfate in suppressing life-threatening ventricular arrhythmias have not been adequately studied.

Described regimens have generally been similar to the regimen described just above for the prophylaxis of symptomatic atrial fibrillation/flutter. Where possible, therapy should be guided by the results of programmed electrical stimulation and/or Holter monitoring with exercise.

HOW SUPPLIED

Quinidex Extentabs tablets are 300 mg, white, sugar-coated, round tablets marked with "QUINIDEX" and "AHR".

Storage: Store tablets at controlled room temperature, 20-25°C (68-77°F).
Dispense in well-closed, light-resistant container.

PRODUCT LISTING - RATED THERAPEUTICALLY EQUIVALENT

Tablet - Oral - 200 mg

Qty	Price	Product	NDC
25's	$9.36	GENERIC, Pd-Rx Pharmaceuticals	55289-0222-97
30's	$6.38	GENERIC, Heartland Healthcare Services	61392-0776-30
30's	$6.38	GENERIC, Heartland Healthcare Services	61392-0776-39
31's	$6.59	GENERIC, Heartland Healthcare Services	61392-0776-31
32's	$6.80	GENERIC, Heartland Healthcare Services	61392-0776-32
45's	$9.56	GENERIC, Heartland Healthcare Services	61392-0776-45
60's	$12.75	GENERIC, Heartland Healthcare Services	61392-0776-60
90's	$19.13	GENERIC, Heartland Healthcare Services	61392-0776-90
100's	$4.25	GENERIC, Global Pharmaceutical Corporation	00115-4380-01
100's	$11.10	GENERIC, Interstate Drug Exchange Inc	00814-6520-14
100's	$11.27	GENERIC, Moore, H.L. Drug Exchange Inc	00839-5063-06
100's	$11.65	GENERIC, Ivax Corporation	00182-0144-01
100's	$12.56	GENERIC, Aligen Independent Laboratories Inc	00405-4916-01
100's	$13.22	GENERIC, Auro Pharmaceutical	55829-0463-10
100's	$15.00	GENERIC, Raway Pharmacal Inc	00686-0031-20
100's	$17.76	GENERIC, Roxane Laboratories Inc	00054-8733-25
100's	$17.91	GENERIC, Major Pharmaceuticals Inc	00904-2201-61
100's	$20.10	GENERIC, Watson/Schein Pharmaceuticals Inc	00364-0229-01
100's	$20.10	GENERIC, Watson/Schein Pharmaceuticals Inc	00591-5438-01
100's	$20.10	GENERIC, Mutual Pharmaceutical Co Inc	53489-0461-01
100's	$20.79	GENERIC, Major Pharmaceuticals Inc	00904-2201-60
100's	$21.00	GENERIC, Eon Labs Manufacturing Inc	00185-4346-01

Tablet - Oral - 300 mg

Qty	Price	Product	NDC
30's	$10.25	GENERIC, Heartland Healthcare Services	61392-0777-30
30's	$10.25	GENERIC, Heartland Healthcare Services	61392-0777-39
31's	$10.59	GENERIC, Heartland Healthcare Services	61392-0777-31
32's	$10.93	GENERIC, Heartland Healthcare Services	61392-0777-32
45's	$15.37	GENERIC, Heartland Healthcare Services	61392-0777-45
60's	$20.50	GENERIC, Heartland Healthcare Services	61392-0777-60
90's	$30.74	GENERIC, Heartland Healthcare Services	61392-0777-90
100's	$18.62	GENERIC, Moore, H.L. Drug Exchange Inc	00839-6605-06
100's	$18.70	GENERIC, Qualitest Products Inc	00603-5595-21
100's	$20.00	GENERIC, Ivax Corporation	00182-1724-01
100's	$20.18	GENERIC, Interstate Drug Exchange Inc	00814-6521-14
100's	$20.32	GENERIC, Aligen Independent Laboratories Inc	00405-4917-01
100's	$23.20	GENERIC, Ivax Corporation	00182-1724-89
100's	$23.23	GENERIC, Watson/Rugby Laboratories Inc	00536-4429-01
100's	$23.23	GENERIC, Geneva Pharmaceuticals	00781-1902-01
100's	$23.95	GENERIC, Geneva Pharmaceuticals	00781-1902-13
100's	$26.01	GENERIC, Auro Pharmaceutical	55829-0464-10
100's	$32.22	GENERIC, Roxane Laboratories Inc	00054-4735-25
100's	$34.16	GENERIC, Roxane Laboratories Inc	00054-8735-25
100's	$36.07	GENERIC, Mutual Pharmaceutical Co Inc	53489-0460-01
100's	$38.68	GENERIC, Watson/Schein Pharmaceuticals Inc	00364-0582-01
100's	$39.60	GENERIC, Major Pharmaceuticals Inc	00904-2203-60
100's	$40.00	GENERIC, Eon Labs Manufacturing Inc	00185-1047-01
100's	$66.81	GENERIC, Moore, H.L. Drug Exchange Inc	00839-7949-06

Tablet, Extended Release - Oral - 300 mg

Qty	Price	Product	NDC
30's	$35.31	QUINIDEX EXTENTABS, Physicians Total Care	54868-2740-03
90's	$103.58	QUINIDEX EXTENTABS, Physicians Total Care	54868-2740-01
100's	$64.85	GENERIC, Qualitest Products Inc	00603-5596-21
100's	$70.73	GENERIC, Ivax Corporation	00182-1997-01
100's	$74.53	GENERIC, Esi Lederle Generics	59911-5895-01
100's	$87.84	GENERIC, Teva Pharmaceuticals Usa	00093-9175-01
100's	$114.63	QUINIDEX EXTENTABS, Esi Lederle Generics	00031-6649-63
250's	$178.21	GENERIC, Esi Lederle Generics	59911-5895-02
250's	$217.98	GENERIC, Teva Pharmaceuticals Usa	00093-9175-52
250's	$286.56	QUINIDEX EXTENTABS, Esi Lederle Generics	00031-6649-67

PRODUCT LISTING - EQUIVALENTS NOT AVAILABLE

Tablet - Oral - 200 mg

Qty	Price	Product	NDC
30's	$5.83	GENERIC, Physicians Total Care	54868-0047-03
100's	$11.95	GENERIC, Cmc-Consolidated Midland Corporation	00223-1560-01
100's	$12.98	GENERIC, Allscripts Pharmaceutical Company	54569-0497-00

Tablet - Oral - 300 mg

Qty	Price	Product	NDC
100's	$19.93	GENERIC, Physicians Total Care	54868-0898-01
100's	$38.68	GENERIC, Watson/Schein Pharmaceuticals Inc	00591-5454-01

Quinine Sulfate *(002168)*

Categories: Malaria; Pregnancy Category X; FDA Pre 1938 Drugs; WHO Formulary
Drug Classes: Antiprotozoals
Brand Names: Qm-260; Quin-Amino; Quinaminoph; **Quinamm**; Quinasul; Quindan; Quinite; Quiphile
Foreign Brand Availability: Biquinate (Australia); Genin (Thailand); Kinin (Denmark; Sweden); Kininh (Germany); Myoquin (Australia); Q200 (New-Zealand); Q300 (New-Zealand); Quinbisu (Australia); Quinate (Australia); Quinimax (Benin; Burkina-Faso; Ethiopia; Gambia; Ghana; Guinea; Ivory-Coast; Kenya; Liberia; Malawi; Mali; Mauritania; Mauritius; Morocco; Niger; Nigeria; Senegal; Seychelles; Sierra-Leone; Sudan; Tanzania; Tunia; Uganda; Zambia; Zimbabwe); Quinoctal (Australia); Quinsul (Australia)
Cost of Therapy: $2.12 (Malaria Treatment; Generic Capsules; 325 mg; 6 capsules/day; 7 day supply)

DESCRIPTION

Quinine sulfate is available as tablets or capsules for oral administration. Each tablet contains 260 mg quinine sulfate. *Also Contains, as Inactive Ingredients:* Corn starch, pregelatinized starch, sodium starch glycolate, sucrose, and zinc stearate.

Neuromuscular agent.

Quinine sulfate occurs as a white, crystalline powder, which darkens on exposure to light. It is odorless and has a persistent, very bitter taste. It is slightly soluble in water, alcohol, chloroform, and ether.

Storage: Store at controlled room temperature, 25-30°C (77-86°F).

CLINICAL PHARMACOLOGY

Quinine sulfate is effective as a malarial suppressant and in control of overt clinical attacks. Its primary action is schizontocidal. No lethal effect is exerted on sporozoites or preerythrocitic tissue forms.

Quinine sulfate is readily absorbed when given orally. Absorption occurs mainly from the upper part of the small intestine, and is almost complete even in patients with marked diarrhea.

The cinchona alkaloids in large measure are metabolically degraded in the body, especially in the liver; less than 5% of an administered dose is excreted unaltered in the urine. It is reported that there is no accumulation of the drugs in the body upon continued administration. The metabolic degradation products are excreted in the urine, where many of them have been identified as hydroxy derivatives, but small amounts also appear in the feces, gastric juice, bile, and saliva. Renal excretion of quinine sulfate is twice as rapid when the urine is acidic as when it is alkaline, due to the greater tubular reabsorption of the alkaloidal base that occurs in an alkaline media. Excretion is also limited by the binding of a large fraction of cinchona alkaloids to plasma proteins.

Peak plasma concentrations of cinchona alkaloids occur within 1-3 hours after a single oral dose. The half-life is 4-5 hours. After chronic administration of total daily doses of 1 g of drug, the average plasma quinine sulfate concentration is approximately 7 μg/ml. After termination of quinine sulfate therapy, the plasma level falls rapidly and only a negligible concentration is detectable after 24 hours.

A large fraction (approximately 70%) of the plasma quinine sulfate is bound to proteins. This explains in part why the concentration of the alkaloid in cerebrospinal fluid is only 2-5% of that in the plasma. However, it can traverse the placental membrane and readily reach fetal tissues.

Tinnitus and impairment of hearing rarely should occur at plasma quinine sulfate concentrations of less than 10 μg/ml. While this level would not be anticipated from use of 1 or 2 tablets of quinine sulfate daily, an occasional patient may have some evidence of cinchonism on this dosage, such as tinnitus. (See WARNINGS.)

INDICATIONS AND USAGE

For the treatment of malaria as a supplement to other antimalarial drugs (*e.g.*, with primaquine in relapsing vivax malaria) or the treatment of malaria due to strains of *P. falciparum* resistant to chloroquine and other antimalarial drugs.

CONTRAINDICATIONS

Quinine sulfate may cause fetal harm when administered to a pregnant woman. Congenital malformations in the human have been reported with the use of quinine sulfate, primarily with large doses (up to 30 g) for attempted abortion. In about half of these reports, the malformation was deafness related to auditory nerve hypoplasia. Among the other abnormalities reported were limb anomalies, visceral defects, and visual changes. In animal tests, teratogenic effects were found in rabbits and guinea pigs and were absent in mice, rats, dogs, and monkeys. Quinine sulfate is contraindicated in women who are or may become pregnant. If this drug is used during pregnancy, or if the patient becomes pregnant while taking this drug, the patient should be apprised of the potential hazard to the fetus.

Q

Because of the quinine content, quinine sulfate is contraindicated in patients with known quinine hypersensitivity and in patients with glucose-6-phosphate dehydrogenase (G-6-PD) deficiency.

Since thrombocytopenic purpura may follow the administration of quinine sulfate in highly sensitive patients, a history of this occurrence associated with previous quinine sulfate ingestion contraindicates its further use. Recovery usually occurs following withdrawal of the medication and appropriate therapy.

This drug should not be used in patients with tinnitus or optic neuritis or in patients with a history of blackwater fever.

WARNINGS

Repeated doses or overdosage of quinine sulfate in some individuals may precipitate a cluster of symptoms referred to as cinchonism. Such symptoms, in the mildest form, include ringing in the ears, headache, nausea, and slightly disturbed vision; however, when medication is continued or after large single doses, symptoms also involve the gastrointestinal tract, the nervous and cardiovascular systems, and the skin.

Hemolysis (with the potential for hemolytic anemia) has been associated with a G-6-PD deficiency in patients taking quinine sulfate. Quinine sulfate should be stopped immediately if evidence of hemolysis appears.

If symptoms occur, drug should be discontinued and supportive measures instituted.

PRECAUTIONS

GENERAL

Quinine sulfate should be discontinued if there is any evidence of hypersensitivity. (See CONTRAINDICATIONS.) Cutaneous flushing, pruritus, skin rashes, fever, gastric distress, dyspnea, ringing in the ears, and visual impairment are the usual expressions of hypersensitivity, particularly if only small doses of quinine sulfate have been taken. Extreme flushing of the skin accompanied by intense, generalized pruritus is the most common form. Hemoglobinuria and asthma from quinine sulfate are rare types of idiosyncrasy.

In patients with atrial fibrillation, the administration of quinine sulfate requires the same precautions as those for quinidine. (See DRUG INTERACTIONS.)

DRUG/LABORATORY TEST INTERACTIONS

Quinine sulfate may produce an elevated value for urinary 17-ketogenic steroids when the Zimmerman method is used.

CARCINOGENESIS, MUTAGENESIS, AND IMPAIRMENT OF FERTILITY

A study of quinine sulfate administered in drinking water (0.1%) to rats for periods up to 20 months showed no evidence of neoplastic changes.

Mutation studies of quinine (dihydrochloride) in male and female mice gave negative results by the micronucleus test. Intraperitoneal injections (0.5 mM/kg) were given twice, 24 hours apart. Direct *Salmonella typhimurium* tests were negative; when mammalian liver homogenate was added, positive results were found.

No information relating to the effect of quinine sulfate upon fertility in animal or in man has been found.

PREGNANCY CATEGORY X

See CONTRAINDICATIONS.

Nonteratogenic Effects

Because quinine sulfate crosses the placenta in humans, the potential for fetal effects is present. Stillbirths in mothers taking quinine sulfate have been reported in which no obvious cause for the fetal deaths was shown. Quinine sulfate in toxic amounts has been associated with abortion. Whether this action is always due to direct effect on the uterus is questionable.

Q

NURSING MOTHERS

Caution should be exercised when quinine sulfate is given to nursing women because quinine sulfate is excreted in breast milk (in small amounts).

DRUG INTERACTIONS

Increased plasma levels of digoxin and digitoxin have been demonstrated in individuals after concomitant quinine administration. Because of possible similar effects from use of quinine sulfate, it is recommended that plasma levels of digoxin and digitoxin be determined for those individuals taking these drugs and quinine sulfate concomitantly.

Concurrent use of aluminum-containing antacids may delay or decrease absorption of quinine sulfate.

Cinchona alkaloids, including quinine sulfate, have the potential to depress the hepatic enzyme system that synthesizes the vitamin K-dependent factors. The resulting hypoprothrombinemic effect may enhance the action of warfarin and other oral anticoagulants.

The effects of neuromuscular blocking agents (particularly pancuronium, succinylcholine, and tubocurarine) may be potentiated with quinine sulfate, and result in respiratory difficulties.

Urinary alkalizers (such as acetazolamide and sodium bicarbonate) may increase quinine sulfate blood levels with potential for toxicity.

ADVERSE REACTIONS

The following adverse reactions have been reported with quinine sulfate in therapeutic or excessive dosage. (Individual or multiple symptoms may represent cinchonism or hypersensitivity.)

Hematologic: Acute hemolysis, thrombocytopenic purpura, agranulocytosis, hypoprothrombinemia.

CNS: Visual disturbances, including blurred vision with scotomata, photophobia, diplopia, diminished visual fields, and disturbed color vision; tinnitus, dizziness, deafness, and vertigo; headache, nausea, vomiting, fever, apprehension, restlessness, confusion, and syncope.

Dermatologic/Allergic: Cutaneous rashes (urticarial, the most frequent type of allergic reaction, papular, or scarlatinal), pruritus, flushing of the skin, sweating, occasional edema of the face.

Respiratory: Asthmatic symptoms.

Cardiovascular: Anginal symptoms.

Gastrointestinal: Nausea and vomiting (may be CNS-related), epigastric pain.

DOSAGE AND ADMINISTRATION

Tablets: One tablet upon retiring. If needed, 2 tablets may be taken nightly—1 following the evening meal and 1 upon retiring.

Capsules: In adults, for use as a component of a malarial suppressant regimen, 2 capsules 3 times per day for 7 days.

After several consecutive nights in which recumbency leg cramps do not occur, quinine sulfatemay be discontinued in order to determine whether continued therapy is needed.

PRODUCT LISTING - RATED THERAPEUTICALLY EQUIVALENT

Size	Price	Manufacturer	NDC
Capsule - Oral - 325 mg			
100's	$15.15	GENERIC, Watson Laboratories Inc	52544-0716-01
Tablet - Oral - 260 mg			
100's	$14.58	GENERIC, Watson Laboratories Inc	52544-0715-01

PRODUCT LISTING - EQUIVALENTS NOT AVAILABLE

Size	Price	Manufacturer	NDC
Capsule - Oral - 200 mg			
100's	$10.52	GENERIC, Moore, H.L. Drug Exchange Inc	00839-5116-06
100's	$10.66	GENERIC, Geneva Pharmaceuticals	00781-2995-01
100's	$14.50	GENERIC, Major Pharmaceuticals Inc	00904-2723-60
100's	$17.50	GENERIC, Cmc-Consolidated Midland Corporation	00223-1559-01
100's	$55.62	GENERIC, Ivax Corporation	00172-4171-60
Capsule - Oral - 325 mg			
24's	$5.14	GENERIC, Parmed Pharmaceuticals Inc	00349-2196-24
30's	$5.35	GENERIC, Allscripts Pharmaceutical Company	54569-2096-00
30's	$8.00	GENERIC, Mutual/United Research Laboratories	00677-0123-07
30's	$27.10	GENERIC, Mutual/United Research Laboratories	00677-1647-07
30's	$27.10	GENERIC, Mutual/United Research Laboratories	53489-0221-07
100's	$5.05	GENERIC, Global Pharmaceutical Corporation	00115-1374-01
100's	$7.49	GENERIC, Advance Biofactures Corporation	17714-0033-01
100's	$8.20	GENERIC, Aligen Independent Laboratories Inc	00405-4922-01
100's	$12.49	GENERIC, Global Source Management	59618-0760-15
100's	$13.50	GENERIC, C.O. Truxton Inc	00463-2019-01
100's	$13.50	GENERIC, Interstate Drug Exchange Inc	00814-6525-14
100's	$14.50	GENERIC, Cmc-Consolidated Midland Corporation	00223-1561-01
100's	$15.00	GENERIC, Mutual/United Research Laboratories	00677-0123-01
100's	$15.29	GENERIC, Major Pharmaceuticals Inc	00904-5398-60
100's	$15.95	GENERIC, Eon Labs Manufacturing Inc	00185-1303-01
100's	$16.50	GENERIC, West Ward Pharmaceutical Corporation	00143-3260-01
100's	$16.99	GENERIC, Physicians Total Care	54868-2858-00
100's	$17.84	GENERIC, Udl Laboratories Inc	51079-0559-20
100's	$18.51	GENERIC, Qualitest Products Inc	00603-5620-21
100's	$19.37	GENERIC, Moore, H.L. Drug Exchange Inc	00839-5117-06
100's	$19.50	GENERIC, Major Pharmaceuticals Inc	00904-2184-60
100's	$20.48	GENERIC, Qualitest Products Inc	00603-5621-21
100's	$25.00	GENERIC, West Ward Pharmaceutical Corporation	00143-3260-25
100's	$31.51	GENERIC, Watson Laboratories Inc	00591-0716-01
100's	$52.60	GENERIC, R.I.D. Inc Distributor	54807-0621-01
100's	$77.54	GENERIC, Ivax Corporation	00172-4172-60
100's	$90.34	GENERIC, Qualitest Products Inc	00603-5622-21
100's	$90.34	GENERIC, Mutual/United Research Laboratories	00677-1647-01
100's	$90.34	GENERIC, Mutual Pharmaceutical Co Inc	53489-0221-01
Tablet - Oral - 260 mg			
25's	$7.20	GENERIC, Pd-Rx Pharmaceuticals	55289-0243-97
30's	$6.00	GENERIC, Medirex Inc	57480-0488-06
31 x 10	$76.73	GENERIC, Vangard Labs	00615-1579-53
31 x 10	$76.73	GENERIC, Vangard Labs	00615-1579-63
100's	$9.95	GENERIC, Eon Labs Manufacturing Inc	00185-0988-01
100's	$10.12	GENERIC, Qualitest Products Inc	00603-5619-21
100's	$10.45	GENERIC, Major Pharmaceuticals Inc	00904-0564-60
100's	$10.45	GENERIC, Major Pharmaceuticals Inc	00904-0604-60
100's	$10.48	GENERIC, Aligen Independent Laboratories Inc	00405-4923-01
100's	$10.91	GENERIC, Vintage Pharmaceuticals Inc	00254-5401-28
100's	$11.54	GENERIC, Moore, H.L. Drug Exchange Inc	00839-6504-06
100's	$11.75	GENERIC, Mutual Pharmaceutical Co Inc	53489-0462-01
100's	$11.93	GENERIC, Interstate Drug Exchange Inc	00814-6527-14
100's	$12.53	GENERIC, Vita-Rx Corporation	49727-0411-02
100's	$14.17	GENERIC, Ivax Corporation	50732-0670-01
100's	$15.35	GENERIC, Physicians Total Care	54868-3652-00
100's	$19.41	GENERIC, Udl Laboratories Inc	51079-0545-20
100's	$20.99	GENERIC, Major Pharmaceuticals Inc	00904-0564-61

100's	$22.50	GENERIC, Interpharm Inc	53746-0250-01
100's	$70.11	GENERIC, Ivax Corporation	00172-3001-60
100's	$79.20	GENERIC, Watson Laboratories Inc	00591-0715-01
250's	$24.50	GENERIC, Eon Labs Manufacturing Inc	00185-0988-52
250's	$24.55	GENERIC, Major Pharmaceuticals Inc	00904-0564-70

Rabeprazole Sodium (003442)

For related information, see the comparative table section in Appendix A.

Categories: Esophagitis, erosive; Gastroesophageal Reflux Disease; Ulcer, duodenal; Zollinger-Ellison syndrome; FDA Approved 1999 Sept; Pregnancy Category B
Drug Classes: Gastrointestinals; Proton pump inhibitors
Brand Names: **Aciphex**
Foreign Brand Availability: Pariet (Australia; Colombia; France; Germany; Indonesia; Mexico; Peru; Philippines; South-Africa; Taiwan; Thailand)
Cost of Therapy: $128.26 (GERD; Aciphex; 20 mg; 1 tablet/day; 30 day supply)
$384.78 (Zollinger-Ellison Syndrome; Aciphex; 20 mg; 3 tablets/day; 30 day supply)

DESCRIPTION

The active ingredient in Aciphex delayed-release tablets is rabeprazole sodium, a substituted benzimidazole that inhibits gastric acid secretion. Rabeprazole sodium is known chemically as 2-[[[4-(3-methoxypropoxy)-3-methyl-2-pyridinyl]-methyl]sulfinyl]-1*H*-benzimidazole sodium salt. It has an empirical formula of $C_{18}H_{20}N_3NaO_3S$ and a molecular weight of 381.43. Rabeprazole sodium is a white to slightly yellowish-white solid. It is very soluble in water and methanol, freely soluble in ethanol, chloroform and ethyl acetate and insoluble in ether and n-hexane. The stability of rabeprazole sodium is a function of pH; it is rapidly degraded in acid media, and is more stable under alkaline conditions.

Aciphex is available for oral administration as delayed-release, enteric-coated tablets containing 20 mg of rabeprazole sodium. Inactive ingredients are carnauba wax, crospovidone, diacetylated monoglycerides, ethylcellulose, hydroxypropl cellulose, hypromellose phthalate, magnesium stearate, mannitol, sodium hydroxide, sodium stearyl fumarate, talc, titanium dioxide, and yellow ferric oxide as a coloring agent.

CLINICAL PHARMACOLOGY

PHARMACOKINETICS AND METABOLISM

Rabeprazole sodium delayed-release tablets are enteric-coated to allow rabeprazole sodium, which is acid labile, to pass through the stomach relatively intact. After oral administration of 20 mg rabeprazole sodium, peak plasma concentrations (C_{max}) of rabeprazole occur over a range of 2.0-5.0 hours (T_{max}). The rabeprazole C_{max} and AUC are linear over an oral dose range of 10-40 mg. There is no appreciable accumulation when doses of 10-40 mg are administered every 24 hours; the pharmacokinetics of rabeprazole are not altered by multiple dosing. The plasma half-life ranges from 1-2 hours.

Absorption

Absolute bioavailability for a 20 mg oral tablet of rabeprazole [compared to intravenous (IV) administration] is approximately 52%. When rabeprazole is administered with a high fat meal, its T_{max} is variable and may delay its absorption up to 4 hours or longer, however, the C_{max} and the extent of rabeprazole absorption (AUC) are not significantly altered. Thus rabeprazole may be taken without regard to timing of meals.

Distribution

Rabeprazole is 96.3% bound to human plasma proteins.

Metabolism

Rabeprazole is extensively metabolized. The thioether and sulphone are the primary metabolites measured in human plasma. These metabolites were not observed to have significant antisecretory activity. *In vitro* studies have demonstrated that rabeprazole is metabolized in the liver primarily by cytochromes P450 3A (CYP3A) to a sulphone metabolite and cytochrome P450 2C19 (CYP2C19) to desmethyl rabeprazole. The thioether metabolite is formed non-enzymatically by reduction of rabeprazole. CYP2C19 exhibits a known genetic polymorphism due to its deficiency in some sub-populations (*e.g.,* 3-5% of Caucasians and 17-20% of Asians). Rabeprazole metabolism is slow in these sub-populations, therefore, they are referred to as poor metabolizers of the drug.

Elimination

Following a single 20 mg oral dose of ^{14}C-labeled rabeprazole, approximately 90% of the drug was eliminated in the urine, primarily as thioether carboxylic acid; its glucuronide, and mercapturic acid metabolites. The remainder of the dose was recovered in the feces. Total recovery of radioactivity was 99.8%. No unchanged rabeprazole was recovered in the urine or feces.

SPECIAL POPULATIONS

Geriatric

In 20 healthy elderly subjects administered 20 mg rabeprazole once daily for 7 days, AUC values approximately doubled and the C_{max} increased by 60% compared to values in a parallel younger control group. There was no evidence of drug accumulation after once daily administration (see PRECAUTIONS).

Pediatric

The pharmacokinetics of rabeprazole in pediatric patients under the age of 18 years have not been studied.

Gender and Race

In analyses adjusted for body mass and height, rabeprazole pharmacokinetics showed no clinically significant differences between male and female subjects. In studies that used different formulations of rabeprazole, AUC(0-∞) values for healthy Japanese men were approximately 50-60% greater than values derived from pooled data from healthy men in the US.

Renal Disease

In 10 patients with stable end-stage renal disease requiring maintenance hemodialysis (creatinine clearance ≤5 ml/min/1.73 m^2), no clinically significant differences were observed in the pharmacokinetics of rabeprazole after a single 20 mg oral dose when compared to 10 healthy volunteers.

Hepatic Disease

In a single dose study of 10 patients with chronic mild to moderate compensated cirrhosis of the liver who were administered a 20 mg dose of rabeprazole, AUC(0-24) was approximately doubled, the elimination half-life was 2- to 3-fold higher, and total body clearance was decreased to less than half compared to values in healthy men.

In a multiple dose study of 12 patients with mild to moderate hepatic impairment administered 20 mg rabeprazole once daily for 8 days, AUC(0-∞) and C_{max} values increased approximately 20% compared to values in healthy age- and gender-matched subjects. These increases were not statistically significant.

No information exists on rabeprazole disposition in patients with severe hepatic impairment. Please refer to DOSAGE AND ADMINISTRATION for information on dosage adjustment in patients with hepatic impairment.

COMBINED ADMINISTRATION WITH ANTIMICROBIALS

Sixteen (16) healthy volunteers genotyped as extensive metabolizers with respect to CYP2C19 were given 20 mg rabeprazole sodium, 1000 mg amoxicillin, 500 mg clarithromycin, or all 3 drugs in a four-way crossover study. Each of the 4 regimens was administered twice daily for 6 days. The AUC and C_{max} for clarithromycin and amoxicillin were not different following combined administration compared to values following single administration. However, the rabeprazole AUC and C_{max} increased by 11% and 34%, respectively, following combined administration. The AUC and C_{max} for 14-hydroxyclarithromycin (active metabolite of clarithromycin) also increased by 42% and 46%, respectively. This increase in exposure to rabeprazole and 14-hydroxyclarithromycin is not expected to produce safety concerns.

PHARMACODYNAMICS

Mechanism of Action

Rabeprazole belongs to a class of antisecretory compounds (substituted benzimidazole proton-pump inhibitors) that do not exhibit anticholinergic or histamine H_2-receptor antagonist properties, but suppress gastric acid secretion by inhibiting the gastric H^+, K^+ATPase at the secretory surface of the gastric parietal cell. Because this enzyme is regarded as the acid (proton) pump within the parietal cell, rabeprazole has been characterized as a gastric proton-pump inhibitor. Rabeprazole blocks the final step of gastric acid secretion.

In gastric parietal cells, rabeprazole is protonated, accumulates, and is transformed to an active sulfenamide. When studied *in vitro,* rabeprazole is chemically activated at pH 1.2 with a half-life of 78 seconds. It inhibits acid transport in porcine gastric vesicles with a half-life of 90 seconds.

Antisecretory Activity

The anti-secretory effect begins within 1 hour after oral administration of 20 mg rabeprazole sodium. The median inhibitory effect of rabeprazole sodium on 24 hour gastric acidity is 88% of maximal after the first dose. Rabeprazole sodium 20 mg inhibits basal and peptone meal-stimulated acid secretion versus placebo by 86% and 95%, respectively, and increases the percent of a 24 hour period that the gastric pH >3 from 10% to 65% (see TABLE 1). This relatively prolonged pharmacodynamic action compared to the short pharmacokinetic half-life (1-2 hours) reflects the sustained inactivation of the H^+, K^+ATPase.

TABLE 1 *Gastric Acid Parameters — Rabeprazole Sodium Versus Placebo After 7 Days of Once Daily Dosing*

Parameter	Rabeprazole Sodium (20 mg qd)	Placebo
Basal acid output (mmol/h)	0.4*	2.8
Stimulated acid output (mmol/h)	0.6*	13.3
% Time gastric pH >3	65*	10

* p <0.01 versus placebo.

Compared to placebo, rabeprazole sodium, 10, 20, and 40 mg, administered once daily for 7 days significantly decreased intragastric acidity with all doses for each of 4 meal-related intervals and the 24 hour time period overall. In this study, there were no statistically significant differences between doses; however, there was a significant dose-related decrease in intragastric acidity. The ability of rabeprazole to cause a dose-related decrease in mean intragastric acidity is shown in TABLE 2.

After administration of 20 mg rabeprazole sodium once daily for 8 days, the mean percent of time that gastric pH >3 or gastric pH >4 after a single dose (Day 1) and multiple doses (Day 8) was significantly greater than placebo (see TABLE 3). The decrease in gastric acidity and the increase in gastric pH observed with 20 mg rabeprazole sodium administered once daily for 8 days were compared to the same parameters for placebo, as shown in TABLE 3.

Effects on Esophageal Acid Exposure

In patients with gastroesophageal reflux disease (GERD) and moderate to severe esophageal acid exposure, rabeprazole sodium 20 and 40 mg/day decreased 24 hour esophageal acid

R

TABLE 2 *AUC Acidity (mmol·h/L) — Rabeprazole Sodium Versus Placebo on Day 7 of Once Daily Dosing (mean ± SD)*

AUC Interval (hours)	Treatment: 10 mg RBP (n=24)	20 mg RBP (n=24)	40 mg RBP (n=24)	Placebo (n=24)
08:00-13:00	19.6 ± 21.5*	12.9 ± 23*	7.6 ± 14.7*	91.1 ± 39.7
13:00-19:00	5.6 ± 9.7*	8.3 ± 29.8*	1.3 ± 5.2*	95.5 ± 48.7
19:00-22:00	0.1 ± 0.1*	0.1 ± 0.06*	0.0 ± 0.02*	11.9 ± 12.5
22:00-08:00	129.2 ± 84*	109.6 ± 67.2*	76.9 ± 58.4*	479.9 ± 165
AUC(0-24h)	155.5 ± 90.6*	130.9 ± 81*	85.8 ± 64.3*	678.5 ± 216

* p <0.001 versus placebo.

TABLE 3 *Gastric Acid Parameters — Rabeprazole Sodium Once Daily Dosing Versus Placebo on Day 1 and Day 8*

Parameter	Rabeprazole Sodium 20 mg qd Day 1	Rabeprazole Sodium 20 mg qd Day 8	Placebo Day 1	Placebo Day 8
Mean AUC(0-24) acidity	340.8*	176.9*	925.5	862.4
Median trough pH (23 h)†	3.77	3.51	1.27	1.38
% Time gastric pH >3‡	54.6*	68.7*	19.1	21.7
% Time gastric pH >4‡	44.1*	60.3*	7.6	11.0

* p <0.001 versus placebo.
† No inferential statistics conducted for this parameter.
‡ Gastric pH was measured every hour over a 24 hour period.

exposure. After 7 days of treatment, the percentage of time that esophageal pH <4 decreased from baselines of 24.7% for 20 mg and 23.7% for 40 mg, to 5.1% and 2.0%, respectively. Normalization of 24 hour intraesophageal acid exposure was correlated to gastric pH >4 for at least 35% of the 24 hour period; this level was achieved in 90% of subjects receiving rabeprazole sodium 20 mg and in 100% of subjects receiving rabeprazole sodium 40 mg. With rabeprazole sodium 20 and 40 mg/day, significant effects on gastric and esophageal pH were noted after 1 day of treatment, and more pronounced after 7 days of treatment.

Effects on Serum Gastrin

In patients given daily doses of rabeprazole sodium for up to 8 weeks to treat ulcerative or erosive esophagitis and in patients treated for up to 52 weeks to prevent recurrence of disease the median fasting gastrin level increased in a dose-related manner. The group median values stayed within the normal range.

In a group of subjects treated daily with rabeprazole sodium 20 mg for 4 weeks a doubling of mean serum gastrin concentrations were observed. Approximately 35% of these treated subjects developed serum gastrin concentrations above the upper limit of normal. In a study of CYP2C19 genotyped subjects in Japan, poor metabolizers developed statistically significantly higher serum gastrin concentrations than extensive metabolizers.

Effects on Enterochromaffin-Like (ECL) Cells

Increased serum gastrin secondary to antisecretory agents stimulates proliferation of gastric ECL cells which, over time, may result in ECL cell hyperplasia in rats and mice and gastric carcinoids in rats, especially in females (see PRECAUTIONS, Carcinogenesis, Mutagenesis, and Impairment of Fertility).

In over 400 patients treated with rabeprazole sodium (10 or 20 mg/day) for up to 1 year, the incidence of ECL cell hyperplasia increased with time and dose, which is consistent with the pharmacological action of the proton-pump inhibitor. No patient developed the adenomatoid, dysplastic or neoplastic changes of ECL cells in the gastric mucosa. No patient developed the carcinoid tumors observed in rats.

Endocrine Effects

Studies in humans for up to 1 year have not revealed clinically significant effects on the endocrine system. In healthy male volunteers treated with rabeprazole sodium for 13 days, no clinically relevant changes have been detected in the following endocrine parameters examined: 17 β-estradiol, thyroid stimulating hormone, tri-iodothyronine, thyroxine, thyroxine-binding protein, parathyroid hormone, insulin, glucagon, renin, aldosterone, follicle-stimulating hormone, luteotrophic hormone, prolactin, somatotrophic hormone, dehydroepiandrosterone, cortisol-binding globulin, and urinary 6β-hydroxycortisol, serum testosterone, and circadian cortisol profile.

Other Effects

In humans treated with rabeprazole sodium for up to 1 year, no systemic effects have been observed on the central nervous, lymphoid, hematopoietic, renal, hepatic, cardiovascular, or respiratory systems. No data are available on long-term treatment with rabeprazole sodium and ocular effects.

MICROBIOLOGY

Rabeprazole sodium, amoxicillin and clarithromycin as a 3 drug regimen has been shown to be active against most strains of *Helicobacter pylori in vitro*and in clinical infections as described in INDICATIONS AND USAGE.

HELICOBACTER PYLORI

Susceptibility testing of *H. pylori* isolates was performed for amoxicilin and clarithromycin using agar dilution methodology[1], and minimum inhibitory concentrations (MICs) were determined. The clarithromycin and amoxicillin MIC values should be interpreted according to the criteria in TABLE 4.

TABLE 4

Clarithromycin MIC*	Interpretation
≤0.25 μg/ml	Susceptible (S)
0.5 μg/ml	Intermediate (I)
≥1.0 μg/ml	Resistant (R)
Amoxicillin MIC*†	**Interpretation**
≤0.25 μg/ml	Susceptible (S)

* These are breakpoints for the agar dilution methodology and they should not be used to interpret results using alternative methods.
† There were not enough organisms with MICs >0.25 μg/ml to determine a resistance breakpoint.

Standardized susceptibility test procedures require the use of laboratory control microorganisms to control the technical aspects of the laboratory procedures. Standard clarithromycin and amoxicillin powders should provide the following MIC values shown in TABLE 5.

TABLE 5

Microorganism	Antimicrobial Agent	MIC (μg/ml)*
H. pylori ATCC 43504	Clarithromycin	0.015 - 0.12
H. pylori ATCC 43504	Amoxicillin	0.015 - 0.12

* These are quality control ranges for the agar dilution methodology and they should be used to control test results obtained using alternative methods.

INCIDENCE OF ANTIBIOTIC-RESISTANT ORGANISMS AMONG CLINICAL ISOLATES

Pretreatment Resistance

Clarithromycin pretreatment resistance rate (MIC ≥1 μg/ml) to *H. pylori* was 9% (51/560) at baseline in all treatment groups combined. A total of >99% (558/560) of patients had *H. pylori* isolates which were considered to be susceptible (MIC ≤0.25 μg/ml) to amoxicillin at baseline. Two patients had baseline *H. pylori* isolates with an amoxicillin MIC of 0.5 μg/ml.

Clarithromycin Susceptibility Test Results and Clinical/Bacteriologic Outcomes

For the US multicenter study, the baseline *H. pylori* clarithromycin susceptibility results and the *H. pylori* eradication results post-treatment are shown in TABLE 6.

TABLE 6 *Clarithromycin Susceptibility Test Results and Clinical/Bacteriologic Outcomes* for a 3 Drug Regimen*

Clarithromycin Pretreatment Results	*H. pylori* negative — eradicated	*H. pylori* positive — persistant Post-Treatment Susceptibility Results: S‡	I‡	R‡	No MIC
7 Days of RAC Therapy					
Susceptible‡ 129	103	2	0	1	23
Intermediate‡ 0	0	0	0	0	0
Resistant‡ 16	5	2	1	4	4
10 Days of RAC Therapy					
Susceptible‡ 133	111	3	1	2	16
Intermediate‡ 0	0	0	0	0	0
Resistant‡ 9	1	0	0	5	3

* Includes only patients with pre-treatment and post-treatment clarithromycin susceptibility test results.
† Rabeprazole 20 mg twice daily, amoxicillin 1000 mg twice daily, and clarithromycin 500 mg twice daily for 7 or 10 days.
‡ Susceptible (S) MIC ≤0.25 μg/ml, Intermediate (I) MIC = 0.5 μg/ml, Resistant (R) MIC ≥1 μg/ml.

Patients with persistent *H. pylori* infection following rabeprazole, amoxicillin, and clarithromycin therapy will likely have clarithromycin resistant clinical isolates. Therefore, clarithromycin susceptibility testing should be done when possible. If resistance of clarithromycin is demonstrated or susceptibility testing is not possible, alternative antimicrobial therapy should be instituted.

Amoxicillin Susceptibilty Test Results and Clinical/Bacteriological Outcomes

In the US, multicenter Study 604, a total of >99% (558/560) of patients had *H. pylori* isolates which were considered to be susceptible (MIC ≤0.25 μg/ml) to amoxicillin at baseline. The other 2 patients had baseline *H. pylori* isolates with an amoxicillin MIC of 0.5 μg/ml, and both isolates were clarithromycin-resistant at baseline; in one case the *H. pylori* was eradicated. In the 7 and 10 day treatment groups 75% (107/145) and 79% (112/142), respectively, of the patients who had pretreatment amoxicillin susceptible MICs (≤0.25 μg/ml) were eradicated of *H. pylori.* No patients developed amoxicillin-resistant *H. pylori* during therapy.

INDICATIONS AND USAGE

HEALING OF EROSIVE OR ULCERATIVE GASTROESOPHAGEAL REFLUX DISEASE (GERD)

Rabeprazole sodium is indicated for short-term (4-8 weeks) treatment in the healing and symptomatic relief of erosive or ulcerative gastroesophageal reflux disease (GERD). For those patients who have not healed after 8 weeks of treatment, an additional 8 week course of rabeprazole sodium may be considered.

MAINTENANCE OF HEALING OF EROSIVE OR ULCERATIVE GASTROESOPHAGEAL REFLUX DISEASE (GERD)

Rabeprazole sodium is indicated for maintaining healing and reduction in relapse rates of heartburn symptoms in patients with erosive or ulcerative gastroesophageal reflux disease (GERD Maintenance). Controlled studies do not extend beyond 12 months.

TREATMENT OF SYMPTOMATIC GASTROESOPHAGEAL REFLUX DISEASE (GERD)

Rabeprazole sodium is indicated for the treatment of daytime and nighttime heartburn and other symptoms associated with GERD.

HEALING OF DUODENAL ULCERS

Rabeprazole sodium is indicated for short-term (up to 4 weeks) treatment in the healing and symptomatic relief of duodenal ulcers. Most patients heal within 4 weeks.

HELICOBACTER PYLORI ERADICATION TO REDUCE THE RISK OF DUODENAL ULCER RECURRENCE

Rabeprazole sodium in combination with amoxicillin and clarithromycin as a 3 drug regimen, is indicated for the treatment of patients with *H. pylori* infection and duodenal ulcer disease (active or history within the past 5 years) to eradicate *H. pylori.* Eradication of *H. pylori* has been shown to reduce the risk of duodenal ulcer recurrence. (See DOSAGE AND ADMINISTRATION.)

In patients who fail therapy, susceptibility testing should be done. If resistance to clarithromycin is demonstrated or susceptibility testing is not possible, alternative antimicrobial therapy should be instituted. (See CLINICAL PHARMACOLOGY, Microbiology, and the clarithromycin package insert, CLINICAL PHARMACOLOGY, Microbiology.

TREATMENT OF PATHOLOGICAL HYPERSECRETORY CONDITIONS, INCLUDING ZOLLINGER-ELLISON SYNDROME

Rabeprazole sodium is indicated for the long-term treatment of pathological hypersecretory conditions, including Zollinger-Ellison syndrome.

NON-FDA APPROVED INDICATIONS

Rabeprazole is also used for gastric ulcer, and duodenal ulcer maintenance, although not FDA-approved.

CONTRAINDICATIONS

Rabeprazole is contraindicated in patients with known hypersensitivity to rabeprazole, substituted benzimidazoles or to any component of the formulation.

Clarithromycin is contraindicated in patients with known hypersensitivity to any macrolide antibiotic.

Concomitant administration of clarithromycin with pimozide and cisapride is contraindicated. There have been post-marketing reports of drug interaction when clarithromycin and/or erythromycin are co-administered with pimozide resulting in cardiac arrhythmias (QT prolongation, venticular tachycardia, ventricular fibrillation, and torsade de pointes) most likely due to inhibition of hepatic metabolism of pimozide by erythromycin and clarithromycin. Fatalities have been reported. (Please refer to full prescribing information for clarthromycin.)

Amoxicillin is contraindicated in patients with a known hypersensitivity to any penicillin. (Please refer to full prescribing information for amoxicillin.)

WARNINGS

CLARITHROMYCIN SHOULD NOT BE USED IN PREGNANT WOMEN EXCEPT IN CLINICAL CIRCUMSTANCES WHERE NO ALTERNATIVE THERAPY IS APPROPRIATE. If pregnancy occurs while taking clarithromycin, the patient should be apprised of the potential hazard to the fetus. (See WARNINGS in prescribing information for clarithromycin.)

AMOXICILLIN

Serious and occasionally fatal hypersensitivity (anaphylactic) reactions have been reported in patients on penicillin therapy. These reactions are more likely to occur in individuals with a history of penicillin hypersensitivity and/or a history of sensitivity to multiple allergens.

There have been well documented reports of individuals with a history of penicillin hypersensitivity reactions who have experienced severe hypersensitivity reactions when treated with a cephalosporin. Before initiating therapy with any penicillin, careful inquiry should be made concerning previous hypersensitivity reactions to penicillin, cephalosporin, and other allergens. If an allergic reaction occurs, amoxicillin should be discontinued and the appropriate therapy instituted. (See WARNINGS in prescribing information for amoxicillin.)

SERIOUS ANAPHYLACTIC REACTIONS REQUIRE IMMEDIATE EMERGENCY TREATMENT WITH EPINEPHRINE, OXYGEN, IV STEROIDS, AND AIRWAY MANAGEMENT, INCLUDING INTUBATION, SHOULD ALSO BE ADMINISTERED AS INDICATED.

Pseudomembranous colitis has been reported with nearly all antibacterial agents, including clarithromycin and amoxicillin, and may range in severity from mild to life threatening. Therefore, it is important to consider this diagnosis in patients who present with diarrhea subsequent to the administration of antibacterial agents.

Treatment with antibacterial agents alters the normal flora of the colon and may permit overgrowth of clostridia. Studies indicate that a toxin produced by *Clostridium difficile* is a primary cause of "antibiotic-associated colitis".

After the diagnosis of pseudomembranous colitis has been established, therapeutic measures should be initiated. Mild cases of pseudomembranous colitis usually respond to discontinuation of the drug alone. In moderate to severe cases, consideration should be given to management with fluid and electrolytes, protein supplementation, and treatment with an antibacterial drug clinically effective against *Clostridium difficile* colitis.

PRECAUTIONS

GENERAL

Symptomatic response to therapy with rabeprazole does not preclude the presence of gastric malignancy.

Patients with healed GERD were treated for up to 40 months with rabeprazole and monitored with serial gastric biopsies. Patients without *H. pylori* infection (221 of 326 patients) had no clinically important pathologic changes in the gastric mucosa. Patients with *H. pylori* infection at baseline (105 of 326 patients) had mild or moderate inflammation in the gastric body or mild inflammation in the gastric antrum. Patients with mild grades of infection or inflammation in the gastric body tended to change to moderate, whereas those graded moderate at baseline tended to remain stable. Patients with mild grades of infection or inflammation in the gastric antrum tended to remain stable. At baseline 8% of patients had atrophy of glands in the gastric body and 15% had atrophy in the gastric antrum. At endpoint, 15% of patients had atrophy of glands in the gastric body and 11% had atrophy in the gastric antrum. Approximately 4% of patients had intestinal metaplasia at some point during follow-up, but no consistent changes were seen.

Steady state interactions of rabeprazole and warfarin have not been adequately evaluated in patients. There have been reports of increased INR and prothrombin time in patients receiving a proton pump inhibitor and warfarin concomitantly. Increases in INR and prothrombin time may lead to abnormal bleeding and even death. Patients treated with a proton pump inhibitor and warfarin concomitantly may need to be monitored for increases in INR and prothrombin time.

INFORMATION FOR THE PATIENT

Patients should be cautioned that rabeprazole sodium delayed-release tablets should be swallowed whole. The tablets should not be chewed, crushed, or split. Rabeprazole can be taken with or without food.

CARCINOGENESIS, MUTAGENESIS, AND IMPAIRMENT OF FERTILITY

In an 88/104 week carcinogenicity study in CD-1 mice, rabeprazole at oral doses up to 100 mg/kg/day did not produce any increased tumor occurrence. The highest tested dose produced a systemic exposure to rabeprazole (AUC) of 1.40 μg·h/ml which is 1.6 times the human exposure [plasma AUC(0-∞) = 0.88 μg·h/ml] at the recommended dose for GERD (20 mg/day). In a 104 week carcinogenicity study in Sprague-Dawley rats, males were treated with oral doses of 5, 15, 30, and 60 mg/kg/day and females with 5, 15, 30, 60, and 120 mg/kg/day. Rabeprazole produced gastric enterochromaffin-like (ECL) cell hyperplasia in male and female rats and ECL cell carcinoid tumors in female rats at all doses including the lowest tested dose. The lowest dose (5 mg/kg/day) produced a systemic exposure to rabeprazole (AUC) of about 0.1 μg·h/ml which is about 0.1 times the human exposure at the recommended dose for GERD. In male rats, no treatment related tumors were observed at doses up to 60 mg/kg/day producing a rabeprazole plasma exposure (AUC) of about 0.2 μg·h/ml (0.2 times the human exposure at the recommended dose for GERD).

Rabeprazole was positive in the Ames test, the Chinese hamster ovary cell (CHO/HGPRT) forward gene mutation test and the mouse lymphoma cell (L5178Y/TK+/-) forward gene mutation test. Its demethylated-metabolite was also positive in the Ames test. Rabeprazole was negative in the *in vitro* Chinese hamster lung cell chromosome aberration test, the *in vivo* mouse micronucleus test, and the *in vivo* and *ex vivo* rat hepatocyte unscheduled DNA synthesis (UDS) tests.

Rabeprazole at intravenous (IV) doses up to 30 mg/kg/day (plasma AUC of 8.8 μg·h/ml, about 10 times the human exposure at the recommended dose for GERD) was found to have no effect on fertility and reproductive performance of male and female rats.

PREGNANCY, TERATOGENIC EFFECTS, PREGNANCY CATEGORY B

Teratology studies have been performed in rats at IV doses up to 50 mg/kg/day (plasma AUC of 11.8 μg·h/ml, about 13 times the human exposure at the recommended dose for GERD) and rabbits at IV doses up to 30 mg/kg/day (plasma AUC of 7.3 μg·h/ml, about 8 times the human exposure at the recommended dose for GERD) and have revealed no evidence of impaired fertility or harm to the fetus due to rabeprazole. There are, however, no adequate and well-controlled studies in pregnant women. Because animal reproduction studies are not always predictive of human response, this drug should be used during pregnancy only if clearly needed.

NURSING MOTHERS

Following IV administration of ^{14}C-labeled rabeprazole to lactating rats, radioactivity in milk reached levels that were 2- to 7-fold higher than levels in the blood. It is not known if unmetabolized rabeprazole is excreted in human breast milk. Administration of rabeprazole to rats in late gestation and during lactation at doses of 400 mg/kg/day (about 195 times the human dose based on mg/m^2) resulted in decreases in body weight gain of the pups. Since many drugs are excreted in milk, and because of the potential for adverse reactions to nursing infants from rabeprazole, a decision should be made to discontinue nursing or discontinue the drug, taking into account the importance of the drug to the mother.

PEDIATRIC USE

The safety and effectiveness of rabeprazole in pediatric patients have not been established.

USE IN WOMEN

Duodenal ulcer and erosive esophagitis healing rates in women are similar to those in men. Adverse events and laboratory test abnormalities in women occurred at rates similar to those in men.

GERIATRIC USE

Of the total number of subjects in clinical studies of rabeprazole sodium, 19% were 65 years and over, while 4% were 75 years and over. No overall differences in safety or effectiveness were observed between these subjects and younger subjects, and other reported clinical experience has not identified differences in responses between the elderly and younger patients, but greater sensitivity of some older individuals cannot be ruled out.

DRUG INTERACTIONS

Rabeprazole is metabolized by the cytochrome P450 (CYP450) drug metabolizing enzyme system. Studies in healthy subjects have shown that rabeprazole does not have clinically significant interactions with other drugs metabolized by the CYP450 system, such as warfarin and theophylline given as single oral doses, diazepam as a single IV dose, and phenytoin given as a single IV dose (with supplemental oral dosing). Steady state interactions of rabeprazole and other drugs metabolized by this enzyme system have not been studied in patients. There have been reports of increased INR and prothrombin time in patients receiving proton pump inhibitors, including rabeprazole, and warfarin concomitantly. Increases in INR and prothrombin time may lead to abnormal bleeding and even death.

In vitro incubations employing human liver microsomes indicated that rabeprazole inhibited cyclosporine metabolism with an IC_{50} of 62 μmol, a concentration that is over 50 times higher than the C_{max} in healthy volunteers following 14 days of dosing with 20 mg of rabeprazole. This degree of inhibition is similar to that by omeprazole at equivalent concentrations.

Rabeprazole produces sustained inhibition of gastric acid secretion. An interaction with compounds which are dependent on gastric pH for absorption may occur due to the magnitude of acid suppression observed with rabeprazole. For example, in normal subjects, co-administration of rabeprazole 20 mg qd resulted in an approximately 30% decrease in the bioavailability of ketoconazole and increases in the AUC and C_{max} for digoxin of 19% and 29%, respectively. Therefore, patients may need to be monitored when such drugs are taken concomitantly with rabeprazole. Co-administration of rabeprazole and antacids produced no clinically relevant changes in plasma rabeprazole concentrations.

In a clinical study in Japan evaluating rabeprazole in patients categorized by CYP2C19 genotype (n=6 per genotype category), gastric acid suppression was higher in poor metabolizers as compared to extensive metabolizers. This could be due to higher rabeprazole plasma levels in poor metabolizers. Whether or not interactions of rabeprazole sodium with other drugs metabolized by CYP2C19 would be different between extensive metabolizers and poor metabolizers has not been studied.

COMBINED ADMINISTRATION WITH CLARITHROMYCIN

Combined administration consisting of rabeprazole, amoxicillin, and clarithromycin resulted in increases in plasma concentrations of rabeprazole and 14-hydroxyclaithromycin. (See CLINICAL PHARMACOLOGY, Combination Therapy With Antimicrobials.)

Concomitant administration of clarithromycin with pimozide and cisapride is contraindicated. (See PRECAUTIONS in prescribing information for clarithromycin.) (See PRECAUTIONS in prescribing information for amoxicillin.)

ADVERSE REACTIONS

Worldwide, over 2900 patients have been treated with rabeprazole in Phase 2-3 clinical trials involving various dosages and durations of treatment. In general, rabeprazole treatment has been well-tolerated in both short- and long-term trials. The adverse events rates were generally similar between the 10 and 20 mg doses.

INCIDENCE IN CONTROLLED NORTH AMERICAN AND EUROPEAN CLINICAL TRIALS

In an analysis of adverse events assessed as possibly or probably related to treatment appearing in greater than 1% of rabeprazole sodium patients and appearing with greater frequency than placebo in controlled North American and European trials, the incidence of headache was 2.4% (n=1552) for rabeprazole sodium versus 1.6% (n=258) for placebo.

In short- and long-term studies, the following adverse events, regardless of causality, were reported in rabeprazole sodium-treated patients. *Rare* events are those reported in ≤1/1000 patients.

Body as a Whole: Asthenia, fever, allergic reaction, chills, malaise, chest pain substernal, neck rigidity, photosensitivity reaction. *Rare:* Abdomen enlarged, face edema, hangover effect.

Cardiovascular System: Hypertension, myocardial infarct, electrocardiogram abnormal, migraine, syncope, angina pectoris, bundle branch block, palpitation, sinus bradycardia, tachycardia. *Rare:* Bradycardia, pulmonary embolus, supraventricular tachycardia, thrombophlebitis, vasodilation, QTC prolongation and ventricular tachycardia.

Digestive System: Diarrhea, nausea, abdominal pain, vomiting, dyspepsia, flatulence, constipation, dry mouth, eructation, gastroenteritis, rectal hemorrhage, melena, anorexia, cholelithiasis, mouth ulceration, stomatitis, dysphagia, gingivitis, cholecystitis, increased appetite, abnormal stools, colitis, esophagitis, glossitis, pancreatitis, proctitis. *Rare:* Bloody diarrhea, cholangitis, duodenitis, gastrointestinal hemorrhage, hepatic encephalopathy, hepatitis, hepatoma, liver fatty deposit, salivary gland enlargement, thirst.

Endocrine System: Hyperthyroidism, hypothyroidism.

Hemic and Lymphatic System: Anemia, ecchymosis, lymphadenopathy, hypochromic anemia.

Metabolic and Nutritional Disorders: Peripheral edema, edema, weight gain, gout, dehydration, weight loss.

Musculoskeletal System: Myalgia, arthritis, leg cramps, bone pain, arthrosis, bursitis. *Rare:* Twitching.

Nervous System: Insomnia, anxiety, dizziness, depression, nervousness, somnolence, hypertonia, neuralgia, vertigo, convulsion, abnormal dreams, libido decreased, neuropathy, paresthesia, tremor. *Rare:* Agitation, amnesia, confusion, extrapyramidal syndrome, hyperkinesia.

Respiratory System: Dyspnea, asthma, epistaxis, laryngitis, hiccup, hyperventilation. *Rare:* Apnea, hypoventilation.

Skin and Appendages: Rash, pruritus, sweating, urticaria, alopecia. *Rare:* Dry skin, herpes zoster, psoriasis, skin discoloration.

Special Senses: Cataract, amblyopia, glaucoma, dry eyes, abnormal vision, tinnitus, otitis media. *Rare:* Corneal opacity, blurry vision, diplopia, deafness, eye pain, retinal degeneration, strabismus.

Urogenital System: Cystitis, urinary frequency, dysmenorrhea, dysuria, kidney calculus, metrorrhagia, polyuria. *Rare:* Breast enlargement, hematuria, impotence, leukorrhea, menorrhagia, orchitis, urinary incontinence.

Laboratory Values

The following changes in laboratory parameters were reported as adverse events: Abnormal platelets, albuminuria, creatine phosphokinase increased, erythrocytes abnormal, hypercholesteremia, hyperglycemia, hyperlipemia, hypokalemia, hyponatremia, leukocytosis, leukorrhea, liver function tests abnormal, prostatic specific antigen increase, SGPT increased, urine abnormality, WBC abnormal.

In controlled clinical studies, 3/1456 (0.2%) patients treated with rabeprazole and 2/237 (0.8%) patients treated with placebo developed treatment-emergent abnormalities (which were either new on study or present at study entry with an increase of 1.25 × baseline value) in SGOT (AST), SGPT (ALT), or both. None of the 3 rabeprazole patients experienced chills, fever, right upper quadrant pain, nausea or jaundice.

Combination Treatment With Amoxicillin and Clarithromycin

In clinical trials using combination therapy with rabeprazole plus amoxicillin and clarithromycin (RAC), no adverse events unique to this drug combination were observed. In the US multicenter study, the most frequently reported drug related adverse events for patients who received RAC therapy for 7 or 10 days were diarrhea (8% and 7%) and taste perversion (6% and 10%), respectively.

No clinically significant laboratory abnormalities particular to the drug combinations were observed.

For more information on adverse events or laboratory changes with amoxicillin or clarithromycin, refer to their respective package prescribing information, ADVERSE REACTIONS sections.

Post-Marketing Adverse Events

Additional adverse events reported from worldwide marketing experience with rabeprazole sodium are: Sudden death, coma and hyperammonenia, jaundice, rhabdomyolysis, disorientation and delirium, anaphylaxis, angioedema, bullous and other drug eruptions of the skin, interstitial pneumonia, interstitial nephritis, and TSH elevations. In most instances, the relationship to rabeprazole sodium was unclear. In addition, agranulocytosis, hemolytic anemia, leukopenia, pancytopenia, and thrombocytopenia have been reported. Increases in prothrombin time/INR in patients treated with concomitant warfarin have been reported.

DOSAGE AND ADMINISTRATION

HEALING OF EROSIVE OR ULCERATIVE GASTROESOPHAGEAL REFLUX DISEASE (GERD)

The recommended adult oral dose is 1 rabeprazole sodium 20 mg delayed-release tablet to be taken once daily for 4-8 weeks. (See INDICATIONS AND USAGE.) For those patients who have not healed after 8 weeks of treatment, an additional 8 week course of rabeprazole sodium may be considered.

MAINTENANCE OF HEALING OF EROSIVE OR ULCERATIVE GASTROESOPHAGEAL REFLUX DISEASE (GERD MAINTENANCE)

The recommended adult oral dose is 1 rabeprazole sodium 20 mg delayed-release tablet to be taken once daily. (See INDICATIONS AND USAGE.)

TREATMENT OF SYMPTOMATIC GASTROESOPHAGEAL REFLUX DISEASE (GERD MAINTENANCE)

The recommended adult oral dose is 1 rabeprazole sodium 20 mg delayed-release tablet to be taken once daily for 4 weeks. (See INDICATIONS AND USAGE). If symptoms do not resolve completely after 4 weeks, an additional course of treatment may be considered.

HEALING OF DUODENAL ULCERS

The recommended adult oral dose is 1 rabeprazole sodium 20 mg delayed-release tablet to be taken once daily after the morning meal for a period up to 4 weeks. (See INDICATIONS AND USAGE.) Most patients with duodenal ulcer heal within 4 weeks. A few patients may require additional therapy to achieve healing.

TABLE 14 *Helicobacter pylori Eradication to Reduce the Risk of Duodenal Ulcer Recurrence: 3 Drug Regimen**

Rabeprazole Sodium	20 mg	Twice daily for 7 days
Amoxicillin	1000 mg	Twice daily for 7 days
Clarithromycin	500 mg	Twice daily for 7 days

* It is important that patients comply with the full 7 day regimen.
All three medications should be taken twice daily with the morning and evening meals.

TREATMENT OF PATHOLOGICAL HYPERSECRETORY CONDITIONS INCLUDING ZOLLINGER-ELLISON SYNDROME

The dosage of rabeprazole sodium in patients with pathologic hypersecretory conditions varies with the individual patient. The recommended adult oral starting dose is 60 mg once a day. Doses should be adjusted to individual patient needs and should continue for as long as clinically indicated. Some patients may require divided doses. Doses up to 100 mg qd and 60 mg bid have been administered. Some patients with Zollinger-Ellison syndrome have been treated continuously with rabeprazole sodium for up to 1 year.

No dosage adjustment is necessary in elderly patients, in patients with renal disease or in patients with mild to moderate hepatic impairment. Administration of rabeprazole to patients with mild to moderate liver impairment resulted in increased exposure and decreased elimination. Due to the lack of clinical data on rabeprazole in patients with severe hepatic impairment, caution should be exercised in those patients.

Rabeprazole sodium should be swallowed whole. The tablets should not be chewed, crushed, or split. Rabeprazole sodium delayed-release tablets can be taken with or without food.

HOW SUPPLIED

Aciphex 20 mg is supplied as delayed-release light yellow enteric-coated tablets. The name and strength, in mg, ("ACIPHEX 20") is imprinted on one side.
Storage: Store at 25°C (77°F); excursions permitted to 15-30°C (59-86°F). Protect from moisture.

PRODUCT LISTING - EQUIVALENTS NOT AVAILABLE

Tablet, Extended Release - Oral - 20 mg

30's	$113.99	ACIPHEX, Allscripts Pharmaceutical Company	54569-4980-00
30's	$124.38	ACIPHEX, Physicians Total Care	54868-4185-00
30's	$128.26	ACIPHEX, Southwood Pharmaceuticals Inc	58016-0597-30
30's	$133.65	ACIPHEX, Janssen Pharmaceuticals	62856-0243-30
60's	$256.52	ACIPHEX, Southwood Pharmaceuticals Inc	58016-0597-60
90's	$384.78	ACIPHEX, Southwood Pharmaceuticals Inc	58016-0597-90
90's	$400.94	ACIPHEX, Janssen Pharmaceuticals	62856-0243-90
100's	$427.53	ACIPHEX, Southwood Pharmaceuticals Inc	58016-0597-00
100's	$445.48	ACIPHEX, Janssen Pharmaceuticals	62856-0243-41

Rabies Immune Globulin (002172)

For complete prescribing information, refer to the CD-ROM included with the book.

Categories: Rabies; Pregnancy Category C; FDA Pre 1938 Drugs; WHO Formulary
Drug Classes: Antivirals; Immune globulins
Brand Names: **Hyperab**; Imogam Rabies
Foreign Brand Availability: Bayer Bayrab Rabies Immune Globulin (Philippines); Bayrab (Canada); Imogam (Australia); Imogan Rabia (Spain); Rabigam (South-Africa); Rabuman Berna (Philippines; Thailand)

DESCRIPTION

Rabies Immune Globulin (Human), (RIGH), is a sterile solution of antirabies immunoglobulin for intramuscular administration. This product is prepared from human plasma. It is prepared by cold alcohol fractionation from the plasma of donors hyperimmunized with rabies vaccine. RIGH is a 15%-18% solution of human protein stabilized in 0.21-0.32 M glycine. The pH of the solution has been adjusted to 6.4-7.2 with sodium carbonate. RIGH contains the mercurial preservative sodium ethylmercurithiosalicylate (thimerosal), 80-120 µg/ml as measured by mercury assay. The product is standardized against the US Standard Rabies Immune Globulin to contain an average potency value of 150 IU/ml. The US unit of potency is equivalent to the international unit (IU) for rabies antibody.

STORAGE

RIGH should be stored under refrigeration (2-8°C, 35-46°F). Solution that has been frozen should not be used.

INDICATIONS AND USAGE

Rabies vaccine and Rabies Immune Globulin (Human), (RIGH), should be given to all persons suspected of exposure to rabies with one exception: persons who have been previously immunized with rabies vaccine and have a confirmed adequate rabies antibody titer should receive only vaccine. RIGH should be administered as promptly as possible after exposure, but can be administered up to the eighth day after the first dose of vaccine is given.

Recommendations for use of passive and active immunization after exposure to an animal suspected of having rabies have been detailed by the US Public Health Service Immunization Practices Advisory Committee (ACIP).[17]

Every exposure to possible rabies infection must be individually evaluated. The following factors should be considered before specific antirabies treatment is initiated.

SPECIES OF BITING ANIMAL

Carnivorous wild animals (especially skunks, foxes, coyotes, raccoons, and bobcats) and bats are the animals most commonly infected with rabies and have caused most of the indigenous cases of human rabies in the US since 1960.[18] Unless the animal is tested and shown not to be rabid, postexposure prophylaxis should be initiated upon bite or nonbite exposure to these animals (See INDICATIONS AND USAGE, Type of Exposure). If treatment has been initiated and subsequent testing in a competent laboratory shows the exposing animal is not rabid, treatment can be discontinued.

In the US, the likelihood that a domestic dog or cat is infected with rabies varies from region to region; hence, the need for postexposure prophylaxis also varies. However, in most of Asia and all of Africa and Latin America, the dog remains the major source of human exposure; exposures to dogs in such countries represent a special threat. Travelers to those countries should be aware that >50% of the rabies cases among humans in the US result from exposure to dogs outside the US.

Rodents (such as squirrels, hamsters, guinea pigs, gerbils, chipmunks, rats, and mice) and lagomorphs (including rabbits and hares) are rarely found to be infected with rabies and have not been known to cause human rabies in the US. However, from 1971 through 1988, woodchucks accounted for 70% of the 179 cases of rabies among rodents reported to CDC.[19] In these cases, the state or local health department should be consulted before a decision is made to initiate postexposure antirabies prophylaxis.

CIRCUMSTANCES OF BITING INCIDENT

An unprovoked attack is more likely to mean that the animal is rabid. (Bites during attempts to feed or handle an apparently healthy animal may generally be regarded as provoked.)

TYPE OF EXPOSURE

Rabies is transmitted only when the virus is introduced into open cuts or wounds in skin or mucous membranes. If there has been no exposure (as described in this section), postexposure treatment is not necessary. Thus, the likelihood that rabies infection will result from exposure to a rabid animal varies with the nature and extent of the exposure. Two categories of exposure should be considered:

Bite

Any penetration of the skin by teeth. Bites to the face and hands carry the highest risk, but the site of the bite should not influence the decision to begin treatment.[20]

Nonbite

Scratches, abrasions, open wounds or mucous membranes contaminated with saliva or any potentially infectious material, such as brain tissue, from a rabid animal constitute nonbite exposures. If the material containing the virus is dry, the virus can be considered noninfectious. Casual contact, such as petting a rabid animal and contact with the blood, urine, or feces (*e.g.*, guano) of a rabid animal, does not constitute an exposure and is not an indication for prophylaxis. Instances of airborne rabies have been reported rarely. Adherence to respiratory precautions will minimize the risk of airborne exposure.[21]

The only documented cases of rabies from human-to-human transmission have occurred in patients who received corneas transplanted from persons who died of rabies undiagnosed at the time of death. Stringent guidelines for acceptance of donor corneas have reduced this risk.

Bite and nonbite exposures from humans with rabies theoretically could transmit rabies, although no cases of rabies acquired this way have been documented.

VACCINATION STATUS OF BITING ANIMAL

A properly immunized animal has only a minimal chance of developing rabies and transmitting the virus.

PRESENCE OF RABIES IN REGION

If adequate laboratory and field records indicate that there is no rabies infection in a domestic species within a given region, local health officials are justified in considering this in making recommendations on antirabies treatment following a bite by that particular species. Such officials should be consulted for current interpretations.

RABIES POSTEXPOSURE PROPHYLAXIS

The following recommendations are only a guide. In applying them, take into account the animal species involved, the circumstances of the bite or other exposure, the vaccination status of the animal, and presence of rabies in the region. Local or state public health officials should be consulted if questions arise about the need for rabies prophylaxis.

Local Treatment of Wounds

Immediate and thorough washing of all bite wounds and scratches with soap and water is perhaps the most effective measure for preventing rabies. In experimental animals, simple local wound cleansing has been shown to reduce markedly the likelihood of rabies.

Tetanus prophylaxis and measures to control bacterial infection should be given as indicated.

Active Immunization

Active immunization should be initiated as soon as possible after exposure (within 24 hours). Many dosage schedules have been evaluated for the currently available rabies vaccines and their respective manufacturers' literature should be consulted.

Passive Immunization

A combination of active and passive immunization (vaccine and immune globulin) is considered the acceptable postexposure prophylaxis except for those persons who have been previously immunized with rabies vaccine and who have documented adequate rabies antibody titer. These individuals should receive vaccine only. For passive immunization, Rabies Immune Globulin (Human) is preferred over antirabies serum, equine.[16,17] It is recommended both for treatment of all bites by animals suspected of having rabies and for nonbite exposure inflicted by animals suspected of being rabid. Rabies Immune Globulin (Human) should be used in conjunction with rabies vaccine and can be administered through the seventh day after the first dose of vaccine is given. Beyond the seventh day, Rabies Immune Globulin (Human) is not indicated since an antibody response to cell culture vaccine is presumed to have occurred.

CONTRAINDICATIONS

None known.

WARNINGS

Rabies Immune Globulin (Human), (RIGH), should be given with caution to patients with a history of prior systemic allergic reactions following the administration of human immunoglobulin preparations or in patients who are known to have had an allergic response to thimerosal.

The attending physician who wishes to administer RIGH to persons with isolated immunoglobulin A (IgA) deficiency must weigh the benefits of immunization against the potential risks of hypersensitivity reactions. Such persons have increased potential for developing antibodies to IgA and could have anaphylactic reactions to subsequent administration of blood products that contain IgA.[22]

As with all preparations administered by the intramuscular route, bleeding complications may be encountered in patients with thrombocytopenia or other bleeding disorders.

DOSAGE AND ADMINISTRATION

The recommended dose for RIGH is 20 IU/kg (0.133 ml/kg) of body weight given preferably at the time of the first vaccine dose.[8,9] It may also be given through the seventh day after the first dose of vaccine is given. If anatomically feasible, up to one-half the dose of RIGH should be thoroughly infiltrated in the area around the wound and the rest should be

R

TABLE 1 *Rabies Postexposure Prophylaxis Guide*[17]

Animal Species	Condition of Animal at Time of Attack	Treatment of Exposed Person*
Dog and cat	Healthy and available for 10 days of observation	None, unless animal develops rabies†
	Rabid or suspected rabid	RIGH‡ and HDCV
	Unknown (escaped)	Consult public health officials
Skunk, bat, fox, coyote, raccoon, bobcat, and other carnivores; woodchuck	Regard as rabid unless geographic area is known to be free of rabies or proven negative by laboratory tests§	RIGH‡ and HDCV
Livestock, rodents, and lagomorphs (rabbits and hares)	Consider individually. Local and state public health officials should be consulted on questions about the need for rabies prophylaxis. In most geographical areas bites of squirrels, hamsters, guinea pigs, gerbils, chipmunks, rats, mice, other rodents, rabbits, and hares almost never call for antirabies prophylaxis.	

* ALL BITES AND WOUNDS SHOULD IMMEDIATELY BE THOROUGHLY CLEANSED WITH SOAP AND WATER. If antirabies treatment is indicated, both Rabies Immune Globulin (Human) [RIGH] and human diploid cell rabies vaccine (HDCV) should be given as soon as possible, REGARDLESS of the interval from exposure.

† During the usual holding period of 10 days, begin treatment with RIGH and vaccine (HDCV) at first sign of rabies in a dog or cat that has bitten someone. The symptomatic animal should be killed immediately and tested.

‡ If RIGH is not available, use antirabies serum, equine (ARS). Do not use more than the recommended dosage.

§ The animal should be killed and tested as soon as possible. Holding for observation is not recommended. Discontinue vaccine if immunofluorescence test results of the animal are negative.

administered intramuscularly in the gluteal area. Because of risk of injury to the sciatic nerve, the central region of the gluteal area MUST be avoided; only the upper, outer quadrant should be used.[23] Rabies Immune Globulin (Human), (RIGH), should never be administered in the same syringe or into the same anatomical site as vaccine.

Parenteral drug products should be inspected visually for particulate matter and discoloration prior to administration, whenever solution and container permit.

PRODUCT LISTING - EQUIVALENTS NOT AVAILABLE

Solution - Intramuscular - 150 IU/ml

Size	Price	Product	NDC
2 ml	$87.50	HYPERAB, Bayer	00026-0608-02
2 ml	$90.00	HYPERAB, Bayer	00192-0608-02
2 ml	$164.44	IMOGAM RABIES, Aventis Pharmaceuticals	49281-0190-20
2 ml	$1199.99	BAYRAB, Bayer	00026-0618-02
10 ml	$345.00	HYPERAB, Bayer	00026-0608-10
10 ml	$360.00	HYPERAB, Bayer	00192-0608-10
10 ml	$750.00	BAYRAB, Allscripts Pharmaceutical Company	54569-4799-00
10 ml	$822.20	IMOGAM RABIES, Aventis Pharmaceuticals	49281-0190-10
10 ml	$1199.99	BAYRAB, Bayer	00026-0618-10

Rabies Vaccine *(002173)*

For complete prescribing information, refer to the CD-ROM included with the book.

Categories: Immunization, rabies; FDA Pre 1938 Drugs; Pregnancy Category C; WHO Formulary
Drug Classes: Vaccines
Brand Names: Imovax Rabies; **RabAvert**
Foreign Brand Availability: Berirab P (Philippines); Imovax Rabbia (Italy); Lyssavac N Berna (Ecuador; Hong-Kong; Malaysia; Peru; Philippines; Thailand); Rabies-Imovax (Finland; Sweden); Rabipur (Austria; Czech-Republic; England; Germany; India; Ireland; Israel); Rabuman Berna (Ecuador); Rasilvax (Italy); Vacuna Antirrabica Humana (Colombia)

DESCRIPTION

Rabies vaccine is a sterile freeze-dried vaccine obtained by growing the fixed-virus strain Flury LEP in primary cultures of chicken fibroblasts. The strain Flury LEP was obtained from American Type Culture Collection as the 59th egg passage. The growth medium for propagation of the virus is a synthetic cell culture medium with the addition of human albumin, polygeline (processed bovine gelatin) and antibiotics. The virus is inactivated with, β-propiolactone, and further processed by zonal centrifugation in a sucrose density-gradient. The vaccine is lyophilized after addition of a stabilizer solution which consists of buffered polygeline and potassium glutamate. One dose of reconstituted vaccine contains less than 12 mg polygeline (processed bovine gelatin), 1 mg potassium glutamate and 0.3 mg sodium EDTA. Small quantities of bovine serum are used in the cell culture process. Testing of the product components and excipients using currently available methods has not detected any adventitious agents. Further, bovine components originate only from source countries known to be free of bovine spongioform encephalopathy. Minimal amounts of chicken protein may be present in the final product; ovalbumin content is less than 3 ng/dose (1 ml), based on ELISA. Antibiotics (neomycin, chlortetracycline, amphotericin B) added during cell and virus propagation are largely removed during subsequent steps in the manufacturing process. In the final vaccine, neomycin is present at <1 μg, chlortetracycline at <20 ng, and amphotericin B at <2 ng per dose. Rabies vaccine is intended for intra muscular (IM) injection. The vaccine contains no preservative and should be used immediately after reconstitution with the supplied diluent (Water For Injection). The potency of the final product is determined by the NIH mouse potency test using the US reference standard. The potency of 1 dose (1.0 ml) rabies vaccine is at least 2.5 IU of rabies antigen. Rabies vaccine is a white, freeze-dried vaccine for reconstitution with the diluent prior to use; the reconstituted vaccine is a clear to slightly opaque, colorless suspension.

INDICATIONS AND USAGE

Rabies vaccine is indicated for pre-exposure immunization, in both primary series and booster dose, and for post exposure prophylaxis against rabies.

There are no data on the interchangeable use of different rabies vaccines in a single pre- or post-exposure series.

Therefore the vaccine from a single manufacturer should be used for the complete series whenever possible. If vaccines from other manufacturers are administered during the immunization series, an adequate antibody response should be confirmed by appropriate serologic tests. However, for booster immunization, rabies vaccine was shown to elicit satisfactory antibody level responses in 41 persons who received a primary series with HDCV[3,10].

PRE-EXPOSURE IMMUNIZATION

See TABLE 1.

Pre-Exposure Immunization Schedule

Pre-exposure immunization consists of three doses of rabies vaccine 1.0 ml, intramuscularly (deltoid region), one each on days 0,7, and 21 or 28[23] (see also TABLE 1 for criteria for pre-exposure immunization).

Pre-exposure immunization should be offered to persons in high-risk groups, such as veterinarians, animal handlers, wildlife officers, certain laboratory workers, and persons spending time in foreign countries where rabies is endemic. Persons whose activities bring them into contact with potentially rabid dogs, cats, foxes, skunks, bats, or other species at risk of having rabies should also be considered for pre-exposure prophylaxis.

Pre-exposure immunization is given for several reasons. First, it may provide protection to persons with inapparent exposure to rabies. Second, it may protect persons whose post-exposure therapy might be expected to be delayed. Finally, although it does not eliminate the need for prompt therapy after a rabies exposure, it simplifies therapy by eliminating the need for globulin and decreasing the number of doses of vaccine needed. This is of particular importance for persons at high risk of being exposed in countries where the available rabies immunizing products may carry a higher risk of adverse reactions.

In some instances, pre-exposure immunization should be boosted periodically in an effort to provide continuous protection (see TABLE 1); each booster immunization consists of a single dose. Serum antibody determinations before and after booster immunization may be helpful in determining both the need for a booster dose and the timing of such a dose.

TABLE 1 *Criteria for Pre-Exposure Immunization*

Risk Category and Nature of Risk	Typical Populations	Pre-exposure regimen
Continuous Virus present continuously, often in high concentrations. Aerolsol, mucous membrane, bite, or nonbite exposures may go unrecognized.	Rabies reserch lab workers,* rabies biologics production workers.	Primary course. Serologic testing every 6 months; booster vaccination when antibody level falls below acceptable level.*
Frequent Exposure usually episodic, with source recognized, but exposure may also be unrecognized. Aerosol, mucous membrane, bite or nonbite exposure.	Rabies diagnostic lab workers,* spelunkers, veterinarians and staff, and animal-control and wildlife workers in rabies enzootic areas. Travelers visiting foreign areas of enzootic rabies for more than 30 days.	Piamry course. Booster vaccination or serologic testing every 2 years.†
Infrequent (greater than population-at-large). Exposure nearly always episodic with source recognized. Mucous membrane, bite, or nonbite exposure.	Veterinarians and animal-control and wildlife workers in areas of low rabies enzooticity. Veterinary students.	Primary course. No routine booster vaccination or serologic testing.†
Rare (population-at-large). Exposures always episodic. Mucous membrane, or bite with source unrecognized.	US population-at-large, including individuals in rabies epizootic areas.	No vaccination necessary.

Adapted from the recommendations of the Immunization Practices Advisory Committee (ACIP) on rabies prevention. MMWR, 1991;40 (Suppl. RR-3): 1-19.

* Judgment of relative risk and extra monitoring of vaccination status of laboratory workers is the responsibility of the laboratory supervisor (see US Department of Health and Human Service's Biosafety in Microbiological and Biomedical Laboratories, 1984).

† Minimal acceptable antibody level is complete virus neutralization at a 1:5 serum dilution by RFFIT. Booster dose should be administered if the titer falls below this level.

POST-EXPOSURE IMMUNIZATION

See TABLE 2.

The following recommendations are only a guide. In applying them, take into account the animal species involved, the circumstances of the bite or other exposure, the immunization status of the animal, and presence of rabies in the region (as outlined in TABLE 2). Local or state public health officials should be consulted if questions arise about the need for rabies prophylaxis [23].

In the US, the following factors should be considered before antirabies treatment is initiated.

TABLE 2 *Rabies Post-Exposure Prophylaxis Guide (Advisory Committee on Immunization Practices [ACIP])* [23]

Animal type	Evaluation and disposition of animal	Post-exposure prophylaxis recommendations
Dogs and cats		
	Healthy and available for 10 days observation	Should not begin prophylaxis unless animal develops symptoms of rabies*
	Rabid or suspected rabid	Immediate Immunization
	Unknown (escaped)	Consult public health officials
Skunks, raccoons, bats, foxes, and most other carnivores; woodchucks		
	Regarded as rabid unless geographic area is known to be free of rabies or until animal proven negative by laboratory tests†	Immediate Immunization
Livestock, rodents, and lagomorphs (rabbits and hares)		
	Consider individually	Consult public health officials. Bites of squirrels, hamsters, guinea pigs, gerbils, chipmunks, rats, mice, other rodents, rabbits, and hares almost never require antirabies treatment

* During the 10 day holding period, begin treatment with HRIG and RabAvert rabies vaccine at first sign of rabies in a dog or cat that has bitten someone. The symptomatic animal should be killed immediately and tested.

† The animal should be killed and tested as soon as possible. Holding for observation is not recommended. Discontinue vaccine if immunofluorescence test results of the animal are negative.

Species of Biting Animal

Carnivorous wild animals (especially skunks, raccoons, foxes and coyotes) and bats are the animals most commonly infected with rabies and have caused most of the indigenous cases of human rabies in the US since 1960. Unless an animal is tested and shown not to be rabid, post-exposure prophylaxis should be initiated upon bite or nonbite exposure to the animals. (See definition in "Type of Exposure" below) If treatment has been initiated and subsequent testing in a qualified laboratory shows the exposing animal is not rabid, treatment can be discontinued[23].

The likelihood that a domestic dog or cat is infected with rabies varies from region to region; hence the need for post-exposure prophylaxis also varies[23].

Rodents (such as squirrels, hamsters, guinea pigs, gerbils, chipmunks, rats, and mice) and lagomorphs (including rabbits and hares) are rarely found to be infected with rabies and have not been known to cause human rabies in the US. In these cases, the state or local health department should be consulted before a decision is made to initiate post-exposure antirabies prophylaxis[23].

Circumstances of Biting Incident

An UNPROVOKED attack is more likely than a provoked attack to indicate the animal is rabid. Bites inflicted on a person attempting to feed or handle an apparently healthy animal should generally be regarded as PROVOKED.

Type of Exposure

Rabies is transmitted by introducing the virus into open cuts or wounds in skin or via mucous membranes. The likelihood of rabies infection varies with the nature and extent of exposure. Two categories of exposure should be considered:

Bite: Any penetration of the skin by teeth. Bites to the face and hands carry the highest risk, but the site of the bite should not influence the decision to begin treatment [23].

Nonbite: Scratches, abrasions, open wounds, or mucous membranes contaminated with saliva or other potentially infectious material, such as brain tissue, from a rabid animal. Casual contact, such as petting a rabid animal (without a bite or nonbite exposure as described above), does not constitute an exposure and is not an indication for prophylaxis. There have been two instances of airborne rabies acquired in laboratories and two probable airborne rabies cases acquired in a bat-infested cave in Texas[23].

The only documented cases for rabies from human-to-human transmission occurred in four patients in the US and overseas who received corneas transplanted from persons who died of rabies undiagnosed at the time of death[2]. Stringent guidelines for acceptance of donor corneas should reduce this risk.

Bite and nonbite exposure from humans with rabies theoretically could transmit rabies, although no cases of rabies acquired this way have been documented. Each potential exposure to human rabies should be carefully evaluated to minimize unnecessary rabies prophylaxis [23].

Post-Exposure Immunization Schedule

The essential components of rabies post-exposure prophylaxis are prompt local treatment of wounds and immunization, including administration, in most instances of both globulin and vaccine (TABLE 2).

A complete course of post-exposure immunization for previously unvaccinated adults and children consists of a total of 5 doses, each 1.0 ml: one IM injection on each of days 0, 3, 7, 14 and 28.

1. Local Treatment of Wounds

Immediate and thorough washing of all bite wounds and scratches with soap and water is an important measure for preventing rabies. In animal studies, simple local wound cleansing has been shown to reduce markedly the likelihood of rabies. Whenever possible, bite injuries should not be sutured to avoid further and/or deeper contamination. Tetanus prophylaxis and measures to control bacteria infection should be given as indicated[23].

2. Specific Treatment of Rabies

The injection schedule for post-exposure prophylaxis depends on whether the patient has had or has not had previous immunization against rabies. For persons who have not previously been immunized against rabies, the schedule consists of an initial injection IM of HRIG exactly 20 IU per kilogram body weight in total. If anatomically feasible, up to half of the dose of HRIG should be thoroughly infiltrated in and around the wound(s) and the remainder should be administered IM in the-gluteal region. HRIG is administered only once (for specific instructions for HRIG use, see the product package insert). The HRIG injection is followed by a series of 5 individual injections of rabies vaccine (1.0 ml each) given IM on days 0, 3, 7, 14 and 28. Administration of HRIG and rabies vaccine should be given at separate sites using separate syringes. Post-exposure rabies prophylaxis should begin the same day exposure occurred or as soon after exposure as possible. The combined use of HRIG and rabies vaccine is recommended for both bite and non-bite exposures, regardless of the interval between exposure and initiation of treatment.

In the event that HRIG is not readily available for the initiation of treatment, it can be given through the seventh day after administration of the first dose of vaccine. HRIG is not indicated beyond the seventh day because an antibody response to rabies vaccine is presumed to have begun by that time[23].

The sooner treatment is begun after exposure, the better. However, there have been instances in which the decision to begin treatment was made as late as 6 months or longer after exposure due to delay in recognition that an exposure had occurred. Post-exposure antirabies immunization should always include administration of both passive antibody and immunization with the exception of persons who have previously received complete immunization regimens (pre-exposure or post-exposure) with a cell culture vaccine, or persons who have been immunized with other types of vaccines and have had documented rabies antibody titers. Persons who have previously received rabies immunization should receive 2 IM doses of rabies vaccine: 1 on day 0 and another on day 3. They should not be given HRIG.

3. Treatment Outside the US

If post-exposure immunization is begun outside the US with regimens or products that are not used in the US, it may be desirable to provide additional treatment when the patient reaches the US State or local health departments should be contacted for specific advice in such cases [23].

CONTRAINDICATIONS

In view of the almost invariably fatal outcome of rabies, there is no contraindication to post-exposure immunization.

However, if an alternative product (*e.g.*, HDCV or Rabies Vaccine Absorbed [RVA]) is not available, care should be taken if the vaccine is to be administered to persons known to be sensitive to processed bovine gelatin, chicken protein, neomycin, chlortetracycline and amphotericin B in trace amounts, which may be present in the vaccine and may cause an allergic reaction in such individuals.

WARNINGS

Serious systemic anaphylactic reactions have been reported and neuroparalytic events have been reported in temporal association with rabies vaccine administration. Against the background of 11.8 million doses distributed worldwide as of June 30, 1995, 10 cases of encephalitis (1 death) or meningitis, 7 cases of transient paralysis (including 2 cases of Guillain-Barré Syndrome), 1 case of myelitis, 1 case of retrobulbar neuritis, and 2 cases of suspected multiple sclerosis have been temporally associated with the use of rabies vaccine. Also 2 cases of anaphylactic shock have been reported. Such events pose a dilemma for the attending physician. A patient's risk of developing rabies must be carefully considered, however, before deciding to discontinue immunization.

RABIES VACCINE MUST NOT BE USED SUBCUTANEOUSLY OR INTRADERMALLY!

Rabies vaccine must be injected intramuscularly. For adults, the deltoid area is the preferred site of immunization; for small children, administration into the anterolateral zone of the thigh is preferred. The use of the gluteal region should be avoided, since administration in this area may result in lower neutralizing antibody titers [2].

DO NOT INJECT INTRAVASCULARLY!

Unintentional intravascular injection may result in systemic reactions, including shock. Immediate measures include catecholamines, volume replacement, high doses of corticosteroids, and oxygen.

Development of active immunity after vaccination may be impaired in immune-compromised individuals.

DOSAGE AND ADMINISTRATION

The individual dose is 1 ml, given intramuscularly.

Administer in adults by IM injection into the deltoid muscle or, in the case of small children, into the anterolateral zone of the thigh. The gluteal area should be avoided for vaccine injections, since administration in this area may result in lower neutralizing antibody titers. Care should be taken to avoid injection into or near blood vessels and nerves. After aspiration, if blood or any suspicious discoloration appears in the syringe, do not inject but discard contents and repeat procedure using a new dose of vaccine, at a different site.

INSTRUCTIONS FOR RECONSTITUTING RABIES VACCINE

Using the longer of the 2 needles supplied, transfer the entire contents of the diluent vial into the vaccine vial. Mix gently to avoid foaming. The white, freeze-dried vaccine dissolves to give a clear or slightly opaque suspension. Withdraw the total amount of dissolved vaccine into the syringe and replace the long needle with the smaller needle for IM injection. The reconstituted vaccine should be used immediately.

Parenteral drug products should be inspected visually for particulate matter and discoloration prior to administration. If either of these conditions exists, the vaccine should not be administered. A separate, sterile syringe and needle or a sterile disposable unit should be used for each patient to prevent transmission of hepatitis and other infectious agents from person to person. Needles should not be recapped and should be properly disposed of. No

R

data are available regarding the concurrent administration of rabies vaccine with other vaccines.

PEDIATRIC USE

Children and adults receive the same dose of 1 ml, given IM.

Only limited data on the safety and efficacy of rabies vaccine in the pediatric age group are available. However, in four studies some pre-exposure and post-exposure experience has been gained [17,31, 32,33].

Pre-Exposure

Pre-exposure administration of rabies vaccine in 11 Thai children from the age of 2 years and older resulted in antibody levels higher than 0.5 IU/ml on day 14 in all children [32]. In another study in Mexico, 15/21 children aged 7-18 years had antibody titers of ≥0.5 IU/ml on day 14, and all 21 children had antibody titers of ≥0.5 IU/ml on day 30. Only mild local pain was noted in approximately one-quarter of the children [33].

Post-Exposure

In a 10 year serosurveillance study, rabies vaccine has been administered to 91 children aged 1-5 years and 436 children and adolescents aged 6-20 years [17]. The vaccine was effective in both age groups. None of these patients developed rabies.

One (1) newborn has received rabies vaccine on an immunization schedule of days 0, 3, 7,14 and 30; the antibody concentration on day 37 was 2.34 IU/ml. There were no clinically significant adverse events[31].

PRE-EXPOSURE DOSAGE

1. Primary Immunization: In the US, the Advisory Committee on Immunization Practices (ACIP) recommends three injections of 1.0 ml each: one injection on day 0 and one on day 7, and one either on day 21 or 28 (for criteria for pre-exposure immunization, see TABLE 1).

2. Booster Immunization: The individual booster dose is 1 ml, given intramuscularly. Booster immunization is given to persons who have received previous rabies immunization and remain at increased risk of rabies exposure by reasons of occupation.

Persons who work with live rabies virus in research laboratories or vaccine production facilities (continuous-risk category: see TABLE 1) should have a serum sample tested for rabies antibodies every 6 months. Booster doses of vaccine should be given to maintain a serum titer >1:5 serum dilution by the RFFIT.

The frequent-risk category includes other laboratory workers such as those doing rabies diagnostic testing, spelunkers, veterinarians and staff, animal-control and wildlife officers in areas where rabies is epizootic, and international travelers living or visiting (for >30 days) in areas where canine rabies is endemic. Persons among this group should have a serum sample tested for rabies antibodies every 2 years and, if the titer is less than complete neutralization at 1:5 serum dilution by RFFIT, should have a booster dose of vaccine. Alternatively, a booster can be administered in the absence of a titer determination.

Veterinarians and animal-control and wildlife officers working in areas of low rabies enzooticity (infrequent exposure group) do not require routine pre-exposure booster doses of rabies vaccine after completion of a full primary pre-exposure immunization scheme (TABLE 1).

POST-EXPOSURE DOSAGE

Immunization should begin as soon as possible after exposure. A complete course of immunization consists of a total of 5 injections of 1 ml each: one injection on each of days 0, 3, 7,14 and 28 in conjunction with the administration of HRIG on day 0. For children, see Pediatric Use.

Begin with the administration of HRIG. Give 20 IU/kg body weight.

This formula is applicable to all age groups, including children. The recommended dosage of HRIG should not exceed 20 IU/kg body weight because it may otherwise interfere with active antibody production. Since vaccine-induced antibody appears within 1 week, HRIG is not indicated more than 7 days after initiating post-exposure immunization with rabies vaccine. If possible, up to one-half the dose of HRIG should be thoroughly infiltrated in the area around the wound and the rest should be administered IM, in a different site from the rabies vaccine, preferably in the gluteal area.

Because the antibody response following the recommended immunization regimen with rabies vaccine has been satisfactory, routine post-immunization serologic testing is not recommended. Serologic testing is indicated in unusual circumstances, as when the patient is known to be immunosuppressed. Contact state health department or CDC for recommendations.

POST-EXPOSURE THERAPY OF PREVIOUSLY IMMUNIZED PERSONS

When rabies exposure occurs in an immunized person who was vaccinated according to the recommended regimen with rabies vaccine or other tissue culture vaccines or who had previously demonstrated rabies antibody, that person should receive two IM doses (1.0 ml each) of rabies vaccine: one immediately and one 3 days later. HRIG should not be given in these cases. Persons should be considered to have been immunized previously if they received pre- or post-exposure prophylaxis with rabies vaccine or other tissue culture vaccines or have been documented to have had an adequate antibody response to duck embryo rabies vaccine. If the immune status of a previously vaccinated person is not known, full primary post-exposure antirabies treatment (HRIG plus 5 doses of vaccine) may be necessary. In such cases, if antibodies can be demonstrated in a serum sample collected before vaccine is given, treatment can be discontinued after at least 2 doses of vaccine.

PRODUCT LISTING - EQUIVALENTS NOT AVAILABLE

Powder For Injection - Intramuscular - Strength n/a

1's	$144.06	RABAVERT, Chiron Therapeutics	53905-0501-01
1's	$146.10	RABAVERT, Physicians Total Care	54868-4340-00
1's	$160.59	IMOVAX RABIES, Aventis Pharmaceuticals	49281-0250-10

Suspension - Intradermal - Strength n/a

1's	$90.63	IMOVAX RABIES I.D., Allscripts Pharmaceutical Company	54569-4314-00
1's	$118.25	IMOVAX RABIES I.D., Aventis Pharmaceuticals	49281-0251-20

Raloxifene Hydrochloride *(003370)*

Categories: Osteoporosis; FDA Approved 1997 Dec; Pregnancy Category X
Drug Classes: Estrogen receptor modulators, selective; Hormones/hormone modifiers
Brand Names: Evista
Foreign Brand Availability: Bonmax (India); Celvista (Thailand); Optruma (Austria; Belgium; Bulgaria; Czech-Republic; Denmark; England; Finland; France; Germany; Greece; Hungary; Ireland; Italy; Netherlands; Norway; Poland; Portugal; Slovenia; Spain; Sweden; Switzerland; Turkey)
Cost of Therapy: $77.63 (Osteoporosis; Evista; 60 mg; 1 tablet/day; 30 day supply)

DESCRIPTION

Raloxifene hydrochloride is a selective estrogen receptor modulator (SERM) that belongs to the benzothiophene class of compounds.

The chemical designation is methanone, [6-hydroxy-2-(4-hydroxyphenyl)benzo[*b*]thien-3-yl]-[4-[2-(1-piperidinyl)ethoxy]phenyl]-, hydrochloride. Raloxifene hydrochloride (HCl) has the empirical formula $C_{28}H_{27}NO_4S$-HCl, which corresponds to a molecular weight of 510.05. Raloxifene HCl is an off-white to pale-yellow solid that is very slightly soluble in water.

Evista is supplied in a tablet dosage form for oral administration. Each Evista tablet contains 60 mg of raloxifene HCl, which is the molar equivalent of 55.71 mg of free base. Inactive ingredients include anhydrous lactose, carnauba wax, crospovidone, FD&C blue no. 2 aluminum lake, hydroxypropyl methylcellulose, lactose monohydrate, magnesium stearate, modified pharmaceutical glaze, polyethylene glycol, polysorbate 80, povidone, propylene glycol, and titanium dioxide.

CLINICAL PHARMACOLOGY

MECHANISM OF ACTION

Decreases in estrogen levels after oophorectomy or menopause lead to increases in bone resorption and accelerated bone loss. Bone is initially lost rapidly because the compensatory increase in bone formation is inadequate to offset resorptive losses. In addition to loss of estrogen, this imbalance between resorption and formation may be due to age-related impairment of osteoblasts or their precursors. In some women, these changes will eventually lead to decreased bone mass, osteoporosis, and increased risk for fractures, particularly of the spine, hip, and wrist. Vertebral fractures are the most common type of osteoporotic fracture in postmenopausal women.

The biological actions of raloxifene are largely mediated through binding to estrogen receptors. This binding results in activation of certain estrogenic pathways and blockade of others. Thus, raloxifene is a SERM.

Raloxifene decreases resorption of bone and reduces biochemical markers of bone turnover to the premenopausal range. These effects on bone are manifested as reductions in the serum and urine levels of bone turnover markers, decreases in bone resorption based on radiocalcium kinetics studies, increases in bone mineral density (BMD) and decreases in incidence of fractures. Raloxifene also has effects on lipid metabolism. Raloxifene decreases total and LDL cholesterol levels but does not increase triglyceride levels (see PRECAUTIONS). It does not change total HDL cholesterol levels. Preclinical data demonstrate that raloxifene is an estrogen antagonist in uterine and breast tissues. Clinical trial data (through a median of 42 months) suggest that raloxifene HCl lacks estrogen-like effects on the uterus and breast tissue.

PHARMACOKINETICS

The disposition of raloxifene has been evaluated in more than 3000 postmenopausal women in selected raloxifene osteoporosis treatment and prevention clinical trials using a population approach. Pharmacokinetic data were also obtained in conventional pharmacology studies in 292 postmenopausal women. Raloxifene exhibits high within-subject variability (approximately 30% coefficient of variation) of most pharmacokinetic parameters. TABLE 1 summarizes the pharmacokinetic parameters of raloxifene.

Absorption

Raloxifene is absorbed rapidly after oral administration. Approximately 60% of an oral dose is absorbed, but presystemic glucuronide conjugation is extensive. Absolute bioavailability of raloxifene is 2.0%. The time to reach average maximum plasma concentration and bioavailability are functions of systemic interconversion and enterohepatic cycling of raloxifene and its glucuronide metabolites.

Administration of raloxifene HCl with a standardized, high-fat meal increases the absorption of raloxifene (C_{max} 28% and AUC 16%), but does not lead to clinically meaningful changes in systemic exposure. Raloxifene HCl can be administered without regard to meals.

Distribution

Following oral administration of single doses ranging from 30-150 mg of raloxifene HCl, the apparent volume of distribution is 2348 L/kg and is not dose dependent.

Raloxifene and the monoglucuronide conjugates are highly (95%) bound to plasma proteins. Raloxifene binds to both albumin and α1-acid glycoprotein, but not to sex-steroid binding globulin.

Metabolism

Biotransformation and disposition of raloxifene in humans have been determined following oral administration of ^{14}C-labeled raloxifene. Raloxifene undergoes extensive first-pass metabolism to the glucuronide conjugates: raloxifene-4′-glucuronide, raloxifene-6-glucuronide, and raloxifene-6,4′-diglucuronide. No other metabolites have been detected, providing strong evidence that raloxifene is not metabolized by cytochrome P450 pathways. Unconjugated raloxifene comprises less than 1% of the total radiolabeled material in plasma. The terminal log-linear portions of the plasma concentration curves for raloxifene and the glucuronides are generally parallel. This is consistent with interconversion of raloxifene and the glucuronide metabolites.

Following intravenous administration, raloxifene is cleared at a rate approximating hepatic blood flow. Apparent oral clearance is 44.1 L/kg·h. Raloxifene and its glucuronide conjugates are interconverted by reversible systemic metabolism and enterohepatic cycling, thereby prolonging its plasma elimination half-life to 27.7 hours after oral dosing.

Results from single oral doses of raloxifene predict multiple-dose pharmacokinetics. Following chronic dosing, clearance ranges from 40-60 L/kg·h. Increasing doses of raloxifene HCl (ranging from 30-150 mg) result in slightly less than a proportional increase in the area under the plasma time concentration curve (AUC).

Excretion

Raloxifene is primarily excreted in feces, and less than 0.2% is excreted unchanged in urine. Less than 6% of the raloxifene dose is eliminated in urine as glucuronide conjugates.

TABLE 1 *Summary of Raloxifene Pharmacokinetic Parameters in the Healthy Postmenopausal Woman*

	C_{max}* (ng/ml)/(mg/kg)	$T_{½}$ (h)	AUC (0-∞)* (ng·h/ml)/(mg/kg)	CL/F (L/kg·h)	V/F (L/kg)
Single Dose					
Mean	0.50	27.7	27.2	44.1	2348
CV (%)	52	10.7-273†	44	46	52
Multiple Dose					
Mean	1.36	32.5	24.2	47.4	2853
CV (%)	37	15.8-86.6†	36	41	56

Abbreviations: C_{max} = maximum plasma concentration, $T_{½}$ = half-life, AUC = area under the curve, CL = clearance, V = volume of distribution, F = bioavailability, CV = coefficient of variation.
* Data normalized for dose in mg and body weight in kg.
† Range of observed half-life.

Special Populations

Geriatric

No differences in raloxifene pharmacokinetics were detected with regard to age (range 42-84 years).

Pediatric

The pharmacokinetics of raloxifene have not been evaluated in a pediatric population.

Gender

Total extent of exposure and oral clearance, normalized for lean body weight, are not significantly different between age-matched female and male volunteers.

Race

Pharmacokinetic differences due to race have been studied in 1712 women including 97.5% Caucasian, 1.0% Asian, 0.7% Hispanic, and 0.5% Black in the osteoporosis treatment trial and in 1053 women including 93.5% Caucasian, 4.3% Hispanic, 1.2% Asian, and 0.5% Black in the osteoporosis prevention trials. There were no discernible differences in raloxifene plasma concentrations among these groups; however, the influence of race cannot be conclusively determined.

Renal Insufficiency

Since negligible amounts of raloxifene are eliminated in urine, a study in patients with renal insufficiency was not conducted. In the osteoporosis treatment and prevention trials, raloxifene and metabolite concentrations in women with estimated creatinine clearance as low as 21 ml/min are similar to women with normal creatinine clearance.

Hepatic Dysfunction

Raloxifene was studied, as a single dose, in Child-Pugh Class A patients with cirrhosis and total serum bilirubin ranging from 0.6-2.0 mg/dl. Plasma raloxifene concentrations were approximately 2.5 times higher than in controls and correlated with bilirubin concentrations. Safety and efficacy have not been evaluated further in patients with hepatic insufficiency (see WARNINGS).

Drug-Drug Interactions

Clinically significant drug-drug interactions are discussed in DRUG INTERACTIONS.

Ampicillin and Amoxicillin

Peak concentrations of raloxifene and the overall extent of absorption are reduced 28% and 14%, respectively, with co-administration of ampicillin. These reductions are consistent with decreased enterohepatic cycling associated with antibiotic reduction of enteric bacteria. However, the systemic exposure and the elimination rate of raloxifene were not affected. Therefore, raloxifene HCl can be concurrently administered with ampicillin. In the osteoporosis treatment trial, co-administration of amoxicillin had no discernable differences in plasma raloxifene concentrations.

Antacids

Concurrent administration of calcium carbonate or aluminum and magnesium hydroxide-containing antacids does not affect the systemic exposure of raloxifene.

Corticosteroids

The chronic administration of raloxifene in postmenopausal women has no effect on the pharmacokinetics of methylprednisolone given as a single oral dose.

Cholestyramine

See DRUG INTERACTIONS.

Cyclosporine

The co-administration of raloxifene HCl with cyclosporine has not been evaluated.

Digoxin

Raloxifene has no effect on the pharmacokinetics of digoxin.

Warfarin

See DRUG INTERACTIONS.

INDICATIONS AND USAGE

Raloxifene HCl is indicated for the treatment and prevention of osteoporosis in postmenopausal women.

For either osteoporosis treatment or prevention, supplemental calcium and/or vitamin D should be added to the diet if daily intake is inadequate.

Postmenopausal osteoporosis may be diagnosed by history or radiographic documentation of osteoporotic fracture, bone mineral densitometry, or physical signs of vertebral crush fractures (*e.g.*, height loss, dorsal kyphosis).

No single clinical finding or test result can quantify risk of postmenopausal osteoporosis with certainty. However, clinical assessment can help to identify women at increased risk. Widely accepted risk factors include Caucasian or Asian descent, slender body build, early estrogen deficiency, smoking, alcohol consumption, low calcium diet, sedentary lifestyle, and family history of osteoporosis. Evidence of increased bone turnover from serum and urine markers and low bone mass (*e.g.*, at least 1 standard deviation below the mean for healthy, young adult women) as determined by densitometric techniques are also predictive. The greater the number of clinical risk factors, the greater the probability of developing postmenopausal osteoporosis.

NON-FDA APPROVED INDICATIONS

Results from osteoporosis prevention studies in postmenopausal women demonstrate that raloxifene reduces the incidence of estrogen receptor-positive breast cancers and may decrease or not increase the risk of endometrial cancer. Long term results are under study. Clinical studies will evaluate raloxifene as a chemopreventive agent for premenopausal women at high risk for developing breast cancer.

CONTRAINDICATIONS

Raloxifene HCl is contraindicated in lactating women or women who are or may become pregnant. Raloxifene HCl may cause fetal harm when administered to a pregnant woman. In rabbit studies, abortion and a low rate of fetal heart anomalies (ventricular septal defects) occurred in rabbits at doses ≥0.1 mg/kg (≥0.04 times the human dose based on surface area, mg/m^2), and hydrocephaly was observed in fetuses at doses ≥10 mg/kg (≥4 times the human dose based on surface area, mg/m^2). In rat studies, retardation of fetal development and developmental abnormalities (wavy ribs, kidney cavitation) occurred at doses ≥1 mg/kg (≥0.2 times the human dose based on surface area, mg/m^2). Treatment of rats at doses of 0.1 to 10 mg/kg (0.02-1.6 times the human dose based on surface area, mg/m^2) during gestation and lactation produced effects that included delayed and disrupted parturition; decreased neonatal survival and altered physical development; sex- and age-specific reductions in growth and changes in pituitary hormone content; and decreased lymphoid compartment size in offspring. At 10 mg/kg, raloxifene disrupted parturition which resulted in maternal and progeny death and morbidity. Effects in adult offspring (4 months of age) included uterine hypoplasia and reduced fertility; however, no ovarian or vaginal pathology was observed. The patient should be apprised of the potential hazard to the fetus if this drug is used during pregnancy, or if the patient becomes pregnant while taking this drug.

Raloxifene HCl is contraindicated in women with active or past history of venous thromboembolic events, including deep vein thrombosis, pulmonary embolism, and retinal vein thrombosis.

Raloxifene HCl is contraindicated in women known to be hypersensitive to raloxifene or other constituents of the tablets.

WARNINGS

VENOUS THROMBOEMBOLISM

In clinical trials, raloxifene HCl-treated women had an increased risk of venous thromboembolism (deep vein thrombosis and pulmonary embolism). Other venous thromboembolic events could also occur. A less serious event, superficial thrombophlebitis, also has been reported more frequently with raloxifene HCl. The greatest risk for deep vein thrombosis and pulmonary embolism occurs during the first 4 months of treatment, and the magnitude of risk appears to be similar to the reported risk associated with use of hormone replacement therapy. Because immobilization increases the risk for venous thromboembolic events independent of therapy, raloxifene HCl should be discontinued at least 72 hours prior to and during prolonged immobilization (*e.g.*, post-surgical recovery, prolonged bed rest), and raloxifene HCl therapy should be resumed only after the patient is fully ambulatory. In addition, women taking raloxifene HCl should be advised to move about periodically during prolonged travel. The risk-benefit balance should be considered in women at risk of thromboembolic disease for other reasons, such as congestive heart failure, superficial thrombophlebitis and active malignancy.

PREMENOPAUSAL USE

There is no indication for premenopausal use of raloxifene HCl. Safety of raloxifene HCl in premenopausal women has not been established and its use is not recommended (see CONTRAINDICATIONS).

R

HEPATIC DYSFUNCTION

Raloxifene was studied, as a single dose, in Child-Pugh Class A patients with cirrhosis and serum total bilirubin ranging from 0.6-2.0 mg/dl. Plasma raloxifene concentrations were approximately 2.5 times higher than in controls and correlated with total bilirubin concentrations. Safety and efficacy have not been evaluated further in patients with severe hepatic insufficiency.

PRECAUTIONS

GENERAL

Concurrent Estrogen Therapy

The concurrent use of raloxifene HCl and systemic estrogen or hormone replacement therapy (ERT or HRT) has not been studied in prospective clinical trials and therefore concomitant use of raloxifene HCl with systemic estrogens is not recommended.

Lipid Metabolism

Raloxifene HCl lowers serum total and LDL cholesterol by 6-11%, but does not affect serum concentrations of total HDL cholesterol or triglycerides. These effects should be taken into account in therapeutic decisions for patients who may require therapy for hyperlipidemia.

Limited clinical data suggest that some women with a history of marked hypertriglyceridemia (>5.6 mmol/L or >500 mg/dl) in response to treatment with oral estrogen or estrogen plus progestin may develop increased levels of triglycerides when treated with raloxifene HCl. Women with this medical history should have serum triglycerides monitored when taking raloxifene HCl.

Concurrent use of raloxifene HCl and lipid-lowering agents has not been studied.

Endometrium

Raloxifene HCl has not been associated with endometrial proliferation (see ADVERSE REACTIONS). Unexplained uterine bleeding should be investigated as clinically indicated.

Breast

Raloxifene HCl has not been associated with breast enlargement, breast pain, or an increased risk of breast cancer (see ADVERSE REACTIONS). Any unexplained breast abnormality occurring during raloxifene HCl therapy should be investigated.

History of Breast Cancer

Raloxifene HCl has not been adequately studied in women with a prior history of breast cancer.

Use in Men

Safety and efficacy have not been evaluated in men.

INFORMATION FOR THE PATIENT

For safe and effective use of raloxifene HCl, the physician should inform patients about the following:

Patient immobilization: Raloxifene HCl should be discontinued at least 72 hours prior to and during prolonged immobilization (*e.g.*, post-surgical recovery, prolonged bed rest), and patients should be advised to avoid prolonged restrictions of movement during travel because of the increased risk of venous thromboembolic events.

Hot flashes or flushes: Raloxifene HCl may increase the incidence of hot flashes and is not effective in reducing hot flashes or flushes associated with estrogen deficiency. In some asymptomatic patients, hot flashes may occur upon beginning raloxifene HCl therapy.

Other osteoporosis treatment and prevention measures: Patients should be instructed to take supplemental calcium and/or vitamin D, if daily dietary intake is inadequate. Weight-bearing exercise should be considered along with the modification of certain behavioral factors, such as cigarette smoking, and/or alcohol consumption, if these factors exist.

Physicians should instruct their patients to read the patient package insert before starting therapy with raloxifene HCl and to re-read it each time the prescription is renewed.

CARCINOGENESIS, MUTAGENESIS, AND IMPAIRMENT OF FERTILITY

Carcinogenesis

In a 21 month carcinogenicity study in mice, there was an increased incidence of ovarian tumors in female animals given 9-242 mg/kg, which included benign and malignant tumors of granulosa/theca cell origin and benign tumors of epithelial cell origin. Systemic exposure (AUC) of raloxifene in this group was 0.3 to 34 times that in postmenopausal women administered a 60 mg dose. There was also an increased incidence of testicular interstitial cell tumors and prostatic adenomas and adenocarcinomas in male mice given 41 or 210 mg/kg (4.7 or 24 times the AUC in humans), and prostatic leiomyoblastoma in male mice given 210 mg/kg.

In a 2 year carcinogenicity study in rats, an increased incidence in ovarian tumors of granulosa/theca cell origin was observed in female rats given 279 mg/kg (approximately 400 times the AUC in humans). The female rodents in these studies were treated during their reproductive lives when their ovaries were functional and responsive to hormonal stimulation.

Mutagenesis

Raloxifene HCl was not genotoxic in any of the following test systems: the Ames test for bacterial mutagenesis with and without metabolic activation, the unscheduled DNA synthesis assay in rat hepatocytes, the mouse lymphoma assay for mammalian cell mutation, the chromosomal aberration assay in Chinese hamster ovary cells, the *in vivo* sister chromatid exchange assay in Chinese hamsters, and the *in vivo* micronucleus test in mice.

Impairment of Fertility

When male and female rats were given daily doses ≥5 mg/kg (≥0.8 times the human dose based on surface area, mg/m^2) prior to and during mating, no pregnancies occurred. In male rats, daily doses up to 100 mg/kg (16 times the human dose based on surface area, mg/m^2) for at least 2 weeks did not affect sperm production or quality, or reproductive performance. In female rats, at doses of 0.1 to 10 mg/kg/day (0.02-1.6 times the human dose based on surface area, mg/m^2), raloxifene disrupted estrous cycles and inhibited ovulation. These effects of raloxifene were reversible. In another study in rats in which raloxifene was given during the preimplantation period at doses ≥0.1 mg/kg (≥0.02 times the human dose based on surface area, mg/m^2), raloxifene delayed and disrupted embryo implantation resulting in prolonged gestation and reduced litter size. The reproductive and developmental effects observed in animals are consistent with the estrogen receptor activity of raloxifene.

PREGNANCY CATEGORY X

Raloxifene HCl should not be used in women who are or may become pregnant (see CONTRAINDICATIONS).

NURSING MOTHERS

Raloxifene HCl should not be used by lactating women (see CONTRAINDICATIONS). It is not known whether raloxifene is excreted in human milk.

PEDIATRIC USE

Raloxifene HCl should not be used in pediatric patients.

GERIATRIC USE

In the osteoporosis treatment trial of 7705 postmenopausal women, 4621 women were considered geriatric (greater than 65 years old). Of these, 845 women were greater than 75 years old. Safety and efficacy in older and younger postmenopausal women in the osteoporosis treatment trial appeared to be comparable.

DRUG INTERACTIONS

CHOLESTYRAMINE

Cholestyramine, an anion exchange resin, causes a 60% reduction in the absorption and enterohepatic cycling of raloxifene after a single dose. Co-administration of cholestyramine with raloxifene HCl is not recommended. Although not specifically studied, it is anticipated that other anion exchange resins would have a similar effect.

WARFARIN

In vitro, raloxifene did not interact with the binding of warfarin. The co-administration of raloxifene HCl and warfarin, a coumarin derivative, has been assessed in a single dose study. In this study, raloxifene had no effect on the pharmacokinetics of warfarin. However, a 10% decrease in prothrombin time was observed in the single-dose study. If raloxifene HCl is given concurrently with warfarin or other coumarin derivatives, prothrombin time should be monitored more closely when starting or stopping therapy with raloxifene HCl. In the osteoporosis treatment trial, there were no clinically relevant effects of warfarin co-administration on plasma concentrations of raloxifene.

OTHER HIGHLY PROTEIN-BOUND DRUGS

Raloxifene is more than 95% bound to plasma proteins. Other highly protein-bound drugs should not cause clinically relevant changes in raloxifene HCl plasma concentrations. Furthermore, in the osteoporosis treatment trial, there were no clinically relevant effects of co-administration of other highly protein-bound drugs (*e.g.*, gemfibrozil) on plasma concentrations of raloxifene. *In vitro,* raloxifene did not interact with the binding of phenytoin, tamoxifen, or warfarin (see above). Although not examined, raloxifene HCl might affect the protein binding of other drugs and should be used with caution with certain other highly protein-bound drugs such as diazepam, diazoxide and lidocaine.

ADVERSE REACTIONS

ADVERSE EVENTS IN THE OSTEOPOROSIS TREATMENT CLINICAL TRIAL

The safety of raloxifene in the treatment of osteoporosis was assessed in a large (7705 patients) multinational placebo-controlled trial. Duration of treatment was 36 months and 5129 postmenopausal women were exposed to raloxifene (2557 received 60 mg/day and 2572 received 120 mg/day).

The majority of adverse events occurring during the study were mild and generally did not require discontinuation of therapy.

Therapy was discontinued due to an adverse event in 10.9% of raloxifene HCl-treated women and 8.8% of placebo-treated women. Common adverse events considered to be related to raloxifene HCl therapy were hot flashes and leg cramps. Hot flashes were most commonly reported during the first 6 months of treatment and were not different from placebo thereafter.

ADVERSE EVENTS IN PLACEBO-CONTROLLED CLINICAL TRIALS TO SUPPORT THE OSTEOPOROSIS PREVENTION INDICATION

The safety of raloxifene has been assessed primarily in 12 Phase 2 and Phase 3 studies with placebo, estrogen, and estrogen-progestin replacement therapy (HRT) control groups. The duration of treatment ranged from 2-30 months and 2036 women were exposed to raloxifene (371 patients received 10-50 mg/day, 828 received 60 mg/day, and 837 received from 120-600 mg/day).

The majority of adverse events occurring during clinical trials were mild and generally did not require discontinuation of therapy.

Therapy was discontinued due to an adverse event in 11.4% of 581 raloxifene HCl-treated women and 12.2% of 584 placebo-treated women. Common adverse events considered to be drug-related were hot flashes and leg cramps (see TABLE 6). The first occurrence of hot flashes was most commonly reported during the first 6 months of treatment. Discontinuation rates due to hot flashes did not differ significantly between raloxifene HCl and placebo groups (1.7% and 2.2%, respectively).

TABLE 6 lists adverse events occurring in either the osteoporosis treatment or the prevention placebo-controlled clinical trial databases at a frequency ≥2.0% in either group and in more raloxifene HCl-treated women than in placebo-treated women. Adverse events are shown without attribution of causality.

TABLE 6 *Adverse Events Occurring in Placebo-Controlled Osteoporosis Clinical Trials at a Frequency ≥2.0% and in More Raloxifene HCl-Treated (60 mg Once Daily) Women Than Placebo-Treated Women*

	Treatment		Prevention	
	Raloxifene HCl	Placebo	Raloxifene HCl	Placebo
Body System	n=2557	n=2576	n=581	n=584
Body as a Whole				
Infection	A	A	15.1%	14.6%
Flu syndrome	13.5%	11.4%	14.6%	13.5%
Headache	9.2%	8.5%	A	A
Leg cramps	7.0%	3.7%	5.9%	1.9%
Chest pain	A	A	4.0%	3.6%
Fever	3.9%	3.8%	3.1%	2.6%
Cardiovascular System				
Hot flashes	9.7%	6.4%	24.6%	18.3%
Migraine	A	A	2.4%	2.1%
Syncope	2.3%	2.1%	B	B
Varicose vein	2.2%	1.5%	A	A
Digestive System				
Nausea	8.3%	7.8%	8.8%	8.6%
Diarrhea	7.2%	6.9%	A	A
Dyspepsia	A	A	5.9%	5.8%
Vomiting	4.8%	4.3%	3.4%	3.3%
Flatulence	A	A	3.1%	2.4%
Gastrointestinal disorder	A	A	3.3%	2.1%
Gastroenteritis	B	B	2.6%	2.1%
Metabolic and Nutritional				
Weight gain	A	A	8.8%	6.8%
Peripheral edema	5.2%	4.4%	3.3%	1.9%
Musculoskeletal System				
Arthralgia	15.5%	14.0%	10.7%	10.1%
Myalgia	A	A	7.7%	6.2%
Arthritis	A	A	4.0%	3.6%
Tendon disorder	3.6%	3.1%	A	A
Nervous System				
Depression	A	A	6.4%	6.0%
Insomnia	A	A	5.5%	4.3%
Vertigo	4.1%	3.7%	A	A
Neuralgia	2.4%	1.9%	B	B
Hypesthesia	2.1%	2.0%	B	B
Respiratory System				
Sinusitis	7.9%	7.5%	10.3%	6.5%
Rhinitis	10.2%	10.1%	A	A
Bronchitis	9.5%	8.6%	A	A
Pharyngitis	5.3%	5.1%	7.6%	7.2%
Cough increased	9.3%	9.2%	6.0%	5.7%
Pneumonia	A	A	2.6%	1.5%
Laryngitis	B	B	2.2%	1.4%
Skin and Appendages				
Rash	A	A	5.5%	3.8%
Sweating	2.5%	2.0%	3.1%	1.7%
Special Senses				
Conjunctivitis	2.2%	1.7%	A	A
Urogenital System				
Vaginitis	A	A	4.3%	3.6%
Urinary tract infection	A	A	4.0%	3.9%
Cystitis	4.6%	4.5%	3.3%	3.1%
Leukorrhea	A	A	3.3%	1.7%
Uterine disorder*†	3.3%	2.3%	A	A
Endometrial disorder*	B	B	3.1%	1.9%
Vaginal hemorrhage	2.5%	2.4%	A	A
Urinary tract disorder	2.5%	2.1%	A	A

A Placebo incidence greater than or equal to raloxifene HCl incidence.
B Less than 2% incidence and more frequent with raloxifene HCl.
* Treatment-emergent uterine-related adverse event, including only patients with an intact uterus: Prevention Trials: raloxifene HCl, n=354, placebo, n=364; Treatment Trial: raloxifene HCl, n=1948, placebo, n=1999.
† Actual terms most frequently referred to endometrial fluid.

COMPARISON OF RALOXIFENE HCl AND HORMONE REPLACEMENT THERAPY ADVERSE EVENTS

Raloxifene HCl was compared with estrogen-progestin replacement therapy (HRT) in three clinical trials for prevention of osteoporosis. TABLE 7 shows adverse events occurring more frequently in one treatment group and at an incidence ≥2.0% in any group. Adverse events are shown without attribution of causality.

LABORATORY CHANGES

The following changes in analyte concentrations are commonly observed during raloxifene HCl therapy: increased apolipoprotein A1; and reduced serum total cholesterol, LDL cholesterol, fibrinogen, apolipoprotein B, and lipoprotein (a). Raloxifene HCl modestly increases hormone-binding globulin concentrations, including sex steroid-binding globulin, thyroxine-binding globulin, and corticosteroid-binding globulin with corresponding increases in measured total hormone concentrations. There is no evidence that these changes in hormone-binding globulin concentrations affect concentrations of the corresponding free hormones.

There were small decreases in serum total calcium, inorganic phosphate, total protein, and albumin which were generally of lesser magnitude than decreases observed during ERT/HRT. Platelet count was also decreased slightly and was not different from ERT.

ADDITIONAL SAFETY INFORMATION

Incidences of estrogen-dependent carcinoma of the endometrium and breast are being evaluated across all completed and ongoing clinical trials involving 17,151 patients, of which at least 10,850 women have received at least one dose of raloxifene. These trials provided over 21,000 person-years of raloxifene exposure with a maximum exposure of 58 months.

Endometrium: Compared to placebo, raloxifene did not increase the risk of endometrial cancer.

Breast: Compared to placebo, raloxifene did not increase the risk of breast cancer.

TABLE 7 *Adverse Events Reported in the Clinical Trials for Osteoporosis Prevention With Raloxifene HCl (60 mg Once Daily) and Continuous Combined or Cyclic Estrogen Plus Progestin (HRT) at an Incidence ≥2.0% in any Treatment Group**

Adverse Event	Raloxifene HCl (n=317)	HRT-Continuous Combined‡ (n=96)	HRT-Cyclic§ (n=219)
Urogenital			
Breast pain	4.4%	37.5%	29.7%
Vaginal bleeding†	6.2%	64.2%	88.5%
Digestive			
Flatulence	1.6%	12.5%	6.4%
Cardiovascular			
Hot flashes	28.7%	3.1%	5.9%
Body as a Whole			
Infection	11.0%	0%	6.8%
Abdominal pain	6.6%	10.4%	18.7%
Chest pain	2.8%	0%	0.5%

* These data are from both blinded and open-label studies.
† Treatment-emergent uterine-related adverse event, including only patients with an intact uterus: raloxifene HCl, n=290, HRT-Continuous Combined, n=67, HRT-Cyclic, n=217.
‡ Continuous Combined HRT = 0.625 mg conjugated estrogens plus 2.5 mg medroxyprogesterone acetate.
§ Cyclic HRT = 0.625 mg conjugated estrogens for 28 days with concomitant 5 mg medroxyprogesterone acetate or 0.15 mg norgestrel on days 1-14 or 17-28.

POSTINTRODUCTION REPORTS

Adverse events reported since market introduction include: very rarely — retinal vein occlusion.

DOSAGE AND ADMINISTRATION

The recommended dosage is one 60 mg raloxifene HCl tablet daily which may be administered any time of day without regard to meals.

ANIMAL PHARMACOLOGY

The skeletal effects of raloxifene treatment were assessed in ovariectomized rats and monkeys. In rats, raloxifene prevented increased bone resorption and bone loss after ovariectomy. There were positive effects of raloxifene on bone strength, but the effects varied with time. Cynomolgus monkeys were treated with raloxifene or conjugated estrogens for 2 years. In terms of bone cycles, this is equivalent to approximately 6 years in humans. Raloxifene and estrogen suppressed bone turnover, and increased BMD in the lumbar spine and in the central cancellous bone of the proximal tibia. In this animal model, there was a positive correlation between vertebral compressive breaking force and BMD of the lumbar spine.

Histologic examination of bone from rats and monkeys treated with raloxifene showed no evidence of woven bone, marrow fibrosis, or mineralization defects.

These results are consistent with data from human studies of radiocalcium kinetics and markers of bone metabolism, and are consistent with the action of raloxifene HCl as a skeletal antiresorptive agent.

HOW SUPPLIED

Evista 60 mg tablets are white, elliptical, and film coated. They are imprinted on one side with "LILLY" and the tablet code "4165" in edible blue ink.

Storage: Store at controlled room temperature, 20-25°C (68-77°F).

PRODUCT LISTING - EQUIVALENTS NOT AVAILABLE

Tablet - Oral - 60 mg

30's	$63.38	EVISTA, Allscripts Pharmaceutical Company	54569-4628-00
30's	$77.63	EVISTA, Lilly, Eli and Company	00002-4165-30
100's	$258.76	EVISTA, Lilly, Eli and Company	00002-4165-02

Ramipril (003032)

For related information, see the comparative table section in Appendix A.

Categories: Myocardial infarction, prophylaxis; Stroke, prophylaxis; Heart failure, congestive; Hypertension, essential; Pregnancy Category D; FDA Approved 1991 Jan
Drug Classes: Angiotensin converting enzyme inhibitors
Brand Names: Altace
Foreign Brand Availability: Cardace (India); Corpril (Thailand); Delix (Germany); Hytren (Austria); Pramace (Sweden); Quark (Italy); Ramace (Australia; Belgium; Denmark; Finland; Korea; Mexico; Netherlands; Philippines; South-Africa; Thailand); Triatec (Denmark; France; Greece; Indonesia; Ireland; Italy; Portugal; Sweden; Switzerland); Tritace (Australia; Austria; Bahamas; Barbados; Belgium; Belize; Benin; Bermuda; Burkina-Faso; Colombia; Costa-Rica; Curacao; Czech-Republic; Denmark; Dominican-Republic; Ecuador; El-Salvador; England; Ethiopia; Gambia; Ghana; Guatemala; Guinea; Guyana; Honduras; Hong-Kong; Ireland; Ivory-Coast; Jamaica; Kenya; Korea; Liberia; Malawi; Mali; Mauritania; Mauritius; Mexico; Morocco; Netherland-Antilles; Netherlands; Nicaragua; Niger; Nigeria; Panama; Philippines; Senegal; Seychelles; Sierra-Leone; South-Africa; Sudan; Surinam; Taiwan; Tanzania; Trinidad; Tunia; Uganda; Zambia; Zimbabwe); Unipril (Italy); Vesdil (Germany)
Cost of Therapy: $37.88 (Hypertension; Altace; 2.5 mg; 1 capsule/day; 30 day supply)

WARNING

USE IN PREGNANCY

When used in pregnancy during the second and third trimesters, ACE inhibitors can cause injury and even death to the developing fetus. When pregnancy is detected, ramipril should be discontinued as soon as possible. (See WARNINGS, Fetal/Neonatal Morbidity and Mortality.)

DESCRIPTION

Ramipril is a 2-aza-bicyclo[3.3.0]-octane-3-carboxylic acid derivative. It is a white, crystalline substance soluble in polar organic solvents and buffered aqueous solutions. Ramipril melts between 105°C and 112°C.

Ramipril's chemical name is (2*S*,3a*S*,6a*S*)-1[(*S*)-*N*-[(*S*)-1-Carboxy-3-phenylpropyl]alanyl]octahydrocyclopenta[*b*]pyrrole-2-carboxylic acid, 1-ethyl ester.

Its empiric formula is $C_{23}H_{32}N_2O_5$, and its molecular weight is 416.5.

Ramiprilat, the diacid metabolite of ramipril, is a non-sulfhydryl angiotensin converting enzyme inhibitor. Ramipril is converted to ramiprilat by hepatic cleavage of the ester group.

Altace is supplied as hard shell capsules for oral administration containing 1.25, 2.5, 5, and 10 mg of ramipril. The inactive ingredients present are pregelatinized starch, gelatin, and titanium dioxide. The 1.25 mg capsule shell contains yellow iron oxide, the 2.5 mg capsule shell contains D&C yellow no. 10 and FD&C red no. 40, the 5 mg capsule shell contains FD&C blue no. 1 and FD&C red no. 40, and the 10 mg capsule shell contains FD&C blue no. 1.

CLINICAL PHARMACOLOGY

MECHANISM OF ACTION

Ramipril and ramiprilat inhibit angiotensin-converting enzyme (ACE) in human subjects and animals. ACE is a peptidyl dipeptidase that catalyzes the conversion of angiotensin I to the vasoconstrictor substance, angiotensin II. Angiotensin II also stimulates aldosterone secretion by the adrenal cortex. Inhibition of ACE results in decreased plasma angiotensin II, which leads to decreased vasopressor activity and to decreased aldosterone secretion. The latter decrease may result in a small increase of serum potassium. In hypertensive patients with normal renal function treated with ramipril alone for up to 56 weeks, approximately 4% of patients during the trial has an abnormally high serum potassium and an increase from baseline greater than 0.75 mEq/L, and none of the patients had an abnormally low potassium and a decrease from baseline greater than 0.75 mEq/L. In the same study, approximately 2% of patients treated with ramipril and hydrochlorothiazide for up to 56 weeks had abnormally high potassium values and an increase from baseline of 0.75 mEq/L or greater, and approximately 2% had abnormally low values and decreases from baseline of 0.75 mEq/L or greater. (See PRECAUTIONS.) Removal of angiotensin II negative feedback on renin secretion leads to increased plasma renin activity.

R

The effect of ramipril on hypertension appears to result at least in part from inhibition of both tissue and circulating ACE activity, thereby reducing angiotensin II formation in tissue and plasma.

ACE is identical to kininase, an enzyme that degrades bradykinin. Whether increased levels of bradykinin, a potent vasodepressor peptide, play a role in the therapeutic effects of ramipril remains to be elucidated.

While the mechanism through which ramipril lowers blood pressure is believed to be primarily suppression of the renin-angiotensin-aldosterone system, ramipril has an antihypertensive effect even in patients with low-renin hypertension. Although ramipril was antihypertensive in all races studied, black hypertensive patients (usually a low renin-hypertensive population) had a smaller average response to monotherapy than non-black patients.

PHARMACOKINETICS AND METABOLISM

Following oral administration of ramipril, peak plasma concentrations of ramipril are reached within 1 hour. The extent of absorption is at least 50-60% and is not significantly influenced by the presence of food in the GI tract, although the rate of absorption is reduced.

In a trial in which subjects received ramipril capsules or the contents of identical capsules dissolved in water, dissolved in apple juice, or suspended in apple sauce, serum ramiprilat levels were essentially unrelated to the use or nonuse of the concomitant liquid or food.

Cleavage of the ester group (primarily in the liver) converts ramipril to its active diacid metabolite, ramiprilat. Peak plasma concentrations of ramiprilat are reached 2-4 hours after drug intake. The serum protein binding of ramipril is about 73% and that of ramiprilat about 56%; *in vitro*, these percentages are independent of concentration over the range of 0.01 to 10 µg/ml.

Ramipril is almost completely metabolized to ramiprilat, which has about 6 times the ACE inhibitory activity of ramipril, and to the diketopiperazine ester, the diketopiperazine acid, and the glucuronides of ramipril and ramiprilat, all of which are inactive. After oral administration of ramipril, about 60% of the parent drug and its metabolites are eliminated in the urine, and about 40% is found in the feces. Drug recovered in the feces may represent both biliary excretion of metabolites and/or unabsorbed drug, however the proportion of a dose eliminated by the bile has not been determined. Less than 2% of the administered dose is recovered in urine as unchanged ramipril.

Blood concentrations of ramipril and ramiprilat increase with increased dose, but are not strictly dose-proportional. The 24 hour AUC for ramiprilat, however, is dose-proportional over the 2.5-20 mg dose range. The absolute bioavailabilities of ramipril and ramiprilat were 28% and 44%, respectively, when 5 mg of oral ramipril was compared with the same dose of ramipril given intravenously.

Plasma concentrations of ramiprilat decline in a triphasic manner (initial rapid decline, apparent elimination phase, terminal elimination phase). The initial rapid decline, which represents distribution of the drug into a large peripheral compartment and subsequent binding to both plasma and tissue ACE, has a half-life of 2-4 hours. Because of its potent binding to ACE and slow dissociation from the enzyme, ramiprilat shows two elimination phases. The apparent elimination phase corresponds to the clearance of free ramiprilat and has a half-life of 9-18 hours. The terminal elimination phase has a prolonged half-life (>50 hours) and probably represents the binding/dissociation kinetics of the ramiprilat/ACE complex. It does not contribute to the accumulation of the drug. After multiple daily doses of ramipril 5-10 mg, the half-life of ramiprilat concentrations within the therapeutic range was 13-17 hours.

After once-daily dosing, steady-state plasma concentrations of ramiprilat are reached by the fourth dose. Steady-state concentrations of ramiprilat are somewhat higher than those seen after the first dose of ramipril, especially at low doses (2.5 mg), but the difference is clinically insignificant.

In patients with creatinine clearance less than 40 ml/min/1.73 m^2, peak levels of ramiprilat are approximately doubled, and trough levels may be as much as quintupled. In multiple-dose regimens, the total exposure to ramiprilat (AUC) in these patients is 3-4 times as large as it is in patients with normal renal function who receive similar doses.

The urinary excretion of ramipril, ramiprilat, and their metabolites is reduced in patients with impaired renal function. Compared to normal subjects, patients with creatinine clearance less than 40 ml/min/1.73 m^2 had higher peak and trough ramiprilat levels and slightly longer times to peak concentrations. (See DOSAGE AND ADMINISTRATION.)

In patients with impaired liver function, the metabolism of ramipril to ramiprilat appears to be slowed, possibly because of diminished activity of hepatic esterases, and plasma ramipril levels in these patients are increased about 3-fold. Peak concentrations of ramiprilat in these patients, however, are not different from those seen in subjects with normal hepatic function, and the effect of a given dose on plasma ACE activity does not vary with hepatic function.

PHARMACODYNAMICS

Single doses of ramipril of 2.5-20 mg produce approximately 60-80% inhibition of ACE activity 4 hours after dosing with approximately 40-60% inhibition after 24 hours. Multiple oral doses of ramipril of 2.0 mg or more cause plasma ACE activity to fall by more than 90% 4 hours after dosing, with over 80% inhibition of ACE activity remaining 24 hours after dosing. The more prolonged effect of even small multiple doses presumably reflects saturation of ACE binding sites by ramiprilat and relatively slow release from those sites.

PHARMACODYNAMICS AND CLINICAL EFFECTS

Reduction in Risk of Myocardial Infarction, Stroke, and Death From Cardiovascular Causes

The Heart Outcomes Prevention Evaluation study (HOPE study) was a large, multi-center, randomized, placebo controlled, 2 × 2 factorial design, double-blind study conducted in 9541 patients (4645 on ramipril) who were 55 years or older and considered at high risk of developing a major cardiovascular event because of a history of coronary artery disease, stroke, peripheral vascular disease, or diabetes that was accompanied by at least one other cardiovascular risk factor (hypertension, elevated total cholesterol levels, low HDL levels, cigarette smoking, or documented microalbuminuria). Patients were either normotensive or under treatment with other antihypertensive agents. Patients were excluded if they had clinical heart failure or were known to have a low ejection fraction (<0.40). This study was designed to examine the long-term (mean of 5 years) effects of ramipril (10 mg orally once a day) on the combined endpoint of myocardial infarction, stroke or death from cardiovascular causes.

The HOPE study results showed that ramipril (10 mg/day) significantly reduced the rate of myocardial infarction, stroke or death from cardiovascular causes (651/4645 vs 826/4652, relative risk 0.78), as well as the rates of the 3 components of the combined endpoint.

This effect was evident after about 1 year of treatment.

TABLE 1

Outcome	Ramipril (n=4645)	Placebo (n=4652)	Relative Risk (95% CI) P-Value
Combined End-Point			
MI, stroke, or death from CV cause	651 (14.0%)	826 (17.8%)	0.78 (0.70-0.86) P=0.0001
Component End-Point			
Death from cardiovascular causes	282 (6.1%)	377 (8.1%)	0.74 (0.64-0.87) P=0.0002
Myocardial infarction	459 (9.9%)	570 (12.3%)	0.80 (0.70-0.90) P=0.0003
Stroke	156 (3.4%)	226 (4.9%)	0.68 (0.56-0.84) P=0.0002
Overall Mortality			
Death from any cause	482 (10.4%)	569 (12.2%)	0.84 (0.75-0.95) P=0.005

Ramipril was effective in different demographic subgroups, (*i.e.*, gender, age), subgroups defined by underlying disease (*e.g.*, cardiovascular disease, hypertension), and subgroups defined by concomitant medication. There were insufficient data to determine whether or not ramipril was equally effective in ethnic subgroups.

This study was designed with a prespecified substudy in diabetics with at least one other cardiovascular risk factor. Effects of ramipril on the combined endpoint and its components were similar in diabetics (n=3577) to those in the overall study population.

TABLE 2

Outcome	Ramipril (n=1808)	Placebo (n=1769)	Relative Risk Reduction (95% CI)
Combined End-Point			
MI, stroke, or death from CV cause	277 (15.3%)	351 (19.8%)	0.25 (0.12-0.36) P=0.0004
Component End-Point			
Death from cardiovascular causes	112 (6.2%)	172 (9.7%)	0.37 (0.21-0.51) P=0.0001
Myocardial infarction	185 (10.2%)	229 (12,9%)	0.22 (0.06-0.36) P=0.01
Stroke	76 (4.2%)	108 (6.1%)	0.33 (0.10-0.50) P=0.007

The benefits of ramipril were observed among patients who were taking aspirin or other anti-platelet agents, beta-blockers, and lipid-lowering agents as well as diuretics and calcium channel blockers.

Hypertension

Administration of ramipril to patients with mild to moderate hypertension results in a reduction of both supine and standing blood pressure to about the same extent with no compensatory tachycardia. Symptomatic postural hypotension is infrequent, although it can occur in patients who are salt- and/or volume-depleted. (See WARNINGS.) Use of ramipril in combination with thiazide diuretics gives a blood pressure lowering effect greater than that seen with either agent alone.

In single-dose studies, doses of 5-20 mg of ramipril lowered blood pressure within 1-2 hours, with peak reductions achieved 3-6 hours after dosing. The antihypertensive effect of a single dose persisted for 24 hours. In longer term (4-12 weeks) controlled studies, once-daily doses of 2.5-10 mg were similar in their effect, lowering supine or standing systolic and diastolic blood pressures 24 hours after dosing by about 6/4 mm Hg more than placebo. In comparisons of peak versus trough effect, the trough effect represented about 50-60% of the peak response. In a titration study comparing divided (bid) versus qd treatment, the divided regimen was superior, indicating that for some patients the antihypertensive effect with once-daily dosing is not adequately maintained. (See DOSAGE AND ADMINISTRATION.)

In most trials, the antihypertensive effect of ramipril increased during the first several weeks of repeated measurements. The antihypertensive effect of ramipril has been shown to continue during long-term therapy for at least 2 years. Abrupt withdrawal of ramipril has not resulted in a rapid increase in blood pressure.

Ramipril has been compared with other ACE inhibitors, beta-blockers, and thiazide diuretics. It was approximately as effective as other ACE inhibitors and as atenolol. In both caucasians and blacks, hydrochlorothiazide (25 or 50 mg) was significantly more effective than ramipril.

Except for thiazides, no formal interaction studies of ramipril with other antihypertensive agents have been carried out. Limited experience in controlled and uncontrolled trials combining ramipril with a calcium channel blocker, a loop diuretic, or triple therapy (beta-blocker, vasodilator, and a diuretic) indicate no unusual drug-drug interactions. Other ACE inhibitors have had less than additive effects with beta adrenergic blockers, presumably because both drugs lower blood pressure by inhibiting parts of the renin-angiotensin system.

Ramipril was less effective in blacks than in caucasians. The effectiveness of ramipril was not influenced by age, sex, or weight.

In a baseline controlled study of 10 patients with mild essential hypertension, blood pressure reduction was accompanied by a 15% increase in renal blood flow. In healthy volunteers, glomerular filtration rate was unchanged.

Heart Failure Post-Myocardial Infarction

Ramipril was studied in the Acute Infarction Ramipril Efficacy (AIRE) trial. This was a multinational (mainly European) 161-center, 2006-patient, double-blind, randomized, parallel-group study comparing ramipril to placebo in stable patients, 2-9 days after an acute myocardial infarction (MI), who had shown clinical signs of congestive heart failure (CHF) at any time after the MI. Patients in severe (NYHA class IV) heart failure, patients with unstable angina, patients with heart failure of congenital or valvular etiology, and patients with contraindications to ACE inhibitors were all excluded. The majority of patients had received thrombolytic therapy at the time of the index infarction, and the average time between infarction and initiation of treatment was 5 days.

Patients randomized to ramipril treatment were given an initial dose of 2.5 mg twice daily. If the initial regimen caused undue hypotension, the dose was reduced to 1.25 mg, but in either event doses were titrated upward (as tolerated) to a target regimen (achieved in 77% of patients randomized to ramipril) of 5 mg twice daily. Patients were then followed for an average of 15 months (range 6-46).

The use of ramipril was associated with a 27% reduction (p=0.002), in the risk of death from any cause; about 90% of the deaths that occurred were cardiovascular, mainly sudden death. The risks of progression to severe heart failure and of CHF-related hospitalization were also reduced, by 23% (p=0.017) and 26% (p=0.011), respectively. The benefits of ramipril therapy were seen in both genders, and they were not affected by the exact timing of the initiation of therapy, but older patients may have had a greater benefit than those under 65. The benefits were seen in patients on, and not on, various concomitant medications; at the time of randomization these included aspirin (about 80% of patients), diuretics (about 60%), organic nitrates (about 55%), beta-blockers (about 20%), calcium channel blockers (about 15%), and digoxin (about 12%).

INDICATIONS AND USAGE

REDUCTION IN RISK OF MYOCARDIAL INFARCTION, STROKE, AND DEATH FROM CARDIOVASCULAR CAUSES

Ramipril is indicated in patients 55 years or older at high risk of developing a major cardiovascular event because of a history of coronary artery disease, stroke, peripheral vascular disease, or diabetes that is accompanied by at least one other cardiovascular risk factor (hypertension, elevated total cholesterol levels, low HDL levels, cigarette smoking, or documented microalbuminuria), to reduce the risk of myocardial infarction, stroke, or death from cardiovascular causes. Ramipril can be used in addition to other needed treatment (such as antihypertensive, antiplatelet or lipid-lowering therapy).

HYPERTENSION

Ramipril is indicated for the treatment of hypertension. It may be used alone or in combination with thiazide diuretics.

In using ramipril, consideration should be given to the fact that another angiotensin converting enzyme inhibitor, captopril, has caused agranulocytosis, particularly in patients with renal impairment or collagen-vascular disease. Available data are insufficient to show that ramipril does not have a similar risk. (See WARNINGS.)

In considering use of ramipril, it should be noted that in controlled trials ACE inhibitors have an effect on blood pressure that is less in black patients than in non-blacks. In addition, ACE inhibitors (for which adequate data are available) cause a higher rate of angioedema in black than in non-black patients (see WARNINGS, Angioedema).

HEART FAILURE POST-MYOCARDIAL INFARCTION

Ramipril is indicated in stable patients who have demonstrated clinical signs of congestive heart failure within the first few days after sustaining acute myocardial infarction. Administration of ramipril to such patients has been shown to decrease the risk of death (principally cardiovascular death) and to decrease the risks of failure-related hospitalization and progression to severe/resistant heart failure. (See CLINICAL PHARMACOLOGY, Heart Failure Post-Myocardial Infarction for details and limitations of the survival trial.)

NON-FDA APPROVED INDICATIONS

Some ACE inhibitors have been shown to decrease proteinuria and preserve renal function in patients with hypertension and diabetes mellitus to a greater extent than other antihypertensive agents. More recently, ACE inhibitors have been shown to decrease the progression of nephropathy in normotensive patients with diabetes mellitus Type 2.

CONTRAINDICATIONS

Ramipril is contraindicated in patients who are hypersensitive to this product or any other angiotensin converting enzyme inhibitor (*e.g.*, a patient who has experienced angioedema during therapy with any other ACE inhibitor).

WARNINGS

ANAPHYLACTOID AND POSSIBLY RELATED REACTIONS

Presumably because angiotensin-converting enzyme inhibitors affect the metabolism of eicosanoids and polypeptides, including endogenous bradykinin, patients receiving ACE inhibitors (including ramipril) may be subject to a variety of adverse reactions, some of them serious.

ANGIOEDEMA

Patients with a history of angioedema unrelated to ACE inhibitor therapy may be at increased risk of angioedema while receiving an ACE inhibitor. (See also CONTRAINDICATIONS.)

Angioedema of the face, extremities, lips, tongue, glottis, and larynx has been reported in patients treated with angiotensin converting enzyme inhibitors. Angioedema associated with laryngeal edema can be fatal. If laryngeal stridor or angioedema of the face, tongue, or glottis occurs, treatment with ramipril should be discontinued and appropriate therapy instituted immediately. **When there is involvement of the tongue, glottis, or larynx, likely to cause airway obstruction, appropriate therapy, *e.g.*, subcutaneous epinephrine solution 1:1000 (0.3-0.5 ml) should be promptly administered. (See ADVERSE REACTIONS.)**

In a large US postmarketing study, angioedema (defined as reports of angio, face, larynx, tongue, or throat edema) was reported in 3/1523 (0.20%) of black patients and in 8/8680 (0.09%) of white patients. These rates were not different statistically.

ANAPHYLACTOID REACTIONS DURING DESENSITIZATION

Two (2) patients undergoing desensitizing treatment with hymenoptera venom while receiving ACE inhibitors sustained life-threatening anaphylactoid reactions. In the same patients, these reactions were avoided when ACE inhibitors were temporarily withheld, but they reappeared upon inadvertent rechallenge.

ANAPHYLACTOID REACTIONS DURING MEMBRANE EXPOSURE

Anaphylactoid reactions have been reported in patients dialyzed with high-flux membranes and treated concomitantly with an ACE inhibitor. Anaphylactoid reactions have also been reported in patients undergoing low-density lipoprotein apheresis with dextran sulfate absorption.

HYPOTENSION

Ramipril can cause symptomatic hypotension, after either the initial dose or a later dose when the dosage has been increased. Like other ACE inhibitors, ramipril has been only rarely associated with hypotension in uncomplicated hypertensive patients. Symptomatic hypotension is most likely to occur in patients who have been volume- and/or salt-depleted as a result of prolonged diuretic therapy, dietary salt restriction, dialysis, diarrhea, or vomiting. Volume and/or salt depletion should be corrected before initiating therapy with ramipril.

In patients with congestive heart failure, with or without associated renal insufficiency, ACE inhibitor therapy may cause excessive hypotension, which may be associated with oliguria or azotemia and, rarely, with acute renal failure and death. In such patients, ramipril therapy should be started under close medical supervision; they should be followed closely for the first 2 weeks of treatment and whenever the dose of ramipril or diuretic is increased.

If hypotension occurs, the patient should be placed in a supine position and, if necessary, treated with intravenous infusion of physiological saline. Ramipril treatment usually can be continued following restoration of blood pressure and volume.

HEPATIC FAILURE

Rarely, ACE inhibitors have been associated with a syndrome that starts with cholestatic jaundice and progresses to fulminant hepatic necrosis and (sometimes) death. The mechanism of this syndrome is not understood. Patients receiving ACE inhibitors who develop jaundice or marked elevations of hepatic enzymes should discontinue the ACE inhibitor and receive appropriate medical follow-up.

NEUTROPENIA/AGRANULOCYTOSIS

As with other ACE inhibitors, rarely, a mild - in isolated cases severe - reduction in the red blood cell count and hemoglobin content, white blood cell or platelet count may develop. In isolated cases, agranulocytosis, pancytopenia, and bone marrow depression may occur. Hematological reactions to ACE inhibitors are more likely to occur in patients with collagen vascular disease (*e.g.,* systemic lupus erythematosus, scleroderma) and renal impairment. Monitoring of white blood cell counts should be considered in patients with collagen-vascular disease, especially if the disease is associated with impaired renal function.

FETAL/NEONATAL MORBIDITY AND MORTALITY

ACE inhibitors can cause fetal and neonatal morbidity and death when administered to pregnant women. Several dozen cases have been reported in the world literature. When pregnancy is detected, ACE inhibitors should be discontinued as soon as possible.

The use of ACE inhibitors during the second and third trimesters of pregnancy has been associated with fetal and neonatal injury, including hypotension, neonatal skull hypoplasia, anuria, reversible or irreversible renal failure, and death. Oligohydramnios has also been reported, presumably resulting from decreased fetal renal function; oligohydramnios in this setting has been associated with fetal limb contractures, craniofacial deformation, and hypoplastic lung development. Prematurity, intrauterine growth retardation, and patent ductus arteriosus have also been reported, although it is not clear whether these occurrences were due to the ACE inhibitor exposure.

These adverse effects do not appear to have resulted from intrauterine ACE inhibitor exposure that has been limited to the first trimester. Mothers whose embryos and fetuses are exposed to ACE inhibitors only during the first trimester should be so informed. Nonetheless, when patients become pregnant, physicians should make every effort to discontinue the use of ramipril as soon as possible.

Rarely (probably less often than once in every 1000 pregnancies), no alternative to ACE inhibitors will be found. In these rare cases, the mothers should be apprised of the potential hazards to their fetuses, and serial ultrasound examinations should be performed to assess the intraamniotic environment.

If oligohydramnios is observed, ramipril should be discontinued unless it is considered life-saving for the mother. Contraction stress testing (CST), a non-stress test (NST), or biophysical profiling (BPP) may be appropriate, depending upon the week of pregnancy. Patients and physicians should be aware, however, that oligohydramnios may not appear until after the fetus has sustained irreversible injury.

Infants with histories of *in utero* exposure to ACE inhibitors should be closely observed for hypotension, oliguria, and hyperkalemia. If oliguria occurs, attention should be directed toward support of blood pressure and renal perfusion. Exchange transfusion or dialysis may be required as means of reversing hypotension and/or substituting for disordered renal function. Ramipril which crosses the placenta can be removed from the neonatal circulation by these means, but limited experience has not shown that such removal is central to the treatment of these infants.

No teratogenic effects of ramipril were seen in studies of pregnant rats, rabbits, and cynomolgus monkeys. On a body surface area basis, the doses used were up to approximately 400 times (in rats and monkeys) and 2 times (in rabbits) the recommended human dose.

PRECAUTIONS

IMPAIRED RENAL FUNCTION

As a consequence of inhibiting the renin-angiotensin-aldosterone system, changes in renal function may be anticipated in susceptible individuals. In patients with severe congestive heart failure whose renal function may depend on the activity of the renin-angiotensin-aldosterone system, treatment with angiotensin converting enzyme inhibitors, including ramipril, may be associated with oliguria and/or progressive azotemia and (rarely) with acute renal failure and/or death.

In hypertensive patients with unilateral or bilateral renal artery stenosis, increases in blood urea nitrogen and serum creatinine may occur. Experience with another angiotensin converting enzyme inhibitor suggests that these increases are usually reversible upon discontinuation of ramipril and/or diuretic therapy. In such patients renal function should be monitored during the first few weeks of therapy. Some hypertensive patients with no apparent pre-existing renal vascular disease have developed increases in blood urea nitrogen and serum creatinine, usually minor and transient, especially when ramipril has been given concomitantly with a diuretic. This is more likely to occur in patients with pre-existing renal impairment. Dosage reduction of ramipril and/or discontinuation of the diuretic may be required.

Evaluation of the hypertensive patient should always include assessment of renal function. (See DOSAGE AND ADMINISTRATION.)

HYPERKALEMIA

In clinical trials, hyperkalemia (serum potassium greater than 5.7 mEq/L) occurred in approximately 1% of hypertensive patients receiving ramipril. In most cases, these were isolated values, which resolved despite continued therapy. None of these patients was discontinued from the trials because of hyperkalemia. Risk factors for the development of hyperkalemia include renal insufficiency, diabetes mellitus, and the concomitant use of potassium-sparing diuretics, potassium supplements, and/or potassium-containing salt substitutes, which should be used cautiously, if at all, with ramipril. (See DRUG INTERACTIONS.)

COUGH

Presumably due to the inhibition of the degradation of endogenous bradykinin, persistent nonproductive cough has been reported with all ACE inhibitors, always resolving after discontinuation of therapy. ACE inhibitor-induced cough should be considered in the differential diagnosis of cough.

IMPAIRED LIVER FUNCTION

Since ramipril is primarily metabolized by hepatic esterases to its active moiety, ramiprilat, patients with impaired liver function could develop markedly elevated plasma levels of ramipril. No formal pharmacokinetic studies have been carried out in hypertensive patients with impaired liver function. However, since the renin-angiotensin system may be activated in patients with severe liver cirrhosis and/or ascites, particular caution should be exercised in treating these patients.

SURGERY/ANESTHESIA

In patients undergoing surgery or during anesthesia with agents that produce hypotension, ramipril may block angiotensin II formation that would otherwise occur secondary to compensatory renin release. Hypotension that occurs as a result of this mechanism can be corrected by volume expansion.

INFORMATION FOR THE PATIENT

Pregnancy

Female patients of childbearing age should be told about the consequences of second- and third-trimester exposure to ACE inhibitors, and they should also be told that these consequences do not appear to have resulted from intrauterine ACE inhibitor exposure that has been limited to the first trimester. These patients should be asked to report pregnancies to their physicians as soon as possible.

Angioedema

Angioedema, including laryngeal edema, can occur with treatment with ACE inhibitors, especially following the first dose. Patients should be so advised and told to report immediately any signs or symptoms suggesting angioedema (swelling of face, eyes, lips, or tongue, or difficulty in breathing) and to take no more drug until they have consulted with the prescribing physician.

Symptomatic Hypotension

Patients should be cautioned that lightheadedness can occur, especially during the first days of therapy, and it should be reported. Patients should be told that if syncope occurs, ramipril should be discontinued until the physician has been consulted.

All patients should be cautioned that inadequate fluid intake or excessive perspiration, diarrhea, or vomiting can lead to an excessive fall in blood pressure, with the same consequences of lightheadedness and possible syncope.

Hyperkalemia

Patients should be told not to use salt substitutes containing potassium without consulting their physician.

Neutropenia

Patients should be told to promptly report any indication of infection (*e.g.,* sore throat, fever), which could be a sign of neutropenia.

CARCINOGENESIS, MUTAGENESIS, AND IMPAIRMENT OF FERTILITY

No evidence of a tumorigenic effect was found when ramipril was given by gavage to rats for up to 24 months at doses of up to 500 mg/kg/day or to mice for up to 18 months at doses of up to 1000 mg/kg/day. (For either species, these doses are about 200 times the maximum recommended human dose when compared on the basis of body surface area.) No mutagenic activity was detected in the Ames test in bacteria, the micronucleus test in mice, unscheduled DNA synthesis in a human cell line, or a forward gene-mutation assay in a Chinese hamster ovary cell line. Several metabolites and degradation products of ramipril were also negative in the Ames test. A study in rats with dosages as great as 500 mg/kg/day did not produce adverse effects on fertility.

PREGNANCY CATEGORIES C (FIRST TRIMESTER) AND D (SECOND AND THIRD TRIMESTERS)

See WARNINGS, Fetal/Neonatal Morbidity and Mortality.

NURSING MOTHERS

Ingestion of single 10 mg oral dose of ramipril resulted in undetectable amounts of ramipril and its metabolites in breast milk. However, because multiple doses may produce low milk concentrations that are not predictable from single doses, women receiving ramipril should not breast feed.

GERIATRIC USE

Of the total number of patients who received ramipril in US clinical studies of ramipril 11.0% were 65 and over while 0.2% were 75 and over. No overall differences in effectiveness or safety were observed between these patients and younger patients, and other reported clinical experience has not identified differences in responses between the elderly and younger patients, but greater sensitivity of some older individuals cannot be ruled out.

One pharmacokinetic study conducted in hospitalized elderly patients indicated that peak ramiprilat levels and area under the plasma concentration time curve (AUC) for ramiprilat are higher in older patients.

PEDIATRIC USE

Safety and effectiveness in pediatric patients have not been established.

DRUG INTERACTIONS

With nonsteroidal anti-inflammatory agents: Rarely, concomitant treatment with ACE inhibitors and nonsteroidal anti-inflammatory agents have been associated with worsening of renal failure and an increase in serum potassium.

With diuretics: Patients on diuretics, especially those in whom diuretic therapy was recently instituted, may occasionally experience an excessive reduction of blood pressure after initiation of therapy with ramipril. The possibility of hypotensive effects with ramipril can be minimized by either discontinuing the diuretic or increasing the salt intake prior to initiation of treatment with ramipril. If this is not possible, the starting dose should be reduced. (See DOSAGE AND ADMINISTRATION.)

With potassium supplements and potassium-sparing diuretics: Ramipril can attenuate potassium loss caused by thiazide diuretics. Potassium-sparing diuretics (spironolactone, amiloride, triamterene, and others) or potassium supplements can increase the risk of hyperkalemia. Therefore, if concomitant use of such agents is indicated, they should be given with caution, and the patient's serum potassium should be monitored frequently.

With lithium: Increased serum lithium levels and symptoms of lithium toxicity have been reported in patients receiving ACE inhibitors during therapy with lithium. These drugs should be coadministered with caution, and frequent monitoring of serum lithium levels is recommended. If a diuretic is also used, the risk of lithium toxicity may be increased.

Other: Neither ramipril nor its metabolites have been found to interact with food, digoxin, antacid, furosemide, cimetidine, indomethacin, and simvastatin. The combination of ramipril and propranolol showed no adverse effects on dynamic parameters (blood pressure and heart rate). The coadministration of ramipril and warfarin did not adversely affect the anticoagulant effects of the latter drug. Additionally, coadministration of ramipril with phenprocoumon did not affect minimum phenprocoumon levels or interfere with the subjects' state of anti-coagulation.

ADVERSE REACTIONS

HYPERTENSION

Ramipril has been evaluated for safety in over 4000 patients with hypertension; of these, 1230 patients were studied in US controlled trials, and 1107 were studied in foreign controlled trials. Almost 700 of these patients were treated for at least 1 year. The overall incidence of reported adverse events was similar in ramipril and placebo patients. The most frequent clinical side effects (possibly or probably related to study drug) reported by patients receiving ramipril in US placebo-controlled trials were: headache (5.4%), "dizziness" (2.2%) and fatigue or asthenia (2.0%), but only the last was more common in ramipril patients than in patients given placebo. Generally, the side effects were mild and transient, and there was no relation to total dosage within the range of 1.25 to 20 mg. Discontinuation of therapy because of a side effect was required in approximately 3% of US patients treated with ramipril. The most common reasons for discontinuation were: cough (1.0%), "dizziness" (0.5%), and impotence (0.4%).

Of observed side effects considered possibly or probably related to study drug that occurred in US placebo-controlled trials in more than 1% of patients treated with ramipril, only asthenia (fatigue) was more common on ramipril than placebo (2% vs 1%). (See TABLE 3.)

TABLE 3 *Patients in US Placebo Controlled Studies*

	Ramipril (n=651)		Placebo (n=286)	
Asthenia (fatigue)	13	2%	2	1%

In placebo-controlled trials, there was also an excess of upper respiratory infection and flu syndrome in the ramipril group, not attributed at that time to ramipril. As these studies were carried out before the relationship of cough to ACE inhibitors was recognized, some of these events may represent ramipril-induced cough. In a later 1 year study, increased cough was seen in almost 12% of ramipril patients, with about 4% of patients requiring discontinuation of treatment.

HEART FAILURE POST-MYOCARDIAL INFARCTION

Adverse reactions (except laboratory abnormalities) considered possibly/probably related to study drug that occurred in more than 1% of patients and more frequently on ramipril are shown in TABLE 4. The incidences represent the experiences from the AIRE study. The follow-up time was between 6 and 46 months for this study.

HOPE STUDY

Safety data in the HOPE trial were collected as reasons for discontinuation or temporary interruption of treatment. The incidence of cough was similar to that seen in the AIRE trial. The rate of angioedema was the same as in previous clinical trials (see WARNINGS).

OTHER ADVERSE EXPERIENCES

Other adverse experiences reported in controlled clinical trials (in less than 1% of ramipril patients), or rarer events seen in postmarketing experience, include the following (in some, a causal relationship to drug use is uncertain); events not likely to be drug related and minor events have been omitted.

Body as a Whole: Anaphylactoid reactions. (See WARNINGS.)

Cardiovascular: Symptomatic hypotension (reported in 0.5% of patients in US trials) (see WARNINGS and PRECAUTIONS), syncope and palpitations.

TABLE 4 *Percentage of Patients With Adverse Events Possibly/Probably Related to Study Drug — Placebo-Controlled (AIRE) Mortality Study*

Adverse Event	Ramipril (n=1004)	Placebo (n=982)
Hypotension	11%	5%
Cough increased	8%	4%
Dizziness	4%	3%
Angina pectoris	3%	2%
Nausea	2%	1%
Postural hypotension	2%	1%
Syncope	2%	1%
Vomiting	2%	0.5%
Vertigo	2%	0.7%
Abnormal kidney function	1%	0.5%
Diarrhea	1%	0.4%

TABLE 5

	Ramipril (n=4645)	Placebo (n=4652)
Discontinuation at any time	34%	32%
Permanent discontinuation	29%	28%
Reasons for stopping:		
Cough	7%	2%
Hypotension or dizziness	1.9%	1.5%
Angioedema	0.3%	0.1%

Hematologic: Pancytopenia, hemolytic anemia and thrombocytopenia.

Renal: Some hypertensive patients with no apparent pre-existing renal disease have developed minor, usually transient, increases in blood urea nitrogen and serum creatinine when taking ramipril, particularly when ramipril was given concomitantly with a diuretic. (See WARNINGS.)

Angioneurotic Edema: Angioneurotic edema has been reported in 0.3% of patients in US clinical trials. (See WARNINGS.)

Gastrointestinal: Pancreatitis, abdominal pain (sometimes with enzyme changes suggesting pancreatitis), anorexia, constipation, diarrhea, dry mouth, dyspepsia, dysphagia, gastroenteritis, hepatitis, increased salivation and taste disturbance.

Dermatologic: Apparent hypersensitivity reactions (manifested by urticaria, pruritus, or rash, with or without fever), erythema multiforme, pemphigus, photosensitivity, purpura, pemphigoid, Stevens-Johnson syndrome, toxic epidermal necrolysis, and onycholysis.

Neurologic and Psychiatric: Anxiety, amnesia, convulsions, depression, hearing loss, insomnia, nervousness, neuralgia, neuropathy, paresthesia, somnolence, tinnitus, tremor, vertigo, and vision disturbances.

Miscellaneous: As with other ACE inhibitors, a symptom complex has been reported which may include a positive ANA, an elevated erythrocyte sedimentation rate, arthralgia/arthritis, myalgia, fever, vasculitis, eosinophilia, photosensitivity, rash and other dermatologic manifestations. Additionally, as with other ACE inhibitors, eosinophilic pneumonitis has been reported.

Fetal/Neonatal Morbidity and Mortality: **See WARNINGS, Fetal/Neonatal Morbidity and Mortality.**

Other: Arthralgia, arthritis, dyspnea, edema, epistaxis, impotence, increased sweating, malaise, myalgia, and weight gain.

CLINICAL LABORATORY TEST FINDINGS

Creatinine and Blood Urea Nitrogen: Increases in creatinine levels occurred in 1.2% of patients receiving ramipril alone, and in 1.5% of patients receiving ramipril and a diuretic. Increases in blood urea nitrogen levels occurred in 0.5% of patients receiving ramipril alone and in 3% of patients receiving ramipril with a diuretic. None of these increases required discontinuation of treatment. Increases in these laboratory values are more likely to occur in patients with renal insufficiency or those pretreated with a diuretic and, based on experience with other ACE inhibitors, would be expected to be especially likely in patients with renal artery stenosis. (See WARNINGS and PRECAUTIONS.) Since ramipril decreases aldosterone secretion, elevation of serum potassium can occur. Potassium supplements and potassium-sparing diuretics should be given with caution, and the patient's serum potassium should be monitored frequently. (See WARNINGS and PRECAUTIONS.)

Hemoglobin and Hematocrit: Decreases in hemoglobin or hematocrit (a low value and a decrease of 5 g/dl or 5% respectively) were rare, occurring in 0.4% of patients receiving ramipril alone and in 1.5% of patients receiving ramipril plus a diuretic. No US patients discontinued treatment because of decreases in hemoglobin or hematocrit.

Other (causal relationships unknown): Clinically important changes in standard laboratory tests were rarely associated with ramipril administration. Elevations of liver enzymes, serum bilirubin, uric acid, and blood glucose have been reported, as have cases of hyponatremia and scattered incidents of leukopenia, eosinophilia, and proteinuria. In US trials, less than 0.2% of patients discontinued treatment for laboratory abnormalities; all of these were cases of proteinuria or abnormal liver-function tests.

DOSAGE AND ADMINISTRATION

Blood pressure decreases associated with any dose of ramipril depend, in part, on the presence or absence of volume depletion (*e.g.*, past and current diuretic use) or the presence or absence of renal artery stenosis. If such circumstances are suspected to be present, the initial starting dose should be 1.25 mg once daily.

R

REDUCTION IN RISK OF MYOCARDIAL INFARCTION, STROKE, AND DEATH FROM CARDIOVASCULAR CAUSES

Ramipril should be given at an initial dose of 2.5 mg, once a day for 1 week, 5 mg, once a day for the next 3 weeks, and then increased as tolerated, to a maintenance dose of 10 mg, once a day. If the patient is hypertensive or recently post-myocardial infarction, it can also be given as a divided dose.

HYPERTENSION

The recommended initial dose for patients not receiving a diuretic is 2.5 mg once a day. Dosage should be adjusted according to the blood pressure response. The usual maintenance dosage range is 2.5 to 20 mg/day administered as a single dose or in 2 equally divided doses. In some patients treated once daily, the antihypertensive effect may diminish toward the end of the dosing interval. In such patients, an increase in dosage or twice daily administration should be considered. If blood pressure is not controlled with ramipril alone, a diuretic can be added.

HEART FAILURE POST-MYOCARDIAL INFARCTION

For the treatment of post-infarction patients who have shown signs of congestive failure, the recommended starting dose of ramipril is 2.5 mg twice daily (5 mg/day). A patient who becomes hypotensive at this dose may be switched to 1.25 mg twice daily, and after 1 week at the starting dose, patients should then be titrated (if tolerated) toward a target dose of 5 mg twice daily, with dosage increases being about 3 weeks apart.

After the initial dose of ramipril, the patient should be observed under medical supervision for at least 2 hours and until blood pressure has stabilized for at least an additional hour. (See WARNINGS and DRUG INTERACTIONS.) If possible, the dose of any concomitant diuretic should be reduced which may diminish the likelihood of hypotension. The appearance of hypotension after the initial dose of ramipril does not preclude subsequent careful dose titration with the drug, following effective management of the hypotension.

The ramipril capsule is usually swallowed whole. The ramipril capsule can also be opened and the contents sprinkled on a small amount (about 4 oz) of apple sauce or mixed in 4 oz (120 ml) of water or apple juice. To be sure that ramipril is not lost when such a mixture is used, the mixture should be consumed in its entirety. The described mixtures can be pre-prepared and stored for up to 24 hours at room temperature or up to 48 hours under refrigeration.

Concomitant administration of ramipril with potassium supplements, potassium salt substitutes, or potassium-sparing diuretics can lead to increases of serum potassium. (See PRECAUTIONS.)

In patients who are currently being treated with a diuretic, symptomatic hypotension occasionally can occur following the initial dose of ramipril. To reduce the likelihood of hypotension, the diuretic should, if possible, be discontinued 2-3 days prior to beginning therapy with ramipril. (See WARNINGS.) Then, if blood pressure is not controlled with ramipril alone, diuretic therapy should be resumed.

If the diuretic cannot be discontinued, an initial dose of 1.25 mg ramipril should be used to avoid excess hypotension.

DOSAGE ADJUSTMENT IN RENAL IMPAIRMENT

In patients with creatinine clearance <40 ml/min/1.73 m^2 (serum creatinine approximately >2.5 mg/dl) doses only 25% of those normally used should be expected to induce full therapeutic levels of ramiprilat. (See CLINICAL PHARMACOLOGY.)

Hypertension

For patients with hypertension and renal impairment, the recommended initial dose is 1.25 mg ramipril once daily. Dosage may be titrated upward until blood pressure is controlled or to a maximum total daily dose of 5 mg.

Heart Failure Post-Myocardial Infarction

For patients with heart failure and renal impairment, the recommended initial dose is 1.25 mg ramipril once daily. The dose may be increased to 1.25 mg bid and up to a maximum dose of 2.5 mg bid depending upon clinical response and tolerability.

R

HOW SUPPLIED

Altace is available in the following potencies:

1.25 mg Capsules: Yellow, hard gelatin capsules.
2.5 mg Capsules: Orange, hard gelatin capsules.
5 mg Capsules: Red, hard gelatin capsules.
10 mg Capsules: Process blue, hard gelatin capsules.

Storage: Dispense in well-closed container with safety closure.
Store at controlled room temperature (59-86°F).

PRODUCT LISTING - EQUIVALENTS NOT AVAILABLE

Capsule - Oral - 1.25 mg

100's	$84.33	ALTACE, Monarch Pharmaceuticals Inc	61570-0110-56
100's	$105.00	ALTACE, Monarch Pharmaceuticals Inc	61570-0110-01

Capsule - Oral - 2.5 mg

30's	$27.48	ALTACE, Allscripts Pharmaceutical Company	54569-3713-00
30's	$34.07	ALTACE, Physicians Total Care	54868-2644-01
100's	$126.25	ALTACE, Monarch Pharmaceuticals Inc	61570-0111-01
100's	$126.25	ALTACE, Monarch Pharmaceuticals Inc	61570-0111-56

Capsule - Oral - 5 mg

30's	$32.43	ALTACE, Allscripts Pharmaceutical Company	54569-3714-00
30's	$36.40	ALTACE, Physicians Total Care	54868-2645-01
100's	$111.46	ALTACE, Physicians Total Care	54868-2645-00
100's	$137.50	ALTACE, Monarch Pharmaceuticals Inc	61570-0112-01
100's	$137.50	ALTACE, Monarch Pharmaceuticals Inc	61570-0112-56

Capsule - Oral - 10 mg

30's	$36.60	ALTACE, Physicians Total Care	54868-3846-00
100's	$168.75	ALTACE, Monarch Pharmaceuticals Inc	61570-0120-01

Ranitidine Hydrochloride *(002174)*

For related information, see the comparative table section in Appendix A.

Categories: Esophagitis, erosive; Gastroesophageal Reflux Disease; Mastocytosis, systemic; Ulcer, duodenal; Ulcer, gastric; Zollinger-Ellison syndrome; Pregnancy Category B; FDA Approved 1983 Jun

Drug Classes: Antihistamines, H2; Gastrointestinals

Brand Names: **Zantac**

Foreign Brand Availability: Acidex (Argentina); Aciloc (India); Acloral (Mexico); Acran (Indonesia); Aldin (India); Anistal (Mexico); Antagonin (Benin; Burkina-Faso; Ethiopia; Gambia; Ghana; Guinea; Ivory-Coast; Kenya; Liberia; Malawi; Mali; Mauritania; Mauritius; Morocco; Niger; Nigeria; Senegal; Seychelles; Sierra-Leone; Sudan; Tanzania; Tunia; Uganda; Zambia; Zimbabwe); Apo-Ranitidine (Canada; New-Zealand); Atural (Peru); Ausran (Australia); Avintac (Mexico); Axoban (Japan); Azantac (France; Mexico); Consec (India); Coralen (Spain); Cygran (Philippines); Duractin (Korea); Eltidine (Korea); Eu-Ran (Philippines); Ezopta (Greece); Galidrin (Mexico); Gastrial (Argentina); Gastridin (Indonesia); Gastrosedol (Argentina); Hexer (Indonesia); Histac (Benin; Burkina-Faso; Ethiopia; Gambia; Ghana; Guinea; India; Ivory-Coast; Kenya; Liberia; Malawi; Mali; Mauritania; Mauritius; Morocco; Niger; Nigeria; Senegal; Seychelles; Sierra-Leone; Singapore; Sudan; Tanzania; Thailand; Tunia; Uganda; Zambia; Zimbabwe); Histak (South-Africa); Hyzan (Singapore); Incid (Philippines); Iqfadina (Mexico); Kemoranin (Indonesia); Kiradin (Taiwan); Lydin (India); Microtid (Mexico); Nadine (Bahrain; Cyprus; Egypt; Iran; Iraq; Jordan; Kuwait; Lebanon; Libya; Oman; Qatar; Republic-of-Yemen; Saudi-Arabia; Syria; United-Arab-Emirates); Neoceptin-R (Benin; Burkina-Faso; Ethiopia; Gambia; Ghana; Guinea; Ivory-Coast; Kenya; Liberia; Malawi; Mali; Mauritania; Mauritius; Morocco; Niger; Nigeria; Senegal; Seychelles; Sierra-Leone; Singapore; Sudan; Tanzania; Tunia; Uganda; Zambia; Zimbabwe); Novo-ranidine (Hong-Kong); Pilorex (Peru); Ponaltin (Korea); Ptinolin (Greece); Quantor (Spain); Quicran (Taiwan); Radinat (Ecuador); Radine (Philippines); Ranacid (Norway); Rancet (Colombia); Randin (Bahrain; Cyprus; Egypt; Iran; Iraq; Jordan; Kuwait; Lebanon; Libya; Oman; Qatar; Republic-of-Yemen; Saudi-Arabia; Syria; United-Arab-Emirates); Rani 2 (Australia); Ranial (India); Raniben (Italy); Ranidil (Italy); Ranidine (Thailand); Ranihexal (Australia); Ranimex (Finland); Ranin (Indonesia); Raniogas (Colombia); Raniplex (France); Ranisen (Mexico); Ranitab (Philippines); Ranital (Slovenia); Ranitax (Peru); Ranitin (Bahrain; Republic-Of-Yemen); Ranolta (Hong-Kong); Rantac (Bahrain; Cyprus; Egypt; India; Iran; Iraq; Jordan; Kuwait; Lebanon; Libya; Oman; Qatar; Republic-of-Yemen; Saudi-Arabia; Syria; United-Arab-Emirates); Rantacid (Finland); Rantin (Indonesia); Ratic (Thailand); Raticina (Argentina); Raxide (Philippines); R-Loc (Benin; Burkina-Faso; Ethiopia; Gambia; Ghana; Guinea; Ivory-Coast; Kenya; Liberia; Malawi; Mali; Mauritania; Mauritius; Morocco; Niger; Nigeria; Senegal; Seychelles; Sierra-Leone; Sudan; Tanzania; Tunia; Uganda; Zambia; Zimbabwe); Rolan (Bahrain; Cyprus; Egypt; Iran; Iraq; Jordan; Kuwait; Lebanon; Libya; Oman; Qatar; Republic-of-Yemen; Saudi-Arabia; Syria; United-Arab-Emirates); Rosimol (Argentina); RND (Taiwan); Simetac (Hong-Kong); Sostril (Germany); Taural (Argentina; Costa-Rica; Dominican-Republic; Ecuador; El-Salvador; Guatemala; Honduras; Nicaragua; Panama); Terodul (Mexico); Ulcaid (South-Africa); Ulceran (Peru); Ulceranin (Indonesia); Ulcex (Italy); Ulcin (Philippines); Ulsal (Austria); Ultak (South-Africa); Urantac (Korea); Verlost (Greece); Vesyca (Taiwan); Vizerul (Argentina); Weichilin (Taiwan); Weidos (Taiwan); Xanidine (Singapore; Thailand); Zantab (Israel); Zantac FR (Philippines); Zantac Relief (New-Zealand); Zantadin (Indonesia); Zantic (Germany; Switzerland); Zinetac (India)

Cost of Therapy: $99.20 (GERD; Zantac; 150 mg; 2 tablets/day; 30 day supply)
$11.89 (GERD; Generic Tablets; 150 mg; 2 tablets/day; 30 day supply)
$112.02 (Duodenal Ulcer; Zantac; 300 mg; 1 tablet/day; 30 day supply)
$77.00 (Duodenal Ulcer; Generic Tablets; 300 mg; 1 tablet/day; 30 day supply)

IM-IV

DESCRIPTION

The active ingredient in Zantac injection and injection premixed is ranitidine hydrochloride (HCl), a histamine H_2-receptor antagonist. Chemically it is N[2-[[[5-[(dimethylamino)methyl]-2-furanyl]methyl]thio]ethyl]-N'-methyl-2-nitro-1,1-ethenediamine, hydrochloride.

The empirical formula is $C_{13}H_{22}N_4O_3S{\cdot}HCl$, representing a molecular weight of 350.87.

Ranitidine HCl is a white to pale yellow, granular substance that is soluble in water.

Zantac injection is a clear, colorless to yellow, nonpyrogenic liquid. The yellow color of the liquid tends to intensify without adversely affecting potency. The pH of the injection solution is 6.7-7.3.

STERILE INJECTION FOR INTRAMUSCULAR OR INTRAVENOUS ADMINISTRATION

Each 1 ml of aqueous solution contains ranitidine 25 mg (as the hydrochloride); phenol 5 mg as preservative; and 0.96 mg of monobasic potassium phosphate and 2.4 mg of dibasic sodium phosphate as buffers.

STERILE, PREMIXED SOLUTION FOR INTRAVENOUS ADMINISTRATION IN SINGLE-DOSE, FLEXIBLE PLASTIC CONTAINERS

Each 50 ml contains ranitidine HCl equivalent to 50 mg of ranitidine, sodium chloride 225 mg, and citric acid 15 mg and dibasic sodium phosphate 90 mg as buffers in water for injection. It contains no preservatives. The osmolarity of this solution is 180 mOsm/L (approx.), and the pH is 6.7-7.3.

The flexible plastic container is fabricated from a specially formulated, nonplasticized, thermoplastic co-polyester (CR3). Water can permeate from inside the container into the overwrap but not in amounts sufficient to affect the solution significantly. Solutions inside the plastic container also can leach out certain of the chemical components in very small amounts before the expiration period is attained. However, the safety of the plastic has been confirmed by tests in animals according to USP biological standards for plastic containers.

CLINICAL PHARMACOLOGY

Ranitidine HCl is a competitive, reversible inhibitor of the action of histamine at the histamine H_2-receptors, including receptors on the gastric cells. Ranitidine HCl does not lower serum Ca^{++} in hypercalcemic states. Ranitidine HCl is not an anticholinergic agent.

PHARMACOKINETICS

Absorption

Ranitidine HCl is absorbed very rapidly after intramuscular (IM) injection. Mean peak levels of 576 ng/ml occur within 15 minutes or less following a 50 mg IM dose. Absorption from IM sites is virtually complete, with a bioavailability of 90-100% compared with intravenous (IV) administration. Following oral administration, the bioavailability of ranitidine HCl tablets is 50%.

Distribution

The volume of distribution is about 1.4 L/kg. Serum protein binding averages 15%.

Metabolism

In humans, the N-oxide is the principal metabolite in the urine; however, this amounts to <4% of the dose. Other metabolites are the S-oxide (1%) and the desmethyl ranitidine (1%). The remainder of the administered dose is found in the stool. Studies in patients with hepatic dysfunction (compensated cirrhosis) indicate that there are minor, but clinically insignificant, alterations in ranitidine half-life, distribution, clearance, and bioavailability.

Excretion

Following IV injection, approximately 70% of the dose is recovered in the urine as unchanged drug. Renal clearance averages 530 ml/min, with a total clearance of 760 ml/min. The elimination half-life is 2.0-2.5 hours.

Four patients with clinically significant renal function impairment (creatinine clearance 25-35 ml/min) administered 50 mg of ranitidine intravenously had an average plasma half-life of 4.8 hours, a ranitidine clearance of 29 ml/min, and a volume of distribution of 1.76 L/kg. In general, these parameters appear to be altered in proportion to creatinine clearance (see DOSAGE AND ADMINISTRATION).

Geriatrics

The plasma half-life is prolonged and total clearance is reduced in the elderly population due to a decrease in renal function. The elimination half-life is 3.1 hours (see PRECAUTIONS, Geriatric Use and DOSAGE AND ADMINISTRATION, Dosage Adjustment for Patients With Impaired Renal Function).

Pediatrics

There are no significant differences in the pharmacokinetic parameter values for ranitidine in pediatric patients (from 1 month up to 16 years of age) and healthy adults when correction is made for body weight. The pharmacokinetics of ranitidine HCl in pediatric patients are summarized in TABLE 1.

***TABLE 1** Ranitidine Pharmacokinetics in Pediatric Patients Following IV Dosing*

Population (age)	n	Dose (mg/kg)	T½ (h)	Vd (L/kg)	CLp (ml/min/kg)
Peptic Ulcer Disease					
(<6 years)	6	1.25 or 2.5	2.2	1.29	11.41
(6-11.9 years)	11	1.25 or 2.5	2.1	1.14	8.96
(>12 years)	6	1.25 or 2.5	1.7	0.98	9.89
Adults	6	2.5	1.9	1.04	8.77
Peptic Ulcer Disease (3.5-16 years)	12	0.13-0.80	1.8	2.3	795 ml/min/1.73 m^2
Children in Intensive Care (1 day-12.6 years)	17	1.0	2.4	2	11.7
Neonates Receiving ECMO	12	2	6.6	1.8	4.3

T½ = Terminal half-life; CLp = Plasma clearance of ranitidine.
ECMO = extracorporeal membrane oxygenation.

Plasma clearance in neonatal patients (less than 1 month of age) receiving ECMO was considerably lower (3-4 ml/min/kg) than observed in children or adults. The elimination half-life in neonates averages 6.6 hours as compared to approximately 2 hours in adults and pediatric patients.

PHARMACODYNAMICS

Serum concentrations necessary to inhibit 50% of stimulated gastric acid secretion are estimated to be 36-94 ng/ml. Following single IV or IM 50 mg doses, serum concentrations of ranitidine HCl are in this range for 6-8 hours.

ANTISECRETORY ACTIVITY

Effects on Acid Secretion

Ranitidine HCl injection inhibits basal gastric acid secretion as well as gastric acid secretion stimulated by betazole and pentagastrin, as shown in TABLE 2.

***TABLE 2** Effect of Intravenous Ranitidine HCl on Gastric Acid Secretion*

	Time After Dose, h	% Inhibition of Gastric Acid Output by Intravenous Dose 20 mg	60 mg	100 mg
Betazole	Up to 2	93%	99%	99%
Pentagastrin	Up to 3	47%	66%	77%

In a group of 10 known hypersecretors, ranitidine plasma levels of 71, 180, and 376 ng/ml inhibited basal acid secretion by 76%, 90%, and 99.5%, respectively.

It appears that basal- and betazole-stimulated secretions are most sensitive to inhibition by ranitidine HCl, while pentagastrin-stimulated secretion is more difficult to suppress.

Effects on Other Gastrointestinal Secretions

Pepsin: Ranitidine HCl does not affect pepsin secretion. Total pepsin output is reduced in proportion to the decrease in volume of gastric juice.

Intrinsic Factor: Ranitidine HCl has no significant effect on pentagastrin-stimulated intrinsic factor secretion.

Serum Gastrin: Ranitidine HCl has little or no effect on fasting or postprandial serum gastrin.

Other Pharmacologic Actions:

Gastric Bacterial Flora: Increase in nitrate-reducing organisms, significance not known.

Prolactin Levels: No effect in recommended oral or intravenous (IV) dosage, but small, transient, dose-related increases in serum prolactin have been reported after IV bolus injections of 100 mg or more.

Other Pituitary Hormones: No effect on serum gonadotropins, TSH, or GH. Possible impairment of vasopressin release.

No change in cortisol, aldosterone, androgen, or estrogen levels.

No antiandrogenic action.

No effect on count, motility, or morphology of sperm.

Pediatrics

The ranitidine concentration necessary to suppress basal acid secretion by at least 90% has been reported to be 40-60 ng/ml in pediatric patients with duodenal or gastric ulcers.

In a study of 20 critically ill pediatric patients receiving ranitidine IV at 1 mg/kg every 6 hours, 10 patients with a baseline pH ≥4 maintained this baseline throughout the study. Eight (8) of the remaining 10 patients with a baseline of pH ≤2 achieved pH ≥4 throughout varying periods after dosing. It should be noted, however, that because these pharmacodynamic parameters were assessed in critically ill pediatric patients, the data should be interpreted with caution when dosing recommendations are made for a less seriously ill pediatric population.

In another small study of neonatal patients (n=5) receiving ECMO, gastric pH <4 pretreatment increased to >4 after a 2 mg/kg dose and remained above 4 for at least 15 hours.

INDICATIONS AND USAGE

Ranitidine HCl injection and injection premixed are indicated in some hospitalized patients with pathological hypersecretory conditions or intractable duodenal ulcers, or as an alternative to the oral dosage form for short-term use in patients who are unable to take oral medication.

NON-FDA APPROVED INDICATIONS

While not FDA approved indications, ranitidine is also used in the management of upper gastrointestinal bleeding and for stress ulcer prophylaxis in the ICU.

CONTRAINDICATIONS

Ranitidine HCl injection and injection premixed are contraindicated for patients known to have hypersensitivity to the drug.

PRECAUTIONS

GENERAL

Symptomatic response to therapy with ranitidine HCl does not preclude the presence of gastric malignancy.

Since ranitidine HCl is excreted primarily by the kidney, dosage should be adjusted in patients with impaired renal function (see DOSAGE AND ADMINISTRATION). Caution should be observed in patients with hepatic dysfunction since ranitidine HCl is metabolized in the liver.

In controlled studies in normal volunteers, elevations in SGPT have been observed when H_2-antagonists have been administered intravenously at greater than recommended dosages for 5 days or longer. Therefore, it seems prudent in patients receiving IV ranitidine at dosages ≥100 mg qid for periods of 5 days or longer to monitor SGPT daily (from day 5) for the remainder of IV therapy.

Bradycardia in association with rapid administration of ranitidine HCl injection has been reported rarely, usually in patients with factors predisposing to cardiac rhythm disturbances. Recommended rates of administration should not be exceeded (see DOSAGE AND ADMINISTRATION).

Rare reports suggest that ranitidine HCl may precipitate acute porphyric attacks in patients with acute porphyria. Ranitidine HCl should therefore be avoided in patients with a history of acute porphyria.

LABORATORY TESTS

False-positive tests for urine protein with Multistix may occur during therapy with ranitidine HCl, and therefore testing with sulfosalicylic acid is recommended.

CARCINOGENESIS, MUTAGENESIS, AND IMPAIRMENT OF FERTILITY

There was no indication of tumorigenic or carcinogenic effects in life-span studies in mice and rats at oral dosages up to 2000 mg/kg/day.

Ranitidine was not mutagenic in standard bacterial tests (*Salmonella, Escherichia coli*) for mutagenicity at concentrations up to the maximum recommended for these assays.

In a dominant lethal assay, a single oral dose of 1000 mg/kg to male rats was without effect on the outcome of two matings per week for the next 9 weeks.

PREGNANCY, TERATOGENIC EFFECTS, PREGNANCY CATEGORY B

Reproduction studies have been performed in rats and rabbits at oral doses up to 160 times the human oral dose and have revealed no evidence of impaired fertility or harm to the fetus due to ranitidine HCl. There are, however, no adequate and well-controlled studies in pregnant women. Because animal reproduction studies are not always predictive of human response, this drug should be used during pregnancy only if clearly needed.

NURSING MOTHERS

Ranitidine HCl is secreted in human milk. Caution should be exercised when ranitidine HCl is administered to a nursing mother.

PEDIATRIC USE

The safety and effectiveness of ranitidine HCl injection have been established in the age-group of 1 month to 16 years for the treatment of duodenal ulcer. Use of ranitidine HCl in this age-group is supported by adequate and well-controlled studies in adults, as well as additional pharmacokinetic data in pediatric patients, and an analysis of the published literature.

Safety and effectiveness in pediatric patients for the treatment of pathological hypersecretory conditions have not been established.

Limited data in neonatal patients (less than 1 month of age) receiving ECMO suggest that ranitidine HCl may be useful and safe for increasing gastric pH for patients at risk of gastrointestinal hemorrhage.

GERIATRIC USE

Clinical studies of ranitidine HCl injection did not include sufficient numbers of subjects aged 65 and over to determine whether they responded differently from younger subjects. However, in clinical studies of oral formulations of ranitidine HCl, of the total number of subjects enrolled in US and foreign controlled clinical trials, for which there were subgroup anaylses, 4197 were 65 and over, while 899 were 75 and older. No overall differences in safety or effectiveness were observed between these subjects and younger subjects, and other reported clinical experience has not identified differences in responses between the elderly and younger patients, but greater sensitivity of some older individuals cannot be ruled out.

This drug is known to be substantially excreted by the kidneys and the risk of toxic reactions to this drug may be greater in patients with impaired renal function. Because elderly patients are more likely to have decreased renal function, caution should be exercised in dose selection, and it may be useful to monitor renal function (see CLINICAL PHARMACOLOGY, Pharmacokinetics, Geriatrics and DOSAGE AND ADMINISTRATION, Dosage Adjustment for Patients With Impaired Renal Function).

DRUG INTERACTIONS

Although ranitidine HCl has been reported to bind weakly to cytochrome P-450 *in vitro,* recommended doses of the drug do not inhibit the action of the cytochrome P-450-linked oxygenase enzymes in the liver. However, there have been isolated reports of drug interactions that suggest that ranitidine HCl may affect the bioavailability of certain drugs by some mechanism as yet unidentified (*e.g.,* a pH-dependent effect on absorption or a change in volume of distribution).

Increased or decreased prothrombin times have been reported during concurrent use of ranitidine and warfarin. However, in human pharmacokinetic studies with dosages of ranitidine up to 400 mg/day, no interaction occurred; ranitidine had no effect on warfarin clearance or prothrombin time. The possibility of an interaction with warfarin at dosages of ranitidine higher than 400 mg/day has not been investigated.

In a ranitidine-triazolam drug-drug interaction study, triazolam plasma concentrations were higher during bid dosing of ranitidine than triazolam given alone. The mean area under the triazolam concentration-time curve (AUC) values, in 18- to 60–year–old subjects were 10% and 28% higher following administration of 75 mg and 150 mg ranitidine tablets, respectively, than triazolam given alone. In subjects older than 60 years of age, the mean AUC values were approximately 30% higher following administration of 75 and 150 mg ranitidine tablets. It appears that there were no changes in pharmacokinetics of triazolam and α-hydroxytriazolam, a major metabolite, and in their elimination. Reduced gastric acidity due to ranitidine may have resulted in an increase in the availability of triazolam. The clinical significance of this triazolam and ranitidine pharmacokinetic interaction is unknown.

ADVERSE REACTIONS

Transient pain at the site of IM injection has been reported. Transient local burning or itching has been reported with IV administration of ranitidine HCl.

The following have been reported as events in clinical trials or in the routine management of patients treated with oral or parenteral ranitidine HCl. The relationship to therapy with ranitidine HCl has been unclear in many cases. Headache, sometimes severe, seems to be related to administration of ranitidine HCl.

Central Nervous System: Rarely, malaise, dizziness, somnolence, insomnia, and vertigo. Rare cases of reversible mental confusion, agitation, depression, and hallucinations have been reported, predominantly in severely ill elderly patients. Rare cases of reversible blurred vision suggestive of a change in accommodation have been reported. Rare reports of reversible involuntary motor disturbances have been received.

Cardiovascular: As with other H_2-blockers, rare reports of arrhythmias such as tachycardia, bradycardia, asystole, atrioventricular block, and premature ventricular beats.

Gastrointestinal: Constipation, diarrhea, nausea/vomiting, abdominal discomfort/pain, and rare reports of pancreatitis.

Hepatic: In normal volunteers, SGPT values were increased to at least twice the pretreatment levels in 6 of 12 subjects receiving 100 mg qid intravenously for 7 days, and in 4 of 24 subjects receiving 50 mg qid intravenously for 5 days. There have been occasional reports of hepatocellular, cholestatic, or mixed hepatitis, with or without jaundice. In such circumstances, ranitidine should be immediately discontinued. These events are usually reversible, but in rare circumstances death has occurred. Rare cases of hepatic failure have also been reported.

Musculoskeletal: Rare reports of arthralgias and myalgias.

Hematologic: Blood count changes (leukopenia, granulocytopenia, and thrombocytopenia) have occurred in a few patients. These were usually reversible. Rare cases of agranulocytosis, pancytopenia, sometimes with marrow hypoplasia, and aplastic anemia and exceedingly rare cases of acquired immune hemolytic anemia have been reported.

Endocrine: Controlled studies in animals and humans have shown no stimulation of any pituitary hormone by ranitidine HCl and no antiandrogenic activity, and cimetidine-induced gynecomastia and impotence in hypersecretory patients have resolved when ranitidine HCl has been substituted. However, occasional cases of gynecomastia, impotence, and loss of libido have been reported in male patients receiving ranitidine HCl, but the incidence did not differ from that in the general population.

Integumentary: Rash, including rare cases of erythema multiforme. Rarely cases of alopecia and vasculitis.

Other: Rare cases of hypersensitivity reactions (*e.g.,* bronchospasm, fever, rash, eosinophilia), anaphylaxis, angioneurotic edema, and small increases in serum creatinine.

DOSAGE AND ADMINISTRATION

PARENTERAL ADMINISTRATION

In some hospitalized patients with pathological hypersecretory conditions or intractable duodenal ulcers, or in patients who are unable to take oral medication, ranitidine HCl may be administered parenterally according to the following recommendations:

Intramuscular Injection

50 mg (2 ml) every 6-8 hours. (No dilution necessary.)

Intermittent Intravenous Injection

Intermittent Bolus

50 mg (2 ml) every 6-8 hours. Dilute ranitidine HCl injection, 50 mg, in 0.9% sodium chloride injection or other compatible IV solution (see Stability) to a concentration no greater than 2.5 mg/ml (20 ml). Inject at a rate no greater than 4 ml/min (5 minutes).

Intermittent Infusion

50 mg (2 ml) every 6-8 hours. Dilute ranitidine HCl injection, 50 mg, in 5% dextrose injection or other compatible IV solution (see Stability) to a concentration no greater than 0.5 mg/ml (100 ml). Infuse at a rate no greater than 5-7 ml/min (15-20 minutes).

Ranitidine HCl injection premixed solution, 50 mg, in 0.45% sodium chloride, 50 ml, requires no dilution and should be infused over 15-20 minutes.

In some patients it may be necessary to increase dosage. When this is necessary, the increases should be made by more frequent administration of the dose, but generally should not exceed 400 mg/day.

Continuous Intravenous Infusion

Add ranitidine HCl injection to 5% dextrose injection or other compatible IV solution (see Stability). Deliver at a rate of 6.25 mg/h (*e.g.,* 150 mg [6 ml] of ranitidine HCl injection in 250 ml of 5% dextrose injection at 10.7 ml/h).

For Zollinger-Ellison patients, dilute ranitidine HCl injection in 5% dextrose injection or other compatible IV solution (see Stability) to a concentration no greater than 2.5 mg/ml. Start the infusion at a rate of 1.0 mg/kg/h. If after 4 hours either a measured gastric acid output is >10 mEq/h or the patient becomes symptomatic, the dose should be adjusted upward in 0.5 mg/kg/h increments, and the acid output should be remeasured. Dosages up to 2.5 mg/kg/h and infusion rates as high as 220 mg/h have been used.

PEDIATRIC USE

While limited data exist on the administration of IV ranitidine to children, the recommended dose in pediatric patients is for a total daily dose of 2-4 mg/kg, to be divided and administered every 6-8 hours, up to a maximum of 50 mg given every 6-8 hours. This recommendation is derived from adult clinical studies and pharmacokinetic data in pediatric patients. Limited data in neonatal patients (less than 1 month of age) receiving ECMO have shown that a dose of 2 mg/kg is usually sufficient to increase gastric pH to >4 for at least 15 hours. Therefore, doses of 2 mg/kg given every 12-24 hours or as a continuous infusion should be considered.

RANITIDINE HCl INJECTION PREMIXED IN FLEXIBLE PLASTIC CONTAINERS

Instructions for Use

To Open

Tear outer wrap at notch and remove solution container. Check for minute leaks by squeezing container firmly. If leaks are found, discard unit as sterility may be impaired.

Caution

Ranitidine HCl injection premixed in flexible plastic containers is to be administered by slow IV drip infusion only. **Additives should not be introduced into this solution.** If used with a primary IV fluid system, the primary solution should be discontinued during ranitidine HCl injection premixed infusion.

Do not administer unless solution is clear and container is undamaged.

Warning

Do not use flexible plastic container in series connections.

DOSAGE ADJUSTMENT FOR PATIENTS WITH IMPAIRED RENAL FUNCTION

The administration of ranitidine as a continuous infusion has not been evaluated in patients with impaired renal function. On the basis of experience with a group of subjects with severely impaired renal function treated with ranitidine HCl, the recommended dosage in patients with a creatinine clearance <50 ml/min is 50 mg every 18-24 hours. Should the patient's condition require, the frequency of dosing may be increased to every 12 hours or even further with caution. Hemodialysis reduces the level of circulating ranitidine. Ideally, the dosing schedule should be adjusted so that the timing of a scheduled dose coincides with the end of hemodialysis.

Elderly patients are more likely to have decreased renal function, therefore caution should be exercised in dose selection, and it may be useful to monitor renal function (see CLINICAL PHARMACOLOGY, Pharmacokinetics, Geriatrics and PRECAUTIONS, Geriatric Use).

STABILITY

Undiluted, ranitidine HCl injection tends to exhibit a yellow color that may intensify over time without adversely affecting potency. Ranitidine HCl injection is stable for 48 hours at room temperature when added to or diluted with most commonly used IV solutions, *e.g.,* 0.9% sodium chloride injection, 5% dextrose injection, 10% dextrose injection, lactated Ringer's injection, or 5% sodium bicarbonate injection.

Ranitidine HCl injection premixed in flexible plastic containers is sterile through the expiration date on the label when stored under recommended conditions.

Note: Parenteral drug products should be inspected visually for particulate matter and discoloration before administration whenever solution and container permit.

HOW SUPPLIED

ZANTAC INJECTION

Zantac injection, 25 mg/ml, containing phenol 0.5% as preservative, is available in 2 ml single-dose vials and 6 ml multidose vials.

Storage

Store between 4 and 30°C (39 and 86°F). Protect from light.

ZANTAC INJECTION PREMIXED

Zantac injection premixed, 50 mg/50 ml, in 0.45% sodium chloride, is available as a sterile, premixed solution for IV administration in single-dose, flexible plastic containers. It contains no preservatives.

Storage

Store between 2 and 25°C (36 and 77°F). Protect from light.

Exposure of pharmaceutical products to heat should be minimized. Avoid excessive heat; however, brief exposure up to 40°C does not adversely affect the product. Protect from freezing.

ORAL

DESCRIPTION

The active ingredient in Zantac 150 tablets, 300 tablets, 150 Efferdose tablets, 150 Efferdose granules, and syrup is ranitidine hydrochloride (HCl), a histamine H_2-receptor antagonist. Chemically it is N[2-[[[5-[(dimethylamino)methyl]-2-furanyl]methyl]thio]ethyl]-N′-methyl-2-nitro-1,1-ethenediamine, HCl.

The empirical formula is $C_{13}H_{22}N_4O_3S{\cdot}HCl$, representing a molecular weight of 350.87.

Ranitidine HCl is a white to pale yellow, granular substance that is soluble in water. It has a slightly bitter taste and sulfurlike odor.

TABLETS

Each Zantac 150 tablet for oral administration contains 168 mg of ranitidine HCl equivalent to 150 mg of ranitidine. Each tablet also contains the inactive ingredients FD&C yellow no. 6 aluminum lake, hydroxypropyl methylcellulose, magnesium stearate, microcrystalline cellulose, titanium dioxide, triacetin, and yellow iron oxide.

Each Zantac 300 tablet for oral administration contains 336 mg of ranitidine HCl equivalent to 300 mg of ranitidine. Each tablet also contains the inactive ingredients croscarmellose sodium, D&C yellow no. 10 aluminum lake, hydroxypropyl methylcellulose, magnesium stearate, microcrystalline cellulose, titanium dioxide, and triacetin.

EFFERDOSE TABLETS AND GRANULES

Zantac 150 Efferdose tablets and Zantac 150 Efferdose granules for oral administration are effervescent formulations of ranitidine that must be dissolved in water before use. Each individual tablet or the contents of a packet contain 168 mg of ranitidine HCl equivalent to 150 mg of ranitidine and the following inactive ingredients: aspartame, monosodium citrate anhydrous, povidone, and sodium bicarbonate. Each tablet also contains sodium benzoate. The total sodium content of each tablet is 183.12 mg (7.96 mEq) per 150 mg of ranitidine, and the total sodium content of each packet of granules is 173.54 mg (7.55 mEq) per 150 mg of ranitidine.

SYRUP

Each 1 ml of Zantac syrup contains 16.8 mg of ranitidine HCl equivalent to 15 mg of ranitidine. Zantac syrup also contains the inactive ingredients alcohol (7.5%), butylparaben, dibasic sodium phosphate, hydroxypropyl methylcellulose, peppermint flavor, monobasic potassium phosphate, propylparaben, purified water, saccharin sodium, sodium chloride, and sorbitol.

CLINICAL PHARMACOLOGY

Ranitidine HCl is a competitive, reversible inhibitor of the action of histamine at the histamine H_2-receptors, including receptors on the gastric cells. Ranitidine HCl does not lower serum Ca^{++} in hypercalcemic states. Ranitidine HCl is not an anticholinergic agent.

PHARMACOKINETICS

Absorption

Ranitidine HCl is 50% absorbed after oral administration, compared to an intravenous (IV) injection with mean peak levels of 440-545 ng/ml occurring 2-3 hours after a 150 mg dose. The syrup and Efferdose formulations are bioequivalent to the tablets. Absorption is not significantly impaired by the administration of food or antacids. Propantheline slightly delays and increases peak blood levels of ranitidine HCl, probably by delaying gastric emptying and transit time. In one study, simultaneous administration of high-potency antacid (150 mmol) in fasting subjects has been reported to decrease the absorption of ranitidine HCl.

Distribution

The volume of distribution is about 1.4 L/kg. Serum protein binding averages 15%.

Metabolism

In humans, the N-oxide is the principal metabolite in the urine; however, this amounts to <4% of the dose. Other metabolites are the S-oxide (1%) and the desmethyl ranitidine (1%). The remainder of the administered dose is found in the stool. Studies in patients with hepatic dysfunction (compensated cirrhosis) indicate that there are minor, but clinically insignificant, alterations in ranitidine half-life, distribution, clearance, and bioavailability.

Excretion

The principal route of excretion is the urine, with approximately 30% of the orally administered dose collected in the urine as unchanged drug in 24 hours. Renal clearance is about 410 ml/min, indicating active tubular excretion. The elimination half-life is 2.5 to 3 hours. Four patients with clinically significant renal function impairment (creatinine clearance 25-35 ml/min) administered 50 mg of ranitidine intravenously had an average plasma half-life of 4.8 hours, a ranitidine clearance of 29 ml/min, and a volume of distribution of 1.76 L/kg. In general, these parameters appear to be altered in proportion to creatinine clearance (see DOSAGE AND ADMINISTRATION).

Geriatrics

The plasma half-life is prolonged and total clearance is reduced in the elderly population due to a decrease in renal function. The elimination half-life is 3-4 hours. Peak levels average 526 ng/ml following a 150 mg twice daily dose and occur in about 3 hours (see PRECAUTIONS, Geriatric Use and DOSAGE AND ADMINISTRATION, Dosage Adjustment for Patients With Impaired Renal Function).

Pediatrics

There are no significant differences in the pharmacokinetic parameter values for ranitidine in pediatric patients (from 1 month up to 16 years of age) and healthy adults when correction is made for body weight. The average bioavailability of ranitidine given orally to pediatric patients is 48% which is comparable to the bioavailability of ranitidine in the adult population. All other pharmacokinetic parameter values ($T_{½}$, Vd, and CL) are similar to those observed with intravenous ranitidine use in pediatric patients. Estimates of C_{max} and T_{max} are displayed in TABLE 5.

TABLE 5 *Ranitidine Pharmacokinetics in Pediatric Patients Following Oral Dosing*

Population (age)	n	Dosage Form (dose)	C_{max} (ng/ml)	T_{max} (h)
Gastric or duodenal ulcer (3.5 to 16 years)	12	Tablets (1-2 mg/kg)	54-492	2.0
Otherwise healthy requiring ranitidine HCl (0.7 to 14 years, single dose)	10	Syrup (2 mg/kg)	244	1.61
Otherwise healthy requiring ranitidine HCl (0.7 to 14 years, multiple dose)	10	Syrup (2 mg/kg)	320	1.66

Plasma clearance measured in 2 neonatal patients (less than 1 month of age) was considerably lower (3 ml/min/kg) than children or adults and is likely due to reduced renal function observed in this population.

PHARMACODYNAMICS

Serum concentrations necessary to inhibit 50% of stimulated gastric acid secretion are estimated to be 36-94 ng/ml. Following a single oral dose of 150 mg, serum concentrations of ranitidine HCl are in this range up to 12 hours. However, blood levels bear no consistent relationship to dose or degree of acid inhibition.

In a pharmacodynamic comparison of the Efferdose with the ranitidine HCl tablets, during the first hour after administration, the Efferdose tablet formulation gave a significantly higher intragastric pH, by approximately 1 pH unit, compared to the ranitidine HCl tablets.

Antisecretory Activity

Effects on Acid Secretion

Ranitidine HCl inhibits both daytime and nocturnal basal gastric acid secretions as well as gastric acid secretion stimulated by food, betazole, and pentagastrin, as shown in TABLE 6.

It appears that basal-, nocturnal-, and betazole-stimulated secretions are most sensitive to inhibition by ranitidine HCl, responding almost completely to doses of 100 mg or less, while pentagastrin- and food-stimulated secretions are more difficult to suppress.

TABLE 6 *Effect of Oral Ranitidine HCl on Gastric Acid Secretion*

	Time After Dose, h	% Inhibition of Gastric Acid Output by Dose 75-80 mg	100 mg	150 mg	200 mg
Basal	Up to 4		99%	95%	
Nocturnal	Up to 13	95%	96%	92%	
Betazole	Up to 3		97%	99%	
Pentagastrin	Up to 5	58%	72%	72%	80%
Meal	Up to 3		73%	79%	95%

Effects on Other Gastrointestinal Secretions

Pepsin: Oral ranitidine HCl does not affect pepsin secretion. Total pepsin output is reduced in proportion to the decrease in volume of gastric juice.

Intrinsic Factor: Oral ranitidine HCl has no significant effect on pentagastrin-stimulated intrinsic factor secretion.

Serum Gastrin: Ranitidine HCl has little or no effect on fasting or postprandial serum gastrin.

Other Pharmacologic Actions:

Gastric Bacterial Flora: Increase in nitrate-reducing organisms, significance not known.

Prolactin Levels: No effect in recommended oral or intravenous (IV) dosage, but small, transient, dose-related increases in serum prolactin have been reported after IV bolus injections of 100 mg or more.

Other Pituitary Hormones: No effect on serum gonadotropins, TSH, or GH. Possible impairment of vasopressin release.

No change in cortisol, aldosterone, androgen, or estrogen levels.

R

No antiandrogenic action.
No effect on count, motility, or morphology of sperm.

Pediatrics

Oral doses of 6-10 mg/kg/day in 2 or 3 divided doses maintain gastric pH >4 throughout most of the dosing interval.

INDICATIONS AND USAGE

Ranitidine HCl is indicated in:

Short-term treatment of active duodenal ulcer. Most patients heal within 4 weeks. Studies available to date have not assessed the safety of ranitidine in uncomplicated duodenal ulcer for periods of more than 8 weeks.

Maintenance therapy for duodenal ulcer patients at reduced dosage after healing of acute ulcers. No placebo-controlled comparative studies have been carried out for periods of longer than 1 year.

The treatment of pathological hypersecretory conditions (*e.g.*, Zollinger-Ellison syndrome and systemic mastocytosis).

Short-term treatment of active, benign gastric ulcer. Most patients heal within 6 weeks and the usefulness of further treatment has not been demonstrated. Studies available to date have not assessed the safety of ranitidine in uncomplicated, benign gastric ulcer for periods of more than 6 weeks.

Maintenance therapy for gastric ulcer patients at reduced dosage after healing of acute ulcers. Placebo-controlled studies have been carried out for 1 year.

Treatment of GERD. Symptomatic relief commonly occurs within 24 hours after starting therapy with ranitidine HCl 150 mg bid.

Treatment of endoscopically diagnosed erosive esophagitis. Symptomatic relief of heartburn commonly occurs within 24 hours of therapy initiation with ranitidine HCl 150 mg qid.

Maintenance of healing of erosive esophagitis. Placebo-controlled trials have been carried out for 48 weeks.

Concomitant antacids should be given as needed for pain relief to patients with active duodenal ulcer; active, benign gastric ulcer; hypersecretory states; GERD; and erosive esophagitis.

CONTRAINDICATIONS

Ranitidine HCl is contraindicated for patients known to have hypersensitivity to the drug or any of the ingredients (see PRECAUTIONS).

PRECAUTIONS

GENERAL

Symptomatic response to therapy with ranitidine HCl does not preclude the presence of gastric malignancy.

Since ranitidine HCl is excreted primarily by the kidney, dosage should be adjusted in patients with impaired renal function (see DOSAGE AND ADMINISTRATION). Caution should be observed in patients with hepatic dysfunction since ranitidine HCl is metabolized in the liver.

Rare reports suggest that ranitidine HCl may precipitate acute porphyric attacks in patients with acute porphyria. Ranitidine HCl should therefore be avoided in patients with a history of acute porphyria.

INFORMATION FOR THE PATIENT

Phenylketonurics: Ranitidine HCl 150 Efferdose tablets and 150 Efferdose granules contain phenylalanine 16.84 mg/150 mg of ranitidine.

LABORATORY TESTS

False-positive tests for urine protein with Multistix may occur during ranitidine HCl therapy, and therefore testing with sulfosalicylic acid is recommended.

CARCINOGENESIS, MUTAGENESIS, AND IMPAIRMENT OF FERTILITY

There was no indication of tumorigenic or carcinogenic effects in life-span studies in mice and rats at dosages up to 2000 mg/kg/day.

Ranitidine was not mutagenic in standard bacterial tests (*Salmonella, Escherichia coli*) for mutagenicity at concentrations up to the maximum recommended for these assays.

In a dominant lethal assay, a single oral dose of 1000 mg/kg to male rats was without effect on the outcome of two matings per week for the next 9 weeks.

PREGNANCY, TERATOGENIC EFFECTS, PREGNANCY CATEGORY B

Reproduction studies have been performed in rats and rabbits at doses up to 160 times the human dose and have revealed no evidence of impaired fertility or harm to the fetus due to ranitidine HCl. There are, however, no adequate and well-controlled studies in pregnant women. Because animal reproduction studies are not always predictive of human response, this drug should be used during pregnancy only if clearly needed.

NURSING MOTHERS

Ranitidine HCl is secreted in human milk. Caution should be exercised when ranitidine HCl is administered to a nursing mother.

PEDIATRIC USE

The safety and effectiveness of ranitidine HCl have been established in the age-group of 1 month to 16 years for the treatment of duodenal and gastric ulcers, gastroesophageal reflux disease and erosive esophagitis, and the maintenance of healed duodenal and gastric ulcer. Use of ranitidine HCl in this age-group is supported by adequate and well-controlled studies in adults, as well as additional pharmacokinetic data in pediatric patients and an analysis of the published literature.

Safety and effectiveness in pediatric patients for the treatment of pathological hypersecretory conditions or the maintenance of healing of erosive esophagitis have not been established.

Safety and effectiveness in neonates (less than 1 month of age) have not been established (see CLINICAL PHARMACOLOGY, Pharmacokinetics, Pediatrics).

GERIATRIC USE

Of the total number of subjects enrolled in US and foreign controlled clinical trials of oral formulations of ranitidine HCl, for which there were subgroup anaylses, 4197 were 65 and over, while 899 were 75 and older. No overall differences in safety or effectiveness were observed between these subjects and younger subjects, and other reported clinical experience has not identified differences in responses between the elderly and younger patients, but greater sensitivity of some older individuals cannot be ruled out.

This drug is known to be substantially excreted by the kidneys and the risk of toxic reactions to this drug may be greater in patients with impaired renal function. Because elderly patients are more likely to have decreased renal function, caution should be exercised in dose selection, and it may be useful to monitor renal function (see CLINICAL PHARMACOLOGY, Pharmacokinetics, Geriatrics and DOSAGE AND ADMINISTRATION, Dosage Adjustment for Patients With Impaired Renal Function).

DRUG INTERACTIONS

Although ranitidine HCl has been reported to bind weakly to cytochrome P-450 *in vitro*, recommended doses of the drug do not inhibit the action of the cytochrome P-450-linked oxygenase enzymes in the liver. However, there have been isolated reports of drug interactions that suggest that ranitidine HCl may affect the bioavailability of certain drugs by some mechanism as yet unidentified (*e.g.*, a pH-dependent effect on absorption or a change in volume of distribution).

Increased or decreased prothrombin times have been reported during concurrent use of ranitidine and warfarin. However, in human pharmacokinetic studies with dosages of ranitidine up to 400 mg/day, no interaction occurred; ranitidine had no effect on warfarin clearance or prothrombin time. The possibility of an interaction with warfarin at dosages of ranitidine higher than 400 mg/day has not been investigated.

In a ranitidine-triazolam drug-drug interaction study, triazolam plasma concentrations were higher during bid dosing of ranitidine than triazolam given alone. The mean area under the triazolam concentration-time curve (AUC) values in 18- to 60-year-old subjects were 10% and 28% higher following administration of 75 and 150 mg ranitidine tablets, respectively, than triazolam given alone. In subjects older than 60 years of age, the mean AUC values were approximately 30% higher following administration of 75 and 150 mg ranitidine tablets. It appears that there were no changes in pharmacokinetics of triazolam and α-hydroxytriazolam, a major metabolite, and in their elimination. Reduced gastric acidity due to ranitidine may have resulted in an increase in the availability of triazolam. The clinical significance of this triazolam and ranitidine pharmacokinetic interaction is unknown.

ADVERSE REACTIONS

The following have been reported as events in clinical trials or in the routine management of patients treated with ranitidine HCl. The relationship to therapy with ranitidine HCl has been unclear in many cases. Headache, sometimes severe, seems to be related to administration of ranitidine HCl.

Central Nervous System: Rarely, malaise, dizziness, somnolence, insomnia, and vertigo. Rare cases of reversible mental confusion, agitation, depression, and hallucinations have been reported, predominantly in severely ill elderly patients. Rare cases of reversible blurred vision suggestive of a change in accommodation have been reported. Rare reports of reversible involuntary motor disturbances have been received.

Cardiovascular: As with other H_2-blockers, rare reports of arrhythmias such as tachycardia, bradycardia, atrioventricular block, and premature ventricular beats.

Gastrointestinal: Constipation, diarrhea, nausea/vomiting, abdominal discomfort/pain, and rare reports of pancreatitis.

Hepatic: There have been occasional reports of hepatocellular, cholestatic, or mixed hepatitis, with or without jaundice. In such circumstances, ranitidine should be immediately discontinued. These events are usually reversible, but in rare circumstances death has occurred. Rare cases of hepatic failure have also been reported. In normal volunteers, SGPT values were increased to at least twice the pretreatment levels in 6 of 12 subjects receiving 100 mg qid intravenously for 7 days, and in 4 of 24 subjects receiving 50 mg qid intravenously for 5 days.

Musculoskeletal: Rare reports of arthralgias and myalgias.

Hematologic: Blood count changes (leukopenia, granulocytopenia, and thrombocytopenia) have occurred in a few patients. These were usually reversible. Rare cases of agranulocytosis, pancytopenia, sometimes with marrow hypoplasia, and aplastic anemia and exceedingly rare cases of acquired immune hemolytic anemia have been reported.

Endocrine: Controlled studies in animals and man have shown no stimulation of any pituitary hormone by ranitidine HCl and no antiandrogenic activity, and cimetidine-induced gynecomastia and impotence in hypersecretory patients have resolved when ranitidine HCl has been substituted. However, occasional cases of gynecomastia, impotence, and loss of libido have been reported in male patients receiving ranitidine HCl, but the incidence did not differ from that in the general population.

Integumentary: Rash, including rare cases of erythema multiforme. Rarely cases of alopecia and vasculitis.

Other: Rare cases of hypersensitivity reactions (*e.g.*, bronchospasm, fever, rash, eosinophilia), anaphylaxis, angioneurotic edema, and small increases in serum creatinine.

DOSAGE AND ADMINISTRATION

ACTIVE DUODENAL ULCER

The current recommended adult oral dosage of ranitidine HCl for duodenal ulcer is 150 mg or 10 ml (2 teaspoonfuls equivalent to 150 mg of ranitidine) twice daily. An alternative dosage of 300 mg or 20 ml (4 teaspoonfuls equivalent to 300 mg of ranitidine) once daily after the evening meal or at bedtime can be used for patients in whom dosing convenience is important. The advantages of one treatment regimen compared to the other in a particular patient population have yet to be demonstrated. Smaller doses have been shown to be equally effective in inhibiting gastric acid secretion in US studies, and several foreign trials have shown that 100 mg twice daily is as effective as the 150 mg dose.

Antacid should be given as needed for relief of pain (see CLINICAL PHARMACOLOGY, Pharmacokinetics).

MAINTENANCE OF HEALING OF DUODENAL ULCERS

The current recommended adult oral dosage is 150 mg or 10 ml (2 teaspoonfuls equivalent to 150 mg of ranitidine) at bedtime.

PATHOLOGICAL HYPERSECRETORY CONDITIONS (SUCH AS ZOLLINGER-ELLISON SYNDROME)

The current recommended adult oral dosage is 150 mg or 10 ml (2 teaspoonfuls equivalent to 150 mg of ranitidine) twice a day. In some patients it may be necessary to administer ranitidine HCl 150 mg doses more frequently. Dosages should be adjusted to individual patient needs, and should continue as long as clinically indicated. Dosages up to 6 g/day have been employed in patients with severe disease.

BENIGN GASTRIC ULCER

The current recommended adult oral dosage is 150 mg or 10 ml (2 teaspoonfuls equivalent to 150 mg of ranitidine) twice a day.

MAINTENANCE OF HEALING OF GASTRIC ULCERS

The current recommended adult oral dosage is 150 mg or 10 ml (2 teaspoonfuls equivalent to 150 mg of ranitidine) at bedtime.

GERD

The current recommended adult oral dosage is 150 mg or 10 ml (2 teaspoonfuls equivalent to 150 mg of ranitidine) twice a day.

EROSIVE ESOPHAGITIS

The current recommended adult oral dosage is 150 mg or 10 ml (2 teaspoonfuls equivalent to 150 mg of ranitidine) 4 times a day.

MAINTENANCE OF HEALING OF EROSIVE ESOPHAGITIS

The current recommended adult oral dosage is 150 mg or 10 ml (2 teaspoonfuls equivalent to 150 mg of ranitidine) twice a day.

PEDIATRIC USE

The safety and effectiveness of ranitidine HCl have been established in the age-group of 1 month to 16 years. There is insufficient information about the pharmacokinetics of ranitidine HCl in neonatal patients (less than 1 month of age) to make dosing recommendations.

Treatment of Duodenal and Gastric Ulcers

The recommended oral dose for the treatment of active duodenal and gastric ulcers is 2-4 mg/kg/day twice daily to a maximum of 300 mg/day. This recommendation is derived from adult clinical studies and pharmacokinetic data in pediatric patients.

Maintenance of Healing of Duodenal and Gastric Ulcers

The recommended oral dose for the maintenance of healing of duodenal and gastric ulcers is 2-4 mg/kg once daily to a maximum of 150 mg/day. This recommendation is derived from adult clinical studies and pharmacokinetic data in pediatric patients.

Treatment of GERD and Erosive Esophagitis

Although limited data exist for these conditions in pediatric patients, published literature supports a dosage of 5-10 mg/kg/day, usually given as 2 divided doses.

DOSAGE ADJUSTMENT FOR PATIENTS WITH IMPAIRED RENAL FUNCTION

On the basis of experience with a group of subjects with severely impaired renal function treated with ranitidine HCl, the recommended dosage in patients with a creatinine clearance <50 ml/min is 150 mg or 10 ml (2 teaspoonfuls equivalent to 150 mg of ranitidine) every 24 hours. Should the patient's condition require, the frequency of dosing may be increased to every 12 hours or even further with caution. Hemodialysis reduces the level of circulating ranitidine. Ideally, the dosing schedule should be adjusted so that the timing of a scheduled dose coincides with the end of hemodialysis.

Elderly patients are more likely to have decreased renal function, therefore caution should be exercised in dose selection, and it may be useful to monitor renal function (see CLINICAL PHARMACOLOGY, Pharmacokinetics, Geriatrics and PRECAUTIONS, Geriatric Use).

HOW SUPPLIED

ZANTAC TABLETS

Zantac 150 Tablets (ranitidine HCl equivalent to 150 mg of ranitidine) are peach, film-coated, five-sided tablets embossed with "ZANTAC 150" on one side and "Glaxo" on the other.

Zantac 300 Tablets (ranitidine HCl equivalent to 300 mg of ranitidine) are yellow, film-coated, capsule-shaped tablets embossed with "ZANTAC 300" on one side and "Glaxo" on the other.

Storage: Store between 15 and 30°C (59 and 86°F) in a dry place. Protect from light. Replace cap securely after each opening.

ZANTAC EFFERDOSE TABLETS AND GRANULES

Zantac 150 Efferdose Tablets (ranitidine HCl equivalent to 150 mg of ranitidine) are white to pale yellow, round, flat-faced, bevel-edged tablets embossed with "ZANTAC 150" on one side and "427" on the other. They are packaged individually in foil.

Zantac 150 Efferdose Granules (ranitidine HCl equivalent to 150 mg of ranitidine) are white to pale yellow granules. Each 150 mg dose of granules (approximately 1.44 g) is packaged in individual foil packets.

Storage: Store between 2 and 30°C (36 and 86°F).

ZANTAC SYRUP

Zantac Syrup, a clear, peppermint-flavored liquid, contains 16.8 mg of ranitidine HCl equivalent to 15 mg of ranitidine per 1 ml (75 mg/5 ml) in bottles of 16 fluid oz (1 pint).

Storage: Store between 4 and 25°C (39 and 77°F). Dispense in tight, light-resistant containers.

PRODUCT LISTING - RATED THERAPEUTICALLY EQUIVALENT

Package	Price	Product, Manufacturer	NDC
Capsule - Oral - 150 mg			
60's	$91.27	GENERIC, Geneva Pharmaceuticals	00781-2855-60
60's	$91.27	GENERIC, Par Pharmaceutical Inc	49884-0647-02
60's	$102.00	GENERIC, Par Pharmaceutical Inc	49884-0757-02
Capsule - Oral - 300 mg			
10's	$32.00	GENERIC, Southwood Pharmaceuticals Inc	58016-0570-10
14's	$44.80	GENERIC, Southwood Pharmaceuticals Inc	58016-0570-14
15's	$48.00	GENERIC, Southwood Pharmaceuticals Inc	58016-0570-15
20's	$65.00	GENERIC, Southwood Pharmaceuticals Inc	58016-0570-20
21's	$67.20	GENERIC, Southwood Pharmaceuticals Inc	58016-0570-21
28's	$89.60	GENERIC, Southwood Pharmaceuticals Inc	58016-0570-28
30's	$82.30	GENERIC, Geneva Pharmaceuticals	00781-2865-31
30's	$82.30	GENERIC, Par Pharmaceutical Inc	49884-0648-11
30's	$92.00	GENERIC, Par Pharmaceutical Inc	49884-0758-11
30's	$96.00	GENERIC, Southwood Pharmaceuticals Inc	58016-0570-30
40's	$128.00	GENERIC, Southwood Pharmaceuticals Inc	58016-0570-40
50's	$160.00	GENERIC, Southwood Pharmaceuticals Inc	58016-0570-50
56's	$179.20	GENERIC, Southwood Pharmaceuticals Inc	58016-0570-56
60's	$192.00	GENERIC, Southwood Pharmaceuticals Inc	58016-0570-60
90's	$288.00	GENERIC, Southwood Pharmaceuticals Inc	58016-0570-90
100's	$266.12	GENERIC, Par Pharmaceutical Inc	49884-0648-01
100's	$320.00	GENERIC, Southwood Pharmaceuticals Inc	58016-0570-00
120's	$384.00	GENERIC, Southwood Pharmaceuticals Inc	58016-0570-02
Tablet - Oral - 150 mg			
6's	$6.63	GENERIC, Pd-Rx Pharmaceuticals	55289-0319-06
6's	$14.75	GENERIC, Pharma Pac	52959-0325-06
10's	$18.90	GENERIC, Compumed Pharmaceuticals	00403-2341-10
14's	$8.10	GENERIC, Pd-Rx Pharmaceuticals	55289-0319-14
14's	$25.18	ZANTAC 150, Allscripts Pharmaceutical Company	54569-0445-00
14's	$27.45	GENERIC, Compumed Pharmaceuticals	00403-2341-14
14's	$29.87	GENERIC, Quality Care Pharmaceuticals Inc	60346-0729-14
14's	$39.08	GENERIC, Pd-Rx Pharmaceuticals	55289-0551-14
14's	$39.12	GENERIC, Pharma Pac	52959-0325-14
15's	$41.08	GENERIC, Pharma Pac	52959-0325-15
20's	$8.94	GENERIC, Pd-Rx Pharmaceuticals	55289-0319-20
20's	$35.75	GENERIC, St. Mary'S Mpp	60760-0025-20
20's	$35.97	ZANTAC 150, Allscripts Pharmaceutical Company	54569-0445-01
25's	$29.45	GENERIC, Pd-Rx Pharmaceuticals	55289-0319-97
25's	$62.02	GENERIC, Pd-Rx Pharmaceuticals	55289-0551-97
28's	$10.20	GENERIC, Pd-Rx Pharmaceuticals	55289-0319-28
28's	$67.20	ZANTAC 150, Pharma Pac	52959-0325-28
28's	$69.61	GENERIC, Pd-Rx Pharmaceuticals	55289-0551-28
30's	$10.94	GENERIC, Pd-Rx Pharmaceuticals	55289-0319-30
30's	$50.35	GENERIC, Compumed Pharmaceuticals	00403-2341-30
30's	$53.95	ZANTAC 150, Allscripts Pharmaceutical Company	54569-0445-02
30's	$62.19	GENERIC, Pharma Pac	52959-0325-30
30's	$65.26	GENERIC, Physicians Total Care	54868-0323-02
31 x 10	$489.71	GENERIC, Vangard Labs	00615-4513-53
31 x 10	$489.71	GENERIC, Vangard Labs	00615-4513-63
40's	$86.61	GENERIC, Physicians Total Care	54868-0323-07
50's	$93.02	GENERIC, Physicians Total Care	54868-0323-04
60's	$29.70	GENERIC, Pd-Rx Pharmaceuticals	55289-0319-60
60's	$88.80	GENERIC, Teva Pharmaceuticals Usa	00093-8544-06
60's	$88.80	GENERIC, Geneva Pharmaceuticals	00781-1883-60
60's	$88.80	GENERIC, Apotex Usa Inc	60505-0025-04
60's	$89.28	GENERIC, Roxane Laboratories Inc	00054-4853-21
60's	$89.28	GENERIC, Eon Labs Manufacturing Inc	00185-0135-60
60's	$89.28	GENERIC, Dixon-Shane Inc	17236-0741-60
60's	$90.29	GENERIC, Major Pharmaceuticals Inc	00904-5261-52
60's	$90.80	GENERIC, Mylan Pharmaceuticals Inc	00378-3252-91
60's	$92.30	GENERIC, Compumed Pharmaceuticals	00403-2341-71
60's	$95.30	GENERIC, Watson Laboratories Inc	00591-0760-60
60's	$95.30	GENERIC, Par Pharmaceutical Inc	49884-0544-02
60's	$95.30	GENERIC, Watson Laboratories Inc	52544-0760-60
60's	$95.30	GENERIC, Ranbaxy Laboratories	63304-0745-60
60's	$95.30	GENERIC, Ranbaxy Laboratories	63304-0770-60
60's	$104.71	GENERIC, Physicians Total Care	54868-0323-01
60's	$107.90	ZANTAC 150, Allscripts Pharmaceutical Company	54569-0445-03
60's	$123.40	ZANTAC 150, Glaxosmithkline	00173-0344-42
60's	$136.09	GENERIC, Pharma Pac	52959-0325-60
90's	$148.80	GENERIC, Allscripts Pharmaceutical Company	54569-8503-01
90's	$157.28	GENERIC, Physicians Total Care	54868-0323-00
100's	$34.11	FEDERAL UPPER LIMIT, H.C.F.A. F F P	99999-2174-02
100's	$148.00	GENERIC, Teva Pharmaceuticals Usa	00093-8544-01
100's	$148.00	GENERIC, Geneva Pharmaceuticals	00781-1883-01
100's	$148.00	GENERIC, Novopharm Usa Inc	55953-0544-40
100's	$148.78	GENERIC, Mylan Pharmaceuticals Inc	00378-3252-01
100's	$148.78	GENERIC, Dixon-Shane Inc	17236-0741-01
100's	$148.80	GENERIC, Eon Labs Manufacturing Inc	00185-0135-01
100's	$148.81	GENERIC, Ranbaxy Laboratories	63304-0745-01
100's	$150.85	GENERIC, Geneva Pharmaceuticals	00781-1883-13
100's	$155.85	GENERIC, Compumed Pharmaceuticals	00403-2341-01
100's	$156.20	GENERIC, Par Pharmaceutical Inc	49884-0544-01
100's	$156.20	GENERIC, Apotex Usa Inc	60505-0025-06

100's	$156.20	GENERIC, Ranbaxy Laboratories	63304-0770-01
100's	$156.22	GENERIC, Major Pharmaceuticals Inc	00904-5261-61
100's	$174.70	GENERIC, Physicians Total Care	54868-0323-06
100's	$208.70	ZANTAC 150, Glaxosmithkline	00173-0344-47
180's	$35.68	GENERIC, Golden State Medical	60429-0704-18
180's	$297.60	GENERIC, Allscripts Pharmaceutical Company	54569-8503-00
180's	$297.61	ZANTAC 150, Glaxosmithkline	00173-0344-16
180's	$370.16	ZANTAC 150, Glaxosmithkline	00173-0344-17

Tablet - Oral - 300 mg

7's	$34.02	GENERIC, Pd-Rx Pharmaceuticals	55289-0539-07
10's	$30.15	GENERIC, Pharma Pac	52959-0201-10
14's	$68.05	GENERIC, Pd-Rx Pharmaceuticals	55289-0539-14
15's	$41.28	GENERIC, Allscripts Pharmaceutical Company	54569-4508-00
15's	$47.44	GENERIC, Pharma Pac	52959-0201-15
15's	$48.64	ZANTAC 300, Allscripts Pharmaceutical Company	54569-0444-04
15's	$48.90	GENERIC, Pharma Pac	52959-0526-15
30's	$9.54	FEDERAL UPPER LIMIT, H.C.F.A. F F P	99999-2174-03
30's	$18.30	GENERIC, Pd-Rx Pharmaceuticals	55289-0505-30
30's	$80.60	GENERIC, Teva Pharmaceuticals Usa	00093-8547-56
30's	$80.60	GENERIC, Geneva Pharmaceuticals	00781-1884-31
30's	$80.60	GENERIC, Major Pharmaceuticals Inc	00904-5262-46
30's	$80.60	GENERIC, Teva Pharmaceuticals Usa	55953-0547-27
30's	$80.60	GENERIC, Apotex Usa Inc	60505-0026-02
30's	$81.04	GENERIC, Dixon-Shane Inc	17236-0742-30
30's	$81.05	GENERIC, Eon Labs Manufacturing Inc	00185-0136-30
30's	$82.42	GENERIC, Allscripts Pharmaceutical Company	54569-4508-01
30's	$83.74	GENERIC, Major Pharmaceuticals Inc	00904-5262-47
30's	$87.90	GENERIC, Mylan Pharmaceuticals Inc	00378-3254-93
30's	$87.90	GENERIC, Watson Laboratories Inc	00591-0761-30
30's	$87.90	GENERIC, Par Pharmaceutical Inc	49884-0545-11
30's	$87.90	GENERIC, Watson/Rugby Laboratories Inc	52544-0761-30
30's	$87.90	GENERIC, Ranbaxy Laboratories	63304-0746-30
30's	$87.90	GENERIC, Ranbaxy Laboratories	63304-0771-30
30's	$97.27	ZANTAC 300, Allscripts Pharmaceutical Company	54569-0444-01
30's	$112.01	ZANTAC 300, Glaxosmithkline	00173-0393-40
30's	$116.90	GENERIC, Physicians Total Care	54868-0324-01
60's	$194.54	ZANTAC 300, Allscripts Pharmaceutical Company	54569-0444-03
90's	$270.18	GENERIC, Allscripts Pharmaceutical Company	54569-8546-00
100's	$268.70	GENERIC, Teva Pharmaceuticals Usa	00093-8547-01
100's	$270.00	GENERIC, Dixon-Shane Inc	17236-0742-01
100's	$270.13	GENERIC, Mylan Pharmaceuticals Inc	00378-3254-01
100's	$270.18	GENERIC, Eon Labs Manufacturing Inc	00185-0136-01
100's	$270.19	GENERIC, Roxane Laboratories Inc	00054-4854-25
100's	$271.96	GENERIC, Geneva Pharmaceuticals	00781-1884-13
100's	$273.00	GENERIC, Watson/Rugby Laboratories Inc	52544-0761-01
100's	$286.70	GENERIC, Par Pharmaceutical Inc	49884-0545-01
100's	$286.70	GENERIC, Apotex Usa Inc	60505-0026-03
100's	$286.70	GENERIC, Ranbaxy Laboratories	63304-0771-01
100's	$333.97	ZANTAC 300, Glaxosmithkline	00173-0393-47
250's	$641.68	GENERIC, Eon Labs Manufacturing Inc	00185-0136-52
250's	$650.00	GENERIC, Dixon-Shane Inc	17236-0742-25
250's	$671.75	GENERIC, Teva Pharmaceuticals Usa	00093-8547-52
250's	$671.75	GENERIC, Geneva Pharmaceuticals	00781-1884-25
250's	$671.75	GENERIC, Novopharm Usa Inc	55953-0547-58
250's	$671.75	GENERIC, Apotex Usa Inc	60505-0026-07
250's	$675.48	GENERIC, Ranbaxy Laboratories	63304-0771-04
250's	$697.00	GENERIC, Par Pharmaceutical Inc	49884-0545-04
250's	$697.29	GENERIC, Major Pharmaceuticals Inc	00904-5262-70
250's	$933.51	ZANTAC 300, Glaxosmithkline	00173-0393-06

R

PRODUCT LISTING - EQUIVALENTS NOT AVAILABLE

Granule, Effervescent - Oral - 150 mg

60's	$110.89	ZANTAC EFFERDOSE, Glaxosmithkline	00173-0451-01

Solution - Injectable - 25 mg/ml

2 ml x 10	$39.90	ZANTAC, Glaxosmithkline	00173-0362-38
6 ml	$9.26	ZANTAC, Glaxosmithkline	00173-0363-01
40 ml	$60.54	ZANTAC, Glaxosmithkline	00173-0363-00

Solution - Intravenous - 1 mg/ml

50 ml x 24	$141.84	ZANTAC, Glaxosmithkline	00173-0441-00

Syrup - Oral - 15 mg/ml

10 ml x 50	$473.00	GENERIC, Alpharma Uspd Makers Of Barre and Nmc	50962-0203-60
480 ml	$200.16	ZANTAC, Allscripts Pharmaceutical Company	54569-4996-00
480 ml	$236.76	ZANTAC, Glaxosmithkline	00173-0383-54

Tablet - Oral - 150 mg

1's	$3.41	GENERIC, Prescript Pharmaceuticals	00247-0211-01
2's	$3.46	GENERIC, Prescript Pharmaceuticals	00247-0211-02
3's	$3.52	GENERIC, Prescript Pharmaceuticals	00247-0211-03
4's	$3.56	GENERIC, Prescript Pharmaceuticals	00247-0211-04
4's	$6.05	GENERIC, Allscripts Pharmaceutical Company	54569-4507-04
6's	$3.67	GENERIC, Prescript Pharmaceuticals	00247-0211-06
6's	$9.07	GENERIC, Allscripts Pharmaceutical Company	54569-4507-03
6's	$24.26	GENERIC, Pharma Pac	52959-0502-06
10's	$3.88	GENERIC, Prescript Pharmaceuticals	00247-0211-10
14's	$4.09	GENERIC, Prescript Pharmaceuticals	00247-0211-14
14's	$49.19	GENERIC, Pharma Pac	52959-0502-14
15's	$4.15	GENERIC, Prescript Pharmaceuticals	00247-0211-15
15's	$46.83	GENERIC, Southwood Pharmaceuticals Inc	58016-0345-15
15's	$51.64	GENERIC, Pharma Pac	52959-0502-15
20's	$4.41	GENERIC, Prescript Pharmaceuticals	00247-0211-20
20's	$30.22	GENERIC, Allscripts Pharmaceutical Company	54569-4507-02
20's	$62.45	GENERIC, Southwood Pharmaceuticals Inc	58016-0345-20
21's	$65.56	GENERIC, Southwood Pharmaceuticals Inc	58016-0345-21
28's	$4.84	GENERIC, Prescript Pharmaceuticals	00247-0211-28
28's	$84.97	GENERIC, Pharma Pac	52959-0502-28
28's	$87.42	GENERIC, Southwood Pharmaceuticals Inc	58016-0345-28
30's	$4.28	GENERIC, Physicians Total Care	54868-4048-02
30's	$4.94	GENERIC, Prescript Pharmaceuticals	00247-0211-30
30's	$45.41	GENERIC, Allscripts Pharmaceutical Company	54569-4507-00
30's	$91.04	GENERIC, Pharma Pac	52959-0502-30
30's	$93.67	GENERIC, Southwood Pharmaceuticals Inc	58016-0345-30
30's	$95.69	GENERIC, Nucare Pharmaceuticals Inc	66267-0188-30
40's	$124.89	GENERIC, Southwood Pharmaceuticals Inc	58016-0345-40
50's	$156.11	GENERIC, Southwood Pharmaceuticals Inc	58016-0345-50
56's	$175.00	GENERIC, Southwood Pharmaceuticals Inc	58016-0345-56
60's	$6.53	GENERIC, Prescript Pharmaceuticals	00247-0211-60
60's	$10.72	GENERIC, Physicians Total Care	54868-4048-00
60's	$89.28	GENERIC, Watson/Schein Pharmaceuticals Inc	00364-2633-06
60's	$90.66	GENERIC, Allscripts Pharmaceutical Company	54569-4507-01
60's	$95.30	GENERIC, Ranbaxy Laboratories	63304-0838-60
60's	$178.19	GENERIC, Pharma Pac	52959-0502-60
60's	$187.39	GENERIC, Southwood Pharmaceuticals Inc	58016-0345-60
80's	$249.78	GENERIC, Southwood Pharmaceuticals Inc	58016-0345-80
90's	$134.20	GENERIC, Pharmaceutical Corporation Of America	51655-0881-26
90's	$281.00	GENERIC, Southwood Pharmaceuticals Inc	58016-0345-90
100's	$8.65	GENERIC, Prescript Pharmaceuticals	00247-0211-00
100's	$10.49	GENERIC, Physicians Total Care	54868-4048-01
100's	$89.10	GENERIC, Par Pharmaceutical Inc	49884-5444-02
100's	$148.78	GENERIC, Watson/Schein Pharmaceuticals Inc	00364-2633-01
100's	$158.60	GENERIC, Udl Laboratories Inc	51079-0879-20
100's	$312.23	GENERIC, Southwood Pharmaceuticals Inc	58016-0345-00

Tablet - Oral - 300 mg

30's	$81.04	GENERIC, Watson/Schein Pharmaceuticals Inc	00364-2634-30
30's	$87.90	GENERIC, Ranbaxy Laboratories	63304-0839-30
250's	$671.75	GENERIC, Watson/Schein Pharmaceuticals Inc	00364-2634-04

Tablet, Effervescent - Oral - 150 mg

60's	$110.89	ZANTAC EFFERDOSE, Glaxosmithkline	00173-0427-02

Rauwolfia Serpentina *(002176)*

Categories: Hypertension, essential; Psychosis; Schizophrenia; Pregnancy Category C; FDA Approval Pre 1982
Drug Classes: Antiadrenergics, peripheral
Brand Names: Rauwolfemms
Cost of Therapy: $1.06 (Hypertension; Generic Tablets; 100 mg; 2 tablets/day; 30 day supply)

DESCRIPTION

Powdered rauwolfia serpentina is a hypotensive agent prepared from the whole root of *Rauwolfia serpentina* Benth. The powder contains not less than 0.15% and not more than 0.2% of reserpine-rescinnamine group alkaloids, calculated as reserpine.

CLINICAL PHARMACOLOGY

Rauwolfia serpentina probably produces its antihypertensive effects through depletion of tissue stores of catecholamines (epinephrine and norepinephrine) from peripheral sites. By contrast, its sedative and tranquilizing properties are thought to be related to depletion of 5-hydroxytryptamine from the brain. Rauwolfia serpentina is characterized by slow onset of action and sustained effect. Both its cardiovascular and central nervous system effects may persist following withdrawal of the drug.

INDICATIONS AND USAGE

Mild essential hypertension; also useful as adjunctive therapy with other antihypertensive agents in the more severe forms of hypertension. Relief of symptoms in agitated psychotic states (*e.g.,* schizophrenia), primarily in those individuals unable to tolerate phenothiazine derivatives or those who also require antihypertensive medication.

CONTRAINDICATIONS

Demonstrated hypersensitivity to rauwolfia, mental depression (especially with suicidal tendencies), active peptic ulcer, ulcerative colitis, and in patients receiving electroconvulsive therapy.

WARNINGS

Extreme caution should be exercised in treating patients with a history of mental depression. Discontinue the drug at first sign of despondency, early morning insomnia, loss of appetite, impotence, or self-deprecation. Drug-induced depression may persist for several months after drug withdrawal and may be severe enough to result in suicide.

In co-therapy, MAO inhibitors should be avoided or used with extreme caution.

Usage in Pregnancy: The safety or rauwolfia preparations for use during pregnancy or lactation has not been established; therefore, the drug should be used in pregnant patients or in women of childbearing potential only when, in the judgement of the physician, it is es-

sential to the welfare of the patient. Increased respiratory tract secretions, nasal congestion, cyanosis, and anorexia may occur in infants born to rauwolfia-treated mothers since the drug crosses the placental barrier and appears in cord blood.
Usage in Nursing: Rauwolfia appears in breast milk.

PRECAUTIONS

Because rauwolfia preparations increase gastrointestinal motility and secretion, this drug should be used cautiously in patients with a history of peptic ulcer, ulcerative colitis, or gallstones (biliary colic may be precipitated). Patients on high dosage should be checked regularly for possible reactivation of peptic ulcer. Caution should be used when treating hypertensive patients with renal insufficiency since they adjust poorly to lowered blood pressure levels.

Use rauwolfia serpentina cautiously with digitalis and quinidine since cardiac arrhythmias have occurred with rauwolfia preparations.

Preoperative withdrawal of rauwolfia serpentina does not assure that circulatory instability will not occur. It is important that the anesthesiologist be aware of the patient's drug intake and consider this in the overall management since hypotension has occurred in patients receiving rauwolfia preparations. Anticholinergic and/or adrenergic drugs (*e.g.*, metaraminol, norepinephrine) have been employed to treat adverse vagocirculatory effects.

Animal tumorigenicity: Rodent studies have shown that reserpine is an animal tumorigen, causing an increased incidence of mammary fibroadenomas in female mice, malignant tumors of the seminal vesicles in male mice, and malignant adrenal medullary tumors in male rats. These findings arose in 2 year studies in which the drug was administered in the feed at concentrations of 5 and 10 ppm—about 100 to 300 times the usual human dose. The breast neoplasms are though to be related to reserpine's prolactin-elevating effect. Several other prolactin-elevating drugs have also been associated with an increased incidence of mammary neoplasia in rodents.

The extent to which these findings indicate a risk to humans in uncertain. Tissue culture experiments show that about one-third of human breast tumors are prolactin-dependent in vitro, a factor of considerable importance if the use of the drug is contemplated in a patient with previously detected breast cancer.

The possibility of an increased risk of breast cancer in reserpine users has been studied extensively; however, non firm conclusion has emerged. Although a few epidemiologic studies have suggested a slightly increased risk (less than twofold in all studies except one) in women who have used reserpine, other studies of generally similar design have not confirmed this. Epidemiologic studies conducted using other drug's (neuroleptic agents) that, like reserpine, increase prolactin levels and therefore would be considered rodent mammary carcinogens, have not shown an association between chronic administration of the drug and human mammary tumorigenesis. While long-term clinical observation has not suggested such an association, the available evidence is considered too limited to be conclusive at this time. An association of reserpine intake with pheochromocytoma or tumors of the seminal vesicles has not been explored.

ADVERSE REACTIONS

Gastrointestinal: Hypersecretion, nausea, vomiting, anorexia, and diarrhea.
Central Nervous System: Drowsiness, depression, nervousness, paradoxical anxiety, nightmares, rare Parkinsonian syndrome and other extrapyramidal tract symptoms, and CNS sensitization manifested by dull sensorium deafness, glaucoma, uveitis, and optic atrophy.
Cardiovascular: Angina-like symptoms, arrhythmias (particularly when used concurrently with digitalis or quinidine), and bradycardia.
Other: Nasal congestion (frequent), pruritus, rash, dryness of mouth, dizziness, headache, dyspnea, syncope, epistaxis, purpura and other hematologic reactions, impotence or decreased libido, dysuria, muscular aches, conjunctival injection, weight gain, breast engorgement, pseudolactation, and gynecomastia have been reported. These reactions are usually reversible and usually disappear after the drug is discontinued.
Water retention with edema in patients with hypertensive vascular disease may occur rarely, but the condition generally clears with cessation of therapy, or with the administration of a diuretic agent.

DOSAGE AND ADMINISTRATION

For adults, the average oral dose is 200 to 400 mg daily, given in divided doses in the morning and evening. Higher doses should be used cautiously because serious mental depression and other side effects may be considerably increased. (Orally, 200 to 300 mg of powdered whole root is equivalent to 0.5 mg of reserpine.) Maintenance doses may vary from 50 to 300 mg per day given as a single dose or as two divided doses. Concomitant use of rauwolfia serpentina and ganglionic blocking agents, guanethidine, veratrum, hydralazine, methyldopa, chlorthalidone, or thiazides necessitates careful titration of dosage with each agent.

PRODUCT LISTING - RATED NOT THERAPEUTICALLY EQUIVALENT

Tablet - Oral - 50 mg

100's	$0.90	GENERIC, Global Pharmaceutical Corporation	00115-4400-01

Tablet - Oral - 100 mg

100's	$1.06	GENERIC, Global Pharmaceutical Corporation	00115-4404-01

PRODUCT LISTING - EQUIVALENTS NOT AVAILABLE

Liquid - Oral - 1X

50 ml	$7.50	GENERIC, Weleda Inc	55946-0373-15

Remifentanil Hydrochloride *(003300)*

For complete prescribing information, refer to the CD-ROM included with the book.

For related information, see the comparative table section in Appendix A.

Categories: Anesthesia, adjunct; DEA Class CII; FDA Approved 1996 Sep; Pregnancy Category C
Drug Classes: Analgesics, narcotic; Anesthetics, general
Brand Names: **Ultiva**

DESCRIPTION

Remifentanil hydrochloride for injection is a μ-opioid agonist chemically designated as a 3-[4-methoxycarbonyl-4-[(1-oxopropyl)phenylamino]-1-piperidine]propanoic acid methyl ester, hydrochloride salt, $C_{20}H_{28}N_2O_5 \cdot HCl$, with a molecular weight of 412.91.

Ultiva is a sterile, nonpyrogenic, preservative-free, white to off-white lyophilized powder for intravenous (IV) administration after reconstitution and dilution. Each vial contains 1, 2, or 5 mg of remifentanil base; 15 mg glycine; and hydrochloric acid to buffer the solutions to a nominal pH of 3 after reconstitution. When reconstituted as directed, solutions of Ultiva are clear and colorless and contain remifentanil HCl equivalent to 1 mg/ml of remifentanil base. The pH of reconstituted solutions of Ultiva ranges from 2.5-3.5. Remifentanil hydrochloride has a pKa of 7.07. Remifentanil HCl has an n-octanol:water partition coefficient of 17.9 at pH 7.3.
Storage: Store Ultiva at 2-25°C (36-77°F).

INDICATIONS AND USAGE

Remifentanil HCl is indicated for IV administration:

As an analgesic agent for use during the induction and maintenance of general anesthesia for inpatient and outpatient procedures, and for continuation as an analgesic into the immediate postoperative period under the direct supervision of an anesthesia practitioner in a postoperative anesthesia care unit or intensive care setting.

As an analgesic component of monitored anesthesia care.

CONTRAINDICATIONS

Due to the presence of glycine in the formulation, remifentanil HCl is contraindicated for epidural or intrathecal administration. Remifentanil HCl is also contraindicated in patients with known hypersensitivity to fentanyl analogs.

WARNINGS

Continuous infusions of remifentanil HCl should be administered only by an infusion device. **IV bolus administration of remifentanil HCl should be used only during the maintenance of general anesthesia.** In nonintubated patients, single doses of remifentanil HCl should be administered over 30-60 seconds.

Interruption of an infusion of remifentanil HCl will result in rapid offset of effect. Rapid clearance and lack of drug accumulation result in rapid dissipation of respiratory depressant and analgesic effects upon discontinuation of remifentanil HCl at recommended doses. Discontinuation of an infusion of remifentanil HCl should be preceded by the establishment of adequate postoperative analgesia.

Injections of remifentanil HCl should be made into IV tubing at or close to the venous cannula. Upon discontinuation of remifentanil HCl, the IV tubing should be cleared to prevent the inadvertent administration of remifentanil HCl at a later point in time. **Failure to adequately clear the IV tubing to remove residual remifentanil HCl has been associated with the appearance of respiratory depression, apnea, and muscle rigidity upon the administration of additional fluids or medications through the same IV tubing.**

USE OF REMIFENTANIL HCL IS ASSOCIATED WITH APNEA AND RESPIRATORY DEPRESSION. REMIFENTANIL HCL SHOULD BE ADMINISTERED ONLY BY PERSONS SPECIFICALLY TRAINED IN THE USE OF ANESTHETIC DRUGS AND THE MANAGEMENT OF THE RESPIRATORY EFFECTS OF POTENT OPIOIDS, INCLUDING RESPIRATORY AND CARDIAC RESUSCITATION OF PATIENTS IN THE AGE GROUP BEING TREATED. SUCH TRAINING MUST INCLUDE THE ESTABLISHMENT AND MAINTENANCE OF A PATENT AIRWAY AND ASSISTED VENTILATION.

REMIFENTANIL HCL SHOULD NOT BE USED IN DIAGNOSTIC OR THERAPEUTIC PROCEDURES OUTSIDE THE MONITORED ANESTHESIA CARE SETTING. PATIENTS RECEIVING MONITORED ANESTHESIA CARE SHOULD BE CONTINUOUSLY MONITORED BY PERSONS NOT INVOLVED IN THE CONDUCT OF THE SURGICAL OR DIAGNOSTIC PROCEDURE. OXYGEN SATURATION SHOULD BE MONITORED ON A CONTINUOUS BASIS.

RESUSCITATIVE AND INTUBATION EQUIPMENT, OXYGEN, AND AN OPIOID ANTAGONIST MUST BE READILY AVAILABLE.

Respiratory depression in spontaneously breathing patients is generally managed by decreasing the rate of the infusion of remifentanil HCl by 50% or by temporarily discontinuing the infusion.

Skeletal muscle rigidity can be caused by remifentanil HCl and is related to the dose and speed of administration. Remifentanil HCl may cause chest wall rigidity (inability to ventilate) after single doses of >1 μg/kg administered over 30-60 seconds, or after infusion rates >0.1 μg/kg/min. Single doses <1 μg/kg may cause chest wall rigidity when given concurrently with a continuous infusion of remifentanil HCl.

Muscle rigidity induced by remifentanil HCl should be managed in the context of the patient's clinical condition. Muscle rigidity occurring during the induction of anesthesia should be treated by the administration of a neuromuscular blocking agent and the concurrent induction medications.

Muscle rigidity seen during the use of remifentanil HCl in spontaneously breathing patients may be treated by stopping or decreasing the rate of administration of remifentanil HCl. Resolution of muscle rigidity after discontinuing the infusion of remifentanil HCl oc-

R

curs within minutes. In the case of life-threatening muscle rigidity, a rapid onset neuromuscular blocker or naloxone may be administered.

Remifentanil HCl should not be administered into the same IV tubing with blood due to potential inactivation by nonspecific esterases in blood products.

DOSAGE AND ADMINISTRATION

Remifentanil HCl is for IV use only. **Continuous infusions of remifentanil HCl should be administered only by an infusion device. The injection site should be close to the venous cannula and all IV tubing should be cleared at the time of discontinuation of infusion.**

DURING GENERAL ANESTHESIA

Remifentanil HCl is not recommended as the sole agent in general anesthesia because loss of consciousness cannot be assured and because of a high incidence of apnea, muscle rigidity, and tachycardia. Remifentanil HCl is synergistic with other anesthetics; therefore, clinicians may need to reduce doses of thiopental, propofol, isoflurane, and midazolam by up to 75% with the coadministration of remifentanil HCl. The administration of remifentanil HCl must be individualized based on the patient's response.

TABLE 6 summarizes the recommended doses in adult patients, predominately ASA physical status I, II, or III. Recommendations for maintenance anesthesia with nitrous oxide also apply to pediatric patients ≥2 years.

TABLE 6 *Dosing Guidlines — General Anesthesia and Continuing as an Analgesic into the Postoperative Care Unit or Intensive Care Setting**

	Continuous IV Infusion of Remifentanil HCl (µg/kg/min)	Infusion Dose Range of Remifentanil HCl (µg/kg/min)	Supplemental IV Bolus Dose of Remifentanil HCl (µg/kg)
Induction of Anesthesia (through intubation)	0.5-1*	—	—
Maintenance of anesthesia with:			
Nitrous oxide (66%)	0.4	0.1-2	1
Isoflurane (0.4-1.5 MAC)	0.25	0.05-2	1
Propofol (100-200 µg/kg/min)	0.25	0.05-2	1
Continuation as an analgesic into the immediate postoperative period	0.1	0.025-0.2	not recommended

* An initial dose of 1 µg/kg may be administered over 30 to 60 seconds.

During Induction of Anesthesia

Remifentanil HCl should be administered at an infusion rate of 0.5-1 µg/kg/min with a hypnotic or volatile agent for the induction of anesthesia. If endotracheal intubation is to occur less than 8 minutes after the start of the infusion of remifentanil HCl, then an initial dose of 1 µg/kg may be administered over 30 to 60 seconds.

During Maintenance of Anesthesia

After endotracheal intubation, the infusion rate of remifentanil HCl should be decreased in accordance with the dosing guidelines in TABLE 6. Due to the fast onset and short duration of action of remifentanil HCl, the rate of administration during anesthesia can be titrated upward in 25-100% increments or downward in 25-50% decrements every 2-5 minutes to attain the desired level of µ-opioid effect. In response to light anesthesia or transient episodes of intense surgical stress, supplemental bolus doses of 1 µg/kg may be administered every 2-5 minutes. At infusion rates >1 µg/kg/min, increases in the concomitant anesthetic agents should be considered to increase the depth of anesthesia.

Continuation as an Analgesic into the Immediate Postoperative Period Under the Direct Supervision of an Anesthesia Practitioner

Infusions of remifentanil HCl may be continued into the immediate postoperative period for select patients for whom later transition to longer acting analgesics may be desired. The use of bolus injections of remifentanil HCl to treat pain during the postoperative period is not recommended. When used as an IV analgesic in the immediate postoperative period, remifentanil HCl should be initially administered by continuous infusion at a rate of 0.1 µg/kg/min. The infusion rate may be adjusted every 5 minutes in 0.025 µg/kg/min increments to balance the patient's level of analgesia and respiratory rate. Infusion rates greater than 0.2 µg/kg/min are associated with respiratory depression (respiratory rate less than 8 breaths/min).

Guidelines for Discontinuation

Upon discontinuation of remifentanil HCl, the IV tubing should be cleared to prevent the inadvertent administration of remifentanil HCl at a later time.

Due to the rapid offset of action of remifentanil HCl, no residual analgesic activity will be present within 5-10 minutes after discontinuation. For patients undergoing surgical procedures where postoperative pain is generally anticipated, alternative analgesics should be administered prior to discontinuation of remifentanil HCl. The choice of analgesic should be appropriate for the patient's surgical procedure and the level of follow-up care.

ANALGESIC COMPONENT OF MONITORED ANESTHESIA CARE

It is strongly recommended that supplemental oxygen be supplied to the patient whenever remifentanil HCl is administered.

TABLE 7 summarizes the recommended doses for monitored anesthesia care in adult patients, predominately ASA physical status I, II or III.

TABLE 7 *Dosing Guidelines-Monitored Anesthesia Care*

Method/Timing	Remifentanil HCl Alone	Remifentanil HCl + 2 mg Midazolam
Single IV Dose		
Given 90 seconds before local anesthetic	1 µg/kg over 30 to 60 seconds	0.5 µg/kg over 30 to 60 seconds
Continuous IV Infusion		
Beginning 5 minutes before local anesthetic	0.1 µg/kg/min	0.05 µg/kg/min
After local anesthetic	0.05 µg/kg/min (Range: 0.025-0.2 µg/kg/min)	0.025 µg/kg/min (Range: 0.025-0.2 µg/kg/min)

Single Dose

A single IV dose of 0.5-1 µg/kg over 30-60 seconds of remifentanil HCl may be given 90 seconds before the placement of the local or regional anesthetic block.

Continuous Infusion

When used alone as an IV analgesic component of monitored anesthesia care, remifentanil HCl should be initially administered by continuous infusion at a rate of 0.1 µg/kg/min beginning 5 minutes before placement of the local or regional anesthetic block. **Because of the risk for hypoventilation, the infusion rate of remifentanil HCl should be decreased to 0.05 µg/kg/min following placement of the block.** Thereafter, rate adjustments of 0.025 µg/kg/min at 5 minute intervals may be used to balance the patient's level of analgesia and respiratory rate. Rates greater than 0.2 µg/kg/min are generally associated with respiratory depression (respiratory rates less than 8 breaths/min). **Bolus doses of remifentanil HCl administered simultaneously with a continuous infusion of remifentanil HCl to spontaneously breathing patients are not recommended.**

INDIVIDUALIZATION OF DOSAGE

Use in Geriatric Patients: The starting doses of remifentanil HCl should be decreased by 50% in elderly patients (>65 years). Remifentanil HCl should then be cautiously titrated to effect.

Use in Pediatric Patients: No data are available on the use of remifentanil HCl in pediatric patients under 2 years of age. The same doses (per kg) as adults are recommended for pediatric patients 2 years of age and older.

Use in Obese Patients: The starting doses of remifentanil HCl should be based on ideal body weight (IBW) in obese patients (greater than 30% over their IBW).

Preanesthetic Medication: The need for premedication and the choice of anesthetic agents must be individualized. In clinical studies, patients who received remifentanil HCl frequently received a benzodiazepine premedication.

Continuous IV infusions of remifentanil HCl should be administered only by an infusion device. Infusion rates of remifentanil HCl can be individualized for each patient using TABLE 8.

TABLE 8 *IV Infusion Rates of Remifentanil HCl (ml/kg/h)*

Drug Delivery Rate	Infusion Delivery Rate (ml/kg/h)		
(µg/kg/min)	25 µg/ml	50 µg/ml	250 µg/ml
0.0125	0.03	0.015	not recommended
0.025	0.06	0.03	not recommended
0.05	0.12	0.06	0.012
0.075	0.18	0.09	0.018
0.1	0.24	0.12	0.024
0.15	0.36	0.18	0.036
0.2	0.48	0.24	0.048
0.25	0.6	0.3	0.06
0.5	1.2	0.6	0.12
0.75	1.8	0.9	0.18
1.0	2.4	1.2	0.24
1.25	3.0	1.5	0.3
1.5	3.6	1.8	0.36
1.75	4.2	2.1	0.42
2.0	4.8	2.4	0.48

When remifentanil HCl is used as an analgesic component of monitored analgesia care or for pediatric patients ≥2 years of age, a final concentration of 25 µg/ml is recommended.

COMPATIBILITY AND STABILITY

Reconstitution and Dilution Prior to Administration: Remifentanil HCl is stable for 24 hours at room temperature after reconstitution and further dilution to concentrations of 20-250 µg/ml with the IV fluids listed below.

- Sterile water for injection
- 5% dextrose injection
- 5% dextrose and 0.9% sodium chloride injection
- 0.9% sodium chloride injection
- 0.45% sodium chloride injection
- Lactated ringer's and 5% dextrose injection

Remifentanil HCl is stable for 4 hours at room temperature after reconstitution and further dilution to concentrations of 20-250 µg/ml with lactated Ringer's injection.

Remifentanil HCl has been shown to be compatible with these IV fluids when coadministered into a running IV administration set.

Compatibility with other therapeutic agents: Remifentanil HCl has been shown to be compatible with Diprivan (propofol) injection when coadministered into a running IV administration set. The compatibility of remifentanil HCl with other therapeutic agents has not been evaluated.

R

Incompatibilities: Nonspecific esterases in blood products may lead to the hydrolysis of remifentanil to its carboxylic acid metabolite. Therefore, administration of remifentanil HCl into the same IV tubing with blood is not recommended.

Note: Parenteral drug products should be inspected visually for particulate matter and discoloration prior to administration whenever solution and container permit. Product should be a clear, colorless liquid after reconstitution and free of visible particulate matter.

Remifentanil HCl does not contain any antimicrobial preservative and thus care must be taken to assure the sterility of prepared solutions.

PRODUCT LISTING - EQUIVALENTS NOT AVAILABLE

Powder For Injection - Intravenous - 1 mg
10's $121.72 ULTIVA, Abbott Pharmaceutical 00074-4498-03
Powder For Injection - Intravenous - 2 mg
10's $255.88 ULTIVA, Abbott Pharmaceutical 00074-4504-05
Powder For Injection - Intravenous - 5 mg
10's $605.98 ULTIVA, Abbott Pharmaceutical 00074-4507-10

Repaglinide *(003378)*

For related information, see the comparative table section in Appendix A.

Categories: Diabetes mellitus; Pregnancy Category C; FDA Approved 1997 Jan
Drug Classes: Antidiabetic agents; Meglitinides
Brand Names: **Prandin**
Foreign Brand Availability: NovoNorm (Australia; Austria; Bahrain; Belgium; Benin; Bulgaria; Burkina-Faso; Colombia; Cyprus; Czech-Republic; Denmark; Egypt; England; Ethiopia; Finland; France; Gambia; Germany; Ghana; Greece; Guinea; Hong-Kong; Hungary; Indonesia; Iran; Iraq; Ireland; Israel; Italy; Ivory-Coast; Jordan; Kenya; Kuwait; Lebanon; Liberia; Libya; Malawi; Mali; Mauritania; Mauritius; Morocco; Netherlands; Niger; Nigeria; Norway; Oman; Philippines; Poland; Portugal; Qatar; Republic-of-Yemen; Saudi-Arabia; Senegal; Seychelles; Sierra-Leone; Slovenia; South-Africa; Spain; Sudan; Sweden; Switzerland; Syria; Taiwan; Tanzania; Thailand; Tunia; Turkey; Uganda; United-Arab-Emirates; Zambia; Zimbabwe); Rapilan (India)
Cost of Therapy: $91.29 (Diabetes Mellitus; Prandin; 0.5 mg; 3 tablets/day; 30 day supply)

DESCRIPTION

Repaglinide is an oral blood glucose-lowering drug of the meglitinide class used in the management of Type 2 diabetes mellitus (also known as non-insulin dependent diabetes mellitus or NIDDM). Repaglinide, S(+)2-ethoxy-4(2((3-methyl-1-(2-(1-piperidinyl)phenyl)-butyl)amino)-2-oxoethyl) benzoic acid, is chemically unrelated to the oral sulfonylurea insulin secretagogues.

Repaglinide is a white to off-white powder with molecular formula $C_{27}H_{36}N_2O_4$ and a molecular weight of 452.6. Prandin tablets contain 0.5, 1, or 2 mg of repaglinide. In addition each tablet contains the following inactive ingredients: calcium hydrogen phosphate (anhydrous), microcrystalline cellulose, maize starch, polacrilin potassium, providone, glycerol (85%), magnesium stearate, meglumine, and poloxamer. The 1 mg and 2 mg tablets contain iron oxides (yellow and red, respectively) as coloring agents.

CLINICAL PHARMACOLOGY

MECHANISM OF ACTION

Repaglinide lowers blood glucose levels by stimulating the release of insulin from the pancreas. This action is dependent upon functioning beta (β) cells in the pancreatic islets. Insulin release is glucose-dependent and diminishes at low glucose concentrations.

Repaglinide closes ATP-dependent potassium channels in the β-cell membrane by binding at characterizable sites. This potassium channel blockade depolarizes the β-cell, which leads to an opening of calcium channels. The resulting increased calcium influx induces insulin secretion. The ion channel mechanism is highly tissue selective with low affinity for heart and skeletal muscle.

PHARMACOKINETICS

Absorption

After oral administration, repaglinide is rapidly and completely absorbed from the gastrointestinal tract. After single and multiple oral doses in healthy subjects or in patients, peak plasma drug levels (C_{max}) occur within 1 hour (T_{max}). Repaglinide is rapidly eliminated from the blood stream with a half-life of approximately 1 hour. The mean absolute bioavailability is 56%. When repaglinide was given with food, the mean T_{max} was not changed, but the mean C_{max} and AUC (area under the time/plasma concentration curve) were decreased 20% and 12.4%, respectively.

Distribution

After intravenous (IV) dosing in healthy subjects, the volume of distribution at steady state (Vss) was 31 L, and the total body clearance (CL) was 38 L/h. Protein binding and binding to human serum albumin was greater than 98%.

Metabolism

Repaglinide is completely metabolized by oxidative biotransformation and direct conjugation with glucuronic acid after either an IV or oral dose. The major metabolites are an oxidized dicarboxylic acid (M2), the aromatic amine (M1), and the acyl glucuronide (M7). The cytochrome P-450 enzyme system, specifically 3A4, has been shown to be involved in the N-dealkylation of repaglinide to M2 and the further oxidation to M1. Metabolites do not contribute to the glucose-lowering effect of repaglinide.

Excretion

Within 96 hours after dosing with ^{14}C-repaglinide as a single, oral dose, approximately 90% of the radiolabel was recovered in the feces and approximately 8% in the urine. Only 0.1% of the dose is cleared in the urine as parent compound. The major metabolite (M2) accounted for 60% of the administered dose. Less than 2% of parent drug was recovered in feces.

Pharmacokinetic Parameters

The pharmacokinetic parameters of repaglinide obtained from a single-dose, crossover study in healthy subjects and from a multiple-dose, parallel, dose-proportionality (0.5, 1, 2 and 4 mg) study in patients with Type 2 diabetes are summarized in TABLE 1.

TABLE 1

Parameter	Patients With Type 2 Diabetes*
Dose	**AUC(0-24h) Mean ±SD (ng/ml·h):**
0.5 mg	68.9 ± 154.4
1 mg	125.8 ± 129.8
2 mg	152.4 ± 89.6
4 mg	447.4 ± 211.3
Dose	**$C_{max\ 0\text{-}5h}$ Mean ±SD (ng/ml):**
0.5 mg	9.8 ± 10.2
1 mg	18.3 ± 9.1
2 mg	26.0 ± 13.0
4 mg	65.8 ± 30.1
Dose	**$T_{max\ 0\text{-}5h}$ Means (SD):**
0.5-4 mg	1.0-1.4 (0.3-0.5) h
Dose	**T½ Means (Ind Range):**
0.5-4 mg	1.0-1.4 (0.4-8.0) h
Parameter	**Healthy Subjects**
CL based on IV	38 ± 16 L/h
Vss based on IV	31 ± 12 L
AbsBio	56 ± 9%

* Dosed preprandially with three meals.
CL = Total body clearance.
Vss = Volume of distribution at steady state.
AbsBio = Absolute bioavailability.

These data indicate that repaglinide did not accumulate in serum. Clearance of oral repaglinide did not change over the 0.5 to 4 mg dose range, indicating a linear relationship between dose and plasma drug levels.

Variability of Exposure

Repaglinide AUC after multiple doses of 0.25 to 4 mg with each meal varies over a wide range. The intra-individual and inter-individual coefficients of variation were 36% and 69%, respectively. AUC over the therapeutic dose range included 69-1005 ng/ml·h, but AUC exposure up to 5417 ng/ml·h was reached in dose escalation studies without apparent adverse consequences.

SPECIAL POPULATIONS

Geriatric

Healthy volunteers were treated with a regimen of 2 mg taken before each of 3 meals. There were no significant differences in repaglinide pharmacokinetics between the group of patients <65 years of age and a comparably sized group of patients ≥65 years of age. (See PRECAUTIONS, Geriatric Use.)

Pediatric

No studies have been performed in pediatric patients.

Gender

A comparison of pharmacokinetics in males and females showed the AUC over the 0.5 to 4 mg dose range to be 15-70% higher in females with Type 2 diabetes. This difference was not reflected in the frequency of hypoglycemic episodes (male: 16%; female: 17%) or other adverse events. With respect to gender, no change in general dosage recommendation is indicated since dosage for each patient should be individualized to achieve optimal clinical response.

Race

No pharmacokinetic studies to assess the effects of race have been performed, but in a US 1 year study in patients with Type 2 diabetes, the blood glucose-lowering effect was comparable between Caucasians (n=297) and African-Americans (n=33). In a US dose-response study, there was no apparent difference in exposure (AUC) between Caucasians (n=74) and Hispanics (n=33).

Renal Insufficiency

Single-dose and steady-state pharmacokinetics of repaglinide were compared between patients with Type 2 diabetes and normal renal function (CRCL >80 ml/min), mild to moderate renal function impairment (CRCL = 40-80 ml/min), and severe renal function impairment (CRCL = 20-40 ml/min). Both AUC and C_{max} of repaglinide were similar in patients with normal and mild to moderately impaired renal function (mean values 56.7 ng/ml·h vs 57.2 ng/ml·h and 37.5 ng/ml vs 37.7 ng/ml, respectively.) Patients with severely reduced renal function had elevated mean AUC and C_{max} values (98.0 ng/ml·h and 50.7 ng/ml, respectively), but this study showed only a weak correlation between repaglinide levels and creatinine clearance. Initial dose adjustment does not appear to be necessary for patients with mild to moderate renal dysfunction. **However, patients with Type 2 diabetes who have *severe* renal function impairment should initiate repaglinide therapy with the 0.5 mg dose — subsequently, patients should be carefully titrated. Studies were not conducted in patients with creatinine clearances below 20 ml/min or patients with renal failure requiring hemodialysis.**

Hepatic Insufficiency

A single-dose, open-label study was conducted in 12 healthy subjects and 12 patients with chronic liver disease (CLD) classified by Child-Pugh scale and caffeine clearance. Patients with moderate to severe impairment of liver function had higher and more prolonged serum concentrations of both total and unbound repaglinide than healthy subjects ($AUC_{healthy}$: 91.6 ng/ml·h; $AUC_{CLD\ patients}$: 368.9 ng/ml·h; $C_{max,\ healthy}$: 46.7 ng/ml; $C_{max,\ CLD\ patients}$: 105.4 ng/ml). AUC was statistically correlated with caffeine clearance. No difference in

R

glucose profiles was observed across patient groups. Patients with impaired liver function may be exposed to higher concentrations of repaglinide and its associated metabolites than would patients with normal liver function receiving usual doses. Therefore, **repaglinide should be used cautiously in patients with impaired liver function. Longer intervals between dose adjustments should be utilized to allow full assessment of response.**

DRUG-DRUG INTERACTIONS

Drug interaction studies performed in healthy volunteers show that repaglinide had no clinically relevant effect on the pharmacokinetic properties of digoxin, theophylline, or warfarin. Co-administration of cimetidine with repaglinide did not significantly alter the absorption and disposition of repaglinide.

Additionally, the following drugs were studied in healthy volunteers with co-administration of repaglinide. Listed below are the results:

Ketoconazole: Co-administration of 200 mg ketoconazole and a single dose of 2 mg repaglinide (after 4 days of once daily ketoconazole 200 mg) resulted in a 15% and 16% increase in repaglinide AUC and C_{max}, respectively. The increases were from 20.2 to 23.5 ng/ml for C_{max} and from 38.9 to 44.9 ng/ml·h for AUC.

Rifampin: Co-administration of 600 mg rifampin and a single dose of 4 mg repaglinide (after 6 days of once daily rifampin 600 mg) resulted in a 32% and 26% decrease in repaglinide AUC and C_{max}, respectively. The decreases were from 40.4 to 29.7 ng/ml for C_{max} and from 56.8 to 38.7 ng/ml·h for AUC.

Levonorgestrel & Ethinyl Estradiol: Co-administration of a combination tablet of 0.15 mg levonorgestrel and 0.03 mg ethinyl estradiol administered once daily for 21 days with 2 mg repaglinide administered 3 times daily (days 1-4) and a single dose on Day 5 resulted in 20% increases in repaglinide, levonorgestrel, and ethinyl estradiol C_{max}. The increase in repaglinide C_{max} was from 40.5 to 47.4 ng/ml. Ethinyl estradiol AUC parameters were increased by 20%, while repaglinide and levonorgestrel AUC values remained unchanged.

Simvastatin: Co-administration of 20 mg simvastatin and a single dose of 2 mg repaglinide (after 4 days of once daily simvastatin 20 mg and 3 times daily repaglinide 2 mg) resulted in a 26% increase in repaglinide C_{max} from 23.6 to 29.7 ng/ml. AUC was unchanged.

Nifedipine: Co-administration of 10 mg nifedipine with a single dose of 2 mg repaglinide (after 4 days of 3 times daily nifedipine 10 mg and 3 times daily repaglinide 2 mg) resulted in unchanged AUC and C_{max} values for both drugs.

Clarithromycin: Co-administration of 250 mg clarithromycin and a single dose of 0.25 mg repaglinide (after 4 days of twice daily clarithromycin 250 mg) resulted in a 40% and 67% increase in repaglinide AUC and C_{max}, respectively. The increase in AUC was from 5.3 ng/ml·h to 7.5 ng/ml·h and the increase in C_{max} was from 4.4 to 7.3 ng/ml.

INDICATIONS AND USAGE

Repaglinide is indicated as an adjunct to diet and exercise to lower the blood glucose in patients with Type 2 diabetes mellitus (NIDDM) whose hyperglycemia cannot be controlled satisfactorily by diet and exercise alone.

Repaglinide is also indicated for combination therapy use (with metformin or thiazolidinediones) to lower blood glucose in patients whose hyperglycemia cannot be controlled by diet and exercise plus monotherapy with any of the following agents: metformin, sulfonylureas, repaglinide, or thiazolidinediones. If glucose control has not been achieved after a suitable trial of combination therapy, consideration should be given to discontinuing these drugs and using insulin. Judgments should be based on regular clinical and laboratory evaluations.

In initiating treatment for patients with Type 2 diabetes, diet and exercise should be emphasized as the primary form of treatment. Caloric restriction, weight loss, and exercise are essential in the obese diabetic patient. Proper dietary management and exercise alone may be effective in controlling the blood glucose and symptoms of hyperglycemia. In addition to regular physical activity, cardiovascular risk factors should be identified and corrective measures taken where possible.

R

If this treatment program fails to reduce symptoms and/or blood glucose, the use of an oral blood glucose-lowering agent or insulin should be considered. Use of repaglinide must be viewed by both the physician and patient as a treatment in addition to diet, and not as a substitute for diet or as a convenient mechanism for avoiding dietary restraint. Furthermore, loss of blood glucose control on diet alone may be transient, thus requiring only short-term administration of repaglinide.

During maintenance programs, repaglinide should be discontinued if satisfactory lowering of blood glucose is no longer achieved. Judgments should be based on regular clinical and laboratory evaluations.

In considering the use of repaglinide or other antidiabetic therapies, it should be recognized that blood glucose control in Type 2 diabetes has not been definitely established to be effective in preventing the long-term cardiovascular complications of diabetes. However, in patients with Type 1 diabetes, the Diabetes Control and Complications Trial (DCCT) demonstrated that improved glycemic control, as reflected by HbA_{1c} and fasting glucose levels, was associated with a reduction in the diabetic complications retinopathy, neuropathy, and nephropathy.

CONTRAINDICATIONS

Repaglinide is contraindicated in patients with:

- Diabetic ketoacidosis, with or without coma. This condition should be treated with insulin.
- Type 1 diabetes.
- Known hypersensitivity to the drug or its inactive ingredients.

PRECAUTIONS

GENERAL

Hypoglycemia

All oral blood glucose-lowering drugs are capable of producing hypoglycemia. Proper patient selection, dosage, and instructions to the patients are important to avoid hypoglycemic episodes. Hepatic insufficiency may cause elevated repaglinide blood levels and may diminish gluconeogenic capacity, both of which increase the risk of serious hypoglycemia. Elderly, debilitated, or malnourished patients, and those with adrenal, pituitary, hepatic or severe renal insufficiency may be particularly susceptible to the hypoglycemic action of glucose-lowering drugs.

Hypoglycemia may be difficult to recognize in the elderly and in people taking beta-adrenergic blocking drugs. Hypoglycemia is more likely to occur when caloric intake is deficient, after severe or prolonged exercise, when alcohol is ingested, or when more than one glucose-lowering drug is used.

The frequency of hypoglycemia is greater in patients with Type 2 diabetes who have not been previously treated with oral blood glucose-lowering drugs (naive) or whose HbA_{1c} is less than 8%. Repaglinide should be administered with meals to lessen the risk of hypoglycemia.

Loss of Control of Blood Glucose

When a patient stabilized on any diabetic regimen is exposed to stress such as fever, trauma, infection, or surgery, a loss of glycemic control may occur. At such times, it may be necessary to discontinue repaglinide and administer insulin. The effectiveness of any hypoglycemic drug in lowering blood glucose to a desired level decreases in many patients over a period of time, which may be due to progression of the severity of diabetes or to diminished responsiveness to the drug. This phenomenon is known as secondary failure, to distinguish it from primary failure in which the drug is ineffective in an individual patient when the drug is first given. Adequate adjustment of dose and adherence to diet should be assessed before classifying a patient as a secondary failure.

INFORMATION FOR THE PATIENT

Patients should be informed of the potential risks and advantages of repaglinide and of alternative modes of therapy. They should also be informed about the importance of adherence to dietary instructions, of a regular exercise program, and of regular testing of blood glucose and HbA_{1c}. The risks of hypoglycemia, its symptoms and treatment, and conditions that predispose to its development and concomitant administration of other glucose-lowering drugs should be explained to patients and responsible family members. Primary and secondary failure should also be explained.

Patients should be instructed to take repaglinide before meals (2, 3, or 4 times a day preprandially). Doses are usually taken within 15 minutes of the meal but time may vary from immediately preceding the meal to as long as 30 minutes before the meal. **Patients who skip a meal (or add an extra meal) should be instructed to skip (or add) a dose for that meal.**

LABORATORY TESTS

Response to all diabetic therapies should be monitored by periodic measurements of fasting blood glucose and glycosylated hemoglobin levels with a goal of decreasing these levels towards the normal range. During dose adjustment, fasting glucose can be used to determine the therapeutic response. Thereafter, both glucose and glycosylated hemoglobin should be monitored. Glycosylated hemoglobin may be especially useful for evaluating long-term glycemic control. Postprandial glucose level testing may be clinically helpful in patients whose pre-meal blood glucose levels are satisfactory but whose overall glycemic control (HbA_{1c}) is inadequate.

CARCINOGENESIS, MUTAGENESIS, AND IMPAIRMENT OF FERTILITY

Long-term carcinogenicity studies were performed for 104 weeks at doses up to and including 120 mg/kg body weight/day (rats) and 500 mg/kg body weight/day (mice) or approximately 60 and 125 times clinical exposure, respectively, on a mg/m^2 basis. No evidence of carcinogenicity was found in mice or female rats. In male rats, there was an increased incidence of benign adenomas of the thyroid and liver. The relevance of these findings to humans is unclear. The no-effect doses for these observations in male rats were 30 mg/kg body weight/day for thyroid tumors and 60 mg/kg body weight/day for liver tumors, which are over 15 and 30 times, respectively, clinical exposure on a mg/m^2 basis.

Repaglinide was non-genotoxic in a battery of *in vivo* and *in vitro* studies: Bacterial mutagenesis (Ames test), *in vitro* forward cell mutation assay in V79 cells (HGPRT), *in vitro* chromosomal aberration assay in human lymphocytes, unscheduled and replicating DNA synthesis in rat liver, and *in vivo* mouse and rat micronucleus tests.

Fertility of male and female rats was unaffected by repaglinide administration at doses up to 80 mg/kg body weight/day (females) and 300 mg/kg body weight/day (males); over 40 times clinical exposure on a mg/m^2 basis.

PREGNANCY CATEGORY C

Teratogenic Effects

Safety in pregnant women has not been established. Repaglinide was not teratogenic in rats or rabbits at doses 40 times (rats) and approximately 0.8 times (rabbit) clinical exposure (on a mg/m^2 basis) throughout pregnancy. Because animal reproduction studies are not always predictive of human response, repaglinide should be used during pregnancy only if it is clearly needed.

Because recent information suggests that abnormal blood glucose levels during pregnancy are associated with a higher incidence of congenital abnormalities, many experts recommend that insulin be used during pregnancy to maintain blood glucose levels as close to normal as possible.

Nonteratogenic Effects

Offspring of rat dams exposed to repaglinide at 15 times clinical exposure on a mg/m^2 basis during days 17-22 of gestation and during lactation developed nonteratogenic skeletal deformities consisting of shortening, thickening, and bending of the humerus during the postnatal period. This effect was not seen at doses up to 2.5 times clinical exposure (on a mg/m^2 basis) on days 1-22 of pregnancy or at higher doses given during days 1-16 of pregnancy. Relevant human exposure has not occurred to date and therefore the safety of repaglinide administration throughout pregnancy or lactation cannot be established.

NURSING MOTHERS

In rat reproduction studies, measurable levels of repaglinide were detected in the breast milk of the dams and lowered blood glucose levels were observed in the pups. Cross fostering studies indicated that skeletal changes (see Pregnancy Category C, Nonteratogenic Effects) could be induced in control pups nursed by treated dams, although this occurred to a lesser degree than those pups treated *in utero*. Although it is not known whether repaglinide is excreted in human milk some oral agents are known to be excreted by this route. Because the potential for hypoglycemia in nursing infants may exist, and because of the effects on nursing animals, a decision should be made as to whether repaglinide should be discontinued in nursing mothers, or if mothers should discontinue nursing. If repaglinide is discontinued and if diet alone is inadequate for controlling blood glucose, insulin therapy should be considered.

PEDIATRIC USE

No studies have been performed in pediatric patients.

GERIATRIC USE

In repaglinide clinical studies of 24 weeks or greater duration, 415 patients were over 65 years of age. In 1 year, active-controlled trials, no differences were seen in effectiveness or adverse events between these subjects and those less than 65 other than the expected age-related increase in cardiovascular events observed for repaglinide and comparator drugs. There was no increase in frequency or severity of hypoglycemia in older subjects. Other reported clinical experience has not identified differences in responses between the elderly and younger patients, but greater sensitivity of some older individuals to repaglinide therapy cannot be ruled out.

DRUG INTERACTIONS

In vitro data indicate that repaglinide metabolism may be inhibited by antifungal agents like ketoconazole and miconazole, and antibacterial agents like erythromycin (cytochrome P450 enzyme system 3A4 inhibitors). Drugs that induce the cytochrome P450 enzyme system 3A4 may increase repaglinide metabolism; such drugs include rifampin, barbiturates, and carbamezapine. See CLINICAL PHARMACOLOGY, Drug-Drug Interactions.

In vivo data from a study that evaluated the co-administration of a cytochrome P450 enzyme inhibitor, clarithromycin, with repaglinide resulted in a clinically significant increase in repaglinide plasma levels. This increase in repaglinide plasma levels may necessitate a repaglinide dose adjustment. See CLINICAL PHARMACOLOGY, Drug-Drug Interactions.

The hypoglycemic action of oral blood glucose-lowering agents may be potentiated by certain drugs including nonsteroidal anti-inflammatory agents and other drugs that are highly protein bound, salicylates, sulfonamides, chloramphenicol, coumarins, probenecid, monoamine oxidase inhibitors, and beta adrenergic blocking agents. When such drugs are administered to a patient receiving oral blood glucose-lowering agents, the patient should be observed closely for hypoglycemia. When such drugs are withdrawn from a patient receiving oral blood glucose-lowering agents, the patient should be observed closely for loss of glycemic control.

Certain drugs tend to produce hyperglycemia and may lead to loss of glycemic control. These drugs include the thiazides and other diuretics, corticosteroids, phenothiazines, thyroid products, estrogens, oral contraceptives, phenytoin, nicotinic acid, sympathomimetics, calcium channel blocking drugs, and isoniazid. When these drugs are administered to a patient receiving oral blood glucose-lowering agents, the patient should be observed for loss of glycemic control. When these drugs are withdrawn from a patient receiving oral blood glucose-lowering agents, the patient should be observed closely for hypoglycemia.

ADVERSE REACTIONS

Hypoglycemia: See PRECAUTIONS.

Repaglinide has been administered to 2931 individuals during clinical trials. Approximately 1500 of these individuals with Type 2 diabetes have been treated for at least 3 months, 1000 for at least 6 months, and 800 for at least 1 year. The majority of these individuals (1228) received repaglinide in one of five 1 year, active-controlled trials. The comparator drugs in these 1 year trials were oral sulfonylurea drugs (SU) including glyburide and glipizide. Over 1 year, 13% of repaglinide patients were discontinued due to adverse events, as were 14% of SU patients. The most common adverse events leading to withdrawal were hyperglycemia, hypoglycemia, and related symptoms (see PRECAUTIONS). Mild or moderate hypoglycemia occurred in 16% of repaglinide patients, 20% of glyburide patients, and 19% of glipizide patients.

TABLE 5 lists common adverse events for repaglinide patients compared to both placebo (in trials 12-24 weeks duration) and to glyburide and glipizide in 1 year trials. The adverse event profile of repaglinide was generally comparable to that for sulfonylurea drugs (SU).

TABLE 5 *Commonly Reported Adverse Events (% of Patients)**

	Placebo Controlled Studies		Active Controlled Studies	
	Repaglinide	Placebo	Repaglinide	SU
Event	n=352	n=108	n=1228	n=498
Metabolic				
Hypoglycemia	31%	7%	16%	20%
Respiratory				
URI	16%	8%	10%	10%
Sinusitis	6%	2%	3%	4%
Rhinitis	3%	3%	7%	8%
Bronchitis	2%	1%	6%	7%
Gastrointestinal				
Nausea	5%	5%	3%	2%
Diarrhea	5%	2%	4%	6%
Constipation	3%	2%	2%	3%
Vomiting	3%	3%	2%	1%
Dyspepsia	2%	2%	4%	2%
Musculoskeletal				
Arthralgia	6%	3%	3%	4%
Back pain	5%	4%	6%	7%
Other				
Headache	11%	10%	9%	8%
Paresthesia	3%	3%	2%	1%
Chest pain	3%	1%	2%	1%
Urinary tract infection	2%	1%	3%	3%
Tooth disorder	2%	0%	<1%	<1%
Allergy	2%	0%	1%	<1%

* Events ≥2% for the repaglinide group in the placebo-controlled studies and ≥ events in the placebo group.

Cardiovascular events also occur commonly in patients with Type 2 diabetes. In 1 year comparator trials, the incidence of individual events was not greater than 1% except for chest pain (1.8%) and angina (1.8%). The individual incidence of other cardiovascular events (hypertension, abnormal EKG, myocardial infarction, arrhythmias, and palpitations) was ≤1% and not different for repaglinide and the comparator drugs.

The incidence of serious cardiovascular adverse events added together, including ischemia, was slightly higher for repaglinide (4%) than for sulfonylurea drugs (3%) in controlled comparator clinical trials. In 1 year controlled trials, repaglinide treatment was not associated with excess mortality rates compared to rates observed with other oral hypoglycemic agent therapies.

TABLE 6 *Summary of Serious Cardiovascular Events (% of Total Patients With Events)*

	Repaglinide	SU*
Total exposed	1228	498
Serious CV events	4%	3%
Cardiac ischemic events	2%	2%
Deaths due to CV events	0.5%	0.4%

* Glyburide and glypizide.

INFREQUENT ADVERSE EVENTS (<1% OF PATIENTS)

Less common adverse clinical or laboratory events observed in clinical trials included elevated liver enzymes, thrombocytopenia, leukopenia, and anaphylactoid reactions (1 patient).

COMBINATION THERAPY WITH THIAZOLIDINEDIONES

During 24 week treatment clinical trials of repaglinide-rosiglitazone or repaglinide-pioglitazone combination therapy (a total of 250 patients in combination therapy), hypoglycemia (blood glucose <50 mg/dl) occurred in 7% of combination therapy patients in comparison to 7% for repaglinide monotherapy, and 2% for thiazolidinedione monotherapy.

Peripheral edema was reported in 12 out of 250 repaglinide-thiazolidinedione combination therapy patients and 3 out of 124 thiazolidinedione monotherapy patients, with no cases reported in these trials for repaglinide monotherapy. When corrected for dropout rates of the treatment groups, the percentage of patients having events of peripheral edema per 24 weeks of treatment were 5% for repaglinide-thiazolidinedione combination therapy, and 4% for thiazolidinedione monotherapy. There were reports in 2 of 250 patients (0.8%) treated with repaglinide-thiazolidinedione therapy of episodes of edema with congestive heart failure. Both patients had a prior history of coronary artery disease and recovered after treatment with diuretic agents. No comparable cases in the monotherapy treatment groups were reported.

Mean change in weight from baseline was +4.9 kg for repaglinide-thiazolidinedione therapy. There were no patients on repaglinide-thiazolidinedione combination therapy who had elevations of liver transaminases (defined as 3 times the upper limit of normal levels).

Although no causal relationship has been established, postmarketing experience includes reports of the following rare adverse events: alopecia, hemolytic anemia, pancreatitis, Stevens-Johnson Syndrome, and severe hepatic dysfunction.

DOSAGE AND ADMINISTRATION

There is no fixed dosage regimen for the management of Type 2 diabetes with repaglinide.

The patient's blood glucose should be monitored periodically to determine the minimum effective dose for the patient; to detect primary failure, *i.e.*, inadequate lowering of blood glucose at the maximum recommended dose of medication; and to detect secondary failure, *i.e.*, loss of an adequate blood glucose-lowering response after an initial period of effectiveness. Glycosylated hemoglobin levels are of value in monitoring the patient's longer term response to therapy.

Short-term administration of repaglinide may be sufficient during periods of transient loss of control in patients usually well controlled on diet.

Repaglinide doses are usually taken within 15 minutes of the meal but time may vary from immediately preceding the meal to as long as 30 minutes before the meal.

STARTING DOSE

For patients not previously treated or whose HbA_{1c} is <8%, the starting dose should be 0.5 mg with each meal. For patients previously treated with blood glucose-lowering drugs and whose HbA_{1c} is ≥8%, the initial dose is 1 or 2 mg with each meal preprandially (see previous paragraph).

DOSE ADJUSTMENT

Dosing adjustments should be determined by blood glucose response, usually fasting blood glucose. Postprandial glucose levels testing may be clinically helpful in patients whose pre-meal blood glucose levels are satisfactory but whose overall glycemic control (HbA_{1c}) is inadequate. The preprandial dose should be doubled up to 4 mg with each meal until satisfactory blood glucose response is achieved. At least 1 week should elapse to assess response after each dose adjustment.

R

The recommended dose range is 0.5 to 4 mg taken with meals. Repaglinide may be dosed preprandially 2, 3, or 4 times a day in response to changes in the patient's meal pattern. The maximum recommended daily dose is 16 mg.

PATIENT MANAGEMENT

Long-term efficacy should be monitored by measurement of HbA_{1c} levels approximately every 3 months. Failure to follow an appropriate dosage regimen may precipitate hypoglycemia or hyperglycemia. Patients who do not adhere to their prescribed dietary and drug regimen are more prone to exhibit unsatisfactory response to therapy including hypoglycemia. When hypoglycemia occurs in patients taking a combination of repaglinide and a thiazolidinedione or repaglinide and metformin, the dose of repaglinide should be reduced.

PATIENTS RECEIVING OTHER ORAL HYPOGLYCEMIC AGENTS

When repaglinide is used to replace therapy with other oral hypoglycemic agents, repaglinide may be started on the day after the final dose is given. Patients should then be observed carefully for hypoglycemia due to potential overlapping of drug effects. When transferred from longer half-life sulfonylurea agents (*e.g.*, chlorpropamide) to repaglinide, close monitoring may be indicated for up to 1 week or longer.

COMBINATION THERAPY

If repaglinide monotherapy does not result in adequate glycemic control, metformin or a thiazolidinedione may be added. If metformin or thiazolidinedione monotherapy does not provide adequate control, repaglinide may be added. The starting dose and dose adjustments for repaglinide combination therapy is the same as for repaglinide monotherapy. The dose of each drug should be carefully adjusted to determine the minimal dose required to achieve the desired pharmacologic effect. Failure to do so could result in an increase in the incidence of hypoglycemic episodes. Appropriate monitoring of FPG and HbA_{1c} measurements should be used to ensure that the patient is not subjected to excessive drug exposure or increased probability of secondary drug failure.

HOW SUPPLIED

Prandin tablets are supplied as unscored, biconvex tablets available in 0.5 mg (white), 1 mg (yellow) and 2 mg (peach) strengths. Tablets are embossed with the Novo Nordisk (Apis) bull symbol and colored to indicate strength.
Storage: Do not store above 25°C (77°F). Protect from moisture. Keep bottles tightly closed. Dispense in tight containers with safety closures.

PRODUCT LISTING - EQUIVALENTS NOT AVAILABLE

Tablet - Oral - 0.5 mg

100's	$101.43	PRANDIN, Novo Nordisk Pharmaceuticals Inc	00169-0081-81

Tablet - Oral - 1 mg

100's	$101.43	PRANDIN, Novo Nordisk Pharmaceuticals Inc	00169-0082-81

Tablet - Oral - 2 mg

100's	$101.43	PRANDIN, Novo Nordisk Pharmaceuticals Inc	00169-0084-81

Reserpine (002179)

Categories: Hypertension, essential; Psychosis; Schizophrenia; Pregnancy Category C; FDA Approved 1955 Jun; WHO Formulary
Drug Classes: Antiadrenergics, peripheral
Foreign Brand Availability: Maviserpin (Mexico); Rauserpine (Taiwan); Rauverid (Philippines); Serpasil (Canada; Indonesia); Serpasol (Spain)
Cost of Therapy: $1.05 (Hypertension; Generic Tablets; 0.25 mg; 1 tablets/day; 30 day supply)

R

DESCRIPTION

Reserpine is an antihypertensive, available as 0.1 and 0.25 mg tablets for oral administration. Its chemical name is methyl 18β- hydroxy-11, 17α- dimethoxy-3β,20α-yohimban-16β-carboxylate 3,4,5- trimethoxybenzoate (ester).

Reserpine, a pure crystalline alkaloid of rauwolfia, is a white or pale buff to slightly yellowish, odorless crystalline powder. It darkens slowly on exposure to light, but more rapidly when in solution. It is insoluble in water, freely soluble in acetic acid and in chloroform, slightly soluble in benzene, and very slightly soluble in alcohol and in ether. It molecular weight is 608.69.
Inactive Ingredients: Lactose, magnesium stearate, polyethylene glycol, starch, sucrose, talc, and tragacanth (0.1 mg tablets).

CLINICAL PHARMACOLOGY

Reserpine depletes stores of catecholamines and 5-hydroxytryptamine in many organs, including the brain and adrenal medulla. Most of its pharmacological effects have been attributed to this action. Depletion is slower and less complete in the adrenal medulla than in other tissues.

The depression of sympathetic nerve function results in a decreased heart rate and a lowering of arterial blood pressure. The sedative and tranquilizing properties of Reserpine are thought to be related to depletion of catecholamines and 5-hydroxytryptamine from the brain.

Reserpine, like other rauwolfia compounds, is characterized by slow onset of action and sustained effects. Both cardiovascular and central nervous system effects may persist for a period of time following withdrawal of the drug.

Mean maximum plasma levels of 1.54 ng/ml were attained after a median of 3.5 hours in 6 normal subjects receiving a single oral dose of four 0.25 mg reserpine tablets. Bioavailability was approximately 50% of that of a corresponding intravenous dose. Plasma levels of reserpine after intravenous administration declined with a mean half-life of 33 hours. Reserpine is extensively bound (96%) to plasma proteins. No definitive studies on the human metabolism of reserpine have been made.

INDICATIONS AND USAGE

Mild essential hypertension; also useful as adjunctive therapy with other antihypertensive agents in the more severe forms of hypertension; relief of symptoms in agitated psychotic states (*e.g.*, schizophrenia), primarily in those individuals unable to tolerate phenothiazine derivatives or in those who also require antihypertensive medication.

NON-FDA APPROVED INDICATIONS

Reserpine has also been used for the treatment of cerebral vasospasm, migraines, Raynaud's syndrome, reflex sympathetic dystrophy (intravenous), refractory depression, tardive dyskinesia, and thyrotoxic crisis; however, none of these uses are approved by the FDA.

CONTRAINDICATIONS

Known hypersensitivity, mental depression or history of mental depression (especially with suicidal tendencies), active peptic ulcer, ulcerative colitis, and patients receiving electroconvulsive therapy.

WARNINGS

Reserpine may cause mental depression. Recognition of depression may be difficult because this condition may often be disguised by somatic complaints. The drug should be discontinued at first signs of depression such as despondency, early morning insomnia, loss of appetite, impotence, or self-deprecation. Drug-induced depression may persist for several months after drug withdrawal and may be severe enough to result in suicide.

PRECAUTIONS

GENERAL

Since Reserpine increases gastrointestinal motility and secretion, it should be used cautiously in patients with a history of peptic ulcer, ulcerative colitis, or gallstones (biliary colic may be precipitated).

Caution should be exercised when treating hypertensive patients with renal insufficiency, since they adjust poorly to lowered blood pressure levels.

Preoperative withdrawal of reserpine does not assure that circulatory instability will not occur. It is important that the anesthesiologist be aware of the patient's drug intake and consider this in the overall management, since hypotension has occurred in patients receiving rauwolfia preparations. Anticholinergic and/or adrenergic drugs (*e.g.*, metaraminol, norepinephrine) have been employed to treat adverse vagocircularory effects.

INFORMATION FOR THE PATIENT

Patients should be informed of possible side effects and advised to take the mediation regularly and continuously as directed.

CARCINOGENESIS, MUTAGENESIS, AND IMPAIRMENT OF FERTILITY

Animal Tumorigenicity

Rodent studies have shown that reserpine is an animal tumorigen, causing an increased incidence of mammary fibroadenomas in female mice, malignant tumors of the seminal vesicles in male mice, and malignant adrenal medullary tumors in male rats. These findings arose in 2 year studies in which the drug was administered in the feed at concentrations of 5 and 10 ppm — about 100-300 times the usual human dose. The breast neoplasms are thought to be related to reserpine's prolactin elevating effect. Several other prolactin-elevating drugs have also been associated with an increased incidence of mammary neoplasia in rodents.

The extent to which these findings indicate a risk to humans is uncertain. Tissue culture experiments show that about one-third of human breast tumors are prolactin-dependent *in vitro*, a factor of considerable importance if the use of the drug is contemplated in a patient with previously detected breast cancer. The possibility of an increased risk of breast cancer in reserpine users has been studied extensively; however, no firm conclusion has emerged. Although a few epidemiologic studies have suggested a slightly increased risk (less than twofold in all studies except one) in women who have used reserpine, other studies of generally similar design ave not confirmed this. Epidemiologic studies conducted using other drugs (neuroleptic agents) that, like reserpine, increase prolactin levels and therefore would be considered rodent mammary carcinogens have not shown an association between chronic administration of the drug and human mammary tumorigenesis. While long-term clinical observation has not suggested such an association, the available evidence is considered too limited to be conclusive at this time. An association of reserpine intake with pheochromocytoma or tumors of the seminal vesicles has not been explored.

PREGNANCY CATEGORY C

Reserpine administered parenterally has been shown to be teratogenic in rats at doses up to 2 mg/kg and to have an embryocidal effect in guinea pigs given dosages of 0.5 mg daily.

There are no adequate and well-controlled studies of reserpine in pregnant women. Reserpine should be used during pregnancy only if the potential benefit justifies the potential risk to the fetus.
Nonteratogenic Effects: Reserpine crosses the placental barrier, and increased respiratory tract secretions, nasal congestion, cyanosis, and anorexia may occur in neonates of reserpine-treated mothers.

NURSING MOTHERS

Reserpine is excreted in maternal breast milk, and increased respiratory tract secretions, nasal congestion, cyanosis, and anorexia may occur in breast-fed infants. Because of the potential for adverse reactions in nursing infants and the potential for adverse reactions in nursing infants and the potential for tumorigenicity shown for reserpine in animal studies, a decision should be made whether to discontinue nursing or to discontinue the drug, taking into account the importance of the drug to the mother.

PEDIATRIC USE

Safety and effectiveness in children have not been established by means of controlled clinical trials, although there is experience with the use of reserpine in children. (See DOSAGE AND ADMINISTRATION.) Because of adverse effects such as emotional depression and lability, sedation, and stuffy nose, reserpine is not usually recommended as a step-2 drug in the treatment of hypertension in children.

DRUG INTERACTIONS

MAO inhibitors should be avoided or used with extreme caution.

Reserpine should be used cautiously with digitalis and quinidine, since cardiac arrhythmias have occurred with rauwolfia preparations.

Concurrent use of reserpine with other antihypertensive agents necessitates careful titration of dosage with each agent.

Concurrent use of tricyclic antidepressants may decrease the antihypertensive effect of reserpine (see CONTRAINDICATIONS.)

Concurrent use of reserpine and direct or indirect-acting sympathomimetics should be closely monitored. The action of direct-acting amines (epinephrine, isoproterenol, phenylephrine, metaraminol) may be prolonged when given to patients taking reserpine. The action of indirect acting amines (ephedrine, tyramine, amphetamines) is inhibited.

ADVERSE REACTIONS

The following adverse reactions have been observed with rauwolfia preparations, but there has not been enough systematic collection of data to support an estimate of their frequency. Consequently the reactions are categorized by organ systems and are listed in decreasing order of severity and not frequency.

Digestive: Vomiting, diarrhea, nausea, anorexia, dryness of mouth, hypersecretion.

Cardiovascular: Arrhythmias (particularly when used concurrently with digitalis or quinidine), syncope, angina-like symptoms, bradycardia, edema.

Respiratory: Dyspnea, epistaxis, nasal congestion.

Neurologic: Rare parkinsonian syndrome and other extrapyramidal tract symptoms; dizziness; headache; paradoxical anxiety; depression; nervousness; night-mares; dull sensorium; drowsiness.

Musculoskeletal: Muscular aches.

Genitourinary: Pseudolactation, impotence, dysuria, gynecomastia, decreased libido, breast engorgement.

Metabolic: Weight gain.

Special Senses: Deafness, optic atrophy, glaucoma, uveitis, conjunctival injection.

Hypersensitive Reactions: Purpura, rash, pruritus.

DOSAGE AND ADMINISTRATION

HYPERTENSION

In the average patient not receiving other antihypertensive agents, the usual initial dosage is 0.5 mg daily for 1 or 2 weeks. For maintenance, reduce to 0.1 to 0.25 mg daily. Higher dosages should be used cautiously, because occurrence of serious mental depression and other side effects may increase considerably.

PSYCHIATRIC DISORDERS

The initial dosage is 0.5 mg daily, but may range from 0.1-1.0 mg. Adjust dosage upward or downward according to the patient's response.

CHILDREN

Reserpine is not recommended for use in children (see PRECAUTIONS, Pediatric Use). If it is to be used in treating a child, the usual recommended starting dose is 20 μg/kg daily. The maximum recommended dose is 0.25 mg (total) daily.

Protect from light. Dispense in tight, light-resistant container.

PRODUCT LISTING - RATED NOT THERAPEUTICALLY EQUIVALENT

Tablet - Oral - 0.1 mg

100's	$2.95	GENERIC, Cmc-Consolidated Midland Corporation	00223-1590-01
100's	$29.28	GENERIC, Physicians Total Care	54868-1972-01
100's	$31.76	GENERIC, Eon Labs Manufacturing Inc	00185-0032-01

Tablet - Oral - 0.25 mg

60's	$2.71	GENERIC, Quality Care Pharmaceuticals Inc	60346-0809-60
90's	$6.00	GENERIC, Quality Care Pharmaceuticals Inc	60346-0809-90
100's	$3.50	GENERIC, Cmc-Consolidated Midland Corporation	00223-1591-01
100's	$45.11	GENERIC, Eon Labs Manufacturing Inc	00185-0134-01

PRODUCT LISTING - EQUIVALENTS NOT AVAILABLE

Tablet - Oral - 0.25 mg

100's	$32.13	GENERIC, Allscripts Pharmaceutical Company	54569-0597-00

Respiratory Syncytial Virus Immune Globulin (003188)

For complete prescribing information, refer to the CD-ROM included with the book.

Categories: Immunization, respiratory syncytial virus; FDA Approved 1996 Jan; Pregnancy Category C; Orphan Drugs
Drug Classes: Immune globulins
Brand Names: **RespiGam**; Respivir
HCFA JCODE(S): J1565 50 mg IV

DESCRIPTION

RespiGam, Respiratory Syncytial Virus Immune Globulin Intravenous (Human) (RSV-IGIV) is a sterile liquid immunoglobulin G containing neutralizing antibody to Respiratory Syncytial Virus (RSV). Each lot of RSV-IGIV meets the minimum potency specifications when compared to the validated Reference Standard. The globulin is stabilized with 5% sucrose and 1% Albumin (Human). RSV-IGIV contains no preservative. The immunoglobulin is purified from pooled adult human plasma selected for high titers of neutralizing antibody against RSV using a proprietary patented screening assay.[1] Source material for fractionated may be obtained from another US-licensed manufacturer. Pooled plasma is fractionated by ethanol precipitation of the proteins according to Cohn Method 6 and Oncley Method 9, with additional steps to yield a product suitable for intravenous administration. A widely utilized solvent-detergent viral inactivation process is used to decrease the possibility of transmission of bloodborne pathogens.[2] Certain manufacturing operations may be performed by other firms. Each milliliter contains 50 ± 10 mg immunoglobulin, primarily IgG, and trace amounts of IgA and IgM; 50 mg sucrose; and 10 mg Albumin (Human). The sodium content is 20-30 mEq/L, *i.e.,* 1.0-1.5 mEq/50 ml. The solution should appear colorless and translucent.

INDICATIONS AND USAGE

Respiratory Syncytial Virus Immune Globulin Intravenous (Human) (RSV-IGIV) is indicated for the prevention of serious lower respiratory tract infection caused by RSV in children under 24 months of age with bronchopulmonary dysplasia (BPD) or a history of premature birth (≤35 weeks gestation). RSV-IGIV has been demonstrated to be safe and effective in reducing the incidence and duration of RSV hospitalization and the severity of RSV illness in these high risk infants.

CONTRAINDICATIONS

RSV-IGIV should not be used in patients with a history of a severe prior reaction associated with the administration of RSV-IGIV or other human immunoglobulin preparations. Patients with selective IgA deficiency have the potential for developing antibodies to IgA and could have anaphylactic or allergic reactions to subsequent administration of blood products that contain IgA, including RSV-IGIV.

WARNINGS

Infants with underlying pulmonary disease may be sensitive to extra fluid volume. Infusion of RSV-IGIV, particularly in children with BPD, may precipitate symptoms of fluid overload. Overall, 8.4% of participants (1% premature and 13% BPD) received new or extra diuretics during the period 24 hours before through 48 hours after at least one of their infusions in the Prevent trial. The reason for this use was not recorded (*e.g.,* prophylaxis, treatment, or part of routine care during a clinical visit). RSV-IGIV-related fluid overload was reported in 3 patients (1.2%) and RSV-IGIV-related respiratory distress was reported in 4 patients (1.6%); all had underlying BPD. With the exception of 1 child with respiratory distress (part of an acute allergic reaction) for whom RSV-IGIV was discontinued, these children were managed with diuretics and/or modification of the infusion rate and went on to receive subsequent infusions. Complications related to fluid volume were recorded as a reason for incomplete or prolonged infusion in 2.0% of children receiving RSV-IGIV (2.5% BPD and 1.1% premature) and in 1.5% of children receiving placebo in the Prevent trial. Children with clinically apparent fluid overload should not be infused with RSV-IGIV.

RSV-IGIV should be administered cautiously (see DOSAGE AND ADMINISTRATION). During administration, a patient's vital signs should be monitored frequently, and a patient should be observed for increases in heart rate, respiratory rate, retractions, and rales. **A loop diuretic such as furosemide or bumetanide should be available for management of fluid overload.**

Severe reactions, such as anaphylaxis or angioneurotic edema, have been reported in association with intravenous immunoglobulins even in patients not known to be sensitive to human immunoglobulins or blood products. Serious allergic reaction was noted in 2 patients in the Prevent trial. These reactions were manifest as an acute episode of cyanosis, mottling and fever in 1 patient and respiratory distress in the other. The rate of allergic reaction appears to be low and consistent with rates observed for other Immune Globulin Intravenous (Human)[IGIV] products. **If hypotension, anaphylaxis, or severe allergic reaction occurs, discontinue infusion and administer epinephrine (1:1000), as required.**

The safety and efficacy of RSV-IGIV in children with CHD has not been established. Although equivalent proportions of children in the RSV-IGIV and control groups in the CARDIAC trial had adverse events, a larger number of RSV-IGIV recipients had severe or life-threatening adverse events. These events were most frequently observed in infants with CHD with right to left shunts who underwent cardiac surgery.

DOSAGE AND ADMINISTRATION

The maximum recommended total dosage per monthly infusion is 750 mg/kg, administered according to the schedule shown in TABLE 3.

Administer RSV-IGIV intravenously at 1.5 ml/kg/h for 15 minutes. It the clinical condition does not contraindicate a higher rate, increase the rate to 3.0 ml/kg/h for 15 minutes and finally increase to a maximum rate of 6.0 ml/kg/h. DO NOT EXCEED THIS RATE OF

R

TABLE 3

Time After Start of Infusion	Rate of Infusion (ml per kg of body mass per hour)
0-15 minutes	1.5 ml/kg/h
15-30 minutes	3.0 ml/kg/h
30 minutes to end of infusion	6.0 ml/kg/h

ADMINISTRATION. Monitor the patient closely during and after each rate change. In especially ill children with BPD, slower rates of infusion may be indicated.

A physician may want to consider factors such as other clinical illness, how well the child has grown and the risk of exposure from siblings or daycare when determining whether to use RSV-IGIV. Respiratory Syncytial Virus Immune Globulin Intravenous (Human) (RSV-IGIV). The first dose should be administered prior to commencement of the RSV season and subsequent doses should be administered monthly throughout the RSV season in order to maintain protection. In the Northern Hemisphere the RSV season typically commences in November and runs through April. Children should be infused from early November through April, unless RSV activity begins earlier or persists later in a community. It is recommended that RSV-IGIV be administered separately from other drugs or medications that the patient may be receiving. It is recommended that children infected with RSV continue to receive monthly doses of RSV-IGIV for the duration of the RSV season.

INFUSION

Infusion should begin within 6 hours and should be completed within 12 hours after the single-use vial is entered. The patient's vital signs and cardiopulmonary status should be assessed prior to infusion, before each rate increase, and thereafter at 30-minute intervals until 30 minutes following completion of the infusion. RSV-IGIV should be administered through an intravenous line using a constant infusion pump (*i.e.*, IVAC pump or equivalent). Predilution of RSV-IGIV before infusion is not recommended. If possible, RSV-IGIV should be administered through a separate intravenous line, although it may be "piggy-backed" into a pre-existing line if that line contains one of the following dextrose solutions (with or without sodium chloride): 2.5, 5, 10, or 20% dextrose in water. If a pre-existing line must be used, the RSV-IGIV should not be diluted more than 1:2 with any other of the above-named solutions. Admixtures of RSV-IGIV with any other solutions have not been evaluated. While filters are not necessary, an in-line filter with a pore size larger than 15 micrometers may be used for the infusion of RSV-IGIV.

To prevent the transmission of hepatitis viruses or infectious agents from one person to another, sterile disposable syringes and needles should be used. Do not reuse syringes and needles.

PRODUCT LISTING - EQUIVALENTS NOT AVAILABLE

Solution - Intravenous - 50 mg/ml

50 ml $859.59   RESPIGAM, Medimmune Inc   60574-2101-01

Reteplase (003334)

Categories: Myocardial infarction; Pregnancy Category C; FDA Approved 1996 Nov
Drug Classes: Thrombolytics
Brand Names: Retavase
Foreign Brand Availability: Rapilysin (Australia; Austria; Belgium; Bulgaria; Czech-Republic; Denmark; England; Finland; France; Germany; Greece; Hungary; Ireland; Italy; Netherlands; New-Zealand; Norway; Poland; Portugal; Slovenia; Spain; Sweden; Switzerland; Turkey)
HCFA JCODE(S): J2994 37.6 mg IV

R

DESCRIPTION

Reteplase is a non-glycosylated deletion mutein of tissue plasminogen activator (tPA), containing the kringle 2 and the protease domains of human tPA. Reteplase contains 355 of the 527 amino acids of native tPA (amino acids 1-3 and 176-527). Reteplase is produced by recombinant DNA technology in *E. coli.* The protein is isolated as inactive inclusion bodies from *E. coli,* converted into its active form by an *in vitro* folding process and purified by chromatographic separation. The molecular weight of reteplase is 39,571 daltons.

Potency is expressed in units (U) using a reference standard which is specific for reteplase and is not comparable with units used for other thrombolytic agents.

Reteplase is a sterile, white lyophilized powder for intravenous bolus injection after reconstitution with sterile water for injection. Following reconstitution, the pH is 6.0 ± 0.3. Retavase is supplied as a 10.4 U vial to ensure sufficient drug for administration of each 10 U dose. Each single-use vial contains: reteplase 18.1 mg, tranexamic acid 8.32 mg, dipotassium hydrogen phosphate 136.24 mg, phosphoric acid 51.27 mg, sucrose 364.0 mg, polysorbate 80 5.20 mg.

CLINICAL PHARMACOLOGY

GENERAL

Reteplase is a recombinant plasminogen activator which catalyzes the cleavage of endogenous plasminogen to generate plasmin. Plasmin in turn degrades the fibrin matrix of the thrombus, thereby exerting its thrombolytic action.[1,2] In a controlled trial, 35 of 56 patients treated for an acute myocardial infarction (AMI) had a decrease in fibrinogen levels to below 100 mg/dl by 2 hours following the administration of reteplase as a double-bolus intravenous injection (10 + 10 U) in which 10 U (17.4 mg) was followed 30 minutes later by a second bolus of 10 U (17.4 mg).[3] The mean fibrinogen level returned to the baseline value by 48 hours.

PHARMACOKINETICS

Based on the measurement of thrombolytic activity, reteplase is cleared from plasma at a rate of 250-450 ml/min, with an effective half-life of 13-16 minutes. Reteplase is cleared primarily by the liver and kidney.

INDICATIONS AND USAGE

Reteplase is indicated for the use in the management of acute myocardial infarction (AMI) in adults for the improvement of ventricular function following AMI, the reduction of the incidence of congestive heart failure and the reduction of mortality associated with AMI. Treatment should be initiated as soon as possible after the onset of AMI symptoms (see CLINICAL PHARMACOLOGY).

NON-FDA APPROVED INDICATIONS

In the SPEED (GUSTO-4 Pilot) trial, reduced-dose reteplase was used in conjunction with the glycoprotein IIb/IIIa inhibitor abciximab in patients undergoing percutaneous coronary intervention (PCI) as treatment for acute myocardial infarction (AMI) with ST segment elevation. Currently, this combination use remains unapproved by the FDA.

CONTRAINDICATIONS

Because thrombolytic therapy increases the risk of bleeding, reteplase is contraindicated in the following situations:

- **Active internal bleeding**
- **History of cerebrovascular accident**
- **Recent intracranial or intraspinal surgery or trauma (see WARNINGS)**
- **Intracranial neoplasm, arteriovenous malformation, or aneurysm**
- **Known bleeding diathesis**
- **Severe uncontrolled hypertension**

WARNINGS

BLEEDING

The most common complication encountered during reteplase therapy is bleeding. The sites of bleeding include both internal bleeding sites (intracranial, retroperitoneal, gastrointestinal, genitourinary, or respiratory) and superficial bleeding sites (venous cutdowns, arterial punctures, sites of recent surgical intervention). The concomitant use of heparin anticoagulation may contribute to bleeding. In clinical trials some of the hemorrhage episodes occurred 1 or more days after the effects of reteplase had dissipated, but while heparin therapy was continuing.

As fibrin is lysed during reteplase therapy, bleeding from recent puncture sites may occur. Therefore, thrombolytic therapy requires careful attention to all potential bleeding sites (including catheter insertion sites, arterial and venous puncture sites, cutdown sites, and needle puncture sites). Noncompressible arterial puncture must be avoided and internal jugular and subclavian venous punctures should be avoided to minimize bleeding from noncompressible sites.

Should an arterial puncture be necessary during the administration of reteplase, it is preferable to use an upper extremity vessel that is accessible to natural compression. Pressure should be applied for at least 30 minutes, a pressure dressing applied, and the puncture site checked frequently for evidence of bleeding.

Intramuscular injections and nonessential handling of the patient should be avoided during treatment with reteplase. Venipunctures should be performed carefully and only as required.

Should serious bleeding (not controllable by local pressure) occur, concomitant anticoagulant therapy should be terminated immediately. In addition, the second bolus of reteplase should not be given if serious bleeding occurs before it is administered.

Each patient being considered for therapy with reteplase should be carefully evaluated and anticipated benefits weighed against the potential risks associated with therapy.

In the following conditions, the risks of reteplase therapy may be increased and should be weighed against the anticipated benefits:

- Recent major surgery (*e.g.*, coronary artery bypass graft, obstetrical delivery, organ biopsy)
- Previous puncture of noncompressible vessels
- Cerebrovascular disease
- Recent gastrointestinal or genitourinary bleeding
- Recent trauma
- ***Hypertension:*** Systolic BP ≥180 mm Hg and/or diastolic BP ≥110 mm Hg
- High likelihood of left heart thrombus *e.g.*, mitral stonosis with atrial fibrillation
- Acute pericarditis
- Subacute bacterial endocarditis
- Hemostatic defects including those secondary to severe hepatic or renal disease
- Severe hepatic or renal dysfunction
- Pregnancy
- Diabetic hemorrhagic retinopathy or other hemorrhagic ophthalmic conditions
- Septic thrombophlebitis or occluded AV cannula at a seriously infected site
- Advanced age
- Patients currently receiving oral anticoagulants *e.g.*, warfarin sodium
- Any other condition in which bleeding constitutes a significant hazard or would be particularly difficult to manage because of its location

CHOLESTEROL EMBOLIZATION

Cholesterol embolism has been reported rarely in patients treated with thrombolytic agents; the true incidence is unknown. This serious condition, which can be lethal, is also associated with invasive vascular procedures (*e.g.*, cardiac catheterization, angiography, vascular surgery) and/or anticoagulant therapy. Clinical features of cholesterol embolism may include livedo reticularis, "purple toe" syndrome, acute renal failure, gangrenous digits, hypertension, pancreatitis, myocardial infarction, cerebral infarction, spinal cord infarction, retinal artery occlusion, bowel infarction, and rhabdomyolysis

ARRHYTHMIAS

Coronary thrombolysis may result in arrhythmias associated with reperfusion. These arrhythmias (such as sinus bradycardia, accelerated idioventricular rhythm, ventricular premature depolarizations, ventricular tachycardia) are not different from those often seen in the ordinary course of acute myocardial infarction and should be managed with standard antiarrhythmic measures. It is recommended that antiarrhythmic therapy for bradycardia and/or ventricular irritability be available when reteplase is administered.

PRECAUTIONS

GENERAL

Standard management of myocardial infarction should be implemented concomitantly with reteplase treatment. Arterial and venous punctures should be minimized (see WARNINGS). In addition, the second bolus of reteplase should not be given if serious bleeding occurs before it is administered. In the event of serious bleeding, any concomitant heparin should be terminated immediately. Heparin effects can be reversed by protamine.

READMINISTRATION

There is no experience with patients receiving repeat courses of therapy with reteplase. Reteplase did not induce the formation of reteplase specific antibodies in any of the approximately 2400 patients who were tested for antibody formation in clinical trials. If an anaphylactoid reaction occurs, the second bolus of reteplase should not be given, and appropriate therapy should be initiated.

DRUG/LABORATORY TEST INTERACTIONS

Administration of reteplase may cause decreases in plasminogen and fibrinogen. During reteplase therapy, if coagulation test and/or measurements of fibrinolytic activity are performed, the results may be unreliable unless specific precautions are taken to prevent *in vitro* artifacts. Reteplase is an enzyme that when present in blood in pharmacologic concentrations remains active under *in vitro* conditions. This can lead to degradation of fibrinogen in blood samples removed for analysis. Collection of blood samples in the presence of PPACK (chloromethylketone) at 2 μM concentrations was used in clinical trials to prevent *in vitro* fibrinolytic artifacts.[6]

USE OF ANTITHROMBOTICS

Heparin and aspirin have been administered concomitantly with and following the administration of reteplase in the management of acute myocardial infarction. Because heparin, aspirin, or reteplase may cause bleeding complications, careful monitoring for bleeding is advised, especially at arterial puncture sites.

CARCINOGENESIS, MUTAGENESIS, AND IMPAIRMENT OF FERTILITY

Long-term studies in animals have not been performed to evaluate the carcinogenic potential of reteplase. Studies to determine mutagenicity, chromosomal aberrations, gene mutations, and micronuclei induction were negative at all concentrations tested. Reproductive toxicity studies in rats revealed no effects on fertility at doses up to 15 times the human dose (4.31 U/kg).

PREGNANCY CATEGORY C

Reteplase has been shown to have an abortifacient effect in rabbits when given in doses 3 times the human dose (0.86 U/kg). Reproduction studies performed in rats at doses up to 15 times the human dose (4.31 U/kg) revealed no evidence of fetal anomalies; however, reteplase administered to pregnant rabbits resulted in hemorrhaging in the genital tract, leading to abortions in mid-gestation. There are no adequate and well-controlled studies in pregnant women. The most common complication of thrombolytic therapy is bleeding and certain conditions, including pregnancy, can increase this risk. Reteplase should be used during pregnancy only if the potential benefit justifies the potential risk to the fetus.

NURSING MOTHERS

It is not known whether reteplase is excreted in human milk. Because many drugs are excreted in human milk, caution should be exercised when reteplase is administered to a nursing woman.

PEDIATRIC USE

Safety and effectiveness in pediatric patients have not been established.

DRUG INTERACTIONS

The interaction of reteplase with other cardioactive drugs has not been studied. In addition to bleeding associated with heparin and vitamin K antagonists, drugs that alter platelet function (such as aspirin, dipyridamole, and abciximab) may increase the risk of bleeding if administered prior to or after reteplase therapy.

ADVERSE REACTIONS

BLEEDING

The most frequent adverse reaction associated with reteplase is bleeding (see WARNINGS). The types of bleeding events associated with thrombolytic therapy may be broadly categorized as either intracranial hemorrhage or other types of hemorrhage.

- ***Intracranial Hemorrhage:*** (See CLINICAL PHARMACOLOGY) In the INJECT clinical trial the rate of in-hospital, intracranial hemorrhage among all patients treated with reteplase was 0.8% (23 of 2965 patients). As seen with reteplase and other thrombolytic agents, the risk for intracranial hemorrhage is increased in patients with advanced age or with elevated blood pressure.
- ***Other Types of Hemorrhage:*** The incidence of other types of bleeding events in clinical studies of reteplase varied depending upon the use of arterial catherization or other invasive procedures and whether the study was performed in Europe or the US. The overall incidence of any bleeding event in patients treated with reteplase in clinical studies (n=3805) was 21.1%. The rates for bleeding events, regardless of severity, for the 10 + 10 U reteplase regimen from controlled clinical studies are summarized in TABLE 3.

TABLE 3 *Reteplase Hemorrhage Rates*

	INJECT	RAPID 1 and RAPID 2	
	Europe	US	Europe
Bleeding Site	(n=2965)	(n=210)	(n=113)
Injection site*	4.6%	48.6%	19.5%
Gastrointestinal	2.5%	9.0%	1.8%
Genitourinary	1.6%	9.5%	0.9%
Anemia, site unknown	2.6%	1.4%	0.9%

* Includes the arterial catheterization site (all patients in the RAPID studies underwent arterial catheterization).

In these studies the severity and sites of bleeding events were comparable for reteplase and the comparison thrombolytic agents.

Should serious bleeding in a critical location (intracranial, gastrointestinal, retroperitoneal, pericardial) occur, any concomitant heparin should be terminated immediately. In addition, the second bolus of reteplase should not be given if the serious bleeding occurs before it is administered. Death and permanent disability are not uncommonly reported in patients who have experienced stroke (including intracranial bleeding) and other serious bleeding episodes.

Fibrin which is part of the hemostatic plug formed at needle puncture sites will be lysed during reteplase therapy. Therefore, reteplase therapy requires careful attention to potential bleeding sites (*e.g.*, catheter insertion sites, arterial puncture sites).

ALLERGIC REACTIONS

Among the 2965 patients receiving reteplase in the INJECT trial, serious allergic reactions were noted in 3 patients, with 1 patient experiencing dyspnea and hypotension. No anaphylactoid reactions were observed among the 3856 patients treated with reteplase in initial clinical trials. In an ongoing clinical trial two anaphylactoid reactions have been reported among approximately 2500 patients receiving reteplase.

OTHER ADVERSE REACTIONS

Patients adminsitered reteplase as treatment for myocardial infarction have experienced many events which are frequent sequelae of myocardial infarction and may or may not be attributable to reteplase therapy. These events include cardiogenic shock, arrhythmias (*e.g.*, sinus bradycardia, accelerated idioventricular rhythm, ventricular premature depolarization, supraventricular tachycardia, ventricular tachycardia, ventricular fibrillation), AV block, pulmonary edema, heart failure, cardiac arrest, recurrent ischemia, reinfarction, myocardial rupture, mitral regurgitation, pericardial effusion, pericarditis, cardiac tamponade, venous thrombosis and embolism, and electromechanical dissociation. These events can be life-threatening and may lead to death. Other adverse events have been reported, including nausea and/or vomiting, hypotension, and fever.

DOSAGE AND ADMINISTRATION

Reteplase is for intravenous administration only. Reteplase is administered as a 10 + 10 U double-bolus injection. Two 10 unit bolus injections are required for a complete treatment. Each bolus is administered as an intravenous injection over 2 minutes. The second bolus is given 30 minutes after initiation of the first bolus injection. Each bolus injection should be given via an intravenous line in which no other medication is being simultaneously injected or infused. No other medication should be added to the injection solution containing reteplase. There is no experience with patients receiving repeat courses of therapy with reteplase. **Heparin and reteplase are incompatible when combined in solution.** Do not administer heparin and reteplase simultaneously in the same intravenous line. If reteplase is to be injected through an intravenous line containg heparin, a normal saline or 5% dextrose (D5W) solution should be flushed through the line prior to and following the reteplase injection.

Although the value of anticoagulants and antiplatelet drugs during and following administration of reteplase has not been studied, heparin has been administered concomitantly in more than 99% of patients. Aspirin has been given either during and/or following heparin treatment. Studies assessing the safety and efficacy of reteplase without adjunctive therapy with heparin and aspirin have not been performed.

HOW SUPPLIED

Retavase is supplied as a sterile, preservative-free, lyophilized powder in 10.4 U (equivalent to 18.1 mg reteplase) vials without a vacuum, in a kit with components for reconstitution. **Storage:** Store the kit containing retaplase at 2-25°C (36-77°F). Kit should remain sealed until use to protect the lyophilisate from exposure to light. Do not use beyond expiration date printed on the kit.

PRODUCT LISTING - EQUIVALENTS NOT AVAILABLE

Kit - Intravenous - 10.8 U

1's $1375.00	RETAVASE, Centocor Inc	57894-0040-02
2's $2640.00	RETAVASE, Centocor Inc	57894-0040-01

R

Rho (D) Immune Globulin *(002184)*

For complete prescribing information, refer to the CD-ROM included with the book.

Categories: Anemia, hemolytic, prevention; Transfusion; Pregnancy Category C; FDA Pre 1938 Drugs; Orphan Drugs; WHO Formulary
Drug Classes: Immune globulins
Brand Names: Gamulin Rh; **Hyprho-D**; Mini-Gamulin Rh; Rhesonativ; Winrho Sd
Foreign Brand Availability: Anti Rho (D) (Mexico); Bay Rho-D (Israel); Cutter Hyperab (Hong-Kong); Cutter Hyprho-D (Hong-Kong); IGRHO (Israel); Natead (France); Partobulin (Czech-Republic; Hong-Kong; Italy; Korea); Partogloman (Austria); Probi RHO (D) (Mexico); Rhesogam (Germany); Rhesogamma (Sweden); Rhesugam (South-Africa); Rhesuman (Belgium; Greece; India; Italy; Spain; Switzerland); Rhesuman Berna (Colombia; Hong-Kong; Israel; Malaysia; Peru; Thailand); Rhogam (Belgium; Hong-Kong); WinRho SDF (New-Zealand)
HCFA JCODE(S): J2790 1 dose package IM

DESCRIPTION

$Rh_o(D)$ Immune Globulin (Human) Gamulin Rh, is a sterile immunoglobulin solution containing $Rh_o(D)$ antibodies for intramuscular use only. It is obtained by alcohol fractionation of plasma from human blood donors, concentrated and standardized to give a total globulin content of 11.5 ± 1.5%. All lots are assayed for $Rh_o(D)$ antibody content by a serological method (anti-globulin titer). The $Rh_o(D)$ antibody level in each vial or syringe of Gamulin Rh is equal to or greater than that of the Office of Biologics Research and Review Reference $Rh_o(D)$ Immune Globulin (Human). This dose has been shown to effectively inhibit the immunizing potential of up to 15 ml of Rh-positive packed red blood cells.

The final product contains 0.3 molar glycine as a stabilizer and 0.01% thimerosal (mercury derivative) as a preservative.

Mini-Gamulin Rh: Mini-Gamulin Rh contains one-sixth the quantity of $Rh_o(D)$ Immune Globulin (Human). The contents of one vial or syringe of Mini-Gamulin Rh will suppress the immunizing potential of 5 ml of whole blood or 2.5 ml of packed red blood cells.

INDICATIONS AND USAGE

GAMULIN RH

Full Term Delivery

$Rh_o(D)$ Immune Globulin (Human) Gamulin Rh is used to prevent sensitization to the $Rh_o(D)$ factor and thus to prevent hemolytic disease of the newborn (Erythroblastosis fetalis) in a pregnancy that follows the injection of Gamulin Rh. It effectively suppresses the immune response of non-sensitized Rh-negative mothers after delivery of an Rh-positive infant.

Criteria for an Rh-incompatible pregnancy requiring administration of: $Rh_o(D)$ Immune Globulin (Human) Gamulin Rh are:

- The mother must be $Rh_o(D)$ negative.
- The mother should not have been previously sensitized to the $Rh_o(D)$ factor.
- The infant must be $Rh_o(D)$ positive and direct antiglobulin negative.

Other Obstetric Conditions

Gamulin Rh should be administered to all non-sensitized Rh-negative women after spontaneous or induced abortions after ruptured tubal pregnancies, amniocentesis, and other abdominal trauma, or any occurrence of transplacental hemorrhage unless the blood type of the fetus has been determined to be $Rh_o(D)$ negative.

If $Rh_o(D)$ Immune Globulin (Human) Gamulin Rh is administered antepartum, it is essential that the mother receive another dose of Gamulin Rh after the delivery of an $Rh_o(D)$ positive infant.

NOTE: In a case of abortion or ectopic pregnancy when Rh typing of the fetus is not possible, the fetus must be assumed to be $Rh_o(D)$ positive. In such an instance the patient should be considered a candidate for administration of $Rh_o(D)$ Immune Globulin (Human) Gamulin Rh.

If the father can be determined to be $Rh_o(D)$ negative, Gamulin Rh need not be given.

Gamulin Rh should be given within 72 hours following an Rh-incompatible delivery, miscarriage or abortion.

Transfusions

Gamulin Rh can be used to prevent $Rh_o(D)$ sensitization in $Rh_o(D)$ negative patients accidentally transfused with $Rh_o(D)$ positive RBC or blood components containing RBC.

It should be administered within 72 hours following an Rh-incompatible transfusion.

MINI-GAMULIN RH

Rh sensitization may occur in nonsensitized $Rh_o(D)$ negative women following transplacental hemorrhage resulting from spontaneous or induced abortions. sensitization occurs more frequently in women undergoing induced abortions than those aborting spontaneously.

$Rh_o(D)$ Immune Globulin, at the dosage level contained in one vial or syringe of Mini-Gamulin Rh prevents the formation of anti-$Rh_o(D)$ antibodies in nonsensitized $Rh_o(D)$ negative women who receive $Rh_o(D)$ positive blood during transplacental hemorrhage resulting from spontaneous or induced abortion up to 12 weeks' gestation.

For spontaneous or induced abortions occurring after 12 weeks' gestation, an appropriate dose of standard $Rh_o(D)$ Immune Globulin (Gamulin Rh) sufficient to suppress the immunizing potential of ml of Rh-positive packed red blood cells, should be given.

NOTE: Mini-Gamulin Rh Prophylaxis is not indicated if the fetus or the father can be determined to be Rh negative. If Rh typing of the fetus is not possible, the fetus must be assumed to be $Rh_o(D)$ positive and the patient should be considered a candidate for treatment.

Mini-Gamulin Rh should be administered promptly following spontaneous or induced abortion. If prompt administration is not possible, Mini-Gamulin Rh should be given within 72 hours following termination of the pregnancy. However, if Mini-Gamulin is not given within this time period, administration of this product should be considered.

CONTRAINDICATIONS

None known.

WARNINGS

Gamulin Rh: Gamulin Rh must not be given to the $Rh_o(D)$ positive postpartum infant. Do not give intravenously.Mini-Gamulin Rh: Do not inject intravenously.

DOSAGE AND ADMINISTRATION

GAMULIN RH

Preadministration Laboratory Procedure

Infant: Immediately postpartum determine the infant's blood group (ABO $Rh_o(D)$) and perform a direct antiglobulin test. Umbilical cord, venous or capillary blood may be used.
Mother: Confirm that the mother is $Rh_o(D)$ negative.

Dosage

Postpartum Prophylaxis Miscarriage, Abortion, or Ectopic Pregnancy

One vial or syringe of $Rh_o(D)$ Immune Globulin (Human) Gamulin Rh is sufficient to prevent maternal sensitization to the Rh factor if the fetal packed red blood cell volume which entered the mother's blood due to fetomaternal hemorrhage is less than 15 ml (30 ml of whole blood). When the fetomaternal hemorrhage exceeds 15 ml of packed cells or 30 ml of whole blood, more than one vial or syringe of Gamulin Rh should be administered.

Antepartum Prophylaxis

The contents of one vial or syringe of Gamulin Rh injected intramuscularly at 28 weeks gestation and the contents of one vial or syringe within 72 hours after an Rh incompatible delivery is highly effective in preventing Rh iso-immunization during pregnancy.

To determine the number of vials or syringes required, the volume of packed fetal red blood cells must be determined by an approved laboratory assay, such as the Kleihauer-Betke Acid Elution Technic or the Clayton Modification. The volume of fetomaternal hemorrhage divided by 2 gives the volume of packed fetal red blood cells in the maternal blood. The number of vials or syringes of Gamulin Rh to be administered is determined by dividing the volume (ml) of packed red blood cells by 15.

Transfusion Accidents

The number of vials or syringes of $Rh_o(D)$ Immune Globulin (Human) Gamulin Rh to be administered is dependent on the volume of packed red cells or whole blood transfused. The method to determine the number of vials or syringes of Gamulin Rh required to prevent sensitization is outlined below. If the dose calculation results in a fraction, administer the next whole number of vials or syringes of Gamulin Rh.

Procedure

Multiply the volume (in ml) of Rh-positive whole blood administered by the hematocrit of the donor unit. This value equals the volume of packed red blood cells transfused.

Divide the volume (in ml) of packed red blood cells by 15 to obtain the number of vials or syringes of Gamulin Rh to be administered.

Administration

Single Vial or Syringe Dose: Inject intramuscularly the entire contents of the vial or syringe of $Rh_o(D)$ Immune Globulin (Human) Gamulin Rh.

Multiple Vial or Syringe Dose: The contents of the total number of vials or syringes may be injected as a divided dose at different injection sites at the same time or the total dosage may be divided and injected at intervals provided the total dosage to be given is injected within 72 hours postpartum or after a transfusion accident.

This product should be administered within 72 hours after Rh-incompatible delivery or transfusion.

Do not inject intravenously.

Parenteral drug products should be inspected visually for particulate matter and discoloration prior to administration, whenever solution and container permit.

Storage: Keep refrigerated at 2-8°C (36-46°F). Do not freeze.

MINI-GAMULIN RH

Do not inject intravenously

The contents of one vial or syringe of Mini-Gamulin Rh provides protection from Rh immunization for women with transplacental hemorrhage resulting from spontaneous or induced abortion up to 12 weeks' gestation. Inject intramuscularly the entire contents of the vial or syringe.

Mini-Gamulin Rh should be administered promptly following spontaneous or induced abortion. If prompt administration is not possible, Mini-Gamulin Rh should be given 72 hours following termination of pregnancy.

Parenteral drug products should be inspected visually for particulate matter and discoloration prior to administration whenever solution and container permit.

PRODUCT LISTING - EQUIVALENTS NOT AVAILABLE

Powder For Injection - Injectable - 120 mcg

1's	$146.35	WINRHO SDF, Nabi	60492-0021-01

Powder For Injection - Injectable - 300 mcg

1's	$324.50	WINRHO SDF, Nabi	60492-0023-01

Powder For Injection - Injectable - 1000 mcg

1's	$1081.50	WINRHO SDF, Nabi	60492-0024-01

Powder For Injection - Intramuscular - 300 mcg

1's	$240.00	BAYRHO-D, Bayer	00026-0631-01

Solution - Intramuscular - Strength n/a

0.17 ml x 10	$268.75	HYPRHO-D MINI-DOSE, Bayer	00192-0621-05
1 ml	$45.00	HYPRHO-D MINI-DOSE, Bayer	00192-0621-01
1 ml x 5	$140.00	MICRHOGAM, Ortho-Clinical Diagnostics Inc	00562-8080-80
1 ml x 5	$725.00	RHOGAM, Ortho-Clinical Diagnostics Inc	00562-7807-05

1 ml x 10	$450.00	HYPRHO-D MINI-DOSE, Bayer	00192-0621-10
1 ml x 10	$450.00	HYPRHO-D MINI-DOSE, Bayer	00192-0621-22
1 ml x 25	$850.20	MICRHOGAM, Ortho-Clinical Diagnostics Inc	00562-8080-82
1 ml x 25	$1471.50	RHOGAM, Ortho-Clinical Diagnostics Inc	00562-8070-20
1 ml x 25	$3625.00	RHOGAM, Ortho-Clinical Diagnostics Inc	00562-7807-25
1 ml x 100	$181.19	RHOGAM, Ortho-Clinical Diagnostics Inc	00562-8070-90
Solution - Intramuscular - 50 mcg/ml			
1 ml x 5	$269.50	MICRHOGAM, Ortho-Clinical Diagnostics Inc	00562-7808-05
1 ml x 25	$1225.00	MICRHOGAM, Ortho-Clinical Diagnostics Inc	00562-7808-25
1 ml x 25	$1347.50	MICRHOGAM, Ortho-Clinical Diagnostics Inc	00562-7808-26
Solution - Intramuscular - 300 mcg/ml			
0.17 ml x 10	$366.00	BAYRHO-D, Bayer	00026-0631-06
0.17 ml x 10	$388.80	BAYRHO-D, Bayer	00026-0631-05
1 ml	$100.00	BAYRHO-D, Bayer	00026-0631-15
1 ml	$110.00	BAYRHO-D, Bayer	00026-0631-02
1 ml x 5	$725.00	GENERIC, Ortho-Clinical Diagnostics Inc	00562-7807-06
5 ml x 10	$378.00	BAYRHO-D, Allscripts Pharmaceutical Company	54569-4396-00

Ribavirin *(002186)*

Categories: Infection, respiratory syncytial virus; Hepatitis C; Pregnancy Category X; FDA Approved 1985 Dec
Drug Classes: Antivirals
Brand Names: Copegus; Rebetol; **Virazole**
Foreign Brand Availability: Cotronak (Germany); Desiken (Mexico); Virazin (Korea)

INHALATION

WARNING

USE OF AEROSOLIZED RIBAVIRIN IN PATIENTS REQUIRING MECHANICAL VENTILATOR ASSISTANCE SHOULD BE UNDERTAKEN ONLY BY PHYSICIANS AND SUPPORT STAFF FAMILIAR WITH THE SPECIFIC VENTILATOR BEING USED AND THIS MODE OF ADMINISTRATION OF THE DRUG. STRICT ATTENTION MUST BE PAID TO PROCEDURES THAT HAVE BEEN SHOWN TO MINIMIZE THE ACCUMULATION OF DRUG PRECIPITATE, WHICH CAN RESULT IN MECHANICAL VENTILATOR DYSFUNCTION AND ASSOCIATED INCREASED PULMONARY PRESSURES. (SEE WARNINGS.)

SUDDEN DETERIORATION OF RESPIRATORY FUNCTION HAS BEEN ASSOCIATED WITH INITIATION OF AEROSOLIZED RIBAVIRIN USE IN INFANTS. RESPIRATORY FUNCTION SHOULD BE CAREFULLY MONITORED DURING TREATMENT. IF INITIATION OF AEROSOLIZED RIBIVIRIN TREATMENT APPEARS TO PRODUCE SUDDEN DETERIORATION OF RESPIRATORY FUNCTION, TREATMENT SHOULD BE STOPPED AND REINSTITUTED ONLY WITH EXTREME CAUTION, CONTINUOUS MONITORING AND CONSIDERATION OF CONCOMITANT ADMINISTRATION OF BRONCHODILATORS. (SEE WARNINGS.)

RIBIVIRIN IS NOT INDICATED FOR USE IN ADULTS. PHYSICIANS AND PATIENTS SHOULD BE AWARE THAT RIBAVIRIN HAS BEEN SHOWN TO PRODUCE TESTICULAR LESIONS IN RODENTS AND TO BE TERATOGENIC IN ALL ANIMAL SPECIES IN WHICH ADEQUATE STUDIES HAVE BEEN CONDUCTED (RODENTS AND RABBITS). (SEE CONTRAINDICATIONS.)

DESCRIPTION

Ribavirin is a synthetic, nucleoside with antiviral activity. Virazole for inhalation solution is a sterile, lyophilized powder to be reconstituted for aerosol administration. Each 100 ml glass vial contains 6 g of ribavirin, and when reconstituted to the recommended volume of 300 ml with sterile water for injection or sterile water for inhalation (no preservatives added), will contain 20 mg of ribavirin/ml, pH approximately 5.5. Aerosolization is to be carried out in a Small Particle Aerosol Generator (SPAG-2) nebulizer only.

Ribavirin is 1-beta-D-ribofuranosyl-1H-1,2,4-triazole-3-carboxamide.

Ribavirin is a stable, white crystalline compound with a maximum solubility in water of 142 mg/ml at 25°C and with only a slight solubility in ethanol. The empirical formula is $C_8H_{12}N_4O_5$ and the molecular weight is 244.21.

CLINICAL PHARMACOLOGY

MECHANISM OF ACTION

In cell cultures the inhibitory activity of ribavirin for respiratory syncytial virus (RSV) is selective. The mechanism of action is unknown. Reversal of the *in vitro* antiviral activity by guanosine or xanthosine suggests ribavirin may act as an analogue of these cellular metabolites.

MICROBIOLOGY

Ribavirin has demonstrated antiviral activity against RSV *in vitro*[1] and experimentally infected cotton rats.[2] Several clinical isolates of RSV were evaluated for ribavirin susceptibility by plaque reduction in tissue culture. Plaques were reduced 85-98% by 16 µg/ml; however, results may vary with the test system. The development of resistance has not been evaluated *in vitro* or in clinical trials.

In addition to the above, ribavirin has been shown to have an *in vitro* activity against influenza A and B viruses and herpes simplex virus, but the clinical significance of these data is unknown.

IMMUNOLOGIC EFFECTS

Neutralizing antibody responses to RSV were decreased in aerosolized ribavirin treated infants compared to placebo treated infants.[3] One study also showed that RSV-specific IgE antibody in bronchial secretions was decreased in patients treated with aerosolized ribavirin. In rats, ribavirin administration resulted in lymphoid atrophy of the thymus, spleen, and lymph nodes. Humoral immunity was reduced in guinea pigs and ferrets. Cellular immunity was also mildly depressed in animal studies. The clinical significance of these observations is unknown.

PHARMACOKINETICS

Assay for ribavirin in human materials is by a radioimmunoassay which detects ribavirin and at least one metabolite.

Virazole brand of ribavirin, when administered by aerosol, is absorbed systematically. Four pediatric patients inhaling ribavirin aerosol administered by face mask for 2.5 hours each day for 3 days had plasma concentrations ranging from 0.44-1.55 µM, with a mean concentration of 0.76 µM. The plasma half-life was reported to be 9.5 hours. Three pediatric patients inhaling aerosolized ribavirin administered by face mask or mist tent for 20 hours each day for 5 days had plasma concentrations ranging from 1.5-14.3 µM, with a mean concentration of 6.8 µM.

The bioavailability of aerosolized ribavirin is unknown and may depend on the mode of aerosol delivery. After aerosol treatment, peak plasma concentrations of ribavirin are 85-98% less than the concentration that reduced RSV plaque formation in tissue culture. After aerosol treatment, respiratory tract secretions are likely to contain ribavirin in concentrations many fold higher than those required to reduce plaque formation. However, RSV is an intracellular virus and it is unknown whether plasma concentrations or respiratory secretion concentrations of the drug better reflect intracellular concentrations in the respiratory tract.

In man, rats, and rhesus monkeys, accumulation of ribavirin and/or metabolites in the red blood cells has been noted, plateauing in red cells in man in about 4 days and gradually declining with an apparent half-life of 40 days (the half-life of erythrocytes). The extent of accumulation of ribavirin following inhalation therapy is not well defined.

INDICATIONS AND USAGE

Ribavirin is indicated for the treatment of hospitalized infants and young children with severe lower respiratory tract infections due to respiratory syncytial virus. Treatment early in the course of severe lower respiratory tract infection may be necessary to achieve efficacy.

Only severe RSV lower respiratory tract infection should be treated with ribavirin. The vast majority of infants and children with RSV infection have disease that is mild, self-limited, and does not require hospitalization or antiviral treatment. Many children with mild lower respiratory tract involvement will require shorter hospitalization than would be required for a full course of ribavirin aerosol (3-7 days) and should not be treated with the drug. Thus the decision to treat with ribavirin should be based on the severity of the RSV infection. The presence of an underlying condition such as prematurity, immunosuppression or cardiopulmonary disease may increase the severity of clinical manifestations and complications of RSV infection.

Use of aerosolized ribavirin in patients requiring mechanical ventilator assistance should be undertaken only by physicians and support staff familiar with this mode of administration and the specific ventilator being used (see WARNINGS and DOSAGE AND ADMINISTRATION).

DIAGNOSIS

RSV infection should be documented by a rapid diagnostic method such as demonstration of viral antigen in respiratory tract secretions by immunofluorescence [3,4] or ELISA[5] before or during the first 24 hours of treatment. Treatment may be initiated while awaiting rapid diagnostic test results. However, treatment should not be continued without documentation of RSV infection. Non-culture antigen detection techniques may have false positives or false negative results. Assessment of the clinical situation, the time of year and other parameters may warrant reevaluation of the laboratory diagnosis.

CONTRAINDICATIONS

Ribavirin is contraindicated in individuals who have shown hypersensitivity to the drug or its components, and in women who are or may become pregnant during exposure to the drug. Ribavirin has demonstrated significant teratogenic and/or embryocidal potential in all animal species in which adequate studies have been conducted (rodents and rabbits). Therefore, although clinical studies have not been performed, it should be assumed that ribavirin may cause fetal harm in humans. Studies in which the drug has been administered systematically demonstrate that ribavirin is concentrated in the red blood cells and persists for the life of the erythrocyte.

WARNINGS

SUDDEN DETERIORATION OF RESPIRATORY FUNCTION HAS BEEN ASSOCIATED WITH INITIATION OF AEROSOLIZED RIBAVIRIN USE IN INFANTS. Respiratory function should be carefully monitored during treatment. If initiation of aerosolized ribavirin treatment appears to produce sudden deterioration of respiratory function, treatment should be stopped and reinstituted only with extreme caution, continuous monitoring, and consideration of concomitant administration of bronchodilators.

USE WITH MECHANICAL VENTILATORS

USE OF AEROSOLIZED RIBAVIRIN IN PATIENTS REQUIRING MECHANICAL VENTILATOR ASSISTANCE SHOULD BE UNDERTAKEN ONLY BY PHYSICIANS AND SUPPORT STAFF FAMILIAR WITH THIS MODE OF ADMINISTRATION AND THE SPECIFIC VENTILATOR BEING USED. Strict attention must be paid to procedures that have been shown to minimize the accumulation of drug precipitate, which can result in mechanical ventilator dysfunction and associated increased pulmonary pressures. These procedures include the use of bacteria filters in series in the expiratory limb of the ventilator circuit with frequent changes (every 4 hours), water column pressure release valves to indicate elevated ventilator pressures, frequent monitoring of these devices and verification that ribavirin crystals have not accumulated within the ventilator circuitry, and frequent suctioning and monitoring of the patient.

Those administering aerosolized ribavirin in conjunction with mechanical ventilator use should be thoroughly familiar with detailed descriptions of these procedures as outlined in the SPAG-2 manual.

PRECAUTIONS

GENERAL

Patients with severe lower respiratory tract infection due to respiratory syncytial virus require optimum monitoring and attention to respiratory and fluid status (see SPAG-2 manual).

CARCINOGENESIS AND MUTAGENESIS

Ribavirin increased the incidence of cell transformations and mutations in mouse Balb/c 3T3 (fibroblasts) and L5178Y (lymphoma) cells at concentrations of 0.015 and 0.03-5.0 mg/ml, respectively (without metabolic activation). Modest increases in mutation rates (3-4×) were observed at concentrations between 3.75-10.0 mg/ml in L5178Y cells *in vitro* with the addition of a metabolic activation fraction. In the mouse micronucleus assay, ribavirin was clastogenic at intravenous doses of 20-200 mg/kg, (estimated human equivalent of 1.67-16.7 mg/kg, based on body surface area adjustment for a 60 kg adult). Ribavirin was not mutagenic in a dominant lethal assay in rats at intraperitoneal doses between 50-200 mg/kg when administered for 5 days (estimated human equivalent of 7.14-28.6 mg/kg, based on body surface area adjustment; see CLINICAL PHARMACOLOGY, Pharmacokinetics).

In vivo carcinogenicity studies with ribavirin are incomplete. However, results of a chronic feeding study with ribavirin in rats, at doses of 16-100 mg/kg/day (estimated human equivalent of 2.3-14.3 mg/kg/day, based on body surface area adjustment for the adult), suggest that ribavirin may induce benign mammary, pancreatic, pituitary and adrenal tumors. Preliminary results of 2 oral gavage oncogenicity studies in the mouse and rat [18-24 months; doses of 20-75 and 10-40 mg/kg/day, respectively (estimated human equivalent of 1.67-6.25 and 1.43-5.71 mg/kg/day, respectively, based on body surface area adjustment for the adult)] are inconclusive as to the carcinogenic potential of ribavirin (see CLINICAL PHARMACOLOGY, Pharmacokinetics). However, these studies have demonstrated a relationship between chronic ribavirin exposure and increased incidences of vascular lesions (microscopic hemorrhages in mice) and retinal degeneration (in rats).

IMPAIRMENT OF FERTILITY

The fertility of ribavirin-treated animals (male or female) has not been fully investigated. However, in the mouse, administration of ribavirin at doses between 35-150 mg/kg/day (estimated human equivalent of 2.92-12.5 mg/kg/day, based on body surface area adjustment for the adult) resulted in significant seminiferous tubule atrophy, decreased sperm concentrations, and increased numbers of sperm with abnormal morphology. Partial recovery of sperm production was apparent 3-6 months following dose cessation in several additional toxicology studies, ribavirin has been shown to cause testicular lesions (tubular atrophy) in adult rats at oral dose levels as low as 16 mg/kg/day (estimated human equivalent of 2.29 mg/kg/day, based on body surface area adjustment; see CLINICAL PHARMACOLOGY, Pharmacokinetics). Lower doses were not tested. The reproductive capacity of treated male animals has not been studied.

PREGNANCY CATEGORY X

Ribavirin has demonstrated significant teratogenic and/or embryocidial potential in all animal species in which adequate studies have been conducted. Teratogenic effects were evident after single oral doses of 2.5 mg/kg or greater in the hamster, and after daily oral doses of 0.3 and 1.0 mg/kg in the rabbit and rat, respectively (estimated human equivalent doses of 0.12 and 0.14 mg/kg, based on body surface area adjustment for the adult). Malformations of the skull, palate, eye, jaw, limbs, skeleton, and gastrointestinal tract were noted. The incidence and severity of teratogenic effects increased with escalation of the drug dose. Survival of fetuses and offspring was reduced. Ribavirin caused embryolethality in the rabbit at daily oral dose levels as low as 1 mg/kg. No teratogenic effects were evident in the rabbit and rat administered daily oral doses of 0.1 and 0.3 mg/kg, respectively with estimated human equivalent doses of 0.01 and 0.04 mg/kg, based on body surface area adjustment (see CLINICAL PHARMACOLOGY, Pharmacokinetics). These doses are considered to define the "No Observable Teratogenic Effects Level" (NOTEL) for ribavirin in the rabbit and rat.

Following oral administration of ribavirin in the pregnant rat (1.0 mg/kg) and rabbit (0.3 mg/kg) mean plasma levels of drug ranged from 0.10-0.20 μM [0.024-0.049 μg/ml] at 1 hour after dosing, to undetectable levels at 24 hours. At 1 hour following the administration of 0.3 or 0.1 mg/kg in the rat and rabbit (NOTEL), respectively, mean plasma levels of drug in both species were near or below the limit of detection (0.05 μM; see CLINICAL PHARMACOLOGY, Pharmacokinetics).

Although clinical studies have not been performed, ribavirin may cause fetal harm in humans. As noted previously, ribavirin is concentrated in red blood cells and persists for the life of the cell. Thus the terminal half-life for the systemic elimination of ribavirin is essentially that of the half-life of circulating erythrocytes. The minimum interval following exposure to ribavirin before pregnancy may be safely initiated is unknown (see CONTRAINDICATIONS; WARNINGS; and PRECAUTIONS, Information for Health Care Personnel).

NURSING MOTHERS

Ribavirin has been shown to be toxic to lactating animals and their offspring. It is not known if ribavirin is excreted in human milk.

INFORMATION FOR HEALTH CARE PERSONNEL

Health care workers directly providing care to patients receiving aerosolized ribavirin should be aware that ribavirin has been shown to be teratogenic in all animal species in which adequate studies have been conducted (rodents and rabbits). Although no reports of teratogenesis in offspring of mothers who were exposed to aerosolized ribavirin during pregnancy have been confirmed, no controlled studies have been conducted in pregnant women. Studies of environmental exposure in treatment settings have shown that the drug can disperse into the immediate bedside area during routine patient care activities with highest ambient levels closest to the patient and extremely low levels outside of the immediate bedside area. Adverse reactions resulting from actual occupational exposure in adults are described below (see ADVERSE REACTIONS, Adverse Events in Health Care Workers). Some studies have documented ambient drug concentrations at the bedside that could potentially lead to systemic exposures above those considered safe for exposure during pregnancy (1/1000 of the NOTEL dose in the most sensitive animal species).[7-9]

A 1992 study conducted by the National Institute of Occupational Safety and Health (NIOSH) demonstrated measurable urine levels of ribavirin in health care workers exposed to aerosol in the course of direct patient care.[7] Levels were lowest in workers caring for infants receiving aerosolized ribavirin with mechanical ventilation and highest in those caring for patients being administered the drug via an oxygen tent or hood. This study employed a more sensitive assay to evaluate ribavirin levels in urine than was available for several previous studies of environmental exposure that failed to detect measurable ribavirin levels in exposed workers. Creatinine adjusted urine levels in the NIOSH study ranged from less than 0.001-0.140 μM of ribavirin/gram of creatine in exposed workers. However, the relationship between urinary ribavirin levels exposed workers, plasma levels in animal studies, and the specific risk of teratogenesis in exposed pregnant women is unknown.

It is good practice to avoid unnecessary occupational exposure to chemicals wherever possible. Hospitals are encouraged to conduct training programs to minimize potential occupational exposure to ribavirin. Health care workers who are pregnant should consider avoiding direct care of patients receiving aerosolized ribavirin. If close patient contact cannot be avoided, precautions to limit exposure should be taken. These include administration of ribavirin in negative pressure rooms; adequate room ventilation (at least 6 air exchanges/hour); the use of ribavirin aerosol scavenging devices; turning off the SPAG-2 device for 5-10 minutes prior to prolonged patient contact; and wearing appropriately fitted respirator masks. Surgical masks do not provide adequate filtration of ribavirin particles. Further information is available from NIOSH's Hazard Evaluation and Technical Assistance Branch and additional recommendations have been published in an Aerosol Consensus Statement by the American Respiratory Care Foundation and the American Association for Respiratory Care.[10]

DRUG INTERACTIONS

Clinical studies of interactions of Virazole with other drugs commonly used to treat infants with RSV infections, such as digoxin, bronchodilators, other antiviral agents, antibiotics or antimetabolites, have not been conducted. Interference by Virazole with laboratory tests has not been evaluated.

ADVERSE REACTIONS

The description of adverse reactions is based on events from clinical studies (approximately 200 patients) conducted prior to 1986, and the controlled trial of aerosolized ribavirin conducted in 1989-1990. Additional data from spontaneous postmarketing reports of adverse events in individual patients have been available since 1986.

DEATHS

Deaths during or shortly after treatment with aerosolized ribavirin have been reported in 20 cases of patients treated with ribavirin (12 of these patients were being treated for RSV infections). Several cases have been characterized as "possibly related" to ribavirin by the treating physician; these were in infants who experienced worsening respiratory status related to bronchospasm while being treated with the drug. Several other cases have been attributed to mechanical ventilator malfunction in which ribavirin precipitation within the ventilator apparatus led to excessively high pulmonary pressures and diminished oxygenation. In these cases the monitoring procedures described in the current package insert were not employed (see WARNINGS and DOSAGE AND ADMINISTRATION).

PULMONARY AND CARDIOVASCULAR

Pulmonary function significantly deteriorated during aerosolized ribavirin treatment in 6 of 6 adults with chronic obstructive lung disease and in 4 of 6 asthmatic adults. Dyspnea and chest soreness were also reported in the latter group. Minor abnormalities in pulmonary function were also seen in healthy adult volunteers.

In the original study population of approximately 200 infants who received aerosolized ribavirin, several serious adverse events occurred in severely ill infants with life-threatening underlying diseases, many of whom required assisted ventilation. The role of ribavirin in these events is indeterminate. Since the drugs approval in 1986, additional reports of similar serious, though non-fatal, events have been filed infrequently. Events associated with aerosolized ribavirin use have included the following:

- ***Pulmonary:*** Worsening of respiratory status, bronchospasm, pulmonary edema, hypoventilation, cyanosis, dyspnea, bacterial pneumonia, pneumothorax, apnea, atelectasis, ventilator dependence.
- ***Cardiovascular:*** Cardiac arrest, hypotension, bradycardia, digitalis toxicity. Bigeminy, bradycardia and tachycardia have been described in patients with underlying congenital heart disease.

Some subjects requiring assisted ventilation experienced serious difficulties, due to inadequate ventilation and gas exchange. Precipitation of drug within the ventilatory apparatus, including the endotracheal tube, has resulted in increased positive end expiratory pressure and increased positive inspiratory pressure. Accumulation of fluid in tubing ("rain out") has also been noted. Measures to avoid these complications should be followed carefully (see DOSAGE AND ADMINISTRATION).

HEMATOLOGIC

Although anemia was not reported with use of aerosolized ribavirin in controlled clinical trials, most infants treated with the aerosol have not been evaluated 1-2 weeks post-treatment when anemia is likely to occur. Anemia has been shown to occur frequently with experimental oral and intravenous ribavirin in humans. Also, cases of anemia (type unspecified), reticulocytosis and hemolytic anemia associated with aerosolized ribavirin use have been reported through postmarketing reporting systems. All have been reversible with discontinuation of the drug.

OTHER

Rash and conjunctivitis have been associated with the use of aerosolized ribavirin. These usually resolve within hours of discontinuing therapy. Seizures and asthenia associated with experimental intravenous ribavirin therapy have also been reported.

ADVERSE EVENTS IN HEALTH CARE WORKERS

Studies of environmental exposure to aerosolized ribavirin in health care workers administering care to patients receiving the drug have not detected adverse signs or symptoms related to exposure. However, 152 health care workers have reported experiencing adverse events through postmarketing surveillance. Nearly all were in individuals providing direct care to infants receiving aerosolized ribavirin. Of 358 events from these 152 individual health care worker reports, the most common signs and symptoms were headache (51% of reports), conjunctivitis (32%), and rhinitis, nausea, rash, dizziness, pharyngitis, or lacrimation (10-20% each). Several cases of bronchospasm and/or chest pain were also reported, usually individuals with known underlying reactive airway disease. Several case reports of damage to contact lenses after prolonged close exposure to aerosolized ribavirin have been reported. Most signs and symptoms reported as having occurred in exposed health care workers resolved within minutes to hours of discontinuing close exposure to aerosolized ribavirin (see PRECAUTIONS, Information for Health Care Personnel).

The symptoms of RSV in adults can include headache, conjunctivitis, sore throat and/or cough, fever, hoarseness, nasal congestion and wheezing, although RSV infections in adults are typically mild and transient. Such infections represent a potential hazard to uninfected hospital patients. It is unknown whether certain symptoms cited in reports from health care workers were due to exposure to the drug or infection with RSV. Hospitals should implement appropriate infection control procedures.

DOSAGE AND ADMINISTRATION

BEFORE USE, READ THOROUGHLY THE ICN SMALL PARTICLE AEROSOL GENERATOR SPAG-2 OPERATORS MANUAL FOR SMALL PARTICLE AEROSOL GENERATOR OPERATING INSTRUCTIONS. AEROSOLIZED RIBAVIRIN SHOULD NOT BE ADMINISTERED WITH ANY OTHER AEROSOL GENERATING DEVICE.

The recommended treatment regimen is 20 mg/ml ribavirin as the starting solution in the drug reservoir of the SPAG-2 unit, with continuous aerosol administration for 12-18 hours/day for 3-7 days. Using the recommended drug concentration of 20 mg/ml the average aerosol concentration for a 12 hour delivery period would be 190 μg/L of air. Aerosolized ribavirin should not be administered in a mixture for combined aerosolization or simultaneously with other aerosolized medications.

NON-MECHANICALLY VENTILATED INFANTS

Ribavirin should be delivered to an infant oxygen hood from the SPAG-2 aerosol generator. Administration by face mask or oxygen tent may be necessary if a hood cannot be employed (see SPAG-2 manual). However, the volume and condensation area are larger in a tent and this may alter delivery dynamics of the drug.

MECHANICALLY VENTILATED INFANTS

The recommended dose and administration schedule for infants who require mechanical ventilation is the same as for those who do not. Either a pressure or volume cycle ventilator may be used in conjunction with the SPAG-2. In either case, patients should have their endotracheal tubes suctioned every 1-2 hours, and their pulmonary pressures monitored frequently (every 2-4 hours). For both pressure and volume ventilators, heated wire connective tubing bacteria filters in series in the expiratory limb of the system (which must be changed frequently, *i.e.,* every 4 hours) must be used to minimize the risk of ribavirin precipitation in the system and the subsequent risk of ventilator dysfunction. Water column pressure release valves should be used in the ventilator circuit for pressure cycled ventilators, and may be utilized with volume cycled ventilators (see SPAG-2 manual for detailed instructions).

METHOD OF PREPARATION

Virazole brand of ribavirin is supplied as 6 g of lyophilized powder/100 ml vial for aerosol administration only. By sterile technique, reconstitute drug with a minimum of 75 ml of **sterile water for injection or inhalation** in the original 100 ml glass vial. Shake well. Transfer to the clean, sterilized 500 ml SPAG-2 reservoir and further dilute to a final volume of 300 ml with sterile water for injection or inhalation. The final concentration should be 20 mg/ml. **Important:** THIS water should NOT have had any antimicrobial agent or other substance added. The solution should be inspected visually for particulate matter and discoloration prior to administration. Solutions that have been placed in the SPAG-2 unit should be discarded at least every 24 hours and when the liquid level is low before adding newly reconstituted solution.

ANIMAL PHARMACOLOGY

ANIMAL TOXICOLOGY

Ribavirin, when administered orally or as an aerosol, produced cardiac lesions in mice, rats, and monkeys when given at doses of 30, 36 and 120 mg/kg or greater for 4 weeks or more (estimated human equivalent doses of 4.8, 12.3 and 111.4 mg/kg for a 5 kg child, or 2.5, 5.1 and 40 mg/kg for 60 kg adult, based on body surface area adjustment). Aerosolized ribavirin administered to developing ferrets at 60 mg/kg for 10-30 days resulted in inflammatory and possibly emphysematous changes in the lungs. Proliferative changes were seen in the lungs following exposure at 131 mg/kg for 30 days. The significance of these findings to human administration is unknown.

HOW SUPPLIED

Virazole (ribavirin for inhalation solution) is supplied in 100 ml glass vials with 6 g of sterile, lyophilized drug which is to be reconstituted with 300 ml sterile water for injection or sterile water for inhalation (no preservatives added) and administered only by a small particle aerosol generator (SPAG-2).

Storage: Vials containing the lyophilized drug powder should be stored in a dry place at 15-25°C (59-78°F). Reconstituted solutions may be stored, under sterile conditions, at room temperature (20-30°C, 68-86°F) for 24 hours. Solutions which have been placed in the SPAG-2 unit should be discarded at least every 24 hours.

ORAL

WARNING

Note: The trade names have been used throughout this monograph for clarity.

REBETOL

- **Ribavirin monotherapy is not effective for the treatment of chronic hepatitis C virus infection and should not be used alone for this indication. (See WARNINGS.)**
- **The primary toxicity of ribavirin is hemolytic anemia. The anemia associated with ribavirin therapy may result in worsening of cardiac disease that has lead to fatal and nonfatal myocardial infarctions. Patients with a history of significant or unstable cardiac disease should not be treated with ribavirin. (See WARNINGS, ADVERSE REACTIONS, and DOSAGE AND ADMINISTRATION.)**
- **Significant teratogenic and/or embryocidal effects have been demonstrated in all animal species exposed to ribavirin. In addition, ribavivin has a multiple-dose half-life of 12 days, and so it may persist in nonplasma compartments for as long as 6 months. Therefore, ribavirin therapy is contraindicated in women who are pregnant and in the male partners of women who are pregnant. Extreme care must be taken to avoid pregnancy during therapy and for 6 months after completion of treatment in both female patients and in female partners of male patients who are taking ribavirin therapy. At least 2 reliable forms of effective contraception must be utilized during treatment and during the 6 month post-treatment follow-up period. (See CONTRAINDICATIONS; WARNINGS; and PRECAUTIONS: Information for the Patient and Pregnancy Category X.)**

COPEGUS

Ribavirin monotherapy is not effective for the treatment of chronic hepatitis C virus infection and should not be used alone for this indication (see WARNINGS).

The primary clinical toxicity of ribavirin is hemolytic anemia. The anemia associated with ribavirin therapy may result in worsening of cardiac disease that has led to fatal and nonfatal myocardial infarctions. Patients with a history of significant or unstable cardiac disease should not be treated with ribavirin (see WARNINGS, ADVERSE REACTIONS, and DOSAGE AND ADMINISTRATION).

Significant teratogenic and/or embryocidal effects have been demonstrated in all animal species exposed to ribavirin. In addition, ribavirin has a multiple dose half-life of 12 days, and it may persist in non-plasma compartments for as long as 6 months. Ribavirin therapy is contraindicated in women who are pregnant and in the male partners of women who are pregnant. Extreme care must be taken to avoid pregnancy during therapy and for 6 months after completion of treatment in both female patients and in female partners of male patients who are taking ribavirin therapy. At least 2 reliable forms of effective contraception must be utilized during treatment and during the 6 month post-treatment follow-up period (see CONTRAINDICATIONS; WARNINGS; and PRECAUTIONS: Information for the Patient and Pregnancy Category X).

DESCRIPTION

REBETOL

Rebetol is Schering Corporation's brand name for ribavirin, a nucleoside analog. The chemical name of ribavirin is 1-β-D-ribofuranosyl-1*H*-1,2,4-triazole-3-carboxamide.

Ribavirin is a white, crystalline powder. It is freely soluble in water and slightly soluble in anhydrous alcohol. The empirical formula is $C_8H_{12}N_4O_5$ and the molecular weight is 244.21.

Rebetol capsules consist of a white powder in a white, opaque, gelatin capsule. Each capsule contains 200 mg ribavirin and the inactive ingredients microcrystalline cellulose, lactose monohydrate, croscarmellose sodium, and magnesium stearate. The capsule shell consists of gelatin, sodium lauryl sulfate, silicon dioxide, and titanium dioxide. The capsule is printed with edible blue pharmaceutical ink which is made of shellac, anhydrous ethyl alcohol, isopropyl alcohol, n-butyl alcohol, propylene glycol, ammonium hydroxide, and FD&C blue no. 2 aluminum lake.

COPEGUS

Copegus, the Hoffmann-La Roche brand name for ribavirin, is a nucleoside analogue with antiviral activity. The chemical name of ribavirin is 1-β-D-ribofuranosyl-1*H*-1,2,4-triazole-3-carboxamide.

The empirical formula of ribavirin is $C_8H_{12}N_4O_5$ and the molecular weight is 244.2. Ribavirin is a white to off-white powder. It is freely soluble in water and slightly soluble in anhydrous alcohol.

Copegus is available as a light pink to pink colored, flat, ovalshaped, film-coated tablet for oral administration. Each tablet contains 200 mg of ribavirin and the following inactive ingredients: pregelatinized starch, microcrystalline cellulose, sodium starch glycolate, corn starch, and magnesium stearate. The coating of the tablet contains Chromatone-P or Opadry Pink (made by using hydroxypropyl methyl cellulose, talc, titanium dioxide, synthetic yellow iron oxide, and synthetic red iron oxide), ethyl cellulose (ECD-30), and triacetin.

CLINICAL PHARMACOLOGY

REBETOL

Mechanism of Action

The mechanism of inhibition of hepatitis C virus (HCV) RNA by combination therapy with interferon products has not been established.

Pharmacokinetics

Ribavirin

Single- and multiple-dose pharmacokinetic properties in adults with chronic hepatitis C are summarized in TABLE 1. Ribavirin was rapidly and extensively absorbed following oral administration. However, due to first-pass metabolism, the absolute bioavailability averaged 64% (44%). There was a linear relationship between dose and AUC(tf) (AUC from time zero to last measurable concentration) following single doses of 200-1200 mg ribavirin. The relationship between dose and C_{max} was curvilinear, tending to asymptote above single doses of 400-600 mg.

Upon multiple oral dosing, based on AUC(12h), a 6-fold accumulation of ribavirin was observed in plasma. Following oral dosing with 600 mg bid, steady-state was reached by approximately 4 weeks, with mean steady-state plasma concentrations of 2200 (37%) ng/ml. Upon discontinuation of dosing, the mean half-life was 298 (30%) hours, which probably reflects slow elimination from nonplasma compartments.

Effect of Food on Absorption of Ribavirin

Both AUC(tf) and C_{max} increased by 70% when ribavirin capsules were administered with a high-fat meal (841 kcal, 53.8 g fat, 31.6 g protein, and 57.4 g carbohydrate) in a single-dose pharmacokinetic study. There are insufficient data to address the clinical relevance of these results. Clinical efficacy studies with Rebetol/Intron A were conducted without instructions with respect to food consumption. During clinical studies with Rebetol/PegIntron, all subjects were instructed to take Rebetol capsules with food. (See DOSAGE AND ADMINISTRATION.)

Effect of Antacid on Absorption of Ribavirin

Coadministration with an antacid containing magnesium, aluminum, and simethicone resulted in a 14% decrease in mean ribavirin AUC(tf). The clinical relevance of results from this single-dose study is unknown.

TABLE 1 *Mean (% CV) Pharmacokinetic Parameters for Rebetol When Administered Individually to Adults With Chronic Hepatitis C*

	Rebetol (n=12)	
	Single Dose	**Multiple Dose**
Parameter	**600 mg**	**600 mg bid**
T_{max} (h)	1.7 (46)*	3 (60)
C_{max} (ng/ml)	782 (37)	3,680 (85)
AUC(tf) (ng·h/ml)	13,400 (48)	228,000 (25)
T½ (h)	43.6 (47)	298 (30)
Apparent volume of distribution (L)	2,825 (9)†	
Apparent clearance (L/h)	38.2 (40)	
Absolute bioavailability	64% (44)‡	

* n=11.
† Data obtained from a single-dose pharmacokinetic study using ^{14}C labeled ribavirin; n=5.
‡ n=6.

Ribavirin transport into nonplasma compartments has been most extensively studied in red blood cells, and has been identified to be primarily via an e_s-type equilibrative nucleoside transporter. This type of transporter is present on virtually all cell types and may account for the extensive volume of distribution. Ribavirin does not bind to plasma proteins.

Ribavirin has two pathways of metabolism: (i) a reversible phosphorylation pathway in nucleated cells; and (ii) a degradative pathway involving deribosylation and amide hydrolysis to yield a triazole carboxylic acid metabolite. Ribavirin and its triazole carboxamide and triazole carboxylic acid metabolites are excreted renally. After oral administration of 600 mg of ^{14}C-ribavirin, approximately 61% and 12% of the radioactivity was eliminated in the urine and feces, respectively, in 336 hours. Unchanged ribavirin accounted for 17% of the administered dose.

Results of *in vitro* studies using both human and rat liver microsome preparations indicated little or no cytochrome P450 enzyme-mediated metabolism of ribavirin, with minimal potential for P450 enzyme-based drug interactions.

No pharmacokinetic interactions were noted between interferon alfa-2b injection and ribavirin capsules in a multiple-dose pharmacokinetic study.

Special Populations

Renal Dysfunction

The pharmacokinetics of ribavirin were assessed after administration of a single oral dose (400 mg) of ribavirin to non HCV-infected subjects with varying degrees of renal dysfunction. The mean AUC(tf) value was 3-fold greater in subjects with creatinine clearance values between 10-30 ml/min when compared to control subjects (creatinine clearance >90 ml/min). In subjects with creatinine clearance values between 30-60 ml/min, AUC(tf) was 2-fold greater when compared to control subjects. The increased AUC(tf) appears to be due to reduction of renal and non-renal clearance in these patients. Phase 3 efficacy trials included subjects with creatinine clearance values >50 ml/min. The multiple dose pharmacokinetics of ribavirin cannot be accurately predicted in patients with renal dysfunction. Ribavirin is not effectively removed by hemodialysis. Patients with creatinine clearance <50 ml/min should not be treated with ribavirin (see WARNINGS).

Hepatic Dysfunction

The effect of hepatic dysfunction was assessed after a single oral dose of ribavirin (600 mg). The mean AUC(tf) values were not significantly different in subjects with mild, moderate, or severe hepatic dysfunction (Child-Pugh Classification A, B, or C), when compared to control subjects. However, the mean C_{max} values increased with severity of hepatic dysfunction and was 2-fold greater in subjects with severe hepatic dysfunction when compared to control subjects.

Pediatric Patients

Pharmacokinetic evaluations in pediatric subjects have not been performed.

Elderly Patients

Pharmacokinetic evaluations in elderly subjects have not been performed.

Gender

There were no clinically significant pharmacokinetic differences noted in a single-dose study of 18 male and 18 female subjects.

****In this section of the label, numbers in parenthesis indicate % coefficient of variation.***

COPEGUS

Mechanism of Action

Ribavirin is a synthetic nucleoside analogue. The mechanism by which the combination of ribavirin and an interferon product exerts its effects against the hepatitis C virus has not been fully established.

Pharmacokinetics

Multiple dose ribavirin pharmacokinetic data are available for HCV patients who received ribavirin in combination with peginterferon alfa-2a. Following administration of 1200 mg/day with food for 12 weeks mean ± SD (n=39; body weight >75 kg) AUC(0-12h) was 25,361 ± 7,110 ng·h/ml and C_{max} was 2,748 ± 818 ng/ml. The average time to reach C_{max} was 2 hours. Trough ribavirin plasma concentrations following 12 weeks of dosing with food were 1662 + 545 ng/ml in HCV infected patients who received 800 mg/day (n=89), and 2112 ± 810 ng/ml in patients who received 1200 mg/day (n=75; body weight >75 kg).

The terminal half-life of ribavirin following administration of a single oral dose of Copegus is about 120-170 hours. The total apparent clearance following administration of a single oral dose of Copegus is about 26 L/h. There is extensive accumulation of ribavirin after multiple dosing (twice daily) such that the C_{max} at steady state was 4-fold higher than that of a single dose.

Effect of Food on Absorption of Ribavirin

Bioavailability of a single oral dose of ribavirin was increased by coadministration with a high-fat meal. The absorption was slowed (T_{max} was doubled) and the AUC(0-192h) and C_{max} increased by 42% and 66%, respectively, when Copegus was taken with a high-fat meal compared with fasting conditions (see PRECAUTIONS and DOSAGE AND ADMINISTRATION).

Elimination and Metabolism

The contribution of renal and hepatic pathways to ribavirin elimination after administration of Copegus is not known. *In vitro* studies indicate that ribavirin is not a substrate of CYP450 enzymes.

Special Populations

Race

There were insufficient numbers of non-Caucasian subjects studied to adequately determine potential pharmacokinetic differences between populations.

Renal Dysfunction

The pharmacokinetics of ribavirin following administration of Copegus have not been studied in patients with renal impairment and there are limited data from clinical trials on administration of Copegus in patients with creatinine clearance <50 ml/min. Therefore, patients with creatinine clearance <50 ml/min should not be treated with Copegus (see WARNINGS and DOSAGE AND ADMINISTRATION).

Hepatic Impairment

The effect of hepatic impairment on the pharmacokinetics of ribavirin following administration of Copegus has not been evaluated. The clinical trials of Copegus were restricted to patients with Child-Pugh class A disease.

Pediatric Patients

Pharmacokinetic evaluations in pediatric patients have not been performed.

Elderly Patients

Pharmacokinetic evaluations in elderly patients have not been performed.

Gender

Ribavirin pharmacokinetics, when corrected for weight, are similar in male and female patients.

Drug Interactions

In vitro studies indicate that ribavirin does not inhibit CYP450 enzymes.

Nucleoside Analogues

Ribavirin has been shown *in vitro* to inhibit phosphorylation of zidovudine and stavudine which could lead to decreased antiretroviral activity. Exposure to didanosine or its active metabolite (dideoxyadenosine 5′-triphosphate) is increased when didanosine is coadministered with ribavirin, which could cause or worsen clinical toxicities (see DRUG INTERACTIONS).

INDICATIONS AND USAGE

REBETOL

Rebetol capsules are indicated in combination with Intron A (interferon alfa-2b, recombinant) injection for the treatment of chronic hepatitis C in patients with compensated liver disease previously untreated with alpha interferon or who have relapsed following alpha interferon therapy.

Rebetol capsules are indicated in combination with Peg-Intron (peginterferon alfa-2b, recombinant) injection for the treatment of chronic hepatitis C in patients with compensated liver disease who have not been previously treated with interferon alpha and are at least 18 years of age.

The safety and efficacy of Rebetol capsules with interferons other than Intron A or Peg-Intron products have not been established.

COPEGUS

Copegus in combination with Pegasys (peginterferon alfa-2a) is indicated for the treatment of adults with chronic hepatitis C virus infection who have compensated liver disease and have not been previously treated with interferon alpha. Patients in whom efficacy was demonstrated included patients with compensated liver disease and histological evidence of cirrhosis (Child-Pugh class A).

CONTRAINDICATIONS

REBETOL

Pregnancy

Rebetol capsules may cause birth defects and/or death of the exposed fetus. Rebetol therapy is contraindicated for use in women who are pregnant or in men whose female partners are pregnant. (See WARNINGS and PRECAUTIONS: Information for the Patient and Pregnancy Category X.)

Rebetol capsules are contraindicated in patients with a history of hypersensitivity to ribavirin or any component of the capsule.

Patients with autoimmune hepatitis must not be treated with combination Rebetol/Intron A therapy because using these medicines can make the hepatitis worse.

Patients with hemoglobinopathies (*e.g.,* thalassemia major, sickle-cell anemia) should not be treated with Rebetol capsules.

COPEGUS

Copegus is contraindicated in:

- Patients with known hypersensitivity to Copegus or to any component of the tablet.
- Women who are pregnant.
- Men whose female partners are pregnant.
- Patients with hemoglobinopathies (*e.g.,* thalassemia major or sickle-cell anemia).

Copegus and Pegasys combination therapy is contraindicated in patients with:

- Autoimmune hepatitis.
- Hepatic decompensation (Child-Pugh class B and C) before or during treatment.

WARNINGS

REBETOL

Based on results of clinical trials ribavirin monotherapy is not effective for the treatment of chronic hepatitis C virus infection; therefore, Rebetol capsules must not be used alone. The safety and efficacy of Rebetol capsules have only been established when used together with Intron A as Rebetron combination therapy or with Peg-Intron Injection.

There are significant adverse events caused by Rebetol/Intron A or Peg-Intron therapy, including severe depression and suicidal ideation, hemolytic anemia, suppression of bone marrow function, autoimmune and infectious disorders, pulmonary dysfunction, pancreatitis, and diabetes. The Rebetron combination therapy and Peg-Intron package inserts should be reviewed in their entirety prior to initiation of combination treatment for additional safety information.

Pregnancy

Rebetol capsules may cause birth defects and/or death of the exposed fetus. Extreme care must be taken to avoid pregnancy in female patients and in female partners of male patients. Rebetol has demonstrated significant teratogenic and/or embryocidal effects in all animal species in which adequate studies have been conducted. These effects occurred at doses as low as one-twentieth of the recommended human dose of ribavirin. REBETOL THERAPY SHOULD NOT BE STARTED UNTIL A REPORT OF A NEGATIVE PREGNANCY TEST HAS BEEN OBTAINED IMMEDIATELY PRIOR TO PLANNED INITIATION OF THERAPY. Patients should be instructed to use at least 2 forms of effective contraception during treatment and during the 6 month period after treatment has been stopped based on multiple dose half-life of ribavirin of 12 days. Pregnancy testing should occur monthly during Rebetol therapy and for 6 months after therapy has stopped (see CONTRAINDICATIONS and PRECAUTIONS: Information for the Patient and Pregnancy Category X).

Anemia

The primary toxicity of ribavirin is hemolytic anemia, which was observed in approximately 10% of Rebetol/Intron A-treated patients in clinical trials (see ADVERSE REACTIONS, Laboratory Values, Hemoglobin). The anemia associated with Rebetol capsules occurs within 1-2 weeks of initiation of therapy. BECAUSE THE INITIAL DROP IN HEMOGLOBIN MAY BE SIGNIFICANT, IT IS ADVISED THAT HEMOGLOBIN OR HEMATOCRIT BE OBTAINED PRETREATMENT AND AT WEEK 2 AND WEEK 4 OF THERAPY, OR MORE FREQUENTLY IF CLINICALLY INDICATED. Patients should then be followed as clinically appropriate.

Fatal and nonfatal myocardial infarctions have been reported in patients with anemia caused by ribavirin. Patients should be assessed for underlying cardiac disease before initiation of ribavirin therapy. Patients with pre-existing cardiac disease should have electrocardiograms administered before treatment, and should be appropriately monitored during therapy. If there is any deterioration of cardiovascular status, therapy should be suspended or discontinued. (See DOSAGE AND ADMINISTRATION, Dose Modification.) Because cardiac disease may be worsened by drug induced anemia, patients with a history of significant or unstable cardiac disease should not use Rebetol. (See ADVERSE REACTIONS.)

Rebetol and Intron A or Peg-Intron therapy should be suspended in patients with signs and symptoms of pancreatitis and discontinued in patients with confirmed pancreatitis.

Rebetol should not be used in patients with creatinine clearance <50 ml/min. (See CLINICAL PHARMACOLOGY, Pharmacokinetics, Special Populations.)

COPEGUS

Copegus must not be used alone because ribavirin monotherapy is not effective for the treatment of chronic hepatitis C virus infection. The safety and efficacy of Copegus have only been established when used together with Pegasys (pegylated interferon alfa-2a, recombinant).

Copegus and Pegasys should be discontinued in patients who develop evidence of hepatic decompensation during treatment.

There are significant adverse events caused by Copegus/Pegasys therapy, including severe depression and suicidal ideation, hemolytic anemia, suppression of bone marrow function, autoimmune and infectious disorders, pulmonary dysfunction, pancreatitis, and diabetes. The Pegasys package insert and Medication Guide should be reviewed in their entirety prior to initiation of combination treatment for additional safety information.

General

Treatment with Copegus and Pegasys should be administered under the guidance of a qualified physician and may lead to moderate to severe adverse experiences requiring dose reduction, temporary dose cessation or discontinuation of therapy.

Pregnancy

Ribavirin may cause birth defects and/or death of the exposed fetus. Extreme care must be taken to avoid pregnancy in female patients and in female partners of male patients. Ribavirin has demonstrated significant teratogenic and/or embryocidal effects in all animal species in which adequate studies have been conducted. These effects occurred at doses as low as one-twentieth of the recommended human dose of ribavirin. COPEGUS THERAPY SHOULD NOT BE STARTED UNLESS A REPORT OF A NEGATIVE PREGNANCY TEST HAS BEEN OBTAINED IMMEDIATELY PRIOR TO PLANNED INITIATION OF THERAPY. Patients should be instructed to use at least 2 forms of effective contraception during treatment and for at least 6 months after treatment has been stopped. Pregnancy testing should occur monthly during Copegus therapy and for 6 months after therapy has stopped (see CONTRAINDICATIONS and PRECAUTIONS: Information for the Patient and Pregnancy Category X).

Anemia

The primary toxicity of ribavirin is hemolytic anemia (hemoglobin <10 g/dl), which was observed in approximately 13% of Copegus and Pegasys treated patients in clinical trials (see PRECAUTIONS, Laboratory Tests). The anemia associated with Copegus occurs within 1-2 weeks of initiation of therapy. BECAUSE THE INITIAL DROP IN HEMOGLOBIN MAY BE SIGNIFICANT, IT IS ADVISED THAT HEMOGLOBIN OR HEMATOCRIT BE OBTAINED PRETREATMENT AND AT WEEK 2 AND WEEK 4 OF THERAPY OR MORE FREQUENTLY IF CLINICALLY INDICATED. Patients should then be followed as clinically appropriate.

Fatal and nonfatal myocardial infarctions have been reported in patients with anemia caused by ribavirin. Patients should be assessed for underlying cardiac disease before initiation of ribavirin therapy. Patients with pre-existing cardiac disease should have electrocardiograms administered before treatment, and should be appropriately monitored during therapy. If there is any deterioration of cardiovascular status, therapy should be suspended or discontinued (see TABLE 15). Because cardiac disease may be worsened by drug induced anemia, patients with a history of significant or unstable cardiac disease should not use Copegus (see ADVERSE REACTIONS).

Pulmonary

Pulmonary symptoms, including dyspnea, pulmonary infiltrates, pneumonitis and occasional cases of fatal pneumonia, have been reported during therapy with ribavirin and interferon. In addition, sarcoidosis or the exacerbation of sarcoidosis has been reported. If there is evidence of pulmonary infiltrates or pulmonary function impairment, the patient should be closely monitored, and if appropriate, combination Copegus/Pegasys treatment should be discontinued.

Other

Copegus and Pegasys therapy should be suspended in patients with signs and symptoms of pancreatitis, and discontinued in patients with confirmed pancreatitis.

Copegus should not be used in patients with creatinine clearance <50 ml/min (see CLINICAL PHARMACOLOGY, Special Populations).

Copegus must be discontinued immediately and appropriate medical therapy instituted if an acute hypersensitivity reaction (*e.g.,* urticaria, angioedema, bronchoconstriction, anaphylaxis) develops. Transient rashes do not necessitate interruption of treatment.

PRECAUTIONS

REBETOL

The safety and efficacy of Rebetol/Intron A and Peg-Intron therapy for the treatment of HIV infection, adenovirus, RSV, parainfluenza, or influenza infections have not been established. Rebetol capsules should not be used for these indications. Please consult the Virazole for inhalation section if ribavirin inhalation therapy is being considered.

The safety and efficacy of Rebetol/Intron A therapy has not been established in liver or other organ transplant patients, patients with decompensated liver disease due to hepatitis C infection, patients who are nonresponders to interferon therapy, or patients coinfected with HBV or HIV.

R

Information for the Patient

Patients must be informed that Rebetol capsules may cause birth defects and/or death of the exposed fetus. Rebetol must not be used by women who are pregnant or by men whose female partners are pregnant. Extreme care must be taken to avoid pregnancy in female patients and in female partners of male patients taking Rebetol. Rebetol should not be initiated until a report of a negative pregnancy test has been obtained immediately prior to initiation of therapy. Patients must perform a pregnancy test monthly during therapy and for 6 months posttherapy. Women of childbearing potential must be counseled about use of effective contraception (2 reliable forms) prior to initiating therapy. Patients (male and female) must be advised of the teratogenic/embryocidal risks and must be instructed to practice effective contraception during Rebetol and for 6 months post therapy. Patients (male and female) should be advised to notify the physician immediately in the event of a pregnancy. (See CONTRAINDICATIONS and WARNINGS.)

If pregnancy does occur during treatment or during 6 months posttherapy, the patient must be advised of the teratogenic risk of Rebetol therapy to the fetus. Patients, or partners of patients, should immediately report any pregnancy that occurs during treatment or within 6 months after treatment cessation to their physician. Physicians should report such cases by calling 1-800-727-7064.

Patients receiving Rebetol capsules should be informed of the benefits and risks associated with treatment, directed in its appropriate use, and referred to the patient **Medication Guide.** Patients should be informed that the effect of treatment of hepatitis C infection on transmission is not known, and that appropriate precautions to prevent transmission of the hepatitis C virus should be taken.

The most common adverse experience occurring with Rebetol capsules is anemia, which may be severe. (See ADVERSE REACTIONS.) Patients should be advised that laboratory evaluations are required prior to starting therapy and periodically thereafter. (See Laboratory Tests.) It is advised that patients be well hydrated, especially during the initial stages of treatment.

Laboratory Tests

The following laboratory tests are recommended for all patients treated with Rebetol capsules, prior to beginning treatment and then periodically thereafter.

Standard Hematologic Tests: Including hemoglobin [pretreatment, Week 2 and Week 4 of therapy, and as clinically appropriate (see WARNINGS)], complete and differential white blood cell counts, and platelet count.

Blood Chemistries: Liver function tests and TSH.

Pregnancy: Including monthly monitoring for women of childbearing potential.

ECG: See WARNINGS.

Carcinogenesis, Mutagenesis, and Impairment of Fertility

Adequate studies to assess the carcinogenic potential of ribavirin in animals have not been conducted. However, ribavirin is a nucleoside analogue that has produced positive findings in multiple *in vitro* and animal *in vivo* genotoxicity assays, and should be considered a potential carcinogen. Further studies to assess the carcinogenic potential of ribavirin in animals are ongoing.

Ribavirin demonstrated increased incidences of mutation and cell transformation in multiple genotoxicity assays. Ribavirin was active in the Balb/3T3 *In Vitro* Cell Transformation Assay. Mutagenic activity was observed in the mouse lymphoma assay, and at doses of 20-200 mg/kg (estimated human equivalent of 1.67-16.7 mg/kg, based on body surface area adjustment for a 60 kg adult; 0.1 to 1 × the maximum recommended human 24 hour dose of ribavirin) in a mouse micronucleus assay. A dominant lethal assay in rats was negative, indicating that if mutations occurred in rats they were not transmitted through male gametes.

Impairment of Fertility

Ribavirin demonstrated significant embryocidal and/or teratogenic effects at doses well below the recommended human dose in all animal species in which adequate studies have been conducted.

Fertile women and partners of fertile women should not receive Rebetol unless the patient and his/her partner are using effective contraception (2 reliable forms). Based on a multiple dose half-life ($T_{1/2}$) of ribavirin of 12 days, effective contraception must be utilized for 6 months posttherapy (*e.g.,* 15 half-lives of clearance for ribavirin).

Rebetol should be used with caution in fertile men. In studies in mice to evaluate the time course and reversibility of ribavirin-induced testicular degeneration at doses of 15-150 mg/kg/day (estimated human equivalent of 1.25-12.5 mg/kg/day, based on body surface area adjustment for a 60 kg adult; 0.1-0.8 × the maximum human 24 hour dose of ribavirin) administered for 3 or 6 months, abnormalities in sperm occurred. Upon cessation of treatment, essentially total recovery from ribavirin-induced testicular toxicity was apparent within 1 or 2 spermatogenesis cycles.

Animal Toxicology

Long-term studies in the mouse and rat [18-24 months; doses of 20-75 and 10-40 mg/kg/day, respectively (estimated human equivalent doses of 1.67-6.25 and 1.43-5.71 mg/kg/day, respectively, based on body surface area adjustment for a 60 kg adult; approximately 0.1-0.4 × the maximum human 24 hour dose of ribavirin)] have demonstrated a relationship between chronic ribavirin exposure and increased incidences of vascular lesions (microscopic hemorrhages) in mice. In rats, retinal degeneration occurred in controls, but the incidence was increased in ribavirin-treated rats.

Pregnancy Category X

See CONTRAINDICATIONS.

Ribavirin produced significant embryocidal and/or teratogenic effects in all animal species in which adequate studies have been conducted. Malformations of the skull, palate, eye, jaw, limbs, skeleton, and gastrointestinal tract were noted. The incidence and severity of teratogenic effects increased with escalation of the drug dose. Survival of fetuses and offspring was reduced. In conventional embryotoxicity/teratogenicity studies in rats and rabbits, observed no effect dose levels were well below those for proposed clinical use (0.3 mg/kg/day for both the rat and rabbit; approximately 0.06 × the recommended human 24 hour dose of ribavirin). No maternal toxicity or effects on offspring were observed in a peri/postnatal toxicity study in rats dosed orally at up to 1 mg/kg/day (estimated human equivalent dose of 0.17 mg/kg based on body surface area adjustment for a 60 kg adult; approximately 0.01 × the maximum recommended human 24 hour dose of ribavirin).

Treatment and Post-Treatment — Potential Risk to the Fetus

Ribavirin is known to accumulate in intracellular components from where it is cleared very slowly. It is not known whether ribavirin contained in sperm will exert a potential teratogenic effect upon fertilization of the ova. In a study in rats, it was concluded that dominant lethality was not induced by ribavirin at doses up to 200 mg/kg for 5 days (estimated human equivalent doses of 7.14-28.6 mg/kg, based on body surface area adjustment for a 60 kg adult; up to 1.7 × the maximum recommended human dose of ribavirin). However, because of the potential human teratogenic effects of ribavirin, male patients should be advised to take every precaution to avoid risk of pregnancy for their female partners.

Women of childbearing potential should not receive Rebetol unless they are using effective contraception (2 reliable forms) during the therapy period. In addition, effective contraception should be utilized for 6 months posttherapy based on a multiple-dose half-life ($T_{1/2}$) of ribavirin of 12 days. Male patients and their female partners must practice effective contraception (2 reliable forms) during treatment with Rebetol and for the 6 month posttherapy period (*e.g.,* 15 half-lives for ribavirin clearance from the body).

If pregnancy occurs in a patient or partner of a patient during treatment or during the 6 months after treatment cessation, physicians should report such cases by calling 1-800-727-7064.

Nursing Mothers

It is not known whether Rebetol is excreted in human milk. Because of the potential for serious adverse reactions from the drug in nursing infants, a decision should be made whether to discontinue nursing or to delay or discontinue Rebetol.

Geriatric Use

Clinical studies of Rebetol/Intron A or Peg-Intron therapy did not include sufficient numbers of subjects aged 65 and over to determine if they respond differently from younger subjects.

Rebetol is known to be substantially excreted by the kidney, and the risk of toxic reactions to this drug may be greater in patients with impaired renal function. Because elderly patients often have decreased renal function, care should be taken in dose selection. Renal function should be monitored and dosage adjustments should be made accordingly. Rebetol should not be used in patients with creatinine clearance <50 ml/min (see WARNINGS).

In general, Rebetol capsules should be administered to elderly patients cautiously, starting at the lower end of the dosing range, reflecting the greater frequency of decreased hepatic and/or cardiac function, and of concomitant disease or other drug therapy. In clinical trials, elderly subjects had a higher frequency of anemia (67%) than did younger patients (28%). (See WARNINGS.)

Pediatric Use

Safety and effectiveness in pediatric patients have not been established.

COPEGUS

The safety and efficacy of Copegus and Pegasys therapy for the treatment of HIV infection, adenovirus, RSV, parainfluenza or influenza infections have not been established. Copegus should not be used for these indications. Ribavirin for inhalation has a separate package insert, which should be consulted if ribavirin inhalation therapy is being considered.

The safety and efficacy of Copegus and Pegasys therapy have not been established in liver or other organ transplant patients, patients with decompensated liver disease due to hepatitis C virus infection, patients who are non-responders to interferon therapy or patients coinfected with HBV or HIV.

Information for the Patient

Patients must be informed that ribavirin may cause birth defects and/or death of the exposed fetus. Copegus therapy must not be used by women who are pregnant or by men whose female partners are pregnant. Extreme care must be taken to avoid pregnancy in female patients and in female partners of male patients taking Copegus therapy and for 6 months posttherapy. Copegus therapy should not be initiated until a report of a negative pregnancy test has been obtained immediately prior to initiation of therapy. Patients must perform a pregnancy test monthly during therapy and for 6 months posttherapy.

Female patients of childbearing potential and male patients with female partners of childbearing potential must be advised of the teratogenic/embryocidal risks and must be instructed to practice effective contraception during Copegus therapy and for 6 months posttherapy. Patients should be advised to notify the physician immediately in the event of a pregnancy (see CONTRAINDICATIONS and WARNINGS).

To monitor maternal-fetal outcomes of pregnant women exposed to Copegus, the Copegus Pregnancy Registry has been established. Physicians and patients are strongly encouraged to register by calling 1-800-526-6367.

The most common adverse event associated with ribavirin is anemia, which may be severe (see ADVERSE REACTIONS). Patients should be advised that laboratory evaluations are required prior to starting Copegus therapy and periodically thereafter (see Laboratory Tests). It is advised that patients be well hydrated, especially during the initial stages of treatment.

Patients who develop dizziness, confusion, somnolence, and fatigue should be cautioned to avoid driving or operating machinery.

Patients should be informed regarding the potential benefits and risks attendant to the use of Copegus. Instructions on appropriate use should be given, including review of the contents of the enclosed **Medication Guide,** which is not a disclosure of all or possible adverse effects.

Patients should be advised to take Copegus with food.

Laboratory Tests

Before beginning Copegus therapy, standard hematological and biochemical laboratory tests must be conducted for all patients. Pregnancy screening for women of childbearing potential must be done.

After initiation of therapy, hematological tests should be performed at 2 weeks and 4 weeks and biochemical tests should be performed at 4 weeks. Additional testing should be performed periodically during therapy. Monthly pregnancy testing should be done during combination therapy and for 6 months after discontinuing therapy.

The entrance criteria used for the clinical studies of Copegus and Pegasys combination therapy may be considered as a guideline to acceptable baseline values for initiation of treatment:

- Platelet count ≥90,000 cells/mm^3.
- Absolute neutrophil count (ANC) ≥1500 cells/mm^3.
- TSH and T4 within normal limits or adequately controlled thyroid function.
- ECG (see WARNINGS).

The maximum drop in hemoglobin usually occurred during the first 8 weeks of initiation of Copegus therapy. Because of this initial acute drop in hemoglobin, it is advised that a complete blood count should be obtained pretreatment and at Week 2 and Week 4 of therapy or more frequently if clinically indicated. Additional testing should be performed periodically during therapy. Patients should then be followed as clinically appropriate.

Carcinogenesis, Mutagenesis, and Impairment of Fertility

Carcinogenesis

The carcinogenic potential of ribavirin has not been fully determined. In a p53 ± mouse carcinogenicity study at doses up to the maximum tolerated dose of 100 mg/kg/day, ribavirin was not oncogenic. However, on a body surface area basis, this dose was 0.5 times maximum recommended human 24 hour dose of ribavirin. A study to assess the carcinogenic potential of ribavirin in rats is ongoing.

Mutagenesis

Ribavirin demonstrated mutagenic activity in the *in vitro* mouse lymphoma assay. No clastogenic activity was observed in an *in vivo* mouse micronucleus assay at doses up to 2000 mg/kg. However, results from studies published in the literature show clastogenic activity in the *in vivo* mouse micronucleus assay at oral doses up to 2000 mg/kg. A dominant lethal assay in rats was negative, indicating that if mutations occurred in rats they were not transmitted through male gametes. However, potential carcinogenic risk to humans cannot be excluded.

Impairment of Fertility

In a fertility study in rats, ribavirin showed a marginal reduction in sperm counts at the dose of 100 mg/kg/day with no effect on fertility. Upon cessation of treatment, total recovery occurred after 1 spermatogenesis cycle. Abnormalities in sperm were observed in studies in mice designed to evaluate the time course and reversibility of ribavirin-induced testicular degeneration at doses of 15-150 mg/kg/day (approximately 0.1-0.8 times the maximum recommended human 24 hour dose of ribavirin) administered for 3-6 months. Upon cessation of treatment, essentially total recovery from ribavirin-induced testicular toxicity was apparent within 1 or 2 spermatogenic cycles.

Female patients of childbearing potential and male patients with female partners of childbearing potential should not receive Copegus unless the patient and his/her partner are using effective contraception (2 reliable forms). Based on a multiple dose half-life ($T_{1/2}$) of ribavirin of 12 days, effective contraception must be utilized for 6 months posttherapy (*i.e.,* 15 halflives of clearance for ribavirin).

No reproductive toxicology studies have been performed using Pegasys in combination with Copegus. However, peginterferon alfa-2a and ribavirin when administered separately, each has adverse effects on reproduction. It should be assumed that the effects produced by either agent alone would also be caused by the combination of the two agents.

Pregnancy Category X

See CONTRAINDICATIONS.

Ribavirin produced significant embryocidal and/or teratogenic effects in all animal species in which adequate studies have been conducted. Malformations of the skull, palate, eye, jaw, limbs, skeleton, and gastrointestinal tract were noted. The incidence and severity of teratogenic effects increased with escalation of the drug dose. Survival of fetuses and offspring was reduced.

In conventional embryotoxicity/teratogenicity studies in rats and rabbits, observed no effect dose levels were well below those for proposed clinical use (0.3 mg/kg/day for both the rat and rabbit; approximately 0.06 times the recommended human 24 hour dose of ribavirin). No maternal toxicity or effects on offspring were observed in a peri/postnatal toxicity study in rats dosed orally at up to 1 mg/kg/day (approximately 0.01 times the maximum recommended human 24 hour dose of ribavirin).

Treatment and Post-Treatment — Potential Risk to the Fetus

Ribavirin is known to accumulate in intracellular components from where it is cleared very slowly. It is not known whether ribavirin is contained in sperm, and if so, will exert a potential teratogenic effect upon fertilization of the ova. In a study in rats, it was concluded that dominant lethality was not induced by ribavirin at doses up to 200 mg/kg for 5 days (up to 1.7 times the maximum recommended human dose of ribavirin). However, because of the potential human teratogenic effects of ribavirin, male patients should be advised to take every precaution to avoid risk of pregnancy for their female partners.

Copegus should not be used by pregnant women or by men whose female partners are pregnant. Female patients of childbearing potential and male patients with female partners of childbearing potential should not receive Copegus unless the patient and his/her partner are using effective contraception (2 reliable forms) during therapy and for 6 months post-therapy.

To monitor maternal-fetal outcomes of pregnant women exposed to Copegus, the Copegus Pregnancy Registry has been established. Physicians and patients are strongly encouraged to register by calling 1-800-526-6367.

Animal Toxicology

Long-term study in the mouse and rat (18-24 months; dose 20-75 and 10-40 mg/kg/day, respectively (approximately 0.1-0.4 times the maximum human daily dose of ribavirin) have demonstrated a relationship between chronic ribavirin exposure and an increased incidence of vascular lesions (microscopic hemorrhages) in mice. In rats, retinal degeneration occurred in controls, but the incidence was increased in ribavirin-treated rats.

Nursing Mothers

It is not known whether ribavirin is excreted in human milk. Because many drugs are excreted in human milk and to avoid any potential for serious adverse reactions in nursing infants from ribavirin, a decision should be made either to discontinue nursing or therapy with Copegus, based on the importance of the therapy to the mother.

Pediatric Use

Safety and effectiveness of Copegus have not been established in patients below the age of 18.

Geriatric Use

Clinical studies of Copegus and Pegasys did not include sufficient numbers of subjects aged 65 or over to determine whether they respond differently from younger subjects. Specific pharmacokinetic evaluations for ribavirin in the elderly have not been performed. The risk of toxic reactions to this drug may be greater in patients with impaired renal function. Copegus should not be administered to patients with creatinine clearance <50 ml/min (see CLINICAL PHARMACOLOGY, Special Populations).

Effect of Gender

No clinically significant differences in the pharmacokinetics of ribavirin were observed between male and female subjects.

DRUG INTERACTIONS

Results from a pharmacokinetic sub-study demonstrated no pharmacokinetic interaction between Pegasys (peginterferon alfa-2a) and ribavirin.

NUCLEOSIDE ANALOGUES

Didanosine

Coadministration of Copegus and didanosine is not recommended. Reports of fatal hepatic failure, as well as peripheral neuropathy, pancreatitis, and symptomatic hyperlactatemia/lactic acidosis have been reported in clinical trials (see CLINICAL PHARMACOLOGY, Drug Interactions).

Stavudine and Zidovudine

Ribavirin can antagonize the *in vitro* antiviral activity of stavudine and zidovudine against HIV. Therefore, concomitant use of ribavirin with either of these drugs should be avoided (see CLINICAL PHARMACOLOGY, Drug Interactions).

ADVERSE REACTIONS

REBETOL

The primary toxicity of ribavirin is hemolytic anemia. Reductions in hemoglobin levels occurred within the first 1-2 weeks of oral therapy. (See WARNINGS.) Cardiac and pulmonary events associated with anemia occurred in approximately 10% of patients. (See WARNINGS.)

Rebetol/Intron A Combination Therapy

In clinical trials, 19% and 6% of previously untreated and relapse patients, respectively, discontinued therapy due to adverse events in the combination arms compared to 13% and 3% in the interferon arms. Selected treatment-emergent adverse events that occurred in the US studies with ≥5% incidence are provided in TABLE 7A and TABLE 7B by treatment group. In general, the selected treatment-emergent adverse events reported with lower incidence in the international studies as compared to the US studies with the exception of asthenia, influenza-like symptoms, nervousness, and pruritus.

In addition, the following spontaneous adverse events have been reported during the marketing surveillance of Rebetol/Intron A therapy: Hearing disorder and vertigo.

Rebetol/Peg-Intron Combination Therapy

Overall, in clinical trials, 14% of patients receiving Rebetol in combination with Peg-Intron, discontinued therapy compared with 13% treated with Rebetol in combination with Intron A. The most common reasons for discontinuation of therapy were related to psychiatric, systemic (*e.g.,* fatigue, headache), or gastrointestinal adverse events. Adverse events that occurred in clinical trial at >5% incidence are provided in TABLE 8A and TABLE 8B by treatment group.

Laboratory Values

Rebetol/Intron A Combination Therapy

Changes in selected hematologic values (hemoglobin, white blood cells, neutrophils, and platelets) during therapy are described below. (See TABLE 9A and TABLE 9B.)

Hemoglobin

Hemoglobin decreases among patients receiving Rebetol therapy began at Week 1, with stabilization by Week 4. In previously untreated patients treated for 48 weeks the mean maximum decrease from baseline was 3.1 g/dl in the US study and 2.9 g/dl in the International study. In relapse patients the mean maximum decrease from baseline was 2.8 g/dl in the US study and 2.6 g/dl in the International study. Hemoglobin values returned to pretreatment levels within 4-8 weeks of cessation of therapy in most patients.

Bilirubin and Uric Acid

Increases in both bilirubin and uric acid, associated with hemolysis, were noted in clinical trials. Most were moderate biochemical changes and were reversed within 4 weeks after treatment discontinuation. This observation occurs most frequently in patients with a previous diagnosis of Gilbert's syndrome. This has not been associated with hepatic dysfunction or clinical morbidity.

TABLE 7A *Selected Treatment-Emergent Adverse Events — US Previously Untreated Study*

Patients Reporting Adverse Events*	24 Weeks of Treatment Intron A + Rebetol (n=228)	24 Weeks of Treatment Intron A + Placebo (n=231)	48 Weeks of Treatment Intron A + Rebetol (n=228)	48 Weeks of Treatment Intron A + Placebo (n=225)
Application Site Disorders				
Injection site inflammation	13%	10%	12%	14%
Injection site reaction	7%	9%	8%	9%
Body as a Whole — General Disorders				
Headache	63%	63%	66%	67%
Fatigue	68%	62%	70%	72%
Rigors	40%	32%	42%	39%
Fever	37%	35%	41%	40%
Influenza-like symptoms	14%	18%	18%	20%
Asthenia	9%	4%	9%	9%
Chest pain	5%	4%	9%	8%
Central & Peripheral Nervous System Disorders				
Dizziness	17%	15%	23%	19%
Gastrointestinal System Disorders				
Nausea	38%	35%	46%	33%
Anorexia	27%	16%	25%	19%
Dyspepsia	14%	6%	16%	9%
Vomiting	11%	10%	9%	13%
Musculoskeletal System Disorders				
Myalgia	61%	57%	64%	63%
Arthralgia	30%	27%	33%	36%
Musculoskeletal pain	20%	26%	28%	32%
Psychiatric Disorders				
Insomnia	39%	27%	39%	30%
Irritability	23%	19%	32%	27%
Depression	32%	25%	36%	37%
Emotional lability	7%	6%	11%	8%
Concentration impaired	11%	14%	14%	14%
Nervousness	4%	2%	4%	4%
Respiratory System Disorders				
Dyspnea	19%	9%	18%	10%
Sinusitis	9%	7%	10%	14%
Skin and Appendages Disorders				
Alopecia	28%	27%	32%	28%
Rash	20%	9%	28%	8%
Pruritus	21%	9%	19%	8%
Special Senses, Other Disorders				
Taste perversion	7%	4%	8%	4%

* Patients reporting 1 or more adverse events. A patient may have reported more than 1 adverse event within a body system/organ class category.

TABLE 7B *Selected Treatment-Emergent Adverse Events — US Relapse Study*

Patients Reporting Adverse Events*	24 Weeks of Treatment Intron A + Rebetol (n=77)	24 Weeks of Treatment Intron A + Placebo (n=76)
Application Site Disorders		
Injection site inflammation	6%	8%
Injection site reaction	5%	3%
Body as a Whole — General Disorders		
Headache	66%	68%
Fatigue	60%	53%
Rigors	43%	37%
Fever	32%	36%
Influenza-like symptoms	13%	13%
Asthenia	10%	4%
Chest pain	6%	7%
Central & Peripheral Nervous System Disorders		
Dizziness	26%	21%
Gastrointestinal System Disorders		
Nausea	47%	33%
Anorexia	21%	14%
Dyspepsia	16%	9%
Vomiting	12%	8%
Musculoskeletal System Disorders		
Myalgia	61%	58%
Arthralgia	29%	29%
Musculoskeletal pain	22%	28%
Psychiatric Disorders		
Insomnia	26%	25%
Irritability	25%	20%
Depression	23%	14%
Emotional lability	12%	8%
Concentration impaired	10%	12%
Nervousness	5%	4%
Respiratory System Disorders		
Dyspnea	17%	12%
Sinusitis	12%	7%
Skin and Appendages Disorders		
Alopecia	27%	26%
Rash	21%	5%
Pruritus	13%	4%
Special Senses, Other Disorders		
Taste perversion	6%	5%

* Patients reporting 1 or more adverse events. A patient may have reported more than 1 adverse event within a body system/organ class category.

TABLE 8A *Adverse Events Occurring in >5% of Patients (% of Patients Reporting Adverse Events*)*

Adverse Events	PEG-Intron 1.5 μg/kg /Rebetol (n=511)	Intron A/Rebetol (n=505)
Application Site		
Injection site inflammation	25%	18%
Injection site reaction	58%	36%
Autonomic Nervous System		
Mouth dry	12%	8%
Sweating increased	11%	7%
Flushing	4%	3%
Body as a Whole		
Fatigue/asthenia	66%	63%
Headache	62%	58%
Rigors	48%	41%
Fever	46%	33%
Weight decrease	29%	20%
RUQ pain	12%	6%
Chest pain	8%	7%
Malaise	4%	6%
Central/Peripheral Nervous System		
Dizziness	21%	17%
Endocrine		
Hypothyroidism	5%	4%
Gastrointestinal		
Nausea	43%	33%
Anorexia	32%	27%
Diarrhea	22%	17%
Vomiting	14%	12%
Abdominal pain	13%	13%
Dyspepsia	9%	8%
Constipation	5%	5%
Hematologic Disorders		
Neutropenia	26%	14%
Anemia	12%	17%
Leukopenia	6%	5%
Thrombocytopenia	5%	2%
Liver and Biliary System		
Hepatomegaly	4%	4%

* Patients reporting 1 or more adverse events. A patient may have reported more than 1 adverse event within a body system/organ class category.

Rebetol/Peg-Intron Combination Therapy

Changes in selected hematologic values (hemoglobin, white blood cells, neutrophils, and platelets) during therapy are described below. (See TABLE 10.)

Hemoglobin

Rebetol induced a decrease in hemoglobin levels in approximately two-thirds of patients. Hemoglobin levels decreased to <11 g/dl in about 30% of patients. Severe anemia (<8 g/dl) occurred in <1% of patients. Dose modification was required in 9 and 13% of patients in the Peg-Intron/Rebetol and Intron A/Rebetol groups.

Bilirubin and Uric

In the Rebetol/Peg-Intron combination trial 10-14% of patients developed hyperbilirubenemia and 33-38% developed hyperuricemia in association with hemolysis. Six patients developed mild to moderate gout.

COPEGUS

Pegasys in combination with Copegus causes a broad variety of serious adverse reactions (see BOXED WARNING and WARNINGS). In all studies, 1 or more serious adverse reactions occurred in 10% of patients receiving Pegasys in combination with Copegus.

The most common life-threatening or fatal events induced or aggravated by Pegasys and Copegus were depression, suicide, relapse of drug abuse/overdose, and bacterial infections; each occurred at a frequency of <1%.

Nearly all patients in clinical trials experienced 1 or more adverse events. The most commonly reported adverse reactions were psychiatric reactions, including depression, irritability, anxiety, and flu-like symptoms such as fatigue, pyrexia, myalgia, headache and rigors.

Ten percent (10%) of patients receiving 48 weeks of therapy with Pegasys in combination with Copegus discontinued therapy. The most common reasons for discontinuation of therapy were psychiatric, flu-like syndrome (*e.g.,* lethargy, fatigue, headache), dermatologic and gastrointestinal disorders.

The most common reason for dose modification in patients receiving combination therapy was for laboratory abnormalities; neutropenia (20%) and thrombocytopenia (4%) for Pegasys and anemia (22%) for Copegus.

Pegasys dose was reduced in 12% of patients receiving 1000-1200 mg Copegus for 48 weeks and in 7% of patients receiving 800 mg Copegus for 24 weeks. Copegus dose was reduced in 21% of patients receiving 1000-1200 mg Copegus for 48 weeks and 12% in patients receiving 800 mg Copegus for 24 weeks.

Because clinical trials are conducted under widely varying and controlled conditions, adverse reaction rates observed in clinical trials of a drug cannot be directly compared to rates in the clinical trials of another drug. Also, the adverse event rates listed here may not predict the rates observed in a broader patient population in clinical practice.

Patients treated for 24 weeks with Pegasys and 800 mg Copegus were observed to have lower incidence of serious adverse events (3% vs 10%), hemoglobin <10 g/dl (3% vs 15%), dose modification of Pegasys (30% vs 36%) and Copegus (19% vs 38%) and of withdrawal from treatment (5% vs 15%) compared to patients treated for 48 weeks with Pegasys and

TABLE 8B *Adverse Events Occurring in >5% of Patients (% of Patients Reporting Adverse Events*)*

Adverse Events	PEG-Intron 1.5 µg/kg /Rebetol (n=511)	Intron A/Rebetol (n=505)
Musculoskeletal		
Myalgia	56%	50%
Arthralgia	34%	28%
Musculoskeletal pain	21%	19%
Psychiatric		
Insomnia	40%	41%
Depression	31%	34%
Anxiety/emotional lability/irritability	47%	47%
Concentration impaired	17%	21%
Agitation	8%	5%
Nervousness	6%	6%
Reproductive, Female		
Menstrual disorder	7%	6%
Resistance Mechanism		
Infection viral	12%	12%
Infection fungal	6%	1%
Respiratory System		
Dyspnea	26%	24%
Coughing	23%	16%
Pharyngitis	12%	13%
Rhinitis	8%	6%
Sinusitis	6%	5%
Skin and Appendages		
Alopecia	36%	32%
Pruritus	29%	28%
Rash	24%	23%
Skin dry	24%	23%
Special Senses, Other		
Taste perversion	9%	4%
Vision Disorders		
Vision blurred	5%	6%
Conjunctivitis	4%	5%

* Patients reporting 1 or more adverse events. A patient may have reported more than 1 adverse event within a body system/organ class category.

TABLE 9A *Selected Hematologic Values During Treatment With Ribavirin Plus Interferon alfa-2b, Recombinant — US Previously Untreated Study*

	24 Weeks of Treatment Intron A + Rebetol (n=228)	24 Weeks Intron A + Placebo (n=231)	48 Weeks of Treatment Intron A + Rebetol (n=228)	48 Weeks Intron A + Placebo (n=225)
Hemoglobin (g/dl)				
9.5-10.9	24%	1%	32%	1%
8.0-9.4	5%	0%	4%	0%
6.5-7.9	0%	0%	0%	0.4%
<6.5	0%	0%	0%	0%
Leukocytes (× 10^9/L)				
2.0-2.9	40%	20%	38%	23%
1.5-1.9	4%	1%	9%	2%
1.0-1.4	0.9%	0%	2%	0%
<1.0	0%	0%	0%	0%
Neutrophils (× 10^9/L)				
1.0-1.49	30%	32%	31%	44%
0.75-0.99	14%	15%	14%	11%
0.5-0.74	9%	9%	14%	7%
<0.5	11%	8%	11%	5%
Platelets (× 10^9/L)				
70-99	9%	11%	11%	14%
50-69	2%	3%	2%	3%
30-49	0%	0.4%	0%	0.4%
<30	0.9%	0%	1%	0.9%
Total Bilirubin (mg/dl)				
1.5-3.0	27%	13%	32%	13%
3.1-6.0	0.9%	0.4%	2%	0%
6.1-12.0	0%	0%	0.4%	0%
>12.0	0%	0%	0%	0%

1000 or 1200 mg Copegus. On the other hand the overall incidence of adverse events appeared to be similar in the two treatment groups.

The most common serious adverse event (3%) was bacterial infection (*e.g.*, sepsis, osteomyelitis, endocarditis, pyelonephritis, pneumonia). Other SAEs occurred at a frequency of <1% and included: suicide, suicidal ideation, psychosis, aggression, anxiety, drug abuse and drug overdose, angina, hepatic dysfunction, fatty liver, cholangitis, arrhythmia, diabetes mellitus, autoimmune phenomena (*e.g.*, hyperthyroidism, hypothyroidism, sarcoidosis, systemic lupus erythematosis, rheumatoid arthritis) peripheral neuropathy, aplastic anemia, peptic ulcer, gastrointestinal bleeding, pancreatitis, colitis, corneal ulcer, pulmonary embolism, coma, myositis, and cerebral hemorrhage.

Laboratory Test Values

Anemia due to hemolysis is the most significant toxicity of ribavirin therapy. Anemia (hemoglobin <10 g/dl) was observed in 13% of Copegus and Pegasys combination-treated patients in clinical trials. The maximum drop in hemoglobin occurred during the first 8 weeks of initiation of ribavirin therapy (see DOSAGE AND ADMINISTRATION, Dose Modification).

TABLE 9B *Selected Hematologic Values During Treatment With Ribavirin Plus Interferon alfa-2b, Recombinant — US Relapse Study*

	24 Weeks of Treatment Intron A + Rebetol (n=77)	Intron A + Placebo (n=76)
Hemoglobin (g/dl)		
9.5-10.9	21%	3%
8.0-9.4	4%	0%
6.5-7.9	0%	0%
<6.5	0%	0%
Leukocytes (× 10^9/L)		
2.0-2.9	45%	26%
1.5-1.9	5%	3%
1.0-1.4	0%	0%
<1.0	0%	0%
Neutrophils (× 10^9/L)		
1.0-1.49	42%	34%
0.75-0.99	16%	18%
0.5-0.74	8%	4%
<0.5	5%	8%
Platelets (× 10^9/L)		
70-99	6%	12%
50-69	0%	5%
30-49	0%	0%
<30	0%	0%
Total Bilirubin (mg/dl)		
1.5-3.0	21%	7%
3.1-6.0	3%	0%
6.1-12.0	0%	0%
>12.0	0%	0%

TABLE 10 *Selected Hematologic Values During Treatment With Rebetol Plus Peg-Intron*

	Peg-Intron + Rebetol (n=511)	Intron A + Rebetol (n=505)
Hemoglobin		
9.5-10.9 g/dl	26	27
8.0-9.4 g/dl	3	3
6.5-7.9 g/dl	0.2	0.2
<6.5 g/dl	0	0
Leukocytes (× 10^9/L)		
2.0-2.9	46	41
1.5-1.9	24	8
1.0-1.4	5	1
<1.0	0	0
Neutrophils (× 10^9/L)		
1.0-1.49	33	37
0.75-0.99	25	13
0.5-0.74	18	7
<0.5	4	2
Platelets (× 10^9/L)		
70-99	15	5
50-69	3	0.8
30-49	0.2	0.2
<30	0	0
Total Bilirubin		
1.5-3.0 mg/dl	10	13
3.1-6.0 mg/dl	0.6	0.2
6.1-12.0 mg/dl	0	0.2
>12.0 mg/dl	0	0
ALT (SGPT)		
2 × Baseline	0.6	0.2
2.1-5 × Baseline	3	1
5.1-10 × Baseline	0	0
>10 × Baseline	0	0

DOSAGE AND ADMINISTRATION

REBETOL

See CLINICAL PHARMACOLOGY, Pharmacokinetics, Special Populations and WARNINGS.

Rebetol/Intron A Combination Therapy

The recommended dose of Rebetol capsules depends on the patient's body weight. The recommended doses of Rebetol is provided in TABLE 12.

The recommended duration of treatment for patients previously untreated with interferon is 24-48 weeks. The duration of treatment should be individualized to the patient depending on baseline disease characteristics, response to therapy, and tolerability of the regimen (see ADVERSE REACTIONS). After 24 weeks of treatment virologic response should be assessed. Treatment discontinuation should be considered in any patient who has not achieved an HCV RNA below the limit of detection of the assay by 24 weeks. There are no safety and efficacy data on treatment for longer than 48 weeks in the previously untreated patient population.

In patients who relapse following interferon therapy, the recommended duration of treatment is 24 weeks. There are no safety and efficacy data on treatment for longer than 24 weeks in the relapse patient population.

Rebetol may be administered without regard to food, but should be administered in a consistent manner with respect to food intake. (See CLINICAL PHARMACOLOGY.)

R

TABLE 11 *Adverse Reactions Occurring in ≥5% of Patients in Hepatitis C Clinical Trials (Study NV15801*)*

Body System	Pegasys 180 μg + Copegus 1000 or 1200 mg 48 Weeks (n=451)	Intron A + Rebetol 1000 or 1200 mg 48 Weeks (n=443)
Application Site Disorders		
Injection site reaction	23%	16%
Endocrine Disorders		
Hypothyroidism	4%	5%
Flu-Like Symptoms and Signs		
Fatigue/asthenia	65%	68%
Pyrexia	41%	55%
Rigors	25%	37%
Pain	10%	9%
Gastrointestinal		
Nausea/vomiting	25%	29%
Diarrhea	11%	10%
Abdominal pain	8%	9%
Dry mouth	4%	7%
Dyspepsia	6%	5%
Hematologic†		
Lymphopenia	14%	12%
Anemia	11%	11%
Neutropenia	27%	8%
Thrombocytopenia	5%	<1%
Metabolic and Nutritional		
Anorexia	24%	26%
Weight decrease	10%	10%
Musculoskeletal, Connective Tissue and Bone		
Myalgia	40%	49%
Arthralgia	22%	23%
Back pain	5%	5%
Neurological		
Headache	43%	49%
Dizziness (excluding vertigo)	14%	14%
Memory impairment	6%	5%
Psychiatric		
Irritability/anxiety/nervousness	33%	38%
Insomnia	30%	37%
Depression	20%	28%
Concentration impairment	10%	13%
Mood alteration	5%	6%
Resistance Mechanism Disorders		
Overall	12%	10%
Respiratory, Thoracic and Mediastinal		
Dyspnea	13%	14%
Cough	10%	7%
Dyspnea exertional	4%	7%
Skin and Subcutaneous Tissue		
Alopecia	28%	33%
Pruritus	19%	18%
Dermatitis	16%	13%
Dry skin	10%	13%
Rash	8%	5%
Sweating increased	6%	5%
Eczema	5%	4%
Visual Disorders		
Vision blurred	5%	2%

* Described as Study 4 in the Pegasys package insert.
† Severe hematologic abnormalities.

TABLE 12 *Recommended Dosing*

Body Weight	Rebetol Capsules
≤75 kg	2 × 200 mg capsules AM, 3 × 200 mg capsules PM daily po
>75 kg	3 × 200 mg capsules AM, 3 × 200 mg capsules PM daily po

Rebetol/Peg-Intron Combination Therapy

The recommended dose of Rebetol capsules is 800 mg/day in 2 divided doses: two capsules (400 mg) in the morning with food and two capsules (400 mg) with in the evening with food.

Dose Modification

See TABLE 13.

If severe adverse reactions or laboratory abnormalities develop during combination Rebetol/Intron A therapy the dose should be modified, or discontinued if appropriate, until the adverse reactions abate. If intolerance persists after dose adjustment, Rebetol/Intron A therapy should be discontinued.

Rebetol should not be used in patients with creatinine clearance <50 ml/min. (See WARNINGS and CLINICAL PHARMACOLOGY, Pharmacokinetics, Special Populations.)

Rebetol should be administered with caution to patients with pre-existing cardiac disease. Patients should be assessed before commencement of therapy and should be appropriately monitored during therapy. If there is any deterioration of cardiovascular status, therapy should be stopped. (See WARNINGS.)

For patients with a history of stable cardiovascular disease, a permanent dose reduction is required if the hemoglobin decreases by ≥2 g/dl during any 4 week period. In addition, for these cardiac history patients, if the hemoglobin remains <12 g/dl after 4 weeks on a reduced dose, the patient should discontinue combination Rebetol/Intron A therapy.

It is recommended that a patient whose hemoglobin level falls below 10 g/dl have his/her Rebetol dose reduced to 600 mg daily (1 × 200 mg capsule AM, 2 × 200 mg capsules PM). A patient whose hemoglobin level falls below 8.5 g/dl should be permanently discontinued from Rebetol therapy. (See WARNINGS.)

TABLE 13 *Guidelines for Dose Modifications and Discontinuation for Anemia*

	Dose Reduction Rebetol — 600 mg daily	Permanent Discontinuation of Rebetol Treatment
Hemoglobin		
No cardiac history	<10 g/dl	<8.5 g/dl
Cardiac history patients	≥2 g/dl decrease during any 4 week period during treatment	<12 g/dl after 4 weeks of dose reduction

COPEGUS

The recommended dose of Copegus tablets is provided in TABLE 14. The recommended duration of treatment for patients previously untreated with ribavirin and interferon is 24-48 weeks.

The daily dose of Copegus is 800-1200 mg administered orally in 2 divided doses. The dose should be individualized to the patient depending on baseline disease characteristics (*e.g.,* genotype), response to therapy, and tolerability of the regimen (see TABLE 14).

In the pivotal clinical trials, patients were instructed to take Copegus with food; therefore, patients are advised to take Copegus with food.

TABLE 14 *Pegasys and Copegus Dosing Recommendations*

Genotype	Pegasys Dose	Copegus Dose	Duration
Genotype 1, 4	180 μg	<75 kg = 1000 mg	48 weeks
		≥75 kg = 1200 mg	48 weeks
Genotype 2, 3	180 μg	800 mg	24 weeks

Genotypes non-1 showed no increased response to treatment beyond 24 weeks.
Data on genotypes 5 and 6 are insufficient for dosing recommendations.

Dose Modification

If severe adverse reactions or laboratory abnormalities develop during combination Copegus/Pegasys therapy, the dose should be modified or discontinued, if appropriate, until the adverse reactions abate. If intolerance persists after dose adjustment, Copegus/Pegasys therapy should be discontinued.

Copegus should be administered with caution to patients with pre-existing cardiac disease (see TABLE 15). Patients should be assessed before commencement of therapy and should be appropriately monitored during therapy. If there is any deterioration of cardiovascular status, therapy should be stopped (see WARNINGS).

TABLE 15 *Copegus Dosage Modification Guidelines*

Laboratory Values	Reduce Only Copegus Dose to 600 mg/day* if:	Discontinue Copegus if:
Hemoglobin in patients with no cardiac disease	<10 g/dl	<8.5 g/dl
Hemoglobin in patients with history of stable cardiac disease	≥2 g/dl decrease in hemoglobin during any 4 week period treatment	<12 g/dl despite 4 weeks at reduced dose

* One 200 mg tablet in the morning and two 200 mg tablets in the evening.

Once Copegus has been withheld due to either a laboratory abnormality or clinical manifestation, an attempt may be made to restart Copegus at 600 mg daily and further increase the dose to 800 mg daily depending upon the physician's judgment. However, it is not recommended that Copegus be increased to its original assigned dose (1000-1200 mg).

Renal Impairment

Copegus should not be used in patients with creatinine clearance <50 ml/min (see WARNINGS and CLINICAL PHARMACOLOGY, Special Populations).

HOW SUPPLIED

REBETOL

Rebetol 200 mg capsules are white, opaque capsules with "REBETOL", "200 mg", and the Schering Corporation logo imprinted on the capsule shell.

Storage: The bottle of Rebetol capsules should be stored at 25°C (77°F); excursions are permitted between 15 and 30°C (59 and 86°F).

COPEGUS

Copegus is available as tablets for oral administration. Each tablet contains 200 mg of ribavirin and is light pink to pink colored, flat, ovalshaped, film-coated, and engraved with "RIB 200" on one side and "ROCHE" on the other side.

Storage Conditions

Store the Copegus tablets bottle at 25°C (77°F); excursions are permitted between 15° and 30°C (59° and 86°F). Keep bottle tightly closed.

PRODUCT LISTING - EQUIVALENTS NOT AVAILABLE

Capsule - Oral - 200 mg

42's	$463.59	REBETOL, Schering-Plough	00085-1327-04
56's	$618.11	REBETOL, Schering-Plough	00085-1351-05
70's	$772.65	REBETOL, Schering-Plough	00085-1385-07
84's	$927.18	REBETOL, Schering-Plough	00085-1194-03

Powder For Reconstitution - Inhalation - 6 Gm

4's	$5499.38	VIRAZOLE, Icn Pharmaceuticals Inc	00187-0007-01
4's	$5499.38	VIRAZOLE, Icn Pharmaceuticals Inc	53095-0007-14

4's $5664.36 VIRAZOLE, Icn Pharmaceuticals Inc 00187-0007-14
Tablet - Oral - 200 mg
168's $1063.38 COPEGUS, Roche Laboratories 00004-0086-94

Rifabutin *(003135)*

Categories: Mycobacterium avium complex; FDA Approved 1992 Dec; Pregnancy Category B; Orphan Drugs
Drug Classes: Antimycobacterials
Brand Names: Ansamycin; **Mycobutin**
Foreign Brand Availability: Alfacid (Germany); Ansatidine (France)
Cost of Therapy: $232.68 (Mycobacterium Avium Complex; Mycobutin; 150 mg; 2 capsules/day; 30 day supply)

DESCRIPTION

Rifabutin is an antimycobacterial agent. It is a semisynthetic ansamycin antibiotic derived from rifamycin S. Mycobutin capsules for oral administration contain 150 mg of rifabutin per capsule, along with the inactive ingredients microcrystalline cellulose, magnesium stearate, red iron oxide, silica gel, sodium lauryl sulfate, titanium dioxide, and edible white ink.

The chemical name for rifabutin is 1',4-didehydro-1-deoxy-1,4-dihydro-5'- (2-methylpropyl)-1- oxorifamycin XIV (Chemical Abstracts Service, 9th Collective Index) or (9*S*, 12*E*, 14*S*, 15*R*, 16*S*, 17*R*, 18*R*, 19*R*, 20*S*, 21*S*, 22*E*, 24*Z*)-6,16, 18,20 -tetrahydroxy-1'-isobutyl-14-methoxy- 7, 9, 15, 17, 19, 21, 25-heptamethyl-spiro [9,4-(epoxypentadeca[1, 11, 13]trienimino)-2*H*-furo[2',3':7,8]naphth[1,2-*d*]imidazole-2,4'-piperidine]-5,10,26-(3*H*,9*H*)-trione-16-acetate. Rifabutin has a molecular formula of $C_{46}H_{62}N_4O_{11}$, a molecular weight of 847.02.

Rifabutin is a red-violet powder soluble in chloroform and methanol, sparingly soluble in ethanol, and very slightly soluble in water (0.19 mg/ml). Its log P value (the base 10 logarithm of the partition coefficient between n-octanol and water) is 3.2 (n-octanol/water).

CLINICAL PHARMACOLOGY

PHARMACOKINETICS

Following a single oral dose of 300 mg to 9 healthy adult volunteers, rifabutin was readily absorbed from the gastrointestinal tract with mean (±SD) peak plasma levels (C_{max}) of 375 (±267) ng/ml (range: 141-1033 ng/ml) attained in 3.3 (±0.9) hours (T_{max} range: 2-4 hours). Plasma concentrations post-C_{max} declined in an apparent biphasic manner. Kinetic dose-proportionality has been established over the 300-600 mg dose range in 9 healthy adult volunteers (crossover design) and in 16 early symptomatic human immunodeficiency virus (HIV)-positive patients over a 300-900 mg dose range. Rifabutin was slowly eliminated from plasma in 7 healthy adult volunteers, presumably because of *distribution-limited elimination*, with a mean terminal half-life of 45 (±17) hours (range: 16-69 hours). Although the systemic levels of rifabutin following multiple dosing decreased by 38%, its terminal half-life remained unchanged. Rifabutin, due to its high lipophilicity, demonstrates a high propensity for distribution and intracellular tissue uptake. Estimates of apparent steady-state distribution volume (9.3 ± 1.5 L/kg) in 5 HIV-positive patients, following IV dosing, exceed total body water by approximately fifteenfold. Substantially higher intracellular tissue levels than those seen in plasma have been observed in both rat and man. The lung to plasma concentration ratio, obtained at 12 hours, was found to be approximately 6.5 in 4 surgical patients administered an oral dose. Mean rifabutin steady-state trough levels ($C_{p,min}^{ss}$; 24 hour post-dose) ranged from 50-65 ng/ml in HIV-positive patients and in healthy adult volunteers. About 85% of the drug is bound in a concentration-independent manner to plasma proteins over a concentration range of 0.05-1 µg/ml. Binding does not appear to be influenced by renal or hepatic dysfunction.

Mean systemic clearance (CL_s/F) in healthy adult volunteers following a single oral dose was 0.69 (±0.32) L/h/kg (range: 0.46-1.34 L/h/kg). Renal and biliary clearance of unchanged drug each contribute approximately 5% to CL_s/F. About 30% of the dose is excreted in the feces. A mass-balance study in 3 healthy adult volunteers with ^{14}C-labeled drug has shown that 53% of the oral dose was excreted in the urine, primarily as metabolites. Of the five metabolites that have been identified, 25-O-desacetyl and 31-hydroxy are the most predominant, and show a plasma metabolite:parent area under the curve ratio of 0.10 and 0.07, respectively. The former has an activity equal to the parent drug and contributes up to 10% to the total antimicrobial activity.

Absolute bioavailability assessed in 5 HIV-positive patients, who received both oral and IV doses, averaged 20%. Total recovery of radioactivity in the urine indicates that at least 53% of the orally administered rifabutin dose is absorbed from the GI tract. The bioavailability of rifabutin from the capsule dosage form, relative to a solution, was 85% in 12 healthy adult volunteers. High-fat meals slow the rate without influencing the extent of absorption from the capsule dosage form. The overall pharmacokinetics of rifabutin are modified only slightly by alterations in hepatic function or age. Rifabutin steady-state kinetics in early symptomatic HIV-positive patients are similar to healthy volunteers. Compared to healthy volunteers, steady-state kinetics of rifabutin are more variable in elderly patients (>70 years) and in symptomatic HIV-positive patients. Somewhat reduced drug distribution and faster elimination of rifabutin in patients with compromised renal function may result in decreased drug concentrations. The clinical implications of this are unknown.

No rifabutin disposition information is currently available in children or adolescents under 18 years of age.

MICROBIOLOGY

Mechanism of Action

Rifabutin inhibits DNA-dependent RNA polymerase in susceptible strains of *Escherichia coli* and *Bacillus subtilis* but not in mammalian cells. In resistant strains of *E. coli*, rifabutin, like rifampin, did not inhibit this enzyme. It is not known whether rifabutin inhibits DNA-dependent RNA polymerase in *Mycobacterium avium* or in *M. intracellulare* which comprise *M. avium* complex (MAC).

Susceptibility Testing

In vitro susceptibility testing methods and diagnostic products used for determining minimum inhibitory concentration (MIC) values against *M. avium* complex (MAC) organisms have not been standardized. Breakpoints to determine whether clinical isolates of MAC and other mycobacterial species are susceptible or resistant to rifabutin have not been established.

In Vitro Studies

Rifabutin has demonstrated *in vitro* activity against *M. avium* complex (MAC) organisms isolated from both HIV-positive and HIV-negative people. While gene probe techniques may be used to identify these two organisms, many reported studies did not distinguish between these two species. The vast majority of isolates from MAC-infected, HIV-positive people are *M. avium*, whereas in HIV-negative people, about 40% of the MAC isolates are *M. intracellulare*.

Various *in vitro* methodologies employing broth or solid media, with and without polysorbate 80 (Tween 80), have been used to determine rifabutin MIC values for mycobacterial species. In general, MIC values determined in broth are several fold lower than that observed with methods employing solid media. Utilization of polysorbate 80 in these assays had been shown to further lower MIC values. However, MIC values were substantially higher for egg based compared to agar based solid media.

Rifabutin activity against 211 MAC isolates from HIV-positive people was evaluated *in vitro* utilizing a radiometric broth and an agar dilution method. Results showed that 78% and 82% of these isolates had MIC_{99} values of ≤0.25 µg/ml and ≤1.0 µg/ml, respectively, when evaluated by these two methods. Rifabutin was also shown to be active against phagocytized, *M. avium* complex in a mouse macrophage cell culture model.

Rifabutin has *in vitro* activity against many strains of*Mycobacterium tuberculosis*. In one study, utilizing the radiometric broth method, each of 17 and 20 rifampin-naive clinical isolates tested from the United States and Taiwan, respectively, were shown to be susceptible to rifabutin concentrations of ≤0.125 µg/ml.

Cross-resistance between rifampin and rifabutin is commonly observed with *M. tuberculosis* and *M. avium* complex isolates. Isolates of *M. tuberculosis* resistant to rifampin are likely to be resistant to rifabutin. Rifampicin and rifabutin MIC_{99} values against 523 isolates of *M. avium* complex were determined utilizing the agar dilution method.[1] (See TABLE 1.)

Rifabutin *in vitro* MIC_{99} values of ≤0.5 µg/ml, determined by the agar dilution method, for *M. kansasii*, *M. gordonae*, and *M. marinum* have been reported; however, the clinical significance of these results is unknown.

TABLE 1 *Susceptibility of M. avium Complex Strains to Rifampin and Rifabutin*

Susceptibility to Rifampin (µg/ml)	Number of Strains	% of Strains Susceptible/Resistant to Different Concentrations of Rifabutin (µg/ml)				
		Susceptible to 0.5	Resistant to 0.5 only	Resistant to 1.0	Resistant to 2.0
Susceptible to 1.0	30	100.0%	0.0%	0.0%	0.0%
Resistant to 1.0 only	163	88.3%	11.7%	0.0%	0.0%
Resistant to 5.0	105	38.0%	57.1%	2.9%	2.0%
Resistant to 10.0	225	20.0%	50.2%	19.6%	10.2%
TOTAL	523	49.5%	36.7%	9.0%	4.8%

INDICATIONS AND USAGE

Rifabutin is indicated for the prevention of disseminated *Mycobacterium avium* complex (MAC) disease in patients with advanced HIV infection.

NON-FDA APPROVED INDICATIONS

Rifabutin is also used an alternative to rifampin in the treatment of Mycobacterium tuberculosis in HIV infected persons who are taking certain antiretroviral agents concomitantly. In addition, rifabutin is recommended by the US Public Health Service/Infectious Diseases Society of America Prevention of Opportunistic Infections in Persons Infected with HIV Working Group as an alternative agent to rifampin for chemoprophylaxis of tuberculosis.

CONTRAINDICATIONS

Rifabutin is contraindicated in patients who have had clinically significant hypersensitivity to this drug, or to any other rifamycins.

WARNINGS

Rifabutin must not be administered for MAC prophylaxis to patients with active tuberculosis. Tuberculosis in HIV-positive patients is common and may present with atypical or extrapulmonary findings. Patients are likely to have a nonreactive purified protein derivative (PPD) despite active disease. In addition to chest X-ray and sputum culture, the following studies may be useful in the diagnosis of tuberculosis in the HIV-positive patient: blood culture, urine culture, or biopsy of a suspicious lymph node.

Patients who develop complaints consistent with active tuberculosis while on prophylaxis with rifabutin should be evaluated immediately, so that those with active disease may be given an effective combination regimen of anti-tuberculosis medications. Administration of single-agent rifabutin to patients with active tuberculosis is likely to lead to the development of tuberculosis that is resistant both to rifabutin and to rifampin.

There is no evidence that rifabutin is effective prophylaxis against *M. tuberculosis*. Patients requiring prophylaxis against both *M. tuberculosis* and *Mycobacterium avium* complex may be given isoniazid and rifabutin concurrently.

PRECAUTIONS

Because treatment with rifabutin may be associated with neutropenia, and more rarely thrombocytopenia, physicians should consider obtaining hematologic studies periodically in patients receiving rifabutin prophylaxis.

R

INFORMATION FOR THE PATIENT

Patients should be advised of the signs and symptoms of both MAC and tuberculosis, and should be instructed to consult their physicians if they develop new complaints consistent with either of these diseases. In addition, since rifabutin may rarely be associated with myositis and uveitis, patients should be advised to notify their physicians if they develop signs or symptoms suggesting either of these disorders.

Urine, feces, saliva, sputum, perspiration, tears, and skin may be colored brown-orange with rifabutin and some of its metabolites. Soft contact lenses may be permanently stained. Patients to be treated with rifabutin should be made aware of these possibilities.

CARCINOGENESIS, MUTAGENESIS, AND IMPAIRMENT OF FERTILITY

Long term carcinogenicity studies were conducted with rifabutin in mice and in rats. Rifabutin was not carcinogenic in mice at doses up to 180 mg/kg/day, or approximately 36 times the recommended human daily dose. Rifabutin was not carcinogenic in the rat at doses up to 60 mg/kg/day, about 12 times the recommended human dose.

Rifabutin was not mutagenic in the bacterial mutation assay (Ames Test) using both rifabutin-susceptible and resistant strains. Rifabutin was not mutagenic in *Schizosaccharomyces pombe* P_1 and was not genotoxic in V-79 Chinese hamster cells, human lymphocytes *in vitro*, or mouse bone marrow cells *in vivo*.

Fertility was impaired in male rats given 160 mg/kg (32 times the recommended human daily dose).

PREGNANCY CATEGORY B

Reproduction studies have been carried out in rats and rabbits given rifabutin using dose levels up to 200 mg/kg (40 times the recommended human daily dose). No teratogenicity was observed in either species. In rats, given 200 mg/kg/day, there was a decrease in fetal viability. In rats, at 40 mg/kg/day (8 times the recommended human daily dose), rifabutin caused an increase in fetal skeletal variants. In rabbits, at 80 mg/kg/day (16 times the recommended human daily dose), rifabutin caused maternotoxicity and increase in fetal skeletal anomalies. There are no adequate and well-controlled studies in pregnant women. Because animal reproduction studies are not always predictive of human response, rifabutin should be used in pregnant women only if the potential benefit justifies the potential risk to the fetus.

NURSING MOTHERS

It is not known whether rifabutin is excreted in human milk. Because many drugs are excreted in human milk and because of the potential for serious adverse reactions in nursing infants, a decision should be made whether to discontinue nursing or discontinue the drug, taking into account the importance of the drug to the mother.

PEDIATRIC USE

Safety and effectiveness of rifabutin for prophylaxis of MAC in children have not been established. Limited safety data are available from treatment use in 22 HIV-positive children with MAC who received rifabutin in combination with at least two other antimycobacterials for periods from 1-183 weeks. Mean doses (mg/kg) for these children were: 18.5 (range 15.0-25.0) for infants 1 year of age; 8.6 (range 4.4-18.8) for children 2-10 years of age; and 4.0 (range 2.8-5.4) for adolescents 14-16 years of age. There is no evidence that doses greater than 5 mg/kg daily are useful. Adverse experiences were similar to those observed in the adult population, and included leukopenia, neutropenia, and rash. Doses of rifabutin may be administered mixed with foods such as applesauce.

DRUG INTERACTIONS

In 10 healthy adult volunteers and 8 HIV-positive patients, steady-state plasma levels of zidovudine (ZDV), an antiretroviral agent which is metabolized mainly through glucuronidation, were decreased after repeated rifabutin dosing; the mean decrease in C_{max} and AUC was decreased by 48% and 32%, respectively. *In vitro* studies have demonstrated that rifabutin does not affect the inhibition of HIV by ZDV.

Steady-state kinetics in 12 HIV-positive patients show that both the rate and extent of systemic availability of didanosine (DDI), was not altered after repeated dosing of rifabutin.

Rifabutin has liver enzyme-inducing properties. The related drug rifampin is known to reduce the activity of a number of other drugs, including dapsone, narcotics (including methadone), anticoagulants, corticosteroids, cyclosporine, cardiac glycoside preparations, quinidine, oral contraceptives, oral hypoglycemic agents (sulfonylureas), and analgesics. Rifampin has also been reported to decrease the effects of concurrently administered ketoconazole, barbiturates, diazepam, verapamil, beta-adrenergic blockers, clofibrate, progestins, disopyramide, mexiletine, theophylline, chloramphenicol, and anticonvulsants. Because of the structural similarity of rifabutin and rifampin, rifabutin may be expected to have some effect on these drugs as well. However, unlike rifampin, rifabutin appears not to affect the acetylation of isoniazid. When rifabutin was compared with rifampin in a study with 8 healthy normal volunteers, rifabutin appeared to be a less potent enzyme inducer than rifampin. The significance of this finding for clinical drug interactions is not known. Dosage adjustment of drugs listed above may be necessary if they are given concurrently with rifabutin. Patients using oral contraceptives should consider changing to nonhormonal methods of birth control.

ADVERSE REACTIONS

Rifabutin was generally well tolerated in the controlled clinical trials. Discontinuation of therapy due to an adverse event was required in 16% of patients receiving rifabutin compared to 8% of patients receiving placebo in these trials. Primary reasons for discontinuation of rifabutin were rash (4% of treated patients), gastrointestinal intolerance (3%), and neutropenia (2%).

TABLE 2 enumerates adverse experiences that occurred at a frequency of 1% or greater, among the patients treated with rifabutin in studies 023 and 027.

CLINICAL ADVERSE EVENTS REPORTED IN <1% OF PATIENTS WHO RECEIVED RIFABUTIN

Considering data from the 023 and 027 pivotal trials, and from other clinical studies, rifabutin appears to be a likely cause of the following adverse events which occurred in less than 1% of treated patients: flu-like syndrome, hepatitis, hemolysis, arthralgia, myositis, chest pressure or pain with dyspnea, and skin discoloration.

TABLE 2 *Clinical Adverse Experiences Reported in ≥1% of Patients Treated With Rifabutin*

Adverse Event	Rifabutin (n=566)	Placebo (n=580)
Body as a Whole		
Abdominal pain	4%	3%
Asthenia	1%	1%
Chest pain	1%	1%
Fever	2%	1%
Headache	3%	5%
Pain	1%	2%
Digestive System		
Anorexia	2%	2%
Diarrhea	3%	3%
Dyspepsia	3%	1%
Eructation	3%	1%
Flatulence	2%	1%
Nausea	6%	5%
Nausea and vomiting	3%	2%
Vomiting	1%	1%
Musculoskeletal System		
Myalgia	2%	1%
Nervous System		
Insomnia	1%	1%
Skin and Appendages		
Rash	11%	8%
Special Senses		
Taste perversion	3%	1%
Urogenital System		
Discolored urine	30%	6%

The following adverse events have occurred in more than 1 patient receiving rifabutin, but an etiologic role has not been established: seizure, paresthesia, aphasia, confusion, and non-specific T wave changes on electrocardiogram.

When rifabutin was administered at doses from 1050-2400 mg/day, generalized arthralgia and uveitis were reported. These adverse experiences abated when rifabutin was discontinued.

TABLE 3 enumerates the changes in laboratory values that were considered as laboratory abnormalities in studies 023 and 027.

TABLE 3 *Percentage of Patients With Laboratory Abnormalities*

Laboratory Abnormalities	Rifabutin (n=566)	Placebo (n=580)
Chemistry		
Increased alkaline phosphatase*	<1%	3%
Increased SGOT†	7%	12%
Increased SGPT†	9%	11%
Hematology		
Anemia‡	6%	7%
Eosinophilia	1%	1%
Leukopenia§	17%	16%
Neutropenia¤	25%	20%
Thrombocytopenia¶	5%	4%

Includes Grade 3 or 4 Toxicities as Specified:
* All values >450 U/L.
† All values >150 U/L.
‡ All hemoglobin values < 8.0 g/dl.
§ All WBC values <1500/mm^3.
¤ All ANC values <750/mm^3.
¶ All platelet count values < 50,000/mm^3.

The incidence of neutropenia in patients treated with rifabutin was significantly greater than in patients treated with placebo (p=0.03). Although thrombocytopenia was not significantly more common among rifabutin treated patients in these trials, rifabutin has been clearly linked to thrombocytopenia in rare cases. One (1) patient in study 023 developed thrombotic thrombocytopenic purpura, which was attributed to rifabutin.

Uveitis is rare when rifabutin is used as a single agent at 300 mg/day for prophylaxis of MAC in HIV-infected persons, even with the concomitant use of fluconazole and/or macrolide antibiotics. However, if higher doses of rifabutin are administered in combination with these agents, the incidence of uveitis is higher.

Patients who developed uveitis had mild to severe symptoms that resolved after treatment with corticosteroids and/or mydriatic eye drops; in some severe cases, however, resolution of symptoms occurred after several weeks.

When uveitis occurs, temporary discontinuance of rifabutin and ophthalmologic evaluation are recommended. In most mild cases, rifabutin may be restarted; however, if signs or symptoms recur, use of rifabutin should be discontinued.[2]

DOSAGE AND ADMINISTRATION

It is recommended that 300 mg of rifabutin be administered once daily. For those patients with propensity to nausea, vomiting, or other gastrointestinal upset, administration of rifabutin at doses of 150 mg twice daily taken with food may be useful.

ANIMAL PHARMACOLOGY

Liver abnormalities, (increased bilirubin and liver weight), occurred in all species tested, in rats at doses 5 times, in monkeys at doses 8 times, and in mice at doses 6 times the recommended human daily dose. Testicular atrophy occurred in baboons at doses 4 times the recommended human dose, and in rats at doses 40 times the recommended human daily dose.

HOW SUPPLIED

Mycobutin is supplied as hard gelatin capsules having an opaque red-brown cap and body, imprinted with "MYCOBUTIN/PHARMACIA" in white ink, each containing 150 mg of rifabutin.

Storage: Keep tightly closed and dispense in a tight container. Store at controlled room temperature, 15-30°C (59-86°F).

PRODUCT LISTING - EQUIVALENTS NOT AVAILABLE

Capsule - Oral - 150 mg

50's	$198.86	MYCOBUTIN, Physicians Total Care	54868-2841-00
60's	$238.39	MYCOBUTIN, Physicians Total Care	54868-2841-01
100's	$387.80	MYCOBUTIN, Allscripts Pharmaceutical Company	54569-3878-00
100's	$395.95	MYCOBUTIN, Physicians Total Care	54868-2841-02
100's	$628.83	MYCOBUTIN, Pharmacia and Upjohn	00013-5301-17

Rifampin *(002188)*

Categories: Meningococcal carrier state; Tuberculosis; Pregnancy Category C; FDA Approved 1971 May; WHO Formulary; Orphan Drugs

Drug Classes: Antimycobacterials

Brand Names: **Rifadin**; Rifamate; Rifampicin; Rimactane

Foreign Brand Availability: Eremfat (Germany); Finamicina (Mexico); Kalrifam (Indonesia); Manorifcin (Thailand); Medifam (Philippines); Prolung (Indonesia); Ramfin (Malaysia; Thailand); Ramicin (Indonesia); Rifa (Germany); Rifacilin (India); Rifadine (Belgium; France); Rifagen (Spain); Rifaldin (Spain); Rifamax (Philippines); Rifapiam (Italy); Rifarad (Bahrain; Benin; Burkina-Faso; Cyprus; Egypt; Ethiopia; Gambia; Ghana; Guinea; Iran; Iraq; Ivory-Coast; Jordan; Kenya; Kuwait; Lebanon; Liberia; Libya; Malawi; Mali; Mauritania; Mauritius; Morocco; Niger; Nigeria; Oman; Qatar; Republic-of-Yemen; Saudi-Arabia; Senegal; Seychelles; Sierra-Leone; Sudan; Syria; Tanzania; Tunia; Uganda; United-Arab-Emirates; Zambia; Zimbabwe); Rifasynt (Hong-Kong); Rifcin (South-Africa); Rifodex (Korea); Rifoldin (Austria; Switzerland); Rimactan (Austria; Belgium; Bulgaria; Colombia; Denmark; Ecuador; France; Germany; Israel; Italy; Mexico; Netherlands; Norway; Peru; Spain; Sweden; Switzerland); Rimpacin (Bahrain; Benin; Burkina-Faso; Cyprus; Egypt; Ethiopia; Gambia; Ghana; Guinea; Iran; Iraq; Ivory-Coast; Jordan; Kenya; Kuwait; Lebanon; Liberia; Libya; Malawi; Mali; Mauritania; Mauritius; Morocco; Niger; Nigeria; Oman; Qatar; Republic-of-Yemen; Saudi-Arabia; Senegal; Seychelles; Sierra-Leone; Sudan; Syria; Tanzania; Tunia; Uganda; United-Arab-Emirates; Zambia; Zimbabwe); Rimpin (India); Rimycin (Australia); Ripin (Taiwan); Ripolin (Taiwan); Rofact (Canada)

Cost of Therapy: $134.32 (Tuberculosis; Rifadin; 300 mg; 2 capsules/day; 30 day supply)
$80.46 (Tuberculosis; Generic Capsules; 300 mg; 2 capsules/day; 30 day supply)

DESCRIPTION

Rifadin capsules for oral administration contain 150 mg or 300 mg rifampin per capsule. *The 150 mg and 300 mg capsules also contain, as inactive ingredients:* Corn starch, D&C red no. 28, FD&C blue no. 1, FD&C red no. 40, gelatin, magnesium stearate, and titanium dioxide.

Rifadin IV contains rifampin 600 mg, sodium formaldehyde sulfoxylate 10 mg, and sodium hydroxide to adjust pH.

Rifampin is a semisynthetic antibiotic derivative of rifamycin SV. Rifampin is a red-brown crystalline powder very slightly soluble in water at neutral pH, freely soluble in chloroform, soluble in ethyl acetate and in methanol. Its molecular weight is 822.95 and its chemical formula is $C_{43}H_{58}N_4O_{12}$. The chemical name for rifampin is either: 3-[[(4-Methyl-1-piperazinyl)imino]methyl]rifamycin or 5,6,9,17,19,21-hexahydroxy-23-methoxy-2,4,12,16,20,22-heptamethyl-8-[N-(4-methyl-1-piperazinyl)formimidoyl]-2,7-(epoxypentadeca [1,11,13]trienimino)naphtho[2,1-*b*]furan-1,11(2H)-dione 21-acetate.

CLINICAL PHARMACOLOGY

ORAL ADMINISTRATION

Rifampin is readily absorbed from the gastrointestinal tract. Peak serum concentrations in healthy adults and pediatric populations vary widely from individual to individual. Following a single 600 mg oral dose of rifampin in healthy adults, the peak serum concentration averages 7 μg/ml but may vary from 4-32 μg/ml. Absorption of rifampin is reduced by about 30% when the drug is ingested with food.

Rifampin is widely distributed throughout the body. It is present in effective concentrations in many organs and body fluids, including cerebrospinal fluid. Rifampin is about 80% protein bound. Most of the unbound fraction is not ionized and, therefore, diffuses freely into tissues.

In healthy adults, the mean biological half-life of rifampin in serum averages 3.35 ± 0.66 hours after a 600 mg oral dose, with increases up to 5.08 ± 2.45 hours reported after a 900 mg dose. With repeated administration, the half-life decreases and reaches average values of approximately 2-3 hours. The half-life does not differ in patients with renal failure at doses not exceeding 600 mg daily, and consequently, no dosage adjustment is required. Following a single 900 mg oral dose of rifampin in patients with varying degrees of renal insufficiency, the mean half-life increased from 3.6 hours in healthy adults to 5.0, 7.3, and 11.0 hours in patients with glomerular filtration rates of 30-50 ml/min, less than 30 ml/min, and in anuric patients, respectively. Refer to WARNINGS for information regarding patients with hepatic insufficiency.

Rifampin is rapidly eliminated in the bile, and an enterohepatic circulation ensues. During this process, rifampin undergoes progressive deacetylation so that nearly all the drug in the bile is in this form in about 6 hours. This metabolite is microbiologically active. Intestinal reabsorption is reduced by deacetylation, and elimination is facilitated. Up to 30% of a dose is excreted in the urine, with about half of this being unchanged drug.

INTRAVENOUS ADMINISTRATION

After intravenous administration of a 300 or 600 mg dose of rifampin infused over 30 minutes to healthy male volunteers (n=12), mean peak plasma concentrations were 9.0 ± 3.0 and 17.5 ± 5.0 μg/ml, respectively. Total body clearances after the 300 and 600 mg IV doses were 0.19 ± 0.06 and 0.14 ± 0.03 L/hr/kg, respectively. Volumes of distribution at steady state were 0.66 ± 0.14 and 0.64 ± 0.11 L/kg for the 300 and 600 mg IV doses, respectively. After intravenous administration of 300 or 600 mg doses, rifampin plasma concentrations in these volunteers remained detectable for 8 and 12 hours, respectively (see TABLE 1).

TABLE 1 *Plasma Concentrations (mean ± standard deviation, μg/ml)*

Rifampin Dosage IV	30 min	1 hr	2 hr	4 hr	8 hr	12 hr
300 mg	8.9 ± 2.9	4.9 ± 1.3	4.0 ± 1.3	2.5 ± 1.0	1.1 ± 0.6	<0.4
600 mg	17.4 ± 5.1	11.7 ± 2.8	9.4 ± 2.3	6.4 ± 1.7	3.5 ± 1.4	1.2 ± 0.6

Plasma concentrations after the 600 mg dose, which were disproportionately higher (up to 30% greater than expected) than those found after the 300 mg dose, indicated that the elimination of larger doses was not as rapid.

After repeated once-a-day infusions (3 hour duration) of 600 mg in patients (n=5) for 7 days, concentrations of IV rifampin decreased from 5.81 ± 3.38 μg/ml 8 hours after the infusion on day 1 to 2.6 ± 1.88 μg/ml 8 hours after the infusion on day 7.

Rifampin is widely distributed throughout the body. It is present in effective concentrations in many organs and body fluids, including cerebrospinal fluid. Rifampin is about 80% protein bound. Most of the unbound fraction is not ionized and therefore diffuses freely into tissues.

Rifampin is rapidly eliminated in the bile and undergoes progressive enterohepatic circulation and deacetylation to the primary metabolite, 25-desacetyl-rifampin. This metabolite is microbiologically active. Less than 30% of the dose is excreted in the urine as rifampin or metabolites. Serum concentrations do not differ in patients with renal failure at a studied dose of 300 mg and consequently, no dosage adjustment is required.

PEDIATRICS

Oral Administration

In one study, pediatric patients 6-58 months old were given rifampin suspended in simple syrup or as dry powder mixed with applesauce at a dose of 10 mg/kg body weight. Peak serum concentrations of 10.7 ± 3.7 and 11.5 ± 5.1 μg/ml were obtained 1 hour after preprandial ingestion of the drug suspension and the applesauce mixture, respectively. After the administration of either preparation, the T½ of rifampin averaged 2.9 hours. It should be noted that in other studies in pediatric populations, at doses of 10 mg/kg body weight, mean peak serum concentrations of 3.5-15 μg/ml have been reported.

Intravenous Administration

In pediatric patients 0.25 to 12.8 years old (n=12), the mean peak serum concentration of rifampin at the end of a 30 minute infusion of approximately 300 mg/m² was 25.9 ± 1.3 μg/ml; individual peak concentrations 1-4 days after initiation of therapy ranged from 11.7-41.5 μg/ml; individual peak concentrations 5-14 days after initiation of therapy were 13.6-37.4 μg/ml. The individual serum half-life of rifampin changed from 1.04-3.81 hours early in therapy to 1.17-3.19 hours 5-14 days after therapy was initiated.

MICROBIOLOGY

Rifampin inhibits DNA-dependent RNA polymerase activity in susceptible cells. Specifically, it interacts with bacterial RNA polymerase but does not inhibit the mammalian enzyme. Rifampin at therapeutic levels has demonstrated bactericidal activity against both intracellular and extracellular *Mycobacterium tuberculosis* organisms.

Organisms resistant to rifampin are likely to be resistant to other rifamycins.

Rifampin has bactericidal activity against slow and intermittently growing *M tuberculosis* organisms. It also has significant activity against *Neisseria meningitidis* isolates (see INDICATIONS AND USAGE).

In the treatment of both tuberculosis and the meningococcal carrier state (see INDICATIONS AND USAGE), the small number of resistant cells present within large populations of susceptible cells can rapidly become predominant. In addition, resistance to rifampin has been determined to occur as single-step mutations of the DNA-dependent RNA polymerase. Since resistance can emerge rapidly, appropriate susceptibility tests should be performed in the event of persistent positive cultures.

Rifampin has been shown to be active against most strains of the following microorganisms, both *in vitro* and in clinical infections as described in INDICATIONS AND USAGE.

Aerobic Gram-Negative Microorganisms: *Neisseria meningitidis.*

"Other" Microorganisms: *Mycobacterium tuberculosis.*

The following *in vitro* data are available, but their clinical significance is unknown.

Rifampin exhibits *in vitro* activity against most strains of the following microorganisms; however, the safety and effectiveness of rifampin in treating clinical infections due to these microorganisms have not been established in adequate and well-controlled trials.

Aerobic Gram-Positive Microorganisms: *Staphylococcus aureus* (including Methicillin-Resistant *S. aureus*/MRSA), *Staphylococcus epidermidis.*

Aerobic Gram-Negative Microorganisms: *Haemophilus influenzae.*

"Other" Microorganisms: *Mycobacterium leprae.*

B-lactamase production should have no effect on rifampin activity.

SUSCEPTIBILITY TESTING

Prior to initiation of therapy, appropriate specimens should be collected for identification of the infecting organism and *in vitro* susceptibility tests.

In vitro Testing For Mycobacterium tuberculosis Isolates

Two standardized *in vitro* susceptibility methods are available for testing rifampin against *M tuberculosis* organisms. The agar proportion method (CDC or NCCLS[1] M24-P) utilizes Middlebrook 7H10 medium impregnated with rifampin at a final concentration of 1.0 μg/ml to determine drug resistance. After three weeks of incubation MIC_{99} values are calculated by comparing the quantity of organisms growing in the medium containing drug to the control cultures. Mycobacterial growth in the presence of drug, of at least 1% of the growth in the control culture, indicates resistance.

The radiometric broth method employs the BACTEC 460 machine to compare the growth index from untreated control cultures to cultures grown in the presence of 2.0 μg/ml of rifampin. Strict adherence to the manufacturer's instructions for sample processing and data interpretation is required for this assay.

R

Susceptibility test results obtained by the two different methods can only be compared if the appropriate rifampin concentration is used for each test method as indicated above. Both procedures require the use of *M tuberculosis* H37Rv ATCC 27294 as a control organism.

The clinical relevance of *in vitro* susceptibility test results for mycobacterial species other than *M tuberculosis* using either the radiometric or the proportion method has not been determined.

In vitro Testing For Neisseria meningitidis Isolates

Dilution Techniques

Quantitative methods that are used to determine minimum inhibitory concentrations provide reproducible estimates of the susceptibility of bacteria to antimicrobial compounds. One such standardized procedure uses a standardized dilution method[2,4] (broth, agar, or microdilution) or equivalent with rifampin powder. The MIC values obtained should be interpreted according to the criteria for *Neisseria meningitidis* as shown in TABLE 2.

TABLE 2

MIC (µg/ml)	Interpretation
≤1	(S) Susceptible
2	(I) Intermediate
≥4	(R) Resistant

A report of "susceptible" indicates that the pathogen is likely to be inhibited by usually achievable concentrations of the antimicrobial compound in the blood. A report of "intermediate" indicates that the result should be considered equivocal, and if the microorganism is not fully susceptible to alternative, clinically feasible drugs, the test should be repeated. This category implies possible clinical applicability in body sites where the drug is physiologically concentrated or in situations where the maximum acceptable dose of drug can be used. This category also provides a buffer zone that prevents small uncontrolled technical factors from causing major discrepancies in interpretation. A report of "resistant" indicates that usually achievable concentrations of the antimicrobial compound in the blood are unlikely to be inhibitory and that other therapy should be selected.

Measurement of MIC or minimum bactericidal concentrations (MBC) and achieved antimicrobial compound concentrations may be appropriate to guide therapy in some infections.

Standardized susceptibility test procedures require the use of laboratory control microorganisms. The use of these microorganisms does not imply clinical efficacy (see INDICATIONS AND USAGE); they are used to control the technical aspects of the laboratory procedures. Standard rifampin powder should give the MIC values as shown in TABLE 3.

Diffusion Techniques

TABLE 3

Microorganism		MIC (µg/ml)
Staphylococcus aureus	ATCC 29213	0.008-0.06
Enterococcus faecalis	ATCC 29212	1-4
Escherichia coli	ATCC 25922	8-32
Pseudomonas aeruginosa	ATCC 27853	32-64
Haemophilus influenzae	ATCC 49247	0.25-1

Quantitative methods that require measurement of zone diameters provide reproducible estimates of the susceptibility of bacteria to antimicrobial compounds. One such standardized procedure[3,4] that has been recommended for use with disks to test the susceptibility of microorganisms to rifampin uses the 5 µg rifampin disk. Interpretation involves correlation of the diameter obtained in the disk test with the MIC for rifampin.

Reports from the laboratory providing results of the standard single-disk susceptibility test with a 5 µg rifampin disk should be interpreted according to the criteria for *Neisseria meningitidis* as shown in TABLE 4.

TABLE 4

Zone Diameter (mm)	Interpretation
≥20	(S) Susceptible
17-19	(I) Intermediate
≤16	(R) Resistant

Interpretation should be as stated above for results using dilution techniques.

As with standard dilution techniques, diffusion methods require the use of laboratory control microorganisms. The use of these microorganisms does not imply clinical efficacy (see INDICATIONS AND USAGE); they are used to control the technical aspects of the laboratory procedures. The 5 µg rifampin disk should provide the zone diameters in these quality control strains as shown in TABLE 5.

TABLE 5

Microorganism		Zone Diameter (mm)
S. aureus	ATCC 25923	26-34
E. coli	ATCC 25922	8-10
H. influenzae	ATCC 49247	22-30

INDICATIONS AND USAGE

In the treatment of both tuberculosis and the meningococcal carrier state, the small number of resistant cells present within large populations of susceptible cells can rapidly become the predominant type. Bacteriologic cultures should be obtained before the start of therapy to confirm the susceptibility of the organism to rifampin and they should be repeated throughout therapy to monitor the response to treatment. Since resistance can emerge rapidly, susceptibility tests should be performed in the event of persistent positive cultures during the course of treatment. If test results show resistance to rifampin and the patient is not responding to therapy, the drug regimen should be modified.

TUBERCULOSIS

Rifampin is indicated in the treatment of all forms of tuberculosis.

A three-drug regimen consisting of rifampin, isoniazid, and pyrazinamide (*e.g.*, Rifater) is recommended in the initial phase of short-course therapy which is usually continued for 2 months. The Advisory Council for the Elimination of Tuberculosis, the American Thoracic Society, and Centers for Disease Control and Prevention recommend that either streptomycin or ethambutol be added as a fourth drug in a regimen containing isoniazid (INH), rifampin, and pyrazinamide for initial treatment of tuberculosis unless the likelihood of INH resistance is very low. The need for a fourth drug should be reassessed when the results of susceptibility testing are known. If community rates of INH resistance are currently less than 4%, an initial treatment regimen with less than four drugs may be considered.

Following the initial phase, treatment should be continued with rifampin and isoniazid (*e.g.*, Rifamate) for at least 4 months. Treatment should be continued for longer if the patient is still sputum or culture positive, if resistant organisms are present, or if the patient is HIV positive.

Rifampin IV is indicated for the initial treatment and retreatment of tuberculosis when the drug cannot be taken by mouth.

MENINGOCOCCAL CARRIERS

Rifampin is indicated for the treatment of asymptomatic carriers of *Neisseria meningitidis* to eliminate meningococci from the nasopharynx. **Rifampin is not indicated for the treatment of meningococcal infection because of the possibility of the rapid emergence of resistant organisms.** (See WARNINGS.)

Rifampin should not be used indiscriminately, and therefore, diagnostic laboratory procedures, including serotyping and susceptibility testing, should be performed for establishment of the carrier state and the correct treatment. So that the usefulness of rifampin in the treatment of asymptomatic meningococcal carriers is preserved, the drug should be used only when the risk of meningococcal disease is high.

CONTRAINDICATIONS

Rifampin is contraindicated in patients with a history of hypersensitivity to any of the rifamycins. (See WARNINGS.)

WARNINGS

Rifampin has been shown to produce liver dysfunction. Fatalities associated with jaundice have occurred in patients with liver disease and in patients taking rifampin with other hepatotoxic agents. Patients with impaired liver function should be given rifampin only in cases of necessity and then with caution and under strict medical supervision. In these patients, careful monitoring of liver function, especially SGPT/ALT and SGOT/AST should be carried out prior to therapy and then every 2-4 weeks during therapy. If signs of hepatocellular damage occur, rifampin should be withdrawn.

In some cases, hyperbilirubinemia resulting from competition between rifampin and bilirubin for excretory pathways of the liver at the cell level can occur in the early days of treatment. An isolated report showing a moderate rise in bilirubin and/or transaminase level is not in itself an indication for interrupting treatment; rather, the decision should be made after repeating the tests, noting trends in the levels, and considering them in conjunction with the patient's clinical condition.

Rifampin has enzyme-inducing properties, including induction of delta amino levulinic acid synthetase. Isolated reports have associated porphyria exacerbation with rifampin administration.

The possibility of rapid emergence of resistant meningococci restricts the use of rifampin to short-term treatment of the asymptomatic carrier state. **Rifampin is not to be used for the treatment of meningococcal disease.**

PRECAUTIONS

GENERAL

For the treatment of tuberculosis, rifampin is usually administered on a daily basis. Doses of rifampin greater than 600 mg given once or twice weekly have resulted in a higher incidence of adverse reactions, including the "flu syndrome" (fever, chills and malaise), hematopoietic reactions (leukopenia, thrombocytopenia, or acute hemolytic anemia), cutaneous, gastrointestinal, and hepatic reactions, shortness of breath, shock, anaphylaxis, and renal failure. Recent studies indicate that regimens using twice-weekly doses of rifampin 600 mg plus isoniazid 15 mg/kg are much better tolerated.

Intermittent therapy may be used if the patient cannot (or will not) self-administer drugs on a daily basis. Patients on intermittent therapy should be closely monitored for compliance and cautioned against intentional or accidental interruption of prescribed therapy, because of the increased risk of serious adverse reactions.

Rifampin has enzyme induction properties that can enhance the metabolism of endogenous substrates including adrenal hormones, thyroid hormones, and vitamin D. Rifampin and isoniazid have been reported to alter vitamin D metabolism. In some cases, reduced levels of circulating 25-hydroxy vitamin D and 1,25-dihydroxy vitamin D have been accompanied by reduced serum calcium and phosphate, and elevated parathyroid hormone.

Rifampin IV

For intravenous infusion only. Must not be administered by intramuscular or subcutaneous route. Avoid extravasation during injection: local irritation and inflammation due to extravascular infiltration of the infusion have been observed. If these occur, the infusion should be discontinued and restarted at another site.

INFORMATION FOR THE PATIENT

The patient should be told that rifampin may produce a reddish coloration of the urine, sweat, sputum, and tears, and the patient should be forewarned of this. Soft contact lenses may be permanently stained.

R

The patient should be advised that the reliability of oral or other systemic hormonal contraceptives may be affected; consideration should be given to using alternative contraceptive measures.

Patients should be instructed to take rifampin either 1 hour before or 2 hours after a meal with a full glass of water.

Patients should be instructed to notify their physicians promptly if they experience any of the following: fever, loss of appetite, malaise, nausea and vomiting, darkened urine, yellowish discoloration of the skin and eyes, and pain or swelling of the joints.

Compliance with the full course of therapy must be emphasized, and the importance of not missing any doses must be stressed.

LABORATORY TESTS

A complete blood count (CBC) and liver function tests should be obtained prior to instituting therapy and periodically throughout the course of therapy. Because of a possible transient rise in transaminase and bilrubin values, blood for baseline clinical chemistries should be obtained before rifampin dosing.

DRUG/LABORATORY TEST INTERACTIONS

Therapeutic levels of rifampin have been shown to inhibit standard microbiological assays for serum folate and vitamin B_{12}. Thus, alternate assay methods should be considered. Transient abnormalities in liver function tests (*e.g.,* elevation in serum bilirubin, alkaline phosphatase, and serum transaminases) and reduced biliary excretion of contrast media used for visualization of the gallbladder have also been observed. Therefore, these tests should be performed before the morning dose of rifampin.

CARCINOGENESIS, MUTAGENESIS, AND IMPAIRMENT OF FERTILITY

There are no known human data on long-term potential for carcinogenicity, mutagenicity, or impairment of fertility. A few cases of accelerated growth of lung carcinoma have been reported in man, but a causal relationship with the drug has not been established. An increase in the incidence of hepatomas in female mice (of a strain known to be particularly susceptible to the spontaneous development of hepatomas) was observed when rifampin was administered in doses 2-10 times the average daily human dose for 60 weeks, followed by an observation period of 46 weeks. No evidence of carcinogenicity was found in male mice of the same strain, mice of a different strain, or rats under similar experimental conditions.

Rifampin has been reported to possess immunosuppressive potential in rabbits, mice, rats, guinea pigs, human lymphocytes *in vitro*, and humans. Antitumor activity *in vitro* has also been shown with rifampin.

There was no evidence of mutagenicity in bacteria, *Drosophila melanogaster*, or mice. An increase in chromotid breaks was noted when whole blood cell cultures were treated with rifampin. Increased frequency of chromosomal aberrations was observed *in vitro* in lymphocytes obtained from patients treated with combinations of rifampin, isoniazid, and pyrazinamide and combinations of streptomycin, rifampin, isoniazid, and pyrazinamide.

PREGNANCY, TERATOGENIC EFFECTS, PREGNANCY CATEGORY C

Rifampin has been shown to be teratogenic in rodents given oral doses of rifampin 15-25 times the human dose. Although rifampin has been reported to cross the placental barrier and appear in cord blood, the effect of rifampin, alone or in combination with other antituberculosis drugs, on the human fetus is not known. Neonates of rifampin-treated mothers should be carefully observed for any evidence of adverse effects. Isolated cases of fetal malformations have been reported; however, there are no adequate and well-controlled studies in pregnant women. Rifampin should be used during pregnancy only if the potential benefit justifies the potential risk to the fetus. Rifampin in oral doses of 150-250 mg/kg produced teratogenic effects in mice and rats. Malformations were primarily cleft palate in the mouse and spina bifida in the rat. The incidence of these anomalies was dose-dependent. When rifampin was given to pregnant rabbits in doses up to 20 times the usual daily human dose, imperfect osteogenesis and embryotoxicity were reported.

PREGNANCY, NONTERATOGENIC EFFECTS

When administered during the last few weeks of pregnancy, rifampin can cause post-natal hemorrhages in the mother and infant for which treatment with vitamin K may be indicated.

NURSING MOTHERS

Because of the potential for tumorigenicity shown for rifampin in animal studies, a decision should be made whether to discontinue nursing or discontinue the drug, taking into account the importance of the drug to the mother.

PEDIATRIC USE

See CLINICAL PHARMACOLOGY, Pediatrics; see also DOSAGE AND ADMINISTRATION.

DRUG INTERACTIONS

ENZYME INDUCTION

Rifampin is known to induce certain cytochrome P-450 enzymes. Administration of rifampin with drugs that undergo biotransformation through these metabolic pathways may accelerate elimination of coadministered drugs. To maintain optimum therapeutic blood levels, dosages of drugs metabolized by these enzymes may require adjustment when starting or stopping concomitantly administered rifampin.

Rifampin has been reported to accelerate the metabolism of the following drugs: Anticonvulsants (*e.g.,* phenytoin), antiarrhythmics (*e.g.,* disopyramide, mexiletine, quinidine, tocainide), oral anticoagulants, antifungals (*e.g.,* fluconazole, itraconazole, ketoconazole), barbiturates, beta-blockers, calcium channel blockers (*e.g.,* diltiazem, nifedipine, verapamil), chloramphenicol, corticosteroids, cyclosporine, cardiac glycoside preparations, clofibrate, oral or other systemic hormonal contraceptives, dapsone, diazepam, doxycycline, fluoroquinolones (*e.g.,* ciprofloxacin), haloperidol, oral hypoglycemic agents (sulfonylureas), levothyroxine, methadone, narcotic analgesics, nortriptyline, progestins, tacrolimus, theophylline and zidovudine. It may be necessary to adjust the dosages of these drugs if they are given concurrently with rifampin.

Patients using oral or other systemic hormonal contraceptives should be advised to change to nonhormonal methods of birth control during rifampin therapy.

Rifampin has been observed to increase the requirements for anticoagulant drugs of the coumarin type. In patients receiving anticoagulants and rifampin concurrently, it is recommended that the prothrombin time be performed daily or as frequently as necessary to establish and maintain the required dose of anticoagulant.

Diabetes may become more difficult to control.

Concurrent use of ketoconazole and rifampin has resulted in decreased serum concentrations of both drugs. Concurrent use of rifampin and enalapril has resulted in decreased concentrations of enalaprilat, the active metabolite of enalapril. Dosage adjustments should be made if indicated by the patient's clinical condition.

OTHER INTERACTIONS

Concomitant antacid administration may reduce the absorption of rifampin. Daily doses of rifampin should be given at least 1 hour before the ingestion of antacids.

Probenecid and cotrimoxazole have been reported to increase the blood level of rifampin.

When rifampin is given concomitantly with either halothane or isoniazid, the potential for hepatotoxicity is increased. The concomitant use of rifampin and halothane should be avoided. Patients receiving both rifampin and isoniazid should be monitored close for hepatotoxicity.

Plasma concentrations of sulfapyridine may be reduced following the concomitant administration of sulfasalazine and rifampin. This finding may be the result of alteration in the colonic bacteria responsible for the reduction of sulfasalazine to sulfapyridine and mesalamine.

ADVERSE REACTIONS

Gastrointestinal: Heartburn, epigastric distress, anorexia, nausea, vomiting, jaundice, flatulence, cramps, and diarrhea have been noted in some patients. Although *Clostridium difficile* has been shown *in vitro* to be sensitive to rifampin, pseudomembranous colitis has been reported with the use of rifampin (and other broad spectrum antibiotics). Therefore, it is important to consider this diagnosis in patients who develop diarrhea in association with antibiotic use. Rarely, hepatitis or a shock-like syndrome with hepatic involvement and abnormal liver function tests has been reported.

Hematologic: Thrombocytopenia has occurred primarily with high dose intermittent therapy, but has also been noted after resumption of interrupted treatment. It rarely occurs during well supervised daily therapy. This effect is reversible if the drug is discontinued as soon as purpura occurs. Cerebral hemorrhage and fatalities have been reported when rifampin administration has been continued or resumed after the appearance of purpura.

Rare reports of disseminated intravascular coagulation have been observed.

Transient leukopenia, hemolytic anemia, and decreased hemoglobin have been observed.

Central Nervous System: Headache, fever, drowsiness, fatigue, ataxia, dizziness, inability to concentrate, mental confusion, behavioral changes, muscular weakness, pains in extremities, and generalized numbness have been observed.

Rare reports of myopathy have also been observed.

Ocular: Visual disturbances have been observed.

Endocrine: Menstrual disturbances have been observed.

Rare reports of adrenal insufficiency in patients with compromised adrenal function have been observed.

Renal: Elevations in BUN and serum uric acid have been reported. Rarely, hemolysis, hemoglobinuria, hematuria, interstitial nephritis, acute tubular necrosis, renal insufficiency, and acute renal failure have been noted. These are generally considered to be hypersensitivity reactions. They usually occur during intermittent therapy or when treatment is resumed following intentional or accidental interruption of a daily dosage regimen, and are reversible when rifampin is discontinued and appropriate therapy instituted.

Dermatologic: Cutaneous reactions are mild and self-limiting and do not appear to be hypersensitivity reactions. Typically, they consist of flushing and itching with or without a rash. More serious cutaneous reactions which may be due to hypersensitivity occur but are uncommon.

Hypersensitivity Reactions: Occasionally, pruritus, urticaria, rash, pemphigoid reaction, erythema multiforme including Stevens-Johnson Syndrome, toxic epidermal necrolysis, vasculitis, eosinophilia, sore mouth, sore tongue, and conjunctivitis have been observed.

Anaphylaxis has been reported rarely.

Miscellaneous: Edema of the face and extremities has been reported. Other reactions reported to have occurred with intermittent dosage regimens include "flu syndrome" (such as episodes of fever, chills, headache, dizziness, and bone pain), shortness of breath, wheezing, decrease in blood pressure and shock. The "flu syndrome" may also appear if rifampin is taken irregularly by the patient or if daily administration is resumed after a drug free interval.

DOSAGE AND ADMINISTRATION

Rifampin can be administered by the oral route or by IV infusion (see INDICATIONS AND USAGE).

See CLINICAL PHARMACOLOGY for dosing information in patients with renal failure.

TUBERCULOSIS

Adults: 600 mg in a single daily administration, oral or IV.

Pediatric Patients: 10-20 mg/kg, not to exceed 600 mg/day, oral or IV.

It is recommended that oral rifampin be administered once daily, either 1 hour before or 2 hours after a meal with a full glass of water.

Rifampin is indicated in the treatment of all forms of tuberculosis. A three-drug regimen consisting of rifampin, isoniazid, and pyrazinamide (*e.g.,* Rifater) is recommended in the

R

initial phase of short-course therapy which is usually continued for 2 months. The Advisory Council for the Elimination of Tuberculosis, the American Thoracic Society, and the Centers for Disease Control and Prevention recommend that either streptomycin or ethambutol be added as a fourth drug in a regimen containing isoniazid (INH), rifampin and pyrazinamide for initial treatment of tuberculosis unless the likelihood of INH resistance is very low. The need for a fourth drug should be reassessed when the results of susceptibility testing are known. If community rates of INH resistance are currently less than 4%, an initial treatment regimen with less than four drugs may be considered.

Following the initial phase, treatment should be continued with rifampin and isoniazid (*e.g.,* Rifamate) for at least 4 months. Treatment should be continued for longer if the patient is still sputum or culture positive, if resistant organisms are present, or if the patient is HIV positive.

PREPARATION OF SOLUTION FOR IV INFUSION

Reconstitute the lyophilized powder by transferring 10 ml of sterile water for injection to a vial containing 600 mg of rifampin for injection. Swirl vial gently to completely dissolve the antibiotic. The reconstituted solution contains 60 mg rifampin per ml and is stable at room temperature for 24 hours. Prior to administration, withdraw from the reconstituted solution a volume equivalent to the amount of rifampin calculated to be administered and add to 500 ml of infusion medium. Mix well and infuse at a rate allowing for complete infusion within 3 hours. Alternatively, the amount of rifampin calculated to be administered may be added to 100 ml of infusion medium and infused in 30 minutes.

Dilutions in dextrose 5% for injection (D5W) are stable at room temperature for up to 4 hours and should be prepared and used within this time. Precipitation of rifampin from the infusion solution may occur beyond this time. Dilutions in normal saline are stable at room temperature for up to 24 hours and should be prepared and used within this time. Other infusion solutions are not recommended.

MENINGOCOCCAL CARRIERS

Adults: For adults, it is recommended that 600 mg rifampin be administered twice daily for two days.

Pediatric Patients: Pediatric patients 1 month of age or older: 10 mg/kg (not to exceed 600 mg per dose) every 12 hours for 2 days.

Pediatric Patients Under 1 Month of Age: 5 mg/kg every 12 hours for 2 days.

PREPARATION OF EXTEMPORANEOUS ORAL SUSPENSION

For pediatric and adult patients in whom capsule swallowing is difficult or where lower doses are needed, a liquid suspension may be prepared as follows:

Rifampin 1% w/v suspension (10 mg/ml) can be compounded using one of three syrups: Simple syrup, Syrpalta syrup, or raspberry syrup.

1. Empty the contents of four rifampin 300 mg capsules or eight rifampin 150 mg capsules onto a piece of weighing paper.
2. If necessary, gently crush the capsule contents with a spatula to produce a fine powder.
3. Transfer the rifampin powder blend to a 4-ounce amber glass or plastic (high density polyethylene [HDPE], polypropylene, or polycarbonate) prescription bottle.
4. Rinse the paper and spatula with 20 ml of one of the above-mentioned syrups, and add the rinse to the bottle. Shake vigorously.
5. Add 100 ml of syrup to the bottle and shake vigorously.

This compounding procedure results in a 1% w/v suspension containing 10 mg rifampin/ml. Stability studies indicate that the suspension is stable when stored at room temperature (25 ± 3°C) or in a refrigerator (2-8°C) for 4 weeks. This extemporaneously prepared suspension must be shaken well prior to administration.

HOW SUPPLIED

TABLETS

Rifadin 150 mg Capsules: Maroon and scarlet capsules imprinted "RIFADIN 150."

Rifadin 300 mg Capsules: Maroon and scarlet capsules imprinted "RIFADIN 300."

Storage: Keep tightly closed. Store in a dry place. Avoid excessive heat.

R

IV

Storage: Avoid excessive heat (temperatures above 40°C or 104°F). Protect from light.

PRODUCT LISTING - RATED THERAPEUTICALLY EQUIVALENT

Capsule - Oral - 150 mg

10's	$18.99	RIFADIN, Pharma Pac	52959-0461-10
30's	$40.23	GENERIC, Eon Labs Manufacturing Inc	00185-0801-30
30's	$47.38	RIFADIN, Aventis Pharmaceuticals	00068-0510-30

Capsule - Oral - 300 mg

8's	$21.18	GENERIC, Pd-Rx Pharmaceuticals	55289-0386-08
25's	$49.50	GENERIC, Udl Laboratories Inc	51079-0890-19
30's	$48.85	GENERIC, Heartland Healthcare Services	61392-0146-30
30's	$48.85	GENERIC, Heartland Healthcare Services	61392-0146-39
30's	$57.02	GENERIC, Eon Labs Manufacturing Inc	00185-0799-30
30's	$67.16	RIFADIN, Aventis Pharmaceuticals	00068-0508-30
30's	$75.13	RIFADIN, Physicians Total Care	54868-2901-02
31's	$50.48	GENERIC, Heartland Healthcare Services	61392-0146-31
32's	$52.11	GENERIC, Heartland Healthcare Services	61392-0146-32
45's	$73.27	GENERIC, Heartland Healthcare Services	61392-0146-45
60's	$97.70	GENERIC, Heartland Healthcare Services	61392-0146-60
60's	$113.99	GENERIC, Eon Labs Manufacturing Inc	00185-0799-60
60's	$126.72	RIFADIN, Allscripts Pharmaceutical Company	54569-8618-00
60's	$134.26	RIFADIN, Aventis Pharmaceuticals	00068-0508-60
60's	$137.64	RIMACTANE, Physicians Total Care	54868-2484-00
60's	$142.04	RIFADIN, Physicians Total Care	54868-2901-01
90's	$146.55	GENERIC, Heartland Healthcare Services	61392-0146-90
100's	$134.10	GENERIC, Eon Labs Manufacturing Inc	00185-0801-01
100's	$190.08	GENERIC, Eon Labs Manufacturing Inc	00185-0799-01
100's	$193.32	RIFAMPIN, Geneva Pharmaceuticals	00781-2077-01
100's	$210.94	GENERIC, Udl Laboratories Inc	51079-0890-20
100's	$223.87	RIFADIN, Aventis Pharmaceuticals	00068-0508-61

Powder For Injection - Intravenous - 600 mg

1's	$77.50	GENERIC, Bedford Laboratories	55390-0123-01

PRODUCT LISTING - EQUIVALENTS NOT AVAILABLE

Capsule - Oral - 300 mg

10's	$27.50	GENERIC, Pharma Pac	52959-0653-10
30's	$47.29	GENERIC, Versapharm Inc	61748-0018-30
30's	$75.00	GENERIC, Pharma Pac	52959-0653-30
100's	$157.16	GENERIC, Versapharm Inc	61748-0018-01

Powder For Injection - Intravenous - 600 mg

1's	$90.28	RIFADIN IV, Aventis Pharmaceuticals	00068-0597-01

Rifapentine *(003403)*

Categories: Tuberculosis; FDA Approved 1998 Jun; Pregnancy Category C; Orphan Drugs
Drug Classes: Antimycobacterials
Brand Names: Priftin
Cost of Therapy: $87.96 (Tuberculosis; Priftin; 150 mg; 8 tablets/week; 28 day supply)

DESCRIPTION

Priftin (rifapentine) for oral administration contains 150 mg of the active ingredient rifapentine per tablet.

The 150 mg tablets also contain, as inactive ingredients: calcium stearate, disodium EDTA, FD&C blue no. 2 aluminum lake, hydroxypropyl cellulose, hydroxypropyl methylcellulose, microcrystalline cellulose, polyethylene glycol, pregelatinized starch, propylene glycol, sodium ascorbate, sodium lauryl sulfate, sodium starch glycolate, synthetic red iron oxide, and titanium dioxide.

Rifapentine is a rifamycin derivative antibiotic and has a similar profile of microbiological activity to rifampin (rifampicin). The molecular weight is 877.04.

The molecular formula is $C_{47}H_{64}N_4O_{12}$.

The chemical name for rifapentine is rifamycin, 3-[[(4-cyclopentyl-1-piperazinyl)imino]methyl]- or 3-[N-(4-Cyclopentyl-1-piperazinyl)formimidoyl] rifamycin or 5,6,9,17,19,21-hexahydroxy-23-methoxy-2,4,12,16,18,20,22 heptamethyl-8-[N-(4-cyclopentyl-l-piperazinyl)-formimidoyl]-2,7-(epoxypentadeca[1,11,13]trienimino)naphtho[2,1-b]furan-1,11(2H)dione 21-acetate.

CLINICAL PHARMACOLOGY

PHARMACOKINETICS

Absorption

The absolute bioavailability of rifapentine has not been determined. The relative bioavailability (with an oral solution as a reference) of rifapentine after a single 600 mg dose to healthy adult volunteers was 70%. The maximum concentrations were achieved from 5-6 hours after administration of the 600 mg rifapentine dose. Food (850 total calories: 33 g protein, 55 g fat and 58 g carbohydrate) increased AUC(0-∞) and C_{max} by 43% and 44%, respectively over that observed when administered under fasting conditions. When oral doses of rifapentine were administered once daily or once every 72 hours to healthy volunteers for 10 days, single dose AUC(0-∞) value of rifapentine was similar to its steady-state AUCss(0-24h) or AUCss(0-72h) values, suggesting no significant auto-induction effect on steady-state pharmacokinetics of rifapentine. Steady-state conditions were achieved by Day 10 following daily administration of rifapentine 600 mg. The pharmacokinetic characteristics of rifapentine and 25-desacetyl rifapentine (active metabolite) on Day 10 following oral administration of 600 mg rifapentine every 72 hours to healthy volunteers are contained in TABLE 1.

TABLE 1 *Pharmacokinetics of Rifapentine and 25-Desacetyl Rifapentine in Healthy Volunteers*

Parameter	Rifapentine Mean ± SD (n=12)	25-desacetyl Rifapentine Mean ± SD (n=12)
C_{max} (μg/ml)	15.05 ± 4.62	6.26 ± 2.06
AUC(0-72h)(μg·h/ml)	319.54 ± 91.52	215.88 ± 85.96
T½ (h)	13.19 ± 1.38	13.35 ± 2.67
T_{max} (h)	4.83 ± 1.80	11.25 ± 2.73
Clpo (L/h)	2.03 ± 0.60	—

Distribution

In a population pharmacokinetic analysis in 351 tuberculosis patients who received 600 mg rifapentine in combination with isoniazid, pyrazinamide and ethambutol, the estimated apparent volume of distribution was 70.2 ± 9.1 L. In healthy volunteers, rifapentine and 25-desacetyl rifapentine were 97.7% and 93.2% bound to plasma proteins, respectively. Rifapentine was mainly bound to albumin. Similar extent of protein binding was observed in healthy volunteers, asymptomatic HIV-infected subjects and hepatically impaired subjects.

Metabolism/Excretion

Following a single 600 mg oral dose of radiolabelled rifapentine to healthy volunteers (n=4), 87% of the total ^{14}C rifapentine was recovered in the urine (17%) and feces (70%). Greater than 80% of the total ^{14}C rifapentine dose was excreted from the body within 7 days. Rifapentine was hydrolyzed by an esterase enzyme to form a microbiologically active 25-desacetyl rifapentine. Rifapentine and 25-desacetyl rifapentine accounted for 99% of the total radioactivity in plasma. Plasma AUC(0-∞) and C_{max} values of the 25-desacetyl rifapentine metabolite were one-half and one-third those of the rifapentine, respectively. Based upon relative *in vitro* activities and AUC(0-∞) values, rifapentine and 25-desacetyl rifapentine potentially contributes 62% and 38% to the clinical activities against *M. tuberculosis*, respectively.

Special Populations

Gender

In a population pharmacokinetics analysis of sparse blood samples obtained from 351 tuberculosis patients who received 600 mg rifapentine in combination with isoniazid, pyrazinamide and ethambutol, the estimated apparent oral clearance of rifapentine for males and females was 2.51 ± 0.14 L/h and 1.69 ± 0.41 L/h, respectively. The clinical significance of the difference in the estimated apparent oral clearance is not known.

Elderly

Following oral administration of a single 600 mg dose of rifapentine to elderly (≥65 years) male healthy volunteers (n=14), the pharmacokinetics of rifapentine and 25-desacetyl metabolite were similar to that observed for young (18-45 years) healthy male volunteers (n=20).

Pediatric (adolescents)

In a pharmacokinetics study of rifapentine in healthy adolescents (age 12-15), 600 mg rifapentine was administered to those weighing ≥45 kg (n=10) and 450 mg was administered to those weighing <45 kg (n=2). The pharmacokinetics of rifapentine were similar to those observed in healthy adults.

Renal Impaired Patients

The pharmacokinetics of rifapentine have not been evaluated in renal impaired patients. Although only about 17% of an administered dose is excreted via the kidneys, the clinical significance of impaired renal function on the disposition of rifapentine and its 25-desacetyl metabolite is not known.

Hepatic Impaired Patients

Following oral administration of a single 600 mg dose of rifapentine to mild to severe hepatic impaired patients (n=15), the pharmacokinetics of rifapentine and 25-desacetyl metabolite were similar in patients with various degrees of hepatic impairment and to that observed in another study for healthy volunteers (n=12). Since the elimination of these agents are primarily via the liver, the clinical significance of impaired hepatic function on the disposition of rifapentine and its 25-desacetyl metabolite is not known.

Asymptomatic HIV-Infected Volunteers

Following oral administration of a single 600 mg dose of rifapentine to asymptomatic HIV-infected volunteers (n=15) under fasting conditions, mean C_{max} and AUC(0-∞) of rifapentine were lower (20-32%) than that observed in other studies in healthy volunteers (n=55). In a cross-study comparision, mean C_{max} and AUC values of the 25-desacetyl metabolite of rifapentine, when compared to healthy volunteers were higher (6-21%) in one study (n=20), but lower (15-16%) in a different study (n=40). The clinical significance of this observation is not known. Food (850 total calories: 33 g protein, 55 g fat, and 58 g carbohydrate) increases the mean AUC and C_{max} of rifapentine observed under fasting conditions in asymptomatic HIV-infected volunteers by about 51% and 53%, respectively.

MICROBIOLOGY

Mechanism of Action

Rifapentine, a cyclopentyl rifamycin, inhibits DNA-dependent RNA polymerase in susceptible strains of *Mycobacterium tuberculosis* but not in mammalian cells. At therapeutic levels, rifapentine exhibits bactericidal activity against both intracellular and extracellular *M. tuberculosis* organisms. Both rifapentine and the 25-desacetyl metabolite accumulate in human monocyte-derived macrophages with intracellular/extracellular ratios of approximately 24:1 and 7:1, respectively.

Resistance Development

In the treatment of tuberculosis (see INDICATIONS AND USAGE), a small number of resistant cells present within large populations of susceptible cells can rapidly become predominant. Rifapentine resistance development in *M. tuberculosis* strains is principally due to one of several single point mutations that occur in the rpoB portion of the gene coding for the beta subunit of the DNA-dependent RNA polymerase. The incidence of rifapentine resistant mutants in an otherwise susceptible population of *M. tuberculosis* strains is approximately 1 in 10^7 to 10^8 bacilli. Due to the potential for resistance development to rifapentine, appropriate susceptibility tests should be performed in the event of persistently positive cultures.

M. tuberculosis organisms resistant to other rifamycins are likely to be resistant to rifapentine. A high level of cross resistance between rifampin and rifapentine has been demonstrated with *M. tuberculosis* strains. Cross resistance does not appear between rifapentine and non-rifamycin antimycobacterial agents such as isoniazid and streptomycin.

In Vitro Activity of Rifapentine Against M. tuberculosis

Rifapentine and its 25-desacetyl metabolite have demonstrated *in vitro* activity against rifamycin-susceptible strains of *Mycobacterium tuberculosis* including cidal activity against phagocytized *M. tuberculosis* organisms grown in activated human macrophages.

In vitro results indicate that rifapentine MIC values for *M. tuberculosis* organisms are influenced by study conditions. Rifapentine MIC values were substantially increased employing egg-based medium compared to liquid or agar-based solid media. The addition of Tween 80 in these assays has been shown to lower MIC values for rifamycin compounds.

In mouse infection studies a therapeutic effect, in terms of enhanced survival time or reduction of organ bioburden, has been observed in *M. tuberculosis*-infected animals treated with various intermittent rifapentine-containing regimens. Animal studies have shown that the activity of rifapentine is influenced by dose and frequency of administration.

Susceptibility Testing for Mycobacterium tuberculosis

Breakpoints to determine whether clinical isolates of *M. tuberculosis* are susceptible or resistant to rifapentine have not been established. The clinical relevance of rifapentine *in vitro* susceptibility test results for other mycobacterial species has not been determined.

INDICATIONS AND USAGE

Rifapentine is indicated for the treatment of pulmonary tuberculosis. Rifapentine must always be used in conjunction with at least 1 other antituberculosis drug to which the isolate is susceptible. In the intensive phase of the short-course treatment of pulmonary tuberculosis, rifapentine should be administered twice weekly for 2 months, with an interval of no less than 3 days (72 hours) between doses, as part of an appropriate regimen which includes daily companion drugs. It may also be necessary to add either streptomycin or ethambutol until the results of susceptibility testing are known. *Compliance with all drugs in the Intensive Phase (i.e., rifapentine, isoniazid, pyrazinamide, ethambutol or streptomycin) is imperative to assure early sputum conversion and protection against relapse.* Following the intensive phase, Continuation Phase treatment should be continued with rifapentine for 4 months. During this phase, rifapentine should be administered on a once-weekly basis in combination with an appropriate antituberculous agent for susceptible organisms (see DOSAGE AND ADMINISTRATION).

In the treatment of tuberculosis, the small number of resistant cells present within large populations of susceptible cells can rapidly become the predominant type. Consequently, clinical samples for mycobacterial culture and susceptibility testing should be obtained prior to the initiation of therapy, as well as during treatment to monitor therapeutic response. The susceptibility of *M. tuberculosis* organisms to isoniazid, rifampin, pyrazinamide, ethambutol, rifapentine and other appropriate agents should be measured. If test results show resistance to any of these drugs and the patient is not responding to therapy, the drug regimen should be modified.

CONTRAINDICATIONS

This product is contraindicated in patients with a history of hypersensitivity to any of the rifamycins (*e.g.*, rifampin and rifabutin).

WARNINGS

Poor compliance with the dosage regimen, particularly the daily administered non-rifamycin drugs in the Intensive Phase, was associated with late sputum conversion and a high relapse rate in the rifapentine arm of Clinical Study 008. Therefore, compliance with the full course of therapy must be emphasized, and the importance of not missing any doses must be stressed. (See PRECAUTIONS and DOSAGE AND ADMINISTRATION.)

Since antituberculous multidrug treatments, including the rifamycin class, are associated with serious hepatic events, patients with abnormal liver tests and/or liver disease should only be given rifapentine in cases of necessity and then with caution and under strict medical supervision. In these patients, careful monitoring of liver tests (especially serum transaminases) should be carried out prior to therapy and then every 2-4 weeks during therapy. If signs of liver disease occur or worsen, rifapentine should be discontinued. Hepatotoxicity of other antituberculosis drugs (*e.g.*, isoniazid, pyrazinamide) used in combination with rifapentine should also be taken into account.

Hyperbilirubinemia resulting from competition for excretory pathways between rifapentine and bilirubin cannot be excluded since competition between the related drug frifampin and bilirubin can occur. An isolated report showing a moderate rise in bilirubin and/or transaminase level is not in itself an indication for interrupting treatment; rather, the decision should be made after repeating the tests, noting trends in the levels and considering them in conjunction with the patient's clinical condition. Pseudomembranous colitis has been reported to occur with various antibiotics, including other rifamycins. Diarrhea, particularly if severe and/or persistent, occurring during treatment or in the initial weeks following treatment may be symptomatic of *Clostridium difficile*-associated disease, the most severe form of which is pseudomembranous colitis. If pseudomembranous colitis is suspected, rifapentine should be stopped immediately and the patient should be treated with supportive and specific treatment without delay (*e.g.*, oral vancomycin). Products inhibiting peristalsis are contraindicated in this clinical situation. Experience in HIV-infected patients is limited. In an ongoing CDC TB trial, 5 out of 30 HIV-infected patients randomized to once weekly rifapentine (plus INH) in the Continuation Phase who completed treatment, relapsed. Four of these patients developed rifampin mono-resistant (RMR) TB. Each RMR patient had late-stage HIV infection, low CD4 counts and extrapulmonary disease, and documented coadministration of antifungal azoles.[1] These findings are consistent with the literature in which an emergence of RMR TB in HIV-infected TB patients has been reported in recent years. Further study in this sub-population is warranted. As with other antituberculous treatments, when rifapentine is used in HIV-infected patients, a more aggressive regimen should be employed (*e.g.*, more frequent dosing). Based on results to date of the CDC trial (see above), once weekly dosing during the Continuous Phase of treatment is not recommended at this time.

Because rifapentine has been shown to increase indinavir metabolism (see DRUG INTERACTIONS), it should be used with extreme caution, if at all, in patients who are also taking protease inhibitors.

PRECAUTIONS

GENERAL

Rifapentine may produce a predominately red-orange discoloration of body tissues and CR fluids (*e.g.*, skin, teeth, tongue, urine, feces, saliva, sputum, tears, sweat, and cerebrospinal fluid).

Contact lenses or dentures may become permanently stained.

Rifapentine should not be used in patients with porphyria. Rifampin has enzyme-inducing properties, including induction of delta amino levulinic acid synthetase. Isolated reports have associated porphyria exacerbation with rifampin administration. Based on these isolated reports with rifampin, it may be assumed that rifapentine has a similar effect.

INFORMATION FOR THE PATIENT

The patient should be told that rifapentine may produce a reddish coloration of the urine, sweat, sputum, tears, and breast milk and the patient should be forewarned that contact lenses or dentures may be permanently stained. The patient should be advised that the reliability of oral or other systemic hormonal contraceptives may be affected; consideration should be given to using alternative contraceptive measures. For those patients with a propensity to nausea, vomiting, or gastrointestinal upset, administration of rifapentine with food may be useful. Patients should be instructed to notify their physician promptly if they experience any of the following: fever, loss of appetite, malaise, nausea and vomiting, darkened urine, yellowish discoloration of the skin and eyes, and pain or swelling of the joints. Compliance with the full course of therapy must be emphasized, and the importance of not missing any doses of the daily administered companion medications in the Intensive Phase must be stressed. (See DOSAGE AND ADMINISTRATION and WARNINGS.)

LABORATORY TESTS

Adults treated for tuberculosis with rifapentine should have baseline measurements of hepatic enzymes, bilirubin, a complete blood count, and a platelet count (or estimate).

Patients should be seen at least monthly during therapy and should be specifically questioned concerning symptoms associated with adverse reactions.

All patients with abnormalities should have follow-up, including laboratory testing, if necessary. Routine laboratory monitoring for toxicity in people with normal baseline measurements is generally not necessary.

Therapeutic concentration of rifampin have been shown to inhibit standard microbiological assays for serum folate and vitamin B_{12}. Similar drug-laboratory interactions should be considered for rifapentine; thus, alternative assay methods should be considered.

CARCINOGENESIS, MUTAGENESIS, AND IMPAIRMENT OF FERTILITY

Carcinogenicity studies with rifapentine have not been completed. Rifapentine was negative in the following genotoxicity tests: *in vitro* gene mutation assay in bacteria (Ames test); *in vitro* point mutation test in *Aspergillus-nidulans; in vitro* gene conversion assay in *Saccharomyces cerevisiae;* host-mediated (mouse) gene conversion assay with *Saccharomyces cerevisiae; in vitro* Chinese hamster ovary cell/hypoxanthine-guanine-phosphoribosyl transferase (CHO/HGPRT) forward mutation assay; *in vitro* chromosomal aberration assay utilizing rat lymphocytes; and *in vivo* mouse bone marrow micronucleus assay. The 25-desacetyl metabolite of rifapentine was also negative in the *in vitro* gene mutation assay in bacteria (Ames test), the *in vitro* Chinese hamster ovary cell/hypoxanthine-guanine-phosphoribosyl transferase (CHO/HGPRT) forward mutation assay, and the *in vivo* mouse bone marrow micronucleus assay. This metabolite did induce chromosomal aberrations in an *in vitro* chromosomal aberration assay. Fertility and reproductive performance were not affected by oral administration of rifapentine to male and female rats at doses of up to one-third of the human dose (based on body surface area conversions).

PREGNANCY, TERATOGENIC EFFECTS, PREGNANCY CATEGORY C

Rifapentine has been shown to be teratogenic in rats and rabbits. In rats, when given in doses 0.6 times the human dose (based on body surface area comparisons) during the period of organogenesis, pups showed cleft palates, right aortic arch and increased incidence of delayed ossification and increased number of ribs. Rabbits treated with drug at doses between 0.3 and 1.3 times the human dose (based on body surface area comparison) displayed major malformations including ovarian-agenesis, pes varus, arhinia, microphthalmia and irregularities of the ossified facial tissues (4 of 321 examined fetuses).

Nonteratogenic Effects

In rats, rifapentine administration was associated with increased resorption rate and post-implantation loss, decreased mean fetus weight, increased number of stillborn pups and slightly increased mortality during lactation. Rabbits given 1.3 times the human dose (based on body surface area comparisons) showed higher post-implantation losses and an increased incidence of stillborn pups.

When rifapentine was administered at 0.3 times the human dose (based on body surface area comparisons) to mated female rats late in gestation (from Day 15 of gestation to Day 21 postpartum), pup weights and gestational survival (live pups born/pups born) were reduced compared to controls.

Pregnancy — Human Experience

There are no adequate and well-controlled studies in pregnant women. In Clinical Study 008, 6 patients randomized to rifapentine became pregnant; 2 had normal deliveries; 2 had first trimester spontaneous abortions, 1 had an elective abortion and 1 patient was lost to follow-up. Of the 2 patients who spontaneously aborted, co-morbid conditions of ethanol abuse in 1 and HIV infection in the other were noted.

When administered during the last few weeks of pregnancy, rifampin can cause postnatal hemorrhages in the mother and infant for which treatment with vitamin K may be indicated. Thus, patients and infants who receive rifapentine during the last few weeks of pregnancy should have appropriate clotting parameters evaluated.

Rifapentine should be used during pregnancy only if the potential benefit justifies the potential risk to the fetus.

NURSING MOTHERS

It is not known whether rifapentine is excreted in human milk. Because many drugs are excreted in human milk and because of the potential for serious adverse reactions in nursing infants, a decision should be made whether to discontinue nursing or discontinue the drug, taking into account the importance of the drug to the mother. Since rifapentine may produce a red-orange discoloration of body fluids, there is a potential for discoloration of breast milk.

PEDIATRIC USE

The safety and effectiveness of rifapentine in pediatric patients under the age of 12 have not been established. A pharmacokinetic study was conducted in 12- to 15-year-old healthy volunteers. (See CLINICAL PHARMACOLOGY, Pharmacokinetics, Special Populations, for pharmacokinetic information.)

GERIATRIC USE

Clinical studies of rifapentine did not include sufficient numbers of subjects aged 65 and over to determine whether they respond differently from younger subjects. Other reported clinical experience has not identified differences in responses between the elderly and younger patients. In general, dose selection for an elderly patient should be cautious, usually starting at the low end of the dosing range, reflecting the greater frequency of decreased hepatic, renal, or cardiac function and of concomitant disease or other drug therapy. (See CLINICAL PHARMACOLOGY, Pharmacokinetics, Special Populations, Elderly.)

DRUG INTERACTIONS

RIFAPENTINE-INDINAVIR INTERACTION

In a study in which 600 mg rifapentine was administered twice weekly for 14 days followed by rifapentine twice weekly plus 800 mg indinavir 3 times a day for an additional 14 days, indinavir C_{max} decreased by 55% while AUC reduced by 70%. Clearance of indinavir increased by 3-fold in the presence of rifapentine while half-life did not change. But when indinavir was administered for 14 days followed by coadministration with rifapentine for an additional 14 days, indinavir did not affect the pharmacokinetics of rifapentine. Rifapentine should be used with extreme caution, if at all, in patients who are also taking protease inhibitors. (See WARNINGS and DOSAGE AND ADMINISTRATION.)

Rifapentine is an inducer of cytochromes P4503A4 and P4502C8/9. Therefore, rifapentine may increase the metabolism of other coadministered drugs that are metabolized by these enzymes. Induction of enzyme activities by rifapentine occurred within 4 days after the first dose. Enzyme activities returned to baseline levels 14 days after discontinuing rifapentine. In addition, the magnitude of enzyme induction by rifapentine was dose and dosing frequency dependent; less enzyme induction occurred when 600 mg oral doses of rifapentine were given once every 72 hours versus daily. *In vitro* and *in vivo* enzyme induction studies have suggested rifapentine induction potential may be less than rifampin but more potent than rifabutin. Rifampin has been reported to accelerate the metabolism and may reduce the activity of the following drugs; hence, rifapentine may also increase the metabolism and decrease the activity of these drugs. Dosage adjustments of the following drugs or of drugs metabolized by cytochrome P4503A4 or P4502C8/9 may be necessary if they are given concurrently with rifapentine. Patients using oral or other systemic hormonal contraceptives should be advised to change to nonhormonal methods of birth control.

- ***Anticonvulsants:*** *e.g.,* phenytoin.
- ***Antiarrhythmics:*** *e.g.,* disopyramide, mexiletine, quinidine, tocainide.
- ***Antibiotics:*** *e.g.,* chloramphenicol, clarithromycin, dapsone, doxycycline, fluoroquinolones (such as ciprofloxacin).
- ***Oral Anticoagulants:*** *e.g.,* warfarin.
- ***Antifungals:*** *e.g.,* fluconazole, itraconazole, ketoconazole.
- ***Barbiturates.***
- ***Benzodiazepines:*** *e.g.,* diazepam.
- ***Beta-Blockers, Calcium Channel Blockers:*** *e.g.,* diltiazem, nifedipine, verapamil.
- ***Corticosteroids.***
- ***Cardiac Glycoside Preparations.***
- ***Clofibrate.***
- ***Oral or Other Systemic Hormonal Contraceptives.***
- ***Haloperidol.***
- ***HIV Protease Inhibitors:*** *e.g.,* indinavir, ritonavir, nelfinavir, saquinavir (see Rifapentine-Indinavir Interaction).
- ***Oral Hypoglycemic Agents:*** *e.g.,* sulfonylureas.
- ***Immunosuppressants:*** *e.g.,* cyclosporine, tacrolimus.
- ***Levothyroxine.***
- ***Narcotic Analgesics:*** *e.g.,* methadone.
- ***Progestins.***
- ***Quinine.***
- ***Reverse Transcriptase Inhibitors:*** *e.g.,* delavirdine, zidovudine.
- ***Sildenafil.***
- ***Theophylline.***
- ***Tricyclic Antidepressants:*** *e.g.,* amitriptyline, nortriptyline.

The conversion of rifapentine to 25-desacetyl rifapentine is mediated by an esterase enzyme. There is minimal potential for rifapentine metabolism to be inhibited or induced by another drug, or for rifapentine to inhibit the metabolism of another drug based upon the characteristics of the esterase enzymes. Rifapentine does not induce its own metabolism. Since rifapentine is highly bound to albumin, drug displacement interactions may also occur.

In Clinical Study 008 patients were advised to take rifapentine at least 1 hour before or 2 hours after ingestion of antacids.

ADVERSE REACTIONS

The investigators in the tuberculosis treatment clinical trial (Study 008) assessed the causality of adverse events as definitely, probably, possibly, unlikely or not related to 1 of the 2 drug regimens tested. TABLE 4A and TABLE 4B present treatment-related adverse events deemed by the investigators to be at least possibly related to any of the 4 drugs in the regimens (rifapentine/rifampin, isoniazid, pyrazinamide, or ethambutol) which occurred in ≥1% of patients. Hyperuricemia was the most frequently reported event that was assessed as treatment related and was most likely related to the pyrazinamide since no cases were reported in the Continuation Phase when this drug was no longer included in the treatment regimen.

Treatment-related adverse events of moderate or severe intensity in <1% of the rifapentine combination therapy patients in Study 008 are presented below by body system.

- ***Hepatic & Biliary:*** Bilirubinemia, hepatitis.
- ***Dermatologic:*** Urticaria, skin discoloration.
- ***Hematologic:*** Thrombocytopenia, neutrophilia, leukocytosis, purpura, hematoma.
- ***Metabolic & Nutritional:*** Hyperkalemia, hypovolemia, alkaline phosphatase increased, LDH increased.
- ***Body as a Whole — General:*** Peripheral edema, fatigue.
- ***Gastrointestinal:*** Constipation, esophagitis, gastritis, pancreatitis.

TABLE 4A *Treatment-Related Adverse Events Occurring in ≥1% of the Patients in Study 008*

	Intensive Phase*		Continuation Phase†	
	Rifapentine Combination	Rifampin Combination	Rifapentine Combination	Rifampin Combination
Preferred Term	(n=361)	(n=361)	(n=321)	(n=307)
Hyperuricemia	78 (21.6%)	55 (15.2%)	0	0
ALT increased	12 (3.3%)	17 (4.7%)	6 (1.9%)	7 (2.3%)
AST increased	11 (3.0%)	16 (4.4%)	5 (1.6%)	7 (2.3%)
Neutropenia	7 (1.9%)	9 (2.5%)	12 (3.7%)	9 (2.9%)
Pyuria	11 (3.0%)	10 (2.8%)	6 (1.9%)	3 (1.0%)
Proteinuria	15 (4.2%)	10 (2.8%)	2 (0.6%)	1 (0.3%)
Hematuria	10 (2.8%)	12 (3.3%)	4 (1.2%)	4 (1.3%)
Lymphopenia	14 (3.9%)	13 (3.6%)	3 (0.9%)	1 (0.3%)
Urinary casts	11 (3.0%)	3 (0.8%)	4 (1.2%)	0
Rash	9 (2.5%)	19 (5.3%)	4 (1.2%)	3 (1.0%)
Pruritus	8 (2.2%)	15 (4.2%)	1 (0.3%)	1 (0.3%)
Acne	5 (1.4%)	3 (0.8%)	2 (0.6%)	1 (0.3%)
Anorexia	6 (1.7%)	8 (2.2%)	3 (0.9%)	4 (1.3%)
Anemia	7 (1.9%)	9 (2.5%)	2 (0.6%)	1 (0.3%)
Leukopenia	4 (1.1%)	4 (1.1%)	3 (0.9%)	5 (1.6%)
Arthralgia	9 (2.5%)	7 (1.9%)	0	0
Pain	7 (1.9%)	5 (1.4%)	0	1 (0.3%)
Nausea	7 (1.9%)	2 (0.6%)	0	1 (0.3%)
Vomiting	4 (1.1%)	6 (1.7%)	1 (0.3%)	1 (0.3%)
Headache	3 (0.8%)	4 (1.1%)	1 (0.3%)	3 (1.0%)
Dyspepsia	3 (0.8%)	5 (1.4%)	2 (0.6%)	3 (1.0%)
Hypertension	3 (0.8%)	0	1 (0.3%)	1 (0.3%)
Dizziness	4 (1.1%)	0	0	1 (0.3%)
Thrombocytosis	4 (1.1%)	2 (0.6%)	0	0
Diarrhea	4 (1.1%)	0	0	0
Rash maculopapular	4 (1.1%)	3 (0.8%)	0	0
Hemoptysis	2 (0.6%)	0	2 (0.6%)	0

Note: ≥1% refers to rifapentine in the TOTAL columns in TABLE 4B.
Note: A patient may have experienced the same adverse event more than once during the course of the study, therefore, patient counts across the columns above may not equal the patient counts in the TOTAL columns in TABLE 4B.
* Intensive Phase consisted of therapy with either rifapentine or rifampin combined with isoniazid, pyrazinamide, and ethambutol administered daily (rifapentine twice weekly) for 60 days.
† Continuation Phase consisted of therapy with either rifapentine or rifampin combined with isoniazid for 120 days. Rifapentine patients were dosed once weekly; rifampin patients were dosed twice weekly. Events recorded in this phase includes those reported up to 3 months after Continuation Phase therapy was completed.

TABLE 4B *Treatment-Related Adverse Events Occurring in ≥1% of the Patients in Study 008*

	Total	
	Rifapentine Combination	Rifampin Combination
Preferred Term	(n=361)	(n=361)
Hyperuricemia	78 (21.5%)	55 (15.2%)
ALT increased	18 (5.0%)	24 (6.6%)
AST increased	15 (4.2%)	23 (6.4%)
Neutropenia	18 (5.0%)	18 (5.0%)
Pyuria	14 (3.9%)	12 (3.3%)
Proteinuria	17 (4.7%)	11 (3.0%)
Hematuria	13 (3.6%)	15 (4.2%)
Lymphopenia	16 (4.4%)	14 (3.9%)
Urinary casts	14 (3.9%)	3 (0.8%)
Rash	13 (3.6%)	21 (5.8%)
Pruritus	9 (2.5%)	16 (4.4%)
Acne	7 (1.9%)	4 (1.1%)
Anorexia	8 (2.2%)	10 (2.8%)
Anemia	9 (2.5%)	10 (2.8%)
Leukopenia	7 (1.9%)	8 (2.2%)
Arthralgia	9 (2.5%)	7 (1.9%)
Pain	7 (1.9%)	6 (1.7%)
Nausea	7 (1.9%)	3 (0.8%)
Vomiting	5 (1.4%)	7 (1.9%)
Headache	4 (1.1%)	7 (1.9%)
Dyspepsia	4 (1.1%)	8 (2.2%)
Hypertension	4 (1.1%)	1 (0.3%)
Dizziness	4 (1.1%)	1 (0.3%)
Thrombocytosis	4 (1.1%)	2 (0.6%)
Diarrhea	4 (1.1%)	0
Rash maculopapular	4 (1.1%)	3 (0.8%)
Hemoptysis	4 (1.1%)	0

Note: ≥1% refers to rifapentine in the TOTAL columns above.
Note: A patient may have experienced the same adverse event more than once during the course of the study, therefore, patient counts across the columns in TABLE 4A may not equal the patient counts in the TOTAL columns above.

Musculoskeletal: Gout, arthrosis.
Psychiatric: Aggressive reaction.

Three patients (2 rifampin combination therapy patients and 1 rifapentine combination therapy patient) were discontinued in the Intensive Phase as a result of hepatitis with increased liver function tests (ALT, AST, LDH, and bilirubin). Concomitant medications for all 3 patients included isoniazid, pyrazinamide, ethambutol, and pyridoxine. The 2 rifampin patients and 1 rifapentine patient recovered without sequelae.

Twenty-two (22) deaths occurred in Study 008 (11 in the rifampin combination therapy group and 11 in the rifapentine combination therapy group). None of the deaths were attributed to study medication. In the study, 18/361 (5.0%) rifampin combination therapy patients discontinued the study due to an adverse event compared to 11/361 (3.0%) rifapentine combination therapy patients.

The overall occurrence rate of treatment-related adverse events was higher in males with the rifapentine combination regimen (50%) versus the rifampin combination regiment (43%), while in females the overall rate was greater in the rifampin combination group (68%) compared to the rifapentine combination group (59%). However, there were higher frequencies of treatment-related hematuria and ALT increases for female patients in both treatment groups compared to those for male patients.

Adverse events associated with rifampin may occur with rifapentine: Effects of enzyme induction to increase metabolism resulting in decreased concentration of endogenous substrates, including adrenal hormones, thyroid hormones, and vitamin D.

DOSAGE AND ADMINISTRATION

Rifapentine should not be used alone, in initial treatment or in retreatment of pulmonary tuberculosis. In the intensive phase of short-course therapy which is to continue for 2 months, 600 mg (four 150 mg tablets) of rifapentine should be given twice weekly with an interval of not less than 3 days (72 hours) between doses. For those patients with propensity to nausea, vomiting or gastrointestinal upset, administration of rifapentine with food may be useful. In the Intensive Phase, rifapentine must be administered in combination as part of an appropriate regimen which includes daily companion drugs. *Compliance with all drugs in the Intensive Phase (i.e., rifapentine, isoniazid, pyrazinamide, ethambutol, or streptomycin), especially on days when rifapentine is not administered, is imperative to assure early sputum conversion and protection against relapse.* The advisory Council for the Elimination of Tuberculosis, the American Thoracic Society and the Centers for Disease Control and Prevention also recommend that either streptomycin or ethambutol be added to the regimen unless the likelihood of isoniazid resistance is very low. The need for streptomycin or ethambutol should be reassessed when the results of susceptibility testing are known. An initial treatment regimen with less than 4 drugs may be considered if there is little possibility of drug resistance (that is, less than 4% primary resistance to isoniazid in the community, and the patient has had no previous treatment with antituberculosis medications, is not from a country with a high prevalence of drug resistance, and has no known exposure to a drug-resistant case).[2]

Following the intensive phase, treatment should be continued with rifapentine once weekly for 4 months in combination with isoniazid or an appropriate agent for susceptible organisms. If the patient is still sputum smear or culture positive, if resistant organisms are present, or if the patient is HIV positive, follow the ATS/CDC treatments guidelines.[2]

Concomitant administration of pyridoxine (vitamin B_6) is recommended in the malnourished, in those predisposed to neuropathy (*e.g.,* alcoholics and diabetics), and in adolescents.

The above recommendations apply to patients with drug-susceptible organisms. Patients with drug-resistant organisms may require longer duration treatment with other drug regimens.

HOW SUPPLIED

Priftin (rifapentine) 150 mg round normal convex dark-pink film-coated tablets debossed "Priftin" on top and "150" on the bottom.

Storage: Store at 25°C (77°F); excursions permitted 15-30°C (59-86°F). Protect from excessive heat and humidity.

PRODUCT LISTING - EQUIVALENTS NOT AVAILABLE

Tablet - Oral - 150 mg

32's	$87.96	PRIFTIN, Aventis Pharmaceuticals	00088-2100-03

Riluzole *(003281)*

R

For complete prescribing information, refer to the CD-ROM included with the book.

Categories: Amyotrophic lateral sclerosis; Pregnancy Category C; FDA Approved 1995 Dec; Orphan Drugs
Drug Classes: Neuroprotectives
Brand Names: Rilutek
Cost of Therapy: $926.71 (Amytrophic Lateral Sclerosis; Rilutek; 50 mg; 2 tablets/day; 30 day supply)

DESCRIPTION

Riluzole is a member of the benzothiazole class. Chemically, riluzole is 2-amino-6-(trifluoromethoxylbenzothiazole). Its molecular formula is $C_8H_5F_3N_2OS$ and its molecular weight is 234.2.

Riluzole is a white to slightly yellow powder that is very soluble in dimethylformamide, dimethylsulfoxide and methanol, freely soluble in dichloromethane, sparingly soluble in 0.1 N HCl and very slightly soluble in water and in 0.1 N NaOH.

Rilutek Inactive Ingredients: *Core:* Anhydrous dibasic calcium phosphate; microcrystalline cellulose; anhydrous colloidal silica; magnesium stearate; croscarmellose sodium. *Film Coating:* Hydroxypropyl methylcellulose; polyethylene glycol 6000; titanium dioxide

INDICATIONS AND USAGE

Riluzole is indicated for the treatment of patients with amyotrophic lateral sclerosis (ALS). Riluzole extends survival and/or time to tracheostomy.

CONTRAINDICATIONS

Riluzole is contraindicated in patients who have a history of severe hypersensitivity reactions to riluzole or any of the tablet components.

WARNINGS

LIVER INJURY/MONITORING LIVER CHEMISTRIES

Riluzole should be prescribed with care in patients with current evidence or history of abnormal liver function indicated by significant abnormalities in serum transaminase (ALT/SGPT; AST/SGOT), bilirubin, and/or gamma-glutemate transferase (GGT) levels (see DOSAGE AND ADMINISTRATION). Baseline elevations of several LFTs (especially elevated bilirubin) should preclude the use of riluzole.

Riluzole, even in patients without a prior history of liver disease, causes serum aminotransferase elevations. Experience in almost 800 ALS patients indicates that about 50% of riluzole-treated patients will experience at least one ALT/SGPT level above the upper limit of normal, about 8% will have elevations >3 times ULN, and about 2% of patients will have elevations >5 times ULN. A single non-ALS patient with epilepsy treated with concomitant carbamazepine and phenobarbital experienced marked, rapid elevations of liver enzymes with jaundice (ALT 26 times ULN, AST 17 times ULN, and bilirubin 11 times ULN) 4 months after starting riluzole; these returned to normal 7 weeks after treatment discontinuation.

Maximum increases in serum ALT usually occurred within 3 months after the start of riluzole therapy and were usually transient when <5 times ULN. In trials, if ALT levels were <5 times ULN, treatment continued and ALT levels usually returned to below 2 times ULN within 2-6 months. Treatment in studies was discontinued, however, if ALT levels exceeded 5 times ULN, so that there is no experience with continued treatment of ALS patients once ALT values exceed 5 times ULN. There were rare instances of jaundice.

Liver chemistries should be monitored.

NEUTROPENIA

Among approximately 4000 patients given riluzole for ALS, there were 3 cases of marked neutropenia (absolute neutrophil count less than 500/mm^3), all seen within the first 2 months of riluzole treatment. In one case, neutrophil counts rose on continued treatment. In a second case, neutrophil counts rose after therapy was stopped. A third case was more complex, with marked anemia as well as neutropenia and the etiology of both is uncertain. Patients should be warned to report any febrile illness to their physicians. The report of a febrile illness should prompt treating physicians to check white blood cell counts.

DOSAGE AND ADMINISTRATION

The recommended dose for riluzole is 50 mg every 12 hours. No increased benefit can be expected from higher daily doses, but adverse events are increased.

Riluzole tablets should be taken at least an hour before, or 2 hours after, a meal to avoid a food-related decrease in bioavailability.

SPECIAL POPULATIONS

Patients With Impaired Renal or Hepatic Function: Studies have not yet been completed in these populations (see WARNINGS).

PRODUCT LISTING - EQUIVALENTS NOT AVAILABLE

Tablet - Oral - 50 mg

60's $926.71 RILUTEK, Aventis Pharmaceuticals 00075-7700-60

Risedronate Sodium *(003387)*

Categories: Paget's disease; FDA Approved 1998 Mar; Pregnancy Category C
Drug Classes: Bisphosphonates
Brand Names: Actonel
Cost of Therapy: $71.21 (Osteoporosis; Actonel; 5 mg; 1 tablet/day; 30 day supply)
$498.49 (Paget's Disease; Actonel; 30 mg; 1 tablet/day; 30 day supply)

R

DESCRIPTION

Risedronate sodium is a pyridinyl bisphosphonate that inhibits osteoclast-mediated bone resorption and modulates bone metabolism. Each Actonel tablet for oral administration contains the equivalent of 5, 30, or 35 mg of anhydrous risedronate sodium in the form of the hemi-pentahydrate with small amounts of monohydrate. The empirical formula for risedronate sodium hemi-pentahydrate is $C_7H_{10}NO_7P_2Na{\cdot}2.5H_2O$. The chemical name of risedronate sodium is [1-hydroxy-2-(3-pyridinyl)ethylidene]bis[phosphonic acid] monosodium salt.

Molecular weight: *Anhydrous:* 305.10. *Hemi-pentahydrate:* 350.13.

Risedronate sodium is a fine, white to off-white, odorless, crystalline powder. It is soluble in water and in aqueous solutions, and essentially insoluble in common organic solvents.

Inactive ingredients: Crospovidone, ferric oxide red (35 mg tablets only), ferric oxide yellow (5 and 35 mg tablets only), hydroxypropyl cellulose, hydroxypropyl methylcellulose, lactose monohydrate, magnesium stearate, microcrystalline cellulose, polyethylene glycol, silicon dioxide, titanium dioxide.

CLINICAL PHARMACOLOGY

MECHANISM OF ACTION

Risedronate sodium has an affinity for hydroxyapatite crystals in bone and acts as an antiresorptive agent. At the cellular level, risedronate sodium inhibits osteoclasts. The osteoclasts adhere normally to the bone surface, but show evidence of reduced active resorption (*e.g.*, lack of ruffled border). Histomorphometry in rats, dogs, and minipigs showed that risedronate sodium treatment reduces bone turnover (activation frequency, *i.e.*, the rate at which bone remodeling sites are activated) and bone resorption at remodeling sites.

PHARMACOKINETICS

Absorption

Absorption after an oral dose is relatively rapid (T_{max}~1 hour) and occurs throughout the upper gastrointestinal tract. The fraction of the dose absorbed is independent of dose over the range studied (single dose, 2.5 to 30 mg; multiple dose, 2.5 to 5 mg). Steady-state conditions in the serum are observed within 57 days of daily dosing. Mean absolute oral bioavailability of the 30 mg tablet is 0.63% (90% CI: 0.54-0.75%) and is comparable to a solution. The extent of absorption of a 30 mg dose (three, 10 mg tablets) when administered 0.5 hours before breakfast is reduced by 55% compared to dosing in the fasting state (no food or drink for 10 hours prior to or 4 hours after dosing). Dosing 1 hour prior to breakfast reduces the extent of absorption by 30% compared to dosing in the fasting state. Dosing either 0.5 hours prior to breakfast or 2 hours after dinner (evening meal) results in a similar extent of absorption. Risedronate sodium is effective when administered at least 30 minutes before breakfast.

Distribution

The mean steady-state volume of distribution is 6.3 L/kg in humans. Human plasma protein binding of drug is about 24%. Preclinical studies in rats and dogs dosed intravenously with single doses of [^{14}C] risedronate indicate that approximately 60% of the dose is distributed to bone. The remainder of the dose is excreted in the urine. After multiple oral dosing in rats, the uptake of risedronate in soft tissues was in the range of 0.001-0.01%.

Metabolism

There is no evidence of systemic metabolism of risedronate.

Elimination

Approximately half of the absorbed dose is excreted in urine within 24 hours, and 85% of an intravenous dose is recovered in the urine over 28 days. Mean renal clearance is 105 ml/min (CV=34%) and mean total clearance is 122 ml/min (CV=19%), with the difference primarily reflecting nonrenal clearance or clearance due to adsorption to bone. The renal clearance is not concentration dependent, and there is a linear relationship between renal clearance and creatinine clearance. Unabsorbed drug is eliminated unchanged in feces. Once risedronate is absorbed, the serum concentration-time profile is multiphasic, with an initial half-life of about 1.5 hours and a terminal exponential half-life of 480 hours. This terminal half-life is hypothesized to represent the dissociation of risedronate from the surface of bone.

SPECIAL POPULATIONS

Pediatric

Risedronate pharmacokinetics have not been studied in patients <18 years of age.

Gender

Bioavailability and pharmacokinetics following oral administration were similar in men and women.

Geriatric

Bioavailability and disposition are similar in elderly (>60 years of age) and younger subjects. No dosage adjustment is necessary.

Race

Pharmacokinetic differences due to race have not been studied.

Renal Insufficiency

Risedronate is excreted unchanged primarily via the kidney. As compared to persons with normal renal function, the renal clearance of risedronate was decreased by about 70% in patients with creatinine clearance of approximately 30 ml/min. Risedronate sodium is not recommended for use in patients with severe renal impairment (creatinine clearance <30 ml/min) because of lack of clinical experience. No dosage adjustment is necessary in patients with a creatinine clearance ≥30 ml/min.

Hepatic Insufficiency

No studies have been performed to assess risedronate's safety or efficacy in patients with hepatic impairment. Risedronate is not metabolized in rat, dog, and human liver preparations. Insignificant amounts (<0.1% of intravenous dose) of drug are excreted in the bile in rats. Therefore, dosage adjustment is unlikely to be needed in patients with hepatic impairment.

PHARMACODYNAMICS

Treatment and Prevention of Osteoporosis in Postmenopausal Women

Osteoporosis is characterized by decreased bone mass and increased fracture risk, most commonly at the spine, hip, and wrist.

The diagnosis can be confirmed by the finding of low bone mass, evidence of fracture on x-ray, a history of osteoporotic fracture, or height loss or kyphosis indicative of vertebral fracture. Osteoporosis occurs in both men and women but is more common among women following menopause. In healthy humans, bone formation and resorption are closely linked; old bone is resorbed and replaced by newly-formed bone. In postmenopausal osteoporosis, bone resorption exceeds bone formation, leading to bone loss and increased risk of bone fracture. After menopause, the risk of fractures of the spine and hip increases; approximately 40% of 50- year-old women will experience an osteoporosis-related fracture during their remaining lifetimes. After experiencing 1 osteoporosis-related fracture, the risk of future fracture increases 5-fold compared to the risk among a non-fractured population.

Risedronate sodium treatment decreases the elevated rate of bone turnover that is typically seen in postmenopausal osteoporosis. In clinical trials, administration of risedronate sodium to postmenopausal women resulted in decreases in biochemical markers of bone turnover, including urinary deoxypyridinoline/creatinine and urinary collagen cross-linked N-telopeptide (markers of bone resorption) and serum bone specific alkaline phosphatase (a marker of bone formation). At the 5 mg dose, decreases in deoxypyridinoline/creatinine were evident within 14 days of treatment. Changes in bone formation markers were observed later than changes in resorption markers, as expected, due to the coupled nature of bone resorption and bone formation; decreases in bone specific alkaline phosphatase of about 20% were evident within 3 months of treatment. Bone turnover markers reached a nadir of about 40% below baseline values by the sixth month of treatment and remained stable with continued treatment for up to 3 years. Bone turnover is decreased as early as 14 days and maximally within about 6 months of treatment, with achievement of a new steady-state that more nearly approximates the rate of bone turnover seen in premenopausal women. In a 1 year study comparing daily versus weekly oral dosing regimens of risedronate sodium for the treatment of osteoporosis in postmenopausal women, risedronate sodium 5 mg daily and risedronate sodium 35 mg once a week decreased urinary collagen cross-linked N-telopeptide by 60% and 61%, respectively. In addition, serum bone-specific alkaline phosphatase was also reduced by 42% and 41% in the risedronate sodium 5 mg daily and risedronate sodium 35 mg once a week groups, respectively. Risedronate sodium is not an estrogen and does not have the benefits and risks of estrogen therapy.

As a result of the inhibition of bone resorption, asymptomatic and usually transient decreases from baseline in serum calcium (<1%) and serum phosphate (<3%) and compensatory increases in serum PTH levels (<30%) were observed within 6 months in patients in osteoporosis clinical trials. There were no significant differences in serum calcium, phosphate, or PTH levels between the risedronate sodium and placebo groups at 3 years. In a 1 year study comparing daily versus weekly oral dosing regimens of risedronate sodium in postmenopausal women, the mean changes from baseline at 12 months were similar between the risedronate sodium 5 mg daily and risedronate sodium 35 mg once a week groups, respectively, for serum calcium (0.4% and 0.7%), phosphate (-3.8% and -2.6%) and PTH (6.4% and 4.2%).

Glucocorticoid-Induced Osteoporosis

Sustained use of glucocorticoids is commonly associated with development of osteoporosis and resulting fractures (especially vertebral, hip, and rib). It occurs both in males and females of all ages. The relative risk of a hip fracture in patients on >7.5 mg/day prednisone is more than doubled (RR=2.27); the relative risk of vertebral fracture is increased 5-fold (RR=5.18). Bone loss occurs most rapidly during the first 6 months of therapy with persistent but slowing bone loss for as long as glucocorticoid therapy continues. Osteoporosis occurs as a result of inhibited bone formation and increased bone resorption resulting in net bone loss. Risedronate sodium decreases bone resorption without directly inhibiting bone formation.

In two 1 year clinical trials in the treatment and prevention of glucocorticoid-induced osteoporosis, risedronate sodium 5 mg decreased urinary collagen cross-linked N-telopeptide (a marker of bone resorption), and serum bone specific alkaline phosphatase (a marker of bone formation) by 50-55% and 25-30%, respectively, within 3-6 months after initiation of therapy.

Paget's Disease

Paget's disease of bone is a chronic, focal skeletal disorder characterized by greatly increased and disordered bone remodeling. Excessive osteoclastic bone resorption is followed by osteoblastic new bone formation, leading to the replacement of the normal bone architecture by disorganized, enlarged, and weakened bone structure.

Clinical manifestations of Paget's disease range from no symptoms to severe bone pain, bone deformity, pathological fractures, and neurological disorders. Serum alkaline phosphatase, the most frequently used biochemical marker of disease activity, provides an objective measure of disease severity and response to therapy.

In pagetic patients treated with risedronate sodium 30 mg/day for 2 months, bone turnover returned to normal in a majority of patients as evidenced by significant reductions in serum alkaline phosphatase (a marker of bone formation) and in urinary hydroxyproline/creatinine and deoxypyridinoline/creatinine, (markers of bone resorption). Radiographic structural changes of bone lesions, especially improvement of a majority of lesions with an osteolytic front in weight-bearing bones, were also observed after risedronate sodium treatment. In addition, histomorphometric data provide further support that risedronate sodium can lead to a more normal bone structure in these patients.

Radiographs taken at baseline and after 6 months from patients treated with risedronate sodium 30 mg daily demonstrate that risedronate sodium decreases the extent of osteolysis in both the appendicular and axial skeleton. Osteolytic lesions in the lower extremities improved or were unchanged in 15/16 (94%) of assessed patients; 9/16 (56%) patients showed clear improvement in osteolytic lesions. No evidence of new fractures was observed.

INDICATIONS AND USAGE

POSTMENOPAUSAL OSTEOPOROSIS

Risedronate sodium is indicated for the treatment and prevention of osteoporosis in postmenopausal women.

Treatment of Osteoporosis

In postmenopausal women with osteoporosis, risedronate sodium increases BMD and reduces the incidence of vertebral fractures and a composite endpoint of nonvertebral osteoporosis-related fractures. Osteoporosis may be confirmed by the presence or history of osteoporotic fracture, or by the finding of low bone mass (for example, at least 2 SD below the premenopausal mean).

Prevention of Osteoporosis

Risedronate sodium may be considered in postmenopausal women who are at risk of developing osteoporosis and for whom the desired clinical outcome is to maintain bone mass and to reduce the risk of fracture.

Factors such as family history of osteoporosis, previous fracture, smoking, BMD (at least 1 SD below the premenopausal mean), high bone turnover, thin body frame, Caucasian or Asian race, and early menopause are associated with an increased risk of developing osteoporosis and fractures. The presence of these risk factors may be important when considering the use of risedronate sodium for prevention of osteoporosis.

GLUCOCORTICOID-INDUCED OSTEOPOROSIS

Risedronate sodium is indicated for the prevention and treatment of glucocorticoid-induced osteoporosis in men and women who are either initiating or continuing systemic glucocorticoid treatment (daily dosage equivalent to 7.5 mg or greater of prednisone) for chronic diseases. Patients treated with glucocorticoids should receive adequate amounts of calcium and vitamin D.

PAGET'S DISEASE

Risedronate sodium is indicated for treatment of Paget's disease of bone (osteitis deformans). Treatment is indicated in patients with Paget's disease of bone (1) who have a level of serum alkaline phosphatase (SAP) at least 2 times the upper limit of normal, or (2) who are symptomatic, or (3) who are at risk for future complications from their disease, to induce remission (normalization of serum alkaline phosphatase).

NON-FDA APPROVED INDICATIONS

Bisphosphonates are also used in the treatment of hypercalcemia of malignancy, breast cancer or multiple myeloma associated osteolytic bone disease.

CONTRAINDICATIONS

- Hypocalcemia. (See PRECAUTIONS, General.)
- Known hypersensitivity to any component of this product.
- Inability to stand or sit upright for at least 30 minutes.

WARNINGS

Bisphosphonates may cause upper gastrointestinal disorders such as dysphagia, esophagitis, and esophageal or gastric ulcer (see PRECAUTIONS).

PRECAUTIONS

GENERAL

Hypocalcemia and other disturbances of bone and mineral metabolism should be effectively treated before starting risedronate sodium therapy. Adequate intake of calcium and vitamin D is important in all patients, especially patients with Paget's disease in whom bone turnover is significantly elevated. Risedronate sodium is not recommended for use in patients with severe renal impairment (creatinine clearance <30 ml/min).

Bisphosphonates have been associated with gastrointestinal disorders such as dysphagia, esophagitis, and esophageal or gastric ulcers. This association has been reported for bisphosphonates in postmarketing experience, but has not been found in most pre-approval clinical trials, including those conducted with risedronate sodium. Patients should be advised that taking the medication according to the instructions is important to minimize the risk of these events. They should take risedronate sodium with sufficient plain water (6-8 oz) to facilitate delivery to the stomach, and should not lie down for 30 minutes after taking the drug.

GLUCOCORTICOID-INDUCED OSTEOPOROSIS

The risk versus benefit of risedronate sodium for the prevention and treatment of glucocorticoid-induced osteoporosis at daily doses of glucocorticoids <7.5 mg of prednisone or equivalent has not been established. Before initiating treatment, the hormonal status of both men and women should be ascertained and appropriate replacement considered.

The efficacy of risedronate sodium for this indication has been established in studies of 1 year's duration. The efficacy of risedronate sodium beyond 1 year has not been studied.

INFORMATION FOR THE PATIENT

The patient should be informed to pay particular attention to the dosing instructions as clinical benefits may be compromised by failure to take the drug according to instructions. Specifically, risedronate sodium should be taken at least 30 minutes before the first food or drink of the day other than water.

To facilitate delivery to the stomach, and thus reduce the potential for esophageal irritation, patients should take risedronate sodium while in an upright position (sitting or standing) with a full glass of plain water (6-8 oz). Patients should not lie down for 30 minutes after taking the medication (see PRECAUTIONS, General). Patients should not chew or suck on the tablet because of a potential for oropharyngeal irritation.

Patients should be instructed that if they develop symptoms of esophageal disease (such as difficulty or pain upon swallowing, retrosternal pain or severe persistent or worsening heartburn) they should consult their physician before continuing risedronate sodium.

Patients should be instructed that if they miss a dose of risedronate sodium 35 mg once a week, they should take 1 tablet on the morning after they remember and return to taking 1 tablet once a week, as originally scheduled on their chosen day. Patients should not take 2 tablets on the same day.

Patients should receive supplemental calcium and vitamin D if dietary intake is inadequate (see PRECAUTIONS, General). Calcium supplements or calcium-, aluminum-, and magnesium-containing medications may interfere with the absorption of risedronate sodium and should be taken at a different time of the day, as with food.

Weight-bearing exercise should be considered along with the modification of certain behavioral factors, such as excessive cigarette smoking, and/or alcohol consumption, if these factors exist.

Physicians should instruct their patients to read the Patient Information before starting therapy with risedronate sodium 5 or 35 mg and to re-read it each time the prescription is renewed.

DRUG/LABORATORY TEST INTERACTIONS

Bisphosphonates are known to interfere with the use of bone-imaging agents. Specific studies with risedronate sodium have not been performed.

CARCINOGENESIS, MUTAGENESIS, AND IMPAIRMENT OF FERTILITY

Carcinogenesis

In a 104 week carcinogenicity study, rats were administered daily oral doses up to 24 mg/kg/day (approximately 7.7 times the maximum recommended human daily dose of 30 mg based on surface area, mg/m^2). There were no significant drug-induced tumor findings in male or female rats. The high dose male group of 24 mg/kg/day was terminated early in the study (week 93) due to excessive toxicity, and data from this group were not included in the statistical evaluation of the study results. In an 80 week carcinogenicity study, mice were administered daily oral doses up to 32 mg/kg/day (approximately 6.4 times the 30 mg/day human dose based on surface area, mg/m^2). There were no significant drug-induced tumor findings in male or female mice.

Mutagenesis

Risedronate did not exhibit genetic toxicity in the following assays: *In vitro* bacterial mutagenesis in *Salmonella* and *E. coli* (Ames assay), mammalian cell mutagenesis in CHO/HGPRT assay, unscheduled DNA synthesis in rat hepatocytes and an assessment of chromosomal aberrations *in vivo* in rat bone marrow. Risedronate was positive in a chromosomal aberration assay in CHO cells at highly cytotoxic concentrations (>675 μg/ml, survival of 6-7%). When the assay was repeated at doses exhibiting appropriate cell survival (29%), there was no evidence of chromosomal damage.

Impairment of Fertility

In female rats, ovulation was inhibited at an oral dose of 16 mg/kg/day (approximately 5.2 times the 30 mg/day human dose based on surface area, mg/m^2). Decreased implantation was noted in female rats treated with ≥7 mg/kg/day (approximately 2.3 times the 30 mg/day human dose based on surface area, mg/m^2). In male rats, testicular and epididymal atrophy and inflammation were noted at 40 mg/kg/day (approximately 13 times the 30 mg/day human dose based on surface area, mg/m^2). Testicular atrophy was also noted in male rats after 13 weeks of treatment at oral doses of 16 mg/kg/day (approximately 5.2 times the 30 mg/day human dose based on surface area, mg/m^2). There was moderate-to-severe spermatid maturation block after 13 weeks in male dogs at an oral dose of 8 mg/kg/day (approximately 8 times the 30 mg/day human dose based on surface area, mg/m^2). These findings tended to increase in severity with increased dose and exposure time.

PREGNANCY CATEGORY C

Survival of neonates was decreased in rats treated during gestation with oral doses ≥16 mg/kg/day (approximately 5.2 times the 30 mg/day human dose based on surface area, mg/m^2). Body weight was decreased in neonates from dams treated with 80 mg/kg (approximately 26 times the 30 mg/day human dose based on surface area, mg/m^2). In rats treated during gestation, the number of fetuses exhibiting incomplete ossification of sternebrae or skull was statistically significantly increased at 7.1 mg/kg/day (approximately 2.3 times the 30 mg/day human dose based on surface area, mg/m^2). Both incomplete ossification and unossified sternebrae were increased in rats treated with oral doses ≥16 mg/kg/day (approximately 5.2 times the 30 mg/day human dose based on surface area, mg/m^2). A low incidence of cleft palate was observed in fetuses from female rats treated with oral doses ≥3.2 mg/kg/day (approximately 1 time the 30 mg/day human dose based on surface area, mg/m^2). The relevance of this finding to human use of risedronate sodium is unclear. No significant fetal ossification effects were seen in rabbits treated with oral doses up to 10 mg/kg/day during gestation (approximately 6.7 times the 30 mg/day human dose based on surface area, mg/m^2). However, in rabbits treated with 10 mg/kg/day, 1 of 14 litters were aborted and 1 of 14 litters were delivered prematurely.

Similar to other bisphosphonates, treatment during mating and gestation with doses as low as 3.2 mg/kg/day (approximately 1 time the 30 mg/day human dose based on surface area, mg/m^2) has resulted in periparturient hypocalcemia and mortality in pregnant rats allowed to deliver.

There are no adequate and well-controlled studies of risedronate sodium in pregnant women. Risedronate sodium should be used during pregnancy only if the potential benefit justifies the potential risk to the mother and fetus.

NURSING MOTHERS

Risedronate was detected in feeding pups exposed to lactating rats for a 24 hour period post-dosing, indicating a small degree of lacteal transfer. It is not known whether risedronate is excreted in human milk. Because many drugs are excreted in human milk and because of the potential for serious adverse reactions in nursing infants from bisphosphonates, a decision should be made whether to discontinue nursing or to discontinue the drug, taking into account the importance of the drug to the mother.

PEDIATRIC USE

Safety and effectiveness in pediatric patients have not been established.

GERIATRIC USE

Of the patients receiving risedronate sodium in postmenopausal osteoporosis studies, 43% were between 65 and 75 years of age, and 17% were over 75. The corresponding proportions were 26% and 11% in glucocorticoid-induced osteoporosis trials, and 40% and 26% in Paget's disease trials. No overall differences in efficacy or safety were observed between these patients and younger patients but greater sensitivity of some older individuals cannot be ruled out.

USE IN MEN

Safety and effectiveness have been demonstrated in clinical studies in men receiving risedronate sodium both for Paget's disease and for treatment and prevention of glucocorticoid-induced osteoporosis. However, the safety and effectiveness in men for osteoporosis due to other causes have not been established.

DRUG INTERACTIONS

No specific drug-drug interaction studies were performed. Risedronate is not metabolized and does not induce or inhibit hepatic microsomal drug-metabolizing enzymes (Cytochrome P450).

Calcium Supplements/Antacids: Coadministration of risedronate sodium and calcium, antacids, or oral medications containing divalent cations will interfere with the absorption of risedronate sodium.

Hormone Replacement Therapy: One study of about 500 early postmenopausal women has been conducted to date in which treatment with risedronate sodium (5 mg/day) plus estrogen replacement therapy was compared with estrogen replacement therapy alone. Exposure to study drugs was approximately 12-18 months and the primary endpoint was change in BMD. If considered appropriate, risedronate sodium may be used concomitantly with hormone replacement therapy.

Aspirin/Nonsteroidal Anti-Inflammatory Drugs (NSAIDs): Of over 5700 patients enrolled in the risedronate sodium Phase 3 osteoporosis studies, aspirin use was reported by 31% of patients, 24% of whom were regular users (3 or more days/week). Forty-eight percent (48%) of patients reported NSAID use, 21% of whom were regular users. Among regular aspirin or NSAID users, the incidence of upper gastrointestinal adverse experiences in risedronate sodium-treated patients (24.5%) was similar to that in placebo-treated patients (24.8%).

H_2 Blockers and Proton Pump Inhibitors (PPIs): Of over 5700 patients enrolled in the Risedronate sodium Phase 3 osteoporosis studies, 21% used H_2 blockers and/or PPIs. Among these patients, the incidence of upper gastrointestinal adverse experiences in the risedronate sodium-treated patients was similar to that in placebo-treated patients.

ADVERSE REACTIONS

OSTEOPOROSIS

Risedronate sodium has been studied in over 5700 patients enrolled in the Phase 3 glucocorticoid-induced osteoporosis clinical trials and in postmenopausal osteoporosis trials of up to 3 years duration. The overall adverse event profile of risedronate sodium 5 mg in these studies was similar to that of placebo. Most adverse events were either mild or moderate and did not lead to discontinuation from the study. The incidence of serious adverse events in the placebo group was 24.9% and in the risedronate sodium 5 mg group was 26.3%. The percentage of patients who withdrew from the study due to adverse events was 14.4% and 13.5% for the placebo and risedronate sodium 5 mg groups, respectively. TABLE 5 lists adverse events from the Phase 3 osteoporosis trials reported in >2% of patients and in more risedronate sodium-treated patients than placebo-treated patients. Adverse events are shown without attribution of causality.

TABLE 5 *Adverse Events Occurring at a Frequency >2% and in More Risedronate Sodium-Treated Patients Than Placebo-Treated Patients Combined Phase 3 Osteoporosis Trials*

Body System	Placebo (n=1914)	Risedronate Sodium 5 mg (n=1916)
Body as a Whole		
Infection	29.7%	29.9%
Back pain	23.6%	26.1%
Pain	13.1%	13.6%
Abdominal pain	9.4%	11.6%
Neck pain	4.5%	5.3%
Asthenia	4.3%	5.1%
Chest pain	4.9%	5.0%
Neoplasm	3.0%	3.3%
Hernia	2.5%	2.9%
Cardiovascular		
Hypertension	9.0%	10.0%
Cardiovascular disorder	1.7%	2.5%
Angina pectoris	2.4%	2.5%
Digestive		
Nausea	10.7%	10.9%
Diarrhea	9.6%	10.6%
Flatulence	4.2%	4.6%
Gastritis	2.3%	2.5%
Gastrointestinal disorder	2.1%	2.3%
Rectal disorder	1.9%	2.2%
Tooth disorder	2.0%	2.1%
Hemic and Lymphatic		
Ecchymosis	4.0%	4.3%
Anemia	1.9%	2.4%
Musculoskeletal		
Arthralgia	21.1%	23.7%
Joint disorder	5.4%	6.8%
Myalgia	6.3%	6.6%
Bone pain	4.3%	4.6%
Bone disorder	3.2%	4.0%
Leg cramps	2.6%	3.5%
Bursitis	2.9%	3.0%
Tendon disorder	2.5%	3.0%
Nervous		
Depression	6.2%	6.8%
Dizziness	5.4%	6.4%
Insomnia	4.5%	4.7%
Anxiety	3.0%	4.3%
Neuralgia	3.5%	3.8%
Vertigo	3.2%	3.3%
Hypertonia	2.1%	2.2%
Paresthesia	1.8%	2.1%
Respiratory		
Pharyngitis	5.0%	5.8%
Rhinitis	5.0%	5.7%
Dyspnea	3.2%	3.8%
Pneumonia	2.6%	3.1%
Skin and Appendages		
Rash	7.2%	7.7%
Pruritus	2.2%	3.0%
Skin carcinoma	1.8%	2.0%
Special Senses		
Cataract	5.4%	5.9%
Conjuctivitis	2.8%	3.1%
Otitis media	2.4%	2.5%
Urogenital		
Urinary tract infection	9.7%	10.9%
Cystitis	3.5%	4.1%

Duodenitis and glossitis have been reported uncommonly (0.1 to 1%). There have been rare reports (<0.1%) of abnormal liver function tests.

Laboratory Test Findings

Asymptomatic and small decreases were observed in serum calcium and phosphorus levels. Overall, mean decreases of 0.8% in serum calcium and of 2.7% in phosphorus were observed at 6 months in patients receiving risedronate sodium. Throughout the Phase 3 studies, serum calcium levels below 8 mg/dl were observed in 18 patients, 9 (0.5%) in each treatment arm (risedronate sodium and placebo). Serum phosphorus levels below 2 mg/dl were observed in 14 patients, 11 (0.6%) treated with risedronate sodium and 3 (0.2%) treated with placebo.

Endoscopic Findings

Risedronate sodium clinical studies enrolled over 5700 patients, many with pre-existing gastrointestinal disease and concomitant use of NSAIDs or aspirin. Investigators were encouraged to perform endoscopies in any patients with moderate-to-severe gastrointestinal complaints, while maintaining the blind. These endoscopies were ultimately performed on equal numbers of patients between the treated and placebo groups [75 (14.5%) placebo; 75 (11.9%) risedronate sodium]. Across treatment groups, the percentage of patients with normal esophageal, gastric, and duodenal mucosa on endoscopy was similar (20% placebo, 21% risedronate sodium). The number of patients who withdrew from the studies due to the event prompting endoscopy was similar across treatment groups. Positive findings on endoscopy were also generally comparable across treatment groups. There was a higher number of reports of mild duodenitis in the risedronate sodium group, however there were more duodenal ulcers in the placebo group. Clinically important findings (perforations, ulcers, or bleeding) among this symptomatic population were similar between groups (51% placebo; 39% risedronate sodium).

Once-a-Week Dosing

In a 1 year, double-blind, multicenter study comparing risedronate sodium 5 mg daily and risedronate sodium 35 mg once a week in postmenopausal women, the overall safety and tolerability profiles of the 2 oral dosing regimens were similar. TABLE 6 lists the adverse events in ≥2% of patients from this trial. Events are shown without attribution of causality.

PAGET'S DISEASE

TABLE 6 *Adverse Events Occurring in ≥2% of Patients of Either Treatment Group in the Daily Versus Weekly Osteoporosis Treatment Study in Postmenopausal Women*

Body System	5 mg Daily Risedronate Sodium (n=480)	35 mg Weekly Risedronate Sodium (n=485)
Body as a Whole		
Infection	19.0%	20.6%
Accidental injury	10.6%	10.7%
Pain	7.7%	9.9%
Back pain	9.2%	8.7%
Flu syndrome	7.1%	8.5%
Abdominal pain	7.3%	7.6%
Headache	7.3%	7.2%
Overdose	6.9%	6.8%
Asthenia	3.5%	5.4%
Chest pain	2.3%	2.7%
Allergic reaction	1.9%	2.5%
Neoplasm	0.8%	2.1%
Neck pain	2.7%	1.2%
Cardiovascular System		
Hypertension	5.8%	4.9%
Syncope	0.6%	2.1%
Vasodilatation	2.3%	1.4%
Digestive System		
Constipation	12.5%	12.2%
Dyspepsia	6.9%	7.6%
Nausea	8.5%	6.2%
Diarrhea	6.3%	4.9%
Gastroenteritis	3.8%	3.5%
Flatulence	3.3%	3.1%
Colitis	0.8%	2.5%
Gastrointestinal disorder	1.9%	2.5%
Vomiting	1.9%	2.5%
Dry mouth	2.5%	1.4%
Metabolic and Nutritional Disorders		
Peripheral edema	4.2%	1.6%
Musculoskeletal System		
Arthralgia	11.5%	14.2%
Traumatic bone fracture	5.0%	6.4%
Myalgia	4.6%	6.2%
Arthritis	4.8%	4.1%
Bursitis	1.3%	2.5%
Bone pain	2.9%	1.4%
Nervous System		
Dizziness	5.8%	4.9%
Anxiety	0.6%	2.7%
Depression	2.3%	2.3%
Vertigo	2.1%	1.6%
Respiratory System		
Bronchitis	2.3%	4.9%
Sinusitis	4.6%	4.5%
Pharyngitis	4.6%	2.9%
Cough increased	3.1%	2.5%
Pneumonia	0.8%	2.5%
Rhinitis	2.3%	2.1%
Skin and Appendages		
Rash	3.1%	4.1%
Pruritus	1.9%	2.3%
Special Senses		
Cataract	2.9%	1.9%
Urogenital System		
Urinary tract infection	2.9%	5.2%

Risedronate sodium has been studied in 392 patients with Paget's disease of bone. As in trials of risedronate sodium for other indications, the adverse experiences reported in the Paget's disease trials have generally been mild or moderate, have not required discontinuation of treatment, and have not appeared to be related to patient age, gender, or race.

In a double-blind, active-controlled study, the adverse event profile was similar for risedronate sodium and etidronate disodium: 6.6% (4/61) of patients treated with risedronate sodium 30 mg/day for 2 months discontinued treatment due to adverse events, compared with 8.2% (5/61) of patients treated with etidronate disodium 400 mg/day for 6 months.

TABLE 7 *Adverse Events Reported in ≥2% of Risedronate Sodium-Treated Patients* in Phase 3 Paget's Disease Trials*

Body System	30 mg/day × 2 months Risedronate Sodium (n=61)	400 mg/day × 6 months Etidronate Disodium (n=61)
Body as a Whole		
Flu syndrome	9.8%	1.6%
Chest pain	6.6%	3.3%
Asthenia	4.9%	0%
Neoplasm	3.3%	1.6%
Gastrointestinal		
Diarrhea	19.7%	14.8%
Abdominal pain	11.5%	8.2%
Nausea	9.8%	9.8%
Constipation	6.6%	8.2%
Belching	3.3%	1.6%
Colitis	3.3%	3.3%
Metabolic & Nutritional Disorders		
Peripheral edema	8.2%	6.6%
Musculoskeletal		
Arthralgia	32.8%	29.5%
Bone pain	4.9%	4.9%
Leg cramps	3.3%	3.3%
Myasthenia	3.3%	0%
Nervous		
Headache	18.0%	16.4%
Dizziness	6.6%	4.9%
Respiratory		
Bronchitis	3.3%	4.9%
Sinusitis	4.9%	1.6%
Skin and Appendages		
Rash	11.5%	8.2%
Special Senses		
Amblyopia	3.3%	3.3%
Tinnitus	3.3%	3.3%
Dry eye	3.3%	0%

* Considered to be possibly or probably causally related in at least 1 patient.

Three patients that received risedronate sodium 30 mg/day experienced acute iritis in 1 supportive study. All 3 patients recovered from their events; however, in 1 of these patients, the event recurred during risedronate sodium treatment and again during treatment with pamidronate. All patients were effectively treated with topical steroids.

DOSAGE AND ADMINISTRATION

Risedronate sodium should be taken at least 30 minutes before the first food or drink of the day other than water.

To facilitate delivery to the stomach, risedronate sodium should be swallowed while the patient is in an upright position and with a full glass of plain water (6-8 oz). Patients should not lie down for 30 minutes after taking the medication (see PRECAUTIONS, General).

Patients should receive supplemental calcium and vitamin D if dietary intake is inadequate (see PRECAUTIONS, General). Calcium supplements and calcium-, aluminum-, and magnesium-containing medications may interfere with the absorption of risedronate sodium and should be taken at a different time of the day. Risedronate sodium is not recommended for use in patients with severe renal impairment (creatinine clearance <30 ml/min). No dosage adjustment is necessary in patients with a creatinine clearance ≥30 ml/min or in the elderly.

TREATMENT OF POSTMENOPAUSAL OSTEOPOROSIS

See INDICATIONS AND USAGE.

The recommended regimen is:

One 5 mg tablet orally, taken daily; or

One 35 mg tablet orally, taken once a week.

PREVENTION OF POSTMENOPAUSAL OSTEOPOROSIS

See INDICATIONS AND USAGE.

The recommended regimen is one 5 mg tablet orally, taken daily.

Alternatively, one 35 mg tablet orally, taken once a week may be considered.

TREATMENT AND PREVENTION OF GLUCOCORTICOID-INDUCED OSTEOPOROSIS

See INDICATIONS AND USAGE.

The recommended regimen is:

One 5 mg tablet orally, taken daily.

PAGET'S DISEASE

See INDICATIONS AND USAGE.

The recommended treatment regimen is 30 mg orally once daily for 2 months. Retreatment may be considered (following post-treatment observation of at least 2 months) if relapse occurs, or if treatment fails to normalize serum alkaline phosphatase. For retreatment, the dose and duration of therapy are the same as for initial treatment. No data are available on more than 1 course of retreatment.

R

ANIMAL PHARMACOLOGY

Risedronate demonstrated potent anti-osteoclast, antiresorptive activity in ovariectomized rats and minipigs. Bone mass and biomechanical strength were increased dose-dependently at oral doses up to 4 and 25 times the human recommended oral dose of 5 mg based on surface area, (mg/m^2) for rats and minipigs, respectively. Risedronate treatment maintained the positive correlation between BMD and bone strength and did not have a negative effect on bone structure or mineralization. In intact dogs, risedronate induced positive bone balance at the level of the bone remodeling unit at oral doses ranging from 0.35-1.4 times the human 5 mg dose based on surface area (mg/m^2).

In dogs treated with an oral dose of 1 mg/kg/day (approximately 5 times the human 5 mg dose based on surface area, mg/m^2), risedronate caused a delay in fracture healing of the radius. The observed delay in fracture healing is similar to other bisphosphonates. This effect did not occur at a dose of 0.1 mg/kg/day (approximately 0.5 times the human 5 mg dose based on surface area, mg/m^2).

The Schenk rat assay, based on histologic examination of the epiphyses of growing rats after drug treatment, demonstrated that risedronate did not interfere with bone mineralization even at the highest dose tested (5 mg/kg/day, subcutaneously), which was approximately 3500 times the lowest antiresorptive dose (1.5 µg/kg/day in this model) and approximately 8 times the human 5 mg dose based on surface area, (mg/m^2). This indicates that risedronate sodium administered at the therapeutic dose is unlikely to induce osteomalacia.

HOW SUPPLIED

Actonel is supplied as follows:

5 mg: Film-coated, oval, yellow tablets with "RSN" on 1 face and "5 mg" on the other.
30 mg: Film-coated, oval, white tablets with "RSN" on 1 face and "30 mg" on the other.
35 mg: Film-coated, oval, orange tablets with "RSN" on 1 face and "35 mg" on the other.

Storage: Store at controlled room temperature 20-25°C (68-77°F).

PRODUCT LISTING - EQUIVALENTS NOT AVAILABLE

Tablet - Oral - 5 mg

30's	$71.21	ACTONEL, Procter and Gamble Pharmaceuticals	00149-0471-01

Tablet - Oral - 30 mg

30's	$498.49	ACTONEL, Procter and Gamble Pharmaceuticals	00149-0470-01

Tablet - Oral - 35 mg

4's	$66.46	ACTONEL, Procter and Gamble Pharmaceuticals	00149-0472-01

Risperidone *(003165)*

Categories: Psychosis; Schizophrenia; FDA Approved 1993 Dec; Pregnancy Category C
Drug Classes: Antipsychotics
Brand Names: Risperdal
Foreign Brand Availability: Neripros (Indonesia); Noprenia (Indonesia); Risperdal Consta (England; Ireland; New-Zealand); Rispid (India); Rizodal (Indonesia); Tractal (Colombia); Zofredal (Indonesia)
Cost of Therapy: $219.03 (Schizophrenia; Risperdal; 4 mg; 1 tablet/day; 30 day supply)
$319.13 (Schizophrenia; Risperdal; 2 mg; 2 tablets/day; 30 day supply)

DESCRIPTION

Risperdal is a psychotropic agent belonging to the chemical class of benzisoxazole derivatives. The chemical designation is 3-[2-[4-(6-fluoro-1,2-benzisoxazol-3-yl)-1-piperidinyl]ethyl]-6,7,8,9-tetrahydro- 2-methyl-4H-pyrido[1,2-a]pyrimidin-4-one. Its molecular formula is $C_{23}H_{27}FN_4O_2$ and its molecular weight is 410.49.

Risperidone is a white to slightly beige powder. It is practically insoluble in water, freely soluble in methylene chloride, and soluble in methanol and 0.1 N HCl.

Risperdal tablets are available in 0.25 mg (dark yellow), 0.5 mg (red-brown), 1 mg (white), 2 mg (orange), 3 mg (yellow), and 4 mg (green) strengths. Inactive ingredients are colloidal silicon dioxide, hydroxypropyl methylcellulose, lactose, magnesium stearate, microcrystalline cellulose, propylene glycol, sodium lauryl sulfate, and starch (corn). Tablets of 0.25, 0.5, 2, 3, and 4 mg also contain talc and titanium dioxide. The 0.25 mg tablets contain yellow iron oxide; the 0.5 mg tablets contain red iron oxide; the 2 mg tablets contain FD&C yellow no. 6 aluminum lake; the 3 mg and 4 mg tablets contain D&C yellow no. 10; the 4 mg tablets contain FD&C blue no. 2 aluminum lake.

Risperdal is also available as a 1 mg/ml oral solution. The inactive ingredients for this solution are tartaric acid, benzoic acid, sodium hydroxide, and purified water.

Risperdal M-TAB orally disintegrating tablets are available in 0.5 mg, 1.0 mg, and 2.0 mg strengths and are light coral in color.

Risperdal M-TAB orally disintegrating tablets contain the following inactive ingredients: Amberlite resin, gelatin, mannitol, glycine, simethicone, carbomer, sodium hydroxide, aspartame, red ferric oxide, and peppermint oil.

CLINICAL PHARMACOLOGY

PHARMACODYNAMICS

The mechanism of action of risperidone, as with other drugs used to treat schizophrenia, is unknown. However, it has been proposed that the drug's therapeutic activity in schizophrenia is mediated through a combination of dopamine Type 2 (D_2) and serotonin Type 2 ($5HT_2$) receptor antagonism. Antagonism at receptors other than D_2 and $5HT_2$ may explain some of the other effects of risperidone.

Risperidone is a selective monoaminergic antagonist with high affinity (Ki of 0.12-7.3 nM) for the serotonin Type 2 ($5HT_2$), dopamine Type 2 (D_2), α_1 and α_2 adrenergic, and H_1 histaminergic receptors. Risperidone acts as an antagonist at other receptors, but with lower potency. Risperidone has low to moderate affinity (Ki of 47-253 nM) for the serotonin $5HT_{1C}$, $5HT_{1D}$, and $5HT_{1A}$ receptors, weak affinity (Ki of 620-800 nM) for the dopamine D1 and haloperidol-sensitive sigma site, and no affinity (when tested at concentrations $>10^{-5}$ M) for cholinergic muscarinic or β_1 and β_2 adrenergic receptors.

PHARMACOKINETICS

Absorption

Risperidone is well absorbed. The absolute oral bioavailability of risperidone is 70% (CV = 25%). The relative oral bioavailability of risperidone from a tablet is 94% (CV = 10%) when compared to a solution.

Pharmacokinetic studies showed that risperidone orally disintegrating tablets are bioequivalent to risperidone tablets.

Plasma concentrations of risperidone, its major metabolite, 9-hydroxyrisperidone, and risperidone plus 9-hydroxyrisperidone are dose proportional over the dosing range of 1-16 mg daily (0.5-8 mg bid). Following oral administration of solution or tablet, mean peak plasma concentrations of risperidone occurred at about 1 hour. Peak concentrations of 9-hydroxyrisperidone occurred at about 3 hours in extensive metabolizers, and 17 hours in poor metabolizers. Steady-state concentrations of risperidone are reached in 1 day in extensive metabolizers and would be expected to reach steady state in about 5 days in poor metabolizers. Steady-state concentrations of 9-hydroxyrisperidone are reached in 5-6 days (measured in extensive metabolizers).

Food Effect

Food does not affect either the rate or extent of absorption of risperidone. Thus, risperidone can be given with or without meals.

Distribution

Risperidone is rapidly distributed. The volume of distribution is 1-2 L/kg. In plasma, risperidone is bound to albumin and α_1-acid glycoprotein. The plasma protein binding of risperidone is 90%, and that of its major metabolite, 9-hydroxyrisperidone, is 77%. Neither risperidone nor 9-hydroxyrisperidone displaces each other from plasma binding sites. High therapeutic concentrations of sulfamethazine (100 µg/ml), warfarin (10 µg/ml), and carbamazepine (10 µg/ml) caused only a slight increase in the free fraction of risperidone at 10 ng/ml and 9-hydroxyrisperidone at 50 ng/ml, changes of unknown clinical significance.

Metabolism

Risperidone is extensively metabolized in the liver. The main metabolic pathway is through hydroxylation of risperidone to 9-hydrox-yrisperidone by the enzyme, CYP 2D6. A minor metabolic pathway is through *N*-dealkylation. The main metabolite, 9-hydroxyrisperidone, has similar pharmacological activity as risperidone. Consequently, the clinical effect of the drug (*i.e.,* the active moiety) results from the combined concentrations of risperidone plus 9-hydroxyrisperidone.

CYP 2D6, also called debrisoquin hydroxylase, is the enzyme responsible for metabolism of many neuroleptics, antidepressants, antiarrhythmics, and other drugs. CYP 2D6 is subject to genetic polymorphism (about 6-8% of Caucasians, and a very low percentage of Asians, have little or no activity and are "poor metabolizers") and to inhibition by a variety of substrates and some non-substrates, notably quinidine. Extensive CYP 2D6 metabolizers convert risperidone rapidly into 9-hydroxyrisperidone, whereas poor CYP 2D6 metabolizers convert it much more slowly. Although extensive metabolizers have lower risperidone and higher 9-hydroxyrisperidone concentrations than poor metabolizers, the pharmacokinetics of the active moiety, after single and multiple doses, are similar in extensive and poor metabolizers.

Risperidone could be subject to two kinds of drug-drug interactions (see DRUG INTERACTIONS). First, inhibitors of CYP 2D6 interfere with conversion of risperidone to 9-hydroxyrisperidone. This occurs with quinidine, giving essentially all recipients a risperidone pharmacokinetic profile typical of poor metabolizers. The therapeutic benefits and adverse effects of risperidone in patients receiving quinidine have not been evaluated, but observations in a modest number ($n \sim 70$) of poor metabolizers given risperidone do not suggest important differences between poor and extensive metabolizers. Second, coadministration of known enzyme inducers (*e.g.,* phenytoin, rifampin, and phenobarbital) with risperidone may cause a decrease in the combined plasma concentrations of risperidone and 9-hydroxyrisperidone. It would also be possible for risperidone to interfere with metabolism of other drugs metabolized by CYP 2D6. Relatively weak binding of risperidone to the enzyme suggests this is unlikely.

Excretion

Risperidone and its metabolites are eliminated via the urine and, to a much lesser extent, via the feces. As illustrated by a mass balance study of a single 1 mg oral dose of ^{14}C-risperidone administered as solution to 3 healthy male volunteers, total recovery of radioactivity at 1 week was 84%, including 70% in the urine and 14% in the feces.

The apparent half-life of risperidone was 3 hours (CV = 30%) in extensive metabolizers and 20 hours (CV = 40%) in poor metabolizers. The apparent half-life of 9-hydroxyrisperidone was about 21 hours (CV = 20%) in extensive metabolizers and 30 hours (CV=25%) in poor metabolizers. The pharmacokinetics of the active moiety, after single and multiple doses, were similar in extensive and poor metabolizers, with an overall mean elimination half-life of about 20 hours.

SPECIAL POPULATIONS

Renal Impairment

In patients with moderate to severe renal disease, clearance of the sum of risperidone and its active metabolite decreased by 60% compared to young healthy subjects. Risperidone doses should be reduced in patients with renal disease (see PRECAUTIONS and DOSAGE AND ADMINISTRATION).

Hepatic Impairment

While the pharmacokinetics of risperidone in subjects with liver disease were comparable to those in young healthy subjects, the mean free fraction of risperidone in plasma was increased by about 35% because of the diminished concentration of both albumin and α_1-acid glycoprotein. Risperidone doses should be reduced in patients with liver disease (see PRECAUTIONS and DOSAGE AND ADMINISTRATION).

Elderly
In healthy elderly subjects renal clearance of both risperidone and 9-hydroxyrisperidone was decreased, and elimination half-lives were prolonged compared to young healthy subjects. Dosing should be modified accordingly in the elderly patients (see DOSAGE AND ADMINISTRATION).

Race and Gender Effects
No specific pharmacokinetic study was conducted to investigate race and gender effects, but a population pharmacokinetic analysis did not identify important differences in the disposition of risperidone due to gender (whether corrected for body weight or not) or race.

INDICATIONS AND USAGE

Risperidone is indicated for the treatment of schizophrenia.

The efficacy of risperidone in schizophrenia was established in short-term (6-8 weeks) controlled trials of schizophrenic inpatients (see CLINICAL PHARMACOLOGY).

The efficacy of risperidone in delaying relapse was demonstrated in schizophrenic patients who had been clinically stable for at least 4 weeks before initiation of treatment with risperidone or an active comparator and who were then observed for relapse during a period of 1-2 years. Nevertheless, the physician who elects to use risperidone for extended periods should periodically re-evaluate the long-term usefulness of the drug for the individual patient (see DOSAGE AND ADMINISTRATION).

NON-FDA APPROVED INDICATIONS

Risperidone has also been reported to be effective in decreasing the severity of stuttering, controlling agitation in patients with dementia, catatonia, and in the treatment of aggressive behavior in children with Tourette's syndrome. However, these uses have not been approved by the FDA and further clinical trials are needed before the drug can be recommended for these indications.

CONTRAINDICATIONS

Risperidone is contraindicated in patients with a known hypersensitivity to the product.

WARNINGS

NEUROLEPTIC MALIGNANT SYNDROME (NMS)

A potentially fatal symptom complex sometimes referred to as Neuroleptic Malignant Syndrome (NMS) has been reported in association with antipsychotic drugs. Clinical manifestations of NMS are hyperpyrexia, muscle rigidity, altered mental status, and evidence of autonomic instability (irregular pulse or blood pressure, tachycardia, diaphoresis, and cardiac dysrhythmia). Additional signs may include elevated creatine phosphokinase, myoglobinuria (rhabdomyolysis), and acute renal failure.

The diagnostic evaluation of patients with this syndrome is complicated. In arriving at a diagnosis, it is important to identify cases in which the clinical presentation includes both serious medical illness (*e.g.*, pneumonia, systemic infection, etc.) and untreated or inadequately treated extrapyramidal signs and symptoms (EPS). Other important considerations in the differential diagnosis include central anticholinergic toxicity, heat stroke, drug fever, and primary central nervous system pathology.

The management of NMS should include: (1) immediate discontinuation of antipsychotic drugs and other drugs not essential to concurrent therapy; (2) intensive symptomatic treatment and medical monitoring; and (3) treatment of any concomitant serious medical problems for which specific treatments are available. There is no general agreement about specific pharmacological treatment regimens for uncomplicated NMS.

If a patient requires antipsychotic drug treatment after recovery from NMS, the potential reintroduction of drug therapy should be carefully considered. The patient should be carefully monitored, since recurrences of NMS have been reported.

TARDIVE DYSKINESIA

A syndrome of potentially irreversible, involuntary, dyskinetic movements may develop in patients treated with antipsychotic drugs. Although the prevalence of the syndrome appears to be highest among the elderly, especially elderly women, it is impossible to rely upon prevalence estimates to predict, at the inception of antipsychotic treatment, which patients are likely to develop the syndrome. Whether antipsychotic drug products differ in their potential to cause tardive dyskinesia is unknown.

The risk of developing tardive dyskinesia and the likelihood that it will become irreversible are believed to increase as the duration of treatment and the total cumulative dose of antipsychotic drugs administered to the patient increase. However, the syndrome can develop, although much less commonly, after relatively brief treatment periods at low doses.

There is no known treatment for established cases of tardive dyskinesia, although the syndrome may remit, partially or completely, if antipsychotic treatment is withdrawn. Antipsychotic treatment, itself, however, may suppress (or partially suppress) the signs and symptoms of the syndrome and thereby may possibly mask the underlying process. The effect that symptomatic suppression has upon the long-term course of the syndrome is unknown.

Given these considerations, risperidone should be prescribed in a manner that is most likely to minimize the occurrence of tardive dyskinesia. Chronic antipsychotic treatment should generally be reserved for patients who suffer from a chronic illness that (1) is known to respond to antipsychotic drugs, and (2) for whom alternative, equally effective, but potentially less harmful treatments are not available or appropriate. In patients who do require chronic treatment, the smallest dose and the shortest duration of treatment producing a satisfactory clinical response should be sought. The need for continued treatment should be reassessed periodically.

If signs and symptoms of tardive dyskinesia appear in a patient treated on risperidone, drug discontinuation should be considered. However, some patients may require treatment with risperidone despite the presence of the syndrome.

CEREBROVASCULAR ADVERSE EVENTS, INCLUDING STROKE, IN ELDERLY PATIENTS WITH DEMENTIA

Cerebrovascular adverse events (*e.g.*, stroke, transient ischemic attack), including fatalities, were reported in patients (mean age 85 years; range 73-97) in trials of risperidone in elderly patients with dementia-related psychosis. In placebo-controlled trials, there was a significantly higher incidence of cerebrovascular adverse events in patients treated with risperidone compared to patients treated with placebo. Risperidone has not been shown to be safe or effective in the treatment of patients with dementia-related psychosis.

POTENTIAL FOR PROARRHYTHMIC EFFECTS

Risperidone and/or 9-hydroxyrisperidone appear to lengthen the QT interval in some patients, although there is no average increase in treated patients, even at 12-16 mg/day, well above the recommended dose. Other drugs that prolong the QT interval have been associated with the occurrence of torsades de pointes, a life-threatening arrhythmia. Bradycardia, electrolyte imbalance, concomitant use with other drugs that prolong QT, or the presence of congenital prolongation in QT can increase the risk for occurrence of this arrhythmia.

PRECAUTIONS

GENERAL

Orthostatic Hypotension
Risperidone may induce orthostatic hypotension associated with dizziness, tachycardia, and in some patients, syncope, especially during the initial dose-titration period, probably reflecting its alpha-adrenergic antagonistic properties. Syncope was reported in 0.2% (6/2607) of risperidone-treated patients in Phase 2-3 studies. The risk of orthostatic hypotension and syncope may be minimized by limiting the initial dose to 2 mg total (either qd or 1 mg bid) in normal adults and 0.5 mg bid in the elderly and patients with renal or hepatic impairment (see DOSAGE AND ADMINISTRATION). Monitoring of orthostatic vital signs should be considered in patients for whom this is of concern. A dose reduction should be considered if hypotension occurs. Risperidone should be used with particular caution in patients with known cardiovascular disease (history of myocardial infarction or ischemia, heart failure, or conduction abnormalities), cerebrovascular disease, and conditions which would predispose patients to hypotension, *e.g.*, dehydration and hypovolemia. Clinically significant hypotension has been observed with concomitant use of risperidone and antihypertensive medication.

Seizures
During premarketing testing, seizures occurred in 0.3% (9/2607) of risperidone-treated patients, two in association with hyponatremia. Risperidone should be used cautiously in patients with a history of seizures.

Dysphagia
Esophageal dysmotility and aspiration have been associated with antipsychotic drug use. Aspiration pneumonia is a common cause of morbidity and mortality in patients with advanced Alzheimer's dementia. Risperidone and other antipsychotic drugs should be used cautiously in patients at risk for aspiration pneumonia.

Hyperprolactinemia
As with other drugs that antagonize dopamine D_2 receptors, risperidone elevates prolactin levels and the elevation persists during chronic administration. Tissue culture experiments indicate that approximately one-third of human breast cancers are prolactin dependent *in vitro*, a factor of potential importance if the prescription of these drugs is contemplated in a patient with previously detected breast cancer. Although disturbances such as galactorrhea, amenorrhea, gynecomastia, and impotence have been reported with prolactin-elevating compounds, the clinical significance of elevated serum prolactin levels is unknown for most patients. As is common with compounds which increase prolactin release, an increase in pituitary gland, mammary gland, and pancreatic islet cell hyperplasia and/or neoplasia was observed in the risperidone carcinogenicity studies conducted in mice and rats (see Carcinogenesis). However, neither clinical studies nor epidemiologic studies conducted to date have shown an association between chronic administration of this class of drugs and tumorigenesis in humans; the available evidence is considered too limited to be conclusive at this time.

Potential for Cognitive and Motor Impairment
Somnolence was a commonly reported adverse event associated with risperidone treatment, especially when ascertained by direct questioning of patients. This adverse event is dose-related, and in a study utilizing a checklist to detect adverse events, 41% of the high dose patients (risperidone 16 mg/day) reported somnolence compared to 16% of placebo patients. Direct questioning is more sensitive for detecting adverse events than spontaneous reporting, by which 8% of risperidone 16 mg/day patients and 1% of placebo patients reported somnolence as an adverse event. Since risperidone has the potential to impair judgment, thinking, or motor skills, patients should be cautioned about operating hazardous machinery, including automobiles, until they are reasonably certain that risperidone therapy does not affect them adversely.

Priapism
Rare cases of priapism have been reported. While the relationship of the events to risperidone use has not been established, other drugs with α-adrenergic blocking effects have been reported to induce priapism, and it is possible that risperidone may share this capacity. Severe priapism may require surgical intervention.

Thrombotic Thrombocytopenic Purpura (TTP)
A single case of TTP was reported in a 28-year-old female patient receiving risperidone in a large, open premarketing experience (approximately 1300 patients). She experienced jaundice, fever, and bruising, but eventually recovered after receiving plasmapheresis. The relationship to risperidone therapy is unknown.

R

Antiemetic Effect

Risperidone has an antiemetic effect in animals; this effect may also occur in humans, and may mask signs and symptoms of overdosage with certain drugs or of conditions such as intestinal obstruction, Reye's syndrome, and brain tumor.

Body Temperature Regulation

Disruption of body temperature regulation has been attributed to antipsychotic agents. Both hyperthermia and hypothermia have been reported in association with oral risperidone use. Caution is advised when prescribing for patients who will be exposed to temperature extremes.

Suicide

The possibility of a suicide attempt is inherent in schizophrenia, and close supervision of high-risk patients should accompany drug therapy. Prescriptions for risperidone should be written for the smallest quantity of tablets, consistent with good patient management, in order to reduce the risk of overdose.

Use in Patients With Concomitant Illness

Clinical experience with risperidone in patients with certain concomitant systemic illnesses is limited. Caution is advisable in using risperidone in patients with diseases or conditions that could affect metabolism or hemodynamic responses.

Risperidone has not been evaluated or used to any appreciable extent in patients with a recent history of myocardial infarction or unstable heart disease. Patients with these diagnoses were excluded from clinical studies during the product's premarket testing. The electrocardiograms of approximately 380 patients who received risperidone and 120 patients who received placebo in two double-blind, placebo-controlled trials were evaluated and the data revealed one finding of potential concern, *i.e.,* 8 patients taking risperidone whose baseline QTc interval was less than 450 msec were observed to have QTc intervals greater than 450 msec during treatment; no such prolongations were seen in the smaller placebo group. There were 3 such episodes in the approximately 125 patients who received haloperidol. Because of the risks of orthostatic hypotension and QT prolongation, caution should be observed in cardiac patients (see WARNINGS and PRECAUTIONS).

Increased plasma concentrations of risperidone and 9-hydroxyrisperidone occur in patients with severe renal impairment (creatinine clearance <30 ml/min/1.73 m^2), and an increase in the free fraction of risperidone is seen in patients with severe hepatic impairment. A lower starting dose should be used in such patients (see DOSAGE AND ADMINISTRATION).

INFORMATION FOR THE PATIENT

Physicians are advised to discuss the following issues with patients for whom they prescribe risperidone:

- **Orthostatic hypotension:** Patients should be advised of the risk of orthostatic hypotension, especially during the period of initial dose titration.
- **Interference with cognitive and motor performance:** Since risperidone has the potential to impair judgment, thinking, or motor skills, patients should be cautioned about operating hazardous machinery, including automobiles, until they are reasonably certain that risperidone therapy does not affect them adversely.
- **Pregnancy:** Patients should be advised to notify their physician if they become pregnant or intend to become pregnant during therapy.
- **Nursing:** Patients should be advised not to breast-feed an infant if they are taking risperidone.
- **Concomitant medication:** Patients should be advised to inform their physicians if they are taking, or plan to take, any prescription or over-the-counter drugs, since there is a potential for interactions.
- **Alcohol:** Patients should be advised to avoid alcohol while taking risperidone.
- **Phenylketonurics:** Phenylalanine is a component of aspartame. Each 2 mg risperidone orally disintegrating tablet contains 0.56 mg phenylalanine; each 1 mg risperidone orally disintegrating tablet contains 0.28 mg phenylalanine; and each 0.5 mg risperidone orally disintegrating tablet contains 0.14 mg phenylalanine.

LABORATORY TESTS

No specific laboratory tests are recommended.

CARCINOGENESIS, MUTAGENESIS, AND IMPAIRMENT OF FERTILITY

Carcinogenesis

Carcinogenicity studies were conducted in Swiss albino mice and Wistar rats. Risperidone was administered in the diet at doses of 0.63, 2.5, and 10 mg/kg for 18 months to mice and for 25 months to rats. These doses are equivalent to 2.4, 9.4, and 37.5 times the maximum recommended human dose (MRHD) (16 mg/day) on a mg/kg basis or 0.2, 0.75, and 3 times the MRHD (mice) or 0.4, 1.5, and 6 times the MRHD (rats) on a mg/m^2 basis. A maximum tolerated dose was not achieved in male mice. There were statistically significant increases in pituitary gland adenomas, endocrine pancreas adenomas, and mammary gland adenocarcinomas. TABLE 1 summarizes the multiples of the human dose on a mg/m^2 (mg/kg) basis at which these tumors occurred.

Antipsychotic drugs have been shown to chronically elevate prolactin levels in rodents. Serum prolactin levels were not measured during the risperidone carcinogenicity studies; however, measurements during subchronic toxicity studies showed that risperidone elevated serum prolactin levels 5- to 6-fold in mice and rats at the same doses used in the carcinogenicity studies. An increase in mammary, pituitary, and endocrine pancreas neoplasms has been found in rodents after chronic administration of other antipsychotic drugs and is considered to be prolactin-mediated. The relevance for human risk of the findings of prolactin-mediated endocrine tumors in rodents is unknown (see Hyperprolactinemia).

Mutagenesis

No evidence of mutagenic potential for risperidone was found in the Ames reverse mutation test, mouse lymphoma assay, *in vitro* rat hepatocyte DNA-repair assay, *in vivo* micronucleus test in mice, the sex-linked recessive lethal test in *Drosophila,* or the chromosomal aberration test in human lymphocytes or Chinese hamster cells.

TABLE 1

Tumor Type	Species	Sex	Multiples of Maximum Human Dose in mg/m^2 (mg/kg): Lowest Effect Level	Highest No-Effect Level
Pituitary adenomas	mouse	female	0.75 (9.4)	0.2 (2.4)
Endocrine pancreas adenomas	rat	male	1.5 (9.4)	0.4 (2.4)
Mammary gland adenocarcinomas	mouse	female	0.2 (2.4)	none
	rat	female	0.4 (2.4)	none
	rat	male	6 (37.5)	1.5 (9.4)
Mammary gland neoplasms, total	rat	male	1.5 (9.4)	0.4 (2.4)

Impairment of Fertility

Risperidone (0.16-5 mg/kg) was shown to impair mating, but not fertility, in Wistar rats in three reproductive studies (two Segment I and a multigenerational study) at doses 0.1-3 times the maximum recommended human dose MRHD) on a mg/m^2 basis. The effect appeared to be in females, since impaired mating behavior was not noted in the Segment I study in which males only were treated. In a subchronic study in Beagle dogs in which risperidone was administered at doses of 0.31-5 mg/kg, sperm motility and concentration were decreased at doses 0.6-10 times the MRHD on a mg/m^2 basis. Dose-related decreases were also noted in serum testosterone at the same doses. Serum testosterone and sperm parameters partially recovered, but remained decreased after treatment was discontinued. No no-effect doses were noted in either rat or dog.

PREGNANCY CATEGORY C

The teratogenic potential of risperidone was studied in three Segment II studies in Sprague-Dawley and Wistar rats (0.63-10 mg/kg or 0.4-6 times the MRHD on a mg/m^2 basis) and in one Segment II study in New Zealand rabbits (0.31-5 mg/kg or 0.4-6 times the MRHD on a mg/m^2 basis). The incidence of malformations was not increased compared to control in offspring of rats or rabbits given 0.4-6 times the MRHD on a mg/m^2 basis. In three reproductive studies in rats (two Segment III and a multigenerational study), there was an increase in pup deaths during the first 4 days of lactation at doses of 0.16-5 mg/kg or 0.1-3 times the MRHD on a mg/m^2 basis. It is not known whether these deaths were due to a direct effect on the fetuses or pups or to effects on the dams.

There was no no-effect dose for increased rat pup mortality. In one Segment III study, there was an increase in stillborn rat pups at a dose of 2.5 mg/kg or 1.5 times the MRHD on a mg/m^2 basis. In a cross-fostering study in Wistar rats, toxic effects on the fetus or pups, as evidenced by a decrease in the number of live pups and an increase in the number of dead pups at birth (Day 0), and a decrease in birth weight in pups of drug-treated dams were observed. In addition, there was an increase in deaths by Day 1 among pups of drug-treated dams, regardless of whether or not the pups were cross-fostered. Risperidone also appeared to impair maternal behavior in that pup body weight gain and survival (from Day 1-4 of lactation) were reduced in pups born to control but reared by drug-treated dams. These effects were all noted at the 1 dose of risperidone tested, *i.e.,* 5 mg/kg or 3 times the MRHD on a mg/m^2 basis.

Placental transfer of risperidone occurs in rat pups. There are no adequate and well-controlled studies in pregnant women. However, there was one report of a case of agenesis of the corpus callosum in an infant exposed to risperidone in utero. The causal relationship to risperidone therapy is unknown.

Risperidone should be used during pregnancy only if the potential benefit justifies the potential risk to the fetus.

LABOR AND DELIVERY

The effect of risperidone on labor and delivery in humans is unknown.

NURSING MOTHERS

In animal studies, risperidone and 9-hydroxyrisperidone are excreted in milk. Risperidone and 9-hydroxyrisperidone are also excreted in human breast milk. Therefore, women receiving risperidone should not breast-feed.

PEDIATRIC USE

Safety and effectiveness in children have not been established.

GERIATRIC USE

Clinical studies of risperidone did not include sufficient numbers of patients aged 65 and over to determine whether or not they respond differently than younger patients. Other reported clinical experience has not identified differences in responses between elderly and younger patients. In general, a lower starting dose recommended for an elderly patient, reflecting a decreased pharmacokinetic clearance in the elderly, as well a greater frequency of decreased hepatic, renal, or cardiac function, and of concomitant disease or other drug therapy (see CLINICAL PHARMACOLOGY and DOSAGE AND ADMINISTRATION). While elderly patients exhibit a greater tendency to orthostatic hypotension, its risk in the elderly may be minimized by limiting initial dose to 0.5 mg bid followed by careful titration (see PRECAUTIONS). Monitoring of orthostatic vital signs should be considered in patients for whom this is of concern.

This drug is substantially excreted by the kidneys, and the risk of toxic reactions to this drug may be greater patients with impaired renal function. Because elderly patients are more likely to have decreased renal function, care should be taken in dose selection, and it may be useful to monitor renal function (see DOSAGE AND ADMINISTRATION).

DRUG INTERACTIONS

The interactions of risperidone and other drugs have not been systematically evaluated. Given the primary CNS effects of risperidone, caution should be used when risperidone is taken in combination with other centrally acting drugs and alcohol.

Because of its potential for inducing hypotension, risperidone may enhance the hypotensive effects of other therapeutic agents with this potential.

Risperidone may antagonize the effects of levodopa and dopamine agonists.

Chronic administration of clozapine with risperidone may decrease the clearance of risperidone.

CARBAMAZEPINE AND OTHER ENZYME INDUCERS

In a drug interaction study in schizophrenic patients, 11 subjects received risperidone titrated to 6 mg/day for 3 weeks, followed by concurrent administration of carbamazepine for an additional 3 weeks. During coadministration, the plasma concentrations of risperidone and its pharmacologically active metabolite, 9-hydroxyrisperidone, were decreased by about 50%. Plasma concentrations of carbamazepine did not appear to be affected. The dose of risperidone may need to be titrated accordingly for patients receiving carbamazepine, particularly during initiation or discontinuation of carbamazepine therapy. Coadministration of other known enzyme inducers (*e.g.*, phenytoin, rifampin, and phenobarbital) with risperidone may cause similar decreases in the combined plasma concentrations of risperidone and 9-hydroxyrisperidone, which could lead to decreased efficacy of risperidone treatment.

FLUOXETINE

Fluoxetine (20 mg qd) has been shown to increase the plasma concentration of risperidone 2.5- to 2.8-fold, while the plasma concentration of 9-hydroxyrisperidone was not affected. When concomitant fluoxetine is initiated or discontinued, the physician should re-evaluate the dosing of risperidone. The effects of discontinuation of concomitant fluoxetine therapy on the pharmacokinetics of risperidone and 9-hydroxyrisperidone have not been studied.

LITHIUM

Repeated oral doses of risperidone (3 mg bid) did not affect the exposure (AUC) or peak plasma concentrations (C_{max}) of lithium (n=13).

VALPROATE

Repeated oral doses of risperidone (4 mg qd) did not affect the pre-dose or average plasma concentrations exposure (AUC) of valproate (1000 mg/day in three divided doses) compared to placebo (n=21). However, there was a 20% increase in valproate peak plasma concentration (C_{max}) after concomitant administration of risperidone.

DRUGS THAT INHIBIT CYP 2D6 AND OTHER CYP ISOZYMES

Risperidone is metabolized to 9-hydroxyrisperidone by CYP 2D6, an enzyme that is polymorphic in the population and that can be inhibited by a variety of psychotropic and other drugs (see CLINICAL PHARMACOLOGY). Drug interactions that reduce the metabolism of risperidone to 9-hydroxyrisperidone would increase the plasma concentrations of risperidone and lower the concentrations of 9-hydroxyrisperidone. Analysis of clinical studies involving a modest number of poor metabolizers (n~70) does not suggest that poor and extensive metabolizers have different rates of adverse effects. No comparison of effectiveness in the two groups has been made.

In vitro studies showed that drugs metabolized by other CYP isozymes, including 1A1, 1A2, 2C9, MP, and 3A4, are only weak inhibitors of risperidone metabolism.

DRUGS METABOLIZED BY CYP 2D6

In vitro studies indicate that risperidone is a relatively weak inhibitor of CYP 2D6. Therefore, risperidone is not expected to substantially inhibit the clearance of drugs that are metabolized by this enzymatic pathway. However, clinical data to confirm this expectation are not available.

ADVERSE REACTIONS

ASSOCIATED WITH DISCONTINUATION OF TREATMENT

Approximately 9% (244/2607) of risperidone (risperidone)-treated patients in Phase 2-3 studies discontinued treatment due to an adverse event, compared with about 7% on placebo and 10% on active control drugs. The more common events (≥0.3%) associated with discontinuation and considered to be possibly or probably drug-related are shown in TABLE 2.

TABLE 2

Adverse Event	Risperidone	Placebo
Extrapyramidal symptoms	2.1%	0%
Dizziness	0.7%	0%
Hyperkinesia	0.6%	0%
Somnlence	0.5%	0%
Nausea	0.3%	0%

Suicide attempt was associated with discontinuation in 1.2% of risperidone-treated patients compared 0.6% of placebo patients, but, given the almost 40-fold greater exposure time in risperidone compared placebo patients, it is unlikely that suicide attempt is a risperidone related adverse event (see PRECAUTIONS). Discontinuation for extrapyramidal symptoms was 0% in placebo patients, but 3.8% active-control patients in the Phase 2-3 trials.

INCIDENCE IN CONTROLLED TRIALS

Commonly Observed Adverse Events in Controlled Clinical Trials

In two 6-8 week placebo-controlled trials, spontaneously-reported, treatment-emergent adverse events with an incidence of 5% or greater in at least one of the risperidone groups and at least twice that of placebo were: anxiety, somnolence, extrapyramidal symptoms, dizziness, constipation, nausea, dyspepsia, rhinitis, rash, and tachycardia.

Adverse events were also elicited in one of these two trials (*i.e.*, in the fixed-dose trial comparing risperidone at doses of 2, 6, 10, and 16 mg/day with placebo) utilizing a checklist for detecting adverse events, a method that is more sensitive than spontaneous reporting. By this method, the following additional common and drug-related adverse events occurred at an incidence of at least 5% and twice the rate of placebo: increased dream activity, increased duration of sleep, accommodation disturbances, reduced salivation, micturition disturbances, diarrhea, weight gain, menorrhagia, diminished sexual desire, erectile dysfunction, ejaculatory dysfunction, and orgastic dysfunction.

Adverse Events Occurring at an Incidence of 1% or More Among Risperidone-Treated Patients

TABLE 3 enumerates adverse events that occurred at an incidence of 1% or more, and were at least frequent among risperidone-treated patients treated at doses of ≤10 mg/day than among placebo-treated patients in the pooled results of two 6-8 week controlled trials. Patients received risperidone doses of 2, 6, 10, or 16 mg/day in the dose comparison trial, or up to a maximum dose of 10 mg/day in the titration study. TABLE 3 shows the percentage of patients in each dose group (≤10 mg/day or 16 mg/day) who spontaneously reported at least one episode of an event at some time during their treatment. Patients given doses of 2, 6, or 10 mg did not differ materially in these rates. Reported adverse events were classified using the World Health Organization preferred terms.

The prescriber should be aware that these figures cannot be used to predict the incidence of side effects in course of usual medical practice where patient characteristics and other factors differ from those which prevailed in this clinical trial. Similarly, the cited frequencies cannot be compared with figures obtained from other clinical investigations involving different treatments, uses and investigators. The cited figures, however, do provide the prescribing physician with some basis for estimating the relative contribution of drug and non-drug factors to the side effect incidence rate in the population studied.

***TABLE 3** Incidence of Treatment-Emergent Adverse Events in 6-8 Week Controlled Clinical Trials**

Body System	Risperidone		
Preferred Term	≤10 mg/day (n=324)	16 mg/day (n=77)	Placebo (n=142)
Psychiatric			
Insomnia	26%	23%	19%
Agitation	22%	26%	20%
Anxiety	12%	20%	9%
Somnolence	3%	8%	1%
Aggressive reaction	1%	3%	1%
Central and Peripheral Nervous System			
Extrapyramidal symptoms†	17%	34%	16%
Headache	14%	12%	12%
Dizziness	4%	7%	1%
Gastrointestinal			
Constipation	7%	13%	3%
Nausea	6%	4%	3%
Dyspepsia	5%	10%	4%
Vomiting	5%	7%	4%
Abdominal pain	4%	1%	0%
Saliva increased	2%	0%	1%
Toothache	2%	0%	0%
Respiratory System			
Rhinitis	10%	8%	4%
Coughing	3%	3%	1%
Sinusitis	2%	1%	1%
Pharyngitis	2%	3%	0%
Dyspnea	1%	0%	0%
Body as a Whole — General			
Back pain	2%	0%	1%
Chest pain	2%	3%	1%
Fever	2%	3%	0%
Dermatological			
Rash	2%	5%	1%
Dry skin	2%	4%	0%
Seborrhea	1%	0%	0%
Infections			
Upper respiratory	3%	3%	1%
Visual			
Abnormal vision	2%	1%	1%
Musculoskeletal			
Arthralgia	2%	3%	0%
Cardiovascular			
Tachycardia	3%	5%	0%

* Events reported by at least 1% of patients treated with risperidone ≤10 mg/day are included, and are rounded to the nearest %. Comparative rates for risperidone 16 mg/day and placebo are provided as well. Events for which the risperidone incidence (in both dose groups) was equal to or less than placebo are not listed in the table, but included the following: nervousness, injury, and fungal infection.

† Includes tremor, dystonia, hypokinesia, hypertonia, hyperkinesia, oculogyric crisis, ataxia, abnormal gait, involuntary muscle contractions, hyporeflexia, akathisia, and extrapyramidal disorders. Although the incidence of "extrapyramidal symptoms" does not appear to differ for the "10 mg/day" group and placebo, the data for individual dose groups in fixed dose trials do suggest a dose/response relationship (see Dose Dependency of Adverse Events).

Dose Dependency of Adverse Events

Extrapyramidal Symptoms

Data from two fixed-dose trials provided evidence of dose-relatedness for extrapyramidal symptoms associated with risperidone treatment.

Two methods were used to measure EPS in an 8 week trial comparing 4 fixed doses of risperidone (2, 6, 10, and 16 mg/day), including (1) a parkinsonism score (mean change from baseline) from the Extrapyramidal Symptom Rating Scale, and (2) incidence of spontaneous complaints of EPS (see TABLE 4).

Similar methods were used to measure extrapyramidal symptoms (EPS) in an 8 week trial comparing 5 fixed doses of risperidone (1, 4, 8, 12, and 16 mg/day) (see TABLE 5).

Other Adverse Events

Adverse event data elicited by a checklist for side effects from a large study comparing 5 fixed doses of risperidone (1, 4, 8, 12, and 16 mg/day) were explored for dose-relatedness

R

TABLE 4

Dose Groups	Parkinsonism	EPS Incidence
Placebo	1.2	13%
Ris 2	0.9	13%
Ris 6	1.8	16%
Ris 10	2.4	20%
Ris 16	2.6	31%

TABLE 5

Dose Groups	Parkinsonism	EPS Incidence
Ris 1	0.6	7%
Ris 4	1.7	12%
Ris 8	2.4	18%
Ris 12	2.9	18%
Ris 16	4.1	21%

of adverse events. A Cochran-Armitage Test for trend in these data revealed a positive trend ($p < 0.05$) for the following adverse events: sleepiness, increased duration of sleep, accommodation disturbances, orthostatic dizziness, palpitations, weight gain, erectile dysfunction, ejaculatory dysfunction, orgastic dysfunction, asthenia/lassitude/increased fatigability, and increased pigmentation.

Vital Sign Changes

Risperidone is associated with orthostatic hypotension and tachycardia (see PRECAUTIONS).

Weight Changes

The proportions of risperidone and placebo-treated patients meeting a weight gain criterion of ≥7% of body weight were compared in a pool of 6-8 week, placebo-controlled trials, revealing a statistically significantly greater incidence of weight gain for risperidone (18%) compared to placebo (9%).

Laboratory Changes

A between-group comparison for 6-8 week placebo-controlled trials revealed no statistically significant risperidone/placebo differences in the proportions of patients experiencing potentially important changes in routine serum chemistry, hematology, or urinalysis parameters. Similarly, there were no risperidone/placebo differences in the incidence of discontinuations for changes in serum chemistry, hematology, or urinalysis. However, risperidone administration was associated with increases in serum prolactin (see PRECAUTIONS).

ECG Changes

The electrocardiograms of approximately 380 patients who received risperidone and 120 patients who received placebo in two double-blind, placebo-controlled trials were evaluated and revealed one finding of potential concern; *i.e.,* 8 patients taking risperidone whose baseline QTc interval was less than 450 msec were observed to have QTc intervals greater than 450 msec during treatment (see WARNINGS). Changes of this type were not seen among about 120 placebo patients, but were seen in patients receiving haloperidol (3/126).

OTHER EVENTS OBSERVED DURING THE PREMARKETING EVALUATION OF RISPERIDONE

During its premarketing assessment, multiple doses of risperidone were administered to 2607 patients in Phase 2 and 3 studies. The conditions and duration of exposure to risperidone varied greatly, and included (in overlapping categories) open-label and double-blind studies, uncontrolled and controlled studies, inpatient and outpatient studies, fixed-dose and titration studies, and short-term or longer-term exposure. In most studies, untoward events associated with this exposure were obtained by spontaneous report and recorded by clinical investigators using terminology of their own choosing. Consequently, it is not possible to provide a meaningful estimate of the proportion of individuals experiencing adverse events without first grouping similar types of untoward events into a smaller number of standardized event categories. In two large studies, adverse events were also elicited utilizing the UKU (direct questioning) side effect rating scale, and these events were not further categorized using standard terminology. (**Note:** These events are marked with an asterisk in the listings that follow.)

In the listings that follow, spontaneously reported adverse events were classified using WHO preferred terms. The frequencies presented, therefore, represent the proportion of the 2607 patients exposed to multiple doses of risperidone who experienced an event of the type cited on at least one occasion while receiving risperidone. All reported events are included, except those already listed in TABLE 3, those events for which a drug cause was remote, and those event terms which were so general as to be uninformative. It is important to emphasize that, although the events reported occurred during treatment with risperidone, they were not necessarily caused by it.

Events are further categorized by body system and listed in order of decreasing frequency according to the following definitions: *frequent* adverse events are those occurring in at least 1/100 patients (only those not already listed in the tabulated results from placebo-controlled trials appear in this listing); *infrequent* adverse events are those occurring in 1/100 to 1/1000 patients; *rare* events are those occurring in fewer than 1/1000 patients.

Psychiatric Disorders: *Frequent:* Increased dream activity,* diminished sexual desire,* nervousness. *Infrequent:* Impaired concentration, depression, apathy, catatonic reaction, euphoria, increased libido, amnesia. *Rare:* Emotional lability, nightmares, delirium, withdrawal syndrome, yawning.

Central and Peripheral Nervous System Disorders: *Frequent:* Increased sleep duration.* *Infrequent:* Dysarthria, vertigo, stupor, paraesthesia, confusion. *Rare:* Aphasia, cholinergic syndrome, hypoesthesia, tongue paralysis, leg cramps, torticollis, hypotonia, coma, migraine, hyperreflexia, choreoathetosis.

Gastrointestinal Disorders: *Frequent:* Anorexia, reduced salivation.* *Infrequent:* Flatulence, diarrhea, increased appetite, stomatitis, melena, dysphagia, hemorrhoids, gastritis. *Rare:* Fecal incontinence, eructation, gastroesophageal reflux, gastroenteritis, esophagitis, tongue discoloration, cholelithiasis, tongue edema, diverticulitis, gingivitis, discolored feces, GI hemorrhage, hematemesis.

Body as a Whole/General Disorders: *Frequent:* Fatigue. *Infrequent:* Edema, rigors, malaise, influenza-like symptoms. *Rare:* Pallor, enlarged abdomen, allergic reaction, ascites, sarcoidosis, flushing.

Respiratory System Disorders: *Infrequent:* Hyperventilation, bronchospasm, pneumonia, stridor. *Rare:* Asthma, increased sputum, aspiration.

Skin and Appendage Disorders: *Frequent:* Increased pigmentation,* photosensitivity.* *Infrequent:* Increased sweating, acne, decreased sweating, alopecia, hyperkeratosis, pruritus, skin exfoliation. *Rare:* Bullous eruption, skin ulceration, aggravated psoriasis, furunculosis, verruca, dermatitis lichenoid, hypertrichosis, genital pruritus, urticaria.

Cardiovascular Disorders: *Infrequent:* Palpitation, hypertension, hypotension, AV block, myocardial infarction. *Rare:* Ventricular tachycardia, angina pectoris, premature atrial contractions, T wave inversions, ventricular extrasystoles, ST depression, myocarditis.

Vision Disorders: *Infrequent:* Abnormal accommodation, xerophthalmia. *Rare:* Diplopia, eye pain, blepharitis, photopsia, photophobia, abnormal lacrimation.

Metabolic and Nutritional Disorders: *Infrequent:* Hyponatremia, weight increase, creatine phosphokinase increase, thirst, weight decrease, diabetes mellitus. *Rare:* Decreased serum iron, cachexia, dehydration, hypokalemia, hypoproteinemia, hyperphosphatemia, hypertriglyceridemia, hyperuricemia, hypoglycemia.

Urinary System Disorders: *Frequent:* Polyuria/polydipsia.* *Infrequent:* Urinary incontinence, hematuria, dysuria. *Rare:* Urinary retention, cystitis, renal insufficiency.

Musculoskeletal System Disorders: *Infrequent:* Myalgia. *Rare:* Arthrosis, synostosis, bursitis, arthritis, skeletal pain.

Reproductive Disorders, Female: *Frequent:* Menorrhagia,* orgastic dysfunction,* dry vagina.* *Infrequent:* Nonpuerperal lactation, amenorrhea, female breast pain, leukorrhea, mastitis, dysmenorrhea, female perineal pain, intermenstrual bleeding, vaginal hemorrhage.

Liver and Biliary System Disorders: *Infrequent:* Increased SGOT, increased SGPT. *Rare:* Hepatic failure, cholestatic hepatitis, cholecystitis, cholelithiasis, hepatitis, hepatocellular damage.

Platelet, Bleeding, and Clotting Disorders: *Infrequent:* Epistaxis, purpura. *Rare:* Hemorrhage, superficial phlebitis, thrombophlebitis, thrombocytopenia.

Hearing and Vestibular Disorders: *Rare:* Tinnitus, hyperacusis, decreased hearing.

Red Blood Cell Disorders: *Infrequent:* Anemia, hypochromic anemia. *Rare:* Normocytic anemia.

Reproductive Disorders, Male: *Frequent:* Erectile dysfunction.* *Infrequent:* Ejaculation failure.

White Cell and Resistance Disorders: *Rare:* Leukocytosis, lymphadenopathy, leucopenia, Pelger-Huet anomaly.

Endocrine Disorders: *Rare:* Gynecomastia, male breast pain, antidiuretic hormone disorder.

Special Senses: *Rare:* Bitter taste.

*Incidence based on elicited reports.

POST-INTRODUCTION REPORTS

Adverse events reported since market introduction which were temporally (but not necessarily causally) related to risperidone therapy, include the following: anaphylactic reaction, angioedema, apnea, atrial fibrillation, cerebrovascular disorder, including cerebrovascular accident, hyperglycemia, diabetes mellitus aggravated, including diabetic ketoacidosis, intestinal obstruction, jaundice, mania, pancreatitis, Parkinson's disease aggravated, pulmonary embolism. There have been rare reports of sudden death and/or cardiopulmonary arrest in patients receiving risperidone. A causal relationship with risperidone has not been established. It is important to note that sudden and unexpected death may occur in psychotic patients whether they remain untreated or whether they are treated with other antipsychotic drugs.

DOSAGE AND ADMINISTRATION

USUAL INITIAL DOSE

Risperidone can be administered on either a bid or a qd schedule. In early clinical trials, risperidone was generally administered at 1 mg bid initially, with increases in increments of 1 mg bid on the second and third day, as tolerated, to a target dose of 3 mg bid by the third day. Subsequent controlled trials have indicated that total daily risperidone doses of up to 8 mg on a qd regimen are also safe and effective. However, regardless of which regimen is employed, in some patients a slower titration may be medically appropriate. Further dosage adjustments, if indicated, should generally occur at intervals of not less than 1 week, since steady state for the active metabolite would not be achieved for approximately 1 week in the typical patient. When dosage adjustments are necessary, small dose increments/decrements of 1-2 mg are recommended.

Efficacy in schizophrenia was demonstrated in a dose range of 4-16 mg/day in the clinical trials supporting effectiveness of risperidone; however, maximal effect was generally seen in a range of 4-8 mg/day. Doses above 6 mg/day for bid dosing were not demonstrated to be more efficacious than lower doses, were associated with more extrapyramidal symptoms and other adverse effects, and are not generally recommended. In a single study supporting qd dosing, the efficacy results were generally stronger for 8 mg than for 4 mg. The safety of doses above 16 mg/day has not been evaluated in clinical trials.

PEDIATRIC USE

Safety and effectiveness of risperidone in pediatric patients have not been established.

DOSING IN SPECIAL POPULATIONS

The recommended initial dose is 0.5 mg bid in patients who are elderly or debilitated, patients with severe renal or hepatic impairment, and patients either predisposed to hypotension or for whom hypotension would pose a risk. Dosage increases in these patients should

R

be in increments of no more than 0.5 mg bid. Increases to dosages above 1.5 mg bid should generally occur at intervals of at least 1 week. In some patients, slower titration may be medically appropriate.

Elderly or debilitated patients, and patients with renal impairment, may have less ability to eliminate risperidone than normal adults. Patients with impaired hepatic function may have increases in the free fraction of risperidone, possibly resulting in an enhanced effect (see CLINICAL PHARMACOLOGY). Patients with a predisposition to hypotensive reactions or for whom such reactions would pose a particular risk likewise need to be titrated cautiously and carefully monitored (see PRECAUTIONS). If a once-a-day dosing regimen in the elderly or debilitated patient is being considered, it is recommended that the patient be titrated on a twice-a-day regimen for 2-3 days at the target dose. Subsequent switches to a once-a-day dosing regimen can be done thereafter.

DIRECTIONS FOR USE OF RISPERIDONE ORALLY DISINTEGRATING TABLETS

Risperidone orally disintegrating tablets are supplied in blister packs of 4 tablet units each.

Tablet Accessing

Do not open the blister until ready to administer. For single tablet removal, separate 1 of the 4 blister units by tearing apart at the perforations. Bend the corner where indicated. Peel back foil to expose the tablet. DO NOT push the tablet through the foil because this could damage the tablet.

Tablet Administration

Using dry hands, remove the tablet from the blister unit and immediately place the entire risperidone orally disintegrating tablet on the tongue. The risperidone orally disintegrating tablet should be consumed immediately, as the tablet cannot be stored once removed from the blister unit. Risperidone orally disintegrating tablets disintegrate in the mouth within seconds and can be swallowed subsequently with or without liquid. Patients should not attempt to split or to chew the tablet.

MAINTENANCE THERAPY

While there is no body of evidence available to answer the question of how long the schizophrenic patient treated with risperidone should remain on it, the effectiveness of risperidone 2-8 mg/day at delaying relapse was demonstrated in a controlled trial in patients who had been clinically stable for at least 4 weeks and were then followed for a period of 1-2 years. In this trial, risperidone was administered on a qd schedule, at 1 mg qd initially, with increases to 2 mg qd on the second day, and to a target dose of 4 mg qd on the third day. Nevertheless, patients should be periodically reassessed to determine the need for maintenance treatment with an appropriate dose.

REINITIATION OF TREATMENT IN PATIENTS PREVIOUSLY DISCONTINUED

Although there are no data to specifically address reinitiation of treatment, it is recommended that when restarting patients who have had an interval off risperidone, the initial titration schedule should be followed.

SWITCHING FROM OTHER ANTIPSYCHOTICS

There are no systematically collected data to specifically address switching schizophrenic patients from other antipsychotics to risperidone, or concerning concomitant administration with other antipsychotics. While immediate discontinuation of the previous antipsychotic treatment may be acceptable for some schizophrenic patients, more gradual discontinuation may be most appropriate for others. In all cases, the period of overlapping antipsychotic administration should be minimized. When switching schizophrenic patients from depot antipsychotics, if medically appropriate, initiate risperidone therapy in place of the next scheduled injection. The need for continuing existing EPS medication should be re-evaluated periodically.

HOW SUPPLIED

RISPERDAL TABLETS

0.25 mg: Dark yellow tablet imprinted "JANSSEN" and "Ris" and "0.25".
0.5 mg: Red-brown tablet imprinted "JANSSEN" and "Ris" and "0.5".
1 mg: White tablet imprinted "JANSSEN" and "R" and "1".
2 mg: Orange tablet imprinted "JANSSEN" and "R" and "2".
3 mg: Yellow tablet imprinted "JANSSEN" and "R" and "3".
4 mg: Green tablet imprinted "JANSSEN" and "R" and "4".

Storage and Handling

Risperdal tablets should be stored at controlled room temperature 15-25°C (59-77°F). Protect from light and moisture.

Keep out of reach of children.

RISPERDAL ORAL SOLUTION

Risperdal 1 mg/ml oral solution is supplied in 30 ml bottles with a calibrated (in milligrams and milliliters) pipette. The minimum calibrated volume is 0.25 ml, while the maximum calibrated volume is 3 ml.

Tests indicate that Risperdal oral solution is compatible in the following beverages: water, coffee, orange juice, and low-fat milk; it is NOT compatible with either cola or tea, however.

Storage and Handling

Risperdal 1 mg/ml oral solution should be stored at controlled room temperature 15-25°C (59-77°F). Protect from light and freezing.

Keep out of reach of children.

RISPERDAL M-TAB ORALLY DISINTEGRATING TABLETS

0.5 mg: Light coral, round, biconvex tablets etched on one side with "R0.5".
1 mg: Light coral, square, biconvex tablets etched on one side with "R1".
2 mg: Light coral, round, biconvex tablets etched on one side with "R2".

Storage and Handling

Risperdal M-TAB orally disintegrating tablets should be stored at controlled room temperature 15-25°C (59-77°F).

Keep out of reach of children.

PRODUCT LISTING - EQUIVALENTS NOT AVAILABLE

Form	Quantity	Price	Product, Company	NDC
Solution - Oral - 1 mg/ml				
	30 ml	$118.29	RISPERDAL, Janssen Pharmaceuticals	50458-0305-03
Tablet - Oral - 0.25 mg				
	60's	$152.00	RISPERDAL, Janssen Pharmaceuticals	50458-0301-06
	60's	$184.85	RISPERDAL, Janssen Pharmaceuticals	50458-0301-04
Tablet - Oral - 0.5 mg				
	60's	$191.73	RISPERDAL, Janssen Pharmaceuticals	50458-0302-06
Tablet - Oral - 1 mg				
	60's	$198.16	RISPERDAL, Janssen Pharmaceuticals	50458-0300-06
	100's	$330.19	RISPERDAL, Janssen Pharmaceuticals	50458-0300-01
Tablet - Oral - 2 mg				
	30's	$150.00	RISPERDAL, Physicians Total Care	54868-3513-01
	60's	$256.53	RISPERDAL, Physicians Total Care	54868-3513-02
	60's	$319.13	RISPERDAL, Janssen Pharmaceuticals	50458-0320-06
	100's	$531.84	RISPERDAL, Janssen Pharmaceuticals	50458-0320-01
Tablet - Oral - 3 mg				
	60's	$385.88	RISPERDAL, Janssen Pharmaceuticals	50458-0330-06
	100's	$643.13	RISPERDAL, Janssen Pharmaceuticals	50458-0330-01
Tablet - Oral - 4 mg				
	60's	$438.05	RISPERDAL, Physicians Total Care	54868-3515-00
	60's	$508.50	RISPERDAL, Janssen Pharmaceuticals	50458-0350-06
	100's	$847.46	RISPERDAL, Janssen Pharmaceuticals	50458-0350-01

Ritodrine Hydrochloride *(002190)*

For complete prescribing information, refer to the CD-ROM included with the book.

Categories: Labor, premature; Pregnancy Category B; FDA Approved 1980 Dec
Drug Classes: Adrenergic agonists; Relaxants, uterine
Brand Names: Yutopar
Foreign Brand Availability: Anpo (Taiwan); Fetodrin (Taiwan); Miolene (Italy); Pre-Par (Belgium; Czech-Republic; Germany; Netherlands; Spain); Ritopar (Israel); Utemerin (Japan); Utopar (Denmark; Finland; Norway)

DESCRIPTION

Yutopar contains the betamimetic (beta sympathomimetic amine) ritodrine HCl. Yutopar is a clear, colorless, sterile, aqueous solution, each milliliter contains either 10 or 15 mg of ritodrine HCl, 4.35 mg of acetic acid, 2.4 mg of sodium hydroxide, 1 mg of sodium metabisulfite, and 2.9 mg of sodium chloride in water for injection. Hydrochloric acid and/or additional sodium hydroxide is used to adjust pH. Filled under nitrogen.

FOR INTRAVENOUS USE ONLY. MUST BE DILUTED BEFORE USE. SEE DOSAGE AND ADMINISTRATION INSTRUCTIONS. DO NOT USE IF INJECTION IS DISCOLORED OR CONTAINS A PRECIPITATE.

Ritodrine HCl is a white, odorless crystalline powder, freely soluble in water, with a melting point between 196-205°C. The chemical name of ritodrine HCl is erythro-p-hydroxy-α-[1- [(p-hydroxyphenethyl)-amino]ethyl] benzyl alcohol hydrochloride.

INDICATIONS AND USAGE

Ritodrine HCl is indicated for the management of preterm labor in suitable patients.

Administered intravenously, the drug will decrease uterine activity and thus prolong gestation in the majority of such patients. Additional acute episodes may be treated by repeating the intravenous infusion. The incidence of neonatal mortality and respiratory distress syndrome increases when the normal gestation period is shortened.

Since successful inhibition of labor is more likely with early treatment, therapy with ritodrine HCl should be instituted as soon as the diagnosis of preterm labor is established and contraindications ruled out in pregnancies of 20 or more weeks gestation. The efficacy and safety of ritodrine HCl in advanced labor, that is, when cervical dilatation is more than 4 cm or effacement is more than 80%, have not been established.

CONTRAINDICATIONS

Ritodrine HCl is contraindicated before the 20th week of pregnancy.

Ritodrine HCl is also contraindicated in those conditions of the mother or fetus in which continuation of pregnancy is hazardous; specific contraindications include:

1. Antepartum hemorrhage which demands immediate delivery.
2. Eclampsia and severe preeclampsia.
3. Intrauterine fetal death.
4. Chorioamnionitis.
5. Maternal cardiac disease.
6. Pulmonary hypertension.
7. Maternal hyperthyroidism.
8. Uncontrolled maternal diabetes mellitus.
9. Pre-existing maternal medical conditions that would be seriously affected by the known pharmacologic properties of a betamimetic drug; such as: hypovolemia, cardiac arrhythmias associated with tachycardia or digitalis intoxication, uncontrolled hypertension, pheochromocytoma, bronchial asthma already treated by betamimetics and/or steroids.
10. Known hypersensitivity to any component of the product.

WARNINGS

Maternal pulmonary edema has been reported in patients treated with ritodrine HCl, sometimes after delivery. It has occurred more often when patients were treated concomitantly with corticosteroids. Maternal death

R

Cont'd
from this condition has been reported with or without corticosteroids given concomitantly with drugs of this class.

Patients so treated must be closely monitored in the hospital. The patient's state of hydration should be carefully monitored; fluid overload must be avoided (see DOSAGE AND ADMINISTRATION). Intravenous fluid loading may be aggravated by the use of betamimetics with or without corticosteroids and may turn into manifest circulatory overloading with subsequent pulmonary edema. If pulmonary edema develops during administration, the drug should be discontinued. Edema should be managed by conventional means.

Intravenous administration of ritodrine HCl should be supervised by persons having knowledge of the pharmacology of the drug and who are qualified to identify and manage complications of drug administration and pregnancy. Beta-adrenergic drugs increase cardiac output, and even in a normal healthy heart this added myocardial oxygen demand can sometimes lead to myocardial ischemia. Complications may include: myocardial necrosis, which may result in death; arrhythmias, including premature atrial and ventricular contractions, ventricular tachycardia, and bundle branch block; anginal pain, with or without ECG changes. Because cardiovascular responses are common and more pronounced during intravenous administration of ritodrine HCl, cardiovascular effects, including maternal pulse rate and blood pressure and fetal heart rate, should be closely monitored. Care should be exercised for maternal signs and symptoms of pulmonary edema. A persistent high tachycardia (over 140 beats per minute) may be one of the signs of impending pulmonary edema with drugs of this class. Occult cardiac disease may be unmasked with the use of ritodrine HCl. If the patient complains of chest pain or tightness of chest, the drug should be temporarily discontinued and an ECG should be done as soon as possible.

The drug should not be administered to patients with mild to moderate preeclampsia, hypertension, or diabetes unless the attending physician considers that the benefits clearly outweigh the risks.

Ritodrine HCl injection contains sodium metabisulfite, a sulfite that may cause allergic-type reactions including anaphylactic symptoms and life-threatening or less severe asthmatic episodes in certain susceptible people. The overall prevalence of sulfite sensitivity in the general population in unknown and probably low. Sulfite sensitivity is seen more frequently in asthmatic than in nonasthmatic people.

DOSAGE AND ADMINISTRATION

The optimum dose of ritodrine HCl is determined by a clinical balance of uterine response and unwanted effects.

INTRAVENOUS THERAPY

Do not use intravenous ritodrine HCl if the solution is discolored or contains any precipitate or particulate matter.

Ritodrine HCl Injection should be used promptly after preparation, but in no case after 48 hours of preparation.

Method of Administration

To minimize the risks of hypotension, the patient should be maintained in the left lateral position throughout infusion and careful attention given to her state of hydration, but fluid overload must be avoided.

For appropriate control and dose titration, a controlled infusion device is recommended to adjust the rate of flow in drops/minute. An IV microdrop chamber (60 drops/ml) can provide a convenient range of infusion rates within the recommended dose range for ritodrine HCl.

Recommended Dilution

150 mg ritodrine HCl in 500 ml fluid yielding a final concentration of 0.3 mg/ml*. Ritodrine for intravenous infusion should be diluted with 5% w/v dextrose solution. Because of the increased probability of pulmonary edema, saline diluents such as:

0.9% w/v sodium chloride solution.
Compound sodium chloride solution (Ringer's solution).
Hartmann's solution, should be reserved for cases where dextrose solution is medically undesirable, *e.g.,* diabetes mellitus.

* In those cases where fluid restriction is medically desirable, a more concentrated solution may be prepared.

Intravenous therapy should be started as soon as possible after diagnosis. The usual initial dose is 0.05 mg/minute (0.17 ml/min, 10 drops/min using a microdrip chamber at the recommended dilution), to be gradually increased by 0.05 mg/min (0.17 ml/min, 10 drops/min using a microdrip chamber at the recommended dilution) every 10 minutes until the desired result is obtained, or the maternal heart rate reaches 130 beats per minute. The effective dosage usually lies between 0.15 and 0.35 mg/minute (0.50-1.17 ml/min, 30-70 drops/min using a microdrip chamber at the recommended dilution).

Frequent monitoring of maternal uterine contractions, heart rate, and blood pressure, and of fetal heart rate is required, with dosage individually titrated according to response. If other drugs need to be given intravenously, the use of "piggyback" or other site of intravenous administration permits the continued independent control of the rate of infusion of the ritodrine HCl.

The infusion should generally be continued for between 12 and 24 hours after uterine contractions cease. With the recommended dilution, the maximum volume of fluid that might be administered after 12 hours at the highest dose (0.35 mg/min) will be approximately 840 ml.

The amount of IV fluids administered and the rate of administration should be monitored to avoid circulatory fluid overload (over-hydration).

Recurrence of unwanted preterm labor may be treated with repeated infusion of ritodrine HCl.

Storage: Store at room temperature, preferably below 30°C (86°F). Protect from excessive heat.

PRODUCT LISTING - RATED THERAPEUTICALLY EQUIVALENT

Solution - Intravenous - 5%;30 mg/100 ml
500 ml x 6 $772.50 GENERIC, Abbott Pharmaceutical 00074-7001-03

Solution - Intravenous - 10 mg/ml
5 ml x 10 $1063.50 YUTOPAR, Astra-Zeneca Pharmaceuticals 00186-0599-03

Solution - Intravenous - 15 mg/ml
10 ml $183.14 YUTOPAR, Astra-Zeneca Pharmaceuticals 00186-0597-12
10 ml x 10 $179.68 YUTOPAR, Astra-Zeneca Pharmaceuticals 00186-0644-01

Ritonavir *(003251)*

For related information, see the comparative table section in Appendix A.

Categories: Infection, human immunodeficiency virus; FDA Approved 1996 Mar; Pregnancy Category B; WHO Formulary
Drug Classes: Antivirals; Protease inhibitors
Brand Names: Norvir
Cost of Therapy: $333.91 (HIV; Norvir; 100 mg; 6 capsules/day; 30 day supply)

WARNING

COADMINISTRATION OF RITONAVIR WITH CERTAIN NONSEDATING ANTIHISTAMINES, SEDATIVE HYPNOTICS, ANTIARRHYTHMICS, OR ERGOT ALKALOID PREPARATIONS MAY RESULT IN POTENTIALLY SERIOUS AND/OR LIFE-THREATENING ADVERSE EVENTS DUE TO POSSIBLE EFFECTS OF RITONAVIR ON THE HEPATIC METABOLISM OF CERTAIN DRUGS. SEE CONTRAINDICATIONS AND PRECAUTIONS.

DESCRIPTION

Ritonavir is an inhibitor of HIV protease with activity against the Human Immunodeficiency Virus (HIV).

Ritonavir is chemically designated as 10-Hydroxy-2-methyl-5-(1-methylethyl)-1-[2-(1-methylethyl)-4-thiazolyl]-3,6-dioxo-8,11-bis (phenylmethyl)-2,4,7,12-tetraazatridecan-13-oic acid, 5-thiazolylmethyl ester, [5S-(5R*,8R*,10R*,11R*)]. Its molecular formula is $C_{37}H_{48}N_6O_5S_2$, and its molecular weight is 720.95.

Ritonavir is a white-to-light-tan powder. Ritonavir has a bitter metallic taste. It is freely soluble in methanol and ethanol, soluble in isopropanol and practically insoluble in water.

Norvir soft gelatin capsules are available for oral administration in a strength of 100 mg ritonavir with the following inactive ingredients: Butylated hydroxytoluene, ethanol, gelatin, iron oxide, oleic acid, polyoxyl 35 castor oil, and titanium dioxide.

Norvir oral solution is available for oral administration as 80 mg/ml of ritonavir in a peppermint and caramel flavored vehicle. Each 8 oz bottle contains 19.2 g of ritonavir. Norvir oral solution also contains ethanol, water, polyoxyl 35 castor oil, propylene glycol, anhydrous citric acid to adjust pH, saccharin sodium, peppermint oil, creamy caramel flavoring, and FD&C yellow no. 6.

CLINICAL PHARMACOLOGY

MICROBIOLOGY

Mechanism of Action

Ritonavir is a peptidomimetic inhibitor of both the HIV-1 and HIV-2 proteases. Inhibition of HIV protease renders the enzyme incapable of processing the *gag-pol* polyprotein precursor which leads to production of non-infectious immature HIV particles.

Antiviral Activity In Vitro

The activity of ritonavir was assessed *in vitro* in acutely infected lymphoblastoid cell lines and in peripheral blood lymphocytes. The concentration of drug that inhibits 50% (EC_{50}) of viral replication ranged from 3.8 to 153 nM depending upon the HIV-1 isolate and the cells employed. The average EC_{50} for low passage clinical isolates was 22 nM (n=13). In MT_4 cells, ritonavir demonstrated additive effects against HIV-1 in combination with either zidovudine (ZDV) or didanosine (ddI). Studies which measured cytotoxicity of ritonavir on several cell lines showed that >20 μM was required to inhibit cellular growth by 50% resulting in an *in vitro* therapeutic index of at least 1000.

Resistance

HIV-1 isolates with reduced susceptibility to ritonavir have been selected *in vitro.* Genotypic analysis of these isolates showed mutations in the HIV protease gene at amino acid positions 84 (Ile to Val), 82 (Val to Phe), 71 (Ala to Val), and 46 (Met to Ile). Phenotypic (n=18) and genotypic (n=44) changes in HIV isolates from selected patients treated with ritonavir were monitored in Phase 1/2 trials over a period of 3-32 weeks. Mutations associated with the HIV viral protease in isolates obtained from 41 patients appeared to occur in a stepwise and ordered fashion; in sequence, these mutations were position 82 (Val to Ala/Phe), 54 (Ile to Val), 71 (Ala to Val/Thr), and 36 (Ile to Leu), followed by combinations of mutations at an additional 5 specific amino acid positions. Of 18 patients for which both phenotypic and genotypic analysis were performed on free virus isolated from plasma, 12 showed reduced susceptibility to ritonavir *in vitro.* All 18 patients possessed one or more mutations in the viral protease gene. The 82 mutation appeared to be necessary but not sufficient to confer phenotypic resistance. Phenotypic resistance was defined as a ≥5-fold decrease in viral sensitivity *in vitro* from baseline. The clinical relevance of phenotypic and genotypic changes associated with ritonavir therapy has not been established.

Cross-Resistance to Other Antiretrovirals

Among protease inhibitors variable cross-resistance has been recognized. Serial HIV isolates obtained from 6 patients during ritonavir therapy showed a decrease in ritonavir susceptibility *in vitro* but did not demonstrate a concordant decrease in susceptibility to saquinavir *in vitro* when compared to matched baseline isolates. However, isolates from 2 of these patients demonstrated decreased susceptibility to indinavir *in vitro* (8-fold). Isolates from 5 patients were also tested for cross-resistance to amprenavir and nelfinavir; isolates from 2 patients had a decrease in susceptibility to nelfinavir (12- to 14-fold), and none to amprenavir. Cross-resistance between ritonavir and reverse transcriptase inhibitors is un-

R

likely because of the different enzyme targets involved. One ZDV-resistant HIV isolate tested *in vitro* retained full susceptibility to ritonavir.

PHARMACOKINETICS

The pharmacokinetics of ritonavir have been studied in healthy volunteers and HIV-infected patients (CD4 ≥50 cells/μl). See TABLE 1 for ritonavir pharmacokinetic characteristics.

Absorption

The absolute bioavailability of ritonavir has not been determined. After a 600 mg dose of oral solution, peak concentrations of ritonavir were achieved approximately 2 and 4 hours after dosing under fasting and non-fasting (514 kcal; 9% fat, 12% protein, and 79% carbohydrate) conditions, respectively.

Effect of Food on Oral Absorption

When the oral solution was given under non-fasting conditions, peak ritonavir concentrations decreased 23% and the extent of absorption decreased 7% relative to fasting conditions. Dilution of the oral solution, within 1 hour of administration, with 240 ml of chocolate milk, Advera or Ensure did not significantly affect the extent and rate of ritonavir absorption. After a single 600 mg dose under non-fasting conditions, in two separate studies, the soft gelatin capsule (n=57) and oral solution (n=18) formulations yielded mean ±SD areas under the plasma concentration-time curve (AUCs) of 121.7 ± 53.8 and 129.0 ± 39.3 μg·h/ml, respectively. Relative to fasting conditions, the extent of absorption of ritonavir from the soft gelatin capsule formulation was 13% higher when administered with a meal (615 kcal; 14.5% fat, 9% protein, and 76% carbohydrate).

Metabolism

Nearly all of the plasma radioactivity after a single oral 600 mg dose of ^{14}C-ritonavir oral solution (n=5) was attributed to unchanged ritonavir. Five (5) ritonavir metabolites have been identified in human urine and feces. The isopropylthiazole oxidation metabolite (M-2) is the major metabolite and has antiviral activity similar to that of parent drug; however, the concentrations of this metabolite in plasma are low. *In vitro* studies utilizing human liver microsomes have demonstrated that cytochrome P450 3A (CYP3A) is the major isoform involved in ritonavir metabolism, although CYP2D6 also contributes to the formation of M-2.

Elimination

In a study of 5 subjects receiving a 600 mg dose of ^{14}C-ritonavir oral solution, 11.3 ± 2.8% of the dose was excreted into the urine, with 3.5 ± 1.8% of the dose excreted as unchanged parent drug. In that study, 86.4 ± 2.9% of the dose was excreted in the feces with 33.8 ± 10.8% of the dose excreted as unchanged parent drug. Upon multiple dosing, ritonavir accumulation is less than predicted from a single dose possibly due to a time and dose-related increase in clearance.

TABLE 1 *Ritonavir Pharmacokinetic Characteristics*

Parameter	n	Values (Mean ±SD)
C_{max} SS*	10	11.2 ± 3.6 μg/ml
C_{trough} SS*	10	3.7 ± 2.6 μg/ml
$V_β/F$†	91	0.41 ± 0.25 L/kg
$T_{½}$		3-5 h
CL/F SS*	10	8.8 ± 3.2 L/h
CL/F†	91	4.6 ± 1.6 L/h
CLR	62	<0.1 L/h
RBC/Plasma ratio		0.14
Percent bound‡		98-99%

* SS = steady state; patients taking ritonavir 600 mg q12h.
† Single ritonavir 600 mg dose.
‡ Primarily bound to human serum albumin and alpha-1 acid glycoprotein over the ritonavir concentration range of 0.01 to 30 μg/ml.

Special Populations

Gender, Race, and Age

No age-related pharmacokinetic differences have been observed in adult patients (18-63 years). Ritonavir pharmacokinetics have not been studied in older patients. A study of ritonavir pharmacokinetics in healthy males and females showed no statistically significant differences in the pharmacokinetics of ritonavir. Pharmacokinetic differences due to race have not been identified.

Pediatric Patients

The pharmacokinetic profile of ritonavir in pediatric patients below the age of 2 years has not been established. Steady-state pharmacokinetics were evaluated in 37 HIV-infected patients ages 2-14 years receiving doses ranging from 250-400 mg/m^2 bid. Across dose groups, ritonavir steady-state oral clearance (CL/F/m^2) was approximately 1.5 times faster in pediatric patients than in adult subjects. Ritonavir concentrations obtained after 350-400 mg/m^2 twice daily in pediatric patients were comparable to those obtained in adults receiving 600 mg (approximately 330 mg/m^2) twice daily.

Renal Insufficiency

Ritonavir pharmacokinetics have not been studied in patients with renal insufficiency; however, since renal clearance is negligible, a decrease in total body clearance is not expected in patients with renal insufficiency.

Hepatic Insufficiency

In 6 HIV-infected adult subjects with mild hepatic insufficiency dosed with ritonavir 400 mg bid, ritonavir exposures were similar to control subjects dosed with 500 mg bid. Adequate pharmacokinetic data are not available for patients with moderate hepatic impairment. Protein binding of ritonavir was not statistically significantly affected by mild or moderately impaired hepatic function (see PRECAUTIONS and DOSAGE AND ADMINISTRATION).

Drug-Drug Interactions

See also CONTRAINDICATIONS, WARNINGS, and DRUG INTERACTIONS.

TABLE 2 summarizes the effects on AUC and C_{max}, with 95% confidence intervals (95% CI), of coadministration of ritonavir with a variety of drugs. For information about clinical recommendations see DRUG INTERACTIONS.

TABLE 2 *Drug Interactions (see DRUG INTERACTIONS, Established Drug Interactions: Alteration in Dose or Regimen Recommended Based on Drug Interaction Studies)*

Coadministered Drug	Ritonavir Dosage	n	AUC % (95% CI)	C_{max} % (95% CI)
Pharmacokinetic Parameters for Ritonavir in the Presence of the Coadminstered Drug				
Clarithromycin 500 mg q12h, 4 days	200 mg q8h, 4 days	22	inc 12% (2, 23%)	inc 15% (2, 28%)
Didanosine 200 mg q12h, 4 days	600 mg q12h, 4 days	12	NC	NC
Fluconazole 400 mg single dose, day 1; 200 mg daily, 4 days	200 mg q6h, 4 days	8	inc 12% (5, 20%)	inc 15% (7, 22%)
Fluoxetine 30 mg q12h, 8 days	600 mg single dose, 1 day	16	inc 19% (7, 34%)	NC
Ketoconazole 200 mg daily, 7 days	500 mg q12h, 10 days	12	inc 18% (-3, 52%)	inc 10% (-11, 36%)
Rifampin 600 or 300 mg daily, 10 days	500 mg q12h, 20 days	7,9*	dec 35% (7, 55%)	dec 25% (-5, 46%)
Zidovudine 200 mg q8h, 4 days	300 mg q6h, 4 days	10	NC	NC
Pharmacokinetic Parameters for Coadminstered Drug in the Presence of Ritonavir				
Alprazolam 1 mg single dose	500 mg q12h, 10 days	12	dec 12% (-5, 30%)	dec 16% (5, 27%)
Clarithromycin 500 mg q12h, 4 days	200 mg q8h, 4 days	22	inc 77% (56, 103%)	inc 31% (15, 51%)
14-OH clarithromycin metabolite			dec 100%	dec 99%
Desipramine 100 mg, single dose	500 mg q12h, 12 days	14	inc 145% (103, 211%)	inc 22% (12, 35%)
2-OH desipramine metabolite			dec 15% (3, 26%)	dec 67% (62, 72%)
Didanosine 200 mg q12h, 4 days	600 mg q12h, 4 days	12	dec 13% (0, 23%)	dec 16% (5, 26%)
Ethinyl estradiol 50 μg single dose	500 mg q12h, 16 days	23	dec 40% (31, 49%)	dec 32% (24, 39%)
Indinavir 400 mg q12h day 14†	400 mg q12h, 15 days	10	inc 6% (-14, 29%)	dec 51% (40, 61%)
Indinavir 400 mg q12h day 15†	400 mg q12h, 15 days	10	dec 7% (-25, 16%)	dec 62% (52, 70%)
Ketoconazole 200 mg daily, 7 days	500 mg q12h, 10 days	12	inc 3.4-fold (2.8, 4.3×)	inc 55% (40, 72%)
Meperidine 50 mg oral single dose	500 mg q12h, 10 days	8	dec 62% (59, 65%)	dec 59% (42, 72%)
Normeperidine metabolite		6	inc 47% (-24, 345%)	inc 87% (42, 147%)
Methadone 5 mg single dose‡	500 mg q12h, 15 days	11	dec 36% (16, 52%)	dec 38% (28, 46%)
Rifabutin 150 mg daily, 16 days	500 mg q12h, 10 days	5,11*	inc 4-fold (2.8, 6.1×)	inc 2.5-fold (1.9, 3.4×)
25-O-desacetyl rifabutin metabolite			inc 35-fold (25, 78×)	inc 16-fold (14, 20×)
Saquinavir 400 mg bid steady-state§	400 mg bid steady-state	7	inc 17-fold (9, 31×)	inc 14-fold (7, 28×)
Sildenafil 100 mg single dose	500 mg bid, 8 days	28	inc 11-fold	inc 4-fold
Sulfamethoxazole 800 mg, single dose¤	500 mg q12h, 12 days	15	inc 20% (16, 23%)	NC
Theophylline 3 mg/kg q8h, 15 days	500 mg q12h, 10 days	13,11*	dec 43% (42, 45%)	dec 32% (29, 34%)
Trimethoprim 160 mg, single dose¤	500 mg q12h, 12 days	15	inc 20% (3, 43%)	NC
Zidovudine 200 mg q8h, 4 days	300 mg q6h, 4 days	9	dec 25% (15, 34%)	dec 27% (4, 45%)

* Parallel group design; entries are subjects receiving combination and control regimens, respectively.
† Ritonavir and indinavir were coadministered for 15 days; day 14 doses were administered after a 15%-fat breakfast (757 kcal) and 9%-fat evening snack (236 kcal), and day 15 doses were administered after a 15%-fat breakfast (757 kcal) and 32%-fat dinner (815 kcal). Indinavir C_{min} was also increased 4-fold. Effects were assessed relative to an indinavir 800 mg q8h regimen under fasting conditions.
‡ Effects were assessed on a dose-normalized comparison to a methadone 20 mg single dose.
§ Comparison to a standard saquinavir HGC 600 mg tid regimen (n=114). Saquinavir C_{min} was 0.48 ± 0.36 μg/ml for 400/400 mg bid compared to below quantifiable limits for saquinavir HGC 600 mg tid.
¤ Sulfamethoxazole and trimethoprim taken as single combination tablet.
inc Indicates increase.
dec Indicates decrease.
NC Indicates no change.

INDICATIONS AND USAGE

Ritonavir is indicated in combination with other antiretroviral agents for the treatment of HIV-infection. This indication is based on the results from a study in patients with advanced HIV disease that showed a reduction in both mortality and AIDS-defining clinical events for

R

patients who received ritonavir either alone or in combination with nucleoside analogues. Median duration of follow-up in this study was 13.5 months.

CONTRAINDICATIONS

Ritonavir is contraindicated in patients with known hypersensitivity to ritonavir or any of its ingredients.

Coadministration of ritonavir is contraindicated with the drugs listed in TABLE 3 (also see TABLE 4) because competition for primarily CYP3A by ritonavir could result in inhibition of the metabolism of these drugs and create the potential for serious and/or life-threatening reactions such as cardiac arrhythmias, prolonged or increased sedation, and respiratory depression.

Postmarketing reports indicate that coadministration of ritonavir with ergotamine or dihydroergotamine has been associated with acute ergot toxicity characterized by peripheral vasospasm and ischemia of the extremities.

***TABLE 3** Drugs That Are Contraindicated With Ritonavir*

Drug Class	Drugs Within Class That Are CONTRAINDICATED With Ritonavir
Antiarrhythmics	Amiodarone, bepridil, flecainide, propafenone, quinidine
Antihistamines	Astemizole, terfenadine
Ergot derivatives	Dihydroergotamine, ergonovine, ergotamine, methylergonovine
GI motility agent	Cisapride
Neuroleptic	Pimozide
Sedative/hypnotics	Midazolam, triazolam

WARNINGS

ALERT: Find out about medicines that should NOT be taken with ritonavir. This statement is included on the product's bottle label.

DRUG INTERACTIONS

Ritonavir is an inhibitor of cytochrome P450 3A (CYP3A) both *in vitro* and *in vivo*. Ritonaivr also inhibits CYP2D6 *in vitro*, but to a lesser extent than CYP3A. Coadministration of ritonavir and drugs primarily metabolized by CYP3A or CYP2D6 may result in increased plasma concentrations of other drugs that could increase or prolong its therapeutic and adverse effects (see CLINICAL PHARMACOLOGY, Pharmacokinetics, Drug-Drug Interactions; DRUG INTERACTIONS, Established Drug Interactions: Alteration in Dose or Regimen Recommended Based on Drug Interaction Studies; TABLE 3; TABLE 4; TABLE 5; and TABLE 6.

The magnitude of the interactions and therapeutic consequences between ritonavir and the drugs listed in TABLE 5 and TABLE 6 cannot be predicted with any certainty. When coadministering ritonavir with any agent listed in TABLE 5 and TABLE 6, special attention is warranted. Refer to DRUG INTERACTIONS, Established Drug Interactions: Alteration in Dose or Regimen Recommended Based on Drug Interaction Studies; TABLE 5; and TABLE 6 for additional information.

Cardiac and neurologic events have been reported with ritonavir when coadministered with disopyramide, mexiletine, nefazodone, fluoxetine and beta blockers. The possibility of drug interaction cannot be excluded.

Particular caution should be used when prescribing sildenafil in patients receiving ritonavir. Coadministration of ritonavir with sildenafil is expected to substantially increase sildenafil concentrations (11-fold increase in AUC) and may result in an increase in sildenafil-associated adverse events, including hypotension, syncope, visual changes, and prolonged erection (see DRUG INTERACTIONS, Established Drug Interactions: Alteration in Dose or Regimen Recommended Based on Drug Interaction Studies and the complete prescribing information for sildenafil).

Concomitant use of ritonavir with lovastatin or simvastatin is not recommended. Caution should be exercised if HIV protease inhibitors, including ritonavir, are used concurrently with other HMG-CoA reductase inhibitors that are also metabolized by the CYP3A4 pathway (*e.g.*, atorvastatin or cerivastatin). The risk of myopathy including rhabdomyolysis may be increased when HIV protease inhibitors, including ritonavir, are used in combination with these drugs.

Concomitant use of ritonavir, and St. John's wort (hypericum perforatum) or products containing St. John's wort is not recommended. Coadministration of protease inhibitors, including ritonavir, with St. John's wort is expected to substantially decrease protease inhibitor concentrations and may result in sub-optimal levels of ritonavir and lead to loss of virologic response and possible resistance to ritonavir or to the class of protease inhibitors.

ALLERGIC REACTIONS

Allergic reactions including urticaria, mild skin eruptions, bronchospasm, and angioedema have been reported. Rare cases of anaphylaxis and Stevens-Johnson syndrome have also been reported.

HEPATIC REACTIONS

Hepatic transaminase elevations exceeding 5 times the upper limit of normal, clinical hepatitis, and jaundice have occurred in patients receiving ritonavir alone or in combination with other antiretroviral drugs (see TABLE 8A and TABLE 8B). There may be an increased risk for transaminase elevations in patients with underlying hepatitis B or C. Therefore, caution should be exercised when administering ritonavir to patients with pre-existing liver diseases, liver enzyme abnormalities, or hepatitis. Increased AST/ALT monitoring should be considered in these patients, especially during the first 3 months of ritonavir treatment.

There have been postmarketing reports of hepatic dysfunction, including some fatalities. These have generally occurred in patients taking multiple concomitant medications and/or with advanced AIDS.

PANCREATITIS

Pancreatitis has been observed in patients receiving ritonavir therapy, including those who developed hypertriglyceridemia. In some cases fatalities have been observed. Patients with advanced HIV disease may be at increased risk of elevated triglycerides and pancreatitis.

Pancreatitis should be considered if clinical symptoms (nausea, vomiting, abdominal pain) or abnormalities in laboratory values (such as increased serum lipase or amylase values) suggestive of pancreatitis should occur. Patients who exhibit these signs or symptoms should be evaluated and ritonavir therapy should be discontinued if a diagnosis of pancreatitis is made.

DIABETES MELLITUS/HYPERGLYCEMIA

New onset diabetes mellitus, exacerbation of pre-existing diabetes mellitus, and hyperglycemia have been reported during postmarketing surveillance in HIV-infected patients receiving protease inhibitor therapy. Some patients required either initiation or dose adjustments of insulin or oral hypoglycemic agents for treatment of these events. In some cases, diabetic ketoacidosis has occurred. In those patients who discontinued protease inhibitor therapy, hyperglycemia persisted in some cases. Because these events have been reported voluntarily during clinical practice, estimates of frequency cannot be made and a causal relationship between protease inhibitor therapy and these events has not been established.

PRECAUTIONS

GENERAL

Ritonavir is principally metabolized by the liver. Therefore, caution should be exercised when administering this drug to patients with impaired hepatic function (see WARNINGS; CLINICAL PHARMACOLOGY, Pharmacokinetics, Special Populations, Hepatic Insufficiency; and DOSAGE AND ADMINISTRATION, Dose Adjustment in Hepatic Insufficiency).

RESISTANCE/CROSS-RESISTANCE

Varying degrees of cross-resistance among protease inhibitors have been observed. Continued administration of ritonavir therapy following loss of viral suppression may increase the likelihood of cross-resistance to other protease inhibitors (see CLINICAL PHARMACOLOGY, Microbiology).

HEMOPHILIA

There have been reports of increased bleeding, including spontaneous skin hematomas and hemarthrosis, in patients with hemophilia Type A and B treated with protease inhibitors. In some patients additional factor VIII was given. In more than half of the reported cases, treatment with protease inhibitors was continued or reintroduced. A causal relationship has not been established.

FAT REDISTRIBUTION

Redistribution/accumulation of body fat including central obesity, dorsocervical fat enlargement (buffalo hump), peripheral wasting, breast enlargement, and "cushingoid appearance" have been observed in patients receiving antiretroviral therapy. The mechanism and long-term consequences of these events are currently unknown. A causal relationship has not been established.

LIPID DISORDERS

Treatment with ritonavir therapy alone or in combination with saquinavir has resulted in substantial increases in the concentration of total triglycerides and cholesterol. Triglyceride and cholesterol testing should be performed prior to initiating ritonavir therapy and at periodic intervals during therapy. Lipid disorders should be managed as clinically appropriate. See TABLE 5 for additional information on potential drug interactions with ritonavir and HMG CoA reductase inhibitors.

INFORMATION FOR THE PATIENT

A statement to patients and health care providers is included on the product's bottle label: **ALERT: Find out about medicines that should NOT be taken with ritonavir.** A Patient Package Insert (PPI) for ritonavir is available for patient information.

Patients should be informed that ritonavir is not a cure for HIV infection and that they may continue to acquire illnesses associated with advanced HIV infection, including opportunistic infections.

Patients should be told that the long-term effects of ritonavir are unknown at this time. They should be informed that ritonavir therapy has not been shown to reduce the risk of transmitting HIV to others through sexual contact or blood contamination.

Patients should be advised to take ritonavir with food, if possible.

Patients should be informed to take ritonavir every day as prescribed. Patients should not alter the dose or discontinue ritonavir without consulting their doctor. If a dose is missed, patients should take the next dose as soon as possible. However, if a dose is skipped, the patient should not double the next dose.

Patients should be informed that redistribution or accumulation of body fat may occur in patients receiving antiretroviral therapy and that the cause and long-term health effects of these conditions are not known at this time.

Ritonavir may interact with some drugs; therefore, patients should be advised to report to their doctor the use of any other prescription, non-prescription medication or herbal products, particularly St. John's wort.

LABORATORY TESTS

Ritonavir has been shown to increase triglycerides, cholesterol, SGOT (AST), SGPT (ALT), GGT, CPK, and uric acid. Appropriate laboratory testing should be performed prior to initiating ritonavir therapy and at periodic intervals or if any clinical signs or symptoms occur during therapy. For comprehensive information concerning laboratory test alterations associated with nucleoside analogues, physicians should refer to the complete product information for each of these drugs.

CARCINOGENESIS AND MUTAGENESIS

Carcinogenicity studies in mice and rats have been carried out on ritonavir. In male mice, at levels of 50, 100, or 200 mg/kg/day, there was a dose dependent increase in the incidence of both adenomas and combined adenomas and carcinomas in the liver. Based on AUC measurements, the exposure at the high dose was approximately 0.3-fold for males that of the exposure in humans with the recommended therapeutic dose (600 mg bid). There were no carcinogenic effects seen in females at the dosages tested. The exposure at the high dose was approximately 0.6-fold for the females that of the exposure in humans. In rats dosed at levels of 7, 15, or 30 mg/kg/day there were no carcinogenic effects. In this study, the exposure at the high dose was approximately 6% that of the exposure in humans with the recommended therapeutic dose. Based on the exposures achieved in the animal studies, the significance of the observed effects is not known. However, ritonavir was found to be negative for mutagenic or clastogenic activity in a battery of *in vitro* and *in vivo* assays including the Ames bacterial reverse mutation assay using *S. typhimurium* and *E. coli,* the mouse lymphoma assay, the mouse micronucleus test and chromosomal aberration assays in human lymphocytes.

PREGNANCY, FERTILITY, AND REPRODUCTION: PREGNANCY CATEGORY B

Ritonavir produced no effects on fertility in rats at drug exposures approximately 40% (male) and 60% (female) of that achieved with the proposed therapeutic dose. Higher dosages were not feasible due to hepatic toxicity.

No treatment-related malformations were observed when ritonavir was administered to pregnant rats or rabbits. Developmental toxicity observed in rats (early resorptions, decreased fetal body weight and ossification delays and developmental variations) occurred at a maternally toxic dosage at an exposure equivalent to approximately 30% of that achieved with the proposed therapeutic dose. A slight increase in the incidence of cryptorchidism was also noted in rats at an exposure approximately 22% of that achieved with the proposed therapeutic dose.

Developmental toxicity observed in rabbits (resorptions, decreased litter size and decreased fetal weights) also occurred at a maternally toxic dosage equivalent to 1.8 times the proposed therapeutic dose based on a body surface area conversion factor.

There are, however, no adequate and well-controlled studies in pregnant women. Because animal reproduction studies are not always predictive of human response, this drug should be used during pregnancy only if clearly needed.

Antiretroviral Pregnancy Registry: To monitor maternal-fetal outcomes of pregnant women exposed to ritonavir, an Antiretroviral Pregnancy Registry has been established. Physicians are encouraged to register patients by calling 1-800-258-4263.

NURSING MOTHERS

The Centers for Disease Control and Prevention recommend that HIV-infected mothers not breast-feed their infants to avoid risking postnatal transmission of HIV. It is not known whether ritonavir is secreted in human milk. Because of both the potential for HIV transmission and the potential for serious adverse reactions in nursing infants, mothers should be instructed **not to breast-feed if they are receiving ritonavir.**

PEDIATRIC USE

The safety and pharmacokinetic profile of ritonavir in pediatric patients below the age of 2 years have not been established. In HIV-infected patients age 2-16 years, the adverse event profile seen during a clinical trial and postmarketing experience was similar to that for adult patients. The evaluation of the antiviral activity of ritonavir in pediatric patients in clinical trials is ongoing.

GERIATRIC USE

Clinical studies of ritonavir did not include sufficient numbers of subjects aged 65 and over to determine whether they respond differently from younger subjects. In general, dose selection for an elderly patient should be cautious, usually starting at the low end of the dosing range, reflecting the greater frequency of decreased hepatic, renal or cardiac function, and of concomitant disease or other drug therapy.

DRUG INTERACTIONS

Ritonavir has been found to be an inhibitor of cytochrome P450 3A (CYP3A) both *in vitro* and *in vivo* (TABLE 2). Agents that are extensively metabolized by CYP3A and have high first pass metabolism appear to be the most susceptible to large increases in AUC (>3-fold) when coadministered with ritonavir. Ritonavir also inhibits CYP2D6 to a lesser extent. Coadministration of substrates of CYP2D6 with ritonavir could result in increases (up to 2-fold) in the AUC of the other agent, possibly requiring a proportional dosage reduction. Ritonavir also appears to induce CYP3A as well as other enzymes, including glucuronosyl transferase, CYP1A2, and possibly CYP2C9.

Drugs that are contraindicated specifically due to the expected magnitude of interaction and potential for serious adverse events are listed both in TABLE 3 and TABLE 4.

Those drug interactions that have been established based on drug interaction studies are listed with the pharmacokinetic results in TABLE 2. The clinical recommendations based on the results of these studies are listed in Established Drug Interactions: Alteration in Dose or Regimen Recommended Based on Drug Interaction Studies.

A systematic review of over 200 medications prescribed to HIV-infected patients was performed to identify potential drug interactions with ritonavir.[2] There are a number of agents in which CYP3A or CYP2D6 partially contribute to the metabolism of the agent. In these cases, the magnitude of the interaction and therapeutic consequences cannot be predicted with any certainty.

When coadministering ritonavir with calcium channel blockers, immunosuppressants, some HMG-CoA reductase inhibitors (see WARNINGS, Drug Interactions), some steroids, or other substrates of CYP3A, or most antidepressants, certain antiarrhythmics, and some narcotic analgesics which are partially mediated by CYP2D6 metabolism, it is possible that substantial increases in concentrations of these other agents may occur, possibly requiring a dosage reduction (>50%); examples are listed in TABLE 5.

When coadministering ritonavir with any agent having a narrow therapeutic margin, such as anticoagulants, anticonvulsants, and antiarrhythmics, special attention is warranted. With some agents, the metabolism may be induced, resulting in decreased concentrations (see TABLE 6).

TABLE 4 *Drugs That Should Not Be Coadministered With Ritonavir*

Drug Class: Drug Name	Clinical Comment
Antiarrhythmics: amiodarone, bepridil, flecainide, propafenone, quinidine	CONTRAINDICATED due to potential for serious and/or life-threatening reactions such as cardiac arrhythmias.
Antihistamines: astemizole, terfenadine	CONTRAINDICATED due to potential for serious and/or life-threatening reactions such as cardiac arrhythmias.
Ergot derivatives: dihydroergotamine, ergonovine, ergotamine, methylergonovine	CONTRAINDICATED due to potential for serious and/or life-threatening reactions such as acute ergot toxicity characterized by peripheral vasospasm and ischemia of the extremities and other tissues.
GI motility agent: cisapride	CONTRAINDICATED due to potential for serious and/or life-threatening reactions such as cardiac arrhythmias.
Herbal Products: St. John's wort (hypericum perforatum)	May lead to loss of virologic response and possible resistance to ritonavir or to the class of protease inhibitors.
HMG-CoA reductase inhibitors: lovastatin, simvastatin	Potential for serious reactions such as risk of myopathy including rhabdomyolysis.
Neuroleptic: pimozide	CONTRAINDICATED due to the potential for serious and/or life-threatening reactions such as cardiac arrhythmias.
Sedative/hypnotics: midazolam, triazolam	CONTRAINDICATED due to potential for serious and/or life-threatening reactions such as prolonged or increased sedation or respiratory depression.

ESTABLISHED DRUG INTERACTIONS: ALTERATION IN DOSE OR REGIMEN RECOMMENDED BASED ON DRUG INTERACTION STUDIES

See TABLE 2 for magnitude of interaction.

HIV-Antiviral Agents

HIV Protease Inhibitor

Indinavir

Effect: *When coadministered with reduced doses of indinavir and ritonavir:* Increases indinavir concentration (no change to AUC, decreases C_{max}, increases C_{min}).

Clinical Comment:

Alterations in concentrations are noted when reduced doses of indinavir are coadministered with ritonavir.

Appropriate doses for this combination, with respect to efficacy and safety, have not been established.

Saquinavir

Effect: *When coadministered with reduced doses of saquinavir and ritonavir:* Increases saquinavir concentration (increases AUC, increases C_{max}, increases C_{min}).

Clinical Comment: When used in combination therapy for up to 24 weeks, doses of 400 mg bid of ritonavir and saquinavir were better tolerated than the higher doses of the combination. Saquinavir plasma concentrations achieved with saquinavir mesylate (400 mg bid) and ritonavir (400 mg bid) are similar to those achieved with saquinavir (400 mg bid) and ritonavir (400 mg bid).

Nucleoside Reverse Transcriptase Inhibitor

Didanosine

Clinical Comment: Dosing of didanosine and ritonavir should be separated by 2.5 hours to avoid formulation incompatibility.

Other Agents

Anesthetic

Meperidine

Effect: Decreases meperidine concentration; increases normeperidine concentration (metabolite).

Clinical Comment: Dosage increase and long-term use of meperidine with ritonavir are not recommended due to the increased concentrations of the metabolite normeperidine which has both analgesic activity and CNS stimulant activity (*e.g.,* seizures).

Antialcoholics

Disulfiram/Metronidazole

Clinical Comment: Ritonavir formulations contain alcohol, which can produce disulfiram-like reactions when coadministered with disulfiram or other drugs that produce this reaction (*e.g.,* metronidazole).

Antidepressant

Desipramine

Effect: Increases desipramine concentration.

Clinical Comment: Dosage reduction and concentration monitoring of desipramine is recommended.

Antifungal

Ketoconazole

Effect: Increases ketoconazole concentration.

Clinical Comment: High doses of ketoconazole (>200 mg/day) are not recommended.

Anti-Infective

Clarithromycin

Effect: Increases clarithromycin concentration.

Clinical Comment:

For patients with renal impairment the following dosage adjustments should be considered:

- For patients with CLCR 30-60 ml/min the dose of clarithromycin should be reduced by 50%.
- For patients with CLCR <30 ml/min the dose of clarithromycin should be decreased by 75%.

No dose adjustment for patients with normal renal function is necessary.

Antimycobacterial

Rifabutin

Effect: Increases rifabutin and rifabutin metabolite concentration.

Clinical Comment: Dosage reduction of rifabutin by at least three-quarters of the usual dose of 300 mg/day is recommended (*e.g.*, 150 mg every other day or 3 times a week). Further dosage reduction may be necessary.

Rifampin

Effect: Decreases ritonavir concentration.

Clinical Comment: May lead to loss of virologic response. Alternate antimycobacterial agents such as rifabutin should be considered (see Rifabutin, for dose reduction recommendations).

Bronchodilator

Theophylline

Effect: Decreases theophylline concentration.

Clinical Comment: Increased dosage of theophylline may be required; therapeutic monitoring should be considered.

Erectile Dysfunction

Sildenafil

Effect: Increases sildenafil concentration.

Clinical Comment: Sildenafil should not exceed a maximum single dose of 25 mg in a 48 hour period in patients receiving concomitant ritonavir therapy (see WARNINGS).

Narcotic Analgesic

Methadone

Effect: Decreases methadone concentration.

Clinical Comment: Dosage increase of methadone may be considered.

Oral Contraceptive

Ethinyl Estradiol

Effect: Decreases ethinyl estradiol concentration.

Clinical Comment: Dosage increase or alternate contraceptive measures should be considered.

TABLE 5 *Predicted Drug Interactions: Use With Caution, Dose Decrease of Coadministered Drug May Be Needed (see WARNINGS)*

Examples of drugs in which plasma concentrations may be increased by coadministration with ritonavir

Drug Class	Examples of Drugs
Analgesics, narcotic	Tramadol, propoxyphene
Antiarrhythmics	Disopyramide, lidocaine, mexilitine
Anticonvulsants	Carbamazepine, clonazepam, ethosuximide
Antidepressants	Bupropion, nefazodone, selective serotonin reuptake inhibitors (SSRIs), tricyclics
Antiemetics	Dronabinol
Antiparasitics	Quinine
β-blockers	Metoprolol, timolol
Calcium channel blockers	Diltiazem, nifedipine, verapamil
Hypolipidemics, HMG CoA reductase inhibitors*	Atorvastatin, cerivastatin†
Immunosuppressants	Cyclosporine, tacrolimus, rapamycin
Neuroleptics	Perphenazine, risperidone, thioridazine
Sedative/hypnotics	Clorazepate, diazepam, estazolam, flurazepam, zolpidem
Steroids	Dexamethasone, prednisone
Stimulants	Methamphetamine

* Coadministration with lovastatin and simvastatin is not recommended (see WARNINGS, Drug Interactions).

† Use lowest possible dose of atorvastatin or cerivastatin with careful monitoring or consider HMG-CoA reductase inhibitor such as pravastatin or fluvastatin.

TABLE 6 *Predicted Drug Interactions: Use With Caution, Dose Increase of Coadministered Drug May Be Needed (see WARNINGS)*

Examples of drugs in which plasma concentrations may be decreased by coadministration with ritonavir

Drug Class	Examples of Drugs
Anticoagulants	Warfarin
Anticonvulsants	Phenytoin, divalproex, lamotrigine
Antiparasitics	Atovaquone

POSTMARKETING EXPERIENCE WITH DRUGS LISTED IN TABLE 5

Cardiac and neurologic events have been reported when ritonavir has been coadministered with disopyramide, mexiletine, nefazodone, fluoxetine, and beta blockers. The possibility of drug interaction cannot be excluded.

ADVERSE REACTIONS

The safety of ritonavir alone and in combination with nucleoside analogues was studied in 1270 patients. TABLE 7A lists treatment-emergent adverse events (at least possibly related and of at least moderate intensity) that occurred in 2% or greater of patients receiving ritonavir alone or in combination with nucleosides in Study 245 or Study 247 and in combination with saquinavir in ongoing Study 462. In that study, 141 protease inhibitor-naive, HIV-infected patients with mean baseline CD4 of 300 cells/μl were randomized to 1 of 4 regimens of ritonavir + saquinavir, including ritonavir 400 mg bid + saquinavir 400 mg bid. Overall the most frequently reported clinical adverse events, other than asthenia, among patients receiving ritonavir were gastrointestinal and neurological disturbances including nausea, diarrhea, vomiting, anorexia, abdominal pain, taste perversion, and circumoral and peripheral paresthesias. Similar adverse event profiles were reported in patients receiving ritonavir in other trials.

TABLE 7A *Percentage of Patients With Treatment-Emergent Adverse Events* of Moderate or Severe Intensity Occurring in ≥2% of Patients Receiving Ritonavir*

	Study 245: Naive Patients†		
Adverse Events	**Ritonavir + ZDV n=116**	**Ritonavir n=117**	**ZDV n=119**
Body as a Whole			
Abdominal pain	5.2%	6.0%	5.9%
Asthenia	28.4%	10.3%	11.8%
Fever	1.7%	0.9%	1.7%
Headache	7.8%	6.0%	6.7%
Malaise	5.2%	1.7%	3.4%
Pain (unspecified)	0.9%	1.7%	0.8%
Cardiovascular			
Syncope	0.9%	1.7%	0.8%
Vasodilation	3.4%	1.7%	0.8%
Digestive			
Anorexia	8.6%	1.7%	4.2%
Constipation	3.4%	0.0%	0.8%
Diarrhea	25.0%	15.4%	2.5%
Dyspepsia	2.6%	0.0%	1.7%
Fecal incontinence	0.0%	0.0%	0.0%
Flatulence	2.6%	0.9%	1.7%
Local throat irritation	0.9%	1.7%	0.8%
Nausea	46.6%	25.6%	26.1%
Vomiting	23.3%	13.7%	12.6%
Metabolic and Nutritional			
Weight loss	0.0%	0.0%	0.0%
Musculoskeletal			
Arthralgia	0.0%	0.0%	0.0%
Myalgia	1.7%	1.7%	0.8%
Nervous			
Anxiety	0.9%	0.0%	0.8%
Circumoral paresthesia	5.2%	3.4%	0.0%
Confusion	0.0%	0.9%	0.0%
Depression	1.7%	1.7%	2.5%
Dizziness	5.2%	2.6%	3.4%
Insomnia	3.4%	2.6%	0.8%
Paresthesia	5.2%	2.6%	0.0%
Peripheral paresthesia	0.0%	6.0%	0.8%
Somnolence	2.6%	2.6%	0.0%
Thinking abnormal	2.6%	0.0%	0.8%
Respiratory			
Pharyngitis	0.9%	2.6%	0.0%
Skin and Appendages			
Rash	0.9%	0.0%	0.8%
Sweating	3.4%	2.6%	1.7%
Special Senses			
Taste perversion	17.2%	11.1%	8.4%
Urogenital			
Nocturia	0.0%	0.0%	0.0%

* Includes those adverse events at least possibly related to study drug or of unknown relationship and excludes concurrent HIV conditions.

† The median duration of treatment for patients randomized to regimens containing ritonavir in Study 245 was 9.1 months.

Adverse events occurring in less than 2% of patients receiving ritonavir in all Phase 2/Phase 3 studies and considered at least possibly related or of unknown relationship to treatment and of at least moderate intensity are listed below by body system.

Body as a Whole: Abdomen enlarged, accidental injury, allergic reaction, back pain, cachexia, chest pain, chills, facial edema, facial pain, flu syndrome, hormone level altered, hypothermia, kidney pain, neck pain, neck rigidity, pelvic pain, photosensitivity reaction, and substernal chest pain.

Cardiovascular System: Cardiovascular disorder, cerebral ischemia, cerebral venous thrombosis, hypertension, hypotension, migraine, myocardial infarct, palpitation, peripheral vascular disorder, phlebitis, postural hypotension, tachycardia and vasospasm.

Digestive System: Abnormal stools, bloody diarrhea, cheilitis, cholestatic jaundice, colitis, dry mouth, dysphagia, eructation, esophageal ulcer, esophagitis, gastritis, gastroenteritis, gastrointestinal disorder, gastrointestinal hemorrhage, gingivitis, hepatic coma, hepatitis, hepatomegaly, hepatosplenomegaly, ileus, liver damage, melena, mouth ulcer, pancreatitis, pseudomembranous colitis, rectal disorder, rectal hemorrhage, sialadenitis, stomatitis, tenesmus, thirst, tongue edema, and ulcerative colitis.

Endocrine System: Adrenal cortex insufficiency and diabetes mellitus.

Hemic and Lymphatic System: Acute myeloblastic leukemia, anemia, ecchymosis, leukopenia, lymphadenopathy, lymphocytosis, myeloproliferative disorder, and thrombocytopenia.

Metabolic and Nutritional Disorders: Albuminuria, alcohol intolerance, avitaminosis, BUN increased, dehydration, edema, enzymatic abnormality, glycosuria, gout, hypercholesteremia, peripheral edema, and xanthomatosis.

Musculoskeletal System: Arthritis, arthrosis, bone disorder, bone pain, extraocular palsy, joint disorder, leg cramps, muscle cramps, muscle weakness, myositis, and twitching.

Nervous System: Abnormal dreams, abnormal gait, agitation, amnesia, aphasia, ataxia, coma, convulsion, dementia, depersonalization, diplopia, emotional lability, euphoria, grand mal convulsion, hallucinations, hyperesthesia, hyperkinesia, hypesthesia, incoordination, libido decreased, manic reaction, nervousness, neuralgia, neuropathy, paralysis, peripheral neuropathic pain, peripheral neuropathy, peripheral sen-

TABLE 7B *Percentage of Patients With Treatment-Emergent Adverse Events* of Moderate or Severe Intensity Occurring in ≥2% of Patients Receiving Ritonavir*

	Study 247: Advanced Patients†		Study 462: PI-Naive Patients‡
	Ritonavir	Placebo	Ritonavir + Saquinavir
Adverse Events	n=541	n=545	n=141
Body as a Whole			
Abdominal pain	8.3%	5.1%	2.1%
Asthenia	15.3%	6.4%	16.3%
Fever	5.0%	2.4%	0.7%
Headache	6.5%	5.7%	4.3%
Malaise	0.7%	0.2%	2.8%
Pain (unspecified)	2.2%	1.8%	4.3%
Cardiovascular			
Syncope	0.6%	0.0%	2.1%
Vasodilation	1.7%	0.0%	3.5%
Digestive			
Anorexia	7.8%	4.2%	4.3%
Constipation	0.2%	0.4%	1.4%
Diarrhea	23.3%	7.9%	22.7%
Dyspepsia	5.9%	1.5%	0.7%
Fecal incontinence	0.0%	0.0%	2.8%
Flatulence	1.7%	0.7%	3.5%
Local throat irritation	2.8%	0.4%	1.4%
Nausea	29.8%	8.4%	18.4%
Vomiting	17.4%	4.4%	7.1%
Metabolic and Nutritional			
Weight loss	2.4%	1.7%	0.0%
Musculoskeletal			
Arthralgia	1.7%	0.7%	2.1%
Myalgia	2.4%	1.1%	2.1%
Nervous			
Anxiety	1.7%	0.9%	2.1%
Circumoral paresthesia	6.7%	0.4%	6.4%
Confusion	0.6%	0.6%	2.1%
Depression	1.7%	0.7%	7.1%
Dizziness	3.9%	1.1%	8.5%
Insomnia	2.0%	1.8%	2.8%
Paresthesia	3.0%	0.4%	2.1%
Peripheral paresthesia	5.0%	1.1%	5.7%
Somnolence	2.4%	0.2%	0.0%
Thinking abnormal	0.9%	0.4%	0.0%
Respiratory			
Pharyngitis	0.4%	0.4%	1.4%
Skin and Appendages			
Rash	3.5%	1.5%	0.7%
Sweating	1.7%	1.1%	2.8%
Special Senses			
Taste perversion	7.0%	2.2%	5.0%
Urogenital			
Nocturia	0.2%	0.0%	2.8%

* Includes those adverse events at least possibly related to study drug or of unknown relationship and excludes concurrent HIV conditions.
† The median duration of treatment for patients randomized to regimens containing ritonavir in Study 247 was 9.4 months.
‡ The median duration of treatment for patients in ongoing Study 462 was 48 weeks.

sory neuropathy, personality disorder, sleep disorder, speech disorder, stupor, subdural hematoma, tremor, urinary retention, vertigo, and vestibular disorder.

Respiratory System: Asthma, bronchitis, dyspnea, epistaxis, hiccup, hypoventilation, increased cough, interstitial pneumonia, larynx edema, lung disorder, rhinitis, and sinusitis.

Skin and Appendages: Acne, contact dermatitis, dry skin, eczema, erythema multiforme, exfoliative dermatitis, folliculitis, fungal dermatitis, furunculosis, maculopapular rash, molluscum contagiosum, onychomycosis, pruritus, psoriasis, pustular rash, seborrhea, skin discoloration, skin disorder, skin hypertrophy, skin melanoma, urticaria, and vesiculobullous rash.

Special Senses: Abnormal electro-oculogram, abnormal electroretinogram, abnormal vision, amblyopia/blurred vision, blepharitis, conjunctivitis, ear pain, eye disorder, eye pain, hearing impairment, increased cerumen, iritis, parosmia, photophobia, taste loss, tinnitus, uveitis, visual field defect, and vitreous disorder.

Urogenital System: Acute kidney failure, breast pain, cystitis, dysuria, hematuria, impotence, kidney calculus, kidney failure, kidney function abnormal, kidney pain, menorrhagia, penis disorder, polyuria, urethritis, urinary frequency, urinary tract infection, and vaginitis.

POSTMARKETING EXPERIENCE

There have been postmarketing reports of seizure. Cause and effect relationship has not been established.

Dehydration, usually associated with gastrointestinal symptoms, and sometimes resulting in hypotension, syncope, or renal insufficiency has been reported. Syncope, orthostatic hypotension, and renal insufficiency have also been reported without known dehydration.

Redistribution/accumulation of body fat has been reported (see PRECAUTIONS, Fat Redistribution). There have been reports of increased bleeding in patients with hemophilia A or B (see PRECAUTIONS, Hemophilia).

LABORATORY ABNORMALITIES

TABLE 8A and TABLE 8B show the percentage of patients who developed marked laboratory abnormalities.

TABLE 8A *Percentage of Patients, by Study and Treatment Group, With Chemistry and Hematology Abnormalities Occurring in >3% of Patients Receiving Ritonavir*

		Study 245: Naive Patients		
Variable	Limit	Ritonavir + ZDV	Ritonavir	ZDV
Chemistry	**High**			
Cholesterol	>240 mg/dl	30.7%	44.8%	9.3%
CPK	>1000 IU/L	9.6%	12.1%	11.0%
GGT	>300 IU/L	1.8%	5.2%	1.7%
SGOT (AST)	>180 IU/L	5.3%	9.5%	2.5%
SGPT (ALT)	>215 IU/L	5.3%	7.8%	3.4%
Triglycerides	>800 mg/dl	9.6%	17.2%	3.4%
Triglycerides	>1500 mg/dl	1.8%	2.6%	—
Triglycerides, fasting	>1500 mg/dl	1.5%	1.3%	—
Uric acid	>12 mg/dl	—	—	—
Hematology	**Low**			
Hematocrit	<30%	2.6%	—	0.8%
Hemoglobin	<8.0 g/dl	0.9%	—	—
Neutrophils	$\leq 0.5 \times 10^9$/L	—	—	—
RBC	$<3.0 \times 10^{12}$/L	1.8%	—	5.9%
WBC	$<2.5 \times 10^9$/L	—	0.9%	6.8%

— Indicates no events reported.

TABLE 8B *Percentage of Patients, by Study and Treatment Group, With Chemistry and Hematology Abnormalities Occurring in >3% of Patients Receiving Ritonavir*

		Study 247: Advanced Patients		Study 462: PI-Naive Patients
Variable	Limit	Ritonavir	Placebo	Ritonavir + Saquinavir
Chemistry	**High**			
Cholesterol	>240 mg/dl	36.5%	8.0%	65.2%
CPK	>1000 IU/L	9.1%	6.3%	9.9%
GGT	>300 IU/L	19.6%	11.3%	9.2%
SGOT (AST)	>180 IU/L	6.4%	7.0%	7.8%
SGPT (ALT)	>215 IU/L	8.5%	4.4%	9.2%
Triglycerides	>800 mg/dl	33.6%	9.4%	23.4%
Triglycerides	>1500 mg/dl	12.6%	0.4%	11.3%
Triglycerides, fasting	>1500 mg/dl	9.9%	0.3%	—
Uric acid	>12 mg/dl	3.8%	0.2%	1.4%
Hematology	**Low**			
Hematocrit	<30%	17.3%	22.0%	0.7%
Hemoglobin	<8.0 g/dl	3.8%	3.9%	—
Neutrophils	$\leq 0.5 \times 10^9$/L	6.0%	8.3%	—
RBC	$<3.0 \times 10^{12}$/L	18.6%	24.4%	—
WBC	$<2.5 \times 10^9$/L	36.9%	59.4%	3.5%

— Indicates no events reported.

DOSAGE AND ADMINISTRATION

Ritonavir is administered orally. It is recommended that ritonavir be taken with meals if possible. Patients may improve the taste of ritonavir oral solution by mixing with chocolate milk, Ensure, or Advera within 1 hour of dosing. The effects of antacids on the absorption of ritonavir have not been studied.

ADULTS

Recommended Dosage

The recommended dosage of ritonavir is 600 mg twice daily by mouth. Use of a dose titration schedule may help to reduce treatment-emergent adverse events while maintaining appropriate ritonavir plasma levels. Ritonavir should be started at no less than 300 mg twice daily and increased at 2-3 day intervals by 100 mg twice daily.

Concomitant Therapy

If saquinavir and ritonavir are used in combination, the dosage of saquinavir should be reduced to 400 mg twice daily. The optimum dosage of ritonavir (400 or 600 mg twice daily), in combination with saquinavir, has not been determined; however, the combination regimen was better tolerated in patients who received ritonavir 400 mg twice daily.

PEDIATRIC PATIENTS

Ritonavir should be used in combination with other antiretroviral agents (see General Dosing Guidelines). The recommended dosage of ritonavir is 400 mg/m^2 twice daily by mouth and should not exceed 600 mg twice daily. Ritonavir should be started at 250 mg/m^2 and increased at 2-3 day intervals by 50 mg/m^2 twice daily. If patients do not tolerate 400 mg/m^2 twice daily due to adverse events, the highest tolerated dose may be used for maintenance therapy in combination with other antiretroviral agents; however, alternative therapy should be considered. When possible, dose should be administered using a calibrated dosing syringe.

DOSE ADJUSTMENT IN HEPATIC INSUFFICIENCY

The ritonavir dose does not need to be adjusted in patients with mild hepatic impairment. At this time, there are insufficient data in patients with moderate to severe hepatic impairment; therefore, ritonavir should be used with caution in this patient population (see CLINICAL PHARMACOLOGY, Pharmacokinetics, Special Populations, Hepatic Insufficiency and PRECAUTIONS.

TABLE 9 *Pediatric Dosage Guidelines*[1]

Body Surface Area* (m^2)	Twice Daily Dose (mg/m^2) 250 ml (mg)	300 ml (mg)	350 ml (mg)	400 ml (mg)
0.25	0.8 (62.5)	0.9 (75)	1.1 (87.5)	1.25 (100)
0.50	1.6 (125)	1.9 (150)	2.2 (175)	2.5 (200)
1.00	3.1 (250)	3.75 (300)	4.4 (350)	5 (400)
1.25	3.9 (312.5)	4.7 (375)	5.5 (437.5)	6.25 (500)
1.50	4.7 (375)	5.6 (450)	6.6 (525)	7.5 (600)

* Body surface area can be calculated with the following equation: BSA (m^2) = {[Ht (cm) × Wt (kg)] ÷ 3600}½

GENERAL DOSING GUIDELINES

Patients should be aware that frequently observed adverse events, such as mild to moderate gastrointestinal disturbances and paraesthesias, may diminish as therapy is continued. In addition, patients initiating combination regimens with ritonavir and nucleosides may improve gastrointestinal tolerance by initiating ritonavir alone and subsequently adding nucleosides before completing 2 weeks of ritonavir monotherapy.

HOW SUPPLIED

NORVIR SOFT GELATIN CAPSULES

Norvir soft gelatin capsules are white capsules imprinted with the Abbott corporate logo, "100" and the Abbo-Code "DS".

Storage

Store soft gelatin capsules in the refrigerator between 2-8°C (36-46°F) until dispensed. Refrigeration of Norvir soft gelatin capsules by the patient is recommended, but not required if used within 30 days and stored below 25°C (77°F). Protect from light. Avoid exposure to excessive heat.

NORVIR ORAL SOLUTION

Norvir oral solution is an orange-colored liquid, supplied in amber-colored, multi-dose bottles containing 600 mg ritonavir per 7.5 ml marked dosage cup (80 mg/ml).

Storage

Store Norvir oral solution at room temperature 20-25°C (68-77°F). Do not refrigerate. Shake well before each use. Use by product expiration date.

Product should be stored and dispensed in the original container.

Avoid exposure to excessive heat. Keep cap tightly closed.

PRODUCT LISTING - EQUIVALENTS NOT AVAILABLE

Capsule - Oral - 100 mg

84's	$155.83	NORVIR, Abbott Pharmaceutical	00074-9492-54
120's	$257.17	NORVIR SOFT GELATIN, Abbott Pharmaceutical	00074-6633-22
168's	$311.65	NORVIR, Abbott Pharmaceutical	00074-9492-02
168's	$322.31	NORVIR, Physicians Total Care	54868-3782-00

Solution - Oral - 80 mg/ml

240 ml	$335.14	NORVIR, Allscripts Pharmaceutical Company	54569-4613-00
240 ml	$360.05	NORVIR, Abbott Pharmaceutical	00074-1940-63

R

Rituximab *(003377)*

Categories: Lymphoma, non-Hodgkin's; FDA Approved 1997 Nov; Pregnancy Category C; Orphan Drugs
Drug Classes: Antineoplastics, monoclonal antibodies; Monoclonal antibodies
Brand Names: Rituxan
Foreign Brand Availability: Mabthera (Australia; Austria; Belgium; Benin; Bulgaria; Burkina-Faso; Colombia; Czech-Republic; Denmark; England; Ethiopia; Finland; France; Gambia; Germany; Ghana; Greece; Guinea; Hong-Kong; Hungary; Ireland; Israel; Italy; Ivory-Coast; Kenya; Liberia; Malawi; Mali; Mauritania; Mauritius; Mexico; Morocco; Netherlands; New-Zealand; Niger; Nigeria; Norway; Philippines; Poland; Portugal; Senegal; Seychelles; Sierra-Leone; Singapore; Slovenia; Spain; Sudan; Sweden; Switzerland; Tanzania; Tunia; Turkey; Uganda; Zambia; Zimbabwe)

WARNING

Fatal Infusion Reactions

Deaths within 24 hours of rituximab infusion have been reported. These fatal reactions followed an infusion reaction complex which included hypoxia, pulmonary infiltrates, acute respiratory distress syndrome, myocardial infarction, ventricular fibrillation or cardiogenic shock. Approximately 80% of fatal infusion reactions occurred in association with the first infusion. (See WARNINGS and ADVERSE REACTIONS.)

Patients who develop severe infusion reactions should have rituximab infusion discontinued and receive medical treatment.

Tumor Lysis Syndrome (TLS)

Acute renal failure requiring dialysis with instances of fatal outcome has been reported in the setting of TLS following treatment with rituximab. (See WARNINGS.)

Severe Mucocutaneous Reactions

Severe mucocutaneous reactions, some with fatal outcome, have been reported in association with rituximab treatment. (See WARNINGS and ADVERSE REACTIONS.)

DESCRIPTION

The Rituxan (rituximab) antibody is a genetically engineered chimeric murine/human monoclonal antibody directed against the CD20 antigen found on the surface of normal and malignant B lymphocytes. The antibody is an IgG_1 kappa immunoglobulin containing murine light- and heavy-chain variable region sequences and human constant region sequences. Rituximab is composed of two heavy chains of 451 amino acids and two light chains of 213 amino acids (based on cDNA analysis) and has an approximate molecular weight of 145 kD. Rituximab has a binding affinity for the CD20 antigen of approximately 8.0 nM.

The chimeric anti-CD20 antibody is produced by mammalian cell (Chinese Hamster Ovary) suspension culture in a nutrient medium containing the antibiotic gentamicin. Gentamicin is not detectable in the final product. The anti-CD20 antibody is purified by affinity and ion exchange chromatography. The purification process includes specific viral inactivation and removal procedures. Rituximab drug product is manufactured from either bulk drug substance manufactured by Genentech, Inc. (US License No. 1048) or utilizing formulated bulk rituximab supplied by IDEC Pharmaceuticals Corporation (US License No. 1235) under a shared manufacturing arrangement.

Rituxan is a sterile, clear, colorless, preservative-free liquid concentrate for intravenous (IV) administration. Rituxan is supplied at a concentration of 10 mg/ml in either 100 mg (10 ml) or 500 mg (50 ml) single-use vials. The product is formulated for IV administration in 9.0 mg/ml sodium chloride, 7.35 mg/ml sodium citrate dihydrate, 0.7 mg/ml polysorbate 80, and sterile water for injection. The pH is adjusted to 6.5.

CLINICAL PHARMACOLOGY

GENERAL

Rituximab binds specifically to the antigen CD20 (human B-lymphocyte-restricted differentiation antigen, Bp35), a hydrophobic transmembrane protein with a molecular weight of approximately 35 kD located on pre-B and mature B lymphocytes.[1,2] The antigen is also expressed on >90% of B-cell non-Hodgkin's lymphomas (NHL),[3] but is not found on hematopoietic stem cells, pro-B cells, normal plasma cells or other normal tissues.[4] CD20 regulates an early step(s) in the activation process for cell cycle initiation and differentiation,[4] and possibly functions as a calcium ion channel.[5] CD20 is not shed from the cell surface and does not internalize upon antibody binding.[6] Free CD20 antigen is not found in the circulation.[2]

PRECLINICAL PHARMACOLOGY AND TOXICOLOGY

Mechanism of Action

The Fab domain of rituximab binds to the CD20 antigen on B lymphocytes, and the Fc domain recruits immune effector functions to mediate B-cell lysis *in vitro*. Possible mechanisms of cell lysis include complement-dependent cytotoxicity (CDC)[7] and antibody-dependent cell mediated cytotoxicity (ADCC). The antibody has been shown to induce apoptosis in the DHL-4 human B-cell lymphoma line.[8]

Normal Tissue Cross-Reactivity

Rituximab binding was observed on lymphoid cells in the thymus, the white pulp of the spleen, and a majority of B lymphocytes in peripheral blood and lymph nodes. Little or no binding was observed in the non-lymphoid tissues examined.

HUMAN PHARMACOKINETICS/PHARMACODYNAMICS

In patients given single doses at 10, 50, 100, 250 or 500 mg/m^2 as an IV infusion, serum levels and the half-life of rituximab were proportional to dose.[9] In 14 patients given 375 mg/m^2 as an IV infusion for 4 weekly doses, the mean serum half-life was 76.3 hours (range, 31.5-152.6 hours) after the first infusion and 205.8 hours (range, 83.9-407.0 hours); after the fourth infusion.[10-12] The wide range of half-lives may reflect the variable tumor burden among patients and the changes in CD20-positive (normal and malignant) B-cell populations upon repeated administrations.

Rituximab at a dose of 375 mg/m^2 was administered as an IV infusion at weekly intervals for 4 doses to 203 patients naive to rituximab. The mean C_{max} following the fourth infusion was 486 µg/ml (range, 77.5-996.6 µg/ml). The peak and trough serum levels of rituximab were inversely correlated with baseline values for the number of circulating CD20 positive B cells and measures of disease burden. Median steady-state serum levels were higher for responders compared with nonresponders; however, no difference was found in the rate of elimination as measured by serum half-life. Serum levels were higher in patients with International Working Formulation (IWF) subtypes B, C, and D as compared with those with subtype A. Rituximab was detectable in the serum of patients 3-6 months after completion of treatment.

Rituximab at a dose of 375 mg/m^2 was administered as an IV infusion at weekly intervals for 8 doses to 37 patients. The mean C_{max} after 8 infusions was 550 µg/ml (range, 171-1177 µg/ml). The mean C_{max} increased with each successive infusion through the eighth infusion (TABLE 1).

TABLE 1 *Rituximab C_{max} Values*

Infusion Number	Mean C_{max} (µg/ml)	Range (µg/ml)
1	242.6	16.1-581.9
2	357.5	106.8-948.6
3	381.3	110.5-731.2
4	460.0	138.0-835.8
5	475.3	156.0-929.1
6	515.4	152.7-865.2
7	544.6	187.0-936.8
8	550.0	170.6-1177.0

The pharmacokinetic profile of rituximab when administered as 6 infusions of 375 mg/m^2 in combination with 6 cycles of CHOP chemotherapy was similar to that seen with rituximab alone.

Administration of rituximab resulted in a rapid and sustained depletion of circulating and tissue-based B cells. Lymph node biopsies performed 14 days after therapy showed a decrease in the percentage of B cells in 7 of 8 patients who had received single doses of rituximab >100 mg/m^2.[9] Among the 166 patients in the pivotal study, circulating B cells (measured as CD19-positive cells) were depleted within the first 3 doses with sustained depletion for up to 6-9 months post-treatment in 83% of patients. Of the responding patients assessed (n=80), 1% failed to show significant depletion of CD19-positive cells after the third infusion of rituximab as compared to 19% of the nonresponding patients. B-cell recovery began at approximately 6 months following completion of treatment. Median B-cell levels returned to normal by 12 months following completion of treatment.

There were sustained and statistically significant reductions in both IgM and IgG serum levels observed from 5-11 months following rituximab administration. However, only 14% of patients had reductions in IgM and/or IgG serum levels, resulting in values below the normal range.

INDICATIONS AND USAGE

Rituximab is indicated for the treatment of patients with relapsed or refractory, low-grade or follicular, CD20-positive, B-cell non-Hodgkin's lymphoma.

NON-FDA APPROVED INDICATIONS

The drug is also used in the treatment of chronic lymphocytic leukemia. One study has reported the drug to be effective in the first-line therapy of patients with low-grade non-Hodgkin's lymphoma. A very small study (n=3) on the treatment of cutaneous B-cell lymphoma has reported complete and lasting remission for up to more than one year. However, these uses have not been approved by the FDA and further clinical trials are needed.

CONTRAINDICATIONS

Rituximab is contraindicated in patients with known anaphylaxis or IgE-mediated hypersensitivity to murine proteins or to any component of this product. (See WARNINGS.)

WARNINGS

See BOXED WARNING.

SEVERE INFUSION REACTIONS

See BOXED WARNING, ADVERSE REACTIONS and Hypersensitivity Reactions.

Rituximab has caused severe infusion reactions. In some cases, these reactions were fatal. These severe reactions typically occurred during the first infusion with time to onset of 30-120 minutes. Signs and symptoms of severe infusion reactions may include hypotension, angioedema, hypoxia or bronchospasm, and may require interruption of rituximab administration. The most severe manifestations and sequelae include pulmonary infiltrates, acute respiratory distress syndrome, myocardial infarction, ventricular fibrillation, and cardiogenic shock. In the reported cases, the following factors were more frequently associated with fatal outcomes: female gender, pulmonary infiltrates, and chronic lymphocytic leukemia or mantle cell lymphoma.

Management of Severe Infusion Reactions

The rituximab infusion should be interrupted for severe reactions and supportive care measures instituted as medically indicated (*e.g.,* intravenous fluids, vasopressors, oxygen, bronchodilators, diphenhydramine, and acetaminophen). In most cases, the infusion can be resumed at a 50% reduction in rate (*e.g.,* from 100 mg/h to 50 mg/h) when symptoms have completely resolved. Patients requiring close monitoring during first and all subsequent infusions include those with pre-existing cardiac and pulmonary conditions, those with prior clinically significant cardiopulmonary adverse events and those with high numbers of circulating malignant cells (≥25,000/mm^3) with or without evidence of high tumor burden.

TUMOR LYSIS SYNDROME (TLS)

See BOXED WARNING and ADVERSE REACTIONS.

Rapid reduction in tumor volume followed by acute renal failure, hyperkalemia, hypocalcemia, hyperuricemia, or hyperphosphatasemia, have been reported within 12-24 hours after the first rituximab infusion. Rare instances of fatal outcome have been reported in the setting of TLS following treatment with rituximab. The risks of TLS appear to be greater in patients with high numbers of circulating malignant cells (≥25,000/mm^3) or high tumor burden. Prophylaxis for TLS should be considered for patients at high risk. Correction of electrolyte abnormalities, monitoring of renal function and fluid balance, and administration of supportive care, including dialysis, should be initiated as indicated. Following complete resolution of the complications of TLS, rituximab has been tolerated when re-administered in conjunction with prophylactic therapy for TLS in a limited number of cases.

HYPERSENSITIVITY REACTIONS

Rituximab has been associated with hypersensitivity reactions (non-IgE-mediated reactions) which may respond to adjustments in the infusion rate and in medical management. Hypotension, bronchospasm, and angioedema have occurred in association with rituximab infusion (see Severe Infusion Reactions). Rituximab infusion should be interrupted for severe hypersensitivity reactions and can be resumed at a 50% reduction in rate (*e.g.,* from 100 mg/h to 50 mg/h) when symptoms have completely resolved. Treatment of these symptoms with diphenhydramine and acetaminophen is recommended; additional treatment with bronchodilators or IV saline may be indicated. In most cases, patients who have experienced non-life-threatening hypersensitivity reactions have been able to complete the full course of therapy. (See DOSAGE AND ADMINISTRATION.) Medications for the treatment of hypersensitivity reactions, *e.g.,* epinephrine, antihistamines and corticosteroids, should be available for immediate use in the event of a reaction during administration.

CARDIOVASCULAR

Infusions should be discontinued in the event of serious or life-threatening cardiac arrhythmias. Patients who develop clinically significant arrhythmias should undergo cardiac monitoring during and after subsequent infusions of rituximab. Patients with pre-existing cardiac conditions including arrhythmias and angina have had recurrences of these events during rituximab therapy and should be monitored throughout the infusion and immediate post-infusion period.

RENAL

Rituximab administration has been associated with severe renal toxicity including acute renal failure requiring dialysis and in some cases, has led to a fatal outcome. Renal toxicity has occurred in patients with high numbers of circulating malignant cells (>25,000/mm^3) or high tumor burden who experience tumor lysis syndrome (see Tumor Lysis Syndrome) and in patients administered concomitant cisplatin therapy during clinical trials. The combination of cisplatin and rituximab is not an approved treatment regimen. If this combination is used in clinical trials *extreme caution* should be exercised; patients should be monitored closely for signs of renal failure. Discontinuation of rituximab should be considered for those with rising serum creatinine or oliguria.

SEVERE MUCOCUTANEOUS REACTIONS

See BOXED WARNING and ADVERSE REACTIONS.

Mucocutaneous reactions, some with fatal outcome, have been reported in patients treated with rituximab. These reports include paraneoplastic pemphigus (an uncommon disorder which is a manifestation of the patient's underlying malignancy),[16] Stevens-Johnson syndrome, lichenoid dermatitis, vesiculobullous dermatitis, and toxic epidermal necrolysis. The onset of the reaction in the reported cases has varied from 1-13 weeks following rituximab exposure. Patients experiencing a severe mucocutaneous reaction should not receive any further infusions and seek prompt medical evaluation. Skin biopsy may help to distinguish among different mucocutaneous reactions and guide subsequent treatment. The safety of readministration of rituximab to patients with any of these mucocutaneous reactions has not been determined.

PRECAUTIONS

LABORATORY MONITORING

Because rituximab targets all CD20-positive B lymphocytes, malignant and nonmalignant, complete blood counts (CBC) and platelet counts should be obtained at regular intervals during rituximab therapy and more frequently in patients who develop cytopenias (see ADVERSE REACTIONS). The duration of cytopenias caused by rituximab can extend well beyond the treatment period.

DRUG/LABORATORY INTERACTIONS

There have been no formal drug interaction studies performed with rituximab. However, renal toxicity was seen with this drug in combination with cisplatin in clinical trials. (See WARNINGS, Renal.)

HACA FORMATION

Human antichimeric antibody (HACA) was detected in 4 of 356 patients and 3 had an objective clinical response. The data reflect the percentage of patients whose test results were considered positive for antibodies to rituximab using an enzyme-linked immunosorbant assay (limit of detection = 7 ng/ml). The observed incidence of antibody positivity in an assay is highly dependent on the sensitivity and specificity of the assay and may be influenced by several factors including sample handling, concomitant medications, and underlying disease. For these reasons, comparison of the incidence of antibodies to rituximab with the incidence of antibodies to other products may be misleading.

IMMUNIZATION

The safety of immunization with live viral vaccines following rituximab therapy has not been studied. The ability to generate a primary or anamnestic humoral response to vaccination is currently being studied.

CARCINOGENESIS, MUTAGENESIS, AND IMPAIRMENT OF FERTILITY

No long-term animal studies have been performed to establish the carcinogenic or mutagenic potential of rituximab, or to determine its effects on fertility in males or females. Individuals of childbearing potential should use effective contraceptive methods during treatment and for up to 12 months following rituximab therapy.

PREGNANCY CATEGORY C

Animal reproduction studies have not been conducted with rituximab. It is not known whether rituximab can cause fetal harm when administered to a pregnant woman or whether it can affect reproductive capacity. Human IgG is known to pass the placental barrier, and thus may potentially cause fetal B-cell depletion; therefore, rituximab should be given to a pregnant woman only if clearly needed.

NURSING MOTHERS

It is not known whether rituximab is excreted in human milk. Because human IgG is excreted in human milk and the potential for absorption and immunosuppression in the infant is unknown, women should be advised to discontinue nursing until circulating drug levels are no longer detectable. (See CLINICAL PHARMACOLOGY.)

PEDIATRIC USE

The safety and effectiveness of rituximab in pediatric patients have not been established.

GERIATRIC USE

Among the 331 patients enrolled in clinical studies of single agent rituximab, 24% were 65-75 years old and 5% were 75 years old and older. The overall response rates were higher in older (age ≥65 years) vs younger (age <65 years) patients (52% vs 44%, respectively). However, the median duration of response, based on Kaplan-Meier estimates, was shorter in older versus younger patients: 10.1 months (range, 1.9 to 36.5+) vs 11.4 months (range, 2.1 to 42.1+), respectively. This shorter duration of response was not statistically significant. Adverse reactions, including incidence, severity and type of adverse reaction were similar between older and younger patients.

ADVERSE REACTIONS

The most serious adverse reactions caused by rituximab include infusion reactions, tumor lysis syndrome, mucocutaneous reactions, hypersensitivity reactions, cardiac arrhythmias and angina, and renal failure. Please refer to BOXED WARNING and WARNINGS for detailed descriptions of these reactions. Infusion reactions and lymphopenia are the most commonly occurring adverse reactions.

Because clinical trials are conducted under widely varying conditions, adverse reaction rates observed in the clinical trials of a drug cannot be directly compared to rates in the clinical trials of another drug and may not reflect the rates observed in practice. The adverse reaction information from clinical trials does, however, provide a basis for identifying the adverse events that appear to be related to drug use and for approximating rates.

Additional adverse reactions have been identified during postmarketing use of rituximab. Because these reactions are reported voluntarily from a population of uncertain size, it is not always possible to reliably estimate their frequency or establish a causal relationship to rituximab exposure. Decisions to include these reactions in labeling are typically based on one or more of the following factors: (1) seriousness of the reaction, (2) frequency of reporting, or (3) strength of causal connection to rituximab.

Where specific percentages are noted, these data are based on 356 patients treated in nonrandomized, single-arm studies of rituximab administered as a single agent. Most patients received rituximab 375 mg/m^2 weekly for 4 doses. These include 39 patients with bulky disease (lesions ≥10 cm) and 60 patients who received more than 1 course of rituximab. Thirty-seven (37) patients received 375 mg/m^2 for 8 doses and 25 patients received doses other than 375 mg/m^2 for 4 doses and up to 500 mg/m^2 single dose in the Phase 1 setting. Adverse events of greater severity are referred to as "Grade 3 and 4 events" defined by the commonly used National Cancer Institute Common Toxicity Criteria.[17]

TABLE 3 *Incidence of Adverse Events ≥5% of Patients in Clinical Trials (n=356)**

	All Grades	Grades 3 and 4
Any Adverse Events	**99%**	**57%**
Body as a Whole	**86%**	**10%**
Fever	53%	1%
Chills	33%	3%
Infection	31%	4%
Asthenia	26%	1%
Headache	19%	1%
Abdominal pain	14%	1%
Pain	12%	1%
Back pain	10%	1%
Throat irritation	9%	0%
Flushing	5%	0%
Cardiovascular System	**25%**	**3%**
Hypotension	10%	1%
Hypertension	6%	1%
Digestive System	**37%**	**2%**
Nausea	23%	1%
Diarrhea	10%	1%
Vomiting	10%	1%
Hemic and Lymphatic System	**67%**	**48%**
Lymphopenia	48%	40%
Leukopenia	14%	4%
Neutropenia	14%	6%
Thrombocytopenia	12%	2%
Anemia	8%	3%
Metabolic and Nutritional Disorders	**38%**	**3%**
Angioedema	11%	1%
Hyperglycemia	9%	1%
Peripheral edema	8%	0%
LDH increase	7%	0%
Musculoskeletal System	**26%**	**3%**
Myalgia	10%	1%
Arthralgia	10%	1%
Nervous System	**32%**	**1%**
Dizziness	10%	1%
Anxiety	5%	1%
Respiratory System	**38%**	**4%**
Increased cough	13%	1%
Rhinitis	12%	1%
Bronchospasm	8%	1%
Dyspnea	7%	1%
Sinusitis	6%	0%
Skin and Appendages	**44%**	**2%**
Night sweats	15%	1%
Rash	15%	1%
Pruritus	14%	1%
Urticaria	8%	1%

* Adverse events were followed for a period of 12 months following rituximab therapy.

RISK FACTORS ASSOCIATED WITH INCREASED RATES OF ADVERSE EVENTS

Administration of rituximab weekly for 8 doses resulted in higher rates of Grade 3 and 4 adverse events[17] overall (70%) compared with administration weekly for 4 doses (57%). The incidence of Grade 3 or 4 adverse events was similar in patients retreated with rituximab compared with initial treatment (58% and 57%, respectively). The incidence of the following clinically significant adverse events was higher in patients with bulky disease (lesions ≥10 cm) (n=39) versus patients with lesions <10 cm (n=195): abdominal pain, anemia, dyspnea, hypotension, and neutropenia.

INFUSION REACTIONS

See BOXED WARNING and WARNINGS.

Mild to moderate infusion reactions consisting of fever and chills/rigors occurred in the majority of patients during the first rituximab infusion. Other frequent infusion reaction symptoms included nausea, pruritus, angioedema, asthenia, hypotension, headache, bronchospasm, throat irritation, rhinitis, urticaria, rash, vomiting, myalgia, dizziness, and hypertension. These reactions generally occurred within 30-120 minutes of beginning the first infusion, and resolved with slowing or interruption of the rituximab infusion and with supportive care (diphenhydramine, acetaminophen, IV saline, and vasopressors). In an analysis of data from 356 patients with relapsed or refractory, low-grade NHL who received 4 (n=319) or 8 (n=37) weekly infusions of rituximab, the incidence of infusion reactions was highest during the first infusion (77%) and decreased with each subsequent infusion (30% with fourth infusion and 14% with eighth infusion).

INFECTIOUS EVENTS

Rituximab induced B-cell depletion in 70-80% of patients and was associated with decreased serum immunoglobulins in a minority of patients; the lymphopenia lasted a median of 14 days (range, 1-588 days). Infectious events occurred in 31% of patients: 19% of patients had bacterial infections, 10% had viral infections, 1% had fungal infections, and 6% were unknown infections. Incidence is not additive because a single patient may have had more than one type of infection. Serious infectious events (Grade 3 or 4),[17] including sepsis, occurred in 2% of patients.

HEMATOLOGIC EVENTS

Grade 3 and 4 cytopenias[17] were reported in 12% of patients treated with rituximab; these include: lymphopenia (40%), neutropenia (6%), leukopenia (4%), anemia (3%), and thrombocytopenia (2%). The median duration of lymphopenia was 14 days (range, 1-588 days) and of neutropenia was 13 days (range, 2-116 days). A single occurrence of transient aplastic anemia (pure red cell aplasia) and two occurrences of hemolytic anemia following rituximab therapy were reported. In addition, there have been rare postmarketing reports of prolonged pancytopenia and marrow hypoplasia.

CARDIAC EVENTS

See BOXED WARNING.

Grade 3 or 4 cardiac-related events include hypotension. Rare, fatal cardiac failure with symptomatic onset weeks after rituximab has also been reported. Patients who develop clinically significant cardiopulmonary events should have rituximab infusion discontinued.

PULMONARY EVENTS

See BOXED WARNING.

135 patients (38%) experienced pulmonary events. The most common respiratory system adverse events experienced were increased cough, rhinitis, bronchospasm, dyspnea, and sinusitis. Three pulmonary events have been reported in temporal association with rituximab infusion as a single agent: acute bronchospasm, acute pneumonitis presenting 1-4 weeks post-rituximab infusion, and bronchiolitis obliterans. One case of bronchiolitis obliterans was associated with progressive pulmonary symptoms and culminated in death several months following the last rituximab infusion. The safety of resumption or continued administration of rituximab in patients with pneumonitis or bronchiolitis obliterans is unknown.

IMMUNE/AUTOIMMUNE EVENTS

Immune/autoimmune events have been reported, including uveitis, optic neuritis in a patient with systemic vasculitis, pleuritis in a patient with a lupus-like syndrome, serum sickness with polyarticular arthritis, and vasculitis with rash.

LESS COMMONLY OBSERVED EVENTS

In clinical trials, <5% and >1% of the patients experienced the following events regardless of causality assessment: agitation, anorexia, arthritis, conjunctivitis, depression, dyspepsia, edema, hyperkinesia, hypertonia, hypesthesia, hypoglycemia, injection site pain, insomnia, lacrimation disorder, malaise, nervousness, neuritis, neuropathy, paresthesia, somnolence, vertigo, weight decrease.

DOSAGE AND ADMINISTRATION

Initial Therapy: Rituximab is given at 375 mg/m^2 IV infusion once weekly for 4 or 8 doses.

Retreatment Therapy: Patients who subsequently develop progressive disease may be safely retreated with rituximab 375 mg/m^2 IV infusion once weekly for 4 doses. Currently there are limited data concerning more than 2 courses.

RITUXIMAB AS A COMPONENT OF IBRITUMOMAB TIUXETAN THERAPEUTIC REGIMEN

As a required component of the ibritumomab tiuxetan therapeutic regimen, rituximab 250 mg/m^2 should be infused within 4 hours prior to the administration of Indium-111- (In-111-) ibritumomab tiuxetan and within 4 hours prior to the administration of Yttrium-90- (Y-90-) ibritumomab tiuxetan. Administration of rituximab and In-111-ibritumomab tiuxetan should precede rituximab and Y-90-ibritumomab tiuxetan by 7-9 days. Refer to the ibritumomab tiuxetan package insert for full prescribing information regarding the ibritumomab tiuxetan therapeutic regimen.

Rituximab may be administered in an outpatient setting. **DO NOT ADMINISTER AS AN INTRAVENOUS PUSH OR BOLUS. (See Administration.)**

INSTRUCTIONS FOR ADMINISTRATION

Preparation for Administration

Use appropriate aseptic technique. Withdraw the necessary amount of rituximab and dilute to a final concentration of 1-4 mg/ml into an infusion bag containing either 0.9% sodium chloride, or 5% dextrose in water. Gently invert the bag to mix the solution. Discard any unused portion left in the vial. Parenteral drug products should be inspected visually for particulate matter and discoloration prior to administration.

Rituximab solutions for infusion may be stored at 2-8°C (36-46°F) for 24 hours. Rituximab solutions for infusion have been shown to be stable for an additional 24 hours at room temperature. However, since rituximab solutions do not contain a preservative, diluted solutions should be stored refrigerated (2-8°C). No incompatibilities between rituximab and polyvinylchloride or polyethylene bags have been observed.

Administration

DO NOT ADMINISTER AS AN INTRAVENOUS PUSH OR BOLUS. Infusion and hypersensitivity reactions may occur (see BOXED WARNING, WARNINGS, and ADVERSE REACTIONS). Premedication consisting of acetaminophen and diphenhydramine should be considered before each infusion of rituximab. Premedication may attenuate infusion reactions. Since transient hypotension may occur during rituximab infusion, consideration should be given to withholding antihypertensive medications 12 hours prior to rituximab infusion.

First Infusion: The rituximab solution for infusion should be administered intravenously at an initial rate of 50 mg/h. Rituximab should not be mixed or diluted with other drugs. If hypersensitivity or infusion reactions do not occur, escalate the infusion rate in 50 mg/h increments every 30 minutes, to a maximum of 400 mg/h. If a hypersensitivity (non-IgE-mediated) or an infusion reaction develops, the infusion should be temporarily slowed or interrupted (see BOXED WARNING and WARNINGS). The infusion can continue at one-half the previous rate upon improvement of patient symptoms.

Subsequent Infusions: If the patient tolerated the first infusion well, subsequent rituximab infusions can be administered at an initial rate of 100 mg/h, and increased by 100 mg/h increments at 30 minute intervals, to a maximum of 400 mg/h as tolerated. If the patient did not tolerate the first infusion well, follow the guidelines under First Infusion.

STABILITY AND STORAGE

Rituximab vials are stable at 2-8°C (36-46°F). Do not use beyond expiration date stamped on carton. Rituximab vials should be protected from direct sunlight. Refer to Preparation for Administration for information on the stability and storage of solutions of rituximab diluted for infusion.

HOW SUPPLIED

Rituxan is supplied as 100 and 500 mg of sterile, preservative-free, single-use vials.
Single unit 100 mg carton: Contains one 10 ml vial of Rituxan (10 mg/ml).
Single unit 500 mg carton: Contains one 50 ml vial of Rituxan (10 mg/ml).

PRODUCT LISTING - EQUIVALENTS NOT AVAILABLE

Solution - Intravenous - 10 mg/ml

10 ml	$527.50	RITUXAN, Genentech	50242-0051-21
50 ml	$2637.52	RITUXAN, Genentech	50242-0053-06

Rivastigmine Tartrate *(003484)*

Categories: Alzheimer's disease; FDA Approved 2000 Apr; Pregnancy Category B
Drug Classes: Cholinesterase inhibitors
Foreign Brand Availability: Exelon (Australia; Austria; Belgium; Bulgaria; Colombia; Czech-Republic; Denmark; England; Finland; France; Germany; Greece; Hong-Kong; Hungary; India; Indonesia; Ireland; Israel; Italy; Mexico; Netherlands; New-Zealand; Norway; Peru; Philippines; Poland; Portugal; Slovenia; South-Africa; Spain; Sweden; Switzerland; Taiwan; Thailand; Turkey); Prometax (Austria; Belgium; Bulgaria; Czech-Republic; Denmark; England; Finland; France; Germany; Greece; Hungary; Ireland; Italy; Netherlands; Norway; Poland; Portugal; Slovenia; Spain; Sweden; Switzerland; Turkey)
Cost of Therapy: $153.74 (Alzheimer's Disease; Exelon; 3 mg; 2 capsules/day; 30 day supply)

DESCRIPTION

Exelon (rivastigmine tartrate) is a reversible cholinesterase inhibitor and is known chemically as (S)-N-Ethyl-N-methyl-3-[1-(dimethylamino)ethyl]-phenyl carbamate hydrogen-(2R,3R)-tartrate. Rivastigmine tartrate is commonly referred to in the pharmacological literature as SDZ ENA 713 or ENA 713. It has an empirical formula of $C_{14}H_{22}N_2O_2 \cdot C_4H_6O_6$ (hydrogen tartrate salt-hta salt) and a molecular weight of 400.43 (hta salt). Rivastigmine tartrate is a white to off-white, fine crystalline powder that is very soluble in water, soluble in ethanol and acetonitrile, slightly soluble in n-octanol and very slightly soluble in ethyl acetate. The distribution coefficient at 37°C in n-octanol/phosphate buffer solution pH 7 is 3.0.

CAPSULES

Exelon is supplied as capsules containing rivastigmine tartrate, equivalent to 1.5, 3, 4.5 and 6 mg of rivastigmine base for oral administration. Inactive ingredients are hydroxypropyl methylcellulose, magnesium stearate, microcrystalline cellulose, and silicon dioxide. Each hard-gelatin capsule contains gelatin, titanium dioxide, and red and/or yellow iron oxides.

ORAL SOLUTION

Exelon oral solution is supplied as a solution containing rivastigmine tartrate, equivalent to 2 mg/ml of rivastigmine base for oral administration. Inactive ingredients are citric acid, D&C yellow no. 10, purified water, sodium benzoate, and sodium citrate.

CLINICAL PHARMACOLOGY

MECHANISM OF ACTION

Pathological changes in dementia of the Alzheimer type involve cholinergic neuronal pathways that project from the basal forebrain to the cerebral cortex and hippocampus. These pathways are thought to be intricately involved in memory, attention, learning, and other cognitive processes. While the precise mechanism of rivastigmine's action is unknown, it is postulated to exert its therapeutic effect by enhancing cholinergic function. This is accomplished by increasing the concentration of acetylcholine through reversible inhibition of its hydrolysis by cholinesterase. If this proposed mechanism is correct, rivastigmine tartrate's effect may lessen as the disease process advances and fewer cholinergic neurons remain functionally intact. There is no evidence that rivastigmine alters the course of the underlying dementing process. After a 6 mg dose of rivastigmine, anticholinesterase activity is present in CSF for about 10 hours, with a maximum inhibition of about 60% five hours after dosing.

PHARMACOKINETICS

Rivastigmine is well absorbed with absolute bioavailability of about 40% (3 mg dose). It shows linear pharmacokinetics up to 3 mg bid but is non-linear at higher doses. Doubling the dose from 3-6 mg bid results in a 3-fold increase in AUC. The elimination half-life is about 1.5 hours, with most elimination as metabolites via the urine.

Absorption

Rivastigmine is rapidly and completely absorbed. Peak plasma concentrations are reached in approximately 1 hour. Absolute bioavailability after a 3 mg dose is about 36%. Administration of rivastigmine tartrate with food delays absorption (T_{max}) by 90 minutes, lowers C_{max} by approximately 30% and increases AUC by approximately 30%.

Distribution

Rivastigmine is widely distributed throughout the body with a volume of distribution in the range of 1.8-2.7 L/kg. Rivastigmine penetrates the blood brain barrier, reaching CSF peak concentrations in 1.4-2.6 hours. Mean AUC(1-12h) ratio of CSF/plasma averaged 40 ± 0.5% following 1-6 mg bid doses.

Rivastigmine is about 40% bound to plasma proteins at concentrations of 1-400 ng/ml, which cover the therapeutic concentration range. Rivastigmine distributes equally between blood and plasma with a blood-to-plasma partition ratio of 0.9 at concentrations ranging from 1-400 ng/ml.

Metabolism

Rivastigmine is rapidly and extensively metabolized, primarily via cholinesterase-mediated hydrolysis to the decarbamylated metabolite. Based on evidence from *in vitro* and animal studies the major cytochrome P450 isozymes are minimally involved in rivastigmine metabolism. Consistent with these observations is the finding that no drug interactions related to cytochrome P450 have been observed in humans (see Drug-Drug Interactions).

Elimination

The major pathway of elimination is via the kidneys. Following administration of ^{14}C-rivastigmine to 6 healthy volunteers total recovery of radioactivity over 120 hours was 97% in urine and 0.4% in feces. No parent drug was detected in urine. The sulfate conjugate of the decarbamylated metabolite is the major component excreted in urine and represents 40% of the dose. Mean oral clearance of rivastigmine is 1.8 ± 0.6 L/min after 6 mg bid.

SPECIAL POPULATIONS

Hepatic Disease

Following a single 3 mg dose, mean oral clearance of rivastigmine was 60% lower in hepatically impaired patients (n=10, biopsy proven) than in healthy subjects (n=10). After multiple 6 mg bid oral dosing, the mean clearance of rivastigmine was 65% lower in mild (n=7, Child-Pugh score 5-6) and moderate (n=3, Child-Pugh score 7-9) hepatically impaired patients (biopsy proven, liver cirrhosis) than in healthy subjects (n=10). Dosage adjustment is not necessary in hepatically impaired patients as the dose of drug is individually titrated to tolerability.

Renal Disease

Following a single 3 mg dose, mean oral clearance of rivastigmine is 64% lower in moderately impaired renal patients (n=8, GFR=10-50 ml/min) than in healthy subjects (n=10, GFR ≥60 ml/min); CL/F=1.7 L/min (cv=45%) and 4.8 L/min (cv=80%), respectively. In severely impaired renal patients (n=8, GFR <10 ml/min), mean oral clearance of rivastigmine is 43% higher than in healthy subjects (n=10, GFR ≥60 ml/min); CL/F=6.9 L/min and 4.8 L/min, respectively. For unexplained reasons, the severely impaired renal patients had a higher clearance of rivastigmine than moderately impaired patients. However, dosage adjustment may not be necessary in renally impaired patients as the dose of the drug is individually titrated to tolerability.

Age

Following a single 2.5 mg oral dose to elderly volunteers (>60 years of age, n=24) and younger volunteers (n=24), mean oral clearance of rivastigmine was 30% lower in elderly (7 L/min) than in younger subjects (10 L/min).

Gender and Race

No specific pharmacokinetic study was conducted to investigate the effect of gender and race on the disposition of rivastigmine tartrate, but a population pharmacokinetic analysis indicates that gender (n=277 males and 348 females) and race (n=575 White, 34 Black, 4 Asian, and 12 Other) did not affect the clearance of rivastigmine tartrate.

Nicotine Use

Population PK analysis showed that nicotine use increases the oral clearance of rivastigmine by 23% (n=75 smokers and 549 nonsmokers).

DRUG-DRUG INTERACTIONS

Effect of Rivastigmine Tartrate on the Metabolism of Other Drugs

Rivastigmine is primarily metabolized through hydrolysis by esterases. Minimal metabolism occurs via the major cytochrome P450 isoenzymes. Based on *in vitro* studies, no pharmacokinetic drug interactions with drugs metabolized by the following isoenzyme systems are expected: CYP1A2, CYP2D6, CYP3A4/5, CYP2E1, CYP2C9, CYP2C8, or CYP2C19.

No pharmacokinetic interaction was observed between rivastigmine and digoxin, warfarin, diazepam, or fluoxetine in studies in healthy volunteers. The elevation of prothrombin time induced by warfarin is not affected by administration of rivastigmine tartrate.

Effect of Other Drugs on the Metabolism of Rivastigmine Tartrate

Drugs that induce or inhibit CYP450 metabolism are not expected to alter the metabolism of rivastigmine. Single dose pharmacokinetic studies demonstrated that the metabolism of rivastigmine is not significantly affected by concurrent administration of digoxin, warfarin, diazepam, or fluoxetine.

R

Population PK analysis with a database of 625 patients showed that the pharmacokinetics of rivastigmine were not influenced by commonly prescribed medications such as antacids (n=77), antihypertensives (n=72), β-blockers (n=42), calcium channel blockers (n=75), antidiabetics (n=21), non-steroidal anti-inflammatory drugs (n=79), estrogens (n=70), salicylate analgesics (n=177), antianginals (n=35), and antihistamines (n=15). In addition, in clinical trials, no increased risk of clinically relevant untoward effects was observed in patients treated concomitantly with rivastigmine tartrate and these agents.

INDICATIONS AND USAGE

Rivastigmine tartrate is indicated for the treatment of mild to moderate dementia of the Alzheimer's type.

CONTRAINDICATIONS

Rivastigmine tartrate is contraindicated in patients with known hypersensitivity to rivastigmine, other carbamate derivatives or other components of the formulation (see DESCRIPTION).

WARNINGS

GASTROINTESTINAL ADVERSE REACTIONS

Rivastigmine tartrate use is associated with significant gastrointestinal adverse reactions, including nausea and vomiting, anorexia, and weight loss. For this reason, patients should always be started at a dose of 1.5 mg bid and titrated to their maintenance dose. If treatment is interrupted for longer than several days, treatment should be reinitiated with the lowest daily dose (see DOSAGE AND ADMINISTRATION) to reduce the possibility of severe vomiting and its potentially serious sequelae (*e.g.,* there has been one post-marketing report of severe vomiting with esophageal rupture following inappropriate reinitiation of treatment with a 4.5 mg dose after 8 weeks of treatment interruption).

Nausea and Vomiting

In the controlled clinical trials, 47% of the patients treated with a rivastigmine tartrate dose in the therapeutic range of 6-12 mg/day (n=1189) developed nausea (compared with 12% in placebo). A total of 31% of rivastigmine tartrate-treated patients developed at least one episode of vomiting (compared with 6% for placebo). The rate of vomiting was higher during the titration phase (24% vs 3% for placebo) than in the maintenance phase (14% vs 3% for placebo). The rates were higher in women than men. Five percent (5%) of patients discontinued for vomiting, compared to less than 1% for patients on placebo. Vomiting was severe in 2% of rivastigmine tartrate-treated patients and was rated as mild or moderate each in 14% of patients. The rate of nausea was higher during the titration phase (43% vs 9% for placebo) than in the maintenance phase (17% vs 4% for placebo).

Weight Loss

In the controlled trials, approximately 26% of women on high doses of rivastigmine tartrate (greater than 9 mg/day) had weight loss of equal to or greater than 7% of their baseline weight compared to 6% in the placebo-treated patients. About 18% of the males in the high dose group experienced a similar degree of weight loss compared to 4% in placebo-treated patients. It is not clear how much of the weight loss was associated with anorexia, nausea, vomiting, and the diarrhea associated with the drug.

Anorexia

In the controlled clinical trials, of the patients treated with an rivastigmine tartrate dose of 6-12 mg/day, 17% developed anorexia compared to 3% of the placebo patients. Neither the time course or the severity of the anorexia is known.

Peptic Ulcers/Gastrointestinal Bleeding

Because of their pharmacological action, cholinesterase inhibitors may be expected to increase gastric acid secretion due to increased cholinergic activity. Therefore, patients should be monitored closely for symptoms of active or occult gastrointestinal bleeding, especially those at increased risk for developing ulcers, *e.g.,* those with a history of ulcer disease or those receiving concurrent nonsteroidal anti-inflammatory drugs (NSAIDS). Clinical studies of rivastigmine tartrate have shown no significant increase, relative to placebo, in the incidence of either peptic ulcer disease or gastrointestinal bleeding.

ANESTHESIA

Rivastigmine tartrate as a cholinesterase inhibitor, is likely to exaggerate succinylcholine-type muscle relaxation during anesthesia.

CARDIOVASCULAR CONDITIONS

Drugs that increase cholinergic activity may have vagotonic effects on heart rate (*e.g.,* bradycardia). The potential for this action may be particularly important to patients with "sick sinus syndrome" or other supraventricular cardiac conduction conditions. In clinical trials, rivastigmine tartrate was not associated with any increased incidence of cardiovascular adverse events, heart rate or blood pressure changes, or ECG abnormalities. Syncopal episodes have been reported in 3% of patients receiving 6-12 mg/day of rivastigmine tartrate, compared to 2% of placebo patients.

GENITOURINARY

Although this was not observed in clinical trials of rivastigmine tartrate, drugs that increase cholinergic activity may cause urinary obstruction.

NEUROLOGICAL CONDITIONS

Seizures: Drugs that increase cholinergic activity are believed to have some potential for causing seizures. However, seizure activity also may be a manifestation of Alzheimer's disease.

PULMONARY CONDITIONS

Like other drugs that increase cholinergic activity, rivastigmine tartrate should be used with care in patients with a history of asthma or obstructive pulmonary disease.

PRECAUTIONS

INFORMATION FOR THE PATIENT AND CAREGIVERS

Caregivers should be advised of the high incidence of nausea and vomiting associated with the use of the drug along with the possibility of anorexia and weight loss. Caregivers should be encouraged to monitor for these adverse events and inform the physician if they occur. It is critical to inform caregivers that if therapy has been interrupted for more than several days, the next dose should not be administered until they have discussed this with the physician.

Oral Solution

Caregivers should be instructed in the correct procedure for administering rivastigmine tartrate oral solution. In addition, they should be informed of the existence of an Instruction Sheet (included with the product) describing how the solution is to be administered. They should be urged to read this sheet prior to administering rivastigmine tartrate oral solution. Caregivers should direct questions about the administration of the solution to either their physician or pharmacist.

CARCINOGENESIS, MUTAGENESIS, AND IMPAIRMENT OF FERTILITY

In carcinogenicity studies conducted at dose levels up to 1.1 mg base/kg/day in rats and 1.6 mg base/kg/day in mice, rivastigmine was not carcinogenic. These dose levels are approximately 0.9 times and 0.7 times the maximum recommended human daily dose of 12 mg/day on a mg/m^2 basis.

Rivastigmine was clastogenic in two *in vitro* assays in the presence, but not the absence, of metabolic activation. It caused structural chromosomal aberrations in V79 Chinese hamster lung cells and both structural and numerical (polyploidy) chromosomal aberrations in human peripheral blood lymphocytes. Rivastigmine was not genotoxic in three *in vitro* assays: the Ames test, the unscheduled DNA synthesis (UDS) test in rat hepatocytes (a test for induction of DNA repair synthesis), and the HGPRT test in V79 Chinese hamster cells. Rivastigmine was not clastogenic in the *in vivo* mouse micronucleus test.

Rivastigmine had no effect on fertility or reproductive performance in the rat at dose levels up to 1.1 mg base/kg/day. This dose is approximately 0.9 times the maximum recommended human daily dose of 12 mg/day on a mg/m^2 basis.

PREGNANCY CATEGORY B

Reproduction studies conducted in pregnant rats at doses up to 2.3 mg base/kg/day (approximately 2 times the maximum recommended human dose on a mg/m^2 basis) and in pregnant rabbits at doses up to 2.3 mg base/kg/day (approximately 4 times the maximum recommended human dose on a mg/m^2 basis) revealed no evidence of teratogenicity. Studies in rats showed slightly decreased fetal/pup weights, usually at doses causing some maternal toxicity; decreased weights were seen at doses which were several fold lower than the maximum recommended human dose on a mg/m^2 basis. There are no adequate or well-controlled studies in pregnant women. Because animal reproduction studies are not always predictive of human response, rivastigmine tartrate should be used during pregnancy only if the potential benefit justifies the potential risk to the fetus.

NURSING MOTHERS

It is not known whether rivastigmine is excreted in human breast milk. Rivastigmine tartrate has no indication for use in nursing mothers.

PEDIATRIC USE

There are no adequate and well-controlled trials documenting the safety and efficacy of rivastigmine tartrate in any illness occurring in children.

DRUG INTERACTIONS

EFFECT OF RIVASTIGMINE TARTRATE ON THE METABOLISM OF OTHER DRUGS

Rivastigmine is primarily metabolized through hydrolysis by esterases. Minimal metabolism occurs via the major cytochrome P450 isoenzymes. Based on *in vitro* studies, no pharmacokinetic drug interactions with drugs metabolized by the following isoenzyme systems are expected: CYP1A2, CYP2D6, CYP3A4/5, CYP2E1, CYP2C9, CYP2C8, or CYP2C19.

No pharmacokinetic interaction was observed between rivastigmine and digoxin, warfarin, diazepam, or fluoxetine in studies in healthy volunteers. The elevation of prothrombin time induced by warfarin is not affected by administration of rivastigmine tartrate.

EFFECT OF OTHER DRUGS ON THE METABOLISM OF RIVASTIGMINE TARTRATE

Drugs that induce or inhibit CYP450 metabolism are not expected to alter the metabolism of rivastigmine. Single dose pharmacokinetic studies demonstrated that the metabolism of rivastigmine is not significantly affected by concurrent administration of digoxin, warfarin, diazepam, or fluoxetine.

Population PK analysis with a database of 625 patients showed that the pharmacokinetics of rivastigmine were not influenced by commonly prescribed medications such as antacids (n=77), antihypertensives (n=72), β-blockers (n=42), calcium channel blockers (n=75), antidiabetics (n=21), nonsteroidal anti-inflammatory drugs (n=79), estrogens (n=70), salicylate analgesics (n=177), antianginals (n=35), and antihistamines (n=15).

USE WITH ANTICHOLINERGICS

Because of their mechanism of action, cholinesterase inhibitors have the potential to interfere with the activity of anticholinergic medications.

USE WITH CHOLINOMIMETICS AND OTHER CHOLINESTERASE INHIBITORS

A synergistic effect may be expected when cholinesterase inhibitors are given concurrently with succinylcholine, similar neuromuscular blocking agents or cholinergic agonists such as bethanechol.

ADVERSE REACTIONS

ADVERSE EVENTS LEADING TO DISCONTINUATION

The rate of discontinuation due to adverse events in controlled clinical trials of rivastigmine tartrate was 15% for patients receiving 6-12 mg/day compared to 5% for patients on placebo during forced weekly dose titration. While on a maintenance dose, the rates were 6% for patients on rivastigmine tartrate compared to 4% for those on placebo.

The most common adverse events leading to discontinuation, defined as those occurring in at least 2% of patients and at twice the incidence seen in placebo patients, are shown in TABLE 3A and TABLE 3B.

***TABLE 3A** Most Frequent Adverse Events Leading to Withdrawal From Clinical Trials During Titration and Maintenance in Patients Receiving 6-12 mg/day Rivastigmine Tartrate Using a Forced Dose Titration*

	Titration		Maintenance	
		Rivastigmine Tartrate		Rivastigmine Tartrate
	Placebo	≥6-12 mg/day	Placebo	≥6-12 mg/day
Study Phase	(n=868)	(n=1189)	(n=788)	(n=987)
Event/% Discontinuing				
Nausea	<1	8	<1	1
Vomiting	<1	4	<1	1
Anorexia	0	2	<1	1
Dizziness	<1	2	<1	1

***TABLE 3B** Most Frequent Adverse Events Leading to Withdrawal From Clinical Trials During Titration and Maintenance in Patients Receiving 6-12 mg/day Rivastigmine Tartrate Using a Forced Dose Titration*

	Overall	
	Placebo	Rivastigmine Tartrate ≥6-12 mg/day
Study Phase	(n=868)	(n=1189)
Event/% Discontinuing		
Nausea	1	8
Vomiting	<1	5
Anorexia	<1	3
Dizziness	<1	2

MOST FREQUENT ADVERSE CLINICAL EVENTS SEEN IN ASSOCIATION WITH THE USE OF RIVASTIGMINE TARTRATE

The most common adverse events, defined as those occurring at a frequency of at least 5% and twice the placebo rate, are largely predicted by rivastigmine tartrate's cholinergic effects. These include nausea, vomiting, anorexia, dyspepsia, and asthenia.

Gastrointestinal Adverse Reactions

Rivastigmine tartrate use is associated with significant nausea, vomiting, and weight loss (see WARNINGS).

ADVERSE EVENTS REPORTED IN CONTROLLED TRIALS

TABLE 4 lists treatment emergent signs and symptoms that were reported in at least 2% of patients in placebo-controlled trials and for which the rate of occurrence was greater for patients treated with rivastigmine tartrate doses of 6-12 mg/day than for those treated with placebo. The prescriber should be aware that these figures cannot be used to predict the frequency of adverse events in the course of usual medical practice when patient characteristics and other factors may differ from those prevailing during clinical studies. Similarly, the cited frequencies cannot be directly compared with figures obtained from other clinical investigations involving different treatments, uses, or investigators. An inspection of these frequencies, however, does provide the prescriber with one basis by which to estimate the relative contribution of drug and non-drug factors to the adverse event incidences in the population studied.

In general, adverse reactions were less frequent later in the course of treatment.

No systematic effect of race or age could be determined on the incidence of adverse events in the controlled studies. Nausea, vomiting, and weight loss were more frequent in women than men.

Other adverse events observed at a rate of 2% or more on rivastigmine tartrate 6-12 mg/day but at a greater or equal rate on placebo were chest pain, peripheral edema, vertigo, back pain, arthralgia, pain, bone fracture, agitation, nervousness, delusion, paranoid reaction, upper respiratory tract infections, infection (general), coughing, pharyngitis, bronchitis, rash (general), urinary incontinence.

***TABLE 4** Adverse Events Reported in Controlled Clinical Trials in at Least 2% of Patients Receiving Rivastigmine Tartrate (6-12 mg/day) and at a Higher Frequency Than Placebo-Treated Patients*

Body System/	Placebo	Rivastigmine Tartrate*
Adverse Event	(n=868)	(n=1189)
Percent of Patients With any Adverse Event	79%	92%
Autonomic Nervous System		
Sweating increased	1%	4%
Syncope	2%	3%
Body as a Whole		
Accidental trauma	9%	10%
Fatigue	5%	9%
Asthenia	2%	6%
Malaise	2%	5%
Influenza-like symptoms	2%	3%
Weight decrease	<1%	3%
Cardiovascular Disorders, General		
Hypertension	2%	3%
Central and Peripheral Nervous System		
Dizziness	11%	21%
Headache	12%	17%
Somnolence	3%	5%
Tremor	1%	4%
Gastrointestinal System		
Nausea	12%	47%
Vomiting	6%	31%
Diarrhea	11%	19%
Anorexia	3%	17%
Abdominal pain	6%	13%
Dyspepsia	4%	9%
Constipation	4%	5%
Flatulence	2%	4%
Eructation	1%	2%
Psychiatric Disorders		
Insomnia	7%	9%
Confusion	7%	8%
Depression	4%	6%
Anxiety	3%	5%
Hallucination	3%	4%
Aggressive reaction	2%	3%
Resistance Mechanism Disorders		
Urinary tract infection	6%	7%
Respiratory System		
Rhinitis	3%	4%

* 6-12 mg/day.

OTHER ADVERSE EVENTS OBSERVED DURING CLINICAL TRIALS

Rivastigmine tartrate has been administered to over 5297 individuals during clinical trials worldwide. Of these, 4326 patients have been treated for at least 3 months, 3407 patients have been treated for at least 6 months, 2150 patients have been treated for 1 year, 1250 have been treated for 2 years, and 168 have been treated for over 3 years. With regard to exposure to the highest dose, 2809 patients were exposed to doses of 10-12 mg, 2615 patients treated for 3 months, 2328 patients treated for 6 months, 1378 patients treated for 1 year, 917 patients treated for 2 years, and 129 treated for over 3 years.

Treatment emergent signs and symptoms that occurred during 8 controlled clinical trials and 9 open-label trials in North America, Western Europe, Australia, South Africa, and Japan were recorded as adverse events by the clinical investigators using terminology of their own choosing. To provide an overall estimate of the proportion of individuals having similar types of events, the events were grouped into a smaller number of standardized categories using a modified WHO dictionary, and event frequencies were calculated across all studies. These categories are used in the listing below. The frequencies represent the proportion of 5297 patients from these trials who experienced that event while receiving rivastigmine tartrate. All adverse events occurring in at least 6 patients (approximately 0.1%) are included, except for those already listed elsewhere in labeling, WHO terms too general to be informative, relatively minor events, or events unlikely to be drug caused. Events are classified by body system and listed using the following definitions: *Frequent adverse events:* Those occurring in at least 1/100 patients; *Infrequent adverse events:* Those occurring in 1/100 to 1/1000 patients. These adverse events are not necessarily related to rivastigmine tartrate treatment and in most cases were observed at a similar frequency in placebo-treated patients in the controlled studies.

Autonomic Nervous System: *Infrequent:* Cold clammy skin, dry mouth, flushing, increased saliva.

Body as a Whole: *Frequent:* Accidental trauma, fever, edema, allergy, hot flushes, rigors; *Infrequent:* Edema periorbital or facial, hypothermia, edema, feeling cold, halitosis.

Cardiovascular System: *Frequent:* Hypotension, postural hypotension, cardiac failure.

Central and Peripheral Nervous System: *Frequent:* Abnormal gait, ataxia, paraesthesia, convulsions; *Infrequent:* Paresis, apraxia, aphasia, dysphonia, hyperkinesia, hyperreflexia, hypertonia, hypoesthesia, hypokinesia, migraine, neuralgia, nystagmus, peripheral neuropathy.

Endocrine System: *Infrequent:* Goiter, hypothyroidism.

Gastrointestinal System: *Frequent:* Fecal incontinence, gastritis; *Infrequent:* Dysphagia, esophagitis, gastric ulcer, gastritis, gastroesophageal reflux, GI hemorrhage, hernia, intestinal obstruction, melena, rectal hemorrhage, gastroenteritis, ulcerative stomatitis, duodenal ulcer, hematemesis, gingivitis, tenesmus, pancreatitis, colitis, glossitis.

Hearing and Vestibular Disorders: *Frequent:* Tinnitus.

Heart Rate and Rhythm Disorders: *Frequent:* Atrial fibrillation, bradycardia, palpitation; *Infrequent:* AV block, bundle branch block, sick sinus syndrome, cardiac arrest, supraventricular tachycardia, extrasystoles, tachycardia.

Liver and Biliary System Disorders: *Infrequent:* Abnormal hepatic function, cholecystitis.

Metabolic and Nutritional Disorders: *Frequent:* Dehydration, hypokalemia; *Infrequent:* Diabetes mellitus, gout, hypercholesterolemia, hyperlipemia, hypoglycemia, cachexia, thirst, hyperglycemia, hyponatremia.

Musculoskeletal Disorders: *Frequent:* Arthritis, leg cramps, myalgia; *Infrequent:* Cramps, hernia, muscle weakness.

Myo-, Endo-, Pericardial and Valve Disorders: *Frequent:* Angina pectoris, myocardial infarction.

Platelet, Bleeding, and Clotting Disorders: *Frequent:* Epistaxis; *Infrequent:* Hematoma, thrombocytopenia, purpura.

Psychiatric Disorders: *Frequent:* Paranoid reaction, confusion; *Infrequent:* Abnormal dreaming, amnesia, apathy, delirium, dementia, depersonalization, emotional labil-

R

ity, impaired concentration, decreased libido, personality disorder, suicide attempt, increased libido, neurosis, suicidal ideation, psychosis.

Red Blood Cell Disorders: *Frequent:* Anemia; *Infrequent:* Hypochromic anemia.

Reproductive Disorders (female & male): *Infrequent:* Breast pain, impotence, atrophic vaginitis.

Resistance Mechanism Disorders: *Infrequent:* Cellulitis, cystitis, herpes simplex, otitis media.

Respiratory System: *Infrequent:* Bronchospasm, laryngitis, apnea.

Skin and Appendages: *Frequent:* Rashes of various kinds (maculopapular, eczema, bullous, exfoliative, psoriaform, erythematous); *Infrequent:* Alopecia, skin ulceration, urticaria, dermatitis contact.

Special Senses: *Infrequent:* Perversion of taste, loss of taste.

Urinary System Disorders: *Frequent:* Hematuria; *Infrequent:* Albuminuria, oliguria, acute renal failure, dysuria, micturition urgency, nocturia, polyuria, renal calculus, urinary retention.

Vascular (extracardiac) Disorders: *Infrequent:* Hemorrhoids, peripheral ischemia, pulmonary embolism, thrombosis, thrombophlebitis deep, aneurysm, hemorrhage intracranial.

Vision Disorders: *Frequent:* Cataract; *Infrequent:* Conjunctival hemorrhage, blepharitis, diplopia, eye pain, glaucoma.

White Cell and Resistance Disorders: *Infrequent:* Lymphadenopathy, leukocytosis.

POST-INTRODUCTION REPORTS

Voluntary reports of adverse events temporally associated with rivastigmine tartrate that have been received since market introduction that are not listed above, and that may or may not be causally related to the drug include the following:

Skin Appendages: Stevens-Johnson syndrome.

DOSAGE AND ADMINISTRATION

The dosage of rivastigmine tartrate shown to be effective in controlled clinical trials is 6-12 mg/day, given as twice a day dosing (daily doses of 3-6 mg bid). There is evidence from the clinical trials that doses at the higher end of this range may be more beneficial.

The starting dose of rivastigmine tartrate is 1.5 mg bid. If this dose is well tolerated, after a minimum of 2 weeks of treatment, the dose may be increased to 3 mg bid. Subsequent increases to 4.5 and 6 mg bid should be attempted after a minimum of 2 weeks at the previous dose. If adverse effects (*e.g.*, nausea, vomiting, abdominal pain, loss of appetite) cause intolerance during treatment, the patient should be instructed to discontinue treatment for several doses and then restart at the same or next lower dose level. If treatment is interrupted for longer than several days, treatment should be reinitiated with the lowest daily dose and titrated as described above (see WARNINGS). The maximum dose is 6 mg bid (12 mg/day).

Rivastigmine tartrate should be taken with meals in divided doses in the morning and evening.

ORAL SOLUTION

Recommendations for Administration

Caregivers should be instructed in the correct procedure for administering rivastigmine tartrate oral solution. In addition, they should be directed to the Instruction Sheet (included with the product) describing how the solution is to be administered. Caregivers should direct questions about the administration of the solution to either their physician or pharmacist (see PRECAUTIONS, Information for the Patient and Caregivers).

Patients should be instructed to remove the oral dosing syringe provided in its protective case, and using the provided syringe, withdraw the prescribed amount of rivastigmine tartrate oral solution from the container. Each dose of rivastigmine tartrate oral solution may be swallowed directly from the syringe or first mixed with a small glass of water, cold fruit juice, or soda. Patients should be instructed to stir and drink the mixture.

Rivastigmine tartrate oral solution and rivastigmine tartrate capsules may be interchanged at equal doses.

R

HOW SUPPLIED

EXELON CAPSULES

Exelon capsules equivalent to 1.5, 3, 4.5, or 6 mg of rivastigmine base are available as follows:

1.5 mg: Yellow; "Exelon 1.5 mg" is printed in red on the body of the capsule.

3.0 mg: Orange; "Exelon 3 mg" is printed in red on the body of the capsule.

4.5 mg: Red; "Exelon 4.5 mg" is printed in white on the body of the capsule.

6.0 mg: Orange and red; "Exelon 6 mg" is printed in red on the body of the capsule.

Storage: Store below 25°C (77°F) in a tight container.

EXELON ORAL SOLUTION

Exelon oral solution is supplied as 120 ml of a clear, yellow solution (2 mg/ml base) in a 4 oz Type III amber glass bottle with a child-resistant 28 mm cap, 0.5 mm foam liner, dip tube, and self-aligning plug. The oral solution is packaged with a dispenser set which consists of an assembled oral dosing syringe that allows dispensing a maximum volume of 3 ml corresponding to a 6 mg dose, with a plastic tube container.

Storage: Store below 25°C (77°F) in an upright position and protect from freezing.

When Exelon oral solution is combined with cold fruit juice or soda, the mixture is stable at room temperature for up to 4 hours.

PRODUCT LISTING - EQUIVALENTS NOT AVAILABLE

Capsule - Oral - 1.5 mg

60's	$153.74	EXELON, Novartis Pharmaceuticals	00078-0323-44
100's	$256.24	EXELON, Novartis Pharmaceuticals	00078-0323-06

Capsule - Oral - 3 mg

60's	$153.74	EXELON, Novartis Pharmaceuticals	00078-0324-44
100's	$256.24	EXELON, Novartis Pharmaceuticals	00078-0324-06

Capsule - Oral - 4.5 mg

60's	$153.74	EXELON, Novartis Pharmaceuticals	00078-0325-44
100's	$256.24	EXELON, Novartis Pharmaceuticals	00078-0325-06

Capsule - Oral - 6 mg

60's	$153.74	EXELON, Novartis Pharmaceuticals	00078-0326-44
100's	$256.24	EXELON, Novartis Pharmaceuticals	00078-0326-06

Solution - Oral - 2 mg/ml

120 ml	$283.05	EXELON, Novartis Pharmaceuticals	00078-0339-31

Rizatriptan Benzoate *(003411)*

For related information, see the comparative table section in Appendix A.

Categories: Headache, migraine; FDA Approved 1998 Jun; Pregnancy Category C
Drug Classes: Serotonin receptor agonists
Brand Names: **Maxalt**; Rizalt
Cost of Therapy: $17.94 (Migraine Headache; Maxalt; 5 mg; 1 tablet/day; 1 day supply)
$17.94 (Migraine Headache; Maxalt-MLT; 5 mg; 1 tablet/day; 1 day supply)

DESCRIPTION

Note: The trade names have been used throughout this monograph for clarity.

Maxalt contains rizatriptan benzoate, a selective 5-hydroxytryptamine$_{1B/1D}$ (5-HT$_{1B/1D}$) receptor agonist.

Rizatriptan benzoate is described chemically as: *N,N*-dimethyl-5-(1*H*-1,2,4-triazol-1-ylmethyl)-1*H*-indole-3-ethanamine monobenzoate.

Its empirical formula is $C_{15}H_{19}N_5 \cdot C_7H_6O_2$, representing a molecular weight of the free base of 269.4. Rizatriptan benzoate is a white to off-white, crystalline solid that is soluble in water at about 42 mg/ml (expressed as free base) at 25°C.

Maxalt tablets and Maxalt-MLT orally disintegrating tablets are available for oral administration in strengths of 5 and 10 mg (corresponding to 7.265 or 14.53 mg of the benzoate salt, respectively). Each compressed tablet contains the following inactive ingredients: lactose monohydrate, microcrystalline cellulose, pregelatinized starch, ferric oxide (red), and magnesium stearate.

Each lyophilized orally disintegrating tablet contains the following inactive ingredients: gelatin, mannitol, glycine, aspartame, and peppermint flavor.

CLINICAL PHARMACOLOGY

MECHANISM OF ACTION

Rizatriptan binds with high affinity to human cloned 5-HT$_{1B}$ and 5-HT$_{1D}$ receptors. Rizatriptan has weak affinity for other 5-HT$_1$ receptor subtypes (5-HT$_{1A}$, 5-HT$_{1E}$, 5-HT$_{1F}$) and the 5-HT$_7$ receptor, but has no significant activity at 5-HT$_2$, 5-HT$_3$, alpha- and beta-adrenergic, dopaminergic, histaminergic, muscarinic or benzodiazepine receptors.

Current theories on the etiology of migraine headache suggest that symptoms are due to local cranial vasodilatation and/or to the release of vasoactive and pro-inflammatory peptides from sensory nerve endings in an activated trigeminal system. The therapeutic activity of rizatriptan in migraine can most likely be attributed to agonist effects at 5-HT$_{1B/1D}$ receptors on the extracerebral, intracranial blood vessels that become dilated during a migraine attack and on nerve terminals in the trigeminal system. Activation of these receptors results in cranial vessel constriction, inhibition of neuropeptide release and reduced transmission in trigeminal pain pathways.

PHARMACOKINETICS

Rizatriptan is completely absorbed following oral administration. The mean oral absolute bioavailability of the Maxalt tablet is about 45%, and mean peak plasma concentrations (C_{max}) are reached in approximately 1-1.5 hours (T_{max}). The presence of a migraine headache did not appear to affect the absorption or pharmacokinetics of rizatriptan. Food has no significant effect on the bioavailability of rizatriptan but delays the time to reach peak concentration by an hour. In clinical trials, Maxalt was administered without regard to food. The plasma half-life of rizatriptan in males and females averages 2-3 hours.

The bioavailability and C_{max} of rizatriptan were similar following administration of Maxalt tablets and Maxalt-MLT orally disintegrating tablets, but the rate of absorption is somewhat slower with Maxalt-MLT, with T_{max} averaging 1.6-2.5 hours. AUC of rizatriptan is approximately 30% higher in females than in males. No accumulation occurred on multiple dosing.

The mean volume of distribution is approximately 140 L in male subjects and 110 L in female subjects. Rizatriptan is minimally bound (14%) to plasma proteins.

The primary route of rizatriptan metabolism is via oxidative deamination by monoamine oxidase-A (MAO-A) to the indole acetic acid metabolite, which is not active at the 5-HT$_{1B/1D}$ receptor. N-monodesmethyl-rizatriptan, a metabolite with activity similar to that of parent compound at the 5-HT$_{1B/1D}$ receptor, is formed to a minor degree. Plasma concentrations of N-monodesmethyl-rizatriptan are approximately 14% of those of parent compound, and it is eliminated at a similar rate. Other minor metabolites, the N-oxide, the 6-hydroxy compound, and the sulfate conjugate of the 6-hydroxy metabolite are not active at the 5-HT$_{1B/1D}$ receptor.

The total radioactivity of the administered dose recovered over 120 hours in urine and feces was 82% and 12%, respectively, following a single 10 mg oral administration of ^{14}C-rizatriptan. Following oral administration of ^{14}C-rizatriptan, rizatriptan accounted for about 17% of circulating plasma radioactivity. Approximately 14% of an oral dose is excreted in urine as unchanged rizatriptan while 51% is excreted as indole acetic acid metabolite, indicating substantial first pass metabolism.

Cytochrome P450 Isoforms

Rizatriptan is not an inhibitor of the activities of human liver cytochrome P450 isoforms 3A4/5, 1A2, 2C9, 2C19, or 2E1; rizatriptan is a competitive inhibitor (Ki = 1400 nM) of cytochrome P450 2D6, but only at high, clinically irrelevant concentrations.

SPECIAL POPULATIONS

Age

Rizatriptan pharmacokinetics in healthy elderly non-migraineur volunteers (age 65-77 years) were similar to those in younger non-migraineur volunteers (age 18-45 years).

Gender

The mean AUC(0-∞) and C_{max} of rizatriptan (10 mg orally) were about 30% and 11% higher in females as compared to males, respectively, while T_{max} occurred at approximately the same time.

Hepatic Impairment

Following oral administration in patients with hepatic impairment caused by mild to moderate alcoholic cirrhosis of the liver, plasma concentrations of rizatriptan were similar in patients with mild hepatic insufficiency compared to a control group of healthy subjects; plasma concentrations of rizatriptan were approximately 30% greater in patients with moderate hepatic insufficiency. (See PRECAUTIONS.)

Renal Impairment

In patients with renal impairment (creatinine clearance 10-60 ml/min/1.73 m^2), the AUC(0-∞) of rizatriptan was not significantly different from that in healthy subjects. In hemodialysis patients, (creatinine clearance <2 ml/min/1.73 m^2), however, the AUC for rizatriptan was approximately 44% greater than that in patients with normal renal function. (See PRECAUTIONS.)

Race

Pharmacokinetic data revealed no significant differences between African American and Caucasian subjects.

DRUG INTERACTIONS

See also DRUG INTERACTIONS.

Monoamine Oxidase Inhibitors

Rizatriptan is principally metabolized via monoamine oxidase, 'A' subtype (MAO-A). Plasma concentrations of rizatriptan may be increased by drugs that are selective MAO-A inhibitors (*e.g.*, moclobemide) or nonselective MAO inhibitors [type A and B] (*e.g.*, isocarboxazid, phenelzine, tranylcypromine, and pargyline). In a drug interaction study, when Maxalt 10 mg was administered to subjects (n=12) receiving concomitant therapy with the selective, reversible MAO-A inhibitor, moclobemide 150 mg tid, there were mean increases in rizatriptan AUC and C_{max} of 119% and 41% respectively; and the AUC of the active N-monodesmethyl metabolite of rizatriptan was increased more than 400%. The interaction would be expected to be greater with irreversible MAO inhibitors. No pharmacokinetic interaction is anticipated in patients receiving selective MAO-B inhibitors. (See CONTRAINDICATIONS and DRUG INTERACTIONS.)

Propranolol

In a study of concurrent administration of propranolol 240 mg/day and a single dose of rizatriptan 10 mg in healthy subjects (n=11), mean plasma AUC for rizatriptan was increased by 70% during propranolol administration, and a 4-fold increase was observed in 1 subject. The AUC of the active N-monodesmethyl metabolite of rizatriptan was not affected by propranolol. (See PRECAUTIONS and DOSAGE AND ADMINISTRATION.)

Nadolol/Metoprolol

In a drug interactions study, effects of multiple doses of nadolol 80 mg or metoprolol 100 mg every 12 hours on the pharmacokinetics of a single dose of 10 mg rizatriptan were evaluated in healthy subjects (n=12). No pharmacokinetic interactions were observed.

Paroxetine

In a study of the interaction between the selective serotonin reuptake inhibitor (SSRI) paroxetine 20 mg/day for 2 weeks and a single dose of Maxalt 10 mg in healthy subjects (n=12), neither the plasma concentrations of rizatriptan nor its safety profile were affected by paroxetine.

Oral Contraceptives

In a study of concurrent administration of an oral contraceptive during 6 days of administration of Maxalt (10-30 mg/day) in healthy female volunteers (n=18), rizatriptan did not affect plasma concentrations of ethinyl estradiol or norethindrone.

INDICATIONS AND USAGE

Maxalt is indicated for the acute treatment of migraine attacks with or without aura in adults.

Maxalt is not intended for the prophylactic therapy of migraine or for use in the management of hemiplegic or basilar migraine (see CONTRAINDICATIONS). Safety and effectiveness of Maxalt have not been established for cluster headache, which is present in an older, predominantly male population.

CONTRAINDICATIONS

Maxalt should not be given to patients with ischemic heart disease (*e.g.*, angina pectoris, history of myocardial infarction, or documented silent ischemia) or to patients who have symptoms or findings consistent with ischemic heart disease, coronary artery vasospasm, including Prinzmetal's variant angina, or other significant underlying cardiovascular disease (see WARNINGS).

Because Maxalt may increase blood pressure, it should not be given to patients with uncontrolled hypertension (see WARNINGS).

Maxalt should not be used within 24 hours of treatment with another 5-HT_1 agonist, or an ergotamine-containing or ergot-type medication like dihydroergotamine or methysergide.

Maxalt should not be administered to patients with hemiplegic or basilar migraine.

Concurrent administration of MAO inhibitors or use of rizatriptan within 2 weeks of discontinuation of MAO inhibitor therapy is contraindicated (see CLINICAL PHARMACOLOGY, Drug Interactions andDRUG INTERACTIONS).

Maxalt is contraindicated in patients who are hypersensitive to rizatriptan or any of its inactive ingredients.

WARNINGS

Maxalt should only be used where a clear diagnosis of migraine has been established.

RISK OF MYOCARDIAL ISCHEMIA AND/OR INFARCTION AND OTHER ADVERSE CARDIAC EVENTS

Because of the potential of this class of compounds (5-$HT_{1B/1D}$ agonists) to cause coronary vasospasm, Maxalt should not be given to patients with documented ischemic or vasospastic coronary artery disease (see CONTRAINDICATIONS). It is strongly recommended that rizatriptan not be given to patients in whom unrecognized coronary artery disease (CAD) is predicted by the presence of risk factors (*e.g.*, hypertension, hypercholesterolemia, smoker, obesity, diabetes, strong family history of CAD, female with surgical or physiological menopause, or male over 40 years of age) unless a cardiovascular evaluation provides satisfactory clinical evidence that the patient is reasonably free of coronary artery and ischemic myocardial disease or other significant underlying cardiovascular disease. The sensitivity of cardiac diagnostic procedures to detect cardiovascular disease or predisposition to coronary artery vasospasm is modest, at best. If, during the cardiovascular evaluation, the patient's medical history, electrocardiographic or other investigations reveal findings indicative of, or consistent with, coronary artery vasospasm or myocardial ischemia, rizatriptan should not be administered (see CONTRAINDICATIONS).

For patients with risk factors predictive of CAD, who are determined to have a satisfactory cardiovascular evaluation, it is strongly recommended that administration of the first dose of rizatriptan take place in the setting of a physician's office or similar medically staffed and equipped facility unless the patient has previously received rizatriptan. Because cardiac ischemia can occur in the absence of clinical symptoms, consideration should be given to obtaining on the first occasion of use an electrocardiogram (ECG) during the interval immediately following Maxalt, in these patients with risk factors.

It is recommended that patients who are intermittent long-term users of Maxalt and who have or acquire risk factors predictive of CAD, as described above, undergo periodic interval cardiovascular evaluation as they continue to use Maxalt.

The systematic approach described above is intended to reduce the likelihood that patients with unrecognized cardiovascular disease will be inadvertently exposed to rizatriptan.

CARDIAC EVENTS AND FATALITIES ASSOCIATED WITH 5-HT_1 AGONISTS

Serious adverse cardiac events, including acute myocardial infarction, have been reported within a few hours following the administration of rizatriptan. Life-threatening disturbances of cardiac rhythm and death have been reported within a few hours following the administration of other 5-HT_1 agonists. Considering the extent of use of 5-HT_1 agonists in patients with migraine, the incidence of these events is extremely low. Maxalt can cause coronary vasospasm. Because of the close proximity of the events to Maxalt use, a causal relationship cannot be excluded. In the cases where there has been known underlying coronary artery disease, the relationship is uncertain.

PREMARKETING EXPERIENCE WITH RIZATRIPTAN

Among the 3700 patients with migraine who participated in premarketing clinical trials of Maxalt, 1 patient was reported to have chest pain with possible ischemic ECG changes following a single dose of 10 mg.

POSTMARKETING EXPERIENCE WITH RIZATRIPTAN

Serious cardiovascular events have been reported in association with the use of Maxalt. The uncontrolled nature of postmarketing surveillance, however, makes it impossible to determine definitively the proportion of the reported cases that were actually caused by rizatriptan or to reliably assess causation in individual cases.

CEREBROVASCULAR EVENTS AND FATALITIES ASSOCIATED WITH 5-HT_1 AGONISTS

Cerebral hemorrhage, subarachnoid hemorrhage, stroke, and other cerebrovascular events have been reported in patients treated with 5-HT_1 agonists; and some have resulted in fatalities. In a number of cases, it appears possible that the cerebrovascular events were primary, the agonist having been administered in the incorrect belief that the symptoms experienced were a consequence of migraine, when they were not. It should be noted that patients with migraine may be at increased risk of certain cerebrovascular events (*e.g.*, stroke, hemorrhage, transient ischemic attack).

OTHER VASOSPASM-RELATED EVENTS

5-HT_1 agonists may cause vasospastic reactions other than coronary artery vasospasm. Both peripheral vascular ischemia and colonic ischemia with abdominal pain and bloody diarrhea have been reported with 5-HT_1 agonists.

INCREASE IN BLOOD PRESSURE

Significant elevation in blood pressure, including hypertensive crisis, has been reported on rare occasions in patients receiving 5-HT_1 agonists with and without a history of hypertension. In healthy young male and female subjects who received maximal doses of Maxalt (10 mg every 2 hours for 3 doses), slight increases in blood pressure (approximately 2-3 mm Hg) were observed. Rizatriptan is contraindicated in patients with uncontrolled hypertension (see CONTRAINDICATIONS).

An 18% increase in mean pulmonary artery pressure was seen following dosing with another 5-HT_1 agonist in a study evaluating subjects undergoing cardiac catheterization.

R

PRECAUTIONS

GENERAL

As with other $5\text{-HT}_{1B/1D}$ agonists, sensations of tightness, pain, pressure, and heaviness have been reported after treatment with Maxalt in the precordium, throat, neck and jaw. These events have not been associated with arrhythmias or definite ischemic ECG changes in clinical trials (1 patient experienced chest pain with possible ischemic ECG changes). Because drugs in this class may cause coronary artery vasospasm, patients who experience signs or symptoms suggestive of angina following dosing should be evaluated for the presence of CAD or a predisposition to Prinzmetal's variant angina before receiving additional doses of medication, and should be monitored electrocardiographically if dosing is resumed and similar symptoms recur. Similarly, patients who experience other symptoms or signs suggestive of decreased arterial flow, such as ischemic bowel syndrome or Raynaud's syndrome following the use of any 5-HT_1 agonist are candidates for further evaluation (see WARNINGS).

Rizatriptan should also be administered with caution to patients with diseases that may alter the absorption, metabolism, or excretion of drugs (see CLINICAL PHARMACOLOGY, Special Populations).

Renally Impaired Patients

Rizatriptan should be used with caution in dialysis patients due to a decrease in the clearance of rizatriptan (see CLINICAL PHARMACOLOGY, Special Populations).

Hepatically Impaired Patients

Rizatriptan should be used with caution in patients with moderate hepatic insufficiency due to an increase in plasma concentrations of approximately 30% (see CLINICAL PHARMACOLOGY, Special Populations).

For a given attack, if a patient has no response to the first dose of rizatriptan, the diagnosis of migraine should be reconsidered before administration of a second dose.

BINDING TO MELANIN-CONTAINING TISSUES

The propensity for rizatriptan to bind melanin has not been investigated. Based on its chemical properties, rizatriptan may bind to melanin and accumulate in melanin rich tissue (*e.g.,* eye) over time. This raises the possibility that rizatriptan could cause toxicity in these tissues after extended use. There were, however, no adverse ophthalmologic changes related to treatment with rizatriptan in the 1 year dog toxicity study. Although no systematic monitoring of ophthalmologic function was undertaken in clinical trials, and no specific recommendations for ophthalmologic monitoring are offered, prescribers should be aware of the possibility of long-term ophthalmologic effects.

PHENYLKETONURICS

Phenylketonuric patients should be informed that Maxalt-MLT orally disintegrating tablets contain phenylalanine (a component of aspartame). Each 5 mg orally disintegrating tablet contains 1.05 mg phenylalanine, and each 10 mg orally disintegrating tablet contains 2.10 mg phenylalanine.

INFORMATION FOR THE PATIENT

Migraine or treatment with Maxalt may cause somnolence in some patients. Dizziness has also been reported in some patients receiving Maxalt. Patients should, therefore, evaluate their ability to perform complex tasks during migraine attacks and after administration of Maxalt.

Physicians should instruct their patients to read the patient package insert distributed with the prescription before taking Maxalt.

MAXALT-MLT ORALLY DISINTEGRATING TABLETS

Patients should be instructed not to remove the blister from the outer pouch until just prior to dosing. The blister pack should then be peeled open with dry hands and the orally disintegrating tablet placed on the tongue, where it will dissolve and be swallowed with the saliva.

R

LABORATORY TESTS

No specific laboratory tests are recommended for monitoring patients prior to and/or after treatment with Maxalt.

DRUG/LABORATORY TEST INTERACTIONS

Maxalt is not known to interfere with commonly employed clinical laboratory tests.

CARCINOGENESIS, MUTAGENESIS, AND IMPAIRMENT OF FERTILITY

Carcinogenesis

The lifetime carcinogenic potential of rizatriptan was evaluated in a 100 week study in mice and a 106 week study in rats at oral gavage doses of up to 125 mg/kg/day. Exposure data were not obtained in those studies, but plasma AUCs of parent drug measured in other studies after 5 and 21 weeks of oral dosing in mice and rats, respectively, indicate that the exposures to parent drug at the highest dose level in the carcinogenicity studies would have been approximately 150 times (mice) and 240 times (rats) average AUCs measured in humans after three 10 mg doses, the maximum recommended total daily dose. There was no evidence of an increase in tumor incidence related to rizatriptan in either species.

Mutagenesis

Rizatriptan, with and without metabolic activation, was neither mutagenic, nor clastogenic in a battery of *in vitro* and *in vivo* genetic toxicity studies, including: the microbial mutagenesis (Ames) assay, the *in vitro* mammalian cell mutagenesis assay in V-79 Chinese hamster lung cells, the *in vitro* alkaline elution assay in rat hepatocytes, the *in vitro* chromosomal aberration assay in Chinese hamster ovary cells and the *in vivo* chromosomal aberration assay in mouse bone marrow.

Impairment of Fertility

In a fertility study in rats, altered estrus cyclicity and delays in time to mating were observed in females treated orally with 100 mg/kg/day rizatriptan. Plasma drug exposure (AUC) at this dose was approximately 225 times the exposure in humans receiving the maximum recommended daily dose (MRDD) of 30 mg. The no-effect dose was 10 mg/kg/day (approximately 15 times the human exposure at the MRDD). There were no other fertility-related effects in the female rats. There was no impairment of fertility or reproductive performance in male rats treated with up to 250 mg/kg/day (approximately 550 times the human exposure at the MRDD).

PREGNANCY CATEGORY C

In a general reproductive study in rats, birth weights and pre- and post-weaning weight gain were reduced in the offspring of females treated prior to and during mating and throughout gestation and lactation with doses of 10 and 100 mg/kg/day. Maternal drug exposures (AUC) at these doses were approximately 15 and 225 times, respectively, the exposure in humans receiving the maximum recommended daily dose (MRDD) of 30 mg. In a pre- and post-natal developmental toxicity study in rats, an increase in mortality of the offspring at birth and for the first 3 days after birth, a decrease in pre-and post-weaning weight gain, and decreased performance in a passive avoidance test (which indicates a decrease in learning capacity of the offspring) were observed at doses of 100 and 250 mg/kg/day. The no-effect dose for all of these effects was 5 mg/kg/day, approximately 7.5 times the exposure in humans receiving the MRDD. With doses of 100 and 250 mg/kg/day, the decreases in average weight of both the male and female offspring persisted into adulthood. All of these effects on the offspring in both reproductive toxicity studies occurred in the absence of any apparent maternal toxicity.

In embryofetal development studies, no teratogenic effects were observed when pregnant rats and rabbits were administered doses of 100 and 50 mg/kg/day, respectively, during organogenesis. Fetal weights were decreased in conjunction with decreased maternal weight gain at the highest doses (maternal exposures approximately 225 and 115 times the human exposure at the MRDD in rats and rabbits, respectively). The developmental no-effect dose in these studies was 10 mg/kg/day in both rats and rabbits (maternal exposures approximately 15 times human exposure at the MRDD). Toxicokinetic studies demonstrated placental transfer of drug in both species.

There are no adequate and well-controlled studies in pregnant women; therefore, rizatriptan should be used during pregnancy only if the potential benefit justifies the potential risk to the fetus.

Merck & Co., Inc. maintains a registry to monitor the pregnancy outcomes of women exposed to Maxalt while pregnant. Healthcare providers are encouraged to report any prenatal exposure to Maxalt by calling the Pregnancy Registry at 800-986-8999.

NURSING MOTHERS

It is not known whether this drug is excreted in human milk. Because many drugs are excreted in human milk, caution should be exercised when Maxalt is administered to women who are breast-feeding. Rizatriptan is extensively excreted in rat milk, at a level of 5-fold or greater than maternal plasma levels.

PEDIATRIC USE

Safety and effectiveness of rizatriptan in pediatric patients have not been established; therefore, Maxalt is not recommended for use in patients under 18 years of age.

The efficacy of Maxalt tablets (5 mg) in patients aged 12-17 years was not established in a randomized placebo-controlled trial of 291 adolescent migraineurs. Adverse events observed were similar in nature to those reported in clinical trials in adults. Postmarketing experience with other triptans includes a limited number of reports that describe pediatric patients who have experienced clinically serious adverse events that are similar in nature to those reported rarely in adults. The long-term safety of rizatriptan in pediatric patients has not been studied.

GERIATRIC USE

The pharmacokinetics of rizatriptan were similar in elderly (aged ≥65 years) and in younger adults. Because migraine occurs infrequently in the elderly, clinical experience with Maxalt is limited in such patients. In clinical trials, there were no apparent differences in efficacy or in overall adverse experience rates between patients under 65 years of age and those 65 and above (n=17).

DRUG INTERACTIONS

See also CLINICAL PHARMACOLOGY, Drug Interactions.

Propranolol: Rizatriptan 5 mg should be used in patients taking propranolol, as propranolol has been shown to increase the plasma concentrations of rizatriptan by 70% (see CLINICAL PHARMACOLOGY, Drug Interations and DOSAGE AND ADMINISTRATION).

Ergot-Containing Drugs: Ergot-containing drugs have been reported to cause prolonged vasospastic reactions. Because there is a theoretical basis that these effects may be additive, use of ergotamine-containing or ergot-type medications (like dihydroergotamine or methysergide) and rizatriptan within 24 hours is contraindicated (see CONTRAINDICATIONS).

Other 5-HT$_1$ Agonists: The administration of rizatriptan with other 5-HT_1 agonists has not been evaluated in migraine patients. Because their vasospastic effects may be additive, coadministration of rizatriptan and other 5-HT_1 agonists within 24 hours of each other is not recommended (see CONTRAINDICATIONS).

Selective Serotonin Reuptake Inhibitors (SSRIs): SSRIs (*e.g.,* fluoxetine, fluvoxamine, paroxetine, sertraline) have been reported, rarely, to cause weakness, hyperreflexia, and incoordination when coadministered with 5-HT_1 agonists. If concomitant treatment with rizatriptan and an SSRI is clinically warranted, appropriate observation of the patient is advised. No clinical or pharmacokinetic interactions were observed when Maxalt 10 mg was administered with paroxetine.

Monoamine Oxidase Inhibitors: Rizatriptan should not be administered to patients taking MAO-A inhibitors and nonselective MAO inhibitors; it has been shown that moclobemide (a specific MAO-A inhibitor) increased the systemic exposure of rizatriptan and its metabolite (see CLINICAL PHARMACOLOGY, Drug Interactions and CONTRAINDICATIONS).

ADVERSE REACTIONS

Serious cardiac events, including some that have been fatal, have occurred following use of 5-HT$_1$ agonists. These events are extremely rare and most have been reported in patients with risk factors predictive of CAD. Events reported have included coronary artery vasospasm, transient myocardial ischemia, myocardial infarction, ventricular tachycardia, and ventricular fibrillation (see CONTRAINDICATIONS, WARNINGS, and PRECAUTIONS).

INCIDENCE IN CONTROLLED CLINICAL TRIALS

Adverse experiences to rizatriptan were assessed in controlled clinical trials that included over 3700 patients who received single or multiple doses of Maxalt tablets. The most common adverse events during treatment with Maxalt were asthenia/fatigue, somnolence, pain/pressure sensation and dizziness. These events appeared to be dose related. In long term extension studies where patients were allowed to treat multiple attacks for up to 1 year, 4% (59 out of 1525 patients) withdrew because of adverse experiences.

TABLE 3 lists the adverse events regardless of drug relationship (incidence ≥2% and greater than placebo) after a single dose of Maxalt. The events cited reflect experience gained under closely monitored conditions of clinical trials in a highly selected patient population. In actual clinical practice or in other clinical trials, these frequency estimates may not apply, as the conditions of use, reporting behavior, and the kinds of patients treated may differ.

TABLE 3 *Incidence (≥2% and greater than placebo) of Adverse Experiences After a Single Dose of Maxalt Tablets or Placebo*

	Maxalt		
	5 mg	10 mg	Placebo
Adverse Experiences	(n=977)	(n=1167)	(n=627)
Atypical Sensations	4%	5%	4%
Paresthesia	3%	4%	<2%
Pain and Other Pressure Sensations	6%	9%	3%
Chest pain:			
Tightness/pressure and/or heaviness	<2%	3%	1%
Neck/throat/jaw:			
Pain/tightness/pressure	<2%	2%	1%
Regional pain:			
Tightness/pressure/heaviness	<1%	2%	0%
Pain, location unspecified	3%	3%	<2%
Digestive	9%	13%	8%
Dry mouth	3%	3%	1%
Nausea	4%	6%	4%
Neurological	14%	20%	11%
Dizziness	4%	9%	5%
Headache	<2%	2%	<1%
Somnolence	4%	8%	4%
Other			
Asthenia/fatigue	4%	7%	2%

Maxalt was generally well-tolerated. Adverse experiences were typically mild in intensity and were transient. The frequencies of adverse experiences in clinical trials did not increase when up to 3 doses were taken within 24 hours. Adverse event frequencies were also unchanged by concomitant use of drugs commonly taken for migraine prophylaxis (including propranolol), oral contraceptives, or analgesics. The incidences of adverse experiences were not affected by age or gender. There were insufficient data to assess the impact of race on the incidence of adverse events.

OTHER EVENTS OBSERVED IN ASSOCIATION WITH THE ADMINISTRATION OF MAXALT

In the section that follows, the frequencies of less commonly reported adverse clinical events are presented. Because the reports include events observed in open studies, the role of Maxalt in their causation cannot be reliably determined. Furthermore, variability associated with adverse event reporting, the terminology used to describe adverse events, etc., limit the value of the quantitative frequency estimates provided. Event frequencies are calculated as the number of patients who used Maxalt (n=3716) and reported an event divided by the total number of patients exposed to Maxalt. All reported events are included, except those already listed in TABLE 3, those too general to be informative, and those not reasonably associated with the use of the drug. Events are further classified within body system categories and enumerated in order of decreasing frequency using the following definitions: *frequent* adverse events are those defined as those occurring in at least (>)1/100 patients; *infrequent* adverse experiences are those occurring in 1/100 to 1/1000 patients; and *rare* adverse experiences are those occurring in fewer than 1/1000 patients.

General: *Infrequent:* Chills, heat sensitivity, facial edema, hangover effect, and abdominal distention. *Rare:* Fever, orthostatic effects, syncope and edema/swelling.

Atypical Sensations: *Frequent:* Warm/cold sensations.

Cardiovascular: *Frequent:* Palpitation. *Infrequent:* Tachycardia, cold extremities, hypertension, arrhythmia, and bradycardia. *Rare:* Angina pectoris.

Digestive: *Frequent:* Diarrhea and vomiting. *Infrequent:* Dyspepsia, thirst, acid regurgitation, dysphagia, constipation, flatulence, and tongue edema. *Rare:* Anorexia, appetite increase, gastritis, paralysis (tongue), and eructation.

Metabolic: *Infrequent:* Dehydration.

Musculoskeletal: *Infrequent:* Muscle weakness, stiffness, myalgia, muscle cramp, musculoskeletal pain, arthralgia, and muscle spasm.

Neurological/Psychiatric: *Frequent:* Hypesthesia, mental acuity decreased, euphoria and tremor. *Infrequent:* Nervousness, vertigo, insomnia, anxiety, depression, disorientation, ataxia, dysarthria, confusion, dream abnormality, gait abnormality, irritability, memory impairment, agitation and hyperesthesia. *Rare:* Dysesthesia, depersonalization, akinesia/bradykinesia, apprehension, hyperkinesia, hypersomnia, and hyporeflexia.

Respiratory: *Frequent:* Dyspnea. *Infrequent:* Pharyngitis, irritation (nasal), congestion (nasal), dry throat, upper respiratory infection, yawning, respiratory congestion (nasal), dry nose, epistaxis, and sinus disorder. *Rare:* Cough, hiccups, hoarseness, rhinorrhea, sneezing, tachypnea, and pharyngeal edema.

Special Senses: *Infrequent:* Blurred vision, tinnitus, dry eyes, burning eye, eye pain, eye irritation, ear pain, and tearing. *Rare:* Hyperacusis, smell perversion, photophobia, photopsia, itching eye, and eye swelling.

Skin and Skin Appendage: *Frequent:* Flushing. *Infrequent:* Sweating, pruritus, rash, and urticaria. *Rare:* Erythema, acne, and photosensitivity.

Urogenital System: *Frequent:* Hot flashes. *Infrequent:* Urinary frequency, polyuria, and menstruation disorder. *Rare:* Dysuria.

The adverse experience profile seen with Maxalt-MLT orally disintegrating tablets was similar to that seen with Maxalt tablets.

POSTMARKETING EXPERIENCE

The following section enumerates potentially important adverse events that have occurred in clinical practice and which have been reported spontaneously to various surveillance systems. The events enumerated represent reports arising from both domestic and non-domestic use of rizatriptan. The events enumerated include all except those already listed in the ADVERSE REACTIONS section above or those too general to be informative. Because the reports cite events reported spontaneously from worldwide postmarketing experience, frequency of events and the role of rizatriptan in their causation cannot be reliably determined.

Cardiovascular: Myocardial ischemia, myocardial infarction (see WARNINGS).

Cerebrovascular: Stroke.

Special Senses: Dysgeusia.

General: *Hypersensitivity:* Angioedema (*e.g.,* facial edema, tongue swelling, pharyngeal edema), wheezing, toxic epidermal necrolysis.

DOSAGE AND ADMINISTRATION

In controlled clinical trials, single doses of 5 and 10 mg of Maxalt tablets or Maxalt-MLT were effective for the acute treatment of migraines in adults. There is evidence that the 10 mg dose may provide a greater effect than the 5 mg dose. Individuals may vary in response to doses of Maxalt tablets. The choice of dose should therefore be made on an individual basis, weighing the possible benefit of the 10 mg dose with the potential risk for increased adverse events.

REDOSING

Doses should be separated by at least 2 hours; no more than 30 mg should be taken in any 24 hour period.

The safety of treating, on average, more than 4 headaches in a 30 day period has not been established.

PATIENTS RECEIVING PROPRANOLOL

In patients receiving propranolol, the 5 mg dose of Maxalt should be used, up to a maximum of 3 doses in any 24 hour period. (See CLINICAL PHARMACOLOGY, Drug Interactions.)

For Maxalt-MLT orally disintegrating tablets, administration with liquid is not necessary. The orally disintegrating tablet is packaged in a blister within an outer aluminum pouch. Patients should be instructed not to remove the blister from the outer pouch until just prior to dosing. The blister pack should then be peeled open with dry hands and the orally disintegrating tablet placed on the tongue, where it will dissolve and be swallowed with the saliva.

HOW SUPPLIED

MAXALT TABLETS

5 mg: Pale pink, capsule-shaped, compressed tablets coded "MRK" on one side and "266" on the other.

10 mg: Pale pink, capsule-shaped, compressed tablets coded "MAXALT" on one side and "MRK 267" on the other.

Storage: Store Maxalt Tablets at room temperature, 15-30°C (59-86°F). Dispense in a tight container, if product is subdivided.

MAXALT-MLT ORALLY DISINTEGRATING TABLETS

5 mg: White to off-white, round lyophilized orally disintegrating tablets debossed with a modified triangle on one side, and measuring 10.0-11.5 mm (side-to-side) with a peppermint flavor. Each orally disintegrating tablet is individually packaged in a blister inside an aluminum pouch (sachet).

10 mg: White to off-white, round lyophilized orally disintegrating tablets debossed with a modified square on one side, and measuring 12.0-13.8 mm (side-to-side) with a peppermint flavor. Each orally disintegrating tablet is individually packaged in a blister inside an aluminum pouch (sachet).

Storage: Store Maxalt-MLT Orally Disintegrating Tablets at room temperature, 15-30°C (59-86°F). The patient should be instructed not to remove the blister from the outer aluminum pouch until the patient is ready to consume the orally disintegrating tablet inside.

PRODUCT LISTING - EQUIVALENTS NOT AVAILABLE

Tablet - Oral - 5 mg

6's	$107.63	MAXALT, Merck & Company Inc	00006-0266-06

Tablet - Oral - 10 mg

6's	$92.90	MAXALT, Southwood Pharmaceuticals Inc	58016-5712-06
6's	$107.63	MAXALT, Merck & Company Inc	00006-0267-06

Tablet, Disintegrating - Oral - 5 mg

6's	$107.63	MAXALT-MLT, Merck & Company Inc	00006-3800-06

Tablet, Disintegrating - Oral - 10 mg

6's	$107.63	MAXALT-MLT, Merck & Company Inc	00006-3801-06

Rofecoxib (003435)

For related information, see the comparative table section in Appendix A.

Categories: Arthritis, osteoarthritis; Arthritis, rheumatoid; Dysmenorrhea; Pain, moderate to severe; FDA Approved 1999 May; Pregnancy Category C
Drug Classes: Analgesics, non-narcotic; COX-2 inhibitors; Nonsteroidal anti-inflammatory drugs
Brand Names: Vioxx
Foreign Brand Availability: Alfof (India); Dolib (India); Flanax (Colombia); Rhuma-Cure (Bahrain; Cyprus; Egypt; Iran; Iraq; Jordan; Kuwait; Lebanon; Libya; Oman; Qatar; Republic-of-Yemen; Saudi-Arabia; Syria; United-Arab-Emirates); Rofetab (India); Rofiz Gel (India); Sivoz (Colombia); Toroxx MT (Republic-Of-Yemen); Vioxx Forte (Israel)
Cost of Therapy: $86.27 (Osteoarthritis; Vioxx; 12.5 mg; 1 tablet/day; 30 day supply)
$78.70 (Rheumatoid Arthritis; Vioxx; 25 mg; 1 Tablet/day; 30 day supply)
$20.09 (Pain; Vioxx; 50 mg; 1 Tablet/day; 5 day supply)

DESCRIPTION

Note: The trade name has been used throughout this monograph for clarity.

Vioxx (rofecoxib) is described chemically as 4-[4-(methylsulfonyl)phenyl]-3-phenyl-2(*5H*)-furanone.

Rofecoxib is a white to off-white to light yellow powder. It is sparingly soluble in acetone, slightly soluble in methanol and isopropyl acetate, very slightly soluble in ethanol, practically insoluble in octanol, and insoluble in water. The empirical formula for rofecoxib is $C_{17}H_{14}O_4S$, and the molecular weight is 314.36.

Each tablet of Vioxx for oral administration contains either 12.5, 25, or 50 mg of rofecoxib and the following inactive ingredients: croscarmellose sodium, hydroxypropyl cellulose, lactose, magnesium stearate, microcrystalline cellulose, and yellow ferric oxide. The 50 mg tablets also contain red ferric oxide.

Each 5 ml of the oral suspension contains either 12.5 or 25 mg of rofecoxib and the following inactive ingredients: citric acid (monohydrate), sodium citrate (dihydrate), sorbitol solution, strawberry flavor, xanthan gum, and purified water. Added as preservatives are sodium methylparaben 0.13% and sodium propylparaben 0.02%.

CLINICAL PHARMACOLOGY

MECHANISM OF ACTION

Vioxx is a nonsteroidal anti-inflammatory drug (NSAID) that exhibits anti-inflammatory, analgesic, and antipyretic activities in animal models. The mechanism of action of Vioxx is believed to be due to inhibition of prostaglandin synthesis, via inhibition of cyclooxygenase-2 (COX-2). At therapeutic concentrations in humans, Vioxx does not inhibit the cyclooxygenase-1 (COX-1) isoenzyme.

PHARMACOKINETICS

Absorption

The mean oral bioavailability of Vioxx at therapeutically recommended doses of 12.5, 25, and 50 mg is approximately 93%. The area under the curve (AUC) and peak plasma level (C_{max}) following a single 25 mg dose were 3286 (±843) ng·h/ml and 207 (±111) ng/ml, respectively. Both C_{max} and AUC are roughly dose proportional across the clinical dose range. At doses greater than 50 mg, there is a less than proportional increase in C_{max} and AUC, which is thought to be due to the low solubility of the drug in aqueous media. The plasma concentration-time profile exhibited multiple peaks. The median time to maximal concentration (T_{max}), as assessed in nine pharmacokinetic studies, is 2-3 hours. Individual T_{max} values in these studies ranged between 2-9 hours. This may not reflect rate of absorption as T_{max} may occur as a secondary peak in some individuals. With multiple dosing, steady-state conditions are reached by Day 4. The AUC(0-24h) and C_{max} at steady state after multiple doses of 25 mg rofecoxib was 4018 (±1140) ng·h/ml and 321 (±104) ng/ml, respectively. The accumulation factor based on geometric means was 1.67.

Vioxx tablets 12.5 mg and 25 mg are bioequivalent to Vioxx oral suspension 12.5 mg/5 ml and 25 mg/5 ml, respectively.

R

Food and Antacid Effects

Food had no significant effect on either the peak plasma concentration (C_{max}) or extent of absorption (AUC) of rofecoxib when Vioxx tablets were taken with a high fat meal. The time to peak plasma concentration (T_{max}), however, was delayed by 1-2 hours. The food effect on the suspension formulation has not been studied. Vioxx tablets can be administered without regard to timing of meals.

There was a 13% and 8% decrease in AUC when Vioxx was administered with calcium carbonate antacid and magnesium/aluminum antacid to elderly subjects, respectively. There was an approximate 20% decrease in C_{max} of rofecoxib with either antacid.

Distribution

Rofecoxib is approximately 87% bound to human plasma protein over the range of concentrations of 0.05 to 25 µg/ml. The apparent volume of distribution at steady state (Vdss) is approximately 91 L following a 12.5 mg dose and 86 L following a 25 mg dose.

Rofecoxib has been shown to cross the placenta in rats and rabbits, and the blood-brain barrier in rats.

Metabolism

Metabolism of rofecoxib is primarily mediated through reduction by cytosolic enzymes. The principal metabolic products are the *cis*-dihydro and *trans*-dihydro derivatives of rofecoxib, which account for nearly 56% of recovered radioactivity in the urine. An additional 8.8% of the dose was recovered as the glucuronide of the hydroxy derivative, a product of oxidative metabolism. The biotransformation of rofecoxib and this metabolite is reversible in humans to a limited extent (<5%). These metabolites are inactive as COX-1 or COX-2 inhibitors.

Cytochrome P450 plays a minor role in metabolism of rofecoxib. Inhibition of CYP 3A activity by administration of ketoconazole 400 mg daily does not affect rofecoxib disposition. However, induction of general hepatic metabolic activity by administration of the non-specific inducer rifampin 600 mg daily produces a 50% decrease in rofecoxib plasma concentrations. (Also see DRUG INTERACTIONS.)

Excretion

Rofecoxib is eliminated predominantly by hepatic metabolism with little (<1%) unchanged drug recovered in the urine. Following a single radiolabeled dose of 125 mg, approximately 72% of the dose was excreted into the urine as metabolites and 14% in the feces as unchanged drug.

The plasma clearance after 12.5 and 25 mg doses was approximately 141 and 120 ml/min, respectively. Higher plasma clearance was observed at doses below the therapeutic range, suggesting the presence of a saturable route of metabolism (*i.e.*, non-linear elimination). The effective half-life (based on steady-state levels) was approximately 17 hours.

SPECIAL POPULATIONS

Gender

The pharmacokinetics of rofecoxib are comparable in men and women.

Geriatric

After a single dose of 25 mg Vioxx in elderly subjects (over 65 years old) a 34% increase in AUC was observed as compared to the young subjects. Dosage adjustment in the elderly is not necessary; however, therapy with Vioxx should be initiated at the lowest recommended dose.

Pediatric

Vioxx has not been investigated in patients below 18 years of age.

Race

Meta-analysis of pharmacokinetic studies has suggested a slightly (10-15%) higher AUC of rofecoxib in Blacks and Hispanics as compared to Caucasians. No dosage adjustment is necessary on the basis of race.

Hepatic Insufficiency

A single-dose pharmacokinetic study in mild (Child-Pugh score ≤6) hepatic insufficiency patients indicated that rofecoxib AUC was similar between these patients and healthy subjects. A pharmacokinetic study in patients with moderate (Child-Pugh score 7-9) hepatic insufficiency indicated that mean rofecoxib plasma concentrations were higher (mean AUC: 55%; mean C_{max}: 53%) relative to healthy subjects. Patients with severe hepatic insufficiency have not been studied.

Renal Insufficiency

In a study (n=6) of patients with end stage renal disease undergoing dialysis, peak rofecoxib plasma levels and AUC declined 18% and 9%, respectively, when dialysis occurred 4 hours after dosing. When dialysis occurred 48 hours after dosing, the elimination profile of rofecoxib was unchanged. While renal insufficiency does not influence the pharmacokinetics of rofecoxib, use of Vioxx in advanced renal disease is not recommended. (See WARNINGS, Advanced Renal Disease.)

DRUG INTERACTIONS

Also see DRUG INTERACTIONS.

General

In human studies the potential for rofecoxib to inhibit or induce CYP 3A4 activity was investigated in studies using the intravenous erythromycin breath test and the oral midazolam test. No significant difference in erythromycin demethylation was observed with rofecoxib (75 mg daily) compared to placebo, indicating no induction of hepatic CYP 3A4. A 30% reduction of the AUC of midazolam was observed with rofecoxib (25 mg daily). This reduction is most likely due to increased first pass metabolism through induction of intestinal CYP 3A4 by rofecoxib. *In vitro* studies in rat hepatocytes also suggest that rofecoxib might be a mild inducer for CYP 3A4.

Drug interaction studies with the recommended doses of rofecoxib have identified potentially significant interactions with rifampin, theophylline, and warfarin. Patients receiving these agents with Vioxx should be appropriately monitored. Drug interaction studies do not support the potential for clinically important interactions between antacids or cimetidine with rofecoxib. Similar to experience with other nonsteroidal anti-inflammatory drugs (NSAIDs), studies with rofecoxib suggest the potential for interaction with ACE inhibitors. The effects of rofecoxib on the pharmacokinetics and/or pharmacodynamics of ketoconazole, prednisone/prednisolone, oral contraceptives, and digoxin have been studied *in vivo* and clinically important interactions have not been found.

INDICATIONS AND USAGE

Vioxx is indicated:

For relief of the signs and symptoms of osteoarthritis.
For relief of the signs and symptoms of rheumatoid arthritis in adults.
For the management of acute pain in adults.
For the treatment of primary dysmenorrhea.

CONTRAINDICATIONS

Vioxx is contraindicated in patients with known hypersensitivity to rofecoxib or any other component of Vioxx.

Vioxx should not be given to patients who have experienced asthma, urticaria, or allergic-type reactions after taking aspirin or other NSAIDs. Severe, rarely fatal, anaphylactic-like reactions to NSAIDs have been reported in such patients (see WARNINGS, Anaphylactoid Reactions and PRECAUTIONS, Preexisting Asthma).

WARNINGS

GASTROINTESTINAL (GI) EFFECTS — RISK OF GI ULCERATION, BLEEDING, AND PERFORATION

Serious gastrointestinal toxicity such as bleeding, ulceration, and perforation of the stomach, small intestine or large intestine, can occur at any time, with or without warning symptoms, in patients treated with nonsteroidal anti-inflammatory drugs (NSAIDs). Minor upper gastrointestinal problems, such as dyspepsia, are common and may also occur at any time during NSAID therapy. Therefore, physicians and patients should remain alert for ulceration and bleeding, even in the absence of previous GI tract symptoms. Patients should be informed about the signs and/or symptoms of serious GI toxicity and the steps to take if they occur. The utility of periodic laboratory monitoring has not been demonstrated, nor has it been adequately assessed. Only 1 in 5 patients who develop a serious upper GI adverse event on NSAID therapy is symptomatic. It has been demonstrated that upper GI ulcers, gross bleeding or perforation, caused by NSAIDs, appear to occur in approximately 1% of patients treated for 3-6 months, and in about 2-4% of patients treated for 1 year. These trends continue thus, increasing the likelihood of developing a serious GI event at some time during the course of therapy. However, even short-term therapy is not without risk.

Although the risk of GI toxicity is not completely eliminated with Vioxx, the results of the Vioxx GI outcomes research (VIGOR) study demonstrate that in patients treated with Vioxx, the risk of GI toxicity with Vioxx 50 mg once daily is significantly less than with naproxen 500 mg twice daily.

NSAIDs should be prescribed with extreme caution in patients with a prior history of ulcer disease or gastrointestinal bleeding. Most spontaneous reports of fatal GI events are in elderly or debilitated patients and therefore special care should be taken in treating this population. **To minimize the potential risk for an adverse GI event, the lowest effective dose should be used for the shortest possible duration.** For high risk patients, alternate therapies that do not involve NSAIDs should be considered.

Previous studies have shown that patients with a *prior history of peptic ulcer disease and/or gastrointestinal bleeding* and who use NSAIDs, have a greater than 10-fold higher risk for developing a GI bleed than patients with neither of these risk factors. In addition to a past history of ulcer disease, pharmacoepidemiological studies have identified several other co-therapies or co-morbid conditions that may increase the risk for GI bleeding such as: treatment with oral corticosteroids, treatment with anticoagulants, longer duration of NSAID therapy, smoking, alcoholism, older age, and poor general health status.

ANAPHYLACTOID REACTIONS

As with NSAIDs in general, anaphylactoid reactions have occurred in patients without known prior exposure to Vioxx. In post-marketing experience, rare cases of anaphylactic/anaphylactoid reactions and angioedema have been reported in patients receiving Vioxx. Vioxx should not be given to patients with the aspirin triad. This symptom complex typically occurs in asthmatic patients who experience rhinitis with or without nasal polyps, or who exhibit severe, potentially fatal bronchospasm after taking aspirin or other NSAIDs (see CONTRAINDICATIONS and PRECAUTIONS, Preexisting Asthma). Emergency help should be sought in cases where an anaphylactoid reaction occurs.

ADVANCED RENAL DISEASE

Treatment with Vioxx is not recommended in patients with advanced renal disease. If Vioxx therapy must be initiated, close monitoring of the patient's kidney function is advisable (see PRECAUTIONS, Renal Effects).

PREGNANCY

In late pregnancy Vioxx should be avoided because it may cause premature closure of the ductus arteriosus.

PRECAUTIONS

GENERAL

Vioxx cannot be expected to substitute for corticosteroids or to treat corticosteroid insufficiency. Abrupt discontinuation of corticosteroids may lead to exacerbation of corticosteroid-responsive illness. Patients on prolonged corticosteroid therapy should have their therapy tapered slowly if a decision is made to discontinue corticosteroids.

The pharmacological activity of Vioxx in reducing inflammation, and possibly fever, may diminish the utility of these diagnostic signs in detecting infectious complications of presumed noninfectious, painful conditions.

CARDIOVASCULAR EFFECTS

The information below should be taken into consideration and caution should be exercised when Vioxx is used in patients with a medical history of ischemic heart disease.

In VIGOR, a study in 8076 patients (mean age 58; Vioxx n=4047, naproxen n=4029) with a median duration of exposure of 9 months, the risk of developing a serious cardiovascular thrombotic event was significantly higher in patients treated with Vioxx 50 mg once daily (n=45) as compared to patients treated with naproxen 500 mg twice daily (n=19). In VIGOR, mortality due to cardiovascular thrombotic events (7 vs 6, Vioxx vs naproxen, respectively) was similar between the treatment groups. In a placebo-controlled database derived from 2 studies with a total of 2142 elderly patients (mean age 75; Vioxx n=1067, placebo n=1075) with a median duration of exposure of approximately 14 months, the number of patients with serious cardiovascular thrombotic events was 21 vs 35 for patients treated with Vioxx 25 mg once daily versus placebo, respectively. In these same 2 placebo-controlled studies, mortality due to cardiovascular thrombotic events was 8 vs 3 for Vioxx versus placebo, respectively. The significance of the cardiovascular findings from these 3 studies (VIGOR and 2 placebo-controlled studies) is unknown. Prospective studies specifically designed to compare the incidence of serious CV events in patients taking Vioxx versus NSAID comparators or placebo have not been performed.

Because of its lack of platelet effects, Vioxx is not a substitute for aspirin for cardiovascular prophylaxis. Therefore, in patients taking Vioxx, antiplatelet therapies should not be discontinued and should be considered in patients with an indication for cardiovascular prophylaxis. (See DRUG INTERACTIONS, Aspirin.) Prospective, long-term studies on concomitant administration of Vioxx and aspirin evaluating cardiovascular outcomes have not been conducted.

FLUID RETENTION, EDEMA, AND HYPERTENSION

Fluid retention, edema, and hypertension have been reported in some patients taking Vioxx. In clinical trials of Vioxx at daily doses of 25 mg in patients with rheumatoid arthritis the incidence of hypertension was twice as high in patients treated with Vioxx as compared to patients treated with naproxen 1000 mg daily. Clinical trials with Vioxx at daily doses of 12.5 and 25 mg in patients with osteoarthritis have shown effects on hypertension and edema similar to those observed with comparator NSAIDs; these occurred with an increased frequency with chronic use of Vioxx at daily doses of 50 mg. (See ADVERSE REACTIONS.) Vioxx should be used with caution, and should be introduced at the lowest recommended dose in patients with fluid retention, hypertension, or heart failure.

RENAL EFFECTS

Long-term administration of NSAIDs has resulted in renal papillary necrosis and other renal injury. Renal toxicity has also been seen in patients in whom renal prostaglandins have a compensatory role in the maintenance of renal perfusion. In these patients, administration of a nonsteroidal anti-inflammatory drug may cause a dose-dependent reduction in prostaglandin formation and, secondarily, in renal blood flow, which may precipitate overt renal decompensation. Patients at greatest risk of this reaction are those with impaired renal function, heart failure, liver dysfunction, those taking diuretics and ACE inhibitors, and the elderly. Discontinuation of NSAID therapy is usually followed by recovery to the pretreatment state.

Caution should be used when initiating treatment with Vioxx in patients with considerable dehydration. It is advisable to rehydrate patients first and then start therapy with Vioxx. Caution is also recommended in patients with pre-existing kidney disease (see WARNINGS, Advanced Renal Disease).

HEPATIC EFFECTS

Borderline elevations of one or more liver tests may occur in up to 15% of patients taking NSAIDs, and notable elevations of ALT or AST (approximately 3 or more times the upper limit of normal) have been reported in approximately 1% of patients in clinical trials with NSAIDs. These laboratory abnormalities may progress, may remain unchanged, or may be transient with continuing therapy. Rare cases of severe hepatic reactions, including jaundice and fatal fulminant hepatitis, liver necrosis and hepatic failure (some with fatal outcome) have been reported with NSAIDs, including Vioxx. In controlled clinical trials of Vioxx, the incidence of borderline elevations of liver tests at doses of 12.5 and 25 mg daily was comparable to the incidence observed with ibuprofen and lower than that observed with diclofenac. In placebo-controlled trials, approximately 0.5% of patients taking rofecoxib (12.5 or 25 mg qd) and 0.1% of patients taking placebo had notable elevations of ALT or AST.

A patient with symptoms and/or signs suggesting liver dysfunction, or in whom an abnormal liver test has occurred, should be monitored carefully for evidence of the development of a more severe hepatic reaction while on therapy with Vioxx. Use of Vioxx is not recommended in patients with severe hepatic insufficiency (see CLINICAL PHARMACOLOGY, Special Populations). If clinical signs and symptoms consistent with liver disease develop, or if systemic manifestations occur (*e.g.,* eosinophilia, rash, etc.), Vioxx should be discontinued.

HEMATOLOGICAL EFFECTS

Anemia is sometimes seen in patients receiving Vioxx. In placebo-controlled trials, there were no significant differences observed between Vioxx and placebo in clinical reports of anemia. Patients on long-term treatment with Vioxx should have their hemoglobin or hematocrit checked if they exhibit any signs or symptoms of anemia or blood loss. Vioxx does not generally affect platelet counts, prothrombin time (PT), or partial thromboplastin time (PTT), and does not inhibit platelet aggregation at indicated dosages.

PREEXISTING ASTHMA

Patients with asthma may have aspirin-sensitive asthma. The use of aspirin in patients with aspirin-sensitive asthma has been associated with severe bronchospasm which can be fatal. Since cross reactivity, including bronchospasm, between aspirin and other nonsteroidal anti-inflammatory drugs has been reported in such aspirin-sensitive patients, Vioxx should not be administered to patients with this form of aspirin sensitivity and should be used with caution in patients with preexisting asthma.

INFORMATION FOR THE PATIENT

Physicians should instruct their patients to read the patient package insert before starting therapy with Vioxx and to reread it each time the prescription is renewed in case any information has changed.

Vioxx can cause discomfort and, rarely, more serious side effects, such as gastrointestinal bleeding, which may result in hospitalization and even fatal outcomes. Although serious GI tract ulcerations and bleeding can occur without warning symptoms, patients should be alert for the signs and symptoms of ulcerations and bleeding, and should ask for medical advice when observing any indicative signs or symptoms. Patients should be apprised of the importance of this follow-up. For additional gastrointestinal safety information see WARNINGS, Gastrointestinal (GI) Effects — Risk of GI Ulceration, Bleeding, and Perforation. Patients should be informed that Vioxx is not a substitute for aspirin for cardiovascular prophylaxis because of its lack of effect on platelets. For additional cardiovascular safety information see PRECAUTIONS, Cardiovascular Effects.

Patients should promptly report signs or symptoms of gastrointestinal ulceration or bleeding, skin rash, unexplained weight gain, edema or chest pain to their physicians.

Patients should be informed of the warning signs and symptoms of hepatotoxicity (*e.g.,* nausea, fatigue, lethargy, pruritus, jaundice, right upper quadrant tenderness, and "flu-like" symptoms). If these occur, patients should be instructed to stop therapy and seek immediate medical therapy.

Patients should also be instructed to seek immediate emergency help in the case of an anaphylactoid reaction (see WARNINGS).

R

In late pregnancy Vioxx should be avoided because it may cause premature closure of the ductus arteriosus.

LABORATORY TESTS

Because serious GI tract ulcerations and bleeding can occur without warning symptoms, physicians should monitor for signs or symptoms of GI bleeding.

CARCINOGENESIS, MUTAGENESIS, AND IMPAIRMENT OF FERTILITY

Rofecoxib was not carcinogenic in mice given oral doses up to 30 mg/kg (male) and 60 mg/kg (female) [approximately 5- and 2-fold the human exposure at 25 and 50 mg daily based on AUC(0-24h)] and in male and female rats given oral doses up to 8 mg/kg [approximately 6- and 2-fold the human exposure at 25 and 50 mg daily based on AUC(0-24h)] for 2 years.

Rofecoxib was not mutagenic in an Ames test or in a V-79 mammalian cell mutagenesis assay, nor clastogenic in a chromosome aberration assay in Chinese hamster ovary (CHO) cells, in an *in vitro* and an *in vivo* alkaline elution assay, or in an *in vivo* chromosomal aberration test in mouse bone marrow.

Rofecoxib did not impair male fertility in rats at oral doses up to 100 mg/kg [approximately 20- and 7-fold human exposure at 25 and 50 mg daily based on the AUC(0-24h)] and rofecoxib had no effect on fertility in female rats at doses up to 30 mg/kg [approximately 19- and 7-fold human exposure at 25 and 50 mg daily based on AUC(0-24h)].

PREGNANCY

Teratogenic Effects: Pregnancy Category C

Rofecoxib was not teratogenic in rats at doses up to 50 mg/kg/day [approximately 28- and 10-fold human exposure at 25 and 50 mg daily based on AUC(0-24h)]. There was a slight, non-statistically significant increase in the overall incidence of vertebral malformations only in the rabbit at doses of 50 mg/kg/day [approximately 1- or <1-fold human exposure at 25 and 50 mg daily based on AUC(0-24h)]. There are no studies in pregnant women. Vioxx should be used during pregnancy only if the potential benefit justifies the potential risk to the fetus.

Nonteratogenic Effects

Rofecoxib produced peri-implantation and post-implantation losses and reduced embryo/fetal survival in rats and rabbits at oral doses ≥10 and ≥75 mg/kg/day, respectively [approximately 9- and 3-fold [rats] and 2- and <1-fold (rabbits) human exposure based on the AUC(0-24h) at 25 and 50 mg daily]. These changes are expected with inhibition of prostaglandin synthesis and are not the result of permanent alteration of female reproductive function. There was an increase in the incidence of postnatal pup mortality in rats at ≥5 mg/kg/day [approximately 5- and 2-fold human exposure at 25 and 50 mg daily based on AUC(0-24h)]. In studies in pregnant rats administered single doses of rofecoxib, there was a treatment-related decrease in the diameter of the ductus arteriosus at all doses used [3-300 mg/kg: 3 mg/kg is approximately 2- and <1-fold human exposure at 25 or 50 mg daily based on AUC(0-24h)]. As with other drugs known to inhibit prostaglandin synthesis, use of Vioxx during the third trimester of pregnancy should be avoided.

LABOR AND DELIVERY

Rofecoxib produced no evidence of significantly delayed labor or parturition in females at doses 15 mg/kg in rats [approximately 10- and 3-fold human exposure as measured by the AUC(0-24h) at 25 and 50 mg]. The effects of Vioxx on labor and delivery in pregnant women are unknown.

Merck & Co., Inc. maintains a registry to monitor the pregnancy outcomes of women exposed to Vioxx while pregnant. Healthcare providers are encouraged to report any prenatal exposure to Vioxx by calling the **Pregnancy Registry at 800-986-8999.**

NURSING MOTHERS

Rofecoxib is excreted in the milk of lactating rats at concentrations similar to those in plasma. There was an increase in pup mortality and a decrease in pup body weight following exposure of pups to milk from dams administered Vioxx during lactation. The dose tested represents an approximate 18- and 6-fold human exposure at 25 and 50 mg based on AUC(0-24h). It is not known whether this drug is excreted in human milk. Because many drugs are excreted in human milk and because of the potential for serious adverse reactions in nursing infants from Vioxx, a decision should be made whether to discontinue nursing or to discontinue the drug, taking into account the importance of the drug to the mother.

R

PEDIATRIC USE

Safety and effectiveness in pediatric patients below the age of 18 years have not been evaluated.

GERIATRIC USE

Of the patients who received Vioxx in osteoarthritis clinical trials, 1455 were 65 years of age or older. This included 460 patients who were 75 years or older, and in one of these studies, 174 patients who were 80 years or older. No substantial differences in safety and effectiveness were observed between these subjects and younger subjects. Greater sensitivity of some older individuals cannot be ruled out. As with other NSAIDs, including those that selectively inhibit COX-2, there have been more spontaneous postmarketing reports of fatal GI events and acute renal failure in the elderly than in younger patients. Dosage adjustment in the elderly is not necessary; however, therapy with Vioxx should be initiated at the lowest recommended dose.

DRUG INTERACTIONS

ACE inhibitors: Reports suggest that NSAIDs may diminish the antihypertensive effect of Angiotensin Converting Enzyme (ACE) inhibitors. In patients with mild to moderate hypertension, administration of 25 mg daily of Vioxx with the ACE inhibitor benazepril, 10-40 mg for 4 weeks, was associated with an average increase in mean arterial pressure of about 3 mm Hg compared to ACE inhibitor alone. This interaction should be given consideration in patients taking Vioxx concomitantly with ACE inhibitors.

Aspirin: Concomitant administration of low-dose aspirin with Vioxx may result in an increased rate of GI ulceration or other complications, compared to use of Vioxx alone. At steady state, Vioxx 50 mg once daily had no effect on the anti-platelet activity of low-dose (81 mg once daily) aspirin, as assessed by *ex vivo* platelet aggregation and serum TXB_2 generation in clotting blood. Because of its lack of platelet effects, Vioxx is not a substitute for aspirin for cardiovascular prophylaxis. Therefore, in patients taking Vioxx, antiplatelet therapies should not be discontinued and should be considered in patients with an indication for cardiovascular prophylaxis. (See PRECAUTIONS, Cardiovascular Effects.) Prospective, long-term studies on concomitant administration of Vioxx and aspirin have not been conducted.

Cimetidine: Co-administration with high doses of cimetidine [800 mg twice daily] increased the C_{max} of rofecoxib by 21%, the AUC(0-120h) by 23% and the $T_{1/2}$ by 15%. These small changes are not clinically significant and no dose adjustment is necessary.

Digoxin: Rofecoxib 75 mg once daily for 11 days does not alter the plasma concentration profile or renal elimination of digoxin after a single 0.5 mg oral dose.

Furosemide: Clinical studies, as well as post-marketing observations, have shown that NSAIDs can reduce the natriuretic effect of furosemide and thiazides in some patients. This response has been attributed to inhibition of renal prostaglandin synthesis.

Ketoconazole: Ketoconazole 400 mg daily did not have any clinically important effect on the pharmacokinetics of rofecoxib.

Lithium: NSAIDs have produced an elevation of plasma lithium levels and a reduction in renal lithium clearance. In post-marketing experience there have been reports of increases in plasma lithium levels. Thus, when Vioxx and lithium are administered concurrently, subjects should be observed carefully for signs of lithium toxicity.

Methotrexate: Vioxx 12.5, 25, and 50 mg, each dose administered once daily for 7 days, had no effect on the plasma concentration of methotrexate as measured by AUC(0-24h) in patients receiving single weekly methotrexate doses of 7.5 to 20 mg for rheumatoid arthritis. At higher than recommended doses, Vioxx 75 mg administered once daily for 10 days increased plasma concentrations by 23% as measured by AUC(0-24h) in patients receiving methotrexate 7.5 to 15 mg/week for rheumatoid arthritis. At 24 hours postdose, a similar proportion of patients treated with methotrexate alone (94%) and subsequently treated with methotrexate co-administered with 75 mg of rofecoxib (88%) had methotrexate plasma concentrations below the measurable limit (5 ng/ml). Standard monitoring of methotrexate-related toxicity should be continued if Vioxx and methotrexate are administered concomitantly.

Oral Contraceptives: Rofecoxib did not have any clinically important effect on the pharmacokinetics of ethinyl estradiol and norethindrone.

Prednisone/Prednisolone: Rofecoxib did not have any clinically important effect on the pharmacokinetics of prednisolone or prednisone.

Rifampin: Co-administration of Vioxx with rifampin 600 mg daily, a potent inducer of hepatic metabolism, produced an approximate 50% decrease in rofecoxib plasma concentrations. Therefore, a starting daily dose of 25 mg of Vioxx should be considered for the treatment of osteoarthritis when Vioxx is co-administered with potent inducers of hepatic metabolism.

Theophylline: Vioxx 12.5, 25, and 50 mg administered once daily for 7 days increased plasma theophylline concentrations [AUC(0-∞)] by 38-60% in healthy subjects administered a single 300 mg dose of theophylline. Adequate monitoring of theophylline plasma concentrations should be considered when therapy with Vioxx is initiated or changed in patients receiving theophylline.

These data suggest that rofecoxib may produce a modest inhibition of cytochrome P450 (CYP) 1A2. Therefore, there is a potential for an interaction with other drugs that are metabolized by CYP1A2 (*e.g.*, amitriptyline, tacrine, and zileuton).

Warfarin: Anticoagulant activity should be monitored, particularly in the first few days after initiating or changing Vioxx therapy in patients receiving warfarin or similar agents, since these patients are at an increased risk of bleeding complications. In single and multiple dose studies in healthy subjects receiving both warfarin and rofecoxib, prothrombin time (measured as INR) was increased by approximately 8% to 11%. In post-marketing experience, bleeding events have been reported, predominantly in the elderly, in association with increases in prothrombin time in patients receiving Vioxx concurrently with warfarin.

ADVERSE REACTIONS

OSTEOARTHRITIS

Approximately 3600 patients with osteoarthritis were treated with Vioxx; approximately 1400 patients received Vioxx for 6 months or longer and approximately 800 patients for 1 year or longer. TABLE 4 lists all adverse events, regardless of causality, occurring in at least 2% of patients receiving Vioxx in nine controlled studies of 6 week to 6 month duration conducted in patients with OA at the therapeutically recommended doses (12.5 and 25 mg), which included a placebo and/or positive control group.

In the OA studies, the following spontaneous adverse events occurred in >0.1% to 1.9% of patients treated with Vioxx regardless of causality:

Body as a Whole: Abdominal distension, abdominal tenderness, abscess, chest pain, chills, contusion, cyst, diaphragmatic hernia, fever, fluid retention, flushing, fungal infection, infection, laceration, pain, pelvic pain, peripheral edema, postoperative pain, syncope, trauma, upper extremity edema, viral syndrome.

Cardiovascular System: Angina pectoris, atrial fibrillation, bradycardia, hematoma, irregular heartbeat, palpitation, premature ventricular contraction, tachycardia, venous insufficiency.

Digestive System: Acid reflux, aphthous stomatitis, constipation, dental caries, dental pain, digestive gas symptoms, dry mouth, duodenal disorder, dysgeusia, esophagitis, flatulence, gastric disorder, gastritis, gastroenteritis, hematochezia, hemorrhoids, infectious gastroenteritis, oral infection, oral lesion, oral ulcer, vomiting.

TABLE 4 *Clinical Adverse Experiences Occurring in ≥2.0% of Patients Treated With Rofecoxib in OA Clinical Trials*

	Placebo	Rofecoxib 12.5 or 25 mg daily	Ibuprofen 2400 mg daily	Diclofenac 150 mg daily
	(n=783)	(n=2829)	(n=847)	(n=498)
Body as a Whole/Site Unspecified				
Abdominal pain	4.1%	3.4%	4.6%	5.8%
Asthenia/fatigue	1.0%	2.2%	2.0%	2.6%
Dizziness	2.2%	3.0%	2.7%	3.4%
Influenza-like disease	3.1%	2.9%	1.5%	3.2%
Lower extremity edema	1.1%	3.7%	3.8%	3.4%
Upper respiratory infection	7.8%	8.5%	5.8%	8.2%
Cardiovascular System				
Hypertension	1.3%	3.5%	3.0%	1.6%
Digestive System				
Diarrhea	6.8%	6.5%	7.1%	10.6%
Dyspepsia	2.7%	3.5%	4.7%	4.0%
Epigastric discomfort	2.8%	3.8%	9.2%	5.4%
Heartburn	3.6%	4.2%	5.2%	4.6%
Nausea	2.9%	5.2%	7.1%	7.4%
Eyes, Ears, Nose, and Throat				
Sinusitis	2.0%	2.7%	1.8%	2.4%
Musculoskeletal System				
Back pain	1.9%	2.5%	1.4%	2.8%
Nervous System				
Headache	7.5%	4.7%	6.1%	8.0%
Respiratory System				
Bronchitis	0.8%	2.0%	1.4%	3.2%
Urogenital System				
Urinary tract infection	2.7%	2.8%	2.5%	3.6%

Eyes, Ears, Nose, and Throat: Allergic rhinitis, blurred vision, cerumen impaction, conjunctivitis, dry throat, epistaxis, laryngitis, nasal congestion, nasal secretion, ophthalmic injection, otic pain, otitis, otitis media, pharyngitis, tinnitus, tonsillitis.

Immune System: Allergy, hypersensitivity, insect bite reaction.

Metabolism and Nutrition: Appetite change, hypercholesterolemia, weight gain.

Musculoskeletal System: Ankle sprain, arm pain, arthralgia, back strain, bursitis, cartilage trauma, joint swelling, muscular cramp, muscular disorder, muscular weakness, musculoskeletal pain, musculoskeletal stiffness, myalgia, osteoarthritis, tendinitis, traumatic arthropathy, wrist fracture.

Nervous System: Hypesthesia, insomnia, median nerve neuropathy, migraine, muscular spasm, paresthesia, sciatica, somnolence, vertigo.

Psychiatric: Anxiety, depression, mental acuity decreased.

Respiratory System: Asthma, cough, dyspnea, pneumonia, pulmonary congestion, respiratory infection.

Skin and Skin Appendages: Abrasion, alopecia, atopic dermatitis, basal cell carcinoma, blister, cellulitis, contact dermatitis, herpes simplex, herpes zoster, nail unit disorder, perspiration, pruritus, rash, skin erythema, urticaria, xerosis.

Urogenital System: Breast mass, cystitis, dysuria, menopausal symptoms, menstrual disorder, nocturia, urinary retention, vaginitis.

The following serious adverse events have been reported rarely (estimated <0.1%) in patients taking Vioxx, regardless of causality. Cases reported only in the post-marketing experience are indicated in italics.

Cardiovascular: Cerebrovascular accident, congestive heart failure, deep venous thrombosis, myocardial infarction, *pulmonary edema,* pulmonary embolism, transient ischemic attack, unstable angina.

Gastrointestinal: Cholecystitis, colitis, colonic malignant neoplasm, *duodenal perforation,* duodenal ulcer, *esophageal ulcer, gastric perforation, gastric ulcer,* gastrointestinal bleeding, *hepatic failure, hepatitis,* intestinal obstruction, *jaundice,* pancreatitis.

Hemic and Lymphatic: *Agranulocytosis, leukopenia,* lymphoma, *thrombocytopenia.*

Immune System: *Anaphylactic/anaphylactoid reaction, angioedema, bronchospasm, hypersensitivity vasculitis.*

Metabolism and Nutrition: *Hyponatremia.*

Nervous System: *Aseptic meningitis.*

Psychiatric: *Confusion, hallucinations.*

Skin and Skin Appendages: *Severe skin reactions, including Stevens-Johnson syndrome and toxic epidermal necrolysis.*

Urogenital System: *Acute renal failure,* breast malignant neoplasm, *hyperkalemia, interstitial nephritis,* prostatic malignant neoplasm, urolithiasis, *worsening chronic renal failure.*

In 1 year controlled clinical trials and in extension studies for up to 86 weeks (approximately 800 patients treated with Vioxx for 1 year or longer), the adverse experience profile was qualitatively similar to that observed in studies of shorter duration.

RHEUMATOID ARTHRITIS

Approximately 1100 patients were treated with Vioxx in the Phase 3 rheumatoid arthritis efficacy studies. These studies included extensions of up to 1 year. The adverse experience profile was generally similar to that reported in the osteoarthritis studies. In studies of at least 3 months, the incidence of hypertension in RA patients receiving the 25 mg once daily dose of Vioxx was 10.0% and the incidence of hypertension in patients receiving naproxen 500 mg twice daily was 4.7%.

ANALGESIA, INCLUDING PRIMARY DYSMENORRHEA

Approximately 1000 patients were treated with Vioxx in analgesia studies. All patients in post-dental surgery pain studies received only a single dose of study medication. Patients in primary dysmenorrhea studies may have taken up to 3 daily doses of Vioxx, and those in the post-orthopedic surgery pain study were prescribed 5 daily doses of Vioxx.

The adverse experience profile in the analgesia studies was generally similar to those reported in the osteoarthritis studies. The following additional adverse experience, which occurred at an incidence of at least 2% of patients treated with Vioxx, was observed in the post-dental pain surgery studies: post-dental extraction alveolitis (dry socket).

CLINICAL STUDIES IN OA AND RA WITH VIOXX 50 MG (TWICE THE HIGHEST DOSE RECOMMENDED FOR CHRONIC USE)

In OA and RA clinical trials which contained Vioxx 12.5 or 25 mg as well as Vioxx 50 mg, Vioxx 50 mg qd was associated with a higher incidence of gastrointestinal symptoms (abdominal pain, epigastric pain, heartburn, nausea and vomiting), lower extremity edema, hypertension, serious* adverse experiences and discontinuation due to clinical adverse experiences compared to the recommended chronic doses of 12.5 and 25 mg (see DOSAGE AND ADMINISTRATION).

*Adverse experience that resulted in death, permanent or substantial disability, hospitalization, congenital anomaly, or cancer, was immediately life threatening, was due to an overdose, or was thought by the investigator to require intervention to prevent one of the above outcomes.

DOSAGE AND ADMINISTRATION

Vioxx is administered orally. The lowest dose of Vioxx should be sought for each patient.

OSTEOARTHRITIS

The recommended starting dose of Vioxx is 12.5 mg once daily. Some patients may receive additional benefit by increasing the dose to 25 mg once daily. The maximum recommended daily dose is 25 mg.

RHEUMATOID ARTHRITIS

The recommended dose is 25 mg once daily. The maximum recommended daily dose is 25 mg.

MANAGEMENT OF ACUTE PAIN AND TREATMENT OF PRIMARY DYSMENORRHEA

The recommended dose of Vioxx is 50 mg once daily. The maximum recommended daily dose is 50 mg. Use of Vioxx for more than 5 days in management of pain has not been studied. Chronic use of Vioxx 50 mg daily is not recommended. (See ADVERSE REACTIONS, Clinical Studies in OA and RA With Vioxx 50 mg.)

HEPATIC INSUFFICIENCY

Because of significant increases in both AUC and C_{max}, patients with moderate hepatic impairment (Child-Pugh score: 7-9) should be treated with the lowest possible dose (see CLINICAL PHARMACOLOGY, Special Populations).

Vioxx tablets may be taken with or without food.

ORAL SUSPENSION

Vioxx oral suspension 12.5 mg/5 ml or 25 mg/5 ml may be substituted for Vioxx tablets 12.5 or 25 mg, respectively, in any of the above indications. Shake before using.

HOW SUPPLIED

VIOXX TABLETS

Vioxx tablets are available in:

12.5 mg: Cream/off-white, round, shallow cup tablets engraved "MRK 74" on one side and "VIOXX" on the other.

25 mg: Yellow, round tablets engraved "MRK 110" on one side and "VIOXX" on the other.

50 mg: Orange, round tablets engraved "MRK 114" on one side and "VIOXX" on the other.

Storage: Store at 25°C (77°F), excursions permitted to 15-30°C (59-86°F).

VIOXX ORAL SUSPENSION

Vioxx oral suspension is available in:

12.5 mg/5 ml as an opaque, white to faint yellow suspension with a strawberry flavor that is easily resuspended upon shaking.

25 mg/5 ml as an opaque, white to faint yellow suspension with a strawberry flavor that is easily resuspended upon shaking.

Storage: Store at 25°C (77°F), excursions permitted to 15-30°C (59-86°F).

PRODUCT LISTING - EQUIVALENTS NOT AVAILABLE

Suspension - Oral - 12.5 mg/5 ml			
150 ml	$128.13	VIOXX, Merck & Company Inc	00006-3784-64
Suspension - Oral - 25 mg/5 ml			
150 ml	$128.13	VIOXX, Merck & Company Inc	00006-3785-64
Tablet - Oral - 12.5 mg			
7's	$17.68	VIOXX, Allscripts Pharmaceutical Company	54569-4758-01
15's	$49.43	VIOXX, Pharma Pac	52959-0548-15
20's	$63.59	VIOXX, Pharma Pac	52959-0548-20
21's	$66.53	VIOXX, Pharma Pac	52959-0548-21
28's	$85.77	VIOXX, Pharma Pac	52959-0548-28
30's	$75.75	VIOXX, Allscripts Pharmaceutical Company	54569-4758-00
30's	$86.28	VIOXX, Merck & Company Inc	00006-0074-31
30's	$86.73	VIOXX, Physicians Total Care	54868-4148-00
30's	$92.05	VIOXX, Pharma Pac	52959-0548-30
100's	$287.56	VIOXX, Merck & Company Inc	00006-0074-28
100's	$287.56	VIOXX, Merck & Company Inc	00006-0074-68
Tablet - Oral - 25 mg			
6's	$18.29	VIOXX, Physicians Total Care	54868-4116-02
10's	$26.23	VIOXX, Southwood Pharmaceuticals Inc	58016-0449-10

R

10's	$29.69	VIOXX, Physicians Total Care	54868-4116-00
10's	$39.62	VIOXX, Pd-Rx Pharmaceuticals	55289-0480-10
10's	$51.36	VIOXX, Pharma Pac	52959-0549-10
14's	$35.35	VIOXX, Allscripts Pharmaceutical Company	54569-4759-01
14's	$36.73	VIOXX, Southwood Pharmaceuticals Inc	58016-0449-14
14's	$62.85	VIOXX, Pd-Rx Pharmaceuticals	55289-0480-14
14's	$71.67	VIOXX, Pharma Pac	52959-0549-14
15's	$39.35	VIOXX, Southwood Pharmaceuticals Inc	58016-0449-15
15's	$76.62	VIOXX, Pharma Pac	52959-0549-15
20's	$52.47	VIOXX, Southwood Pharmaceuticals Inc	58016-0449-20
20's	$72.05	VIOXX, Pd-Rx Pharmaceuticals	55289-0480-20
20's	$95.94	VIOXX, Pharma Pac	52959-0549-20
21's	$99.29	VIOXX, Pharma Pac	52959-0549-21
30's	$75.75	VIOXX, Allscripts Pharmaceutical Company	54569-4759-00
30's	$78.70	VIOXX, Southwood Pharmaceuticals Inc	58016-0449-30
30's	$86.28	VIOXX, Merck & Company Inc	00006-0110-31
30's	$86.73	VIOXX, Physicians Total Care	54868-4116-01
30's	$89.25	VIOXX, St. Mary'S Mpp	60760-0011-30
30's	$107.90	VIOXX, Pharma Pac	52959-0549-30
40's	$135.32	VIOXX, Pharma Pac	52959-0549-40
60's	$157.40	VIOXX, Southwood Pharmaceuticals Inc	58016-0449-60
60's	$199.10	VIOXX, Pharma Pac	52959-0549-60
100's	$262.33	VIOXX, Southwood Pharmaceuticals Inc	58016-0449-00
100's	$287.56	VIOXX, Merck & Company Inc	00006-0110-28
100's	$287.56	VIOXX, Merck & Company Inc	00006-0110-68
Tablet - Oral - 50 mg			
5's	$18.44	VIOXX, Allscripts Pharmaceutical Company	54569-4940-00
7's	$40.25	VIOXX, Pharma Pac	52959-0495-07
10's	$40.19	VIOXX, Southwood Pharmaceuticals Inc	58016-0487-10
10's	$53.99	VIOXX, Pd-Rx Pharmaceuticals	55289-0538-10
10's	$56.60	VIOXX, Pharma Pac	52959-0495-10
14's	$77.14	VIOXX, Pharma Pac	52959-0495-14
15's	$55.31	VIOXX, Allscripts Pharmaceutical Company	54569-4940-01
15's	$60.28	VIOXX, Southwood Pharmaceuticals Inc	58016-0487-15
15's	$82.50	VIOXX, Pharma Pac	52959-0495-15
20's	$80.37	VIOXX, Southwood Pharmaceuticals Inc	58016-0487-20
20's	$84.47	VIOXX, Physicians Total Care	54868-4210-01
28's	$154.16	VIOXX, Pd-Rx Pharmaceuticals	55289-0538-28
30's	$119.18	VIOXX, Physicians Total Care	54868-4210-00
30's	$120.56	VIOXX, Southwood Pharmaceuticals Inc	58016-0487-30
30's	$159.00	VIOXX, Pharma Pac	52959-0495-30
40's	$160.75	VIOXX, Southwood Pharmaceuticals Inc	58016-0487-40
60's	$241.12	VIOXX, Southwood Pharmaceuticals Inc	58016-0487-60
90's	$361.68	VIOXX, Southwood Pharmaceuticals Inc	58016-0487-90
100's	$401.87	VIOXX, Southwood Pharmaceuticals Inc	58016-0487-00
100's	$419.96	VIOXX, Merck & Company Inc	00006-0114-28
100's	$419.96	VIOXX, Merck & Company Inc	00006-0114-68

Ropinirole Hydrochloride *(003358)*

Categories: Parkinson's disease; FDA Approved 1997 Sep; Pregnancy Category C
Drug Classes: Antiparkinson agents; Dopaminergics
Brand Names: Requip
Cost of Therapy: $118.16 (Parkinsonism; Requip; 1 mg; 3 tablets/day; 30 day supply)

R

DESCRIPTION

Ropinirole HCl, an orally administered anti-Parkinsonian drug, is a non-ergoline dopamine agonist. It is the hydrochloride salt of 4-[2-(dipropylamino)ethyl]-1,3-dihydro-2H-indol-2-one monohydrochloride and has an empirical formula of $C_{16}H_{24}N_2O \cdot HCl$. The molecular weight is 296.84 (260.38 as the free base).

Ropinirole HCl is a white to pale greenish-yellow powder with a melting range of 243-250°C and a solubility of 133 mg/ml in water.

Each pentagonal film-coated Tiltab tablet with beveled edges contains ropinirole HCl equivalent to ropinirole, 0.25, 0.5, 1, 2, or 5 mg. Inactive ingredients consist of: croscarmellose sodium, hydrous lactose, magnesium stearate, microcrystalline cellulose, and one or more of the following: FD&C blue no. 2 aluminum lake, FD&C yellow no. 6 aluminum lake, hydroxypropyl methylcellulose, iron oxides, polyethylene glycol, polysorbate 80, titanium dioxide.

CLINICAL PHARMACOLOGY

MECHANISM OF ACTION

Ropinirole HCl is a non-ergoline dopamine agonist with high relative *in vitro* specificity and full intrinsic activity at the D_2 and D_3 dopamine receptor subtypes, binding with higher affinity to D_3 than to D_2 or D_4 receptor subtypes. The relevance of D_3 receptor binding in Parkinson's disease is unknown.

Ropinirole has moderate *in vitro* affinity for opioid receptors. Ropinirole and its metabolites have negligible *in vitro* affinity for dopamine D_1, 5-HT_1, 5-HT_2, benzodiazepine, GABA, muscarinic, alpha$_1$-, alpha$_2$-, and beta-adrenoreceptors.

The precise mechanism of action of ropinirole HCl as a treatment for Parkinson's disease is unknown, although it is believed to be due to stimulation of post-synaptic dopamine D_2-type receptors within the caudate-putamen in the brain. This conclusion is supported by studies that show that ropinirole improves motor function in various animal models of Parkinson's disease. In particular, ropinirole attenuates the motor deficits induced by lesioning the ascending nigrostriatal dopaminergic pathway with the neurotoxin 1-methyl-4-phenyl-1,2,3,6-tetrahydropyridine (MPTP) in primates.

CLINICAL PHARMACOLOGY STUDIES

In healthy normotensive subjects, single oral doses of ropinirole HCl in the range 0.01-2.5 mg had little or no effect on supine blood pressure and pulse rates. Upon standing, ropinirole HCl caused decreases in systolic and diastolic blood pressure at doses above 0.25 mg. In some subjects, these changes were associated with the emergence of orthostatic symptoms, bradycardia and, in one case, transient sinus arrest with syncope. The effect of repeat dosing and slow titration of ropinirole HCl was not studied in healthy volunteers.

The mechanism of ropinirole HCl-induced postural hypotension is presumed to be due to a D_2-mediated blunting of the noradrenergic response to standing and subsequent decrease in peripheral vascular resistance. Nausea is a common concomitant of orthostatic signs and symptoms.

At oral doses as low as 0.2 mg, ropinirole HCl suppressed serum prolactin concentrations in healthy male volunteers.

Ropinirole HCl had no dose-related effect on ECG wave form and rhythm in young healthy male volunteers in the range of 0.01-2.5 mg.

PHARMACOKINETICS

Absorption, Distribution, Metabolism, and Elimination

Ropinirole is rapidly absorbed after oral administration, reaching peak concentration in approximately 1-2 hours. In clinical studies, over 88% of a radiolabeled dose was recovered in urine and the absolute bioavailability was 55%, indicating a first pass effect. Relative bioavailability from a tablet compared to an oral solution is 85%. Food does not affect the extent of absorption of ropinirole, although its T_{max} is increased by 2.5 hours when the drug is taken with a meal. The clearance of ropinirole after oral administration to patients if 47 L/h (cv=45%) and its elimination half-life is approximately 6 hours. Ropinirole is extensively metabolized by the liver to inactive metabolites and displays linear kinetics over the therapeutic dosing range of 1-8 mg tid. Steady-state concentrations are expected to be achieved within 2 days of dosing. Accumulation upon multiple dosing is predictive from single dosing.

Ropinirole is widely distributed throughout the body, with an apparent volume of distribution of 7.5 L/kg (cv=32%). It is up to 40% bound to plasma proteins and has a blood-to-plasma ratio of 1:1.

The major metabolic pathways are N-despropylation and hydroxylation to form the inactive N-despropyl and hydroxy metabolites. *In vitro* studies indicate that the major cytochrome P450 isozyme involved in the metabolism of ropinirole is CYP1A2, an enzyme known to be stimulated by smoking and omeprazole, and inhibited by, for example, fluvoxamine, mexiletine, and the older fluoroquinolones, such as ciprofloxacin and norfloxacin. The N-despropyl metabolite is converted to carbamyl glucuronide, carboxylic acid, and N-despropyl hydroxy metabolites. The hydroxy metabolite of ropinirole is rapidly glucuronidated. Less than 10% of the administered dose is excreted as unchanged drug in urine. N-despropyl ropinirole is the predominant metabolite found in urine (40%), followed by the carboxylic acid metabolite (10%), and the glucuronide of the hydroxy metabolite (10%).

P450 Interaction

In vitro metabolism studies showed that CYP1A2 was the major enzyme responsible for the metabolism of ropinirole. There is thus the potential for inhibitors or substrates of this enzyme to alter its clearance when coadministered with ropinirole. Therefore, if therapy with a drug known to be a potent inhibitor of CYP1A2 is stopped or started during treatment with ropinirole HCl, adjustment of the ropinirole HCl dose may be required.

Population Subgroups

Because therapy with ropinirole HCl is initiated at a subtherapeutic dosage and gradually titrated upward according to clinical tolerability to obtain the optimum therapeutic effect, adjustment of the initial dose based on gender, weight or age is not necessary.

Age: Oral clearance of ropinirole is reduced by 30% in patients above 65 years of age compared to younger patients. Dosage adjustment is not necessary in the elderly (above 65 years) as the dose of ropinirole is to be individually titrated to clinical response.

Gender: Female and male patients showed similar oral clearance.

Race: The influence of race on the pharmacokinetics of ropinirole has not been evaluated.

Cigarette Smoking: The effect of smoking on the oral clearance of ropinirole has not been evaluated. Smoking is expected to increase the clearance of ropinirole since CYP1A2 is known to be induced by smoking.

Renal Impairment: Based on population pharmacokinetic analysis, no difference was observed in the pharmacokinetics of ropinirole in patients with moderate renal impairment (creatinine clearance between 30-50 ml/min) compared to an age-matched population with creatinine clearance above 50 ml/min. Therefore, no dosage adjustment is necessary in moderately renally impaired patients. The use of ropinirole HCl in patients with severe renal impairment has not been studied. The effect of hemodialysis on drug removal is not known, but because of the relatively high apparent volume of distribution of ropinirole (525 L), the removal of the drug by hemodialysis is unlikely.

Hepatic Impairment: The pharmacokinetics of ropinirole have not been studied in hepatically impaired patients. These patients may have higher plasma levels and lower clearance of the drug than patients with normal hepatic function. The drug should be titrated with caution in this population.

Other Diseases: Population pharmacokinetic analysis revealed no change in the oral clearance of ropinirole in patients with concomitant diseases, such as hypertension, depression, osteoporosis/arthritis, and insomnia, compared to patients with Parkinson's disease only.

INDICATIONS AND USAGE

Ropinirole HCl is indicated for the treatment of the signs and symptoms of idiopathic Parkinson's disease.

The effectiveness of ropinirole HCl was demonstrated in randomized, controlled trials in patients with early Parkinson's disease who were not receiving concomitant levodopa therapy as well as in patients with advanced disease on concomitant levodopa.

CONTRAINDICATIONS

Ropinirole HCl is contraindicated for patients known to have hypersensitivity to the product.

WARNINGS

FALLING ASLEEP DURING ACTIVITIES OF DAILY LIVING

Patients treated with ropinirole HCl have reported falling asleep while engaged in activities of daily living, including the operation of motor vehicles which sometimes resulted in accidents. Although many of these patients reported somnolence while on ropinirole HCl, some perceived that they had no warning signs such as excessive drowsiness, and believed that they were alert immediately prior to the event. Some of these events have been reported as late as 1 year after initiation of treatment.

Somnolence is a common occurrence in patients receiving ropinirole HCl. Many clinical experts believe that falling asleep while engaged in activities of daily living always occurs in a setting of pre-existing somnolence although patients may not give such a history. For this reason, prescribers should continually reassess patients for drowsiness or sleepiness especially since some of the events occur well after the start of treatment. Prescribers should also be aware that patients may not acknowledge drowsiness or sleepiness until directly questioned about drowsiness or sleepiness during specific activities.

Before initiating treatment with ropinirole HCl, patients should be advised of the potential to develop drowsiness and specifically asked about factors that may increase the risk with ropinirole HCl such as concomitant sedating medications, the presence of sleep disorders, and concomitant medications that increase ropinirole plasma levels (*e.g.*, ciprofloxacin; see DRUG INTERACTIONS). If a patient develops significant daytime sleepiness or episodes of falling asleep during activities that require active participation (*e.g.*, conversations, eating, etc.), ropinirole HCl should ordinarily be discontinued. See DOSAGE AND ADMINISTRATION for guidance in discontinuing ropinirole HCl. If a decision is made to continue ropinirole HCl, patients should be advised to not drive and to avoid other potentially dangerous activities. There is insufficient information to establish that dose reduction will eliminate episodes of falling asleep while engaged in activities of daily living.

SYNCOPE

Syncope, sometimes associated with bradycardia, was observed in association with ropinirole in both early Parkinson's disease (without levodopa) patients and advanced Parkinson's disease (with levodopa) patients. In the two double-blind placebo-controlled studies of ropinirole HCl in patients with Parkinson's disease who were not being treated with levodopa, 11.5% (18 of 157) of patients on ropinirole HCl had syncope compared to 1.4% (2 of 147) of patients on placebo. Most of these cases occurred more than 4 weeks after initiation of therapy with ropinirole HCl, and were usually associated with a recent increase in dose.

Of 208 patients being treated with both levodopa and ropinirole HCl, in placebo-controlled advanced Parkinson's disease trials, there were reports of syncope in 6 (2.9%) compared to 2 of 120 (1.7%) of placebo/levodopa patients.

Because the studies of ropinirole HCl excluded patients with significant cardiovascular disease, it is not known to what extent the estimated incidence figures apply to Parkinson's disease patients as a whole. Therefore, patients with severe cardiovascular disease should be treated with caution.

Two (2) of 47 Parkinson's disease patient volunteers enrolled in Phase 1 studies had syncope following a 1 mg dose. In Phase 1 studies including 110 healthy volunteers, 1 patient developed hypotension, bradycardia, and sinus arrest of 26 seconds accompanied by syncope; the patient recovered spontaneously without intervention. One other healthy volunteer reported syncope.

SYMPTOMATIC HYPOTENSION

Dopamine agonists, in clinical studies and clinical experience, appear to impair the systemic regulation of blood pressure, with resulting postural hypotension, especially during dose escalation. Parkinson's disease patients, in addition, appear to have an impaired capacity to respond to a postural challenge. For these reasons, Parkinson's patients being treated with dopaminergic agonists ordinarily (1) require careful monitoring for signs and symptoms of postural hypotension, especially during dose escalation; and (2) should be informed of this risk (see PRECAUTIONS, Information for the Patient).

Although the clinical trials were not designed to systematically monitor blood pressure, there were individual reported cases of postural hypotension in early Parkinson's disease (without levodopa) ropinirole-treated patients. Most of these cases occurred more than 4 weeks after initiation of therapy with ropinirole HCl, and were usually associated with a recent increase in dose.

In Phase 1 studies of ropinirole HCl that included 110 healthy volunteers, 9 subjects had documented symptomatic postural hypotension. These episodes appeared mainly at doses above 0.8 mg and these doses are higher than the starting doses recommended for Parkinson's disease patients. In 8 of these 9 individuals, the hypotension was accompanied by bradycardia, but did not develop into syncope. (See Syncope.) None of these events resulted in death or hospitalization.

One (1) of 47 Parkinson's disease patient volunteers enrolled in Phase 1 studies had documented hypotension following a 2 mg dose on two occasions.

HALLUCINATIONS

In double-blind, placebo-controlled, early therapy studies in patients with Parkinson's disease who were not treated with levodopa, 5.2% (8 of 157) of patients treated with ropinirole HCl reported hallucinations, compared to 1.4% of patients on placebo (2 of 147). Among those patients receiving both ropinirole HCl and levodopa, in advanced Parkinson's disease (with levodopa) studies, 10.1% (21 of 208) were reported to experience hallucinations, compared to 4.2% (5 of 120) of patients treated with placebo and levodopa.

Hallucinations were of sufficient severity to cause discontinuation of treatment in 1.3% of the early Parkinson's disease (without levodopa) patients and 1.9% of the advanced Parkinson's disease (with levodopa) patients compared to 0% and 1.7% of placebo patients, respectively.

PRECAUTIONS

GENERAL

Dyskinesia

Ropinirole HCl may potentiate the dopaminergic side effects of levodopa and may cause and/or exacerbate pre-existing dyskinesia. Decreasing the dose of levodopa may ameliorate this side effect.

Renal and Hepatic

No dosage adjustment is needed in patients with mild to moderate renal impairment (creatinine clearance of 30-50 ml/min). Because the use of ropinirole HCl in patients with severe renal or hepatic impairment has not been studied, administration of ropinirole HCl to such patients should be carried out with caution.

Events Reported With Dopaminergic Therapy

Withdrawal Emergent Hyperpyrexia and Confusion

Although not reported with ropinirole HCl, a symptom complex resembling the neuroleptic malignant syndrome (characterized by elevated temperature, muscular rigidity, altered consciousness, and autonomic instability), with no other obvious etiology, has been reported in association with rapid dose reduction, withdrawal of, or changes in anti-Parkinsonian therapy.

Fibrotic Complications

Cases of retroperitoneal fibrosis, pulmonary infiltrates, pleural effusion, and pleural thickening have been reported in some patients treated with ergot-derived dopaminergic agents. While these complications may resolve when the drug is discontinued, complete resolution does not always occur.

Although these adverse events are believed to be related to the ergoline structure of these compounds, whether other, nonergot derived dopamine agonists can cause them is unknown.

In the ropinirole HCl development program, a 69 year old man with obstructive lung disease was treated with ropinirole HCl for 16 months and developed pleural thickening and effusion accompanied by lower extremity edema, cardiomegaly, pleuritic pain, and shortness of breath. Pleural biopsy demonstrated chronic inflammation and sclerosis. The effusion resolved after medical therapy and discontinuation of ropinirole HCl. The patient was lost to follow-up. The relationship of these events to ropinirole HCl (ropinirole HCl) cannot be established.

Retinal Pathology in Albino Rats

Retinal degeneration was observed in albino rats in the 2 year carcinogenicity study at all doses tested (equivalent to 0.6-20 times the maximum recommended human dose on a mg/m^2 basis), but was statistically significant at the highest dose (50 mg/kg/day). Additional studies to further evaluate the specific pathology (*e.g.*, loss of photoreceptor cells) have not been performed. Similar changes were not observed in a 2 year carcinogenicity study in albino mice or in rats or monkeys treated for 1 year.

The potential significance of this effect in humans has not been established, but cannot be disregarded because disruption of a mechanism that is universally present in vertebrates (*e.g.*, disk shedding) may be involved.

Binding to Melanin

Ropinirole HCl binds to melanin-containing tissues (*i.e.*, eyes, skin) in pigmented rats. After a single dose, long-term retention of drug was demonstrated, with a half-life in the eye of 20 days. It is not known if ropinirole HCl accumulates in these tissues over time.

INFORMATION FOR THE PATIENT

Patients should be instructed to take ropinirole HCl only as prescribed.

Ropinirole HCl can be taken with or without food. Since ingestion with food reduces the maximum concentration (C_{max}) of ropinirole HCl, patients should be advised that taking ropinirole HCl with food may reduce the occurrence of nausea. However, this has not been established in controlled clinical trials.

Patients should be informed that hallucinations can occur, and that the elderly are at a higher risk than younger patients with Parkinson's disease.

Patients should be advised that they may develop postural (orthostatic) hypotension with or without symptoms such as dizziness, nausea, syncope, and sometimes sweating. Hypotension and/or orthostatic symptoms may occur more frequently during initial therapy or with an increase in dose at any time (cases have been seen after weeks of treatment). Accordingly, patients should be cautioned against rising rapidly after sitting or lying down, especially if they have been doing so for prolonged periods, and especially at the initiation of treatment with ropinirole HCl.

Patients should be alerted to the potential sedating effects associated with ropinirole HCl including somnolence and the possibility of falling asleep while engaged in activities of daily living. Since somnolence is a frequent adverse event with potentially serious consequences, patients should neither drive a car nor engage in other potentially dangerous activities until they have gained sufficient experience with ropinirole HCl to gauge whether or not it affects their mental and/or motor performance adversely. Patients should be advised that if increased somnolence or episodes of falling asleep during activities of daily living (*e.g.*, watching television, passenger in a car, etc.) are experienced at any time during treatment, they should not drive or participate in potentially dangerous activities until they have contacted their physician. Because of possible additive effects, caution should be advised when patients are taking other sedating medications or alcohol in combination with ropinirole HCl and when taking concomitant medications that increase plasma levels of ropinirole (*e.g.*, ciprofloxacin).

Because of the possible additive sedative effects, caution should also be used when patients are taking alcohol or other CNS depressants (*e.g.*, benzodiazepines, antipsychotics, antidepressants, etc.) in combination with ropinirole HCl.

R

Because of the possibility that ropinirole may be excreted in breast milk, patients should be advised to notify their physicians if they intend to breast-feed or are breast-feeding an infant.

Because ropinirole has been shown to have adverse effects on embryo-fetal development, including teratogenic effects, in animals, and because experience in humans is limited, patients should be advised to notify their physician if they become pregnant or intend to become pregnant during therapy (see Pregnancy Category C).

CARCINOGENESIS, MUTAGENESIS, AND IMPAIRMENT OF FERTILITY

Two (2) year carcinogenicity studies were conducted in Charles River CD-1 mice at doses of 5, 15, and 50 mg/kg/day and in Sprague-Dawley rats at doses of 1.5, 15, and 50 mg/kg/day (top doses equivalent to 10 times and 20 times, respectively, the maximum recommended human dose of 24 mg/day on a mg/m^2 basis). In the male rat, there was a significant increase in testicular Leydig cell adenomas at all doses tested, *i.e.*, ≥1.5 mg/kg (0.6 times the maximum recommended human dose on a mg/m^2 basis). This finding is of questionable significance because the endocrine mechanisms believed to be involved in the production of Leydig cell hyperplasia and adenomas in rats are not relevant to humans. In the female mouse, there was an increase in benign uterine endometrial polyps at a dose of 50 mg/kg/day (10 times the maximum recommended human dose on a mg/m^2 basis).

Ropinirole was not mutagenic or clastogenic in the *in vitro* Ames test, the *in vitro* chromosome aberration test in human lymphocytes, the *in vitro* mouse lymphoma (L1578Y cells) assay, and the *in vivo* mouse micronucleus test.

When administered to female rats prior to and during mating and throughout pregnancy, ropinirole caused disruption of implantation at doses of 20 mg/kg/day (8 times the maximum recommended human dose on a mg/m^2 basis) or greater. This effect is thought to be due to the prolactin-lowering effect of ropinirole. In humans, chorionic gonadotropin, not prolactin, is essential for implantation. In rat studies using low doses (5 mg/kg) during the prolactin-dependent phase of early pregnancy (gestation days 0-8), ropinirole did not affect female fertility at dosages up to 100 mg/kg/day (40 times the maximum recommended human dose on a mg/m^2 basis). No effect on male fertility was observed in rats at dosages up to 125 mg/kg/day (50 times the maximum recommended human dose on a mg/m^2 basis).

PREGNANCY CATEGORY C

In animal reproduction studies, ropinirole has been shown to have adverse effects on embryo-fetal development, including teratogenic effects. Ropinirole given to pregnant rats during organogenesis (20 mg/kg on gestation days 6 and 7 followed by 20, 60, 90, 120, or 150 mg/kg on gestation days 8 through 15) resulted in decreased fetal body weight at 60 mg/kg/day, increased fetal death at 90 mg/kg/day, and digital malformations at 150 mg/kg/day (24, 36 and 60 times the maximum recommended clinical dose on a mg/m^2 basis, respectively). The combined administration of ropinirole (10 mg/kg/day; 8 times the maximum recommended human dose on a mg/m^2 basis) and levodopa (250 mg/kg/day) to pregnant rabbits during organogenesis produced a greater incidence and severity of fetal malformations (primarily digit defects) than were seen in the offspring of rabbits treated with levodopa alone. No indication of an effect on development of the conceptus was observed in rabbits when a maternally toxic dose of ropinirole was administered alone (20 mg/kg/day: 16 times the maximum recommended human dose on a mg/m^2 basis). In a perinatal-postnatal study in rats, 10 mg/kg/day (4 times the maximum recommended human dose on a mg/m^2 basis) of ropinirole impaired growth and development of nursing offspring and altered neurological development of female offspring.

There are no adequate and well-controlled studies using ropinirole in pregnant women. Ropinirole HCl should be used during pregnancy only if the potential benefit outweighs the potential risk to the fetus.

NURSING MOTHERS

Ropinirole HCl inhibits prolactin secretion in humans and could potentially inhibit lactation.

Studies in rats have shown that ropinirole HCl and/or its metabolite(s) is excreted in breast milk. It is not known whether this drug is excreted in human milk. Because many drugs are excreted in human milk and because of the potential for serious adverse reactions in nursing infants from ropinirole HCl, a decision should be made whether to discontinue nursing or to discontinue the drug, taking into account the importance of the drug to the mother.

R

PEDIATRIC USE

Safety and effectiveness in the pediatric population have not been established.

DRUG INTERACTIONS

P450 INTERACTION

In vitro metabolism studies showed that CYP1A2 was the major enzyme responsible for the metabolism of ropinirole. There is thus the potential for substrates or inhibitors of this enzyme when coadministered with ropinirole to alter its clearance. Therefore, if therapy with a drug known to be a potent inhibitor of CYP1A2 is stopped or started during treatment with ropinirole HCl, adjustment of the ropinirole HCl dose may be required.

LEVODOPA

Co-administration of carbidopa + levodopa (Sinemet 10/100 mg bid) with ropinirole (2.0 mg tid) had no effect on the steady-state pharmacokinetics of ropinirole (n=28 patients). Oral administration of ropinirole HCl 2.0 mg tid increased mean steady-state C_{max} of levodopa by 20% but its AUC was unaffected (n=23 patients).

DIGOXIN

Co-administration of ropinirole HCl (2.0 mg tid) with digoxin (0.125-0.25 mg qd) did not alter the steady-state pharmacokinetics of digoxin in 10 patients.

THEOPHYLLINE

Administration of theophylline (300 mg bid, a substrate of CYP1A2) did not alter the steady-state pharmacokinetics of ropinirole (2 mg tid) in 12 patients with Parkinson's disease. Ropinirole (2 mg tid) did not alter the pharmacokinetics of theophylline (5 mg/kg IV) in 12 patients with Parkinson's disease.

CIPROFLOXACIN

Co-administration of ciprofloxacin (500 mg bid), an inhibitor of CYP1A2, with ropinirole (2 mg tid) increased ropinirole AUC by 84% on average, and C_{max} by 60% (n=12 patients).

ESTROGENS

Population pharmacokinetic analysis revealed that estrogens (mainly ethinylestradiol: intake 0.6-3 mg over a 4 month to 23 year period) reduced the oral clearance of ropinirole by 36% in 16 patients. Dosage adjustment may not be needed for ropinirole HCl in patients on estrogen therapy because patients must be carefully titrated with ropinirole to tolerance or adequate effect. However, if estrogen therapy is stopped or started during treatment with ropinirole HCl, then adjustment of the ropinirole HCl dose may be required.

DOPAMINE ANTAGONISTS

Since ropinirole is a dopamine agonist, it is possible that dopamine antagonists, such as neuroleptics (phenothiazines, butyrophenones, thioxanthenes) or metoclopramide, may diminish the effectiveness of ropinirole HCl. Patients with major psychotic disorders, treated with neuroleptics, should only be treated with dopamine agonists if the potential benefits outweigh the risks.

Population analysis showed that commonly administered drugs, *e.g.*, selegiline, amantadine, tricyclic antidepressants, benzodiazepines, ibuprofen, thiazides, antihistamines, and anticholinergics did not affect the oral clearance of ropinirole.

ADVERSE REACTIONS

During the pre-marketing development of ropinirole HCl, patients received ropinirole HCl either without levodopa (early Parkinson's disease studies) or as concomitant therapy with levodopa (advanced Parkinson's disease studies). Because these 2 populations may have differential risks for various adverse events, this section will, in general, present adverse event data for these 2 populations separately.

EARLY PARKINSON'S DISEASE (WITHOUT LEVODOPA)

The most commonly observed adverse events (>5%) in the double-blind, placebo-controlled early Parkinson's disease trials associated with the use of ropinirole HCl (n=157) not seen at an equivalent frequency among the placebo-treated patients (n=147) were, in order of decreasing incidence: nausea, dizziness, somnolence, headache, vomiting, syncope, fatigue, dyspepsia, viral infection, constipation, pain, increased sweating, asthenia, dependent/leg edema, orthostatic symptoms, abdominal pain, pharyngitis, confusion, hallucinations, urinary tract infections, and abnormal vision.

Approximately 24% of 157 ropinirole HCl-treated patients who participated in the double-blind, placebo-controlled early Parkinson's disease (without levodopa) trials discontinued treatment due to adverse events compared to 13% of 147 patients who received placebo. The adverse events most commonly causing discontinuation of treatment by ropinirole HCl-treated patients were: nausea (6.4%), dizziness (3.8%), aggravated Parkinson's disease (1.3%), hallucinations (1.3%), somnolence (1.3%), vomiting (1.3%), and headache (1.3%). Of these, hallucinations appear to be dose-related. While other adverse events leading to discontinuation may be dose-related, the titration design utilized in these trials precluded an adequate assessment of the dose response. For example, in the larger of the 2 trials, the difference in the rate of discontinuations emerged only after 10 weeks of treatment, suggesting, although not proving, that the effect could be related to dose.

Adverse Event Incidence in Controlled Clinical Studies

TABLE 1 lists treatment-emergent adverse events that occurred in ≥2% of patients with early Parkinson's disease (without levodopa) treated with ropinirole HCl participating in the double-blind, placebo-controlled studies and were numerically more common in the ropinirole HCl group. In these studies, either ropinirole HCl or placebo was used as early therapy (*i.e.*, without levodopa).

The prescriber should be aware that these figures cannot be used to predict the incidence of adverse events in the course of usual medical practice where patient characteristics and other factors differ from those that prevailed in the clinical studies. Similarly, the cited frequencies cannot be compared with figures obtained from other clinical investigations involving different treatments, uses and investigators. However, the cited figures do provide the prescribing physician with some basis for estimating the relative contribution of drug and non-drug factors to the adverse-events incidence rate in the population studied.

Other events reported by 1% or more of early Parkinson's disease (without levodopa) patients treated with ropinirole HCl, but that were equally or more frequent in the placebo group were: headache, upper respiratory infection, insomnia, arthralgia, tremor, back pain, anxiety, dyskinesias, aggravated Parkinsonism, depression, falls, myalgia, leg cramps, paresthesias, nervousness, diarrhea, arthritis, hot flushes, weight loss, rash, cough, hyperglycemia, muscle spasm, arthrosis, abnormal dreams, dystonia, increased salivation, bradycardia, gout, basal cell carcinoma, gingivitis, hematuria, and rigors.

Among the treatment-emergent adverse events in patients treated with ropinirole HCl, hallucinations appear to be dose-related.

The incidence of adverse events was not materially different between women and men.

ADVANCED PARKINSON'S DISEASE (WITH LEVODOPA)

The most commonly observed adverse events (>5%), in the double-blind, placebo-controlled advanced Parkinson's disease (with levodopa) trials associated with the use of ropinirole HCl (n=208) as an adjunct to levodopa not seen at an equivalent frequency among the placebo-treated patients (n=120) were, in order of decreasing incidence: dyskinesias, nausea, dizziness, aggravated Parkinsonism, somnolence, headache, insomnia, injury, hallucinations, falls, abdominal pain, upper respiratory infection, confusion, increased sweating, vomiting, viral infection, increased drug level, arthralgia, tremor, anxiety, urinary tract infection, constipation, dry mouth, pain, hypokinesia, and paresthesia.

Approximately 24% of 208 patients who received ropinirole HCl in the double-blind, placebo-controlled advanced Parkinson's disease (with levodopa) trials discontinued treatment due to adverse events compared to 18% of 120 patients who received placebo. The

TABLE 1 *Treatment-Emergent Adverse Event* Incidence in Double-Blind, Placebo-Controlled Early Parkinson's Disease (without levodopa) Trials*

Events ≥2% of Patients Treated With Ropinirole HCl and Numerically More Frequent Than the Placebo Group

	Ropinirole Hydrochloride n=157	Placebo n=147
Autonomic Nervous System		
Flushing	3%	1%
Dry mouth	5%	3%
Increased sweating	6%	4%
Body as a Whole		
Asthenia	6%	1%
Chest Pain	4%	2%
Dependent edema	6%	3%
Leg edema	7%	1%
Fatigue	11%	4%
Malaise	3%	1%
Pain	8%	4%
Cardiovascular General		
Hypertension	5%	3%
Hypotension	2%	0%
Orthostatic symptoms	6%	5%
Syncope	12%	1%
Central/Peripheral Nervous System		
Dizziness	40%	22%
Hyperkinesia	2%	1%
Hypesthesia	4%	2%
Vertigo	2%	0%
Gastrointestinal System		
Abdominal pain	6%	3%
Anorexia	4%	1%
Dyspepsia	10%	5%
Flatulence	3%	1%
Nausea	60%	22%
Vomiting	12%	7%
Heart Rate/Rhythm		
Extrasystoles	2%	1%
Atrial fibrillation	2%	0%
Palpitation	3%	2%
Tachycardia	2%	0%
Metabolic/Nutritional		
Increased alkaline phosphatase	3%	1%
Psychiatric		
Amnesia	3%	1%
Impaired concentration	2%	0%
Confusion	5%	1%
Hallucination	5%	1%
Somnolence	40%	6%
Yawning	3%	0%
Reproductive Male		
Impotence	3%	1%
Resistance Mechanism		
Viral infection	11%	3%
Respiratory System		
Bronchitis	3%	1%
Dyspnea	3%	0%
Pharyngitis	6%	4%
Rhinitis	4%	3%
Sinusitis	4%	3%
Urinary System		
Urinary tract infection	5%	4%
Vascular Extracardiac		
Peripheral ischemia	3%	0%
Vision		
Eye abnormality	3%	1%
Abnormal vision	6%	3%
Xerophthalmia	2%	0%

* Patients may have reported multiple adverse experiences during the study or at discontinuation; thus, patients may be included in more than one category.

TABLE 2 *Treatment-Emergent Adverse Event* Incidence in Double-Blind, Placebo-Controlled Advanced Parkinson's Disease (with levodopa) Trials*

Events ≥2% of Patients Treated With Ropinirole HCl and Numerically More Frequent Than the Placebo Group

	Ropinirole Hydrochloride n=208	Placebo n=120
Autonomic Nervous System		
Dry mouth	5%	1%
Increased sweating	7%	2%
Body as a Whole		
Increased drug level	7%	3%
Pain	5%	3%
Cardiovascular General		
Hypotension	2%	1%
Syncope	3%	2%
Central/Peripheral Nervous System		
Dizziness	26%	16%
Dyskinesia	34%	13%
Falls	10%	7%
Headache	17%	12%
Hypokinesia	5%	4%
Paresis	3%	0%
Paresthesia	5%	3%
Tremor	6%	3%
Gastrointestinal System		
Abdominal pain	9%	8%
Constipation	6%	3%
Diarrhea	5%	3%
Dysphagia	2%	1%
Flatulence	2%	1%
Nausea	30%	18%
Increased saliva	2%	1%
Vomiting	7%	4%
Metabolic/Nutritional		
Weight decrease	2%	1%
Musculoskeletal System		
Arthralgia	7%	5%
Arthritis	3%	1%
Psychiatric		
Amnesia	5%	1%
Anxiety	6%	3%
Confusion	9%	2%
Abnormal dreaming	3%	2%
Hallucination	10%	4%
Nervousness	5%	3%
Somnolence	20%	8%
Red Blood Cell		
Anemia	2%	0%
Resistance Mechanism		
Upper respiratory tract infection	9%	8%
Respiratory System		
Dyspnea	3%	2%
Urinary System		
Pyuria	2%	1%
Urinary incontinence	2%	1%
Urinary tract infection	6%	3%
Vision		
Diplopia	2%	1%

* Patients may have reported multiple adverse experiences during the study or at discontinuation; thus, patients may be included in more than one category.

events most commonly (≥1%) causing discontinuation of treatment by ropinirole-treated patients were: dizziness (2.9%), dyskinesias (2.4%), vomiting (2.4%), confusion (2.4%), nausea (1.9%), hallucinations (1.9%), anxiety (1.9%), and increased sweating (1.4%). Of these, hallucinations and dyskinesias appear to be dose-related.

Adverse Event Incidence in Controlled Clinical Studies

TABLE 2 lists treatment-emergent adverse events that occurred in ≥2% of patients with advanced Parkinson's disease (with levodopa) treated with ropinirole HCl who participated in the double-blind, placebo-controlled studies and were numerically more common in the ropinirole HCl group. In these studies, either ropinirole HCl or placebo was used as an adjunct to levodopa. Adverse events were usually mild or moderate in intensity.

The prescriber should be aware that these figures cannot be used to predict the incidence of adverse events in the course of usual medical practice where patient characteristics and other factors differ from those that prevailed in the clinical studies. Similarly, the cited frequencies cannot be compared with figures obtained from other clinical investigations involving different treatments, uses, and investigators. However, the cited figures do provide the prescribing physician with some basis for estimating the relative contribution of drug and non-drug factors to the adverse-events incidence rate in the population studied.

Other events reported by 1% or more of patients treated with both ropinirole HCl and levodopa, but equally or more frequent in the placebo/levodopa group were: myocardial infarction, orthostatic symptoms, virus infections, asthenia, dyspepsia, myalgia, back pain, depression, leg cramps, fatigue, rhinitis, chest pain, hematuria, vertigo, tinnitus, leg edema, hot flushes, abnormal gait, hyperkinesia, and pharyngitis.

Among the treatment-emergent adverse events in patients treated with ropinirole HCl, hallucinations and dyskinesias appear to be dose-related.

OTHER ADVERSE EVENTS OBSERVED DURING ALL PHASE 2/3 CLINICAL TRIALS

Ropinirole HCl has been administered to 1599 individuals in clinical trials. During these trials, all adverse events were recorded by the clinical investigators using terminology of their own choosing. To provide a meaningful estimate of the proportion of individuals having adverse events, similar types of events were grouped into a smaller number of standardized categories using modified WHOART dictionary terminology. These categories are used in the listing below. The frequencies presented represent the proportion of the 1599 individuals exposed to ropinirole HCl who experienced events of the type cited on at least one occasion while receiving ropinirole HCl. All reported events that occurred at least twice (or once for serious or potentially serious events), except those already listed above, trivial events, and terms too vague to be meaningful are included, without regard to determination of a causal relationship to ropinirole HCl, except that events very unlikely to be drug-related have been deleted.

Events are further classified within body system categories and enumerated in order of decreasing frequency using the following definitions: *Frequent* adverse events are defined as those occurring in at least 1/100 patients and *infrequent* adverse events are those occurring in 1/100 to 1/1000 patients and *rare* events are those occurring in fewer than 1/1000 patients.

Body as a Whole: *Infrequent:* Cellulitis, peripheral edema, fever, influenza-like symptoms, enlarged abdomen, precordial chest pain, and generalized edema; *Rare:* Ascites.

Cardiovascular: *Infrequent:* Cardiac failure, bradycardia, tachycardia, supraventricular tachycardia, angina pectoris, bundle branch block, cardiac arrest, cardiomegaly, aneurysm, mitral insufficiency; *Rare:* Ventricular tachycardia.

Central/Peripheral Nervous System: *Frequent:* Neuralgia; *Infrequent:* Involuntary muscle contractions, hypertonia, dysphonia, abnormal coordination, extrapyramidal disorder, migraine, choreoathetosis, coma, stupor, aphasia, convulsions, hypotonia, peripheral neuropathy, paralysis; *Rare:* Grand mal convulsions, hemiparesis, hemiplegia.

Endocrine: *Infrequent:* Hypothyroidism, gynecomastia, hyperthyroidism; *Rare:* Goiter, SIADH.

Gastrointestinal: *Infrequent:* Increased hepatic enzymes, bilirubinemia, cholecystitis, cholelithiasis colitis, dysphagia, periodontitis, fecal incontinence, gastroesophageal reflux, hemorrhoids, toothache, eructation, gastritis, esophagitis, hiccups, diverticulitis, duodenal ulcer, gastric ulcer, melena, duodenitis, gastrointestinal hemorrhage, glossitis, rectal hemorrhage, pancreatitis, stomatitis and ulcerative stomatitis, tongue edema; *Rare:* Biliary pain, hemorrhagic gastritis, hematemesis, salivary duct obstruction.

Hematologic: *Infrequent:* Purpura, thrombocytopenia, hematoma, vitamin B12 deficiency, hypochromic anemia, eosinophilia, leukocytosis, leukopenia, lymphocytosis, lymphopenia, lymphedema.

Metabolic/Nutritional: *Frequent:* Increased BUN; *Infrequent:* Hypoglycemia, increased alkaline phosphatase, increased LDH, weight increase, hyperphosphatemia, hyperuricemia, diabetes mellitus, glycosuria, hypokalemia, hypercholesterolemia, hyperkalemia, acidosis, hyponatremia, thirst, increased CPK, dehydration; *Rare:* Hypochloremia.

Musculoskeletal: *Infrequent:* Aggravated arthritis, tendinitis, osteoporosis, bursitis, polymyalgia rheumatica, muscle weakness, skeletal pain, torticollis; *Rare:* Dupuytren's contracture requiring surgery.

Neoplasm: *Infrequent:* Malignant breast neoplasm; *Rare:* Bladder carcinoma, benign brain neoplasm, esophageal carcinoma, malignant laryngeal neoplasm, lipoma, rectal carcinoma, uterine neoplasm.

Psychiatric: *Infrequent:* Increased libido, agitation, apathy, impaired concentration, depersonalization, paranoid reaction, personality disorder, euphoria, delirium, dementia, delusion, emotional lability, decreased libido, manic reaction, somnambulism, aggressive reaction, neurosis; *Rare:* Suicide attempt.

Genito-urinary: *Infrequent:* Amenorrhea, vaginal hemorrhage, penile disorder, prostatic disorder, balanoposthitis, epididymitis, perineal pain, dysuria, micturition frequency, albuminuria, nocturia, polyuria, renal calculus; *Rare:* Breast enlargement, mastitis, uterine hemorrhage, ejaculation disorder, Peyronie's Disease, pyelonephritis, acute renal failure, uremia.

Resistance Mechanism: *Infrequent:* Herpes zoster, otitis media, sepsis, abscess, herpes simplex, fungal infection, genital moniliasis.

Respiratory: *Infrequent:* Asthma, epistaxis, laryngitis, pleurisy, pulmonary edema.

Skin/Appendage: *Infrequent:* Pruritus, dermatitis, eczema, skin ulceration, alopecia, skin hypertrophy, skin discoloration, urticaria, fungal dermatitis, furunculosis, hyperkeratosis, photosensitivity reaction, psoriasis, maculopapular rash, psoriaform rash, seborrhea.

Special Senses: *Infrequent:* Tinnitus, earache, decreased hearing, abnormal lacrimation, conjunctivitis, blepharitis, glaucoma, abnormal accommodation, blepharospasm, eye pain, photophobia; *Rare:* Scotoma.

Vascular Extracardiac: *Infrequent:* Varicose veins, phlebitis, peripheral gangrene; *Rare:* Limb embolism, pulmonary embolism, gangrene, subarachnoid hemorrhage, deep thrombophlebitis, leg thrombophlebitis, thrombosis.

FALLING ASLEEP DURING ACTIVITIES OF DAILY LIVING

Patients treated with ropinirole HCl have reported falling asleep while engaged in activities of daily living, including operation of a motor vehicle which sometimes resulted in accidents (see WARNINGS).

DOSAGE AND ADMINISTRATION

In all clinical studies, dosage was initiated at a subtherapeutic level and gradually titrated to therapeutic response. The dosage should be increased to achieve a maximum therapeutic effect, balanced against the principal side effects of nausea, dizziness, somnolence, and dyskinesia.

Ropinirole HCl should be taken 3 times daily. Ropinirole HCl can be taken with or without food. Since ingestion with food reduces the maximum concentration (C_{max}) of ropinirole HCl, patients should be advised that taking ropinirole HCl with food may reduce the occurrence of nausea. However, this has not been established in controlled clinical trials.

The recommended starting dose is 0.25 mg three times daily. Based on individual patient response, dosage should then be titrated with weekly increments as described in TABLE 3. After week 4, if necessary, daily dosage may be increased by 1.5 mg/day on a weekly basis up to a dose of 9 mg/day, and then by up to 3 mg/day weekly to a total dose of 24 mg/day.

Doses greater than 24 mg/day have not been tested in clinical trials.

TABLE 3 *Ascending-Dose Schedule of Ropinirole HCl*

Week	Dosage	Total Daily Dose
1	0.25 mg three times daily	0.75 mg
2	0.5 mg three times daily	1.5 mg
3	0.75 mg three times daily	2.25 mg
4	1.0 mg three times daily	3.0 mg

When ropinirole HCl is administered as adjunct therapy to levodopa, the concurrent dose of levodopa may be decreased gradually as tolerated. Levodopa dosage reduction was allowed during the advanced Parkinson's disease (with levodopa) study if dyskinesias or other dopaminergic effects occurred. Overall, reduction of levodopa dose was sustained in 87% of ropinirole-treated patients and in 57% of patients on placebo. On average the levodopa dose was reduced by 31% in ropinirole-treated patients.

Ropinirole HCl should be discontinued gradually over a 7 day period. The frequency of administration should be reduced from 3 times daily to twice daily for 4 days. For the remaining 3 days, the frequency should be reduced to once daily prior to complete withdrawal of ropinirole HCl.

HOW SUPPLIED

Requip Tablets: Each pentagonal film-coated Tiltab tablet with beveled edges contains ropinirole HCl as follows:

0.25 mg: White imprinted with "SB" and "4890".
0.5 mg: Yellow imprinted with "SB" and "4891".
1.0 mg: Green imprinted with "SB" and "4892".
2.0 mg: Pale yellowish pink imprinted with "SB" and "4893".
4.0 mg: Pale brown imprinted with "SB" and "4896".
5.0 mg: Blue imprinted with "SB" and "4894".

Storage: Protect from light and moisture. Close container tightly after each use. Store at controlled room temperature 20-25°C (68-77°F).

PRODUCT LISTING - EQUIVALENTS NOT AVAILABLE

Tablet - Oral - 0.25 mg			
30's	$26.63	REQUIP, Glaxosmithkline	00007-4890-14
100's	$131.29	REQUIP, Glaxosmithkline	00007-4890-20
Tablet - Oral - 0.5 mg			
30's	$26.63	REQUIP, Glaxosmithkline	00007-4891-14
100's	$131.29	REQUIP, Glaxosmithkline	00007-4891-20
Tablet - Oral - 1 mg			
30's	$30.50	REQUIP, Glaxosmithkline	00007-4892-14
100's	$131.29	REQUIP, Glaxosmithkline	00007-4892-20
Tablet - Oral - 2 mg			
30's	$30.50	REQUIP, Glaxosmithkline	00007-4893-14
100's	$134.05	REQUIP, Glaxosmithkline	00007-4893-20
Tablet - Oral - 3 mg			
100's	$234.45	REQUIP, Glaxosmithkline	00007-4895-20
Tablet - Oral - 4 mg			
100's	$234.45	REQUIP, Glaxosmithkline	00007-4896-20
Tablet - Oral - 5 mg			
30's	$53.25	REQUIP, Glaxosmithkline	00007-4894-14
100's	$234.45	REQUIP, Glaxosmithkline	00007-4894-20

Ropivacaine Hydrochloride *(003305)*

For complete prescribing information, refer to the CD-ROM included with the book.

Categories: Anesthesia, local; Anesthesia, regional; Pregnancy Category B; FDA Approved 1996 Sep
Drug Classes: Anesthetics, local
Brand Names: **Naropin**
Foreign Brand Availability: Narop (Israel; Sweden); Naropeine (France)

DESCRIPTION

Naropin injection contains ropivacaine HCl which is a member of the amino amide class of local anesthetics. Naropin injection is a sterile, isotonic solution that contains the enantiomerically pure drug substance, sodium chloride for isotonicity and water for injection. Sodium hydroxide and/or hydrochloric acid may be used for pH adjustment. It is administered parenterally.

Ropivacaine HCl is chemically described as S-(-)-1-propyl-2',6'-pipecoloxylidide hydrochloride monohydrate. The drug substance is a white crystalline powder, with a molecular formula of $C_{17}H_{26}N_2O{\cdot}HCl{\cdot}H_2O$, molecular weight of 328.89.

At 25°C ropivacaine HCl has a solubility of 53.8 mg/ml in water, a distribution ratio between n-octanol and phosphate buffer at pH 7.4 of 14:1 and a pKa of 8.07 in 0.1 M KCl solution. The pKa of ropivacaine is approximately the same as bupivacaine (8.1) and is similar to that of mepivacaine (7.7). However, ropivacaine has an intermediate degree of lipid solubility compared to bupivacaine and mepivacaine.

Naropin injection is preservative-free and is available in single dose containers in 2.0 (0.2%), 5.0 (0.5%), 7.5 (0.75%) and 10.0 mg/ml (1.0%) concentrations. The specific gravity of Naropin injection solutions range from 1.002 to 1.005 at 25°C.

INDICATIONS AND USAGE

Ropivacaine HCl is indicated for the production of local or regional anesthesia for surgery and for acute pain management.

Surgical Anesthesia: Epidural block for surgery including cesarean section; major nerve block; local infiltration.

Acute Pain Management: Epidural continuous infusion or intermittent bolus, *e.g.*, postoperative or labor; local infiltration.

CONTRAINDICATIONS

Ropivacaine HCl is contraindicated in patients with a known hypersensitivity to ropivacaine or to any local anesthetic agent of the amide type.

WARNINGS

IN PERFORMING ROPIVACAINE HCl BLOCKS, UNINTENDED INTRAVENOUS INJECTION IS POSSIBLE AND MAY RESULT IN CARDIAC ARRHYTHMIA OR CARDIAC ARREST. THE POTENTIAL FOR SUCCESSFUL RESUSCITATION HAS NOT BEEN STUDIED IN HUMANS. ROPIVACAINE HCl SHOULD BE ADMINISTERED IN INCREMENTAL DOSES. IT IS NOT RECOMMENDED FOR EMERGENCY SITUATIONS, WHERE A FAST ONSET OF SURGICAL ANESTHESIA IS NECESSARY. HISTORICALLY, PREGNANT PATIENTS WERE REPORTED TO HAVE A HIGH RISK FOR CARDIAC ARRHYTHMIAS, CARDIAC/CIRCULATORY ARREST AND DEATH WHEN 0.75% BUPIVACAINE (ANOTHER MEMBER OF THE AMINO AMIDE CLASS OF LOCAL ANESTHETICS) WAS INADVERTENTLY RAPIDLY INJECTED INTRAVENOUSLY.

LOCAL ANESTHETICS SHOULD ONLY BE ADMINISTERED BY CLINICIANS WHO ARE WELL VERSED IN THE DIAGNOSIS AND MANAGEMENT OF DOSE-RELATED TOXICITY AND OTHER ACUTE EMERGENCIES WHICH MIGHT ARISE

FROM THE BLOCK TO BE EMPLOYED, AND THEN ONLY AFTER INSURING THE **IMMEDIATE (WITHOUT DELAY)** AVAILABILITY OF OXYGEN, OTHER RESUSCITATIVE DRUGS, CARDIOPULMONARY RESUSCITATIVE EQUIPMENT, AND THE PERSONNEL RESOURCES NEEDED FOR PROPER MANAGEMENT OF TOXIC REACTIONS AND RELATED EMERGENCIES. DELAY IN PROPER MANAGEMENT OF DOSE-RELATED TOXICITY, UNDERVENTILATION FROM ANY CAUSE, AND/OR ALTERED SENSITIVITY MAY LEAD TO THE DEVELOPMENT OF ACIDOSIS, CARDIAC ARREST AND, POSSIBLY, DEATH. SOLUTIONS OF ROPIVACAINE HCl SHOULD NOT BE USED FOR THE PRODUCTION OF OBSTETRICAL PARACERVICAL BLOCK ANESTHESIA, RETROBULBAR BLOCK, OR SPINAL ANESTHESIA (SUBARACHNOID BLOCK) DUE TO INSUFFICIENT DATA TO SUPPORT SUCH USE. INTRAVENOUS REGIONAL ANESTHESIA (BIER BLOCK) SHOULD NOT BE PERFORMED DUE TO A LACK OF CLINICAL EXPERIENCE AND THE RISK OF ATTAINING TOXIC BLOOD LEVELS OF ROPIVACAINE.

It is essential that aspiration for blood, or cerebrospinal fluid (where applicable), be done prior to injecting any local anesthetic, both the original dose and all subsequent doses, to avoid intravascular or subarachnoid injection. However, a negative aspiration does *not* ensure against an intravascular or subarachnoid injection.

A well-known risk of epidural anesthesia may be an unintentional subarachnoid injection of local anesthetic. Two clinical studies have been performed to verify the safety of ropivacaine HCl at a volume of 3 ml injected into the subarachnoid space since this dose represents an incremental epidural volume that could be unintentionally injected. The 15 and 22.5 mg doses injected resulted in sensory levels as high as T5 and T4, respectively. Anesthesia to pinprick started in the sacral dermatomes in 2-3 minutes, extended to the T10 level in 10-13 minutes and lasted for approximately 2 hours. The results of these two clinical studies showed that a 3 ml dose did not produce any serious adverse events when spinal anesthesia blockade was achieved. Ropivacaine HCl should be used with caution in patients receiving other local anesthetics or agents structurally related to amide-type local anesthetics, since the toxic effects of these drugs are additive.

DOSAGE AND ADMINISTRATION

The rapid injection of a large volume of local anesthetic solution should be avoided and fractional (incremental) doses should always be used. The smallest dose and concentration required to produce the desired result should be administered.

The dose of any local anesthetic administered varies with the anesthetic procedure, the area to be anesthetized, the vascularity of the tissues, the number of neuronal segments to be blocked, the depth of anesthesia and degree of muscle relaxation required, the duration of anesthesia desired, individual tolerance, and the physical condition of the patient. Patients in poor general condition due to aging or other compromising factors such as partial or complete heart conduction block, advanced liver disease or severe renal dysfunction require special attention although regional anesthesia is frequently indicated in these patients. To reduce the risk of potentially serious adverse reactions, attempts should be made to optimize the patient's condition before major blocks are performed, and the dosage should be adjusted accordingly.

TABLE 7 *Dosage Recommendations*

	Conc mg/ml (%)	Volume ml	Dose mg	Onset min	Duration hours
Surgical Anesthesia					
Lumbar Epidural	5.0 (0.5%)	15-30	75-150	15-30	2-4
Administration	7.5 (0.75%)	15-25	113-188	10-20	3-5
Surgery	10.0 (1.0%)	15-20	150-200	10-20	4-6
Lumbar Epidural	5.0 (0.5%)	20-30	100-150	15-25	2-4
Administration	7.5 (0.75%)	15-20	113-150	10-20	3-5
Cesarean section					
Thoracic Epidural	5.0 (0.5%)	5-15	25-75	10-20	N/A
Administration	7.5 (0.75%)	5-15	38-113	10-20	N/A
Surgery					
Major Nerve Block	5.0 (0.5%)	35-50	175-250	15-30	5-8
(*e.g.*, brachial plexus block)	7.5 (0.75%)	10-40	75-300	10-25	6-10
Field Block (*e.g.*, minor nerve blocks and infiltration)	5.0 (0.5%)	1-40	5-200	1-15	2-6
Labor Pain Management					
Lumbar Epidural Administration					
Initial dose	2.0 (0.2%)	10-20	20-40	10-15	0.5-1.5
Continuous infusion*	2.0 (0.2%)	6-14 ml/h	12-28 mg/h	N/A	N/A
Incremental injection (top-up)*	2.0 (0.2%)	10-15 ml/h	20-30 mg/h	N/A	N/A
Postoperative Pain Management					
Lumbar Epidural Administration					
Continuous infusion†	2.0 (0.2%)	6-14 ml/h	12-28 mg/h	N/A	N/A
Thoracic Epidural Administration	2.0 (0.2%)	6-14 ml/h	12-28 mg/h	N/A	N/A
Continuous infusion†	2.0 (0.2%)	1-100	2-200	1-5	2-6
Infiltration(*e.g.*, minor nerve block)	5.0 (0.5%)	1-40	5-200	1-5	2-6

* Median dose of 21 mg/h was administered by continuous infusion or by incremental injections (top-ups) over a median delivery time of 5.5 hours.

† Cumulative doses up to 770 mg of ropivacaine HCl over 24 hours (intraoperative block plus postoperative infusion); continuous epidural infusion at rates up to 28 mg/h for 72 hours have been well tolerated in adults, *i.e.*, 2016 mg plus surgical dose of approximately 100-150 mg as top-up.

N/A = Not Applicable.

Use an adequate test dose (3-5 ml of a short acting local anesthetic solution containing epinephrine) prior to induction of complete block. This test dose should be repeated if the patient is moved in such a fashion as to have displaced the epidural catheter. Allow adequate time for onset of anesthesia following administration of each test dose.

Parenteral drug products should be inspected visually for particulate matter and discoloration prior to administration, whenever solution and container permit. Solutions which are discolored or which contain particulate matter should not be administered.

The doses in TABLE 7 are those considered to be necessary to produce a successful block and should be regarded as guidelines for use in adults. Individual variations in onset and duration occur. The figures reflect the expected average dose range needed. For other local anesthetic techniques standard current textbooks should be consulted.

When prolonged blocks are used, either through continuous infusion or through repeated bolus administration, the risks of reaching a toxic plasma concentration or inducing local neural injury must be considered. Experience to date indicates that a cumulative dose of up to 770 mg ropivacaine HCl administered over 24 hours is well tolerated in adults when used for postoperative pain management: *i.e.*, 2016 mg. Caution should be exercised when administering ropivacaine HCl for prolonged periods of time, *e.g.*, >70 hours in debilitated patients.

For treatment of postoperative pain, the following technique can be recommended: If regional anesthesia was not used intraoperatively, then an initial epidural block with 5-7 ml ropivacaine HCl is induced via an epidural catheter. Analgesia is maintained with an infusion of ropivacaine HCl, 2 mg/ml (0.2%). Clinical studies have demonstrated that infusion rates of 6-14 ml (12-28 mg) per hour provide adequate analgesia with nonprogressive motor block. With this technique a significant reduction in the need for opioids was demonstrated. Clinical experience supports the use of ropivacaine HCl epidural infusions for up to 72 hours.

PRODUCT LISTING - EQUIVALENTS NOT AVAILABLE

Package	Price	Product	NDC
Solution - Injectable - 0.2%			
10 ml x 5	$16.32	NAROPIN, Astra-Zeneca Pharmaceuticals	00186-0859-44
10 ml x 10	$20.84	NAROPIN, Astra-Zeneca Pharmaceuticals	00186-0859-81
20 ml x 5	$32.70	NAROPIN POLYAMP, Astra-Zeneca Pharmaceuticals	00186-0859-54
20 ml x 10	$33.77	NAROPIN, Astra-Zeneca Pharmaceuticals	00186-0859-91
Solution - Injectable - 0.5%			
10 ml x 5	$26.15	GENERIC, Astra-Zeneca Pharmaceuticals	00186-0863-44
20 ml x 5	$44.83	NAROPIN, Astra-Zeneca Pharmaceuticals	00186-0863-57
20 ml x 5	$45.14	GENERIC, Astra-Zeneca Pharmaceuticals	00186-0863-54
30 ml	$13.45	NAROPIN, Astra-Zeneca Pharmaceuticals	00186-0863-61
30 ml x 5	$74.40	NAROPIN, Astra-Zeneca Pharmaceuticals	00186-0863-69
Solution - Injectable - 0.75%			
10 ml x 5	$29.55	NAROPIN SDV, Astra-Zeneca Pharmaceuticals	00186-0867-47
10 ml x 5	$31.00	NAROPIN SDV, Astra-Zeneca Pharmaceuticals	00186-0867-44
20 ml x 5	$59.80	NAROPIN, Astra-Zeneca Pharmaceuticals	00186-0867-54
Solution - Injectable - 1%			
10 ml x 5	$35.88	NAROPIN POLYAMP, Astra-Zeneca Pharmaceuticals	00186-0868-44
20 ml x 5	$71.50	NAROPIN, Astra-Zeneca Pharmaceuticals	00186-0868-54

Rosiglitazone Maleate *(003437)*

For related information, see the comparative table section in Appendix A.

Categories: Diabetes mellitus; FDA Approved 1999 May; Pregnancy Category C
Drug Classes: Antidiabetic agents; Thiazolidinediones
Brand Names: **Avandia**
Foreign Brand Availability: Nyracta (Austria; Belgium; Bulgaria; Czech-Republic; Denmark; England; Finland; France; Germany; Greece; Hungary; Ireland; Italy; Netherlands; Norway; Poland; Portugal; Slovenia; Spain; Sweden; Switzerland; Turkey); Rezult (India); Rosi (Israel); Venvia (Austria; Belgium; Bulgaria; Czech-Republic; Denmark; England; Finland; France; Germany; Greece; Hungary; Ireland; Italy; Netherlands; Norway; Poland; Portugal; Slovenia; Spain; Sweden; Switzerland; Turkey)
Cost of Therapy: $83.23 (Diabetes mellitus; Avandia; 4 mg; 1 tablet/day; 30 day supply)

DESCRIPTION

Avandia (rosiglitazone maleate) is an oral antidiabetic agent which acts primarily by increasing insulin sensitivity. Avandia is used in the management of Type 2 diabetes mellitus (also known as non-insulin-dependent diabetes mellitus [NIDDM] or adult-onset diabetes). Avandia improves glycemic control while reducing circulating insulin levels.

Pharmacological studies in animal models indicate that rosiglitazone improves sensitivity to insulin in muscle and adipose tissue and inhibits hepatic gluconeogenesis. Rosiglitazone maleate is not chemically or functionally related to the sulfonylureas, the biguanides, or the alpha-glucosidase inhibitors.

Chemically, rosiglitazone maleate is (±)-5-[[4-[2-(methyl-2-pyridinylamino)ethoxy]-phenyl]methyl]-2,4-thiazolidinedione,(*Z*)-2-butenedioate(1:1) with a molecular weight of 473.52 (357.44 free base). The molecule has a single chiral center and is present as a racemate. Due to rapid interconversion, the enantiomers are functionally indistinguishable.

The molecular formula is $C_{18}H_{19}N_3O_3S{\cdot}C_4H_4O_4$. Rosiglitazone maleate is a white to off-white solid with a melting point range of 122-123°C. The pKa values of rosiglitazone maleate are 6.8 and 6.1. It is readily soluble in ethanol and a buffered aqueous solution with pH of 2.3; solubility decreases with increasing pH in the physiological range.

Each pentagonal film-coated Tiltab tablet contains rosiglitazone maleate equivalent to rosiglitazone, 2, 4, or 8 mg, for oral administration. Inactive ingredients are: hypromellose 2910, lactose monohydrate, magnesium stearate, microcrystalline cellulose, polyethylene glycol 3000, sodium starch glycolate, titanium dioxide, triacetin, and 1 or more of the following: synthetic red and yellow iron oxides and talc.

CLINICAL PHARMACOLOGY

MECHANISM OF ACTION

Rosiglitazone, a member of the thiazolidinedione class of antidiabetic agents, improves glycemic control by improving insulin sensitivity. Rosiglitazone is a highly selective and potent agonist for the peroxisome proliferator-activated receptor-gamma (PPARγ). In humans, PPAR receptors are found in key target tissues for insulin action such as adipose tissue, skeletal muscle, and liver. Activation of PPARγ nuclear receptors regulates the transcription of insulin-responsive genes involved in the control of glucose production, transport, and utilization. In addition, PPARγ-responsive genes also participate in the regulation of fatty acid metabolism.

Insulin resistance is a common feature characterizing the pathogenesis of Type 2 diabetes. The antidiabetic activity of rosiglitazone has been demonstrated in animal models of Type 2 diabetes in which hyperglycemia and/or impaired glucose tolerance is a consequence of insulin resistance in target tissues. Rosiglitazone reduces blood glucose concentrations and reduces hyperinsulinemia in the ob/ob obese mouse, db/db diabetic mouse, and fa/fa fatty Zucker rat.

In animal models, rosiglitazone's antidiabetic activity was shown to be mediated by increased sensitivity to insulin's action in the liver, muscle, and adipose tissues. The expression of the insulin-regulated glucose transporter GLUT-4 was increased in adipose tissue. Rosiglitazone did not induce hypoglycemia in animal models of Type 2 diabetes and/or impaired glucose tolerance.

PHARMACOKINETICS AND DRUG METABOLISM

Maximum plasma concentration (C_{max}) and the area under the curve (AUC) of rosiglitazone increase in a dose-proportional manner over the therapeutic dose range (TABLE 1). The elimination half-life is 3-4 hours and is independent of dose.

TABLE 1 *Mean (SD) Pharmacokinetic Parameters for Rosiglitazone Following Single Oral Doses (n=32)*

	Fasting			Fed
Parameter	1 mg	2 mg	8 mg	8 mg
AUC(0-∞) [ng·h/ml]	358 (112)	733 (184)	2971 (730)	2890 (795)
C_{max} [ng/ml]	76 (13)	156 (42)	598 (117)	432 (92)
Half-life [h]	3.16 (0.72)	3.15 (0.39)	3.37 (0.63)	3.59 (0.70)
CL/F* [L/h]	3.03 (0.87)	2.89 (0.71)	2.85 (0.69)	2.97 (0.81)

* CL/F = Oral Clearance.

ABSORPTION

The absolute bioavailability of rosiglitazone is 99%. Peak plasma concentrations are observed about 1 hour after dosing. Administration of rosiglitazone with food resulted in no change in overall exposure (AUC), but there was an approximately 28% decrease in C_{max} and a delay in T_{max} (1.75 hours). These changes are not likely to be clinically significant; therefore, rosiglitazone maleate may be administered with or without food.

DISTRIBUTION

The mean (CV%) oral volume of distribution (Vss/F) of rosiglitazone is approximately 17.6 L (30%), based on a population pharmacokinetic analysis. Rosiglitazone is approximately 99.8% bound to plasma proteins, primarily albumin.

METABOLISM

Rosiglitazone is extensively metabolized with no unchanged drug excreted in the urine. The major routes of metabolism were N-demethylation and hydroxylation, followed by conjugation with sulfate and glucuronic acid. All the circulating metabolites are considerably less potent than parent and, therefore, are not expected to contribute to the insulin-sensitizing activity of rosiglitazone.

In vitro data demonstrate that rosiglitazone is predominantly metabolized by Cytochrome P450 (CYP) isoenzyme 2C8, with CYP2C9 contributing as a minor pathway.

EXCRETION

Following oral or intravenous (IV) administration of [^{14}C]rosiglitazone maleate, approximately 64% and 23% of the dose was eliminated in the urine and in the feces, respectively. The plasma half-life of [^{14}C]related material ranged from 103 to 158 hours.

POPULATION PHARMACOKINETICS IN PATIENTS WITH TYPE 2 DIABETES

Population pharmacokinetic analyses from three large clinical trials including 642 men and 405 women with Type 2 diabetes (aged 35-80 years) showed that the pharmacokinetics of rosiglitazone are not influenced by age, race, smoking, or alcohol consumption. Both oral clearance (CL/F) and oral steady-state volume of distribution (Vss/F) were shown to increase with increases in body weight. Over the weight range observed in these analyses (50-150 kg), the range of predicted CL/F and Vss/F values varied by <1.7-fold and <2.3-fold, respectively. Additionally, rosiglitazone CL/F was shown to be influenced by both weight and gender, being lower (about 15%) in female patients.

SPECIAL POPULATIONS

Age

Results of the population pharmacokinetic analysis (n=716 <65 years; n=331 ≥65 years) showed that age does not significantly affect the pharmacokinetics of rosiglitazone.

Gender

Results of the population pharmacokinetics analysis showed that the mean oral clearance of rosiglitazone in female patients (n=405) was approximately 6% lower compared to male patients of the same body weight (n=642).

As monotherapy and in combination with metformin, rosiglitazone maleate improved glycemic control in both males and females. In metformin combination studies, efficacy was demonstrated with no gender differences in glycemic response.

In monotherapy studies, a greater therapeutic response was observed in females; however, in more obese patients, gender differences were less evident. For a given body mass index (BMI), females tend to have a greater fat mass than males. Since the molecular target PPARγ is expressed in adipose tissues, this differentiating characteristic may account, at least in part, for the greater response to rosiglitazone maleate in females. Since therapy should be individualized, no dose adjustments are necessary based on gender alone.

Hepatic Impairment

Unbound oral clearance of rosiglitazone was significantly lower in patients with moderate to severe liver disease (Child-Pugh Class B/C) compared to healthy subjects. As a result, unbound C_{max} and AUC(0-∞) were increased 2- and 3-fold, respectively. Elimination half-life for rosiglitazone was about 2 hours longer in patients with liver disease, compared to healthy subjects.

Therapy with rosiglitazone maleate should not be initiated if the patient exhibits clinical evidence of active liver disease or increased serum transaminase levels (ALT >2.5 times upper limit of normal) at baseline (see PRECAUTIONS, General, Hepatic Effects).

Renal Impairment

There are no clinically relevant differences in the pharmacokinetics of rosiglitazone in patients with mild to severe renal impairment or in hemodialysis-dependent patients compared to subjects with normal renal function. No dosage adjustment is therefore required in such patients receiving rosiglitazone maleate. Since metformin is contraindicated in patients with renal impairment, coadministration of metformin with rosiglitazone maleate is contraindicated in these patients.

Race

Results of a population pharmacokinetic analysis including subjects of Caucasian, Black, and other ethnic origins indicate that race has no influence on the pharmacokinetics of rosiglitazone.

Pediatric Use

The safety and effectiveness of rosiglitazone maleate in pediatric patients have not been established.

INDICATIONS AND USAGE

Rosiglitazone maleate is indicated as an adjunct to diet and exercise to improve glycemic control in patients with Type 2 diabetes mellitus. Rosiglitazone maleate is indicated as monotherapy. Rosiglitazone maleate is also indicated for use in combination with a sulfonylurea or metformin, or insulin when diet, exercise, and a single agent do not result in adequate glycemic control. For patients inadequately controlled with a maximum dose of a sulfonylurea or metformin, rosiglitazone maleate should be added to, rather than substituted for, a sulfonylurea or metformin.

Management of Type 2 diabetes should include diet control. Caloric restriction, weight loss, and exercise are essential for the proper treatment of the diabetic patient because they help improve insulin sensitivity. This is important not only in the primary treatment of Type 2 diabetes, but also in maintaining the efficacy of drug therapy. Prior to initiation of therapy with rosiglitazone maleate, secondary causes of poor glycemic control, *e.g.*, infection, should be investigated and treated.

CONTRAINDICATIONS

Rosiglitazone maleate is contraindicated in patients with known hypersensitivity to this product or any of its components.

WARNINGS

CARDIAC FAILURE AND OTHER CARDIAC EFFECTS

Rosiglitazone maleate, like other thiazolidinediones, alone or in combination with other antidiabetic agents, can cause fluid retention, which may exacerbate or lead to heart failure. Patients should be observed for signs and symptoms of heart failure. Patients should be observed for signs and symptoms of heart failure. In combination with insulin, thiazolidinediones may also increase the risk of other cardiovascular adverse events. Rosiglitazone maleate should be discontinued if any deterioration in cardiac status occurs.

In three 26-week trials in patients with Type 2 diabetes, 216 received 4 mg of rosiglitazone maleate plus insulin, 322 received 8 mg of rosiglitazone maleate plus insulin, and 338 received insulin alone. These trials included patients with long-standing diabetes and a high prevalence of pre-existing medical conditions, including peripheral neuropathy, retinopathy, ischemic heart disease, vascular disease, and congestive heart failure. In these clinical studies an increased incidence of edema, cardiac failure, and other cardiovascular adverse events was seen in patients on rosiglitazone maleate and insulin combination therapy compared to insulin and placebo. Patients who experienced cardiovascular events were on average older and had a longer duration of diabetes. These cardiovascular events were noted at both the 4 and 8 mg daily doses of rosiglitazone maleate. In this population, however, it was not possible to determine specific risk factors that could be used to identify all patients at risk of heart failure and other cardiovascular events on combination therapy. Three (3) of 10 patients who developed cardiac failure on combination therapy during the double blind part of the studies had no known prior evidence of congestive heart failure, or pre-existing cardiac condition.

In a double-blind study in Type 2 diabetes patients with chronic renal failure (112 received 4 or 8 mg of rosiglitazone maleate plus insulin and 108 received insulin control), there was no difference in cardiovascular adverse events with rosiglitazone maleate in combination with insulin compared to insulin control.

Patients treated with combination rosiglitazone maleate and insulin should be monitored for cardiovascular adverse events. This combination therapy should be discontinued in patients who do not respond as manifested by a reduction in HbA1c or insulin dose after 4-5 months of therapy or who develop any significant adverse events (see ADVERSE REACTIONS).

PRECAUTIONS

GENERAL

Due to its mechanism of action, rosiglitazone maleate is active only in the presence of endogenous insulin. Therefore, rosiglitazone maleate should not be used in patients with Type 1 diabetes or for the treatment of diabetic ketoacidosis.

Hypoglycemia

Patients receiving rosiglitazone maleate in combination with other hypoglycemic agents may be at risk for hypoglycemia, and a reduction in the dose of the concomitant agent may be necessary.

Edema

Rosiglitazone maleate should be used with caution in patients with edema. In a clinical study in healthy volunteers who received rosiglitazone maleate 8 mg once daily for 8 weeks, there was a statistically significant increase in median plasma volume compared to placebo.

Since thiazolidinediones, including rosiglitazone, can cause fluid retention, which can exacerbate or lead to congestive heart failure, rosiglitazone maleate should be used with caution in patients at risk for heart failure. Patients should be monitored for signs and symptoms of heart failure (see WARNINGS, Cardiac Failure and Other Cardiac Effects; and PRECAUTIONS, Information for the Patient).

In controlled clinical trials of patients with Type 2 diabetes, mild to moderate edema was reported in patients treated with rosiglitazone maleate, and may be dose related. Patients with ongoing edema are more likely to have adverse events associated with edema if started on combination therapy with insulin and rosiglitazone maleate (see ADVERSE REACTIONS).

Weight Gain

Dose-related weight gain was seen with rosiglitazone maleate alone and in combination with other hypoglycemic agents (see TABLE 6A and TABLE 6B). The mechanism of weight gain is unclear but probably involves a combination of fluid retention and fat accumulation.

In postmarketing experience, there have been rare reports of unusually rapid increases in weight and increases in excess of that generally observed in clinical trials. Patients who experience such increases should be assessed for fluid accumulation and volume-Hyprelated events such as excessive edema and congestive heart failure.

***TABLE 6A** Weight Changes (kg) From Baseline During Clinical Trials With Rosiglitazone Maleate*

	Duration	Control Group	Median*
Monotherapy			
	26 weeks	Placebo	-0.9 (-2.8, 0.9)
	52 weeks	Sulfonylurea	2.0 (0, 4.0)
Combination Therapy			
Sulfonylurea	26 weeks	Sulfonylurea	0 (-1.3, 1.2)
Metformin	26 weeks	Metformin	-1.4 (-3.2, 0.2)
Insulin	26 weeks	Insulin	0.9 (-0.5, 2.7)

* (25th, 75th percentile).

***TABLE 6B** Weight Changes (kg) From Baseline During Clinical Trials With Rosiglitazone Maleate*

			Rosiglitazone Maleate	
			4 mg	8 mg
	Duration	Control Group	Median*	
Monotherapy				
	26 weeks	Placebo	1.0 (-0.9, 3.6)	3.1 (1.1, 5.8)
	52 weeks	Sulfonylurea	2.0 (-0.6, 4.0)	2.6 (0, 5.3)
Combination Therapy				
Sulfonylurea	26 weeks	Sulfonylurea	1.8 (0, 3.1)	—
Metformin	26 weeks	Metformin	0.8 (-1.0, 2.6)	2.1 (0, 4.3)
Insulin	26 weeks	Insulin	4.1 (1.4, 6.3)	5.4 (3.4, 7.3)

* (25th, 75th percentile).

Hematologic

Across all controlled clinical studies, decreases in hemoglobin and hematocrit (mean decreases in individual studies ≤1.0 g/dl and ≤3.3%, respectively) were observed for rosiglitazone maleate alone and in combination with other hypoglycemic agents. The changes occurred primarily during the first 3 months following initiation of therapy with rosiglitazone maleate or following a dose increase in rosiglitazone maleate. White blood cell counts also decreased slightly in patients treated with rosiglitazone maleate. The observed changes may be related to the increased plasma volume observed with treatment with rosiglitazone maleate and may be dose related (see ADVERSE REACTIONS, Laboratory Abnormalities, Hematologic).

Ovulation

Therapy with rosiglitazone maleate, like other thiazolidinediones, may result in ovulation in some premenopausal anovulatory women. As a result, these patients may be at an increased risk for pregnancy while taking rosiglitazone maleate (see Pregnancy Category C). Thus, adequate contraception in premenopausal women should be recommended. This possible effect has not been specifically investigated in clinical studies so the frequency of this occurrence is not known.

Although hormonal imbalance has been seen in preclinical studies (see Carcinogenesis, Mutagenesis, and Impairment of Fertility), the clinical significance of this finding is not known. If unexpected menstrual dysfunction occurs, the benefits of continued therapy with rosiglitazone maleate should be reviewed.

Hepatic Effects

Another drug of the thiazolidinedione class, troglitazone, was associated with idiosyncratic hepatotoxicity, and very rare cases of liver failure, liver transplants, and death were reported during clinical use. In pre-approval controlled clinical trials in patients with Type 2 diabetes, troglitazone was more frequently associated with clinically significant elevations in liver enzymes (ALT >3 times upper limit of normal) compared to placebo. Very rare cases of reversible jaundice were also reported.

In pre-approval clinical studies in 4598 patients treated with rosiglitazone maleate, encompassing approximately 3600 patient years of exposure, there was no signal of drug-induced hepatotoxicity or elevation of ALT levels. In the pre-approval controlled trials, 0.2% of patients treated with rosiglitazone maleate had elevations in ALT >3 times the upper limit of normal compared to 0.2% on placebo and 0.5% on active comparators. The ALT elevations in patients treated with rosiglitazone maleate were reversible and were not clearly causally related to therapy with rosiglitazone maleate.

In postmarketing experience with rosiglitazone maleate, reports of hepatitis and of hepatic enzyme elevations to 3 or more times the upper limit of normal have been received. Very rarely, these reports have involved hepatic failure with and without fatal outcome, although causality has not been established. Rosiglitazone is structurally related to troglitazone, a thiazolidinedione no longer marketed in the US, which was associated with idiosyncratic hepatotoxicity and rare cases of liver failure, liver transplants, and death during clinical use. Pending the availability of the results of additional large, long-term controlled clinical trials and additional postmarketing safety data, it is recommended that patients treated with rosiglitazone maleate undergo periodic monitoring of liver enzymes.

Liver enzymes should be checked prior to the initiation of therapy with rosiglitazone maleate in all patients. Therapy with rosiglitazone maleate should not be initiated in patients with increased baseline liver enzyme levels (ALT >2.5 times upper limit of normal). In patients with normal baseline liver enzymes, following initiation of therapy with rosiglitazone maleate, it is recommended that liver enzymes be monitored every 2 months for the first 12 months, and periodically thereafter. Patients with mildly elevated liver enzymes (ALT levels ≤2.5 times upper limit of normal) at baseline or during therapy with rosiglitazone maleate should be evaluated to determine the cause of the liver enzyme elevation. Initiation of, or continuation of, therapy with rosiglitazone maleate in patients with mild liver enzyme elevations should proceed with caution and include close clinical follow-up, including more frequent liver enzyme monitoring, to determine if the liver enzyme elevations resolve or worsen. If at any time ALT levels increase to >3 times the upper limit of normal in patients on therapy with rosiglitazone maleate, liver enzyme levels should be rechecked as soon as possible. If ALT levels remain >3 times the upper limit of normal, therapy with rosiglitazone maleate should be discontinued.

There are no data available from clinical trials to evaluate the safety of rosiglitazone maleate in patients who experienced liver abnormalities, hepatic dysfunction, or jaundice while on troglitazone. Rosiglitazone maleate should not be used in patients who experienced jaundice while taking troglitazone.

If any patient develops symptoms suggesting hepatic dysfunction, which may include unexplained nausea, vomiting, abdominal pain, fatigue, anorexia and/or dark urine, liver enzymes should be checked. The decision whether to continue the patient on therapy with rosiglitazone maleate should be guided by clinical judgment pending laboratory evaluations. If jaundice is observed, drug therapy should be discontinued.

LABORATORY TESTS

Periodic fasting blood glucose and HbA1c measurements should be performed to monitor therapeutic response.

Liver enzyme monitoring is recommended prior to initiation of therapy with rosiglitazone maleate in all patients and periodically thereafter (see Hepatic Effects and ADVERSE REACTIONS, Laboratory Abnormalities, Serum Transaminase Levels).

INFORMATION FOR THE PATIENT

Patients should be informed of the following:

Management of Type 2 diabetes should include diet control. Caloric restriction, weight loss, and exercise are essential for the proper treatment of the diabetic patient because they help improve insulin sensitivity. This is important not only in the primary treatment of Type 2 diabetes, but in maintaining the efficacy of drug therapy.

It is important to adhere to dietary instructions and to regularly have blood glucose and glycosylated hemoglobin tested. Patients should be advised that it can take 2 weeks to see a reduction in blood glucose and 2-3 months to see full effect. Patients should be informed that blood will be drawn to check their liver function prior to the start of therapy and every 2 months for the first 12 months, and periodically thereafter. Patients with unexplained symptoms of nausea, vomiting, abdominal pain, fatigue, anorexia, or dark urine should immediately report these symptoms to their physician. Patients who experience an unusually rapid increase in weight or edema or who develop shortness of breath or other symptoms of heart failure while on rosiglitazone maleate should immediately report these symptoms to their physician.

Rosiglitazone maleate can be taken with or without meals.

When using rosiglitazone maleate in combination with other hypoglycemic agents, the risk of hypoglycemia, its symptoms and treatment, and conditions that predispose to its development should be explained to patients and their family members.

Therapy with rosiglitazone maleate, like other thiazolidinediones, may result in ovulation in some premenopausal anovulatory women. As a result, these patients may be at an increased risk for pregnancy while taking rosiglitazone maleate (see Pregnancy Category C). Thus, adequate contraception in premenopausal women should be recommended. This possible effect has not been specifically investigated in clinical studies so the frequency of this occurrence is not known.

CARCINOGENESIS, MUTAGENESIS, AND IMPAIRMENT OF FERTILITY

Carcinogenesis

A 2 year carcinogenicity study was conducted in Charles River CD-1 mice at doses of 0.4, 1.5, and 6 mg/kg/day in the diet (highest dose equivalent to approximately 12 times human AUC at the maximum recommended human daily dose). Sprague-Dawley rats were dosed for 2 years by oral gavage at doses of 0.05, 0.3, and 2 mg/kg/day (highest dose equivalent

R

to approximately 10 and 20 times human AUC at the maximum recommended human daily dose for male and female rats, respectively).

Rosiglitazone was not carcinogenic in the mouse. There was an increase in incidence of adipose hyperplasia in the mouse at doses ≥1.5 mg/kg/day (approximately 2 times human AUC at the maximum recommended human daily dose). In rats, there was a significant increase in the incidence of benign adipose tissue tumors (lipomas) at doses ≥0.3 mg/kg/day (approximately 2 times human AUC at the maximum recommended human daily dose). These proliferative changes in both species are considered due to the persistent pharmacological overstimulation of adipose tissue.

Mutagenesis

Rosiglitazone was not mutagenic or clastogenic in the *in vitro* bacterial assays for gene mutation, the *in vitro* chromosome aberration test in human lymphocytes, the *in vivo* mouse micronucleus test, and the *in vivo/in vitro* rat UDS assay. There was a small (about 2-fold) increase in mutation in the *in vitro* mouse lymphoma assay in the presence of metabolic activation.

Impairment of Fertility

Rosiglitazone had no effects on mating or fertility of male rats given up to 40 mg/kg/day (approximately 116 times human AUC at the maximum recommended human daily dose). Rosiglitazone altered estrous cyclicity (2 mg/kg/day) and reduced fertility (40 mg/kg/day) of female rats in association with lower plasma levels of progesterone and estradiol (approximately 20 and 200 times human AUC at the maximum recommended human daily dose, respectively). No such effects were noted at 0.2 mg/kg/day (approximately 3 times human AUC at the maximum recommended human daily dose). In monkeys, rosiglitazone (0.6 and 4.6 mg/kg/day; approximately 3 and 15 times human AUC at the maximum recommended human daily dose, respectively) diminished the follicular phase rise in serum estradiol with consequential reduction in the luteinizing hormone surge, lower luteal phase progesterone levels, and amenorrhea. The mechanism for these effects appears to be direct inhibition of ovarian steroidogenesis.

ANIMAL TOXICOLOGY

Heart weights were increased in mice (3 mg/kg/day), rats (5 mg/kg/day), and dogs (2 mg/kg/day) with rosiglitazone treatments (approximately 5, 22, and 2 times human AUC at the maximum recommended human daily dose, respectively). Morphometric measurement indicated that there was hypertrophy in cardiac ventricular tissues, which may be due to increased heart work as a result of plasma volume expansion.

PREGNANCY CATEGORY C

There was no effect on implantation or the embryo with rosiglitazone treatment during early pregnancy in rats, but treatment during mid-late gestation was associated with fetal death and growth retardation in both rats and rabbits. Teratogenicity was not observed at doses up to 3 mg/kg in rats and 100 mg/kg in rabbits (approximately 20 and 75 times human AUC at the maximum recommended human daily dose, respectively). Rosiglitazone caused placental pathology in rats (3 mg/kg/day). Treatment of rats during gestation through lactation reduced litter size, neonatal viability, and postnatal growth, with growth retardation reversible after puberty. For effects on the placenta, embryo/fetus, and offspring, the no-effect dose was 0.2 mg/kg/day in rats and 15 mg/kg/day in rabbits. These no-effect levels are approximately 4 times human AUC at the maximum recommended human daily dose.

There are no adequate and well-controlled studies in pregnant women. Rosiglitazone maleate should not be used during pregnancy unless the potential benefit justifies the potential risk to the fetus.

Because current information strongly suggests that abnormal blood glucose levels during pregnancy are associated with a higher incidence of congenital anomalies as well as increased neonatal morbidity and mortality, most experts recommend that insulin monotherapy be used during pregnancy to maintain blood glucose levels as close to normal as possible.

LABOR AND DELIVERY

The effect of rosiglitazone on labor and delivery in humans is not known.

NURSING MOTHERS

Drug-related material was detected in milk from lactating rats. It is not known whether rosiglitazone maleate is excreted in human milk. Because many drugs are excreted in human milk, rosiglitazone maleate should not be administered to a nursing woman.

DRUG INTERACTIONS

DRUGS METABOLIZED BY CYTOCHROME P450

In vitro drug metabolism studies suggest that rosiglitazone does not inhibit any of the major P450 enzymes at clinically relevant concentrations. *In vitro* data demonstrate that rosiglitazone is predominantly metabolized by CYP2C8, and to a lesser extent, 2C9.

Rosiglitazone maleate (4 mg twice daily) was shown to have no clinically relevant effect on the pharmacokinetics of nifedipine and oral contraceptives (ethinylestradiol and norethindrone), which are predominantly metabolized by CYP3A4.

Glyburide: Rosiglitazone maleate (2 mg twice daily) taken concomitantly with glyburide (3.75 to 10 mg/day) for 7 days did not alter the mean steady-state 24 hour plasma glucose concentrations in diabetic patients stabilized on glyburide therapy.

Metformin: Concurrent administration of rosiglitazone maleate (2 mg twice daily) and metformin (500 mg twice daily) in healthy volunteers for 4 days had no effect on the steady-state pharmacokinetics of either metformin or rosiglitazone.

Acarbose: Coadministration of acarbose (100 mg three times daily) for 7 days in healthy volunteers had no clinically relevant effect on the pharmacokinetics of a single oral dose of rosiglitazone maleate.

Digoxin: Repeat oral dosing of rosiglitazone maleate (8 mg once daily) for 14 days did not alter the steady-state pharmacokinetics of digoxin (0.375 mg once daily) in healthy volunteers.

Warfarin: Repeat dosing with rosiglitazone maleate had no clinically relevant effect on the steady-state pharmacokinetics of warfarin enantiomers.

Ethanol: A single administration of a moderate amount of alcohol did not increase the risk of acute hypoglycemia in Type 2 diabetes mellitus patients treated with rosiglitazone maleate.

Ranitidine: Pretreatment with ranitidine (150 mg twice daily for 4 days) did not alter the pharmacokinetics of either single oral or IV doses of rosiglitazone in healthy volunteers. These results suggest that the absorption of oral rosiglitazone is not altered in conditions accompanied by increases in gastrointestinal pH.

ADVERSE REACTIONS

In clinical trials, approximately 4600 patients with Type 2 diabetes have been treated with rosiglitazone maleate; 3300 patients were treated for 6 months or longer and 2000 patients were treated for 12 months or longer.

TRIALS OF ROSIGLITAZONE MALEATE AS MONOTHERAPY AND IN COMBINATION WITH OTHER HYPOGLYCEMIC AGENTS

The incidence and types of adverse events reported in clinical trials of rosiglitazone maleate as monotherapy are shown in TABLE 7.

TABLE 7 *Adverse Events (≥5% in any treatment group) Reported by Patients in Double-Blind Clinical Trials With Rosiglitazone Maleate as Monotherapy*

Preferred Term	Rosiglitazone Maleate* n=2526	Placebo n=601	Metformin n=225	Sulfonylureas† n=626
Upper respiratory tract infection	9.9%	8.7%	8.9%	7.3%
Injury	7.6%	4.3%	7.6%	6.1%
Headache	5.9%	5.0%	8.9%	5.4%
Back pain	4.0%	3.8%	4.0%	5.0%
Hyperglycemia	3.9%	5.7%	4.4%	8.1%
Fatigue	3.6%	5.0%	4.0%	1.9%
Sinusitis	3.2%	4.5%	5.3%	3.0%
Diarrhea	2.3%	3.3%	15.6%	3.0%
Hypoglycemia	0.6%	0.2%	1.3%	5.9%

* Monotherapy.
† Includes patients receiving glyburide (n=514), gliclazide (n=91) or glipizide (n=21).

There were a small number of patients treated with rosiglitazone maleate who had adverse events of anemia and edema. Overall, these events were generally mild to moderate in severity and usually did not require discontinuation of treatment with rosiglitazone maleate.

In double-blind studies, anemia was reported in 1.9% of patients receiving rosiglitazone maleate compared to 0.7% on placebo, 0.6% on sulfonylureas and 2.2% on metformin. Edema was reported in 4.8% of patients receiving rosiglitazone maleate compared to 1.3% on placebo, 1.0% on sulfonylureas, and 2.2% on metformin. Overall, the types of adverse experiences reported when rosiglitazone maleate was used in combination with a sulfonylurea or metformin were similar to those during monotherapy with rosiglitazone maleate. Reports of anemia (7.1%) were greater in patients treated with a combination of rosiglitazone maleate and metformin compared to monotherapy with rosiglitazone maleate or in combination with a sulfonylurea.

Lower pre-treatment hemoglobin/hematocrit levels in patients enrolled in the metformin combination clinical trials may have contributed to the higher reporting rate of anemia in these studies (see Laboratory Abnormalities, Hematologic).

In 26 week double-blind studies, edema was reported with higher frequency in the rosiglitazone maleate plus insulin combination trials (insulin, 5.4%; and rosiglitazone maleate in combination with insulin, 14.7%). Reports of new onset or exacerbation of congestive heart failure occurred at rates of 1% for insulin alone, and 2% (4 mg) and 3% (8 mg) for insulin in combination with rosiglitazone maleate (see WARNINGS, Cardiac Failure and Other Cardiac Effects).

In postmarketing experience with rosiglitazone maleate, adverse events potentially related to volume expansion (*e.g.*, congestive heart failure, pulmonary edema, and pleural effusions) have been reported.

Hypoglycemia was the most frequently reported adverse event in the fixed-dose insulin combination trials, although few patients withdrew for hypoglycemia (4 of 408 for rosiglitazone maleate plus insulin and 1 of 203 for insulin alone). Rates of hypoglycemia, confirmed by capillary blood glucose concentration ≤50 mg/dl, were 6% for insulin alone and 12% (4 mg) and 14% (8 mg) for insulin in combination with rosiglitazone maleate.

LABORATORY ABNORMALITIES

Hematologic

Decreases in mean hemoglobin and hematocrit occurred in a dose-related fashion in patients treated with rosiglitazone maleate (mean decreases in individual studies up to 1.0 g/dl hemoglobin and up to 3.3% hematocrit). The time course and magnitude of decreases were similar in patients treated with a combination of rosiglitazone maleate and other hypoglycemic agents or rosiglitazone maleate monotherapy. Pre-treatment levels of hemoglobin and hematocrit were lower in patients in metformin combination studies and may have contributed to the higher reporting rate of anemia. White blood cell counts also decreased slightly in patients treated with rosiglitazone maleate. Decreases in hematologic parameters may be related to increased plasma volume observed with treatment with rosiglitazone maleate.

Lipids

Changes in serum lipids have been observed following treatment with rosiglitazone maleate.

Serum Transaminase Levels

In clinical studies in 4598 patients treated with rosiglitazone maleate encompassing approximately 3600 patient years of exposure, there was no evidence of drug-induced hepatotoxicity or elevated ALT levels.

In controlled trials, 0.2% of patients treated with rosiglitazone maleate had reversible elevations in ALT >3 times the upper limit of normal compared to 0.2% on placebo and 0.5% on active comparators. Hyperbilirubinemia was found in 0.3% of patients treated with rosiglitazone maleate compared with 0.9% treated with placebo and 1% in patients treated with active comparators.

In the clinical program including long-term, open-label experience, the rate per 100 patient years exposure of ALT increase to >3 times the upper limit of normal was 0.35 for patients treated with rosiglitazone maleate, 0.59 for placebo-treated patients, and 0.78 for patients treated with active comparator agents.

In pre-approval clinical trials, there were no cases of idiosyncratic drug reactions leading to hepatic failure. In postmarketing experience with rosiglitazone maleate, reports of hepatic enzyme elevations 3 or more times the upper limit of normal and hepatitis have been received (see PRECAUTIONS, General, Hepatic Effects).

DOSAGE AND ADMINISTRATION

The management of antidiabetic therapy should be individualized. Rosiglitazone maleate may be administered either at a starting dose of 4 mg as a single daily dose or divided and administered in the morning and evening. For patients who respond inadequately following 8-12 weeks of treatment, as determined by reduction in FPG, the dose may be increased to 8 mg daily as monotherapy or in combination with metformin. Rosiglitazone maleate may be taken with or without food.

MONOTHERAPY

The usual starting dose of rosiglitazone maleate is 4 mg administered either as a single dose once daily or in divided doses twice daily. In clinical trials, the 4 mg twice daily regimen resulted in the greatest reduction in FPG and HbA1c.

COMBINATION THERAPY

When rosiglitazone maleate is added to existing therapy, the current dose of sulfonylurea, metformin, or insulin can be continued upon initiation of rosiglitazone maleate therapy.

Sulfonylurea

When used in combination with sulfonylurea, the recommended dose of rosiglitazone maleate is 4 mg administered as either a single dose once daily or in divided doses twice daily. If patients report hypoglycemia, the dose of the sulfonylurea should be decreased.

Metformin

The usual starting dose of rosiglitazone maleate in combination with metformin is 4 mg administered as either a single dose once daily or in divided doses twice daily. It is unlikely that the dose of metformin will require adjustment due to hypoglycemia during combination therapy with rosiglitazone maleate.

Insulin

For patients stabilized on insulin, the insulin dose should be continued upon initiation of therapy with rosiglitazone maleate. Rosiglitazone maleate should be dosed at 4 mg daily. Doses of rosiglitazone maleate greater than 4 mg daily in combination with insulin are not currently indicated. It is recommended that the insulin dose be decreased by 10-25% if the patient reports hypoglycemia or if FPG concentrations decrease to less than 100 mg/dl. Further adjustments should be individualized based on glucose-lowering response.

MAXIMUM RECOMMENDED DOSE

The dose of rosiglitazone maleate should not exceed 8 mg daily, as a single dose or divided twice daily. The 8 mg daily dose has been shown to be safe and effective in clinical studies as monotherapy and in combination with metformin. Doses of rosiglitazone maleate greater than 4 mg daily in combination with a sulfonylurea have not been studied in adequate and well-controlled clinical trials. Doses of rosiglitazone maleate greater than 4 mg daily in combination with insulin are not currently indicated.

Rosiglitazone maleate may be taken with or without food.

No dosage adjustments are required for the elderly.

No dosage adjustment is necessary when rosiglitazone maleate is used as monotherapy in patients with renal impairment. Since metformin is contraindicated in such patients, concomitant administration of metformin and rosiglitazone maleate is also contraindicated in patients with renal impairment.

Therapy with rosiglitazone maleate should not be initiated if the patient exhibits clinical evidence of active liver disease or increased serum transaminase levels (ALT >2.5 times upper limit of normal at start of therapy) (see PRECAUTIONS, General, Hepatic Effects; and CLINICAL PHARMACOLOGY, Special Populations, Hepatic Impairment). Liver enzyme monitoring is recommended in all patients prior to initiation of therapy with rosiglitazone maleate and periodically thereafter (see PRECAUTIONS, General, Hepatic Effects).

There are no data on the use of rosiglitazone maleate in patients younger than 18 years; therefore, use of rosiglitazone maleate in pediatric patients is not recommended.

HOW SUPPLIED

AVANDIA TABLETS

Each pentagonal film-coated Tiltab tablet contains rosiglitazone as the maleate as follows:

2 mg: Pink, debossed with "SB" on one side and "2" on the other.

4 mg: Orange, debossed with "SB" on one side and "4" on the other.

8 mg: Red-brown, debossed with "SB" on one side and "8" on the other.

Storage: Store at 25°C (77°F); excursions 15-30°C (59-86°F). Dispense in a tight, light-resistant container.

PRODUCT LISTING - EQUIVALENTS NOT AVAILABLE

Tablet - Oral - 2 mg			
30's	$54.38	AVANDIA, Allscripts Pharmaceutical Company	54569-4801-00
60's	$108.75	AVANDIA, Glaxosmithkline	00029-3358-18
60's	$119.89	AVANDIA, Glaxosmithkline	00029-3158-18
Tablet - Oral - 4 mg			
30's	$75.00	AVANDIA, Allscripts Pharmaceutical Company	54569-4802-00
30's	$83.23	AVANDIA, Glaxosmithkline	00029-3159-13
30's	$85.29	AVANDIA, Physicians Total Care	54868-4198-00
60's	$166.45	AVANDIA, Glaxosmithkline	00029-3159-18
100's	$277.44	AVANDIA, Glaxosmithkline	00029-3159-20
Tablet - Oral - 8 mg			
30's	$136.88	AVANDIA, Allscripts Pharmaceutical Company	54569-4803-00
30's	$154.03	AVANDIA, Glaxosmithkline	00029-3160-13
100's	$513.33	AVANDIA, Glaxosmithkline	00029-3160-20

Rubella Virus Vaccine Live *(002196)*

For complete prescribing information, refer to the CD-ROM included with the book.

Categories: Immunization, rubella; Pregnancy Category C; FDA Pre 1938 Drugs; WHO Formulary
Drug Classes: Vaccines
Brand Names: **Meruvax II**
Foreign Brand Availability: Cendevax (Benin; Burkina-Faso; Ethiopia; Gambia; Ghana; Guinea; Ivory-Coast; Kenya; Liberia; Malawi; Mali; Mauritania; Mauritius; Morocco; Niger; Nigeria; Senegal; Seychelles; Sierra-Leone; Sudan; Tanzania; Tunia; Uganda; Zambia; Zimbabwe); Ervevax (Australia; Austria; Bulgaria; Czech-Republic; England; Germany; Italy; Malaysia; Netherlands; Philippines; Switzerland; Taiwan; Thailand); Gunevax (Philippines; Thailand); Rubavax (England); Rubeaten (Austria; Czech-Republic; Greece; Italy; Spain; Switzerland); Rubeaten Berna (Malaysia; Philippines; South-Africa; Taiwan; Thailand); Rudivax (Malaysia; Taiwan)

DESCRIPTION

Meruvax II (rubella virus vaccine live) is a live virus vaccine for immunization against rubella (German measles).

Meruvax II is a sterile lyophilized preparation of the Wistar Institute RA 27/3 strain of live attenuated rubella virus. The virus was adapted to and propagated in human diploid cell (WI-38) culture.[1-2]

The reconstituted vaccine is for subcutaneous administration. When reconstituted as directed, the dose for injection is 0.5 ml and contains not less than the equivalent of 1,000 $TCID_{50}$ (tissue culture infectious doses) of the US Reference Rubella Virus. Each dose also contains approximately 25 µg of neomycin. The product contains no preservative. Sorbitol and hydrolyzed gelatin are added as stabilizers.

STORAGE

It is recommended that the vaccine be used as soon as possible after reconstitution. Protect vaccine from light at all times, since such exposure may inactivate the virus. Store reconstituted vaccine in the vaccine vial in a dark place at 2-8°C (36-46°F) and discard if not used within 8 hours.

INDICATIONS AND USAGE

(This section is based, in part, on the recommendation for rubella vaccine use of the Immunitazation Practices Advisory Committee (AICP), MMWR Report: 33 (22): 301-310, 315-318, June 8, 1984).

CHILDREN BETWEEN 12 MONTHS OF AGE AND PUBERTY

Meruvax II is indicated for immunization against rubella (German measles) in persons from 12 months of age to puberty. A booster is not needed. It is not recommended for infants younger than 12 months because they may retain maternal rubella neutralizing antibodies that may interfere with the immune response. Children in kindergarten and the first grades of elementary school deserve priority for vaccination because often they are epidemiologically the major source of virus dissemination in the community. A history of rubella illness is usually not reliable enough to exclude children from immunization.

Previously unimmunized children of susceptible pregnant women should receive live attenuated rubella vaccine, because an immunized child will be less likely to acquire natural rubella and introduce the virus into the household.

ADOLESCENT AND ADULT MALES

Vaccination of adolescent or adult males may be a useful procedure in preventing or controlling outbreaks of rubella in circumscribed population groups (*e.g.*, military bases and schools).

NON-PREGNANT ADOLESCENT AND ADULT FEMALES

Immunization of susceptible non-pregnant adolescent and adult females of childbearing age with live attenuated rubella virus vaccine is indicated if certain precautions are observed. Vaccinating susceptible postpubertal females confers individual protection against subsequently acquiring rubella infection during pregnancy, which in turn prevents infection of the fetus and consequent congenital rubella injury.[17]

Women of childbearing age should be advised not to become pregnant for 3 months after vaccination and should be informed of the reason for this precaution.*

It is recommended that rubella susceptibility be determined by serologic testing prior to immunization.† If immune, as evidenced by a specific rubella antibody titer of 1:8 or greater (hemagglutination-inhibition test), vaccination is unnecessary. Congenital malformations do occur in up to 7% of all live births.[18] Their chance appearance after vaccination could lead to misinterpretation of the cause, particularly if the prior rubella-immune status of vaccinees is unknown.

Postpubertal females should be informed of the frequent occurrence of generally self-limited arthralgia and/or arthritis beginning 2-4 weeks after vaccination.

POSTPARTUM WOMEN

It has been found convenient in many instances to vaccinate rubella susceptible women in the immediate postpartum period.

INTERNATIONAL TRAVELERS

Individuals planning travel outside the US, if not immune can acquire measles, mumps or rubella and import these diseases to the US. Therefore, prior to International travel, individuals known to be susceptible to one or more of these diseases can receive either a single antigen vaccine (measles, mumps or rubella), or a combined antigen vaccine as appropriate. However, M-M-R II (Measles Mumps, and Rubella Virus Vaccine Live) is preferred for persons likely to be susceptible to mumps and rubella; and if single-antigen measles vaccine is not readily available, travelers should receive M-M-R II (Measles, Mumps, and Rubella Virus Vaccine Live) regardless of their immune status to mumps or rubella.[19-21]

REVACCINATION

Children vaccinated when younger than 12 months of age should be revaccinated. Based on available evidence, there is no reason to routinely revaccinate persons who were vaccinated originally when 12 months of age or older. However, persons should be revaccinated if there is evidence to suggest that initial immunization was ineffective.

USE WITH OTHER VACCINES

Routine administration of DTP (diphtheria, tetanus, pertussis) and/or OPV (oral poliovirus vaccine) concomitantly with measles, mumps and rubella vaccines is not recommended because there are insufficient data relating to the simultaneous administration of these antigens. However, the American Academy of Pediatrics has noted that in some circumstances, particularly when the patient may not return, some practitioners prefer to administer all these antigens on a single day. If done, separate sites and syringes should be used for DTP and Meruvax II.[22]

Meruvax II should not be given less than 1 month before or after administration of other virus vaccines.

***NOTE:** The Immunization Practices Advisory Committee (ACIP) has recommended "In view of the importance of protecting this age group against rubella, reasonable precautions in a rubella immunization program include asking females if they are pregnant, excluding those who say they are, and explaining the theoretical risks to the others."[17]

†NOTE: The Immunization Practices Advisory Committee (ACIP) has stated "When practical, and when reliable laboratory services are available, potential vaccinees of childbearing age can have serologic tests to determine susceptibility to rubella.... However, routinely performing serologic tests for all females of childbearing age to determine susceptibility so that vaccine is given only to proven susceptibles is expensive and has been ineffective in some areas. Accordingly, the ACIP believes that rubella vaccination of a woman who is not known to be pregnant and has no history of vaccination is justifiable without serologic testing."[17]

CONTRAINDICATIONS

Do not give Meruvax II to pregnant females; the possible effects of the vaccine on fetal development are unknown at this time. If vaccination of postpubertal females is undertaken, pregnancy should be avoided for 3 months following vaccination

Anaphylactic or anaphylactoid reactions to neomycin (each dose of reconstituted vaccine contains approximately 25 µg of neomycin).

Any febrile respiratory illness or other active febrile infection.

Active untreated tuberculosis.

Patients receiving immunosuppressive therapy. This contraindication does not apply to patients who are receiving corticosteroids as replacement therapy, *e.g.,* for Addison's disease.

Individuals with blood dyscrasias, leukemia, lymphomas of any type, or other malignant neoplasms affecting the bone marrow or lymphatic systems.

Primary and acquired immunodeficiency states, including patients who are immunosuppressed in association with AIDS or other clinical manifestations of infection with human immunodeficiency viruses;[23,24] cellular immune deficiencies; and hypogammaglobulinemic and dysgammaglobulinemic states.

Individuals with a family history of congenital or hereditary immunodeficiency, until the immune competence of the potential vaccine recipient is demonstrated.[25]

DOSAGE AND ADMINISTRATION

FOR SUBCUTANEOUS ADMINISTRATION

Do not inject intravenously.

The dosage of vaccine is the same for all persons. Inject the total volume of the single dose vial (about 0.5 ml) or 0.5 ml of the multiple dose vial of reconstituted vaccine subcutaneously, preferably into the outer aspect of upper arm. **Do not give immune globulin (IG) concurrently with Meruvax II.**

To insure that there is no loss of potency during shipment, the vaccine must be maintained at a temperature of 10°C (50°F) or less.

Before reconstitution, store Meruvax II at 2-8°C (36-46°F). Protect from light.

CAUTION: A sterile syringe free of preservatives, antiseptics, and detergents should be used for each injection and/or reconstitution of the vaccine because these substances may inactivate the live virus vaccine. A 25 gauge, 5/8" needle is recommended.

To reconstitute, use only the diluent supplied, since it is free of preservatives or other antiviral substances which might inactivate the vaccine.

SINGLE DOSE VIAL

First withdraw the entire volume of diluent into the syringe to be used for reconstitution. Inject all the diluent in the syringe into the vial of lyophilized vaccine, and agitate to mix thoroughly. Withdraw the entire contents into a syringe and inject the total volume of restored vaccine subcutaneously.

It is important to use a separate sterile syringe and needle for each individual patient to prevent transmission of hepatitis B and other infectious agents from 1 person to another.

10 DOSE VIAL (AVAILABLE ONLY TO GOVERNMENT AGENCIES/INSTITUTIONS)

Withdraw the entire contents (7 ml) of the diluent vial into the sterile syringe to be used for reconstitution, and introduce into the 10 dose vial of lyophilized vaccine. Agitate to ensure thorough mixing. The outer labeling suggests "For Jet Injector or Syringe Use". Use with separate sterile syringes is permitted for containers of 10 doses or less. The vaccine and diluent do not contain preservatives; therefore, the user must recognize the potential contamination hazards and exercise special precautions to protect the sterility and potency of the product. The use of aseptic techniques and proper storage prior to and after restoration of the vaccine and subsequent withdrawal of the individual doses is essential. Use 0.5 ml of the reconstituted vaccine for subcutaneous injection.

It is important to use a separate sterile syringe and needle for each individual patient to prevent transmission of hepatitis B and other infectious agents from 1 person to another.

50 DOSE VIAL (AVAILABLE ONLY TO GOVERNMENT AGENCIES/INSTITUTIONS)

Withdraw the entire contents (30 ml) of diluent vial into the sterile syringe to be used for reconstitution and introduce into the 50 dose vial of lyophilized vaccine. Agitate to ensure thorough mixing. With full aseptic precautions, attach the vial to the sterilized multidose jet injector apparatus. Use 0.5 ml of the reconstituted vaccine for subcutaneous injection.

Each dose contains not less than the equivalent of 1000 $TCID_{50}$ of the US Reference Rubella Virus.

Parenteral drug products should be inspected visually for particulate matter and discoloration prior to administration. Meruvax II, when reconstituted, is clear yellow.

PRODUCT LISTING - EQUIVALENTS NOT AVAILABLE

Powder For Injection - Subcutaneous - Strength n/a

1's	$20.64	MERUVAX II, Merck & Company Inc	00006-4747-00
10's	$176.16	MERUVAX II, Merck & Company Inc	00006-4673-00

Salmeterol Xinafoate (003156)

For related information, see the comparative table section in Appendix A.

Categories: Asthma; Bronchospasm, exercise-induced; Chronic obstructive pulmonary disease; FDA Approved 1994 Feb; Pregnancy Category C; Patent Expiration 2012 Jan

Drug Classes: Adrenergic agonists; Bronchodilators

Brand Names: **Serevent**; Servent

Foreign Brand Availability: Aeromax (Germany); Salmeter (India); Seretide (Philippines); Serevent Inhaler and Disks (Australia); Serobid (India); Zamitrel (Mexico)

Cost of Therapy: $66.84 (Asthma; Serevent Aerosol; 21 µg/inh;13 g; 4 inhalations/day; 30 day supply)
$72.58 (Asthma; Serevent Diskus; 50 µg/inh; 2 inhalations/day; 30 day supply)

DESCRIPTION

SEREVENT INHALATION AEROSOL

Bronchodilator Aerosol.

For Oral Inhalation Only.

Serevent (salmeterol xinafoate) Inhalation Aerosol contains salmeterol xinafoate as the racemic form of the 1-hydroxy-2-naphthoic acid salt of salmeterol. The active component of the formulation is salmeterol base, a highly selective $beta_2$-adrenergic bronchodilator. The chemical name of salmeterol xinafoate is 4-hydroxy-α^1-[[[6-(4-phenylbutoxy) hexyl]amino]methyl]-1,3-benzenedimethanol, 1-hydroxy-2-naphthalenecarboxylate.

The molecular weight of salmeterol xinafoate is 603.8, and the empirical formula is $C_{25}H_{37}NO_4{\cdot}C_{11}H_8O_3$. Salmeterol xinafoate is a white to off-white powder. It is freely soluble in methanol; slightly soluble in ethanol, chloroform, and isopropanol; and sparingly soluble in water.

Serevent Inhalation Aerosol is a pressurized, metered-dose aerosol unit for oral inhalation. It contains a microcrystalline suspension of salmeterol xinafoate in a mixture of 2 chlorofluorocarbon propellants (trichlorofluoromethane and dichlorodifluoromethane) with lecithin. 36.25 µg of salmeterol xinafoate is equivalent to 25 µg of salmeterol base. Each actuation delivers 25 µg of salmeterol base (as salmeterol xinafoate) from the valve and 21 µg of salmeterol base (as salmeterol xinafoate) from the actuator. Each 6.5 g canister provides 60 inhalations and each 13 g canister provides 120 inhalations.

SEREVENT DISKUS INHALATION POWDER

FOR ORAL INHALATION ONLY.

Serevent Diskus (salmeterol xinafoate inhalation powder) contains salmeterol xinafoate as the racemic form of the 1-hydroxy-2-naphthoic acid salt of salmeterol. The active component of the formulation is salmeterol base, a highly selective $beta_2$-adrenergic bronchodilator. The chemical name of salmeterol xinafoate is 4-hydroxy-α^1-[[[6-(4-phenylbutoxy)hexyl]amino]methyl]-1,3-benzenedimethanol, 1-hydroxy-2-naphthalenecarboxylate.

Salmeterol xinafoate is a white to off-white powder with a molecular weight of 603.8, and the empirical formula is $C_{25}H_{37}NO_4{\cdot}C_{11}H_8O_3$. It is freely soluble in methanol; slightly soluble in ethanol, chloroform, and isopropanol; and sparingly soluble in water.

Serevent Diskus is a specially designed plastic inhalation delivery system containing a double-foil blister strip of a powder formulation of salmeterol xinafoate intended for oral inhalation only. The Diskus, which is the delivery component, is an integral part of the drug product. Each blister on the double-foil strip within the unit contains 50 µg of salmeterol administered as the salmeterol xinafoate salt in 12.5 mg of formulation containing lactose. After a blister containing medication is opened by activating the Diskus, the medication is dispersed into the airstream created by the patient inhaling through the mouthpiece.

Under standardized *in vitro* test conditions, Serevent Diskus delivers 47 μg when tested at a flow rate of 60 L/min for 2 seconds. In adult patients with obstructive lung disease and severely compromised lung function (mean forced expiratory volume in 1 second [FEV_1] 20-30% of predicted), mean peak inspiratory flow (PIF) through a Diskus was 82.4 L/min (range, 46.1-115.3 L/min).

The actual amount of drug delivered to the lung will depend on patient factors, such as inspiratory flow profile.

CLINICAL PHARMACOLOGY

SEREVENT INHALATION AEROSOL

Mechanism of Action

Salmeterol is a long-acting beta-adrenergic agonist. *In vitro* studies and *in vivo* pharmacologic studies demonstrate that salmeterol is selective for $beta_2$-adrenoceptors compared with isoproterenol, which has approximately equal agonist activity on $beta_1$- and $beta_2$-adrenoceptors. *In vitro* studies show salmeterol to be at least 50 times more selective for $beta_2$-adrenoceptors than albuterol. Although $beta_2$-adrenoceptors are the predominant adrenergic receptors in bronchial smooth muscle and $beta_1$-adrenoceptors are the predominant receptors in the heart, there are also $beta_2$-adrenoceptors in the human heart comprising 10-50% of the total beta-adrenoceptors. The precise function of these is not yet established, but they raise the possibility that even highly selective $beta_2$-agonists may have cardiac effects.

The pharmacologic effects of $beta_2$-adrenoceptor agonist drugs, including salmeterol, are at least in part attributable to stimulation of intracellular adenyl cyclase, the enzyme that catalyzes the conversion of adenosine triphosphate (ATP) to cyclic-3′,5′-adenosine monophosphate (cyclic AMP). Increased cyclic AMP levels cause relaxation of bronchial smooth muscle and inhibition of release of mediators of immediate hypersensitivity from cells, especially from mast cells.

In vitro tests show that salmeterol is a potent and long-lasting inhibitor of the release of mast cell mediators, such as histamine, leukotrienes, and prostaglandin D_2, from human lung. Salmeterol inhibits histamine-induced plasma protein extravasation and inhibits platelet activating factor-induced eosinophil accumulation in the lungs of guinea pigs when administered by the inhaled route. In humans, single doses of salmeterol attenuate allergen-induced bronchial hyper-responsiveness.

Pharmacokinetics

Salmeterol xinafoate, an ionic salt, dissociates in solution so that the salmeterol and 1-hydroxy-2-naphthoic acid (xinafoate) moieties are absorbed, distributed, metabolized, and excreted independently. Salmeterol acts locally in the lung; therefore, plasma levels do not predict therapeutic effect.

Absorption

Because of the small therapeutic dose, systemic levels of salmeterol are low or undetectable after inhalation of recommended doses (42 μg of salmeterol inhalation aerosol twice daily). Following chronic administration of an inhaled dose of 42 μg twice daily, salmeterol was detected in plasma within 5-10 minutes in 6 asthmatic patients; plasma concentrations were very low, with peak concentrations of 150 pg/ml and no accumulation with repeated doses. Larger inhaled doses gave approximately proportionally increased blood levels. In these patients, a second peak concentration of 115 pg/ml occurred at about 45 minutes, probably due to absorption of the swallowed portion of the dose (most of the dose delivered by a metered-dose inhaler is swallowed).

Distribution

Binding of salmeterol to human plasma proteins averages 96% *in vitro* over the concentration range of 8 to 7722 ng of salmeterol base per milliliter, much higher than those achieved following therapeutic doses of salmeterol.

Metabolism

Salmeterol base is extensively metabolized by hydroxylation, with subsequent elimination predominantly in the feces. No significant amount of unchanged salmeterol base was detected in either urine or feces.

Excretion

In 2 healthy subjects who received 1 mg of radiolabeled salmeterol (as salmeterol xinafoate) orally, approximately 25% and 60% of the radiolabeled salmeterol was eliminated in urine and feces, respectively, over a period of 7 days. The terminal elimination half-life was about 5.5 hours (1 volunteer only).

The xinafoate moiety has no apparent pharmacologic activity. The xinafoate moiety is highly protein bound (>99%) and has a long elimination half-life of 11 days.

Special Populations

The pharmacokinetics of salmeterol base has not been studied in elderly patients or in patients with hepatic or renal impairment. Since salmeterol is predominantly cleared by hepatic metabolism, liver function impairment may lead to accumulation of salmeterol in plasma. Therefore, patients with hepatic disease should be closely monitored.

Pharmacodynamics

Inhaled salmeterol, like other beta-adrenergic agonist drugs, can in some patients produce dose-related cardiovascular effects and effects on blood glucose and/or serum potassium (see PRECAUTIONS, Serevent Inhalation Aerosol). The cardiovascular effects (heart rate, blood pressure) associated with salmeterol occur with similar frequency, and are of similar type and severity, as those noted following albuterol administration.

The effects of rising doses of salmeterol and standard inhaled doses of albuterol were studied in volunteers and in patients with asthma. Salmeterol doses up to 84 μg administered as inhalation aerosol resulted in heart rate increases of 3-16 beats/min, about the same as albuterol dosed at 180 μg by inhalation aerosol (4-10 beats/min). In 2 double-blind asthma studies, patients receiving either 42 μg of salmeterol inhalation aerosol twice daily (n=81) or 180 μg of albuterol inhalation aerosol 4 times daily (n=80) underwent continuous electrocardiographic monitoring during four 24 hour periods; no clinically significant dysrhythmias were noted. Continuous electrocardiographic monitoring was also performed in 2 double-blind studies in COPD patients (see ADVERSE REACTIONS, Serevent Inhalation Aerosol).

Studies in laboratory animals (minipigs, rodents, and dogs) have demonstrated the occurrence of cardiac arrhythmias and sudden death (with histologic evidence of myocardial necrosis) when beta-agonists and methylxanthines are administered concurrently. The clinical significance of these findings is unknown.

SEREVENT DISKUS INHALATION POWDER

Mechanism of Action

Salmeterol is a selective, long-acting beta-adrenergic agonist. *In vitro* studies and *in vivo* pharmacologic studies demonstrate that salmeterol is selective for $beta_2$-adrenoceptors compared with isoproterenol, which has approximately equal agonist activity on $beta_1$- and $beta_2$-adrenoceptors. *In vitro* studies show salmeterol to be at least 50 times more selective for $beta_2$-adrenoceptors than albuterol. Although $beta_2$-adrenoceptors are the predominant adrenergic receptors in bronchial smooth muscle and $beta_1$-adrenoceptors are the predominant receptors in the heart, there are also $beta_2$-adrenoceptors in the human heart comprising 10-50% of the total beta-adrenoceptors. The precise function of these receptors has not been established, but they raise the possibility that even highly selective $beta_2$-agonists may have cardiac effects.

The pharmacologic effects of $beta_2$-adrenoceptor agonist drugs, including salmeterol, are at least in part attributable to stimulation of intracellular adenyl cyclase, the enzyme that catalyzes the conversion of adenosine triphosphate (ATP) to cyclic-3′,5′-adenosine monophosphate (cyclic AMP). Increased cyclic AMP levels cause relaxation of bronchial smooth muscle and inhibition of release of mediators of immediate hypersensitivity from cells, especially from mast cells.

In vitro tests show that salmeterol is a potent and long-lasting inhibitor of the release of mast cell mediators, such as histamine, leukotrienes, and prostaglandin D_2, from human lung. Salmeterol inhibits histamine-induced plasma protein extravasation and inhibits platelet-activating factor-induced eosinophil accumulation in the lungs of guinea pigs when administered by the inhaled route. In humans, single doses of salmeterol administered via inhalation aerosol attenuate allergen-induced bronchial hyper-responsiveness.

Pharmacokinetics

Salmeterol xinafoate, an ionic salt, dissociates in solution so that the salmeterol and 1-hydroxy-2-naphthoic acid (xinafoate) moieties are absorbed, distributed, metabolized, and excreted independently. Salmeterol acts locally in the lung; therefore, plasma levels do not predict therapeutic effect.

Absorption

Because of the small therapeutic dose, systemic levels of salmeterol are low or undetectable after inhalation of recommended doses (50 μg of salmeterol inhalation powder twice daily). Following chronic administration of an inhaled dose of 50 μg of salmeterol inhalation powder twice daily, salmeterol was detected in plasma within 5-45 minutes in 7 patients with asthma; plasma concentrations were very low, with mean peak concentrations of 167 pg/ml at 20 minutes and no accumulation with repeated doses.

Distribution

The percentage of salmeterol bound to human plasma proteins averages 96% *in vitro* over the concentration range of 8 to 7722 ng of salmeterol base per milliliter, much higher concentrations than those achieved following therapeutic doses of salmeterol.

Metabolism

Salmeterol base is extensively metabolized by hydroxylation, with subsequent elimination predominantly in the feces. No significant amount of unchanged salmeterol base has been detected in either urine or feces.

Elimination

In 2 healthy subjects who received 1 mg of radiolabeled salmeterol (as salmeterol xinafoate) orally, approximately 25% and 60% of the radiolabeled salmeterol was eliminated in urine and feces, respectively, over a period of 7 days. The terminal elimination half-life was about 5.5 hours (1 volunteer only).

The xinafoate moiety has no apparent pharmacologic activity. The xinafoate moiety is highly protein bound ((99%) and has a long elimination half-life of 11 days.

Special Populations

The pharmacokinetics of salmeterol base has not been studied in elderly patients nor in patients with hepatic or renal impairment. Since salmeterol is predominantly cleared by hepatic metabolism, liver function impairment may lead to accumulation of salmeterol in plasma. Therefore, patients with hepatic disease should be closely monitored.

Pharmacodynamics

Inhaled salmeterol, like other beta-adrenergic agonist drugs, can in some patients produce dose-related cardiovascular effects and effects on blood glucose and/or serum potassium (see PRECAUTIONS, Serevent Diskus Inhalation Powder). The cardiovascular effects (heart rate, blood pressure) associated with salmeterol inhalation aerosol occur with similar frequency, and are of similar type and severity, as those noted following albuterol administration.

The effects of rising doses of salmeterol and standard inhaled doses of albuterol were studied in volunteers and in patients with asthma. Salmeterol doses up to 84 μg administered as inhalation aerosol resulted in heart rate increases of 3-16 beats/min, about the same as albuterol dosed at 180 μg by inhalation aerosol (4-10 beats/min). Adolescent and adult patients receiving 50 μg doses of salmeterol inhalation powder (n=60) underwent continuous electrocardiographic monitoring during two 12 hour periods after the first dose and after 1 month of therapy, and no clinically significant dysrhythmias were noted. Also, pediatric patients receiving 50 μg doses of salmeterol inhalation powder (n=67) underwent continu-

S

ous electrocardiographic monitoring during two 12 hour periods after the first dose and after 3 months of therapy, and no clinically significant dysrhythmias were noted.

In 24 week clinical studies in patients with chronic obstructive pulmonary disease (COPD), the incidence of clinically significant abnormalities on the predose electrocardiograms (ECGs) at Weeks 12 and 24 in patients who received salmeterol 50 µg was not different compared with placebo.

No effect of treatment with salmeterol 50 µg was observed on pulse rate and systolic and diastolic blood pressure in a subset of patients with COPD who underwent 12 hour serial vital sign measurements after the first dose (n=91) and after 12 weeks of therapy (n=74). Median changes from baseline in pulse rate and systolic and diastolic blood pressure were similar for patients receiving either salmeterol or placebo (see ADVERSE REACTIONS, Serevent Diskus Inhalation Powder).

Studies in laboratory animals (minipigs, rodents, and dogs) have demonstrated the occurrence of cardiac arrhythmias and sudden death (with histologic evidence of myocardial necrosis) when beta-agonists and methylxanthines are administered concurrently. The clinical significance of these findings is unknown.

INDICATIONS AND USAGE

SEREVENT INHALATION AEROSOL

Asthma

Serevent Inhalation Aerosol is indicated for long-term, twice-daily (morning and evening) administration in the maintenance treatment of asthma and in the prevention of bronchospasm in patients 12 years of age and older with reversible obstructive airway disease, including patients with symptoms of nocturnal asthma, who require regular treatment with inhaled, short-acting beta$_2$-agonists. It should not be used in patients whose asthma can be managed by occasional use of inhaled, short-acting beta$_2$-agonists.

Serevent Inhalation Aerosol may be used alone or in combination with inhaled or systemic corticosteroid therapy.

Serevent Inhalation Aerosol is also indicated for prevention of exercise-induced bronchospasm in patients 12 years of age and older.

COPD

Serevent Inhalation Aerosol is indicated for long-term, twice daily (morning and evening) administration in the maintenance treatment of bronchospasm associated with COPD (including emphysema and chronic bronchitis).

SEREVENT DISKUS INHALATION POWDER

Asthma

Serevent Diskus is indicated for long-term, twice-daily (morning and evening) administration in the maintenance treatment of asthma and in the prevention of bronchospasm in patients 4 years of age and older with reversible obstructive airway disease, including patients with symptoms of nocturnal asthma, who require regular treatment with inhaled, short-acting beta$_2$-agonists. It is not indicated for patients whose asthma can be managed by occasional use of inhaled, short-acting beta$_2$-agonists.

Serevent Diskus is also indicated for prevention of exercise-induced bronchospasm in patients 4 years of age and older.

Serevent Diskus may be used alone or in combination with inhaled or systemic corticosteroid therapy.

Chronic Obstructive Pulmonary Disease (COPD)

Serevent Diskus is indicated for the long-term, twice-daily (morning and evening) administration in the maintenance treatment of bronchospasm associated with COPD (including emphysema and chronic bronchitis).

CONTRAINDICATIONS

SEREVENT INHALATION AEROSOL

Serevent Inhalation Aerosol is contraindicated in patients with a history of hypersensitivity to salmeterol or any of its components.

SEREVENT DISKUS INHALATION POWDER

Serevent Diskus is contraindicated in patients with a history of hypersensitivity to salmeterol or any other component of the drug product.

WARNINGS

SEREVENT INHALATION AEROSOL

IMPORTANT INFORMATION: SEREVENT INHALATION AEROSOL SHOULD NOT BE INITIATED IN PATIENTS WITH SIGNIFICANTLY WORSENING OR ACUTELY DETERIORATING ASTHMA, WHICH MAY BE A LIFE-THREATENING CONDITION. Serious acute respiratory events, including fatalities, have been reported, both in the US and worldwide, when Serevent Inhalation Aerosol has been initiated in this situation.

Although it is not possible from these reports to determine whether Serevent Inhalation Aerosol contributed to these adverse events or simply failed to relieve the deteriorating asthma, the use of Serevent Inhalation Aerosol in this setting is inappropriate.

SEREVENT INHALATION AEROSOL SHOULD NOT BE USED TO TREAT ACUTE SYMPTOMS. It is crucial to inform patients of this and prescribe an inhaled, short-acting beta$_2$-agonist for this purpose as well as warn them that increasing inhaled beta$_2$-agonist use is a signal of deteriorating asthma.

SEREVENT INHALATION AEROSOL IS NOT A SUBSTITUTE FOR INHALED OR ORAL CORTICOSTEROIDS. Corticosteroids should not be stopped or reduced when Serevent Inhalation Aerosol is initiated. (See PRECAUTIONS, Serevent Inhalation Aerosol, Information for the Patient and the accompanying PATIENT'S INSTRUCTIONS FOR USE.)

Do Not Introduce Serevent Inhalation Aerosol as a Treatment for Acutely Deteriorating Asthma: Serevent Inhalation Aerosol is intended for the maintenance treatment of asthma (see INDICATIONS AND USAGE, Serevent Inhalation Aerosol) and should not be introduced in acutely deteriorating asthma, which is a potentially life-threatening condition. There are no data demonstrating that Serevent Inhalation Aerosol provides greater efficacy than or additional efficacy to inhaled, short-acting beta$_2$-agonists in patients with worsening asthma. Serious acute respiratory events, including fatalities, have been reported, both in the US and worldwide, in patients receiving Serevent Inhalation Aerosol. In most cases, these have occurred in patients with severe asthma (*e.g.,* patients with a history of corticosteroid dependence, low pulmonary function, intubation, mechanical ventilation, frequent hospitalizations, or previous life-threatening acute asthma exacerbations) and/or in some patients in whom asthma has been acutely deteriorating (*e.g.,* unresponsive to usual medications; increasing need for inhaled, short-acting beta$_2$-agonists; increasing need for systemic corticosteroids; significant increase in symptoms; recent emergency room visits; sudden or progressive deterioration in pulmonary function). However, they have occurred in a few patients with less severe asthma as well. It was not possible from these reports to determine whether Serevent Inhalation Aerosol contributed to these events or simply failed to relieve the deteriorating asthma.

Do Not Use Serevent Inhalation Aerosol to Treat Acute Symptoms: An inhaled, short-acting beta$_2$-agonist, not Serevent Inhalation Aerosol, should be used to relieve acute asthma or COPD symptoms. When prescribing Serevent Inhalation Aerosol, the physician must also provide the patient with an inhaled, short-acting beta$_2$-agonist (*e.g.,* albuterol) for treatment of symptoms that occur acutely, despite regular twice-daily (morning and evening) use of Serevent Inhalation Aerosol.

When beginning treatment with Serevent Inhalation Aerosol, patients who have been taking inhaled, short-acting beta$_2$-agonists on a regular basis (*e.g.,* 4 times a day) should be instructed to discontinue the regular use of these drugs and use them only for symptomatic relief of acute asthma or COPD symptoms (see PRECAUTIONS, Serevent Inhalation Aerosol, Information for the Patient).

Watch for Increasing Use of Inhaled, Short-Acting beta$_2$-Agonists, Which Is a Marker of Deteriorating Asthma: Asthma may deteriorate acutely over a period of hours or chronically over several days or longer. If the patient's inhaled, short-acting beta$_2$-agonist becomes less effective or the patient needs more inhalations than usual, this may be a marker of destabilization of asthma. In this setting, the patient requires immediate reevaluation with reassessment of the treatment regimen, giving special consideration to the possible need for corticosteroids. If the patient uses 4 or more inhalations per day of an inhaled, short-acting beta$_2$-agonist for 2 or more consecutive days, or if more than 1 canister (200 inhalations per canister) of inhaled, short-acting beta$_2$-agonist is used in an 8 week period in conjunction with Serevent Inhalation Aerosol, then the patient should consult the physician for reevaluation. **Increasing the daily dosage of Serevent Inhalation Aerosol in this situation is not appropriate. Serevent Inhalation Aerosol should not be used more frequently than twice daily (morning and evening) at the recommended dose of 2 inhalations.**

Do Not Use Serevent Inhalation Aerosol as a Substitute for Oral or Inhaled Corticosteroids: The use of beta-adrenergic agonist bronchodilators alone may not be adequate to control asthma in many patients. Early consideration should be given to adding anti-inflammatory agents, *e.g.,* corticosteroids. There are no data demonstrating that Serevent Inhalation Aerosol has a clinical anti-inflammatory effect and could be expected to take the place of corticosteroids. Patients who already require oral or inhaled corticosteroids for treatment of asthma should be continued on this type of treatment even if they feel better as a result of initiating Serevent Inhalation Aerosol. Any change in corticosteroid dosage should be made ONLY after clinical evaluation (see PRECAUTIONS, Serevent Inhalation Aerosol, Information for the Patient).

Do Not Exceed Recommended Dosage: As with other inhaled beta$_2$-adrenergic drugs, Serevent Inhalation Aerosol should not be used more often or at higher doses than recommended. Fatalities have been reported in association with excessive use of inhaled sympathomimetic drugs. Large doses of inhaled or oral salmeterol (12-20 times the recommended dose) have been associated with clinically significant prolongation of the QTc interval, which has the potential for producing ventricular arrhythmias.

Paradoxical Bronchospasm: Serevent Inhalation Aerosol can produce paradoxical bronchospasm, which may be life threatening. If paradoxical bronchospasm occurs, Serevent Inhalation Aerosol should be discontinued immediately and alternative therapy instituted. It should be recognized that paradoxical bronchospasm, when associated with inhaled formulations, frequently occurs with the first use of a new canister or vial.

Immediate Hypersensitivity Reactions: Immediate hypersensitivity reactions may occur after administration of Serevent Inhalation Aerosol, as demonstrated by rare cases of urticaria, angioedema, rash, and bronchospasm.

Upper Airway Symptoms: Symptoms of laryngeal spasm, irritation, or swelling, such as stridor and choking, have been reported rarely in patients receiving Serevent Inhalation Aerosol.

Serevent Inhalation Aerosol, like all other beta-adrenergic agonists, can produce a clinically significant cardiovascular effect in some patients as measured by pulse rate, blood pressure, and/or symptoms. Although such effects are uncommon after administration of Serevent Inhalation Aerosol at recommended doses, if they occur, the drug may need to be discontinued. In addition, beta-agonists have been reported to produce electrocardiogram (ECG) changes, such as flattening of the T wave, prolongation of the QTc interval, and ST segment depression. The clinical significance of these findings is unknown. Therefore, Serevent Inhalation Aerosol, like all sympathomimetic amines, should be used with caution in patients with cardiovascular disorders, especially coronary insufficiency, cardiac arrhythmias, and hypertension.

SEREVENT DISKUS INHALATION POWDER

IMPORTANT INFORMATION: SEREVENT DISKUS SHOULD NOT BE INITIATED IN PATIENTS WITH SIGNIFICANTLY WORSENING OR ACUTELY DETERIORATING ASTHMA, WHICH MAY BE A LIFE-THREATENING CONDITION. Serious acute respiratory events, including fatalities, have been re-

ported both in the US and worldwide when Serevent has been initiated in this situation.

Although it is not possible from these reports to determine whether Serevent contributed to these adverse events or simply failed to relieve the deteriorating asthma, the use of Serevent Diskus in this setting is inappropriate.

SEREVENT DISKUS SHOULD NOT BE USED TO TREAT ACUTE SYMPTOMS. It is crucial to inform patients of this and prescribe an inhaled, short-acting beta$_2$-agonist for this purpose as well as warn them that increasing inhaled beta$_2$-agonist use is a signal of deteriorating asthma.

SEREVENT DISKUS IS NOT A SUBSTITUTE FOR INHALED OR ORAL CORTICOSTEROIDS. Corticosteroids should not be stopped or reduced when Serevent Diskus is initiated.

(See PRECAUTIONS, Serevent Diskus Inhalation Powder, Information for the Patient and the accompanying Patient's Instructions for Use.)

Do Not Introduce Serevent Diskus as a Treatment for Acutely Deteriorating Asthma: Serevent Diskus is intended for the maintenance treatment of asthma (see INDICATIONS AND USAGE, Serevent Diskus Inhalation Powder) and should not be introduced in acutely deteriorating asthma, which is a potentially life-threatening condition. There are no data demonstrating that Serevent Diskus provides greater efficacy than or additional efficacy to inhaled, short-acting beta$_2$-agonists in patients with worsening asthma. Serious acute respiratory events, including fatalities, have been reported both in the US and worldwide in patients receiving Serevent. In most cases, these have occurred in patients with severe asthma (*e.g.*, patients with a history of corticosteroid dependence, low pulmonary function, intubation, mechanical ventilation, frequent hospitalizations, or previous life-threatening acute asthma exacerbations) and/or in some patients in whom asthma has been acutely deteriorating (*e.g.*, unresponsive to usual medications; increasing need for inhaled, short-acting beta$_2$-agonists; increasing need for systemic corticosteroids; significant increase in symptoms; recent emergency room visits; sudden or progressive deterioration in pulmonary function). However, they have occurred in a few patients with less severe asthma as well. It was not possible from these reports to determine whether Serevent contributed to these events or simply failed to relieve the deteriorating asthma.

Do Not Use Serevent Diskus to Treat Acute Symptoms: An inhaled, short-acting beta$_2$-agonist, not Serevent Diskus, should be used to relieve acute asthma or COPD symptoms. When prescribing Serevent Diskus, the physician must also provide the patient with an inhaled, short-acting beta$_2$-agonist (*e.g.*, albuterol) for treatment of symptoms that occur acutely, despite regular twice-daily (morning and evening) use of Serevent Diskus.

When beginning treatment with Serevent Diskus, patients who have been taking inhaled, short-acting beta$_2$-agonists on a regular basis (*e.g.*, 4 times a day) should be instructed to discontinue the regular use of these drugs and use them only for symptomatic relief of acute asthma or COPD symptoms (see PRECAUTIONS, Serevent Diskus Inhalation Powder, Information for the Patient).

Watch for Increasing Use of Inhaled, Short-Acting beta$_2$-Agonists, Which Is a Marker of Deteriorating Asthma or COPD: The patient's condition may deteriorate acutely over a period of hours or chronically over several days or longer. If the patient's inhaled, short-acting beta$_2$-agonist becomes less effective or the patient needs more inhalations than usual, or the patient develops a significant decrease in PEF or lung function, these may be markers of destabilization of their disease. In this setting, the patient requires immediate reevaluation with reassessment of the treatment regimen, giving special consideration to the possible need for corticosteroids. If the patient uses 4 or more inhalations per day of an inhaled, short-acting beta$_2$-agonist for 2 or more consecutive days, or if more than 1 canister (200 inhalations per canister) of inhaled, short-acting beta$_2$-agonist is used in an 8 week period in conjunction with Serevent Diskus, then the patient should consult the physician for reevaluation. **Increasing the daily dosage of Serevent Diskus in this situation is not appropriate. Serevent Diskus should not be used more frequently than twice daily (morning and evening) at the recommended dose of 1 inhalation.**

Do Not Use Serevent Diskus as a Substitute for Oral or Inhaled Corticosteroids: The use of beta-adrenergic agonist bronchodilators alone may not be adequate to control asthma in many patients. Early consideration should be given to adding anti-inflammatory agents, *e.g.*, corticosteroids. There are no data demonstrating that Serevent Diskus has a clinical anti-inflammatory effect and could be expected to take the place of corticosteroids. Patients who already require oral or inhaled corticosteroids for treatment of asthma should be continued on a suitable dose to maintain clinical stability even if they feel better as a result of initiating Serevent Diskus. Any change in corticosteroid dosage should be made ONLY after clinical evaluation (see PRECAUTIONS, Serevent Diskus Inhalation Powder, Information for the Patient).

Do Not Exceed Recommended Dosage: As with other inhaled beta$_2$-adrenergic drugs, Serevent Diskus should not be used more often or at higher doses than recommended. Fatalities have been reported in association with excessive use of inhaled sympathomimetic drugs. Large doses of inhaled or oral salmeterol (12-20 times the recommended dose) have been associated with clinically significant prolongation of the QTc interval, which has the potential for producing ventricular arrhythmias.

Paradoxical Bronchospasm: As with other inhaled asthma and COPD medications, Serevent Diskus can produce paradoxical bronchospasm, which may be life threatening. If paradoxical bronchospasm occurs following dosing with Serevent Diskus, it should be treated with a short-acting, inhaled bronchodilator; Serevent Diskus should be discontinued immediately; and alternative therapy should be instituted.

Immediate Hypersensitivity Reactions: Immediate hypersensitivity reactions may occur after administration of Serevent Diskus, as demonstrated by cases of urticaria, angioedema, rash, and bronchospasm.

Upper Airway Symptoms: Symptoms of laryngeal spasm, irritation, or swelling, such as stridor and choking, have been reported in patients receiving Serevent Diskus.

Cardiovascular Disorders: Serevent Diskus, like all sympathomimetic amines, should be used with caution in patients with cardiovascular disorders, especially coronary insufficiency, cardiac arrhythmias, and hypertension. Serevent Diskus, like all other beta-adrenergic agonists, can produce a clinically significant cardiovascular effect in some patients as measured by pulse rate, blood pressure, and/or symptoms. Although such effects are uncommon after administration of Serevent Diskus at recommended doses, if they occur, the drug may need to be discontinued. In addition, beta-agonists have been reported to produce electrocardiogram (ECG) changes, such as flattening of the T wave, prolongation of the QTc interval, and ST segment depression. The clinical significance of these findings is unknown.

PRECAUTIONS

SEREVENT INHALATION AEROSOL

General

Use With Spacer or Other Devices: The safety and effectiveness of Serevent Inhalation Aerosol when used with a spacer or other devices have not been adequately studied.

Cardiovascular and Other Effects: No effect on the cardiovascular system is usually seen after the administration of inhaled salmeterol in recommended doses, but the cardiovascular and central nervous system effects seen with all sympathomimetic drugs (*e.g.*, increased blood pressure, heart rate, excitement) can occur after use of salmeterol and may require discontinuation of the drug. Salmeterol, like all sympathomimetic amines, should be used with caution in patients with cardiovascular disorders, especially coronary insufficiency, cardiac arrhythmias, and hypertension; in patients with convulsive disorders or thyrotoxicosis; and in patients who are unusually responsive to sympathomimetic amines.

As has been described with other beta-adrenergic agonist bronchodilators, clinically significant changes in systolic and/or diastolic blood pressure, pulse rate, and electrocardiograms have been seen infrequently in individual patients in controlled clinical studies with salmeterol.

Metabolic Effects: Doses of the related beta$_2$-adrenoceptor agonist albuterol, when administered intravenously, have been reported to aggravate preexisting diabetes mellitus and ketoacidosis. No effects on glucose have been seen with Serevent Inhalation Aerosol at recommended doses. Beta-adrenergic agonist medications may produce significant hypokalemia in some patients, possibly through intracellular shunting, which has the potential to produce adverse cardiovascular effects. The decrease is usually transient, not requiring supplementation.

Clinically significant changes in blood glucose and/or serum potassium were seen rarely during clinical studies with long-term administration of Serevent Inhalation Aerosol at recommended doses.

Information for the Patient

See illustrated PATIENT'S INSTRUCTIONS FOR USE. **SHAKE WELL BEFORE USING.**

It is important that patients understand how to use Serevent Inhalation Aerosol appropriately and how it should be used in relation to other asthma or COPD medications they are taking. Patients should be given the following information:

Shake well before using.

The action of Serevent Inhalation Aerosol may last up to 12 hours or longer. The recommended dosage (2 inhalations twice daily, morning and evening) should not be exceeded.

Serevent Inhalation Aerosol is not meant to relieve acute asthma or COPD symptoms and extra doses should not be used for that purpose. Acute symptoms should be treated with an inhaled, short-acting beta$_2$-agonist such as albuterol (the physician should provide the patient with such medication and instruct the patient in how it should be used).

Patients should not stop Serevent therapy for COPD without physician/provider guidance since symptoms may recur after discontinuation.

The physician should be notified immediately if any of the following situations occur, which may be a sign of seriously worsening asthma.

- Decreasing effectiveness of inhaled, short-acting beta$_2$-agonists.
- Need for more inhalations than usual of inhaled, short-acting beta$_2$-agonists.
- Use of 4 or more inhalations per day of a short-acting beta$_2$-agonist for 2 or more days consecutively.
- Use of more than one 200 inhalation canister of an inhaled, short-acting beta$_2$-agonist (*e.g.*, albuterol) in an 8 week period.

Serevent Inhalation Aerosol should not be used as a substitute for oral or inhaled corticosteroids. The dosage of these medications should not be changed and they should not be stopped without consulting the physician, even if the patient feels better after initiating treatment with Serevent Inhalation Aerosol.

Patients should be cautioned regarding common adverse cardiovascular effects, such as palpitations, chest pain, rapid heart rate, tremor, or nervousness.

In patients receiving Serevent Inhalation Aerosol, other inhaled medications should be used only as directed by the physician.

When using Serevent Inhalation Aerosol to prevent exercise-induced bronchospasm, patients should take the dose at least 30-60 minutes before exercise.

If you are pregnant or nursing, contact your physician about use of Serevent Inhalation Aerosol.

Effective and safe use of Serevent Inhalation Aerosol includes an understanding of the way that it should be administered.

Carcinogenesis, Mutagenesis, and Impairment of Fertility

In an 18 month oral carcinogenicity study in CD-mice, salmeterol xinafoate at oral doses of 1.4 mg/kg and above (approximately 9 times the maximum recommended daily inhalation dose in adults based on comparison of the areas under the plasma concentration versus time curves [AUCs]) caused dose-related increases in the incidence of smooth muscle hyperplasia, cystic glandular hyperplasia, leiomyomas of the uterus, and cysts in the ovaries. The incidence of leiomyosarcomas was not statistically significant. No tumors were seen at 0.2 mg/kg (comparable to the maximum recommended human daily inhalation dose in adults based on comparison of the AUCs).

In a 24 month inhalation and oral carcinogenicity study in Sprague Dawley rats, salmeterol caused dose-related increases in the incidence of mesovarian leiomyomas and ovarian

S

cysts at inhalation and oral doses of 0.68 mg/kg/day and above (approximately 55 times the maximum recommended human daily inhalation dose in adults on a mg/m^2 basis). No tumors were seen at 0.21 mg/kg/day (approximately 15 times the maximum recommended human daily inhalation dose in adults on a mg/m^2 basis). These findings in rodents are similar to those reported previously for other beta-adrenergic agonist drugs. The relevance of these findings to human use is unknown.

Salmeterol xinafoate produced no detectable or reproducible increases in microbial and mammalian gene mutation *in vitro*. No clastogenic activity occurred *in vitro* in human lymphocytes or *in vivo* in a rat micronucleus test. No effects on fertility were identified in male and female rats treated orally with salmeterol xinafoate at doses up to 2 mg/kg (approximately 160 times the maximum recommended human daily inhalation dose in adults on a mg/m^2 basis).

Pregnancy, Teratogenic Effects, Pregnancy Category C

No teratogenic effects occurred in the rat at oral doses up to 2 mg/kg (approximately 160 times the maximum recommended human daily inhalation dose in adults on a mg/m^2 basis). In pregnant Dutch rabbits administered oral doses of 1 mg/kg and above (approximately 20 times the maximum recommended human daily inhalation dose in adults based on the comparison of the AUCs), salmeterol xinafoate exhibited fetal toxic effects characteristically resulting from beta-adrenoceptor stimulation; these included precocious eyelid openings, cleft palate, sternebral fusion, limb and paw flexures, and delayed ossification of the frontal cranial bones. No significant effects occurred at an oral dose of 0.6 mg/kg (approximately 10 times the maximum recommended human daily inhalation dose in adults based on comparison of the AUCs).

New Zealand White rabbits were less sensitive since only delayed ossification of the frontal cranial bones was seen at oral doses of 10 mg/kg (approximately 1600 times the maximum recommended human daily inhalation dose on a mg/m^2 basis). Extensive use of other beta-agonists has provided no evidence that these class effects in animals are relevant to use in humans. There are no adequate and well-controlled studies with Serevent Inhalation Aerosol in pregnant women. Serevent Inhalation Aerosol should be used during pregnancy only if the potential benefit justifies the potential risk to the fetus.

Use in Labor and Delivery

There are no well-controlled human studies that have investigated effects of salmeterol on preterm labor or labor at term. Because of the potential for beta-agonist interference with uterine contractility, use of Serevent Inhalation Aerosol for prevention of bronchospasm during labor should be restricted to those patients in whom the benefits clearly outweigh the risks.

Nursing Mothers

Plasma levels of salmeterol after inhaled therapeutic doses are very low. In rats, salmeterol xinafoate is excreted in milk. However, since there is no experience with use of Serevent Inhalation Aerosol by nursing mothers, a decision should be made whether to discontinue nursing or to discontinue the drug, taking into account the importance of the drug to the mother. Caution should be exercised when salmeterol xinafoate is administered to a nursing woman.

Pediatric Use

The safety and effectiveness of Serevent Inhalation Aerosol in children younger than 12 years of age have not been established.

Geriatric Use

Of the total number of patients who received Serevent Inhalation Aerosol in all asthma clinical studies, 241 were 65 years of age and older. Geriatric patients (65 years and older) with reversible obstructive airway disease were evaluated in 4 well-controlled studies of 3 weeks' to 3 months' duration. Two placebo-controlled, crossover studies evaluated twice-daily dosing with salmeterol for 21-28 days in 45 patients. An additional 75 geriatric patients were treated with salmeterol for 3 months in 2 large parallel group, multicenter studies. These 120 patients experienced increases in AM and PM peak expiratory flow rate and decreases in diurnal variation in peak expiratory flow rate similar to responses seen in the total populations of the 2 latter studies. The adverse event type and frequency in geriatric patients were not different from those of the total populations studied.

In 2 large, randomized, double-blind, placebo-controlled 3 month studies involving patients with COPD, 133 patients using Serevent Inhalation Aerosol were 65 years and older. These patients experienced similar improvements in FEV_1 as observed for patients younger than 65.

No apparent differences in the efficacy and safety of Serevent Inhalation Aerosol were observed when geriatric patients were compared with younger patients in asthma and COPD clinical trials. As with other $beta_2$-agonists, however, special caution should be observed when using Serevent Inhalation Aerosol in geriatric patients who have concomitant cardiovascular disease that could be adversely affected by this class of drug. Based on available data, no adjustment of salmeterol dosage in geriatric patients is warranted.

SEREVENT DISKUS INHALATION POWDER

General

Cardiovascular and Other Effects

No effect on the cardiovascular system is usually seen after the administration of inhaled salmeterol at recommended doses, but the cardiovascular and central nervous system effects seen with all sympathomimetic drugs (*e.g.*, increased blood pressure, heart rate, excitement) can occur after use of salmeterol and may require discontinuation of the drug. Salmeterol, like all sympathomimetic amines, should be used with caution in patients with cardiovascular disorders, especially coronary insufficiency, cardiac arrhythmias, and hypertension; in patients with convulsive disorders or thyrotoxicosis; and in patients who are unusually responsive to sympathomimetic amines.

As has been described with other beta-adrenergic agonist bronchodilators, clinically significant changes in systolic and/or diastolic blood pressure, pulse rate, and electrocardiograms have been seen infrequently in individual patients in controlled clinical studies with salmeterol.

Metabolic Effects

Doses of the related $beta_2$-adrenoceptor agonist albuterol, when administered intravenously, have been reported to aggravate preexisting diabetes mellitus and ketoacidosis. Beta-adrenergic agonist medications may produce significant hypokalemia in some patients, possibly through intracellular shunting, which has the potential to produce adverse cardiovascular effects. The decrease in serum potassium is usually transient, not requiring supplementation.

Clinically significant changes in blood glucose and/or serum potassium were seen rarely during clinical studies with long-term administration of salmeterol at recommended doses.

Information for the Patient

Patients being treated with Serevent Diskus should receive the following information and instructions. This information is intended to aid them in the safe and effective use of this medication. It is not a disclosure of all possible adverse or intended effects.

It is important that patients understand how to use the Diskus appropriately and how to use Serevent Diskus in relation to other asthma or COPD medications they are taking. Patients should be given the following information:

The action of Serevent Diskus may last up to 12 hours or longer. The recommended dosage (1 inhalation twice daily, morning and evening) should not be exceeded.

Serevent Diskus is not meant to relieve acute asthma or COPD symptoms and extra doses should not be used for that purpose. Acute symptoms should be treated with an inhaled, short-acting bronchodilator (the physician should provide the patient with such medication and instruct the patient in how it should be used).

Patients should not stop therapy with Serevent Diskus without physician/provider guidance since symptoms may worsen after discontinuation.

When used for the treatment of EIB, 1 inhalation of Serevent Diskus should be taken 30 minutes before exercise.

- Additional doses of Serevent should not be used for 12 hours.
- Patients who are receiving Serevent Diskus twice daily should not use additional Serevent for prevention of EIB.

The physician should be notified immediately if any of the following situations occur, which may be a sign of seriously worsening asthma or COPD:

- Decreasing effectiveness of inhaled, short-acting $beta_2$-agonists,
- Need for more inhalations than usual of inhaled, short-acting $beta_2$-agonists,
- Significant decrease in PEF or lung function as outlined by the physician,
- Use of 4 or more inhalations per day of a short-acting $beta_2$-agonist for 2 or more days consecutively,
- Use of more than 1 canister (200 inhalations per canister) of an inhaled, short-acting $beta_2$-agonist in an 8 week period.

Serevent Diskus should not be used as a substitute for oral or inhaled corticosteroids. The dosage of these medications should not be changed and they should not be stopped without consulting the physician, even if the patient feels better after initiating treatment with Serevent Diskus.

Patients should be cautioned regarding adverse effects associated with $beta_2$-agonists, such as palpitations, chest pain, rapid heart rate, tremor, or nervousness.

When patients are prescribed Serevent Diskus, other medications for asthma and COPD should be used only as directed by the physician.

Serevent Diskus should not be used with a spacer device.

If you are pregnant or nursing, contact your physician about the use of Serevent Diskus.

Effective and safe use of Serevent Diskus includes an understanding of the way that it should be used:

- Never exhale into the Diskus.
- Never attempt to take the Diskus apart.
- Always activate and use the Diskus in a level, horizontal position.
- Never wash the mouthpiece or any part of the Diskus. KEEP IT DRY.
- Always keep the Diskus in a dry place.
- Discard **6 weeks** after removal from the moisture-protective foil overwrap pouch or after all blisters have been used (when the dose indicator reads "0"), whichever comes first.

For the proper use of Serevent Diskus and to attain maximum benefit, the patient should read and follow carefully the Patient's Instructions for Use accompanying the product.

Carcinogenesis, Mutagenesis, and Impairment of Fertility

In an 18 month carcinogenicity study in CD-mice, salmeterol xinafoate at oral doses of 1.4 mg/kg and above (approximately 20 times the maximum recommended daily inhalation dose in adults and children based on comparison of the area under the plasma concentration versus time curves [AUCs]) caused a dose-related increase in the incidence of smooth muscle hyperplasia, cystic glandular hyperplasia, leiomyomas of the uterus, and cysts in the ovaries. The incidence of leiomyosarcomas was not statistically significant. No tumors were seen at 0.2 mg/kg (approximately 3 times the maximum recommended daily inhalation doses in adults and children based on comparison of the AUCs).

In a 24 month oral and inhalation carcinogenicity study in Sprague Dawley rats, salmeterol caused a dose-related increase in the incidence of mesovarian leiomyomas and ovarian cysts at doses of 0.68 mg/kg and above (approximately 55 times the maximum recommended daily inhalation dose in adults and approximately 25 times the maximum recommended daily inhalation dose in children on a mg/m^2 basis). No tumors were seen at 0.21 mg/kg (approximately 15 times the maximum recommended daily inhalation dose in adults and approximately 8 times the maximum recommended daily inhalation dose in children on a mg/m^2 basis). These findings in rodents are similar to those reported previously for other beta-adrenergic agonist drugs. The relevance of these findings to human use is unknown.

Salmeterol produced no detectable or reproducible increases in microbial and mammalian gene mutation *in vitro*. No clastogenic activity occurred *in vitro* in human lymphocytes or *in vivo* in a rat micronucleus test. No effects on fertility were identified in male and female rats treated with salmeterol at oral doses up to 2 mg/kg (approximately 160 times the maximum recommended daily inhalation dose in adults on a mg/m^2 basis).

Pregnancy, Teratogenic Effects, Pregnancy Category C

No teratogenic effects occurred in rats at oral doses up to 2 mg/kg (approximately 160 times the maximum recommended daily inhalation dose in adults on a mg/m^2 basis). In pregnant Dutch rabbits administered oral doses of 1 mg/kg and above (approximately 50 times the maximum recommended daily inhalation dose in adults based on comparison of the AUCs), salmeterol exhibited fetal toxic effects characteristically resulting from beta-adrenoceptor stimulation. These included precocious eyelid openings, cleft palate, sternebral fusion, limb and paw flexures, and delayed ossification of the frontal cranial bones. No significant effects occurred at an oral dose of 0.6 mg/kg (approximately 20 times the maximum recommended daily inhalation dose in adults based on comparison of the AUCs).

New Zealand White rabbits were less sensitive since only delayed ossification of the frontal bones was seen at an oral dose of 10 mg/kg (approximately 1600 times the maximum recommended daily inhalation dose in adults on a mg/m^2 basis). Extensive use of other beta-agonists has provided no evidence that these class effects in animals are relevant to their use in humans. There are no adequate and well-controlled studies with Serevent Diskus in pregnant women. Serevent Diskus should be used during pregnancy only if the potential benefit justifies the potential risk to the fetus.

Salmeterol xinafoate crossed the placenta following oral administration of 10 mg/kg to mice and rats (approximately 410 and 810 times, respectively, the maximum recommended daily inhalation dose in adults on a mg/m^2 basis).

Use in Labor and Delivery

There are no well-controlled human studies that have investigated effects of salmeterol on preterm labor or labor at term. Because of the potential for beta-agonist interference with uterine contractility, use of Serevent Diskus during labor should be restricted to those patients in whom the benefits clearly outweigh the risks.

Nursing Mothers

Plasma levels of salmeterol after inhaled therapeutic doses are very low. In rats, salmeterol xinafoate is excreted in the milk. However, since there are no data from controlled trials on the use of salmeterol by nursing mothers, a decision should be made whether to discontinue nursing or to discontinue Serevent Diskus, taking into account the importance of Serevent Diskus to the mother. Caution should be exercised when Serevent Diskus is administered to a nursing woman.

Pediatric Use

The safety and efficacy of salmeterol inhalation powder has been evaluated in over 2500 patients aged 4-11 years with asthma, 346 of whom were administered salmeterol inhalation powder for 1 year. Based on available data, no adjustment of salmeterol dosage in pediatric patients is warranted for either asthma or EIB (see DOSAGE AND ADMINISTRATION, Serevent Diskus Inhalation Powder).

In 2 randomized, double-blind, controlled clinical trials of 12 weeks' duration, salmeterol 50 µg powder was administered to 211 pediatric asthma patients who did and who did not receive concurrent inhaled corticosteroids. The efficacy of salmeterol inhalation powder was demonstrated over the 12 week treatment period with respect to PEF and FEV_1. Salmeterol inhalation powder was effective in demographic subgroups (gender and age) of the population. Salmeterol was effective when coadministered with other inhaled asthma medications, such as short-acting bronchodilators and inhaled corticosteroids. Salmeterol inhalation powder was well tolerated in the pediatric population, and there were no safety issues identified specific to the administration of salmeterol inhalation powder to pediatric patients.

In 2 randomized studies in children 4-11 years old with asthma and EIB, a single 50 µg dose of salmeterol inhalation powder prevented EIB when dosed 30 minutes prior to exercise, with protection lasting up to 11.5 hours in repeat testing following this single dose in many patients.

Geriatric Use

Of the total number of adolescent and adult patients with asthma who received salmeterol inhalation powder in chronic dosing clinical trials, 209 were 65 years of age and older. Of the total number of patients with COPD who received salmeterol inhalation powder in chronic dosing clinical trials, 167 were 65 years of age or older and 45 were 75 years of age or older. No apparent differences in the safety of Serevent inhalation powder were observed when geriatric patients were compared with younger patients in clinical trials. As with other $beta_2$-agonists, however, special caution should be observed when using Serevent Diskus in geriatric patients who have concomitant cardiovascular disease that could be adversely affected by this class of drug. Data from the trials in patients with COPD suggested a greater effect on FEV_1 of salmeterol inhalation powder in the <65 years age-group, as compared with the ≥ 65 years age-group. However, based on available data, no adjustment of salmeterol dosage in geriatric patients is warranted.

DRUG INTERACTIONS

SEREVENT INHALATION AEROSOL

Short-Acting Beta-Agonists

In the two 3 month, repetitive-dose clinical asthma trials (n=184), the mean daily need for additional $beta_2$-agonist use was 1 to 1½ inhalations per day, but some patients used more. Eight percent (8%) of patients used at least 8 inhalations per day at least on 1 occasion. Six percent (6%) used 9-12 inhalations at least once. There were 15 patients (8%) who averaged over 4 inhalations per day. Four of these used an average of 8-11 inhalations per day. In these 15 patients there was no observed increase in frequency of cardiovascular adverse events. The safety of concomitant use of more than 8 inhalations per day of short-acting $beta_2$-agonists with Serevent Inhalation Aerosol has not been established. In 15 patients who experienced worsening of asthma while receiving Serevent Inhalation Aerosol, nebulized albuterol (1 dose in most) led to improvement in FEV_1 and no increase in occurrence of cardiovascular adverse events.

Monoamine Oxidase Inhibitors and Tricyclic Antidepressants

Salmeterol should be administered with extreme caution to patients being treated with monoamine oxidase inhibitors or tricyclic antidepressants, or within 2 weeks of discontinuation of such agents, because the action of salmeterol on the vascular system may be potentiated by these agents.

Corticosteroids and Cromoglycate

In clinical trials, inhaled corticosteroids and/or inhaled cromolyn sodium did not alter the safety profile of Serevent Inhalation Aerosol when administered concurrently.

Methylxanthines

The concurrent use of intravenously or orally administered methylxanthines (*e.g.*, aminophylline, theophylline) by patients receiving Serevent Inhalation Aerosol has not been completely evaluated. In 1 clinical asthma trial, 87 patients receiving Serevent Inhalation Aerosol 42 µg twice daily concurrently with a theophylline product had adverse event rates similar to those in 71 patients receiving Serevent Inhalation Aerosol without theophylline. Resting heart rates were slightly higher in the patients on theophylline but were little affected by Serevent Inhalation Aerosol therapy.

Beta-adrenergic receptor blocking agents not only block the pulmonary effect of beta-agonists, such as Serevent Inhalation Aerosol, but may also produce severe bronchospasm in asthmatic patients. Therefore, patients with asthma should not normally be treated with beta-blockers. However, under certain circumstances, *e.g.*, as prophylaxis after myocardial infarction, there may be no acceptable alternatives to the use of beta-adrenergic blocking agents in patients with asthma. In this setting, cardioselective beta-blockers could be considered, although they should be administered with caution.

The ECG changes and/or hypokalemia that may result from the administration of nonpotassium-sparing diuretics (such as loop or thiazide diuretics) can be acutely worsened by beta-agonists, especially when the recommended dose of the beta-agonist is exceeded. Although the clinical significance of these effects is not known, caution is advised in the coadministration of beta-agonists with nonpotassium-sparing diuretics.

SEREVENT DISKUS INHALATION POWDER

Short-Acting Beta-Agonists

In the two 12 week, repetitive-dose adolescent and adult clinical trials in patients with asthma (n=149), the mean daily need for additional $beta_2$-agonist in patients using salmeterol inhalation powder was approximately 1½ inhalations/day. Twenty-six percent (26%) of the patients in these trials used between 8 and 24 inhalations of short-acting beta-agonist per day on 1 or more occasions. Nine percent (9%) of the patients in these trials averaged over 4 inhalations/day over the course of the 12 week trials. No increase in frequency of cardiovascular events was observed among the 3 patients who averaged 8-11 inhalations per day; however, the safety of concomitant use of more than 8 inhalations per day of short-acting $beta_2$-agonist with salmeterol inhalation powder has not been established. In 29 patients who experienced worsening of asthma while receiving salmeterol inhalation powder during these trials, albuterol therapy administered via either nebulizer or inhalation aerosol (1 dose in most cases) led to improvement in FEV_1 and no increase in occurrence of cardiovascular adverse events.

In 2 clinical trials in patients with COPD, the mean daily need for additional $beta_2$-agonist for patients using salmeterol inhalation powder was approximately 4 inhalations/day. Twenty-four percent (24%) of the patients using salmeterol inhalation powder in these trials averaged 6 or more inhalations of albuterol per day over the course of the 24 week trials. No increase in frequency of cardiovascular events was observed among patients who averaged 6 or more inhalations per day.

Monoamine Oxidase Inhibitors and Tricyclic Antidepressants

Salmeterol should be administered with extreme caution to patients being treated with monoamine oxidase inhibitors or tricyclic antidepressants, or within 2 weeks of discontinuation of such agents, because the action of salmeterol on the vascular system may be potentiated by these agents.

Corticosteroids and Cromoglycate

In clinical trials, inhaled corticosteroids and/or inhaled cromolyn sodium did not alter the safety profile of salmeterol when administered concurrently.

Methylxanthines

The concurrent use of intravenously or orally administered methylxanthines (*e.g.*, aminophylline, theophylline) by patients receiving salmeterol has not been completely evaluated. In 1 clinical asthma trial, 87 patients receiving Serevent Inhalation Aerosol 42 µg twice daily concurrently with a theophylline product had adverse event rates similar to those in 71 patients receiving Serevent Inhalation Aerosol without theophylline. Resting heart rates were slightly higher in the patients on theophylline but were little affected by therapy with Serevent Inhalation Aerosol.

In 2 clinical trials in patients with COPD, 39 subjects receiving salmeterol inhalation powder concurrently with a theophylline product had adverse event rates similar to those in 302 patients receiving salmeterol inhalation powder without theophylline. Based on the available data, the concomitant administration of methylxanthines with salmeterol inhalation powder did not alter the observed adverse event profile.

Beta-Adrenergic Receptor Blocking Agents

Beta-blockers not only block the pulmonary effect of beta-agonists, such as Serevent Diskus, but may also produce severe bronchospasm in patients with asthma or COPD. Therefore, patients with asthma or COPD should not normally be treated with beta-blockers. However, under certain circumstances, *e.g.*, as prophylaxis after myocardial infarction, there may be no acceptable alternatives to the use of beta-adrenergic blocking agents in patients with asthma or COPD. In this setting, cardioselective beta-blockers could be considered, although they should be administered with caution.

S

Diuretics

The ECG changes and/or hypokalemia that may result from the administration of nonpotassium-sparing diuretics (such as loop or thiazide diuretics) can be acutely worsened by beta-agonists, especially when the recommended dose of the beta-agonist is exceeded. Although the clinical significance of these effects is not known, caution is advised in the coadministration of beta-agonists with nonpotassium-sparing diuretics.

ADVERSE REACTIONS

SEREVENT INHALATION AEROSOL

Adverse reactions to salmeterol are similar in nature to reactions to other selective beta$_2$-adrenoceptor agonists, *i.e.*, tachycardia; palpitations; immediate hypersensitivity reactions, including urticaria, angioedema, rash, bronchospasm (see WARNINGS, Serevent Inhalation Aerosol); headache; tremor; nervousness; and paradoxical bronchospasm (see WARNINGS, Serevent Inhalation Aerosol).

Asthma

Two multicenter, 12 week, controlled studies have evaluated twice-daily doses of Serevent Inhalation Aerosol in patients 12 years of age and older with asthma. TABLE 5 reports the incidence of adverse events in these 2 studies.

TABLE 5 *Adverse Experience Incidence in 2 Large 12 Week Asthma Clinical Trials**

Adverse Event Type	Placebo (n=187)	Serevent Inhalation Aerosol 42 µg Twice Daily (n=184)	Albuterol Inhalation Aerosol 180 µg 4 Times Daily (n=185)
Ear, Nose, and Throat			
Upper respiratory tract infection	13%	14%	16%*
Nasopharyngitis	12%	14%	11%
Disease of nasal cavity/sinus	4%	6%	1%
Sinus headache	2%	4%	<1%
Gastrointestinal			
Stomachache	0%	4%	0%
Neurological			
Headache	23%	28%	27%
Tremor	2%	4%	3%
Respiratory			
Cough	6%	7%	3%
Lower respiratory infection	2%	4%	2%

* The only adverse experience classified as serious was 1 case of upper respiratory tract infection in a patient treated with albuterol.

TABLE 5 includes all events (whether considered drug-related or nondrug-related by the investigator) that occurred at a rate of over 3% in the Serevent Inhalation Aerosol treatment group and were more common in the Serevent Inhalation Aerosol group than in the placebo group.

Pharyngitis, allergic rhinitis, dizziness/giddiness, and influenza occurred at 3% or more but were equally common on placebo. Other events occurring in the Serevent Inhalation Aerosol treatment group at a frequency of 1-3% were as follows:

Cardiovascular: Tachycardia, palpitations.

Ear, Nose, and Throat: Rhinitis, laryngitis.

Gastrointestinal: Nausea, viral gastroenteritis, nausea and vomiting, diarrhea, abdominal pain.

Hypersensitivity: Urticaria.

Mouth and Teeth: Dental pain.

Musculoskeletal: Pain in joint, back pain, muscle cramp/contraction, myalgia/myositis, muscular soreness.

Neurological: Nervousness, malaise/fatigue.

Respiratory: Tracheitis/bronchitis.

Skin: Rash/skin eruption.

Urogenital: Dysmenorrhea.

Data from small dose-response studies show an apparent dose relationship for tremor, nervousness, and palpitations.

In clinical trials evaluating concurrent therapy of salmeterol with inhaled corticosteroids, adverse events were consistent with those previously reported for salmeterol, or might otherwise be expected with the use of inhaled corticosteroids.

COPD

Two multicenter, 12 week, controlled studies have evaluated twice-daily doses of Serevent Inhalation Aerosol in patients with COPD. TABLE 6 reports the incidence of adverse events in these 2 studies.

TABLE 6 includes all events (whether considered drug-related or nondrug-related by the investigator) that occurred at a rate of over 3% in the Serevent Inhalation Aerosol treatment group and were more common in the Serevent Inhalation Aerosol group than in the placebo group.

Common cold, rhinorrhea, bronchitis, cough, exacerbation of chest congestion, chest pain, and dizziness occurred at 3% or more but were equally common on placebo. Other events occurring in the Serevent Inhalation Aerosol treatment group at a frequency of 1-3% were as follows:

Ear, Nose, and Throat: Cold symptoms, earache, epistaxis, nasal congestion, nasal sinus congestion, sneezing.

Gastrointestinal: Nausea, dyspepsia, gastric pain, gastric upset, abdominal pain, constipation, heartburn, oral candidiasis, xerostomia, vomiting, surgical removal of tooth.

TABLE 6 *Adverse Experience Incidence in 2 Large 12 Week COPD Clinical Trials*

Adverse Event Type	Placebo (n=278)	Serevent Inhalation Aerosol 42 µg Twice Daily (n=267)	Ipratropium Inhalation Aerosol 36 µg 4 Times Daily (n=271)
Ear, Nose, and Throat			
Upper respiratory tract infection	7%	9%	9%
Sore throat	3%	8%	6%
Nasal sinus infection	1%	4%	2%
Gastrointestinal			
Diarrhea	3%	5%	4%
Musculoskeletal			
Back pain	3%	4%	3%
Neurological			
Headache	10%	12%	8%
Respiratory			
Chest congestion	3%	4%	3%

Musculoskeletal: Leg cramps, myalgia, neck pain, pain in arm, shoulder pain, muscle injury of neck.

Neurological: Insomnia, sinus headache.

Non-Site Specific: Fatigue, fever, pain in body, discomfort in chest.

Respiratory: Acute bronchitis, dyspnea, influenza, lower respiratory tract infection, pneumonia, respiratory tract infection, shortness of breath, wheezing.

Urogenital: Urinary tract infection.

Electrocardiographic Monitoring in Patients With COPD

Continuous electrocardiographic (Holter) monitoring was performed on 284 patients in 2 large COPD clinical trials during five 24 hour periods. No cases of sustained ventricular tachycardia were observed. At baseline, non-sustained, asymptomatic ventricular tachycardia was recorded for 7 (7.1%), 8 (9.4%), and 3 (3.0%) patients in the placebo, Serevent, and ipratropium groups, respectively. During treatment, nonsustained, asymptomatic ventricular tachycardia that represented a clinically significant change from baseline was reported for 11 (11.6%), 15 (18.3%), and 20 (20.8%) patients receiving placebo, Serevent, and ipratropium, respectively. Four of these cases of ventricular tachycardia were reported as adverse events (1 placebo, 3 Serevent) by 1 investigator based upon review of Holter data. One case of ventricular tachycardia was observed during ECG evaluation of chest pain (ipratropium) and reported as an adverse event.

Observed During Clinical Practice

In extensive US and worldwide postmarketing experience, serious exacerbations of asthma, including some that have been fatal, have been reported. In most cases, these have occurred in patients with severe asthma and/or in some patients in whom asthma has been acutely deteriorating (see WARNINGS, Serevent Inhalation Aerosol, Do Not Introduce Serevent Inhalation Aerosol as a Treatment for Acutely Deteriorating Asthma), but they have occurred in a few patients with less severe asthma as well. It was not possible from these reports to determine whether Serevent Inhalation Aerosol contributed to these events or simply failed to relieve the deteriorating asthma.

The following events have also been identified during postapproval use of Serevent in clinical practice. Because they are reported voluntarily from a population of unknown size, estimates of frequency cannot be made. These events have been chosen for inclusion due to a combination of their seriousness, frequency of reporting, or potential causal connection to Serevent.

Respiratory: Rare reports of upper airway symptoms of laryngeal spasm, irritation, or swelling such as stridor or choking; oropharyngeal irritation.

Cardiovascular: Hypertension, arrhythmias (including atrial fibrillation, supraventricular tachycardia, extrasystoles).

SEREVENT DISKUS INHALATION POWDER

Adverse reactions to salmeterol are similar in nature to reactions to other selective beta$_2$-adrenoceptor agonists, *i.e.*, tachycardia; palpitations; immediate hypersensitivity reactions, including urticaria, angioedema, rash, bronchospasm (see WARNINGS, Serevent Diskus Inhalation Powder); headache; tremor; nervousness; and paradoxical bronchospasm (see WARNINGS, Serevent Diskus Inhalation Powder).

Asthma

Two multicenter, 12 week, controlled studies have evaluated twice-daily doses of salmeterol inhalation powder in patients 12 years of age and older with asthma. TABLE 7 reports the incidence of adverse experiences in these 2 studies.

TABLE 7 includes all experiences (whether considered drug-related or nondrug-related by the investigator) that occurred at a rate of 3% or greater in the group receiving salmeterol inhalation powder and were more common than in the placebo group.

Pharyngitis, sinusitis, upper respiratory tract infection, and cough occurred at ≥3% but were more common in the placebo group. However, throat irritation has been described at rates exceeding that of placebo in other controlled clinical trials.

Other adverse experiences that occurred in the group receiving salmeterol inhalation powder in these studies with an incidence of 1-3% and that occurred at a greater incidence than with placebo were:

Ear, Nose, and Throat: Sinus headache.

Gastrointestinal: Nausea.

Mouth and Teeth: Oral mucosal abnormality.

Musculoskeletal: Pain in joint.

Neurological: Sleep disturbance, paresthesia.

Skin: Contact dermatitis, eczema.

Miscellaneous: Localized aches and pains, pyrexia of unknown origin.

TABLE 7 *Adverse Experience Incidence in Two 12 Week Adolescent and Adult Clinical Trials in Patients With Asthma*

Adverse Experience Type	Placebo (n=152)	Salmeterol Inhalation Powder 50 µg Twice Daily (n=149)	Albuterol Inhalation Aerosol 180 µg 4 Times Daily (n=150)
Ear, Nose, and Throat			
Nasal/sinus congestion, pallor	6%	9%	8%
Rhinitis	4%	5%	4%
Neurological			
Headache	9%	13%	12%
Respiratory			
Asthma	1%	3%	<1%
Tracheitis/bronchitis	4%	7%	3%
Influenza	2%	5%	5%

Two multicenter, 12 week, controlled studies have evaluated twice-daily doses of salmeterol inhalation powder in patients aged 4-11 years with asthma. TABLE 8 includes all experiences (whether considered drug-related or nondrug-related by the investigator) that occurred at a rate of 3% or greater in the group receiving salmeterol inhalation powder and were more common than in the placebo group.

TABLE 8 *Adverse Experience Incidence in Two 12 Week Pediatric Clinical Trials in Patients With Asthma*

Adverse Experience Type	Placebo (n=215)	Salmeterol Inhalation Powder 50 µg Twice Daily (n=211)	Albuterol Inhalation Powder 200 µg 4 Times Daily (n=115)
Ear, Nose and Throat			
Ear signs and symptoms	3%	4%	9%
Pharyngitis	3%	6%	3%
Neurological			
Headache	14%	17%	20%
Respiratory			
Asthma	2%	4%	<1%
Skin			
Skin rashes	3%	4%	2%
Urticaria	0%	3%	2%

The following experiences were reported at an incidence of 1-2% (3-4 patients) in the salmeterol group and with a higher incidence than in the albuterol and placebo groups: gastrointestinal signs and symptoms, lower respiratory signs and symptoms, photodermatitis, and arthralgia and articular rheumatism.

In clinical trials evaluating concurrent therapy of salmeterol with inhaled corticosteroids, adverse experiences were consistent with those previously reported for salmeterol, or might otherwise be expected with the used of inhaled corticosteroids.

Chronic Obstructive Pulmonary Disease (COPD)

Two multicenter, 24 week, controlled studies have evaluated twice-daily doses of salmeterol inhalation powder administered via the Diskus in patients with COPD. For presentation (TABLE 9), the placebo data from a third trial, identical in design, patient entrance criteria, and overall conduct but comparing fluticasone propionate with placebo, were integrated with the placebo data from these 2 studies (total n=341 for salmeterol and 576 for placebo).

Other experiences occurring in the group treated with salmeterol inhalation powder that occurred at a frequency of 1% to <3% and were more common than in the placebo group were as follows:

Endocrine and Metabolic: Hyperglycemia.
Eye: Keratitis and conjunctivitis.
Gastrointestinal: Candidiasis mouth/throat, dyspeptic symptoms, hyposalivation, dental discomfort and pain, gastrointestinal infections.
Lower Respiratory: Lower respiratory signs and symptoms.
Musculoskeletal: Arthralgia and articular rheumatism; muscle pain; bone and skeletal pain; musculoskeletal inflammation; muscle stiffness, tightness, and rigidity.
Neurology: Migraines.
Non-Site Specific: Pain, edema and swelling.
Psychiatry: Anxiety.
Skin: Skin rashes.

Observed During Clinical Practice

In addition to adverse experiences reported from clinical trials, the following experiences have been identified during postapproval use of salmeterol. Because they are reported voluntarily from a population of unknown size, estimates of frequency cannot be made. These experiences have been chosen for inclusion due either their seriousness, frequency of reporting, or causal connection to salmeterol or a combination of these factors.

In extensive US and worldwide postmarketing experience with salmeterol, serious exacerbations of asthma, including some that have been fatal, have been reported. In most cases, these have occurred in patients with severe asthma and/or in some patients in whom asthma has been acutely deteriorating (see WARNINGS, Serevent Diskus Inhalation Powder, Do Not Introduce Serevent Diskus as a Treatment for Acutely Deteriorating Asthma), but they have also occurred in a few patients with less severe asthma. It was not possible from these reports to determine whether salmeterol contributed to these events or simply failed to relieve the deteriorating asthma.

TABLE 9 *Adverse Experiences With ≥3% Incidence in US Controlled Clinical Trials With Salmeterol Inhalation Powder in Patients With Chronic Obstructive Pulmonary Disease* *

Adverse Experience Type	Placebo (n=576)	Salmeterol Inhalation Powder 50 µg Twice Daily (n=341)
Cardiovascular		
Hypertension	2%	4%
Ear, nose, and throat		
Throat irritation	6%	7%
Nasal congestion/blockage	3%	4%
Sinusitis	2%	4%
Ear signs and symptoms	1%	3%
Gastrointestinal		
Nausea and vomiting	3%	3%
Lower Respiratory		
Cough	4%	5%
Rhinitis	2%	4%
Viral respiratory infection	4%	5%
Musculoskeletal		
Musculoskeletal pain	10%	12%
Muscle cramps and spasms	1%	3%
Neurological		
Headache	11%	14%
Dizziness	2%	4%
Average duration of exposure	128.9 days	138.5 days

* TABLE 9 includes all events (whether considered drug-related or nondrug-related by the investigator) that occurred at a rate of 3% or greater in the group treated with salmeterol inhalation powder and were more common in the group treated with salmeterol inhalation powder than in the placebo group.

Respiratory: Reports of upper airway symptoms of laryngeal spasm, irritation, or swelling such as stridor or choking; oropharyngeal irritation.
Cardiovascular: Arrhythmias (including atrial fibrillation, supraventricular tachycardia, extrasystoles), and anaphylaxis.

DOSAGE AND ADMINISTRATION

SEREVENT INHALATION AEROSOL

Serevent Inhalation Aerosol should be administered by the orally inhaled route only (see Patient's Instructions for Use). It is recommended to "test spray" Serevent Inhalation Aerosol into the air 4 times before using for the first time and in cases where the aerosol has not been used for a prolonged period of time (*i.e.,* more than 4 weeks).

Asthma

For maintenance of bronchodilatation and prevention of symptoms of asthma, including the symptoms of nocturnal asthma, the usual dosage for patients 12 years of age and older is 2 inhalations (42 µg) twice daily (morning and evening, approximately 12 hours apart). Adverse effects are more likely to occur with higher doses of salmeterol, and more frequent administration or administration of a larger number of inhalations is not recommended.

To gain full therapeutic benefit, Serevent Inhalation Aerosol should be administered twice daily (morning and evening) in the treatment of reversible airway obstruction.

If a previously effective dosage regimen fails to provide the usual response, medical advice should be sought immediately as this is often a sign of destabilization of asthma. Under these circumstances, the therapeutic regimen should be re-evaluated and additional therapeutic options, such as inhaled or systemic corticosteroids, should be considered. If symptoms arise in the period between doses, an inhaled, short-acting beta$_2$-agonist should be taken for immediate relief.

COPD

For maintenance treatment of bronchospasm associated with COPD (including chronic bronchitis and emphysema), the usual dosage for adults is 2 inhalations (42 µg) twice daily (morning and evening, approximately 12 hours apart).

Prevention of Exercise-Induced Bronchospasm

Two inhalations at least 30-60 minutes before exercise have been shown to protect against exercise-induced bronchospasm in many patients for up to 12 hours. Additional doses of Serevent Inhalation Aerosol should not be used for 12 hours after the administration of this drug. Patients who are receiving Serevent Inhalation Aerosol twice daily (morning and evening) should not use additional Serevent Inhalation Aerosol for prevention of exercise-induced bronchospasm. If this dose is not effective, other appropriate therapy for exercise-induced bronchospasm should be considered.

Geriatric Use

In studies where geriatric patients (65 years of age or older, see PRECAUTIONS, Serevent Inhalation Aerosol) have been treated with Serevent Inhalation Aerosol, efficacy and safety of 42 µg given twice daily (morning and evening) did not differ from that in younger patients. Consequently, no dosage adjustment is recommended.

SEREVENT DISKUS INHALATION POWDER

Serevent Diskus should be administered by the orally inhaled route only (see Patient's Instructions for Use). The patient must not exhale into the Diskus and the Diskus should only be activated and used in a level, horizontal position.

Asthma

For maintenance of bronchodilatation and prevention of symptoms of asthma, including the symptoms of nocturnal asthma, the usual dosage for adults and children 4 years of age and older is 1 inhalation (50 µg) twice daily (morning and evening, approximately 12 hours apart). If a previously effective dosage regimen fails to provide the usual response, medical

S

advice should be sought immediately as this is often a sign of destabilization of asthma. Under these circumstances, the therapeutic regimen should be reevaluated and additional therapeutic options, such as inhaled or systemic corticosteroids, should be considered. If symptoms arise in the period between doses, an inhaled, short-acting beta$_2$-agonist should be taken for immediate relief.

Chronic Obstructive Pulmonary Disease (COPD)

For maintenance treatment of bronchospasm associated with COPD (including chronic bronchitis and emphysema), the usual dosage for adults is 1 inhalation (50 µg) twice daily (morning and evening, approximately 12 hours apart).

For both asthma and COPD, adverse effects are more likely to occur with higher doses of salmeterol, and more frequent administration or administration of a larger number of inhalations is not recommended.

To gain full therapeutic benefit, Serevent Diskus should be administered twice daily (morning and evening) in the treatment of reversible airway obstruction.

Geriatric Use

Based on available data for Serevent Diskus, no dosage adjustment is recommended.

Prevention of Exercise-Induced Bronchospasm (EIB)

One inhalation of Serevent Diskus at least 30 minutes before exercise has been shown to protect patients against EIB. When used intermittently as needed for prevention of EIB, this protection may last up to 9 hours in adolescents and adults and up to 12 hours in patients 4-11 years of age. Additional doses of Serevent should not be used for 12 hours after the administration of this drug. Patients who are receiving Serevent Diskus twice daily should not use additional Serevent for prevention of EIB. If regular, twice-daily dosing is not effective in preventing EIB, other appropriate therapy for EIB should be considered.

HOW SUPPLIED

SEREVENT INHALATION AEROSOL

Serevent Inhalation Aerosol is supplied in 13 g canisters containing 120 metered actuations in boxes of 1. Each actuation delivers 25 µg of salmeterol base (as salmeterol xinafoate) from the valve and 21 µg of salmeterol base (as salmeterol xinafoate) from the actuator. Each canister is supplied with a green plastic actuator with a teal-colored strapcap and patient's instructions. Also available, Serevent Inhalation Aerosol Refill, a 13 g canister only with patient's instructions.

Serevent Inhalation Aerosol is also supplied in a pack that consists of a 6.5 g canister containing 60 metered actuations in boxes of 1. Each actuation delivers 25 µg of salmeterol base (as salmeterol xinafoate) from the valve and 21 µg of salmeterol base from the actuator (as salmeterol xinafoate). Each canister is supplied with a green plastic actuator with a teal-colored strapcap and patient's instructions.

For use with Serevent Inhalation Aerosol actuator only. The green actuator with Serevent Inhalation Aerosol should not be used with other aerosol medications, and actuators from other aerosol medications should not be used with a Serevent Inhalation Aerosol canister.

The correct amount of medication in each inhalation cannot be assured after 120 actuations from the 13 g canister or 60 actuations from the 6.5 g canister even though the canister is not completely empty. The canister should be discarded when the labeled number of actuations has been used.

Storage: Store between 15 and 30°C (59 and 86°F). Store canister with nozzle end down. Protect from freezing temperatures and direct sunlight.

Avoid spraying in eyes. Contents under pressure. Do not puncture or incinerate. Do not store at temperatures above 120°F. Keep out of reach of children. As with most inhaled medications in aerosol canisters, the therapeutic effect of this medication may decrease when the canister is cold; for best results, the canister should be at room temperature before use. Shake well before using.

Note: The indented statement below is required by the Federal government's Clean Air Act for all products containing or manufactured with chlorofluorocarbons (CFCs).

> *WARNING:* Contains trichlorofluoromethane and dichlorodifluoromethane, substances which harm public health and environment by destroying ozone in the upper atmosphere.

A notice similar to the above WARNING has been placed in the patient information leaflet of this product pursuant to EPA regulations. The patient's warning states that the patient should consult his or her physician if there are questions about alternatives.

SEREVENT DISKUS INHALATION POWDER

Serevent Diskus is supplied as a disposable, teal green-colored unit containing 60 blisters. The drug product is packaged within a teal green-colored, plastic-coated, moisture-protective foil pouch.

Serevent Diskus is also supplied in an institutional pack of 1 teal green-colored, disposable unit containing 28 blisters. The drug product is packaged within a teal green-colored, plastic-coated, moisture-protective foil pouch.

Storage: Store at controlled room temperature, 20-25°C (68-77°F) in a dry place away from direct heat or sunlight. Keep out of reach of children. Serevent Diskus should be discarded 6 weeks after removal from the moisture-protective foil overwrap pouch or after all blisters have been used (when the dose indicator reads "0"), whichever comes first. The Diskus is not reusable. Do not attempt to take the Diskus apart.

PRODUCT LISTING - EQUIVALENTS NOT AVAILABLE

Aerosol - Inhalation - 21 mcg

13 gm	$84.49	SEREVENT, Glaxosmithkline	00173-0465-00

Aerosol with Adapter - Inhalation - 21 mcg

6 gm	$54.25	SEREVENT, Glaxosmithkline	00173-0467-00
13 gm	$66.84	SEREVENT, Allscripts Pharmaceutical Company	54569-3855-00
13 gm	$73.39	SEREVENT, Physicians Total Care	54868-3702-00
13 gm	$87.51	SEREVENT, Glaxosmithkline	00173-0464-00

Powder - Inhalation - 50 mcg

28's	$47.23	SEREVENT DISKUS, Glaxosmithkline	00173-0520-00
60's	$72.58	SEREVENT DISKUS, Allscripts Pharmaceutical Company	54569-4867-00
60's	$87.51	SEREVENT DISKUS, Glaxosmithkline	00173-0521-00

Salsalate (002206)

For related information, see the comparative table section in Appendix A.

Categories: Arthritis, osteoarthritis; Arthritis, rheumatoid; Pregnancy Category C; FDA Pre 1938 Drugs
Drug Classes: Analgesics, non-narcotic; Salicylates
Brand Names: Amigesic; Anaflex 750; Artha-G; Carsalate; Diagen; **Disalcid**; Marthritic; Mono-Gesic; Ro-Salcid; Salflex; Salgesic; Salicylsalicylic Acid; Salsitab
Foreign Brand Availability: Atisuril (Spain); Disal (Korea; Taiwan); Disalgesic (Germany); Salina (Japan); Saril (Korea); Umbradol (Spain)
Cost of Therapy: $39.51 (Osteoarthritis; Salflex; 500 mg; 6 tablets/day; 30 day supply)
$21.78 (Osteoarthritis; Generic Tablets; 500 mg; 6 tablets/day; 30 day supply)
$39.90 (Osteoarthritis; Salflex; 750 mg; 4 tablets/day; 30 day supply)
$16.20 (Osteoarthritis; Generic Tablets; 750 mg; 4 tablets/day; 30 day supply)

DESCRIPTION

Salsalate is a nonsteroidal anti-inflammatory agent for oral administration. Chemically, salsalate (salicylsalicylic acid or 2-hydroxybenzoic acid, 2-carboxyphenyl ester) is a dimer of salicylic acid.

Each Disalcid capsule contains 500 mg salsalate. *Inactive Ingredients:* Colloidal silicon dioxide, gelatin, magnesium stearate, pregelatinized starch, corn starch, titanium dioxide, FD&C blue no. 1, and D&C yellow no. 10.

Each Disalcid tablet contains 500 mg or 750 mg salsalate. *Inactive Ingredients:* Croscarmellose, hydroxypropyl methylcellulose, magnesium stearate, microcrystalline cellulose, polyethylene glycol, polysorbate 80, propylene glycol, talc, titanium dioxide, FD&C blue no. 1, and D&C yellow no. 10.

CLINICAL PHARMACOLOGY

Salsalate is insoluble in acid gastric fluids (<0.1 mg/ml at pH 1.0), but readily soluble in the small intestine where it is partially hydrolyzed to two molecules of salicylic acid. A significant portion of the parent compound is absorbed unchanged and undergoes rapid esterase hydrolysis in the body; its half-life is about one hour. About 13% is excreted through the kidneys as a glucuronide conjugate of the parent compound, the remainder as salicylic acid and its metabolites. Thus, the amount of salicylic acid available from salsalate is about 15% less than from aspirin, when the two drugs are administered on a salicylic acid molar equivalent basis (3.6 g salsalate/5 g aspirin). Salicylic acid biotransformation is saturated at anti-inflammatory doses of salsalate. Such capacity-limited biotransformation results in an increase in the half-life of salicylic acid from 3.5 to 16 or more hours. Thus, dosing with salsalate twice a day will satisfactorily maintain blood levels within the desired therapeutic range (10-30 mg/100 ml) throughout the 12 hour intervals. Therapeutic blood levels continue for up to 16 hours after the last dose. The parent compound does not show capacity-limited biotransformation, nor does it accumulate in the plasma on multiple dosing. Food slows the absorption of all salicylates including salsalate.

The mode of anti-inflammatory action of salsalate and other nonsteroidal anti-inflammatory drugs is not fully defined. Although salicylic acid (the primary metabolite of salsalate) is a weak inhibitor of prostaglandin synthesis *in vitro,* salsalate appears to selectively inhibit prostaglandin synthesis *in vivo,*[1] providing anti-inflammatory activity equivalent to aspirin [2] and indomethacin.[3] Unlike aspirin, salsalate does not inhibit platelet aggregation.[4]

The usefulness of salicylic acid, the active *in vivo* product of salsalate, in the treatment of arthritic disorders has been established.[5,6] In contrast to aspirin, salsalate causes no greater fecal gastrointestinal blood loss than placebo.[7]

INDICATIONS AND USAGE

Salsalate is indicated for relief of the signs and symptoms of rheumatoid arthritis, osteoarthritis and related rheumatic disorders.

CONTRAINDICATIONS

Salsalate is contraindicated in patients hypersensitive to salsalate.

WARNINGS

Reye's Syndrome may develop in individuals who have chicken pox, influenza, or flu symptoms. Some studies suggest a possible association between the development of Reye's Syndrome and the use of medicines containing salicylate or aspirin. Salsalate contains a salicylate and therefore is not recommended for use in patients with chicken pox, influenza, or flu symptoms.

PRECAUTIONS

GENERAL

Patients on treatment with salsalate should be warned not to take other salicylates so as to avoid potentially toxic concentrations. Great care should be exercised when salsalate is prescribed in the presence of chronic renal insufficiency or peptic ulcer disease. Protein binding of salicylic acid can be influenced by nutritional status, competitive binding of other drugs, and fluctuations in serum proteins caused by disease (rheumatoid arthritis, etc.).

Although cross reactivity, including bronchospasm, has been reported occasionally with non-acetylated salicylates, including salsalate, in aspirin-sensitive patients,[8,9] salsalate is less likely than aspirin to induce asthma in such patients.[10]

LABORATORY TESTS

Plasma salicylic acid concentrations should be periodically monitored during long-term treatment with salsalate to aid maintenance of therapeutically effective levels: 10-30 mg/100 ml. Toxic manifestations are not usually seen until plasma concentrations exceed 30 mg/100 ml. Urinary pH should also be regularly monitored: sudden acidification, as from pH 6.5-5.5, can double the plasma level, resulting in toxicity.

DRUG/LABORATORY TEST INTERACTIONS

Salicylate competes with thyroid hormone for binding to plasma proteins, which may be reflected in a depressed plasma T_4 value in some patients; thyroid function and basal metabolism are unaffected.

CARCINOGENESIS

No long-term animal studies have been performed with salsalate to evaluate its carcinogenic potential.

PREGNANCY CATEGORY C

Salsalate and salicylic acid have been shown to be teratogenic and embryocidal in rats when given in doses 4-5 times the usual human dose. These effects were not observed at doses twice as great as the usual human dose. There are no adequate and well-controlled studies in pregnant women. Salsalate should be used during pregnancy only if the potential benefit justifies the potential risk to the fetus.

LABOR AND DELIVERY

There exist no adequate and well-controlled studies in pregnant women. Although adverse effects on mother or infant have not been reported with salsalate use during labor, caution is advised when anti-inflammatory dosage is involved. However, other salicylates have been associated with prolonged gestation and labor, maternal and neonatal bleeding sequelae, potentiation of narcotic and barbiturate effects (respiratory or cardiac arrest in the mother), delivery problems and stillbirth.

NURSING MOTHERS

It is not known whether salsalate per se is excreted in human milk; salicylic acid, the primary metabolite of salsalate, has been shown to appear in human milk in concentrations approximating the maternal blood level. Thus, the infant of a mother on salsalate therapy might ingest in mother's milk 30-80% as much salicylate per kg body weight as the mother is taking. Accordingly, caution should be exercised when salsalate is administered to a nursing woman.

PEDIATRIC USE

Safety and effectiveness of salsalate use in pediatric patients have not been established. (See WARNINGS.)

DRUG INTERACTIONS

Salicylates antagonize the uricosuric action of drugs used to treat gout. ASPIRIN AND OTHER SALICYLATE DRUGS WILL BE ADDITIVE TO SALSALATE AND MAY INCREASE PLASMA CONCENTRATIONS OF SALICYLIC ACID TO TOXIC LEVELS. Drugs and foods that raise urine pH will increase renal clearance and urinary excretion of salicylic acid, thus lowering plasma levels; acidifying drugs or foods will decrease urinary excretion and increase plasma levels. Salicylates given concomitantly with anticoagulant drugs may predispose to systemic bleeding. Salicylates may enhance the hypoglycemic effect of oral antidiabetic drugs of the sulfonylurea class. Salicylate competes with a number of drugs for protein binding sites, notably penicillin, thiopental, thyroxine, triiodothyronine, phenytoin, sulfinpyrazone, naproxen, warfarin, methotrexate, and possibly corticosteroids.

ADVERSE REACTIONS

In two well-controlled clinical trials (n=280 patients), the following reversible adverse experience characteristic of salicylates were most commonly reported with salsalate, listed in descending order of frequency: tinnitus, nausea, hearing impairment, rash, and vertigo. These common symptoms of salicylates, *i.e.,* tinnitus or reversible hearing impairment, are often used as a guide to therapy.

Although cause-and-effect relationships have not been established, spontaneous reports over a ten-year period have include the following additional medically significant adverse experiences: abdominal pain, abnormal hepatic function, anaphylactic shock, angioedema, bronchospasm, decreased creatinine clearance, diarrhea, G.I. bleeding, hepatitis, hypotension, nephritis, and urticaria.

DOSAGE AND ADMINISTRATION

ADULTS

The usual dosage is 3000 mg daily, given in divided doses as follows: 1) two doses of two 750 mg tablets: 2) two doses of three 500 mg tablets/capsules; or 3) three doses of two 500 mg tablets/capsules. Some patients, *e.g.,* the elderly, may require a lower dosage to achieve therapeutic blood concentrations and to avoid the more common side effects such as auditory.

Alleviation of symptoms is gradual, and full benefit may not be evidence for 3-4 days, when plasma salicylate levels have achieved steady state. There is no evidence for development of tissue tolerance (tachyphylaxis), but salicylate therapy may induce increased activity of metabolizing liver enzymes, causing a greater rate of salicyluric acid production and excretion, with a resultant increase in dosage requirement for maintenance of therapeutic serum salicylate levels.

CHILDREN

Dosage recommendations and indications for salsalate use in children have not been established.

HOW SUPPLIED

Disalcid 500 mg Capsule: Aqua/white capsule printed with Disalcid/3M.

Disalcid 500 mg Tablet: Aqua, film coated, round, bisected tablet embossed with "DISALCID" on one side and "3M" on the other side.

Disalcid 750 mg Tablet: Aqua, film coated, capsule shaped, bisected tablet embossed with "DISALCID" 750 on one side and "3M" on the other side.

Storage: Store at controlled room temperature 15-30°C (59-86°F).

PRODUCT LISTING - RATED THERAPEUTICALLY EQUIVALENT

Tablet - Oral - 750 mg

100's	$31.35	GENERIC, Major Pharmaceuticals Inc	00904-5407-60

PRODUCT LISTING - EQUIVALENTS NOT AVAILABLE

Capsule - Oral - 500 mg

100's	$65.58	DISALCID, 3M Pharmaceuticals	00089-0148-10

Tablet - Oral - 500 mg

10's	$4.27	GENERIC, Southwood Pharmaceuticals Inc	58016-0219-10
12's	$5.13	GENERIC, Southwood Pharmaceuticals Inc	58016-0219-12
15's	$6.42	GENERIC, Southwood Pharmaceuticals Inc	58016-0219-15
15's	$13.26	DISALCID, Pd-Rx Pharmaceuticals	55289-0244-15
20's	$4.25	GENERIC, Allscripts Pharmaceutical Company	54569-2544-01
20's	$8.56	GENERIC, Southwood Pharmaceuticals Inc	58016-0219-20
20's	$18.38	DISALCID, Pd-Rx Pharmaceuticals	55289-0244-20
28's	$7.35	GENERIC, Pd-Rx Pharmaceuticals	55289-0275-28
28's	$11.97	GENERIC, Southwood Pharmaceuticals Inc	58016-0219-28
28's	$14.14	GENERIC, Alpharma Uspd Makers Of Barre and Nmc	63874-0479-28
30's	$6.38	GENERIC, Allscripts Pharmaceutical Company	54569-2544-00
30's	$7.95	GENERIC, Pd-Rx Pharmaceuticals	55289-0275-30
30's	$12.83	GENERIC, Southwood Pharmaceuticals Inc	58016-0219-30
30's	$14.63	GENERIC, Alpharma Uspd Makers Of Barre and Nmc	63874-0479-30
40's	$10.80	GENERIC, Alpharma Uspd Makers Of Barre and Nmc	63874-0479-40
40's	$10.83	GENERIC, Pharma Pac	52959-0394-40
60's	$6.90	GENERIC, Pd-Rx Pharmaceuticals	55289-0275-60
60's	$12.75	GENERIC, Allscripts Pharmaceutical Company	54569-2544-02
60's	$15.21	GENERIC, Pharma Pac	52959-0394-60
100's	$12.10	GENERIC, Major Pharmaceuticals Inc	00904-1250-60
100's	$12.10	GENERIC, Major Pharmaceuticals Inc	00904-1253-60
100's	$13.59	GENERIC, Caraco Pharmaceutical Laboratories	57664-0103-08
100's	$16.80	GENERIC, Economed Pharmaceuticals Inc	38130-0711-01
100's	$17.70	GENERIC, Trinity Technologies Corporation	61355-0404-10
100's	$18.99	GENERIC, Mutual Pharmaceutical Co Inc	53489-0465-01
100's	$20.77	GENERIC, Invamed Inc	52189-0243-24
100's	$20.99	GENERIC, Able Laboratories Inc	53265-0132-10
100's	$21.00	GENERIC, Interpharm Inc	53746-0276-01
100's	$21.12	GENERIC, Eon Labs Manufacturing Inc	00185-0693-01
100's	$21.25	GENERIC, Eon Labs Manufacturing Inc	00185-0761-01
100's	$21.25	GENERIC, Eon Labs Manufacturing Inc	00185-0856-01
100's	$21.25	GENERIC, Aligen Independent Laboratories Inc	00405-4934-01
100's	$21.25	GENERIC, Sidmak Laboratories Inc	50111-0390-01
100's	$21.25	GENERIC, Martec Pharmaceuticals Inc	52555-0560-01
100's	$21.25	GENERIC, Martec Pharmaceuticals Inc	52555-0629-01
100's	$21.26	GENERIC, Moore, H.L. Drug Exchange Inc	00839-7167-06
100's	$21.95	SALFLEX, Carnrick Laboratories Inc	00086-0071-10
100's	$21.95	GENERIC, Major Pharmaceuticals Inc	00904-5072-60
100's	$24.95	GENERIC, Amide Pharmaceutical Inc	52152-0019-02
100's	$25.02	GENERIC, Alpharma Uspd Makers Of Barre and Nmc	00472-0132-10
100's	$25.02	GENERIC, Boca Pharmacal Inc	64376-0507-01
100's	$26.15	GENERIC, Ivax Corporation	00182-1802-89
100's	$29.94	GENERIC, Vintage Pharmaceuticals Inc	00254-5811-28
100's	$29.94	GENERIC, Qualitest Products Inc	00603-5754-21
100's	$29.95	GENERIC, Geneva Pharmaceuticals	00781-1108-01
100's	$30.18	GENERIC, R.I.D. Inc Distributor	54807-0140-01
100's	$33.28	GENERIC, Major Pharmaceuticals Inc	00904-1250-61
100's	$36.28	GENERIC, Mutual/United Research Laboratories	00677-1024-01
100's	$42.78	GENERIC, Southwood Pharmaceuticals Inc	58016-0219-00

Tablet - Oral - 750 mg

10's	$5.48	GENERIC, Southwood Pharmaceuticals Inc	58016-0221-10
12's	$3.36	GENERIC, Allscripts Pharmaceutical Company	54569-1712-05
12's	$6.57	GENERIC, Southwood Pharmaceuticals Inc	58016-0221-12
14's	$7.67	GENERIC, Southwood Pharmaceuticals Inc	58016-0221-14
15's	$8.22	GENERIC, Southwood Pharmaceuticals Inc	58016-0221-15
20's	$6.09	SALFLEX, Pharmaceutical Corporation Of America	51655-0592-52
20's	$7.28	GENERIC, Pd-Rx Pharmaceuticals	55289-0844-20
20's	$10.96	GENERIC, Southwood Pharmaceuticals Inc	58016-0221-20
21's	$10.96	GENERIC, Southwood Pharmaceuticals Inc	58016-0221-21
24's	$13.15	GENERIC, Southwood Pharmaceuticals Inc	58016-0221-24
24's	$24.95	GENERIC, Pharma Pac	52959-0332-24
28's	$7.84	GENERIC, Allscripts Pharmaceutical Company	54569-1712-01
28's	$15.34	GENERIC, Southwood Pharmaceuticals Inc	58016-0221-28
28's	$16.21	GENERIC, Alpharma Uspd Makers Of Barre and Nmc	63874-0308-28
28's	$27.93	GENERIC, Pharma Pac	52959-0332-28
30's	$5.86	GENERIC, Physicians Total Care	54868-0088-04
30's	$8.40	GENERIC, Allscripts Pharmaceutical Company	54569-1712-04
30's	$9.08	GENERIC, Pd-Rx Pharmaceuticals	55289-0844-30
30's	$16.43	GENERIC, Southwood Pharmaceuticals Inc	58016-0221-30

30's	$16.98	GENERIC, Alpharma Uspd Makers Of Barre and Nmc	63874-0308-30
30's	$28.56	DISALCID, Pd-Rx Pharmaceuticals	55289-0069-30
30's	$29.16	GENERIC, Pharma Pac	52959-0332-30
40's	$7.26	GENERIC, Physicians Total Care	54868-0088-06
40's	$10.40	GENERIC, Pd-Rx Pharmaceuticals	55289-0844-40
40's	$11.20	GENERIC, Allscripts Pharmaceutical Company	54569-1712-00
40's	$21.91	GENERIC, Southwood Pharmaceuticals Inc	58016-0221-40
40's	$22.03	GENERIC, Alpharma Uspd Makers Of Barre and Nmc	63874-0308-40
40's	$30.58	DISALCID, Pd-Rx Pharmaceuticals	55289-0069-40
40's	$35.42	GENERIC, Pharma Pac	52959-0332-40
60's	$16.80	SALFLEX, Pharmaceutical Corporation Of America	51655-0592-25
60's	$16.80	GENERIC, Allscripts Pharmaceutical Company	54569-1712-03
60's	$25.20	GENERIC, St. Mary'S Mpp	60760-0391-60
60's	$32.87	GENERIC, Southwood Pharmaceuticals Inc	58016-0221-60
60's	$45.78	GENERIC, Pharma Pac	52959-0332-60
90's	$49.77	GENERIC, Pharma Pac	52959-0332-90
100's	$13.50	GENERIC, Interstate Drug Exchange Inc	00814-6791-14
100's	$13.50	GENERIC, Major Pharmaceuticals Inc	00904-1251-60
100's	$13.50	GENERIC, Major Pharmaceuticals Inc	00904-1254-60
100's	$14.81	GENERIC, Physicians Total Care	54868-0088-01
100's	$15.12	GENERIC, Caraco Pharmaceutical Laboratories	57664-0105-08
100's	$15.12	GENERIC, Caraco Pharmaceutical Laboratories	57664-0184-08
100's	$22.16	GENERIC, Martec Pharmaceuticals Inc	52555-0561-01
100's	$22.25	GENERIC, Blansett Pharmacal Company Inc	51674-0013-01
100's	$23.50	GENERIC, Trinity Technologies Corporation	61355-0405-10
100's	$26.56	GENERIC, Invamed Inc	52189-0244-24
100's	$26.88	GENERIC, Marnel Pharmaceuticals Inc	00682-0810-01
100's	$27.00	GENERIC, Interpharm Inc	53746-0277-01
100's	$27.95	GENERIC, Major Pharmaceuticals Inc	00904-5073-60
100's	$27.95	GENERIC, Mutual Pharmaceutical Co Inc	53489-0466-01
100's	$27.98	GENERIC, Eon Labs Manufacturing Inc	00185-0694-01
100's	$27.98	GENERIC, Eon Labs Manufacturing Inc	00185-0762-01
100's	$27.98	GENERIC, Eon Labs Manufacturing Inc	00185-0857-01
100's	$28.00	GENERIC, Aligen Independent Laboratories Inc	00405-4935-01
100's	$28.00	GENERIC, Sidmak Laboratories Inc	50111-0391-01
100's	$28.00	GENERIC, Martec Pharmaceuticals Inc	52555-0630-01
100's	$28.00	GENERIC, Allscripts Pharmaceutical Company	54569-1712-02
100's	$28.01	GENERIC, Moore, H.L. Drug Exchange Inc	00839-7168-06
100's	$30.00	GENERIC, Ivax Corporation	00182-1803-89
100's	$30.95	GENERIC, Amide Pharmaceutical Inc	52152-0020-02
100's	$31.65	GENERIC, Boca Pharmacal Inc	64376-0508-01
100's	$32.03	GENERIC, Alpharma Uspd Makers Of Barre and Nmc	00472-0133-10
100's	$33.25	SALFLEX, Carnrick Laboratories Inc	00086-0072-10
100's	$34.94	GENERIC, Able Laboratories Inc	53265-0133-10
100's	$35.94	GENERIC, Vintage Pharmaceuticals Inc	00254-5812-28
100's	$35.94	GENERIC, Qualitest Products Inc	00603-5755-21
100's	$37.20	GENERIC, St. Mary'S Mpp	60760-0391-00
100's	$39.94	GENERIC, Major Pharmaceuticals Inc	00904-1251-61
100's	$40.36	GENERIC, Schwarz Pharma	00131-2164-37
100's	$42.25	GENERIC, Mutual/United Research Laboratories	00677-1025-01
100's	$42.43	GENERIC, R.I.D. Inc Distributor	54807-0141-01
100's	$54.78	GENERIC, Southwood Pharmaceuticals Inc	58016-0221-00
100's	$55.36	GENERIC, Alpharma Uspd Makers Of Barre and Nmc	63874-0308-10

S

Saquinavir (003365)

For related information, see the comparative table section in Appendix A.

Categories: Infection, human immunodeficiency virus; FDA Approved 1997 Nov; Pregnancy Category B; WHO Formulary
Drug Classes: Antivirals; Protease inhibitors
Brand Names: Fortovase
Cost of Therapy: $751.02 (HIV; Fortovase; 200mg; 18 capsules/day; 30 day supply)

DESCRIPTION

Note: The trade name has been used throughout this monograph for clarity.
Fortovase brand of saquinavir is an inhibitor of the human immunodeficiency virus (HIV) protease. Fortovase is available as beige, opaque, soft gelatin capsules for oral administration in a 200 mg strength (as saquinavir free base). Each capsule also contains the inactive ingredients medium chain mono- and diglycerides, povidone and dl-alpha tocopherol. Each capsule shell contains gelatin and glycerol 85% with the following colorants: red iron oxide, yellow iron oxide and titanium dioxide. The chemical name for saquinavir is N-tert-butyl-decahydro-2-[2(R)-hydroxy-4-phenyl-3(S)-[[N-(2-quinolylcarbonyl)-L-asparaginyl]amino]butyl]-(4aS,8aS)-isoquinoline-3(S)-carboxamide which has a molecular formula $C_{38}H_{50}N_6O_5$ and a molecular weight of 670.86.

Saquinavir is a white to off-white powder and is insoluble in aqueous medium at 25°C.

CLINICAL PHARMACOLOGY

MICROBIOLOGY

Mechanism of Action

Saquinavir is an inhibitor of HIV protease. HIV protease is an enzyme required for the proteolytic cleavage of viral polyprotein precursors into individual functional proteins found in infectious HIV. Saquinavir is a peptide-like substrate analogue that binds to the protease active site and inhibits the activity of the enzyme. Saquinavir inhibition prevents cleavage of the viral polyproteins resulting in the formation of immature noninfectious virus particles.

Antiviral Activity In Vitro

In vitro antiviral activity of saquinavir was assessed in lymphoblastoid and monocytic cell lines and in peripheral blood lymphocytes. Saquinavir inhibited HIV activity in both acutely and chronically infected cells. IC_{50} and IC_{90} values (50 and 90% inhibitory concentrations) were in the range of 1-30 nM and 5-80 nM, respectively; however, these concentrations may be altered in the presence of human plasma due to protein binding of saquinavir. In cell culture saquinavir demonstrated additive to synergistic effects against HIV in double- and triple-combination regimens with reverse transcriptase inhibitors zidovudine, zalcitabine, didanosine, lamivudine, stavudine and nevirapine, without enhanced cytotoxicity. The relationship between *in vitro* susceptibility of HIV to saquinavir and inhibition of HIV replication in humans has not been established.

Drug Resistance

HIV isolates with reduced susceptibility to saquinavir (4-fold or greater increase in IC_{50} from baseline; *i.e.*, phenotypic resistance) have been selected *in vitro*. Genotypic analyses of these HIV isolates showed several mutations in the HIV-protease gene but only those at codons 48 (Gly→Val) and/or 90 (Leu→Met) were consistently associated with saquinavir resistance.

Isolates from selected patients with loss of antiviral activity and prolonged (range: 24-147 weeks) therapy with Invirase (alone or in combination with nucleoside analogues) showed reduced susceptibility to saquinavir. Genotypic analysis of these isolates showed that mutations at amino acid positions 48 and/or 90 of the HIV-protease gene were most consistently associated with saquinavir resistance. Other mutations in the protease gene were also observed. Mutations at codons 48 and 90 have not been detected in isolates from protease inhibitor naive patients.

In a study (NV15107) of treatment-experienced patients receiving Fortovase monotherapy (1200 mg tid) for 8 weeks followed by antiretroviral combination therapy for a period of 4-48 weeks (median 32 weeks), 10 of 32 patients showed genotypic changes associated with reduced susceptibility to saquinavir. However, for resistance evaluation virus could not be recovered from 11 of 32 patients.

In a study (NV15355) of treatment-naive patients receiving Fortovase in combination with 2 nucleoside analogues for a period of 16 weeks, 1 of 28 patient isolates showed genotypic changes at codon 71 and 90 in the HIV-protease gene.

Cross-Resistance

Among protease inhibitors variable cross-resistance has been recognized. Analysis of saquinavir-resistant isolates from patients following prolonged (24-147 weeks) therapy with Invirase showed that a majority of patients had resistance to at least 1 of 4 other protease inhibitors (indinavir, nelfinavir, ritonavir, 141W94).

PHARMACOKINETICS

The pharmacokinetic properties of saquinavir when administered as Fortovase have been evaluated in healthy volunteers (n=207) and HIV-infected patients (n=91) after single-oral doses (range: 300-1200 mg) and multiple-oral doses (range: 400-1200 mg tid). The disposition properties of saquinavir have been studied in healthy volunteers after intravenous doses of 6, 12, 36 or 72 mg (n=21).

Absorption and Bioavailability in Adults

Following multiple dosing of Fortovase (1200 mg tid) in HIV-infected patients in study NV15107, the mean steady-state area under the plasma concentration versus time curve (AUC) at week 3 was 7249 ng·h/ml (n=31) compared to 866 ng·h/ml (n=10) following multiple dosing with 600 mg tid of Invirase (TABLE 1). Preliminary results from a pharmacokinetic substudy of NV15182 showed a mean saquinavir AUC of 3485 (CV 66%) ng·h/ml (n=11) in patients sampled between weeks 61-69 of therapy (see PRECAUTIONS, General). While this mean AUC value was lower than that of the week 3 steady-state value for Fortovase (1200 mg tid) from study NV15107, it remained higher than the mean AUC value for Invirase in study NV15107.

TABLE 1 *Mean AUC(8) in Patients Treated With Fortovase and Invirase (Week 3)*

Treatment	n	AUC(8) (ng·h/ml)	±SD
Fortovase 1200 mg tid	31	7249	±6174
Invirase 600 mg tid	10	866	±533

The absolute bioavailability of saquinavir administered as Fortovase has not been assessed. However, following single 600 mg doses, the relative bioavailability of saquinavir as Fortovase compared to saquinavir administered as Invirase was estimated as 331% (95% CI 207-530%). The absolute bioavailability of saquinavir administered as Invirase averaged 4% (CV 73%, range 1-9%) in 8 healthy volunteers who received a single 600 mg dose of Invirase following a high-fat breakfast (48 g protein, 60 g carbohydrate, 57 g fat; 1006 kcal). In healthy volunteers receiving single doses of Fortovase (300-1200 mg) and in HIV-infected patients receiving multiple doses of Fortovase (400-1200 mg tid), a greater than dose-proportional increase in saquinavir plasma concentrations has been observed.

Comparison of pharmacokinetic parameters between single- and multiple-dose studies shows that following multiple dosing of Fortovase (1200 mg tid) in healthy male volunteers (n=18), the steady-state AUC was 80% (95% CI 22-176%) higher than that observed after a single 1200 mg dose (n=30).

HIV-infected patients administered Fortovase (1200 mg tid) had AUC and maximum plasma concentration (C_{max}) values approximately twice those observed in healthy volunteers receiving the same treatment regimen. The mean AUC values at week 1 were 4159 (CV 88%) and 8839 (CV 82%) ng·h/ml, and C_{max} values were 1420 (CV 81%) and 2477 (CV 76%) ng/ml for healthy volunteers and HIV-infected patients, respectively.

Food Effect

The mean 12 hour AUC after a single 800 mg oral dose of saquinavir in healthy volunteers (n=12) was increased from 167 ng·h/ml (CV 45%), under fasting conditions, to 1120 ng·h/ml (CV 54%) when Fortovase was given with breakfast (48 g protein, 60 g carbohydrate, 57 g fat; 1006 kcal).

Distribution in Adults

The mean steady-state volume of distribution following intravenous administration of a 12 mg dose of saquinavir (n=8) was 700 L (CV 39%), suggesting saquinavir partitions into tissues. It has been shown that saquinavir, up to 30 μg/ml is approximately 97% bound to plasma proteins.

Metabolism and Elimination in Adults

In vitro studies using human liver microsomes have shown that the metabolism of saquinavir is cytochrome P450 mediated with the specific isoenzyme, CYP3A4, responsible for more than 90% of the hepatic metabolism. Based on *in vitro* studies, saquinavir is rapidly metabolized to a range of mono- and di-hydroxylated inactive compounds. In a mass balance study using 600 mg ^{14}C-saquinavir mesylate (n=8), 88% and 1% of the orally administered radioactivity was recovered in feces and urine, respectively, within 5 days of dosing. In an additional 4 subjects administered 10.5 mg ^{14}C-saquinavir intravenously, 81% and 3% of the intravenously administered radioactivity was recovered in feces and urine, respectively, within 5 days of dosing. In mass balance studies, 13% of circulating radioactivity in plasma was attributed to unchanged drug after oral administration and the remainder attributed to saquinavir metabolites. Following intravenous administration, 66% of circulating radioactivity was attributed to unchanged drug and the remainder attributed to saquinavir metabolites, suggesting that saquinavir undergoes extensive first-pass metabolism.

Systemic clearance of saquinavir was rapid, 1.14 L/h/kg (CV 12%) after intravenous doses of 6, 36 and 72 mg. The mean residence time of saquinavir was 7 hours (n=8).

SPECIAL POPULATIONS

Hepatic or Renal Impairment

Saquinavir pharmacokinetics in patients with hepatic or renal insufficiency has not been investigated (see PRECAUTIONS). Only 1% of saquinavir is excreted in the urine, so the impact of renal impairment on saquinavir elimination should be minimal.

Gender, Race and Age

The effect of gender was investigated in healthy volunteers receiving single 1200 mg doses of Fortovase (n=12 females, 18 males). No effect of gender was apparent on the pharmacokinetics of saquinavir in this study.

The effect of race on the pharmacokinetics of saquinavir when administered as Fortovase is unknown.

The pharmacokinetics of saquinavir when administered as Fortovase has not been investigated in patients >65 years of age or in pediatric patients (<16 years of age).

DRUG INTERACTIONS

See DRUG INTERACTIONS.

Several drug interaction studies have been completed with both Invirase and Fortovase. Results from studies conducted with Invirase may not be applicable to Fortovase. TABLE 2 summarizes the effect of Fortovase on the geometric mean AUC and C_{max} of coadministered drugs. TABLE 3A and TABLE 3B summarize the effect of coadministered drugs on the geometric mean AUC and C_{max} of saquinavir.

For information regarding clinical recommendations, see DRUG INTERACTIONS.

TABLE 2 *Effect of Fortovase on the Pharmacokinetics of Coadministered Drugs*

Coadministered Drug	Fortovase Dose	n	% Change for Coadministered Drug: AUC (95% CI)	C_{max} (95% CI)
Clarithromycin 500 mg bid × 7 days	1200 mg tid × 7 days	12V		
Clarithromycin			inc 45% (17-81%)	inc 39% (10-76%)
14-OH clarithromycin metabolite			dec 24% (5-40%)	dec 34% (14-50%)
Nelfinavir 750 mg single dose	1200 mg tid × 4 days	14P	inc 18% (5-33%)	NC
Ritonavir 400 mg bid × 14 days	400 mg bid × 14 days	8V	NC	NC
Sildenafil 100 mg single dose	1200 mg tid × 8 days	27V	inc 210% (150-300%)	inc 140% (80-230%)
Terfenadine 60 mg bid × 11 days*	1200 mg tid × 4 days	12V		
Terfenadine			inc 368% (257-514%)	inc 253% (164-373%)
Terfenadine acid metabolite			inc 120% (89-156%)	inc 93% (59-133%)

inc Denotes an average increase in exposure by the percentage indicated.
dec Denotes an average decrease in exposure by the percentage indicated.
NC Denotes no statistically significant change in exposure was observed.
* Fortovase should not be coadministered with terfenadine (see DRUG INTERACTIONS).
P Patient.
V Healthy volunteers.

TABLE 3A *Effect of Coadministered Drugs on Fortovase Pharmacokinetics*

Coadministered Drug	Fortovase Dose	n	% Change for Saquinavir: AUC (95% CI)	C_{max} (95% CI)
Clarithromycin 500 mg bid × 7 days	1200 mg tid × 7 days	12V	inc 177% (108-269%)	inc 187% (105-300%)
Indinavir 800 mg q8h × 2 days	800 mg single dose	6V	inc 620% (273-1288%)	inc 551% (320-908%)
	1200 mg single dose	6V	inc 364% (190-644%)	inc 299% (138-568%)
Nelfinavir 750 mg × 4 days	1200 mg single dose	14P	inc 392% (271-553%)	inc 179% (105-280%)
Ritonavir 400 mg bid × 14 days*	400 mg bid × 14 days†	8V	inc 121% (7-359%)	inc 64%‡

inc Denotes an average increase in exposure by the percentage indicated.
* When ritonavir was combined with the same dose of either Invirase or Fortovase, actual mean plasma exposures [AUC(12), 18.2 μg·h/ml, 20.0 μg·h/ml, respectively] were not significantly different.
† Compared to standard Fortovase 1200 mg tid regimen (n=33).
‡ Did not reach statistical significance.
P Patient.
V Healthy volunteers.

INDICATIONS AND USAGE

Fortovase is indicated for use in combination with other antiretroviral agents for the treatment of HIV infection. This indication is based on a study that showed a reduction in both mortality and AIDS-defining clinical events for patients who received Invirase in combination with zalcitabine compared to patients who received either zalcitabine or Invirase alone. This indication is also based on studies that showed increased saquinavir concentrations and improved antiviral activity for Fortovase 1200 mg tid compared to Invirase 600 mg tid.

CONTRAINDICATIONS

Fortovase is contraindicated in patients with clinically significant hypersensitivity to saquinavir or to any of the components contained in the capsule.

Fortovase should not be administered concurrently with terfenadine, cisapride, astemizole, triazolam, midazolam or ergot derivatives, because competition for CYP3A by saquinavir could result in inhibition of the metabolism of these drugs and create the potential for serious and/or life-threatening reactions such as cardiac arrhythmias or prolonged sedation (see DRUG INTERACTIONS).

WARNINGS

ALERT: Find out about medicines that should not be taken with Fortovase. This statement is included on the product's bottle label.

New onset diabetes mellitus, exacerbation of pre-existing diabetes mellitus and hyperglycemia have been reported during postmarketing surveillance in HIV-infected patients receiving protease-inhibitor therapy. Some patients required either initiation or dose adjustments of insulin or oral hypoglycemic agents for the treatment of these events. In some cases diabetic ketoacidosis has occurred. In those patients who discontinued protease-inhibitor therapy, hyperglycemia persisted in some cases. Because these events have been reported voluntarily during clinical practice, estimates of frequency cannot be made and a causal relationship between protease-inhibitor therapy and these events has not been established.

Concomitant use of Fortovase with lovastatin or simvastatin is not recommended. Caution should be exercised if HIV protease inhibitors, including Fortovase, are used concurrently with other HMG-CoA reductase inhibitors that are also metabolized by the CYP3A4 pathway (*e.g.*, atorvastatin, or cerivastatin). Since increased concentrations of statins can, in rare cases, cause severe adverse events such as myopathy including rhabdomyolysis, this risk may be increased when HIV protease inhibitors, including saquinavir, are used in combination with these drugs.

Concomitant use of Fortovase and St. John's wort (hypericum perforatum) or products containing St. John's wort is not recommended. Coadministration of protease inhibitors, including Fortovase, with St. John's wort is expected to substantially decrease protease inhibitor concentrations and may result in sub-optimal levels of Fortovase and lead to loss of virologic response and possible resistance to Fortovase or to the class of protease inhibitors.

PRECAUTIONS

GENERAL

Fortovase soft gelatin capsules and Invirase capsules are not bioequivalent and cannot be used interchangeably. Only Fortovase should be used for the initiation of saquinavir therapy (see DOSAGE AND ADMINISTRATION) since Fortovase soft gelatin capsules provide greater bioavailability and efficacy than Invirase capsules. For patients taking Invirase capsules with a viral load below the limit of quantification, a switch to Fortovase is recommended to maintain a virologic response. For patients taking Invirase capsules who have not had an adequate response or are failing therapy, if saquinavir resistance is clinically suspected, then Fortovase should not be used. If resistance to saquinavir is not clinically suspected, a switch to Fortovase may be considered.

If a serious or severe toxicity occurs during treatment with Fortovase, Fortovase should be interrupted until the etiology of the event is identified or the toxicity resolves. At that time, resumption of treatment with full-dose Fortovase may be considered.

Preliminary results from a pharmacokinetic substudy of NV15182 from patients sampled between weeks 61-69 of treatment showed that the mean saquinavir AUC was lower than

S

TABLE 3B *Effect of Coadministered Drugs on Invirase Pharmacokinetics*

Coadministered Drug	Invirase Dose	n	% Change for Saquinavir AUC (95% CI)	C_{max} (95% CI)
Delavirdine 400 mg tid × 14 days	600 mg tid × 21 days	13V	inc 5-fold	Not available
Ketoconazole 200 mg qd × 6 days	600 mg tid × 6 days	12V	inc 30% (58-235%)	inc 147% (53-298%)
Nevirapine 200 mg bid × 21 days	600 mg tid × 7 days	23P	dec 24% (1-42%)	dec 28% (1-47%)
Ranitidine 150 mg × 2 doses	600 mg single dose	12V	inc 67%‡	inc 74% (16-161%)
Rifabutin 300 mg qd × 14 days	600 mg tid × 14 days	12P	dec 43% (29-53%)	dec 30%‡
Rifampin 600 mg qd × 7 days	600 mg tid × 14 days	12V	dec 84% (79-88%)	dec 79% (68-86%)
Ritonavir 400 mg bid steady state*	400 mg bid steady state†	7P	inc 1587% (808-3034%)	inc 1277% (577-2702%)
Zalcitabine (ddC) 0.75 mg tid × 7 days	600 mg tid × 7 days	27P	NC	NC
Zidovudine (ZDV) 200 mg tid × >7 days	600 mg tid >7 days	20P	NC	NC

inc Denotes an average increase in exposure by the percentage indicated.
dec Denotes an average decrease in exposure by the percentage indicated.
NC Denotes no statistically significant change in exposure was observed.
* When ritonavir was combined with the same dose of either Invirase or Fortovase, actual mean plasma exposures [AUC(12), 18.2 μg·h/ml, 20.0 μg·h/ml, respectively] were not significantly different.
† Compared to standard Invirase 600 mg tid regimen (n=114).
‡ Did not reach statistical significance.
P Patient.
V Healthy volunteers.

the week 3 mean AUC from study NV15107. However, the mean AUC of saquinavir at week 61-69 remained higher than the mean AUC of Invirase in study NV15107 (see CLINICAL PHARMACOLOGY, Pharmacokinetics). The clinical significance of this finding is unknown.

Hepatic Insufficiency

Saquinavir is principally metabolized by the liver. Therefore, caution should be exercised when administering Fortovase to patients with hepatic insufficiency since patients with baseline liver function tests >5 times the upper limit of normal were not included in clinical studies. Although a causal relationship has not been established, there have been reports of exacerbation of chronic liver dysfunction, including portal hypertension, in patients with underlying hepatitis B or C, cirrhosis or other underlying liver abnormalities.

Hemophilia

There have been reports of spontaneous bleeding in patients with hemophilia A and B treated with protease inhibitors. In some patients additional factor VIII was required. In the majority of reported cases treatment with protease inhibitors was continued or restarted. A causal relationship between protease-inhibitor therapy and these episodes has not been established.

Fat Redistribution

Redistribution/accumulation of body fat including central obesity, dorsocervical fat enlargement (buffalo hump), peripheral wasting, breast enlargement and "cushingoid appearance" have been observed in patients receiving protease inhibitors. A causal relationship between protease inhibitor therapy and these events has not been established and the long-term consequences are currently unknown.

S

RESISTANCE/CROSS-RESISTANCE

Varying degrees of cross-resistance among protease inhibitors have been observed. Continued administration of saquinavir therapy following loss of viral suppression may increase the likelihood of cross-resistance to other protease inhibitors (see CLINICAL PHARMACOLOGY, Microbiology).

INFORMATION FOR THE PATIENT

A statement to patients and health care providers is included on the product's bottle label: **ALERT: Find out about medicines that should NOT be taken with Fortovase.** A Patient Package Insert (PPI) for Fortovase is available for patient information.

Patients should be informed that any change from Invirase to Fortovase should be made only under the supervision of a physician.

Patients should be informed that Fortovase is not a cure for HIV infection and that they may continue to contract illnesses associated with advanced HIV infection, including opportunistic infections. They should be informed that Fortovase therapy has not been shown to reduce the risk of transmitting HIV to others through sexual contact or blood contamination.

Fortovase may interact with some drugs; therefore, patients should be advised to report to their physician the use of any other prescription, nonprescription medication, or herbal products, particularly St. John's wort.

Patients should be informed that redistribution or accumulation of body fat may occur in patients receiving protease inhibitors and that the cause and long-term health effects of these conditions are not known at this time.

Patients should be advised that Fortovase should be taken within 2 hours after a full meal (see CLINICAL PHARMACOLOGY, Pharmacokinetics). Patients should be advised of the importance of taking their medication every day, as prescribed, to achieve maximum benefit. Patients should not alter the dose or discontinue therapy without consulting their physician. If a dose is missed, patients should take the next dose as soon as possible. However, the patient should not double the next dose.

Patients should be told that the long-term effects of Fortovase are unknown at this time.

Patients should be informed that refrigerated (2-8°C, 36-46°F) capsules of Fortovase remain stable until the expiration date printed on the label. Once brought to room temperature [at or below 25°C (77°F)], capsules should be used within 3 months.

LABORATORY TESTS

Clinical chemistry tests should be performed prior to initiating Fortovase therapy and at appropriate intervals thereafter. Elevated nonfasting triglyceride levels have been observed in patients in saquinavir trials. Triglyceride levels should be periodically monitored during therapy. For comprehensive information concerning laboratory test alterations associated with use of other antiretroviral therapies, physicians should refer to the complete product information for these drugs.

CARCINOGENESIS, MUTAGENESIS, AND IMPAIRMENT OF FERTILITY

Carcinogenesis

Carcinogenicity studies in rats and mice have not yet been completed.

Mutagenesis

Mutagenicity and genotoxicity studies, with and without metabolic activation where appropriate, have shown that saquinavir has no mutagenic activity *in vitro* in either bacterial (Ames test) or mammalian cells (Chinese hamster lung V79/HPRT test). Saquinavir does not induce chromosomal damage *in vivo* in the mouse micronucleus assay or *in vitro* in human peripheral blood lymphocytes and does not induce primary DNA damage *in vitro* in the unscheduled DNA synthesis test.

Impairment of Fertility

Fertility and reproductive performance were not affected in rats at plasma exposures (AUC values) approximately 50% of those achieved in humans at the recommended dose.

PREGNANCY, TERATOGENIC EFFECTS, PREGNANCY CATEGORY B

Reproduction studies conducted with saquinavir in rats have shown no embryotoxicity or teratogenicity at plasma exposures (AUC values) approximately 50% of those achieved in humans at the recommended dose or in rabbits at plasma exposures approximately 40% of those achieved at the recommended clinical dose of Fortovase. Distribution studies in these species showed that placental transfer of saquinavir is low (less than 5% of maternal plasma concentrations).

Studies in rats indicated that exposure to saquinavir from late pregnancy through lactation at plasma concentrations (AUC values) approximately 50% of those achieved in humans at the recommended dose of Fortovase had no effect on the survival, growth and development of offspring to weaning. Because animal reproduction studies are not always predictive of human response, Fortovase should only be used during pregnancy after taking into account the importance of the drug to the mother. Presently, there are no reports of women receiving Fortovase in clinical trials who became pregnant.

Antiretroviral Pregnancy Registry: To monitor maternal-fetal outcomes of pregnant women exposed to antiretroviral medications, including Fortovase, an Antiretroviral Pregnancy Registry has been established. Physicians are encouraged to register patients by calling 1-800-258-4263.

NURSING MOTHERS

The Centers for Disease Control and Prevention recommend that HIV-infected mothers not breastfeed their infants to avoid risking postnatal transmission of HIV. It is not known whether saquinavir is excreted in human milk. Because of both the potential for HIV transmission and the potential for serious adverse reactions in nursing infants, **mothers should be instructed not to breastfeed if they are receiving antiretroviral medications, including Fortovase.**

PEDIATRIC USE

Safety and effectiveness of Fortovase in HIV-infected pediatric patients younger than 16 years of age have not been established.

GERIATRIC USE

Clinical studies of Fortovase did not include sufficient numbers of subjects aged 65 and over to determine whether they respond differently from younger subjects. In general, caution should be taken when dosing Fortovase in elderly patients due to the greater frequency of decreased hepatic, renal, or cardiac function, and of concomitant disease or other drug therapy.

DRUG INTERACTIONS

Several drug interaction studies have been completed with both Invirase and Fortovase. Observations from drug interaction studies with Invirase may not be predictive for Fortovase.

Drugs that should not be coadministered with Fortovase:

Antihistamines: Astemizole, terfenadine.
Antimigraine: Ergot derivatives.
GI motility agents: Cisapride.
Sedatives/hypnotics: Midazolam, triazolam.

Clinically significant drug interactions which decrease saquinavir plasma concentrations:

HIV non-nucleoside reverse transcriptase inhibitors: Nevirapine*.
Antimycobacterial agents: Rifabutin*, rifampin*.

Clinically significant drug interactions which increase saquinavir plasma concentrations:

Antibiotics: Clarithromycin.†

HIV protease inhibitors: Indinavir†, ritonavir†, nelfinavir†.

HIV non-nucleoside reverse transcriptase inhibitors: Delavirdine*.

Antifungal agents: Ketoconazole*.

Other potential drug interactions‡:

Anticonvulsants: *Carbamazepine, Phenobarbital, Phenytoin:* May decrease saquinavir plasma concentrations.

Corticosteriods: *Dexamethasone:* May decrease saquinavir plasma concentrations.

*Studied with Invirase. †Studied with Fortovase. ‡This list is not all inclusive.

ANTIBIOTICS

Clarithromycin

Coadministration of clarithromycin with Fortovase resulted in a 177% increase in saquinavir plasma AUC, a 45% increase in clarithromycin AUC and a 24% decrease in clarithromycin 14-OH metabolite AUC.

ANTIHISTAMINES

Terfenadine

Coadministration of terfenadine with Fortovase resulted in increased terfenadine plasma levels; therefore, Fortovase should not be administered concurrently with terfenadine because of the potential for serious and/or life-threatening cardiac arrhythmias.

Astemizole

Because a similar interaction to that seen with terfenadine is likely from the coadministration of Fortovase and astemizole, Fortovase should not be administered concurrently with astemizole.

ERECTILE DYSFUNCTION AGENTS

Sildenafil

In a study performed in healthy male volunteers, coadministration of saquinavir, a CYP3A4 inhibitor, at steady state (1200 mg tid) with sildenafil (100 mg single dose) resulted in a 140% increase in sildenafil C_{max} and a 210% increase in sildenafil AUC. Sildenafil had no effect on saquinavir pharmacokinetics. When sildenafil is administered concomitantly with saquinavir a starting dose of 25 mg of sildenafil should be considered.

HIV PROTEASE INHIBITORS

Indinavir

Coadministration of indinavir with Fortovase (1200 mg single dose) resulted in a 364% increase in saquinavir plasma AUC. Currently, there are no safety and efficacy data available from the use of this combination.

Nelfinavir

Coadministration of nelfinavir with Fortovase resulted in an 18% increase in nelfinavir plasma AUC and a 392% increase in saquinavir plasma AUC. Currently, there are no safety and efficacy data available from the use of this combination.

Ritonavir

Following approximately 4 weeks of a combination regimen of saquinavir (400 or 600 mg bid) and ritonavir (400 or 600 mg bid) in HIV-infected patients, saquinavir AUC values were at least 17-fold greater than historical AUC values from patients who received saquinavir 600 mg tid without ritonavir. When used in combination therapy for up to 24 weeks, doses greater than 400 mg bid of either ritonavir or saquinavir were associated with an increase in adverse events. Plasma exposures achieved with Invirase (400 mg bid) and ritonavir (400 mg bid) are similar to those achieved with Fortovase (400 mg bid) and ritonavir (400 mg bid).

HIV REVERSE TRANSCRIPTASE INHIBITORS

Based on known metabolic pathways and routes of elimination for nucleoside reverse transcriptase inhibitors, no interaction with saquinavir is expected.

HIV NON-NUCLEOSIDE REVERSE TRANSCRIPTASE INHIBITORS

Delavirdine

Coadministration of delavirdine with Invirase resulted in a 5-fold increase in saquinavir plasma AUC. Currently there are limited safety and no efficacy data available from the use of this combination. In a small, preliminary study, hepatocellular enzyme elevations occurred in 13% of subjects during the first several weeks of the delavirdine and saquinavir combination (6% Grade 3 or 4). Hepatocellular changes should be monitored frequently if this combination is prescribed.

Nevirapine

Coadministration of nevirapine with Invirase resulted in a 24% decrease in saquinavir plasma AUC. Currently, there are no safety and efficacy data available from the use of this combination.

ANTIFUNGAL AGENTS

Ketoconazole

Coadministration of ketoconazole with Invirase resulted in a 130% increase in saquinavir plasma AUC.

ANTIMYCOBACTERIAL AGENTS

Rifabutin

Coadministration of rifabutin with Invirase resulted in a 43% decrease in saquinavir plasma AUC. Physicians should consider using an alternative to rifabutin when a patient is taking Fortovase.

Rifampin

Coadministration of rifampin with Invirase resulted in an 84% decrease in saquinavir plasma AUC. Physicians should consider using an alternative to rifampin when a patient is taking Fortovase.

H_2 ANTAGONISTS

Ranitidine

Little or no change in the pharmacokinetics of Invirase was observed when coadministered with ranitidine. No significant interaction would be expected between Fortovase and ranitidine.

GI MOTILITY AGENTS

Cisapride

Although no interaction study has been conducted, cisapride should not be administered concurrently with Fortovase because of the potential for serious and/or life-threatening cardiac arrhythmias.

ADVERSE REACTIONS

See PRECAUTIONS.

The safety of Fortovase was studied in more than 500 patients who received the drug either alone or in combination with other antiretroviral agents. The majority of treatment-related adverse events were of mild intensity. The most frequently reported treatment-emergent adverse events among patients receiving Fortovase in combination with other antiretroviral agents were diarrhea, nausea, abdominal discomfort and dyspepsia.

Clinical adverse events of at least moderate intensity which occurred in ≥2% of patients in studies NV15182 and NV15355 are summarized in TABLE 4. The median duration of treatment in studies NV15182 and NV15355 were 52 and 18 weeks, respectively. In NV15182, more than 300 patients were on treatment for approximately 1 year.

Fortovase did not appear to alter the pattern, frequency or severity of known major toxicities associated with the use of nucleoside analogues. Physicians should refer to the complete product information for other antiretroviral agents as appropriate for drug-associated adverse reactions to these other agents.

Rare occurrences of the following serious adverse experiences have been reported during clinical trials of Fortovase and/or Invirase and were considered at least possibly related to use of study drugs: confusion, ataxia and weakness; seizures; headache; acute myelobastic leukemia; hemolytic anemia; thrombocytopenia; thrombocytopenia and intracranial hemorrhage leading to death; attempted suicide; Stevens-Johnson syndrome; bullous skin eruption and polyarthritis; severe cutaneous reaction associated with increased liver function tests; isolated elevation of transaminases; exacerbation of chronic liver disease with Grade 4 elevated liver function tests, jaundice, ascites, and right and left upper quadrant abdominal pain; pancreatitis leading to death; intestinal obstruction; portal hypertension; thrombophlebitis; peripheral vasoconstriction; drug fever; nephrolithiasis; and acute renal insufficiency.

TABLE 5 summarizes the percentage of patients with marked laboratory abnormalities in study NV15182 and NV15355 (median duration of treatment was 52 and 18 weeks, respectively). In study NV15182, by 48 weeks <1% of patients discontinued treatment due to laboratory abnormalities.

TABLE 4 *Percentage of Patients With Treatment-Emergent Adverse Events* of at Least Moderate Intensity, Occuring in ≥2% of Patients*

	NV15182 (48 weeks)	NV15355 (16 weeks) Naive Patients	
	Fortovase + TOC†	Invirase + 2 RTIs‡	Fortovase + 2 RTIs‡
Adverse Event	n=442	n=81	n=90
Gastrointestinal			
Diarrhea	19.9%	12.3%	15.6%
Nausea	10.6%	13.6%	17.8%
Abdominal discomfort	8.6%	4.9%	13.3%
Dyspepsia	8.4%	—	8.9%
Flatulence	5.7%	7.4%	12.2%
Vomiting	2.9%	1.2%	4.4%
Abdominal pain	2.3%	1.2%	7.8%
Constipation	—	—	3.3%
Body as a Whole			
Fatigue	4.8%	6.2%	6.7%
Central and Peripheral Nervous System			
Headaches	5.0%	4.9%	8.9%
Psychiatric Disorders			
Depression	2.7%	—	—
Insomnia	—	1.2%	5.6%
Anxiety	—	2.5%	2.2%
Libido disorder	—	—	2.2%
Special Senses Disorders			
Taste alteration	—	1.2%	4.4%
Musculoskeletal Disorders			
Pain	—	3.7%	3.3%
Dermatologic Disorders			
Eczema	—	2.5%	—
Rash	—	2.5%	—
Verruca	—	—	2.2%

* Includes adverse events at least possibly related to study drug or of unknown intensity and/or relationship to treatment (corresponding to ACTG Grade 3 and 4).
† Antiretroviral Treatment of Choice.
‡ Reverse Transcriptase Inhibitor.

Additional marked lab abnormalities have been observed with Invirase. These include: calcium (low), phosphate (low), potassium (low), sodium (low).

MONOTHERAPY AND COMBINATION STUDIES

Other clinical adverse experiences of any intensity, at least remotely related to Fortovase and Invirase, including those in <2% of patients, are listed below by body system.

S

TABLE 5 *Percentage of Patients With Marked Laboratory Abnormalities**

	Limit	NV15182 (48 weeks) Fortovase + TOC† n=442	NV15355 (16 weeks) Naive Patients Invirase + 2 RTIs‡ n=81	Fortovase + 2 RTIs‡ n=90
Biochemistry				
Alkaline phosphatase	>5 × ULN§	0.5%	0.0%	0.0%
Calcium (high)	>12.5 mg/dl	0.2%	0.0%	0.0%
Creatine kinase	>4 × ULN§	7.8%	0.0%	4.8%
Gamma GT	>5 × ULN§	5.7%	2.6%	7.1%
Glucose (low)	<40 mg/dl	6.4%	2.5%	3.5%
Glucose (high)	>250 mg/dl	1.4%	1.3%	1.2%
Phosphate	<1.5 mg/dl	0.5%	0.0%	0.0%
Potassium (high)	>6.5 mEq/L	2.7%	0.0%	1.2%
Serum amylase	>2 × ULN§	1.9%	ND	ND
SGOT (AST)	>5 × ULN§	4.1%	0.0%	1.2%
SGPT (ALT)	>5 × ULN§	5.7%	1.3%	2.3%
Sodium (high)	>157 mEq/L	0.7%	0.0%	0.0%
Total bilirubin	>2.5 × ULN§	1.6%	0.0%	0.0%
Hematology				
Hemoglobin	<7.0 g/dl	0.7%	0.0%	1.2%
Absolute neutrophil count	<750 mm^3	2.9%	2.9%	1.2%
Platelets	<50,000 mm^3	0.9%	2.5%	0.0%

* ACTG Grade 3 or above.
† Antiretroviral Treatment of Choice.
‡ Reverse Transcriptase Inhibitor.
§ ULN=Upper limit of normal range.
ND Not Done.

Autonomic Nervous System: Mouth dry, night sweats, sweating increased.

Body as a Whole: Allergic reaction, anorexia, appetite decreased, appetite disturbances, asthenia, chest pain, edema, fever, intoxication, malaise, olfactory disorder, pain body, pain pelvic, retrosternal pain, shivering, trauma, wasting syndrome, weakness generalized, weight decrease, redistribution/accumulation of body fat (see PRECAUTIONS, Fat Redistribution).

Cardiovascular/Cerebrovascular: Cyanosis, heart murmur, heart rate disorder, heart valve disorder, hypertension, hypotension, stroke, syncope, vein distended.

Central and Peripheral Nervous System: Ataxia, cerebral hemorrhage, confusion, convulsions, dizziness, dysarthria, dysesthesia, hyperesthesia, hyperreflexia, hyporeflexia, light-headed feeling, myelopolyradiculoneuritis, neuropathy, numbness extremities, numbness face, paresis, paresthesia, peripheral neuropathy, poliomyelitis, prickly sensation, progressive multifocal leukoencephalopathy, spasms, tremor, unconsciousness.

Dermatologic: Acne, alopecia, chalazion, dermatitis, dermatitis seborrheic, erythema, folliculitis, furunculosis, hair changes, hot flushes, nail disorder, papillomatosis, papular rash, photosensitivity reaction, pigment changes skin, parasites external, pruritus, psoriasis, rash maculopapular, rash pruritic, red face, skin disorder, skin nodule, skin syndrome, skin ulceration, urticaria, verruca, xeroderma.

Endocrine/Metabolic: Dehydration, diabetes mellitus, hyperglycemia, hypoglycemia, hypothyroidism, thirst, triglyceride increase, weight increase.

Gastrointestinal: Abdominal distention, bowel movements frequent, buccal mucosa ulceration, canker sores oral, cheilitis, colic abdominal, dysphagia, esophageal ulceration, esophagitis, eructation, fecal incontinence, feces bloodstained, feces discolored, gastralgia, gastritis, gastroesophageal reflux, gastrointestinal inflammation, gingivitis, glossitis, hemorrhage rectum, hemorrhoids, infectious diarrhea, melena, painful defecation, parotid disorder, pruritus ani, pyrosis, salivary glands disorder, stomach upset, stomatitis, taste unpleasant, toothache, tooth disorder, ulcer gastrointestinal.

Hematologic: Anemia, neutropenia, pancytopenia, splenomegaly.

Liver and Biliary: Cholangitis sclerosing, cholelithiasis, hepatitis, hepatomegaly, hepatosplenomegaly, jaundice, liver enzyme disorder, pancreatitis.

Musculoskeletal: Arthralgia, arthritis, back pain, cramps leg, cramps muscle, lumbago, musculoskeletal disorders, myalgia, myopathy, pain facial, pain jaw, pain leg, pain musculoskeletal, stiffness, tissue changes.

Neoplasm: Kaposi's sarcoma, tumor.

Platelet, Bleeding, Clotting: Bleeding dermal, hemorrhage, microhemorrhages, thrombocytopenia.

Psychiatric: Agitation, amnesia, anxiety attack, behavior disturbances, dreaming excessive, euphoria, hallucination, intellectual ability reduced, irritability, lethargy, overdose effect, psychic disorder, psychosis, somnolence, speech disorder.

Reproductive System: Epididymitis, erectile impotence, impotence, menstrual disorder, menstrual irregularity, penis disorder, prostate enlarged, vaginal discharge.

Resistance Mechanism: Abscess, angina tonsillaris, candidiasis, cellulitis, herpes simplex, herpes zoster, infection bacterial, infection mycotic, infection staphylococcal, infestation parasitic, influenza, lymphadenopathy, molluscum contagiosum, moniliasis.

Respiratory: Asthma bronchial, bronchitis, cough, dyspnea, epistaxis, hemoptysis, laryngitis, pharyngitis, pneumonia, pulmonary disease, respiratory disorder, rhinitis, rhinitis allergic atopic, sinusitis, upper respiratory tract infection.

Special Senses: Blepharitis, conjunctivitis, cytomegalovirus retinitis, dry eye syndrome, earache, ear pressure, eye irritation, hearing decreased, otitis, taste unpleasant, tinnitus, visual disturbance, xerophthalmia.

Urinary System: Micturition disorder, nocturia, renal calculus, renal colic, urinary tract bleeding, urinary tract infection.

DOSAGE AND ADMINISTRATION

Fortovase soft gelatin capsules and Invirase capsules are not bioequivalent and cannot be used interchangeably. When using saquinavir as part of an antiviral regimen Fortovase is the recommended formulation. In rare circumstances, Invirase may be considered if it is to be combined with antiretrovirals that significantly inhibit saquinavir's metabolism (see CLINICAL PHARMACOLOGY, Drug Interactions).

The recommended dose of Fortovase is six 200 mg capsules orally, 3 times a day (1200 mg tid). Fortovase should be taken with a meal or up to 2 hours after a meal. When used in combination with nucleoside analogues, the dosage of Fortovase should not be reduced as this will lead to greater than dose proportional decreases in saquinavir plasma levels.

Patients should be advised that Fortovase, like other protease inhibitors, is recommended for use in combination with active antiretroviral therapy. Greater activity has been observed when new antiretroviral therapies are begun at the same time as Fortovase. As with all protease inhibitors, adherence to the prescribed regimen is strongly recommended. Concomitant therapy should be based on a patient's prior drug exposure.

MONITORING OF PATIENTS

Clinical chemistry tests should be performed prior to initiating Fortovase therapy and at appropriate intervals thereafter. For comprehensive patient monitoring recommendations for other antiretroviral therapies, physicians should refer to the complete product information for these drugs.

DOSE ADJUSTMENT FOR COMBINATION THERAPY WITH FORTOVASE

For toxicities that may be associated with Fortovase, the drug should be interrupted. For recipients of combination therapy with Fortovase and other antiretroviral agents, dose adjustment of the other antiretroviral agents should be based on the known toxicity profile of the individual drug. Physicians should refer to the complete product information for these drugs for comprehensive dose adjustment recommendations and drug-associated adverse reactions.

HOW SUPPLIED

Fortovase 200 mg capsules are beige, opaque, soft gelatin capsules with "ROCHE" and "0246" imprinted on the capsule shell.

STORAGE

The capsules should be refrigerated at 2-8°C (36-46°F) in tightly closed bottles until dispensed.

For patient use, refrigerated (2-8°C, 36-46°F) capsules of Fortovase remain stable until the expiration date printed on the label. Once brought to room temperature [at or below 25°C (77°F)], capsules should be used within 3 months.

Saquinavir Mesylate (003250)

For related information, see the comparative table section in Appendix A.

Categories: Infection, human immunodeficiency virus; FDA Approved 1995 Dec; Pregnancy Category B
Drug Classes: Antivirals; Protease inhibitors
Brand Names: Invirase
Foreign Brand Availability: Invi-rase (South-Africa)
Cost of Therapy: $320.93 (HIV; Invirase; 200 mg; 9 capsules/day; 30 day supply)

WARNING

Note: The trade name has been used throughout this monograph for clarity.

Invirase (saquinavir mesylate) capsules and Fortovase (saquinavir) soft gelatin capsules are not bioequivalent and cannot be used interchangeably. When using saquinavir as part of an antiviral regimen Fortovase is the recommended formulation. In rare circumstances, Invirase may be considered if it is to be combined with antiretrovirals that significantly inhibit saquinavir's metabolism (see CLINICAL PHARMACOLOGY, Drug Interactions).

DESCRIPTION

Invirase brand of saquinavir mesylate is an inhibitor of the human immunodeficiency virus (HIV) protease. Invirase is available as light brown and green, opaque hard gelatin capsules for oral administration in a 200 mg strength (as saquinavir free base). Each capsule also contains the inactive ingredients lactose, microcrystalline cellulose, povidone K30, sodium starch glycolate, talc and magnesium stearate. Each capsule shell contains gelatin and water with the following dye systems: red iron oxide, yellow iron oxide, black iron oxide, FD&C blue no. 2 and titanium dioxide. The chemical name for saquinavir mesylate is N-tert-butyl-decahydro-2-[2(R)-hydroxy-4-phenyl-3(S)-[[N-(2-quinolylcarbonyl)-L-asparaginyl]amino]butyl]-(4aS,8aS)-isoquinoline-3(S)-carboxamide methanesulfonate with a molecular formula $C_{38}H_{50}N_6O_5 \cdot CH_4O_3S$ and a molecular weight of 766.96. The molecular weight of the free base is 670.86.

Saquinavir mesylate is a white to off-white, very fine powder with an aqueous solubility of 2.22 mg/ml at 25°C.

CLINICAL PHARMACOLOGY

MECHANISM OF ACTION

HIV protease cleaves viral polyprotein precursors to generate functional proteins in HIV-infected cells. The cleavage of viral polyprotein precursors is essential for maturation of infectious virus. Saquinavir mesylate, henceforth referred to as saquinavir, is a synthetic peptide-like substrate analogue that inhibits the activity of HIV protease and prevents the cleavage of viral polyproteins.

MICROBIOLOGY

Antiviral Activity In Vitro

The *in vitro* antiviral activity of saquinavir was assessed in lymphoblastoid and monocytic cell lines and in peripheral blood lymphocytes. Saquinavir inhibited HIV activity in both acutely and chronically infected cells. IC_{50} values (50% inhibitory concentration) were in the range of 1-30 nM. In cell culture saquinavir demonstrated additive to synergistic effects against HIV in double- and triple-combination regimens with reverse transcriptase inhibitors zidovudine (ZDV), zalcitabine (ddC) and didanosine (ddI), without enhanced cytotoxicity.

Resistance

HIV isolates with reduced susceptibility to saquinavir have been selected *in vitro*. Genotypic analyses of these isolates showed substitution mutations in the HIV protease at amino acid positions 48 (Glycine to Valine) and 90 (Leucine to Methionine).

Phenotypic and genotypic changes in HIV isolates from patients treated with saquinavir were also monitored in Phase 1/2 clinical trials. Phenotypic changes were defined as a 10-fold decrease in sensitivity from baseline. Two viral protease mutations (L90M and/or G48V, the former predominating) were found in virus from treated, but not untreated, patients. The incidence across studies of phenotypic and genotypic changes in the subsets of patients studied for a period of 16-74 weeks (median observation time approximately 1 year) is shown in TABLE 1. However, the clinical relevance of phenotypic and genotypic changes associated with saquinavir therapy has not been established.

TABLE 1 *Frequency of Genotypic and Phenotypic Changes in Selected Patients Treated With Saquinavir*

	Genotypic*		Phenotypic†	
	24 Week	1 Year	24 Week	1 Year
Monotherapy	3/8 (38%)	15/33 (45%)	2/22 (9%)	5/11 (45%)
Combination therapy	5/30 (17%)	16/52 (31%)	0/23 (0%)	11/29 (38%)

* Double mutation (G48V and L90M) has occurred in 2 of 33 patients receiving monotherapy. The double mutation has not occurred with combination therapy.
† Phenotypic changes have been defined as at least a 10-fold change in sensitivity relative to baseline. In a few patients genotypic and phenotypic changes were unrelated.

Cross-Resistance to Other Antiretrovirals

The potential for HIV cross-resistance between protease inhibitors has not been fully explored. Therefore, it is unknown what effect saquinavir therapy will have on the activity of subsequent protease inhibitors. Cross-resistance between saquinavir and reverse transcriptase inhibitors is unlikely because of the different enzyme targets involved. ZDV-resistant HIV isolates have been shown to be sensitive to saquinavir *in vitro*.

PHARMACOKINETICS

The pharmacokinetic properties of saquinavir have been evaluated in healthy volunteers (n=351) and HIV-infected patients (n=270) after single and multiple oral doses of 25, 75, 200, and 600 mg tid and in healthy volunteers after intravenous doses of 6, 12, 36, or 72 mg (n=21).

Absorption and Bioavailability in Adults

Following multiple dosing (600 mg tid) in HIV-infected patients (n=30), the steady-state area under the plasma concentration versus time curve (AUC) was 2.5 times (95% CI 1.6-3.8) higher than that observed after a single dose. HIV-infected patients administered saquinavir 600 mg tid, with the instructions to take saquinavir after a meal or substantial snack, had AUC and maximum plasma concentration (C_{max}) values which were about twice those observed in healthy volunteers receiving the same treatment regimen (TABLE 2).

TABLE 2 *Mean (%CV) AUC and C_{max} in Patients and Healthy Volunteers*

	AUC(8) (dose interval) (ng·h/ml)	C_{max} (ng/ml)
Healthy volunteers (n=6)	359.0 (46)	90.39 (49)
Patients (n=113)	757.2 (84)	253.3 (99)

Absolute bioavailability averaged 4% (CV 73%, range: 1-9%) in 8 healthy volunteers who received a single 600 mg dose (3 × 200 mg) of saquinavir following a high fat breakfast (48 g protein, 60 g carbohydrate, 57 g fat; 1006 kcal). The low bioavailability is thought to be due to a combination of incomplete absorption and extensive first-pass metabolism.

Food Effect

The mean 24 hour AUC after a single 600 mg oral dose (6 × 100 mg) in healthy volunteers (n=6) was increased from 24 ng·h/ml (CV 33%), under fasting conditions, to 161 ng·h/ml (CV 35%) when saquinavir was given following a high fat breakfast (48 g protein, 60 g carbohydrate, 57 g fat; 1006 kcal). Saquinavir 24 hour AUC and C_{max} (n=6) following the administration of a higher calorie meal (943 kcal, 54 g fat) were on average 2 times higher than after a lower calorie, lower fat meal (355 kcal, 8 g fat). The effect of food has been shown to persist for up to 2 hours.

Distribution in Adults

The mean steady-state volume of distribution following intravenous administration of a 12 mg dose of saquinavir (n=8) was 700 L (CV 39%), suggesting saquinavir partitions into tissues. Saquinavir was approximately 98% bound to plasma proteins over a concentration range of 15-700 ng/ml. In 2 patients receiving saquinavir 600 mg tid, cerebrospinal fluid concentrations were negligible when compared to concentrations from matching plasma samples.

Metabolism and Elimination in Adults

In vitro studies using human liver microsomes have shown that the metabolism of saquinavir is cytochrome P450 mediated with the specific isoenzyme, CYP3A4, responsible for more than 90% of the hepatic metabolism. Based on *in vitro* studies, saquinavir is rapidly metabolized to a range of mono- and di-hydroxylated inactive compounds. In a mass balance study using 600 mg ^{14}C-saquinavir (n=8), 88% and 1% of the orally administered radioactivity, was recovered in feces and urine, respectively, within 5 days of dosing. In an additional 4 subjects administered 10.5 mg ^{14}C-saquinavir intravenously, 81% and 3% of the intravenously administered radioactivity was recovered in feces and urine, respectively, within 5 days of dosing. In mass balance studies, 13% of circulating radioactivity in plasma was attributed to unchanged drug after oral administration and the remainder attributed to saquinavir metabolites. Following intravenous administration, 66% of circulating radioactivity was attributed to unchanged drug and the remainder attributed to saquinavir metabolites, suggesting that saquinavir undergoes extensive first-pass metabolism. Systemic clearance of saquinavir was rapid, 1.14 L/h/kg (CV 12%) after intravenous doses of 6, 36, and 72 mg. The mean residence time of saquinavir was 7 hours (n=8).

Special Populations

Hepatic or Renal Impairment

Saquinavir pharmacokinetics in patients with hepatic or renal insufficiency has not been investigated (see PRECAUTIONS).

Gender, Race, and Age

Pharmacokinetic data were available for 17 women in the Phase 1/2 studies. Pooled data did not reveal an apparent effect of gender on the pharmacokinetics of saquinavir.

The effect of race on the pharmacokinetics of saquinavir has not been evaluated, due to the small numbers of minorities for whom pharmacokinetic data were available.

Saquinavir pharmacokinetics has not been investigated in patients >65 years of age or in pediatric patients (<16 years).

Drug Interactions

Hivid and ZDV

Concomitant use of Invirase with Hivid (zalcitabine, ddC) and ZDV has been studied (as triple combination) in adults. Pharmacokinetic data suggest that the absorption, metabolism and elimination of each of these drugs are unchanged when they are used together.

Nelfinavir

In 14 HIV-positive patients, coadministration of nelfinavir (750 mg) with saquinavir (given as Fortovase, 1200 mg) resulted in an 18% (95% CI 5-33%) increase in nelfinavir plasma AUC and a 392% (95% CI 271-553%) increase in saquinavir plasma AUC (see DRUG INTERACTIONS).

Ritonavir

Following approximately 4 weeks of a combination regimen of saquinavir (400 or 600 mg bid) and ritonavir (400 or 600 mg bid) in HIV-positive patients, saquinavir AUC and C_{max} values increased at least 17-fold (95% CI 9- to 31-fold) and 14-fold, respectively (see DRUG INTERACTIONS).

Delavirdine

In 13 healthy volunteers, coadministration of saquinavir (600 mg tid) with delavirdine (400 mg tid) resulted in a 5-fold increase in saquinavir AUC. In 7 healthy volunteers, coadministration of saquinavir (600 mg tid) with delavirdine (400 mg tid) resulted in a 15% ± 16% decrease in delavirdine AUC (see DRUG INTERACTIONS).

Nevirapine

In 23 HIV-positive patients, coadministration of saquinavir (600 mg tid) with nevirapine (200 mg bid) resulted in a 24% (95% CI 1-42%) and 28% (95% CI 1-47%) decrease in saquinavir plasma AUC and C_{max}, respectively (see DRUG INTERACTIONS).

Ketoconazole

Concomitant administration of ketoconazole (200 mg qd) and saquinavir (600 mg tid) to 12 healthy volunteers resulted in steady-state saquinavir AUC and C_{max} values which were 3 times those seen with saquinavir alone. No dose adjustment is required when the 2 drugs are coadministered at the doses studied. Ketoconazole pharmacokinetics was unaffected by coadministration with saquinavir.

Rifampin

Coadministration of rifampin (600 mg qd) and saquinavir (600 mg tid) to 12 healthy volunteers decreased the steady-state AUC and C_{max} of saquinavir by approximately 80%.

Rifabutin

Preliminary data from 12 HIV-infected patients indicate that the steady-state AUC of saquinavir (600 mg tid) was decreased by 40% when saquinavir was coadministered with rifabutin (300 mg qd).

INDICATIONS AND USAGE

Invirase in combination with other antiretroviral agents is indicated for the treatment of HIV infection. This indication is based on results from studies of surrogate marker responses and from a clinical study that showed a reduction in both mortality and AIDS-defining clinical events for patients who received Invirase in combination with Hivid compared to patients who received either Hivid or Invirase alone.

CONTRAINDICATIONS

Invirase is contraindicated in patients with clinically significant hypersensitivity to saquinavir or to any of the components contained in the capsule.

Invirase should not be administered concurrently with terfenadine, cisapride, astemizole, triazolam, midazolam or ergot derivatives. Inhibition of CYP3A4 by saquinavir could result in elevated plasma concentrations of these drugs, potentially causing serious or life-threatening reactions.

WARNINGS

ALERT: Find out about medicines that should not be taken with Invirase. This statement is included on the product's bottle label.

New onset diabetes mellitus, exacerbation of preexisting diabetes mellitus and hyperglycemia have been reported during postmarketing surveillance in HIV-infected patients receiving protease inhibitor therapy. Some patients required either initiation or dose adjustments of insulin or oral hypoglycemic agents for treatment of these events. In some cases diabetic ketoacidosis has occurred. In those patients who discontinued protease inhibitor therapy, hyperglycemia persisted in some cases. Because these events have been reported voluntarily during clinical practice, estimates of frequency cannot be made and a causal relationship between protease inhibitor therapy and these events has not been established.

Concomitant use of Invirase with lovastatin or simvastatin is not recommended. Caution should be exercised if HIV protease inhibitors, including Invirase, are used concurrently with other HMG-CoA reductase inhibitors that are also metabolized by the CYP3A4 pathway (*e.g.*, atorvastatin, or cerivastatin). Since increased concentrations of statins can, in rare cases, cause severe adverse events such as myopathy including rhabdomyolysis, this risk may be increased when HIV protease inhibitors, including saquinavir, are used in combination with these drugs.

Concomitant use of Invirase and St. John's wort (hypericum perforatum) or products containing St. John's wort is not recommended. Coadministration of protease inhibitors, including Invirase, with St. John's wort is expected to substantially decrease protease inhibitor concentrations and may result in sub-optimal levels of Invirase and lead to loss of virologic response and possible resistance to Invirase or to the class of protease inhibitors.

PRECAUTIONS

GENERAL

Invirase (saquinavir mesylate) capsules and Fortovase (saquinavir) soft gelatin capsules are not bioequivalent and cannot be used interchangeably. Only Fortovase should be used for the initiation of saquinavir therapy (see DOSAGE AND ADMINISTRATION) since Fortovase soft gelatin capsules provide greater bioavailability and efficacy than Invirase capsules. For patients taking Invirase capsules with a viral load below the limit of quantification, a switch to Fortovase is recommended to maintain a virologic response. For patients taking Invirase capsules who have not had an adequate response or are failing therapy, if saquinavir resistance is clinically suspected, then Fortovase should not be used. If resistance to saquinavir is not clinically suspected, a switch to Fortovase may be considered.

The safety profile of Invirase in children younger than 16 years has not been established.

If a serious or severe toxicity occurs during treatment with Invirase, Invirase should be interrupted until the etiology of the event is identified or the toxicity resolves. At that time, resumption of treatment with full-dose Invirase may be considered. For nucleoside analogues used in combination with Invirase, physicians should refer to the complete prescribing information for these drugs for dose adjustment recommendations and for information regarding drug-associated adverse reactions.

Caution should be exercised when administering Invirase to patients with hepatic insufficiency since patients with baseline liver function tests >5 times the upper limit of normal were not included in clinical studies. Although a causal relationship has not been established, exacerbation of chronic liver dysfunction, including portal hypertension, has been reported in patients with underlying hepatitis B or C, cirrhosis or other underlying liver abnormalities.

There have been reports of spontaneous bleeding in patients with hemophilia A and B treated with protease inhibitors. In some patients additional factor VIII was required. In the majority of reported cases treatment with protease inhibitors was continued or restarted. A causal relationship between protease inhibitor therapy and these episodes has not been established.

Fat Redistribution

Redistribution/accumulation of body fat including central obesity, dorsocervical fat enlargement (buffalo hump), peripheral wasting, breast enlargement, and "cushingoid appearance" have been observed in patients receiving protease inhibitors. A causal relationship between protease inhibitor therapy and these events has not been established and the long-term consequences are currently unknown.

RESISTANCE/CROSS-RESISTANCE

The potential for HIV cross-resistance between protease inhibitors has not been fully explored. Therefore, it is unknown what effect saquinavir therapy will have on the activity of subsequent protease inhibitors (see CLINICAL PHARMACOLOGY, Microbiology).

INFORMATION FOR THE PATIENT

A statement to patients and health care providers is included on the product's bottle label: *ALERT:* **Find out about medicines that should NOT be taken with Invirase.**

Invirase may interact with some drugs; therefore, patients should be advised to report to their doctor the use of any other prescription, non-prescription medication, or herbal products, particularly St. John's wort.

Patients should be informed that Invirase is not a cure for HIV infection and that they may continue to acquire illnesses associated with advanced HIV infection, including opportunistic infections. Patients should be advised that Invirase should be used only in combination with an active nucleoside analogue regimen.

Patients should be informed that redistribution or accumulation of body fat may occur in patients receiving protease inhibitors and that the cause and long-term health effects of these conditions are not known at this time.

Patients should be told that the long-term effects of Invirase are unknown at this time. They should be informed that Invirase therapy has not been shown to reduce the risk of transmitting HIV to others through sexual contact or blood contamination.

Patients should be advised that Invirase should be taken within 2 hours after a full meal (see CLINICAL PHARMACOLOGY, Pharmacokinetics). When Invirase is taken without food, concentrations of saquinavir in the blood are substantially reduced and may result in no antiviral activity.

LABORATORY TESTS

Clinical chemistry tests should be performed prior to initiating Invirase therapy and at appropriate intervals thereafter. For comprehensive information concerning laboratory test alterations associated with use of individual nucleoside analogues, physicians should refer to the complete prescribing information for these drugs.

CARCINOGENESIS, MUTAGENESIS, AND IMPAIRMENT OF FERTILITY

Carcinogenesis

Carcinogenicity studies in rats and mice have not yet been completed.

Mutagenesis

Mutagenicity and genotoxicity studies, with and without metabolic activation where appropriate, have shown that saquinavir has no mutagenic activity *in vitro* in either bacterial (Ames test) or mammalian cells (Chinese hamster lung V79/HPRT test). Saquinavir does not induce chromosomal damage *in vivo* in the mouse micronucleus assay or *in vitro* in human peripheral blood lymphocytes, and does not induce primary DNA damage *in vitro* in the unscheduled DNA synthesis test.

Impairment of Fertility

Fertility and reproductive performance were not affected in rats at plasma exposures (AUC values) up to 5 times those achieved in humans at the recommended dose.

PREGNANCY, TERATOGENIC EFFECTS, PREGNANCY CATEGORY B

Reproduction studies conducted with saquinavir in rats have shown no embryotoxicity or teratogenicity at plasma exposures (AUC values) up to 5 times those achieved in humans at the recommended dose or in rabbits at plasma exposures 4 times those achieved at the recommended clinical dose. Studies in rats indicated that exposure to saquinavir from late pregnancy through lactation at plasma concentrations (AUC values) up to 5 times those achieved in humans at the recommended dose had no effect on the survival, growth and development of offspring to weaning. Because animal reproduction studies are not always predictive of human response, Invirase should be used during pregnancy after taking into account the importance of the drug to the mother. Presently, there are no reports of infants being born after women receiving Invirase in clinical trials became pregnant.

Antiretroviral Pregnancy Registry: To monitor maternal-fetal outcomes of pregnant women exposed to antiretroviral medications, including Invirase, an Antiretroviral Pregnancy Registry has been established. Physicians are encouraged to register patients by calling 1-800-258-4263.

NURSING MOTHERS

The Centers for Disease Control and Prevention recommend that HIV-infected mothers not breastfeed their infants to avoid risking postnatal transmission of HIV. It is not known whether saquinavir is excreted in human milk. Because of both the potential for HIV transmission and the potential for serious adverse reactions in nursing infants, **mothers should be instructed not to breastfeed if they are receiving antiretroviral medications, including Invirase.**

PEDIATRIC USE

Safety and effectiveness of Invirase in HIV-infected pediatric patients younger than 16 years of age have not been established.

GERIATRIC USE

Clinical studies of Invirase did not include sufficient numbers of subjects aged 65 and over to determine whether they respond differently from younger subjects. In general, caution should be taken when dosing Invirase in elderly patients due to the greater frequency of decreased hepatic, renal, or cardiac function, and of concomitant disease or other drug therapy.

DRUG INTERACTIONS

METABOLIC ENZYME INDUCERS

Invirase should not be administered concomitantly with rifampin, since rifampin decreases saquinavir concentrations by 80% (see CLINICAL PHARMACOLOGY, Pharmacokinetics). Rifabutin also substantially reduces saquinavir plasma concentrations by 40%. Other drugs that induce CYP3A4 (*e.g.*, phenobarbital, phenytoin, dexamethasone, carbamazepine) may also reduce saquinavir plasma concentrations. If therapy with such drugs is warranted, physicians should consider using alternatives when a patient is taking Invirase.

OTHER POTENTIAL INTERACTIONS

Coadministration of terfenadine, astemizole or cisapride with drugs that are known to be potent inhibitors of the cytochrome P4503A pathway (*i.e.*, ketoconazole, itraconazole, etc.) may lead to elevated plasma concentrations of terfenadine, astemizole or cisapride, which may in turn prolong QT intervals leading to rare cases of serious cardiovascular adverse events. Although Invirase is not a strong inhibitor of cytochrome P4503A, pharmacokinetic interaction studies with Invirase and terfenadine, astemizole or cisapride have not been conducted. Physicians should use alternatives to terfenadine, astemizole or cisapride when a patient is taking Invirase. Other compounds that are substrates of CYP3A4 (*e.g.*, calcium channel blockers, clindamycin, dapsone, quinidine, triazolam) may have elevated plasma concentrations when coadministered with Invirase; therefore, patients should be monitored for toxicities associated with such drugs.

ANTI-HIV COMPOUNDS

Nelfinavir

Coadministration of nelfinavir with saquinavir (given as Fortovase, 1200 mg) resulted in an 18% increase in nelfinavir plasma AUC and a 4-fold increase in saquinavir plasma AUC. If used in combination with saquinavir hard gelatin capsules at the recommended dose of 600 mg tid, no dose adjustments are needed. Currently, there are no safety and efficacy data available from the use of this combination.

Ritonavir

Following approximately 4 weeks of a combination regimen of saquinavir (400 or 600 mg bid) and ritonavir (400 or 600 mg bid) in HIV-positive patients, saquinavir AUC values were at least 17-fold greater than historical AUC values from patients who received saquinavir 600 mg tid without ritonavir. When used in combination therapy for up to 24 weeks, doses greater than 400 mg bid of either ritonavir or saquinavir were associated with an increase in adverse events.

Delavirdine

Saquinavir AUC increased 5-fold when delavirdine (400 mg tid) and saquinavir (600 mg tid) were administered in combination. Currently, there are limited safety and no efficacy data available from the use of this combination. In a small, preliminary study, hepatocellular enzyme elevations occurred in 15% of subjects during the first several weeks of the delavirdine and saquinavir combination (6% Grade 3 or 4). Hepatocellular enzymes (ALT/AST) should be monitored frequently if this combination is prescribed.

Nevirapine

Coadministration of nevirapine with Invirase resulted in a 24% decrease in saquinavir plasma AUC. Currently, there are no safety and efficacy data available from the use of this combination.

ERECTILE DYSFUNCTION AGENTS

Sildenafil

In a study performed in healthy male volunteers, coadministration of saquinavir, a CYP3A4 inhibitor, at steady state (1200 mg tid) with sildenafil (100 mg single dose) resulted in a 140% increase in sildenafil C_{max} and a 210% increase in sildenafil AUC. Sildenafil had no effect on saquinavir pharmacokinetics. When sildenafil is administered concomitantly with saquinavir a starting dose of 25 mg of sildenafil should be considered.

ADVERSE REACTIONS

See PRECAUTIONS.

The safety of Invirase was studied in patients who received the drug either alone or in combination with ZDV and/or Hivid (zalcitabine, ddC). The majority of adverse events were of mild intensity. The most frequently reported adverse events among patients receiving Invirase (excluding those toxicities known to be associated with ZDV and Hivid when used in combinations) were diarrhea, abdominal discomfort, and nausea.

Invirase did not alter the pattern, frequency, or severity of known major toxicities associated with the use of Hivid and/or ZVD. Physicians should refer to the complete prescribing information for these drugs (or other antiretroviral agents as appropriate) for drug-associated adverse reactions to other nucleoside analogues.

In an open-label protocol, NV15114, in which 33 patients received treatment with Invirase, ZDV and lamivudine for 4-16 weeks, no unexpected toxicities were reported.

TABLE 4A and TABLE 4B list clinical adverse events that occurred in ≥2% of patients receiving Invirase 600 mg tid alone or in combination with ZDV and/or Hivid in two trials. Median duration of treatment in NV14255/ACTG229 (triple-combination study) was 48 weeks; median duration of treatment in NV14256 (double-combination study) was approximately 1 year.

TABLE 4A *Percentage of Patients, by Study Arm, With Clinical Adverse Experiences Considered At Least Possibly Related to Study Drug or of Unknown Relationship and of Moderate, Severe, or Life-Threatening Intensity, Occurring in ≥2% of Patients in NV14255/ACTG229*

Adverse Event	SAQ+ZDV n=99	SAQ+ddC+ZDV n=98	ddC+ZDV n=100
Gastrointestinal			
Diarrhea	3.0%	1.0%	—
Abdominal discomfort	2.0%	3.1%	4.0%
Nausea	—	3.1%	3.0%
Dyspepsia	1.0%	1.0%	2.0%
Abdominal pain	2.0%	1.0%	2.0%
Mucosa damage	—	—	4.0%
Buccal mucosa ulceration	—	2.0%	2.0%
Central and Peripheral Nervous System			
Headache	2.0%	2.0%	2.0%
Paresthesia	2.0%	3.1%	4.0%
Extremity numbness	2.0%	1.0%	4.0%
Dizziness	—	2.0%	1.0%
Peripheral neuropathy	—	1.0%	2.0%
Body as a Whole			
Asthenia	6.1%	9.2%	10.0%
Appetite disturbances	—	1.0%	2.0%
Skin and Appendages			
Rash	—	—	3.0%
Pruritus	—	—	2.0%
Musculoskeletal Disorders			
Musculoskeletal pain	2.0%	2.0%	4.0%
Myalgia	1.0%	—	3.0%

— Indicates no events reported.

TABLE 4B *Percentage of Patients, by Study Arm, With Clinical Adverse Experiences Considered At Least Possibly Related to Study Drug or of Unknown Relationship and of Moderate, Severe, or Life-Threatening Intensity, Occurring in ≥2% of Patients in N14256*

Adverse Event	ddC n=325	SAQ n=327	SAQ+ddC n=318
Gastrointestinal			
Diarrhea	0.9%	4.9%	4.4%
Abdominal discomfort	0.9%	0.9%	0.9%
Nausea	1.5%	2.4%	0.9%
Dyspepsia	0.6%	0.9%	0.9%
Abdominal pain	0.6%	1.2%	0.3%
Mucosa damage	—	—	0.3%
Buccal mucosa ulceration	6.2%	2.1%	3.8%
Central and Peripheral Nervous System			
Headache	3.4%	2.4%	0.9%
Paresthesia	1.2%	0.3%	0.3%
Extremity numbness	1.5%	0.6%	0.9%
Dizziness	—	0.3%	—
Peripheral neuropathy	11.4%	3.1%	11.3%
Body as a Whole			
Asthenia	—	0.3%	—
Appetite disturbances	—	—	—
Skin and Appendages			
Rash	1.5%	2.1%	1.3%
Pruritus	—	0.6%	—
Musculoskeletal Disorders			
Musculoskeletal pain	0.6%	0.6%	0.6%
Myalgia	0.6%	0.3%	0.3%

— Indicates no events reported.

Rare occurrences of the following serious adverse experiences have been reported during clinical trials of Invirase and were considered at least possibly related to use of study drugs: Confusion, ataxia and weakness; acute myeloblastic leukemia; hemolytic anemia; attempted suicide; Stevens-Johnson syndrome; seizures; severe cutaneous reaction associated with increased liver function tests; isolated elevation of transaminases; thrombophlebitis; headache; thrombocytopenia; exacerbation of chronic liver disease with Grade 4 elevated liver function tests, jaundice, ascites, and right and left upper quadrant abdominal pain; drug fever; bullous skin eruption and polyarthritis; pancreatitis leading to death; nephrolithiasis; thrombocytopenia and intracranial hemorrhage leading to death; peripheral vasoconstriction; portal hypertension; intestinal obstruction. These events were reported from a database of >6000 patients. Over 100 patients on saquinavir therapy have been followed for >2 years.

TABLE 5A and TABLE 5B show the percentage of patients with marked laboratory abnormalities in studies NV14255/ACTG229 and NV14256. Marked laboratory abnormalities are defined as a Grade 3 or 4 abnormality in a patient with a normal baseline value or a Grade 4 abnormality in a patient with a Grade 1 abnormality at baseline (ACTG Grading System).

TABLE 5A *Percentage of Patients, by Treatment Group, With Marked Laboratory Abnormalities* in NV14255/ACTG229*

	SAQ+ZDV n=99	SAQ+ddC+ZDV n=98	ddC+ZDV n=100
Biochemistry			
Calcium (high)	1%	0%	0%
Calcium (low)	—	—	—
Creatine phosphokinase (high)	10%	12%	7%
Glucose (high)	0%	0%	0%
Glucose (low)	0%	0%	0%
Phosphate (low)	2%	1%	0%
Potassium (high)	0%	0%	0%
Potassium (low)	0%	0%	0%
Serum amylase (high)	2%	1%	1%
SGOT (AST) (high)	2%	2%	0%
SGPT (ALT) (high)	0%	3%	1%
Sodium (high)	—	—	—
Sodium (low)	—	—	—
Total bilirubin (high)	1%	0%	0%
Uric acid	0%	0%	1%
Hematology			
Neutrophils (low)	2%	2%	8%
Hemoglobin (low)	0%	0%	1%
Platelets (low)	0%	0%	2%

* Marked Laboratory Abnormality defined as a shift from Grade 0 to at least Grade 3 or from Grade 1 to Grade 4 (ACTG Grading System).

MONOTHERAPY AND COMBINATION STUDIES

Other clinical adverse experiences of any intensity, at least remotely related to Invirase, including those in <2% of patients on arms containing Invirase in studies NV14255/ACTG229 and NV14256, and those in smaller clinical trials, are listed below by body system.

Body as a Whole: Allergic reaction, anorexia, chest pain, edema, fatigue, fever, intoxication, parasites external, retrosternal pain, shivering, wasting syndrome, weakness generalized, weight decrease, redistribution/accumulation of body fat (see PRECAUTIONS, Fat Redistribution).

Cardiovascular: Cyanosis, heart murmur, heart valve disorder, hypertension, hypotension, syncope, vein distended.

Endocrine/Metabolic: Dehydration, diabetes mellitus, dry eye syndrome, hyperglycemia, weight increase, xerophthalmia.

Gastrointestinal: Cheilitis, colic abdominal, constipation, dyspepsia, dysphagia, esophagitis, eructation, feces bloodstained, feces discolored, flatulence, gastralgia, gastri-

S

TABLE 5B *Percentage of Patients, by Treatment Group, With Marked Laboratory Abnormalities* in N14256*

	ddC n=325	SAQ n=327	SAQ+ddC n=318
Biochemistry			
Calcium (high)	<1%	0%	0%
Calcium (low)	<1%	<1%	0%
Creatine phosphokinase (high)	6%	3%	7%
Glucose (high)	<1%	1%	1%
Glucose (low)	5%	5%	5%
Phosphate (low)	0%	<1%	<1%
Potassium (high)	2%	2%	3%
Potassium (low)	0%	1%	0%
Serum amylase (high)	2%	1%	1%
SGOT (AST) (high)	2%	2%	3%
SGPT (ALT) (high)	2%	2%	2%
Sodium (high)	0%	0%	<1%
Sodium (low)	0%	<1%	0%
Total bilirubin (high)	0%	<1%	1%
Uric acid	NA	NA	NA
Hematology			
Neutrophils (low)	1%	1%	1%
Hemoglobin (low)	<1%	<1%	0%
Platelets (low)	1%	1%	<1%

* Marked Laboratory Abnormality defined as a shift from Grade 0 to at least Grade 3 or from Grade 1 to Grade 4 (ACTG Grading System).
NA Not assessed.

tis, gastrointestinal inflammation, gingivitis, glossitis, hemorrhage rectum, hemorrhoids, hepatitis, hepatomegaly, hepatosplenomegaly, infectious diarrhea, jaundice, liver enzyme disorder, melena, pain pelvic, painful defecation, pancreatitis, parotid disorder, salivary glands disorder, stomach upset, stomatitis, toothache, tooth disorder, vomiting.

Hematologic: Anemia, bleeding dermal, microhemorrhages, neutropenia, pancytopenia, splenomegaly, thrombocytopenia.

Musculoskeletal: Arthralgia, arthritis, back pain, cramps leg, cramps muscle, creatine phosphokinase increased, musculoskeletal disorders, stiffness, tissue changes, trauma.

Neurological: Ataxia, bowel movements frequent, confusion, convulsions, dysarthria, dysesthesia, heart rate disorder, hyperesthesia, hyperreflexia, hyporeflexia, lightheaded feeling, mouth dry, myelopolyradiculoneuritis, numbness face, pain facial, paresis, poliomyelitis, prickly sensation, progressive multifocal leukoencephalopathy, spasms, tremor, unconsciousness.

Psychological: Agitation, amnesia, anxiety, anxiety attack, depression, dreaming excessive, euphoria, hallucination, insomnia, intellectual ability reduced, irritability, lethargy, libido disorder, overdose effect, psychic disorder, psychosis, somnolence, speech disorder, suicide attempt.

Reproductive System: Impotence, prostate enlarged, vaginal discharge.

Resistance Mechanism: Abscess, angina tonsillaris, candidiasis, cellulitis, herpes simplex, herpes zoster, infection bacterial, infection mycotic, infection staphylococcal, influenza, lymphadenopathy, moniliasis, tumor.

Respiratory: Bronchitis, cough, dyspnea, epistaxis, hemoptysis, laryngitis, pharyngitis, pneumonia, pulmonary disease, respiratory disorder, rhinitis, sinusitis, upper respiratory tract infection.

Skin and Appendages: Acne, alopecia, chalazion, dermatitis, dermatitis seborrheic, eczema, erythema, folliculitis, furunculosis, hair changes, hot flushes, nail disorder, night sweats, papillomatosis, photosensitivity reaction, pigment changes skin, rash maculopapular, skin disorder, skin nodule, skin ulceration, sweating increased, urticaria, verruca, xeroderma.

Special Senses: Blepharitis, earache, ear pressure, eye irritation, hearing decreased, otitis, taste alteration, tinnitus, visual disturbance.

Urinary System: Micturition disorder, renal calculus, urinary tract bleeding, urinary tract infection.

S

DOSAGE AND ADMINISTRATION

Invirase (saquinavir mesylate) capsules and Fortovase (saquinavir) soft gelatin capsules are not bioequivalent and cannot be used interchangeably. When using saquinavir as part of an antiviral regimen Fortovase is the recommended formulation. In rare circumstances, Invirase may be considered if it is to be combined with antiretrovirals that significantly inhibit saquinavir's metabolism (see CLINICAL PHARMACOLOGY, Drug Interactions).

The recommended dose for Invirase in combination with a nucleoside analogue is three 200 mg capsules 3 times daily taken within 2 hours after a full meal. Please refer to the complete prescribing information for each of the nucleoside analogues for the recommended doses of these agents.

Invirase should be used only in combination with an active antiretroviral nucleoside analogue regimen. Concomitant therapy should be based on a patient's prior drug exposure.

MONITORING OF PATIENTS

Clinical chemistry tests should be performed prior to initiating Invirase therapy and at appropriate intervals thereafter. For comprehensive patient monitoring recommendations for other nucleoside analogues, physicians should refer to the complete prescribing information for these drugs.

DOSE ADJUSTMENT FOR COMBINATION THERAPY WITH INVIRASE

For toxicities that may be associated with Invirase, the drug should be interrupted. Invirase at doses less than 600 mg tid are not recommended since lower doses have not shown antiviral activity. For recipients of combination therapy with Invirase and nucleoside analogues, dose adjustment of the nucleoside analogue should be based on the known toxicity profile of the individual drug. Physicians should refer to the complete prescribing information for these drugs for comprehensive dose adjustment recommendations and drug-associated adverse reactions of nucleoside analogues.

HOW SUPPLIED

Invirase 200 mg capsules are light brown and green opaque capsules with "ROCHE" and "0245" imprinted on the capsule shell.

Storage: The capsules should be stored at 15-30°C (59-86°F) in tightly closed bottles.

PRODUCT LISTING - EQUIVALENTS NOT AVAILABLE

Capsule - Oral - Mesylate 200 mg

9's	$24.70	INVIRASE, Quality Care Pharmaceuticals Inc	60346-1018-09
27's	$72.57	INVIRASE, Quality Care Pharmaceuticals Inc	60346-1018-02
180's	$213.95	INVIRASE, Allscripts Pharmaceutical Company	54569-4563-01
270's	$622.07	INVIRASE, Allscripts Pharmaceutical Company	54569-4242-01
270's	$636.20	INVIRASE, Physicians Total Care	54868-3699-00
270's	$673.91	INVIRASE, Roche Laboratories	00004-0245-15

Capsule - Oral - 200 mg

180's	$250.34	FORTOVASE, Roche Laboratories	00004-0246-48

Sargramostim *(003050)*

Categories: Leukapheresis, adjunct; Leukemia, acute myelogenous, adjunct; Transplantation, bone marrow, adjunct; Pregnancy Category C; Recombinant DNA Origin; FDA Approved 1991 Mar; Orphan Drugs
Drug Classes: Hematopoietic agents
Brand Names: GM-CSF; Granulocyte Macrophage-Colony Stimulating Factor; **Leukine**; Prokine
Foreign Brand Availability: Leucogen (Korea)
HCFA JCODE(S): J2820 250 µg IV

DESCRIPTION

Leukine is a recombinant human granulocyte-macrophage colony stimulating factor (rhu GM-CSF) produced by recombinant DNA technology in a yeast (*S. cerevisiae*) expression system. GM-CSF is a hematopoietic growth factor which stimulates proliferation and differentiation of hematopoietic progenitor cells. Leukine is a glycoprotein of 127 amino acids characterized by 3 primary molecular species having molecular masses of 19,500, 16,800, and 15,500 daltons. The amino acid sequence of Leukine differs from the natural human GM-CSF by a substitution of leucine at position 23, and the carbohydrate moiety may be different from the native protein. Sargramostim has been selected as the proper name for yeast-derived rhu GM-CSF.

Leukine liquid is a sterile, clear, colorless, preserved (1.1% benzyl alcohol) injectible solution (500 µg/ml). Lyophilized Leukine is a sterile, white, preservative-free powder (250 and 500 µg). Lyophilized Leukine requires reconstitution with 1 ml sterile water for injection or 1 ml bacteriostatic water for injection. Both Leukine liquid and reconstituted lyophilized Leukine are suitable for sucutaneous injection or intravenous infusion. Each vial of Leukine liquid contains 500 µg (2.8×10^6 IU) sargramostim; 40 mg mannitol, 10 mg sucrose, and 1.2 mg tromethamine, sterile water for injection, and 1.1% benzyl acohol. Each vial of lyophilized Leukine contains either 250 µg (1.4×10^6 IU) or 500 µg (2.8×10^6 IU) sargramostim, 40 mg mannitol, 10 mg sucrose, and 1.2 mg tromethamine. Biological potency is expressed in International Units as tested against the WHO First International Reference Standard. The specific activity of sargramostim is approximately 5.6×10^6 IU/mg.

Storage: The sterile, preserved, injectable solution; the sterile powder; the reconstituted solution; and the diluted solution for injection should be refrigerated at 2-8°C (36-46°F). Do not freeze or shake. Do not use beyond the expiration date printed on the vial.

CLINICAL PHARMACOLOGY

GENERAL

GM-CSF belongs to a group of growth factors termed colony stimulating factors which support survival, clonal expansion, and differentiation of hematopoietic progenitor cells. GM-CSF induces partially committed progenitor cells to divide and differentiate in the granulocyte-macrophage pathways.

GM-CSF is also capable of activating mature granulocytes and macrophages. GM-CSF is a multilineage factor and, in addition to dose-dependent effects on the myelomonocytic lineage, can promote the proliferation of megakaryocytic and erythroid progenitors.[1] However, other factors are required to induce complete maturation in these two lineages. The various cellular responses (*i.e.*, division, maturation, activation) are induced through GM-CSF binding to specific receptors expressed on the cell surface of target cells.[2]

IN VITRO STUDIES OF SARGRAMOSTIM IN HUMAN CELLS

The biological activity of GM-CSF is species-specific. Consequently, *in vitro* studies have been performed on human cells to characterize the pharmacological activity of sargramostim. *In vitro* exposure of human bone marrow cells to sargramostim at concentrations ranging from 1-100 ng/ml results in the proliferation of hematopoietic progenitors and in the formation of pure granulocyte, pure macrophage, and mixed granulocyte-macrophage colonies.[3] Chemotactic, anti-fungal, and anti-parasitic[4] activities of granulocytes and monocytes are increased by exposure to sargramostim *in vitro*. Sargramostim increases the cytotoxicity of monocytes toward certain neoplastic cell lines[3] and activates polymorphonuclear neutrophils to inhibit the growth of tumor cells.

IN VIVO PRIMATE STUDIES OF SARGRAMOSTIM

Pharmacology/toxicology studies of sargramostim were performed in cynomolgus monkeys. An acute toxicity study revealed an absence of treatment-related toxicity following a single IV bolus injection at a dose of 300 µg/kg. Two subacute studies were performed using IV injection (maximum dose 200 µg/kg/day × 14 days) and subcutaneous injection (maximum dose 200 µg/kg/day × 28 days). No major visceral organ toxicity was documented. Notable histopathology findings included increased cellularity in hematologic organs, and heart and lung tissues. A dose-dependent increase in leukocyte count, which consisted primarily of segmented neutrophils, occurred during the dosing period; increases in monocytes, basophils, eosinophils, and lymphocytes were also noted. Leukocyte counts decreased to pretreatment values over a 1-2 week recovery period.

PHARMACOKINETICS

Pharmacokinetic profiles have been analyzed in controlled studies of 24 normal male volunteers. Liquid and lyophilized sargramostim, at the recommended dose of 250 µg/m^2, have been determined to bioequivalent based on the statistical evaluation of AUC.[5]

When sargramostim (either liquid or lyophilized) was administered IV over 2 hours to normal volunteers, the mean beta half-life was approximately 60 minutes. Peak concentrations of GM-CSF were observed in blood samples obtained during or immediately after completion of sargramostim infusion. For sargramostim liquid, the mean maximum concentration (C_{max}) was 5.0 ng/ml, the mean clearance rate was approximately 420 ml/min/m^2 and the mean AUC $_{(0\text{-}inf)}$ was 640 ng/ml·min. Corresponding results for lyophilized sargramostim in the same subjects were mean C_{max} of 5.4 ng/ml, mean clearance rate of 431 ml/min/m^2, and mean AUC $_{(0\text{-}inf)}$ of 677 ng/ml·min. GM-CSF was last detected in blood samples obtained at 3 or 6 hours.

When sargramostim (either liquid or lyophilized) was administered SC to normal volunteers, GM-CSF was detected in the serum at 15 minutes, the first sample point. The mean beta half-life was approximately 162 minutes. Peak levels occurred at 1-3 hours post injection, and sargramostim remained detectable for up to 6 hours after injection. The mean C_{max} was 1.5 ng/ml. For sargramostim liquid, the mean clearance was 549 ml/min/m^2 and the mean AUC $_{(0\text{-}inf)}$ was 549 ng/ml·min. For lyophilized sargramostim, the mean clearance was 529 ml/min/m^2 and the mean AUC $_{(0\text{-}inf)}$ was 501 ng/ml·min.

ANTIBODY FORMATION

Serum samples collected before and after sargramostim treatment from 214 patients with a variety of underlying diseases have been examined for the presence of antibodies. Neutralizing antibodies were detected in 5 of 214 patients (2.3%) after receiving sargramostim by continuous IV infusion (3 patients) or subcutaneous injection (2 patients) for 28-84 days in multiple courses. All 5 patients had impaired hematopoiesis before the administration of sargramostim and, consequently, the effect of the development of anti-GM-CSF antibodies on normal hematopoiesis could not be assessed. Drug-induced neutropenia, neutralization of endogenous GM-CSF activity, and diminution of the therapeutic effect of sargramostim secondary to formation of neutralizing antibody remain a theoretical possibility.

INDICATIONS AND USAGE

USE FOLLOWING INDUCTION CHEMOTHERAPY IN ACUTE MYELOGENOUS LEUKEMIA

Sargramostim is indicated for use following induction chemotherapy in older adult patients with acute myelogenous leukemia (AML) to shorten time to neutrophil recovery and to reduce the incidence of severe and life-threatening infections and infections resulting in death. The safety and efficacy of sargramostim have not been assessed in patients with AML under 55 years of age.

The term acute myelogenous leukemia, also referred to as acute non-lymphocytic leukemia (ANLL), encompasses a heterogenous group of leukemias arising from various nonlymphoid cell lines which have been defined morphologically by the French-American-British (FAB) system of classification.

USE IN MOBILIZATION AND FOLLOWING TRANSPLANTATION OF AUTOLOGOUS PERIPHERAL BLOOD PROGENITOR CELLS

Sargramostim is indicated for the mobilization of hematopoietic progenitor cells into peripheral blood for collection by leukapheresis. Mobilization allows for the collection of increased numbers of progenitor cells capable of engraftment as compared with collection without mobilization. After myeloablative chemotherapy, the transplantation of an increased number of progenitor cells can lead to more rapid engraftment, which may result in a decreased need for supportive care. Myeloid reconstitution is further accelerated by administration of sargramostim following peripheral blood progenitor cell transplantation.

USE IN MYELOID RECONSTITUTION AFTER AUTOLOGOUS BONE MARROW TRANSPLANTATION

Sargramostim is indicated for acceleration of myeloid recovery in patients with non-Hodgkin's lymphoma (NHL), acute lymphoblastic leukemia (ALL), and Hodgkin's disease undergoing autologous bone marrow transplantation (BMT). After autologous BMT in patients with NHL, ALL, or Hodgkin's disease, sargramostim has been found to be safe and effective in accelerating myeloid engraftment, decreasing median duration of antibiotic administration, reducing the median duration of infectious episodes and shortening the median duration of hospitalization. Hematologic response to sargramostim can be detected by complete blood count (CBC) with differential performed twice per week.

USE IN MYELOID RECONSTITUTION AFTER ALLOGENEIC BONE MARROW TRANSPLANTATION

Sargramostim is indicated for acceleration of myeloid recovery in patients undergoing allogeneic BMT from HLA-matched related donors. Sargramostim has been found to be safe and effective in accelerating myeloid engraftment, reducing the incidence of bacteremia and other culture positive infections, and shortening the median duration of hospitalization.

USE IN BONE MARROW TRANSPLANTATION FAILURE OR ENGRAFTMENT DELAY

Sargramostim is indicated in patients who have undergone allogenic or autologous bone marrow transplantation (BMT) in whom engraftment is delayed or has failed. Sargramostim has been found to be safe and effective in prolonging survival of patients who are experiencing graft failure or engraftment delay, in the presence or absence of infection, following autologous or allogeneic BMT. Survival benefit may be relatively greater in those patients who demonstrate one or more of the following characteristics: autologous BMT failure or engraftment delay, no previous total body irradiation, malignancy other than leukemia or a multiple organ failure (MOF) score ≤2. Hematologic response to sargramostim can be detected by complete blood count (CBC) with differential performed twice per week.

NON-FDA APPROVED INDICATIONS

Although not FDA approved, sargramostim has been used in myelodysplastic syndromes, aplastic anemia, and in patients with AIDS or zidovudine-associated neutropenia.

CONTRAINDICATIONS

Sargramostim is Contraindicated:

1. In patients with excessive leukemic myeloid blasts in the bone marrow or peripheral blood (≥ 10%).
2. In patients with known hypersensitivity to GM-CSF, yeast-derived products, or any component of the product.
3. For concomitant use with chemotherapy and radiotherapy. Due to the potential sensitivity of rapidly dividing hematopoietic progenitor cells, sargramostin should not be administered simultaneously with cytotoxic chemotherapy or radiotherapy or within 24 hours preceding or following chemotherapy or radiotherapy. In one controlled study, patients with small cell lung cancer received sargramostin and concurrent thoracic radiotherapy and chemotherapy or the identical radiotherapy and chemotherapy without sargramostin. The patients randomized to sargramostin had significantly higher adverse events, inlcuding higher mortality and a higher incidence of grade 3 and 4 infections and grade 3 and 4 thrombocytopenia.[11]

WARNINGS

PEDIATRIC USE

Benzyl alcohol is a constituent of sargramostim liquid and bacteriostatic water for injection diluent. Benzyl alcohol has been reported to be associated with a fatal "Gasping Syndrome" in premature infants. **Liquid solutions containing benzyl alcohol (including sargramostim liquid) or lyophilized sargramostim reconstituted with bacteriostatic water for injection (0.9% benzyl alcohol) should not be adminstered to neonates** (see PRECAUTIONS and DOSAGE AND ADMINISTRATION).

FLUID RETENTION:

Edema, capillary leak syndrome, pleural and/or pericardial effusion have been reported in patients after sargramostim administration. In 156 patients enrolled in placebo-controlled studies using sargramostim at a dose of 250 µg/m^2/day by 2 hour IV infusion, the reported incidence of fluid retention (sargramostim versus placebo) were as follows: peripheral edema, 11% vs 7%; pleural effusion, 1% vs 0%; and pericardial effusion, 4% vs 1%. Capillary leak syndrome was not observed in this limited number of studies; based on other uncontrolled studies and reports from users of marketed sargramostim, incidence is estimated to be less than 1%. In patients with preexisting pleural and pericardial effusions, administration of sargramostim may aggravate fluid retention; however, fluid retention associated with or worsened by sargramostim has been reversible after interruption or dose reduction of sargramostim with or without diuretic therapy. Sargramostim should be used with caution in patients with preexisting fluid retention, pulmonary infiltrates or congestive heart failure.

RESPIRATORY SYMPTOMS

Sequestration of granulocytes in the pulmonary circulation has been documented following sargramostim infusion,[12] and dyspnea has been reported occasionally in patients treated with sargramostim. Special attention should be given to respiratory symptoms during or immediately following sargramostim infusion, especially in patients with preexisting lung disease. In patients displaying dyspnea during sargramostim administration, the rate of infusion should be reduced by half. If respiratory symptoms worsen despite infusion rate reduction, the infusion should be discontinued. Subsequent IV infusions may administered following the standard dose schedule with careful monitoring. Sargramostim should be administered with caution in patients with hypoxia.

CARDIOVASCULAR SYMPTOMS

Occasional transient supraventricular arrhythmia has been reported in uncontrolled studies during sargramostim administration, particularly in patients with a previous history of cardiac arrhythmia. However, these arrhythmias have been reversible after discontinuation of sargramostim. Sargramostim should be used with caution in patients with preexisting cardiac disease.

RENAL AND HEPATIC DYSFUNCTION

In some patients with preexisting renal or hepatic dysfunction enrolled in uncontrolled clinical trials, administration of sargramostim has induced elevation of serum creatinine or bilirubin and hepatic enzymes. Dose reduction or interruption of sargramostim administration has resulted in a decrease to pretreatment values. However, in controlled clinical trials the incidences of renal and hepatic dysfunction were comparable between sargramostim (250 µg/m^2/day by 2 hour IV infusion) and placebo-treated patients. Monitoring of renal and hepatic function in patients displaying renal or hepatic dysfunction prior to initiation of treatment is recommended at least every other week during sargramostim administration.

PRECAUTIONS

GENERAL

Parenteral administration of recombinant proteins should be attended by appropriate precautions in case an allergic or untoward reaction occurs. Serious allergic or anaphylactic reactions have been reported. If any serious allergic or anaphylactic reaction occurs, sargramostim therapy should immediately be discontinued and appropriate therapy initiated (see WARNINGS).

Rarely, hypotension with flushing and syncope has been reported following the first administration of sargramostim. These signs have resolved with symptomatic treatment and usually do not recur with subsequent doses in the same cycle of treatment.

Stimulation of marrow precursors with sargramostim may result in a rapid rise in white blood cell (WBC) count. If the ANC exceeds 20,000 cells/mm^3 or if the platelet count exceeds 500,000/mm^3, sargramostim administration should be interrupted or the dose reduced by half. The decision to reduce the dose or interrupt treatment should be based on the clinical condition of the patient. Excessive blood counts have returned to normal or baseline levels within 3-7 days following cessation of sargramostim therapy. Twice weekly monitoring of CBC with differential (including examination for the presence of blast cells) should be performed to preclude development of excessive counts.

GROWTH FACTOR POTENTIAL

Sargramostim is a growth factor that primarily stimulates normal myeloid precursors. However, the possibility that sargramostim can act as a growth factor for any tumor type, particularly myeloid malignancies, cannot be excluded. Because of the possibility of tumor growth potentiation, precaution should be exercised when using this drug in any malignancy with myeloid characteristics.

Should disease progression be detected during sargramostim treatment, sargramostim therapy should be discontinued.

Sargramostim has been administered to patients with myelodysplastic syndromes (MDS) in uncontrolled studies without evidence of increased relapse rates.[13-15] Controlled studies have not been performed in patients with MDS.

USE IN PATIENTS RECEIVING PURGED BONE MARROW:

Sargramostim is effective in accelerating myeloid recovery in patients receiving bone marrow purged by anti-B lymphocyte monoclonal antibodies. Data obtained from uncontrolled studies suggest that if *in vitro* marrow purging with chemical agents causes a significant decrease in the number of responsive hematopoietic progenitors, the patient may not respond to sargramostim. When the bone marrow purging process preserves a sufficient number of progenitors (>1.2 × 10^4/kg), a beneficial effect of sargramostim on myeloid engraftment has been reported.[16]

USE IN PATIENTS PREVIOUSLY EXPOSED TO INTENSIVE CHEMOTHERAPY/ RADIOTHERAPY

In patients who before autologous BMT, have received extensive radiotherapy to hematopoietic sites for the treatment of primary disease in the abdomen or chest, or have been exposed to multiple myelotoxic agents (alkylating agents, anthracycline antibiotics and antimetabolites), the effect of sargramostim on myeloid reconstitution may be limited.

USE IN PATIENTS WITH MALIGNANCY UNDEROING SARGRAMOSTIM-MOBILIZED PBPC COLLECTION

When using sargramostim to mobilize PBPC, the limited *in vitro* data suggest that tumor cells may be released and reinfused into the patient in the leukapheresis product. The effect of reinfusion of tumor cells has not been well studied and the data are inconclusive.

PATIENT MONITORING

Sargramostim can induce variable increases in WBC and/or platelet counts. In order to avoid potential complications of excessive leukocytosis (WBC >50,000 cells/mm^3; ANC >20,000 cells/mm^3), a CBC is recommended twice per week during sargramostim therapy. Monitoring of renal and hepatic function in patients displaying renal or hepatic dysfunction prior to initiation of treatment is recommended at least biweekly during sargramostim administration. Body weight and hydration status should be carefully monitored during sargramostim administration.

CARCINOGENESIS, MUTAGENESIS, AND IMPAIRMENT OF FERTILITY

Animal studies have not been conducted with sargramostim to evaluate the carcinogenic potential or the effect on fertility.

PREGNANCY CATEGORY C

Animal reproduction studies have not been conducted with sargramostim. It is not known whether sargramostim can cause fetal harm when administered to a pregnant woman or can affect reproductive capability. Sargramostim should be given to a pregnant woman only if clearly needed.

NURSING MOTHERS

It is not known whether sargramostin is excreted in human milk. Because many drugs are excreted in human milk, sargramostim should be administered to a nursing woman only if clearly needed.

PEDIATRIC USE

Safety and effectiveness in pediatric patients have not been established; however, available safety data indicate that sargramostin does not exhibit any greater toxicity in pediatric patients than adults. A total of 124 pediatric subjects between the ages of 4 months and 18 years have been treated with sargramostim in clinical trials at doses ranging from 60-1000 μg/m^2/day intravenously and 4-1500 μg/m^2/day subcutaneously. In 53 pediatric patients enrolled in controlled studies at a dose of 250 μg/m^2/day by 2 hour IV infusion, the type and frequency of adverse events were comparable to those reported for the adult population. **Liquid solutions containing benzyl alcohol (including sargramostim liquid) or lyophilized sargramostim reconstituted with bacteriostatic water for injection (0.9% benzyl alcohol) should not be adminstered to neonates (see WARNINGS.)**

DRUG INTERACTIONS

Interactions between sargramostim and other drugs have not been fully evaluated. Drugs which may potentiate the myeloproliferative effects of sargramostim, such as lithium and corticosteroids, should be used with caution.

ADVERSE REACTIONS

AUTOLOGUS AND ALLOGENIC BONE MARROW TRANSPLANTATION

Sargramostim is generally well tolerated. In 3 placebo-controlled studies enrolling a total of 156 patients after autologous BMT or peripheral blood progenitor cell transplantation, events reported in at least 10% of patients who received IV sargramostim or placebo were as reported in TABLE 6.

TABLE 6 *Percent of AuBMT Patients Reporting Events*

Events by Body System	Sargramostim (n=79)	Placebo (n=77)
Body, General		
Fever	95%	96%
Mucous membrane disorder	75%	78%
Asthenia	66%	51%
Malaise	57%	51%
Sepsis	11%	14%
Digestive System		
Nausea	90%	96%
Diarrhea	89%	82%
Vomiting	85%	90%
Anorexia	54%	58%
GI disorder	37%	47%
GI hemorrhage	27%	33%
Stomatitis	24%	29%
Liver damage	13%	14%
Skin and Appendages		
Alopecia	73%	74%
Rash	44%	38%
Metabolic/Nutritional Disorder		
Edema	34%	35%
Peripheral edema	11%	7%
Respiratory		
Dyspnea	28%	31%
Lung disorder	20%	23%
Hemic and Lympatic System		
Blood dyscrasia	25%	27%
Cardiovascular System		
Hemorrhage	23%	30%
Urogenital System		
Urinary tract disorder	14%	13%
Kidney function abnormal	8%	10%
Nervous System		
CNS disorder	11%	16%

No significant differences were observed between sargramostim and placebo-treated patients in the type or frequency of laboratory abnormalities, including renal and hepatic parameters. In some patients with preexisting renal or hepatic dysfunction enrolled in uncontrolled clinical trials, administration of sargramostin has induced elevation of serum creatinine or bilirubin and hepatic enzymes (see WARNINGS). In addition, there was no significant difference in relapse rate and 24 month survival between the sargramostim and placebo-treated patients.

In the placebo-controlled trial of 109 patients after allogeneic BMT, events reported in at least 10% of patients who received IV sargramostim or placebo were as reported in TABLE 7.

There were no significant differences in the incidence or severity of GVHD, relapse rates, and survival between sargramostim and placebo-treated patients.

Adverse events observed for the patients treated with sargramostim in the historically controlled BMT failure study were similar to those reported in the placebo-controlled studies. In addition, headache (26%), pericardial effusion (25%), arthralgia (21%), and myalgia (18%) were also reported in patients treated with sargramostim in the graft failure study.

In uncontrolled Phase I/II studies with sargramostim in 215 patients, the most frequent adverse events were fever, asthenia, headache, bone pain, chills, and myalgia. These systemic events were generally mild or moderate and were usually prevented or reversed by the administration of analgesics and antipyretics such as acetaminophen. In these uncontrolled trials, other infrequent events reported were dyspnea, peripheral edema, and rash.

Reports of events occurring with marketed sargramostim include arrhythmia, eosinophilia, hypotension, injection site reactions, pain (including abdominal, back, chest, and joint pain), tachycardia, thrombosis, and transient liver function abnormalities.

In patients with preexisting edema, capillary leak syndrome, pleural and/or pericardial effusion, administration of sargramostim may aggravate fluid retention (see WARNINGS). Body weight and hydration status should be carefully monitored during sargramostim administration.

Adverse events observed in pediatric patients in controlled studies were comparable to those observed in adult patients.

ACUTE MYELOGENOUS LEUKEMIA

Adverse events reported in at least 10% of patients who received sargramostim or placebo were as reported in TABLE 8.

Nearly all patients reported leukopenia, thrombocytopenia, and anemia. The frequency and type of adverse events observed following induction were similar between sargramostim and placebo groups. The only significant difference in the rates of these adverse events was an increase in skin associated events in the sargramostim group (p=0.002). No significant differences were observed in laboratory results, renal or hepatic toxicity. No significant differences were observed between the sargramostim- and placebo-treated patients for adverse events following consolidation. There was no significant difference in response rate or relapse rate.

In a historically controlled study of 86 patients with acute myelogenous leukemia (AML), the sargramostim treated group exhibited an increased incidence of weight gain (p=0.007), low serum proteins and prolonged prothrombin time (p=0.02) when compared to the control group. Two sargramostim treated patients had progressive increase in circulating monocytes and promonocytes and blasts in the marrow which reversed when sargramostim was discontinued. The historical control group exhibited an increased incidence of cardiac events

S

TABLE 7 *Percent of Allogeneic BMT Patients Reporting Events*

Events by Body System	Sargramostim (n=53)	Placebo (n=56)
Body, General		
Fever	77%	80%
Abdominal pain	38%	23%
Headache	36%	36%
Chills	25%	20%
Pain	17%	36%
Asthenia	17%	20%
Chest pain	15%	9%
Back pain	9%	18%
Digestive System		
Diarrhea	81%	66%
Nausea	70%	66%
Vomiting	70%	57%
Stomatitis	62%	63%
Anorexia	51%	57%
Dyspepsia	17%	20%
Hematemesis	13%	7%
Dysphagia	11%	7%
GI hemorrhage	11%	5%
Constipation	8%	11%
Skin and Appendages		
Rash	70%	73%
Alopecia	45%	45%
Pruritus	23%	13%
Musculo-Skeletal System		
Bone pain	21%	5%
Arthralgia	11%	4%
Special Senses		
Eye hemorrhage	11%	0%
Cardiovascular System		
Hypertension	34%	32%
Tachycardia	11%	9%
Metabolic /Nutritional Disorders		
Bilirubinemia	30%	27%
Hyperglycemia	25%	23%
Peripheral edema	15%	21%
Increased creatinine	15%	14%
Hypomagnesemia	15%	9%
Increased SGPT	13%	16%
Edema	13%	11%
Increased alk. phosphatase	8%	14%
Respiratory System		
Pharyngitis	23%	13%
Epistaxis	17%	16%
Dyspnea	15%	14%
Rhinitis	11%	14%
Hemic and Lymphatic System		
Thrombocytopenia	19%	34%
Leukopenia	17%	29%
Petechia	6%	11%
Agranulocytosis	6%	11%
Urogenital System		
Hematuria	9%	21%
Nervous System		
Paresthesia	11%	13%
Insomnia	11%	9%
Anxiety	11%	2%
Laboratory Abnormalities*		
High glucose	41%	49%
Low albumin	27%	36%
High BUN	23%	17%
Low calcium	2%	7%
High cholesterol	17%	8%

* Grade 3 and 4 laboratory abnormalities only. Denominators may vary due to missing laboratory measurements.

(p=0.018), liver function abnormalities (p=0.008), and neurocortical hemorrhagic events (p=0.025).[15]

DOSAGE AND ADMINISTRATION

NEUTROPHIL RECOVERY FOLLOWING CHEMOTHERAPY IN ACUTE MYELOGENOUS LEUKEMIA

The recommended dose is 250 μg/m²/day administered intravenously over a 4 hour period starting approximately on day 11 or 4 days following the completion of induction chemotherapy, if the day 10 bone marrow is hypoplastic with <5% blasts. Sargramostim should be continued until an ANC >1500/mm³ for consecutive days or a maximum of 42 days. If a second cycle of induction chemotherapy is necessary, sargramostim should be administered approximately 4 days after the completion of chemotherapy if the bone marrow is hypoplastic with <5% blasts. Sargramostim should be discontinued immediately if leukemic regrowth occurs. If a severe adverse reaction occurs, the dose can be reduced by 50%, or temporarily discontinued until the reaction abates.

In order to avoid potential complications of excessive leukocytosis (WBC >50,000 cells/mm³ ANC >20,000 cells/mm³), a CBC with differential is recommended twice per week during sargramostim therapy. Sargramostim treatment should be interrupted or the dose reduced by half if the ANC exceeds >20,000 cells/mm³.

MOBILIZATION OF PERIPHERAL BLOOD PROGENITOR CELLS

The recommended dose is 250 μg/m²/day administered IV over 24 hours or SC once daily. Dosing should continue at the same dose through the period of PBPC collection. The optimal schedule for PBPC collection has not been established. In clinical studies, collection of PBPC was usually begun by day 5 and performed daily until protocol specified targets were achieved. If WBC >50,000 cells/mm³, the sargramostim dose should be reduced by 50%. If adequate numbers of progenitor cells are not collected, other mobilization therapy should be considered.

TABLE 8 *Percent of AML Patients Reporting Event*

Events by Body System	Sargramostim (n=52)	Placebo (n=47)
Body, General		
Fever (no infection)	81%	74%
Infection	65%	68%
Weight loss	37%%	28%
Weight gain	8%	21%
Chills	19%	26%
Allergy	12%	15%
Sweats	6%	13%
Digestive System		
Nausea	58%	55%
Liver	77%	83%
Diarrhea	52%	53%
Vomiting	46%	34%
Stomatitis	42%	43%
Anorexia	13%	11%
Abdominal distention	4%	13%
Skin and Appendages		
Skin	77%	45%
Alopecia	37%	51%
Metabolic/Nutritional Disorder		
Metabolic	58%	49%
Edema	25%	23%
Respiratory System		
Pulmonary	48%	64%
Hemic and Lymphatic System		
Coagulation	19%	21%
Cardiovascular System		
Hemorrhage	29%	43%
Hypertension	25%	32%
Cardiac	23%	32%
Hypotension	13%	26%
Urogenital System		
GU	50%	57%
Nervous System		
Neuro-clinical	42%	53%
Neuro-motor	25%	26%
Neuro-psych	15%	26%
Neuro-sensory	6%	11%

POST PERIPHERAL BLOOD PROGENITOR CELL TRANSPLANTATION

The recommended dose is 250 μg/m²/day administered IV over 24 hours or SC once daily beginning immediately following infusion of progenitor cells and continuing until an ANC>1500 cells/mm³ for 3 consecutive days is attained.

MYELOID RECONSTITUTION AFTER AUTOLOGOUS OR ALLOGENEIC BONE MARROW TRANSPLANTATION

The recommended dose is 250 μg/m²/day administered IV over a 2 hour period beginning 2-4 hours after bone marrow infusion, and not less than 24 hours after the last dose of chemotherapy or radiotherapy. Patients should not receive sargramostim until the post marrow infusion ANC is less than 500 cells/mm³. Sargramostim should be continued until an ANC >1500 cells/mm³ for 3 consecutive days is attained. If a severe adverse reaction occurs, the dose can be reduced by 50% or temporarily discontined until the reaction abates. Sargramostim should be discontinued immediately if blast cells appear or disease progression occurs.

In order to avoid potential complications of excessive leukocytosis (WBC>50,000 cells/mm³, ANC>20,000 cells/mm³), a CBC with differential is recommended twice per week during sargramostin therapy. Sargramostin treatment should be interrupted or the dose reduced by 50% if the ANC exceeds 20,000/mm³.

BONE MARROW TRANSPLANTATION FAILURE OR ENGRAFTMENT DELAY

The recommended dose is 250 μg/m²/day for 14 days as a 2 hour IV infusion. The dose can be repeated after 7 days off therapy if engraftment still has not occurred. If engraftment still has not occurred, a third course of 500 μg/m²/day for 14 days may be tried after another 7 days off therapy. If there is still no improvement, it is unlikely that further dose escalation will be beneficial. If a severe adverse reaction occurs, the dose can be reduced by 50% or temporarily discontinued until the reaction abates. Sargramostim should be discontinued immediately if blast cells appear or disease progression occurs.

In order to avoid potential complications of excessive leukocytosis (WBC >50,000 cells/mm³, ANC >20,000 cells/mm³) a CBC with differential is recommended twice per week during sargramostim therapy. Sargramostim treatment should be interrupted or the dose reduced by half if the ANC exceeds 20,000 cells/mm³.

Preparation of Sargramostim:

1. Sargramostim liquid is a preserved (1.1% benzyl alcohol), sterile, injectable solution. Lyophilized sargramostim is a sterile, white, preservative-free, lyophilized powder. Both sargramostim liquid and reconstituted lyophilized sargramostim are suitable for SC injection and IV infusion. Lyophilized sargramostim requires reconstitution with 1 ml sterile water for injection, or 1 ml bacteriostatic water for injection. The sargramostim liquid injectable and reconstituted lyophilized sargramostim solutions are clear, colorless, isotonic solutions.
2. Once the vial has been entered, sargramostim liquid may be stored for up to 20 days at 2-8°C. Discard any remaining solution after 20 days.
3. Lyophilized sargramostim (250 μg or 500 μg vials) should be reconstituted aseptically with 1.0 ml of diluent. The contents of vials reconstituted with different diluents should not be mixed together. *Sterile Water for Injection (Without Preservative):* Lyophilized sargramostim vials contain no antibacterial preservative, and therefore solutions prepared with sterile water for injection should be adminstered as soon as possible, and within 6 hours following reconstitution and/or dilution for IV infusion. the vial should not be re-entered or reused. Do not save any unused portion for administration more than 6 hours following reconstitution. *Bacteriostatic Water for Injection (0.9% Benzyl Alcohol):* Reconstituted solutions prepared with bacteriostatic water for injection (0.9% ben-

S

zyl alcohol) may be stored for up to 20 days at 2-8°C prior to use. Discard reconstituted solution after 20 days. Previously reconstituted solutions mixed with freshly reconstituted solutions must be administered within 6 hours following mixing. **Preparations containing benzyl alcohol (including sargramostim liquid and lyophilized sargramostim reconstituted with bacteriostatic water for injection) should not be used in neonates (see WARNINGS).**

4. During reconstitution of lyophilized sargramostim the diluent should be directed at the side of the vial and contents gently swirled to avoid foaming during dissolution. Avoid excessive or vigorous agitation; do not shake.
5. Sargramostim should be used for SC injection without further dilution. Dilution for IV infusion should be performed in 0.9% sodium chloride injection. If the final concentration of sargramostim is below 10 μg/ml, Albumin (Human) at a final concentration of 0.1% should be added to the saline prior to addition of sargramostim to prevent adsorption to the components of the drug delivery system. To obtain a final concentration of 0.1% Albumin (Human) per 1 ml 0.9% sodium chloride injection (*eg.*, use 1 ml 5% Albumin [Human] in 50 ml 0.9% sodium chloride injection.)
6. An in-line membrane filter should not be used for intravenous infusion of sargramostim.
7. Store sargramostim liquid and reconstituted lyophilized sargramostim solutions under refrigeration at 2-8°C (36-46°F); do not freeze.
8. In the absence of compatibility and stability information, no other medication should be added to infusion solutions containing sargramostin. Use only 0.9% sodium chloride injection to prepare IV infusion solutions.
9. Aseptic technique should be employed in the preparation of all sargramostin solutions. To assure correct concentration following reconstitution, care should be exercised to eliminate any air bubbles from the needle hub of the syringe used to prepare the diluent. Parental drug products should be inspected visually for particulate matter and discoloration prior to administration whenever solution and container permit.

PRODUCT LISTING - EQUIVALENTS NOT AVAILABLE

Powder For Injection - Intravenous - 250 mcg

1's	$117.79	LEUKINE, Immunex Corporation	58406-0002-01
5's	$764.75	LEUKINE, Immunex Corporation	58406-0002-33

Solution - Intravenous - 500 mcg/ml

1 ml	$252.06	LEUKINE, Immunex Corporation	58406-0050-14
1 ml x 5	$1529.55	LEUKINE, Immunex Corporation	58406-0050-30

Scopolamine *(002213)*

Categories: Cycloplegia induction; Delirium tremens; Diverticulitis; Dysentery; Gastrointestinal spasm; Iridocyclitis; Irritable bowel syndrome; Motion sickness; Mydriasis induction; Nausea; Paralysis Agitans; Parkinsonism, postencephalitic; Preanesthesia; Sedation; Spasticity; Vomiting; Pregnancy Category C

Drug Classes: Anticholinergics; Antiemetics/antivertigo; Cycloplegics; Gastrointestinals; Mydriatics; Ophthalmics; Preanesthetics; Sedatives/hypnotics

Brand Names: Isopto Hyoscine; Minims Hyoscine Hydrobromide; Scopoderm; Transderm Scop

Foreign Brand Availability: Kimite-patch (Korea); Scopoderm Depotplast (Norway); Scopoderm TTS (Austria; Bulgaria; China; England; France; Germany; Netherlands; New-Zealand; Switzerland; Taiwan); Transcop (Italy); Transderm-V (Canada)

Cost of Therapy: $10.49 (Parkinson's Disease; Scopace; 0.4 mg; 1 tablet/day; 30 day supply)

IM-IV-SC

DESCRIPTION

FOR INTRAMUSCULAR, INTRAVENOUS OR SUBCUTANEOUS USE

Protect From Light

Opaque covering needed until contents used

Scopolamine hydrobromide injection is a sterile solution of scopolamine hydrobromide ($C_{17}H_{21}NO_4 \cdot HBr \cdot 3H_2O$) in water for injection. The injection is preserved with methylparaben 0.18% and propylparaben 0.02%. Scopolamine hydrobromide injection is intended for intramuscular, intravenous and subcutaneous use. The pH (3.5-6.5) is adjusted with hydrobromic acid if necessary.

CLINICAL PHARMACOLOGY

Scopolamine hydrobromide is one of the major antimuscarinic agents that inhibit the action of acetylcholine (ACh) on autonomic effectors innervated by postganglionic cholinergic nerves as well as on smooth muscles that lack cholinergic innervation. It exerts little effects on the actions of ACh at nicotinic receptor sites such as autonomic ganglia. The major action of this antimuscarinic agent is a surmountable antagonism to ACh and other muscarinic agents.

As compared with atropine, scopolamine differs only quantitatively in antimuscarinic actions. Scopolamine has a stronger action on the iris, ciliary body and certain secretory glands such as salivary, bronchial and sweat. Scopolamine, in therapeutic doses, normally causes drowsiness, euphoria, amnesia, fatigue and dreamless sleep with a reduction in rapid-eye-movement sleep. However, the same doses occasionally cause excitement, restlessness, hallucinations or delirium, especially in the presence of severe pain. Scopolamine depresses the EEG arousal response to photo-stimulation. It is more potent than atropine on the antitremor activity (parkinsonism) in animals induced by surgical lesions. Scopolamine is effective in preventing motion sickness by acting on the maculae of the utricle and saccule.

Scopolamine, although less potent than atropine, has been used frequently in preanesthetic medication for the purpose of inhibiting the secretions of the nose, mouth, pharynx and bronchi and reduces the occurrence of laryngospasm during general anesthesia. Scopolamine is less potent in the decrease of cardiac rate, but not in the changes of blood pressure or cardiac output. Like other antimuscarinic agents, scopolamine has been used widely in the treatment of peptic ulcers and as an antispasmodic agent for GI disorders. This is due to the fact that scopolamine reduces salivary secretion, the gastric secretion (both the volume and acid content), and also it inhibits the motor activity of the stomach, duodenum, jejunum, ileum and colon, characterized by a decrease in tone, amplitude and frequency of peristaltic contractions.

INDICATIONS AND USAGE

Scopolamine hydrobromide injection is indicated as a sedative and tranquilizing depressant to the central nervous system. In its peripheral actions, scopolamine differs from atropine in that it is a stronger blocking agent for the iris, ciliary body and salivary, bronchial and sweat glands but is weaker in its action on the heart (in which it is incapable of exerting actions in tolerated doses), the intestinal tract and bronchial musculature.

In addition to the usual uses for antimuscarinic drugs, scopolamine is employed for its central depressant actions as a sedative. Frequently it is given as a preanesthetic medicament for both its sedative-tranquilizing and antisecretory actions. It is an effective antiemetic. It is used in maniacal states, in delirium tremens and in obstetrics. As a mydriatic and cycloplegic, it has a somewhat shorter duration (3-7 days) and intraocular pressure is affected less markedly than with atropine.

CONTRAINDICATIONS

Scopolamine hydrobromide is contraindicated in patients with narrow-angle glaucoma, since administration of the drug could raise the intraocular pressure to dangerous levels. However, this will not happen for side-angle glaucoma patients. Repeated administration of scopolamine to a patient with chronic lung disease is considered to be potentially hazardous. Patients hypersensitive to belladonna or to barbiturates may be hypersensitive to scopolamine hydrobromide.

WARNINGS

Addiction does not occur, although vomiting, malaise, sweating and salivation have been reported in patients with parkinsonism upon sudden withdrawal of large doses of scopolamine. Scopolamine is one of the most important drugs of the belladonna group from the standpoint of poisoning; infants and young children are especially susceptible to the belladonna alkaloids. Scopolamine is usually stated more toxic than atropine. Idiosyncrasy is more common with scopolamine than with atropine and ordinary therapeutic doses sometimes cause alarming reactions.

PRECAUTIONS

GENERAL

If there is mydriasis and photophobia, dark glasses should be worn. Appropriate dosage precautions must be taken with infants, children, persons with mongolism, brain damage, spasticity, or light irides. Elevated intraocular pressure, urinary difficulty and retention and constipation are more probable in elderly persons. Men with prostatic hypertrophy should especially be monitored for urinary function. Because of the tachycardic effects of the drugs, care must be exercised when tachycardia, other tachyarrhythmias, coronary heart disease, congestive heart disease or hyperthyroidism preexist. Persons with hypertension may experience both exaggerated orthostatic hypotension and tachycardia. Similarly, autonomic neuropathy requires caution. Persons with a history of allergies or bronchial asthma will show a higher than normal incidence of hypersensitivity reactions.

LABORATORY TESTS

Barbiturates may increase bromosulfonphthalein (BSP) levels; administration is not recommended during the 24 hours preceding the test.

PREGNANCY CATEGORY C

Scopolamine hydrobromide can pass the placental barrier; the threat to the fetus *in utero* is unknown, but use during pregnancy may cause respiratory depression in the neonate and may contribute to neonatal hemorrhage due to reduction in vitamin K-dependent clotting factors in the neonate.

Scopolamine should be used during pregnancy only if the potential benefit justifies the potential risk to the fetus.

NURSING MOTHERS

Problems in humans have not been documented; however, risk-benefit must be considered since barbiturates and belladonna alkaloids are excreted in breast milk.

DRUG INTERACTIONS

Other drugs, such as phenothiazines, tricyclic antidepressants, certain antihistamines, meperidine, etc., which have weak antimuscarinic activity, may considerably intensify the effects of antimuscarinic drugs. Aluminum- and magnesium trisillicate-containing antacids have been shown to decrease the absorption of some antimuscarinic drugs and may possibly do so with all of them.

ADVERSE REACTIONS

With nearly all antimuscarinic drugs, dry mouth is the first and dry skin is the second most common side effect. Thirst and difficulty swallowing occur when the mouth and esophagus become sufficiently dry; chronic dry mouth also fosters dental caries. Suppression of sweating causes reflexive flushing and heat intolerance and can result in heat exhaustion or heat stroke in a hot environment; it also contributes to the hyperthermia seen in intoxication. Mydriasis frequently occurs, especially with scopolamine; photophobia and blurring of vision are consequences of mydriasis. Cycloplegia (which exacerbates blurred vision) occurs approximately concomitantly with mydriasis, but usually higher doses are required. In susceptible persons, especially the elderly, cycloplegia may contribute to an elevation of intraocular pressure. Difficulty in urination and urinary retention may occur. Tachycardia is a common side effect. Constipation, even bowel stasis, may occur.

In the larger therapeutic doses, scopolamine may cause dizziness, restlessness, tremors, fatigue and locomotor difficulties.

DOSAGE AND ADMINISTRATION

ADULTS

For obstetric amnesia or preoperative sedation, 0.32-0.65 mg (320-650 μg).

For sedation or tranquilization, 0.6 mg (600 μg) 3 or 4 times a day.

Subcutaneous, as an antiemetic, 0.6 to 1 mg.

S

PEDIATRIC

Age 6 months to 3 years, 0.1-0.15 mg (100-150 μg).

Age 3-6 years, 0.2-0.3 mg (200-300 μg).

Subcutaneous, as antiemetic, 0.006 mg (6 μg) per kg.

TABLE 1 *Dosage Equivalents*

1 mg (1000 μg)/ml		
1 mg	(1000 μg)	1 ml
0.8 mg	(800 μg)	0.8 ml
0.6 mg	(600 μg)	0.6 ml
0.5 mg	(500 μg)	0.5 ml
0.4 mg	(400 μg)	0.4 ml
0.3 mg	(300 μg)	0.3 ml
0.2 mg	(200 μg)	0.2 ml
0.1 mg	(100 μg)	0.1 ml
0.4 mg (400 μg)/ml		
0.4 mg	(400 μg)	1 ml
0.3 mg	(300 μg)	0.75 ml
0.25 mg	(250 μg)	0.63 ml
0.2 mg	(200 μg)	0.50 ml
0.15 mg	(150 μg)	0.38 ml

Belladonna alkaloids provide a therapeutic effect in about 1 or 2 hours with a duration of about 4 hours.

Geriatric and debilitated patients may respond to the usual doses with excitement, agitation, drowsiness or confusion; lower doses may be required in such patients.

Close supervision is recommended for infants, blondes, mongoloids and children with spastic paralysis or brain damage, since an increased responsiveness to belladonna alkaloids has been reported in these patients and dosage adjustments are often required.

Administration of belladonna alkaloids and barbiturates 30-60 minutes before meals is recommended to maximize absorption and, when issued for reducing stomach acid formation, to allow its effect to coincide better with antacid administration following the meal.

Parenteral drug products should be inspected visually for particulate matter prior to administration, whenever solution and container permit.

HOW SUPPLIED

Scopolamine hydrobromide injection is supplied in multiple dose vials, preserved, in the following volumes: 0.4 mg/ml (1 ml in a 2 ml vial) and 1 mg/ml (1 ml in a 2 ml vial). **PROTECT FROM LIGHT.**

Use only if solution is clear and seal intact.

Storage: Store at controlled room temperature 15-30°C (59-86°F).

OPHTHALMIC

DESCRIPTION

Scopolamine hydrobromide is an anticholinergic prepared as a sterile topical ophthalmic solution.

Established name: Scopolamine hydrobromide.

Chemical name: Benzeneacetic acid, α-(hydroxy-methyl)-,9-methyl-3-oxa-9-azatricyclo[3.3.1.$0^{2,4}$]non-7-yl ester, hydrobromide, trihydrate, (7(*S*)-(1α,2β,4β,5α,7β))-.

Each ml contains: *Active:* Scopolamine hydrobromide 0.25%. *Preservative:* Benzalkonium chloride 0.01%. *Vehicle:* Hydroxypropyl methylcellulose 0.5%. *Inactive:* Sodium chloride, glacial acetic acid, sodium acetate (to adjust pH), purified water.

CLINICAL PHARMACOLOGY

This anticholinergic preparation blocks the responses of the sphincter muscle of the ciliary body to cholinergic stimulation, producing pupillary dilation (mydriasis) and paralysis of accommodation (cycloplegia).

INDICATIONS AND USAGE

For mydriasis and cycloplegia in diagnostic procedures. For some pre- and postoperative states when a mydriatic and cycloplegic is needed in the treatment of iridocyclitis.

CONTRAINDICATIONS

Contraindicated in persons with primary glaucoma or a tendency toward glaucoma, *e.g.,* narrow anterior chamber angle; and in those showing hypersensitivity to any component of this preparation.

WARNINGS

Do not touch dropper tip to any surface, as this may contaminate the solution. For topical use only — not for injection. In infants and small children, use with extreme caution.

PRECAUTIONS

To avoid excessive absorption, the lacrimal sac should be compressed by digital pressure for 2-3 minutes after instillation. To avoid inducing angle closure glaucoma, an estimation of the depth of the angle of the anterior chamber should be made.

Patient warning: Patient should be advised not to drive or engage in other hazardous activities when drowsy or while pupils are dilated. Patient may experience sensitivity to light and should protect eyes in bright illumination during dilation. Parents should be warned not to get this preparation in their child's mouth and to wash their own hands and the child's hands following administration.

ADVERSE REACTIONS

Prolonged use may produce local irritation, characterized by follicular conjunctivitis, vascular congestion, edema, exudate, and an eczematoid dermatitis. Somnolence, dryness of the mouth, or visual hallucinations may occur.

DOSAGE AND ADMINISTRATION

For refraction, administer 1 or 2 drops topically in the eye(s) 1 hour before refracting. For uveitis, administer 1 or 2 drops topically in the eye(s) up to 4 times daily.

HOW SUPPLIED

Isopto Hyoscine is available in 5 ml and 15 ml plastic Drop-Tainer dispensers.

Storage: Store at 46–80°F. Protect from light.

ORAL

DESCRIPTION

The hydrobromide of an alkaloid, l-scopolamine (hyoscine), this compound combines the base (scopine) with D-tropic acid. Obtained from plants of the Solanaceae family, it is one of the belladonna alkaloids related to atropine. It is freely soluble in water (1:1.5) and soluble in alcohol (1:20).

Scopolamine, an anticholinergic drug, is a primary central depressant with marked sedative and tranquilizing properties; like atropine, it is a mydriatic.

Scopolamine hydrobromide occurs as colorless or white crystals or as white granular powder. It is odorless and slightly efflorescent in dry air.

Each Scopace tablet contains 0.4 mg scopolamine hydrobromide.

The chemical name of scopolamine hydrobromide is [6β,7β-epoxy-1αH,5αH-tropan-3α-ol(-)-tropate (ester) hydrobromide; hyoscine hydrobromide].

CLINICAL PHARMACOLOGY

The official variety of levoscopolamine is paralyzant to peripheral ends of the parasympathetic nerves, acting in this respect like atropine, although less powerfully. It dilates the pupil, causes dryness of the throat and skin, accelerates heart action, etc. As a mydriatic, it is much quicker and less lasting in its effects than atropine and is used to paralyze accommodation in correcting errors of refraction. It differs strikingly from atropine, however, in that it does not stimulate the medullary centers and therefore does not increase respiration or elevate blood pressure; also, it frequently appears to act as a cerebral depressant and tends to promote sleep. In some persons, the sleep it produces is attended with a kind of low muttering delirium recalling the mental confusion seen in atropine poisoning; this effect may be observed in a patient with pain. A striking effect of large doses of scopolamine is the loss of memory for events which happened while the patient was under the influence of the drug. It has been reported that scopolamine has slight analgesic properties and greatly as morphine or urethan. In large doses, it is depressant to the respiratory center and, apparently, also in some degree to motor ganglia of the spinal cord.

INDICATIONS AND USAGE

Scopolamine soluble tablets are used as an anticholinergic central-nervous system depressant; in the symptomatic treatment of postencephalitic parkinsonism and paralysis agitans; in spastic states; and, locally as a substitute for atropine in ophthalmology.

Scopolamine soluble tablets inhibit excessive motility and hypertonus of the gastrointestinal tract in such conditions as the irritable colon syndrome, mild dysentery, diverticulitis, pylorospasm, and cardiospasm. It may also prevent motion sickness.

CONTRAINDICATIONS

Scopolamine ophthalmic solution is contraindicated in the presence of narrow-angle glaucoma, prostatic hypertrophy, and pyloric obstruction. It should not be administered to patients with impaired renal or hepatic function or to those who have an idiosyncrasy to anticholinergic drugs.

WARNINGS

Since drowsiness, disorientation, and confusion may occur with the use of scopolamine, patients should be warned of the possibility and cautioned against engaging in activities that require mental alertness, such as driving a motor vehicle or operating dangerous machinery.

PRECAUTIONS

GENERAL

Use with caution in patients with cardiac disease and in the elderly.

PREGNANCY CATEGORY C

Animal reproductions studies have not been conducted with scopolamine hydrobromide. It is also not known whether the drug can cause fetal harm when administered to a pregnant woman or can affect reproduction capacity. Scopolamine hydrobromide should be given to a pregnant woman only if clearly needed.

NURSING MOTHERS

It is not known whether this drug is excreted in human milk. Because many drugs are excreted in human milk, caution should be exercised when scopolamine hydrobromide is administered to a nursing woman.

USAGE IN CHILDREN

Safety and effectiveness in children have not been established.

DRUG INTERACTIONS

Scopolamine should be used with care in patients taking drugs, including alcohol, capable of causing CNS effects. Special attention should be given to drugs having anticholinergic properties, *e.g.,* belladonna alkaloids, antihistamines (including meclizine), and antidepressants.

ADVERSE REACTIONS

Side effects are similar to those of atropine *i.e.,* dry mouth, flushing, tachycardia, mydriasis, blurred vision, or urinary retention.

In susceptible individuals, there may be dryness of the skin and other signs and symptoms typical of anticholinergic drugs.

Many persons are excessively susceptible to scopolamine, and toxic symptoms may occur; such symptoms are often very alarming. There are marked disturbances of the intellect, ranging from complete disorientation to an active delirium resembling that encountered in atropine poisoning. Many cases present marked somnolence, but in others this may be lacking. At times the pupils are dilated, the pulse rate is accelerated, and there is dryness of the mouth with a husky quality of the voice apparently due to laryngeal paralysis; these symptoms are often absent or very mild.

DOSAGE AND ADMINISTRATION

The dosage range for scopolamine is 0.4-0.8 mg. The dosage may be cautiously increased in parkinsonism and spastic states.

HOW SUPPLIED

SCOPOLAMINE HYDROBROMIDE, SOLUBLE TABLETS 0.4 MG

Tablet identification: White, imprinted "HOPE", "301".

Storage: Store at controlled room temperature 15-30°C (59-86°F).

TRANSDERMAL

DESCRIPTION

The Transderm Scop (transdermal scopolamine) system is a circular flat patch designed for continuous release of scopolamine following application to an area of intact skin on the head, behind the ear. Each system contains 1.5 mg of scopolamine base. Scopolamine is a-(hydroxymethyl) benzeneacetic acid 9-methyl-3-oxa-9-azatricyclo[3.3.1.02,4] non-7-yl ester. The empirical formula is $C_{17}H_{21}NO_4$.

Scopolamine is a viscous liquid that has a molecular weight of 303.35 and a pKa of 7.55-7.81. The Transderm Scop system is a film 0.2 mm thick and 2.5 cm^2, with four layers. Proceeding from the visible surface towards the surface attached to the skin, these layers are: (1) a backing layer of tan-colored, aluminized, polyester film; (2) a drug reservoir of scopolamine, light mineral oil, and polyisobutylene; (3) a microporous polypropylene membrane that controls the rate of delivery of scopolamine from the system to the skin surface; and (4) an adhesive formulation of mineral oil, polyisobutylene, and scopolamine. A protective peel strip of siliconized polyester, which covers the adhesive layer, is removed before the system is used. The inactive components, light mineral oil (12.4 mg) and polyisobutylene (11.4 mg), are not released from the system.

CLINICAL PHARMACOLOGY

PHARMACOLOGY

The sole active agent of Transderm Scop is scopolamine, a belladonna alkaloid with well-known pharmacological properties. It is an anticholinergic agent which acts: (1) as a competitive inhibitor at postganglionic muscarinic receptor sites of the parasympathetic nervous system, and (2) on smooth muscles that respond to acetylcholine but lack cholinergic innervation. It has been suggested that scopolamine acts in the central nervous system (CNS) by blocking cholinergic transmission from the vestibular nuclei to higher centers in the CNS and from the reticular formation to the vomiting center.[1,2] Scopolamine can inhibit the secretion of saliva and sweat, decrease gastrointestinal secretions and motility, cause drowsiness, dilate the pupils, increase heart rate, and depress motor function.[2]

PHARMACOKINETICS

Scopolamine's activity is due to the parent drug. The pharmacokinetics of scopolamine delivered via the system are due to the characteristics of both the drug and dosage form. The system is programmed to deliver *in vivo* approximately 1.0 mg of scopolamine at an approximately constant rate to the systemic circulation over 3 days. Upon application to the post-auricular skin, an initial priming dose of scopolamine is released from the adhesive layer to saturate skin binding sites. The subsequent delivery of scopolamine to the blood is determined by the rate controlling membrane and is designed to produce stable plasma levels in a therapeutic range. Following removal of the used system, there is some degree of continued systemic absorption of scopolamine bound in the skin layers.

Absorption

Scopolamine is well-absorbed percutaneously. Following application to the skin behind the ear, circulating plasma levels are detected within 4 hours with peak levels being obtained, on average, within 24 hours. The average plasma concentration produced is 87 pg/ml for free scopolamine and 354 pg/ml for total scopolamine (free + conjugates).

Distribution

The distribution of scopolamine is not well characterized. It crosses the placenta and the blood brain barrier and may be reversibly bound to plasma proteins.

Metabolism

Although not well characterized, scopolamine is extensively metabolized and conjugated with less than 5% of the total dose appearing unchanged in the urine.

Elimination

The exact elimination pattern of scopolamine has not been determined. Following patch removal, plasma levels decline in a log linear fashion with an observed half-life of 9.5 hours. Less than 10% of the total dose is excreted in the urine as parent and metabolites over 108 hours.

INDICATIONS AND USAGE

Transdermal scopolamine is indicated in adults for prevention of nausea and vomiting associated with motion sickness and recovery from anesthesia and surgery. The patch should be applied only to skin in the postauricular area.

NON-FDA APPROVED INDICATIONS

The scopolamine transdermal patch has also been used alone or with other antiemetic agents to prevent chemotherapy-induced nausea and vomiting, as well as to control symptoms of vertigo, although these indications are not approved by the FDA.

CONTRAINDICATIONS

Transdermal scopolamine is contraindicated in persons who are hypersensitive to the drug scopolamine or to other belladonna alkaloids, or to any ingredient or component in the formulation or delivery system, or in patients with angle-closure (narrow angle) glaucoma.

WARNINGS

Glaucoma therapy in patients with chronic open-angle (wide-angle) glaucoma should be monitored and may need to be adjusted during transdermal scopolamine use, as the mydriatic effect of scopolamine may cause an increase in intraocular pressure. Transdermal scopolamine should not be used in children and should be used with caution in the elderly. See PRECAUTIONS. Since drowsiness, disorientation, and confusion may occur with the use of scopolamine, patients should be warned of the possibility and cautioned against engaging in activities that require mental alertness, such as driving a motor vehicle or operating dangerous machinery. Rarely, idiosyncratic reactions may occur with ordinary therapeutic doses of scopolamine. The most serious of these that have been reported are: acute toxic psychosis, including confusion, agitation, rambling speech, hallucinations, paranoid behaviors, and delusions.

PRECAUTIONS

GENERAL

Scopolamine should be used with caution in patients with pyloric obstruction or urinary bladder neck obstruction. Caution should be exercised when administering an antiemetic or antimuscarinic drug to patients suspected of having intestinal obstruction.

Transdermal scopolamine should be used with caution in the elderly or in individuals with impaired liver or kidney functions because of the increased likelihood of CNS effects.

Caution should be exercised in patients with a history of seizures or psychosis, since scopolamine can potentially aggravate both disorders.

INFORMATION FOR THE PATIENT

Since scopolamine can cause temporary dilation of the pupils and blurred vision if it comes in contact with the eyes, patients should be strongly advised to wash their hands thoroughly with soap and water immediately after handling the patch. In addition, it is important that used patches be disposed of properly to avoid contact with children or pets.

Patients should be advised to remove the patch immediately and promptly contact a physician in the unlikely event that they experience symptoms of acute narrow-angle glaucoma (pain and reddening of the eyes, accompanied by dilated pupils). Patients should also be instructed to remove the patch if they develop any difficulties in urinating.

Patients who expect to participate in underwater sports should be cautioned regarding the potentially disorienting effects of scopolamine. A patient brochure is available.

LABORATORY TEST INTERACTIONS

Scopolamine will interfere with the gastric secretion test.

CARCINOGENESIS, MUTAGENESIS, AND IMPAIRMENT OF FERTILITY

No long-term studies in animals have been completed to evaluate the carcinogenic potential of scopolamine. The mutagenic potential of scopolamine has not been evaluated. Fertility studies were performed in female rats and revealed no evidence of impaired fertility or harm to the fetus due to scopolamine hydrobromide administered by daily subcutaneous injection. Maternal body weights were reduced in the highest-dose group (plasma level approximately 500 times the level achieved in humans using a transdermal system).

PREGNANCY CATEGORY C

Teratogenic studies were performed in pregnant rats and rabbits with scopolamine hydrobromide administered by daily intravenous injection. No adverse effects were recorded in rats. Scopolamine hydrobromide has been shown to have a marginal embryotoxic effect in rabbits when administered by daily intravenous injection at doses producing plasma levels approximately 100 times the level achieved in humans using a transdermal system. During a clinical study among women undergoing cesarean section treated with transdermal scopolamine in conjunction with epidural anesthesia and opiate analgesia, no evidence of CNS depression was found in the newborns. There are no other adequate and well-controlled studies in pregnant women. Other than in the adjunctive use for delivery by cesarean section, transdermal scopolamine should be used in pregnancy only if the potential benefit justifies the potential risk to the fetus.

NURSING MOTHERS

Because scopolamine is excreted in human milk, caution should be exercised when transdermal scopolamine is administered to a nursing woman.

LABOR AND DELIVERY

Scopolamine administered parenterally at higher doses than the dose delivered by transdermal scopolamine does not increase the duration of labor, nor does it affect uterine contractions. Scopolamine does cross the placenta.

PEDIATRIC USE

The safety and effectiveness of transdermal scopolamine in children has not been established. Children are particularly susceptible to the side effects of belladonna alkaloids. Transdermal scopolamine should not be used in children because it is not known whether this system will release an amount of scopolamine that could produce serious adverse effects in children.

DRUG INTERACTIONS

The absorption of oral medications may be decreased during the concurrent use of scopolamine because of decreased gastric motility and delayed gastric emptying.

Scopolamine should be used with care in patients taking other drugs that are capable of causing CNS effects such as sedatives, tranquilizers, or alcohol. Special attention should be paid to potential interactions with drugs having anticholinergic properties; *e.g.,* other belladonna alkaloids, antihistamines (including meclizine), tricyclic antidepressants, and muscle relaxants.

ADVERSE REACTIONS

The adverse reactions for transdermal scopolamine are provided separately for patients with motion sickness and with post-operative nausea and vomiting.

MOTION SICKNESS

In motion sickness clinical studies of transdermal scopolamine, the most frequent adverse reaction was dryness of the mouth. This occurred in about two-thirds of patients on drug. A less frequent adverse drug reaction was drowsiness, which occurred in less than one-sixth of patients on drug. Transient impairment of eye accommodation, including blurred vision and dilation of the pupils, was also observed.

POST-OPERATIVE NAUSEA AND VOMITING

In a total of five clinical studies in which transdermal scopolamine was administered perioperatively to a total of 461 patients and safety was assessed, dry mouth was the most frequently reported adverse drug experience, which occurred in approximately 29% of patients on drug. Dizziness was reported by approximately 12% of patients on drug.[7]

POSTMARKETING AND OTHER EXPERIENCE

In addition to the adverse experiences reported during clinical testing of transdermal scopolamine, the following are spontaneously reported adverse events from postmarketing experience. Because the reports cite events reported spontaneously from worldwide postmarketing experience, frequency of events and the role of transdermal scopolamine in their causation cannot be reliably determined: acute angle-closure (narrow-angle) glaucoma; confusion; difficulty urinating; dry, itchy, or conjunctival injection of eyes; restlessness; hallucinations; memory disturbances; rashes and erythema; and transient changes in heart rate.

DRUG WITHDRAWAL/POST-REMOVAL SYMPTOMS

Symptoms such as dizziness, nausea, vomiting, and headache occur following abrupt discontinuation of antimuscarinics. Similar symptoms, including disturbances of equilibrium, have been reported in some patients following discontinuation of the use of the transdermal scopolamine system. These symptoms usually do not appear until 24 hours or more after the patch has been removed. Some symptoms may be related to adaptation from a motion environment to a motion-free environment. More serious symptoms including muscle weakness, bradycardia and hypotension may occur following discontinuation of transdermal scopolamine.

DOSAGE AND ADMINISTRATION

INITIATION OF THERAPY

To prevent the nausea and vomiting associated with motion sickness, one transdermal scopolamine patch (programmed to deliver approximately 1.0 mg of scopolamine over 3 days) should be applied to the hairless area behind one ear at least 4 hours before the antiemetic effect is required. To prevent post operative nausea and vomiting, the patch should be applied the evening before scheduled surgery. To minimize exposure of the newborn baby to the drug, apply the patch 1 hour prior to cesarean section. Only one patch should be worn at any time. Do not cut the patch.

HANDLING

After the patch is applied on dry skin behind the ear, the hands should be washed thoroughly with soap and water and dried. Upon removal, the patch should be discarded. To prevent any traces of scopolamine from coming into direct contact with the eyes, the hands and the application site should be washed thoroughly with soap and water and dried. (A patient brochure is available.)

CONTINUATION OF THERAPY

Should the patch become displaced, it should be discarded, and a fresh one placed on the hairless area behind the other ear. For motion sickness, if therapy is required for longer than 3 days, the first patch should be removed and a fresh one placed on the hairless area behind the other ear. For perioperative use, the patch should be kept in place for 24 hours following surgery at which time it should be removed and discarded.

HOW SUPPLIED

The Transderm Scop system is a tan-colored circular patch, 2.5 cm^2, on a clear, oversized, hexagonal peel strip, which is removed prior to use.

Each Transderm Scop system contains 1.5 mg of scopolamine and is programmed to deliver *in vivo* approximately 1.0 mg of scopolamine over 3 days. Transderm Scop is available in packages of 4 patches. Each patch is foil wrapped. Patient instructions are included. **Storage:** The system should be stored at controlled room temperature between 20 and 25°C (68 and 77°F).

PRODUCT LISTING - RATED THERAPEUTICALLY EQUIVALENT

Solution - Injectable - 0.4 mg/ml

1 ml x 25	$49.50	GENERIC, American Pharmaceutical Partners	63323-0268-01

PRODUCT LISTING - EQUIVALENTS NOT AVAILABLE

Film, Extended Release - Transdermal - 1.5 mg			
4's	$18.21	TRANSDERM-SCOP, Physicians Total Care	54868-2803-01
4's	$20.21	TRANSDERM-SCOP, Allscripts Pharmaceutical Company	54569-0367-00
4's	$24.94	TRANSDERM-SCOP, Novartis Pharmaceuticals	00067-4345-04
24's	$149.70	TRANSDERM-SCOP, Novartis Consumer Health	00067-4346-24
Solution - Injectable - 0.4 mg/ml			
1 ml x 25	$44.00	GENERIC, American Pharmaceutical Partners	63323-0268-25
Solution - Injectable - 1 mg/ml			
1 ml x 25	$31.50	GENERIC, Cmc-Consolidated Midland Corporation	00223-8414-25
1 ml x 25	$44.00	GENERIC, American Pharmaceutical Partners	63323-0270-01
Solution - Ophthalmic - 0.25%			
5 ml	$15.56	ISOPTO HYOSCINE, Southwood Pharmaceuticals Inc	58016-6473-01
5 ml	$17.06	ISOPTO HYOSCINE, Allscripts Pharmaceutical Company	54569-2971-00
5 ml	$17.46	ISOPTO HYOSCINE, Physicians Total Care	54868-0658-01
5 ml	$20.13	ISOPTO HYOSCINE, Alcon Laboratories Inc	00998-0331-05
15 ml	$27.69	ISOPTO HYOSCINE, Alcon Laboratories Inc	00998-0331-15
Tablet - Oral - 0.4 mg			
100's	$34.95	GENERIC, Hope Pharmaceuticals	60267-0301-00

Secobarbital Sodium *(002216)*

Categories: Anesthesia, adjunct; Insomnia; Pregnancy Category D; DEA Class CII; FDA Approval Pre 1982
Drug Classes: Barbiturates; Preanesthetics; Sedatives/hypnotics
Brand Names: Immenoctal; Novosecobarb; Seconal; **Seconal Sodium**; Sodium Secobarbital
Cost of Therapy: $3.17 (Insomnia; Seconal; 100 mg; 1 capsule/day; 14 day supply)
HCFA JCODE(S): J2860 up to 250 mg IM, IV

DESCRIPTION

WARNING: MAY BE HABIT-FORMING.

The barbiturates are nonselective central-nervous-system (CNS) depressants that are primarily used as sedative-hypnotics. In subhypnotic doses, they are also used as anticonvulsants. The barbiturates and their sodium salts are subject to control under the Federal Controlled Substances Act.

Secobarbital sodium is a barbituric acid derivative and occurs as a white, odorless, bitter powder that is very soluble in water, soluble in alcohol, and practically insoluble in ether. Chemically, the drug is sodium 5-allyl-5-(1-methylbutyl)barbiturate, with the empirical formula $C_{12}H_{17}N_2NaO_3$. Its molecular weight is 260.27.

Each Seconal Sodium capsule contains 100 mg (0.38 mmol) of secobarbital sodium. These products also contain cornstarch, D&C yellow no. 10, FD&C red no. 3, gelatin, magnesium stearate, silicone, and other inactive ingredients.

CLINICAL PHARMACOLOGY

Barbiturates are capable of producing all levels of CNS mood alteration, from excitation to mild sedation, hypnosis, and deep coma. Overdosage can produce death. In high enough therapeutic doses, barbiturates induce anesthesia. Barbiturates depress the sensory cortex, decrease motor activity, alter cerebellar function, and produce drowsiness, sedation, and hypnosis.

Barbiturate-induced sleep differs from physiologic sleep. Sleep laboratory studies have demonstrated that barbiturates reduce the amount of time spent in the rapid eye movement (REM) phase, or dreaming stage of sleep. Also, Stages III and IV sleep are decreased. Following abrupt cessation of regularly used barbiturates, patients may experience markedly increased dreaming, nightmares, and/or insomnia. Therefore, withdrawal of a single therapeutic dose over 5 or 6 days has been recommended to lessen the REM rebound and disturbed sleep that contribute to drug withdrawal syndrome (for example, decreasing the dose from 3 to 2 doses a day for 1 week).

In studies, secobarbital sodium and pentobarbital sodium have been found to lose most of their effectiveness for both inducing and maintaining sleep by the end of 2 weeks of continued drug administration, even with the use of multiple doses. As with secobarbital sodium and pentobarbital sodium, other barbiturates (including amobarbital) might be expected to lose their effectiveness for inducing and maintaining sleep after about 2 weeks. The short-, intermediate-, and to a lesser degree, long-acting barbiturates have been widely prescribed for treating insomnia. Although the clinical literature abounds with claims that the short-acting barbiturates are superior for producing sleep whereas the intermediate-acting compounds are more effective in maintaining sleep, controlled studies have failed to demonstrate these differential effects. Therefore, as sleep medications, the barbiturates are of limited value beyond short-term use.

Barbiturates have little analgesic action at subanesthetic doses. Rather, in subanesthetic doses, these drugs may increase the reaction to painful stimuli. All barbiturates exhibit anticonvulsant activity in anesthetic doses. However, of the drugs in this class, only phenobarbital, mephobarbital, and metharbital are effective as oral anticonvulsants in subhypnotic doses.

Barbiturates are respiratory depressants, and the degree of depression is dependent on the dose. With hypnotic doses, respiratory depression is similar to that which occurs during physiologic sleep accompanied by a slight decrease in blood pressure and heart rate.

S

Studies in laboratory animals have shown that barbiturates cause reduction in the tone and contractility of the uterus, ureters, and urinary bladder. However, concentrations of the drugs required to produce this effect in humans are not reached with sedative-hypnotic doses.

Barbiturates do not impair normal hepatic function, but have been shown to induce liver microsomal enzymes, thus increasing and/or altering the metabolism of barbiturates and other drugs (see DRUG INTERACTIONS).

Pharmacokinetics: Barbiturates are absorbed in varying degrees following oral or parenteral administration. The salts are more rapidly absorbed than are the acids. The rate of absorption is increased if the sodium salt is ingested as a dilute solution or taken on an empty stomach.

Duration of action, which is related to the rate at which barbiturates are redistributed throughout the body, varies among persons and in the same person from time to time.

Secobarbital sodium is classified as a short-acting barbiturate when taken orally. Its onset of action is 10-15 minutes and its duration of action ranges from 3-4 hours.

Barbiturates are weak acids that are absorbed and rapidly distributed to all tissues and fluids, with high concentrations in the brain, liver, and kidneys. Lipid solubility of the barbiturates is the dominant factor in their distribution within the body. The more lipid soluble the barbiturate, the more rapidly it penetrates all tissues of the body. Barbiturates are bound to plasma and tissue proteins to a varying degree, with the degree of binding increasing directly as a function of lipid solubility.

Phenobarbital has the lowest lipid solubility, lowest plasma binding, lowest brain protein binding, the longest delay in onset of activity, and the longest duration of action. At the opposite extreme is secobarbital, which has the highest lipid solubility, highest plasma protein binding, highest brain protein binding, the shortest delay in onset of activity, and the shortest duration of action. The plasma half-life for secobarbital sodium in adults ranges between 15-40 hours, with a mean of 28 hours. No data are available for pediatric patients and newborns.

Barbiturates are metabolized primarily by the hepatic microsomal enzyme system, and the metabolic products are excreted in the urine and, less commonly, in the feces. The excretion of unmetabolized barbiturate is 1 feature that distinguishes the long-acting category from those belonging to other categories, which are almost entirely metabolized. The inactive metabolites of the barbiturates are excreted as conjugates of glucuronic acid.

INDICATIONS AND USAGE

A. Hypnotic, for the short-term treatment of insomnia, since barbiturates appear to lose their effectiveness for sleep induction and sleep maintenance after 2 weeks (see CLINICAL PHARMACOLOGY).

B. Preanesthetic.

CONTRAINDICATIONS

Secobarbital sodium is contraindicated in patients who are hypersensitive to barbiturates. It is also contraindicated in patients with a history of manifest or latent porphyria, marked impairment of liver function, or respiratory disease in which dyspnea or obstruction is evident.

WARNINGS

HABIT-FORMING

Secobarbital sodium may be habit-forming. Tolerance and psychologic and physical dependence may occur with continued use (see CLINICAL PHARMACOLOGY, Pharmacokinetics). Patients who have psychologic dependence on barbiturates may increase the dosage or decrease the dosage interval without consulting a physician and subsequently may develop a physical dependence on barbiturates. To minimize the possibility of overdosage or development of dependence, the prescribing and dispensing of sedative-hypnotic barbiturates should be limited to the amount required for the interval until the next appointment. The abrupt cessation after prolonged use in a person who is dependent on the drug may result in withdrawal symptoms, including delirium, convulsions, and possibly death. Barbituates should be withdrawn gradually from any patient known to be taking excessive doses over long periods.

ACUTE OR CHRONIC PAIN

Caution should be exercised when barbiturates are administered to patients with acute or chronic pain, because paradoxical excitement could be induced or important symptoms could be masked.

USAGE IN PREGNANCY

Barbiturates can cause fetal harm when administered to a pregnant woman. Retrospective, case-controlled studies have suggested that there may be a connection between the maternal consumption of barbiturates and a higher than expected incidence of fetal abnormalities. Barbituates readily cross the placental barrier and are distributed throughout fetal tissues; the highest concentrations are found in the placenta, liver, and brain. Fetal blood levels aproach maternal blood levels following parenteral administration.

Withdrawal symptoms occur in infants born to women who receive secobarbital sodium throughout the last trimester of pregnancy (see DRUG ABUSE AND DEPENDENCE). If secobarbital sodium is used during pregnancy or if the patient becomes pregnant while taking this drug, the patient should be apprised of the potential hazard to the fetus.

SYNERGISTIC EFFECTS

The concomitant use of alcohol or other CNS depressants may produce additive CNS-depressant effects.

PRECAUTIONS

GENERAL

Barbiturates may be habit-forming. Tolerance and psychologic and physical dependence may occur with continuing use. Barbiturates should be administered with caution, if at all, to patients who are mentally depressed, have suicidal tendencies, or have a history of drug abuse.

Elderly or debilitated patients may react to barbiturates with marked excitement, depression, or confusion. In some persons, especially pediatric patients, barbiturates repeatedly produce excitement rather then depression.

In patients with hepatic damage, barbiturates should be administered with caution and initially in reduced doses. Barbiturates should not be administered to patients showing the premonitory signs of hepatic coma.

INFORMATION FOR PATIENTS

The following information should be given to patients receiving secobarbital sodium:

1. The use of secobarbital sodium carries with it an associated risk of psychologic and/or physical dependence. The patient should be warned against increasing the dose of the drug without consulting a physician.
2. Secobarbital sodium may impair the mental and/or physical abilities required for the performance of potentially hazardous tasks, such as driving a car or operating machinery. The patient should be cautioned accordingly.
3. Alcohol should not be consumed while taking secobarbital sodium. The concurrent use of secobarbital sodium with other CNS depressants (*e.g.,* alcohol, narcotics, tranquilizers, and antihistamines) may result in additional CNS-depressant effects.

LABORATORY TESTS

Prolonged therapy with barbiturates should be accompanied by periodic laboratory evaluation of organic systems, including hematopoietic, renal, and hepatic systems (see PRECAUTIONS, General, and ADVERSE REACTIONS).

CARCINOGENESIS

Animal Data

Phenobarbital sodium is carcinogenic in mice and rats after lifetime administration. In mice, it produced benign and malignant liver cell tumors. In rats, benign liver cell tumors were observed very late in life.

Human Data

In a 29 year epidemiologic study of 9136 patients who were treated on an anticonvulsant protocol that included phenobarbital, results indicated a higher then normal incidence of hepatic carcinoma. Previously, some of these patients had been treated with thorotrast, a drug that is known to produce hepatic carcinomas. Thus, this study did not provide sufficient evidence that phenobarbital sodium is carcinogenic in humans.

A retrospective study of 84 pediatric patients with brain tumors matched to 73 normal controls and 78 cancer controls (malignant disease other than brain tumors) suggested an association between exposure to barbiturates prenatally and an increased incidence of brain tumors.

PREGNANCY CATEGORY D

Teratogenic Effects

See WARNINGS, Use in Pregnancy.

Nonteratogenic Effects

Reports of infants suffering from long-term barbiturate exposure *in utero* included the acute withdrawal syndrome of seizures and hyperirritability from birth to a delayed onset of up to 14 days.

LABOR AND DELIVERY

Hypnotic doses of barbiturates do not appear to impair uterine activity significantly during labor. Full anesthetic doses of barbiturates decrease the force and frequency of uterine contractions. Administration of sedative-hypnotic barbiturates to the mother during labor may result in respiratory depression in the newborn. Premature infants are particularly susceptible to the depressant effects of barbiturates. If barbiturates are used during labor and delivery, resuscitation equipment should be available.

Data are not available to evaluate the effect of barbiturates when forceps delivery or other intervention is necessary or to determine the effect of barbiturates on the later growth, development, and functional maturity of the pediatric patient.

NURSING MOTHERS

Caution should be exercised when secobarbital sodium is administered to a nursing woman, because small amounts of barbiturates are excreted in the milk.

PEDIATRIC USE

See DOSAGE AND ADMINISTRATION

DRUG INTERACTIONS

Most reports of clinically significant drug interactions occurring with the barbiturates have involved phenobarbital. However, the application of these data to other barbiturates appears valid and warrants serial blood level determinations of the relevant drugs when there are multiple therapies.

ANTICOAGULANTS

Phenobarbital lowers the plasma levels of dicumarol and causes a decrease in anticoagulant activity as measured by the prothrombin time. Barbiturates can induce hepatic microsomal enzymes, resulting in increased metabolism and decreased anticoagulant response of oral anticoagulants (*e.g.,* warfarin, acenocoumarol, dicumarol, and phenprocoumon). Patients stabilized on anticoagulant therapy may require dosage adjustments if barbiturates are added to or withdrawn from their dosage regimen.

CORTICOSTEROIDS

Barbiturates appear to enhance the metabolism of exogenous corticosteroids, probably through the induction of hepatic microsomal enzymes. Patients stabilized on corticosteroid therapy may require dosage adjustments if barbiturates are added to or withdrawn from their dosage regimen.

GRISEOFULVIN

Phenobarbital appears to interfere with the absorption of orally administered griseofulvin, thus decreasing its blood level. The effect of the resultant decreased blood levels of griseofulvin on therapeutic response has not been established. However, it would be preferable to avoid concomitant administration of these drugs.

DOXYCYCLINE

Phenobarbital has been shown to shorten the half-life of doxycycline for as long as 2 weeks after barbiturate therapy is discontinued.

This mechanism is probably through the induction of hepatic microsomal enzymes that metabolize the antibiotic. If barbiturates and doxycycline are administered concurrently, the clinical response to doxycycline should be monitored closely.

PHENYTOIN, SODIUM VALPROATE, VALPROIC ACID

The effect of barbiturates on the metabolism of phenytoin appears to be variable. Some investigators report an accelerating effect, whereas others report no effect. Because the effect of barbiturates on the metabolism of phenytoin is not predictable, phenytoin and barbiturate blood levels should be monitored more frequently if these drugs are given concurrently. Sodium valproate and valproic acid increase the secobarbital sodium blood levels; therefore, secobarbital sodium blood levels should be monitored closely and appropriate dosage adjustments made as clinically indicated.

CNS DEPRESSANTS

The concomitant use of other CNS depressants, including other sedatives or hypnotics, antihistamines, tranquilizers, or alcohol, may produce additive depressant effects.

MONOAMINE OXIDASE INHIBITORS (MAOIS)

MAOIs prolong the effects of barbiturates, probably because metabolism of the barbiturate is inhibited.

ESTRADIOL, ESTRONE, PROGESTERONE, AND OTHER STEROIDAL HORMONES

Pretreatment with or concurrent administration of phenobarbital may decrease the effect of estradiol by increasing its metabolism. There have been reports of patients treated with antiepileptic drugs (*e.g.*, phenobarbital) who become pregnant while taking oral contraceptives. An alternate contraceptive method might be suggested to women taking barbiturates.

ADVERSE REACTIONS

The following adverse reactions and their incidences were compiled from surveillance of thousands of hospitalized patients who received barbiturates. Because such patients may be less aware of some of the milder adverse effects of barbiturates, the incidence of these reactions may be somewhat higher in fully ambulatory patients.

MORE THAN 1 IN 100 PATIENTS

The most common adverse reaction estimated to occur at a rate of 1-3 patients per 100 is the following:

Nervous System: Somnolence.

LESS THAN 1 IN 100 PATIENTS

Adverse reactions estimated to occur at a rate of less than 1 in 100 patients are listed below, grouped by organ system and by decreasing order of occurrence:

Nervous System: Agitation, confusion, hyperkinesia, ataxia, CNS depression, nightmares, nervousness, psychiatric disturbance, hallucinations, insomnia, anxiety, dizziness, abnormality in thinking

Respiratory System: Hypoventilation, apnea.

Cardiovascular System: Bradycardia, hypotension, syncope.

Digestive System: Nausea, vomiting, constipation.

Other Reported Reactions: Headache, injection site reactions, hypersensitivity reactions (angioedema, skin rashes, exfoliative dermatitis), fever, liver damage, megaloblastic anemia following chronic phenobarbital use.

DOSAGE AND ADMINISTRATION

Dosage of barbiturates must be individualized with full knowledge of their particular characteristics. Factors of consideration are the patient's age, weight, and condition.

Adults: As a hypnotic, 100 mg at bedtime. Preoperatively, 200-300 mg 1-2 hours before surgery.

Pediatric Patients: Preoperatively, 2-6 mg/kg, with a maximum dosage of 100 mg.

Special Patient Population: Dosage should be reduced in the elderly or debilitated because these patients may be more sensitive to barbiturates. Dosage should be reduced for patients with impaired renal function or hepatic disease.

HOW SUPPLIED

Seconal Sodium is supplied as orange capsules: 100 mg (No. 240)

Store at controlled room temperature, 15-30°C (59-86°F). Dispense in a tight container.

PRODUCT LISTING - RATED THERAPEUTICALLY EQUIVALENT

Capsule - Oral - 100 mg

100's	$22.64	SECONAL SODIUM, Lilly, Eli and Company	00002-0640-02
100's	$27.57	SECONAL SODIUM, Lilly, Eli and Company	00002-0640-33
100's	$83.68	SECONAL SODIUM, Ddn/Obergfel	63304-0679-80

PRODUCT LISTING - EQUIVALENTS NOT AVAILABLE

Capsule - Oral - 100 mg

100's	$79.78	SECONAL SODIUM, Ddn/Obergfel	63304-0679-01

Selegiline Hydrochloride *(002218)*

Categories: Parkinson's disease; Pregnancy Category C; FDA Approved 1989 Jun; Orphan Drugs

Drug Classes: Antiparkinson agents; Dopaminergics

Brand Names: Alzene; Carbex; Deprenyl; **Eldepryl**

Foreign Brand Availability: Apo-Selegiline (New-Zealand); Elegelin (Thailand); Julab (Hong-Kong; Thailand); Julegil (Malaysia); Jumex (Austria; China; Hong-Kong; Hungary; Indonesia; Israel; Italy; Korea; Malaysia; Philippines; Thailand); Jumexal (Costa-Rica; El-Salvador; Guatemala; Honduras; Nicaragua; Panama; Switzerland; Taiwan); Kinline (Thailand); MAO-B (Korea); MAOtil (Germany); Movergan (Germany); Niar (Mexico); Otrasel (France); Plurimen (Spain); Procythol (Greece); Sedicel (Colombia); Sefmex (Hong-Kong); Selegil (Colombia; Peru); Selegos (Hong-Kong; Singapore); Selgene (Australia; New-Zealand; Thailand); Selgin (India); Xilopar (Germany); Zelapar (Philippines)

Cost of Therapy: $162.00 (Parkinsonism; Eldepryl; 5 mg; 2 tablets/day; 30 day supply)
$122.40 (Parkinsonism; Generic Tablets; 5 mg; 2 tablets/day; 30 day supply)

DESCRIPTION

Selegiline hydrochloride is a levorotatory acetylenic derivative of phenethylamine. It is commonly referred to in the clinical and pharmacological literature as L-deprenyl.

The chemical name is: (R)-(-)-N,2-dimethyl-N-2- propynylphenethylamine hydrochloride. It is a white to near white crystalline powder, freely soluble in water, chloroform, and methanol. The molecular formula is $C_{13}H_{17}N\text{·}HCl$and has a molecular weight of 223.75.

Each Eldepryl white, shield shaped, unscored tablet, debossed on one side with "S" and "5" on the other side, contains 5 mg selegiline hydrochloride. Inactive ingredients are citric acid, lactose, magnesium stearate, and microcrystalline cellulose.

Each Carbex tablet for oral administration contains 5 mg selegiline hydrochloride and the following inactive ingredients: corn starch, lactose monohydrate, magnesium stearate, povidone, and talc.

CLINICAL PHARMACOLOGY

The mechanisms accounting for selegiline's beneficial adjunctive action in the treatment of Parkinson's disease are not fully understood. Inhibition of monoamine oxidase, type B, activity is generally considered to be of primary importance; in addition, there is evidence that selegiline may act through other mechanisms to increase dopaminergic activity.

Selegiline is best known as an irreversible inhibitor of monoamine oxidase (MAO), an intracellular enzyme associated with the outer membrane of mitochondria. Selegiline inhibits MAO by acting as a 'suicide' substrate for the enzyme; that is, it is converted by MAO to an active moiety which combines irreversibly with the active site and/or the enzyme's essential FAD cofactor. Because selegiline has greater affinity for type B than for type A active sites, it can serve as a selective inhibitor of MAO type B if it is administered at the recommended dose.

MAOs are widely distributed throughout the body; their concentration is especially high in liver, kidney, stomach, intestinal wall, and brain. MAOs are currently subclassified into two types, A and B, which differ in their substrate specificity and tissue distribution. In humans, intestinal MAO is predominantly type A, while most of that in brain is type B.

In CNS neurons, MAO plays an important role in the catabolism of catecholamines (dopamine, norepinephrine and epinephrine) and serotonin. MAOs are also important in the catabolism of various exogenous amines found in a variety of foods and drugs. MAO in the GI tract and liver (primarily type A), for example, is thought to provide vital protection from exogenous amines (*e.g.*, tyramine) that have the capacity, if absorbed intact, to cause a 'hypertensive crisis,' the so-called 'cheese reaction.' (If large amounts of certain exogenous amines gain access to the systemic circulation [*e.g.*, from fermented cheese, red wine, herring, over-the-counter cough/cold medications, etc.] they are taken up by adrenergic neurons and displace norepinephrine from storage sites within membrane bound vesicles. Subsequent release of the displaced norepinephrine causes the rise in systemic blood pressure, etc.)

In theory, therefore, because MAO A of the gut is not inhibited, patients treated with selegiline at a dose of 10 mg a day can take medications containing pharmacologically active amines and consume tyramine-containing foods without risk of uncontrolled hypertension. However, one case of hypertensive crisis has been reported in a patient taking the recommended dose of selegiline and a sympathomimetic medication (ephedrine). The pathophysiology of the 'cheese reaction' is complicated and, in addition to its ability to inhibit MAO B selectively, selegiline's relative freedom from this reaction has been attributed to an ability to prevent tyramine and other indirect acting sympathomimetrics from displacing norepinephrine from adrenergic neurons.

However, until the pathophysiology of the cheese reaction is more completely understood, it seems prudent to assume that selegiline can only be used safely without dietary restrictions at doses where it presumably selectively inhibits MAO B (*e.g.*, 10 mg/day). **In short, attention to the dose dependent nature of selegiline's selectivity is critical if it is to be used without elaborate restrictions being placed on diet and concomitant drug use although, as noted above, a case of hypertensive crisis has been reported at the recommended dose.** (See WARNINGS and PRECAUTIONS.)

It is important to be aware that selegiline may have pharmacological effects unrelated to MAO B inhibition. As noted above, there is some evidence that it may increase dopaminergic activity by other mechanisms, including interfering with dopamine re-uptake at the synapse. Effects resulting from selegiline administration may also be mediated through its metabolites. Two of its three principal metabolites, amphetamine and methamphetamine, have pharmacological actions of their own; they interfere with neuronal uptake and enhance release of several neurotransmitters (*e.g.*, norepinephrine, dopamine, serotonin). However, the extent to which these metabolites contribute to the effects of selegiline are unknown.

RATIONALE FOR THE USE OF A SELECTIVE MONOAMINE OXIDASE TYPE B INHIBITOR IN PARKINSON'S DISEASE

Many of the prominent symptoms of Parkinson's disease are due to a deficiency of striatal dopamine that is the consequence of a progressive degeneration and loss of a population of dopaminergic neurons which originate in the substantia nigra of the midbrain and project to the basal ganglia or striatum. Early in the course of Parkinson's, the deficit in the capacity of these neurons to synthesize dopamine can be overcome by administration of exogenous

S

levodopa, usually given in combination with a peripheral decarboxylase inhibitor (carbidopa).

With the passage of time, due to the progression of the disease and/or the effect of sustained treatment, the efficacy and quality of the therapeutic response to levodopa diminishes. Thus, after several years of levodopa treatment, the response, for a given dose of levodopa, is shorter, has less predictable onset and offset (*i.e.*, there is "wearing off"), and is often accompanied by side effects (*e.g.*, dyskinesia, akinesias, on-off phenomena, freezing, etc.).

This deteriorating response is currently interpreted as a manifestation of the inability of the ever decreasing population of intact nigrostriatal neurons to synthesize and release adequate amounts of dopamine.

MAO B inhibition may be useful in this setting because, by blocking the catabolism of dopamine, it would increase the net amount of dopamine available (*i.e.*, it would increase the pool of dopamine). Whether or not this mechanism or an alternative one actually accounts for the observed beneficial effects of adjunctive selegiline is unknown.

Selegiline's benefit in Parkinson's disease has only been documented as an adjunct to levodopa/carbidopa. Whether or not it might be effective as a sole treatment is unknown, but past attempts to treat Parkinson's disease with non-selective MAOI monotherapy are reported to have been unsuccessful. It is important to note that attempts to treat Parkinsonian patients with combinations of levodopa and currently marketed non-selective MAO inhibitors were abandoned because of multiple side effects including hypertension, increase in involuntary movement, and toxic delirium.

PHARMACOKINETIC INFORMATION (ABSORPTION, DISTRIBUTION, METABOLISM AND ELIMINATION — ADME)

Only preliminary information about the details of the pharmacokinetics of selegiline and its metabolites is available.

Data obtained in a study of 12 healthy subjects that was intended to examine the effects of selegiline on the ADME of an oral hypoglycemic agent, however, provides some information. Following the oral administration of a single dose of 10 mg of selegiline hydrochloride to these subjects, serum levels of intact selegiline were below the limit of detection (less than 10 ng/ml). Three metabolites, N-desmethyldeprenyl, the major metabolite (mean half-life 2.0 hours), amphetamine (mean half- life 17.7 hours), and methamphetamine (mean half-life 20.5 hours), were found in serum and urine. Over a period of 48 hours, 45% of the dose administered appeared in the urine as these 3 metabolites.

In an extension of this study intended to examine the effects of steady state conditions, the same subjects were given a 10 mg dose of selegiline hydrochloride for 7 consecutive days. Under these conditions, the mean trough serum levels for amphetamine were 3.5 ng/ml and 8.0 ng/ml for methamphetamine; trough levels of N-desmethyldeprenyl were below the levels of detection.

The rate of MAO B regeneration following discontinuation of treatment has not been quantitated. It is this rate, dependent upon *de novo* protein synthesis, which seems likely to determine how fast normal MAO B activity can be restored.

INDICATIONS AND USAGE

Selegiline hydrochloride is indicated as an adjunct in the management of Parkinsonian patients being treated with levodopa/carbidopa who exhibit deterioration in the quality of their response to this therapy. There is no evidence from controlled clinical studies that selegiline has any beneficial effect in the absence of concurrent levodopa therapy.

Evidence supporting this claim was obtained in randomized controlled clinical investigations that compared the effects of added selegiline or placebo in patients receiving levodopa/carbidopa. Selegiline was significantly superior to placebo on all three principal outcome measures employed; change from baseline in daily levodopa/carbidopa dose, the amount of 'off' time, and patient self-rating of treatment success. Beneficial effects were also observed on other measures of treatment success (*e.g.*, measures of reduced end of dose akinesia, decreased tremor and sialorrhea, improved speech and dressing ability and improved overall disability as assessed by walking and comparison to previous state).

NON-FDA APPROVED INDICATIONS

Selegiline has shown efficacy as initial therapy and monotherapy in the treatment of Parkinson's Disease, in the treatment of dementia of the Alzheimer type, and in the treatment of narcolepsy. However, these uses are not approved by the FDA and further clinical studies are needed.

S

CONTRAINDICATIONS

Selegiline hydrochloride is contraindicated in patients with a known hypersensitivity to this drug.

Selegiline hydrochloride is contraindicated for use with meperidine. This contraindication is often extended to other opioids. (See DRUG INTERACTIONS.)

WARNINGS

Selegiline should not be used at daily doses exceeding those recommended (10 mg/day) because of the risks associated with non-selective inhibition of MAO. (See CLINICAL PHARMACOLOGY.)

The selectivity of selegiline for MAO B may not be absolute even at the recommended daily dose of 10 mg a day and selectivity is further diminished with increasing daily doses. The precise dose at which selegiline becomes a non-selective inhibitor of all MAO is unknown, but may be in the range of 30-40 mg a day.

Severe CNS toxicity associated with hyperpyrexia and death have been reported with the combination of tricyclic antidepressants and non-selective MAOIs (phenelzine, tranylcypromine). A similar reaction has been reported for a patient on amitriptyline and selegiline. Another patient receiving protriptyline and selegiline developed tremors, agitation, and restlessness followed by unresponsiveness and death 2 weeks after selegiline was added. Related adverse events including hypertension, syncope, asystole, diaphoresis, seizures, changes in behavioral and mental status, and muscular rigidity have also been reported in some patients receiving selegiline and various tricyclic antidepressants.

Serious, sometimes fatal, reactions with signs and symptoms that may include hyperthermia, rigidity, myoclonus, autonomic instability with rapid fluctuations of the vital signs, and mental status changes that include extreme agitation progressing to delirium and coma have been reported with patients receiving a combination of fluoxetine hydrochloride and non-selective MAOIs. Similar signs have been reported in some patients on the combination of selegiline (10 mg a day) and selective serotonin reuptake inhibitors including fluoxetine, sertraline, and paroxetine.

Since the mechanisms of these reactions are not fully understood, it seems prudent, in general, to avoid the combination of selegiline and tricyclic antidepressants as well as selegiline and selective serotonin reuptake inhibitors. At least 14 days should elapse between discontinuation of selegiline and initiation of treatment with a tricyclic antidepressant or selective serotonin reuptake inhibitors. Because of the long half lives of fluoxetine and its active metabolite, at least 5 weeks (perhaps longer, especially if fluoxetine has been prescribed chronically and/or at higher doses) should elapse between discontinuation of fluoxetine and initiation of treatment with selegiline.

PRECAUTIONS

GENERAL

Some patients given selegiline may experience an exacerbation of levodopa associated side effects, presumably due to the increased amounts of dopamine reacting with super-sensitive post-synaptic receptors. These effects may often be mitigated by reducing the dose of levodopa/carbidopa by approximately 10-30%.

The decision to prescribe selegiline should take into consideration that the MAO system of enzymes is complex and incompletely understood and there is only a limited amount of carefully documented clinical experience with selegiline. Consequently, the full spectrum of possible responses to selegiline may not have been observed in pre-marketing evaluation of the drug. It is advisable, therefore, to observe patients closely for atypical responses.

INFORMATION FOR THE PATIENT

Patients should be advised of the possible need to reduce levodopa dosage after the initiation of selegiline hydrochloride therapy.

Patients (or their families if the patient is incompetent) should be advised not to exceed the daily recommended dose of 10 mg. The risk of using higher daily doses of selegiline should be explained, and a brief description of the 'cheese reaction' provided. While hypertensive reactions with selegiline associated with dietary influences have not been reported, documented experience is limited.

Consequently, it may be useful to inform patients (or their families) about the signs and symptoms associated with MAOI induced hypertensive reactions. In particular, patients should be urged to report, immediately, any severe headache or other atypical or unusual symptoms not previously experienced.

LABORATORY TESTS

No specific laboratory tests are deemed essential for the management of patients on selegiline hydrochloride. Periodic routine evaluation of all patients, however, is appropriate.

CARCINOGENESIS, MUTAGENESIS, AND IMPAIRMENT OF FERTILITY

Assessement of the carcinogenic potential of selegiline in mice and rats is ongoing.

Selegiline did not induce mutations or chromosomal damage when tested in the bacterial mutation assay in *Salmonella typhimurium* and an *in vivo* chromosomal aberration assay. While these studies provide some resurrance that selegiline is not mutagenic or clastogenic, they are not definitive because of methodological limitations. No definitive *in vitro* chromosomal aberration or *in vitro* mammalian gene mutation assays have been performed.

The effect of selegiline on fertility has not been adequately assessed.

PREGNANCY, TERATOGENIC EFFECTS, PREGNANCY CATEGORY C

No teratogenic effects were observed in a study of embryo-fetal development in Sprague-Dawley rats at oral doses of 4, 12, and 36 mg/kg or 4, 12, and 35 times the human therapeutic dose on a mg/m^2 basis. No teratogenic effects were observed in a study of embryo-fetal development in New Zealand White rabbits at oral doses of 5, 25, and 50 mg/kg or 10, 48, and 95 times the human therapeutic dose on a mg/m^2 basis; however, in this study, the number of litters produced at the 2 higher doses was less than recommended for assessing teratogenic potential. In the rat study, increases in total resorptions and percent post-implantation loss, and a decrease in the number of live fetuses per dam occurred at the highest dose tested. In a peri- postnatal development study in Sprague-Dawley rats oral doses of 4, 16, and 64 mg/kg or 4, 15, and 62 times the human therapeutic dose on a mg/m^2 basis, an increase in the numbers if stillbirths and decrease in the number of pups per dam, pup survival, and pup body weight (at birth and throughout the lactation period) were observed at the 2 highest doses. At the highest dose tested, no pups born alive survived to Day 4 postpartum. Postnatal development at the highest dose tested in dams could not be evaluated because of the lack of surviving pups. The reproductive performance of the untreated offspring was not assessed.

There are no adequate and well-controlled studies in pregnant women. Selegiline should be used during pregnancy only if the potential benefit justifies the potential risk to the fetus.

NURSING MOTHERS

It is not known whether selegiline hydrochloride is excreted in human milk. Because many drugs are excreted in human milk, consideration should be given to discontinuing the use of all but absolutely essential drug treatments in nursing women.

PEDIATRIC USE

The effects of selegiline hydrochloride in pediatric patients have not been evaluated.

DRUG INTERACTIONS

The occurrence of stupor, muscular rigidity, severe agitation, and elevated temperature has been reported in some patients receiving the combination of selegiline and meperidine. Symptoms usually resolve over days when the combination is discontinued. This is typical of the interaction of meperidine and MAOIs. Other serious reactions (including severe agitation, hallucinations, and death) have been reported in patients receiving this combination (see CONTRAINDICATIONS). Severe toxicity has also been reported in patients receiving the combination of tricyclic antidepressants and selegiline hydrochloride and selective serotonin reuptake inhibitors and selegiline hydrochloride. (See WARNINGS for details.)

ADVERSE REACTIONS

INTRODUCTION

The number of patients who received selegiline in prospectively monitored pre-marketing studies is limited. While other sources of information about the use of selegiline are available (*e.g.*, literature reports, foreign post-marketing reports, etc.) they do not provide the kind of information necessary to estimate the incidence of adverse events. Thus, overall incidence figures for adverse reactions associated with the use of selegiline cannot be provided. Many of the adverse reactions seen have also been reported as symptoms of dopamine excess.

Moreover, the importance and severity of various reactions reported often cannot be ascertained. One index of relative importance, however, is whether or not a reaction caused treatment discontinuation. In prospective pre-marketing studies, the following events led, in decreasing order of frequency, to discontinuation of treatment with selegiline: nausea, hallucinations, confusion, depression, loss of balance, insomnia, orthostatic hypotension, increased akinetic involuntary movements, agitation, arrhythmia, bradykinesia, chorea, delusions, hypertension, new or increased angina pectoris, and syncope. Events reported only once as a cause of discontinuation are ankle edema, anxiety, burning lips/mouth, constipation, drowsiness/lethargy, dystonia, excess perspiration, increased freezing, gastrointestinal bleeding, hair loss, increased tremor, nervousness, weakness, and weight loss.

Experience with selegiline hydrochloride obtained in parallel, placebo controlled, randomized studies provides only a limited basis for estimates of adverse reaction rates. The following reactions that occurred with greater frequency among the 49 patients assigned to selegiline as compared to the 50 patients assigned to placebo in the only parallel, placebo controlled trial performed in patients with Parkinson's disease are shown in TABLE 1. None of these adverse reactions led to a discontinuation of treatment.

TABLE 1 *Incidence Of Treatment-Emergent Adverse Experiences In The Placebo-Controlled Clinical Trial*

	Number of Patients Reporting Events	
	Selegiline HCl	Placebo
Adverse Event	n=49	n=50
Nausea	10	3
Dizziness/lightheaded/fainting	7	1
Abdominal pain	4	2
Confusion	3	0
Hallucinations	3	1
Dry mouth	3	1
Vivid dreams	2	0
Dyskinesias	2	5
Headache	2	1
The following events were reported once in either or both groups:		
Ache, generalized	1	0
Anxiety/tension	1	1
Anemia	0	1
Diarrhea	1	0
Hair loss	0	1
Insomnia	1	1
Lethargy	1	0
Leg pain	1	0
Low back pain	1	0
Malaise	0	1
Palpitations	1	0
Urinary retention	1	0
Weight loss	1	0

In all prospectively monitored investigations, enrolling approximately 920 patients, the following adverse events, classified by body system, were reported.

Central Nervous System: *Motor/Coordination/Extrapyramidal:* increased tremor, chorea, loss of balance, restlessness, blepharospasm, increased bradykinesia, facial grimace, falling down, heavy leg, muscle twitch,* myoclonic jerks,* stiff neck, tardive dyskinesia, dystonic symptoms, dyskinesia, involuntary movements, freezing, festination, increased apraxia, muscle cramps. *Mental Status/Behavioral/Psychiatric:* hallucinations, dizziness, confusion, anxiety, depression, drowsiness, behavior/mood change, dreams/nightmares, tiredness, delusions, disorientation, lightheadedness, impaired memory,* increased energy,* transient high,* hollow feeling, lethargy/malaise, apathy, overstimulation, vertigo, personality change, sleep disturbance, restlessness, weakness, transient irritability. *Pain/Altered Sensation:* headache, back pain, leg pain, tinnitus, migraine, supraorbital pain, throat burning, generalized ache, chills, numbness of toes/fingers, taste disturbance.

Autonomic Nervous System: Dry mouth, blurred vision, sexual dysfunction.

Cardiovascular: Orthostatic hypotension, hypertension, arrhythmia, palpitations, new or increased angina pectoris, hypotension, tachycardia, peripheral edema, sinus bradycardia, syncope.

Gastrointestinal: Nausea/vomiting, constipation, weight loss, anorexia, poor appetite, dysphagia, diarrhea, heartburn, rectal bleeding, bruxism,* gastrointestinal bleeding (exacerbation of preexisting ulcer disease).

Genitourinary/Gynecologic/Endocrine: Slow urination, transient anorgasmia,* nocturia, prostatic hypertrophy, urinary hesitancy, urinary retention, decreased penile sensation,* urinary frequency.

Skin and Appendages: Increased sweating, diaphoresis, facial hair, hair loss, hematoma, rash, photosensitivity.

Miscellaneous: Asthma, diplopia, shortness of breath, speech affected.

*Indicates events reported only at doses greater than 10 mg/day.

POSTMARKETING REPORTS

The following experiences were described in spontaneous post-marketing reports. These reports do not provide sufficient information to establish a clear causal relationship with the use of selegiline hydrochloride.

CNS: Seizure in dialyzed chronic renal failure patient on concomitant medications.

DOSAGE AND ADMINISTRATION

Selegiline hydrochloride is intended for administration to Parkinsonian patients receiving levodopa/carbidopa therapy who demonstrate a deteriorating response to this treatment. The recommended regimen for the administration of selegiline hydrochloride is 10 mg per day administered as divided doses of 5 mg each taken at breakfast and lunch. There is no evidence that additional benefit will be obtained from the administration of higher doses. Moreover, higher doses should ordinarily be avoided because of the increased risk of side effects.

After 2-3 days of selegiline treatment, an attempt may be made to reduce the dose of levodopa/carbidopa. A reduction of 10-30% was achieved with the typical participant in the domestic placebo controlled trials who was assigned to selegiline treatment. Further reductions of levodopa/carbidopa may be possible during continued selegiline therapy.

HOW SUPPLIED

Eldepryl tablets are available containing 5 mg of selegiline hydrochloride. Each white, shield shaped, unscored tablet is debossed with "S" on one side and "5" on the other side.

Carbex 5 mg tablets are white, oval tablets; debossed with E620 on one side and plain on the other.

Storage: Store at controlled room temperature, 15-30°C (59-86°F).

PRODUCT LISTING - RATED THERAPEUTICALLY EQUIVALENT

Capsule - Oral - 5 mg			
30's	$93.15	GENERIC, Udl Laboratories Inc	51079-0887-03
60's	$138.10	GENERIC, Apotex Usa Inc	60505-0055-01
Tablet - Oral - 5 mg			
31 x 10	$681.96	GENERIC, Vangard Labs	00615-4516-53
31 x 10	$681.96	GENERIC, Vangard Labs	00615-4516-63
60's	$45.95	FEDERAL UPPER LIMIT, H.C.F.A. F F P	99999-2218-01
60's	$109.90	ATAPRYL, Athena Neurosciences Inc	59075-0660-60
60's	$114.40	GENERIC, Dupont Pharmaceuticals	00056-0408-60
60's	$122.45	GENERIC, Stason Pharmaceuticals Inc	60763-0102-03
60's	$122.45	GENERIC, Boscogen Inc	62033-0102-03
60's	$126.10	GENERIC, Major Pharmaceuticals Inc	00904-5266-52
60's	$126.10	GENERIC, Apotex Usa Inc	60505-3438-03
60's	$126.10	GENERIC, Apotex Usa Inc	60505-3438-04
60's	$138.24	GENERIC, Par Pharmaceutical Inc	49884-0610-02
60's	$138.24	GENERIC, Watson Laboratories Inc	52544-0136-60
60's	$138.24	GENERIC, Watson/Rugby Laboratories Inc	52544-0137-60
60's	$138.24	GENERIC, Esi Lederle Generics	59911-5886-01
60's	$145.80	GENERIC, Endo Laboratories Llc	60951-0620-60
100's	$208.82	GENERIC, Vangard Labs	00615-4516-29

PRODUCT LISTING - EQUIVALENTS NOT AVAILABLE

Capsule - Oral - 5 mg			
60's	$162.00	ELDEPRYL, Somerset Pharmaceuticals Inc	39506-0022-60
Tablet - Oral - 5 mg			
60's	$122.40	GENERIC, Bristol-Myers Squibb	59772-0908-10

Sertraline Hydrochloride *(003087)*

For related information, see the comparative table section in Appendix A.

Categories: Depression; Obsessive compulsive disorder; Panic disorder; Posttraumatic stress disorder; Premenstrual dysphoric disorder; Pregnancy Category C; FDA Approved 1991 Dec

Drug Classes: Antidepressants, serotonin specific reuptake inhibitors

Brand Names: Lustral; **Zoloft**

Foreign Brand Availability: Altruline (Mexico); Aremis (Spain); Atruline (Costa-Rica; El-Salvador; Guatemala; Honduras; Nicaragua; Panama); Besitran (Spain); Dominum (Colombia; Peru); Fatral (Indonesia); Gladem (Austria; Germany); Lesefer (Colombia); Nudep (Indonesia); Serlain (Belgium); Sertranex (Bahrain; Colombia; Cyprus; Egypt; Iran; Iraq; Israel; Jordan; Kuwait; Lebanon; Libya; Oman; Qatar; Republic-of-Yemen; Saudi-Arabia; Syria; United-Arab-Emirates); Sertranquil (Colombia); Sosser (Colombia); Zolof (Colombia); Zosert (India)

Cost of Therapy: $69.15 (Depression; Zoloft; 50 mg; 1 tablet/day; 30 day supply)

DESCRIPTION

Note: The trade name has been used throughout this monograph for clarity.

Zoloft (sertraline hydrochloride) is a selective serotonin reuptake inhibitor (SSRI) for oral administration. It has a molecular weight of 342.7. Sertraline hydrochloride has the following chemical name: (1S-cis)-4-(3,4-dichlorophenyl)-1,2,3,4-tetrahydro-N-methyl-1-naphthalenamine hydrochloride. The empirical formula is $C_{17}H_{17}NCl_2 \cdot HCl$.

Sertraline hydrochloride is a white crystalline powder that is slightly soluble in water and isopropyl alcohol, and sparingly soluble in ethanol.

ZOLOFT TABLETS

Zoloft is supplied for oral administration as scored tablets containing sertraline hydrochloride equivalent to 25, 50 and 100 mg of sertraline and the following inactive ingredients: dibasic calcium phosphate dihydrate, D&C yellow no. 10 aluminum lake (in 25 mg tablet), FD&C blue no. 1 aluminum lake (in 25 mg tablet), FD&C red no. 40 aluminum lake (in 25 mg tablet), FD&C blue no. 2 aluminum lake (in 50 mg tablet), hydroxypropyl cellulose, hydroxypropyl methylcellulose, magnesium stearate, microcrystalline cellulose, polyethylene glycol, polysorbate 80, sodium starch glycolate, synthetic yellow iron oxide (in 100 mg tablet), and titanium dioxide.

ZOLOFT ORAL CONCENTRATE

Zoloft oral concentrate is available in a multidose 60 ml bottle. Each ml of solution contains sertraline hydrochloride equivalent to 20 mg of sertraline. The solution contains the following inactive ingredients: glycerin, alcohol (12%), menthol, butylated hydroxytoluene (BHT). The oral concentrate must be diluted prior to administration (see PRECAUTIONS, Information for the Patient and DOSAGE AND ADMINISTRATION).

CLINICAL PHARMACOLOGY

PHARMACODYNAMICS

The mechanism of action of sertraline is presumed to be linked to its inhibition of CNS neuronal uptake of serotonin (5HT). Studies at clinically relevant doses in man have demonstrated that sertraline blocks the uptake of serotonin into human platelets. *In vitro* studies in animals also suggest that sertraline is a potent and selective inhibitor of neuronal serotonin reuptake and has only very weak effects on norepinephrine and dopamine neuronal reuptake. *In vitro* studies have shown that sertraline has no significant affinity for adrenergic ($alpha_1$, $alpha_2$, beta), cholinergic, GABA, dopaminergic, histaminergic, serotonergic ($5HT_{1A}$, $5HT_{1B}$, $5HT_2$), or benzodiazepine receptors; antagonism of such receptors has been hypothesized to be associated with various anticholinergic, sedative, and cardiovascular effects for other psychotropic drugs. The chronic administration of sertraline was found in animals to downregulate brain norepinephrine receptors, as has been observed with other drugs effective in the treatment of major depressive disorder. Sertraline does not inhibit monoamine oxidase.

PHARMACOKINETICS

Systemic Bioavailability

In man, following oral once-daily dosing over the range of 50-200 mg for 14 days, mean peak plasma concentrations (C_{max}) of sertraline occurred between 4.5-8.4 hours post-dosing. The average terminal elimination half-life of plasma sertraline is about 26 hours. Based on this pharmacokinetic parameter, steady-state sertraline plasma levels should be achieved after approximately 1 week of once-daily dosing. Linear dose-proportional pharmacokinetics were demonstrated in a single dose study in which the C_{max} and area under the plasma concentration time curve (AUC) of sertraline were proportional to dose over a range of 50-200 mg. Consistent with the terminal elimination half-life, there is an approximately 2-fold accumulation, compared to a single dose, of sertraline with repeated dosing over a 50-200 mg dose range. The single dose bioavailability of sertraline tablets is approximately equal to an equivalent dose of solution.

In a relative bioavailability study comparing the pharmacokinetics of 100 mg sertraline as the oral solution to a 100 mg sertraline tablet in 16 healthy adults, the solution to tablet ratio of geometric mean AUC and C_{max} values were 114.8% and 120.6%, respectively. 90% confidence intervals (CI) were within the range of 80-125% with the exception of the upper 90% CI limit for C_{max} which was 126.5%.

The effects of food on the bioavailability of the sertraline tablet and oral concentrate were studied in subjects administered a single dose with and without food. For the tablet, AUC was slightly increased when drug was administered with food but the C_{max} was 25% greater, while the time to reach peak plasma concentration (T_{max}) decreased from 8 hours post-dosing to 5.5 hours. For the oral concentrate, T_{max} was slightly prolonged from 5.9 hours to 7.0 hours with food.

Metabolism

Sertraline undergoes extensive first pass metabolism. The principal initial pathway of metabolism for sertraline is N-demethylation. N-desmethylsertraline has a plasma terminal elimination half-life of 62-104 hours. Both *in vitro* biochemical and *in vivo* pharmacological testing have shown N-desmethylsertraline to be substantially less active than sertraline. Both sertraline and N-desmethylsertraline undergo oxidative deamination and subsequent reduction, hydroxylation, and glucuronide conjugation. In a study of radiolabeled sertraline involving 2 healthy male subjects, sertraline accounted for less than 5% of the plasma radioactivity. About 40-45% of the administered radioactivity was recovered in urine in 9 days. Unchanged sertraline was not detectable in the urine. For the same period, about 40-45% of the administered radioactivity was accounted for in feces, including 12-14% unchanged sertraline.

Desmethylsertraline exhibits time-related, dose dependent increases in AUC(0-24h), C_{max} and C_{min}, with about a 5- to 9-fold increase in these pharmacokinetic parameters between Day 1 and Day 14.

Protein Binding

In vitro protein binding studies performed with radiolabeled ^3H-sertraline showed that sertraline is highly bound to serum proteins (98%) in the range of 20-500 ng/ml. However, at up to 300 and 200 ng/ml concentrations, respectively, sertraline and N-desmethylsertraline did not alter the plasma protein binding of two other highly protein bound drugs, viz., warfarin and propranolol (see PRECAUTIONS).

Pediatric Pharmacokinetics

Sertraline pharmacokinetics were evaluated in a group of 61 pediatric patients (29 aged 6-12 years, 32 aged 13-17 years) with a DSM-III-R diagnosis of major depressive disorder or obsessive-compulsive disorder. Patients included both males (n=28) and females (n=33). During 42 days of chronic sertraline dosing, sertraline was titrated up to 200 mg/day and maintained at that dose for a minimum of 11 days. On the final day of sertraline 200 mg/day, the 6- to 12-year-old group exhibited a mean sertraline AUC(0-24h) of 3107 ng-h/ml, mean C_{max} of 165 ng/ml, and mean half-life of 26.2 hours. The 13- to 17-year-old group exhibited a mean sertraline AUC(0-24h) of 2296 ng·h/ml, mean C_{max} of 123 ng/ml, and mean half-life of 27.8 hours. Higher plasma levels in the 6- to 12-year-old group were largely attributable to patients with lower body weights. No gender associated differences were observed. By comparison, a group of 22 separately studied adults between 18 and 45 years of age (11 male, 11 female) received 30 days of 200 mg/day sertraline and exhibited a mean sertraline AUC(0-24h) of 2570 ng·h/ml, mean C_{max} of 142 ng/ml, and mean half-life of 27.2 hours. Relative to the adults, both the 6- to 12-year-olds and the 13- to 17-year-olds showed about 22% lower AUC(0-24h) and C_{max} values when plasma concentration was adjusted for weight. These data suggest that pediatric patients metabolize sertraline with slightly greater efficiency than adults. Nevertheless, lower doses may be advisable for pediatric patients given their lower body weights, especially in very young patients, in order to avoid excessive plasma levels (see DOSAGE AND ADMINISTRATION).

Age

Sertraline plasma clearance in a group of 16 (8 male, 8 female) elderly patients treated for 14 days at a dose of 100 mg/day was approximately 40% lower than in a similarly studied group of younger (25-32 years old) individuals. Steady-state, therefore, should be achieved after 2-3 weeks in older patients. The same study showed a decreased clearance of desmethylsertraline in older males, but not in older females.

Liver Disease

As might be predicted from its primary site of metabolism, liver impairment can affect the elimination of sertraline. In patients with chronic mild liver impairment (n=10, 8 patients with Child-Pugh scores of 5-6 and 2 patients with Child-Pugh scores of 7-8) who received 50 mg sertraline per day maintained for 21 days, sertraline clearance was reduced, resulting in approximately 3-fold greater exposure compared to age-matched volunteers with no hepatic impairment (n=10). The exposure to desmethylsertraline was approximately 2-fold greater compared to age-matched volunteers with no hepatic impairment. There were no significant differences in plasma protein binding observed between the two groups. The effects of sertraline in patients with moderate and severe hepatic impairment have not been studied. The results suggest that the use of sertraline in patients with liver disease must be approached with caution. If sertraline is administered to patients with liver impairment, a lower or less frequent dose should be used (see PRECAUTIONS and DOSAGE AND ADMINISTRATION).

Renal Disease

Sertraline is extensively metabolized and excretion of unchanged drug in urine is a minor route of elimination. In volunteers with mild to moderate (CLCR = 30-60 ml/min), moderate to severe (CLCR = 10-29 ml/min) or severe (receiving hemodialysis) renal impairment (n=10 each group), the pharmacokinetics and protein binding of 200 mg sertraline per day maintained for 21 days were not altered compared to age-matched volunteers (n=12) with no renal impairment. Thus sertraline multiple dose pharmacokinetics appear to be unaffected by renal impairment (see PRECAUTIONS).

INDICATIONS AND USAGE

MAJOR DEPRESSIVE DISORDER

Zoloft is indicated for the treatment of major depressive disorder.

The efficacy of Zoloft in the treatment of a major depressive episode was established in 6-8 week controlled trials of outpatients whose diagnoses corresponded most closely to the DSM-III category of major depressive disorder.

A major depressive episode implies a prominent and relatively persistent depressed or dysphoric mood that usually interferes with daily functioning (nearly every day for at least 2 weeks); it should include at least 4 of the following 8 symptoms: change in appetite, change in sleep, psychomotor agitation or retardation, loss of interest in usual activities or decrease in sexual drive, increased fatigue, feelings of guilt or worthlessness, slowed thinking or impaired concentration, and a suicide attempt or suicidal ideation.

The antidepressant action of Zoloft in hospitalized depressed patients has not been adequately studied.

The efficacy of Zoloft in maintaining an antidepressant response for up to 44 weeks following 8 weeks of open-label acute treatment (52 weeks total) was demonstrated in a placebo-controlled trial. The usefulness of the drug in patients receiving Zoloft for extended periods should be reevaluated periodically.

OBSESSIVE-COMPULSIVE DISORDER

Zoloft is indicated for the treatment of obsessions and compulsions in patients with obsessive-compulsive disorder (OCD), as defined in the DSM-III-R; *i.e.*, the obsessions or compulsions cause marked distress, are time-consuming, or significantly interfere with social or occupational functioning.

The efficacy of Zoloft was established in 12 week trials with obsessive-compulsive outpatients having diagnoses of obsessive-compulsive disorder as defined according to DSM-III or DSM-III-R criteria.

Obsessive-compulsive disorder is characterized by recurrent and persistent ideas, thoughts, impulses, or images (obsessions) that are ego-dystonic and/or repetitive, purposeful, and intentional behaviors (compulsions) that are recognized by the person as excessive or unreasonable.

The efficacy of Zoloft in maintaining a response, in patients with OCD who responded during a 52 week treatment phase while taking Zoloft and were then observed for relapse during a period of up to 28 weeks, was demonstrated in a placebo-controlled trial. Nevertheless, the physician who elects to use Zoloft for extended periods should periodically re-evaluate the long-term usefulness of the drug for the individual patient (see DOSAGE AND ADMINISTRATION).

PANIC DISORDER

Zoloft is indicated for the treatment of panic disorder, with or without agoraphobia, as defined in DSM-IV. Panic disorder is characterized by the occurrence of unexpected panic attacks and associated concern about having additional attacks, worry about the implications or consequences of the attacks, and/or a significant change in behavior related to the attacks.

The efficacy of Zoloft was established in three 10-12 week trials in panic disorder patients whose diagnoses corresponded to the DSM-III-R category of panic disorder.

Panic disorder (DSM-IV) is characterized by recurrent unexpected panic attacks, *i.e.*, a discrete period of intense fear or discomfort in which four (or more) of the following symptoms develop abruptly and reach a peak within 10 minutes: (1) palpitations, pounding heart, or accelerated heart rate; (2) sweating; (3) trembling or shaking; (4) sensations of shortness of breath or smothering; (5) feeling of choking; (6) chest pain or discomfort; (7) nausea or abdominal distress; (8) feeling dizzy, unsteady, lightheaded, or faint; (9) derealization (feelings of unreality) or depersonalization (being detached from oneself); (10) fear of losing control; (11) fear of dying; (12) paresthesias (numbness or tingling sensations); (13) chills or hot flushes.

The efficacy of Zoloft in maintaining a response, in patients with panic disorder who responded during a 52 week treatment phase while taking Zoloft and were then observed for relapse during a period of up to 28 weeks, was demonstrated in a placebo-controlled trial. Nevertheless, the physician who elects to use Zoloft for extended periods should periodically re-evaluate the long-term usefulness of the drug for the individual patient (see DOSAGE AND ADMINISTRATION).

POSTTRAUMATIC STRESS DISORDER (PTSD)

Zoloft is indicated for the treatment of posttraumatic stress disorder.

The efficacy of Zoloft in the treatment of PTSD was established in two 12 week placebo-controlled trials of outpatients whose diagnosis met criteria for the DSM-III-R category of PTSD.

PTSD, as defined by DSM-III-R/IV, requires exposure to a traumatic event that involved actual or threatened death or serious injury, or threat to the physical integrity of self or others, and a response which involves intense fear, helplessness, or horror. Symptoms that occur as a result of exposure to the traumatic event include reexperiencing of the event in the form of intrusive thoughts, flashbacks or dreams, and intense psychological distress and physiological reactivity on exposure to cues to the event; avoidance of situations reminiscent of the traumatic event, inability to recall details of the event, and/or numbing of general responsiveness manifested as diminished interest in significant activities, estrangement from others, restricted range of affect, or sense of foreshortened future; and symptoms of autonomic arousal including hypervigilance, exaggerated startle response, sleep disturbance, impaired concentration, and irritability or outbursts of anger. A PTSD diagnosis requires that the symptoms are present for at least a month and that they cause clinically significant distress or impairment in social, occupational, or other important areas of functioning.

The efficacy of Zoloft in maintaining a response in patients with PTSD for up to 28 weeks following 24 weeks of open-label treatment was demonstrated in a placebo-controlled trial. Nevertheless, the physician who elects to use Zoloft for extended periods should periodically re-evaluate the long-term usefulness of the drug for the individual patient (see DOSAGE AND ADMINISTRATION).

PREMENSTRUAL DYSPHORIC DISORDER (PMDD)

Zoloft is indicated for the treatment of premenstrual dysphoric disorder (PMDD).

The efficacy of Zoloft in the treatment of PMDD was established in two placebo-controlled trials of female outpatients treated for 3 menstrual cycles who met criteria for the DSM-III-R/IV category of PMDD.

The essential features of PMDD include markedly depressed mood, anxiety or tension, affective lability, and persistent anger or irritability. Other features include decreased interest in activities, difficulty concentrating, lack of energy, change in appetite or sleep, and feeling out of control. Physical symptoms associated with PMDD include breast tenderness, headache, joint and muscle pain, bloating, and weight gain. These symptoms occur regularly during the luteal phase and remit within a few days following onset of menses; the disturbance markedly interferes with work or school or with usual social activities and relationship with others. In making the diagnosis, care should be taken to rule out other cyclical mood disorders that may be exacerbated by treatment with an antidepressant.

The effectiveness of Zoloft in long-term use, that is, for more than 3 menstrual cycles, has not been systematically evaluated in controlled trials. Therefore, the physician who elects to use Zoloft for extended periods should periodically re-evaluate the long-term usefulness of the drug for the individual patient (see DOSAGE AND ADMINISTRATION).

NON-FDA APPROVED INDICATIONS

Sertraline and other SSRIs may also have clinical utility in a number of other disorders including eating disorders, substance abuse, headaches, and social phobia, although none of these uses is approved by the FDA for sertraline. One study (n=310) concluded that sertraline is effective in the treatment of dysthymia without concurrent major depression. Another study (n=30) concluded that the use of sertraline in patients with unexplained chest pain of noncardiac origin produced clinically significant reduction of daily pain. However, these uses also have not been approved by the FDA and further clinical trials are needed.

CONTRAINDICATIONS

ALL DOSAGE FORMS OF ZOLOFT

Concomitant use in patients taking monoamine oxidase inhibitors (MAOIs) is contraindicated (see WARNINGS). Concomitant use in patients taking pimozide is contraindicated (see PRECAUTIONS).

Zoloft is contraindicated in patients with a hypersensitivity to sertraline or any of the inactive ingredients in Zoloft.

ORAL CONCENTRATE

Zoloft oral concentrate is contraindicated with disulfiram due to the alcohol content of the concentrate.

WARNINGS

Cases of serious sometimes fatal reactions have been reported in patients receiving Zoloft, a selective serotonin reuptake inhibitor (SSRI), in combination with a monoamine oxidase inhibitor (MAOI). Symptoms of a drug interaction between an SSRI and an MAOI include: hyperthermia, rigidity, myoclonus, autonomic instability with possible rapid fluctuations of vital signs, mental status changes that include confusion, irritability, and extreme agitation progressing to delirium and coma. These reactions have also been reported in patients who have recently discontinued an SSRI and have been started on an MAOI. Some cases presented with features resembling neuroleptic malignant syndrome. Therefore, Zoloft should not be used in combination with an MAOI, or within 14 days of discontinuing treatment with an MAOI. Similarly, at least 14 days should be allowed after stopping Zoloft before starting an MAOI.

PRECAUTIONS

GENERAL

Activation of Mania/Hypomania

During premarketing testing, hypomania or mania occurred in approximately 0.4% of Zoloft treated patients.

Weight Loss

Significant weight loss may be an undesirable result of treatment with sertraline for some patients, but on average, patients in controlled trials had minimal, 1-2 lb weight loss, versus smaller changes on placebo. Only rarely have sertraline patients been discontinued for weight loss.

Seizure

Zoloft has not been evaluated in patients with a seizure disorder. These patients were excluded from clinical studies during the product's premarket testing. No seizures were observed among approximately 3000 patients treated with Zoloft in the development program for major depressive disorder. However, 4 patients out of approximately 1800 (220 <18 years of age) exposed during the development program for obsessive-compulsive disorder experienced seizures, representing a crude incidence of 0.2%. Three of these patients were adolescents, 2 with a seizure disorder and 1 with a family history of seizure disorder, none of whom were receiving anticonvulsant medication. Accordingly, Zoloft should be introduced with care in patients with a seizure disorder.

Suicide

The possibility of a suicide attempt is inherent in major depressive disorder and may persist until significant remission occurs. Close supervision of high risk patients should accompany initial drug therapy. Prescriptions for Zoloft should be written for the smallest quantity of tablets consistent with good patient management, in order to reduce the risk of overdose.

Because of the well-established comorbidity between OCD and major depressive disorder, panic disorder and major depressive disorder, and PTSD and major depressive disorder, and PMDD and major depressive disorder, the same precautions observed when treating patients with major depressive disorder should be observed when treating patients with OCD, panic disorder, PTSD or PMDD.

Weak Uricosuric Effect

Zoloft is associated with a mean decrease in serum uric acid of approximately 7%. The clinical significance of this weak uricosuric effect is unknown.

Use in Patients With Concomitant Illness

Clinical experience with Zoloft in patients with certain concomitant systemic illness is limited. Caution is advisable in using Zoloft in patients with diseases or conditions that could affect metabolism or hemodynamic responses.

Zoloft has not been evaluated or used to any appreciable extent in patients with a recent history of myocardial infarction or unstable heart disease. Patients with these diagnoses were excluded from clinical studies during the product's premarket testing. However, the electrocardiograms of 774 patients who received Zoloft in double-blind trials were evaluated and the data indicate that Zoloft is not associated with the development of significant ECG abnormalities.

Zoloft is extensively metabolized by the liver. In patients with chronic mild liver impairment, sertraline clearance was reduced, resulting in increased AUC, C_{max} and elimination half-life. The effects of sertraline in patients with moderate and severe hepatic impairment have not been studied. The use of sertraline in patients with liver disease must be approached with caution. If sertraline is administered to patients with liver impairment, a lower or less frequent dose should be used (see CLINICAL PHARMACOLOGY and DOSAGE AND ADMINISTRATION).

Since Zoloft is extensively metabolized, excretion of unchanged drug in urine is a minor route of elimination. A clinical study comparing sertraline pharmacokinetics in healthy volunteers to that in patients with renal impairment ranging from mild to severe (requiring dialysis) indicated that the pharmacokinetics and protein binding are unaffected by renal disease. Based on the pharmacokinetic results, there is no need for dosage adjustment in patients with renal impairment (see CLINICAL PHARMACOLOGY).

Interference With Cognitive and Motor Performance

In controlled studies, Zoloft did not cause sedation and did not interfere with psychomotor performance. (See Information for the Patient.)

Hyponatremia

Several cases of hyponatremia have been reported and appeared to be reversible when Zoloft was discontinued. Some cases were possibly due to the syndrome of inappropriate antidiuretic hormone secretion. The majority of these occurrences have been in elderly individuals, some in patients taking diuretics or who were otherwise volume depleted.

Platelet Function

There have been rare reports of altered platelet function and/or abnormal results from laboratory studies in patients taking Zoloft. While there have been reports of abnormal bleeding or purpura in several patients taking Zoloft, it is unclear whether Zoloft had a causative role.

INFORMATION FOR THE PATIENT

Physicians are advised to discuss the following issues with patients for whom they prescribe Zoloft:

Patients should be told that although Zoloft has not been shown to impair the ability of normal subjects to perform tasks requiring complex motor and mental skills in laboratory experiments, drugs that act upon the central nervous system may affect some individuals adversely. Therefore, patients should be told that until they learn how they respond to Zoloft they should be careful doing activities when they need to be alert, such as driving a car or operating machinery.

Patients should be told that although Zoloft has not been shown in experiments with normal subjects to increase the mental and motor skill impairments caused by alcohol, the concomitant use of Zoloft and alcohol is not advised.

Patients should be told that while no adverse interaction of Zoloft with over-the-counter (OTC) drug products is known to occur, the potential for interaction exists. Thus, the use of any OTC product should be initiated cautiously according to the directions of use given for the OTC product.

Patients should be advised to notify their physician if they become pregnant or intend to become pregnant during therapy.

Patients should be advised to notify their physician if they are breast feeding an infant.

Zoloft oral concentrate is contraindicated with disulfiram due to the alcohol content of the concentrate.

Zoloft oral concentrate contains 20 mg/ml of sertraline (as the hydrochloride) as the active ingredient and 12% alcohol. Zoloft oral concentrate must be diluted before use. Just before taking, use the dropper provided to remove the required amount of Zoloft oral concentrate and mix with 4 oz (½ cup) of water, ginger ale, lemon/lime soda, lemonade, or orange juice ONLY. Do not mix Zoloft oral concentrate with anything other than the liquids listed. The dose should be taken immediately after mixing. Do not mix in advance. At times, a slight haze may appear after mixing; this is normal. Note that caution should be exercised for persons with latex sensitivity, as the dropper dispenser contains dry natural rubber.

LABORATORY TESTS

None.

CARCINOGENESIS

Lifetime carcinogenicity studies were carried out in CD-1 mice and Long-Evans rats at doses up to 40 mg/kg/day. These doses correspond to 1 times (mice) and 2 times (rats) the maximum recommended human dose (MRHD) on a mg/m^2 basis. There was a dose-related increase of liver adenomas in male mice receiving sertraline at 10-40 mg/kg (0.25-1.0 times the MRHD on a mg/m^2 basis). No increase was seen in female mice or in rats of either sex receiving the same treatments, nor was there an increase in hepatocellular carcinomas. Liver adenomas have a variable rate of spontaneous occurrence in the CD-1 mouse and are of unknown significance to humans. There was an increase in follicular adenomas of the thyroid in female rats receiving sertraline at 40 mg/kg (2 times the MRHD on a mg/m^2 basis); this was not accompanied by thyroid hyperplasia. While there was an increase in uterine adenocarcinomas in rats receiving sertraline at 10-40 mg/kg (0.5-2.0 times the MRHD on a mg/m^2 basis) compared to placebo controls, this effect was not clearly drug related.

MUTAGENESIS

Sertraline had no genotoxic effects, with or without metabolic activation, based on the following assays: bacterial mutation assay; mouse lymphoma mutation assay; and tests for cytogenetic aberrations *in vivo* in mouse bone marrow and *in vitro* in human lymphocytes.

IMPAIRMENT OF FERTILITY

A decrease in fertility was seen in one of two rat studies at a dose of 80 mg/kg (4 times the maximum recommended human dose on a mg/m^2 basis).

PREGNANCY CATEGORY C

Reproduction studies have been performed in rats and rabbits at doses up to 80 mg/kg/day and 40 mg/kg/day, respectively. These doses correspond to approximately 4 times the maximum recommended human dose (MRHD) on a mg/m^2 basis. There was no evidence of teratogenicity at any dose level. When pregnant rats and rabbits were given sertraline during the period of organogenesis, delayed ossification was observed in fetuses at doses of 10 mg/kg (0.5 times the MRHD on a mg/m^2 basis) in rats and 40 mg/kg (4 times the MRHD on a mg/m^2 basis) in rabbits. When female rats received sertraline during the last third of gestation and throughout lactation, there was an increase in the number of stillborn pups and in the number of pups dying during the first 4 days after birth. Pup body weights were also decreased during the first 4 days after birth. These effects occurred at a dose of 20 mg/kg (1 times the MRHD on a mg/m^2 basis). The no effect dose for rat pup mortality was 10 mg/kg (0.5 times the MRHD on a mg/m^2 basis). The decrease in pup survival was shown to be due to *in utero* exposure to sertraline. The clinical significance of these effects is unknown. There are no adequate and well-controlled studies in pregnant women. Zoloft should be used during pregnancy only if the potential benefit justifies the potential risk to the fetus.

LABOR AND DELIVERY

The effect of Zoloft on labor and delivery in humans is unknown.

NURSING MOTHERS

It is not known whether, and if so in what amount, sertraline or its metabolites are excreted in human milk. Because many drugs are excreted in human milk, caution should be exercised when Zoloft is administered to a nursing woman.

PEDIATRIC USE

The efficacy of Zoloft for the treatment of obsessive-compulsive disorder was demonstrated in a 12 week, multicenter, placebo-controlled study with 187 outpatients ages 6-17. The efficacy of Zoloft in pediatric patients with major depressive disorder, panic disorder, PTSD or PMDD has not been systematically evaluated.

The safety of Zoloft use in children and adolescents, ages 6-18, was evaluated in a 12 week, multicenter, placebo-controlled study with 187 outpatients, ages 6-17, and in a flexible dose, 52 week open extension study of 137 patients, ages 6-18, who had completed the initial 12 week, double-blind, placebo-controlled study. Zoloft was administered at doses of either 25 mg/day (children, ages 6-12) or 50 mg/day (adolescents, ages 13-18) and then titrated in weekly 25 mg/day or 50 mg/day increments, respectively, to a maximum dose of 200 mg/day based upon clinical response. The mean dose for completers was 157 mg/day. In the acute 12 week pediatric study and in the 52 week study, Zoloft had an adverse event profile generally similar to that observed in adults.

Sertraline pharmacokinetics were evaluated in 61 pediatric patients between 6 and 18 years of age with major depressive disorder and/or OCD and revealed similar drug exposures to those of adults when plasma concentration was adjusted for weight (see CLINICAL PHARMACOLOGY, Pharmacokinetics).

More than 250 patients with major depressive disorder and/or OCD between 6 and 18 years of age have received Zoloft in clinical trials. The adverse event profile observed in these patients was generally similar to that observed in adult studies with Zoloft (see ADVERSE REACTIONS). As with other SSRIs, decreased appetite and weight loss have been observed in association with the use of Zoloft. Consequently, regular monitoring of weight and growth is recommended if treatment of a child with an SSRI is to be continued long term. Safety and effectiveness in pediatric patients below the age of 6 have not been established.

The risks, if any, that may be associated with the use of Zoloft beyond 1 year in children and adolescents with OCD have not been systematically assessed. The prescriber should be mindful that the evidence relied upon to conclude that sertraline is safe for use in children and adolescents derives from clinical studies that were 12-52 weeks in duration and from the extrapolation of experience gained with adult patients. In particular, there are no studies that directly evaluate the effects of long-term sertraline use on the growth, development, and maturation of children and adolescents. Although there is no affirmative finding to suggest that sertraline possesses a capacity to adversely affect growth, development or maturation, the absence of such findings is not compelling evidence of the absence of the potential of sertraline to have adverse effects in chronic use.

GERIATRIC USE

US geriatric clinical studies of Zoloft in major depressive disorder included 663 Zoloft-treated subjects ≥65 years of age, of those, 180 were ≥75 years of age. No overall differences in the pattern of adverse reactions were observed in the geriatric clinical trial subjects relative to those reported in younger subjects (see ADVERSE REACTIONS), and other reported experience has not identified differences in safety patterns between the elderly and younger subjects. As with all medications, greater sensitivity of some older individuals cannot be ruled out. There were 947 subjects in placebo-controlled geriatric clinical studies of Zoloft in major depressive disorder. No overall differences in the pattern of efficacy were observed in the geriatric clinical trial subjects relative to those reported in younger subjects.

Other Adverse Events in Geriatric Patients

In 354 geriatric subjects treated with Zoloft in placebo-controlled trials, the overall profile of adverse events was generally similar to that shown in TABLE 1A, TABLE 1B, and TABLE 2. Urinary tract infection was the only adverse event not appearing in TABLE 1A, TABLE 1B, and TABLE 2 and reported at an incidence of at least 2% and at a rate greater than placebo in placebo-controlled trials.

As with other SSRIs, Zoloft has been associated with cases of clinically significant hyponatremia in elderly patients (see General, Hyponatremia).

DRUG INTERACTIONS

POTENTIAL EFFECTS OF COADMINISTRATION OF DRUGS HIGHLY BOUND TO PLASMA PROTEINS

Because sertraline is tightly bound to plasma protein, the administration of Zoloft to a patient taking another drug which is tightly bound to protein (*e.g.,* warfarin, digitoxin) may cause a shift in plasma concentrations potentially resulting in an adverse effect. Conversely, adverse effects may result from displacement of protein bound Zoloft by other tightly bound drugs.

In a study comparing prothrombin time AUC(0-120h) following dosing with warfarin (0.75 mg/kg) before and after 21 days of dosing with either Zoloft (50-200 mg/day) or placebo, there was a mean increase in prothrombin time of 8% relative to baseline for Zoloft compared to a 1% decrease for placebo ($p < 0.02$). The normalization of prothrombin time for the Zoloft group was delayed compared to the placebo group. The clinical significance of this change is unknown. Accordingly, prothrombin time should be carefully monitored when Zoloft therapy is initiated or stopped.

CIMETIDINE

In a study assessing disposition of Zoloft (100 mg) on the second of 8 days of cimetidine administration (800 mg daily), there were significant increases in Zoloft mean AUC (50%), C_{max} (24%) and half-life (26%) compared to the placebo group. The clinical significance of these changes is unknown.

CNS ACTIVE DRUGS

In a study comparing the disposition of intravenously administered diazepam before and after 21 days of dosing with either Zoloft (50-200 mg/day escalating dose) or placebo, there was a 32% decrease relative to baseline in diazepam clearance for the Zoloft group compared to a 19% decrease relative to baseline for the placebo group ($p < 0.03$). There was a 23% increase in T_{max} for desmethyldiazepam in the Zoloft group compared to a 20% decrease in the placebo group ($p < 0.03$). The clinical significance of these changes is unknown.

In a placebo-controlled trial in normal volunteers, the administration of two doses of Zoloft did not significantly alter steady-state lithium levels or the renal clearance of lithium.

Nonetheless, at this time, it is recommended that plasma lithium levels be monitored following initiation of Zoloft therapy with appropriate adjustments to the lithium dose.

In a controlled study of a single dose (2 mg) of pimozide, 200 mg sertraline (qd) co-administration to steady state was associated with a mean increase in pimozide AUC and C_{max} of about 40%, but was not associated with any changes in EKG. Since the highest recommended pimozide dose (10 mg) has not been evaluated in combination with sertraline, the effect on QT interval and PK parameters at doses higher than 2 mg at this time are not known. While the mechanism of this interaction is unknown, due to the narrow therapeutic index of pimozide and due to the interaction noted at a low dose of pimozide, concomitant administration of Zoloft and pimozide should be contraindicated (see CONTRAINDICATIONS).

The risk of using Zoloft in combination with other CNS active drugs has not been systematically evaluated. Consequently, caution is advised if the concomitant administration of Zoloft and such drugs is required.

There is limited controlled experience regarding the optimal timing of switching from other drugs effective in the treatment of major depressive disorder, obsessive-compulsive disorder, panic disorder, posttraumatic stress disorder and premenstrual dysphoric disorder to Zoloft. Care and prudent medical judgment should be exercised when switching, particularly from long-acting agents. The duration of an appropriate washout period which should intervene before switching from one selective serotonin reuptake inhibitor (SSRI) to another has not been established.

MONOAMINE OXIDASE INHIBITORS

See CONTRAINDICATIONS and WARNINGS.

DRUGS METABOLIZED BY P450 3A4

In two separate *in vivo* interaction studies, sertraline was co-administered with cytochrome P450 3A4 substrates, terfenadine or carbamazepine, under steady-state conditions. The results of these studies demonstrated that sertraline co-administration did not increase plasma concentrations of terfenadine or carbamazepine. These data suggest that sertraline's extent of inhibition of P450 3A4 activity is not likely to be of clinical significance. In three separate *in vivo* interaction studies, sertraline was co-administered with cytochrome P450 3A4 substrates, terfenadine, carbamazepine, or cisapride under steady-state conditions. The results of these studies indicated that sertraline did not increase plasma concentrations of terfenadine, carbamazepine, or cisapride. These data indicate that sertraline's extent of inhibition of P450 3A4 activity is not likely to be of clinical significance. Results of the interaction study with cisapride indicate that sertraline 200 mg (qd) induces the metabolism of cisapride (cisapride AUC and C_{max} were reduced by about 35%).

DRUGS METABOLIZED BY P450 2D6

Many drugs effective in the treatment of major depressive disorder, *e.g.*, the SSRIs, including sertraline, and most tricyclic antidepressant drugs effective in the treatment of major depressive disorder inhibit the biochemical activity of the drug metabolizing isozyme cytochrome P450 2D6 (debrisoquin hydroxylase), and, thus, may increase the plasma concentrations of co-administered drugs that are metabolized by P450 2D6. The drugs for which this potential interaction is of greatest concern are those metabolized primarily by 2D6 and which have a narrow therapeutic index, *e.g.*, the tricyclic antidepressant drugs effective in the treatment of major depressive disorder and the Type 1C antiarrhythmics propafenone and flecainide. The extent to which this interaction is an important clinical problem depends on the extent of the inhibition of P450 2D6 by the antidepressant and the therapeutic index of the co-administered drug. There is variability among the drugs effective in the treatment of major depressive disorder in the extent of clinically important 2D6 inhibition, and in fact sertraline at lower doses has a less prominent inhibitory effect on 2D6 than some others in the class. Nevertheless, even sertraline has the potential for clinically important 2D6 inhibition. Consequently, concomitant use of a drug metabolized by P450 2D6 with Zoloft may require lower doses than usually prescribed for the other drug. Furthermore, whenever Zoloft is withdrawn from co-therapy, an increased dose of the co-administered drug may be required [see Tricyclic Antidepressant Drugs Effective in the Treatment of Major Depressive Disorder (TCAs)].

SUMATRIPTAN

There have been rare postmarketing reports describing patients with weakness, hyperreflexia, and incoordination following the use of a selective serotonin reuptake inhibitor (SSRI) and sumatriptan. If concomitant treatment with sumatriptan and an SSRI (*e.g.*, citalopram, fluoxetine, fluvoxamine, paroxetine, sertraline) is clinically warranted, appropriate observation of the patient is advised.

TRICYCLIC ANTIDEPRESSANT DRUGS EFFECTIVE IN THE TREATMENT OF MAJOR DEPRESSIVE DISORDER (TCAS)

The extent to which SSRI-TCA interactions may pose clinical problems will depend on the degree of inhibition and the pharmacokinetics of the SSRI involved. Nevertheless, caution is indicated in the co-administration of TCAs with Zoloft, because sertraline may inhibit TCA metabolism. Plasma TCA concentrations may need to be monitored, and the dose of TCA may need to be reduced, if a TCA is co-administered with Zoloft (see Drugs Metabolized by P450 2D6).

HYPOGLYCEMIC DRUGS

In a placebo-controlled trial in normal volunteers, administration of Zoloft for 22 days (including 200 mg/day for the final 13 days) caused a statistically significant 16% decrease from baseline in the clearance of tolbutamide following an intravenous 1000 mg dose. Zoloft administration did not noticeably change either the plasma protein binding or the apparent volume of distribution of tolbutamide, suggesting that the decreased clearance was due to a change in the metabolism of the drug. The clinical significance of this decrease in tolbutamide clearance is unknown.

ATENOLOL

Zoloft (100 mg) when administered to 10 healthy male subjects had no effect on the beta-adrenergic blocking ability of atenolol.

DIGOXIN

In a placebo-controlled trial in normal volunteers, administration of Zoloft for 17 days (including 200 mg/day for the last 10 days) did not change serum digoxin levels or digoxin renal clearance.

MICROSOMAL ENZYME INDUCTION

Preclinical studies have shown Zoloft to induce hepatic microsomal enzymes. In clinical studies, Zoloft was shown to induce hepatic enzymes minimally as determined by a small (5%) but statistically significant decrease in antipyrine half-life following administration of 200 mg/day for 21 days. This small change in antipyrine half-life reflects a clinically insignificant change in hepatic metabolism.

ELECTROCONVULSIVE THERAPY

There are no clinical studies establishing the risks or benefits of the combined use of electroconvulsive therapy (ECT) and Zoloft.

ALCOHOL

Although Zoloft did not potentiate the cognitive and psychomotor effects of alcohol in experiments with normal subjects, the concomitant use of Zoloft and alcohol is not recommended.

ADVERSE REACTIONS

During its premarketing assessment, multiple doses of Zoloft were administered to over 4000 adult subjects as of February 26, 1998. The conditions and duration of exposure to Zoloft varied greatly, and included (in overlapping categories) clinical pharmacology studies, open and double-blind studies, uncontrolled and controlled studies, inpatient and outpatient studies, fixed-dose and titration studies, and studies for multiple indications, including major depressive disorder, OCD, panic disorder, PTSD and PMDD.

Untoward events associated with this exposure were recorded by clinical investigators using terminology of their own choosing. Consequently, it is not possible to provide a meaningful estimate of the proportion of individuals experiencing adverse events without first grouping similar types of untoward events into a smaller number of standardized event categories.

In the tabulations that follow, a World Health Organization dictionary of terminology has been used to classify reported adverse events. The frequencies presented, therefore, represent the proportion of the over 4000 adult individuals exposed to multiple doses of Zoloft who experienced a treatment-emergent adverse event of the type cited on at least one occasion while receiving Zoloft. An event was considered treatment-emergent if it occurred for the first time or worsened while receiving therapy following baseline evaluation. It is important to emphasize that events reported during therapy were not necessarily caused by it.

The prescriber should be aware that the figures in the tables and tabulations cannot be used to predict the incidence of side effects in the course of usual medical practice where patient characteristics and other factors differ from those that prevailed in the clinical trials. Similarly, the cited frequencies cannot be compared with figures obtained from other clinical investigations involving different treatments, uses, and investigators. The cited figures, however, do provide the prescribing physician with some basis for estimating the relative contribution of drug and nondrug factors to the side effect incidence rate in the population studied.

INCIDENCE IN PLACEBO-CONTROLLED TRIALS

TABLE 1A, TABLE 1B, and TABLE 1C enumerate the most common treatment-emergent adverse events associated with the use of Zoloft (incidence of at least 5% for Zoloft and at least twice that for placebo within at least one of the indications) for the treatment of adult patients with major depressive disorder/other*, OCD, panic disorder, PTSD and PMDD in placebo-controlled clinical trials. Most patients in major depressive disorder/other*, OCD, panic disorder, and PTSD studies received doses of 50-200 mg/day. Patients in the PMDD study with daily dosing throughout the menstrual cycle received doses of 50-150 mg/day, and in the PMDD study with dosing during the luteal phase of the menstrual cycle received doses of 50-100 mg/day. TABLE 2 enumerates treatment-emergent adverse events that occurred in 2% or more of adult patients treated with Zoloft and with incidence greater than placebo who participated in controlled clinical trials comparing Zoloft with placebo in the treatment of major depressive disorder/other*, OCD, panic disorder, PTSD and PMDD. TABLE 2 provides combined data for the pool of studies that are provided separately by indication in TABLE 1A, TABLE 1B and TABLE 1C.

ASSOCIATED WITH DISCONTINUATION IN PLACEBO-CONTROLLED CLINICAL TRIALS

The adverse events associated with discontinuation of Zoloft treatment (incidence at least twice that for placebo and at least 1% for Zoloft in clinical trials) in major depressive disorder/other*, OCD, panic disorder, PTSD and PMDD are listed below.

Major Depressive Disorder/Other*, OCD, Panic Disorder, PTSD, and PMDD Combined (n=2455): Diarrhea (2%), dizziness (1%), ejaculation failure† (1%), headache (1%), insomnia (2%), nausea (3%), somnolence (1%).

Major Depressive Disorder/Other* (n=861): Agitation (1%), diarrhea (2%), dry mouth (1%), ejaculation failure† (1%), headache (2%), insomnia (1%), nausea (4%), somnolence (1%), tremor (2%).

OCD (n=533): Diarrhea (2%), dizziness (1%), ejaculation failure† (1%), insomnia (3%), nausea (3%), somnolence (2%).

Panic Disorder (n=430): Agitation (2%), diarrhea (1%), dyspepsia (1%), ejaculation failure† (2%), insomnia (2%), nausea (3%), nervousness (2%), somnolence (2%).

PTSD (n=374): Headache (1%), nausea (2%).

PMDD Daily Dosing (n=121): Diarrhea (2%), nausea (2%), nervousness (2%).

PMDD Luteal Phase Dosing (n=136): Hot flushes (1%), insomnia (1%), nausea (1%), palpitation (1%).

* Major depressive disorder and other premarketing controlled trials.

† Primarily ejaculatory delay. Denominator used was for male patients only (n=271 major depressive disorder/other*; n=296 OCD; n=216 panic disorder; n=130 PTSD; No male patients in PMDD studies).

MALE AND FEMALE SEXUAL DYSFUNCTION WITH SSRIS

Although changes in sexual desire, sexual performance and sexual satisfaction often occur as manifestations of a psychiatric disorder, they may also be a consequence of pharmacologic treatment. In particular, some evidence suggests that selective serotonin reuptake inhibitors (SSRIs) can cause such untoward sexual experiences. Reliable estimates of the incidence and severity of untoward experiences involving sexual desire, performance and

S

TABLE 1A *Most Common Treatment-Emergent Adverse Events: Incidence in Placebo-Controlled Clinical Trials*

Body System / Adverse Event	Major Depressive Disorder/Other* Zoloft (n=861)	Major Depressive Disorder/Other* Placebo (n=853)	OCD Zoloft (n=533)	OCD Placebo (n=373)
Autonomic Nervous System Disorders				
Ejaculation failure†	7%	<1%	17%	2%
Mouth dry	16%	9%	14%	9%
Sweating increased	8%	3%	6%	1%
Central & Peripheral Nervous System Disorders				
Somnolence	13%	6%	15%	8%
Tremor	11%	3%	8%	1%
General				
Fatigue	11%	8%	14%	10%
Pain	1%	2%	3%	1%
Gastrointestinal Disorders				
Abdominal pain	2%	2%	5%	5%
Anorexia	3%	2%	11%	2%
Constipation	8%	6%	6%	4%
Diarrhea/loose stools	18%	9%	24%	10%
Dyspepsia	6%	3%	10%	4%
Nausea	26%	12%	30%	11%
Psychiatric Disorders				
Agitation	6%	4%	6%	3%
Insomnia	16%	9%	28%	12%
Libido decreased	1%	<1%	11%	2%

* Major depressive disorder and other premarketing controlled trials.
† Primarily ejaculatory delay. Denominator used was for male patients only (n=271 Zoloft major depressive disorder/other*; n=271 placebo major depressive disorder/other*; n=296 Zoloft OCD; n=219 placebo OCD.

TABLE 1B *Most Common Treatment-Emergent Adverse Events: Incidence in Placebo-Controlled Clinical Trials*

Body System / Adverse Event	Panic Disorder Zoloft (n=430)	Panic Disorder Placebo (n=275)	PTSD Zoloft (n=374)	PTSD Placebo (n=376)
Autonomic Nervous System Disorders				
Ejaculation failure*	19%	1%	11%	1%
Mouth dry	15%	10%	11%	6%
Sweating increased	5%	1%	4%	2%
Central & Peripheral Nervous System Disorders				
Somnolence	15%	9%	13%	9%
Tremor	5%	1%	5%	1%
General				
Fatigue	11%	6%	10%	5%
Pain	3%	3%	4%	6
Gastrointestinal Disorders				
Abdominal pain	6%	7%	6%	5%
Anorexia	7%	2%	8%	2%
Constipation	7%	3%	3%	3%
Diarrhea/loose stools	20%	9%	24%	15%
Dyspepsia	10%	8%	6%	6%
Nausea	29%	18%	21%	11%
Psychiatric Disorders				
Agitation	6%	2%	5%	5%
Insomnia	25%	18%	20%	11%
Libido decreased	7%	1%	7%	2%

* Primarily ejaculatory delay. Denominator used was for male patients only (n=216 Zoloft panic disorder; n=134 placebo panic disorder; n=130 Zoloft PTSD).

satisfaction are difficult to obtain, however, in part because patients and physicians may be reluctant to discuss them. Accordingly, estimates of the incidence of untoward sexual experience and performance cited in product labeling, are likely to underestimate their actual incidence.

TABLE 3 displays the incidence of sexual side effects reported by at least 2% of patients taking Zoloft in placebo-controlled trials.

There are no adequate and well-controlled studies examining sexual dysfunction with sertraline treatment.

Priapism has been reported with all SSRIs.

While it is difficult to know the precise risk of sexual dysfunction associated with the use of SSRIs, physicians should routinely inquire about such possible side effects.

OTHER ADVERSE EVENTS IN PEDIATRIC PATIENTS

In approximately n=250 pediatric patients treated with Zoloft, the overall profile of adverse events was generally similar to that seen in adult studies, as shown in TABLE 1A, TABLE 1B, and TABLE 2. However, the following adverse events, not appearing in TABLE 1A, TABLE 1B, and TABLE 2, were reported at an incidence of at least 2% and occurred at a rate of at least twice the placebo rate in a controlled trial (n=187): hyperkinesia, twitching, fever, malaise, purpura, weight decrease, concentration impaired, manic reaction, emotional lability, thinking abnormal, and epistaxis.

OTHER EVENTS OBSERVED DURING THE PREMARKETING EVALUATION OF ZOLOFT

Following is a list of treatment-emergent adverse events reported during premarketing assessment of Zoloft in clinical trials (over 4000 adult subjects) except those already listed in the previous tables or elsewhere in labeling.

TABLE 1C *Most Common Treatment-Emergent Adverse Events: Incidence in Placebo-Controlled Clinical Trials*

Body System / Adverse Event	PMDD Daily Dosing Zoloft (n=121)	PMDD Daily Dosing Placebo (n=122)	PMDD Luteal Phase Dosing* Zoloft (n=136)	PMDD Luteal Phase Dosing* Placebo (n=127)
Autonomic Nervous System Disorders				
Mouth dry	6%	3%	10%	3%
Sweating increased	6%	<1%	3%	0%
Central & Peripheral Nervous System Disorders				
Somnolence	7%	<1%	2%	0%
Tremor	2%	0%	<1%	<1%
General				
Fatigue	16%	7%	10%	<1%
Pain	6%	<1%	3%	2%
Gastrointestinal Disorders				
Abdominal pain	7%	<1%	3%	3%
Anorexia	3%	2%	5%	0%
Constipation	2%	3%	1%	2%
Diarrhea/loose stools	13%	3%	13%	7%
Dyspepsia	7%	2%	7%	3%
Nausea	23%	9%	13%	3%
Psychiatric Disorders				
Agitation	2%	<1%	1%	0%
Insomnia	17%	11%	12%	10%
Libido decreased	11%	2%	4%	2%

* The luteal phase and daily dosing PMDD trials were not designed for making direct comparisons between the two dosing regimens. Therefore, a comparison between the two dosing regimens of the PMDD trials of incidence rates shown in TABLE 1C should be avoided.

TABLE 2 *Treatment-Emergent Adverse Events: Incidence In Placebo-Controlled Clinical Trials — Major Depressive Disorder/Other*, OCD, Panic Disorder, PTSD and PMDD Combined*

Body System / Adverse Event	Zoloft (n=2455)	Placebo (n=2126)
Autonomic Nervous System Disorders		
Ejaculation failure†	14%	1%
Mouth dry	14%	8%
Sweating increased	6%	2%
Central & Peripheral Nervous System Disorders		
Somnolence	13%	7%
Dizziness	11%	7%
Headache	25%	23%
Paresthesia	2%	1%
Tremor	7%	1%
Disorders of Skin and Appendages		
Rash	3%	2%
Gastrointestinal Disorders		
Abdominal pain	4%	4%
Anorexia	6%	2%
Constipation	6%	4%
Diarrhea/loose stools	20%	10%
Dyspepsia	8%	4%
Flatulence	4%	3%
Nausea	26%	12%
Vomiting	4%	2%
General		
Fatigue	12%	7%
Hot flushes	2%	1%
Psychiatric Disorders		
Agitation	5%	3%
Anxiety	4%	3%
Insomnia	21%	11%
Libido decreased	6%	1%
Nervousness	5%	4%
Respiratory System Disorders		
Pharyngitis	3%	2%
Special Senses		
Vision abnormal	3%	2%

* Major depressive disorder and other premarketing controlled trials.
† Primarily ejaculatory delay. Denominator used was for male patients only (n=913 Zoloft; n=773 placebo).

TABLE 3

	Treatment Zoloft	Treatment Placebo
Ejaculation Failure (primarily Delayed Ejaculation)		
n (males only)	913	773
Incidence	14%	1%
Decreased Libido		
n (males and females)	2455	2126
Incidence	6%	1%

In the tabulations that follow, a World Health Organization dictionary of terminology has been used to classify reported adverse events. The frequencies presented, therefore, represent the proportion of the over 4000 adult individuals exposed to multiple doses of Zoloft who experienced an event of the type cited on at least one occasion while receiving Zoloft. All events are included except those already listed in the previous tables or elsewhere in labeling and those reported in terms so general as to be uninformative and those for which a causal relationship to Zoloft treatment seemed remote. It is important to emphasize that although the events reported occurred during treatment with Zoloft, they were not necessarily caused by it.

Events are further categorized by body system and listed in order of decreasing frequency according to the following definitions: *frequent* adverse events are those occurring on one or more occasions in at least 1/100 patients; *infrequent* adverse events are those occurring in 1/100 to 1/1000 patients; *rare* events are those occurring in fewer than 1/1000 patients. Events of major clinical importance are also described in PRECAUTIONS.

Autonomic Nervous System Disorders: *Frequent:* Impotence; *Infrequent:* Flushing, increased saliva, cold clammy skin, mydriasis; *Rare:* Pallor, glaucoma, priapism, vasodilation.

Body as a Whole — General Disorders: *Rare:* Allergic reaction, allergy.

Cardiovascular: *Frequent:* Palpitations, chest pain; *Infrequent:* Hypertension, tachycardia, postural dizziness, postural hypotension, periorbital edema, peripheral edema, hypotension, peripheral ischemia, syncope, edema, dependent edema; *Rare:* Precordial chest pain, substernal chest pain, aggravated hypertension, myocardial infarction, cerebrovascular disorder.

Central and Peripheral Nervous System Disorders: *Frequent:* Hypertonia, hypoesthesia; *Infrequent:* Twitching, confusion, hyperkinesia, vertigo, ataxia, migraine, abnormal coordination, hyperesthesia, leg cramps, abnormal gait, nystagmus, hypokinesia; *Rare:* Dysphonia, coma, dyskinesia, hypotonia, ptosis, choreoathetosis, hyporeflexia.

Disorders of Skin and Appendages: *Infrequent:* Pruritus, acne, urticaria, alopecia, dry skin, erythematous rash, photosensitivity reaction, maculopapular rash; *Rare:* Follicular rash, eczema, dermatitis, contact dermatitis, bullous eruption, hypertrichosis, skin discoloration, pustular rash.

Endocrine Disorders: *Rare:* Exophthalmos, gynecomastia.

Gastrointestinal Disorders: *Frequent:* Appetite increased; *Infrequent:* Dysphagia, tooth caries aggravated, eructation, esophagitis, gastroenteritis; *Rare:* Melena, glossitis, gum hyperplasia, hiccup, stomatitis, tenesmus, colitis, diverticulitis, fecal incontinence, gastritis, rectum hemorrhage, hemorrhagic peptic ulcer, proctitis, ulcerative stomatitis, tongue edema, tongue ulceration.

General: *Frequent:* Back pain, asthenia, malaise, weight increase; *Infrequent:* Fever, rigors, generalized edema; *Rare:* Face edema, aphthous stomatitis.

Hearing and Vestibular Disorders: *Rare:* Hyperacusis, labyrinthine disorder.

Hematopoietic and Lymphatic: *Rare:* Anemia, anterior chamber eye hemorrhage.

Liver and Biliary System Disorders: *Rare:* Abnormal hepatic function.

Metabolic and Nutritional Disorders: *Infrequent:* Thirst; *Rare:* Hypoglycemia, hypoglycemia reaction.

Musculoskeletal System Disorders: *Frequent:* Myalgia; *Infrequent:* Arthralgia, dystonia, arthrosis, muscle cramps, muscle weakness.

Psychiatric Disorders: *Frequent:* Yawning, other male sexual dysfunction, other female sexual dysfunction; *Infrequent:* Depression, amnesia, paroniria, teeth-grinding, emotional lability, apathy, abnormal dreams, euphoria, paranoid reaction, hallucination, aggressive reaction, aggravated depression, delusions; *Rare:* Withdrawal syndrome, suicide ideation, libido increased, somnambulism, illusion.

Reproductive: *Infrequent:* Menstrual disorder, dysmenorrhea, intermenstrual bleeding, vaginal hemorrhage, amenorrhea, leukorrhea; *Rare:* Female breast pain, menorrhagia, balanoposthitis, breast enlargement, atrophic vaginitis, acute female mastitis.

Respiratory System Disorders: *Frequent:* Rhinitis; *Infrequent:* Coughing, dyspnea, upper respiratory tract infection, epistaxis, bronchospasm, sinusitis; *Rare:* Hyperventilation, bradypnea, stridor, apnea, bronchitis, hemoptysis, hypoventilation, laryngismus, laryngitis.

Special Senses: *Frequent:* Tinnitus; *Infrequent:* Conjunctivitis, earache, eye pain, abnormal accommodation; *Rare:* Xerophthalmia, photophobia, diplopia, abnormal lacrimation, scotoma, visual field defect.

Urinary System Disorders: *Infrequent:* Micturition frequency, polyuria, urinary retention, dysuria, nocturia, urinary incontinence; *Rare:* Cystitis, oliguria, pyelonephritis, hematuria, renal pain, strangury.

LABORATORY TESTS

In man, asymptomatic elevations in serum transaminases (SGOT [or AST] and SGPT [or ALT]) have been reported infrequently (approximately 0.8%) in association with Zoloft administration. These hepatic enzyme elevations usually occurred within the first 1-9 weeks of drug treatment and promptly diminished upon drug discontinuation.

Zoloft therapy was associated with small mean increases in total cholesterol (approximately 3%) and triglycerides (approximately 5%), and a small mean decrease in serum uric acid (approximately 7%) of no apparent clinical importance.

The safety profile observed with Zoloft treatment in patients with major depressive disorder, OCD, panic disorder and PTSD is similar.

OTHER EVENTS OBSERVED DURING THE POSTMARKETING EVALUATION OF ZOLOFT

Reports of adverse events temporally associated with Zoloft that have been received since market introduction, that are not listed above and that may have no causal relationship with the drug, include the following: Acute renal failure, anaphylactoid reaction, angioedema, blindness, optic neuritis, cataract, increased coagulation times, bradycardia, AV block, atrial arrhythmias, QT-interval prolongation, ventricular tachycardia (including torsade de pointes-type arrhythmias), hypothyroidism, agranulocytosis, aplastic anemia and pancytopenia, leukopenia, thrombocytopenia, lupus-like syndrome, serum sickness, hyperglycemia, galactorrhea, hyperprolactinemia, neuroleptic malignant syndrome-like events, extrapyramidal symptoms, oculogyric crisis, serotonin syndrome, psychosis, pulmonary hypertension, severe skin reactions, which potentially can be fatal, such as Stevens-Johnson syndrome, vasculitis, photosensitivity and other severe cutaneous disorders, rare reports of pancreatitis, and liver events — clinical features (which in the majority of cases appeared to be reversible with discontinuation of Zoloft) occurring in 1 or more patients include: elevated enzymes, increased bilirubin, hepatomegaly, hepatitis, jaundice, abdominal pain, vomiting, liver failure and death.

DOSAGE AND ADMINISTRATION

INITIAL TREATMENT

Dosage for Adults

Major Depressive Disorder and Obsessive-Compulsive Disorder

Zoloft treatment should be administered at a dose of 50 mg once daily.

Panic Disorder and Posttraumatic Stress Disorder

Zoloft treatment should be initiated with a dose of 25 mg once daily. After 1 week, the dose should be increased to 50 mg once daily.

While a relationship between dose and effect has not been established for major depressive disorder, OCD, panic disorder, or PTSD, patients were dosed in a range of 50-200 mg/day in the clinical trials demonstrating the effectiveness of Zoloft for the treatment of these indications. Consequently, a dose of 50 mg, administered once daily, is recommended as the initial dose. Patients not responding to a 50 mg dose may benefit from dose increases up to a maximum of 200 mg/day. Given the 24 hour elimination half-life of Zoloft, dose changes should not occur at intervals of less than 1 week.

Premenstrual Dysphoric Disorder

Zoloft treatment should be initiated with a dose of 50 mg/day, either daily throughout the menstrual cycle or limited to the luteal phase of the menstrual cycle, depending on physician assessment.

While a relationship between dose and effect has not been established for PMDD, patients were dosed in the range of 50-150 mg/day with dose increases at the onset of each new menstrual cycle. Patients not responding to a 50 mg/day dose may benefit from dose increases (at 50 mg increments/menstrual cycle) up to 150 mg/day when dosing daily throughout the menstrual cycle, or 100 mg/day when dosing during the luteal phase of the menstrual cycle. If a 100 mg/day dose has been established with luteal phase dosing, a 50 mg/day titration step for 3 days should be utilized at the beginning of each luteal phase dosing period.

Zoloft should be administered once daily, either in the morning or evening.

Dosage for Pediatric Population (Children and Adolescents)

Obsessive-Compulsive Disorder

Zoloft treatment should be initiated with a dose of 25 mg once daily in children (ages 6-12) and at a dose of 50 mg once daily in adolescents (ages 13-17).

While a relationship between dose and effect has not been established for OCD, patients were dosed in a range of 25-200 mg/day in the clinical trials demonstrating the effectiveness of Zoloft for pediatric patients (6-17 years) with OCD. Patients not responding to an initial dose of 25 or 50 mg/day may benefit from dose increases up to a maximum of 200 mg/day. For children with OCD, their generally lower body weights compared to adults should be taken into consideration in advancing the dose, in order to avoid excess dosing. Given the 24 hour elimination half-life of Zoloft, dose changes should not occur at intervals of less than 1 week.

Zoloft should be administered once daily, either in the morning or evening.

DOSAGE FOR HEPATICALLY IMPAIRED PATIENTS

The use of sertraline in patients with liver disease should be approached with caution. The effects of sertraline in patients with moderate and severe hepatic impairment have not been studied. If sertraline is administered to patients with liver impairment, a lower or less frequent dose should be used (see CLINICAL PHARMACOLOGY and PRECAUTIONS).

MAINTENANCE/CONTINUATION/EXTENDED TREATMENT

Major Depressive Disorder

It is generally agreed that acute episodes of major depressive disorder require several months or longer of sustained pharmacologic therapy beyond response to the acute episode. Systematic evaluation of Zoloft has demonstrated that its antidepressant efficacy is maintained for periods of up to 44 weeks following 8 weeks of initial treatment at a dose of 50-200 mg/day (mean dose of 70 mg/day). It is not known whether the dose of Zoloft needed for maintenance treatment is identical to the dose needed to achieve an initial response. Patients should be periodically reassessed to determine the need for maintenance treatment.

Posttraumatic Stress Disorder

It is generally agreed that PTSD requires several months or longer of sustained pharmacological therapy beyond response to initial treatment. Systematic evaluation of Zoloft has demonstrated that its efficacy in PTSD is maintained for periods of up to 28 weeks following 24 weeks of treatment at a dose of 50-200 mg/day. It is not known whether the dose of Zoloft needed for maintenance treatment is identical to the dose needed to achieve an initial response. Patients should be periodically reassessed to determine the need for maintenance treatment.

Obsessive-Compulsive Disorder and Panic Disorder

It is generally agreed that OCD and panic disorder require several months or longer of sustained pharmacological therapy beyond response to initial treatment. Systematic evaluation of continuing Zoloft for periods of up to 28 weeks in patients with OCD and panic disorder who have responded while taking Zoloft during initial treatment phases of 24-52 weeks of treatment at a dose range of 50-200 mg/day has demonstrated a benefit of such maintenance treatment. It is not known whether the dose of Zoloft needed for maintenance treatment is identical to the dose needed to achieve an initial response. Nevertheless, patients should be periodically reassessed to determine the need for maintenance treatment.

Premenstrual Dysphoric Disorder

The effectiveness of Zoloft in long-term use, that is, for more than 3 menstrual cycles, has not been systematically evaluated in controlled trials. However, as women commonly report that symptoms worsen with age until relieved by the onset of menopause, it is reasonable to consider continuation of a responding patient. Dosage adjustments, which may include changes between dosage regimens (*e.g.*, daily throughout the menstrual cycle versus during

S

the luteal phase of the menstrual cycle), may be needed to maintain the patient on the lowest effective dosage and patients should be periodically reassessed to determine the need for continued treatment.

Switching Patients to or From a Monoamine Oxidase Inhibitor

At least 14 days should elapse between discontinuation of an MAOI and initiation of therapy with Zoloft. In addition, at least 14 days should be allowed after stopping Zoloft before starting an MAOI (see CONTRAINDICATIONS and WARNINGS).

ZOLOFT ORAL CONCENTRATE

Zoloft oral concentrate contains 20 mg/ml of sertraline (as the hydrochloride) as the active ingredient and 12% alcohol. Zoloft oral concentrate must be diluted before use. Just before taking, use the dropper provided to remove the required amount of Zoloft oral concentrate and mix with 4 oz (½ cup) of water, ginger ale, lemon/lime soda, lemonade or orange juice ONLY. Do not mix Zoloft oral concentrate with anything other than the liquids listed. The dose should be taken immediately after mixing. Do not mix in advance. At times, a slight haze may appear after mixing; this is normal. Note that caution should be exercised for patients with latex sensitivity, as the dropper dispenser contains dry natural rubber.

Zoloft oral concentrate is contraindicated with disulfiram due to the alcohol content of the concentrate.

HOW SUPPLIED

ZOLOFT TABLETS

Zoloft capsular-shaped scored tablets, containing sertraline hydrochloride equivalent to 25, 50 and 100 mg of sertraline are available as follows:

25 mg: Light green film coated tablets engraved on one side with "ZOLOFT" and on the other side scored and engraved with "25 mg".

50 mg: Light blue film coated tablets engraved on one side with "ZOLOFT" and on the other side scored and engraved with "50 mg".

100 mg: Light yellow film coated tablets engraved on one side with "ZOLOFT" and on the other side scored and engraved with "100 mg".

Storage: Store at 25°C (77°F); excursions permitted to15-30°C (59-86°F).

ZOLOFT ORAL CONCENTRATE

Zoloft oral concentrate is a clear, colorless solution with a menthol scent containing sertraline hydrochloride equivalent to 20 mg of sertraline per ml and 12% alcohol. It is supplied with an accompanying calibrated dropper.

Storage: Store at 25°C (77°F); excursions permitted to 15-30°C (59-86°F).

PRODUCT LISTING - EQUIVALENTS NOT AVAILABLE

Concentrate - Oral - 20 mg/ml

60 ml	$62.73	ZOLOFT, Pfizer U.S. Pharmaceuticals	00049-4940-23

Tablet - Oral - 25 mg

7's	$15.87	ZOLOFT, Allscripts Pharmaceutical Company	54569-4529-00
14's	$31.75	ZOLOFT, Allscripts Pharmaceutical Company	54569-4529-01
30's	$68.03	ZOLOFT, Allscripts Pharmaceutical Company	54569-4529-02
30's	$75.62	ZOLOFT, Southwood Pharmaceuticals Inc	58016-0664-30
50's	$132.34	ZOLOFT, Pfizer U.S. Pharmaceuticals	00049-4960-50
60's	$151.24	ZOLOFT, Southwood Pharmaceuticals Inc	58016-0664-60
90's	$226.86	ZOLOFT, Southwood Pharmaceuticals Inc	58016-0664-90
100's	$252.07	GENERIC, Southwood Pharmaceuticals Inc	58016-0664-00

Tablet - Oral - 50 mg

3's	$11.38	ZOLOFT, Prescript Pharmaceuticals	00247-0675-03
7's	$16.39	ZOLOFT, Allscripts Pharmaceutical Company	54569-3724-05
7's	$22.07	ZOLOFT, Prescript Pharmaceuticals	00247-0675-07
8's	$24.74	ZOLOFT, Prescript Pharmaceuticals	00247-0675-08
14's	$30.18	ZOLOFT, Allscripts Pharmaceutical Company	54569-3724-03
14's	$40.64	ZOLOFT, Cheshire Drugs	55175-2714-04
14's	$40.79	ZOLOFT, Prescript Pharmaceuticals	00247-0675-14
14's	$42.65	ZOLOFT, Pharma Pac	52959-0361-14
15's	$35.13	ZOLOFT, Allscripts Pharmaceutical Company	54569-3724-04
15's	$35.67	ZOLOFT, Physicians Total Care	54868-2192-03
20's	$49.87	ZOLOFT, Physicians Total Care	54868-2192-04
30's	$61.00	ZOLOFT, Compumed Pharmaceuticals	00403-4721-30
30's	$64.67	ZOLOFT, Allscripts Pharmaceutical Company	54569-3724-00
30's	$70.12	ZOLOFT, Cheshire Drugs	55175-2714-03
30's	$70.15	ZOLOFT, Physicians Total Care	54868-2192-01
30's	$72.50	ZOLOFT, Southwood Pharmaceuticals Inc	58016-0366-30
30's	$81.96	ZOLOFT, Quality Care Pharmaceuticals Inc	60346-0516-30
30's	$83.55	ZOLOFT, Prescript Pharmaceuticals	00247-0675-30
30's	$84.97	ZOLOFT, Pharma Pac	52959-0361-30
30's	$91.77	ZOLOFT, Pd-Rx Pharmaceuticals	55289-0409-30
50's	$135.70	ZOLOFT, Quality Care Pharmaceuticals Inc	60346-0516-50
60's	$129.33	ZOLOFT, Allscripts Pharmaceutical Company	54569-3724-02
60's	$140.27	ZOLOFT, Cheshire Drugs	55175-2714-06
60's	$145.00	ZOLOFT, Southwood Pharmaceuticals Inc	58016-0366-60
60's	$174.97	ZOLOFT, Pd-Rx Pharmaceuticals	55289-0409-60
90's	$181.98	ZOLOFT, Allscripts Pharmaceutical Company	54569-8579-00
90's	$243.98	ZOLOFT, Prescript Pharmaceuticals	00247-0675-90
100's	$215.55	ZOLOFT, Allscripts Pharmaceutical Company	54569-3724-01
100's	$230.51	ZOLOFT, Physicians Total Care	54868-2192-00
100's	$241.67	ZOLOFT, Southwood Pharmaceuticals Inc	58016-0366-00
100's	$264.68	ZOLOFT, Pfizer U.S. Pharmaceuticals	00049-4900-41
100's	$264.68	ZOLOFT, Pfizer U.S. Pharmaceuticals	00049-4900-66
100's	$315.00	ZOLOFT, Pharma Pac	52959-0361-00

Tablet - Oral - 100 mg

3's	$11.38	ZOLOFT, Prescript Pharmaceuticals	00247-0371-03
6's	$19.40	ZOLOFT, Prescript Pharmaceuticals	00247-0371-06
7's	$22.07	ZOLOFT, Prescript Pharmaceuticals	00247-0371-07
10's	$30.09	ZOLOFT, Prescript Pharmaceuticals	00247-0371-10
14's	$33.73	ZOLOFT, Allscripts Pharmaceutical Company	54569-3575-01
14's	$40.79	ZOLOFT, Prescript Pharmaceuticals	00247-0371-14
15's	$35.63	ZOLOFT, Physicians Total Care	54868-2637-01
15's	$36.14	ZOLOFT, Allscripts Pharmaceutical Company	54569-3575-03
15's	$49.24	ZOLOFT, Quality Care Pharmaceuticals Inc	60346-0707-15
15's	$58.14	ZOLOFT, Pd-Rx Pharmaceuticals	55289-0550-15
20's	$51.27	ZOLOFT, Physicians Total Care	54868-2637-04
28's	$70.12	ZOLOFT, Cheshire Drugs	55175-2716-08
28's	$78.21	ZOLOFT, Prescript Pharmaceuticals	00247-0371-28
30's	$59.45	ZOLOFT, Compumed Pharmaceuticals	00403-4321-30
30's	$67.73	ZOLOFT, Southwood Pharmaceuticals Inc	58016-0137-30
30's	$72.29	ZOLOFT, Allscripts Pharmaceutical Company	54569-3575-02
30's	$76.33	ZOLOFT, Physicians Total Care	54868-2637-00
30's	$83.55	ZOLOFT, Prescript Pharmaceuticals	00247-0371-30
30's	$97.57	ZOLOFT, Quality Care Pharmaceuticals Inc	60346-0707-30
45's	$123.66	ZOLOFT, Prescript Pharmaceuticals	00247-0371-45
50's	$137.04	ZOLOFT, Prescript Pharmaceuticals	00247-0371-50
60's	$135.46	ZOLOFT, Southwood Pharmaceuticals Inc	58016-0137-60
60's	$163.76	ZOLOFT, Prescript Pharmaceuticals	00247-0371-60
100's	$198.50	ZOLOFT, Compumed Pharmaceuticals	00403-4321-01
100's	$237.16	ZOLOFT, Physicians Total Care	54868-2637-03
100's	$240.95	ZOLOFT, Allscripts Pharmaceutical Company	54569-3575-00
100's	$264.68	ZOLOFT, Pfizer U.S. Pharmaceuticals	00049-4910-41
100's	$264.68	ZOLOFT, Pfizer U.S. Pharmaceuticals	00049-4910-66

Sevelamer Hydrochloride *(003422)*

For complete prescribing information, refer to the CD-ROM included with the book.

Categories: Hyperphosphatemia; FDA Approved 1998 Oct; Pregnancy Category C
Drug Classes: Metabolics
Brand Names: Renagel
Cost of Therapy: $127.92 (Hyperphosphatemia; Renagel; 403 mg; 6 capsules/day; 30 day supply)
$123.26 (Hyperphosphatemia; Renagel; 400 mg; 6 tablets/day; 30 day supply)

DESCRIPTION

The active ingredient in Renagel capsules and tablets is sevelamer hydrochloride (HCl), a polymeric phosphate binder intended for oral administration. Sevelamer hydrochloride is poly(allylamine hydrochloride) crosslinked with epichlorohydrin in which 40% of the amines are protonated. It is known chemically as poly(allylamine-co-N,N′-diallyl-1,3-diamino-2-hydroxypropane) hydrochloride. Sevelamer hydrochloride is hydrophilic but insoluble in water.

The primary amine groups are derived directly from poly(allylamine hydrochloride). The crosslinking groups consist of two secondary amine groups derived from poly(allylamine hydrochloride) and one molecule of epichlorohydrin.

TABLETS

Each film-coated tablet of Renagel contains either 800 or 400 mg of sevelamer hydrochloride on an anhydrous basis. The inactive ingredients are hydroxypropyl methylcellulose, diacetylated monoglyceride, colloidal silicon dioxide, and stearic acid. The tablet imprint contains iron oxide black ink.

CAPSULES

Each hard-gelatin capsule of Renagel contains 403 mg of sevelamer hydrochloride on an anhydrous basis. The inactive ingredients are colloidal silicon dioxide and stearic acid. The capsule and imprint contain titanium dioxide and indigo carmine ink.

INDICATIONS AND USAGE

Sevelamer hydrochloride is indicated for the reduction of serum phosphorus in patients with end-stage renal disease (ESRD). The safety and efficacy of sevelamer hydrochloride in ESRD patients who are not on hemodialysis have not been studied. In hemodialysis patients, sevelamer hydrochloride decreases the incidence of hypercalcemic episodes relative to patients on calcium acetate treatment.

CONTRAINDICATIONS

Sevelamer hydrochloride is contraindicated in patients with hypophosphatemia or bowel obstruction. It is also contraindicated in patients known to be hypersensitive to sevelamer hydrochloride or any of its constituents.

DOSAGE AND ADMINISTRATION

DOSAGE RECOMMENDATION

Patients Not Taking a Phosphate Binder

The recommended starting dose of sevelamer hydrochloride is 800-1600 mg, which can be administered as 1-2 sevelamer hydrochloride 800 mg tablets, 2-4 sevelamer hydrochloride 400 mg tablets, or 2-4 sevelamer hydrochloride capsules with each meal, based on serum phosphorus level (see TABLE 3).

TABLE 3 *Starting Dose for Patients Not Taking a Phosphate Binder*

Serum Phosphorus	Sevelamer 800 mg	Sevelamer HCl 400 mg
>6.0 and <7.5 mg/dl	1*	2†
≥7.5 and <9.0 mg/dl	2*	3†
≥9.0 mg/dl	2*	4†

* Number of tablets to be taken 3 times daily with meals.
† Number of capsules to be taken 3 times daily with meals.

Patients Switching From Calcium Acetate

In a study in 84 ESRD patients on hemodialysis, a similar reduction in serum phosphorus was seen with equivalent doses (mg for mg) of sevelamer capsules and calcium acetate (see TABLE 4).

TABLE 4 *Starting Dose for Patients Switching From Calcium Acetate to Sevelamer HCl*

Calcium Acetate 667 mg	Sevelamer 800 mg	Sevelamer HCl 400 mg
1	1*	2†
2	2*	3†
3	3*	5†

* Number of tablets per meals.
† Number of tablets or capsules per meal.

Dose Titration for all Patients Taking Sevelamer Hydrochloride

The dosage should be gradually adjusted based on the serum phosphorus concentration with a goal of lowering serum phosphorus to 6 mg/dl or less. The dose may be increased or decreased by 1 tablet or capsule per meal at 2 week intervals, as necessary. TABLE 5 gives a dose titration guideline. The average dose in Phase 3 clinical trials was 4 capsules (403 mg) per meal. The maximum dose studied was 10 capsules per meal (the equivalent of 5 sevelamer HCl mg tablets per meal or 10 sevelamer HCl 400 mg tablets per meal).

TABLE 5 *Dose Titration Guideline*

Serum Phosphorus	Sevelamer HCl Dose
>6 mg/dl	Increase 1 tablet/capsule per meal at 2 week intervals
3.5-6 mg/dl	Maintain current dose
<3.5 mg/dl	Decrease 1 tablet/capsule per meal

Drug interaction studies have demonstrated that sevelamer hydrochloride capsules have no effect on the bioavailability of digoxin, warfarin, enalapril, or metoprolol. When administering any oral drug for which alteration in blood levels could have a clinically significant effect on safety or efficacy, the drug should be administered at least 1 hour before or 3 hours after sevelamer hydrochloride, or the physician should consider monitoring blood levels of the drug.

PRODUCT LISTING - EQUIVALENTS NOT AVAILABLE

Capsule - Oral - 403 mg
200's $142.13 RENAGEL, Genzyme Corporation 58468-4709-01
Tablet - Oral - 800 mg
180's $246.51 RENAGEL, Genzyme Corporation 58468-0021-01

Sibutramine Hydrochloride *(003372)*

Categories: Obesity, exogenous; Pregnancy Category C; FDA Approved 1997 Dec
Drug Classes: Anorexiants; Stimulants, central nervous system
Brand Names: Meridia
Foreign Brand Availability: Ectiva (Mexico); Plenty (Colombia); Reductil (Australia; Bahrain; Colombia; Cyprus; Egypt; England; Germany; Hong-Kong; Iran; Iraq; Ireland; Israel; Jordan; Korea; Kuwait; Lebanon; Libya; Mexico; New-Zealand; Oman; Peru; Philippines; Qatar; Republic-of-Yemen; Saudi-Arabia; Singapore; South-Africa; Syria; Thailand; United-Arab-Emirates); Sibutral (France); Sibutrex (India)
Cost of Therapy: $89.61 (Weight Loss; Meridia; 10 mg; 1 capsule/day; 30 day supply)

DESCRIPTION

Meridia (sibutramine hydrochloride monohydrate) is an orally administered agent for the treatment of obesity. Chemically, the active ingredient is a racemic mixture of the (+) and (−) enantiomers of cyclobutanemethanamine, 1-(4-chlorophenyl)-*N,N*-dimethyl-α-(2-methylpropyl)-, hydrochloride, monohydrate, and has an empirical formula of $C_{17}H_{29}Cl_2NO$. Its molecular weight is 334.33.

Sibutramine hydrochloride monohydrate is a white to cream crystalline powder with a solubility of 2.9 mg/ml in pH 5.2 water. Its octanol:water partition coefficient is 30.9 at pH 5.0.

Each Meridia capsule contains 5, 10, and 15 mg of sibutramine hydrochloride monohydrate. It also contains as inactive ingredients: lactose monohydrate; microcrystalline cellulose; colloidal silicon dioxide; and magnesium stearate in a hard-gelatin capsule [which contains titanium dioxide; gelatin; FD&C blue no. 2 (5 and 10 mg capsules only); D&C yellow no. 10 (5 and 15 mg capsules only), and other inactive ingredients].

CLINICAL PHARMACOLOGY

MODE OF ACTION

Sibutramine produces its therapeutic effects by norepinephrine, serotonin and dopamine reuptake inhibition. Sibutramine and its major pharmacologically active metabolites (M_1 and M_2) do not act via release of monoamines.

PHARMACODYNAMICS

Sibutramine exerts its pharmacological actions predominantly via its secondary (M_1) and primary (M_2) amine metabolites. The parent compound, sibutramine, is a potent inhibitor of serotonin (5-hydroxytryptamine, 5-HT) and norepinephrine reuptake *in vivo*, but not *in vitro*. However, metabolites M_1 and M_2 inhibit the reuptake of these neurotransmitters both *in vitro* and *in vivo*.

In human brain tissue, M_1 and M_2 also inhibit dopamine reuptake *in vitro*, but with ~3-fold lower potency than for the reuptake inhibition of serotonin or norepinephrine.

TABLE 1 *Potencies of Sibutramine, M_1 and M_2 as In Vitro Inhibitors of Monoamine Reuptake in Human Brain — Potency to Inhibit Monoamine Reuptake (Ki; nM)*

	Serotonin	Norepinephrine	Dopamine
Sibutramine	298	5451	943
M_1	15	20	49
M_2	20	15	45

A study using plasma samples taken from sibutramine-treated volunteers showed monoamine reuptake inhibition of norepinephrine >serotonin >dopamine; maximum inhibitions were norepinephrine = 73%, serotonin = 54% and dopamine = 16%.

Sibutramine and its metabolites (M_1 and M_2) are not serotonin, norepinephrine or dopamine releasing agents. Following chronic administration of sibutramine to rats, no depletion of brain monoamines has been observed.

Sibutramine, M_1 and M_2 exhibit no evidence of anticholinergic or antihistaminergic actions. In addition, receptor binding profiles show that sibutramine, M_1 and M_2 have low affinity for serotonin (5-HT_1, 5-HT_{1A}, 5-HT_{1B}, 5-HT_{2A}, 5-HT_{2C}), norepinephrine (β, β_1, β_3, α_1 and α_2), dopamine (D_1 and D_2), benzodiazepine, and glutamate (NMDA) receptors. These compounds also lack monoamine oxidase inhibitory activity *in vitro* and *in vivo*.

PHARMACOKINETICS

Absorption

Sibutramine is rapidly absorbed from the GI tract (T_{max} of 1.2 hours) following oral administration and undergoes extensive first-pass metabolism in the liver (oral clearance of 1750 L/h and half-life of 1.1 hours) to form the pharmacologically active mono- and di-desmethyl metabolites M_1 and M_2. Peak plasma concentrations of M_1 and M_2 are reached within 3-4 hours. On the basis of mass balance studies, on average, at least 77% of a single oral dose of sibutramine is absorbed. The absolute bioavailability of sibutramine has not been determined.

Distribution

Radiolabeled studies in animals indicated rapid and extensive distribution into tissues: highest concentrations of radiolabeled material were found in the eliminating organs, liver and kidney. *In vitro*, sibutramine, M_1 and M_2 are extensively bound (97%, 94% and 94%, respectively) to human plasma proteins at plasma concentrations seen following therapeutic doses.

Metabolism

Sibutramine is metabolized in the liver principally by the cytochrome P450(3A4) isoenzyme, to desmethyl metabolites, M_1 and M_2. These active metabolites are further metabolized by hydroxylation and conjugation to pharmacologically inactive metabolites, M_5 and M_6. Following oral administration of radiolabeled sibutramine, essentially all of the peak radiolabeled material in plasma was accounted for by unchanged sibutramine (3%), M_1 (6%), M_2 (12%), M_5 (52%), and M_6 (27%).

M_1 and M_2 plasma concentrations reached steady-state within 4 days of dosing and were approximately 2-fold higher than following a single dose. The elimination half-lives of M_1 and M_2, 14 and 16 hours, respectively, were unchanged following repeated dosing.

Excretion

Approximately 85% (range 68-95%) of a single orally administered radiolabeled dose was excreted in urine and feces over a 15 day collection period with the majority of the dose (77%) excreted in the urine. Major metabolites in urine were M_5 and M_6; unchanged sibutramine, M_1, and M_2 were not detected. The primary route of excretion for M_1 and M_2 is hepatic metabolism and for M_5 and M_6 is renal excretion.

S

TABLE 2A *Mean (%CV) and 95% Confidence Intervals of Pharmacokinetic Parameters — (Dose = 15 mg)*

Study Population	C_{max} (ng/ml)	T_{max} (h)
Metabolite M_1		
Target Population:		
Obese subjects (n=18)	4.0 (42) 3.2-4.8	3.6 (28) 3.1-4.1
Special Population:		
Moderate hepatic impairment (n=12)	2.2 (36) 1.8-2.7	3.3 (33) 2.7-3.9
Metabolite M_2		
Target Population:		
Obese subjects (n=18)	6.4 (28) 5.6-7.2	3.5 (17) 3.2-3.8
Special Population:		
Moderate hepatic impairment (n=12)	4.3 (37) 3.4-5.2	3.8 (34) 3.1-4.5

Calculated only up to 24 hours for M_1.

TABLE 2B *Mean (%CV) and 95% Confidence Intervals of Pharmacokinetic Parameters — (Dose = 15 mg)*

Study Population	AUC* (ng·h/ml)	T½ (h)
Metabolite M_1		
Target Population:		
Obese subjects (n=18)	25.5 (63) 18.1-32.9	—
Special Population:		
Moderate hepatic impairment (n=12)	18.7 (65) 11.9-25.5	—
Metabolite M_2		
Target Population:		
Obese subjects (n=18)	92.1 (26) 81.2-103	17.2 (58) 12.5-21.8
Special Population:		
Moderate hepatic impairment (n=12)	90.5 (27) 76.9-104	22.7 (30) 18.9-26.5

* Calculated only up to 24 hours for M_1.

Effect of Food

Administration of a single 20 mg dose of sibutramine with a standard breakfast resulted in reduced peak M_1 and M_2 concentrations (by 27% and 32%, respectively) and delayed the time to peak by approximately 3 hours. However, the AUCs of M_1 and M_2 were not significantly altered.

Special Populations

Geriatric

Plasma concentrations of M_1 and M_2 were similar between elderly (ages 61-77 years) and young (ages 19-30 years) subjects following a single 15 mg oral sibutramine dose. Plasma concentrations of the inactive metabolites M_5 and M_6 were higher in the elderly; these differences are not likely to be of clinical significance. In general, dose selection for an elderly patient should be cautious, reflecting the greater frequency of decreased hepatic, renal, or cardiac function, and of concomitant disease or other drug therapy.

Pediatric

The safety and effectiveness of sibutramine hydrochloride monohydrate capsules in pediatric patients under 16 years old have not been established.

Gender

Pooled pharmacokinetic parameters from 54 young, healthy volunteers (37 males and 17 females) receiving a 15 mg oral dose of sibutramine showed the mean C_{max} and AUC of M_1 and M_2 to be slightly ($\leq$19% and $\leq$36%, respectively) higher in females than males. Somewhat higher steady-state trough plasma levels were observed in female obese patients from a large clinical efficacy trial. However, these differences are not likely to be of clinical significance. Dosage adjustment based upon the gender of a patient is not necessary (see DOSAGE AND ADMINISTRATION).

Race

The relationship between race and steady-state trough M_1 and M_2 plasma concentrations was examined in a clinical trial in obese patients. A trend towards higher concentrations in Black patients over Caucasian patients was noted for M_1 and M_2. However, these differences are not considered to be of clinical significance.

Renal Insufficiency

The effect of renal disease has not been studied. However, since sibutramine and its active metabolites M_1 and M_2 are eliminated by hepatic metabolism, renal disease is unlikely to have a significant effect on their disposition. Elimination of the inactive metabolites M_5 and M_6, which are renally excreted, may be affected in this population. Sibutramine hydrochloride monohydrate should not be used in patients with severe renal impairment.

Hepatic Insufficiency

In 12 patients with moderate hepatic impairment receiving a single 15 mg oral dose of sibutramine, the combined AUCs of M_1 and M_2 were increased by 24% compared to healthy subjects while M_5 and M_6 plasma concentrations were unchanged. The observed differences in M_1 and M_2 concentrations do not warrant dosage adjustment in patients with mild to moderate hepatic impairment. Sibutramine hydrochloride monohydrate should not be used in patients with severe hepatic dysfunction.

INDICATIONS AND USAGE

Sibutramine hydrochloride monohydrate capsules are indicated for the management of obesity, including weight loss and maintenance of weight loss, and should be used in conjunction with a reduced calorie diet. Sibutramine hydrochloride monohydrate is recommended for obese patients with an initial body mass index $\geq$30 kg/m^2, or $\geq$27 kg/m^2 in the presence of other risk factors (*e.g.,* hypertension, diabetes, dyslipidemia).

BMI is calculated by taking the patient's weight, in kg, and dividing by the patient's height, in meters, squared. Metric conversions are as follows: lb ÷ 2.2 = kg; inches × 0.0254 = meters.

CONTRAINDICATIONS

Sibutramine hydrochloride monohydrate capsules are contraindicated in patients receiving monoamine oxidase inhibitors (MAOIs) (see WARNINGS).

Sibutramine hydrochloride monohydrate is contraindicated in patients with hypersensitivity to sibutramine or any of the inactive ingredients of sibutramine hydrochloride monohydrate.

Sibutramine hydrochloride monohydrate is contraindicated in patients who have anorexia nervosa.

Sibutramine hydrochloride monohydrate is contraindicated in patients taking other centrally acting appetite suppressant drugs.

WARNINGS

BLOOD PRESSURE AND PULSE

SIBUTRAMINE HYDROCHLORIDE MONOHYDRATE SUBSTANTIALLY INCREASES BLOOD PRESSURE IN SOME PATIENTS. REGULAR MONITORING OF BLOOD PRESSURE IS REQUIRED WHEN PRESCRIBING SIBUTRAMINE HYDROCHLORIDE MONOHYDRATE.

In placebo-controlled obesity studies, sibutramine hydrochloride monohydrate 5-20 mg once daily was associated with mean increases in systolic and diastolic blood pressure of approximately 1-3 mm Hg relative to placebo, and with mean increases in pulse rate relative to placebo of approximately 4-5 beats/min. Larger increases were seen in some patients, particularly when therapy with sibutramine hydrochloride monohydrate was initiated at the higher doses (see TABLE 6). In pre-marketing placebo-controlled obesity studies, 0.4% of patients treated with sibutramine hydrochloride monohydrate were discontinued for hypertension (SBP $\geq$160 mm Hg or DBP $\geq$95 mm Hg), compared with 0.4% in the placebo group, and 0.4% of patients treated with sibutramine hydrochloride monohydrate were discontinued for tachycardia (pulse rate $\geq$100 bpm), compared with 0.1% in the placebo group. Blood pressure and pulse should be measured prior to starting therapy with sibutramine hydrochloride monohydrate and should be monitored at regular intervals thereafter. For patients who experience a sustained increase in blood pressure or pulse rate while receiving sibutramine hydrochloride monohydrate, either dose reduction or discontinuation should be considered. Sibutramine hydrochloride monohydrate should be given with caution to those patients with a history of hypertension (see DOSAGE AND ADMINISTRATION), and should not be given to patients with uncontrolled or poorly controlled hypertension.

TABLE 6 *Percent Outliers in Studies 1 and 2*

Dose (mg)	% Outliers* SBP	DBP	Pulse
Placebo	9%	7%	12%
5 mg	6%	20%	16%
10 mg	12%	15%	28%
15 mg	13%	17%	24%
20 mg	14%	22%	37%

* Outlier defined as increase from baseline of $\geq$15 mm Hg for 3 consecutive visits (SBP), $\geq$10 mm Hg for 3 consecutive visits (DBP), or pulse $\geq$10 bpm for 3 consecutive visits.

POTENTIAL INTERACTION WITH MONOAMINE OXIDASE INHIBITORS

Sibutramine hydrochloride monohydrate is a norepinephrine, serotonin and dopamine reuptake inhibitor and should not be used concomitantly with MAOIs (see DRUG INTERACTIONS). There should be at least a 2 week interval after stopping MAOIs before commencing treatment with sibutramine hydrochloride monohydrate. Similarly, there should be at least a 2 week interval after stopping sibutramine hydrochloride monohydrate before starting treatment with MAOIs.

CONCOMITANT CARDIOVASCULAR DISEASE

Treatment with sibutramine hydrochloride monohydrate has been associated with increases in heart rate and/or blood pressure. Therefore, sibutramine hydrochloride monohydrate should not be used in patients with a history of coronary artery disease, congestive heart failure, arrhythmias, or stroke.

GLAUCOMA

Because sibutramine hydrochloride monohydrate can cause mydriasis, it should be used with caution in patients with narrow angle glaucoma.

MISCELLANEOUS

Organic causes of obesity (*e.g.,* untreated hypothyroidism) should be excluded before prescribing sibutramine hydrochloride monohydrate.

PRECAUTIONS

PULMONARY HYPERTENSION

Certain centrally-acting weight loss agents that cause release of serotonin from nerve terminals have been associated with pulmonary hypertension (PPH), a rare but lethal disease. In premarketing clinical studies, no cases of PPH have been reported with sibutramine hydrochloride monohydrate capsules. Because of the low incidence of this disease in the underlying population, however, it is not known whether or not sibutramine hydrochloride monohydrate may cause this disease.

SEIZURES

During premarketing testing, seizures were reported in <0.1% of sibutramine hydrochloride monohydrate treated patients. Sibutramine hydrochloride monohydrate should be used cautiously in patients with a history of seizures. It should be discontinued in any patient who develops seizures.

GALLSTONES

Weight loss can precipitate or exacerbate gallstone formation.

RENAL/HEPATIC DYSFUNCTION

Patients with severe renal impairment or severe hepatic dysfunction have not been systematically studied; sibutramine hydrochloride monohydrate should therefore not be used in such patients.

INTERFERENCE WITH COGNITIVE AND MOTOR PERFORMANCE

Although sibutramine did not affect psychomotor or cognitive performance in healthy volunteers, any CNS active drug has the potential to impair judgment, thinking or motor skills.

INFORMATION FOR THE PATIENT

Physicians should instruct their patients to read the patient package insert before starting therapy with sibutramine hydrochloride monohydrate and to reread it each time the prescription is renewed.

Physicians should also discuss with their patients any part of the package insert that is relevant to them. In particular, the importance of keeping appointments for follow-up visits should be emphasized.

Patients should be advised to notify their physician if they develop a rash, hives, or other allergic reactions.

Patients should be advised to inform their physicians if they are taking, or plan to take, any prescription or over-the-counter drugs, especially weight-reducing agents, decongestants, antidepressants, cough suppressants, lithium, dihydroergotamine, sumatriptan, or tryptophan, since there is a potential for interactions.

Patients should be reminded of the importance of having their blood pressure and pulse monitored at regular intervals.

CARCINOGENESIS, MUTAGENESIS, AND IMPAIRMENT OF FERTILITY

Carcinogenesis

Sibutramine was administered in the diet to mice (1.25, 5, or 20 mg/kg/day) and rats (1, 3, or 9 mg/kg/day) for 2 years generating combined maximum plasma AUCs of the two major active metabolites equivalent to 0.4 and 16 times, respectively, those following a daily human dose of 15 mg. There was no evidence of carcinogenicity in mice or in female rats. In male rats there was a higher incidence of benign tumors of the testicular interstitial cells; such tumors are commonly seen in rats and are hormonally mediated. The relevance of these tumors to humans is not known.

Mutagenicity

Sibutramine was not mutagenic in the Ames test, *in vitro* Chinese hamster V79 cell mutation assay, *in vitro* clastogenicity assay in human lymphocytes or micronucleus assay in mice. Its two major active metabolites were found to have equivocal bacterial mutagenic activity in the Ames test. However, both metabolites gave consistently negative results in the *in vitro* Chinese hamster V79 cell mutation assay, *in vitro* clastogenicity assay in human lymphocytes, *in vitro* DNA-repair assay in HeLa cells, micronucleus assay in mice and *in vivo* unscheduled DNA-synthesis assay in rat hepatocytes.

Impairment of Fertility

In rats, there were no effects on fertility at doses generating combined plasma AUCs of the two major active metabolites up to 32 times those following a human dose of 15 mg. At 13 times the human combined AUC, there was maternal toxicity, and the dams' nest-building behavior was impaired, leading to a higher incidence of perinatal mortality; there was no effect at approximately 4 times the human combined AUC.

PREGNANCY, TERATOGENIC EFFECTS, PREGNANCY CATEGORY C

Radiolabeled studies in animals indicated that tissue distribution was unaffected by pregnancy, with relatively low transfer to the fetus. In rats, there was no evidence of teratogenicity at doses of 1, 3, or 10 mg/kg/day generating combined plasma AUCs of the two major active metabolites up to approximately 32 times those following human dose of 15 mg. In rabbits dosed at 3, 15, or 75 mg/kg/day, plasma AUCs greater than approximately 5 times those following the human dose of 15 mg caused maternal toxicity. At markedly toxic doses, Dutch Belted rabbits had a slightly higher than control incidence of pups with a broad short snout, short rounded pinnae, short tail and, in some, shorter thickened long bones in the limbs; at comparably high doses in New Zealand White rabbits, one study showed a slightly higher than control incidence of pups with cardiovascular anomalies while a second study showed a lower incidence than in the control group.

No adequate and well controlled studies with sibutramine hydrochloride monohydrate capsules have been conducted in pregnant women. The use of sibutramine hydrochloride monohydrate during pregnancy is not recommended. Women of child-bearing potential should employ adequate contraception while taking sibutramine hydrochloride monohydrate. Patients should be advised to notify their physician if they become pregnant or intend to become pregnant during therapy.

NURSING MOTHERS

It is not known whether sibutramine or its metabolites are excreted in human milk. Sibutramine hydrochloride monohydrate is not recommended for use in nursing mothers. Patients should be advised to notify their physician if they are breast-feeding.

PEDIATRIC USE

The safety and effectiveness of sibutramine hydrochloride monohydrate in pediatric patients under 16 years of age have not been established.

GERIATRIC USE

Clinical studies of sibutramine hydrochloride monohydrate did not include sufficient numbers of patients aged 65 and over to determine whether they respond differently from younger patients. In general, dose selection for an elderly patient should be cautious, reflecting the greater frequency of decreased hepatic, renal, or cardiac function, and of concomitant disease or other drug therapy. Pharmacokinetics in elderly patients are discussed in CLINICAL PHARMACOLOGY.

DRUG INTERACTIONS

CNS ACTIVE DRUGS

The use of sibutramine hydrochloride monohydrate capsules in combination with other CNS-active drugs, particularly serotonergic agents, has not been systematically evaluated. Consequently, caution is advised if the concomitant administration of sibutramine hydrochloride monohydrate with other centrally-acting drugs is indicated (see CONTRAINDICATIONS and WARNINGS).

In patients receiving monoamine oxidase inhibitors (MAOIs) (*e.g.*, phenelzine, selegiline) in combination with serotonergic agents (*e.g.*, fluoxetine, fluvoxamine, paroxetine, sertraline, venlafaxine), there have been reports of serious, sometimes fatal, reactions ("serotonin syndrome;" see below). Because sibutramine hydrochloride monohydrate inhibits serotonin reuptake, sibutramine hydrochloride monohydrate should not be used concomitantly with a MAOI (see CONTRAINDICATIONS). At least 2 weeks should elapse between discontinuation of a MAOI and initiation of treatment with sibutramine hydrochloride monohydrate. Similarly, at least 2 weeks should elapse between discontinuation of sibutramine hydrochloride monohydrate and initiation of treatment with a MAOI.

The rare, but serious, constellation of symptoms termed "serotonin syndrome" has also been reported with the concomitant use of selective serotonin reuptake inhibitors and agents for migraine therapy, such as sumatriptan succinate and dihydroergotamine, certain opioids, such as dextromethorphan, meperidine, pentazocine and fentanyl, lithium, or tryptophan. Serotonin syndrome has also been reported with the concomitant use of two serotonin reuptake inhibitors. The syndrome requires immediate medical attention and may include one or more of the following symptoms: excitement, hypomania, restlessness, loss of consciousness, confusion, disorientation, anxiety, agitation, motor weakness, myoclonus, tremor, hemiballismus, hyperreflexia, ataxia, dysarthria, incoordination, hyperthermia, shivering, pupillary dilation, diaphoresis, emesis, and tachycardia.

Because sibutramine hydrochloride monohydrate inhibits serotonin reuptake, in general, it should not be administered with other serotonergic agents such as those listed above. However, if such a combination is clinically indicated, appropriate observation of the patient is warranted.

DRUGS THAT MAY RAISE BLOOD PRESSURE AND/OR HEART RATE

Concomitant use of sibutramine hydrochloride monohydrate and other agents that may raise blood pressure or heart rate have not been evaluated. These include certain decongestants, cough, cold, and allergy medications that contain agents such as ephedrine, or pseudoephedrine. Caution should be used when prescribing sibutramine hydrochloride monohydrate to patients who use these medications.

DRUGS THAT INHIBIT CYTOCHROME P450(3A4) METABOLISM

In vitro studies indicated that the cytochrome P450(3A4)-mediated metabolism of sibutramine was inhibited by ketoconazole and to a lesser extent by erythromycin. Clinical interaction trials were conducted on these substrates. The potential for such interactions is described below.

Ketoconazole

Concomitant administration of 200 mg doses of ketoconazole twice daily and 20 mg sibutramine once daily for 7 days in 12 uncomplicated obese subjects resulted in moderate increases in AUC and C_{max} of 58% and 36% for M_1 and of 20% and 19% for M_2, respectively.

Erythromycin

The steady-state pharmacokinetics of sibutramine and metabolites M_1 and M_2 were evaluated in 12 uncomplicated obese subjects following concomitant administration of 500 mg of erythromycin 3 times daily and 20 mg of sibutramine once daily for 7 days. Concomitant erythromycin resulted in small increases in the AUC (less than 14%) for M_1 and M_2. A small reduction in C_{max} for M_1 (11%) and a slight increase in C_{max} for M_2 (10%) were observed.

CIMETIDINE

Concomitant administration of cimetidine 400 mg twice daily and sibutramine 15 mg once daily for 7 days in 12 volunteers resulted in small increases in combined (M_1 and M_2) plasma C_{max} (3.4%) and AUC (7.3%); these differences are unlikely to be of clinical significance.

ALCOHOL

In a double-blind, placebo-controlled, crossover study in 19 volunteers, administration of a single dose of ethanol (0.5 ml/kg) together with 20 mg of sibutramine resulted in no psychomotor interactions of clinical significance between alcohol and sibutramine. However, the concomitant use of sibutramine hydrochloride monohydrate capsules and excess alcohol is not recommended.

ORAL CONTRACEPTIVES

The suppression of ovulation by oral contraceptives was not inhibited by sibutramine hydrochloride monohydrate. In a crossover study, 12 healthy female volunteers on oral steroid contraceptives received placebo in one period and 15 mg sibutramine in another period over the course of 8 weeks. No clinically significant systemic interaction was observed; therefore, no requirement for alternative contraceptive precautions are needed when patients taking oral contraceptives are concurrently prescribed sibutramine.

DRUGS HIGHLY BOUND TO PLASMA PROTEINS

Although sibutramine and its active metabolites M_1 and M_2 are extensively bound to plasma proteins (≥94%), the low therapeutic concentrations and basic characteristics of these compounds make them unlikely to result in clinically significant protein binding interactions with other highly protein bound drugs such as warfarin and phenytoin. *In vitro* protein binding interaction studies have not been conducted.

ADVERSE REACTIONS

In placebo-controlled studies, 9% of patients treated with sibutramine hydrochloride monohydrate (n=2068) and 7% of patients treated with placebo (n=884) withdrew for adverse events.

In placebo-controlled studies, the most common events were dry mouth, anorexia, insomnia, constipation and headache. Adverse events in these studies occurring in ≥1% of sibutramine hydrochloride monohydrate treated patients and more frequently than in the placebo group are shown in TABLE 7.

S

TABLE 7

Body System/Adverse Event	Obese Patients in Placebo-Controlled Studies: Sibutramine HCl Monohydrate (n=2068)	Placebo (n=884)
Body as a Whole		
Headache	30.3%	18.6%
Back pain	8.2%	5.5%
Flu syndrome	8.2%	5.8%
Injury accident	5.9%	4.1%
Asthenia	5.9%	5.3%
Abdominal pain	4.5%	3.6%
Chest pain	1.8%	1.2%
Neck pain	1.6%	1.1%
Allergic reaction	1.5%	0.8%
Cardiovascular System		
Tachycardia	2.6%	0.6%
Vasodilation	2.4%	0.9%
Migraine	2.4%	2.0%
Hypertension/increased blood pressure	2.1%	0.9%
Palpitation	2.0%	0.8%
Digestive System		
Anorexia	13.0%	3.5%
Constipation	11.5%	6.0%
Increased appetite	8.7%	2.7%
Nausea	5.9%	2.8%
Dyspepsia	5.0%	2.6%
Gastritis	1.7%	1.2%
Vomiting	1.5%	1.4%
Rectal disorder	1.2%	0.5%
Metabolic & Nutritional		
Thirst	1.7%	0.9%
Generalized edema	1.2%	0.8%
Musculoskeletal System		
Arthralgia	5.9%	5.0%
Myalgia	1.9%	1.1%
Tenosynovitis	1.2%	0.5%
Joint disorder	1.1%	0.6%
Nervous System		
Dry mouth	17.2%	4.2%
Insomnia	10.7%	4.5%
Dizziness	7.0%	3.4%
Nervousness	5.2%	2.9%
Anxiety	4.5%	3.4%
Depression	4.3%	2.5%
Paresthesia	2.0%	0.5%
Somnolence	1.7%	0.9%
CNS stimulation	1.5%	0.5%
Emotional lability	1.3%	0.6%
Respiratory System		
Rhinitis	10.2%	7.1%
Pharyngitis	10.0%	8.4%
Sinusitis	5.0%	2.6%
Cough increase	3.8%	3.3%
Laryngitis	1.3%	0.9%
Skin & Appendages		
Rash	3.8%	2.5%
Sweating	2.5%	0.9%
Herpes simplex	1.3%	1.0%
Acne	1.0%	0.8%
Special Senses		
Taste perversion	2.2%	0.8%
Ear disorder	1.7%	0.9%
Ear pain	1.1%	0.7%
Urogenital System		
Dysmenorrhea	3.5%	1.4%
Urinary tract infection	2.3%	2.0%
Vaginal monilia	1.2%	0.5%
Metrorrhagia	1.0%	0.8%

The following additional adverse events were reported in ≥1% of all patients who received sibutramine hydrochloride monohydrate capsules in controlled and uncontrolled pre-marketing studies:

Body as a Whole: Fever.
Digestive System: Diarrhea, flatulence, gastroenteritis, tooth disorder.
Metabolic and Nutritional: Peripheral edema.
Musculoskeletal System: Arthritis.
Nervous System: Agitation, leg cramps, hypertonia, thinking abnormal.
Respiratory System: Bronchitis, dyspnea.
Skin and Appendages: Pruritus.
Special Senses: Amblyopia.
Urogenital System: Menstrual disorder.

OTHER NOTABLE ADVERSE EVENTS

Postmarketing Report

Voluntary reports of adverse events temporally associated with the use of sibutramine hydrochloride monohydrate are listed below. It is important to emphasize that although these events occurred during treatment with sibutramine hydrochloride monohydrate, they may have no causal relationship with the drug. Obesity itself, concurrent disease states/risk factors, or weight reduction may be associated with an increased risk for some of these events:

Abnormal dreams, abnormal ejaculation, abnormal gait, abnormal vision, alopecia, amnesia, anaphylactic shock, anaphylactoid reaction, anemia, anger, angina pectoris, arthrosis, atrial fibrillation, blurred vision, bursitis, cerebrovascular accident, chest pressure, chest tightness, cholecystitis, cholelithiasis, concentration impaired, confusion, congestive heart failure, depression aggravated, dermatitis, dry eye, duodenal ulcer, epistaxis, eructation, eye pain, facial edema, gastrointestinal hemorrhage, Gilles de la Tourette's syndrome, goiter, heart arrest, heart rate decreased, hematuria, hyperglycemia, hyperthyroidism, hypesthesia, hypoglycemia, hypothyroidism, impotence, increased intraocular pressure, increased salivation, increased urinary frequency, intestinal obstruction, leukopenia, libido decreased, libido increased, limb pain, lymphadenopathy, manic reaction, micturition difficulty, mood changes, mouth ulcer, myocardial infarction, nasal congestion, nightmares, otitis externa, otitis media, petechiae, photosensitivity (eyes), photosensitivity (skin), respiratory disorder, serotonin syndrome, short term memory loss, speech disorder, stomach ulcer, sudden unexplained death, supraventricular tachycardia, syncope, thrombocytopenia, tinnitus, edema, torsade de pointes, transient ischemic attack, tremor, twitch, urticaria vascular headache, ventricular tachycardia, ventricular extrasystoles, ventricular fibrillation, vertigo, yawn.

Seizures: Convulsions were reported as an adverse event in 3 of 2068 (0.1%) sibutramine hydrochloride monohydrate treated patients and in none of 884 placebo-treated patients in placebo-controlled premarketing obesity studies. Two (2) of the 3 patients with seizures had potentially predisposing factors (1 had a prior history of epilepsy; 1 had a subsequent diagnosis of brain tumor). The incidence in all subjects who received sibutramine hydrochloride monohydrate (3 of 4588 subjects) was less than 0.1%.

Ecchymosis/Bleeding Disorders: Ecchymosis (bruising) was observed in 0.7% of sibutramine hydrochloride monohydrate capsules treated patients and in 0.2% of placebo-treated patients in premarketing placebo-controlled obesity studies. One (1) patient had prolonged bleeding of a small amount which occurred during minor facial surgery. Sibutramine hydrochloride monohydrate may have an effect on platelet function due to its effect on serotonin uptake.

Interstitial Nephritis: Acute interstitial nephritis (confirmed by biopsy) was reported in 1 obese patient receiving sibutramine hydrochloride monohydrate during premarketing studies. After discontinuation of the medication, dialysis and oral corticosteroids were administered; renal function normalized. The patient made a full recovery.

Altered Laboratory Findings: Abnormal liver function tests, including increases in AST, ALT, GGT, LDH, alkaline phosphatase and bilirubin, were reported as adverse events in 1.6% of sibutramine hydrochloride monohydrate-treated obese patients in placebo-controlled trials compared with 0.8% of placebo patients. In these studies, potentially clinically significant values (total bilirubin ≥2 mg/dl; ALT, AST, GGT, LDH, or alkaline phosphatase ≥3 times upper limit of normal) occurred in 0% (alkaline phosphatase) to 0.6% (ALT) of the sibutramine hydrochloride monohydrate treated patients and in none of the placebo-treated patients. Abnormal values tended to be sporadic, often diminished with continued treatment, and did not show a clear dose-response relationship.

DOSAGE AND ADMINISTRATION

The recommended starting dose of sibutramine hydrochloride monohydrate capsules are 10 mg administered once daily with or without food. If there is inadequate weight loss, the dose may be titrated after 4 weeks to a total of 15 mg once daily. The 5 mg dose should be reserved for patients who do not tolerate the 10 mg dose. Blood pressure and heart rate changes should be taken into account when making decisions regarding dose titration (see PRECAUTIONS).

Doses above 15 mg daily are not recommended. In most of the clinical trials, sibutramine hydrochloride monohydrate was given in the morning.

Analysis of numerous variables has indicated that approximately 60% of patients who lose at least 4 lb in the first 4 weeks of treatment with a given dose of sibutramine hydrochloride monohydrate in combination with a reduced-calorie diet lose at least 5% (placebo-subtracted) of their initial body weight by the end of 6 months to 1 year of treatment on that dose of sibutramine hydrochloride monohydrate. Conversely, approximately, 80% of patients who do not lose at least 4 lb in the first 4 weeks of treatment with a given dose of sibutramine hydrochloride monohydrate do not lose at least 5% (placebo-subtracted) of their initial body weight by the end of 6 months to 1 year of treatment on that dose. If a patient has not lost at least 4 lb in the first 4 weeks of treatment, the physician should consider reevaluation of therapy which may include increasing the dose or discontinuation of sibutramine hydrochloride monohydrate.

The safety and effectiveness of sibutramine hydrochloride monohydrate, as demonstrated in double-blind, placebo-controlled trials, have not been determined beyond 2 years at this time.

HOW SUPPLIED

Meridia capsules contain 5, 10, or 15 mg sibutramine hydrochloride monohydrate and are supplied as follows:

5 mg: Blue/yellow capsules imprinted with "MERIDIA" on the cap and "-5-" on the body.

10 mg: Blue/white capsules imprinted with "MERIDIA" on the cap and "-10-" on the body.

15 mg: Yellow/white capsules imprinted with "MERIDIA" on the cap and "-15-" on the body.

Storage: Store at 2-5°C (77°F); excursions permitted to 15-30°C (59-86°F). Protect capsules from heat and moisture. Dispense in a tight, light-resistant container.

PRODUCT LISTING - EQUIVALENTS NOT AVAILABLE

Capsule - Oral - 5 mg

100's	$313.76	MERIDIA, Knoll Pharmaceutical Company	00048-0605-01
100's	$321.63	MERIDIA, Abbott Pharmaceutical	00074-2456-13

Capsule - Oral - 10 mg

100's	$298.70	MERIDIA, Knoll Pharmaceutical Company	00048-0610-01
100's	$321.63	MERIDIA, Abbott Pharmaceutical	00074-2457-13

Capsule - Oral - 15 mg

100's	$386.25	MERIDIA, Knoll Pharmaceutical Company	00048-0615-01
100's	$415.88	MERIDIA, Abbott Pharmaceutical	00074-2458-13

Sildenafil Citrate *(003400)*

Categories: Erectile dysfunction; FDA Approved 1998 Mar; Pregnancy Category B
Drug Classes: Impotence agents
Brand Names: Viagra
Foreign Brand Availability: Aphrodil (Bahrain; Cyprus; Egypt; Iran; Iraq; Jordan; Kuwait; Lebanon; Libya; Oman; Qatar; Republic-of-Yemen; Saudi-Arabia; Syria; United-Arab-Emirates); Edegra (India); Ejertol (Colombia); Erilin (Colombia); Eroxim (Colombia); Patrex (Austria; Belgium; Bulgaria; Czech-Republic; Denmark; England; Finland; France; Germany; Greece; Hungary; Ireland; Italy; Netherlands; Norway; Poland; Portugal; Slovenia; Spain; Sweden; Switzerland; Turkey); Penegra (Benin; Burkina-Faso; Ethiopia; Gambia; Ghana; Guinea; India; Ivory-Coast; Kenya; Liberia; Malawi; Mali; Mauritania; Mauritius; Morocco; Niger; Nigeria; Senegal; Seychelles; Sierra-Leone; Sudan; Tanzania; Tunia; Uganda; Zambia; Zimbabwe); Vigain (Bahrain; Cyprus; Egypt; Iran; Iraq; Jordan; Kuwait; Lebanon; Libya; Oman; Qatar; Republic-of-Yemen; Saudi-Arabia; Syria; United-Arab-Emirates); Zwagra (Bahrain; Cyprus; Egypt; Iran; Iraq; Jordan; Kuwait; Lebanon; Libya; Oman; Qatar; Republic-of-Yemen; Saudi-Arabia; Syria; United-Arab-Emirates)
Cost of Therapy: $303.79 (Erectile Dysfunction; Viagra; 50 mg; 1 tablet/day; 30 day supply)

DESCRIPTION

Viagra, an oral therapy for erectile dysfunction, is the citrate salt of sildenafil, a selective inhibitor of cyclic guanosine monophosphate (cGMP)-specific phosphodiesterase type 5 (PDE5).

Sildenafil citrate is designated chemically as 1-[[3-(6,7-dihydro-1-methyl-7-oxo-3-propyl-1*H*-pyrazolo[4,3-*d*]pyrimidin-5-yl)-4-ethoxyphenyl]sulfonyl]-4-methylpiperazine citrate.

Sildenafil citrate is a white to off-white crystalline powder with a solubility of 3.5 mg/ml in water and a molecular weight of 666.7. Viagra is formulated as blue, film-coated, rounded-diamond-shaped tablets equivalent to 25, 50, and 100 mg of sildenafil for oral administration. In addition to the active ingredient, sildenafil citrate, each tablet contains the following inactive ingredients: microcrystalline cellulose, anhydrous dibasic calcium phosphate, croscarmellose sodium, magnesium stearate, hydroxypropyl methylcellulose, titanium dioxide, lactose, triacetin, and FD&C blue no. 2 aluminum lake.

CLINICAL PHARMACOLOGY

MECHANISM OF ACTION

The physiologic mechanism of erection of the penis involves release of nitric oxide (NO) in the corpus cavernosum during sexual stimulation. NO then activates the enzyme guanylate cyclase, which results in increased levels of cGMP, producing smooth muscle relaxation in the corpus cavernosum and allowing inflow of blood. Sildenafil has no direct relaxant effect on isolated human corpus cavernosum, but enhances the effect of NO by inhibiting PDE5, which is responsible for degradation of cGMP in the corpus cavernosum. When sexual stimulation causes local release of NO, inhibition of PDE5 by sildenafil causes increased levels of cGMP in the corpus cavernosum, resulting in smooth muscle relaxation and inflow of blood to the corpus cavernosum. Sildenafil at recommended doses has no effect in the absence of sexual stimulation.

Studies *in vitro* have shown that sildenafil is selective for PDE5. Its effect is more potent on PDE5 than on other known phosphodiesterases (10-fold for PDE6, >80-fold for PDE1, >700-fold for PDE2, PDE3, PDE4, PDE7, PDE8, PDE9, PDE10, and PDE11). The approximately 4000-fold selectivity for PDE5 versus PDE3 is important because PDE3 is involved in the control of cardiac contractility. Sildenafil is only about 10-fold as potent for PDE5 compared to PDE6, an enzyme found in the retina which is involved in the phototransduction pathway of the retina. This lower selectivity is thought to be the basis for abnormalities related to color vision observed with higher doses or plasma levels (see Pharmacodynamics).

In addition to human corpus cavernosum smooth muscle, PDE5 is also found in lower concentrations in other tissues including platelets, vascular and visceral smooth muscle, and skeletal muscle. The inhibition of PDE5 in these tissues by sildenafil may be the basis for the enhanced platelet antiaggregatory activity of nitric oxide observed *in vitro*, an inhibition of platelet thrombus formation *in vivo* and peripheral arterial-venous dilatation *in vivo*.

PHARMACOKINETICS AND METABOLISM

Sildenafil citrate is rapidly absorbed after oral administration, with absolute bioavailability of about 40%. Its pharmacokinetics are dose-proportional over the recommended dose range. It is eliminated predominantly by hepatic metabolism (mainly cytochrome P450 3A4) and is converted to an active metabolite with properties similar to the parent, sildenafil. The concomitant use of potent cytochrome P450 3A4 inhibitors (*e.g.*, erythromycin, ketoconazole, itraconazole) as well as the nonspecific CYP inhibitor, cimetidine, is associated with increased plasma levels of sildenafil (see DOSAGE AND ADMINISTRATION). Both sildenafil and the metabolite have terminal half lives of about 4 hours.

ABSORPTION AND DISTRIBUTION

Sildenafil citrate is rapidly absorbed. Maximum observed plasma concentrations are reached within 30-120 minutes (median 60 minutes) of oral dosing in the fasted state. When sildenafil citrate is taken with a high fat meal, the rate of absorption is reduced, with a mean delay in T_{max} of 60 minutes and a mean reduction in C_{max} of 29%. The mean steady state volume of distribution (Vss) for sildenafil is 105 L, indicating distribution into the tissues. Sildenafil and its major circulating N-desmethyl metabolite are both approximately 96% bound to plasma proteins. Protein binding is independent of total drug concentrations.

Based upon measurements of sildenafil in semen of healthy volunteers 90 minutes after dosing, less than 0.001% of the administered dose may appear in the semen of patients.

METABOLISM AND EXCRETION

Sildenafil is cleared predominantly by the CYP3A4 (major route) and CYP2C9 (minor route) hepatic microsomal isoenzymes. The major circulating metabolite results from N-desmethylation of sildenafil, and is itself further metabolized. This metabolite has a PDE selectivity profile similar to sildenafil and an *in vitro* potency for PDE5 approximately 50% of the parent drug. Plasma concentrations of this metabolite are approximately 40% of those seen for sildenafil, so that the metabolite accounts for about 20% of sildenafil's pharmacologic effects.

After either oral or intravenous administration, sildenafil is excreted as metabolites predominantly in the feces (approximately 80% of administered oral dose) and to a lesser extent in the urine (approximately 13% of the administered oral dose). Similar values for pharmacokinetic parameters were seen in normal volunteers and in the patient population, using a population pharmacokinetic approach.

PHARMACOKINETICS IN SPECIAL POPULATIONS

Geriatrics

Healthy elderly volunteers (65 years or over) had a reduced clearance of sildenafil, with free plasma concentrations approximately 40% greater than those seen in healthy younger volunteers (18-45 years).

Renal Insufficiency

In volunteers with mild (CLCR = 50-80 ml/min) and moderate (CLCR = 30-49 ml/min) renal impairment, the pharmacokinetics of a single oral dose of sildenafil citrate (50 mg) were not altered. In volunteers with severe (CLCR = <30 ml/min) renal impairment, sildenafil clearance was reduced, resulting in approximately doubling of AUC and C_{max} compared to age-matched volunteers with no renal impairment.

Hepatic Insufficiency

In volunteers with hepatic cirrhosis (Child-Pugh A and B), sildenafil clearance was reduced, resulting in increases in AUC (84%) and C_{max} (47%) compared to age-matched volunteers with no hepatic impairment.

Therefore, age >65, hepatic impairment and severe renal impairment are associated with increased plasma levels of sildenafil. A starting oral dose of 25 mg should be considered in those patients (see DOSAGE AND ADMINISTRATION).

PHARMACODYNAMICS

Effects of Sildenafil Citrate on Erectile Response

In eight double-blind, placebo-controlled crossover studies of patients with either organic or psychogenic erectile dysfunction, sexual stimulation resulted in improved erections, as assessed by an objective measurement of hardness and duration of erections (RigiScan), after sildenafil citrate administration compared with placebo. Most studies assessed the efficacy of sildenafil citrate approximately 60 minutes post dose. The erectile response, as assessed by RigiScan, generally increased with increasing sildenafil dose and plasma concentration. The time course of effect was examined in one study, showing an effect for up to 4 hours but the response was diminished compared to 2 hours.

Effects of Sildenafil Citrate on Blood Pressure

Single oral doses of sildenafil (100 mg) administered to healthy volunteers produced decreases in supine blood pressure (mean maximum decrease in systolic/diastolic blood pressure of 8.4/5.5 mm Hg). The decrease in blood pressure was most notable approximately 1-2 hours after dosing, and was not different than placebo at 8 hours. Similar effects on blood pressure were noted with 25, 50, and 100 mg of sildenafil citrate, therefore the effects are not related to dose or plasma levels within this dosage range. Larger effects were recorded among patients receiving concomitant nitrates (see CONTRAINDICATIONS).

Effects of Sildenafil Citrate on Cardiac Parameters

Single oral doses of sildenafil up to 100 mg produced no clinically relevant changes in the ECGs of normal male volunteers.

Studies have produced relevant data on the effects of sildenafil citrate on cardiac output. In one small, open-label, uncontrolled pilot study, 8 patients with stable ischemic heart disease underwent Swan-Ganz catheterization. A total dose of 40 mg sildenafil was administered by 4 intravenous infusions.

The results from this pilot study are shown in TABLE 1A and TABLE 1B; the mean resting systolic and diastolic blood pressures decreased by 7 and 10% compared to baseline in these patients. Mean resting values for right atrial pressure, pulmonary artery pressure, pulmonary artery occluded pressure, and cardiac output decreased by 28%, 28%, 20%, and 7% respectively. Even though this total dosage produced plasma sildenafil concentrations which were approximately 2-5 times higher than the mean maximum plasma concentrations following a single oral dose of 100 mg in healthy male volunteers, the hemodynamic response to exercise was preserved in these patients.

TABLE 1A *Hemodynamic Data in Patients With Stable Ischemic Heart Disease After IV Administration of 40 mg Sildenafil: At Rest*

Means ±SD	Baseline (B2)		Sildenafil (D1)	
PAOP (mm Hg)	n=8	8.1 ± 5.1	n=8	6.5 ± 4.3
Mean PAP (mm Hg)	n=8	16.7 ± 4	n=8	12.1 ± 3.9
Mean RAP (mm Hg)	n=7	5.7 ± 3.7	n=8	4.1 ± 3.7
Systolic SAP (mm Hg)	n=8	150.4 ± 12.4	n=8	140.6 ± 16.5
Diastolic SAP (mm Hg)	n=8	73.6 ± 7.8	n=8	65.9 ± 10
Cardiac output (L/min)	n=8	5.6 ± 0.9	n=8	5.2 ± 1.1
Heart rate (bpm)	n=8	67 ± 11.1	n=8	66.9 ± 12

TABLE 1B *Hemodynamic Data in Patients With Stable Ischemic Heart Disease After IV Administration of 40 mg Sildenafil: After 4 Minutes of Exercise*

Means ±SD	Baseline		Sildenafil	
PAOP (mm Hg)	n=8	36.0 ± 13.7	n=8	27.8 ± 15.3
Mean PAP (mm Hg)	n=8	39.4 ± 12.9	n=8	31.7 ± 13.2
Systolic SAP (mm Hg)	n=8	199.5 ± 37.4	n=8	187.8 ± 30.0
Diastolic SAP (mm Hg)	n=8	84.6 ± 9.7	n=8	79.5 ± 9.4
Cardiac output (L/min)	n=8	11.5 ± 2.4	n=8	10.2 ± 3.5
Heart rate (bpm)	n=8	101.9 ± 11.6	n=8	99.0 ± 20.4

In a double-blind study, 144 patients with erectile dysfunction and chronic stable angina limited by exercise, not receiving chronic oral nitrates, were randomized to a single dose of placebo or sildenafil citrate 100 mg 1 hour prior to exercise testing. The primary endpoint was time to limiting angina in the evaluable cohort. The mean times (adjusted for baseline) to onset of limiting angina were 423.6 and 403.7 seconds for sildenafil (n=70) and placebo, respectively. These results demonstrated that the effect of sildenafil citrate on the primary endpoint was statistically non-inferior to placebo.

Effects of Sildenafil Citrate on Vision

At single oral doses of 100 and 200 mg, transient dose-related impairment of color discrimination (blue/green) was detected using the Farnsworth-Munsell 100-hue test, with peak effects near the time of peak plasma levels. This finding is consistent with the inhibition of PDE6, which is involved in phototransduction in the retina. An evaluation of visual function at doses up to twice the maximum recommended dose revealed no effects of sildenafil citrate on visual acuity, intraocular pressure, or pupillometry.

INDICATIONS AND USAGE

Sildenafil citrate is indicated for the treatment of erectile dysfunction.

NON-FDA APPROVED INDICATIONS

Although not uses approved by the FDA, sildenafil has been studied for use as a diagnostic aid in evaluating erectile dysfunction arising from vascular insufficiency, as well as treatment for sexual arousal disorder in premenopausal women.

CONTRAINDICATIONS

Consistent with its known effects on the nitric oxide/cGMP pathway (see CLINICAL PHARMACOLOGY), sildenafil citrate was shown to potentiate the hypotensive effects of nitrates, and its administration to patients who are using organic nitrates, either regularly and/or intermittently, in any form is therefore contraindicated.

After patients have taken sildenafil citrate, it is unknown when nitrates, if necessary, can be safely administered. Based on the pharmacokinetic profile of a single 100 mg oral dose given to healthy normal volunteers, the plasma levels of sildenafil at 24 hours post dose are approximately 2 ng/ml (compared to peak plasma levels of approximately 440 ng/ml) (see CLINICAL PHARMACOLOGY, Pharmacokinetics and Metabolism). In the following patients: age >65, hepatic impairment (*e.g.,* cirrhosis), severe renal impairment (*e.g.,* creatinine clearance <30 ml/min), and concomitant use of potent cytochrome P450 3A4 inhibitors (erythromycin), plasma levels of sildenafil at 24 hours post dose have been found to be 3-8 times higher than those seen in healthy volunteers. Although plasma levels of sildenafil at 24 hours post dose are much lower than at peak concentration, it is unknown whether nitrates can be safely coadministered at this time point.

Sildenafil citrate is contraindicated in patients with a known hypersensitivity to any component of the tablet.

WARNINGS

There is a potential for cardiac risk of sexual activity in patients with preexisting cardiovascular disease. Therefore, treatments for erectile dysfunction, including sildenafil citrate, should not be generally used in men for whom sexual activity is inadvisable because of their underlying cardiovascular status.

Sildenafil citrate has systemic vasodilatory properties that resulted in transient decreases in supine blood pressure in healthy volunteers (mean maximum decrease of 8.4/5.5 mm Hg), (see CLINICAL PHARMACOLOGY, Pharmacodynamics). While this normally would be expected to be of little consequence in most patients, prior to prescribing sildenafil citrate, physicians should carefully consider whether their patients with underlying cardiovascular disease could be affected adversely by such vasodilatory effects, especially in combination with sexual activity.

Patients with the following underlying conditions can be particularly sensitive to the actions of vasodilators including sildenafil citrate — those with left ventricular outflow obstruction (*e.g.,* aortic stenosis, idiopathic hypertrophic subaortic stenosis) and those with severely impaired autonomic control of blood pressure.

There is no controlled clinical data on the safety or efficacy of sildenafil citrate in the following groups; if prescribed, this should be done with caution:

- Patients who have suffered a myocardial infarction, stroke, or life-threatening arrhythmia within the last 6 months.
- Patients with resting hypotension (BP <90/50) or hypertension (BP >170/110).
- Patients with cardiac failure or coronary artery disease causing unstable angina.
- Patients with retinitis pigmentosa (a minority of these patients have genetic disorders of retinal phosphodiesterases).

Prolonged erection greater than 4 hours and priapism (painful erections greater than 6 hours in duration) have been reported infrequently since market approval of sildenafil citrate. In the event of an erection that persists longer than 4 hours, the patient should seek immediate medical assistance. If priapism is not treated immediately, penile tissue damage and permanent loss of potency could result.

The concomitant administration of the protease inhibitor ritonavir substantially increases serum concentrations of sildenafil **(11-fold increase in AUC).** If sildenafil citrate is prescribed to patients taking ritonavir, caution should be used. Data from subjects exposed to high systemic levels of sildenafil are limited. Visual disturbances occurred more commonly at higher levels of sildenafil exposure. Decreased blood pressure, syncope, and prolonged erection were reported in some healthy volunteers exposed to high doses of sildenafil (200-800 mg). To decrease the chance of adverse events in patients taking ritonavir, a decrease in sildenafil dosage is recommended (see DRUG INTERACTIONS,ADVERSE REACTIONS, and DOSAGE AND ADMINISTRATION).

PRECAUTIONS

GENERAL

The evaluation of erectile dysfunction should include a determination of potential underlying causes and the identification of appropriate treatment following a complete medical assessment.

Before prescribing sildenafil citrate, it is important to note the following:

Patients on multiple antihypertensive medications were included in the pivotal clinical trials for sildenafil citrate. In a separate drug interaction study, when amlodipine 5 or 10 mg, and sildenafil citrate 100 mg were orally administered concomitantly to hypertensive patients mean additional blood pressure reduction of 8 mm Hg systolic and 7 mm Hg diastolic were noted (see DRUG INTERACTIONS).

When the alpha blocker doxazosin (4 mg) and sildenafil citrate (25 mg) were administered simultaneously to patients with benign prostatic hyperplasia (BPH), mean additional reductions of supine blood pressure of 7 mm Hg systolic and 7 mm Hg diastolic were observed. When higher doses of sildenafil citrate and doxazosin (4 mg) were administered simultaneously, there were infrequent reports of patients who experienced symptomatic postural hypotension within 1-4 hours of dosing. Simultaneous administration of sildenafil citrate to patients taking alpha-blocker therapy may lead to symptomatic hypotension in some patients. Therefore, sildenafil citrate doses above 25 mg should not be taken within 4 hours of taking an alpha-blocker.

The safety of sildenafil citrate is unknown in patients with bleeding disorders and patients with active peptic ulceration.

Sildenafil citrate should be used with caution in patients with anatomical deformation of the penis (such as angulation, cavernosal fibrosis or Peyronie's disease), or in patients who have conditions which may predispose them to priapism (such as sickle cell anemia, multiple myeloma, or leukemia).

The safety and efficacy of combinations of sildenafil citrate with other treatments for erectile dysfunction have not been studied. Therefore, the use of such combinations is not recommended.

In humans, sildenafil citrate has no effect on bleeding time when taken alone or with aspirin. *In vitro* studies with human platelets indicate that sildenafil potentiates the antiaggregatory effect of sodium nitroprusside (a nitric oxide donor). The combination of heparin and sildenafil citrate had an additive effect on bleeding time in the anesthetized rabbit, but this interaction has not been studied in humans.

INFORMATION FOR THE PATIENT

Physicians should discuss with patients the contraindication of sildenafil citrate with regular and/or intermittent use of organic nitrates.

Physicians should discuss with patients the potential cardiac risk of sexual activity in patients with preexisting cardiovascular risk factors. Patients who experience symptoms (*e.g.,* angina pectoris, dizziness, nausea) upon initiation of sexual activity should be advised to refrain from further activity and should discuss the episode with their physician.

Physicians should warn patients that prolonged erections greater than 4 hours and priapism (painful erections greater than 6 hours in duration) have been reported infrequently since market approval of sildenafil citrate. In the event of an erection that persists longer than 4 hours, the patient should seek immediate medical assistance. If priapism is not treated immediately, penile tissue damage and permanent loss of potency may result.

Physicians should advise patients that simultaneous administration of sildenafil citrate doses above 25 mg and an alpha-blocker may lead to symptomatic hypotension in some patients. Therefore, sildenafil citrate doses above 25 mg should not be taken within 4 hours of taking an alpha-blocker.

The use of sildenafil citrate offers no protection against sexually transmitted diseases. Counseling of patients about the protective measures necessary to guard against sexually transmitted diseases, including the Human Immunodeficiency Virus (HIV), may be considered.

CARCINOGENESIS, MUTAGENESIS, AND IMPAIRMENT OF FERTILITY

Sildenafil was not carcinogenic when administered to rats for 24 months at a dose resulting in total systemic drug exposure (AUCs) for unbound sildenafil and its major metabolite of 29 and 42 times, for male and female rats, respectively, the exposures observed in human males given the Maximum Recommended Human Dose (MRHD) of 100 mg. Sildenafil was not carcinogenic when administered to mice for 18-21 months at dosages up to the Maximum Tolerated Dose (MTD) of 10 mg/kg/day, approximately 0.6 times the MRHD on a mg/m^2 basis.

Sildenafil was negative in *in vitro* bacterial and Chinese hamster ovary cell assays to detect mutagenicity, and *in vitro* human lymphocytes and *in vivo* mouse micronucleus assays to detect clastogenicity.

There was no impairment of fertility in rats given sildenafil up to 60 mg/kg/day for 36 days to females and 102 days to males, a dose producing an AUC value of more than 25 times the human male AUC.

There was no effect on sperm motility or morphology after single 100 mg oral doses of sildenafil citrate in healthy volunteers.

PREGNANCY, NURSING MOTHERS, AND PEDIATRIC USE

Sildenafil citrate is not indicated for use in newborns, children, or women.

PREGNANCY CATEGORY B

No evidence of teratogenicity, embryotoxicity or fetotoxicity was observed in rats and rabbits which received up to 200 mg/kg/day during organogenesis. These doses represent, respectively, about 20 and 40 times the MRHD on a mg/m^2 basis in a 50 kg subject. In the rat pre- and postnatal development study, the no observed adverse effect dose was 30 mg/kg/day given for 36 days. In the nonpregnant rat the AUC at this dose was about 20 times human AUC. There are no adequate and well-controlled studies of sildenafil in pregnant women.

GERIATRIC USE

Healthy elderly volunteers (65 years or over) had a reduced clearance of sildenafil (see CLINICAL PHARMACOLOGY, Pharmacokinetics in Special Populations). Since higher plasma levels may increase both the efficacy and incidence of adverse events, a starting dose of 25 mg should be considered (see DOSAGE AND ADMINISTRATION).

DRUG INTERACTIONS

EFFECTS OF OTHER DRUGS ON SILDENAFIL CITRATE

In Vitro Studies: Sildenafil metabolism is principally mediated by the cytochrome P450 (CYP) isoforms 3A4 (major route) and 2C9 (minor route). Therefore, inhibitors of these isoenzymes may reduce sildenafil clearance.

In Vivo Studies: Cimetidine (800 mg), a nonspecific CYP inhibitor, caused a 56% increase in plasma sildenafil concentrations when coadministered with sildenafil citrate (50 mg) to healthy volunteers.

When a single 100 mg dose of sildenafil citrate was administered with erythromycin, a specific CYP3A4 inhibitor, at steady state (500 mg bid for 5 days), there was a 182% increase in sildenafil systemic exposure (AUC). In addition, in a study performed in healthy male volunteers, coadministration of the HIV protease inhibitor saquinavir, also a CYP3A4 inhibitor, at steady state (1200 mg tid) with sildenafil citrate (100 mg single dose) resulted in a 140% increase in sildenafil C_{max} and a 210% increase in sildenafil AUC. Sildenafil citrate had no effect on saquinavir pharmacokinetics. Stronger CYP3A4 inhibitors such as ketoconazole or itraconazole would be expected to have still greater effects, and population data from patients in clinical trials did indicate a reduction in sildenafil clearance when it was coadministered with CYP3A4 inhibitors (such as ketoconazole, erythromycin, or cimetidine) (see DOSAGE AND ADMINISTRATION).

In another study of healthy male volunteers, coadministration with the HIV protease inhibitor ritonavir, which is a highly potent P450 inhibitor, at steady state (500 mg bid) with sildenafil citrate (100 mg single dose) resulted in a 300% (4-fold) increase in sildenafil C_{max} and a 1000% (11-fold) increase in sildenafil plasma AUC. At 24 hours the plasma levels of sildenafil were still approximately 200 ng/ml, compared to approximately 5 ng/ml when sildenafil was dosed alone. This is consistent with ritonavir's marked effects on a broad range of P450 substrates. Sildenafil citrate had no effect on ritonavir pharmacokinetics (see DOSAGE AND ADMINISTRATION).

Although the interaction between other protease inhibitors and sildenafil has not been studied, their concomitant use is expected to increase sildenafil levels.

It can be expected that concomitant administration of CYP3A4 inducers, such as rifampin, will decrease plasma levels of sildenafil.

Single doses of antacid (magnesium hydroxide/aluminum hydroxide) did not affect the bioavailability of sildenafil citrate.

Pharmacokinetic data from patients in clinical trials showed no effect on sildenafil pharmacokinetics of CYP2C9 inhibitors (such as tolbutamide, warfarin), CYP2D6 inhibitors (such as selective serotonin reuptake inhibitors, tricyclic antidepressants), thiazide and related diuretics, ACE inhibitors, and calcium channel blockers. The AUC of the active metabolite, N-desmethyl sildenafil, was increased 62% by loop and potassium-sparing diuretics and 102% by nonspecific beta-blockers. These effects on the metabolite are not expected to be of clinical consequence.

EFFECTS OF SILDENAFIL CITRATE ON OTHER DRUGS

In Vitro Studies: Sildenafil is a weak inhibitor of the cytochrome P450 isoforms 1A2, 2C9, 2C19, 2D6, 2E1, and 3A4 (IC50 >150 μM). Given sildenafil peak plasma concentrations of approximately 1 μM after recommended doses, it is unlikely that sildenafil citrate will alter the clearance of substrates of these isoenzymes.

In Vivo Studies: When sildenafil citrate 100 mg oral was coadministered with amlodipine, 5 or 10 mg oral, to hypertensive patients, the mean additional reduction on supine blood pressure was 8 mm Hg systolic and 7 mm Hg diastolic.

No significant interactions were shown with tolbutamide (250 mg) or warfarin (40 mg), both of which are metabolized by CYP2C9.

Sildenafil citrate (50 mg) did not potentiate the increase in bleeding time caused by aspirin (150 mg).

Sildenafil citrate (50 mg) did not potentiate the hypotensive effect of alcohol in healthy volunteers with mean maximum blood alcohol levels of 0.08%.

In a study of healthy male volunteers, sildenafil (100 mg) did not affect the steady state pharmacokinetics of the HIV protease inhibitors, saquinavir and ritonavir, both of which are CYP3A4 substrates.

ADVERSE REACTIONS

PRE-MARKETING EXPERIENCE

Sildenafil citrate was administered to over 3700 patients (aged 19-87 years) during clinical trials worldwide. Over 550 patients were treated for longer than 1 year.

In placebo-controlled clinical studies, the discontinuation rate due to adverse events for sildenafil citrate (2.5%) was not significantly different from placebo (2.3%). The adverse events were generally transient and mild to moderate in nature.

In trials of all designs, adverse events reported by patients receiving sildenafil citrate were generally similar. In fixed-dose studies the incidence of some adverse events increased with dose. The nature of the adverse events in flexible-dose studies, which more closely reflects the recommended dosage regimen, was similar to that for fixed-dose studies.

When sildenafil citrate was taken as recommended (on an as-needed basis) in flexible-dose, placebo-controlled clinical trials, the adverse events in TABLE 2 were reported.

TABLE 2 *Adverse Events Reported by ≥2% of Patients Treated With Sildenafil Citrate and More Frequent on Drug Than Placebo in PRN Flexible-Dose Phase 2/3 Studies*

	Percentage of Patients Reporting Event	
	Sildenafil Citrate	Placebo
Adverse Event	n=734	n=725
Headache	16%	4%
Flushing	10%	1%
Dyspepsia	7%	2%
Nasal congestion	4%	2%
Urinary tract infection	3%	2%
Abnormal vision*	3%	0%
Diarrhea	3%	1%
Dizziness	2%	1%
Rash	2%	1%

* Abnormal vision: mild and transient, predominantly color tinge to vision, but also increased sensitivity to light or blurred vision. In these studies, only 1 patient discontinued due to abnormal vision.

Other adverse reactions occurred at a rate of >2%, but equally common on placebo: Respiratory tract infection, back pain, flu syndrome, and arthralgia.

In fixed-dose studies, dyspepsia (17%) and abnormal vision (11%) were more common at 100 mg than at lower doses. At doses above the recommended dose range, adverse events were similar to those detailed above but generally were reported more frequently.

The following events occurred in <2% of patients in controlled clinical trials; a causal relationship to sildenafil citrate is uncertain. Reported events include those with a plausible relation to drug use; omitted are minor events and reports too imprecise to be meaningful:

Body as a Whole: Face edema, photosensitivity reaction, shock, asthenia, pain, chills, accidental fall, abdominal pain, allergic reaction, chest pain, accidental injury.

Cardiovascular: Angina pectoris, AV block, migraine, syncope, tachycardia, palpitation, hypotension, postural hypotension, myocardial ischemia, cerebral thrombosis, cardiac arrest, heart failure, abnormal electrocardiogram, cardiomyopathy.

Digestive: Vomiting, glossitis, colitis, dysphagia, gastritis, gastroenteritis, esophagitis, stomatitis, dry mouth, liver function tests abnormal, rectal hemorrhage, gingivitis.

Hemic and Lymphatic: Anemia and leukopenia.

Metabolic and Nutritional: Thirst, edema, gout, unstable diabetes, hyperglycemia, peripheral edema, hyperuricemia, hypoglycemic reaction, hypernatremia.

Musculoskeletal: Arthritis, arthrosis, myalgia, tendon rupture, tenosynovitis, bone pain, myasthenia, synovitis.

Nervous: Ataxia, hypertonia, neuralgia, neuropathy, paresthesia, tremor, vertigo, depression, insomnia, somnolence, abnormal dreams, reflexes decreased, hypesthesia.

Respiratory: Asthma, dyspnea, laryngitis, pharyngitis, sinusitis, bronchitis, sputum increased, cough increased.

Skin and Appendages: Urticaria, herpes simplex, pruritus, sweating, skin ulcer, contact dermatitis, exfoliative dermatitis.

Special Senses: Mydriasis, conjunctivitis, photophobia, tinnitus, eye pain, deafness, ear pain, eye hemorrhage, cataract, dry eyes.

Urogenital: Cystitis, nocturia, urinary frequency, breast enlargement, urinary incontinence, abnormal ejaculation, genital edema and anorgasmia.

POST-MARKETING EXPERIENCE

Cardiovascular and Cerebrovascular

Serious cardiovascular, crerebrovascular, and vascular events, including myocardial infarction, sudden cardiac death, ventricular arrhythmia, cerebrovascular hemorrhage, transient ischemic attack, hypertension, subarachnoid and intracerebral hemorrhages, and pulmonary hemorrhage have been reported post-marketing in temporal association with the use of sildenafil citrate. Most, but not all, of these patients had preexisting cardiovascular risk factors. Many of these events were reported to occur during or shortly after sexual activity, and a few were reported to occur shortly after the use of sildenafil citrate without sexual activity. Others were reported to have occurred hours to days after the use of sildenafil citrate and sexual activity. It is not possible to determine whether these events are related directly to sildenafil citrate, to sexual activity, to the patient's underlying cardiovascular disease, to a combination of these factors, or to other factors (see WARNINGS for further important cardiovascular information).

Other Events

Other events reported post-marketing to have been observed in temporal association with sildenafil citrate and not listed in Pre-Marketing Experience include:

Nervous: Seizure and anxiety.

Urogenital: Prolonged erection, priapism (see WARNINGS) and hematuria.

Special Senses: Diplopia, temporary vision loss/decreased vision, ocular redness or bloodshot appearance, ocular burning, ocular swelling/pressure, increased intraocular pressure, retinal vascular disease or bleeding, vitreous detachment/traction, paramacular edema and epistaxis.

DOSAGE AND ADMINISTRATION

For most patients, the recommended dose is 50 mg taken, as needed, approximately 1 hour before sexual activity. However, sildenafil citrate may be taken anywhere from 4 hours to 0.5 hour before sexual activity. Based on effectiveness and toleration, the dose may be increased to a maximum recommended dose of 100 mg or decreased to 25 mg. The maximum recommended dosing frequency is once per day.

The following factors are associated with increased plasma levels of sildenafil: Age >65 (40% increase in AUC), hepatic impairment (*e.g.*, cirrhosis, 80%), severe renal impairment (creatinine clearance <30 ml/min, 100%), and concomitant use of potent cytochrome P450 3A4 inhibitors [ketoconazole, itraconazole, erythromycin (182%), saquinavir (210%)]. Since higher plasma levels may increase both the efficacy and incidence of adverse events, a starting dose of 25 mg should be considered in these patients.

Ritonavir greatly increased the systemic level of sildenafil in a study of healthy non-HIV infected volunteers (11-fold increase in AUC, see DRUG INTERACTIONS). Based on these pharmacokinetic data, it is recommended not to exceed a maximum single dose of 25 mg of sildenafil citrate in a 48 hour period.

Sildenafil citrate was shown to potentiate the hypotensive effects of nitrates and its administration in patients who use nitric oxide donors or nitrates in any form is therfore contraindicated.

Simultaneous administration of sildenafil citrate doses above 25 mg and an alpha-blocker may lead to symptomatic hypotension in some patients. Doses of 50 mg or 100 mg of sildenafil citrate should not be taken within 4 hours of alpha-blocker administration. A 25 mg dose of sildenafil citrate may be taken at any time.

S

HOW SUPPLIED

Viagra is supplied as blue, film-coated, rounded-diamond-shaped tablets containing sildenafil citrate equivalent to the nominally indicated amount of sildenafil as follows:

25 mg: Imprinted "VGR25" on obverse side, "PFIZER" on reverse.

50 mg: Imprinted "VGR50" on obverse side, "PFIZER" on reverse.

100 mg: Imprinted "VGR100" on obverse side, "PFIZER" on reverse.

Recommended Storage: Store at 25°C (77°F); excursions permitted to 15-30°C (59-86°F).

PRODUCT LISTING - EQUIVALENTS NOT AVAILABLE

Qty	Price	Product	NDC
Tablet - Oral - 25 mg			
10's	$90.21	VIAGRA, Allscripts Pharmaceutical Company	54569-4568-00
30's	$303.79	VIAGRA, Pfizer U.S. Pharmaceuticals	00069-4200-30
Tablet - Oral - 50 mg			
5's	$45.11	VIAGRA, Allscripts Pharmaceutical Company	54569-4569-01
5's	$52.12	VIAGRA, Physicians Total Care	54868-4084-00
6's	$54.13	VIAGRA, Allscripts Pharmaceutical Company	54569-4569-03
8's	$72.17	VIAGRA, Allscripts Pharmaceutical Company	54569-4569-04
10's	$90.21	VIAGRA, Allscripts Pharmaceutical Company	54569-4569-00
30's	$270.64	VIAGRA, Allscripts Pharmaceutical Company	54569-4569-02
30's	$303.79	VIAGRA, Pfizer U.S. Pharmaceuticals	00069-4210-30
100's	$1012.63	VIAGRA, Pfizer U.S. Pharmaceuticals	00069-4210-66
Tablet - Oral - 100 mg			
6's	$54.13	VIAGRA, Allscripts Pharmaceutical Company	54569-4570-02
10's	$90.21	VIAGRA, Allscripts Pharmaceutical Company	54569-4570-00
10's	$126.65	VIAGRA, Pd-Rx Pharmaceuticals	55289-0523-10
30's	$270.64	VIAGRA, Allscripts Pharmaceutical Company	54569-4570-01
30's	$303.79	VIAGRA, Pfizer U.S. Pharmaceuticals	00069-4220-30
100's	$1012.63	VIAGRA, Pfizer U.S. Pharmaceuticals	00069-4220-66

Simvastatin *(003088)*

For related information, see the comparative table section in Appendix A.

Categories: Coronary heart disease, prevention; Hypercholesterolemia; Hyperlipidemia; Myocardial infarction, prophylaxis; Stroke, prophylaxis; Pregnancy Category X; FDA Approved 1991 Dec

Drug Classes: Antihyperlipidemics; HMG CoA reductase inhibitors

Brand Names: Zocor

Foreign Brand Availability: Bestatin (Thailand); Cholestat (Indonesia); Colastatina (Colombia); Denan (Germany); Ethicol (Indonesia); Eucor (Thailand); Kolestevan (Costa-Rica); Lipex (Australia); Lipinorm (Indonesia); Liponorm (Italy); Lipovas (Japan); Lodales (France); Normofat (Indonesia); Nor-Vastina (El-Salvador); Rechol (Indonesia); Simbado (Indonesia); Simchol (Indonesia); Simcor (Indonesia); Simovil (Israel); Simvacor (Israel); Simvatin (Bahrain; Cyprus; Egypt; Iran; Iraq; Jordan; Kuwait; Lebanon; Libya; Oman; Qatar; Republic-of-Yemen; Saudi-Arabia; Syria; United-Arab-Emirates); Simvor (Singapore; Thailand); Simvotin (India); Sinvacor (Italy); Sivastin (Italy); Statin (Colombia); Valemia (Indonesia); Vasotenal (Peru); Vazim (Indonesia); Zimmex (Thailand); Zocord (Austria; Sweden); Zocor Forte (Germany); Zovast (Indonesia)

Cost of Therapy: $123.98 (Hypercholesterolemia; Zocor; 20 mg; 1 tablet/day; 30 day supply)

DESCRIPTION

Zocor (simvastatin) is a lipid-lowering agent that is derived synthetically from a fermentation product of *Aspergillus terreus.* After oral ingestion, simvastatin, which is an inactive lactone, is hydrolyzed to the corresponding β-hydroxyacid form. This is an inhibitor of 3-hydroxy-3-methylglutaryl-coenzyme A (HMG-CoA) reductase. This enzyme catalyzes the conversion of HMG-CoA to mevalonate, which is an early and rate-limiting step in the biosynthesis of cholesterol.

Simvastatin is butanoic acid, 2,2-dimethyl-,1,2,3,7,8,8a-hexahydro-3,7-dimethyl-8-[2-(tetrahydro-4-hydroxy-6-oxo-2*H*-pyran-2-yl)-ethyl]-1-naphthalenyl ester,[1*S*-[1α,3α,7β,8β(2*S**,4*S**),-8aβ]]. The empirical formula of simvastatin is $C_{25}H_{38}O_5$ and its molecular weight is 418.57.

Simvastatin is a white to off-white, nonhygroscopic, crystalline powder that is practically insoluble in water, and freely soluble in chloroform, methanol and ethanol.

Zocor tablets for oral administration contain either 5, 10, 20, 40, or 80 mg of simvastatin and the following inactive ingredients: cellulose, hydroxypropyl cellulose, hydroxypropyl methylcellulose, iron oxides, lactose, magnesium stearate, starch, talc, titanium dioxide and other ingredients. Butylated hydroxyanisole is added as a preservative.

CLINICAL PHARMACOLOGY

The involvement of low-density lipoprotein cholesterol (LDL-C) in atherogenesis has been well-documented in clinical and pathological studies, as well as in many animal experiments. Epidemiological studies have established that elevated plasma levels of total cholesterol (total-C), LDL-C, and apolipoprotein B (Apo B) promote human atherosclerosis and are risk factors for developing cardiovascular disease, while increased levels of high-density lipoprotein cholesterol (HDL-C) and its transport complex, Apo A-I, are associated with decreased cardiovascular risk. High plasma triglycerides (TG) and cholesterol-enriched TG-rich lipoproteins, including very-low-density lipoproteins (VLDL), intermediate-density lipoproteins (IDL), and remnants, can also promote atherosclerosis. Elevated plasma TG are frequently found in a triad with low HDL-C and small LDL particles, as well as in association with non-lipid metabolic risk factors for CHD. As such, total plasma TG has not consistently been shown to be an independent risk factor for CHD. Furthermore, the independent effect of raising HDL-C or lowering TG on the risk of coronary and cardiovascular morbidity and mortality has not been determined.

In the Scandinavian Simvastatin Survival Study (4S), the effect of improving lipoprotein levels with simvastatin on total mortality was assessed in 4444 patients with CHD and baseline total cholesterol (total-C) 212-309 mg/dl (5.5-8.0 mmol/L). The patients were followed for a median of 5.4 years. In this multicenter, randomized, double-blind, placebo-controlled study, simvastatin significantly reduced the risk of mortality by 30% (11.5% vs 8.2%, placebo versus simvastatin); of CHD mortality by 42% (8.5% vs 5.0%); and of having a hospital-verified non-fatal myocardial infarction by 37% (19.6% vs 12.9%). Furthermore, simvastatin significantly reduced the risk for undergoing myocardial revascularization procedures (coronary artery bypass grafting or percutaneous transluminal coronary angioplasty) by 37% (17.2% vs 11.4%).

Simvastatin has been shown to reduce both normal and elevated LDL-C concentrations. LDL is formed from very-low-density lipoprotein (VLDL) and is catabolized predominantly by the high-affinity LDL receptor. The mechanism of the LDL-lowering effect of simvastatin may involve both reduction of VLDL cholesterol concentration, and induction of the LDL receptor, leading to reduced production and/or increased catabolism of LDL-C. Apo B also falls substantially during treatment with simvastatin. As each LDL particle contains 1 molecule of Apo B, and since in patients with predominant elevations in LDL-C (without accompanying elevation in VLDL) little Apo B is found in other lipoproteins, this strongly suggests that simvastatin does not merely cause cholesterol to be lost from LDL, but also reduces the concentration of circulating LDL particles. In addition, simvastatin reduces VLDL and TG and increases HDL-C. The effects of simvastatin on Lp(a), fibrinogen, and certain other independent biochemical risk markers for CHD are unknown.

Simvastatin is a specific inhibitor of HMG-CoA reductase, the enzyme that catalyzes the conversion of HMG-CoA to mevalonate. The conversion of HMG-CoA to mevalonate is an early step in the biosynthetic pathway for cholesterol.

PHARMACOKINETICS

Simvastatin is a lactone that is readily hydrolyzed *in vivo* to the corresponding β-hydroxyacid, a potent inhibitor of HMG-CoA reductase. Inhibition of HMG-CoA reductase is the basis for an assay in pharmacokinetic studies of the β-hydroxyacid metabolites (active inhibitors) and, following base hydrolysis, active plus latent inhibitors (total inhibitors) in plasma following administration of simvastatin.

Following an oral dose of ^{14}C-labeled simvastatin in man, 13% of the dose was excreted in urine and 60% in feces. The latter represents absorbed drug equivalents excreted in bile, as well as any unabsorbed drug. Plasma concentrations of total radioactivity (simvastatin plus ^{14}C-metabolites) peaked at 4 hours and declined rapidly to about 10% of peak by 12 hours postdose. Absorption of simvastatin, estimated relative to an IV reference dose, in each of 2 animal species tested, averaged about 85% of an oral dose. In animal studies, after oral dosing, simvastatin achieved substantially higher concentrations in the liver than in non-target tissues. Simvastatin undergoes extensive first-pass extraction in the liver, its primary site of action, with subsequent excretion of drug equivalents in the bile. As a consequence of extensive hepatic extraction of simvastatin (estimated to be >60% in man), the availability of drug to the general circulation is low. In a single-dose study in 9 healthy subjects, it was estimated that less than 5% of an oral dose of simvastatin reaches the general circulation as active inhibitors. Following administration of simvastatin tablets, the coefficient of variation, based on between-subject variability, was approximately 48% for the area under the concentration-time curve (AUC) for total inhibitory activity in the general circulation.

Both simvastatin and its β-hydroxyacid metabolite are highly bound (approximately 95%) to human plasma proteins. Animal studies have not been performed to determine whether simvastatin crosses the blood-brain and placental barriers. However, when radiolabeled simvastatin was administered to rats, simvastatin-derived radioactivity crossed the blood-brain barrier.

The major active metabolites of simvastatin present in human plasma are the β-hydroxyacid of simvastatin and its 6′-hydroxy, 6′-hydroxymethyl, and 6′-exomethylene derivatives. Peak plasma concentrations of both active and total inhibitors were attained within 1.3-2.4 hours postdose. While the recommended therapeutic dose range is 5-80 mg/day, there was no substantial deviation from linearity of AUC of inhibitors in the general circulation with an increase in dose to as high as 120 mg. Relative to the fasting state, the plasma profile of inhibitors was not affected when simvastatin was administered immediately before an American Heart Association recommended low-fat meal.

In a study including 16 elderly patients between 70-78 years of age who received simvastatin 40 mg/day, the mean plasma level of HMG-CoA reductase inhibitory activity was increased approximately 45% compared with 18 patients between 18-30 years of age. Clinical study experience in the elderly (n=1522), suggests that there were no overall differences in safety between elderly and younger patients (see PRECAUTIONS,Geriatric Use).

Kinetic studies with another reductase inhibitor, having a similar principal route of elimination, have suggested that for a given dose level higher systemic exposure may be achieved in patients with severe renal insufficiency (as measured by creatinine clearance).

In a study of 12 healthy volunteers, simvastatin at the 80 mg dose had no effect on the metabolism of the probe cytochrome P450 isoform 3A4 (CYP3A4) substrates midazolam and erythromycin. This indicates that simvastatin is not an inhibitor of CYP3A4, and, therefore, is not expected to affect the plasma levels of other drugs metabolized by CYP3A4.

The risk of myopathy is increased by high levels of HMG-CoA reductase inhibitory activity in plasma. Potent inhibitors of CYP3A4 can raise the plasma levels of HMG-CoA reductase inhibitory activity and increase the risk of myopathy (see WARNINGS, Myopathy/Rhabdomyolysis and DRUG INTERACTIONS).

Simvastatin is a substrate for CYP3A4 (see DRUG INTERACTIONS). Grapefruit juice contains 1 or more components that inhibit CYP3A4 and can increase the plasma concentrations of drugs metabolized by CYP3A4. In 1 study[1], 10 subjects consumed 200 ml of double-strength grapefruit juice (1 can of frozen concentrate diluted with 1 rather than 3 cans of water) 3 times daily for 2 days and an additional 200 ml double-strength grapefruit juice together with and 30 and 90 minutes following a single dose of 60 mg simvastatin on the third day. This regimen of grapefruit juice resulted in mean increases in the concentration (as measured by the area under the concentration-time curve) of active and total HMG-CoA reductase inhibitory activity [measured using a radioenzyme inhibition assay both

S

before (for active inhibitors) and after (for total inhibitors) base hydrolysis] of 2.4-fold and 3.6-fold, respectively, and of simvastatin and its β-hydroxyacid metabolite [measured using a chemical assay — liquid chromatography/tandem mass spectrometry] of 16-fold and 7-fold, respectively. In a second study, 16 subjects consumed one 8 oz glass of single-strength grapefruit juice (1 can of frozen concentrate diluted with 3 cans of water) with breakfast for 3 consecutive days and a single dose of 20 mg simvastatin in the evening of the third day. This regimen of grapefruit juice resulted in a mean increase in the plasma concentration (as measured by the area under the concentration-time curve) of active and total HMG-CoA reductase inhibitory activity [using a validated enzyme inhibition assay different from that used in the first[1] study, both before (for active inhibitors) and after (for total inhibitors) base hydrolysis] of 1.13-fold and 1.18-fold, respectively, and of simvastatin and its β-hydroxyacid metabolite [measured using a chemical assay — liquid chromatography/tandem mass spectrometry] of 1.88-fold and 1.31-fold, respectively. The effect of amounts of grapefruit juice between those used in these 2 studies on simvastatin pharmacokinetics has not been studied.

INDICATIONS AND USAGE

Therapy with lipid-altering agents should be considered in those individuals at increased risk for atherosclerosis-related clinical events as a function of cholesterol level, the presence of CHD, or other risk factors. Lipid-altering agents should be used in addition to a diet restricted in saturated fat and cholesterol when the response to diet and other nonpharmacological measures alone has been inadequate (see TABLE 6).

CORONARY HEART DISEASE

In patients with coronary heart disease and hypercholesterolemia, simvastatin is indicated to:

- Reduce the risk of total mortality by reducing coronary death.
- Reduce the risk of non-fatal myocardial infarction.
- Reduce the risk for undergoing myocardial revascularization procedures.
- Reduce the risk of stroke or transient ischemic attack.

HYPERLIPIDEMIA

- Simvastatin is indicated to reduce elevated total-C, LDL-C, Apo B, and TG, and to increase HDL-C in patients with primary hypercholesterolemia (heterozygous familial and nonfamilial) and mixed dyslipidemia (Fredrickson Types IIa and IIb [see TABLE 5]).
- Simvastatin is indicated for the treatment of patients with hypertriglyceridemia (Fredrickson Type IV hyperlipidemia).
- Simvastatin is indicated for the treatment of patients with primary dysbetalipoproteinemia (Fredrickson Type III hyperlipidemia).
- Simvastatin is also indicated to reduce total-C and LDL-C in patients with homozygous familial hypercholesterolemia as an adjunct to other lipid-lowering treatments (*e.g.*, LDL apheresis) or if such treatments are unavailable.

TABLE 5 *Classification of Hyperlipoproteinemias*

Type	Lipoproteins Elevated	Lipid Elevations: Major	Minor
I (rare)	Chylomicrons	TG	C*
IIa	LDL	C	—
IIb	LDL, VLDL	C	TG
III (rare)	IDL	C/TG	—
IV	VLDL	TG	C*
V (rare)	Chylomicrons, VLDL	TG	C*

C = cholesterol, TG = triglycerides, LDL = low-density lipoprotein, VLDL = very-low-density lipoprotein, IDL = intermediate-density lipoprotein.
* Increases or no change.

ADOLESCENT PATIENTS WITH HETEROZYGOUS FAMILIAL HYPERCHOLESTEROLEMIA (HEFH)

Simvastatin is indicated as an adjunct to diet to reduce total-C, LDL-C, and Apo B levels in adolescent boys and girls who are at least 1 year post-menarche, 10-17 years of age, with heterozygous familial hypercholesterolemia, if after an adequate trial of diet therapy the following findings are present:

LDL cholesterol remains ≥190 mg/dl; or
LDL cholesterol remains ≥160 mg/dl and

- There is a positive family history of premature cardiovascular disease (CVD) or
- Two or more other CVD risk factors are present in the adolescent patient.

The minimum goal of treatment in pediatric and adolescent patients is to achieve a mean LDL-C <130 mg/dl. The optimal age at which to initiate lipid-lowering therapy to decrease the risk of symptomatic adulthood CAD has not been determined.

GENERAL RECOMMENDATIONS

Prior to initiating therapy with simvastatin, secondary causes for hypercholesterolemia (*e.g.*, poorly controlled diabetes mellitus, hypothyroidism, nephrotic syndrome, dysproteinemias, obstructive liver disease, other drug therapy, alcoholism) should be excluded, and a lipid profile performed to measure total-C, HDL-C, and TG. For patients with TG less than 400 mg/dl (<4.5 mmol/L), LDL-C can be estimated using the following equation:

LDL-C = total-C - [(0.20 × TG) + HDL-C]

For TG levels >400 mg/dl (>4.5 mmol/L), this equation is less accurate and LDL-C concentrations should be determined by ultracentrifugation. In many hypertriglyceridemic patients, LDL-C may be low or normal despite elevated total-C. In such cases, simvastatin is not indicated.

Lipid determinations should be performed at intervals of no less than 4 weeks and dosage adjusted according to the patient's response to therapy.

The NCEP Treatment Guidelines are summarized in TABLE 6.

TABLE 6 *NCEP Treatment Guidelines: LDL-C Goals and Cutpoints for Therapeutic Lifestyle Changes and Drug Therapy in Different Risk Categories*

Risk Category	LDL Goal	LDL Level at Which to: Initiate Therapeutic Lifestyle Changes	Consider Drug Therapy
CHD* or CHD risk equivalents (10 year risk >20%)	<100 mg/dl	≥100 mg/dl	≥130 mg/dl (100-129: drug optional)†
2+ Risk factors (10 year risk ≤20%)	<130 mg/dl	≥130 mg/dl	10 year risk 10-20%: ≥130 mg/dl; 10 year risk <10%: ≥160 mg/dl
0-1 Risk factor‡	<160 mg/dl	≥160 mg/dl	≥190 mg/dl (160-189: LDL-lowering drug optional)

* CHD, coronary heart disease.
† Some authorities recommend use of LDL-lowering drugs in this category if an LDL-C level of <100 mg/dl cannot be achieved by therapeutic lifestyle changes. Others prefer use of drugs that primarily modify triglycerides and HDL-C, *e.g.*, nicotinic acid or fibrate. Clinical judgment also may call for deferring drug therapy in this subcategory.
‡ Almost all people with 0-1 risk factor have a 10 year risk <10%; thus, 10 year risk assessment in people with 0-1 risk factor is not necessary.

After the LDL-C goal has been achieved, if the TG is still ≥200 mg/dl, non-HDL-C (total-C minus HDL-C) becomes a secondary target of therapy. Non-HDL-C goals are set 30 mg/dl higher than LDL-C goals for each risk category.

At the time of hospitalization for an acute coronary event, consideration can be given to initiating drug therapy at discharge if the LDL-C is ≥130 mg/dl (see TABLE 6).

The NCEP classification of cholesterol levels in pediatric patients with a familial history of either hypercholesterolemia or premature cardiovascular disease is summarized in TABLE 7.

TABLE 7 *NCEP Classification of Cholesterol Levels in Pediatric Patients With a Familial History of Either HeFH or Premature CVD*

Category	Total-C	LDL-C
Acceptable	<170 mg/dl	<110 mg/dl
Borderline	170-199 mg/dl	110-129 mg/dl
High	≥200 mg/dl	≥130 mg/dl

Since the goal of treatment is to lower LDL-C, the NCEP recommends that LDL-C levels be used to initiate and assess treatment response. Only if LDL-C levels are not available, should the total-C be used to monitor therapy.

Simvastatin is indicated to reduce elevated LDL-C and TG levels in patients with Type IIb hyperlipidemia (where hypercholesterolemia is the major abnormality). However, it has not been studied in conditions where the major abnormality is elevation of chylomicrons (*i.e.*, hyperlipidemia Fredrickson Types I and V) (see TABLE 5).

CONTRAINDICATIONS

Hypersensitivity to any component of this medication.

Active liver disease or unexplained persistent elevations of serum transaminases (see WARNINGS).

PREGNANCY AND LACTATION

Atherosclerosis is a chronic process and the discontinuation of lipid-lowering drugs during pregnancy should have little impact on the outcome of long-term therapy of primary hypercholesterolemia. Moreover, cholesterol and other products of the cholesterol biosynthesis pathway are essential components for fetal development, including synthesis of steroids and cell membranes. Because of the ability of inhibitors of HMG-CoA reductase such as simvastatin to decrease the synthesis of cholesterol and possibly other products of the cholesterol biosynthesis pathway, simvastatin is contraindicated during pregnancy and in nursing mothers. **Simvastatin should be administered to women of childbearing age only when such patients are highly unlikely to conceive.** If the patient becomes pregnant while taking this drug, simvastatin should be discontinued immediately and the patient should be apprised of the potential hazard to the fetus (see PRECAUTIONS, Pregnancy Category X).

WARNINGS

MYOPATHY/RHABDOMYOLYSIS

Simvastatin, like other inhibitors of HMG-CoA reductase, occasionally causes myopathy manifested as muscle pain, tenderness or weakness with creatine kinase (CK) above 10× the upper limit of normal (ULN). Myopathy sometimes takes the form of rhabdomyolysis with or without acute renal failure secondary to myoglobinuria, and rare fatalities have occurred. The risk of myopathy is increased by high levels of HMG-CoA reductase inhibitory activity in plasma.

The risk of myopathy/rhabdomyolysis is increased by concomitant use of simvastatin with the following:

Potent inhibitors of CYP3A4: **Cyclosporine, itraconazole, ketoconazole, erythromycin, clarithromycin, HIV protease inhibitors, nefazodone, or large quantities of grapefruit juice (>1 quart daily), particularly with higher doses of simvastatin** (see DRUG INTERACTIONS, CYP3A4 Interactions).

Lipid-lowering drugs that can cause myopathy when given alone: **Gemfibrozil, other fibrates, or lipid-lowering doses (≥1 g/day) of niacin, particularly with higher doses of simvastatin** (see CLINICAL PHARMACOLOGY, Pharmacokinetics and DRUG INTERACTIONS, Interactions With Lipid-Lowering Drugs That Can Cause Myopathy When Given Alone).

Other drugs: **Amiodarone or verapamil with higher doses of simvastatin** (see DRUG INTERACTIONS, Other Drug Interactions). In an ongoing clinical trial, myopathy has been reported in 6% of patients receiving simvastatin 80 mg and

S

amiodarone. In an analysis of clinical trials involving 25,248 patients treated with simvastatin 20-80 mg, the incidence of myopathy was higher in patients receiving verapamil and simvastatin (4/635; 0.63%) than in patients taking simvastatin without a calcium channel blocker (13/21,224; 0.061%).

The risk of myopathy/rhabdomyolysis is dose related. The incidence in clinical trials, in which patients were carefully monitored and some interacting drugs were excluded, has been approximately 0.02% at 20 mg, 0.07% at 40 mg and 0.3% at 80 mg.

Consequently:

Use of simvastatin concomitantly with itraconazole, ketoconazole, erythromycin, clarithromycin, HIV protease inhibitors, nefazodone, or large quantities of grapefruit juice (>1 quart daily) should be avoided. If treatment with itraconazole, ketoconazole, erythromycin, or clarithromycin is unavoidable, therapy with simvastatin should be suspended during the course of treatment. Concomitant use with other medicines labeled as having a potent inhibitory effect on CYP3A4 at therapeutic doses should be avoided unless the benefits of combined therapy outweigh the increased risk.

The dose of simvastatin should not exceed 10 mg daily in patients receiving concomitant medication with cyclosporine, gemfibrozil, other fibrates or lipid-lowering doses (≥1 g/day) of niacin. The combined use of simvastatin with fibrates or niacin should be avoided unless the benefit of further alteration in lipid levels is likely to outweigh the increased risk of this drug combination. Addition of these drugs to simvastatin typically provides little additional reduction in LDL-C, but further reductions of TG and further increases in HDL-C may be obtained.

The dose of simvastatin should not exceed 20 mg daily in patients receiving concomitant medication with amiodarone or verapamil. The combined use of simvastatin at doses higher than 20 mg daily with amiodarone or verapamil should be avoided unless the clinical benefit is likely to outweigh the increased risk of myopathy.

All patients starting therapy with simvastatin, or whose dose of simvastatin is being increased, should be advised of the risk of myopathy and told to report promptly any unexplained muscle pain, tenderness or weakness. Simvastatin therapy should be discontinued immediately if myopathy is diagnosed or suspected. The presence of these symptoms, and/or a CK level >10 times the ULN indicates myopathy. In most cases, when patients were promptly discontinued from treatment, muscle symptoms and CK increases resolved. Periodic CK determinations may be considered in patients starting therapy with simvastatin or whose dose is being increased, but there is no assurance that such monitoring will prevent myopathy.

Many of the patients who have developed rhabdomyolysis on therapy with simvastatin have had complicated medical histories, including renal insufficiency usually as a consequence of long-standing diabetes mellitus. Such patients merit closer monitoring. Therapy with simvastatin should be temporarily stopped a few days prior to elective major surgery and when any major medical or surgical condition supervenes.

LIVER DYSFUNCTION

Persistent increases (to more than 3× the ULN) in serum transaminases have occurred in approximately 1% of patients who received simvastatin in clinical studies. When drug treatment was interrupted or discontinued in these patients, the transaminase levels usually fell slowly to pretreatment levels. The increases were not associated with jaundice or other clinical signs or symptoms. There was no evidence of hypersensitivity.

In 4S, the number of patients with more than 1 transaminase elevation to >3× ULN, over the course of the study, was not significantly different between the simvastatin and placebo groups (14 [0.7%] vs 12 [0.6%]). Elevated transaminases resulted in the discontinuation of 8 patients from therapy in the simvastatin group (n=2221) and 5 in the placebo group (n=2223). Of the 1986 simvastatin treated patients in 4S with normal liver function tests (LFTs) at baseline, only 8 (0.4%) developed consecutive LFT elevations to >3× ULN and/or were discontinued due to transaminase elevations during the 5.4 years (median follow-up) of the study. Among these 8 patients, 5 initially developed these abnormalities within the first year. All of the patients in this study received a starting dose of 20 mg of simvastatin; 37% were titrated to 40 mg.

In 2 controlled clinical studies in 1105 patients, the 12 month incidence of persistent hepatic transaminase elevation without regard to drug relationship was 0.9% and 2.1% at the 40 and 80 mg dose, respectively. No patients developed persistent liver function abnormalities following the initial 6 months of treatment at a given dose.

It is recommended that liver function tests be performed before the initiation of treatment, and periodically thereafter (*e.g.,* semiannually) for the first year of treatment or until 1 year after the last elevation in dose. Patients titrated to the 80 mg dose should receive an additional test at 3 months. Patients who develop increased transaminase levels should be monitored with a second liver function evaluation to confirm the finding and be followed thereafter with frequent liver function tests until the abnormality(ies) return to normal. Should an increase in AST or ALT of 3× ULN or greater persist, withdrawal of therapy with simvastatin is recommended.

The drug should be used with caution in patients who consume substantial quantities of alcohol and/or have a past history of liver disease. Active liver diseases or unexplained transaminase elevations are contraindications to the use of simvastatin.

As with other lipid-lowering agents, moderate (less than 3× ULN) elevations of serum transaminases have been reported following therapy with simvastatin. These changes appeared soon after initiation of therapy with simvastatin, were often transient, were not accompanied by any symptoms and did not require interruption of treatment.

PRECAUTIONS

GENERAL

Simvastatin may cause elevation of CK and transaminase levels (see WARNINGS and ADVERSE REACTIONS). This should be considered in the differential diagnosis of chest pain in a patient on therapy with simvastatin.

INFORMATION FOR THE PATIENT

Patients should be advised about substances they should not take concomitantly with simvastatin and be advised to report promptly unexplained muscle pain, tenderness, or weakness (see list below and WARNINGS, Myopathy/Rhabdomyolysis). Patients should also be advised to inform other physicians prescribing a new medication that they are taking simvastatin.

CNS TOXICITY

Optic nerve degeneration was seen in clinically normal dogs treated with simvastatin for 14 weeks at 180 mg/kg/day, a dose that produced mean plasma drug levels about 12 times higher than the mean plasma drug level in humans taking 80 mg/day.

A chemically similar drug in this class also produced optic nerve degeneration (Wallerian degeneration of retinogeniculate fibers) in clinically normal dogs in a dose-dependent fashion starting at 60 mg/kg/day, a dose that produced mean plasma drug levels about 30 times higher than the mean plasma drug level in humans taking the highest recommended dose (as measured by total enzyme inhibitory activity). This same drug also produced vestibulocochlear Wallerian-like degeneration and retinal ganglion cell chromatolysis in dogs treated for 14 weeks at 180 mg/kg/day, a dose that resulted in a mean plasma drug level similar to that seen with the 60 mg/kg/day dose.

CNS vascular lesions, characterized by perivascular hemorrhage and edema, mononuclear cell infiltration of perivascular spaces, perivascular fibrin deposits and necrosis of small vessels were seen in dogs treated with simvastatin at a dose of 360 mg/kg/day, a dose that produced mean plasma drug levels that were about 14 times higher than the mean plasma drug levels in humans taking 80 mg/day. Similar CNS vascular lesions have been observed with several other drugs of this class.

There were cataracts in female rats after 2 years of treatment with 50 and 100 mg/kg/day (22 and 25 times the human AUC at 80 mg/day, respectively) and in dogs after 3 months at 90 mg/kg/day (19 times) and at 2 years at 50 mg/kg/day (5 times).

CARCINOGENESIS, MUTAGENESIS, AND IMPAIRMENT OF FERTILITY

In a 72 week carcinogenicity study, mice were administered daily doses of simvastatin of 25, 100, and 400 mg/kg body weight, which resulted in mean plasma drug levels approximately 1, 4, and 8 times higher than the mean human plasma drug level, respectively (as total inhibitory activity based on AUC) after an 80 mg oral dose. Liver carcinomas were significantly increased in high-dose females and mid- and high-dose males with a maximum incidence of 90% in males. The incidence of adenomas of the liver was significantly increased in mid- and high-dose females. Drug treatment also significantly increased the incidence of lung adenomas in mid- and high-dose males and females. Adenomas of the Harderian gland (a gland of the eye of rodents) were significantly higher in high-dose mice than in controls. No evidence of a tumorigenic effect was observed at 25 mg/kg/day.

In a separate 92 week carcinogenicity study in mice at doses up to 25 mg/kg/day, no evidence of a tumorigenic effect was observed (mean plasma drug levels were 1 times higher than humans given 80 mg simvastatin as measured by AUC).

In a 2 year study in rats at 25 mg/kg/day, there was a statistically significant increase in the incidence of thyroid follicular adenomas in female rats exposed to approximately 11 times higher levels of simvastatin than in humans given 80 mg simvastatin (as measured by AUC).

A second 2 year rat carcinogenicity study with doses of 50 and 100 mg/kg/day produced hepatocellular adenomas and carcinomas (in female rats at both doses and in males at 100 mg/kg/day). Thyroid follicular cell adenomas were increased in males and females at both doses; thyroid follicular cell carcinomas were increased in females at 100 mg/kg/day. The increased incidence of thyroid neoplasms appears to be consistent with findings from other HMG-CoA reductase inhibitors. These treatment levels represented plasma drug levels (AUC) of approximately 7 and 15 times (males) and 22 and 25 times (females) the mean human plasma drug exposure after an 80 mg daily dose.

No evidence of mutagenicity was observed in a microbial mutagenicity (Ames) test with or without rat or mouse liver metabolic activation. In addition, no evidence of damage to genetic material was noted in an *in vitro* alkaline elution assay using rat hepatocytes, a V-79 mammalian cell forward mutation study, an *in vitro* chromosome aberration study in CHO cells, or an *in vivo* chromosomal aberration assay in mouse bone marrow.

There was decreased fertility in male rats treated with simvastatin for 34 weeks at 25 mg/kg body weight (4 times the maximum human exposure level, based on AUC, in patients receiving 80 mg/day); however, this effect was not observed during a subsequent fertility study in which simvastatin was administered at this same dose level to male rats for 11 weeks (the entire cycle of spermatogenesis including epididymal maturation). No microscopic changes were observed in the testes of rats from either study. At 180 mg/kg/day, (which produces exposure levels 22 times higher than those in humans taking 80 mg/day based on surface area, mg/m^2), seminiferous tubule degeneration (necrosis and loss of spermatogenic epithelium) was observed. In dogs, there was drug-related testicular atrophy, decreased spermatogenesis, spermatocytic degeneration and giant cell formation at 10 mg/kg/day, (approximately 2 times the human exposure, based on AUC, at 80 mg/day). The clinical significance of these findings is unclear.

PREGNANCY CATEGORY X

See CONTRAINDICATIONS.

Safety in pregnant women has not been established.

Simvastatin was not teratogenic in rats at doses of 25 mg/kg/day or in rabbits at doses up to 10 mg/kg daily. These doses resulted in 3 times (rat) or 3 times (rabbit) the human exposure based on mg/m^2 surface area. However, in studies with another structurally-related HMG-CoA reductase inhibitor, skeletal malformations were observed in rats and mice.

Rare reports of congenital anomalies have been received following intrauterine exposure to HMG-CoA reductase inhibitors. In a review[2] of approximately 100 prospectively followed pregnancies in women exposed to simvastatin or another structurally related HMG-CoA reductase inhibitor, the incidences of congenital anomalies, spontaneous abortions and fetal deaths/stillbirths did not exceed what would be expected in the general population. The number of cases is adequate only to exclude a 3- to 4-fold increase in congenital anomalies over the background incidence. In 89% of the prospectively followed pregnancies, drug treatment was initiated prior to pregnancy and was discontinued at some point in the first trimester when pregnancy was identified. As safety in pregnant women has not been established and there is no apparent benefit to therapy with simvastatin during pregnancy (see CONTRAINDICATIONS), treatment should be immediately discontinued as soon as pregnancy is recognized. Simvastatin should be administered to women of child-bearing potential only when such patients are highly unlikely to conceive and have been informed of the potential hazards.

NURSING MOTHERS

It is not known whether simvastatin is excreted in human milk. Because a small amount of another drug in this class is excreted in human milk and because of the potential for serious adverse reactions in nursing infants, women taking simvastatin should not nurse their infants (see CONTRAINDICATIONS).

PEDIATRIC USE

Safety and effectiveness of simvastatin in patients 10-17 years of age with heterozygous familial hypercholesterolemia have been evaluated in a controlled clinical trial in adolescent boys and in girls who were at least 1 year post-menarche. Patients treated with simvastatin had an adverse experience profile generally similar to that of patients treated with placebo. Doses greater than 40 mg have not been studied in this population. In this limited controlled study, there was no detectable effect on growth or sexual maturation in the adolescent boys or girls, or any effect on menstrual cycle length in girls. See ADVERSE REACTIONS, Adolescent Patients and DOSAGE AND ADMINISTRATION, Dosage in Adolescents (10-17 years of age) with Heterozygous Familial Hypercholesterolemia. Adolescent females should be counseled on appropriate contraceptive methods while on simvastatin therapy (see CONTRAINDICATIONS and PRECAUTIONS, Pregnancy Category X). Simvastatin has not been studied in patients younger than 10 years of age, nor in premenarchal girls.

GERIATRIC USE

A pharmacokinetic study with simvastatin showed the mean plasma level of HMG-CoA reductase inhibitory activity to be approximately 45% higher in elderly patients between 70-78 years of age compared with patients between 18-30 years of age. In 4S and other large clinical studies conducted with simvastatin, 22% of patients were elderly (1522 of 6985 patients were ≥65 years). Simvastatin significantly reduced total mortality and CHD mortality in elderly patients with a history of CHD (see CLINICAL PHARMACOLOGY). Lipid-lowering efficacy was at least as great in elderly patients compared with younger patients, and there were no overall differences in safety over the 20-80 mg/day dosage range.

DRUG INTERACTIONS

CYP3A4 INTERACTIONS

Simvastatin is metabolized by CYP3A4 but has no CYP3A4 inhibitory activity; therefore it is not expected to affect the plasma concentrations of other drugs metabolized by CYP3A4. Potent inhibitors of CYP3A4 (below) increase the risk of myopathy by reducing the elimination of simvastatin.

See WARNINGS, Myopathy/Rhabdomyolysis; and CLINICAL PHARMACOLOGY, Pharmacokinetics.

Itraconazole
Ketoconazole
Erythromycin
Clarithromycin
HIV protease inhibitors
Nefazodone
Cyclosporine
Large quantities of grapefruit juice (>1 quart daily)

INTERACTIONS WITH LIPID-LOWERING DRUGS THAT CAN CAUSE MYOPATHY WHEN GIVEN ALONE

The risk of myopathy is also increased by the following lipid-lowering drugs that are not potent CYP3A4 inhibitors, but which can cause myopathy when given alone.

See WARNINGS, Myopathy/Rhabdomyolysis.

Gemfibrozil
Other fibrates
Niacin (nicotinic acid) (>1 g/day)

OTHER DRUG INTERACTIONS

Amiodarone or Verapamil: The risk of myopathy/rhabdomyolysis is increased by concomitant administration of amiodarone or verapamil (see WARNINGS, Myopathy/Rhabdomyolysis).

Propranolol: In healthy male volunteers there was a significant decrease in mean C_{max}, but no change in AUC, for simvastatin total and active inhibitors with concomitant administration of single doses of simvastatin and propranolol. The clinical relevance of this finding is unclear. The pharmacokinetics of the enantiomers of propranolol were not affected.

Digoxin: Concomitant administration of a single dose of digoxin in healthy male volunteers receiving simvastatin resulted in a slight elevation (less than 0.3 ng/ml) in digoxin concentrations in plasma (as measured by a radioimmunoassay) compared to concomitant administration of placebo and digoxin. Patients taking digoxin should be monitored appropriately when simvastatin is initiated.

Warfarin: In 2 clinical studies, 1 in normal volunteers and the other in hypercholesterolemic patients, simvastatin 20-40 mg/day modestly potentiated the effect of coumarin anticoagulants: the prothrombin time, reported as International Normalized Ratio (INR), increased from a baseline of 1.7-1.8 and from 2.6-3.4 in the volunteer and patient studies, respectively. With other reductase inhibitors, clinically evident bleeding and/or increased prothrombin time has been reported in a few patients taking coumarin anticoagulants concomitantly. In such patients, prothrombin time should be determined before starting simvastatin and frequently enough during early therapy to insure that no significant alteration of prothrombin time occurs. Once a stable prothrombin time has been documented, prothrombin times can be monitored at the intervals usually recommended for patients on coumarin anticoagulants. If the dose of simvastatin is changed or discontinued, the same procedure should be repeated. Simvastatin therapy has not been associated with bleeding or with changes in prothrombin time in patients not taking anticoagulants.

ADVERSE REACTIONS

In the pre-marketing controlled clinical studies and their open extensions (2423 patients with mean duration of follow-up of approximately 18 months), 1.4% of patients were discontinued due to adverse experiences attributable to simvastatin. Adverse reactions have usually been mild and transient. Simvastatin has been evaluated for serious adverse reactions in more than 21,000 patients and is generally well tolerated.

CLINICAL ADVERSE EXPERIENCES IN ADULTS

Adverse experiences occurring at an incidence of 1% or greater in patients treated with simvastatin, regardless of causality, in controlled clinical studies are shown in TABLE 8.

TABLE 8 *Adverse Experiences in Clinical Studies — Incidence 1% or Greater, Regardless of Causality*

	Simvastatin (n=1583)	Placebo (n=157)	Cholestyramine (n=179)
Body as a Whole			
Abdominal pain	3.2%	3.2%	8.9%
Asthenia	1.6%	2.5%	1.1%
Gastrointestinal			
Constipation	2.3%	1.3%	29.1%
Diarrhea	1.9%	2.5%	7.8%
Dyspepsia	1.1%	—	4.5%
Flatulence	1.9%	1.3%	14.5%
Nausea	1.3%	1.9%	10.1%
Nervous System/Psychiatric			
Headache	3.5%	5.1%	4.5%
Respiratory			
Upper respiratory infection	2.1%	1.9%	3.4%

SCANDINAVIAN SIMVASTATIN SURVIVAL STUDY

Clinical Adverse Experiences

In 4S involving 4444 patients treated with 20-40 mg/day of simvastatin (n=2221) or placebo (n=2223), the safety and tolerability profiles were comparable between groups over the median 5.4 years of the study. The clinical adverse experiences reported as possibly, probably, or definitely drug-related in ≥0.5% in either treatment group are shown in TABLE 9.

The following effects have been reported with drugs in this class. Not all the effects listed below have necessarily been associated with simvastatin therapy.

TABLE 9 *Drug-Related Clinical Adverse Experiences in 4S — Incidence 0.5% or Greater*

	Simvastatin (n=2221)	Placebo (n=2223)
Body as a Whole		
Abdominal pain	0.9%	0.9%
Gastrointestinal		
Diarrhea	0.5%	0.3%
Dyspepsia	0.6%	0.5%
Flatulence	0.9%	0.7%
Nausea	0.4%	0.6%
Musculoskeletal		
Myalgia	1.2%	1.3%
Skin		
Eczema	0.8%	0.8%
Pruritus	0.5%	0.4%
Rash	0.6%	0.6%
Special Senses		
Cataract	0.5%	0.8%

Skeletal: Muscle cramps, myalgia, myopathy, rhabdomyolysis, arthralgias.

Neurological: Dysfunction of certain cranial nerves (including alteration of taste, impairment of extra-ocular movement, facial paresis), tremor, dizziness, vertigo, memory loss, paresthesia, peripheral neuropathy, peripheral nerve palsy, psychic disturbances, anxiety, insomnia, depression.

Hypersensitivity Reactions: *An apparent hypersensitivity syndrome has been reported rarely which has included 1 or more of the following features:* Anaphylaxis, angioedema, lupus erythematous-like syndrome, polymyalgia rheumatica, dermatomyositis, vasculitis, purpura, thrombocytopenia, leukopenia, hemolytic anemia, positive ANA, ESR increase, eosinophilia, arthritis, arthralgia, urticaria, asthenia, photosensitivity, fever, chills, flushing, malaise, dyspnea, toxic epidermal necrolysis, erythema multiforme, including Stevens-Johnson syndrome.

Gastrointestinal: Pancreatitis, hepatitis, including chronic active hepatitis, cholestatic jaundice, fatty change in liver, and, rarely, cirrhosis, fulminant hepatic necrosis, and hepatoma; anorexia, vomiting.

Skin: Alopecia, pruritus. A variety of skin changes (*e.g.*, nodules, discoloration, dryness of skin/mucous membranes, changes to hair/nails) have been reported.

Reproductive: Gynecomastia, loss of libido, erectile dysfunction.

Eye: Progression of cataracts (lens opacities), ophthalmoplegia.

Laboratory Abnormalities: Elevated transaminases, alkaline phosphatase, γ-glutamyl transpeptidase, and bilirubin; thyroid function abnormalities.

LABORATORY TESTS

Marked persistent increases of serum transaminases have been noted (see WARNINGS, Liver Dysfunction). About 5% of patients had elevations of CK levels of 3 or more times the normal value on 1 or more occasions. This was attributable to the noncardiac fraction of CK. Muscle pain or dysfunction usually was not reported (see WARNINGS, Myopathy/Rhabdomyolysis).

CONCOMITANT LIPID-LOWERING THERAPY

In controlled clinical studies in which simvastatin was administered concomitantly with cholestyramine, no adverse reactions peculiar to this concomitant treatment were observed. The adverse reactions that occurred were limited to those reported previously with simvastatin or cholestyramine. The combined use of simvastatin at doses exceeding 10 mg/day with gemfibrozil, other fibrates or lipid-lowering doses (≥1 g/day) of niacin should be avoided (see WARNINGS, Myopathy/Rhabdomyolysis).

ADOLESCENT PATIENTS (AGES 10-17 YEARS)

In a 48 week controlled study in adolescent boys and girls who were at least 1 year post-menarche, 10-17 years of age with heterozygous familial hypercholesterolemia (n=175), the safety and tolerability profile of the group treated with simvastatin (10-40 mg daily) was generally similar to that of the group treated with placebo, with the most common adverse experiences observed in both groups being upper respiratory infection, headache, abdominal pain, and nausea (see PRECAUTIONS, Pediatric Use).

DOSAGE AND ADMINISTRATION

The patient should be placed on a standard cholesterol-lowering diet before receiving simvastatin and should continue on this diet during treatment with simvastatin. The dosage should be individualized according to the baseline LDL-C level, the recommended goal of therapy (see TABLE 6), and the patient's response. The dosage range is 5-80 mg/day.

The recommended usual starting dose is 20 mg once a day in the evening. Patients who require a large reduction in LDL-C (more than 45%) may be started at 40 mg/day in the evening. Adjustments of dosage should be made at intervals of 4 weeks or more. See below for dosage recommendations for patients receiving concomitant therapy with cyclosporine, fibrates or niacin, and for those with severe renal insufficiency.

DOSAGE IN PATIENTS WITH HOMOZYGOUS FAMILIAL HYPERCHOLESTEROLEMIA

Based on the results of a controlled clinical study, the recommended dosage for patients with homozygous familial hypercholesterolemia is simvastatin 40 mg/day in the evening or 80 mg/day in 3 divided doses of 20 mg, 20 mg, and an evening dose of 40 mg. Simvastatin should be used as an adjunct to other lipid-lowering treatments (*e.g.*, LDL apheresis) in these patients or if such treatments are unavailable.

DOSAGE IN ADOLESCENTS (10-17 YEARS OF AGE) WITH HETEROZYGOUS FAMILIAL HYPERCHOLESTEROLEMIA

The recommended usual starting dose is 10 mg once a day in the evening. The recommended dosing range is 10-40 mg/day; the maximum recommended dose is 40 mg/day. Doses should be individualized according to the recommended goal of therapy (see NCEP Pediatric Panel Guidelines[3] and CLINICAL PHARMACOLOGY). Adjustments should be made at intervals of 4 weeks or more.

DOSAGE IN PATIENTS TAKING CYCLOSPORINE

In patients taking cyclosporine concomitantly with simvastatin (see WARNINGS, Myopathy/Rhabdomyolysis), therapy should begin with 5 mg/day and should not exceed 10 mg/day.

DOSAGE IN PATIENTS TAKING AMIODARONE OR VERAPAMIL

In patients taking amiodarone or verapamil concomitantly with simvastatin, the dose should not exceed 20 mg/day (see WARNINGS, Myopathy/Rhabdomyolysis and DRUG INTERACTIONS, Other Drug Interactions).

CONCOMITANT LIPID-LOWERING THERAPY

Simvastatin is effective alone or when used concomitantly with bile-acid sequestrants. If simvastatin is used in combination with gemfibrozil, other fibrates or lipid-lowering doses (≥1 g/day) of niacin, the dose of simvastatin should not exceed 10 mg/day (see WARNINGS, Myopathy/Rhabdomyolysis and DRUG INTERACTIONS).

DOSAGE IN PATIENTS WITH RENAL INSUFFICIENCY

Because simvastatin does not undergo significant renal excretion, modification of dosage should not be necessary in patients with mild to moderate renal insufficiency. However, caution should be exercised when simvastatin is administered to patients with severe renal insufficiency; such patients should be started at 5 mg/day and be closely monitored (see CLINICAL PHARMACOLOGY, Pharmacokinetics and WARNINGS, Myopathy/Rhabdomyolysis).

HOW SUPPLIED

Zocor tablets are available as follows:

5 mg: Zocor 5 mg tablets are buff, shield-shaped, film-coated tablets, coded "MSD 726" on 1 side and "ZOCOR" on the other.

10 mg: Zocor 10 mg tablets are peach, shield-shaped, film-coated tablets, coded "MSD 735" on 1 side and "ZOCOR" on the other.

20 mg: Zocor 20 mg tablets are tan, shield-shaped, film-coated tablets, coded "MSD 740" on 1 side and "ZOCOR" on the other.

40 mg: Zocor 40 mg tablets are brick red, shield-shaped, film-coated tablets, coded "MSD 749" on 1 side and "ZOCOR" on the other.

80 mg: Zocor 80 mg tablets are brick red, capsule-shaped, film-coated tablets, coded "543" on 1 side and "80" on the other.

Storage: Store between 5-30°C (41-86°F).

PRODUCT LISTING - EQUIVALENTS NOT AVAILABLE

Tablet - Oral - 5 mg

30's	$58.84	ZOCOR, Merck & Company Inc	00006-0726-31
60's	$106.84	ZOCOR, Merck & Company Inc	00006-0726-61
90's	$176.49	ZOCOR, Merck & Company Inc	00006-0726-54
100's	$196.09	ZOCOR, Merck & Company Inc	00006-0726-28

Tablet - Oral - 10 mg

7's	$13.67	ZOCOR, Allscripts Pharmaceutical Company	54569-4180-00
30's	$60.87	ZOCOR, Allscripts Pharmaceutical Company	54569-4180-01
30's	$67.33	ZOCOR, Physicians Total Care	54868-2639-01
30's	$71.25	ZOCOR, Southwood Pharmaceuticals Inc	58016-0364-30
30's	$78.85	ZOCOR, Merck & Company Inc	00006-0735-31
60's	$142.50	ZOCOR, Southwood Pharmaceuticals Inc	58016-0364-60
60's	$143.20	ZOCOR, Merck & Company Inc	00006-0735-61
90's	$213.75	ZOCOR, Southwood Pharmaceuticals Inc	58016-0364-90
90's	$236.54	ZOCOR, Merck & Company Inc	00006-0735-54
100's	$237.50	ZOCOR, Southwood Pharmaceuticals Inc	58016-0364-00
100's	$262.81	ZOCOR, Merck & Company Inc	00006-0735-28

Tablet - Oral - 20 mg

30's	$114.42	ZOCOR, Physicians Total Care	54868-3104-00
30's	$119.30	ZOCOR, Allscripts Pharmaceutical Company	54569-4403-00
30's	$123.98	ZOCOR, Southwood Pharmaceuticals Inc	58016-0385-30
30's	$137.56	ZOCOR, Merck & Company Inc	00006-0740-31
60's	$247.95	ZOCOR, Southwood Pharmaceuticals Inc	58016-0385-60
60's	$249.80	ZOCOR, Merck & Company Inc	00006-0740-61
90's	$371.93	ZOCOR, Southwood Pharmaceuticals Inc	58016-0385-90
90's	$412.66	ZOCOR, Merck & Company Inc	00006-0740-54
100's	$413.25	ZOCOR, Southwood Pharmaceuticals Inc	58016-0385-00
100's	$458.51	ZOCOR, Merck & Company Inc	00006-0740-28

Tablet - Oral - 40 mg

30's	$106.17	ZOCOR, Allscripts Pharmaceutical Company	54569-4404-00
30's	$123.98	ZOCOR, Southwood Pharmaceuticals Inc	58016-0365-30
30's	$128.42	ZOCOR, Physicians Total Care	54868-4157-00
30's	$137.56	ZOCOR, Merck & Company Inc	00006-0749-31
60's	$247.95	ZOCOR, Southwood Pharmaceuticals Inc	58016-0365-60
60's	$249.80	ZOCOR, Merck & Company Inc	00006-0749-61
90's	$371.93	ZOCOR, Southwood Pharmaceuticals Inc	58016-0365-90
90's	$412.66	ZOCOR, Merck & Company Inc	00006-0749-54
100's	$413.25	ZOCOR, Southwood Pharmaceuticals Inc	58016-0365-00
100's	$458.51	ZOCOR, Merck & Company Inc	00006-0749-28

Tablet - Oral - 80 mg

15's	$68.54	ZOCOR, Physicians Total Care	54868-4181-00
30's	$137.56	ZOCOR, Merck & Company Inc	00006-0543-31
60's	$249.80	ZOCOR, Merck & Company Inc	00006-0543-61
90's	$412.66	ZOCOR, Merck & Company Inc	00006-0543-54
100's	$458.51	ZOCOR, Merck & Company Inc	00006-0543-28

Sirolimus *(003451)*

Categories: Rejection, renal transplant, prophylaxis; FDA Approved 1999 Sept; Pregnancy Category C
Drug Classes: Immunosuppressives
Foreign Brand Availability: Rapamune (Austria; Belgium; Bulgaria; Colombia; Czech-Republic; Denmark; England; Finland; France; Germany; Greece; Hungary; Ireland; Israel; Italy; Mexico; Netherlands; New-Zealand; Norway; Poland; Portugal; Slovenia; Spain; Sweden; Switzerland; Turkey)
Cost of Therapy: $450.00 (Transplant Rejection; Rapamune Oral Solution; 1 mg/ml; 60 ml; 2 ml/day; 30 day supply)
$450.00 (Transplant Rejection; Rapamune; 1 mg; 2 tablets/day; 30 day supply)

WARNING

Increased susceptibility to infection and the possible development of lymphoma may result from immunosuppression. Only physicians experienced in immunosuppressive therapy and management of renal transplant patients should use sirolimus. Patients receiving the drug should be managed in facilities equipped and staffed with adequate laboratory and supportive medical resources. The physician responsible for maintenance therapy should have complete information requisite for the follow-up of the patient.

DESCRIPTION

Sirolimus is an immunosuppressive agent. Sirolimus is a macrocyclic lactone produced by *Streptomyces hygroscopicus.* The chemical name of sirolimus (also known as rapamycin) is (3*S*,6*R*,7*E*,9*R*,10*R*,12*R*,14*S*,15*E*,17*E*,19*E*,21*S*,23*S*,26*R*,27*R*,34a*S*)-9,10,12,13,14,21,22,23,24,25,26,27,32,33,34,34a-hexadecahydro-9,27-dihydroxy-3-[(1*R*)-2-[(1*S*,3*R*,4*R*)-4-hydroxy-3-methoxycyclohexyl]-1-methylethyl]-10,21-dimethoxy-6,8,12,14,20,26-hexamethyl-23,27-epoxy-3*H*-pyrido[2,1-c][1,4] oxaazacyclohentriacontine-1,5,11,28,29 (4*H*,6*H*,31*H*)-pentone. Its molecular formula is $C_{51}H_{79}NO_{13}$ and its molecular weight is 914.2.

Sirolimus is a white to off-white powder and is insoluble in water, but freely soluble in benzyl alcohol, chloroform, acetone, and acetonitrile.

Rapamune is available for administration as an oral solution containing 1 mg/ml sirolimus and as a white, triangular-shaped tablet containing 1 mg sirolimus, and as a yellow to beige triangular-shaped tablet containing 2 mg sirolimus.

The inactive ingredients in Rapamune oral solution are Phosal 50 PG (phosphatidylcholine, propylene glycol, mono- and di-glycerides, ethanol, soy fatty acids, and ascorbyl palmitate) and polysorbate 80. Rapamune oral solution contains 1.5-2.5% ethanol.

The inactive ingredients in Rapamune tablets include sucrose, lactose, polyethylene glycol 8000, calcium sulfate, microcrystalline cellulose, pharmaceutical glaze, talc, titanium

S

dioxide, magnesium stearate, povidone, poloxamer 188, polyethylene glycol 20,000, glyceryl monooleate, carnauba wax, and other ingredients. The 2 mg dosage strength also contains iron oxide yellow 10 and iron oxide brown 70.

CLINICAL PHARMACOLOGY

MECHANISM OF ACTION

Sirolimus inhibits T lymphocyte activation and proliferation that occurs in response to antigenic and cytokine (Interleukin [IL]-2, IL-4, and IL-15) stimulation by a mechanism that is distinct from that of other immunosuppressants. Sirolimus also inhibits antibody production. In cells, sirolimus binds to the immunophilin, FK Binding Protein-12 (FKBP-12), to generate an immunosuppressive complex. The sirolimus:FKBP-12 complex has no effect on calcineurin activity. This complex binds to and inhibits the activation of the mammalian Target Of Rapamycin (mTOR), a key regulatory kinase. This inhibition suppresses cytokine-driven T-cell proliferation, inhibiting the progression from the G_1 to the S phase of the cell cycle.

Studies in experimental models show that sirolimus prolongs allograft (kidney, heart, skin, islet, small bowel, pancreatico-duodenal, and bone marrow) survival in mice, rats, pigs, and/or primates. Sirolimus reverses acute rejection of heart and kidney allografts in rats and prolonged the graft survival in presensitized rats. In some studies, the immunosuppressive effect of sirolimus lasted up to 6 months after discontinuation of therapy. This tolerization effect is alloantigen specific.

In rodent models of autoimmune disease, sirolimus suppresses immune-mediated events associated with systemic lupus erythematosus, collagen-induced arthritis, autoimmune Type 1 diabetes, autoimmune myocarditis, experimental allergic encephalomyelitis, graft-versus-host disease, and autoimmune uveoretinitis.

PHARMACOKINETICS

Sirolimus pharmacokinetic activity has been determined following oral administration in healthy subjects, pediatric dialysis patients, hepatically-impaired patients, and renal transplant patients.

Absorption

Following administration of sirolimus oral solution, sirolimus is rapidly absorbed, with a mean time-to-peak concentration (T^{max}) of approximately 1 hour after a single dose in healthy subjects and approximately 2 hours after multiple oral doses in renal transplant recipients. The systemic availability of sirolimus was estimated to be approximately 14% after the administration of sirolimus oral solution. The mean bioavailability of sirolimus after administration of the tablet is about 27% higher relative to the oral solution. Sirolimus oral tablets are not bioequivalent to the oral solution; however, clinical equivalence has been demonstrated at the 2 mg dose level. (See DOSAGE AND ADMINISTRATION.) Sirolimus concentrations, following the administration of sirolimus oral solution to stable renal transplant patients, are dose proportional between 3 and 12 mg/m^2.

Food Effects

In 22 healthy volunteers receiving sirolimus oral solution, a high-fat meal (861.8 kcal, 54.9% kcal from fat) altered the bioavailability characteristics of sirolimus. Compared with fasting, a 34% decrease in the peak blood sirolimus concentration (C_{max}), a 3.5-fold increase in the time-to-peak concentration (T_{max}), and a 35% increase in total exposure (AUC) was observed. After administration of sirolimus tablets and a high-fat meal in 24 healthy volunteers, C_{max}, T_{max}, and AUC showed increases of 65%, 32%, and 23%, respectively. To minimize variability, both sirolimus oral solution and tablets should be taken consistently with or without food (see DOSAGE AND ADMINISTRATION).

Distribution

The mean (±SD) blood-to-plasma ratio of sirolimus was 36 (±17.9) in stable renal allograft recipients, indicating that sirolimus is extensively partitioned into formed blood elements. The mean volume of distribution (Vss/F) of sirolimus is 12 ± 7.52 L/kg. Sirolimus is extensively bound (approximately 92%) to human plasma proteins. In man, the binding of sirolimus was shown mainly to be associated with serum albumin (97%), α_1-acid glycoprotein, and lipoproteins.

Metabolism

Sirolimus is a substrate for both cytochrome P450 3A4 (CYP3A4) and P-glycoprotein. Sirolimus is extensively metabolized by O-demethylation and/or hydroxylation. Seven (7) major metabolites, including hydroxy, demethyl, and hydroxydemethyl, are identifiable in whole blood. Some of these metabolites are also detectable in plasma, fecal, and urine samples. Glucuronide and sulfate conjugates are not present in any of the biologic matrices. Sirolimus is the major component in human whole blood and contributes to more than 90% of the immunosuppressive activity.

Excretion

After a single dose of [^{14}C]sirolimus in healthy volunteers, the majority (91%) of radioactivity was recovered from the feces, and only a minor amount (2.2%) was excreted in urine.

Pharmacokinetics in Renal Transplant Patients

Sirolimus Oral Solution

Pharmacokinetic parameters for sirolimus oral solution given daily in combination with cyclosporine and corticosteroids in renal transplant patients are summarized in TABLE 1 based on data collected at Months 1, 3, and 6 after transplantation. There were no significant differences in any of these parameters with respect to treatment group or month.

Whole blood sirolimus trough concentrations (mean ± SD), as measured by immunoassay, for the 2 mg/day and 5 mg/day dose groups were 8.6 ± 4.0 ng/ml (n=226) and 17.3 ± 7.4 ng/ml (n=219), respectively. Whole blood trough sirolimus concentrations, as measured by LC/MS/MS, were significantly correlated (r^2 = 0.96) with AUC(τ,ss). Upon repeated twice daily administration without an initial loading dose in a multiple-dose study, the average trough concentration of sirolimus increases approximately 2- to 3-fold over the initial 6 days of therapy at which time steady-state is reached. A loading dose of 3 times the maintenance dose will provide near steady-state concentrations within 1 day in most patients. The mean ± SD terminal elimination half-life (T½) of sirolimus after multiple dosing in stable renal transplant patients was estimated to be about 62 ± 16 hours.

TABLE 1 *Sirolimus Pharmacokinetic Parameters (Mean ± SD) in Renal Transplant Patients (Multiple Dose Oral Solution)*†*

n	Dose (mg)	$C_{max,ss}$‡ (ng/ml)	$T_{max,ss}$ (h)	AUC(τ,ss)‡ (ng·h/ml)	CL/F/WT§ (ml/h/kg)
19	2	12.2 ± 6.2	3.01 ± 2.40	158 ± 70	182 ± 72
23	5	37.4 ± 21	1.84 ± 1.30	396 ± 193	221 ± 143

* Sirolimus administered 4 hours after cyclosporine oral solution (MODIFIED) (*e.g.*, Neoral oral solution) and/or cyclosporine capsules (MODIFIED) (*e.g.*, Neoral soft gelatin capsules).
† As measured by the Liquid Chromatographic/Tandem Mass Spectrometric Method (LC/MS/MS).
‡ These parameters were dose normalized prior to the statistical comparison.
§ CL/F/WT = oral dose clearance.

Sirolimus Tablets

Pharmacokinetic parameters for sirolimus tablets administered daily in combination with cyclosporine and corticosteroids in renal transplant patients are summarized in TABLE 2 based on data collected at Months 1 and 3 after transplantation.

TABLE 2 *Sirolimus Pharmacokinetic Parameters (Mean ± SD) in Renal Transplant Patients (Multiple Dose Tablets)*†*

n	Dose (2 mg/day)	$C_{max,ss}$‡ (ng/ml)	$T_{max,ss}$ (h)	AUC(τ,ss)‡ (ng·h/ml)	CL/F/WT§ (ml/h/kg)
17	Oral solution	14.4 ± 5.3	2.12 ± 0.84	194 ± 78	173 ± 50
13	Tablets	15.0 ± 4.9	3.46 ± 2.40	230 ± 67	139 ± 63

* Sirolimus administered 4 hours after cyclosporine oral solution (MODIFIED) (*e.g.*, Neoral oral solution) and/or cyclosporine capsules (MODIFIED) (*e.g.*, Neoral soft gelatin capsules).
† As measured by the Liquid Chromatographic/Tandem Mass Spectrometric Method (LC/MS/MS).
‡ These parameters were dose normalized prior to the statistical comparison.
§ CL/F/WT = oral dose clearance.

Whole blood sirolimus trough concentrations (mean ± SD), as measured by immunoassay, for the 2 mg oral solution and 2 mg tablets over 6 months, were 8.9 ± 4.4 ng/ml (n=172) and 9.5 ± 3.9 ng/ml (n=179), respectively. Whole blood trough sirolimus concentrations, as measured by LC/MS/MS, were significantly correlated (r^2 = 0.85) with AUC(τ,ss). Mean whole blood sirolimus trough concentrations in patients receiving either sirolimus oral solution or tablets with a loading dose of 3 times the maintenance dose achieved steady-state concentrations within 24 hours after the start of dose administration.

Average sirolimus doses and sirolimus whole blood trough concentrations for tablets administered daily in combination with cyclosporine and following cyclosporine withdrawal, in combination with corticosteroids in renal transplant patients are summarized in TABLE 3.

TABLE 3 *Average Sirolimus Doses and Sirolimus Trough Concentrations (Mean ± SD) in Renal Transplant Patients After Multiple Dose Tablet Administration*

	Sirolimus With Cyclosporine Therapy*	Sirolimus Following Cyclosporine Withdrawal*
Sirolimus Dose (mg/day)		
Months 4-12	2.1 ± 0.7	8.2 ± 4.2
Months 12-24	2.0 ± 0.8	6.4 ± 3.0
Sirolimus C_{min}, (ng/ml)†		
Months 4-12	10.7 ± 3.8	23.3 ± 5.0
Months 12-24	11.2 ± 4.1	22.5 ± 4.8

* 215 patients were randomized to each group.
† Expressed by immunoassay and equivalence.

The withdrawal of cyclosporine and concurrent increases in sirolimus trough concentrations to steady-state required approximately 6 weeks. Larger sirolimus doses were required due to the absence of the inhibition of sirolimus metabolism and transport by cyclosporine and to achieve higher target concentrations during concentration-controlled administration following cyclosporine withdrawal.

SPECIAL POPULATIONS

Hepatic Impairment

Sirolimus (15 mg) was administered as a single oral dose to 18 subjects with normal hepatic function and to 18 patients with Child-Pugh classification A or B hepatic impairment, in which hepatic impairment was primary and not related to an underlying systemic disease. TABLE 4 shows the mean ± SD pharmacokinetic parameters following the administration of sirolimus oral solution.

Compared with the values in the normal hepatic group, the hepatic impairment group had higher mean values for sirolimus AUC (61%) and T½ (43%) and had lower mean values for sirolimus CL/F/WT (33%). The mean T½ increased from 79 ± 12 hours in subjects with normal hepatic function to 113 ± 41 hours in patients with impaired hepatic function. The rate of absorption of sirolimus was not altered by hepatic disease, as evidenced by C_{max} and T_{max} values. However, hepatic diseases with varying etiologies may show different effects and the pharmacokinetics of sirolimus in patients with severe hepatic dysfunction is unknown. Dosage adjustment is recommended for patients with mild to moderate hepatic impairment (see DOSAGE AND ADMINISTRATION).

S

TABLE 4 *Sirolimus Pharmacokinetic Parameters (Mean ± SD) in 18 Healthy Subjects and 18 Patients With Hepatic Impairment (15 mg Single Dose — Oral Solution)*

Population	$C_{max,ss}$* (ng/ml)	T_{max} (h)	AUC(0-∞) (ng·h/ml)	CL/F/WT (ml/h/kg)
Healthy subjects	78.2 ± 18.3	0.82 ± 0.17	970 ± 272	215 ± 76
Hepatic impairment	77.9 ± 23.1	0.84 ± 0.17	1567 ± 616	144 ± 62

* As measured by LC/MS/MS.

Renal Impairment
The effect of renal impairment on the pharmacokinetics of sirolimus is not known. However, there is minimal (2.2%) renal excretion of the drug or its metabolites.

Pediatric
Limited pharmacokinetic data are available in pediatric patients. TABLE 5 summarizes pharmacokinetic data obtained in pediatric dialysis patients with chronically impaired renal function.

TABLE 5 *Sirolimus Pharmacokinetic Parameters (Mean ± SD) in Pediatric Patients With Stable Chronic Renal Failure Maintained on Hemodialysis or Peritoneal Dialysis (1, 3, 9, 15 mg/m² Single Dose)*

Age Group	n	T_{max} (h)	$T_{½}$ (h)	CL/F/WT (ml/h/kg)
5-11 years	9	1.1 ± 0.5	71 ± 40	580 ± 450
12-18 years	11	0.79 ± 0.17	55 ± 18	450 ± 232

Geriatric
Clinical studies of sirolimus did not include a sufficient number of patients >65 years of age to determine whether they will respond differently than younger patients. After the administration of sirolimus oral solution, sirolimus trough concentration data in 35 renal transplant patients >65 years of age were similar to those in the adult population (n=822) 18-65 years of age. Similar results were obtained after the administration of sirolimus tablets to 12 renal transplant patients >65 years of age compared with adults (n=167) 18-65 years of age.

Gender
After the administration of sirolimus oral solution, sirolimus oral dose clearance in males was 12% lower than that in females; male subjects had a significantly longer $T_{½}$ than did female subjects (72.3 hours versus 61.3 hours). A similar trend in the effect of gender on sirolimus oral dose clearance and $T_{½}$ was observed after the administration of sirolimus tablets. Dose adjustments based on gender are not recommended.

Race
In large Phase 3 trials (Studies 1 and 2) using sirolimus oral solution and cyclosporine oral solution (MODIFIED) (*e.g.*, Neoral oral solution) and/or cyclosporine capsules (MODIFIED) (*e.g.*, Neoral soft gelatin capsules), there were no significant differences in mean trough sirolimus concentrations over time between black (n=139) and non-black (n=724) patients during the first 6 months after transplantation at sirolimus doses of 2 and 5 mg/day. Similarly, after administration of sirolimus tablets (2 mg/day) in a Phase 3 trial, mean sirolimus trough concentrations over 6 months were not significantly different among black (n=51) and non-black (n=128) patients.

INDICATIONS AND USAGE

Sirolimus is indicated for the prophylaxis of organ rejection in patients receiving renal transplants. It is recommended that sirolimus be used initially in a regimen with cyclosporine and corticosteroids. In patients at low to moderate immunological risk cyclosporine should be withdrawn 2-4 months after transplantation and sirolimus dose should be increased to reach recommended blood concentrations (see DOSAGE AND ADMINISTRATION).

The safety and efficacy of cyclosporine withdrawal in high-risk patients have not been adequately studied and it is therefore not recommended. This includes patients with Banff grade III acute rejection or vascular rejection prior to cyclosporine withdrawal, those who are dialysis-dependent, or with serum creatinine >4.5 mg/dl, black patients, re-transplants, multi-organ transplants, patients with high panel of reactive antibodies.

CONTRAINDICATIONS

Sirolimus is contraindicated in patients with a hypersensitivity to sirolimus or its derivatives or any component of the drug product.

WARNINGS

Increased susceptibility to infection and the possible development of lymphoma and other malignancies, particularly of the skin, may result from immunosuppression (see ADVERSE REACTIONS). Oversuppression of the immune system can also increase susceptibility to infection including opportunistic infections, fatal infections, and sepsis. Only physicians experienced in immunosuppressive therapy and management of organ transplant patients should use sirolimus. Patients receiving the drug should be managed in facilities equipped and staffed with adequate laboratory and supportive medical resources. The physician responsible for maintenance therapy should have complete information requisite for the follow-up of the patient.

As usual for patients with increased risk for skin cancer, exposure to sunlight and UV light should be limited by wearing protective clothing and using sunscreen with a high protection factor.

Increased serum cholesterol and triglycerides, that may require treatment, occurred more frequently in patients treated with sirolimus compared to azathioprine or placebo controls (see PRECAUTIONS).

In Studies 1 and 2, from Month 6 through Months 24 and 36, respectively, mean serum creatinine was increased and mean glomerular filtration rate was decreased in patients treated with sirolimus and cyclosporine compared with those treated with cyclosporine and placebo or azathioprine controls. The rate of decline in renal function was greater in patients receiving sirolimus and cyclosporine compared with control therapies.

Renal function should be closely monitored during the administration of sirolimus in combination with cyclosporine since long-term administration can be associated with deterioration of renal function. Appropriate adjustment of the immunosuppression regimen, including discontinuation of sirolimus and/or cyclosporine, should be considered in patients with elevated or increasing serum creatinine levels. Caution should be exercised when using other drugs which are known to impair renal function. In patients at low to moderate immunological risk continuation of combination therapy with cyclosporine beyond 4 months following transplantation should only be considered when the benefits outweigh the risks of this combination for the individual patients (see PRECAUTIONS).

In clinical trials, sirolimus has been administered concurrently with corticosteroids and with the following formulations of cyclosporine:

Sandimmune injection (cyclosporine injection)
Sandimmune oral solution (cyclosporine oral solution)
Sandimmune soft gelatin capsules (cyclosporine capsules)
Neoral soft gelatin capsules [cyclosporine capsules (MODIFIED)]
Neoral oral solution [cyclosporine oral solution (MODIFIED)]

The efficacy and safety of the use of sirolimus in combination with other immunosuppressive agents has not been determined.

Liver Transplantation — Excess Mortality, Graft Loss, and Hepatic Artery Thrombosis (HAT)

The use of sirolimus in combination with tacrolimus was associated with excess mortality and graft loss in a study in *de novo* liver transplant recipients. Many of these patients had evidence of infection at or near the time of death.

In this and another study in *de novo* liver transplant recipients, the use of sirolimus in combination with cyclosporine or tacrolimus was associated with an increase in HAT; most cases of HAT occurred within 30 days post-transplantation and most led to graft loss or death.

Lung Transplantation — Bronchial Anastomotic Dehiscence

Cases of bronchial anastomotic dehiscence, most fatal, have been reported in *de novo* lung transplant patients when sirolimus has been used as part of an immunosuppressive regimen.

The safety and efficacy of sirolimus as immunosuppressive therapy have not been established in liver or lung transplant patients, and therefore, such use is not recommended.

PRECAUTIONS

GENERAL

Sirolimus is intended for oral administration only.

Lymphocele, a known surgical complication of renal transplantation, occurred significantly more often in a dose-related fashion in patients treated with sirolimus. Appropriate post-operative measures should be considered to minimize this complication.

Lipids
The use of sirolimus in renal transplant patients was associated with increased serum cholesterol and triglycerides that may require treatment.

In Studies 1 and 2, in *de novo* renal transplant recipients who began the study with normal, fasting, total serum cholesterol (<200 mg/dl) or normal, fasting, total serum triglycerides (<200 mg/dl), there was an increased incidence of hypercholesterolemia (fasting serum cholesterol >240 mg/dl) or hypertriglyceridemia (fasting serum triglycerides >500 mg/dl), respectively, in patients receiving both sirolimus 2 and 5 mg compared with azathioprine and placebo controls.

Treatment of new-onset hypercholesterolemia with lipid-lowering agents was required in 42-52% of patients enrolled in the sirolimus arms of Studies 1 and 2 compared with 16% of patients in the placebo arm and 22% of patients in the azathioprine arm.

In Study 4 during the prerandomization period, mean fasting serum cholesterol and triglyceride values rapidly increased, and peaked at 2 months with mean cholesterol values >240 mg/dl and triglycerides >250 mg/dl. After randomization mean cholesterol and triglyceride values remained higher in the cyclosporine withdrawal arm compared to the sirolimus and cyclosporine combination.

Renal transplant patients have a higher prevalence of clinically significant hyperlipidemia. Accordingly, the risk/benefit should be carefully considered in patients with established hyperlipidemia before initiating an immunosuppressive regimen including sirolimus.

Any patient who is administered sirolimus should be monitored for hyperlipidemia using laboratory tests and if hyperlipidemia is detected, subsequent interventions such as diet, exercise, and lipid-lowering agents, as outlined by the National Cholesterol Education Program guidelines, should be initiated.

In clinical trials, the concomitant administration of sirolimus and HMG-CoA reductase inhibitors and/or fibrates appeared to be well tolerated.

During sirolimus therapy with cyclosporine, patients administered an HMG-CoA reductase inhibitor and/or fibrate should be monitored for the possible development of rhabdomyolysis and other adverse effects as described in the respective labeling for these agents.

Renal Function
Patients treated with cyclosporine and sirolimus were noted to have higher serum creatinine levels and lower glomerular filtration rates compared with patients treated with cyclosporine and placebo or azathioprine controls (Studies 1 and 2). The rate of decline in renal function in these studies was greater in patients receiving sirolimus and cyclosporine compared with control therapies. In patients at low to moderate immunological risk continuation of combination therapy with cyclosporine beyond 4 months following transplantation should only be considered when the benefits outweigh the risks of this combination for the individual patient (see WARNINGS).

S

Renal function should be monitored during the administration of sirolimus in combination with cyclosporine. Appropriate adjustment of the immunosuppression regimen, including discontinuation of sirolimus and/or cyclosporine, should be considered in patients with elevated or increasing serum creatinine levels. Caution should be exercised when using agents (*e.g.*, aminoglycosides, and amphotericin B) that are known to have a deleterious effect on renal function.

Antimicrobial Prophylaxis

Cases of *Pneumocystis carinii* pneumonia have been reported in patients not receiving antimicrobial prophylaxis. Therefore, antimicrobial prophylaxis for *Pneumocystis carinii* pneumonia should be administered for 1 year following transplantation.

Cytomegalovirus (CMV) prophylaxis is recommended for 3 months after transplantation, particularly for patients at increased risk for CMV disease.

Interstitial Lung Disease

Cases of interstitial lung disease (including pneumonitis, and infrequently bronchiolitis obliterans organizing pneumonia [BOOP] and pulmonary fibrosis), some fatal, with no identified infectious etiology have occurred in patients receiving immunosuppressive regimens including sirolimus. In some cases, the interstitial lung disease has resolved upon discontinuation or dose reduction of sirolimus. The risk may be increased as the trough sirolimus concentration increases (see ADVERSE REACTIONS).

INFORMATION FOR THE PATIENT

Patients should be given complete dosage instructions (see Patient Instructions that are distributed with the prescription). Women of childbearing potential should be informed of the potential risks during pregnancy and that they should use effective contraception prior to initiation of sirolimus therapy, during sirolimus therapy and for 12 weeks after sirolimus therapy has been stopped (see Pregnancy Category C).

Patients should be told that exposure to sunlight and UV light should be limited by wearing protective clothing and using a sunscreen with a high protection factor because of the increased risk for skin cancer (see WARNINGS).

LABORATORY TESTS

Whole blood sirolimus concentrations should be monitored in patients receiving concentration-controlled sirolimus. Monitoring is also necessary in patients likely to have altered drug metabolism, in patients ≥13 years who weigh less than 40 kg, in patients with hepatic impairment, and during concurrent administration of potent CYP3A4 inducers and inhibitors (see DRUG INTERACTIONS).

DRUG/LABORATORY TEST INTERACTIONS

There are no studies on the interactions of sirolimus in commonly employed clinical laboratory tests.

CARCINOGENESIS, MUTAGENESIS, AND IMPAIRMENT OF FERTILITY

Sirolimus was not genotoxic in the *in vitro* bacterial reverse mutation assay, the Chinese hamster ovary cell chromosomal aberration assay, the mouse lymphoma cell forward mutation assay, or the *in vivo* mouse micronucleus assay.

Carcinogenicity studies were conducted in mice and rats. In an 86 week female mouse study at dosages of 0, 12.5, 25 and 50/6 (dosage lowered from 50 to 6 mg/kg/day at Week 31 due to infection secondary to immunosuppression) there was a statistically significant increase in malignant lymphoma at all dose levels (approximately 16-135 times the clinical doses adjusted for body surface area) compared with controls. In a second mouse study at dosages of 0, 1, 3 and 6 mg/kg (approximately 3-16 times the clinical dose adjusted for body surface area), hepatocellular adenoma and carcinoma (males), were considered sirolimus related. In the 104 week rat study at dosages of 0, 0.05, 0.1, and 0.2 mg/kg/day (approximately 0.4 to 1 times the clinical dose adjusted for body surface area), there was a statistically significant increased incidence of testicular adenoma in the 0.2 mg/kg/day group.

There was no effect on fertility in female rats following the administration of sirolimus at dosages up to 0.5 mg/kg (approximately 1-3 times the clinical doses adjusted for body surface area). In male rats, there was no significant difference in fertility rate compared to controls at a dosage of 2 mg/kg (approximately 4-11 times the clinical doses adjusted for body surface area). Reductions in testicular weights and/or histological lesions (*e.g.*, tubular atrophy and tubular giant cells) were observed in rats following dosages of 0.65 mg/kg (approximately 1-3 times the clinical doses adjusted for body surface area) and above and in a monkey study at 0.1 mg/kg (approximately 0.4 to 1 times the clinical doses adjusted for body surface area) and above. Sperm counts were reduced in male rats following the administration of sirolimus for 13 weeks at a dosage of 6 mg/kg (approximately 12-32 times the clinical doses adjusted for body surface area), but showed improvement by 3 months after dosing was stopped.

PREGNANCY CATEGORY C

Sirolimus was embryo/feto toxic in rats at dosages of 0.1 mg/kg and above (approximately 0.2-0.5 the clinical doses adjusted for body surface area). Embryo/feto toxicity was manifested as mortality and reduced fetal weights (with associated delays in skeletal ossification). However, no teratogenesis was evident. In combination with cyclosporine, rats had increased embryo/feto mortality compared with sirolimus alone. There were no effects on rabbit development at the maternally toxic dosage of 0.05 mg/kg (approximately 0.3-0.8 times the clinical doses adjusted for body surface area). There are no adequate and well controlled studies in pregnant women. Effective contraception must be initiated before sirolimus therapy, during sirolimus therapy, and for 12 weeks after sirolimus therapy has been stopped. Sirolimus should be used during pregnancy only if the potential benefit outweighs the potential risk to the embryo/fetus.

USE DURING LACTATION

Sirolimus is excreted in trace amounts in milk of lactating rats. It is not known whether sirolimus is excreted in human milk. The pharmacokinetic and safety profiles of sirolimus in infants are not known. Because many drugs are excreted in human milk and because of the potential for adverse reactions in nursing infants from sirolimus, a decision should be made whether to discontinue nursing or to discontinue the drug, taking into account the importance of the drug to the mother.

PEDIATRIC USE

The safety and efficacy of sirolimus in pediatric patients below the age of 13 years have not been established.

GERIATRIC USE

Clinical studies of sirolimus oral solution or tablets did not include sufficient numbers of patients aged 65 years and over to determine whether safety and efficacy differ in this population from younger patients. Data pertaining to sirolimus trough concentrations suggest that dose adjustments based upon age in geriatric renal patients are not necessary.

DRUG INTERACTIONS

Sirolimus is known to be a substrate for both cytochrome CYP3A4 and P-glycoprotein. The pharmacokinetic interaction between sirolimus and concomitantly administered drugs is discussed below. Drug interaction studies have not been conducted with drugs other than those described below.

CYCLOSPORINE CAPSULES MODIFIED

Sirolimus Oral Solution

In a single dose drug-drug interaction study, 24 healthy volunteers were administered 10 mg sirolimus either simultaneously or 4 hours after a 300 mg dose of Neoral soft gelatin capsules [cyclosporine capsules (MODIFIED)]. For simultaneous administration, the mean C_{max} and AUC of sirolimus were increased by 116% and 230%, respectively, relative to administration of sirolimus alone. However, when given 4 hours after Neoral soft gelatin capsules [cyclosporine capsules (MODIFIED)] administration, sirolimus C_{max} and AUC were increased by 37% and 80%, respectively, compared with administration of sirolimus alone.

Mean cyclosporine C_{max} and AUC were not significantly affected when sirolimus was given simultaneously or when administered 4 hours after Neoral soft gelatin capsules [cyclosporine capsules (MODIFIED)]. However, after multiple-dose administration of sirolimus given 4 hours after Neoral in renal post-transplant patients over 6 months, cyclosporine oral-dose clearance was reduced, and lower doses of Neoral soft gelatin capsules [cyclosporine capsules (MODIFIED)] were needed to maintain target cyclosporine concentration.

Sirolimus Tablets

In a single-dose drug-drug interaction study, 24 healthy volunteers were administered 10 mg sirolimus either simultaneously or 4 hours after a 300 mg dose of Neoral soft gelatin capsules [cyclosporine capsules (MODIFIED)]. For simultaneous administration, mean C_{max} and AUC were increased by 512% and 148%, respectively, relative to administration of sirolimus alone. However, when given 4 hours after cyclosporine administration, sirolimus C_{max} and AUC were both increased by only 33% compared with administration of sirolimus alone.

Because of the effect of cyclosporine capsules (MODIFIED), it is recommended that sirolimus should be taken 4 hours after administration of cyclosporine oral solution (MODIFIED) and/or cyclosporine capsules (MODIFIED), (see DOSAGE AND ADMINISTRATION).

CYCLOSPORINE ORAL SOLUTION

In a multiple-dose study in 150 psoriasis patients, sirolimus 0.5, 1.5, and 3 mg/m^2/day was administered simultaneously with Sandimmune oral solution (cyclosporine oral solution) 1.25 mg/kg/day. The increase in average sirolimus trough concentrations ranged between 67-86% relative to when sirolimus was administered without cyclosporine. The intersubject variability (%CV) for sirolimus trough concentrations ranged from 39.7-68.7%. There was no significant effect of multiple-dose sirolimus on cyclosporine trough concentrations following Sandimmune oral solution (cyclosporine oral solution) administration. However, the %CV was higher (range 85.9-165%) than those from previous studies.

Sandimmune oral solution (cyclosporine oral solution) is not bioequivalent to Neoral oral solution (cyclosporine oral solution MODIFIED), and should not be used interchangeably. Although there is no published data comparing Sandimmune oral solution (cyclosporine oral solution) to SangCya oral solution [cyclosporine oral solution (MODIFIED)], they should not be used interchangeably. Likewise, Sandimmune soft gelatin capsules (cyclosporine capsules) are not bioequivalent to Neoral soft gelatin capsules [cyclosporine capsules (MODIFIED)] and should not be used interchangeably.

DILTIAZEM

The simultaneous oral administration of 10 mg of sirolimus oral solution and 120 mg of diltiazem to 18 healthy volunteers significantly affected the bioavailability of sirolimus. Sirolimus C_{max}, T_{max}, and AUC were increased 1.4-, 1.3-, and 1.6-fold, respectively. Sirolimus did not affect the pharmacokinetics of either diltiazem or its metabolites desacetyldiltiazem and desmethyldiltiazem. If diltiazem is administered, sirolimus should be monitored and a dose adjustment may be necessary.

KETOCONAZOLE

Multiple-dose ketoconazole administration significantly affected the rate and extent of absorption and sirolimus exposure after administration of sirolimus oral solution, as reflected by increases in sirolimus C_{max}, T_{max}, and AUC of 4.3-fold, 38%, and 10.9-fold, respectively. However, the terminal $T_{1/2}$ of sirolimus was not changed. Single-dose sirolimus did not affect steady-state 12 hour plasma ketoconazole concentrations. It is recommended that sirolimus oral solution and oral tablets should not be administered with ketoconazole.

RIFAMPIN

Pretreatment of 14 healthy volunteers with multiple doses of rifampin, 600 mg daily for 14 days, followed by a single 20 mg dose of sirolimus, greatly increased sirolimus oral-dose clearance by 5.5-fold (range = 2.8 to 10), which represents mean decreases in AUC and C_{max} of about 82% and 71%, respectively. In patients where rifampin is indicated, alternative therapeutic agents with less enzyme induction potential should be considered.

DRUGS WHICH MAY BE COADMINISTERED WITHOUT DOSE ADJUSTMENT

Clinically significant pharmacokinetic drug-drug interactions were not observed in studies of drugs listed below. A synopsis of the type of study performed for each drug is provided. Sirolimus and these drugs may be coadministered without dose adjustments.

Acyclovir: Acyclovir, 200 mg, was administered once daily for 3 days followed by a single 10 mg dose of sirolimus oral solution on Day 3 in 20 adult healthy volunteers.

Digoxin: Digoxin, 0.25 mg, was administered daily for 8 days and a single 10 mg dose of sirolimus oral solution was given on Day 8 to 24 healthy volunteers.

Glyburide: A single 5 mg dose of glyburide and a single 10 mg dose of sirolimus oral solution were administered to 24 healthy volunteers. Sirolimus did not affect the hypoglycemic action of glyburide.

Nifedipine: A single 60 mg dose of nifedipine and a single 10 mg dose of sirolimus oral solution were administered to 24 healthy volunteers.

Ethinyl Estradiol; Norgestrel: Sirolimus oral solution, 2 mg, was given daily for 7 days to 21 healthy female volunteers on ethinyl estradiol; norgestrel.

Prednisolone: Pharmacokinetic information was obtained from 42 stable renal transplant patients receiving daily doses of prednisone (5-20 mg/day) and either single or multiple doses of sirolimus oral solution (0.5-5 mg/m^2 q12h).

Sulfamethoxazole; Trimethoprim: A single oral dose of sulfamethoxazole (400 mg)/ trimethoprim (80 mg) was given to 15 renal transplant patients receiving daily oral doses of sirolimus (8-25 mg/m^2).

OTHER DRUG INTERACTIONS

Sirolimus is extensively metabolized by the CYP3A4 isoenzyme in the gut wall and liver. Therefore, absorption and the subsequent elimination of systemically absorbed sirolimus may be influenced by drugs that affect this isoenzyme. Inhibitors of CYP3A4 may decrease the metabolism of sirolimus and increase sirolimus concentrations, while inducers of CYP3A4 may increase the metabolism of sirolimus and decrease sirolimus concentrations.

Drugs that may increase sirolimus blood concentrations include:

Calcium Channel Blockers: Nicardipine, verapamil.
Antifungal Agents: Clotrimazole, fluconazole, itraconazole.
Macrolide Antibiotics: Clarithromycin, erythromycin, troleandomycin.
Gastrointestinal Prokinetic Agents: Cisapride, metoclopramide.
Other Drugs: Bromocriptine, cimetidine, danazol, HIV-protease inhibitors (*e.g.*, ritonavir, indinavir).

Drugs that may decrease sirolimus concentrations include:

Anticonvulsants: Carbamazepine, phenobarbital, phenytoin.
Antibiotics: Rifabutin, rifapentine.

This list is not all inclusive.

Care should be exercised when drugs or other substances that are metabolized by CYP3A4 are administered concomitantly with sirolimus. Grapefruit juice reduces CYP3A4-mediated metabolism of sirolimus and must not be used for dilution (see DOSAGE AND ADMINISTRATION).

Herbal Preparations

St. John's Wort (*hypericum perforatum*) induces CYP3A4 and P-glycoprotein. Since sirolimus is a substrate for both cytochrome CYP3A4 and P-glycoprotein, there is the potential that the use of St. John's Wort in patients receiving sirolimus could result in reduced sirolimus levels.

Vaccination

Immunosuppressants may affect response to vaccination. Therefore, during treatment with sirolimus, vaccination may be less effective. The use of live vaccines should be avoided; live vaccines may include, but are not limited to measles, mumps, rubella, oral polio, BCG, yellow fever, varicella, and TY21a typhoid.

ADVERSE REACTIONS

SIROLIMUS ORAL SOLUTION

The incidence of adverse reactions was determined in two randomized, double-blind, multicenter controlled trials in which 499 renal transplant patients received sirolimus oral solution 2 mg/day, 477 received sirolimus oral solution 5 mg/day, 160 received azathioprine, and 124 received placebo. All patients were treated with cyclosporine and corticosteroids. Data (≥12 months post-transplant) presented in TABLE 16 show the adverse reactions that occurred in any treatment group with an incidence of ≥20%.

Specific adverse reactions associated with the administration of sirolimus oral solution occurred at a significantly higher frequency than with the respective control group. For both sirolimus oral solution 2 and 5 mg/day these include hypercholesterolemia, hyperlipemia, hypertension, and rash; for sirolimus oral solution 2 mg/day acne; and for sirolimus oral solution 5 mg/day anemia, arthralgia, diarrhea, hypokalemia, and thrombocytopenia. The elevations of triglycerides and cholesterol and decreases in platelets and hemoglobin occurred in a dose-related manner in patients receiving sirolimus.

Patients maintained on sirolimus oral solution 5 mg/day, when compared with patients on sirolimus oral solution 2 mg/day, demonstrated an increased incidence of the following adverse events: Anemia, leukopenia, thrombocytopenia, hypokalemia, hyperlipemia, fever, and diarrhea.

In general, adverse events related to the administration of sirolimus were dependent on dose/concentration.

With longer term follow-up, the adverse event profile remained similar. Some new events became significantly different among the treatment groups. For events which occurred at a frequency of ≥20% by 24 months for Study 1 and 36 months for Study 2, only the incidence of edema became significantly higher in both sirolimus groups as compared with the control group. The incidence of headache became significantly more common in the sirolimus 5 mg/day group as compared with control therapy.

At 24 months for Study 1, the following treatment-emergent infections were significantly different among the treatment groups: Bronchitis, Herpes simplex, pneumonia, pyelonephritis, and upper respiratory infections. In each instance, the incidence was highest in the sirolimus 5 mg/day group, lower in the sirolimus 2 mg/day group and lowest in the azathioprine group. Except for upper respiratory infections in the sirolimus 5 mg/day cohort, the remainder of events occurred with a frequency of <20%.

***TABLE 16** Adverse Events Occurring at a Frequency of ≥20% in Any Treatment Group in Prevention of Acute Renal Rejection Trials (%) at ≥12 Months Post-Transplantation for Studies 1 and 2**

	Sirolimus Oral Solution				Azathioprine	
	2 mg/day		5 mg/day		2-3 mg/kg/day	Placebo
Body System	Study 1	Study 2	Study 1	Study 2	Study 1	Study 2
Adverse Event	(n=281)	(n=218)	(n=269)	(n=208)	(n=160)	(n=124)
Body as a Whole						
Abdominal pain	28%	29%	30%	36%	29%	30%
Asthenia	38%	22%	40%	28%	37%	28%
Back pain	16%	23%	26%	22%	23%	20%
Chest pain	16%	18%	19%	24%	16%	19%
Fever	27%	23%	33%	34%	33%	35%
Headache	23%	34%	27%	34%	21%	31%
Pain	24%	33%	29%	29%	30%	25%
Cardiovascular System						
Hypertension	43%	45%	39%	49%	29%	48%
Digestive System						
Constipation	28%	36%	34%	38%	37%	31%
Diarrhea	32%	25%	42%	35%	28%	27%
Dyspepsia	17%	23%	23%	25%	24%	34%
Nausea	31%	25%	36%	31%	39%	29%
Vomiting	21%	19%	25%	25%	31%	21%
Hemic and Lymphatic System						
Anemia	27%	23%	37%	33%	29%	21%
Leukopenia	9%	9%	15%	13%	20%	8%
Thrombocytopenia	13%	14%	20%	30%	9%	9%
Metabolic and Nutritional						
Creatinine increased	35%	39%	37%	40%	28%	38%
Edema	24%	20%	16%	18%	23%	15%
Hypercholesteremia †	38%	43%	42%	46%	33%	23%
Hyperkalemia	15%	17%	12%	14%	24%	27%
Hyperlipemia †	38%	45%	44%	57%	28%	23%
Hypokalemia	17%	11%	21%	17%	11%	9%
Hypophosphatemia	20%	15%	23%	19%	20%	19%
Peripheral edema	60%	54%	64%	58%	58%	48%
Weight gain	21%	11%	15%	8%	19%	15%
Musculoskeletal System						
Arthralgia	25%	25%	27%	31%	21%	18%
Nervous System						
Insomnia	14%	13%	22%	14%	18%	8%
Tremor	31%	21%	30%	22%	28%	19%
Respiratory System						
Dyspnea	22%	24%	28%	30%	23%	30%
Pharyngitis	17%	16%	16%	21%	17%	22%
Upper respiratory infection	20%	26%	24%	23%	13%	23%
Skin and Appendages						
Acne	31%	22%	20%	22%	17%	19%
Rash	12%	10%	13%	20%	6%	6%
Urogenital System						
Urinary tract infection	20%	26%	23%	33%	31%	26%

* Patients received cyclosporine and corticosteroids.
† See WARNINGS and PRECAUTIONS.

At 36 months in Study 2 only the incidence of treatment-emergent Herpes simplex was significantly different among the treatment groups, being higher in the sirolimus 5 mg/day group than either of the other groups.

TABLE 17 summarizes the incidence of malignancies in the two controlled trials for the prevention of acute rejection. At 24 (Study 1) and 36 months (Study 2) there were no significant differences among treatment groups.

***TABLE 17** Incidence (%) of Malignancies in Studies 1 (24 Months) and Study 2 (36 Months) Post-Transplant*†*

	Sirolimus Oral Solution				Azathioprine	
	2 mg/day		5 mg/day		2-3 mg/kg/day	Placebo
	Study 1	Study 2	Study 1	Study 2	Study 1	Study 2
Malignancy	(n=284)	(n=227)	(n=274)	(n=219)	(n=161)	(n=130)
Lymphoma/ lymphoproliferative disease	0.7%	1.8%	1.1%	3.2%	0.6%	0.8%
Skin Carcinoma						
Any squamous cell‡	0.4%	2.7%	2.2%	0.9%	3.8%	3.0%
Any basal cell‡	0.7%	2.2%	1.5%	1.8%	2.5%	5.3%
Melanoma	0.0%	0.4%	0.0%	1.4%	0.0%	0.0%
Miscellaneous/not speicified	0.0%	0.0%	0.0%	0.0%	0.0%	0.8%
Total	**1.1%**	**4.4%**	**3.3%**	**4.1%**	**4.3%**	**7.7%**
Other Malignancy	**1.1%**	**2.2%**	**1.5%**	**1.4%**	**0.6%**	**2.3%**

* Patients received cyclosporine and corticosteroids.
† Includes patients who prematurely discontinued treatment.
‡ Patients may be counted in more than one category.

Among the adverse events that were reported at a rate of ≥3% and <20% at 12 months, the following were more prominent in patients maintained on sirolimus 5 mg/day, when compared to patients on sirolimus 2 mg/day: Epistaxis, lymphocele, insomnia, thrombotic thrombocytopenic purpura (hemolytic-uremic syndrome), skin ulcer, increased LDH, hypotension, facial edema.

The following adverse events were reported with ≥3% and <20% incidence in patients in any sirolimus treatment group in the two controlled clinical trials for the prevention of acute rejection:

Body as a Whole: Abdomen enlarged, abscess, ascites, cellulitis, chills, face edema, flu syndrome, generalized edema, hernia, *Herpes zoster* infection, lymphocele, malaise, pelvic pain, peritonitis, sepsis.

Cardiovascular System: Atrial fibrillation, congestive heart failure, hemorrhage, hypervolemia, hypotension, palpitation, peripheral vascular disorder, postural hypotension, syncope, tachycardia, thrombophlebitis, thrombosis, vasodilatation.

Digestive System: Anorexia, dysphagia, eructation, esophagitis, flatulence, gastritis, gastroenteritis, gingivitis, gum hyperplasia, ileus, liver function tests abnormal, mouth ulceration, oral moniliasis, stomatitis.

Endocrine System: Cushing's syndrome, diabetes mellitus, glycosuria.

Hemic and Lymphatic System: Ecchymosis, leukocytosis, lymphadenopathy, polycythemia, thrombotic thrombocytopenic purpura (hemolytic-uremic syndrome).

Metabolic and Nutritional: Acidosis, alkaline phosphatase increased, BUN increased, creatine phosphokinase increased, dehydration, healing abnormal, hypercalcemia, hyperglycemia, hyperphosphatemia, hypocalcemia, hypoglycemia, hypomagnesemia, hyponatremia, lactic dehydrogenase increased, AST/SGOT increased, ALT/SGPT increased, weight loss.

Musculoskeletal System: Arthrosis, bone necrosis, leg cramps, myalgia, osteoporosis, tetany.

Nervous System: Anxiety, confusion, depression, dizziness, emotional lability, hypertonia, hypesthesia, hypotonia, insomnia, neuropathy, paresthesia, somnolence.

Respiratory System: Asthma, atelectasis, bronchitis, cough increased, epistaxis, hypoxia, lung edema, pleural effusion, pneumonia, rhinitis, sinusitis.

Skin and Appendages: Fungal dermatitis, hirsutism, pruritus, skin hypertrophy, skin ulcer, sweating.

Special Senses: Abnormal vision, cataract, conjunctivitis, deafness, ear pain, otitis media, tinnitus.

Urogenital System: Albuminuria, bladder pain, dysuria, hematuria, hydronephrosis, impotence, kidney pain, kidney tubular necrosis, nocturia, oliguria, pyelonephritis, pyuria, scrotal edema, testis disorder, toxic nephropathy, urinary frequency, urinary incontinence, urinary retention.

Less frequently occurring adverse events included: Mycobacterial infections, Epstein-Barr virus infections, and pancreatitis.

Among the events which were reported at an incidence of ≥3% and <20% by 24 months for Study 1 and 36 months for Study 2, tachycardia and Cushing's syndrome were reported significantly more commonly in both sirolimus groups as compared with the control therapy. Events that were reported more commonly in the sirolimus 5 mg/day group than either the sirolimus 2 mg/day group and/or control group were: abnormal healing, bone necrosis, chills, congestive heart failure, dysuria, hernia, hirsutism, urinary frequency, and lymphadenopathy.

SIROLIMUS TABLETS

The safety profile of the tablet did not differ from that of the oral solution formulation. The incidence of adverse reactions up to 12 months was determined in a randomized, multicenter controlled trial (Study 3) in which 229 renal transplant patients received sirolimus oral solution 2 mg once daily and 228 patients received sirolimus tablets 2 mg once daily. All patients were treated with cyclosporine and corticosteroids. The adverse reactions that occurred in either treatment group with an incidence of ≥20% in Study 3 are similar to those reported for Studies 1 and 2. There was no notable difference in the incidence of these adverse events between treatment groups (oral solution versus tablets) in Study 3, with the exception of acne, which occurred more frequently in the oral solution group, and tremor which occurred more frequently in the tablet group, particularly in Black patients.

The adverse events that occurred in patients with an incidence of ≥3% and <20% in either treatment group in Study 3 were similar to those reported in Studies 1 and 2. There was no notable difference in the incidence of these adverse events between treatment groups (oral solution versus tablets) in Study 3, with the exception of hypertonia, which occurred more frequently in the oral solution group and diabetes mellitus which occurred more frequently in the tablet group. Hispanic patients in the tablet group experienced hyperglycemia more frequently than Hispanic patients in the oral solution group. In Study 3 alone, menorrhagia, metrorrhagia, and polyuria occurred with an incidence of ≥3% and <20%.

The clinically important opportunistic or common transplant-related infections were identical in all three studies and the incidences of these infections were similar in Study 3 compared with Studies 1 and 2. The incidence rates of these infections were not significantly different between the oral solution and tablet treatment groups in Study 3.

In Study 3 (at 12 months), there were 2 cases of lymphoma/lymphoproliferative disorder in the oral solution treatment group (0.8%) and 2 reported cases of lymphoma/lymphoproliferative disorder in the tablet treatment group (0.8%). These differences were not statistically significant and were similar to the incidences observed in Studies 1 and 2.

SIROLIMUS FOLLOWING CYCLOSPORINE WITHDRAWAL

The incidence of adverse reactions was determined through 36 months in a randomized, multicenter controlled trial (Study 4) in which 215 renal transplant patients received sirolimus as a maintenance regimen following cyclosporine withdrawal and 215 patients received sirolimus with cyclosporine therapy. All patients were treated with corticosteroids. The safety profile prior to randomization (start of cyclosporine withdrawal) was similar to that of the 2 mg sirolimus groups in Studies 1, 2, and 3. Following randomization (at 3 months) patients who had cyclosporine eliminated from their therapy experienced significantly higher incidences of abnormal liver function tests (including increased AST/SGOT and increased ALT/SGPT), hypokalemia, thrombocytopenia, abnormal healing, ileus, and rectal disorder. Conversely, the incidence of hypertension, cyclosporine toxicity, increased creatinine, abnormal kidney function, toxic nephropathy, edema, hyperkalemia, hyperuricemia, and gum hyperplasia was significantly higher in patients who remained on cyclosporine than those who had cyclosporine withdrawn from therapy. Mean systolic and diastolic blood pressure improved significantly following cyclosporine withdrawal.

In Study 4, at 36 months, the incidence of Herpes zoster infection was significantly lower in patients receiving sirolimus following cyclosporine withdrawal compared with patients who continued to receive sirolimus and cyclosporine.

The incidence of malignancies in Study 4 is presented in TABLE 18. In Study 4, the incidence of lymphoma/lymphoproliferative disease was similar in all treatment groups. The overall incidence of malignancy was higher in patients receiving sirolimus plus cyclosporine compared with patients who had cyclosporine withdrawn.

TABLE 18 *Incidence (%) of Malignancies in Study 4 at 36 Months Post-Transplant*†*

Malignancy	Nonrandomized (n=95)	Sirolimus With Cyclosporine Therapy (n=215)	Sirolimus Following Cyclosprorine Withdrawal (n=215)
Lymphoma/ lymphoproliferative disease	**1.1%**	**1.4%**	**0.5%**
Skin Carcinoma			
Any squamous cell‡	1.1%	1.9%	2.3%
Any basel cell‡	3.2%	4.7%	2.3%
Melanoma	0.0%	0.5%	0.0%
Miscellaneous/not specified	1.1%	0.9%	0.0%
Total	**4.2%**	**6.5%**	**3.7%**
Other Malignancy	**1.1%**	**3.3%**	**1.4%**

* Patients received cyclosporine and corticosteroids.
† Includes patients who prematurely discontinued treatment.
‡ Patients may be counted in more than one category.

OTHER CLINICAL EXPERIENCE

Cases of interstitial lung disease (including pneumonitis, and infrequently bronchiolitis obliterans organizing pneumonia [BOOP] and pulmonary fibrosis), some fatal, with no identified infectious etiology have occurred in patients receiving immunosuppressive regimens including sirolimus. In some cases, the interstitial lung disease has resolved upon discontinuation or dose reduction of sirolimus. The risk may be increased as the sirolimus trough concentration increases (see PRECAUTIONS).

There have been rare reports of pancytopenia.

Hepatotoxicity has been reported, including fatal hepatic necrosis with elevated sirolimus trough levels.

Abnormal healing following transplant surgery has been reported, including fascial dehiscence and anastomatic disruption (*e.g.*, wound, vascular, airway, ureteral, biliary).

DOSAGE AND ADMINISTRATION

It is recommended that sirolimus oral solution and tablets be used initially in a regimen with cyclosporine and corticosteroids. Cyclosporine withdrawal is recommended 2-4 months after transplantation in patients at low to moderate immunological risk.

The safety and efficacy of cyclosporine withdrawal in high-risk patients have not been adequately studied and it is therefore not recommended. This includes patients with Banff grade III acute rejection or vascular rejection prior to cyclosporine withdrawal, those who are dialysis-dependent, or with serum creatinine >4.5 mg/dl, black patients, re-transplants, multi-organ transplants, patients with high panel of reactive antibodies (see INDICATIONS AND USAGE).

Two mg (2 mg) of sirolimus oral solution has been demonstrated to be clinically equivalent to 2 mg sirolimus oral tablets and hence, are interchangeable on a mg to mg basis. However, it is not known if higher doses of sirolimus oral solution are clinically equivalent to higher doses of tablets on a mg to mg basis. (See CLINICAL PHARMACOLOGY, Pharmacokinetics, Absorption.) Sirolimus is to be administered orally once daily.

SIROLIMUS AND CYCLOSPORINE COMBINATION THERAPY

The initial dose of sirolimus should be administered as soon as possible after transplantation. For *de novo* transplant recipients, a loading dose of sirolimus of 3 times the maintenance dose should be given. A daily maintenance dose of 2 mg is recommended for use in renal transplant patients, with a loading dose of 6 mg. Although a daily maintenance dose of 5 mg, with a loading dose of 15 mg was used in clinical trials of the oral solution and was shown to be safe and effective, no efficacy advantage over the 2 mg dose could be established for renal transplant patients. Patients receiving 2 mg of sirolimus oral solution per day demonstrated an overall better safety profile than did patients receiving 5 mg of sirolimus oral solution per day.

SIROLIMUS FOLLOWING CYCLOSPORINE WITHDRAWAL

Initially, patients considered for cyclosporine withdrawal should be receiving sirolimus and cyclosporine combination therapy. At 2-4 months following transplantation, cyclosporine should be progressively discontinued over 4-8 weeks and the sirolimus dose should be adjusted to obtain whole blood trough concentrations within the range of 12-24 ng/ml (chromatographic method). Therapeutic drug monitoring should not be the sole basis for adjusting sirolimus therapy. Careful attention should be made to clinical signs/symptoms, tissue biopsy, and laboratory parameters. Cyclosporine inhibits the metabolism and transport of sirolimus, and consequently, sirolimus concentrations will decrease when cyclosporine is discontinued unless the sirolimus dose is increased. The sirolimus dose will need to be approximately 4-fold higher to account for both the absence of the pharmacokinetic interaction (approximately 2-fold increase) and the augmented immunosuppressive requirement in the absence of cyclosporine (approximately 2-fold increase).

Frequent sirolimus dose adjustments based on non-steady-state sirolimus concentrations can lead to overdosing or underdosing because sirolimus has a long half-life. Once sirolimus maintenance dose is adjusted, patients should be retained on the new maintenance dose at least for 7-14 days before further dosage adjustment with concentration monitoring. In most patients dose adjustments can be based on simple proportion: new sirolimus dose = current dose × (target concentration / current concentration). A loading dose should be considered in addition to a new maintenance dose when it is necessary to considerably increase sirolimus trough concentrations: sirolimus loading dose = 3 × (new maintenance dose — current maintenance dose). The maximum sirolimus dose administered on any day should not exceed 40 mg. If an estimated daily dose exceeds 40 mg due to the addition of a loading dose, the loading dose should be administered over 2 days. Sirolimus trough concentrations should be monitored at least 3-4 days after a loading dose(s).

To minimize the variability of exposure to sirolimus, this drug should be taken consistently with or without food. Grapefruit juice reduces CYP3A4-mediated metabolism of sirolimus and must not be administered with sirolimus or used for dilution.

It is recommended that sirolimus be taken 4 hours after administration of cyclosporine oral solution (MODIFIED) and/or cyclosporine capsules (MODIFIED).

DOSE ADJUSTMENT

The initial dosage in patients ≥13 years who weigh less than 40 kg should be adjusted, based on body surface area, to 1 mg/m²/day. The loading dose should be 3 mg/m².

It is recommended that the maintenance dose of sirolimus be reduced by approximately one-third in patients with hepatic impairment. It is not necessary to modify the sirolimus loading dose. Dosage need not be adjusted because of impaired renal function.

BLOOD CONCENTRATION MONITORING

Whole blood trough concentrations of sirolimus should be monitored in patients receiving concentration-controlled sirolimus. Monitoring is also necessary in pediatric patients, in patients with hepatic impairment, during concurrent administration of strong CYP3A4 and/or p-glycoprotein inducers and inhibitors, and/or if cyclosporine dosage is markedly changed or discontinued (see DOSAGE AND ADMINISTRATION).

In controlled clinical trials with concomitant cyclosporine (Studies 1 and 2), mean sirolimus whole blood trough concentrations through Month 12 following transplantation, as measured by immunoassay, were 9 ng/ml (range 4.5-14 ng/ml [10th to 90th percentile]) for the 2 mg/day treatment group, and 17 ng/ml (range 10-28 ng/ml [10th to 90th percentile]) for the 5 mg/day dose.

In a controlled clinical trial with cyclosporine withdrawal (Study 4), the mean sirolimus whole blood trough concentrations during Months 4 through 12 following transplantation, as measured by immunoassay, were 10.7 ng/ml (range 6.3-16.0 ng/ml [10th to 90th percentile]) in the concomitant sirolimus and cyclosporine treatment group (n=205) and were 23.3 ng/ml (range 17.0-29.0 ng/ml [10th to 90th percentile]) in the cyclosporine withdrawal treatment group (n=200).

Results from other assays may differ from those with an immunoassay. On average, chromatographic methods (HPLC UV or LC/MS/MS) yield results that are approximately 20% lower than the immunoassay for whole blood concentration determinations. Adjustments to the targeted range should be made according to the assay utilized to determine sirolimus trough concentrations. Therefore, comparison between concentrations in the published literature and an individual patient concentration using current assays must be made with detailed knowledge of the assay methods employed. A discussion of the different assay methods is contained in *Clinical Therapeutics*, Volume 22, Supplement B, April 2000.

INSTRUCTIONS FOR DILUTION AND ADMINISTRATION OF SIROLIMUS ORAL SOLUTION

Bottles

The amber oral dose syringe should be used to withdraw the prescribed amount of sirolimus oral solution from the bottle. Empty the correct amount of sirolimus from the syringe into only a glass or plastic container holding at least two (2) ounces (¼ cup, 60 ml) of water or orange juice. No other liquids, including grapefruit juice, should be used for dilution. Stir vigorously and drink at once. Refill the container with an additional volume (minimum of four [4] ounces [½ cup, 120 ml]) of water or orange juice, stir vigorously, and drink at once.

Pouches

When using the pouch, squeeze the entire contents of the pouch into only a glass or plastic container holding at least two (2) ounces (¼ cup, 60 ml) of water or orange juice. No other liquids, including grapefruit juice, should be used for dilution. Stir vigorously and drink at once. Refill the container with an additional volume (minimum of four [4] ounces [½ cup, 120 ml]) of water or orange juice, stir vigorously, and drink at once.

Handling and Disposal

Since sirolimus is not absorbed through the skin, there are no special precautions. However, if direct contact with the skin or mucous membranes occurs, wash thoroughly with soap and water; rinse eyes with plain water.

HOW SUPPLIED

RAPAMUNE ORAL SOLUTION

Rapamune oral solution is supplied at a concentration of 1 mg/ml in 2 oz (60 ml fill) and 5 oz (150 ml fill) amber glass bottles.

Rapamune oral solution is also supplied in 1, 2, or 5 ml laminated aluminum pouches.

RAPAMUNE TABLETS

Rapamune tablets are available as:

1 mg: White, trangular-shaped tablets marked "RAPAMUNE 1 mg" on one side.

2 mg: Yellow to beige triangular-shaped tablets marked "RAPAMUNE 2 mg" on one side.

STORAGE

Rapamune oral solution bottles and pouches should be stored protected from light and refrigerated at 2-8°C (36-46°F). Once the bottle is opened, the contents should be used within 1 month. If necessary, the patient may store both the pouches and the bottles at room temperatures up to 25°C (77°F) for a short period of time (*e.g.*, up to 24 hours for the pouches and not more than 15 days for the bottles).

An amber syringe and cap are provided for dosing and the product may be kept in the syringe for a maximum of 24 hours at room temperatures up to 25°C (77°F) or refrigerated at 2-8°C (36-46°F). The syringe should be discarded after one use. After dilution, the preparation should be used immediately.

Rapamune oral solution provided in bottles may develop a slight haze when refrigerated. If such a haze occurs allow the product to stand at room temperature and shake gently until the haze disappears. The presence of this haze does not affect the quality of the product.

Rapamune tablets should be stored at 20-25°C (68-77°F). Use cartons to protect blister cards and strips from light. Dispense in a tight, light-resistant container.

PRODUCT LISTING - EQUIVALENTS NOT AVAILABLE

Solution - Oral - 1 mg/ml
60 ml $450.00 RAPAMUNE, Wyeth-Ayerst Laboratories 00008-1030-06
Tablet - Oral - 1 mg
100's $750.00 RAPAMUNE, Wyeth-Ayerst Laboratories 00008-1031-05
100's $750.00 RAPAMUNE, Wyeth-Ayerst Laboratories 00008-1031-10
Tablet - Oral - 2 mg
100's $1500.00 RAPAMUNE, Wyeth-Ayerst Laboratories 00008-1032-05

Sodium Ferric Gluconate *(003431)*

For complete prescribing information, refer to the CD-ROM included with the book.

Categories: Anemia, iron-deficiency; FDA Approved 1999 Feb; Pregnancy Category B
Drug Classes: Hematinics; Vitamins/minerals
Brand Names: Ferrlecit

DESCRIPTION

Sodium ferric gluconate complex in sucrose injection is a stable macromolecular complex with an apparent molecular weight on gel chromatography of 289,000-440,000 daltons. The macromolecular complex is negatively charged at alkaline pH and is present in solution with sodium cations. The product has a deep red color indicative of ferric oxide linkages.

Each ampule of 5 ml of Ferrlecit for intravenous injection contains 62.5 mg (12.5 mg/ml) of elemental iron as the sodium salt of a ferric ion carbohydrate complex in an alkaline aqueous solution with approximately 20% sucrose w/v (195 mg/ml) in water for injection, pH 7.7-9.7.

Each ml contains 9 mg of benzyl alcohol as an inactive ingredient.
Therapeutic Class: Hematinic.

INDICATIONS AND USAGE

Sodium ferric gluconate is indicated for treatment of iron deficiency anemia in patients undergoing chronic hemodialysis who are receiving supplemental epoetin therapy.

CONTRAINDICATIONS

- All anemias not associated with iron deficiency.
- Hypersensitivity to sodium ferric gluconate or any of its inactive components.
- Evidence of iron overload.

WARNINGS

Hypersensitivity reactions have been reported with injectable iron products.

DOSAGE AND ADMINISTRATION

The dosage of sodium ferric gluconate is expressed in terms of mg of elemental iron. Each 5 ml ampule contains 62.5 mg of elemental iron (12.5 mg/ml).

The recommended dosage of sodium ferric gluconate for the repletion treatment of iron deficiency in hemodialysis patients is 10 ml of sodium ferric gluconate (125 mg of elemental iron). Sodium ferric gluconate may be diluted in 100 ml of 0.9% sodium chloride administered by intravenous infusion over 1 hour. Sodium ferric gluconate may also be administered undiluted as a slow IV injection (at a rate of up to 12.5 mg/min). Most patients will require a minimum cumulative dose of 1.0 g of elemental iron, administered over eight sessions at sequential dialysis treatments, to achieve a favorable hemoglobin or hematocrit response. Patients may continue to require therapy with intravenous iron at the lowest dose necessary to maintain target levels of hemoglobin, hematocrit, and laboratory parameters of iron storage within acceptable limits. Sodium ferric gluconate has been administered at sequential dialysis sessions by infusion or by slow IV injection during the dialysis session itself.

Note: Do not mix sodium ferric gluconate with other medications, or add to parenteral nutrition solutions for intravenous infusion. The compatibility of sodium ferric gluconate with intravenous infusion vehicles other than 0.9% sodium chloride has not been evaluated. Parenteral drug products should be inspected visually for particulate matter and discoloration before administration, whenever the solution and container permit.
If diluted in saline, use immediately after dilution.

PRODUCT LISTING - RATED THERAPEUTICALLY EQUIVALENT

Solution - Intravenous - 12.5 mg/ml
5 ml x 10 $430.00 FERRLECIT, Watson/Schein Pharmaceuticals Inc 00364-2791-23

PRODUCT LISTING - EQUIVALENTS NOT AVAILABLE

Solution - Intravenous - 12.5 mg/ml
5 ml x 10 $430.00 FERRLECIT, Watson Laboratories Inc 52544-0922-26

Sodium Fluoride (002244)

Categories: Caries, dental, prevention; FDA Pre 1938 Drugs; WHO Formulary
Drug Classes: Dental preparations; Vitamins/minerals
Brand Names: Acidulated Phosphate Fluoride; Altaflor; Audifluor; Fluorabon; Fluorineed; Fluorinse; Fluoritab; Fluorodex; Flura; Karidium; Karigel; Liqui-Flur; **Luride**; Nafrinse; Neutracare; Pediaflor; Perio Med; Pharmaflur; Phos-Flur; Phosphate Fluoride; Prevident; Prevident 5000 Plus; Thera-Flur; Zymafluor
Foreign Brand Availability: Fluoen (Israel); Fluor-A-Day (Canada); Fluoravit (Mexico); Flurets (Australia); Ossin (Colombia); Pedi-Dent (Canada); Teeth Tough (Israel); Vinafluor (Indonesia)

DESCRIPTION

ORAL RINSE

Sodium fluoride oral rinse is acidulated phosphate sodium fluoride and is an oral rinse/supplement. Each teaspoonful (5 ml) contains 1.0 mg fluoride ion (F-) from 2.2 mg sodium fluoride (NaF), in a 0.1 Molar phosphate solution at pH 4, for use as a dental caries preventive in children. Cherry, cool mint, bubble gum, grape - sugar and saccharin free. Cinnamon - contains saccharin, but is sugar free.

DENTAL RINSE

Sodium fluoride dental rinse provides 0.2% sodium fluoride in a mint-flavored, neutral aqueous solution containing 6% alcohol. For weekly use as caries preventive.

BRUSH-ON GEL

Self-topical neutral fluoride containing 1.1% sodium fluoride for use as a dental caries preventive in children and adults. This prescription product is not a dentifrice.

GEL-DROPS

Sodium fluoride (acidulated) gel-drops contain 0.5% fluoride ion (F-) from 1.1% sodium fluoride (NaF) in a lime-flavored aqueous solution containing 0.1 Molar Phosphate at pH 4.5. For daily self-topical use as a dental caries preventive. This form of this drug (neutral) also contains 0.5% fluoride ion (F-) from 1.1% NaF, but with no acid phosphate, nor artificial flavor or color, at neutral pH.

DROPS/TABLETS

Each ml contains 0.5 mg fluoride ion (F-) from 1.1 mg sodium fluoride (NaF). For use as a dental caries preventive in children. Sugar free. Saccharin-free.

Sodium fluoride lozenge-type chewable tablets for use as a dental caries preventive in children. Sugar free. Saccharin-free. Erythrosine (FD&C red no. 3) Free. Each 0.25 mg F tablet (quarter-strength) contains 0.25 mg F from 0.55 mg NaF. Each 0.5 mg F tablet (half-strength) contains 0.5 mg F from 1.1 mg NaF. Each 1.0 mg F tablet (full-strength) contains 1.0 mg F from 2.2 mg NaF. Each *SF* 0.25 mg F tablet (SF for Special Formula: no artificial color or flavor) contains 0.25 mg F from 0.55 mg NaF.

CLINICAL PHARMACOLOGY

ORAL RINSE AND DROPS/TABLETS

Sodium fluoride acts systemically, before tooth eruption and topically, post-eruption, by increasing tooth resistance to acid dissolution, by promoting remineralization, and by inhibiting the cariogenic microbial process. Acidulation provides greater topical fluoride uptake by dental enamel than neutral solutions. Phosphate protects enamel from demineralization by the acidulated formulation (common ion effect).

DENTAL RINSE

Topical application of sodium fluoride increases tooth resistance to acid dissolution, promotes remineralization, and inhibits the cariogenic microbial process.

BRUSH-ON GEL/GEL DROPS

Frequent topical applications to the teeth with preparations having a relatively high fluoride content increase tooth resistance to acid dissolution and enhance penetration of the fluoride ion into tooth enamel.

INDICATIONS AND USAGE

ORAL RINSE

It has been well established that ingestion of fluoridated drinking water (1 ppm F) during the period of tooth development results in a significant decrease in the incidence of dental caries. This oral rinse was developed to provide topical and systemic fluoride use as a supplement (rinse-and-swallow) in children age 3 and older living in areas where the water fluoride level does not exceed 0.6 ppm. Sodium fluoride oral rinse provides benefits as a topical fluoride dental rinse only (rinse-and-expectorate) for children age 6 and older. Pioneering clinical studies on sodium fluoride oral rinse were published by Frankel *et al.* and Aasenden *et al.* in 1972.

DENTAL RINSE

It has been established that weekly rinsing with a neutral 0.2% sodium fluoride solution protects against dental caries in children. Prevident Rinse was developed to provide a ready-to-use, flavored preparation for convenient administration and favorable compliance.

BRUSH-ON GEL

It is well established that 1.1% sodium fluoride is safe and extraordinarily effective as a caries preventive when applied frequently with mouthpiece applicators. Sodium fluoride Brush-on Gel in a squeeze-tube is a particularly convenient dosage form which permits the application of a thin ribbon of gel onto a tooth brush as well as a mouth-piece tray.

GEL-DROPS

It is well established that 1.1% sodium fluoride is a safe and effective caries preventive when applied frequently with mouthpiece applicators. Pioneering clinical studies with this form of sodium fluoride in school children were conducted by Englander et al.

Both neutral and acidulated phosphate fluoride gels have been effective in controlling rampant dental decay which frequently follows xerostomia-producing radiotherapy of tumors in the head and neck region.

DROPS/TABLETS

It has been well established that ingestion of fluoridated drinking water (1 ppm F) during the period of tooth development results in a significant decrease in the incidence of dental caries. These forms were developed to provide systemic fluoride use as a supplement in children age 6 months to 3 years living in areas where the water fluoride level does not exceed 0.3 ppm and in children age 3-16 years living in areas where the water fluoride level does not exceed 0.6 ppm.

CONTRAINDICATIONS

ORAL RINSE

DO NOT SWALLOW in areas where the F-content of drinking water exceeds 0.6 ppm, nor in children under the age of 3.

DENTAL RINSE/BRUSH-ON GEL/GEL DROPS

None. (May be used whether drinking water is fluoridated or not, since **topical** fluoride cannot produce fluorosis).

DROPS/TABLETS

These forms are contraindicated in areas where the drinking water exceeds 0.6 ppm F and in pediatric patients under 6 months of age. The 1 mg F strength tablet is contraindicated where the drinking water exceeds 0.3 ppm F. The 0.5 mg tablets should not be administered to pediatric patients under the age of 3, and the 1 mg tablets should not be administered to pediatric patients under the age of 6.

WARNINGS

ORAL RINSE

Do not use as rinse in children under age 6. Do not use as a supplement in children under age 3, nor in areas where the drinking water exceeds 0.6 ppm F. As in the case of all medications, keep out of reach of infants and children.

DENTAL RINSE

DO NOT SWALLOW. Do not use in children under age 6, since younger children frequently cannot perform the rinse process without significant swallowing. As in the case of all medications, keep out of reach of children.

BRUSH-ON GEL/GEL DROPS

As with all medications, keep out of reach of children. Not to be used in children under 6. The fruit sherbet flavor of the brush-on gel contains FD&C yellow no. 6.

DROPS/TABLETS

(See CONTRAINDICATIONS.) As in the case of all medications, keep out of reach of infants and children. The 0.5 mg/ml F drops and orange 1.0 mg F tablets contain FD&C yellow no. 6.

PRECAUTIONS

Oral Rinse: Incompatibility of systemic fluoride with dairy foods has been reported due to formation of calcium fluoride which is poorly absorbed.
Dental Rinse: Not for systemic use. (Each 5 ml contains 4.5 mg fluoride ion).
Gel-Drops: Laboratory tests indicate that the use of acidulated fluoride may cause dulling of porcelain and ceramic restorations. Therefore, the neutral formulation of this form of sodium fluoride is recommended for this type of patient.
Drops/Tablets: Incompatibility of fluoride with dairy foods has been reported due to formation of calcium fluoride which is poorly absorbed.

ADVERSE REACTIONS

Oral Rinse and Drops/Tablets: Allergic reactions and other idiosyncrasies have been rarely reported.
Dental Rinse/Gel Drops: In patients with mucositis, gingival tissues may be hypersensitive to flavor or alcohol present in formulation or to the acidity.

DOSAGE AND ADMINISTRATION

ORAL RINSE

As a Daily Dental Rinse

Pediatric patients age 6-12, use 5 ml (1 teaspoonful); pediatric patients age 12 and over, use 10 ml (2 teaspoonful). After thoroughly brushing teeth, preferably at bedtime, rinse vigorously around and between teeth for 1 minute, then expectorate.

As a Daily Supplement

In areas where the drinking water contains less than 0.3 ppm F: pediatric patients age 3-6, rinse with half a teaspoonful (2.5 ml) and swallow; age 6-16, rinse with 1 teaspoonful (5 ml) and swallow. When drinking water contains 0.3-0.6 ppm F, inclusive, reduce dosage to half a teaspoonful (2.5 ml) for age 6-16; do not use in age 3-6 when water is partially fluoridated (0.3-0.6 ppm F). Dental Rinse

Children ages 6-12, 1 teaspoonful (5 ml); over age 12, 2 teaspoonfuls (10 ml). Once a week, preferably at bedtime after thoroughly brushing the teeth, rinse vigorously around and between teeth for 1 minute then expectorate. DO NOT SWALLOW. For maximum benefit, do not eat, drink, or rinse mouth for at least 30 minutes afterwards.

GEL-DROPS

Age 6 and older. For daily use with applicators supplied by the dentist. Apply 4-8 drops as required to cover inner surface of each applicator. Spread gel-drops with tip of bottle. Place applicators over upper and lower teeth at the same time. Bite down lightly for 6 minutes. Remove applicators and rinse mouth. Clean applicators with cold water.

S

BRUSH-ON GEL

After brushing with toothpaste, rinse as usual. Adults and children 6 years of age and older. Apply a thin ribbon of gel to the teeth with a toothbrush or mouthtrays, for at least 1 minute, preferably at bedtime. After use, adults expectorate gel. For best results, do not eat, drink or rinse for 30 minutes. Children age 6-16, expectorate gel and rinse mouth thoroughly.

DROPS/TABLETS

Adjustable dose gives you the flexibility to prescribe optimal DAILY dosage (based on age and F content of water) as shown in TABLE 1.

TABLE 1

F- Content of Drinking Water	Daily Dosage (Fluoride Ion)* Birth to Age 2	Age 2-3	Age 3 and Over
Less than 0.3 ppm	0.25 mg tab or 2 drops	0.5 mg tab or 4 drops	1.0 mg tab or 8 drops
0.3-0.7 ppm	one-half above dosage		
over 0.7 ppm	Fluoride dietary supplements contraindicated		

PRODUCT LISTING - RATED THERAPEUTICALLY EQUIVALENT

Liquid - Oral - 0.25 mg/Drop

23 ml	$2.16	FLUORITAB, Fluoritab Corporation	00288-5523-23
24 ml	$2.75	FLURA-DROPS, Kirkman Sales Company	58223-0684-24

Solution - Oral - 0.5 mg/ml

19 ml	$2.17	FLUORITAB, Fluoritab Corporation	00288-0002-01

Tablet - Oral - 1 mg

100's	$1.88	FLUORITAB, Fluoritab Corporation	00288-0003-01
100's	$1.88	FLUORITAB, Fluoritab Corporation	00288-0005-01
100's	$1.88	FLUORITAB, Fluoritab Corporation	00288-0007-01
100's	$1.88	FLUORITAB, Fluoritab Corporation	00288-2204-01

Tablet, Chewable - Oral - 0.25 mg

100's	$2.16	FLUORITAB, Fluoritab Corporation	00288-5509-01
100's	$2.16	FLUORITAB, Fluoritab Corporation	00288-5510-01

Tablet, Chewable - Oral - 0.5 mg

100's	$2.16	FLUORITAB, Fluoritab Corporation	00288-1106-01
100's	$2.16	FLUORITAB, Fluoritab Corporation	00288-1107-01
100's	$2.16	FLUORITAB, Fluoritab Corporation	00288-1108-01

Tablet, Chewable - Oral - 1 mg

100's	$4.34	FLUORITAB, Fluoritab Corporation	00288-2201-01

PRODUCT LISTING - EQUIVALENTS NOT AVAILABLE

Cream - Topical - 1.1%

54 gm	$7.99	ETHEDENT , Ethex Corporation	58177-0835-37

Gel - Topical - 0.4%

120 gm x 12	$72.03	STANIMAX GEL, Sdi Laboratories Inc	58640-4020-01
121.90 gm	$7.75	GENERIC, Omnii International	48878-4020-03
121.90 gm	$7.75	GENERIC, Omnii International	48878-4070-03
121.90 gm	$7.75	GENERIC, Omnii International	48878-4080-03
129 gm	$7.75	GENERIC, Omnii International	48878-4021-03
129 gm	$7.75	GENERIC, Omnii International	48878-4031-03
129 gm	$7.75	GENERIC, Omnii International	48878-4051-03
129 gm	$7.75	GENERIC, Omnii International	48878-4061-03
129 gm	$8.50	GENERIC, Omnii International	48878-4041-03
210 gm	$5.00	GENERIC, Dunhall Pharmaceuticals Inc	00217-3010-30
210 gm	$5.00	GENERIC, Dunhall Pharmaceuticals Inc	00217-3020-30
210 gm	$5.00	GENERIC, Dunhall Pharmaceuticals Inc	00217-3030-30
210 gm	$5.00	GENERIC, Dunhall Pharmaceuticals Inc	00217-3040-30
210 gm	$5.00	GENERIC, Dunhall Pharmaceuticals Inc	00217-3050-30
210 gm	$5.00	GENERIC, Dunhall Pharmaceuticals Inc	00217-3060-30

Gel - Topical - 1%

60 gm	$9.88	GENERIC, Emerson Laboratories	00802-3923-92

Gel - Topical - 1.1%

24 ml	$5.62	THERA-FLUR-N, Colgate Oral Pharmaceuticals Inc	00126-0196-54
51 gm	$8.30	APF GEL, Cypress Pharmaceutical Inc	60258-0153-01
51 gm	$8.30	APF GEL, Cypress Pharmaceutical Inc	60258-0154-01
56 gm	$8.23	GENERIC, Cypress Pharmaceutical Inc	60258-0151-01
56 gm	$8.88	PREVIDENT, Colgate Oral Pharmaceuticals Inc	00126-0089-02
56 gm	$8.88	PREVIDENT, Colgate Oral Pharmaceuticals Inc	00126-0289-02
56 gm	$9.25	PREVIDENT, Colgate Oral Pharmaceuticals Inc	00126-0088-02
56 gm	$9.25	PREVIDENT, Colgate Oral Pharmaceuticals Inc	00126-0288-02
56 gm	$9.25	PREVIDENT, Colgate Oral Pharmaceuticals Inc	00126-0290-02
56 gm	$9.27	PHOS-FLUR, Colgate Oral Pharmaceuticals Inc	00126-0130-66
56 gm	$9.27	PHOS-FLUR, Colgate Oral Pharmaceuticals Inc	00126-0131-66
56 gm	$9.37	PREVIDENT, Colgate Oral Pharmaceuticals Inc	00126-0288-66
60 gm	$4.78	NEUTRACARE MINT GEL, Oral B Laboratories	00041-0241-22
60 gm	$11.04	PREVIDENT, Physicians Total Care	54868-3030-00

Kit - Topical - 0.14%;1.09%;0.4%

204.50 ml	$17.81	GEL-KAM SENSITIVITY THERAPY, Colgate Oral Pharmaceuticals Inc	00126-0253-00

Liquid - Oral - 0.125 mg/Drop

30 ml	$2.10	FLURA-DROPS, Kirkman Sales Company	58223-0684-30
30 ml	$5.28	GENERIC, Pharmascience Laboratories	51817-0656-61
30 ml	$7.70	GENERIC, Southwood Pharmaceuticals Inc	58016-9077-01
30 ml	$8.50	GENERIC, Tri Med Laboratories Inc	55654-0014-02
50 ml	$5.10	GENERIC, Vintage Pharmaceuticals Inc	00254-9430-48
50 ml	$5.10	GENERIC, Qualitest Products Inc	00603-1244-47

Liquid - Oral - 0.25 mg/0.6 ml

60 ml	$3.13	FLUORABON, Perry Medical Products	11763-0524-20

Lozenge - Oral - 1 mg

60's	$7.25	GENERIC, Pharmascience Laboratories	51817-0672-16
90's	$21.00	GENERIC, Dreir Pharmaceutical	64061-0115-90

Paste - Topical - 1.1%

51 gm	$8.33	GENERIC, Cypress Pharmaceutical Inc	60258-0150-01
51 gm	$9.38	PREVIDENT 5000 PLUS, Allscripts Pharmaceutical Company	54569-4862-00
56 gm	$9.00	PREVIDENT 5000 PLUS, Colgate Oral Pharmaceuticals Inc	00126-0287-02
56 gm	$9.37	PREVIDENT 5000 PLUS, Colgate Oral Pharmaceuticals Inc	00126-0287-66
56 gm x 2	$17.06	PREVIDENT 5000 PLUS, Colgate Oral Pharmaceuticals Inc	00126-0287-33
60 gm	$9.01	GENERIC, Omnii International	48878-3100-06

Solution - Oral - 0.5 mg/ml

50 ml	$6.53	GENERIC, Liquipharm Inc	54198-0171-50
50 ml	$7.00	GENERIC, Hi-Tech Pharmacal Company Inc	50383-0656-50
50 ml	$8.06	GENERIC, Watson/Rugby Laboratories Inc	00536-1998-80
50 ml	$8.15	GENERIC, Teva Pharmaceuticals Usa	00093-9654-57
50 ml	$9.06	LURIDE, Colgate Oral Pharmaceuticals Inc	00126-0002-62
50 ml	$10.40	GENERIC, Altaire Pharmaceuticals Inc	59390-0041-23
50 ml	$15.46	PEDIAFLOR DROPS, Abbott Pharmaceutical	00074-0101-50

Solution - Oral - 1 mg/ml

30 ml	$4.25	GENERIC, Major Pharmaceuticals Inc	00904-1127-30
30 ml	$6.30	GENERIC, Ivax Corporation	00182-6133-66
60 ml	$8.52	KARIDIUM, Colgate Oral Pharmaceuticals Inc	00273-0102-02

Solution - Topical - 0.02%

240 ml	$1.65	GENERIC, Orachem Pharmaceuticals	10733-0569-08
480 ml	$9.75	PHOS-FLUR, Colgate Oral Pharmaceuticals Inc	00126-0135-16
480 ml	$9.75	PHOS-FLUR, Colgate Oral Pharmaceuticals Inc	00126-0138-16
480 ml	$9.75	PHOS-FLUR, Colgate Oral Pharmaceuticals Inc	00126-0139-16
500 ml	$7.55	GENERIC, Liquipharm Inc	54198-0108-16
500 ml	$7.55	GENERIC, Liquipharm Inc	54198-0109-16
500 ml	$7.55	GENERIC, Liquipharm Inc	54198-0172-16
500 ml	$7.55	GENERIC, Liquipharm Inc	54198-0179-16
500 ml	$9.30	PHOS-FLUR, Colgate Oral Pharmaceuticals Inc	00126-0151-46
500 ml	$9.75	PHOS-FLUR, Colgate Oral Pharmaceuticals Inc	00126-0135-46
500 ml	$9.75	PHOS-FLUR, Colgate Oral Pharmaceuticals Inc	00126-0138-46
500 ml	$9.75	PHOS-FLUR, Colgate Oral Pharmaceuticals Inc	00126-0139-46
500 ml	$9.75	PHOS-FLUR, Colgate Oral Pharmaceuticals Inc	00126-0144-46

Solution - Topical - 0.2%

250 ml	$6.63	PREVIDENT DENTAL RINSE, Colgate Oral Pharmaceuticals Inc	00126-0179-99
480 ml	$7.49	FLUORINSE, Oral B Laboratories	00041-0350-07
480 ml	$7.49	FLUORINSE, Oral B Laboratories	00041-0351-07
500 ml	$6.30	GENERIC, Moore, H.L. Drug Exchange Inc	00839-7484-79

Solution - Topical - 0.63%

283 ml	$15.75	GEL-KAM, Colgate Oral Pharmaceuticals Inc	00126-2310-02
283 ml	$15.75	GEL-KAM, Colgate Oral Pharmaceuticals Inc	00126-2310-68
283 ml	$15.75	GEL-KAM, Colgate Oral Pharmaceuticals Inc	00126-2312-02
283 ml	$15.75	GEL-KAM, Colgate Oral Pharmaceuticals Inc	00126-2312-68
300 ml	$6.00	GENERIC, Dunhall Pharmaceuticals Inc	00217-3315-35
300 ml	$6.00	GENERIC, Dunhall Pharmaceuticals Inc	00217-3316-35
300 ml	$9.07	GENERIC, Omnii International	48878-3316-00
300 ml	$9.75	GENERIC, Omnii International	48878-3315-00
300 ml	$9.75	GENERIC, Omnii International	48878-3317-00
300 ml	$14.10	GENERIC, Cypress Pharmaceutical Inc	60258-0159-10
300 ml x 24	$152.40	GENERIC, Sdi Laboratories Inc	58640-4010-01

Swab - Topical - 0.14%;1.09%;0.4%

0.75 gm x 12	$12.50	GEL-KAM DENTINBLOC, Colgate Oral Pharmaceuticals Inc	00126-2381-12

Tablet - Oral - 1 mg

100's	$0.59	GENERIC, Global Pharmaceutical Corporation	00115-4631-01
100's	$1.25	GENERIC, Kirkman Sales Company	58223-0671-01
100's	$2.50	GENERIC, Cmc-Consolidated Midland Corporation	00223-1773-01
180's	$5.50	KARIDIUM, Colgate Oral Pharmaceuticals Inc	00273-0101-01

Tablet, Chewable - Oral - 0.25 mg

100's	$2.16	FLUORITAB, Fluoritab Corporation	00288-5511-01
120's	$6.06	LURIDE, Allscripts Pharmaceutical Company	54569-1254-00

120's	$6.29	GENERIC, Qualitest Products Inc	00603-3621-22
120's	$6.38	GENERIC, Pharmascience Laboratories	51817-0602-16
120's	$6.65	GENERIC, Ethex Corporation	58177-0432-40
120's	$7.40	LURIDE, Colgate Oral Pharmaceuticals Inc	00126-0186-21
120's	$7.43	LURIDE-SF, Colgate Oral Pharmaceuticals Inc	00126-0009-21
Tablet, Chewable - Oral - 0.5 mg			
15's	$2.89	GENERIC, Southwood Pharmaceuticals Inc	58016-0900-50
30's	$0.40	GENERIC, Allscripts Pharmaceutical Company	54569-2870-02
100's	$1.34	GENERIC, Allscripts Pharmaceutical Company	54569-2870-01
100's	$1.98	GENERIC, Perry Medical Products	11763-0217-01
100's	$4.23	GENERIC, Southwood Pharmaceuticals Inc	58016-0900-00
120's	$1.65	NAFRINSE, Orachem Pharmaceuticals	10733-0765-04
120's	$6.38	GENERIC, Pharmascience Laboratories	51817-0611-16
120's	$6.65	GENERIC, Ethex Corporation	58177-0433-40
120's	$7.40	LURIDE, Colgate Oral Pharmaceuticals Inc	00126-0014-21
Tablet, Chewable - Oral - 1 mg			
30's	$0.47	GENERIC, Allscripts Pharmaceutical Company	54569-2871-03
100's	$1.50	FLURA-LOZ, Kirkman Sales Company	58223-0672-01
100's	$1.56	GENERIC, Allscripts Pharmaceutical Company	54569-2871-01
100's	$1.86	FLUORABON, Perry Medical Products	11763-0532-01
100's	$2.25	FLUORABON, Perry Medical Products	11763-0525-01
100's	$2.25	FLUORABON, Perry Medical Products	11763-0526-01
100's	$4.84	GENERIC, Southwood Pharmaceuticals Inc	58016-0978-00
120's	$1.65	NAFRINSE, Orachem Pharmaceuticals	10733-0567-05
120's	$3.55	GENERIC, Allscripts Pharmaceutical Company	54569-2871-00
120's	$5.28	GENERIC, Pd-Rx Pharmaceuticals	55289-0676-98
120's	$6.38	GENERIC, Pharmascience Laboratories	51817-0622-16
120's	$6.65	GENERIC, Ethex Corporation	58177-0434-40
120's	$7.39	LURIDE, Colgate Oral Pharmaceuticals Inc	00126-0006-21
120's	$7.39	LURIDE, Colgate Oral Pharmaceuticals Inc	00126-0143-21
120's	$7.40	LURIDE, Colgate Oral Pharmaceuticals Inc	00126-0007-21

Sodium Oxybate *(003563)*

Categories: Narcolepsy; Pregnancy Category B; FDA Approved 2002 Jul; Orphan Drugs
Drug Classes: Depressants, central nervous system
Brand Names: **Xyrem**

WARNING

Note: The trade name was used throughout this monograph for clarity.

Central nervous system depressant with abuse potential. Should not be used with alcohol or other CNS depressants.

Sodium oxybate is GHB, a known drug of abuse. Abuse has been associated with some important central nervous system (CNS) adverse events (including death). Even at recommended doses, use has been associated with confusion, depression and other neuropsychiatric events. Reports of respiratory depression occurred in clinical trials. Almost all of the patients who received sodium oxybate during clinical trials were receiving CNS stimulants; whether this affected respiration during the night is unknown. Xyrem is available only through restricted distribution, the Xyrem Success Program, by calling 1-866-XYREM88 (1-866-997-3688).

Important CNS adverse events associated with abuse of GHB include seizure, respiratory depression and profound decreases in level of consciousness, with instances of coma and death. For events that occurred outside of clinical trials, in people taking GHB for recreational purposes, the circumstances surrounding the events are often unclear (*e.g.,* dose of GHB taken, the nature and amount of alcohol or any concomitant drugs).

Under the Xyrem Success Program, Xyrem is made available to prescribers through a single centralized pharmacy and with the following procedures: (1) The prescriber must contact the centralized pharmacy (1-866-XYREM88), which will provide the prescriber with educational materials explaining the risks and proper use of sodium oxybate, and the details of the program. (2) Once the prescriber has read the materials and returned the necessary form, the pharmacy will ship educational materials to the patient. (3) Once it is documented that the patient has read the materials, the drug will be shipped to the patient. The Xyrem Success Program also includes provisions for detailed surveillance of the patients (patients are to be seen no less frequently than every 3 months and physicians are expected to report all serious adverse events to the manufacturer) and information to help minimize the risks of inadvertent use by others. (See WARNINGS.)

DESCRIPTION

Xyrem (sodium oxybate) is a central nervous system depressant with anti-cataplectic activity in patients with narcolepsy. Sodium oxybate is intended for oral administration. The chemical name for sodium oxybate is sodium 4-hydroxybutyrate. The molecular formula is $C_4H_7NaO_3$ and the molecular weight is 126.09 g/mole.

Sodium oxybate is a white to off-white, crystalline powder that is very soluble in aqueous solutions. Xyrem oral solution contains 500 mg of sodium oxybate/ml of USP purified water, neutralized to pH 7.5 with malic acid.

CLINICAL PHARMACOLOGY

MECHANISM OF ACTION

The precise mechanism by which sodium oxybate produces an effect on cataplexy is unknown.

PHARMACOKINETICS

Sodium oxybate is rapidly but incompletely absorbed after oral administration; absorption is delayed and decreased by a high fat meal. It is eliminated mainly by metabolism with a half-life of 0.5 to 1 hour. Pharmacokinetics are nonlinear with blood levels increasing 3.7-fold as dose is doubled from 4.5 to 9 g. The pharmacokinetics are not altered with repeat dosing.

Absorption

Sodium oxybate is absorbed rapidly following oral administration with an absolute bioavailability of about 25%. The average peak plasma concentrations (1st and 2nd peak) following administration of a 9 g daily dose divided into 2 equivalent doses given 4 hours apart were 78 and 142 μg/ml, respectively. The average time to peak plasma concentration (T_{max}) ranged from 0.5-1.25 hours in eight pharmacokinetic studies. Following oral administration, the plasma levels of sodium oxybate increase more than proportionally with increasing dose. Single doses greater than 4.5 g have not been studied. Administration of sodium oxybate immediately after a high fat meal resulted in delayed absorption (average T_{max} increased from 0.75 h to 2.0 h) and a reduction in peak plasma level (C_{max}) by a mean of 58% and of systemic exposure (AUC) by 37%.

Distribution

Sodium oxybate is a hydrophilic compound with an apparent volume of distribution averaging 190-384 ml/kg. At sodium oxybate concentrations ranging from 3-300 μg/ml, less than 1% is bound to plasma proteins.

Metabolism

Animal studies indicate that metabolism is the major elimination pathway for sodium oxybate, producing carbon dioxide and water via the tricarboxylic acid (Krebs) cycle and secondarily by beta-oxidation. The primary pathway involves a cytosolic $NADP^+$-linked enzyme, GHB dehydrogenase, that catalyses the conversion of sodium oxybate to succinic semialdehyde, which is then biotransformed to succinic acid by the enzyme succinic semialdehyde dehydrogenase. Succinic acid enters the Krebs cycle where it is metabolized to carbon dioxide and water. A second mitochondrial oxidoreductase enzyme, a transhydrogenase, also catalyses the conversion to succinic semialdehyde in the presence of α-ketoglutarate. An alternate pathway of biotransformation involves β-oxidation via 3,4-dihydroxybutyrate to carbon dioxide and water. No active metabolites have been identified.

Studies *in vitro* with pooled human liver microsomes indicate that sodium oxybate does not significantly inhibit the activities of the human isoenzymes: CYP1A2, CYP2C9, CYP2C19, CYP2D6, CYP2E1, or CYP3A up to the concentration of 3 mM (378 μg/ml). These levels are considerably higher than levels achieved with therapeutic doses.

Elimination

The clearance of sodium oxybate is almost entirely by biotransformation to carbon dioxide, which is then eliminated by expiration. On average, less than 5% of unchanged drug appears in human urine within 6-8 hours after dosing. Fecal excretion is negligible.

SPECIAL POPULATIONS

Geriatric

The pharmacokinetics of sodium oxybate in patients greater than the age of 65 years have not been studied.

Pediatric

The pharmacokinetics of sodium oxybate in pediatric patients under the age of 18 years have not been studied.

Gender

In a study of 18 female and 18 male healthy adult volunteers, no gender differences were detected in the pharmacokinetics of sodium oxybate following a single oral dose of 4.5 g.

Race

There are insufficient data to evaluate any pharmacokinetic differences among races.

Renal Disease

Because the kidney does not have a significant role in the excretion of sodium oxybate, no pharmacokinetic study in patients with renal dysfunction has been conducted; no effect of renal function on sodium oxybate pharmacokinetics would be expected.

Hepatic Disease

Sodium oxybate undergoes significant presystemic (hepatic first-pass) metabolism. The kinetics of sodium oxybate in 16 cirrhotic patients, half without ascites, (Child's Class A) and half with ascites (Child's Class C) were compared to the kinetics in 8 healthy adults after a single oral dose of 25 mg/kg. AUC values were double in the cirrhotic patients, with apparent oral clearance reduced from 9.1 in healthy adults to 4.5 and 4.1 ml/min/kg in Class A and Class C patients, respectively. Elimination half-life was significantly longer in Class C and Class A patients than in control subjects (mean $T_{1/2}$ of 59 and 32 vs 22 minutes). It is prudent to reduce the starting dose of sodium oxybate by one-half in patients with liver dysfunction (see DOSAGE AND ADMINISTRATION).

Drug-Drug Interaction

Drug interaction studies in healthy adults demonstrated no pharmacokinetic interactions between sodium oxybate and protriptyline HCl, zolpidem tartrate, and modafinil. However, pharmacodynamic interactions with these drugs cannot be ruled out.

INDICATIONS AND USAGE

Xyrem (sodium oxybate) oral solution is indicated for the treatment of cataplexy in patients with narcolepsy.

In Xyrem clinical trials, approximately 80% of patients maintained concomitant stimulant use (see BOXED WARNING).

S

CONTRAINDICATIONS

Sodium oxybate is contraindicated in patients being treated with sedative hypnotic agents.

Sodium oxybate is contraindicated in patients with succinic semialdehyde dehydrogenase deficiency. This rare disorder is an inborn error of metabolism variably characterized by mental retardation, hypotonia, and ataxia.

WARNINGS

SEE BOXED WARNING.

Due to the rapid onset of its CNS depressant effects, sodium oxybate should only be ingested at bedtime, and while in bed. For at least 6 hours after ingesting sodium oxybate, patients must not engage in hazardous occupations or activities requiring complete mental alertness or motor coordination, such as operating machinery, driving a motor vehicle, or flying an airplane. When patients first start taking Xyrem or any other sleep medicine, until they know whether the medicine will still have some carryover effect on them the next day, they should use extreme care while driving a car, operating heavy machinery, or performing any other task that could be dangerous or requires full mental alertness.

The combined use of alcohol (ethanol) with sodium oxybate may result in potentiation of the central nervous system-depressant effects of sodium oxybate and alcohol. Therefore, patients should be warned strongly against the use of any alcoholic beverages in conjunction with sodium oxybate. Sodium oxybate should not be used in combination with sedative hypnotics or other CNS depressants.

CENTRAL NERVOUS SYSTEM DEPRESSION/RESPIRATORY DEPRESSION

Sodium oxybate is a CNS depressant with the potential to impair respiratory drive, especially in patients with already-compromised respiratory function. In overdoses, life-threatening respiratory depression has been reported. In clinical trials 2 subjects had profound CNS depression. A 39-year-old woman, a healthy volunteer received a single 4.5 g dose of sodium oxybate after fasting for 10 hours. An hour later, while asleep, she developed decreased respiration and was treated with an oxygen mask. An hour later, this event recurred. She also vomited and had fecal incontinence. In another case, a 64-year-old narcoleptic man was found unresponsive on the floor on day 170 of treatment with sodium oxybate at a total daily dose of 4.5 g/day. He was taken to an emergency room where he was intubated. He improved and was able to return home later the same day. Two other patients discontinued sodium oxybate because of severe difficulty breathing and an increase in obstructive sleep apnea.

The respiratory depressant effects of Xyrem, at recommended doses, were assessed in 21 patients with narcolepsy, and no dose-related changes in oxygen saturation were demonstrated in the group as a whole. One of these patients had significant concomitant pulmonary illness, and 4 of the 21 had moderate-to-severe sleep apnea. One of the 4 patients with sleep apnea had significant worsening of the apnea/hypopnea index during treatment, but worsening did not increase at higher doses. Another patient discontinued treatment because of a perceived increase in clinical apnea events. Caution should be observed if Xyrem is prescribed to patients with compromised respiratory function. Prescribers should be aware that sleep apnea has been reported with a high incidence (even 50%) in some cohorts of narcoleptic patients.

CONFUSION/NEUROPSYCHIATRIC ADVERSE EVENTS

During clinical trials, 7% of patients treated with sodium oxybate experienced confusion. Fewer than 1% of patients discontinued the drug because of confusion. Confusion was reported at all recommended doses from 6-9 g/day. In a controlled trial where patients were randomized to fixed total daily doses of 3, 6, and 9 g/day or placebo, a dose-response relationship for confusion was demonstrated with 17% of patients at 9 g/day experiencing confusion. In all cases, the confusion resolved soon after termination of treatment. In the majority of cases, confusion resolved with continued treatment. However, patients treated with Xyrem who become confused should be evaluated fully, and appropriate intervention considered on an individual basis.

Other neuropsychiatric events included psychosis, paranoia, hallucinations, and agitation. The emergence of thought disorders and/or behavior abnormalities when patients are treated with sodium oxybate requires careful and immediate evaluation.

DEPRESSION

In clinical trials, 6% of patients treated with sodium oxybate reported depressive symptoms. In the majority of cases, no change in sodium oxybate treatment was required. Three patients (<1%) discontinued because of depressive symptoms. In the controlled clinical trial where patients were randomized to fixed doses of 3, 6, 9 g/day or placebo, there was a single event of depression at the 3 g/day dose.

Among patients with a previous history of depressive psychiatric disorder, there were 2 suicides and 1 attempted suicide recorded in the 448 patient dataset. Of the 2 suicides, 1 patient used sodium oxybate in conjunction with other drugs. Sodium oxybate was not involved in the second suicide. Sodium oxybate was the only drug involved in the attempted suicide. A fourth patient without a previous history of depression attempted suicide by taking an overdose of a drug other than sodium oxybate.

The emergence of depression when patients are treated with Xyrem requires careful and immediate evaluation. Patients with a previous history of a depressive illness and/or suicide attempt should be monitored especially carefully for the emergence of depressive symptoms while taking Xyrem.

USAGE IN THE ELDERLY

There is very limited experience with sodium oxybate in the elderly. Therefore, elderly patients should be monitored closely for impaired motor and/or cognitive function when taking sodium oxybate.

PRECAUTIONS

INCONTINENCE

During clinical trials, 9% of narcoleptic patients treated with sodium oxybate experienced either a single episode or sporadic nocturnal urinary incontinence and <1% experienced a single episode of nocturnal fecal incontinence. Less than 1% of patients discontinued as a result of incontinence. Incontinence has been reported at all doses tested.

In a controlled trial where patients were randomized to fixed total daily doses of 3, 6, and 9 g/day or placebo, a dose-response relationship for urinary incontinence was demonstrated with 14% of patients at 9 g/day experiencing urinary incontinence. In the same trial, 1 patient experienced fecal incontinence at a dose of 9 g/day and discontinued treatment as a result.

If a patient experiences urinary or fecal incontinence during Xyrem therapy, the prescriber should consider pursuing investigations to rule out underlying etiologies, including worsening sleep apnea or nocturnal seizures, although there is no evidence to suggest that incontinence has been associated with seizures in patients being treated with Xyrem.

SLEEPWALKING

The term "sleepwalking" in this section refers to confused behavior occurring at night and, at times, associated with wandering. It is unclear if some or all of these episodes correspond to true somnambulism, which is a parasomnia occurring during non-REM sleep, or to any other specific medical disorder. Sleepwalking was reported in 7% of 448 patients treated in clinical trials with sodium oxybate. In sodium oxybate-treated patients <1% discontinued due to sleepwalking. In controlled trials of up to 4 weeks duration, the incidence of sleepwalking was 1% in both placebo and sodium oxybate-treated patients. Sleepwalking was reported by 32% of patients treated with sodium oxybate for periods up to 16 years in one independent uncontrolled trial. Fewer than 1% of the patients discontinued due to sleepwalking. Five instances of significant injury or potential injury were associated with sleepwalking during a clinical trial of sodium oxybate including a fall, clothing set on fire while attempting to smoke, attempted ingestion of nail polish remover, and overdose of oxybate. Therefore, episodes of sleepwalking should be fully evaluated and appropriate interventions considered.

SODIUM INTAKE

Daily sodium intake in patients taking sodium oxybate ranges from 0.5 g (for a 3 g sodium oxybate dose) to 1.6 g (for a 9 g sodium oxybate dose). This should be considered in patients with heart failure, hypertension or compromised renal function.

HEPATIC INSUFFICIENCY

Patients with compromised liver function will have an increased elimination half-life and systemic exposure to sodium oxybate. (See CLINICAL PHARMACOLOGY, Pharmacokinetics.) The starting dose should therefore be decreased by one-half in such patients, and response to dose increments monitored closely (see DOSAGE AND ADMINISTRATION).

RENAL INSUFFICIENCY

No studies have been conducted in patients with renal failure. Because less than 5% of sodium oxybate is excreted via the kidney, no dose adjustment should be necessary in patients with renal impairment. The sodium load associated with administration of sodium oxybate should be considered in patients with renal insufficiency.

INFORMATION FOR THE PATIENT

The Xyrem Patient Success Program includes detailed information about the safe and proper use of sodium oxybate, as well as information to help the patient prevent accidental use or abuse of sodium oxybate by others. Patients must confirm that they have read the materials before the first prescription will be filled. Prescribers will discuss the details of the program and the treatment (including the procedure for preparing the dose to be administered) prior to the initiation of treatment. Patients should also be informed that they must be seen by the prescriber frequently during the course of their treatment, and that a detailed account of the adverse reactions they may have experienced will be taken. Food significantly decreases the bioavailability of sodium oxybate (see CLINICAL PHARMACOLOGY, Pharmacokinetics). Whether sodium oxybate is taken in the fed or fasted state may affect both the efficacy and safety of sodium oxybate for a given patient. Patients should be made aware of this and try to take the first dose several hours after a meal. Patients should be informed that sodium oxybate is associated with urinary and, less frequently, fecal incontinence. Patients should be instructed to lie down and sleep after each dose of sodium oxybate, and not to take sodium oxybate at any time other than at night, immediately before bedtime and again 2.5 to 4 hours later. Patients should be instructed that they should not take alcohol or other sedative hypnotics with sodium oxybate.

For additional information, patients should see the Medication Guide for Xyrem.

LABORATORY TESTS

Laboratory tests are not required to monitor patient response or adverse events resulting from sodium oxybate administration.

In an open-label trial of long term exposure to sodium oxybate, which extended as long as 16 years for some patients, 30% (26/87) of patients tested had at least one positive antinuclear antibody (ANA) test. Of the 26, 17 patients had multiple positive ANA tests over time. The clinical course of these patients was not always clearly recorded, but 1 patient was clearly diagnosed with rheumatoid arthritis at the time of the first recorded positive ANA test.

CARCINOGENESIS, MUTAGENESIS, AND IMPAIRMENT OF FERTILITY

Oral carcinogenicity studies have been conducted in rats and mice with gamma-butyrolactone, a compound that is metabolized to sodium oxybate *in vivo*, with no clear evidence of carcinogenic potential. Plasma levels (AUC) of sodium oxybate achieved in these studies were estimated to be approximately 1/2 (mice and female rats) and 1/10 (male rats) those seen in humans receiving the maximum recommended daily dose of sodium oxybate.

Sodium oxybate was negative in the Ames microbial mutagen test, an *in vitro* chromosomal aberration assay in CHO cells, and an *in vivo* rat micronucleus assay.

Sodium oxybate did not impair fertility in rats at doses up to 1000 mg/kg (approximately equal to the maximum recommended human daily dose on a mg/m^2 basis).

PREGNANCY CATEGORY B

Reproduction studies conducted in pregnant rats at doses up to 1000 mg/kg (approximately equal to the maximum recommended human daily dose on a mg/m^2 basis) and in pregnant rabbits at doses up to 1200 mg/kg (approximately 3 times the maximum recommended human daily dose on a mg/m^2 basis) revealed no evidence of teratogenicity. In a study in which rats were given sodium oxybate from day 6 of gestation through day 21 post-partum, slight decreases in pup and maternal weight gains were seen at 1000 mg/kg; there were no drug effects on other developmental parameters. There are, however, no adequate and well-controlled studies in pregnant women. Because animal reproduction studies are not always predictive of human response, this drug should be used during pregnancy only if clearly needed.

LABOR AND DELIVERY

Sodium oxybate has not been studied in labor or delivery. In obstetric anesthesia using an injectable formulation of sodium oxybate newborns had stable cardiovascular and respiratory measures but were very sleepy, causing a slight decrease in Apgar scores. There was a fall in the rate of uterine contractions 20 minutes after injection. Placental transfer is rapid, but umbilical vein levels of sodium oxybate were no more than 25% of the maternal concentration. No sodium oxybate was detected in the infant's blood 30 minutes after delivery. Elimination curves of sodium oxybate between a 2-day-old infant and a 15-year-old patient were similar. Subsequent effects of sodium oxybate on later growth, development and maturation in humans are unknown.

NURSING MOTHERS

It is not known whether sodium oxybate is excreted in human milk. Because many drugs are excreted in human milk, caution should be exercised when sodium oxybate is administered to a nursing woman.

PEDIATRIC USE

Safety and effectiveness in patients under 16 years of age have not been established.

RACE AND GENDER EFFECTS

There were too few non-Caucasian patients to permit evaluation of racial effects on safety or efficacy. More than 90% of the subjects in clinical trials were Caucasian.

The database was 58% female. No important differences in safety or efficacy of Xyrem were noted between men and women. The overall percentage of patients with at least 1 adverse event was slightly higher in women (80%) than in men (69%). The incidence of serious adverse events and discontinuations due to adverse events were similar in both men and women.

DRUG INTERACTIONS

Interactions between sodium oxybate and 3 drugs commonly used in patients with narcolepsy (zolpidem tartrate, protriptyline HCl, and modafinil) have been evaluated in formal studies. Sodium oxybate, in combination with these drugs, produced no significant pharmacokinetic changes for either drug (see CLINICAL PHARMACOLOGY, Pharmacokinetics). However, pharmacodynamic interactions cannot be ruled out. Nonetheless, sodium oxybate should not be used in combination with sedative hypnotics or other CNS depressants.

In animal models, sodium oxybate and depressant drug combinations generally gave greater central depressant effects than did either drug alone. Concomitant administration to animals of sodium oxybate and benzodiazepines, barbiturates, or ethanol increases sleep duration. In primates, sodium oxybate blood levels were elevated with phenytoin pretreatment and reduced with L-Dopa, ethosuximide, and trimethadione.

ADVERSE REACTIONS

A total of 448 narcoleptic patients were exposed to sodium oxybate in clinical trials. The most commonly observed adverse events associated with the use of sodium oxybate were:

Headache 25%, nausea 21%, dizziness 17%, pain 16%, somnolence 13%, pharyngitis 11%, infection 10%, viral infection 10%, flu syndrome 9%, accidental injury 9%, diarrhea 8%, urinary incontinence 8%, vomiting 8%, rhinitis 8%, asthenia 8%, sinusitis 7%, nervousness 7%, back pain 7%, confusion 7%, sleepwalking 7%, depression 6%, dyspepsia 6%, abdominal pain 6%, abnormal dreams 6%, insomnia 5%.

Two deaths occurred in these clinical trials, both from drug overdoses. Both of these deaths resulted from ingestion of multiple drugs, including sodium oxybate in 1 patient.

In these clinical trials, 13% of patients discontinued because of adverse events.

The most frequent reasons for discontinuation (>1%) were nausea 2% and headache 1%.

Approximately 6% of patients receiving sodium oxybate in 3 controlled clinical trials (n=147) withdrew due to an adverse event, compared to 1% receiving placebo (n=79). The reasons for discontinuation that occurred more frequently in sodium oxybate-treated patients than placebo-treated patients were: nausea 3%, somnolence 2% and confusion 1%. Amnesia, asthenia, chest pain, dizziness, dyspnea, fecal incontinence, hallucinations, headache, hyperkinesia, paranoid reaction, thinking abnormal, vertigo, and vomiting each caused discontinuation in a single patient.

INCIDENCE IN CONTROLLED CLINICAL TRIALS

Most Commonly Reported Adverse Events in Controlled Clinical Trials

The most commonly reported adverse events associated with the use of sodium oxybate and occurring with at least 5% greater frequency than seen in placebo-treated patients were dizziness (23%), headache (20%), nausea (16%), pain (12%), sleep disorder (9%), confusion (7%), infection (7%), vomiting (6%), and urinary incontinence (5%). These incidences are based on combined data from Trial 1 and two smaller randomized, double-blind, placebo-controlled, cross-over trials (n=181).

Trial 1, the parallel-group, placebo-controlled trial, used 3 fixed doses of sodium oxybate (3, 6, and 9 g). In that trial, dizziness, nausea, urinary incontinence, and vomiting were more common at higher doses, with the majority of events occurring in the 6 and 9 g dose groups.

Adverse Events With an Incidence of at Least 6% (2 events) in 1 or More Treatment Groups in Trial 1

TABLE 2 lists the incidence of treatment emergent adverse events in Trial 1. Events have been included for which there are at least 2 episodes in the considered drug group and for which the incidence in at least 1 dosage group is greater on drug than placebo.

The prescriber should be aware that data provided below cannot be used to predict the incidence of adverse experiences during the course of usual medical practice where patient characteristics and other factors may differ from those occurring during clinical trials. Similarly, the cited frequencies cannot be compared with figures obtained from other clinical investigations involving different treatments, uses, and investigators. However, the cited figures do provide the prescribing physician with some basis for estimating the relative contribution of drug and non-drug factors to the adverse event incidence rate in the population studied.

TABLE 2 *Incidence (%) of Treatment-Emergent Adverse Events in Trial 1*

Body System	Placebo	Sodium Oxybate Dose		
		3 g	6 g	9 g
Preferred Term	(n=34)	(n=34)	(n=33)	(n=35)
Body as a Whole				
Asthenia	1 (3%)	0 (0%)	2 (6%)	0 (0%)
Flu syndrome	0 (0%)	1 (3%)	0 (0%)	2 (6%)
Headache	7 (21%)	3 (9%)	5 (15%)	11 (31%)
Infection	1 (3%)	3 (9%)	5 (15%)	0 (0%)
Infection viral	1 (3%)	1 (3%)	3 (9%)	0 (0%)
Pain	2 (6%)	3 (9%)	4 (12%)	7 (20%)
Digestive System				
Diarrhea	0 (0%)	0 (0%)	2 (6%)	2 (6%)
Dyspepsia	2 (6%)	0 (0%)	3 (9%)	2 (6%)
Nausea	2 (6%)	2 (6%)	5 (15%)	12 (34%)
Nausea and vomiting	0 (0%)	0 (0%)	2 (6%)	2 (6%)
Vomiting	0 (0%)	0 (0%)	2 (6%)	4 (11%)
Musculoskeletal System				
Myasthenia	0 (0%)	2 (6%)	1 (3%)	0 (0%)
Nervous System				
Amnesia	0 (0%)	1 (3%)	0 (0%)	2 (6%)
Anxiety	1 (3%)	1 (3%)	0 (0%)	2 (6%)
Confusion	1 (3%)	3 (9%)	1 (3%)	5 (14%)
Dizziness	2 (6%)	8 (24%)	10 (30%)	12 (34%)
Dream abnormal	0 (0%)	0 (0%)	3 (9%)	1 (3%)
Hypertension	1 (3%)	0 (0%)	2 (6%)	0 (0%)
Hypesthesia	0 (0%)	2 (6%)	0 (0%)	0 (0%)
Sleep disorder	1 (3%)	2 (6%)	4 (12%)	5 (14%)
Somnolence	4 (12%)	5 (15%)	4 (12%)	5 (14%)
Thinking abnormal	0 (0%)	1 (3%)	0 (0%)	2 (6%)
Skin				
Increased sweating	0 (0%)	1 (3%)	1 (3%)	4 (11%)
Special Senses				
Amblyopia	1 (3%)	2 (6%)	0 (0%)	0 (0%)
Tinnitus	0 (0%)	2 (6%)	0 (0%)	0 (0%)
Urogenital System				
Dysmenorrhea	1 (3%)	1 (3%)	0 (0%)	2 (6%)
Incontinence urine	0 (0%)	0 (0%)	2 (6%)	5 (14%)

Other Adverse Events Observed During All Clinical Trials

During clinical trials sodium oxybate was administered to 448 patients with narcolepsy, and 125 healthy volunteers. A total of 150 patients received 9 g/day, the maximum recommended dose. A total of 223 patients received sodium oxybate for at least 1 year. To establish the rate of adverse events, data from all subjects receiving any dose of sodium oxybate were pooled. All adverse events reported by at least 2 people are included except for those already listed elsewhere in the labeling, terms too general to be informative, or events unlikely to be drug induced. Events are classified by body system and listed under the following definitions: *frequent* adverse events (those occurring in at least 1/100 people); *infrequent* events (those occurring in 1/100-1/1000 people). These events are not necessarily related to sodium oxybate treatment.

Body as a Whole: *Frequent:* Allergic reaction, chills; *Infrequent:* Abdomen enlarged, hangover effect, neck rigidity.

Cardiovascular System: *Infrequent:* Syncope.

Digestive System: *Frequent:* Anorexia, constipation; *Infrequent:* Mouth ulceration, stomatitis.

Hemic and Lymphatic System: *Infrequent:* Anemia, ecchymosis, leukocytosis, lymphadenopathy, polycythemia.

Metabolic and Nutritional: *Frequent:* Alkaline phosphatase increased, edema, hypercholesteremia, hypocalcemia, weight gain; *Infrequent:* Bilirubinemia, creatinine increased, dehydration, hyperglycemia, hypernatremia, hyperuricemia, SGOT increased, SGPT increased, thirst.

Musculoskeletal System: *Frequent:* Arthritis, leg cramps, myalgia.

Nervous System: *Frequent:* Agitation, ataxia, convulsion, stupor, tremor; *Infrequent:* Akathisia, apathy, coma, depersonalization, euphoria, hypertonia, libido decreased, myoclonus, neuralgia, paralysis.

Respiratory System: *Frequent:* Dyspnea; *Infrequent:* Apnea, epistaxis, hiccup.

Skin and Appendages: *Frequent:* Acne, alopecia, rash; *Infrequent:* Contact dermatitis, urticaria.

Special Senses: *Infrequent:* Taste loss.

Urogenital System: *Frequent:* Albuminuria, cystitis, hematuria, metrorrhagia, urinary frequency; *Infrequent:* Urinary urgency.

DOSAGE AND ADMINISTRATION

Xyrem is required to be taken at bedtime while in bed and again 2.5 to 4 hours later. The recommended starting dose is 4.5 g/day divided into 2 equal doses of 2.25 g. The starting dosage can then be increased to a maximum of 9 g/day in increments of 1.5 g/day (0.75 g/dose). Two weeks are recommended between dosage increases to evaluate clinical re-

S

sponse and minimize adverse effects. Xyrem is effective at doses of 6-9 g/day. The efficacy and safety of Xyrem at doses higher than 9 g/day have not been investigated, and doses greater than 9 g/day ordinarily should not be administered.

Prepare both doses of Xyrem prior to bedtime. Each dose of Xyrem must be diluted with 2 oz (60 ml, ¼ cup, or 4 tablespoons) of water in the child resistant dosing cups provided prior to ingestion. The first dose is to be taken at bedtime while in bed and the second taken 2.5 to 4 hours later while sitting in bed. Patients will probably need to set an alarm to awaken for the second dose. The second dose must be prepared prior to ingesting the first dose, and should be placed in close proximity to the patient's bed. After ingesting each dose patients should then lie down and remain in bed.

Because food significantly reduces the bioavailability of sodium oxybate, the patient should try to eat well before (several hours) going to sleep and taking the first dose of sodium oxybate. Patients should try to minimize variability in the timing of dosing in relation to meals.

HEPATIC INSUFFICIENCY

Patients with compromised liver function will have increased elimination half-life and systemic exposure along with reduced clearance (see CLINICAL PHARMACOLOGY, Pharmacokinetics). As a result, the starting dose should be decreased by one-half and dose increments should be titrated to effect while closely monitoring potential adverse events.

PREPARATION AND ADMINISTRATION PRECAUTIONS

Each bottle of Xyrem is provided with a child resistant cap and 2 dosing cups with child resistant caps.

Care should be taken to prevent access to this medication by children and pets. See the Medication Guide for a complete description.

HANDLING AND DISPOSAL

Xyrem is a Schedule III drug under the Controlled Substances Act. Xyrem should be handled according to state and federal regulations. It is safe to dispose of Xyrem oral solution down the sanitary sewer.

CAUTION

Federal law prohibits the transfer of this drug to any person other than the patient for whom it was prescribed.

HOW SUPPLIED

Xyrem (sodium oxybate) is a clear to slightly opalescent oral solution. It is supplied in kits containing 1 bottle of Xyrem, a press-in-bottle-adaptor, a 10 ml oral measuring device (plastic syringe), a Medication Guide, a professional insert, and two 90 ml dosing cups with child resistant caps. Each amber oval PET bottle contains 180 ml of Xyrem oral solution at a concentration of 500 mg/ml and is sealed with a child resistant cap.

Each tamper evident single unit carton contains one 180 ml bottle (500 mg/ml) of Xyrem, 1 press-in-bottle-adaptor, 1 oral dispensing syringe, and 2 dosing cups with child resistant cap.

STORAGE

Store at 25°C (77°F); excursions permitted up to 15-30°C (59-86°F).

Solutions prepared following dilution should be consumed within 24 hours to minimize bacterial growth and contamination.

Sodium Polystyrene Sulfonate *(002258)*

Categories: Hyperkalemia; Pregnancy Category C; FDA Approval Pre 1982
Drug Classes: Resins
Brand Names: **Kayexalate**; Resonium; Sps
Foreign Brand Availability: Resinsodio (Spain); Resonium A (Australia; Austria; England; Germany; Hong-Kong; Hungary; Ireland; Netherlands; New-Zealand; Switzerland; Taiwan)

S

DESCRIPTION

Sodium polystyrene sulfonate is a benzene, diethenyl-, polymer with ethenylbenzene, sulfonated, sodium salt.

The drug is a light brown to brown finely ground, powdered form of sodium polystyrene sulfonate, a cation-exchange resin prepared in the sodium phase with an *in vitro* exchange capacity of approximately 3.1 mEq (*in vivo* approximately 1 mEq) of potassium per gram. The sodium content is approximately 100 mg (4.1 mEq) per gram of the drug. It can be administered orally or in an enema.

STORAGE

Store at room temperature.

Sodium polystyrene sulfonate should not be heated for to do so may alter the exchange properties of the resin.

CLINICAL PHARMACOLOGY

As the resin passes along the intestine or is retained in the colon after administration by enema, the sodium ions are partially released and are replaced by potassium ions. For the most part, this action occurs in the large intestine, which excretes potassium ions to a greater degree than does the small intestine. The efficiency of this process is limited and unpredictably variable. It commonly approximates the order of 33% but the range is so large that definitive indices of electrolyte balance must be clearly monitored. Metabolic data are unavailable.

INDICATIONS AND USAGE

Sodium polystyrene sulfonate is indicated for the treatment of hyperkalemia.

NON-FDA APPROVED INDICATIONS

A pilot study demonstrated that sodium polystyrene sulfonate may be useful in the treatment of lithium toxicity via increased clearance of lithium, but larger studies are needed before dosing recommendations can be made.

CONTRAINDICATIONS

Sodium polystyrene sulfonate is contraindicated in patients with hypokalemia or those patients who are hypersensitive to it.

WARNINGS

ALTERNATIVE THERAPY IN SEVERE HYPERKALEMIA

Since effective lowering of serum potassium with sodium polystyrene sulfonate may take hours to days, treatment with this drug alone may be insufficient to rapidly correct severe hyperkalemia associated with states of rapid tissue breakdown (*e.g.*, burns and renal failure) or hyperkalemia so marked as to constitute a medical emergency. Therefore, other definitive measures, including dialysis, should always be considered and may be imperative.

HYPOKALEMIA

Serious potassium deficiency can occur from therapy with sodium polystyrene sulfonate. The effect must be carefully controlled by frequent serum potassium determinations within each 24 hour period. Since intracellular potassium deficiency is not always reflected by serum potassium levels, the level at which treatment with sodium polystyrene sulfonate should be discontinued must be determined individually for each patient. Important aids in making this determination are the patient's clinical condition and electrocardiogram. Early clinical signs of severe hypokalemia include a pattern of irritable confusion and delayed thought processes. Electrocardiographically, severe hypokalemia is often associated with a lengthened Q-T interval, widening, flattening, or inversion of the T wave, and prominent U waves. Also, cardiac arrhythmias may occur, such as premature atrial, nodal, and ventricular contractions, and supraventricular and ventricular tachycardias. The toxic effects of digitalis are likely to be exaggerated. Marked hypokalemia can also be manifested by severe muscle weakness, at times extending into frank paralysis.

ELECTROLYTE DISTURBANCES

Like all cation-exchange resins, sodium polystyrene sulfonate is not totally selective (for potassium) in its actions, and small amounts of other cations such as magnesium and calcium can also be lost during treatment. Accordingly, patients receiving sodium polystyrene sulfonate should be monitored for all applicable electrolyte disturbances.

SYSTEMIC ALKALOSIS

Systemic alkalosis has been reported after cation-exchange resins were administered orally in combination with nonabsorbable cation-donating antacids and laxatives such as magnesium hydroxide and aluminum carbonate. Magnesium hydroxide should not be administered with sodium polystyrene sulfonate. One case of grand mal seizure has been reported in a patient with chronic hypocalcemia of renal failure who was given sodium polystyrene sulfonate with magnesium hydroxide as laxative. (See DRUG INTERACTIONS.)

PRECAUTIONS

Caution is advised when sodium polystyrene sulfonate is administered to patients who cannot tolerate even a small increase in sodium loads (*i.e.*, severe congestive heart failure, severe hypertension, or marked edema). In such instances compensatory restriction of sodium intake from other sources may be indicated.

If constipation occurs, patients should be treated with sorbitol (from 10-20 ml of 70% syrup every 2 hours or as needed to produce one or two watery stools daily), a measure which also reduces any tendency to fecal impaction.

CARCINOGENESIS, MUTAGENESIS, AND IMPAIRMENT OF FERTILITY

Studies have not been performed.

PREGNANCY CATEGORY C

Animal reproduction studies have not been conducted with sodium polystyrene sulfonate. It is also not known whether sodium polystyrene sulfonate can cause fetal harm when administered to a pregnant woman or can affect reproduction capacity. Sodium polystyrene sulfonate should be given to a pregnant woman only if clearly needed.

NURSING MOTHERS

It is not known whether this drug is excreted in human milk. Because many drugs are excreted in human milk, caution should be exercised when sodium polystyrene sulfonate is administered to a nursing woman.

DRUG INTERACTIONS

ANTACIDS

The simultaneous oral administration of sodium polystyrene sulfonate with nonabsorbable cation-donating antacids and laxatives may reduce the resin's potassium exchange capability.

Systemic alkalosis has been reported after cation-exchange resins were administered orally in combination with nonabsorbable cation-donating antacids and laxatives such as magnesium hydroxide and aluminum carbonate. Magnesium hydroxide should not be administered with sodium polystyrene sulfonate. One case of grand mal seizure has been reported in a patient with chronic hypocalcemia of renal failure who was given sodium polystyrene sulfonate with magnesium hydroxide as a laxative.

Intestinal obstruction due to concretions of aluminum hydroxide when used in combination with sodium polystyrene sulfonate has been reported.

DIGITALIS

The toxic effects of digitalis on the heart, especially various ventricular arrhythmias and A-V nodal dissociation, are likely to be exaggerated by hypokalemia, even in the face of serum digoxin concentrations in the "normal range". (See WARNINGS.)

ADVERSE REACTIONS

Sodium polystyrene sulfonate may cause some degree of gastric irritation. Anorexia, nausea, vomiting, and constipation may occur especially if high doses are given. Also, hypokalemia, hypocalcemia, and significant sodium retention may occur. Occasionally diarrhea develops. Large doses in elderly individuals may cause fecal impaction (see PRECAUTIONS.) This effect may be obviated through usage of the resin in enemas as described under DOSAGE AND ADMINISTRATION. Rare instances of colonic necrosis have been reported. Intestinal obstruction due to concretions of aluminum hydroxide, when used in combination with sodium polystyrene sulfonate, has been reported.

DOSAGE AND ADMINISTRATION

Suspension of this drug should be freshly prepared and not stored beyond 24 hours.

The average daily adult dose of the resin is 15-60 g. This is best provided by administering 15 g (approximately 4 *level* teaspoons) of sodium polystyrene sulfonate 1-4 times daily. One (1) g of sodium polystyrene sulfonate contains 4.1 mEq of sodium; 1 level teaspoon contains approximately 3.5 g of sodium polystyrene sulfonate and 15 mEq of sodium. (A heaping teaspoon may contain as much as 10-12 g of sodium polystyrene sulfonate.) Since the *in vivo* efficiency of sodium-potassium exchange resins is approximately 33%, about one-third of the resin's actual sodium content is being delivered to the body.

In smaller children and infants, lower doses should be employed by using as a guide a rate of 1 mEq of potassium per gram of resin as the basis for calculation.

Each dose should be given as a suspension in a small quantity of water or, for greater palatability, in syrup. The amount of fluid usually ranges from 20-100 ml, depending on the dose, or may be simply determined by allowing 3-4 ml per gram of resin. Sorbitol may be administered in order to combat constipation.

The resin may be introduced into the stomach through a plastic tube and, if desired, mixed with a diet appropriate for a patient in renal failure.

The resin may also be given, although with less effective results, in an enema consisting (for adults) of 30-50 g every 6 hours. Each dose is administered as a warm emulsion (at body temperature) in 100 ml of aqueous vehicle, such as sorbitol. The emulsion should be agitated gently during administration. The enema should be retained as long as possible and followed by a cleansing enema.

After an initial cleansing enema, a soft, large size (French 28) rubber tube is inserted into the rectum for a distance of about 20 cm, with the tip well into the sigmoid colon, and taped in place. The resin is then suspended in the appropriate amount of aqueous vehicle at body temperature and introduced by gravity, while the particles are kept in suspension by stirring. The suspension is flushed with 50 ml or 100 ml of fluid, following which the tube is clamped and left in place. If back leakage occurs, the hips are elevated on pillows or a knee-chest position is taken temporarily. A somewhat thicker suspension may be used, but care should be taken that no paste is formed, because the latter has a greatly reduced exchange surface and will be particularly ineffective if deposited in the rectal ampulla. The suspension is kept in the sigmoid colon for several hours, if possible. Then, the colon is irrigated with nonsodium containing solution at body temperature in order to remove the resin. Two (2) quarts of flushing solution may be necessary. The returns are drained constantly through a Y tube connection. Particular attention should be paid to this cleansing enema when sorbitol has been used.

The intensity and duration of therapy depend upon the severity and resistance of hyperkalemia.

PRODUCT LISTING - RATED THERAPEUTICALLY EQUIVALENT

Enema - Rectal - 15 Gm/60 ml

120 ml	$19.67	GENERIC, Roxane Laboratories Inc	00054-8815-01
200 ml	$29.00	GENERIC, Roxane Laboratories Inc	00054-8817-55

Suspension - Oral - 15 Gm/60 ml

60 ml x 10	$58.50	GENERIC, Carolina Medical Products Company	46287-0006-60
60 ml x 10	$86.50	GENERIC, Roxane Laboratories Inc	00054-8816-11
120 ml x 6	$11.55	GENERIC, Carolina Medical Products Company	46287-0006-04
480 ml	$30.95	GENERIC, Carolina Medical Products Company	46287-0006-01
500 ml	$47.86	GENERIC, Roxane Laboratories Inc	00054-3805-63

Sotalol Hydrochloride (003089)

For related information, see the comparative table section in Appendix A.

Categories: Arrhythmia, atrial fibrillation; Arrhythmia, atrial flutter; Arrhythmia, ventricular; Tachycardia, ventricular; FDA Approved 1992 Oct; Pregnancy Category B; Orphan Drugs
Drug Classes: Antiadrenergics, beta blocking; Antiarrhythmics, class III
Brand Names: **Betapace**; Sotacor
Foreign Brand Availability: Beta-Cardone (England); Betacor (Bahrain; Cyprus; Egypt; Iran; Iraq; Jordan; Kuwait; Lebanon; Libya; Oman; Qatar; Republic-of-Yemen; Saudi-Arabia; Syria; United-Arab-Emirates); Betades (Italy); Cardol (Australia); Favorex (Germany); Jutalex (Germany); Rentibloc (Korea); Solavert (Australia); Sotab (Australia); Sotahexal (Australia; Germany; South-Africa); Sotalex (Belgium; France; Germany; Greece; Italy; Philippines; Portugal; Switzerland); Sotapor (Spain)
Cost of Therapy: $184.61 (Arrhythmia; Betapace; 80 mg; 2 tablets/day; 30 day supply)
$140.81 (Arrhythmia; Generic Tablets; 80 mg; 2 tablets/day; 30 day supply)

WARNING

Note: The brand names Betapace (for ventricular arrhythmias) and Betapace AF (for atrial arrhythmias) will be used throughout this monograph for clarification.

Betapace

To minimize the risk of induced arrhythmia, patients initiated or re-initiated on Betapace should be placed for a minimum of 3 days (on their maintenance dose) in a facility that can provide cardiac

WARNING — *Cont'd*

resuscitation and continuous electrocardiographic monitoring. Creatinine clearance should be calculated prior to dosing. For detailed instructions regarding dose selection and special cautions for people with renal impairment, see DOSAGE AND ADMINISTRATION. Sotalol is also indicated for the maintenance of normal sinus rhythm [delay in time to recurrence of atrial fibrillation/atrial flutter(AFIB/AFL)] in patients with symptomatic AFIB/AFL who are currently in sinus rhythm and is marketed under the brand name Betapace AF. Betapace is not approved for the AFIB/AFL indication and should not be substituted for Betapace AF because only Betapace AF is distributed with a patient package insert that is appropriate for patients with AFIB/AFL.

Betapace AF

To minimize the risk of induced arrhythmia, patients initiated or re-initiated on Betapace AF should be placed for a minimum of 3 days (on their maintenance dose) in a facility that can provide cardiac resuscitation, continuous electrocardiographic monitoring and calculations of creatinine clearance. For detailed instructions regarding dose selection and special cautions for people with renal impairment, see DOSAGE AND ADMINISTRATION. Sotalol is also indicated for the treatment of documented life-threatening ventricular arrhythmias and is marketed under the brand name Betapace. Betapace, however, should not be substituted for Betapace AF because of significant differences in labeling (*i.e.,* patient package insert, dosing administration and safety information).

DESCRIPTION

BETAPACE

Betapace (sotalol hydrochloride), is an antiarrhythmic drug with Class II (beta-adrenoreceptor blocking) and Class III (cardiac action potential duration prolongation) properties. It is supplied as a light-blue, capsule-shaped tablet for oral administration. Sotalol hydrochloride is a white, crystalline solid with a molecular weight of 308.8. It is hydrophilic, soluble in water, propylene glycol and ethanol, but is only slightly soluble in chloroform. Chemically, sotalol hydrochloride is d,l-*N*-[4-[l-hydroxy-2-[(l-methylethyl)amino]ethyl]phenyl]methane-sulfonamide monohydrochloride. The molecular formula is $C_{12}H_{20}N_2O_3S{\cdot}HCl$.

Betapace tablets contain the following inactive ingredients: Microcrystalline cellulose, lactose, starch, stearic acid, magnesium stearate, colloidal silicon dioxide, and FD&C blue color no. 2 (aluminum lake, conc.).

BETAPACE AF

Betapace (sotalol hydrochloride), is an antiarrhythmic drug with Class II (beta-adrenoreceptor blocking) and Class III (cardiac action potential duration prolongation) properties. It is supplied as a white, capsule-shaped tablet for oral administration. Sotalol hydrochloride is a white, crystalline solid with a molecular weight of 308.8. It is hydrophilic, soluble in water, propylene glycol and ethanol, but is only slightly soluble in chloroform. Chemically, sotalol hydrochloride is d,l-N-[4-[l-hydroxy-2-[(l-methylethyl)amino]ethyl]phenyl]methane-sulfonamide monohydrochloride. The molecular formula is $C_{12}H_{20}N_2O_3S{\cdot}HCl$.

Betapace AF tablets contain the following inactive ingredients: Microcrystalline cellulose, lactose, starch, stearic acid, magnesium stearate, and colloidal silicon dioxide.

CLINICAL PHARMACOLOGY

BETAPACE

Mechanism of Action

Betapace (sotalol HCl) has both beta-adrenoreceptor blocking (Vaughan Williams Class II) and cardiac action potential duration prolongation (Vaughan Williams Class III) antiarrhythmic properties. Betapace (sotalol HCl) is a racemic mixture of d- and l-sotalol. Both isomers have similar Class III antiarrhythmic effects, while the l-isomer is responsible for virtually all of the beta-blocking activity. The beta-blocking effect of sotalol is non-cardioselective, half maximal at about 80 mg/day and maximal at doses between 320 and 640 mg/day. Sotalol does not have partial agonist or membrane stabilizing activity. Although significant beta-blockade occurs at oral doses as low as 25 mg, significant Class III effects are seen only at daily doses of 160 mg and above.

Electrophysiology

Sotalol HCl prolongs the plateau phase of the cardiac action potential in the isolated myocyte, as well as in isolated tissue preparations of ventricular or atrial muscle (Class III activity). In intact animals it slows heart rate, slows AV nodal conduction and increases the refractory periods of atrial and ventricular muscle and conduction tissue.

In man, the Class II (beta-blockade) electrophysiological effects of Betapace are manifested by increased sinus cycle length (slowed heart rate), decreased AV nodal conduction and increased AV nodal refractoriness. The Class III electrophysiological effects in man include prolongation of the atrial and ventricular monophasic action potentials, and effective refractory period prolongation of atrial muscle, ventricular muscle, and atrioventricular accessory pathways (where present) in both the anterograde and retrograde directions. With oral doses of 160-640 mg/day, the surface ECG shows dose-related mean increases of 40-100 milliseconds in QT and 10-40 milliseconds in QTc. (See WARNINGS for description of relationship between QTc and torsade de pointes type arrhythmias.) No significant alteration in QRS interval is observed.

In a small study (n=25) of patients with implanted defibrillators treated concurrently with Betapace, the average defibrillatory threshold was 6 joules (range 2-15 joules) compared to a mean of 16 joules for a non-randomized comparative group primarily receiving amiodarone.

Hemodynamics

In a study of systemic hemodynamic function measured invasively in 12 patients with a mean LV ejection fraction of 37% and ventricular tachycardia (9 sustained and 3 non-sustained), a median dose of 160 mg twice daily of Betapace produced a 28% reduction in heart rate and a 24% decrease in cardiac index at 2 hours post dosing at steady-state. Concurrently, systemic vascular resistance and stroke volume showed non-significant increases

S

of 25% and 8%, respectively. Pulmonary capillary wedge pressure increased significantly from 6.4 mm Hg to 11.8 mm Hg in the 11 patients who completed the study. One patient was discontinued because of worsening congestive heart failure. Mean arterial pressure, mean pulmonary artery pressure and stroke work index did not significantly change. Exercise and isoproterenol induced tachycardia are antagonized by Betapace, and total peripheral resistance increases by a small amount.

In hypertensive patients, Betapace (sotalol HCl) produces significant reductions in both systolic and diastolic blood pressures. Although Betapace (sotalol HCl) is usually well-tolerated hemodynamically, caution should be exercised in patients with marginal cardiac compensation as deterioration in cardiac performance may occur. (See WARNINGS, Congestive Heart Failure.)

Pharmacokinetics

In healthy subjects, the oral bioavailability of Betapace (sotalol HCl) is 90-100%. After oral administration, peak plasma concentrations are reached in 2.5 to 4 hours, and steady-state plasma concentrations are attained within 2-3 days (*i.e.*, after 5-6 doses when administered twice daily). Over the dosage range 160-640 mg/day Betapace (sotalol HCl) displays dose proportionality with respect to plasma concentrations. Distribution occurs to a central (plasma) and to a peripheral compartment, with a mean elimination half-life of 12 hours. Dosing every 12 hours results in trough plasma concentrations which are approximately one-half of those at peak.

Betapace (sotalol HCl) does not bind to plasma proteins and is not metabolized. Betapace (sotalol HCl) shows very little intersubject variability in plasma levels. The pharmacokinetics of the d and l enantiomers of sotalol are essentially identical. Betapace (sotalol HCl) crosses the blood brain barrier poorly. Excretion is predominantly via the kidney in the unchanged form, and therefore lower doses are necessary in conditions of renal impairment (see DOSAGE AND ADMINISTRATION). Age per se does not significantly alter the pharmacokinetics of Betapace, but impaired renal function in geriatric patients can increase the terminal elimination half-life, resulting in increased drug accumulation. The absorption of Betapace (sotalol HCl) was reduced by approximately 20% compared to fasting when it was administered with a standard meal. Since Betapace (sotalol HCl) is not subject to first-pass metabolism, patients with hepatic impairment show no alteration in clearance of Betapace.

BETAPACE AF

Mechanism of Action

Betapace AF (sotalol HCl) has both beta-adrenoreceptor blocking (Vaughan Williams Class II) and cardiac action potential duration prolongation (Vaughan Williams Class III) antiarrhythmic properties. Betapace AF (sotalol HCl) is a racemic mixture of d- and l-sotalol. Both isomers have similar Class III antiarrhythmic effects, while the l-isomer is responsible for virtually all of the beta-blocking activity. The beta-blocking effect of sotalol is non-cardioselective, half maximal at about 80 mg/day and maximal at doses between 320 and 640 mg/day. Sotalol does not have partial agonist or membrane stabilizing activity. Although significant beta-blockade occurs at oral doses as low as 25 mg, significant Class III effects are seen only at daily doses of 160 mg and above.

In children, a Class III electrophysiologic effect can be seen at daily doses of 210 mg/m^2 body surface area (BSA). A reduction of the resting heart rate due to the beta-blocking effect of sotalol is observed at daily doses $\geq$90 mg/m^2 in children.

Electrophysiology

Sotalol HCl prolongs the plateau phase of the cardiac action potential in the isolated myocyte, as well as in isolated tissue preparations of ventricular or atrial muscle (Class III activity). In intact animals it slows heart rate, slows AV nodal conduction and increases the refractory periods of atrial and ventricular muscle and conduction tissue.

In man, the Class II (beta-blockade) electrophysiological effects of Betapace AF are manifested by increased sinus cycle length (slowed heart rate), decreased AV nodal conduction and increased AV nodal refractoriness. The Class III electrophysiological effects in man include prolongation of the atrial and ventricular monophasic action potentials, and effective refractory period prolongation of atrial muscle, ventricular muscle, and atrio-ventricular accessory pathways (where present) in both the anterograde and retrograde directions. With oral doses of 160-640 mg/day, the surface ECG shows dose-related mean increases of 40-100 milliseconds in QT and 10-40 milliseconds in QTc. In a study of patients with atrial fibrillation (AFIB)/flutter (AFIB/AFL) receiving three different oral doses of Betapace AF given q12h (or q24h in patients with a reduced creatinine clearance), mean increases in QT intervals measured from 12-lead ECGs of 25 milliseconds, 40 milliseconds and 54 milliseconds were found in the 80 mg, 120 mg and 160 mg dose groups, respectively. (See WARNINGS for description of relationship between QTc and torsade de pointes type arrhythmias.) No significant alteration in QRS interval is observed.

S

In a small study (n=25) of patients with implanted defibrillators treated concurrently with sotalol the average defibrillatory threshold was 6 joules (range 2-15 joules) compared to a mean of 16 joules for a non-randomized comparative group primarily receiving amiodarone.

In a dose-response trial comparing three dose levels of Betapace AF, 80, 120, and 160 mg with placebo given q12h (or q24h in patients with a reduced renal creatinine clearance) for the prevention of recurrence of symptomatic atrial fibrillation (AFIB)/flutter (AFL), the mean ventricular rate during recurrence of AFIB/AFL was 125, 107, 110 and 99 beats/min in the placebo, 80 mg, 120 mg and 160 mg dose groups, respectively ($p < 0.017$ for each sotalol dose group versus placebo). In another placebo controlled trial in which Betapace AF was titrated to a dose between 160 and 320 mg/day in patients with chronic AFIB, the mean ventricular rate during recurrence of AFIB was 107 and 84 beats/min in the placebo and Betapace AF groups, respectively ($p < 0.001$).

Twenty-five (25) children in an unblinded, multicenter trial with supraventricular (SVT) and/or ventricular (VT) tachyarrhythmias, aged between 3 days and 12 years (mostly neonates and infants), received an ascending titration regimen with daily doses of 30, 90 and 210 mg/m^2 with dosing every 8 hours for a total of 9 doses. During steady-state, the respective average increases above baseline of the QTc interval, in milliseconds (%), were 2 (+1%), 14 (+4%) and 29 (+7%) milliseconds at the 3 dose levels. The respective mean maximum increases above baseline of the QTc interval, in milliseconds (%), were 23 (+6%), 36 (+9%) and 55 (+14%) milliseconds at the 3 dose levels. The steady-state percent increases in the RR interval were 3, 9 and 12%. The smallest children (BSA <0.33 m^2) showed a tendency for larger Class III effects (QTc) and an increased frequency of prolongations of the QTc interval as compared with the larger children (BSA 0.33 m^2). The beta-blocking effects also tended to be greater in the smaller children (BSA <0.33 m^2). Both the Class III and beta-blocking effects of sotalol were linearly related with the plasma concentrations.

Hemodynamics

In a study of systemic hemodynamic function measured invasively in 12 patients with a mean LV ejection fraction of 37% and ventricular tachycardia (9 sustained and 3 non-sustained), a median dose of 160 mg twice daily of sotalol produced a 28% reduction in heart rate and a 24% decrease in cardiac index at 2 hours post dosing at steady-state. Concurrently, systemic vascular resistance and stroke volume showed non-significant increases of 25% and 8%, respectively. Pulmonary capillary wedge pressure increased significantly from 6.4 mm Hg to 11.8 mm Hg in the 11 patients who completed the study. One patient was discontinued because of worsening congestive heart failure. Mean arterial pressure, mean pulmonary artery pressure and stroke work index did not significantly change. Exercise and isoproterenol induced tachycardia are antagonized by sotalol, and total peripheral resistance increases by a small amount.

In hypertensive patients, sotalol produces significant reductions in both systolic and diastolic blood pressures. Although sotalol is usually well-tolerated hemodynamically, caution should be exercised in patients with marginal cardiac compensation as deterioration in cardiac performance may occur. (See WARNINGS, Congestive Heart Failure.)

Pharmacokinetics

In healthy subjects, the oral bioavailability of sotalol is 90-100%. After oral administration, peak plasma concentrations are reached in 2.5 to 4 hours, and steady-state plasma concentrations are attained within 2-3 days (*i.e.*, after 5-6 doses when administered twice daily). Over the dosage range 160-640 mg/day sotalol displays dose proportionality with respect to plasma concentrations. Distribution occurs to a central (plasma) and to a peripheral compartment, with a mean elimination half-life of 12 hours. Dosing every 12 hours results in trough plasma concentrations which are approximately one-half of those at peak.

Sotalol does not bind to plasma proteins and is not metabolized. Sotalol shows very little intersubject variability in plasma levels. The pharmacokinetics of the d and l enantiomers of sotalol are essentially identical. Sotalol crosses the blood brain barrier poorly. Excretion is predominantly via the kidney in the unchanged form, and therefore lower doses are necessary in conditions of renal impairment (see DOSAGE AND ADMINISTRATION). Age per se does not significantly alter the pharmacokinetics of sotalol, but impaired renal function in geriatric patients can increase the terminal elimination half-life, resulting in increased drug accumulation. The absorption of sotalol was reduced by approximately 20% compared to fasting when it was administered with a standard meal. Since sotalol is not subject to first-pass metabolism, patients with hepatic impairment show no alteration in clearance of sotalol.

The combined analysis of two unblinded, multicenter trials (a single dose and a multiple dose study) with 59 children, aged between 3 days and 12 years, showed the pharmacokinetics of sotalol to be first order. A daily dose of 30 mg/m^2 of sotalol was administered in the single dose study and daily doses of 30, 90 and 210 mg/m^2 were administered q8h in the multi-dose study. After rapid absorption with peak levels occurring on average between 2-3 hours following administration, sotalol was eliminated with a mean half life of 9.5 hours. Steady-state was reached after 1-2 days. The average peak to trough concentration ratio was 2. BSA was the most important covariate and more relevant than age for the pharmacokinetics of sotalol. The smallest children (BSA <0.33 m^2) exhibited a greater drug exposure (+59%) than the larger children who showed a uniform drug concentration profile. The intersubject variation for oral clearance was 22%.

INDICATIONS AND USAGE

BETAPACE

Oral Betapace (sotalol HCl) is indicated for the treatment of documented ventricular arrhythmias, such as sustained ventricular tachycardia, that in the judgment of the physician are life-threatening. Because of the proarrhythmic effects of Betapace (see WARNINGS), including a 1.5 to 2% rate of torsade de pointes or new VT/VF in patients with either NSVT or supraventricular arrhythmias, its use in patients with less severe arrhythmias, even if the patients are symptomatic, is generally not recommended. Treatment of patients with asymptomatic ventricular premature contractions should be avoided. Initiation of Betapace treatment or increasing doses, as with other antiarrhythmic agents used to treat life-threatening arrhythmias, should be carried out in the hospital. The response to treatment should then be evaluated by a suitable method (*e.g.*, PES or Holter monitoring) prior to continuing the patient on chronic therapy. Various approaches have been used to determine the response to antiarrhythmic therapy, including Betapace.

In the ESVEM Trial, response by Holter monitoring was tentatively defined as 100% suppression of ventricular tachycardia, 90% suppression of non-sustained VT, 80% suppression of paired VPCs, and 75% suppression of total VPCs in patients who had at least 10 VPCs/hour at baseline; this tentative response was confirmed if VT lasting 5 or more beats was not observed during treadmill exercise testing using a standard Bruce protocol. The PES protocol utilized a maximum of three extrastimuli at three pacing cycle lengths and two right ventricular pacing sites. Response by PES was defined as prevention of induction of the following: (1) monomorphic VT lasting over 15 seconds; (2) non-sustained polymorphic VT containing more than 15 beats of monomorphic VT in patients with a history of monomorphic VT; (3) polymorphic VT or VF greater than 15 beats in patients with VF or a history of aborted sudden death without monomorphic VT; and (4) two episodes of polymorphic VT or VF of greater than 15 beats in a patient presenting with monomorphic VT. Sustained VT or NSVT producing hypotension during the final treadmill test was considered a drug failure. In a multicenter open-label long-term study of Betapace in patients with life-threatening ventricular arrhythmias which had proven refractory to other antiarrhythmic medications, response by Holter monitoring was defined as in ESVEM. Response by PES was defined as non-inducibility of sustained VT by at least double extrastimuli delivered at a pacing cycle length of 400 milliseconds. Overall survival and arrhythmia recurrence rates in this study were similar to those seen in ESVEM, although there was no comparative group to allow a definitive assessment of outcome.

Antiarrhythmic drugs have not been shown to enhance survival in patients with ventricular arrhythmias.

Sotalol is also indicated for the maintenance of normal sinus rhythm [delay in time to recurrence of atrial fibrillation/atrial flutter (AFIB/AFL)] in patients with symptomatic AFIB/AFL who are currently in sinus rhythm and is marketed under the brand name Betapace AF. Betapace is not approved for the AFIB/AFL indication and should not be substituted for Betapace AF because only Betapace AF is distributed with a patient package insert that is appropriate for patients with AFIB/AFL.

BETAPACE AF

Betapace AF is indicated for the maintenance of normal sinus rhythm [delay in time to recurrence of atrial fibrillation/atrial flutter (AFIB/AFL)] in patients with symptomatic AFIB/AFL who are currently in sinus rhythm. Because Betapace AF can cause life-threatening ventricular arrhythmias, it should be reserved for patients in whom AFIB/AFL is highly symptomatic. Patients with paroxysmal AFIB/AFL that is easily reversed (by Valsalva maneuver, for example) should usually not be given Betapace AF (see WARNINGS).

In general, antiarrhythmic therapy for AFIB/AFL aims to prolong the time in normal sinus rhythm. Recurrence is expected in some patients.

Sotalol is also indicated for the treatment of documented life-threatening ventricular arrhythmias and is marketed under the brand name Betapace (sotalol HCl). Betapace, however, must not be substituted for Betapace AF because of significant differences in labeling (*i.e.*, patient package insert, dosing administration and safety information).

CONTRAINDICATIONS

BETAPACE

Betapace (sotalol HCl) is contraindicated in patients with bronchial asthma, sinus bradycardia, second and third degree AV block, unless a functioning pacemaker is present, congenital or acquired long QT syndromes, cardiogenic shock, uncontrolled congestive heart failure, and previous evidence of hypersensitivity to Betapace.

BETAPACE AF

Betapace AF (sotalol HCl) is contraindicated in patients with sinus bradycardia (<50 bpm during waking hours), sick sinus syndrome or second and third degree AV block (unless a functioning pacemaker is present), congenital or acquired long QT syndromes, baseline QT interval >450 milliseconds, cardiogenic shock, uncontrolled heart failure, hypokalemia (<4 mEq/L), creatinine clearance <40 ml/min, bronchial asthma and previous evidence of hypersensitivity to sotalol.

WARNINGS

BETAPACE

Mortality

The National Heart, Lung, and Blood Institute's Cardiac Arrhythmia Suppression Trial I (CAST I) was a long-term, multi-center, double-blind study in patients with asymptomatic, non-life-threatening ventricular arrhythmias, 1-103 weeks after acute myocardial infarction. Patients in CAST I were randomized to receive placebo or individually optimized doses of encainide, flecainide, or moricizine. The Cardiac Arrhythmia Suppression Trial II (CAST II) was similar, except that the recruited patients had had their index infarction 4-90 days before randomization, patients with left ventricular ejection fractions greater than 40% were not admitted, and the randomized regimens were limited to placebo and moricizine.

CAST I was discontinued after an average time-on-treatment of 10 months, and CAST II was discontinued after an average time-on-treatment of 18 months. As compared to placebo treatment, all three active therapies were associated with increases in short-term (14 day) mortality, and encainide and flecainide were associated with significant increases in longer-term mortality as well. The longer-term mortality rate associated with moricizine treatment could not be statistically distinguished from that associated with placebo.

The applicability of these results to other populations (*e.g.*, those without recent myocardial infarction) and to other than Class I antiarrhythmic agents is uncertain. Betapace (sotalol HCl) is devoid of Class I effects, and in a large (n=1456) controlled trial in patients with a recent myocardial infarction, who did not necessarily have ventricular arrhythmias, Betapace did not produce increased mortality at doses up to 320 mg/day. On the other hand, in the large post-infarction study using a non-titrated initial dose of 320 mg once daily and in a second small randomized trial in high-risk post-infarction patients treated with high doses (320 mg bid), there have been suggestions of an excess of early sudden deaths.

Proarrhythmia

Like other antiarrhythmic agents, Betapace can provoke new or worsened ventricular arrhythmias in some patients, including sustained ventricular tachycardia or ventricular fibrillation, with potentially fatal consequences. Because of its effect on cardiac repolarization (QTc interval prolongation), torsade de pointes, a polymorphic ventricular tachycardia with prolongation of the QT interval and a shifting electrical axis is the most common form of proarrhythmia associated with Betapace, occurring in about 4% of high risk (history of sustained VT/VF) patients. The risk of torsade de pointes progressively increases with prolongation of the QT interval, and is worsened also by reduction in heart rate and reduction in serum potassium. (See Electrolyte Disturbances.)

Because of the variable temporal recurrence of arrhythmias, it is not always possible to distinguish between a new or aggravated arrhythmic event and the patient's underlying rhythm disorder. (Note, however, that torsade de pointes is usually a drug-induced arrhythmia in people with an initially normal QTc.) Thus, the incidence of drug-related events cannot be precisely determined, so that the occurrence rates provided must be considered approximations. Note also that drug-induced arrhythmias may often not be identified, particularly if they occur long after starting the drug, due to less frequent monitoring. It is clear from the NIH-sponsored CAST (see WARNINGS, Mortality) that some antiarrhythmic drugs can cause increased sudden death mortality, presumably due to new arrhythmias or asystole, that do not appear early in treatment but that represent a sustained increased risk.

Overall in clinical trials with sotalol, 4.3% of 3257 patients experienced a new or worsened ventricular arrhythmia. Of this 4.3%, there was new or worsened sustained ventricular tachycardia in approximately 1% of patients and torsade de pointes in 2.4%. Additionally, in approximately 1% of patients, deaths were considered possibly drug-related; such cases, although difficult to evaluate, may have been associated with proarrhythmic events. **In patients with a history of sustained ventricular tachycardia, the incidence of torsade de pointes was 4% and worsened VT in about 1%; in patients with other, less serious, ventricular arrhythmias and supraventricular arrhythmias, the incidence of torsade de pointes was 1% and 1.4%, respectively.**

Torsade de pointes arrhythmias were dose related, as is the prolongation of QT(QTc) interval, as shown in TABLE 5.

TABLE 5 *Percent Incidence of Torsade de Pointes and Mean QTc Interval by Dose for Patients With Sustained VT/VF*

Daily Dose	Incidence of Torsade de Pointes	Mean QTc* (msec)
80 mg	0.0 (69)	463 (17)
160 mg	0.5 (832)	467 (181)
320 mg	1.6 (836)	473 (344)
480 mg	4.4 (459)	483 (234)
640 mg	3.7 (324)	490 (185)
>640 mg	5.8 (103)	512 (62)

* Highest on-therapy value.
() Number of patients assessed.

In addition to dose and presence of sustained VT, other risk factors for torsade de pointes were gender (females had a higher incidence), excessive prolongation of the QTc interval (see TABLE 6) and history of cardiomegaly or congestive heart failure. Patients with sustained ventricular tachycardia and a history of congestive heart failure appear to have the highest risk for serious proarrhythmia (7%). Of the patients experiencing torsade de pointes, approximately two-thirds spontaneously reverted to their baseline rhythm. The others were either converted electrically (D/C cardioversion or overdrive pacing) or treated with other drugs. It is not possible to determine whether some sudden deaths represented episodes of torsade de pointes, but in some instances sudden death did follow a documented episode of torsade de pointes. Although Betapace therapy was discontinued in most patients experiencing torsade de pointes, 17% were continued on a lower dose. Nonetheless, Betapace should be used with particular caution if the QTc is greater than 500 milliseconds on-therapy and serious consideration should be given to reducing the dose or discontinuing therapy when the QTc exceeds 550 milliseconds. Due to the multiple risk-factors associated with torsade de pointes, however, caution should be exercised regardless of the QTc interval. TABLE 6 relates the incidence of torsade de pointes to on-therapy QTc and change in QTc from baseline. It should be noted, however, that the highest on-therapy QTc was in many cases the one obtained at the time of the torsade de pointes event, so that the table overstates the predictive value of a high QTc.

TABLE 6 *Relationship Between QTc Interval Prolongation and Torsade de Pointes (TdP)*

On-Therapy QTc Interval (msec)	Incidence of TdP	Changes in QTc Intervals From Baseline (msec)	Incidence of TdP
Less than 500	1.3% (1787)	Less than 65	1.6% (1516)
500-525	3.4% (236)	65-80	3.2% (158)
525-550	5.6% (125)	80-100	4.1% (146)
>550	10.8% (157)	100-130	5.2% (115)
		>130	7.1% (99)

() Number of patients assessed.

Proarrhythmic events must be anticipated not only on initiating therapy, but with every upward dose adjustment. Proarrhythmic events most often occur within 7 days of initiating therapy or of an increase in dose; 75% of serious proarrhythmias (torsade de pointes and worsened VT) occurred within 7 days of initiating Betapace therapy, while 60% of such events occurred within 3 days of initiation or a dosage change. Initiating therapy at 80 mg bid with gradual upward dose titration and appropriate evaluations for efficacy (*e.g.*, PES or Holter) and safety (*e.g.*, QT interval, heart rate and electrolytes) prior to dose escalation, should reduce the risk of proarrhythmia. Avoiding excessive accumulation of sotalol in patients with diminished renal function, by appropriate dose reduction, should also reduce the risk of proarrhythmia (see DOSAGE AND ADMINISTRATION).

Congestive Heart Failure

Sympathetic stimulation is necessary in supporting circulatory function in congestive heart failure, and beta-blockade carries the potential hazard of further depressing myocardial contractility and precipitating more severe failure. In patients who have congestive heart failure controlled by digitalis and/or diuretics, Betapace should be administered cautiously. Both digitalis and sotalol slow AV conduction. As with all beta-blockers, caution is advised when initiating therapy in patients with any evidence of left ventricular dysfunction. In premarketing studies, new or worsened congestive heart failure (CHF) occurred in 3.3% (n=3257) of patients and led to discontinuation in approximately 1% of patients receiving Betapace. The incidence was higher in patients presenting with sustained ventricular tachycardia/fibrillation (4.6%, n=1363), or a prior history of heart failure (7.3%, n=696). Based on a life-table analysis, the 1 year incidence of new or worsened CHF was 3% in patients without a prior history and 10% in patients with a prior history of CHF. NYHA Classification was also closely associated to the incidence of new or worsened heart failure while receiving Betapace (1.8% in 1395 Class I patients, 4.9% in 1254 Class II patients and 6.1% in 278 Class III or IV patients).

Electrolyte Disturbances

Betapace should not be used in patients with hypokalemia or hypomagnesemia prior to correction of imbalance, as these conditions can exaggerate the degree of QT prolongation, and increase the potential for torsade de pointes. Special attention should be given to electrolyte and acid-base balance in patients experiencing severe or prolonged diarrhea or patients receiving concomitant diuretic drugs.

Conduction Disturbances

Excessive prolongation of the QT interval (>550 milliseconds) can promote serious arrhythmias and should be avoided (see Proarrhythmias). Sinus bradycardia (heart rate less than 50 bpm) occurred in 13% of patients receiving Betapace in clinical trials, and led to discontinuation in about 3% of patients. Bradycardia itself increases the risk of torsade de pointes. Sinus pause, sinus arrest and sinus node dysfunction occur in less than 1% of patients. The incidence of 2nd- or 3rd-degree AV block is approximately 1%.

Recent Acute MI

Betapace can be used safely and effectively in the long-term treatment of life-threatening ventricular arrhythmias following a myocardial infarction. However, experience in the use of Betapace to treat cardiac arrhythmias in the early phase of recovery from acute MI is limited and at least at high initial doses is not reassuring. (See Mortality.) In the first 2 weeks post-MI caution is advised and careful dose titration is especially important, particularly in patients with markedly impaired ventricular function.

NOTE: The following warnings are related to the beta-blocking activity of Betapace.

Abrupt Withdrawal

Hypersensitivity to catecholamines has been observed in patients withdrawn from beta-blocker therapy. Occasional cases of exacerbation of angina pectoris, arrhythmias and, in some cases, myocardial infarction have been reported after abrupt discontinuation of beta-blocker therapy. Therefore, it is prudent when discontinuing chronically administered Betapace, particularly in patients with ischemic heart disease, to carefully monitor the patient and consider the temporary use of an alternate beta-blocker if appropriate. If possible, the dosage of Betapace should be gradually reduced over a period of 1-2 weeks. If angina or acute coronary insufficiency develops, appropriate therapy should be instituted promptly. Patients should be warned against interruption or discontinuation of therapy without the physician's advice. Because coronary artery disease is common and may be unrecognized in patients receiving Betapace, abrupt discontinuation in patients with arrhythmias may unmask latent coronary insufficiency.

Non-Allergic Bronchospasm (e.g., chronic bronchitis and emphysema)

PATIENTS WITH BRONCHOSPASTIC DISEASES SHOULD IN GENERAL NOT RECEIVE BETA-BLOCKERS. It is prudent, if Betapace (sotalol HCl) is to be administered, to use the smallest effective dose, so that inhibition of bronchodilation produced by endogenous or exogenous catecholamine stimulation of beta$_2$ receptors may be minimized.

Anaphylaxis

While taking beta-blockers, patients with a history of anaphylactic reaction to a variety of allergens may have a more severe reaction on repeated challenge, either accidental, diagnostic or therapeutic. Such patients may be unresponsive to the usual doses of epinephrine used to treat the allergic reaction.

Anesthesia

The management of patients undergoing major surgery who are being treated with beta-blockers is controversial. Protracted severe hypotension and difficulty in restoring and maintaining normal cardiac rhythm after anesthesia have been reported in patients receiving beta-blockers.

Diabetes

In patients with diabetes (especially labile diabetes) or with a history of episodes of spontaneous hypoglycemia, Betapace should be given with caution since beta-blockade may mask some important premonitory signs of acute hypoglycemia; *e.g.*, tachycardia.

S

Sick Sinus Syndrome

Betapace should be used only with extreme caution in patients with sick sinus syndrome associated with symptomatic arrhythmias, because it may cause sinus bradycardia, sinus pauses or sinus arrest.

Thyrotoxicosis

Beta-blockade may mask certain clinical signs (*e.g.*, tachycardia) of hyperthyroidism. Patients suspected of developing thyrotoxicosis should be managed carefully to avoid abrupt withdrawal of beta-blockade which might be followed by an exacerbation of symptoms of hyperthyroidism, including thyroid storm.

BETAPACE AF

Ventricular Arrhythmia

Betapace AF (sotalol) can cause serious ventricular arrhythmias, primarily torsade de pointes (TdP) type ventricular tachycardia, a polymorphic ventricular tachycardia associated with QT interval prolongation. QT interval prolongation is directly related to the dose of Betapace AF. Factors such as reduced creatinine clearance, gender (female) and larger doses increase the risk of TdP. The risk of TdP can be reduced by adjustment of the Betapace AF dose according to creatinine clearance and by monitoring the ECG for excessive increases in the QT interval.

Treatment with Betapace AF must therefore be started only in patients observed for a minimum of 3 days on their maintenance dose in a facility that can provide electrocardiographic monitoring and in the presence of personnel trained in the management of serious ventricular arrhythmias. Calculation of the creatinine clearance must precede administration of the first dose of Betapace AF. For detailed instructions regarding dose selection, see DOSAGE AND ADMINISTRATION.

Proarrhythmia in Atrial Fibrillation/Atrial Flutter Patients

In eight controlled trials of patients with AFIB/AFL and other supraventricular arrhythmias (n=659) there were 4 cases of torsade de pointes reported (0.6%) during the controlled phase of treatment with Betapace AF. The incidence of torsade de pointes was significantly lower in those patients receiving total daily doses of 320 mg or less (0.3%), as summarized in TABLE 7. Both patients who had torsade de pointes in the group receiving >320 mg/day were receiving 640 mg/day. In the group receiving 320 mg daily, one case of TdP occurred at a daily dose of 320 mg on day 4 of treatment and one case occurred on a daily dose of 160 mg on day 1 of treatment.

***TABLE 7** Incidence of Torsade de Pointes in Controlled Trials of AFIB and Other Supraventricular Arrhythmias*

		Torsade de Pointes n (%)
Betapace AF (Daily Dose)		
Any Dose	(n=659)	4 (0.6%)
>320 mg/day	(n=62)	2 (3.2%)
≤320 mg/day	(n=597)	2 (0.3%)
≤240 mg/day	(n=340)	1 (0.3%)
Placebo	(n=358)	0

Prolongation of the QT interval is dose related, increasing from baseline an average of 25, 40, and 50 milliseconds in the 80, 120, and 160 mg groups, respectively, in the clinical dose-response study. In this clinical trial Betapace AF treatment was not initiated if the QT interval was greater than 450 milliseconds and during therapy the dose was reduced or discontinued if the QT interval was ≥520 milliseconds.

Experience in patients with ventricular arrhythmias is also pertinent to the risk of torsade de pointes in patients with AFIB/AFL (see below).

Proarrhythmia in Ventricular Arrhythmia Patients

See Betapace (sotalol HCl) Package Insert.

In patients with a history of sustained ventricular tachycardia, the incidence of torsade de pointes during sotalol treatment was 4% and worsened VT in about 1%; in patients with other less serious ventricular arrhythmias the incidence of torsade de pointes was 1% and new or worsened VT in about 0.7%. Additionally, in approximately 1% of patients, deaths were considered possibly drug related; such cases, although difficult to evaluate, may have been associated with proarrhythmic events.

Torsade de pointes arrhythmias in patients with VT/VF were dose related, as was the prolongation of QT (QTc) interval, as shown in TABLE 8.

***TABLE 8** Percent Incidence of Torsade de Pointes and Mean QTc Interval by Dose for Patients With Sustained VT/VF*

Daily Dose	Incidence of Torsade de Pointes	Mean QTc* (msec)
80 mg	0 (69)	463 (17)
160 mg	0.5 (832)	467 (181)
320 mg	1.6 (835)	473 (344)
480 mg	4.4 (459)	483 (234)
640 mg	3.7 (324)	490 (185)
>640 mg	5.8 (103)	512 (62)

* Highest on-therapy value.
() Number of patients assessed.

TABLE 9 relates the incidence of torsade de pointes to on-therapy QTc and change in QTc from baseline. It should be noted, however, that the highest on-therapy QTc was in many cases the one obtained at the time of the torsade de pointes event, so that the table overstates the predictive value of a high QTc.

***TABLE 9** Relationship Between QTc Interval Prolongation and Torsade de Pointes (TdP)*

On-Therapy QTc Interval	Incidence of TdP	Change in QTc Interval From Baseline	Incidence of TdP
Less than 500 msec	1.3% (1787)	Less than 65 msec	1.6% (1516)
500-525 msec	3.4% (236)	65-80 msec	3.2% (158)
525-550 msec	5.6% (125)	80-100 msec	4.1% (146)
>550 msec	10.8% (157)	100-130 msec	5.2% (115)
		>130 msec	7.1% (99)

() Number of patients assessed.

In addition to dose and presence of sustained VT, other risk factors for torsade de pointes were gender (females had a higher incidence), excessive prolongation of the QTc interval and history of cardiomegaly or congestive heart failure. Patients with sustained ventricular tachycardia and a history of congestive heart failure appear to have the highest risk for serious proarrhythmia (7%). Of the ventricular arrhythmia patients experiencing torsade de pointes, approximately two-thirds spontaneously reverted to their baseline rhythm. The others were either converted electrically (D/C cardioversion or overdrive pacing) or treated with other drugs. It is not possible to determine whether some sudden deaths represented episodes of torsade de pointes, but in some instances sudden death did follow a documented episode of torsade de pointes. Although sotalol therapy was discontinued in most patients experiencing torsade de pointes, 17% were continued on a lower dose.

Use With Drugs That Prolong QT Interval and Antiarrhythmic Agents

The use of Betapace AF in conjunction with other drugs that prolong the QT interval has not been studied and is not recommended. Such drugs include many antiarrhythmics, some phenothiazines, bepridil, tricyclic antidepressants, certain oral macrolides. Class I or Class III antiarrhythmic agents should be withheld for at least three half-lives prior to dosing with Betapace AF. In clinical trials, Betapace AF was not administered to patients previously treated with oral amiodarone for >1 month in the previous 3 months. Class Ia antiarrhythmic drugs, such as disopyramide, quinidine and procainamide and other Class III drugs (*e.g.*, amiodarone) are not recommended as concomitant therapy with Betapace AF, because of their potential to prolong refractoriness (see WARNINGS). There is only limited experience with the concomitant use of Class Ib or Ic antiarrhythmics.

Congestive Heart Failure

Sympathetic stimulation is necessary in supporting circulatory function in congestive heart failure, and beta-blockade carries the potential hazard of further depressing myocardial contractility and precipitating more severe failure. In patients who have heart failure controlled by digitalis and/or diuretics, Betapace AF should be administered cautiously. Both digitalis and sotalol slow AV conduction. As with all beta-blockers, caution is advised when initiating therapy in patients with any evidence of left ventricular dysfunction. In a pooled data base of four placebo-controlled AFIB/AFL and PSVT studies, new or worsening CHF occurred during therapy with Betapace AF in 5 (1.2%) of 415 patients. In these studies patients with uncontrolled heart failure were excluded (*i.e.*, NYHA Functional Classes III or IV). In other premarketing sotalol studies, new or worsened congestive heart failure (CHF) occurred in 3.3% (n=3257) of patients and led to discontinuation in approximately 1% of patients receiving sotalol. The incidence was higher in patients presenting with sustained ventricular tachycardia/fibrillation (4.6%, n=1363), or a prior history of heart failure (7.3%, n=696). Based on a life-table analysis, the 1 year incidence of new or worsened CHF was 3% in patients without a prior history and 10% in patients with a prior history of CHF. NYHA Classification was also closely associated to the incidence of new or worsened heart failure while receiving sotalol (1.8% in 1395 Class I patients, 4.9% in 1254 Class II patients and 6.1% in 278 Class III or IV patients).

Electrolyte Disturbances

Betapace AF should not be used in patients with hypokalemia or hypomagnesemia prior to correction of imbalance, as these conditions can exaggerate the degree of QT prolongation, and increase the potential for torsade de pointes. Special attention should be given to electrolyte and acid-base balance in patients experiencing severe or prolonged diarrhea or patients receiving concomitant diuretic drugs.

Bradycardia/Heart Block

The incidence of bradycardia (as determined by the investigators) in the supraventricular arrhythmia population treated with Betapace AF (n=415) was 13%, and led to discontinuation in 2.4% of patients. Bradycardia itself increases the risk of torsade de pointes.

Recent Acute MI

Sotalol has been used in a controlled trial following an acute myocardial infarction without evidence of increased mortality. Although specific studies of its use in treating atrial arrhythmias after infarction have not been conducted, the usual precautions regarding heart failure, avoidance of hypokalemia, bradycardia or prolonged QT interval apply.

Note: The following warnings are related to the beta-blocking activity of Betapace AF.

Abrupt Withdrawal

Hypersensitivity to catecholamines has been observed in patients withdrawn from beta-blocker therapy. Occasional cases of exacerbation of angina pectoris, arrhythmias and, in some cases, myocardial infarction have been reported after abrupt discontinuation of beta-blocker therapy. Therefore, it is prudent when discontinuing chronically administered Betapace AF, particularly in patients with ischemic heart disease, to carefully monitor the patient and consider the temporary use of an alternate beta-blocker if appropriate. If possible, the dosage of Betapace AF should be gradually reduced over a period of 1-2 weeks. If angina or acute coronary insufficiency develops, appropriate therapy should be instituted promptly. Patients should be warned against interruption or discontinuation of therapy without the physician's advice. Because coronary artery disease is common and may be unrecognized in patients receiving Betapace AF, abrupt discontinuation in patients with arrhythmias may unmask latent coronary insufficiency.

Non-Allergic Bronchospasm (e.g., chronic bronchitis and emphysema)

PATIENTS WITH BRONCHOSPASTIC DISEASES SHOULD IN GENERAL NOT RECEIVE BETA-BLOCKERS. It is prudent, if Betapace AF (sotalol HCl) is to be administered, to use the smallest effective dose, so that inhibition of bronchodilation produced by endogenous or exogenous catecholamine stimulation of $beta_2$ receptors may be minimized.

Anaphylaxis

While taking beta-blockers, patients with a history of anaphylactic reaction to a variety of allergens may have a more severe reaction on repeated challenge, either accidental, diagnostic or therapeutic. Such patients may be unresponsive to the usual doses of epinephrine used to treat the allergic reaction.

Anesthesia

The management of patients undergoing major surgery who are being treated with beta-blockers is controversial. Protracted severe hypotension and difficulty in restoring and maintaining normal cardiac rhythm after anesthesia have been reported in patients receiving beta-blockers.

Diabetes

In patients with diabetes (especially labile diabetes) or with a history of episodes of spontaneous hypoglycemia, Betapace AF should be given with caution since beta-blockade may mask some important premonitory signs of acute hypoglycemia; *e.g.*, tachycardia.

Sick Sinus Syndrome

Betapace AF should be used only with extreme caution in patients with sick sinus syndrome associated with symptomatic arrhythmias, because it may cause sinus bradycardia, sinus pauses or sinus arrest. In patients with AFIB and sinus node dysfunction, the risk of torsade de pointes with Betapace AF therapy is increased, especially after cardioversion. Bradycardia following cardioversion in these patients is associated with QTc interval prolongation which is augmented due to the reverse use dependence of the Class III effects of Betapace AF. Patients with AFIB/AFL associated with the sick sinus syndrome may be treated with Betapace AF if they have an implanted pacemaker for control of bradycardia symptoms.

Thyrotoxicosis

Beta-blockade may mask certain clinical signs (*e.g.*, tachycardia) of hyperthyroidism. Patients suspected of developing thyrotoxicosis should be managed carefully to avoid abrupt withdrawal of beta-blockade which might be followed by an exacerbation of symptoms of hyperthyroidism, including thyroid storm. The beta-blocking effects of Betapace AF may be useful in controlling heart rate in AFIB associated with thyrotoxicosis but no study has been conducted to evaluate this.

PRECAUTIONS

BETAPACE

Renal Impairment

Betapace (sotalol HCl) is mainly eliminated via the kidneys through glomerular filtration and to a small degree by tubular secretion. There is a direct relationship between renal function, as measured by serum creatinine or creatinine clearance, and the elimination rate of Betapace. Guidance for dosing in conditions of renal impairment can be found under DOSAGE AND ADMINISTRATION.

Drug/Laboratory Test Interactions

The presence of sotalol in the urine may result in falsely elevated levels of urinary metanephrine when measured by fluorimetric or photometric methods. In screening patients suspected of having a pheochromocytoma and being treated with sotalol, a specific method, such as a high performance liquid chromatographic assay with solid phase extraction (*e.g.*, J. Chromatogr. 385:241, 1987) should be employed in determining levels of catecholamines.

Carcinogenesis, Mutagenesis, and Impairment of Fertility

No evidence of carcinogenic potential was observed in rats during a 24 month study at 137-275 mg/kg/day (approximately 30 times the maximum recommended human oral dose (MRHD) as mg/kg or 5 times the MRHD as mg/m^2) or in mice, during a 24 month study at 4141-7122 mg/kg/day (approximately 450-750 times the MRHD as mg/kg or 36-63 times the MRHD as mg/m^2).

Sotalol has not been evaluated in any specific assay of mutagenicity or clastogenicity.

No significant reduction in fertility occurred in rats at oral doses of 1000 mg/kg/day (approximately 100 times the MRHD as mg/kg or 9 times the MRHD as mg/m^2) prior to mating, except for a small reduction in the number of offspring per litter.

Pregnancy Category B

Reproduction studies in rats and rabbits during organogenesis at 100 and 22 times the MRHD as mg/kg (9 and 7 times the MRHD as mg/m^2), respectively, did not reveal any teratogenic potential associated with sotalol HCl. In rabbits, a high dose of sotalol HCl (160 mg/kg/day) at 16 times the MRHD as mg/kg (6 times the MRHD as mg/m^2) produced a slight increase in fetal death likely due to maternal toxicity. Eight times the maximum dose (80 mg/kg/day or 3 times the MRHD as mg/m^2) did not result in an increased incidence of fetal deaths. In rats, 1000 mg/kg/day sotalol HCl, 100 times the MRHD (18 times the MRHD as mg/m^2), increased the number of early resorptions, while at 14 times the maximum dose (2.5 times the MRHD as mg/m^2), no increase in early resorptions was noted. However, animal reproduction studies are not always predictive of human response.

Although there are no adequate and well-controlled studies in pregnant women, sotalol HCl has been shown to cross the placenta, and is found in amniotic fluid. There has been a report of subnormal birth weight with Betapace. Therefore, Betapace should be used during pregnancy only if the potential benefit outweighs the potential risk.

Nursing Mothers

Sotalol is excreted in the milk of laboratory animals and has been reported to be present in human milk. Because of the potential for adverse reactions in nursing infants from Betapace, a decision should be made whether to discontinue nursing or to discontinue the drug, taking into account the importance of the drug to the mother.

Pediatric Use

The safety and effectiveness of Betapace in children have not been established.

BETAPACE AF

Renal Impairment

Betapace AF (sotalol HCl) is eliminated principally via the kidneys through glomerular filtration and to a small degree by tubular secretion. There is a direct relationship between renal function, as measured by serum creatinine or creatinine clearance, and the elimination rate of Betapace AF. Guidance for dosing in conditions of renal impairment can be found under DOSAGE AND ADMINISTRATION.

Information for the Patient

Please refer to the patient information distributed with the prescription.

Prior to initiation of Betapace AF therapy, the patient should be advised to read the patient package insert and reread it each time therapy is renewed. The patient should be fully instructed on the need for compliance with the recommended dosing of Betapace AF, the potential interactions with drugs that prolong the QT interval and other antiarrhythmics, and the need for periodic monitoring of QT and renal function to minimize the risk of serious abnormal rhythms.

S

Medications and Supplements

Assessment of patients' medication history should include all over-counter, prescription and herbal/natural preparations with emphasis on preparations that may affect the pharmacodynamics of Betapace AF such as other cardiac antiarrhythmic drugs, some phenothiazines, bepridil, tricyclic antidepressants and oral macrolides (see WARNINGS and WARNINGS, Use With Drugs That Prolong QT Interval and Antiarrhythmic Agents). Patients should be instructed to notify their health care providers of any change in over-the-counter, prescription or supplement use. If a patient is hospitalized or is prescribed a new medication for any condition, the patient must inform the health care provider of ongoing Betapace AF therapy. Patients should also check with their health care provider and/or pharmacist prior to taking a new over-the-counter medicine.

Electrolyte Imbalance

If patients experience symptoms that may be associated with altered electrolyte balance, such as excessive or prolonged diarrhea, sweating, or vomiting, or loss of appetite or thirst, these conditions should be immediately reported to their health care provider.

Dosing Schedule

Patients should be instructed NOT to double the next dose if a dose is missed. The next dose should be taken at the usual time.

Drug/Laboratory Test Interactions

The presence of sotalol in the urine may result in falsely elevated levels of urinary metanephrine when measured by fluorimetric or photometric methods. In screening patients suspected of having a pheochromocytoma and being treated with sotalol, a specific method, such as a high performance liquid chromatographic assay with solid phase extraction (*e.g.*, J. Chromatogr. 385:241, 1987) should be employed in determining levels of catecholamines.

Carcinogenesis, Mutagenesis, and Impairment of Fertility

No evidence of carcinogenic potential was observed in rats during a 24 month study at 137-275 mg/kg/day (approximately 30 times the maximum recommended human oral dose (MRHD) as mg/kg or 5 times the MRHD as mg/m^2) or in mice, during a 24 month study at 4141-7122 mg/kg/day (approximately 450-750 times the MRHD as mg/kg or 36-63 times the MRHD as mg/m^2).

Sotalol has not been evaluated in any specific assay of mutagenicity or clastogenicity.

No significant reduction in fertility occurred in rats at oral doses of 1000 mg/kg/day (approximately 100 times the MRHD as mg/kg or 9 times the MRHD as mg/m^2) prior to mating, except for a small reduction in the number of offspring per litter.

Pregnancy Category B

Reproduction studies in rats and rabbits during organogenesis at 100 and 22 times the MRHD as mg/kg (9 and 7 times the MRHD as mg/m^2), respectively, did not reveal any teratogenic potential associated with sotalol HCl. In rabbits, a high dose of sotalol HCl (160 mg/kg/day) at 16 times the MRHD as mg/kg (6 times the MRHD as mg/m^2) produced a slight increase in fetal death likely due to maternal toxicity. Eight times the maximum dose (80 mg/kg/day or 3 times the MRHD as mg/m^2) did not result in an increased incidence of fetal deaths. In rats, 1000 mg/kg/day sotalol HCl, 100 times the MRHD (18 times the MRHD as mg/m^2), increased the number of early resorptions, while at 14 times the maximum dose (2.5 times the MRHD as mg/m^2), no increase in early resorptions was noted. However, animal reproduction studies are not always predictive of human response.

Although there are no adequate and well-controlled studies in pregnant women, sotalol HCl has been shown to cross the placenta, and is found in amniotic fluid. There has been a report of subnormal birth weight with sotalol. Therefore, Betapace AF should be used during pregnancy only if the potential benefit outweighs the potential risk.

Nursing Mothers

Sotalol is excreted in the milk of laboratory animals and has been reported to be present in human milk. Because of the potential for adverse reactions in nursing infants from Betapace AF, a decision should be made whether to discontinue nursing or to discontinue the drug, taking into account the importance of the drug to the mother.

Pediatric Use

The safety and effectiveness of Betapace AF in children have not been established. However, the Class III electrophysiologic and beta-blocking effects, the pharmacokinetics, and the relationship between the effects (QTc interval and resting heart rate) and drug concentrations have been evaluated in children aged between 3 days and 12 year old. (See CLINICAL PHARMACOLOGY.)

DRUG INTERACTIONS

BETAPACE

Drugs undergoing CYP450 metabolism: Sotalol is primarily eliminated by renal excretion; therefore, drugs that are metabolized by CYP450 are not expected to alter the pharmacokinetics of sotalol. Sotalol is not expected to inhibit or induce any CYP450 enzymes, therefore, it is not expected to alter the PK of drugs that are metabolized by these enzymes.

Antiarrhythmics: Class Ia antiarrhythmic drugs, such as disopyramide, quinidine and procainamide and other Class III drugs (*e.g.*, amiodarone) are not recommended as concomitant therapy with Betapace, because of their potential to prolong refractoriness (see WARNINGS). There is only limited experience with the concomitant use of Class Ib or Ic antiarrhythmics. Additive Class II effects would also be anticipated with the use of other beta-blocking agents concomitantly with Betapace.

Digoxin: Single and multiple doses of Betapace do not substantially affect serum digoxin levels. Proarrhythmic events were more common in Betapace treated patients also receiving digoxin; it is not clear whether this represents an interaction or is related to the presence of CHF, a known risk factor for proarrhythmia, in the patients receiving digoxin.

Calcium blocking drugs: Betapace should be administered with caution in conjunction with calcium blocking drugs because of possible additive effects on atrioventricular conduction or ventricular function. Additionally, concomitant use of these drugs may have additive effects on blood pressure, possibly leading to hypotension.

Catecholamine-depleting agents: Concomitant use of catecholamine-depleting drugs, such as reserpine and guanethidine, with a beta-blocker may produce an excessive reduction of resting sympathetic nervous tone. Patients treated with Betapace plus a catecholamine depletor should therefore be closely monitored for evidence of hypotension and or marked bradycardia which may produce syncope.

Insulin and oral antidiabetics: Hyperglycemia may occur, and the dosage of insulin or antidiabetic drugs may require adjustment. Symptoms of hypoglycemia may be masked.

Beta-2-receptor stimulants: Beta-agonists such as salbutamol, terbutaline and isoprenaline may have to be administered in increased dosages when used concomitantly with Betapace.

Clonidine: Beta-blocking drugs may potentiate the rebound hypertension sometimes observed after discontinuation of clonidine; therefore, caution is advised when discontinuing clonidine in patients receiving Betapace.

Other: No pharmacokinetic interactions were observed with hydrochlorothiazide or warfarin.

Antacids: Administration of Betapace within 2 hours of antacids containing aluminum oxide and magnesium hydroxide should be avoided because it may result in a reduction in C_{max} and AUC of 26% and 20%, respectively and consequently in a 25% reduction in the bradycardic effect at rest. Administration of the antacid 2 hours after Betapace has no effect on the pharmacokinetics or pharmacodynamics of sotalol.

Drugs prolonging the QT interval: Betapace should be administered with caution in conjunction with other drugs known to prolong the QT interval such as Class I and Class III antiarrhythmic agents, phenothiazines, tricyclic antidepressants, astemizole, bepridil, certain oral macrolides, and certain quinolone antibiotics (see WARNINGS).

BETAPACE AF

Drugs undergoing CYP450 metabolism: Sotalol is primarily eliminated by renal excretion; therefore, drugs that are metabolized by CYP450 are not expected to alter the pharmacokinetics of sotalol.

Digoxin: Proarrhythmic events were more common in sotalol treated patients also receiving digoxin; it is not clear whether this represents an interaction or is related to the presence of CHF, a known risk factor for proarrhythmia, in the patients receiving digoxin.

Calcium blocking drugs: Betapace AF should be administered with caution in conjunction with calcium blocking drugs because of possible additive effects on atrioventricular conduction or ventricular function. Additionally, concomitant use of these drugs may have additive effects on blood pressure, possibly leading to hypotension.

Catecholamine-depleting agents: Concomitant use of catecholamine-depleting drugs, such as reserpine and guanethidine, with a beta-blocker may produce an excessive reduction of resting sympathetic nervous tone. Patients treated with Betapace AF plus a catecholamine depletor should therefore be closely monitored for evidence of hypotension and or marked bradycardia which may produce syncope.

Insulin and oral antidiabetics: Hyperglycemia may occur, and the dosage of insulin or antidiabetic drugs may require adjustment. Symptoms of hypoglycemia may be masked.

Beta-2-receptor stimulants: Beta-agonists such as salbutamol, terbutaline and isoprenaline may have to be administered in increased dosages when used concomitantly with Betapace AF.

Clonidine: Beta-blocking drugs may potentiate the rebound hypertension sometimes observed after discontinuation of clonidine; therefore, caution is advised when discontinuing clonidine in patients receiving Betapace AF.

Other: No pharmacokinetic interactions were observed with hydrochlorothiazide or warfarin.

Antacids: Administration of Betapace AF within 2 hours of antacids containing aluminum oxide and magnesium hydroxide should be avoided because it may result in a reduction in C_{max} and AUC of 26% and 20%, respectively and consequently in a 25% reduction in the bradycardic effect at rest. Administration of the antacid 2 hours after Betapace AF has no effect on the pharmacokinetics or pharmacodynamics of sotalol.

ADVERSE REACTIONS

BETAPACE

During premarketing trials, 3186 patients with cardiac arrhythmias (1363 with sustained ventricular tachycardia) received oral Betapace, of whom 2451 received the drug for at least 2 weeks. The most important adverse effects are torsade de pointes and other serious new ventricular arrhythmias (see WARNINGS), occurring at rates of almost 4% and 1%, respectively, in the VT/VF population. Overall, discontinuation because of unacceptable side-effects was necessary in 17% of all patients in clinical trials, and in 13% of patients treated for at least 2 weeks. The most common adverse reactions leading to discontinuation of Betapace are as follows: fatigue 4%, bradycardia (less than 50 bpm) 3%, dyspnea 3%, proarrhythmia 3%, asthenia 2%, and dizziness 2%. Occasional reports of elevated serum liver enzymes have occurred with Betapace therapy but no cause and effect relationship has been established. One case of peripheral neuropathy which resolved on discontinuation of Betapace and recurred when the patient was rechallenged with the drug was reported in an early dose tolerance study. Elevated blood glucose levels and increased insulin requirements can occur in diabetic patients.

TABLE 10 lists as a function of dosage the most common (incidence of 2% or greater) adverse events, regardless of relationship to therapy and the percent of patients discontinued due to the event, as collected from clinical trials involving 1292 patients with sustained VT/VF.

TABLE 10 *Incidence (%) of Adverse Events and Discontinuations*

Body System	Daily Dose (mg) 160 n=832	240 n=263	320 n=835	480 n=459	640 n=324	Any Dose* n=1292	Patients Discontinued n=1292
Body as a Whole							
Infection	1%	2%	2%	2%	3%	4%	<1%
Fever	1%	2%	3%	2%	2%	4%	<1%
Localized pain	1%	1%	2%	2%	2%	3%	<1%
Cardiovascular							
Dyspnea	5%	8%	11%	15%	15%	21%	2%
Bradycardia	8%	8%	9%	7%	5%	16%	2%
Chest pain	4%	3%	10%	10%	14%	16%	<1%
Palpitation	3%	3%	8%	9%	12%	14%	<1%
Edema	2%	2%	5%	3%	5%	8%	1%
ECG abnormal	4%	2%	4%	2%	2%	7%	1%
Hypotension	3%	4%	3%	2%	3%	6%	2%
Proarrhythmia	<1%	<1%	2%	4%	5%	5%	3%
Syncope	1%	1%	3%	2%	5%	5%	1%
Heart failure	2%	3%	2%	2%	2%	5%	1%
Presyncope	1%	2%	2%	4%	3%	4%	<1%
Peripheral vascular disorder	1%	2%	1%	1%	2%	3%	<1%
Cardiovascular disorder	1%	<1%	2%	2%	2%	3%	<1%
Vasodilation	1%	<1%	1%	2%	1%	3%	<1%
AICD discharge	<1%	2%	2%	2%	2%	3%	<1%
Hypertension	<1%	1%	1%	1%	2%	2%	<1%
Nervous							
Fatigue	5%	8%	12%	12%	13%	20%	2%
Dizziness	7%	6%	11%	11%	14%	20%	1%
Asthenia	4%	5%	7%	8%	10%	13%	1%
Light-headed	4%	3%	6%	6%	9%	12%	1%
Headache	3%	2%	4%	4%	4%	8%	<1%
Sleep-problem	1%	1%	5%	5%	6%	8%	<1%
Perspiration	1%	2%	3%	4%	5%	6%	<1%
Altered consciousness	2%	3%	1%	2%	3%	4%	<1%
Depression	1%	2%	2%	2%	3%	4%	<1%
Paresthesia	1%	1%	2%	3%	2%	4%	<1%
Anxiety	2%	2%	2%	3%	2%	4%	<1%
Mood change	<1%	<1%	1%	3%	2%	3%	<1%
Appetite disorder	1%	2%	2%	1%	3%	3%	<1%
Stroke	<1%	<1%	1%	1%	<1%	1%	<1%
Digestive							
Nausea/vomiting	5%	4%	4%	6%	6%	10%	1%
Diarrhea	2%	3%	3%	3%	5%	7%	<1%
Dyspepsia	2%	3%	3%	3%	3%	6%	<1%
Abdominal pain	<1%	<1%	2%	2%	2%	3%	<1%
Colon problem	2%	1%	1%	<1%	2%	3%	<1%
Flatulence	1%	<1%	1%	1%	2%	2%	<1%
Respiratory							
Pulmonary problem	3%	3%	5%	3%	4%	8%	<1%
Upper respiratory tract problem	1%	1%	3%	4%	3%	5%	<1%
Asthma	1%	<1%	1%	1%	1%	2%	<1%
Urogenital							
Genitourinary disorder	1%	0%	1%	1%	2%	3%	<1%
Sexual dysfunction	<1%	1%	1%	1%	3%	2%	<1%
Metabolic							
Abnormal lab value	1%	2%	3%	2%	1%	4%	<1%
Weight change	1%	1%	1%	<1%	2%	2%	<1%
Musculoskeletal							
Extremity pain	2%	2%	4%	5%	3%	7%	<1%
Back pain	1%	<1%	2%	2%	2%	3%	<1%
Skin and Appendages							
Rash	2%	3%	2%	3%	4%	5%	<1%
Hematologic							
Bleeding	1%	<1%	1%	<1%	2%	2%	<1%
Special Senses							
Visual problem	1%	1%	2%	4%	5%	5%	<1%

* Because patients are counted at each dose level tested, the Any Dose column cannot be determined by adding across the doses.

Potential Adverse Effects

Foreign marketing experience with sotalol HCl shows an adverse experience profile similar to that described above from clinical trials. Voluntary reports since introduction include rare reports (less than 1 report per 10,000 patients) of: emotional lability, slightly clouded sensorium, incoordination, vertigo, paralysis, thrombocytopenia, eosinophilia, leukopenia, photosensitivity reaction, fever, pulmonary edema, hyperlipidemia, myalgia, pruritis, alopecia.

The oculomucocutaneous syndrome associated with the beta-blocker practolol has not been associated with Betapace during investigational use and foreign marketing experience.

BETAPACE AF

Adverse events that are clearly related to Betapace AF are those which are typical of its Class II (beta-blocking) and Class III (cardiac action potential duration prolongation) effects. The common documented beta-blocking adverse events (bradycardia, dyspnea, and fatigue) and Class III effects (QT interval prolongation) are dose related.

In a pooled clinical trial population consisting of four placebo-controlled studies with 275 patients with AFIB/AFL treated with 160-320 mg doses of Betapace AF, the following adverse events were reported at a rate of 2% or more in the 160-240 mg treated patients and greater than the rate in placebo patients (see TABLE 11). The data are presented by incidence of events in the Betapace AF and placebo groups by body system and daily dose. No significant irreversible non-cardiac end-organ toxicity was observed.

TABLE 11 *Incidence (%) of Common Adverse Events (≥2% in the 160-240 mg group and more frequent than on placebo) in Four Placebo-Controlled Studies of Patients With AFIB/AFL*

Body System / Adverse Event (Preferred Term)	Placebo n=282	Betapace AF Total Daily Dose 160-240 n=153	>240-320 n=122
Cardiovascular			
Abnormality ECG	0.4%	3.3%	2.5%
Angina pectoris	1.1%	2.0%	1.6%
Bradycardia	2.5%	13.1%	12.3%
Chest pain cardiac/non-anginal	4.6%	4.6%	2.5%
Disturbance rhythm atrial	2.1%	2.0%	1.6%
Disturbance rhythm subjective	9.9%	9.8%	7.4%
Gastrointestinal			
Appetite decreased	0.4%	2.0%	1.6%
Diarrhea	2.1%	5.2%	5.7%
Distention abdomen	0.4%	0.7%	2.5%
Dyspepsia/heartburn	1.8%	2.0%	2.5%
Nausea/vomiting	5.3%	7.8%	5.7%
Pain abdomen	2.5%	3.9%	2.5%
General			
Fatigue	8.5%	19.6%	18.9%
Fever	0.7%	0.7%	3.3%
Hyperhidrosis	3.2%	5.2%	4.9%
Influenza	0.4%	2.0%	0.8%
Sensation cold	0.7%	2.0%	2.5%
Weakness	3.2%	5.2%	4.9%
Musculoskeletal/Connective Tissue			
Pain chest musculoskeletal	1.4%	2.0%	2.5%
Pain musculoskeletal	2.8%	2.6%	4.1%
Nervous System			
Dizziness	12.4%	16.3%	13.1%
Headache	5.3%	3.3%	11.5%
Insomnia	1.1%	2.6%	4.1%
Respiratory			
Cough	2.5%	3.3%	2.5%
Dyspnea	7.4%	9.2%	9.8%
Infection upper respiratory	1.1%	2.6%	3.3%
Tracheobronchitis	0.7%	0.7%	3.3%
Special Senses			
Disturbance vision	0.7%	2.6%	0.8%

Overall, discontinuation because of unacceptable adverse events was necessary in 17% of the patients, and occurred in 10% of patients less than 2 weeks after starting treatment. The most common adverse events leading to discontinuation of Betapace AF were: fatigue 4.6%, bradycardia 2.4%, proarrhythmia 2.2%, dyspnea 2%, and QT interval prolongation 1.4%.

In clinical trials involving 1292 patients with sustained VT/VF, the common adverse events (occurring in ≥2% of patients) were similar to those described for the AFIB/AFL population.

Occasional reports of elevated serum liver enzymes have occurred with sotalol therapy but no cause and effect relationship has been established. One case of peripheral neuropathy, which resolved on discontinuation of sotalol and recurred when the patient was rechallenged with the drug, was reported in an early dose tolerance study. Elevated blood glucose levels and increased insulin requirements can occur in diabetic patients.

In an unblinded multicenter trial of 25 pediatric patients with SVT and/or VT receiving daily doses of 30, 90 and 210 mg/m^2 with dosing every 8 hours for a total of 9 doses, no torsade de pointes or other serious new arrhythmias were observed. One (1) patient, receiving 30 mg/m^2 daily, was discontinued because of increased frequency of sinus pauses/bradycardia. Additional cardiovascular AEs were seen at the 90 and 210 mg/m^2 daily dose levels. They included QT prolongations (2 patients), sinus pauses/bradycardia (1 patient), increased severity of atrial flutter and reported chest pain (1 patient). Values for QTc ≥525 milliseconds were seen in 2 patients at the 210 mg/m^2 daily dose level. Serious adverse events including death, torsades de pointe, other proarrhythmias, high-degree A-V blocks and bradycardia have been reported in infants and/or children.

Potential Adverse Effects

Foreign marketing experience with sotalol HCl shows an adverse experience profile similar to that described above from clinical trials. Voluntary reports since introduction also include rare reports of: emotional lability, slightly clouded sensorium, incoordination, vertigo, paralysis, thrombocytopenia, eosinophilia, leukopenia, photosensitivity reaction, fever, pulmonary edema, hyperlipidemia, myalgia, pruritus, alopecia.

The oculomucocutaneous syndrome associated with the beta-blocker practolol has not been associated with Betapace AF during investigational use and foreign marketing experience.

DOSAGE AND ADMINISTRATION

BETAPACE

As with other antiarrhythmic agents, Betapace should be initiated and doses increased in a hospital with facilities for cardiac rhythm monitoring and assessment (see INDICATIONS AND USAGE). Betapace should be administered only after appropriate clinical assessment (see INDICATIONS AND USAGE), and the dosage of Betapace must be individualized for each patient on the basis of therapeutic response and tolerance. Proarrhythmic events can occur not only at initiation of therapy, but also with each upward dosage adjustment.

Dosage of Betapace should be adjusted gradually, allowing 3 days between dosing increments in order to attain steady-state plasma concentrations, and to allow monitoring of QT intervals. Graded dose adjustment will help prevent the usage of doses which are higher than necessary to control the arrhythmia. The recommended initial dose is 80 mg twice daily. This dose may be increased, if necessary, after appropriate evaluation to 240 or 320 mg/day (120-160 mg twice daily). In most patients, a therapeutic response is obtained at a total daily dose of 160-320 mg/day, given in 2 or 3 divided doses. Some patients with life-threatening refractory ventricular arrhythmias may require doses as high as 480-640 mg/day; however, these doses should only be prescribed when the potential benefit outweighs the increased risk of adverse events, in particular proarrhythmia. Because of the long terminal elimination half-life of Betapace, dosing on more than a bid regimen is usually not necessary.

Dosage in Renal Impairment

Because sotalol is excreted predominantly in urine and its terminal elimination half-life is prolonged in conditions of renal impairment, the dosing interval (time between divided doses) of sotalol should be modified (when creatinine clearance is lower than 60 ml/min) according to TABLE 12.

TABLE 12

Creatinine Clearance	Dosing* Interval
>60 ml/min	12 hours
30-59 ml/min	24 hours
10-29 ml/min	36-48 hours
<10 ml/min	Dose should be individualized

* The initial dose of 80 mg and subsequent doses should be administered at these intervals. See following paragraph for dosage escalations.

Since the terminal elimination half-life of Betapace (sotalol HCl) is increased in patients with renal impairment, a longer duration of dosing is required to reach steady-state. Dose escalations in renal impairment should be done after administration of at least 5-6 doses at appropriate intervals (see TABLE 12).

Extreme caution should be exercised in the use of sotalol in patients with renal failure undergoing hemodialysis. The half-life of sotalol is prolonged (up to 69 hours) in anuric patients. Sotalol, however, can be partly removed by dialysis with subsequent partial rebound in concentrations when dialysis is completed. Both safety (heart rate, QT interval) and efficacy (arrhythmia control) must be closely monitored.

Transfer to Betapace

Before starting Betapace, previous antiarrhythmic therapy should generally be withdrawn under careful monitoring for a minimum of 2-3 plasma half-lives if the patient's clinical condition permits (see DRUG INTERACTIONS). Treatment has been initiated in some patients receiving IV lidocaine without ill effect. After discontinuation of amiodarone, Betapace should not be initiated until the QT interval is normalized (see WARNINGS).

Transfer to Betapace AF From Betapace

Patients with a history of symptomatic AFIB/AFL who are currently receiving Betapace for the maintenance of normal sinus rhythm should be transferred to Betapace AF because of the significant differences in labeling (*i.e.,* patient package insert for Betapace AF, dosing administration, and safety information).

BETAPACE AF
Dosing and Administration in Adults

Therapy with Betapace AF must be initiated (and, if necessary, titrated) in a setting that provides continuous electrocardiographic (ECG) monitoring and in the presence of personnel trained in the management of serious ventricular arrhythmias. Patients should continue to be monitored in this way for a minimum of 3 days on the maintenance dose. In addition, patients should not be discharged within 12 hours of electrical or pharmacological conversion to normal sinus rhythm.

The QT interval is used to determine patient eligibility for Betapace AF treatment and for monitoring safety during treatment. The baseline QT interval must be ≤450 milliseconds in order for a patient to be started on Betapace AF therapy. During initiation and titration, the QT interval should be monitored 2-4 hours after each dose. If the QT interval prolongs to 500 milliseconds or greater, the dose must be reduced or the drug discontinued.

The dose of Betapace AF must be individualized according to creatinine clearance. In patients with a creatinine clearance >60 ml/min Betapace AF is administered twice daily (bid) while in those with a creatinine clearance between 40 and 60 ml/min, the dose is administered once daily (qd). In patients with a creatinine clearance less than 40 ml/min Betapace AF is contraindicated. The recommended initial dose of Betapace AF is 80 mg and is initiated as shown in the dosing algorithm described below. The 80 mg dose can be titrated upward to 120 mg during initial hospitalization or after discharge on 80 mg in the event of recurrence, by rehospitalization and repeating the same steps used during the initiation of therapy (see Upward Titration of Dose).

Patients with atrial fibrillation should be anticoagulated according to usual medical practice. Hypokalemia should be corrected before initiation of Betapace AF therapy (see WARNINGS, Ventricular Arrhythmia).

Patients to be discharged on Betapace AF therapy from an in-patient setting should have an adequate supply of Betapace AF to allow uninterrupted therapy until the patient can fill a Betapace AF prescription.

Initiation of Betapace AF Therapy

Step 1

Electrocardiographic Assessment: Prior to administration of the first dose, the QT interval must be determined using an average of 5 beats. If the baseline QT is greater than 450 milliseconds (JT ≥330 milliseconds if QRS over 100 milliseconds), Betapace AF is contraindicated.

Step 2

Calculation of Creatinine Clearance: Prior to the administration of the first dose, the patient's creatinine clearance should be calculated using the following formula:

Creatinine clearance (male) = [(140-age) × body weight in kg] ÷ [72 × serum creatinine (mg/dl)]

Creatinine clearance (female) = [(140-age) × body weight in kg × 0.85] ÷ [72 × serum creatinine (mg/dl)]

When serum creatinine is given in μmol/L, divide the value by 88.4 (1 mg/dl = 88.4 μmol/L).

Step 3

Starting Dose: The starting dose of Betapace AF is 80 mg twice daily (bid) if the creatinine clearance is >60 ml/min, and 80 mg once daily (qd) if the creatinine clearance is 40-60 ml/min. If the creatinine clearance is <40 ml/min Betapace AF is contraindicated.

Step 4

Administer the appropriate daily dose of Betapace AF and begin continuous ECG monitoring with QT interval measurements 2-4 hours after each dose.

Step 5

If the 80 mg dose level is tolerated and the QT interval remains <500 milliseconds after at least 3 days (after 5 or 6 doses if patient receiving qd dosing), the patient can be discharged. Alternatively, during hospitalization, the dose can be increased to 120 mg bid and the patient followed for 3 days on this dose (followed for 5 or 6 doses if patient receiving qd doses).

Upward Titration of Dose

If the 80 mg dose level (given bid or qd depending upon the creatinine clearance) does not reduce the frequency of relapses of AFIB/AFL and is tolerated without excessive QT interval prolongation (*i.e.,* ≥520 milliseconds), the dose level may be increased to 120 mg (bid or qd depending upon the creatinine clearance). As proarrhythmic events can occur not only at initiation of therapy, but also with each upward dosage adjustment, Steps 2 through 5 used during initiation of Betapace AF therapy should be followed when increasing the dose level. In the US multicenter dose-response study, the 120 mg dose (bid or qd) was found to be the most effective in prolonging the time to ECG documented symptomatic recurrence of AFIB/AFL. If the 120 mg dose does not reduce the frequency of early relapse of AFIB/AFL and is tolerated without excessive QT interval prolongation (≥520 milliseconds), an increase to 160 mg (bid or qd depending upon the creatinine clearance can be considered. Steps 2 through 5 used during the initiation of therapy should be used again to introduce such an increase.

Maintenance of Betapace AF Therapy

Renal function and QT should be re-evaluated regularly if medically warranted. If QT is 520 milliseconds or greater (JT 430 milliseconds or greater if QRS is >100 milliseconds), the dose of Betapace AF therapy should be reduced and patients should be carefully monitored until QT returns to less than 520 milliseconds. If the QT interval is ≥520 milliseconds while on the lowest maintenance dose level (80 mg) the drug should be discontinued. If renal function deteriorates, reduce the daily dose in half by administering the drug once daily as described in Initiation of Betapace AF Therapy, Step 3.

Special Considerations

The maximum recommended dose in patients with a calculated creatinine clearance greater than 60 ml/min is 160 mg bid, doses greater than 160 mg bid have been associated with an increased incidence of torsade de pointes and are not recommended. A patient who misses a dose should NOT double the next dose. The next dose should be taken at the usual time.

Dosing and Administration in Children

As in adults the following precautionary measures should be considered when initiating sotalol treatment in children: Initiation of treatment in the hospital after appropriate clinical assessment; individualized regimen as appropriate; gradual increase of doses if required; careful assessment of therapeutic response and tolerability; and frequent monitoring of the QTc interval and heart rate.

For children aged about 2 years and greater, with normal renal function, doses normalized for body surface area are appropriate for both initial and incremental dosing. Since the Class III potency in children (see CLINICAL PHARMACOLOGY) is not very different from that in adults, reaching plasma concentrations that occur within the adult dose range is an appropriate guide. From pediatric pharmacokinetic data the following is recommended.

For initiation of treatment, 30 mg/m^2 three times a day (90 mg/m^2 total daily dose) is approximately equivalent to the initial 160 mg total daily dose for adults. Subsequent titration to a maximum of 60 mg/m^2 (approximately equivalent to the 360 mg total daily dose for adults) can then occur. Titration should be guided by clinical response, heart rate and QTc, with increased dosing being preferably carried out in-hospital. At least 36 hours should be allowed between dose increments to attain steady state plasma concentrations of sotalol in patients with age-adjusted normal renal function.

For children aged about 2 years or younger the above pediatric dosage should be reduced by a factor that depends heavily upon age. **(Refer to manufacturer's insert for detailed information.)**

For a child aged 20 months, the dosing suggested for children with normal renal function aged 2 years or greater should be multiplied by about 0.97; the initial starting dose would be (30 × 0.97) = 29.1 mg/m^2, administered 3 times daily. For a child aged 1 month, the starting dose should be multiplied by 0.68; the initial starting dose would be (30 × 0.68) = 20 mg/m^2, administered 3 times daily. For a child aged about 1 week, the initial starting dose should be multiplied by 0.3; the starting dose would be (30 × 0.3) = 9 mg/m^2. Similar calculations should be made for increased doses as titration proceeds. Since the half-life of sotalol decreases with decreasing age (below about 2 years), time to steady state will also increase. Thus, in neonates the time to steady state may be as long as a week or longer.

In all children, individualization of dosage is required. As in adults Betapace (sotalol HCl should be used with particular caution in children if the QTC is greater than 500 milliseconds on therapy and serious consideration should be given to reducing the dose or discontinuing therapy when QTC exceeds 550 milliseconds.

The use of Betapace (sotalol HCl) in children with renal impairment has not been investigated. Sotalol elimination is predominantly via the kidney in the unchanged form. Use of sotalol in any age group with decreased renal function should be at lower doses or at increased intervals between doses. Monitoring of heart rate and QTC is more important and it will take much longer to reach steady state with any dose and/or frequency of administration.

Transfer to Betapace AF From Betapace

Patients with a history of symptomatic AFIB/AFL who are currently receiving Betapace for the maintenance of normal sinus rhythm should be transferred to Betapace AF because of the significant differences in labeling (*i.e.,* patient information distributed with prescription, dosing administration, and safety information).

Transfer to Betapace AF From Other Antiarrhythmic Agents

Before starting Betapace AF, previous antiarrhythmic therapy should generally be withdrawn under careful monitoring for a minimum of 2-3 plasma half-lives if the patient's clinical condition permits (see DRUG INTERACTIONS). Treatment has been initiated in some patients receiving IV lidocaine without ill effect. After discontinuation of amiodarone, Betapace AF should not be initiated until the QT interval is normalized (see WARNINGS).

Preparation of Extemporaneous Oral Solution

Betapace AF syrup 5 mg/ml can be compounded using simple syrup containing 0.1% sodium benzoate (syrup) available from Humco Laboratories as follows:

1. Measure 120 ml of simple syrup.
2. Transfer the syrup to a 6 ounce amber plastic (polyethylene terephthalate [PET]) prescription bottle. *NOTE:* An oversized bottle is used to allow for a headspace, so that there will be more effective mixing during shaking of the bottle.
3. Add 5 Betapace AF 120 mg tablets to the bottle. These tablets are added intact; it is not necessary to crush the tablets. *NOTE:* The addition of the tablets can also be done first. The tablets can also be crushed if preferred. If the tablets are crushed, care should be taken to transfer the entire quantity of tablet powder into the bottle containing the syrup.
4. Shake the bottle to wet the entire surface of the tablets. If the tablets have been crushed, shake the bottle until the endpoint is achieved.
5. Allow the tablets to hydrate for approximately 2 hours.
6. After at least 2 hours have elapsed; shake the bottle intermittently over the course of at least another 2 hours until the tablets are completely disintegrated. *NOTE:* The tablets can be allowed to hydrate overnight to simplify the disintegration process.

The endpoint is achieved when a dispersion of fine particles in the syrup is obtained.

This compounding procedure results in a solution containing 5 mg/ml of sotalol HCl. The fine solid particles are the water-insoluble inactive ingredients of the tablets.

This extemporaneously prepared oral solution of sotalol HCl (with suspended inactive particles) must be shaken well prior to administration. This is to ensure that the amount of inactive solid particles per dose remains constant throughout the duration of use.

Stability studies indicate that the suspension is stable when stored at controlled room temperature (15-30°C/59-86°F) and ambient humidity for 3 months.

HOW SUPPLIED

BETAPACE

Betapace is supplied in capsule-shaped light-blue scored tablets imprinted with the strengths "80 mg", "120 mg", "160 mg", or "240 mg" and "BETAPACE".

Storage: Store at 25°C (77°F) with excursions permitted between 15-30°C (59-86°F).

BETAPACE AF

Betapace AF is supplied in capsule-shaped white scored tablets imprinted with the strengths "80 mg", "120 mg", or "160 mg" and "BERLEX".

Storage: Store at 25°C (77°F) with excursions permitted between 15-30°C (59-86°F).

PRODUCT LISTING - RATED THERAPEUTICALLY EQUIVALENT

Tablet - Oral - 80 mg

30's	$73.94	GENERIC, Mutual/United Research Laboratories	00677-1709-07
60's	$140.85	GENERIC, Mutual/United Research Laboratories	00677-1709-06
100's	$234.69	GENERIC, Global Pharmaceutical Corporation	00115-2711-01
100's	$234.72	GENERIC, Teva Pharmaceuticals Usa	00093-1061-01
100's	$234.72	GENERIC, Par Pharmaceutical Inc	49884-0582-01
100's	$241.98	GENERIC, Upsher-Smith Laboratories Inc	00245-0012-11
100's	$244.72	GENERIC, Watson Laboratories Inc	52544-0654-01
100's	$256.28	GENERIC, Eon Labs Manufacturing Inc	00185-0171-01
100's	$256.28	GENERIC, Mutual/United Research Laboratories	00677-1709-01
100's	$260.89	GENERIC, Upsher-Smith Laboratories Inc	00245-0012-01
100's	$307.69	BETAPACE, Berlex Laboratories	50419-0105-10

Tablet - Oral - 120 mg

100's	$313.09	GENERIC, Global Pharmaceutical Corporation	00115-2722-01
100's	$313.14	GENERIC, Teva Pharmaceuticals Usa	00093-1060-01
100's	$313.14	GENERIC, Par Pharmaceutical Inc	49884-0583-01
100's	$321.98	GENERIC, Upsher-Smith Laboratories Inc	00245-0013-11
100's	$326.48	GENERIC, Watson Laboratories Inc	52544-0665-01
100's	$341.89	GENERIC, Eon Labs Manufacturing Inc	00185-0170-01
100's	$341.89	GENERIC, Mutual/United Research Laboratories	00677-1710-01
100's	$346.39	GENERIC, Upsher-Smith Laboratories Inc	00245-0013-01
100's	$410.50	BETAPACE, Berlex Laboratories	50419-0109-10

Tablet - Oral - 160 mg

100's	$391.49	GENERIC, Global Pharmaceutical Corporation	00115-2733-01
100's	$391.50	GENERIC, Teva Pharmaceuticals Usa	00093-1062-01
100's	$391.50	GENERIC, Par Pharmaceutical Inc	49884-0584-01
100's	$403.70	GENERIC, Upsher-Smith Laboratories Inc	00245-0014-11
100's	$408.18	GENERIC, Watson Laboratories Inc	52544-0655-01
100's	$427.45	GENERIC, Eon Labs Manufacturing Inc	00185-0177-01
100's	$430.98	GENERIC, Upsher-Smith Laboratories Inc	00245-0014-01
100's	$513.25	BETAPACE, Berlex Laboratories	50419-0106-10

Tablet - Oral - 240 mg

30's	$160.32	GENERIC, Mutual/United Research Laboratories	00677-1712-07
60's	$316.90	GENERIC, Mutual/United Research Laboratories	00677-1712-06
100's	$480.15	GENERIC, Mutual/United Research Laboratories	00677-1712-01
100's	$508.89	GENERIC, Global Pharmaceutical Corporation	00115-2744-01
100's	$508.95	GENERIC, Teva Pharmaceuticals Usa	00093-1063-01
100's	$508.95	GENERIC, Par Pharmaceutical Inc	49884-0585-01
100's	$524.51	GENERIC, Watson Laboratories Inc	52544-0656-01
100's	$524.77	GENERIC, Upsher-Smith Laboratories Inc	00245-0015-11
100's	$555.64	GENERIC, Eon Labs Manufacturing Inc	00185-0174-01
100's	$559.97	GENERIC, Upsher-Smith Laboratories Inc	00245-0015-01
100's	$667.13	BETAPACE, Berlex Laboratories	50419-0107-10

PRODUCT LISTING - EQUIVALENTS NOT AVAILABLE

Tablet - Oral - 80 mg

60's	$159.31	BETAPACE AF, Berlex Laboratories	50419-0115-06
100's	$270.38	BETAPACE AF, Berlex Laboratories	50419-0115-11
100's	$313.25	BETAPACE, Berlex Laboratories	50419-0105-11

Tablet - Oral - 120 mg

60's	$187.88	GENERIC, Mutual/United Research Laboratories	00677-1710-06
60's	$212.50	BETAPACE AF, Berlex Laboratories	50419-0119-06
100's	$325.94	BETAPACE AF, Berlex Laboratories	50419-0119-11
100's	$399.88	BETAPACE, Berlex Laboratories	50419-0109-11

Tablet - Oral - 160 mg

60's	$234.90	GENERIC, Mutual/United Research Laboratories	00677-1711-06
60's	$265.81	BETAPACE AF, Berlex Laboratories	50419-0116-06
100's	$406.38	BETAPACE AF, Berlex Laboratories	50419-0116-11
100's	$427.45	GENERIC, Mutual/United Research Laboratories	00677-1711-01
100's	$498.63	BETAPACE, Berlex Laboratories	50419-0106-11

Tablet - Oral - 240 mg

100's	$492.37	BETAPACE, Berlex Laboratories	50419-0107-11

Sparfloxacin *(003324)*

For related information, see the comparative table section in Appendix A.

Categories: Bronchitis, chronic, acute exacerbation; Infection, lower respiratory tract; Pneumonia, community-acquired; Pregnancy Category C; FDA Approved 1997 Jan
Drug Classes: Antibiotics, quinolones
Brand Names: **Zagam**
Foreign Brand Availability: Newspar (Indonesia); Resflox (Indonesia); Spara (China; Japan; Korea); Spardac (India); Sparlox (India); Sparos (Indonesia); Sparx (Benin; Burkina-Faso; Ethiopia; Gambia; Ghana; Guinea; Ivory-Coast; Kenya; Liberia; Malawi; Mali; Mauritania; Mauritius; Morocco; Niger; Nigeria; Senegal; Seychelles; Sierra-Leone; Sudan; Tanzania; Tunia; Uganda; Zambia; Zimbabwe); Torospar (India); Wanflox (Indonesia)
Cost of Therapy: $73.52 (Infection; Zagam; 200 mg; 1 tablet/day; 10 day supply)

DESCRIPTION

Sparfloxacin is a synthetic broad-spectrum antimicrobial agent for oral administration. Sparfloxacin, an aminodifluoroquinolone, is 5-Amino-1-cyclopropyl-7-(*cis*-3,5-dimethyl-1-piperazinyl)-6,8-difluoro-1,4-dihydro-4-oxo-3-quinolinecarboxylic acid. Its empirical formula is $C_{19}H_{22}F_2N_4O_3$.

Sparfloxacin has a molecular weight of 392.41. It occurs as a yellow crystalline powder. It is sparingly soluble in glacial acetic acid or chloroform, very slightly soluble in ethanol (95%), and practically insoluble in water and ether. It dissolves in dilute acetic acid or 0.1 N sodium hydroxide.

Zagam is available as a 200 mg round, white film-coated tablet. Each 200 mg tablet contains the following inactive ingredients: microcrystalline cellulose, corn starch, L-hydroxypropylcellulose, magnesium stearate, and colloidal silicone dioxide. The film coating contains: methylhydroxypropylcellulose, polyethylene glycol 6000, and titanium dioxide.

CLINICAL PHARMACOLOGY

ABSORPTION

Sparfloxacin is well absorbed following oral administration with an absolute oral bioavailability of 92%. The mean maximum plasma sparfloxacin concentration following a single 400 mg oral dose was approximately 1.3 (±0.2) μg/ml. The area under the curve (mean AUC(0→∞) following a single 400 mg oral dose was approximately 34 (±6.8) μg·h/ml.

Steady-state plasma concentration was achieved on the first day by giving a loading dose that was double the daily dose. Mean (±SD) pharmacokinetic parameters observed for the 24 hour dosing interval with the recommended dosing regimen are shown in TABLE 1.

Maximum plasma concentrations for the initial oral 400 mg loading dose were typically achieved between 3-6 hours following administration with a mean value of approximately

S

TABLE 1

Dosing Regimen (mg/day)	Peak C_{max} (µg/ml)	Trough C_{24} (µg/ml)	AUC(0→24) (h·µg/ml)
400 mg loading dose (day 1)	1.3 (±0.2)	0.5 (±0.1)	20.6 (±3.1)
200 mg q24 hours (steady-state)	1.1 (±0.1)	0.5 (±0.1)	18.7 (±2.6)

4 hours. Maximum plasma concentrations for a 200 mg dose were also achieved between 3-6 hours after administration with a mean of about 4 hours.

Oral absorption of sparfloxacin is unaffected by administration with milk or food, including high fat meals. Concurrent administration of antacids containing magnesium hydroxide and aluminum hydroxide reduces the oral bioavailability of sparfloxacin by as much as 50%. (See PRECAUTIONS, Information for the Patient, and DRUG INTERACTIONS.)

DISTRIBUTION

Upon reaching general circulation, sparfloxacin distributes well into the body, as reflected by the large mean steady-state volume of distribution (Vdss) of 3.9 (±0.8) L/kg. Sparfloxacin exhibits low plasma protein binding in serum at about 45%.

Sparfloxacin penetrates well into body fluids and tissues. Results of tissue and body fluid distribution studies demonstrated that oral administration of sparfloxacin produces sustained concentrations and that sparfloxacin concentrations in lower respiratory tract tissues and fluids generally exceed the corresponding plasma concentrations. The concentration of sparfloxacin in respiratory tissues (pulmonary parenchyma, bronchial wall, and bronchial mucosa) at 2-6 hours following standard oral dosing was approximately 3-6 times greater than the corresponding concentration in plasma. Concentrations in these respiratory tissues increase at up to 24 hours following dosing. Sparfloxacin is also highly concentrated into alveolar macrophages compared to plasma. Tissue or fluid to plasma sparfloxacin concentration ratios for respiratory tissues and fluids are found in TABLE 2.

TABLE 2 *Tissue to Plasma Sparfloxacin Concentration Mean Ratio (%CV)**

Respiratory Tissues and Fluids	n value†	Time of Collection Postdose 2-6 hour	12-24 hour
Alveolar macrophage	6/5	51.8 (88.7%)	68.1 (47.9%)
Epithelial lining fluid	10/10	12.3 (26.7%)	17.6 (35.3%)
Pulmonary parenchyma	8/7	5.9 (15.0%)	15.8 (32.0%)
Bronchial wall	8/7	2.8 (16.0%)	5.7 (25.0%)
Bronchial mucosa	6/5	2.7 (11.5%)	3.1 (11.6%)

* % CV (percent coefficient of variation)
† For tissues with two values, the first n is for 2-6 hours and the second n is for 12-24 hours.

Mean pleural effusion to plasma concentration ratios were 0.34 and 0.69 at 4 and 20 hours postdose, respectively.

METABOLISM

Sparfloxacin is metabolized by the liver, primarily by phase II glucuronidation, to form a glucuronide conjugate. Its metabolism does not utilize or interfere with cytochrome-mediated oxidation, in particular cytochrome P450.

EXCRETION

The total body clearance and renal clearance of sparfloxacin were 11.4 (±3.5) and 1.5 (±0.5) L/h, respectively. Sparfloxacin is excreted in both the feces (50%) and urine (50%). Approximately 10% of an orally administered dose is excreted in the urine as unchanged drug in patients with normal renal function. Following a 400 mg loading dose of sparfloxacin, the mean urine concentration 4 hours postdose was in excess of 12.0 µg/ml, and measurable concentrations of active drug persisted through 6 days for subjects with normal renal function.

S

The terminal elimination phase half-life ($T_{1/2}$) of sparfloxacin in plasma generally varies between 16 and 30 hours, with a mean $T_{1/2}$ of approximately 20 hours. The $T_{1/2}$ is independent of the administered dose, suggesting that sparfloxacin elimination kinetics are linear.

SPECIAL POPULATIONS

Geriatric

The pharmacokinetics of sparfloxacin are not altered in the elderly with normal renal function.

Pediatric

The pharmacokinetics of sparfloxacin in pediatric subjects have not been studied.

Gender

There are no gender differences in the pharmacokinetics of sparfloxacin.

Renal Insufficiency

In patients with renal impairment (creatinine clearance <50 ml/min), the terminal elimination half-life of sparfloxacin is lengthened. Single or multiple doses of sparfloxacin in patients with varying degrees of renal impairment typically produce plasma concentrations that are twice those observed in subjects with normal renal function. (See PRECAUTIONS, General and DOSAGE AND ADMINISTRATION.)

Hepatic Insufficiency

The pharmacokinetics of sparfloxacin are not altered in patients with mild or moderate hepatic impairment without cholestasis.

MICROBIOLOGY

Sparfloxacin has *in vitro* activity against a wide range of gram-negative and gram-positive microorganisms. Sparfloxacin exerts its antibacterial activity by inhibiting DNA gyrase, a bacterial topoisomerase. DNA gyrase is an essential enzyme which controls DNA topology and assists in DNA replication, repair, deactivation, and transcription.

Quinolones differ in chemical structure and mode of action from β-lactam antibiotics. Quinolones may, therefore, be active against bacteria resistant to β-lactam antibiotics.

Although cross-resistance has been observed between sparfloxacin and other fluoroquinolones, some microorganisms resistant to other fluoroquinolones may be susceptible to sparfloxacin.

In vitro tests show that the combination of sparfloxacin and rifampin is antagonistic against *Staphylococcus aureus*.

Sparfloxacin has been shown to be active against most strains of the following microorganisms, both *in vitro* and in clinical infections as described in INDICATIONS AND USAGE.

Aerobic Gram-Positive Microorganisms:
Staphylococcus aureus
Streptococcus pneumoniae, (penicillin-susceptible strains)

Aerobic Gram-Negative Microorganisms:
Enterobacter cloacae
Haemophilus influenzae
Haemophilus parainfluenzae
Klebsiella pneumoniae
Moraxella catarrhalis

Other Microorganisms:
Chlamydia pneumoniae
Mycoplasma pneumoniae

The following *in vitro* data are available, **but their clinical significance is unknown.**

Sparfloxacin exhibits *in vitro* minimal inhibitory concentrations (MICs) of 1 µg/ml or less against most (≥90%) strains of the following microorganisms; however, the safety and effectiveness of sparfloxacin in treating clinical infections due to these microorganisms have not been established in adequate and well controlled clinical trials.

Aerobic Gram-Positive Microorganisms:
Streptococcus agalactiae
Streptococcus pneumoniae, (penicillin-resistant strains)
Streptococcus pyogenes
Viridans group streptococci

Aerobic Gram-Negative Microorganisms:
Acinetobacter anitratus
Acinetobacter lwoffi
Citrobacter diversus
Enterobacter aerogenes
Klebsiella oxytoca
Legionella pneumophila
Morganella morganii
Proteus mirabilis
Proteus vulgaris

SUSCEPTIBILITY TESTING

Dilution Techniques

Quantitative methods are used to determine antimicrobial minimal inhibitory concentrations (MICs). These MICs provide estimates of the susceptibility of bacteria to antimicrobial compounds. The MICs should be determined using a standardized procedure. Standardized procedures are based on a dilution method[1] (broth or agar) or equivalent with standardized inoculum concentrations and standardized concentrations of sparfloxacin powder. The MIC values should be interpreted according to the criteria in TABLE 3.

TABLE 3 *For Testing Aerobic Microorganisms Other Than Haemophilus influenzae, Haemophilus parainfluenzae and Streptococcus pneumoniae*

MIC (µg/ml)	Interpretation
≤1	Susceptible (S)
2	Intermediate (I)
≥4	Resistant (R)

TABLE 4 *For Testing Haemophilus influenzae and Haemophilus parainfluenzae**

MIC (µg/ml)	Interpretation
≤0.25	Susceptible (S)

* These interpretive standards are applicable only to broth microdilution susceptibility testing with *Haemophilus influenzae* and *Haemophilus parainfluenzae* using Haemophilus Test Medium[1].

The current absence of data on resistant strains precludes defining any categories other than "Susceptible". Strains yielding MIC results suggestive of a "nonsusceptible" category should be submitted to a reference laboratory for further testing.

TABLE 5 *For Testing Streptococcus Pneumoniae**

MIC (µg/ml)	Interpretation
≤0.5	Susceptible

* These interpretive standards are applicable only to broth microdilution susceptibility tests using cation-adjusted Mueller-Hinton broth with 2-5% lysed horse blood.

The current absence of data on resistant strains precludes defining any categories other than "Susceptible". Strains yielding MIC results suggestive of a "nonsusceptible" category should be submitted to a reference laboratory for further testing.

A report of "Susceptible" indicates that the pathogen is likely to be inhibited if the antimicrobial compound in the blood reaches the concentration usually achievable. A report of "Intermediate" indicates that the result should be considered equivocal, and, if the microorganism is not fully susceptible to alternative, clinically feasible drugs, the test should be repeated. This category implies possible clinical applicability in body sites where the drug is physiologically concentrated or in situations where a high dosage of drug can be used. This category also provides a buffer zone which prevents small uncontrolled technical factors from causing major discrepancies in interpretation. A report of "Resistant" indicates that the pathogen is not likely to be inhibited if the antimicrobial compound in the blood reaches the concentration usually achievable; other therapy should be selected.

Standardized susceptibility test procedures require the use of laboratory control microorganisms to control the technical aspects of the laboratory procedures. Standard sparfloxacin powder should provide the MIC values found in TABLE 6.

TABLE 6

Microorganism	MIC Range (μg/ml)
Enterococcus faecalis ATCC 29212	0.12-0.5
Escherichia coli ATCC 25922	0.004-0.016
Haemophilus influenzae ATCC 49247*	0.004-0.016
Staphylococcus aureaus ATCC 29213	0.03-0.12
Streptococcus pneumoniae ATCC 49619†	0.12-0.5

* This quality control range is applicable to only *H. influenzae* ATCC 49247 tested by a broth microdilution procedure using Haemophilus Test Medium (HTM).[1]

† This quality control range is applicable to only *S. pneumoniae* ATCC 49619 tested by a broth microdilution procedure using cation-adjusted Mueller-Hinton broth with 2-5% lysed horse blood.

Diffusion Techniques

Quantitative methods that require measurement of zone diameters also provide reproducible estimates of the susceptibility of bacteria to antimicrobial compounds. One such standardized procedure[2] requires the use of standardized inoculum concentrations. This procedure uses paper disks impregnated with 5 μg sparfloxacin to test the susceptibility of microorganisms to sparfloxacin.

Reports from the laboratory providing results of the standard single-disk susceptibility test with a 5 μg sparfloxacin disk should be interpreted according to the criteria in TABLE 7.

TABLE 7 *For Aerobic Microorganisms Other Than Haemophilus influenzae, Haemophilus parainfluenzae, and Streptococcus pneumoniae*

Zone Diameter (mm)	Interpretation
≥19	Susceptible (S)
16-18	Intermediate (I)
≤15	Resistant (R)

Haemophilus influenzae and *Haemophilus parainfluenzae* should not be tested by diffusion techniques. An MIC should be determined for these isolates.

TABLE 8 *For Streptococcus pneumoniae**

Zone Diameter	Interpretation
≥19	Susceptible (S)

* These zone diameter standards for *Streptococcus pneumoniae* apply only to tests performed using Mueller-Hinton agar supplemented with 5% sheep blood and incubated in 5% CO_2.

The current absence of data on resistant strains precludes any category other than "Susceptible". Strains yielding zone diameter results suggestive of a "nonsusceptible" category should be submitted to a reference laboratory for further testing.

Interpretation should be as stated above for results using dilution techniques. Interpretation involves correlation of the diameter obtained in the disk test with the MIC for sparfloxacin.

As with standard dilution techniques, diffusion methods require the use of laboratory control microorganisms that are used to control the technical aspects of the laboratory procedures. For the diffusion technique, the 5 μg sparfloxacin disk should provide the zone diameters in these laboratory quality control strains found in TABLE 9.

TABLE 9

Microorganism	Zone Diameter (mm)
Escherichia coli ATCC 25922	30-38
Staphylococcus areus ATCC 25923	27-33
Streptococcus pneumoniae ATCC 49619*	21-27

* These quality control limits apply to tests conducted with *S. pneumoniae* ATCC 49619 using Mueller-Hinton agar supplemented with 5% sheep blood incubated in 5% CO_2.

INDICATIONS AND USAGE

Sparfloxacin is indicated for the treatment of adults (≥18 years of age) with the following infections caused by susceptible strains of the designated microorganisms:

Community-Acquired Pneumonia: Caused by *Chlamydia pneumoniae, Haemophilus influenzae, Haemophilus parainfluenzae, Moraxella catarrhalis, Mycoplasma pneumoniae,* or *Streptococcus pneumoniae.*

Acute Bacterial Exacerbations of Chronic Bronchitis: Caused by *Chlamydia pneumoniae, Enterobacter cloacae, Haemophilus influenzae, Haemophilus parainfluenzae, Klebsiella pneumoniae, Moraxella catarrhalis, Staphylococcus aureus,* or *Streptococcus pneumoniae.*

Appropriate culture and susceptibility tests should be performed before treatment in order to isolate and identify organisms causing the infection and to determine their susceptibility to sparfloxacin. Therapy with sparfloxacin may be initiated before results of these tests are known; once results become available, appropriate therapy should be selected. Culture and susceptibility testing performed periodically during therapy will provide information on the continued susceptibility of the pathogen to the antimicrobial agent and also on the possible emergence of bacterial resistance.

CONTRAINDICATIONS

Sparfloxacin is contraindicated for individuals with a history of hypersensitivity or photosensitivity reactions.

Torsade de pointes has been reported in patients receiving sparfloxacin concomitantly with disopyramide and amiodarone. Consequently, sparfloxacin is contraindicated for individuals receiving these drugs as well as other QTc-prolonging antiarrhythmic drugs reported to cause torsade de pointes, such as class Ia antiarrhythmic agents (*e.g.,* quinidine, procainamide), class III antiarrhythmic agents (*e.g.,* sotalol), and bepridil. Sparfloxacin is contraindicated in patients with known QTc prolongation or in patients being treated concomitantly with medications known to produce an increase in the QTc interval and/or torsade de pointes (*e.g.,* terfenadine). (See WARNINGS and PRECAUTIONS.)

It is essential to avoid exposure to the sun, bright natural light, and UV rays throughout the entire duration of treatment and for 5 days after treatment is stopped. Sparfloxacin is contraindicated in patients whose life-style or employment will not permit compliance with required safety precautions concerning phototoxicity. (See WARNINGS and PRECAUTIONS.)

WARNINGS

MODERATE TO SEVERE PHOTOTOXIC REACTIONS HAVE OCCURRED IN PATIENTS EXPOSED TO DIRECT OR INDIRECT SUNLIGHT OR TO ARTIFICIAL ULTRAVIOLET LIGHT (*e.g.,* SUNLAMPS) DURING OR FOLLOWING TREATMENT. THESE REACTIONS HAVE ALSO OCCURRED IN PATIENTS EXPOSED TO SHADED OR DIFFUSE LIGHT, INCLUDING EXPOSURE THROUGH GLASS OR DURING CLOUDY WEATHER. PATIENTS SHOULD BE ADVISED TO DISCONTINUE SPARFLOXACIN THERAPY AT THE FIRST SIGNS OR SYMPTOMS OF A PHOTOTOXICITY REACTION SUCH AS A SENSATION OF SKIN BURNING, REDNESS, SWELLING, BLISTERS, RASH, ITCHING, OR DERMATITIS.

The overall incidence of drug related phototoxicity in the 1585 patients who received sparfloxacin during clinical trials with recommended dosage was 7.9% (n=126). Phototoxicity ranged from mild 4.1% (n=65) to moderate 3.3% (n=52) to severe 0.6% (n=9), with severe defined as involving at least significant curtailment of normal daily activity. The frequency of phototoxicity reactions characterized by blister formation was 0.8% (n=13) of which 3 were severe. The discontinuation rate due to phototoxicity independent of drug relationship was 1.1% (n=17).

As with some other types of phototoxicity, there is the potential for exacerbation of the reaction on reexposure to sunlight or artificial ultraviolet light prior to complete recovery from the reaction. In a few cases, recovery from phototoxicity reactions was prolonged for several weeks. In rare cases, reactions have recurred up to several weeks after stopping sparfloxacin therapy.

EXPOSURE TO DIRECT AND INDIRECT SUNLIGHT (EVEN WHEN USING SUNSCREENS OR SUNBLOCKS) SHOULD BE AVOIDED WHILE TAKING SPARFLOXACIN AND FOR 5 DAYS FOLLOWLNG THERAPY. SPARFLOXACIN THERAPY SHOULD BE DISCONTINUED IMMEDIATELY AT THE FIRST SIGNS OR SYMPTOMS OF PHOTOTOXICITY.

These phototoxic reactions have occurred with and without the use of sunscreens or sunblocks and have been associated with a single dose of sparfloxacin. However, a study in healthy volunteers has demonstrated that some sunscreen products, specifically those active in blocking UVA spectrum wavelengths (those containing the active ingredients octocrylene or Parsol 1789), can moderate the photosensitizing effect of sparfloxacin. However, many over-the-counter sunscreens do not provide adequate UVA protection.

Increases in the QTc interval have been observed in healthy volunteers treated with sparfloxacin. After a single loading dose of 400 mg, a mean increase in QTc interval of 11 msec (2.9%) is seen; at steady-state the mean increase is 7 msec (1.9%). The magnitude of the QTc effect does not increase with repeated administration, and the QTc returns to baseline within 48 hours of the last dose. In clinical trials involving 1489 patients with a baseline QTc measurement, the mean prolongation at steady-state was 10 msec (2.5%); 0.7% of patients had a QTc interval greater than 500 msec; however, no arrhythmic effects were seen.

THE SAFETY AND EFFECTIVENESS OF SPARFLOXACIN IN CHILDREN, ADOLESCENTS (UNDER THE AGE OF 18 YEARS), PREGNANT WOMEN, AND LACTATING WOMEN HAVE NOT BEEN ESTABLISHED. (See PRECAUTIONS: Pregnancy, Teratogenic Effects, Pregnancy Category C, Nursing Mothers; and Pediatric Use.)

Sparfloxacin has been shown to cause arthropathy in immature dogs when given in oral doses of 25 mg/kg/day (approximately 1.9 times the highest human dose on a mg/m^2 basis) for 7 consecutive days. Examination of the weight-bearing joints of the dogs revealed small erosive lesions of the cartilage. Other quinolones also produce erosions of cartilage of weight-bearing joints and other signs of arthropathy in immature animals of various species.

Convulsions and toxic psychoses have been reported in patients receiving quinolones, including sparfloxacin. Quinolones may also cause increased intracranial pressure and central nervous system stimulation which may lead to tremors, restlessness/agitation, anxiety/nervousness, lightheadedness, confusion, hallucinations, paranoia, depression, nightmares, insomnia, and, rarely, suicidal thoughts or acts. These reactions may occur following the first dose. If these reactions occur in patients receiving sparfloxacin, the drug should be

S

discontinued and appropriate measures instituted. As with other quinolones, sparfloxacin should be used with caution in patients with a known or suspected CNS disorder that may predispose to seizures or lower the seizure threshold (*e.g.,* severe cerebral arteriosclerosis, epilepsy) or in the presence of other risk factors that may predispose to seizures or lower the seizure threshold (*e.g.,* certain drug therapy, renal dysfunction). Cases of seizure associated with hypoglycemia have been reported. (See PRECAUTIONS: General, Information for the Patient; DRUG INTERACTIONS; and ADVERSE REACTIONS.)

Serious and occasionally fatal hypersensitivity (including anaphylactoid or anaphylactic) reactions, some following the first dose, have been reported in patients receiving quinolones. Some reactions were accompanied by cardiovascular collapse, hypotension/shock, seizure, loss of consciousness, tingling, angioedema (including tongue, laryngeal, throat, or facial edema), airway obstruction (including bronchosyasm, shortness of breath, and acute respiratory distress), dyspnea, urticaria, and/or itching. Only a few patients had a history of previous hypersensitivity reactions. If an allergic reaction to sparfloxacin occurs, the drug should be discontinued immediately. Serious acute hypersensitivity reactions may require immediate treatment with epinephrine, and other resuscitative measures including oxygen, intravenous fluids, antihistamines, corticosteroids, pressor amines, and airway management, including intubation, as clinically indicated.

Serious and sometimes fatal events, some due to hypersensitivity, and some due to uncertain etiology, have been reported rarely in patients receiving therapy with quinolones. These events may be severe and generally occur following the administration of multiple doses. Clinical manifestations may include one or more of the following: fever, rash or severe dermatologic reactions (*e.g.,* toxic epidermal necrolysis, Stevens-Johnson Syndrome); vasculitis; arthralgia; myalgia; serum sickness; allergic pneumonitis; interstitial nephritis; acute renal insufficiency or failure; hepatitis; jaundice; acute hepatic necrosis or failure; anemia, including hemolytic and aplastic; thrombocytopenia, including thrombotic thrombocytopenic purpura; leukopenia; agranulocytosis; pancytopenia; and/or other hematologic abnormalities. The drug should be discontinued immediately at the first appearance of a skin rash or any other sign of hypersensitivity and supportive measures instituted. (See PRECAUTIONS, Information for the Patient and ADVERSE REACTIONS.)

Pseudomembranous colitis has been reported with nearly all antibacterial agents, including sparfloxacin, and may range in severity from mild to life-threatening. Therefore, it is important to consider this diagnosis in patients who present with diarrhea subsequent to the administration of antibacterial agents.

Treatment with antibacterial agents alters the normal flora of the colon and may permit overgrowth of clostridia. Studies indicate that a toxin produced by *Clostridium difficile* is one primary cause of "antibiotic-associated colitis".

After the diagnosis of pseudomembranous colitis has been established, therapeutic measures should be initiated. Mild cases of pseudomembranous colitis usually respond to drug discontinuation alone. In moderate to severe cases, consideration should be given to management with fluids and electrolytes, protein supplementation, and treatment with an antibacterial drug clinically effective against *C. difficile* colitis.

Ruptures of the shoulder, hand, and Achilles tendons that required surgical repair or resulted in prolonged disability have been reported with sparfloxacin and other quinolones. Sparfloxacin should be discontinued if the patient experiences pain, inflammation, or rupture of a tendon. Patients should rest and refrain from exercise until the diagnosis of tendonitis or tendon rupture has been confidently excluded. Tendon rupture can occur at any time during or after therapy with sparfloxacin.

PRECAUTIONS

GENERAL

Adequate hydration of patients receiving sparfloxacin should be maintained to prevent the formation of a highly concentrated urine.

Administer sparfloxacin with caution in the presence of renal insufficiency. Careful clinical observation and appropriate laboratory studies should be performed prior to and during therapy since elimination of sparfloxacin may be reduced. Adjustment of the dosage regimen is necessary for patients with impaired renal function-creatinine clearance <50 ml/min. (See CLINICAL PHARMACOLOGY and DOSAGE AND ADMINISTRATION.)

Avoid the concomitant prescription of medications known to prolong the QTc interval, (*e.g.,* erythromycin, terfenadine, astemizole, cisapride, pentamidine, tricyclic antidepressants, some antipsychotics including phenothiazines). (See CONTRAINDICATIONS.) Sparfloxacin is not recommended for use in patients with pro-arrhythmic conditions (*e.g.,* hypokalemia, significant bradycardia, congestive heart failure, myocardial ischemia, and atrial fibrillation).

Moderate to severe phototoxicity reactions have been observed in patients exposed to direct sunlight while receiving drugs in this class. Excessive exposure to sunlight should be avoided. In clinical trials with sparfloxacin, phototoxicity was observed in approximately 7% of patients. Therapy should be discontinued if phototoxicity (*e.g.,* a skin eruption) occurs.

As with other quinolones, sparfloxacin should be used with caution in any patient with a known or suspected CNS disorder that may predispose to seizures or lower the seizure threshold (*e.g.,* severe cerebral arteriosclerosis, epilepsy) or in the presence of other risk factors that may predispose to seizures or lower the seizure threshold (*e.g.,* certain drug therapy, renal dysfunction). (See WARNINGS and DRUG INTERACTIONS.)

INFORMATION FOR THE PATIENT

Patients should be advised:

- To avoid exposure to direct or indirect sunlight (including through glass, while using sunscreens and sunblocks, reflected sunlight, and cloudy weather) and exposure to artificial ultraviolet light (*e.g.,* sunlamps) during treatment with sparfloxacin and for 5 days after therapy. If brief exposure to the sun cannot be avoided, patients should cover as much of their skin as possible with clothing.
- To discontinue sparfloxacin therapy at the first sign or symptom of phototoxicity reaction such as a sensation of skin burning, redness, swelling, blisters, rash, itching or dermatitis.
- That a patient who has experienced a phototoxic reaction with sparfloxacin should also be advised to avoid further exposure to sunlight and artificial ultraviolet light until the phototoxicity reaction has resolved and he or she has completely recovered from the reaction or for 5 days whichever is longer. In rare cases, reactions have recurred up to several weeks after stopping sparfloxacin therapy.
- That sparfloxacin may cause neurologic adverse effects (*e.g.,* dizziness, lightheadedness) and that patients should know how they react to sparfloxacin before they operate an automobile or machinery or engage in other activities requiring mental alertness and coordination (see WARNINGS and ADVERSE REACTIONS).
- To discontinue treatment and inform their physician if they experience pain, inflammation, or rupture of a tendon, and to rest and refrain from exercise until the diagnosis of tendonitis or tendon rupture has been confidently excluded.
- That sparfloxacin can be taken with food or milk or caffeine-containing products.
- That mineral supplements or vitamins with iron, or zinc, or calcium may be taken 4 hours after sparfloxacin administration.
- That sucralfate or magnesium- and aluminum-containing antacids may be taken 4 hours after sparfloxacin administration (see DRUG INTERACTIONS).
- That sparfloxacin may be associated with hypersensitivity reactions, even following the first dose, and to discontinue the drug at the first sign of a skin rash or other allergic reaction.
- To drink fluids liberally.

DRUG/LABORATORY TEST INTERACTIONS

Sparfloxacin therapy may produce false-negative culture results for *Mycobacterium tuberculosis* by suppression of mycobacterial growth.

CARCINOGENESIS, MUTAGENESIS, AND IMPAIRMENT OF FERTILITY

Carcinogenesis

Sparfloxacin was not carcinogenic in mice or rats when administered for 104 weeks at daily oral doses 3.5-6.2 times greater than the maximum human dose (400 mg), respectively, based upon mg/m^2. These doses corresponded to plasma concentrations approximately equal to (mice) and 2.2 times greater than (rats) maximum human plasma concentrations.

Mutagenesis

Sparfloxacin was not mutagenic in *Salmonella typhimurium* TA98, TA100, TA1535, or TA1537, in *Escherichia coli* strain WP2 uvrA, nor in Chinese hamster lung cells. Sparfloxacin and other quinolones have been shown to be mutagenic in *Salmonella typhimurium* strain TA102 and to induce DNA repair in *Escherichia coli,* perhaps due to their inhibitory effect on bacterial DNA gyrase. Sparfloxacin induced chromosomal aberrations in Chinese hamster lung cells *in vitro* at cytotoxic concentrations; however, no increase in chromosomal aberrations or micronuclei in bone marrow cells was observed after sparfloxacin was administered orally to mice.

Impairment of Fertility

Sparfloxacin had no effect on the fertility or reproductive performance of male or female rats at oral doses up to 15.4 times the maximum human dose (400 mg) based upon mg/m^2 (equivalent to approximately 12 times the maximum human plasma concentration).

PREGNANCY, TERATOGENIC EFFECTS, PREGNANCY CATEGORY C

Reproduction studies performed in rats, rabbits, and monkeys at oral doses 6.2, 4.4, and 2.6 times higher than the maximum human dose, respectively, based upon mg/m^2 (corresponding to plasma concentrations 4.5- and 6.5-fold higher than in humans in the monkey and rat, respectively) did not reveal any evidence of teratogenic effects. At these doses, sparfloxacin was clearly maternally toxic to the rabbit and monkey with evidence of slight maternal toxicity observed in the rat. When administered to pregnant rats at clearly maternally toxic doses ($\geq$9.3 times the maximum human dose based upon mg/m^2), sparfloxacin induced a dose-dependent increase in the incidence of fetuses with ventricular septal defects. Among the three species tested, this effect was specific to the rat. There are, however, no adequate and well controlled studies in pregnant women. Sparfloxacin should be used during pregnancy only if the potential benefit justifies the potential risk to the fetus. (See WARNINGS.)

NURSING MOTHERS

Sparfloxacin is excreted in human milk. Because of the potential for serious adverse reactions in infants nursing from mothers taking sparfloxacin, a decision should be made whether to discontinue nursing or to discontinue the drug, taking into account the importance of the drug to the mother. (See WARNINGS.)

PEDIATRIC USE

Safety and effectiveness have not been established in patients below the age of 18 years. Quinolones, including sparfloxacin, cause arthropathy and osteochondrosis in juvenile animals of several species. (See WARNINGS.)

DRUG INTERACTIONS

Digoxin: Sparfloxacin has no effect on the pharmacokinetics of digoxin.

Methylxanthines: Sparfloxacin does not increase plasma theophylline concentrations. Since there is no interaction with theophylline, interaction with other methylxanthines such as caffeine is unlikely.

Warfarin: Sparfloxacin does not increase the anti-coagulant effect of warfarin.

Cimetidine: Cimetidine does not affect the pharmacokinetics of sparfloxacin.

Antacids and Sucralfate: Aluminum and magnesium cations in antacids and sucralfate form chelation complexes with sparfloxacin. The oral bioavailability of sparfloxacin is reduced when an aluminum magnesium suspension is administered between 2 hours before and 2 hours after sparfloxacin administration. The oral bioavailability of sparfloxacin is not reduced when the aluminum-magnesium suspension is administered 4 hours following sparfloxacin administration.

Zinc/Iron Salts: Absorption of quinolones is reduced significantly by these preparations. These products may be taken 4 hours after sparfloxacin administration.

Probenecid: Probenecid does not alter the pharmacokinetics of sparfloxacin.

ADVERSE REACTIONS

In clinical trials, most of the adverse events were mild to moderate in severity and transient in nature. During clinical investigations with the recommended dosage, 1585 patients received sparfloxacin and 1331 patients received a comparator. The discontinuation rate due to adverse events was 6.6% for sparfloxacin versus 5.6% for cefaclor, 14.8% for erythromycin, 8.9% for ciprofloxacin, 7.4% for ofloxacin, and 8.3% for clarithromycin.

The most frequently reported events (remotely, possibly, or probably drug related with an incidence of ≥1%) among sparfloxacin treated patients in the US Phase 3 clinical trials with the recommended dosage were: Photosensitivity reaction (7.9%), diarrhea (4.6%), nausea (4.3%), headache (4.2%), dyspepsia (2.3%), dizziness (2.0%), insomnia (1.9%), abdominal pain (1.8%), pruritus (1.8%), taste perversion (1.4%), and QTc interval prolongation (1.3%), vomiting (1.3%), flatulence (1.1%) and vasodilatation (1.0%).

In US Phase 3 clinical trials of shorter treatment duration than the recommended dosage, the most frequently reported events (incidence ≥1%, remotely, possibly, or probably drug related) were: Headache (8.1%), nausea (7.6%), dizziness (3.8%), photosensitivity reaction (3.6%), pruritus (3.3%), diarrhea (3.2%), vaginal moniliasis (2.8%), abdominal pain (2.4%), asthenia (1.7%), dyspepsia (1.6%), somnolence (1.5%), dry mouth (1.4%), and rash (1.1%).

Additional possibly or probably related events that occurred in less than 1% of all patients enrolled in US Phase 3 clinical trials are listed below:

Body as a Whole: Fever, chest pain, generalized pain, allergic reaction, cellulitis, back pain, chills, face edema, malaise, accidental injury, anaphylactoid reaction, infection, mucous membrane disorder, neck pain, rheumatoid arthritis.

Cardiovascular: Palpitation, electrocardiogram abnormal, hypertension, tachycardia, sinus bradycardia, PR interval shortened, angina pectoris, arrhythmia, atrial fibrillation, atrial flutter, complete AV block, first degree AV block, second degree AV block, cardiovascular disorder, hemorrhage, migraine, peripheral vascular disorder, supraventricular extrasystoles, ventricular extrasystoles, postural hypotension.

Gastrointestinal: Constipation, anorexia, gingivitis, oral moniliasis, stomatitis, tongue disorder, tooth disorder, gastroenteritis, increased appetite, mouth ulceration, flatulence, vomiting.

Hematologic: Cyanosis, ecchymosis, lymphadenopathy.

Metabolism: Gout, peripheral edema, thirst.

Musculoskeletal: Arthralgia, arthritis, joint disorder, myalgia;

Central Nervous System: Paresthesia, hypesthesia, nervousness, somnolence, abnormal dreams, dry mouth, depression, tremor, anxiety, confusion, hallucinations, hyperesthesia, hyperkinesia, sleep disorder, hypokinesia, vertigo, abnormal gait, agitation, lightheadedness, emotional lability, euphoria, abnormal thinking, amnesia, twitching.

Respiratory: Asthma, epistaxis, pneumonia, rhinitis, pharyngitis, bronchitis, hemoptysis, sinusitis, cough increased, dyspnea, laryngismus, lung disorder, pleural disorder.

Skin/Hypersensitivity: Rash, maculopapular rash, dry skin, herpes simplex, sweating, urticaria, vesiculobullous rash, exfoliative dermatitis, acne, alopecia, angioedema, contact dermatitis, fungal dermatitis, furunculosis, pustular rash, skin discoloration, herpes zoster, petechial rash.

Special Senses: Ear pain, amblyopia, photophobia, tinnitus, conjunctivitis, diplopia, abnormality of accommodation, blepharitis, ear disorder, eye pain, lacrimation disorder, otitis media.

Urogenital: Vaginitis, dysuria, breast pain, dysmenorrhea, hematuria, menorrhagia, nocturia, polyuria, urinary tract infection, kidney pain, leukorrhea, metrorrhagia, vulvovaginal disorder.

LABORATORY CHANGES

In the US Phase 3 clinical trials, with the recommended dosage, the most frequently (incidence ≥1%) reported changes in laboratory parameters listed as adverse events, regardless of relationship to drug, were: Elevated ALT (SGPT) (2.0%), AST (SGOT) (2.3%) and white blood cells (1.1%).

Increases for the following laboratory tests were reported in less than 1% of all patients enrolled in clinical trials: alkaline phosphatase, serum amylase, aPTT, blood urea nitrogen, calcium, creatinine, eosinophils, serum lipase, monocytes, neutrophils, total bilirubin, urine glucose, urine protein, urine red blood cells, and urine white blood cells.

Decreases for the following laboratory tests were reported in less than 1% of all patients enrolled in clinical trials: albumin, creatinine clearance, hematocrit, hemoglobin, lymphocytes, phosphorus, red blood cells, and sodium.

Increases and decreases for the following laboratory tests were reported in less than 1% of all patients in clinical trials: blood glucose, platelets, potassium, and white blood cells.

POSTMARKETING ADVERSE EVENTS

The following are additional adverse events (regardless of relationship to drug) reported from worldwide postmarketing experience with sparfloxacin or other quinolones: acidosis, acute renal failure, agranulocytosis, albuminuria, anaphylactic shock, angioedema, anosmia, ataxia, bullous eruption, candiduria, cardiopulmonary arrest, cerebral thrombosis, convulsions, crystalluria, dysgeusia, dysphasia, ebrious feeling, embolism, erythema nodosum, exacerbation of myasthenia gravis, gastralgia, hemolytic anemia, hepatic necrosis, hepatitis, hiccough, hyperpigmentation, interstitial nephritis, interstitial pneumonia, intestinal perforation, jaundice, laryngeal or pulmonary edema, manic reaction, numbness, nystagmus, painful oral mucosa, pancreatitis, phobia, prolongation of prothrombin time, pseudomembranous colitis, Quincke's edema, renal calculi, rhabdomyolysis, sensory disturbance, Stevens-Johnson syndrome, squamous cell carcinoma, tendonitis, tendon rupture, tremor, thrombocytopenia, thrombocytopenia purpura, toxic epidermal necrolysis, toxic psychosis, urinary retention, uveitis, vaginal candidiasis, vasculitis.

Laboratory Changes

Elevation of serum triglycerides, serum cholesterol, blood glucose, serum potassium, decrease in WBC counts, RBC counts, hemoglobin level, hematocrit level, thrombocyte counts, elevation in GOT, GPT, ALP, LDH, γ-GTP, total bilirubin.

DOSAGE AND ADMINISTRATION

Sparfloxacin can be taken with or without food.

The recommended daily dose of sparfloxacin in patients with normal renal function is two 200 mg tablets taken on the first day as a loading dose. Thereafter, one 200 mg tablet should be taken every 24 hours for a total of 10 days of therapy (11 tablets).

The recommended daily dose of sparfloxacin in patients with renal impairment (creatinine clearance <50 ml/min) is two 200 mg tablets taken on the first day as a loading dose. Thereafter, one 200 mg tablet should be taken every 48 hours for a total of 9 days of therapy (6 tablets).

Store at controlled room temperature 20-25°C (68-77°F).

ANIMAL PHARMACOLOGY

Sparfloxacin and other quinolones have been shown to cause arthropathy in juvenile animals of most species tested. (See WARNINGS.)

Sparfloxacin had no convulsive activity in mice when administered alone or in combination with the nonsteroidal anti-inflammatory agents ketoprofen, or naproxen.

PRODUCT LISTING - EQUIVALENTS NOT AVAILABLE

Tablet - Oral - 200 mg

11's	$73.58	ZAGAM RESPIPAC, Bertek Pharmaceuticals Inc	62794-0011-11
55's	$367.62	ZAGAM, Bertek Pharmaceuticals Inc	62794-0011-55

Spironolactone *(002269)*

Categories: Adenoma, adrenal; Ascites; Edema; Hyperaldosteronism, primary; Hyperplasia, adrenal; Hypertension, essential; Hypokalemia; FDA Approved 1983 Dec; Pregnancy Category D; WHO Formulary

Drug Classes: Diuretics, potassium sparing

Brand Names: **Aldactone**

Foreign Brand Availability: Adultmin (Japan); Aldospirone (Israel); Almatol (Taiwan); Berlactone (Thailand); Diram (Japan); Flumach (France); Hypazon (Japan); Idrolattone (Italy); Merabis (Japan); Novospiroton (Canada); Osyrol (Germany; Japan); Pirolacton (Japan); Pondactone (Thailand); Resacton (Japan); Spiractin (Australia; South-Africa); Spirix (Denmark; Finland; Norway; Sweden); Spiroctan (England; France; Netherlands; Switzerland); Spirolacton (Indonesia); Spirolang (Italy); Spiron (Denmark); Spirone (Peru); Spironex (Thailand); Spirono-Isis (Germany); Spironol (Israel); Spirotone (New-Zealand); Tensin (South-Africa); Xenalon Lactabs (Dominican-Republic); Youlactone (Japan)

Cost of Therapy: $40.91 (Hypertension; Aldactone; 25 mg; 2 tablets/day; 30 day supply)
$3.75 (Hypertension; Generic Tablets; 25 mg; 2 tablets/day; 30 day supply)

WARNING

Spironolactone has been shown to be a tumorigen in chronic toxicity studies in rats (see PRECAUTIONS). Spironolactone should be used only in those conditions described in INDICATIONS AND USAGE. Unnecessary use of this drug should be avoided.

DESCRIPTION

Spironolactone oral tablets contain 25, 50, or 100 mg of the aldosterone antagonist spironolactone, 17-hydroxy-7*alpha*-mercapto-3-oxo-17*alpha*-pregn-4-ene -21-carboxylic acid *gamma*-lactone acetate.

Spironolactone is practically insoluble in water, soluble in alcohol, and freely soluble in benzene and in chloroform.

Inactive ingredients include calcium sulfate, corn starch, flavor, hydroxypropyl methylcellulose, iron oxide, magnesium stearate, polyethylene glycol, povidone, and titanium dioxide.

CLINICAL PHARMACOLOGY

MECHANISM OF ACTION

Spironolactone is a specific pharmacologic antagonist of aldosterone, acting primarily through competitive binding of receptors at the aldosterone-dependent sodium-potassium exchange site in the distal convoluted renal tubule. Spironolactone causes increased amounts of sodium and water to be excreted, while potassium is retained. Spironolactone acts both as a diuretic and as an antihypertensive drug by this mechanism. It may be given alone or with other diuretic agents which act more proximally in the renal tubule.

Aldosterone Antagonist Activity

Increased levels of the mineralocorticoid, aldosterone, are present in primary and secondary hyperaldosteronism. Edematous states in which secondary aldosteronism is usually involved include congestive heart failure, hepatic cirrhosis, and the nephrotic syndrome. By competing with aldosterone for receptor sites, spironolactone provides effective therapy for the edema and ascites in those conditions. Spironolactone counteracts secondary aldosteronism induced by the volume depletion and associated sodium loss caused by active diuretic therapy.

Spironolactone is effective in lowering the systolic and diastolic blood pressure in patients with primary hyperaldosteronism. It is also effective in most cases of essential hypertension, despite the fact that aldosterone secretion may be within normal limits in benign essential hypertension.

Through its action in antagonizing the effect of aldosterone, spironolactone inhibits the exchange of sodium for potassium in the distal renal tubule and helps to prevent potassium loss.

Spironolactone has not been demonstrated to elevate serum uric acid, to precipitate gout, or to alter carbohydrate metabolism.

PHARMACOKINETICS

Spironolactone is rapidly and extensively metabolized. Sulfur-containing products are the predominant metabolites and are thought to be primarily responsible, together with spirono-

S

lactone, for the therapeutic effects of the drug. The following pharmacokinetic data found in TABLE 1 were obtained from 12 healthy volunteers following administration of 100 mg of spironolactone film-coated tablets daily for 15 days. On the 15th day, spironolactone was given immediately after a low-fat breakfast and blood was drawn thereafter.

TABLE 1

	Accumulation Factor: AUC (0-24 h, day 15)/ AUC (0-24 h, day 1)	Mean Peak Serum Concentration	Mean (SD) Post-Steady State Half-Life
7-*alpha*-(thiomethyl) spirolactone (TMS)	1.25	391 ng/ml at 3.2 h	13.8 h (6.4) (terminal)
6-*beta*-hydroxy-7-*alpha*-(thiomethyl) spirolactone (HTMS)	1.50	125 ng/ml at 5.1 h	15.0 h (4.0) (terminal)
Canrenone (C)	1.41	181 ng/ml at 4.3 h	16.5 h (6.3) (terminal)
Spironolactone	1.30	80 ng/ml at 2.6 h	Approximately 1.4 h (0.5) (*beta* half-life)

The pharmacological activity of spironolactone metabolites in man is not known. However, in the adrenalectomized rat the antimineralocorticoid activities of the metabolites C, TMS, and HTMS, relative to spironolactone, were 1.10, 1.28, and 0.32, respectively. Relative to spironolactone, their binding affinities to the aldosterone receptors in rat kidney slices were 0.19, 0.86, and 0.06, respectively.

In humans the potencies of TMS and 7-*alpha*-thiospirolactone in reversing the effects of the synthetic mineralocorticoid, fludrocortisone, on urinary electrolyte composition were 0.33 and 0.26, respectively, relative to spironolactone. However, since the serum concentrations of these steroids were not determined, their incomplete absorption and/or first-pass metabolism could not be ruled out as a reason for their reduced *in vivo* activities.

Spironolactone and its metbolites are more than 90% bound to plasma proteins. The metabolites are excreted primarily in the urine and secondarily in bile.

The effect food on spironolactone absorption (two 100 mg spironolactone tablets) was assessed in a single dose study of 9 healthy, drug-free volunteers. Food increased the bioavailability of unmetabolized spironolactone by almost 100%. The clinical importance of this finding is not known.

INDICATIONS AND USAGE

Spironolactone is indicated in the management of:

Primary Hyperaldosteronism: For establishing the diagnosis of primary hyperaldosteronism by therapeutic trial.

- Short-term preoperative treatment of patients with primary hyperaldosteronism.
- Long-term maintenance therapy for patients with discrete aldosterone-producing adrenal adenomas who are judged to be poor operative risks or who decline surgery.
- Long-term maintenance therapy for patients with bilateral micro- or macronodular adrenal hyperplasia (idiopathic hyperaldosteronism).

Edematous Conditions for Patients With:

- ***Congestive Heart Failure:*** For the management of edema and sodium retention when the patient is only partially responsive to, or is intolerant of, other therapeutic measures. Spironolactone is also indicated for patients with congestive heart failure taking digitalis when other therapies are considered inappropriate.
- ***Cirrhosis of the Liver Accompanied by Edema and/or Ascites:*** Spironolactone levels may be exceptionally high in this condition. Spironolactone is indicated for maintenance therapy together with bed rest and the restriction of fluid and sodium.
- ***The Nephrotic Syndrome:*** For nephrotic patients when treatment of the underlying disease, restriction of fluid and sodium intake, and the use of other diuretics do not provide on adequate response.

ESSENTIAL HYPERTENSION

Usually in combination with other drugs, spironolactone is indicated for patients who cannot be treated adequately with other agents or for whom other agents are considered inappropriate.

HYPOKALEMIA

For the treatment of patients with hypokalemia when other measures are considered inappropriate or inadequate. Spironolactone is also indicated for the prophylaxis of hypokalemia in patients taking digitalis when other measures are considered inadequate or inappropriate.

USAGE IN PREGNANCY

The routine uses of diuretics in an otherwise healthy woman is inappropriate and exposes mother and fetus to unnecessary hazard. Diuretics do not prevent development of toxemia of pregnancy, and there is no satisfactory evidence that they are useful in the treatment of developing toxemia.

Edema during pregnancy may arise from pathologic causes or from the physiologic and mechanical consequences of pregnancy.

Spironolactone is indicated in pregnancy when edema is due to pathologic causes just as it is in the absence of pregnancy (however, see PRECAUTIONS). Dependent edema in pregnancy, resulting from restriction of venous return by the expanded uterus, is properly treated through elevation of the lower extremities and use of support hose; use of diuretics to lower intravascular volume in this case is unsupported and unnecessary. There is hypervolemia during normal pregnancy which is not harmful to either the fetus or the mother (in the absence of cardiovascular disease), but which is associated with edema, including generalized edema, in the majority of pregnant women. If this edema produces discomfort, increased recumbency will often provide relief. In rare instances, this edema may cause extreme discomfort which is not relieved by rest. In these cases, a short course of diuretics may provide relief and may be appropriate.

NON-FDA APPROVED INDICATIONS

Due to its antiandrogenic properties, spironolactone is used without FDA approval for the treatment of hirsutism, female acne, and familial male precocious puberty.

CONTRAINDICATIONS

Spironolactone is contraindicated for patients with anuria, acute renal insufficiency, significant impairment of renal excretory function, or hyperkalemia.

WARNINGS

Potassium supplementation, either in the form of medication or as a diet rich in potassium, should not ordinarily be given in association with spironolactone therapy. Excessive potassium intake may cause hyperkalemia in patients receiving spironolactone (see PRECAUTIONS, General). Spironolactone should not be administered concurrently with other potassium-sparing diuretics. Spironolactone, when used with ACE inhibitors or indomethacin, even in the presence of a diuretic, has been associatd with severe hyperkalemia. Extreme caution should be exercised when spironolactone is given concomitantly with these drugs.

Spironolactone should be used with caution in patients with impaired hepatic function because minor alterations of fluid and electrolyte balance may precipitate hepatic coma.

Lithium generally should not be given with diuretics (see DRUG INTERACTIONS).

PRECAUTIONS

GENERAL

All patients receiving diuretic therapy should be observed for evidence of fluid or electrolyte imbalance, *e.g.,* hypomagnesemia, hyponatremia, hypochloremic alkalosis, and hyperkalemia.

Serum and urine electrolyte determinations are particularly important when the patient is vomiting excessively or receiving parenteral fluids. Warning signs or symptoms of fluid and electrolyte imbalance, irrespective of cause, include dryness of the mouth, thirst, weakness, lethargy, drowsiness, restlessness, muscle pains or cramps, muscular fatigue, hypotension, oliguria, tachycardia, and gastrointestinal disturbances such as nausea and vomiting. Hyperkalemia may occur in patients with impaired renal function or excessive potassium intake and can cause cardiac irregularities, which may be fatal. Consequently, no potassium supplement should ordinarily be given with spironolactone.

Concomitant administration of potassium-sparing diuretics and ACE inhibitors or nonsteroidal anti-inflammatory drugs (NSAIDs), *e.g.,* indomethacin, has been associated with severe hyperkalemia.

If hyperkalemia is suspected (warning signs include paresthesia, muscle weakness, fatigue, flaccid paralysis of the extremities, bradycardia and shock) an electrocardiogram (ECG) should be obtained. However, it is important to monitor serum potassium levels because mild hyperkalemia may not be associated with ECG changes.

If hyperkalemia is present, spironolactone should be discontinued immediately. With severe hyperkalemia, the clinical situation dictates the procedures to be employed. These include the intravenous administration of calcium chloride solution, sodium bicarbonate solution and/or the oral or parenteral administration of glucose with a rapid-acting insulin preparation. These are temporary measures to be repeated as required. Cationic exchange resins such as sodium polystyrene sulfonate may be orally or rectally administered. Persistent hyperkalemia may require dialysis.

Reversible hyperchloremic metabolic acidosis, usually in association with hyperkalemia, has been reported to occur in some patients with decompensated hepatic cirrhosis, even in the presence of normal renal function.

Dilutional hyponatremia, manifested by dryness of the mouth, thirst, lethargy, and drowsiness, and confirmed by a low serum sodium level, may be caused or aggravated, especially when spironolactone is administered in combination with other diuretics, and dilutional hyponatremia may occur in edematous patients in hot weather; appropriate therapy is water restriction rather than administration of sodium, except in rare instances when the hyponatremia is life-threatening.

Spironolactone therapy may cause a transient elevation of BUN, especially in patients with preexisting renal impairment. Spironolactone may cause mild acidosis.

Gynecomastia may develop in association with the use of spironolactone; physicians should be alert to its possible onset. The development of gynecomastia appears to be related to both dosage level and duration of therapy and is normally reversible when spironolactone is discontinued. In rare instances some breast enlargement may persist when spironolactone is discontinued.

INFORMATION FOR THE PATIENT

Patients who receive spironolactone should be advised to avoid potassium supplements and foods containing high levels of potassium including salt substitutes.

LABORATORY TESTS

Periodic determination of serum electrolytes to detect possible electrolyte imbalance should be done at appropriate intervals, particularly in the elderly and those with significant renal or hepatic impairments.

DRUG/LABORATORY TEST INTERACTIONS

Several reports of possible interference with digoxin radioimmunoassays by spironolactone, or its metabolites, have appeared in the literature. Neither the extent nor the potential clinical significance of its interference (which may be assay-specific) has been fully established.

CARCINOGENESIS, MUTAGENESIS, AND IMPAIRMENT OF FERTILITY

Carcinogenesis, mutagenesis, impairment of fertility: Orally administered spironolactone has been shown to be a tumorigen in dietary administration studies performed in rats, with its proliferative effects manifested on endocrine organs and the liver. In an 18 month study using doses of about 50, 150 and 500 mg/kg/day, there were statistically significant increases in benign adenomas of the thyroid and testes and, in male rats, a dose-related increase in proliferative changes in the liver (including hepatocytomegaly and hyperplastic nodules). In a 24 month study in which the same strain of rat was administered doses of

S

about 10, 30, 100 and 150 mg spironolactone/kg/day, the range of proliferative effects included significant increases in hepatocellular adenomas and testicular interstitial cell tumors in males, and significant increases in thyroid follicular cell adenomas and carcinomas in both sexes. There was also a statistically significant, but not dose-related, increase in benign uterine endometrial stromal polyps in females. A dose-related (above 20 mg/kg/day) incidence of myelocytic leukemia was observed in rats fed daily doses of potassium canrenoate (a compound chemically similar to spironolactone and whose primary metabolite, canrenone, is also a major product of spironolactone in man) for a period of 1 year. In 2 year studies in the rat, oral administration of potassium canrenoate was associated with myelocytic leukemia and hepatic, thyroid, testicular and mammary tumors.

Neither spironolactone nor potassium canrenoate produced mutagenic effects in tests using bacteria or yeast. In the absence of metabolic activation, neither spironolactone nor potassium canrenoate has been shown to be mutagenic in mammalian tests *in vitro*. In the presence of metabolic activation, spironolactone has been reported to be negative in some mammalian mutagenicity tests *in vitro* and inconclusive (but slightly positive) for mutagenicity in other mammalian tests *in vitro*. In the presence of metabolic activation, potassium canrenoate has been reported to test positive for mutagenicity in some mammalian tests *in vitro*, inconclusive in others, and negative in still others.

In a 3-litter reproduction study in which female rats received dietary doses of 15 and 50 mg spironolactone/kg/day, there were no effects on mating and fertility, but there was a small increase in incidence of stillborn pups at 50 mg/kg/day. When injected into female rats (100 mg/kg/day for 7 days, i.p.), spironolactone was found to increase the length of the estrous cycle by prolonging diestrus during treatment and inducing constant diestrus during a 2 week posttreatment observation period. These effects were associated with retarded ovarian follicle development and a reduction in circulating estrogen levels, which would be expected to impair mating, fertility and fecundity. Spironolactone (100 mg/kg/day), administered i.p. to female mice during a 2 week cohabitation period with untreated males, decreased the number of mated mice that conceived (effect shown to be caused by an inhibition of ovulation) and decreased the number of implanted embryos in those that became pregnant (effect shown to be caused by an inhibition of implantation), and at 200 mg/kg, also increased the latency period to mating.

PREGNANCY, TERATOGENIC EFFECTS, PREGNANCY CATEGORY C

Teratology studies with spironolactone have been carried out in mice and rabbits at doses of up to 20 mg/kg/day. On a body surface area basis, this dose in the mouse is substantially below the maximum recommended human dose and, in the rabbit, approximates the maximum recommended human dose. No teratogenic or other embryotoxic effects were observed in mice, but the 20 mg/kg dose caused an increased rate of resorption and a lower number of live fetuses in rabbits. Because of its anti-androgenic activity and the requirement of testosterone for male morphogenesis, spironolactone may have the potential for adversely affecting sex differentiation of the male during embryogenesis. When administered to rats at 200 mg/kg/day between gestation days 13 and 21 (late embryogenesis and fetal development), feminization of male fetuses was observed. Offspring exposed during late pregnancy to 50 and 100 mg/kg/day doses of spironolactone exhibited changes in the reproductive tract including dose-dependent decreases in weights of the ventral prostate and seminal vesicle in males, ovaries and uteri that were enlarged in females, and other indications of endocrine dysfunction, that persisted into adulthood. There are no adequate and well-controlled studies with spironolactone in pregnant women. Spironolactone has known endocrine effects in animals including progestational and antiandrogenic effects. The antiandrogenic effects can result in apparent estrogenic side effects in humans, such as gynecomastia. Therefore, the use of spironolactone in pregnant women requires that the anticipated benefit be weighed against the possible hazards to the fetus.

NURSING MOTHERS

Canrenone, a major (and active) metabolite of spironolactone, appears in human breast milk. Because spironolactone has been found to be tumorigenic in rats, a decision should be made whether to discontinue the drug, taking into account the importance of the drug to the mother. If use of the drug is deemed essential, an alternative method of infant feeding should be instituted.

PEDIATRIC USE

Safety and effectiveness in pediatric patients have not been established.

DRUG INTERACTIONS

ACE Inhibitors: Concomitant administration of ACE inhibitors with potassium-sparing diuretics has been associated with severe hyperkalemia.

Alcohol, Barbiturates, or Narcotics: Potentiation of orthostatic hypotension may occur.

Corticosteroids, ACTH: Intensified electrolyte depletion, particularly hypokalemia, may occur.

Pressor Amines (e.g., norepinephrine): Spironolactone reduces the vascular responsiveness to norepinephrine. Therefore, caution should be exercised in the management of patients subjected to regional or general anesthesia while they are being treated with spironolactone.

Skeletal Muscle Relaxants, Nondepolarizing (e.g., tubocurarine): Possible increased responsiveness to the muscle relaxant may result.

Lithium: Lithium generally should not be given with diuretics. Diuretic agents reduce the renal clearance of lithium and add a high risk of lithium toxicity.

Nonsteroidal Anti-inflammatory Drugs (NSAIDs): In some patients, the administration of an NSAID can reduce the diuretic, natriuretic, and antihypertensive effect of loop, potassium-sparing and thiazide diuretics. Combination of NSAIDs, (*e.g.*, indomethacin, with potassium-sparing diuretics) has been associated with severe hyperkalemia. Therefore, when spironolactone and NSAIDs are used concomitantly, the patient should be observed closely to determine if the desired effect of the diuretic is obtained.

Digoxin: Spironolactone has been shown to increase the half-life of digoxin. This may result in increased serum digoxin levels and subsequent digitalis toxicity. It may be necessary to reduce the maintenance and digitalization doses when spironolactone is administered, and the patient should be carefully monitored to avoid over- or underdigitalization.

ADVERSE REACTIONS

The following adverse reactions have been reported and, within each category (body system), are listed in order of decreasing severity.

Digestive: Gastric bleeding, ulceration, gastritis, diarrhea and cramping, nausea, vomiting.

Endocrine: Gynecomastia (see PRECAUTIONS), inability to achieve or maintain erection, irregular menses or amenorrhea, postmenopausal bleeding. Carcinoma of the breast has been reported in patients taking spironolactone but a cause and effect relationship has not been established.

Hematologic: Agranulocytosis.

Hypersensitivity: Fever, urticaria, maculopapular or erythematous cutaneous eruptions, anaphylactic reactions, vasculitis.

Nervous System/Psychiatric: Mental confusion, ataxia, headache, drowsiness, lethargy.

Liver/Biliary: A very few cases of mixed cholestatic/hepatocellular toxicity, with 1 reported fatality, have been reported with spironolactone administration.

DOSAGE AND ADMINISTRATION

PRIMARY HYPERALDOSTERONISM

Spironolactone may be employed as an initial diagnostic measure to provide presumptive evidence of primary hyperaldosteronism while patients are on normal diets.

Long Test: Spironolactone is administered at a daily dosage of 400 mg for 3-4 weeks. Correction of hyperkalemia and of hypertension provides presumptive evidence for the diagnosis of primary hyperaldosteronism.

Short Test: Spironolactone is administered at a daily dosage of 400 mg for 4 days. If serum potassium increases during spironolactone administration but drops when spironolactone is discontinued, a presumptive diagnosis of primary hyperaldosteronism should be considered.

After the diagnosis of hyperaldosteronism has been established by more definitive testing procedures, spironolactone may be administered in doses of 100-400 mg daily in preparation for surgery. For patients who are considered unsuitable for surgery, spironolactone may be employed for long-term maintenance therapy at the lowest effective dosage determined for the individual patient.

EDEMA IN ADULTS

Congestive Heart Failure, Hepatic Cirrhosis or Nephrotic Syndrome

An initial daily dosage of 100 mg of spironolactone administered in either single or divided doses is recommended, but may range from 25-200 mg daily. When given as the sole agent for diuresis, spironolactone should be continued for at least 5 days at the initial dosage level, after which it may be adjusted to the optimal therapeutic or maintenance level administered in either single or divided daily doses. If, after 5 days, an adequate diuretic response to spironolactone has not occurred, a second diuretic which acts more proximally in the renal tubule may be added to the regimen. Because of the additive effect of spironolactone when administered concurrently with such diuretics, an enhanced diuresis usually begins on the first day of combined treatment; combined therapy is indicated when more rapid diuresis is desired. The dosage of spironolactone should remain unchanged when other diuretic therapy is added.

ESSENTIAL HYPERTENSION

For adults, an initial daily dosage of 50-100 mg of spironolactone administered in either single or divided doses is recommended. Spironolactone may also be given with diuretics which act more proximally in the renal tubule or with other antihypertensive agents. Treatment with spironolactone should be continued for at least 2 weeks, since the maximum response may not occur before this time. Subsequently, dosage should be adjusted according to the response of the patient.

HYPOKALEMIA

Spironolactone in a dosage ranging from 25-100 mg daily is useful in treating a diuretic-induced hypokalemia, when oral potassium supplements or other potassium-sparing regimens are considered inappropriate.

HOW SUPPLIED

Aldactone 25-mg Tablets: Round, light yellow, film coated, with "SEARLE" and "1001" debossed on one side and "ALDACTONE" and "25" on the other side.

Aldactone 50-mg Tablets: Oval, light orange, scored, film coated, with "SEARLE" and "1041" debossed on the scored side and "ALDACTONE" and "50" on the other side.

Aldactone 100-mg Tablets: Round, peach colored, scored, film coated, with "SEARLE" and "1031" debossed on the scored side and "ALDACTONE" and "100' on the other side.

Storage: Store below25°C (77°F).

PRODUCT LISTING - RATED THERAPEUTICALLY EQUIVALENT

Tablet - Oral - 25 mg

25's	$4.32	GENERIC, Udl Laboratories Inc	51079-0103-19
25's	$28.25	GENERIC, Pd-Rx Pharmaceuticals	55289-0507-97
30's	$6.00	GENERIC, Heartland Healthcare Services	61392-0161-30
30's	$6.00	GENERIC, Heartland Healthcare Services	61392-0161-39
30's	$10.88	GENERIC, Pd-Rx Pharmaceuticals	55289-0507-30
30's	$13.82	GENERIC, Mutual/United Research Laboratories	00677-0625-07
31 x 10	$116.48	GENERIC, Vangard Labs	00615-1535-53
31 x 10	$116.48	GENERIC, Vangard Labs	00615-1535-63
31's	$6.20	GENERIC, Heartland Healthcare Services	61392-0161-31
32's	$6.40	GENERIC, Heartland Healthcare Services	61392-0161-32
45's	$9.00	GENERIC, Heartland Healthcare Services	61392-0161-45
60's	$12.00	GENERIC, Heartland Healthcare Services	61392-0161-60

60's	$27.84	GENERIC, Mutual/United Research Laboratories	00677-0625-06
90's	$18.00	GENERIC, Heartland Healthcare Services	61392-0161-90
100's	$5.13	GENERIC, Us Trading Corporation	56126-0304-11
100's	$6.25	GENERIC, Cmc-Consolidated Midland Corporation	00223-1724-01
100's	$6.53	GENERIC, Interstate Drug Exchange Inc	00814-7120-14
100's	$7.57	GENERIC, Aligen Independent Laboratories Inc	00405-4940-01
100's	$7.61	GENERIC, Caremark Inc	00339-5355-12
100's	$7.95	GENERIC, Raway Pharmacal Inc	00686-0103-20
100's	$8.17	GENERIC, Moore, H.L. Drug Exchange Inc	00839-6330-06
100's	$9.18	GENERIC, Purepac Pharmaceutical Company	00228-2388-10
100's	$9.35	GENERIC, Ivax Corporation	00182-1157-01
100's	$16.64	GENERIC, Auro Pharmaceutical	55829-0471-10
100's	$20.00	GENERIC, Geneva Pharmaceuticals	00781-1599-13
100's	$21.87	GENERIC, Pd-Rx Pharmaceuticals	55289-0507-01
100's	$30.00	FEDERAL UPPER LIMIT, H.C.F.A. F F P	99999-2269-01
100's	$34.06	GENERIC, Major Pharmaceuticals Inc	00904-0343-60
100's	$42.75	GENERIC, Udl Laboratories Inc	51079-0103-20
100's	$45.90	GENERIC, Mylan Pharmaceuticals Inc	00378-2146-01
100's	$45.92	GENERIC, Geneva Pharmaceuticals	00781-1599-01
100's	$45.94	GENERIC, Qualitest Products Inc	00603-5766-21
100's	$45.94	GENERIC, Mutual/United Research Laboratories	00677-0625-01
100's	$45.94	GENERIC, Mutual Pharmaceutical Co Inc	53489-0143-01
100's	$68.18	ALDACTONE, Searle	00025-1001-31
200 x 5	$375.73	GENERIC, Vangard Labs	00615-1535-43
250's	$12.90	GENERIC, Major Pharmaceuticals Inc	00904-0343-70

Tablet - Oral - 50 mg

30's	$24.90	GENERIC, Mutual/United Research Laboratories	00677-1707-07
30's	$31.11	GENERIC, Physicians Total Care	54868-3087-00
60's	$49.95	GENERIC, Mutual/United Research Laboratories	00677-1707-06
100's	$81.57	GENERIC, Purepac Pharmaceutical Company	00228-2672-11
100's	$81.59	GENERIC, Mutual/United Research Laboratories	00677-1707-01
100's	$81.59	GENERIC, Mutual Pharmaceutical Co Inc	53489-0328-01
100's	$88.12	GENERIC, Udl Laboratories Inc	51079-0979-20
100's	$119.74	ALDACTONE, Searle	00025-1041-31
100's	$125.40	ALDACTONE, Searle	00025-1041-34

Tablet - Oral - 100 mg

30's	$43.80	GENERIC, Mutual/United Research Laboratories	00677-1708-07
60's	$88.10	GENERIC, Mutual/United Research Laboratories	00677-1708-06
100's	$142.28	GENERIC, Mutual/United Research Laboratories	00677-1708-01
100's	$142.28	GENERIC, Mutual Pharmaceutical Co Inc	53489-0329-01
100's	$142.43	GENERIC, Purepac Pharmaceutical Company	00228-2673-11
100's	$147.74	GENERIC, Udl Laboratories Inc	51079-0980-20
100's	$200.75	ALDACTONE, Searle	00025-1031-31
100's	$210.50	ALDACTONE, Searle	00025-1031-34
100's	$649.80	GENERIC, Mutual/United Research Laboratories	00677-1708-05

PRODUCT LISTING - EQUIVALENTS NOT AVAILABLE

Tablet - Oral - 25 mg

30's	$3.29	GENERIC, Physicians Total Care	54868-0700-01
30's	$11.85	GENERIC, Allscripts Pharmaceutical Company	54569-0505-01
50's	$4.59	GENERIC, Physicians Total Care	54868-0700-02
60's	$5.25	GENERIC, Physicians Total Care	54868-0700-05
60's	$23.69	GENERIC, Allscripts Pharmaceutical Company	54569-0505-03
100's	$7.85	GENERIC, Physicians Total Care	54868-0700-00
100's	$39.49	GENERIC, Allscripts Pharmaceutical Company	54569-0505-00
100's	$46.01	GENERIC, Greenstone Limited	59762-5011-01
120's	$9.16	GENERIC, Physicians Total Care	54868-0700-04

Tablet - Oral - 50 mg

100's	$81.72	GENERIC, Greenstone Limited	59762-5012-01

Tablet - Oral - 100 mg

100's	$142.49	GENERIC, Greenstone Limited	59762-5013-01

S

Stavudine *(003209)*

For related information, see the comparative table section in Appendix A.

Categories: Infection, human immunodeficiency virus; Pregnancy Category C; FDA Approved 1994 Jun; WHO Formulary
Drug Classes: Antivirals; Nucleoside reverse transcriptase inhibitors
Brand Names: d4T; Zerit
Foreign Brand Availability: Stavir (India)
Cost of Therapy: $329.93 (HIV; Zerit; 40 mg; 2 capsules/day; 30 day supply)

WARNING

LACTIC ACIDOSIS AND SEVERE HEPATOMEGALY WITH STEATOSIS, INCLUDING FATAL CASES, HAVE BEEN REPORTED WITH THE USE OF NUCLEOSIDE ANALOGUES ALONE OR IN COMBINATION, INCLUDING STAVUDINE AND OTHER ANTIRETROVIRALS. FATAL LACTIC ACIDOSIS HAS BEEN REPORTED IN PREGNANT WOMEN WHO RECEIVED THE COMBINATION OF STAVUDINE AND DIDANOSINE WITH OTHER ANTIRETROVIRAL AGENTS. THE COMBINATION OF STAVUDINE AND DIDANOSINE SHOULD BE USED WITH CAUTION DURING PREGNANCY AND IS RECOMMENDED ONLY IF THE POTENTIAL BENEFIT CLEARLY OUTWEIGHS THE POTENTIAL RISK (SEE WARNINGS AND PRECAUTIONS, Pregnancy Category C).

FATAL AND NONFATAL PANCREATITIS HAVE OCCURRED DURING THERAPY WHEN STAVUDINE WAS PART OF A COMBINATION REGIMEN THAT INCLUDED DIDANOSINE, WITH OR WITHOUT HYDROXYUREA, IN BOTH TREATMENT-NAIVE AND TREATMENT-EXPERIENCED PATIENTS, REGARDLESS OF DEGREE OF IMMUNOSUPPRESSION (SEE WARNINGS).

DESCRIPTION

Stavudine (d4T) is a synthetic thymidine nucleoside analogue, active against the Human Immunodeficiency Virus (HIV).

Zerit Capsules: Zerit capsules are supplied for oral administration in strengths of 15, 20, 30, and 40 mg of stavudine. Each capsule also contains inactive ingredients microcrystalline cellulose, sodium starch glycolate, lactose, and magnesium stearate. The hard gelatin shell consists of gelatin, silicon dioxide, sodium lauryl sulfate, titanium dioxide, and iron oxides.

Zerit for Oral Solution: Zerit for oral solution is supplied as a dye-free, fruit-flavored powder in bottles with child-resistant closures providing 200 ml of a 1 mg/ml stavudine solution upon constitution with water per label instructions. The powder for oral solution contains the following inactive ingredients: methylparaben, propylparaben, sodium carboxymethylcellulose, sucrose, and antifoaming and flavoring agents.

The chemical name for stavudine is 2′,3′-didehydro-3′-deoxythymidine.

Stavudine is a white to off-white crystalline solid with the molecular formula $C_{10}H_{12}N_2O_4$ and a molecular weight of 224.2. The solubility of stavudine at 23°C is approximately 83 mg/ml in water and 30 mg/ml in propylene glycol. The n-octanol/water partition coefficient of stavudine at 23°C is 0.144.

CLINICAL PHARMACOLOGY

MICROBIOLOGY

Mechanism of Action

Stavudine, a nucleoside analogue of thymidine, inhibits the replication of HIV in human cells *in vitro.* Stavudine is phosphorylated by cellular kinases to the active metabolite stavudine triphosphate. Stavudine triphosphate inhibits the activity of HIV reverse transcriptase both by competing with the natural substrate deoxythymidine triphosphate (Ki=0.0083-0.032 μM), and by its incorporation into viral DNA causing a termination of DNA chain elongation because stavudine lacks the essential 3′-OH group. Stavudine triphosphate inhibits cellular DNA polymerase beta and gamma, and markedly reduces the synthesis of mitochondrial DNA.

In Vitro HIV Susceptibility

The *in vitro* antiviral activity of stavudine was measured in peripheral blood mononuclear cells, monocytic cells, and lymphoblastoid cell lines. The concentration of drug necessary to inhibit viral replication by 50% (ED_{50}) ranged from 0.009 to 4 μM against laboratory and clinical isolates of HIV-1. Stavudine had additive and synergistic activity in combination with didanosine and zalcitabine, respectively, *in vitro.* Stavudine combined with zidovudine had additive or antagonistic activity *in vitro* depending upon the molar ratios of the agents tested. The relationship between *in vitro* susceptibility of HIV to stavudine and the inhibition of HIV replication in humans has not been established.

Drug-Resistance

HIV isolates with reduced susceptibility to stavudine have been selected *in vitro* and were also obtained from patients treated with stavudine. Phenotypic analysis of HIV isolates from stavudine-treated patients revealed, in 3 of 20 paired isolates, a 4- to 12-fold decrease in susceptibility to stavudine *in vitro.* The genetic basis for these susceptibility changes has not been identified. The clinical relevance of changes in stavudine susceptibility has not been established.

Cross-Resistance

Five of 11 stavudine post-treatment isolates developed moderate resistance to zidovudine (9- to 176-fold) and 3 of those 11 isolates developed moderate resistance to didanosine (7- to 29-fold). The clinical relevance of these findings is unknown.

PHARMACOKINETICS IN ADULTS

The pharmacokinetics of stavudine have been evaluated in HIV-infected adult and pediatric patients (see TABLE 1). Peak plasma concentrations (C_{max}) and area under the plasma concentration-time curve (AUC) increased in proportion to dose after both single and multiple doses ranging from 0.03 to 4 mg/kg. There was no significant accumulation of stavudine with repeated administration every 6, 8, or 12 hours.

Absorption

Following oral administration, stavudine is rapidly absorbed, with peak plasma concentrations occurring within 1 hour after dosing. The systemic exposure to stavudine is the same following administration as capsules or solution.

Distribution

Binding of stavudine to serum proteins was negligible over the concentration range of 0.01-11.4 µg/ml. Stavudine distributes equally between red blood cells and plasma.

Metabolism

The metabolic fate of stavudine has not been elucidated in humans.

Excretion

Renal elimination accounted for about 40% of the overall clearance regardless of the route of administration. The mean renal clearance was about twice the average endogenous creatine clearance, indicating active tubular secretion in addition to glomerular filtration.

***TABLE 1** Mean ±SD Pharmacokinetic Parameters of Stavudine in Adult and Pediatric HIV-Infected Patients*

Parameter	Adult Patients	n	Pediatric Patients	n
Oral bioavailability (F)	86.4 ± 18.2%	25	76.9 ± 31.7%	20
Volume of distribution* (VD)	58 ± 21 L	44	18.5 ± 9.2 L/m^2	21
Apparent oral volume of distribution† (VD/F)	66 ± 22 L	71	not determined	—
Ratio of CSF:plasma concentrations (as %)‡	not determined	—	59 ± 35%	8
Total body clearance* (CL)	8.3 ± 2.3 ml/min/kg	44	247 ± 94 ml/min/m^2	21
Apparent oral clearance† (CL/F)	8.0 ± 2.6 ml/min/kg	113	333 ± 87 ml/min/m^2	20
Elimination half-life (T½) IV dose*	1.15 ± 0.35 h	44	1.11 ± 0.28 h	21
Elimination half-life (T½), oral dose†	1.44 ± 0.30 h	115	0.96 ± 0.26 h	20
Urinary recovery of stavudine (% of dose)	39 ± 23%	88	34 ± 16%	19

* Following 1 hour IV infusion.
† Following single oral dose.
‡ Following multiple oral doses.

SPECIAL POPULATIONS

Pediatric

For pharmacokinetic properties of stavudine in pediatric patients see TABLE 1.

Renal Insufficiency

Data from two studies indicated that the apparent oral clearance of stavudine decreased and the terminal elimination half-life increased as creatinine clearance decreased (see TABLE 2). C_{max} and T_{max} were not significantly altered by renal insufficiency. The mean ±SD hemodialysis clearance value of stavudine was 120 ± 18 ml/min (n=12); the mean ±SD percentage of the stavudine dose recovered in the dialysate, timed to occur between 2-6 hours post-dose, was 31 ± 5%. Based on these observations, it is recommended that stavudine dosage be modified in patients with reduced creatinine clearance and in patients receiving maintenance hemodialysis (see DOSAGE AND ADMINISTRATION).

***TABLE 2** Mean ±SD Pharmacokinetic Parameter Values — Single 40 mg Oral Dose of Stavudine*

	Creatinine Clearance (ml/min)			
	>50	26-50	9-25	Hemodialysis Patients*
	(n=10)	(n=5)	(n=5)	(n=11)
CLCR (ml/min)	104 ± 28	41 ± 5	17 ± 3	NA
CL/F (ml/min)	335 ± 57	191 ± 39	116 ± 25	105 ± 17
CLR (ml/min)	167 ± 65	73 ± 18	17 ± 3	NA
T½(h)	1.7 ± 0.4	3.5 ± 2.5	4.6 ± 0.9	5.4 ± 1.4

CLCR Creatine clearance.
CL/F Apparent oral clearance.
CLR Renal clearance.
T½ Terminal elimination half-life.
NA Not applicable.
* Determined while patients were off dialysis.

Hepatic Insufficiency

Stavudine pharmacokinetics were not altered in 5 non-HIV-infected patients with hepatic impairment secondary to cirrhosis (Child-Pugh classification B or C) following the administration of a single 40 mg dose.

Geriatric

Stavudine pharmacokinetics have not been studied in patients >65 years of age. (See PRECAUTIONS, Geriatric Use.)

Gender

A population pharmacokinetic analysis of stavudine concentrations collected during a controlled clinical study in HIV-infected patients showed no clinically important differences between males (n=291) and females (n=27).

Race

A population pharmacokinetic analysis of stavudine concentrations collected during a controlled clinical study in HIV-infected patients (233 Caucasian, 39 African American, 41 Hispanic, 1 Asian, and 4 Other) showed no clinically important differences associated with race.

Drug Interactions

Drug interaction studies have demonstrated that there are no clinically significant interactions between stavudine and the following: didanosine, lamivudine, or nelfinavir.

Zidovudine may competitively inhibit the intracellular phosphorylation of stavudine. Therefore, use of zidovudine in combination with stavudine is not recommended.

INDICATIONS AND USAGE

Stavudine, in combination with other antiretroviral agents, is indicated for the treatment of HIV-1 infection.

CONTRAINDICATIONS

Stavudine is contraindicated in patients with clinically significant hypersensitivity to stavudine or to any of the components contained in the formulation.

WARNINGS

LACTIC ACIDOSIS/SEVERE HEPATOMEGALY WITH STEATOSIS/HEPATIC FAILURE

Lactic acidosis and severe hepatomegaly with steatosis, including fatal cases, have been reported with the use of nucleoside analogues alone or in combination, including stavudine and other antiretrovirals. Although relative rates of lactic acidosis have not been assessed in prospective well-controlled trials, longitudinal cohort and retrospective studies suggest that this infrequent event may be more often associated with antiretroviral combinations containing stavudine. Female gender, obesity, and prolonged nucleoside exposure may be risk factors. Fatal lactic acidosis has been reported in pregnant women who received the combination of stavudine and didanosine with other antiretroviral agents. The combination of stavudine and didanosine should be used with caution during pregnancy and is recommended only if the potential benefit clearly outweighs the potential risk (see PRECAUTIONS, Pregnancy Category C).

Particular caution should be exercised when administering stavudine to any patient with known risk factors for liver disease; however, cases of lactic acidosis have also been reported in patients with no known risk factors. Generalized fatigue, digestive symptoms (nausea, vomiting, abdominal pain, and sudden unexplained weight loss); respiratory symptoms (tachypnea and dyspnea); or neurologic symptoms (including motor weakness, see Neurologic Symptoms) might be indicative of lactic acidosis development.

Treatment with stavudine should be suspended in any patient who develops clinical or laboratory findings suggestive of lactic acidosis or pronounced hepatotoxicity (which may include heptomegaly and steatosis even in the absence of marked transaminase elevations).

An increased risk of hepatotoxicity may occur in patients treated with stavudine in combination with didanosine and hydroxyurea compared to when stavudine is used alone. Deaths attributed to hepatotoxicity have occurred in patients receiving this combination. Patients treated with this combination should be closely monitored for signs of liver toxicity.

NEUROLOGIC SYMPTOMS

Motor weakness has been reported rarely in patients receiving combination antiretroviral therapy including stavudine. Most of these cases occurred in the setting of lactic acidosis. The evolution of motor weakness may mimic the clinical presentation of Guillain-Barré syndrome (including respiratory failure). Symptoms may continue or worsen following discontinuation of therapy.

Peripheral neuropathy, manifested by numbness, tingling, or pain in the hands or feet, has been reported in patients receiving stavudine therapy. Peripheral neuropathy has occurred more frequently in patients with advanced HIV disease, a history of neuropathy, or concurrent neurotoxic drug therapy, including didanosine (see ADVERSE REACTIONS).

PANCREATITIS

Fatal and nonfatal pancreatitis have occurred during therapy when stavudine was part of a combination regimen that included didanosine, with or without hydroxyurea, in both treatment-naive and treatment-experienced patients, regardless of degree of immunosuppression. The combination of stavudine and didanosine (with or without hydroxyurea) and any other agents that are toxic to the pancreas should be suspended in patients with suspected pancreatitis. Reinstitution of stavudine after a confirmed diagnosis of pancreatitis should be undertaken with particular caution and close patient monitoring. The new regimen should contain neither didanosine nor hydroxyurea.

PRECAUTIONS

FAT REDISTRIBUTION

Redistribution/accumulation of body fat including central obesity, dorsocervical fat enlargement (buffalo hump), peripheral wasting, facial wasting, breast enlargement, and "cushingoid appearance" have been observed in patients receiving antiretroviral therapy. The mechanism and longterm consequences of these events are currently unknown. A causal relationship has not been established.

INFORMATION FOR THE PATIENT

See Patient Information Leaflet received with the prescription.

Patients should be informed of the importance of early recognition of symptoms of lactic acidosis, which include abdominal discomfort, nausea, vomiting, fatigue, dyspnea, and motor weakness. Patients in whom these symptoms develop should seek medical attention immediately. Discontinuation of stavudine therapy may be required.

Patients should be informed that an important toxicity of stavudine is peripheral neuropathy. Patients should be aware that peripheral neuropathy is manifested by numbness, tingling, or pain in hands or feet, and that these symptoms should be reported to their physicians. Patients should be counseled that peripheral neuropathy occurs with greatest frequency in patients who have advanced HIV disease or a history of peripheral neuropathy, and that dose modification and/or discontinuation of stavudine may be required if toxicity develops.

Caregivers of young children receiving stavudine therapy should be instructed regarding detection and reporting of peripheral neuropathy.

Patients should be informed that when stavudine is used in combination with other agents with similar toxicities, the incidence of adverse events may be higher than when stavudine is used alone. An increased risk of pancreatitis, which may be fatal, may occur in patients treated with the combination of stavudine and didanosine, with or without hydroxyurea. Patients treated with this combination should be closely monitored for symptoms of pancreatitis. An increased risk of hepatotoxicity, which may be fatal, may occur in patients treated with stavudine in combination with didanosine and hydroxyurea. Patients treated with this combination should be closely monitored for signs of liver toxicity.

Patients should be informed that stavudine is not a cure for HIV infection, and that they may continue to acquire illnesses associated with HIV infection, including opportunistic infections. Patients should be advised to remain under the care of a physician when using stavudine. They should be advised that stavudine therapy has not been shown to reduce the risk of transmission of HIV to others through sexual contact or blood contamination. Patients should be informed that the long-term effects of stavudine are unknown at this time.

Patients should be informed that the Centers for Disease Control and Prevention (CDC) recommend that HIV-infected mothers not nurse newborn infants to reduce the risk of postnatal transmission of HIV infection.

Patients should be informed that redistribution or accumulation of body fat may occur in patients receiving antiretroviral therapy and that the cause and long-term health effects of these conditions are not known at this time.

CARCINOGENESIS, MUTAGENESIS, AND IMPAIRMENT OF FERTILITY

In 2 year carcinogenicity studies in mice and rats, stavudine was noncarcinogenic at doses which produced exposures (AUC) 39 and 168 times, respectively, human exposure at the recommended clinical dose. Benign and malignant liver tumors in mice and rats and malignant urinary bladder tumors in male rats occurred at levels of exposure, 250 (mice) and 732 (rats) times human exposure at the recommended clinical dose.

Stavudine was not mutagenic in the Ames, *E. coli* reverse mutation, or the CHO/HGPRT mammalian cell forward gene mutation assays, with and without metabolic activation. Stavudine produced positive results in the *in vitro* human lymphocyte clastogenesis and mouse fibroblast assays, and in the *in vivo* mouse micronucleus test. In the *in vitro* assays, stavudine elevated the frequency of chromosome aberrations in human lymphocytes (concentrations of 25-250 μg/ml, without metabolic activation) and increased the frequency of transformed foci in mouse fibroblast cells (concentrations of 25-2500 μg/ml, with and without metabolic activation). In the *in vivo* micronucleus assay, stavudine was clastogenic in bone marrow cells following oral stavudine administration to mice at dosages of 600-2000 mg/kg/day for 3 days.

No evidence of impaired fertility was seen in rats with exposures (based on C_{max}) up to 216 times that observed following a clinical dosage of 1 mg/kg/day.

PREGNANCY CATEGORY C

Reproduction studies have been performed in rats and rabbits with exposures (based on C_{max}) up to 399 and 183 times, respectively, of that seen at a clinical dosage of 1 mg/kg/day and have revealed no evidence of teratogenicity. The incidence in fetuses of a common skeletal variation, unossified or incomplete ossification of sternebra, was increased in rats at 399 times human exposure, while no effect was observed at 216 times human exposure. A slight post-implantation loss was noted at 216 times the human exposure with no effect noted at approximately 135 times the human exposure. An increase in early rat neonatal mortality (birth to 4 days of age) occurred at 399 times the human exposure, while survival of neonates was unaffected at approximately 135 times the human exposure. A study in rats showed that stavudine is transferred to the fetus through the placenta. The concentration in fetal tissue was approximately one-half the concentration in maternal plasma. Animal reproduction studies are not always predictive of human response.

There are no adequate and well-controlled studies of stavudine in pregnant women. Stavudine should be used during pregnancy only if the potential benefit justifies the potential risk.

Fatal lactic acidosis has been reported in pregnant women who received the combination of stavudine and didanosine with other antiretroviral agents. It is unclear if pregnancy augments the risk of lactic acidosis/hepatic steatosis syndrome reported in nonpregnant individuals receiving nucleoside analogues (see WARNINGS, Lactic Acidosis/Severe Hepatomegaly With Steatosis/Hepatic Failure). **The combination of stavudine and didanosine should be used with caution during pregnancy and is recommended only if the potential benefit clearly outweighs the potential risk.** Healthcare providers caring for HIV-infected pregnant women receiving stavudine should be alert for early diagnosis of lactic acidosis/hepatic steatosis syndrome.

Antiretroviral Pregnancy Registry: To monitor maternal-fetal outcomes of pregnant women exposed to stavudine and other antiretroviral agents, an Antiretroviral Pregnancy Registry has been established. Physicians are encouraged to register patients by calling 1-800-258-4263.

NURSING MOTHERS

The Centers for Disease Control and Prevention recommend that HIV-infected mothers not breast-feed their infants to avoid risking postnatal transmission of HIV. Studies in lactating rats demonstrated that stavudine is excreted in milk. Although it is not known whether stavudine is excreted in human milk, there exists the potential for adverse effects from stavudine in nursing infants. Because of both the potential for HIV transmission and the potential for serious adverse reactions in nursing infants, **mothers should be instructed not to breast-feed if they are receiving stavudine.**

PEDIATRIC USE

Use of stavudine in pediatric patients is supported by evidence from adequate and well-controlled studies of stavudine in adults with additional pharmacokinetic and safety data in pediatric patients.

Adverse events that were reported to occur in 105 pediatric patients receiving stavudine 2 mg/kg/day for a median of 6.4 months in study ACTG 240 were generally similar to those reported in adults.

Stavudine pharmacokinetics have been evaluated in 25 HIV-infected pediatric patients ranging in age from 5 weeks to 15 years and in weight from 2-43 kg after IV or oral administration of single doses and twice daily regimens (see TABLE 1).

GERIATRIC USE

Clinical studies of stavudine did not include sufficient numbers of patients aged 65 years and over to determine whether they respond differently than younger patients. Greater sensitivity of some older individuals to the effects of stavudine cannot be ruled out.

In a monotherapy Expanded Access Program for patients with advanced HIV infection, peripheral neuropathy or peripheral neuropathic symptoms were observed in 15 of 40 (38%) elderly patients receiving 40 mg twice daily and 8 of 51 (16%) elderly patients receiving 20 mg twice daily. Of the approximately 12,000 patients enrolled in the Expanded Access Program, peripheral neuropathy or peripheral neuropathic symptoms developed in 30% of patients receiving 40 mg twice daily and 25% of patients receiving 20 mg twice daily. Elderly patients should be closely monitored for signs and symptoms of peripheral neuropathy.

Stavudine is known to be substantially excreted by the kidney, and the risk of toxic reactions to this drug may be greater in patients with impaired renal function. Because elderly patients are more likely to have decreased renal function, it may be useful to monitor renal function. Dose adjustment is recommended for patients with renal impairment (see DOSAGE AND ADMINISTRATION, Dosage Adjustment).

DRUG INTERACTIONS

Zidovudine may competitively inhibit the intracellular phosphorylation of stavudine. Therefore, use of zidovudine in combination with stavudine is not recommended (see CLINICAL PHARMACOLOGY).

ADVERSE REACTIONS

ADULTS

Fatal lactic acidosis has occurred in patients treated with stavudine in combination with other antiretroviral agents. Patients with suspected lactic acidosis should immediately suspend therapy with stavudine. Permanent discontinuation of stavudine should be considered for patients with confirmed lactic acidosis.

Stavudine therapy has rarely been associated with motor weakness, occurring predominantly in the setting of lactic acidosis. If motor weakness develops, stavudine should be discontinued.

Stavudine therapy has also been associated with peripheral sensory neuropathy, which can be severe, is dose related, and occurs more frequently in patients being treated with neurotoxic drug therapy, including didanosine, in patients with advanced HIV infection, or in patients who have previously experienced peripheral neuropathy.

Patients should be monitored for the development of neuropathy, which is usually manifested by numbness, tingling, or pain in the feet or hands. Stavudine-related peripheral neuropathy may resolve if therapy is withdrawn promptly. In some cases, symptoms may worsen temporarily following discontinuation of therapy. If symptoms resolve completely, patients may tolerate resumption of treatment at one-half the dose (see DOSAGE AND ADMINISTRATION). If neuropathy recurs after resumption, permanent discontinuation of stavudine should be considered.

When stavudine is used in combination with other agents with similar toxicities, the incidence of adverse events may be higher than when stavudine is used alone. Pancreatitis, peripheral neuropathy, and liver function abnormalities occur more frequently in patients treated with the combination of stavudine and didanosine, with or without hydroxyurea. Fatal pancreatitis and hepatotoxicity may occur more frequently in patients treated with stavudine in combination with didanosine and hydroxyurea (see WARNINGS and PRECAUTIONS).

Selected clinical adverse events that occurred in adult patients receiving stavudine in a controlled monotherapy study (Study AI455-019) are provided in TABLE 3.

TABLE 3 *Selected Clinical Adverse Events in Study AI455-019* (Monotherapy)*

Adverse Events	Stavudine (40 mg twice daily) (n=412)	Zidovudine (200 mg three times daily) (n=402)
Headache	54%	49%
Diarrhea	50%	44%
Peripheral neurologic symptoms/neuropathy	52%	39%
Rash	40%	35%
Nausea and vomiting	39%	44%

* Median duration of stavudine therapy = 79 weeks; median duration of zidovudine therapy = 53 weeks.

Pancreatitis was observed in 3 of the 412 adult patients who received stavudine in a controlled monotherapy study.

Selected clinical adverse events that occurred in antiretroviral naive adult patients receiving stavudine from two controlled combination studies are provided in TABLE 4A and TABLE 4B.

Pancreatitis resulting in death was observed in patients treated with stavudine plus didanosine, with or without hydroxyurea, in controlled clinical studies and in postmarketing reports.

TABLE 4A *Selected Clinical Adverse Events in the START 1 Study (Combination Therapy)*

Adverse Events	Stavudine + Lamivudine + Indinavir (n=100)*	Zidovudine + Lamivudine + Indinavir (n=102)
Nausea	43%	63%
Diarrhea	34%	16%
Headache	25%	26%
Rash	18%	13%
Vomiting	18%	33%
Peripheral neurologic symptoms/neuropathy	8%	7%

* Duration of stavudine therapy = 48 weeks.

TABLE 4B *Selected Clinical Adverse Events in the START 2* Study (Combination Therapy)*

Adverse Events	Stavudine + Didanosine + Indinavir (n=102)†	Zidovudine + Lamivudine + Indinavir (n=103)
Nausea	53%	67%
Diarrhea	45%	39%
Headache	46%	37%
Rash	30%	18%
Vomiting	30%	35%
Peripheral neurologic symptoms/neuropathy	21%	10%

* START 2 compared two triple-combination regimens in 205 treatment-naive patients. Patients received either stavudine (40 mg twice daily) plus didanosine plus indinavir or zidovudine plus lamivudine plus indinavir.
† Duration of stavudine therapy = 48 weeks.

Selected laboratory abnormalities reported in a controlled monotherapy study (Study AI455-019) are provided in TABLE 5.

TABLE 5 *Selected Adult Laboratory Abnormalities in Study AI455-019*†*

Parameter	Stavudine (40 mg twice daily) (n=412)	Zidovudine (200 mg three times daily) (n=402)
AST (SGOT) (>5.0 × ULN)	11%	10%
ALT (SGPT) (>5.0 × ULN)	13%	11%
Amylase (≥1.4 × ULN)	14%	13%

* Data presented for patients for whom laboratory evaluations were performed.
† Median duration of stavudine therapy = 79 weeks; median duration of zidovudine therapy = 53 weeks.
ULN = Upper limit of normal.

Selected laboratory abnormalities reported in two controlled combination studies are provided in TABLE 6A and TABLE 6B and TABLE 7A and TABLE 7B.

TABLE 6A *Selected Laboratory Abnormalities in the START 1 Study (Grades 3-4)*

Parameter	Stavudine + Lamivudine + Indinavir (n=100)	Zidovudine + Lamivudine + Indinavir (n=102)
Bilirubin (>2.6 × ULN)	7%	6%
SGOT (AST) (>5 × ULN)	5%	2%
SGPT (ALT) (>5 × ULN)	6%	2%
GGT (>5 × ULN)	2%	2%
Lipase (>2 × ULN)	6%	3%
Amylase (>2 × ULN)	4%	<1%

ULN = Upper limit of normal.

TABLE 6B *Selected Laboratory Abnormalities in the START 2 Study (Grades 3-4)*

Parameter	Stavudine + Didanosine + Indinavir (n=102)	Zidovudine + Lamivudine + Indinavir (n=103)
Bilirubin (>2.6 × ULN)	16%	8%
SGOT (AST) (>5 × ULN)	7%	7%
SGPT (ALT) (>5 × ULN)	8%	5%
GGT (>5 × ULN)	5%	2%
Lipase (>2 × ULN)	5%	5%
Amylase (>2 × ULN)	8%	2%

ULN = Upper limit of normal.

OBSERVED DURING CLINICAL PRACTICE

The following events have been identified during postapproval use of stavudine. Because they are reported voluntarily from a population of unknown size, estimates of frequency cannot be made. These events have been chosen for inclusion due to their seriousness, frequency of reporting, causal connection to stavudine, or a combination of these factors.

TABLE 7A *Selected Laboratory Abnormalities in the START 1 Study (All Grades)*

Parameter	Stavudine + Lamivudine + Indinavir (n=100)	Zidovudine + Lamivudine + Indinavir (n=102)
Total bilirubin	65%	60%
SGOT (AST)	42%	20%
SGPT (ALT)	40%	20%
GGT	15%	8%
Lipase	27%	12%
Amylase	21%	19%

TABLE 7B *Selected Laboratory Abnormalities in the START 2 Study (All Grades)*

Parameter	Stavudine + Didanosine + Indinavir (n=102)	Zidovudine + Lamivudine + Indinavir (n=103)
Total bilirubin	68%	55%
SGOT (AST)	53%	20%
SGPT (ALT)	50%	18%
GGT	28%	12%
Lipase	26%	19%
Amylase	31%	17%

Body as a Whole: Abdominal pain, allergic reaction, chills/fever, and redistribution/accumulation of body fat (see PRECAUTIONS, Fat Redistribution).
Digestive Disorders: Anorexia.
Exocrine Gland Disorders: Pancreatitis [including fatal cases (see WARNINGS)].
Hematologic Disorders: Anemia, leukopenia, and thrombocytopenia.
Liver: Lactic acidosis and hepatic steatosis (see WARNINGS), hepatitis and liver failure.
Musculoskeletal: Myalgia.
Nervous System: Insomnia, severe motor weakness (most often reported in the setting of lactic acidosis, see WARNINGS).

PEDIATRIC PATIENTS

Adverse reactions and serious laboratory abnormalities in pediatric patients were similar in type and frequency to those seen in adult patients.

DOSAGE AND ADMINISTRATION

The interval between doses of stavudine should be 12 hours. Stavudine may be taken without regard to meals.

ADULTS

The recommended dose based on body weight is as follows:
40 mg twice daily for patients ≥60 kg.
30 mg twice daily for patients <60 kg.

PEDIATRICS

The recommended dose for pediatric patients weighing less than 30 kg is 1 mg/kg/dose, given every 12 hours. Pediatric patients weighing 30 kg or greater should receive the recommended adult dosage.

DOSAGE ADJUSTMENT

Patients should be monitored for the development of peripheral neuropathy, which is usually manifested by numbness, tingling, or pain in the feet or hands. These symptoms may be difficult to detect in young children (see WARNINGS). If these symptoms develop during treatment, stavudine therapy should be interrupted. Symptoms may resolve if therapy is withdrawn promptly. In some cases, symptoms may worsen temporarily following discontinuation of therapy. If symptoms resolve completely, patients may tolerate resumption of treatment at one-half the recommended dose:
20 mg twice daily for patients ≥60 kg.
15 mg twice daily for patients <60 kg.

If peripheral neuropathy recurs after resumption of stavudine, permanent discontinuation should be considered.

Renal Impairment

Stavudine may be administered to adult patients with impaired renal function with adjustment in dose as shown in TABLE 8.

TABLE 8 *Recommended Dosage Adjustment for Renal Impairment*

Creatinine Clearance	Recommended Stavudine Dose by Patient Weight ≥60 kg	<60 kg
>50 ml/min	40 mg every 12 hours	30 mg every 12 hours
26-50 ml/min	20 mg every 12 hours	15 mg every 12 hours
10-25 ml/min	20 mg every 24 hours	15 mg every 24 hours

Since urinary excretion is also a major route of elimination of stavudine in pediatric patients, the clearance of stavudine may be altered in children with renal impairment. Although there are insufficient data to recommend a specific dose adjustment of stavudine in this patient population, a reduction in the dose and/or an increase in the interval between doses should be considered.

S

Hemodialysis Patients
The recommended dose is 20 mg every 24 hours (≥60 kg) or 15 mg every 24 hours (<60 kg), administered after the completion of hemodialysis and at the same time of day on non-dialysis days.

HOW SUPPLIED

ZERIT CAPSULES
Zerit capsules are available in the following strengths and configurations:

15 mg: Light yellow and dark red capsules, marked with "BMS 1964" and "15" in black ink.
20 mg: Light brown capsules, marked with "BMS 1965" and "20" in black ink.
30 mg: Light orange and dark orange capsules, with "BMS 1966" and "30" in black ink.
40 mg: Dark orange capsules, marked with "BMS 1967" and "40" in black ink.

Storage: Store in tightly closed containers at controlled room temperature, 15-30°C (59-86°F).

ZERIT FOR ORAL SOLUTION
Zerit for Oral Solution is a dye-free, fruit-flavored powder that provides 1 mg of stavudine per ml of solution upon constitution with water. Directions for solution preparation are included on the product label. Zerit for Oral Solution is available in child-resistant containers that provide 200 ml of solution after constitution with water.
Storage: Store protected from excessive moisture and stored in tightly closed containers at controlled room temperature, 15-30°C (59-86°F). After constitution, store tightly closed containers in a refrigerator, 2-8°C (36-46°F). Discard any unused portion after 30 days.

PRODUCT LISTING - EQUIVALENTS NOT AVAILABLE

Capsule - Oral - 15 mg			
60's	$293.36	ZERIT, Physicians Total Care	54868-3360-00
60's	$308.82	ZERIT, Bristol-Myers Squibb	00003-1964-01
Capsule - Oral - 20 mg			
60's	$305.05	ZERIT, Physicians Total Care	54868-3353-00
60's	$321.14	ZERIT, Bristol-Myers Squibb	00003-1965-01
Capsule - Oral - 30 mg			
60's	$305.90	ZERIT, Allscripts Pharmaceutical Company	54569-4053-00
60's	$323.98	ZERIT, Physicians Total Care	54868-3448-00
60's	$341.11	ZERIT, Bristol-Myers Squibb	00003-1966-01
Capsule - Oral - 40 mg			
6's	$29.67	ZERIT, Allscripts Pharmaceutical Company	54569-4054-01
30's	$171.36	ZERIT, Physicians Total Care	54868-3352-01
60's	$311.54	ZERIT, Allscripts Pharmaceutical Company	54569-4054-00
60's	$329.93	ZERIT, Physicians Total Care	54868-3352-00
60's	$347.40	ZERIT, Bristol-Myers Squibb	00003-1967-01
Powder For Reconstitution - Oral - 1 mg/ml			
200 ml	$64.51	ZERIT, Bristol-Myers Squibb	00003-1968-01

Streptokinase *(002276)*

Categories: Embolism, arterial; Embolism, pulmonary; Myocardial infarction; Occlusion, arteriovenous cannula; Thrombosis, arterial; Thrombosis, coronary artery; Thrombosis, deep vein; Pregnancy Category C; FDA Pre 1938 Drugs; WHO Formulary
Drug Classes: Thrombolytics
Brand Names: Kabikinase; **Streptase**
Foreign Brand Availability: K-Nase (Korea); Zykinase (India)
HCFA JCODE(S): J2995 per 250,000 IU IV

DESCRIPTION

Streptase is a sterile, purified preparation of a bacterial protein elaborated by group C β-hemolytic streptococci. It is supplied as a lyophilized white powder containing 25 mg cross-linked gelatin polypeptides, 25 mg sodium L-glutamate, sodium hydroxide to adjust pH, and 100 mg albumin (human) per vial or infusion bottle as stabilizers. The preparation contains no preservatives and is intended for intravenous and intracoronary administration.

CLINICAL PHARMACOLOGY

Streptokinase acts with plasminogen to produce an "activator complex" that converts plasminogen to the proteolytic enzyme plasmin. The $t_{1/2}$ of the activator complex is about 23 minutes; the complex is inactivated, in part, by antistreptococcal antibodies. The mechanism by which dissociated streptokinase is eliminated is clearance by sites in the liver; however, no metabolites of streptokinase have been identified. Plasmin degrades fibrin clots as well as fibrinogen and other plasma proteins. Plasmin is inactivated by circulating inhibitors, such as α-2-plasmin inhibitor or α-2-macroglobulin. These inhibitors are rapidly consumed at high doses of streptokinase.

Intravenous infusion of streptokinase is followed by increased fibrinolytic activity, which decreases plasma fibrinogen levels for 24-36 hours. The decrease in plasma fibrinogen in associated with decreases in plasma and blood viscosity and red blood cell aggregation. The hyperfibrinolytic effect disappears within a few hours after discontinuation, but a prolonged thrombin time may persist for up to 24 hours due to the decrease in plasma levels of fibrinogen and an increase in the amount of circulating fibrin(ogen) degradation products (FDP). Depending upon the dosage and duration of infusion of streptokinase, the thrombin time will decrease to less than 2 times the normal control value within 4 hours, and return to normal by 24 hours.

Intravenous administration has been shown to reduce blood pressure and total peripheral resistance with a corresponding reduction in cardiac afterload. These expected responses were not studied with the intracoronary administration of streptokinase. The quantitative benefit has not been evaluated.

Variable amounts of circulating antistreptokinase antibody are present in individuals as a result of recent streptococcal infections. The recommended dosage schedule usually obviates the need for antibody titration.

Two very large, randomized, placebo-controlled studies[1, 2] involving almost 30,000 patients have demonstrated that a 60 minute intravenous infusion of 1,500,000 IU of streptokinase significantly reduces mortality following a myocardial infarction. One of these studies also evaluated concomitant oral administration of low dose aspirin (160 mg/d over 1 month).

In the GISSI study, the reduction in mortality was time dependent. There was a 47% reduction in mortality among patients treated within 1 hour of the onset of chest pain, a 23% reduction among patients treated within 3 hours, and a 17% reduction among patients treated between 3 and 6 hours. There was also a reduction in mortality in patients treated between 6 and 12 hours from the onset of symptoms, but the reduction was not statistically significant.

In the ISIS-2 study the reduction in mortality was also time dependent. If streptokinase and aspirin were administered within the first hour after symptom onset, the reduction in mortality was 44%. The reduction in the odds of death in patients treated within 4 hours was 53% for the combination of streptokinase and aspirin, and 35% for streptokinase alone. However, the reduction was still significant when treatment was started 5-24 hours after symptom onset: 33% for the combined therapy and 17% for streptokinase alone. Overall, in the 0-24 hour time period there was a 42% reduction in the odds of death with combined treatment (streptokinase and aspirin) versus placebo ($2p<0.00001$) and a 25% reduction in the odds of death with streptokinase alone versus placebo ($2p<0.00001$).

One of eight smaller studies using a similar dosing schedule showed a statistically significant reduction in mortality. When all of these studies were pooled, the overall decrease in mortality was approximately 23%. Results from pooling several studies using different dosages with long term infusion corroborate these observations.

In addition, studies measuring left ventricular ejection fraction (LVEF) at discharge showed the mean LVEFs were approximately 3-6 percentage points higher in the streptokinase group than in the control group. This difference was statistically significant in some of the studies.[3,4] Furthermore, some studies reported greater improvement in LVEF among patients treated within 3 hours than in patients treated later.

Results from a randomized controlled trial in over 11,000 patients show that, following treatment with IV streptokinase, there is a reduction in the number of patients with clinical congestive heart failure during the 14-21 day in-hospital period. Clinical congestive heart failure occurred in 12.8% of streptokinase-treated patients compared with 15% of the control patients ($p=0.001$).[1]

The rate of reocclusion of the infarct-related vessel has been reported to be approximately 15-20%. The rate of reocclusion depends on dosage, additional anticoagulant therapy and residual stenosis. When the reinfarctions were evaluated in studies involving 8800 streptokinase-treated patients, the overall rate was 3.8% (range 2-15%). In over 8500 control patients, the rate of reinfarction was 2.4%. However, the ISIS-2 study showed that an increase in reinfarction was avoided when streptokinase was combined with lose dose aspirin. The rate of reinfarction in the combination group was 1.8% vs 1.9% in the group given aspirin alone.

Streptokinase, administered by the intracoronary route has resulted in thrombolysis usually within 1 hour, and ensuing reperfusion results in improvement of cardiac function, and reduction of mortality.[5,6] LVEF was increased in patients treated with streptokinase when compared to patients treated with conventional therapy. When the initial LVEF was low, the streptokinase-treated patients showed greater improvement than did the controls. Spontaneous reperfusion is known to occur and has been observed with angiography at various time points after infarction. Data from one study show that 73% of streptokinase-treated patients and 47% of the placebo-allocated patients reperfused during hospitalization.

Studies with thrombolytic therapy for pulmonary embolism show no significant difference in lung perfusion scan between the thrombolysis group and the heparin group at 1 year follow-up. However, measurements of pulmonary capillary blood volumes and diffusing capacities at 2 weeks and 1 year after therapy indicate that a more complete resolution of thrombotic obstruction and normalization of pulmonary physiology was achieved with thrombolytic therapy, thus preventing the long term sequelae of pulmonary hypertension and pulmonary failure.[7]

The long term benefit of streptokinase therapy for deep vein thrombosis (DVT) has been evaluated venographically.[8] The combined results of five randomized studies show no residual thrombotic material in 60-75% of patients treated with streptokinase versus only 10% of those treated with heparin. Thrombolytic therapy also preserves venous valve function in a majority of cases, thus avoiding the pathologic venous changes that produce the clinical post-phlebitic syndrome which occurs in 90% of the DVT patients treated with heparin.

There is a time-related decrease in effectiveness when streptokinase is used in the management of peripheral arterial thromboembolism. When administered 3-10 days after onset of obstruction, rates of clearance of 50-75% were reported.

INDICATIONS AND USAGE

ACUTE EVOLVING TRANSMURAL MYOCARDIAL INFARCTION
Streptokinase is indicated for use in the management of acute myocardial infarction (AMI) in adults, the lysis of intracoronary thrombi, for the improvement of ventricular function, and the reduction of mortality associated with AMI, when administered by either the intravenous or the intracoronary route, as well as for the reduction of infarct size and congestive heart failure associated with AMI when administered by the intravenous route. Earlier administration of streptokinase is correlated with greater clinical benefit. (See CLINICAL PHARMACOLOGY.)

PULMONARY EMBOLISM
Streptokinase is indicated for the lysis of objectively diagnosed (angiography or lung scan) pulmonary emboli, involving obstruction of blood flow to a lobe or multiple segments, with or without unstable hemodynamics.

DEEP VEIN THROMBOSIS
Streptokinase is indicated for the lysis of objectively diagnosed (preferably ascending venography), acute, extensive thrombi of the deep veins such as those involving the popliteal and more proximal vessels.

ARTERIAL THROMBOSIS OR EMBOLISM

Streptokinase is indicated for the lysis of acute arterial thrombi and emboli. Streptokinase is not indicated for arterial emboli originating from the left side of the heart due to the risk of new embolic phenomena such as cerebral embolism.

OCCLUSION OF ARTERIOVENOUS CANNULAE

Streptokinase is indicated as an alternative to surgical revision for clearing totally or partially occluded arteriovenous cannulae when acceptable flow cannot be achieved.

NON-FDA APPROVED INDICATIONS

Although not FDA approved, intrapleural streptokinase has been used successfully in a limited number of patients for treatment of pleural effusions and empyemas.

CONTRAINDICATIONS

Because thrombolytic therapy increases the risk of bleeding, streptokinase is contraindicated in the following situations:

- Active internal bleeding.
- Recent (within 2 months) cerebrovascular accident, intracranial or intraspinal surgery (see WARNINGS).
- Intracranial neoplasm.
- Severe uncontrolled hypertension.

Streptokinase should not be administered to patients having experienced severe allergic reaction to the product.

WARNINGS

BLEEDING

Following intravenous high-dose brief-duration streptokinase therapy in acute myocardial infarction, severe bleeding complications requiring transfusion are extremely rare (0.3-0.5%), and combined therapy with low dose aspirin does not appear to increase the risk of major bleeding. The addition of aspirin to streptokinase may cause a slight increase in the risk of minor bleeding (3.1% without aspirin versus 3.9% with).[2]

Streptokinase will cause lysis of hemostatic fibrin deposits such as those occurring at sites of needle punctures, particularly when infused over several hours, and bleeding may occur from such sites. In order to minimize the risk of bleeding during treatment with streptokinase, venipunctures and physical handling of the patient should be performed carefully and as infrequently as possible, and intramuscular injections must be avoided.

Should arterial puncture be necessary during intravenous therapy, upper extremity vessels are preferable. Pressure should be applied for at least 30 minutes, a pressure dressing applied, and the puncture site checked frequently for evidence of bleeding.

In the following conditions, the risks of therapy may be increased and should be weighed against the anticipated benefits.

- Recent (within 10 days) major surgery, obstetrical delivery, organ biopsy, previous puncture of noncompressible vessels.
- Recent (within 10 days) serious gastrointestinal bleeding.
- Recent (within 10 days) trauma including cardiopulmonary resuscitation.
- Hypertension: systolic BP >180 mm Hg and/or diastolic BP >110 mm Hg.
- High likelihood of left heart thrombus, *e.g.,* mitral stenosis with atrial fibrillation.
- Subacute bacterial endocarditis.
- Hemostatic defects including those secondary to severe hepatic or renal disease.
- Pregnancy.
- Age >75 years.
- Cerebrovascular disease.
- Diabetic hemorrhagic retinopathy.
- Septic thrombophlebitis or occluded AV cannula at seriously infected site.
- Any other condition in which bleeding constitutes a significant hazard or would be particularly difficult to manage because of its location.

Should serious spontaneous bleeding (not controllable by local pressure) occur, the infusion of streptokinase should be terminated immediately and treatment instituted as described under ADVERSE REACTIONS.

Bleeding into the pericardium, sometimes associated with myocardial rupture, has been seen in individual cases and has resulted in fatalities.

ARRHYTHMIAS

Rapid lysis of coronary thrombi has been shown to cause reperfusion atrial or ventricular dysrhythmias requiring immediate treatment. Careful monitoring for arrhythmia is recommended during and immediately following administration of streptokinase for acute myocardial infarction. Occasionally, tachycardia and bradycardia have been observed.

HYPOTENSION

Hypotension, sometimes severe, not secondary to bleeding or anaphylaxis has been observed during intravenous streptokinase infusion in 1-10% of patients. Patients should be monitored closely and, should symptomatic or alarming hypotension occur, appropriate treatment should be administered. This treatment may include a decrease in the intravenous streptokinase infusion rate. Smaller hypotensive effects are common and have not required treatment.

CHOLESTEROL EMBOLISM

Cholesterol embolism has been reported rarely in patients treated with all types of thrombolytic agents; the true incidence is unknown. This serious condition, which can be lethal, is also associated with invasive vascular procedures (*e.g.,* cardiac catheterization, angiography, vascular surgery) and/or anticoagulant therapy. Clinical features of cholesterol embolism may include livedo reticularis, "purple toe" syndrome, acute renal failure, gangrenous digits, hypertension, pancreatitis, myocardial infarction, cerebral infarction, spinal cord infarction, retinal artery occlusion, bowel infarction, and rhabdomyolysis.

OTHER

Non-cardiogenic pulmonary edema has been reported rarely in patients treated with streptokinase. The risk of this appears greatest in patients who have large myocardial infarctions and are undergoing thrombolytic therapy by the intracoronary route.

Rarely, polyneuropathy has been temporally related to the use of streptokinase, with some cases described as Guillain Barré Syndrome.

Should pulmonary embolism or recurrent pulmonary embolism occur during streptokinase therapy, the originally planned course of treatment should be completed in an attempt to lyse the embolus. While pulmonary embolism may occasionally occur during streptokinase treatment, the incidence is no greater than when patients are treated with heparin alone. In addition to pulmonary embolism, embolization to other sites during streptokinase treatment has been observed.

PRECAUTIONS

GENERAL

There have been rare cares where streptokinase has been administered for suspected AMI subsequently diagnosed as pancreatitis. Fatalities have occurred under these circumstances.

Repeated Administration

Because of the increased likelihood of resistance due to antistreptokinase antibody, streptokinase may not be effective if administered between 5 days and 12 months of prior streptokinase or anistreplase administration, or streptococcal infections, such as streptococcal pharyngitis, acute rheumatic fever, or acute glomerulonephritis secondary to a streptococcal infection.

LABORATORY TESTS

Intravenous or Intracoronary Infusion for Myocardial Infarction

Intravenous administration of streptokinase will cause marked decreases in plasminogen and fibrinogen and increases in thrombin time (TT), activated partial thromboplastin time (APTT), and prothrombin time (PT), which usually normalize within 12-24 hours. These changes may also occur in some patients with intracoronary administration of streptokinase.

Intravenous Infusion for Other Indications

Before commencing thrombolytic therapy, it is desirable to obtain an activated partial thromboplastin time (APTT), a prothrombin time (PT), a thrombin time (TT), or fibrinogen levels, and a hematocrit and platelet count. If heparin has been given, it should be discontinued and the TT or APTT should be less than twice the normal control value before thrombolytic therapy is started.

During the infusion, decreases in plasminogen and fibrinogen levels and an increase in the level of FDP (the latter two causing a prolongation in the clotting times of coagulation tests) will generally confirm the existence of a lytic state. Therefore, lytic therapy can be confirmed by performing the TT, APTT, PT, or fibrinogen levels approximately 4 hours after initiation of therapy.

If heparin is to be (re)instituted following the streptokinase infusion, the TT or APTT should be less than twice the normal control value (see prescribing information for heparin).

PREGNANCY CATEGORY C

Animal reproduction studies have not been conducted with streptokinase. It is also not known whether streptokinase can cause fetal harm when administered to a pregnant woman or can affect reproduction capacity. Streptokinase should be given to a pregnant woman only if clearly needed.

PEDIATRIC USE

Safety and effectiveness in pediatric patients have not been established.

DRUG INTERACTIONS

The interaction of streptokinase with other drugs has not been well studied.

USE OF ANTICOAGULANTS AND ANTIPLATELET AGENTS

Streptokinase alone or in combination with antiplatelet agents and anticoagulants, may cause bleeding complications. Therefore, careful monitoring is advised. In the treatment of acute MI, aspirin, when not otherwise contraindicated, should be administered with streptokinase (See Anticoagulation and Antiplatelets After Treatment for Myocardial Infarction).

ANTICOAGULATION AND ANTIPLATELETS AFTER TREATMENT FOR MYOCARDIAL INFARCTION

In the treatment of acute myocardial infarction, the use of aspirin has been shown to reduce the incidence of reinfarction and stroke. The addition of aspirin to streptokinase causes a minimal increase in the risk of minor bleeding (3.9% vs 3.1%), but does not appear to increase the incidence of major bleeding (see ADVERSE REACTIONS).[2] The use of anticoagulants following administration of streptokinase increases the risk of bleeding, but has not yet been shown to be of unequivocal clinical benefit. Therefore, whereas the use of aspirin is recommended unless otherwise contraindicated, the use of anticoagulants should be decided by the treating physician.

ANTICOAGULATION AFTER IV TREATMENT FOR OTHER INDICATIONS

Continuous intravenous infusion of heparin, without a loading dose, has been recommended following termination of streptokinase infusion for treatment of pulmonary embolism or deep vein thrombosis to prevent rethrombosis. The effect of streptokinase on thrombin time (TT) and activated partial thromboplastin time (APTT) will usually diminish within 3-4 hours after streptokinase therapy, and heparin therapy without a loading dose can be initiated when the TT or the APTT is less than twice the normal control value.

ADVERSE REACTIONS

The following adverse reactions have been associated with intravenous therapy and may also occur with intracoronary artery infusion:

Bleeding: The reported incidence of bleeding (major or minor) has varied widely depending on the indication, dose, route and duration of administration, and concomitant therapy.

Minor bleeding can be anticipated mainly at invaded or disturbed sites. If such bleeding occurs, local measures should be taken to control the bleeding.

Severe internal bleeding involving gastrointestinal (including hepatic bleeding), genitourinary, retroperitoneal, or intracerebral sites has occurred and has resulted in fatalities. In the treatment of acute myocardial infarction with intravenous streptokinase, the GISSI and ISIS-2 studies reported a rate of major bleeding (requiring transfusion) of 0.3-0.5%. However, rates as high as 16% have been reported in studies which required administration of anticoagulants and invasive procedures.

Major bleed rates are difficult to determine for other dosages and patient populations because of the different dosing and intervals of infusions. The rates reported appear to be within the ranges reported for intravenous administration in acute myocardial infarction.

Should uncontrollable bleeding occur, streptokinase infusion should be terminated immediately, rather than slowing the rate of administration of or reducing the dose of streptokinase. If necessary, bleeding can be reversed and blood loss effectively managed with appropriate replacement therapy. Although the use of aminocaproic acid in humans as an antidote for streptokinase has not been documented, it may be considered in an emergency situation.

Allergic Reactions: Fever and shivering, occurring in 1-4% of patients,[1,2] are the most commonly reported allergic reactions with intravenous use of streptokinase in acute myocardial infarction. Anaphylactic and anaphylactoid reactions ranging in severity from minor breathing difficulty to bronchospasm, periorbital swelling or angioneurotic edema have been observed rarely. Other milder allergic effects such as urticaria, itching, flushing, nausea, headache and musculoskeletal pain have also been observed, as have delayed hypersensitivity reactions such as vasculitis and interstitial nephritis. Anaphylactic shock is very rare, having been reported in 0-0.1% of patients.[1,2,4]

Mild or moderate allergic reactions may be managed with concomitant antihistamine and/or corticosteroid therapy. Severe allergic reactions require immediate discontinuation of streptokinase, with adrenergic, antihistamine, and/or corticosteroid agents administered intravenously as required.

Respiratory: There have been reports of repiratory depression in patients receiving streptokinase. In some cases, it was not possible to determine whether the respiratory depression was associated with streptokinase or was a symptom of the underlying process. If respiratory depression is associated with streptokinase, the occurrence is believed to be rare.

Other Adverse Reactions: Transient elevations of serum transaminases have been observed. The source of these enzyme rises and their clinical significance is not fully understood.

There have been reports in the literature of cases of back pain associated with the use of streptokinase. In most cases the pain developed during streptokinase intravenous infusion and ceased within minutes of discontinuation of the infusion.

DOSAGE AND ADMINISTRATION

ACUTE EVOLVING TRANSMURAL MYOCARDIAL INFARCTION

Administer streptokinase as soon as possible after onset of symptoms. The greatest benefit in mortality reduction was observed when streptokinase was administered within 4 hours, but statistically significant benefits has been reported up to 24 hours (see CLINICAL PHARMACOLOGY). (See TABLE 1.)

TABLE 1

Route	Total Dose	Dosage/Duration
Intravenous infusion	1,500,000 IU	1,500,000 IU within 60 min
Intracoronary infusion	140,000 IU	20,000 IU by bolus followed by 2000 IU/min for 60 min

PULMONARY EMBOLISM, DEEP VEIN THROMBOSIS, ARTERIAL THROMBOSIS OR EMBOLISM

Streptokinase treatment should be instituted as soon as possible after onset of the thrombotic event, preferably within 7 days. Any delay in instituting lytic therapy to evaluate the effect of heparin therapy decreases the potential for optimal efficacy. Since human exposure to streptococci is common, antibodies to streptokinase are prevalent. Thus, a loading dose of streptokinase sufficient to neutralize these antibodies is required. A dose of 250,000 IU of streptokinase infused into a peripheral vein over 30 minutes has been found appropriate in over 90% of patients. Furthermore, if the thrombin time or any other parameter of lysis after 4 hours of therapy is not significantly different from the normal control level, discontinue streptokinase because excessive resistance is present (see TABLE 2).

TABLE 2

Indication	Loading Dose	IV Infusion Dosage/Duration
Pulmonary Embolism	250,000 IU/30 min	100,000 IU/h for 24 h (72 hours if concurrent DVT is suspected).
Deep Vein Thrombosis	250,000 IU/30 min	100,000 IU/h for 72 hours
Arterial Thrombosis or Embolism	250,000 IU/30 min	100,000 IU/h for 24-72 hours

ARTERIOVENOUS CANNULAE OCCLUSION

Before using streptokinase, an attempt should be made to clear the cannula by careful syringe technique, using heparinized saline solution. If adequate flow is not re-established, streptokinase may be employed. Allow the effect of any pretreatment anticoagulants to diminish. Instill 250,000 IU streptokinase in 2 ml of solution into each occluded limb of the cannula slowly. Clamp off cannula limb(s) for 2 hours. Observe the patient closely for possible adverse effects. After treatment, aspirate contents of infused cannula limb(s), flush with saline, reconnect cannula.

RECONSTITUTION AND DILUTION

The protein nature and lyophilized form of streptokinase require careful reconstitution and dilution. Slight flocculation (described as thin translucent fibers) of reconstituted streptokinase occurred occasionally during clinical trials but did not interfere with the safe use of the solution. The following reconstitution and dilution procedures are recommended:

Vials and Infusion Bottles:

1. Slowly add 5 ml sodium chloride injection or 5% dextrose injection to the streptokinase vial, directing the diluent at the side of the vacuum-packed vial rather than into the drug powder.
2. Roll and tilt the vial gently to reconstitute. Avoid shaking. (Shaking may cause foaming.) (If necessary, total volume may be increased to a maximum of 500 ml in glass or 50 ml in plastic containers, and the infusion pump rate in TABLE 3 should be adjusted accordingly.) To facilitate setting the infusion pump rate, a total volume of 45 ml, or a multiple thereof, is recommended.
3. Withdraw the entire reconstituted contents of the vial; slowly and carefully dilute further to a total volume as recommended in TABLE 3. Avoid shaking and agitation on dilution.
4. When diluting the 1,500,000 IU infusion bottle (50 ml), slowly add 5 ml sodium chloride injection or 5% dextrose injection, directing it at the side of the bottle rather than into the drug powder. Roll and tilt the bottle gently to reconstitute. Avoid shaking as it may cause foaming. Add an additional 40 ml of diluent to the bottle, avoiding shaking and agitation. (Total volume = 45 ml). Administer by infusion pump at the rate indicated in TABLE 3.
5. Parenteral drug products should be inspected visually for particulate matter and discoloration prior to administration. (The albumin [human] may impart a slightly yellow color to the solution.)
6. The reconstituted solution can be filtered through a 0.8 µm or larger pore size filter.
7. Because streptokinase contains no preservatives, it should be reconstituted immediately before use. The solution may be used for direct intravenous administration within 8 hours following reconstitution if stored at 2-8°C (36-46°F).
8. Do not add other medication to the container of streptokinase.
9. Unused reconstituted drug should be discarded.

TABLE 3 *Suggested Dilutions and Infusion Rates*

Dosage	Vial Size (IU)	Total Solution Volume	Infusion Rate
I. Acute Myocardial Infarction			
A. Intravenous infusion	1,500,000	45 ml	Infuse 45 ml within 60 min
B. Intracoronary infusion	250,000	125 ml	
1. 20,000 IU bolus			1. Loading Dose of 10 ml
2. 2000 IU/min for 60 minutes			2. Then 60 ml/h
II. Pulmonary Embolism, Deep Vein Thrombosis, Arterial Thrombosis or Embolism			
Intravenouslion			
A. 1. 250,000 IU loading dose over 30 minutes	1,500,000	90 ml	1. Infuse 30 ml/h for 30 minutes
2. 100,000 IU/h maintenance dose			2. Infuse 6 ml/h
B. SAME	1,500,000 infusion bottle	45 ml	1. 15 ml/h for 30 minutes 2. Infuse 3 ml/h

FOR USE IN ARTERIOVENOUS CANNULAE

Slowly reconstitute the contents of 250,000 IU streptokinase vacuum-packed vial with 2 ml sodium chloride injection or 5% dextrose injection.

HOW SUPPLIED

Streptase is supplied as a lyophilized white powder in 50 ml infusion bottles (1,500,000 IU) or in 6.5 ml vials with a color-coded label corresponding to the amount of purified streptokinase in each vial.

Storage: Store unopened vials at controlled room temperature (15-30°C or 59-86°F).

PRODUCT LISTING - RATED THERAPEUTICALLY EQUIVALENT

Powder For Injection - Injectable - 250000 IU

1's	$138.90	STREPTASE, Astra-Zeneca Pharmaceuticals	00186-1770-01

Powder For Injection - Injectable - 750000 IU

1's	$306.58	STREPTASE, Astra-Zeneca Pharmaceuticals	00186-1771-01

Powder For Injection - Injectable - 1500000 IU

1's	$613.18	STREPTASE, Astra-Zeneca Pharmaceuticals	00186-1773-01

PRODUCT LISTING - EQUIVALENTS NOT AVAILABLE

Powder For Injection - Injectable - 250000 IU

1's	$93.75	STREPTASE, Aventis Pharmaceuticals	00053-1770-01
1's	$127.83	KABIKINASE, Pharmacia and Upjohn	00013-0110-59

Powder For Injection - Injectable - 750000 IU

1 x 6	$2188.75	KABIKINASE, Pharmacia and Upjohn	00016-0119-35
1's	$362.15	KABIKINASE, Pharmacia and Upjohn	00013-0119-35

Powder For Injection - Injectable - 1500000 IU

1 x 6	$4120.00	KABIKINASE, Pharmacia and Upjohn	00016-0111-75
1's	$562.50	GENERIC, Aventis Pharmaceuticals	00053-1773-01
1's	$566.74	STREPTASE, Astra-Zeneca Pharmaceuticals	00186-1774-01
1's	$681.70	KABIKINASE, Pharmacia and Upjohn	00013-0111-75

Streptozocin *(002278)*

For complete prescribing information, refer to the CD-ROM included with the book.

Categories: Carcinoma, pancreatic; Pregnancy Category D; FDA Approved 1982 May
Drug Classes: Antineoplastics, alkylating agents
Brand Names: Zanosar
HCFA JCODE(S): J9320 1 gm IV

WARNING

Streptozocin sterile powder should be administered under the supervision of a physician experienced in the use of cancer chemotherapeutic agents.

A patient need not be hospitalized but should have access to a facility with laboratory and supportive resources sufficient to monitor drug tolerance and to protect and maintain a patient compromised by drug toxicity. Renal toxicity is dose-related and cumulative and may be severe or fatal. Other major toxicities are nausea and vomiting which may be severe and at times treatment-limiting. In addition, liver dysfunction, diarrhea, and hematological changes have been observed in some patients. Streptozocin is mutagenic. When administered parenterally, it has been found to be tumorigenic or carcinogenic in some rodents.

The physician must judge the possible benefit to his patient against the known toxic effects of this drug in considering the advisability of therapy with streptozocin. The physician should be familiar with the following text before making his judgement and beginning treatment.

DESCRIPTION

Each vial of Zanosar sterile powder contains 1 g of the active ingredient streptozocin 2-deoxy-2[[(methylnitrosoamino)carbonyl]amino]-α(and β)-D-glucopyranose and 220 mg citric acid anhydrous. Streptozocin is available as a sterile, pale yellow, freeze-dried preparation for intravenous administration. The pH was adjusted with sodium hydroxide. When reconstituted as directed, the pH of the solution will be between 3.5 and 4.5. Streptozocin is a synthetic antineoplastic agent that is chemically related to other nitrosoureas used in cancer chemotherapy. Streptozocin is an ivory-colored crystalline powder with a molecular weight of 265.2. It is very soluble in water or physiological saline and is soluble in alcohol.
Storage: Unopened vials of Zanosar should be stored at refrigeration temperatures (2-8°C) and protected from light (preferably stored in carton).

INDICATIONS AND USAGE

Streptozocin sterile powder is indicated in the treatment of metastatic islet cell carcinoma of the pancreas. Responses have been obtained with both functional and nonfunctional carcinomas. Because of its inherent renal toxicity, therapy with this drug should be limited to patients with symptomatic or progressive metastatic disease.

WARNINGS

RENAL TOXICITY

Many patients treated with streptozocin sterile powder have experienced renal toxicity, as evidenced by azotemia, anuria hypophosphatemia, glycosuria, and renal tubular acidosis. **Such toxicity is dose-related and cumulative and may be severe or fatal.** Renal function must be monitored before and after each course of therapy. Serial urinalysis, blood urea nitrogen, plasma creatinine, serum electrolytes, and creatinine clearance should be obtained prior to, at least weekly during, and for 4 weeks after drug administration. Serial urinalysis is particularly important for the early detection of proteinuria and should be quantitated with a 24 hour collection when proteinuria is detected. Mild proteinuria is one of the first signs of renal toxicity and may herald further deterioration of renal function. Reduction of the dose of streptozocin or discontinuation of treatment is suggested in the presence of significant renal toxicity. Adequate hydration may help reduce the risk of nephrotoxicity to renal tubular epithelium by decreasing renal and urinary concentration of the drug and its metabolites.

Use of streptozocin in patients with preexisting renal disease requires a judgment by the physician of potential benefit as opposed to the known risk of serious renal damage.

This drug should not be used in combination with or concomitantly with other potential nephrotoxins.

When exposed dermally, some rats developed benign tumors at the site of application of streptozocin. Consequently, streptozocin may pose a carcinogenic hazard following topical exposure if not properly handled (see DOSAGE AND ADMINISTRATION).

See additional warnings in BOXED WARNING.

DOSAGE AND ADMINISTRATION

Streptozocin sterile powder should be administered intravenously by rapid injection or short/prolonged infusion. It is not active orally. Although it has been administered intra-arterially, this is not recommended pending further evaluation of the possibility that adverse renal effects may be evoked more rapidly by this route of administration.

Two different dosage schedules have been employed successfully with streptozocin.

DAILY SCHEDULE

The recommended dose for daily intravenous administration is 500 mg/m^2 of body surface area for 5 consecutive days every 6 weeks until maximum benefit or until treatment-limiting toxicity is observed. Dose escalation on this schedule is not recommended.

WEEKLY SCHEDULE

The recommended initial dose for weekly intravenous administration is 1000 mg/m^2 of body surface area at weekly intervals for the first 2 courses (weeks). In subsequent courses, drug doses may be escalated in patients who have not achieved a therapeutic response and who have not experienced significant toxicity with the previous course of treatment. However, A SINGLE DOSE OF 1500 mg/m^2 BODY SURFACE AREA SHOULD NOT BE EXCEEDED as a greater dose may cause azotemia. When administrated on this schedule, the median time to onset of response is about 17 days and the median time to maximum response is about 35 days. The median **total** dose to onset of response is about 2000 mg/m^2 body surface area and the median **total** dose to maximum response is about 4000 mg/m^2 body surface area.

The ideal duration of maintenance therapy with streptozocin has not yet been clearly established for either of the above schedules.

For patients with functional tumors, serial monitoring of fasting insulin levels allows a determination of biochemical response to therapy. For patients with either functional or nonfunctional tumors, response to therapy can be determined by measurable reductions of tumor size (reduction of organomegaly, masses, or lymph nodes).

Reconstitute streptozocin with 9.5 ml of dextrose injection or 0.9% sodium chloride injection. The resulting pale-gold solution will contain 100 mg of streptozocin and 22 mg of citric acid per ml. Where more dilute infusion solutions are desirable, further dilution in the above vehicles is recommended. The total storage time for streptozocin after it has been placed in solution should not exceed 12 hours. This product contains no preservatives and is not intended as a multiple-dose vial.

Caution in the handling and preparation of the powder and solution should be exercised, and the use of gloves is recommended. If streptozocin sterile powder or a solution prepared from streptozocin contacts the skin or mucosae, immediately wash the affected area with soap and water.

Procedures for proper handling and disposal of anticancer drugs should be considered. Several guidelines on this subject have been published.[4-9] There is no general agreement that all of the procedures recommended in the guidelines are necessary or appropriate.

PRODUCT LISTING - EQUIVALENTS NOT AVAILABLE

Powder For Injection - Intravenous - 1 Gm

1's $143.90 ZANOSAR, Pharmacia and Upjohn 00009-0844-01

Sucralfate *(002280)*

Categories: Ulcer, duodenal; Pregnancy Category B; FDA Approved 1981 Oct
Drug Classes: Cytoprotectives; Gastrointestinals
Brand Names: Carafate
Foreign Brand Availability: Adopilon (Japan); Alsucral (Czech-Republic; Finland; Portugal; Singapore); Andapsin (Sweden); Antepsin (Argentina; Denmark; Ecuador; England; Finland; Ireland; Italy; Norway); Bisma (Japan); Dolisec (Greece); Hexagastron (Denmark); Inpepsa (Indonesia); Iselpin (Philippines); Keal (France; Taiwan); Melicide (Greece); Neciblok (Indonesia); Peptonorm (Greece); Succosa (Finland; Sweden); Sucrabest (Germany); Sucralbene (Hungary); Sucralfin (Italy); Sucramal (Italy); Sulcran (Peru); Sulcrate (Canada); Treceptan (Chile; Ecuador); Ufarene (Greece); Ulcar (Benin; Burkina-Faso; Ethiopia; France; Gambia; Ghana; Guinea; Ivory-Coast; Kenya; Liberia; Malawi; Mali; Mauritania; Mauritius; Morocco; Niger; Nigeria; Senegal; Seychelles; Sierra-Leone; Sudan; Tanzania; Tunia; Uganda; Zambia; Zimbabwe); Ulcekon (India); Ulcerlmin (Japan; Korea); Ulcertec (Singapore); Ulcogant (Austria; Belgium; Costa-Rica; Czech-Republic; Dominican-Republic; El-Salvador; Germany; Guatemala; Honduras; Hungary; Netherlands; Nicaragua; Panama; Peru; Switzerland); Ulcyte (Australia); Ulsaheal (Bahrain; Iraq; Jordan); Ulsanic (Hong-Kong; Israel; South-Africa; Thailand); Ulsidex Forte (Indonesia); Unival (Mexico); Urbal (Spain); Yuwan S (Japan)
Cost of Therapy: $121.02 (Duodenal Ulcer; Carafate; 1 g; 4/day; 30 day supply)
$82.92 (Duodenal Ulcer; Generic Tablets; 1 g; 4 tablets/day; 30 day supply)

DESCRIPTION

Sucralfate is an α-D-glucopyranoside, β-D-fructofuranosyl-, octakis-(hydrogen sulfate), aluminum complex.

Carafate tablets for oral administration contain 1 g of sucralfate. *Also contain:* D&C red no. 30 Lake, FD&C blue no. 1 lake, magnesium stearate, microcrystalline cellulose, and starch.

Carafate suspension for oral administration contains 1 g of sucralfate per 10 ml. *Carafate suspension also contains:* Colloidal silicon dioxide, FD&C red no. 40, flavor, glycerin, methylcellulose, methylparaben, microcrystalline cellulose, purified water, simethicone, and sorbitol solution.
Therapeutic Category: Antiulcer.

CLINICAL PHARMACOLOGY

Sucralfate is only minimally absorbed from the gastrointestinal tract. The small amounts of the sulfated disaccharide that are absorbed are excreted primarily in the urine.

Although the mechanism of sucralfate's ability to accelerate healing of duodenal ulcers remains to be fully defined, it is known that it exerts its effect through a local, rather than systemic, action. The following observations also appear pertinent:

1. Studies in human subjects and with animal models of ulcer disease have shown that sucralfate forms an ulcer-adherent complex with proteinaceous exudate at the ulcer site.
2. *In vitro*, a sucralfate-albumin film provides a barrier to diffusion of hydrogen ions.
3. In human subjects, sucralfate given in doses recommended for ulcer therapy inhibits pepsin activity in gastric juice by 32%.
4. *In vitro*, sucralfate adsorbs bile salts.

These observations suggest that sucralfate's antiulcer activity is the result of formation of an ulcer-adherent complex that covers the ulcer site and protects it against further attack by acid, pepsin, and bile salts. There are approximately 14-16 mEq of acid-neutralizing capacity per 1-g dose of sucralfate.

INDICATIONS AND USAGE

Tablets:

- Short-term treatment (up to 8 weeks) of active duodenal ulcer. While healing with sucralfate may occur during the first week or two, treatment should be continued for 4-8 weeks unless healing has been demonstrated by x-ray or endoscopic examination.
- Maintenance therapy for duodenal ulcer patients at reduced dosage after healing of acute ulcers.

Suspension: Sucralfate suspension is indicated in the short-term (up to 8 weeks) treatment of active duodenal ulcer.

NON-FDA APPROVED INDICATIONS

While not FDA approved indications, sucralfate is also used in the treatment of gastric ulcer, the prophylaxis of stress ulcer, the treatment of gastroesophageal reflux disease, the management of hyperphosphatemia in renal failure, chemotherapy and radiation-induced mucositis, and in triple therapy for duodenal ulcer treatment and H. Pylori eradication.

CONTRAINDICATIONS

There are no known contraindications to the use of sucralfate.

PRECAUTIONS

GENERAL

Duodenal ulcer is a chronic, recurrent disease. While short-term treatment with sucralfate can result in complete healing of the ulcer, a successful course of treatment with sucralfate should not be expected to alter the posthealing frequency or severity of duodenal ulceration.

Special Populations

Chronic Renal Failure and Dialysis Patients

When sucralfate is administered orally, small amounts of aluminum are absorbed from the gastrointestinal tract. Concomitant use of sucralfate with other products that contain aluminum, such as aluminum-containing antacids, may increase the total body burden of aluminum. Patients with normal renal function receiving the recommended doses of sucralfate and aluminum-containing products adequately excrete aluminum in the urine. Patients with chronic renal failure or those receiving dialysis have impaired excretion of absorbed aluminum. In addition, aluminum does not cross dialysis membranes because it is bound to albumin and transferrin plasma proteins. Aluminum accumulation and toxicity (aluminum osteodystrophy, osteomalacia, encephalopathy) have been described in patients with renal impairment. Sucralfate should be used with caution in patients with chronic renal failure.

CARCINOGENESIS, MUTAGENESIS, AND IMPAIRMENT OF FERTILITY

Chronic oral toxicity studies of 24 months' duration were conducted in mice and rats at doses up to 1 g/kg (12 times the human dose). There was no evidence of drug-related tumorigenicity. A reproduction study in rats at doses up to 38 times the human dose did not reveal any indication of fertility impairment. Mutagenicity studies were not conducted.

PREGNANCY, TERATOGENIC EFFECTS, PREGNANCY CATEGORY B

Teratogenicity studies have been performed in mice, rats, and rabbits at doses up to 50 times the human dose and have revealed no evidence of harm to the fetus due to sucralfate. There are, however, no adequate and well-controlled studies in pregnant women. Because animal reproduction studies are not always predictive of human response, this drug should be used during pregnancy only if clearly needed.

NURSING MOTHERS

It is not known whether this drug is excreted in human milk. Because many drugs are excreted in human milk, caution should be exercised when sucralfate is administered to a nursing woman.

PEDIATRIC USE

Safety and effectiveness in pediatric patients have not been established.

DRUG INTERACTIONS

Some studies have shown that simultaneous sucralfate administration in healthy volunteers reduced the extent of absorption (bioavailability) of single doses of the following: cimetidine, digoxin, fluoroquinolone antibiotics, ketoconazole, I-thyroxine, phenytoin, quinidine, ranitidine, tetracycline, and theophylline. Subtherapeutic prothrombin times with concomitant warfarin and sucralfate therapy have been reported in spontaneous and published case reports. However, two clinical studies have demonstrated no change in either serum warfarin concentration or prothrombin time with the addition of sucralfate to chronic warfarin therapy.

The mechanism of these interactions appears to be nonsystemic in nature, presumably resulting from sucralfate binding to the concomitant agent in the gastrointestinal tract. In all cases studied to date (cimetidine, ciprofloxacin, digoxin, norfloxacin, ofloxacin, and ranitidine), dosing the concomitant medication 2 hours before sucralfate eliminated the interaction. Because of the potential of sucralfate to alter the absorption of some drugs, sucralfate should be administered separately from other drugs when alterations in bioavailability are felt to be critical. In these cases, patients should be monitored appropriately.

ADVERSE REACTIONS

Adverse reactions to sucralfate in clinical trials were minor and only rarely led to discontinuation of the drug. In studies involving over 2700 patients treated with sucralfate tablets, adverse effects were reported in 129 (4.7%).

Constipation was the most frequent complaint (2%). Other adverse effects reported in less than 0.5% of the patients are listed below by body system:

- ***Gastrointestinal:*** Diarrhea, nausea, vomiting, gastric discomfort, indigestion, flatulence, dry mouth.
- ***Dermatologic:*** Pruritus, rash.
- ***Nervous System:*** Dizziness, insomnia, sleepiness, vertigo.
- ***Other:*** Back pain, headache.

Postmarketing reports of hypersensitivity reactions, including urticaria (hives), angioedema, respiratory difficulty, rhinitis, laryngospasm, and facial swelling have been reported in patients receiving sucralfate tablets. Similar events were reported with sucralfate suspension. However, a causal relationship has not been established.

Bezoars have been reported in patients treated with sucralfate. The majority of patients had underlying medical conditions that may predispose to bezoar formation (such as delayed gastric emptying) or were receiving concomitant enteral tube feedings.

Inadvertent injection of insoluble sucralfate and its insoluble excipients has led to fatal complications, including pulmonary and cerebral emboli. Sucralfate is **not** intended for intravenous administration.

DOSAGE AND ADMINISTRATION

ACTIVE DUODENAL ULCER

The recommended adult oral dosage for duodenal ulcer is 1 g four times a day on an empty stomach.

Antacids may be prescribed as needed for relief of pain but should not be taken within one-half hour before or after sucralfate.

While healing with sucralfate may occur during the first week or two, treatment should be continued for 4-8 weeks unless healing has been demonstrated by x-ray or endoscopic examination.

MAINTENANCE THERAPY

Tablets: The recommended adult oral dosage is 1 g twice a day.

HOW SUPPLIED

Tablets: Carafate 1-g tablets are light pink, scored, oblong tablets embossed with Carafate on one side and 1712 on the other.

Suspension: Carafate suspension 1 g/10 ml is a pink suspension.

Shake Well Before Using. Store at controlled room temperature 15-30°C (59- 86°F). Avoid freezing.

PRODUCT LISTING - RATED THERAPEUTICALLY EQUIVALENT

Tablet - Oral - 1 Gm

20's	$20.58	CARAFATE, Allscripts Pharmaceutical Company	54569-0422-00
20's	$24.33	CARAFATE, Pd-Rx Pharmaceuticals	55289-0968-20
25 x 30	$577.28	GENERIC, Sky Pharmaceuticals Packaging, Inc	63739-0261-03
25's	$20.35	GENERIC, Udl Laboratories Inc	51079-0871-19
30's	$33.90	CARAFATE, Pharma Pac	52959-0052-30
31 x 10	$238.85	GENERIC, Vangard Labs	00615-4517-53
31 x 10	$238.85	GENERIC, Vangard Labs	00615-4517-63
60's	$43.77	GENERIC, Allscripts Pharmaceutical Company	54569-4446-00
60's	$61.75	CARAFATE, Physicians Total Care	54868-0312-05
100's	$69.10	GENERIC, Major Pharmaceuticals Inc	00904-5438-60
100's	$70.80	GENERIC, Qualitest Products Inc	00603-5773-21
100's	$70.92	GENERIC, Watson/Rugby Laboratories Inc	00536-1127-01
100's	$70.92	GENERIC, Watson Laboratories Inc	52544-0780-01
100's	$72.94	GENERIC, Martec Pharmaceuticals Inc	52555-0057-01
100's	$72.94	GENERIC, Warrick Pharmaceuticals Corporation	59930-1532-01
100's	$72.95	GENERIC, Teva Pharmaceuticals Usa	00093-2210-01
100's	$77.06	GENERIC, Udl Laboratories Inc	51079-0871-20
100's	$84.60	GENERIC, Eon Labs Manufacturing Inc	00185-2100-01
100's	$100.85	CARAFATE, Aventis Pharmaceuticals	00088-1712-47
100's	$109.08	CARAFATE, Aventis Pharmaceuticals	00088-1712-49
120's	$114.86	CARAFATE, Aventis Pharmaceuticals	00088-1712-53
120's	$129.42	CARAFATE, Physicians Total Care	54868-0312-02
200 x 5	$770.48	GENERIC, Vangard Labs	00615-4517-43

Tablet - Oral - 1 gm

100's	$36.90	FEDERAL UPPER LIMIT, H.C.F.A. F F P	99999-2280-01

PRODUCT LISTING - EQUIVALENTS NOT AVAILABLE

Suspension - Oral - 1 Gm/10 ml

10 ml x 50	$110.00	GENERIC, Alpharma Uspd Makers Of Barre and Nmc	50962-0875-60
414 ml	$42.10	CARAFATE, Aventis Pharmaceuticals	00088-1700-15
420 ml	$40.82	CARAFATE, Physicians Total Care	54868-3735-00

Tablet - Oral - 1 Gm

30's	$20.19	GENERIC, Physicians Total Care	54868-3933-00
100's	$72.95	GENERIC, Dixon-Shane Inc	17236-0546-01
120's	$87.54	GENERIC, Allscripts Pharmaceutical Company	54569-4446-02

Sufentanil Citrate (002281)

For complete prescribing information, refer to the CD-ROM included with the book.

For related information, see the comparative table section in Appendix A.

Categories: Anesthesia, general; Anesthesia, general, adjunct; Pain, subdural; Pregnancy Category C; DEA Class CII; FDA Approved 1984 May
Drug Classes: Analgesics, narcotic; Anesthetics, general
Brand Names: Sufenta
Foreign Brand Availability: Sufenta Forte (South-Africa)

DESCRIPTION

Sufenta (sufentanil citrate) is a potent opioid analgesic chemically designated as N-[4-(methoxymethyl)-1-[2-(2-thienyl)ethyl]-4- piperidinyl]-N-phenylpropanamide 2-hydroxy-1,2,3-propanetricarboxylate (1:1) with a molecular weight of 578.68.

Sufenta is a sterile, preservative free, aqueous solution containing sufentanil citrate equivalent to 50 μg/ml of sufentanil base for intravenous injection. The solution has a pH range of 3.5-6.0.

INDICATIONS AND USAGE

Sufentanil citrate is indicated for intravenous administration:

as an analgesic adjunct in the maintenance of balanced general anesthesia in patients who are intubated and ventilated.

as a primary anesthetic agent for the induction and maintenance of anesthesia with 100% oxygen in patients undergoing major surgical procedures, in patients who are intubated and ventilated, such as cardiovascular surgery or neurosurgical procedures in the sitting position, to provide favorable and cerebral oxygen balance or when extended postoperative ventilation is anticipated.

Sufentanil citrate is indicated for epidural administration asa an analgesic combined with low dose bupivacaine, usually 12.5 mg per administration, during labor and vaginal delivery.

SEE DOSAGE AND ADMINISTRATION FOR MORE COMPLETE INFORMATION ON THE USE OF SUFENTANIL CITRATE.

CONTRAINDICATIONS

Sufentanil citrate is contraindicated in patients with known hypersensitivity to the drug.

WARNINGS

SUFENTANIL CITRATE SHOULD BE ADMINISTERED ONLY BY PERSONS SPECIFICALLY TRAINED IN THE USE OF INTRAVENOUS ANESTHETICS AND MANAGEMENT OF THE RESPIRATORY EFFECTS OF POTENT OPIOIDS.

AN OPIOID ANTAGONIST, RESUSCITATIVE AND INTUBATION EQUIPMENT AND OXYGEN SHOULD BE READILY AVAILABLE.

PRIOR TO CATHETER INSERTION, THE PHYSICIAN SHOULD BE FAMILIAR WITH PATIENT CONDITIONS (SUCH AS INFECTION AT THE SITE, BLEEDING DIATHESIS, ANTICOAGULANT THERAPY, ETC.) WHICH CALL FOR SPECIAL EVALUATION OF THE BENEFIT VERSUS RISK POTENTIAL.

INTRAVENOUS USE

Intravenous administration or unintentional intravascular injection during epidural administration of sufentanil citrate may cause skeletal muscle rigidity, particularly of the truncal muscles. The incidence and severity of muscle rigidity is dose related. Administration of sufentanil citrate may produce muscular rigidity with a more rapid onset of action than that seen with fentanyl. Sufentanil citrate may produce muscular rigidity that involves the skeletal muscles of the neck and extremities. As with fentanyl, muscular rigidity has been reported to occur or recur infrequently in the extended postoperative period. The incidence of muscular rigidity associated with intravenous sufentanil citrate can be reduced by: 1) administration of up to ¼ of the full paralyzing dose of a non- depolarizing neuromuscular blocking agent just prior to administration of sufentanil citrate at dosages of up to 8 μg/kg, 2) administration of a full paralyzing dose of a neuromuscular blocking agent following loss of consciousness when sufentanil citrate is used in anesthetic dosages (above 8 μg/kg) titrated by slow intravenous infusion, or, 3) simultaneous administration of sufentanil citrate and a full paralyzing dose of a neuromuscular blocking agent when sufentanil citrate is used in rapidly administered anesthetic dosages (above 8 μg/kg).

The neuromuscular blocking agents used should be compatible with the patient's cardiovascular status. Adequate facilities should be available for post-operative monitoring and ventilation of patients administered sufentanil citrate. It is essential that these facilities be fully equipped to handle all degrees of respiratory depression.

DOSAGE AND ADMINISTRATION

The dosage of sufentanil citrate should be individualized in each case according to body weight, physical status, underlying pathological condition, use of other drugs, and type of surgical procedure and anesthesia. In obese patients (more than 20% above ideal total body weight), the dosage of sufentanil citrate should be determined on the basis of lean body weight. Dosage should be reduced in elderly and debilitated patients.

Vital signs should be monitored routinely.

Parenteral drug products should be inspected visually for particulate matter and discoloration prior to administration, whenever solution and container permit.

INTRAVENOUS USE

Sufentanil citrate may be administered intravenously by slow injection or infusion 1) in doses of up to 8 μg/kg as an analgesic adjunct to general anesthesia, and 2) in doses ≥8 μg/kg as a primary anesthetic agent for induction and maintenance of anesthesia. If benzodiazepines, barbiturates, inhalation agents, other opioids or other central nervous system depressants are used concomitantly, the dose of sufentanil citrate and/or these agents should be reduced. In all cases dosage should be titrated to individual patient response.

Usage in Children

For induction and maintenance of anesthesia in children less than 12 years of age undergoing cardiovascular surgery, an anesthetic dose of 10-25 μg/kg administered with 100% oxygen is generally recommended. Supplemental dosages of up to 25-50 μg are recommended for maintenance, based on response to initial dose and as determined by changes in vital signs indicating surgical stress or lightening of anesthesia.

Premedication

The selection of preanesthetic medications should be based upon the needs of the individual patient.

Neuromuscular Blocking Agents

The neuromuscular blocking agent selected should be compatible with the patient's condition, taking into account the hemodynamic effects of a particular muscle relaxant and the degree of skeletal muscle relaxation required (see WARNINGS).

ANALGESIC DOSAGES

Total Dosage

Total dosage requirements of 1 μg/kg/h or less are recommended

Incremental or Infusion: 1-2 μg/kg

(Expected duration of anesthesia 1-2 hours). Approximately 75% or more of the total calculated sufentanil citrate dosage may be administered prior to intubation by either slow injection or infusion titrated to individual patient response. Dosage in this range generally administered with nitrous oxide/oxygen in patients undergoing general surgery in which endotracheal intubation and mechanical ventilation are required.

MAINTENANCE DOSAGE

Maintenance Dosage

Total dosage requirements of 1 μg/kg/h or less are recommended

Incremental: 10-25 μg (0.2-0.5 ml)

May be administered in increments as needed when movement and/or changes in vital signs indicate surgical stress or lightening of analgesia. Supplemental dosages should be individualized and adjusted to remaining operative time anticipated.

Infusion

Sufentanil citrate may be administered as an intermittent or continuous infusion as needed in response to signs of lightening of analgesia. In absence of signs of lightening of analgesia infusion rates should always be adjusted downward until there is some response to surgical stimulation. Maintenance infusion rates should be adjusted based upon the induction dose of sufentanil citrate so that the total dose does not exceed 1 μg/kg/h of expected surgical time. Dosage should be individualized and adjusted to remaining operative time anticipated.

ANALGESIC DOSAGES

Total Dosage

Total dosage requirements of 1 μg/kg/h or less are recommended

Incremental or Infusion: 2-8 μg/kg

(Expected duration of anesthesia 2-8 hours). Approximately 75% or less of the total calculated sufentanil citrate dosage may be administered by slow injection or infusion prior to intubation, titrated to individual patient response. Dosages in this range are generally administered with nitrous oxide/oxygen in patients undergoing more complicated major surgical procedures in which endotracheal intubation and mechanical ventilation are required. At dosages in this range, sufentanil citrate has been shown to provide some attenuation of sympathetic reflex activity in response to surgical stimuli, provide hemodynamic stability, and provide relatively rapid recovery.

MAINTENANCE DOSAGE

Maintenance Dosage

Total dosage requirements of 1 μg/kg/h or less are recommended

Incremental

10-50 μg (0.2 ml) may be administered in increments as needed when movement and/or changes in vital signs indicate surgical stress or lightening of analgesia. Supplemental dosages should be individualized and adjusted to remaining operative time anticipated.

Infusion

Sufentanil citrate may be administered as an intermittent or continuous infusion as needed in response to signs of lightening of analgesia. In the absence of signs of lightening of analgesia, infusion rates should always be adjusted downward until there is some response to surgical stimulation. Maintenance infusion rates should be adjusted based upon the induction dose of sufentanil citrate so that the total dose does not exceed 1 μg/kg/h of expected surgical time. Dosage should be individualized and adjusted to remaining operative time anticipated.

ANESTHETIC DOSAGES - TOTAL DOSAGE

Incremental or Infusion: 8-30 μg/kg (anesthetic doses)

At this anesthetic dosage range sufentanil citrate is generally administered as a slow injection, as an infusion, or as an injection followed by an infusion. Sufentanil citrate with 100% oxygen and a muscle relaxant has been found to produce sleep at dosages ≥8 μg/kg and to maintain a deep level of anesthesia without the use of additional anesthetic agents. The addition of N_2O to these dosages will reduce systolic blood pressure. At dosages in this range of up to 25 μg/kg, catecholamine release is attenuated. Dosages of 25-30 μg/kg have been shown to block sympathetic responses including catecholamine release. High doses are indicated in patients undergoing major surgical procedures, in which endotracheal intubation and mechanical ventilation are required, such as cardiovascular surgery and neurosurgery in the sitting position with maintenance of favorable myocardial and cerebral oxygen balance. Postoperative observation is essential and postoperative mechanical ventilation may be required at the higher dosage range due to extended postoperative respiratory depression. Dosage should be titrated to individual patient response.

ANESTHETIC DOSAGES — MAINTENANCE DOSAGE

Incremental

Depending on the initial dose, maintenance doses of 0.5-10 μg/kg may be administered by slow injection in anticipation of surgical stress such as incision, sternotomy or cardiopulmonary bypass.

Infusion

Sufentanil citrate may be administered by continuous or intermittent infusion as needed in response to signs of lightening of anesthesia. In the absence of lightening of anesthesia, infusion rates should be adjusted downward until there is some response to surgical stimulation. The maintenance infusion rate for sufentanil citrate should be based upon the induction dose so that the total dose for the procedure does not exceed 30 μg/kg.

In patients administered high doses of sufentanil citrate, it is essential that qualified personnel and adequate facilities are available for the management of postoperative respiratory depression.

Also see WARNINGS section.

For purposes of administering small volumes of sufentanil citrate accurately, the use of a tuberculin syringe or equivalent is recommended.

EPIDURAL USE IN LABOR AND DELIVERY

Proper placement of the needle or catheter in the epidural space should be verified before sufentanil citrate is injected to assure that unintentional intravascular or intrathecal administration does not occur. unintentional intravascular injection of sufentanil citrate could result in a potentially serious overdose, including acute truncal muscular rigidity and apnea. Unintentional intrathecal injection of the full sufentanil, bupivacaine epidural doses and volume could produce effects of high spinal anesthesia including prolonged paralysis and delayed recovery. If analgesia is inadequate, the placement and integrity of the catheter should be verified prior to the administration of any additional epidural medication. Sufentanil citrate should be administered by slow injection. Respiration should be closely monitored following each administration of an epidural injection of sufentanil citrate.

Dosage for Labor and Delivery

The recommended dosage is sufentanil citrate 10-15 µg administered with 10 ml bupivacaine 0.125% with or without epinephrine. Sufentanil citrate and bupivacaine should be mixed together before administration. Doses can be repeated twice (for a total of 3 doses) at not less than 1 hour intervals until delivery.

PRODUCT LISTING - RATED THERAPEUTICALLY EQUIVALENT

Solution - Intravenous - 50 mcg/ml

Size	Price	Product	NDC
1 ml x 10	$63.65	GENERIC, Abbott Pharmaceutical	00074-3380-31
1 ml x 10	$112.50	GENERIC, Baxter Pharmaceutical Products, Inc	10019-0050-43
1 ml x 10	$113.88	GENERIC, Esi Lederle Generics	00641-5141-33
1 ml x 10	$113.90	GENERIC, Esi Lederle Generics	00641-1141-33
1 ml x 10	$116.61	GENERIC, Abbott Pharmaceutical	00074-3382-21
1 ml x 10	$146.50	SUFENTA, Taylor Pharmaceuticals	11098-0050-01
2 ml x 10	$111.74	GENERIC, Abbott Pharmaceutical	00074-3380-32
2 ml x 10	$200.00	GENERIC, Baxter Pharmaceutical Products, Inc	10019-0050-21
2 ml x 10	$203.89	GENERIC, Esi Lederle Generics	00641-5142-33
2 ml x 10	$203.90	GENERIC, Esi Lederle Generics	00641-1142-33
2 ml x 10	$206.51	GENERIC, Abbott Pharmaceutical	00074-3382-22
2 ml x 10	$259.80	SUFENTA, Taylor Pharmaceuticals	11098-0050-02
5 ml x 10	$239.52	GENERIC, Abbott Pharmaceutical	00074-3380-35
5 ml x 10	$244.98	GENERIC, Abbott Pharmaceutical	00074-3382-25
5 ml x 10	$423.10	GENERIC, Esi Lederle Generics	00641-1143-33
5 ml x 10	$423.13	GENERIC, Esi Lederle Generics	00641-5143-33
5 ml x 10	$539.80	SUFENTA, Taylor Pharmaceuticals	11098-0050-05

Sulconazole Nitrate *(002282)*

Categories: Tinea corporis; Tinea cruris; Tinea pedis; Tinea versicolor; Pregnancy Category C; FDA Approved 1989 Feb
Drug Classes: Antifungals, topical; Dermatologics
Brand Names: Exelderm; Sulcosyn
Foreign Brand Availability: Suldisyn (Greece)
Cost of Therapy: $12.56 (Fungal Infection; Exelderm Cream; 1%; 15 g; 2 applications/day; variable day supply)

DESCRIPTION

Sulconazole nitrate is a white to off-white crystalline powder with a molecular weight of 460.77. It is freely soluble in pyridine: slightly soluble in ethanol, acetone, and chloroform: and very slightly soluble in water. It has a melting point of about 130°C.

Exelderm (sulconazole nitrate) Cream 1.0% and Exelderm (sulconazole nitrate) Solution 1.0% is a broad-spectrum antifungal agent intended for topical application. Sulconazole nitrate, the active ingredient in Exelderm Cream, is an imidazole derivative with in vitro antifungal and antiyeast activity. Its chemical name is (±)-1-(2.4-dichloro-β-((p-chlorobenzyl)-thio)-phenethyl) imidazole mononitrate.

Exelderm Cream contains sulconazole nitrate 10 mg/g in an emollient cream base consisting of propylene glycol, stearyl alcohol, isopropyl myristate, cetyl alcohol, polysorbate 60, sorbitan monostearate, glyceryl stearate (and) PEG-100 stearate, ascorbyl palmitate, and purified water, with sodium hydroxide and/or nitric acid added to adjust the pH.

Exelderm Solution contains sulconazole nitrate 10 mg/ml in a solution consisting of propylene glycol, poloxamer 407, polysorbate 20, butylated hydroxyanisole, and purified water, with sodium hydroxide and, if necessary, nitric acid added to adjust the pH.

Storage: Avoid excessive heat, above 40°C (104°F).

CLINICAL PHARMACOLOGY

Sulconazole nitrate is an imidazole derivative with broad-spectrum antifungal activity that inhibits the growth in vitro of the common pathogenic dermatophytes including *Trichophyton rubrum, Trichophyton mentagrophytes, Epidermophyton floccosum* and *Microsporum canis*. It also inhibits (*in vitro*) the organism responsible for tinea versicolor, *Malassezia furfur*. Sulconazole nitrate has been shown to be active *in vitro* against the following microorganisms, although clinical efficacy has not been established:*Candida albicans* and certain gram positive bacteria.

A modified Draize test showed no allergic contact dermatitis and a phototoxicity study showed no phototoxic or photoallergic reaction to sulconazole nitrate cream. Maximization tests with sulconazole nitrate cream showed no evidence of contact sensitization or irritation.

INDICATIONS AND USAGE

Sulconazole nitrate cream, 1.0% is an antifungal agent indicated for the treatment of tinea pedis (athlete's foot), tinea cruris, and tinea corporis caused by *Trichophyton rubrum, Trichophyton mentagrophytes, Epidermophyton floccosum,* and *Microsporum canis,** and for the treatment of tinea versicolor.

CONTRAINDICATIONS

Sulconazole nitrate cream, 1.0% is contraindicated in patients who have a history of hypersensitivity to any of its ingredients.

PRECAUTIONS

GENERAL

Sulconazole nitrate cream, 1.0% is for external use only. Avoid contact with the eyes. If irritation develops, the cream should be discontinued and appropriate therapy instituted.

INFORMATION FOR THE PATIENT

Patients should be told to use sulconazole nitrate cream as directed by the physician, to use it externally only, and to avoid contact with he eyes.

CARCINOGENESIS, MUTAGENESIS, AND IMPAIRMENT OF FERTILITY

Long-term animal studies to determine carcinogenic potential have not been performed. In vitro studies have shown no mutagenic activity.

PREGNANCY CATEGORY C

There are no adequate and well controlled studies in pregnant women. Sulconazole nitrate should be used during pregnancy only if clearly needed. Sulconazole nitrate has been shown to be embryotoxic in rats when given in doses of 125 times the adult human dose (in mg/kg). The drug was not teratogenic in rats or rabbits at oral doses of 50 mg/kg/day.

Sulconazole nitrate given orally to rats at a dose 125 times the human dose resulted in prolonged gestation and dystocia. Several females died during the prenatal period, most likely due to labor complications.

NURSING MOTHERS

It is not known whether sulconazole nitrate is excreted in human milk. Caution should be exercised when sulconazole nitrate is administered to an nursing woman.

PEDIATRIC USE

Safety and effectiveness in children have not been established.

ADVERSE REACTIONS

There were no systemic effects and only infrequent cutaneous adverse reactions in 1185 patient treated with sulconazole nitrate cream in controlled clinical trials. Approximately 3% of these patients reported itching, 3% burning or stinging, and 1% redness. These complaints did not usually interfere with treatment.

DOSAGE AND ADMINISTRATION

CREAM

A small amount of cream should be gently massaged into the affected and surrounding skin areas once or twice daily, except in tinea pedis, where administration should be twice daily.

Early relief of symptoms is experienced by the majority of patients and clinical improvement may be seen fairly soon after treatment is begun; however, tinea corporis/cruris and tinea versicolor should be treated for 3 weeks and tinea pedis for 4 weeks to reduce the possibility of recurrence.

If significant clinical improvement is not seen after 4-6 weeks of treatment, an alternate diagnosis should be considered.

SOLUTION

A small amount of the solution should be gently massaged into the affected and surrounding skin areas once or twice daily.

Symptomatic relief usually occurs within a few days after starting sulconazole nitrate solution, 1.0% and clinical improvement usually occurs within one week. To reduce the possibility of recurrence, tinea cruris, tinea corporis, and tinea versicolor should be treated for 3 weeks.

If significant clinical improvement is not seen after 4 weeks of treatment, an alternate diagnosis should be considered.

*Efficacy for this organism in the organ system was studied in fewer than ten infections.

PRODUCT LISTING - EQUIVALENTS NOT AVAILABLE

Size	Price	Product	NDC
Cream - Topical - 1%			
15 gm	$12.56	EXELDERM, Bristol-Myers Squibb	00072-8200-15
30 gm	$22.10	EXELDERM, Bristol-Myers Squibb	00072-8200-30
60 gm	$36.64	EXELDERM, Bristol-Myers Squibb	00072-8200-60
Solution - Topical - 1%			
30 ml	$27.05	EXELDERM, Bristol-Myers Squibb	00072-8400-30

Sulfacetamide Sodium *(002284)*

Categories: Conjunctivitis, infectious; Trachoma; Pregnancy Category C; FDA Approved 1946 Aug

Drug Classes: Antibiotics, sulfonamides; Anti-infectives, ophthalmic; Ophthalmics

Brand Names: Ak-Sulf; Bleph-10; Cetamide; Colirio Sulfacetamido Kriya; Dayto-Sulf; I-Sulfacet; Infa-Sulf; Isopto Cetamide; **Klaron**; Lersa; Ocu-Sul; Ocusulf; Ophthacet; Optin; Sebizon; **Sodium Sulamyd**; Sodium Sulfacetamide; Spectro-Sulf; Storz-Sulf; Sulf-10; Sulfac; Sulfacel-15; Sulfacet Sodium; Sulfair; Sulfamide; Sulten-10

Foreign Brand Availability: Acetopt (Australia; New-Zealand; Philippines); Albucid (Bahamas; Bahrain; Barbados; Belize; Benin; Bermuda; Burkina-Faso; Curacao; Cyprus; Egypt; Ethiopia; Gambia; Germany; Ghana; Guinea; Guyana; India; Indonesia; Iran; Iraq; Ivory-Coast; Jamaica; Jordan; Kenya; Kuwait; Lebanon; Liberia; Libya; Malawi; Mali; Mauritania; Mauritius; Morocco; Netherland-Antilles; Niger; Nigeria; Oman; Puerto-Rico; Qatar; Republic-of-Yemen; Saudi-Arabia; Senegal; Seychelles; Sierra-Leone; Sudan; Surinam; Syria; Tanzania; Trinidad; Tunia; Uganda; United-Arab-Emirates; Zambia; Zimbabwe); Antebor (Belgium; France; Switzerland); Beocid Puroptal (Austria); Blef-10 (Colombia; Ecuador; Peru); Blef 10 con Lagrifilm (Mexico); Blef-30 (Colombia); Bleph-30 (Bahrain; Cyprus; Egypt; Iran; Iraq; Jordan; Kuwait; Lebanon; Libya; Oman; Qatar; Republic-of-Yemen; Saudi-Arabia; Syria; United-Arab-Emirates); Bleph Liquifilm (New-Zealand); Cetazin (Austria); Covosulf (South-Africa); Dansemid (Indonesia); Isopto Cetamida (Ecuador); Locula (India); Optamide (Australia); Optisol (Israel); Prontamid (Italy); Spersacet (Hong-Kong; Switzerland); Sul 10 (Mexico); Sulfableph (Germany); Sulfacetamid Ofteno al 10% (Costa-Rica; Dominican-Republic; El-Salvador; Guatemala; Honduras; Mexico; Nicaragua; Panama); Sulfacid (Israel); Sulfa 10 (Belgium); Sulfex (Hong-Kong); Sulop (Peru); Sulphacalyre (Bahamas; Barbados; Belize; Bermuda; Curacao; Guyana; Jamaica; Netherland-Antilles; Puerto-Rico; Surinam; Trinidad)

OPHTHALMIC

DESCRIPTION

Sulfacetamide sodium ophthalmic solution is a sterile, topical anti-bacterial agent for ophthalmic use.

Chemical name: *N*-Sulfanilylacetamide monosodium salt monohydrate.

The plastic squeeze bottle contains: *Active:* Sulfacetamide sodium 10% (100 mg/ml). *Preservative:* Thimerosal 0.1 mg/ml. *Inactives:* Boric acid, hydroxypropyl methylcellulose 2208 (4000 cps) 1.0 mg/ml, sodium thiosulfate and purified water. Sodium carbonate anhydrous and/or hydrochloric acid to adjust pH (7.0-7.4) when necessary.

The dropperettes applicator contains: *Active:* Sulfacetamide sodium 10% (100 mg/ml). *Preservative:* Thimerosal 0.05 mg/ml. *Inactives:* Boric acid, sodium thiosulfate and purified water. Sodium carbonate anhydrous and/or hydrochloric acid to adjust pH (7.0-7.4) when necessary.

STORAGE

KEEP BOTTLE TIGHTLY CLOSED.

Store at controlled room temperature 15-30°C (59-86°F).

Sulfonamide solutions darken on prolonged standing and exposure to heat and light. Do not use if solution has darkened. Yellowishness does not affect activity.

CLINICAL PHARMACOLOGY

MICROBIOLOGY

The sulfonamides are bacteriostatic agents and the spectrum of activity is similar for all. Sulfonamides inhibit bacterial synthesis of dihydrofolic acid by preventing the condensation of the pteridine with aminobenzoic acid through competitive inhibition of the enzyme dihydropteroate synthetase. Resistant strains have altered dihydropteroate synthetase with reduced affinity for sulfonamides or produce increased quantities of aminobenzoic acid.

Topically applied sulfonamides do not provide adequate coverage against susceptible strains of the following common bacterial eye pathogens: *Escherichia coli, Staphylococcus aureus, Streptococcus pneumoniae, Streptococcus* (viridans group), *Haemophilus influenzae, Klebsiella species,* and *Enterobacter* species.

Topically applied sulfonamides do not provide adequate coverage against *Neisseria* species, *Serratia marcescens* and *Pseudomonas aeruginosa.* A significant percentage of staphylococcal isolates are completely resistant to sulfa drugs.

INDICATIONS AND USAGE

For the treatment of conjunctivitis and other superficial ocular infections due to susceptible microorganisms and as an adjunctive in systemic sulfonamide therapy of trachoma:

Escherichia coli, Staphylococcus aureus, Streptococcus pneumoniae, Streptococcus (viridans group), *Haemophilus influenzae, Klebsiella* species, and *Enterobacter* species.

Topically applied sulfonamides do not provide adequate coverage against *Neisseria* species, *Serratia marcescens* and *Pseudomonas aeruginosa.* A significant percentage of staphylococcal isolates are completely resistant sulfa drugs.

CONTRAINDICATIONS

Hypersensitivity to sulfonamides or to any ingredient of the preparation.

WARNINGS

FOR TOPICAL EYE USE ONLY — NOT FOR INJECTION. FATALITIES HAVE OCCURRED, ALTHOUGH RARELY, DUE TO SEVERE REACTIONS TO SULFONAMIDES INCLUDING STEVENS-JOHNSON SYNDROME, TOXIC EPIDERMAL NECROLYSIS, FULMINANT HEPATIC NECROSIS, AGRANULOCYTOSIS, APLASTIC ANEMIA AND OTHER BLOOD DYSCRASIAS. Sensitizations may recur when a sulfonamide is readministered, irrespective of the route of administration. Sensitivity reactions have been reported in individuals with no prior history of sulfonamide hypersensitivity. At the first sign of hypersensitivity, skin rash or other serious reaction, discontinue use of this preparation.

PRECAUTIONS

GENERAL

Prolonged use of topical anti-bacterial agents may give rise to overgrowth of nonsusceptible organisms including fungi. Bacterial resistance to sulfonamides may also develop.

The effectiveness of sulfonamides may be reduced by the paraminobenzoic acid present in purulent exudates.

Sensitization may recur when a sulfonamide is readministered irrespective of the route of administration, and cross-sensitivity between different sulfonamides may occur.

At the first sign of hypersensitivity, increase in purulent discharge, or aggravation of inflammation or pain, the patient should discontinue use of the medication and consult a physician (see WARNINGS).

INFORMATION FOR THE PATIENT

To avoid contamination, do not touch tip of container to eye, eyelid or any surface.

CARCINOGENESIS, MUTAGENESIS, AND IMPAIRMENT OF FERTILITY

No studies have been conducted in animals or in humans to evaluate the possibility of these effects with ocularly administered sulfacetamide. Rats appear to be especially susceptible to the goitrogenic effects of sulfonamides, and long-term oral administration of sulfonamides has resulted in thyroid malignancies in these animals.

PREGNANCY CATEGORY C

Animal reproduction studies have not been conducted with sulfonamide ophthalmic preparations. Kernicterus may occur in the newborn as a result of treatment of a pregnant woman at term with orally administered sulfonamides. There are no adequate and well controlled studies of sulfonamide ophthalmic preparation in pregnant women and it is not known whether topically applied sulfonamides can cause fetal harm when administered to a pregnant woman. This product should be used in pregnancy only if the potential benefit justifies the potential risk to the fetus.

NURSING MOTHERS

Systemically administered sulfonamides are capable of producing kernicterus in infants of lactating women. Because of the potential for the development of kernicterus in neonates, a decision should be made whether to discontinue nursing or discontinue the drug taking into account the importance of the drug to the mother.

PEDIATRIC USE

Safety and effectiveness in children below the age of 2 months have not been established.

ADVERSE REACTIONS

Bacterial and fungal corneal ulcers have developed during treatment with sulfonamide ophthalmic preparations.

The most frequently reported reactions are local irritation, stinging and burning. Less commonly reported reactions include non-specific conjunctivitis, conjunctival hyperemia, secondary infections and allergic reactions.

Fatalities have occurred, although rarely, due to severe reactions to sulfonamides including Stevens-Johnson syndrome, toxic epidermal necrolysis, fulminant hepatic necrosis, agranulocytosis, aplastic anemia, and other blood dyscrasias (see WARNINGS).

DOSAGE AND ADMINISTRATION

FOR CONJUNCTIVITIS AND OTHER SUPERFICIAL OCULAR INFECTIONS

Instill 1 or 2 drops into the conjunctival sac(s) every 2 or 3 hours initially. Dosages may be tapered by increasing the time interval between doses as the condition responds. The usual duration if treatment is 7-10 days.

FOR TRACHOMA

Instill 2 drops into the conjunctival sac(s) of the affected eye(s) every 2 hours. Topical administration must be accompanied by systemic administration.

TOPICAL

DESCRIPTION

Each ml of Klaron lotion, 10%, contains 100 mg of sodium sulfacetamide in a vehicle consisting of purified water; propylene glycol; lauramide DEA (and) diethanolamine; polyethylene glycol 400, monolaurate; hydroxyethyl cellulose; sodium chloride; sodium metabisulfite; methylparaben; xanthan gum; EDTA and simethicone.

Sodium sulfacetamide is a sulfonamide with antibacterial activity. Chemically, sodium sulfacetamide is N′-[(4-aminophenyl)sulfonyl]-acetamide, monosodium salt, monohydrate.

CLINICAL PHARMACOLOGY

The most widely accepted mechanism of action of sulfonamides is the Woods-Fildes theory, based on sulfonamides acting as a competitive inhibitor of para-aminobenzoic acid (PABA) utilization, an essential component for bacterial growth. While absorption through intact skin in humans has not been determined, *in vitro* studies with human cadaver skin indicated a percutaneous absorption of about 4%. Sodium sulfacetamide is readily absorbed from the gastrointestinal tract when taken orally and excreted in the urine largely unchanged. The biological half-life has been reported to be between 7-13 hours.

INDICATIONS AND USAGE

Sodium sulfacetamide lotion, 10%, is indicated in the topical treatment of *acne vulgaris.*

CONTRAINDICATIONS

Sodium sulfacetamide lotion, 10%, is contraindicated for use by patients having known hypersensitivity to sulfonamides or any other component of this preparation (see WARNINGS).

WARNINGS

Fatalities have occurred, although rarely, due to severe reactions to sulfonamides including Stevens-Johnson syndrome, toxic epidermal necrolysis, fulminant hepatic necrosis, agranulocytosis, aplastic anemia, and other blood dyscrasias. Hypersensitivity reactions may occur when a sulfonamide is readministered, irrespective of the route of administration. Sensitiv-

S

ity reactions have been reported in individuals with no prior history of sulfonamide hypersensitivity. At the first sign of hypersensitivity, skin rash or other reactions, discontinue use of this preparation (see ADVERSE REACTIONS).

Sodium sulfacetamide lotion, 10%, contains sodium metabisulfite, a sulfite that may cause allergic-type reactions including anaphylactic symptoms and life-threatening or less severe asthmatic episodes in certain susceptible people. The overall prevalence of sulfite sensitivity in the general population is unknown and probably low. Sulfite sensitivity is seen more frequently in asthmatic than in non-asthmatic people (see CONTRAINDICATIONS).

PRECAUTIONS

GENERAL

For external use only. Keep away from eyes. If irritation develops, use of the product should be discontinued and appropriate therapy instituted. Patients should be carefully observed for possible local irritation or sensitization during long-term therapy. Hypersensitivity reactions may occur when a sulfonamide is readministered irrespective of the route of administration, and cross-sensitivity between different sulfonamides may occur. Sodium sulfacetamide can cause reddening and scaling of the skin. Particular caution should be employed if areas of involved skin to be treated are denuded or abraded.

Keep out of the reach of children.

CARCINOGENESIS, MUTAGENESIS, AND IMPAIRMENT OF FERTILITY

Long-term studies in animals have not been performed to evaluate carcinogenic potential.

PREGNANCY CATEGORY C

Animal reproduction studies have not been conducted with sodium sulfacetamide lotion, 10%. It is also not known whether sodium sulfacetamide lotion, 10%, can cause fetal harm when administered to a pregnant woman or can affect reproduction capacity. Sodium sulfacetamide lotion, 10%, should be given to a pregnant woman only if clearly needed.

Kernicterus may occur in the newborn as a result of treatment of a pregnant woman at term with orally administered sulfonamide. There are no adequate and well controlled studies of sodium sulfacetamide lotion, 10%, in pregnant women, and it is not known whether topically applied sulfonamides can cause fetal harm when administered to a pregnant woman.

NURSING MOTHERS

It is not known whether sodium sulfacetamide is excreted in the human milk following topical use of sodium sulfacetamide lotion, 10%. Systemically administered sulfonamides are capable of producing kernicterus in the infants of lactating women. Small amounts of orally administered sulfonamides have been reported to be eliminated in human milk. Because many drugs are excreted in human milk, caution should be exercised in prescribing for nursing women.

PEDIATRIC USE

Safety and effectiveness in pediatric patients under the age of 12 have not been established.

ADVERSE REACTIONS

In controlled clinical trials for the management of *acne vulgaris*, the occurrence of adverse reactions associated with the use of sodium sulfacetamide lotion, 10%, was infrequent and restricted to local events. The total incidence of adverse reactions reported in these studies was less than 2%. Only 1 of the 105 patients treated with sodium sulfacetamide lotion, 10%, had adverse reactions of erythema, itching and edema. It has been reported that sodium sulfacetamide may cause local irritation, stinging and burning. While the irritation may be transient, occasionally, the use of medication has to be discontinued.

DOSAGE AND ADMINISTRATION

Apply a thin film to affected areas twice daily.

HOW SUPPLIED

Klaron Lotion, 10% (sodium sulfacetamide lotion) comes in 2 and 4 fl oz bottles. Shake well before using.

Storage: Store at controlled room temperature 20-20°C (68-77°F). Keep tightly closed.

S

PRODUCT LISTING - RATED THERAPEUTICALLY EQUIVALENT

Ointment - Ophthalmic - 10%

3 gm	$2.32	GENERIC, Bausch and Lomb	24208-0770-02
3.50 gm	$2.70	GENERIC, Moore, H.L. Drug Exchange Inc	00839-5501-43
3.50 gm	$3.39	GENERIC, Akorn Inc	17478-0227-35
3.50 gm	$8.10	GENERIC, Fougera	00168-0079-38
3.50 gm	$16.25	BLEPH-10, Allergan Inc	00023-0311-04
3.50 gm	$16.25	CETAMIDE, Allscripts Pharmaceutical Company	54569-3235-00
3.50 gm	$19.31	SODIUM SULAMYD, Schering Corporation	00085-0066-03
3.50 gm	$19.31	SODIUM SULAMYD, Allscripts Pharmaceutical Company	54569-0876-00

Solution - Ophthalmic - 10%

1 ml x 12	$27.69	GENERIC, Ciba Vision Ophthalmics	00058-0786-12
1 ml x 12	$35.42	GENERIC, Ciba Vision Ophthalmics	58768-0732-12
2 ml	$2.25	GENERIC, Miza Pharmaceutcials Dba Optopics Laboratories Corporation	52238-0650-02
2 ml	$2.93	GENERIC, Akorn Inc	17478-0221-20
2.50 ml	$4.08	BLEPH-10, Allergan Inc	11980-0011-03
5 ml	$1.08	GENERIC, Miza Pharmaceutcials Dba Optopics Laboratories Corporation	52238-0650-05
5 ml	$3.15	GENERIC, Akorn Inc	17478-0221-10
5 ml	$16.35	BLEPH-10, Allscripts Pharmaceutical Company	54569-1208-00
5 ml	$18.71	BLEPH-10, Allergan Inc	11980-0011-05
5 ml	$22.99	BLEPH-10, Pharma Pac	52959-0272-00
5 ml x 25	$444.00	SODIUM SULAMYD, Schering Corporation	00085-0946-03
15 ml	$1.85	GENERIC, Logen	00820-0104-25
15 ml	$2.30	FEDERAL UPPER LIMIT, H.C.F.A. F F P	99999-2284-06
15 ml	$2.48	SODIUM SULAMYD, Interstate Drug Exchange Inc	00814-7063-42
15 ml	$2.50	GENERIC, Qualitest Products Inc	00603-7280-41
15 ml	$2.56	GENERIC, Roberts/Hauck Pharmaceutical Corporation	43797-0324-21
15 ml	$2.75	GENERIC, Cmc-Consolidated Midland Corporation	00223-6710-15
15 ml	$2.82	GENERIC, Moore, H.L. Drug Exchange Inc	00839-5523-31
15 ml	$3.30	GENERIC, Major Pharmaceuticals Inc	00904-2728-35
15 ml	$3.50	GENERIC, Ivax Corporation	00182-0671-64
15 ml	$3.50	GENERIC, Aligen Independent Laboratories Inc	00405-6135-15
15 ml	$3.53	GENERIC, Akorn Inc	17478-0221-12
15 ml	$3.55	GENERIC, Geneva Pharmaceuticals	00781-7120-85
15 ml	$3.90	GENERIC, Watson/Schein Pharmaceuticals Inc	00364-7136-72
15 ml	$4.20	GENERIC, Miza Pharmaceutcials Dba Optopics Laboratories Corporation	52238-0650-15
15 ml	$5.05	GENERIC, Falcon Pharmaceuticals, Ltd.	61314-0701-01
15 ml	$5.08	GENERIC, Fougera	00168-0220-15
15 ml	$5.08	GENERIC, Mutual/United Research Laboratories	00677-0917-30
15 ml	$5.08	GENERIC, Bausch and Lomb	24208-0418-15
15 ml	$5.08	GENERIC, Bausch and Lomb	24208-0670-04
15 ml	$7.06	GENERIC, Ocusoft	54799-0782-15
15 ml	$22.86	BLEPH-10, Allergan Inc	11980-0011-15
15 ml	$23.58	SODIUM SULAMYD, Schering Corporation	00085-0946-06
15 ml	$24.00	BLEPH-10, Pharma Pac	52959-0272-01
15 ml	$24.41	SODIUM SULAMYD, Allscripts Pharmaceutical Company	54569-0880-00
15 ml	$31.79	SODIUM SULAMYD, Physicians Total Care	54868-0273-00
24 ml	$27.00	GENERIC, Bausch and Lomb	24208-0670-59

Solution - Ophthalmic - 15%

2 ml	$4.72	GENERIC, Alcon Laboratories Inc	00065-0731-12
5 ml	$14.00	ISOPTO CETAMIDE, Alcon Laboratories Inc	00998-0522-05

Solution - Ophthalmic - 30%

15 ml	$5.26	GENERIC, Aligen Independent Laboratories Inc	00405-6137-15
15 ml	$6.30	GENERIC, Qualitest Products Inc	00603-7281-41
15 ml	$6.50	GENERIC, Cmc-Consolidated Midland Corporation	00223-6711-15
15 ml	$25.01	SODIUM SULAMYD, Schering Corporation	00085-0717-06

PRODUCT LISTING - EQUIVALENTS NOT AVAILABLE

Lotion - Topical - 10%

59 ml	$52.21	KLARON, Aventis Pharmaceuticals	00066-7500-02
85 ml	$23.72	SEBIZON, Schering Corporation	00085-0600-05
120 ml	$104.16	KLARON, Aventis Pharmaceuticals	00066-7500-04

Ointment - Ophthalmic - 10%

3 gm	$5.14	GENERIC, Prescript Pharmaceuticals	00247-0113-81
3.50 gm	$1.65	OCU-SUL 10, Ocumed Inc	51944-3500-00
3.50 gm	$2.70	GENERIC, Raway Pharmacal Inc	00686-0771-35
3.50 gm	$2.75	GENERIC, Cmc-Consolidated Midland Corporation	00223-4430-03
3.50 gm	$10.20	GENERIC, Allscripts Pharmaceutical Company	54569-1192-00
3.50 gm	$14.86	GENERIC, Southwood Pharmaceuticals Inc	58016-6063-01
3.50 gm	$16.75	GENERIC, Pharma Pac	52959-1358-03
3.50 gm	$23.09	GENERIC, Pharma Pac	52959-0572-03
4 gm	$2.99	GENERIC, Physicians Total Care	54868-1955-00
4 gm	$17.53	GENERIC, Alpharma Uspd Makers Of Barre and Nmc	63874-0157-04

Soap - Topical - 10%

170 ml	$38.25	OVACE, Healthpoint	00064-4000-06
340 ml	$70.13	OVACE, Healthpoint	00064-4000-12

Solution - Ophthalmic - 10%

2 ml	$2.25	GENERIC, Apotex Usa Inc	60505-7551-01
15 ml	$1.80	OCU-SUL 10, Ocumed Inc	51944-4405-02
15 ml	$2.95	GENERIC, Raway Pharmacal Inc	00686-0670-04
15 ml	$2.95	GENERIC, Apotex Usa Inc	60505-7551-05
15 ml	$2.98	GENERIC, Physicians Total Care	54868-0727-01
15 ml	$4.21	GENERIC, Allscripts Pharmaceutical Company	54569-1186-00
15 ml	$4.51	GENERIC, Dhs Inc	55887-0886-15
15 ml	$4.96	GENERIC, Prescript Pharmaceuticals	00247-0016-15
15 ml	$17.33	GENERIC, Alpharma Uspd Makers Of Barre and Nmc	63874-0136-15
15 ml	$17.75	GENERIC, Southwood Pharmaceuticals Inc	58016-6064-15
15 ml	$21.94	GENERIC, Southwood Pharmaceuticals Inc	58016-6064-01
15 ml	$31.75	GENERIC, Pharma Pac	52959-0117-00

Solution - Ophthalmic - 15%

15 ml	$2.10	OCU-SUL 15, Ocumed Inc	51944-4400-02

Solution - Ophthalmic - 30%

15 ml	$2.40	OCU-SUL 30, Ocumed Inc	51944-4430-02
15 ml	$4.75	GENERIC, Cmc-Consolidated Midland Corporation	00223-0000-00

Sulfadiazine (002286)

For related information, see the comparative table section in Appendix A.

Categories: Chancroid; Conjunctivitis, infectious; Infection, ear, middle; Infection, urinary tract; Malaria; Meningitis; Meningococcal carrier state; Nocardiosis; Toxoplasmosis; Trachoma; Pregnancy Category C; FDA Approved 1994 Jul; Orphan Drugs; WHO Formulary
Drug Classes: Antibiotics, sulfonamides
Brand Names: Microsulfon; Sulfadiazine Sodium
Cost of Therapy: $11.05 (Infection; Generic Tablets; 500 mg; 4 tablets/day; 7 day supply)

DESCRIPTION

Sulfadiazine is an oral sulfonamide anti-bacterial agent.

Each tablet, for oral administration, contains 500 mg sulfadiazine. In addition, each tablet contains the following inactive ingredients: croscarmellose sodium, docusate sodium, microcrystalline cellulose, povidone, sodium benzoate, sodium starch glycolate and stearic acid.

Sulfadiazine occurs as a white or slightly yellow powder. It is odorless, or nearly so, and slowly darkens on exposure to light. It is practically insoluble in water and slightly soluble in alcohol. The chemical name of sulfadiazine is N^1-2-pyrimidinyl sulfanilamide. The molecular formula is $C_{10}H_{10}N_4O_2S$. It has a molecular weight of 250.27.

Most sulfonamides slowly darken on exposure to light.

CLINICAL PHARMACOLOGY

The systemic sulfonamides are bacteriostatic agents having a similar spectrum of activity. Sulfonamides competitively inhibit bacterial synthesis of folic acid (pteroylglutamic acid) from aminobenzoic acid. Resistant strains are capable of utilizing folic acid precursors or preformed folic acid.

Sulfonamides exist in the blood in 3 forms — free, conjugated (acetylated and possibly others), and protein bound. The free form is considered to be the therapeutically active one.

Sulfadiazine given orally is readily absorbed from the gastrointestinal tract. After a single 2 g oral dose, a peak of 6.04 mg/100 ml is reached in 4 hours; of this, 4.65 mg/100 ml is free drug.

When a dose of 100 mg/kg of body weight is given initially and followed by 50 mg/kg every 6 hours, blood levels of free sulfadiazine are about 7 mg/100 ml. Protein binding is 38-48%.

Sulfadiazine diffuses into the cerebrospinal fluid; free drug reaches 32-65% of blood levels and total drug 40-60%.

Sulfadiazine is excreted largely in the urine, where concentrations are 10-25 times greater than serum levels. Approximately 10% of a single oral dose is excreted in the first 6 hours, 50% within 24 hours, and 60-85% in 48-72 hours. Of the amount excreted in the urine, 15%-40% is in the acetyl form.

INDICATIONS AND USAGE

Sulfadiazine tablets are indicated in the following conditions:

- Chancroid.
- Trachoma.
- Inclusion conjunctivitis.
- Nocardiosis.
- Urinary tract infections (primarily pyelonephritis, pyelitis, and cystitis) in the absence of obstructive uropathy or foreign bodies, when these infections are caused by susceptible strains of the following organisms: *Escherichia coli, Klebsiella species, Enterobacter species, Staphylococcus aureus, Proteus mirabilis,* and *P. vulgaris.* Sulfadiazine should be used for urinary tract infections only after use of more soluble sulfonamides has been unsuccessful.
- Toxoplasmosis, as adjunctive therapy with pyrimethamine. Malaria due to chloroquine-resistant strains of *Plasmodium falciparum,* when used as an adjunctive therapy.
- Prophylaxis of meningococcal meningitis when sulfonamide-sensitive group A strains are known to prevail in family groups or larger closed populations (the prophylactic usefulness of sulfonamides when group B or C infections are prevalent is not proved and may be harmful in closed population groups.)
- Meningococcal meningitis, when the organism has been demonstrated to be susceptible.
- Acute otitis media due to *Haemophilus influenzae,* when used concomitantly with adequate doses of penicillin.
- Prophylaxis against recurrences of rheumatic fever, as an alternative to penicillin.
- *H. influenzae meningitis,* as an adjunctive therapy with parenteral streptomycin.

IMPORTANT NOTES

In vitro sulfonamide susceptibility tests are not always reliable. The test must be carefully coordinated with bacteriologic and clinical response. When the patient is already taking sulfonamides, follow-up cultures should have aminobenzoic acid added to the culture media.

Currently, the increasing frequency of resistant organisms limits the usefulness of antibacterial agents, including the sulfonamides, especially in the treatment of recurrent and complicated urinary tract infections.

Wide variation in blood levels may result with identical doses. Blood levels should be measured in patients receiving sulfonamides for serious infections. Free sulfonamide blood levels of 5-15 mg per 100 ml may be considered therapeutically effective for most infections, and blood levels of 12-15 mg per 100 ml may be considered optimal for serious infections. Twenty mg per 100 ml should be the maximum total sulfonamide level, since adverse reactions occur more frequently above this level.

CONTRAINDICATIONS

Sulfadiazine is contraindicated in the following circumstances: hypersensitivity to sulfonamides.

In infants less than 2 months of age (except as adjunctive therapy with pyrimethamine in the treatment of congenital toxoplasmosis).

In pregnancy at term and during the nursing period, because sulfonamides cross the placenta and are excreted in breast milk and may cause kernicterus.

WARNINGS

The sulfonamides should not be used for the treatment of group A beta-hemolytic streptococcal infections. In an established infection, they will not eradicate the streptococcus and, therefore, will not prevent sequelae such as rheumatic fever and glomerulonephritis.

Deaths associated with the administration of sulfonamides have been reported from hypersensitivity reactions, agranulocytosis, aplastic anemia, and other blood dyscrasias.

The presence of such clinical signs as sore throat, fever, pallor, purpura, or jaundice may be early indications of serious blood disorders.

The frequency of renal complications is considerably lower in patients receiving the more soluble sulfonamides.

PRECAUTIONS

GENERAL

Sulfonamides should be given with caution to patients with impaired renal of hepatic function and to those with severe allergy or bronchial asthma.

Hemolysis may occur in individuals deficient in glucose-6-phosphate dehydrogenase. This reaction is dose related.

Adequate fluid intake must be maintained in order to prevent crystalluria and stone formation.

INFORMATION FOR THE PATIENT

Patients should be instructed to drink an 8 ounce glass of water with each dose of medication and at frequent intervals throughout the day. Caution patients to report promptly the onset of sore throat, fever, pallor, purpura, or jaundice when taking this drug, since these may be early indications of serious blood disorders.

LABORATORY TESTS

Complete blood counts and urinalyses with careful microscopic examinations should be done frequently in patients receiving sulfonamides.

CARCINOGENESIS, MUTAGENESIS, AND IMPAIRMENT OF FERTILITY

The sulfonamides bear certain chemical similarities to some goitrogens. Rats appear to be especially susceptible to the goitrogenic effects of sulfonamides, and long-term administration has produced thyroid malignancies in rats.

PREGNANCY, TERATOGENIC EFFECTS, PREGNANCY CATEGORY C

The safe use of sulfonamides in pregnancy has not been established. The teratogenic potential of most sulfonamides has not been thoroughly investigated in either animals or humans. However, a significant increase in the incidence of cleft palate and other bony abnormalities in offspring has been observed when certain sulfonamides of the short, intermediate, and long acting types were given to pregnant rats and mice in high oral doses (7-25 times the human therapeutic dose).

NURSING MOTHERS

Sulfadiazine is contraindicated for use in nursing mothers because the sulfonamides cross the placenta, are excreted in breast milk and may cause kernicterus.

Because of the potential for serious adverse reactions in nursing infants from sulfadiazine, a decision should be made whether to discontinue nursing or to discontinue the drug, taking into account the importance of the drug to the mother. See CONTRAINDICATIONS.

PEDIATRIC USE

Sulfadiazine is contraindicated in infants less than 2 months of age (except as adjunctive therapy with pyrimethamine in the treatment of congenital toxoplasmosis). See CONTRAINDICATIONS and DOSAGE AND ADMINISTRATION.

S

ADVERSE REACTIONS

Blood Dyscrasias: Agranulocytosis, aplastic anemia, thrombocytopenia, leukopenia, hemolytic anemia, purpura, hypothrombinemia, and methemoglobinemia.

Allergic Reactions: Erythema multiforme (Stevens-Johnson syndrome), generalized skin eruptions, epidermal necrolysis, urticaria, serum sickness, pruritus, exfoliative dermatitis, anaphylactoid reactions, periorbital edema, conjunctival and scleral injection, photosensitization, arthralgia, allergic myocarditis, drug fever, and chills.

Gastrointestinal Reactions: Nausea, emesis, abdominal pains, hepatitis, diarrhea, anorexia, pancreatitis, and stomatitis.

C.N.S. Reactions: Headache, peripheral neuritis, mental depression, convulsions, ataxia, hallucinations, tinnitus, vertigo, and insomnia.

Renal: Crystalluria, stone formation, toxic nephrosis with oliguria and anuria; periarteritis nodosa and lupus erythematosus phenomenon have been noted.

Miscellaneous Reactions: The sulfonamides bear certain chemical similarities to some goitrogens, diuretics (acetazolamide and the thiazides), and oral hypoglycemic agents. Goiter production, diuresis, and hypoglycemia have occurred rarely in patients receiving sulfonamides. Cross-sensitivity may exist with these agents.

DOSAGE AND ADMINISTRATION

SYSTEMIC SULFONAMIDES ARE CONTRAINDICATED IN INFANTS UNDER 2 MONTHS OF AGE except as adjunctive therapy with pyrimethamine in the treatment of congenital toxoplasmosis.

USAGE DOSAGE FOR INFANTS OVER 2 MONTHS OF AGE AND CHILDREN

Initially, one-half the 24 hour dose. Maintenance, 150 mg/kg or 4 g/m², divided into 4-6 doses, every 24 hours, with a maximum of 6 g every 24 hours. Rheumatic fever prophylaxis, under 30 kg (66 pounds), 500 mg every 24 hours; over 30 kg (66 pounds), 1 g every 24 hours.

USUAL ADULT DOSAGE

Initially, 2-4 g. Maintenance, 2-4 g, divided into 3-6 doses, every 24 hours.

HOW SUPPLIED

Sulfadiazine 500 mg Tablets: White, unscored, capsule-shaped tablets, imprinted 757 and are available in bottles of 100 and 1000.

Storage: Store at controlled room temperature 15-30°C (59-86°F).

Dispense in a tight, light-resistant container.

PRODUCT LISTING - RATED THERAPEUTICALLY EQUIVALENT

Tablet - Oral - 500 mg

100's	$39.47	GENERIC, Aligen Independent Laboratories Inc	00405-4955-01
100's	$43.89	GENERIC, Ivax Corporation	00182-1996-01
100's	$50.25	GENERIC, Major Pharmaceuticals Inc	00904-2543-60
100's	$130.53	GENERIC, Udl Laboratories Inc	51079-0840-20
100's	$144.26	GENERIC, Eon Labs Manufacturing Inc	00185-0757-01

PRODUCT LISTING - EQUIVALENTS NOT AVAILABLE

Tablet - Oral - 500 mg

100's	$49.75	GENERIC, Major Pharmaceuticals Inc	00904-7870-60

Sulfamethoxazole; Trimethoprim *(002289)*

For related information, see the comparative table section in Appendix A.

Categories: Bronchitis, chronic, acute exacerbation; Diarrhea, travelers'; Infection, ear, middle; Infection, lower respiratory tract; Infection, urinary tract; Pneumonia, pneumocystis carinii; Shigellosis; Pregnancy Category C; FDA Approval Pre 1982; WHO Formulary

Drug Classes: Antibiotics, folate antagonists; Antibiotics, sulfonamides

***Brand Names:* Bactrim**; Bethaprim; Co-Trimoxizole; Cotrim; Septra; Smz-Tmp; Sulfamar; Sulfamethoprim; Sulfamethoxazole Trimethoprim; Sulfaprim; Sulfatrim; Sulfoxaprim; Sulmeprim; Sultrex; Tmp Smx; Triazole; Trimeth/Sulfa; Trisulfam; Trizole; Uro-D S; Urobactrim; Uroplus

Foreign Brand Availability: Abacin (Italy); Abactrim (Spain); Alcorim-F (India); Anitrim (Mexico); Antrimox (Ireland); Apo-Sulfatrim (Canada); Bacidal (Philippines); Bacin (Hong-Kong; Malaysia; Thailand); Bacticel (Argentina); Bactifor (Spain); Bactoprim (Indonesia); Bactramin (Japan); Bactrim DS (Australia; India); Bactrim Forte (Austria; Bulgaria; Costa-Rica; Czech-Republic; Dominican-Republic; El-Salvador; Finland; France; Guatemala; Honduras; Nicaragua; Panama; Portugal; Sweden); Bactrimel (Greece; Netherlands); Baktar (Japan); Bencole (South-Africa); Briscotrim (South-Africa); Chemitrim (Hong-Kong); Chemoprim (Thailand); Cipaprim (Peru); Cipaprim Forte (Peru); Colizole (India); Colizole DS (India); Comox (England); Conprim (Thailand); Cosig Forte (Australia); Cotribase (Philippines); Cotrim-Diolan (Bahrain; Cyprus; Egypt; Iran; Iraq; Jordan; Kuwait; Lebanon; Libya; Oman; Qatar; Republic-of-Yemen; Saudi-Arabia; Syria; United-Arab-Emirates); Cotrimel (Hong-Kong); Cotrix (Bahrain; Cyprus; Egypt; Iran; Iraq; Jordan; Kuwait; Lebanon; Libya; Oman; Qatar; Republic-of-Yemen; Saudi-Arabia; Syria; United-Arab-Emirates); Cozole (Philippines); Diseptyl (Israel); Duocide (Taiwan); Duratrimet (Germany); Ectaprim (Mexico); Epitrim (Bahrain; Cyprus; Egypt; Iran; Iraq; Jordan; Kuwait; Lebanon; Libya; Oman; Qatar; Republic-of-Yemen; Saudi-Arabia; Syria; United-Arab-Emirates); Esbesul (Slovenia); Espectrin (Brazil); Eusaprim (Austria; Belgium; Finland; France; Germany; Italy; Netherlands; Norway; Sweden; Switzerland); Eutrim (Mexico); Fectrim (England); Fermagex (Philippines); Gantaprim (Italy); Gantrim (Italy); Hulin (Spain); Kemocid (Indonesia); Kemotrim (Indonesia); Ikaprim (Indonesia); Infectrim (Peru); Isobac (Mexico); Isotrim (Italy); Kepinol (Germany); Lagatrim (Bahamas; Bahrain; Barbados; Belize; Benin; Bermuda; Burkina-Faso; Curacao; Cyprus; Egypt; Ethiopia; Gambia; Ghana; Guinea; Guyana; Iran; Iraq; Ivory-Coast; Jamaica; Jordan; Kenya; Kuwait; Lebanon; Liberia; Libya; Malawi; Mali; Mauritania; Mauritius; Morocco; Netherland-Antilles; Niger; Nigeria; Oman; Qatar; Republic-of-Yemen; Saudi-Arabia; Senegal; Seychelles; Sierra-Leone; Sudan; Surinam; Syria; Tanzania; Trinidad; Tunia; Uganda; United-Arab-Emirates; Zambia; Zimbabwe); Lagatrim Forte (Bahamas; Barbados; Belize; Benin; Bermuda; Burkina-Faso; Curacao; Ethiopia; Gambia; Ghana; Guinea; Guyana; Ivory-Coast; Jamaica; Kenya; Liberia; Malawi; Mali; Mauritania; Mauritius; Morocco; Netherland-Antilles; Niger; Nigeria; Senegal; Seychelles; Sierra-Leone; Sudan; Surinam; Tanzania; Trinidad; Tunia; Uganda; Zambia; Zimbabwe); Lastrim (Thailand); Leprim (Philippines); Lescot (Argentina); Medixin (Italy); Mezenol (South-Africa); Microtrim (Germany); Missile (Argentina); Moxalas (Indonesia); M-Trim (Thailand); Nopil (Bahrain; Cyprus; Ecuador; Egypt; Iran; Iraq; Jordan; Kuwait; Lebanon; Libya; Oman; Qatar; Republic-of-Yemen; Saudi-Arabia; Syria; United-Arab-Emirates); Novotrimel (Canada); Omsat (Benin; Burkina-Faso; Ethiopia; Gambia; Germany; Ghana; Guinea; Ivory-Coast; Kenya; Liberia; Malawi; Mali; Mauritania; Mauritius; Morocco; Niger; Nigeria; Senegal; Seychelles; Sierra-Leone; Sudan; Tanzania; Tunia; Uganda; Zambia; Zimbabwe); Oriprim DS (Kenya; Tanzania; Uganda; Zimbabwe); Oxaprim (Italy; Japan); Piltrim (Philippines); Plurisul Forte (Peru); Purbal (South-Africa); Resprim (Australia; Israel); Resprim Forte (Australia); Salvatrim (Dominican-Republic; El-Salvador; Honduras; Panama); Septran (Costa-Rica; Dominican-Republic; El-Salvador; Honduras; India; Panama; South-Africa; Uruguay); Septrin (Argentina; Australia; Bahrain; Benin; Burkina-Faso; Colombia; Cyprus; Egypt; England; Ethiopia; Gambia; Ghana; Guinea; Hong-Kong; Indonesia; Iran; Iraq; Ivory-Coast; Jordan; Kenya; Korea; Kuwait; Lebanon; Liberia; Libya; Malawi; Malaysia; Mali; Mauritania; Mauritius; Mexico; Morocco; Niger; Nigeria; Oman; Peru; Philippines; Qatar; Republic-of-Yemen; Saudi-Arabia; Senegal; Seychelles; Sierra-Leone; Spain; Sudan; Syria; Taiwan; Tanzania; Tunia; Uganda; United-Arab-Emirates; Zambia; Zimbabwe); Septrin DS (Hong-Kong; Thailand); Septrin Familia (Mexico); Septrin Forte (Australia); Septrin S (Thailand); Servitrim (Mexico); Sigaprim (Germany); Sinotrim (Korea); Stopan (Japan); Sugaprim (India); Sulfacet (Germany); Sulfinam (Colombia); Sulfotrimin (Germany); Sulthrim (Colombia); Sumetropin (Peru); Suprim (Peru); Suprin (Italy); TMS (Germany); Trim (Italy; South-Africa); Trimel (New-Zealand); Trimephar (Philippines); Trimesulf F (Colombia); Trimetox (Mexico); Trimezol (Ecuador); Trimezole (Indonesia); Trimox (Thailand); Trimoxis (Philippines); Trisul (New-Zealand); Trisulcom (Philippines); Trizakim (Mexico); Ulfaprim (Indonesia); Unitrizole (Philippines); Xeroprim (South-Africa); Zamboprim (Philippines); Zultrop (Indonesia); Zultrop Forte (Indonesia)

Cost of Therapy: $39.37 (Infection; Bactrim; 400 mg; 80 mg; 4 tablets/day; 10 day supply)
$44.28 (Infection; Septra; 400 mg; 80 mg; 4 tablets/day; 10 day supply)
$3.50 (Infection; Generic Tablets; 400 mg; 80 mg; 4 tablets/day; 10 day supply)
$32.30 (Infection; Bactrim DS; 800 mg; 160 mg; 2 tablets/day; 10 day supply)
$1.82 (Infection; Generic DS Tablets; 800 mg; 160 mg; 2 mg/day; 10 day supply)

IV-INFUSION

DESCRIPTION

Bactrim (trimethoprim and sulfamethoxazole) IV infusion, a sterile solution for intravenous infusion only, is a synthetic antibacterial combination product. Each 5 ml contains 80 mg trimethoprim (16 mg/ml) and 400 mg sulfamethoxazole (80 mg/ml) compounded with 40% propylene glycol, 10% ethyl alcohol and 0.3% diethanolamine; 1% benzyl alcohol and 0.1% sodium metabisulfite added as preservatives, water for injection, and pH adjusted to approximately 10 with sodium hydroxide.

Trimethoprim is 2,4-diamino-5-(3,4,5-trimethoxybenzyl)pyrimidine. It is a white to light yellow, odorless, bitter compound with a molecular weight of 290.3.

Sulfamethoxazole is N^1-(5-methyl-3-isoxazolyl)sulfanilamide. It is an almost white, odorless, tasteless compound with a molecular weight of 253.28.

CLINICAL PHARMACOLOGY

Following a 1 hour intravenous infusion of a single dose of 160 mg trimethoprim and 800 mg sulfamethoxazole to 11 patients whose weight ranged from 105–165 lb (mean, 143 lb), the peak plasma concentrations of trimethoprim and sulfamethoxazole were 3.4 ± 0.3 μg/ml and 46.3 ± 2.7 μg/ml, respectively. Following repeated intravenous administration of the same dose at 8 hour intervals, the mean plasma concentrations just prior to and immediately after each infusion at steady state were 5.6 ± 0.6 μg/ml and 8.8 ± 0.9 μg/ml for trimethoprim and 70.6 ± 7.3 μg/ml and 105.6 ± 10.9 μg/ml for sulfamethoxazole. The mean plasma half-life was 11.3 ± 0.7 hours for trimethoprim and 12.8 ± 1.8 hours for sulfamethoxazole. All of these 11 patients had normal renal function, and their ages ranged from 17–78 years (median, 60 years).[1]

Pharmacokinetic studies in children and adults suggest an age-dependent half-life of trimethoprim, as indicated in TABLE 1.[2]

TABLE 1

Age (years)	No. of Patients	Mean TMP Half-life (h)
<1	2	7.67
1-10	9	5.49
10-20	5	8.19
20-63	6	12.82

Patients with severely impaired renal function exhibit an increase in the half-lives of both components, requiring dosage regimen adjustment (see DOSAGE AND ADMINISTRATION).

Both trimethoprim and sulfamethoxazole exist in the blood as unbound, protein-bound and metabolized forms; sulfamethoxazole also exists as the conjugated form. The metabolism of sulfamethoxazole occurs predominately by N_4-acetylation, although the glucuronide conjugate has been identified. The principal metabolites of trimethoprim are the 1- and 3-oxides and the 3′- and 4′-hydroxy derivatives. The free forms of trimethoprim and sulfamethoxazole are considered to be the therapeutically active forms. Approximately 44% of trimethoprim and 70% of sulfamethoxazole are bound to plasma proteins. The presence of 10 mg percent sulfamethoxazole in plasma decreases the protein binding of trimethoprim by an insignificant degree; trimethoprim does not influence the protein binding of sulfamethoxazole.

Excretion of trimethoprim and sulfamethoxazole is primarily by the kidneys through both glomerular filtration and tubular secretion. Urine concentrations of both trimethoprim and sulfamethoxazole are considerably higher than are the concentrations in the blood. The percent of dose excreted in urine over a 12 hour period following the intravenous administration of the first dose of 240 mg of trimethoprim and 1200 mg of sulfamethoxazole on day 1 ranged from 17–42.4% as free trimethoprim; 7–12.7% as free sulfamethoxazole; and 36.7–56% as total (free plus the N_4-acetylated metabolite) sulfamethoxazole. When administered together as a combination product, neither trimethoprim nor sulfamethoxazole affects the urinary excretion pattern of the other. Both trimethoprim and sulfamethoxazole distribute to sputum and vaginal fluid; trimethoprim also distributes to bronchial secretions, and both pass the placental barrier and are excreted in breast milk.

MICROBIOLOGY

Sulfamethoxazole inhibits bacterial synthesis of dihydrofolic acid by competing with *para*-aminobenzoic acid (PABA). Trimethoprim blocks the production of tetrahydrofolic acid from dihydrofolic acid by binding to and reversibly inhibiting the required enzyme, dihydrofolate reductase. Thus, sulfamethoxazole; trimethoprim blocks two consecutive steps in the biosynthesis of nucleic acids and proteins essential to many bacteria.

In vitro studies have shown that bacterial resistance develops more slowly with sulfamethoxazole; trimethoprim than with either trimethoprim or sulfamethoxazole alone.

In vitro serial dilution tests have shown that the spectrum of antibacterial activity of sulfamethoxazole; trimethoprim includes common bacterial pathogens with the exception of *Pseudomonas aeruginosa*. The following organisms are usually susceptible: *Escherichia coli, Klebsiella* species, *Enterobacter* species, *Morganella morganii, Proteus mirabilis,* indole-positive *Proteus* species including *Proteus vulgaris, Haemophilus influenzae* (including ampicillin-resistant strains), *Streptococcus pneumoniae, Shigella flexneri* and *Shigella sonnei.* It should be noted, however, that there are little clinical data on the use of sulfamethoxazole; trimethoprim IV infusion in serious systemic infections due to *Haemophilus influenzae* and *Streptococcus pneumoniae.*

The recommended quantitative disc susceptibility method may be used for estimating the susceptibility of bacteria to sulfamethoxazole; trimethoprim.[3,4] With this procedure, a report from the laboratory of "Susceptible to trimethoprim and sulfamethoxazole" indicates that the infection is likely to respond to therapy with sulfamethoxazole; trimethoprim. If the infection is confined to the urine, a report of "Intermediate susceptibility to trimethoprim and sulfamethoxazole" also indicates that the infection is likely to respond. A report of "Resistant to trimethoprim and sulfamethoxazole" indicates that the infection is unlikely to respond to therapy with sulfamethoxazole; trimethoprim.

INDICATIONS AND USAGE

PNEUMOCYSTIS CARINII PNEUMONIA

Sulfamethoxazole; trimethoprim IV infusion is indicated in the treatment of *Pneumocystis carinii* pneumonia in children and adults.

TABLE 2 *Representative Minimum Inhibitory Concentration Values for Sulfamethoxazole; Trimethoprim-Susceptible Organisms (MIC — μg/ml)*

			TMP/SMX (1:20)	
Bacteria	**TMP alone**	**SMX alone**	**TMP**	**SMX**
Escherichia coli	0.05–1.5	1.0–245	0.05–0.5	0.95–9.5
Proteus species (indole positive)	0.5–5.0	7.35–300	0.05–1.5	0.95–28.5
Morganella morganii	0.5–5.0	7.35–300	0.05–1.5	0.95–28.5
Proteus mirabilis	0.5–1.5	7.35–30	0.05–0.15	0.95–2.85
Klebsiella species	0.15–5.0	2.45–245	0.05–1.5	0.95–28.5
Enterobacter species	0.15–5.0	2.45–245	0.05–1.5	0.95–28.5
Haemophilus influenzae	0.15–1.5	2.85–95	0.015–0.15	0.285–2.85
Streptococcus pneumoniae	0.15–1.5	7.35–24.5	0.05–0.15	0.95–2.85
*Shigella flexneri**	<0.01–0.04	<0.16–>320	<0.002–0.03	0.04–0.625
*Shigella sonnei**	0.02–0.08	0.625–>320	0.004–0.06	0.08–1.25

TMP = trimethoprim
SMX = sulfamethoxazole
* Rudoy RC, Nelson JD, Haltalin KC. Antimicrob Agents Chemother. May 1974;5:439-443.

SHIGELLOSIS

Sulfamethoxazole; trimethoprim IV infusion is indicated in the treatment of enteritis caused by susceptible strains of *Shigella flexneri* and *Shigella sonnei* in children and adults.

URINARY TRACT INFECTIONS

Sulfamethoxazole; trimethoprim IV infusion is indicated in the treatment of severe or complicated urinary tract infections due to susceptible strains of *Escherichia coli, Klebsiella* species, *Enterobacter* species, *Morganella morganii* and *Proteus* species when oral administration of sulfamethoxazole; trimethoprim is not feasible and when the organism is not susceptible to single-agent antibacterials effective in the urinary tract.

Although appropriate culture and susceptibility studies should be performed, therapy may be started while awaiting the results of these studies.

CONTRAINDICATIONS

Sulfamethoxazole; trimethoprim is contraindicated in patients with a known hypersensitivity to trimethoprim or sulfonamides and in patients with documented megaloblastic anemia due to folate deficiency. Sulfamethoxazole; trimethoprim is also contraindicated in pregnant patients and nursing mothers, because sulfonamides pass the placenta and are excreted in the milk and may cause kernicterus. Sulfamethoxazole; trimethoprim is contraindicated in infants less than 2 months of age.

WARNINGS

FATALITIES ASSOCIATED WITH THE ADMINISTRATION OF SULFONAMIDES, ALTHOUGH RARE, HAVE OCCURRED DUE TO SEVERE REACTIONS, INCLUDING STEVENS-JOHNSON SYNDROME, TOXIC EPIDERMAL NECROLYSIS, FULMINANT HEPATIC NECROSIS, AGRANULOCYTOSIS, APLASTIC ANEMIA AND OTHER BLOOD DYSCRASIAS.

SULFAMETHOXAZOLE; TRIMETHOPRIM SHOULD BE DISCONTINUED AT THE FIRST APPEARANCE OF SKIN RASH OR ANY SIGN OF ADVERSE REACTION. Clinical signs, such as rash, sore throat, fever, arthralgia, cough, shortness of breath, pallor, purpura or jaundice may be early indications of serious reactions. In rare instances a skin rash may be followed by more severe reactions, such as Stevens-Johnson syndrome, toxic epidermal necrolysis, hepatic necrosis or serious blood disorder. Complete blood counts should be done frequently in patients receiving sulfonamides.

SULFAMETHOXAZOLE; TRIMETHOPRIM SHOULD NOT BE USED IN THE TREATMENT OF STREPTOCOCCAL PHARYNGITIS. Clinical studies have documented that patients with group A beta-hemolytic streptococcal tonsillopharyngitis have a greater incidence of bacteriologic failure when treated with sulfamethoxazole; trimethoprim than do those patients treated with penicillin, as evidenced by failure to eradicate this organism from the tonsillopharyngeal area.

Sulfamethoxazole; trimethoprim IV infusion contains sodium metabisulfite, a sulfite that may cause allergic-type reactions, including anaphylactic symptoms and life-threatening or less severe asthmatic episodes in certain susceptible people. The overall prevalence of sulfite sensitivity in the general population is unknown and probably low. Sulfite sensitivity is seen more frequently in asthmatic than in nonasthmatic people.

PRECAUTIONS

GENERAL

Sulfamethoxazole; trimethoprim should be given with caution to patients with impaired renal or hepatic function, to those with possible folate deficiency (*e.g.*, the elderly, chronic alcoholics, patients receiving anticonvulsant therapy, patients with malabsorption syndrome, and patients in malnutrition states) and to those with severe allergies or bronchial asthma. In glucose-6-phosphate dehydrogenase deficient individuals, hemolysis may occur. This reaction is frequently dose-related.

Local irritation and inflammation due to extravascular infiltration of the infusion have been observed with sulfamethoxazole; trimethoprim IV infusion. If these occur the infusion should be discontinued and restarted at another site.

USE IN THE ELDERLY

There may be an increased risk of severe adverse reactions in elderly patients, particularly when complicating conditions exist, *e.g.*, impaired kidney and/or liver function, or concomitant use of other drugs. Severe skin reactions, generalized bone marrow suppression (see WARNINGS and ADVERSE REACTIONS) or a specific decrease in platelets (with or without purpura) are the most frequently reported severe adverse reactions in elderly patients. In those concurrently receiving certain diuretics, primarily thiazides, an increased incidence of thrombocytopenia with purpura has been reported. Appropriate dosage adjustments should be made for patients with impaired kidney function (see DOSAGE AND ADMINISTRATION).

USE IN THE TREATMENT OF PNEUMOCYSTIS CARINII PNEUMONIA IN PATIENTS WITH ACQUIRED IMMUNODEFICIENCY SYNDROME (AIDS)

AIDS patients may not tolerate or respond to sulfamethoxazole; trimethoprim in the same manner as non-AIDS patients. The incidence of side effects, particularly rash, fever, leukopenia, and elevated aminotransferase (transaminase) values, with sulfamethoxazole; trimethoprim therapy in AIDS patients who are being treated for *Pneumocystis carinii* pneumonia has been reported to be greatly increased compared with the incidence normally associated with the use of sulfamethoxazole; trimethoprim in non-AIDS patients.

LABORATORY TESTS

Appropriate culture and susceptibility studies should be performed before and throughout treatment. Complete blood counts should be done frequently in patients receiving sulfamethoxazole; trimethoprim; if a significant reduction in the count of any formed blood element is noted, sulfamethoxazole; trimethoprim should be discontinued. Urinalyses with careful microscopic examination and renal function tests should be performed during therapy, particularly for those patients with impaired renal function.

DRUG/LABORATORY TEST INTERACTIONS

Sulfamethoxazole; trimethoprim, specifically the trimethoprim component, can interfere with a serum methotrexate assay as determined by the competitive binding protein technique (CBPA) when a bacterial dihydrofolate reductase is used as the binding protein. No interference occurs, however, if methotrexate is measured by a radioimmunoassay (RIA).

The presence of trimethoprim and sulfamethoxazole may also interfere with the Jaffé alkaline picrate reaction assay for creatinine, resulting in overestimations of about 10% in the range of normal values.

CARCINOGENESIS, MUTAGENESIS, AND IMPAIRMENT OF FERTILITY

Carcinogenesis

Long-term studies in animals to evaluate carcinogenic potential have not been conducted with sulfamethoxazole; trimethoprim IV infusion.

Mutagenesis

Bacterial mutagenic studies have not been performed with sulfamethoxazole and trimethoprim in combination. Trimethoprim was demonstrated to be nonmutagenic in the Ames assay. No chromosomal damage was observed in human leukocytes cultured *in vitro* with sulfamethoxazole and trimethoprim alone or in combination; the concentrations used exceeded blood levels of these compounds following therapy with sulfamethoxazole; trimethoprim. Observations of leukocytes obtained from patients treated with sulfamethoxazole; trimethoprim revealed no chromosomal abnormalities.

Impairment of Fertility

Sulfamethoxazole; trimethoprim IV infusion has not been studied in animals for evidence of impairment of fertility. However, studies in rats at oral dosages as high as 70 mg/kg trimethoprim plus 350 mg/kg sulfamethoxazole daily showed no adverse effects on fertility or general reproductive performance.

PREGNANCY

Teratogenic Effects, Pregnancy Category C

In rats, oral doses of 533 mg/kg sulfamethoxazole or 200 mg/kg trimethoprim produced teratological effects manifested mainly as cleft palates.

The highest dose which did not cause cleft palates in rats was 512 mg/kg sulfamethoxazole or 192 mg/kg trimethoprim when administered separately. In two studies in rats, no teratology was observed when 512 mg/kg of sulfamethoxazole was used in combination with 128 mg/kg of trimethoprim. In one study, however, cleft palates were observed in 1 litter out of 9 when 355 mg/kg of sulfamethoxazole was used in combination with 88 mg/kg of trimethoprim.

In some rabbit studies, an overall increase in fetal loss (dead and resorbed and malformed conceptuses) was associated with doses of trimethoprim 6 times the human therapeutic dose.

While there are no large, well-controlled studies on the use of trimethoprim and sulfamethoxazole in pregnant women, Brumfitt and Pursell,[5] in a retrospective study, reported the outcome of 186 pregnancies during which the mother received either placebo or oral trimethoprim and sulfamethoxazole. The incidence of congenital abnormalities was 4.5% (3 of 66) in those who received placebo and 3.3% (4 of 120) in those receiving trimethoprim and sulfamethoxazole. There were no abnormalities in the 10 children whose mothers received the drug during the first trimester. In a separate survey, Brumfitt and Pursell also found no congenital abnormalities in 35 children whose mothers had received oral trimethoprim and sulfamethoxazole at the time of conception or shortly thereafter.

Because trimethoprim and sulfamethoxazole may interfere with folic acid metabolism, sulfamethoxazole; trimethoprim IV infusion should be used during pregnancy only if the potential benefit justifies the potential risk to the fetus.

Nonteratogenic Effects

See CONTRAINDICATIONS.

NURSING MOTHERS

See CONTRAINDICATIONS.

PEDIATRIC USE

Sulfamethoxazole; trimethoprim IV infusion is not recommended for infants younger than 2 months of age (see CONTRAINDICATIONS).

DRUG INTERACTIONS

In elderly patients concurrently receiving certain diuretics, primarily thiazides, an increased incidence of thrombocytopenia with purpura has been reported.

S

It has been reported that sulfamethoxazole; trimethoprim may prolong the prothrombin time in patients who are receiving the anticoagulant warfarin. This interaction should be kept in mind when sulfamethoxazole; trimethoprim is given to patients already on anticoagulant therapy, and the coagulation time should be reassessed.

Sulfamethoxazole; trimethoprim may inhibit the hepatic metabolism of phenytoin. Sulfamethoxazole; trimethoprim, given at a common clinical dosage, increased the phenytoin half-life by 39% and decreased the phenytoin metabolic clearance rate by 27%. When administering these drugs concurrently, one should be alert for possible excessive phenytoin effect.

Sulfonamides can also displace methotrexate from plasma protein binding sites, thus increasing free methotrexate concentrations.

ADVERSE REACTIONS

The most common adverse effects are gastrointestinal disturbances (nausea, vomiting, anorexia) and allergic skin reactions (such as rash and urticaria). **FATALITIES ASSOCIATED WITH THE ADMINISTRATION OF SULFONAMIDES, ALTHOUGH RARE, HAVE OCCURRED DUE TO SEVERE REACTIONS, INCLUDING STEVENS-JOHNSON SYNDROME, TOXIC EPIDERMAL NECROLYSIS, FULMINANT HEPATIC NECROSIS, AGRANULOCYTOSIS, APLASTIC ANEMIA AND OTHER BLOOD DYSCRASIAS (SEE WARNINGS).** Local reaction, pain and slight irritation on IV administration are infrequent. Thrombophlebitis has rarely been observed.

Hematologic: Agranulocytosis, aplastic anemia, thrombocytopenia, leukopenia, neutropenia, hemolytic anemia, megaloblastic anemia, hypoprothrombinemia, methemoglobinemia, eosinophilia.

Allergic Reactions: Stevens-Johnson syndrome, toxic epidermal necrolysis, anaphylaxis, allergic myocarditis, erythema multiforme, exfoliative dermatitis, angioedema, drug fever, chills. Henoch-Schoenlein purpura, serum sickness-like syndrome, generalized allergic reactions, generalized skin eruptions, conjunctival and scleral injection, photosensitivity, pruritus, urticaria and rash. In addition, periarteritis nodosa and systemic lupus erythematosus have been reported.

Gastrointestinal: Hepatitis (including cholestatic jaundice and hepatic necrosis), elevation of serum transaminase and bilirubin, pseudomembranous enterocolitis, pancreatitis, stomatitis, glossitis, nausea, emesis, abdominal pain, diarrhea, anorexia.

Genitourinary: Renal failure, interstitial nephritis, BUN and serum creatinine elevation, toxic nephrosis with oliguria and anuria, and crystalluria.

Neurologic: Aseptic meningitis, convulsions, peripheral neuritis, ataxia, vertigo, tinnitus, headache.

Psychiatric: Hallucinations, depression, apathy, nervousness.

Endocrine: The sulfonamides bear certain chemical similarities to some goitrogens, diuretics (acetazolamide and the thiazides) and oral hypoglycemic agents. Cross-sensitivity may exist with these agents. Diuresis and hypoglycemia have occurred rarely in patients receiving sulfonamides.

Musculoskeletal: Arthralgia and myalgia.

Respiratory: Pulmonary infiltrates.

Miscellaneous: Weakness, fatigue, insomnia.

DOSAGE AND ADMINISTRATION

CONTRAINDICATED IN INFANTS LESS THAN 2 MONTHS OF AGE.

CAUTION — SULFAMETHOXAZOLE; TRIMETHOPRIM IV INFUSION MUST BE DILUTED IN 5% DEXTROSE IN WATER SOLUTION PRIOR TO ADMINISTRATION. DO NOT MIX SULFAMETHOXAZOLE; TRIMETHOPRIM IV INFUSION WITH OTHER DRUGS OR SOLUTIONS. RAPID INFUSION OR BOLUS INJECTION MUST BE AVOIDED.

DOSAGE

Children and Adults

Pneumocystis Carinii Pneumonia

Total daily dose is 15–20 mg/kg (based on the trimethoprim component) given in 3 or 4 equally divided doses every 6–8 hours for up to 14 days. One investigator noted that a total daily dose of 10–15 mg/kg was sufficient in 10 adult patients with normal renal function.[6]

Severe Urinary Tract Infections and Shigellosis

Total daily dose is 8–10 mg/kg (based on the trimethoprim component) given in 2–4 equally divided doses every 6, 8 or 12 hours for up to 14 days for severe urinary tract infections and 5 days for shigellosis. The maximum recommended daily dose is 60 ml per day.

FOR PATIENTS WITH IMPAIRED RENAL FUNCTION

When renal function is impaired, a reduced dosage should be employed (see TABLE 3).

TABLE 3 *Dosage for Patients With Impaired Renal Function*

Creatine Clearance (ml/min)	Recommended Dosage Regimen
Above 30	Usual standard regimen
15-30	½ the usual regimen
Below 15	Use not recommended

ADMINISTRATION

The solution should be given by intravenous infusion over a period of 60–90 minutes. Rapid infusion or bolus injection must be avoided. Sulfamethoxazole; trimethoprim IV infusion should not be given intramuscularly.

ANIMAL PHARMACOLOGY

The LD_{50} of sulfamethoxazole; trimethoprim IV infusion in mice is 700 mg/kg or 7.3 ml/kg; in rats and rabbits the LD_{50} is >500 mg/kg or >5.2 ml/kg. The vehicle produced the same LD_{50} in each of these species as the active drug.

The signs and symptoms noted in mice, rats and rabbits with sulfamethoxazole; trimethoprim IV infusion or its vehicle at the high IV doses used in acute toxicity studies included ataxia, decreased motor activity, loss of righting reflex, tremors or convulsions, and/or respiratory depression.

HOW SUPPLIED

10 ml Vials: Containing 160 mg trimethoprim (16 mg/ml) and 800 mg sulfamethoxazole (80 mg/ml) for infusion with 5% dextrose in water.

30 ml Multidose Vials: Each 5 ml containing 80 mg trimethoprim (16 mg/ml) and 400 mg sulfamethoxazole (80 mg/ml) for infusion with 5% dextrose in water.

Storage: STORE AT ROOM TEMPERATURE (15-30°C or 59 -86°F). DO NOT REFRIGERATE.

ORAL

DESCRIPTION

Bactrim (trimethoprim and sulfamethoxazole) is a synthetic antibacterial combination product available in DS (double strength) tablets, tablets and pediatric suspension for oral administration.

DS Tablet: Each DS tablet contains 160 mg trimethoprim and 800 mg sulfamethoxazole plus magnesium stearate, pregelatinized starch and sodium starch glycolate.

Tablet: Each tablet contains 80 mg trimethoprim and 400 mg sulfamethoxazole plus magnesium stearate, pregelatinized starch, sodium starch glycolate, FD&C blue no. 1 lake, FD&C yellow no. 6 lake and D&C yellow no. 10 lake.

Pediatric Suspension: Each teaspoonful (5 ml) of the pediatric suspension contains 40 mg trimethoprim and 200 mg sulfamethoxazole in a vehicle containing 0.3% alcohol, edetate disodium, glycerin, microcrystalline cellulose, parabens (methyl and propyl), polysorbate 80, saccharin sodium, simethicone, sorbitol, sucrose, FD&C yellow no. 6, FD&C red no. 40, flavors and water.

Trimethoprim is 2,4-diamino-5-(3,4,5 trimethoxybenzyl)pyrimidine; the molecular formula is $C_{14}H_{18}N_4O_3$. It is a white to light yellow, odorless, bitter compound with a molecular weight of 290.3.

Sulfamethoxazole is N^1-(5-methyl-3-isoxazolyl)sulfanilamide; the molecular formula is $C_{10}H_{11}N_3O_3S$. It is almost white, odorless, tasteless compound with a molecular weight of 253.28.

CLINICAL PHARMACOLOGY

Sulfamethoxazole; trimethoprim is rapidly absorbed following oral administration. Both sulfamethoxazole and trimethoprim exist in the blood as unbound, protein-bound and metabolized forms; sulfamethoxazole also exists as the conjugated form. The metabolism of sulfamethoxazole occurs predominately by N_4-acetylation, although the glucuronide conjugate has been identified. The principal metabolites of trimethoprim are the 1- and 3-oxides and the 3′- and 4′-hydroxy derivatives. The free forms of sulfamethoxazole and trimethoprim are considered to be the therapeutically active forms. Approximately 44% of trimethoprim and 70% of sulfamethoxazole are bound to plasma proteins. The presence of 10 mg percent sulfamethoxazole in plasma decreases the protein binding of trimethoprim by an insignificant degree; trimethoprim does not influence the protein binding of sulfamethoxazole.

Peak blood levels for the individual components occur 1–4 hours after oral administration. The mean serum half-lives of sulfamethoxazole and trimethoprim are 10 and 8–10 hours, respectively. However, patients with severely impaired renal function exhibit an increase in the half-lives of both components, requiring dosage regimen adjustment (see DOSAGE AND ADMINISTRATION). Detectable amounts of trimethoprim and sulfamethoxazole are present in the blood 24 hours after drug administration. During administration of 160 mg trimethoprim and 800 mg sulfamethoxazole bid, the mean steady-state plasma concentration of trimethoprim was 1.72 μg/ml. The steady-state mean plasma levels of free and total sulfamethoxazole were 57.4 μg/ml and 68.0 μg/ml, respectively. These steady-state levels were achieved after three days of drug administration.[1]

Excretion of sulfamethoxazole and trimethoprim is primarily by the kidneys through both glomerular filtration and tubular secretion. Urine concentrations of both sulfamethoxazole and trimethoprim are considerably higher than are the concentrations in the blood. The average percentage of the dose recovered in urine from 0–72 hours after a single oral dose of sulfamethoxazole; trimethoprim is 84.5% for total sulfonamide and 66.8% for free trimethoprim. Thirty percent (30%) of the total sulfonamide is excreted as free sulfamethoxazole, with the remaining as N_4-acetylated metabolite.[2] when administered together as sulfamethoxazole; trimethoprim, neither sulfamethoxazole nor trimethoprim affects the urinary excretion pattern of the other.

Both trimethoprim and sulfamethoxazole distribute to sputum, vaginal fluid and middle ear fluid; trimethoprim also distributes to bronchial secretion, and both pass the placental barrier and are excreted in human milk.

MICROBIOLOGY

Trimethoprim blocks the production of tetrahydrofolic acid from dihydrofolic acid by binding to and reversibly inhibiting the required enzyme, dihydrofolate reductase. Sulfamethoxazole inhibits bacterial synthesis of dihydrofolic acid by competing with *para*-aminobenzoic acid (paba). Thus, trimethoprim and sulfamethoxazole blocks two consecutive steps in the biosynthesis of nucleic acids and proteins essential to many bacteria.

In vitro studies have shown that bacterial resistance develops more slowly with both trimethoprim and sulfamethoxazole in combination than with either trimethoprim or sulfamethoxazole alone.

Trimethoprim and sulfamethoxazole have been shown to be active against most strains of the following microorganisms, both *in vitro* and in clinical infections as described in INDICATIONS AND USAGE.

Aerobic Gram-Positive Microorganisms:

Streptococcus pneumoniae.

Aerobic Gram-Negative Microorganisms:

Escherichia coli (including susceptible enterotoxigenic strains implicated in traveler's diarrhea).

Klebsiella species.
Enterobacter species.
Haemophilus influenzae.
Morganella morganii.
Proteus mirabilis.
Proteus vulgaris.
Shigella flexneri.[3]
Shigella sonnei.[3]

Other Organisms:

Pneumocystis carinii.

Susceptibility Testing Methods

Dilution Techniques

Quantitative methods are used to determine antimicrobial Minimum Inhibitory Concentrations (MICs). These MICs provide estimates of the susceptibility of bacteria to antimicrobial compounds. The MICs should be determined using a standardized procedure. Standardized procedures are based on a dilution method[4] *(broth or agar) or equivalent with standardized inoculum concentrations and standardized concentrations of trimethoprim/sulfamethoxazole powder. The MIC values should be interpreted according to the following criteria:*

For testing *Enterobacteriaceae* (see TABLE 4).

TABLE 4

MIC (µg/ml)	Interpretation
≤2/38	Susceptible (S)
≥4/76	Resistant (R)

When testing either *Haemophilus influenzae** or *Streptococcus pneumoniae†* (see TABLE 5).

TABLE 5

MIC (µg/ml)	Interpretation†
≤0.5/9.5	Susceptible (S)
1/19 — 2/38	Intermediate (I)
≥4/76	Resistant (R)

* These interpretative standards are applicable only to broth microdilution susceptibility tests with *Haemophilus influenzae* using *Haemophilus* Test Medium (HTM).[4]
† These interpretative standards are applicable only to broth microdilution susceptibility tests with *Haemophilus influenzae* using *Haemophilus* Test Medium (HTM).[4]

A report of "Susceptible" indicated that the pathogen is likely to be inhibited if the antimicrobial compound in the blood reaches the concentrations usually achievable. A report of "Intermediate" indicates that the result should be considered equivocal, and, if the microorganism is not fully susceptible to alternative, clinically feasible drugs, the test should be repeated. This category implies possible clinical applicability in body sites where the drug is physiologically concentrated or in situations where high dosage of drug can be used. This category also provides a buffer zone which prevents small uncontrolled technical factors from causing major discrepancies in interpretation. A report of "Resistant" indicates that the pathogen is not likely to be inhibited if the antimicrobial compound in the blood reaches the concentrations usually achievable; other therapy should be selected.

Quality Control

Standardized susceptibility test procedures require the use of laboratory control microorganisms to control the technical aspects of the laboratory procedures. Standard trimethoprim/sulfamethoxazole powder should provide the range of values listed in TABLE 6.

TABLE 6

Microorganism		MIC (µg/ml)
Escherichia coli	ATCC 25922	≤0.5/9.5
*Haemophilus influenzae**	ATCC 49247	0.03/0.59 — 0.25/4.75
Streptococcus pneumoniae†	ATCC 49619	0.12/2.4 — 1/19

* This quality control range is applicable only to *Haemophilus influenzae* ATCC 49247 tested by broth microdilution procedure using *Haemophilus* Test Medium (HTM).[4]
† This quality control range is applicable to tests performed by the broth microdilution method only using cation-adjusted Mueller-Hinton broth with 2–5% lysed horse blood.[4]

Diffusion Techniques

Quantitative methods that require measurement of zone diameters also provide reproducible estimates of the susceptibility of bacteria to antimicrobial compounds. One such standardized procedure[5] requires the use of standardized inoculum concentrations. This procedure uses paper disks impregnated with 1.25/23.75 µg of trimethoprim/sulfamethoxazole to test the susceptibility of microorganisms to trimethoprim/sulfamethoxazole.

Reports from the laboratory providing results of the standard single-disk susceptibility test with a 1.25/23.75 µg of trimethoprim/sulfamethoxazole disk should be interpreted according to the following criteria:

For testing either *Enterobacteriaceae* or *Haemophilus influenzae** (see TABLE 7).

When testing *Streptococcus pneumoniae** (see TABLE 8).

Interpretation should be as stated above for results using dilution techniques. Interpretation involves correlation of the diameter obtained in the disk test with the MIC for trimethoprim/sulfamethoxazole.

As with standardized dilution techniques, diffusion methods require the use of laboratory control microorganisms that are used to control the technical aspects of the laboratory procedures. For the diffusion technique, the 1.25/23.75 µg trimethoprim/sulfamethoxazole disk* should provide the zone diameters listed in TABLE 9 in these laboratory test quality control strains.

TABLE 7

Zone Diameter (mm)	Interpretation
≥16	Susceptible (S)
11–15	Intermediate (I)
≤10	Resistant (R)

* These zone diameter standards are applicable only for disk diffusion testing with *Haemophilus influenzae* and *Haemophilus* Test Medium (HTM).[5]

TABLE 8

Zone Diameter (mm)	Interpretation
≥19	Susceptible (S)
16–18	Intermediate (I)
≤15	Resistant (R)

* These zone diameter interpretative standards are applicable only to tests performed using Mueller-Hinton agar supplemented with 5% defibrinated sheep blood when incubated in 5% CO_2.[5]

TABLE 9

Microorganism		Zone Diameter Ranges (mm)
Escherichia coli	ATCC 25922	24–32
Haemophilus influenzae†	ATCC 49247	24–32
Streptococcus pneumoniae‡	ATCC 49619	20–28

* Mueller-Hinton agar should be checked for excessive levels of thymidine or thymine. To determine whether Mueller-Hinton medium has sufficiently low levels of thymidine and thymine, an *Enterococcus faecalis* (ATCC 29212 or ATCC 33186) may be tested with trimethoprim/sulfamethoxazole disks. A zone of inhibition ≥20 mm that is essentially free of fine colonies indicates a sufficiently low level of thymidine and thymine.
† This quality control range is applicable only to *Haemophilus influenzae* ATCC 49247 tested by a disk diffusion procedure using *Haemophilus* Test Medium (HTM).[5]
‡ This quality control range is applicable only to tests performed by disk diffusion using Mueller-Hinton agar supplemented with 5% defibrinated sheep blood when incubated in 5% CO_2.[5]

INDICATIONS AND USAGE

URINARY TRACT INFECTIONS

For the treatment of urinary tract infections due to susceptible strains of the following organisms: *Escherichia coli, Klebsiella* species, *Enterobacter* species, *Morganella morganii, Proteus mirabilis* and *Proteus vulgaris.* It is recommended that initial episodes of uncomplicated urinary tract infections be treated with a single effective antibacterial agent rather than the combination.

ACUTE OTITIS MEDIA

For the treatment of acute otitis media in pediatric patients due to susceptible strains of *Streptococcus pneumoniae* or *Haemophilus influenzae* when in the judgment of the physician sulfamethoxazole; trimethoprim offers some advantage over the use of other antimicrobial agents. To date, there are limited data on the safety of repeated use of sulfamethoxazole; trimethoprim in pediatric patients under 2 years of age. Sulfamethoxazole; trimethoprim is not indicated for prophylactic or prolonged administration in otitis media at any age.

ACUTE EXACERBATIONS OF CHRONIC BRONCHITIS IN ADULTS

For the treatment of acute exacerbations of chronic bronchitis due to susceptible strains of *Streptococcus pneumoniae* or *Haemophilus influenzae* when in the judgment of the physician sulfamethoxazole; trimethoprim offers some advantage over the use of a single antimicrobial agent.

SHIGELLOSIS

For the treatment of enteritis caused by susceptible strains of *Shigella flexneri* and *Shigella sonnei* when antibacterial therapy is indicated.

PNEUMOCYSTIS CARINII PNEUMONIA

For the treatment of documented *Pneumocystis carinii* pneumonia and for prophylaxis against *Pneumocystis carinii* pneumonia in individuals who are immunosuppressed and considered to be at an increased risk of developing *Pneumocystis carinii* pneumonia.

TRAVELER'S DIARRHEA IN ADULTS

For the treatment of traveler's diarrhea due to susceptible strains of enterotoxigenic *E. coli.*

CONTRAINDICATIONS

Sulfamethoxazole; trimethoprim is contraindicated in patients with a known hypersensitivity to trimethoprim or sulfonamides and in patients with documented megaloblastic anemia due to folate deficiency. Sulfamethoxazole; trimethoprim is also contraindicated in pregnant patients and nursing mothers, because sulfonamides pass the placenta and are excreted in the milk and may cause kernicterus. Sulfamethoxazole; trimethoprim is contraindicated in pediatric patients less than 2 months of age. Sulfamethoxazole; trimethoprim is also contraindicated in patients with marked hepatic damage or with severe renal insufficiency when renal function status cannot be monitored.

S

WARNINGS

FATALITIES ASSOCIATED WITH THE ADMINISTRATION OF SULFONAMIDES, ALTHOUGH RARE, HAVE OCCURRED DUE TO SEVERE REACTIONS INCLUDING STEVENS-JOHNSON SYNDROME, TOXIC EPIDERMAL NECROLYSIS, FULMINANT HEPATIC NECROSIS, AGRANULOCYTOSIS, APLASTIC ANEMIA AND OTHER BLOOD DYSCRASIAS.

SULFONAMIDES, INCLUDING SULFONAMIDE-CONTAINING PRODUCTS SUCH AS TRIMETHOPRIM/SULFAMETHOXAZOLE, SHOULD BE DISCONTINUED AT THE FIRST APPEARANCE OF SKIN RASH OR ANY SIGN OF ADVERSE REACTION. In rare instances, a skin rash may be followed by a more severe reaction, such as Stevens-Johnson syndrome, toxic epidermal necrolysis, hepatic necrosis, and serious blood disorders (see PRECAUTIONS).

Clinical signs such as rash, sore throat, fever, arthralgia, pallor, purpura, or jaundice may be early indications of serious reactions.

Cough, shortness of breath, and pulmonary infiltrates are hypersensitivity reactions of the respiratory tract that have been reported in association with sulfonamide treatment.

The sulfonamides should not be used for the treatment of group A beta-hemolytic streptococcal infections. In an established infection, they will not eradicate the streptococcus and, therefore, will not prevent sequelae such as rheumatic fever.

Pseudomembranous colitis has been reported with nearly all antibacterial agents, including trimethoprim/sulfamethoxazole, and may range in severity from mild to life-threatening. Therefore, it is important to consider this diagnosis in patients who present with diarrhea subsequent to the administration of antibacterial agents.

Treatment with antibacterial agents alters the normal flora of the colon and may permit overgrowth of clostridia. Studies indicate that a toxin produced by *Clostridium difficile* is one primary cause of "antibiotic-associated colitis".

After the diagnosis of pseudomembranous colitis has been established, therapeutic measures should be initiated. Mild cases of pseudomembranous colitis usually respond to drug discontinuation alone. In moderate to severe cases, consideration should be given to management with fluids and electrolytes, protein supplementation, and treatment with an antibacterial drug effective against *C. difficile.*

PRECAUTIONS

GENERAL

Sulfamethoxazole; trimethoprim should be given with caution to patients with impaired renal or hepatic function, to those with possible folate deficiency (*e.g.*, the elderly, chronic alcoholics, patients receiving anticonvulsant therapy, patients with malabsorption syndrome, and patients in malnutrition states) and to those with severe allergies or bronchial asthma. In glucose-6-phosphate dehydrogenase deficient individuals, hemolysis may occur. This reaction is frequently dose-related (see CLINICAL PHARMACOLOGY and DOSAGE AND ADMINISTRATION).

Cases of hypoglycemia in non-diabetic patients treated with sulfamethoxazole; trimethoprim are seen rarely, usually occurring after a few days of therapy. Patients with renal dysfunction, liver disease, malnutrition or those receiving high doses of sulfamethoxazole; trimethoprim are particularly at risk.

Hematological changes indicative of folic acid deficiency may occur in elderly patients or in patients with preexisting folic acid deficiency or kidney failure. These effects are reversible by folinic acid therapy.

Trimethoprim has been noted to impair phenylalanine metabolism, but this is of no significance in phenylketonuric patients on appropriate dietary restriction.

As with all drugs containing sulfonamides, caution is advisable in patients with porphyria or thyroid dysfunction.

USE IN THE ELDERLY

There may be an increased risk of severe adverse reactions in elderly patients, particularly when complicating conditions exist, *e.g.*, impaired kidney and/or liver function, or concomitant use of other drugs. Severe skin reactions, generalized bone marrow suppression (see WARNINGS and ADVERSE REACTIONS) or a specific decrease in platelets (with or without purpura) are the most frequently reported severe adverse reactions in elderly patients. In those concurrently receiving certain diuretics, primarily thiazides, an increased incidence of thrombocytopenia with purpura has been reported. Appropriate dosage adjustments should be made for patients with impaired kidney function and duration of use should be as short as possible to minimize risks of undesired reactions (see DOSAGE AND ADMINISTRATION). The trimethoprim component of sulfamethoxazole; trimethoprim may cause hyperkalemia when administered to patients with underlying disorders of potassium metabolism, with renal insufficiency, or when given concomitantly with drugs known to induce hyperkalemia. Close monitoring of serum potassium is warranted in these patients. Discontinuation of sulfamethoxazole; trimethoprim treatment is recommended to help lower potassium serum levels.

USE IN THE TREATMENT OF AND PROPHYLAXIS FOR PNEUMOCYSTIS CARINII PNEUMONIA IN PATIENTS WITH ACQUIRED IMMUNODEFICIENCY SYNDROME (AIDS)

AIDS patients may not tolerate or respond to sulfamethoxazole; trimethoprim in the same manner as non-AIDS patients. The incidence of side effects, particularly rash, fever, leukopenia and elevated aminotransferase (transaminase) values, with sulfamethoxazole; trimethoprim therapy in AIDS patients who are being treated for *Pneumocystis carinii* pneumonia has been reported to be greatly increased compared with the incidence normally associated with the use of sulfamethoxazole; trimethoprim in non-AIDS patients. The incidence of hyperkalemia appears to be increased in AIDS patients receiving sulfamethoxazole; trimethoprim. Adverse effects are generally less severe in patients receiving sulfamethoxazole; trimethoprim for prophylaxis. A history of mild intolerance to sulfamethoxazole; trimethoprim in AIDS patients does not appear to predict intolerance of subsequent secondary prophylaxis.6 However, if a patient develops skin rash or any sign of adverse reaction, therapy with sulfamethoxazole; trimethoprim should be reevaluated (see WARNINGS).

High dosage of trimethoprim, as used in patients with *Pneumocystis carinii* pneumonia, induces a progressive but reversible increase of serum potassium concentrations in a substantial number of patients. Even treatment with recommended doses may cause hyperkalemia when trimethoprim is administered to patients with underlying disorders of potassium metabolism, with renal insufficiency, or if drugs known to induce hyperkalemia are given concomitantly. Close monitoring of serum potassium is warranted in these patients.

During treatment, adequate fluid intake and urinary output should be ensured to prevent crystalluria. Patients who are "slow acetylators" may be more prone to idiosyncratic reactions to sulfonamides.

INFORMATION FOR THE PATIENT

Patients should be instructed to maintain an adequate fluid intake in order to prevent crystalluria and stone formation.

LABORATORY TESTS

Complete blood counts should be done frequently in patients receiving sulfamethoxazole; trimethoprim; if a significant reduction in the count of any formed blood element is noted, sulfamethoxazole; trimethoprim should be discontinued. Urinalyses with careful microscopic examination and renal function tests should be performed during therapy, particularly for those patients with impaired renal function.

DRUG/LABORATORY TEST INTERACTIONS

Sulfamethoxazole; trimethoprim, specifically the trimethoprim component, can interfere with a serum methotrexate assay as determined by the competitive binding protein technique (CBPA) when a bacterial dihydrofolate reductase is used as the binding protein. No interference occurs, however, if methotrexate is measured by a radioimmunoassay (RIA).

The presence of trimethoprim and sulfamethoxazole may also interfere with the Jaffé alkaline picrate reaction assay for creatinine, resulting in overestimations of about 10% in the range of normal values.

CARCINOGENESIS, MUTAGENESIS, AND IMPAIRMENT OF FERTILITY

Carcinogenesis

Long-term studies in animals to evaluate carcinogenic potential have not been conducted with sulfamethoxazole; trimethoprim.

Mutagenesis

Bacterial mutagenic studies have not been performed with sulfamethoxazole and trimethoprim in combination. Trimethoprim was demonstrated to be nonmutagenic in the Ames assay. No chromosomal damage was observed in human leukocytes cultured *in vitro* with sulfamethoxazole and trimethoprim alone or in combination; the concentrations used exceeded blood levels of these compounds following therapy with sulfamethoxazole; trimethoprim. Observations of leukocytes obtained from patients treated with sulfamethoxazole; trimethoprim revealed no chromosomal abnormalities.

Impairment of Fertility

No adverse effects on fertility or general reproductive performance were observed in rats given oral dosages as high as 70 mg/kg/day trimethoprim plus 350 mg/kg/day sulfamethoxazole. These doses are 10.9-fold higher than the recommended human dose for trimethoprim and sulfamethoxazole.

PREGNANCY CATEGORY C

Teratogenic Effects

In rats, oral doses of 533 mg/kg sulfamethoxazole (16.7-fold higher than the recommended human dose) or 200 mg/kg trimethoprim (31.3-fold higher than the recommended human dose) produced teratologic effects manifested mainly as cleft palates.

The highest dose which did not cause cleft palates in rats was 512 mg/kg sulfamethoxazole (16-fold higher than the recommended human dose) or 192 mg/kg trimethoprim (30-fold higher than the recommended human dose) when administered separately. In two studies in rats, no teratology was observed when 512 mg/kg of sulfamethoxazole (16-fold higher than the recommended human dose) was used in combination with 128 mg/kg of trimethoprim (20-fold higher than the recommended human dose). In one study, however, cleft palates were observed in 1 litter out of 9 when 355 mg/kg of sulfamethoxazole (11.1-fold higher than the recommended human dose) was used in combination with 88 mg/kg of trimethoprim (13.8-fold higher than the recommended human dose).

In some rabbit studies, an overall increase in fetal loss (dead and resorbed and malformed conceptuses) was associated with doses of trimethoprim 6 times the human therapeutic dose.

While there are no large, well-controlled studies on the use of trimethoprim and sulfamethoxazole in pregnant women, Brumfitt and Pursell,[7] in a retrospective study, reported the outcome of 186 pregnancies during which the mother received either placebo or trimethoprim and sulfamethoxazole. The incidence of congenital abnormalities was 4.5% (3 of 66) in those who received placebo and 3.3% (4 of 120) in those receiving trimethoprim and sulfamethoxazole. There were no abnormalities in the 10 children whose mothers received the drug during the first trimester. In a separate survey, Brumfitt and Pursell also found no congenital abnormalities in 35 children whose mothers had received oral trimethoprim and sulfamethoxazole at the time of conception or shortly thereafter.

Because trimethoprim and sulfamethoxazole may interfere with folic acid metabolism, sulfamethoxazole; trimethoprim should be used during pregnancy only if the potential benefit justifies the potential risk to the fetus.

Nonteratogenic Effects

See CONTRAINDICATIONS.

NURSING MOTHERS

See CONTRAINDICATIONS.

PEDIATRIC USE

Sulfamethoxazole; trimethoprim is not recommended for pediatric patients younger than 2 months of age (see INDICATIONS AND USAGE and CONTRAINDICATIONS).

DRUG INTERACTIONS

In elderly patients concurrently receiving certain diuretics, primarily thiazides, an increased incidence of thrombocytopenia with purpura has been reported.

It has been reported that sulfamethoxazole; trimethoprim may prolong the prothrombin time in patients who are receiving the anticoagulant warfarin. This interaction should be kept in mind when sulfamethoxazole; trimethoprim is given to patients already on anticoagulant therapy, and the coagulation time should be reassessed.

Sulfamethoxazole; trimethoprim may inhibit the hepatic metabolism of phenytoin. Sulfamethoxazole; trimethoprim, given at a common clinical dosage, increased the phenytoin half-life by 39% and decreased the phenytoin metabolic clearance rate by 27%. When administering these drugs concurrently, one should be alert for possible excessive phenytoin effect.

Sulfonamides can also displace methotrexate from plasma protein binding sites and can compete with the renal transport of methotrexate, thus increasing free methotrexate concentrations.

There have been reports of marked but reversible nephrotoxicity with coadministration of sulfamethoxazole; trimethoprim and cyclosporine in renal transplant recipients.

Increased digoxin blood levels can occur with concomitant sulfamethoxazole; trimethoprim therapy, especially in elderly patients. Serum digoxin levels should be monitored.

Increased sulfamethoxazole blood levels may occur in patients who are also receiving indomethacin.

Occasional reports suggest that patients receiving pyrimethamine as malaria prophylaxis in doses exceeding 25 mg weekly may develop megaloblastic anemia if sulfamethoxazole; trimethoprim is prescribed.

The efficacy of tricyclic antidepressants can decrease when coadministered with sulfamethoxazole; trimethoprim.

Like other sulfonamide-containing drugs, sulfamethoxazole; trimethoprim potentiates the effect of oral hypoglycemics.

In the literature, a single case of toxic delirium has been reported after concomitant intake of trimethoprim/sulfamethoxazole and amantadine.

ADVERSE REACTIONS

The most common adverse effects are gastrointestinal disturbances (nausea, vomiting, anorexia) and allergic skin reactions (such as rash and urticaria). **FATALITIES ASSOCIATED WITH THE ADMINISTRATION OF SULFONAMIDES, ALTHOUGH RARE, HAVE OCCURRED DUE TO SEVERE REACTIONS, INCLUDING STEVENS-JOHNSON SYNDROME, TOXIC EPIDERMAL NECROLYSIS, FULMINANT HEPATIC NECROSIS, AGRANULOCYTOSIS, APLASTIC ANEMIA AND OTHER BLOOD DYSCRASIAS (SEE WARNINGS).**

Hematologic: Agranulocytosis, aplastic anemia, thrombocytopenia, leukopenia, neutropenia, hemolytic anemia, megaloblastic anemia, hypoprothrombinemia, methemoglobinemia, eosinophilia, pancytopenia, purpura.

Allergic Reactions: Stevens-Johnson syndrome, toxic epidermal necrolysis, anaphylaxis, allergic myocarditis, erythema multiforme, exfoliative dermatitis, angioedema, drug fever, chills, Henoch-Schoenlein purpura, serum sickness-like syndrome, generalized allergic reactions, generalized skin eruptions, photosensitivity, conjunctival and scleral injection, pruritus, urticaria and rash. In addition, periarteritis nodosa and systemic lupus erythematosus have been reported.

Gastrointestinal: Hepatitis (including cholestatic jaundice and hepatic necrosis), elevation of serum transaminase and bilirubin, pseudomembranous enterocolitis, pancreatitis, stomatitis, glossitis, nausea, emesis, abdominal pain, diarrhea, anorexia.

Genitourinary: Renal failure, interstitial nephritis, BUN and serum creatinine elevation, toxic nephrosis with oliguria and anuria, crystalluria and nephrotoxicity in association with cyclosporine.

Metabolic and Nutritional: Hyperkalemia (see PRECAUTIONS, Use in the Elderly and PRECAUTIONS, Use in the Treatment of and Prophylaxis for Pneumocystis carinii Pneumonia in Patients With Acquired Immunodeficiency Syndrome [AIDS])..

Neurologic: Aseptic meningitis, convulsions, peripheral neuritis, ataxia, vertigo, tinnitus, headache.

Psychiatric: Hallucinations, depression, apathy, nervousness.

Endocrine: The sulfonamides bear certain chemical similarities to some goitrogens, diuretics (acetazolamide and the thiazides) and oral hypoglycemic agents. Cross-sensitivity may exist with these agents. Diuresis and hypoglycemia have occurred rarely in patients receiving sulfonamides.

Musculoskeletal: Arthralgia and myalgia. Isolated cases of rhabdomyolysis have been reported with sulfamethoxazole; trimethoprim, mainly in AIDS patients.

Respiratory: Cough, shortness of breath, and pulmonary infiltrates (see WARNINGS).

Miscellaneous: Weakness, fatigue, insomnia.

DOSAGE AND ADMINISTRATION

Not recommended for use in pediatric patients less than 2 months of age.

URINARY TRACT INFECTIONS AND SHIGELLOSIS IN ADULTS AND PEDIATRIC PATIENTS, AND ACUTE OTITIS MEDIA IN PEDIATRIC PATIENTS

Adults

The usual adult dosage in the treatment of urinary tract infections is 1 sulfamethoxazole; trimethoprim DS (double strength) tablet, 2 sulfamethoxazole; trimethoprim tablets or 4 teaspoonfuls (20 ml) of sulfamethoxazole; trimethoprim pediatric suspension every 12 hours for 10–14 days. An identical daily dosage is used for 5 days in the treatment of shigellosis.

Pediatric Patients

The recommended dose for pediatric patients with urinary tract infections or acute otitis media is 8 mg/kg trimethoprim and 40 mg/kg sulfamethoxazole per 24 hours, given in two divided doses every 12 hours for 10 days. An identical daily dosage is used for 5 days in the treatment of shigellosis. TABLE 10 is a guideline for the attainment of this dosage.

TABLE 10 *Pediatric Patients 2 Months of Age or Older*

Weight		Dose — Every 12 hours	
lb	kg	Teaspoonfuls	Tablets
22	10	1 (5 ml)	—
44	20	2 (10 ml)	1
66	30	3 (15 ml)	1½
88	40	4 (20 ml)	2 (or 1 DS tablet)

FOR PATIENTS WITH IMPAIRED RENAL FUNCTION

When renal function is impaired, a reduced dosage should be employed (see TABLE 11).

TABLE 11 *Dosage for Patients With Impaired Renal Function*

Creatinine Clearance (ml/min)	Recommended Dosage Regimen
Above 30	Usual standard regimen
15-30	½ the usual regimen
Below 1[5]	Use not recommended

ACUTE EXACERBATIONS OF CHRONIC BRONCHITIS IN ADULTS

The usual adult dosage in the treatment of acute exacerbations of chronic bronchitis is 1 sulfamethoxazole; trimethoprim DS (double strength) tablet, 2 sulfamethoxazole; trimethoprim tablets or 4 teaspoonfuls (20 ml) of sulfamethoxazole; trimethoprim pediatric suspension every 12 hours for 14 days.

PNEUMOCYSTIS CARINII PNEUMONIA

Treatment

Adults and Pediatric Patients

The recommended dosage for treatment of patients with documented *Pneumocystis carinii* pneumonia is 15–20 mg/kg trimethoprim and 75–100 mg/kg sulfamethoxazole per 24 hours given in equally divided doses every 6 hours for 14–21 days.[8] TABLE 12 is a guideline for the upper limit of this dosage.

TABLE 12 *Dosage for Patients With Pneumocystis carinii Pneumonia*

Weight		Dose — every 6 hours	
lb	kg	Teaspoonfuls	Tablets
18	8	1 (5 ml)	—
35	16	2 (10 ml)	1
53	24	3 (15 ml)	1½
70	32	4 (20 ml)	2 (or 1 DS tablet)
88	40	5 (25 ml)	2½
106	48	6 (30 ml)	3 (or 1½ DS tablets)
141	64	8 (40 ml)	4 (or 2 DS tablets)
176	80	10 (50 ml)	5 (or 2½ DS tablets)

For the lower limit dose (15 mg/kg trimethoprim and 75 mg/kg sulfamethoxazole per 24 hours) administer 75% of the dose in TABLE 12.

Prophylaxis

Adults

The recommended dosage for prophylaxis in adults is 1 sulfamethoxazole; trimethoprim DS (double strength) tablet daily.[9]

Pediatric Patients

For pediatric patients, the recommended dose is 150 mg/m^2/day trimethoprim with 750 mg/m^2/day sulfamethoxazole given orally in equally divided doses twice a day, on 3 consecutive days per week. The total daily dose should not exceed 320 mg trimethoprim and 1600 mg sulfamethoxazole.[10] TABLE 13 is a guideline for the attainment of this dosage in pediatric patients.

TABLE 13

Body Surface Area	Dose — Every 12 Hours	
(m^2)	Teaspoonfuls	Tablets
0.26	½ (2.5 ml)	—
0.53	1 (5 ml)	½
1.06	2 (10 ml)	1

TRAVELER'S DIARRHEA IN ADULTS

For the treatment of traveler's diarrhea, the usual adult dosage is 1 sulfamethoxazole; trimethoprim DS (double strength) tablet; 2 sulfamethoxazole; trimethoprim tablets or 4 teaspoonfuls (20 ml) of pediatric suspension every 12 hours for 5 days.

HOW SUPPLIED

TABLETS

DS (Double Strength) Tablets: White, notched, capsule shaped, containing 160 mg trimethoprim and 800 mg sulfamethoxazole. *Imprint on Tablets:* (front) "BACTRIM-DS"; (back) "ROCHE".

S

Tablets: Light green, scored, capsule shaped, containing 80 mg trimethoprim and 400 mg sulfamethoxazole. *Imprint on Tablets:* (front) "BACTRIM"; (back) "ROCHE".
Storage: STORE AT 15-30°C (59-86°F) IN A DRY PLACE AND PROTECTED FROM LIGHT.

PEDIATRIC SUSPENSION

Pediatric Suspension: Pink, cherry flavored, containing 40 mg trimethoprim and 200 mg sulfamethoxazole per teaspoonful (5 ml).
Storage: STORE AT 15-30°C (59-86°F) AND PROTECT FROM LIGHT.

PRODUCT LISTING - RATED THERAPEUTICALLY EQUIVALENT

Solution - Intravenous - 16 mg;80 mg/ml

Size	Price	Product, Manufacturer	NDC
5 ml x 10	$41.30	GENERIC, Gensia Sicor Pharmaceuticals Inc	00703-9503-03
5 ml x 10	$53.00	SEPTRA I.V., Monarch Pharmaceuticals Inc	61570-0056-10
5 ml x 10	$64.75	GENERIC, Esi Lederle Generics	00641-2764-43
10 ml x 10	$87.10	GENERIC, Gensia Sicor Pharmaceuticals Inc	00703-9514-03
10 ml x 10	$103.84	SEPTRA INFUSION, Monarch Pharmaceuticals Inc	61570-0054-10
10 ml x 10	$126.91	GENERIC, Esi Lederle Generics	00641-2765-43
20 ml x 10	$192.80	SEPTRA I.V., Monarch Pharmaceuticals Inc	61570-0055-10
30 ml	$19.49	GENERIC, Gensia Sicor Pharmaceuticals Inc	00703-9526-01
30 ml	$35.35	GENERIC, Esi Lederle Generics	00641-2766-41

Suspension - Oral - 40 mg;200 mg/5 ml

Size	Price	Product, Manufacturer	NDC
20 ml x 50	$56.00	GENERIC, Xactdose Inc	50962-0302-20
20 ml x 50	$65.00	GENERIC, Raway Pharmacal Inc	00686-0638-10
20 ml x 50	$83.50	SULFATRIM PEDIATRIC, Alpharma Uspd Makers Of Barre and Nmc	50962-0302-60
20 ml x 100	$172.66	GENERIC, Alpharma Uspd Makers Of Barre and Nmc	50962-0302-61
100 ml	$7.86	SULFATRIM PEDIATRIC, Alpharma Uspd Makers Of Barre and Nmc	63874-0150-10
100 ml	$7.90	SULFATRIM PEDIATRIC, Allscripts Pharmaceutical Company	54569-1017-00
100 ml	$12.63	SULFATRIM PEDIATRIC, Alpharma Uspd Makers Of Barre and Nmc	00472-1285-33
100 ml	$12.63	SEPTRA, Allscripts Pharmaceutical Company	54569-0179-00
100 ml	$12.63	SEPTRA, Allscripts Pharmaceutical Company	54569-4005-01
100 ml	$14.85	SEPTRA, Physicians Total Care	54868-1420-01
100 ml	$75.75	SEPTRA, Monarch Pharmaceuticals Inc	61570-0050-11
150 ml	$8.15	SULFATRIM PEDIATRIC, Alpharma Uspd Makers Of Barre and Nmc	00472-1285-06
150 ml	$8.15	SULFATRIM PEDIATRIC, Allscripts Pharmaceutical Company	54569-4918-00
200 ml	$8.75	SULFATRIM PEDIATRIC, Alpharma Uspd Makers Of Barre and Nmc	00472-1285-09
200 ml	$8.75	SULFATRIM PEDIATRIC, Allscripts Pharmaceutical Company	54569-4898-00
473 ml	$14.45	GENERIC, Teva Pharmaceuticals Usa	00093-0562-16
473 ml	$58.10	GENERIC, Hi-Tech Pharmacal Company Inc	50383-0823-16
473 ml	$64.54	SEPTRA, Monarch Pharmaceuticals Inc	61570-0050-16
473 ml	$64.54	SEPTRA, Monarch Pharmaceuticals Inc	61570-0051-16
480 ml	$9.75	GENERIC, Raway Pharmacal Inc	00686-6100-38
480 ml	$10.98	GENERIC, Watson/Schein Pharmaceuticals Inc	00364-2076-16
480 ml	$11.70	GENERIC, Mutual/United Research Laboratories	00677-0841-33
480 ml	$11.71	GENERIC, Moore, H.L. Drug Exchange Inc	00839-7709-69
480 ml	$11.95	BETHAPRIM, Major Pharmaceuticals Inc	00904-0405-16
480 ml	$12.27	GENERIC, Geneva Pharmaceuticals	00781-6062-16
480 ml	$12.27	GENERIC, Geneva Pharmaceuticals	00781-6063-16
480 ml	$12.30	GENERIC, Ivax Corporation	00182-1559-40
480 ml	$12.34	GENERIC, Moore, H.L. Drug Exchange Inc	00839-6699-69
480 ml	$12.34	GENERIC, Moore, H.L. Drug Exchange Inc	00839-6718-69
480 ml	$13.34	GENERIC, Aligen Independent Laboratories Inc	00405-3675-16
480 ml	$13.51	SULFATRIM PEDIATRIC, Alpharma Uspd Makers Of Barre and Nmc	63874-0150-20
480 ml	$14.44	SULFATRIM SUSPENSION, Mutual/United Research Laboratories	00677-0840-33
480 ml	$14.93	BETHAPRIM PEDIATRIC, Major Pharmaceuticals Inc	00904-0406-16
480 ml	$16.40	GENERIC, Watson/Rugby Laboratories Inc	00536-1725-85
480 ml	$35.90	SULFATRIM PEDIATRIC, Qualitest Products Inc	00603-1687-58
480 ml	$35.90	SULFATRIM, Qualitest Products Inc	00603-1688-58
480 ml	$52.19	BACTRIM PEDIATRIC, Roche Laboratories	00004-1033-28
480 ml	$57.95	SULFATRIM, Alpharma Uspd Makers Of Barre and Nmc	00472-1284-16
480 ml	$57.95	SULFATRIM PEDIATRIC, Alpharma Uspd Makers Of Barre and Nmc	00472-1285-16
480 ml	$58.10	GENERIC, Hi-Tech Pharmacal Company Inc	50383-0824-16

Suspension - Oral - 200 mg/5 ml;40 mg/5 ml

Size	Price	Product, Manufacturer	NDC
480 ml	$11.23	FEDERAL UPPER LIMIT, H.C.F.A. F F P	99999-2289-16

Tablet - Oral - 80 mg;400 mg

Size	Price	Product, Manufacturer	NDC
10's	$3.00	GENERIC, Pd-Rx Pharmaceuticals	55289-0457-10
12's	$3.60	GENERIC, Pd-Rx Pharmaceuticals	55289-0457-12
20's	$6.69	GENERIC, Pd-Rx Pharmaceuticals	55289-0457-20
20's	$13.28	GENERIC, Allscripts Pharmaceutical Company	54569-0269-00
20's	$13.56	GENERIC, Mutual/United Research Laboratories	00677-0783-60
30's	$12.28	GENERIC, Heartland Healthcare Services	61392-0782-30
30's	$12.28	GENERIC, Heartland Healthcare Services	61392-0782-39
31's	$12.69	GENERIC, Heartland Healthcare Services	61392-0782-31
32's	$13.10	GENERIC, Heartland Healthcare Services	61392-0782-32
45's	$18.42	GENERIC, Heartland Healthcare Services	61392-0782-45
60's	$24.56	GENERIC, Heartland Healthcare Services	61392-0782-60
90's	$36.85	GENERIC, Heartland Healthcare Services	61392-0782-90
100's	$7.92	GENERIC, Us Trading Corporation	56126-0139-11
100's	$8.75	GENERIC, Raway Pharmacal Inc	00686-2130-09
100's	$11.93	GENERIC, Interstate Drug Exchange Inc	00814-7239-14
100's	$12.14	GENERIC, Roxane Laboratories Inc	00054-4800-25
100's	$12.69	UROPLUS, Shionogi Usa Inc	45809-0910-11
100's	$13.40	GENERIC, Major Pharmaceuticals Inc	00904-2726-61
100's	$13.85	GENERIC, Major Pharmaceuticals Inc	00904-2726-60
100's	$15.12	GENERIC, Auro Pharmaceutical	55829-0485-10
100's	$15.50	GENERIC, Raway Pharmacal Inc	00686-0171-13
100's	$16.70	GENERIC, Roxane Laboratories Inc	00054-8800-25
100's	$18.95	GENERIC, Martec Pharmaceuticals Inc	52555-0341-01
100's	$21.50	GENERIC, Watson/Rugby Laboratories Inc	00536-4692-01
100's	$23.24	GENERIC, Ivax Corporation	00182-1478-01
100's	$24.00	GENERIC, Aligen Independent Laboratories Inc	00405-4928-01
100's	$28.00	GENERIC, Geneva Pharmaceuticals	00781-1062-13
100's	$28.00	GENERIC, Medirex Inc	57480-0436-01
100's	$31.44	GENERIC, American Health Packaging	62584-0856-01
100's	$40.94	GENERIC, Vangard Labs	00615-0171-13
100's	$66.40	GENERIC, Teva Pharmaceuticals Usa	00093-0088-01
100's	$66.45	GENERIC, Mutual Pharmaceutical Co Inc	53489-0145-01
100's	$84.65	GENERIC, Watson/Schein Pharmaceuticals Inc	00364-2068-90
100's	$98.42	BACTRIM, Roche Laboratories	00004-0050-01
100's	$102.54	BACTRIM, Women First Healthcare	64248-0004-10
100's	$110.69	SEPTRA, Monarch Pharmaceuticals Inc	61570-0052-01

Tablet - Oral - 160 mg;800 mg

Size	Price	Product, Manufacturer	NDC
1's	$4.79	BACTRIM DS, Prescript Pharmaceuticals	00247-0360-01
2's	$2.03	GENERIC, Pd-Rx Pharmaceuticals	55289-0241-02
2's	$7.20	GENERIC, Allscripts Pharmaceutical Company	54569-2986-00
4's	$2.90	GENERIC, Pd-Rx Pharmaceuticals	55289-0241-04
6's	$5.90	GENERIC, Pd-Rx Pharmaceuticals	55289-0241-06
10's	$5.64	GENERIC, Pd-Rx Pharmaceuticals	55289-0241-10
10's	$17.65	BACTRIM DS, Prescript Pharmaceuticals	00247-0360-10
14's	$7.90	GENERIC, Pd-Rx Pharmaceuticals	55289-0241-14
14's	$9.87	GENERIC, Golden State Medical	60429-0170-14
14's	$23.36	BACTRIM DS, Prescript Pharmaceuticals	00247-0360-14
15's	$8.46	GENERIC, Pd-Rx Pharmaceuticals	55289-0241-15
20's	$4.70	GENERIC, Pd-Rx Pharmaceuticals	58864-0478-20
20's	$4.83	UROPLUS DS, Shionogi Usa Inc	45809-0911-24
20's	$11.28	GENERIC, Pd-Rx Pharmaceuticals	55289-0241-20
20's	$13.00	GENERIC, St. Mary'S Mpp	60760-0069-20
20's	$13.89	GENERIC, Golden State Medical	60429-0170-20
20's	$22.25	GENERIC, Mutual/United Research Laboratories	00677-0784-60
20's	$24.00	SEPTRA DS, Prescript Pharmaceuticals	00247-0397-20
20's	$31.94	BACTRIM DS, Prescript Pharmaceuticals	00247-0360-20
20's	$33.66	BACTRIM DS, Physicians Total Care	54868-0337-00
20's	$36.00	GENERIC, Major Pharmaceuticals Inc	00904-2725-95
20's	$37.80	SEPTRA DS, Monarch Pharmaceuticals Inc	61570-0053-20
25's	$15.00	GENERIC, Pd-Rx Pharmaceuticals	55289-0241-97
28's	$7.52	UROPLUS DS, Shionogi Usa Inc	45809-0911-25
28's	$7.52	UROPLUS DS, Shionogi Usa Inc	45809-0911-26
28's	$15.80	GENERIC, Pd-Rx Pharmaceuticals	55289-0241-28
30's	$26.85	GENERIC, Heartland Healthcare Services	61392-0783-30
30's	$26.85	GENERIC, Heartland Healthcare Services	61392-0783-39
30's	$60.00	GENERIC, Udl Laboratories Inc	51079-0128-90
31 x 10	$204.99	GENERIC, Vangard Labs	00615-0170-53
31 x 10	$204.99	GENERIC, Vangard Labs	00615-0170-63
31's	$27.75	GENERIC, Heartland Healthcare Services	61392-0783-31
32's	$28.64	GENERIC, Heartland Healthcare Services	61392-0783-32
45's	$40.28	GENERIC, Heartland Healthcare Services	61392-0783-45
60's	$33.84	GENERIC, Pd-Rx Pharmaceuticals	55289-0241-60
60's	$53.71	GENERIC, Heartland Healthcare Services	61392-0783-60
90's	$80.56	GENERIC, Heartland Healthcare Services	61392-0783-90
100's	$9.09	GENERIC, Bristol-Myers Squibb	00003-0171-50
100's	$9.80	GENERIC, Us Trading Corporation	56126-0140-11
100's	$11.00	GENERIC, Raway Pharmacal Inc	00686-2132-09
100's	$15.95	GENERIC, Roxane Laboratories Inc	00054-4801-25
100's	$16.28	GENERIC, Interstate Drug Exchange Inc	00814-7240-14
100's	$17.39	UROPLUS DS, Shionogi Usa Inc	45809-0911-21
100's	$18.13	GENERIC, Geneva Pharmaceuticals	00781-1063-01
100's	$18.23	GENERIC, Roxane Laboratories Inc	00054-8801-25
100's	$19.80	GENERIC, Pd-Rx Pharmaceuticals	55289-0241-17
100's	$27.38	GENERIC, Auro Pharmaceutical	55829-0486-10
100's	$28.96	GENERIC, Moore, H.L. Drug Exchange Inc	00839-6406-06
100's	$29.95	GENERIC, Raway Pharmacal Inc	00686-0170-13

S

Qty	Price	Description	NDC
100's	$34.00	GENERIC, Parmed Pharmaceuticals Inc	00349-2336-01
100's	$36.00	GENERIC, Geneva Pharmaceuticals	00781-1063-13
100's	$37.10	GENERIC, American Health Packaging	62584-0857-01
100's	$38.14	GENERIC, Ivax Corporation	00182-1408-01
100's	$39.00	GENERIC, Aligen Independent Laboratories Inc	00405-4929-01
100's	$39.00	GENERIC, Martec Pharmaceuticals Inc	52555-0342-01
100's	$64.13	GENERIC, Vangard Labs	00615-0170-13
100's	$108.49	GENERIC, Major Pharmaceuticals Inc	00904-2725-60
100's	$108.99	GENERIC, Watson/Schein Pharmaceuticals Inc	00364-2069-01
100's	$109.02	GENERIC, Mutual Pharmaceutical Co Inc	53489-0146-01
100's	$114.20	GENERIC, Major Pharmaceuticals Inc	00904-2725-61
100's	$114.56	GENERIC, Watson/Schein Pharmaceuticals Inc	00364-2069-90
100's	$115.43	GENERIC, Teva Pharmaceuticals Usa	00093-0089-01
100's	$144.12	GENERIC, Eon Labs Manufacturing Inc	00185-0112-01
100's	$161.48	BACTRIM DS, Roche Laboratories	00004-0117-01
100's	$172.94	SEPTRA DS, Monarch Pharmaceuticals Inc	61570-0053-01
100's	$185.04	BACTRIM DS, Women First Healthcare	64248-0117-10
250's	$271.48	BACTRIM DS, Roche Laboratories	00004-0117-04
Tablet - Oral - 400 mg;80 mg			
100's	$13.25	FEDERAL UPPER LIMIT, H.C.F.A. F F P	99999-2289-06
Tablet - Oral - 800 mg;160 mg			
100's	$15.90	FEDERAL UPPER LIMIT, H.C.F.A. F F P	99999-2289-11

PRODUCT LISTING - EQUIVALENTS NOT AVAILABLE

Qty	Price	Description	NDC
Suspension - Oral - 40 mg;200 mg/5 ml			
5 ml	$3.47	GENERIC, Prescript Pharmaceuticals	00247-0096-05
20 ml	$3.80	GENERIC, Prescript Pharmaceuticals	00247-0096-20
30 ml	$4.04	GENERIC, Prescript Pharmaceuticals	00247-0096-30
50 ml	$3.35	GENERIC, Southwood Pharmaceuticals Inc	58016-0164-10
50 ml	$4.48	GENERIC, Prescript Pharmaceuticals	00247-0096-50
60 ml	$4.71	GENERIC, Prescript Pharmaceuticals	00247-0096-60
90 ml	$5.39	GENERIC, Prescript Pharmaceuticals	00247-0096-90
100 ml	$5.27	GENERIC, Physicians Total Care	54868-0276-01
100 ml	$5.60	GENERIC, Southwood Pharmaceuticals Inc	58016-0164-20
100 ml	$5.61	GENERIC, Prescript Pharmaceuticals	00247-0096-00
100 ml	$6.05	GENERIC, Pharma Pac	52959-1023-05
118 ml	$6.02	GENERIC, Prescript Pharmaceuticals	00247-0096-52
120 ml	$6.07	GENERIC, Prescript Pharmaceuticals	00247-0096-77
120 ml	$6.73	GENERIC, Southwood Pharmaceuticals Inc	58016-0164-24
120 ml	$7.05	GENERIC, Pharma Pac	52959-1023-07
150 ml	$4.74	GENERIC, Allscripts Pharmaceutical Company	54569-4003-02
150 ml	$6.75	GENERIC, Prescript Pharmaceuticals	00247-0096-78
150 ml	$7.59	GENERIC, Southwood Pharmaceuticals Inc	58016-0164-30
150 ml	$7.99	GENERIC, Pharma Pac	52959-1023-09
180 ml	$7.42	GENERIC, Prescript Pharmaceuticals	00247-0096-59
180 ml	$8.37	GENERIC, Southwood Pharmaceuticals Inc	58016-0164-36
180 ml	$8.74	GENERIC, Pharma Pac	52959-1023-01
200 ml	$6.33	GENERIC, Allscripts Pharmaceutical Company	54569-4003-01
200 ml	$7.88	GENERIC, Prescript Pharmaceuticals	00247-0096-79
200 ml	$8.74	GENERIC, Southwood Pharmaceuticals Inc	58016-0164-40
200 ml	$9.26	GENERIC, Pharma Pac	52959-1023-03
240 ml	$8.79	GENERIC, Prescript Pharmaceuticals	00247-0096-95
240 ml	$9.44	GENERIC, Southwood Pharmaceuticals Inc	58016-0164-48
300 ml	$10.14	GENERIC, Prescript Pharmaceuticals	00247-0096-33
400 ml	$12.41	GENERIC, Prescript Pharmaceuticals	00247-0096-49
473 ml	$14.06	GENERIC, Prescript Pharmaceuticals	00247-0096-38
Tablet - Oral - 80 mg;400 mg			
20's	$6.22	GENERIC, Southwood Pharmaceuticals Inc	58016-0171-20
30's	$7.12	GENERIC, Southwood Pharmaceuticals Inc	58016-0171-30
Tablet - Oral - 160 mg;800 mg			
1's	$3.45	GENERIC, Prescript Pharmaceuticals	00247-0063-01
2's	$3.54	GENERIC, Prescript Pharmaceuticals	00247-0063-02
3's	$3.64	GENERIC, Prescript Pharmaceuticals	00247-0063-03
4's	$3.73	GENERIC, Prescript Pharmaceuticals	00247-0063-04
5's	$7.20	GENERIC, Allscripts Pharmaceutical Company	54569-2986-04
6's	$3.91	GENERIC, Prescript Pharmaceuticals	00247-0063-06
6's	$4.36	GENERIC, Pharmaceutical Corporation Of America	51655-0112-87
6's	$8.08	GENERIC, Southwood Pharmaceuticals Inc	58016-0109-06
6's	$8.52	GENERIC, Pharma Pac	52959-0144-06
7's	$4.00	GENERIC, Prescript Pharmaceuticals	00247-0063-07
7's	$9.43	GENERIC, Southwood Pharmaceuticals Inc	58016-0109-07
8's	$4.09	GENERIC, Prescript Pharmaceuticals	00247-0063-08
10's	$3.90	GENERIC, Ampharco Inc	59015-0459-01
10's	$4.02	GENERIC, Physicians Total Care	54868-0021-06
10's	$4.28	GENERIC, Prescript Pharmaceuticals	00247-0063-10
10's	$12.48	GENERIC, Alpharma Uspd Makers Of Barre and Nmc	63874-0118-10
10's	$13.47	GENERIC, Southwood Pharmaceuticals Inc	58016-0109-10
10's	$13.56	GENERIC, Pharma Pac	52959-0144-10
10's	$14.41	GENERIC, Allscripts Pharmaceutical Company	54569-0075-00
12's	$4.47	GENERIC, Prescript Pharmaceuticals	00247-0063-12
12's	$16.16	GENERIC, Southwood Pharmaceuticals Inc	58016-0109-12
12's	$17.29	GENERIC, Allscripts Pharmaceutical Company	54569-2986-05
14's	$4.65	GENERIC, Prescript Pharmaceuticals	00247-0063-14
14's	$8.84	GENERIC, Pharmaceutical Corporation Of America	51655-0112-84
14's	$17.68	GENERIC, Alpharma Uspd Makers Of Barre and Nmc	63874-0118-14
14's	$18.47	GENERIC, Pharma Pac	52959-0144-14
14's	$18.86	GENERIC, Southwood Pharmaceuticals Inc	58016-0109-14
15's	$4.74	GENERIC, Prescript Pharmaceuticals	00247-0063-15
15's	$5.20	GENERIC, Physicians Total Care	54868-0021-05
15's	$20.20	GENERIC, Southwood Pharmaceuticals Inc	58016-0109-15
16's	$4.84	GENERIC, Prescript Pharmaceuticals	00247-0063-16
18's	$24.24	GENERIC, Southwood Pharmaceuticals Inc	58016-0109-18
20's	$5.21	GENERIC, Prescript Pharmaceuticals	00247-0063-20
20's	$6.38	GENERIC, Physicians Total Care	54868-0021-01
20's	$12.20	GENERIC, Pharmaceutical Corporation Of America	51655-0112-52
20's	$23.92	GENERIC, Alpharma Uspd Makers Of Barre and Nmc	63874-0118-20
20's	$25.69	GENERIC, Pharma Pac	52959-0144-20
20's	$26.94	GENERIC, Southwood Pharmaceuticals Inc	58016-0109-20
21's	$26.62	GENERIC, Pharma Pac	52959-0144-21
21's	$28.28	GENERIC, Southwood Pharmaceuticals Inc	58016-0109-21
24's	$32.32	GENERIC, Southwood Pharmaceuticals Inc	58016-0109-24
28's	$5.95	GENERIC, Prescript Pharmaceuticals	00247-0063-28
28's	$16.68	GENERIC, Pharmaceutical Corporation Of America	51655-0112-29
28's	$35.52	GENERIC, Pharma Pac	52959-0144-28
28's	$37.71	GENERIC, Southwood Pharmaceuticals Inc	58016-0109-28
30's	$6.13	GENERIC, Prescript Pharmaceuticals	00247-0063-30
30's	$8.47	GENERIC, Physicians Total Care	54868-0021-07
30's	$17.80	GENERIC, Pharmaceutical Corporation Of America	51655-0112-24
30's	$37.74	GENERIC, Pharma Pac	52959-0144-30
30's	$40.40	GENERIC, Southwood Pharmaceuticals Inc	58016-0109-30
40's	$53.87	GENERIC, Southwood Pharmaceuticals Inc	58016-0109-40
42's	$7.25	GENERIC, Prescript Pharmaceuticals	00247-0063-42
50's	$67.34	GENERIC, Southwood Pharmaceuticals Inc	58016-0109-50
60's	$8.92	GENERIC, Prescript Pharmaceuticals	00247-0063-60
60's	$15.81	GENERIC, Physicians Total Care	54868-0021-04
60's	$34.60	GENERIC, Pharmaceutical Corporation Of America	51655-0112-25
60's	$80.81	GENERIC, Southwood Pharmaceuticals Inc	58016-0109-60
80's	$107.74	GENERIC, Southwood Pharmaceuticals Inc	58016-0109-80
98's	$49.68	GENERIC, Prescript Pharmaceuticals	00247-0063-98
100's	$12.62	GENERIC, Prescript Pharmaceuticals	00247-0063-00
100's	$24.40	GENERIC, Physicians Total Care	54868-0021-00
100's	$134.68	GENERIC, Southwood Pharmaceuticals Inc	58016-0109-00

Sulfasalazine *(002292)*

Categories: Colitis, ulcerative; Pregnancy Category B; FDA Approved 1950 Jun; WHO Formulary
Drug Classes: Disease modifying antirheumatic drugs; Gastrointestinals; Salicylates
Brand Names: Azaline; **Azulfidine**
Foreign Brand Availability: Colo-Pleon (Germany); Disalazin (Peru); Pleon RA (Germany); Pyralin EN (Australia); Rosulfant (Colombia); Salazopirina (Portugal); Salazopyrin (Australia; Austria; Bahrain; Canada; China; Cyprus; Denmark; Egypt; England; Finland; Hungary; India; Iran; Iraq; Israel; Italy; Japan; Jordan; Kuwait; Lebanon; Libya; Norway; Oman; Qatar; Republic-of-Yemen; Saudi-Arabia; South-Africa; Sweden; Switzerland; Syria; United-Arab-Emirates); Salazopyrin-EN (Australia; Canada; Colombia; England; Finland; Hong-Kong; India; Israel; Italy; Korea; Malaysia; New-Zealand; Norway; South-Africa; Sweden; Taiwan; Thailand); Salazopyrin Entabs (Bahrain; Cyprus; Denmark; Egypt; Iran; Iraq; Jordan; Kuwait; Lebanon; Libya; Oman; Qatar; Republic-of-Yemen; Saudi-Arabia; Syria; United-Arab-Emirates); Salazopyrina (Spain); Salazopyrine (Belgium; France; Netherlands); Salazopyrine EC (Belgium); Saridine (Thailand); Sulcolon (Indonesia); Sulfazine (Ireland); Zopyrin (Korea)
Cost of Therapy: $70.02 (Ulcerative Colitis; Azulfidine; 500 mg; 6 tablets/day; 30 day supply)
$22.95 (Ulcerative Colitis; Generic Tablets; 500 mg; 6 tablets/day; 30 day supply)
$83.88 (Ulcerative Colitis; Azulfidine En-Tabs; 500 mg; 6 tablets/day; 30 day supply)
$55.92 (Rheumatoid Arthritis; Azulfidine En-Tabs; 500 mg; 4 tablets/day; 30 day supply)

DESCRIPTION

Azulfidine EN-tabs tablets contain sulfasalazine, formulated in a delayed-release tablet (enteric-coated), 500 mg, for oral administration.

Azulfidine EN-tabs tablets are film coated with cellulose acetate phthalate to retard disintegration of the tablet in the stomach and reduce potential irritation of the gastric mucosa.

Therapeutic Classification: Anti-inflammatory agent and/or immunomodulatory agent.
Chemical Designation: 5-([p-(2-pyridylsulfamoyl)phenyl]azo) salicylic acid.
Molecular Formula: $C_{18}H_{14}N_4O_5S$.

CLINICAL PHARMACOLOGY

PHARMACODYNAMICS

The mode of action of sulfasalazine (SSZ) or its metabolites, 5-aminosalicylic acid (5-ASA) and sulfapyridine (SP), is still under investigation, but may be related to the anti-inflammatory and/or immunomodulatory properties that have been observed in animal and *in vitro* models, to its affinity for connective tissue, and/or to the relatively high concentration it reaches in serous fluids, the liver, and intestinal walls, as demonstrated in autoradiographic studies in animals. In ulcerative colitis, clinical studies utilizing rectal administration of SSZ, SP, and 5-ASA have indicated that the major therapeutic action may reside in the 5-ASA moiety. The relative contribution of the parent drug and the major metabolites in rheumatoid arthritis is unknown.

PHARMACOKINETICS

In vivo studies have indicated that the absolute bioavailability of orally administered SSZ is less than 15% for parent drug. In the intestine, SSZ is metabolized by intestinal bacteria to SP and 5-ASA. Of the two species, SP is relatively well absorbed from the intestine and highly metabolized, while 5-ASA is much less well absorbed.

S

Absorption

Following oral administration of 1 g of SSZ to 9 healthy males, less than 15% of a dose of SSZ is absorbed as parent drug. Detectable serum concentrations of SSZ have been found in healthy subjects within 90 minutes after the ingestion. Maximum concentrations of SSZ occur between 3 and 12 hours post-ingestion, with the mean peak concentration (6 μg/ml) occurring at 6 hours.

In comparison, peak plasma levels of both SP and 5-ASA occur approximately 10 hours after dosing. This longer time to peak is indicative of gastrointestinal transit to the lower intestine, where bacteria-mediated metabolism occurs. SP apparently is well absorbed from the colon, with an estimated bioavailability of 60%. In this same study, 5-ASA is much less well absorbed from the gastrointestinal tract, with an estimated bioavailability of 10-30%.

Distribution

Following intravenous injection, the calculated volume of distribution (Vdss) for SSZ was 7.5 ± 1.6 L. SSZ is highly bound to albumin (>99.3%), while SP is only about 70% bound to albumin. Acetylsulfapyridine (AcSP), the principal metabolite of SP, is approximately 90% bound to plasma proteins.

Metabolism

As mentioned above, SSZ is metabolized by intestinal bacteria to SP and 5-ASA. Approximately 15% of a dose of SSZ is absorbed as parent and is metabolized to some extent in the liver to the same two species. The observed plasma half-life for intravenous sulfasalazine is 7.6 ± 3.4 hours. The primary route of metabolism of SP is via acetylation to form AcSP. The rate of metabolism of SP to AcSP is dependent upon acetylator phenotype. In fast acetylators, the mean plasma half-life of SP is 10.4 hours, while in slow acetylators it is 14.8 hours. SP can also be metabolized to 5-hydroxy-sulfapyridine (SPOH) and N-acetyl-5-hydroxy-sulfapyridine. 5-ASA is primarily metabolized in both the liver and intestine to N-acetyl-5-aminosalicylic acid via a non-acetylation phenotype dependent route. Due to low plasma levels produced by 5-ASA after oral administration, reliable estimates of plasma half-life are not possible.

Excretion

Absorbed SP and 5-ASA and their metabolites are primarily eliminated in the urine either as free metabolites or as glucuronide conjugates. The majority of 5-ASA stays within the colonic lumen and is excreted as 5-ASA and acetyl-5-ASA with the feces. The calculated clearance of SSZ following intravenous administration was 1 L/h. Renal clearance was estimated to account for 37% of total clearance.

SPECIAL POPULATIONS

Elderly

Elderly patients with rheumatoid arthritis showed a prolonged plasma half-life for SSZ, SP, and their metabolites. The clinical impact of this is unknown.

Pediatric

Small studies have been reported in the literature in children down to the age of 4 years with ulcerative colitis and inflammatory bowel disease. In these populations, relative to adults, the pharmacokinetics of SSZ and SP correlated poorly with either age or dose. To date, comparative pharmacokinetic trials have not been conducted to determine whether or not significant pharmacokinetic differences exist between children with juvenile rheumatoid arthritis and adults with rheumatoid arthritis.

Acetylator Status

The metabolism of SP to AcSP is mediated by polymorphic enzymes such that two distinct populations of slow and fast metabolizers exist. Approximately 60% of the Caucasian population can be classified as belonging to the slow acetylator phenotype. These subjects will display a prolonged plasma half-life for SP (14.8 hours vs 10.4 hours) and an accumulation of higher plasma levels of SP than fast acetylators. The clinical implication of this is unclear; however, in a small pharmacokinetic trial where acetylator status was determined, subjects who were slow acetylators of SP showed a higher incidence of adverse events.

Gender

Gender appears not to have an effect on either the rate or the pattern of metabolites of SSZ, SP, or 5-ASA.

INDICATIONS AND USAGE

Sulfasalazine tablets are indicated:

In the treatment of mild to moderate ulcerative colitis, and as adjunctive therapy in severe ulcerative colitis.

For the prolongation of the remission period between acute attacks of ulcerative colitis.

In the treatment of patients with rheumatoid arthritis who have responded inadequately to salicylates or other nonsteroidal anti-inflammatory drugs (*e.g.,* an insufficient therapeutic response to, or intolerance of, an adequate trial of full doses of one or more nonsteroidal anti-inflammatory drugs).

In the treatment of pediatric patients with polyarticular-course[1] juvenile rheumatoid arthritis who have responded inadequately to salicylates or other nonsteroidal anti-inflammatory drugs.

Sulfasalazine delayed-release tablets are particularly indicated in patients with ulcerative colitis who cannot take uncoated sulfasalazine tablets because of gastrointestinal intolerance, and in whom there is evidence that this intolerance is not primarily the result of high blood levels of sulfapyridine and its metabolites, *e.g.,* patients experiencing nausea and vomiting with the first few doses of the drug, or patients in whom a reduction in dosage does not alleviate the adverse gastrointestinal effects.

In patients with rheumatoid arthritis or juvenile rheumatoid arthritis, rest and physiotherapy as indicated should be continued. Unlike anti-inflammatory drugs, sulfasalazine delayed-release tablets do not produce an immediate response. Concurrent treatment with analgesics and/or nonsteroidal anti-inflammatory drugs is recommended at least until the effect of sulfasalazine delayed-release tablets is apparent.

CONTRAINDICATIONS

Sulfasalazine tablets are contraindicated in:

Hypersensitivity to sulfasalazine, its metabolites, sulfonamides or salicylates.

Patients with intestinal or urinary obstruction.

Patients with porphyria, as the sulfonamides have been reported to precipitate an acute attack.

WARNINGS

Only after critical appraisal should sulfasalazine tablets be given to patients with hepatic or renal damage or blood dyscrasias. Deaths associated with the administration of sulfasalazine have been reported from hypersensitivity reactions, agranulocytosis, aplastic anemia, other blood dyscrasias, renal and liver damage, irreversible neuromuscular and central nervous system changes, and fibrosing alveolitis. The presence of clinical signs such as sore throat, fever, pallor, purpura, or jaundice may be indications of serious blood disorders. Complete blood counts, as well as urinalysis with careful microscopic examination, should be done frequently in patients receiving sulfasalazine tablets (see PRECAUTIONS, Laboratory Tests). Oligospermia and infertility have been observed in men treated with sulfasalazine; however, withdrawal of the drug appears to reverse these effects.

PRECAUTIONS

GENERAL

Sulfasalazine tablets should be given with caution to patients with severe allergy or bronchial asthma. Adequate fluid intake must be maintained in order to prevent crystalluria and stone formation. Patients with glucose-6-phosphate dehydrogenase deficiency should be observed closely for signs of hemolytic anemia. This reaction is frequently dose related. If toxic or hypersensitivity reactions occur, sulfasalazine tablets should be discontinued immediately.

Isolated instances have been reported when sulfasalazine delayed-release tablets have passed undisintegrated. If this is observed, the administration of sulfasalazine delayed-release tablets should be discontinued immediately.

INFORMATION FOR THE PATIENT

Patients should be informed of the possibility of adverse effects and of the need for careful medical supervision. The occurrence of sore throat, fever, pallor, purpura, or jaundice may indicate a serious blood disorder. Should any of these occur, the patient should seek medical advice.

Patients should be instructed to take sulfasalazine tablets in evenly divided doses, preferably after meals, and to swallow the tablets whole. Additionally, patients should be advised that sulfasalazine may produce an orange-yellow discoloration of the urine or skin.

Ulcerative Colitis

Patients with ulcerative colitis should be made aware that ulcerative colitis rarely remits completely, and that the risk of relapse can be substantially reduced by continued administration of sulfasalazine delayed-release tablets at a maintenance dosage.

Rheumatoid Arthritis

Rheumatoid arthritis rarely remits. Therefore, continued administration of sulfasalazine delayed-release tablets is indicated. Patients requiring sulfasalazine should follow up with their physicians to determine the need for continued administration.

LABORATORY TESTS

Complete blood counts, including differential white cell count and liver function tests, should be performed before starting sulfasalazine tablets and every second week during the first 3 months of therapy. During the second 3 months, the same tests should be done once monthly and, thereafter, once every 3 months and as clinically indicated. Urinalysis and an assessment of renal function should also be done periodically during treatment with sulfasalazine tablets.

The determination of serum sulfapyridine levels may be useful since concentrations greater than 50 μg/ml appear to be associated with an increased incidence of adverse reactions.

DRUG/LABORATORY TEST INTERACTIONS

The presence of sulfasalazine or its metabolites in body fluids has not been reported to interfere with laboratory test procedures.

CARCINOGENESIS, MUTAGENESIS, AND IMPAIRMENT OF FERTILITY

Two year oral carcinogenicity studies were conducted in male and female F344/N rats and B6C3F1 mice. Sulfasalazine was tested at 84 (496 mg/m^2), 168 (991 mg/m^2), and 337.5 (1991 mg/m^2) mg/kg/day doses in rats. A statistically significant increase in the incidence of urinary bladder transitional cell papillomas was observed in male rats. In female rats, 2 (4%) of the 337.5 mg/kg rats had transitional cell papilloma of the kidney. The increased incidence of neoplasms in the urinary bladder and kidney of rats was also associated with an increase in the renal calculi formation and hyperplasia of transitional cell epithelium. For the mouse study, sulfasalazine was tested at 675 (2025 mg/m^2), 1350 (4050 mg/m^2), and 2700 (8100 mg/m^2) mg/kg/day. The incidence of hepatocellular adenoma or carcinoma in male and female mice was significantly greater than the control at all doses tested.

Sulfasalazine did not show mutagenicity in the bacterial reverse mutation assay (Ames test) or in the L51784 mouse lymphoma cell assay at the HGPRT gene. However, sulfasalazine showed equivocal mutagenic response in the micronucleus assay of mouse and rat bone marrow and mouse peripheral RBC and in the sister chromatid exchange, chromosomal aberration, and micronucleus assays in lymphocytes obtained from humans.

Impairment of male fertility was observed in reproductive studies performed in rats at a dose of 800 mg/kg/day (4800 mg/m^2). Oligospermia and infertility have been described in men treated with sulfasalazine. Withdrawal of the drug appears to reverse these effects.

PREGNANCY CATEGORY B

Teratogenic Effects

Reproduction studies have been performed in rats and rabbits at doses up to 6 times the human dose and have revealed no evidence of impaired female fertility or harm to the fetus due to sulfasalazine. There are, however, no adequate and well-controlled studies in pregnant women. Because animal reproduction studies are not always predictive of human response, this drug should be used during pregnancy only if clearly needed.

A national survey evaluated the outcome of pregnancies associated with inflammatory bowel disease (IBD). In 186 pregnancies in women treated with sulfasalazine alone or sulfasalazine and concomitant steroid therapy, the incidence of fetal morbidity and mortality was comparable both to that of 245 untreated IBD pregnancies, and to pregnancies in the general population.[2]

A study of 1455 pregnancies associated with exposure to sulfonamides, including sulfasalazine, indicated that this group of drugs did not appear to be associated with fetal malformation.[3] A review of the medical literature covering 1155 pregnancies in women with ulcerative colitis suggested that the outcome was similar to that expected in the general population.[4]

No clinical studies have been performed to evaluate the effect of sulfasalazine on the growth development and functional maturation of children whose mothers received the drug during pregnancy.

Nonteratogenic Effects

Sulfasalazine and sulfapyridine pass the placental barrier. Although sulfapyridine has been shown to have poor bilirubin-displacing capacity, the potential for kernicterus in newborns should be kept in mind.

A case of agranulocytosis has been reported in an infant whose mother was taking both sulfasalazine and prednisone throughout pregnancy.

NURSING MOTHERS

Caution should be exercised when sulfasalazine tablets are administered to a nursing mother. Sulfonamides are excreted in the milk. In the newborn, they compete with bilirubin for binding sites on the plasma proteins and may cause kernicterus. Insignificant amounts of uncleaved sulfasalazine have been found in milk, whereas the sulfapyridine levels in milk are about 30-60% of those in the maternal serum. Sulfapyridine has been shown to have a poor bilirubin-displacing capacity.

PEDIATRIC USE

The safety and effectiveness of sulfasalazine delayed-release tablets in pediatric patients below the age of 2 years with ulcerative colitis have not been established.

The safety and effectiveness of sulfasalazine delayed-release tablets for the treatment of the signs and symptoms of polyarticular-course juvenile rheumatoid arthritis in pediatric patients aged 6-16 years is supported by evidence from adequate and well-controlled studies in adult rheumatoid arthritis patients. The extrapolation from adults with rheumatoid arthritis to children with polyarticular-course juvenile rheumatoid arthritis is based on similarities in disease and response to therapy between these two patient populations. Published studies support the extrapolation of safety and effectiveness for sulfasalazine to polyarticular-course juvenile rheumatoid arthritis[1,5] (see ADVERSE REACTIONS).

It has been reported that the frequency of adverse events in patients with systemic-course of juvenile arthritis is high.[6] Use in children with systemic-course juvenile rheumatoid arthritis has frequently resulted in a serum sickness-like reaction.[5] This reaction is often severe and presents as fever, nausea, vomiting, headache, rash, and abnormal liver function tests. Treatment of systemic-course juvenile rheumatoid arthritis with sulfasalazine is not recommended.

DRUG INTERACTIONS

Reduced absorption of folic acid and digoxin have been reported when those agents were administered concomitantly with sulfasalazine.

When daily doses of sulfasalazine 2 g and weekly doses of methotrexate 7.5 mg were coadministered to 15 rheumatoid arthritis patients in a drug-drug interaction study, the pharmacokinetic disposition of the drugs was not altered.

Daily doses of sulfasalazine 2 g (maximum 3 g) and weekly doses of methotrexate 7.5 mg (maximum 15 mg) were administered alone or in combination to 310 rheumatoid arthritis patients in two controlled 52 week clinical studies. The overall toxicity profile of the combination revealed an increased incidence of gastrointestinal adverse events, especially nausea, when compared to the incidence associated with either drug administered alone.

ADVERSE REACTIONS

The most common adverse reactions associated with sulfasalazine in ulcerative colitis are anorexia, headache, nausea, vomiting, gastric distress, and apparently reversible oligospermia. These occur in about one-third of the patients. Less frequent adverse reactions are pruritus, urticaria, rash, fever, Heinz body anemia, hemolytic anemia, and cyanosis, which may occur at a frequency of 1 in 30 patients or less. Experience suggests that with a daily dosage of 4 g or more, or total serum sulfapyridine levels above 50 μg/ml, the incidence of adverse reactions tends to increase.

Similar adverse reactions are associated with sulfasalazine use in adult rheumatoid arthritis, although there was a greater incidence of some reactions. In rheumatoid arthritis studies, the following common adverse reactions were noted: nausea (19%), dyspepsia (13%), rash (13%), headache (9%), abdominal pain (8%), vomiting (8%), fever (5%), dizziness (4%), pruritus (4%), abnormal liver function tests (4%), leukopenia (3%), and thrombocytopenia (1%). One report[7] showed a 10% rate of immunoglobulin suppression, which was slowly reversible and rarely accompanied by clinical findings.

In general, the adverse reactions in juvenile rheumatoid arthritis patients are similar to those seen in patients with adult rheumatoid arthritis except for a high frequency of serum sickness-like syndrome in systemic-course juvenile rheumatoid arthritis (see PRECAUTIONS, Pediatric Use). One clinical trial showed an approximate 10% rate of immunoglobulin suppression.[1]

Although the listing which follows includes a few adverse reactions which have not been reported with this specific drug, the pharmacological similarities among the sulfonamides require that each of these reactions be considered when sulfasalazine tablets are administered.

Less common or rare adverse reactions include:

Blood Dyscrasias: Aplastic anemia, agranulocytosis, megaloblastic (macrocytic) anemia, purpura, hypoprothrombinemia, methemoglobinemia, congenital neutropenia, and myelodysplastic syndrome.

Hypersensitivity Reactions: Erythema multiforme (Stevens-Johnson syndrome), exfoliative dermatitis, epidermal necrolysis (Lyell's syndrome) with corneal damage, anaphylaxis, serum sickness syndrome, pneumonitis with or without eosinophilia, vasculitis, fibrosing alveolitis, pleuritis, pericarditis with or without tamponade, allergic myocarditis, polyarteritis nodosa, lupus erythematosus-like syndrome, hepatitis and hepatic necrosis with or without immune complexes, fulminant hepatitis, sometimes leading to liver transplantation, parapsoriasis varioliformis acuta (Mucha-Haberman syndrome), rhabdomyolysis, photosensitization, arthralgia, periorbital edema, conjunctival and scleral injection, and alopecia.

Gastrointestinal Reactions: Hepatitis, pancreatitis, bloody diarrhea, impaired folic acid absorption, impaired digoxin absorption, diarrhea, and neutropenic enterocolitis.

Central Nervous System Reactions: Transverse myelitis, convulsions, meningitis, transient lesions of the posterior spinal column, cauda equina syndrome, Guillain-Barre syndrome, peripheral neuropathy, mental depression, vertigo, hearing loss, insomnia, ataxia, hallucinations, tinnitus, and drowsiness.

Renal Reactions: Toxic nephrosis with oliguria and anuria, nephritis, nephrotic syndrome, urinary tract infections, hematuria, crystalluria, proteinuria, and hemolytic-uremic syndrome.

Other Reactions: Urine discoloration and skin discoloration.

The sulfonamides bear certain chemical similarities to some goitrogens, diuretics (acetazolamide and the thiazides), and oral hypoglycemic agents. Goiter production, diuresis, and hypoglycemia have occurred rarely in patients receiving sulfonamides. Cross-sensitivity may exist with these agents. Rats appear to be especially susceptible to the goitrogenic effects of sulfonamides, and long-term administration has produced thyroid malignancies in this species.

POSTMARKETING REPORTS

The following events have been identified during post-approval use of products which contain (or are metabolized to) mesalamine in clinical practice. Because they are reported voluntarily from a population of unknown size, estimates of frequency cannot be made. These events have been chosen for inclusion due to a combination of seriousness, frequency of reporting, or potential causal connection to mesalamine.

Gastrointestinal

Reports of hepatotoxicity, including elevated liver function tests (SGOT/AST, SGPT/ALT, GGT, LDH, alkaline phosphatase, bilirubin), jaundice, cholestatic jaundice, cirrhosis, and possible hepatocellular damage including liver necrosis and liver failure. Some of these cases were fatal. One case of Kawasaki-like syndrome, which included hepatic function changes, was also reported.

DOSAGE AND ADMINISTRATION

The dosage of sulfasalazine tablets should be adjusted to each individual's response and tolerance.

Patients should be instructed to take sulfasalazine delayed-release tablets in evenly divided doses, preferably after meals, and to swallow the tablets whole.

ULCERATIVE COLITIS

Initial Therapy

Adults

3-4 g daily in evenly divided doses with dosage intervals not exceeding 8 hours. It may be advisable to initiate therapy with a lower dosage, *e.g.*, 1-2 g daily, to reduce possible gastrointestinal intolerance. If daily doses exceeding 4 g are required to achieve the desired therapeutic effect, the increased risk of toxicity should be kept in mind.

Children, 6 Years of Age and Older

40-60 mg/kg of body weight in each 24 hour period, divided into 3-6 doses.

Maintenance Therapy

Adults

2 g daily.

Children, 6 Years of Age and Older

30 mg/kg of body weight in each 24 hour period, divided into 4 doses. The response of acute ulcerative colitis to sulfasalazine delayed-release tablets can be evaluated by clinical criteria, including the presence of fever, weight changes, and degree and frequency of diarrhea and bleeding, as well as by sigmoidoscopy and the evaluation of biopsy samples. It is often necessary to continue medication even when clinical symptoms, including diarrhea, have been controlled. When endoscopic examination confirms satisfactory improvement, dosage of sulfasalazine should be reduced to a maintenance level. If diarrhea recurs, dosage should be increased to previously effective levels.

Sulfasalazine delayed-release tablets are particularly indicated in patients who cannot take uncoated sulfasalazine tablets because of gastrointestinal intolerance (*e.g.*, anorexia, nausea). If symptoms of gastric intolerance (anorexia, nausea, vomiting, etc.) occur after the first few doses of sulfasalazine delayed-release tablets, they are probably due to increased serum levels of total sulfapyridine, and may be alleviated by having the daily dose of sulfasalazine delayed-release tablets and subsequently increasing it gradually over several days. If gastric intolerance continues, the drug should be stopped for 5-7 days, then reintroduced at a lower daily dose.

ADULT RHEUMATOID ARTHRITIS

2 g daily in 2 evenly divided doses. It is advisable to initiate therapy with a lower dosage of sulfasalazine delayed-release tablets, *e.g.*, 0.5-1.0 g daily, to reduce possible gastrointestinal intolerance. A suggested dosing schedule is given in TABLE 1.

In rheumatoid arthritis, the effect of sulfasalazine delayed-release tablets can be assessed by the degree of improvement in the number and extent of actively inflamed joints. A therapeutic response has been observed as early as 4 weeks after starting therapy with sulfasalazine delayed-release tablets, but treatment for 12 weeks may be required in some patients before clinical benefit is noted. Consideration can be given to increasing the daily dose of sulfasalazine delayed-release tablets to 3 g if the clinical response after 12 weeks is inadequate. Careful monitoring is recommended for doses over 2 g/day.

TABLE 1 *Suggested Dosing Schedule for Adult Rheumatoid Arthritis*

Week of Treatment	Number of Sulfasalazine Extended-Release Tablets	
	Morning	Evening
1	—	One
2	One	One
3	One	Two
4	Two	Two

JUVENILE RHEUMATOID ARTHRITIS — POLYARTICULAR COURSE

Children, 6 Years of Age and Older

30-50 mg/kg of body weight daily in 2 evenly divided doses. Typically, the maximum dose is 2 g/day. To reduce possible gastrointestinal intolerance, begin with a quarter to a third of the planned maintenance dose and increase weekly until reaching the maintenance dose at 1 month.

Some patients may be sensitive to treatment with sulfasalazine. Various desensitization-like regimens have been reported to be effective in 34 of 53 patients,[8] 7 of 8 patients,[9] and 19 of 20 patients.[10] These regimens suggest starting with a total daily dose of 50-250 mg sulfasalazine initially, and doubling it every 4-7 days until the desired therapeutic level is achieved. If the symptoms of sensitivity recur, sulfasalazine delayed-release tablets should be discontinued. Desensitization should not be attempted in patients who have a history of agranulocytosis, or who have experienced an anaphylactoid reaction while previously receiving sulfasalazine.

HOW SUPPLIED

Azulfidine EN-tabs tablets, 500 mg, are elliptical, gold-colored, film enteric-coated tablets, monogrammed "102" on one side and "KPh" on the other.

Storage: Store at 25°C (77°F); excursions permitted to 15-30°C (59-86°F).

PRODUCT LISTING - RATED THERAPEUTICALLY EQUIVALENT

Tablet - Oral - 500 mg

30's	$4.32	GENERIC, Heartland Healthcare Services	61392-0147-30
30's	$4.32	GENERIC, Heartland Healthcare Services	61392-0147-39
30's	$4.44	GENERIC, Allscripts Pharmaceutical Company	54569-0313-03
31's	$4.46	GENERIC, Heartland Healthcare Services	61392-0147-31
32's	$4.60	GENERIC, Heartland Healthcare Services	61392-0147-32
45's	$6.48	GENERIC, Heartland Healthcare Services	61392-0147-45
50's	$3.51	GENERIC, Circle Pharmaceuticals Inc	00659-0106-05
60's	$8.63	GENERIC, Heartland Healthcare Services	61392-0147-60
90's	$12.95	GENERIC, Heartland Healthcare Services	61392-0147-90
100's	$10.74	GENERIC, Us Trading Corporation	56126-0306-11
100's	$12.75	GENERIC, Cmc-Consolidated Midland Corporation	00223-1727-01
100's	$14.40	GENERIC, Ivax Corporation	00182-1016-01
100's	$14.93	GENERIC, Interstate Drug Exchange Inc	00814-7230-14
100's	$15.55	GENERIC, Aligen Independent Laboratories Inc	00405-4956-01
100's	$17.57	FEDERAL UPPER LIMIT, H.C.F.A. F F P	99999-2292-01
100's	$20.08	GENERIC, Qualitest Products Inc	00603-5802-21
100's	$20.08	GENERIC, Allscripts Pharmaceutical Company	54569-0313-01
100's	$24.25	GENERIC, Greenstone Limited	59762-5000-01
100's	$25.49	GENERIC, Qualitest Products Inc	00603-5801-21
100's	$25.49	GENERIC, Major Pharmaceuticals Inc	00904-1152-60
100's	$25.49	GENERIC, Mutual Pharmaceutical Co Inc	53489-0147-01
100's	$25.50	GENERIC, Watson Laboratories Inc	00591-0796-01
100's	$25.50	GENERIC, Watson Laboratories Inc	52544-0796-01
100's	$38.90	AZULFIDINE, Pharmacia and Upjohn	00013-0101-01

Tablet, Enteric Coated - Oral - 500 mg

100's	$38.42	GENERIC, Vintage Pharmaceuticals Inc	00254-5905-28
100's	$38.42	GENERIC, Qualitest Products Inc	00603-5803-21
100's	$46.60	AZULFIDINE EN-TABS, Pharmacia and Upjohn	00013-0102-01

PRODUCT LISTING - EQUIVALENTS NOT AVAILABLE

Tablet - Oral - 500 mg

10's	$5.25	GENERIC, Pd-Rx Pharmaceuticals	55289-0176-10
40's	$8.78	GENERIC, Pd-Rx Pharmaceuticals	55289-0176-40
50's	$8.16	GENERIC, Physicians Total Care	54868-1138-00

Sulfisoxazole (002294)

For related information, see the comparative table section in Appendix A.

Categories: Chancroid; Conjunctivitis, infectious; Infection, ear, middle; Infection, urinary tract; Meningitis; Meningococcal carrier state; Nocardiosis; Toxoplasmosis; Trachoma; Pregnancy Category C; FDA Approved 1974 Mar

Drug Classes: Antibiotics, sulfonamides

Brand Names: Gantrisin; Gulfasin; Isoxazine; Lipo Gantrisin; Novosoxazole; Oxazole; Sosol; Soxa; Sulfalar; Sulfazin; Sulfazole; Sulphafurazole; Sulsoxin; Thiasin; Truxazole; Urazole

Cost of Therapy: $2.68 (Infection; Generic Tablets; 500 mg; 8 tablets/day; 10 day supply)

DESCRIPTION

Sulfisoxazole is an antibacterial sulfonamide available in tablets, pediatric suspension and syrup for oral administration. Each tablet contains 0.5 g sulfisoxazole with corn starch, gelatin, lactose and magnesium stearate. Each teaspoonful (5 ml) of the pediatric suspension contains the equivalent of approximately 0.5 g sulfisoxazole in the form of acetyl sulfisoxazole in a vehicle containing 0.3% alcohol, carboxymethylcellulose (sodium), citric acid, methylcellulose, parabens (methyl and propyl), partial invert sugar, sodium citrate, sorbitan monolaurate, sucrose, flavors and water. Each teaspoonful (5 ml) of the syrup contains the equivalent of approximately 0.5 g sulfisoxazole in the form of acetyl sulfisoxazole in a vehicle containing 0.9% alcohol, benzoic acid, carrageenan, citric acid, cocoa, sodium citrate, sorbitan monolaurate, sucrose, flavors and water.

Sulfisoxazole is N^1-(3,4-dimethyl-5-isoxazolyl) sulfanilamide. It is a white to slightly yellowish, odorless, slightly bitter, crystalline powder that is soluble in alcohol and very slightly soluble in water. Sulfisoxazole has a molecular weight of 267.30.

Acetyl sulfisoxazole, the tasteless form of sulfisoxazole, is N^1-acetyl sulfisoxazole and must be distinguished from N^4-acetyl sulfisoxazole, which is a metabolite of sulfisoxazole. Acetyl sulfisoxazole is a white or slightly yellow, crystalline powder that is slightly soluble in alcohol and practically insoluble in water. Acetyl sulfisoxazole has a molecular weight of 309.34.

CLINICAL PHARMACOLOGY

Following oral administration, sulfisoxazole is rapidly and completely absorbed; the small intestine is the major site of absorption, but some of the drug is absorbed from the stomach. Sulfisoxazole exists in the blood as unbound, protein-bound and conjugated forms. Sulfisoxazole is metabolized primarily by acetylation and oxidation in the liver. The free form is considered to be the therapeutically active form. Approximately 85% of sulfisoxazole is bound to plasma proteins, primarily to albumin; of the unbound portion, 65-72% is in the nonacetylated form.

Maximum plasma concentrations of intact sulfisoxazole following a single 2-g oral dose of sulfisoxazole to healthy adult volunteers ranged from 127-211 µg/ml (mean, 169 µg/ml) and the time of peak plasma concentration ranged from 1-4 hours (mean, 2.5 hours). The half-life of elimination of sulfisoxazole ranged from 4.6-7.8 hours after oral administration. The elimination of sulfisoxazole has been shown to be slower in elderly subjects (63-75 years) with diminished renal function (creatinine clearance, 37-68 ml/min).[1] After multiple dose oral administration of 500 mg qid to healthy volunteers, the average steady-state plasma concentrations of intact sulfisoxazole ranged from 49.9-88.8 µg/ml (mean, 63.4 µg/ml).[2]

Wide variation in blood levels may result following identical doses of a sulfonamide. Blood levels should be measured in patients receiving sulfonamides at the higher recommended doses or being treated for serious infections. Free sulfonamide blood levels of 50-150 µg/ml may be considered therapeutically effective for most infections, with blood levels of 120-150 µg/ml being optimal for serious infections. The maximum sulfonamide level should not exceed 200 µg/ml, since adverse reactions occur more frequently above this concentration.

N^1-acetyl sulfisoxazole is metabolized to sulfisoxazole by digestive enzymes in the gastrointestinal tract and is absorbed as sulfisoxazole. This enzymatic splitting is presumed to be responsible for slower absorption and lower peak blood concentrations than are attained following administration of an equal oral dose of sulfisoxazole. With continued administration of acetyl sulfisoxazole, blood concentrations approximate those of sulfisoxazole. Following a single 4-g dose of acetyl sulfisoxazole to healthy volunteers, maximum plasma concentrations of sulfisoxazole ranged from 122-282 µg/ml (mean, 181 µg/ml) for the pediatric suspension and from 101-202 µg/ml (mean, 144 µg/ml) for the syrup, and occurred between 2 and 6 hours postadministration. The half-lives of elimination from plasma ranged from 5.4-7.4 and from 5.9-8.5 hours, respectively.

Sulfisoxazole and acetylated metabolites are excreted primarily by the kidneys through glomerular filtration. Concentrations of sulfisoxazole are considerably higher in the urine than in the blood. The mean urinary excretion recovery following oral administration of sulfisoxazole is 97% within 48 hours, of which 52% is intact drug, with the remaining as the N^4-acetylated metabolite. Following administration of acetyl sulfisoxazole syrup or suspension, approximately 58% is excreted in the urine as total drug within 72 hours.

Sulfisoxazole is distributed only in extracellular body water. It is excreted in human milk. It readily crosses the placental barrier and enters into fetal circulation and also crosses the blood-brain barrier. In healthy subjects, cerebrospinal fluid concentrations of sulfisoxazole vary; in patients with meningitis, however, concentrations of free drug as high as 94 µg/ml have been reported.

MICROBIOLOGY

The sulfonamides are bacteriostatic agents and the spectrum of activity is similar for all. Sulfonamides inhibit bacterial synthesis of dihydrofolic acid by preventing the condensation of the pteridine with aminobenzoic acid through competitive inhibition of the enzyme dihydropteroate synthetase. Resistant strains have altered dihydropteroate synthetase with reduced affinity for sulfonamides or produce increased quantities of aminobenzoic acid.

SUSCEPTIBILITY TESTING

Diffusion Techniques

Quantitative methods that require measurement of zone diameters give the most precise estimate of the susceptibility of bacteria to antimicrobial agents. One such standard procedure[3] which has been recommended for use with disks to test susceptibility of organisms to sulfisoxazole uses the 250 or 300 µg sulfisoxazole disk. Interpretation involves the correlation of the diameter obtained in the disk test with the minimum inhibitory concentration (MIC) for sulfisoxazole.

Reports from the laboratory giving results of the standard single-disk susceptibility test with a 250 or 300 µg sulfisoxazole disk should be interpreted according to the following criteria:

TABLE 1

Zone Diameter (mm)	Interpretation
≥17	Susceptible
13-16	Moderately Susceptible
≤12	Resistant

A report of "susceptible" indicates that the pathogen is likely to be inhibited by generally achievable blood levels. A report of "moderately susceptible" suggests that the organism would be susceptible if high dosage is used or if the infection is confined to tissues and fluids in which high antimicrobial levels are attained. A report of "resistant" indicates that achievable concentrations are unlikely to be inhibitory, and other therapy should be selected.

Standardized procedures require the use of laboratory control organisms. The 250 or 300 µg sulfisoxazole disk should give the following zone diameters:

TABLE 2

Organism	Zone Diameter (mm)
E. coli ATCC 25922	16-26 mm
S. aureus ATCC 25923	24-34 mm

Dilution Techniques

Use a standard dilution method[4] (broth, agar, microdilution) or equivalent with sulfisoxazole powder. The MIC values obtained should be interpreted according to the following criteria:

TABLE 3

MIC (µg/ml)	Interpretation
≤256	Susceptible
≥512	Resistant

As with standard diffusion techniques, dilution methods require the use of laboratory control organisms. Dilutions of standard sulfisoxazole powder should provide the following MIC values:

TABLE 4

Organism	MIC/(µg/ml)
S. aureus ATCC 29213	32-128
E. faecalis ATCC 29212	32-128
E. coli ATCC 25922	8-32

INDICATIONS AND USAGE

Acute, recurrent or chronic urinary tract infections (primarily pyelonephritis, pyelitis and cystitis) due to susceptible organisms (usually *Escherichia coli, Klebsiella-Enterobacter,* staphylococcus, *Proteus mirabilis* and, less frequently,*Proteus vulgaris*) in the absence of obstructive uropathy or foreign bodies.

Meningococcal meningitis where the organism has been demonstrated to be susceptible. *Haemophilus influenzae* meningitis as adjunctive therapy with parenteral streptomycin.

Meningococcal meningitis prophylaxis when sulfonamide-sensitive group A strains are known to prevail in family groups or larger closed populations. (The prophylactic usefulness of sulfonamides when group B or C infections are prevalent has not been proven and in closed population groups may be harmful.)

Acute otitis media due to *Haemophilus influenzae* when used concomitantly with adequate doses of penicillin or erythromycin (see appropriate labeling for prescribing information).

Trachoma. Inclusion conjunctivitis. Nocardiosis. Chancroid. Toxoplasmosis as adjunctive therapy with pyrimethamine. Malaria due to chloroquine-resistant strains of *Plasmodium falciparum,* when used as adjunctive therapy.

Currently, the increasing frequency of resistant organisms is a limitation of the usefulness of antibacterial agents including the sulfonamides, especially in the treatment of chronic and recurrent urinary tract infections.

Important Note: *In vitro* sulfonamide susceptibility tests are not always reliable. The test must be carefully coordinated with bacteriologic and clinical response. When the patient is already taking sulfonamides, follow-up cultures should have aminobenzoic acid added to the culture media.

CONTRAINDICATIONS

Sulfisoxazole is contraindicated in the following patient populations: patients with a known hypersensitivity to sulfonamides; children younger than 2 months (except in the treatment of congenital toxoplasmosis as adjunctive therapy with pyrimethamine); pregnant women *at term*; and mothers nursing infants less than 2 months of age.

Use in pregnant women at term, in children less than 2 months of age and in mothers nursing infants less than 2 months of age is contraindicated because sulfonamides may promote kernicterus in the newborn by displacing bilirubin from plasma proteins.

WARNINGS

FATALITIES ASSOCIATED WITH THE ADMINISTRATION OF SULFONAMIDES, ALTHOUGH RARE, HAVE OCCURRED DUE TO SEVERE REACTIONS, INCLUDING STEVENS-JOHNSON SYNDROME, TOXIC EPIDERMAL NECROLYSIS, FULMINANT HEPATIC NECROSIS, AGRANULOCYTOSIS, APLASTIC ANEMIA AND OTHER BLOOD DYSCRASIAS.

SULFONAMIDES, INCLUDING SULFISOXAZOLE, SHOULD BE DISCONTINUED AT THE FIRST APPEARANCE OF SKIN RASH OR ANY SIGN OF AN ADVERSE REACTION. In rare instances, a skin rash may be followed by more severe reactions such as Stevens-Johnson syndrome, toxic epidermal necrolysis, hepatic necrosis and serious blood disorders. (See PRECAUTIONS.)

Clinical signs such as rash, sore throat, fever, arthralgia, pallor, purpura or jaundice may be early indications of serious reactions.

Cough, shortness of breath and pulmonary infiltrates are hypersensitivity reactions of the respiratory tract that have been reported in association with sulfonamide treatment.

The sulfonamides should not be used for the treatment of group A beta-hemolytic streptococcal infections. In an established infection, they will not eradicate the streptococcus, and therefore, will not prevent sequelae such as rheumatic fever.

Pseudomembranous colitis has been reported with nearly all antibacterial agents, including sulfisoxazole, and may range in severity from mild to life-threatening. Therefore, it is important to consider this diagnosis in patients who present with diarrhea subsequent to the administration of antibacterial agents.

Treatment with antibacterial agents alters the normal flora of the colon and may permit overgrowth of clostridia. Studies indicate that toxin produced by *Clostridium difficile* is one primary cause of "antibiotic-associated colitis."

After the diagnosis of pseudomembranous colitis has been established, therapeutic measures should be initiated. Mild cases of pseudomembranous colitis usually respond to drug discontinuation alone. In moderate to severe cases, consideration should be given to management with fluids and electrolytes, protein supplementation, and treatment with an antibacterial drug clinically effective against *C. difficile* colitis.

PRECAUTIONS

GENERAL

Sulfonamides should be given with caution to patients with impaired renal or hepatic function and to those with severe allergy or bronchial asthma. In glucose-6-phosphate dehydrogenase-deficient individuals, hemolysis may occur; this reaction is frequently dose-related.

The frequency of resistant organisms limits the usefulness of antibacterial agents, including the sulfonamides, as sole therapy in the treatment of urinary tract infections. Since sulfonamides are bacteriostatic and not bactericidal, a complete course of therapy is needed to prevent immediate regrowth and the development of resistant uropathogens.

INFORMATION FOR THE PATIENT

Patients should maintain an adequate fluid intake to prevent crystalluria and stone formation.

LABORATORY TESTS

Complete blood counts should be done frequently in patients receiving sulfonamides. If a significant reduction in the count of any formed blood element is noted, sulfisoxazole should be discontinued. Urinalyses with careful microscopic examination and renal function tests should be performed during therapy, particularly for those patients with impaired renal function. Blood levels should be measured in patients receiving a sulfonamide for serious infections. (See INDICATIONS AND USAGE.)

CARCINOGENESIS, MUTAGENESIS, AND IMPAIRMENT OF FERTILITY

Carcinogenesis

Sulfisoxazole was not carcinogenic in either sex when administered by gavage for 103 weeks at dosages up to approximately 18 times the highest recommended human daily dose or to rats at 4 times the highest recommended human daily dose. Rats appear to be especially susceptible to the goitrogenic effects of sulfonamides and long-term administration of sulfonamides has resulted in thyroid malignancies in this species.

Mutagenesis

There are no studies available that adequately evaluate the mutagenic potential of sulfisoxazole. Ames mutagenic assays have not been performed with sulfisoxazole. However, sulfisoxazole was not observed to be mutagenic in *E. coli* Sd-4-73 when tested in the absence of a metabolic activating system.

Impairment of Fertility

Sulfisoxazole has not undergone adequate trials relating to impairment of fertility. In a reproduction study in rats given 7 times the highest recommended human dose per day of sulfisoxazole, no effects were observed regarding mating behavior, conception rate or fertility index (percent pregnant).

PREGNANCY CATEGORY C

Teratogenic Effects

At dosages 7 times the highest recommended human daily dose, sulfisoxazole was not teratogenic in either rats or rabbits. However, in two other teratogenicity studies, cleft palates developed in both rats and mice, and skeletal defects were also observed in rats after administration of 9 times the highest recommended human daily dose of sulfisoxazole.

There are no adequate and well-controlled studies of sulfisoxazole in pregnant women. Sulfisoxazole should be used during pregnancy only if the potential benefit justifies the potential risk to the fetus.

S

Nonteratogenic Effects
Kernicterus may occur in the newborn as a result of treatment of a pregnant woman *at term* with sulfonamides. (See CONTRAINDICATIONS.)

NURSING MOTHERS
Sulfisoxazole is excreted in human milk. Because of the potential for the development of kernicterus in neonates due to the displacement of bilirubin from plasma proteins by sulfisoxazole, a decision should be made whether to discontinue nursing or discontinue the drug taking into account the importance of the drug to the mother. (See CONTRAINDICATIONS.)

PEDIATRIC USE
Sulfisoxazole is not recommended for use in infants younger than 2 months of age except in the treatment of congenital toxoplasmosis as adjunctive therapy with pyrimethamine. (See CONTRAINDICATIONS.)

DRUG INTERACTIONS

It has been reported that sulfisoxazole may prolong the prothrombin time in patients who are receiving the anticoagulant warfarin. This interaction should be kept in mind when sulfisoxazole is given to patients already on anticoagulant therapy, and prothrombin time or other suitable coagulation test should be monitored.

It has been proposed that sulfisoxazole competes with thiopental for plasma protein binding. In one study involving 48 patients, intravenous sulfisoxazole reduced the amount of thiopental required for anesthesia and shortened the awakening time. It is not known whether chronic oral doses of sulfisoxazole would have a similar effect. Until more is known about this interaction, physicians should be aware that patients receiving sulfisoxazole might require less thiopental for anesthesia.

Sulfonamides can displace methotrexate from plasma protein-binding sites, thus increasing free methotrexate concentrations. Studies in man have shown sulfisoxazole infusions to decrease plasma protein-bound methotrexate by one-fourth.

Sulfisoxazole can also potentiate the blood sugar lowering activity of sulfonylureas, as well as cause hypoglycemia by itself.

ADVERSE REACTIONS

The listing that follows includes adverse reactions both that have been reported with sulfisoxazole and some which have not been reported with this specific drug; however, the pharmacologic similarities among the sulfonamides require that each of the reactions be considered with the administration of any of the sulfisoxazole dosage forms.

Allergic/Dermatologic: Anaphylaxis, erythema multiforme (Stevens- Johnson syndrome), toxic epidermal necrolysis, exfoliative dermatitis, angioedema, arteritis and vasculitis, allergic myocarditis, serum sickness, rash, urticaria, pruritus, photosensitivity, and conjunctival and scleral injection, generalized allergic reactions and generalized skin eruptions. In addition, periarteritis nodosa and systemic lupus erythematosus have been reported. (See WARNINGS.)

Cardiovascular: Tachycardia, palpitations, syncope, cyanosis.

Endocrine: The sulfonamides bear certain chemical similarities to some goitrogens, diuretics (acetazolamide and thiazides) and oral hypoglycemia agents. Cross-sensitivity may exist with these agents. Development of goiter, diuresis and hypoglycemia have occurred rarely in patients receiving sulfonamides.

Gastrointestinal: Hepatitis, hepatocellular necrosis, jaundice, pseudomembranous colitis, nausea, emesis, anorexia, abdominal pain, diarrhea, gastrointestinal hemorrhage, melena, flatulence, glossitis, stomatitis, salivary gland enlargement, pancreatitis.

Onset of pseudomembranous colitis symptoms may occur during or after treatment with sulfisoxazole. (See WARNINGS.)

Sulfisoxazole has been reported to cause increased elevations of liver-associated enzymes in patients with hepatitis.

Genitourinary: Crystalluria, hematuria, BUN and creatine elevations, nephritis and toxic nephrosis with oliguria and anuria. Acute renal failure and urinary retention have also been reported. The frequency of renal complications, commonly associated with some sulfonamides, is lower in patients receiving the more soluble sulfonamides such as sulfisoxazole.

Hematologic: Leukopenia, agranulocytosis, aplastic anemia, thrombocytopenia, purpura, hemolyticanemia, anemia, eosinophilia, clotting disorders including hypoprothrombinemia, and hypofibrinogenemia, sulfhemoglobinemia, methemoglobinemia.

Musculoskeletal: Arthralgia, myalgia.

Neurologic: Headache, dizziness, peripheral neuritis, paresthesia, convulsions, tinnitus, vertigo, ataxia, intracranial hypertension.

Psychiatric: Psychosis, hallucination, disorientation, depression, anxiety, apathy.

Respiratory: Cough, shortness of breath, pulmonary infiltrates. (See WARNINGS.)

Vascular: Angioedema, arteritis, vasculitis.

Miscellaneous: Edema (including periorbital), pyrexia, drowsiness, weakness, fatigue, lassitude, rigors, flushing, hearing loss, insomnia, pneumonitis, chills.

DOSAGE AND ADMINISTRATION

Systemic sulfonamides are contraindicated in infants under 2 months of age, except in the treatment of congenital toxoplasmosis as adjunctive therapy with pyrimethamine.

Usual Dose for Infants over 2 Months of Age and Children: *Initial Dose:* One-half of the 24-hour dose. *Maintenance Dose:* 150 mg/kg/24 hours or 4 g/M^2/24 hours—dose to be divided into 4-6 doses/24 hours. The maximum dose should not exceed 6 g/24 hours.

Usual Adult Dose: *Initial Dose:* 2-4 g. *Maintenance Dose:* 4-8 g/24 hours, divided in 4-6 doses/24 hours.

PRODUCT LISTING - RATED THERAPEUTICALLY EQUIVALENT

Tablet - Oral - 500 mg

12's	$7.56	GENERIC, Pd-Rx Pharmaceuticals	55289-0776-12
28's	$11.64	GENERIC, Pd-Rx Pharmaceuticals	55289-0776-28
30's	$12.15	GENERIC, Pd-Rx Pharmaceuticals	55289-0776-30
40's	$14.63	GENERIC, Pd-Rx Pharmaceuticals	55289-0776-40
56's	$18.78	GENERIC, Pd-Rx Pharmaceuticals	55289-0776-56
80's	$4.50	GENERIC, Circle Pharmaceuticals Inc	00659-0120-80
80's	$11.16	GENERIC, Allscripts Pharmaceutical Company	54569-0231-02
80's	$24.90	GENERIC, Pd-Rx Pharmaceuticals	55289-0776-80
100's	$3.35	GENERIC, Global Pharmaceutical Corporation	00115-4747-01
100's	$8.50	GENERIC, Cmc-Consolidated Midland Corporation	00223-1980-01
100's	$12.15	GENERIC, Moore, H.L. Drug Exchange Inc	00839-1649-06
100's	$13.08	GENERIC, Aligen Independent Laboratories Inc	00405-4971-01
100's	$13.15	GENERIC, Martec Pharmaceuticals Inc	52555-0323-01
100's	$13.45	GENERIC, Major Pharmaceuticals Inc	00904-2218-60
100's	$13.95	GENERIC, Geneva Pharmaceuticals	00781-1015-01
100's	$51.70	GENERIC, Ivax Corporation	00172-2218-60

PRODUCT LISTING - EQUIVALENTS NOT AVAILABLE

Solution - Ophthalmic - 4%			
15 ml	$9.44	GANTRISIN OPHTHALMIC, Roche Laboratories	00004-1702-39
15 ml	$9.63	GANTRISIN OPHTHALMIC, Allscripts Pharmaceutical Company	54569-4018-00
15 ml	$15.76	GANTRISIN OPHTHALMIC, Cheshire Drugs	55175-0355-05
Suspension - Oral - 500 mg/5 ml			
100 ml	$13.18	GANTRISIN, Southwood Pharmaceuticals Inc	58016-0132-20
473 ml	$47.94	GANTRISIN PEDIATRIC, Roche Laboratories	00004-1003-28
480 ml	$42.22	GANTRISIN PEDIATRIC, Allscripts Pharmaceutical Company	54569-4013-00
Tablet - Oral - 500 mg			
20's	$4.94	GENERIC, Prescript Pharmaceuticals	00247-0364-20
40's	$6.53	GENERIC, Prescript Pharmaceuticals	00247-0364-40
56's	$7.80	GENERIC, Prescript Pharmaceuticals	00247-0364-56
80's	$21.45	GENERIC, Physicians Total Care	54868-1535-00
84's	$10.02	GENERIC, Prescript Pharmaceuticals	00247-0364-84

Sulindac *(002298)*

Categories: Ankylosing spondylitis; Arthritis, gouty; Arthritis, osteoarthritis; Arthritis, rheumatoid; Bursitis, subacromial; Tendonitis, supraspinatus; FDA Approved 1978 Sep; Pregnancy Category B; Pregnancy Category D, 3rd Trimester
Drug Classes: Analgesics, non-narcotic; Nonsteroidal anti-inflammatory drugs
Brand Names: Clinoril
Foreign Brand Availability: Aclin (Australia; Hong-Kong; Malaysia); Aflodac (Italy); Algocetil (Italy); Apo-Sulin (Canada); Arthrocine (France); Cenlidac (Taiwan); Clidol (Korea); Citireuma (Italy); Copal (Mexico); Daclin (New-Zealand); Dometon (Taiwan); Imbaron (China); Kenalin (Mexico); Klimacobal (Greece); Norilafin (Greece); Novo-Sundac (Canada); Sulen (Italy); Sulic (Italy); Sulindaco Lisan (Costa-Rica); Sulindal (Spain); Sulindec (Taiwan); Sulinol (Italy); Suloril (Taiwan); Sulreuma (Italy); Zirofalen (Greece)
Cost of Therapy: $73.52 (Osteoarthritis; Clinoril; 150 mg; 2 tablets/day; 30 day supply)
$17.89 (Osteoarthritis; Generic Tablets; 150 mg; 2 tablets/day; 30 day supply)

DESCRIPTION

Sulindac is a non-steroidal, anti-inflammatory indene derivative designated chemically as (Z)-5-fluoro-2-methyl-1-[[*p*-(methylsulfinyl)phenyl]methylene]-1*H*-indene-3-acetic acid. It is not a salicylate, pyrazolone or propionic acid derivative. Its empirical formula is $C_{20}H_{17}FO_3S$, with a molecular weight of 356.42. Sulindac, a yellow crystalline compound, is a weak organic acid practically insoluble in water below pH 4.5, but very soluble as the sodium salt or in buffers of pH 6 or higher.

Clinoril (sulindac) is available in 150 and 200 mg tablets for oral administration. Each tablet contains the following inactive ingredients: cellulose, magnesium stearate, starch.

Following absorption, sulindac undergoes two major biotransformations — reversible reduction to the sulfide metabolite, and irreversible oxidation to the sulfone metabolite. Available evidence indicates that the biological activity resides with the sulfide metabolite.

CLINICAL PHARMACOLOGY

Sulindac is a non-steroidal anti-inflammatory drug, also possessing analgesic and antipyretic activities. Its mode of action, like that of other non-steroidal, anti-inflammatory agents, is not known; however, its therapeutic action is not due to pituitary-adrenal stimulation. Inhibition of prostaglandin synthesis by the sulfide metabolite may be involved in the anti-inflammatory action of sulindac.

Sulindac is approximately 90% absorbed in man after oral administration. The peak plasma concentrations of the biologically active sulfide metabolite are achieved in about 2 hours when sulindac is administered in the fasting state, and in about 3-4 hours when sulindac is administered with food. The mean half-life of sulindac is 7.8 hours while the mean half-life of the sulfide metabolite is 16.4 hours. Sustained plasma levels of the sulfide metabolite are consistent with a prolonged anti-inflammatory action which is the rationale for a twice per day dosage schedule.

Sulindac and its sulfone metabolite undergo extensive enterohepatic circulation relative to the sulfide metabolite in animals. Studies in man have also demonstrated that recirculation of the parent drug, sulindac, and its sulfone metabolite, is more extensive than that of the active sulfide metabolite. The active sulfide metabolite accounts for less than 6% of the total intestinal exposure to sulindac and its metabolites.

The primary route of excretion in man is via the urine as both sulindac and its sulfone metabolite (free and glucuronide conjugates). Approximately 50% of the administered dose is excreted in the urine, with the conjugated sulfone metabolite accounting for the major portion. Less than 1% of the administered dose of sulindac appears in the urine as the sulfide metabolite. Approximately 25% is found in the feces, primarily as the sulfone and sulfide metabolites.

The bioavailability of sulindac, as assessed by urinary excretion, was not changed by concomitant administration of an antacid containing magnesium hydroxide 200 mg and aluminum hydroxide 225 mg/5 ml.

Because sulindac is excreted in the urine primarily as biologically inactive forms, it may possibly affect renal function to a lesser extent than other non-steroidal anti-inflammatory drugs, however, renal adverse experiences have been reported with sulindac (see ADVERSE REACTIONS). In a study of patients with chronic glomerular disease treated with therapeutic doses of sulindac, no effect was demonstrated on renal blood flow, glomerular filtration rate, or urinary excretion of prostaglandin E_2 and the primary metabolite of prostacyclin, 6-keto-$PGF_{1\alpha}$. However, in other studies in healthy volunteers and patients with liver disease, sulindac was found to blunt the renal responses to intravenous furosemide, *i.e.*, the diuresis, natriuresis, increments in plasma renin activity and urinary excretion of prostaglandins. These observations may represent a differentiation of the effects of sulindac on renal functions based on differences in pathogenesis of the renal prostaglandin dependence associated with differing dose-response relationships of different NSAIDs to the various renal functions influenced by prostaglandins. These observations need further clarification and in the interim, sulindac should be used with caution in patients whose renal function may be impaired (see PRECAUTIONS).

In healthy men, the average fecal blood loss, measured over a 2 week period during administration of 400 mg/day of sulindac, was similar to that for placebo, and was statistically significantly less than that resulting from 4800 mg/day of aspirin.

In controlled clinical studies sulindac was evaluated in the following five conditions:

Osteoarthritis: In patients with osteoarthritis of the hip and knee, the anti-inflammatory and analgesic activity of sulindac was demonstrated by clinical measurements that included: assessments by both patient and investigator of overall response; decrease in disease activity as assessed by both patient and investigator; improvement in ARA Functional Class; relief of night pain; improvement in overall evaluation of pain, including pain on weight bearing and pain on active and passive motion; improvement in joint mobility, range of motion, and functional activities; decreased swelling and tenderness; and decreased duration of stiffness following prolonged inactivity.

In clinical studies in which dosages were adjusted according to patient needs, sulindac 200-400 mg daily was shown to be comparable in effectiveness to aspirin 2400-4800 mg daily. Sulindac was generally well tolerated, and patients on it had a lower overall incidence of total adverse effects, of milder gastrointestinal reactions, and of tinnitus than did patients on aspirin. (See ADVERSE REACTIONS.)

Rheumatoid Arthritis: In patients with rheumatoid arthritis, the anti-inflammatory and analgesic activity of sulindac was demonstrated by clinical measurements that included: assessments by both patients and investigator of overall; response decrease in disease activity as assessed by both patient and investigator; reduction in overall joint pain; reduction in duration and severity of morning stiffness; reduction in day and night pain; decrease in time required to walk 50 feet; decrease in general pain as measured on a visual analog scale; improvement in the Ritchie articular index; decrease in proximal interphalangeal joint size; improvement in ARA Functional Class; increase in grip strength; reduction in painful joint count and score; reduction in swollen joint count and score; and increased flexion and extension of the wrist.

In clinical studies in which dosages were adjusted according to patient needs, sulindac 300-400 mg daily was shown to be comparable in effectiveness to aspirin 3600-4800 mg daily. Sulindac was generally well tolerated, and patients on it had a lower overall incidence of total adverse effects, of milder gastrointestinal reactions, and of tinnitus than did patients on aspirin. (See ADVERSE REACTIONS.)

In patients with rheumatoid arthritis, sulindac may be used in combination with gold salts at usual dosage levels. In clinical studies, sulindac added to the regimen of gold salts usually resulted in additional symptomatic relief but did not alter the course of the underlying disease.

Ankylosing Spondylitis: In patients with ankylosing spondylitis, the anti-inflammatory and analgesic activity of sulindac was demonstrated by clinical measurements that included: assessments by both patient and investigator of overall response; decrease in disease activity as assessed by both patient and investigator; improvement in ARA Functional Class; improvement in patient and investigator evaluation of spinal pain, tenderness and/or spasm; reduction in the duration of morning stiffness; increase in the time to onset of fatigue; relief of night pain; increase in chest expansion; and increase in spinal mobility evaluated by fingers-to-floor distance, occiput to wall distance, the Schober Test, and the Wright Modification of the Schober Test. In a clinical study in which dosages were adjusted according to patient need, sulindac 200-400 mg daily was as effective as indomethacin 75-150 mg daily. In a second study, sulindac 300-400 mg daily was comparable in effectiveness to phenylbutazone 400-600 mg daily. Sulindac was better tolerated than phenylbutazone. (See ADVERSE REACTIONS.)

Acute Painful Shoulder (acute subacromial bursitis/supraspinatus tendinitis): In patients with acute painful shoulder (acute subacromial bursitis/supraspinatus tendinitis), the anti-inflammatory and analgesic activity of sulindac was demonstrated by clinical measurements that included: assessments by both patient and investigator of overall response; relief of night pain, spontaneous pain, and pain on active motion; decrease in local tenderness; and improvement in range of motion measured by abduction, and internal and external rotation. In clinical studies in acute painful shoulder, sulindac 300-400 mg daily and oxyphenbutazone 400-600 mg daily were shown to be equally effective and well tolerated.

Acute Gouty Arthritis: In patients with acute gouty arthritis, the anti-inflammatory and analgesic activity of sulindac was demonstrated by clinical measurements that included: assessments by both the patient and investigator of overall response; relief of weight-bearing pain; relief of pain at rest and on active and passive motion; decrease in tenderness; reduction in warmth and swelling; increase in range of motion; and improvement in ability to function. In clinical studies, sulindac at 400 mg daily and phenylbutazone at 600 mg daily were shown to be equally effective. In these short-term studies in which reduction of dosage was permitted according to response, both drugs were equally well tolerated.

INDICATIONS AND USAGE

Sulindac is indicated for acute or long-term use in the relief of signs and symptoms of the following:

1. Osteoarthritis
2. Rheumatoid arthritis*
3. Ankylosing spondylitis
4. Acute painful shoulder (acute subacromial bursitis/supraspinatus tendinitis)
5. Acute gouty arthritis

*The safety and effectiveness of Sulindac have not been established in rheumatoid arthritis patients who are designated in the American Rheumatism Association classification as Functional Class IV (incapacitated, largely or wholly bedridden, or confined to wheelchair; little or no self-care).

CONTRAINDICATIONS

Sulindac should not be used in:

Patients who are hypersensitive to this product.

Patients in whom acute asthmatic attacks, urticaria, or rhinitis are precipitated by aspirin or other non-steroidal anti-inflammatory agents.

WARNINGS

GASTROINTESTINAL EFFECTS

Peptic ulceration and gastrointestinal bleeding have been reported in patients receiving sulindac. Fatalities have occurred. Gastrointestinal bleeding is associated with higher morbidity and mortality in patients acutely ill with other conditions, the elderly, and patients with hemorrhagic disorders. In patients with active gastrointestinal bleeding or an active peptic ulcer, an appropriate ulcer regimen should be instituted, and the physician must weigh the benefits of therapy with sulindac against possible hazards, and careful monitor the patient's progress. When sulindac is given to patients with history of either upper or lower gastrointestinal tract disease, it should be given under close supervision and only after consulting the ADVERSE REACTIONS section.

RISK OF GL ULCERATIONS, BLEEDING AND PERFORATION WITH NSAID THERAPY

Serious gastrointestinal toxicity such as bleeding, ulceration, and perforation, can occur at any time, with or without warning symptoms, in patient treated chronically with NSAID therapy. Although minor upper gastrointestinal problems, such as dyspepsia, are common, usually developing early therapy, physicians should remain alert for ulceration and bleeding in patient treated chronically with NSAIDs even in the absence of previous Gl tract symptoms. In patients observed in clinical trials of several months to 2 years duration, symptomatic upper Gl ulcers, gross bleeding or perforation appear to occur in approximately 1% of patients treated for 3-6 months, and about 2-4% of patients treated for 1 year. Physicians should inform patients about the signs and/or symptoms of serious Gl toxicity and what steps to take if they occur.

Studies to date have not identified any subset of patients not at risk on developing peptic ulceration and bleeding. Except for a prior history of serious Gl events and other risk factors known to be associated with peptic ulcer disease, such as alcoholism, smoking, etc., no risk factors (*e.g.*, age, sex) have been associated with increased risk. Elderly or debilitated patients seem to tolerate ulceration or bleeding less well than other individuals and most spontaneous reports of fatal Gl events are in this population. Studies to date are inconclusive concerning the relative risk of various NSAIDs in causing such reactions. High doses of any NSAID probably carry a greater risk of these reactions, although controlled clinical trials showing this do not exist in most cases. In considering the use of relatively large doses (within the recommended dosage range), sufficient benefit should be anticipated to offset the potential increased risk of Gl toxicity.

HYPERSENSITIVITY

Rarely, fever and other evidence of hypersensitivity (see ADVERSE REACTIONS) including abnormalities in one or more liver function tests and severe skin reactions have occurred during therapy with sulindac. Fatalities have occurred in these patients. Hepatitis, jaundice, or both, with or without fever may occur usually within the first 1-3 months of therapy. Determinations of liver function should be considered whenever a patient on therapy with sulindac develops unexplained fever, rash or other dermatologic reactions or constitutional symptoms. If unexplained fever or other evidence of hypersensitivity occurs, therapy with sulindac should be discontinued. The elevated temperature and abnormalities in liver function caused by sulindac characteristically have reverted to normal after discontinuation of therapy. Administration of sulindac should not be reinstituted in such patients.

HEPATIC EFFECTS

In addition to hypersensitivity reactions involving the liver, in some patients the findings are consistent with those of cholestatic hepatitis. As with other non-steroidal anti-inflammatory drugs, borderline elevations of one or more liver tests without any other signs and symptoms may occur in up to 15% of patients. These abnormalities may progress, may remain essentially unchanged, or may be transient with continued therapy. The SGPT (ALT) test is probably the most sensitive indicator of liver dysfunction. Meaningful (3 times the upper limit of normal) elevations of SGPT or SGOT (AST) occurred in controlled clinical trials in less than 1% of patients. A patient with symptoms and/or signs suggesting liver dysfunction, or in whom an abnormal liver test has occurred, should be evaluated for evidence of the development of more severe hepatic reaction while on therapy with sulindac. Although such reactions as described above are rare, if abnormal liver tests persist or worsen, if clinical signs and symptoms consistent with liver disease develop, or if systemic manifestations occur (*e.g.*, eosinophilia, rash, etc.), sulindac should be discontinued.

In clinical trials with sulindac, the use of doses of 600 mg/day has been associated with an increased incidence of mild liver test abnormalities (see DOSAGE AND ADMINISTRATION for maximum dosage recommendation).

S

PRECAUTIONS

GENERAL

Non-steroidal anti-inflammatory drugs, including sulindac, may mask the usual signs and symptoms of infection. Therefore, the physician must be continually on alert and should use the drug with extra care in the presence of existing infection.

Although sulindac has less effect on platelet function and bleeding time than aspirin, it is an inhibitor of platelet function; therefore, patients who may be adversely affected should be carefully observed when sulindac is administered.

Pancreatitis has been reported in patients receiving sulindac (see ADVERSE REACTIONS). Should pancreatitis be suspected, the drug should be discontinued and not restarted, supportive medical therapy instituted, and the patient monitored closely with appropriate laboratory studies (*e.g.*, serum and urine amylase, amylase/creatinine clearance ratio, electrolytes, serum calcium, glucose, lipase, etc.). A search for other causes of pancreatitis as well as those conditions which mimic pancreatitis should be conducted.

Because of reports of adverse eye findings with non-steroidal anti-inflammatory agents, it is recommended that patients who develop eye complaints during treatment with sulindac have ophthalmologic studies.

In patients with poor liver function, delayed, elevated and prolonged circulating levels of the sulfide and sulfone metabolites may occur. Such patients should be monitored closely; a reduction of daily dosage may be required.

Edema has been observed in some patients taking sulindac. Therefore, as with other non-steroidal anti-inflammatory drugs, sulindac should be used with caution in patients with compromised cardiac function, hypertension, or other conditions predisposing to fluid retention.

Sulindac may allow a reduction in dosage or the elimination of chronic corticosteroid therapy in some patients with rheumatoid arthritis. However, it is generally necessary to reduce corticosteroids gradually over several months in order to avoid an exacerbation of disease or signs and symptoms of adrenal insufficiency. Abrupt withdrawal of chronic corticosteroid treatment is generally not recommended even when patients have had a serious complication of chronic corticosteroid therapy.

RENAL EFFECTS

As with other non-steroidal anti-inflammatory drugs, long term administration of sulindac to animals has resulted in renal papillary necrosis and other abnormal renal pathology. In humans, there have been reports of acute interstitial nephritis with hematuria, proteinuria, and occasionally nephrotic syndrome.

A second form of renal toxicity has been seen in patients with prerenal and renal conditions leading to a reduction in renal blood flow or blood volume, where the renal prostaglandins have a supportive role in the maintenance of renal perfusion. In these patients administration of an NSAID may cause a dose dependent reduction in prostaglandin formation and may precipitate overt renal decompensation. Sulindac may affect renal function less than other NSAIDs in patients with chronic glomerular renal disease (see CLINICAL PHARMACOLOGY). Until these observations are better understood and clarified, however, and because renal adverse experiences have been reported with sulindac (see ADVERSE REACTIONS), caution should be exercised when administering the drug to patients with conditions associated with increased risk of the effects of non-steroidal anti-inflammatory drugs on renal function, such as those with renal or hepatic dysfunction, diabetes mellitus, advanced age, extracellular volume depletion from any cause, congestive heart failure, septicemia, pyelonephritis, or concomitant use of any nephrotoxic drug. Discontinuation of NSAID therapy is typically followed by recovery to the pretreatment state.

Since sulindac is eliminated primarily by the kidneys, patients with significantly impaired renal function should be closely monitored; a lower daily dosage should be anticipated to avoid excessive drug accumulation.

Sulindac metabolites have been reported rarely as the major or a minor component in renal stones in association with other calculus components. Sulindac should be used with caution in patients with a history of renal lithiasis, and they should be kept well hydrated while receiving sulindac.

INFORMATION FOR THE PATIENT

Sulindac, like other drugs of its class, is not free of side effects. The side effects of these drugs can cause discomfort and, rarely, there are more serious side effects such as gastrointestinal bleeding, which may result in hospitalization and even fatal outcomes.

NSAIDs (Non-steroidal Anti-inflammatory Drugs) are often essential agents in the management of arthritis, but they also may be commonly employed for conditions which are less serious.

Physicians may wish to discuss with their patients the potential risks (see WARNINGS, PRECAUTIONS, and ADVERSE REACTIONS) and likely benefits of NSAID treatment, particularly when the drugs are used for less serious conditions where treatment without NSAIDs may represent an acceptable alternative to both the patient and physician.

LABORATORY TESTS

Because serious GI tract ulceration and bleeding can occur without warning symptoms, physicians should follow chronically treated patients for the signs and symptoms of ulceration and bleeding and should inform them of the importance of this follow-up (see WARNINGS, Risk of GI Ulcerations, Bleeding and Perforation with NSAID Therapy).

PREGNANCY

Sulindac is not recommended for use in pregnant women, since safety for use has not been established. The known effects of drugs of this class on the human fetus during the third trimester of include: constriction of the ductus arteriosus prenatally, tricuspid incompetence, and pulmonary hypertension; non-closure of the ductus arteriosus postnatally which may be resistant to medical management; myocardial degenerative changes, platelet dysfunction with resultant bleeding, intracranial bleeding, renal dysfunction or failure, renal injury/dysgenesis which may result in prolonged or permanent renal failure, oligohydramnios, gastrointestinal bleeding or perforation, and increased risk of necrotizing enterocolitis.

In reproduction studies in the rat, a decrease in average fetal weight and an increase in numbers of dead pups were observed on the first day of the postpartum period at dosage levels of 20 and 40 mg/kg/day (2½ and 5 times the usual maximum daily dose in humans), although there was no adverse effect on the survival and growth during the remainder of the postpartum period. Sulindac prolongs the duration of gestation in rats, as do other compounds of this class which also may cause dystocia and delayed parturition in pregnant animals. Visceral and skeletal malformations observed in low incidence among rabbits in some teratology studies did not occur at the same dosage levels in repeat studies, nor at a higher dosage level in the same species.

NURSING MOTHERS

Nursing should not be undertaken while a patient is on sulindac. It is not known whether sulindac is secreted in human milk; however, it is secreted in the milk of lactating rats.

PEDIATRIC USE

Safety and effectiveness in children have not been established.

GERIATRIC USE

As with any NSAID, caution should be exercised in treating the elderly (65 years and older) since advancing age appears to increase the possibility of adverse reactions. Elderly patients seem to tolerate ulceration or bleeding less well than other individuals and many spontaneous reports of fatal GI events are in this population (see WARNINGS, Gastrointestinal Effects and Risk of GI Ulcerations, Bleeding and Perforation with NSAID Therapy).

This drug is known to be substantially excreted by the kidney and the risk of toxic reactions to this drug may be greater in patients with impaired renal function. Because elderly patients are more likely to have decreased renal function, care should be taken in dose selection and it may be useful to monitor renal function (see Renal Effects).

DRUG INTERACTIONS

DMSO should not be used with sulindac. Concomitant administration has been reported to reduce the plasma levels of the active sulfide metabolite and potentially reduce efficacy. In addition, this combination has been reported to cause peripheral neuropathy.

Although sulindac and its sulfide metabolite are highly bound to protein, studies in which sulindac was given at a dose of 400 mg daily, have shown no clinically significant interaction with oral anticoagulants or oral hypoglycemic agents. However, patients should be monitored carefully until it is certain that no change in their anticoagulant or hypoglycemic dosage is required. Special attention should be paid to patients taking higher doses than those recommended and to patients with renal impairment or other metabolic defects that might increase sulindac blood levels.

The concomitant administration of aspirin with sulindac significantly depressed the plasma levels of the active sulfide metabolite. A double-blind study compared the safety and efficacy of sulindac 300 or 400 mg daily given alone or with aspirin 2.4 g/day for the treatment of osteoarthritis. The addition of aspirin did not alter the types of clinical or laboratory adverse experiences for sulindac; however, the combination showed an increase in the incidence of gastrointestinal adverse experiences. Since the addition of aspirin did not have a favorable effect on the therapeutic response to sulindac, the combination is not recommended.

The concomitant use of sulindac with other NSAIDs is not recommended due to the increased possibility of gastrointestinal toxicity, with little or no increase in efficacy.

Caution should be used if sulindac is administered concomitantly with methotrexate. Non-steroidal anti-inflammatory drugs have been reported to decrease the tubular secretion of methotrexate and to potentiate its toxicity.

Administration of non-steroidal anti-inflammatory drugs concomitantly with cyclosporine has been associated with an increase in cyclosporine-induced toxicity, possibly due to decreased synthesis of renal prostacyclin. NSAIDs should be used with caution in patients taking cyclosporine, and renal function should be carefully monitored.

The concomitant administration of sulindac and diflunisal in normal volunteers resulted in lowering of the plasma levels of the active sulindac sulfide metabolite by approximately one-third.

Probenecid given concomitantly with sulindac had only a slight effect on plasma sulfide levels, while plasma levels of sulindac and sulfone were increased. Sulindac was shown to produce a modest reduction in the uricosuric action of probenecid, which probably is not significant under most circumstances.

Neither propoxyphene hydrochloride nor acetaminophen had any effect on the plasma levels of sulindac or its sulfide metabolite.

ADVERSE REACTIONS

The following adverse reactions were reported in clinical trials or have been reported since the drug was marketed. The probability exists of a causal relationship between sulindac and these adverse reactions. The adverse reactions which have been observed in clinical trials encompass observations in 1865 patients, including 232 observed for at least 48 weeks.

Incidence Greater Than 1%

Gastrointestinal: The most frequent types of adverse reactions occurring with sulindac are gastrointestinal; these include gastrointestinal pain (10%), dyspepsia*, nausea* with or without vomiting, diarrhea*, constipation*, flatulence, anorexia and gastrointestinal cramps.

Dermatologic: Rash*, pruritus.

Central Nervous System: Dizziness*, headache*, nervousness.

Special Senses: Tinnitus.

Miscellaneous: Edema (see PRECAUTIONS).

*Incidence between 3% and 9%. Those reactions occurring in 1-3% of patients are not marked with an asterisk.

INCIDENCE LESS THAN 1 IN 100

Gastrointestinal: Gastritis, gastroenteritis or colitis. Peptic ulcer and gastrointestinal bleeding have been reported. GI perforation and intestinal strictures (diaphragms) have been reported rarely.

Liver function abnormalities; jaundice, sometimes with fever; cholestasis; hepatitis; hepatic failure.

There have been rare reports of sulindac metabolites in common bile duct "sludge" and in bilary calculi in patients with symptoms of cholecystitis who underwent a cholecystectomy.

Pancreatitis (see PRECAUTIONS).

Ageusia; glossitis.

Dermatologic: Stomatitis, sore or dry mucous membranes, alopecia, photosensitivity.

Erythema multiforme, toxic epidermal necrolysis, Stevens-Johnson syndrome, and exfoliative dermatitis have been reported.

Cardiovascular: Congestive heart failure, especially in patients with marginal cardiac function; palpitation; hypertension.

Hematologic: Thrombocytopenia; ecchymosis; purpura; leukopenia; agranulocytosis; neutropenia; bone marrow depression, including aplastic anemia; hemolytic anemia; increased prothrombin time in patients on oral anticoagulants (see PRECAUTIONS).

Genitourinary: Urine discoloration; dysuria; vaginal bleeding; hematuria; proteinuria; crystalluria; renal impairment, including renal failure; interstitial nephritis; nephrotic syndrome.

Renal calculi containing sulindac metabolites have been observed rarely.

Metabolic: Hyperkalemia.

Musculoskeletal: Muscle weakness.

Psychiatric: Depression; psychic disturbances including acute psychosis.

Nervous System: Vertigo; insomnia; somnolence; paresthesia; convulsions; syncope; aseptic meningitis.

Special Senses: Blurred vision; visual disturbances; decreased hearing; metallic or bitter taste.

Respiratory: Epistaxis.

Hypersensitivity Reactions: Anaphylaxis; angioneurotic edema; bronchial spasm; dyspnea.

Hypersensitivity vasculitis.

A potentially fatal apparent hypersensitivity syndrome has been reported. This syndrome may include constitutional symptoms (fever, chills, diaphoresis, flushing), cutaneous findings (rash or other dermatologic reactions—see above), conjunctivitis, involvement of major organs (changes in liver function including hepatic failure, jaundice, pancreatitis, pneumonitis with or without pleural effusion, leukopenia, leukocytosis, eosinophilia, disseminated intravascular coagulation, anemia, renal impairment, including renal failure), and other less specific findings (adenitis, arthralgia, arthritis, myalgia, fatigue, malaise, hypotension, chest pain, tachycardia).

CAUSAL RELATIONSHIP UNKNOWN

A rare occurrence of fulminant necrotizing fasciitis, particularly in association with Group A β- hemolytic streptococcus has been described in persons treated with non-steroidal anti-inflammatory agents, sometimes with fatal outcome (see also PRECAUTIONS, General).

Other reactions have been reported in clinical trials or since the drug was marketed, but occurred under circumstances where a causal relationship could not be established. However, in these rarely reported events, that possibility cannot be excluded. Therefore, these observations are listed to serve as alerting information to physicians.

Cardiovascular: Arrhythmia.

Metabolic: Hyperglycemia.

Nervous System: Neuritis.

Special Senses: Disturbances of the retina and its vasculature.

Miscellaneous: Gynecomastia.

DOSAGE AND ADMINISTRATION

Sulindac should be administered orally twice a day with food. The maximum dosage is 400 mg/day. Dosages above 400 mg/day are not recommended.

In osteoarthritis, rheumatoid arthritis, and ankylosing spondylitis, the recommended starting dosage is 150 mg twice a day. The dosage may be lowered or raised depending on the response.

A prompt response (within 1 week) can be expected in about one-half of patients with osteoarthritis, ankylosing spondylitis, and rheumatoid arthritis. Others may require longer to respond.

In acute painful shoulder (acute subacromial bursitis/supraspinatus tendinitis) and acute gouty arthritis, the recommended dosage is 200 mg twice a day. After a satisfactory response has been achieved, the dosage may be reduced according to the response. In acute painful shoulder, therapy for 7-14 days is usually adequate. In acute gouty arthritis, therapy for 7 days is usually adequate.

HOW SUPPLIED

Clinoril 150 mg are bright yellow, hexagon-shaped, compressed tablets, coded "MSD 941" on one side and "CLINORIL" on the other.

Clinoril 200 mg are bright yellow, hexagon-shaped, scored, compressed tablets, coded "MSD 942" on one side and "CLINORIL" on the other.

PRODUCT LISTING - RATED THERAPEUTICALLY EQUIVALENT

Tablet - Oral - 150 mg

Qty	Price	Product	NDC
14's	$6.48	GENERIC, Pd-Rx Pharmaceuticals	55289-0541-14
15's	$27.55	CLINORIL, Pd-Rx Pharmaceuticals	55289-0387-15
30's	$13.88	GENERIC, Pd-Rx Pharmaceuticals	55289-0541-30
30's	$26.28	GENERIC, Heartland Healthcare Services	61392-0784-30
30's	$26.28	GENERIC, Heartland Healthcare Services	61392-0784-39
31's	$27.16	GENERIC, Heartland Healthcare Services	61392-0784-31
32's	$28.03	GENERIC, Heartland Healthcare Services	61392-0784-32
45's	$39.42	GENERIC, Heartland Healthcare Services	61392-0784-45
60's	$52.56	GENERIC, Heartland Healthcare Services	61392-0784-60
60's	$62.98	GENERIC, Mutual/United Research Laboratories	00677-1173-06
90's	$78.84	GENERIC, Heartland Healthcare Services	61392-0784-90
100's	$26.25	FEDERAL UPPER LIMIT, H.C.F.A. F F P	99999-2298-02
100's	$36.00	GENERIC, Raway Pharmacal Inc	00686-0666-20
100's	$68.48	GENERIC, Major Pharmaceuticals Inc	00904-3378-61
100's	$70.00	GENERIC, Aligen Independent Laboratories Inc	00405-4973-01
100's	$75.53	GENERIC, Moore, H.L. Drug Exchange Inc	00839-7621-06
100's	$78.35	GENERIC, West Point Pharma	59591-0170-68
100's	$82.95	GENERIC, Ivax Corporation	00182-1705-01
100's	$83.98	GENERIC, Watson/Rugby Laboratories Inc	00536-4621-01
100's	$83.98	GENERIC, Geneva Pharmaceuticals	00781-1811-01
100's	$84.40	GENERIC, Endo Laboratories Llc	60951-0780-70
100's	$87.59	GENERIC, Watson/Schein Pharmaceuticals Inc	00364-2441-90
100's	$87.60	GENERIC, Geneva Pharmaceuticals	00781-1811-13
100's	$87.60	GENERIC, Medirex Inc	57480-0399-01
100's	$93.50	GENERIC, Mylan Pharmaceuticals Inc	00378-0427-01
100's	$98.20	GENERIC, Qualitest Products Inc	00603-5872-21
100's	$98.21	GENERIC, Watson/Schein Pharmaceuticals Inc	00364-2441-01
100's	$98.21	GENERIC, Mutual/United Research Laboratories	00677-1173-01
100's	$98.21	GENERIC, Mutual Pharmaceutical Co Inc	53489-0478-01
100's	$101.15	GENERIC, Udl Laboratories Inc	51079-0666-20
100's	$102.93	GENERIC, Major Pharmaceuticals Inc	00904-3378-60
100's	$122.54	CLINORIL, Merck & Company Inc	00006-0941-68

Tablet - Oral - 200 mg

Qty	Price	Product	NDC
10's	$10.65	GENERIC, Pd-Rx Pharmaceuticals	55289-0930-10
14's	$11.72	GENERIC, Pd-Rx Pharmaceuticals	55289-0930-14
14's	$20.10	CLINORIL, Allscripts Pharmaceutical Company	54569-0268-05
14's	$21.14	GENERIC, Prescript Pharmaceuticals	00247-0392-14
15's	$28.86	CLINORIL, Pd-Rx Pharmaceuticals	55289-0434-15
20's	$14.30	GENERIC, Pd-Rx Pharmaceuticals	55289-0930-20
30's	$32.03	GENERIC, Heartland Healthcare Services	61392-0785-30
30's	$32.03	GENERIC, Heartland Healthcare Services	61392-0785-39
30's	$41.47	GENERIC, Prescript Pharmaceuticals	00247-0392-30
30's	$43.07	CLINORIL, Allscripts Pharmaceutical Company	54569-0268-01
31's	$33.10	GENERIC, Heartland Healthcare Services	61392-0785-31
32's	$34.17	GENERIC, Heartland Healthcare Services	61392-0785-32
40's	$45.98	GENERIC, St. Mary'S Mpp	60760-0424-40
45's	$48.05	GENERIC, Heartland Healthcare Services	61392-0785-45
60's	$64.07	GENERIC, Heartland Healthcare Services	61392-0785-60
60's	$71.00	GENERIC, Golden State Medical	60429-0172-60
60's	$72.45	GENERIC, Mutual/United Research Laboratories	00677-1174-06
90's	$96.10	GENERIC, Heartland Healthcare Services	61392-0785-90
100's	$34.94	FEDERAL UPPER LIMIT, H.C.F.A. F F P	99999-2298-05
100's	$39.00	GENERIC, Raway Pharmacal Inc	00686-0667-20
100's	$83.47	GENERIC, Major Pharmaceuticals Inc	00904-3379-61
100's	$87.90	GENERIC, Aligen Independent Laboratories Inc	00405-4974-01
100's	$93.49	GENERIC, Moore, H.L. Drug Exchange Inc	00839-7622-06
100's	$95.75	GENERIC, West Point Pharma	59591-0154-68
100's	$96.50	GENERIC, Major Pharmaceuticals Inc	00904-3379-60
100's	$106.70	GENERIC, Geneva Pharmaceuticals	00781-1812-01
100's	$106.75	GENERIC, Ivax Corporation	00182-1706-01
100's	$106.75	GENERIC, Ivax Corporation	00182-1721-01
100's	$106.75	GENERIC, Medirex Inc	57480-0400-01
100's	$106.95	GENERIC, Geneva Pharmaceuticals	00781-1812-13
100's	$107.28	GENERIC, Endo Laboratories Llc	60951-0781-70
100's	$114.90	GENERIC, Mylan Pharmaceuticals Inc	00378-0531-01
100's	$120.59	GENERIC, Qualitest Products Inc	00603-5873-21
100's	$120.69	GENERIC, Watson/Schein Pharmaceuticals Inc	00364-2442-01
100's	$120.69	GENERIC, Watson/Schein Pharmaceuticals Inc	00591-5660-01
100's	$120.69	GENERIC, Mutual/United Research Laboratories	00677-1174-01
100's	$120.69	GENERIC, Mutual Pharmaceutical Co Inc	53489-0479-01
100's	$124.22	GENERIC, Udl Laboratories Inc	51079-0667-20
100's	$150.59	CLINORIL, Merck & Company Inc	00006-0942-68

PRODUCT LISTING - EQUIVALENTS NOT AVAILABLE

Tablet - Oral - 150 mg

Qty	Price	Product	NDC
10's	$8.76	GENERIC, Allscripts Pharmaceutical Company	54569-3336-00
12's	$11.55	GENERIC, Southwood Pharmaceuticals Inc	58016-0743-12
14's	$7.06	GENERIC, Prescript Pharmaceuticals	00247-0037-14
15's	$7.33	GENERIC, Prescript Pharmaceuticals	00247-0037-15
15's	$13.14	GENERIC, Allscripts Pharmaceutical Company	54569-3336-02
15's	$14.43	GENERIC, Southwood Pharmaceuticals Inc	58016-0743-15
15's	$19.03	GENERIC, Alpharma Uspd Makers Of Barre and Nmc	63874-0349-15
20's	$8.65	GENERIC, Prescript Pharmaceuticals	00247-0037-20
20's	$19.24	GENERIC, Southwood Pharmaceuticals Inc	58016-0743-20
20's	$25.01	GENERIC, Alpharma Uspd Makers Of Barre and Nmc	63874-0349-20
20's	$25.31	GENERIC, Pharma Pac	52959-0196-20
21's	$8.92	GENERIC, Prescript Pharmaceuticals	00247-0037-21
30's	$11.29	GENERIC, Prescript Pharmaceuticals	00247-0037-30
30's	$28.86	GENERIC, Southwood Pharmaceuticals Inc	58016-0743-30
30's	$34.15	GENERIC, Alpharma Uspd Makers Of Barre and Nmc	63874-0349-30

S

Qty	Price	Description	NDC
60's	$19.24	GENERIC, Prescript Pharmaceuticals	00247-0037-60
60's	$21.68	GENERIC, Physicians Total Care	54868-0879-00
60's	$63.79	GENERIC, Pharma Pac	52959-0196-60
90's	$27.18	GENERIC, Prescript Pharmaceuticals	00247-0037-90
100's	$29.82	GENERIC, Prescript Pharmaceuticals	00247-0037-00
100's	$96.20	GENERIC, Southwood Pharmaceuticals Inc	58016-0743-00
100's	$99.78	GENERIC, Alpharma Uspd Makers Of Barre and Nmc	63874-0349-10
118's	$34.59	GENERIC, Prescript Pharmaceuticals	00247-0037-52
180's	$51.00	GENERIC, Prescript Pharmaceuticals	00247-0037-59
Tablet - Oral - 200 mg			
10's	$6.53	GENERIC, Prescript Pharmaceuticals	00247-0376-10
12's	$14.22	GENERIC, Southwood Pharmaceuticals Inc	58016-0294-12
14's	$7.80	GENERIC, Prescript Pharmaceuticals	00247-0376-14
14's	$16.09	GENERIC, Allscripts Pharmaceutical Company	54569-4032-00
14's	$29.25	GENERIC, Pharma Pac	52959-0195-14
15's	$8.12	GENERIC, Prescript Pharmaceuticals	00247-0376-15
15's	$16.09	GENERIC, Allscripts Pharmaceutical Company	54569-4032-03
15's	$17.77	GENERIC, Southwood Pharmaceuticals Inc	58016-0294-15
15's	$20.73	GENERIC, Alpharma Uspd Makers Of Barre and Nmc	63874-0350-15
15's	$30.71	GENERIC, Pharma Pac	52959-0195-15
20's	$9.71	GENERIC, Prescript Pharmaceuticals	00247-0376-20
20's	$21.46	GENERIC, Allscripts Pharmaceutical Company	54569-4032-05
20's	$23.70	GENERIC, Southwood Pharmaceuticals Inc	58016-0294-20
20's	$26.57	GENERIC, Alpharma Uspd Makers Of Barre and Nmc	63874-0350-20
20's	$38.85	GENERIC, Pharma Pac	52959-0195-20
28's	$33.18	GENERIC, Southwood Pharmaceuticals Inc	58016-0294-28
28's	$52.63	GENERIC, Pharma Pac	52959-0195-28
30's	$12.88	GENERIC, Prescript Pharmaceuticals	00247-0376-30
30's	$32.18	GENERIC, Allscripts Pharmaceutical Company	54569-4032-01
30's	$35.55	GENERIC, Southwood Pharmaceuticals Inc	58016-0294-30
30's	$37.76	GENERIC, Alpharma Uspd Makers Of Barre and Nmc	63874-0350-30
30's	$55.13	GENERIC, Pharma Pac	52959-0195-30
40's	$47.40	GENERIC, Southwood Pharmaceuticals Inc	58016-0294-40
60's	$22.41	GENERIC, Prescript Pharmaceuticals	00247-0376-60
60's	$27.87	GENERIC, Physicians Total Care	54868-1118-01
60's	$71.10	GENERIC, Southwood Pharmaceuticals Inc	58016-0294-60
60's	$94.82	GENERIC, Pharma Pac	52959-0195-60
100's	$118.50	GENERIC, Southwood Pharmaceuticals Inc	58016-0294-00
100's	$120.38	GENERIC, Alpharma Uspd Makers Of Barre and Nmc	63874-0350-10

Sumatriptan Succinate *(003090)*

For related information, see the comparative table section in Appendix A.

Categories: Headache, migraine; Pregnancy Category C; FDA Approved 1992 Dec
Drug Classes: Serotonin receptor agonists
Brand Names: Imigran; **Imitrex**
Foreign Brand Availability: Cetatrex (Indonesia); Imigrane (France); Imiject (France); Migragesin (Colombia); Migranol (Bahrain; Cyprus; Egypt; Iran; Iraq; Jordan; Kuwait; Lebanon; Libya; Oman; Qatar; Republic-of-Yemen; Saudi-Arabia; Syria; United-Arab-Emirates); Sumitrex (India); Suvalan (Australia)
Cost of Therapy: $13.57 (Migraine Headache; Imitrex; 50 mg; 1 tablet/day; 1 day supply)
$85.12 (Migraine Headache; Imitrex; 6 mg/0.5 ml; 1 injection; 1 day supply)
HCFA JCODE(S): J3030 6 mg SC

ORAL

DESCRIPTION

Imitrex tablets contain sumatriptan (as the succinate), a selective 5-hydroxytryptamine$_1$ receptor subtype agonist. Sumatriptan succinate is chemically designated as 3-[2-(dimethylamino)ethyl]-N-methyl-indole-5-methanesulfonamide succinate (1:1).

The empirical formula is $C_{14}H_{21}N_3O_2S{\cdot}C_4H_6O_4$, representing a molecular weight of 413.5. Sumatriptan succinate is a white to off-white powder that is readily soluble in water and in saline. Each Imitrex tablet for oral administration contains 35, 70, or 140 mg of sumatriptan succinate equivalent to 25, 50, or 100 mg of sumatriptan, respectively. Each tablet also contains the inactive ingredients croscarmellose sodium, iron oxide (100 mg tablet only), lactose, magnesium stearate, microcrystalline cellulose, and titanium dioxide.

CLINICAL PHARMACOLOGY

MECHANISM OF ACTION

Sumatriptan is an agonist for a vascular 5-hydroxytryptamine$_1$ receptor subtype (probably a member of the 5-HT$_{1D}$ family) having only a weak affinity for 5-HT$_{1A}$, 5-HT$_{5A}$, and 5-HT$_7$ receptors and no significant affinity (as measured using standard radioligand binding assays) or pharmacological activity at 5-HT$_2$, 5-HT$_3$, or 5-HT$_4$ receptor subtypes or at alpha$_1$-, alpha$_2$-, or beta-adrenergic; dopamine$_1$; dopamine$_2$; muscarinic; or benzodiazepine receptors.

The vascular 5-HT$_1$ receptor subtype that sumatriptan activates is present on cranial arteries in both dog and primate, on the human basilar artery, and in the vasculature of human dura mater and mediates vasoconstriction. This action in humans correlates with the relief of migraine headache. In addition to causing vasoconstriction, experimental data from animal studies show that sumatriptan also activates 5-HT$_1$ receptors on peripheral terminals of the trigeminal nerve innervating cranial blood vessels. Such an action may also contribute to the antimigrainous effect of sumatriptan in humans.

In the anesthetized dog, sumatriptan selectively reduces the carotid arterial blood flow with little or no effect on arterial blood pressure or total peripheral resistance. In the cat, sumatriptan selectively constricts the carotid arteriovenous anastomoses while having little effect on blood flow or resistance in cerebral or extracerebral tissues.

PHARMACOKINETICS

The mean maximum concentration following oral dosing with 25 mg is 18 ng/ml (range, 7-47 ng/ml) and 51 ng/ml (range, 28-100 ng/ml) following oral dosing with 100 mg of sumatriptan. This compares with a C_{max} of 5 and 16 ng/ml following dosing with a 5 and 20 mg intranasal dose, respectively. The mean C_{max} following a 6 mg subcutaneous injection is 71 ng/ml (range, 49-110 ng/ml). The bioavailability is approximately 15%, primarily due to presystemic metabolism and partly due to incomplete absorption. The C_{max} is similar during a migraine attack and during a migraine-free period, but the T_{max} is slightly later during the attack, approximately 2.5 hours compared to 2.0 hours. When given as a single dose, sumatriptan displays dose proportionality in its extent of absorption (area under the curve [AUC]) over the dose range of 25-200 mg, but the C_{max} after 100 mg is approximately 25% less than expected (based on the 25 mg dose). Food has no significant effect on the bioavailability of sumatriptan, but delays the T_{max} slightly (by about 0.5 hours).

Plasma protein binding is low (14-21%). The effect of sumatriptan on the protein binding of other drugs has not been evaluated, but would be expected to be minor, given the low rate of protein binding. The apparent volume of distribution is 2.4 L/kg.

The elimination half-life of sumatriptan is approximately 2.5 hours. Radiolabeled ^{14}C-sumatriptan administered orally is largely renally excreted (about 60%) with about 40% found in the feces. Most of the radiolabeled compound excreted in the urine is the major metabolite, indole acetic acid (IAA), which is inactive, or the IAA glucuronide. Only 3% of the dose can be recovered as unchanged sumatriptan.

In vitro studies with human microsomes suggest that sumatriptan is metabolized by monoamine oxidase (MAO), predominantly the A isoenzyme, and inhibitors of that enzyme may alter sumatriptan pharmacokinetics to increase systemic exposure. No significant effect was seen with an MAO-B inhibitor (see CONTRAINDICATIONS, WARNINGS, and DRUG INTERACTIONS).

SPECIAL POPULATIONS

Renal Impairment

The effect of renal impairment on the pharmacokinetics of sumatriptan has not been examined, but little clinical effect would be expected as sumatriptan is largely metabolized to an inactive substance.

Hepatic Impairment

The liver plays an important role in the presystemic clearance of orally administered sumatriptan. Accordingly, the bioavailability of sumatriptan following oral administration may be markedly increased in patients with liver disease. In 1 small study of hepatically impaired patients (n=8) matched for sex, age, and weight with healthy subjects, the hepatically impaired patients had an approximately 70% increase in AUC and C_{max} and a T_{max} 40 minutes earlier compared to the healthy subjects (see DOSAGE AND ADMINISTRATION).

Age

The pharmacokinetics of oral sumatriptan in the elderly (mean age, 72 years; 2 males and 4 females) and in patients with migraine (mean age, 38 years, 25 males and 155 females) were similar to that in healthy male subjects (mean age, 30 years) (see PRECAUTIONS, Geriatric Use).

Gender

In a study comparing females to males, no pharmacokinetic differences were observed between genders for AUC, C_{max}, T_{max} and half-life.

Race

The systemic clearance and C_{max} of sumatriptan were similar in black (n=34) and Caucasian (n=38) healthy male subjects.

DRUG INTERACTIONS

Monoamine Oxidase Inhibitors (MAOI)

Treatment with MAO-A inhibitors generally leads to an increase of sumatriptan plasma levels (see CONTRAINDICATIONS and PRECAUTIONS).

Due to gut and hepatic metabolic first-pass effects, the increase of systemic exposure after coadministration of an MAO-A inhibitor with oral sumatriptan is greater than after coadministration of the MAOI with subcutaneous sumatriptan. In a study of 14 healthy females, pretreatment with an MAO-A inhibitor decreased the clearance of subcutaneous sumatriptan. Under the conditions of this experiment, the result was a 2-fold increase in the area under the sumatriptan plasma concentration × time curve (AUC), corresponding to a 40% increase in elimination half-life. This interaction was not evident with an MAO-B inhibitor.

A small study evaluating the effect of pretreatment with an MAO-A inhibitor on the bioavailability from a 25 mg oral sumatriptan tablet resulted in an approximately 7-fold increase in systemic exposure.

Alcohol

Alcohol consumed 30 minutes prior to sumatriptan ingestion had no effect on the pharmacokinetics of sumatriptan.

INDICATIONS AND USAGE

Sumatriptan succinate tablets are indicated for the acute treatment of migraine attacks with or without aura in adults.

Sumatriptan succinate tablets are not intended for the prophylactic therapy of migraine or for use in the management of hemiplegic or basilar migraine (see CONTRAINDICA-

TIONS). Safety and effectiveness of sumatriptan succinate tablets have not been established for cluster headache, which is present in an older, predominantly male population.

CONTRAINDICATIONS

Sumatriptan succinate tablets should not be given to patients with history, symptoms, or signs of ischemic cardiac, cerebrovascular, or peripheral vascular syndromes. In addition, patients with other significant underlying cardiovascular diseases should not receive sumatriptan succinate tablets. Ischemic cardiac syndromes include, but are not limited to, angina pectoris of any type (*e.g.,* stable angina of effort and vasospastic forms of angina such as the Prinzmetal variant), all forms of myocardial infarction, and silent myocardial ischemia. Cerebrovascular syndromes include, but are not limited to, strokes of any type as well as transient ischemic attacks. Peripheral vascular disease includes, but is not limited to, ischemic bowel disease (see WARNINGS).

Because sumatriptan succinate tablets may increase blood pressure, they should not be given to patients with uncontrolled hypertension.

Concurrent administration of MAO-A inhibitors or use within 2 weeks of discontinuation of MAO-A inhibitor therapy is contraindicated (see CLINICAL PHARMACOLOGY, Drug Interactions and DRUG INTERACTIONS).

Sumatriptan succinate tablets should not be administered to patients with hemiplegic or basilar migraine.

Sumatriptan succinate tablets and any ergotamine-containing or ergot-type medication (like dihydroergotamine or methysergide) should not be used within 24 hours of each other, nor should sumatriptan succinate and another 5-HT$_1$ agonist.

Sumatriptan succinate tablets are contraindicated in patients with hypersensitivity to sumatriptan or any of their components.

Sumatriptan succinate tablets are contraindicated in patients with severe hepatic impairment.

WARNINGS

Sumatriptan succinate tablets should only be used where a clear diagnosis of migraine headache has been established.

RISK OF MYOCARDIAL ISCHEMIA AND/OR INFARCTION AND OTHER ADVERSE CARDIAC EVENTS

Sumatriptan should not be given to patients with documented ischemic or vasospastic coronary artery disease (CAD) (see CONTRAINDICATIONS). It is strongly recommended that sumatriptan not be given to patients in whom unrecognized CAD is predicted by the presence of risk factors (*e.g.,* hypertension, hypercholesterolemia, smoker, obesity, diabetes, strong family history of CAD, female with surgical or physiological menopause, or male over 40 years of age) unless a cardiovascular evaluation provides satisfactory clinical evidence that the patient is reasonably free of coronary artery and ischemic myocardial disease or other significant underlying cardiovascular disease. The sensitivity of cardiac diagnostic procedures to detect cardiovascular disease or predisposition to coronary artery vasospasm is modest, at best. If, during the cardiovascular evaluation, the patient's medical history or electrocardiographic investigations reveal findings indicative of, or consistent with, coronary artery vasospasm or myocardial ischemia, sumatriptan should not be administered (see CONTRAINDICATIONS).

For patients with risk factors predictive of CAD, who are determined to have a satisfactory cardiovascular evaluation, it is strongly recommended that administration of the first dose of sumatriptan tablets take place in the setting of a physician's office or similar medically staffed and equipped facility unless the patient has previously received sumatriptan. Because cardiac ischemia can occur in the absence of clinical symptoms, consideration should be given to obtaining on the first occasion of use an electrocardiogram (ECG) during the interval immediately following sumatriptan succinate tablets, in these patients with risk factors.

It is recommended that patients who are intermittent long-term users of sumatriptan and who have or acquire risk factors predictive of CAD, as described above, undergo periodic interval cardiovascular evaluation as they continue to use sumatriptan.

The systematic approach described above is intended to reduce the likelihood that patients with unrecognized cardiovascular disease will be inadvertently exposed to sumatriptan.

DRUG-ASSOCIATED CARDIAC EVENTS AND FATALITIES

Serious adverse cardiac events, including acute myocardial infarction, life-threatening disturbances of cardiac rhythm, and death have been reported within a few hours following the administration of sumatriptan succinate injection or tablets. Considering the extent of use of sumatriptan in patients with migraine, the incidence of these events is extremely low.

The fact that sumatriptan can cause coronary vasospasm, that some of these events have occurred in patients with no prior cardiac disease history and with documented absence of CAD, and the close proximity of the events to sumatriptan use support the conclusion that some of these cases were caused by the drug. In many cases, however, where there has been known underlying coronary artery disease, the relationship is uncertain.

Premarketing Experience With Sumatriptan

Of 6348 patients with migraine who participated in premarketing controlled and uncontrolled clinical trials of oral sumatriptan, 2 experienced clinical adverse events shortly after receiving oral sumatriptan that may have reflected coronary vasospasm. Neither of these adverse events was associated with a serious clinical outcome.

Among the more than 1900 patients with migraine who participated in premarketing controlled clinical trials of subcutaneous sumatriptan, there were 8 patients who sustained clinical events during or shortly after receiving sumatriptan that may have reflected coronary artery vasospasm. Six (6) of these 8 patients had ECG changes consistent with transient ischemia, but without accompanying clinical symptoms or signs. Of these 8 patients, 4 had either findings suggestive of CAD or risk factors predictive of CAD prior to study enrollment.

Among approximately 4000 patients with migraine who participated in premarketing controlled and uncontrolled clinical trials of sumatriptan nasal spray, 1 patient experienced an asymptomatic subendocardial infarction possibly subsequent to a coronary vasospastic event.

Postmarketing Experience With Sumatriptan

Serious cardiovascular events, some resulting in death, have been reported in association with the use of sumatriptan succinate injection or tablets. The uncontrolled nature of postmarketing surveillance, however, makes it impossible to determine definitively the proportion of the reported cases that were actually caused by sumatriptan or to reliably assess causation in individual cases. On clinical grounds, the longer the latency between the administration of sumatriptan succinate and the onset of the clinical event, the less likely the association is to be causative. Accordingly, interest has focused on events beginning within 1 hour of the administration of sumatriptan succinate.

Cardiac events that have been observed to have onset within 1 hour of sumatriptan administration include: Coronary artery vasospasm, transient ischemia, myocardial infarction, ventricular tachycardia and ventricular fibrillation, cardiac arrest, and death.

Some of these events occurred in patients who had no findings of CAD and appear to represent consequences of coronary artery vasospasm. However, among domestic reports of serious cardiac events within 1 hour of sumatriptan administration, almost all of the patients had risk factors predictive of CAD and the presence of significant underlying CAD was established in most cases (see CONTRAINDICATIONS).

DRUG-ASSOCIATED CEREBROVASCULAR EVENTS AND FATALITIES

Cerebral hemorrhage, subarachnoid hemorrhage, stroke, and other cerebrovascular events have been reported in patients treated with oral or subcutaneous sumatriptan, and some have resulted in fatalities. The relationship of sumatriptan to these events is uncertain. In a number of cases, it appears possible that the cerebrovascular events were primary, sumatriptan having been administered in the incorrect belief that the symptoms experienced were a consequence of migraine when they were not. As with other acute migraine therapies, before treating headaches in patients not previously diagnosed as migraineurs, and in migraineurs who present with atypical symptoms, care should be taken to exclude other potentially serious neurological conditions. It should also be noted that patients with migraine may be at increased risk of certain cerebrovascular events (*e.g.,* cerebrovascular accident, transient ischemic attack).

OTHER VASOSPASM-RELATED EVENTS

Sumatriptan may cause vasospastic reactions other than coronary artery vasospasm. Both peripheral vascular ischemia and colonic ischemia with abdominal pain and bloody diarrhea have been reported.

INCREASE IN BLOOD PRESSURE

Significant elevation in blood pressure, including hypertensive crisis, has been reported on rare occasions in patients with and without a history of hypertension. Sumatriptan is contraindicated in patients with uncontrolled hypertension (see CONTRAINDICATIONS). Sumatriptan should be administered with caution to patients with controlled hypertension as transient increases in blood pressure and peripheral vascular resistance have been observed in a small proportion of patients.

CONCOMITANT DRUG USE

In patients taking MAO-A inhibitors, sumatriptan plasma levels attained after treatment with recommended doses are 7-fold higher following oral administration than those obtained under other conditions. Accordingly, the coadministration of sumatriptan succinate tablets and an MAO-A inhibitor is contraindicated (see CLINICAL PHARMACOLOGY and CONTRAINDICATIONS).

HYPERSENSITIVITY

Hypersensitivity (anaphylaxis/anaphylactoid) reactions have occurred on rare occasions in patients receiving sumatriptan. Such reactions can be life threatening or fatal. In general, hypersensitivity reactions to drugs are more likely to occur in individuals with a history of sensitivity to multiple allergens (see CONTRAINDICATIONS).

PRECAUTIONS

GENERAL

Chest discomfort and jaw or neck tightness have been reported following use of sumatriptan succinate tablets and have also been reported infrequently following administration of sumatriptan nasal spray. Chest, jaw, or neck tightness is relatively common after administration of sumatriptan succinate injection. Only rarely have these symptoms been associated with ischemic ECG changes. However, because sumatriptan may cause coronary artery vasospasm, patients who experience signs or symptoms suggestive of angina following sumatriptan should be evaluated for the presence of CAD or a predisposition to Prinzmetal variant angina before receiving additional doses of sumatriptan, and should be monitored electrocardiographically if dosing is resumed and similar symptoms recur. Similarly, patients who experience other symptoms or signs suggestive of decreased arterial flow, such as ischemic bowel syndrome or Raynaud syndrome following sumatriptan should be evaluated for atherosclerosis or predisposition to vasospasm (see WARNINGS).

Sumatriptan succinate should also be administered with caution to patients with diseases that may alter the absorption, metabolism, or excretion of drugs, such as impaired hepatic or renal function.

There have been rare reports of seizure following administration of sumatriptan. Sumatriptan should be used with caution in patients with a history of epilepsy or structural brain lesions that lower their seizure threshold.

Care should be taken to exclude other potentially serious neurologic conditions before treating headache in patients not previously diagnosed with migraine headache or who experience a headache that is atypical for them. There have been rare reports where patients received sumatriptan for severe headaches that were subsequently shown to have been secondary to an evolving neurologic lesion (see WARNINGS).

For a given attack, if a patient does not respond to the first dose of sumatriptan, the diagnosis of migraine should be reconsidered before administration of a second dose.

S

BINDING TO MELANIN-CONTAINING TISSUES

In rats treated with a single subcutaneous dose (0.5 mg/kg) or oral dose (2 mg/kg) of radiolabeled sumatriptan, the elimination half-life of radioactivity from the eye was 15 and 23 days, respectively, suggesting that sumatriptan and/or its metabolites bind to the melanin of the eye. Because there could be an accumulation in melanin-rich tissues over time, this raises the possibility that sumatriptan could cause toxicity in these tissues after extended use. However, no effects on the retina related to treatment with sumatriptan were noted in any of the oral or subcutaneous toxicity studies. Although no systematic monitoring of ophthalmologic function was undertaken in clinical trials, and no specific recommendations for ophthalmologic monitoring are offered, prescribers should be aware of the possibility of long-term ophthalmologic effects.

CORNEAL OPACITIES

Sumatriptan causes corneal opacities and defects in the corneal epithelium in dogs; this raises the possibility that these changes may occur in humans. While patients were not systematically evaluated for these changes in clinical trials, and no specific recommendations for monitoring are being offered, prescribers should be aware of the possibility of these changes (see ANIMAL PHARMACOLOGY).

INFORMATION FOR THE PATIENT

See the Patient Information that is distributed with the prescription for complete instructions.

LABORATORY TESTS

No specific laboratory tests are recommended for monitoring patients prior to and/or after treatment with sumatriptan.

DRUG/LABORATORY TEST INTERACTIONS

Sumatriptan succinate tablets are not known to interfere with commonly employed clinical laboratory tests.

CARCINOGENESIS, MUTAGENESIS, AND IMPAIRMENT OF FERTILITY

Carcinogenesis

In carcinogenicity studies, rats and mice were given sumatriptan by oral gavage (rats, 104 weeks), or drinking water (mice, 78 weeks). Average exposures achieved in mice receiving the highest dose (target dose of 160 mg/kg/day) were approximately 40 times the exposure attained in humans after the maximum recommended single oral dose of 100 mg. The highest dose administered to rats (160 mg/kg/day, reduced from 360 mg/kg/day during week 21) was approximately 15 times the maximum recommended single human oral dose of 100 mg on a mg/m^2 basis. There was no evidence of an increase in tumors in either species related to sumatriptan administration.

Mutagenesis

Sumatriptan was not mutagenic in the presence or absence of metabolic activation when tested in 2 gene mutation assays (the Ames test and the *in vitro* mammalian Chinese hamster V79/HGPRT assay). In 2 cytogenetics assays (the *in vitro* human lymphocyte assay and the *in vivo* rat micronucleus assay) sumatriptan was not associated with clastogenic activity.

Impairment of Fertility

In a study in which male and female rats were dosed daily with oral sumatriptan prior to and throughout the mating period, there was a treatment-related decrease in fertility secondary to a decrease in mating in animals treated with 50 and 500 mg/kg/day. The highest no-effect dose for this finding was 5 mg/kg/day, or approximately one-half of the maximum recommended single human oral dose of 100 mg on a mg/m^2 basis. It is not clear whether the problem is associated with treatment of the males or females or both combined. In a similar study by the subcutaneous route there was no evidence of impaired fertility at 60 mg/kg/day, the maximum dose tested, which is equivalent to approximately 6 times the maximum recommended single human oral dose of 100 mg on a mg/m^2 basis.

S

PREGNANCY CATEGORY C

In reproductive toxicity studies in rats and rabbits, oral treatment with sumatriptan was associated with embryolethality, fetal abnormalities, and pup mortality. When administered by the intravenous (IV) route to rabbits, sumatriptan has been shown to be embryolethal. There are no adequate and well-controlled studies in pregnant women. Therefore, sumatriptan succinate tablets should be used during pregnancy only if the potential benefit justifies the potential risk to the fetus. In assessing this information, the following findings should be considered.

Embryolethality

When given orally or intravenously to pregnant rabbits daily throughout the period of organogenesis, sumatriptan caused embryolethality at doses at or close to those producing maternal toxicity. In the oral studies this dose was 100 mg/kg/day, and in the intravenous studies this dose was 2.0 mg/kg/day. The mechanism of the embryolethality is not known. The highest no-effect dose for embryolethality by the oral route was 50 mg/kg/day, which is approximately 9 times the maximum single recommended human oral dose of 100 mg on a mg/m^2 basis. By the IV route, the highest no-effect dose was 0.75 mg/kg/day, or approximately one-tenth of the maximum single recommended human oral dose of 100 mg on a mg/m^2 basis.

The IV administration of sumatriptan to pregnant rats throughout organogenesis at 12.5 mg/kg/day, the maximum dose tested, did not cause embryolethality. This dose is equivalent to the maximum single recommended human oral dose of 100 mg on a mg/m^2 basis. Additionally, in a study in rats given subcutaneous sumatriptan daily prior to and throughout pregnancy at 60 mg/kg/day, the maximum dose tested, there was no evidence of increased embryo/fetal lethality. This dose is equivalent to approximately 6 times the maximum recommended single human oral dose of 100 mg on a mg/m^2 basis.

Teratogenicity

Oral treatment of pregnant rats with sumatriptan during the period of organogenesis resulted in an increased incidence of blood vessel abnormalities (cervicothoracic and umbilical) at doses of approximately 250 mg/kg/day or higher. The highest no-effect dose was approximately 60 mg/kg/day, which is approximately 6 times the maximum single recommended human oral dose of 100 mg on a mg/m^2 basis. Oral treatment of pregnant rabbits with sumatriptan during the period of organogenesis resulted in an increased incidence of cervicothoracic vascular and skeletal abnormalities. The highest no-effect dose for these effects was 15 mg/kg/day, or approximately 3 times the maximum single recommended human oral dose of 100 mg on a mg/m^2 basis.

A study in which rats were dosed daily with oral sumatriptan prior to and throughout gestation demonstrated embryo/fetal toxicity (decreased body weight, decreased ossification, increased incidence of rib variations) and an increased incidence of a syndrome of malformations (short tail/short body and vertebral disorganization) at 500 mg/kg/day. The highest no-effect dose was 50 mg/kg/day, or approximately 5 times the maximum single recommended human oral dose of 100 mg on a mg/m^2 basis. In a study in rats dosed daily with subcutaneous sumatriptan prior to and throughout pregnancy, at a dose of 60 mg/kg/day, the maximum dose tested, there was no evidence of teratogenicity. This dose is equivalent to approximately 6 times the maximum recommended single human oral dose of 100 mg on a mg/m^2 basis.

Pup Deaths

Oral treatment of pregnant rats with sumatriptan during the period of organogenesis resulted in a decrease in pup survival between birth and postnatal day 4 at doses of approximately 250 mg/kg/day or higher. The highest no-effect dose for this effect was approximately 60 mg/kg/day, or 6 times the maximum single recommended human oral dose of 100 mg on a mg/m^2 basis.

Oral treatment of pregnant rats with sumatriptan from gestational day 17 through postnatal day 21 demonstrated a decrease in pup survival measured at postnatal days 2, 4, and 20 at the dose of 1000 mg/kg/day. The highest no-effect dose for this finding was 100 mg/kg/day, approximately 10 times the maximum single recommended human oral dose of 100 mg on a mg/m^2 basis. In a similar study in rats by the subcutaneous route there was no increase in pup death at 81 mg/kg/day, the highest dose tested, which is equivalent to 8 times the maximum single recommended human oral dose of 100 mg on a mg/m^2 basis.

To monitor fetal outcomes of pregnant women exposed to sumatriptan succinate, GlaxoSmithKline maintains a Sumatriptan Pregnancy Registry. Physicians are encouraged to register patients by calling 800-336-2176.

NURSING MOTHERS

Sumatriptan is excreted in human breast milk. Therefore, caution should be exercised when considering the administration of sumatriptan succinate tablets to a nursing woman.

PEDIATRIC USE

Safety and effectiveness of sumatriptan succinate tablets in pediatric patients have not been established.

Completed placebo-controlled clinical trials evaluating oral sumatriptan (25-100 mg) in pediatric patients aged 12-17 years enrolled a total of 701 adolescent migraineurs. These studies did not establish the efficacy of oral sumatriptan compared to placebo in the treatment of migraine in adolescents. Adverse events observed in these clinical trials were similar in nature to those reported in clinical trials in adults. The frequency of all adverse events in these patients appeared to be both dose- and age-dependent, with younger patients reporting events more commonly than older adolescents. Postmarketing experience includes a limited number of reports that describe pediatric patients who have experienced adverse events, some clinically serious, after use of subcutaneous sumatriptan and/or oral sumatriptan. These reports include events similar in nature to those reported rarely in adults. A myocardial infarct has been reported in a 14-year-old male following the use of oral sumatriptan; clinical signs occurred within 1 day of drug administration. Since clinical data to determine the frequency of serious adverse events in pediatric patients who might receive injectable, oral, or intranasal sumatriptan are not presently available, the use of sumatriptan in patients aged younger than 18 years is not recommended.

GERIATRIC USE

The use of sumatriptan in elderly patients is not recommended because elderly patients are more likely to have decreased hepatic function, they are at higher risk for CAD, and blood pressure increases may be more pronounced in the elderly (see WARNINGS).

DRUG INTERACTIONS

Ergot-containing drugs have been reported to cause prolonged vasospastic reactions. Because there is a theoretical basis that these effects may be additive, use of ergotamine-containing or ergot-type medications (like dihydroergotamine or methysergide) and sumatriptan within 24 hours of each other should be avoided (see CONTRAINDICATIONS).

MAO-A inhibitors reduce sumatriptan clearance, significantly increasing systemic exposure. Therefore, the use of sumatriptan succinate tablets in patients receiving MAO-A inhibitors is contraindicated (see CLINICAL PHARMACOLOGY and CONTRAINDICATIONS).

Selective serotonin reuptake inhibitors (SSRIs) (*e.g.*, fluoxetine, fluvoxamine, paroxetine, sertraline) have been reported, rarely, to cause weakness, hyperreflexia, and incoordination when coadministered with sumatriptan. If concomitant treatment with sumatriptan and an SSRI is clinically warranted, appropriate observation of the patient is advised.

ADVERSE REACTIONS

Serious cardiac events, including some that have been fatal, have occurred following the use of sumatriptan succinate injection or tablets. These events are extremely rare and most have been reported in patients with risk factors predictive of CAD. Events reported have included coronary artery vasospasm, transient myocardial ischemia, myocardial infarction, ventricular tachycardia, and ventricular fibrillation (see CONTRAINDICATIONS, WARNINGS, and PRECAUTIONS).

Significant hypertensive episodes, including hypertensive crises, have been reported on rare occasions in patients with or without a history of hypertension (see WARNINGS).

INCIDENCE IN CONTROLLED CLINICAL TRIALS

TABLE 2 lists adverse events that occurred in placebo-controlled clinical trials in patients who took at least 1 dose of study drug. Only events that occurred at a frequency of 2% or more in any group treated with sumatriptan succinate tablets and were more frequent in that group than in the placebo group are included in TABLE 2. The events cited reflect experience gained under closely monitored conditions of clinical trials in a highly selected patient population. In actual clinical practice or in other clinical trials, these frequency estimates may not apply, as the conditions of use, reporting behavior, and the kinds of patients treated may differ.

TABLE 2 *Treatment-Emergent Adverse Events Reported by at Least 2% of Patients in Controlled Migraine Trials**

		Sumatriptan Succinate Tablets		
	Placebo	25 mg	50 mg	100 mg
Adverse Event Type	(n=309)	(n=417)	(n=771)	(n=437)
Atypical Sensations	4%	5%	6%	6%
Paresthesia (all types)	2%	3%	5%	3%
Sensation warm/cold	2%	3%	2%	3%
Pain and Other Pressure Sensations	4%	6%	6%	8%
Chest — pain/tightness/ pressure and/or heaviness	1%	1%	2%	2%
Neck/throat/jaw — pain/ tightness/pressure	<1%	<1%	2%	3%
Pain — location specified	1%	2%	1%	1%
Other — pressure/ tightness/heaviness	2%	1%	1%	3%
Neurological				
Vertigo	<1%	<1%	<1%	2%
Other				
Malaise/fatigue	<1%	2%	2%	3%

* Events that occurred at a frequency of 2% or more in the group treated with sumatriptan succinate tablets and that occurred more frequently in that group than the placebo group.

Other events that occurred in more than 1% of patients receiving sumatriptan succinate tablets and at least as often on placebo included nausea and/or vomiting, migraine, headache, hyposalivation, dizziness, and drowsiness/sleepiness.

Sumatriptan succinate tablets are generally well tolerated. Across all doses, most adverse reactions were mild and transient and did not lead to long-lasting effects. The incidence of adverse events in controlled clinical trials was not affected by gender or age of the patients. There were insufficient data to assess the impact of race on the incidence of adverse events.

OTHER EVENTS OBSERVED IN ASSOCIATION WITH THE ADMINISTRATION OF SUMATRIPTAN SUCCINATE TABLETS

In the paragraphs that follow, the frequencies of less commonly reported adverse clinical events are presented. Because the reports include events observed in open and uncontrolled studies, the role of sumatriptan succinate tablets in their causation cannot be reliably determined. Furthermore, variability associated with adverse event reporting, the terminology used to describe adverse events, etc., limit the value of quantitative frequency estimates provided. Event frequencies are calculated as the number of patients who used sumatriptan succinate tablets (25, 50, or 100 mg) and reported an event divided by the total number of patients (n=6348) exposed to sumatriptan succinate tablets. All reported events are included except those already listed in TABLE 2, those too general to be informative, and those not reasonably associated with the use of the drug. Events are further classified within body system categories and enumerated in order of decreasing frequency using the following definitions: *frequent* adverse events are defined as those occurring in at least 1/100 patients; *infrequent* adverse events are those occurring in 1/100 to 1/1000 patients; and *rare* adverse events are those occurring in fewer than 1/1000 patients.

Atypical Sensations: *Frequent:* Burning sensation and numbness. *Infrequent:* Tight feeling in head. *Rare:* Dysesthesia.

Cardiovascular: *Frequent:* Palpitations, syncope, decreased blood pressure, and increased blood pressure. *Infrequent:* Arrhythmia, changes in ECG, hypertension, hypotension, pallor, pulsating sensations, and tachycardia. *Rare:* Angina, atherosclerosis, bradycardia, cerebral ischemia, cerebrovascular lesion, heart block, peripheral cyanosis, thrombosis, transient myocardial ischemia, and vasodilation.

Ear, Nose, and Throat: *Frequent:* Sinusitis; tinnitus; allergic rhinitis; upper respiratory inflammation; ear, nose, and throat hemorrhage; external otitis; hearing loss; nasal inflammation; and sensitivity to noise. *Infrequent:* Hearing disturbances and otalgia. *Rare:* Feeling of fullness in the ear(s).

Endocrine and Metabolic: *Infrequent:* Thirst. *Rare:* Elevated thyrotropin stimulating hormone (TSH) levels; galactorrhea; hyperglycemia; hypoglycemia; hypothyroidism; polydipsia; weight gain; weight loss; endocrine cysts, lumps, and masses; and fluid disturbances.

Eye: *Rare:* Disorders of sclera, mydriasis, blindness and low vision, visual disturbances, eye edema and swelling, eye irritation and itching, accommodation disorders, external ocular muscle disorders, eye hemorrhage, eye pain, and keratitis and conjunctivitis.

Gastrointestinal: *Frequent:* Diarrhea and gastric symptoms. *Infrequent:* Constipation, dysphagia, and gastroesophageal reflux. *Rare:* Gastrointestinal bleeding, hematemesis, melena, peptic ulcer, gastrointestinal pain, dyspeptic symptoms, dental pain, feelings of gastrointestinal pressure, gastroesophageal reflux, gastritis, gastroenteritis, hypersalivation, abdominal distention, oral itching and irritation, salivary gland swelling, and swallowing disorders.

Hematological Disorders: *Rare:* Anemia.

Musculoskeletal: *Frequent:* Myalgia. *Infrequent:* Muscle cramps. *Rare:* Tetany; muscle atrophy, weakness, and tiredness; arthralgia and articular rheumatitis; acquired musculoskeletal deformity; muscle stiffness, tightness, and rigidity; and musculoskeletal inflammation.

Neurological: *Frequent:* Phonophobia and photophobia. *Infrequent:* Confusion, depression, difficulty concentrating, disturbance of smell, dysarthria, euphoria, facial pain, heat sensitivity, incoordination, lacrimation, monoplegia, sleep disturbance, shivering, syncope, and tremor. *Rare:* Aggressiveness, apathy, bradylogia, cluster headache, convulsions, decreased appetite, drug abuse, dystonic reaction, facial paralysis, hallucinations, hunger, hyperesthesia, hysteria, increased alertness, memory disturbance, neuralgia, paralysis, personality change, phobia, radiculopathy, rigidity, suicide, twitching, agitation, anxiety, depressive disorders, detachment, motor dysfunction, neurotic disorders, psychomotor disorders, taste disturbances, and raised intracranial pressure.

Respiratory: *Frequent:* Dyspnea. *Infrequent:* Asthma. *Rare:* Hiccoughs, breathing disorders, cough, and bronchitis.

Skin: *Frequent:* Sweating. *Infrequent:* Erythema, pruritus, rash, and skin tenderness. *Rare:* Dry/scaly skin, tightness of skin, wrinkling of skin, eczema, seborrheic dermatitis, and skin nodules.

Breasts: *Infrequent:* Tenderness. *Rare:* Nipple discharge; breast swelling; cysts, lumps, and masses of breasts; and primary malignant breast neoplasm.

Urogenital: *Infrequent:* Dysmenorrhea, increased urination, and intermenstrual bleeding. *Rare:* Abortion and hematuria, urinary frequency, bladder inflammation, micturition disorders, urethritis, urinary infections, menstruation symptoms, abnormal menstrual cycle, inflammation of fallopian tubes, and menstrual cycle symptoms.

Miscellaneous: *Frequent:* Hypersensitivity. *Infrequent:* Fever, fluid retention, and overdose. *Rare:* Edema, hematoma, lymphadenopathy, speech disturbance, voice disturbances, contusions.

OTHER EVENTS OBSERVED IN THE CLINICAL DEVELOPMENT OF SUMATRIPTAN SUCCINATE

The following adverse events occurred in clinical trials with sumatriptan succinate injection and nasal spray. Because the reports include events observed in open and uncontrolled studies, the role of sumatriptan succinate in their causation cannot be reliably determined. All reported events are included except those already listed, those too general to be informative, and those not reasonably associated with the use of the drug.

Atypical Sensations: Feeling strange, prickling sensation, tingling, and hot sensation.

Cardiovascular: Abdominal aortic aneurysm, abnormal pulse, flushing, phlebitis, Raynaud syndrome, and various transient ECG changes (nonspecific ST or T wave changes, prolongation of PR or QTc intervals, sinus arrhythmia, nonsustained ventricular premature beats, isolated junctional ectopic beats, atrial ectopic beats, delayed activation of the right ventricle).

Chest Symptoms: Chest discomfort.

Endocrine and Metabolic: Dehydration.

Ear, Nose, and Throat: Disorder/discomfort nasal cavity and sinuses, ear infection, Meniere disease, and throat discomfort.

Eye: Vision alterations.

Gastrointestinal: Abdominal discomfort, colitis, disturbance of liver function tests, flatulence/eructation, gallstones, intestinal obstruction, pancreatitis, and retching.

Injection Site Reaction

Miscellaneous: Difficulty in walking, hypersensitivity to various agents, jaw discomfort, miscellaneous laboratory abnormalities, "serotonin agonist effect," swelling of the extremities, and swelling of the face.

Mouth and Teeth: Disorder of mouth and tongue (*e.g.,* burning of tongue, numbness of tongue, dry mouth).

Musculoskeletal: Arthritis, backache, intervertebral disc disorder, neck pain/stiffness, need to flex calf muscles, and various joint disturbances (pain, stiffness, swelling, ache).

Neurological: Bad/unusual taste, chills, diplegia, disturbance of emotions, sedation, globus hystericus, intoxication, myoclonia, neoplasm of pituitary, relaxation, sensation of lightness, simultaneous hot and cold sensations, stinging sensations, stress, tickling sensations, transient hemiplegia, and yawning.

Respiratory: Influenza and diseases of the lower respiratory tract and lower respiratory tract infection.

Skin: Skin eruption, herpes, and peeling of the skin.

Urogenital: Disorder of breasts, endometriosis, and renal calculus.

POSTMARKETING EXPERIENCE (REPORTS FOR SUBCUTANEOUS OR ORAL SUMATRIPTAN)

The following section enumerates potentially important adverse events that have occurred in clinical practice and that have been reported spontaneously to various surveillance systems. The events enumerated represent reports arising from both domestic and nondomestic use of oral or subcutaneous dosage forms of sumatriptan. The events enumerated include all except those already listed in ADVERSE REACTIONS or those too general to be informative. Because the reports cite events reported spontaneously from worldwide postmarketing experience, frequency of events and the role of sumatriptan in their causation cannot be reliably determined. It is assumed, however, that systemic reactions following sumatriptan use are likely to be similar regardless of route of administration.

Blood: Hemolytic anemia, pancytopenia, thrombocytopenia.

Cardiovascular: Atrial fibrillation, cardiomyopathy, colonic ischemia (see WARNINGS), Prinzmetal variant angina, pulmonary embolism, shock, thrombophlebitis.

Ear, Nose, and Throat: Deafness.

Eye: Ischemic optic neuropathy, retinal artery occlusion, retinal vein thrombosis, loss of vision.

Gastrointestinal: Ischemic colitis with rectal bleeding (see WARNINGS), xerostomia.

Hepatic: Elevated liver function tests.
Neurological: Central nervous system vasculitis, cerebrovascular accident, dysphasia, subarachnoid hemorrhage.
Non-Site Specific: Angioneurotic edema, cyanosis, death (see WARNINGS), temporal arteritis.
Psychiatry: Panic disorder.
Respiratory: Bronchospasm in patients with and without a history of asthma.
Skin: Exacerbation of sunburn, hypersensitivity reactions (allergic vasculitis, erythema, pruritus, rash, shortness of breath, urticaria; in addition, severe anaphylaxis/anaphylactoid reactions have been reported [see WARNINGS]), photosensitivity.
Urogenital: Acute renal failure.

DOSAGE AND ADMINISTRATION

In controlled clinical trials, single doses of 25, 50, or 100 mg of sumatriptan succinate tablets were effective for the acute treatment of migraine in adults. There is evidence that doses of 50 and 100 mg may provide a greater effect than 25 mg. There is also evidence that doses of 100 mg do not provide a greater effect than 50 mg. Individuals may vary in response to doses of sumatriptan succinate tablets. The choice of dose should therefore be made on an individual basis, weighing the possible benefit of a higher dose with the potential for a greater risk of adverse events.

If the headache returns or the patient has a partial response to the initial dose, the dose may be repeated after 2 hours, not to exceed a total daily dose of 200 mg. If a headache returns following an initial treatment with sumatriptan succinate injection, additional single sumatriptan succinate tablets (up to 100 mg/day) may be given with an interval of at least 2 hours between tablet doses. The safety of treating an average of more than 4 headaches in a 30 day period has not been established.

Because of the potential of MAO-A inhibitors to cause unpredictable elevations in the bioavailability of oral sumatriptan, their combined use is contraindicated (see CONTRAINDICATIONS).

Hepatic disease/functional impairment may also cause unpredictable elevations in the bioavailability of orally administered sumatriptan. Consequently, if treatment is deemed advisable in the presence of liver disease, the maximum single dose should in general not exceed 50 mg (see CLINICAL PHARMACOLOGY for the basis of this recommendation).

ANIMAL PHARMACOLOGY

CORNEAL OPACITIES

Dogs receiving oral sumatriptan developed corneal opacities and defects in the corneal epithelium. Corneal opacities were seen at the lowest dosage tested, 2 mg/kg/day, and were present after 1 month of treatment. Defects in the corneal epithelium were noted in a 60 week study. Earlier examinations for these toxicities were not conducted and no-effect doses were not established; however, the relative exposure at the lowest dose tested was approximately 5 times the human exposure after a 100 mg oral dose. There is evidence of alterations in corneal appearance on the first day of intranasal dosing to dogs. Changes were noted at the lowest dose tested, which was approximately one-half the maximum single human oral dose of 100 mg on a mg/m^2 basis.

HOW SUPPLIED

IMITREX TABLETS

Imitrex tablets, 25, 50, and 100 mg of sumatriptan (base) as the succinate.

25 mg: White, round, film-coated tablets embossed with "I" on one side and "25" on the other.
50 mg: White, triangular-shaped, film-coated tablets embossed with "IMITREX" on one side and "50" on the other.
100 mg: Pink, triangular-shaped, film-coated tablets embossed with "IMITREX" on one side and "100" on the other.

Storage: Store between 2 and 30°C (36 and 86°F).

SUBCUTANEOUS

DESCRIPTION

Sumatriptan succinate injection is a selective 5-hydroxytryptamine$_1$ receptor subtype agonist. Sumatriptan succinate is chemically designated as 3-[2-(dimethylamino)ethyl]-N-methyl-indole-5-methanesulfonamide succinate (1:1).

The empirical formula is $C_{14}H_{21}N_3O_2S{\cdot}C_4H_6O_4$, representing a molecular weight of 413.5.

Sumatriptan succinate is a white to off-white powder that is readily soluble in water and in saline.

Imitrex injection is a clear, colorless to pale yellow, sterile, nonpyrogenic solution for subcutaneous injection. Each 0.5 ml of solution contains 6 mg of sumatriptan (base) as the succinate salt and 3.5 mg of sodium chloride in water for injection. The pH range of the solution is approximately 4.2-5.3. The osmolality of the injection is 291 mOsmol.

CLINICAL PHARMACOLOGY

MECHANISM OF ACTION

Sumatriptan has been demonstrated to be a selective agonist for a vascular 5-hydroxytryptamine$_1$ receptor subtype (probably a member of the 5-HT_{1D} family) with no significant affinity (as measured using standard radioligand binding assays) or pharmacological activity at 5-HT_2, 5-HT_3 receptor subtypes or at alpha$_1$-, alpha$_2$-, or beta-adrenergic; dopamine$_1$; dopamine$_2$; muscarinic; or benzodiazepine receptors.

The vascular 5-HT_1 receptor subtype to which sumatriptan binds selectively, and through which it presumably exerts its antimigrainous effect, has been shown to be present on cranial arteries in both dog and primate, on the human basilar artery, and in the vasculature of the isolated dura mater of humans. In these tissues, sumatriptan activates this receptor to cause vasoconstriction, an action in humans correlating with the relief of migraine and cluster headache. In the anesthetized dog, sumatriptan selectively reduces the carotid arterial blood flow with little or no effect on arterial blood pressure or total peripheral resistance. In the cat, sumatriptan selectively constricts the carotid arteriovenous anastomoses while having little effect on blood flow or resistance in cerebral or extracerebral tissues.

CORNEAL OPACITIES

Dogs receiving oral sumatriptan developed corneal opacities and defects in the corneal epithelium. Corneal opacities were seen at the lowest dosage tested, 2 mg/kg/day, and were present after 1 month of treatment. Defects in the corneal epithelium were noted in a 60 week study. Earlier examinations for these toxicities were not conducted and no-effect doses were not established; however, the relative exposure at the lowest dose tested was approximately 5 times the human exposure after a 100 mg oral dose or 3 times the human exposure after a 6 mg subcutaneous dose.

MELANIN BINDING

In rats with a single subcutaneous dose (0.5 mg/kg) of radiolabeled sumatriptan, the elimination half-life of radioactivity from the eye was 15 days, suggesting that sumatriptan and its metabolites bind to the melanin of the eye. The clinical significance of this binding is unknown.

PHARMACOKINETICS

Pharmacokinetic parameters following a 6 mg subcutaneous injection into the deltoid area of the arm in 9 males *(mean age, 33 years; mean weight, 77 kg)* were systemic clearance: 1194 ± 149 ml/min *(mean ±SD)*, distribution half-life: 15 ± 2 minutes, terminal half-life: 115 ± 19 minutes, and volume of distribution central compartment: 50 ± 8 liters. Of this dose, 22% ± 4% was excreted in the urine as unchanged sumatriptan and 38% ± 7% as the indole acetic acid metabolite.

After a single 6 mg subcutaneous manual injection into the deltoid area of the arm in 18 healthy males *(age, 24 ± 6 years; weight, 70 kg)*, the maximum serum concentration (C_{max}) was *(mean ± standard deviation)* 74 ± 15 ng/ml and the time to peak concentration (T_{max}) was 12 minutes after injection *(range, 5-20 minutes)*. In this study, the same dose injected subcutaneously in the thigh gave a C_{max} of 61 ± 15 ng/ml by manual injection versus 52 ± 15 ng/ml by autoinjector techniques. The T_{max} or amount absorbed was not significantly altered by either the site or technique of injection.

The bioavailability of sumatriptan via subcutaneous site injection to 18 healthy male subjects was 97% ± 16% of that obtained following IV injection. Protein binding, determined by equilibrium dialysis over the concentration of 10-1000 ng/ml, is low, approximately 14-21%. The effect of sumatriptan on protein binding of other drugs has not yet been evaluated.

SPECIAL POPULATIONS

Renal Impairment

The effect of renal impairment on the pharmacokinetics of sumatriptan has not been examined, but little clinical effect would be expected as sumatriptan is largely metabolized to an inactive substance.

Hepatic Impairment

The effect of hepatic disease on the pharmacokinetics of subcutaneously and orally administered sumatriptan has been evaluated. There were no statistically significant differences in the pharmacokinetics of subcutaneously administered sumatriptan in hepatically impaired patients compared to healthy controls. However, the liver plays an important role in the presystemic clearance of orally administered sumatriptan. Accordingly, the bioavailability of sumatriptan following oral administration may be markedly increased in patients with liver disease. In 1 small study of hepatically impaired patients (n=8) matched for sex, age, and weight with healthy subjects, the hepatically impaired patients had an approximately 70% increase in AUC and C_{max} and a T_{max} 40 minutes earlier compared to the healthy subjects.

Age

The pharmacokinetics of sumatriptan in the elderly *(mean age, 72 years; 2 males and 4 females)* and in patients with migraine *(mean age, 38 years; 25 males and 155 females)* were similar to that in healthy male subjects *(mean age, 30 years)* (see PRECAUTIONS, Geriatric Use).

Race

The systemic clearance and C_{max} of sumatriptan were similar in black (n=34) and Caucasian (n=38) healthy male subjects.

DRUG INTERACTIONS

MAO Inhibitors

In vitro studies with human microsomes suggest that sumatriptan is metabolized by monoamine oxidase (MAO), predominantly the A isoenzyme. In a study of 14 healthy females, pretreatment with MAO-A inhibitor decreased the clearance of sumatriptan. Under the conditions of this experiment, the result was a 2-fold increase in the area under the sumatriptan plasma concentration × time curve (AUC), corresponding to a 40% increase in elimination half-life. No significant effect was seen with an MAO-B inhibitor.

PHARMACODYNAMICS

Typical physiologic responses:

Blood Pressure: See WARNINGS.
Peripheral (small) Arteries: In healthy volunteers (n=18), a study evaluating the effects of sumatriptan on peripheral (small vessel) arterial reactivity failed to detect a clinically significant increase in peripheral resistance.
Heart Rate: Transient increases in blood pressure observed in some patients in clinical studies carried out during sumatriptan's development as a treatment for migraine were not accompanied by any clinically significant changes in heart rate.
Respiratory Rate: Experience gained during the clinical development of sumatriptan as a treatment for migraine failed to detect an effect of the drug on respiratory rate.

S

INDICATIONS AND USAGE

Sumatriptan succinate injection is indicated for (1) the acute treatment of migraine attacks with or without aura and; (2) the acute treatment of cluster headache episodes.

Sumatriptan succinate injection is not for use in the management of hemiplegic or basilar migraine (see CONTRAINDICATIONS).

CONTRAINDICATIONS

Sumatriptan succinate injection should not be given intravenously because of its potential to cause coronary vasospasm.

Sumatriptan succinate injection should not be given to patients with history, symptoms, or signs of ischemic cardiac, cerebrovascular, or peripheral vascular syndromes. In addition, patients with other significant underlying cardiovascular diseases should not receive sumatriptan succinate tablets. Ischemic cardiac syndromes include, but are not limited to, angina pectoris of any type (*e.g.,* stable angina of effort and vasospastic forms of angina such as the Prinzmetal variant), all forms of myocardial infarction, and silent myocardial ischemia. Cerebrovascular syndromes include, but are not limited to, strokes of any type as well as transient ischemic attacks. Peripheral vascular disease includes, but is not limited to, ischemic bowel disease (see WARNINGS).

Because sumatriptan succinate injection may increase blood pressure, it should not be given to patients with uncontrolled hypertension.

Sumatriptan succinate injection and any ergotamine-containing or ergot-type medication (like dihydroergotamine or methysergide) should not be used within 24 hours of each other, nor should sumatriptan succinate injection and another 5-HT$_1$ agonist.

Sumatriptan succinate injection should not be administered to patients with hemiplegic or basilar migraine.

Sumatriptan succinate injection is contraindicated in patients with hypersensitivity to sumatriptan or any of its components.

Sumatriptan succinate injection is contraindicated in patients with severe hepatic impairment.

WARNINGS

Sumatriptan succinate injection should only be used where a clear diagnosis of migraine or cluster headache has been established. The prescriber should be aware that cluster headache patients often possess 1 or more predictive risk factors for coronary artery disease (CAD).

RISK OF MYOCARDIAL ISCHEMIA AND/OR INFARCTION AND OTHER ADVERSE CARDIAC EVENTS

Sumatriptan should not be given to patients with documented ischemic or vasospastic CAD (see CONTRAINDICATIONS). It is strongly recommended that sumatriptan not be given to patients in whom unrecognized CAD is predicted by the presence of risk factors (*e.g.,* hypertension, hypercholesterolemia, smoker, obesity, diabetes, strong family history of CAD, female with surgical or physiological menopause, or male over 40 years of age) unless a cardiovascular evaluation provides satisfactory clinical evidence that the patient is reasonably free of coronary artery and ischemic myocardial disease or other significant underlying cardiovascular disease. The sensitivity of cardiac diagnostic procedures to detect cardiovascular disease or predisposition to coronary artery vasospasm is modest, at best. If, during the cardiovascular evaluation, the patient's medical history or electrocardiographic investigations reveal findings indicative of or consistent with coronary artery vasospasm or myocardial ischemia, sumatriptan should not be administered (see CONTRAINDICATIONS).

For patients with risk factors predictive of CAD who are determined to have a satisfactory cardiovascular evaluation, it is strongly recommended that administration of the first dose of sumatriptan injection take place in the setting of a physician's office or similar medically staffed and equipped facility. Because cardiac ischemia can occur in the absence of clinical symptoms, consideration should be given to obtaining on the first occasion of use an ECG during the interval immediately following sumatriptan succinate injection, in these patients with risk factors.

It is recommended that patients who are intermittent long-term users of sumatriptan and who have or acquire risk factors predictive of CAD, as described above, undergo periodic interval cardiovascular evaluation as they continue to use sumatriptan. In considering this recommendation for periodic cardiovascular evaluation, it is noted that patients with cluster headache are predominantly male and over 40 years of age, which are risk factors for CAD.

The systematic approach described above is intended to reduce the likelihood that patients with unrecognized cardiovascular disease will be inadvertently exposed to sumatriptan.

DRUG-ASSOCIATED CARDIAC EVENTS AND FATALITIES

Serious adverse cardiac events, including acute myocardial infarction, life-threatening disturbances of cardiac rhythm, and death have been reported within a few hours following the administration of sumatriptan succinate injection or tablets. Considering the extent of use of sumatriptan in patients with migraine, the incidence of these events is extremely low.

The fact that sumatriptan can cause coronary vasospasm, that some of these events have occurred in patients with no prior cardiac disease history and with documented absence of CAD, and the close proximity of the events to sumatriptan use support the conclusion that some of these cases were caused by the drug. In many cases, however, where there has been known underlying CAD, the relationship is uncertain.

Premarketing Experience With Sumatriptan

Among the more than 1900 patients with migraine who participated in premarketing controlled clinical trials of subcutaneous sumatriptan, there were 8 patients who sustained clinical events during or shortly after receiving sumatriptan that may have reflected coronary artery vasospasm. Six (6) of these 8 patients had ECG changes consistent with transient ischemia, but without accompanying clinical symptoms or signs. Of these 8 patients, 4 had either findings suggestive of CAD or risk factors predictive of CAD prior to study enrollment.

Of 6348 patients with migraine who participated in premarketing controlled and uncontrolled clinical trials of oral sumatriptan, 2 experienced clinical adverse events shortly after receiving oral sumatriptan that may have reflected coronary vasospasm. Neither of these adverse events was associated with a serious clinical outcome.

Among approximately 4000 patients with migraine who participated in premarketing controlled and uncontrolled clinical trials of sumatriptan nasal spray, 1 patient experienced an asymptomatic subendocardial infarction possibly subsequent to a coronary vasospastic event.

Postmarketing Experience With Sumatriptan

Serious cardiovascular events, some resulting in death, have been reported in association with the use of sumatriptan succinate injection or tablets. The uncontrolled nature of postmarketing surveillance, however, makes it impossible to determine definitively the proportion of the reported cases that were actually caused by sumatriptan or to reliably assess causation in individual cases. On clinical grounds, the longer the latency between the administration of sumatriptan succinate and the onset of the clinical event, the less likely the association is to be causative. Accordingly, interest has focused on events beginning within 1 hour of the administration of sumatriptan succinate.

Cardiac events that have been observed to have onset within 1 hour of sumatriptan administration include: coronary artery vasospasm, transient ischemia, myocardial infarction, ventricular tachycardia and ventricular fibrillation, cardiac arrest, and death.

Some of these events occurred in patients who had no findings of CAD and appear to represent consequences of coronary artery vasospasm. However, among domestic reports of serious cardiac events within 1 hour of sumatriptan administration, the majority had risk factors predictive of CAD and the presence of significant underlying CAD was established in most cases (see CONTRAINDICATIONS).

DRUG-ASSOCIATED CEREBROVASCULAR EVENTS AND FATALITIES

Cerebral hemorrhage, subarachnoid hemorrhage, stroke, and other cerebrovascular events have been reported in patients treated with oral or subcutaneous sumatriptan, and some have resulted in fatalities. The relationship of sumatriptan to these events is uncertain. In a number of cases, it appears possible that the cerebrovascular events were primary, sumatriptan having been administered in the incorrect belief that the symptoms experienced were a consequence of migraine when they were not. As with other acute migraine therapies, before treating headaches in patients not previously diagnosed as migraineurs, and in migraineurs who present with atypical symptoms, care should be taken to exclude other potentially serious neurological conditions. It should also be noted that patients with migraine may be at increased risk of certain cerebrovascular events (*e.g.,* cerebrovascular accident, transient ischemic attack).

OTHER VASOSPASM-RELATED EVENTS

Sumatriptan may cause vasospastic reactions other than coronary artery vasospasm. Both peripheral vascular ischemia and colonic ischemia with abdominal pain and bloody diarrhea have been reported.

INCREASE IN BLOOD PRESSURE

Significant elevation in blood pressure, including hypertensive crisis, has been reported on rare occasions in patients with and without a history of hypertension. Sumatriptan is contraindicated in patients with uncontrolled hypertension (see CONTRAINDICATIONS). Sumatriptan should be administered with caution to patients with controlled hypertension as transient increases in blood pressure and peripheral vascular resistance have been observed in a small proportion of patients.

CONCOMITANT DRUG USE

In patients taking MAO-A inhibitors, sumatriptan plasma levels attained after treatment with recommended doses are nearly double those obtained under other conditions. Accordingly, the coadministration of sumatriptan and an MAO-A inhibitor is not generally recommended. If such therapy is clinically warranted, however, suitable dose adjustment and appropriate observation of the patient is advised (see CLINICAL PHARMACOLOGY).

USE IN WOMEN OF CHILDBEARING POTENTIAL

See PRECAUTIONS.

HYPERSENSITIVITY

Hypersensitivity (anaphylaxis/anaphylactoid) reactions have occurred on rare occasions in patients receiving sumatriptan. Such reactions can be life threatening or fatal. In general, hypersensitivity reactions to drugs are more likely to occur in individuals with a history of sensitivity to multiple allergens (see CONTRAINDICATIONS).

PRECAUTIONS

GENERAL

Chest, jaw, or neck tightness is relatively common after administration of sumatriptan succinate injection. Chest discomfort and jaw or neck tightness has been reported following use of sumatriptan succinate tablets and has also been reported infrequently following the administration of sumatriptan nasal spray. Only rarely have these symptoms been associated with ischemic ECG changes. However, because sumatriptan may cause coronary artery vasospasm, patients who experience signs or symptoms suggestive of angina following sumatriptan should be evaluated for the presence of CAD or a predisposition to Prinzmetal variant angina before receiving additional doses of sumatriptan and should be monitored electrocardiographically if dosing is resumed and similar symptoms recur. Similarly, patients who experience other symptoms or signs suggestive of decreased arterial flow, such as ischemic bowel syndrome or Raynaud syndrome, following sumatriptan should be evaluated for atherosclerosis or predisposition to vasospasm (see WARNINGS).

Sumatriptan succinate should also be administered with caution to patients with diseases that may alter the absorption, metabolism, or excretion of drugs, such as impaired hepatic or renal function.

S

There have been rare reports of seizure following administration of sumatriptan. Sumatriptan should be used with caution in patients with a history of epilepsy or structural brain lesions that lower their seizure threshold.

Care should be taken to exclude other potentially serious neurologic conditions before treating headache in patients not previously diagnosed with migraine or cluster headache or who experience a headache that is atypical for them. There have been rare reports where patients received sumatriptan for severe headaches that were subsequently shown to have been secondary to an evolving neurologic lesion (see WARNINGS). For a given attack, if a patient does not respond to the first dose of sumatriptan, the diagnosis of migraine or cluster headache should be reconsidered before administration of a second dose.

BINDING TO MELANIN-CONTAINING TISSUES

Because sumatriptan binds to melanin, it could accumulate in melanin-rich tissues (such as the eye) over time. This raises the possibility that sumatriptan could cause toxicity in these tissues after extended use. However, no effects on the retina related to treatment with sumatriptan were noted in any of the toxicity studies. Although no systematic monitoring of ophthalmologic function was undertaken in clinical trials, and no specific recommendations for ophthalmologic function was undertaken in clinical trials, and no specific recommendations for ophthalmologic monitoring are offered, prescribers should be aware of the possibility of long-term ophthalmologic effects (see CLINICAL PHARMACOLOGY).

CORNEAL OPACITIES

Sumatriptan causes corneal opacities and defects in the corneal epithelium in dogs; this raises the possibility that these changes may occur in humans. While patients were not systematically evaluated for these changes in clinical trials, and no specific recommendations for monitoring are being offered, prescribers should be aware of the possibility of these changes (see CLINICAL PHARMACOLOGY).

Patients who are advised to self-administer sumatriptan succinate injection in medically unsupervised situations should receive instruction on the proper use of the product from the physician or other suitably qualified health care professional prior to doing so for the first time.

INFORMATION FOR THE PATIENT

With the autoinjector, the needle penetrates approximately ¼ of an inch (5-6 mm). Since the injection is intended to be given subcutaneously, intramuscular or intravascular delivery should be avoided. Patients should be directed to use injection sites with an adequate skin and subcutaneous thickness to accommodate the length of the needle. See the Patient Information that is distributed with the prescription for complete instructions.

LABORATORY TESTS

No specific laboratory tests are recommended for monitoring patients prior to and/or after treatment with sumatriptan.

DRUG/LABORATORY TEST INTERACTIONS

Sumatriptan succinate is not known to interfere with commonly employed clinical laboratory tests.

CARCINOGENESIS, MUTAGENESIS, AND IMPAIRMENT OF FERTILITY

In carcinogenicity studies, rats and mice were given sumatriptan by oral gavage (rats, 104 weeks), or drinking water (mice, 78 weeks). Average exposures achieved in mice receiving the highest dose were approximately 110 times the exposure attained in humans after the maximum recommended single dose of 6 mg. The highest dose to rats was approximately 260 times the maximum single dose of 6 mg on a mg/m^2 basis. There was no evidence of an increase in tumors in either species related to sumatriptan administration.

Sumatriptan was not mutagenic in the presence or absence of metabolic activation when tested in 2 gene mutation assays (the Ames test and the *in vitro* mammalian Chinese hamster V79/HGPRT assay). In 2 cytogenetics assays (the *in vitro* human lymphocyte assay and the *in vivo* rat micronucleus assay) sumatriptan was not associated with clastogenic activity.

A fertility study (Segment I) by the subcutaneous route, during which male and female rats were dosed daily with sumatriptan prior to and throughout the mating period, has shown no evidence of impaired fertility at doses equivalent to approximately 100 times the maximum recommended single human dose of 6 mg on a mg/m^2 basis. However, following oral administration, a treatment-related decrease in fertility, secondary to a decrease in mating, was seen for rats treated with 50 and 500 mg/kg/day. The no-effect dose for this finding was approximately 8 times the maximum recommended single human dose of 6 mg on a mg/m^2 basis. It is not clear whether the problem is associated with the treatment of males or females or both.

PREGNANCY CATEGORY C

Sumatriptan has been shown to be embryolethal in rabbits when given daily at a dose approximately equivalent to the maximum recommended single human subcutaneous dose of 6 mg on a mg/m^2 basis. There is no evidence that establishes that sumatriptan is a human teratogen; however, there are no adequate and well-controlled studies in pregnant women. Sumatriptan succinate injection should be used during pregnancy only if the potential benefit justifies the potential risk to the fetus.

In assessing this information, the following additional findings should be considered.

Embryolethality

When given intravenously to pregnant rabbits daily throughout the period of organogenesis, sumatriptan caused embryolethality at doses at or close to those producing maternal toxicity. The mechanism of the embryolethality is not known. These doses were approximately equivalent to the maximum single human dose of 6 mg on a mg/m^2 basis.

The IV administration of sumatriptan to pregnant rats throughout organogenesis at doses that are approximately 20 times a human dose of 6 mg on a mg/m^2 basis, did not cause embryolethality. Additionally, in a study of pregnant rats given subcutaneous sumatriptan daily prior to and throughout pregnancy, there was no evidence of increased embryo/fetal lethality.

Teratogenicity

Term fetuses from Dutch Stride rabbits treated during organogenesis with oral sumatriptan exhibited an increased incidence of cervicothoracic vascular and skeletal abnormalities. The functional significance of these abnormalities is not known. The highest no-effect dose for these effects was 15 mg/kg/day, approximately 50 times the maximum single dose of 6 mg on a mg/m^2 basis.

In a study in rats dosed daily with subcutaneous sumatriptan prior to and throughout pregnancy, there was no evidence of teratogenicity.

To monitor fetal outcomes of pregnant women exposed to sumatriptan succinate, GlaxoSmithKline maintains a Sumatriptan Pregnancy Registry. Physicians are encouraged to register patients by calling 800-336-2176.

NURSING MOTHERS

Sumatriptan is excreted in human breast milk. Therefore, caution should be exercised when considering the administration of sumatriptan succinate injection to a nursing woman.

PEDIATRIC USE

Safety and effectiveness of sumatriptan succinate injection in pediatric patients have not been established.

Completed placebo-controlled clinical trials evaluating oral sumatriptan (25-100 mg) in pediatric patients aged 12-17 years enrolled a total of 701 adolescent migraineurs. These studies did not establish the efficacy of oral sumatriptan compared to placebo in the treatment of migraine in adolescents. Adverse events observed in these clinical trials were similar in nature to those reported in clinical trials in adults. The frequency of all adverse events in these patients appeared to be both dose- and age-dependent, with younger patients reporting events more commonly than older adolescents. Postmarketing experience includes a limited number of reports that describe pediatric patients who have experienced adverse events, some clinically serious, after use of subcutaneous sumatriptan and/or oral sumatriptan. These reports include events similar in nature to those reported rarely in adults. A myocardial infarct has been reported in a 14-year-old male following the use of oral sumatriptan; clinical signs occurred within 1 day of drug administration. Since clinical data to determine the frequency of serious adverse events in pediatric patients who might receive injectable, oral, or intranasal sumatriptan are not presently available, the use of sumatriptan in patients aged younger than 18 years is not recommended.

GERIATRIC USE

The use of sumatriptan in elderly patients is not recommended because elderly patients are more likely to have decreased hepatic function, they are at higher risk for CAD, and blood pressure increases may be more pronounced in the elderly (see WARNINGS).

DRUG INTERACTIONS

There is no evidence that concomitant use of migraine prophylactic medications has any effect on the efficacy of sumatriptan. In two Phase 3 trials in the US, a retrospective analysis of 282 patients who had been using prophylactic drugs (verapamil n=63, amitriptyline n=57, propranolol n=94, for 45 other drugs n=123) were compared to those who had not used prophylaxis (n=452). There were no differences in relief rates at 60 minutes postdose for sumatriptan succinate injection, whether or not prophylactic medications were used.

Ergot-containing drugs have been reported to cause prolonged vasospastic reactions. Because there is a theoretical basis that these effects may be additive, use of ergotamine-containing or ergot-type medications (like dihydroergotamine or methysergide) and sumatriptan within 24 hours of each other should be avoided (see CONTRAINDICATIONS).

MAO-A inhibitors reduce sumatriptan clearance, significantly increasing systemic exposure. Therefore, the use of sumatriptan in patients receiving MAO-A inhibitors is not ordinarily recommended. If the clinical situation warrants the combined use of sumatriptan and an MAOI, the dose of sumatriptan employed should be reduced (see CLINICAL PHARMACOLOGY and WARNINGS).

Selective serotonin reuptake inhibitors (SSRIs) (*e.g.,* fluoxetine, fluvoxamine, paroxetine, sertraline) have been reported, rarely, to cause weakness, hyperreflexia, and incoordination when coadministered with sumatriptan. If concomitant treatment with sumatriptan and an SSRI is clinically warranted, appropriate observation of the patient is advised.

ADVERSE REACTIONS

Serious cardiac events, including some that have been fatal, have occurred following use of sumatriptan succinate injection or tablets. These events are extremely rare and most have been reported in patients with risk factors predictive of CAD. Events reported have included coronary artery vasospasm, transient myocardial ischemia, myocardial infarction, ventricular tachycardia, and ventricular fibrillation (see CONTRAINDICATIONS, WARNINGS, and PRECAUTIONS).

Significant hypertensive episodes, including hypertensive crises, have been reported on rare occasions in patients with or without a history of hypertension (see WARNINGS).

Among patients in clinical trials of subcutaneous sumatriptan succinate injection (n=6218), up to 3.5% of patients withdrew for reasons related to adverse events.

INCIDENCE IN CONTROLLED CLINICAL TRIALS OF MIGRAINE HEADACHE

TABLE 6 lists adverse events that occurred in 2 large US, Phase 3, placebo-controlled clinical trials in migraine patients following either a single dose of sumatriptan succinate injection or placebo. Only events that occurred at a frequency of 1% or more in groups treated with sumatriptan succinate injection and were at least as frequent as in the placebo group are included in TABLE 6.

The sum of the percentages cited is greater than 100% because patients may experience more than 1 type of adverse event. Only events that occurred at a frequency of 1% or more in groups treated with sumatriptan succinate injection and were at least as frequent as in the placebo groups are included.

The incidence of adverse events in controlled clinical trials was not affected by gender or age of the patients. There was insufficient data to assess the impact of race on the incidence of adverse events.

S

TABLE 6 *Treatment-Emergent Adverse Experience Incidence in 2 Large Placebo-Controlled Migrane Clinical Trials — Events Reported by at Least 1% of Sumatriptan Succinate Injection Patients*

Adverse Event Type	Sumatriptan Succinate Injection 6 mg sc n=547	Placebo n=370
Atypical Sensations	42.0%	9.2%
Tingling	13.5%	3.0%
Warm/hot sensation	10.8%	3.5%
Burning sensation	7.5%	0.3%
Feeling of heaviness	7.3%	1.1%
Pressure sensation	7.1%	1.6%
Feeling of tightness	5.1%	0.3%
Numbness	4.6%	2.2%
Feeling strange	2.2%	0.3%
Tight feeling in head	2.2%	0.3%
Cold sensation	1.1%	0.5%
Cardiovascular		
Flushing	6.6%	2.4%
Chest Discomfort	4.5%	1.4%
Tightness in chest	2.7%	0.5%
Pressure in chest	1.8%	0.3%
Ear, Nose, and Throat		
Throat discomfort	3.3%	0.5%
Discomfort: nasal cavity/sinuses	2.2%	0.3%
Eye		
Vision alterations	1.1%	0.0
Gastrointestinal		
Abdominal discomfort	1.3%	0.8%
Dysphagia	1.1%	0.0
Injection Site Reaction	58.7%	23.8%
Miscellaneous		
Jaw discomfort	1.8%	0.0
Mouth and Teeth		
Discomfort of mouth/tongue	4.9%	4.6%
Musculoskeletal		
Weakness	4.9%	0.3%
Neck pain/stiffness	4.8%	0.5%
Myalgia	1.8%	0.5%
Muscle cramp(s)	1.1%	0.0%
Neurological		
Dizziness/vertigo	11.9%	4.3%
Drowsiness/sedation	2.7%	2.2%
Headache	2.2%	0.3%
Anxiety	1.1%	0.5%
Malaise/fatigue	1.1%	0.8%
Skin		
Sweating	1.6%	1.1%

INCIDENCE IN CONTROLLED CLINICAL TRIALS OF CLUSTER HEADACHE

In the controlled clinical trials assessing sumatriptan's efficacy as a treatment for cluster headache, no new significant adverse events associated with the use of sumatriptan were detected that had not already been identified in association with the drug's use in migraine.

Overall, the frequency of adverse events reported in the studies of cluster headache were generally lower. Exceptions include reports of paresthesia (5% sumatriptan succinate, 0% placebo), nausea and vomiting (4% sumatriptan succinate, 0% placebo), and bronchospasm (1% sumatriptan succinate, 0% placebo).

OTHER EVENTS OBSERVED IN ASSOCIATION WITH THE ADMINISTRATION OF SUMATRIPTAN SUCCINATE INJECTION

In the paragraphs that follow, the frequencies of less commonly reported adverse clinical events are presented. Because the reports include events observed in open and uncontrolled studies, the role of sumatriptan succinate injection in their causation cannot be reliably determined. Furthermore, variability associated with adverse event reporting, the terminology used to describe adverse events, etc., limit the value of the quantitative frequency estimates provided.

Event frequencies are calculated as the number of patients reporting an event divided by the total number of patients (n=6218) exposed to subcutaneous sumatriptan succinate injection. All reported events are included except those already listed in TABLE 6, those too general to be informative, and those not reasonably associated with the use of the drug. Events are further classified within body system categories and enumerated in order of decreasing frequency using the following definitions: *frequent* adverse events are defined as those occurring in at least 1/100 patients; *infrequent* adverse events are those occurring in 1/100 to 1/1000 patients; and *rare* adverse events are those occurring in fewer than 1/1000 patients.

Cardiovascular: *Infrequent:* Hypertension, hypotension, bradycardia, tachycardia, palpitations, pulsating sensations, various transient ECG changes (nonspecific ST or T wave changes, prolongation of PR or QTc intervals, sinus arrhythmia, nonsustained ventricular premature beats, isolated junctional ectopic beats, atrial ectopic beats, delayed activation of the right ventricle), and syncope. *Rare:* Pallor, arrhythmia, abnormal pulse, vasodilation, and Raynaud syndrome.

Endocrine and Metabolic: *Infrequent:* Thirst. *Rare:* Polydipsia and dehydration.

Eye: *Infrequent:* Irritation of the eye.

Gastrointestinal: *Infrequent:* Gastroesophageal reflux, diarrhea, and disturbances of liver function tests. *Rare:* Peptic ulcer, retching, flatulence/eructation, and gallstones.

Musculoskeletal: *Infrequent:* Various joint disturbances (pain, stiffness, swelling, ache). *Rare:* Muscle stiffness, need to flex calf muscles, backache, muscle tiredness, and swelling of the extremities.

Neurological: *Infrequent:* Mental confusion, euphoria, agitation, relaxation, chills, sensation of lightness, tremor, shivering, disturbances of taste, prickling sensations, paresthesia, stinging sensations, facial pain, photophobia, and lacrimation. *Rare:* Transient hemiplegia, hysteria, globus hystericus, intoxication, depression, myoclonia, monoplegia/diplegia, sleep disturbance, difficulties in concentration, disturbances of smell, hyperesthesia, dysesthesia, simultaneous hot and cold sensations, tickling sensations, dysarthria, yawning, reduced appetite, hunger, and dystonia.

Respiratory: *Infrequent:* Dyspnea. *Rare:* Influenza, diseases of the lower respiratory tract, and hiccoughs.

Skin: *Infrequent:* Erythema, pruritus, and skin rashes and eruptions. *Rare:* Skin tenderness.

Urogenital: *Rare:* Dysuria, frequency, dysmenorrhea, and renal calculus.

Miscellaneous: *Infrequent:* Miscellaneous laboratory abnormalities, including minor disturbances in liver function tests, "serotonin," and hypersensitivity to various agents. *Rare:* Fever.

OTHER EVENTS OBSERVED IN THE CLINICAL DEVELOPMENT OF SUMATRIPTAN SUCCINATE

The following adverse events occurred in clinical trials with sumatriptan succinate tablets and nasal spray. Because the reports include events observed in open and uncontrolled studies, the role of sumatriptan succinate in their causation cannot be reliably determined. All reported events are included except those already listed, those too general to be informative, and those not reasonably associated with the use of the drug.

Breasts: Breast swelling, cysts, disorder of breasts, lumps, masses of breasts, nipple discharge, primary malignant breast neoplasm, and tenderness.

Cardiovascular: Abdominal aortic aneurysm, angina, atherosclerosis, cerebral ischemia, cerebrovascular lesion, heart block, peripheral cyanosis, phlebitis, thrombosis, and transient myocardial ischemia.

Ear, Nose, and Throat: Allergic rhinitis; disorder of nasal cavity/sinuses; ear, nose, and throat hemorrhage; ear infection; external otitis; feeling of fullness in the ear(s); hearing disturbances; hearing loss; Meniere disease; nasal inflammation; otalgia; sensitivity to noise; sinusitis; tinnitus; and upper respiratory inflammation.

Endocrine and Metabolic: Elevated thyrotropin stimulating hormone (TSH) levels; endocrine cysts, lumps, and masses; fluid disturbances; galactorrhea; hyperglycemia; hypoglycemia; hypothyroidism; weight gain; and weight loss.

Eye: Accommodation disorders, blindness and low vision, conjunctivitis, disorders of sclera, external ocular muscle disorders, eye edema and swelling, eye hemorrhage, eye itching, eye pain, keratitis, mydriasis, and visual disturbances.

Gastrointestinal: Abdominal distention, colitis, constipation, dental pain, dyspeptic symptoms, feelings of gastrointestinal pressure, gastric symptoms, gastritis, gastroenteritis, gastrointestinal bleeding, gastrointestinal pain, hematemesis, hypersalivation, hyposalivation, intestinal obstruction, melena, nausea and/or vomiting, oral itching and irritation, pancreatitis, salivary gland swelling, and swallowing disorders.

Hematological Disorders: Anemia.

Mouth and Teeth: Disorder of mouth and tongue (*e.g.*, burning of tongue, numbness of tongue, dry mouth).

Musculoskeletal: Acquired musculoskeletal deformity, arthralgia and articular rheumatitis, arthritis, intervertebral disc disorder, muscle atrophy, muscle tightness and rigidity, musculoskeletal inflammation, and tetany.

Neurological: Apathy, aggressiveness, bad/unusual taste, bradylogia, cluster headache, convulsions, depressive disorders, detachment, disturbance of emotions, drug abuse, facial paralysis, hallucinations, heat sensitivity, incoordination, increased alertness, memory disturbance, migraine, motor dysfunction, neoplasm of pituitary, neuralgia, neurotic disorders, paralysis, personality change, phobia, phonophobia, psychomotor disorders, radiculopathy, raised intracranial pressure, rigidity, stress, syncope, suicide, and twitching.

Respiratory: Asthma, breathing disorders, bronchitis, cough, and lower respiratory tract infection.

Skin: Dry/scaly skin, eczema, herpes, seborrheic dermatitis, skin nodules, tightness of skin, and wrinkling of skin.

Urogenital: Abnormal menstrual cycle, abortion, bladder inflammation, endometriosis, hematuria, increased urination, inflammation of fallopian tubes, intermenstrual bleeding, menstruation symptoms, micturition disorders, urethritis, and urinary infections.

Miscellaneous: Contusions, difficulty in walking, edema, hematoma, hypersensitivity, fever, fluid retention, lymphadenopathy, overdose, speech disturbance, swelling of extremities, swelling of face, and voice disturbances.

Pain and Other Pressure Sensations: Chest pain and/or heaviness, neck/throat/jaw pain/tightness/pressure, and pain (location specified).

POSTMARKETING EXPERIENCE (REPORTS FOR SUBCUTANEOUS OR ORAL SUMATRIPTAN)

The following section enumerates potentially important adverse events that have occurred in clinical practice and that have been reported spontaneously to various surveillance systems. The events enumerated represent reports arising from both domestic and nondomestic use of oral or subcutaneous dosage forms of sumatriptan. The events enumerated include all except those already listed in ADVERSE REACTIONS or those too general to be informative. Because the reports cite events reported spontaneously from worldwide postmarketing experience, frequency of events and the role of sumatriptan succinate injection in their causation cannot be reliably determined. It is assumed, however, that systemic reactions following sumatriptan use are likely to be similar regardless of route of administration.

Blood: Hemolytic anemia, pancytopenia, thrombocytopenia.

Cardiovascular: Atrial fibrillation, cardiomyopathy, colonic ischemia (see WARNINGS), Prinzmetal variant angina, pulmonary embolism, shock, thrombophlebitis.

Ear, Nose, and Throat: Deafness.

Eye: Ischemic optic neuropathy, retinal artery occlusion, retinal vein thrombosis, loss of vision.

Gastrointestinal: Ischemic colitis with rectal bleeding (see WARNINGS), xerostomia.

Hepatic: Elevated liver function tests.

S

Neurological: Central nervous system vasculitis, cerebrovascular accident, dysphasia, subarachnoid hemorrhage.
Non-Site Specific: Angioneurotic edema, cyanosis, death (see WARNINGS), temporal arteritis.
Psychiatry: Panic disorder.
Respiratory: Bronchospasm in patients with and without a history of asthma.
Skin: Exacerbation of sunburn, hypersensitivity reactions (allergic vasculitis, erythema, pruritus, rash, shortness of breath, urticaria; in addition, severe anaphylaxis/anaphylactoid reactions have been reported [see WARNINGS]), photosensitivity. Following subcutaneous administration of sumatriptan, pain, redness, stinging, induration, swelling, contusion, subcutaneous bleeding, and, on rare occasions, lipoatrophy (depression in the skin) or lipohypertrophy (enlargement or thickening of tissue) have been reported.
Urogenital: Acute renal failure.

DOSAGE AND ADMINISTRATION

The maximum single recommended adult dose of sumatriptan succinate injection is 6 mg injected subcutaneously. Controlled clinical trials have failed to show that clear benefit is associated with the administration of a second 6 mg dose in patients who have failed to respond to a first injection.

The maximum recommended dose that may be given in 24 hours is two 6 mg injections separated by at least 1 hour. Although the recommended dose is 6 mg, if side effects are dose limiting, then lower doses may be used (see CLINICAL PHARMACOLOGY). In patients receiving MAO inhibitors, decreased doses of sumatriptan should be considered (see WARNINGS and CLINICAL PHARMACOLOGY). In patients receiving doses lower than 6 mg, only the single-dose vial dosage form should be used. An autoinjection device is available for use with 6 mg prefilled syringe cartridges to facilitate self-administration in patients in whom this dose is deemed necessary. With this device, the needle penetrates approximately ¼ inch (5-6 mm). Since the injection is intended to be given subcutaneously, intramuscular or intravascular delivery should be avoided. Patients should be directed to use injection sites with an adequate skin and subcutaneous thickness to accomodate the length of the needle.

Parenteral drug products should be inspected visually for particulate matter and discoloration before administration whenever solution and container permit.

HOW SUPPLIED

Imitrex injection 6 mg (12 mg/ml) containing sumatriptan (base) as the succinate salt is supplied as a clear, colorless to pale yellow, sterile, nonpyrogenic solution.
Storage: Store between 2 and 30°C (36 and 86°F). Protect from light.

INTRANASAL

DESCRIPTION

Sumatriptan is a selective 5-hydroxytryptamine$_1$ receptor subtype agonist. Sumatriptan is chemically designated as 3-[2-(dimethylamino)ethyl]-N-methyl-1H-indole-5-methanesulfonamide.

The empirical formula is $C_{14}H_{21}N_3O_2S$, representing a molecular weight of 295.4. Sumatriptan is a white to off-white powder that is readily soluble in water and in saline. Each Imitrex nasal spray contains 5 or 20 mg of sumatriptan in a 100 µl unit dose aqueous buffered solution containing monobasic potassium phosphate, anhydrous dibasic sodium phosphate, sulfuric acid, sodium hydroxide, and purified water. The pH of the solution is approximately 5.5. The osmolality of the solution is 372 or 742 mOsmol for the 5 and 20 mg Imitrex nasal spray, respectively.

CLINICAL PHARMACOLOGY

MECHANISM OF ACTION

Sumatriptan is an agonist for a vascular 5-hydroxytryptamine$_1$ receptor subtype (probably a member of the 5-HT_{1D} family) having only a weak affinity for 5-HT_{1A}, 5-HT_{5A}, and 5-HT_7 receptors and no significant affinity (as measured using standard radioligand binding assays) or pharmacological activity at 5-HT_2, 5-HT_3, or 5-HT_4 receptor subtypes or at alpha$_1$-, alpha$_2$-, or beta-adrenergic; dopamine$_1$; dopamine$_2$; muscarinic; or benzodiazepine receptors.

The vascular 5-HT_1 receptor subtype that sumatriptan activates is present on cranial arteries in both dog and primate, on the human basilar artery, and in the vasculature of human dura mater and mediates vasoconstriction. This action in humans correlates with the relief of migraine headache. In addition to causing vasoconstriction, experimental data from animal studies show that sumatriptan also activates 5-HT_1 receptors on peripheral terminals of the trigeminal nerve innervating cranial blood vessels. Such an action may contribute to the antimigrainous effect of sumatriptan in humans.

In the anesthetized dog, sumatriptan selectively reduces the carotid arterial blood flow with little or no effect on arterial blood pressure or total peripheral resistance. In the cat, sumatriptan selectively constricts the carotid arteriovenous anastomoses while having little effect on blood flow or resistance in cerebral or extracerebral tissues.

PHARMACOKINETICS

In a study of 20 female volunteers, the mean maximum concentration following a 5 and 20 mg intranasal dose was 5 and 16 ng/ml, respectively. The mean C_{max} following a 6 mg subcutaneous injection is 71 ng/ml (range, 49-110 ng/ml). The mean C_{max} is 18 ng/ml (range, 7-47 ng/ml) following oral dosing with 25 mg and 51 ng/ml (range, 28-100 ng/ml) following oral dosing with 100 mg of sumatriptan. In a study of 24 male volunteers, the bioavailability relative to subcutaneous injection was low, approximately 17%, primarily due to presystemic metabolism and partly due to incomplete absorption.

Protein binding, determined by equilibrium dialysis over the concentration range of 10-1000 ng/ml, is low, approximately 14-21%. The effect of sumatriptan on the protein binding of other drugs has not been evaluated, but would be expected to be minor, given the low rate of protein binding. The mean volume of distribution after subcutaneous dosing is 2.7 L/kg and the total plasma clearance is approximately 1200 ml/min.

The elimination half-life of sumatriptan administered as a nasal spray is approximately 2 hours, similar to the half-life seen after subcutaneous injection. Only 3% of the dose is excreted in the urine as unchanged sumatriptan; 42% of the dose is excreted as the major metabolite, the indole acetic acid analogue of sumatriptan.

Clinical and pharmacokinetic data indicate that administration of two 5 mg doses, 1 dose in each nostril, is equivalent to administration of a single 10 mg dose in 1 nostril.

SPECIAL POPULATIONS

Renal Impairment

The effect of renal impairment on the pharmacokinetics of sumatriptan has not been examined, but little clinical effect would be expected as sumatriptan is largely metabolized to an inactive substance.

Hepatic Impairment

The effect of hepatic disease on the pharmacokinetics of subcutaneously and orally administered sumatriptan has been evaluated, but the intranasal dosage form has not been studied in hepatic impairment. There were no statistically significant differences in the pharmacokinetics of subcutaneously administered sumatriptan in hepatically impaired patients compared to healthy controls. However, the liver plays an important role in the presystemic clearance of orally administered sumatriptan. In 1 small study involving oral sumatriptan in hepatically impaired patients (n=8) matched for sex, age, and weight with healthy subjects, the hepatically impaired patients had an approximately 70% increase in AUC and C_{max} and a T_{max} 40 minutes earlier compared to the healthy subjects. The bioavailability of nasally absorbed sumatriptan following intranasal administration, which would not undergo first-pass metabolism, should not be altered in hepatically impaired patients. The bioavailability of the swallowed portion of the intranasal sumatriptan dose has not been determined, but would be increased in these patients. The swallowed intranasal dose is small, however, compared to the usual oral dose, so that its impact should be minimal.

Age

The pharmacokinetics of oral sumatriptan in the elderly (mean age, 72 years; 2 males and 4 females) and in patients with migraine (mean age, 38 years; 25 males and 155 females) were similar to that in healthy male subjects (mean age, 30 years). Intranasal sumatriptan has not been evaluated for age differences (see PRECAUTIONS, Geriatric Use).

Race

The systemic clearance and C_{max} of sumatriptan were similar in black (n=34) and Caucasian (n=38) healthy male subjects. Intranasal sumatriptan has not been evaluated for race differences.

DRUG INTERACTIONS

Monoamine Oxidase Inhibitors (MAOIs)

Treatment with MAOIs generally leads to an increase of sumatriptan plasma levels (see CONTRAINDICATIONS and PRECAUTIONS).

MAOI interaction studies have not been performed with intranasal sumatriptan. Due to gut and hepatic metabolic first-pass effects, the increase of systemic exposure after coadministration of an MAO-A inhibitor with oral sumatriptan is greater than after coadministration of the MAOI with subcutaneous sumatriptan. The effects of an MAOI on systemic exposure after intranasal sumatriptan would be expected to be greater than the effect after subcutaneous sumatriptan but smaller than the effect after oral sumatriptan because only swallowed drug would be subject to first-pass effects.

In a study of 14 healthy females, pretreatment with an MAO-A inhibitor decreased the clearance of subcutaneous sumatriptan. Under the conditions of this experiment, the result was a 2-fold increase in the area under the sumatriptan plasma concentration × time curve (AUC), corresponding to a 40% increase in elimination half-life. This interaction was not evident with an MAO-B inhibitor.

A small study evaluating the effect of pretreatment with an MAO-A inhibitor on the bioavailability from a 25 mg oral sumatriptan tablet resulted in an approximately 7-fold increase in systemic exposure.

Xylometazoline

An *in vivo* drug interaction study indicated that 3 drops of xylometazoline (0.1% w/v), a decongestant, administered 15 minutes prior to a 20 mg nasal dose of sumatriptan did not alter the pharmacokinetics of sumatriptan.

INDICATIONS AND USAGE

Sumatriptan nasal spray is indicated for the acute treatment of migraine attacks with or without aura in adults.

Sumatriptan nasal spray is not intended for the prophylactic therapy of migraine or for use in the management of hemiplegic or basilar migraine (see CONTRAINDICATIONS). Safety and effectiveness of sumatriptan nasal spray have not been established for cluster headache, which is present in an older, predominantly male population.

CONTRAINDICATIONS

Sumatriptan nasal spray should not be given to patients with history, symptoms, or signs of ischemic cardiac, cerebrovascular, or peripheral vascular syndromes. In addition, patients with other significant underlying cardiovascular diseases should not receive sumatriptan nasal spray. Ischemic cardiac syndromes include, but are not limited to, angina pectoris of any type (*e.g.*, stable angina of effort and vasospastic forms of angina such as the Prinzmetal variant), all forms of myocardial ischemia. Cerebrovascular syndromes include, but are not limited to, strokes of any type as well as transient ischemic attacks. Peripheral vascular disease includes, but it not limited to, ischemic bowel disease (see WARNINGS).

Because sumatriptan nasal spray may increase blood pressure, it should not be given to patients with uncontrolled hypertension.

Concurrent administration of MAO-A inhibitors or use within 2 weeks of discontinuation of MAO-A inhibitor therapy is contraindicated (see CLINICAL PHARMACOLOGY, Drug Interactions and DRUG INTERACTIONS).

S

Sumatriptan nasal spray and any ergotamine-containing or ergot-type medication (like dihydroergotamine or methysergide) should not be used within 24 hours of each other, nor should sumatriptan nasal spray and another 5-HT_1 agonist.

Sumatriptan nasal spray should not be administered to patients with hemiplegic or basilar migraine.

Sumatriptan nasal spray is contraindicated in patients with hypersensitivity to sumatriptan or any of its components.

Sumatriptan nasal spray is contraindicated in patients with severe hepatic impairment.

WARNINGS

Sumatriptan nasal spray should only be used where a clear diagnosis of migraine headache has been established.

RISK OF MYOCARDIAL ISCHEMIA AND/OR INFARCTION AND OTHER ADVERSE CARDIAC EVENTS

Sumatriptan should not be given to patients with documented ischemic or vasospastic coronary artery disease (CAD) (see CONTRAINDICATIONS). It is strongly recommended that sumatriptan not be given to patients in whom unrecognized CAD is predicted by the presence of risk factors (*e.g.,* hypertension, hypercholesterolemia, smoker, obesity, diabetes, strong family history of CAD, female with surgical or physiological menopause, or male over 40 years of age) unless a cardiovascular evaluation provides satisfactory clinical evidence that the patient is reasonably free of coronary artery and ischemic myocardial disease or other significant underlying cardiovascular disease. The sensitivity of cardiac diagnostic procedures to detect cardiovascular disease or predisposition to coronary artery vasospasm is modest, at best. If, during the cardiovascular evaluation, the patient's medical history or electrocardiographic investigations reveal findings indicative of, or consistent with, coronary artery vasospasm or myocardial ischemia, sumatriptan should not be administered (see CONTRAINDICATIONS).

For patients with risk factors predictive of CAD, who are determined to have a satisfactory cardiovascular evaluation, it is strongly recommended that administration of the first dose of sumatriptan nasal spray take place in the setting of a physician's office or similar medically staffed and equipped facility unless the patient has previously received sumatriptan. Because cardiac ischemia can occur in the absence of clinical symptoms, consideration should be given to obtaining on the first occasion of use an ECG during the interval immediately following sumatriptan nasal spray, in these patients with risk factors.

It is recommended that patients who are intermittent long-term users of sumatriptan and who have or acquire risk factors predictive of CAD, as described above, undergo periodic interval cardiovascular evaluation as they continue to use sumatriptan.

The systematic approach described above is intended to reduce the likelihood that patients with unrecognized cardiovascular disease will be inadvertently exposed to sumatriptan.

DRUG-ASSOCIATED CARDIAC EVENTS AND FATALITIES

Serious adverse cardiac events, including acute myocardial infarction, life-threatening disturbances of cardiac rhythm, and death have been reported within a few hours following the administration of sumatriptan succinate injection or tablets. Considering the extent of use of sumatriptan in patients with migraine, the incidence of these events is extremely low.

The fact that sumatriptan can cause coronary vasospasm, that some of these events have occurred in patients with no prior cardiac disease history and with documented absence of CAD, and the close proximity of the events to sumatriptan use support the conclusion that some of these cases were caused by the drug. In many cases, however, where there has been known underlying coronary artery disease, the relationship is uncertain.

Premarketing Experience With Sumatriptan

Among approximately 4000 patients with migraine who participated in premarketing controlled and uncontrolled clinical trials of sumatriptan nasal spray, 1 patient experienced an asymptomatic subendocardial infarction possibly subsequent to a coronary vasospastic event.

Of 6348 patients with migraine who participated in premarketing controlled and uncontrolled clinical trials of oral sumatriptan, 2 experienced clinical adverse events shortly after receiving oral sumatriptan that may have reflected coronary vasospasm. Neither of these adverse events was associated with a serious clinical outcome.

Among the more than 1900 patients with migraine who participated in premarketing controlled clinical trials of subcutaneous sumatriptan, there were 8 patients who sustained clinical events during or shortly after receiving sumatriptan that may have reflected coronary artery vasospasm. Six (6) of these 8 patients had ECG changes consistent with transient ischemia, but without accompanying clinical symptoms or signs. Of these 8 patients, 4 had either findings suggestive of CAD or risk factors predictive of CAD prior to study enrollment.

Postmarketing Experience With Sumatriptan

Serious cardiovascular events, some resulting in death, have been reported in association with the use of sumatriptan succinate injection or tablets. The uncontrolled nature of postmarketing surveillance, however, makes it impossible to determine definitively the proportion of the reported cases that were actually caused by sumatriptan or to reliably assess causation in individual cases. On clinical grounds, the longer the latency between the administration of sumatriptan and the onset of the clinical event, the less likely the association is to be causative. Accordingly, interest has focused on events beginning within 1 hour of the administration of sumatriptan.

Cardiac events that have been observed to have onset within 1 hour of sumatriptan administration include: coronary artery vasospasm, transient ischemia, myocardial infarction, ventricular tachycardia and ventricular fibrillation, cardiac arrest, and death.

Some of these events occurred in patients who had no findings of CAD and appear to represent consequences of coronary artery vasospasm. However, among domestic reports of serious cardiac events within 1 hour of sumatriptan administration, almost all of the patients had risk factors predictive of CAD and the presence of significant underlying CAD was established in most cases (see CONTRAINDICATIONS).

DRUG-ASSOCIATED CEREBROVASCULAR EVENTS AND FATALITIES

Cerebral hemorrhage, subarachnoid hemorrhage, stroke, and other cerebrovascular events have been reported in patients treated with oral or subcutaneous sumatriptan, and some have resulted in fatalities. The relationship of sumatriptan to these events is uncertain. In a number of cases, it appears possible that the cerebrovascular events were primary, sumatriptan having been administered in the incorrect belief that the symptoms experienced were a consequence of migraine when they were not. As with other acute migraine therapies, before treating headaches in patients not previously diagnosed as migraineurs, and in migraineurs who present with atypical symptoms, care should be taken to exclude other potentially serious neurological conditions. It should also be noted that patients with migraine may be at increased risk of certain cerebrovascular events (*e.g.,* cerebrovascular accident, transient ischemic attack).

OTHER VASOSPASM-RELATED EVENTS

Sumatriptan may cause vasospastic reactions other than coronary artery vasospasm. Both peripheral vascular ischemia and colonic ischemia with abdominal pain and bloody diarrhea have been reported.

INCREASE IN BLOOD PRESSURE

Significant elevation in blood pressure, including hypertensive crisis, has been reported on rare occasions in patients with and without a history of hypertension. Sumatriptan is contraindicated in patients with uncontrolled hypertension (see CONTRAINDICATIONS). Sumatriptan should be administered with caution to patients with controlled hypertension as transient increases in blood pressure and peripheral vascular resistance have been observed in a small proportion of patients.

LOCAL IRRITATION

Of the 3378 patients using the nasal spray (5, 10, or 20 mg doses) on 1 or 2 occasions in controlled clinical studies, approximately 5% noted irritation in the nose and throat. Irritative symptoms such as burning, numbness, paresthesia, discharge, and pain or soreness were noted to be severe in about 1% of patients treated. The symptoms were transient and in approximately 60% of the cases, the symptoms resolved in less than 2 hours. Limited examinations of the nose and throat did not reveal any clinically noticeable injury in these patients. The consequences of extended and repeated use of sumatriptan nasal spray on the nasal and/or respiratory mucosa have not been systematically evaluated in patients.

No increase in the incidence of local irritation was observed in patients using sumatriptan nasal spray repeatedly for up to 1 year.

In inhalation studies in rats dosed daily for up to 1 month at exposures as low as one-half the maximum daily human exposure (based on dose per surface area of nasal cavity), epithelial hyperplasia (with and without keratinization) and squamous metaplasia were observed in the larynx at all doses tested. These changes were partially reversible after a 2 week drug-free period. When dogs were dosed daily with various formulations by intranasal instillation for up to 13 weeks at exposures of 2-4 times the maximum daily human exposure (based on dose per surface area of nasal cavity), respiratory and nasal mucosa exhibited evidence of epithelial hyperplasia, focal squamous metaplasia, granulomata, bronchitis, and fibrosing alveolitis. A no-effect dose was not established. The changes observed in both species are not considered to be signs of either preneoplastic or neoplastic transformation.

Local effects on nasal and respiratory tissues after chronic intranasal dosing in animals have not been studied.

CONCOMITANT DRUG USE

In patients taking MAO-A inhibitors, sumatriptan plasma levels attained after treatment with recommended doses are 2-fold (following subcutaneous administration) to 7-fold (following oral administration) higher than those obtained under other conditions. Accordingly, the coadministration of sumatriptan nasal spray and an MAO-A inhibitor is contraindicated (see CLINICAL PHARMACOLOGY and CONTRAINDICATIONS).

HYPERSENSITIVITY

Hypersensitivity (anaphylaxis/anaphylactoid) reactions have occurred on rare occasions in patients receiving sumatriptan. Such reactions can be life threatening or fatal. In general, hypersensitivity reactions to drugs are more likely to occur in individuals with a history of sensitivity to multiple allergens (see CONTRAINDICATIONS).

PRECAUTIONS

GENERAL

Chest discomfort and jaw or neck tightness have been reported infrequently following the administration of sumatriptan nasal spray and have also been reported following use of sumatriptan tablets. Chest, jaw, or neck tightness is relatively common after administration of sumatriptan succinate injection. Only rarely have these symptoms been associated with ischemic ECG changes. However, because sumatriptan may cause coronary artery vasospasm, patients who experience signs or symptoms suggestive of angina following sumatriptan should be evaluated for the presence of CAD or a predisposition to Prinzmetal variant angina before receiving additional doses of sumatriptan, and should be monitored electrocardiographically if dosing is resumed and similar symptoms recur. Similarly, patients who experience other symptoms or signs suggestive of decreased arterial flow, such as ischemic bowel syndrome or Raynaud syndrome following sumatriptan should be evaluated for atherosclerosis or predisposition to vasospasm (see WARNINGS).

Sumatriptan nasal spray should also be administered with caution to patients with diseases that may alter the absorption, metabolism, or excretion of drugs, such as impaired hepatic or renal function.

There have been rare reports of seizure following administration of sumatriptan. Sumatriptan should be used with caution in patients with a history of epilepsy or structural brain lesions that lower their seizure threshold.

Care should be taken to exclude other potentially serious neurologic conditions before treating headache in patients not previously diagnosed with migraine headache or who experience a headache that is atypical for them. There have been rare reports where patients received sumatriptan for severe headaches that were subsequently shown to have been secondary to an evolving neurologic lesion (see WARNINGS).

For a given attack, if a patient does not respond to the first dose of sumatriptan, the diagnosis of migraine headache should be reconsidered before administration of a second dose.

BINDING TO MELANIN-CONTAINING TISSUES

In rats treated with a single subcutaneous dose (0.5 mg/kg) or oral dose (2 mg/kg) of radiolabeled sumatriptan, the elimination half-life of radioactivity from the eye was 15 and 23 days, respectively, suggesting that sumatriptan and/or its metabolites bind to the melanin of the eye. Comparable studies were not performed by the intranasal route. Because there could be an accumulation in melanin-rich tissues over time, this raises the possibility that sumatriptan could cause toxicity in these tissues after extended use. However, no effects on the retina related to treatment with sumatriptan were noted in any of the oral or subcutaneous toxicity studies. Although no systematic monitoring of ophthalmologic function was undertaken in clinical trials, and no specific recommendations for ophthalmologic monitoring are offered, prescribers should be aware of the possibility of long-term ophthalmologic effects.

CORNEAL OPACITIES

Sumatriptan causes corneal opacities and defects in the corneal epithelium in dogs; this raises the possibility that these changes may occur in humans. While patients were not systematically evaluated for these changes in clinical trials, and no specific recommendations for monitoring are being offered, prescribers should be aware of the possibility of these changes (see ANIMAL PHARMACOLOGY).

INFORMATION FOR THE PATIENT

See the Patient Information that is distributed with the prescription for additional information for patients.

LABORATORY TESTS

No specific laboratory tests are recommended for monitoring patients prior to and/or after treatment with sumatriptan.

DRUG/LABORATORY TEST INTERACTIONS

Sumatriptan nasal spray is not known to interfere with commonly employed clinical laboratory tests.

CARCINOGENESIS, MUTAGENESIS, AND IMPAIRMENT OF FERTILITY

Carcinogenesis

In carcinogenicity studies, rats and mice were given sumatriptan by oral gavage (rats, 104 weeks), or drinking water (mice, 78 weeks). Average exposures achieved in mice receiving the highest dose (target dose of 160 mg/kg/day) were approximately 184 times the exposure attained in humans after the maximum recommended single intranasal dose of 20 mg. The highest dose administered to rats (160 mg/kg/day, reduced from 360 mg/kg/day during week 21) was approximately 78 times the maximum recommended single intranasal dose of 20 mg on a mg/m^2 basis. There was no evidence of an increase in tumors in either species related to sumatriptan administration. Local effects on nasal and respiratory tissue after chronic intranasal dosing in animals have not been evaluated (see WARNINGS).

Mutagenesis

Sumatriptan was not mutagenic in the presence or absence of metabolic activation when tested in 2 gene mutation assays (the Ames test and the *in vitro* mammalian Chinese hamster V79/HGPRT assay). In 2 cytogenetics assays (the *in vitro* human lymphocyte assay and the *in vivo* rat micronucleus assay) sumatriptan was not associated with clastogenic activity.

Impairment of Fertility

In a study in which male and female rats were dosed daily with oral sumatriptan prior to and throughout the mating period, there was a treatment-related decrease in fertility secondary to a decrease in mating in animals treated with 50 and 500 mg/kg/day. The highest no-effect dose for this finding was 5 mg/kg/day, or approximately twice the maximum recommended single human intranasal dose of 20 mg on a mg/m^2 basis. It is not clear whether the problem is associated with treatment of the males or females or both combined. In a similar study by the subcutaneous route there was no evidence of impaired fertility at 60 mg/kg/day, the maximum dose tested, which is equivalent to approximately 29 times the maximum recommended single human intranasal dose of 20 mg on a mg/m^2 basis. Fertility studies, in which sumatriptan was administered by the intranasal route, were not conducted.

PREGNANCY CATEGORY C

In reproductive toxicity studies in rats and rabbits, oral treatment with sumatriptan was associated with embryolethality, fetal abnormalities, and pup mortality. When administered by the IV route to rabbits, sumatriptan has been shown to be embryolethal. Reproductive toxicity studies for sumatriptan by the intranasal route have not been conducted.

There are no adequate and well-controlled studies in pregnant women. Therefore, sumatriptan nasal spray should be used during pregnancy only if the potential benefit justifies the potential risk to the fetus. In assessing this information, the following findings should be considered.

Embryolethality

When given orally or intravenously to pregnant rabbits daily throughout the period of organogenesis, sumatriptan caused embryolethality at doses at or close to those producing maternal toxicity. In the oral studies this dose was 100 mg/kg/day, and in the intravenous studies this dose was 2.0 mg/kg/day. The mechanism of the embryolethality is not known. The highest no-effect dose for embryolethality by the oral route was 50 mg/kg/day, which is approximately 48 times the maximum single recommended human intranasal dose of 20 mg on a mg/m^2 basis. By the IV route, the highest no-effect dose was 0.75 mg/kg/day, or approximately 0.7 times the maximum single recommended human intranasal dose of 20 mg on a mg/m^2 basis.

The IV administration of sumatriptan to pregnant rats throughout organogenesis at 12.5 mg/kg/day, the maximum dose tested, did not cause embryolethality. This dose is approximately 6 times the maximum single recommended human intranasal dose of 20 mg on a mg/m^2 basis. Additionally, in a study in rats given subcutaneous sumatriptan daily, prior to and throughout pregnancy, at 60 mg/kg/day, the maximum dose tested, there was no evidence of increased embryo/fetal lethality. This dose is equivalent to approximately 29 times the maximum recommended single human intranasal dose of 20 mg on a mg/m^2 basis.

Teratogenicity

Oral treatment of pregnant rats with sumatriptan during the period of organogenesis resulted in an increased incidence of blood vessel abnormalities (cervicothoracic and umbilical) at doses of approximately 250 mg/kg/day or higher. The highest no-effect dose was approximately 60 mg/kg/day, which is approximately 29 times the maximum single recommended human intranasal dose of 20 mg on a mg/m^2 basis. Oral treatment of pregnant rabbits with sumatriptan during the period of organogenesis resulted in an increased incidence of cervicothoracic vascular and skeletal abnormalities. The highest no-effect dose for these effects was 15 mg/kg/day, or approximately 14 times the maximum single recommended human intranasal dose of 20 mg on a mg/m^2 basis.

A study in which rats were dosed daily with oral sumatriptan prior to and throughout gestation demonstrated embryo/fetal toxicity (decreased body weight, decreased ossification, increased incidence of rib variations) and an increased incidence of a syndrome of malformations (short tail/short body and vertebral disorganization) at 500 mg/kg/day. The highest no-effect dose was 50 mg/kg/day, or approximately 24 times the maximum single recommended human intranasal dose of 20 mg on a mg/m^2 basis. In a study in rats dosed daily with subcutaneous sumatriptan prior to and throughout pregnancy, at a dose of 60 mg/kg/day, the maximum dose tested, there was no evidence of teratogenicity. This dose is equivalent to approximately 29 times the maximum recommended single human intranasal dose of 20 mg on a mg/m^2 basis.

Pup Deaths

Oral treatment of pregnant rats with sumatriptan during the period of organogenesis resulted in a decrease in pup survival between birth and postnatal day 4 at doses of approximately 250 mg/kg/day or higher. The highest no-effect dose for this effect was approximately 60 mg/kg/day, or 29 times the maximum single recommended human intranasal dose of 20 mg on a mg/m^2 basis.

Oral treatment of pregnant rats with sumatriptan from gestational day 17 through postnatal day 21 demonstrated a decrease in pup survival measured at postnatal days 2, 4, and 20 at the dose of 1000 mg/kg/day. The highest no-effect dose for this finding was 100 mg/kg/day, approximately 49 times the maximum single recommended human intranasal dose of 20 mg on a mg/m^2 basis. In a similar study in rats by the subcutaneous route there was no increase in pup death at 81 mg/kg/day, the highest dose tested, which is equivalent to 40 times the maximum single recommended human intranasal dose of 20 mg on a mg/m^2 basis.

To monitor fetal outcomes of pregnant women exposed to sumatriptan, GlaxoSmithKline maintains a Sumatriptan Pregnancy Registry. Physicians are encouraged to register patients by calling 800-336-2176.

NURSING MOTHERS

Sumatriptan is excreted in human breast milk. Therefore, caution should be exercised when considering the administration of sumatriptan nasal spray to a nursing woman.

PEDIATRIC USE

Safety and effectiveness of sumatriptan nasal spray in pediatric patients have not been established.

Completed placebo-controlled clinical trials evaluating oral sumatriptan (25-100 mg) in pediatric patients aged 12-17 years enrolled a total of 701 adolescent migraineurs. These studies did not establish the efficacy of oral sumatriptan compared to placebo in the treatment of migraine in adolescents. Adverse events observed in these clinical trials were similar in nature to those reported in clinical trials in adults. The frequency of all adverse events in these patients appeared to be both dose- and age-dependent, with younger patients reporting events more commonly than older adolescents. Postmarketing experience includes a limited number of reports that describe pediatric patients who have experienced adverse events, some clinically serious, after use of subcutaneous sumatriptan and/or oral sumatriptan. These reports include events similar in nature to those reported rarely in adults. A myocardial infarct has been reported in a 14-year-old male following the use of oral sumatriptan; clinical signs occurred within 1 day of drug administration. Since clinical data to determine the frequency of serious adverse events in pediatric patients who might receive injectable, oral, or intranasal sumatriptan are not presently available, the use of sumatriptan in patients aged younger than 18 years is not recommended.

GERIATRIC USE

The use of sumatriptan in elderly patients is not recommended because elderly patients are more likely to have decreased hepatic function, they are at higher risk for CAD, and blood pressure increases may be more pronounced in the elderly (see WARNINGS).

DRUG INTERACTIONS

Ergot-containing drugs have been reported to cause prolonged vasospastic reactions. Because there is a theoretical basis that these effects may be additive, use of ergotamine-containing or ergot-type medications (like dihydroergotamine or methysergide) and sumatriptan within 24 hours of each other should be avoided (see CONTRAINDICATIONS).

MAO-A inhibitors reduce sumatriptan clearance, significantly increasing systemic exposure. Therefore, the use of sumatriptan nasal spray in patients receiving MAO-A inhibitors is contraindicated (see CLINICAL PHARMACOLOGY and CONTRAINDICATIONS).

Selective serotonin reuptake inhibitors (SSRIs) (*e.g.,* fluoxetine, fluvoxamine, paroxetine, sertraline) have been reported, rarely, to cause weakness, hyperreflexia, and incoordination when coadministered with sumatriptan. If concomitant treatment with sumatriptan and an SSRI is clinically warranted, appropriate observation of the patient is advised.

ADVERSE REACTIONS

Serious cardiac events, including some that have been fatal, have occurred following the use of sumatriptan succinate injection or tablets. These events are extremely rare and most have been reported in patients with risk factors predictive of CAD. Events reported have included coronary artery vasospasm, transient myocardial ischemia, myocardial infarction, ventricular tachycardia, and ventricular fibrillation (see CONTRAINDICATIONS, WARNINGS, and PRECAUTIONS).

Significant hypertensive episodes, including hypertensive crises, have been reported on rare occasions in patients with or without a history of hypertension (see WARNINGS).

INCIDENCE IN CONTROLLED CLINICAL TRIALS

Among 3653 patients treated with sumatriptan nasal spray in active- and placebo-controlled clinical trials, less than 0.4% of patients withdrew for reasons related to adverse events. TABLE 8 lists adverse events that occurred in worldwide placebo-controlled trials in 3419 migraineurs. The events cited reflect experience gained under closely monitored conditions of clinical trials in a highly selected patient population. In actual clinical practice or in other clinical trials, these frequency estimates may not apply, as the conditions of use, reporting behavior, and the kinds of patients treated may differ.

Only events that occurred at a frequency of 1% or more in the sumatriptan nasal spray 20 mg treatment group and were more frequent in that group than in the placebo group are included in TABLE 8 .

TABLE 8 *Treatment-Emergent Adverse Events Reported by at Least 1% of Patients in Controlled Migraine Trials*

Adverse Event	Placebo (n=704)	Sumatriptan 5 mg (n=496)	Sumatriptan 10 mg (n=1007)	Sumatriptan 20 mg (n=1212)
Atypical Sensations				
Burning sensation	0.1%	0.4%	0.6%	1.4%
Ear, Nose, and Throat				
Disorder/discomfort of nasal cavity/sinuses	2.4%	2.8%	2.5%	3.8%
Throat discomfort	0.9%	0.8%	1.8%	2.4%
Gastrointestinal				
Nausea and/or vomiting	11.3%	12.2%	11.0%	13.5%
Neurological				
Bad/unusual taste	1.7%	13.5%	19.3%	24.5%
Dizziness/vertigo	0.9%	1.0%	1.7%	1.4%

Phonophobia also occurred in more than 1% of patients but was more frequent on placebo.

Sumatriptan nasal spray is generally well tolerated. Across all doses, most adverse reactions were mild and transient and did not lead to long-lasting effects. The incidence of adverse events in controlled clinical trials was not affected by gender, weight, or age of the patients; use of prophylactic medications; or presence of aura. There were insufficient data to assess the impact of race on the incidence of adverse events.

OTHER EVENTS OBSERVED IN ASSOCIATION WITH THE ADMINISTRATION OF SUMATRIPTAN NASAL SPRAY

In the paragraphs that follow, the frequencies of less commonly reported adverse clinical events are presented. Because the reports include events observed in open and uncontrolled studies, the role of sumatriptan nasal spray in their causation cannot be reliably determined. Furthermore, variability associated with adverse event reporting, the terminology used to describe the adverse events, etc., limit the value of the quantitative frequency estimates provided. Event frequencies are calculated as the number of patients who used sumatriptan nasal spray (5, 10, or 20 mg in controlled and uncontrolled trials) and reported an event divided by the total number of patients (n=3711) exposed to sumatriptan nasal spray. All reported events are included except those already listed in TABLE 8, those too general to be informative, and those not reasonably associated with the use of the drug. Events are further classified within body system categories and enumerated in order of decreasing frequency using the following definitions: *infrequent* adverse events are those occurring in 1/100 to 1/1000 patients; and *rare* adverse events are those occurring in fewer than 1/1000 patients.

Atypical Sensations: *Infrequent:* Tingling, warm/hot sensation, numbness, pressure sensation, feeling strange, feeling of heaviness, feeling of tightness, paresthesia, cold sensation, and tight feeling in head. *Rare:* Dysesthesia and prickling sensation.

Cardiovascular: *Infrequent:* Flushing and hypertension (see WARNINGS), palpitations, tachycardia, changes in ECG, and arrhythmia (see WARNINGS and PRECAUTIONS). *Rare:* Abdominal aortic aneurysm, hypotension, bradycardia, pallor, and phlebitis.

Chest Symptoms: *Infrequent:* Chest tightness, chest discomfort, and chest pressure/heaviness (see PRECAUTIONS, General).

Ear, Nose, and Throat: *Infrequent:* Disturbance of hearing and ear infection. *Rare:* Otalgia and Meniere disease.

Endocrine and Metabolic: *Infrequent:* Thirst. *Rare:* Galactorrhea, hypothyroidism, and weight loss.

Eye: *Infrequent:* Irritation of eyes and visual disturbance.

Gastrointestinal: *Infrequent:* Abdominal discomfort, diarrhea, dysphagia, and gastroesophogeal reflux. *Rare:* Constipation, flatulence/eructation, hematemesis, intestinal obstruction, melena, gastroenteritis, colitis, hemorrhage of gastrointestinal tract, and pancreatitis.

Mouth and Teeth: *Infrequent:* Disorder of mouth and tongue (*e.g.*, burning of tongue, numbness of tongue, dry mouth).

Musculoskeletal: *Infrequent:* Neck pain/stiffness, backache, weakness, joint symptoms, arthritis, and myalgia. *Rare:* Muscle cramps, tetany, intervertebral disc disorder, and muscle stiffness.

Neurological: *Infrequent:* Drowsiness/sedation, anxiety, sleep disturbances, tremors, syncope, shivers, chills, depression, agitation, sensation of lightness, and mental confusion. *Rare:* Difficulty concentrating, hunger, lacrimation, memory disturbances, monoplegia/diplegia, apathy, disturbance of smell, disturbance of emotions, dysarthria, facial pain, intoxication, stress, decreased appetite, difficulty coordinating, euphoria, and neoplasm of pituitary.

Respiratory: *Infrequent:* Dyspnea and lower respiratory tract infection; *Rare:* Asthma.

Skin: *Infrequent:* Rash/skin eruption, pruritus, and erythema. *Rare:* Herpes, swelling of face, sweating, and peeling of skin.

Urogenital: *Infrequent:* Dysuria, disorder of breasts, and dysmenorrhea. *Rare:* Endometriosis and increased urination.

Miscellaneous: *Infrequent:* Cough, edema, and fever. *Rare:* Hypersensitivity, swelling of extremities, voice disturbances, difficulty in walking, and lymphadenopathy.

OTHER EVENTS OBSERVED IN THE CLINICAL DEVELOPMENT OF SUMATRIPTAN

The following adverse events occurred in clinical trials with sumatriptan succinate injection and tablets. Because the reports include events observed in open and uncontrolled studies, the role of sumatriptan in their causation cannot be reliably determined. All reported events are included except those already listed, those too general to be informative, and those not reasonably associated with the use of the drug.

Breasts: Breast swelling, cysts, lumps, and masses of breasts; nipple discharge; primary malignant breast neoplasm; and tenderness.

Cardiovascular: Abnormal pulse, angina, atherosclerosis, cerebral ischemia, cerebrovascular lesion, heart block, peripheral cyanosis, pulsating sensations, Raynaud syndrome, thrombosis, transient myocardial ischemia, various transient ECG changes (nonspecific ST or T wave changes, prolongation of PR or QTc intervals, sinus arrhythmia, nonsustained ventricular premature beats, isolated junctional ectopic beats, atrial ectopic beats, delayed activation of the right ventricle), and vasodilation.

Ear, Nose, and Throat: Allergic rhinitis; ear, nose, and throat hemorrhage; external otitis; feeling of fullness in the ear(s); hearing disturbances; hearing loss; nasal inflammation; sensitivity to noise; sinusitis; tinnitus; and upper respiratory inflammation.

Endocrine and Metabolic: Dehydration; endocrine cysts, lumps, and masses; elevated thyrotropin stimulating hormone (TSH) levels; fluid disturbances; hyperglycemia; hypoglycemia; polydipsia; and weight gain.

Eye: Accommodation disorders, blindness and low vision, conjunctivitis, disorders of sclera, external ocular muscle disorders, eye edema and swelling, eye itching, eye hemorrhage, eye pain, keratitis, mydriasis, and vision alterations.

Gastrointestinal: Abdominal distention, dental pain, disturbances of liver function tests, dyspeptic symptoms, feelings of gastrointestinal pressure, gallstones, gastric symptoms, gastritis, gastrointestinal pain, hypersalivation, hyposalivation, oral itching and irritation, peptic ulcer, retching, salivary gland swelling, and swallowing disorders.

Hematological Disorders: Anemia.

Injection Site Reaction

Miscellaneous: Contusions, fluid retention, hematoma, hypersensitivity to various agents, jaw discomfort, miscellaneous laboratory abnormalities, overdose, "serotonin agonist effect," and speech disturbance.

Musculoskeletal: Acquired musculoskeletal deformity, arthralgia and articular rheumatitis, muscle atrophy, muscle tiredness, musculoskeletal inflammation, need to flex calf muscles, rigidity, tightness, and various joint disturbances (pain, stiffness, swelling, ache).

Neurological: Aggressiveness, bradylogia, cluster headache, convulsions, detachment, disturbances of taste, drug abuse, dystonia, facial paralysis, globus hystericus, hallucinations, headache, heat sensitivity, hyperesthesia, hysteria, increased alertness, malaise/fatigue, migraine, motor dysfunction, myoclonia, neuralgia, neurotic disorders, paralysis, personality change, phobia, photophobia, psychomotor disorders, radiculopathy, raised intracranial pressure, relaxation, stinging sensations, transient hemiplegia, simultaneous hot and cold sensations, suicide, tickling sensations, twitching, and yawning.

Pain and Other Pressure Sensations: Chest pain, neck tightness/pressure, throat/jaw pain/tightness/pressure, and pain (location specified).

Respiratory: Breathing disorders, bronchitis, diseases of the lower respiratory tract, hiccoughs, and influenza.

Skin: Dry/scaly skin, eczema, seborrheic dermatitis, skin nodules, skin tenderness, tightness of skin, and wrinkling of skin.

Urogenital: Abortion, abnormal menstrual cycle, bladder inflammation, hematuria, inflammation of fallopian tubes, intermenstrual bleeding, menstruation symptoms, micturition disorders, renal calculus, urethritis, urinary frequency, and urinary infections.

POSTMARKETING EXPERIENCE (REPORTS FOR SUBCUTANEOUS OR ORAL SUMATRIPTAN)

The following section enumerates potentially important adverse events that have occurred in clinical practice and that have been reported spontaneously to various surveillance systems. The events enumerated represent reports arising from both domestic and nondomestic use of oral or subcutaneous dosage forms of sumatriptan. The events enumerated include all except those already listed in ADVERSE REACTIONS above or those too general to be informative. Because the reports cite events reported spontaneously from worldwide postmarketing experience, frequency of events and the role of sumatriptan in their causation cannot be reliably determined. It is assumed, however, that systemic reactions following sumatriptan use are likely to be similar regardless of route of administration.

S

Blood: Hemolytic anemia, pancytopenia, thrombocytopenia.
Cardiovascular: Atrial fibrillation, cardiomyopathy, colonic ischemia (see WARNINGS), Prinzmetal variant angina, pulmonary embolism, shock, thrombophlebitis.
Ear, Nose, and Throat: Deafness.
Eye: Ischemic optic neuropathy, retinal artery occlusion, retinal vein thrombosis, loss of vision.
Gastrointestinal: Ischemic colitis with rectal bleeding (see WARNINGS), xerostomia.
Hepatic: Elevated liver function tests.
Neurological: Central nervous system vasculitis, cerebrovascular accident, dysphasia, subarachnoid hemorrhage.
Non-Site Specific: Angioneurotic edema, cyanosis, death (see WARNINGS), temporal arteritis.
Psychiatry: Panic disorder.
Respiratory: Bronchospasm in patients with and without a history of asthma.
Skin: Exacerbation of sunburn, hypersensitivity reactions (allergic vasculitis, erythema, pruritus, rash, shortness of breath, urticaria; in addition, severe anaphylaxis/anaphylactoid reactions have been reported [see WARNINGS]), photosensitivity.
Urogenital: Acute renal failure.

DOSAGE AND ADMINISTRATION

In controlled clinical trials, single doses of 5, 10, or 20 mg of sumatriptan nasal spray administered into 1 nostril were effective for the acute treatment of migraine in adults. A greater proportion of patients had headache response following a 20 mg dose than following a 5 or 10 mg dose. Individuals may vary in response to doses of sumatriptan nasal spray. The choice of dose should therefore be made on an individual basis, weighing the possible benefit of the 20 mg dose with the potential for a greater risk of adverse events. A 10 mg dose may be achieved by the administration of a single 5 mg dose in each nostril. There is evidence that doses above 20 mg do not provide a greater effect than 20 mg.

If the headache returns, the dose may be repeated once after 2 hours, not to exceed a total daily dose of 40 mg. The safety of treating an average of more than 4 headaches in a 30 day period has not been established.

ANIMAL PHARMACOLOGY

CORNEAL OPACITIES

Dogs receiving oral sumatriptan developed corneal opacities and defects in the corneal epithelium. Corneal opacities were seen at the lowest dosage tested, 2 mg/kg/day, and were present after 1 month of treatment. Defects in the corneal epithelium were noted in a 60 week study. Earlier examinations for these toxicities were not conducted and no-effect doses were not established; however, the relative exposure at the lowest dose tested was approximately 5 times the human exposure after a 100 mg oral dose or 3 times the human exposure after a 6 mg subcutaneous dose or 22 times the human exposure after a single 20 mg intranasal dose. There is evidence of alterations in corneal appearance on the first day of intranasal dosing to dogs. Changes were noted at the lowest dose tested, which was approximately 2 times the maximum single human intranasal dose of 20 mg on a mg/m^2 basis.

HOW SUPPLIED

Imitrex Nasal Spray 5 and 20 mg are available in nasal spray devices. Each unit dose spray supplied 5 and 20 mg, respectively, of sumatriptan.
Storage: Store between 2-30°C (36-86°F). Protect from light.

PRODUCT LISTING - EQUIVALENTS NOT AVAILABLE

Kit - Subcutaneous - 6 mg/0.5 ml			
1's	$85.12	IMITREX, Allscripts Pharmaceutical Company	54569-3705-00
1's	$95.44	IMITREX, Physicians Total Care	54868-3180-00
1's	$100.73	IMITREX STATDOSE, Physicians Total Care	54868-3959-00
1's	$104.02	IMITREX STATDOSE, Physicians Total Care	54868-3960-00
1's	$104.20	IMITREX STATDOSE, Allscripts Pharmaceutical Company	54569-4505-00
1's	$117.88	IMITREX, Glaxosmithkline	00173-0449-01
1's	$129.43	IMITREX STATDOSE, Glaxosmithkline	00173-0479-00
Solution - Subcutaneous - 6 mg/0.5 ml			
0.50 ml	$116.69	IMITREX, Physicians Total Care	54868-3181-00
0.50 ml	$122.59	IMITREX STATDOSE, Glaxosmithkline	00173-0478-00
0.50 ml x 2	$39.04	IMITREX, Physicians Total Care	54868-2652-00
0.50 ml x 2	$80.63	IMITREX, Allscripts Pharmaceutical Company	54569-3706-00
0.50 ml x 2	$103.62	IMITREX STATDOSE, Allscripts Pharmaceutical Company	54569-4511-00
0.50 ml x 5	$184.75	IMITREX, Compumed Pharmaceuticals	00403-4713-18
0.50 ml x 5	$198.55	IMITREX, Allscripts Pharmaceutical Company	54569-3704-00
0.50 ml x 5	$301.90	IMITREX, Glaxosmithkline	00173-0449-02
Spray - Nasal - 5 mg			
6's	$155.08	IMITREX NASAL, Glaxosmithkline	00173-0524-00
Spray - Nasal - 20 mg			
6's	$155.08	IMITREX NASAL, Glaxosmithkline	00173-0523-00
Tablet - Oral - 25 mg			
9's	$96.66	IMITREX, Cheshire Drugs	55175-4055-09
9's	$100.25	IMITREX, Compumed Pharmaceuticals	00403-0639-09
9's	$107.72	IMITREX, Allscripts Pharmaceutical Company	54569-4190-00
9's	$110.92	IMITREX, Pharma Pac	52559-0422-09
9's	$120.28	IMITREX, Physicians Total Care	54868-3777-00
9's	$144.20	IMITREX, Pharma Pac	52959-0422-09
9's	$172.05	IMITREX, Southwood Pharmaceuticals Inc	58016-0246-09
9's	$180.65	IMITREX, Glaxosmithkline	00173-0460-02
Tablet - Oral - 50 mg			
9's	$122.17	IMITREX, Allscripts Pharmaceutical Company	54569-4191-00
9's	$137.29	IMITREX, Physicians Total Care	54868-3852-00
9's	$151.26	IMITREX, Southwood Pharmaceuticals Inc	58016-5574-09
9's	$152.80	IMITREX, Pharma Pac	52959-0477-09
9's	$160.75	IMITREX, Glaxosmithkline	00173-0459-00
Tablet - Oral - 100 mg			
9's	$154.56	IMITREX, Glaxosmithkline	00173-0450-03

Tacrine Hydrochloride *(003091)*

Categories: Alzheimer's disease; FDA Approved 1993 Sep; Pregnancy Category C
Drug Classes: Cholinesterase inhibitors
Brand Names: **Cognex**; THA
Cost of Therapy: $175.02 (Alzheimer's Disease; Cognex; 10 mg; 4 capsules/day; 30 day supply)
$175.02 (Alzheimer's Disease; Cognex; 40 mg; 4 capsules/day; 30 day supply)

DESCRIPTION

Tacrine hydrochloride is a reversible cholinesterase inhibitor, known chemically as 1,2,3,4-tetrahydro-9-acridinamine monohydrochloride monohydrate. Tacrine hydrochloride is commonly referred to in the clinical and pharmacological literature as THA. It has an empirical formula of $C_{13}H_{14}N_2 \cdot H_2O$ and a molecular weight of 252.74.

Tacrine hydrochloride is a white solid and is freely soluble in distilled water, 0.1N hydrochloric acid, acetate buffer (pH 4.0), phosphate buffer (pH 7.0-7.4), methanol, dimethylsulfoxide (DMSO), ethanol, and propylene glycol. The compound is sparingly soluble in linoleic acid and PEG 400.

Each capsule of Cognex contains tacrine as the hydrochloride. Inactive ingredients are hydrous lactose, magnesium stearate, and microcrystalline cellulose. The hard gelatin capsules contain gelatin; silicon dioxide; sodium lauryl sulfate; and the following dyes: 10 mg: D&C yellow no. 10, FD&C green no. 3, titanium dioxide; 20 mg: D&C yellow no. 10, FD&C blue no. 1, titanium dioxide; 30 mg: D&C yellow no. 10, FD&C blue no. 1 , FD&C red no. 40, titanium dioxide; 40 mg: D&C yellow no. 10, FD&C blue no. 1, FD&C red no. 40, D&C red no. 28; titanium dioxide.

Each 10, 20, 30, and 40 mg Cognex capsule for oral administration contains 12.75, 25.50, 38.25, and 51.00 mg of tacrine HCl respectively.

CLINICAL PHARMACOLOGY

Although widespread degeneration of multiple CNS neuronal systems eventually occurs, early pathological changes in Alzheimer's Disease involve, in a relatively selective manner, cholinergic neuronal pathways that project from the basal forebrain to the cerebral cortex and hippocampus. The resulting deficiency of cortical acetylcholine is believed to account for some the clinical manifestations of mild to moderate dementia. Tacrine, an orally bioavailable, centrally active, reversible cholinesterase inhibitor, presumably acts by elevating acetylcholine concentrations in the cerebral cortex by slowing the degradation of acetylcholine released by still intact cholinergic neurons. If this theoretical mechanism of action is correct, tacrine's effects may lessen as the disease process advances and fewer cholinergic neurons remain functionally intact. There is no evidence that tacrine alters the course of the underlying dementing process.

CLINICAL PHARMACOKINETICS (ABSORPTION, DISTRIBUTION, METABOLISM, AND ELIMINATION)

Absorption

Tacrine HCl is rapidly absorbed after oral administration; maximal plasma concentrations occur with 1-2 hours. The rate and extent of tacrine absorption following administration of tacrine capsules and solution are virtually indistinguishable. Absolute bioavailability of tacrine is approximately 17 (SD ± 13)%. Food reduces tacrine bioavailability by approximately 30-40%; however, there is no food effect if tacrine is administered at least an hour before meals. The effect of achlorhydria on the absorption of tacrine is unknown.

Distribution

Mean volume of distribution of tacrine is approximately 349 (SD ± 193) L. Tacrine is about 55% bound to plasma proteins. The extent and degree of tacrine's distribution within various body compartments has not been systematically studied. However, 336 hours after the administration of a single radiolabeled dose, approximately 25% of the radiolabeled dose, approximately 25% of the radiolabel was not recovered in a mass balance study, suggesting the possibility that tacrine and/or one or more of its metabolites may be retained.

Metabolism

Tacrine is extensively metabolized by the cytochrome P450 system to multiple metabolites, not all of which have been identified. The vast majority of radiolabeled species present in the plasma following a single dose of ^{14}C radiolabeled tacrine are unidentified (*i.e.*, only 5% of radioactivity in plasma has been identified (tacrine and 3-hydroxylated metabolites 1-,2-, and 4-hydroxytacrine)).

Studies utilizing human liver preparations demonstrated that cytochrome P450 1A2 is the principal isozyme involved in tacrine metabolism. These findings are consistent with the observation that tacrine and/or one of its metabolite inhibits the metabolism of theophylline in humans (see DRUG INTERACTIONS, Theophylline.) Results from a study utilizing quinidine to inhibit cytochrome P450 IID6 indicate that tacrine is not metabolized extensively by this enzyme system.

Following aromatic ring hydroxylation, tacrine metabolites undergo glucuronidation. Whether tacrine and/or its metabolites undergo biliary excretion or entero-hepatic circulation is unknown.

Special Populations:

Age

Based on poled pharmacokinetic studies (n=192), there is no clinically relevant influence of age (50-84 years) on tacrine clearance.

Gender

Average tacrine plasma concentrations are approximately 50% higher in females than in males. This is not explained by differences in body surface area or elimination half-life. The difference is probably due to higher systemic availability after oral dosing and may reflect the known lower activity of cytochrome P450 IA2 in women.

Race

The effect of race on tacrine clearance has not been studied.

Smoking

Mean plasma tacrine concentrations in current smokers are approximately one-third the concentrations in nonsmoker. Cigarette smoking is known to induce cytochrome P450 IA2.

Renal Disease

Renal disease does not appear to affect the clearance of tacrine.

Liver Disease

Although studies in patients with liver disease have not been done, it is likely that functional hepatic impairment will reduce the clearance of tacrine and its metabolites.

Presystemic Clearance/Elimination/Excretion

Tacrine undergoes presystemic clearance (*i.e.,* first pass metabolism). The extent of this first pass metabolism depends upon the dose of tacrine administered. Because the enzyme system involved can be saturated at relatively low doses, a larger fraction of a high dose of tacrine will escape first pass elimination than of a smaller dose. Thus, when a 40 mg daily dose is increased by 40 mg, the average plasma concentration will be increased by 6 ng/ml. However, when a daily dose of 80 or 120 mg is increased by 40 mg, the increment in average plasma concentration is approximately 10 ng/ml.

Elimination of tacrine from the plasma, however, is not dose dependent (*i.e.,* the half-life is independent of dose or plasma concentration). The elimination half-life is approximately 2-4 hours. Following initiation of therapy or a change in daily dose, steady state tacrine plasma concentration should be attained with 24-36 hours.

INDICATIONS AND USAGE

Tacrine hydrochloride is indicated for the treatment of mild to moderate dementia of the Alzheimer's type.

Evidence of tacrine HCl's effectiveness in the treatment of dementia of the Alzheimer's type derives from results of two adequate and well-controlled clinical investigations that compared tacrine and placebo on both a performance based measure of cognition and clinician's global assessment of change.

NON-FDA APPROVED INDICATIONS

Tacrine has also been used to reverse postoperative sedation, prolong the muscle relaxation effect of succinylcholine, and treat myasthenia gravis, tricyclic antidepressant overdose, barbiturate overdose, tardive dyskinesia, and chronic severe pain (as an adjunct to morphine). However, none of these uses is approved by the FDA and no standard dosage recommendations are available for these uses.

CONTRAINDICATIONS

Tacrine HCl is contraindicated in patients with known hypersensitivity to tacrine or acridine derivatives.

Tacrine HCl is contraindicated in patients previously treated with tacrine HCl who developed treatment-associated jaundice confirmed by elevated total bilirubin greater than 3.0 mg/dl.

WARNINGS

ANESTHESIA

Tacrine HCl, as a cholinesterase inhibitor, is likely to exaggerate succinylcholine-type muscle relaxation during anesthesia.

CARDIOVASCULAR CONDITIONS

Because of its cholinomimetic action, tacrine HCl may have vagotonic effects on the heart rate (*e.g.,* bradycardia). This action may be particularly important to patients with conduction abnormalities, bradyarrhythmia, or a sick sinus syndrome.

GASTROINTESTINAL DISEASE AND DYSFUNCTION

Tacrine HCl is an inhibitor of cholinesterase and may be expected to increase gastric acid secretion due to increased cholinergic activity. Therefore, patients at increased risk for developing ulcers — *e.g.,* those with a history of ulcer disease or those receiving concurrent nonsteroidal anti- inflammatory drugs (NSAIDs) — should be monitored closely for symptoms of active or occult gastrointestinal bleeding.

Tacrine HCl, also as a predictable consequence of its pharmacological properties, can cause nausea, vomiting, and loose stools at recommended doses.

LIVER DYSFUNCTION

Tacrine HCl should be prescribed with care in patients with concurrent evidence or history of abnormal liver function indicated by significant abnormalities in serum transanimase (ALT/SGPT, AST/SGOT), bilirubin, and gamma-glutamyl transpeptidase (GGT) levels (see PRECAUTIONS and DOSAGE AND ADMINISTRATION).

The use of tacrine in patients without a prior history of liver disease is commonly associated with serum transanimase elevations, some to levels ordinarily considered to indicate clinically important hepatic injury (see TABLE 2.)

Experience gained in more than 8000 patients who received tacrine in clinical studies and the treatment IND program indicated that if tacrine is promptly withdrawn following detection of these elevations, clinically evident signs and symptoms of liver injury are rare.

Long-term follow up of patients who experience transanimase elevations, however, is limited and it is impossible, therefore, to exclude, with certainty, the possibility of chronic sequelae.

CONTROLLED CLINICAL TRIALS, TREATMENT IND AND POST-MARKETING EXPERIENCE

Experience with tacrine in controlled trials and in a large, less closely monitored experience (a treatment IND) is summarized below:

Clinically Evident Liver Toxicity

One of more than 8000 patients exposed to tacrine in clinical studies and the treatment IND program had documented elevated bilirubin (5.3 X Upper Limit of Normal, ULN) and jaundice with transanimase levels (AST/SGOT) nearly 20 X ULN.

Rare cases of liver toxicity associated with jaundice, raised serum bilirubin, pyrexia, hepatitis and liver failure have been reported in post-marketing experience. Most of these cases have been reversible but some deaths have occured. Since there was multiple pathology including infection, gallstones and carcinoma it was not possible to clearly establish the relationship to tacrine HCl treatment.

Blood Chemistry Signs of Liver Injury

Experience from the 30 week clinical study (described earlier) provides a representative estimate of the frequency of ALT/SGPT elevations expected for patients whose transaminase levels were monitored weekly and who receive tacrine HCl according to the recommended regimen for dose introduction and titration (TABLE 2). A dosing regimen employing a more rapid escalation of the daily dose of tacrine, or less frequent monitoring of liver chemistries, may be associated with more serious clinical events (see Monitoring of Liver Function and the Management of the Patient Who Develops Transanimase Elevations.)

***TABLE 2** Cumulative Incidence of ALT/SGPT Elevations Based on Maximum Values During the 30 week Study (number and % of patients)*

Maximum ALT	Males n=229	Females n=250	Total n=479
Within Normal Limits	121 (53)	100 (40)	221 (46)
>ULN	108 (47)	150 (60)	258 (54)
>2 times ULN	77 (34)	104 (42)	181 (38)
>3 times ULN	58 (25)	81 (32)	139 (29)
>10 times ULN	12 (5)	19 (8)	31 (6)
>20 times ULN	3 (1)	6 (2)	9 (2)

Experience in 2446 patients who participated in all clinical trials, including the 30 week study, indicated approximately 50% of patients treated with tacrine HCl can be expected to have at least 1 ALT/SGPT level above ULN; approximately 25% of patients are likely to develop elevations >3 X ULN, and about 7% of patients may develop elevations >10 X ULN. Data collected from the treatment IND program were consistent with those obtained during clinical studies, and showed 3% of 5665 patients experiencing an ALT/SGPT elevation >10 X ULN.

In clinical trials where transanimases were monitored weekly, the median time to onset of the first ALT/SGPT elevation above ULN was approximately 6 weeks, with maximum ALT/SGPT occurring 1 week later, even in instances when tacrine HCl treatment was stopped. Under the conditions of forced slow upwards dose titration (increases of 40 mg a day every 6 weeks) employed in clinical studies, 95% of transanimase elevations >3 X ULN occurred within the first 18 weeks of tacrine HCl therapy, and 99% of the 10-fold elevations occurred by the 12th week and on not more than 80 mg; note, however, that for most patients ALT was monitored weekly and tacrine HCl was stopped when liver enzymes exceeded 3 X ULN. A total of 276 patients were monitored for ALT/SGPT levels every other week in two double-blind clinical studies, an open-label study, and amended treatment IND. The incidence, severity, time to onset, peak and recovery of ALT/SGPT levels were similar to weekly monitoring. With less frequent monitoring or the less stringent discontinuation criteria recommended below (see DOSAGE AND ADMINISTRATION), it is possible that marked elevations might be more common. It must also be appreciated that experience with prolonged exposure to the high dose (160 mg/day) is limited. In all cases, transanimase levels returned to within normal limits upon discontinuation of tacrine HCl treatment or following dosage reduction, usually within 4-6 weeks.

This relatively benign experience may be the consequence of careful laboratory monitoring that facilitated the discontinuation of patients early on after the onset of their transanimase elevations. Consequently, frequent monitoring of serum transanimase levels is recommended (see DOSAGE AND ADMINISTRATION, WARNINGS, Liver Dysfunction, Monitoring of Liver Function and the Management of the Patient Who Develops Transanimase Elevations and PRECAUTIONS, Laboratory Tests).

Liver Biopsy Experience

Liver biopsy results in 7 patients who received tacrine (1 in a Parke-Davis sponsored study and 6 in studies reported in the literature) revealed hepatocellular necrosis in 6 patients, and granulomatous changes in the seventh. In all cases, liver function tests returned to normal with no evidence of persisting hepatic dysfunction.

Experience With the Rechallenge of Patients With Transanimase Elevations Following Recovery

Two hundred and twelve (212) patients among the 866 patients assigned to tacrine in the 12 and 30 week studies were withdrawn because they developed transanimase elevations >3 X ULN. One hundred and forty-five of these patients were subsequently rechallenged. During

T

their initial exposure to tacrine, 20 of these 145 had experienced initial elevations >10 times ULN, while the remainder had experienced elevations between 3 and 10 X ULN.

Upon rechallenge with an initial dose of 40 mg/day, only 48 (33%) of the 145 patients developed transanimase elevations greater than 3 X ULN. Of these patients, 44 had elevations that were between 3 and 10 X ULN and 4 had elevations that were >10 X ULN.

The mean time to onset of elevations occurred earlier on rechallenge than on initial exposure (22 versus 48 days). Of the 145 patients rechallenged, 127 (88%) were able to continue tacrine HCl treatment, and 91 of these 127 patients titrated to doses higher than those associated with the initial transanimase elevation.

Predictors of the Risk of Transanimase Elevations: The incidence of transanimase elevations is higher among females. There are no other known predictors of the risk of hepatocellular injury.

MONITORING OF LIVER FUNCTION AND THE MANAGEMENT OF THE PATIENT WHO DEVELOPS TRANSANIMASE ELEVATIONS

See also DOSAGE AND ADMINISTRATIONand PRECAUTIONS, Laboratory Tests.

Blood Chemistries

Serum transanimase levels (specifically ALT/SGPT) should be monitored every other week for at least the first 16 weeks following initiation of tacrine HCl treatment, after which monitoring may be decreased to monthly for 2 months and every 3 months thereafter. For patients who develope ALT/SGPT elevations greater than two times the upper limit of normal, the dose and monitoring regimen should be monitored as described in Table 4 (See DOSAGE AND ADMINISTRATION.)

A full monitoring sequence should be repeated in the event that a patient suspends treatment with tacrine for more than 4 weeks.

If transanimase elevations occur, the dose of tacrine HCl should be modified according to the table shown in DOSAGE AND ADMINISTRATION.

Rechallenge

Patients with clinical jaundice confirmed by a significant elevations in total bilirubin (>3 mg/dl) and/or those exhibiting clinical signs and/or symptoms of hypersensitivity (*e.g.*, rash or fever) in association with ALT/SGPT elevations should immediately and permanently discontinue tacrine HCl and not be rechallenged. Other patients who are required to discontinue tacrine HCl treatment because of transanimase elevations may be rechallenged once transanimase levels return to within normal limits. (See DOSAGE AND ADMINISTRATION.)

Rechallenge of patients with transanimase elevations less than 10 X ULN has not resulted in serious liver injury. However, because experience in the rechallenge of patients who had elevation greater than 10 X ULN is limited, the risks associated with the rechallenge of these patients are not well characterized. Careful, frequent (weekly) monitoring of serum ALT should be undertaken when rechallenging such patients.

If rechallenged, patients should be given an initial dose of 40 mg/day (10 mg QID) and transanimase levels monitored weekly. If, after 6 weeks on 40 mg/day,the patient is tolerating the dosage with no unacceptable elevations in transanimases, recommended dose-titration and transanimase monitoring may be resumed. Weekly monitoring of the ALT/SGPT levels should continue for a total of 16 weeks after which monitoring may be decreased to monthly for 2 months and every 3 months thereafter.

Liver Biopsy

Liver biopsy is not indicated in cases of uncomplicated transanimase elevation.

GENITOURINARY

Cholinomimetics may cause bladder outflow obstruction.

NEUROLOGICAL CONDITIONS

Seizures: Cholinomimetics are believed to have some potential to cause generalized convulsions; seizure activity may, however, also be a manifestation of Alzheimer's Disease.

Sudden Worsening of the Degree of Cognitive Impairment: Worsening of cognitive function has been reported following abrupt discontinuation of tacrine HCl or after a large reduction in total daily dose (80 mg/day or more).

PULMONARY CONDITIONS

Because of its cholinomimetic action, tacrine HCl should be prescribed with care to patients with a history of asthma.

T

PRECAUTIONS

GENERAL

Liver Injury: See WARNINGS.

HEMATOLOGY

An absolute neutrophil count (ANC) less than 500/μl occurred in 4 patients who received tacrine HCl (tacrine HCl) during the course of clinical trials. Three (3) of the 4 patients had concurrent medical conditions commonly associated with a low ANC; 2 of these patients remained on tacrine HCl. The fourth patient, who had a history of hypersensitivity (penicillin allergy), withdrew from the study as a result of a rash and also developed an ANC <500/μl, which returned to normal; this patient was not rechallenged and, therefore, the role played by tacrine HCl in this reaction is unknown.

Six (6) patients had an absolute neutrophil count ≤1500/μl, associated with an elevation of ALT/SGPT.

The total clinical experience in more than 8000 patients does not indicate a clear association between tacrine HCl treatment and serious white blood cell abnormalities.

INFORMATION FOR PATIENTS AND CAREGIVERS

Patients and caregivers should be advised that the effect of tacrine HCl therapy is thought to depend upon its administration at regular intervals, as directed.

The caregiver should be divided about the possibility of adverse effects. Two types should be distinguished: (1) those occurring in close temporal association with the initiation of treatment or an increase in dose (*e.g.*, nausea, vomiting, loose stools, diarrhea, etc) and (2) those with a delayed onset (*e.g.*, rash, jaundice, changes in the color of stool - black, very dark or light (*i.e.*, alcoholic)).

Patients and caregivers should be encouraged to inform the physician about the emergence of new events or any increase in the severity of existing adverse clinical events.

Caregivers should be advised that abrupt discontinuation of tacrine HCl or a large reduction in total daily dose (80 mg/day or more) may cause a decline in cognitive function and behavioral disturbances. Unsupervised increases in the dose of tacrine may also have serious consequences. Consequently, changes in dose should not be undertaken in the absence of direct instruction of a physician.

LABORATORY TESTS

(See WARNINGS, Liver Dysfunctionand DOSAGE AND ADMINISTRATION.) Serum transanimase levels (specifically ALT/SGPT) should be monitored in patients given tacrine HCl (see WARNINGS, Liver Dysfunction.)

CARCINOGENESIS, MUTAGENESIS, AND IMPAIRMENT OF FERTILITY

Tacrine was mutagenic to bacteria in the Ames test. Unscheduled DNA synthesis was induced in rat and mouse hepatocytes *in vitro*. Results of cytogenic (chromosomal aberration) studies were equivocal. Tacrine was not mutagenic in an *in vitro* mammalian mutation test. Overall, the results of these tests, along with the fact that tacrine belongs to a chemical class (acridines) containing some members which are animal carcinogens, suggest that tacrine may be carcinogenic.

Studies of the effects of tacrine on fertility have not been performed.

PREGNANCY CATEGORY C

Animal reproduction studies have not been conducted with tacrine. It is also not known whether tacrine HCl can cause fetal harm when administered to a pregnant woman or can affect reproductive capacity.

NURSING MOTHERS

It is not known whether this drug is excreted in human milk.

PEDIATRIC USE

There are no adequate and well-controlled trials to document the safety and efficacy of tacrine in any dementing illness occurring in children.

DRUG INTERACTIONS

DRUG-DRUG INTERACTIONS

Possible Metabolic Basis for Interactions

Tacrine is primarily eliminated by hepatic metabolism via cytochrome P450 drug metabolizing enzymes. Drug-drug interactions may occur when tacrine HCl is given concurrently with agents such as theophylline that undergo extensive metabolism via cytochrome P450 IA2.

***Theophylline:* Coadministration of tacrine with theophylline increased theophylline elimination half-life and average plasma theophylline concentrations by approximately 2-fold. Therefore, monitoring of plasma theophylline concentrations and appropriate reduction of theophylline dose are recommended in patients receiving tacrine and theophylline concurrently. The effect of theophylline on tacrine pharmacokinetics has not been assessed.**

Cimetidine: Cimetidine increased the Cmax and AUC of tacrine by approximately 54% and 64% respectively.

Anticholinergics: Because of its mechanism of action, tacrine HCl has the potential to interfere with the activity of anticholinergic medications.

Cholinomimetics and Cholinesterase Inhibitors: A synergistic effect is expected when tacrine HCl is given concurrently with succinylcholine (see WARNINGS), cholinesterase inhibitors, or cholinergic agonists such as bethanechol.

Other Interactions: Rate and extent of tacrine absorption were not influenced by the coadministration of an antacid containing magnesium and aluminum. Tacrine had no major effect on digoxin or diazepam pharmacokinetics or the anticoagulant activity of warfarin.

ADVERSE REACTIONS

COMMON ADVERSE EVENTS LEADING TO DISCONTINUATION

In clinical trials, approximately 17% of the 2706 patients who received tacrine HCl and 5% of the 1886 patients who received placebo withdrew permanently because of adverse events. It should be noted that some the placebo-treated patients were exposed to tacrine HCl prior to receiving placebo due to the variety of study designs used, including crossover studies. Transanimase elevations were the most common reason for withdrawals during tacrine HCl treatment (8% of all tacrine HCl-treated patients, or 212 of 456 patients withdrawn). The controlled clinical trial protocols required that any patient with an ALT/SGPT elevation >3 X ULN be withdrawn, because of concern about potential hepatotoxicity. Apart from withdrawals due to transanimase elevations, 244 patients (9%) withdrew for adverse events while receiving tacrine HCl.

Other adverse events that most frequently led to the withdrawal of tacrine-treated patients in clinical trials were nausea and/or vomiting (1.5%), agitation (0.9%), rash (0.7%), anorexia (0.7%), and confusion (0.5%). These adverse events also most frequently led to the withdrawal of placebo-treated patients, although lower frequencies (0.1-0.2%).

MOST FREQUENT ADVERSE CLINICAL EVENTS SEEN IN ASSOCIATION WITH THE USE OF TACRINE

The events identified here are those that occurred at an absolute incidence of at least 5% of patients treated with tacrine HCl, and at a rate at least 2-fold higher in patients treated with tacrine HCl than placebo.

The most common adverse events associated with the use of tacrine HCl were elevated transanimases, nausea and/or vomiting, diarrhea, dyspepsia, myalgia, anorexia, and ataxia. Of these events, nausea and/or vomiting, diarrhea, dyspepsia and anorexia appeared to be dose-dependent.

ADVERSE EVENTS REPORTED IN CONTROLLED TRIALS

The events cited in the table below (TABLE 3) reflect experience gained under closely monitored conditions of clinical trials with a highly selected patient population. In actual clinical practice or in other clinical trials, these frequency estimates may not apply, as the conditions of use, reporting behavior, and the kinds of patients treated may differ.

TABLE 3 lists treatment-emergent signs and symptoms that occurred in at least 2% of patients with Alzheimer's Disease in placebo-controlled trials and who received the recommended regimen for dose introduction and titration of tacrine HCl (see DOSAGE AND ADMINISTRATION).

TABLE 3 *Adverse Events Occurring in at Least 2% of Patients Receiving Tacrine HCl Using the Recommended Regimen for Dose Introduction and Titration in Controlled Clinical Trials*

	Number (%) of Patients	
Body System/Adverse Events	**Tacrine HCl n=634**	**Placebo n=342**
Laboratory Deviations		
Elevated transanimase*	184 (29)	5 (20)
Body As A Whole		
Headache	67 (11)	52 (15)
Fatigue	26 (4)	9 (3)
Chest pain	24 (4)	18 (5)
Weight decrease	21 (3)	4 (1)
Back pain	15 (2)	14 (4)
Asthenia	15 (2)	7 (2)
Digestive System		
Nausea and/or vomiting	178 (28)	29 (9)
Diarrhea	99 (16)	18 (5)
Dyspepsia	57 (9)	22 (6)
Anorexia	54 (9)	11 (3)
Abdominal pain	48 (8)	24 (7)
Flatulence	22 (4)	5 (2)
Constipation	24 (4)	8 (2)
Hemic And Lymphatic System		
Purpura	15 (2)	8 (2)
Musculoskeletal System		
Myalgia	54 (9)	18 (5)
Nervous System		
Dizziness	73 (12)	39 (11)
Confusion	42 (7)	24 (7)
Ataxia	36 (6)	12 (4)
Insomnia	37 (6)	18 (5)
Somnolence	22 (4)	11 (3)
Tremor	14 (2)	2 (<1)
Psychological Function		
Agitation	43 (7)	20 (9)
Depression	22 (4)	14 (4)
Thinking abnormal	17 (3)	14 (4)
Anxiety	16 (3)	7 (2)
Hallucination	15 (2)	12 (4)
Hostility	15 (2)	5 (2)
Respiratory System		
Rhinitis	51 (8)	22 (6)
Upper respiratory infection	18 (3)	11 (3)
Coughing	17 (3)	18 (5)
Skin And Appendages		
Rash†	46 (7)	18 (5)
Facial flushing, skin flushing	16 (3)	3 (<1)
Urogenital System		
Urination frequency	21 (3)	12 (4)
Urinary tract infection	21 (3)	20 (6)
Urinary incontinence	16 (3)	9 (3)

* ALT or AST value of approximately 3 X ULN or greater or that resulted in a change in patient management.
† Included COSTART terms: rash, rash-erythematous, rash-maculopapular, urticaria, petechial rash, rash-vesiculobullous, and pruritus.

OTHER ADVERSE EVENTS OBSERVED DURING ALL CLINICAL TRIALS

Tacrine HCl has been administered to 2706 individuals during clinical trials. A total of 1471 patients were treated for at least 3 months, 1137 for at least 6 months, and 773 for at least 1 year. Any untoward reactions that occurred during these trials were recorded as adverse events by the clinical investigators using terminology of their own choosing. To provide a meaningful estimate of the proportion of individuals having similar types of events, the events were grouped into a smaller number of standardized categories using a modified COSTART dictionary. These categories are used in the listing below. The frequencies represent the proportion of the 2706 individuals exposed to tacrine HCl who experienced that event while receiving tacrine HCl. All adverse events are included except those already listed on the previous table and those COSTART terms too general to be informative. Events are further classified by body system categories and listed using the following definitions: *frequent* adverse events are defined as those occurring in at least 1/100 patients; *infrequent* adverse events are those occurring in 1/100 to 1/1000 patients; and *rare* adverse events are those occurring in less than 1/1000 patients. These adverse events are not necessarily related to tacrine HCl treatment. Only rare adverse events deemed to be potentially important are included.

Body as a Whole: *Frequent:* Chill, fever, malaise, peripheral edema. *Infrequent:* Face edema, dehydration, weight increase, cachexia, edema (generalized), lipoma. *Rare:* Heat exhaustion, sepsis, cholinergic crisis, death.

Cardiovascular System: *Frequent:* Hypotension, hypertension.*Infrequent:* Heart failure, myocardial infarction, angina pectoris, cerebrovascular accident, transient ischemic attack, phlebitis, venous insufficiency, abdominal aortic aneurysm, atrial fibrillation or flutter, palpitation, tachycardia, bradycardia, pulmonary embolus, migraine, hypercholesterolemia. *Rare:* Heart arrest, premature atrial contractions, A-V block, bundle branch block.

Digestive System: *Infrequent:* Glossitis, gingivitis, mouth or throat dry, stomatitis, increased salivation, dysphagia, esophagitis, gastritis, gastroenteritis, GI hemorrhage, stomach ulcer, hiatal hernia, hemorrhoids, stools bloody, diverticulitis, fecal impaction, fecal incontinence, hemorrhage (rectum), cholelithiasis, cholecystitis, increased appetite. *Rare:* Duodenal ulcer, bowel obstruction.

Endocrine System: *Infrequent:* Diabetes. *Rare:* Hyperthyroid, hypothyroid.

Hemic and Lymphatic: *Infrequent:* Anemia, lymphadenopathy. *Rare:* Leukopenia, thrombocytopenia, hemolysis, pancytopenia.

Musculoskeletal: *Frequent:* Fracture, arthralgia, arthritis, hypertonia. *Infrequent:* Osteoporosis, tendinitis, bursitis, gout. *Rare:* Myopathy.

Nervous System: *Frequent:* Convulsions , vertigo, syncope, hyperkinesia, paresthesia. *Infrequent:* Dreaming abnormal, dysarthria, aphasia, amnesia, wandering, twitching, hypesthesia, delirium, paralysis, bradykinesia, movement disorder, cogwheel rigidity, paresis, neuritis, hemiplegia, Parkinson's disease, neuropathy, extrapyramidal syndrome, reflexes decreased/absent. *Rare:* Tardive dyskinesia, dysesthesia, dystonia, encephalitis, coma, apraxia, oculogyric crisis, akathisia, oral facial dyskinesia, Bell's palsy, exacerbation of Parkinson's disease.

Psychobiologic Function: *Frequent:* Nervousness.*Infrequent:* Apathy, increased libido, paranoia, neurosis.*Rare:* Suicidal, psychosis, hysteria.

Respiratory System: *Frequent:* Pharyngitis, sinusitis, bronchitis, pneumonia, dyspnea. *Infrequent:* Epistaxis, chest congestion, asthma, hyperventilation, lower respiratory infection. *Rare:* Hemoptysis, lung edema, lung cancer, acute epiglottis.

Skin and Appendages: *Frequent:* Sweating increased. *Infrequent:* Acne, alopecia, dermatitis eczema, skin dry, herpes zoster, psoriasis, cellulitis, cyst, furunculosis, herpes simplex, hyperkeratosis, basal cell carcinoma, skin cancer. *Rare:* Desquamation, seborrhea, squamous cell carcinoma, ulcer (skin), skin necrosis, melanoma.

Urogenital System: *Infrequent:* Hematuria, renal stone, kidney function, glycosuria, dysuria, polyuria, nocturia, pyuria, cystitis, urinary retention, urination urgency, vaginal hemorrhage, pruritus (genital), breast pain, impotence, prostate cancer. *Rare:* Bladder tumor, renal tumor, renal failure, urinary obstruction, breast cancer, epididymitis, carcinoma (ovary).

Special Senses: *Frequent:* Conjunctivitis. *Infrequent:* Cataract, eyes dry, eye pain, visual field defect, diplopia, amblyopia, glaucoma, hordeolum, deafness, earache, tinnitus, inner ear infection, otitis media, unusual taste. *Rare:* Vision loss, ptosis, blepharitis, labyrinthitis, inner ear disturbance.

POSTINTRODUCTION REPORTS

Voluntary reports of adverse events temporally with tacrine HCl that have been received since market introduction, that are not listed above, and that may have no causal relationship with the drug include the following: pancreatitis, perforated duodenal ulcer.

DOSAGE AND ADMINISTRATION

The recommendations for dose titration are base on experience from clinical trials. The rate of dose of escalation may be slowed if a patient is intolerant to the titration schedule recommended below. It is not advisable, however, to accelerate the dose incrementation plan.

Following initiation of therapy, or any dosage increase, patients should be observed carefully for adverse effects. Tacrine HCl should be taken between meals whenever possible; however, if minor GI upset occurs, tacrine HCl may be taken with meals to improve tolerability. Taking tacrine HCl with meals can be expected to reduce plasma levels by approximately 30-40%.

INITIATION OF TREATMENT

The initial dose of tacrine hydrochloride is 40 mg/day (10 mg qid). This dose should be maintained for a minimum of 4 weeks with every other week monitoring of transaminase levels beginning 4 weeks after initiation of treatment. It is important that the dose not be increased during this period because of the potential for delayed onset of transaminase elevations.

DOSE TITRATION

Following 4 weeks of treatment at 40 mg/day (10 mg qid), the dose of tacrine HCl should then be increased to 80 mg/day (20 mg qid), providing there are no significant transanimase elevations and the patient is tolerating treatment. Patients should be titrated to higher doses (120 and 160 mg/day, in divided doses on a qid schedule) at 4 week intervals on the basis of tolerance.

DOSE ADJUSTMENT

Serum ALT/SGOT should be monitored every other week for at least week 4 to week 16 following initiation of treatment, after which monitoring may be decreased to every 3 months. For patients who develope ALT/SGPT elevations greater than two times the upper limit of normal, the dose and monitoring regimen should be modified as described in TABLE 4.

A full monitoring and dose titration sequence must be repeated in the event that a patient suspends treatment with tacrine for more than 4 weeks.

RECHALLENGE

Patients who are required to discontinue tacrine HCl treatment because of transanimase elevations may be rechallenged once transanimase levels return to within normal limits.

Rechallenge of patients exposed to transanimase elevations less than 10 X ULN has not resulted in serious liver injury. However, because experience in the rechallenge of patients who had elevations greater than 10 X ULN is limited, the risks associated with the rechallenge of these patients are not well characterized. Careful, frequent (weekly) monitoring of serum ALT should be undertaken when rechallenging such patients.

T

TABLE 4 *Recommended Dose Regimen Modification in Response to Transanimase Elevations*

ALT/SGPT Level	Treatment and Monitoring Regimen
≤2 X ULN	Continue treatment according to recommended titration and monitoring schedule.
>2 to ≤3 X ULN	Continue treatment according to recommended titration. Monitor ALT/SGPT levels weekly until levels return to normal limits.
>3 to ≤5 X ULN	Reduce the daily dose of tacrine HCl by 40 mg/day. Monitor ALT/SGPT levels weekly. Resume dose titration and every other week monitoring when the levels of the ALT/SGPT return to normal limits.
>5 X ULN	Stop tacrine HCl treatment. Monitor the patient closely for signs and symptoms associated with hepatitis and follow ALT/SGPT levels until within normal limits. See Rechallenge section below.

Experience is limited with patients with ALT >10 X ULN. The risk of rechallenge must be considered against demonstrated clinical benefit.
Patients with clinical jaundice confirmed by a significant elevation in total bilirubin (>3 mg/dl) and/or symptoms of hypersensitivity (*e.g.,* rash or fever) in association with ALT/SGPT elevations should immediately and permanently discontinue tacrine HCl and not be rechallenged.

If rechallenged, patients should be given an initial dose of 40 mg/day (10 mg QID) and transanimase levels monitored weekly. If, after 6 weeks on 40 mg/day, the patient is tolerating the dosage with no unacceptable elevations in transanimases, recommended dose-titration and transaminase monitoring may be resumed. Weekly monitoring of the ALT/SGPT levels should continue for a total of 16 weeks after which monitoring may be decreased to monthly for 2 months and every 3 months thereafter.

HOW SUPPLIED

Cognex is supplied as capsules of tacrine hydrochloride containing 10, 20, 30, 40 mg of tacrine. The capsule logo is Cognex, with the strength printed underneath and the colors as follows:

10 mg: Yellow/dark green
20 mg: Yellow/light blue
30 mg: Yellow/swedish orange
40 mg: Yellow/lavender

Storage: Store at controlled room temperature 15-30°C (59-86°F) away from moisture.

PRODUCT LISTING - EQUIVALENTS NOT AVAILABLE

Capsule - Oral - 10 mg
120's $175.02 COGNEX, First Horizon Pharmaceutical Corporation 59630-0190-12

Capsule - Oral - 20 mg
120's $175.02 COGNEX, First Horizon Pharmaceutical Corporation 59630-0191-12

Capsule - Oral - 30 mg
120's $175.02 COGNEX, First Horizon Pharmaceutical Corporation 59630-0192-12

Capsule - Oral - 40 mg
120's $175.02 COGNEX, First Horizon Pharmaceutical Corporation 59630-0193-12

Tacrolimus *(003138)*

Categories: Dermatitis, atopic; Rejection, liver transplant, prophylaxis; Rejection, renal transplant, prophylaxis; FDA Approved 1994 Apr; Pregnancy Category C
Drug Classes: Dermatologics; Immunosuppressives
Brand Names: Prograf; FK-506
Foreign Brand Availability: Protopic (England; France; Hong-Kong; Ireland)
Cost of Therapy: $1115.30 (Transplant Rejection; Prograf; 5 mg; 2 capsules/day; 30 day supply)
HCFA JCODE(S): J7507 per 1 mg ORAL; J7508 per 5 mg ORAL

T

ORAL

WARNING

Note: This information refers to tacrolimus capsules and injection.

Increased susceptibility to infection and the possible development of lymphoma may result from immunosuppression. Only physicians experienced in immunosuppressive therapy and management of organ transplant patients should prescribe tacrolimus capsules and injection. Patients receiving the drug should be managed in facilities equipped and staffed with adequate laboratory and supportive medical resources. The physician responsible for maintenance therapy should have complete information requisite for the follow-up of the patient.

DESCRIPTION

Prograf is available for oral administration as capsules (tacrolimus capsules) containing the equivalent of 0.5, 1, or 5 mg of anhydrous tacrolimus. Inactive ingredients include lactose, hydroxypropyl methylcellulose, croscarmellose sodium, and magnesium stearate. The 0.5 mg capsule shell contains gelatin, titanium dioxide and ferric oxide, the 1 mg capsule shell contains gelatin and titanium dioxide, and the 5 mg capsule shell contains gelatin, titanium dioxide and ferric oxide.

Prograf is also available as a sterile solution (tacrolimus injection) containing the equivalent of 5 mg anhydrous tacrolimus in 1 ml for administration by intravenous (IV) infusion only. Each ml contains polyoxyl 60 hydrogenated castor oil (HCO-60), 200 mg, and dehydrated alcohol, 80.0% v/v. Prograf injection must be diluted with 0.9% sodium chloride injection or 5% dextrose injection before use.

Tacrolimus, previously known as FK506, is the active ingredient in Prograf. Tacrolimus is a macrolide immunosuppressant produced by *Streptomyces tsukubaensis.* Chemically, tacrolimus is designated as [3*S*-[3*R**[*E*(1*S**,3*S**,4*S**)],4*S**,5*R**,8*S**,9*E*,12*R**,14*R**,15*S**,16*R**,18*S**,19*S**,26a*R**]]-5,6,8,11,12,13,14,15,16,17,18,19,24,25,26,26a-hexadecahydro-5,19-dihydroxy-3-[2-(4-hydroxy-3-methoxycyclohexyl)-1-methylethenyl]-14,16-dimethoxy-4,10,12,18-tetramethyl-8-(2-propenyl)-15,19-epoxy-3H-pyrido[2,1-*c*][1,4] oxaazacyclotricosine-1,7,20,21(4H,23H)-tetrone, monohydrate.

Tacrolimus has an empirical formula of $C_{44}H_{69}NO_{12}{\cdot}H_2O$ and a formula weight of 822.05. Tacrolimus appears as white crystals or crystalline powder. It is practically insoluble in water, freely soluble in ethanol, and very soluble in methanol and chloroform.

CLINICAL PHARMACOLOGY

MECHANISM OF ACTION

Tacrolimus prolongs the survival of the host and transplanted graft in animal transplant models of liver, kidney, heart, bone marrow, small bowel and pancreas, lung and trachea, skin, cornea, and limb.

In animals, tacrolimus has been demonstrated to suppress some humoral immunity and, to a greater extent, cell-mediated reactions such as allograft rejection, delayed type hypersensitivity, collagen- induced arthritis, experimental allergic encephalomyelitis, and graft versus host disease.

Tacrolimus inhibits T-lymphocyte activation, although the exact mechanism of action is not known. Experimental evidence suggests that tacrolimus binds to an intracellular protein, FKBP-12. A complex of tacrolimus-FKBP-12, calcium, calmodulin, and calcineurin is then formed and the phosphatase activity of calcineurin inhibited. This effect may prevent the dephosphorylation and translocation of nuclear factor of activated T-cells (NF-AT), a nuclear component thought to initiate gene transcription for the formation of lymphokines (such as interleukin-2, gamma interferon). The net result is the inhibition of T-lymphocyte activation (*i.e.,* immunosuppression).

PHARMACOKINETICS

Tacrolimus activity is primarily due to the parent drug. The pharmacokinetic parameters (mean ±SD) of tacrolimus have been determined following intravenous (IV) and oral (po) administration in healthy volunteers, and in kidney transplant and liver transplant patients. (See TABLE 1.)

TABLE 1

Route (Dose)	C_{max} (ng/ml)	T_{max} (h)	AUC (ng·h/ml)	T½ (h)	CL (L/h/kg)	V (L/kg)
Healthy Volunteers						
IV (0.025 mg/kg/4h) (n=8)	—	—	598* ± 125	34.2 ± 7.7	0.040 ± 0.009	1.91 ± 0.31
po (5 mg) (n=16)	29.7 ± 7.2	1.6 ± 0.7	243† ± 73	34.8 ± 11.4	0.041§ ± 0.008	1.94§ ± 0.53
Kidney Transplant Patients (n=26)						
IV (0.02 mg/kg/12h)	—	—	294‡ ± 262	18.8 ± 16.7	0.083 ± 0.050	1.41 ± 0.66
po (0.2 mg/kg/day)	19.2 ± 10.3	3.0	203‡ ± 42	NA	NA	NA
po (0.3 mg/kg/day)	24.2 ± 15.8	1.5	288‡ ± 93	NA	NA	NA
Liver Transplant Patients (n=17)						
IV (0.05 mg/kg/12h)	—	—	3300‡ ± 2130	11.7 ± 3.9	0.053 ± 0.017	0.85 ± 0.30
po (0.3 mg/kg/day)	68.5 ± 30.0	2.3 ± 1.5	519‡ ± 179	NA	NA	NA

* AUC(0-120).
† AUC(0-72).
‡ AUC(0-∞).
§ Corrected for individual bioavailability.
— Not applicable.
NA Not available.

Due to intersubject variability in tacrolimus pharmacokinetics, individualization of dosing regimen is necessary for optimal therapy. (See DOSAGE AND ADMINISTRATION.) Pharmacokinetic data indicate that whole blood concentrations rather than plasma concentrations serve as the more appropriate sampling compartment to describe tacrolimus pharmacokinetics.

Absorption

Absorption of tacrolimus from the gastrointestinal tract after oral administration is incomplete and variable. The absolute bioavailability of tacrolimus was 17 ± 10% in adult kidney transplant patients (n=26), 22 ± 6% in adult liver transplant patients (n=17), and 18 ± 5% in healthy volunteers (n=16).

A single dose study conducted in 32 healthy volunteers established the bioequivalence of the 1 and 5 mg capsules. Another single dose study in 32 healthy volunteers established the bioequivalence of the 0.5 and 1 mg capsules. Tacrolimus maximum blood concentration (C_{max}) and area under the curve (AUC) appeared to increase in a dose-proportional fashion in 18 fasted healthy volunteers receiving a single oral dose of 3, 7 and 10 mg.

In 18 kidney transplant patients, tacrolimus trough concentrations from 3-30 ng/ml measured at 10-12 hours post-dose (C_{min}) correlated well with the AUC (correlation coefficient 0.93). In 24 liver transplant patients over a concentration range of 10-60 ng/ml, the correlation coefficient was 0.94.

Food Effects

The rate and extent of tacrolimus absorption were greatest under fasted conditions. The presence and composition of food decreased both the rate and extent of tacrolimus absorption when administered to 15 healthy volunteers.

The effect was most pronounced with a high-fat meal (848 kcal, 46% fat): mean AUC and C_{max} were decreased 37% and 77%, respectively; T_{max} was lengthened 5-fold. A high-carbohydrate meal (668 kcal, 85% carbohydrate) decreased mean AUC and mean C_{max} by 28% and 65%, respectively.

In healthy volunteers (n=16), the time of the meal also affected tacrolimus bioavailability. When given immediately following the meal, mean C_{max} was reduced 71%, and mean AUC was reduced 39%, relative to the fasted condition. When administered 1.5 hours following the meal, mean C_{max} was reduced 63%, and mean AUC was reduced 39%, relative to the fasted condition.

In 11 liver transplant patients, tacrolimus administered 15 minutes after a high-fat (400 kcal, 34% fat) breakfast, resulted in decreased AUC (27 ± 18%) and C_{max} (50 ± 19%), as compared to a fasted state.

Distribution

The plasma protein binding of tacrolimus is approximately 99% and is independent of concentration over a range of 5-50 ng/ml. Tacrolimus is bound mainly to albumin and alpha-1-acid glycoprotein, and has a high level of association with erythrocytes. The distribution of tacrolimus between whole blood and plasma depends on several factors, such as hematocrit, temperature at the time of plasma separation, drug concentration, and plasma protein concentration. In a US study, the ratio of whole blood concentration to plasma concentration averaged 35 (range 12-67).

Metabolism

Tacrolimus is extensively metabolized by the mixed-function oxidase system, primarily the cytochrome P-450 system (CYP3A). A metabolic pathway leading to the formation of 8 possible metabolites has been proposed. Demethylation and hydroxylation were identified as the primary mechanisms of biotransformation *in vitro*. The major metabolite identified in incubations with human liver microsomes is 13-demethyl tacrolimus. In *in vitro* studies, a 31-demethyl metabolite has been reported to have the same activity as tacrolimus.

Excretion

The mean clearance following IV administration of tacrolimus is 0.040, 0.083 and 0.053 L/h/kg in healthy volunteers, adult kidney transplant patients and adult liver transplant patients, respectively. In man, less than 1% of the dose administered is excreted unchanged in urine.

In a mass balance study of IV administered radiolabeled tacrolimus to 6 healthy volunteers, the mean recovery of radiolabel was 77.8 ± 12.7%. Fecal elimination accounted for 92.4 ± 1.0% and the elimination half-life based on radioactivity was 48.1 ± 15.9 hours whereas it was 43.5 ± 11.6 hours based on tacrolimus concentrations. The mean clearance of radiolabel was 0.029 ± 0.015 L/h/kg and clearance of tacrolimus was 0.029 ± 0.009 L/h/kg. When administered po, the mean recovery of the radiolabel was 94.9 ± 30.7%. Fecal elimination accounted for 92.6 ± 30.7%, urinary elimination accounted for 2.3 ± 1.1% and the elimination half-life based on radioactivity was 31.9 ± 10.5 hours whereas it was 48.4 ± 12.3 hours based on tacrolimus concentrations. The mean clearance of radiolabel was 0.226 ± 0.116 L/h/kg and clearance of tacrolimus 0.172 ± 0.088 L/h/kg.

SPECIAL POPULATIONS

Pediatric

Pharmacokinetics of tacrolimus have been studied in liver transplantation patients, 0.7-13.2 years of age. Following IV administration of a 0.037 mg/kg/day dose to 12 pediatric patients, mean terminal half-life, volume of distribution and clearance were 11.5 ± 3.8 hours, 2.6 ± 2.1 L/kg and 0.138 ± 0.071 L/h/kg, respectively. Following oral administration to 9 patients, mean AUC and C_{max} were 337 ± 167 ng·h/ml and 43.4 ± 27.9 ng/ml, respectively. The absolute bioavailability was 31 ± 21%.

Whole blood trough concentrations from 31 patients less than 12 years old showed that pediatric patients needed higher doses than adults to achieve similar tacrolimus trough concentrations. (See DOSAGE AND ADMINISTRATION.)

Renal and Hepatic Insufficiency

The mean pharmacokinetic parameters for tacrolimus following single administrations to patients with renal and hepatic impairment are given in TABLE 2.

Renal Insufficiency

Tacrolimus pharmacokinetics following a single IV administration were determined in 12 patients (7 not on dialysis and 5 on dialysis, serum creatinine of 3.9 ± 1.6 and 12.0 ± 2.4 mg/dl, respectively) prior to their kidney transplant. The pharmacokinetic parameters obtained were similar for both groups.

The mean clearance of tacrolimus in patients with renal dysfunction was similar to that in normal volunteers (see TABLE 2).

Hepatic Insufficiency

Tacrolimus pharmacokinetics have been determined in 6 patients with mild hepatic dysfunction (mean Pugh score: 6.2) following single IV and oral administrations. The mean clearance of tacrolimus in patients with mild hepatic dysfunction was not substantially different from that in normal volunteers (see TABLE 2). Tacrolimus pharmacokinetics were studied in 6 patients with severe hepatic dysfunction (mean Pugh score: >10). The mean clearance was substantially lower in patients with severe hepatic dysfunction, irrespective of the route of administration.

TABLE 2

Dose	AUC(0-t) (ng·h/ml)	T½ (hours)	V (L/kg)	Cl (L/h/kg)
Renal Impairment (n=12)				
0.02 mg/kg/4h IV	393 ± 123 (t=60 h)	26.3 ± 9.2	1.07 ± 0.20	0.038 ± 0.014
Mild Hepatic Impairment (n=6)				
0.02 mg/kg/4h IV	367 ± 107 (t=72 h)	60.6 ± 9.2 Range: 27.8-141	3.1 ± 1.6	0.042 ± 0.02
7.7 mg po	488 ± 320 (t=72 h)	66.1 ± 43.8 Range: 29.5-138	3.7 ± 4.7*	0.034 ± 0.019*
Severe Hepatic Impairment (n=6, IV) (n=5, po†)				
0.02 mg/kg/4h IV (n=2)	762 ± 204 (t=120 h)	198 ± 158 Range:81-436	3.9 ± 1.0	0.017 ± 0.013
0.01 mg/kg/8h IV (n=4)	289 ± 117 (t=144 h)			
8 mg po (n=1)	658 (t=120 h)	119 ± 35 Range: 85-178	3.1 ± 3.4*	0.016 ± 0.011*
5 mg po (n=4)	533 ± 156 (t=144 h)			
4 mg po (n=1)				

* Corrected for bioavailability.
† 1 patient did not receive the po dose.

Race

A formal study to evaluate the pharmacokinetic disposition of tacrolimus in Black transplant patients has not been conducted. However, a retrospective comparison of Black and Caucasian kidney transplant patients indicated that Black patients required higher tacrolimus doses to attain similar trough concentrations. (See DOSAGE AND ADMINISTRATION.)

Gender

A formal study to evaluate the effect of gender on tacrolimus pharmacokinetics has not been conducted, however, there was no difference in dosing by gender in the kidney transplant trial. A retrospective comparison of pharmacokinetics in healthy volunteers, and in kidney and liver transplant patients indicated no gender-based differences.

INDICATIONS AND USAGE

Tacrolimus is indicated for the prophylaxis of organ rejection in patients receiving allogeneic liver or kidney transplants. It is recommended that tacrolimus be used concomitantly with adrenal corticosteroids. Because of the risk of anaphylaxis, tacrolimus injection should be reserved for patients unable to take tacrolimus capsules orally.

CONTRAINDICATIONS

Tacrolimus is contraindicated in patients with a hypersensitivity to tacrolimus. Tacrolimus injection is contraindicated in patients with a hypersensitivity to HCO-60 (polyoxyl 60 hydrogenated castor oil).

WARNINGS

See BOXED WARNING.

Insulin-dependent post-transplant diabetes mellitus (PTDM) was reported in 20% of tacrolimus-treated kidney transplant patients without pretransplant history of diabetes mellitus in the Phase 3 study (see TABLE 3 and TABLE 4). The median time to onset of PTDM was 68 days. Insulin dependence was reversible in 15% of these PTDM patients at 1 year and in 50% at 2 years post-transplant. Black and Hispanic kidney transplant patients were at an increased risk of development of PTDM.

TABLE 3 *Incidence of Post-Transplant Diabetes Mellitus and Insulin Use at 2 Years in Kidney Transplant Recipients in the Phase 3 Study*

Status of PTDM*	Tacrolimus	CBIR
Patients without pretransplant history of diabetes mellitus	151	151
New onset PTDM*, 1st year	30/151 (20%)	6/151 (4%)
Still insulin dependent at 1 year in those without prior history of diabetes	25/151 (17%)	5/151 (3%)
New onset PTDM* post 1 year	1	0
Patients with PTDM* at 2 years	16/151 (11%)	5/151 (3%)

* Use of insulin for 30 or more consecutive days, with <5 day gap, without a prior history of insulin dependent diabetes mellitus or non-insulin dependent diabetes mellitus.

Insulin-dependent post-transplant diabetes mellitus was reported in 18% and 11% of tacrolimus-treated liver transplant patients and was reversible in 45% and 31% of these patients at 1 year post-transplant, in the US and European randomized studies, respectively (see TABLE 5). Hyperglycemia was associated with the use of tacrolimus in 47% and 33% of liver transplant recipients in the US and European randomized studies, respectively, and may require treatment (see ADVERSE REACTIONS).

Tacrolimus can cause neurotoxicity and nephrotoxicity, particularly when used in high doses. Nephrotoxicity was reported in approximately 52% of kidney transplantation patients

TABLE 4 *Development of Post-Transplant Diabetes Mellitus by Race and by Treatment Group During First Year Post-Kidney Transplantation in the Phase 3 Study*

	Tacrolimus		CBIR	
Patient Race	No. of Patients at Risk	Patients Who Developed PTDM*	No. of Patients at Risk	Patients Who Developed PTDM*
Black	41	15 (37%)	36	3 (8%)
Hispanic	17	5 (29%)	18	1 (6%)
Caucasian	82	10 (12%)	87	1 (1%)
Other	11	0 (0%)	10	1 (10%)
Total	151	30 (20%)	151	6 (4%)

* Use of insulin for 30 or more consecutive days, with <5 day gap, without a prior history of insulin dependent diabetes mellitus or non-insulin dependent diabetes mellitus.

TABLE 5 *Incidence of Post-Transplant Diabetes Mellitus and Insulin Use at 1 Year in Liver Transplant Recipients*

	US Study		European Study	
Status of PTDM*	Tacrolimus	CBIR	Tacrolimus	CBIR
Patients at risk†	239	236	239	249
New onset PTDM*	42 (18%)	30 (13%)	26 (11%)	12 (5%)
Patients still on insulin at 1 year	23 (10%)	19 (8%)	18 (8%)	6 (2%)

* Use of insulin for 30 or more consecutive days, with <5 day gap, without a prior history of insulin dependent diabetes mellitus or non-insulin dependent diabetes mellitus.
† Patients without pretransplant history of diabetes mellitus.

and in 40% and 36% of liver transplantation patients receiving tacrolimus in the US and European randomized trials, respectively (see ADVERSE REACTIONS). More overt nephrotoxicity is seen early after transplantation, characterized by increasing serum creatinine and a decrease in urine output. Patients with impaired renal function should be monitored closely as the dosage of tacrolimus may need to be reduced. In patients with persistent elevations of serum creatinine who are unresponsive to dosage adjustments, consideration should be given to changing to another immunosuppressive therapy. Care should be taken in using tacrolimus with other nephrotoxic drugs. **In particular, to avoid excess nephrotoxicity, tacrolimus should not be used simultaneously with cyclosporine. Tacrolimus or cyclosporine should be discontinued at least 24 hours prior to initiating the other. In the presence of elevated tacrolimus or cyclosporine concentrations, dosing with the other drug usually should be further delayed.**

Mild to severe hyperkalemia was reported in 31% of kidney transplant recipients and in 45% and 13% of liver transplant recipients treated with tacrolimus in the US and European randomized trials, respectively, and may require treatment (see ADVERSE REACTIONS). **Serum potassium levels should be monitored and potassium-sparing diuretics should not be used during tacrolimus therapy (see PRECAUTIONS).**

Neurotoxicity, including tremor, headache, and other changes in motor function, mental status, and sensory function were reported in approximately 55% of liver transplant recipients in the two randomized studies. Tremor occurred more often in tacrolimus-treated kidney transplant patients (54%) compared to cyclosporine-treated patients. The incidence of other neurological events in kidney transplant patients was similar in the two treatment groups (see ADVERSE REACTIONS). Tremor and headache have been associated with high whole-blood concentrations of tacrolimus and may respond to dosage adjustment. Seizures have occurred in adult and pediatric patients receiving tacrolimus (see ADVERSE REACTIONS). Coma and delirium also have been associated with high plasma concentrations of tacrolimus.

As in patients receiving other immunosuppressants, patients receiving tacrolimus are at increased risk of developing lymphomas and other malignancies, particularly of the skin. The risk appears to be related to the intensity and duration of immunosuppression rather than to the use of any specific agent. A lymphoproliferative disorder (LPD) related to Epstein-Barr Virus (EBV) infection has been reported in immunosuppressed organ transplant recipients. The risk of LPD appears greatest in young children who are at risk for primary EBV infection while immunosuppressed or who are switched to tacrolimus following long-term immunosuppression therapy. Because of the danger of oversuppression of the immune system which can increase susceptibility to infection, combination immunosuppressant therapy should be used with caution.

A few patients receiving tacrolimus injection have experienced anaphylactic reactions. Although the exact cause of these reactions is not known, other drugs with castor oil derivatives in the formulation have been associated with anaphylaxis in a small percentage of patients. Because of this potential risk of anaphylaxis, tacrolimus injection should be reserved for patients who are unable to take tacrolimus capsules.

Patients receiving tacrolimus injection should be under continuous observation for at least the first 30 minutes following the start of the infusion and at frequent intervals thereafter. If signs or symptoms of anaphylaxis occur, the infusion should be stopped. An aqueous solution of epinephrine should be available at the bedside as well as a source of oxygen.

PRECAUTIONS

GENERAL

Hypertension is a common adverse effect of tacrolimus therapy (see ADVERSE REACTIONS). Mild or moderate hypertension is more frequently reported than severe hypertension. Antihypertensive therapy may be required; the control of blood pressure can be accomplished with any of the common antihypertensive agents. Since tacrolimus may cause hyperkalemia, potassium-sparing diuretics should be avoided. While calcium-channel blocking agents can be effective in treating tacrolimus-associated hypertension, care should be taken since interference with tacrolimus metabolism may require a dosage reduction (see DRUG INTERACTIONS).

RENALLY AND HEPATICALLY IMPAIRED PATIENTS

For patients with renal insufficiency some evidence suggests that lower doses should be used (see CLINICAL PHARMACOLOGY and DOSAGE AND ADMINISTRATION).

The use of tacrolimus in liver transplant recipients experiencing post-transplant hepatic impairment may be associated with increased risk of developing renal insufficiency related to high whole-blood levels of tacrolimus. These patients should be monitored closely and dosage adjustments should be considered. Some evidence suggests that lower doses should be used in these patients (see DOSAGE AND ADMINISTRATION).

MYOCARDIAL HYPERTROPHY

Myocardial hypertrophy has been reported in association with the administration of tacrolimus, and is generally manifested by echocardiographically demonstrated concentric increases in left ventricular posterior wall and interventricular septum thickness. Hypertrophy has been observed in infants, children and adults. This condition appears reversible in most cases following dose reduction or discontinuance of therapy. In a group of 20 patients with pre- and post-treatment echocardiograms who showed evidence of myocardial hypertrophy, mean tacrolimus whole-blood concentrations during the period prior to diagnosis of myocardial hypertrophy ranged from 11-53 ng/ml in infants (n=10, age 0.4 to 2 years), 4-46 ng/ml in children (n=7, age 2-15 years) and 11-24 ng/ml in adults (n=3, age 37-53 years).

In patients who develop renal failure or clinical manifestations of ventricular dysfunction while receiving tacrolimus therapy, echocardiographic evaluation should be considered. If myocardial hypertrophy is diagnosed, dosage reduction or discontinuation of tacrolimus should be considered.

INFORMATION FOR THE PATIENT

Patients should be informed of the need for repeated appropriate laboratory tests while they are receiving tacrolimus. They should be given complete dosage instructions, advised of the potential risks during pregnancy, and informed of the increased risk of neoplasia. Patients should be informed that changes in dosage should not be undertaken without first consulting their physician.

Patients should be informed that tacrolimus can cause diabetes mellitus and should be advised of the need to see their physician if they develop frequent urination, increased thirst or hunger.

LABORATORY TESTS

Serum creatinine, potassium, and fasting glucose should be assessed regularly. Routine monitoring of metabolic and hematologic systems should be performed as clinically warranted.

CARCINOGENESIS, MUTAGENESIS, AND IMPAIRMENT OF FERTILITY

An increased incidence of malignancy is a recognized complication of immunosuppression in recipients of organ transplants. The most common forms of neoplasms are non-Hodgkin's lymphomas and carcinomas of the skin. As with other immunosuppressive therapies, the risk of malignancies in tacrolimus recipients may be higher than in the normal, healthy population. Lymphoproliferative disorders associated with Epstein-Barr Virus infection have been seen. It has been reported that reduction or discontinuation of immunosuppression may cause the lesions to regress.

No evidence of genotoxicity was seen in bacterial (*Salmonella* and *E. coli*) or mammalian (Chinese hamster lung-derived cells) *in vitro* assays of mutagenicity, the *in vitro* CHO/HGPRT assay of mutagenicity, or *in vivo* clastogenicity assays performed in mice; tacrolimus did not cause unscheduled DNA synthesis in rodent hepatocytes.

Carcinogenicity studies were carried out in male and female rats and mice. In the 80 week mouse study and in the 104 week rat study no relationship of tumor incidence to tacrolimus dosage was found. The highest doses used in the mouse and rat studies were 0.8-2.5 times (mice) and 3.5-7.1 times (rats) the recommended clinical dose range of 0.1-0.2 mg/kg/day when corrected for body surface area.

No impairment of fertility was demonstrated in studies of male and female rats. Tacrolimus, given orally at 1.0 mg/kg (0.7-1.4 times the recommended clinical dose range of 0.1-0.2 mg/kg/day based on body surface area corrections) to male and female rats, prior to and during mating, as well as to dams during gestation and lactation, was associated with embryolethality and with adverse effects on female reproduction. Effects on female reproductive function (parturition) and embryolethal effects were indicated by a higher rate of pre-implantation loss and increased numbers of undelivered and nonviable pups. When given at 3.2 mg/kg (2.3-4.6 times the recommended clinical dose range based on body surface area correction), tacrolimus was associated with maternal and paternal toxicity as well as reproductive toxicity including marked adverse effects on estrus cycles, parturition, pup viability, and pup malformations.

PREGNANCY CATEGORY C

In reproduction studies in rats and rabbits, adverse effects on the fetus were observed mainly at dose levels that were toxic to dams. Tacrolimus at oral doses of 0.32 and 1.0 mg/kg during organogenesis in rabbits was associated with maternal toxicity as well as an increase in incidence of abortions; these doses are equivalent to 0.5-1 times and 1.6-3.3 times the recommended clinical dose range (0.1-0.2 mg/kg) based on body surface area corrections. At the higher dose only, an increased incidence of malformations and developmental variations was also seen. Tacrolimus, at oral doses of 3.2 mg/kg during organogenesis in rats, was associated with maternal toxicity and caused an increase in late resorptions, decreased numbers of live births, and decreased pup weight and viability. Tacrolimus, given orally at 1.0 and 3.2 mg/kg (equivalent to 0.7-1.4 times and 2.3-4.6 times the recommended clinical dose range based on body surface area corrections) to pregnant rats after organogenesis and during lactation, was associated with reduced pup weights.

No reduction in male or female fertility was evident.

There are no adequate and well-controlled studies in pregnant women. Tacrolimus is transferred across the placenta. The use of tacrolimus during pregnancy has been associated with neonatal hyperkalemia and renal dysfunction. Tacrolimus should be used during pregnancy only if the potential benefit to the mother justifies potential risk to the fetus.

NURSING MOTHERS

Since tacrolimus is excreted in human milk, nursing should be avoided.

PEDIATRIC PATIENTS

Experience with tacrolimus in pediatric kidney transplant patients is limited. Successful liver transplants have been performed in pediatric patients (ages up to 16 years) using tacrolimus. Two randomized active-controlled trials of tacrolimus in primary liver transplantation included 56 pediatric patients. Thirty-one (31) patients were randomized to tacrolimus-based and 25 to cyclosporine-based therapies. Additionally, a minimum of 122 pediatric patients were studied in an uncontrolled trial of tacrolimus in living related donor liver transplantation. Pediatric patients generally required higher doses of tacrolimus to maintain blood trough concentrations of tacrolimus similar to adult patients (see DOSAGE AND ADMINISTRATION).

DRUG INTERACTIONS

Due to the potential for additive or synergistic impairment of renal function, care should be taken when administering tacrolimus with drugs that may be associated with renal dysfunction. These include, but are not limited to, aminoglycosides, amphotericin B, and cisplatin. Initial clinical experience with the coadministration of tacrolimus and cyclosporine resulted in additive/synergistic nephrotoxicity. Patients switched from cyclosporine to tacrolimus should receive the first tacrolimus dose no sooner than 24 hours after the last cyclosporine dose. Dosing may be further delayed in the presence of elevated cyclosporine levels.

DRUGS THAT MAY ALTER TACROLIMUS CONCENTRATIONS

Since tacrolimus is metabolized mainly by the CYP3A enzyme systems, substances known to inhibit these enzymes may decrease the metabolism or increase the bioavailability of tacrolimus as indicated by increased whole blood or plasma concentrations. Drugs known to induce these enzyme systems may result in an increased metabolism of tacrolimus or decreased bioavailability as indicated by decreased whole blood or plasma concentrations. Monitoring of blood concentrations and appropriate dosage adjustments are essential when such drugs are used concomitantly.

Drugs that may increase tacrolimus blood concentrations (this list is not all inclusive):

Calcium Channel Blockers: Diltiazem, nicardipine, nifedipine, verapamil.
Antifungal Agents: Clotrimazole, fluconazole, itraconazole, ketoconazole.
Macrolide Antibiotics: Clarithromycin, erythromycin, troleandomycin.
Gastrointestinal Prokinetic Agents: Cisapride, metoclopramide.
Other Drugs: Bromocriptine, cimetidine, cyclosporine, danazol, ethinyl estradiol, methylprednisolone, omeprazole, protease inhibitors, nefazodone.

In a study of 6 normal volunteers, a significant increase in tacrolimus oral bioavailability (14 ± 5% vs 30 ± 8%) was observed with concomitant ketoconazole administration (200 mg). The apparent oral clearance of tacrolimus during ketoconazole administration was significantly decreased compared to tacrolimus alone (0.430 ± 0.129 L/h/kg vs 0.148 ± 0.043 L/h/kg). Overall, IV clearance of tacrolimus was not significantly changed by ketoconazole coadministration, although it was highly variable between patients.

Drugs that may decrease tacrolimus blood concentrations (this list is not all inclusive):

Anticonvulsants: Carbamazepine, phenobarbital, phenytoin.
Antibiotics: Rifabutin, rifampin.
Herbal Preparations: St. John's Wort

St. John's Wort (hypericum perforatum) induces CYP3A4 and P-glycoprotein. Since tacrolimus is a substrate for CYP3A4, there is the potential that the use of St. John's Wort in patients receiving tacrolimus could result in reduced tacrolimus levels.

In a study of 6 normal volunteers, a significant decrease in tacrolimus oral bioavailability (14 ± 6% vs 7 ± 3%) was observed with concomitant rifampin administration (600 mg). In addition, there was a significant increase in tacrolimus clearance (0.036 ± 0.008 L/h/kg vs 0.053 ± 0.010 L/h/kg) with concomitant rifampin administration.

Interaction studies with drugs used in HIV therapy have not been conducted. However, care should be exercised when drugs that are nephrotoxic (*e.g.,* ganciclovir) or that are metabolized by CYP3A (*e.g.,* ritonavir) are administered concomitantly with tacrolimus. Tacrolimus may affect the pharmacokinetics of other drugs (*e.g.,* phenytoin) and increase their concentration. Grapefruit juice affects CYP3A-mediated metabolism and should be avoided (see DOSAGE AND ADMINISTRATION).

OTHER DRUG INTERACTIONS

Immunosuppressants may affect vaccination. Therefore, during treatment with tacrolimus, vaccination may be less effective. The use of live vaccines should be avoided; live vaccines may include, but are not limited to measles, mumps, rubella, oral polio, BCG, yellow fever, and TY 21a typhoid.[1]

ADVERSE REACTIONS

LIVER TRANSPLANTATION

The principal adverse reactions of tacrolimus are tremor, headache, diarrhea, hypertension, nausea, and renal dysfunction. These occur with oral and IV administration of tacrolimus and may respond to a reduction in dosing. Diarrhea was sometimes associated with other gastrointestinal complaints such as nausea and vomiting.

Hyperkalemia and hypomagnesemia have occurred in patients receiving tacrolimus therapy. Hyperglycemia has been noted in many patients; some may require insulin therapy (see WARNINGS).

The incidence of adverse events was determined in two randomized comparative liver transplant trials among 514 patients receiving tacrolimus and steroids and 515 patients receiving a cyclosporine-based regimen (CBIR). The proportion of patients reporting more than one adverse event was 99.8% in the tacrolimus group and 99.6% in the CBIR group. Precautions must be taken when comparing the incidence of adverse events in the US study to that in the European study. The 12 month post-transplant information from the US study and from the European study is presented in TABLE 6. The two studies also included different patient populations and patients were treated with immunosuppressive regimens of differing intensities. Adverse events reported in ≥15% in tacrolimus patients (combined study results) are presented in TABLE 6 for the two controlled trials in liver transplantation.

***TABLE 6** Liver Transplantation — Adverse Events Occurring in ≥15% of Tacrolimus-Treated Patients*

	US Study		European Study	
	Tacrolimus (n=250)	CBIR (n=250)	Tacrolimus (n=264)	CBIR (n=265)
Nervous System				
Headache*	64%	60%	37%	26%
Tremor*	56%	46%	48%	32%
Insomnia	64%	68%	32%	23%
Paresthesia	40%	30%	17%	17%
Gastrointestinal				
Diarrhea	72%	47%	37%	27%
Nausea	46%	37%	32%	27%
Constipation	24%	27%	23%	21%
LFT abnormal	36%	30%	6%	5%
Anorexia	34%	24%	7%	5%
Vomiting	27%	15%	14%	11%
Cardiovascular				
Hypertension†	47%	56%	38%	43%
Urogenital				
Kidney function abnormal*	40%	27%	36%	23%
Creatinine increased*	39%	25%	24%	19%
BUN increased*	30%	22%	12%	9%
Urinary tract infection	16%	18%	21%	19%
Oliguria	18%	15%	19%	12%
Metabolic and Nutritional				
Hyperkalemia*	45%	26%	13%	9%
Hypokalemia	29%	34%	13%	16%
Hyperglycemia*	47%	38%	33%	22%
Hypomagnesemia	48%	45%	16%	9%
Hemic and Lymphatic				
Anemia	47%	38%	5%	1%
Leukocytosis	32%	26%	8%	8%
Thrombocytopenia	24%	20%	14%	19%
Miscellaneous				
Abdominal pain	59%	54%	29%	22%
Pain	63%	57%	24%	22%
Fever	48%	56%	19%	22%
Asthenia	52%	48%	11%	7%
Back pain	30%	29%	17%	17%
Ascites	27%	22%	7%	8%
Peripheral edema	26%	26%	12%	14%
Respiratory System				
Pleural effusion	30%	32%	36%	35%
Atelectasis	28%	30%	5%	4%
Dyspnea	9%	23%	5%	4%
Skin and Appendages				
Pruritus	36%	20%	15%	7%
Rash	24%	19%	10%	4%

* See WARNINGS.
† See PRECAUTIONS.

Less frequently observed adverse reactions in both liver transplantation and kidney transplantation patients are described in Less Frequently Reported Adverse Reactions.

KIDNEY TRANSPLANTATION

The most common adverse reactions reported were infection, tremor, hypertension, decreased renal function, constipation, diarrhea, headache, abdominal pain, and insomnia.

Adverse events that occurred in ≥15% of tacrolimus-treated kidney transplant patients are presented in TABLE 7.

Less frequently observed adverse reactions in both liver transplantation and kidney transplantation patients are described in Less Frequently Reported Adverse Reactions.

LESS FREQUENTLY REPORTED ADVERSE REACTIONS

The following adverse events were reported in the range of 3% to less than 15% incidence in either liver or kidney transplant recipients who were treated with tacrolimus in the Phase 3 comparative trials.

Nervous System: See WARNINGS. Abnormal dreams, agitation, amnesia, anxiety, confusion, convulsion, depression, dizziness, emotional lability, encephalopathy, hallucinations, hypertonia, incoordination, myoclonus, nervousness, neuropathy, psychosis, somnolence, thinking abnormal.
Special Senses: Abnormal vision, amblyopia, ear pain, otitis media, tinnitus.
Gastrointestinal: Anorexia, cholangitis, cholestatic jaundice, dyspepsia, dysphagia, esophagitis, flatulence, gastritis, gastrointestinal hemorrhage, GGT increase, GI perforation, hepatitis, ileus, increased appetite, jaundice, liver damage, liver function test abnormal, oral moniliasis, rectal disorder, stomatitis.
Cardiovascular: Angina pectoris, chest pain, deep thrombophlebitis, abnormal ECG, hemorrhage, hypotension, postural hypotension, peripheral vascular disorder, phlebitis, tachycardia, thrombosis, vasodilatation.
Urogenital: See WARNINGS. Albuminuria, cystitis, dysuria, hematuria, hydronephrosis, kidney failure, kidney tubular necrosis, nocturia, pyuria, toxic nephropathy, oliguria, urinary frequency, urinary incontinence, vaginitis.
Metabolic/Nutritional: Acidosis, alkaline phosphatase increased, alkalosis, ALT (SGPT) increased, AST (SGOT) increased, bicarbonate decreased, bilirubinemia, BUN increased, dehydration, GGT increased, healing abnormal, hypercalcemia, hypercholesterolemia, hyperlipemia, hyperphosphatemia, hyperuricemia, hyperv-

T

TABLE 7 *Kidney Transplantation — Adverse Events Occurring in ≥15% of Tacrolimus-Treated Patients*

	Tacrolimus (n=205)	CBIR (n=207)
Nervous System		
Tremor*	54%	34%
Headache*	44%	38%
Insomnia	32%	30%
Paresthesia	23%	16%
Dizziness	19%	16%
Gastrointestinal		
Diarrhea	44%	41%
Nausea	38%	36%
Constipation	35%	43%
Vomiting	29%	23%
Dyspepsia	28%	20%
Cardiovascular		
Hypertension†	50%	52%
Chest pain	19%	13%
Urogenital		
Creatinine increased*	45%	42%
Urinary tract infection	34%	35%
Metabolic and Nutritional		
Hypophosphatemia	49%	53%
Hypomagnesemia	34%	17%
Hyperlipemia	31%	38%
Hyperkalemia*	31%	32%
Diabetes mellitus*	24%	9%
Hypokalemia	22%	25%
Hyperglycemia*	22%	16%
Edema	18%	19%
Hemic and Lymphatic		
Anemia	30%	24%
Leukopenia	15%	17%
Miscellaneous		
Infection	45%	49%
Peripheral edema	36%	48%
Asthenia	34%	30%
Abdominal pain	33%	31%
Pain	32%	30%
Fever	29%	29%
Back pain	24%	20%
Respiratory System		
Dyspnea	22%	18%
Cough increased	18%	15%
Musculoskeletal		
Arthralgia	25%	24%
Skin		
Rash	17%	12%
Pruritus	15%	7%

* See WARNINGS.
† See PRECAUTIONS.

olemia, hypocalcemia, hypoglycemia, hyponatremia, hypophosphatemia, hypoproteinemia, lactic dehydrogenase increase, weight gain.

Endocrine: See PRECAUTIONS. Cushing's syndrome, diabetes mellitus.

Hemic/Lymphatic: Coagulation disorder, ecchymosis, hypochromic anemia, leukocytosis, leukopenia, polycythemia, prothrombin decreased, serum iron decreased, thrombocytopenia.

Miscellaneous: Abdomen enlarged, abscess, accidental injury, allergic reaction, cellulitis, chills, flu syndrome, generalized edema, hernia, peritonitis, photosensitivity reaction, sepsis.

Musculoskeletal: Arthralgia, cramps, generalized spasm, joint disorder, leg cramps, myalgia, myasthenia, osteoporosis.

Respiratory: Asthma, bronchitis, cough increased, lung disorder, pneumothorax, pulmonary edema, pharyngitis, pneumonia, respiratory disorder, rhinitis, sinusitis, voice alteration.

Skin: Acne, alopecia, exfoliative dermatitis, fungal dermatitis, herpes simplex, hirsutism, skin discoloration, skin disorder, skin ulcer, sweating.

The overall safety profile of the tacrolimus-mycophenolate mofetil Phase 4 study did not differ from the safety profile of the Phase 3 kidney study.

T

POSTMARKETING

The following have been reported: Increased amylase including pancreatitis, hearing loss including deafness, leukoencephalopathy, thrombocytopenic purpura, hemolytic-uremic syndrome, acute renal failure, Stevens-Johnson syndrome, stomach ulcer, glycosuria, cardiac arrhythmia, and gastroenteritis.

There have been rare spontaneous reports of myocardial hypertrophy associated with clinically manifested ventricular dysfunction in patients receiving tacrolimus therapy (see PRECAUTIONS, Myocardial Hypertrophy).

DOSAGE AND ADMINISTRATION

TACROLIMUS INJECTION

For IV Infusion Only.

Note: Anaphylactic reactions have occurred with injectables containing castor oil derivatives. See WARNINGS.

In patients unable to take oral tacrolimus capsules, therapy may be initiated with tacrolimus injection. The initial dose of tacrolimus should be administered no sooner than 6 hours after transplantation. The recommended starting dose of tacrolimus injection is 0.03-0.05 mg/kg/day as a continuous IV infusion. Adult patients should receive doses at the lower end of the dosing range. Concomitant adrenal corticosteroid therapy is recommended early post-transplantation. Continuous IV infusion of tacrolimus injection should be continued only until the patient can tolerate oral administration of tacrolimus capsules.

Preparation for Administration/Stability

Tacrolimus injection must be diluted with 0.9% sodium chloride injection or 5% dextrose injection to a concentration between 0.004 and 0.02 mg/ml prior to use. Diluted infusion solution should be stored in glass or polyethylene containers and should be discarded after 24 hours. The diluted infusion solution should not be stored in a PVC container due to decreased stability and the potential for extraction of phthalates. In situations where more dilute solutions are utilized (*e.g.*, pediatric dosing, etc.), PVC-free tubing should likewise be used to minimize the potential for significant drug adsorption onto the tubing. Parenteral drug products should be inspected visually for particulate matter and discoloration prior to administration, whenever solution and container permit. Due to the chemical instability of tacrolimus in alkaline media, tacrolimus injection should not be mixed or co-infused with solutions of pH 9 or greater (*e.g.*, ganciclovir or acyclovir).

TACROLIMUS CAPSULES

TABLE 8 *Summary of Initial Oral Dosage Recommendations and Typical Whole Blood Trough Concentrations*

Patient Population	Recommended Initial Oral Dose*	Typical Whole Blood Trough Concentrations
Adult kidney transplant patients	0.2 mg/kg/day	month 1-3 : 7-20 ng/ml month 4-12 : 5-15 ng/ml
Adult liver transplant patients	0.10-0.15 mg/kg/day	month 1-12 : 5-20 ng/ml
Pediatric liver transplant patients	0.15-0.20 mg/kg/day	month 1-12 : 5-20 ng/ml

* **Note:** 2 divided doses, q12h.

LIVER TRANSPLANTATION

It is recommended that patients initiate oral therapy with tacrolimus capsules if possible. If IV therapy is necessary, conversion from IV to oral tacrolimus is recommended as soon as oral therapy can be tolerated. This usually occurs within 2-3 days. The initial dose of tacrolimus should be administered no sooner than 6 hours after transplantation. In a patient receiving an IV infusion, the first dose of oral therapy should be given 8-12 hours after discontinuing the IV infusion. The recommended starting oral dose of tacrolimus capsules is 0.10-0.15 mg/kg/day administered in two divided daily doses every 12 hours. Coadministered grapefruit juice has been reported to increase tacrolimus blood trough concentrations in liver transplant patients. (See DRUG INTERACTIONS, Drugs That May Alter Tacrolimus Concentrations.)

Dosing should be titrated based on clinical assessments of rejection and tolerability. Lower tacrolimus dosages may be sufficient as maintenance therapy. Adjunct therapy with adrenal corticosteroids is recommended early post-transplant.

Dosage and typical tacrolimus whole blood trough concentrations are shown in TABLE 8; blood concentration details are described in Blood Concentration Monitoring, Liver Transplantation.

KIDNEY TRANSPLANTATION

The recommended starting oral dose of tacrolimus is 0.2 mg/kg/day administered every 12 hours in 2 divided doses. The initial dose of tacrolimus may be administered within 24 hours of transplantation, but should be delayed until renal function has recovered (as indicated for example by a serum creatinine <4 mg/dl). Black patients may require higher doses to achieve comparable blood concentrations. Dosage and typical tacrolimus whole blood trough concentrations are shown in TABLE 8; blood concentration details are described in Blood Concentration Monitoring, Kidney Transplantation.

The data in kidney transplant patients indicate that the Black patients required a higher dose to attain comparable trough concentrations compared to Caucasian patients.

TABLE 9

Time After Transplant	Caucasian (n=114) Dose (mg/kg)	Caucasian (n=114) Trough Concentrations (ng/ml)	Black (n=56) Dose (mg/kg)	Black (n=56) Trough Concentrations (ng/ml)
Day 7	0.18	12.0	0.23	10.9
Month 1	0.17	12.8	0.26	12.9
Month 6	0.14	11.8	0.24	11.5
Month 12	0.13	10.1	0.19	11.0

PEDIATRIC PATIENTS

Pediatric liver transplantation patients without pre-existing renal or hepatic dysfunction have required and tolerated higher doses than adults to achieve similar blood concentrations. Therefore, it is recommended that therapy be initiated in pediatric patients at a starting IV dose of 0.03-0.05 mg/kg/day and a starting oral dose of 0.15-0.20 mg/kg/day. Dose adjustments may be required. Experience in pediatric kidney transplantation patients is limited.

PATIENTS WITH HEPATIC OR RENAL DYSFUNCTION

Due to the reduced clearance and prolonged half-life, patients with severe hepatic impairment (Pugh ≥10) may require lower doses of tacrolimus. Close monitoring of blood concentrations is warranted.

Due to the potential for nephrotoxicity, patients with renal or hepatic impairment should receive doses at the lowest value of the recommended IV and oral dosing ranges. Further reductions in dose below these ranges may be required. Tacrolimus therapy usually should be delayed up to 48 hours or longer in patients with post-operative oliguria.

CONVERSION FROM ONE IMMUNOSUPPRESSIVE REGIMEN TO ANOTHER

Tacrolimus should not be used simultaneously with cyclosporine. Tacrolimus or cyclosporine should be discontinued at least 24 hours before initiating the other. In the presence of elevated tacrolimus or cyclosporine concentrations, dosing with the other drug usually should be further delayed.

BLOOD CONCENTRATION MONITORING

Monitoring of tacrolimus blood concentrations in conjunction with other laboratory and clinical parameters is considered an essential aid to patient management for the evaluation of rejection, toxicity, dose adjustments and compliance. Factors influencing frequency of monitoring include but are not limited to hepatic or renal dysfunction, the addition or discontinuation of potentially interacting drugs and the post-transplant time. Blood concentration monitoring is not a replacement for renal and liver function monitoring and tissue biopsies.

Two methods have been used for the assay of tacrolimus, a microparticle enzyme immunoassay (MEIA) and an ELISA. Both methods have the same monoclonal antibody for tacrolimus. Comparison of the concentrations in published literature to patient concentrations using the current assays must be made with detailed knowledge of the assay methods and biological matrices employed. Whole blood is the matrix of choice and specimens should be collected into tubes containing ethylene diamine tetraacetic acid (EDTA) anticoagulant. Heparin anti-coagulation is not recommended because of the tendency to form clots on storage. Samples which are not analyzed immediately should be stored at room temperature or in a refrigerator and assayed within 7 days; if samples are to be kept longer they should be deep frozen at -20°C for up to 12 months.

Liver Transplantation

Although there is a lack of direct correlation between tacrolimus concentrations and drug efficacy, data from Phase 2 and 3 studies of liver transplant patients have shown an increasing incidence of adverse events with increasing trough blood concentrations. Most patients are stable when trough whole blood concentrations are maintained between 5-20 ng/ml. Long-term post-transplant patients often are maintained at the low end of this target range.

Data from the US clinical trial show that tacrolimus whole blood concentrations, as measured by ELISA, were most variable during the first week post-transplantation. After this early period, the median trough blood concentrations, measured at intervals from the second week to 1 year post-transplantation, ranged from 9.8-19.4 ng/ml.

Therapeutic Drug Monitoring, 1995, Volume 17, Number 6 contains a consensus document and several position papers regarding the therapeutic monitoring of tacrolimus from the 1995 International Consensus Conference on Immunosuppressive Drugs. Refer to these manuscripts for further discussions of tacrolimus monitoring.

Kidney Transplantation

Data from the Phase 3 study indicates that trough concentrations of tacrolimus in whole blood, as measured by IMx, were most variable during the first week of dosing. During the first 3 months, 80% of the patients maintained trough concentrations between 7-20 ng/ml, and then between 5-15 ng/ml, through 1 year.

The relative risk of toxicity is increased with higher trough concentrations. Therefore, monitoring of whole blood trough concentrations is recommended to assist in the clinical evaluation of toxicity.

HOW SUPPLIED

PROGRAF CAPSULES

Prograf capsules are available as follows:

0.5 mg: Oblong, light yellow, branded with red "0.5 mg" on the capsule cap and the Fujisawa Healthcare logo and "607" on the capsule body.

1 mg: Oblong, white, branded with red "1 mg" on the capsule cap and Fujisawa Healthcare logo and "617" on the capsule body.

5 mg: Oblong, grayish/red, branded with white "5 mg" on the capsule cap and Fujisawa Healthcare logo and "657" on the capsule body.

Store and Dispense: Store at 25°C (77°F); excursions permitted to 15-30°C (59-86°F).

PROGRAF INJECTION

5 mg (for IV infusion only): Supplied as a sterile solution in 1 ml ampules containing the equivalent of 5 mg of anhydrous tacrolimus per ml.

Store and Dispense: Store between 5 and 25°C (41 and 77°F).

TOPICAL

DESCRIPTION

FOR DERMATOLOGIC USE ONLY NOT FOR OPHTHALMIC USE.

Protopic (tacrolimus) ointment contains tacrolimus, a macrolide immunosuppressant produced by *Streptomyces tsukubaensis.* It is for topical dermatologic use only. Chemically, tacrolimus is designated as [3*S*-[3*R**[*E*(1*S**,3*S**,4*S**)],4*S**,5*R**,8*S**,9*E*,12*R**,14*R**,15*S**,16*R**,18*S**,19*S**,26a*R**]]-5,6,8,11,12,13,14,15,16,17,18,19,24,25,26,26a-hexadecahydro-5,19-dihydroxy-3-[2-(4-hydroxy-3-methoxycyclohexyl)-1-methylethenyl]-14,16-dimethoxy-4,10,12,18-tetramethyl-8-(2-propenyl)-15,19-epoxy-3H-pyrido[2,1-*c*][1,4]oxaazacyclotricosine-1,7,20,21(4H,23H)-tetrone, monohydrate.

Tacrolimus has an empirical formula of $C_{44}H_{69}NO_{12}{\cdot}H_2O$ and a formula weight of 822.05. Each gram of Protopic ointment contains (w/w) either 0.03% or 0.1% of tacrolimus in a base of mineral oil, paraffin, propylene carbonate, white petrolatum and white wax.

CLINICAL PHARMACOLOGY

MECHANISM OF ACTION

The mechanism of action of tacrolimus in atopic dermatitis is not known. While the following have been observed, the clinical significance of these observations in atopic dermatitis is not known. It has been demonstrated that tacrolimus inhibits T-lymphocyte activation by first binding to an intracellular protein, FKBP-12. A complex of tacrolimus-FKBP-12, calcium, calmodulin, and calcineurin is then formed and the phosphatase activity of calcineurin is inhibited. This effect has been shown to prevent the dephosphorylation and translocation of nuclear factor of activated T-cells (NF-AT), a nuclear component thought to initiate gene transcription for the formation of lymphokines (such as interleukin-2, gamma interferon). Tacrolimus also inhibits the transcription for genes which encode IL-3, IL-4, IL-5, GM-CSF, and TNF-α, all of which are involved in the early stages of T-cell activation. Additionally, tacrolimus has been shown to inhibit the release of pre-formed mediators from skin mast cells and basophils, and to downregulate the expression of FcεRI on Langerhans cells.

PHARMACOKINETICS

The pooled results from two pharmacokinetic studies in 49 adult atopic dermatitis patients indicate that tacrolimus is absorbed after the topical application of 0.1% tacrolimus ointment. Peak tacrolimus blood concentrations ranged from undetectable to 20 ng/ml after single or multiple doses of 0.1% tacrolimus ointment, with 45 of the 49 patients having peak blood concentrations less than 5 ng/ml. The results from a pharmacokinetic study of 0.1% tacrolimus ointment in 20 pediatric atopic dermatitis patients (ages 6-13 years), show peak tacrolimus blood concentrations below 1.6 ng/ml in all patients.

There was no evidence based on blood concentrations that tacrolimus accumulates systemically upon intermittent topical application for periods of up to 1 year. The absolute bioavailability of topical tacrolimus is unknown. Using IV historical data for comparison, the bioavailability of tacrolimus from tacrolimus ointment in atopic dermatitis patients is less than 0.5%. In adults with an average of 53% BSA treated, exposure (*i.e.,* AUC) of tacrolimus from tacrolimus ointment is approximately 30-fold less than that seen with oral immunosuppressive doses in kidney and liver transplant patients. The lowest tacrolimus blood level at which systemic effects can be observed is not known.

INDICATIONS AND USAGE

Tacrolimus ointment, both 0.03% and 0.1% for adults, and only 0.03% for children aged 2-15 years, is indicated for short-term and intermittent long-term therapy in the treatment of patients with moderate to severe atopic dermatitis in whom the use of alternative, conventional therapies are deemed inadvisable because of potential risks, or in the treatment of patients who are not adequately responsive to or are intolerant of alternative, conventional therapies.

NON-FDA APPROVED INDICATIONS

Tacrolimus topical has been reported to be effective in the treatment of recalcitrant facial erythema and steroid-induced rosacea. However, these uses have not been approved by the FDA and further clinical trials are needed.

CONTRAINDICATIONS

Tacrolimus ointment is contraindicated in patients with a history of hypersensitivity to tacrolimus or any other component of the preparation.

PRECAUTIONS

GENERAL

Studies have not evaluated the safety and efficacy of tacrolimus ointment in the treatment of clinically infected atopic dermatitis. Before commencing treatment with tacrolimus ointment, clinical infections at treatment sites should be cleared.

While patients with atopic dermatitis are predisposed to superficial skin infections including eczema herpeticum (Kaposi's varicelliform eruption), treatment with tacrolimus ointment may be associated with an increased risk of varicella zoster virus infection (chicken pox or shingles), herpes simplex virus infection, or eczema herpeticum. In the presence of these infections, the balance of risks and benefits associated with tacrolimus ointment use should be evaluated.

In clinical studies, 33 cases of lymphadenopathy (0.8%) were reported and were usually related to infections (particularly of the skin) and noted to resolve upon appropriate antibiotic therapy. Of these 33 cases, the majority had either a clear etiology or were known to resolve. Transplant patients receiving immunosuppressive regimens (*e.g.,* systemic tacrolimus) are at increased risk for developing lymphoma; therefore, patients who receive tacrolimus ointment and who develop lymphadenopathy should have the etiology of their lymphadenopathy investigated. In the absence of a clear etiology for the lymphadenopathy, or in the presence of acute infectious mononucleosis, discontinuation of tacrolimus ointment should be considered. Patients who develop lymphadenopathy should be monitored to ensure that the lymphadenopathy resolves.

The enhancement of ultraviolet carcinogenicity is not necessarily dependent on phototoxic mechanisms. Despite the absence of observed phototoxicity in humans (see ADVERSE REACTIONS), tacrolimus ointment shortened the time to skin tumor formation in an animal photocarcinogenicity study (see Carcinogenesis, Mutagenesis, and Impairment of Fertility). Therefore, it is prudent for patients to minimize or avoid natural or artificial sunlight exposure.

The use of tacrolimus ointment may cause local symptoms such as skin burning (burning sensation, stinging, soreness) or pruritus. Localized symptoms are most common during the first few days of tacrolimus ointment application and typically improve as the lesions of atopic dermatitis heal. With tacrolimus ointment 0.1%, 90% of the skin burning events had a duration between 2 minutes and 3 hours (median 15 minutes). Ninety percent (90%) of the pruritus events had a duration between 3 minutes and 10 hours (median 20 minutes).

The use of tacrolimus ointment in patients with Netherton's Syndrome is not recommended due to the potential for increased systemic absorption of tacrolimus. The safety of tacrolimus ointment has not been established in patients with generalized erythroderma.

INFORMATION FOR THE PATIENT

Refer to the Patient Instructions that are distributed with the prescription for complete instructions.

T

Patients using tacrolimus ointment should receive the following information and instructions:

Patients should use tacrolimus ointment as directed by the physician. Tacrolimus ointment is for external use only. As with any topical medication, patients or caregivers should wash hands after application if hands are not an area for treatment.

Patients should minimize or avoid exposure to natural or artificial sunlight (tanning beds or UVA/B treatment) while using tacrolimus ointment.

Patients should not use this medication for any disorder other than that for which it was prescribed.

Patients should report any signs of adverse reactions to their physician.

Before applying tacrolimus ointment after a bath or shower, be sure your skin is completely dry.

CARCINOGENESIS, MUTAGENESIS, AND IMPAIRMENT OF FERTILITY

No evidence of genotoxicity was seen in bacterial (*Salmonella* and *E. coli*) or mammalian (Chinese hamster lung-derived cells) *in vitro* assays of mutagenicity, the *in vitro* CHO/HGPRT assay of mutagenicity, or *in vivo* clastogenicity assays performed in mice. Tacrolimus did not use unscheduled DNA synthesis in rodent hepatocytes.

Oral (feed) carcinogenicity studies have been carried out with systemically administered tacrolimus in male and female rats and mice. In the 80 week mouse study and in the 104 week rat study no relationship of tumor incidence to tacrolimus dosage was found at daily doses up to 3 mg/kg [9 times the maximum recommended human dose (MRHD) based on AUC comparisons] and 5 mg/kg (3 times theMRHD based on AUC comparisons), respectively.

A 104 week dermal carcinogenicity study was performed in mice with tacrolimus ointment (0.03 to 3%), equivalent to tacrolimus doses of 1.1-118 mg/kg/day or 3.3-354 mg/m^2/day. In the study, the incidence of skin tumors was minimal and the topical application of tacrolimus was not associated with skin tumor formation under ambient room lighting. However, a statistically significant elevation in the incidence of pleomorphic lymphoma in high dose male (25/50) and female animals (27/50) and in the incidence of undifferentiated lymphoma in high dose female animals (13/50) was noted in the mouse dermal carcinogenicity study. Lymphomas were noted in the mouse dermal carcinogenicity study at a daily dose of 3.5 mg/kg (0.1% tacrolimus ointment) (26 times MRHD based on AUC comparisons). No drug-related tumors were noted in the mouse dermal carcinogenicity study at a daily dose of 1.1 mg/kg (0.03% tacrolimus ointment) (10 times MRHD based on AUC comparisons).

In a 52 week photocarcinogenicity study, the median time to onset of skin tumor formation was decreased in hairless mice following chronic topical dosing with concurrent exposure to UV radiation (40 weeks of treatment followed by 12 weeks of observation) with tacrolimus ointment at ≥0.1% tacrolimus.

Reproductive toxicology studies were not performed with topical tacrolimus. In studies of oral tacrolimus no impairment of fertility was seen in male and female rats. Tacrolimus, given orally at 1.0 mg/kg (0.12 times MRHD based on body surface area [BSA]) to male and female rats, prior to and during mating, as well as to dams during gestation and lactation, was associated with embryolethality and with adverse effects on female reproduction. Effects on female reproductive function (parturition) and embryolethal effects were indicated by a higher rate of pre-implantation loss and increased numbers of undelivered and nonviable pups. When given at 3.2 mg/kg (0.43 times MRHD based on BSA), tacrolimus was associated with maternal and paternal toxicity as well as reproductive toxicity including marked adverse effects on estrus cycles, parturition, pup viability, and pup malformations.

PREGNANCY, TERATOGENIC EFFECTS, PREGNANCY CATEGORY C

There are no adequate and well-controlled studies of topically administered tacrolimus in pregnant women. The experience with tacrolimus ointment when used by pregnant women is too limited to permit assessment of the safety of its use during pregnancy.

Reproduction studies were carried out with systemically administered tacrolimus in rats and rabbits. Adverse effects on the fetus were observed mainly at oral dose levels that were toxic to dams. Tacrolimus at oral doses of 0.32 and 1.0 mg/kg (0.04-0.12 times MRHD based on BSA) during organogenesis in rabbits was associated with maternal toxicity as well as an increase in incidence of abortions. At the higher dose only, an increased incidence of malformations and developmental variations was also seen. Tacrolimus, at oral doses of 3.2 mg/kg during organogenesis in rats, was associated with maternal toxicity and caused an increase in late resorptions, decreased numbers of live births, and decreased pup weight and viability. Tacrolimus, given orally at 1.0 and 3.2 mg/kg (0.04-0.12 times MRHD based on BSA) to pregnant rats after organogenesis and during lactation, was associated with reduced pup weights.

No reduction in male or female fertility was evident.

There are no adequate and well-controlled studies of systemically administered tacrolimus in pregnant women. Tacrolimus is transferred across the placenta. The use of systemically administered tacrolimus during pregnancy has been associated with neonatal hyperkalemia and renal dysfunction. Tacrolimus ointment should be used during pregnancy only if the potential benefit to the mother justifies a potential risk to the fetus.

NURSING MOTHERS

Although systemic absorption of tacrolimus following topical applications of tacrolimus ointment is minimal relative to systemic administration, it is known that tacrolimus is excreted in human milk. Because of the potential for serious adverse reactions in nursing infants from tacrolimus, a decision should be made whether to discontinue nursing or to discontinue the drug, taking into account the importance of the drug to the mother.

PEDIATRIC USE

Tacrolimus ointment 0.03% may be used in pediatric patients 2 years of age and older. Two Phase 3 pediatric studies were conducted involving 606 patients 2-15 years of age: one 12 week randomized vehicle-controlled study and one open-label, 1 year, long-term safety study. Three hundred and thirty (330) of these patients were 2-6 years of age.

The most common adverse events associated with tacrolimus ointment application in pediatric patients were skin burning and pruritus (see ADVERSE REACTIONS). In addition to skin burning and pruritus, the less common events (<5%) of varicella zoster (mostly chicken pox), and vesiculobullous rash were more frequent in patients treated with tacrolimus ointment 0.03% compared to vehicle. In the long-term 1 year safety study involving 255 pediatric patients using tacrolimus ointment, the incidence of adverse events, including infections, did not increase with increased duration of study drug exposure or amount of ointment used. In 491 pediatric patients treated with tacrolimus ointment 3 (0.6%) developed eczema herpeticum. Since the safety and efficacy of tacrolimus ointment have not been established in pediatric patients below 2 years of age, its use in this age group is not recommended.

GERIATRIC USE

Twenty-five (25) patients ≥65 years old received tacrolimus ointment in Phase 3 studies. The adverse event profile for these patients was consistent with that for other adult patients.

DRUG INTERACTIONS

Formal topical drug interaction studies with tacrolimus ointment have not been conducted. Based on its minimal extent of absorption, interactions of tacrolimus ointment with systemically administered drugs are unlikely to occur but cannot be ruled out. The concomitant administration of known CYP3A4 inhibitors in patients with widespread and/or erythrodermic disease should be done with caution. Some examples of such drugs are erythromycin, itraconazole, ketoconazole, fluconazole, calcium channel blockers, and cimetidine.

TABLE 11A *Incidence of Treatment Emergent Adverse Events — Adults*

		Ointment		
Incidence	**Vehicle n=212**	**0.03%* n=210**	**0.1%* n=209**	**0.1%† n=316**
Skin burning‡	26%	46%	58%	47%
Pruritus‡	37%	46%	46%	25%
Flu-like symptoms‡	19%	23%	31%	22%
Allergic reaction	8%	12%	6%	22%
Skin erythema	20%	25%	28%	12%
Headache‡	11%	20%	19%	10%
Skin infection	11%	12%	5%	11%
Fever	4%	4%	1%	2%
Infection	1%	1%	2%	14%
Cough increased	2%	1%	1%	3%
Asthma	4%	6%	4%	5%
Herpes simplex	4%	4%	4%	12%
Eczema herpeticum	0%	1%	1%	2%
Pharyngitis	3%	3%	4%	5%
Accidental injury	4%	3%	6%	4%
Pustular rash	2%	3%	4%	6%
Folliculitis‡	1%	6%	4%	11%
Rhinitis	4%	3%	2%	5%
Otitis media	4%	0%	1%	1%
Sinusitis‡	1%	4%	2%	3%
Diarrhea	3%	3%	4%	4%
Urticaria	3%	3%	6%	5%
Lack of drug effect	1%	1%	0%	10%
Bronchitis	0%	2%	2%	3%
Vomiting	0%	1%	1%	1%
Maculopapular rash	2%	2%	2%	4%
Rash‡	1%	5%	2%	2%
Abdominal pain	3%	1%	1%	1%
Fungal dermatitis	0%	2%	1%	2%
Gastroenteritis	1%	2%	2%	4%
Alcohol intolerance‡	0%	3%	7%	6%
Acne‡	2%	4%	7%	2%
Sunburn	1%	2%	1%	4%
Skin disorder	2%	2%	1%	1%
Conjunctivitis	0%	2%	2%	4%
Pain	1%	2%	1%	4%
Vesiculobullous rash‡	3%	3%	2%	2%
Lymphadenopathy	2%	2%	1%	2%
Nausea	4%	3%	2%	1%
Skin tingling‡	2%	3%	8%	2%
Face edema	2%	2%	1%	3%
Dyspepsia‡	1%	1%	4%	1%
Dry skin	7%	3%	3%	0%
Hyperesthesia‡	1%	3%	7%	3%
Skin neoplasm benign§	1%	1%	1%	2%
Back pain‡	0%	2%	2%	3%
Peripheral edema	2%	4%	3%	2%
Varicella zoster/Herpes zoster‡¤	0%	1%	0%	1%
Contact dermatitis	1%	3%	3%	1%
Asthenia	1%	2%	3%	2%
Pneumonia	0%	1%	1%	1%
Eczema	2%	2%	2%	3%
Insomnia	3%	4%	3%	1%
Exfoliative dermatitis	3%	3%	1%	0%
Dysmenorrhea	2%	4%	4%	0%
Periodontal abscess	1%	0%	1%	3%
Myalgia‡	0%	3%	2%	1%
Cyst‡	0%	1%	3%	0%

* 12 week, randomized, double-blind, Phase 3 studies.
† Open-label studies (up to 1 year).
‡ May be reasonably associated with the use of this drug product.
§ Generally "warts".
¤ Four cases of chicken pox in the pediatric 12 week study; 1 case of "zoster of the lip" in the adult 12 week study; 7 cases of chicken pox and 1 case of shingles in the open-label pediatric study; 2 cases of herpes zoster in the open-label adult study.

T

ADVERSE REACTIONS

No phototoxicity and no photoallergenicity was detected in clinical studies of 12 and 216 normal volunteers, respectively. One (1) out of 198 normal volunteers showed evidence of sensitization in a contact sensitization study.

In three randomized vehicle-controlled studies and two long-term safety studies, 655 and 571 patients respectively, were treated with tacrolimus ointment.

TABLE 11A and TABLE 11B depict the adjusted incidence of adverse events pooled across the 3 identically designed 12 week studies for patients in vehicle, tacrolimus ointment 0.03%, and tacrolimus ointment 0.1% treatment groups, and the unadjusted incidence of adverse events in two 1 year long-term safety studies, regardless of relationship to study drug.

TABLE 11B *Incidence of Treatment Emergent Adverse Events — Pediatric*

		Ointment	
	Vehicle	**0.03%***	**0.1%†**
Incidence	**n=116**	**n=118**	**n=255**
Skin burning‡	29%	43%	26%
Pruritus‡	27%	41%	25%
Flu-like symptoms‡	25%	28%	35%
Allergic Reaction	8%	4%	15%
Skin erythema	13%	12%	9%
Headache‡	8%	5%	18%
Skin infection	14%	10%	11%
Fever	13%	21%	18%
Infection	9%	7%	8%
Cough increased	14%	18%	15%
Asthma	6%	6%	16%
Herpes simplex	2%	0%	5%
Eczema herpeticum	0%	2%	0%
Pharyngitis	11%	6%	10%
Accidental injury	3%	6%	12%
Pustular rash	3%	2%	8%
Folliculitis‡	0%	2%	2%
Rhinitis	2%	6%	5%
Otitis media	6%	12%	7%
Sinusitis‡	8%	3%	7%
Diarrhea	2%	5%	6%
Urticaria	1%	1%	5%
Lack of drug effect	1%	1%	2%
Bronchitis	3%	3%	6%
Vomiting	7%	6%	5%
Maculopapular rash	3%	0%	3%
Rash‡	4%	2%	5%
Abdominal pain	2%	3%	5%
Fungal dermatitis	3%	0%	6%
Gastroenteritis	3%	0%	2%
Alcohol intolerance‡	0%	0%	0%
Acne‡	1%	0%	4%
Sunburn	0%	0%	4%
Skin disorder	1%	4%	4%
Conjunctivitis	2%	1%	2%
Pain	0%	1%	3%
Vesiculobullous rash‡	0%	4%	2%
Lymphadenopathy	0%	3%	3%
Nausea	0%	1%	2%
Skin tingling‡	1%	2%	1%
Face edema	2%	1%	1%
Dyspepsia‡	0%	0%	4%
Dry skin	0%	1%	1%
Hyperesthesia‡	0%	0%	0%
Skin neoplasm benign§	0%	0%	3%
Back pain‡	1%	1%	1%
Peripheral edema	0%	0%	1%
Varicella zoster/Herpes zoster‡¤	0%	5%	3%
Contact dermatitis	3%	4%	1%
Asthenia	0%	0%	1%
Pneumonia	2%	0%	2%
Eczema	0%	0%	0%
Insomnia	1%	1%	0%
Exfoliative dermatitis	0%	0%	2%
Dysmenorrhea	0%	0%	2%
Periodontal abscess	0%	0%	0%
Myalgia‡	0%	0%	0%
Cyst‡	0%	0%	0%

* 12 week, randomized, double-blind, Phase 3 studies.
† Open-label studies (up to 1 year).
‡ May be reasonably associated with the use of this drug product.
§ Generally "warts".
¤ Four cases of chicken pox in the pediatric 12 week study; 1 case of "zoster of the lip" in the adult 12 week study; 7 cases of chicken pox and 1 case of shingles in the open-label pediatric study; 2 cases of herpes zoster in the open-label adult study.

Other adverse events which occurred at an incidence greater than or equal to 1% in any clinical study include: Alopecia, ALT or AST increased, anaphylactoid reaction, angina pectoris, angioedema, anorexia, anxiety, arrhythmia, arthralgia, arthritis, bilirubinemia, breast pain, cellulitis, cerebrovascular accident, cheilitis, chills, constipation, creatinine increased, dehydration, depression, dizziness, dyspnea, ear pain, ecchymosis, edema, epistaxis, exacerbation of untreated area, eye disorder, eye pain, furunculosis, gastritis, hernia, hyperglycemia, hypertension, hypoglycemia, hypoxia, laryngitis, leukocytosis, leukopenia, liver function tests abnormal, lung disorder, malaise, migraine, neck pain, neuritis, palpitations, paresthesia, peripheral vascular disorder, photosensitivity reaction, procedural complication, routine procedure, skin discoloration, sweating, taste perversion, tooth disorder, unintended pregnancy, vaginal moniliasis, vasodilation, and vertigo.

DOSAGE AND ADMINISTRATION

ADULTS

Tacrolimus Ointment 0.03% and 0.1%

Apply a thin layer of tacrolimus ointment 0.03% or 0.1% to the affected skin areas twice daily and rub in gently and completely. Treatment should be continued for 1 week after clearing of signs and symptoms of atopic dermatitis.

The safety of tacrolimus ointment under occlusion which may promote systemic exposure, has not been evaluated. **Tacrolimus ointment 0.03% and 0.1% should not be used with occlusive dressings.**

PEDIATRIC

Tacrolimus Ointment 0.03%

Apply a thin layer of tacrolimus ointment 0.03% to the affected skin areas twice daily and rub in gently and completely. Treatment should be continued for 1 week after clearing of signs and symptoms of atopic dermatitis. The safety of tacrolimus ointment under occlusion, which may promote systemic exposure, has not been evaluated. **Tacrolimus ointment 0.03% should not be used with occlusive dressings.**

HOW SUPPLIED

Protopic Ointment 0.03% is available in 30 and 60 g laminate tubes.

Protopic Ointment 0.1% is available in 30 and 60 g laminate tubes.

Storage: Store at room temperature 25°C (77°F); excursions permitted to 15-30°C (59-86°F).

PRODUCT LISTING - EQUIVALENTS NOT AVAILABLE

Capsule - Oral - 0.5 mg

60's	$116.87	PROGRAF, Fujisawa	00469-0607-67
100's	$227.03	PROGRAF, Fujisawa	00469-0607-73

Capsule - Oral - 1 mg

100's	$318.83	PROGRAF, Fujisawa	00469-0617-10
100's	$325.18	PROGRAF, Fujisawa	00469-0617-71
100's	$368.05	PROGRAF, Fujisawa	00469-0617-11
100's	$375.39	PROGRAF, Fujisawa	00469-0617-73

Capsule - Oral - 5 mg

100's	$1593.96	PROGRAF, Fujisawa	00469-0657-10
100's	$1625.84	PROGRAF, Fujisawa	00469-0657-71
100's	$1840.08	PROGRAF, Fujisawa	00469-0657-11
100's	$1858.83	PROGRAF, Fujisawa	00469-0657-73

Ointment - Topical - 0.03%

30 gm	$59.95	PROTOPIC, Fujisawa	00469-5201-30
60 gm	$119.90	PROTOPIC, Fujisawa	00469-5201-60

Ointment - Topical - 0.1%

30 gm	$64.09	PROTOPIC, Fujisawa	00469-5202-30
60 gm	$128.16	PROTOPIC, Fujisawa	00469-5202-60

Solution - Intravenous - 5 mg/ml

1 ml x 10	$1250.50	PROGRAF, Fujisawa	00469-3016-01

Tamoxifen Citrate *(002306)*

Categories: Carcinoma, breast; Ductal Carcinoma in Situ; Pregnancy Category D; WHO Formulary; FDA Approved 1994 Mar
Drug Classes: Antineoplastics, antiestrogens; Estrogen receptor modulators, selective; Hormones/hormone modifiers
Brand Names: **Nolvadex**
Foreign Brand Availability: Exiphen (El-Salvador; Guatemala; Honduras; Panama); Genox (Australia; New-Zealand); Gynatam (Philippines); Istubol (Canada); Kessar (France; Germany; Greece; Italy; Philippines; South-Africa; Switzerland); Mamofen (India); Moxafen (Bahrain; Cyprus; Egypt; Iran; Iraq; Israel; Jordan; Korea; Kuwait; Lebanon; Libya; Oman; Qatar; Republic-of-Yemen; Saudi-Arabia; Syria; United-Arab-Emirates); Noltam (England); Nolvadex-D (Australia; Hong-Kong; Israel; Malaysia; New-Zealand); Novofen (Bahamas; Barbados; Belize; Bermuda; Curacao; Guyana; Jamaica; Netherland-Antilles; Puerto-Rico; Surinam; Taiwan; Thailand; Trinidad); Oncetam (France); Tadex (Finland; Taiwan); Tamaxin (Denmark; Sweden); Tamifen (Bahrain; Cyprus; Egypt; Indonesia; Iran; Iraq; Jordan; Kuwait; Lebanon; Libya; Oman; Qatar; Republic-of-Yemen; Saudi-Arabia; Syria; United-Arab-Emirates); Tamofen (China; Denmark; England; Finland; Germany; Indonesia; Israel; New-Zealand; Norway; Singapore; Thailand); Tamofene (France); Tamoplex (Netherlands; Peru; Philippines; South-Africa; Switzerland); Tamosin (Australia); Tamoxi (Israel); Tamoxasta (Germany); Tamoxen (Israel); Tamoxsta (Philippines); Taxus (Colombia; Peru); Tecnofen (Mexico); Zitazonium (China; Hong-Kong; Hungary; Philippines; Thailand)
Cost of Therapy: $89.58 (Breast Cancer; Nolvadex; 10 mg; 2 tablets/day; 30 day supply)
$85.18 (Breast Cancer; Generic Tablets; 10 mg; 2 tablets/day; 30 day supply)
$126.41 (Breast Cancer; Nolvadex; 20 mg; 1 tablets/day; 30 day supply)
$113.64 (Breast Cancer; Generic Tablets; 20 mg; 1 tablet/day; 30 day supply)

T

WARNING

For Women With Ductal Carcinoma *In Situ* (DCIS) and Women at High Risk for Breast Cancer: Serious and life-threatening events associated with tamoxifen citrate in the risk reduction setting (women at high risk for cancer and women with DCIS) include uterine malignancies, stroke and pulmonary embolism. Incidence rates for these events were estimated from the NSABP P-1 trial. Uterine malignancies consist of both endometrial adenocarcinoma (incidence rate per 1000 women-years of 2.20 for tamoxifen citrate versus 0.71 for placebo) and uterine sarcoma (incidence rate per 1000 women-years of 0.17 for tamoxifen citrate versus 0.0 for placebo)*. For stroke, the incidence rate per 1000 women-years was 1.43 for tamoxifen citrate versus 1.00 for placebo. For pulmonary embolism, the incidence rate per 1000 women-years was 0.75 for tamoxifen citrate versus 0.25 for placebo.

Some of the strokes, pulmonary emboli, and uterine malignancies were fatal.

Health care providers should discuss the potential benefits versus the potential risks of these serious events with women at high risk of breast cancer and women with DCIS considering tamoxifen citrate to reduce their risk of developing breast cancer.

The benefits of tamoxifen citrate outweigh its risks in women already diagnosed with breast cancer.

***Updated long-term follow-up data (median length of follow-up is 6.9 years) from NSABP P-1 study. See WARNINGS, Effects on the Uterus — Endometrial Cancer and Uterine Sarcoma.**

DESCRIPTION

Nolvadex (tamoxifen citrate) tablets, a nonsteroidal antiestrogen, are for oral administration. Nolvadex tablets are available as:

10 mg Tablets: Each tablet contains 15.2 mg of tamoxifen citrate which is equivalent to 10 mg of tamoxifen.

20 mg Tablets: Each tablet contains 30.4 mg of tamoxifen citrate which is equivalent to 20 mg of tamoxifen.

Inactive Ingredients: Carboxymethylcellulose calcium, magnesium stearate, mannitol and starch.

Chemically, tamoxifen citrate is the trans-isomer of a triphenylethylene derivative. The chemical name is (Z)2-[4-(1,2-diphenyl-1-butenyl)phenoxy]-N,N-dimethylethanamine 2-hydroxy-1,2,3- propanetricarboxylate (1:1). The empirical formula is $C_{32}H_{37}NO_8$.

Tamoxifen citrate has a molecular weight of 563.62, the pKa is 8.85, the equilibrium solubility in water at 37°C is 0.5 mg/ml and in 0.02 N HCl at 37°C, it is 0.2 mg/ml.

CLINICAL PHARMACOLOGY

Tamoxifen citrate is a nonsteroidal agent that has demonstrated potent antiestrogenic properties in animal test systems. The antiestrogenic effects may be related to its ability to compete with estrogen for binding sites in target tissues such as breast. Tamoxifen inhibits the induction of rat mammary carcinoma induced by dimethylbenzanthracene (DMBA) and causes the regression of already established DMBA-induced tumors. In this rat model, tamoxifen appears to exert its antitumor effects by binding the estrogen receptors.

In cytosols derived from human breast adenocarcinomas, tamoxifen competes with estradiol for estrogen receptor protein.

ABSORPTION AND DISTRIBUTION

Following a single oral dose of 20 mg tamoxifen, an average peak plasma concentration of 40 ng/ml (range 35-45 ng/ml) occurred approximately 5 hours after dosing. The decline in plasma concentrations of tamoxifen is biphasic with a terminal elimination half-life of about 5-7 days. The average peak plasma concentration of N-desmethyl tamoxifen is 15 ng/ml (range 10-20 ng/ml). Chronic administration of 10 mg tamoxifen given twice daily for 3 months to patients results in average steady-state plasma concentrations of 120 ng/ml (range 67-183 ng/ml) for tamoxifen and 336 ng/ml (range 148-654 ng/ml) for N-desmethyl tamoxifen. The average steady-state plasma concentrations of tamoxifen and N-desmethyl tamoxifen after administration of 20 mg tamoxifen once daily for 3 months are 122 ng/ml (range 71-183 ng/ml) and 353 ng/ml (range 152-706 ng/ml), respectively. After initiation of therapy, steady state concentrations for tamoxifen are achieved in about 4 weeks and steady-state concentrations for N-desmethyl tamoxifen are achieved in about 8 weeks, suggesting a half-life of approximately 14 days for this metabolite. In a steady-state, crossover study of 10 mg tamoxifen citrate tablets given twice a day versus a 20 mg tamoxifen citrate tablet given once daily, the 20 mg tamoxifen citrate tablet was bioequivalent to the 10 mg tamoxifen citrate tablets.

METABOLISM

Tamoxifen is extensively metabolized after oral administration. N-desmethyl tamoxifen is the major metabolite found in patients' plasma. The biological activity of N-desmethyl tamoxifen appears to be similar to that of tamoxifen. 4-Hydroxytamoxifen and a side chain primary alcohol derivative of tamoxifen have been identified as minor metabolites in plasma. Tamoxifen is a substrate of cytochrome P-450 3A, 2C9 and 2D6, and an inhibitor of P-glycoprotein.

EXCRETION

Studies in women receiving 20 mg of ^{14}C tamoxifen have shown that approximately 65% of the administered dose was excreted from the body over a period of 2 weeks with fecal excretion as the primary route of elimination. The drug is excreted mainly as polar conjugates, with unchanged drug and unconjugated metabolites accounting for less than 30% of the total fecal radioactivity.

SPECIAL POPULATIONS

The effects of age, gender and race on the pharmacokinetics of tamoxifen have not been determined. The effects of reduced liver function on the metabolism and pharmacokinetics of tamoxifen have not been determined.

T

PEDIATRIC PATIENTS

The pharmacokinetics of tamoxifen and N-desmethyl tamoxifen were characterized using a population pharmacokinetic analysis with sparse samples per patient obtained from 27 female pediatric patients aged 2-10 years enrolled in a study designed to evaluate the safety, efficacy, and pharmacokinetics of tamoxifen citrate in treating McCune-Albright Syndrome. Rich data from 2 tamoxifen citrate pharmacokinetic trials in which 59 postmenopausal women with breast cancer completed the studies were included in the analysis to determine the structural pharmacokinetic model for tamoxifen. A one-compartment model provided the best fit to the data.

In pediatric patients, an average steady state peak plasma concentration ($C_{ss,max}$) and AUC were of 187 ng/ml and 4110 ng h/ml, respectively, and $C_{ss,max}$ occurred approximately 8 hours after dosing. Clearance (CL/F) as body weight adjusted in female pediatric patients was approximately 2.3-fold higher than in female breast cancer patients. In the youngest cohort of female pediatric patients (2-6 year olds), CL/F was 2.6-fold higher; in the oldest cohort (7-10.9 year olds) CL/F was approximately 1.9-fold higher. Exposure to N-desmethyl tamoxifen was comparable between the pediatric and adult patients. **The safety and efficacy of tamoxifen citrate for girls aged 2-10 years with McCune-Albright Syndrome and precocious puberty have not been studied beyond 1 year of treatment. The long-term effects of tamoxifen citrate therapy in girls have not been established.** In adults treated with tamoxifen citrate an increase in the incidence of uterine malignancies, stroke and pulmonary embolism has been noted (see BOXED WARNING).

DRUG-DRUG INTERACTIONS

In vitro studies showed that erythromycin, cyclosporin, nifedipine and diltiazem competitively inhibited formation of N-desmethyl tamoxifen with apparent K_i of 20, 1, 45 and 30 μM, respectively. The clinical significance of these *in vitro* studies is unknown.

Tamoxifen reduced the plasma concentration of letrozole by 37% when these drugs were co-administered. Rifampin, a cytochrome P-450 3A4 inducer reduced tamoxifen AUC and C_{max} by 86% and 55%, respectively. Aminoglutethimide reduces tamoxifen and N-desmethyl tamoxifen plasma concentrations. Medroxyprogesterone reduces plasma concentrations of N-desmethyl, but not tamoxifen.

INDICATIONS AND USAGE

METASTATIC BREAST CANCER

Tamoxifen citrate is effective in the treatment of metastatic breast cancer in women and men. In premenopausal women with metastatic breast cancer, tamoxifen citrate is an alternative to oophorectomy or ovarian irradiation. Available evidence indicates that patients whose tumors are estrogen receptor positive are more likely to benefit from tamoxifen citrate therapy.

ADJUVANT TREATMENT OF BREAST CANCER

Tamoxifen citrate is indicated for the treatment of node-positive breast cancer in postmenopausal women following total mastectomy or segmental mastectomy, axillary dissection, and breast irradiation. In some tamoxifen citrate adjuvant studies, most of the benefit to date has been in the subgroup with 4 or more positive axillary nodes.

Tamoxifen citrate is indicated for the treatment of axillary node-negative breast cancer in women following total mastectomy or segmental mastectomy, axillary dissection, and breast irradiation.

The estrogen and progesterone receptor values may help to predict whether adjuvant tamoxifen citrate therapy is likely to be beneficial.

Tamoxifen citrate reduces the occurrence of contralateral breast cancer in patients receiving adjuvant tamoxifen citrate therapy for breast cancer.

DUCTAL CARCINOMA IN SITU (DCIS)

In women with DCIS, following breast surgery and radiation, tamoxifen citrate is indicated to reduce the risk of invasive breast cancer (see BOXED WARNING). The decision regarding therapy with tamoxifen citrate for the reduction in breast cancer incidence should be based upon an individual assessment of the benefits and risks of tamoxifen citrate therapy.

Current data from clinical trials support 5 years of adjuvant tamoxifen citrate therapy for patients with breast cancer.

REDUCTION IN BREAST CANCER INCIDENCE IN HIGH RISK WOMEN

Tamoxifen citrate is indicated to reduce the incidence of breast cancer in women at high risk for breast cancer. This effect was shown in a study of 5 years planned duration with a median follow-up of 4.2 years. Twenty-five percent (25%) of the participants received the drug for 5 years. The longer-term effects are not known. In this study, there was no impact of tamoxifen on overall or breast cancer-related mortality (see BOXED WARNING).

Tamoxifen citrate is indicated for high-risk women. "High risk" is defined as women at least 35 years of age with a 5 year predicted risk of breast cancer ≥1.67%, as calculated by the Gail Model.

Examples of combinations of factors predicting a 5 year risk ≥1.67% are:

Age 35 or older and any of the following combinations of factors:

One first degree relative with a history of breast cancer, 2 or more benign biopsies, and a history of a breast biopsy showing atypical hyperplasia; or

At least 2 first degree relatives with a history of breast cancer, and a personal history of at least 1 breast biopsy; or

LCIS.

Age 40 or older and any of the following combination of factors:

One first degree relative with a history of breast cancer, 2 or more benign biopsies, age at first live birth 25 or older, and age at menarche 11 or younger; or

At least 2 first degree relatives with a history of breast cancer, and age at first live birth 19 or younger; or

One first degree relative with a history of breast cancer, and a personal history of a breast biopsy showing atypical hyperplasia.

Age 45 or older and any of the following combination of factors:

At least 2 first degree relatives with a history of breast cancer and age at first live birth 24 or younger; or

One first degree relative with a history of breast cancer with a personal history of a benign breast biopsy, age at menarche 11 or less and age at first live birth 20 or more.

Age 50 or older and any of the following combination of factors:

At least 2 first degree relatives with a history of breast cancer; or

History of 1 breast biopsy showing atypical hyperplasia, and age at first live birth 30 or older and age at menarche 11 or less; or

History of at least 2 breast biopsies with a history of atypical hyperplasia, and age at first live birth 30 or more.

Age 55 and any of the following combination of factors:

One first degree relative with a history of breast cancer with a personal history of a benign breast biopsy, and age at menarche 11 or less; or

History of at least 2 breast biopsies with a history of atypical hyperplasia, and age at first live birth 20 or older.

Age 60 or older and:

Five year predicted risk of breast cancer ≥1.67%, as calculated by the Gail Model.

For women whose risk factors are not described in the examples, the Gail Model is necessary to estimate absolute breast cancer risk. Health Care Professionals can obtain a Gail Model Risk Assessment Tool by dialing 1-800-544-2007.

There are no data available regarding the effect of tamoxifen citrate on breast cancer incidence in women with inherited mutations (BRCA1, BRCA2).

After an assessment of the risk of developing breast cancer, the decision regarding therapy with tamoxifen citrate for the reduction in breast cancer incidence should be based upon an individual assessment of the benefits and risks of tamoxifen citrate therapy. In the NSABP P-1 trial, tamoxifen citrate treatment lowered the risk of developing breast cancer during the follow-up period of the trial, but did not eliminate breast cancer risk.

NON-FDA APPROVED INDICATIONS

While not FDA approved indications, tamoxifen has also been used for the palliative treatment of hepatocellular carcinoma, and other cancers with estrogen receptors as well as for the treatment of benign breast disease and anovulation. In addition, the efficacy of tamoxifen in retroperitoneal fibrosis, is currently being evaluated.

CONTRAINDICATIONS

Tamoxifen citrate is contraindicated in patients with known hypersensitivity to the drug or any of its ingredients.

Reduction in breast cancer incidence in high risk women and women with DCIS: Tamoxifen citrate is contraindicated in women who require concomitant coumarin-type anticoagulant therapy or in women with a history of deep vein thrombosis or pulmonary embolus.

WARNINGS

EFFECTS IN METASTATIC BREAST CANCER PATIENTS

As with other additive hormonal therapy (estrogens and androgens), hypercalcemia has been reported in some breast cancer patients with bone metastases within a few weeks of starting treatment with tamoxifen citrate. If hypercalcemia does occur, appropriate measures should be taken and, if severe, tamoxifen citrate should be discontinued.

EFFECTS ON THE UTERUS — ENDOMETRIAL CANCER AND UTERINE SARCOMA

An increased incidence of uterine malignancies has been reported in association with tamoxifen citrate treatment. The underlying mechanism is unknown, but may be related to the estrogen-like effect of tamoxifen citrate. Most uterine malignancies seen in association with tamoxifen citrate are classified as adenocarcinoma of the endometrium. However, rare uterine sarcomas, including malignant mixed mullerian tumors, have also been reported. Uterine sarcoma is generally associated with a higher FIGO stage (III/IV) at diagnosis, poorer prognosis, and shorter survival. Uterine sarcoma has been reported to occur more frequently among long-term users (≥2 years) of tamoxifen citrate than non-users. Some of the uterine malignancies (endometrial carcinoma or uterine sarcoma) have been fatal.

In the NSABP P-1 trial, among participants randomized to tamoxifen citrate there was a statistically significant increase in the incidence of endometrial cancer [33 cases of invasive endometrial cancer, compared to 14 cases among participants randomized to placebo (RR=2.48, 95% CI: 1.27-4.92)]. The 33 cases in participants receiving tamoxifen citrate were FIGO Stage I, including 20 IA, 12 IB, and 1 IC endometrial adenocarcinomas. In participants randomized to placebo, 13 were FIGO Stage I (8 IA and 5 IB) and 1 was FIGO Stage IV. Five (5) women on tamoxifen citrate and 1 on placebo received postoperative radiation therapy in addition to surgery. This increase was primarily observed among women at least 50 years of age at the time of randomization [26 cases of invasive endometrial cancer, compared to 6 cases among participants randomized to placebo (RR=4.50, 95% CI: 1.78-13.16)]. Among women ≤49 years of age at the time of randomization there were 7 cases of invasive endometrial cancer, compared to 8 cases among participants randomized to placebo (RR=0.94, 95% CI: 0.28-2.89). If age at the time of diagnosis is considered, there were 4 cases of endometrial cancer among participants ≤49 randomized to tamoxifen citrate compared to 2 among participants randomized to placebo (RR=2.21, 95% CI: 0.4-12.0). For women ≥50 at the time of diagnosis, there were 29 cases among participants randomized to tamoxifen citrate compared to 12 among women on placebo (RR=2.5, 95% CI: 1.3-4.9). The risk ratios were similar in the 2 groups, although fewer events occurred in younger women. Most (29 of 33 cases in the tamoxifen group) endometrial cancers were diagnosed in symptomatic women, although 5 of 33 cases in the tamoxifen citrate group occurred in asymptomatic women. Among women receiving tamoxifen citrate the events appeared between 1 and 61 months (average = 32 months) from the start of treatment.

In an updated review of long-term data (median length of total follow-up is 6.9 years, including blinded follow-up) on 8306 women with an intact uterus at randomization in the NSABP P-1 risk reduction trial, the incidence of both adenocarcinomas and rare uterine sarcomas was increased in women taking tamoxifen citrate. Endometrial adenocarcinoma was reported in 53 women randomized to tamoxifen citrate (52 cases of FIGO Stage I, and 1 Stage III endometrial adenocarcinoma) and 17 women randomized to placebo (16 cases of FIGO Stage I and 1 case of FIGO Stage II endometrial adenocarcinoma) (incidence per 1000 women-years of 2.20 and 0.71, respectively). Some patients received post-operative radiation therapy in addition to surgery. Uterine sarcomas were reported in 4 women randomized to tamoxifen citrate (2 FIGO I, 1 FIGO II, 1 FIGO III. The FIGO I cases were a sarcoma and a MMMT. The FIGO II was a MMMT and the FIGO III was a sarcoma) and 0 patients randomized to placebo (incidence per 1000 women-years of 0.17 and 0.0, respectively). A similar increased incidence in endometrial adenocarcinoma and uterine sarcoma was observed among women receiving tamoxifen citrate in 5 other NSABP clinical trials.

Any patient receiving or who has previously received tamoxifen citrate who reports abnormal vaginal bleeding should be promptly evaluated. Patients receiving or who have previously received tamoxifen citrate should have annual gynecological examinations and they should promptly inform their physicians if they experience any abnormal gynecological symptoms, *e.g.*, menstrual irregularities, abnormal vaginal bleeding, changes in vaginal discharge, or pelvic pain or pressure.

In the P-1 trial, endometrial sampling did not alter the endometrial cancer detection rate compared to women who did not undergo endometrial sampling (0.6% with sampling, 0.5% without sampling) for women with an intact uterus. There are no data to suggest that routine endometrial sampling in asymptomatic women taking tamoxifen citrate to reduce the incidence of breast cancer would be beneficial.

NON-MALIGNANT EFFECTS ON THE UTERUS

An increased incidence of endometrial changes including hyperplasia and polyps have been reported in association with tamoxifen citrate treatment. The incidence and pattern of this increase suggest that the underlying mechanism is related to the estrogenic properties of tamoxifen citrate.

There have been a few reports of endometriosis and uterine fribroids in women receiving tamoxifen citrate. The underlying mechanism may be due to the partial estrogenic effect of tamoxifen citrate. Ovarian cysts have also been observed in a small number of premenopausal patients with advanced breast cancer who have been treated with tamoxifen citrate.

Tamoxifen citrate has been reported to cause menstrual irregularity or amenorrhea.

THROMBOEMBOLIC EFFECTS OF TAMOXIFEN CITRATE

There is evidence of an increased incidence of thromboembolic events, including deep vein thrombosis and pulmonary embolism, during tamoxifen citrate therapy. When tamoxifen citrate is coadministered with chemotherapy, there may be further increase in the incidence of thromboembolic effects. For treatment of breast cancer, the risks and benefits of tamoxifen citrate should be carefully considered in women with a history of thromboembolic events.

Data from the NSABP P-1 trial show that participants receiving tamoxifen citrate without a history of pulmonary emboli (PE) had a statistically significant increase in pulmonary emboli (18-tamoxifen citrate, 6-placebo, RR=3.01, 95% CI: 1.15-9.27). Three of the pulmonary emboli, all in the tamoxifen citrate arm, were fatal. Eighty-seven percent (87%) of the cases of pulmonary embolism occurred in women at least 50 years of age at randomization. Among women receiving tamoxifen citrate, the events appeared between 2 and 60 months (average = 27 months) from the start of treatment.

In this same population, a non-statistically significant increase in deep vein thrombosis (DVT) was seen in the tamoxifen citrate group (30-tamoxifen citrate, 19-placebo; RR=1.59, 95% CI: 0.86-2.98). The same increase in relative risk was seen in women ≤49 and in women ≥50, although fewer events occurred in younger women. Women with thromboembolic events were at risk for a second related event (7 out of 25 women on placebo, 5 out of 48 women on tamoxifen citrate) and were at risk for complications of the event and its treatment (0/25 on placebo, 4/48 on tamoxifen citrate). Among women receiving tamoxifen citrate, deep vein thrombosis events occurred between 2 and 57 months (average = 19 months) from the start of treatment.

There was a non-statisically significant increase in stroke among patients randomized to tamoxifen citrate (24-placebo, 34-tamoxifen citrate; RR=1.42; 95% CI: 0.82-2.51). Six (6) of the 24 strokes in the placebo group were considered hemorrhagic in origin and 10 of the 34 strokes in the tamoxifen citrate group were categorized as hemorrhagic. Seventeen (17) of the 34 strokes in the tamoxifen citrate group were considered occlusive and 7 were considered to be of unknown etiology. Fourteen (14) of the 24 strokes on the placebo arm were reported to be occlusive and 4 of unknown etiology. Among these strokes, 3 strokes in the placebo group and 4 strokes in the tamoxifen citrate group were fatal. Eighty-eight percent (88%) of the strokes occurred in women at least 50 years of age at the time of randomization. Among women receiving tamoxifen citrate, the events occurred between 1 and 63 months (average = 30 months) from the start of treatment.

EFFECTS ON THE LIVER

Liver Cancer

In the Swedish trial using adjuvant tamoxifen citrate 40 mg/day for 2-5 years, 3 cases of liver cancer have been reported in the tamoxifen citrate-treated group versus 1 case in the observation group (see PRECAUTIONS, Carcinogenesis). In other clinical trials evaluating tamoxifen citrate, no other cases of liver cancer have been reported to date.

One case of liver cancer was reported in NSABP P-1 in a participant randomized to tamoxifen citrate.

Non-Malignant Effects

Tamoxifen citrate has been associated with changes in liver enzyme levels, and on rare occasions, a spectrum of more severe liver abnormalities including fatty liver, cholestasis, hepatitis and hepatic necrosis. A few of these serious cases included fatalities. In most reported cases the relationship to tamoxifen citrate is uncertain. However, some positive rechallenges and dechallenges have been reported.

In the NSABP P-1 trial, few Grade 3-4 changes in liver function (SGOT, SGPT, bilirubin, alkaline phosphatase) were observed (10 on placebo and 6 on tamoxifen citrate). Serum lipids were not systematically collected.

OTHER CANCERS

A number of second primary tumors, occuring at sites other than the endometrium, have been reported following the treatment of breast cancer with tamoxifen citrate in clinical trials. Data from the NSABP B-14 and P-1 studies show no increase in other (non-uterine) cancers among patients receiving tamoxifen citrate. Whether an increased risk for other (non-uterine) cancers is associated with tamoxifen citrate is still uncertain and continues to be evaluated.

EFFECTS ON THE EYE

Ocular disturbances, including corneal changes, decrement in color vision perception, retinal vein thrombosis, and retinopathy have been reported in patients receiving tamoxifen citrate. An increased incidence of cataracts and the need for cataract surgery have been reported in patients receiving tamoxifen citrate.

In the NSABP P-1 trial, an increased risk of borderline significance of developing cataracts among those women without cataracts at baseline (540-tamoxifen citrate; 483-placebo; RR=1.13, 95% CI: 1.00-1.28) was observed. Among these same women, tamoxifen citrate was associated with an increased risk of having cataract surgery (101-tamoxifen citrate; 63-placebo; RR=1.62, 95% CI: 1.17-2.25). Among all women on the trial (with or without cataracts at baseline), tamoxifen citrate was associated with an increased risk of having cataract surgery (210-tamoxifen citrate; 129-placebo; RR=1.51, 95% CI: 1.21-1.89). Eye examinations were not required during the study. No other conclusions regarding non-cataract ophthalmic events can be made.

PREGNANCY CATEGORY D

Tamoxifen citrate may cause fetal harm when administered to a pregnant woman. Women should be advised not to become pregnant while taking tamoxifen citrate or within 2 months

T

of discontinuing tamoxifen citrate and should use barrier or nonhormonal contraceptive measures if sexually active. Tamoxifen does not cause infertility, even in the presence of menstrual irregularity. Effects on reproductive functions are expected from the antiestrogenic properties of the drug. In reproductive studies in rats at dose levels equal to or below the human dose, nonteratogenic developmental skeletal changes were seen and were found reversible. In addition, in fertility studies in rats and in teratology studies in rabbits using doses at or below those used in humans, a lower incidence of embryo implantation and a higher incidence of fetal death or retarded *in utero* growth were observed, with slower learning behavior in some rat pups when compared to historical controls. Several pregnant marmosets were dosed with 10 mg/kg/day (about 2-fold the daily maximum recommended human dose on a mg/m^2 basis) during organogenesis or in the last half of pregnancy. No deformations were seen and, although the dose was high enough to terminate pregnancy in some animals, those that did maintain pregnancy showed no evidence of teratogenic malformations.

In rodent models of fetal reproductive tract development, tamoxifen (at doses 0.002- to 2.4-fold the daily maximum recommended human dose on a mg/m^2 basis) caused changes in both sexes that are similar to those caused by estradiol, ethynylestradiol and diethylstilbestrol. Although the clinical relevance of these changes is unknown, some of these changes, especially vaginal adenosis, are similar to those seen in young women who were exposed to diethylstilbestrol *in utero* and who have a 1 in 1000 risk of developing clear-cell adenocarcinoma of the vagina or cervix. To date, *in utero* exposure to tamoxifen has not been shown to cause vaginal adenosis, or clear-cell adenocarcinoma of the vagina or cervix, in young women. However, only a small number of young women have been exposed to tamoxifen *in utero,* and a smaller number have been followed long enough (to age 15-20) to determine whether vaginal or cervical neoplasia could occur as a result of this exposure.

There are no adequate and well-controlled trials of tamoxifen in pregnant women. There have been a small number of reports of vaginal bleeding, spontaneous abortions, birth defects, and fetal deaths in pregnant women. If this drug is used during pregnancy, or the patient becomes pregnant while taking this drug, or within approximately 2 months after discontinuing therapy, the patient should be apprised of the potential risks to the fetus including the potential long-term risk of a DES-like syndrome.

REDUCTION IN BREAST CANCER INCIDENCE IN HIGH RISK WOMEN — PREGNANCY CATEGORY D

For sexually active women of child-bearing potential, tamoxifen citrate therapy should be initiated during menstruation. In women with menstrual irregularity, a negative B-HCG immediately prior to the initiation of therapy is sufficient (see PRECAUTIONS, Information for the Patient, Reduction in Breast Cancer Incidence in High Risk Women).

PRECAUTIONS

GENERAL

Decreases in platelet counts, usually to 50,000-100,000/mm^3, infrequently lower, have been occasionally reported in patients taking tamoxifen citrate for breast cancer. In patients with significant thrombocytopenia, rare hemorrhagic episodes have occurred, but it is uncertain if these episodes are due to tamoxifen citrate therapy. Leukopenia has been observed, sometimes in association with anemia and/or thrombocytopenia. There have been rare reports of neutropenia and pancytopenia in patients receiving tamoxifen citrate; this can sometimes be severe.

In the NSABP P-1 trial, 6 women on tamoxifen citrate and 2 on placebo experienced Grade 3-4 drops in platelet counts ($\leq$50,000/mm^3).

INFORMATION FOR THE PATIENT

Reduction in Invasive Breast Cancer and DCIS in Women With DCIS

Women with DCIS treated with lumpectomy and radiation therapy who are considering tamoxifen citrate to reduce the incidence of a second breast cancer event should assess the risks and benefits of therapy, since treatment with tamoxifen citrate decreased the incidence of invasive breast cancer, but has not been shown to affect survival.

Reduction in Breast Cancer Incidence in High Risk Women

Women who are at high risk for breast cancer can consider taking tamoxifen citrate therapy to reduce the incidence of breast cancer. Whether the benefits of treatment are considered to outweigh the risks depends on a woman's personal health history and on how she weighs the benefits and risks. Tamoxifen citrate therapy to reduce the incidence of breast cancer may therefore not be appropriate for all women at high risk for breast cancer. Women who are considering tamoxifen citrate therapy should consult their health care professional for an assessment of the potential benefits and risks prior to starting therapy for reduction in breast cancer incidence. Women should understand that tamoxifen citrate reduces the incidence of breast cancer, but may not eliminate risk. Tamoxifen citrate decreased the incidence of small estrogen receptor positive tumors, but did not alter the incidence of estrogen receptor negative tumors or larger tumors. In women with breast cancer who are at high risk of developing a second breast cancer, treatment with about 5 years of tamoxifen citrate reduced the annual incidence rate of a second breast cancer by approximately 50%.

Women who are pregnant or who plan to become pregnant should not take tamoxifen citrate to reduce her risk of breast cancer. Effective nonhormonal contraception must be used by all premenopausal women taking tamoxifen citrate and for approximately 2 months after discontinuing therapy if they are sexually active. Tamoxifen does not cause infertility, even in the presence of menstrual irregularity. For sexually active women of child-bearing potential, tamoxifen citrate therapy should be initiated during menstruation. In women with menstrual irregularity, a negative B-HCG immediately prior to the initiation of therapy is sufficient (see WARNINGS, Pregnancy Category D).

Two European trials of tamoxifen to reduce the risk of breast cancer were conducted and showed no difference in the number of breast cancer cases between the tamoxifen and placebo arms. These studies had trial designs that differed from that of NSABP P-1, were smaller than NSABP P-1, and enrolled women at a lower risk for breast cancer than those in P-1.

Monitoring During Tamoxifen Citrate Therapy

Women taking or having previously taken tamoxifen citrate should be instructed to seek prompt medical attention for new breast lumps, vaginal bleeding, gynecologic symptoms (menstrual irregularities, changes in vaginal discharge, or pelvic pain or pressure), symptoms of leg swelling or tenderness, unexplained shortness of breath, or changes in vision. Women should inform all care providers, regardless of the reason for evaluation, that they take tamoxifen citrate.

Women taking tamoxifen citrate to reduce the incidence of breast cancer should have a breast examination, a mammogram, and a gynecologic examination prior to the initiation of therapy. These studies should be repeated at regular intervals while on therapy, in keeping with good medical practice. Women taking tamoxifen citrate as adjuvant breast cancer therapy should follow the same monitoring procedures as for women taking tamoxifen citrate for the reduction in the incidence of breast cancer. Women taking tamoxifen citrate as treatment for metastatic breast cancer should review this monitoring plan with their care provider and select the appropriate modalities and schedule of evaluation.

LABORATORY TESTS

Periodic complete blood counts, including platelet counts and periodic liver function tests should be obtained.

DRUG/LABORATORY TEST INTERACTIONS

During postmarketing surveillance, T_4 elevations were reported for a few postmenopausal patients which may be explained by increases in thyroid-binding globulin. These elevations were not accompanied by clinical hyperthyroidism.

Variations in the karyopyknotic index on vaginal smears and various degrees of estrogen effect on Pap smears have been infrequently seen in postmenopausal patients given tamoxifen citrate.

In the postmarketing experience with tamoxifen citrate, infrequent cases of hyperlipidemias have been reported. Periodic monitoring of plasma triglycerides and cholesterol may be indicated in patients with pre-existing hyperlipidemias. (See ADVERSE REACTIONS, Postmarketing Experience.)

CARCINOGENESIS

A conventional carcinogenesis study in rats at doses of 5, 20, and 35 mg/kg/day (about 1-, 3- and 7-fold the daily maximum recommended human dose on a mg/m^2 basis) administered by oral gavage for up to 2 years revealed a significant increase in hepatocellular carcinoma at all doses. The incidence of these tumors was significantly greater among rats administered 20 or 35 mg/kg/day (69%) compared to those administered 5 mg/kg/day (14%). In a separate study, rats were administered tamoxifen at 45 mg/kg/day (about 9-fold the daily maximum recommended human dose on a mg/m^2 basis); hepatocellular neoplasia was exhibited at 3-6 months.

Granulosa cell ovarian tumors and interstitial cell testicular tumors were observed in 2 separate mouse studies. The mice were administered the trans and racemic forms of tamoxifen for 13-15 months at doses of 5, 20 and 50 mg/kg/day (about ½-, 2- and 5-fold the daily recommended human dose on a mg/m^2 basis).

MUTAGENESIS

No genotoxic potential was found in a conventional battery of *in vivo* and *in vitro* tests with pro- and eukaryotic test systems with drug metabolizing systems. However, increased levels of DNA adducts were observed by ^{32}P post-labeling in DNA from rat liver and cultured human lymphocytes. Tamoxifen also has been found to increase levels of micronucleus formation *in vitro* in human lymphoblastoid cell line (MCL-5). Based on these findings, tamoxifen is genotoxic in rodent and human MCL-5 cells.

IMPAIRMENT OF FERTILITY

Tamoxifen produced impairment of fertility and conception in female rats at doses of 0.04 mg/kg/day (about 0.01-fold the daily maximum recommended human dose on a mg/m^2 basis) when dosed for 2 weeks prior to mating through day 7 of pregnancy. At this dose, fertility and reproductive indices were markedly reduced with total fetal mortality. Fetal mortality was also increased at doses of 0.16 mg/kg/day (about 0.03-fold the daily maximum recommended human dose on a mg/m^2 basis) when female rats were dosed from days 7-17 of pregnancy. Tamoxifen produced abortion, premature delivery and fetal death in rabbits administered doses equal to or greater than 0.125 mg/kg/day (about 0.05-fold the daily maximum recommended human dose on a mg/m^2 basis). There were no teratogenic changes in either rats or rabbits.

PREGNANCY CATEGORY D

See WARNINGS.

NURSING MOTHERS

It is not known whether this drug is excreted in human milk. Because many drugs are excreted in human milk and because of the potential for serious adverse reactions in nursing infants from tamoxifen citrate, a decision should be made whether to discontinue nursing or to discontinue the drug, taking into account the importance of the drug to the mother.

PEDIATRIC USE

The safety and efficacy of tamoxifen citrate for girls aged 2-10 years with McCune-Albright Syndrome and precocious puberty have not been studied beyond 1 year of treatment. The long-term effects of tamoxifen citrate therapy for girls have not been established. In adults treated with tamoxifen citrate, an increase in the incidence of uterine malignancies, stroke and pulmonary embolism has been noted (see BOXED WARNING.

GERIATRIC USE

In the NSABP P-1 trial, the percentage of women at least 65 years of age was 16%. Women at least 70 years of age accounted for 6% of the participants. A reduction in breast cancer incidence was seen among participants in each of the subsets: a total of 28 and 10 invasive breast cancers were seen among participants 65 and older in the placebo and tamoxifen citrate groups, respectively. Across all other outcomes, the results in this subset reflect the results observed in the subset of women at least 50 years of age. No overall differences in tolerability were observed between older and younger patients.

In the NSABP B-24 trial, the percentage of women at least 65 years of age was 23%. Women at least 70 years of age accounted for 10% of participants. A total of 14 and 12 invasive breast cancers were seen among participants 65 and older in the placebo and tamoxifen citrate groups, respectively. This subset is too small to reach any conclusions on efficacy. Across all other endpoints, the results in this subset were comparable to those of younger women enrolled in this trial. No overall differences in tolerability were observed between older and younger patients.

DRUG INTERACTIONS

When tamoxifen citrate is used in combination with coumarin-type anticoagulants, a significant increase in anticoagulant effect may occur. Where such coadministration exists, careful monitoring of the patient's prothrombin time is recommended.

In the NSABP P-1 trial, women who required coumarin-type anticoagulants for any reason were ineligible for participation in the trial (see CONTRAINDICATIONS).

There is an increased risk of thromboembolic events occurring when cytotoxic agents are used in combination with tamoxifen citrate.

Tamoxifen reduced letrozole plasma concentrations by 37%. The effect of tamoxifen on metabolism and excretion of other antineoplastic drugs, such as cyclophosphamide and other drugs that require mixed function oxidases for activation, is not known. Tamoxifen and N-desmethyl tamoxifen plasma concentrations have been shown to be reduced when coadministered with rifampin or aminoglutethimide. Induction of CYP3A4-mediated metabolism is considered to be the mechanism by which these reductions occur; other CYP3A4 inducing agents have not been studied to confirm this effect.

One patient receiving tamoxifen citrate with concomitant phenobarbital exhibited a steady state serum level of tamoxifen lower than that observed for other patients (*i.e.,* 26 ng/ml versus mean value of 122 ng/ml). However, the clinical significance of this finding is not known. Rifampin induced the metabolism of tamoxifen and significantly reduced the plasma concentrations of tamoxifen in 10 patients. Aminoglutethimide reduces tamoxifen and N-desmethyl tamoxifen plasma concentrations. Medroxyprogesterone reduces plasma concentrations of N-desmethyl, but not tamoxifen.

Concomitant bromocriptine therapy has been shown to elevate serum tamoxifen and N-desmethyl tamoxifen.

ADVERSE REACTIONS

Adverse reactions to tamoxifen citrate are relatively mild and rarely severe enough to require discontinuation of treatment in breast cancer patients.

Continued clinical studies have resulted in further information which better indicates the incidence of adverse reactions with tamoxifen citrate as compared to placebo.

METASTATIC BREAST CANCER

Increased bone and tumor pain and, also, local disease flare have occurred, which are sometimes associated with a good tumor response. Patients with increased bone pain may require additional analgesics. Patients with soft tissue disease may have sudden increases in the size of preexisting lesions, sometimes associated with marked erythema within and surrounding the lesions and/or the development of new lesions. When they occur, the bone pain or disease flare are seen shortly after starting tamoxifen citrate and generally subside rapidly.

In patients treated with tamoxifen citrate for metastatic breast cancer, the most frequent adverse reaction to tamoxifen citrate is hot flashes.

Other adverse reactions which are seen infrequently are hypercalcemia, peripheral edema, distaste for food, pruritus vulvae, depression, dizziness, light-headedness, headache, hair thinning and/or partial hair loss, and vaginal dryness.

PREMENOPAUSAL WOMEN

TABLE 5 summarizes the incidence of adverse reactions reported at a frequency of 2% or greater from clinical trials (Ingle, Pritchard, Buchanan) which compared tamoxifen citrate therapy to ovarian ablation in premenopausal patients with metastatic breast cancer.

TABLE 5

Adverse Reactions*	Tamoxifen Citrate All Effects n=104	Ovarian Ablation All Effects n=100
Flush	33%	46%
Amenorrhea	16%	69%
Altered menses	13%	5%
Oligomenorrhea	9%	1%
Bone pain	6%	6%
Menstrual disorder	6%	4%
Nausea	5%	4%
Cough/coughing	4%	1%
Edema	4%	1%
Fatigue	4%	1%
Musculoskeletal pain	3%	0%
Pain	3%	4%
Ovarian cyst(s)	3%	2%
Depression	2%	2%
Abdominal cramps	1%	2%
Anorexia	1%	2%

* Some women had more than 1 adverse reaction.

MALE BREAST CANCER

Tamoxifen citrate is well tolerated in males with breast cancer. Reports from the literature and case reports suggest that the safety profile of tamoxifen citrate in males is similar to that seen in women. Loss of libido and impotence have resulted in discontinuation of tamoxifen therapy in male patients. Also, in oligospermic males treated with tamoxifen, LH, FSH, testosterone and estrogen levels were elevated. No significant clinical changes were reported.

ADJUVANT BREAST CANCER

In the NSABP B-14 study, women with axillary node-negative breast cancer were randomized to 5 years of tamoxifen citrate 20 mg/day or placebo following primary surgery. The reported adverse effects are tabulated in TABLE 6 (mean follow-up of approximately 6.8 years) showing adverse events more common on tamoxifen citrate than on placebo. The incidence of hot flashes (64% vs 48%), vaginal discharge (30% vs 15%), and irregular menses (25% vs 19%) were higher with tamoxifen citrate compared with placebo. All other adverse effects occurred with similar frequency in the 2 treatment groups, with the exception of thrombotic events; a higher incidence was seen in tamoxifen citrate-treated patients (through 5 years, 1.7% vs 0.4%). Two of the patients treated with tamoxifen citrate who had thrombotic events died.

TABLE 6 *NSABP B-14 Study*

Adverse Effect	Tamoxifen Citrate (n=1422)	Placebo (n=1437)
Hot flashes	64%	48%
Fluid retention	32%	30%
Vaginal discharge	30%	15%
Nausea	26%	24%
Irregular menses	25%	19%
Weight loss (>5%)	23%	18%
Skin changes	19%	15%
Increased SGOT	5%	3%
Increased bilirubin	2%	1%
Increased creatinine	2%	1%
Thrombocytopenia*	2%	1%
Thrombotic events		
Deep vein thrombosis	0.8%	0.2%
Pulmonary embolism	0.5%	0.2%
Superficial phlebitis	0.4%	0.0%

* Defined as a platelet count of <100,000/mm³.

In the Eastern Cooperative Oncology Group (ECOG) adjuvant breast cancer trial, tamoxifen citrate or placebo was administered for 2 years to women following mastectomy. When compared to placebo, tamoxifen citrate showed a significantly higher incidence of hot flashes (19% vs 8% for placebo). The incidence of all other adverse reactions was similar in the 2 treatment groups with the exception of thrombocytopenia where the incidence for tamoxifen citrate was 10% vs 3% for placebo, an observation of borderline statistical significance.

In other adjuvant studies, Toronto and Nolvadex Adjuvant Trial Organization (NATO), women received either tamoxifen citrate or no therapy. In the Toronto study, hot flashes were observed in 29% of patients for tamoxifen citrate versus 1% in the untreated group. In the NATO trial, hot flashes and vaginal bleeding were reported in 2.8% and 2.0% of women, respectively, for tamoxifen citrate versus 0.2% for each in the untreated group.

DUCTAL CARCINOMA IN SITU (DCIS)

The type and frequency of adverse events in the NSABP B-24 trial were consistent with those observed in the other adjuvant trials conducted with tamoxifen citrate.

REDUCTION IN BREAST CANCER INCIDENCE IN HIGH RISK WOMEN

In the NSABP P-1 Trial, there was an increase in 5 serious adverse effects in the tamoxifen citrate group: endometrial cancer (33 cases in the tamoxifen citrate group versus 14 in the placebo group); pulmonary embolism (18 cases in the tamoxifen citrate group versus 6 in the placebo group); deep vein thrombosis (30 cases in the tamoxifen citrate group versus 19 in the placebo group); stroke (34 cases in the tamoxifen citrate group versus 24 in the placebo group); cataract formation (540 cases in the tamoxifen citrate group versus 483 in the placebo group) and cataract surgery (101 cases in the tamoxifen citrate group versus 63 in the placebo group) (see WARNINGS).

TABLE 7 presents the adverse events observed in NSABP P-1 by treatment arm. Only adverse events more common on tamoxifen citrate than placebo are shown.

TABLE 7 *NSABP P-1 Trial: All Adverse Events*

	Tamoxifen Citrate (n=6681)	Placebo (n=6707)
Self Reported Symptoms	n=6441*	n=6469*
Hot flashes	80%	68%
Vaginal discharges	55%	35%
Vaginal bleeding	23%	22%
Laboratory Abnormalities	n=6520†	n=6535†
Platelets decreased	0.7%	0.3%
Adverse Effects	n=6492‡	n=6484‡
Other Toxicities		
Mood	11.6%	10.8%
Infection/sepsis	6.0%	5.1%
Constipation	4.4%	3.2%
Alopecia	5.2%	4.4%
Skin	5.6%	4.7%
Allergy	2.5%	2.1%

* Number with quality of life questionnaires.
† Number with treatment follow-up forms.
‡ Number with adverse drug reaction forms.

In the NSABP P-1 trial, 15.0% and 9.7% of participants receiving tamoxifen citrate and placebo therapy, respectively withdrew from the trial for medical reasons. The following are the medical reasons for withdrawing from tamoxifen citrate and placebo therapy, respectively: hot flashes (3.1% vs 1.5%) and vaginal discharge (0.5% vs 0.1%).

In the NSABP P-1 trial, 8.7% and 9.6% of participants receiving tamoxifen citrate and placebo therapy, respectively, withdrew for non-medical reasons.

On the NSABP P-1 trial, hot flashes of any severity occurred in 68% of women on placebo and in 80% of women on tamoxifen citrate. Severe hot flashes occurred in 28% of women on placebo and 45% of women on tamoxifen citrate. Vaginal discharge occurred in 35% and 55% of women on placebo and tamoxifen citrate respectively; and was severe in 4.5% and 12.3% respectively. There was no difference in the incidence of vaginal bleeding between treatment arms.

PEDIATRIC PATIENTS

McCune-Albright Syndrome

Mean uterine volume increased after 6 months of treatment and doubled at the end of the 1 year study. A causal relationship has not been established; however, as an increase in the incidence of endometrial adenocarcinoma and uterine sarcoma has been noted in adults treated with tamoxifen citrate (see BOXED WARNING), continued monitoring of McCune-Albright patients treated with tamoxifen citrate for long-term effects is recommended. **The safety and efficacy of tamoxifen citrate for girls aged 2-10 years with McCune-Albright Syndrome and precocious puberty have not been studied beyond 1 year of treatment. The long-term effects of tamoxifen citrate therapy in girls have not been established.**

POSTMARKETING EXPERIENCE

Less frequently reported adverse reactions are vaginal bleeding, vaginal discharge, menstrual irregularities, skin rash and headaches. Usually these have not been of sufficient severity to require dosage reduction or discontinuation of treatment. Very rare reports of erythema multiforme, Stevens-Johnson syndrome, bullous pemphigoid, interstitial pneumonitis, and rare reports of hypersensitivity reactions including angioedema have been reported with tamoxifen citrate therapy. In some of these cases, the time to onset was more than 1 year. Rarely, elevation of serum triglyceride levels, in some cases with pancreatitis, may be associated with the use of tamoxifen citrate (see PRECAUTIONS, Drug/Laboratory Test Interactions).

DOSAGE AND ADMINISTRATION

For patients with breast cancer, the recommended daily dose is 20-40 mg. Dosages greater than 20 mg/day should be given in divided doses (morning and evening).

In 3 single agent adjuvant studies in women, one 10 mg tamoxifen citrate tablet was administered 2 (ECOG and NATO) or 3 (Toronto) times a day for 2 years. In the NSABP B-14 adjuvant study in women with node-negative breast cancer, one 10 mg tamoxifen citrate tablet was given twice a day for at least 5 years. Results of the B-14 study suggest that continuation of therapy beyond 5 years does not provide additional benefit (see CLINICAL PHARMACOLOGY). In the EBCTCG 1995 overview, the reduction in recurrence and mortality was greater in those studies that used tamoxifen for about 5 years than in those that used tamoxifen for a shorter period of therapy. There was no indication that doses greater than 20 mg/day were more effective. Current data from clinical trials support 5 years of adjuvant tamoxifen citrate therapy for patients with breast cancer.

Ductal Carcinoma In Situ (DCIS): The recommended dose is tamoxifen citrate 20 mg daily for 5 years.

Reduction in Breast Cancer Incidence in High Risk Women: The recommended dose is tamoxifen citrate 20 mg daily for 5 years. There are no data to support the use of tamoxifen citrate other than for 5 years.

HOW SUPPLIED

NOLVADEX TABLETS

10 mg: Contain tamoxifen as the citrate in an amount equivalent to 10 mg of tamoxifen and are round, biconvex, uncoated, white tablets identified with "NOLVADEX 600" debossed on 1 side and a cameo debossed on the other side.

20 mg: Contain tamoxifen as the citrate in an amount equivalent to 20 mg of tamoxifen and are round, biconvex, uncoated, white tablets identified with "NOLVADEX 604" debossed on 1 side and a cameo debossed on the other side.

Storage: Store at controlled room temperature, 20-25°C (68-77°F). Dispense in a well-closed, light-resistant container.

PRODUCT LISTING - RATED THERAPEUTICALLY EQUIVALENT

Tablet - Oral - 10 mg

Qty	Price	Product	NDC
60's	$113.64	TAMOXIFEN CITRATE, Barr Laboratories Inc	00555-0446-09
180's	$340.92	TAMOXIFEN CITRATE, Barr Laboratories Inc	00555-0446-63
250's	$441.08	TAMOXIFEN CITRATE, Barr Laboratories Inc	00555-0446-03

Tablet - Oral - 20 mg

Qty	Price	Product	NDC
30's	$113.64	TAMOXIFEN CITRATE, Barr Laboratories Inc	00555-0904-01
90's	$340.92	TAMOXIFEN CITRATE, Barr Laboratories Inc	00555-0904-14

PRODUCT LISTING - EQUIVALENTS NOT AVAILABLE

Tablet - Oral - 10 mg

Qty	Price	Product	NDC
30's	$86.07	NOLVADEX, Pd-Rx Pharmaceuticals	55289-0585-30
30's	$113.65	GENERIC, Mylan Pharmaceuticals Inc	00378-0274-93
60's	$109.57	GENERIC, Allscripts Pharmaceutical Company	54569-3765-00
60's	$110.63	GENERIC, Southwood Pharmaceuticals Inc	58016-0657-60
60's	$113.10	GENERIC, Ivax Corporation	00172-5656-49
60's	$113.65	GENERIC, Mylan Pharmaceuticals Inc	00378-0144-91
60's	$113.77	GENERIC, Roxane Laboratories Inc	00054-4831-21
60's	$116.98	GENERIC, Astra-Zeneca Pharmaceuticals	00310-0730-60
60's	$126.41	NOLVADEX, Astra-Zeneca Pharmaceuticals	00310-0600-60
100's	$227.54	GENERIC, Roxane Laboratories Inc	00054-8831-25
120's	$247.59	GENERIC, Physicians Total Care	54868-3004-01
180's	$255.54	GENERIC, Allscripts Pharmaceutical Company	54569-8602-00
180's	$268.74	NOLVADEX, Allscripts Pharmaceutical Company	54569-8531-00
180's	$339.40	GENERIC, Ivax Corporation	00172-5656-58
180's	$341.32	GENERIC, Roxane Laboratories Inc	00054-4831-26
180's	$379.24	NOLVADEX, Astra-Zeneca Pharmaceuticals	00310-0600-18
250's	$441.07	NOLVADEX, Astra-Zeneca Pharmaceuticals	00310-0600-25

Tablet - Oral - 20 mg

Qty	Price	Product	NDC
30's	$113.77	GENERIC, Roxane Laboratories Inc	00054-4834-13
30's	$116.98	TAMOXIFEN, Astra-Zeneca Pharmaceuticals	00310-0731-30
30's	$126.41	NOLVADEX, Astra-Zeneca Pharmaceuticals	00310-0604-30
90's	$341.32	GENERIC, Roxane Laboratories Inc	00054-4834-22
90's	$379.24	NOLVADEX, Astra-Zeneca Pharmaceuticals	00310-0604-90
100's	$377.10	GENERIC, Ivax Corporation	00172-5657-60
100's	$378.85	GENERIC, Mylan Pharmaceuticals Inc	00378-0274-01

Tamsulosin Hydrochloride *(003338)*

Categories: Hyperplasia, benign prostatic; Pregnancy Category B; FDA Approved 1997 May
Drug Classes: Antiadrenergics, alpha blocking
Brand Names: Flomax
Foreign Brand Availability: Alna (Germany); Harnal (Indonesia; Korea; Philippines; Thailand); Josir (France); Omnic (Colombia; Denmark; Finland; Germany; Israel; Netherlands; New-Zealand; Peru); Secotex (Colombia; Mexico; Peru)
Cost of Therapy: $60.37 (Benign Prostatic Hyperplasia; Flomax; 0.4 mg; 1 capsule/day; 30 day supply)

DESCRIPTION

Tamsulosin hydrochloride is an antagonist of alpha$_{1A}$ adrenoceptors in the prostate.

Tamsulosin HCl is (-)-(*R*)-5-[2-[[2-(O-ethoxyphenoxy)ethyl]amino]propyl]-2-methoxybenzenesulfonamide, monohydrochloride. Tamsulosin HCl occurs as white crystals that melt with decomposition at approximately 230°C. It is sparingly soluble in water and in methanol, slightly soluble in glacial acetic acid and in ethanol, and practically insoluble in ether.

The empirical formula of tamsulosin HCl is $C_{20}H_{28}N_2O_5S \cdot HCl$. The molecular weight of tamsulosin HCl is 444.98.

Each Flomax capsule for oral administration contains tamsulosin HCl 0.4 mg, and the following inactive ingredients: methacrylic acid copolymer, microcrystalline cellulose, triacetin, polysorbate 80, sodium lauryl sulfate, calcium stearate, talc, FD&C blue no. 2, titanium dioxide, ferric oxide, gelatin, and trace amounts of shellac, industrial methylated spirit 74 OP, n-butyl alcohol, isopropyl alcohol, propylene glycol, dimethylpolysiloxane, and black iron oxide E172.

CLINICAL PHARMACOLOGY

The symptoms associated with benign prostatic hyperplasia (BPH) are related to bladder outlet obstruction, which is comprised of two underlying components: static and dynamic. The static component is related to an increase in prostate size caused, in part, by a proliferation of smooth muscle cells in the prostatic stroma. However, the severity of BPH symptoms and the degree of urethral obstruction do not correlate well with the size of the prostate. The dynamic component is a function of an increase in smooth muscle tone in the prostate and bladder neck leading to constriction of the bladder outlet. Smooth muscle tone is mediated by the sympathetic nervous stimulation of alpha$_1$ adrenoceptors, which are abundant in the prostate, prostatic capsule, prostatic urethra, and bladder neck. Blockade of these adrenoceptors can cause smooth muscles in the bladder neck and prostate to relax, resulting in an improvement in urine flow rate and a reduction in symptoms of BPH.

Tamsulosin, an alpha$_1$ adrenoceptor blocking agent, exhibits selectivity for alpha$_1$ receptors in the human prostate. At least three discrete alpha$_1$-adrenoceptor subtypes have been identified: alpha$_{1A}$, alpha$_{1B}$ and alpha$_{1D}$; their distribution differs between human organs and tissue. Approximately 70% of the alpha$_1$-receptors in human prostate are of the alpha$_{1A}$ subtype.

Tamsulosin HCl capsules are not intended for use as an antihypertensive drug.

PHARMACOKINETICS

The pharmacokinetics of tamsulosin HCl have been evaluated in adult healthy volunteers and patients with BPH after single and/or multiple administration with doses ranging from 0.1 to 1 mg.

Absorption

Absorption of tamsulosin HCl from tamsulosin HCl capsules 0.4 mg is essentially complete (>90%) following oral administration under fasting conditions. Tamsulosin HCl exhibits linear kinetics following single and multiple dosing, with achievement of steady-state concentrations by the fifth day of once-a-day dosing.

Effect of Food

The time to maximum concentration (T_{max}) is reached by 4-5 hours under fasting conditions and by 6-7 hours when tamsulosin HCl capsules are administered with food. Taking tamsulosin HCl capsules under fasted conditions results in a 30% increase in bioavailability (AUC) and 40-70% increase in peak concentrations (C_{max}) compared to fed conditions.

The effects of food on the pharmacokinetics of tamsulosin HCl are consistent regardless of whether a tamsulosin HCl capsule is taken with a light breakfast or a high-fat breakfast (TABLE 1).

TABLE 1 *Mean (±SD) Pharmacokinetic Parameters Following Tamsulosin 0.4 mg or 0.8 mg Once Daily With a Light Breakfast, High-Fat Breakfast, or Fasted*

	0.4 mg, qd*		0.8 mg, qd†		
Pharmacokinetic Parameter	**Light Breakfast**	**Fasted**	**Light Breakfast**	**High-Fat Breakfast**	**Fasted**
C_{min} (ng/ml)	4.0 ± 2.6	3.8 ± 2.5	12.3 ± 6.7	13.5 ± 7.6	13.3 ± 13.3
C_{max} (ng/ml)	10.1 ± 4.8	17.1 ± 17.1	29.8 ± 10.3	29.1 ± 11.0	41.6 ± 15.6
C_{max}/C_{min} Ratio	3.1 ± 1.0	5.3 ± 2.2	2.7 ± 0.7	2.5 ± 0.8	3.6 ± 1.1
T_{max} (h)	6.0	4.0	7.0	6.6	5.0
T½ (h)	—	—	—	—	14.9 ± 3.9
AUC(tgr) (ng·h/ml)	151 ± 81.5	199 ± 94.1	440 ± 195	449 ± 217	557 ± 257

* To healthy volunteers; n=23 (age range 18-32 years)
† To healthy volunteers; n=22 (age range 55-75 years)
C_{min} = Observed minimum concentration; C_{max} = Observed maximum tamsulosin plasma concentration; T_{max} = Median time-to-maximum concentration; T½ = Observed half-life; AUC = Area under the tamsulosin plasma time curve over the dosing interval.

Distribution

The mean steady-state apparent volume of distribution of tamsulosin HCl after intravenous administration to 10 healthy male adults was 16 L, which is suggestive of distribution into extracellular fluids in the body. Additionally, whole body autoradiographic studies in mice and rats and tissue distribution in rats and dogs indicate that tamsulosin HCl is widely distributed to most tissues including kidney, prostate, liver, gall bladder, heart, aorta, and brown fat, and minimally distributed to the brain, spinal cord, and testes. Tamsulosin HCl is extensively bound to human plasma proteins (94-99%), primarily alpha$_1$ acid glycoprotein (AAG), with linear binding over a wide concentration range (20-600 ng/ml). The results of two-way *in vitro* studies indicate that the binding of tamsulosin HCl to human plasma proteins is not affected by amitriptyline, diclofenac, glyburide, simvastatin plus simvastatin-hydroxy acid metabolite, warfarin, diazepam, propranolol, trichlormethiazide, or chlormadinone. Likewise, tamsulosin HCl had no effect on the extent of binding of these drugs.

Metabolism

There is no enantiometric bioconversion from tamsulosin HCl [R(-) isomer] to the S(+) isomer in humans. Tamsulosin HCl is extensively metabolized by cytochrome P450 enzymes in the liver and less than 10% of the dose is excreted in urine unchanged. However, the pharmacokinetic profile of the metabolites in humans has not been established. Additionally, the cytochrome P450 enzymes that primarily catalyze the Phase I metabolism of tamsulosin HCl have not been conclusively identified. Therefore, possible interactions with other cytochrome P450 metabolized compounds cannot be discerned with current information. The metabolites of tamsulosin HCl undergo extensive conjugation to glucuronide or sulfate prior to renal excretion.

Incubations with human liver microsomes showed no evidence of clinically significant metabolic interactions between tamsulosin HCl and amitriptyline, albuterol (beta agonist), glyburide (glibenclamide) and finasteride (5alpha-reductase inhibitor for treatment of BPH). However, results of the *in vitro* testing of the tamsulosin HCl interaction with diclofenac and warfarin were equivocal.

Excretion

On administration of the radiolabeled dose of tamsulosin HCl to 4 healthy volunteers, 97% of the administered radioactivity was recovered, with urine (76%) representing the primary route of excretion compared to feces (21%) over 168 hours. Following intravenous or oral administration of an immediate-release formulation, the elimination half-life of tamsulosin HCl in plasma range from 5-7 hours. Because of absorption rate-controlled pharmacokinetics with tamsulosin HCl capsules, the apparent half-life of tamsulosin HCl is approximately 9-13 hours in healthy volunteers and 14-15 hours in the target population. Tamsulosin HCl undergoes restrictive clearance in humans, with a relatively low systemic clearance (2.88 L/h).

Special Populations

Geriatrics (Age)

Cross-study comparison of tamsulosin HCl capsules overall exposure (AUC) and half-life indicate that the pharmacokinetic disposition of tamsulosin HCl may be slightly prolonged in geriatric males compared to young, healthy male volunteers. Intrinsic clearance is independent of tamsulosin HCl binding to AAG, but diminishes with age, resulting in a 40% overall higher exposure (AUC) in subjects of age 55-75 years compared to subjects of age 20-32 years.

Renal Dysfunction

The pharmacokinetics of tamsulosin HCl have been compared in 6 subjects with mild-moderate (30 ≤CLCR <70 ml/min/1.73 m^2) or moderate-severe (10 ≤CLCR <30 ml/min/1.73 m^2) renal impairment and 6 normal subjects (CLCR <90 ml/min/1.73 m^2). While a change in the overall plasma concentration of tamsulosin HCl was observed as the result of altered binding to AAG, the unbound (active) concentration of tamsulosin HCl, as well as the intrinsic clearance, remained relatively constant. Therefore, patients with renal impairment do not require an adjustment in tamsulosin HCl capsules dosing. However, patients with endstage renal disease (CLCR <10 ml/min/1.73 m^2) have not been studied.

Hepatic Dysfunction

The pharmacokinetics of tamsulosin HCl have been compared in 8 subjects with moderate hepatic dysfunction (Child-Pugh's classification: Grades A and B) and 8 normal subjects. While a change in the overall plasma concentration of tamsulosin HCl was observed as the result of altered binding to AAG, the unbound (active) concentration of tamsulosin HCl does not change significantly with only a modest (32%) change in intrinsic clearance of unbound tamsulosin HCl. Therefore, patients with moderate hepatic dysfunction do not require an adjustment in tamsulosin HCl capsules dosage.

Drug-Drug Interactions

Nifedipine, Atenolol, Enalapril: In three studies in hypertensive subjects (age range 47-79 years) whose blood pressure was controlled with stable doses of nifedipine extended release, atenolol, or enalapril for at least 3 months, tamsulosin HCl capsules 0.4 mg for 7 days followed by tamsulosin HCl capsules 0.8 mg for another 7 days (n=8 per study) resulted in no clinically significant effects on blood pressure and pulse rate compared to placebo (n=4 per study). Therefore, dosage adjustments are not necessary when tamsulosin HCl capsules are administered concomitantly with nifedipine extended release, atenolol, or enalapril.

Warfarin: A definitive drug-drug interaction study between tamsulosin HCl and warfarin was not conducted. Results from limited *in vitro* and *in vivo* studies are inconclusive. Therefore, caution should be exercised with concomitant administration of warfarin and tamsulosin HCl capsules.

Digoxin and Theophylline: In two studies in healthy volunteers (n=10 per study; age range 19-39 years) receiving tamsulosin HCl capsules 0.4 mg/day for 2 days, followed by tamsulosin HCl capsules 0.8 mg/day for 5-8 days, single intravenous doses of digoxin 0.5 mg or theophylline 5 mg/kg resulted in no change in the pharmacokinetics of digoxin or theophylline. Therefore, dosage adjustments are not necessary when a tamsulosin HCl capsule is administered concomitantly with digoxin or theophylline.

Furosemide: The pharmacokinetic and pharmacodynamic interaction between tamsulosin HCl capsules 0.8 mg/day (steady-state) and furosemide 20 mg intravenously (single dose) was evaluated in 10 healthy volunteers (age range 21-40 years). Tamsulosin HCl capsules had no effect on the pharmacodynamics (excretion of electrolytes) of furosemide. While furosemide produced an 11-12% reduction in tamsulosin HCl C_{max} and AUC, these changes are expected to be clinically insignificant and do not require adjustment of the tamsulosin HCl capsules dosage.

Cimetidine: The effects of cimetidine at the highest recommended dose (400 mg every 6 hours for 6 days) on the pharmacokinetics of a single tamsulosin HCl capsule 0.4 mg dose was investigated in 10 healthy volunteers (age range 21-38 years). Treatment with cimetidine resulted in a significant decrease (26%) in the clearance of tamsulosin HCl which resulted in a moderate increase in tamsulosin HCl AUC (44%). Therefore, tamsulosin HCl capsules should be used with caution in combination with cimetidine, particularly at doses higher than 0.4 mg.

INDICATIONS AND USAGE

Tamsulosin HCl capsules are indicated for the treatment of the signs and symptoms of benign prostatic hyperplasia (BPH). Tamsulosin HCl capsules are not indicated for the treatment of hypertension.

CONTRAINDICATIONS

Tamsulosin HCl capsules are contraindicated in patients known to be hypersensitive to tamsulosin HCl or any component of tamsulosin HCl capsules.

WARNINGS

The signs and symptoms of orthostasis (postural hypotension, dizziness and vertigo) were detected more frequently in tamsulosin HCl capsule treated patients than in placebo recipients. As with other alpha-adrenergic blocking agents there is a potential risk of syncope (see ADVERSE REACTIONS).

Patients beginning treatment with tamsulosin HCl capsules should be cautioned to avoid situations where injury could result should syncope occur.

Rarely (probably less than one in fifty thousand patients), tamsulosin, like other alpha$_1$ antagonists, has been associated with priapism (persistent painful penile erection unrelated to sexual activity). Because this condition can lead to permanent impotence if not properly treated, patients must be advised about the seriousness of the condition (see PRECAUTIONS, Information for the Patient).

PRECAUTIONS

GENERAL

Carcinoma of the Prostate

Carcinoma of the prostate and BPH cause many of the same symptoms. These two diseases frequently co-exist. Patients should be evaluated prior to the start of tamsulosin HCl capsules therapy to rule out the presence of carcinoma of the prostate.

INFORMATION FOR THE PATIENT

See the Patient Package Insert that is distributed with the prescription for complete information.

Patients should be told about the possible occurrence of symptoms related to postural hypotension such as dizziness when taking tamsulosin HCl capsules, and they should be cautioned about driving, operating machinery or performing hazardous tasks.

Patients should be advised not to crush, chew or open the tamsulosin HCl capsules.

Patients should be advised about the possibility of priapism as a result of treatment with tamsulosin HCl capsules and other similar medications. Patients should be informed that this reaction is extremely rare, but if not brought to immediate medical attention, can lead to permanent erectile dysfunction (impotence).

LABORATORY TESTS

No laboratory test interactions with tamsulosin HCl capsules are known. Treatment with tamsulosin HCl capsules for up to 12 months had no significant effect on prostate-specific antigen (PSA).

PREGNANCY, TERATOGENIC EFFECTS, PREGNANCY CATEGORY B

Administration of tamsulosin HCl to pregnant female rats at dose levels up to 300 mg/kg/day (approximately 50 times the human therapeutic AUC exposure) revealed no evidence of harm to the fetus. Administration of tamsulosin HCl to pregnant rabbits at dose levels up to 50 mg/kg/day produced no evidence of fetal harm. Tamsulosin HCl capsules are not indicated for use in women.

NURSING MOTHERS

Tamsulosin HCl capsules are not indicated for use in women.

PEDIATRIC USE

Tamsulosin HCl capsules are not indicated for use in pediatric populations.

CARCINOGENESIS, MUTAGENESIS, AND IMPAIRMENT OF FERTILITY

Rats administered doses up to 43 mg/kg/day in males and 52 mg/kg/day in females had no increases in tumor incidence with the exception of a modest increase in the frequency of mammary gland fibroadenomas in female rats receiving doses ≥5.4 mg/kg (P <0.015). The highest doses of tamsulosin HCl evaluated in the rat carcinogenicity study produced systemic exposures (AUC) in rats 3 times the exposures in men receiving the maximum therapeutic dose of 0.8 mg/day.

Mice were administered doses up to 127 mg/kg/day in males and 158 mg/kg/day in females. There were no significant tumor findings in male mice. Female mice treated for 2 years with the two highest doses of 45 and 158 mg/kg/day had statistically significant increases in the incidence of mammary gland fibroadenomas (P <0.0001) and adenocarcinomas (P <0.0075). The highest dose levels of tamsulosin HCl evaluated in the mice carcinogenicity study produced systemic exposures (AUC) in mice 8 times the exposures in men receiving the maximum therapeutic dose of 0.8 mg/day.

The increased incidences of mammary gland neoplasms in female rats and mice were considered secondary to tamsulosin HCl-induced hyperprolactinemia. It is not known if tamsulosin HCl capsules elevate prolactin in humans. The relevance for human risk of the findings of prolactin-mediated endocrine tumors in rodents is not known.

Tamsulosin HCl produced no evidence of mutagenic potential *in vitro* in the Ames reverse mutation test, mouse lymphoma thymidine kinase assay, unscheduled DNA repair synthesis assay, and chromosomal aberration assays in Chinese hamster ovary cells or human lymphocytes. There were no mutagenic effects in the *in vivo* sister chromatid exchange and mouse micronucleus assay.

Studies in rats revealed significantly reduced fertility in males dosed with single or multiple daily doses of 300 mg/kg/day of tamsulosin HCl (AUC exposure in rats about 50 times the human exposure with the maximum therapeutic dose). The mechanism of decreased fertility in male rats is considered to be an effect of the compound on the vaginal plug formation possibly due to changes of semen content or impairment of ejaculation. The effects on fertility were reversible showing improvement by 3 days after a single dose and 4 weeks after multiple dosing. Effects on fertility in males were completely reversed within 9 weeks of discontinuation of multiple dosing. Multiple doses of 10 and 100 mg/kg/day tamsulosin HCl (1/5 and 16 times the anticipated human AUC exposure) did not significantly alter fertility in male rats. Effects of tamsulosin HCl on sperm counts or sperm function have not been evaluated. Studies in females rats revealed significant reductions in fertility after single or multiple dosing with 300 mg/kg/day of the R-isomer or racemic mixture of tamsulosin HCl, respectively. In female rats, the reductions in fertility after single doses were considered to be associated with impairments in fertilization. Multiple dosing with 10 or 100 mg/kg/day of the racemic mixture did not significantly alter fertility in female rats.

DRUG INTERACTIONS

The pharmacokinetic and pharmacodynamic interactions between tamsulosin HCl capsules and other alpha-adrenergic blocking agents have not been determined. However, interactions may be expected and tamsulosin HCl capsules should NOT be used in combination with other alpha-adrenergic blocking agents.

The pharmacokinetic interaction between cimetidine and tamsulosin HCl capsules was investigated. The results indicate significant changes in tamsulosin HCl clearance (26% decrease) and AUC (44% increase). Therefore, tamsulosin HCl capsules should be used with caution in combination with cimetidine, particularly at doses higher than 0.4 mg.

Results from limited *in vitro* and *in vivo* drug-drug interaction studies between tamsulosin HCl and warfarin are inconclusive. Therefore, caution should be exercised with concomitant administration of warfarin and tamsulosin HCl capsules.

(See also CLINICAL PHARMACOLOGY, Pharmacokinetics, Drug-Drug Interactions.)

ADVERSE REACTIONS

The incidence of treatment-emergent adverse events has been ascertained from six short-term US and European placebo-controlled clinical trials in which daily doses of 0.1-0.8 mg tamsulosin HCl capsules were used. These studies evaluated safety in 1783 patients treated with tamsulosin HCl capsules and 798 patients administered placebo. TABLE 3 summarizes the treatment-emergent adverse events that occurred in ≥2% of patients receiving either tamsulosin HCl capsules 0.4 mg, or 0.8 mg and at an incidence numerically higher than that in the placebo group during two 13 week US trials (US92-03A and US93-01) conducted in 1487 men.

TABLE 3 *Treatment Emergent* Adverse Events Occurring in ≥2% of Tamsulosin or Placebo Patients in Two US Short-Term Placebo-Controlled Clinical Studies*

Body Sytem / Adverse Event	Tamsulosin 0.4 mg n=502	Tamsulosin 0.8 mg n=492	Placebo n=493
Body as a Whole			
Headache	97 (19.3%)	104 (21.1%)	99 (20.1%)
Infection	45 (9.0%)	53 (10.8%)	37 (7.5%)
Asthenia	39 (7.8%)	42 (8.5%)	27 (5.5%)
Back pain	35 (7.0%)	41 (8.3%)	27 (5.5%)
Chest pain	20 (4.0%)	20 (4.1%)	18 (3.7%)
Nervous System			
Dizziness	75 (14.9%)	84 (17.1%)	50 (10.1%)
Somnolence	15 (3.0%)	21 (4.3%)	8 (1.6%)
Insomnia	12 (2.4%)	7 (1.4%)	3 (0.6%)
Libido decreased	5 (1.0%)	10 (2.0%)	6 (1.2%)
Respiratory System			
Rhinitis	66 (13.1%)	88 (17.9%)	41 (8.3%)
Pharyngitis	29 (5.8%)	25 (5.1%)	23 (4.7%)
Cough increased	17 (3.4%)	22 (4.5%)	12 (2.4%)
Sinusitis	11 (2.2%)	18 (3.7%)	8 (1.6%)
Digestive System			
Diarrhea	31 (6.2%)	21 (4.3%)	22 (4.5%)
Nausea	13 (2.6%)	19 (3.9%)	16 (3.2%)
Tooth disorder	6 (1.2%)	10 (2.0%)	7 (1.4%)
Urogenital System			
Abnormal ejaculation	42 (8.4%)	89 (18.1%)	1 (0.2%)
Special Senses			
Amblyopia	1 (0.2%)	10 (2.0%)	2 (0.4%)

* A treatment emergent adverse event was defined as any event satisfying one of the following criteria:
The adverse event occurred for the first time after initial dosing with double-blind study medication.
The adverse event was present prior to or at the time of initial dosing with double-blind study medication and subsequently increased in severity during double-blind treatment; OR
The adverse event was present prior to or at the time of initial dosing with double-blind study medication, disappeared completely, and then reappeared during double-blind treatment.

SIGNS AND SYMPTOMS OF ORTHOSTASIS

In the two US studies, symptomatic postural hypotension was reported by 0.2% of patients (1 of 502) in the 0.4 mg group, 0.4% of patients (2 of 492) in the 0.8 mg group, and by no patients in the placebo group. Syncope was reported by 0.2% of patients (1 of 502) in the 0.4 mg group, 0.4% of patients (2 of 492) in the 0.8 mg group and 0.6% of patients (3 of 493) in the placebo group. Dizziness was reported by 15% of patients (75 of 502) in the 0.4 mg group, 17% of patients (84 of 492) in the 0.8 mg group, and 10% of patients (50 of 493) in the placebo group. Vertigo was reported by 0.6% of patients (3 of 502) in the 0.4 mg group, 1% of patients (5 of 492) in the 0.8 mg group and by 0.6% of patients (3 of 493) in the placebo group.

Multiple testing for orthostatic hypotension was conducted in a number of studies. Such a test was considered positive if it met one or more of the following criteria: (1) a decrease in systolic blood pressure of ≥20 mm Hg upon standing from the supine position during the orthostatic tests; (2) a decrease in diastolic blood pressure ≥10 mm Hg upon standing, with the standing diastolic blood pressure <65 mm Hg during the orthostatic test; (3) an increase in pulse rate of ≥20 bpm upon standing with a standing pulse rate ≥100 bpm during the orthostatic test; and (4) the presence of clinical symptoms (faintness, lightheadedness/lightheaded, dizziness, spinning sensation, vertigo, or postural hypotension) upon standing during the orthostatic test.

Following the first dose of double-blind medication in Study 1, a positive orthostatic test result at 4 hours post-dose was observed in 7% of patients (37 of 498) who received tamsulosin HCl capsules 0.4 mg once daily and in 3% of the patients (8 of 253) who received placebo. At 8 hours post-dose, a positive orthostatic test result was observed for 6% of the patients (31 of 498) who received tamsulosin HCl capsules 0.4 mg once daily and 4% (9 of 250) who received placebo (Note: patients in the 0.8 mg group received 0.4 mg once daily for the first week of Study 1).

In Studies 1 and 2, at least one positive orthostatic test result was observed during the course of these studies for 81 of the 502 patients (16%) in the tamsulosin HCl capsules 0.4 mg once daily group, 92 of the 491 patients (19%) in the tamsulosin HCl capsules 0.8 mg once daily group and 54 of the 493 patients (11%) in the placebo group.

Because orthostasis was detected more frequently in tamsulosin HCl capsule-treated patients than in placebo recipients, there is a potential risk of syncope (see WARNINGS).

ABNORMAL EJACULATION

Abnormal ejaculation includes ejaculation failure, ejaculation disorder, retrograde ejaculation and ejaculation decrease. As shown in TABLE 3, abnormal ejaculation was associated with tamsulosin HCl capsules administration and was dose-related in the US studies. Withdrawal from these clinical studies of tamsulosin HCl capsules because of abnormal ejaculation was also dose-dependent with 8 of 492 patients (1.6%) in the 0.8 mg group, and no patients in the 0.4 mg or placebo groups discontinuing treatment due to abnormal ejaculation.

POST-MARKETING EXPERIENCE

Allergic-type reactions such as skin rash, pruritus, angioedema of tongue, lips and face and urticaria have been reported with positive rechallenge in some cases. Priapism has been reported rarely. Infrequent reports of palpitations, constipation and vomiting have been received during the post-marketing period.

DOSAGE AND ADMINISTRATION

Tamsulosin HCl capsules 0.4 mg once daily is recommended as the dose for the treatment of the signs and symptoms of BPH. It should be administered approximately one-half hour following the same meal each day.

For those patients who fail to respond to the 0.4 mg dose after 2-4 weeks of dosing, the dose of tamsulosin HCl capsules can be increased to 0.8 mg once daily. If tamsulosin HCl capsules administration is discontinued or interrupted for several days at either the 0.4 or 0.8 mg dose, therapy should be started again with the 0.4 mg once daily dose.

HOW SUPPLIED

Flomax capsules 0.4 mg are hard gelatin capsules with olive green opaque cap and orange opaque body. The capsules are imprinted on one side with "Flomax 0.4 mg" and on the other side with "BI 58".

Storage: Store at controlled room temperature 20-25°C (68-77°F). Keep Flomax capsules and all medicines out of reach of children.

PRODUCT LISTING - EQUIVALENTS NOT AVAILABLE

Capsule - Oral - 0.4 mg

30's	\$46.70	FLOMAX, Allscripts Pharmaceutical Company	54569-4768-00
100's	\$201.23	FLOMAX, Abbott Pharmaceutical	00597-0058-01

Tazarotene *(003344)*

Categories: Acne vulgaris; Hyperpigmentation, facial; Hypopigmentation, facial; Lentigines, facial; Psoriasis; FDA Approved 1997 Jun; Pregnancy Category X
Drug Classes: Dermatologics; Retinoids
Brand Names: Avage; Tazorac
Foreign Brand Availability: Zorac (England; France; Germany; Ireland; Israel; South-Africa)
Cost of Therapy: \$39.11 (Acne; Tazorac Cream; 0.1%; 15 g; 1 application/day; variable day supply)
\$78.20 (Psoriasis; Tazorac Gel; 0.1%; 30 g; 1 application/day; variable day supply)

DESCRIPTION

Note: The trade names have been used throughout this monograph for clarity.

AVAGE CREAM

FOR TOPICAL USE ONLY. NOT FOR OPHTHALMIC, ORAL, OR INTRAVAGINAL USE.

Avage cream is a white cream and contains the compound tazarotene; this formulation of tazarotene cream is also marketed for the treatment of plaque psoriasis and acne vulgaris as Tazorac cream, 0.1%. Tazarotene is a member of the acetylenic class of retinoids.

The chemical formula is $C_{21}H_{21}NO_2S$, the molecular weight is 351.46, and the chemical name is ethyl 6-[2-(4,4-dimethylthiochroman-6-yl)ethynyl] nicotinate.

Active: Tazarotene 0.1% (w/w).

Preservative: Benzyl alcohol 1.0% (w/w).

Inactives: Carbomer 934P, carbomer 1342, edetate disodium, medium chain triglycerides, mineral oil, purified water, sodium thiosulfate, sorbitan monooleate and sodium hydroxide to adjust the pH.

TAZORAC GEL

FOR DERMATOLOGIC USE ONLY. NOT FOR OPHTHALMIC USE.

Tazorac is a translucent, aqueous gel and contains the compound tazarotene, a member of the acetylenic class of retinoids. It is for topical dermatologic use only. The molecular weight of tazarotene is 351.46, its molecular formula is $C_{21}H_{21}NO_2S$, and its chemical name is ethyl 6-[2-(4,4-dimethylthiochroman-6-yl)-ethynyl] nicotinate.

Active Ingredient: Tazarotene 0.05% or 0.1% (w/w).

Preservative: Benzyl alcohol 1.0% (w/w).

Inactive Ingredients: Ascorbic acid, butylated hydroxyanisole, butylated hydroxytoluene, carbomer 934P, edetate disodium, hexylene glycol, purified water, poloxamer 407, polyethylene glycol 400, polysorbate 40, and tromethamine.

TAZORAC CREAM

FOR TOPICAL USE ONLY. NOT FOR OPHTHALMIC, ORAL, OR INTRAVAGINAL USE.

Tazorac cream is a white cream and contains the compound tazarotene. Tazarotene is a member of the acetylenic class of retinoids. The formula is $C_{21}H_{21}NO_2S$, the molecular weight is 351.46, and the chemical name is ethyl 6-[2-(4,4-dimethylthiochroman-6-yl)ethynyl] nicotinate.

Contains:

Active: Tazarotene 0.05% or 0.1% (w/w).

Preservative: Benzyl alcohol 1.0% (w/w).

Inactives: Carbomer 934P, carbomer 1342, edetate disodium, medium chain triglycerides, mineral oil, purified water, sodium thiosulfate, sorbitan monooleate and sodium hydroxide to adjust the pH.

CLINICAL PHARMACOLOGY

AVAGE CREAM

Tazarotene is a retinoid prodrug which is converted to its active form, the cognate carboxylic acid of tazarotene (AGN 190299), by rapid deesterification in animals and man. AGN 190299 ("tazarotenic acid") binds to all three members of the retinoic acid receptor (RAR) family: RARα, RARβ, and RARγ, but shows relative selectivity for RARβ, and RARγ and may modify gene expression. The clinical significance of these findings is unknown.

The mechanism of tazarotene action in the amelioration of fine wrinkling, facial mottled hypo- and hyperpigmentation, and benign facial lentigines is unknown. A histological study of tazarotene cream 0.1% applied in subjects with fine wrinkling and mottled hyperpigmentation but otherwise normal skin for 24 weeks showed that tazarotene cream was associated with significantly greater proportions of patients who had an increase from baseline in the number of granular cell layers and in epidermal edema. The clinical significance of these changes is unknown.

Pharmacokinetics

Following topical application, tazarotene undergoes esterase hydrolysis to form its active metabolite, tazarotenic acid. Little parent compound could be detected in the plasma. Tazarotenic acid was highly bound to plasma proteins (>99%). Tazarotene and tazarotenic acid were metabolized to sulfoxides, sulfones and other polar metabolites which were eliminated through urinary and fecal pathways. The half-life of tazarotenic acid was approximately 18 hours.

Tazarotene cream 0.1% was topically applied once daily to either the face (6 females and 2 males) or to 15% of body surface area (8 females and 8 males) over 4 weeks in patients with fine wrinkling and mottled hyperpigmentation. In the "face-only" dosing group, the maximum average C_{max} and AUC(0-24h) values of tazarotenic acid occurred on Day 15 with mean ± SD values of C_{max} and AUC(0-24h) of tazarotenic acid being 0.236 ± 0.255 ng/ml (n=8) and 2.44 ± 1.38 ng·h/ml (n=8), respectively. The mean C_{max} and AUC(0-24h) values of tazarotenic acid from patients in the 15% body surface area dosing group were approximately 10 times higher than those from patients in the face-only dosing group. The single highest C_{max} throughout the study period was 3.43 ng/ml on Day 29 from patients in the 15% body surface area dosing group. Gender had no influence on the systemic bioavailability of tazarotenic acid.

Blood samples were collected from one of the two Phase 3 studies to evaluate the systemic exposure following application of tazarotene cream 0.1% once daily for 24 weeks (double-blind period) followed by 28 weeks (open-label) under clinical conditions. The mean plasma tazarotenic acid concentrations following topical treatment with tazarotene cream 0.1% over 52 weeks ranged between 0.092 ± 0.073 ng/ml and 0.127 ± 0.142 ng/ml. The single highest observed tazarotenic acid concentration throughout the 52 week study was 0.705 ng/ml (observed at Week 36). Systemic availability of tazarotenic acid was minimal and remained steady following once daily application of tazarotene cream 0.1% to the faces of patients in the study for up to 52 weeks.

TAZORAC GEL

Tazarotene is a retinoid prodrug which is converted to its active form, the cognate carboxylic acid of tazarotene (AGN 190299), by rapid deesterification in most biological systems. AGN 190299 binds to all three members of the retinoic acid receptor (RAR) family: RARα, RARβ, RARγ, but shows relative selectivity for RARβ, and RARγ and may modify gene expression. The clinical significance of these findings is unknown.

Psoriasis

The mechanism of tazarotene action in psoriasis is not defined. Topical tazarotene blocks induction of mouse epidermal ornithine decarboxylase (ODC) activity, which is associated with cell proliferation and hyperplasia. In cell culture and *in vitro* models of the skin, tazarotene suppresses expression of MRP8, a marker of inflammation present in the epidermis of psoriasis subjects at high levels. In human keratinocyte cultures, it inhibits cornified envelope formation, whose build-up is an element of the psoriatic scale. The clinical significance of these findings is unknown.

Acne

The mechanism of tazarotene action in acne is not defined. Tazarotene inhibited corneocyte accumulation in rhino mouse skin and cross-linked envelope formation in cultured human keratinocytes. The clinical significance of these findings is unknown.

Pharmacokinetics

Following topical application, tazarotene undergoes esterase hydrolysis to form its active metabolite, AGN 190299. Little parent compound could be detected in the plasma. AGN 190299 was highly bound to plasma proteins (>99%). Tazarotene and AGN 190299 were metabolized to sulfoxides, sulfones and other polar metabolites which were eliminated through urinary and fecal pathways. The half-life of AGN 190299 following topical application of tazarotene was similar in normal and psoriatic subjects, approximately 18 hours.

The human *in vivo* studies described below were conducted with tazarotene gel applied topically at approximately 2 mg/cm^2 and left on the skin for 10-12 hours. Both the peak plasma concentration (C_{max}) and area under the plasma concentration time curve (AUC) refer to the active metabolite only.

Two single, topical dose studies were conducted using ^{14}C-tazarotene gel. Systemic absorption, as determined from radioactivity in the excreta, was less than 1% of the applied dose (without occlusion) in 6 psoriatic patients and approximately 5% of the applied dose (under occlusion) in 6 healthy subjects. One non-radiolabeled single-dose study comparing the 0.05% gel to the 0.1% gel in healthy subjects indicated that the C_{max} and AUC were 40% higher for the 0.1% gel.

After 7 days of topical dosing with measured doses of tazarotene 0.1% gel on 20% of the total body surface without occlusion in 24 healthy subjects, the C_{max} was 0.72 ± 0.58 ng/ml (mean ± SD) occurring 9 hours after the last dose, and the AUC(0-24h) was 10.1 ± 7.2 ng·h/ml. Systemic absorption was 0.91 ± 0.67% of the applied dose.

In a 14 day study in 5 psoriatic patients, measured doses of tazarotene 0.1% gel were applied daily by nursing staff to involved skin without occlusion (8-18% of total body surface area; mean ± SD: 13 ± 5%). The C_{max} was 12.0 ± 7.6 ng/ml occurring 6 hours after the final dose, and the AUC(0-24h) was 105 ± 55 ng·h/ml. Systemic absorption was 14.8 ± 7.6% of the applied dose. Extrapolation of these results to represent dosing on 20% of total body surface yielded estimates of C_{max} of 18.9 ± 10.6 ng/ml and AUC(0-24h) of 172 ± 88 ng·h/ml.

An *in vitro* percutaneous absorption study, using radiolabeled drug and freshly excised human skin or human cadaver skin, indicated that approximately 4-5% of the applied dose was in the stratum corneum (tazarotene:AGN 190299 = 5:1) and 2-4% was in the viable epidermis-dermis layer (tazarotene:AGN 190299 = 2:1) 24 hours after topical application of the gel.

TAZORAC CREAM

Tazarotene is a retinoid prodrug which is converted to its active form, the cognate carboxylic acid of tazarotene (AGN 190299), by rapid deesterification in animals and man. AGN 190299 ("tazarotenic acid") binds to all three members of the retinoic acid receptor (RAR) family: RARα, RARβ, and RARγ, but shows relative selectivity for RARβ, and RARγ and may modify gene expression. The clinical significance of these findings is unknown.

Psoriasis

The mechanism of tazarotene action in psoriasis is not defined. Topical tazarotene blocks induction of mouse epidermal ornithine decarboxylase (ODC) activity, which is associated with cell proliferation and hyperplasia. In cell culture and *in vitro* models of skin, tazarotene suppresses expression of MRP8, a marker of inflammation present in the epidermis of psoriasis patients at high levels. In human keratinocyte cultures, it inhibits cornified envelope formation, whose build-up is an element of the psoriatic scale. Tazarotene also induces the expression of a gene which may be a growth suppressor in human keratinocytes and which

T

may inhibit epidermal hyperproliferation in treated plaques. However, the clinical significance of these findings is unknown.

Acne

The mechanism of tazarotene action in acne vulgaris is not defined. However, the basis of tazarotene's therapeutic effect in acne may be due to its anti-hyperproliferative, normalizing-of-differentiation and anti-inflammatory effects. Tazarotene inhibited corneocyte accumulation in rhino mouse skin and cross-linked envelope formation in cultured human keratinocytes. The clinical significance of these findings is unknown.

Pharmacokinetics

Following topical application, tazarotene undergoes esterase hydrolysis to form its active metabolite, tazarotenic acid. Little parent compound could be detected in the plasma. Tazarotenic acid was highly bound to plasma proteins (>99%). Tazarotene and tazarotenic acid were metabolized to sulfoxides, sulfones and other polar metabolites which were eliminated through urinary and fecal pathways. The half-life of tazarotenic acid was approximately 18 hours, following topical application of tazarotene to normal, acne or psoriatic skin.

In a multiple dose study with a once daily dose for 14 consecutive days in 9 psoriatic patients (male = 5; female = 4), measured doses of tazarotene 0.1% cream were applied by medical staff to involved skin without occlusion (5-35% of total body surface area: mean ± SD: 14 ± 11%). The C_{max} of tazarotenic acid was 2.31 ± 2.78 ng/ml occurring 8 hours after the final dose, and the AUC(0-24h) was 31.2 ± 35.2 ng·h/ml on Day 15 in the 5 patients who were administered clinical doses of 2 mg cream/cm^2.

During clinical trials with 0.05% or 0.1% tazarotene cream treatment for plaque psoriasis, 3 out of 139 patients with their systemic exposure monitored had detectable plasma tazarotene concentrations, with the highest value at 0.09 ng/ml. Tazarotenic acid was detected in 78 out of 139 patients (LLOQ = 0.05 ng/ml). Three patients using tazarotene cream 0.1% had plasma tazarotenic acid concentrations greater than 1 ng/ml. The highest value was 2.4 ng/ml. However, because of the variations in the time of blood sampling, the area of psoriasis involvement, and the dose of tazarotene applied, actual maximal plasma levels are unknown.

Tazarotene cream 0.1% was applied once daily to either the face (n=8) or to 15% of body surface area (n=10) of female patients with moderate to severe acne vulgaris. The mean C_{max} and AUC values of tazarotenic acid peaked at Day 15 for both dosing groups during a 29 day treatment period. Mean C_{max} and AUC(0-24h) values of tazarotenic acid from patients in the 15% body surface area dosing group were more than 10 times higher than those from patients in the face-only dosing group. The single highest C_{max} throughout the study period was 1.91 ng/ml on Day 15 in the exaggerated dosing group. In the face-only group, the mean ± SD values of C_{max} and AUC(0-24h) of tazarotenic acid on Day 15 were 0.10 ± 0.06 ng/ml and 1.54 ± 1.01 ng·h/ml, respectively, whereas in the 15% body surface area dosing group, the mean ± SD values of C_{max} and AUC(0-24h) of tazarotenic acid on Day 15 were 1.20 ± 0.41 ng/ml and 17.01 ± 6.15 ng·h/ml, respectively. The steady state pharmacokinetics of tazarotenic acid had been reached by Day 8 in the face-only and by Day 15 in the 15% body surface area dosing groups.

In a Phase 3 clinical trial, tazarotene 0.1% cream was applied once daily for 12 weeks to each of 48 patients (22 females and 26 males) with facial acne vulgaris. The mean ± SD values of plasma tazarotenic acid at Weeks 4 and 8 were 0.078 ± 0.073 ng/ml (n=47) and 0.052 ± 0.037 ng/ml (n=42), respectively. The highest observed individual plasma tazarotenic acid concentration was 0.41 ng/ml at Week 4 from a female patient. The magnitude of plasma tazarotenic acid concentrations appears to be independent of gender, age, and body weight.

INDICATIONS AND USAGE

AVAGE CREAM

To understand fully the indication for this product, please read the entire INDICATIONS AND USAGE section of the labeling.

Avage cream 0.1% is indicated as an adjunctive agent for use in the mitigation (palliation) of facial fine wrinkling, facial mottled hyper- and hypopigmentation, and benign facial lentigines in patients who use comprehensive skin care and sunlight avoidance programs. **AVAGE CREAM 0.1% DOES NOT ELIMINATE or PREVENT WRINKLES, REPAIR SUN-DAMAGED SKIN, REVERSE PHOTOAGING, or RESTORE MORE YOUTHFUL or YOUNGER SKIN.**

Avage cream 0.1% has NOT DEMONSTRATED A MITIGATING EFFECT on significant signs of chronic sunlight exposure such as coarse or deep wrinkling, tactile roughness, telangiectasia, skin laxity, keratinocytic atypia, melanocytic atypia, or dermal elastosis.

Avage cream 0.1% should be used under medical supervision as an adjunct to a comprehensive skin care and sunlight avoidance program that includes the use of effective sunscreens (minimum SPF of 15) and protective clothing.

Neither the safety nor the effectiveness of Avage cream 0.1% for the prevention or treatment of actinic keratoses, skin neoplasms, or lentigo maligna has been established.

Neither the safety nor the efficacy of using Avage cream 0.1% daily for greater than 52 weeks has been established, and daily use beyond 52 weeks has not been systematically and histologically investigated in adequate and well-controlled trials. (See WARNINGS, Avage Cream.)

TAZORAC GEL

Tazorac topical gel 0.05% and 0.1% are indicated for the topical treatment of patients with stable plaque psoriasis of up to 20% body surface area involvement.

Tazorac topical gel 0.1% is also indicated for the topical treatment of patients with facial acne vulgaris of mild to moderate severity.

The efficacy of Tazorac in the treatment of acne previously treated with other retinoids or resistant to oral antibiotics has not been established.

TAZORAC CREAM

Tazorac cream 0.05% and 0.1% are indicated for the topical treatment of patients with plaque psoriasis.

Tazorac cream 0.1% is also indicated for the topical treatment of patients with acne vulgaris.

CONTRAINDICATIONS

AVAGE CREAM

Retinoids may cause fetal harm when administered to a pregnant woman.

In rats, tazarotene 0.05% gel administered **topically** during gestation Days 6-17 at 0.25 mg/kg/day resulted in reduced fetal body weights and reduced skeletal ossification. Rabbits dosed **topically** with 0.25 mg/kg/day tazarotene gel during gestation Days 6-18 were noted with single incidences of known retinoid malformations, including spina bifida, hydrocephaly, and heart anomalies.

Systemic exposure [AUC(0-24h)] to tazarotenic acid at topical doses of 0.25 mg/kg/day tazarotene in a gel formulation in rats and rabbits represented 2.4 and 26 times, respectively, the maximum AUC(0-24h) in patients treated with 2 mg/cm^2 of tazarotene cream 0.1% over 15% body surface area for fine wrinkling and mottled hyperpigmentation.

As with other retinoids, when tazarotene was given **orally** to experimental animals, developmental delays were seen in rats, and teratogenic effects and post-implantation loss were observed in rats and rabbits at doses producing 2.1 and 52 times, respectively, the maximum AUC(0-24h) in patients treated with 2 mg/cm^2 of tazarotene cream 0.1% over 15% body surface area for fine wrinkling and mottled hyperpigmentation.

In a study of the effect of oral tazarotene on fertility and early embryonic development in rats, decreased number of implantation sites, decreased litter size, decreased number of live fetuses, and decreased fetal body weights, all classic developmental effects of retinoids, were observed when female rats were administered 2 mg/kg/day from 15 days before mating through gestation Day 7. A low incidence of retinoid-related malformations at that dose were reported to be related to treatment. That dose produced an AUC(0-24h) that was 6.7 times the maximum AUC(0-24h) in patients treated with 2 mg/cm^2 of tazarotene cream 0.1% over 15% body surface area for signs of fine wrinkling and mottled hyperpigmentation.

Systemic exposure to tazarotenic acid is dependent upon the extent of the body surface area treated. IN PATIENTS TREATED TOPICALLY OVER SUFFICIENT BODY SURFACE AREA, EXPOSURE COULD BE IN THE SAME ORDER OF MAGNITUDE AS IN THESE ORALLY TREATED ANIMALS. As a retinoid, tazarotene is a teratogenic substance, and it is not known what level of exposure is required for teratogenicity in humans. However, there may be less systemic exposure in the treatment of the face alone, due to less surface area for application (see CLINICAL PHARMACOLOGY, Avage Cream, Pharmacokinetics).

There were 13 reported pregnancies in patients who participated in clinical trials for topical tazarotene. Nine (9) of the patients were found to have been treated with topical tazarotene, and the other 4 had been treated with vehicle. One of the patients who was treated with tazarotene cream elected to terminate the pregnancy for non-medical reasons unrelated to treatment. The other 8 pregnant women who were inadvertently exposed to topical tazarotene during clinical trials subsequently delivered apparently healthy babies. As the exact timing and extent of exposure in relation to the gestation times are not certain, the significance of these findings is unknown.

Avage cream is contraindicated in women who are or may become pregnant. If this drug is used during pregnancy, or if the patient becomes pregnant while taking this drug, treatment should be discontinued and the patient apprised of the potential hazard to the fetus. Women of child-bearing potential should be warned of the potential risk and use adequate birth-control measures when Avage cream is used. The possibility that a woman of child-bearing potential is pregnant at the time of institution of therapy should be considered. A negative result for pregnancy test having a sensitivity down to at least 50 mIU/ml for human chorionic gonadotropin (hCG) should be obtained within 2 weeks prior to Avage cream therapy, which should begin during a normal menstrual period (see also PRECAUTIONS, Avage Cream, Pregnancy, Teratogenic Effects, Pregnancy Category X).

Avage cream is contraindicated in individuals who have shown hypersensitivity to any of its components.

TAZORAC GEL

Retinoids may cause fetal harm when administered to a pregnant woman.

In rats, tazarotene 0.05%, administered **topically** during gestation Days 6-17 at 0.25 mg/kg/day (1.5 mg/m^2/day) resulted in reduced fetal body weights and reduced skeletal ossification. Rabbits dosed **topically** with 0.25 mg/kg/day (2.75 mg/m^2 total body surface area/day) tazarotene during gestation Days 6-18 were noted with single incidences of known retinoid malformations, including spina bifida, hydrocephaly, and heart anomalies. As with other retinoids, when tazarotene was given **orally** to experimental animals, development delays were seen in rats, and teratogenic effects and post-implantation fetal loss were seen in rats and rabbits at doses producing 0.7 and 13 times, respectively, the systemic exposure [AUC(0-24h)] in human psoriasis patients, when extrapolated for **topical** treatment of 20% of body surface area. THUS, SYSTEMIC EXPOSURE IN TOPICALLY TREATED PSORIASIS PATIENTS (FOR USE ON UP TO 20% OF BODY SURFACE AREA) COULD BE IN THE SAME ORDER OF MAGNITUDE AS IN THESE ORALLY TREATED ANIMALS.

Systemic exposure anticipated in the treatment of facial acne may be less, due to a more limited area of application.

Six women inadvertently exposed to Tazorac during pregnancy in clinical trials have subsequently delivered healthy babies. As the exact timing and extent of exposure in relation to the gestation time are not certain, the significance of these findings is not known.

Tazorac is contraindicated in women who are or may become pregnant. If this drug is used during pregnancy, or if the patient becomes pregnant while taking this drug, treatment should be discontinued and the patient apprised of the potential hazard to the fetus. Women of child-bearing potential should be warned of the potential risk and use adequate birth-control measures when Tazorac is used. The possibility that a woman of childbearing potential is pregnant at the time of institution of therapy should be considered. A negative result for pregnancy test having a sensitivity down to at least 50 mIU/ml for human chorionic gonadotropin (hCG) should be obtained within 2 weeks prior to Tazorac therapy, which should begin during a normal menstrual period.

Tazarotene is contraindicated in individuals who have shown hypersensitivity to any of its components.

TAZORAC CREAM

Retinoids may cause fetal harm when administered to a pregnant woman.

In rats, tazarotene 0.05% gel administered **topically** during gestation Days 6-17 at 0.25 mg/kg/day resulted in reduced fetal body weights and reduced skeletal ossification. Rabbits dosed **topically** with 0.25 mg/kg/day tazarotene gel during gestation Days 6-18 were noted with single incidences of known retinoid malformations, including spina bifida, hydrocephaly, and heart anomalies.

Systemic exposure AUC(0-24h) to tazarotenic acid at topical doses of 0.25 mg/kg/day tazarotene in a gel formulation in rats and rabbits represented 1.2 and 13 times, respectively, that in a psoriatic patient treated with 0.1% tazarotene cream at 2 mg/cm^2 over 35% body surface area in a controlled pharmacokinetic study, and 4.0 and 44 times the maximum AUC(0-24h) in acne patients treated with 2 mg/cm^2 of tazarotene cream 0.1% over 15% body surface area.

As with other retinoids, when tazarotene was given **orally** to experimental animals, developmental delays were seen in rats; and teratogenic effects and post-implantation loss were observed in rats and rabbits at doses producing 1.1 and 26 times, respectively, the systemic exposure AUC(0-24h) seen in a psoriatic patient treated topically with 0.1% tazarotene cream at 2 mg/cm^2 over 35% body surface area in a controlled pharmacokinetic study and 3.5 and 85 times the maximum AUC(0-24h) in acne patients treated with 2 mg/cm^2 of tazarotene cream 0.1% over 15% body surface area.

In a study of the effect of oral tazarotene on fertility and early embryonic development in rats, decreased number of implantation sites, decreased litter size, decreased number of live fetuses, and decreased fetal body weights, all classic developmental effects of retinoids, were observed when female rats were administered 2 mg/kg/day from 15 days before mating through gestation Day 7. A low incidence of retinoid-related malformations at that dose were reported to be related to treatment. That dose produced an AUC(0-24h) that was 3.4 times that observed in a psoriatic patient treated with 0.1% tazarotene cream at 2 mg/cm^2 over 35% body surface area and 11 times the maximum AUC(0-24h) in acne patients treated with 2 mg/cm^2 of tazarotene cream 0.1% over 15% body surface area.

Systemic exposure to tazarotenic acid is dependent upon the extent of the body surface area treated. IN PATIENTS TREATED TOPICALLY OVER SUFFICIENT BODY SURFACE AREA, EXPOSURE COULD BE IN THE SAME ORDER OF MAGNITUDE AS IN THESE ORALLY TREATED ANIMALS. Although there may be less systemic exposure in the treatment of acne of the face alone due to less surface area for application, tazarotene is a teratogenic substance, and it is not known what level of exposure is required for teratogenicity in humans (see CLINICAL PHARMACOLOGY, Tazorac Cream, Pharmacokinetics).

There were 3 reported pregnancies in patients who participated in the clinical trials on acne with tazarotene cream 0.1%. Two of the patients were found to have been treated with tazarotene cream and the other had been treated with vehicle. One of the patients who was treated with tazarotene cream elected to terminate the pregnancy. The other gave birth to an apparently normal, healthy child at 36 weeks gestation. Seven pregnant women who were inadvertently exposed to topical tazarotene during other clinical trials subsequently delivered healthy babies. As the exact timing and extent of exposure in relation to the gestation times are not certain, the significance of these findings is unknown.

Tazorac cream is contraindicated in women who are or may become pregnant. If this drug is used during pregnancy, or if the patient becomes pregnant while taking this drug, treatment should be discontinued and the patient apprised of the potential hazard to the fetus. Women of child-bearing potential should be warned of the potential risk and use adequate birth-control measures when Tazorac cream is used. The possibility that a woman of child-bearing potential is pregnant at the time of institution of therapy should be considered. A negative result for pregnancy test having a sensitivity down to at least 50 mIU/ml for human chorionic gonadotropin (hCG) should be obtained within 2 weeks prior to Tazorac cream therapy, which should begin during a normal menstrual period (see also PRECAUTIONS, Tazorac Cream, Pregnancy, Teratogenic Effects, Pregnancy Category X).

Tazorac cream is contraindicated in individuals who have shown hypersensitivity to any of its components.

WARNINGS

AVAGE CREAM

Pregnancy Category X

See CONTRAINDICATIONS, Avage Cream. Women of child-bearing potential should be warned of the potential risk and use adequate birth-control measures when Avage cream is used. The possibility that a woman of child-bearing potential is pregnant at the time of institution of therapy should be considered. A negative result for pregnancy test having a sensitivity down to at least 50 mIU/ml for hCG should be obtained within 2 weeks prior to Avage cream therapy, which should begin during a normal menstrual period.

TAZORAC GEL

Pregnancy Category X

See CONTRAINDICATIONS, Tazorac Gel.

Women of childbearing potential should be warned of the potential risk and use adequate birth-control measures when Tazorac is used. The possibility that a woman of childbearing potential is pregnant at the time of institution of therapy should be considered. A negative result for pregnancy test having a sensitivity down to at least 50 mIU/ml for hCG should be obtained within 2 weeks prior to Tazorac therapy, which should begin during a normal menstrual period.

TAZORAC CREAM

Pregnancy Category X

See CONTRAINDICATIONS, Tazorac Cream. Women of childbearing potential should be warned of the potential risk and use adequate birth-control measures when Tazorac cream is used. The possibility that a woman of child-bearing potential is pregnant at the time of institution of therapy should be considered. A negative result for pregnancy test having a sensitivity down to at least 50 mIU/ml for hCG should be obtained within 2 weeks prior to Tazorac cream therapy, which should begin during a normal menstrual period.

PRECAUTIONS

AVAGE CREAM

General

Avage cream should be applied only to the affected areas. For external use only. Avoid contact with eyes and mouth. If contact with eyes occurs, rinse thoroughly with water.

Retinoids should not be used on eczematous skin, as they may cause severe irritation. Because of heightened burning susceptibility, exposure to sunlight (including sunlamps) should be avoided unless deemed medically necessary, and in such cases, exposure should be minimized during the use of Avage cream. Patients must be warned to use sunscreens (minimum SPF of 15) and protective clothing when using Avage cream. Patients with sunburn should be advised not to use Avage cream until fully recovered.

Patients who may have considerable sun exposure due to their occupation and those patients with inherent sensitivity to sunlight should exercise particular caution when using Avage cream and ensure that the precautions outlined in the Information for Patients subsection are observed.

Avage cream should be administered with caution if the patient is also taking drugs known to be photosensitizers (*e.g.*, thiazides, tetracyclines, fluoroquinolones, phenothiazines, sulfonamides) because of the increased possibility of augmented photosensitivity.

Some individuals may experience excessive pruritus, burning, skin redness or peeling. If these effects occur, the medication should either be discontinued until the integrity of the skin is restored, or the dosing should be reduced to an interval the patient can tolerate. However, efficacy at reduced frequency of application has not been established. Weather extremes, such as wind or cold, may be more irritating to patients using Avage cream.

Some facial pigmented lesions are not lentigines, but rather lentigo maligna, a type of melanoma. Facial pigmented lesions of concern should be carefully assessed by a qualified physician (*e.g.*, dermatologist) before application of Avage cream. Lentigo maligna should not be treated with Avage cream.

Information for the Patient

Avage cream 0.1% is to be used as described below when used for treatment of facial fine wrinkling, mottled hypo- and hyperpigmentation, and benign facial lentigines, unless otherwise directed by your physician:

It is for use on the face.

Avoid contact with the eyes and mouth. Avage cream 0.1% may cause severe redness, itching, burning, stinging, and peeling.

Before applying Avage cream 0.1% once per day, gently wash your face with a mild soap. Make sure skin is dry before applying Avage cream 0.1%. Apply only a small pea sized amount (about 1/4 inch or 5 millimeter diameter) of Avage cream 0.1% to your face at 1 time. This should be enough to lightly cover the entire face.

For best results, you are advised that if emollients or moisturizers are used, they can be applied either before or after tazarotene cream, ensuring that the first cream or lotion has absorbed into the skin and dried completely.

In the morning, apply a moisturizing sunscreen, SPF 15 or greater.

Avage cream 0.1% is a serious medication. Do not use Avage cream 0.1% if you are pregnant or attempting to become pregnant. If you become pregnant while using Avage cream 0.1%, please contact your physician immediately.

Avoid sunlight and other medicines that may increase your sensitivity to sunlight. For the mitigation of fine wrinkling, mottled hypo- and hyperpigmentation, and benign facial lentigines, avoidance of excessive sun exposure and the use of sunscreens with protective measures (hat, visor) are recommended.

Avage cream 0.1% does not remove or prevent wrinkles or repair sun-damaged skin.

Please refer to the Patient Package Insert that is included with the prescription for additional patient information.

Carcinogenesis, Mutagenesis, and Impairment of Fertility

A long term study of tazarotene following oral administration of 0.025, 0.050, and 0.125 mg/kg/day to rats showed no indications of increased carcinogenic risks. Based on pharmacokinetic data from a shorter term study in rats, the highest dose of 0.125 mg/kg/day was anticipated to give systemic exposure in the rat equivalent to 1.4 times the maximum AUC(0-24h) in patients treated with 2 mg/cm^2 of tazarotene cream 0.1% over 15% body surface area for fine wrinkling and mottled hyperpigmentation.

In evaluation of photo co-carcinogenicity, median time to onset of tumors was decreased, and the number of tumors increased in hairless mice following chronic topical dosing with intercurrent exposure to ultraviolet radiation at tazarotene concentrations of 0.001%, 0.005%, and 0.01% in a gel formulation for up to 40 weeks.

A long-term topical application study of up to 0.1% tazarotene in a gel formulation in mice terminated at 88 weeks showed that dose levels of 0.05, 0.125, 0.25, and 1.0 mg/kg/day (reduced to 0.5 mg/kg/day for males after 41 weeks due to severe dermal irritation) revealed no apparent carcinogenic effects when compared to vehicle control animals; untreated control animals were not completely evaluated. Systemic exposure (AUC0-12h) at the highest dose was 7.8 times the maximum AUC(0-24h) in patients treated with 2 mg/cm^2 of tazarotene cream 0.1% over 15% body surface area for fine wrinkling and mottled hyperpigmentation.

Tazarotene was found to be non-mutagenic in the Ames assays using *Salmonella* and *E. coli* and did not produce structural chromosomal aberrations in a human lymphocyte assay. Tazarotene was also non-mutagenic in the CHO/HGPRT mammalian cell forward gene mutation assay and was nonclastogenic in the in vivo mouse micronucleus test.

No impairment of fertility occurred in rats when male animals were treated for 70 days prior to mating and female animals were treated for 14 days prior to mating and continuing through gestation and lactation with topical doses of tazarotene gel up to 0.125 mg/kg/day. Based on data from another study, the systemic drug exposure in the rat would be equivalent to 1.2 times the maximum AUC(0-24h) in patients treated with 2 mg/cm^2 of tazarotene cream 0.1% over 15% body surface area for fine wrinkling and mottled hyperpigmentation.

T

No impairment of mating performance or fertility was observed in male rats treated for 70 days prior to mating with oral doses of up to 1.0 mg/kg/day tazarotene. That dose produced an AUC(0-24h) that was 3.7 times the maximum AUC(0-24h) in patients treated with 2 mg/cm^2 of tazarotene cream 0.1% over 15% body surface area for fine wrinkling and mottled hyperpigmentation.

No effect on parameters of mating performance or fertility was observed in female rats treated for 15 days prior to mating and continuing through Day 7 of gestation with oral doses of tazarotene up to 2.0 mg/kg/day. However, there was a significant decrease in the number of estrous stages and an increase in developmental effects at that dose (see CONTRAINDICATIONS, Avage Cream). That dose produced an AUC(0-24h) that was 6.7 times the maximum AUC(0-24h) in patients treated with 2 mg/cm^2 of tazarotene cream 0.1% over 15% body surface area for signs of fine wrinkling and mottled hyperpigmentation.

Reproductive capabilities of F1 animals, including F2 survival and development, were not affected by topical administration of tazarotene gel to female F0 parental rats from gestation Day 16 through lactation Day 20 at the maximum tolerated dose of 0.125 mg/kg/day. Based on data from another study, the systemic drug exposure in the rat would be equivalent to 1.2 times the maximum AUC(0-24h) in patients treated with 2 mg/cm^2 of tazarotene cream 0.1% over 15% body surface area for fine wrinkling and mottled hyperpigmentation.

Pregnancy, Teratogenic Effects, Pregnancy Category X

See CONTRAINDICATIONS, Avage Cream. Women of child-bearing potential should use adequate birth-control measures when Avage cream is used. The possibility that a woman of childbearing potential is pregnant at the time of institution of therapy should be considered. A negative result for pregnancy test having a sensitivity down to at least 50 mIU/ml for hCG should be obtained within 2 weeks prior to Avage cream therapy, which should begin during a normal menstrual period. There are no adequate and well-controlled studies in pregnant women. As a retinoid, tazarotene is a teratogenic substance, and it is not known what level of exposure is required for teratogenicity in humans. However, there may be less systemic exposure in the treatment of the face alone, due to less surface area for application (see CLINICAL PHARMACOLOGY, Avage Cream, Pharmacokinetics).

Nursing Mothers

After single topical doses of ^{14}C-tazarotene gel to the skin of lactating rats, radioactivity was detected in milk, suggesting that there would be transfer of drug-related material to the offspring via milk. It is not known whether this drug is excreted in human milk. Caution should be exercised when tazarotene is administered to a nursing woman.

Pediatric Use

The safety and efficacy of tazarotene cream have not been established in patients under the age of 17 years with facial fine wrinkling, facial mottled hypo- and hyperpigmentation, and benign facial lentigines.

Geriatric Use

In the studies of facial fine wrinkling, facial mottled hypo- and hyperpigmentation, and benign facial lentigines , 44 male patients and 180 female patients out of the total population of 1131 patients were older than 65 years of age. No overall differences in safety or effectiveness were observed between these patients and younger patients, and other clinical experience has not identified differences in responses between the elderly and younger patients, but greater sensitivity of some older individuals cannot be ruled out.

TAZORAC GEL

General

Tazorac should only be applied to the affected areas. For external use only. Avoid contact with eyes, eyelids, and mouth. If contact with eyes occurs, rinse thoroughly with water. The safety of use over more than 20% of body surface area has not been established in psoriasis or acne.

Retinoids should not be used on eczematous skin, as they may cause severe irritation.

Because of heightened burning susceptibility, exposure to sunlight (including sunlamps) should be avoided unless deemed medically necessary, and in such cases, exposure should be minimized during the use of Tazorac. Patients must be warned to use sunscreens (minimum SPF of 15) and protective clothing when using Tazorac. Patients with sunburn should be advised not to use Tazorac until fully recovered. Patients who may have considerable sun exposure due to their occupation and those patients with inherent sensitivity to sunlight should exercise particular caution when using Tazorac and ensure that the precautions outlined in the Information for Patients leaflet that is distributed with the prescription are observed.

Tazorac should be administered with caution if the patient is also taking drugs known to be photosensitizers (*e.g.,* thiazides, tetracyclines, fluoroquinolones, phenothiazines, sulfonamides) because of the increased possibility of augmented photosensitivity.

If pruritus, burning, skin redness or peeling is excessive, the medication should be discontinued until the integrity of the skin is restored.

Weather extremes, such as wind or cold, may be more irritating to patients using Tazorac gel.

Information for the Patient

See the Information for Patients leaflet that is distributed with the prescription.

Carcinogenesis, Mutagenesis, and Impairment of Fertility

Long-term studies of tazarotene following oral administration of 0.025, 0.050, and 0.125 mg/kg/day to rats showed no indications of increased carcinogenic risks. However, in other rat studies, oral doses twice that of the highest dose in the rat carcinogenicity study produced an AUC(0-24h) that was less (0.7 times) than that in topically treated psoriatic patients extrapolated for treatment of 20% of body surface area. In evaluation of photocarcinogenicity, median time to onset of tumors was decreased and the number of tumors increased in hairless mice following chronic topical dosing with intercurrent exposure to ultraviolet radiation at tazarotene concentrations of 0.001%, 0.005%, and 0.01% for up to 40 weeks.

A long-term topical application study in mice terminated at 88 weeks showed that dose levels of 0.05, 0.125, 0.25 and 1.0 mg/kg/day (reduced to 0.5 mg/kg/day for males after 41 weeks due to severe dermal irritation) revealed no apparent carcinogenic effects when compared to vehicle control animals; untreated control animals were not completely evaluated. The AUC(0-12h)s for these doses were 82.7, 137, 183, 136 (males at 1.0/0.5 mg/kg) and 344 ng·h/ml (females at 1.0 mg/kg), respectively. The mean AUC(0-24h) for psoriatic patients was 172 ng·h/ml, extrapolated for 20% total body surface area.

Tazarotene was found to be non-mutagenic in the Ames assay and did not produce structural chromosomal aberrations in a human lymphocyte assay. Tazarotene was also non-mutagenic in the CHO/HPRT mammalian cell forward gene mutation assay and was non-clastogenic in the *in vivo* mouse micronucleus test.

No impairment of fertility occurred in rats when male animals were treated for 70 days prior to mating and female animals were treated for 14 days prior to mating and continuing through gestation and lactation with topical doses of Tazorac gel of up to 0.125 mg/kg/day (0.738 mg/m^2/day).

Reproductive capabilities of F1 animals, including F2 survival and development, were not affected by topical administration of Tazorac gel to female F0 parental rats from gestation Day 16 through lactation Day 20 at the maximum tolerated dose of 0.125 mg/kg/day (0.738 mg/m^2/day).

Pregnancy, Teratogenic Effects, Pregnancy Category X

See CONTRAINDICATIONS, Tazorac Gel. Women of childbearing potential should use adequate birth-control measures when Tazorac is used. The possibility that a woman of childbearing potential is pregnant at the time of institution of therapy should be considered. A negative result for pregnancy test having a sensitivity down to at least 50 mIU/ml for hCG should be obtained within 2 weeks prior to Tazorac therapy, which should begin during a normal menstrual period.

Nursing Mothers

After single topical doses of ^{14}C-tazarotene to the skin of lactating rats, secretion of radioactivity was detected in milk, suggesting that there would be transfer of drug-related material to the offspring via milk. It is not known whether this drug is excreted in human milk. Caution should be exercised when tazarotene is administered to a nursing woman.

Pediatric Use

The safety and efficacy of tazarotene have not been established in pediatric patients under the age of 12 years.

TAZORAC CREAM

General

Tazorac cream should be applied only to the affected areas. For external use only. Avoid contact with eyes, eyelids, and mouth. If contact with eyes occurs, rinse thoroughly with water.

Retinoids should not be used on eczematous skin, as they may cause severe irritation. Because of heightened burning susceptibility, exposure to sunlight (including sunlamps) should be avoided unless deemed medically necessary, and in such cases, exposure should be minimized during the use of Tazorac cream. Patients must be warned to use sunscreens (minimum SPF of 15) and protective clothing when using Tazorac cream. Patients with sunburn should be advised not to use Tazorac cream until fully recovered. Patients who may have considerable sun exposure due to their occupation and those patients with inherent sensitivity to sunlight should exercise particular caution when using Tazorac cream and ensure that the precautions outlined in the Information for Patients leaflet that is distributed with the prescription are observed.

Tazorac cream should be administered with caution if the patient is also taking drugs known to be photosensitizers (*e.g.,* thiazides, tetracyclines, fluoroquinolones, phenothiazines, sulfonamides) because of the increased possibility of augmented photosensitivity.

Some individuals may experience excessive pruritus, burning, skin redness or peeling. If these effects occur, the medication should either be discontinued until the integrity of the skin is restored, or the dosing should be reduced to an interval the patient can tolerate. However, efficacy at reduced frequency of application has not been established. Alternatively, patients with psoriasis who are being treated with the 0.1% concentration can be switched to the lower concentration. Weather extremes, such as wind or cold, may be more irritating to patients using Tazorac cream.

Information for the Patient

See the Information for Patients leaflet that is distributed with the prescription.

Carcinogenesis, Mutagenesis, and Impairment of Fertility

A long term study of tazarotene following oral administration of 0.025, 0.050, and 0.125 mg/kg/day to rats showed no indications of increased carcinogenic risks. Based on pharmacokinetic data from a shorter term study in rats, the highest dose of 0.125 mg/kg/day was anticipated to give systemic exposure in the rat equivalent to 0.6 times that seen in a psoriatic patient treated with 0.1% tazarotene cream at 2 mg/cm^2 over 35% body surface area in a controlled pharmacokinetic study. This estimated systemic exposure in rats was 2.0 times the maximum AUC(0-24h) in acne patients treated with 2 mg/cm^2 of tazarotene cream 0.1% over 15% body surface area.

In evaluation of photo co-carcinogenicity, median time to onset of tumors was decreased, and the number of tumors increased in hairless mice following chronic topical dosing with intercurrent exposure to ultraviolet radiation at tazarotene concentrations of 0.001%, 0.005%, and 0.01% in a gel formulation for up to 40 weeks.

A long-term topical application study of up to 0.1% tazarotene in a gel formulation in mice terminated at 88 weeks showed that dose levels of 0.05, 0.125, 0.25, and 1.0 mg/kg/day (reduced to 0.5 mg/kg/day for males after 41 weeks due to severe dermal irritation) revealed no apparent carcinogenic effects when compared to vehicle control animals; untreated control animals were not completely evaluated. Systemic exposure (AUC0-12h) at the highest dose was 3.9 times that AUC(0-24h) seen in a psoriatic patient treated with 0.1% tazarotene cream at 2 mg/cm^2 over 35% body surface area in a controlled pharmacokinetic study, and 13 times the maximum AUC(0-24h) in acne patients treated with 2 mg/cm^2 of tazarotene cream 0.1% over 15 % body surface area.

Tazarotene was found to be non-mutagenic in the Ames assays using *Salmonella* and *E. coli* and did not produce structural chromosomal aberrations in a human lymphocyte assay. Tazarotene was also non-mutagenic in the CHO/HGPRT mammalian cell forward gene mutation assay and was non-clastogenic in the *in vivo* mouse micronucleus test.

No impairment of fertility occurred in rats when male animals were treated for 70 days prior to mating and female animals were treated for 14 days prior to mating and continuing through gestation and lactation with topical doses of tazarotene gel up to 0.125 mg/kg/day. Based on data from another study, the systemic drug exposure in the rat would be equivalent to 0.6 times that observed in a psoriatic patient treated with 0.1% tazarotene cream at 2 mg/cm^2 over 35% body surface area in a controlled pharmacokinetic study, and 2.0 times the maximum AUC(0-24h) in acne patients treated with 2 mg/cm^2 of tazarotene cream 0.1% over 15% body surface area.

No impairment of mating performance or fertility was observed in male rats treated for 70 days prior to mating with oral doses of up to 1.0 mg/kg/day tazarotene. That dose produced an AUC(0-24h) that was 1.9 times that observed in a psoriatic patient treated with 0.1% tazarotene cream at 2 mg/cm^2 over 35% body surface area, and 6.3 times the maximum AUC(0-24h) in acne patients treated with 2 mg/cm^2 of tazarotene cream 0.1% over 15 % body surface area.

No effect on parameters of mating performance or fertility was observed in female rats treated for 15 days prior to mating and continuing through Day 7 of gestation with oral doses of tazarotene up to 2.0 mg/kg/day. However, there was a significant decrease in the number of estrous stages and an increase in developmental effects at that dose (see CONTRAINDICATIONS, Tazorac Cream). That dose produced an AUC(0-24h) that was 3.4 times that observed in a psoriatic patient treated with 0.1% tazarotene cream at 2 mg/cm^2 over 35% body surface area and 11 times the maximum AUC(0-24h) in acne patients treated with 2 mg/cm^2 of tazarotene cream 0.1% over 15% body surface area.

Reproductive capabilities of F1 animals, including F2 survival and development, were not affected by topical administration of tazarotene gel to female F0 parental rats from gestation Day 16 through lactation day 20 at the maximum tolerated dose of 0.125 mg/kg/day. Based on data from another study, the systemic drug exposure in the rat would be equivalent to 0.6 times that observed in a psoriatic patient treated with 0.1% tazarotene cream at 2 mg/cm^2 over 35% body surface area, and 2.0 times the maximum AUC(0-24h) in acne patients treated with 2 mg/cm^2 of tazarotene cream 0.1% over 15% body surface area.

Pregnancy, Teratogenic Effects, Pregnancy Category X

See CONTRAINDICATIONS, Tazorac Cream. Women of childbearing potential should use adequate birth-control measures when Tazorac cream is used. The possibility that a woman of childbearing potential is pregnant at the time of institution of therapy should be considered. A negative result for pregnancy test having a sensitivity down to at least 50 mIU/ml for hCG should be obtained within 2 weeks prior to Tazorac cream therapy, which should begin during a normal menstrual period. There are no adequate and well-controlled studies in pregnant women. Although there may be less systemic exposure in the treatment of acne of the face alone due to less surface area for application, tazarotene is a teratogenic substance, and it is not known what level of exposure is required for teratogenicity in humans (see CLINICAL PHARMACOLOGY, Tazorac Cream, Pharmacokinetics).

Nursing Mothers

After single topical doses of ^{14}C-tazarotene gel to the skin of lactating rats, radioactivity was detected in milk, suggesting that there would be transfer of drug-related material to the offspring via milk. It is not known whether this drug is excreted in human milk. Caution should be exercised when tazarotene is administered to a nursing woman.

Pediatric Use

The safety and efficacy of tazarotene cream have not been established in patients with psoriasis under the age of 18 years or in patients with acne under the age of 12 years.

Geriatric Use

Of the total number of patients in clinical studies of tazarotene cream for plaque psoriasis, 120 were over the age of 65. No overall differences in safety or effectiveness were observed between these patients and younger patients. Currently there is no other clinical experience on the differences in responses between the elderly and younger patients, but greater sensitivity of some older individuals cannot be ruled out. Tazarotene cream for the treatment of acne has not been clinically tested in persons 65 years of age or older.

DRUG INTERACTIONS

AVAGE CREAM

Concomitant dermatologic medications and cosmetics that have a strong drying effect should be avoided. It is also advisable to "rest" a patient's skin until the effects of such preparations subside before use of Avage cream is begun.

TAZORAC GEL

Concomitant dermatologic medications and cosmetics that have a strong drying effect should be avoided. It is also advisable to "rest" a patient's skin until the effects of such preparations subside before use of Tazorac is begun.

TAZORAC CREAM

Concomitant dermatologic medications and cosmetics that have a strong drying effect should be avoided. It is also advisable to "rest" a patient's skin until the effects of such preparations subside before use of Tazorac cream is begun.

ADVERSE REACTIONS

AVAGE CREAM

In human dermal safety studies, tazarotene 0.05% and 0.1% creams did not induce allergic contact sensitization, phototoxicity or photoallergy.

The most frequent treatment-related adverse reactions (≥5%) reported during the clinical trials with Avage cream 0.1% in the treatment of facial fine wrinkling, mottled hypo- and hyperpigmentation, and benign facial lentigines were limited to the skin. Those occurring in >10%, in descending order, included: desquamation, erythema, burning sensation, and dry skin. Events occurring in ≥1% to ≤10% of patients, in descending order included: skin irritation, pruritus, irritant contact dermatitis, stinging, acne, rash or cheilitis. Common adverse events observed in the clinical trials are presented in TABLE 10.

TABLE 10 *Table of Adverse Events Seen in Clinical Trials With Avage Cream 0.1%*

Adverse Event	Avage n=567	Vehicle n=564
Desquamation	40%	3%
Erythema	34%	3%
Burning sensation	26%	<1%
Dry skin	16%	3%
Irritation skin	10%	1%
Pruritus	10%	1%
Irritant contact dermatitis	8%	1%
Stinging	3%	<1%
Acne	3%	3%
Rash	3%	1%
Cheilitis	1%	0%

A few patients reported adverse events at Week 0; however, for patients who were treated with Avage the highest number of new reports for each adverse event was at Week 2.

When combining data from the two pivotal studies, 5.3% of patients in the tazarotene cream group and 0.9% of patients in the vehicle group discontinued due to adverse events.

Overall, 20/567 (3.5%) patients in the Avage cream 0.1% group and 16/564 (2.8%) patients in the vehicle group reported adverse events (including edema, irritation, and inflammation) directly related to the eye or eyelid. The majority of these conditions were mild.

TAZORAC GEL

Psoriasis

The most frequent adverse events reported with Tazorac 0.05% and 0.1% gels were limited to the skin. Those occurring in 10-30% of patients, in descending order, included pruritus, burning/stinging, erythema, worsening of psoriasis, irritation, and skin pain. Events occurring in 1-10% of patients included rash, desquamation, irritant contact dermatitis, skin inflammation, fissuring, bleeding and dry skin. Increases in "psoriasis worsening" and "sun-induced erythema" were noted in some patients over the 4th to 12th months as compared to the first 3 months of a 1 year study. In general, the incidence of adverse events with Tazorac 0.05% gel was 2-5% lower than that seen with Tazorac 0.1% gel.

Acne

The most frequent adverse events reported with Tazorac 0.1% gel were limited to the skin. Those events occurring in 10-30% of patients, in descending order, included desquamation, burning/stinging, dry skin, erythema and pruritus. Events occurring in 1-10% of patients included irritation, skin pain, fissuring, localized edema and skin discoloration.

In human dermal safety studies, tazarotene 0.05% and 0.1% gels did not induce contact sensitization, phototoxicity or photoallergy.

TAZORAC CREAM

In human dermal safety studies, tazarotene 0.05% and 0.1% creams did not induce allergic contact sensitization, phototoxicity or photoallergy.

Psoriasis

The most frequent adverse events reported with Tazorac 0.05% and 0.1% creams were limited to the skin. Those occurring in 10-23% of patients, in descending order, included pruritus, erythema, and burning. Events occurring in >1 to <10% of patients, in descending order, included irritation, desquamation, stinging, contact dermatitis, dermatitis, eczema, worsening of psoriasis, skin pain, rash, hypertriglyceridemia, dry skin, skin inflammation, and peripheral edema.

Tazarotene cream 0.1% was associated with a somewhat greater degree of local irritation than the 0.05% cream. In general, the rates of irritation adverse events reported during psoriasis studies with Tazorac 0.1% cream were 1-4 percentage points higher than those reported for Tazorac 0.05% cream.

Acne

The most frequent adverse reactions reported during clinical trials with Tazorac cream 0.1% in the treatment of acne, occurring in 10-30% of patients, in descending order included desquamation, dry skin, erythema, and burning sensation. Events occurring in 1-5% of patients included pruritus, irritation, face pain, and stinging.

T

DOSAGE AND ADMINISTRATION

AVAGE CREAM

General

Application may cause excessive irritation in the skin of certain sensitive individuals. In cases where it has been necessary to temporarily discontinue therapy, or the dosing has been reduced to an interval the patient can tolerate, therapy can be resumed, or the frequency of application can be increased as the patient becomes able to tolerate the treatment. Frequency of application should be closely monitored by careful observation of the clinical therapeutic response and skin tolerance. Efficacy has not been established for less than once daily dosing frequencies.

Apply a pea-sized amount once a day at bedtime to lightly cover the entire face including the eyelids if desired. Facial moisturizers may be used as frequently as desired. If any makeup is present it should be removed before applying Avage cream 0.1% to the face. If the face is washed or a bath or shower is taken prior to application, the skin should be dry before applying the cream. If emollients or moisturizers are used, they can be applied either before or after application of tazarotene cream ensuring that the first cream or lotion has absorbed into the skin and has dried completely. Frequency of application should be closely monitored by careful observation of the clinical therapeutic response and skin tolerance. If the frequency of dosing is reduced, it should be noted that efficacy at a reduced frequency of application has not been established. The duration of the mitigating effects on facial fine wrinkling, mottled hypo- and hyperpigmentation, and benign facial lentigines following discontinuation of Avage cream 0.1% has not been studied.

TAZORAC GEL

General

Application may cause a transitory feeling of burning or stinging. If irritation is excessive, application should be discontinued.

For Psoriasis: Apply Tazorac once a day, in the evening, to psoriatic lesions, using enough (2 mg/cm^2) to cover only the lesion with a thin film to no more than 20% of body surface area. If a bath or shower is taken prior to application, the skin should be dry before applying the gel. Because unaffected skin may be more susceptible to irritation, application of tazarotene to these areas should be carefully avoided. Tazorac was investigated for up to 12 months during clinical trials for psoriasis.

For Acne: Cleanse the face gently. After the skin is dry, apply a thin film of Tazorac (2 mg/cm^2) once a day, in the evening, to the skin where acne lesions appear. Use enough to cover the entire affected area. Tazorac was investigated for up to 12 weeks during clinical trials for acne.

TAZORAC CREAM

General

Application may cause excessive irritation in the skin of certain sensitive individuals. In cases where it has been necessary to temporarily discontinue therapy, or the dosing has been reduced to a lower concentration (in patients with psoriasis) or to an interval the patient can tolerate, therapy can be resumed, or the drug concentration or frequency of application can be increased as the patient becomes able to tolerate the treatment. Frequency of application should be closely monitored by careful observation of the clinical therapeutic response and skin tolerance. Efficacy has not been established for less than once daily dosing frequencies.

For Psoriasis

It is recommended that treatment start with Tazorac 0.05% cream, with strength increased to 0.1% if tolerated and medically indicated. Apply Tazorac cream once per day, in the evening, to psoriatic lesions, using enough (2 mg/cm^2) to cover only the lesion with a thin film. If a bath or shower is taken prior to application, the skin should be dry before applying the cream. If emollients are used, they should be applied at least an hour before application of Tazorac cream. Because unaffected skin may be more susceptible to irritation, application of Tazorac cream to these areas should be carefully avoided.

For Acne

Cleanse the face gently. After the skin is dry, apply a thin layer (2 mg/cm^2) of Tazorac cream 0.1% once per day, in the evening, to the skin areas where acne lesions appear. Use enough to cover the entire affected area. Tazorac cream 0.1% was investigated for up to 12 weeks during clinical trials for acne.

HOW SUPPLIED

AVAGE CREAM

Avage cream is available in a concentrations of 0.1%. It is available in a collapsible aluminum tube with a tamper-evident aluminum membrane over the opening and a white polypropylene screw cap, in a 30 g size.

Storage: Store at 25°C (77°F). Excursions permitted from -5 to 30°C (23-86°F).

TAZORAC GEL

Tazorac is available in concentrations of 0.05% and 0.1%. It comes in collapsible aluminum tubes, in 30 and 100 g sizes.

Storage: Tazorac gel should be stored at 25°C (77°F). Excursion permitted to 15-30°C (59-86°F).

TAZORAC CREAM

Tazorac cream is available in concentrations of 0.05% and 0.1%. It is available in a collapsible aluminum tube with a tamper-evident aluminmum membrane over the opening and a white polypropylene screw cap, in 15, 30, and 60 g sizes.

Storage: Store at 25°C (77°F). Excursions permitted from -5 to 30°C (23-86°F).

PRODUCT LISTING - EQUIVALENTS NOT AVAILABLE

Size	Price	Product	NDC
Cream - Topical - 0.05%			
15 gm	$36.80	TAZORAC, Allergan Inc	00023-9155-15
30 gm	$73.60	TAZORAC, Allergan Inc	00023-9155-30
60 gm	$147.20	TAZORAC, Allergan Inc	00023-9155-60
Cream - Topical - 0.1%			
15 gm	$39.11	TAZORAC, Allergan Inc	00023-9156-15
30 gm	$78.20	TAZORAC, Allergan Inc	00023-9156-30
30 gm	$78.20	AVAGE, Allergan Inc	00023-9236-30
60 gm	$156.40	TAZORAC, Allergan Inc	00023-9156-60
Gel - Topical - 0.05%			
30 gm	$73.60	TAZORAC, Allergan Inc	00023-8335-03
100 gm	$245.34	TAZORAC, Allergan Inc	00023-8335-10
Gel - Topical - 0.1%			
30 gm	$78.20	TAZORAC, Allergan Inc	00023-0042-03
100 gm	$260.66	TAZORAC, Allergan Inc	00023-0042-10

Tegaserod Maleate *(003566)*

Categories: Irritable bowel syndrome; Pregnancy Category B; FDA Approved 2002 Jul
Drug Classes: Gastrointestinals; Serotonin receptor agonists
Brand Names: Zelnorm
Foreign Brand Availability: Zelmac (Colombia; Singapore; Thailand)
Cost of Therapy: $153.75 (Irritable Bowel Syndrome; Zelnorm; 6 mg; 2 tablets/day; 30 day supply)

DESCRIPTION

Zelnorm (tegaserod maleate) tablets contain tegaserod as the hydrogen maleate salt. As the maleate salt, tegaserod is chemically designated as 3-(5-methoxy-1H-indol-3-ylmethylene)-N-pentylcarbazimidamide hydrogen maleate. Its empirical formula is $C_{16}H_{23}N_5O{\cdot}C_4H_4O_4$. The molecular weight is 417.47.

Tegaserod as the maleate salt is a white to off-white crystalline powder and is slightly soluble in ethanol and very slightly soluble in water. Each 1.385 mg of tegaserod as the maleate is equivalent to 1 mg of tegaserod. Zelnorm is available for oral use as tablets containing either 2 mg or 6 mg of tegaserod; inactive ingredients are crospovidone, glyceryl monostearate, hydroxypropyl methylcellulose, lactose monohydrate, poloxamer 188, and polyethylene glycol 4000.

CLINICAL PHARMACOLOGY

MECHANISM OF ACTION

Clinical investigations have shown that both motor and sensory functions of the gut appear to be altered in patients suffering from irritable bowel syndrome (IBS). Both the enteric nervous system, which acts to integrate and process information in the gut, and 5-hydroxytryptamine (5-HT, serotonin) are thought to represent key elements in the etiology of IBS. Approximately 95% of serotonin is found throughout the gastrointestinal tract, primarily stored in enterochromaffin cells but also in enteric nerves acting as a neurotransmitter. Serotonin has been shown to be involved in regulating motility, visceral sensitivity and intestinal secretion. Investigations suggest an important role of serotonin Type-4 (5-HT$_4$) receptors in the maintenance of gastrointestinal functions in humans.

Tegaserod is a 5-HT$_4$ receptor partial agonist that binds with high affinity at human 5-HT$_4$ receptors, whereas it has no appreciable affinity for 5-HT$_3$ or dopamine receptors. It has moderate affinity for 5-HT$_1$ receptors. Tegaserod, by acting as an agonist at neuronal 5-HT$_4$ receptors, triggers the release of further neurotransmitters such as calcitonin gene-related peptide from sensory neurons. The activation of 5-HT$_4$ receptors in the gastrointestinal tract stimulates the peristaltic reflex and intestinal secretion, as well as inhibits visceral sensitivity. *In vivo* studies showed that tegaserod enhanced basal motor activity and normalized impaired motility throughout the gastrointestinal tract. In addition, studies demonstrated that tegaserod moderated visceral sensitivity during colorectal distension in animals.

PHARMACOKINETICS

Absorption

Peak plasma concentrations are reached approximately 1 hour after oral dosing. The absolute bioavailability of tegaserod when administered to fasting subjects is approximately 10%. The pharmacokinetics are dose proportional over the 2-12 mg range given twice daily for 5 days. There was no clinically relevant accumulation of tegaserod in plasma when a 6 mg bid dose was given for 5 days. (See DOSAGE AND ADMINISTRATION.)

Food Effects

When the drug is administered with food, the bioavailability of tegaserod is reduced by 40-65% and C_{max} by approximately 20-40%. Similar reductions in plasma concentration occur when tegaserod is administered to subjects within 30 minutes prior to a meal, or 2.5 hours after a meal. T_{max} of tegaserod is prolonged from approximately 1 hour to 2 hours when taken following a meal, but decreased to 0.7 hours when taken 30 minutes prior to a meal.

Distribution

Tegaserod is approximately 98% bound to plasma proteins, predominantly alpha-1-acid glycoprotein. Tegaserod exhibits pronounced distribution into tissues following intravenous dosing with a volume of distribution at steady state of 368 ± 223 L.

Metabolism

Tegaserod is metabolized mainly via two pathways. The first is a presystemic acid catalyzed hydrolysis in the stomach followed by oxidation and conjugation which produces the main metabolite of tegaserod, 5-methoxyindole-3-carboxylic acid glucuronide. The main metabolite has negligible affinity for 5HT$_4$ receptors *in vitro*. In humans, systemic exposure to tegaserod was not altered at neutral gastric pH values. The second metabolic pathway of tegaserod is direct glucuronidation which leads to generation of three isomeric N-glucuronides.

Elimination

The plasma clearance of tegaserod is 77 ± 15 L/h with an estimated terminal half-life (T½) of 11 ± 5 hours following intravenous dosing. Approximately two-thirds of the orally administered dose of tegaserod is excreted unchanged in the feces, with the remaining one-third excreted in the urine, primarily as the main metabolite.

Sub Populations

Patients

The pharmacokinetics of tegaserod in IBS patients are comparable to those in healthy subjects.

Reduced Renal Function

No change in the pharmacokinetics of tegaserod was observed in subjects with severe renal impairment requiring hemodialysis (creatinine clearance 15 ml/min/1.73 m^2). C_{max} and AUC of the main pharmacologically inactive metabolite of tegaserod, 5-methoxy-indole-

3-carboxylic acid glucuronide, increased 2- and 10- fold respectively, in subjects with severe renal impairment compared to healthy controls. No dosage adjustment is required in patients with mild-to-moderate renal impairment. Tegaserod is not recommended in patients with severe renal impairment.

Reduced Hepatic Function

In subjects with mild hepatic impairment, mean AUC was 31% higher and C_{max} 16% higher compared to subjects with normal hepatic function. No dosage adjustment is required in patients with mild impairment, however, caution is recommended when using tegaserod in this patient population. Tegaserod has not adequately been studied in patients with moderate and severe hepatic impairment, and is therefore not recommended in these patients.

Gender

Gender has no effect on the pharmacokinetics of tegaserod.

Race

Data were inadequate to assess the effect of race on the pharmacokinetics of tegaserod.

Age

In a clinical pharmacology study conducted to assess the pharmacokinetics of tegaserod administered to healthy young (18-40 years) and healthy elderly (65-85 years) subjects, peak plasma concentration and exposure were 22% and 40% greater, respectively, in elderly females than young females but still within the variability seen in tegaserod pharmacokinetics in healthy subjects. Based on an analysis across several pharmacokinetic studies in healthy subjects, there is no age effect on the pharmacokinetics of tegaserod when allowing for body weight as a covariate. Therefore, dose adjustment in elderly patients is not necessary.

INDICATIONS AND USAGE

Tegaserod maleate is indicated for the short-term treatment of women with irritable bowel syndrome (IBS) whose primary bowel symptom is constipation.

The safety and effectiveness of tegaserod maleate in men have not been established.

CONTRAINDICATIONS

Tegaserod maleate is contraindicated in those patients with:

- Severe renal impairment.
- Moderate or severe hepatic impairment.
- A history of bowel obstruction, symptomatic gallbladder disease, suspected sphincter of Oddi dysfunction, or abdominal adhesions.
- A known hypersensitivity to the drug or any of its excipients.

PRECAUTIONS

Tegaserod maleate should not be initiated in patients who are currently experiencing or frequently experience diarrhea. (See ADVERSE REACTIONS.) Tegaserod maleate should be discontinued immediately in patients with new or sudden worsening of abdominal pain.

INFORMATION FOR THE PATIENT

Patients should take tegaserod maleate before a meal.

Patients should also be aware of the possible occurrence of diarrhea during therapy. The majority of the tegaserod maleate patients reporting diarrhea had a single episode. In most cases, diarrhea occurred within the first week of treatment. Typically, diarrhea resolved with continued therapy. Patients should consult their physician if they experience severe diarrhea, or if the diarrhea is accompanied by severe cramping, abdominal pain, or dizziness. Patients should not initiate therapy with tegaserod maleate if they are currently experiencing or frequently experience diarrhea. (See ADVERSE REACTIONS.)

Patients should consult their physician if they experience new or worsening abdominal pain.

CARCINOGENESIS, MUTAGENESIS, AND IMPAIRMENT OF FERTILITY

Tegaserod was not carcinogenic in rats given oral dietary doses up to 180 mg/kg/day [approximately 93-111 times the human exposure at 6 mg bid based on plasma AUC(0-24 h)] for 110-124 weeks.

In mice, dietary administration of tegaserod for 104 weeks produced mucosal hyperplasia and adenocarcinoma of small intestine at 600 mg/kg/day [approximately 83-110 times the human exposure at 6 mg bid based on plasma AUC(0-24 h)]. There was no evidence of carcinogenicity at a lower dose of 200 mg/kg/day [approximately 24-35 times the human exposure at 6 mg bid based on plasma AUC(0-24 h)] or 60 mg/kg/day [approximately 3-4 times the human exposure at 6 mg bid based on plasma AUC(0-24 h)].

Tegaserod was not genotoxic in the *in vitro* Chinese hamster lung fibroblast (CHL/V79) cell chromosomal aberration test, the *in vitro* Chinese hamster lung fibroblast (CHL/V79) cell forward mutation test, the *in vitro* rat hepatocyte unscheduled DNA synthesis (UDS) test or the *in vivo* mouse micronucleus test. The results of Ames tests for mutagenicity were equivocal.

Tegaserod at oral doses up to 240 mg/kg/day [approximately 57 times the human exposure at 6 mg bid based on plasma AUC(0-24 h)] in male rats and 150 mg/kg/day [approximately 42 times the human exposure at 6 mg bid based on plasma AUC(0-24 h)] in female rats was found to have no effect on fertility and reproductive performance.

PREGNANCY, TERATOGENIC EFFECTS, PREGNANCY CATEGORY B

Reproduction studies have been performed in rats at oral doses up to 100 mg/kg/day [approximately 15 times the human exposure at 6 mg bid based on plasma AUC(0-24 h)] and rabbits at oral doses up to 120 mg/kg/day [approximately 51 times the human exposure at 6 mg bid based on plasma AUC(0-24 h)] and have revealed no evidence of impaired fertility or harm to the fetus due to tegaserod. Because animal reproduction studies are not always predictive of human response, this drug should be used during pregnancy only if clearly needed.

NURSING MOTHERS

Tegaserod and its metabolites are excreted in the milk of lactating rats with a high milk to plasma ratio. It is not known whether tegaserod is excreted in human milk. Many drugs, which are excreted in human milk, have potential for serious adverse reactions in nursing infants. Based on the potential for tumorigenicity shown for tegaserod in the mouse carcinogenicity study, a decision should be made whether to discontinue nursing or to discontinue the drug, taking into account the importance of the drug to the mother.

PEDIATRIC USE

The safety and effectiveness of tegaserod maleate in pediatric patients below the age of 18 have not been established.

GERIATRIC USE

Of 4035 patients in Phase 3 clinical studies of tegaserod maleate, 290 were at least 65 years of age, while 52 were at least 75 years old. No overall differences in safety was observed between these patients and younger patients with regard to adverse events.

A clinical study conducted to assess the pharmacokinetics of tegaserod in healthy young (18-40 years) versus healthy elderly (65-85 years) subjects did not indicate that a dose adjustment is necessary when administering tegaserod maleate to patients over 65 years old. (See CLINICAL PHARMACOLOGY.)

DRUG INTERACTIONS

In vitro drug-drug interaction data with tegaserod indicated no inhibition of the cytochrome P450 isoenzymes CYP2C8, CYP2C9, CYP2C19, CYP2E1 and CYP3A4, whereas inhibition of CYP1A2 and CYP2D6 could not be excluded. However, *in vivo*, no clinically relevant drug-drug interactions have been observed with dextromethorphan (CYP2D6 prototype substrate), and theophylline (CYP1A2 prototype substrate). There was no effect on the pharmacokinetics of digoxin, oral contraceptives, and warfarin. The main human metabolite of tegaserod hydrogen maleate, 5-methoxyindole-3-carboxylic acid glucuronide, did not inhibit the activity of any of the above cytochrome P450 isoenzymes in *in vitro* tests.

Dextromethorphan: A pharmacokinetic interaction study demonstrated that co-administration of tegaserod and dextromethorphan did not change the pharmacokinetics of either compound to a clinically relevant extent. Dose adjustment of either drug is not necessary when tegaserod is combined with dextromethorphan. Therefore, tegaserod is not expected to alter the pharmacokinetics of drugs metabolized by CYP2D6 (*e.g.*, fluoxetine, omeprazole, captopril).

Theophylline: A pharmacokinetic interaction study demonstrated that co-administration of tegaserod and theophylline did not affect the pharmacokinetics of theophylline. Dose adjustment of theophylline is not necessary when tegaserod is co-administered. Therefore, tegaserod is not expected to alter the pharmacokinetics of drugs metabolized by CYP1A2 (*e.g.*, estradiol, omeprazole).

Digoxin: A pharmacokinetic interaction study with digoxin demonstrated that concomitant administration of tegaserod reduced peak plasma concentration and exposure of digoxin by approximately 15%. This reduction of bioavailability is not considered clinically relevant. When tegaserod is co-administered with digoxin dose adjustment is unlikely to be required.

Warfarin: A pharmacokinetic and pharmacodynamic interaction study with warfarin demonstrated no effect of concomitant administration of tegaserod on warfarin pharmacokinetics and pharmacodynamics. Dose adjustment of warfarin is not necessary when tegaserod is coadministered.

Oral Contraceptives: Co-administration of tegaserod did not affect the steady state pharmacokinetics of ethinylestradiol and reduced peak concentrations and exposure of levonorgestrel by 8%. Tegaserod is not expected to alter the risk of ovulation in subjects taking oral contraceptives. No alteration in oral contraceptive medication is necessary when tegaserod is coadministered.

ADVERSE REACTIONS

In Phase 3 clinical trials in which 2632 patients received tegaserod maleate 6 mg bid or placebo, the following adverse experiences were reported in 1% or more of patients who received tegaserod maleate and occurred more frequently on tegaserod maleate than placebo (see TABLE 2).

TABLE 2 *Adverse Events Occurring in ≥1% of IBS Patients and More Frequently on Tegaserod Maleate Than Placebo*

System Adverse Experience	Tegaserod Maleate 6 mg bid (n=1327)	Placebo (n=1305)
Gastrointestinal System Disorders		
Abdominal pain	12%	11%
Diarrhea	9%	4%
Nausea	8%	7%
Flatulence	6%	5%
Central and Peripheral Nervous System		
Headache	15%	12%
Dizziness	4%	3%
Migraine	2%	1%
Body as a Whole — General Disorders		
Accidental trauma	3%	2%
Leg pain	1%	<1%
Musculoskeletal System Disorders		
Back pain	5%	4%
Arthropathy	2%	1%

Tegaserod maleate was not associated with changes in ECG intervals.

The following adverse events also occurred during treatment with tegaserod maleate:

Tegaserod Maleate-Induced Diarrhea: In the Phase 3 clinical studies, 8.8% of patients receiving tegaserod maleate reported diarrhea as an adverse experience compared to

T

3.8% of patients receiving placebo. The majority of the tegaserod maleate patients reporting diarrhea had a single episode. In most cases, diarrhea occurred within the first week of treatment. Typically, diarrhea resolved with continued therapy. Overall, the discontinuation rate from the studies due to diarrhea was 1.6% among the tegaserod maleate-treated patients. Patients who experience severe diarrhea during therapy with tegaserod maleate should be directed to consult their physician. Diarrhea can be the pharmacologic response to tegaserod maleate.

In two clinical studies of 4-8 weeks duration designed to assess the safety and tolerability of tegaserod maleate in IBS patients with diarrhea as a predominant symptom (n=162), no serious adverse events were observed; 6% of tegaserod maleate-treated patients discontinued treatment due to diarrhea or abdominal pain.

Abdominal Surgeries, Including Cholecystectomy: An increase in abdominal surgeries was observed on tegaserod maleate (9/2965; 0.3%) versus placebo (3/1740; 0.2%) in the Phase 3 clinical studies. The increase was primarily due to a numerical imbalance in cholecystectomies reported in patients treated with tegaserod maleate (5/2965; 0.17%) vs. placebo (1/1740; 0.06%). A causal relationship between abdominal surgeries and tegaserod maleate has not been established.

The following list of adverse events includes those considered possibly related to tegaserod maleate, occurred in at least 2 patients in the Phase 3 clinical trials, and occurred more often on tegaserod maleate than placebo. Also included are those serious adverse events reported in the tegaserod maleate clinical program in at least 2 patients treated with tegaserod maleate, regardless of causality, or any serious adverse event considered possibly related to tegaserod maleate. Although the events reported occurred during treatment with tegaserod maleate, they were not necessarily caused by it.

Body as a Whole: Pain, flushing, facial edema.

Cardiovascular: Hypotension, angina pectoris, syncope, arrhythmia, bundle branch block, supraventricular tachycardia.

Central Nervous System: Vertigo.

Female Reproductive: Ovarian cyst, miscarriage, menorrhagia.

Gastrointestinal: Irritable colon, fecal incontinence, tenesmus, increased appetite, eructation, increased SGOT, increased SGPT, bilirubinemia, cholecystitis, appendicitis, subileus.

Metabolic: Increased creatine phosphokinase.

Musculoskeletal: Back pain, cramps.

Neoplasms: Breast carcinoma.

Psychiatric: Attempted suicide, impaired concentration, emotional lability, increased appetite, sleep disorder, depression.

Respiratory: Asthma.

Skin: Pruritis, increased sweating.

Urinary: Albuminuria, frequent micturition, polyuria, renal pain.

POST MARKETING EXPERIENCE

Voluntary reports of other adverse events occurring with the use of tegaserod maleate include the following: suspected sphincter of Oddi spasm, bile duct stone, and cholecystitis with elevated transaminases.

DOSAGE AND ADMINISTRATION

The recommended dosage of tegaserod maleate is 6 mg taken twice daily orally before meals for 4-6 weeks. For those patients who respond to therapy at 4-6 weeks, an additional 4-6 week course can be considered.

HOW SUPPLIED

Zelnorm is available as whitish to slightly yellowish, marbled, circular flat tablets with a bevelled edge containing 2 mg or 6 mg tegaserod as follows:

2 mg Tablet: White round engraved with "NVR" and "DL".

6 mg Tablet: White round engraved with "NVR" and "EH".

Storage: Store at 25°C (77°F); excursions permitted to 15-30°C (59-86°F). Protect from moisture.

PRODUCT LISTING - EQUIVALENTS NOT AVAILABLE

Tablet - Oral - 2 mg

10 x 6 $153.75 ZELNORM, Novartis Pharmaceuticals 00078-0355-80

Tablet - Oral - 6 mg

10 x 6 $153.75 ZELNORM, Novartis Pharmaceuticals 00078-0356-80

T

Telmisartan *(003425)*

For related information, see the comparative table section in Appendix A.

Categories: Hypertension, essential; FDA Approved 1998 Nov; Pregnancy Category C, 1st Trimester; Pregnancy Category D, 2nd & 3rd Trimesters

Drug Classes: Angiotensin II receptor antagonists

Brand Names: **Micardis**

Foreign Brand Availability: Pritor (Australia; Korea; Mexico; Peru; Philippines)

Cost of Therapy: $45.21 (Hypertension; Micardis; 40 mg; 1 tablet/day; 30 day supply)

WARNING

USE IN PREGNANCY

When used in pregnancy during the second and third trimesters, drugs that act directly on the renin-angiotensin system can cause injury and even death to the developing fetus. When pregnancy is detected, telmisartan tablets should be discontinued as soon as possible. See WARNINGS, Fetal/Neonatal Morbidity and Mortality.

DESCRIPTION

Telmisartan is a nonpeptide angiotensin II receptor (type AT_1) antagonist.

Telmisartan is chemically described as 4′-[(1,4′-dimethyl-2′-propyl[2,6′-bi-1H-benzimidazol]-1′-yl)methyl]-[1,1′-biphenyl]-2-carboxylic acid. Its empirical formula is $C_{33}H_{30}N_4O_2$, its molecular weight is 514.63.

Telmisartan is a white to off-white, odorless crystalline powder. It is practically insoluble in water and in the pH range of 3 to 9, sparingly soluble in strong acid (except insoluble in hydrochloric acid), and soluble in strong base.

Telmisartan is available as tablets for oral administration, containing either 40 mg or 80 mg of telmisartan. The tablets contain the following inactive ingredients: sodium hydroxide, meglumine, povidone, sorbitol, and magnesium stearate. Telmisartan tablets are hygroscopic and require protection from moisture.

CLINICAL PHARMACOLOGY

MECHANISM OF ACTION

Angiotensin II is formed from angiotensin I in a reaction catalyzed by angiotensin-converting enzyme (ACE, kininase II). Angiotensin II is the principal pressor agent of the renin-angiotensin system, with effects that include vasoconstriction, stimulation of synthesis and release of aldosterone, cardiac stimulation, and renal reabsorption of sodium. Telmisartan blocks the vasoconstrictor and aldosterone-secreting effects of angiotensin II by selectively blocking the binding of angiotensin II to the AT_1 receptor in many tissues, such as vascular smooth muscle and the adrenal gland. Its action is therefore independent of the pathways for angiotensin II synthesis.

There is also an AT_2 receptor found in many tissues, but AT_2 is not known to be associated with cardiovascular homeostasis. Telmisartan has much greater affinity (>3000-fold) for the AT_1 receptor than for the AT_2 receptor.

Blockade of the renin-angiotensin system with ACE inhibitors, which inhibit the biosynthesis of angiotensin II from angiotensin I, is widely used in the treatment of hypertension. ACE inhibitors also inhibit the degradation of bradykinin, a reaction also catalyzed by ACE. Because telmisartan does not inhibit ACE (kininase II), it does not affect the response to bradykinin. Whether this difference has clinical relevance is not yet known. Telmisartan does not bind to or block other hormone receptors or ion channels known to be important in cardiovascular regulation.

Blockade of the angiotensin II receptor inhibits the negative regulatory feedback of angiotensin II on renin secretion, but the resulting increased plasma renin activity and angiotensin II circulating levels do not overcome the effect of telmisartan on blood pressure.

PHARMACOKINETICS

General

Following oral administration, peak concentrations (C_{max}) of telmisartan are reached in 0.5-1 hour after dosing. Food slightly reduces the bioavailability of telmisartan, with a reduction in the area under the plasma concentration-time curve (AUC) of about 6% with the 40 mg tablet and about 20% after a 160 mg dose. The absolute bioavailability of telmisartan is dose dependent. At 40 and 160 mg the bioavailability was 42% and 58%, respectively. The pharmacokinetics of orally administered telmisartan are nonlinear over the dose range 20-160 mg, with greater than proportional increases of plasma concentrations (C_{max} and AUC) with increasing doses. Telmisartan shows bi-exponential decay kinetics with a terminal elimination half life of approximately 24 hours. Trough plasma concentrations of telmisartan with once daily dosing are about 10-25% of peak plasma concentrations. Telmisartan has an accumulation index in plasma of 1.5 to 2.0 upon repeated once daily dosing.

Metabolism and Elimination

Following either intravenous or oral administration of ^{14}C-labeled telmisartan, most of the administered dose (>97%) was eliminated unchanged in feces via biliary excretion; only minute amounts were found in the urine (0.91% and 0.49% of total radioactivity, respectively).

Telmisartan is metabolized by conjugation to form a pharmacologically inactive acylglucuronide; the glucuronide of the parent compound is the only metabolite that has been identified in human plasma and urine. After a single dose, the glucuronide represents approximately 11% of the measured radioactivity in plasma. The cytochrome P450 isoenzymes are not involved in the metabolism of telmisartan.

Total plasma clearance of telmisartan is >800 ml/min. Terminal half-life and total clearance appear to be independent of dose.

Distribution

Telmisartan is highly bound to plasma proteins (>99.5%), mainly albumin and α_1-acid glycoprotein. Plasma protein binding is constant over the concentration range achieved with recommended doses. The volume of distribution for telmisartan is approximately 500 L, indicating additional tissue binding.

SPECIAL POPULATIONS

Pediatric

Telmisartan pharmacokinetics have not been investigated in patients <18 years of age.

Geriatric

The pharmacokinetics of telmisartan do not differ between the elderly and those younger than 65 years (see DOSAGE AND ADMINISTRATION).

Gender

Plasma concentrations of telmisartan are generally 2-3 times higher in females than in males. In clinical trials, however, no significant increases in blood pressure response or in the incidence of orthostatic hypotension were found in women. No dosage adjustment is necessary.

Renal Insufficiency

Renal excretion does not contribute to the clearance of telmisartan. Based on modest experience in patients with mild-to-moderate renal impairment (creatinine clearance of 30-80 ml/min, mean clearance approximately 50 ml/min), no dosage adjustment is necessary in patients with decreased renal function. Telmisartan is not removed from blood by hemofiltration (see PRECAUTIONS, and DOSAGE AND ADMINISTRATION).

Hepatic Insufficiency

In patients with hepatic insufficiency, plasma concentrations of telmisartan are increased, and absolute bioavailability approaches 100% (see PRECAUTIONS, and DOSAGE AND ADMINISTRATION).

Drug Interactions:

See DRUG INTERACTIONS.

PHARMACODYNAMICS

In normal volunteers, a dose of telmisartan 80 mg inhibited the pressor response to an intravenous infusion of angiotensin II by about 90% at peak plasma concentrations with approximately 40% inhibition persisting for 24 hours.

Plasma concentration of angiotensin II and plasma renin activity (PRA) increased in a dose-dependent manner after single administration of telmisartan to healthy subjects and repeated administration to hypertensive patients. The once-daily administration of up to 80 mg telmisartan to healthy subjects did not influence plasma aldosterone concentrations. In multiple dose studies with hypertensive patients, there were no clinically significant changes in electrolytes (serum potassium or sodium), or in metabolic function (including serum levels of cholesterol, triglycerides, HDL, LDL, glucose, or uric acid).

In 30 hypertensive patients with normal renal function treated for 8 weeks with telmisartan 80 mg or telmisartan 80 mg in combination with hydrochlorothiazide 12.5 mg, there were no clinically significant changes from baseline in renal blood flow, glomerular filtration rate, filtration fraction, renovascular resistance, or creatinine clearance.

INDICATIONS AND USAGE

Telmisartan is indicated for the treatment of hypertension. It may be used alone or in combination with other antihypertensive agents.

CONTRAINDICATIONS

Telmisartan is contraindicated in patients who are hypersensitive to any component of this product.

WARNINGS

FETAL/NEONATAL MORBIDITY AND MORTALITY

Drugs that act directly on the renin-angiotensin system can cause fetal and neonatal morbidity and death when administered to pregnant women. Several dozen cases have been reported in the world literature in patients who were taking angiotensin converting enzyme inhibitors. When pregnancy is detected, telmisartan tablets should be discontinued as soon as possible.

The use of drugs that act directly on the renin-angiotensin system during the second and third trimesters of pregnancy has been associated with fetal and neonatal injury, including hypotension, neonatal skull hypoplasia, anuria, reversible or irreversible renal failure, and death. Oligohydramnios has also been reported, presumably resulting from decreased fetal renal function; oligohydramnios in this setting has been associated with fetal limb contractures, craniofacial deformation, and hypoplastic lung development. Prematurity, intrauterine growth retardation, and patent ductus arteriosus have also been reported, although it is not clear whether these occurrences were due to exposure to the drug.

These adverse effects do not appear to have resulted from intrauterine drug exposure that has been limited to the first trimester. Mothers whose embryos and fetuses are exposed to an angiotensin II receptor antagonist only during the first trimester should be so informed. Nonetheless, when patients become pregnant, physicians should have the patient discontinue the use of telmisartan tablets as soon as possible.

Rarely (probably less often than once in every thousand pregnancies), no alternative to an angiotensin II receptor antagonist will be found. In these rare cases, the mothers should be apprised of the potential hazards to their fetuses, and serial ultrasound examinations should be performed to assess the intra-amniotic environment.

If oligohydramnios is observed, telmisartan tablets should be discontinued unless they are considered life-saving for the mother. Contraction stress testing (CST), a non-stress test (NTS), or biophysical profiling (BPP) may be appropriate, depending upon the week of pregnancy. Patients and physicians should be aware, however, that oligohydramnios may not appear until after the fetus has sustained irreversible injury.

Infants with histories of *in utero* exposure to an angiotensin II receptor antagonist should be closely observed for hypotension, oliguria, and hyperkalemia. If oliguria occurs, attention should be directed toward support of blood pressure and renal perfusion. Exchange transfusion or dialysis may be required as a means of reversing hypotension and/or substituting for disordered renal function.

There is no clinical experience with the use of telmisartan tablets in pregnant women. No teratogenic effects were observed when telmisartan was administered to pregnant rats at oral doses of up to 50 mg/kg/day and to pregnant rabbits at oral doses up to 45 mg/kg/day. In rabbits, embryolethality associated with maternal toxicity (reduced body weight gain and food consumption) was observed at 45 mg/kg/day [about 6.4 times the maximum recommended human dose (MRHD) of 80 mg on a mg/m^2 basis]. In rats, maternally toxic (reduction in body weight gain and food consumption) telmisartan doses of 15 mg/kg/day (about 1.9 times the MRHD on a mg/m^2 basis), administered during late gestation and lactation, were observed to produce adverse effects in neonates, including reduced viability, low birth weight, delayed maturation, and decreased weight gain. Telmisartan has been shown to be present in rat fetuses during late gestation and in rat milk. The no observed effect doses for developmental toxicity in rats and rabbits, 5 and 15 mg/kg/day, respectively, are about 0.64 and 3.7 times, on a mg/m^2 basis, the maximum recommended human dose of telmisartan (80 mg/day).

HYPOTENSION IN VOLUME-DEPLETED PATIENTS

In patients with an activated renin-angiotensin system, such as volume- and/or salt-depleted patients (*e.g.,* those being treated with high doses of diuretics), symptomatic hypotension may occur after initiation of therapy with telmisartan tablets. This condition should be corrected prior to administration of telmisartan tablets, or treatment should either start under close medical supervision or with a reduced dose of an AII antagonist (this may require use of a drug other than telmisartan as it is not possible to give less than 40 mg at present).

If hypotension does occur, the patient should be placed in the supine position and, if necessary, given an intravenous infusion of normal saline. A transient hypotensive response is not a contraindication to further treatment, which usually can be continued without difficulty once the blood pressure has stabilized.

PRECAUTIONS

GENERAL

Impaired Hepatic Function

As the majority of telmisartan is eliminated by biliary excretion, patients with biliary obstructive disorders or hepatic insufficiency can be expected to have reduced clearance. Telmisartan tablets should be used with caution in these patients, but there is no way to reduce the dose below 40 mg; an alternative treatment can be considered.

Impaired Renal Function

As a consequence of inhibiting the renin-angiotensin-aldosterone system, changes in renal function may be anticipated in susceptible individuals. In patients whose renal function may depend on the activity of the renin-angiotensin-aldosterone system (*e.g.,* patients with severe congestive heart failure), treatment with angiotensin-converting enzyme inhibitors and angiotensin receptor antagonists has been associated with oliguria and/or progressive azotemia and (rarely) with acute renal failure and/or death. Similar results may be anticipated in patients treated with telmisartan tablets.

In studies of ACE inhibitors in patients with unilateral or bilateral renal artery stenosis, increases in serum creatinine or blood urea nitrogen were observed. There has been no long term use of telmisartan tablets in patients with unilateral or bilateral renal artery stenosis but an effect similar to that seen with ACE inhibitors should be anticipated.

INFORMATION FOR THE PATIENT

Pregnancy

Female patients of childbearing age should be told about the consequences of second- and third-trimester exposure to drugs that act on the renin-angiotensin system, and they should also be told that these consequences do not appear to have resulted from intrauterine drug exposure that has been limited to the first trimester. These patients should be asked to report pregnancies to their physicians as soon as possible.

CARCINOGENESIS, MUTAGENESIS, AND IMPAIRMENT OF FERTILITY

There was no evidence of carcinogenicity when telmisartan was administered in the diet to mice and rats for up to 2 years. The highest doses administered to mice (1000 mg/kg/day) and rats (100 mg/kg/day) are, on a mg/m^2 basis, about 59 and 13 times, respectively, the maximum recommended human dose (MRHD) of telmisartan. These same doses have been shown to provide average systemic exposure to telmisartan >100 times and >25 times, respectively, the systemic exposure in humans receiving the MRHD (80 mg/day).

Genotoxicity assays did not reveal any telmisartan-related effects at either the gene or chromosome level. These assays included bacterial mutagenicity tests with Salmonella and *E coli* (Ames), a gene mutation test with Chinese hamster V79 cells, a cytogenetic test with human lymphocytes, and a mouse micronucleus test.

No drug-related effects on the reproductive performance of male and female rats were noted at 100 mg/kg/day (the highest dose administered), about 13 times, on a mg/m^2 basis, the MRHD of telmisartan. This dose in the rat resulted in an average systemic exposure (telmisartan AUC as determined on day 6 of pregnancy) at least 50 times the average systemic exposure in humans at the MRHD (80 mg/day).

PREGNANCY CATEGORY C AND PREGNANCY, TERATOGENIC EFFECTS, PREGNANCY CATEGORY D

See WARNINGS, Fetal/Neonatal Morbidity and Mortality.

NURSING MOTHERS

It is not known whether telmisartan is excreted in human milk, but telmisartan was shown to be present in the milk of lactating rats. Because of the potential for adverse effects on the nursing infant, a decision should be made whether to discontinue nursing or discontinue the drug, taking into account the importance of the drug to the mother.

PEDIATRIC USE

Safety and effectiveness in pediatric patients have not been established.

GERIATRIC USE

Of the total number of patients receiving telmisartan in clinical studies, 551 (18.6%) were 65-74 years of age and 130 (4.4%) were 75 years or older. No overall differences in effectiveness and safety were observed in these patients compared to younger patients and other reported clinical experience has not identified differences in responses between the elderly and younger patients, but greater sensitivity of some older individuals cannot be ruled out.

DRUG INTERACTIONS

Digoxin: When telmisartan was coadministered with digoxin, median increases in digoxin peak plasma concentration (49%) and in trough concentration (20%) were observed. It is, therefore, recommended that digoxin levels be monitored when initiating, adjusting, and discontinuing telmisartan to avoid possible over- or under-digitalization.

Warfarin: Telmisartan administered for 10 days slightly decreased the mean warfarin trough plasma concentration; this decrease did not result in a change in International Normalized Ratio (INR).

T

Other Drugs: Coadministration of telmisartan did not result in a clinically significant interaction with acetaminophen, amlodipine, glibenclamide, hydrochlorothiazide or ibuprofen. Telmisartan is not metabolized by the cytochrome P450 system and had no effects *in vitro* on cytochrome P450 enzymes, except for some inhibition of CYP2C19. Telmisartan is not expected to interact with drugs that inhibit cytochrome P450 enzymes: it is also not expected to interact with drugs metabolized by cytochrome P450 enzymes, except for possible inhibition of the metabolism of drugs metabolized by CYP2C19.

ADVERSE REACTIONS

Telmisartan has been evaluated for safety in more than 3700 patients, including 1900 treated for over 6 months and more than 1300 for over 1 year. Adverse experiences have generally been mild and transient in nature and have only infrequently required discontinuation of therapy.

In placebo-controlled trials involving 1041 patients treated with various doses of telmisartan (20-160 mg) monotherapy for up to 12 weeks, an overall incidence of adverse events similar to that of placebo was observed.

Adverse events occurring at an incidence of 1% or more in patients treated with telmisartan and at a greater rate than in patients treated with placebo, irrespective of their causal association, are presented in TABLE 1.

TABLE 1

	Telmisartan n=1455	Placebo n=380
Upper respiratory tract infection	7%	6%
Back pain	3%	1%
Sinusitis	3%	2%
Diarrhea	3%	2%
Pharyngitis	1%	0%

In addition to the adverse events in TABLE 1, the following events occurred at a rate of 1% but were at least as frequent in the placebo group: influenza-like symptoms, dyspepsia, myalgia, urinary tract infection, abdominal pain, headache, dizziness, pain, fatigue, coughing, hypertension, chest pain, nausea and peripheral edema. Discontinuation of therapy due to adverse events was required in 2.8% of 1455 patients treated with telmisartan tablets and 6.1% of 380 placebo patients in placebo-controlled clinical trials.

The incidence of adverse events was not dose-related and did not correlate with gender, age, or race of patients.

The incidence of cough occurring with telmisartan in six placebo-controlled trials was identical to that noted for placebo-treated patients (1.6%).

In addition to those listed above, adverse events that occurred in more than 0.3% of 3500 patients treated with telmisartan monotherapy in controlled or open trials are listed below. It cannot be determined whether these events were causally related to telmisartan tablets:

Autonomic Nervous System: Impotence, increased sweating, flushing.

Body as a Whole : Allergy, fever, leg pain, malaise.

Cardiovascular: Palpitation, dependent edema, angina pectoris, tachycardia, leg edema, abnormal ECG.

CNS: Insomnia, somnolence, migraine, vertigo, paresthesia, involuntary muscle contractions, hypoaesthesia.

Gastrointestinal: Flatulence, constipation, gastritis, vomiting, dry mouth, hemorrhoids, gastroenteritis, enteritis, gastroesophageal reflux, toothache, non-specific gastrointestinal disorders.

Metabolic: Gout, hypercholesterolemia, diabetes mellitus.

Musculoskeletal: Arthritis, arthralgia, leg cramps.

Psychiatric: Anxiety, depression, nervousness.

Resistance Mechanism: Infection, fungal infection, abscess, otitis media.

Respiratory: Asthma, bronchitis, rhinitis, dyspnea, epistaxis.

Skin: Dermatitis, rash, eczema, pruritus.

Urinary: Micturition frequency, cystitis.

Vascular: Cerebrovascular disorder.

Special Senses: Abnormal vision, conjunctivitis, tinnitus, earache.

A single case of angioedema was reported (among a total of 3781 patients treated with telmisartan).

CLINICAL LABORATORY FINDINGS

In placebo-controlled clinical trials, clinically relevant changes in standard laboratory test parameters were rarely associated with administration of telmisartan tablets.

Hemoglobin: A greater than 2 g/dl decrease in hemoglobin was observed in 0.8% telmisartan patients compared with 0.3% placebo patients. No patients discontinued therapy due to anemia.

Creatinine: A 0.5 mg/dl rise or greater in creatinine was observed in 0.4% telmisartan patients compared with 0.3% placebo patients. One telmisartan-treated patient discontinued therapy due to increases in creatinine and blood urea nitrogen.

Liver Enzymes: Occasional elevations of liver chemistries occurred in patients treated with telmisartan; all marked elevations occurred at a higher frequency with placebo. No telmisartan-treated patients discontinued therapy due to abnormal hepatic function.

DOSAGE AND ADMINISTRATION

Dosage must be individualized. The usual starting dose of telmisartan tablets is 40 mg once a day. Blood pressure response is dose related over the range of 20-80 mg.

Special Populations: Patients with depletion of intravascular volume should have the condition corrected or telmisartan tablets should be initiated under close medical supervision (see WARNINGS, Hypotension in Volume-Depleted Patients). Patients with biliary obstructive disorders or hepatic insufficiency should have treatment started under close medical supervision (see PRECAUTIONS, General: Impaired Hepatic Function, and Impaired Renal Function).

Most of the antihypertensive effect is apparent within 2 weeks and maximal reduction is generally attained after 4 weeks. When additional blood pressure reduction beyond that achieved with 80 mg telmisartan is required, a diuretic may be added.

No initial dosing adjustment is necessary for elderly patients or patients with mild-to-moderate renal impairment. Patients on dialysis may develop orthostatic hypotension; their blood pressure should be closely monitored.

Telmisartan tablets may be administered with other antihypertensive agents.

Telmisartan tablets may be administered with or without food.

HOW SUPPLIED

Micardis is available as white, oblong-shaped, uncoated tablets containing telmisartan 40 or 80 mg. Tablets are marked with the Boehringer Ingelheim logo on one side, and on the other side, with a decorative score and either "51H "or "52H" for the 40 and 80 mg strengths, respectively.

Storage: Store at 25°C (77°F); excursions permitted to 15-30°C (59-86°F). Tablets should not be removed from blisters until immediately before administration.

PRODUCT LISTING - EQUIVALENTS NOT AVAILABLE

Tablet - Oral - 20 mg

28's	$42.20	MICARDIS, Boehringer-Ingelheim	00597-0039-28

Tablet - Oral - 40 mg

28's	$42.20	MICARDIS, Boehringer-Ingelheim	00597-0040-28

Tablet - Oral - 80 mg

28's	$45.85	MICARDIS, Boehringer-Ingelheim	00597-0041-28

Temazepam *(002310)*

Categories: Insomnia; Pregnancy Category X; DEA Class CIV; FDA Approved 1981 Feb
Drug Classes: Benzodiazepines; Sedatives/hypnotics
Brand Names: Euhypnos; Levanxol; Normison; Planum; **Restoril**
Foreign Brand Availability: Cerepax (Argentina); Lenal (Argentina); Levanxene (Argentina)
Cost of Therapy: $27.66 (Insomnia; Restoril; 15 mg; 1 capsule/day; 10 day supply)
$0.75 (Insomnia; Generic Capsules; 15 mg; 1 capsule/day; 10 day supply)

DESCRIPTION

Temazepam is a benzodiazepine hypnotic agent. The chemical name is 7-chloro-1,3-dihydro-3-hydroxy-1-methyl-5-phenyl-2*H*-1,4-benzodiaz epin-2-one.

Temazepam is a white, crystalline substance, very slightly soluble in water and sparingly soluble in alcohol.

Temazepam capsules, 7.5 mg, 15 mg and 30 mg, are for oral administration.

Restoril 15 mg and 30 mg Capsules: *Active Ingredient:* Temazepam

Restoril 7.5 mg Capsules: *Inactive Ingredients:* FD&C blue no. 1, FD&C red no. 3, gelatin, lactose, magnesium stearate, sodium lauryl sulfate, synthetic red ferric oxide, and titanium dioxide. *May Also Include:* Benzyl alcohol, butylparaben, edetate calcium disodium, methylparaben, propylparaben, silicon dioxide, sodium propionate, and another ingredient.

Restoril 15 mg Capsules: *Inactive Ingredients:* FD&C blue no. 1, FD&C red no. 3, gelatin, lactose, magnesium stearate, sodium lauryl sulfate, synthetic red ferric oxide, and titanium dioxide. *May Also Include:* Benzyl alcohol, butylparaben, edetate calcium disodium, methylparaben, propylparaben, silicon dioxide, sodium propionate, and another ingredient.

Restoril 30 mg Capsules: *Inactive Ingredients:* FD&C blue no. 1, FD&C red no. 3, gelatin, lactose, magnesium stearate, sodium lauryl sulfate, and titanium dioxide. *May Also Include:* Benzyl alcohol, butylparaben, edetate calcium disodium, methylparaben, propylparaben, silicon dioxide, sodium propionate, and another ingredient.

CLINICAL PHARMACOLOGY

PHARMACOKINETICS

In a single and multiple dose absorption, distribution, metabolism, and excretion (ADME) study, using ^{3}H labeled drug. Temazepam was well absorbed and found to have minimal (8%) first pass metabolism. There were no active metabolites formed and the only significant metabolite present in blood was the O-conjugate. The unchanged drug was 96% bound to plasma proteins. The blood level decline of the parent drug was biphasic and the short half-life ranging from 0.4-0.6 hours and the terminal half life ranging from 3.5-18.4 hours (mean 8.8 hours), depending on the study population and the method of determination. Metabolites were formed with a half-life of 10 hours and excreted with a half-life of approximately 2 hours. Thus, formation of the major metabolite is the rate limiting step in the biodisposition of temazepam. There is no accumulation of metabolites. A dose-proportional relationship has been established for the area under the plasma concentration/time curve over the 15-30 mg dose range.

Temazepam was completely metabolized through conjugation prior to excretion: 80%-90% of the dose appeared in the urine. The major metabolite was th O-conjugate of temazepam (90%): the O-conjugate of N- desmethyl temazepam was a minor metabolite (7%).

BIOAVAILABILITY, INDUCTION, AND PLASMA LEVELS

Following ingestion of a 30 mg temazepam capsule, measurable plasma concentrations were achieved 10-20 minutes after dosing with peak plasma levels ranging from 666-982 ng/ml (mean 865 ng/ml) occurring approximately 1.2-1.6 hours (mean 1.5 hours) after dosing.

In a 7 day study, in which subjects were given a 30 mg temazepam capsule 1 hour before retiring, steady-state (as measured by the attainment of maximal trough concentrations) was achieved by the third dose. Mean plasma levels of temazepam (for days 2-7) were 260 ± 210 ng/ml at 9 hours and 75 ± 80 ng/ml at 24 hours after dosing. A slight trend toward declining 24 hour plasma levels was seen after day 4 in the study, however, the 24 hour plasma levels were quite variable.

At a dose of 30 mg once-a-day for 8 weeks, no evidence of enzyme induction was found in man.

ELIMINATION RATE OF BENZODIAZEPINE HYPNOTICS AND PROFILE OF COMMON UNTOWARD EFFECTS

The type and duration of unwanted effects during administration of benzodiazepine hypnotics may be influenced by the biologic half-life of the administered drug and for some hypnotics, the half-life of any active metabolites formed. Benzodiazepine hypnotics have a spectrum of half- lives from short (<4 hours) or long (>20 hours). When half-lives are long, drug (and for some drugs their inactive metabolites) may accumulate during periods of nightly administration and may be associated with impairments of cognitive and/or motor performance during waking hours; the possibility of interaction with other psychoactive drugs or alcohol will be enhanced. In contrast, if half-lives are shorter, drug (and for some drug their active metabolites may be accumulate during periods of nightly administration and be associated with impairments of cognitive and/or motor performance during waking hours; the possibility of interaction with other psychotropic drugs or alcohol will be enhanced. In contrast, if half-lives are shorter, drug (and, where appropriate, its active metabolites) will be cleared before the next dose is ingested, and carry-over effects related to excessive sedation or CNS depression should be minimized or absent. However, during nightly use for an extended period , pharmacodynamic tolerance or adaptation to some effects of benzodiazepine hypnotics may develop. If the drug has a short elimination half-life, it is possible that a relative deficiency of the drug, or, if appropriate, its active metabolites (*i.e.,* in relationship to the receptor site) may occur at some point in the interval between each night's use. This sequence of events may account for 2 clinical findings reported to occur after several weeks of nightly use of rapidly eliminated benzodiazepines hypnotics, namely increased wakefulness during the last third of the night, and the appearance of daytime anxiety.

INDICATIONS AND USAGE

Temazepam is indicated for the short-term treatment of insomnia (generally 7-10 days). For patients in whom the drug is used for more than 2-3 weeks, periodic reevaluation is recommended to determine whether there is a continuing need. (See WARNINGS.)

For patients with short-term insomnia, instructions in the prescription should indicate that temazepam should be used for short periods of time (7-10 days).

Temazepam should not be prescribed in quantities exceeding a 1-month supply.

Insomnia is characterized by complaints of difficulty in falling asleep, frequent nocturnal awakenings, and/or early morning awakenings. Both sleep laboratory and outpatient studies provide support for the effectiveness of temazepam administered 30 minutes before bedtime in decreasing sleep latency and improving sleep maintenance in patients with chronic insomnia. In addition, sleep laboratory studies have confirmed similar effects in normal subjects with transient insomnia. (See CLINICAL PHARMACOLOGY.)

CONTRAINDICATIONS

Benzodiazepines may cause fetal damage when administered during pregnancy. An increased risk of congenital malformations associated with the use of diazepam and chlordiazepoxide during the first trimester of pregnancy has been suggested in several studies. Transplacental distribution has resulted in neonatal CNS depression following the ingestion of therapeutic doses of a benzodiazepine hypnotic during the last weeks of pregnancy.

Reproduction studies in animals with temazepam were performed in rats and rabbits. In a perinatal-postnatal study in rats, oral doses of 60 mg/kg/day resulted in increasing nursling mortality. Teratology studies in rats demonstrated increased fetal resorptions at doses of 30 and 120 mg/kg in one study and increased occurrence of rudimentary ribs, which are considered skeletal variants, in a second study at doses of 240 mg/kg or higher. In rabbits, occasional abnormalities such as exencephaly and fusion or asymmetry of ribs were reported without dose relationship. Although these abnormalities were not found in the concurrent control group, they have been reported to occur randomly in historical controls. At doses of 40 mg/kg or higher, there was an increased incidence of the 13th rib variant when compared to the incidence in concurrent and historical controls.

Temazepam is contraindicated in pregnant women. If there is a likelihood of the patient becoming pregnant while receiving temazepam, she should be warned of the potential risk to the fetus. Patients should be instructed to discontinue the drug prior to becoming pregnant. The possibility that a woman of childbearing potential may be pregnant at the time of institution of therapy should be considered.

WARNINGS

Sleep disturbance may be the presenting manifestation of an underlying physical and/or psychiatric disorder. Consequently, a decision to initiate symptomatic treatment of insomnia should only be made after the patient has been carefully evaluated.

The failure of insomnia to remit after 7-10 days of treatment may indicate the presence of a primary psychiatric and/or medical illness.

Worsening of insomnia may be the consequence of an unrecognized psychiatric or physical disorder as may be the emergence of new abnormalities of thinking or behavior. Such abnormalities have also been reported to occur in association with the central nervous system depressant activity, including those of the benzodiazepine class. Some of these changes may be characterized by decreased inhibition, e.g., aggressiveness and extroversion that seem out of character, similar to that seen with alcohol. Other kinds of behavioral changes can also occur, for example, bizarre behavior, agitation, hallucinations, depersonalization, and, in primarily depressed patients, the worsening of depression, including suicidal thinking. In controlled clinical trials involving 1076 patients on temazepam and 783 patients on placebo, reports of hallucinations, agitation, and overstimulation occurred at rates less than 1 in 100 patients. Hallucinations were reported in 2 temazepam patients and 1 temazepam patient; 2 temazepam patients reported overstimulation. There were no reports of worsening of depression or suicidal ideation, aggressiveness, extroversion, bizarre behavior or depersonalization in these controlled clinical trials.

It can rarely determined with certainty whether a particular instance of the abnormal behavior listed above is induced, spontaneous in origin, or a result of an underlying psychiatric or physical disorder. Nonetheless, the emergence of any new behavioral sign or symptom of concern requires careful and immediate evaluation.

Because some of the worrisome adverse effects of benzodiazepines, including temazepam, appear to be dose related (see PRECAUTIONS and DOSAGE AND ADMINISTRATION), it is important to use the lowest possible effective dose. Elderly patients are especially at risk.

Patients receiving temazepam should be cautioned about possible combined effects with alcohol and other CNS depressants. Withdrawal symptoms of the barbiturate type) have occurred after the abrupt discontinuation of benzodiazepines.

PRECAUTIONS

GENERAL

Since the risk of the development of over-sedation, dizziness, confusion, and/or ataxia increases substantially with larger doses of benzodiazepines in elderly and debilitated patients, 7.5 mg of temazepam is recommended as the initial dosage for such patients.

Temazepam should be administered with caution in severely depressed patients or those in whom there is any evidence of latent depression; it should be recognized that suicidal tendencies may be present and protective measures may be necessary.

The usual precautions should be observed in patients with impaired renal or hepatic function and in patients with chronic pulmonary insufficiency.

If temazepam is to be combined with other drugs having known hypnotic properties or CNS-depressant effects, consideration should be given to potential additive effects.

The possibility of a synergistic effect exists with the co-administration of temazepam and diphenhydramine. One case of stillbirth at term has been reported 8 hours after a pregnant patient received temazepam and diphenhydramine. A cause and effect relationship has not yet been determined. (See CONTRAINDICATIONS)

INFORMATION FOR THE PATIENT

The text of a patient package insert is printed at the end of this insert. To assure safe and effective use of temazepam, the information and instructions provided in this patient package insert should be discussed with patients.

LABORATORY TESTS

The usual precautions should be observed in patients with impaired renal or hepatic function and in patients with chronic pulmonary insufficiency. Abnormal liver function tests as well as blood dyscrasias have been reported with benzodiazepines.

CARCINOGENESIS, MUTAGENESIS, AND IMPAIRMENT OF FERTILITY

Carcinogenicity studies were conducted in rats at dietary diazepam doses up to 160 mg/kg/day for 24 months and in mice at dietary dose of 160 mg/kg/day for 18 months. No evidence of carcinogenicity was observed although hyperplastic liver nodules were observed in female mice exposed in female mice exposed to the highest dose. The clinical significance of this finding is not known.

Fertility in male and female rats was not adversely affected by temazepam.

No mutagenicity tests have been done with temazepam.

PREGNANCY CATEGORY X

(See CONTRAINDICATIONS.)

NURSING MOTHERS

It is not known whether this drug is excreted in human milk. Because many drugs are excreted in human milk, caution should be exercised when temazepam is administered to a nursing woman.

PEDIATRIC USE

Safety and effectiveness in children below the age of 18 years have not been established.

ADVERSE REACTIONS

During clinical studies in which 1076 patients received temazepam at bedtime, the drug was well tolerated. Side effects were usually mild and transient. Adverse reactions occurring in 1% or more of patients are presented in TABLE 1.

TABLE 1

	Temazepam % Incidence (n=1076)	Placebo % Incidence (n=783)
Drowsiness	9.1%	5.6%
Headache	8.5%	9.1%
Fatigue	4.8%	4.7%
Nervousness	4.6%	8.2%
Lethargy	4.5%	3.4%
Dizziness	4.5%	3.8%
Nausea	3.1%	3.3%
Hangover	2.5%	1.1%%
Anxiety	2.0%	1.5%
Depression	1.7%	1.8%
Dry Mouth	1.7%	2.2%
Diarrhea	1.7%	1.1%
Abdominal discomfort	1.5%	1.9%
Euphoria	1.5%	0.4%
Weakness	1.4%	0.9%
Confusion	1.3%	0.5%
Blurred vision	1.3%	1.3%
Nightmares	1.2%	1.7%
Vertigo	1.2%	0.8%

The following adverse events have been reported less frequently (0.5-0.9%):

Central Nervous System: Anorexia, ataxia, equilibrium loss, tremor, increased dreaming.

Cardiovascular: Dyspnea, palpitations.

Gastrointestinal: Vomiting.
Musculoskeletal: Backache.
Special Senses: Hyperhidrosis, burning eyes.

Amnesia, hallucinations, horizontal nystagmus, and paradoxical reactions including restlessness, overstimulation and agitation were rare (less than 0.5%).

DOSAGE AND ADMINISTRATION

While the recommended usual adult dose is 15 mg before retiring, 7.5 mg may be sufficient for some patients, and others may need 30 mg. In transient insomnia, a 7.5 mg dose may be sufficient to improve sleep latency. In elderly and/or debilitated patients it is recommended that therapy be initiated with 7.5 mg until individual responses are determined.

PRODUCT LISTING - RATED THERAPEUTICALLY EQUIVALENT

Package	Price	Product, Manufacturer	NDC
Capsule - Oral - 7.5 mg			
100's	$46.67	GENERIC, Creighton Products Corporation	50752-0271-05
100's	$47.99	GENERIC, Creighton Products Corporation	50752-0271-06
100's	$67.18	GENERIC, Geneva Pharmaceuticals	00781-2209-01
Capsule - Oral - 15 mg			
25's	$0.00	RESTORIL, Novartis Pharmaceuticals	00078-0098-13
30's	$14.07	GENERIC, Med-Pro Inc	53978-5016-05
100's	$7.50	GENERIC, Interstate Drug Exchange Inc	00814-7600-14
100's	$12.98	FEDERAL UPPER LIMIT, H.C.F.A. F F P	99999-2310-02
100's	$23.75	GENERIC, Moore, H.L. Drug Exchange Inc	00839-7164-06
100's	$24.20	GENERIC, Martec Pharmaceuticals Inc	52555-0242-01
100's	$25.04	GENERIC, Aligen Independent Laboratories Inc	00405-0185-01
100's	$25.25	GENERIC, Ivax Corporation	00182-1822-01
100's	$26.12	GENERIC, Moore, H.L. Drug Exchange Inc	00839-7899-06
100's	$27.31	GENERIC, Ivax Corporation	00182-1822-89
100's	$28.68	GENERIC, Auro Pharmaceutical	55829-0875-10
100's	$29.40	GENERIC, Major Pharmaceuticals Inc	00904-2810-61
100's	$32.95	GENERIC, Geneva Pharmaceuticals	00781-2201-13
100's	$44.00	GENERIC, Qualitest Products Inc	00603-5895-21
100's	$44.93	GENERIC, Major Pharmaceuticals Inc	00904-2810-60
100's	$69.30	GENERIC, Geneva Pharmaceuticals	00781-2201-01
100's	$71.38	GENERIC, Udl Laboratories Inc	51079-0418-20
100's	$71.38	GENERIC, Udl Laboratories Inc	51079-0418-21
100's	$73.45	GENERIC, Purepac Pharmaceutical Company	00228-2076-10
100's	$73.45	GENERIC, Mylan Pharmaceuticals Inc	00378-4010-01
100's	$76.92	RESTORIL, Novartis Pharmaceuticals	00078-0098-06
100's	$276.55	RESTORIL, Novartis Pharmaceuticals	00078-0098-05
Capsule - Oral - 30 mg			
25's	$0.00	RESTORIL, Novartis Pharmaceuticals	00078-0099-13
30's	$15.92	GENERIC, Med-Pro Inc	53978-5017-05
100's	$8.25	GENERIC, Interstate Drug Exchange Inc	00814-7602-14
100's	$15.60	FEDERAL UPPER LIMIT, H.C.F.A. F F P	99999-2310-05
100's	$25.80	GENERIC, Aligen Independent Laboratories Inc	00405-0186-01
100's	$28.05	GENERIC, Martec Pharmaceuticals Inc	52555-0243-01
100's	$28.75	GENERIC, Ivax Corporation	00182-1823-01
100's	$30.31	GENERIC, Moore, H.L. Drug Exchange Inc	00839-7900-06
100's	$31.84	GENERIC, Auro Pharmaceutical	55829-0876-10
100's	$32.76	GENERIC, Major Pharmaceuticals Inc	00904-2811-61
100's	$39.95	GENERIC, Geneva Pharmaceuticals	00781-2202-13
100's	$48.00	GENERIC, Qualitest Products Inc	00603-5896-21
100's	$50.93	GENERIC, Major Pharmaceuticals Inc	00904-2811-60
100's	$80.90	GENERIC, Geneva Pharmaceuticals	00781-2202-01
100's	$83.33	GENERIC, Udl Laboratories Inc	51079-0419-20
100's	$83.33	GENERIC, Udl Laboratories Inc	51079-0419-21
100's	$85.68	RESTORIL, Novartis Pharmaceuticals	00078-0099-06
100's	$88.45	GENERIC, Purepac Pharmaceutical Company	00228-2077-10
100's	$88.45	GENERIC, Mylan Pharmaceuticals Inc	00378-5050-01
100's	$309.26	RESTORIL, Novartis Pharmaceuticals	00078-0099-05
100's	$309.26	RESTORIL, Mallinckrodt Medical Inc	00406-9917-01

PRODUCT LISTING - EQUIVALENTS NOT AVAILABLE

Package	Price	Product, Manufacturer	NDC
Capsule - Oral - 7.5 mg			
12's	$10.68	GENERIC, Southwood Pharmaceuticals Inc	58016-0515-12
15's	$13.35	GENERIC, Southwood Pharmaceuticals Inc	58016-0515-15
20's	$17.80	GENERIC, Southwood Pharmaceuticals Inc	58016-0515-20
30's	$26.70	GENERIC, Southwood Pharmaceuticals Inc	58016-0515-30
60's	$53.40	GENERIC, Southwood Pharmaceuticals Inc	58016-0515-60
100's	$89.00	GENERIC, Southwood Pharmaceuticals Inc	58016-0515-00
100's	$89.54	RESTORIL, Novartis Pharmaceuticals	00078-0140-05
100's	$92.10	RESTORIL, Novartis Pharmaceuticals	00078-0140-06
100's	$217.68	RESTORIL, Mallinckrodt Medical Inc	00406-9915-01
Capsule - Oral - 15 mg			
2's	$3.49	GENERIC, Prescript Pharmaceuticals	00247-0207-02
4's	$3.65	GENERIC, Prescript Pharmaceuticals	00247-0207-04
5's	$3.72	GENERIC, Prescript Pharmaceuticals	00247-0207-05
8's	$3.94	GENERIC, Prescript Pharmaceuticals	00247-0207-08
12's	$11.03	GENERIC, Southwood Pharmaceuticals Inc	58016-0829-12
15's	$13.79	GENERIC, Southwood Pharmaceuticals Inc	58016-0829-15
20's	$4.81	GENERIC, Prescript Pharmaceuticals	00247-0207-20
20's	$18.38	GENERIC, Southwood Pharmaceuticals Inc	58016-0829-20
30's	$5.54	GENERIC, Prescript Pharmaceuticals	00247-0207-30
30's	$27.57	GENERIC, Southwood Pharmaceuticals Inc	58016-0829-30
60's	$55.14	GENERIC, Southwood Pharmaceuticals Inc	58016-0829-60
100's	$10.64	GENERIC, Prescript Pharmaceuticals	00247-0207-00
100's	$91.90	GENERIC, Southwood Pharmaceuticals Inc	58016-0829-00
100's	$276.55	RESTORIL, Mallinckrodt Medical Inc	00406-9916-01
Capsule - Oral - 30 mg			
12's	$12.34	GENERIC, Southwood Pharmaceuticals Inc	58016-0831-12
15's	$15.42	GENERIC, Southwood Pharmaceuticals Inc	58016-0831-15
20's	$20.56	GENERIC, Southwood Pharmaceuticals Inc	58016-0831-20
28's	$28.78	GENERIC, Southwood Pharmaceuticals Inc	58016-0831-28
30's	$30.84	GENERIC, Southwood Pharmaceuticals Inc	58016-0831-30
60's	$61.68	GENERIC, Southwood Pharmaceuticals Inc	58016-0831-60
100's	$102.80	GENERIC, Southwood Pharmaceuticals Inc	58016-0831-00

Temozolomide *(003444)*

For complete prescribing information, refer to the CD-ROM included with the book.

Categories: Astrocytoma; FDA Approved 1999 Aug; Pregnancy Category D; Orphan Drugs
Drug Classes: Antineoplastics, alkylating agents
Brand Names: Temodar
Foreign Brand Availability: Temodal (Australia; Austria; Bahrain; Belgium; Bulgaria; Canada; Cyprus; Czech-Republic; Denmark; Egypt; England; Finland; France; Germany; Greece; Hungary; Iran; Iraq; Ireland; Israel; Italy; Jordan; Korea; Kuwait; Lebanon; Libya; Mexico; Netherlands; Norway; Oman; Philippines; Poland; Portugal; Qatar; Republic-of-Yemen; Saudi-Arabia; Slovenia; Spain; Sweden; Switzerland; Syria; Turkey; United-Arab-Emirates); Temoxol (South-Africa)

DESCRIPTION

Temodar capsules for oral administration contain temozolomide, an imidazotetrazine derivative. The chemical name of temozolomide is 3,4-dihydro-3-methyl-4-oxoimidazo[5,1-d]-*as*-tetrazine-8-carboxamide.

The material is a white to light tan/light pink powder with a molecular formula of $C_6H_6N_6O_2$ and a molecular weight of 194.15. The molecule is stable at acidic pH (<5), and labile at pH >7, hence Temodar can be administered orally. The prodrug, temozolomide, is rapidly hydrolysed to the active 5-(3-methyltriazen-1-yl)imidazole-4-carboxamide (MTIC) at neutral and alkaline pH values, with hydrolysis taking place even faster at alkaline pH.

Each capsule contains 5, 20, 100, or 250 mg of temozolomide. The inactive ingredients for Temodar capsules are lactose anhydrous, colloidal silicon dioxide, sodium starch glycolate, tartaric acid, and stearic acid. Gelatin capsule shells contain titanium dioxide. The capsules are imprinted with pharmaceutical ink.

Temodar 5 mg: Green imprint contains pharmaceutical grade shellac, anhydrous ethyl alcohol, isopropyl alcohol, n-butyl alcohol, propylene glycol, ammonium hydroxide, titanium dioxide, yellow iron oxide, and FD&C blue no. 2 aluminum lake.

Temodar 20 mg: Brown imprint contains pharmaceutical grade shellac, anhydrous ethyl alcohol, isopropyl alcohol, n-butyl alcohol, propylene glycol, purified water, ammonium hydroxide, potassium hydroxide, titanium dioxide, black iron oxide, yellow iron oxide, brown iron oxide, and red iron oxide.

Temodar 100 mg: Blue imprint contains pharmaceutical glaze (modified) in an ethanol/shellac mixture, isopropyl alcohol, n-butyl alcohol, propylene glycol, titanium dioxide, and FD&C blue no. 2 aluminium lake.

Temodar 250 mg: Black, imprint contains pharmaceutical grade shellac, anhydrous ethyl alcohol, isopropyl alcohol, n-butyl alcohol, propylene glycol, purified water, ammonium hydroxide, potassium hydroxide, and black iron oxide.

INDICATIONS AND USAGE

Temozolomide capsules are indicated for the treatment of adult patients with refractory anaplastic astrocytoma, *i.e.*, patients at first relapse who have experienced disease progression on a drug regimen containing a nitrosourea and procarbazine.

This indication is based on the response rate in the indicated population. No results are available from randomized controlled trials in recurrent anaplastic astrocytoma that demonstrate a clinical benefit resulting from treatment, such as improvement in disease-related symptoms, delayed disease progression, or improved survival.

CONTRAINDICATIONS

Temozolomide capsules are contraindicated in patients who have a history of hypersensitivity reaction to any of its components. Temozolomide is also contraindicated in patients who have a history of hypersensitivity to DTIC, since both drugs are metabolized to MTIC.

WARNINGS

Patients treated with temozolomide capsules may experience myelosuppression. Prior to dosing patients must have an absolute neutrophil count (ANC) $\geq 1.5 \times 10^9$/L and a platelet count $\geq 100 \times 10^9$/L. A complete blood count should be obtained on Day 22 (21 days after the first dose) or within 48 hours of that day, and weekly until the ANC is above 1.5×10^9/L and platelet count exceeds 100×10^9/L. In the clinical trials, if the ANC fell to $<1.0 \times 10^9$/L or the platelet count was $<50 \times 10^9$/L during any cycle, the next cycle was reduced by 50 mg/m^2, but not below 100 mg/m^2. Patients who do not tolerate 100 mg/m^2 should not receive temozolomide capsules. Geriatric patients and women have been shown in clinical trials to have a higher risk of developing myelosuppression. Myelosuppression generally occurred late in the treatment cycle. The median nadirs occurred at 26 days for platelets (range 21-40 days) and 28 days for neutrophils (range 1-44 days). Only 14% (22/158) of patients had a neutrophil nadir and 20% (32/158) of patients had a platelet nadir which may have delayed the start of the next cycle. Neutrophil and platelet counts returned to normal, on average, within 14 days of nadir counts.

PREGNANCY

Temozolomide may cause fetal harm when administered to a pregnant woman. Five consecutive days of oral administration of 75 mg/m^2/day in rats and 150 mg/m^2/day in rabbits during the period of organogenesis (3/8 and 3/4 the maximum recommended human dose, respectively) caused numerous malformations of the external organs, soft tissues, and skeleton in both species. Doses of 150 mg/m^2/day in rats and rabbits also caused embryolethality as indicated by increased resorptions. There are no adequate and well-controlled studies in pregnant women. If this drug is used during pregnancy, or if the patient becomes pregnant while taking this drug, the patient should be apprised of the potential hazard to the fetus. Women of childbearing potential should be advised to avoid becoming pregnant during therapy with temozolomide capsules.

DOSAGE AND ADMINISTRATION

Dosage of temozolomide capsules must be adjusted according to nadir neutrophil and platelet counts in the previous cycle and neutrophil and platelet counts at the time of initiating the next cycle.

For adults the initial dose is 150 mg/m^2 orally once daily for 5 consecutive days per 28 day treatment cycle. For adult patients, if both the nadir and day of dosing (Day 29, Day 1 of next cycle) ANC are $\geq 1.5 \times 10^9$/L (1500/μl) and both the nadir and Day 29, Day 1 of next cycle platelet counts are $\geq 100 \times 10^9$/L (100,000/μl), the temozolomide dose may be increased to 200 mg/m^2/day for 5 consecutive days per 28 day treatment cycle. During treatment, a complete blood count should be obtained on Day 22 (21 days after the first dose) or within 48 hours of that day, and weekly until the ANC is above 1.5×10^9/L (1500/μl) and the platelet count exceeds 100×10^9/L (100,000/μl). The next cycle of temozolomide should not be started until the ANC and platelet count exceed these levels. If the ANC falls to $<1.0 \times 10^9$/L (1000/μl) or the platelet count is $<50 \times 10^9$/L (50,000/μl) during any cycle, the next cycle should be reduced by 50 mg/m^2, but not below 100 mg/m^2, the lowest recommended dose (see TABLE 4) (see WARNINGS).

Temozolomide therapy can be continued until disease progression. In the clinical trial, treatment could be continued for a maximum of 2 years; but the optimum duration of therapy is not known. For temozolomide dosage calculations based on body surface area (BSA), see TABLE 5. For suggested capsule combinations based on daily dose, see TABLE 6.

TABLE 4 *Dosing Modification*

150 mg/m^2/day × 5 day (Starting Dose) or 200 mg/m^2/day × 5 day
↓
Measure Day 22 ANC and platelets
↓
Measure ANC and platelets on Day 29 (Day 1 of next cycle)
↓
Based on lowest counts at either Day 22 or Day 29

↓	↓	↓
ANC <1000/μl or platelets <50,000/μl	ANC 1000-1500/μl or platelets 50,000-100,000/μl	ANC >1500/μl or platelets >100,000/μl
↓	↓	↓
Postpone therapy until ANC >1500/μl and platelets >100,000/μl; reduce dose by 50 mg/m^2/day for subsequent cycle	Postpone therapy until ANC >1500/μl and platelets >100,000/μl; maintain initial dose	Increase dose to, or maintain dose at, 200/mg/m^2/day × 5 days for subsequent cycle

TABLE 5 *Adult Daily Dose Calculations by Body Surface Area (BSA)**

Total BSA	150 mg/m^2 daily	200 mg/m^2 daily
0.5 m^2	75 mg	100 mg
0.6 m^2	90 mg	120 mg
0.7 m^2	105 mg	140 mg
0.8 m^2	120 mg	160 mg
0.9 m^2	135 mg	180 mg
1.0 m^2	150 mg	200 mg
1.1 m^2	165 mg	220 mg
1.2 m^2	180 mg	240 mg
1.3 m^2	195 mg	260 mg
1.4 m^2	210 mg	280 mg
1.5 m^2	225 mg	300 mg
1.6 m^2	240 mg	320 mg
1.7 m^2	255 mg	340 mg
1.8 m^2	270 mg	360 mg
1.9 m^2	285 mg	380 mg
2.0 m^2	300 mg	400 mg
2.1 m^2	315 mg	420 mg
2.2 m^2	330 mg	440 mg
2.3 m^2	345 mg	460 mg
2.4 m^2	360 mg	480 mg
2.5 m^2	375 mg	500 mg

* For 5 consecutive days per 28 day treatment cycle for the initial chemotherapy cycle (150 mg/m^2) and for subsequent chemotherapy cycles (200 mg/m^2) for adult patients whose nadir and day of dosing (Day 29, Day 1 of next cycle) absolute neutrophil count (ANC) is $>1.5 \times 10^9$/L (1500/μl) and whose nadir and Day 29, Day 1 of next cycle platelet count is $>100 \times 10^9$/L (100,000/μl).

Temozolomide capsules were administered under both fasting and non-fasting conditions; however, absorption is affected by food and consistency of administration with respect to food is recommended. There are no dietary restrictions with temozolomide. To reduce nausea and vomiting, temozolomide should be taken on an empty stomach. Bedtime administration may be advised. Antiemetic therapy may be administered prior to and/or following administration of temozolomide capsules.

Temozolomide capsules should not be opened or chewed. They should be swallowed whole with a glass of water.

HANDLING AND DISPOSAL

Temozolomide causes the rapid appearance of malignant tumors in rats. Capsules should not be opened. If capsules are accidentally opened or damaged, rigorous precautions should be taken with the capsule contents to avoid inhalation or contact with the skin or mucous membranes. Procedures for proper handling and disposal of anticancer drugs should be considered.[1-7] Several guidelines on this subject have been published. There is no general agreement that all of the procedures recommended in the guidelines are necessary or appropriate.

TABLE 6 *Suggested Capsule Combinations Based on Daily Dose in Adults*

Total Daily Dose (mg)	Number of Daily Capsules by Strength (mg)			
	250	100	20	5
200	0	2	0	0
205	0	2	0	1
210	0	2	0	2
215	0	2	0	3
220	0	2	1	0
225	0	2	1	1
230	0	2	1	2
235	0	2	1	3
240	0	2	2	0
245	0	2	2	1
250	1	0	0	0
255	1	0	0	1
260	1	0	0	2
265	1	0	0	3
270	1	0	1	0
275	1	0	1	1
280	1	0	1	2
285	1	0	1	3
290	1	0	2	0
295	1	0	2	1
300	0	3	0	0
305	0	3	0	1
310	0	3	0	2
315	0	3	0	3
320	0	3	1	0
325	0	3	1	1
330	1	0	4	0
335	1	0	4	1
340	0	3	2	0
345	0	3	2	1
350	1	1	0	0
355	1	1	0	1
360	1	1	0	2
365	1	1	0	3
370	1	1	1	0
375	1	1	1	1
380	1	1	1	2
385	1	1	1	3
390	1	1	2	0
395	1	1	2	1
400	0	4	0	0
405	0	4	0	1
410	0	4	0	2
415	0	4	0	3
420	0	4	1	0
425	0	4	1	1
430	1	1	4	0
435	0	4	1	3
440	0	4	2	0
445	0	4	2	1
450	1	2	0	0
455	1	2	0	1
460	1	2	0	2
465	1	2	0	3
470	1	2	1	0
475	1	2	1	1
480	1	2	1	2
485	1	2	1	3
490	1	2	2	0
495	1	2	2	1
500	2	0	0	0

PRODUCT LISTING - EQUIVALENTS NOT AVAILABLE

Capsule - Oral - 5 mg

5's	$40.33	TEMODAR, Schering Corporation	00085-1248-01
20's	$161.34	TEMODAR, Schering Corporation	00085-1248-02

Capsule - Oral - 20 mg

5's	$161.34	TEMODAR, Schering Corporation	00085-1244-01
20's	$645.43	TEMODAR, Schering Corporation	00085-1244-02

Capsule - Oral - 100 mg

5's	$806.76	TEMODAR, Schering Corporation	00085-1259-01
20's	$3227.13	TEMODAR, Schering Corporation	00085-1259-02

Capsule - Oral - 250 mg

5's	$2016.95	TEMODAR, Schering Corporation	00085-1252-01
20's	$6890.11	TEMODAR, Schering Corporation	00085-1252-02

Tenecteplase *(003504)*

Categories: Myocardial infarction; FDA Approved 2000 Jun; Pregnancy Category C
Drug Classes: Thrombolytics
Brand Names: **TNKase**
Foreign Brand Availability: Metalyse (Australia; Austria; Bahrain; Belgium; Bulgaria; Cyprus; Czech-Republic; Denmark; Egypt; England; Finland; France; Germany; Greece; Hungary; Iran; Iraq; Ireland; Italy; Jordan; Kuwait; Lebanon; Libya; Netherlands; New-Zealand; Norway; Oman; Poland; Portugal; Qatar; Republic-of-Yemen; Saudi-Arabia; Slovenia; Spain; Sweden; Switzerland; Syria; Taiwan; Turkey; United-Arab-Emirates)

DESCRIPTION

Tenecteplase is a tissue plasminogen activator (tPA) produced by recombinant DNA technology using an established mammalian cell line (Chinese Hamster Ovary cells). Tenecteplase is a 527 amino acid glycoprotein developed by introducing the following modifications to the complementary DNA (cDNA) for natural human tPA: a substitution of

T

threonine 103 with asparagine, and a substitution of asparagine 117 with glutamine, both within the kringle 1 domain, and a tetra-alanine substitution at amino acids 296-299 in the protease domain. Cell culture is carried out in nutrient medium containing the antibiotic gentamicin (65 mg/L). However, the presence of the antibiotic is not detectable in the final product (limit of detection is 0.67 µg/vial). TNKase is a sterile, white to off-white, lyophilized powder for single intravenous (IV) bolus administration after reconstitution with sterile water for injection. Each vial of TNKase nominally contains 52.5 mg tenecteplase, 0.55 g L-arginine, 0.17 g phosphoric acid, and 4.3 mg polysorbate 20, which includes a 5% overfill. Each vial will deliver 50 mg of tenecteplase.

CLINICAL PHARMACOLOGY

GENERAL

Tenecteplase is a modified form of human tissue plasminogen activator (tPA) that binds to fibrin and converts plasminogen to plasmin. In the presence of fibrin, *in vitro* studies demonstrate that tenecteplase conversion of plasminogen to plasmin is increased relative to its conversion in the absence of fibrin. This fibrin specificity decreases systemic activation of plasminogen and the resulting degradation of circulating fibrinogen as compared to a molecule lacking this property. Following administration of 30, 40, or 50 mg of tenecteplase, there are decreases in circulating fibrinogen (4-15%) and plasminogen (11-24%). The clinical significance of fibrin-specificity on safety (*e.g.,* bleeding) or efficacy has not been established. Biological potency is determined by an *in vitro* clot lysis assay and is expressed in tenecteplase-specific units. The specific activity of tenecteplase has been defined as 200 units/mg.

PHARMACOKINETICS

In patients with acute myocardial infarction (AMI), tenecteplase administered as a single bolus exhibits a biphasic disposition from the plasma. Tenecteplase was cleared from the plasma with an initial half-life of 20-24 minutes. The terminal phase half-life of tenecteplase was 90-130 minutes. In 99 of 104 patients treated with tenecteplase, mean plasma clearance ranged from 99-119 ml/min.

The initial volume of distribution is weight related and approximates plasma volume. Liver metabolism is the major clearance mechanism for tenecteplase.

INDICATIONS AND USAGE

Tenecteplase is indicated for use in the reduction of mortality associated with acute myocardial infarction (AMI). Treatment should be initiated as soon as possible after the onset of AMI symptoms.

CONTRAINDICATIONS

Tenecteplase therapy in patients with acute myocardial infarction is contraindicated in the following situations because of an increased risk of bleeding (see WARNINGS):

- **Active internal bleeding.**
- **History of cerebrovascular accident.**
- **Intracranial or intraspinal surgery or trauma within 2 months.**
- **Intracranial neoplasm, arteriovenous malformation, or aneurysm.**
- **Known bleeding diathesis.**
- **Severe uncontrolled hypertension.**

WARNINGS

BLEEDING

The most common complication encountered during tenecteplase therapy is bleeding. The type of bleeding associated with thrombolytic therapy can be divided into two broad categories:

- Internal bleeding, involving intracranial and retroperitoneal sites, or the gastrointestinal, genitourinary, or respiratory tracts.
- Superficial or surface bleeding, observed mainly at vascular puncture and access sites (*e.g.,* venous cutdowns, arterial punctures) or sites of recent surgical intervention.

Should serious bleeding (not controlled by local pressure) occur, any concomitant heparin or antiplatelet agents should be discontinued immediately.

In clinical studies of tenecteplase, patients were treated with both aspirin and heparin. Heparin may contribute to the bleeding risks associated with tenecteplase. The safety of the use of tenecteplase with other antiplatelet agents has not been adequately studied (see DRUG INTERACTIONS). Intramuscular injections and nonessential handling of the patient should be avoided for the first few hours following treatment with tenecteplase. Venipunctures should be performed and monitored carefully.

Should an arterial puncture be necessary during the first few hours following tenecteplase therapy, it is preferable to use an upper extremity vessel that is accessible to manual compression. Pressure should be applied for at least 30 minutes, a pressure dressing applied, and the puncture site checked frequently for evidence of bleeding.

Each patient being considered for therapy with tenecteplase should be carefully evaluated and anticipated benefits weighed against potential risks associated with therapy. In the following conditions, the risk of tenecteplase therapy may be increased and should be weighed against the anticipated benefits:

- Recent major surgery, *e.g.,* coronary artery bypass graft, obstetrical delivery, organ biopsy, previous puncture of noncompressible vessels.
- Cerebrovascular disease.
- Recent gastrointestinal or genitourinary bleeding.
- Recent trauma.
- Hypertension: systolic BP ≥180 mm Hg and/or diastolic BP ≥110 mm Hg.
- High likelihood of left heart thrombus, *e.g.,* mitral stenosis with atrial fibrillation.
- Acute pericarditis.
- Subacute bacterial endocarditis.
- Hemostatic defects, including those secondary to severe hepatic or renal disease.
- Severe hepatic dysfunction.
- Pregnancy.
- Diabetic hemorrhagic retinopathy or other hemorrhagic ophthalmic conditions.
- Septic thrombophlebitis or occluded AV cannula at seriously infected site.
- Advanced age (see PRECAUTIONS, Geriatric Use).
- Patients currently receiving oral anticoagulants, *e.g.,* warfarin sodium.
- Recent administration of GP IIb/IIIa inhibitors.
- Any other condition in which bleeding constitutes a significant hazard or would be particularly difficult to manage because of its location.

CHOLESTEROL EMBOLIZATION

Cholesterol embolism has been reported rarely in patients treated with all types of thrombolytic agents; the true incidence is unknown. This serious condition, which can be lethal, is also associated with invasive vascular procedures (*e.g.,* cardiac catheterization, angiography, vascular surgery) and/or anticoagulant therapy. Clinical features of cholesterol embolism may include livedo reticularis, "purple toe" syndrome, acute renal failure, gangrenous digits, hypertension, pancreatitis, myocardial infarction, cerebral infarction, spinal cord infarction, retinal artery occlusion, bowel infarction, and rhabdomyolysis.

ARRHYTHMIAS

Coronary thrombolysis may result in arrhythmias associated with reperfusion. These arrhythmias (such as sinus bradycardia, accelerated idioventricular rhythm, ventricular premature depolarizations, ventricular tachycardia) are not different from those often seen in the ordinary course of acute myocardial infarction and may be managed with standard antiarrhythmic measures. It is recommended that anti-arrhythmic therapy for bradycardia and/or ventricular irritability be available when tenecteplase is administered.

PRECAUTIONS

GENERAL

Standard management of myocardial infarction should be implemented concomitantly with tenecteplase treatment. Arterial and venous punctures should be minimized. Noncompressible arterial puncture must be avoided and internal jugular and subclavian venous punctures should be avoided to minimize bleeding from the noncompressible sites. In the event of serious bleeding, heparin and antiplatelet agents should be discontinued immediately. Heparin effects can be reversed by protamine.

READMINISTRATION

Readministration of plasminogen activators, including tenecteplase, to patients who have received prior plasminogen activator therapy has not been systematically studied. Three (3) of 487 patients tested for antibody formation to tenecteplase had a positive antibody titer at 30 days. The data reflect the percentage of patients whose test results were considered positive for antibodies to tenecteplase in a radioimmunoprecipitation assay, and are highly dependent on the sensitivity and specificity of the assay. Additionally, the observed incidence of antibody positivity in an assay may be influenced by several factors including sample handling, concomitant medications, and underlying disease. For these reasons, comparison of the incidence of antibodies to tenecteplase with the incidence of antibodies to other products may be misleading. Although sustained antibody formation in patients receiving one dose of tenecteplase has not been documented, readministration should be undertaken with caution. If an anaphylactic reaction occurs, appropriate therapy should be administered.

DRUG/LABORATORY TEST INTERACTIONS

During tenecteplase therapy, results of coagulation tests and/or measures of fibrinolytic activity may be unreliable unless specific precautions are taken to prevent *in vitro* artifacts. Tenecteplase is an enzyme that, when present in blood in pharmacologic concentrations, remains active under *in vitro* conditions. This can lead to degradation of fibrinogen in blood samples removed for analysis.

CARCINOGENESIS, MUTAGENESIS, AND IMPAIRMENT OF FERTILITY

Studies in animals have not been performed to evaluate the carcinogenic potential, mutagenicity, or the effect on fertility.

PREGNANCY CATEGORY C

Tenecteplase has been shown to elicit maternal and embryo toxicity in rabbits given multiple IV administrations. In rabbits administered 0.5, 1.5 and 5.0 mg/kg/day, vaginal hemorrhage resulted in maternal deaths. Subsequent embryonic deaths were secondary to maternal hemorrhage and no fetal anomalies were observed. Tenecteplase does not elicit maternal and embryo toxicity in rabbits following a single IV administration. Thus, in developmental toxicity studies conducted in rabbits, the no observable effect level (NOEL) of a single IV administration of tenecteplase on maternal or developmental toxicity was 5 mg/kg (approximately 8-10 times the human dose). There are no adequate and well-controlled studies in pregnant women. Tenecteplase should be given to pregnant women only if the potential benefits justify the potential risk to the fetus.

NURSING MOTHERS

It is not known if tenecteplase is excreted in human milk. Because many drugs are excreted in human milk, caution should be exercised when tenecteplase is administered to a nursing woman.

PEDIATRIC USE

The safety and effectiveness of tenecteplase in pediatric patients have not been established.

GERIATRIC USE

Of the patients in ASSENT-2 who received tenecteplase, 4958 (59%) were under the age of 65; 2256 (27%) were between the ages of 65 and 74; and 1244 (15%) were 75 and over. The 30 day mortality rates by age were 2.5% in patients under the age of 65, 8.5% in patients between the ages of 65 and 74, and 16.2% in patients age 75 and over. The ICH rates were 0.4% in patients under the age of 65, 1.6% in patients between the ages of 65 and 74, and 1.7% in patients age 75 and over. The rates of any stroke were 1.0% in patients under the age of 65, 2.9% in patients between the ages of 65 and 74, and 3.0% in patients age 75 and over. Major bleeding rates, defined as bleeding requiring blood transfusion or leading to hemodynamic compromise, were 3.1% in patients under the age of 65, 6.4% in patients between the ages of 65 and 74, and 7.7% in patients age 75 and over. In elderly patients, the benefits of tenecteplase on mortality should be carefully weighed against the risk of increased adverse events, including bleeding.

DRUG INTERACTIONS

Formal interaction studies of tenecteplase with other drugs have not been performed. Patients studied in clinical trials of tenecteplase were routinely treated with heparin and aspirin. Anticoagulants (such as heparin and vitamin K antagonists) and drugs that alter platelet function (such as acetylsalicylic acid, dipyridamole, and GP IIb/IIIa inhibitors) may increase the risk of bleeding if administered prior to, during, or after tenecteplase therapy.

ADVERSE REACTIONS

BLEEDING

The most frequent adverse reaction associated with tenecteplase is bleeding (see WARNINGS).

Should serious bleeding occur, concomitant heparin and antiplatelet therapy should be discontinued. Death or permanent disability can occur in patients who experience stroke or serious bleeding episodes.

For tenecteplase-treated patients in ASSENT-2, the incidence of intracranial hemorrhage was 0.9% and any stroke was 1.8%. The incidence of all strokes, including intracranial bleeding, increases with increasing age (see PRECAUTIONS, Geriatric Use).

In the ASSENT-2 study, the following bleeding events were reported (see TABLE 3).

TABLE 3 *ASSENT-2*

Non-ICH Bleeding Events

	Tenecteplase (n=8461)	Accelerated Alteplase, Recombinant (n=8488)	Relative Risk Tenecteplase/Alteplase (95% CI)
Major bleeding*	4.7%	5.9%	0.78 (0.69, 0.89)
Minor bleeding	21.8%	23.0%	0.94 (0.89, 1.00)
Units of transferred blood			
Any	4.3%	5.5%	0.77 (0.67, 0.89)
1-2	2.6%	3.2%	
>2	1.7%	2.2%	

* Major bleeding is defined as bleeding requiring blood transfusion or leading to hemodynamic compromise.

Non-intracranial major bleeding and the need for blood transfusions were lower in patients treated with tenecteplase.

Types of major bleeding reported in 1% or more of the patients were hematoma (1.7%) and gastrointestinal tract (1%). Types of major bleeding reported in less than 1% of the patients were urinary tract, puncture site (including cardiac catheterization site), retroperitoneal, respiratory tract, and unspecified. Types of minor bleeding reported in 1% or more of the patients were hematoma (12.3%), urinary tract (3.7%), puncture site (including cardiac catheterization site) (3.6%), pharyngeal (3.1%), gastrointestinal tract (1.9%), epistaxis (1.5%), and unspecified (1.3%).

ALLERGIC REACTIONS

Allergic-type reactions (*e.g.*, anaphylaxis, angioedema, laryngeal edema, rash, and urticaria) have rarely (<1%) been reported in patients treated with tenecteplase. Anaphylaxis was reported in <0.1% of patients treated with tenecteplase; however, causality was not established. When such reactions occur, they usually respond to conventional therapy.

OTHER ADVERSE REACTIONS

The following adverse reactions have been reported among patients receiving tenecteplase in clinical trials. These reactions are frequent sequelae of the underlying disease, and the effect of tenecteplase on the incidence of these events is unknown.

These events include cardiogenic shock, arrhythmias, atrioventricular block, pulmonary edema, heart failure, cardiac arrest, recurrent myocardial ischemia, myocardial reinfarction, myocardial rupture, cardiac tamponade, pericarditis, pericardial effusion, mitral regurgitation, thrombosis, embolism, and electromechanical dissociation. These events can be life-threatening and may lead to death. Nausea and/or vomiting, hypotension, and fever have also been reported.

DOSAGE AND ADMINISTRATION

DOSAGE

Tenecteplase is for intravenous administration only. The recommended total dose should not exceed 50 mg and is based upon patient weight.

A single bolus dose should be administered over 5 seconds based on patient weight. Treatment should be initiated as soon as possible after the onset of AMI symptoms.

TABLE 4 *Dose Information Table*

Patient Weight	Tenecteplase	Volume Tenecteplase* to be Administered
<60 kg	30 mg	6 ml
≥60 to <70 kg	35 mg	7 ml
≥70 to <80 kg	40 mg	8 ml
≥80 to <90 kg	45 mg	9 ml
≥90 kg	50 mg	10 ml

* From 1 vial of tenecteplase reconstituted with 10 ml sterile water for injection.

The safety and efficacy of tenecteplase has only been investigated with concomitant administration of heparin and aspirin.

HOW SUPPLIED

TNKase is supplied as a sterile, lyophilized powder in a 50 mg vial under partial vacuum.

Stability and Storage: Store lyophilized TNKase at controlled room temperature not to exceed 30°C (86°F) or under refrigeration 2-8°C (36-46°F). Do not use beyond the expiration date stamped on the vial.

PRODUCT LISTING - EQUIVALENTS NOT AVAILABLE

Powder For Injection - Intravenous - 50 mg

1's $2832.50 TNKASE, Genentech 50242-0038-61

Teniposide *(003127)*

Categories: Leukemia, acute lymphoblastic; FDA Approved 1992 Jul; Pregnancy Category D; Orphan Drugs
Drug Classes: Antineoplastics, epipodophyllotoxins
Brand Names: Vumon

WARNING

Teniposide is a cytotoxic drug, which should be administered under the supervision of a qualified physician experienced in the use of cancer chemotherapeutic agents. Appropriate management of therapy and complications is possible only when adequate treatment facilities are readily available.

Severe myelosupression with resulting infection or bleeding may occur. Hypersensitivity reactions, including anaphylaxis-like symptoms, may occur with initial dosing or at repeated exposure to teniposide. Epinephrine, with or without corticosteroids and antihistamines has been employed to alleviate hypersensitivity reaction symptoms.

DESCRIPTION

Vumon (also commonly known as VM-26), is supplied as a sterile nonpyrogenic solution in a nonaqueous medium intended for dilution with a suitable parenteral vehicle prior to intravenous infusion. Vumon is available in 50 mg (5 ml) ampules. Each ml contains 10 mg teniposide, 30 mg benzyl alcohol, 60 mg N,N-dimethylacetamide, 500 mg Cremophor EL (polyoxyethylated castor oil) and 42.7% (V/V) dehydrated alcohol. The pH of the clear solution is adjusted to approximately 5 with maleic acid.

Teniposide is a semisynthetic derivative of podophyllotoxin. The chemical name for teniposide is 4-demethylepipodophyllotoxin 9-(4,6-0-(R)-2- thenylidene-β-D-glucopyranoside). Teniposide differs from etoposide, another podophyllotoxin derivative, by the substitution of a thenylidene group on the glucopyranoside ring.

Teniposide is a white to off-white crystalline powder with the empirical formula $C_{32}H_{32}O_{13}S$ and a molecular weight of 656.66. It is a lipophilic compound with a partition coefficient value (octanol/water) of approximately 100. Teniposide is insoluble in water and ether. It is slightly soluble in methanol and very soluble in acetone and dimethylformamide.

CLINICAL PHARMACOLOGY

Teniposide is a phase-specific cytotoxic drug acting in the late S or early G_2 phase of the cell cycle, thus preventing cells from entering mitosis. Teniposide causes dose-dependent single- and double-stranded breaks in DNA and DNA:protein cross-links. The mechanism of action appears to be related to the inhibition of type II topoisomerase activity since teniposide does not intercalate into DNA or bind strongly to DNA. The cytotoxic effects of teniposide are related to the relative number of double-stranded DNA breaks produced in cells, which are a reflection of the stabilization of a topoisomerase II-DNA intermediate.

Teniposide has a broad spectrum of *in vivo* antitumor activity against murine tumors, including hematologic malignancies and various solid tumors. Notably, teniposide is active against sublines of certain murine leukemias with acquired resistance to cisplatin, doxorubicin, amsacrine, daunorubicin, mitoxantrone or vincristine.

Plasma drug levels declined biexponentially following intravenous infusion (155 mg/m²) over 1 to 2.5 hours) of teniposide given to 8 children (4 - 11 years old) with newly diagnosed acute lymphoblastic leukemia (ALL). The observed average pharmacokinetic parameters and associated coefficients of variation (CV%) based on a two-compartmental model analysis of the data are as follows (TABLE 1):

TABLE 1

Parameter	Mean	CV%
Total body clearance (ml/min/m²)	10.3	25
Volume at steady-state (L/m²)	3.1	30
Terminal half-life (hours)	5.0	44
Volume of central compartment (L/m²)	1.5	36
Rate constant, central to peripheral (1/hours)	0.47	62
Rate constant, peripheral to central (1/hours)	0.42	37

There appears to be some association between an increase in serum alkaline phosphatase or gamma glutamyl-transpeptidase and a decrease in plasma clearance of teniposide. Therefore, caution should be exercised if teniposide is to be administered to patients with hepatic dysfunction.

In adults, at doses of 100-333 mg/m²/day, plasma levels increased linearly with dose. Drug accumulation in adult patients did not occur after daily administration of teniposide for 3 days. In pediatric patients, maximum plasma concentrations (Cmax) after infusions of 137-203 mg/m² over a period of 1-2 hours exceeded 40 μg/ml; by 20-24 hours after infusion plasma levels were generally <2 μg/ml.

Renal clearance of parent teniposide accounts for about 10% of total body clearance. In adults, after intravenous administration of 10 mg/kg or 67 mg/m² of tritium-labeled teniposide, 44% of the radiolabel was recovered in urine (parent drug and metabolites) within

T

120 hours after dosing. From 4-12% of a dose is excreted in urine as parent drug. Fecal excretion of radioactivity within 72 hours after dosing accounted for 0-10% of the dose.

Mean steady-state volumes of distribution range from 8-44 L/m^2 for adults and 3-11 L/m^2 for children. The blood-brain barrier appears to limit diffusion of teniposide into the brain, although in a study in patients with brain tumors, CSF levels of teniposide were higher than CSF levels reported in other studies of patients who did not have brain tumors.

Teniposide is highly protein bound. *In vitro* plasma protein binding of teniposide is >99%. The high affinity of teniposide for plasma proteins may be an important factor in limiting distribution of drug within the body. Steady state volume of distribution of the drug increases with a decrease in plasma albumin levels. Therefore, careful monitoring of children with hypoalbuminemia is indicated during therapy. Levels of teniposide in saliva, CSF and malignant ascites fluid are low relative to simultaneously measured plasma levels.

The pharmacokinetic characteristics of teniposide differ from those of etoposide, another podophyllotoxin. Teniposide is more extensively bound to plasma proteins, and its cellular uptake is greater. Teniposide also has a lower systemic clearance, a longer elimination half-life, and is excreted in the urine as parent drug to a lesser extent than etoposide.

In a study at St. Jude Children's Research Hospital (SJCRH), 9 children with acute lymphocytic leukemia (ALL) failing induction therapy with a cytarabine-containing regimen, were treated with teniposide for injection concentrate plus cytarabine. Three (3) of these patients were induced into complete remission with durations of remissions of 30 weeks, 59 weeks, and 13 years. In another study at SJCRH, 16 children with ALL refractory to vincristine/prednisone-containing regimens were treated with teniposide plus vincristine and prednisone. Three (3) of these patients were induced into complete remission with durations of remission of 5.5, 37, and 73 weeks. In these two studies patients served as their own control based on the premise that long term complete remissions could not be achieved by retreatment with drugs to which they had previously failed to respond.

INDICATIONS AND USAGE

Teniposide, in combination with other approved anticancer agents, is indicated for induction therapy in patients with refractory childhood acute lymphoblastic leukemia.

NON-FDA APPROVED INDICATIONS

The drug has also been reported to have modest activity in the treatment of extensive small cell lung carcinoma. However, this use has not been approved by the FDA and further clinical trials are needed.

CONTRAINDICATIONS

Teniposide is generally contraindicated in patients who have demonstrated a previous hypersensitivity to teniposide and/or Cremophor EL (polyoxyethylated castor oil).

WARNINGS

Teniposide is a potent drug and should be used only by physicians experienced in the administration of cancer chemotherapeutic drugs. Blood counts as well as renal and hepatic function tests should be carefully monitored prior to and during therapy.

Patients being treated with teniposide should be observed frequently for myelosupression both during and after therapy. Dose-limiting bone marrow suppression is the most significant toxicity associated with teniposide therapy. Therefore, the following studies should be obtained at the start of therapy and prior to each subsequent dose of teniposide: hemoglobin, white blood cell count and differential and platelet count. If necessary, repeat bone marrow examination should be performed prior to the decision to continue therapy in the setting of severe myelosupression.

Physicians should be aware of the possible occurrence of a hypersensitivity reaction variably manifested by chills, fever, urticaria, tachycardia, bronchospasm, dyspnea, hypertension or hypotension and facial flushing. This reaction may occur with the first dose of teniposide and may be life threatening if not treated promptly with antihistamines, corticosteroids, epinephrine, intravenous fluids and other supportive measures as clinically indicated. The exact cause of these reactions is unknown. They may be due to the Cremophor EL (polyoxyethylated castor oil) component of the vehicle or to teniposide itself.[1] Patients who have experienced prior hypersensitivity reactions to teniposide are at risk for recurrence of symptoms and should only be retreated with teniposide if the antileukemic benefit already demonstrated clearly outweighs the risk of a probable hypersensitivity reaction for that patient. When a decision is made to retreat a patient with teniposide in spite of an earlier hypersensitivity reaction, the patient should be pretreated with corticosteroids and antihistamines and receive careful clinical observation during and after teniposide infusion. In the clinical experience with teniposide at SJCRH and the National Cancer Institute (NCI), retreatment of patients with prior hypersensitivity reactions has been accomplished using measures described above. To date, there is no evidence to suggest cross-sensitization between teniposide and VePesid.

One episode of sudden death, attributable to probable arrhythmia and intractable hypotension has been reported in an elderly patient receiving teniposide combination therapy for a non leukemic malignancy. (See ADVERSE REACTIONS.) **Patients receiving teniposide treatment should be under continuous observation for at least the first 60 minutes following the start of the infusion and at frequent intervals thereafter. If symptoms or signs of anaphylaxis occur, the infusion should be stopped immediately, followed by the administration of epinephrine, corticosteroids, antihistamines, pressor agents, or volume expanders at the discretion of the physician. An aqueous solution of epinephrine 1:1000 and a source of oxygen should be available at the bedside.**

For parenteral administration, teniposide should be given only by slow intravenous infusion (lasting at least 30-60 minutes) since hypotension has been reported as a possible side-effect of rapid intravenous injection, perhaps due to a direct effect of Cremophor EL.[2,3] If clinically significant hypotension develops, the teniposide infusion should be discontinued. The blood pressure usually normalizes within hours in response to cessation of the infusion and administration of fluids or other supportive therapy as appropriate. If the infusion is restarted, a slower administration rate should be used and the patient should be carefully monitored.

Acute central nervous system depression and hypotension have been observed in patients receiving investigational infusions of high-dose teniposide who were pretreated with antiemetic drugs. The depressant effects of the antiemetic agents and the alcohol content of the teniposide formulation may place patients receiving higher than recommended doses of teniposide at risk for central nervous system depression.

PREGNANCY CATEGORY D

Teniposide may cause fetal harm when administered to a pregnant woman. Teniposide has been shown to be teratogenic and embryotoxic in laboratory animals. In pregnant rats intravenous administration of teniposide, 0.1-3 mg/kg (0.6 - 18 mg/m^2), every second day from day 6 to day 16 post coitum caused dose-related embryotoxicity and teratogenicity. Major anomalies included spinal and rib defects, deformed extremities, anophthalmia and celosomia.

There are no adequate and well-controlled studies in pregnant women. If teniposide for injection concentrate is used during pregnancy, or if the patient become pregnant while receiving this drug, the patient should be apprised of the potential hazard to the fetus. Women of childbearing potential should be advised to avoid becoming pregnant therapy with teniposide.

PRECAUTIONS

GENERAL

In all instances where the use of teniposide is considered for chemotherapy the physician must evaluate the need and usefulness of the drug against the risk of adverse reactions. Most such adverse reactions are reversible if detected early. If severe reactions occur, the drug should be reduced in dosage or discontinued and appropriate corrective measures should be taken according to the clinical judgement of the physician. Reinstitution of teniposide therapy should be carried out with caution, and with adequate consideration of the further need for the drug and alertness as to possible recurrence of toxicity.

Teniposide must be administered as an intravenous infusion, Care should be taken to ensure that the intravenous catheter or needle is in the proper position and functional prior to infusion. Improper administration of teniposide may result in extravasation causing local tissue necrosis and/or thrombophlebitis. In some instances, occlusion of central venous access devices has occurred during 24 hour infusion of teniposide and a concentration of 0.1-0.2 mg/ml. Frequent observation during these infusions is necessary to minimize this risk.[4,5]

LABORATORY TESTS

Periodic complete blood counts and assessments of renal and hepatic function should be done during the course of teniposide treatment. They should be performed prior to therapy and at clinically appropriate intervals during and after therapy. There should be at least one determination of hematologic status prior to therapy with teniposide.

CARCINOGENESIS, MUTAGENESIS, AND IMPAIRMENT OF FERTILITY

Children at SJCRH with ALL in remission who received maintenance therapy with teniposide at weekly or twice weekly doses (plus other chemotherapeutic agents), had a relative risk of developing secondary acute non- lymphocytic leukemia (ANLL) approximately 12 times that of patients treated according to other less intensive schedules.[6] A short course of teniposide or remission-induction and/or consolidation therapy was not associated with an increased risk of secondary ANLL, but the number of patients assessed was small. The potential benefit from teniposide must be weighed on a case by case basis against the potential risk of the induction of a secondary leukemia. The carcinogenicity of teniposide has not been studies in laboratory animals. Compounds with similar mechanisms of action and mutagenicity profiles have been reported to be carcinogenic and teniposide should be considered a potential carcinogen in humans. Teniposide has been shown to be mutagenic in various bacterial and mammalian genetic toxicity tests. These include positive mutagenic effects in the Ames/Salmonella and *B. subtilis* bacterial mutagenicity assays. Teniposide caused gene mutations in both Chinese hamster ovary cells and mouse lymphoma cells and DNA damage as measured by alkaline elution in human lung carcinoma derived cell lines. In addition, teniposide induced aberrations in chromosome structure in primary cultures of human lymphocytes *in vitro* and in L5178y/TK +/- mouse lymphoma cells *in vitro*. Chromosome aberrations were observed *in vivo* in the embryonic tissue of pregnant Swiss albino mice treated with teniposide. Teniposide also caused a dose-related increase in sister-chromatid exchanges in Chinese hamster ovary cells and it has been shown to be embryotoxic and teratogenic in rats receiving teniposide during organogenesis. Treatment of pregnant rats IV with doses between 1.0 and 3.0 mg/kg/day on alternate days from day 6-16 post coitum caused retardation of embryonic development, prenatal mortality and fetal abnormalities.

PREGNANCY CATEGORY D

See WARNINGS.

NURSING MOTHERS

It is not known whether this drug is excreted in human milk. Because many drugs are excreted in human milk and because of the potential for serious adverse reactions in nursing infants, a decision should be made whether to discontinue nursing or to discontinue the drug, taking into account the importance of teniposide therapy to the mother.

PATIENTS WITH DOWN'S SYNDROME

Patients with both Down's Syndrome and leukemia may be especially sensitive to myelosuppressive chemotherapy, therefore, initial dosing with teniposide should be reduced in these patients. It is suggested that the first course of teniposide should be given at half the usual dose. Subsequent courses may be administered at higher dosages depending on the degree of myelosupression and mucositis encountered in earlier courses in an individual patient.

DRUG INTERACTIONS

In a study in which 34 different drugs were tested, therapeutically relevant concentrations of tolbutamide, sodium salicylate and sulfamethizole displaced protein-bound teniposide in fresh human serum to a small but significant extent. Because of the extremely high binding

T

of teniposide to plasma proteins, these small decreases in binding could cause substantial increases in free drug levels in plasma which could result in potentiation of drug toxicity. Therefore, caution should be used in administering teniposide to patients receiving these other agents. There was no change in the plasma kinetic of teniposide when coadministered with methotrexate. However, the plasma clearance of methotrexate was slightly increased. An increase in intracellular levels of methotrexate was observed *in vitro* in the presence of teniposide.

ADVERSE REACTIONS

TABLE 2 presents the incidences of adverse reactions derived from an analysis of data contained within literature reports of 7 studies involving 303 pediatric patients in which teniposide was administered by injection as a single agent in a variety of doses and schedules for a variety of hematologic malignancies and solid tumors. The total number patients evaluable for a given event was not 303 since the individual studies did not address the occurrence of each event listed. Five of these seven studies assessed teniposide activity in hematologic malignancies, such as leukemia. Thus, many of these patients had abnormal hematologic status at start of therapy with teniposide and were expected to develop significant myelosupression as an endpoint of treatment.

HEMATOLOGIC TOXICITY

Teniposide, when used with other chemotherapeutic agents for the treatment of ALL, results in severe myelosuppression. Early onset of profound myelosuppression with delayed recovery can be expected when using the doses and schedules of teniposide necessary for treatment of refractory ALL, since bone marrow hypoplasia is a desired endpoint of therapy. The occurrence of acute non-lymphocytic leukemia (ANLL), with or without a preleukemic phase has been reported in patients treated with teniposide in combination with other antineoplastic agents. See PRECAUTIONS, Carcinogenesis, Mutagenesis, and Impairment of Fertility.

TABLE 2 *Single-Agent Teniposide*

Summary of Toxicity for All Evaluable Pediatric Patients

Toxicity	Incidence in Evaluable Patients
Hematologic Toxicity	
Myelosupression, non-specified	75%
Leukopenia (<3000 WCB/µl)	89%
Neutropenia (<2000 ANC/µl)	95%
Thombocytopenia (<100,000 plt/µl)	85%
Anemia	88%
Non-Hematologic Toxicity	
Mucositis	76%
Diarrhea	33%
Nausea/Vomiting	29%
Infection	12%
Alopecia	9%
Bleeding	5%
Hypersensitivity reactions	5%
Rash	3%
Fever	3%
Hypotension/cardiovascular	3%
Neurotoxicity	<1%
Hepatic dysfunction	<1%
Renal dysfunction	<1%
Metabolic abnormalities	<1%

GASTROINTESTINAL TOXICITY

Nausea and vomiting are the most common gastrointestinal toxicities, having occurred in 29% of evaluable pediatric patients. The severity of this nausea and vomiting is generally mild to moderate.

HYPOTENSION

Transient hypotension following rapid intravenous administration has been reported in 2% of evaluable pediatric patients. One episode of sudden death, attributed too probable arrhythmia and intractable hypotension, has been reported in an elderly patient receiving teniposide for injection concentrate combination therapy for a non-leukemic malignancy.

No other cardiac toxicity or electrocardiographic changes have been documented. No delayed hypotension has been noted.

ALLERGIC REACTIONS

Hypersensitivity reactions characterized by chills, fever, tachycardia, flushing, bronchospasm, dyspnea, and blood pressure changes (hypertension or hypotension) have been reported to occur in approximately 5% of evaluable pediatric patients receiving intravenous teniposide. The incidence of hypersensitivity reactions to teniposide appears to be increased in patients with brain tumors, and in patients with neuroblastoma.[1]

CENTRAL NERVOUS SYSTEM

Acute central nervous system depression and hypotension have been observed in patients receiving investigational infusions of high-dose teniposide who were pretreated with antiemetic drugs. The depressant effects of the antiemetic agents and the alcohol content of the teniposide formulation may place patients receiving higher than recommended doses of teniposide at risk for central nervous system depression.

ALOPECIA

Alopecia, sometimes progressing to total baldness, was observed in 9% of evaluable pediatric patients who received teniposide as single agent therapy. It was usually reversible.

DOSAGE AND ADMINISTRATION

NOTE: Contact of undiluted teniposide for injection concentrate with plastic equipment or devices used to prepare solutions for infusion may result in softening or cracking and possible drug product leakage. this effect has *not* been reported with *diluted solutions* of teniposide.

In order to prevent extraction of the plasticizer DEHP (di(2- ethylhexyl)phtalate), solutions of teniposide for injection concentrate should be prepared in non-DEHP containing LVP container such as glass or Pololefin plastic bags or containers.

Teniposide solutions should be administered with non-DEHP containing IV administration sets.

In one study, childhood ALL patients failing induction therapy with a cytarabine-containing regimen were treated with the combination of teniposide 165 mg/m² and cytarabine 300 mg/m² intravenously, twice weekly for 8-9 doses. In another study, patients with childhood ALL refractory to vincristine/prednisone-containing regimens were treated with the combination of teniposide 250 mg/m² and vincristine 1.5 mg/m² intravenously, weekly for 4-8 weeks and prednisone 40 mg/m² orally × 28 days.

Adequate data in patients with hepatic insufficiency and/or renal insufficiency are lacking, but dose adjustments may be necessary for patients with significant renal or hepatic impairment.

PREPARATION AND ADMINISTRATION PRECAUTIONS

Teniposide is a cytotoxic anticancer drug and as with other potentially toxic compound, caution should be exercised in handling and preparing the solutions of teniposide. Skin reactions associated with accidental exposure to teniposide may occur. The use of gloves is recommended. If teniposide solution contacts the skin, immediately wash the skin thoroughly with soap and water. If teniposide contacts mucous membranes the membranes should be flushed thoroughly with water.

PREPARATION FOR INTRAVENOUS ADMINISTRATION

Teniposide must be diluted with either 5% dextrose injection or 0.9% sodium chloride injection to give final teniposide concentrations of 0.1 mg/ml, 0.2 mg/ml, 0.4 mg/ml or 1.0 mg/ml. Solutions prepared in 5% dextrose injection or 0.9% sodium chloride injection at teniposide concentrations of 0.1 mg/ml, 0.2 mg/ml or 0.4 mg/ml are stable at room temperature for up to 24 hours after preparation. Teniposide solutions prepared at a final teniposide concentration of 1.0 mg/ml should be administered within 4 hours of preparation to reduce the potential for precipitation.

Refrigeration of teniposide solutions is not recommended.

Stability and use times are identical in glass and plastic parenteral solution containers.

Although solutions are chemically stable under the conditions indicated, precipitation of teniposide may occur at the recommended concentrations, especially if the diluted solution is subjected to more agitation than is recommended to prepare the drug solution for parenteral administration.[7] In addition, storage time prior to administration should be minimized and care should be taken to avoid contact of the diluted solution with other drugs or fluids. Parenteral drug products should be inspected visually for particulate matter and discoloration prior to administration whenever solution and container permit. **Precipitation has been reported during 24 hour infusions of teniposide for injection concentrate diluted to teniposide concentrations of 0.1-0.2 mg/ml, resulting in occlusion of central venous access catheters in several patients.[4,5] Heparin solutions can cause precipitation of teniposide, therefore, the administration apparatus should be flushed thoroughly with 5% dextrose injection or 0.9% sodium chloride injection before and after administration of teniposide.[5]**

Hypotension has been reported following rapid bolus intravenous administration; it is recommended that the teniposide solution be administered over at least as 30-60 minute period. **Teniposide should not be given by rapid intravenous injection.**

In a 24 hour study under simulated conditions of actual use of the product relative to dilution strength, diluent and administration rates, dilution at 0.1-1.0 mg/ml were chemically stable for at least 24 hours. Data collected for the presence of the extractable DEHP (di(23- ethylhexyl)phtalate) from PVC containers show that levels increased with time and concentration of the solutions. The data appeared similar for 0.9% sodium chloride injection and 5% dextrose injection. Consequently, the use of PVC containers is not recommended.

Similarly, the use of non-DEHP IV administration sets is recommended. Lipid administration sets or low DEHP containing nitroglycerin sets will keep patients' exposure to DEHP at low levels and are suitable for use. the diluted solutions are chemically and physically compatible with the recommended IV administration sets and LVP containers of up to 24 hours at ambient room temperature and lighting conditions. **Because of the potential for precipitation, compatibility with other drugs, infusion materials or IV pumps cannot be assured.**

Stability: Unopened ampules of teniposide are stable until the date indicated in the package when stored under refrigeration (2-8°C) in the original package. Freezing does not adversely affect the product.

HANDLING AND DISPOSAL

Procedures for proper handling and disposal of anticancer drugs should be considered. Several guidelines on this subject have been published.[8-14] There is no general agreement that all of the procedures recommended in the guidelines are necessary or appropriate.

PRODUCT LISTING - EQUIVALENTS NOT AVAILABLE

Solution - Intravenous - 10 mg/ml

5 ml	$253.29	VUMON, Bristol-Myers Squibb	00015-3075-19
5 ml x 10	$2532.88	VUMON, Bristol-Myers Squibb	00015-3075-97

T

Tenofovir Disoproxil Fumarate (003533)

For related information, see the comparative table section in Appendix A.

Categories: Infection, human immunodeficiency virus; FDA Approved 2001 Oct; Pregnancy Category B
Drug Classes: Antivirals; Nucleotide reverse transcriptase inhibitors
Brand Names: Viread
Cost of Therapy: $432.00 (HIV; Viread; 300 mg; 1 tablet/day; 30 day supply)

WARNING

LACTIC ACIDOSIS AND SEVERE HEPATOMEGALY WITH STEATOSIS, INCLUDING FATAL CASES, HAVE BEEN REPORTED WITH THE USE OF NUCLEOSIDE ANALOGS ALONE OR IN COMBINATION WITH OTHER ANTIRETROVIRALS (SEE WARNINGS).

DESCRIPTION

Viread is the brand name for tenofovir disoproxil fumarate (a prodrug of tenofovir) which is a fumaric acid salt of *bis*-isopropoxycarbonyloxymethyl ester derivative of tenofovir. *In vivo* tenofovir disoproxil fumarate is converted to tenofovir, an acyclic nucleoside phosphonate (nucleotide) analog of adenosine 5′-monophosphate. Tenofovir exhibits activity against HIV reverse transcriptase.

The chemical name of tenofovir disoproxil fumarate is 9-[(*R*)-2-[[bis[[(isopropoxycarbonyl)oxy]methoxy]phosphinyl]methoxy]propyl]adenine fumarate (1:1). It has a molecular formula of $C_{19}H_{30}N_5O_{10}P \cdot C_4H_4O_4$ and a molecular weight of 635.52.

Tenofovir disoproxil fumarate is a white to off-white crystalline powder with a solubility of 13.4 mg/ml in distilled water at 25°C. It has an octanol/phosphate buffer (pH 6.5) partition coefficient (log_p) of 1.25 at 25°C.

Tenofovir disoproxil fumarate tablets are for oral administration. Each tablet contains 300 mg of tenofovir disoproxil fumarate, which is equivalent to 245 mg of tenofovir disoproxil, and the following inactive ingredients: croscarmellose sodium, lactose monohydrate, magnesium stearate, microcrystalline cellulose, and pregelatinized starch. The tablets are coated with a blue colored film (Opadry II Y-30-10671-A) that is made of FD&C blue no. 2 aluminum lake, hydroxypropyl methylcellulose 2910, lactose monohydrate, titanium dioxide, and triacetin.

In this insert, all dosages are expressed in terms of tenofovir disoproxil fumarate except where otherwise noted.

CLINICAL PHARMACOLOGY

MICROBIOLOGY

Mechanism of Action

Tenofovir disoproxil fumarate is an acyclic nucleoside phosphonate diester analog of adenosine monophosphate. Tenofovir disoproxil fumarate requires initial diester hydrolysis for conversion to tenofovir and subsequent phosphorylations by cellular enzymes to form tenofovir diphosphate. Tenofovir diphosphate inhibits the activity of HIV reverse transcriptase by competing with the natural substrate deoxyadenosine 5′-triphosphate and, after incorporation into DNA, by DNA chain termination. Tenofovir diphosphate is a weak inhibitor of mammalian DNA polymerases α, β, and mitochondrial DNA polymerase γ.

Antiviral Activity In Vitro

The *in vitro* antiviral activity of tenofovir against laboratory and clinical isolates of HIV was assessed in lymphoblastoid cell lines, primary monocyte/macrophage cells and peripheral blood lymphocytes. The IC_{50} (50% inhibitory concentrations) for tenofovir was in the range of 0.04 to 8.5 μM. In drug combination studies of tenofovir with nucleoside and non-nucleoside analog inhibitors of HIV reverse transcriptase, and protease inhibitors, additive to synergistic effects were observed. Most of these drug combinations have not been studied in humans.

In Vitro Resistance

HIV isolates with reduced susceptibility to tenofovir have been selected *in vitro*. These viruses expressed a K65R mutation in reverse transcriptase and showed a 3- to 4-fold reduction in susceptibility to tenofovir.

In Vitro Cross-Resistance

Cross-resistance among certain reverse transcriptase inhibitors has been recognized. The *in vitro* activity of tenofovir against HIV-1 strains with zidovudine-associated reverse transcriptase mutations (M41L, D67N, K70R, L210W, T215Y/F or K219Q/E/N) was evaluated. Zidovudine-associated mutations may also confer reductions in susceptibility to other NRTIs and these mutations have been reported to emerge during combination therapy with stavudine and didanosine. In 20 samples that had multiple zidovudine-associated mutations (mean 3), a mean 3.1-fold increase of the IC_{50} of tenofovir was observed (range 0.8-8.4). The K65R mutation is selected both *in vitro* and in some HIV-infected subjects treated with didanosine, zalcitabine, or abacavir; therefore, some cross-resistance may occur in patients who develop this mutation following treatment with these drugs. Multinucleoside resistant HIV-1 with a T69S double insertion mutation in the reverse transcriptase showed reduced susceptibility to tenofovir.

Genotypic and Phenotypic Analyses of Tenofovir Disoproxil Fumarate in Patients With Previous Antiretroviral Therapy (Studies 902 and 907)

In Vivo Resistance

Post baseline genotyping in Studies 902 and 907 showed that 7 of 237 tenofovir disoproxil fumarate-treated patients' HIV (3%) developed the K65R mutation, a mutation selected by tenofovir disoproxil fumarate and other NRTIs *in vitro*. Among tenofovir disoproxil fumarate-treated patients whose HIV developed NRTI-associated mutations, there was continued HIV RNA suppression through 24 weeks. The rate and extent of tenofovir-associated resistance mutations has not been characterized in antiretroviral naïve patients initiating tenofovir disoproxil fumarate treatment.

Phenotypic analyses of HIV isolates after 48 weeks (Study 902, n=30) or 24 weeks (Study 907, n=35) of tenofovir disoproxil fumarate therapy showed no significant changes in tenofovir disoproxil fumarate susceptibility unless the K65R mutation had developed.

PHARMACOKINETICS

The pharmacokinetics of tenofovir disoproxil fumarate have been evaluated in healthy volunteers and HIV-infected individuals. Tenofovir pharmacokinetics are similar between these populations.

Absorption

Tenofovir disoproxil fumarate is a water soluble diester prodrug of the active ingredient tenofovir. The oral bioavailability of tenofovir from tenofovir disoproxil fumarate in fasted patients is approximately 25%. Following oral administration of a single dose of tenofovir disoproxil fumarate 300 mg to HIV-infected patients in the fasted state, maximum serum concentrations (C_{max}) are achieved in 1.0 ± 0.4 hours. C_{max} and AUC values are 296 ± 90 ng/ml and 2287 ± 685 ng·h/ml, respectively.

The pharmacokinetics of tenofovir are dose proportional over a tenofovir disoproxil fumarate dose range of 75-600 mg and are not affected by repeated dosing.

Effects of Food on Oral Absorption

Administration of tenofovir disoproxil fumarate following a high-fat meal (~700 to 1000 kcal containing 40-50% fat) increases the oral bioavailability, with an increase in tenofovir AUC(0-∞) of approximately 40% and an increase in C_{max} of approximately 14%. Food delays the time to tenofovir C_{max} by approximately 1 hour. C_{max} and AUC of tenofovir are 326 ± 119 ng/ml and 3324 ± 1370 ng·h/ml following multiple doses of tenofovir disoproxil fumarate 300 mg once daily in the fed state. Tenofovir disoproxil fumarate should be taken with a meal to enhance the bioavailability of tenofovir.

Distribution

In vitro binding of tenofovir to human plasma or serum proteins is less than 0.7 and 7.2%, respectively, over the tenofovir concentration range 0.01 to 25 μg/ml. The volume of distribution at steady-state is 1.3 ± 0.6 L/kg and 1.2 ± 0.4 L/kg, following intravenous administration of tenofovir 1.0 and 3.0 mg/kg.

Metabolism and Elimination

In vitro studies indicate that neither tenofovir disoproxil nor tenofovir are substrates of CYP450 enzymes.

Following IV administration of tenofovir, approximately 70-80% of the dose is recovered in the urine as unchanged tenofovir within 72 hours of dosing. After multiple oral doses of tenofovir disoproxil fumarate 300 mg once daily (under fed conditions), 32 ± 10% of the administered dose is recovered in urine over 24 hours.

Tenofovir is eliminated by a combination of glomerular filtration and active tubular secretion. There may be competition for elimination with other compounds that are also renally eliminated.

Special Populations

There were insufficient numbers from racial and ethnic groups other than Caucasian to adequately determine potential pharmacokinetic differences among these populations.

Tenofovir pharmacokinetics are similar in male and female patients.

Pharmacokinetic studies have not been performed in children or in the elderly.

The pharmacokinetics of tenofovir have not been studied in patients with hepatic impairment; however, tenofovir and tenofovir disoproxil are not metabolized by liver enzymes, so the impact of liver impairment should be limited. (See PRECAUTIONS, Hepatic Impairment.)

The pharmacokinetics of tenofovir have not been evaluated in patients with renal impairment (creatinine clearance <60 ml/min). Because tenofovir is primarily renally eliminated, tenofovir pharmacokinetics are likely to be affected by renal impairment. (See WARNINGS, Renal Impairment.)

Drug Interactions

At concentrations substantially higher (~300-fold) than those observed *in vivo*, tenofovir did not inhibit *in vitro* drug metabolism mediated by any of the following human CYP450 isoforms: CYP3A4, CYP2D6, CYP2C9 or CYP2E1. However, a small (6%) but statistically significant reduction in metabolism of CYP1A substrate was observed. Based on the results of *in vitro* experiments and the known elimination pathway of tenofovir, the potential for CYP450 mediated interactions involving tenofovir with other medicinal products is low. (See Pharmacokinetics.)

Tenofovir is primarily excreted by the kidneys by a combination of glomerular filtration and active tubular secretion. Co-administration of tenofovir disoproxil fumarate with drugs that are eliminated by active tubular secretion may increase serum concentrations of either tenofovir or the co-administered drug, due to competition for this elimination pathway. Drugs that decrease renal function may also increase serum concentrations of tenofovir.

Tenofovir disoproxil fumarate has been evaluated in healthy volunteers in combination with didanosine, lamivudine, indinavir, efavirenz, and lopinavir/ritonavir. TABLE 1 and TABLE 2 summarize pharmacokinetic effects of co-administered drug on tenofovir pharmacokinetics and effects of tenofovir on the pharmacokinetics of co-administered drug.

INDICATIONS AND USAGE

Tenofovir disoproxil fumarate is indicated in combination with other antiretroviral agents for the treatment of HIV-1 infection. This indication is based on analyses of plasma HIV-1 RNA levels and CD4 cell counts in a controlled study of tenofovir disoproxil fumarate of 24 weeks duration and in a controlled, dose ranging study of tenofovir disoproxil fumarate of 48 weeks duration. Both studies were conducted in treatment experienced adults with evidence of HIV-1 viral replication despite ongoing antiretroviral therapy. Studies in antiret-

T

TABLE 1 *Changes in Pharmacokinetic Parameters for Tenofovir* in the Presence of the Co-Administered Drug*

Co-Administered Drug	Dose of Co-Administered Drug (mg)		% Change of Tenofovir Pharmacokinetic Parameters (90% CI) C_{max}	AUC	C_{min}
Lamivudine	150 twice daily × 7 days	n=15	No effect	No effect	No effect
Didanosine†	250 or 400 once daily × 7 days	n=14	No effect	No effect	No effect
Indinavir	800 three times daily × 7 days	n=13	Inc. 14 (Dec. 3 to Inc. 33)	No effect	No effect
Lopinavir/ Ritonavir	400/100 twice daily × 14 days	n=21	Inc. 31 (Inc. 12 to Inc. 53)	Inc. 34 (Inc. 25 to Inc. 44)	Inc. 29 (Inc. 11 to Inc. 48)
Efavirenz	600 once daily × 14 days	n=29	No effect	No effect	No effect

* Patients received tenofovir disoproxil fumarate 300 mg once daily.
† Buffered formulation.

TABLE 2 *Changes in Pharmacokinetic Parameters for Co-Administered Drug in the Presence of Tenofovir Disoproxil Fumarate 300 mg Once Daily.*

Co-Administered Drug	Dose of Co-Administered Drug (mg)		% Change of Co-Administered Drug Pharmacokinetic Parameters (90% CI) C_{max}	AUC	C_{min}
Lamivudine	150 twice daily × 7 days	n=15	Dec. 24 (Dec. 34 to Dec. 12)	No effect	No effect
Didanosine*	250 or 400 once daily × 7 days	n=14	Inc. 28 (Inc. 11 to Inc. 48)	Inc. 44 (Inc. 31 to Inc. 59)	—
Indinavir	800 three times daily × 7 days	n=12	Dec. 11 (Dec. 30 to Inc. 12)	No effect	No effect
Lopinavir	Lopinavir/ Ritonavir 400/100 twice daily × 14 days	n=21	Dec. 15 (Dec. 23 to Dec. 6)	Dec. 15 (Dec. 22 to Dec. 7)	No effect
Ritonavir 400/ 100 twice	Lopinavir/ Ritonavir daily × 14 days	n=21	Dec. 28 (Dec. 43 to Dec. 9)	Dec. 24 (Dec. 33 to Dec. 13)	Inc. 7 (Dec. 22 to Inc. 37)
Efavirenz	600 once daily × 14 days	n=30	No effect	No effect	No effect

* Buffered formulation. (See PRECAUTIONS.)

roviral naïve patients are ongoing; consequently, the risk-benefit ratio for this population has yet to be determined.

Additional important information regarding the use of tenofovir disoproxil fumarate for the treatment of HIV infection:

There are no study results demonstrating the effect of tenofovir disoproxil fumarate on clinical progression of HIV.

The use of tenofovir disoproxil fumarate should be considered for treating adult patients with HIV strains that are expected to be susceptible to tenofovir as assessed by laboratory testing or treatment history.

CONTRAINDICATIONS

Tenofovir disoproxil fumarate is contraindicated in patients with previously demonstrated hypersensitivity to any of the components of the product.

WARNINGS

LACTIC ACIDOSIS/SEVERE HEPATOMEGALY WITH STEATOSIS

Lactic acidosis and severe hepatomegaly with steatosis, including fatal cases, have been reported with the use of nucleoside analogs alone or in combination with other antiretrovirals. A majority of these cases have been in women. Obesity and prolonged nucleoside exposure may be risk factors. Particular caution should be exercised when administering nucleoside analogs to any patient with known risk factors for liver disease; however, cases have also been reported in patients with no known risk factors. Treatment with tenofovir disoproxil fumarate should be suspended in any patient who develops clinical or laboratory findings suggestive of lactic acidosis or pronounced hepatotoxicity (which may include hepatomegaly and steatosis even in the absence of marked transaminase elevations).

RENAL IMPAIRMENT

Tenofovir is principally eliminated by the kidney. Tenofovir disoproxil fumarate should not be administered to patients with renal insufficiency (creatinine clearance <60 ml/min) until data become available describing the disposition of tenofovir disoproxil fumarate in these patients.

PRECAUTIONS

HEPATIC IMPAIRMENT

The pharmacokinetics of tenofovir have not been studied in patients with hepatic impairment. As tenofovir and tenofovir disoproxil are not metabolized by liver enzymes, the impact of liver impairment should be limited. However, because tenofovir is not entirely renally excreted (70-80%), tenofovir pharmacokinetics may be altered in patients with hepatic insufficiency.

FAT REDISTRIBUTION

Redistribution/accumulation of body fat including central obesity, dorsocervical fat enlargement (buffalo hump), peripheral wasting, facial wasting, breast enlargement, and "cushingoid appearance" have been observed in patients receiving antiretroviral therapy. The mechanism and long-term consequences of these events are currently unknown. A causal relationship has not been established.

CLINICAL MONITORING FOR BONE AND RENAL TOXICITY

It is not known if long term administration of tenofovir disoproxil fumarate (>1 year) will cause bone abnormalities. Therefore if bone abnormalities are suspected then appropriate consultation should be obtained.

Although tenofovir-associated renal toxicity has not been observed in pooled clinical studies for up to 1 year, long term renal effects are unknown. Consideration should be given to monitoring for changes in serum creatinine and serum phosphorus in patients at risk or with a history of renal dysfunction.

CARCINOGENESIS, MUTAGENESIS, AND IMPAIRMENT OF FERTILITY

Long-term carcinogenicity studies of tenofovir disoproxil fumarate in rats and mice are in progress.

Tenofovir disoproxil fumarate was mutagenic in the *in vitro* mouse lymphoma assay and negative in an *in vitro* bacterial mutagenicity test (Ames test). In an *in vivo* mouse micronucleus assay, tenofovir disoproxil fumarate was negative at doses up to 2000 mg/kg when administered to male mice.

There were no effects on fertility, mating performance or early embryonic development when tenofovir disoproxil fumarate was administered at 600 mg/kg/day to male rats for 28 days prior to mating and to female rats for 15 days prior to mating through day 7 of gestation. There was, however, an alteration of the estrous cycle in female rats. A dose of 600 mg/kg/day is equivalent to 10 times the human dose based on body surface area comparisons.

PREGNANCY CATEGORY B

Reproduction studies have been performed in rats and rabbits at doses up to 14 and 19 times the human dose based on body surface area comparisons and revealed no evidence of impaired fertility or harm to the fetus due to tenofovir. There are, however, no adequate and well-controlled studies in pregnant women. Because animal reproduction studies are not always predictive of human response, tenofovir disoproxil fumarate should be used during pregnancy only if clearly needed.

Antiretroviral Pregnancy Registry: To monitor fetal outcomes of pregnant women exposed to tenofovir disoproxil fumarate, an Antiretroviral Pregnancy Registry has been established. Healthcare providers are encouraged to register patients by calling 1-800-258-4263.

NURSING MOTHERS

The Centers for Disease Control and Prevention recommend that HIV-infected mothers not breast-feed their infants to avoid risking postnatal transmission of HIV. Studies in rats have demonstrated that tenofovir is secreted in milk. It is not known whether tenofovir is excreted in human milk. Because of both the potential for HIV transmission and the potential for serious adverse reactions in nursing infants, **mothers should be instructed not to breast-feed if they are receiving tenofovir disoproxil fumarate.**

PEDIATRIC USE

Safety and effectiveness in pediatric patients have not been established.

GERIATRIC USE

Clinical studies of tenofovir disoproxil fumarate did not include sufficient numbers of subjects aged 65 and over to determine whether they respond differently from younger subjects. In general, dose selection for the elderly patient should be cautious, keeping in mind the greater frequency of decreased hepatic, renal, or cardiac function, and of concomitant disease or other drug therapy.

DRUG INTERACTIONS

When administered with tenofovir disoproxil fumarate, C_{max} and AUC of didanosine (administered as the buffered formulation) increased by 28% and 44%, respectively. The mechanism for this interaction is unknown. Although an increased rate of didanosine-associated adverse events has not been observed in pooled clinical studies at this time, long term effects are unknown. Patients taking tenofovir disoproxil fumarate and didanosine concomitantly should be monitored for long term didanosine-associated adverse events. (See CLINICAL PHARMACOLOGY, Pharmacokinetics, Drug Interactions and DOSAGE AND ADMINISTRATION.)

Since tenofovir is primarily eliminated by the kidneys, co-administration of tenofovir disoproxil fumarate with drugs that reduce renal function or compete for active tubular secretion may increase serum concentrations of tenofovir and/or increase the concentrations of other renally eliminated drugs. Some examples include, but are not limited to, cidofovir, acyclovir, valacyclovir, ganciclovir and valganciclovir.

ADVERSE REACTIONS

More than 1000 patients have been treated with tenofovir disoproxil fumarate alone or in combination with other antiretroviral medicinal products for periods of 28 days to 143 weeks in Phase 1-3 clinical trials and a compassionate access study.

Assessment of adverse reactions is based on two studies (902 and 907) in which 653 treatment experienced patients received double-blind treatment with tenofovir disoproxil fumarate 300 mg (n=443) or placebo (n=210) for 24 weeks followed by extended treatment with tenofovir disoproxil fumarate.

TREATMENT-RELATED ADVERSE EVENTS

The most common adverse events that occurred in patients receiving tenofovir disoproxil fumarate with other antiretroviral agents in clinical trials were mild to moderate gastrointestinal events, such as nausea, diarrhea, vomiting and flatulence. Less than 1% of patients discontinued participation in the clinical studies due to gastrointestinal adverse events.

A summary of treatment related adverse events is provided in TABLE 6.

TABLE 6 *Treatment-Related Adverse Events (Grades 1-4) Reported in ≥3% of Tenofovir Disoproxil Fumarate-Treated Patients in the Pooled 902-907 Studies (0-24 weeks)*

	Tenofovir Disoproxil Fumarate 300 mg n=443	Placebo n=210
Nausea	11%	10%
Diarrhea	9%	8%
Asthenia	8%	8%
Headache	6%	7%
Vomiting	5%	2%
Flatulence	4%	0%
Abdominal pain	3%	3%
Anorexia	3%	1%

LABORATORY ABNORMALITIES

Laboratory abnormalities observed in these studies occurred with similar frequency in the tenofovir disoproxil fumarate and placebo treated groups. A summary of Grade 3 and 4 laboratory abnormalities is provided in TABLE 7.

TABLE 7 *Grade 3/4 Laboratory Abnormalities Reported in ≥1% of Tenofovir Disoproxil Fumarate-Treated Patients in the Pooled 902-907 Studies (0-24 weeks)*

	Tenofovir Disoproxil Fumarate 300 mg n=443	Placebo n=210
Number of Patients with Grade 3 or 4 Laboratory Abnormalities	117 (26%)	78 (37%)
Laboratory Abnormalities		
Triglyceride (>750 mg/dl)	37 (8%)	28 (13%)
Creatine kinase (>782 U/L)	53 (12%)	38 (18%)
Serum amylase (>175 U/L)	21 (5%)	14 (7%)
AST (M; >180 U/L) (F: >170 U/L)	16 (4%)	6 (3%)
Urine glucose (3+ or 4+)	12 (3%)	6 (3%)
ALT elevation (M: >215 U/L) (F: >170 U/L)	10 (2%)	4 (2%)
Serum glucose (>250 mg/dl)	8 (2%)	8 (4%)
Neutrophil (<650/mm^3)	6 (1%)	3 (1%)

DOSAGE AND ADMINISTRATION

The dose of tenofovir disoproxil fumarate is 300 mg once daily taken orally with a meal.

Concomitant Administration: Didanosine. When administered with didanosine, tenofovir disoproxil fumarate should be administered 2 hours before or 1 hour after administration of didanosine (see DRUG INTERACTIONS).

ANIMAL PHARMACOLOGY

Tenofovir and tenofovir disoproxil fumarate administered in toxicology studies to rats, dogs and monkeys at exposures (based on AUCs) between 6- and 12-fold those observed in humans caused bone toxicity. In monkeys the bone toxicity was diagnosed as osteomalacia. Osteomalacia observed in monkeys appeared to be reversible upon dose reduction or discontinuation of tenofovir. In rats and dogs, the bone toxicity manifested as reduced bone mineral density. The mechanism(s) underlying bone toxicity is unknown.

Evidence of renal toxicity was noted in 4 animal species. Increases in serum creatinine, BUN, glycosuria, proteinuria, phosphaturia and/or calciuria and decreases in serum phosphate were observed to varying degrees in these animals. These toxicities were noted at exposures (based on AUCs) 2-20 times higher than those observed in humans. The relationship of the renal abnormalities, particularly the phosphaturia, to the bone toxicity is not known.

HOW SUPPLIED

Viread is available as tablets. Each tablet contains 300 mg of tenofovir disoproxil fumarate, which is equivalent to 245 mg of tenofovir disoproxil. The tablets are almond-shaped, light blue film-coated, and debossed with "GILEAD" and "4331" on one side and with "300" on the other side.

Storage: Store at 25°C (77°F), excursions permitted to 15-30°C (59-86°F).

PRODUCT LISTING - EQUIVALENTS NOT AVAILABLE

Tablet - Oral - 300 mg

30's $432.00 VIREAD, Gilead Sciences 61958-0401-01

T

Terazosin Hydrochloride (002311)

Categories: Hyperplasia, benign prostatic; Hypertension, essential; Pregnancy Category C; FDA Approved 1987 Aug
Drug Classes: Antiadrenergics, alpha blocking; Antiadrenergics, peripheral
Brand Names: Hytrin
Foreign Brand Availability: Adecur (Mexico); Conmy (Taiwan); Deflox (Spain); Dysalfa (France); Flotrin (Germany); Heitrin (Germany); Hitrin (Costa-Rica; El-Salvador; Guatemala; Honduras; Nicaragua; Panama); Hydrin (Korea); Hytracin (Japan); Hytrine (France; Korea); Hytrinex (Denmark; Sweden); Itrin (Italy); Kinzosin (Taiwan); Magnurol (Spain); Olyster (India); Teradrin (Taiwan); Teralfa (India); Terapam (Korea); Terasin (Korea); Tructum (Colombia); Vasomet (Japan); Vicard (Austria; Switzerland)
Cost of Therapy: $63.52 (Benign Prostatic Hyperplasia; Hytrin; 2 mg; 1 capsule/day; 30 day supply)
$47.63 (Benign Prostatic Hyperplasia; Generic Capsules; 2 mg; 1 capsule/day; 30 day supply)
$63.52 (Hypertension; Hytrin; 5 mg; 1 capsule/day; 30 day supply)
$48.09 (Hypertension; Generic Capsules; 5 mg; 1 capsule/day; 30 day supply)

DESCRIPTION

Terazosin hydrochloride, an alpha-1-selective adrenoceptor blocking agent, is a quinazoline derivative represented by the following chemical name: (RS)-piperazine, 1-(4-amino-6,7-dimethoxy-2-quinazolinyl)-4-[(tetra-hydro-2-furanyl)carbonyl]-, monohydrochloride, dihydrate. Its molecular formula is $C_{19}H_{25}N_5O_4$·HCl.

Terazosin hydrochloride is a white, crystalline substance freely soluble in water and isotonic saline. It has a molecular weight of 459.93.

HYTRIN CAPSULES

Hytrin capsules for oral administration contain 1, 2, 5, or 10 mg of terazosin hydrochloride.

Inactive Ingredients

1 mg Capsules: Gelatin, glycerin, iron oxide, methylparaben, mineral oil, polyethylene glycol, povidone, propylparaben, titanium dioxide, and vanillin. *2 mg Capsules:* D&C yellow no. 10, gelatin, glycerin, methylparaben, mineral oil, polyethylene glycol, povidone, propylparaben, titanium dioxide, and vanillin. *5 mg Capsules:* D&C red no. 28, FD&C red no. 40, gelatin, glycerin, methylparaben, mineral oil, polyethylene glycol, povidone, propylparaben, titanium dioxide, and vanillin. *10 mg Capsules:* FD&C blue no. 1, gelatin, glycerin, methylparaben, mineral oil, polyethylene glycol, povidone, propylparaben, titanium dioxide, and vanillin.

CLINICAL PHARMACOLOGY

PHARMACODYNAMICS

Benign Prostatic Hyperplasia (BPH)

The symptoms associated with BPH are related to bladder outlet obstruction, which is comprised of two underlying components: a static component and a dynamic component. The static component is a consequence of an increase in prostate size. Over time, the prostate will continue to enlarge. However, clinical studies have demonstrated that the size of the prostate does not correlate with the severity of BPH symptoms or the degree of urinary obstruction. The dynamic component is a function of an increase in smooth muscle tone in the prostate and bladder neck, leading to constriction of the bladder outlet. Smooth muscle tone is mediated by sympathetic nervous stimulation of alpha-1 adrenoceptors, which are abundant in the prostate, prostatic capsule, and bladder neck. The reduction in symptoms and improvement in urine flow rates following administration of terazosin is related to relaxation of smooth muscle produced by blockade of alpha-1 adrenoceptors in the bladder neck and prostate. Because there are relatively few alpha-1 adrenoceptors in the bladder body, terazosin is able to reduce the bladder outlet obstruction without affecting bladder contractility.

Terazosin has been studied in 1222 men with symptomatic BPH. In three placebo-controlled studies, symptom evaluation and uroflowmetric measurements were performed approximately 24 hours following dosing. Symptoms were quantified using the Boyarsky Index. The questionnaire evaluated both obstructive (hesitancy, intermittently, terminal dribbling, impairment of size and force of stream, sensation of incomplete bladder emptying) and irritative (nocturia, daytime frequency, urgency, dysuria) symptoms by rating each of the 9 symptoms from 0-3, for a total score of 27 points. Results from these studies indicated that terazosin statistically significantly improved symptoms and peak urine flow rates over placebo as illustrated in TABLE 1.

TABLE 1

	Symptom Score (Range 0-27)			Peak Flow Rate (ml/sec)		
	n	Mean Baseline	Mean Change (%)	n	Mean Baseline	Mean Change (%)
Study 1 (10 mg)*						
Titration to Fixed Dose (12 wk)						
Placebo	55	9.7	-2.3 (24)	54	10.1	+1.0 (10)
Terazosin	54	10.1	-4.5 (45)†	52	8.8	+3.0 (34)†
Study 2 (2, 5, 10, 20 mg)‡						
Titration to Response (24 wk)						
Placebo	89	12.5	-3.8 (30)	88	8.8	+1.4 (16)
Terazosin	85	12.2	-5.3 (43)†	84	8.4	+2.9 (35)†
Study 3 (1, 2, 5, 10 mg)§						
Titration to Response (24 wk)						
Placebo	74	10.4	-1.1 (11)	74	8.8	+1.2 (14)
Terazosin	73	10.9	-4.6 (42)†	73	8.6	+2.6 (30)†

* Highest dose 10 mg shown.
† Significantly (p ≤0.05) more improvement than placebo.
‡ 23% of patients on 10 mg, 41% of patients on 20 mg.
§ 67% of patients on 10 mg.

In all three studies, both symptom scores and peak urine flow rates showed statistically significant improvement from baseline in patients treated with terazosin from week 2 (or the first clinic visit) and throughout the study duration.

Analysis of the effect of terazosin on individual urinary symptoms demonstrated that, compared to placebo, terazosin significantly improved the symptoms of hesitancy, intermittence, impairment in size and force of urinary stream, sensation of incomplete emptying, terminal dribbling, daytime frequency, and nocturia.

Global assessments of overall urinary function and symptoms were also performed by investigators who were blinded to patient treatment assignment. In studies 1 and 3, patients treated with terazosin had a significantly ($p \leq 0.001$) greater overall improvement compared to placebo-treated patients.

In a short-term study (Study 1), patients were randomized to either 2, 5 or 10 mg of terazosin or placebo. Patients randomized to the 10 mg group achieved a statistically significant response in both symptoms and peak flow rate compared to placebo.

In a long-term, open-label, non-placebo-controlled clinical trial, 181 men were followed for 2 years, and 58 of these men were followed for 30 months. The effect of terazosin on urinary symptom scores and peak flow rates was maintained throughout the study duration.

In this long-term trial, both symptom scores and peak urinary flow rates showed statistically significant improvement suggesting a relaxation of smooth muscle cells.

Although blockade of alpha-1 adrenoceptors also lowers blood pressure in hypertensive patients with increased peripheral vascular resistance, terazosin treatment of normotensive men with BPH did not result in a clinically significant blood pressure lowering effect (TABLE 2).

***TABLE 2** Mean Changes in Blood Pressure From Baseline to Final Visit in All Double-Blind, Placebo-Controlled Studies*

		Normotensive Patients DBP ≤90 mm Hg		Hypertensive Patients DBP >90 mm Hg	
	Group	n	Mean Change	n	Mean Change
SBP (mm Hg)	Placebo	293	-0.1	45	-5.8
	Terazosin	519	-3.3*	65	-14.4*
DBP (mm Hg)	Placebo	293	+0.4	45	-7.1
	Terazosin	519	-2.2*	65	-15.1*

* $p \leq 0.05$ vs placebo

Hypertension

In animals, terazosin causes a decrease in blood pressure by decreasing total peripheral vascular resistance. The vasodilatory hypotensive action of terazosin appears to be produced mainly by blockade of alpha-1-adrenoceptors. Terazosin decreases blood pressure gradually within 15 minutes following oral administration.

Patients in clinical trials of terazosin were administered once daily (the great majority) and twice daily regimens with total doses usually in the range of 5-20 mg/day, and had mild (about 77%, diastolic pressure 95-105 mm Hg) or moderate (23%, diastolic pressure 105-115 mm Hg) hypertension. Because terazosin, like all alpha antagonists, can cause unusually large falls in blood pressure after the first dose or first few doses, the initial dose was 1 mg in virtually all trials, with subsequent titration to a specified fixed dose or titration to some specified blood pressure end point (usually a supine diastolic pressure of 90 mm Hg).

Blood pressure responses were measured at the end of the dosing interval (usually 24 hours) and effects were shown to persist throughout the interval, with the usual supine responses 5-10 mm Hg systolic and 3.5-8 mm Hg diastolic greater than placebo. The responses in the standing position tended to be somewhat larger, by 1-3 mm Hg, although this was not true in all studies. The magnitude of the blood pressure responses was similar to prazosin and less than hydrochlorothiazide (in a single study of hypertensive patients). In measurements 24 hours after dosing, heart rate was unchanged.

Limited measurements of peak response (2-3 hours after dosing) during chronic terazosin administration indicate that it is greater than about twice the trough (24 hour) response, suggesting some attenuation of response at 24 hours, presumably due to a fall in blood terazosin concentrations at the end of the dose interval. The explanation is not established with certainty, however, and is not consistent with the similarity of blood pressure response to once daily and twice daily dosing and with the absence of an observed dose-response relationship over a range of 5-20 mg, *i.e.,* if blood concentrations had fallen to the point of providing less than full effect at 24 hours, a shorter dosing interval or larger dose should have led to increased response.

Further dose response and dose duration studies are being carried out. Blood pressure should be measured at the end of the dose interval; if response is not satisfactory, patients may be tried on a larger dose or twice daily dosing regimen. The latter should also be considered if possible blood pressure-related side effects such as dizziness, palpitations, or orthostatic complaints are seen within a few hours after dosing.

The greater blood pressure effect associated with peak plasma concentrations (first few hours after dosing) appears somewhat more position-dependent (greater in the erect position) than the effect of terazosin at 24 hours and in the erect position. There is also a 6-10 beat per minute increase in heart rate in the first few hours after dosing. During the first 3 hours after dosing 12.5% of patients had a systolic pressure fall of 30 mm Hg or more from supine to standing, or standing systolic pressure below 90 mm Hg with a fall of at least 20 mm Hg compared to 4% of a placebo group.

There was a tendency for patients to gain weight during terazosin therapy. In placebo-controlled monotherapy trials, male and female patients receiving terazosin gained a mean of 1.7 and 2.2 pounds respectively, compared to losses of 0.2 and 1.2 pounds respectively in the placebo group. Both differences were statistically significant.

During controlled clinical trials, patients receiving terazosin monotherapy had a small, but statistically significant, decrease (a 3% fall) compared to placebo in total cholesterol and the combined low-density and very-low-density lipoprotein fractions. No significant changes were observed in high-density lipoprotein fraction and triglycerides compared to placebo.

Analysis of clinical laboratory data following administration of terazosin suggested the possibility of hemodilution based on decreases in hematocrit, hemoglobin, white blood cells, total protein and albumin. Decreases in hematocrit and total protein have been observed with alpha-blockade and are attributed to hemodilution.

PHARMACOKINETICS

Terazosin hydrochloride capsules are essentially completely absorbed in man. Administration of capsules immediately after meals had a minimal effect on the extent of absorption. The time to reach peak plasma concentration, however, was delayed by about 40 minutes. Terazosin has been shown to undergo minimal hepatic first-pass metabolism, and nearly all of the circulating dose is in the form of parent drug. The plasma levels peak about 1 hour after dosing and then decline with a half-life of approximately 12 hours. In a study that evaluated the effect of age on terazosin pharmacokinetics, the mean plasma half-lives were 14 and 11.4 hours for the age group ≥70 years and the age group of 20-39 years, respectively. After oral administration the plasma clearance was decreased by 31.7% in patients 70 years of age or older compared to that in patients 20-39 years of age.

The drug is 90-94% bound to plasma proteins, and binding is constant over the clinically observed concentration range. Approximately 10% of an orally administered dose is excreted as parent drug in the urine, and approximately 20% is excreted in the feces. The remainder is eliminated as metabolites. Impaired renal function had no significant effect on the elimination of terazosin, and dosage adjustment of terazosin to compensate for the drug removal during hemodialysis (approximately 10%) does not appear to be necessary. Overall, approximately 40% of the administered dose is excreted in the urine and approximately 60% in the feces. The disposition of the compound in animals is qualitatively similar to that in man.

INDICATIONS AND USAGE

Terazosin hydrochloride is indicated for the treatment of symptomatic benign prostatic hyperplasia (BPH). There is rapid response, with approximately 70% of patients experiencing an increase in urinary flow and improvement in symptoms of BPH when treated with terazosin hydrochloride. The long-term effects of terazosin hydrochloride on the incidence of surgery, acute urinary obstruction, or other complications of BPH are yet to be determined.

Terazosin hydrochloride is also indicated for the treatment of hypertension. It can be used alone or in combination with other antihypertensive agents such as diuretics or beta-adrenergic blocking agents.

CONTRAINDICATIONS

Terazosin hydrochloride capsules are contraindicated in patients known to be hypersensitive to terazosin hydrochloride.

WARNINGS

SYNCOPE AND "FIRST-DOSE" EFFECT

Terazosin hydrochloride capsules, like other alpha-adrenergic blocking agents, can cause marked lowering of blood pressure, especially postural hypotension, and syncope in association with the first dose or first few days of therapy. A similar effect can be anticipated if therapy is interrupted for several days and then restarted. Syncope has also been reported with other alpha-adrenergic blocking agents in association with rapid dosage increases or the introduction of another antihypertensive drug. Syncope is believed to be due to an excessive postural hypotensive effect, although occasionally the syncopal episode has been preceded by a bout of severe supraventricular tachycardia, with heart rates of 120-160 beats per minute. Additionally, the possibility of the contribution of hemodilution to the symptoms of postural hypotension should be considered.

To decrease the likelihood of syncope or excessive hypotension, treatment should always be initiated with a 1-mg dose of terazosin, given at bedtime. The 2, 5, and 10 mg capsules are not indicated as initial therapy. Dosage should then be increased slowly, according to recommendations (see DOSAGE AND ADMINISTRATION), and additional antihypertensive agents should be added with caution. The patient should be cautioned to avoid situations, such as driving or hazardous tasks, where injury could result should syncope occur during initiation of therapy.

In early investigational studies, where increasing single doses of up to 7.5 mg were given at 3 day intervals, tolerance to the first dose phenomenon did not necessarily develop, and the "first dose" effect could be observed at all doses. Syncopal episodes occurred in 3 of the 14 subjects given terazosin at doses of 2.5, 5, and 7.5 mg, which are higher than the recommended initial dose. In addition, severe orthostatic hypotension (blood pressure falling to 50/0 mm Hg) was seen in 2 others and dizziness, tachycardia, and lightheadedness occurred in most subjects. These adverse effects all occurred within 90 minutes of dosing.

In three placebo-controlled BPH studies 1, 2, and 3 (see CLINICAL PHARMACOLOGY), the incidence of postural hypotension in the terazosin-treated patients was 5.1, 5.2, and 3.7%, respectively.

In multiple-dose clinical trials involving nearly 2000 hypertensive patients treated with terazosin, syncope was reported in about 1% of patients. Syncope was not necessarily associated only with the first dose.

If syncope occurs, the patient should be placed in a recumbent position and treated supportively, as necessary. There is evidence that the orthostatic effect of terazosin is greater, even in chronic use, shortly after dosing. The risk of events is greatest during the initial 7 days of treatment but continues at all time intervals.

PRIAPISM

Rarely (probably less than once in every several thousand patients), terazosin and other α_1-antagonists have been associated with priapism (painful erection, sustained for hours and unrelieved by sexual intercourse or masturbation). Two (2) or 3 dozen cases have been reported. Because this condition can lead to permanent impotence if not promptly treated, patients must be advised about the seriousness of the condition (see PRECAUTIONS, Information for the Patient).

PRECAUTIONS

GENERAL

Prostatic Cancer

Carcinoma of the prostate and BPH cause many of the same symptoms. These two diseases frequently coexist. Therefore, patients thought to have BPH should be examined prior to starting terazosin hydrochloride therapy to rule out the presence of carcinoma of the prostate.

Orthostatic Hypotension

While syncope is the most severe orthostatic effect of terazosin (see WARNINGS), other symptoms of lowered blood pressure such as dizziness, lightheadedness, and palpitations were more common and occurred in some 28% of patients in clinical trials of hypertension. In BPH clinical trials, 21% of the patients experienced one or more of the following: dizziness, hypotension, postural hypotension, syncope, and vertigo. Patients with occupations in which such events represent potential problems should be treated with particular caution.

INFORMATION FOR THE PATIENT

See the prescribing information received with the prescription for further information.)

Patients should be made aware of the possibility of syncopal and orthostatic symptoms, especially at the initiation of therapy, and to avoid driving or hazardous tasks for 12 hours after the first dose, after a dosage increase, and after interruption of therapy when treatment is resumed. They should be cautioned to avoid situations where injury could result should syncope occur during initiation of terazosin therapy. They should also be advised of the need to sit or lie down when symptoms of lowered blood pressure occur, although these symptoms are not always orthostatic, and to be careful when rising from a sitting or lying position. If dizziness, lightheadedness, or palpitations are bothersome they should be reported to the physician so that dose adjustment can be considered.

Patients should also be told that drowsiness or somnolence can occur with terazosin, requiring caution in people who must drive or operate heavy machinery.

Patients should be advised about the possibility of priapism as a result of treatment with terazosin and other similar medications. Patients should know that this reaction to terazosin is extremely rare, but that if it is not brought to immediate medical attention, it can lead to permanent erectile dysfunction (impotence).

LABORATORY TESTS

Small but statistically significant decreases in hematocrit, hemoglobin, white blood cells, total protein, and albumin were observed in controlled clinical trials. These laboratory findings suggested the possibility of hemodilution. Treatment with terazosin for up to 24 months had no significant effect on prostate specific antigen (PSA) levels.

CARCINOGENESIS, MUTAGENESIS, AND IMPAIRMENT OF FERTILITY

Terazosin was devoid of mutagenic potential when evaluated *in vivo* and *in vitro* (the Ames test, *in vivo* cytogenetics, the dominant lethal test in mice, *in vivo* Chinese hamster chromosome aberration test, and V79 forward mutation assay).

Terazosin administered in the feed to rats at doses of 8, 40, and 250 mg/kg/day (70, 350, and 2100 mg/m^2/day) for 2 years was associated with a statistically significant increase in benign adrenal medullary tumors of male rats exposed to the 250 mg/kg dose. This dose is 175 times the maximum recommended human dose of 20 mg (12 mg/m^2). Female rats were unaffected. Terazosin was not oncogenic in mice when administered in feed for 2 years at a maximum tolerated dose of 32 mg/kg/day (110 mg/m^2; 9 times the maximum recommended human dose). The absence of mutagenicity in a battery of tests, of tumorigenicity of any cell type in the mouse carcinogenicity assay, of increased total tumor incidence in either species, and of proliferative adrenal lesions in female rats, suggests a male rat species-specific event. Numerous other diverse pharmaceutical and chemical compounds have also been associated with benign adrenal medullary tumors in male rats without supporting evidence for carcinogenicity in man.

The effect of terazosin on fertility was assessed in a standard fertility/reproductive performance study in which male and female rats were administered oral doses of 8, 30, and 120 mg/kg/day. Four (4) of 20 male rats given 30 mg/kg (240 mg/m^2; 20 times the maximum recommended human dose) and 5 of 19 male rats given 120 mg/kg (960 mg/m^2; 80 times the maximum recommended human dose) failed to sire a litter. Testicular weights and morphology were unaffected by treatment. Vaginal smears at 30 and 120 mg/kg/day, however, appeared to contain less sperm than smears from control matings, and good correlation was reported between sperm count and subsequent pregnancy.

Oral administration of terazosin for 1 or 2 years elicited a statistically significant increase in the incidence of testicular atrophy in rats exposed to 40 and 250 mg/kg/day (29 and 175 times the maximum recommended human dose), but not in rats exposed to 8 mg/kg/day (>6 times the maximum recommended human dose). Testicular atrophy was also observed in dogs dosed with 300 mg/kg/day (>500 times the maximum recommended human dose) for 3 months but not after 1 year when dosed with 20 mg/kg/day (38 times the maximum recommended human dose). This lesion has also been seen with prazosin, another selective-alpha-1 blocking agent.

PREGNANCY CATEGORY C

Teratogenic Effects

Terazosin was not teratogenic in either rats or rabbits when administered oral doses of up to 280 and 60 times, respectively, the maximum recommended human dose. Fetal resorptions occurred in rats dosed with 480 mg/kg/day, approximately 280 times the maximum recommended human dose. Increased fetal resorptions, decreased fetal weight, and an increased number of supernumerary ribs were observed in offspring of rabbits dosed with 60 times the maximum recommended human dose. These findings (in both species) were most likely secondary to maternal toxicity. There are no adequate and well-controlled studies in pregnant women, and the safety of terazosin in pregnancy has not been established. Terazosin hydrochloride is not recommended during pregnancy unless the potential benefit justifies the potential risk to the mother and fetus.

Nonteratogenic Effects

In a peri- and postnatal development study in rats, significantly more pups died in the group dosed with 120 mg/kg/day (>75 times the maximum recommended human dose) than in the control group during the 3-week postpartum period.

NURSING MOTHERS

It is not known whether terazosin is excreted in breast milk. Because many drugs are excreted in breast milk, caution should be exercised when terazosin is administered to a nursing woman.

PEDIATRIC USE

Safety and effectiveness in pediatric patients have not been determined.

DRUG INTERACTIONS

In controlled trials, terazosin has been added to diuretics and several beta-adrenergic blockers; no unexpected interactions were observed. Terazosin has also been used in patients on a variety of concomitant therapies; while these were not formal interaction studies, no interactions were observed. Terazosin has been used concomitantly in at least 50 patients on the following drugs or drug classes:

1. Analgesic/antiinflammatory (*e.g.,* acetaminophen, aspirin, codeine, ibuprofen, indomethacin).
2. Antibiotics (*e.g.,* erythromycin, trimethoprim and sulfamethoxazole).
3. Anticholinergic/sympathomimetics (*e.g.,* phenylephrine HCl, phenylpropanolamine HCl, pseudoephedrine HCl).
4. Antigout (*e.g.,* allopurinol).
5. Antihistamines (*e.g.,* chlorpheniramine).
6. Cardiovascular agents (*e.g.,* atenolol, hydrochlorothiazide, methyclothiazide, propranolol).
7. Corticosteroids.
8. Gastrointestinal agents (*e.g.,* antacids).
9. Hypoglycemics.
10. Sedatives and tranquilizers (*e.g.,* diazepam).

USE WITH OTHER DRUGS

In a study (n=24) where terazosin and verapamil were administered concomitantly, terazosin's mean AUC(0-24) increased 11% after the first verapamil dose, and after 3 weeks of verapamil treatment it increased by 24% with associated increases in C_{max} (25%) and C_{min} (32%) means. Terazosin mean T_{max} decreased from 1.3 hours to 0.8 hours after 3 weeks of verapamil treatment. Statistically significant differences were not found in the verapamil level with and without terazosin. In a study (n=6) where terazosin and captopril were administered concomitantly, plasma disposition of captopril was not influenced by concomitant administration of terazosin and terazosin; maximum plasma concentrations increased linearly with dose at steady state after administration of terazosin plus captopril (see DOSAGE AND ADMINISTRATION).

ADVERSE REACTIONS

BENIGN PROSTATIC HYPERPLASIA

The incidence of treatment-emergent adverse events has been ascertained from clinical trials conducted worldwide. All adverse events reported during these trials were recorded as adverse reactions. The incidence rates presented below are based on combined data from 6 placebo-controlled trials involving once-a-day administration of terazosin at doses ranging from 1-20 mg. TABLE 3 summarizes those adverse events reported for patients in these trials when the incidence rate in the terazosin group was at least 1% and was greater than that for the placebo group, or where the reaction is of clinical interest. Asthenia, postural hypertension, dizziness, somnolence, nasal congestion/rhinitis, and impotence were the only events that were significantly ($p \leq 0.05$) more common in patients receiving terazosin than in patients receiving placebo. The incidence of urinary tract infection was significantly lower in the patients receiving terazosin than in patients receiving placebo. An analysis of the incidence rate of hypotensive adverse events (see PRECAUTIONS) adjusted for the length of drug treatment has shown that the risk of the events is greatest during the initial 7 days of treatment but continues at all time intervals (TABLE 3).

Additional adverse events have been reported, but these are, in general, not distinguishable from symptoms that might have occurred in the absence of exposure to terazosin. The safety profile of patients treated in the long-term open-label study was similar to that observed in the controlled studies.

The adverse events were usually transient and mild to moderate in intensity, but sometimes they were serious enough to interrupt treatment. In the placebo-controlled clinical trials, the rates of premature termination due to adverse events were not statistically different between the placebo and terazosin groups. The adverse events that were bothersome, as judged by their being reported as reasons for discontinuation of therapy by at least 0.5% of the terazosin group and being reported more often than in the placebo group, are shown in (TABLE 4).

HYPERTENSION

The prevalence of adverse reactions has been ascertained from clinical trials conducted primarily in the US. All adverse experiences (events) reported during these trials were recorded as adverse reactions. The prevalence rates presented in TABLE 5 are based on combined data from 14 placebo-controlled trials involving once-a-day administration of terazosin as monotherapy or in combination with other antihypertensive agents, at doses ranging from 1-40 mg. TABLE 5 summarizes those adverse experiences reported for patients in these trials where the prevalence rate in the terazosin group was at least 5%, where the prevalence rate for the terazosin group was at least 2% and greater than the prevalence rate for the placebo group, or where the reaction is of particular interest. Asthenia, blurred vision, dizziness, nasal congestion, nausea, peripheral edema, palpitations and somnolence were the only symptoms that were significantly ($p < 0.05$) more common in patients receiving terazosin than in patients receiving placebo. Similar adverse reaction rates were observed in placebo-controlled monotherapy trials.

TABLE 3 *Adverse Reactions During Placebo-Controlled Trials*

Benign Prostatic Hyperplasia

Body System	Terazosin (n=636)	Placebo (n=360)
Body as a Whole		
Asthenia*	7.4%†	3.3%
Flu syndrome	2.4%	1.7%
Headache	4.9%	5.8%
Cardiovascular System		
Hypotension	0.6%	0.6%
Palpitations	0.9%	1.1%
Postural hypotension	3.9%†	0.8%
Syncope	0.6	0.0
Digestive System		
Nausea	1.7%	1.1%
Metabolic and Nutritional Disorders		
Peripheral edema	0.9%	0.3%
Weight gain	0.5%	0.0%
Nervous System		
Dizziness	9.1%†	4.2%
Somnolence	3.6%†	1.9%
Vertigo	1.4%	0.3%
Respiratory System		
Dyspnea	1.7%	0.8%
Nasal congestion/rhinitis	1.9%†	0.0%
Special Senses		
Blurred vision/amblyopia	1.3%	0.6%
Urogenital System		
Impotence	1.6%†	0.6%
Urinary tract infection	1.3%	3.9%†

* Includes weakness, tiredness, lassitude, and fatigue.
† p ≤0.05 comparison between groups.

TABLE 4 *Discontinuation During Placebo-Controlled Trials*

Benign Prostatic Hyperplasia

Body System	Terazosin (n=636)	Placebo (n=360)
Body As A Whole		
Fever	0.5%	0.0%
Headache	1.1%	0.8%
Cardiovascular System		
Postural hypotension	0.5%	0.0%
Syncope	0.5%	0.0%
Digestive System		
Nausea	0.5%	0.3%
Nervous System		
Dizziness	2.0%	1.1%
Vertigo	0.5%	0.0%
Respiratory System		
Dyspnea	0.5%	0.3%
Special Senses		
Blurred vision/amblyopia	0.6%	0.0%
Urogenital System		
Urinary tract infection	0.5%	0.3%

ADDITIONAL ADVERSE REACTIONS

Addition adverse reactions have been reported, but these are, in general, not distinguishable from symptoms that might have occurred in the absence of exposure to terazosin. The following additional adverse reactions were reported by at least 1% of 1987 patients who received terazosin in controlled- or open-, short- or long-term clinical trials or have been reported during marketing experience:

Body as a Whole: Chest pain, facial edema, fever, abdominal pain, neck pain, shoulder pain.
Cardiovascular System: Arrhythmia, vasodilation.
Digestive System: Constipation, diarrhea, dry mouth, dyspepsia, flatulence, vomiting.
Metabolic/Nutritional Disorders: Gout.
Musculoskeletal System: Arthralgia, arthritis, joint disorder, myalgia.
Nervous System: Anxiety, insomnia.
Respiratory System: Bronchitis, cold symptoms, epistaxis, flu symptoms, increased cough, pharyngitis, rhinitis.
Skin and Appendages: Pruritus, rash, sweating.
Special Senses: Abnormal vision, conjunctivitis, tinnitus.
Urogenital System: Urinary frequency, urinary incontinence primarily reported in post-menopausal women, urinary tract infection.

Postmarketing experience indicates that in rare instances patients may develop allergic reactions, including anaphylaxis, following administration of terazosin hydrochloride.

There have been reports of priapism during postmarketing surveillance.

The adverse reactions were usually mild or moderate in intensity but sometimes were serious enough to interrupt treatment. The adverse reactions that were most bothersome, as judged by their being reported as reasons for discontinuation of therapy by at least 0.5% of the terazosin group and being reported more often than in the placebo group, are shown in TABLE 6.

TABLE 5 *Adverse Reactions During Placebo-Controlled Trials*

Hypertension

Body System	Terazosin (n=859)	Placebo (n=506)
Body as a Whole		
Asthenia*	11.3%†	4.3%
Back pain	2.4%	1.2%
Headache	16.2%	15.8%
Cardiovascular System		
Palpitations	4.3%†	1.2%
Postural hypotension	1.3%	0.4%
Tachycardia	1.9%	1.2%
Digestive System		
Nausea	4.4%†	1.4%
Metabolic and Nutritional Disorders		
Edema	0.9%	0.6%
Peripheral edema	5.5%†	2.4%
Weight gain	0.5%	0.2%
Musculoskeletal System		
Pain-extremities	3.5%	3.0%
Nervous System		
Depression	0.3%	0.2%
Dizziness	19.3%†	7.5%
Libido decreased	0.6%	0.2%
Nervousness	2.3%	1.8%
Paresthesia	2.9%	1.4%
Somnolence	5.4%†	2.6%
Respiratory System		
Dyspnea	3.1%	2.4%
Nasal congestion	5.9%†	3.4%
Sinusitis	2.6%	1.4%
Special Senses		
Blurred vision	1.6%†	0.0%
Urogenital System		
Impotence	1.2%	1.4%

* Includes weakness, tiredness, lassitude, and fatigue.
† Statistically significant at p=0.05 level.

TABLE 6 *Discontinuations During Placebo-Controlled Trials*

Hypertension

Body System	Terazosin (n=859)	Placebo (n=506)
Body as a Whole		
Asthenia	1.6%	0.0%
Headache	1.3%	1.0%
Cardiovascular System		
Palpitations	1.4%	0.2%
Postural hypotension	0.5%	0.0%
Syncope	0.5%	0.2%
Tachycardia	0.6%	0.0%
Digestive System		
Nausea	0.8%	0.0%
Metabolic and Nutritional Disorders		
Peripheral edema	0.6%	0.0%
Nervous System		
Dizziness	3.1%	0.4%
Paresthesia	0.8%	0.2%
Somnolence	0.6%	0.2%
Respiratory System		
Dyspnea	0.9%	0.6%
Nasal congestion	0.6%	0.0%
Special Senses		
Blurred vision	0.6%	0.0%

DOSAGE AND ADMINISTRATION

If terazosin HCl administration is discontinued for several days, therapy should be reinstituted using the initial dosing regimen.

BENIGN PROSTATIC HYPERPLASIA

Initial Dose

1 mg at bedtime is the starting dose for all patients, and this dose should not be exceeded as an initial dose. Patients should be closely followed during initial administration in order to minimize the risk of severe hypotensive response.

Subsequent Doses

The dose should be increased in a stepwise fashion to 2, 5, or 10 mg once daily to achieve the desired improvement of symptoms and/or flow rates. Doses of 10 mg once daily are generally required for the clinical response. Therefore, treatment with 10 mg for a minimum of 4-6 weeks may be required to assess whether a beneficial response has been achieved. Some patients may not achieve a clinical response despite appropriate titration. Although some additional patients responded at a 20 mg daily dose, there was an insufficient number of patients studied to draw definitive conclusions about this dose. There are insufficient data to support the use of higher doses for those patients who show inadequate or no response to 20 mg daily. **If terazosin administration is discontinued for several days or longer, therapy should be reinstituted using the initial dosing regimen.**

Use With Other Drugs

Caution should be observed when terazosin HCl is administered concomitantly with other antihypertensive agents, especially the calcium channel blocker verapamil, to avoid the possibility of developing significant hypotension. When using terazosin HCl and other antihypertensive agents concomitantly, dosage reduction and retitration of either agent may be necessary (see PRECAUTIONS).

HYPERTENSION

The dose of terazosin hydrochloride and the dose interval (12-24 hours) should be adjusted according to the patient's individual blood pressure response. The following is a guide to its administration.

Initial Dose

1 mg at bedtime is the starting dose for all patients, and this dose should not be exceeded. This initial dosing regimen should be strictly observed to minimize the potential for severe hypotensive effects.

Subsequent Doses

The dose may be slowly increased to achieve the desired blood pressure response. The usual recommended dose range is 1-5 mg administered once a day; however, some patients may benefit from doses as high as 20 mg/day. Doses over 20 mg do not appear to provide further blood pressure effect and doses over 40 mg have not been studied. Blood pressure should be monitored at the end of the dosing interval to be sure control is maintained throughout the interval. It may also be helpful to measure blood pressure 2-3 hours after dosing to see if the maximum and minimum responses are similar, and to evaluate symptoms such as dizziness or palpitations, which can result from excessive hypotensive response. If response is substantially diminished at 24 hours an increased dose or use of a twice-daily regimen can be considered. **If terazosin administration is discontinued for several days or longer, therapy should be reinstituted using the initial dosing regimen.** In clinical trials, except for the initial dose, the dose was given in the morning.

Use With Other Drugs

See Benign Prostatic Hyperplasia, Use With Other Drugs.

HOW SUPPLIED

Hytrin capsules (terazosin HCl capsules) are available in four dosage strengths:

1 mg: Grey capsules (imprinted with and the Abbo-Code "HH").
2 mg: Yellow capsules (imprinted with and the Abbo-Code "HY").
5 mg: Red capsules (imprinted with and the Abbo-Code "HK").
10 mg: Blue capsules (imprinted with and the Abbo-Code "HN").

Storage: Store at controlled room temperature between 20-25°C (68-77°F). Protect from light and moisture.

PRODUCT LISTING - RATED THERAPEUTICALLY EQUIVALENT

Capsule - Oral - 1 mg

Qty	Price	Product	NDC
7's	$10.80	HYTRIN, Allscripts Pharmaceutical Company	54569-4196-02
30's	$46.30	HYTRIN, Allscripts Pharmaceutical Company	54569-4196-00
30's	$53.12	HYTRIN, Quality Care Pharmaceuticals Inc	60346-0438-30
30's	$57.07	HYTRIN, Pd-Rx Pharmaceuticals	55289-0194-30
30's	$63.09	HYTRIN, Pd-Rx Pharmaceuticals	55289-0353-30
90's	$144.95	GENERIC, Golden State Medical	60429-0707-90
100's	$154.13	FEDERAL UPPER LIMIT, H.C.F.A. F F P	99999-2311-01
100's	$154.34	HYTRIN, Allscripts Pharmaceutical Company	54569-4196-01
100's	$158.78	GENERIC, Major Pharmaceuticals Inc	00904-5482-60
100's	$160.38	GENERIC, Geneva Pharmaceuticals	00781-2051-01
100's	$160.39	GENERIC, Caremark Inc	00339-6533-12
100's	$160.50	GENERIC, Teva Pharmaceuticals Usa	00093-0760-01
100's	$160.50	GENERIC, Mylan Pharmaceuticals Inc	00378-2260-01
100's	$160.56	GENERIC, Mylan Pharmaceuticals Inc	51079-0936-20
100's	$170.69	GENERIC, Ivax Corporation	00172-4336-60
100's	$172.28	GENERIC, Ivax Corporation	00172-4336-10
100's	$211.73	HYTRIN, Abbott Pharmaceutical	00074-3805-13

Capsule - Oral - 2 mg

Qty	Price	Product	NDC
30's	$43.24	HYTRIN, Physicians Total Care	54868-3842-00
30's	$46.30	HYTRIN, Allscripts Pharmaceutical Company	54569-4111-00
30's	$54.17	HYTRIN, Quality Care Pharmaceuticals Inc	60346-0330-30
30's	$56.23	HYTRIN, Pd-Rx Pharmaceuticals	55289-0042-30
90's	$144.95	GENERIC, Golden State Medical	60429-0708-90
100's	$154.13	FEDERAL UPPER LIMIT, H.C.F.A. F F P	99999-2311-02
100's	$158.78	GENERIC, Major Pharmaceuticals Inc	00904-5483-60
100's	$160.38	GENERIC, Geneva Pharmaceuticals	00781-2052-01
100's	$160.39	GENERIC, Caremark Inc	00339-6534-12
100's	$160.50	GENERIC, Teva Pharmaceuticals Usa	00093-0761-01
100's	$160.50	GENERIC, Mylan Pharmaceuticals Inc	00378-2264-01
100's	$160.56	GENERIC, Udl Laboratories Inc	51079-0937-20
100's	$170.69	GENERIC, Ivax Corporation	00172-4337-60
100's	$172.28	GENERIC, Ivax Corporation	00172-4337-10
100's	$211.73	HYTRIN, Abbott Pharmaceutical	00074-3806-13

Capsule - Oral - 5 mg

Qty	Price	Product	NDC
30's	$37.80	HYTRIN, Compumed Pharmaceuticals	00403-4881-60
30's	$45.12	HYTRIN, Physicians Total Care	54868-3662-00
30's	$46.30	HYTRIN, Allscripts Pharmaceutical Company	54569-4062-01
30's	$56.23	HYTRIN, Pd-Rx Pharmaceuticals	55289-0070-30
90's	$144.95	GENERIC, Golden State Medical	60429-0709-90
100's	$117.40	HYTRIN, Compumed Pharmaceuticals	00403-4881-01
100's	$154.13	FEDERAL UPPER LIMIT, H.C.F.A. F F P	99999-2311-03
100's	$154.34	HYTRIN, Allscripts Pharmaceutical Company	54569-4062-00
100's	$160.38	GENERIC, Geneva Pharmaceuticals	00781-2053-01
100's	$160.39	GENERIC, Caremark Inc	00339-6535-12
100's	$160.50	GENERIC, Teva Pharmaceuticals Usa	00093-0762-01
100's	$160.50	GENERIC, Mylan Pharmaceuticals Inc	00378-2268-01
100's	$160.56	GENERIC, Udl Laboratories Inc	51079-0938-20
100's	$170.69	GENERIC, Ivax Corporation	00172-4338-60
100's	$172.28	GENERIC, Ivax Corporation	00172-4338-10
100's	$208.45	HYTRIN, Abbott Pharmaceutical	00074-3807-11
100's	$211.73	HYTRIN, Abbott Pharmaceutical	00074-3807-13

Capsule - Oral - 10 mg

Qty	Price	Product	NDC
30's	$46.30	HYTRIN, Allscripts Pharmaceutical Company	54569-4051-00
30's	$53.12	HYTRIN, Quality Care Pharmaceuticals Inc	60346-0436-30
90's	$144.95	GENERIC, Physicians Total Care	60429-0710-90
100's	$126.99	HYTRIN, Allscripts Pharmaceutical Company	54569-4051-01
100's	$154.13	FEDERAL UPPER LIMIT, H.C.F.A. F F P	99999-2311-04
100's	$160.38	GENERIC, Geneva Pharmaceuticals	00781-2054-01
100's	$160.39	GENERIC, Caremark Inc	00339-6536-12
100's	$160.50	GENERIC, Teva Pharmaceuticals Usa	00093-0763-01
100's	$160.50	GENERIC, Mylan Pharmaceuticals Inc	00378-1570-01
100's	$160.56	GENERIC, Mylan Pharmaceuticals Inc	51079-0939-20
100's	$170.69	GENERIC, Ivax Corporation	00172-4339-60
100's	$211.73	HYTRIN, Abbott Pharmaceutical	00074-3808-13
100's	$216.51	HYTRIN, Abbott Pharmaceutical	00074-3808-11

Tablet - Oral - 1 mg

Qty	Price	Product	NDC
100's	$160.38	GENERIC, Geneva Pharmaceuticals	00781-1551-01

Tablet - Oral - 2 mg

Qty	Price	Product	NDC
100's	$160.38	GENERIC, Geneva Pharmaceuticals	00781-1561-01

Tablet - Oral - 5 mg

Qty	Price	Product	NDC
100's	$160.38	GENERIC, Geneva Pharmaceuticals	00781-1571-01

Tablet - Oral - 10 mg

Qty	Price	Product	NDC
100's	$160.38	GENERIC, Geneva Pharmaceuticals	00781-1541-01

PRODUCT LISTING - EQUIVALENTS NOT AVAILABLE

Capsule - Oral - 1 mg

Qty	Price	Product	NDC
30's	$48.15	GENERIC, Allscripts Pharmaceutical Company	54569-4873-00
100's	$224.74	HYTRIN, Abbott Pharmaceutical	00074-3805-11

Capsule - Oral - 2 mg

Qty	Price	Product	NDC
30's	$17.39	GENERIC, Physicians Total Care	54868-4247-00
30's	$48.15	GENERIC, Allscripts Pharmaceutical Company	54569-4874-00
100's	$216.51	HYTRIN, Abbott Pharmaceutical	00074-3806-11

Capsule - Oral - 5 mg

Qty	Price	Product	NDC
30's	$17.39	GENERIC, Physicians Total Care	54868-4248-00
30's	$46.65	GENERIC, Southwood Pharmaceuticals Inc	58016-0673-30
30's	$48.15	GENERIC, Allscripts Pharmaceutical Company	54569-4875-00
60's	$93.30	GENERIC, Southwood Pharmaceuticals Inc	58016-0673-60
90's	$139.95	GENERIC, Southwood Pharmaceuticals Inc	58016-0673-90
100's	$155.50	TERAZOSIN HYDROCHLORIDE, Southwood Pharmaceuticals Inc	58016-0673-00

Capsule - Oral - 10 mg

Qty	Price	Product	NDC
30's	$17.39	GENERIC, Physicians Total Care	54868-4249-22
30's	$48.15	GENERIC, Allscripts Pharmaceutical Company	54569-4876-00

Terbinafine Hydrochloride *(003149)*

For related information, see the comparative table section in Appendix A.

Categories: Tinea corporis; Tinea cruris; Tinea pedis; Tinea unguium; Tinea versicolor; FDA Approved 1992 Dec; Pregnancy Category B
Drug Classes: Antifungals; Antifungals, topical; Dermatologics
Brand Names: Lamisil
Foreign Brand Availability: Labijin (Korea); Lamifen (Philippines); Lamisil Dermgel (New-Zealand); Lespo (Korea); Micosil (Korea); Sulmedin (Taiwan); Terbisil (Singapore); Termisil (Indonesia)
Cost of Therapy: $797.62 (Onychomycosis of Toenail; Lamisil; 250 mg; 1 tablet/day; 84 day supply)
$398.81 (Onychomycosis of Fingernail; Lamisil; 250 mg; 1 tablet/day; 42 day supply)

ORAL

DESCRIPTION

Lamisil tablets contain the synthetic allylamine antifungal compound terbinafine hydrochloride.

Chemically, terbinafine hydrochloride is (E)-*N*-(6,6-dimethyl-2-hepten-4-ynyl)-*N*-methyl-1-naphthalenemethanamine hydrochloride. The empirical formula $C_{21}H_{26}ClN$ with a molecular weight of 327.90.

Terbinafine hydrochloride is a white to off-white fine crystalline powder. It is freely soluble in methanol and methylene chloride, soluble in ethanol, and slightly soluble in water.

Each tablet contains: *Active Ingredients:* Terbinafine hydrochloride (equivalent to 250 mg base). *Inactive Ingredients:* Colloidal silicon dioxide, hydroxypropyl methylcellulose, magnesium stearate, microcrystalline cellulose, sodium starch glycolate.

CLINICAL PHARMACOLOGY

PHARMACOKINETICS

Following oral administration, terbinafine is well absorbed (>70%) and the bioavailability of terbinafine HCl tablets as a result of first-pass metabolism is approximately 40%. Peak plasma concentrations of 1 µg/ml appear within 2 hours after a single 250 mg dose; the AUC (area under the curve) is approximately 4.56 µg·h/ml. An increase in the AUC of terbinafine of less than 20% is observed when terbinafine HCl is administered with food. No clinically relevant age-dependent changes in steady-state plasma concentrations of terbinafine have been reported. In patients with renal impairment (creatinine clearance ≤50 ml/min) or hepatic cirrhosis, the clearance of terbinafine is decreased by approximately 50% compared to

T

normal volunteers. No effect of gender on the blood levels of terbinafine was detected in clinical trials. In plasma, terbinafine is >99% bound to plasma proteins and there are no specific binding sites. At steady-state, in comparison to a single dose, the peak concentration of terbinafine is 25% higher and plasma AUC increases by a factor of 2.5; the increase in plasma AUC is consistent with an effective half-life of ~36 hours. Terbinafine is distributed to the sebum and skin. A terminal half-life of 200-400 hours may represent the slow elimination of terbinafine from tissues such as skin and adipose. Prior to excretion, terbinafine is extensively metabolized. No metabolites have been identified that have antifungal activity similar to terbinafine. Approximately 70% of the administered dose is eliminated in the urine.

MICROBIOLOGY

Terbinafine HCl is a synthetic allylamine derivative. Terbinafine HCl is hypothesized to act by inhibiting squalene epoxidase, thus blocking the biosynthesis of ergosterol, an essential component of fungal cell membranes. *In vitro,* mammalian squalene epoxidase is only inhibited at higher (4000-fold) concentrations than is needed for inhibition of the dermatophyte enzyme. Depending on the concentration of the drug and the fungal species test *in vitro,* terbinafine HCl may be fungicidal. However, the clinical significance of *in vitro* data is unknown.

Terbinafine has been shown to be active against most strains of the following microorganisms both *in vitro* and in clinical infections as described in INDICATIONS AND USAGE:

Trichophyton mentagrophytes
Trichophyton rubrum

The following *in vitro* data are available, but their clinical significance is unknown. *In vitro,* terbinafine exhibits satisfactory MICs against most strains of the following microorganisms; however, the safety and efficacy of terbinafine in treating clinical infections due to these microorganisms have not been established in adequate and well-controlled clinical trials:

Candida albicans
Epidermophyton floccosum
Scopulariopsis brevicaulis

INDICATIONS AND USAGE

Terbinafine HCl tablets are indicated for the treatment of onychomycosis of the toenail or fingernail due to dermatophytes (tinea unguium) (see DOSAGE AND ADMINISTRATION).

Prior to initiating treatment, appropriate nail specimens for laboratory testing (KOH preparation, fungal culture, or nail biopsy) should be obtained to confirm the diagnosis of onychomycosis.

CONTRAINDICATIONS

Terbinafine HCl tablets are contraindicated in individuals with hypersensitivity to terbinafine or to any other ingredients of the formulation.

WARNINGS

Rare cases of liver failure, some leading to death or liver transplant, have occurred with the use of terbinafine HCl tablets for the treatment of onychomycosis in individuals with and without pre-existing liver disease.

In the majority of liver cases reported in association with terbinafine HCl use, the patients had serious underlying systemic conditions and an uncertain causal association with terbinafine HCl. The severity of heptic events and/or their outcome may be worse in patients with active or chronic liver disease (see PRECAUTIONS). Treatment with terbinafine HCl tablets should be discontinued if biochemical or clinical evidence of liver injury develops (see PRECAUTIONS). There have been isolated reports of serious skin reactions (*e.g.,* Stevens-Johnson Syndrome and toxic epidermal necrolysis). If progressive skin rash occurs, treatment with terbinafine HCl should be discontinued.

PRECAUTIONS

GENERAL

Terbinafine HCl is not recommended for patients with chronic or active liver disease. Before prescribing terbinafine HCl tablets, pre-existing liver disease should be assessed. Hepatotoxicity may occur in patients with and without pre-existing liver disease. Pretreatment serum transaminase (ALT and AST) tests are advised for all patients before taking terbinafine HCl tablets. Patients prescribed terbinafine HCl tablets should be warned to report immediately to their physician any symptoms of persistent nausea, anorexia, fatigue, vomiting, right upper abdominal pain or jaundice, dark urine or pale stools (see WARNINGS). Patients with these symptoms should discontinue taking oral terbinafine, and the patient's liver function should be immediately evaluated.

In patients with renal impairment (creatinine clearance ≤50 ml/min), the use of terbinafine HCl has not been adequately studied, and therefore, is not recommended (see CLINICAL PHARMACOLOGY, Pharmacokinetics).

Changes in the ocular lens and retina have been reported following the use of terbinafine HCl tablets in controlled trials. The clinical significance of these changes is unknown.

Transient decreases in absolute lymphocyte counts (ALC) have been observed in controlled clinical trials. In placebo-controlled trials, 8/465 terbinafine HCl-treated patients (1.7%) and 3/137 placebo-treated patients (2.2%) had decreases in ALC to below 1000/mm^3 on two or more occasions. The clinical significance of this observation is unknown. However, in patients with known or suspected immunodeficiency, physicians should consider monitoring complete blood counts in individuals using terbinafine HCl therapy for greater than 6 weeks.

Isolated cases of severe neutropenia have been reported. These were reversible upon discontinuation of terbinafine HCl, with or without supportive therapy. If clinical signs and symptoms suggestive of secondary infection occur, a complete blood count should be obtained. If the neutrophil count is ≤1000 cells/mm^3, terbinafine HCl should be discontinued and supportive management started.

CARCINOGENESIS, MUTAGENESIS, AND IMPAIRMENT OF FERTILITY

In a 28 month oral carcinogenicity study in rats, an increase in the incidence of liver tumors was observed in males at the highest dose tested, 69 mg/kg/day [2× the Maximum Recommended Human Dose (MRHD) based on AUC comparisons of the parent terbinafine]; however, even though dose-limiting toxicity was not achieved at the highest tested dose, higher doses were not tested.

The results of a variety of *in vitro* (mutations in *E. coli* and *S. typhimurium,* DNA repair in rat hepatocytes, mutagenicity in Chinese hamster fibroblasts, chromosome aberration and sister chromatid exchanges in Chinese hamster lung cells), and *in vivo* (chromosome aberration in Chinese hamsters, micronucleus test in mice) genotoxicity tests gave no evidence of a mutagenic or clastogenic potential. Oral reproduction studies in rats at doses up to 300 mg/kg/day (approximately 12× the MRHD based on body surface area comparisons, BSA) did not reveal any specific effects on fertility or other reproductive parameters. Intravaginal application of terbinafine HCl at 150 mg/day in pregnant rabbits did not increase the incidence of abortions or premature deliveries nor affect fetal parameters.

PREGNANCY CATEGORY B

Oral reproduction studies have been performed in rabbits and rats at doses up to 300 mg/kg/day (12× to 23× the MRHD, in rabbits and rats, respectively, based on BSA) and have revealed no evidence of impaired fertility or harm to the fetus due to terbinafine. There are, however, no adequate and well-controlled studies in pregnant women.

Because animal reproduction studies are not always predictive of human response, and because treatment of onychomycosis can be postponed until after pregnancy is completed, it is recommended that terbinafine HCl not be initiated during pregnancy.

NURSING MOTHERS

After oral administration, terbinafine is present in breast milk of nursing mothers. The ratio of terbinafine in milk to plasma is 7:1. Treatment with terbinafine HCl is not recommended in nursing mothers.

PEDIATRIC USE

The safety and efficacy of terbinafine HCl have not been established in pediatric patients.

DRUG INTERACTIONS

In vitro studies with human liver microsomes showed that terbinafine does not inhibit the metabolism of tolbutamide, ethinylestradiol, ethoxycoumarin, and cyclosporine. *In vitro* studies have also shown that terbinafine inhibits CYP2D6-mediated metabolism. This may be of clinical relevance for compounds predominantly metabolized by this enzyme, such as tricyclic antidepressants, β-blockers, selective serotonin reuptake inhibitors (SSRIs), and monoamine oxidase inhibitors (MAO-Is) Type B, if they have a narrow therapeutic window.

In vivo drug-drug interaction studies conducted in normal volunteer subjects showed that terbinafine does not affect the clearance of antipyrine, digoxin, and the antihistamine terfenadine. Terbinafine decreases the clearance of intravenously administered caffeine by 19%. Terbinafine increases the clearance of cyclosporine by 15%.

There have been spontaneous reports of increase or decrease in prothrombin times in patients concomitantly taking oral terbinafine and warfarin, however, a causal relationship between terbinafine HCl tablets and these changes has not been established.

Terbinafine clearance is increased 100% by rifampin, a CyP450 enzyme inducer, and decreased 33% by cimetidine, a CyP450 enzyme inhibitor. Terbinafine clearance is unaffected by cyclosporine.

There is no information available from adequate drug-drug interaction studies with the following classes of drugs: Oral contraceptives, hormone replacement therapies, hypoglycemics, theophyllines, phenytoins, thiazide diuretics, beta blockers, and calcium channel blockers.

ADVERSE REACTIONS

The most frequently reported adverse events observed in the three US/Canadian placebo-controlled trials are listed in TABLE 1. The adverse events reported encompass gastrointestinal symptoms (including diarrhea, dyspepsia, and abdominal pain), liver test abnormalities, rashes, urticaria, pruritus, and taste disturbances. In general, the adverse events were mild, transient, and did not lead to discontinuation from study participation.

TABLE 1

	Adverse Event		Discontinuation	
	Terbinafine	Placebo	Terbinafine	Placebo
	n=465	n=137	n=465	n=137
Headache	12.9%	9.5%	0.2%	0.0%
Gastrointestinal Symptoms				
Diarrhea	5.6%	2.9%	0.6%	0.0%
Dyspepsia	4.3%	2.9%	0.4%	0.0%
Abdominal pain	2.4%	1.5%	0.4%	0.0%
Nausea	2.6%	2.9%	0.2%	0.0%
Flatulence	2.2%	2.2%	0.0%	0.0%
Dermatological Symptoms				
Rash	5.6%	2.2%	0.9%	0.7%
Pruritus	2.8%	1.5%	0.2%	0.0%
Urticaria	1.1%	0.0%	0.0%	0.0%
Liver Enzyme Abnormalities*	3.3%	1.4%	0.2%	0.0%
Taste Disturbance	2.8%	0.7%	0.2%	0.0%
Visual Disturbance	1.1%	1.5%	0.9%	0.0%

* Liver enzyme abnormalities ≥2× the upper limit of the normal range.

Rare adverse events, based on worldwide experience with terbinafine HCl tablets use, include: Idiosyncratic and symptomatic hepatic injury and more rarely, cases of liver failure, some leading to death or liver transplant, (see WARNINGS and PRECAUTIONS), serious skin reactions (see WARNINGS), severe neutropenia (see PRECAUTIONS), thrombocytopenia and allergic reactions (including anaphylaxis). Uncommonly, terbinafine

T

HCl may cause taste disturbance (including taste loss) which usually recovers within several weeks after discontinuation of the drug. There have been isolated reports of prolonged (greater than one year) taste disturbance. Rarely, taste disturbances associated with oral terbinafine have been reported to be severe enough to result in decreased food intake leading to significant and unwanted weight loss.

Other adverse reactions which have been reported include malaise, fatigue, vomiting, arthralgia, myalgia, and hair loss.

Clinical adverse effects reported spontaneously since the drug was marketed include altered prothrombin time (prolongation and reduction) in patients concomitantly treated with warfarin and terbinafine HCl tablets and agranulocytosis (very rare).

DOSAGE AND ADMINISTRATION

Terbinafine HCl, one 250 mg tablet, should be taken once daily for 6 weeks by patients with fingernail onychomycosis. Terbinafine HCl, one 250 mg tablet, should be taken once daily for 12 weeks by patients with toenail onychomycosis. The optimal clinical effect is seen some months after mycological cure and cessation of treatment. This is related to the period required for outgrowth of healthy nail.

ANIMAL PHARMACOLOGY

A wide range of *in vivo* studies in mice, rats, dogs, and monkeys, and *in vitro* studies using rat, monkey, and human hepatocytes suggest that peroxisome proliferation in the liver is a rat-specific finding. However, other effects, including increased liver weights and APTT, occurred in dogs and monkeys at doses giving Css trough levels of the parent terbinafine 2-3× those seen in humans at the MRHD. Higher doses were not tested.

HOW SUPPLIED

Lamisil tablets are supplied as white to yellow-tinged white circular, bi-convex, bevelled tablets containing 250 mg of terbinafine imprinted with "LAMISIL" in circular form on one side and code "250" on the other.

Storage: Store tablets below 25°C (77°F); in a tight container. Protect from light.

TOPICAL

DESCRIPTION

CREAM

FOR TOPICAL DERMATOLOGICAL USE ONLY.

NOT FOR OPHTHALMIC, ORAL OR INTRAVAGINAL USE.

Lamisil cream, 1%, contains the synthetic antifungal compound, terbinafine hydrochloride. It is intended for topical dermatologic use only.

Chemically, terbinafine hydrochloride is (E)-*N*-(6,6-dimethyl-2-hepten-4-ynyl)-*N*-methyl-1-naphthalenemethanamine hydrochloride. The compound has the empirical formula $C_{21}H_{26}ClN$ and a molecular weight of 327.90.

Terbinafine hydrochloride is a white to off-white fine crystalline powder. It is freely soluble in methanol and methylene chloride, soluble in ethanol, and slightly soluble in water.

Each gram of Lamisil cream, 1%, contains 10 mg of terbinafine hydrochloride in a white cream base of benzyl alcohol, cetyl alcohol, cetyl palmitate, isopropyl myristate, polysorbate 60, purified water, sodium hydroxide, sorbitan monostearate, and stearyl alcohol.

SOLUTION

FOR TOPICAL DERMATOLOGIC USE ONLY — NOT FOR OPHTHALMIC, ORAL, OR INTRAVAGINAL USE.

Lamisil solution, 1%, contains the synthetic antifungal compound, terbinafine hydrochloride. It is intended for topical dermatologic use only.

Chemically, terbinafine hydrochloride is (E)-N-(6,6-dimethyl-2-hepten-4-ynyl)-N-methyl-1-naphthalenemethanamine hydrochloride. The compound has the empirical formula $C_{21}H_{26}ClN$ and a molecular weight of 327.90.

Terbinafine hydrochloride is a white to off-white fine crystalline powder. It is freely soluble in methanol and methylene chloride, soluble in ethanol, and slightly soluble in water.

Each gram of Lamisil solution, 1%, contains 10 mg of terbinafine hydrochloride in a solution of cetomacrogol 1000, ethanol (28.7%), propylene glycol, and purified water.

CLINICAL PHARMACOLOGY

CREAM

Pharmacokinetics

Following a single application of 100 μL of terbinafine HCl cream (containing 1 mg of ^{14}C-terbinafine) to a 30 cm^2 area of the ventral forearm of 6 healthy subjects, the recovery of radioactivity in urine and feces averaged 3.5% of the administered dose.

In a study of 16 healthy subjects, 8 of whose skin was artificially compromised by stripping the stratum corneum to the viable layer, single and multiple applications (average 0.1 mg/cm^2 bid for 5 days) of terbinafine HCl cream were made to various sites. In this study, systemic absorption was highly variable. The maximum measured plasma concentration of terbinafine was 11.4 ng/ml, and the maximum measured plasma concentration of the demethylated metabolite was 11.0 ng/ml. In many patients there were no detectable plasma levels of either parent compound or metabolite. Urinary excretion accounted for up to 9% of the topically applied dose; the majority excreted less than 4%. No measurement of fecal drug content was performed.

In a study of 10 patients with tinea cruris, once daily application of terbinafine HCl cream for 7 days resulted in plasma concentrations of terbinafine of 0-11 ng/ml on day 7. Plasma concentrations of the metabolites of terbinafine ranged from 11-80 ng/ml in these patients.

Approximately 75% of cutaneously absorbed terbinafine is eliminated in the urine predominantly as metabolites.

Microbiology

Terbinafine HCl is a synthetic allylamine derivative. Terbinafine HCl exerts its antifungal effect by inhibiting squalene epoxidase, a key enzyme in sterol biosynthesis in fungi. This action results in a deficiency in ergosterol and a corresponding accumulation of squalene within the fungal cell and causes fungal cell death.

Terbinafine has been shown to be active against most strains of the following organisms both *in vitro* and in clinical infections at indicated body sites (see INDICATIONS AND USAGE, Cream):

Epidermophyton floccosum
Trichophyton mentagrophytes
Trichophyton rubrum

The following *in vitro* data are available; **however, their clinical significance is unknown.**

Terbinafine exhibits satisfactory *in vitro* MICs against most strains of the following organisms; however, the safety and efficacy of terbinafine in treating clinical infections due to these organisms have not been established in adequate and well-controlled clinical trials:

Microsporum canis
Microsporum gypseum
Microsporum nanum
Trichophyton verrucosum

SOLUTION

Pharmacokinetics

Absorption

In a study of 10 patients with tinea cruris, once daily application of terbinafine HCl solution, 1%, for 7 days (total amount of terbinafine HCl applied averaged 0.8 g) resulted in plasma concentrations of terbinafine of up to 21 ng/ml on Day 7, representing approximately 2% of plasma concentrations achieved with a 250 mg terbinafine HCl tablet. Plasma concentrations of the N-demethylated metabolite of terbinafine ranged up to 14 ng/ml in these patients. In subjects with healthy skin, neither the parent nor the N-demethylated metabolite were detected in the plasma following once daily dosing for 7 days with 0.3 g of 1% terbinafine HCl solution.

Distribution

The skin pharmacokinetics of terbinafine HCl solution, 1%, delivered by spray was compared to the 1% cream in 36 healthy subjects following both single and multiple applications (approximately 5 mg of terbinafine HCl was applied to roughly a 190 cm^2 area on the back). Maximum mean total stratum corneum drug concentrations (C_{max}) averaged 720 and 810 ng/cm^2 on Days 1 and 7, respectively. No significant differences in total stratum corneum AUC (area under the curve), C_{max} and half-life were seen between the 1% spray and the 1% cream after 1 or 7 days of treatment. Similar skin levels of terbinafine are achieved by delivery of terbinafine HCl solution, 1%, from the spray bottle or from application of terbinafine HCl 1% cream.

Metabolism

It is unknown whether or not there is any significant skin metabolism of topically applied terbinafine. Radiolabeled studies with oral dosage forms indicate that terbinafine is highly metabolized into a number of metabolites which undergo conjugation and excretion into the urine. The primary metabolite seen in the urine (10% of the oral dose) is N-demethyl terbinafine.

Elimination

The half-life of terbinafine when absorbed through the skin, regardless of the method of topical administration, is ~21 hours. Approximately 75% of cutaneously absorbed terbinafine is eliminated in the urine, predominately as metabolites.

Microbiology

Terbinafine HCl is a synthetic allylamine derivative. Terbinafine HCl is hypothesized to act by inhibiting the epoxidation of squalene, thus blocking the biosynthesis of ergosterol, an essential component of fungal cell membranes. The allylamine derivatives, like the benzylamines, act at an earlier step in the ergosterol biosynthesis pathway than the azole class of antifungal drugs. Depending on the concentration of the drug and the fungal species tested *in vitro*, terbinafine HCl may be fungicidal. However, the clinical significance of *in vitro* data is unknown.

Terbinafine has been shown to be active against most strains of the following organisms both *in vitro* and in clinical infections as described in INDICATIONS AND USAGE, Solution:

Epidermophyton floccosum
Malassezia furfur
Trichophyton mentagrophytes
Trichophyton rubrum

The following *in vitro* data are available, **but their clinical significance is unknown.** *In vitro*, terbinafine exhibits satisfactory MICs against most strains of the following microorganisms; however, the safety and efficacy of terbinafine in treating clinical infections due to these microorganisms have not been established in adequate and well-controlled clinical trials:

Microsporum canis
Microsporum gypseum
Microsporum nanum
Trichophyton verrucosum

INDICATIONS AND USAGE

CREAM

Terbinafine HCl cream is indicated for the topical treatment of the following dermatologic infections: Interdigital tinea pedis (athlete's foot), tinea cruris (jock itch), or tinea corporis (ringworm) due to *Epidermophyton floccosum, Trichophyton mentagrophytes,* or *Trichophyton rubrum* (see DOSAGE AND ADMINISTRATION, Cream).

Diagnosis of the disease should be confirmed either by direct microscopic examination of scrapings from infected tissue mounted in a solution of potassium hydroxide or by culture.

SOLUTION

Prescription terbinafine HCl solution, 1%, is indicated for the topical treatment of tinea (pityriasis) versicolor due to *Malassezia furfur* (formerly *Pityrosporum ovale*). Diagnosis of disease should be confirmed by direct microscopic examination of scrapings from infected tissue mounted in a solution of potassium hydroxide.

CONTRAINDICATIONS

CREAM

Terbinafine HCl cream is contraindicated in individuals who have known or suspected hypersensitivity to terbinafine or any other of its components.

SOLUTION

Terbinafine HCl solution, 1%. is contraindicated in individuals who have known or suspected hypersensitivity to terbinafine or any other of its components.

WARNINGS

CREAM

Terbinafine HCl cream is not for ophthalmic, oral, or intravaginal use.

SOLUTION

Terbinafine HCl solution, 1%. is not for ophthalmic, oral, or intravaginal use.

PRECAUTIONS

CREAM

General

If irritation or sensitivity develops with the use of terbinafine HCl cream, treatment should be discontinued and appropriate therapy instituted.

Information for the Patient

The patient should be told to:

- Use terbinafine HCl cream as directed by the physician and avoid contact with the eyes, nose, mouth, or other mucous membranes.
- Use the medication for the treatment time recommended by the physician.
- Inform the physician if the area of application shows signs of increased irritation or possible sensitization (redness, itching, burning, blistering, swelling, or oozing).
- Avoid the use of occlusive dressings unless otherwise directed by the physician.

Carcinogenesis, Mutagenesis, and Impairment of Fertility

In a 2 year oral carcinogenicity study in mice, a 4% incidence of splenic hemangiosarcomas and a 6% incidence of leiomyosarcoma-like tumors of the seminal vesicles were observed in males at the highest dose level, 156 mg/kg/day (equivalent to at least 390 times the maximum potential exposure at the recommended human topical dose*). In a carcinogenicity study in rats at the highest dose level, 69 mg/kg/day (equivalent to at least 173 times the maximum potential exposure at the recommended human topical dose*), a 6% incidence of both liver tumors and skin lipomas were observed in males. In rats, the formation of liver tumors was associated with peroxisomal proliferation.

A battery of *in vitro* and *in vivo* genotoxicity tests, including Ames assay, mutagenicity evaluation in Chinese hamster ovarian cells, chromosome aberration test, sister chromatid exchanges, and mouse micronucleus test revealed no evidence for a mutagenic or clastogenic potential for the drug.

Reproductive studies in rats administered up to 300 mg/kg/day orally (equivalent to at least 750 times the maximum potential exposure at the recommended human topical dose*) did not reveal any adverse effects on fertility or other reproductive parameters. Intravaginal mucosal application of terbinafine HCl at 150 mg/day in pregnant rabbits did not increase the incidence of abortions or premature deliveries or affect fetal parameters.

Pregnancy Category B

Oral doses of terbinafine HCl, up to 300 mg/kg/day (equivalent to at least 750 times the maximum potential exposure at the recommended human topical dose*), during organogenesis in rats and rabbits were not teratogenic. Similarly, a subcutaneous study in rats at doses up to 100 mg/kg/day (equivalent to at least 250 times the maximum potential exposure at the recommended human topical dose*) and a percutaneous study in rabbits, including doses up to 150 mg/kg/day (equivalent to at least 350 times the maximum potential exposure at the recommended human topical dose*) did not reveal any teratogenic potential. There are, however, no adequate and well-controlled studies in pregnant women. Because animal reproduction studies are not always predictive of human response, this drug should be used only if clearly indicated during pregnancy.

* The comparisons in Carcinogenesis, Mutagenesis, and Impairment of Fertility and Pregnancy Category B between oral animal doses and maximum potential exposure at the recommended human topical doses are based upon the application to human skin of 0.1 mg of terbinafine/cm^2, the assumption of average human cutaneous exposure of 100 cm^2 [assuming the use of 1 g of terbinafine HCl cream per dose], and the **theoretical** worst case scenario of 100% human cutaneous absorption. At present, comparative animal and human systemic exposure pharmacokinetic data are not available.

Nursing Mothers

After a single **oral** dose of 500 mg of terbinafine HCl to 2 volunteers, the total dose of terbinafine HCl secreted in human milk during the 72 hour post-dosing period was 0.65 mg in one person and 0.15 mg in the other. The total excretion of terbinafine in human milk was 0.13% and 0.03% of the administered dose, respectively. The concentrations of the 1 metabolite measured in the human milk of these 2 volunteers were below the detection limit of the assay used (150 ng/ml of milk).

Because of the small amount of data on human neonatal exposure, a decision should be made whether to discontinue nursing or to discontinue the drug, taking into account the importance of the drug to the mother, as well as the findings of tumors in male mice and rats following **oral** administration of terbinafine HCl and the lack of data on carcinogenicity in neonatal animals.

Nursing mothers should avoid application of terbinafine HCl cream to the breast.

Pediatric Use

Safety and efficacy in children or infants below the age of 12 years have not been established.

SOLUTION

General

Terbinafine HCl solution, 1%, contains 28.7% alcohol. If irritation or sensitivity develops with the use of terbinafine HCl solution, 1%, treatment should be discontinued and appropriate therapy instituted.

Terbinafine HCl solution, 1%, may be irritating to the eyes.

Information for the Patient

The patient should be told to:

- Use terbinafine HCl solution, 1%, as directed by the physician and avoid contact with the eyes, nose, mouth, or other mucous membranes. The spray form should not be used on the face. In case of accidental contact with the eyes, rinse eyes thoroughly with running water and consult a physician if any symptoms persist.
- Apply terbinafine HCl solution, 1%, twice daily.
- Cleanse and dry the affected areas thoroughly before applying terbinafine HCl solution. Sufficient solution should be applied to wet the treatment area(s) thoroughly, and to cover the affected skin and surrounding area.
- Use the medication for the full treatment time (1 week) even though symptoms may have improved.
- Inform the physician if the area of application shows signs of increased irritation or possible sensitization (redness, itching, burning, blistering, swelling, or oozing).
- Notify the physician if there is no improvement after 1 week of treatment.
- Avoid the use of occlusive dressings unless otherwise directed by the physician.

Carcinogenesis, Mutagenesis, and Impairment of Fertility

In a 28 month oral carcinogenicity study in rats, a marginal increase in the incidence of liver tumors was observed in males at the highest dose level, 69 mg/kg/day (in terms of mg/m^2/day equivalent to 34 times the maximum potential exposure at the recommended topical human dose*). There was no dose-related trend, and the mid-dose male rats, 20 mg/kg/day (in terms of mg/m^2/day equivalent to 10 times the maximum potential exposure at the recommended topical human dose*), did not have any tumors. No increased incidence in liver tumors was noted in female rats at dose levels up to 97 mg/kg/day (in terms of mg/m^2/day equivalent to 47 times the maximum potential exposure at the recommended topical human dose*) or in male or female mice treated orally for 23 months at doses up to 156 mg/kg/day (in terms of mg/m^2/day equivalent to 38 times the maximum potential exposure at the recommended topical human dose*).

A wide range of oral *in vivo* studies in mice, rats, dogs, and monkeys, and *in vitro* studies using rat, monkey, and human hepatocytes suggest that the development of liver tumors in the high-dose male rats may be associated with peroxisome proliferation and support the conclusion that this is a rat-specific finding.

The results of a variety of *in vitro* (mutations in *E. coli* and *Salmonella,* DNA repair in rat hepatocytes, mutagenicity in Chinese hamster fibroblasts, chromosome aberration and sister chromatid exchanges in Chinese hamster lung cells) and *in vivo* (chromosome aberration in Chinese hamsters, micronucleus test in mice) genotoxicity tests gave no evidence of a mutagenic or clastogenic potential and demonstrated the absence of tumor-initiating or cell-proliferating activity.

Oral reproduction studies in rats at doses up to 300 mg/kg/day (in terms of mg/m^2/day equivalent to 146 times the maximum potential exposure at the recommended topical human dose*) did not reveal any specific effects on fertility or other reproductive parameters. Intravaginal application of terbinafine HCl at 150 mg/day (in terms of mg/m^2/day equivalent to 165 times the maximum potential exposure at the recommended topical human dose*) in pregnant rabbits did not increase the incidence of abortions, premature deliveries, or fetal abnormalities.

Pregnancy Category B

Oral doses of terbinafine HCl up to 300 mg/kg/day (in terms of mg/m^2/day equivalent to 146 and 329 times the maximum potential exposure at the recommended topical human dose*) during organogenesis in rats and rabbits, respectively, were not teratogenic. Similarly, a subcutaneous study in rats at doses up to 100 mg/kg/day (in terms of mg/m^2/day equivalent to 49 times the maximum potential exposure at the recommended topical human dose*) and a percutaneous study in rabbits, including doses up to 150 mg/kg/day (in terms of mg/m^2/day equivalent to 329 times the maximum potential exposure at the recommended topical human dose*), did not reveal any teratogenic potential. There are, however, no adequate and well-controlled studies in pregnant women. Because animal reproduction studies are not always predictive of human response, terbinafine HCl solution, 1%, should be used only if clearly indicated during pregnancy.

*The comparisons in Carcinogenesis, Mutagenesis, and Impairment of Fertility and Pregnancy Category B between oral animal doses and the maximum potential exposure at the recommended topical human dose are based upon the application to human skin of 0.1 mg of terbinafine/cm^2 twice daily, the assumption of average human cutaneous exposure of 100 cm^2 (assuming the use of 1 g of terbinafine HCl solution/dose), and the theoretical maximum human cutaneous absorption of 100%.

Nursing Mothers

After a single oral dose of 500 mg of terbinafine HCl to 2 volunteers, the total dose of terbinafine secreted in human milk during the 72 hour post-dosing period was 0.65 mg in 1 person and 0.15 mg in the other. The total excretion of terbinafine in human milk was 0.13% and 0.03% of the administered dose, respectively. This 500 mg dose represents about 50 times the percutaneous exposure as described in the previous paragraph. The concentrations

T

of the N-demethylated metabolite measured in the human milk of these 2 volunteers were below the detection limit of the assay used (150 ng/ml of milk).

Because of the small amount of data on human neonatal exposure, a decision should be made whether to discontinue nursing or to discontinue the drug, taking into account the importance of the drug to the mother.

Nursing mothers should avoid application of terbinafine HCl solution, 1%, to the breast.

Pediatric Use

The safety and efficacy of terbinafine HCl solution, 1%, have not been established in pediatric patients.

DRUG INTERACTIONS

CREAM

Potential interactions between terbinafine HCl cream and other drugs have not been systematically evaluated.

SOLUTION

Potential interactions between terbinafine HCl solution, 1%, and other drugs have not been systematically evaluated.

ADVERSE REACTIONS

CREAM

Clinical Trials

In clinical trials, 6 (0.2%) of 2265 patients treated with terbinafine HCl cream discontinued therapy due to adverse events and 52 (2.3%) reported adverse reactions thought to be possibly, probably, or definitely related to drug therapy. These reactions included irritation (1%), burning (0.8%), itching (0.2%), and dryness (0.2%).

SOLUTION

Clinical Trials

For terbinafine HCl solution-treated patients, adverse reactions thought to be possibly, probably, or definitely related to drug therapy included application site reactions (burning or irritation) (1.3%), itching (1.1%), skin exfoliation (1.0%) and erythematous rash (0.9%). In clinical trials with terbinafine HCl solution in dermatophyte infections, 2 (0.2%) of 898 patients treated with terbinafine HCl solution, 1%, and 2 (0.6%) of 306 patients treated with placebo (vehicle) discontinued therapy due to adverse events.

DOSAGE AND ADMINISTRATION

CREAM

In the treatment of interdigital tinea pedis (athlete's foot), terbinafine HCl cream should be applied to cover the affected and immediately surrounding areas twice daily **until clinical signs and symptoms are significantly improved.** In many patients this occurs by Day 7 of drug therapy. The duration of drug therapy should be for a minimum of 1 week and should not exceed 4 weeks. (See the following Note.)

In the treatment of tinea cruris (jock itch) or tinea corporis (ringworm), terbinafine HCl cream should be applied to cover the affected and immediately surrounding areas once or twice daily **until clinical signs and symptoms are significantly improved.** In many patients this occurs by Day 7 of drug therapy. The duration of drug therapy should be for a minimum of 1 week and should not exceed 4 weeks. (See the following Note.)

Note: Many patients treated with shorter durations of therapy (1-2 weeks) continue to improve during the 2-4 weeks after drug therapy has been completed. As a consequence, patients should not be considered therapeutic failures until they have been observed for a period of 2-4 weeks off therapy.

If successful outcome is not achieved during the post-treatment observation period, the diagnosis should be reviewed.

SOLUTION

Terbinafine HCl solution, 1%, is applied twice daily for 1 week. The affected areas should be cleansed and dried thoroughly before applying terbinafine HCl solution, 1%. Sufficient solution should be applied to wet the treatment area(s) thoroughly, and to cover the affected skin and surrounding area. If successful outcome is not achieved during the post treatment period, the diagnosis should be reviewed.

HOW SUPPLIED

SOLUTION

Lamisil solution, 1%, is supplied in a 30 ml pump spray bottle containing 290 mg of terbinafine HCl with a spray-pump assembly, which will also function upside-down, and protective cap.

Storage: Store at 5-25°C (41-77°F); do not refrigerate.

PRODUCT LISTING - EQUIVALENTS NOT AVAILABLE

Cream - Topical - 1%			
15 gm	$32.00	LAMISIL TOPICAL, Southwood Pharmaceuticals Inc	58016-3416-01
15 gm	$32.61	LAMISIL TOPICAL, Allscripts Pharmaceutical Company	54569-4278-00
15 gm	$37.61	LAMISIL TOPICAL, Pharma Pac	52959-0439-15
30 gm	$53.23	LAMISIL TOPICAL, Pharma Pac	52959-0439-30
Solution - Topical - 1%			
30 ml	$7.81	LAMISIL TOPICAL, Novartis Pharmaceuticals	00078-0328-82
30 ml	$8.49	LAMISIL AT ATHLETES FOOT, Novartis Consumer Health	00067-4002-30
Spray - Topical - 1%			
30 ml	$8.49	LAMISIL AT JOCK ITCH, Novartis Consumer Health	00067-4000-01
30 ml	$8.49	LAMISIL AT ATHLETES FOOT, Novartis Consumer Health	00067-4001-30
Tablet - Oral - 250 mg			
14's	$164.93	LAMISIL, Pd-Rx Pharmaceuticals	55289-0513-14
30's	$240.86	LAMISIL, Allscripts Pharmaceutical Company	54569-4406-00
30's	$284.94	LAMISIL, Novartis Pharmaceuticals	00078-0179-15
100's	$949.55	LAMISIL, Novartis Pharmaceuticals	00078-0179-05

Terbutaline Sulfate *(002312)*

Categories: Asthma; Bronchitis, chronic; Emphysema; Pregnancy Category B; FDA Approved 1974 Mar

Drug Classes: Adrenergic agonists; Bronchodilators

Brand Names: Brethaire; Brethancer; Brethine; **Bricanyl**

Foreign Brand Availability: Asmabet (Indonesia); Asthmasian (Thailand); Ataline (Hong-Kong; Malaysia; Thailand); Blucodil (Philippines); Brasmatic (Indonesia); Bricanyl retard (Denmark; Netherlands); Bricasma (Indonesia); Bronchodam (Philippines); Bronco Asmo (Thailand); Bucanil (Singapore); Bucaril (Thailand); Butylin (Hong-Kong); Contimit (Germany); Draconyl (Greece); Glin (Taiwan); Lanterbine SR (Hong-Kong); Nairet (Indonesia); Taziken (Mexico); Terasma (Indonesia); Terbasmin (Italy; Spain); Terbron (Hong-Kong); Terbulin (Israel); Terburop (Colombia); Tismalin (Indonesia); Tolbin (Singapore); Vacanyl (Thailand)

Cost of Therapy: $54.95 (Asthma; Brethine; 5 mg; 3 tablets/day; 30 day supply)

HCFA JCODE(S): J3105 up to 1 mg SC, IV

DESCRIPTION

TABLETS

Terbutaline sulfate tablets for oral administration contain 2.5 or 5 mg of terbutaline sulfate (equivalent to 2.05 and 4.1 mg free base, respectively). Both the 2.5 and 5 mg tablets contain the following inactive ingredients: corn starch (or pregelatinized corn starch), lactose, magnesium stearate, microcrystalline cellulose, and povidone.

Terbutaline sulfate (5-[2-[(1,1-dimethylethyl)amino]-1-hydroxyethyl]-1,3-benzenediol sulfate) is a β-adrenergic agonist bronchodilator.

INJECTION

Terbutaline sulfate subcutaneous injection is a sterile, isotonic solution. Each ml of solution contains 1 mg terbutaline sulfate (equivalent to 0.82 mg free base) and 8.9 mg sodium chloride in water for injection. Hydrochloric acid is used to adjust pH to 3.5. Filled under nitrogen.

Terbutaline sulfate (5-[2-[(1,1-dimethylethyl)amino]-1-hydroxyethyl]-1,3-benzenediol sulfate) is a β- adrenergic agonist bronchodilator.

INHALATION

A metered-dose dispenser containing micronized terbutaline sulfate in a suspension of the following composition (TABLE 1):

TABLE 1

	7.5-ml (10.5-g) Canister
Terbutaline sulfate	0.075 g
Sorbitan trioleate	0.105 g
Trichloromonofluoromethane	2.58 g
Dichlorotetrafluoroethane	2.58 g
Dichlorodifluoromethane	5.16 g

Each actuation delivers 0.20 mg of terbutaline sulfate form the mouthpiece (0.25 mg valve delivery). Each canister provides at least 300 inhalations.

Terbutaline sulfate is a white to gray-white crystalline powder. It is odor less or has a faint odor of acetic acid. It is soluble in water and in 0.1N hydrochloride acid, slightly soluble in methanol, and insoluble in chloroform. Its molecular weight is 548.65.

CLINICAL PHARMACOLOGY

Terbutaline sulfate is a β-adrenergic receptor agonist which has been shown by *in vitro* and *in vivo* pharmacologic studies in animals to exert a preferential effect on β_2-adrenergic receptors, such as those located in bronchial smooth muscle. However, controlled clinical studies of patients who were administered the drug have not revealed a preferential β_2-adrenergic effect.

It has been postulated that β-adrenergic agonists produce many of their pharmacologic effects by activation of adenyl cyclase, the enzyme which catalyzes the conversion of adenosine triphosphate to cyclic adenosine monophosphate.

Terbutaline sulfate tablets have been shown in controlled clinical studies to relieve bronchospasm in chronic obstructive pulmonary disease, such as asthma, chronic bronchitis, and emphysema. This action was manifested by a clinically significant increase in pulmonary function as demonstrated by an increase of 15% or greater in FEV_1 in some patients. A measurable change in pulmonary function usually occurs within 30 minutes following oral administration. The maximum effect usually occurs within 120-180 minutes. There is a clinically significant decrease in airway and pulmonary resistance which persists for at least 4 hours or longer in most patients. Significant bronchodilator action, as measured by various pulmonary function determinations (airway resistance, MMEFR, PEFR) has been demonstrated in studies for periods up to 8 hours in many patients.

Following administration of 0.25 mg by subcutaneous injectin, a measurable change in flow rate is usually observed within 5 minutes, and a clinically significant increase in FEV_1 occurs by 15 minutes following the injection. The maximum effect usually occurs within 30-60 minutes and clinically significant bronchodilator activity has been observed to persist for 90 minutes to 4 hours in most patients. The duration of clinically significant improvement is comparable to that found with equimilligram doses of epinephrine.

Subcutaneously administered terbutaline sulfate shows peak plasma concentration 15-30 minutes after injection (0.5 mg dose, mean peak plasma level 7.6 mg/L). Approximately one-third is metabolized (inactive), the majority of the dose being excreted in urine unchanged. A half-life of 3-4 hours has been reported.

Terbutaline crosses the placenta. After single dose IV administration of terbutaline to 22 women in late pregnancy who were delievered by elective Caesarean section due to clinical reasons, umbilical blood levels of terbutaline were found to range from 11-48% of the maternal blood levels.

Clinical studies have evaluated the effectiveness of oral terbutaline sulfate for periods up to 12 months and the drug continued to produce significant improvement of pulmonary function throughout the period of treatment.

Orally administered terbutaline sulfate is 30-70% absorbed in the GI tract (food reduces bioavailability by one-third). Sixty percent (60%) of the absorbed oral dose is metabolized via first pass conjugation in the gut wall and liver. There are no known active metabolites. After single oral doses, peak concentrations are found 30 minutes to 5 hours after administration. Each mg of orally administered terbutaline sulfate (in fasting adults) produces an average peak serum concentration of approximately 1 mcg/L. Terbutaline has a half-life of 3-4 hours and is excreted in the urine.

Recent studies in laboratory animals (minipigs, rodents, and dogs) recorded the occurrence of cardiac arrhythmias and sudden death (with histologic evidence of myocardial necrosis) when β agonists and methylxanthines were administered concurrently. The significance of these findings when applied to humans is currently unknown.

INDICATIONS AND USAGE

Terbutaline sulfate is indicated as a bronchodilator for the relief of reversible bronchospasm in patients with obstructive airway diseases, such as asthma, bronchitis, and emphysema.

INHALATION

In controlled clinical trials the inset of improvement in pulmonary function was within 15-30 minutes. These studies also showed that maximum improvement in pulmonary function occurred at 120 minutes following 2 inhalations of terbutaline sulfate and that clinically significant improvement (*i.e.,* 15% increase in FEV_1/predicted FEV_1) generally continued for 3-4 hours in most patients. In some studies there was a significant decrease in improvement of pulmonary function noted with continued administration of terbutaline sulfate aerosol. Continued effectiveness of terbutaline sulfate was demonstrated over a 14 week period in some patients in these clinical trials.

Some patients with asthma, in single-dose studies only, have shown a therapeutic response that was still apparent at 6 hours.

NON-FDA APPROVED INDICATIONS

Terbutaline is also commonly used for the treatment of premature labor, although this indication is not approved by the FDA.

CONTRAINDICATIONS

Terbutaline sulfate is contraindicated in patients with a history of hypersensitivity to any of its components or to sympathomimetic amines.

WARNINGS

There have been rare reports of seizures occurring in patients receiving terbutaline, which do not recur when the drug is discontinued and have not been explained on any other basis.

USAGE IN LABOR AND DELIVERY

Terbutaline sulfate is not indicated and should not be used for the management of preterm labor. Serious adverse reactions have been reported following administration of terbutaline sulfate to women in labor. These reports have included transient hypokalemia, pulmonary edema (sometimes after delivery), and hypoglycemia in the mother and/or the neonatal child. Maternal death has been reported with terbutaline sulfate and other drugs of this class.

INHALATION

As with other adrenergic aerosols, the potential for paradoxical bronchospasm (which can be life-threatening) should be kept in mind. If it occurs, the preparation should be discontinued immediately and alternative therapy instituted.

Fatalities have been reported in association with excessive use of inhaled sympathomimetic drugs. The exact cause of death in unknown. As with other beta-adrenergic aerosols, terbutaline sulfate should not be used in excess. Controlled clinical studies and other clinical experience have shown that terbutaline, like other inhaled beta-adrenergic agonists, can produce a significant cardiovascular effect in some patients, as measured by pulse rate, blood pressure, symptoms, and/or ECG changes.

The contents of terbutaline sulfate inhalation are under pressure. Do not puncture the container. Do not use or store it near heat or open flame. Exposure to temperatures above 120°F may cause bursting. Never throw the container into a fire or incinerator. Keep out of children's reach.

PRECAUTIONS

GENERAL

Terbutaline sulfate is a sympathomimetic amine and as such should be used with caution in patients with cardiovascular disorders (including arrhythmias, coronary insufficiency, and hypertension), in patients with hyperthyroidism or diabetes mellitus, history of seizures, or in patients who are unusually responsive to sympathomimetic amines. Age-related differences in the hemodynamic response to β-adrenergic receptor stimulation have been reported.

Patients susceptible to hypokalemia should be monitored because transient early falls in serum potassium levels have been reported with β agonists.

Large doses of intravenous terbutaline sulfate have been reported to aggravate preexisting diabetes and ketoacidosis. The relevance of this observation to the use of terbutaline sulfate tablets is unknown.

Immediate hypersensitivity reactions and exacerbation of bronchospasm have been reported after terbutaline administration.

INFORMATION FOR THE PATIENT

The patient should be advised regarding the potential adverse reactions associated with terbutaline sulfate and that: (1) the action of terbutaline sulfate tablets may last up to 8 hours (terbutaline sulfate inhalation: up to 6 hours) and, therefore, should not be used more frequently than recommended, (2) the number or frequency of doses should not be increased without medical consultation, (3) medical consultation should be sought promptly if symptoms get worse, and (4) other medicines should not be used while taking terbutaline sulfate without consulting the physician.

CARCINOGENESIS, MUTAGENESIS, AND IMPAIRMENT OF FERTILITY

A 2 year, oral carcinogenesis bioassay of terbutaline sulfate (50, 500, 1000, and 2000 mg/kg, corresponding to 167, 1667, 3333, and 6667 times the recommended daily adult oral dose, respectively) in the Sprague-Dawley rat revealed drug-related changes in the female genital system. Females showed dose-related increases in leiomyomas of the mesovarium: 3 (5%) at 50 mg/kg, 17 (28%) at 500 mg/kg, 21 (35%) at 1000 mg/kg, and 23 (38%) at 2000 mg/kg, which were significant at the three highest levels. None occurred in female controls. The incidence of ovarian cysts was significantly elevated at all dose levels except at 2000 mg/kg and hyperplasia of the mesovarium was increased significantly at 500 and 2000 mg/kg. A 21 month oral study of terbutaline sulfate (5, 50, and 200 mg/kg, corresponding to 17, 167, and 667 times the recommended daily adult oral dose, respectively) in the mouse revealed no evidence of carcinogenicity.

Studies of terbutaline sulfate have not been conducted to determine mutagenic potential.

An oral reproduction study of terbutaline sulfate up to 50 mg/kg (corresponding to 167 times the human oral dose) in the rat revealed no adverse effects on fertility.

PREGNANCY, TERATOGENIC EFFECTS, PREGNANCY CATEGORY B

Reproduction studies in mice (up to 1.1 mg/kg subcutaneously, corresponding to 4 times the human oral dose) and in rats and rabbits (up to 50 mg/kg orally, corresponding to 167 times the human oral dose) have revealed no evidence of impaired fertility or harm to the fetus due to terbutaline. There are, however, no adequate and well-controlled studies in pregnant women. Because animal reproduction studies are not always predictive of human response, this drug should be used during pregnancy only if clearly needed.

LABOR AND DELIVERY

The safe use of terbutaline sulfate for the management of preterm labor or for other uses during labor and delivery has not been established and the drug should not be used. (See WARNINGS.)

NURSING MOTHERS

Terbutaline is excreted in breast milk. Caution should be exercised when terbutaline sulfate is administered to a nursing woman.

PEDIATRIC USE

Tablets

The safety and effectiveness of terbutaline oral tablets have been estalished in children 6 years of age and older. Use of terbutaline in this age group is supported by published reports in which oral terbutaline producted significant bronchodilation in children with asthma. In these studies, the adverse event profile largely reflected expected pharmacological effects of beta-adrenergic stimulation such as tachycardia, systolic blood pressure elevation and tremor. The safety and effectiveness of terbutaline oral tablets in children below 6 years of age have not been established.

Injection

The safety and effectiveness of terbutaline subcutaneous injection have been estalished in children 6 years of age and older. Use of terbutaline in this age group is supported by published reports in which subscutaneous terbutaline at doses of 0.006 to 0.01 milligrams per kilogram produced significant bronchodilation in children with asthma. In these studies, the adverse event profile largely reflected expected pharmacological effects of beta-adrenergic stimulation such as tachycardia, systolic blood pressure elevations and tremor. There are no adequate electrocardiographic data evaluating the effect of subcutaneously administered terbutaline in this age group. The safety and effectiveness of terbutaline subcutaneous injection in children below 6 years of age have not been established.

DRUG INTERACTIONS

Other sympathomimetic bronchodilators or epinephrine should not be used concomitantly with terbutaline sulfate, since their combined effect on the cardiovascular system may be deleterious to the patient. This recommendation does not preclude the judicious use of an aerosol bronchodilator of the adrenergic stimulant type in patients receiving terbutaline sulfate tablets. Such concomitant use, however, should be individualized and not given on a routine basis. If regular coadministration is required, alternative therapy should be considered. Terbutaline sulfate should be administered with caution in patients being treated with monoamine oxidase (MAO) inhibitors or tricyclic antidepressants, since the action of terbutaline sulfate on the vascular system may be potentiated.

β-Adrenergic receptor blocking agents not only block the pulmonary effect of terbutaline but may produce severe asthmatic attacks in asthmatic patients. Therefore, patients requiring treatment for both bronchospastic disease and hypertension should be treated with medication other than β-adrenergic blocking agents for hypertension.

ADVERSE REACTIONS

The adverse reactions of terbutaline sulfate are similar to those of other sympathomimetic agents.

The most commonly observed side effects are tremor and nervousness. The frequency of these side effects appear to diminish with continued therapy. Other commonly reported reactions include increased heart rate, palpitations, and dizziness. Other reported reactions include headache, drowsiness, vomiting, nausea, sweating, and muscle cramps. These reactions are generally transient and usually do not require treatment.

T

DOSAGE AND ADMINISTRATION

TABLETS

Adults and Pediatric Patients Over 12 Years of Age

Usual dose is 5 mg three times daily. Dosing may be initiated at 2.5 mg three or four times daily and titrated upward depending on clinical response. A total dose of 15 mg in a 24 hour period should not be exceeded.

Pediatric Patients (6-12 years)

The usual dose of terbutaline oral tablets is 2.5 mg three times daily. If a previously effective dosage regime fails to provide the usual relief, medical advice should be sought immediatley as this is often a sign of seriously worsening asthma which would require reassessment of therapy.

INJECTION

Adults and Pediatric Patients Over 12 Years of Age

The usual subscutaneous dose of terbutaline is 0.25 mg (0.25 ml, 1/4 ampul contents) injected into the lateral deltoid area. If significant improvement does not oiccur by 15-30 minutes, a second dose of 0.25mg may be administered. Any unused portion of the ampul should be discarded immediately. A total dose of 0.5 mg should not be exceeded within a 4 hour period. If a patient fails to respond to a second 0.25 mg (0.25 ml) dose within 15-30 minutes, other therapeutic measures should be considered.

Pediatric Patients (6-12 years)

The usual subcutaneous dose of terbutaline is 0.006-0.01 mg/kg, to a maximum dose of 0.25 mg. If significant clinical improvement does not occur by 15-30 minutes, a second dose may be administered. Any unused portion of the ampul should be discarded immediately. Subsequent doses should not be given within a 4 hour period. If a patient fails to respond to a second dose within 15-30 minutes, other therapeutic measures should be considered.

INHALATION

Adults and Pediatric Patients Over 12 Years of Age

The usual dosage for adults and children 12 years and older is 2 inhalations separated by a 60 second interval, every 4-6 hours. Dosing should not be repeated more often than every 4-6 hours. The use of terbutaline sulfate inhalator can be continued as medically indicated to control recurring bouts of bronchospasm. During this time most patients gain optimal benefit from regular use of the inhaler. Safe usage for periods extending over several years has been documented.

If a previously effective dosage regimen fails to provide the usual relief, medical advice should be sought immediately, as this is often a sign of seriously worsening asthma, which would require reassessment of therapy.

HOW SUPPLIED

TABLETS

2.5 mg Tablets: Round, white, debossed "BRICANYL 2 1/2".
5.0 mg Tablets: Square, white, scored, debossed "BRICANYL 5".
Storage: Store at controlled room temperature 15-30° C (59-86°F)

INJECTION

Each ml size ampul contains 1 ml of solution (1 mg terbutaline sulfate). *NOTE:* 0.25 ml of solution will provide the ususal clinical dose of 0.25 mg.

Parenteral drug products should be inspected visually for particulate matter and discoloration prior to administration, whenever solution and container permit.

Solutions of terbutaline sulfate are sensitive to excessive heat and light. Ampuls should, therefore, be stored at controlled room temperature 15- 30°C (59-86°F) in their original carton to provide protection from light until dispensed. Solutions should not be used if discolored.

T

PRODUCT LISTING - RATED THERAPEUTICALLY EQUIVALENT

Tablet - Oral - 2.5 mg

100's	$38.90	BRETHINE, Novartis Pharmaceuticals	00028-0072-61
100's	$43.22	BRETHINE, Physicians Total Care	54868-2849-01
100's	$43.24	GENERIC, Global Pharmaceutical Corporation	00115-2611-01
100's	$48.15	BRETHINE, Novartis Pharmaceuticals	00028-0072-01

Tablet - Oral - 5 mg

30's	$19.14	BRETHINE, Physicians Total Care	54868-1240-00
100 x 12	$557.16	BRETHINE, Novartis Pharmaceuticals	00028-0105-65
100's	$59.27	BRETHINE, Novartis Pharmaceuticals	00028-0105-61
100's	$61.05	BRETHINE, Physicians Total Care	54868-1240-01
100's	$62.21	GENERIC, Global Pharmaceutical Corporation	00115-2622-01
100's	$69.28	BRETHINE, Novartis Pharmaceuticals	00028-0105-01
200's	$120.93	BRETHINE, Physicians Total Care	54868-1240-02

PRODUCT LISTING - EQUIVALENTS NOT AVAILABLE

Solution - Injectable - 1 mg/ml

1 ml x 10	$311.90	BRETHINE, Novartis Pharmaceuticals	00028-7507-23
1 ml x 100	$3094.00	BRETHINE, Novartis Pharmaceuticals	00028-7507-01

Terconazole *(002313)*

Categories: Vaginitis, secondary to monilia; Vulvovaginitis, secondary to monilia; Pregnancy Category C; FDA Approved 1987 Dec
Drug Classes: Antifungals, topical; Dermatologics
Brand Names: Terazol
Foreign Brand Availability: Fungistat (Mexico); Fungistat 3 (Bahamas; Barbados; Belize; Bermuda; Curacao; Guyana; Jamaica; Netherland-Antilles; Surinam; Trinidad); Fungistat 5 (Colombia; Costa-Rica; Dominican-Republic; El-Salvador; Guatemala; Honduras; Nicaragua; Panama); Gyno-Terazol (Belgium; Israel; Netherlands; Portugal); Gyno-Terazol 3 (Czech-Republic); Terazol 3 (Canada); Terazol 7 (Canada); Tercospor (Germany)
Cost of Therapy: $32.23 (Moniliasis; Terazol 3 Cream; 0.8%; 20 g; 1 applicator/day; 3 day supply)
$26.22 (Moniliasis; Terazol 7 Cream; 0.4%; 45 g; 1 applicator/day; 7 day supply)
$26.22 (Moniliasis; Terazol 3 Suppository; 80 mg; 1 suppository/day; 3 day supply)

DESCRIPTION

VAGINAL CREAM 0.4%, 0.8%

Terazol (terconazole) vaginal cream is a white to off-white, water washable cream for intravaginal administration containing 0.4% or 0.8% of the antifungal agent terconazole, *cis*-1-[*p*-[[2-(2,4-dichlorophenyl)-2-(1*H*-1,2,4-triazol-1-ylmethyl)-1,3-dioxolan-4-yl]methoxy]phenyl]-4-isopropylpiperazine, compounded in a cream base consisting of butylated hydroxyanisole, cetyl alcohol, isopropyl myristate, polysorbate 60, polysorbate 80, propylene glycol, stearyl alcohol, and purified water.

VAGINAL SUPPOSITORIES

Terazol 3 (terconazole) vaginal suppositories are white to off-white suppositories for intravaginal administration containing 80 mg of the antifungal agent terconazole, *cis*-1-[*p*-[[2-(2,4-dichlorophenyl)-2-(1*H*-1,2,4-triazol-1-ylmethyl)-1,3-dioxolan-4-yl] methoxy] phenyl]-4-isopropylpiperazine, in triglycerides derived from coconut and/or palm kernel oil (a base of hydrogenated vegetable oils) and butylated hydroxyanisole. The structual formula is $C_{26}H_{31}Cl_2N_5O_3$.

Terconazole, a triazole derivative, is a white to almost white powder with a molecular weight of 532.47. It is insoluble in water; sparingly soluble in ethanol; and soluble in butanol.

CLINICAL PHARMACOLOGY

Following intravaginal administration of terconazole in humans, absorption ranged from 5-8% in 3 hysterectomized subjects and 12-16% in 2 non-hysterectomized subjects with tubal ligations.

Following daily intravaginal administration of 0.8% terconazole 40 mg (0.8% cream × 5 g) for 7 days to normal humans, plasma concentrations were low and gradually rose to a daily peak (mean of 5.9 ng/ml or 0.006 µg/ml) at 6.6 hours.

Results from similar studies in patients with vulvovaginal candidiasis indicate that the slow rate of absorption, the lack of accumulation, and the mean peak plasma concentration of terconazole was not different from that observed in healthy women. The absorption characteristics of terconazole 0.8% in pregnant or non-pregnant patients with vulvovaginal candidiasis were also similar to those found in normal volunteers.

Following oral (30 mg) administration of ^{14}C-labeled terconazole, the harmonic half-life of elimination from the blood for the parent terconazole was 6.9 hours (range 4.0-11.3). Terconazole is extensively metabolized; the plasma AUC for terconazole compared to the AUC for total radioactivity was 0.6%. Total radioactivity was eliminated from the blood with a harmonic half-life of 52.2 hours (range 44-60). Excretion of radioactivity was both by renal (32-56%) and fecal (47-52%) routes.

In vitro, terconazole is highly protein bound (94.9%) and the degree of binding is independent of drug concentration.

Photosensitivity reactions were observed in some normal volunteers following repeated dermal application of terconazole, 2.0 and 0.8% creams under conditions of filtered artificial ultraviolet light.

Photosensitivity reactions have not been observed in US and foreign clinical trials in patients who were treated with terconazole suppositories or cream (0.4 and 0.8%).

MICROBIOLOGY

Terconazole exhibits fungicidal activity *in vitro* against *Candida albicans.* Antifungal activity also has been demonstrated against other fungi. The MIC values for terconazole against most *Lactobacillus* typically found in the human vagina were ≥128 µg/ml, therefore these beneficial bacteria were not affected by drug treatment.

The exact pharmacologic mode of action of terconazole is uncertain; however, it may exert its antifungal activity by the disruption of normal fungal cell membrane permeability. No resistance to terconazole has developed during successive passages of *C. albicans*.

INDICATIONS AND USAGE

Terconazole vaginal creams (0.4 and 0.8%) and suppositories 80 mg are indicated for the local treatment of vulvovaginal candidiasis (moniliasis). As these products are effective only for vulvovaginitis caused by the genus *Candida,* the diagnosis should be confirmed by KOH smears and/or cultures.

CONTRAINDICATIONS

Patients known to be hypersensitive to terconazole or to any of its components of the cream or suppositories.

WARNINGS

None.

PRECAUTIONS

GENERAL

Discontinue use and do not retreat with terconazole if sensitization, irritation, fever, chills or flu-like symptoms are reported during use.

The base contained in the suppository formulation may interact with certain rubber or latex products, such as those used in vaginal contraceptive diaphragms, therefore concurrent use is not recommended.

LABORATORY TESTS

If there is lack of response to terconazole, appropriate microbiological studies (standard KOH smear and/or cultures) should be repeated to confirm the diagnosis and rule out other pathogens.

CARCINOGENESIS, MUTAGENESIS, AND IMPAIRMENT OF FERTILITY

Carcinogenesis

Studies to determine the carcinogenic potential of terconazole have not been performed.

Mutagenicity

Terconazole was not mutagenic when tested *in vitro* for induction of microbial point mutations (Ames test) or for inducing cellular transformation, or *in vivo* for chromosome breaks (micronucleus test) or dominant lethal mutations in mouse germ cells.

Impairment of Fertility

No impairment of fertility occurred when female rats were administered terconazole orally up to 40 mg/kg/day for a 3 month period.

PREGNANCY, TERATOGENIC EFFECTS, PREGNANCY CATEGORY C

There was no evidence of teratogenicity when terconazole was administered orally up to 40 mg/kg/day (25× the recommended intravaginal human dose of the suppository formulation, 50× the recommended intravaginal dose of the 0.8% vaginal cream formulation, and 100× the intravaginal human dose of the 0.4% vaginal cream formulation) in rats, or 20 mg/kg/day in rabbits, or subcutaneously up to 20 mg/kg/day in rats.

Dosages at or below 10 mg/kg/day produced no embryotoxicity; however, there was a delay in fetal ossification at 10 mg/kg/day in rats. There was some evidence of embryotoxicity in rabbits and rats at 20-40 mg/kg. In rats, this was reflected as a decrease in litter size and number of viable young and reduced fetal weight. There was also delay in ossification and an increased incidence of skeletal variants.

The no-effect dose of 10 mg/kg/day resulted in a mean peak plasma level of terconazole in pregnant rats of 0.176 μg/ml which exceeds by 44 times the mean peak plasma level (0.004 μg/ml) seen in normal subjects after intravaginal administration of terconazole 0.4% vaginal cream, by 30 times the mean peak plasma level (0.006 μg/ml) seen in normal subjects after intravaginal administration of terconazole 0.8% vaginal cream, and by 17 times the mean peak plasma level (0.010 μg/ml) seen in normal subjects after intravaginal administration of terconazole 80 mg vaginal suppository. This safety assessment does not account for possible exposure of the fetus through direct transfer to terconazole from the irritated vagina by diffusion across amniotic membranes.

Since terconazole is absorbed from the human vagina, it should not be used in the first trimester of pregnancy unless the physician considers it essential to the welfare of the patient.

NURSING MOTHERS

It is not known whether this drug is excreted in human milk. Animal studies have shown that rat offspring exposed via the milk of treated (40 mg/kg/orally) dams showed decreased survival during the first few post-partum days, but overall pup weight and weight gain were comparable to or greater than controls throughout lactation. Because many drugs are excreted in human milk, and because of the potential of adverse reaction in nursing infants from terconazole, a decision should be made whether to discontinue nursing or to discontinue the drug, taking into account the importance of the drug to the mother.

PEDIATRIC USE

Safety and efficacy in children have not been established.

GERIATRIC USE

Clinical studies of terconazole did not include sufficient numbers of subjects aged 65 and over to determine whether they respond differently from younger subjects. Other reported clinical experience has not identified differences in responses between the elderly and younger patients.

DRUG INTERACTIONS

Terconazole vaginal cream 0.4% and terconazole vaginal suppositories 80 mg: The therapeutic effect of these products is not affected by oral contraceptive usage.

Terconazole vaginal cream 0.8%: The levels of estradiol (E2) and progesterone did not differ significantly when 0.8% terconazole vaginal cream was administered to healthy female volunteers established on a low dose oral contraceptive.

ADVERSE REACTIONS

VAGINAL CREAM, 0.4%

During controlled clinical studies conducted in the US, 521 patients with vulvovaginal candidiasis were treated with terconazole 0.4% vaginal cream. Based on comparative analyses with placebo, the adverse experiences considered most likely related to terconazole 0.4% vaginal cream were headache (26% vs 17% with placebo) and body pain (2.1% vs 0% with placebo). Vulvovaginal burning (5.2%), itching (2.3%) or irritation (3.1%) occurred less frequently with terconazole 0.4% vaginal cream than with the vehicle placebo. Fever (1.7% vs 0.5% with placebo) and chills (0.4% vs 0.0% with placebo) have also been reported. The therapy-related dropout rate was 1.9%. The adverse drug experience on terconazole most frequently causing discontinuation was vulvovaginal itching (0.6%), which was lower than the incidence for placebo (0.9%).

VAGINAL CREAM, 0.8%

During controlled clinical studies conducted in the US, patients with vulvovaginal candidiasis were treated with terconazole 0.8% vaginal cream for 3 days. Based on comparative analyses with placebo and a standard agent, the adverse experiences considered most likely related to terconazole 0.8% vaginal cream were headache (21% vs 16% with placebo) and dysmenorrhea (6% vs 2% with placebo). Genital complaints in general, and burning and itching in particular, occurred less frequently in the terconazole 0.8% vaginal cream 3 day regimen (5% vs 6%-9% with placebo). Other adverse experiences reported with terconazole 0.8% vaginal cream were abdominal pain (3.4% vs 1% with placebo) and fever (1% vs 0.3% with placebo). The therapy-related dropout rate was 2.0% for the terconazole 0.8% vaginal cream. The adverse drug experience most frequently causing discontinuation of therapy was vulvovaginal itching, 0.7% with the terconazole 0.8% vaginal cream group and 0.3% with the placebo group.

VAGINAL SUPPOSITORIES 80 MG

During controlled clinical studies conducted in the US, 284 patients with vulvovaginal candidiasis were treated with terconazole 80 mg vaginal suppositories. Based on comparative analyses with placebo (295 patients) the adverse experiences considered adverse reactions most likely related to terconazole 80 mg vaginal suppositories were headache (30.3% vs 20.7% with placebo) and pain of the female genitalia (4.2% vs 0.7% with placebo). Adverse reactions that were reported but were not statistically significantly different from placebo were burning (15.2% vs 11.2% with placebo) and body pain (3.9% vs 1.7% with placebo). Fever (2.8% vs 1.4% with placebo) and chills (1.8% vs 0.7% with placebo) have also been reported. The therapy-related dropout rate was 3.5% and the placebo therapy-related dropout rate was 2.7%. The adverse drug experience on terconazole most frequently causing discontinuation was burning (2.5% vs 1.4% with placebo) and pruritus (1.8% vs 1.4% with placebo).

DOSAGE AND ADMINISTRATION

VAGINAL CREAM, 0.4%

One full applicator (5 g) of vaginal cream 20 mg terconazole should be administered intravaginally once daily at bedtime for 7 consecutive days.

VAGINAL CREAM, 0.8%

One full applicator (5 g) of vaginal cream 40 mg terconazole should be administered intravaginally once daily at bedtime for 3 consecutive days.

VAGINAL SUPPOSITORIES 80 MG

One vaginal suppository 80 mg terconazole should be administered intravaginally once daily at bedtime for 3 consecutive days.

Before prescribing another course of therapy, the diagnosis should be reconfirmed by smears and/or cultures and other pathogens commonly associated with vulvovaginitis ruled out. The therapeutic effect of products is not affected by menstruation.

HOW SUPPLIED

TERAZOL VAGINAL CREAM

0.4%: Available in 45 g tubes with an Ortho measured-dose applicator.
0.8%: Available in 20 g tubes with an Ortho measured-dose applicator.
Storage: Store at controlled room temperature 15-30°C (59-86°F).

TERAZOL VAGINAL SUPPOSITORIES

80 mg: Available as 2.5 g elliptically shaped white to off-white suppositories in packages of 3 with a vaginal applicator.
Storage: Store at controlled room temperature 15-30°C (59-86°F).

PRODUCT LISTING - EQUIVALENTS NOT AVAILABLE

Cream - Vaginal - 0.4%			
45 gm	$26.22	TERAZOL 7, Allscripts Pharmaceutical Company	54569-2013-00
45 gm	$33.84	TERAZOL 7, Southwood Pharmaceuticals Inc	58016-3119-01
45 gm	$36.26	TERAZOL 7, Pharma Pac	52959-1161-00
45 gm	$36.39	TERAZOL 7, Physicians Total Care	54868-2862-00
45 gm	$39.13	TERAZOL 7, Janssen Pharmaceuticals	00062-5350-01
45 gm	$40.65	TERAZOL 7, Prescript Pharmaceuticals	00247-0257-45
Cream - Vaginal - 0.8%			
20 gm	$32.23	TERAZOL 3, Allscripts Pharmaceutical Company	54569-3195-00
20 gm	$33.84	TERAZOL 3, Southwood Pharmaceuticals Inc	58016-2021-01
20 gm	$33.84	TERAZOL 3, Southwood Pharmaceuticals Inc	58016-2021-20
20 gm	$36.39	TERAZOL 3, Physicians Total Care	54868-1687-01
20 gm	$38.91	TERAZOL 3, Prescript Pharmaceuticals	00247-0283-20
20 gm	$39.13	TERAZOL 3, Janssen Pharmaceuticals	00062-5356-01
Suppository - Vaginal - 80 mg			
3's	$26.22	TERAZOL 3, Allscripts Pharmaceutical Company	54569-2012-00
3's	$28.94	TERAZOL 3, Southwood Pharmaceuticals Inc	58016-3149-01
3's	$29.80	TERAZOL 3, Pharma Pac	52959-0574-00
3's	$36.39	TERAZOL 3, Physicians Total Care	54868-0515-01
3's	$39.13	TERAZOL 3, Janssen Pharmaceuticals	00062-5351-01
3's	$40.65	TERAZOL 3, Prescript Pharmaceuticals	00247-0256-03

Teriparatide (rDNA origin) *(003579)*

Categories: Osteoporosis; Pregnancy Category C; FDA Approved 2002 Nov
Drug Classes: Hormones/hormone modifiers
Brand Names: Forteo
Cost of Therapy: $466.67 (Osteoporosis; Forteo; 250 µg/ml; 20 µg/day; 30 day supply)

WARNING

In male and female rats, teriparatide caused an increase in the incidence of osteosarcoma (a malignant bone tumor) that was dependent on dose and treatment duration. The effect was observed at systemic exposures to teriparatide ranging from 3-60 times the exposure in humans given a 20 µg dose. Because of the uncertain relevance of the rat osteosarcoma finding to humans, teriparatide should be prescribed only to patients for whom the potential benefits are considered to outweigh the potential risk. Teriparatide should not be prescribed for patients who are at increased baseline risk for osteosarcoma (including those with Paget's disease of bone or unexplained elevations of alkaline phosphatase, open epiphyses, or prior radiation therapy involving the skeleton) (see WARNINGS and PRECAUTIONS, Carcinogenesis, Mutagenesis, and Impairment of Fertility, Carcinogenesis).

DESCRIPTION

Teriparatide (rDNA origin) injection contains recombinant human parathyroid hormone (1-34), [rhPTH(1-34)], which has an identical sequence to the 34 N-terminal amino acids (the biologically active region) of the 84-amino acid human parathyroid hormone.

Teriparatide has a molecular weight of 4117.8 daltons.

Teriparatide (rDNA origin) is manufactured by Eli Lilly and Company using a strain of *Escherichia coli* modified by recombinant DNA technology. Forteo is supplied as a sterile, colorless, clear, isotonic solution in a glass cartridge which is pre-assembled into a disposable pen device for subcutaneous injection. Each prefilled delivery device is filled with 3.3 ml to deliver 3 ml. Each ml contains 250 µg teriparatide (corrected for acetate, chloride, and water content), 0.41 mg glacial acetic acid, 0.10 mg sodium acetate (anhydrous), 45.4 mg mannitol, 3.0 mg metacresol, and water for injection. In addition, hydrochloric acid solution 10% and/or sodium hydroxide solution 10% may have been added to adjust the product to pH 4.

Each cartridge pre-assembled into a pen device delivers 20 µg of teriparatide per dose each day for up to 28 days.

See User Manual: Instructions for Use that accompany the package insert.

CLINICAL PHARMACOLOGY

MECHANISM OF ACTION

Endogenous 84-amino-acid parathyroid hormone (PTH) is the primary regulator of calcium and phosphate metabolism in bone and kidney. Physiological actions of PTH include regulation of bone metabolism, renal tubular reabsorption of calcium and phosphate, and intestinal calcium absorption. The biological actions of PTH and teriparatide are mediated through binding to specific high-affinity cell-surface receptors. Teriparatide and the 34 N-terminal amino acids of PTH bind to these receptors with the same affinity and have the same physiological actions on bone and kidney. Teriparatide is not expected to accumulate in bone or other tissues.

The skeletal effects of teriparatide depend upon the pattern of systemic exposure. Once-daily administration of teriparatide stimulates new bone formation on trabecular and cortical (periosteal and/or endosteal) bone surfaces by preferential stimulation of osteoblastic activity over osteoclastic activity. In monkey studies, teriparatide improved trabecular microarchitecture and increased bone mass and strength by stimulating new bone formation in both cancellous and cortical bone. In humans, the anabolic effects of teriparatide are manifest as an increase in skeletal mass, an increase in markers of bone formation and resorption, and an increase in bone strength. By contrast, continuous excess of endogenous PTH, as occurs in hyperparathyroidism, may be detrimental to the skeleton because bone resorption may be stimulated more than bone formation.

HUMAN PHARMACOKINETICS

Teriparatide is extensively absorbed after subcutaneous injection; the absolute bioavailability is approximately 95% based on pooled data from 20-, 40-, and 80 µg doses. The rates of absorption and elimination are rapid. The peptide reaches peak serum concentrations about 30 minutes after subcutaneous injection of a 20 µg dose and declines to non-quantifiable concentrations within 3 hours.

Systemic clearance of teriparatide (approximately 62 L/h in women and 94 L/h in men) exceeds the rate of normal liver plasma flow, consistent with both hepatic and extra-hepatic clearance. Volume of distribution, following intravenous injection, is approximately 0.12 L/kg. Intersubject variability in systemic clearance and volume of distribution is 25-50%. The half-life of teriparatide in serum is 5 minutes when administered by intravenous injection and approximately 1 hour when administered by subcutaneous injection. The longer half-life following subcutaneous administration reflects the time required for absorption from the injection site.

No metabolism or excretion studies have been performed with teriparatide. However, the mechanisms of metabolism and elimination of PTH(1-34) and intact PTH have been extensively described in published literature. Peripheral metabolism of PTH is believed to occur by non-specific enzymatic mechanisms in the liver followed by excretion via the kidneys.

SPECIAL POPULATIONS

Pediatric

Pharmacokinetic data in pediatric patients are not available (see WARNINGS).

Geriatric

No age-related differences in teriparatide pharmacokinetics were detected (range 31-85 years).

Gender

Although systemic exposure to teriparatide was approximately 20-30% lower in men than women, the recommended dose for both genders is 20 µg/day.

Race

The populations included in the pharmacokinetic analyses were 98.5% Caucasian. The influence of race has not been determined.

Renal Insufficiency

No pharmacokinetic differences were identified in 11 patients with mild or moderate renal insufficiency [creatinine clearance (CrCl) 30-72 ml/min] administered a single dose of teriparatide. In 5 patients with severe renal insufficiency (CrCl <30 ml/min), the AUC and T½ of teriparatide were increased by 73% and 77%, respectively. Maximum serum concentration of teriparatide was not increased. No studies have been performed in patients undergoing dialysis for chronic renal failure (see PRECAUTIONS).

Heart Failure

No clinically relevant pharmacokinetic, blood pressure, or pulse rate differences were identified in 13 patients with stable New York Heart Association Class I to III heart failure after the administration of two 20 µg doses of teriparatide.

Hepatic Insufficiency

Non-specific proteolytic enzymes in the liver (possibly Kupffer cells) cleave PTH(1-34) and PTH(1-84) into fragments that are cleared from the circulation mainly by the kidney. No studies have been performed in patients with hepatic impairment.

DRUG INTERACTIONS

Hydrochlorothiazide

In a study of 20 healthy people, the coadministration of hydrochlorothiazide 25 mg with teriparatide did not affect the serum calcium response to teriparatide 40 µg. The 24 hour urine excretion of calcium was reduced by a clinically unimportant amount (15%). The effect of coadministration of a higher dose of hydrochlorothiazide with teriparatide on serum calcium levels has not been studied.

Furosemide

In a study of 9 healthy people and 17 patients with mild, moderate, or severe renal insufficiency (CrCl 13-72 ml/min), coadministration of intravenous furosemide (20-100 mg) with teriparatide 40 µg resulted in small increases in the serum calcium (2%) and 24 hour urine calcium (37%) responses to teriparatide that did not appear to be clinically important.

HUMAN PHARMACODYNAMICS

Effects on Mineral Metabolism

Teriparatide affects calcium and phosphorus metabolism in a pattern consistent with the known actions of endogenous PTH (*e.g.,* increases serum calcium and decreases serum phosphorus).

Serum Calcium Concentrations

When teriparatide 20 µg is administered once daily, the serum calcium concentration increases transiently, beginning approximately 2 hours after dosing and reaching a maximum concentration between 4 and 6 hours (median increase, 0.4 mg/dl). The serum calcium concentration begins to decline approximately 6 hours after dosing and returns to baseline by 16-24 hours after each dose.

In a clinical study of postmenopausal women with osteoporosis, the median peak serum calcium concentration measured 4-6 hours after dosing with teriparatide 20 µg was 2.42 mmol/L (9.68 mg/dl) at 12 months. The peak serum calcium remained below 2.76 mmol/L (11.0 mg/dl) in >99% of women at each visit. Sustained hypercalcemia was not observed.

In this study, 11.1% of women treated with teriparatide had at least 1 serum calcium value above the upper limit of normal [2.64 mmol/L (10.6 mg/dl)] compared with 1.5% of women treated with placebo. The percentage of women treated with teriparatide whose serum calcium was above the upper limit of normal on consecutive 4-6 hour post-dose measurements was 3.0% compared with 0.2% of women treated with placebo. In these women, calcium supplements and/or teriparatide doses were reduced. The timing of these dose reductions was at the discretion of the investigator. Teriparatide dose adjustments were made at varying intervals after the first observation of increased serum calcium (median 21 weeks). During these intervals, there was no evidence of progressive increases in serum calcium.

In a clinical study of men with either primary or hypogonadal osteoporosis, the effects on serum calcium were similar to those observed in postmenopausal women. The median peak serum calcium concentration measured 4-6 hours after dosing with teriparatide was 2.35 mmol/L (9.44 mg/dl) at 12 months. The peak serum calcium remained below 2.76 mmol/L (11.0 mg/dl) in 98% of men at each visit. Sustained hypercalcemia was not observed.

In this study, 6.0% of men treated with teriparatide daily had at least 1 serum calcium value above the upper limit of normal [2.64 mmol/L (10.6 mg/dl)] compared with none of the men treated with placebo. The percentage of men treated with teriparatide whose serum calcium was above the upper limit of normal on consecutive measurements was 1.3% (2 men) compared with none of the men treated with placebo. Although calcium supplements and/or teriparatide doses could have been reduced in these men, only calcium supplementation was reduced (see PRECAUTIONS and ADVERSE REACTIONS).

In a clinical study of women previously treated for 18-39 months with raloxifene (n=26) or alendronate (n=33), mean serum calcium >12 hours after teriparatide injection was increased by 0.09-0.14 mmol/L (0.36-0.56 mg/dl), after 1-6 months of teriparatide treatment compared with baseline. Of the women pretreated with raloxifene, 3 (11.5%) had a serum calcium >2.76 mmol/L (11.0 mg/dl), and of those pretreated with alendronate, 3 (9.1%) had a serum calcium >2.76 mmol/L (11.0 mg/dl). The highest serum calcium reported was 3.12

mmol/L (12.5 mg/dl). None of the women had symptoms of hypercalcemia. There were no placebo controls in this study.

Urinary Calcium Excretion

In a clinical study of postmenopausal women with osteoporosis who received 1000 mg of supplemental calcium and at least 400 IU of vitamin D, daily teriparatide increased urinary calcium excretion. The median urinary excretion of calcium was 4.8 mmol/day (190 mg/day) at 6 months and 4.2 mmol/day (170 mg/day) at 12 months. These levels were 0.76 mmol/day (30 mg/day) and 0.30 mmol/day (12 mg/day) higher, respectively, than in women treated with placebo. The incidence of hypercalciuria (>7.5 mmol Ca/day or 300 mg/day) was similar in the women treated with teriparatide or placebo.

In a clinical study of men with either primary or hypogonadal osteoporosis who received 1000 mg of supplemental calcium and at least 400 IU of vitamin D, daily teriparatide had inconsistent effects on urinary calcium excretion. The median urinary excretion of calcium was 5.6 mmol/day (220 mg/day) at 1 month and 5.3 mmol/day (210 mg/day) at 6 months. These levels were 0.50 mmol/day (20 mg/day) higher and 0.20 mmol/day (8.0 mg/day) lower, respectively, than in men treated with placebo. The incidence of hypercalciuria (>7.5 mmol Ca/day or 300 mg/day) was similar in the men treated with teriparatide or placebo.

Phosphorus and Vitamin D

In single-dose studies, teriparatide produced transient phosphaturia and mild transient reductions in serum phosphorus concentration. However, hypophosphatemia (<0.74 mmol/L or 2.4 mg/dl) was not observed in clinical trials with teriparatide.

In clinical trials of daily teriparatide, the median serum concentration of 1,25-dihydroxyvitamin D was increased at 12 months by 19% in women and 14% in men, compared with baseline. In the placebo group, this concentration decreased by 2% in women and increased by 5% in men. The median serum 25-hydroxyvitamin D concentration at 12 months was decreased by 19% in women and 10% in men compared with baseline. In the placebo group, this concentration was unchanged in women and increased by 1% in men.

Effects on Markers of Bone Turnover

Daily administration of teriparatide to men and postmenopausal women with osteoporosis in clinical studies stimulated bone formation, as shown by increases in the formation markers serum bone-specific alkaline phosphatase (BSAP) and procollagen I carboxy-terminal propeptide (PICP). Data on biochemical markers of bone turnover were available for the first 12 months of treatment. Peak concentrations of PICP at 1 month of treatment were approximately 41% above baseline, followed by a decline to near-baseline values by 12 months. BSAP concentrations increased by 1 month of treatment and continued to rise more slowly from 6 through 12 months. The maximum increases of BSAP were 45% above baseline in women and 23% in men. After discontinuation of therapy, BSAP concentrations returned toward baseline. The increases in formation markers were accompanied by secondary increases in the markers of bone resorption: urinary N-telopeptide (NTX) and urinary deoxypyridinoline (DPD), consistent with the physiological coupling of bone formation and resorption in skeletal remodeling. Changes in BSAP, NTX, and DPD were lower in men than in women, possibly because of lower systemic exposure to teriparatide in men.

INDICATIONS AND USAGE

Teriparatide is indicated for the treatment of postmenopausal women with osteoporosis who are at high risk for fracture. These include women with a history of osteoporotic fracture, or who have multiple risk factors for fracture, or who have failed or are intolerant of previous osteoporosis therapy, based upon physician assessment (see BOXED WARNING). In postmenopausal women with osteoporosis, teriparatide increases BMD and reduces the risk of vertebral and nonvertebral fractures.

Teriparatide is indicated to increase bone mass in men with primary or hypogonadal osteoporosis who are at high risk for fracture. These include men with a history of osteoporotic fracture, or who have multiple risk factors for fracture, or who have failed or are intolerant to previous osteoporosis therapy, based upon physician assessment (see BOXED WARNING). In men with primary or hypogonadal osteoporosis, teriparatide increases BMD. The effects of teriparatide on risk for fracture in men have not been studied.

- Teriparatide reduces the risk of vertebral fractures in postmenopausal women with osteoporosis.
- Teriparatide reduces the risk of nonvertebral fractures in postmenopausal women with osteoporosis.
- Teriparatide increases vertebral and femoral neck BMD in postmenopausal women with osteoporosis and in men with primary or hypogonadal osteoporosis.
- The effects of teriparatide on fracture risk have not been studied in men.

CONTRAINDICATIONS

Teriparatide should not be given to patients with hypersensitivity to teriparatide or to any of its excipients.

WARNINGS

In male and female rats, teriparatide caused an increase in the incidence of osteosarcoma (a malignant bone tumor) that was dependent on dose and treatment duration (see BOXED WARNING and PRECAUTIONS, Carcinogenesis, Mutagenesis, and Impairment of Fertility, Carcinogenesis).

The following categories of patients have increased baseline risk of osteosarcoma and therefore should not be treated with teriparatide:

Paget's disease of bone: Teriparatide should not be given to patients with Paget's disease of bone. Unexplained elevations of alkaline phosphatase may indicate Paget's disease of bone.

Pediatric populations: Teriparatide has not been studied in pediatric populations. Teriparatide should not be used in pediatric patients or young adults with open epiphyses.

Prior radiation therapy: Patients with a prior history of radiation therapy involving the skeleton should be excluded from treatment with teriparatide.

Patients with bone metastases or a history of skeletal malignancies should be excluded from treatment with teriparatide.

Patients with metabolic bone diseases other than osteoporosis should be excluded from treatment with teriparatide.

Teriparatide has not been studied in patients with pre-existing hypercalcemia. These patients should be excluded from treatment with teriparatide because of the possibility of exacerbating hypercalcemia.

PRECAUTIONS

GENERAL

The safety and efficacy of teriparatide have not been evaluated beyond 2 years of treatment. Consequently, use of the drug for more than 2 years is not recommended.

In clinical trials, the frequency of urolithiasis was similar in patients treated with teriparatide and placebo. However, teriparatide has not been studied in patients with active urolithiasis. If active urolithiasis or pre-existing hypercalcemia are suspected, measurement of urinary calcium excretion should be considered. Teriparatide should be used with caution in patients with active or recent urolithiasis because of the potential to exacerbate this condition.

Hypotension

In short-term clinical pharmacology studies with teriparatide, transient episodes of symptomatic orthostatic hypotension were observed infrequently. Typically, an event began within 4 hours of dosing and spontaneously resolved within a few minutes to a few hours. When transient orthostatic hypotension occurred, it happened within the first several doses, it was relieved by placing the person in a reclining position, and it did not preclude continued treatment.

Concomitant Treatment With Digitalis

In a study of 15 healthy people administered digoxin daily to steady state, a single teriparatide dose did not alter the effect of digoxin on the systolic time interval (from electrocardiographic Q-wave onset to aortic valve closure, a measure of digoxin's calcium-mediated cardiac effect). However, sporadic case reports have suggested that hypercalcemia may predispose patients to digitalis toxicity. Because teriparatide transiently increases serum calcium, teriparatide should be used with caution in patients taking digitalis.

Hepatic, Renal, and Cardiac

Limited information is available to evaluate safety in patients with hepatic, renal, and cardiac disease.

INFORMATION FOR THE PATIENT

For safe and effective use of teriparatide, the physician should inform patients about the following:

General: Patients should read the Medication Guide and pen User Manual before starting therapy with teriparatide and re-read them each time the prescription is renewed.

Osteosarcomas in Rats: Patients should be made aware that teriparatide caused osteosarcomas in rats and that the clinical relevance of these findings is unknown.

Orthostatic Hypotension: Teriparatide should be administered initially under circumstances where the patient can immediately sit or lie down if symptoms occur. Patients should be instructed that if they feel lightheaded or have palpitations after the injection, they should sit or lie down until the symptoms resolve. If symptoms persist or worsen, patients should be instructed to consult a physician before continuing treatment (see PRECAUTIONS, General).

Hypercalcemia: Although symptomatic hypercalcemia was not observed in clinical trials, physicians should instruct patients to contact a health care provider if they develop persistent symptoms of hypercalcemia (*i.e.*, nausea, vomiting, constipation, lethargy, muscle weakness).

Use of the Pen: Patients should be instructed on how to properly use the delivery device (refer to User Manual), properly dispose of needles, and be advised not to share their pens with other patients.

Other Osteoporosis Treatments: Patients should be informed regarding the roles of supplemental calcium and/or vitamin D, weight-bearing exercise, and modification of certain behavioral factors such as cigarette smoking and/or alcohol consumption.

LABORATORY TESTS

Serum Calcium

Teriparatide transiently increases serum calcium, with the maximal effect observed at approximately 4-6 hours post-dose. By 16 hours post-dose, serum calcium generally has returned to or near baseline. These effects should be kept in mind because serum calcium concentrations observed within 16 hours after a dose may reflect the pharmacologic effect of teriparatide. Persistent hypercalcemia was not observed in clinical trials with teriparatide. If persistent hypercalcemia is detected, treatment with teriparatide should be discontinued pending further evaluation of the cause of hypercalcemia.

Patients known to have an underlying hypercalcemic disorder, such as primary hyperparathyroidism, should not be treated with teriparatide (see WARNINGS).

Urinary Calcium

Teriparatide increases urinary calcium excretion, but the frequency of hypercalciuria in clinical trials was similar for patients treated with teriparatide and placebo (see CLINICAL PHARMACOLOGY, Human Pharmacodynamics).

Renal Function

No clinically important adverse renal effects were observed in clinical studies. Assessments included creatinine clearance; measurements of blood urea nitrogen (BUN), creatinine, and electrolytes in serum; urine specific gravity and pH; and examination of urine sediment. Long-term evaluation of patients with severe renal insufficiency, patients undergoing acute or chronic dialysis, or patients who have functioning renal transplants has not been performed.

T

Serum Uric Acid

Teriparatide increases serum uric acid concentrations. In clinical trials, 2.8% of teriparatide patients had serum uric acid concentrations above the upper limit of normal compared with 0.7% of placebo patients. However, the hyperuricemia did not result in an increase in gout, arthralgia, or urolithiasis.

CARCINOGENESIS, MUTAGENESIS, AND IMPAIRMENT OF FERTILITY

Carcinogenesis

Two carcinogenicity bioassays were conducted in Fischer 344 rats. In the first study, male and female rats were given daily subcutaneous teriparatide injections of 5, 30, or 75 μg/kg/day for 24 months from 2 months of age. These doses resulted in systemic exposures that were, respectively, 3, 20, and 60 times higher than the systemic exposure observed in humans following a subcutaneous dose of 20 μg (based on AUC comparison). Teriparatide treatment resulted in a marked dose-related increase in the incidence of osteosarcoma, a rare malignant bone tumor, in both male and female rats. Osteosarcomas were observed at all doses and the incidence reached 40-50% in the high-dose groups. Teriparatide also caused a dose-related increase in osteoblastoma and osteoma in both sexes. No osteosarcomas, osteoblastomas or osteomas were observed in untreated control rats. The bone tumors in rats occurred in association with a large increase in bone mass and focal osteoblast hyperplasia.

The second 2 year study was carried out in order to determine the effect of treatment duration and animal age on the development of bone tumors. Female rats were treated for different periods between 2 and 26 months of age with subcutaneous doses of 5 and 30 μg/kg (equivalent to 3 and 20 times the human exposure at the 20 μg dose, based on AUC comparison). The study showed that the occurrence of osteosarcoma, osteoblastoma and osteoma was dependent upon dose and duration of exposure. Bone tumors were observed when immature 2 month old rats were treated with 30 μg/kg/day for 24 months or with 5 or 30 μg/kg/day for 6 months. Bone tumors were also observed when mature 6 month old rats were treated with 30 μg/kg/day for 6 or 20 months. Tumors were not detected when mature 6 month old rats were treated with 5 μg/kg/day for 6 or 20 months. The results did not demonstrate a difference in susceptibility to bone tumor formation, associated with teriparatide treatment, between mature and immature rats.

The relevance of these rat findings to humans is uncertain.

Mutagenesis

Teriparatide was not genotoxic in any of the following test systems: the Ames test for bacterial mutagenesis; the mouse lymphoma assay for mammalian cell mutation; the chromosomal aberration assay in Chinese hamster ovary cells, with and without metabolic activation; and the in vivo micronucleus test in mice.

Impairment of Fertility

No effects on fertility were observed in male and female rats given subcutaneous teriparatide doses of 30, 100, or 300 μg/kg/day prior to mating and in females continuing through gestation Day 6 (16-160 times the human dose of 20 μg based on surface area, μg/m^2).

PREGNANCY CATEGORY C

In pregnant rats given subcutaneous teriparatide doses up to 1000 μg/kg/day, there were no findings. In pregnant mice given subcutaneous doses of 225 or 1000 μg/kg/day (≥60 times the human dose based on surface area, μg/m^2) from gestation Day 6 through 15, the fetuses showed an increased incidence of skeletal deviations or variations (interrupted rib, extra vertebra or rib).

Developmental effects in a perinatal/postnatal study in pregnant rats given subcutaneous doses of teriparatide from gestation Day 6 through postpartum Day 20 included mild growth retardation in female offspring at doses ≥225 μg/kg/day (≥120 times the human dose based on surface area, μg/m^2), and in male offspring at 1000 μg/kg/day (540 times the human dose based on surface area, μg/m^2). There was also reduced motor activity in both male and female offspring at 1000 μg/kg/day. There were no developmental or reproductive effects in mice or rats at a dose of 30 μg/kg (8 or 16 times the human dose based on surface area, μg/m^2). The effect of teriparatide treatment on human fetal development has not been studied. Teriparatide is not indicated for use in pregnancy.

NURSING MOTHERS

Because teriparatide is indicated for the treatment of osteoporosis in postmenopausal women, it should not be administered to women who are nursing their children. There have been no clinical studies to determine if teriparatide is secreted into breast milk.

PEDIATRIC USE

The safety and efficacy of teriparatide have not been established in pediatric populations. Teriparatide is not indicated for use in pediatric patients (see WARNINGS).

GERIATRIC USE

Of the patients receiving teriparatide in the osteoporosis trial of 1637 postmenopausal women, 75% were 65 years of age and over and 23% were 75 years of age and over. Of the patients receiving teriparatide in the osteoporosis trial of 437 men, 39% were 65 years of age and over and 13% were 75 years of age and over. No significant differences in bone response or adverse reactions were seen in geriatric patients receiving teriparatide as compared with younger patients. Nonetheless, as with many medications, elderly patients may have greater sensitivity to the adverse effects of teriparatide.

ADVERSE REACTIONS

The safety of teriparatide has been evaluated in 24 clinical trials that enrolled over 2800 women and men. Four long-term Phase 3 clinical trials included 1 large placebo-controlled, double-blind, multinational trial with 1637 postmenopausal women; 1 placebo-controlled, double-blind, multinational trial with 437 men; and 2 active-controlled trials including 393 postmenopausal women. Teriparatide doses ranged from 5-100 μg/day in short-term trials and 20-40 μg/day in the other trials. A total of 1943 of the patients studied received teriparatide, including 815 patients at 20 μg/day and 1107 patients at 40 μg/day. In the clinical trials, a total of 1432 patients were treated with teriparatide for 3 months to 2 years, of whom 1137 were treated for greater than 1 year (500 at 20 μg/day and 637 at 40 μg/day). The maximum duration of treatment was 2 years. Adverse events associated with teriparatide usually were mild and generally did not require discontinuation of therapy.

In the two Phase 3 placebo-controlled clinical trials in men and postmenopausal women, early discontinuation due to adverse events occurred in 5.6% of patients assigned to placebo and 7.1% of patients assigned to teriparatide. Reported adverse events that appeared to be increased by teriparatide treatment were dizziness and leg cramps.

TABLE 5 lists adverse events that occurred in the two Phase 3 placebo-controlled clinical trials in men and postmenopausal women at a frequency ≥2.0% in the teriparatide groups and in more teriparatide-treated patients than in placebo-treated patients, without attribution of causality.

TABLE 5 *Percentage of Patients With Adverse Events Reported by at Least 2% of Teriparatide-Treated Patients and in More Teriparatide-Treated Patients Than Placebo-Treated Patients From the Two Principal Osteoporosis Trials in Women and Men**

Event Classification	Teriparatide n=691	Placebo n=691
Body as a Whole		
Pain	21.3%	20.5%
Headache	7.5%	7.4%
Asthenia	8.7%	6.8%
Neck pain	3.0%	2.7%
Cardiovascular		
Hypertension	7.1%	6.8%
Angina pectoris	2.5%	1.6%
Syncope	2.6%	1.4%
Digestive System		
Nausea	8.5%	6.7%
Constipation	5.4%	4.5%
Diarrhea	5.1%	4.6%
Dyspepsia	5.2%	4.1%
Vomiting	3.0%	2.3%
Gastrointestinal disorder	2.3%	2.0%
Tooth disorder	2.0%	1.3%
Musculoskeletal		
Arthralgia	10.1%	8.4%
Leg Cramps	2.6%	1.3%
Nervous System		
Dizziness	8.0%	5.4%
Depression	4.1%	2.7%
Insomnia	4.3%	3.6%
Vertigo	3.8%	2.7%
Respiratory System		
Rhinitis	9.6%	8.8%
Cough increased	6.4%	5.5%
Pharyngitis	5.5%	4.8%
Dyspnea	3.6%	2.6%
Pneumonia	3.9%	3.3%
Skin and Appendages		
Rash	4.9%	4.5%
Sweating	2.2%	1.7%

* Adverse events are shown without attribution of causality.

SERUM CALCIUM

Teriparatide transiently increases serum calcium, with the maximal effect observed at approximately 4-6 hours post-dose. Serum calcium measured at least 16 hours post-dose was not different from pretreatment levels. In clinical trials, the frequency of at least 1 episode of transient hypercalcemia in the 4-6 hours after teriparatide administration was increased from 1.5% of women and none of the men treated with placebo to 11.1% of women and 6.0% of men treated with teriparatide. The number of patients treated with teriparatide whose transient hypercalcemia was verified on consecutive measurements was 3.0% of women and 1.3% of men.

IMMUNOGENICITY

In a large clinical trial, antibodies that cross-reacted with teriparatide were detected in 2.8% of women receiving teriparatide. Generally, antibodies were first detected following 12 months of treatment and diminished after withdrawal of therapy. There was no evidence of hypersensitivity reactions, allergic reactions, effects on serum calcium, or effects on BMD response.

DOSAGE AND ADMINISTRATION

Teriparatide should be administered as a subcutaneous injection into the thigh or abdominal wall. The recommended dosage is 20 μg once a day.

Teriparatide should be administered initially under circumstances in which the patient can sit or lie down if symptoms of orthostatic hypotension occur (see PRECAUTIONS, Information for the Patient).

Teriparatide is a clear and colorless liquid. Do not use if solid particles appear or if the solution is cloudy or colored. The teriparatide pen should not be used past the stated expiration date.

No data are available on the safety or efficacy of intravenous or intramuscular injection of teriparatide.

The safety and efficacy of teriparatide have not been evaluated beyond 2 years of treatment. Consequently, use of the drug for more than 2 years is not recommended.

INSTRUCTIONS FOR PEN USE

Patients and caregivers who administer teriparatide should receive appropriate training and instruction on the proper use of the teriparatide pen from a qualified health professional. It is important to read, understand, and follow the instructions in the teriparatide pen User Manual for priming the pen and dosing. Failure to do so may result in inaccurate dosing. Each teriparatide pen can be used for up to 28 days after the first injection. After the 28 day use period, discard the teriparatide pen, even if it still contains some unused solution. Never share a teriparatide pen.

HOW SUPPLIED

The Forteo pen is available as one 3 ml prefilled pen delivery device.

STORAGE

The Forteo pen should be stored under refrigeration at 2-8°C (36-46°F) at all times. Recap the pen when not in use to protect the cartridge from physical damage and light. During the use period, time out of the refrigerator should be minimized; the dose may be delivered immediately following removal from the refrigerator.

Do not freeze. Do not use Forteo if it has been frozen.

PRODUCT LISTING - EQUIVALENTS NOT AVAILABLE

Device - Subcutaneous - 750 mcg/3 ml

1's $583.34 FORTEO, Lilly, Eli and Company 00002-8971-01

Testolactone *(002317)*

For complete prescribing information, refer to the CD-ROM included with the book.

Categories: Carcinoma, breast; Pregnancy Category C; FDA Approved 1970 May
Drug Classes: Antineoplastics, aromatase inhibitors; Hormones/hormone modifiers
Brand Names: Fludestrin; **Teslac**
Cost of Therapy: $1,342.26 (Breast Cancer; Teslac; 50 mg; 20 tablets/day; 30 day supply)

DESCRIPTION

Teslac is available for oral administration as tablets providing 50 mg testolactone per tablet. Testolactone is a synthetic antineoplastic agent that is structurally distinct from the androgen steroid nucleus in possessing a six-membered lactone ring in place of the usual five-membered carbocyclic D-ring. Testolactone is chemically designated as 13-hydroxy-3-oxo-13,17-secoandrosta-1,4-dien-17-oic acid δ-lactone. The empirical formula is $C_{19}H_{24}O_3$. The molecular weight is 300.40.
Inactive Ingredients: Calcium stearate, cornstarch, gelatin, and lactose.
Testolactone is a white, odorless, crystalline solid, soluble in ethanol and slightly soluble in water.

INDICATIONS AND USAGE

Testolactone is recommended as adjunctive therapy in the palliative treatment of advanced or disseminated breast cancer in postmenopausal women when hormonal therapy is indicated. It may also be used in women who were diagnosed as having had disseminated breast carcinoma when premenopausal, in whom ovarian function has been subsequently terminated.

Testolactone was found to be effective in approximately 15% of patients with advanced or disseminated mammary cancer evaluated according to the following criteria: (1) those with a measurable decrease in size of all demonstrable tumor masses; (2) those in whom more than 50% of non-osseous lesions decreased in size although all bone lesions remained static; and (3) those in whom more than 50% of total lesions improved while the remainder were static.

NON-FDA APPROVED INDICATIONS

When used to treat familial male precocious puberty in one small study (n=9), the combination of spironolactone and testolactone has been reported to restore the growth rate and the rate of bone maturation to normal prepubertal levels, and to control acne, spontaneous erections, and aggressive behavior. However, use of this combination for the treatment of familial male precocious puberty has not been approved by the FDA and a significant amount of additional studies are needed before this combination of drugs can be recommended for this indication.

CONTRAINDICATIONS

Testolactone is contraindicated in the treatment of breast cancer in men and in patients with a history of hypersensitivity to the drug.

DOSAGE AND ADMINISTRATION

The recommended oral dose is 250 mg qid.

In order to evaluate the response, therapy with testolactone should be continued for a minimum of 3 months unless there is active progression of the disease.

PRODUCT LISTING - EQUIVALENTS NOT AVAILABLE

Tablet - Oral - 50 mg

100's $223.71 TESLAC, Bristol-Myers Squibb 00003-0690-50

Testosterone Cypionate *(002319)*

Categories: Hypogonadism, male, hypogonadotropic; Hypogonadism, male, primary; Pregnancy Category X; DEA Class CIII; FDA Approved 1979 Jul
Drug Classes: Androgens; Hormones/hormone modifiers
Brand Names: Andro-Cyp; Andronaq-La; D-Tes; Dep-Andro; **Depo-Testosterone**; Depotest; Dura-Testosterone; Duratest; Med-itest; Shotest; T-Cypionate; Testa-C; Testaspan; Testoject; Testred Cypionate 200; Vigorex; Virilon Im
Foreign Brand Availability: Depot Hormon-M (Taiwan)
HCFA JCODE(S): J1070 up to 100 mg IM; J1080 1 cc, 200 mg IM; J1090 1 cc, 50 mg IM

DESCRIPTION

Depo-Testosterone sterile solution, for intramuscular injection, contains testosterone cypionate which is the oil-soluble 17 (beta)-cyclopentylpropionate ester of the androgenic hormone testosterone.

Testosterone cypionate is a white or creamy white crystalline powder, odorless or nearly so and stable in air. It is insoluble in water, freely soluble in alcohol, chloroform, dioxane, ether, and soluble in vegetable oils.

The chemical name for testosterone cypionate is androst-4-en-3-one, 17-(3-cyclopentyl-1-oxopropoxy)-, (17β)-. Its molecular formula is $C_{27}H_{40}O_3$, and the molecular weight 412.61.

Depo-Testosterone is available in two strengths, 100 mg/ml and 200 mg/ml testosterone cypionate.
Each ml of the 100 mg/ml Solution Contains: *Testosterone Cypionate:* 100 mg. *Benzyl Benzoate:* 0.1 ml.*Cottonseed Oil:* 736 mg.*Benzyl Alcohol (as Preservative):* 9.45 mg.
Each ml of the 200 mg/ml Solution Contains: *Testosterone Cypionate:* 200 mg. *Benzyl Benzoate:* 0.2 ml.*Cottonseed Oil:* 560 mg.*Benzyl Alcohol (as Preservative):* 9.45 mg.
Storage: Vials should be stored at controlled room temperature 20-25°C (68-77°F). Protect from light.

CLINICAL PHARMACOLOGY

Endogenous androgens are responsible for normal growth and development of the male sex organs and for maintenance of secondary sex characteristics. These effects include growth and maturation of the prostate, seminal vesicles, penis, and scrotum; development of male hair distribution, such as beard, pubic, chest, and axillary hair; laryngeal enlargement, vocal cord thickening, and alterations in body musculature and fat distribution. Drugs in this class also cause retention of nitrogen, sodium, potassium, and phosphorous, and decreased urinary excretion of calcium. Androgens have been reported to increase protein anabolism and decrease protein catabolism. Nitrogen balance is improved only when there is sufficient intake of calories and protein.

Androgens are responsible for the growth spurt of adolescence and for eventual termination of linear growth, brought about by fusion of the epiphyseal growth centers. In children, exogenous androgens accelerate linear growth rates, but may cause disproportionate advancement in bone maturation. Use over long periods may result in fusion of the epiphyseal growth centers and termination of the growth process. Androgens have been reported to stimulate production of red blood cells by enhancing production of erythropoietic stimulation factor.

During exogenous administration of androgens, endogenous testosterone release is inhibited through feedback inhibition of pituitary luteinizing hormone (LH). At large doses of exogenous androgens, spermatogenesis may also be suppressed through feedback inhibition of pituitary follicle stimulating hormone (FSH).

There is a lack of substantial evidence that androgens are effective in fractures, surgery, convalescence, and functional uterine bleeding.

PHARMACOKINETICS

Testosterone esters are less polar than free testosterone. Testosterone esters in oil injected intramuscularly are absorbed slowly from the lipid phase; thus, testosterone cypionate can be given at intervals of 2-4 weeks.

Testosterone in plasma is 98% bound to a specific testosterone-estradiol binding globulin, and about 2% is free. Generally, the amount of this sex-hormone binding globulin in the plasma will determine the distribution of testosterone between free and bound forms, and the free testosterone concentration will determine its half-life.

About 90% of a dose of testosterone is excreted in the urine as glucuronic and sulfuric acid conjugates of testosterone and its metabolites; about 6% of a dose is excreted in the feces, mostly in the unconjugated form. Inactivation of testosterone occurs primarily in the liver. Testosterone is metabolized to various 17-keto steroids through two different pathways.

The half-life of testosterone cypionate when injected intramuscularly is approximately 8 days.

In many tissues the activity of testosterone appears to depend on reduction to dihydrotestosterone, which binds to cytosol receptor proteins. The steroid-receptor complex is transported to the nucleus where it initiates transcription events and cellular changes related to androgen action.

INDICATIONS AND USAGE

Testosterone cypionate sterile solution is indicated for replacement therapy in the male in conditions associated with symptoms of deficiency or absence of endogenous testosterone.

1. Primary hypogonadism (congenital or acquired)-testicular failure due to cryptorchidism, bilateral torsion, orchitis, vanishing testis syndrome; or orchidectomy.
2. Hypogonadotropic hypogonadism (congenital or acquired)-idiopathic gonadotropin or LHRH deficiency, or pituitary-hypothalamic injury from tumors, trauma, or radiation.

CONTRAINDICATIONS

1. Known hypersensitivity to the drug.
2. Males with carcinoma of the breast.
3. Males with known or suspected carcinoma of the prostate gland.

T

4. Women who are or who may become pregnant.
5. Patients with serious cardiac, hepatic or renal disease.

WARNINGS

Hypercalcemia may occur in immobilized patients. If this occurs, the drug should be discontinued.

Prolonged use of high doses of androgens (principally the 17-αalkyl-androgens) has been associated with development of hepatic adenomas, hepatocellular carcinoma, and peliosis hepatis—all potentially life-threatening complications.

Geriatric patients treated with androgens may be at an increased risk of developing prostatic hypertrophy and prostatic carcinoma although conclusive evidence to support this concept is lacking.

Edema, with or without congestive heart failure, may be a serious complication in patients with pre-existing cardiac, renal or hepatic disease.

Gynecomastia may develop and occasionally persists in patients being treated for hypogonadism.

This product contains benzyl alcohol. Benzyl alcohol has been reported to be associated with a fatal "Gasping Syndrome" in premature infants.

Androgen therapy should be used cautiously in healthy males with delayed puberty. The effect on bone maturation should be monitored by assessing bone age of the wrist and hand every 6 months. In children, androgen treatment may accelerate bone maturation without producing compensatory gain in linear growth. This adverse effect may result in compromised adult stature. The younger the child the greater the risk of compromising final mature height.

This drug has not been shown to be safe and effective for the enhancement of athletic performance. Because of the potential risk of serious adverse health effects, this drug should not be used for such purpose.

PRECAUTIONS

GENERAL

Patients with benign prostatic hypertrophy may develop acute urethral obstruction. Priapism or excessive sexual stimulation may develop. Oligospermia may occur after prolonged administration or excessive dosage. If any of these effects appear, the androgen should be stopped and if restarted, a lower dosage should be utilized.

Testosterone cypionate should not be used interchangeably with testosterone propionate because of differences in duration of action.

Testosterone cypionate *is not* for intravenous use.

INFORMATION FOR THE PATIENT

Patients should be instructed to report any of the following: nausea, vomiting, changes in skin color, ankle swelling, too frequent or persistent erections of the penis.

LABORATORY TESTS

Hemoglobin and hematocrit levels (to detect polycythemia) should be checked periodically in patients receiving long-term androgen administration.

Serum cholesterol may increase during androgen therapy.

DRUG/LABORATORY TEST INTERACTIONS

Androgens may decrease levels of thyroxine-binding globulin, resulting in decreased total T_4 serum levels and increased resin uptake of T_3 and T_4. Free thyroid hormone levels remain unchanged, however, and there is no clinical evidence of thyroid dysfunction.

CARCINOGENESIS

Animal Data

Testosterone has been tested by subcutaneous injection and implantation in mice and rats. The implant induced cervical-uterine tumors in mice, which metastasized in some cases. There is suggestive evidence that injection of testosterone into some strains of female mice increases their susceptibility to hepatoma. Testosterone is also known to increase the number of tumors and decrease the degree of differentiation of chemically-induced carcinomas of the liver in rats.

Human Data

There are rare reports of hepatocellular carcinoma in patients receiving long-term therapy with androgens in high doses. Withdrawal of the drugs did not lead to regression of the tumors in all cases.

Geriatric patients treated with androgens may be at an increased risk of developing prostatic hypertrophy and prostatic carcinoma although conclusive evidence to support this concept is lacking.

PREGNANCY, TERATOGENIC EFFECTS, PREGNANCY CATEGORY X

See CONTRAINDICATIONS.

NURSING MOTHERS

Testosterone cypionate is not recommended for use in nursing mothers.

PEDIATRIC USE

Safety and effectiveness in pediatric patients below the age of 12 years have not been established.

DRUG INTERACTIONS

Androgens may increase sensitivity to oral anticoagulants. Dosage of the anticoagulant may require reduction in order to maintain satisfactory therapeutic hypoprothrombinemia.

Concurrent administration of oxyphenbutazone and androgens may result in elevated serum levels of oxyphenbutazone.

In diabetic patients, the metabolic effects of androgens may decrease blood glucose and, therefore, insulin requirements.

ADVERSE REACTIONS

The following adverse reactions in the male have occurred with some androgens:

Endocrine and Urogenital: Gynecomastia and excessive frequency and duration of penile erections. Oligospermia may occur at high dosages.

Skin and Appendages: Hirsutism, male pattern of baldness, seborrhea, and acne.

Fluid and Electrolyte Disturbances: Retention of sodium, chloride, water, potassium, calcium, and inorganic phosphates.

Gastrointestinal: Nausea, cholestatic jaundice, alterations in liver function tests, rarely hepatocellular neoplasms, and peliosis hepatis (see WARNINGS).

Hematologic Suppression of clotting factors II, V, VII, and X, bleeding in patients on concomitant anticoagulant therapy, and polycythemia.

Nervous System: Increased or decreased libido, headache, anxiety, depression, and generalized paresthesia.

Allergic: Hypersensitivity, including skin manifestations and anaphylactoid reactions.

Miscellaneous: Inflammation and pain at the site of intramuscular injection.

DOSAGE AND ADMINISTRATION

Testosterone cypionate sterile solution is for intramuscular use only.

It should not be given intravenously. Intramuscular injections should be given deep in the gluteal muscle.

The suggested dosage for testosterone cypionate sterile solution varies depending on the age, sex, and diagnosis of the individual patient. Dosage is adjusted according to the patient's response and the appearance of adverse reactions.

Various dosage regimens have been used to induce pubertal changes in hypogonadal males; some experts have advocated lower dosages initially, gradually increasing the dose as puberty progresses, with or without a decrease to maintenance levels. Other experts emphasize that higher dosages are needed to induce pubertal changes and lower dosages can be used for maintenance after puberty. The chronological and skeletal ages must be taken into consideration, both in determining the initial dose and in adjusting the dose.

For replacement in the hypogonadal male, 50-400 mg should be administered every 2-4 weeks.

Parenteral drug products should be inspected visually for particulate matter and discoloration prior to administration, whenever solution and container permit. Warming and shaking the vial should redissolve any crystals that may have formed during storage at temperatures lower than recommended.

PRODUCT LISTING - RATED THERAPEUTICALLY EQUIVALENT

Solution - Intramuscular - Cypionate 100 mg/ml

10 ml	$15.05	GENERIC, Geneva Pharmaceuticals	00781-3096-70
10 ml	$15.75	GENERIC, Watson/Rugby Laboratories Inc	00536-9480-70
10 ml	$54.23	DEPO-TESTOSTERONE, Pharmacia and Upjohn	00009-0347-02

Solution - Intramuscular - Cypionate 200 mg/ml

1 ml	$22.31	DEPO-TESTOSTERONE, Pharmacia and Upjohn	00009-0417-01
10 ml	$20.75	GENERIC, Geneva Pharmaceuticals	00781-3097-70
10 ml	$103.46	DEPO-TESTOSTERONE, Pharmacia and Upjohn	00009-0417-02

Tetanus Immune Globulin *(002323)*

For complete prescribing information, refer to the CD-ROM included with the book.

Categories: Immunization, tetanus; Pregnancy Category C; FDA Pre 1938 Drugs; WHO Formulary
Drug Classes: Immune globulins
Brand Names: Hyper-Tet; **Hypertet**
Foreign Brand Availability: BayTet (Canada; Israel; Philippines); IG tetano/tetanus immune globulin (Israel; Philippines); Tetabulin (Austria; Hong-Kong; Italy; Korea; Switzerland); Tetabuline (Belgium); Tetagam (Germany; Indonesia; South-Africa); Tetagam-P (Greece); Tetagamma (Italy); Tetaglobulin (Germany); Tetaglobuline (Benin; Burkina-Faso; Ethiopia; Gambia; Ghana; Guinea; Israel; Ivory-Coast; Kenya; Liberia; Malawi; Malaysia; Mali; Mauritania; Mauritius; Morocco; Niger; Nigeria; Philippines; Senegal; Seychelles; Sierra-Leone; Sudan; Tanzania; Thailand; Tunia; Uganda; Zambia; Zimbabwe); Tetagloman (Austria); Tetamyn enzimatico liofilizado (Mexico); Tetanobulin (Taiwan); Tetanogamma (Dominican-Republic); Tetanosson (Greece); Tetuman berna (Hong-Kong; Malaysia; Peru; Philippines; South-Africa)
HCFA JCODE(S): J1670 up to 250 units IM

DESCRIPTION

Tetanus immune globulin (human)—BayTet treated with solvent/detergent is a sterile solution of tetanus hyperimmune immune globulin for intramuscular administration; it contains no preservative. BayTet is prepared by cold ethanol fractionation from the plasma of donors immunized with tetanus toxoid. The immune globulin is isolated from solubilized Cohn Fraction II. The Fraction II solution is adjusted to a final concentration of 0.3% tri-n-butyl phosphate (TNBP) and 0.2% sodium cholate. After the addition of solvent (TNBP) and detergent (sodium cholate), the solution is heated to 30°C and maintained at that temperature for not less than 6 hours. After the viral inactivation step, the reactants are removed by precipitation, filtration and finally ultrafiltration and diafiltration. BayTet is formulated as a 15-18% protein solution at a pH of 6.4-7.2 in 0.21-0.32 M glycine. BayTet is then incubated in the final container for 21-28 days at 20-27°C. The product is standardized against the US Standard Antitoxin and the US Control Tetanus Toxin and contains not less than 250 tetanus antitoxin units per container.

The removal and inactivation of spiked model enveloped and non-enveloped viruses during the manufacturing process for BayTet has been validated in laboratory studies. Human Immunodeficiency Virus, Type 1 (HIV-1), was chosen as the relevant virus for blood products; Bovine Viral Diarrhea Virus (BVDV) was chosen to model Hepatitis C virus; Pseudorabies virus (PRV) was chosen to model Hepatitis B virus and the Herpes viruses; and Reo virus type 3 (Reo) was chosen to model non-enveloped viruses and for its resistance to physical and chemical inactivation. Significant removal of model enveloped and non-

enveloped viruses is achieved at two steps in the Cohn fractionation process leading to the collection of Cohn Fraction II: the precipitation and removal of Fraction III in the processing of Fraction II + IIIW suspension to Effluent III and the filtration step in the processing of Effluent III to Filtrate III. Significant inactivation of enveloped viruses is achieved at the time of treatment of solubilized Cohn Fraction II with TNBP/sodium cholate.
Storage: Store at 2-8°C (36-46°F). Solution that has been frozen should not be used.

INDICATIONS AND USAGE

Tetanus immune globulin is indicated for prophylaxis against tetanus following injury in patients whose immunization is incomplete or uncertain. It is also indicated, although evidence of effectiveness is limited, in the regimen of treatment of active cases of tetanus.[7,8,15]

A thorough attempt must be made to determine whether a patient has completed primary vaccination. Patients with unknown or uncertain previous vaccination histories should be considered to have had no previous tetanus toxoid doses. Persons who had military service since 1941 can be considered to have received at least 1 dose, and although most of them may have completed a primary series of tetanus toxoid, this cannot be assumed for each individual. Patients who have not completed a primary series may require tetanus toxoid and passive immunization at the time of wound cleaning and debridement.[2]

TABLE 1 is a summary guide to tetanus prophylaxis in wound management:

TABLE 1 *Guide to Tetanus Prophylaxis in Wound Management*[2]

History of Tetanus Immunization (Doses)	Clean, Minor Wounds		All Other Wounds*	
	Td†	TIG‡	Td	TIG
Uncertain or less than 3	Yes	No	Yes	Yes
3 or more§	No‖	No	No¶	No

* Such as, but not limited to, wounds contaminated with dirt, feces, soil, and saliva; puncture wounds; avulsions; and wounds resulting from missiles, crushing, burns and frostbite.
† Adult type tetanus and diphtheria toxoids. If the patient is less than 7 years old, DT or DTP is preferred to tetanus toxoid alone. For persons ≥7 years of age, Td is preferred to tetanus toxoid alone. (see DOSAGE AND ADMINISTRATION).
‡ Tetanus Immune Globulin (Human).
§ If only 3 doses of fluid tetanus toxoid have been received, a fourth dose of toxoid, preferably an absorbed toxoid, should be given.
‖ Yes if more than 10 years since the last dose.
¶ Yes if more than 5 years since the last dose. (More frequent boosters are not needed and can accentuate side effects).

CONTRAINDICATIONS

None known.

WARNINGS

Tetanus immune globulin should be given with caution to patients with a history of prior systemic allergic reactions following the administration of human immunoglobulin preparations.

In patients who have severe thrombocytopenia or any coagulation disorder that would contraindicate intramuscular injections, tetanus immune globulin should be given only if the expected benefits outweigh the risks.

DOSAGE AND ADMINISTRATION

ROUTINE PROPHYLACTIC DOSAGE SCHEDULE

Adults and Children 7 Years and Older

Tetanus immune globulin, 250 units should be given by deep intramuscular injection. At the same time, but in a different extremity and with a separate syringe, Tetanus and Diphtheria Toxoids Adsorbed (For Adult Use) (Td) should be administered according to the manufacturer's package insert. Adults with uncertain histories of a complete primary vaccination series should receive a primary series using the combined Td toxoid. To ensure continued protection, booster doses of Td should be given every 10 years.[2]

Children Less Than 7 Years Old

In small children the routine prophylactic dose of tetanus immune globulin may be calculated by the body weight (4.0 units/kg). However, it may be advisable to administer the entire contents of the vial or syringe of tetanus immune globulin (250 units) regardless of the child's size, since theoretically the same amount of toxin will be produced in the child's body by the infecting tetanus organism as it will in an adult's body. At the same time but in a different extremity and with a different syringe, Diphtheria and Tetanus Toxoids and Pertussis Vaccine Adsorbed (DTP) or Diphtheria and Tetanus Toxoids Adsorbed (For Pediatric Use) (DT), if pertussis vaccine is contraindicated, should be administered per the manufacturer's package insert.

NOTE: The single injection of tetanus toxoid only initiates the series for producing active immunity in the recipient. The physician must impress upon the patient the need for further toxoid injections in 1 month and 1 year. Without such, the active immunization series is incomplete. If a contraindication to using tetanus toxoid-containing preparations exists for a person who has not completed a primary series of tetanus toxoid immunization and that person has a wound that is neither clean nor minor, *only* passive immunization should be given using tetanus immune globulin.[2] (See TABLE 1.)

Available evidence indicates that complete primary vaccination with tetanus toxoid provides long lasting protection ≥10 years for most recipients. Consequently, after complete primary tetanus vaccination, boosters—even for wound management—need be given only every 10 years when wounds are minor and uncontaminated. For other wounds, a booster is appropriate if the patient has not received tetanus toxoid within the preceding 5 years. Persons who have received at least 2 doses of tetanus toxoid rapidly develop antibodies.[2] The prophylactic dosage schedule for these patients and for those with incomplete or uncertain immunity is shown in TABLE 1.

Since tetanus is actually a local infection, proper initial wound care is of paramount importance. The use of antitoxin is adjunctive to this procedure. However, in approximately 10% of recent tetanus cases, no wound or other breach in skin or mucous membrane could be implicated.[17]

TREATMENT OF ACTIVE CASES OF TETANUS

Standard therapy for the treatment of ctive tetanus including the use of tetanus immune globulin must be implemented immediately. The dosage should be adjusted according to the severity of the infection.[7,8]

Parenteral drug products should be inspected visually for particulate matter and discoloration prior to administration, whenever solution and container permit. They should not be used if particulate matter and/or discoloration are present.

DIRECTIONS FOR SYRINGE USAGE

1. Remove the prefilled syringe from the package. Lift syringe by barrel, **not** by plunger.
2. Twist the plunger rod clockwise until the threads are seated.
3. With the rubber needle shield secured on the syringe tip, push the plunger rod forward a few millimeters to break any friction seal between the rubber stopper and the glass syringe barrel.
4. Remove the needle shield and expel air bubbles.
5. Proceed with hypodermic needle puncture.
6. Aspirate prior to injection to confirm that the needle is not in a vein or artery.
7. Inject the medication.
8. Withdraw the needle and dispose or destroy it.

PRODUCT LISTING - EQUIVALENTS NOT AVAILABLE

Solution - Intramuscular - 250 U

1 ml	$24.13	HYPER-TET, Bayer	00026-0614-01
1 ml	$25.20	HYPER-TET, Bayer	00192-0614-01
1 ml	$93.60	BAYTET , Bayer	00026-0634-01
1 ml	$108.00	BAYTET , Allscripts Pharmaceutical Company	54569-4398-00
1 ml	$125.00	BAYTET , Bayer	00026-0634-02
1 ml x 10	$252.00	HYPER-TET, Bayer	00192-0614-70
10 ml	$252.00	HYPER-TET, Bayer	00026-0614-70

Tetanus Toxoid *(002324)*

For complete prescribing information, refer to the CD-ROM included with the book.

Categories: Immunization, tetanus; Pregnancy Category C; FDA Pre 1938 Drugs; WHO Formulary
Drug Classes: Vaccines
Brand Names: Tetanus Toxoid Adsorbed
Foreign Brand Availability: Anatetall (Malaysia; Philippines; Thailand); Anatoxal Tetanica Berna (Peru); Clostet (England); TE Anatoxal (Austria); TE Anatoxal Berna (Switzerland); Tetatox (Italy); Tetanol (Benin; Burkina-Faso; Ecuador; Ethiopia; Gambia; Germany; Ghana; Greece; Guinea; Honduras; Ivory-Coast; Kenya; Liberia; Malawi; Mali; Mauritania; Mauritius; Mexico; Morocco; Niger; Nigeria; Senegal; Seychelles; Sierra-Leone; Sudan; Tanzania; Tunia; Uganda; Zambia; Zimbabwe); Tetavax (England; Germany; Hong-Kong; Malaysia; Philippines; South-Africa; Thailand); Tet-Tox (New-Zealand)

DESCRIPTION

Tetanus Toxoid Adsorbed, Aluminum Phosphate Adsorbed, is prepared by growing a suitable strain of Cl. tetani on a protein-free, semisynthetic medium (Appl. Microbiol. *10:*146, 1962). Formaldehyde is used as the toxoiding (detoxifying) agent for tetanus toxin. The final product contains no more than 0.02% free formaldehyde and contains 0.01% thimerosal (mercury derivative) as preservative.

Tetanus Toxoid Adsorbed, is refined by methods which eliminate at least 97% of the nontoxoid nitrogen. Adsorption of purified antigens on an optimal quantity of aluminum phosphate, a mineral adjuvant, prolongs and enhances the antigenic properties by retarding the rate of absorption. The aluminum content of the final product does not exceed 0.85 mg per 0.5 ml dose. During processing, hydrochloric acid and sodium hydroxide are used to adjust the pH. Sodium chloride is added to the finished product to control isotonicity.
Storage: Keep between 2 and 8° C (35 and 46° F)

INDICATIONS AND USAGE

Tetanus Toxoid Adsorbed, Aluminum Phosphate Adsorbed, Wyeth, is indicated for active immunization against tetanus.

CONTRAINDICATIONS

An acute respiratory infection or other active infection is reason for deferring administration of routine primary immunizing or recall (booster) doses but *not* emergency recall (booster) doses. Prolonging the interval between primary immunizing doses, for 6 months or longer, does not interfere with the final immunity. Any dose of tetanus toxoid an individual has received, even a decade earlier, should be counted as 1 of his immunizing injections.[2]

DOSAGE AND ADMINISTRATION

The basic immunizing course for all age groups consists of 2 (primary) doses of 0.5 ml each, given at an interval of 4-8 weeks, followed by a third (reinforcing) dose of 0.5 ml 6-12 months later. The third (reinforcing) dose is an integral part of the basic immunizing course; basic immunization cannot be considered completed until the third dose has been given.[1]
Prolonging the interval between primary immunizing doses, for 6 months or longer, does not interfere with the final immunity. Any dose of tetanus toxoid an individual has received, even a decade earlier, should be counted as 1 of his immunizing injections.[2] Injections should be given intramuscularly, preferably into the deltoid or midlateral muscles of the thigh. The same muscle site should not be injected more than once during the course of basic immunization.

A routine recall (booster) dose of 0.5 ml should be given at 10 year intervals throughout life to maintain immunity.[2-5]

T

In event of injury for which tetanus prophylaxis is indicated, an emergency recall (booster) dose of 0.5 ml should be given:

a. ***For clean, minor wounds:*** if more than TEN (10) years have elapsed since the time of administration of the last recall (booster) dose or the last (reinforcing) dose of the basic immunizing series.

b. ***For all other wounds:*** if more than FIVE (5) years have elapsed since the time of administration of the last recall (booster) dose or the last (reinforcing) dose of the basic immunizing series.

If emergency tetanus prophylaxis is indicated during the period between the second primary dose and the reinforcing dose, a 0.5 ml dose of toxoid should be given. If given before 6 months have elapsed, it should be counted as a primary dose; if given after 6 months, it should be regarded as the reinforcing dose.

A 0.5 ml dose of tetanus toxoid adsorbed *and* an appropriate dose of tetanus immune globulin (human), given with *separate* syringes and at *different* sites, are indicated at time of injury if:

a. The past immunization history with tetanus toxoid or the date of the last recall (booster) dose is unknown or of questionable validity.

b. The interval since the third (reinforcing) dose of the basic immunizing series or the last recall (booster) dose is more than 10 years; *and* a delay of more than 24 hours has occurred between the time of injury and initiation of specific tetanus prophylaxis; *and* the injury is of the type that could readily lead to fulminating tetanus[2] (for example—compound fracture; extensive burn; crushing, penetrating, or massively contaminated wound; injury causing interruption or impairment of the local blood supply).

Individuals who have received no prior injections of tetanus toxoid, or who have received only 1 injection of tetanus toxoid should be given an adequate dose of tetanus immune globulin (human) at time of injury.

TECHNIC FOR INJECTION

Before injection, the skin over the site to be injected should be cleansed and prepared with a suitable germicide. After insertion of the needle, aspirate to help avoid inadvertent injection into a blood vessel. Expel the antigen slowly and terminate the dose with a small bubble of air (0.1-0.2 ml). Do not inject intracutaneously or into superficial subcutaneous tissues.

PRODUCT LISTING - EQUIVALENTS NOT AVAILABLE

Solution - Intramuscular - 4 U/0.5 ml

5 ml	$151.25	GENERIC, Aventis Pharmaceuticals	49281-0800-83
7.50 ml	$28.94	GENERIC, Allscripts Pharmaceutical Company	54569-4928-00
7.50 ml	$226.88	GENERIC, Aventis Pharmaceuticals	49281-0812-84

Solution - Intramuscular - 5 U/0.5 ml

7.50 ml	$46.94	GENERIC, Physicians Total Care	54868-0182-01

Suspension - Intramuscular - 5 U/0.5 ml

0.50 ml	$2.04	GENERIC, Sclavo Inc	42021-0110-19
0.50 ml x 10	$31.41	GENERIC, Allscripts Pharmaceutical Company	54569-2540-00
0.50 ml x 10	$35.93	GENERIC, Allscripts Pharmaceutical Company	54569-3611-00
5 ml	$7.00	GENERIC, Sclavo Inc	42021-0110-23
7.50 ml	$25.00	GENERIC, Aventis Pharmaceuticals	49281-0181-84
7.50 ml	$25.00	GENERIC, Aventis Pharmaceuticals	49281-8128-40

Suspension - Intramuscular - 10 U/0.5 ml

0.50 ml x 10	$30.69	GENERIC, Berna	58337-1301-02
5 ml	$19.79	GENERIC, Berna	58337-1301-01

Tetracaine Hydrochloride *(002325)*

For complete prescribing information, refer to the CD-ROM included with the book.

Categories: Anesthesia, spinal; Pregnancy Category C; FDA Pre 1938 Drugs; WHO Formulary
Drug Classes: Anesthetics, local; Anesthetics, spinal
Brand Names: Ak-T-Caine; Dermacaine; **Pontocaine**; Tetocain
Foreign Brand Availability: Ametop (South-Africa); Pantocain (Indonesia); Tetocaine (Taiwan)

DESCRIPTION

PROLONGED SPINAL ANESTHESIA

Tetracaine hydrochloride is 2-(Dimethylamino)ethyl p-(butylamino) benzoate monohydrochloride.

It is a white crystalline, odorless powder that is readily soluble in water, physiologic saline solution, and dextrose solution.

Tetracaine hydrochloride is a local anesthetic of the ester-linkage type, related to procaine.

Pontocaine hydrochloride is supplied in 2 forms for prolonged spinal anesthesia: niphanoid and 1% solution.

Niphanoid: A sterile, instantly soluble form consisting of a network of extremely fine, highly purified particles, resembling snow.

1% Solution: A sterile, isotonic, isobaric solution, each 1 ml containing 10 mg tetracaine hydrochloride, 6.7 mg sodium chloride, and not more than 2 mg acetone sodium bisulfite. The air in the ampuls has been displaced by nitrogen gas.

The pH is 3.2-6.

These formulations do not contain preservatives.

INDICATIONS AND USAGE

Tetracaine hydrochloride is indicated for the production of spinal anesthesia for procedures requiring 2-3 hours.

CONTRAINDICATIONS

Spinal anesthesia with tetracaine hydrochloride is contraindicated in patients with known hypersensitivity to tetracaine hydrochloride or to drugs of a similar chemical configuration (ester-type local anesthetics), or aminobenzoic acid or its derivatives; and in patients for whom spinal anesthesia as a technique is contraindicated.

The decision as to whether or not spinal anesthesia should be used for an individual patient should be made by the physician after weighing the advantages with the risks and possible complications.

Contraindications to spinal anesthesia as a technique can be found in standard reference texts, and usually include generalized septicemia, infection at the site of injection, certain diseases of the cerebrospinal system, uncontrolled hypotension, etc.

WARNINGS

RESUSCITATIVE EQUIPMENT AND DRUGS SHOULD BE IMMEDIATELY AVAILABLE WHENEVER ANY LOCAL ANESTHETIC DRUG IS USED.

Large doses of local anesthetics should not be used in patients with heartblock.

Reactions resulting in fatality have occurred on rare occasions with the use of local anesthetics, even in the absence of a history of hypersensitivity.

Contains acetone sodium bisulfite, a sulfite that may cause allergic-type reactions including anaphylactic symptoms and life-threatening or less severe asthmatic episodes in certain susceptible people. The overall prevalence of sulfite sensitivity in the general population is unknown and probably low. Sulfite sensitivity is seen more frequently in asthmatic than in nonasthmatic people.

DOSAGE AND ADMINISTRATION

As with all anesthetics, the dosage varies and depends upon the area to be anesthetized, the number of neuronal segments to be blocked, individual tolerance, and the technique of anesthesia. The lowest dosage needed to provide effective anesthesia should be administered. For specific techniques and procedures, refer to standard textbooks.

TABLE 1 *Suggested Dosage For Spinal Anesthesia*

	Using Niphanoid		Using 1% solution		
Extent of anesthesia	Dose of Niphanoid (mg)	Volume of spinal fluid (ml)	Dose of solution (ml)	Volume of spinal fluid (ml)	Site of injection (lumbar interspace)
Perineum	5*	1	0.5 (=5 mg)*	0.5	4th
Perineum and lower extremities	10	2	1.0 (=10 mg)	1.0	3rd or 4th
Up to costal margin	15-20†	3	1.5-2.0 (=15 to 20 mg)†	1.5-2.0	2nd, 3rd, or 4th

* For vaginal delivery (saddle block) from 2-5 mg in dextrose.
† Doses exceeding 15 mg are rarely required and should be used only in exceptional cases. Inject solution at rate of about 1 ml per 5 seconds.

The extent and degree of spinal anesthesia depend upon dosage, specific gravity of the anesthetic solution, volume of solution used, force of the injection, level of puncture, position of the patient during and immediately after injection, etc.

When spinal fluid is added to either the niphanoid or solution, some turbidity results, the degree depending on the pH of the spinal fluid, the temperature of the solution during mixing, as well as the amount of drug and diluent employed. This cloudiness is due to the release of the base from the hydrochloride. Liberation of base (which is completed within the spinal canal) is held to be essential for satisfactory results with any spinal anesthetic.

The specific gravity of spinal fluid at 25°C/ 25°C varies under normal conditions from 1.0063-1.0075. A solution of the instantly soluble form (niphanoid) in spinal fluid has only a slightly greater specific gravity. The 1% concentration in saline solution has a specific gravity of 1.0060-1.0074 at 25°C/25°C.

A hyperbaric solution may be prepared by mixing equal volumes of the 1% solution and dextrose solution 10% (which is available in ampuls of 3 ml).

If the niphanoid form is preferred, it is first dissolved in dextrose solution 10% in a ratio of 1 ml dextrose to 10 mg of the anesthetic. Further dilution is made with an equal volume of spinal fluid. The resulting solution now contains 5% dextrose with 5 mg of anesthetic agent per milliliter.

A hypobaric solution may be prepared by dissolving the niphanoid in sterile water for injection (1 mg per milliliter). The specific gravity of this solution is essentially the same as that of water, 1.000 at 25°C/25°C.

Examine ampuls carefully before use. Do not use solution if crystals, cloudiness, or discoloration is observed.

THESE FORMULATIONS OF TETRACAINE HYDROCHLORIDE DO NOT CONTAIN PRESERVATIVES; THEREFORE, UNUSED PORTIONS SHOULD BE DISCARDED AND THE RECONSTITUTED niphanoid SHOULD BE USED IMMEDIATELY.

STERILIZATION OF AMPULS

The drug in intact ampuls is sterile. The preferred method of destroying bacteria on the exterior of ampuls before opening is heat sterilization (autoclaving). Immersion in antiseptic solution is not recommended.

AUTOCLAVE AT 15-POUND PRESSURE, AT 121°C (250°F), FOR 15 MINUTES. The niphanoid form may also be autoclaved in the same way but may lose its snowlike appearance and tend to adhere to the sides of the ampul. This may slightly decrease the rate at which the drug dissolves but does not interfere with its anesthetic potency.

AUTOCLAVING INCREASES LIKELIHOOD OF CRYSTAL FORMATION. UNUSED AUTOCLAVED AMPULS SHOULD BE DISCARDED. UNDER NO CIRCUM-

STANCE SHOULD UNUSED AMPULS WHICH HAVE BEEN AUTOCLAVED BE RETURNED TO STOCK.

PRODUCT LISTING - EQUIVALENTS NOT AVAILABLE

Size	Price	Product, Manufacturer	NDC
Ointment - Ophthalmic - 0.5%			
3.50 gm	$16.21	PONTOCAINE OPHTHALMIC, Southwood Pharmaceuticals Inc	58016-6453-01
Powder For Injection - Injectable - 20 mg			
100's	$1180.38	PONTOCAINE HCL, Abbott Pharmaceutical	00074-1849-06
Solution - Injectable - 0.2%			
2 ml x 10	$55.25	DEXTROSE-PONTOCAINE HCL, Abbott Pharmaceutical	00074-1872-02
Solution - Injectable - 0.3%			
5 ml x 10	$72.68	DEXTROSE-PONTOCAINE HCL, Abbott Pharmaceutical	00074-1874-05
Solution - Injectable - 1%			
2 ml x 25	$146.25	PONTOCAINE HCL, Abbott Pharmaceutical	00074-1846-02
Solution - Ophthalmic - 0.5%			
1 ml x 12	$29.06	GENERIC, Ciba Vision Ophthalmics	00058-0787-12
1 ml x 12	$35.30	GENERIC, Allscripts Pharmaceutical Company	54569-1659-01
1 ml x 12	$37.92	GENERIC, Ciba Vision Ophthalmics	58768-0787-12
2 ml x 12	$63.00	GENERIC, Alcon Laboratories Inc	00065-0741-12
15 ml	$4.07	GENERIC, Physicians Total Care	54868-0901-00
15 ml	$4.55	GENERIC, Bausch and Lomb	24208-0920-64
15 ml	$4.56	GENERIC, Aligen Independent Laboratories Inc	00405-6139-15
15 ml	$4.82	GENERIC, Allscripts Pharmaceutical Company	54569-1961-00
15 ml	$5.50	GENERIC, Miza Pharmaceutcials Dba Optopics Laboratories Corporation	52238-0914-16
15 ml	$5.74	GENERIC, Prescript Pharmaceuticals	00247-0287-15
15 ml	$5.94	GENERIC, Ocusoft	54799-0502-15
15 ml	$6.20	GENERIC, Prescript Pharmaceuticals	00247-0044-15
15 ml	$16.19	GENERIC, Akorn Inc	17478-0245-12
15 ml	$19.81	GENERIC, Allscripts Pharmaceutical Company	54569-4362-00
15 ml	$21.80	GENERIC, Dhs Inc	55887-0743-15
15 ml	$23.11	GENERIC, Southwood Pharmaceuticals Inc	58016-6098-01
15 ml	$23.99	PONTOCAINE OPHTHALMIC, Abbott Pharmaceutical	00074-1862-01
15 ml	$27.02	GENERIC, Alpharma Uspd Makers Of Barre and Nmc	63874-0909-15
59 ml	$34.43	PONTOCAINE OPHTHALMIC, Abbott Pharmaceutical	00074-1863-01
Solution - Topical - 2%			
30 ml	$14.73	PONTOCAINE, Abbott Pharmaceutical	00074-1866-01
30 ml	$27.00	PONTOCAINE, Compumed Pharmaceuticals	00403-3163-18
120 ml	$70.02	PONTOCAINE, Abbott Pharmaceutical	00074-1866-02

Tetracycline Hydrochloride *(002326)*

Categories: Acne vulgaris; Actinomycosis; Amebiasis, adjunct; Anthrax; Conjunctivitis, infectious; Gonorrhea; Granuloma inguinale; Infection, lower respiratory tract; Infection, upper respiratory tract; Infection, urinary tract; Lymphogranuloma venereum; Ophthalmia neonatorum; Pneumonia; Psittacosis; Q fever; Relapsing fever; Rickettsialpox; Rocky mountain spotted fever; Syphilis; Tick fever; Trachoma; Typhus; Vincent's infection; Yaws; FDA Approved 1953 Nov; WHO Formulary; Pregnancy Category D

Drug Classes: Antibiotics, tetracyclines; Anti-infectives, ophthalmic; Anti-infectives, topical; Dermatologics; Ophthalmics

Brand Names: **Achromycin**; Actisite; Ala-Tet; Biocycline; Bristacycline; Brodspec; Cyclopar; Emtet-500; Nor-Tet; Panmycin; Robitet; Sarocycline; Sumycin; Tega-Cycline; Teline; Tetracap; Tetrachel; Tetracon; Tetracyn; Tetralan; Tetram; Tetramed; Topicycline; Wesmycin

Foreign Brand Availability: Achromycin V (Bahrain; Canada; Cyprus; Egypt; Iran; Iraq; Japan; Jordan; Kuwait; Lebanon; Libya; Oman; Qatar; Republic-of-Yemen; Saudi-Arabia; South-Africa; Syria; United-Arab-Emirates); Acromicina (Argentina; Italy; Mexico); Ambramicina (Italy; Spain); Apo-Tetra (Canada); Apocyclin (Finland); Beatacycline (Singapore); Bristaciclina (Spain); Cadicycline (Benin; Burkina-Faso; Ethiopia; Gambia; Ghana; Guinea; Ivory-Coast; Kenya; Liberia; Malawi; Mali; Mauritania; Mauritius; Morocco; Niger; Nigeria; Senegal; Seychelles; Sierra-Leone; Sudan; Tanzania; Tunia; Uganda; Zambia; Zimbabwe); Calociclina (Italy); Ciclotetryl (Argentina); Combicyclin (Indonesia); Conmycin (Indonesia); Cyclabid (South-Africa); Dhatracin (Malaysia); Dicyclin Forte (India); Dumocyclin (Denmark; Finland); Economycin (England); Enkacyclin (Indonesia); Florocycline (France); Hexacycline (France); Hostaciclina (Ecuador); Hostacyclin (Austria; Greece); Hostacycline (Belgium; Benin; Burkina-Faso; Ethiopia; Gambia; Ghana; Guinea; India; Ivory-Coast; Kenya; Liberia; Malawi; Mali; Mauritania; Mauritius; Morocco; Niger; Nigeria; Philippines; Senegal; Seychelles; Sierra-Leone; Sudan; Tanzania; Tunia; Uganda; Zambia; Zimbabwe); Hostacycline-P (South-Africa); Hydromycin (Thailand); Ibicyn (Taiwan); Ikacycline (Indonesia); Kemoclin (Indonesia); Latycin (Australia; Bahrain; Cyprus; Egypt; Iran; Iraq; Jordan; Kuwait; Lebanon; Libya; Oman; Qatar; Republic-of-Yemen; Saudi-Arabia; Singapore; Syria; United-Arab-Emirates); Lenocin (Thailand); Medocycline (Hong-Kong); Mysteclin (Australia); Novotetra (Canada); Ofticlin (Mexico); Omnaze (Argentina); Orencyclin F-500 (Peru); Oricyclin (Finland); Pantocycline (Thailand); Parenciclina (Mexico); Pervasol (Argentina); Polarcyclin (Finland); Quimocyclar (Mexico); Recycline (Israel); Resteclin (India); Rimatet (Bahamas; Bahrain; Barbados; Belize; Benin; Bermuda; Burkina-Faso; Curacao; Cyprus; Egypt; Ethiopia; Gambia; Ghana; Guinea; Guyana; Iran; Iraq; Ivory-Coast; Jamaica; Jordan; Kenya; Kuwait; Lebanon; Liberia; Libya; Malawi; Mali; Mauritania; Mauritius; Morocco; Netherland-Antilles; Niger; Nigeria; Oman; Qatar; Republic-of-Yemen; Saudi-Arabia; Senegal; Seychelles; Sierra-Leone; Sudan; Surinam; Syria; Tanzania; Trinidad; Tunia; Uganda; United-Arab-Emirates; Zambia; Zimbabwe); Servitet (Malaysia; Thailand); Steclin (Argentina; Germany); Steclin V (South-Africa); Subamycin (India); Tefilin (Germany); Tetra-Atlantis (Mexico); Tetrabioptal (Italy); Tetrablet (Germany); Tetra Central (Thailand); Tetracitro S (Germany); Tetralen (Spain); Tetralim (Thailand); Tetralution (Germany); Tetramig (France); Tetrana (Thailand); Tetranase (Peru); Tetrano (Thailand); Tetrarco (Indonesia; Netherlands); Tetrarco L.A. (Austria); Tetraseptin (Switzerland); Tetrasuiss (Bahamas; Bahrain; Barbados; Belize; Benin; Bermuda; Burkina-Faso; Curacao; Cyprus; Egypt; Ethiopia; Gambia; Ghana; Guinea; Guyana; Iran; Iraq; Ivory-Coast; Jamaica; Jordan; Kenya; Kuwait; Lebanon; Liberia; Libya; Malawi; Mali; Mauritania; Mauritius; Morocco; Netherland-Antilles; Niger; Nigeria; Oman; Qatar; Republic-of-Yemen; Saudi-Arabia; Senegal; Seychelles; Sierra-Leone; Sudan; Surinam; Syria; Taiwan; Tanzania; Trinidad; Tunia; Uganda; United-Arab-Emirates; Zambia; Zimbabwe); Tetrecu (Ecuador); Tetrex (Australia; Bahrain; Cyprus; Egypt; Iran; Iraq; Japan; Jordan; Kuwait; Lebanon; Libya; Mexico; Oman; Qatar; Republic-of-Yemen; Saudi-Arabia; South-Africa; Syria; United-Arab-Emirates); Tevacycline (Israel); Triphacyclin (Switzerland)

Cost of Therapy: $3.31 (Infection; Sumycin; 500 mg; 2 tablets/day; 10 day supply)
$1.09 (Infection; Generic Capsule; 500 mg; 2 capsules/day; 10 day supply)

DESCRIPTION

Tetracycline is a broad-spectrum antibiotic prepared from the cultures of certain streptomyces species. Chemically, tetracycline HCl is: (4*S*-(48,1α,4aα,5aα,6β,12aα))-4-(dimethylamino)-1, 4,4a,5, 5a,6, 11, 12a-octahydro -3,6,10,12,12a-pentahydroxy-6-methyl-1,11-dioxo-2- napthacenecarboxamide monohydrochloride.

CAPSULES

Storage

Store at controlled room temperature, between 15 and 30°C (59 and 86°F).

Dispense in tight, light-resistant container.

TOPICAL SOLUTION

Storage: Tetracycline topical solution should be kept at controlled room temperature 59-86°F (15-30C°) or below.

OPHTHALMIC SUSPENSION

Storage: Store at controlled room temperature 15-30°C (59-86°F).

CLINICAL PHARMACOLOGY

CAPSULES

The tetracyclines are primarily bacteriostatic and are thought to exert their antimicrobial effect by the inhibition of protein synthesis. Tetracyclines are active against a wide range of gram-negative and gram-positive organisms.

The drugs in the tetracycline class have closely similar antimicrobial spectra, and cross-resistance among them is common. Micro-organisms may be considered susceptible if the MIC (minimum inhibitory concentration) is not more than 4.0 μg/ml and intermediate if the MIC is 4.0-12.5 μg/ml.

Susceptibility Testing

A tetracycline disc may be used to determine microbial susceptibility to drugs in the tetracycline class. If the Kirby-Bauer method of disc susceptibility testing is used, a 30 μg tetracycline disc should give a zone of at least 19 mm when tested against a tetracycline-susceptible bacterial strain.

Tetracyclines are readily absorbed and are bound to plasma proteins in varying degree. They are concentrated by the liver in the bile and excreted in the urine and feces at high concentrations and in a biologically active form.

TOPICAL SOLUTION

This form delivers tetracycline to the pilosebaceous apparatus and the adjacent tissues. Tetracycline topical solution reduces inflammatory acne lesions, but its mode of actions is not fully understood.

In clinical studies, use of tetracycline topical solution on the face and neck twice daily delivered to the skin an average dose of 2.9 mg of tetracycline HCl per day. Patients who used the medication twice daily on other acne-involved areas in addition to the face and neck applied an average dose of 4.8 mg of tetracycline HCl per day.

Tetracycline topical solution has been formulated such that the recrystallization properties of the tetracycline on the skin greatly reduce or eliminate the yellow color after associated with topical tetracycline.

T

INDICATIONS AND USAGE

CAPSULES

Tetracycline is indicated in infections caused by the following micro-organisms: Rickettsiae (Rocky Mountain spotted fever, typhus fever and the typhus group, Q fever, rickettsialpox and tick fevers),*Mycoplasma pneumoniae* (PPLO, Eaton Agent), Agents of psittacosis and ornithosis, Agents of lymphogranuloma venereum and granuloma inguinale. The spirochetal agent of relapsing fever (*Borrelia recurrentis*).

The following gram-negative micro-organisms: *Haemophilus ducreyi* (chancroid), *Pasteurella pestis, Pasteurella tularensis, Bartonella bacilliformis, Bacteroides* species, *Vibrio comma* and *Vibrio fetus* and *Brucella*species (in conjunction with streptomycin).

Because many strains of the following groups of micro-organisms have been shown to be resistant to tetracyclines, culture and susceptibility testing are recommended.

Tetracycline is indicated for treatment of infections caused by the following gram-negative micro-organisms, when bacteriologic testing indicates appropriate susceptibility to the drug: *Escherichia coli, Enterobacter aerogenes* (formerly *Aerobacter aerogenes*), *Shigella* species, *Mima* species and *Herellea* species, *Haemophilus influenzae* (respiratory infections) and *Klebsiella* species (respiratory and urinary infections).

Tetracycline is indicated for treatment of infections caused by the following gram-positive micro-organisms when bacteriologic testing indicates appropriate susceptibility to the drug. Streptococcus species: Up to 44% of strains of *Streptococcus pyogenes* and 74% of *Streptococcus faecalis* have been found to be resistant to tetracycline drugs. Therefore, tetracyclines should not be used for streptococcal disease unless the organism has been demonstrated to be sensitive. For upper respiratory infections due to group A beta-hemolytic streptococci, penicillin is the usual drug of choice, including prophylaxis of rheumatic fever. *Diplococcus pneumoniae, Staphylococcus aureus*, skin and soft tissue infections. Tetracyclines are not the drugs of choice in the treatment of any type of staphylococcal infections.

When penicillin is contraindicated, tetracyclines are alternative drugs in the treatment of infections due to: *Neisseria gonorrhoeae, Treponema pallidum* and *Treponema pertenue* (syphilis and yaws), *Listeria monocytogenes, Clostridium* species, *Bacillus anthracis, Fusobacterium fusiforme* (Vincent's infection) and *Actinomyces* species.

In acute intestinal amebiasis, the tetracyclines may be a useful adjunct to amebicides.

In severe acne, the tetracyclines may be useful adjunctive therapy.

Tetracycline HCl is indicated for the treatment of uncomplicated urethral, endocervical or rectal infections in adults caused by *Chlamydia trachomatis.*[1]

Tetracyclines are indicated in the treatment of trachoma, although the infectious agent is not always eliminated, as judged by immunofluorescence.

Inclusion conjunctivitis may be treated with oral tetracyclines or with a combination of oral and topical agents.

TOPICAL SOLUTION

Tetracycline topical solution is indicated in the treatment of acne vulgaris.

OPHTHALMIC SUSPENSION

For the treatment of superficial ocular infections susceptible to tetracycline hydrochloride.

For prophylaxis of ophthalmia neonatorum due to *Neisseria gonorrhoeae* or *Chlamydia trachomatis*. The Center for Disease Control (U.S.P.H.S.) and the Committee on Drugs, the Committee on Fetus and Newborn, and the Committee on Infectious Diseases of the American Academy of Pediatrics recommend 1% silver nitrate solution in single-dose ampoules or single-use tubes of an ophthalmic ointment containing 0.5% erythromycin or 1% tetracycline as "effective and acceptable regimens of prophylaxis of gonococcal ophthalmia neonatorum."[2] (For infants born to mothers with clinically apparent gonorrhea, intravenous or intramuscular injections of aqueous crystalline penicillin G should be given; a single dose of 50,000 units for term infants or 20,00 for infants of low birth weight. Topical prophylaxis alone is inadequate for these infants.[2])

The following organisms have demonstrated susceptibility to tetracycline hydrochloride: *Staphylococcus aureus,, Streptococci* including *Streptococcus pneumoniae, E. coli, Neisseria* species, *Chlamydia trachomatis.*

When treating trachoma a concomitant oral tetracycline is helpful.

Other organisms, not known to cause superficial eye infections, but with demonstrated susceptibility to tetracycline hydrochloride, have been omitted from the above list.

Tetracycline hydrochloride does not provide adequate coverage against: *Haemophilus influenzae, Klebsiella/Enterobacter* species, *Pseudomonas aeruginosa* and *Serratia marcescens.*

T

CONTRAINDICATIONS

This drug is contraindicated in persons who have shown hypersensitivity to any of the tetracyclines or to any of the other ingredients.

WARNINGS

CAPSULES

THE USE OF DRUGS OF THE TETRACYCLINE CLASS DURING TOOTH DEVELOPMENT (LAST HALF OF PREGNANCY, INFANCY AND CHILDHOOD TO THE AGE OF 8 YEARS) MAY CAUSE PERMANENT DISCOLORATION OF THE TEETH (YELLOW-GRAY-BROWN). This adverse reaction is more common during long-term use of the drugs but has been observed following repeated short-term courses. Enamel hypoplasia has also been reported. TETRACYCLINE DRUGS, THEREFORE, SHOULD NOT BE USED IN THIS AGE GROUP UNLESS OTHER DRUGS ARE NOT LIKELY TO BE EFFECTIVE OR ARE CONTRAINDICATED.

If renal impairment exists, even usual oral or parenteral doses may lead to excessive systemic accumulation of the drug and possible liver toxicity. Under such conditions, lower than usual total doses are indicated and, if therapy is prolonged, serum level determinations of the drug may be advisable.

Photosensitivity manifested by an exaggerated sunburn reaction has been observed in some individuals taking tetracyclines. Patients apt to be exposed to direct sunlight or ultraviolet light should be advised that this reaction can occur with tetracycline drugs, and treatment should be discontinued at the first evidence of skin erythema. *NOTE:* Photsensitization reactions have occurred most frequently with democycline, less with chlortetracycline, and very rarely with oxytetracycline and tetracycline.

The anti-anabolic action of the tetracyclines may cause an increase in BUN. While this is not a problem in those with normal renal function, in patients with significantly impaired function, higher serum levels of tetracycline may lead to azotemia, hyperphosphatemia, and acidosis.

Use in Pregnancy

See WARNINGS about use during tooth development.

Results of animal studies indicate that tetracyclines cross the placenta, are found in fetal tissues and can have toxic effects on the developing fetus (often related to retardation of skeletal development). Evidence of embryotoxicity has also been noted in animals treated early in pregnancy.

Usage in Newborns, Infants, and Children

See WARNINGS about use during tooth development.

All tetracyclines form a stable calcium complex in any bone forming tissue. A decrease in the fibula growth rate has been observed in prematures given oral tetracycline in doses of 25 mg/kg every 6 hours. This reaction was shown to be reversible when the drug was discontinued.

Tetracyclines are present in the milk of lactating women who are taking a drug in this class.

TOPICAL SOLUTION

Contains sodium bisulfite, a sulfite that may cause allergic-type reactions including anaphylactic symptoms and life threatening or less severe asthmatic episodes in certain susceptible people. The overall prevalence of sulfite sensitivity in the general population is unknown and probably low. Sulfite sensitivity is seen more frequently in asthmatic than in non-asthmatic people.

PRECAUTIONS

GENERAL

Capsules

As with other antibiotic preparations, use of this drug may result in overgrowth of nonsusceptible organisms, including fungi. If superinfection occurs, the antibiotic should be discontinued and appropriate therapy instituted. *NOTE:* Superinfection of the bowel by staphylococci may be life-threatening.

In venereal diseases when coexistent syphilis is suspected, darkfield examination should be done before treatment is started and the blood serology repeated monthly for at least 4 months.

Because tetracyclines have been shown to depress plasma prothrombin activity, patients who are on anticoagulant therapy may require downward adjustment of their anticoagulant dosage.

In long-term therapy, periodic laboratory evaluation of organ systems, including hematopoietic, renal and hepatic studies should be performed.

All infections due to Group A beta-hemolytic streptococci should be treated for at least 10 days.

Since bacteriostatic drugs may interfere with the bactericidal action of penicillin, it is advisable to avoid giving tetracycline in conjunction with penicillin.

Since sensitivity reactions are more likely to occur in oersons with a history of allergy, asthma, hay fever, or urticaria, the preparation should be used with caution in such individuals.

Topical Solution

This is for external use only and care should be taken to keep it out of the eyes, nose, and mouth.

Ophthalmic Suspension

The use of antibiotics occasionally may result in overgrowth of nonsusceptible organisms. Constant observation of the patient is essential. If new infections appear during therapy, appropriate measures should be taken.

CARCINOGENESIS, MUTAGENESIS, AND IMPAIRMENT OF FERTILITY

Capsules

Long-term animal studies are currently being conducted to determine whether tetracycline HCl has carcinogenic potential. Some related antibiotics (oxytetracycline, minocycline) have shown evidence of oncogenic activity in rats.

In two *in vitro* mammalian cell assay systems (L 51784y mouse lymphoma and Chinese hamster lung cells), there was evidence of mutagenicity at tetracycline HCl concentrations of 60 and 10 μg/ml, respectively.

Tetracycline HCl had no effect on fertility when administered in the diet to the male and female rats at a daily intake of 25 times the human dose.

Topical Solution

A 2 year dermal study in mice has been performed in rats and rabbits at doses of up to 246 times the human dose (assuming the human to be 1.3 ml/40kg/day) and have revealed no evidence of impaired fertility or harm ti the fetus. There are, however, no adequate and well-controlled studies in pregnant women. Because animal reproduction studies are not always predictive of human response, this drug should be used during pregnancy only if clearly needed.

NURSING MOTHERS

It is not known whether tetracycline or any other component of tetracycline topical solution is excreted in human milk. Because many drugs are excreted in human milk, caution should be exercised when tetracycline topical solution is administered to a nursing woman.

PEDIATRIC USE

Safety and effectiveness in children below the age of eleven has not yet been established.

ADVERSE REACTIONS

CAPSULES

Gastrointestinal: Anorexia, epigastric distress, nausea, vomiting, diarrhea, bulky loose stools, stomatitis, sore throat, glossitis, black hairy tongue, dysphagia, hoarseness, enterocolitis, and inflammatory lesions (with monilial overgrowth) in the anogenital region, including proctitus and pruritus ani. These reactions have been caused by both the oral and parenteral administration of tetracyclines.

Skin: Maculopapular and erythematous rashes. Exfoliative dermatitis has been reported but is uncommon. Photosensitivity is discussed above. (See WARNINGS.)

Renal Toxicity: Rise in BUN has been reported and is apparently dose related. (See WARNINGS.)

Hepatic cholestasis has been reported rarely, and is usually associated with high dosage levels of tetracycline.

Hypersensitivity Reactions: urticaria, angioneurotic edema, anaphylaxis, anaphylactoid purpura, pericarditis and exacerbation of systemic lupus erythematosus, and serum sickness-like reactions, as fever, rash, and arthralgia.

Bulging fontanels have been reported in young infants following full therapeutic dosage. This sign disappeared rapidly when the drug was discontinued.

Blood: anemia, hemolytic anemia, thrombocytopenia, thrombocytopenic purpura, neutropenia and eosinophilia have been reported.

Dizziness and heachache have been reported.

When given over prolonged periods, tetracyclines have been reported to produce brown-black microscopic discoloration of thyroid glands. No abnormalities of thyroid function studies are known to occur.

TOPICAL SOLUTION

Among the 838 patients treated with tetracycline topical solution under normal usage conditions during clinical evaluation, there was one instance of severe dermatitis requiring systemic steroid therapy.

About one-third of patients are likely to experience a stinging or burning sensation. The sensation ordinarily lasts no more than a few minutes, and does not occur at every application. There has been no indication that patients experience sufficient discomfort to reduce the frequency of use or to discontinue use of the product.

The kinds of side effects often associated with oral or parenteral administration of tetracyclines (*e.g.*, various gastrointestinal complaints, vaginitis, hematologic abnormalities, manifestations of systemic hypersensitivity reactions, and dental and skeletal disorders) have not been observed with tetracycline topical solution. Because this drug's topical from of administration, it is highly unlikely that such side effects will occur from its use.

OPHTHALMIC SUSPENSION

Dermatitis and allied symptomatology have been reported. If adverse reaction or idiosyncrasy occurs, discontinue medication and institute appropriate therapy.

DOSAGE AND ADMINISTRATION

CAPSULES

Therapy should be continued for at least 24-48 hours after symptoms and fever have subsided.

Concomitant Therapy

Antacids containing aluminum, calcium, or magnesium impair absorption and should not be given to patients taking oral tetracycline.

Food and some dairy products also interfere with absorption. Oral forms of tetracycline should be given 1 hour before or 2 hours after meals. Pediatric oral dosage forms should not be given with milk formulas and should be given at least 1 hour prior to feeding.

In Patients with Renal Impairment

(See WARNINGS.) Total dosage should be decreased by reduction of recommended individual doses and/or by extending time intervals between doses.

In the treatment of streptococcal infections, a therapeutic dose of tetracycline should be administered for at least 10 days.

Adults

Usual daily dose, 1-2 g divided in 2 or 4 equal doses, depending on the severity of the infection.

For Children Above Eight (8) Years of Age

Usual daily dose, 10-20 mg (25-50 mg/kg) per pound of body weight divided in 4 equal doses.

For treatment of brucellosis, 500 mg tetracycline 4 times daily for 3 weeks should be accompanied by streptomycin. 1 gram intramuscularly twice daily the first week, and once daily the second week.

For treatment of syphilis, a total of 30-40 grams in equally divided doses over a period of 10-15 days should be given. Close follow up, including laboratory tests, is recommended.

Treatment of Uncomplicated Gonorrhea

When penicillin is contraindicated, tetracycline may be used for the treatment of both males and females in the following divided dosage schedule: 1.5 grams initially followed by 0.5 grams qid for a total of 9.0 grams.

For treatment of uncomplicated urethral, endocervical, or rectal infections in adults caused by *Chlamydia trachomatis:* 500 mg, by mouth, 4 times a day for at least 7 days.[1]

In cases of severe acne which, in the judgment of the clinician, require long-term treatment, the recommended initial dosage is 2 g daily in the divided doses. When improvement is noted, usually within 1 week, dosage shoulf be gradually reduced to maintenance levels ranging from 125-500 mg daily. In some patients it may be possible to maintain adequate remission of lesions with alternate-day or intermittent therapy. Tetracycline therapy of acne should agument the other standard measures known to be of value.

TOPICAL SOLUTION

It is recommended that tetracycline topical solution be applied generously twice-daily to the entire affected area (not just to the individual lesions) until the skin is thoroughly wet. Instructions to the patient for proper application are provided on the bottle label. Patients may continue their normal use of cosmetics.

Concomitant use with benzoyl peroxide or oral tetracycline has been reported without observed problems.

OPHTHALMIC SUSPENSION

For most susceptible bacterial infections shake well, then gently squeeze the plastic dropper bottle to instill 2 drops in the affected eye, or if necessary, in both eyes, 2 or 4 times daily, or more frequently, depending upon the severity of the infection. Very severe infections may require days of treatment, whereas other cases may be cured by instillation with much less frequency for 48 hours.

In acute and chronic trachoma instill 2 drops in each eye 2-4 times daily. This treatment should be continued for 1-3 months except that certain individual or complicated cases may require a longer duration. A concomitant oral tetracycline is helpful.

For unit dose administration and convenience, the dispenser may be used. Immediately prior to use, simultaneously roll, invert and squeeze dispenser between thumb and fingers. Repeat several times to mix contents well. Use aseptic technique to cut the tip of the dispenser, thereby maintaining sterility. Discard first 2 drops before instilling drops in eye(s). Instill 2 drops in eye(s), then discard dispenser.

PRODUCT LISTING - RATED THERAPEUTICALLY EQUIVALENT

Capsule - Oral - 250 mg			
10's	$2.69	GENERIC, Pd-Rx Pharmaceuticals	55289-0256-10
12's	$3.23	GENERIC, Pd-Rx Pharmaceuticals	55289-0256-12
12's	$4.28	SUMYCIN, Pd-Rx Pharmaceuticals	55289-0494-12
20's	$1.12	SUMYCIN, Allscripts Pharmaceutical Company	54569-5112-00
20's	$3.54	GENERIC, Pd-Rx Pharmaceuticals	55289-0256-20
20's	$5.39	GENERIC, Alpharma Uspd Makers Of Barre and Nmc	63874-0125-20
25's	$5.72	GENERIC, Pd-Rx Pharmaceuticals	55289-0256-97
28's	$1.75	GENERIC, Circle Pharmaceuticals Inc	00659-0101-28
28's	$3.75	GENERIC, Pd-Rx Pharmaceuticals	55289-0256-28
28's	$5.96	GENERIC, Alpharma Uspd Makers Of Barre and Nmc	63874-0125-28
30's	$2.53	SUMYCIN, Physicians Total Care	54868-1047-02
30's	$6.96	GENERIC, Alpharma Uspd Makers Of Barre and Nmc	63874-0125-30
40's	$2.00	GENERIC, Circle Pharmaceuticals Inc	00659-0101-40
40's	$2.98	SUMYCIN, Physicians Total Care	54868-1047-01
40's	$3.42	GENERIC, Pd-Rx Pharmaceuticals	58864-0493-40
40's	$3.90	GENERIC, Pd-Rx Pharmaceuticals	55289-0256-40
40's	$7.88	GENERIC, Alpharma Uspd Makers Of Barre and Nmc	63874-0125-40
60's	$3.88	SUMYCIN, Physicians Total Care	54868-1047-03
60's	$4.50	GENERIC, Pd-Rx Pharmaceuticals	55289-0256-60
90's	$5.23	SUMYCIN, Physicians Total Care	54868-1047-04
90's	$6.50	GENERIC, Pd-Rx Pharmaceuticals	55289-0256-90
100's	$0.54	GENERIC, Global Pharmaceutical Corporation	00115-1405-01
100's	$3.00	GENERIC, C.O. Truxton Inc	00463-5001-01
100's	$4.25	GENERIC, Eon Labs Manufacturing Inc	00185-0670-01
100's	$4.79	GENERIC, Us Trading Corporation	56126-0362-11
100's	$5.10	SUMYCIN, Physicians Total Care	54868-1047-00
100's	$5.63	GENERIC, Interstate Drug Exchange Inc	00814-7755-14
100's	$5.68	GENERIC, Pharmacia and Upjohn	00009-0782-01
100's	$6.11	GENERIC, Auro Pharmaceutical	55829-0696-10
100's	$6.21	GENERIC, Moore, H.L. Drug Exchange Inc	00839-1656-06
100's	$6.27	TETRACAP, Circle Pharmaceuticals Inc	00659-6144-01
100's	$6.31	GENERIC, Aligen Independent Laboratories Inc	00405-4981-01
100's	$6.80	GENERIC, Ivax Corporation	00172-2416-60
100's	$6.80	GENERIC, Pd-Rx Pharmaceuticals	55289-0256-01
100's	$6.81	GENERIC, Major Pharmaceuticals Inc	00904-2416-60
100's	$6.88	GENERIC, Global Pharmaceutical Corporation	00115-1400-01
100's	$6.88	GENERIC, Barr Laboratories Inc	00555-0011-02
100's	$8.24	GENERIC, Ivax Corporation	00182-0112-89
100's	$10.91	GENERIC, Alpharma Uspd Makers Of Barre and Nmc	63874-0125-01
100's	$14.60	GENERIC, Del Ray Laboratories Inc	00316-0142-01
100's	$14.88	GENERIC, Med-Pro Inc	53978-5048-09
120's	$6.44	GENERIC, Pd-Rx Pharmaceuticals	58864-0493-98
120's	$11.85	SUMYCIN, Pd-Rx Pharmaceuticals	55289-0494-98
Capsule - Oral - 500 mg			
10's	$2.82	GENERIC, Pd-Rx Pharmaceuticals	55289-0446-10
12's	$2.94	GENERIC, Pd-Rx Pharmaceuticals	55289-0446-12
16's	$3.02	GENERIC, Pd-Rx Pharmaceuticals	55289-0446-16
20's	$2.25	GENERIC, Allscripts Pharmaceutical Company	54569-2501-04
20's	$3.24	GENERIC, Pd-Rx Pharmaceuticals	55289-0446-20
24's	$7.61	GENERIC, Alpharma Uspd Makers Of Barre and Nmc	63874-0124-24
28's	$2.14	GENERIC, Circle Pharmaceuticals Inc	00659-0102-28
28's	$3.15	GENERIC, Allscripts Pharmaceutical Company	54569-2501-00
28's	$4.28	GENERIC, Pd-Rx Pharmaceuticals	55289-0446-28

T

28's	$7.98	GENERIC, Alpharma Uspd Makers Of Barre and Nmc	63874-0124-28
30's	$2.97	SUMYCIN, Physicians Total Care	54868-1048-01
30's	$4.43	GENERIC, Pd-Rx Pharmaceuticals	55289-0446-30
30's	$8.61	GENERIC, Alpharma Uspd Makers Of Barre and Nmc	63874-0124-30
40's	$3.26	GENERIC, Circle Pharmaceuticals Inc	00659-0102-40
40's	$3.57	SUMYCIN, Physicians Total Care	54868-1048-03
40's	$4.50	GENERIC, Allscripts Pharmaceutical Company	54569-2501-02
40's	$4.73	GENERIC, Pd-Rx Pharmaceuticals	55289-0446-40
40's	$9.51	GENERIC, Alpharma Uspd Makers Of Barre and Nmc	63874-0124-40
56's	$5.15	GENERIC, Allscripts Pharmaceutical Company	54569-2501-06
60's	$4.76	SUMYCIN, Physicians Total Care	54868-1048-02
60's	$5.78	GENERIC, Pd-Rx Pharmaceuticals	55289-0446-60
60's	$6.75	GENERIC, Allscripts Pharmaceutical Company	54569-2501-08
100's	$7.40	GENERIC, Us Trading Corporation	56126-0363-11
100's	$8.42	GENERIC, Purepac Pharmaceutical Company	00228-2406-10
100's	$8.48	GENERIC, Pd-Rx Pharmaceuticals	55289-0446-01
100's	$8.70	GENERIC, Interstate Drug Exchange Inc	00814-7758-14
100's	$8.90	GENERIC, Geneva Pharmaceuticals	00781-2466-01
100's	$8.95	GENERIC, Major Pharmaceuticals Inc	00904-2407-60
100's	$9.08	GENERIC, Global Pharmaceutical Corporation	00115-1402-01
100's	$9.75	FEDERAL UPPER LIMIT, H.C.F.A. F F P	99999-2326-04
100's	$10.20	GENERIC, Aligen Independent Laboratories Inc	00405-4976-01
100's	$10.50	GENERIC, Raway Pharmacal Inc	00686-0162-13
100's	$10.94	GENERIC, Moore, H.L. Drug Exchange Inc	00839-5075-06
100's	$11.04	GENERIC, Auro Pharmaceutical	55829-0697-10
100's	$11.25	GENERIC, Mylan Pharmaceuticals Inc	00378-0102-01
100's	$11.25	GENERIC, Allscripts Pharmaceutical Company	54569-2501-03
100's	$11.80	GENERIC, Ivax Corporation	00172-2407-60
100's	$11.80	GENERIC, Barr Laboratories Inc	00555-0010-02
100's	$14.09	GENERIC, Alpharma Uspd Makers Of Barre and Nmc	63874-0124-01
100's	$16.00	GENERIC, Watson/Schein Pharmaceuticals Inc	00364-2029-90
100's	$19.02	GENERIC, Ivax Corporation	00182-0679-89

Suspension - Oral - 125 mg/5 ml

480 ml	$6.00	GENERIC, C.O. Truxton Inc	00463-5002-16

Tablet - Oral - 250 mg

100's	$8.51	SUMYCIN, Bristol-Myers Squibb	00003-0663-45

Tablet - Oral - 500 mg

100's	$16.57	SUMYCIN, Bristol-Myers Squibb	00003-0603-43

PRODUCT LISTING - EQUIVALENTS NOT AVAILABLE

Capsule - Oral - 250 mg

4's	$3.56	GENERIC, Prescript Pharmaceuticals	00247-0067-04
8's	$1.25	GENERIC, Southwood Pharmaceuticals Inc	58016-0101-08
8's	$3.78	GENERIC, Prescript Pharmaceuticals	00247-0067-08
10's	$1.50	GENERIC, Southwood Pharmaceuticals Inc	58016-0101-10
10's	$3.88	GENERIC, Prescript Pharmaceuticals	00247-0067-10
12's	$1.60	GENERIC, Southwood Pharmaceuticals Inc	58016-0101-12
12's	$3.99	GENERIC, Prescript Pharmaceuticals	00247-0067-12
12's	$5.95	GENERIC, Pharma Pac	52959-0283-12
14's	$1.75	GENERIC, Southwood Pharmaceuticals Inc	58016-0101-14
15's	$2.00	GENERIC, Southwood Pharmaceuticals Inc	58016-0101-15
15's	$4.15	GENERIC, Prescript Pharmaceuticals	00247-0067-15
16's	$1.00	GENERIC, Allscripts Pharmaceutical Company	54569-2279-05
16's	$4.20	GENERIC, Prescript Pharmaceuticals	00247-0067-16
20's	$1.25	GENERIC, Allscripts Pharmaceutical Company	54569-2279-01
20's	$2.02	GENERIC, Southwood Pharmaceuticals Inc	58016-0101-20
20's	$3.23	GENERIC, Physicians Total Care	54868-0024-07
20's	$4.41	GENERIC, Prescript Pharmaceuticals	00247-0067-20
20's	$10.44	GENERIC, Pharma Pac	52959-0283-20
21's	$2.25	GENERIC, Southwood Pharmaceuticals Inc	58016-0101-21
21's	$4.47	GENERIC, Prescript Pharmaceuticals	00247-0067-21
24's	$2.50	GENERIC, Southwood Pharmaceuticals Inc	58016-0101-24
28's	$1.75	GENERIC, Allscripts Pharmaceutical Company	54569-2279-00
28's	$2.23	GENERIC, Pharmaceutical Corporation Of America	51655-0097-29
28's	$2.83	GENERIC, Southwood Pharmaceuticals Inc	58016-0101-28
28's	$4.84	GENERIC, Prescript Pharmaceuticals	00247-0067-28
28's	$8.25	GENERIC, Pharma Pac	52959-0283-28
30's	$1.88	GENERIC, Allscripts Pharmaceutical Company	54569-2279-08
30's	$3.03	GENERIC, Southwood Pharmaceuticals Inc	58016-0101-30
30's	$4.01	GENERIC, Physicians Total Care	54868-0024-03
30's	$4.94	GENERIC, Prescript Pharmaceuticals	00247-0067-30
40's	$2.50	GENERIC, Allscripts Pharmaceutical Company	54569-2279-02
40's	$3.20	GENERIC, Pharmaceutical Corporation Of America	51655-0097-51
40's	$4.04	GENERIC, Southwood Pharmaceuticals Inc	58016-0101-40
40's	$4.78	GENERIC, Physicians Total Care	54868-0024-01
40's	$5.47	GENERIC, Prescript Pharmaceuticals	00247-0067-40
40's	$11.06	GENERIC, Pharma Pac	52959-0283-40
56's	$6.32	GENERIC, Prescript Pharmaceuticals	00247-0067-56
60's	$3.76	GENERIC, Allscripts Pharmaceutical Company	54569-3315-00
60's	$6.12	GENERIC, Southwood Pharmaceuticals Inc	58016-0101-60
60's	$6.34	GENERIC, Physicians Total Care	54868-0024-04
60's	$6.53	GENERIC, Prescript Pharmaceuticals	00247-0067-60
90's	$8.12	GENERIC, Prescript Pharmaceuticals	00247-0067-90
90's	$8.68	GENERIC, Physicians Total Care	54868-0024-08
90's	$9.17	GENERIC, Southwood Pharmaceuticals Inc	58016-0101-90
100's	$6.26	GENERIC, Allscripts Pharmaceutical Company	54569-2279-06
100's	$7.50	GENERIC, Cmc-Consolidated Midland Corporation	00223-1655-01
100's	$8.65	GENERIC, Prescript Pharmaceuticals	00247-0067-00
100's	$9.46	GENERIC, Physicians Total Care	54868-0024-05
100's	$10.10	GENERIC, Southwood Pharmaceuticals Inc	58016-0101-00
100's	$18.96	GENERIC, Pharma Pac	52959-0283-00
118's	$9.60	GENERIC, Prescript Pharmaceuticals	00247-0067-52

Capsule - Oral - 500 mg

4's	$3.73	GENERIC, Prescript Pharmaceuticals	00247-0066-04
10's	$1.09	GENERIC, Southwood Pharmaceuticals Inc	58016-0102-10
12's	$1.31	GENERIC, Southwood Pharmaceuticals Inc	58016-0102-12
12's	$4.47	GENERIC, Prescript Pharmaceuticals	00247-0066-12
14's	$1.53	GENERIC, Southwood Pharmaceuticals Inc	58016-0102-14
14's	$5.80	GENERIC, Pharma Pac	52959-0336-14
15's	$1.64	GENERIC, Southwood Pharmaceuticals Inc	58016-0102-15
20's	$2.18	GENERIC, Southwood Pharmaceuticals Inc	58016-0102-20
20's	$5.21	GENERIC, Prescript Pharmaceuticals	00247-0066-20
20's	$7.71	GENERIC, Pharma Pac	52959-0336-20
21's	$2.29	GENERIC, Southwood Pharmaceuticals Inc	58016-0102-21
21's	$5.29	GENERIC, Prescript Pharmaceuticals	00247-0066-21
24's	$2.62	GENERIC, Southwood Pharmaceuticals Inc	58016-0102-24
28's	$3.05	GENERIC, Southwood Pharmaceuticals Inc	58016-0102-28
28's	$5.95	GENERIC, Prescript Pharmaceuticals	00247-0066-28
28's	$9.24	GENERIC, Pharma Pac	52959-0336-28
30's	$3.27	GENERIC, Southwood Pharmaceuticals Inc	58016-0102-30
30's	$5.27	GENERIC, Physicians Total Care	54868-0025-01
30's	$6.13	GENERIC, Prescript Pharmaceuticals	00247-0066-30
30's	$9.50	GENERIC, Pharma Pac	52959-0336-30
40's	$4.36	GENERIC, Southwood Pharmaceuticals Inc	58016-0102-40
40's	$6.47	GENERIC, Physicians Total Care	54868-0025-03
40's	$7.06	GENERIC, Prescript Pharmaceuticals	00247-0066-40
40's	$11.48	GENERIC, Pharma Pac	52959-0336-40
50's	$5.46	GENERIC, Southwood Pharmaceuticals Inc	58016-0102-50
56's	$14.15	GENERIC, Pharma Pac	52959-0336-56
60's	$6.55	GENERIC, Southwood Pharmaceuticals Inc	58016-0102-60
60's	$8.92	GENERIC, Prescript Pharmaceuticals	00247-0066-60
60's	$16.14	GENERIC, Physicians Total Care	54868-0025-04
90's	$12.47	GENERIC, Physicians Total Care	54868-0025-07
90's	$21.52	GENERIC, Pharma Pac	52959-0336-90
100's	$5.46	GENERIC, Southwood Pharmaceuticals Inc	58016-0102-00
100's	$8.96	EMTET-500, Economed Pharmaceuticals Inc	38130-0203-01
100's	$11.00	GENERIC, Ampharco Inc	59015-0460-02
100's	$12.50	GENERIC, Cmc-Consolidated Midland Corporation	00223-1656-01
100's	$12.62	GENERIC, Prescript Pharmaceuticals	00247-0066-00
100's	$13.67	GENERIC, Physicians Total Care	54868-0025-05

Solution - Topical - 2.2 mg/ml

70 ml	$59.83	TOPICYCLINE, Roberts Pharmaceutical Corporation	54092-0315-70

Suspension - Oral - 125 mg/5 ml

473 ml	$59.63	SUMYCIN, Bristol-Myers Squibb	59772-0815-05
473 ml	$59.64	SUMYCIN, Bristol-Myers Squibb	59772-0815-50
480 ml	$13.98	SUMYCIN, Physicians Total Care	54868-3424-00

Thalidomide *(003413)*

Categories: Erythema nodosum leprosum; FDA Approved 1998 Jul; Pregnancy Category X; Orphan Drugs

Drug Classes: Immunomodulators; Tumor necrosis factor modulators

Brand Names: Thalomid

Cost of Therapy: $1,074.38 (Erythema Nodosum Leprosum; Thalomid; 50 mg; 2 capsules/day; 30 day supply)

WARNING

SEVERE, LIFE-THREATENING HUMAN BIRTH DEFECTS.

IF THALIDOMIDE IS TAKEN DURING PREGNANCY, IT CAN CAUSE SEVERE BIRTH DEFECTS OR DEATH TO AN UNBORN BABY. THALIDOMIDE SHOULD NEVER BE USED BY WOMEN WHO ARE PREGNANT OR WHO COULD BECOME PREGNANT WHILE TAKING THE DRUG. EVEN A SINGLE DOSE [1 CAPSULE (50 mg)] TAKEN BY A PREGNANT WOMAN DURING HER PREGNANCY CAN CAUSE SEVERE BIRTH DEFECTS.

BECAUSE OF THIS TOXICITY AND IN AN EFFORT TO MAKE THE CHANCE OF FETAL EXPOSURE TO THALIDOMIDE AS NEGLIGIBLE AS POSSIBLE, THALIDOMIDE IS APPROVED FOR MARKETING ONLY UNDER A SPECIAL RESTRICTED DISTRIBUTION PROGRAM APPROVED BY THE FOOD AND DRUG ADMINISTRATION. THIS PROGRAM IS CALLED THE "SYSTEM FOR THALIDOMIDE EDUCATION AND PRESCRIBING SAFETY (*S.T.E.P.S.*)".

UNDER THIS RESTRICTED DISTRIBUTION PROGRAM, ONLY PRESCRIBERS AND PHARMACISTS REGISTERED WITH THE PROGRAM ARE ALLOWED TO PRESCRIBE AND DISPENSE THE PRODUCT. IN

WARNING — *Cont'd*

ADDITION, PATIENTS MUST BE ADVISED OF, AGREE TO, AND COMPLY WITH THE REQUIREMENTS OF THE *S.T.E.P.S.* PROGRAM IN ORDER TO RECEIVE PRODUCT.

PLEASE SEE THE FOLLOWING BOXED WARNINGS CONTAINING SPECIAL INFORMATION FOR PRESCRIBERS, FEMALE PATIENTS, AND MALE PATIENTS ABOUT THIS RESTRICTED DISTRIBUTION PROGRAM.

PRESCRIBERS

Thalidomide may be prescribed only by licensed prescribers who are registered in the *S.T.E.P.S.* program and understand the risk of teratogenicity if thalidomide is used during pregnancy.

Major human fetal abnormalities related to thalidomide administration during pregnancy have been documented: amelia (absence of limbs), phocomelia (short limbs), hypoplasticity of the bones, absence of bones, external ear abnormalities (including anotia, micro pinna, small or absent external auditory canals), facial palsy, eye abnormalities (anophthalmos, microphthalmos), and congenital heart defects. Alimentary tract, urinary tract, and genital malformations have also been documented.[1] Mortality at or shortly after birth has been reported at about 40%.[2]

Effective contraception (see CONTRAINDICATIONS) must be used for at least 4 weeks before beginning thalidomide therapy, during thalidomide therapy, and for 4 weeks following discontinuation of thalidomide therapy. Reliable contraception is indicated even where there has been a history of infertility, unless due to hysterectomy or because the patient has been postmenopausal for at least 24 months. Two reliable forms of contraception must be used simultaneously unless continuous abstinence from heterosexual sexual contact is the chosen method. Women of childbearing potential should be referred to a qualified provider of contraceptive methods, if needed. Sexually mature women who have not undergone a hysterectomy or who have not been postmenopausal for at least 24 consecutive months (*i.e.,* who have had menses at some time in the preceding 24 consecutive months) are considered to be women of childbearing potential.

Before starting treatment, women of childbearing potential should have a pregnancy test (sensitivity of at least 50 mIU/ml). The test should be performed within the 24 hours prior to beginning therapy. A prescription for thalidomide for a woman of childbearing potential must not be issued by the prescriber until a written report of a negative pregnancy test has been obtained by the prescriber.

Male Patients: Because thalidomide is present in the semen of patients receiving the drug, males receiving thalidomide must always use a latex condom during any sexual contact with women of childbearing potential.

Once treatment has started, pregnancy testing should occur weekly during the first month of use, then monthly thereafter in women with regular menstrual cycles. If menstrual cycles are irregular, the pregnancy testing should occur every 2 weeks. Pregnancy testing and counseling should be performed if a patient misses her period or if there is any abnormality in menstrual bleeding.

If pregnancy does occur during thalidomide treatment, thalidomide must be discontinued immediately.

Any suspected fetal exposure to thalidomide must be reported immediately to the FDA *via* the MedWATCH number at 1-800-FDA-1088 and also to Celgene Corporation. The patient should be referred to an obstetrician/gynecologist experienced in reproductive toxicity for further evaluation and counseling.

FEMALE PATIENTS

Thalidomide is contraindicated in WOMEN of childbearing potential unless alternative therapies are considered inappropriate AND the patient MEETS ALL OF THE FOLLOWING CONDITIONS (*i.e.,* she is essentially unable to become pregnant while on thalidomide therapy):

She understands and can reliably carry out instructions.

She is capable of complying with the mandatory contraceptive measures, pregnancy testing, patient registration, and patient survey as described in the System for Thalidomide Education and Prescribing Safety (*S.T.E.P.S.*) program.

She has received both oral and written warnings of the hazards of taking thalidomide during pregnancy and of exposing a fetus to the drug.

She has received both oral and written warnings of the risk of possible contraception failure and of the need to use two reliable forms of contraception simultaneously (see CONTRAINDICATIONS), unless continuous abstinence from heterosexual sexual contact is the chosen method. (Sexually mature women who have not undergone a hysterectomy or who have not been postmenopausal for at least 24 consecutive months [*i.e.,* who have had menses at some time in the preceding 24 consecutive months] are considered to be women of childbearing potential.)

She acknowledges, in writing, her understanding of these warnings and of the need for using two reliable methods of contraception for 4 weeks prior to starting thalidomide therapy, during thalidomide therapy, and for 4 weeks after stopping thalidomide therapy.

She has had a negative pregnancy test with a sensitivity of at least 50 mIU/ml, within the 24 hours prior to beginning therapy. (See PRECAUTIONS and CONTRAINDICATIONS.)

If the patient is between 12 and 18 years of age, her parent or legal guardian must have read this material and agreed to ensure compliance with the above.

MALE PATIENTS

Thalidomide is contraindicated in sexually mature MALES unless the PATIENT MEETS ALL OF THE FOLLOWING CONDITIONS:

He understands and can reliably carry out instructions.

He is capable of complying with the mandatory contraceptive measures that are appropriate for men, patient registration, and patient survey as described in the *S.T.E.P.S.* program.

He has received both oral and written warnings of the hazards of taking thalidomide and exposing a fetus to the drug.

He has received both oral and written warnings of the risk of possible contraception failure and of the presence of thalidomide in semen. He has been instructed that he must always use barrier contraception (latex condom) during any sexual contact with women of childbearing potential, even if he has undergone successful vasectomy.

He acknowledges, in writing, his understanding of these warnings and of the need to use barrier contraception (latex condom) during any sexual contact with women of childbearing potential,

WARNING — *Cont'd*

even if he has undergone successful vasectomy. Sexually mature women who have not undergone a hysterectomy or who have not been postmenopausal for at least 24 consecutive months (*i.e.,* who have had menses at some time in the preceding 24 consecutive months) are considered to be women of childbearing potential.

If the patient is between 12 and 18 years of age, his parent or legal guardian must have read this material and agreed to ensure compliance with the above.

DESCRIPTION

Thalidomide, α-(N-phthalimido)glutarimide, is an immunomodulatory agent. The empirical formula for thalidomide is $C_{13}H_{10}N_2O_4$ and the gram molecular weight is 258.2.

Thalidomide is an off-white to white, nearly odorless, crystalline powder that is soluble at 25°C in dimethyl sulfoxide and sparingly soluble in water and ethanol. The glutarimide moiety contains a single asymmetric center and, therefore, may exist in either of two optically active forms designated S-(-) or R-(+). Thalidomide is an equal mixture of the S-(-) and R-(+) forms and, therefore, has a net optical rotation of zero.

Thalomid is available in 50 mg capsules for oral administration. *Active Ingredient:* Thalidomide. *Inactive Ingredients:* Anhydrous lactose, microcrystalline cellulose, polyvinylpyrrolidone, stearic acid, colloidal anhydrous silica, and gelatin.

CLINICAL PHARMACOLOGY

MECHANISM OF ACTION

Thalidomide is an immunomodulatory agent with a spectrum of activity that is not fully characterized. In patients with erythema nodosum leprosum (ENL) the mechanism of action is not fully understood.

Available data from *in vitro* studies and preliminary clinical trials suggest that the immunologic effects of this compound can vary substantially under different conditions, but may be related to suppression of excessive tumor necrosis factor-alpha (TNF-α) production and down-modulation of selected cell surface adhesion molecules involved in leukocyte migration.[3-6] For example, administration of thalidomide has been reported to decrease circulating levels of TNF-α in patients with ENL,[3] however, it has also been shown to increase plasma TNF-α levels in HIV-seropositive patients.[7]

PHARMACOKINETICS AND DRUG METABOLISM

Absorption

The absolute bioavailability of thalidomide from thalidomide capsules has not yet been characterized in human subjects due to its poor aqueous solubility. In studies of both healthy volunteers and subjects with Hansen's disease, the mean time to peak plasma concentrations (T_{max}) of thalidomide ranged from 2.9-5.7 hours indicating that thalidomide is slowly absorbed from the gastrointestinal tract. While the extent of absorption (as measured by area under the curve [AUC]) is proportional to dose in healthy subjects, the observed peak concentration (C_{max}) increased in a less than proportional manner (see TABLE 1). This lack of C_{max} dose proportionality, coupled with the observed increase in T_{max} values, suggests that the poor solubility of thalidomide in aqueous media may be hindering the rate of absorption.

Coadministration of thalidomide with a high fat meal causes minor (<10%) changes in the observed AUC and C_{max} values; however, it causes an increase in T_{max} to approximately 6 hours.

TABLE 1 *Pharmacokinetic Parameter Values for Thalidomide**

Population /Single Dose	AUC(0-∞) (μg·h/ml)	C_{max} (μg/ml)	T_{max} (h)	Half-life (h)
Healthy Subjects (n=14)				
50 mg	4.9 (16%)	0.62 (52%)	2.9 (66%)	5.52 (37%)
200 mg	18.9 (17%)	1.76 (30%)	3.5 (57%)	5.53 (25%)
400 mg	36.4 (26%)	2.82 (28%)	4.3 (37%)	7.29 (36%)
Patients With Hansen's Disease (n=6)				
400 mg	46.4 (44.1%)	3.44 (52.6%)	5.7 (27%)	6.86 (17%)

* Mean (%CV).

Distribution

In human blood plasma, the geometric mean plasma protein binding was 55% and 66%, respectively, for (+)-(R)- and (-)-(S)-thalidomide.[8] In a pharmacokinetic study of thalidomide in HIV-seropositive adult male subjects receiving thalidomide 100 mg/day, thalidomide was detectable in the semen.

Metabolism

At the present time, the exact metabolic route and fate of thalidomide is not known in humans. Thalidomide itself does not appear to be hepatically metabolized to any large extent, but appears to undergo non-enzymatic hydrolysis in plasma to multiple metabolites. In a repeat dose study in which thalidomide 200 mg was administered to 10 healthy females for 18 days, thalidomide displayed similar pharmacokinetic profiles on the first and last day of dosing. This suggests that thalidomide does not induce or inhibit its own metabolism.

Elimination

As indicated in TABLE 1, the mean half-life of elimination ranges from approximately 5-7 hours following a single dose and is not altered upon multiple dosing. As noted in Metabolism, the precise metabolic rate and route of elimination of thalidomide in humans is not known at this time. Thalidomide itself has a renal clearance of 1.15 ml/minute with less than 0.7% of the dose excreted in the urine as unchanged drug. Following a single dose, urinary levels of thalidomide were undetectable 48 hrs after dosing. Although thalidomide is thought to be hydrolyzed to a number of metabolites,[9] only a very small amount (0.02% of the administered dose) of 4-OH-thalidomide was identified in the urine of subjects 12-24 hours after dosing.

T

Pharmacokinetic Data in Special Populations

HIV-Seropositive Subjects: There is no apparent significant difference in measured pharmacokinetic parameter values between healthy human subjects and HIV-seropositive subjects following single dose administration of thalidomide capsules.

Patients With Hansen's Disease: Analysis of data from a small study in Hansen's patients suggests that these patients, relative to healthy subjects, may have an increased bioavailability of thalidomide. The increase is reflected both in an increased area under the curve and in increased peak plasma levels. The clinical significance of this increase is unknown.

Patients With Renal Insufficiency: The pharmacokinetics of thalidomide in patients with renal dysfunction have not been determined.

Patients With Hepatic Disease: The pharmacokinetics of thalidomide in patients with hepatic impairment have not been determined.

Age: Analysis of the data from pharmacokinetic studies in healthy volunteers and patients with Hansen's disease ranging in age from 20-69 years does not reveal any age-related changes.

Pediatric: No pharmacokinetic data are available in subjects below the age of 18 years.

Gender: While a comparative trial of the effects of gender on thalidomide pharmacokinetics has not been conducted, examination of the data for thalidomide does not reveal any significant gender differences in pharmacokinetic parameter values.

Race: Pharmacokinetic differences due to race have not been studied.

INDICATIONS AND USAGE

Thalidomide is indicated for the acute treatment of the cutaneous manifestations of moderate to severe erythema nodosum leprosum (ENL).

Thalidomide is not indicated as monotherapy for such ENL treatment in the presence of moderate to severe neuritis.

Thalidomide is also indicated as maintenance therapy for prevention and suppression of the cutaneous manifestations of ENL recurrence.

NON-FDA APPROVED INDICATIONS

Although not FDA approved, thalidomide has been used to treat wasting associated with AIDS, multiple myeloma, aphthous stomatitis, rheumatoid arthritis, cutaneous lupus erythematosus, Behcet's syndrome, Crohn's disease, and graft versus host disease in bone marrow transplant patients.

CONTRAINDICATIONS

See BOXED WARNING.

PREGNANCY CATEGORY X

Due to its known human teratogenicity, even following a single dose, thalidomide is contraindicated in pregnant women and women capable of becoming pregnant. (See BOXED WARNING.) When there is no alternative treatment, women of childbearing potential may be treated with thalidomide provided adequate precautions are taken to avoid pregnancy. Women must commit either to abstain continuously from heterosexual sexual contact or to use two methods of reliable birth control, including at least one highly effective method (*e.g.,* IUD, hormonal contraception, tubal ligation, or partner's vasectomy) and one additional effective method (*e.g.,* latex condom, diaphragm, or cervical cap), beginning 4 weeks prior to initiating treatment with thalidomide, during therapy with thalidomide, and continuing for 4 weeks following discontinuation of thalidomide therapy. If hormonal or IUD contraception is medically contraindicated (see also DRUG INTERACTIONS), two other effective or highly effective methods may be used.

Women of childbearing potential being treated with thalidomide should have pregnancy testing (sensitivity of at least 50 mIU/ml). The test should be performed within the 24 hours before beginning thalidomide therapy and then weekly during the first month of thalidomide therapy, then monthly thereafter in women with regular menstrual cycles or every 2 weeks in women with irregular menstrual cycles. Pregnancy testing and counseling should be performed if a patient misses her period or if there is any abnormality in menstrual bleeding. If pregnancy occurs during thalidomide treatment, thalidomide must be immediately discontinued. Under these conditions, the patient should be referred to an obstetrician/gynecologist experienced in reproductive toxicity for further evaluation and counseling.

Because thalidomide is present in the semen of patients receiving the drug, males receiving thalidomide must always use a latex condom during any sexual contact with women of childbearing potential.

Thalidomide is contraindicated in patients who have demonstrated hypersensitivity to the drug and its components.

WARNINGS

See BOXED WARNING.

BIRTH DEFECTS

Thalidomide can cause severe birth defects in humans. (See BOXED WARNING and CONTRAINDICATIONS.) Patients should be instructed to take thalidomide only as prescribed and not to share their thalidomide with anyone else. Because thalidomide is present in the semen of patients receiving the drug, males receiving thalidomide must always use a latex condom during any sexual contact with women of childbearing potential.

DROWSINESS AND SOMNOLENCE

Thalidomide frequently causes drowsiness and somnolence. Patients should be instructed to avoid situations where drowsiness may be a problem and not to take other medications that may cause drowsiness without adequate medical advice. Patients should be advised as to the possible impairment of mental and/or physical abilities required for the performance of hazardous tasks, such as driving a car or operating other complex or dangerous machinery.

PERIPHERAL NEUROPATHY

Thalidomide is known to cause nerve damage that may be permanent. Peripheral neuropathy is a common, potentially severe, side effect of treatment with thalidomide that may be irreversible. Peripheral neuropathy generally occurs following chronic use over a period of months, however, reports following relatively short-term use also exist. The correlation with cumulative dose is unclear. Symptoms may occur some time after thalidomide treatment has been stopped and may resolve slowly or not at all. Few reports of neuropathy have arisen in the treatment of ENL despite long-term thalidomide treatment. However, the inability clinically to differentiate thalidomide neuropathy from the neuropathy often seen in Hansen's disease makes it difficult to determine accurately the incidence of thalidomide-related neuropathy in ENL patients treated with thalidomide.

Patients should be examined at monthly intervals for the first 3 months of thalidomide therapy to enable the clinician to detect early signs of neuropathy, which include numbness, tingling or pain in the hands and feet. Patients should be evaluated periodically thereafter during treatment. Patients should be regularly counseled, questioned, and evaluated for signs or symptoms of peripheral neuropathy. Consideration should be given to electrophysiological testing, consisting of measurement of sensory nerve action potential (SNAP) amplitudes at baseline and thereafter every 6 months in an effort to detect asymptomatic neuropathy. If symptoms of drug-induced neuropathy develop, thalidomide should be discontinued immediately to limit further damage, if clinically appropriate. Usually, treatment with thalidomide should only be reinitiated if the neuropathy returns to baseline status. Medications known to be associated with neuropathy should be used with caution in patients receiving thalidomide.

DIZZINESS AND ORTHOSTATIC HYPOTENSION

Patients should also be advised that thalidomide may cause dizziness and orthostatic hypotension and that, therefore, they should sit upright for a few minutes prior to standing up from a recumbent position.

NEUTROPENIA

Decreased white blood cell counts, including neutropenia, have been reported in association with the clinical use of thalidomide. Treatment should not be initiated with an absolute neutrophil count (ANC) of $<750/mm^3$. White blood cell count and differential should be monitored on an ongoing basis, especially in patients who may be more prone to neutropenia, such as patients who are HIV-seropositive. If ANC decreases to below $750/mm^3$ while on treatment, the patient's medication regimen should be re-evaluated and, if the neutropenia persists, consideration should be given to withholding thalidomide if clinically appropriate.

INCREASED HIV-VIRAL LOAD

In a randomized, placebo controlled trial of thalidomide in an HIV-seropositive patient population, plasma HIV RNA levels were found to increase (median change = 0.42 $\log_{10}$ copies HIV RNA/ml, p = 0.04 compared to placebo).[7] A similar trend was observed in a second, unpublished study conducted in patients who were HIV-seropostive.[13] The clinical significance of this increase is unknown. Both studies were conducted prior to availability of highly active antiretroviral therapy. Until the clinical significance of this finding is further understood, in HIV-seropositive patients, viral load should be measured after the first and third months of treatment and every 3 months thereafter.

PRECAUTIONS

HYPERSENSITIVITY

Hypersensitivity to thalidomide has been reported. Signs and symptoms have included the occurrence of erythematous macular rash, possibly associated with fever, tachycardia, and hypotension, and if severe, may necessitate interruption of therapy. If the reaction recurs when dosing is resumed, thalidomide should be discontinued.

BRADYCARDIA

Bradycardia in association with thalidomide use has been reported. At present there have been no reports of bradycardia requiring medical or other intervention. The clinical significance and underlying etiology of the bradycardia noted in some thalidomide-treated patients are presently unknown.

STEVENS-JOHNSON SYNDROME AND TOXIC EPIDERMAL NECROLYSIS

Serious dermatologic reactions including Stevens-Johnson syndrome and toxic epidermal necrolysis, which may be fatal, have been reported. Thalidomide should be discontinued if a skin rash occurs and only resumed following appropriate clinical evaluation. If the rash is exfoliative, purpuric, or bullous or if Stevens-Johnson syndrome or toxic epidermal necrolysis is suspected, use of thalidomide should not be resumed.

SEIZURES

Although not reported from pre-marketing controlled clinical trials, seizures, including grand mal convulsions, have been reported during post-approval use of thalidomide in clinical practice. Because these events are reported voluntarily from a population of unknown size, estimates of frequency cannot be made. Most patients had disorders that may have predisposed them to seizure activity, and it is not currently known whether thalidomide has any epilopeogenic influence. During therapy with thalidomide, patients with a history of seizures or with other risk factors for the development of seizures should be monitored closely for clinical changes that could precipitate acute seizure activity.

INFORMATION FOR THE PATIENT

See BOXED WARNING.

Patients should be instructed about the potential teratogenicity of thalidomide and the precautions that must be taken to preclude fetal exposure as per the *S.T.E.P.S.* program and BOXED WARNING. Patients should be instructed to take thalidomide only as prescribed in compliance with all of the provisions of the *S.T.E.P.S.* Restricted Distribution Program.

Patients should be instructed not to share medication with anyone else.

Patients should be instructed that thalidomide frequently causes drowsiness and somnolence. Patients should be instructed to avoid situations where drowsiness may be a problem and not to take other medications that may cause drowsiness without adequate medical advice. Patients should be advised as to the possible impairment of mental and/or physical abilities required for the performance of hazardous tasks, such as driving a car or operating

T

other complex machinery. Patients should be instructed that thalidomide may potentiate the somnolence caused by alcohol.

Patients should be instructed that thalidomide can cause peripheral neuropathies that may be initially signaled by numbness, tingling, or pain or a burning sensation in the feet or hands. Patients should be instructed to report such occurrences to their prescriber immediately.

Patients should also be instructed that thalidomide may cause dizziness and orthostatic hypotension and that, therefore, they should sit upright for a few minutes prior to standing up from a recumbent position.

Patients should be instructed that they are not permitted to donate blood while taking thalidomide. In addition, male patients should be instructed that they are not permitted to donate sperm while taking thalidomide.

LABORATORY TESTS

Pregnancy Testing

(See BOXED WARNING.) Women of childbearing potential should have pregnancy testing performed (sensitivity of at least 50 mIU/ml). The test should be performed within the 24 hours prior to beginning thalidomide therapy and then weekly during the first month of use, then monthly thereafter in women with regular menstrual cycles or every 2 weeks in women with irregular menstrual cycles. Pregnancy testing should also be performed if a patient misses her period or if there is any abnormality in menstrual bleeding.

Neutropenia

See WARNINGS.

HIV Viral Load

See WARNINGS.

CARCINOGENESIS, MUTAGENESIS, AND IMPAIRMENT OF FERTILITY

Long-term carcinogenicity tests have not been conducted using thalidomide. Thalidomide gave no evidence of mutagenic effects when assayed in *in vitro* bacterial (*Salmonella typhimurium* and *Escherichia coli;* Ames mutagenicity test), *in vitro* mammalian (AS52 Chinese hamster ovary cells; AS52/XPRT mammalian cell forward gene mutation assay) and *in vivo* mammalian (CD-1 mice; *in vivo* micronucleus test) test systems.

Animal studies to characterize the effects of thalidomide on fertility have not been conducted.

PREGNANCY CATEGORY X

See BOXED WARNING and CONTRAINDICATIONS.

Because of the known human teratogenicity of thalidomide, thalidomide is contraindicated in women who are or may become pregnant and who are not using the two required types of birth control or who are not continually abstaining from heterosexual sexual contact. If thalidomide is taken during pregnancy, it can cause severe birth defects or death to an unborn baby. Thalidomide should never be used by women who are pregnant or who could become pregnant while taking the drug. Even a single dose [1 capsule (50 mg)] taken by a pregnant woman can cause birth defects. If pregnancy does occur during treatment, the drug should be immediately discontinued. Under these conditions, the patient should be referred to an obstetrician/gynecologist experienced in reproductive toxicity for further evaluation and counseling. Any suspected fetal exposure to thalidomide must be reported to the FDA *via* the MedWatch program at 1-800-FDA-1088 and also to Celgene Corporation.

Because thalidomide is present in the semen of patients receiving the drug, males receiving thalidomide must always use a latex condom during any sexual contact with women of childbearing potential.

Animal studies to characterize the effects of thalidomide on late stage pregnancy have not been conducted.

NURSING MOTHERS

It is not known whether thalidomide is excreted in human milk. Because many drugs are excreted in human milk and because of the potential for serious adverse reactions in nursing infants from thalidomide, a decision should be made whether to discontinue nursing or to discontinue the drug, taking into account the importance of the drug to the mother.

PEDIATRIC USE

Safety and effectiveness in pediatric patients below the age of 12 years have not been established.

GERIATRIC USE

No systematic studies in geriatric patients have been conducted. Thalidomide has been used in clinical trials in patients up to 90 years of age. Adverse events in patients over the age of 65 years did not appear to differ in kind from those reported for younger individuals.

DRUG INTERACTIONS

Thalidomide has been reported to enhance the sedative activity of barbiturates, alcohol, chlorpromazine, and reserpine.

PERIPHERAL NEUROPATHY

Medications known to be associated with peripheral neuropathy should be used with caution in patients receiving thalidomide.

ORAL CONTRACEPTIVES

In 10 healthy women, the pharmacokinetic profiles of norethindrone and ethinyl estradiol following administration of a single dose containing 1.0 mg of norethindrone acetate and 75 µg of ethinyl estradiol were studied. The results were similar with and without coadministration of thalidomide 200 mg/day to steady-state levels.

IMPORTANT NON-THALIDOMIDE DRUG INTERACTIONS

Drugs That Interfere With Hormonal Contraceptives

Concomitant use of HIV-protease inhibitors, griseofulvin, rifampin, rifabutin, phenytoin, or carbamazepine with hormonal contraceptive agents, may reduce the effectiveness of the contraception. Therefore, women requiring treatment with one or more of these drugs must use two OTHER effective or highly effective methods of contraception or abstain from heterosexual sexual contact.

ADVERSE REACTIONS

The most serious toxicity associated with thalidomide is its documented human teratogenicity. (See BOXED WARNING and CONTRAINDICATIONS.) The risk of severe birth defects, primarily phocomelia or death to the fetus, is extremely high during the critical period of pregnancy. The critical period is estimated, depending on the source of information, to range from 35-50 days after the last menstrual period. The risk of other potentially severe birth defects outside this critical period is unknown, but may be significant. Based on present knowledge, thalidomide must not be used at any time during pregnancy.

Because thalidomide is present in the semen of patients receiving the drug, males receiving thalidomide must always use a latex condom during any sexual contact with women of childbearing potential.

Thalidomide is associated with drowsiness/somnolence, peripheral neuropathy, dizziness/orthostatic hypotension, neutropenia, and HIV viral load increase. (See WARNINGS.)

Hypersensitivity to thalidomide and bradycardia in patients treated with thalidomide have been reported. (See PRECAUTIONS.)

Somnolence, dizziness, and rash are the most commonly observed adverse events associated with the use of thalidomide. Thalidomide has been studied in controlled and uncontrolled clinical trials in patients with ENL and in people who are HIV-seropositive. In addition, thalidomide has been administered investigationally for more than 20 years in numerous indications. Adverse event profiles from these uses are summarized in the sections that follow.

OTHER ADVERSE EVENTS

Due to the nature of the longitudinal data that form the basis of this product's safety evaluation, no determination has been made of the causal relationship between the reported adverse events listed below and thalidomide. These lists are of various adverse events noted by investigators in patients to whom they had administered thalidomide under various conditions.

INCIDENCE IN CONTROLLED CLINICAL TRIALS

TABLE 4 lists treatment-emergent signs and symptoms that occurred in thalidomide-treated patients in controlled clinical trials in ENL. Doses ranged from 50-300 mg/day. All adverse events were mild to moderate in severity, and none resulted in discontinuation. TABLE 4 also lists treatment-emergent adverse events that occurred in at least 3 of the thalidomide-treated HIV-seropositive patients who participated in an 8 week, placebo-controlled clinical trial. Events that were more frequent in the placebo-treated group are not included. (See WARNINGS, PRECAUTIONS, and DRUG INTERACTIONS.)

OTHER ADVERSE EVENTS OBSERVED IN ENL PATIENTS

Thalidomide in doses up to 400 mg/day has been administered investigationally in the US over a 19 year period in 1465 patients with ENL. The published literature describes the treatment of an additional 1678 patients. To provide a meaningful estimate of the proportion of the individuals having adverse events, similar types of events were grouped into a smaller number of standardized categories using a modified COSTART dictionary/terminology. These categories are used in the listing below. All reported events are included except those already listed in TABLE 4. Due to the fact that these data were collected from uncontrolled studies, the incidence rate cannot be determined. As mentioned previously, **no causal relationship between thalidomide and these events can be conclusively determined at this time.** These are reports of all adverse events noted by investigators in patients to whom they had administered thalidomide.

Body as a Whole: Abdomen enlarged, fever, photosensitivity, upper extremity pain.

Cardiovascular System: Bradycardia, hypertension, hypotension, peripheral vascular disorder, tachycardia.

Digestive System: Anorexia, appetite increase/weight gain, dry mouth, dyspepsia, enlarged liver, eructation, flatulence, increased liver function tests, intestinal obstruction, vomiting.

Hemic and Lymphatic: ESR decrease, eosinophilia, granulocytopenia, hypochromic anemia, leukemia, leukocytosis, leukopenia, MCV elevated, RBC abnormal, spleen palpable, thrombocytopenia.

Metabolic and Endocrine: ADH inappropriate, alkaline phosphatase, amyloidosis, bilirubinemia, BUN increased, creatinine increased, cyanosis, diabetes, edema, electrolyte abnormalities, hyperglycemia, hyperkalemia, hyperuricemia, hypocalcemia, hypoproteinemia, LDH increased, phosphorus decreased, SGPT increased.

Muscular Skeletal: Arthritis, bone tenderness, hypertonia, joint disorder, leg cramps, myalgia, myasthenia, periosteal disorder.

Nervous System: Abnormal thinking, agitation, amnesia, anxiety, causalgia, circumoral paresthesia, confusion, depression, euphoria, hyperesthesia, insomnia, nervousness, neuralgia, neuritis, neuropathy, paresthesia, peripheral neuritis, psychosis, vasodilation.

Respiratory System: Cough, emphysema, epistaxis, pulmonary embolus, rales, upper respiratory infection, voice alteration.

Skin and Appendages: Acne, alopecia, dry skin, eczematous rash, exfoliative dermatitis, ichthyosis, perifollicular thickening, skin necrosis, seborrhea, sweating, urticaria, vesiculobullous rash.

Special Senses: Amblyopia, deafness, dry eye, eye pain, tinnitus.

Urogenital: Decreased creatinine clearance, hematuria, orchitis, proteinuria, pyuria, urinary frequency.

TABLE 4 *Summary of Adverse Events (AEs) Reported in Celgene-Sponsored Controlled Clinical Trials*

Body System	All AEs Reported in ENL Patients	AEs Reported in ≥3 HIV-Seropositive Patients		
		Thalidomide (mg/day)		
	50-300 mg/day	100	200	Placebo
Adverse Event	(n=24)	(n=36)	(n=32)	(n=35)
Body as a Whole	16 (66.7%)	18 (50.0%)	19 (59.4%)	13 (37.1%)
Abdominal pain	1 (4.2%)	1 (2.8%)	1 (3.1%)	4 (11.4%)
Accidental injury	1 (4.2%)	2 (5.6%)	0	1 (2.9%)
Asthenia	2 (8.3%)	2 (5.6%)	7 (21.9%)	1 (2.9%)
Back pain	1 (4.2%)	2 (5.6%)	0	0
Chills	1 (4.2%)	0	3 (9.4%)	4 (11.4%)
Facial edema	1 (4.2%)	0	0	0
Fever	0	7 (19.4%)	7 (21.9%)	6 (17.1%)
Headache	3 (12.5%)	6 (16.7%)	6 (18.7%)	4 (11.4%)
Infection	0	3 (8.3%)	2 (6.3%)	1 (2.9%)
Malaise	2 (8.3%)	0	0	0
Neck pain	1 (4.2%)	0	0	0
Neck rigidity	1 (4.2%)	0	0	0
Pain	2 (8.3%)	0	1 (3.1%)	2 (5.7%)
Digestive System	5 (20.8%)	16 (44.4%)	16 (50.0%)	15 (42.9%)
Anorexia	0	1 (2.8%)	3 (9.4%)	2 (5.7%)
Constipation	1 (4.2%)	1 (2.8%)	3 (9.4%)	0
Diarrhea	1 (4.2%)	4 (11.1%)	6 (18.7%)	6 (17.1%)
Dry mouth	0	3 (8.3%)	3 (9.4%)	2 (5.7%)
Flatulence	0	3 (8.3%)	0	2 (5.7%)
Liver function tests multiple abnormalities	0	0	3 (9.4%)	0
Nausea	1 (4.2%)	0	4 (12.5%)	1 (2.9%)
Oral moniliasis	1 (4.2%)	4 (11.1%)	2 (6.3%)	0
Tooth pain	1 (4.2%)	0	0	0
Hemic and Lymphatic	0	8 (22.2%)	13 (40.6%)	10 (28.6%)
Anemia	0	2 (5.6%)	4 (12.5%)	3 (8.6%)
Leukopenia	0	6 (16.7%)	8 (25.0%)	3 (8.6%)
Lymphadenopathy	0	2 (5.6%)	4 (12.5%)	3 (8.6%)
Metabolic and Endocrine Disorders	1 (4.2%)	8 (22.2%)	12 (37.5%)	8 (22.9%)
Edema peripheral	1 (4.2%)	3 (8.3%)	1 (3.1%)	0
Hyperlipemia	0	2 (5.6%)	3 (9.4%)	1 (2.9%)
SGOT increased	0	1 (2.8%)	4 (12.5%)	2 (5.7%)
Nervous System	13 (54.2%)	19 (52.8%)	18 (56.3%)	12 (34.3%)
Agitation	0	0	3 (9.4%)	0
Dizziness	1 (4.2%)	7 (19.4%)	6 (18.7%)	0
Insomnia	0	0	3 (9.4%)	2 (5.7%)
Nervousness	0	1 (2.8%)	3 (9.4%)	0
Neuropathy	0	3 (8.3%)	0	0
Paresthesia	0	2 (5.6%)	5 (15.6%)	4 (11.4%)
Somnolence	9 (37.5%)	13 (36.1%)	12 (37.5%)	4 (11.4%)
Tremor	1 (4.2%)	0	0	0
Vertigo	2 (8.3%)	0	0	0
Respiratory System	3 (12.5%)	9 (25.0%)	6 (18.7%)	9 (25.7%)
Pharyngitis	1 (4.2%)	3 (8.3%)	2 (6.3%)	2 (5.7%)
Rhinitis	1 (4.2%)	0	0	4 (11.4%)
Sinusitis	1 (4.2%)	3 (8.3%)	1 (3.1%)	2 (5.7%)
Skin and Appendages	10 (41.7%)	17 (47.2%)	18 (56.3%)	19 (54.3%)
Acne	0	4 (11.1%)	1 (3.1%)	0
Dermatitis fungal	1 (4.2%)	2 (5.6%)	3 (9.4%)	0
Nail disorder	1 (4.2%)	0	1 (3.1%)	0
Pruritus	2 (8.3%)	1 (2.8%)	2 (6.3%)	2 (5.7%)
Rash	5 (20.8%)	9 (25.0%)	8 (25.0%)	11 (31.4%)
Rash maculo-papular	1 (4.2%)	6 (16.7%)	6 (18.7%)	2 (5.7%)
Sweating	0	0	4 (12.5%)	4 (11.4%)
Urogenital System	2 (8.3%)	6 (16.7%)	2 (6.3%)	4 (11.4%)
Albuminuria	0	3 (8.3%)	1 (3.1%)	2 (5.7%)
Hematuria	0	4 (11.1%)	0	1 (2.9%)
Impotence	2 (8.3%)	1 (2.8%)	0	0

OTHER ADVERSE EVENTS OBSERVED IN HIV-SEROPOSITIVE PATIENTS

In addition to controlled clinical trials, thalidomide has been used in uncontrolled studies in 145 patients. Less frequent adverse events that have been reported in these HIV-seropositive patients treated with thalidomide were grouped into a smaller number of standardized categories using modified COSTART dictionary/terminology and these categories are used in the listing below. Adverse events that have already been included in TABLE 4 and narrative above, or that are too general to be informative are not listed.

Body as a Whole: Ascites, AIDS, allergic reaction, cellulitis, chest pain, chills and fever, cyst, decreased CD4 count, facial edema, flu syndrome, hernia, hormone level altered, moniliasis, photosensitivity reaction, sarcoma, sepsis, viral infection.

Cardiovascular System: Angina pectoris, arrhythmia, atrial fibrillation, bradycardia, cerebral ischemia, cerebrovascular accident, congestive heart failure, deep thrombophlebitis, heart arrest, heart failure, hypertension, hypotension, murmur, myocardial infarct, palpitation, pericarditis, peripheral vascular disorder, postural hypotension, syncope, tachycardia, thrombophlebitis, thrombosis.

Digestive System: Cholangitis, cholestatic jaundice, colitis, dyspepsia, dysphagia, esophagitis, gastroenteritis, gastrointestinal disorder, gastrointestinal hemorrhage, gum disorder, hepatitis, pancreatitis, parotid gland enlargement, periodontitis, stomatitis, tongue discoloration, tooth disorder.

Hemic and Lymphatic: Aplastic anemia, macrocytic anemia, megaloblastic anemia, microcytic anemia.

Metabolic and Endocrine: Avitaminosis, bilirubinemia, dehydration, hypercholesteremia, hypoglycemia, increased alkaline phosphatase, increased lipase, increased serum creatinine, peripheral edema.

Muscular Skeletal: Myalgia, myasthenia.

Nervous System: Abnormal gait, ataxia, decreased libido, decreased reflexes, dementia, dysesthesia, dyskinesia, emotional lability, hostility, hypalgesia, hyperkinesia, incoordination, meningitis, neurologic disorder, tremor, vertigo.

Respiratory System: Apnea, bronchitis, lung disorder, lung edema, pneumonia (including *Pneumocystis carinii* pneumonia), rhinitis.

Skin and Appendages: Angioedema, benign skin neoplasm, eczema, herpes simplex, incomplete Stevens-Johnson syndrome, nail disorder, pruritus, psoriasis, skin discoloration, skin disorder.

Special Senses: Conjunctivitis, eye disorder, lacrimation disorder, retinitis, taste perversion.

OTHER ADVERSE EVENTS IN THE PUBLISHED LITERATURE OR REPORTED FROM OTHER SOURCES

The following additional events have been identified either in the published literature or from spontaneous reports from other sources: acute renal failure, amenorrhea, aphthous stomatitis, bile duct obstruction, carpal tunnel, chronic myelogenous leukemia, diplopia, dysesthesia, dyspnea, enuresis, erythema nodosum, erythroleukemia, foot drop, galactorrhea, gynecomastia, hangover effect, hypomagnesemia, hypothyroidism, lymphedema, lymphopenia, metrorrhagia, migraine, myxedema, nodular sclerosing Hodgkin's disease, nystagmus, oliguria, pancytopenia, petechiae, purpura, Raynaud's syndrome, stomach ulcer, and suicide attempt.

DOSAGE AND ADMINISTRATION

THALIDOMIDE MUST ONLY BE ADMINISTERED IN COMPLIANCE WITH ALL OF THE TERMS OUTLINED IN THE *S.T.E.P.S.* PROGRAM. THALIDOMIDE MAY ONLY BE PRESCRIBED BY PRESCRIBERS REGISTERED WITH THE *S.T.E.P.S.* PROGRAM AND MAY ONLY BE DISPENSED BY PHARMACISTS REGISTERED WITH THE *S.T.E.P.S.* PROGRAM.

Drug prescribing to women of childbearing potential should be contingent upon initial and continued confirmed negative results of pregnancy testing.

For an episode of cutaneous ENL, thalidomide dosing should be initiated at 100-300 mg/day, administered once daily with water, preferably at bedtime and at least 1 hour after the evening meal. Patients weighing less than 50 kg should be started at the low end of the dose range.

In patients with a severe cutaneous ENL reaction, or in those who have previously required higher doses to control the reaction, thalidomide dosing may be initiated at higher doses up to 400 mg/day once daily at bedtime or in divided doses with water, at least 1 hour after meals.

In patients with moderate to severe neuritis associated with a severe ENL reaction, corticosteroids may be started concomitantly with thalidomide. Steroid usage can be tapered and discontinued when the neuritis has ameliorated.

Dosing with thalidomide should usually continue until signs and symptoms of active reaction have subsided, usually a period of at least 2 weeks. Patients may then be tapered off medication in 50 mg decrements every 2-4 weeks.

Patients who have a documented history of requiring prolonged maintenance treatment to prevent the recurrence of cutaneous ENL or who flare during tapering, should be maintained on the minimum dose necessary to control the reaction. Tapering off medication should be attempted every 3-6 months, in decrements of 50 mg every 2-4 weeks.

HOW SUPPLIED

THIS PRODUCT IS ONLY SUPPLIED TO PHARMACISTS REGISTERED WITH THE *S.T.E.P.S.* PROGRAM. See BOXED WARNING.

THALOMID CAPSULES

Thalomid is supplied in hard gelatin, 50 mg capsules [white opaque], imprinted "Celgene" with a "do not get pregnant" logo.

STORAGE AND DISPENSING

Pharmacists Note

BEFORE DISPENSING THALIDOMIDE, YOU MUST ACTIVATE THE AUTHORIZATION NUMBER ON EVERY PRESCRIPTION BY CALLING THE CELGENE CUSTOMER CARE CENTER AT 1-888-4-CELGENE (1-888-423-5436) AND OBTAINING A CONFIRMATION NUMBER. YOU MUST ALSO WRITE THE CONFIRMATION NUMBER ON THE PRESCRIPTION. YOU SHOULD ACCEPT A PRESCRIPTION ONLY IF IT HAS BEEN ISSUED WITHIN THE PREVIOUS 7 DAYS (TELEPHONE PRESCRIPTIONS ARE NOT PERMITTED); DISPENSE NO MORE THAN A 4 WEEK (28 DAY) SUPPLY, WITH NO AUTOMATIC REFILLS; DISPENSE BLISTER PACKS INTACT (CAPSULES CANNOT BE REPACKAGED); DISPENSE SUBSEQUENT PRESCRIPTIONS ONLY IF FEWER THAN 7 DAYS OF THERAPY REMAIN ON THE PREVIOUS PRESCRIPTION; AND EDUCATE ALL STAFF PHARMACISTS ABOUT THE DISPENSING PROCEDURE FOR THALIDOMIDE.

This drug must not be repackaged.

Storage: Store at 15-30°C; 59-86°F. Protect from light.

Rx only and only able to be prescribed and dispensed under the terms of the *S.T.E.P.S.* Restricted Distribution Program.

PRODUCT LISTING - EQUIVALENTS NOT AVAILABLE

Capsule - Oral - 50 mg

14 x 6	$630.00	THALOMID, Celgene Corporation	59572-0105-11
14 x 10	$2290.00	THALOMID, Celgene Corporation	59572-0105-92
28 x 10	$2526.25	THALOMID, Celgene Corporation	59572-0105-13
28 x 10	$5013.75	THALOMID, Celgene Corporation	59572-0105-93

Theophylline *(002329)*

Categories: Asthma; Bronchitis, chronic; Emphysema; Pregnancy Category C; FDA Approved 1979 Apr; WHO Formulary

Drug Classes: Bronchodilators; Xanthine derivatives

Brand Names: Accurbron; Aerolate; Aquaphyllin; Asmalix; Bronkodyl; Constant-T; Elixicon; Elixomin; **Elixophyllin**; Hydro-Spec; Labid; Lanophyllin; Lixolin; Pulmo; Respbid; Slo-Bid; Slo-Phyllin; Solu-Phyllin; Somophyllin; Sustaire; T-Phyl; Theo-24; Theo-Dur; Theo-Time; Theobid; Theochron; Theoclear; Theocontin; Theocot; Theolair; Theomar; Theophyl; Theophylline Anhydrous; Theosol-80; Theospan Sr; Theostat 80; Theovent; Theox; Truxophyllin; Uni-Dur; Uniphyl

Foreign Brand Availability: Aerobin (Germany); Aerodyne Retard (Austria); Afonilum Mite (Germany); Afonilum Forte (Germany); Afonilum Retard (Germany); Almarion (Thailand); Armophylline (France); Asmasalon (Philippines); Asperal-T (Belgium); Austyn (Korea); Bronchoretard (Germany); Bronsolvan (Indonesia); Cronasma (Germany); Deo-Q Syrup (Korea); Ditenaten (Germany); Elixofilina (Mexico; Peru); Euphyllin Retard (Benin; Burkina-Faso; Ethiopia; Gambia; Ghana; Guinea; Ivory-Coast; Kenya; Liberia; Malawi; Mali; Mauritania; Mauritius; Morocco; Niger; Nigeria; Senegal; Seychelles; Sierra-Leone; South-Africa; Sudan; Tanzania; Tunia; Uganda; Zambia; Zimbabwe); Euphylong (Bahrain; Cyprus; Egypt; Hong-Kong; Iran; Iraq; Jordan; Kuwait; Lebanon; Libya; Oman; Qatar; Republic-of-Yemen; Saudi-Arabia; Syria; United-Arab-Emirates); Euphylong Retardkaps (Germany); Euphylong SR (Philippines); Godafilin (Spain); Lasma (Bahrain; Cyprus; Egypt; England; Iran; Iraq; Jordan; Kuwait; Lebanon; Libya; Oman; Qatar; Republic-of-Yemen; Saudi-Arabia; Syria; United-Arab-Emirates); Nefoben (Argentina); Neobiphyllin (China); Neulin-SR (Taiwan); Neulin SA (South-Africa); Nuelin (Australia; Bahamas; Barbados; Belize; Bermuda; Costa-Rica; Curacao; Denmark; Dominican-Republic; El-Salvador; Finland; Guyana; Honduras; Jamaica; Malaysia; Netherland-Antilles; New-Zealand; Norway; Panama; Philippines; Surinam; Trinidad); Nuelin SA (Bahrain; Benin; Burkina-Faso; Costa-Rica; Cyprus; Dominican-Republic; Egypt; El-Salvador; Ethiopia; Gambia; Ghana; Guatemala; Guinea; Honduras; Iran; Iraq; Ivory-Coast; Jordan; Kenya; Kuwait; Lebanon; Liberia; Libya; Malawi; Mali; Mauritania; Mauritius; Morocco; Niger; Nigeria; Oman; Panama; Qatar; Republic-of-Yemen; Saudi-Arabia; Senegal; Seychelles; Sierra-Leone; Sudan; Syria; Tanzania; Tunia; Uganda; United-Arab-Emirates; Zambia; Zimbabwe); Nuelin SR (Australia; Bahrain; Cyprus; Egypt; Hong-Kong; Iran; Iraq; Jordan; Kuwait; Lebanon; Libya; Malaysia; Oman; Qatar; Republic-of-Yemen; Saudi-Arabia; Syria; Thailand; United-Arab-Emirates); Pharphylline (Netherlands); Phylobid (Benin; Burkina-Faso; Ethiopia; Gambia; Ghana; Guinea; India; Ivory-Coast; Kenya; Liberia; Malawi; Mali; Mauritania; Mauritius; Morocco; Niger; Nigeria; Senegal; Seychelles; Sierra-Leone; Sudan; Tanzania; Tunia; Uganda; Zambia; Zimbabwe); Protheo (China); Pulmidur (Austria; Germany); Quibron T SR (Canada; Indonesia); Slo-Theo (Hong-Kong); Solosin (Germany); Somofillina (Italy); Teobid (Colombia); Teoclear (Korea); Teoclear LA (Argentina); Teofilina Retard (Colombia); Teolixir (Spain); Teolong (Mexico); Teosona (Argentina); Theo-2 (Belgium); Theo-Bros (Greece); Theo PA (India); Theolair S (Peru); Theolan (Korea; Taiwan); Theolin (Singapore); Theolin SR (Singapore); Theolong (Japan); Theomax (Spain); Theon (Switzerland); Theoplus (Bulgaria; Singapore; Spain); Theoplus Retard (Austria; Greece); Theospirex Retard (Austria; Switzerland); Theostat LP (France); Theotard (Israel); Theotrim (Israel); Theovent LA (Hong-Kong); Theo von CT (Germany); Tiodilax (Argentina); Tyrex (Peru); Unicontin-400 Continus (India); Unifyl Retard (Switzerland); Uniphyl CR (Korea); Uniphyllin (Taiwan); Uniphyllin Continus (Benin; Burkina-Faso; Ethiopia; Gambia; Ghana; Guinea; Ivory-Coast; Kenya; Liberia; Malawi; Mali; Mauritania; Mauritius; Morocco; Niger; Nigeria; Senegal; Seychelles; Sierra-Leone; Sudan; Tanzania; Tunia; Uganda; Zambia; Zimbabwe); Xanthium (Singapore); Xantivent (Switzerland)

Cost of Therapy: \$24.99 (Asthma; Theo-Dur; 300 mg; 2 tablets/day; 30 day supply)
\$6.14 (Asthma; Generic Extended Release Tablet; 300 mg; 2 tablets/day; 30 day supply)

HCFA JCODE(S): J2810 per 40 mg IV

DESCRIPTION

Theophylline is structurally classified as a methylxanthine. It occurs as a white, odorless, crystalline powder with a bitter taste. Anhydrous theophylline has the chemical name 1H-Purine-2,6-dione,3,7-dihydro-1,3-dimethyl-.

The molecular formula of anhydrous theophylline is $C_7H_8N_4O_2$ with a molecular weight of 180.17. (For products containing theophylline monohydrate, substitute the following: The molecular formula of theophylline monohydrate is $C_7H_8N_4O_2H_2O$ with a molecular weight of 198.18.)

The molecular formula of oxtriphylline is $C_{12}H_{21}N_5O_3$ with a molecular weight of 283.33. Theophylline is a bronchodilator structurally classified as a xanthine derivative.

IMMEDIATE-RELEASE ORAL FORMS

Slo-Phyllin tablets (theophylline tablets) are scored, dye-free tablets providing 100 or 200 mg of theophylline, anhydrous.

Slo-Phyllin 80 mg Syrup (theophylline, anhydrous) is a nonalcoholic, sugar-free solution containing per 15 ml theophylline, anhydrous 80 mg with sodium benzoate, 18 mg and methylparaben, 3 mg added as preservatives.

Both tablets and syrup are intended for oral administration.

Syrup: Syrup inactive ingredients are citric acid, flavors, glycerine, methylparaben, propylene glycol, saccharin sodium, sodium benzoate, sorbitol, purified water.

Tablets: 100 mg inactive ingredients are lactose, magnesium stearate, microcrystalline cellulose, sodium starch glycolate; 200 mg inactive ingredients are magnesium stearate, microcrystalline cellulose, sodium starch glycolate.

SUSTAINED ACTION CAPSULES

Theo-Dur Sprinkle sustained action capsules contain 50, 75, 125, or 200 mg anhydrous theophylline. The inactive ingredients for Theo-Dur Sprinkle are: Ethylcellulose, hydroxypropylcellulose, povidone, and sucrose. Theo-Dur Sprinkle takes the form of long-acting microencapsulated beads within a hard gelatin capsule for oral administration.

The theophylline has been microencapsulated in a proprietary coating of polymers to mask the bitter taste associated with the drug while providing a prolonged effect. The entire contents of a Theo-Dur Sprinkle capsule are intended to be sprinkled on a small amount of soft food immediately prior to ingestion, or it may be swallowed whole. SUBDIVIDING THE CONTENTS OF A CAPSULE IS NOT RECOMMENDED. Each capsule is oversized to allow ease of opening.

Storage: Keep tightly closed. Store at controlled room temperature 15-30°C (59-86°F).

CLINICAL PHARMACOLOGY

MECHANISM OF ACTION

Theophylline has two distinct actions in the airways of patients with reversible obstruction; smooth muscle relaxation (*i.e.*, bronchodilation) and suppression of the response of the airways to stimuli (*i.e.*, non-bronchodilator prophylactic effects). While the mechanisms of action of theophylline are not known with certainty, studies in animals suggest that bronchodilatation is mediated by the inhibition of two isozymes of phosphodiesterase (PDE III and, to a lesser extent, PDE IV) while non-bronchodilator prophylactic actions are probably mediated through one or more different molecular mechanisms, that do not involve inhibition of PDE III or antagonism of adenosine receptors. Some of the adverse effects associated with theophylline appear to be mediated by inhibition of PDE III (*e.g.*, hypotension, tachycardia, headache, and emesis) and adenosine receptor antagonism (*e.g.*, alterations in cerebral blood flow).

Theophylline increases the force of contraction of diaphragmatic muscles. This action appears to be due to enhancement of calcium uptake through an adenosine-mediated channel.

SERUM CONCENTRATION-EFFECT RELATIONSHIP

Bronchodilation occurs over the serum theophylline concentration range of 5-20 μg/ml. Clinically important improvement in symptom control has been found in most studies to require peak serum theophylline concentrations >10 μg/ml, but patients with mild disease may benefit from lower concentrations. At serum theophylline concentrations >20 μg/ml, both the frequency and severity of adverse reactions increase. In general, maintaining peak serum theophylline concentrations between 10 and 15 μg/ml will achieve most of the drug's potential therapeutic benefit while minimizing the risk of serious adverse events.

PHARMACOKINETICS

Overview

Theophylline is rapidly and completely absorbed after oral administration in solution or immediate-release solid oral dosage form. Theophylline does not undergo any appreciable pre-systemic elimination, distributes freely into fat-free tissues and is extensively metabolized in the liver.

The pharmacokinetics of theophylline vary widely among similar patients and cannot be predicted by age, sex, body weight or other demographic characteristics. In addition, certain concurrent illnesses and alterations in normal physiology (see TABLE 1) and co-administration of other drugs (see TABLE 2A and TABLE 2B) can significantly alter the pharmacokinetic characteristics of theophylline. Within-subject variability in metabolism has also been reported in some studies, especially in acutely ill patients. It is, therefore, recommended that serum theophylline concentrations be measured frequently in acutely ill patients (*e.g.*, at 24 hour intervals) and periodically in patients receiving long-term therapy, *e.g.*, at 6-12 month intervals. More frequent measurements should be made in the presence of any condition that may significantly alter theophylline clearance (see PRECAUTIONS, Laboratory Tests).

TABLE 1 *Mean and Range of Total Body Clearance and Half-Life of Theophylline Related to Age and Altered Physiological States**

Population Characteristics	Total Body Clearance† Mean (Range)‡ (ml/kg/min)	Half-life Mean (Range)‡ (hours)
	Age	
Premature Neonates		
Postnatal age 3-15 days	0.29 (0.09-0.49)	30 (17-43)
Postnatal age 25-57 days	0.64 (0.04-1.2)	20 (9.4-30.6)
Term Infants		
Postnatal age 1-2 days	NR§	25.7 (25-26.5)
Postnatal age 3-30 weeks	NR§	11 (6-29)
Children		
1-4 years	1.7 (0.5-2.9)	3.4 (1.2-5.6)
4-12 years	1.6 (0.8-2.4)	NR§
13-15 years	0.9 (0.48-1.3)	NR§
6-17 years	1.4 (0.2-2.6)	3.7 (1.5-5.9)
Adults (16-60 years) otherwise healthy non-smoking asthmatics	0.65 (0.27-1.03)	8.7 (6.1-12.8)
Elderly (>60 years) non-smokers with normal cardiac, liver, and renal function	0.41 (0.21-0.61)	9.8 (1.6-18)
	Concurrent Illness or Altered Physiological State	
Acute pulmonary edema	0.33¤ (0.07-2.45)	19¤ (3.1-82)
COPD >60 years, stable non-smoker >1 year	0.54 (0.44-0.64)	11 (9.4-12.6)
COPD with cor pulmonale	0.48 (0.08-0.88)	NR§
Cystic fibrosis (14-28 years)	1.25 (0.31-2.2)	6.0 (1.8-10.2)
Fever associated with acute viral respiratory illness (children 9-15 years)	NR§	7.0 (1.0-13)
Liver disease		
Cirrhosis	0.31¤ (0.1-0.7)	32¤ (10-56)
Acute hepatitis	0.35 (0.25-0.45)	19.2 (16.6-21.8)
Cholestasis	0.65 (0.25-1.45)	14.4 (5.7-31.8)
Pregnancy		
1st trimester	NR§	8.5 (3.1-13.9)
2nd trimester	NR§	8.8 (3.8-13.8)
3rd trimester	NR§	13.0 (8.4-17.6)
Sepsis with multi-organ failure	0.47 (0.19-1.9)	18.8 (6.3-24.1)
Thyroid disease		
Hypothyroid	0.38 (0.13-0.57)	11.6 (8.2-25)
Hyperthyroid	0.8 (0.68-0.97)	4.5 (3.7-5.6)

* For various North American patient populations from literature reports. Different rates of elimination and consequent dosage requirements have been observed among other peoples.
† Clearance represents the volume of blood completely cleared of theophylline by the liver in one minute. Values listed were generally determined at serum theophylline concentrations <20 μg/ml; clearance may decrease and half-life may increase at higher serum concentrations due to non-linear pharmacokinetics.
‡ Reported range or estimated range (mean ± 2 SD) where actual range not reported.
§ NR = not reported or not reported in a comparable format.
¤ Median.

Note: In addition to the factors listed above, theophylline clearance is increased and half-life decreased by low carbohydrate/high protein diets, parenteral nutrition, and daily consumption of charcoal-broiled beef. A high carbohydrate/low protein diet can decrease the clearance and prolong the half-life of theophylline.

Absorption

Theophylline is rapidly and completely absorbed after oral administration in solution or immediate-release solid oral dosage form. After a single dose of the immediate-release dosage form of 5 mg/kg in adults, a mean peak serum concentration of about 10 μg/ml (range

5-15 μg/ml) can be expected 1-2 hours after the dose. Co-administration of theophylline with food or antacids does not cause clinically significant changes in the absorption of theophylline from immediate-release dosage forms.

Distribution

Once theophylline enters the systemic circulation, about 40% is bound to plasma protein, primarily albumin. Unbound theophylline distributes throughout body water, but distributes poorly into body fat. The apparent volume of distribution of theophylline is approximately 0.45 L/kg (range 0.3-0.7 L/kg) based on ideal body weight. Theophylline passes freely across the placenta, into breast milk and into the cerebrospinal fluid (CSF). Saliva theophylline concentrations approximate unbound serum concentrations, but are not reliable for routine or therapeutic monitoring unless special techniques are used. An increase in the volume of distribution of theophylline, primarily due to reduction in plasma protein binding, occurs in premature neonates, patients with hepatic cirrhosis, uncorrected acidemia, the elderly and in women during the third trimester of pregnancy. In such cases, the patient may show signs of toxicity at total (bound + unbound) serum concentrations of theophylline in the therapeutic range (10-20 μg/ml) due to elevated concentrations of the pharmacologically active unbound drug. Similarly, a patient with decreased theophylline binding may have a sub-therapeutic total drug concentration while the pharmacologically active unbound concentration is in the therapeutic range. If only total serum theophylline concentration is measured, this may lead to an unnecessary and potentially dangerous dose increase. In patients with reduced protein binding, measurement of unbound serum theophylline concentration provides a more reliable means of dosage adjustment than measurement of total serum theophylline concentration. Generally, concentrations of unbound theophylline should be maintained in the range of 6-12 μg/ml.

Metabolism

Following oral dosing, theophylline does not undergo any measurable first-pass elimination. In adults and children beyond 1 year of age, approximately 90% of the dose is metabolized in the liver. Biotransformation takes place through demethylation to 1-methylxanthine and 3-methylxanthine and hydroxylation to 1,3-dimethyluric acid. 1-methylxanthine is further hydroxylated, by xanthine oxidase, to 1-methyluric acid. About 6% of a theophylline dose is N-methylated to caffeine. Theophylline demethylation to 3-methylxanthine is catalyzed by cytochrome P-450 1A2, while cytochromes P-450 2E1 and P-450 3A3 catalyze the hydroxylation to 1,3-dimethyluric acid. Demethylation to 1-methylxanthine appears to be catalyzed either by cytochrome P-450 1A2 or a closely related cytochrome. In neonates, the N-demethylation pathway is absent while the function of the hydroxylation pathway is markedly deficient. The activity of these pathways slowly increases to maximal levels by 1 year of age.

Caffeine and 3-methylxanthine are the only theophylline metabolites with pharmacologic activity. 3-methylxanthine has approximately one tenth the pharmacologic activity of theophylline and serum concentrations in adults with normal renal function are <1 μg/ml. In patients with end-stage renal disease, 3-methylxanthine may accumulate to concentrations that approximate the unmetabolized theophylline concentration. Caffeine concentrations are usually undetectable in adults regardless of renal function. In neonates, caffeine may accumulate to concentrations that approximate the unmetabolized theophylline concentration and thus, exert a pharmacologic effect. Both the N-demethylation and hydroxylation pathways of theophylline biotransformation are capacity-limited. Due to the wide intersubject variability of the rate of theophylline metabolism, non-linearity of elimination may begin in some patients at serum theophylline concentrations <10 μg/ml. Since this non-linearity results in more than proportional changes in serum theophylline concentrations with changes in dose, it is advisable to make increases or decreases in dose in small increments in order to achieve desired changes in serum theophylline concentrations (see TABLE 5). Accurate prediction of dose-dependency of theophylline metabolism in patients *a priori* is not possible, but patients with very high initial clearance rates (*i.e.*, low steady state serum theophylline concentrations at above average doses) have the greatest likelihood of experiencing large changes in serum theophylline concentration in response to dosage changes.

Excretion

In neonates, approximately 50% of the theophylline dose is excreted unchanged in the urine. Beyond the first 3 months of life, approximately 10% of the theophylline dose is excreted unchanged in the urine. The remainder is excreted in the urine mainly as 1,3-dimethyluric acid (35-40%), 1-methyluric acid (20-25%) and 3-methylxanthine (15-20%). Since little theophylline is excreted unchanged in the urine and since active metabolites of theophylline (*i.e.*, caffeine, 3-methylxanthine) do not accumulate to clinically significant levels even in the face of end-stage renal disease, no dosage adjustment for renal insufficiency is necessary in adults and children >3 months of age. In contrast, the large fraction of the theophylline dose excreted in the urine as unchanged theophylline and caffeine in neonates requires careful attention to dose reduction and frequent monitoring of serum theophylline concentrations in neonates with reduced renal function (see WARNINGS).

Serum Concentrations at Steady State

After multiple doses of theophylline, steady state is reached in 30-65 hours (average 40 hours) in adults. At steady state, on a dosage regimen with 6 hour intervals, the expected mean trough concentration is approximately 60% of the mean peak concentration, assuming a mean theophylline half-life of 8 hours. The difference between peak and trough concentrations is larger in patients with more rapid theophylline clearance. In patients with high theophylline clearance and half-lives of about 4-5 hours, such as children age 1-9 years, the trough serum theophylline concentration may be only 30% of peak with a 6 hour dosing interval. In these patients a slow release formulation would allow a longer dosing interval (8-12 hours) with a smaller peak/trough difference.

SPECIAL POPULATIONS

See TABLE 1 for mean clearance and half-life values.

Geriatric

The clearance of theophylline is decreased by an average of 30% in healthy elderly adults (>60 years) compared to healthy young adults. Careful attention to dose reduction and frequent monitoring of serum theophylline concentrations are required in elderly patients (see WARNINGS).

Pediatrics

The clearance of theophylline is very low in neonates (see WARNINGS). Theophylline clearance reaches maximal values by 1 year of age, remains relatively constant until about 9 years of age and then slowly decreases by approximately 50% to adult values at about age 16. Renal excretion of unchanged theophylline in neonates amounts to about 50% of the dose, compared to about 10% in children older than 3 months and in adults. Careful attention to dosage selection and monitoring of serum theophylline concentrations are required in pediatric patients (see WARNINGS and DOSAGE AND ADMINISTRATION).

Gender

Gender differences in theophylline clearance are relatively small and unlikely to be of clinical significance. Significant reduction in theophylline clearance, however, has been reported in women on the 20th day of the menstrual cycle and during the third trimester of pregnancy.

Race

Pharmacokinetic differences in theophylline clearance due to race have not been studied.

Renal Insufficiency

Only a small fraction, *e.g.*, about 10%, of the administered theophylline dose is excreted unchanged in the urine of children greater than 3 months of age and adults. Since little theophylline is excreted unchanged in the urine and since active metabolites of theophylline (*i.e.*, caffeine, 3-methylxanthine) do not accumulate to clinically significant levels even in the face of end-stage renal disease, no dosage adjustment for renal insufficiency is necessary in adults and children >3 months of age. In contrast, approximately 50% of the administered theophylline dose is excreted unchanged in the urine in neonates. Careful attention to dose reduction and frequent monitoring of serum theophylline concentrations are required in neonates with decreased renal function (see WARNINGS).

Hepatic Insufficiency

Theophylline clearance is decreased by 50% or more in patients with hepatic insufficiency (*e.g.*, cirrhosis, acute hepatitis, cholestasis). Careful attention to dose reduction and frequent monitoring of serum theophylline concentrations are required in patients with reduced hepatic function (see WARNINGS).

Congestive Heart Failure (CHF)

Theophylline clearance is decreased by 50% or more in patients with CHF. The extent of reduction in theophylline clearance in patients with CHF appears to be directly correlated to the severity of the cardiac disease. Since theophylline clearance is independent of liver blood flow, the reduction in clearance appears to be due to impaired hepatocyte function rather than reduced perfusion. Careful attention to dose reduction and frequent monitoring of serum theophylline concentrations are required in patients with CHF (see WARNINGS).

Smokers

Tobacco and marijuana smoking appears to increase the clearance of theophylline by induction of metabolic pathways. Theophylline clearance has been shown to increase by approximately 50% in young adult tobacco smokers and by approximately 80% in elderly tobacco smokers compared to non-smoking subjects. Passive smoke exposure has also been shown to increase theophylline clearance by up to 50%. Abstinence from tobacco smoking for 1 week causes a reduction of approximately 40% in theophylline clearance. Careful attention to dose reduction and frequent monitoring of serum theophylline concentrations are required in patients who stop smoking (see WARNINGS). Use of nicotine gum has been shown to have no effect on theophylline clearance.

Fever

Fever, regardless of its underlying cause, can decrease the clearance of theophylline. The magnitude and duration of the fever appear to be directly correlated to the degree of decrease of theophylline clearance. Precise data are lacking, but a temperature of 39°C (102°F) for at least 24 hours is probably required to produce a clinically significant increase in serum theophylline concentrations. Children with rapid rates of theophylline clearance (*i.e.*, those who require a dose that is substantially larger than average [*e.g.*, >22 mg/kg/day] to achieve a therapeutic peak serum theophylline concentration when afebrile) may be at greater risk of toxic effects from decreased clearance during sustained fever. Careful attention to dose reduction and frequent monitoring of serum theophylline concentrations are required in patients with sustained fever (see WARNINGS).

Miscellaneous

Other factors associated with decreased theophylline clearance include the third trimester of pregnancy, sepsis with multiple organ failure, and hypothyroidism. Careful attention to dose reduction and frequent monitoring of serum theophylline concentrations are required in patients with any of these conditions (see WARNINGS). Other factors associated with increased theophylline clearance include hyperthyroidism and cystic fibrosis.

INDICATIONS AND USAGE

Theophylline is indicated for the treatment of the symptoms and reversible airflow obstruction associated with chronic asthma and other chronic lung diseases, *e.g.*, emphysema and chronic bronchitis.

CONTRAINDICATIONS

This product is contraindicated in individuals who have shown hypersensitivity to theophylline or any of the components of the formulation. It is also contraindicated in patients with active peptic ulcer disease, and in individuals with underlying seizure disorders (unless receiving appropriate anti-convulsant medication).

T

WARNINGS

CONCURRENT ILLNESS

Theophylline should be used with extreme caution in patients with the following clinical conditions due to the increased risk of exacerbation of the concurrent condition: Active peptic ulcer disease, seizure disorders, and cardiac arrhythmias (not including bradyarrhythmias).

CONDITIONS THAT REDUCE THEOPHYLLINE CLEARANCE

There are several readily identifiable causes of reduced theophylline clearance. **If the total daily dose is not appropriately reduced in the presence of these risk factors, severe and potentially fatal theophylline toxicity can occur.** Careful consideration must be given to the benefits and risks of theophylline use and the need for more intensive monitoring of serum theophylline concentrations in patients with the following risk factors:

Age: Neonates (term and premature); children <1 year; elderly >60 years.

Concurrent Diseases: Acute pulmonary edema; congestive heart failure; cor-pulmonale; fever ≥102°F for 24 hours or more, or lesser temperature elevations for longer periods; Hypothyroidism; liver disease, cirrhosis, acute hepatitis; reduced renal function in infants <3 months of age; sepsis with multi-organ failure; shock

Cessation of Smoking.

WHEN SIGNS OR SYMPTOMS OF THEOPHYLLINE TOXICITY ARE PRESENT

Whenever a patient receiving theophylline develops nausea or vomiting, particularly repetitive vomiting, or other signs or symptoms consistent with theophylline toxicity (even if another cause may be suspected), additional doses of theophylline should be withheld and a serum theophylline concentration measured immediately. Patients should be instructed not to continue any dosage that causes adverse effects and to withhold subsequent doses until the symptoms have resolved, at which time the clinician may instruct the patient to resume the drug at a lower dosage (see TABLE 5).

Dosage Increases

Increases in the dose of theophylline should not be made in response to an acute exacerbation of symptoms of chronic lung disease since theophylline provides little added benefit to inhaled $beta_2$-selective agonists and systemically administered corticosteroids in this circumstance and increases the risk of adverse effects. A peak steady-state serum theophylline concentration should be measured before increasing the dose in response to persistent chronic symptoms to ascertain whether an increase in dose is safe. Before increasing the theophylline dose on the basis of a low serum concentration, the clinician should consider whether the blood sample was obtained at an appropriate time in relationship to the dose and whether the patient has adhered to the prescribed regimen (see PRECAUTIONS, Laboratory Tests).

As the rate of theophylline clearance may be dose-dependent (*i.e.,* steady-state serum concentrations may increase disproportionately to the increase in dose), an increase in dose based upon a sub-therapeutic serum concentration measurement should be conservative. In general, limiting dose increases to about 25% of the previous total daily dose will reduce the risk of unintended excessive increases in serum theophylline concentration (see TABLE 5).

Serum levels above 20 μg/ml are rarely found after appropriate administration of the recommended doses. However, in individuals in whom theophylline plasma clearance is reduced *for any reason,* even conventional doses may result in increased serum levels and potential toxicity.

Reduced theophylline clearance has been documented in the following readily identifiable groups: (1) patients with impaired liver function; (2) patients over 55 years of age, particularly males and those with chronic lung disease; (3) those with cardiac failure from any cause; (4) patients with sustained high fever; (5) neonates and infants under 1 year of age; and (6) patients taking certain drugs (see DRUG INTERACTIONS). Frequently, such patients have markedly prolonged theophylline serum levels following discontinuation of the drug.

Reduction of dosage and laboratory monitoring is especially appropriate in the above individuals.

Serious side effects such as ventricular arrhythmias, convulsions or even death may appear as the first sign of toxicity without any previous warning. Less serious signs of theophylline toxicity (*i.e.,* nausea and restlessness) may occur frequently when initiating therapy, but are usually transient. When such signs are persistent during maintenance therapy, they are often associated with serum concentrations above 20 μg/ml.

Stated differently, serious toxicity is not reliably preceded by less severe side effects. A serum concentration measurement is the only reliable method of predicting potentially life-threatening toxicity.

Many patients who require theophylline exhibit tachycardia due to their underlying disease process so that the cause/effect relationship to elevated serum theophylline concentrations may not be appreciated.

Theophylline products may cause dysrhythmia and/or worsen pre-existing arrhythmias and any significant change in rate and/or rhythm warrants monitoring and further investigation.

Studies in laboratory animals (minipigs, rodents, and dogs) recorded the occurrence of cardiac arrhythmias and sudden death (with histologic evidence of myocardial necrosis) when beta-agonists and methylxanthines were administered concurrently. The significance of these findings when applied to humans is currently unknown.

PRECAUTIONS

GENERAL

Immediate Release Products

Careful consideration of the various interacting drugs and physiologic conditions that can alter theophylline clearance and require dosage adjustment should occur prior to initiation of theophylline therapy, prior to increases in theophylline dose, and during follow up (see WARNINGS). The dose of theophylline selected for initiation of therapy should be low and, **if tolerated,** increased slowly over a period of a week or longer with the final dose guided by monitoring serum theophylline concentrations and the patient's clinical response (see DOSAGE AND ADMINISTRATION).

Monitoring Serum Theophylline Concentrations

Serum theophylline concentration measurements are readily available and should be used to determine whether the dosage is appropriate. Specifically, the serum theophylline concentration should be measured as follows:

1. When initiating therapy to guide final dosage adjustment after titration.
2. Before making a dose increase to determine whether the serum concentration is sub-therapeutic in a patient who continues to be symptomatic.
3. Whenever signs or symptoms of theophylline toxicity are present.
4. Whenever there is a new illness, worsening of a chronic illness or a change in the patient's treatment regimen that may alter theophylline clearance (*e.g.,* fever >102°F sustained for ≥24 hours, hepatitis, or drugs listed in TABLE 2A and TABLE 2B are added or discontinued).

To guide a dose increase, the blood sample should be obtained at the time of the expected peak serum theophylline concentration; 1-2 hours after a dose of an immediate-release product at steady-state. For most patients, steady-state will be reached after 3 days of dosing when no doses have been missed, no extra doses have been added, and none of the doses have been taken at unequal intervals. A trough concentration (*i.e.,* at the end of the dosing interval) provides no additional useful information and may lead to an inappropriate dose increase since the peak serum theophylline concentration can be 2 or more times greater than the trough concentration with an immediate-release formulation. If the serum sample is drawn more than 2 hours after the dose, the results must be interpreted with caution since the concentration may not be reflective of the peak concentration. In contrast, when signs or symptoms of theophylline toxicity are present, the serum sample should be obtained as soon as possible, analyzed immediately, and the result reported to the clinician without delay. In patients in whom decreased serum protein binding is suspected (*e.g.,* cirrhosis, women during the third trimester of pregnancy), the concentration of unbound theophylline should be measured and the dosage adjusted to achieve an unbound concentration of 6-12 μg/ml.

Saliva concentrations of theophylline cannot be used reliably to adjust dosage without special techniques.

Extended-Release Capsules

THE CONTENTS OF A THEO-DUR SPRINKLE CAPSULE SHOULD NOT BE CHEWED OR CRUSHED.

General

On the average, theophylline half-life is shorter in cigarette and marijuana smokers than in non-smokers, but smokers can have half-lives as long as non-smokers. Theophylline should not be administered concurrently with other xanthine medications. Use with caution in patients with hypoxemia, hypertension or those with history of peptic ulcer. Theophylline preparations should be used cautiously in patients with history of peptic ulcer. Theophylline may occasionally act as a local irritant to the GI tract; although gastrointestinal symptoms are more commonly centrally mediated and associated with serum drug concentrations over 20 μg/ml.

LABORATORY TESTS

Immediate Release Products

As a result of its pharmacological effects, theophylline at serum concentrations within the 10-20 μg/ml range modestly increases plasma glucose (from a mean of 88-98 mg%), uric acid (from a mean of 4-6 mg/dl), free fatty acids (from a mean of 451-800 μeq/l, total cholesterol (from a mean of 140 vs 160 mg/dl), HDL (from a mean of 36-50 mg/dl), HDL/LDL ratio (from a mean of 0.5-0.7), and urinary free cortisol excretion (from a mean of 44-63 μg/24 hours). Theophylline at serum concentrations within the 10-20 μg/ml range may also transiently decrease serum concentrations of triiodothyronine (144 before, 131 after 1 week and 142 ng/dl after 4 weeks of theophylline). The clinical importance of these changes should be weighed against the potential therapeutic benefit of theophylline in individual patients.

INFORMATION FOR THE PATIENT

Immediate Release Products

The patient (or parent/caregiver) should be instructed to seek medical advice whenever nausea, vomiting, persistent headache, insomnia or rapid heart beat occurs during treatment with theophylline, even if another cause is suspected. The patient should be instructed to contact their clinician if they develop a new illness, especially if accompanied by a persistent fever, if they experience worsening of a chronic illness, if they start or stop smoking cigarettes or marijuana, or if another clinician adds a new medication or discontinues a previously prescribed medication. Patients should be instructed to inform all clinicians involved in their care that they are taking theophylline, especially when a medication is being added or deleted from their treatment. Patients should be instructed to not alter the dose, timing of the dose, or frequency of administration without first consulting their clinician. If a dose is missed, the patient should be instructed to take the next dose at the usually scheduled time and to not attempt to make up for the missed dose.

Extended-Release Capsules

This information is intended to aid in the safe and effective use of this medication. It is not a disclosure of all possible adverse or intended effects.

The physician should reinforce the importance of taking only the prescribed dose and the time interval between doses. As with any controlled-release theophylline product, the patient should alert the physician of symptoms occur repeatedly, especially near the end of the dosing interval.

When prescribing administration by the sprinkle method, details of the proper technique should be explained to patient (see DOSAGE AND ADMINISTRATION, Sprinkling Contents on Food).

Patients should be informed of the need to take this drug in the fasting state, and that drug administration should be 1 hour before or 2 hours after meals (see DOSAGE AND ADMINISTRATION).

T

CARCINOGENESIS, MUTAGENESIS, AND IMPAIRMENT OF FERTILITY

Immediate Release Products

Long term carcinogenicity studies have been carried out in mice (oral doses 30-150 mg/kg) and rats (oral doses 5-75 mg/kg). Results are pending.

Theophylline has been studied in Ames salmonella, *in vivo* and *in vitro* cytogenetics, micronucleus and Chinese hamster ovary test systems and has not been shown to be genotoxic.

In a 14 week continuous breeding study, theophylline, administered to mating pairs of B6C3F$_1$ mice at oral doses of 120, 270 and 500 mg/kg (approximately 1.0-3.0 times the human dose on a mg/m^2 basis) impaired fertility, as evidenced by decreases in the number of live pups per litter, decreases in the mean number of litters per fertile pair, and increases in the gestation period at the high dose as well as decreases in the proportion of pups born alive at the mid and high dose. In 13 week toxicity studies, theophylline was administered to F344 rats and B6C3F$_1$ mice at oral doses of 40-300 mg/kg (approximately 2.0 times the human dose on a mg/m^2 basis). At the high dose, systemic toxicity was observed in both species including decreases in testicular weight.

Extended-Release Capsules

Long-term carcinogenicity studies have not been performed with theophylline. Chromosome-breaking activity was detected in human cell cultures at concentrations of theophylline up to 50 times the therapeutic serum concentration in humans. Theophylline was not mutagenic in the dominant lethal assay in male mice given theophylline intraperitoneally in doses up to 30 times the maximum daily human oral dose.

Studies to determine the effect on fertility have not been performed with theophylline.

PREGNANCY CATEGORY C

Immediate Release Products

There are no adequate and well controlled studies in pregnant women. Additionally, there are no teratogenicity studies in non-rodents (*e.g.*, rabbits). Theophylline was not shown to be teratogenic in CD-1 mice at oral doses up to 400 mg/kg, approximately 2.0 times the human dose on a mg/m^2 basis or in CD-1 rats at oral doses up to 260 mg/kg, approximately 3.0 times the recommended human dose on a mg/m^2 basis. At a dose of 220 mg/kg, embryotoxicity was observed in rats in the absence of maternal toxicity.

Extended-Release Capsules

Animal reproduction studies have not been conducted with theophylline. It is not known whether theophylline can cause fetal harm when administered to a pregnant woman or can affect reproduction capacity. Xanthines should be given to a pregnant woman only if clearly needed.

NURSING MOTHERS

Immediate Release Products

Theophylline is excreted into breast milk and may cause irritability or other signs of mild toxicity in nursing human infants. The concentration of theophylline in breast milk is about equivalent to the maternal serum concentration. An infant ingesting a liter of breast milk containing 10-20 µg/ml of theophylline day is likely to receive 10-20 mg of theophylline per day. Serious adverse effects in the infant are unlikely unless the mother has toxic serum theophylline concentrations.

Extended-Release Capsules

Theophylline is distributed into breast milk and may cause irritability or other signs of toxicity in nursing infants. Because of the potential of serious adverse reactions in nursing infants from theophylline, a decision should be made whether to discontinue nursing or to discontinue the drug, taking into account the importance of the drug to the mother.

PEDIATRIC USE

Immediate Release Products

Theophylline is safe and effective for the approved indications in pediatric patients (See INDICATIONS AND USAGE). The maintenance dose of theophylline must be selected with caution in pediatric patients since the rate of theophylline clearance is highly variable across the age range of neonates to adolescents (see CLINICAL PHARMACOLOGY, TABLE 1, WARNINGS, and DOSAGE AND ADMINISTRATION). Due to the immaturity of theophylline metabolic pathways in infants under the age of 1 year, particular attention to dosage selection and frequent monitoring of serum theophylline concentrations are required when theophylline is prescribed to pediatric patients in this age group.

Extended-Release Capsules

Safety and efficacy of Theo-Dur Sprinkle in children under 6 years of age have not been established with this product.

Safety and effectiveness of Theo-Dur Extended-Release Tablets administered:

1. Every 24 hours in children under 12 years of age, have not been established.
2. Every 12 hours in children under 6 years of age, have not been established.

GERIATRIC USE

Elderly patients are at significantly greater risk of experiencing serious toxicity from theophylline than younger patients due to pharmacokinetic and pharmacodynamic changes associated with aging. Theophylline clearance is reduced in patients greater than 60 years of age, resulting in increased serum theophylline concentrations in response to a given theophylline dose. Protein binding may be decreased in the elderly resulting in a larger proportion of the total serum theophylline concentration in the pharmacologically active unbound form. Elderly patients also appear to be more sensitive to the toxic effects of theophylline after chronic overdosage than younger patients. For these reasons, the maximum daily dose of theophylline in patients greater than 60 years of age ordinarily should not exceed 400 mg/day unless the patient continues to be symptomatic and the peak steady state serum theophylline concentration is <10 µg/ml (see DOSAGE AND ADMINISTRATION). Theophylline doses greater than 400 mg/day should be prescribed with caution in elderly patients.

DRUG INTERACTIONS

Theophylline interacts with a wide variety of drugs. The interaction may be pharmacodynamic, *i.e.*, alterations in the therapeutic response to theophylline or another drug or occurrence of adverse effects without a change in serum theophylline concentration. More frequently, however, the interaction is pharmacokinetic, *i.e.*, the rate of theophylline clearance is altered by another drug resulting in increased or decreased serum theophylline concentrations. Theophylline only rarely alters the pharmacokinetics of other drugs.

The drugs listed in TABLE 2A and TABLE 2B have the potential to produce clinically significant pharmacodynamic or pharmacokinetic interactions with theophylline. The information in the "Effect" column of TABLE 2A and TABLE 2B assumes that the interacting drug is being added to a steady-state theophylline regimen. If theophylline is being initiated in a patient who is already taking a drug that inhibits theophylline clearance (*e.g.*, cimetidine, erythromycin), the dose of theophylline required to achieve a therapeutic serum theophylline concentration will be smaller. Conversely, if theophylline is being initiated in a patient who is already taking a drug that enhances theophylline clearance (*e.g.*, rifampin), the dose of theophylline required to achieve a therapeutic serum theophylline concentration will be larger. Discontinuation of a concomitant drug that increases theophylline clearance will result in accumulation of theophylline to potentially toxic levels, unless the theophylline dose is appropriately reduced. Discontinuation of a concomitant drug that inhibits theophylline clearance will result in decreased serum theophylline concentrations, unless the theophylline dose is appropriately increased.

The drugs listed in TABLE 3 have either been documented not to interact with theophylline or do not produce a clinically significant interaction (*i.e.*, <15% change in theophylline clearance).

The listing of drugs in TABLE 2A, TABLE 2B and TABLE 3 are current as of May 1996. New interactions are continuously being reported for theophylline, especially with new chemical entities. **The clinician should not assume that a drug does not interact with theophylline if it is not listed in TABLE 2A and TABLE 2B.** Before addition of a newly available drug in a patient receiving theophylline, the package insert of the new drug and/or the medical literature should be consulted to determine if an interaction between the new drug and theophylline has been reported.

DRUG/FOOD INTERACTIONS

Administration of a single dose of theophylline sustained-release tablets immediately after a high-fat content breakfast (8 ounces of whole milk, 2 fried eggs, 2 bacon strips, 2 ounces of hash browns and 2 slices of buttered toast, which equate to approximately 71 grams of fat and 985 calories) to 35 healthy volunteers resulted in plasma concentrations (for the first 8 hours) of 40-60% of those noted during the fasted state and a delay in the time of peak plasma level (T_{max}) of 17.1 hours in contrast to 5.1 hours observed during the fasted state.

However, when theophylline sustained-release tablets were administered on an every 12 hours schedule for 5 days, no consequential effect on absorption was noted following similar high-fat content breakfast, and the time to peak concentration averaged 5.4 hours. The rate and extent of absorption seen was similar when the drug was taken immediately after, and 2 hours after, a low-fat content breakfast.

The effect of other types and amounts of food, and the pharmacokinetic profile following an evening meal is not presently known.

THE EFFECT OF OTHER DRUGS ON THEOPHYLLINE SERUM CONCENTRATION MEASUREMENTS

Most serum theophylline assays in clinical use are immunoassays which are specific for theophylline. Other xanthines such as caffeine, dyphylline, and pentoxifylline are not detected by these assays. Some drugs (*e.g.*, cefazolin, cephalothin), however, may interfere with certain HPLC techniques. Caffeine and xanthine metabolites in neonates or patients with renal dysfunction may cause the reading from some dry reagent office methods to be higher than the actual serum theophylline concentration.

CESSATION OF SMOKING

Drug Interactions

Adding a drug that inhibits theophylline metabolism (*e.g.*, cimetidine, erythromycin, tacrine) or stopping a concurrently administered drug that enhances theophylline metabolism (*e.g.*, carbamazepine, rifampin). (see TABLE 2A and TABLE 2B).

ADVERSE REACTIONS

Adverse reactions associated with theophylline are generally mild when peak serum theophylline concentrations are <20 µg/ml and mainly consist of transient caffeine-like adverse effects such as nausea, vomiting, headache, and insomnia. When peak serum theophylline concentrations exceed 20 µg/ml, however, theophylline produces a wide range of adverse reactions including persistent vomiting, cardiac arrhythmias, and intractable seizures which can be lethal. The transient caffeine-like adverse reactions occur in about 50% of patients when theophylline therapy is initiated at doses higher than recommended initial doses (*e.g.*, >300 mg/day in adults and >12 mg/kg/day in children beyond >1 year of age). During the initiation of theophylline therapy, caffeine-like adverse effects may transiently alter patient behavior, especially in school age children, but this response rarely persists. Initiation of theophylline therapy at a low dose with subsequent slow titration to a predetermined age-related maximum dose will significantly reduce the frequency of these transient adverse effects (see DOSAGE AND ADMINISTRATION). In a small percentage of patients (<3% of children and <10% of adults) the caffeine-like adverse effects persist during maintenance therapy, even at peak serum theophylline concentrations within the therapeutic range (*i.e.*, 10-20 µg/ml). Dosage reduction may alleviate the caffeine-like adverse effects in these patients, however, persistent adverse effects should result in a reevaluation of the need for continued theophylline therapy and the potential therapeutic benefit of alternative treatment.

Other adverse reactions that have been reported at serum theophylline concentrations <20 µg/ml include diarrhea, irritability, restlessness, fine skeletal muscle tremors, and transient diuresis. In patients with hypoxia secondary to COPD, multifocal atrial tachycardia and flutter have been reported at serum theophylline concentrations ≥15 µg/ml. There have been a few isolated reports of seizures at serum theophylline concentrations <20 µg/ml in patients with an underlying neurological disease or in elderly patients. The occurrence of

T

TABLE 2A *Clinically Significant Drug Interactions with Theophylline**

Drug	Type of Interaction	Effect†
Adenosine	Theophylline blocks adenosine receptors.	Higher doses of adenosine may be required to achieve desired effect.
Alcohol	A single large dose of alcohol (3 ml/kg of whiskey) decreases theophylline clearance for up to 24 hours.	30% increase.
Allopurinol	Decreases theophylline clearance at allopurinol doses ≥600 mg/day.	25% increase.
Aminoglutethimide	Increases theophylline clearance by induction of microsomal enzyme activity.	25% decrease.
Carbamazepine	Similar to aminoglutethimide.	30% decrease.
Cimetidine	Decreases theophylline clearance by inhibiting cytochrome P450 1A2.	70% increase.
Ciprofloxacin	Similar to cimetidine.	40% increase.
Clarithromycin	Similar to erythromycin.	25% increase.
Diazepam	Benzodiazepines increase CNS concentrations of adenosine, a potent CNS depressant, while theophylline blocks adenosine receptors.	Larger diazepam doses may be required to produce desired level of sedation. Discontinuation of theophylline without reduction of diazepam dose may result in respiratory depression.
Disulfiram	Decreases theophylline clearance by inhibiting hydroxylation and demethylation.	50% increase.
Enoxacin	Similar to cimetidine.	300% increase.
Ephedrine	Synergistic CNS effects.	Increased frequency of nausea, nervousness, and insomnia.
Erythromycin	Erythromycin metabolite decreases theophylline clearance by inhibiting cytochrome P450 3A3.	35% increase. Erythromycin steady-state serum concentrations decreased by a similar amount.
Estrogen	Estrogen containing oral contraceptives decrease theophylline clearance in a dose-dependent fashion. The effect of progesterone on theophylline clearance is unknown.	30% increase.
Flurazepam	Similar to diazepam.	Similar to diazepam.
Fluvoxamine	Similar to cimetidine.	Similar to cimetidine.
Halothane	Halothane sensitizes the myocardium to catecholamines, theophylline increases release of endogenous catecholamines.	Increased risk of ventricular arrhythmias.
Interferon, human recombinant alpha-A	Decreases theophylline clearance.	100% increase.
Isoproterenol (IV)	Increases theophylline clearance.	20% decrease.
Ketamine	Pharmacologic.	May lower theophylline seizure threshold.
Lithium	Theophylline increases renal lithium clearance.	Lithium dose required to achieve a therapeutic serum concentration increased an average of 60%.
Lorazepam	Similar to diazepam.	Similar to diazepam.

* Refer to DRUG INTERACTIONS for further information regarding table.
† Average effect on steady state theophylline concentration or other clinical effect for pharmacologic interactions. Individual patients may experience larger changes in serum theophylline concentration than the value listed.

TABLE 2B *Clinically Significant Drug Interactions With Theophylline**

Drug	Type of Interaction	Effect†
Methotrexate (MTX)	Decreases theophylline clearance.	20% increase after low dose MTX, higher dose MTX may have a greater effect.
Mexiletine	Similar to disulfiram.	80% increase.
Midazolam	Similar to diazepam.	Similar to diazepam.
Moricizine	Increases theophylline clearance.	25% decrease.
Pancuronium	Theophylline may antagonize non-depolarizing neuromuscular blocking effects; possibly due to phosphodiesterase inhibition.	Larger dose of pancuronium may be required to achieve neuromuscular blockade.
Pentoxifylline	Decreases theophylline clearance.	30% increase.
Phenobarbital (PB)	Similar to aminoglutethimide.	25% decrease after two weeks of concurrent PB.
Phenytoin	Phenytoin increases theophylline clearance by increasing microsomal enzyme activity. Theophylline decreases phenytoin absorption.	Serum theophylline and phenytoin concentrations decrease about 40%.
Propafenone	Decreases theophylline clearance and pharmacologic interaction.	40% increase. Beta-2 blocking effect may decrease efficacy of theophylline.
Propranolol	Similar to cimetidine and pharmacologic interaction.	100% increase. Beta-2 blocking effect may decrease efficacy of theophylline.
Rifampin	Increases theophylline clearance by increasing cytochrome P450 1A2 and 3A3 activity.	20-40% decrease.
Sulfinpyrazone	Increases theophylline clearance by increasing demethylation and hydroxylation. Decreases renal clearance of theophylline.	20% decrease.
Tacrine	Similar to cimetidine, also increases renal clearance of theophylline.	90% increase.
Thiabendazole	Decreases theophylline clearance.	190% increase.
Ticlopidine	Decreases theophylline clearance.	60% increase.
Troleandomycin	Similar to erythromycin.	33-100% increase depending on troleandomycin dose.
Verapamil	Similar to disulfiram.	20% increase.

* Refer to DRUG INTERACTIONS for further information regarding table.
† Average effect on steady state theophylline concentration or other clinical effect for pharmacologic interactions. Individual patients may experience larger changes in serum theophylline concentration than the value listed.

TABLE 3 *Drugs That Have Been Documented Not to Interact With Theophylline or Drugs That Produce No Clinically Significant Interaction With Theophylline**

Albuterol, systemic and inhaled	Mebendazole
Amoxicillin	Medroxyprogesterone
Ampicillin, with or without sulbactam	Methylprednisolone
Atenolol	Metronidazole
Anithromycin	Metroprolol
Caffeine, dietary ingestion	Nadolol
Cefaclor	Nifedipine
Co-trimoxazole (trimethoprim and sulfamethoxazole)	Nizatidine
Diltiazem	Norfloxacin
Dirithromycin	Ofloxacin
Enflurane	Omeprazole
Famotidine	Prednisone, prednisolone
Felodipine	Ranitidine
Finasteride	Rifabutin
Hydrocortisone	Roxithromycin
Isoflurane	Sorbitol (purgative doses do no inhibit theophylline absorption)
Isoniazid	Sucralfate
Isradipine	Terbutaline, systemic
Influenza vaccine	Terfenadine
Ketoconazole	Tetracycline
Lomefloxacin	Tocainide

* Refer to PRECAUTIONS, Drug Interactions for information regarding table.

seizures in elderly patients with serum theophylline concentrations <20 µg/ml may be secondary to decreased protein binding resulting in a larger proportion of the total serum theophylline concentration in the pharmacologically active unbound form. The clinical characteristics of the seizures reported in patients with serum theophylline concentrations <20 µg/ml have generally been milder than seizures associated with excessive serum theophylline concentrations resulting from an overdose (*i.e.*, they have generally been transient, often stopped without anticonvulsant therapy, and did not result in neurological residua).

DOSAGE AND ADMINISTRATION

IMMEDIATE RELEASE ORAL PRODUCTS

General Considerations

The steady-state peak serum theophylline concentration is a function of the dose, the dosing interval, and the rate of theophylline absorption and clearance in the individual patient. Because of marked individual differences in the rate of theophylline clearance, the dose required to achieve a peak serum theophylline concentration in the 10-20 µg/ml range varies 4-fold among otherwise similar patients in the absence of factors known to alter theophylline clearance (*e.g.*, 400-1600 mg/day in adults <60 years old and 10-36 mg/kg/day in children 1-9 years old). For a given population there is no single theophylline dose that will provide both safe and effective serum concentrations for all patients. Administration of the median theophylline dose required to achieve a therapeutic serum theophylline concentration in a given population may result in either sub-therapeutic or potentially toxic serum theophylline concentrations in individual patients. For example, at a dose of 900 mg/day in adults <60 years or 22 mg/kg/day in children 1-9 years, the steady-state peak serum theophylline concentration will be <10 µg/ml in about 30% of patients, 10-20 µg/ml in about 50% and 20-30 µg/ml in about 20% of patients. **The dose of theophylline must be individualized on the basis of peak serum theophylline concentration measurements in order to achieve a dose that will provide maximum potential benefit with minimal risk of adverse effects.**

Transient caffeine-like adverse effects and excessive serum concentrations in slow metabolizers can be avoided in most patients by starting with a sufficiently low dose and slowly increasing the dose, if judged to be clinically indicated, in small increments. Dose increases should only be made if the previous dosage is well tolerated and at intervals of no less than 3 days to allow serum theophylline concentrations to reach the new steady state. Final dosage adjustment should be guided by serum theophylline concentration measurement (see PRECAUTIONS, Laboratory Tests and TABLE 5). Health care providers should instruct patients and caregivers to discontinue any dosage that causes adverse effects, to withhold the medication until these symptoms are gone and to then resume therapy at a lower, previously tolerated dosage (see WARNINGS).

If the patient's symptoms are well controlled, there are no apparent adverse effects, and no intervening factors that might alter dosage requirements (see WARNINGS and PRECAUTIONS), serum theophylline concentrations should be monitored at 6 month intervals for rapidly growing children and at yearly intervals for all others. In acutely ill patients, serum theophylline concentrations should be monitored at frequent intervals, *e.g.*, every 24 hours.

Theophylline distributes poorly into body fat, therefore, mg/kg dose should be calculated on the basis of ideal body weight.

T

***TABLE 4** Manifestations Of Theophylline Toxicity**

	Percentage of Patients Reported with Sign or Symptom			
	Acute Overdosage (Large Single Ingestion)		Chronic Overdosage (Multiple Excessive Doses)	
	Study 1	Study 2	Study 1	Study 2
Sign/Symptom	(n=157)	(n=14)	(n=92)	(n=102)
Asymptomatic	NR†	0	NR†	6
Gastrointestinal				
Vomiting	73	93	30	61
Abdominal pain	NR†	21	NR†	12
Diarrhea	NR†	0	NR†	14
Hematemesis	NR†	0	NR†	2
Metabolic/Other				
Hypokalemia	85	79	44	43
Hyperglycemia	98	NR†	18	NR†
Acid/base disturbance	34	21	9	5
Rhabdomyolysis	NR†	7	NR†	0
Cardiovascular				
Sinus tachycardia	100	86	100	62
Other supraventricular tachycardias	2	21	12	14
Ventricular premature beats	3	21	10	19
Atrial fibrillation or flutter	1	NR†	12	NR†
Multifocal atrial tachycardia	0	NR†	2	NR†
Ventricular arrhythmias with hemodynamic instability	7	14	40	0
Hypotension/shock	NR†	21	NR†	8
Neurologic				
Nervousness	NR†	64	NR†	21
Tremors	38	29	16	14
Disorientation	NR†	7	NR†	11
Seizures	5	14	14	5
Death	3	21	10	4

* These data are derived from two studies in patients with serum theophylline concentrations >30 μg/ml. In the first study (Study #1 - Shanon, Ann Intern Med 1993;119:1161-67), data were prospectively collected from 249 consecutive cases of theophylline toxicity referred to a regional poison center for consultation. In the second study (Study #2 - Sessler, Am J Med 1990;88:567-76), data were retrospectively collected from 116 cases with serum theophylline concentrations >30 μg/ml among 6000 blood samples obtained for measurement of serum theophylline concentrations in three emergency departments. Differences in the incidence of manifestations of theophylline toxicity between the two studies may reflect sample selection as a result of study design (*e.g.*, in Study #1, 48% of the patients had acute intoxications versus only 10% in Study #2) and different methods of reporting results.

† NR = Not reported in a comparable manner.

The following list contains theophylline dosing titration schema recommended for patients in various age groups and clinical circumstances. TABLE 5 contains recommendations for final theophylline dosage adjustment based on serum theophylline concentrations. **Application of these general dosing recommendations to individual patients must take into account the unique clinical characteristics of each patient. In general, these recommendations should serve as the upper limit for dosage adjustments in order to decrease the risk of potentially serious adverse events associated with unexpected large increases in serum theophylline concentration.**

A. Infants <1 year old:

1. Initial Dosage:

a. Premature Neonates:

i. <24 days postnatal age; 1.0 mg/kg every 12 hours.

ii. ≥24 days postnatal age; 1.5 mg/kg every 12 hours.

b. Full Term Infants and Infants Up to 52 Weeks of Age:

Total daily dose (mg) = [(0.2 × age in weeks)+5.0] × (kg body weight)

i. up to age 26 weeks; divide dose into 3 equal amounts administered at 8 hour intervals.

ii. >26 weeks of age; divide dose into 4 equal amounts administered at 6 hour intervals.

2. ***Final Dosage:*** Adjusted to maintain a peak steady-state serum theophylline concentration of 5-10 μg/ml in neonates and 10-15 μg/ml in older infants (see TABLE 5) Since the time required to reach steady-state is a function of theophylline half-life, up to 5 days may be required to achieve steady-state in a premature neonate while only 2-3 days may be required in a 6 month old infant without other risk factors for impaired clearance in the absence of a loading dose. **If a serum theophylline concentration is obtained before steady-state is achieved, the maintenance dose should not be increased, even if the serum theophylline concentration is <10 μg/ml.**

B. *Children (1-15 years) and Adults (16-60 years) Without Risk Factors for Impaired Clearance:*

C. *Patients With Risk Factors For Impaired Clearance, The Elderly (>60 Years), And Those In Whom It Is Not Feasible To Monitor Serum Theophylline Concentrations:* In children 1-15 years of age, the initial theophylline dose should not exceed 16 mg/kg/day up to a maximum of 400 mg/day in the presence of risk factors for reduced theophylline clearance (see WARNINGS) or if it is not feasible to monitor serum theophylline concentrations. In adolescents ≥16 years and adults, including the elderly, the initial theophylline dose should not exceed 400 mg/day in the presence of risk factors for reduced theophylline clearance (see WARNINGS) or if it is not feasible to monitor serum theophylline concentrations.

***TABLE 5** Dosing Titration (as Anhydrous Theophylline)*†*

Titration Step	Children <45 kg	Children >45 kg and adults
1. Starting Dosage	12-14 mg/kg/day up to a maximum of 300 mg/day divided q8-12 hrs*	300 mg/day divided q8-12 hrs*
2. After 3 days, <u>if tolerated,</u> increase dose to:	16 mg/kg/day up to a maximum of 400 mg/day divided q8-12 hrs*	400 mg/day divided q8-12 hrs*
3. After 3 more days, <u>if tolerated,</u> increase dose to:	20 mg/kg/day up to a maximum of 600 mg/day divided q8-12 hrs*	600 mg/day divided q8-12 hrs*

* Patients with more rapid metabolism, clinically identified by higher than average dose requirements, should receive a smaller dose more frequently to prevent breakthrough symptoms resulting from low trough concentrations before the next dose. A reliably absorbed slow-release formulation will decrease fluctuations and permit longer dosing intervals.

† For products containing theophylline salts, the appropriate dose of the theophylline salt should be substituted for the anhydrous theophylline dose. To calculate the equivalent dose for theophylline salts, divide the anhydrous theophylline dose listed below by 0.8 for aminophylline, by 0.65 for oxtriphylline, and by 0.5 for the calcium salicylate and sodium glycinate salts.

D. *Loading Dose for Acute Bronchodilatation:* An inhaled beta-2 selective agonist, alone or in combination with a systemically administered corticosteroid, is the most effective treatment for acute exacerbations of reversible airways obstruction. Theophylline is a relatively weak bronchodilator, is less effective than an inhaled beta-2 selective agonist and provides no added benefit in the treatment of acute bronchospasm. If an inhaled or parenteral beta agonist is not available, a loading dose of an oral immediate release theophylline can be used as a temporary measure. A single 5 mg/kg dose of theophylline, in a patient who has not received any theophylline in the previous 24 hours, will produce an average peak serum theophylline concentration of 10 μg/ml (range 5-15 μg/ml). If dosing with theophylline is to be continued beyond the loading dose, the guidelines in Sections A.1.b., B.3., or C., above, should be utilized and serum theophylline concentration monitored at 24 hour intervals to adjust final dosage.

***TABLE 6** Final Dosage Adjustment Guided by Serum Theophylline Concentration.*

Peak Serum Concentration	Dosage Adjustment
<9.9 μg/ml	If symptoms are not controlled and current dosage is tolerated, increase dose about 25%. Recheck serum concentration after 3 days for further dosage adjustment
10-14.9 μg/ml	If symptoms are controlled and current dosage is tolerated, maintain dose and recheck serum concentration at 6-12 month intervals.* If symptoms are not controlled and current dosage is tolerated consider adding additional medication(s) to treatment regimen.
15-19.9 μg/ml	Consider 10% decrease in dose to provide greater margin of safety even if current dosage is tolerated.*
20-24.9 μg/ml	Decrease dose by 25% even if no adverse effects are present. Recheck serum concentration after 3 days to guide further dosage adjustment.
25-30 μg/ml	Skip next dose and decrease subsequent doses at least 25% even if no adverse effects are present. Recheck serum concentration after 3 days to guide further dosage adjustment. If symptomatic, consider whether overdose treatment is indicated.
>30 μg/ml	Treat overdose as indicated. If theophylline is subsequently resumed, decrease dose by at least 50% and recheck serum concentration after 3 days to guide further dosage adjustment.

* Dose reduction and/or serum theophylline concentration measurement is indicated whenever adverse effects are present, physiologic abnormalities that can reduce theophylline clearance occur (*e.g.*, sustained fever), or a drug that interacts with theophylline is added or discontinued (see WARNINGS).

SUSTAINED ACTION CAPSULES: SPRINKLING CONTENTS ON FOOD

Theo-Dur Sprinkle may be administered by carefully opening the capsule and sprinkling the beaded contents on a spoonful of soft food such as applesauce or pudding. The soft food should be swallowed immediately without chewing and followed with a glass of cool water or juice to ensure complete swallowing of the beads. It is recommended that the food used should not be hot and should be soft enough to be swallowed without chewing. Any bead/food mixture should be used immediately and not stored for future use. The small amount of food (one spoonful) used to administer the dose will not alter the bioavailability of Theo-Dur Sprinkle; however, the dosing should be at least 1 hour before or 2 hours after a meal. SUBDIVIDING THE CONTENTS OF A CAPSULE IS NOT RECOMMENDED.

DOSAGE GUIDELINES

Because administration of Theo-Dur Sprinkle at the time of food ingestion has been shown to result in significantly lower peak-serum concentrations and reduced extent of absorption (bioavailability). Patients should be instructed to take this medication at least 1 hour before or 2 hours after a meal (see DRUG INTERACTIONS).

Taking Theo-Dur Sprinkle at 12 hour intervals under the above restrictive recommendations in regard to food ingestion may be difficult for the patient to follow. Under such circumstances, consideration should be given to prescribing this drug every 8 hours (giving one-third of the 24 hour dosage requirement with each dose), if this regimen would more easily permit dosing under fasting conditions.

I. *Acute Symptoms:* NOTE: Status asthmaticus should be considered a medical emergency and is defined as that degree of bronchospasm which is not rapidly responsive to usual doses of conventional bronchodilators. Optimal therapy for such patients frequently requires both *additional medication,* Parenterally administered, and *close monitoring,* preferably in an intensive care setting. Theo-Dur Sprinkle is not intended for

T

patients experiencing an acute episode of bronchospasm (associated with asthma, chronic bronchitis, or emphysema). Such patients require rapid relief of symptoms and should be treated with an immediate release or intravenous theophylline preparation (or other bronchodilators) and not with controlled-release products.

II. Chronic Therapy:

A. ***Initiating Therapy with an Immediate-Release Product:*** It is recommended that the appropriate dosage be established sing an immediate-release preparation. Children weighing less than 25 kg should have their daily dosage requirements established with a liquid preparation to permit small dosage increments. Slow clinical titration is generally preferred to help assure acceptance and safety of the medication, and to allow the patient to develop tolerance to transient caffeine-like side effects. Then, if the total 24 hour dose can be given by use of the sustained-release product, the patient can usually be switched to Theo-Dur Sprinkle, giving one-half of the daily dose at 12 hour intervals. Patients who metabolize theophylline rapidly such as the young, smokers, and some nonsmoking adults, are the most likely candidates for dosing at 8 hour intervals. Such patients can generally be identified as having trough-serum concentrations lower than desired for repeatedly exhibiting symptoms near the end of a dosing interval.

B. ***Initiating Therapy with Theo-Dur Sprinkle:*** Alternatively, therapy can be initiated with Theo-Dur Sprinkle since it is available in dosage strengths which permit titration and adjustments of dosage in adults and older children: *Initial Dose:* 16 mg/kg/24 hours or 400 mg/24 hours (whichever is less) of anhydrous theophylline in 2 divided doses, 12 hour intervals. *Increasing Dose:* The above dosage may be increased in approximately 25% increments at 3 day intervals so long as the drug is tolerated; until clinical response is satisfactory or the maximum dose as indicated in Section III is reached. The serum concentration may be checked at these intervals, but at a minimum, should be checked at the end of this adjustment period.

III. *Maintenance Dose of Theophylline Where the Serum Concentration is Not Measured:* See TABLE 5.

WARNING: DO NOT ATTEMPT TO MAINTAIN ANY DOSE THAT IS NOT TOLERATED

TABLE 7 Sustained-Release Capsules Not to Exceed the Following:

		Dose per 12 hours
Age 6-9 years	24 mg/kg/day	12.0 mg/kg
Age 9-12 years	20 mg/kg/day	10.0 mg/kg
Age 12-16 years	18 mg/kg/day	9.0 mg/kg
Age Over 16 years	13 mg/kg/day or 900 mg (WHICHEVER IS LESS)	6.5 mg/kg

IV. *Measurement of Serum Theophylline Concentrations During Chronic Therapy:* If the above maximum doses are to maintained or exceeded, serum theophylline measurement is recommended. The serum sample should be obtained at the time of peak absorption: 1-2 hours after administration for immediate-release products and 5-10 hours after dosing for Theo-Dur Sprinkle. It is important that the patient will have missed no doses during the previous 48 hours and the dosing intervals will have been reasonably typical with no added doses during that time. DOSAGE ADJUSTMENT BASED ON SERUM THEOPHYLLINE CONCENTRATION MEASUREMENTS WHEN THESE INSTRUCTIONS HAVE NOT BEEN FOLLOWED MAY RESULT IN RECOMMENDATIONS THAT PRESENT RISK OF TOXICITY TO THE PATIENT.

V. *Final Adjustment of Dosage:* Caution should be exercised for younger children who cannot complain of minor side effects. Those with cor pulmonale, congestive heart failure, and/or other liver disease may have unusually low dosage requirements and thus may experience toxicity at the maximum dose recommended above. It is important that no patient be maintained on any dosage that is not tolerated. In instructing patients to increase dosage according to the schedule above, they should be instructed not to take a subsequent dose if apparent side effects occur and to resume therapy at a lower dose once adverse effects have disappeared.

TABLE 8 Sustained-Release Capsules

Dosage Adjustment after serum theophylline measurement.

If Serum Theophylline is:		Directions
Within normal limits	10-20 µg/ml	Maintain dosage of tolerated. Recheck serum theophylline concentration at 6-12 month intervals.*
Too high	20-25 µg/ml	Decrease doses by about 10%. Serum theophylline concentrations should be checked until within normal limits. Recheck at 6-12 months.
	25-30 µg/ml	Skip next dose and decrease subsequent doses by about 25%. Serum theophylline concentrations should be checked until within normal limits. Recheck at 6-12 months.
	over 30 µg/ml	Skip next 2 doses and decrease subsequent doses by 50%. Serum theophylline should be checked until within normal limits. Recheck at 6-12 months.
Too low	7.5-10 µg/ml	Increase dose by about 25%.† Serum theophylline concentrations should be checked for guidance in further dosage adjustment. Recheck serum theophylline concentration at 6-12 month intervals.*
	5-7.5	Increase dose by about 25% to the nearest dose increment and recheck serum theophylline for guidance in further dosage adjustment (another increase will probably be needed, but provides a safety check).

* Finer adjustments in dosage may be needed for some patients.
† The total daily dose may need to be administered at more frequent intervals if asthma symptoms occur repeatedly at the end of a dosing interval.

PRODUCT LISTING - RATED THERAPEUTICALLY EQUIVALENT

Size	Price	Product	NDC
Capsule, Extended Release - Oral - 100 mg			
30's	$10.77	SLO-BID GYROCAPS, Pd-Rx Pharmaceuticals	55289-0318-30
60's	$20.64	SLO-BID GYROCAPS, Pd-Rx Pharmaceuticals	55289-0318-60
100's	$19.61	GENERIC, Inwood Laboratories Inc	00258-3637-01
100's	$20.00	GENERIC, Qualitest Products Inc	00603-5949-21
100's	$20.55	GENERIC, Major Pharmaceuticals Inc	00904-7846-60
100's	$22.36	GENERIC, Moore, H.L. Drug Exchange Inc	00839-7885-06
Capsule, Extended Release - Oral - 125 mg			
100's	$25.75	GENERIC, Major Pharmaceuticals Inc	00904-7847-60
100's	$29.74	GENERIC, Moore, H.L. Drug Exchange Inc	00839-7886-06
100's	$36.58	GENERIC, Qualitest Products Inc	00603-5950-21
100's	$36.99	GENERIC, Inwood Laboratories Inc	00258-3638-01
Capsule, Extended Release - Oral - 200 mg			
30's	$20.76	SLO-BID GYROCAPS, Pd-Rx Pharmaceuticals	55289-0751-30
60's	$35.85	SLO-BID GYROCAPS, Pd-Rx Pharmaceuticals	55289-0751-60
100's	$30.70	GENERIC, Major Pharmaceuticals Inc	00904-7848-60
100's	$34.12	GENERIC, Watson/Rugby Laboratories Inc	00536-5633-01
100's	$35.41	GENERIC, Moore, H.L. Drug Exchange Inc	00839-7887-06
100's	$44.03	GENERIC, Inwood Laboratories Inc	00258-3634-01
100's	$44.03	GENERIC, Qualitest Products Inc	00603-5951-21
Capsule, Extended Release - Oral - 300 mg			
60's	$35.91	SLO-BID GYROCAPS, Pd-Rx Pharmaceuticals	55289-0788-60
100's	$36.55	GENERIC, Major Pharmaceuticals Inc	00904-7849-60
100's	$40.63	GENERIC, Watson/Rugby Laboratories Inc	00536-5634-01
100's	$42.17	GENERIC, Moore, H.L. Drug Exchange Inc	00839-7888-06
100's	$51.86	GENERIC, Inwood Laboratories Inc	00258-3625-01
100's	$51.86	GENERIC, Qualitest Products Inc	00603-5952-21
Elixir - Oral - 80 mg/15 ml			
15 ml x 100	$40.00	GENERIC, Roxane Laboratories Inc	00054-8845-04
19 ml x 40	$26.40	GENERIC, Roxane Laboratories Inc	00054-8848-16
30 ml x 100	$48.00	GENERIC, Roxane Laboratories Inc	00054-8846-04
480 ml	$3.84	GENERIC, Moore, H.L. Drug Exchange Inc	00839-5029-69
480 ml	$4.48	GENERIC, Major Pharmaceuticals Inc	00904-1444-16
480 ml	$4.70	GENERIC, Halsey Drug Company Inc	00879-0226-16
480 ml	$5.45	GENERIC, Ivax Corporation	00182-0226-40
480 ml	$5.80	GENERIC, Alpharma Uspd Makers Of Barre and Nmc	00472-1444-16
480 ml	$87.74	ELIXOPHYLLIN, Forest Pharmaceuticals	00456-0644-16
3840 ml	$19.97	GENERIC, Moore, H.L. Drug Exchange Inc	00839-5029-70
3840 ml	$20.74	GENERIC, Halsey Drug Company Inc	00879-0226-28
3840 ml	$20.74	GENERIC, Major Pharmaceuticals Inc	00904-1444-28
3840 ml	$23.62	GENERIC, Alpharma Uspd Makers Of Barre and Nmc	00472-1444-28
3840 ml	$25.34	GENERIC, Ivax Corporation	00182-0226-41
3840 ml	$25.34	GENERIC, Morton Grove Pharmaceuticals Inc	60432-0019-28
3840 ml	$26.11	GENERIC, Geneva Pharmaceuticals	00781-6600-28
Solution - Intravenous - 5%;40 mg/100 ml			
1000 ml x 12	$191.09	GENERIC, Abbott Pharmaceutical	00074-7662-09
Solution - Intravenous - 5%;80 mg/100 ml			
500 ml	$15.16	GENERIC, B. Braun/Mcgaw Inc	00264-9554-10
500 ml x 10	$143.00	GENERIC, B. Braun/Mcgaw Inc	00264-5554-10
500 ml x 18	$181.98	GENERIC, Baxter I.V. Systems Division	00338-0439-03
500 ml x 24	$120.56	GENERIC, Abbott Pharmaceutical	00074-7665-03
1000 ml	$64.00	GENERIC, B. Braun/Mcgaw Inc	00264-9554-00
1000 ml x 10	$164.16	GENERIC, B. Braun/Mcgaw Inc	00264-5554-00
1000 ml x 12	$87.64	GENERIC, Abbott Pharmaceutical	00074-7665-09
1000 ml x 12	$166.17	GENERIC, Baxter I.V. Systems Division	00338-0439-04
Solution - Intravenous - 5%;160 mg/100 ml			
250 ml x 24	$146.21	GENERIC, Abbott Pharmaceutical	00074-7666-62
250 ml x 24	$242.40	GENERIC, Baxter I.V. Systems Division	00338-0441-02
250 ml x 24	$340.80	GENERIC, B. Braun/Mcgaw Inc	00264-9558-20
500 ml	$16.21	GENERIC, B. Braun/Mcgaw Inc	00264-9558-10
500 ml x 10	$119.50	GENERIC, B. Braun/Mcgaw Inc	00264-5558-10
500 ml x 18	$98.10	GENERIC, Baxter I.V. Systems Division	00338-0441-03
500 ml x 24	$164.73	GENERIC, Abbott Pharmaceutical	00074-7666-03
Solution - Intravenous - 5%;200 mg/50 ml			
50 ml x 24	$140.79	GENERIC, Abbott Pharmaceutical	00074-7677-13
50 ml x 24	$226.80	GENERIC, Baxter I.V. Systems Division	00338-0445-41
50 ml x 24	$306.36	GENERIC, B. Braun/Mcgaw Inc	00264-5557-31
Solution - Intravenous - 5%;200 mg/100 ml			
100 ml x 24	$140.79	GENERIC, Abbott Pharmaceutical	00074-7668-23
100 ml x 24	$227.52	GENERIC, Baxter I.V. Systems Division	00338-0443-48
100 ml x 24	$306.24	GENERIC, B. Braun/Mcgaw Inc	00264-5552-32
Solution - Intravenous - 5%;320 mg/100 ml			
250 ml x 24	$150.48	GENERIC, Abbott Pharmaceutical	00074-7705-62
250 ml x 24	$262.80	GENERIC, Baxter I.V. Systems Division	00338-0444-02
Solution - Intravenous - 5%;400 mg/100 ml			
100 ml x 24	$143.93	GENERIC, Abbott Pharmaceutical	00074-7677-23
100 ml x 24	$234.48	GENERIC, Baxter I.V. Systems Division	00338-0445-48
100 ml x 24	$257.04	GENERIC, B. Braun/Mcgaw Inc	00264-5557-32
Solution - Oral - 80 mg/15 ml			
480 ml	$2.50	GENERIC, C.O. Truxton Inc	00463-9031-16
480 ml	$3.50	GENERIC, Cenci, H.R. Labs Inc	00556-0149-16
480 ml	$4.42	GENERIC, Interstate Drug Exchange Inc	00814-7785-82

Package	Price	Brand/Manufacturer	NDC
500 ml	$7.31	GENERIC, Roxane Laboratories Inc	00054-3841-63
3840 ml	$17.66	GENERIC, Cenci, H.R. Labs Inc	00556-0149-28

Tablet - Oral - 100 mg

Package	Price	Brand/Manufacturer	NDC
100's	$8.50	GENERIC, Dixon-Shane Inc	17236-0335-01

Tablet, Extended Release - Oral - 100 mg

Package	Price	Brand/Manufacturer	NDC
30's	$6.83	THEO-DUR, Allscripts Pharmaceutical Company	54569-0318-01
30's	$87.00	GENERIC, Medirex Inc	57480-0365-06
100's	$9.57	FEDERAL UPPER LIMIT, H.C.F.A. F F P	99999-2329-06
100's	$11.19	GENERIC, Moore, H.L. Drug Exchange Inc	00839-6730-06
100's	$11.19	GENERIC, Moore, H.L. Drug Exchange Inc	00839-7705-06
100's	$11.25	GENERIC, Watson/Schein Pharmaceuticals Inc	00364-0680-01
100's	$11.85	GENERIC, Forest Pharmaceuticals	00456-3584-01
100's	$11.85	GENERIC, Dey Laboratories	49502-0431-01
100's	$12.50	GENERIC, Martec Pharmaceuticals Inc	52555-0702-01
100's	$14.70	GENERIC, Parmed Pharmaceuticals Inc	00349-8280-01
100's	$15.48	GENERIC, Forest Pharmaceuticals	00456-4310-01
100's	$18.56	GENERIC, Major Pharmaceuticals Inc	00904-1610-60
100's	$20.35	GENERIC, Ivax Corporation	00182-1589-89
100's	$20.36	GENERIC, Sidmak Laboratories Inc	50111-0483-01
100's	$20.48	GENERIC, Inwood Laboratories Inc	00258-3584-01
100's	$22.75	THEO-DUR, Schering Corporation	00085-0487-01
100's	$23.02	GENERIC, Major Pharmaceuticals Inc	00904-1610-61
100's	$34.10	THEO-DUR, Schering Corporation	00085-0487-81

Tablet, Extended Release - Oral - 200 mg

Package	Price	Brand/Manufacturer	NDC
2's	$3.84	THEO-DUR, Prescript Pharmaceuticals	00247-0070-02
9's	$5.49	THEO-DUR, Prescript Pharmaceuticals	00247-0070-09
10's	$5.74	THEO-DUR, Prescript Pharmaceuticals	00247-0070-10
12's	$6.21	THEO-DUR, Prescript Pharmaceuticals	00247-0070-12
20's	$8.12	THEO-DUR, Prescript Pharmaceuticals	00247-0070-20
30's	$4.31	GENERIC, Pd-Rx Pharmaceuticals	55289-0259-30
30's	$10.45	GENERIC, Heartland Healthcare Services	61392-0016-30
30's	$10.49	THEO-DUR, Prescript Pharmaceuticals	00247-0070-30
30's	$107.80	GENERIC, Medirex Inc	57480-0366-06
45's	$15.67	GENERIC, Heartland Healthcare Services	61392-0016-45
50's	$15.27	THEO-DUR, Prescript Pharmaceuticals	00247-0070-50
60's	$7.37	GENERIC, Parmed Pharmaceuticals Inc	00349-8281-60
60's	$10.05	GENERIC, Pd-Rx Pharmaceuticals	55289-0259-60
60's	$17.65	THEO-DUR, Prescript Pharmaceuticals	00247-0070-60
60's	$20.89	GENERIC, Heartland Healthcare Services	61392-0016-60
60's	$29.04	THEO-DUR, Pd-Rx Pharmaceuticals	55289-0003-60
90's	$24.80	THEO-DUR, Prescript Pharmaceuticals	00247-0070-90
90's	$31.34	GENERIC, Heartland Healthcare Services	61392-0016-90
100's	$7.58	GENERIC, Pd-Rx Pharmaceuticals	55289-0259-01
100's	$16.07	FEDERAL UPPER LIMIT, H.C.F.A. F F P	99999-2329-10
100's	$17.67	GENERIC, Moore, H.L. Drug Exchange Inc	00839-7706-06
100's	$18.65	GENERIC, Forest Pharmaceuticals	00456-3583-01
100's	$18.65	GENERIC, Dixon-Shane Inc	17236-0324-01
100's	$19.00	GENERIC, Warrick Pharmaceuticals Corporation	59930-1660-01
100's	$19.25	GENERIC, Watson/Schein Pharmaceuticals Inc	00364-0681-01
100's	$19.44	GENERIC, Moore, H.L. Drug Exchange Inc	00839-6729-06
100's	$19.95	GENERIC, Martec Pharmaceuticals Inc	52555-0703-01
100's	$20.79	GENERIC, Major Pharmaceuticals Inc	00904-1611-60
100's	$24.80	GENERIC, Forest Pharmaceuticals	00456-4320-01
100's	$27.18	THEO-DUR, Prescript Pharmaceuticals	00247-0070-00
100's	$31.24	GENERIC, Major Pharmaceuticals Inc	00904-1611-61
100's	$32.65	GENERIC, Sidmak Laboratories Inc	50111-0482-01
100's	$32.83	GENERIC, Inwood Laboratories Inc	00258-3583-01
100's	$32.83	GENERIC, Qualitest Products Inc	00603-5945-21
100's	$36.48	THEO-DUR, Schering Corporation	00085-0933-01
100's	$47.41	THEO-DUR, Schering Corporation	00085-0933-81
100's	$62.41	GENERIC, Ivax Corporation	00182-1590-89
118's	$31.47	THEO-DUR, Prescript Pharmaceuticals	00247-0070-52
180's	$49.10	THEO-DUR, Allscripts Pharmaceutical Company	54569-8586-00

Tablet, Extended Release - Oral - 300 mg

Package	Price	Brand/Manufacturer	NDC
2's	$3.96	THEO-DUR, Prescript Pharmaceuticals	00247-0061-02
6's	$1.98	GENERIC, Pd-Rx Pharmaceuticals	55289-0260-06
6's	$4.06	THEO-DUR, Southwood Pharmaceuticals Inc	58016-0477-06
8's	$5.79	THEO-DUR, Prescript Pharmaceuticals	00247-0061-08
20's	$5.78	GENERIC, Pd-Rx Pharmaceuticals	55289-0260-20
20's	$9.45	THEO-DUR, Prescript Pharmaceuticals	00247-0061-20
25's	$7.68	GENERIC, Pd-Rx Pharmaceuticals	55289-0260-97
25's	$18.14	THEO-DUR, Pd-Rx Pharmaceuticals	55289-0155-97
30's	$7.34	GENERIC, Pd-Rx Pharmaceuticals	55289-0260-30
30's	$12.48	THEO-DUR, Prescript Pharmaceuticals	00247-0061-30
30's	$127.80	GENERIC, Medirex Inc	57480-0367-06
50's	$18.58	THEO-DUR, Prescript Pharmaceuticals	00247-0061-50
60's	$7.68	GENERIC, Parmed Pharmaceuticals Inc	00349-8266-60
60's	$11.19	GENERIC, Pd-Rx Pharmaceuticals	55289-0260-60
60's	$21.62	THEO-DUR, Prescript Pharmaceuticals	00247-0061-60
90's	$30.75	THEO-DUR, Prescript Pharmaceuticals	00247-0061-90
100's	$15.93	FEDERAL UPPER LIMIT, H.C.F.A. F F P	99999-2329-14
100's	$18.38	GENERIC, Pd-Rx Pharmaceuticals	55289-0260-01
100's	$21.18	GENERIC, Moore, H.L. Drug Exchange Inc	00839-6693-06
100's	$22.00	GENERIC, Warrick Pharmaceuticals Corporation	59930-1670-01
100's	$22.10	GENERIC, Warner Chilcott Laboratories	00047-0592-24
100's	$22.10	GENERIC, Martec Pharmaceuticals Inc	52555-0704-01
100's	$22.75	GENERIC, Forest Pharmaceuticals	00456-3581-01
100's	$25.03	GENERIC, Major Pharmaceuticals Inc	00904-1612-60
100's	$25.28	GENERIC, Sidmak Laboratories Inc	50111-0459-01
100's	$30.03	GENERIC, Dixon-Shane Inc	17236-0325-01
100's	$31.10	GENERIC, Major Pharmaceuticals Inc	00904-1612-61
100's	$38.98	GENERIC, Inwood Laboratories Inc	00258-3581-01
100's	$38.98	GENERIC, Qualitest Products Inc	00603-5946-21
100's	$40.59	GENERIC, Forest Pharmaceuticals	00456-4330-01
100's	$41.65	THEO-DUR, Allscripts Pharmaceutical Company	54569-0062-02
100's	$43.33	THEO-DUR, Schering Corporation	00085-0584-01
100's	$56.44	THEO-DUR, Schering Corporation	00085-0584-81
100's	$74.91	GENERIC, Ivax Corporation	00182-1400-89
180's	$58.32	THEO-DUR, Allscripts Pharmaceutical Company	54569-8580-00

Tablet, Extended Release - Oral - 400 mg/24 Hours

Package	Price	Brand/Manufacturer	NDC
100's	$110.34	UNI-DUR, Schering Corporation	00085-0694-01

Tablet, Extended Release - Oral - 450 mg

Package	Price	Brand/Manufacturer	NDC
100's	$27.75	GENERIC, Warrick Pharmaceuticals Corporation	59930-1680-01
100's	$28.58	GENERIC, Qualitest Products Inc	00603-5747-21
100's	$31.45	GENERIC, Inwood Laboratories Inc	00258-3614-01
100's	$32.95	GENERIC, Major Pharmaceuticals Inc	00904-1613-60
100's	$33.50	GENERIC, Martec Pharmaceuticals Inc	52555-0705-01
100's	$57.55	GENERIC, Forest Pharmaceuticals	00456-4345-01
100's	$57.55	GENERIC, Forest Pharmaceuticals	00785-4345-01

PRODUCT LISTING - RATED NOT THERAPEUTICALLY EQUIVALENT

Capsule, Extended Release - Oral - 50 mg

Package	Price	Brand/Manufacturer	NDC
30's	$9.53	SLO-BID GYROCAPS, Pd-Rx Pharmaceuticals	55289-0317-30
60's	$19.05	SLO-BID GYROCAPS, Pd-Rx Pharmaceuticals	55289-0317-60

Capsule, Extended Release - Oral - 75 mg

Package	Price	Brand/Manufacturer	NDC
30's	$11.93	SLO-BID GYROCAPS, Pd-Rx Pharmaceuticals	55289-0785-30
60's	$18.06	SLO-BID GYROCAPS, Pd-Rx Pharmaceuticals	55289-0785-60

Capsule, Extended Release - Oral - 100 mg/24 Hours

Package	Price	Brand/Manufacturer	NDC
100's	$45.07	GENERIC, Ucb Pharma Inc	50474-0100-01

Capsule, Extended Release - Oral - 200 mg/24 Hours

Package	Price	Brand/Manufacturer	NDC
100's	$64.91	GENERIC, Ucb Pharma Inc	50474-0200-60
100's	$67.18	GENERIC, Ucb Pharma Inc	50474-0200-01

Capsule, Extended Release - Oral - 300 mg/24 Hours

Package	Price	Brand/Manufacturer	NDC
30's	$19.54	GENERIC, Allscripts Pharmaceutical Company	54569-1666-01
100's	$65.14	GENERIC, Allscripts Pharmaceutical Company	54569-1666-00
100's	$71.33	GENERIC, Ucb Pharma Inc	50474-0300-60
100's	$78.26	GENERIC, Ucb Pharma Inc	50474-0300-01

Capsule, Extended Release - Oral - 400 mg/24 Hours

Package	Price	Brand/Manufacturer	NDC
100's	$116.03	GENERIC, Ucb Pharma Inc	50474-0400-01

Tablet, Extended Release - Oral - 100 mg

Package	Price	Brand/Manufacturer	NDC
100's	$20.48	GENERIC, Qualitest Products Inc	00603-5944-21

Tablet, Extended Release - Oral - 200 mg

Package	Price	Brand/Manufacturer	NDC
100's	$61.71	T-PHYL, Purdue Frederick Company	00034-7102-80

Tablet, Extended Release - Oral - 300 mg

Package	Price	Brand/Manufacturer	NDC
100's	$68.13	QUIBRON-T/SR, Monarch Pharmaceuticals Inc	61570-0019-01

Tablet, Extended Release - Oral - 400 mg/24 Hours

Package	Price	Brand/Manufacturer	NDC
30's	$39.44	UNIPHYL, Pd-Rx Pharmaceuticals	55289-0789-30
60's	$64.10	UNIPHYL, Physicians Total Care	54868-1438-01
100's	$107.94	UNIPHYL, Purdue Frederick Company	00034-7004-80

Tablet, Extended Release - Oral - 600 mg/24 Hours

Package	Price	Brand/Manufacturer	NDC
100's	$129.89	UNI-DUR, Schering Corporation	00085-0814-01
100's	$155.97	UNIPHYL, Purdue Frederick Company	00034-7006-80

PRODUCT LISTING - EQUIVALENTS NOT AVAILABLE

Capsule, Extended Release - Oral - 65 mg

Package	Price	Brand/Manufacturer	NDC
100's	$20.00	AEROLATE III, Fleming and Company	00256-0150-01

Capsule, Extended Release - Oral - 200 mg

Package	Price	Brand/Manufacturer	NDC
30's	$13.25	GENERIC, Pharma Pac	52959-0279-30

Capsule, Extended Release - Oral - 400 mg/24 Hours

Package	Price	Brand/Manufacturer	NDC
100's	$59.33	GENERIC, Ucb Pharma Inc	50474-0400-60

Elixir - Oral - 80 mg/15 ml

Package	Price	Brand/Manufacturer	NDC
118 ml	$6.74	GENERIC, Prescript Pharmaceuticals	00247-0308-52

Tablet - Oral - 100 mg

Package	Price	Brand/Manufacturer	NDC
100's	$13.35	GENERIC, Interstate Drug Exchange Inc	00814-7801-14

Tablet - Oral - 125 mg

Package	Price	Brand/Manufacturer	NDC
100's	$53.19	THEOLAIR, 3M Pharmaceuticals	00089-0342-10

Tablet - Oral - 200 mg

Package	Price	Brand/Manufacturer	NDC
30's	$11.19	SLO-PHYLLIN, Southwood Pharmaceuticals Inc	58016-0683-30

Tablet - Oral - 250 mg

Package	Price	Brand/Manufacturer	NDC
100's	$79.26	THEOLAIR, 3M Pharmaceuticals	00089-0344-10

Tablet - Oral - 300 mg

Package	Price	Brand/Manufacturer	NDC
100's	$54.00	QUIBRON-T, Roberts Pharmaceutical Corporation	54092-0069-01
100's	$60.48	QUIBRON-T, Monarch Pharmaceuticals Inc	61570-0020-01

Tablet, Extended Release - Oral - 100 mg

Package	Price	Brand/Manufacturer	NDC
30's	$3.63	GENERIC, Allscripts Pharmaceutical Company	54569-2032-00

Tablet, Extended Release - Oral - 200 mg

Qty	Price	Product	NDC
14's	$6.49	GENERIC, Cheshire Drugs	55175-4187-04
20's	$7.19	GENERIC, Cheshire Drugs	55175-4187-00
25's	$4.39	GENERIC, Circle Pharmaceuticals Inc	00659-2805-25
30's	$7.72	GENERIC, Allscripts Pharmaceutical Company	54569-2482-01
30's	$8.21	GENERIC, Cheshire Drugs	55175-4187-03
50's	$5.33	GENERIC, Physicians Total Care	54868-0028-03
60's	$6.07	GENERIC, Physicians Total Care	54868-0028-01
60's	$13.70	GENERIC, Allscripts Pharmaceutical Company	54569-2482-00
100's	$9.00	GENERIC, Physicians Total Care	54868-0028-02
100's	$17.94	GENERIC, Qualitest Products Inc	00603-5945-29
100's	$19.35	GENERIC, Interstate Drug Exchange Inc	00814-7802-14
100's	$25.72	GENERIC, Allscripts Pharmaceutical Company	54569-2482-05

Tablet, Extended Release - Oral - 300 mg

Qty	Price	Product	NDC
2's	$3.65	GENERIC, Prescript Pharmaceuticals	00247-0177-02
3's	$3.79	GENERIC, Prescript Pharmaceuticals	00247-0177-03
4's	$3.94	GENERIC, Prescript Pharmaceuticals	00247-0177-04
6's	$4.22	GENERIC, Prescript Pharmaceuticals	00247-0177-06
10's	$4.81	GENERIC, Prescript Pharmaceuticals	00247-0177-10
10's	$6.45	GENERIC, Allscripts Pharmaceutical Company	54569-0065-05
14's	$5.39	GENERIC, Prescript Pharmaceuticals	00247-0177-14
20's	$4.58	GENERIC, Allscripts Pharmaceutical Company	54569-2483-03
20's	$6.27	GENERIC, Prescript Pharmaceuticals	00247-0177-20
30's	$4.24	GENERIC, Physicians Total Care	54868-0029-06
30's	$6.88	GENERIC, Allscripts Pharmaceutical Company	54569-2483-02
30's	$7.72	GENERIC, Prescript Pharmaceuticals	00247-0177-30
30's	$9.85	GENERIC, Allscripts Pharmaceutical Company	54569-0065-01
50's	$5.69	GENERIC, Physicians Total Care	54868-0029-03
60's	$6.81	GENERIC, Physicians Total Care	54868-0029-05
60's	$12.09	GENERIC, Prescript Pharmaceuticals	00247-0177-60
60's	$13.90	GENERIC, Allscripts Pharmaceutical Company	54569-0065-02
60's	$14.71	GENERIC, Allscripts Pharmaceutical Company	54569-2483-00
100's	$10.23	GENERIC, Physicians Total Care	54868-0029-02
100's	$17.92	GENERIC, Prescript Pharmaceuticals	00247-0177-00
100's	$21.90	GENERIC, Qualitest Products Inc	00603-5946-29
100's	$22.92	GENERIC, Allscripts Pharmaceutical Company	54569-2483-01
100's	$25.20	GENERIC, Interstate Drug Exchange Inc	00814-7805-14
100's	$56.00	QUIBRON-T/SR, Roberts Pharmaceutical Corporation	54092-0070-01

Tablet, Extended Release - Oral - 450 mg

Qty	Price	Product	NDC
100's	$33.41	GENERIC, Moore, H.L. Drug Exchange Inc	00839-7651-06
100's	$57.55	THEO-DUR, Schering Corporation	00085-0806-01

Thiabendazole *(002332)*

For complete prescribing information, refer to the CD-ROM included with the book.

Categories: Ascariasis; Enterobiasis; Strongyloidiasis; Trichinosis; Trichuriasis; Uncinariasis; Pregnancy Category C; FDA Approved 1967 Apr
Drug Classes: Antihelmintics
Brand Names: **Mintezol**; Tiabendazole; Triasox
Cost of Therapy: $7.56 (Helminth Infection; Mintezol; 500 mg; 3 tablets/day; 2 day supply)

DESCRIPTION

Mintezol (thiabendazole) is an anthelmintic provided as 500 mg chewable tablets, and as a suspension, containing 500 mg thiabendazole per 5 ml. The suspension also contains sorbic acid 0.1% added as a preservative. Inactive ingredients in the tablets are acacia, calcium phosphate, flavors, lactose, magnesium stearate, mannitol, methylcellulose, and sodium saccharin. Inactive ingredients in the suspension are an antifoam agent, flavors, polysorbate, purified water, sorbitol solution, and tragacanth.

Thiabendazole is a white to off-white odorless powder with a molecular weight of 201.26, which is practically insoluble in water but readily soluble in dilute acid and alkali. Its chemical name is 2-(4-thiazolyl)-1*H*-benzimidazole. The empirical formula is $C_{10}H_7N_3S$.

INDICATIONS AND USAGE

Thiabendazole is indicated for the treatment of:

- Strongyloidiasis (threadworm)
- Cutaneous larva migrans (creeping eruption)
- Visceral larva migrans
- ***Trichinosis:*** Relief of symptoms and fever and a reduction of eosinophilia have followed the use of thiabendazole during the invasion stage of the disease.

Thiabendazole is usually inappropriate as first line therapy for enterobiasis (pinworm). However, when enterobiasis occurs with any of the conditions listed above, additional therapy is not required for most patients.

Thiabendazole should be used only in the following infestations when more specific therapy is not available or cannot be used or when further therapy with a second agent is desirable: Uncinariasis (hookworm: *Necator americanus* and *Ancylostoma duodenale*); Trichuriasis (whipworm); Ascariasis (large roundworm).

CONTRAINDICATIONS

Hypersensitivity to this product.

Thiabendazole is contraindicated as prophylactic treatment for pinworm infestation.

WARNINGS

If hypersensitivity reactions occur, the drug should be discontinued immediately and not be resumed. Erythema multiforme has been associated with thiabendazole therapy; in severe cases (Stevens-Johnson syndrome), fatalities have occurred.

Because CNS side effects may occur quite frequently, activities requiring mental alertness should be avoided.

Jaundice, cholestasis, and parenchymal liver damage have been reported in patients treated with thiabendazole. In rare cases, liver damage has been severe and has led to irreversible hepatic failure.

Abnormal sensation in eyes, xanthopsia, blurred vision, drying of mucous membranes, and Sicca syndrome have been reported in patients treated with thiabendazole. These adverse effects of the eye were in some cases persistent for prolonged intervals which have exceeded 1 year.

Thiabendazole should not usually be used as first line therapy for the treatment of enterobiasis. It should be reserved for use in patients who have experienced allergic reactions, or resistance to other treatments.

DOSAGE AND ADMINISTRATION

The recommended maximum daily dose of thiabendazole is 3 g.

Thiabendazole should be given after meals if possible. Thiabendazole tablets should be chewed before swallowing. Dietary restriction, complementary medications and cleansing enemas are not needed.

The usual dosage schedule for all conditions is 2 doses per day. The dosage is determined by the patient's weight.

A weight-dose chart follows (see TABLE 1).

TABLE 1

Weight	Each Dose	
30 lb	0.25 g (½ tablet)	2.5 ml (½ teaspoon)
50 lb	0.5 g (1 tablet)	5.0 ml (1 teaspoon)
75 lb	0.75 g (1½ tablets)	7.5 ml (1½ teaspoons)
100 lb	1.0 g (2 tablets)	10.0 ml (2 teaspoons)
125 lb	1.25 g (2½ tablets)	12.5 ml (2½ teaspoons)
150 lb & over	1.5 g (3 tablets)	15.0 ml (3 teaspoons)

The regimen for each indication is listed in TABLE 2.

TABLE 2 *Therapeutic Regimens*

Indication	Regimen	Comments
Strongyloidiasis*	2 doses per day for 2 successive days.	A single dose of 20 mg/lb or 50 mg/kg may be employed as an alternative schedule, but a higher incidence of side effects should be expected.
Cutaneous Larva Migrans (Creeping Eruption)	2 doses per day for 2 successive days.	If active lesions are still present 2 days after completion of therapy, a second course is recommended.
Visceral Larva Migrans	2 doses per day for 7 successive days.	Safety and efficacy data on the 7 day treatment course are limited.
Trichinosis*	2 doses per day for 2-4 successive days according to the response of the patient.	The optimal dosage for the treatment of trichinosis has not been established.
Other Indications		
*Intestinal roundworms (including Ascariasis, Uncinariasis and Trichuriasis)	2 doses per day for 2 successive days.	A single dose of 20 mg/lb or 50 mg/kg may be employed as an alternative schedule, but a higher incidence of side effects should be expected.

* Clinical experience with thiabendazole for treatment of each of these conditions in pediatric patients weighing less than 30 lb has been limited.

PRODUCT LISTING - EQUIVALENTS NOT AVAILABLE

Suspension - Oral - 500 mg/5 ml

Qty	Price	Product	NDC
120 ml	$26.32	MINTEZOL, Merck & Company Inc	00006-3331-60

Tablet, Chewable - Oral - 500 mg

Qty	Price	Product	NDC
36's	$45.35	MINTEZOL, Merck & Company Inc	00006-0907-36

T

Thiamine Hydrochloride (002333)

Categories: Beriberi; Deficiency, thiamine; Pregnancy Category A; FDA Approved 1973 Apr; WHO Formulary
Drug Classes: Vitamins/minerals
Brand Names: Actamin; Alivio; Anacrodyne; Benerva; Beneuril; Beneuron; Betabion; **Betalin S**; Betamin; Betatabs; Betaxin; Bevitine; Bewon; Biamine; Dumovit; Invite; Metabolin; Oryzanin; Ottovit; Tiamina; Vitamin B-1; Vitanon; Vitantial

DESCRIPTION

Injection thiamine HCl (thiamine hydrochloride injection) is a sterile solution of thiamine hydrochloride for injection. It has a pH between 2.5 and 4.5. Sodium hydroxide and/or hydrochloric acid may have been added during manufacture to adjust the pH.

Thiamine hydrochloride, or vitamin B1, occurs as small white hygroscopic crystals or crystalline powder that usually has a slight characteristic odor. One g dissolves in about 1 ml of water. Thiamine is rapidly destroyed in neutral or or alkaline solutions but is stable in the dry state. It is reasonably stable to heat in acid solution.

The chemical name of thiamine hydrochloride is 3-(4-amino-2-methylpyrimidal-5-methyl)-4-methyl-5(beta-hydroxyethyl) thiazolium chloride hydrochloride.

$C_{12}H_{17}ClN_4OS$. HCl

Storage: Protect from light. Store in carton until contents have been used. Store at controlled room temperature, 15-30°C (59-86°F).

CLINICAL PHARMACOLOGY

The water-soluble vitamins are widely distributed in both plants and animals. They are absorbed in man by both diffusion and active transport mechanisms. These vitamins are structurally diverse (derivatives of sugar, pyridine, purines, pyrimidine, organic acid complexes, and nucleotide complex) and act as coenzymes, as oxidation-reduction agents, or possibly as mitochondrial agents. Metabolism is rapid, and the excess is excreted in the urine.

Thiamine is distributed in all tissues. The highest concentrations occur in liver, brain, kidney, and heart. When thiamine intake is greatly in excess of need, tissue stores increase 2-3 times. If intake is insufficient, tissues become depleted of their vitamin content. Absorption of thiamine following intramuscular administration is rapid and complete.

Thiamine combines with adenosine triphosphate (ATP) to form thiamine pyrophosphate, also known as carboxylase, a coenzyme. Its role in carbohydrate metabolism is the decarboxylation of pyruvic acid and alpha-ketoacids to acetaldehyde and carbon dioxide. Increased levels of pyruvic acid in the blood indicate vitamin B1 deficiency.

The requirement for thiamine is greater when the carbohydrate content of the diet is raised. Body depletion of vitamin B1 can occur after approximately 3 weeks of total absence of thiamine in the diet.

INDICATIONS AND USAGE

Thiamine hydrochloride injection is effective for the treatment of thiamine deficiency or beriberi. Beriberi may be manifested as the "dry" or the "wet" type.

Parenteral administration is indicated when the oral route is not feasible, as in anorexia, nausea, vomiting, or preoperative and postoperative conditions. It is also indicated when gastrointestinal absorption is impaired, as in the "malabsorption syndrome" (steatorrhea).

CONTRAINDICATIONS

A history of sensitivity to thiamine or to any of the ingredients in thiamine HCl is a contraindication.

WARNINGS

Serious sensitivity reactions can occur. Deaths have resulted from intravenous use. An intradermal test dose is recommended prior to administration in patients suspected of being sensitive to the drug.

PRECAUTIONS

GENERAL

Simple vitamin B1 deficiency is rare. Multiple vitamin deficiencies should be suspected in any case of dietary inadequacy.

INFORMATION FOR THE PATIENT

The patient should be advised as to proper dietary habits during treatment so that relapses will be less likely to occur with reduction in dosage or cessation of injection therapy.

PREGNANCY CATEGORY A

Studies in pregnant women have not shown that thiamine HCl increases the risk of fetal abnormalities if administered during pregnancy. If the drug is used during pregnancy, the possibility of fetal harm appears remote. Because studies cannot rule out the possibility of harm, however, thiamine HCl should be used during pregnancy only if clearly needed.

NURSING MOTHERS

It is not known whether this drug is excreted in human milk. Because many drugs are excreted in human milk, caution should be exercised when thiamine HCl is administered to a nursing woman.

ADVERSE REACTIONS

An occasional individual may develop a sensitivity or intolerance to thiamine, especially after repeated intravenous administration.

Some tenderness and induration may follow intramuscular use. A feeling of warmth, pruritus, urticaria, weakness, sweating, nausea, restlessness, tightness of the throat, angioneurotic edema, cyanosis, pulmonary edema, hemorrhage into the gastrointestinal tract, collapse, and deaths have been recorded.

DOSAGE AND ADMINISTRATION

"Wet" beriberi with myocardial failure must be treated as an emergency cardiac condition by the intravenous route.

In the treatment of beriberi, 10-20 mg of thiamine are given intramuscularly 3 times daily for as long as 2 weeks. An oral therapeutic multivitamin preparation containing 5-10 mg thiamine, administered daily for 1 month, is recommended to achieve body tissue saturation.

Poor dietary habits should be corrected, and an abundant and well-balanced dietary intake should be prescribed.

PRODUCT LISTING - RATED THERAPEUTICALLY EQUIVALENT

Solution - Injectable - 100 mg/ml

1 ml x 10	$21.50	GENERIC, Abbott Pharmaceutical	00074-2174-01
1 ml x 25	$25.00	GENERIC, Esi Lederle Generics	00641-0610-25
2 ml x 25	$59.50	GENERIC, American Pharmaceutical Partners	63323-0013-02
10 ml	$1.70	GENERIC, Major Pharmaceuticals Inc	00904-0944-10
25 ml	$30.00	GENERIC, Cmc-Consolidated Midland Corporation	00223-8680-01
30 ml	$3.50	GENERIC, Keene Pharmaceuticals Inc	00588-5201-90
30 ml	$4.00	GENERIC, C.O. Truxton Inc	00463-1074-30
30 ml	$4.00	GENERIC, Major Pharmaceuticals Inc	00904-0944-30
30 ml	$4.95	GENERIC, Roberts/Hauck Pharmaceutical Corporation	43797-0033-13
30 ml	$5.75	GENERIC, Pasadena Research Laboratories Inc	00418-2541-61
30 ml	$7.75	GENERIC, Ivax Corporation	00182-0567-66

PRODUCT LISTING - EQUIVALENTS NOT AVAILABLE

Solution - Injectable - 100 mg/ml

1 ml x 25	$24.98	GENERIC, Allscripts Pharmaceutical Company	54569-2431-00
1 ml x 25	$25.00	GENERIC, Cmc-Consolidated Midland Corporation	00223-8709-01
1 ml x 100	$98.00	GENERIC, Raway Pharmacal Inc	00686-0610-25
30 ml	$3.97	GENERIC, Mcguff Company	49072-0739-30
30 ml	$5.50	GENERIC, Primedics Laboratories	00684-0148-30
30 ml	$8.50	GENERIC, Cmc-Consolidated Midland Corporation	00223-8711-02

Thioguanine (002339)

For complete prescribing information, refer to the CD-ROM included with the book.

Categories: Leukemia, acute myelogenous; Leukemia, nonlymphocytic; Pregnancy Category D; FDA Approved 1966 Jan
Drug Classes: Antineoplastics, antimetabolites
Brand Names: Tabloid
Foreign Brand Availability: Lanvis (Australia; Bahamas; Bahrain; Barbados; Belgium; Belize; Benin; Bermuda; Bulgaria; Burkina-Faso; Canada; Curacao; Cyprus; Egypt; England; Ethiopia; Finland; France; Gambia; Ghana; Greece; Guinea; Guyana; Hong-Kong; Hungary; Iran; Iraq; Ivory-Coast; Jamaica; Jordan; Kenya; Kuwait; Lebanon; Liberia; Libya; Malawi; Malaysia; Mali; Mauritania; Mauritius; Morocco; Netherland-Antilles; Netherlands; New-Zealand; Niger; Nigeria; Oman; Puerto-Rico; Qatar; Republic-of-Yemen; Saudi-Arabia; Senegal; Seychelles; Sierra-Leone; South-Africa; Sudan; Surinam; Sweden; Switzerland; Syria; Taiwan; Tanzania; Thailand; Trinidad; Tunia; Uganda; United-Arab-Emirates; Zambia; Zimbabwe)
Cost of Therapy: $455.69 (Nonlymphocytic Leukemia; Thioguanine; 40 mg; 3 capsules/day; 30 day supply)

DESCRIPTION

CAUTION: Thioguanine is a potent drug. It should not be used unless a diagnosis of acute nonlymphocytic leukemia has been adequately established and the responsible physician is knowledgeable in assessing response to chemotherapy.

Thioguanine was synthesized and developed by Hitchings, Elion and associates at the Wellcome Research Laboratories. It is one of a large series of purine analogues which interfere with nucleic acid biosynthesis, and has been found active against selected human neoplastic diseases.[1]

Thioguanine, known chemically as 2-amino-1,7-dihydro-6*H*-purine-6-thione, is an analogue of the nucleic acid constituent guanine, and is closely related structurally and functionally to mercaptopurine.

Tabloid is available in tablets for oral administration. Each scored tablet contains 40 mg thioguanine and the inactive ingredients gum acacia, lactose, magnesium stearate, potato starch, and stearic acid.

INDICATIONS AND USAGE

ACUTE NONLYMPHOCYTIC LEUKEMIAS

Thioguanine is indicated for remission induction, remission consolidation, and maintenance therapy of acute nonlymphocytic leukemias.[8,9] The response to this agent depends upon the age of the patient (younger patients faring better than older) and whether thioguanine is used in previously treated or previously untreated patients. Reliance upon thioguanine alone is seldom justified for initial remission induction of acute nonlymphocytic leukemias because combination chemotherapy including thioguanine results in more frequent remission induction and longer duration of remission than thioguanine alone.

OTHER NEOPLASMS

Thioguanine is not effective in chronic lymphocytic leukemia, Hodgkin's lymphoma, multiple myeloma or solid tumors. Although thioguanine is one of several agents with activity in the treatment of the chronic phase of chronic myelogenous leukemia, more objective responses are observed with busulfan, and therefore busulfan is usually regarded as the preferred drug.

NON-FDA APPROVED INDICATIONS

Thioguanine has been tested in studies, and shown to be effective for the treatment of patients with severe psoriasis, in whom other treatment is ineffective or impossible due to side effects. This indication has not been approved by the FDA.

CONTRAINDICATIONS

Thioguanine should not be used in patients whose disease has demonstrated prior resistance to this drug. In animals and humans, there is usually complete cross-resistance between mercaptopurine and thioguanine.

WARNINGS

SINCE DRUGS USED IN CANCER CHEMOTHERAPY ARE POTENTIALLY HAZARDOUS, IT IS RECOMMENDED THAT ONLY PHYSICIANS EXPERIENCED WITH THE RISKS OF THIOGUANINE AND KNOWLEDGEABLE IN THE NATURAL HISTORY OF ACUTE NONLYMPHOCYTIC LEUKEMIAS ADMINISTER THIS DRUG.

The most consistent, dose-related toxicity is bone marrow suppression. This may be manifested by anemia, leukopenia, thrombocytopenia, or any combination of these. Any one of these findings may also reflect progression of the underlying disease. Since thioguanine may have a delayed effect, it is important to withdraw the medication temporarily at the first sign of an abnormally large fall in any of the formed elements of the blood.

There are individuals with an inherited deficiency of the enzyme thiopurine methyltransferase (TPMT) who may be unusually sensitive to the myelosuppressive effects of mercaptopurine and prone to developing rapid bone marrow suppression following the initiation of treatment. This problem could be exacerbated by coadministration with drugs that inhibit TPMT, such as olsalazine, mesalazine, or sulphasalazine.

It is recommended that evaluation of the hemoglobin concentration or hematocrit, total white blood cell count and differential count, and quantitative platelet count be obtained frequently while the patient is on thioguanine therapy. In cases where the cause of fluctuations in the formed elements in the peripheral blood is obscure, bone marrow examination may be useful for the evaluation of marrow status. The decision to increase, decrease, continue, or discontinue a given dosage of thioguanine must be based not only on the absolute hematologic values, but also upon the rapidity with which changes are occurring. In many instances, particularly during the induction phase of acute leukemia, complete blood counts will need to be done more frequently in order to evaluate the effect of the therapy. The dosage of thioguanine may need to be reduced when this agent is combined with other drugs whose primary toxicity is myelosuppression.

Myelosuppression is often unavoidable during the induction phase of adult acute nonlymphocytic leukemias if remission induction is to be successful. Whether or not this demands modification or cessation of dosage depends both upon the response of the underlying disease and a careful consideration of supportive facilities (granulocyte and platelet transfusions) which may be available. Life-threatening infections and bleeding have been observed as consequences of thioguanine-induced granulocytopenia and thrombocytopenia.

The effect of thioguanine on the immunocompetence of patients is unknown.

PREGNANCY CATEGORY D

Drugs such as thioguanine are potential mutagens and teratogens. Thioguanine may cause fetal harm when administered to a pregnant woman. Thioguanine has been shown to be teratogenic in rats when given in doses 5 times the human dose. When given to the rat on the 4th and 5th days of gestation, 13% of surviving placentas did not contain fetuses, and 19% of offspring were malformed or stunted. The malformations noted included generalized edema, cranial defects and general skeletal hypoplasia, hydrocephalus, ventral hernia, situs inversus, and incomplete development of the limbs.[10] There are no adequate and well-controlled studies in pregnant women. If this drug is used during pregnancy, or if the patient becomes pregnant while taking the drug, the patient should be apprised of the potential hazard to the fetus. Women of childbearing potential should be advised to avoid becoming pregnant.

DOSAGE AND ADMINISTRATION

Thioguanine is administered orally. The dosage which will be tolerated and effective varies according to the stage and type of neoplastic process being treated. Because the usual therapies for adult and pediatric acute nonlymphocytic leukemias involve the use of thioguanine with other agents in combination, physicians responsible for administering these therapies should be experienced in the use of cancer chemotherapy and in the chosen protocol.

Ninety-six of 163 (59%) pediatric patients with previously untreated acute nonlymphocytic leukemia obtained complete remission with a multiple-drug protocol including thioguanine, prednisone, cytarabine, cyclophosphamide, and vincristine. Remission was maintained with daily thioguanine, 4 day pulses of cytarabine and cyclophosphamide, and a single dose of vincristine every 28 days. The median duration of remission was 11.5 months.[8]

Fifty-three percent (53%) of previously untreated adults with acute nonlymphocytic leukemias attained remission following use of the combination of thioguanine and cytarabine according to a protocol developed at The Memorial Sloan-Kettering Cancer Center. A median duration of remission of 8.8 months was achieved with the multiple-drug maintenance regimen which included thioguanine.[9]

On those occasions when single-agent chemotherapy with thioguanine may be appropriate, the usual initial dosage for pediatric patients and adults is approximately 2 mg/kg of body weight per day. If, after 4 weeks on this dosage, there is no clinical improvement and no leukocyte or platelet depression, the dosage may be cautiously increased to 3 mg/kg/day. The total daily dose may be given at one time.

The dosage of thioguanine used does not depend on whether or not the patient is receiving allopurinol; **this is in contradistinction to the dosage reduction which is mandatory when mercaptopurine or azathioprine is given simultaneously with allopurinol.**

Procedures for proper handling and disposal of anticancer drugs should be considered. Several guidelines on this subject have been published.[17-23]

There is no general agreement that all of the procedures recommended in the guidelines are necessary or appropriate.

PRODUCT LISTING - EQUIVALENTS NOT AVAILABLE

Tablet - Oral - 40 mg

25's	$126.58	THIOGUANINE, Glaxosmithkline	00173-0880-25

Thiopental Sodium (002340)

For complete prescribing information, refer to the CD-ROM included with the book.

Categories: Anesthesia, general; Anesthesia, induction; Narcoanalysis; Narcosynthesis; Seizures, secondary to anesthesia; Pregnancy Category C; DEA Class CIII; FDA Approved 1959 May; WHO Formulary
Drug Classes: Anesthetics, general; Barbiturates; Sedatives/hypnotics
Brand Names: **Pentothal**
Foreign Brand Availability: Anesthal (India); Hypnostan (Finland); Intraval (Bahamas; Bahrain; Barbados; Belize; Bermuda; Curacao; Cyprus; Egypt; Guyana; Iran; Iraq; Jamaica; Jordan; Kuwait; Lebanon; Libya; Netherland-Antilles; Oman; Qatar; Republic-of-Yemen; Saudi-Arabia; Surinam; Syria; Trinidad; United-Arab-Emirates); Nesdonal (France; Netherlands); Pentothal Sodico (Peru); Pentothal Sodium (Hong-Kong; Indonesia); Sodipental (Colombia; Mexico); Thionyl (Korea); Tiopendal (Bahrain; Cyprus; Egypt; Iran; Iraq; Jordan; Kuwait; Lebanon; Libya; Oman; Qatar; Republic-of-Yemen; Saudi-Arabia; Syria; United-Arab-Emirates); Tiopental Sodico (Colombia; Ecuador); Trapanal (Germany)

DESCRIPTION

WARNING: MAY BE HABIT FORMING.

Thiopental is a thiobarbiturate, the sulfur analogue of sodium pentobarbital.

The drug is prepared as a sterile powder and after reconstitution with an appropriate diluent is administered by the intravenous route.

Thiopental is chemically designated sodium 5-ethyl-5- (1-methylbutyl)-2-thiobarbiturate.

The drug is a yellowish, hygroscopic powder, stabilized with anhydrous sodium carbonate as a buffer (60 mg/g of thiopental sodium).

READY-TO-MIX SYRINGES AND VIALS

(For preparing solutions of thiopental sodium for injection). The following diluents in various container, syringe and vial sizes are provided in Pentothal Kits, Pentothal Ready-to-Mix Syringes and Vials for preparing solutions of thiopental for clinical use:

Sterile water for injection is a sterile, nonpyrogenic preparation of water for injection which contains no bacteriostat, antimicrobial agents or added buffers. The pH is 5.7 (5.0-7.0). Sterile water for injection is a pharmaceutic aid (solvent) for intravenous administration only after addition of a solute.

Water is chemically designated H_2O. 0.9% sodium chloride injection is a sterile, nonpyrogenic, isotonic solution of sodium chloride and water for injection. Each ml contains sodium chloride 9 mg (308 mOsmol/L calc). It contains no bacteriostat, antimicrobial agents or added buffers except for pH adjustment. May contain hydrochloric acid and/or sodium hydroxide for pH adjustment. pH is 5.7 (4.5-7.0). 0.9% sodium chloride injection is an isotonic vehicle for intravenous administration of another solute. Sodium chloride is chemically designated NaCl, a white crystalline compound freely soluble in water. The semi-rigid vial contained in List Nos. 3329, 6418, 6419, 6420 and 6435 is fabricated from a specially formulated polyolefin. It is a copolymer of ethylene and propylene. The safety of the plastic has been confirmed by tests in animals according to biological standards for plastic containers. The container requires no vapor barrier to maintain the proper labeled volume.

INDICATIONS AND USAGE

Thiopental is indicated (1) as the sole anesthetic agent for brief (15 minute) procedures, (2) for induction of anesthesia prior to administration of other anesthetic agents, (3) to supplement regional anesthesia, (4) to provide hypnosis during balanced anesthesia with other agents for analgesia or muscle relaxation, (5) for the control of convulsive states during or following inhalation anesthesia, local anesthesia, or other causes, (6) in neurosurgical patients with increased intracranial pressure, if adequate ventilation is provided, and (7) for narcoanalysis and narcosynthesis in psychiatric disorders.

CONTRAINDICATIONS

Absolute Contraindications:

- Absence of suitable veins for intravenous administration
- Hypersensitivity (allergy) to barbiturates
- Variegate porphyria (South African) or acute intermittent porphyria

Relative Contraindications:

- Severe cardiovascular disease
- Hypotension or shock
- Conditions in which the hypnotic effect may be prolonged or potentiated—excessive premedication, Addison's disease, hepatic or renal dysfunction, myxedema, increased blood urea, severe anemia, asthma, myasthenia gravis
- Status asthmaticus.

Diluents in Pentothal Kits, Ready-to-Mix Syringes or Vials should not be used for fluid or sodium chloride replacement.

WARNINGS

KEEP RESUSCITATIVE AND ENDOTRACHEAL INTUBATION EQUIPMENT AND OXYGEN READILY AVAILABLE. MAINTAIN PATENCY of THE AIRWAY AT ALL TIMES.

THIS DRUG SHOULD BE ADMINISTERED ONLY BY PERSONS QUALIFIED IN THE USE of INTRAVENOUS ANESTHETICS.

Avoid extravasation or intra-arterial injection. WARNING: MAY BE HABIT FORMING.

Intravenous administration of sterile water for injection without a solute may result in hemolysis.

Use aseptic technique for preparing thiopental solutions when using Pentothal Kits, Syringes or Vials and during withdrawal from reconstituted single or multiple-use containers.

Administer only clear reconstituted solutions. Use within 24 hours after reconstitution. Discard unused portions.

T

DOSAGE AND ADMINISTRATION

Thiopental is administered by the intravenous route only. Individual response to the drug is so varied that there can be no fixed dosage. The drug should be titrated against patient requirements as governed by age, sex and body weight. Younger patients require relatively larger doses than middle-aged and elderly persons; the latter metabolize the drug more slowly. Pre-puberty requirements are the same for both sexes, but adult females require less than adult males. Dose is usually proportional to body weight and obese patients require a larger dose than relatively lean persons of the same weight.

PREMEDICATION

Premedication usually consists of atropine or scopolamine to suppress vagal reflexes and inhibit secretions. in addition, a barbiturate or an opiate is often given. Sodium pentobarbital injection (Nembutal) is suggested because it provides a preliminary indication of how the patient will react to barbiturate anesthesia.

Ideally, the peak effect of these medications should be reached shortly before the time of induction.

TEST DOSE

It is advisable to inject a small "test" dose of 25-75 mg (1-3 mL of a 2.5% solution) of thiopental to assess tolerance or unusual sensitivity to thiopental, and pausing to observe patient reaction for at least 60 seconds. If unexpectedly deep anesthesia develops or if respiratory depression occurs, consider these possibilities: (1) the patient may be unusually sensitive to thiopental, (2) the solution may be more concentrated than had been assumed, or (3) the patient may have received too much premedication.

USE IN ANESTHESIA

Moderately slow induction can usually be accomplished in the "average" adult by injection of 50-75 mg (2-3 mL of a 2.5% solution) at intervals of 20-40 seconds, depending on the reaction of the patient. Once anesthesia is established, additional injections of 25-50 mg can be given whenever the patient moves. Slow injection is recommended to minimize respiratory depression and the possibility of overdosage. The smallest dose consistent with attaining the surgical objective is the desired goal. Momentary apnea following each injection is typical, and progressive decrease in the amplitude of respiration appears with increasing dosage. Pulse remains normal or increases slightly and returns to normal. Blood pressure usually falls slightly but returns toward normal.

Muscles usually relax about 30 seconds after unconsciousness is attained, but this may be masked if a skeletal muscle relaxant is used. The tone of jaw muscles is a fairly reliable index.

The pupils may dilate but later contract; sensitivity to light is not usually lost until a level of anesthesia deep enough to permit surgery is attained. Nystagmus and divergent strabismus are characteristic during early stages, but at the level of surgical anesthesia, the eyes are central and fixed. Corneal and conjunctival reflexes disappear during surgical anesthesia.

When thiopental is used for induction in balanced anesthesia with a skeletal muscle relaxant and an inhalation agent, the total dose of thiopental can be estimated and then injected in 2-4 fractional doses. With this technique, brief periods of apnea may occur which may require assisted or controlled pulmonary ventilation. As an initial dose, 210-280 mg (3-4 mg/kg) of thiopental is usually required for rapid induction in the average adult (70 kg). When thiopental is used as the sole anesthetic agent, the desired level of anesthesia can be maintained by injection of small repeated doses as needed or by using a continuous intravenous drip in a 0.2% or 0.4% concentration. (Sterile water should not be used as the diluent in these concentrations, since hemolysis will occur.) With continuous drip, the depth of anesthesia is controlled by adjusting the rate of infusion.

USE IN CONVULSIVE STATES

For the control of convulsive states following anesthesia (inhalation or local) or other causes, 75-125 mg (3-5 ml of a 2.5% solution) should be given as soon as possible after the convulsion begins. Convulsions following the use of a local anesthetic may require 125-250 mg of thiopental given over a 10 minute period. If the convulsion is caused by a local anesthetic, the required dose of thiopental will depend upon the amount of local anesthetic given and its convulsant properties.

USE IN NEUROSURGICAL PATIENTS WITH INCREASED INTRACRANIAL PRESSURE

In neurosurgical patients, intermittent bolus injections of 1.5-3.5 mg/kg of body weight may be given to reduce intraoperative elevations of intracranial pressure, if adequate ventilation is provided.

USE IN PSYCHIATRIC DISORDERS

For narcoanalysis and narcosynthesis in psychiatric disorders, premedication with an anticholinergic agent may precede administration of thiopental. After a test dose, thiopental is injected at a slow rate of 100 mg/min (4 ml/min of a 2.5% solution) with the patient counting backwards from 100. Shortly after counting becomes confused but before actual sleep is produced, the injection is discontinued. Allow the patient to return to a semidrowsy state where conversation is coherent. Alternatively, thiopental may be administered by rapid IV drip using a 0.2% concentration in 5% dextrose and water. At this concentration, the rate of administration should not exceed 50 ml/min.

MANAGEMENT OF SOME COMPLICATIONS

Respiratory Depression (hypoventilation, apnea), which may result from either unusual responsiveness to thiopental or overdosage, is managed as stated above. Thiopental should be considered to have the same potential for producing respiratory depression as an inhalation agent, and patency of the airway must be protected at all times.

Laryngospasm may occur with light thiopental narcosis at intubation, or in the absence of intubation if foreign matter or secretions in the respiratory tract create irritation. Laryngeal and bronchial vagal reflexes can be suppressed, and secretions minimized by giving atropine or scopolamine premedication and a barbiturate or opiate. Use of a skeletal muscle relaxant or positive pressure oxygen will usually relieve laryngospasm. Tracheostomy may be indicated in difficult cases.

Myocardial depression, proportional to the amount of drug in direct contact with the heart, can occur and may cause hypotension, particularly in patients with an unhealthy myocardium.

Arrhythmias may appear if PCO2 is elevated, but they are uncommon with adequate ventilation.

Management of myocardial depression is the same as for overdosage. Thiopental does not sensitize the heart to epinephrine or other sympathomimetic amines.

Extravascular Infiltration should be avoided. Care should be taken to insure that the needle is within the lumen of the vein before injection of thiopental. Extravascular injection may cause chemical irritation of the tissues varying from slight tenderness to venospasm, extensive necrosis and sloughing. This is due primarily to the high alkaline pH (10-11) of clinical concentrations of the drug. If extravasation occurs, the local irritant effects can be reduced by injection of 1% procaine locally to relieve pain and enhance vasodilatation. Local application of heat also may help to increase local circulation and removal of the infiltrate.

Intra-arterial injection can occur inadvertently, especially if an aberrant superficial artery is present at the medial aspect of the antecubital fossa. The area selected for intravenous injection of the drug should be palpated for detection of an underlying pulsating vessel. Accidental intra-arterial injection can cause arteriospasm and severe pain along the course of the artery with blanching of the arm and fingers.

Appropriate corrective measures should be instituted promptly to avoid possible development of gangrene. Any patient complaint of pain warrants stopping the injection. Methods suggested for dealing with this complication vary with the severity of symptoms. The following have been suggested:

1. Dilute the injected thiopental by removing the tourniquet and any restrictive garments.
2. Leave the needle in place, if possible.
3. Inject the artery with a dilute solution of papaverine, 40-80 mg, or 10 mL of 1% procaine, to inhibit smooth muscle spasm.
4. If necessary, perform sympathetic block of the brachial plexus and/or stellate ganglion to relieve pain and assist in opening collateral circulation. Papaverine can be injected into the subclavian artery, if desired.
5. Unless otherwise contraindicated, institute immediate heparinization to prevent thrombus formation.
6. Consider local infiltration of an alpha-adrenergic blocking agent such as phentolamine into the vasospastic area.
7. Provide additional symptomatic treatment as required. Shivering after thiopental anesthesia, manifested by twitching face muscles and occasional progression to tremors of the arms, head, shoulder and body, is a thermal reaction due to increased sensitivity to cold. Shivering appears if the room environment is cold and if a large ventilatory heat loss has been sustained with balanced inhalation anesthesia employing nitrous oxide. Treatment consists of warming the patient with blankets, maintaining room temperature near 22°C (72°F), and administration of chlorpromazine or methylphenidate.

WARNING

The 2.5 g and larger sizes contain adequate medication for several patients.

COMPATIBILITY

Any solution of thiopental with a visible precipitate should not be administered. The stability of thiopental solutions depends upon several factors, including the diluent, temperature of storage and the amount of carbon dioxide from room air that gains access to the solution. Any factor or condition which tends to lower pH (increase acidity) of thiopental solutions will increase the likelihood of precipitation of thiopental acid. Such factors include the use of diluents which are too acidic and the absorption of carbon dioxide which can combine with water to form carbonic acid.

Solutions of succinylcholine, tubocurarine or other drugs which have an acid pH should not be mixed with thiopental solutions. The most stable solutions are those reconstituted in water or isotonic saline, kept under refrigeration and tightly stoppered. The presence or absence of a visible precipitate offers a practical guide to the physical compatibility of prepared solutions of thiopental.

TABLE 2 *Calculations For Various Concentrations*

Concentration Desired		Amounts to Use: Thiopental	Dilutent
0.2%	2 mg/ml	1 g	500 ml
0.4%	4 mg/ml	1 g	250 ml
		2 g	500 ml
2.0%	20 mg/ml	5 g	250 ml
		10 g	500 ml
2.5%	25 mg/ml	1 g	40 ml
		5 g	200 ml
5%	50 mg/ml	1 g	20 ml
		5 g	100 ml

Reconstituted solutions of thiopental should be inspected visually for particulate matter and discoloration, whenever solution and container permit. Thiopental solutions should be administered only by intravenous injection and by individuals experienced in the conduct of intravenous anesthesia.

The volume and choice of diluent for preparing thiopental solutions for clinical use depends on the concentration and vehicle desired. Thiopental Kits provide only sterile water for injection as the diluent for individual or multi-patient use; Thiopental Ready-to-Mix Syringes provide only 0.9% sodium chloride injection as the diluent for individual patient use; vials provide only sterile water for injection as the diluent for individual patient use.

Parenteral drug products should be inspected visually for particulate matter and discoloration prior to administration, whenever solution and container permit.

PRODUCT LISTING - EQUIVALENTS NOT AVAILABLE

Size	Price	Product	NDC
Powder For Injection - Intravenous - 1 Gm			
1's	$17.50	GENERIC, Baxter Pharmaceutical Products, Inc	10019-0253-99
1's	$17.75	GENERIC, Gensia Sicor Pharmaceuticals Inc	00703-2530-01
25's	$139.23	PENTOTHAL, Abbott Pharmaceutical	00074-6431-02
25's	$268.75	PENTOTHAL, Abbott Pharmaceutical	00074-6244-01
25's	$326.86	PENTOTHAL, Abbott Pharmaceutical	00074-6435-01
Powder For Injection - Intravenous - 2.5 Gm			
1's	$10.80	GENERIC, Baxter Pharmaceutical Products, Inc	10019-0252-97
1's	$23.13	GENERIC, Gensia Sicor Pharmaceuticals Inc	00703-2540-01
25's	$693.80	PENTOTHAL, Abbott Pharmaceutical	00074-6260-01
Powder For Injection - Intravenous - 5 Gm			
1's	$33.36	GENERIC, Gensia Sicor Pharmaceuticals Inc	00703-2550-01
1's	$33.75	GENERIC, Baxter Pharmaceutical Products, Inc	10019-0255-98
25's	$1007.59	PENTOTHAL, Abbott Pharmaceutical	00074-6108-01
25's	$1053.31	PENTOTHAL, Abbott Pharmaceutical	00074-6504-01
Powder For Injection - Intravenous - 250 mg			
25's	$128.84	PENTOTHAL, Abbott Pharmaceutical	00074-6418-01
25's	$135.97	PENTOTHAL, Abbott Pharmaceutical	00074-3351-01
25's	$228.60	PENTOTHAL, Abbott Pharmaceutical	00074-6241-03
Powder For Injection - Intravenous - 400 mg			
25's	$141.61	PENTOTHAL, Abbott Pharmaceutical	00074-6419-01
25's	$193.86	PENTOTHAL, Abbott Pharmaceutical	00074-3352-01
25's	$282.30	PENTOTHAL, Abbott Pharmaceutical	00074-6246-03
Powder For Injection - Intravenous - 500 mg			
1's	$8.10	GENERIC, Gensia Sicor Pharmaceuticals Inc	00703-2580-01
1's	$8.13	GENERIC, Baxter Pharmaceutical Products, Inc	10019-0258-96
25's	$148.73	PENTOTHAL, Abbott Pharmaceutical	00074-6420-01
25's	$199.80	PENTOTHAL, Abbott Pharmaceutical	00074-3329-01
25's	$222.66	PENTOTHAL, Abbott Pharmaceutical	00074-3353-01
25's	$318.30	PENTOTHAL, Abbott Pharmaceutical	00074-6243-01
Suspension - Rectal - 400 mg/Gm			
1 ml	$37.50	PENTOTHAL, Abbott Pharmaceutical	00074-7236-04

Thioridazine Hydrochloride *(002341)*

Categories: Behavior disorder; Depression; Psychosis; FDA Approved 1961 Jan; Pregnancy Category C
Drug Classes: Antipsychotics; Phenothiazines
Brand Names: **Mellaril**; Mellaril-S
Foreign Brand Availability: Aldazine (Australia; Malaysia; New-Zealand); Calmaril (Thailand); Mallorol (Sweden); Meleril (Argentina; Colombia; Peru; Spain); Melleretten (Austria; Germany; Italy; Netherlands; Switzerland); Melleril (Austria; Bahrain; Belgium; Benin; Bulgaria; Burkina-Faso; Cyprus; Czech-Republic; Denmark; Egypt; England; Ethiopia; Finland; France; Gambia; Germany; Ghana; Greece; Guinea; Hong-Kong; Hungary; Indonesia; Iran; Iraq; Ireland; Israel; Italy; Ivory-Coast; Japan; Jordan; Kenya; Kuwait; Lebanon; Liberia; Libya; Malawi; Mali; Mauritania; Mauritius; Mexico; Morocco; Netherlands; New-Zealand; Niger; Nigeria; Norway; Oman; Philippines; Portugal; Qatar; Republic-of-Yemen; Saudi-Arabia; Senegal; Seychelles; Sierra-Leone; Slovenia; South-Africa; Spain; Sudan; Switzerland; Syria; Taiwan; Tanzania; Tunia; Turkey; Uganda; United-Arab-Emirates; Zambia; Zimbabwe); Mellerzin (Taiwan); Mepiozin (Japan); Orsanil (Finland); Ridazin (Israel); Ridazine (Thailand); Thiomed (Thailand); Thioril (India); Thiosia (Thailand)
Cost of Therapy: $54.00 (Schizophrenia; Mellaril; 100 mg; 2 tablets/day; 30 day supply)
$8.70 (Schizophrenia; Generic Tablets; 100 mg; 2 tablets/day; 30 day supply)
$8.55 (Depression; Generic Tablets; 25 mg; 3 tablets/day; 30 day supply)

WARNING

THIORIDAZINE HCl HAS BEEN SHOWN TO PROLONG THE QTc INTERVAL IN A DOSE-RELATED MANNER, AND DRUGS WITH THIS POTENTIAL HAVE BEEN ASSOCIATED WITH TORSADES DE POINTES-TYPE ARRHYTHMIAS AND SUDDEN DEATH. DUE TO ITS POTENTIAL FOR SIGNIFICANT, POSSIBLY LIFE-THREATENING, PROARRHYTHMIC EFFECTS, THIORIDAZINE HCl SHOULD BE RESERVED FOR USE IN THE TREATMENT OF SCHIZOPHRENIC PATIENTS WHO FAIL TO SHOW AN ACCEPTABLE RESPONSE TO ADEQUATE COURSES OF TREATMENT WITH OTHER ANTIPSYCHOTIC DRUGS, EITHER BECAUSE OF INSUFFICIENT EFFECTIVENESS OR THE INABILITY TO ACHIEVE AN EFFECTIVE DOSE DUE TO INTOLERABLE ADVERSE EFFECTS FROM THOSE DRUGS. (SEE WARNINGS, CONTRAINDICATIONS, AND INDICATIONS AND USAGE).

DESCRIPTION

Thioridazine HCl is 2-methylmercapto-10-[2-(N-methyl-2-piperidyl)ethyl] phenothiazine.

MELLARIL TABLETS

The active ingredient is thioridazine HCl.

Inactive Ingredients:

10 mg: Acacia, calcium sulfate dihydrate, carnauba wax, D&C yellow no. 10, FD&C blue no. 1, FD&C yellow no. 6, gelatin, lactose, methylparaben, povidone, propylparaben, sodium benzoate, starch, stearic acid, sucrose, synthetic black iron oxide, talc, titanium dioxide, and other ingredients.

15 mg: Acacia, calcium sulfate dihydrate, carnauba wax, D&C red no. 7, gelatin, lactose, methylparaben, povidone, propylparaben, starch, stearic acid, sucrose, synthetic black iron oxide, talc, titanium dioxide, and other ingredients.

25 mg: Acacia, calcium sulfate dihydrate, carnauba wax, gelatin, lactose, methylparaben, povidone, propylparaben, sodium benzoate, starch, stearic acid, sucrose, synthetic black iron oxide, synthetic iron oxide, talc, titanium dioxide, and other ingredients.

50 mg: Acacia, calcium sulfate dihydrate, carnauba wax, gelatin, lactose, sodium benzoate, starch, stearic acid, sucrose, synthetic black iron oxide, talc, titanium dioxide, and other ingredients.

100 mg: Acacia, calcium sulfate dihydrate, carnauba wax, D&C yellow no. 10, FD&C blue no. 1, FD&C blue no. 2, FD&C yellow no. 6, lactose, methylparaben, povidone, propylparaben, sodium benzoate, sorbitol, starch, stearic acid, sucrose, synthetic black iron oxide, talc, titanium dioxide, and other ingredients.

150 mg: Acacia, calcium sulfate dihydrate, carnauba wax, D&C yellow no. 10, FD&C green no. 3, FD&C yellow no. 6, lactose, methylparaben, povidone, propylparaben, sodium benzoate, starch, stearic acid, sucrose, synthetic black iron oxide, talc, titanium dioxide, and other ingredients.

200 mg: Acacia, ammonium calcium alginate, calcium sulfate dihydrate, carnauba wax, colloidal silicon dioxide, D&C red no. 7, lactose, magnesium stearate, methylparaben, povidone, propylparaben, sodium benzoate, starch, stearic acid, sucrose, synthetic black iron oxide, talc, titanium dioxide, and other ingredients.

MELLARIL ORAL SOLUTION (CONCENTRATE)

The active ingredient is thioridazine HCl.

Inactive Ingredients:

30 mg/ml: Alcohol, 3.0%, flavor, methylparaben, propylparaben, purified water, and sorbitol solution. May contain sodium hydroxide or hydrochloric acid to adjust the pH.

100 mg/ml: Alcohol, 4.2%, flavor, glycerin, methylparaben, propylparaben, purified water, sorbitol solution, and sucrose. May contain sodium hydroxide or hydrochloric acid to adjust pH.

MELLARIL ORAL SUSPENSION

Each ml contains thioridazine, equivalent to 5 and 20 mg thioridazine HCl, respectively, as the active ingredient.

Inactive Ingredients:

5 mg/ml: Carbomer 934, flavor, polysorbate 80, purified water, sodium hydroxide, and sucrose.

20 mg/ml: Carbomer 934, D&C yellow no. 10, FD&C yellow no. 6, flavor, polysorbate 80, purified water, sodium hydroxide, and sucrose.

CLINICAL PHARMACOLOGY

The basic pharmacological activity of thioridazine HCl is similar to that of other phenothiazines, but is associated with minimal extrapyramidal stimulation.

However, thioridazine has been shown to prolong the QTc interval in a dose-dependent fashion. This effect may increase the risk of serious, potentially fatal, ventricular arrhythmias, such as torsades de pointes-type arrhythmias. Due to this risk, thioridazine HCl is indicated only for schizophrenic patients who have not been responsive to or cannot tolerate other antipsychotic agents (see WARNINGS and CONTRAINDICATIONS). However, the prescriber should be aware that thioridazine HCl has not been systematically evaluated in controlled trials in treatment refractory schizophrenic patients and its efficacy in such patients is unknown.

INDICATIONS AND USAGE

Thioridazine HCl is indicated for the management of schizophrenic patients who fail to respond adequately to treatment with other antipsychotic drugs. Due to the risk of significant, potentially life-threatening, proarrhythmic effects with thioridazine HCl treatment, thioridazine HCl should be used only in patients who have failed to respond adequately to treatment with appropriate courses of other antipsychotic drugs, either because of insufficient effectiveness or the inability to achieve an effective dose due to intolerable adverse effects from those drugs. Consequently, before initiating treatment with thioridazine HCl, it is strongly recommended that a patient be given at least 2 trials, each with a different antipsychotic drug product, at an adequate dose, and for an adequate duration (see WARNINGS and CONTRAINDICATIONS).

However, the prescriber should be aware that thioridazine HCl has not been systematically evaluated in controlled trials in treatment refractory schizophrenic patients and its efficacy in such patients is unknown.

CONTRAINDICATIONS

Thioridazine HCl use should be avoided in combination with other drugs that are known to prolong the QTc interval and in patients with congenital long QT syndrome or a history of cardiac arrhythmias.

Reduced cytochrome P450 2D6 isozyme activity drugs that inhibit this isozyme (*e.g.*, fluoxetine and paroxetine) and certain other drugs (*e.g.*, fluvoxamine, propranolol, and pindolol) appear to appreciably inhibit the metabolism of thioridazine. The resulting elevated levels of thioridazine would be expected to augment the prolongation of the QTc interval associated with thioridazine HCl and may increase the risk of serious, potentially fatal, cardiac arrhythmias, such as torsades de pointes-type arrhythmias. Such an increased risk may result also from the additive effect of coadministering thioridazine HCl with other agents that prolong the QTc interval. Therefore, thioridazine HCl is contraindicated with these drugs as well as in patients, comprising about 7% of the normal population, who are known to have a genetic defect leading to reduced levels of activity of P450 2D6 (see WARNINGS and PRECAUTIONS).

In common with other phenothiazines, thioridazine HCl is contraindicated in severe central nervous system depression or comatose states from any cause including drug induced central nervous system depression (see WARNINGS). It should also be noted that hypertensive or hypotensive heart disease of extreme degree is a contraindication of phenothiazine administration.

T

WARNINGS

POTENTIAL FOR PROARRHYTHMIC EFFECTS

DUE TO THE POTENTIAL FOR SIGNIFICANT, POSSIBLY LIFE-THREATENING, PROARRHYTHMIC EFFECTS WITH THIORIDAZINE HCl TREATMENT, THIORIDAZINE HCl SHOULD BE RESERVED FOR USE IN THE TREATMENT OF SCHIZOPHRENIC PATIENTS WHO FAIL TO SHOW AN ACCEPTABLE RESPONSE TO ADEQUATE COURSES OF TREATMENT WITH OTHER ANTIPSYCHOTIC DRUGS, EITHER BECAUSE OF INSUFFICIENT EFFECTIVENESS OR THE INABILITY TO ACHIEVE AN EFFECTIVE DOSE DUE TO INTOLERABLE ADVERSE EFFECTS FROM THOSE DRUGS. CONSEQUENTLY, BEFORE INITIATING TREATMENT WITH THIORIDAZINE HCl, IT IS STRONGLY RECOMMENDED THAT A PATIENT BE GIVEN AT LEAST TWO TRIALS, EACH WITH A DIFFERENT ANTIPSYCHOTIC DRUG PRODUCT, AT AN ADEQUATE DOSE, AND FOR AN ADEQUATE DURATION. THIORIDAZINE HCl HAS NOT BEEN SYSTEMATICALLY EVALUATED IN CONTROLLED TRIALS IN THE TREATMENT OF REFRACTORY SCHIZOPHRENIC PATIENTS AND ITS EFFICACY IN SUCH PATIENTS IS UNKNOWN.

A crossover study in 9 healthy males comparing single doses of thioridazine 10 and 50 mg with placebo demonstrated a dose-related prolongation of the QTc interval. The mean maximum increase in QTc interval following the 50 mg dose was about 23 milliseconds; greater prolongation may be observed in the clinical treatment of unscreened patients.

Prolongation of the QTc interval has been associated with the ability to cause torsades de pointes-type arrhythmias, a potentially fatal polymorphic ventricular tachycardia, and sudden death. There are several published case reports of torsades de pointes and sudden death associated with thioridazine treatment. A causal relationship between these events and thioridazine HCl therapy has not been established but, given the ability of thioridazine HCl to prolong the QTc interval, such a relationship is possible.

Certain circumstances may increase the risk of torsades de pointes and/or sudden death in association with the use of drugs that prolong the QTc interval, including (1) bradycardia; (2) hypokalemia; (3) concomitant use of other drugs that prolong the QTc interval; (4) presence of congenital prolongation of the QT interval; and (5) for thioridazine in particular, its use in patients with reduced activity of P450 2D6 or its coadministration with drugs that may inhibit P450 2D6 or by some other mechanism interfere with the clearance of thioridazine (see CONTRAINDICATIONS and PRECAUTIONS).

It is recommended that patients being considered for thioridazine HCl treatment have a baseline ECG performed and serum potassium levels measured. Serum potassium should be normalized before initiating treatment and patients with a QTc interval greater than 450 milliseconds should not receive thioridazine HCl treatment. It may also be useful to periodically monitor ECG's and serum potassium during thioridazine HCl treatment, especially during a period of dose adjustment. Thioridazine HCl should be discontinued in patients who are found to have a QTc interval over 500 milliseconds.

Patients taking thioridazine HCl who experience symptoms that may be associated with the occurrence of torsades de pointes (*e.g.,* dizziness, palpitations, or syncope) may warrant further cardiac evaluation; in particular, Holter monitoring should be considered.

TARDIVE DYSKINESIA

Tardive dyskinesia, a syndrome consisting of potentially irreversible, involuntary, dyskinetic movements may develop in patients treated with antipsychotic drugs. Although the prevalence of the syndrome appears to be highest among the elderly, especially elderly women, it is impossible to rely upon prevalence estimates to predict, at the inception of antipsychotic treatment, which patients are likely to develop the syndrome. Whether antipsychotic drug products differ in their potential to cause tardive dyskinesia is unknown.

Both the risk of developing the syndrome and the likelihood that it will become irreversible are believed to increase as the duration of treatment and the total cumulative dose of antipsychotic drugs administered to the patient increase. However, the syndrome can develop, although much less commonly, after relatively brief treatment periods at low doses.

There is no known treatment for established cases of tardive dyskinesia, although the syndrome may remit, partially or completely, if antipsychotic treatment is withdrawn. Antipsychotic treatment itself, however, may suppress (or partially suppress) the signs and symptoms of the syndrome and thereby may possibly mask the underlying disease process. The effect that symptomatic suppression has upon the long-term course of the syndrome is unknown.

Given these considerations, antipsychotics should be prescribed in a manner that is most likely to minimize the occurrence of tardive dyskinesia. Chronic antipsychotic treatment should generally be reserved for patients who suffer from a chronic illness that, (1) is known to respond to antipsychotic drugs; and, (2) for whom alternative, equally effective, but potentially less harmful treatments are *not* available or appropriate. In patients who do require chronic treatment, the smallest dose and the shortest duration of treatment producing a satisfactory clinical response should be sought. The need for continued treatment should be reassessed periodically.

If signs and symptoms of tardive dyskinesia appear in a patient on antipsychotics, drug discontinuation should be considered. However, some patients may require treatment despite the presence of the syndrome.

(For further information about the description of tardive dyskinesia and its clinical detection, please refer to PRECAUTIONS, Information for the Patient and ADVERSE REACTIONS.)

It has been suggested in regard to phenothiazines in general, that people who have demonstrated a hypersensitivity reaction (*e.g.,* blood dyscrasias, jaundice) to one may be more prone to demonstrate a reaction to others. Attention should be paid to the fact that phenothiazines are capable of potentiating central nervous system depressants (*e.g.,* anesthetics, opiates, alcohol, etc.) as well as atropine and phosphorus insecticides. Physicians should carefully consider benefit versus risk when treating less severe disorders.

Reproductive studies in animals and clinical experience to date have failed to show a teratogenic effect with thioridazine HCl. However, in view of the desirability of keeping the administration of all drugs to a minimum during pregnancy, thioridazine HCl should be given only when the benefits derived from treatment exceed the possible risks to mother and fetus.

NEUROLEPTIC MALIGNANT SYNDROME (NMS)

A potentially fatal symptom complex sometimes referred to as Neuroleptic Malignant Syndrome (NMS) has been reported in association with antipsychotic drugs. Clinical manifestations of NMS are hyperpyrexia, muscle rigidity, altered mental status, and evidence of autonomic instability (irregular pulse or blood pressure, tachycardia, diaphoresis, and cardiac dysrhythmias).

The diagnostic evaluation of patients with this syndrome is complicated. In arriving at a diagnosis, it is important to identify cases where the clinical presentation includes both serious medical illness (*e.g.,* pneumonia, systemic infection, etc.) and untreated or inadequately treated extrapyramidal signs and symptoms (EPS). Other important considerations in the differential diagnosis include central anticholinergic toxicity, heat stroke, drug fever, and primary central nervous system (CNS) pathology.

The management of NMS should include, (1) immediate discontinuation of antipsychotic drugs and other drugs not essential to concurrent therapy; (2) intensive symptomatic treatment and medical monitoring; and (3) treatment of any concomitant serious medical problems for which specific treatments are available. There is no general agreement about specific pharmacological treatment regimens for uncomplicated NMS.

If a patient requires antipsychotic drug treatment after recovery from NMS, the potential reintroduction of drug therapy should be carefully considered. The patient should be carefully monitored, since recurrences of NMS have been reported.

CENTRAL NERVOUS SYSTEM DEPRESSANTS

As in the case of other phenothiazines, thioridazine HCl is capable of potentiating central nervous system depressants (*e.g.,* alcohol, anesthetics, barbiturates, narcotics, opiates, other psychoactive drugs, etc.) as well as atropine and phosphorus insecticides. Severe respiratory depression and respiratory arrest have been reported when a patient was given a phenothiazine and a concomitant high dose of a barbiturate.

PRECAUTIONS

Leukopenia and/or agranulocytosis and convulsive seizures have been reported but are infrequent. In schizophrenic patients with epilepsy, anticonvulsant medication should be maintained during treatment with thioridazine HCl. Pigmentary retinopathy, which has been observed primarily in patients taking larger than recommended doses, is characterized by diminution of visual acuity, brownish coloring of vision, and impairment of night vision; examination of the fundus discloses deposits of pigment. The possibility of this complication may be reduced by remaining within the recommended limits of dosage.

Where patients are participating in activities requiring complete mental alertness (*e.g.,* driving) it is advisable to administer the phenothiazines cautiously and to increase the dosage gradually. Female patients appear to have a greater tendency to orthostatic hypotension than male patients. The administration of epinephrine should be avoided in the treatment of drug-induced hypotension in view of the fact that phenothiazines may induce a reversed epinephrine effect on occasion. Should a vasoconstrictor be required, the most suitable are levarterenol and phenylephrine.

Antipsychotic drugs elevate prolactin levels; the elevation persists during chronic administration. Tissue culture experiments indicate that approximately one-third of human breast cancers are prolactin dependent *in vitro,* a factor of potential importance if the prescription of these drugs is contemplated in a patient with a previously detected breast cancer. Although disturbances such as galactorrhea, amenorrhea, gynecomastia, and impotence have been reported, the clinical significance of elevated serum prolactin levels is unknown for most patients. An increase in mammary neoplasms has been found in rodents after chronic administration of antipsychotic drugs. Neither clinical studies nor epidemiologic studies conducted to date, however, have shown an association between chronic administration of these drugs and mammary tumorigenesis; the available evidence is considered too limited to be conclusive at this time.

INFORMATION FOR THE PATIENT

Patients should be informed that thioridazine HCl has been associated with potentially fatal heart rhythm disturbances. The risk of such events may be increased when certain drugs are given together with thioridazine HCl. Therefore, patients should inform the prescriber that they are receiving thioridazine HCl treatment before taking any new medication.

Given the likelihood that some patients exposed chronically to antipsychotics will develop tardive dyskinesia, it is advised that all patients in whom chronic use is contemplated be given, if possible, full information about this risk. The decision to inform patients and/or their guardians must obviously take into account the clinical circumstances and the competency of the patient to understand the information provided.

PEDIATRIC USE

See DOSAGE AND ADMINISTRATION, Pediatric Patients.

DRUG INTERACTIONS

Reduced cytochrome P450 2D6 isozyme activity, drugs which inhibit this isozyme (*e.g.,* fluoxetine and paroxetine), and certain other drugs (*e.g.,* fluvoxamine, propranolol, and pindolol) appear to appreciably inhibit the metabolism of thioridazine. The resulting elevated levels of thioridazine would be expected to augment the prolongation of the QTc interval associated with thioridazine HCl and may increase the risk of serious, potentially fatal, cardiac arrhythmias, such as torsades de pointes-type arrhythmias. Such an increased risk may result also from the additive effect of coadministering thioridazine HCl with other agents that prolong the QTc interval. Therefore, thioridazine HCl is contraindicated with these drugs as well as in patients, comprising about 7% of the normal population, who are known to have a genetic defect leading to reduced levels of activity of P450 2D6 (see WARNINGS and CONTRAINDICATIONS).

DRUGS THAT INHIBIT CYTOCHROME P450 2D6

In a study of 19 healthy male subjects, which included 6 slow and 13 rapid hydroxylators of debrisoquin, a single 25 mg oral dose of thioridazine produced a 2.4-fold higher C_{max} and a 4.5-fold higher AUC for thioridazine in the slow hydroxylators compared to rapid hydroxylators. The rate of debrisoquin hydroxylation is felt to depend on the level of cytochrome P450 2D6 isozyme activity. Thus, this study suggests that drugs that inhibit P450

2D6 or the presence of reduced activity levels of this isozyme will produce elevated plasma levels of thioridazine. Therefore, the coadministration of drugs that inhibit P450 2D6 with thioridazine HCl and the use of thioridazine HCl in patients known to have reduced activity of P450 2D6 are contraindicated.

DRUGS THAT REDUCE THE CLEARANCE OF THIORIDAZINE HCl THROUGH OTHER MECHANISMS

Fluvoxamine

The effect of fluvoxamine (25 mg bid for 1 week) on thioridazine steady state concentration was evaluated in 10 male in-patients with schizophrenia. Concentrations of thioridazine and its two active metabolites, mesoridazine and sulforidazine, increased 3-fold following coadministration of fluvoxamine. Fluvoxamine and thioridazine HCl should not be coadministered.

Propranolol

Concurrent administration of propranolol (100-800 mg daily) has been reported to produce increases in plasma levels of thioridazine (approximately 50-400%) and its metabolites (approximately 80-300%). Propranolol and thioridazine HCl should not be coadministered.

Pindolol

Concurrent administration of pindolol and thioridazine have resulted in moderate, dose-related increases in the serum levels of thioridazine and two of its metabolites, as well as higher than expected serum pindolol levels. Pindolol and thioridazine HCl should not be coadministered.

DRUGS THAT PROLONG THE QTC INTERVAL

There are no studies of the coadministration of thioridazine HCl and other drugs that prolong the QTc interval. However, it is expected that such coadministration would produce additive prolongation of the QTc interval and, thus, such use is contraindicated.

ADVERSE REACTIONS

In the recommended dosage ranges with thioridazine HCl most side effects are mild and transient.

Central Nervous System: Drowsiness may be encountered on occasion, especially where large doses are given early in treatment. Generally, this effect tends to subside with continued therapy or a reduction in dosage. Pseudoparkinsonism and other extrapyramidal symptoms may occur but are infrequent. Nocturnal confusion, hyperactivity, lethargy, psychotic reactions, restlessness, and headache have been reported but are extremely rare.

Autonomic Nervous System: Dryness of mouth, blurred vision, constipation, nausea, vomiting, diarrhea, nasal stuffiness, and pallor have been seen.

Endocrine System: Galactorrhea, breast engorgement, amenorrhea, inhibition of ejaculation, and peripheral edema have been described.

Skin: Dermatitis and skin eruptions of the urticarial type have been observed infrequently. Photosensitivity is extremely rare.

Cardiovascular System: Thioridazine HCl produces a dose related prolongation of the QTc interval, which is associated with the ability to cause torsades de pointes-type arrhythmias, a potentially fatal polymorphic ventricular tachycardia, and sudden death (see WARNINGS). Both torsades de pointes-type arrhythmias and sudden death have been reported in association with thioridazine HCl. A causal relationship between these events and thioridazine HCl therapy has not been established but, given the ability of thioridazine HCl to prolong the QTc interval, such a relationship is possible. Other ECG changes have been reported (see Phenothiazine Derivatives, Cardiovascular Effects).

Other: Rare cases described as parotid swelling have been reported following administration of thioridazine HCl.

POST INTRODUCTION REPORTS

These are voluntary reports of adverse events temporally associated with thioridazine HCl that were received since marketing, and there may be no causal relationship between thioridazine HCl use and these events: priapism.

PHENOTHIAZINE DERIVATIVES

It should be noted that efficacy, indications, and untoward effects have varied with the different phenothiazines. It has been reported that old age lowers the tolerance for phenothiazines. The most common neurological side effects in these patients are parkinsonism and akathisia. There appears to be an increased risk of agranulocytosis and leukopenia in the geriatric population. The physician should be aware that the following have occurred with one or more phenothiazines and should be considered whenever one of these drugs is used.

Autonomic Reactions

Miosis, obstipation, anorexia, paralytic ileus.

Cutaneous Reactions

Erythema, exfoliative dermatitis, contact dermatitis.

Blood Dyscrasias

Agranulocytosis, leukopenia, eosinophilia, thrombocytopenia, anemia, aplastic anemia, pancytopenia.

Allergic Reactions

Fever, laryngeal edema, angioneurotic edema, asthma.

Hepatotoxicity

Jaundice, biliary stasis.

Cardiovascular Effects

Changes in the terminal portion of the electrocardiogram to include prolongation of the QT interval, depression and inversion of the T wave and the appearance of a wave tentatively identified as a bifid T wave or U wave have been observed in patients receiving the phenothiazines, including thioridazine HCl. To date, these appear to be due to altered repolarization, not related to myocardial damage, and reversible. Nonetheless, significant prolongation of the QT interval has been associated with serious ventricular arrhythmias and sudden death (see WARNINGS). Hypotension, rarely resulting in cardiac arrest, has been reported.

Extrapyramidal Symptoms

Akathisia, agitation, motor restlessness, dystonic reactions, trismus, torticollis, opisthotonus, oculogyric crises, tremor, muscular rigidity, akinesia.

Tardive Dyskinesia

Chronic use of antipsychotics may be associated with the development of tardive dyskinesia. The salient features of this syndrome are described in WARNINGS and subsequently.

The syndrome is characterized by involuntary choreoathetoid movements which variously involve the tongue, face, mouth, lips, or jaw (*e.g.*, protrusion of the tongue, puffing of cheeks, puckering of the mouth, chewing movements), trunk, and extremities. The severity of the syndrome and the degree of impairment produced vary widely.

The syndrome may become clinically recognizable either during treatment, upon dosage reduction, or upon withdrawal of treatment. Movements may decrease in intensity and may disappear altogether if further treatment with antipsychotics is withheld. It is generally believed that reversibility is more likely after short- rather than long-term antipsychotic exposure. Consequently, early detection of tardive dyskinesia is important. To increase the likelihood of detecting the syndrome at the earliest possible time, the dosage of antipsychotic drug should be reduced periodically (if clinically possible) and the patient observed for signs of the disorder. This maneuver is critical, for antipsychotic drugs may mask the signs of the syndrome.

Neuroleptic Malignant Syndrome (NMS)

Chronic use of neuroleptics may be associated with the development of NMS. The salient features of this syndrome are described in WARNINGS and subsequently. Clinical manifestations of NMS are hyperpyrexia, muscle rigidity, altered mental status, and evidence of autonomic instability (irregular pulse or blood pressure, tachycardia, diaphoresis, and cardiac dysrhythmias).

Endocrine Disturbances

Menstrual irregularities, altered libido, gynecomastia, lactation, weight gain, edema. False positive pregnancy tests have been reported.

Urinary Disturbances

Retention, incontinence.

Others

Hyperpyrexia. Behavioral effects suggestive of a paradoxical reaction have been reported. These include excitement, bizarre dreams, aggravation of psychoses, and toxic confusional states. More recently, a peculiar skin-eye syndrome has been recognized as a side effect following long-term treatment with phenothiazines. This reaction is marked by progressive pigmentation of areas of the skin or conjunctiva and/or accompanied by discoloration of the exposed sclera and cornea. Opacities of the anterior lens and cornea described as irregular or stellate in shape have also been reported. Systemic lupus erythematosus-like syndrome.

DOSAGE AND ADMINISTRATION

Since thioridazine HCl is associated with a dose-related prolongation of the QTc interval, which is a potentially life-threatening event, its use should be reserved for schizophrenic patients who fail to respond adequately to treatment with other antipsychotic drugs. Dosage must be individualized and the smallest effective dosage should be determined for each patient (see INDICATIONS AND USAGE and WARNINGS).

ADULTS

The usual starting dose for adult schizophrenic patients is 50-100 mg three times a day, with a gradual increment to a maximum of 800 mg daily if necessary. Once effective control of symptoms has been achieved, the dosage may be reduced gradually to determine the minimum maintenance dose. The total daily dosage ranges from 200-800 mg, divided into 2-4 doses.

PEDIATRIC PATIENTS

For pediatric patients with schizophrenia who are unresponsive to other agents, the recommended initial dose is 0.5 mg/kg/day given in divided doses. Dosage may be increased gradually until optimum therapeutic effect is obtained or the maximum dose of 3 mg/kg/day has been reached.

HOW SUPPLIED

MELLARIL TABLETS

10 mg: Bright chartreuse, coated tablets; triangle with "S" in center imprinted on one side, "78-2'' imprinted on the other side, in black.

15 mg: Pink, coated tablets; triangle with "S" in center imprinted on one side, "78-8'' imprinted on the other side, in black.

25 mg: Light tan, coated tablets; triangle with "S" in center imprinted on one side, "MELLARIL 25'' imprinted on the other side, in black.

50 mg: White, coated tablets; triangle with "S" in center imprinted on one side, "MELLARIL 50'' imprinted on the other side, in black.

100 mg: Light green, coated tablets; triangle with "S" in center imprinted on one side, "MELLARIL 100'' imprinted on the other side, in black.

150 mg: Yellow, coated tablets; triangle with "S" in center imprinted on one side, "MELLARIL 150'' imprinted on the other side, in black.

200 mg: Pink, coated tablets, triangle with "S" in center imprinted on one side, "MELLARIL 200" imprinted on the other side, in black.

Storage: Store at 25°C (77°F); excursions permitted to 15-30°C (59-86°F). Dispense in a tight container.

MELLARIL ORAL SOLUTION (CONCENTRATE)

30 mg/ml: A clear, straw-yellow liquid with a cherry-like odor. Each ml contains 30 mg thioridazine HCl, alcohol, 3.0% by volume.

100 mg/ml: A clear, light-yellow liquid with a strawberry-like odor. Each ml contains 100 mg thioridazine HCl, alcohol, 4.2% by volume.

Storage

Store and dispense below 30°C (86°F); tight, amber glass bottle.

The oral solution (concentrate) may be diluted with distilled water, acidified tap water, or suitable juices. Each dose should be so diluted just prior to administration. Preparation and storage of bulk dilutions is not recommended.

MELLARIL-S ORAL SUSPENSION

5 mg/ml: An off-white suspension with a buttermint taste and a peppermint odor. Each ml contains thioridazine, equivalent to 5 mg thioridazine HCl.

20 mg/ml: A yellow suspension with a buttermint taste and a peppermint odor. Each ml contains thioridazine, equivalent to 20 mg thioridazine HCl.

Storage: Store and dispense below 25°C (77°F); tight, amber glass bottle.

PRODUCT LISTING - RATED THERAPEUTICALLY EQUIVALENT

Concentrate - Oral - 30 mg/ml

Size	Price	Product	NDC
118 ml	$46.54	MELLARIL, Novartis Pharmaceuticals	00078-0001-31
120 ml	$14.50	GENERIC, Raway Pharmacal Inc	00686-0608-14
120 ml	$15.28	GENERIC, Roxane Laboratories Inc	00054-3860-50
120 ml	$15.85	GENERIC, Geneva Pharmaceuticals	00781-6150-04
120 ml	$18.76	GENERIC, Major Pharmaceuticals Inc	00904-1808-20
120 ml	$20.34	GENERIC, Pharmaceutical Assoc Inc Div Beach Products	00121-0661-04

Concentrate - Oral - 100 mg/ml

Size	Price	Product	NDC
118 ml	$50.00	GENERIC, Pharmaceutical Assoc Inc Div Beach Products	00121-0662-04
120 ml	$25.00	GENERIC, Raway Pharmacal Inc	00686-1451-94
120 ml	$36.89	GENERIC, Roxane Laboratories Inc	00054-3861-50
120 ml	$43.05	GENERIC, Alpharma Uspd Makers Of Barre and Nmc	00472-1451-94
120 ml	$43.20	GENERIC, Major Pharmaceuticals Inc	00904-1809-20

Tablet - Oral - 10 mg

Size	Price	Product	NDC
15's	$2.61	GENERIC, Heartland Healthcare Services	61392-0462-15
25's	$8.55	GENERIC, Udl Laboratories Inc	51079-0565-19
30's	$5.23	GENERIC, Heartland Healthcare Services	61392-0462-30
30's	$5.23	GENERIC, Heartland Healthcare Services	61392-0462-39
30's	$30.56	GENERIC, Medirex Inc	57480-0362-06
31 x 10	$96.70	GENERIC, Vangard Labs	00615-2504-53
31's	$5.40	GENERIC, Heartland Healthcare Services	61392-0462-31
32 x 10	$96.70	GENERIC, Vangard Labs	00615-2504-63
32's	$5.58	GENERIC, Heartland Healthcare Services	61392-0462-32
45's	$7.84	GENERIC, Heartland Healthcare Services	61392-0462-45
60's	$10.46	GENERIC, Heartland Healthcare Services	61392-0462-60
60's	$20.54	GENERIC, Mutual/United Research Laboratories	00677-0823-06
90's	$15.69	GENERIC, Heartland Healthcare Services	61392-0462-90
100's	$5.25	GENERIC, Interstate Drug Exchange Inc	00814-7846-14
100's	$5.56	GENERIC, Aligen Independent Laboratories Inc	00405-4993-01
100's	$6.25	GENERIC, Cmc-Consolidated Midland Corporation	00223-2128-01
100's	$8.20	GENERIC, Major Pharmaceuticals Inc	00904-1614-60
100's	$8.20	GENERIC, Major Pharmaceuticals Inc	00904-1793-60
100's	$8.49	GENERIC, Moore, H.L. Drug Exchange Inc	00839-6703-06
100's	$8.75	GENERIC, Raway Pharmacal Inc	00686-0565-20
100's	$13.65	FEDERAL UPPER LIMIT, H.C.F.A. F F P	99999-2341-03
100's	$15.41	GENERIC, Major Pharmaceuticals Inc	00904-1793-61
100's	$15.41	GENERIC, Major Pharmaceuticals Inc	00904-1800-61
100's	$17.36	GENERIC, Us Trading Corporation	56126-0096-11
100's	$17.94	GENERIC, Auro Pharmaceutical	55829-0501-10
100's	$30.56	GENERIC, Major Pharmaceuticals Inc	00904-5240-60
100's	$31.51	GENERIC, Qualitest Products Inc	00603-5992-21
100's	$31.60	GENERIC, Mylan Pharmaceuticals Inc	00378-0612-01
100's	$31.60	GENERIC, Dixon-Shane Inc	17236-0318-01
100's	$33.20	GENERIC, Mutual/United Research Laboratories	00677-0823-01
100's	$33.20	GENERIC, Mutual Pharmaceutical Co Inc	53489-0148-01
100's	$33.25	GENERIC, Geneva Pharmaceuticals	00781-1604-01
100's	$33.96	GENERIC, Geneva Pharmaceuticals	00781-1604-13
100's	$34.20	GENERIC, Udl Laboratories Inc	51079-0565-20
200 x 5	$311.93	GENERIC, Vangard Labs	00615-2504-43

Tablet - Oral - 15 mg

Size	Price	Product	NDC
31 x 10	$113.17	GENERIC, Vangard Labs	00615-2505-53
100's	$4.97	GENERIC, Us Trading Corporation	56126-0097-11
100's	$7.75	GENERIC, Cmc-Consolidated Midland Corporation	00223-2129-01
100's	$10.50	GENERIC, Major Pharmaceuticals Inc	00904-1615-60
100's	$10.50	GENERIC, Major Pharmaceuticals Inc	00904-1794-60
100's	$15.80	GENERIC, Aligen Independent Laboratories Inc	00405-4994-01
100's	$43.17	GENERIC, Geneva Pharmaceuticals	00781-1614-01
100's	$50.79	MELLARIL, Novartis Pharmaceuticals	00078-0008-05
100's	$107.50	GENERIC, Geneva Pharmaceuticals	00781-1614-13

Tablet - Oral - 25 mg

Size	Price	Product	NDC
30's	$7.76	GENERIC, Medirex Inc	57480-0363-06
30's	$12.03	GENERIC, Heartland Healthcare Services	61392-0463-30
30's	$12.03	GENERIC, Heartland Healthcare Services	61392-0463-39
31 x 10	$135.80	GENERIC, Vangard Labs	00615-2506-53
31's	$12.43	GENERIC, Heartland Healthcare Services	61392-0463-31
32 x 10	$135.80	GENERIC, Vangard Labs	00615-2506-63
32's	$12.83	GENERIC, Heartland Healthcare Services	61392-0463-32
45's	$18.05	GENERIC, Heartland Healthcare Services	61392-0463-45
60's	$24.06	GENERIC, Heartland Healthcare Services	61392-0463-60
60's	$28.89	GENERIC, Mutual/United Research Laboratories	00677-0824-06
90's	$36.09	GENERIC, Heartland Healthcare Services	61392-0463-90
100's	$5.54	GENERIC, Us Trading Corporation	56126-0098-11
100's	$7.50	GENERIC, Interstate Drug Exchange Inc	00814-7847-14
100's	$9.50	GENERIC, Cmc-Consolidated Midland Corporation	00223-2130-01
100's	$11.35	GENERIC, Raway Pharmacal Inc	00686-0566-20
100's	$11.60	GENERIC, Major Pharmaceuticals Inc	00904-1616-60
100's	$11.60	GENERIC, Major Pharmaceuticals Inc	00904-1795-60
100's	$13.50	GENERIC, Aligen Independent Laboratories Inc	00405-4995-01
100's	$13.57	GENERIC, Moore, H.L. Drug Exchange Inc	00839-6704-06
100's	$16.91	GENERIC, Major Pharmaceuticals Inc	00904-1795-61
100's	$16.91	GENERIC, Major Pharmaceuticals Inc	00904-1802-61
100's	$17.87	FEDERAL UPPER LIMIT, H.C.F.A. F F P	99999-2341-06
100's	$43.06	GENERIC, Major Pharmaceuticals Inc	00904-5241-60
100's	$44.39	GENERIC, Qualitest Products Inc	00603-5993-21
100's	$44.40	GENERIC, Dixon-Shane Inc	17236-0301-01
100's	$44.45	GENERIC, Mylan Pharmaceuticals Inc	00378-0614-01
100's	$46.70	GENERIC, Mutual/United Research Laboratories	00677-0824-01
100's	$46.70	GENERIC, Mutual Pharmaceutical Co Inc	53489-0149-01
100's	$46.75	GENERIC, Geneva Pharmaceuticals	00781-1624-01
100's	$47.22	GENERIC, Geneva Pharmaceuticals	00781-1624-13
100's	$48.10	GENERIC, Udl Laboratories Inc	51079-0566-20
100's	$60.61	MELLARIL, Novartis Pharmaceuticals	00078-0003-05
200 x 5	$438.06	GENERIC, Vangard Labs	00615-2506-43

Tablet - Oral - 50 mg

Size	Price	Product	NDC
30's	$9.12	GENERIC, Medirex Inc	57480-0364-06
30's	$14.36	GENERIC, Heartland Healthcare Services	61392-0464-30
30's	$14.36	GENERIC, Heartland Healthcare Services	61392-0464-39
31 x 10	$166.15	GENERIC, Vangard Labs	00615-2507-53
31's	$14.83	GENERIC, Heartland Healthcare Services	61392-0464-31
32 x 10	$166.15	GENERIC, Vangard Labs	00615-2507-63
32's	$15.31	GENERIC, Heartland Healthcare Services	61392-0464-32
45's	$21.53	GENERIC, Heartland Healthcare Services	61392-0464-45
60's	$28.71	GENERIC, Heartland Healthcare Services	61392-0464-60
60's	$36.12	GENERIC, Mutual/United Research Laboratories	00677-0825-06
90's	$43.07	GENERIC, Heartland Healthcare Services	61392-0464-90
100's	$6.77	GENERIC, Us Trading Corporation	56126-0099-11
100's	$9.88	GENERIC, Raway Pharmacal Inc	00686-0616-01
100's	$9.90	GENERIC, Interstate Drug Exchange Inc	00814-7848-14
100's	$12.50	GENERIC, Cmc-Consolidated Midland Corporation	00223-2131-01
100's	$12.75	GENERIC, Raway Pharmacal Inc	00686-0567-20
100's	$16.10	GENERIC, Major Pharmaceuticals Inc	00904-1617-60
100's	$16.10	GENERIC, Major Pharmaceuticals Inc	00904-1796-60
100's	$17.20	GENERIC, Aligen Independent Laboratories Inc	00405-4996-01
100's	$19.24	GENERIC, Moore, H.L. Drug Exchange Inc	00839-6705-06
100's	$20.57	GENERIC, Major Pharmaceuticals Inc	00904-1796-61
100's	$20.57	GENERIC, Major Pharmaceuticals Inc	00904-1803-61
100's	$21.22	FEDERAL UPPER LIMIT, H.C.F.A. F F P	99999-2341-08
100's	$53.89	GENERIC, Qualitest Products Inc	00603-5994-21
100's	$53.95	GENERIC, Dixon-Shane Inc	17236-0302-01
100's	$55.57	GENERIC, Major Pharmaceuticals Inc	00904-5242-60
100's	$55.60	GENERIC, Mylan Pharmaceuticals Inc	00378-0616-01
100's	$58.40	GENERIC, Mutual/United Research Laboratories	00677-0825-01
100's	$58.40	GENERIC, Mutual Pharmaceutical Co Inc	53489-0150-01
100's	$58.45	GENERIC, Geneva Pharmaceuticals	00781-1634-01
100's	$60.15	GENERIC, Udl Laboratories Inc	51079-0567-20
100's	$76.65	MELLARIL, Novartis Pharmaceuticals	00078-0004-05
200 x 5	$535.96	GENERIC, Vangard Labs	00615-2507-43

Tablet - Oral - 100 mg

Size	Price	Product	NDC
30's	$16.44	GENERIC, Heartland Healthcare Services	61392-0465-30
30's	$16.44	GENERIC, Heartland Healthcare Services	61392-0465-39
31 x 10	$194.13	GENERIC, Vangard Labs	00615-2508-53
31's	$16.99	GENERIC, Heartland Healthcare Services	61392-0465-31
32's	$17.54	GENERIC, Heartland Healthcare Services	61392-0465-32
45's	$24.66	GENERIC, Heartland Healthcare Services	61392-0465-45
60's	$32.88	GENERIC, Heartland Healthcare Services	61392-0465-60
60's	$41.13	GENERIC, Mutual/United Research Laboratories	00677-0832-06
90's	$49.33	GENERIC, Heartland Healthcare Services	61392-0465-90
100's	$10.74	GENERIC, Us Trading Corporation	56126-0101-11
100's	$14.50	GENERIC, Raway Pharmacal Inc	00686-0618-01
100's	$17.25	GENERIC, Interstate Drug Exchange Inc	00814-7849-14
100's	$17.95	GENERIC, Raway Pharmacal Inc	00686-0580-20
100's	$19.50	GENERIC, Cmc-Consolidated Midland Corporation	00223-2132-01
100's	$21.90	GENERIC, Major Pharmaceuticals Inc	00904-1618-60
100's	$21.90	GENERIC, Major Pharmaceuticals Inc	00904-1797-60

T

100's	$23.36	GENERIC, Moore, H.L. Drug Exchange Inc	00839-6720-06
100's	$24.00	GENERIC, Aligen Independent Laboratories Inc	00405-4997-01
100's	$34.06	GENERIC, Vangard Labs	00615-2508-13
100's	$35.88	GENERIC, Major Pharmaceuticals Inc	00904-1797-61
100's	$35.88	GENERIC, Major Pharmaceuticals Inc	00904-1804-61
100's	$38.25	FEDERAL UPPER LIMIT, H.C.F.A. F F P	99999-2341-11
100's	$63.30	GENERIC, Qualitest Products Inc	00603-5995-21
100's	$63.36	GENERIC, Mylan Pharmaceuticals Inc	00378-0618-01
100's	$63.36	GENERIC, Dixon-Shane Inc	17236-0305-01
100's	$65.62	GENERIC, Geneva Pharmaceuticals	00781-0268-06
100's	$66.50	GENERIC, Mutual/United Research Laboratories	00677-0832-01
100's	$66.50	GENERIC, Mutual Pharmaceutical Co Inc	53489-0500-01
100's	$66.55	GENERIC, Geneva Pharmaceuticals	00781-1644-01
100's	$68.50	GENERIC, Udl Laboratories Inc	51079-0580-20
100's	$90.00	MELLARIL, Novartis Pharmaceuticals	00078-0005-05
200 x 5	$626.22	GENERIC, Vangard Labs	00615-2508-43
Tablet - Oral - 150 mg			
31 x 10	$253.31	GENERIC, Vangard Labs	00615-2509-53
100's	$19.17	GENERIC, Us Trading Corporation	56126-0310-11
100's	$30.00	GENERIC, Cmc-Consolidated Midland Corporation	00223-2133-01
100's	$31.65	GENERIC, Major Pharmaceuticals Inc	00904-7649-60
100's	$34.42	GENERIC, Aligen Independent Laboratories Inc	00405-4998-01
100's	$35.00	GENERIC, Watson/Rugby Laboratories Inc	00536-4654-01
100's	$37.35	GENERIC, Major Pharmaceuticals Inc	00904-1798-61
100's	$37.35	GENERIC, Major Pharmaceuticals Inc	00904-1805-61
100's	$96.63	GENERIC, Geneva Pharmaceuticals	00781-1664-01
Tablet - Oral - 200 mg			
31 x 10	$288.52	GENERIC, Vangard Labs	00615-2510-53
100's	$20.25	GENERIC, Us Trading Corporation	56126-0311-11
100's	$34.50	GENERIC, Cmc-Consolidated Midland Corporation	00223-2134-01
100's	$36.10	GENERIC, Major Pharmaceuticals Inc	00904-1799-60
100's	$41.95	GENERIC, Aligen Independent Laboratories Inc	00405-4999-01
100's	$45.52	GENERIC, Major Pharmaceuticals Inc	00904-1806-61
100's	$49.51	GENERIC, Watson/Schein Pharmaceuticals Inc	00364-0724-01
100's	$110.06	GENERIC, Geneva Pharmaceuticals	00781-1674-01
100's	$115.47	MELLARIL, Novartis Pharmaceuticals	00078-0007-05

PRODUCT LISTING - EQUIVALENTS NOT AVAILABLE

Tablet - Oral - 25 mg			
30's	$3.86	GENERIC, Physicians Total Care	54868-0067-04
60's	$6.05	GENERIC, Physicians Total Care	54868-0067-05
Tablet - Oral - 50 mg			
30's	$7.73	GENERIC, Physicians Total Care	54868-1832-02
100's	$21.98	GENERIC, Physicians Total Care	54868-1832-03
Tablet - Oral - 100 mg			
100's	$16.52	GENERIC, Physicians Total Care	54868-1828-02

Thiotepa *(002342)*

For complete prescribing information, refer to the CD-ROM included with the book.

Categories: Carcinoma, bladder; Carcinoma, breast; Carcinoma, ovarian; Effusion, secondary to neoplasia; Lymphoma, Hodgkin's; Lymphosarcoma; Pregnancy Category D; FDA Approved 1959 Feb
Drug Classes: Antineoplastics, alkylating agents
Brand Names: Triethylenethiophosphoramide
Foreign Brand Availability: Ledertepa (Belgium; Netherlands); Tespamin (Taiwan)
HCFA JCODE(S): J9340 5 mg IV

DESCRIPTION

Thiotepa for injection is an ethylenimine-type compound. It is supplied as a non-pyrogenic, sterile lyophilized powder for intravenous, intracavitary or intravesical administration, containing 15 mg of thiotepa. Thioplex is a synthetic product with antitumor activity. The chemical name for thiotepa is Aziridine, 1, 1′,1″-phosphinothioylidynetris-, or Tris (1-aziridinyl) phosphine sulfide.

Thiotepa has the empirical formula $C_6H_{12}N_3PS$ and a molecular weight of 189.22. When reconstituted with sterile water for injection, the resulting solution has a pH of approximately 5.5-7.5. Thiotepa is stable in alkaline medium and unstable in acid medium.
Storage: Store in refrigerator between 2-8°C (36-46°F). PROTECT FROM LIGHT AT ALL TIMES.

INDICATIONS AND USAGE

Thiotepa has been tried with varying results in the palliation of a wide variety of neoplastic diseases. However, the most consistent results have been seen in the following tumors:

1. Adenocarcinoma of the breast.
2. Adenocarcinoma of the ovary.
3. For controlling intracavitary effusions secondary to diffuse or localized neoplastic diseases of various serosal cavities.
4. For the treatment of superficial papillary carcinoma of the urinary bladder.

While now largely superseded by other treatments, thiotepa has been effective against other lymphomas, such as lymphosarcoma and Hodgkin's disease.

CONTRAINDICATIONS

Thiotepa is contraindicated in patients with a known hypersensitivity (allergy) to this preparation.

Therapy is probably contraindicated in cases of existing hepatic, renal, or bone-marrow damage. However, if the need outweighs the risk in such patients, thiotepa may be used in low dosage, and accompanied by hepatic, renal and hemopoietic function tests.

WARNINGS

Death has occurred after intravesical administration, caused by bone-marrow depression from systematically absorbed drug.

Death from septicemia and hemorrhage has occurred as a direct result of hematopoietic depression by thiotepa.

Thiotepa is highly toxic to the hematopoietic system. A rapidly falling white blood cell or platelet count indicates the necessity for discontinuing or reducing the dosage of thiotepa. Weekly blood and platelet counts are recommended during therapy and for at least 3 weeks after therapy has been discontinued.

Thiotepa can cause fetal harm when administered to a pregnant woman. Thiotepa given by the intraperitoneal (IP) route was teratogenic in mice at doses ≥1 mg/kg (3.2 mg/m^2), approximately 8-fold less than the maximum recommended human therapeutic dose (0.8 mg/kg, 27 mg/m^2), based on body-surface area. Thiotepa given by the IP route was teratogenic in rats at doses ≥3 mg/kg (21 mg/m^2), approximately equal to the maximum recommended human therapeutic dose, based on body-surface area. Thiotepa was lethal to rabbit fetuses at a dose of 3 mg/kg (41 mg/m^2), approximately two times the maximum recommended human therapeutic dose based on body-surface area.

Effective contraception should be used during thiotepa therapy if either the patient or partner is of childbearing potential. There are no adequate and well-controlled studies in pregnant women. If thiotepa is used during pregnancy, or if pregnancy occurs during thiotepa therapy, the patient and partner should be apprised of the potential hazard to the fetus.

Thiotepa is a polyfunctional alkylating agent, capable of cross-linking the DNA within a cell and changing its nature. The replication of the cell is, therefore, altered, and thiotepa may be described as mutagenic. An *in vitro* study has shown that it causes chromosomal aberrations of the chromatid type and that the frequency of induced aberrations increases with the age of the subject.

Like many alkylating agents, thiotepa has been reported to be carcinogenic when administered to laboratory animals. Carcinogenicity is shown most clearly in studies using mice, but there is some evidence of carcinogenicity in man. In patients treated with thiotepa, cases of myelodysplastic syndromes and acute non-lymphocytic leukemia have been reported.

DOSAGE AND ADMINISTRATION

Since absorption from the gastrointestinal tract is variable, thiotepa should not be administered orally.

Dosage must be carefully individualized. A slow response to thiotepa does not necessarily indicate a lack of effect. Therefore, increasing the frequency of dosing may only increase toxicity. After maximum benefit is obtained by initial therapy, it is necessary to continue the patient on maintenance therapy (1 to 4 week intervals). In order to continue optimal effect, maintenance doses should not be administered more frequently than weekly in order to preserve correlation between dose and blood counts.

PREPARATION AND ADMINISTRATION PRECAUTIONS

Thiotepa is a cytotoxic anticancer drug and as with other potentially toxic compounds, caution should be exercised in handling and preparation of thiotepa. Skin reactions associated with accidental exposure to thiotepa may occur. The use of gloves is recommended. If thiotepa solution contacts the skin, immediately wash the skin thoroughly with soap and water. If thiotepa contacts mucous membranes, the membranes should be flushed thoroughly with water.

The reconstituted solution is hypotonic and should be further diluted with sodium chloride injection (0.9% sodium chloride) before use.

When reconstituted with sterile water for injection, solutions of thiotepa should be stored in a refrigerator and used within 8 hours. Reconstituted solutions further diluted with sodium chloride injection should be used immediately.

In order to eliminate haze, solutions should be filtered through a 0.22 micron filter* prior to administration. Filtering does not alter solution potency. Reconstituted solutions should be clear. Solutions that remain opaque or precipitate after filtration should not be used.

*Polysulfone membrane (Gelman's Sterile Aerodisc, Single Use) or triton-free mixed ester of cellulose/PVC (Millipore's MILLEX-GS Filter Unit).

Parenteral drug products should be inspected visually for particulate matter and discoloration prior to administration, whenever solution and container permit.

Initial and Maintenance Doses

Initially the higher dose in the given range is commonly administered. The maintenance dose should be adjusted weekly on the basis of pretreatment control blood counts and subsequent blood counts.

Intravenous Administration

Thiotepa may be given by rapid intravenous administration in doses of 0.3-0.4 mg/kg. Doses should be given at 1 to 4 week intervals.

Intracavitary Administration

The dosage recommended is 0.6-0.8 mg/kg. Administration is usually effected through the same tubing which is used to remove the fluid from the cavity involved.

Intravesical Administration

Patients with papillary carcinoma of the bladder are dehydrated for 8 to 12 hours prior to treatment. Then 60 mg of thiotepa in 30-60 ml of sodium chloride injection is instilled into the bladder by catheter. For maximum effect, the solution should be retained for 2 hours. If the patient finds it impossible to retain 60 ml for 2 hours, the dose may be given in a volume of 30 ml. If desired, the patient may be positioned every 15 minutes for maximum area contact. The usual course of treatment is once a week for 4 weeks. The course may be repeated if necessary, but second and third courses must be given with caution since bone-marrow depression may be increased. Deaths have occurred after intravesical administration, caused by bone-marrow depression from systemically absorbed drug.

Handling and Disposal

Follow safe cytotoxic agent handling procedures. Several guidelines on this subject have been published.[1-6] There is no general agreement that all of the procedures recommended in the guidelines are necessary or appropriate.

PRODUCT LISTING - RATED THERAPEUTICALLY EQUIVALENT

Powder For Injection - Injectable - 15 mg

1's	$123.13	GENERIC, Bedford Laboratories	55390-0030-10

Powder For Injection - Injectable - 30 mg

1's	$296.88	GENERIC, Gensia Sicor Pharmaceuticals Inc	00703-4303-01

PRODUCT LISTING - EQUIVALENTS NOT AVAILABLE

Powder For Injection - Injectable - 15 mg

1's	$123.13	THIOPLEX, Immunex Corporation	58406-0662-01
5's	$742.19	GENERIC, Gensia Sicor Pharmaceuticals Inc	00703-4301-02
6's	$738.75	THIOPLEX, Immunex Corporation	58406-0662-36

Thiothixene *(002343)*

Categories: Psychosis; FDA Approved 1967 Jul; Pregnancy Category C
Drug Classes: Antipsychotics
Brand Names: Navane
Foreign Brand Availability: Onaven (Korea); Orbinamon (Germany); Thixit (New-Zealand)
Cost of Therapy: $79.25 (Schizophrenia; Navane; 10 mg; 2 capsules/day; 30 day supply)
$28.29 (Schizophrenia; Generic Capsules; 10 mg; 2 capsules/day; 30 day supply)
HCFA JCODE(S): J2330 up to 4 mg IM

DESCRIPTION

Navane (thiothixene) is a thioxanthene derivative. Specifically, it is the *cis* isomer of N,N-dimethyl-9-[3-(4-methyl-1-piperazinyl)-propylidene] thioxanthene-2-sulfonamide.

The thioxanthenes differ from the phenothiazines by the replacement of nitrogen in the central ring with a carbon-linked side chain fixed in space in a rigid structural configuration. An N,N-dimethyl sulfonamide functional group is bonded to the thioxanthene nucleus.

Capsules: Inert ingredients for the capsule formulations are: hard gelatin capsules (which contain gelatin and titanium dioxide; may contain yellow 10, yellow 6, blue 1, green 3, red 3, and other inert ingredients); lactose; magnesium stearate; sodium lauryl sulfate; starch.

Oral Concentrate: Inert ingredients for the oral concentrate formulation are: alcohol; cherry flavor; dextrose; passion fruit flavor; sorbitol solution; water.

IM Solution: Inert ingredients for the IM solution formulation are dextrose; benzyl alcohol; and propyl gallate.

CLINICAL PHARMACOLOGY

ACTIONS

Thiothixene is a psychotropic agent of the thioxanthene series. Thiothixene possesses certain chemical and pharmacological similarities to the piperazine phenothiazines and differences from the aliphatic group of phenothiazines.

INDICATIONS AND USAGE

Thiothixene is effective in the management of schizophrenia. Thiothixene has not been evaluated in the management of behavioral complications in patients with mental retardation.

NON-FDA APPROVED INDICATIONS

It has also been used for managing paranoid disorders and depression, although these uses are not FDA approved.

CONTRAINDICATIONS

Thiothixene is contraindicated in patients with circulatory collapse, comatose states, central nervous system depression due to any cause, and blood dyscrasias. Thiothixene is contraindicated in individuals who have shown hypersensitivity to the drug. It is not known whether there is a cross sensitivity between the thioxanthenes and the phenothiazine derivatives, but this possibility should be considered.

WARNINGS

TARDIVE DYSKINESIA

Tardive dyskinesia, a syndrome consisting of potentially irreversible, involuntary, dyskinetic movements may develop in patients treated with antipsychotic drugs. Although the prevalence of the syndrome appears to be highest among the elderly, especially elderly women, it is impossible to rely upon prevalence estimates to predict, at the inception of antipsychotic treatment, which patients are likely to develop the syndrome. Whether antipsychotic drug products differ in their potential to cause tardive dyskinesia is unknown.

Both the risk of developing the syndrome and the likelihood that it will become irreversible are believed to increase as the duration of treatment and the total cumulative dose of antipsychotic drugs administered to the patient increase. However, the syndrome can develop, although much less commonly, after relatively brief treatment periods at low doses.

There is no known treatment for established cases of tardive dyskinesia, although the syndrome may remit, partially or completely, if antipsychotic treatment is withdrawn. Antipsychotic treatment, itself, however, may suppress (or partially suppress) the signs and symptoms of the syndrome and thereby may possibly mask the underlying disease process. The effect that symptomatic suppression has upon the long-term course of the syndrome is unknown.

Given these considerations, antipsychotics should be prescribed in a manner that is most likely to minimize the occurrence of tardive dyskinesia. Chronic antipsychotic treatment should generally be reserved for patients who suffer from a chronic illness that, (1) is known to respond to antipsychotic drugs, and, (2) for whom alternative, equally effective, but potentially less harmful treatments are not available or appropriate. In patients who do require chronic treatment, the smallest dose and the shortest duration of treatment producing a satisfactory clinical response should be sought. The need for continued treatment should be reassessed periodically.

If signs and symptoms of tardive dyskinesia appear in a patient on antipsychotics, drug discontinuation should be considered. However, some patients may require treatment despite the presence of the syndrome.

(For further information about the description of tardive dyskinesia and its clinical detection, please refer to PRECAUTIONS, Information for the Patient, and ADVERSE REACTIONS.)

NEUROLEPTIC MALIGNANT SYNDROME (NMS)

A potentially fatal symptom complex sometimes referred to as Neuroleptic Malignant Syndrome (NMS) has been reported in association with antipsychotic drugs. Clinical manifestations of NMS are hyperpyrexia, muscle rigidity, altered mental status and evidence of autonomic instability (irregular pulse or blood pressure, tachycardia, diaphoresis, and cardiac dysrhythmias).

The diagnostic evaluation of patients with this syndrome is complicated. In arriving at a diagnosis, it is important to identify cases where the clinical presentation includes both serious medical illness (*e.g.*, pneumonia, systemic infection, etc.) and untreated or inadequately treated extrapyramidal signs and symptoms (EPS). Other important considerations in the differential diagnosis include central anticholinergic toxicity, heat stroke, drug fever and primary central nervous system (CNS) pathology.

The management of NMS should include (1) immediate discontinuation of antipsychotic drugs and other drugs not essential to concurrent therapy, (2) intensive symptomatic treatment and medical monitoring, and (3) treatment of any concomitant serious medical problems for which specific treatments are available. There is no general agreement about specific pharmacological treatment regimens for uncomplicated NMS.

If a patient requires antipsychotic drug treatment after recovery from NMS, the potential reintroduction of drug therapy should be carefully considered. The patient should be carefully monitored, since recurrences of NMS have been reported.

USE IN PREGNANCY

Safe use of thiothixene during pregnancy has not been established. Therefore, this drug should be given to pregnant patients only when, in the judgment of the physician, the expected benefits from the treatment exceed the possible risks to mother and fetus. Animal reproduction studies and clinical experience to date have not demonstrated any teratogenic effects.

In the animal reproduction studies with thiothixene, there was some decrease in conception rate and litter size, and an increase in resorption rate in rats and rabbits. Similar findings have been reported with other psychotropic agents. After repeated oral administration of thiothixene to rats (5-15 mg/kg/day), rabbits (3-50 mg/kg/day), and monkeys (1-3 mg/kg/day) before and during gestation, no teratogenic effects were seen.

USE IN CHILDREN

The use of thiothixene in children under 12 years of age is not recommended because safe conditions for its use have not been established.

As is true with many CNS drugs, thiothixene may impair the mental and/or physical abilities required for the performance of potentially hazardous tasks such as driving a car or operating machinery, especially during the first few days of therapy. Therefore, the patient should be cautioned accordingly.

As in the case of other CNS-acting drugs, patients receiving thiothixene should be cautioned about the possible additive effects (which may include hypotension) with CNS depressants and with alcohol.

PRECAUTIONS

An antiemetic effect was observed in animal studies with thiothixene; since this effect may also occur in man, it is possible that thiothixene may mask signs of overdosage of toxic drugs and may obscure conditions such as intestinal obstruction and brain tumor.

In consideration of the known capability of thiothixene and certain other psychotropic drugs to precipitate convulsions, extreme caution should be used in patients with a history of convulsive disorders or those in a state of alcohol withdrawal, since it may lower the convulsive threshold. Although thiothixene potentiates the actions of the barbiturates, the dosage of the anticonvulsant therapy should not be reduced when thiothixene is administered concurrently.

Though exhibiting rather weak anticholinergic properties, thiothixene should be used with caution in patients who might be exposed to extreme heat or who are receiving atropine or related drugs.

Use with caution in patients with cardiovascular disease.

Caution as well as careful adjustment of the dosages is indicated when thiothixene is used in conjunction with other CNS depressants.

Also, careful observation should be made for pigmentary retinopathy and lenticular pigmentation (fine lenticular pigmentation has been noted in a small number of patients treated with thiothixene for prolonged periods). Blood dyscrasias (agranulocytosis, pancytopenia, thrombocytopenic purpura), and liver damage (jaundice, biliary stasis) have been reported with related drugs.

Antipsychotic drugs elevate prolactin levels; the elevation persists during chronic administration. Tissue culture experiments indicate that approximately one-third of human breast cancers are prolactin dependent *in vitro,* a factor of potential importance if the prescription of these drugs is contemplated in a patient with a previously detected breast cancer. Although disturbances such as galactorrhea, amenorrhea, gynecomastia, and impotence have been reported, the clinical significance of elevated serum prolactin levels is unknown for most patients. An increase in mammary neoplasms has been found in rodents after chronic administration of antipsychotic drugs. Neither clinical studies nor epidemiologic studies conducted to date, however, have shown an association between chronic administration of these drugs and mammary tumorigenesis; the available evidence is considered too limited to be conclusive at this time.

INFORMATION FOR THE PATIENT

Given the likelihood that some patients exposed chronically to antipsychotics will develop tardive dyskinesia, it is advised that all patients in whom chronic use is contemplated be given, if possible, full information about this risk. The decision to inform patients and/or their guardians must obviously take into account the clinical circumstances and the competency of the patient to understand the information provided.

Additional Information for IM Solution

As with all IM preparations, thiothixene should be injected well within the body of a relatively large muscle. The preferred sites are the upper outer quadrant of the buttock (*i.e.,* gluteus maximus) and the mid-lateral thigh.

The deltoid area should be used only if well developed such as in certain adults and older children, and then only with caution to avoid radial nerve injury. IM injections should not be made into the lower- and mid-thirds of the upper arm. Aspiration is necessary to help avoid inadvertent injection into a blood vessel.

ADVERSE REACTIONS

NOTE: Not all of the following adverse reactions have been reported with thiothixene. However, since thiothixene has certain chemical and pharmacologic similarities to the phenothiazines, all of the known side effects and toxicity associated with phenothiazine therapy should be borne in mind when thiothixene is used.

CARDIOVASCULAR EFFECTS

Tachycardia, hypotension, lightheadedness, and syncope. In the event hypotension occurs, epinephrine should not be used as a pressor agent since a paradoxical further lowering of blood pressure may result. Nonspecific EKG changes have been observed in some patients receiving thiothixene. These changes are usually reversible and frequently disappear on continued thiothixene therapy. The incidence of these changes is lower than that observed with some phenothiazines. The clinical significance of these changes is not known.

CNS EFFECTS

Drowsiness, usually mild, may occur although it usually subsides with continuation of thiothixene therapy. The incidence of sedation appears similar to that of the piperazine group of phenothiazines but less than that of certain aliphatic phenothiazines. Restlessness, agitation and insomnia have been noted with thiothixene. Seizures and paradoxical exacerbation of psychotic symptoms have occurred with thiothixene infrequently.

Hyperreflexia has been reported in infants delivered from mothers having received structurally related drugs.

In addition, phenothiazine derivatives have been associated with cerebral edema and cerebrospinal fluid abnormalities.

Extrapyramidal symptoms, such as pseudoparkinsonism, akathisia and dystonia have been reported. Management of these extrapyramidal symptoms depends upon the type and severity. Rapid relief of acute symptoms may require the use of an injectable antiparkinson agent. More slowly emerging symptoms may be managed by reducing the dosage of thiothixene and/or administering an oral antiparkinson agent.

PERSISTENT TARDIVE DYSKINESIA

As with all antipsychotic agents, tardive dyskinesia may appear in some patients on long-term therapy or may occur after drug therapy has been discontinued. The syndrome is characterized by rhythmical involuntary movements of the tongue, face, mouth or jaw (*e.g.,* protrusion of tongue, puffing of cheeks, puckering of mouth, chewing movements). Sometimes these may be accompanied by involuntary movements of extremities.

Since early detection of tardive dyskinesia is important, patients should be monitored on an ongoing basis. It has been reported that fine vermicular movement of the tongue may be an early sign of the syndrome. If this or any other presentation of the syndrome is observed, the clinician should consider possible discontinuation of antipsychotic medication. (See WARNINGS.)

HEPATIC EFFECTS

Elevations of serum transaminase and alkaline phosphatase, usually transient, have been infrequently observed in some patients. No clinically confirmed cases of jaundice attributable to thiothixene have been reported.

HEMATOLOGIC EFFECTS

As is true with certain other psychotropic drugs, leukopenia and leucocytosis, which are usually transient, can occur occasionally with thiothixene. Other antipsychotic drugs have been associated with agranulocytosis, eosinophilia, hemolytic anemia, thrombocytopenia and pancytopenia.

ALLERGIC REACTIONS

Rash, pruritus, urticaria, photosensitivity and rare cases of anaphylaxis have been reported with thiothixene. Undue exposure to sunlight should be avoided. Although not experienced with thiothixene, exfoliative dermatitis and contact dermatitis (in nursing personnel) have been reported with certain phenothiazines.

ENDOCRINE DISORDERS

Lactation, moderate breast enlargement and amenorrhea have occurred in a small percentage of females receiving thiothixene. If persistent, this may necessitate a reduction in dosage or the discontinuation of therapy. Phenothiazines have been associated with false positive pregnancy tests, gynecomastia, hypoglycemia, hyperglycemia and glycosuria.

AUTONOMIC EFFECTS

Dry mouth, blurred vision, nasal congestion, constipation, increased sweating, increased salivation and impotence have occurred infrequently with thiothixene therapy. Phenothiazines have been associated with miosis, mydriasis, and adynamic ileus.

OTHER ADVERSE REACTIONS

Hyperpyrexia, anorexia, nausea, vomiting, diarrhea, increase in appetite and weight, weakness or fatigue, polydipsia, and peripheral edema.

Although not reported with thiothixene, evidence indicates there is a relationship between phenothiazine therapy and the occurrence of a systemic lupus erythematosus-like syndrome.

NEUROLEPTIC MALIGNANT SYNDROME (NMS)

Please refer to the text regarding NMS in WARNINGS.

NOTE: Sudden deaths have occasionally been reported in patients who have received certain phenothiazine derivatives. In some cases the cause of death was apparently cardiac arrest or asphyxia due to failure of the cough reflex. In others, the cause could not be determined nor could it be established that death was due to phenothiazine administration.

DOSAGE AND ADMINISTRATION

CAPSULES

Dosage of thiothixene should be individually adjusted depending on the chronicity and severity of the schizophrenia. In general, small doses should be used initially and gradually increased to the optimal effective level, based on patient response.

Some patients have been successfully maintained on once-a-day thiothixene therapy.

The use of thiothixene in children under 12 years of age is not recommended because safe conditions for its use have not been established.

In milder conditions, an initial dose of 2 mg three times daily. If indicated, a subsequent increase to 15 mg/day total daily dose is often effective.

In more severe conditions, an initial dose of 5 mg twice daily.

The usual optimal dose is 20-30 mg daily. If indicated, an increase to 60 mg/day total daily dose is often effective. Exceeding a total daily dose of 60 mg rarely increases the beneficial response.

IM INJECTION

Dosage of thiothixene should be individually adjusted depending on the chronicity and severity of the condition. In general, small doses should be used initially and gradually increased to the optimal effective level, based on patient response. The use of thiothixene in children under 12 years of age is not recommended.

When more rapid control and treatment of acute behavior is desirable, the IM form of thiothixene may be indicated. It is also of benefit where the very nature of the patients's symptomatology, whether acute or chronic, renders oral administration impractical or even impossible.

For the treatment of acute symptomatology or in patients unable or unwilling to take oral medication, the usual dose is 4 mg of thiothixene IM administered 2-4 times daily. Dosage may be increased or decreased depending on response. Most patients are controlled on a total daily dosage of 16-20 mg. The maximum recommended dosage is 30 mg/day. An oral form should supplant the injectable as soon as possible. It may be necessary to adjust the dosage when changing from the IM to the oral dosage forms.

HOW SUPPLIED

CAPSULES

Navane capsules are available in 1, 2, 5, 10, and 20 mg dosage strengths.

ORAL CONCENTRATE

Navane concentrate is available in 120 ml bottles, with an accompanying dropper calibrated at 2, 3, 4, 5, 6, 8, and 10 mg. It is also available in 30 ml bottles, with an accompanying dropper calibrated at 2, 3, 4, and 5 mg. Each ml contains thiothixene hydrochloride equivalent to 5 mg of thiothixene. Contains alcohol 7.0% v/v (small loss unavoidable).

IM SOLUTION

Navane intramuscular for injection is available in amber glass vials. When reconstituted with 2.2 ml of sterile water for injection, each ml contains thiothixene hydrochloride equivalent to 5 mg of thiothixene and 59.6 mg mannitol. The reconstituted solution of Navane IM may be stored for 48 hours at room temperature before discarding.

PRODUCT LISTING - RATED THERAPEUTICALLY EQUIVALENT

Capsule - Oral - 1 mg

30's	$8.64	GENERIC, Heartland Healthcare Services	61392-0788-30
30's	$8.64	GENERIC, Heartland Healthcare Services	61392-0788-39
31's	$8.93	GENERIC, Heartland Healthcare Services	61392-0788-31
32's	$9.22	GENERIC, Heartland Healthcare Services	61392-0788-32
45's	$12.96	GENERIC, Heartland Healthcare Services	61392-0788-45
60's	$17.28	GENERIC, Heartland Healthcare Services	61392-0788-60
90's	$25.92	GENERIC, Heartland Healthcare Services	61392-0788-90
100's	$12.23	GENERIC, Us Trading Corporation	56126-0378-11
100's	$13.29	FEDERAL UPPER LIMIT, H.C.F.A. F F P	99999-2343-01
100's	$15.77	GENERIC, Qualitest Products Inc	00603-6018-21
100's	$16.20	GENERIC, Aligen Independent Laboratories Inc	00405-5004-01
100's	$17.50	GENERIC, Major Pharmaceuticals Inc	00904-2955-60
100's	$17.90	GENERIC, Watson/Rugby Laboratories Inc	00536-4951-01
100's	$21.06	GENERIC, Moore, H.L. Drug Exchange Inc	00839-7288-06
100's	$21.30	GENERIC, Dixon-Shane Inc	17236-0465-01
100's	$21.95	GENERIC, Mylan Pharmaceuticals Inc	00378-1001-01

T

100's	$22.43	GENERIC, Major Pharmaceuticals Inc	00904-2890-60
100's	$23.00	GENERIC, Geneva Pharmaceuticals	00781-2226-01
100's	$23.69	GENERIC, Udl Laboratories Inc	51079-0586-20
100's	$24.92	GENERIC, Major Pharmaceuticals Inc	00904-2955-61
100's	$28.80	GENERIC, Dixon-Shane Inc	17236-0465-11
100's	$28.95	GENERIC, Geneva Pharmaceuticals	00781-2226-13
100's	$45.44	NAVANE, Pfizer U.S. Pharmaceuticals	00049-5710-66
Capsule - Oral - 2 mg			
30's	$11.64	GENERIC, Heartland Healthcare Services	61392-0789-30
30's	$11.64	GENERIC, Heartland Healthcare Services	61392-0789-39
31's	$12.03	GENERIC, Heartland Healthcare Services	61392-0789-31
32's	$12.42	GENERIC, Heartland Healthcare Services	61392-0789-32
45's	$17.46	GENERIC, Heartland Healthcare Services	61392-0789-45
60's	$23.29	GENERIC, Heartland Healthcare Services	61392-0789-60
90's	$34.93	GENERIC, Heartland Healthcare Services	61392-0789-90
100's	$15.02	GENERIC, Us Trading Corporation	56126-0379-11
100's	$18.60	FEDERAL UPPER LIMIT, H.C.F.A. F F P	99999-2343-02
100's	$20.89	GENERIC, Qualitest Products Inc	00603-6019-21
100's	$24.85	GENERIC, Major Pharmaceuticals Inc	00904-2891-60
100's	$24.85	GENERIC, Major Pharmaceuticals Inc	00904-2956-60
100's	$27.54	GENERIC, Moore, H.L. Drug Exchange Inc	00839-7289-06
100's	$27.75	GENERIC, Dixon-Shane Inc	17236-0466-01
100's	$28.95	GENERIC, Mylan Pharmaceuticals Inc	00378-2002-01
100's	$30.40	GENERIC, Geneva Pharmaceuticals	00781-2227-01
100's	$31.31	GENERIC, Udl Laboratories Inc	51079-0587-20
100's	$31.59	GENERIC, Major Pharmaceuticals Inc	00904-2956-61
100's	$38.81	GENERIC, Dixon-Shane Inc	17236-0466-11
100's	$38.85	GENERIC, Geneva Pharmaceuticals	00781-2227-13
100's	$65.38	NAVANE, Pfizer U.S. Pharmaceuticals	00049-5720-66
Capsule - Oral - 5 mg			
30's	$18.23	GENERIC, Heartland Healthcare Services	61392-0790-30
30's	$18.23	GENERIC, Heartland Healthcare Services	61392-0790-39
31's	$18.84	GENERIC, Heartland Healthcare Services	61392-0790-31
32's	$19.44	GENERIC, Heartland Healthcare Services	61392-0790-32
45's	$27.34	GENERIC, Heartland Healthcare Services	61392-0790-45
60's	$36.46	GENERIC, Heartland Healthcare Services	61392-0790-60
90's	$54.68	GENERIC, Heartland Healthcare Services	61392-0790-90
100's	$18.77	GENERIC, Us Trading Corporation	56126-0380-11
100's	$29.63	FEDERAL UPPER LIMIT, H.C.F.A. F F P	99999-2343-05
100's	$36.80	GENERIC, Major Pharmaceuticals Inc	00904-2892-60
100's	$36.80	GENERIC, Major Pharmaceuticals Inc	00904-2957-60
100's	$37.11	GENERIC, Qualitest Products Inc	00603-6020-21
100's	$38.25	GENERIC, Aligen Independent Laboratories Inc	00405-5006-01
100's	$42.46	GENERIC, Moore, H.L. Drug Exchange Inc	00839-7290-06
100's	$42.75	GENERIC, Dixon-Shane Inc	17236-0467-01
100's	$43.95	GENERIC, Mylan Pharmaceuticals Inc	00378-3005-01
100's	$46.10	GENERIC, Geneva Pharmaceuticals	00781-2228-01
100's	$46.59	GENERIC, Major Pharmaceuticals Inc	00904-2957-61
100's	$47.48	GENERIC, Udl Laboratories Inc	51079-0588-20
100's	$60.76	GENERIC, Dixon-Shane Inc	17236-0467-11
100's	$60.80	GENERIC, Geneva Pharmaceuticals	00781-2228-13
100's	$102.24	NAVANE, Pfizer U.S. Pharmaceuticals	00049-5730-66
Capsule - Oral - 10 mg			
30's	$24.02	GENERIC, Heartland Healthcare Services	61392-0791-30
30's	$24.02	GENERIC, Heartland Healthcare Services	61392-0791-39
31's	$24.82	GENERIC, Heartland Healthcare Services	61392-0791-31
32's	$25.63	GENERIC, Heartland Healthcare Services	61392-0791-32
45's	$36.04	GENERIC, Heartland Healthcare Services	61392-0791-45
60's	$48.05	GENERIC, Heartland Healthcare Services	61392-0791-60
90's	$72.07	GENERIC, Heartland Healthcare Services	61392-0791-90
100's	$27.17	GENERIC, Us Trading Corporation	56126-0381-11
100's	$40.65	FEDERAL UPPER LIMIT, H.C.F.A. F F P	99999-2343-08
100's	$47.15	GENERIC, Major Pharmaceuticals Inc	00904-2893-60
100's	$47.15	GENERIC, Major Pharmaceuticals Inc	00904-2958-60
100's	$52.70	GENERIC, Qualitest Products Inc	00603-6021-21
100's	$55.80	GENERIC, Aligen Independent Laboratories Inc	00405-5007-01
100's	$55.95	GENERIC, Watson/Rugby Laboratories Inc	00536-4954-01
100's	$58.25	GENERIC, Major Pharmaceuticals Inc	00904-2958-61
100's	$59.93	GENERIC, Moore, H.L. Drug Exchange Inc	00839-7291-06
100's	$60.15	GENERIC, Dixon-Shane Inc	17236-0468-01
100's	$61.95	GENERIC, Mylan Pharmaceuticals Inc	00378-5010-01
100's	$65.00	GENERIC, Geneva Pharmaceuticals	00781-2229-01
100's	$66.95	GENERIC, Udl Laboratories Inc	51079-0589-20
100's	$80.08	GENERIC, Dixon-Shane Inc	17236-0468-11
100's	$80.10	GENERIC, Geneva Pharmaceuticals	00781-2229-13
100's	$132.08	NAVANE, Pfizer U.S. Pharmaceuticals	00049-5740-66
Capsule - Oral - 20 mg			
100's	$5.07	GENERIC, Us Trading Corporation	56126-0416-11
100's	$197.75	NAVANE, Pfizer U.S. Pharmaceuticals	00049-5770-66
Concentrate - Oral - 5 mg/ml			
30 ml	$11.48	GENERIC, Alpharma Uspd Makers Of Barre and Nmc	00472-1457-91
30 ml	$11.90	GENERIC, Major Pharmaceuticals Inc	00904-2899-30
120 ml	$36.00	GENERIC, Roxane Laboratories Inc	00054-3872-50
120 ml	$38.44	GENERIC, Alpharma Uspd Makers Of Barre and Nmc	00472-1457-94
120 ml	$40.10	GENERIC, Major Pharmaceuticals Inc	00904-2899-20
120 ml	$42.35	GENERIC, Ivax Corporation	00182-6112-71
120 ml	$51.92	GENERIC, Teva Pharmaceuticals Usa	00093-9613-12

PRODUCT LISTING - EQUIVALENTS NOT AVAILABLE

Capsule - Oral - 2 mg			
100's	$11.33	GENERIC, Physicians Total Care	54868-2343-00
Capsule - Oral - 5 mg			
100's	$15.57	GENERIC, Physicians Total Care	54868-2358-00

Tiagabine Hydrochloride *(003354)*

Categories: Seizures, partial; FDA Approved 1997 Sep; Pregnancy Category C
Drug Classes: Anticonvulsants
Brand Names: Gabitril
Foreign Brand Availability: Gabatril (Mexico)
Cost of Therapy: $138.00 (Epilepsy; Gabitril; 16 mg; 2 tablets/day; 30 day supply)

DESCRIPTION

Gabitril is an antiepilepsy drug available as 4, 12, 16, and 20 mg tablets for oral administration. Its chemical name is (-)-(R)-1-[4,4-bis(3-methyl-2-thienyl)-3-butenyl] nipecotic acid hydrochloride, its molecular formula is $C_{20}H_{25}NO_2S_2 \cdot HCl$, and its molecular weight is 412.0. Tiagabine HCl is a white to off-white, odorless, crystalline powder. It is insoluble in heprane, sparingly soluble in water, and soluble in aqueous base.

Gabitril Inactive Ingredients: Ascorbic acid, colloidal silicon dioxide, crospovidone, hydrogenated vegetable oil wax, hydroxypropyl cellulose, hydroxypropyl methylcellulose, lactose, magnesium stearate, microcrystalline cellulose, pregelatinized starch, stearic acid, and titanium dioxide. In addition, individual tablets contain: *4 mg Tablets:* D&C yellow no. 10; *12 mg Tablets:* D&C yellow no. 10 and FD&C blue no. 1; *16 mg Tablets:* D&C blue no. 2; *20 mg Tablets:* D&C red no. 30.

CLINICAL PHARMACOLOGY

MECHANISM OF ACTION

The precise mechanism by which tiagabine exerts its antiseizure effect is unknown, although it is believed to be related to its ability, documented in *in vitro* experiments, to enhance the activity of gamma aminobutyric acid (GABA), the major inhibitory neurotransmitter in the central nervous system. These experiments have shown that tiagabine binds to recognition sites associated with the GABA uptake carrier. It is thought that, by this action, tiagabine blocks GABA uptake into presynaptic neurons, permitting more GABA to be available for receptor binding on the surfaces of post-synaptic. Inhibition of GABA uptake has been shown for synaptosomes, neuronal cell cultures, and glial cell cultures. In rat-derived hippocampal slices, tiagabine has been shown to prolong GABA-mediated inhibitory post-synaptic potentials. Tiagabine increases the amount of GABA available in the extracellular space of the globus pallidus, ventral palladium, and substantia nigra in rats at the ED_{50} and ED_{85} doses for inhibition of pentylenetetrazol (PTZ)-induced tonic seizures. This suggests that tiagabine prevents the propagation of neural impulses that contribute to seizures by a GABA-ergic action.

Tiagabine has shown efficacy in several animal models of seizures. It is effective against the tonic phase of subcutaneous PTZ-induced seizures in mice and rats, seizures induced by the proconvulsant DMCM in mice, audiogenic seizures in genetically epilepsy-prone rats (GEPR), and amygdala-kindled seizures in rats. Tiagabine has little efficacy against maximal electroshock seizures in rats and is only partially effective against subcutaneous PTZ-induced clonic seizures in mice, picrotoxin-induced tonic seizures in the mouse, bicuculline-induced seizures in the rat, and photic seizures in photosensitive baboons. Tiagabine produces a biphasic dose-response curve against PTZ and DMCM-induced convulsions with attenuated effectiveness at higher doses.

Based on *in vitro* binding studies, tiagabine does not significantly inhibit the uptake of dopamine, norepinephrine, serotonin, glutamate, or choline and shows little or no binding to dopamine D1 and D2 muscarinic, serotonin $5HT_{1A}$, $5HT_2$, and $5HT_3$, beta-1 and 2 adrenergic, alpha-1 and alpha-2 adrenergic, histamine H2 and H3, adenosine A_1 and A_2, opiate μ and K_1, NMDA glutamate, and $GABA_A$ receptors at 100μM. It also lacks significant affinity for sodium or calcium channels. Tiagabine binds to histamine H1, serotonin $5HT_{1B}$, benzodiazepine, and chloride channel receptors at concentrations 20 to 400 times those inhibiting the uptake of GABA.

PHARMACOKINETICS

Tiagabine is well absorbed, with food slowing absorption rate but not altering the extent of absorption. Although its elimination half-life is 7 to 9 hours in normal volunteers, it is only 4 to 7 hours in patients receiving hepatic enzyme-inducing drugs (carbamazepine, phenytoin, primidone, and phenobarbital). In clinical trials, most patients were induced.

Absorption and Distribution

Absorption of tiagabine is rapid, with peak plasma concentrations occurring at approximately 45 minutes following an oral dose in the fasting state. Tiagabine is nearly completely absorbed (>95%), with an absolute oral bioavailability of about 90%. A high fat meal decreases the rate (mean T_{max} was prolonged to 2.5 hours, and mean C_{max} was reduced by about 40%) but not the extent (AUC) of tiagabine absorption. In all clinical trials, tiagabine was given with meals.

The pharmacokinetics of tiagabine are linear over the single dose range of 2-24 mg. Following multi-dosing, steady state is achieved within 2 days.

Tiagabine is 96% bound to human plasma proteins, mainly to serum albumin and α1-acid glycoprotein over the concentration range of 10 to 10,000 ng/ml. While the relationship between tiagabine plasma concentrations and clinical response is not currently understood, trough plasma concentrations observed in controlled clinical trials at doses from 30 to 56 mg/day ranged from <1 ng/ml to 234 ng/ml.

Metabolism and Elimination

Although the metabolism of tiagabine has not been fully elucidated, *in vivo* and *in vitro* studies suggest that at least two metabolic pathways for tiagabine have been identified in

T

humans: (1) thiophene ring oxidation leading to the formation of 5-oxo-tiagabine; and (2) glucuronidation. The 5-oxo-tiagabine metabolite does not contribute to the pharmacologic activity of tiagabine.

Based on *in vitro* data, tiagabine is likely to be metabolized primarily by the 3A isoform subfamily of hepatic cytochrome P450 (CYP 3A), although contributions to the metabolism of tiagabine from CYP 1A2, CYP 2D6 or CYP 2C19 have not been excluded.

Approximately 2% of an oral dose of tiagabine is excreted unchanged, with 25% and 63% of the remaining dose excreted into the urine and feces, respectively, primarily as metabolites, at least 2 of which have not been identified. The mean systemic plasma clearance is 109 ml/min (CV=23%) and the average elimination half-life for tiagabine in healthy subjects ranged from 7-9 hours. The elimination half-life decreased by 50 to 65% in hepatic enzyme-induced patients with epilepsy compared to uninduced patients with epilepsy.

A diurnal effect on the pharmacokinetics of tiagabine was observed. Mean steady-state C_{min} values were 40% lower in the evening than in the morning. Tiagabine steady-state AUC values were also found to be 15% lower following the evening tiagabine dose compared to the AUC following the morning dose.

SPECIAL POPULATIONS

Renal Insufficiency

The pharmacokinetics of total and unbound tiagabine were similar in subjects with normal renal function (creatinine clearance >80 ml/min) and in subjects with mild (creatinine clearance 40 to 80 ml/min), moderate (creatinine clearance 20 to 39 ml/min), or severe (creatinine clearance 5 to 19 ml/min) renal impairment. The pharmacokinetics of total and unbound tiagabine were also unaffected in subjects with renal failure requiring hemodialysis.

Hepatic Insufficiency

In patients with moderate hepatic impairment (Child-Pugh Class B), clearance of unbound tiagabine was reduced by about 60%. Patients with impaired liver function may require reduced initial and maintenance doses of tiagabine and/or longer dosing intervals compared to patients with normal hepatic function (see PRECAUTIONS).

Geriatric

The pharmacokinetic profile of tiagabine was similar in healthy elderly and healthy young adults.

Pediatric

Tiagabine has not been investigated in adequate and well-controlled clinical trials in patients below the age of 12. The apparent clearance and volume of distribution of tiagabine per unit body surface area or per kg were fairly similar in 25 children (age: 3 to 10 years) and in adults taking enzyme-inducing antiepilepsy drugs ([AEDS] *e.g.,* carbamazepine or phenytoin). In children who were taking a non-inducing AED (*e.g.,* valproate), the clearance of tiagabine based upon body weight and body surface area was 2- and 1.5-fold higher, respectively, than in uninduced adults with epilepsy.

Gender, Race, and Cigarette Smoking

No specific pharmacokinetic studies were conducted to investigate the effect of gender, race, and cigarette smoking on the disposition of tiagabine. Retrospective pharmacokinetic analyses, however, suggest that there is no clinically important difference between the clearance of tiagabine in males and females, when adjusted for body weight. Population pharmacokinetic analyses indicated that tiagabine clearance values were not significantly different in Caucasian (n=463), Black (n=23), or Hispanic (n=17) patients with epilepsy and that tiagabine clearance values were not significantly affected by tobacco use.

INTERACTIONS WITH OTHER ANTIEPILEPSY DRUGS

The clearance of tiagabine is affected by the co-administration of hepatic enzyme-inducing antiepilepsy drugs. Tiagabine is eliminated more rapidly in patients who have been taking hepatic enzyme-inducing drugs (*e.g.,* carbamazepine, phenytoin, primidone, and phenobarbital) than in patients not receiving such treatment (see DRUG INTERACTIONS).

INDICATIONS AND USAGE

Tiagabine is indicated as adjunctive therapy in adults and children 12 years and older in the treatment of partial seizures.

CONTRAINDICATIONS

Tiagabine is contraindicated in patients who have demonstrated hypersensitivity to the drug or its ingredients.

WARNINGS

WITHDRAWAL SEIZURES

As a rule, antiepilepsy drugs should not be abruptly discontinued because of the possibility of increasing seizure frequency. In a placebo-controlled, double-blind, dose-response study designed, in part, to investigate the capacity of tiagabine to induce withdrawal seizures, study drug was tapered over a 4 week period after 16 weeks of treatment. Patients' seizure frequency during this 4 week withdrawal period was compared to their baseline seizure frequency (before study drug). For each partial seizure type, for all partial seizure types combined, and for secondarily generalized tonic-clonic seizures, more patients experienced increases in their seizure frequencies during the withdrawal period in the three tiagabine groups than in the placebo group. The increase in seizure frequency was not affected by dose. Tiagabine should be withdrawn gradually to minimize the potential of increased seizure frequency, unless safety concerns require a more rapid withdrawal.

COGNITIVE/NEUROPSYCHIATRIC ADVERSE EVENTS

Adverse events most often associated with the use of tiagabine were related to the central nervous system. The most significant of these can be classified into 2 general categories: (1) impaired concentration, speech or language problems, and confusion (effects on thought processes); and (2) somnolence and fatigue (effects on level of consciousness). The majority of these events were mild to moderate. In controlled clinical trials, these events led to discontinuation of treatment with tiagabine in 6% (31 of 494) of patients compared to 2% (5 of 275) of the placebo-treated patients. A total of 1.6% (8 of 494) of the tiagabine treated patients in the controlled trials were hospitalized secondary to the occurrence of these events compared to 0% of the placebo treated patients. Some of these events were dose related and usually began during initial titration.

Patients with a history of spike and wave discharges on EEG have been reported to have exacerbations of their EEG abnormalities associated with these cognitive/neuropsychiatric events. This raises the possibility that these clinical events may, in some cases, be a manifestation of underlying seizure activity (see Laboratory Tests, PRECAUTIONS, EEG). In the documented cases of spike and wave discharges on EEG with cognitive/neuropsychiatric events, patients usually continued tiagabine, but required dosage adjustment.

STATUS EPILEPTICUS

In the three double-blind, placebo-controlled, parallel-group studies (Studies 1, 2, and 3), the incidence of any type of status epilepticus (simple, complex, or generalized tonic-clonic) in patients receiving tiagabine was 0.8% (4 of 494 patients) versus 0.7% (2 of 275 patients) receiving placebo. Among the patients treated with tiagabine across all epilepsy studies (controlled and uncontrolled), 5% had some form of status epilepticus. Of the 5%, 57% of patients experienced complex partial status epilepticus. A critical risk factor for status epilepticus was the presence of a previous history: 33% of patients with a history of status epilepticus had recurrence during tiagabine treatment. Because adequate information about the incidence of status epilepticus in a similar population of patients with epilepsy who have not received treatment with tiagabine is not available, it is impossible to state whether or not treatment with tiagabine is associated with a higher or lower rate of status epilepticus than would be expected to occur in a similar population not treated with tiagabine.

SUDDEN UNEXPECTED DEATH IN EPILEPSY (SUDEP)

There have been as many as 10 cases of sudden unexpected deaths during the clinical development of tiagabine among 2531 patients with epilepsy (3831 patient-years of exposure).

This represents an estimated incidence of 0.0026 deaths per patient-year. This rate is within the range of estimates for the incidence of sudden and unexpected deaths in patients with epilepsy not receiving tiagabine (ranging from 0.0005 for the general population with epilepsy, 0.003 to 0.004 for clinical trial populations similar to that in the clinical development program for tiagabine, to 0.005 for patients with refractory epilepsy). The estimated SUDEP rates in patients receiving tiagabine are also similar to those observed in patients receiving other antiepilepsy drugs, chemically unrelated to tiagabine, that underwent clinical testing in similar populations at about the same time. This evidence suggests that the SUDEP rates reflect population rates, not a drug effect.

PRECAUTIONS

GENERAL

Use in Non-Induced Patients

Virtually all experience with tiagabine has been obtained in patients receiving at least one concomitant enzyme-inducing antiepilepsy drug (AED). Use in non-induced patients (*e.g.,* patients receiving valproate monotherapy) may require lower doses or a slower dose titration of tiagabine for clinical response. Patients taking a combination of inducing and non-inducing drugs (*e.g.,* carbamazepine and valproate) should be considered to be induced.

Generalized Weakness

Moderately severe to incapacitating generalized weakness has been reported following administration of tiagabine in 28 of 2531 (approximately 1%) patients with epilepsy. The weakness resolved in all cases after a reduction in dose or discontinuation of tiagabine.

Binding in the Eye and Other Melanin-Containing Tissues

When dogs received a single dose of radiolabeled tiagabine, there was evidence of residual binding in the retina and uvea after 3 weeks (the latest time point measured). Although not directly measured, melanin binding is suggested. The ability of available tests to detect potentially adverse consequences, if any, of the binding of tiagabine to melanin-containing tissue is unknown and there was no systematic monitoring for relevant ophthalmological changes during the clinical development of tiagabine. However, long- term (up to 1 year) toxicological studies of tiagabine in dogs showed no treatment-related ophthalmoscopic changes and macro- and microscopic examinations of the eye were unremarkable. Accordingly, although there are no specific recommendations for periodic ophthalmologic monitoring, prescribers should be aware of the possibility of long-term ophthalmologic effects.

Use in Hepatically-Impaired Patients

Because the clearance of tiagabine is reduced in patients with liver disease, dosage reduction may be necessary in these patients.

Serious Rash

Four patients treated with tiagabine during the product's premarketing clinical testing developed what were considered to be serious rashes. In 2 patients, the rash was described as maculopapular; in one it was described as vesiculobullous; and in the 4th case, a diagnosis of Stevens Johnson Syndrome was made. In none of the 4 cases is it certain that tiagabine was the primary, or even a contributory, cause of the rash. Nevertheless, drug associated rash can, if extensive and serious, cause irreversible morbidity, even death.

INFORMATION FOR THE PATIENT

Patients should be instructed to take tiagabine only as prescribed.

Patients should be advised that tiagabine may cause dizziness, somnolence, and other symptoms and signs of CNS depression. Accordingly, they should be advised neither to drive nor to operate other complex machinery until they have gained sufficient experience on tiagabine to gauge whether or not it affects their mental and/or motor performance adversely. Because of possible additive depressive effects, caution should also be used when patients are taking other CNS depressants in combination with tiagabine.

Because teratogenic effects were seen in the offspring of rats exposed to maternally toxic doses of tiagabine and because experience in humans is limited, patients should be advised to notify their physicians if they become pregnant or intend to become pregnant during therapy.

Because of the possibility that tiagabine may be excreted in breast milk, patients should be advised to notify those providing care to themselves and their children if they intend to breast-feed or are breast-feeding an infant.

LABORATORY TESTS

Therapeutic Monitoring of Plasma Concentrations of Tiagabine

A therapeutic range for tiagabine plasma concentrations has not been established. In controlled trials, trough plasma concentrations observed among patients randomized to doses of tiagabine that were statistically significantly more effective than placebo ranged from <1 ng/ml to 234 ng/ml (median, 10th and 90th percentiles are 23.7 ng/ml, 5.4 ng/ml, and 69.8 ng/ml, respectively). Because of the potential for pharmacokinetic interactions between tiagabine and drugs that induce or inhibit hepatic metabolizing enzymes, it may be useful to obtain plasma levels of tiagabine before and after changes are made in the therapeutic regimen.

Clinical Chemistry and Hematology

During the development of tiagabine, no systematic abnormalities on routine laboratory testing were noted. Therefore, no specific guidance is offered regarding routine monitoring; the practitioner retains responsibility for determining how best to monitor the patient in his/her care.

EEG

Patients with a history of spike and wave discharges on EEG have been reported to have exacerbations of their EEG abnormalities associated with cognitive/neuropsychiatric events. This raises the possibility that these clinical events may, in some cases, be a manifestation of underlying seizure activity (see WARNINGS, Cognitive/Neuropsychiatric Adverse Events). In the documented cases of spike and wave discharges on EEG with cognitive/neuropsychiatric events, patients usually continued tiagabine, but required dosage adjustment.

CARCINOGENESIS, MUTAGENESIS, AND IMPAIRMENT OF FERTILITY

Carcinogenesis

In rats, a study of the potential carcinogenicity associated with tiagabine HCl administration showed that 200 mg/kg/day (plasma exposure [AUC] 36 to 100 times that at the maximum recommended human dosage [MRHD] of 56 mg/day) for 2 years resulted in small, but statistically significant increases in the incidences of hepatocellular adenomas in females and Leydig cell tumors of the testis in males. The significance of these findings relative to the use of tiagabine in humans is unknown. The no effect dosage for induction of tumors in this study was 100 mg/kg/day (17-50 times the exposure at the MRHD). No statistically significant increases in tumor formation were noted in mice at dosages up to 250 mg/kg/day (20 times the MRHD on a mg/m^2 basis).

Mutagenesis

Tiagabine produced an increase in structural chromosome aberration frequency in human lymphocytes *in vitro* in the absence of metabolic activation. No increase in chromosomal aberration frequencies was demonstrated in this assay in the presence of metabolic activation. No evidence of genetic toxicity was found in the *in vitro* bacterial gene mutation assays, the *in vitro* HGPRT forward mutation assay in Chinese hamster lung cells, the *in vivo* mouse micronucleus test, or an unscheduled DNA synthesis assay.

Impairment of Fertility

Studies of male and female rats administered dosages of tiagabine HCl prior to and during mating, gestation, and lactation have shown no impairment of fertility at doses up to 100 mg/kg/day. This dose represents approximately 16 times the maximum recommended human dose (MRHD) of 56 mg/day, based on body surface area (mg/m^2). Lowered maternal weight gain and decreased viability and growth in the rat pups were found at 100 mg/kg, but not at 20 mg/kg/day (3 times the MRHD on a mg/m^2 basis).

PREGNANCY CATEGORY C

Tiagabine has been shown to have adverse effects on embryo-fetal development, including teratogenic effects, when administered to pregnant rats and rabbits at doses greater than the human therapeutic dose.

An increased incidence of malformed fetuses (various craniofacial, appendicular, and visceral defects) and decreased fetal weights were observed following oral administration of 100 mg/kg/day to pregnant rats during the period of organogenesis. This dose is approximately 16 times the maximum recommended human dose (MRHD) of 56 mg/day, based on body surface area (mg/m^2). Maternal toxicity (transient weight loss/reduced maternal weight gain during gestation) was associated with this dose, but there is no evidence to suggest that the teratogenic effects were secondary to the maternal effects. No adverse maternal or embryo-fetal effects were seen at a dose of 20 mg/kg/day (3 times the MRHD on a mg/m^2 basis).

Decreased maternal weight gain, increased resorption of embryos and increased incidences of fetal variations, but not malformations, were observed when pregnant rabbits were given 25 mg/kg/day (8 times the MRHD on a mg/m^2 basis) during organogenesis. The no effect level for maternal and embryo-fetal toxicity in rabbits was 5 mg/kg/day (equivalent to the MRHD on a mg/m^2 basis).

When female rats were given tiagabine 100 mg/kg/day during late gestation and throughout parturition and lactation, decreased maternal weight gain during gestation, an increase in stillbirths, and decreased postnatal offspring viability and growth were found. There are no adequate and well-controlled studies in pregnant women. Tiagabine should be used during pregnancy only if clearly needed.

T

NURSING MOTHERS

Studies in rats have shown that tiagabine HCl and/or its metabolites are excreted in the milk of that species. Levels of excretion of tiagabine and/or its metabolites in human milk have not been determined and effects on the nursing infant are unknown. Tiagabine should be used in women who are nursing only if the benefits clearly outweigh the risks.

PEDIATRIC USE

Safety and effectiveness in pediatric patients below the age of 12 have not been established. The pharmacokinetics of tiagabine were evaluated in pediatric patients age 3 to 10 years (see CLINICAL PHARMACOLOGY, Pediatric).

GERIATRIC USE

Because few patients over the age of 65 (approximately 20) were exposed to tiagabine during its clinical evaluation, no specific statements about the safety or effectiveness of tiagabine in this age group could be made.

DRUG INTERACTIONS

In evaluating the potential for interactions among co-administered antiepilepsy drugs (AEDs), whether or not an AED induces or does not induce metabolic enzymes is an important consideration. Phenytoin, phenobarbital and carbamazepine are generally classified as enzyme inducers, valproate and gabapentin are not. Tiagabine is considered to be a non-enzyme inducing AED.

The drug interaction data described in this section were obtained from studies involving either healthy subjects or patients with epilepsy.

EFFECTS OF TIAGABINE ON OTHER ANTIEPILEPSY DRUGS (AEDS)

Phenytoin: Tiagabine had no effect on the steady-state plasm concentrations of phenytoin in patients with epilepsy.

Carbamazepine: Tiagabine had no effect on the steady-state plasma concentrations of carbamazepine or its epoxide metabolite in patients with epilepsy.

Valproate: Tiagabine causes a slight decrease (about 10%) in steady-state valproate concentrations.

Phenobarbital or Primidone: No formal pharmacokinetic studies have been performed examining the addition of tiagabine to regimens containing phenobarbital or primidone. The addition of tiagabine in a limited number of patients in three well-controlled studies caused no systematic changes in phenobarbital or primidone concentrations when compared to placebo.

EFFECTS OF OTHER ANTIEPILEPSY DRUGS (AEDS) ON TIAGABINE

Carbamazepine: Population pharmacokinetic analyses indicate that tiagabine clearance is 60% greater in patients taking carbamazepine with or without other enzyme-inducing AEDs.

Phenytoin: Population pharmacokinetic analyses indicate that tiagabine clearance is 60% greater in patients taking phenytoin with or without other enzyme-inducing AEDs.

Phenobarbital or Primidone: Population pharmacokinetic analyses indicate that tiagabine clearance is 60% greater in patients taking phenobarbital or primidone with or without other enzyme-inducing AEDs.

Valproate: The addition of tiagabine to patients taking valproate chronically had no effect on tiagabine pharmacokinetics, but valproate significantly decreased tiagabine binding *in vitro* from 96.3 to 94.8%, which resulted in an increase of approximately 40% in the free tiagabine concentration. The clinical relevance of this *in vitro* finding is unknown.

INTERACTION OF TIAGABINE WITH OTHER DRUGS

Cimetidine: Co-administration of cimetidine (800 mg/day) to patients taking tiagabine chronically had no effect on tiagabine pharmacokinetics.

Theophylline: A single 10 mg dose of tiagabine did not affect the pharmacokinetics of theophylline at steady-state.

Warfarin: No significant difference were observed in the steady-state pharmacokinetics of R-warfarin or S-warfarin with the addition of tiagabine given as a single dose. Prothrombin times were not affected by tiagabine.

Digoxin: Concomitant administration of tiagabine did not affect the steady-state pharmacokinetics of digoxin or the mean daily trough serum level of digoxin.

Ethanol or Triazolam: No significant differences were observed in the pharmacokinetics of triazolam (0.125 mg) and tiagabine (10 mg) when given together as a single dose. The pharmacokinetics of ethanol were not affected by multiple-dose administration of tiagabine. Tiagabine has shown no clinically important potentiation of the pharmacodynamic effects of triazolam or alcohol. Because of the possible additive effects of drugs that may depress the nervous system, ethanol or triazolam should be used cautiously in combination of tiagabine.

Oral Contraceptives: Multiple dose administration of tiagabine (8 mg/day monotherapy) did not alter the pharmacokinetics of oral contraceptives in healthy women of child-bearing age.

Antipyrine: Antipyrine pharmacokinetics were not significantly different before and after tiagabine multiple-dose regimens. This indicates that tiagabine does not cause induction or inhibition of the hepatic microsomal enzyme systems responsible for the metabolism of antipyrine.

ADVERSE REACTIONS

The most commonly observed adverse events in placebo-controlled, parallel-group, add-on epilepsy trials associated with the use of tiagabine in combination with other antiepilepsy drugs not seen at an equivalent frequency among placebo-treated patients were dizziness/light-headedness, asthenia/lack of energy, somnolence, nausea, nervousness/irritability, tremor, abdominal pain, and thinking abnormal/difficulty with concentration or attention.

Approximately 21% of the 2531 patients who received tiagabine in clinical trials of epilepsy discontinued treatment because of an adverse event. The adverse events most commonly associated with discontinuation were dizziness (1.7%), somnolence (1.6%), depression (1.3%), confusion (1.1%), and asthenia (1.1%).

In Studies 1 and 2 (US studies), the double-blind, placebo-controlled, parallel-group, add-on studies, the proportion of patients who discontinued treatment because of adverse events was 11% for the group treated with tiagabine and 6% for the placebo group. The most common adverse events considered the primary reason for discontinuation were confusion (1.2%), somnolence (1.0%), and ataxia (1.0%).

ADVERSE EVENT INCIDENCE IN CONTROLLED CLINICAL TRIALS

TABLE 4 lists treatment-emergent signs and symptoms that occurred in at least 1% of patients treated with tiagabine for epilepsy participating in parallel-group, placebo-controlled trials and were numerically more common in the tiagabine group. In these studies, either tiagabine or placebo was added to the patient's current antiepilepsy drug therapy. Adverse events were usually mild or moderate in intensity.

The prescriber should be aware that these figures, obtained when tiagabine was added to concurrent antiepilepsy drug therapy, cannot be use to predict the frequency of adverse events in the course of usual medical practice when patient characteristics and other factors may differ from those prevailing during clinical studies. Similarly, the cited frequencies cannot be directly compared with figures obtained from other clinical investigation involving different treatments, uses, or investigators. An inspection of these frequencies, however, does provide the prescribing physician with one basis to estimate the relative contribution of drug and non-drug factors to the adverse event incidences in the population studied.

TABLE 4 *Treatment-Emergent Adverse Event† Incidence in Parallel-Group Placebo-Controlled, Add-On Trials*

(Events in at least 1% of patients treated with tiagabine and numerically more frequent than in the placebo group)

Body System COSTART	Tiagabine n=494	Placebo n=275
Body as a Whole		
Abdominal pain	7%	3%
Pain (unspecified)	5%	3%
Cardiovascular		
Vasodilation	2%	1%
Digestive		
Nausea	11%	9%
Diarrhea	7%	3%
Vomiting	7%	4%
Increased appetite	2%	0%
Mouth alceration	1%	0%
Musculoskeletal		
Myasthenia	1%	0%
Nervous System		
Dizziness	27%	15%
Asthenia	20%	14%
Somnolence	18%	15%
Nervousness	10%	3%
Tremor	9%	3%
Diffuculty with concentration/attention*	6%	2%
Insomnia	6%	4%
Ataxia	5%	3%
Confusion	5%	3%
Speech disorder	4%	2%
Difficulty with memory*	4%	3%
Paresthesia	4%	2%
Depression	3%	1%
Emotional lability	3%	2%
Abnormal gait	3%	2%
Hostility	2%	1%
Nystagmus	2%	1%
Language problems*	2%	0%
Agitation	1%	0%
Respiratory System		
Pharyngitis	7%	4%
Cough increased	4%	3%
Skin and Appendages		
Rash	5%	4%
Pruritus	2%	0%

* COSTART term substituted with a more clinically descriptive term
† Patients in these add-on studies were receiving one to three concomitant enzyme-inducing antiepilepsy drugs in addition to tiagabine or placebo. Patients may have reported multiple adverse experiences; thus, patients may be included in more than one category.

Other events reported by 1% or more of patients treated with tiagabine but equally or more frequent in the placebo group were: accidental injury, chest pain, constipation, flu syndrome, rhinitis, anorexia, back pain, dry mouth, flatulence, ecchymosis, twitching, fever, amblyopia, conjunctivitis, urinary tract infection, urinary frequency, infection, dyspepsia, gastroenteritis, nausea and vomiting, myalgia, diplopia, headache, anxiety, acne, sinusitis, and incoordination.

Study 1 was a dose-response study including doses of 32 and 56 mg. TABLE 5 shows adverse events reported at a rate of 5% in at least one tiagabine group and more frequent than in the placebo group. Among these events, tremor, difficulty with concentration/attention, and perhaps asthenia exhibited a positive relationship to dose.

The effects of tiagabine in relation to those of placebo on the incidence of adverse events and the types of adverse events reported were independent of age, weight, and gender. Because only 10% of patients were non-Caucasian in parallel-group, placebo-controlled trials, there is insufficient data to support a statement regarding the distribution of adverse experience reports by race.

TABLE 5 *Treatment-Emergent Adverse Event† in Study 1*

(Events in at least 5% of patients treated with Tiagabine 32 or 56 mg and numerically more frequent than in the placebo group)

Body System COSTART	Tiagabine 56 mg n=57	 32 mg n=88	Placebo n=91
Body as a Whole			
Accidental injury	21%	15%	20%
Infection	19%	10%	12%
Flu syndrome	9%	6%	3%
Pain	7%	2%	3%
Abdominal pain	5%	7%	4%
Digestive			
Diarrhea	2%	10%	6%
Hemic and Lymphatic			
Ecchymosis	0%	6%	1%
Musculoskeletal			
Myalgia	5%	2%	3%
Nervous System			
Dizziness	28%	31%	12%
Asthenia	23%	18%	15%
Tremor	21%	14%	1%
Somnolence	19%	21%	17%
Nervousness	14%	11%	6%
Difficulty with concentration/attention*	14%	7%	3%
Ataxia	9%	6%	6%
Depression	7%	1%	0%
Insomnia	5%	6%	3%
Abnormal gait	5%	5%	3%
Hostility	5%	5%	2%
Respiratory System			
Pharyngitis	7%	8%	6%
Special Senses			
Amblyopia	4%	9%	8%
Urogenital			
Urinary tract infection	5%	0%	2%

* COSTART term substituted with a more clinically descriptive term
† Patients in this study were receiving one to three concomitant enzyme-inducing antiepilepsy drugs in addition to tiagabine or placebo. Patients may have reported multiple adverse experiences; thus, patients may be included in more than one category.

OTHER ADVERSE EVENTS OBSERVED DURING ALL CLINICAL TRIALS

Tiagabine has been administered to 2531 patients during all Phase 2/3 clinical trials, only some of which were placebo-controlled. During these trials, all adverse events were recorded by the clinical investigators using terminology of their own choosing. To provide a meaningful estimate of the proportion of individuals having adverse events, similar types of events were grouped into a smaller number of standardized categories using modified COSTART dictionary terminology. These categories are used in the listing below. The frequencies presented represent the proportion of the 2531 patients exposed to tiagabine who experienced events of the type cited on at least one occasion while receiving tiagabine. All reported events are included except those already listed above, events seen only three times or fewer (unless potentially important), events very unlikely to be drug-related, and those too general to be informative. Events are included without regard to determination of a causal relationship to tiagabine.

Events further classified within body system categories and enumerated in order of decreasing frequency using the following definitions: *frequent* adverse events are defined as those occurring in at least 1/100 patients; *infrequent* adverse events are those occurring in 1/100 to 1/1000 patients; *rare* events are those occurring in fewer than 1/1000 patients.

Body as a Whole: *Frequent:* Allergic reaction, chest pain, chills, cyst, neck pain, and malaise. *Infrequent:* Abscess, cellulitis, facial edema, halitosis, hernia, neck rigidity, neoplasm, pelvic pain, photosensitivity reaction, sepsis, sudden death, and suicide attempt.

Cardiovascular System: *Frequent:* Hypertension, palpitation, syncope, and tachycardia. *Infrequent:* Angina pectoris, cerebral ischemia, electrocardiogram abnormal, hemorrhage, hypotension, myocardial infarct, pallor, peripheral vascular disorder, phlebitis, postural hypotension, and thrombophlebitis.

Digestive System: *Frequent:* Gingivitis and stomatitis. *Infrequent:* Abnormal stools, cholecystitis, cholelithiasis, dysphagia, eructation, esophagitis, fecal incontinence, gastritis, gastrointestinal hemorrhage, glossitis, gum hyperplasia, hepatomegaly, increased salivation, liver function tests abnormal, melena, periodontal abscess, rectal hemorrhage, thirst, tooth caries, and ulcerative stomatitis.

Endocrine System: *Infrequent:* Goiter and hypothyroidism.

Hemic and Lymphatic System: *Frequent:* Lymphadenopathy. *Infrequent:* Anemia, erythrocytes abnormal, leukopenia, petechia, and thrombocytopenia.

Metabolic and Nutritional: *Frequent:* Edema, peripheral edema, weight gain, and weight loss. *Infrequent:* Dehydration, hypercholesteremia, hyperglycemia, hyperlipemia, hypoglycemia, hypokalemia, and hyponatremia.

Musculoskeletal System: *Frequent:* Arthralgia. *Infrequent:* Arthritis, arthrosis, bursitis, generalized spasm, and tendinous contracture.

Nervous System: *Frequent:* Depersonalization, dysarthria, euphoria, hallucination, hyperkinesia, hypertonia, hyperesthesia, hypokinesia, hypotonia, migraine, myoclonus, paranoid reaction, personality disorder, reflexes decreased, stupor, twitching, and vertigo. *Infrequent:* Abnormal dreams, apathy, choreoathetosis, circumoral paresthesia, CNS neoplasm, coma, delusions, dry mouth, dystonia, encephalopathy, hemiplegia, leg cramps, libido increased, libido decreased, movement disorder, neuritis, neurosis, paralysis, peripheral neuritis, psychosis, reflexes increased, and urinary retention.

T

Respiratory System: Frequent: Bronchitis, dyspnea, epistaxis, and pneumonia. *Infrequent:* Apnea, asthma, hemoptysis, hiccups, hyperventilation, laryngitis, respiratory disorder, and voice alteration.

Skin and Appendages: Frequent: Alopecia, dry skin, and sweating. *Infrequent:* Contact dermatitis, eczema, exfoliative dermatitis, furunculosis, herpes simplex, herpes zoster, hirsutism, maculopapular rash, psoriasis, skin benign neoplasm, skin carcinoma, skin discoloration, skin nodules, skin ulcer, subcutaneous nodule, urticaria, and vesiculobullous rash.

Special Senses: Frequent: Abnormal vision, ear pain, otitis media, and tinnitus. *Infrequent:* Blepharitis, blindness, deafness, eye pain, hyperacusis, keratoconjunctivitis, otitis externa, parosmia, photophobia, taste loss, taste perversion, and visual field defect.

Urogenital System: Frequent: Dysmenorrhea, dysuria, metrorrhagia, urinary incontinence, and vaginitis. *Infrequent:* Abortion, amenorrhea, breast enlargement, breast pain, cystitis, fibrocystic breast, hematuria, impotence, kidney failure, menorrhagia, nocturia, papanicolaou smear suspicious, polyuria, pyelonephritis, salpingitis, urethritis, urinary urgency, and vaginal hemorrhage.

DOSAGE AND ADMINISTRATION

Tiagabine is recommended as adjunctive therapy in patients 12 years and older. Tiagabine is given orally and should be taken with food.

Adequate and controlled clinical studies with tiagabine were conducted in patients taking enzyme-inducing AEDs (*e.g.*, phenytoin, carbamazepine, and barbiturates). Patients taking only non-enzyme-inducing AEDs (*e.g.*, valproate, gabapentin, and lamotrigine) may require lower doses or a slower titration of tiagabine for clinical response.

ADULTS AND ADOLESCENTS 12 YEARS OR OLDER

In adolescents 12-18 years old, tiagabine should be initiated at 4 mg once daily. Modification of concomitant antiepilepsy drugs is not necessary, unless clinically indicated. The total daily dose of tiagabine may be increased by 4 mg at the beginning of Week 2. Thereafter, the total daily dose may be increased by 4-8 mg at weekly intervals until clinical response is achieved or up to 32 mg/day. The total daily dose should be given in divided doses 2-4 times daily. Doses above 32 mg/day have been tolerated in a small number of adolescent patients for a relatively short duration.

In adults, tiagabine should be initiated at 4 mg once daily. Modification of concomitant antiepilepsy drugs is not necessary, unless clinically indicated. The total daily dose of tiagabine may be increased by 4-8 mg at weekly intervals until clinical response is achieved or up to 56 mg/day. The total daily dose should be given in divided doses 2-4 times daily. Doses above 56 mg/day have not been systematically evaluated in adequate well-controlled trials.

Experience is limited in patients taking total daily doses above 32 mg/day using twice daily dosing. A typical dosing titration regimen for patients taking enzyme-inducing AEDs is provided in TABLE 6.

TABLE 6 *Typical Dosing Titration Regimen for Patients Taking Enzyme-Inducing AEDs*

Week	Initiation and Titration Schedule	Total Daily Dose
1	Initiate at 4 mg once daily	4 mg/day
2	Increase total daily dose by 4 mg	8 mg/day (in 2 divided doses)
3	Increase total daily dose by 4 mg	12 mg/day (in 3 divided doses)
4	Increase total daily dose by 4 mg	16 mg/day (in 2-4 divided doses)
5	Increase total daily dose by 4-8 mg	20-24 mg/day (in 2-4 divided doses)
6	Increase total daily dose by 4-8 mg	24-32 mg/day (in 2-4 divided doses)
Usual Adult Maintenance Dose: 32-56 mg/day in 2-4 divided doses		

ANIMAL PHARMACOLOGY

In repeat dose toxicology studies, dogs receiving daily oral doses of 5 mg/kg/day or greater experienced unexpected CNS effects throughout the study. These effects occurred acutely and included marked sedation and apparent visual impairment which was characterized by a lack of awareness of objects, failure to fix on and follow moving objects, and absence of a blink reaction. Plasma exposures (AUCs) at 5 mg/kg/day were equal to those in humans receiving the maximum recommended daily human dose of 56 mg/day. The effects were reversible upon cessation of treatment and were not associated with any observed structural abnormality. The implications of these findings for humans are unknown.

HOW SUPPLIED

Gabitril Filmtab tablets are available in four dosage strengths:

4 mg: Yellow, round tablets, debossed with the Abbott symbol on one side and the Abbo-Code FK on the opposite side.

12 mg: Green, ovaloid tablets, debossed with the Abbott symbol on one side and the Abbo-Code FL on the opposite side.

16 mg: Blue, ovaloid tablets, debossed with the Abbott symbol on one side and the Abbo-Code FM on the opposite side.

20 mg: Pink, ovaloid tablets, debossed with the Abbott symbol on one side and the Abbo-Code FN on the opposite side.

Storage: Store tablets at controlled room temperature, between 20-25°C (68-77°F). Protect from light and moisture.

PRODUCT LISTING - EQUIVALENTS NOT AVAILABLE

Tablet - Oral - 2 mg
100's $145.00 GABITRIL, Cephalon, Inc 63459-0402-01
Tablet - Oral - 4 mg
100's $145.00 GABITRIL, Cephalon, Inc 63459-0404-01
Tablet - Oral - 12 mg
100's $194.00 GABITRIL, Cephalon, Inc 63459-0412-01
Tablet - Oral - 16 mg
100's $230.00 GABITRIL, Abbott Pharmaceutical 00074-3960-13
100's $268.00 GABITRIL, Cephalon, Inc 63459-0416-01
Tablet - Oral - 20 mg
100's $218.75 GABITRIL, Abbott Pharmaceutical 00074-3984-13

Ticarcillin Disodium (002352)

For related information, see the comparative table section in Appendix A.

Categories: Abscess, lung; Abscess, pelvic; Bacteremia; Empyema; Endometritis; Infection, intra-abdominal; Infection, lower respiratory tract; Infection, skin and skin structures; Infection, urinary tract; Pelvic inflammatory disease; Peritonitis; Pneumonitis; Salpingitis; Septicemia; FDA Approved 1976 Nov; Pregnancy Category B

Drug Classes: Antibiotics, penicillins

Brand Names: Ticar

Foreign Brand Availability: Ticarcin (Korea); Ticarpen (Czech-Republic; Netherlands; Spain); Triacilline (Belgium)

Cost of Therapy: $456.00 (Infection; Ticar Injection; 3 g; 12 g/day; 10 day supply)

DESCRIPTION

Ticarcillin disodium is a semisynthetic injectable penicillin derived from the penicillin nucleus, 6-aminopenicillanic acid. Chemically, it is *N*-(2-Carboxy-3,3-dimethyl-7-oxo-4-thia-1-azabicyclo[3.2.0]hept-6-yl)-3-thiophenemalonamic acid disodium salt.

It is supplied as a white to pale yellow powder for reconstitution. The reconstituted solution is clear, colorless or pale yellow, having a pH of 6.0-8.0. Ticarcillin is very soluble in water, its solubility is greater than 600 mg/ml.

Storage: Store dry powder at room temperature or below.

CLINICAL PHARMACOLOGY

ACTIONS

Ticarcillin is not absorbed orally, therefore, it must be given intravenously or intramuscularly. Following intramuscular administration, peak serum concentrations occur within ½-1 hour. Somewhat higher and more prolonged serum levels can be achieved with the concurrent administration of probenecid.

The minimum inhibitory concentrations (MICs) for many strains of *Pseudomonas* are relatively high by usual standards; serum levels of 60 μg/ml or greater are required. However, the low degree of toxicity of ticarcillin permits the use of doses large enough to achieve inhibitory levels for these strains in serum or tissues. Other susceptible organisms usually require serum levels in the 10-25 μg/ml range (see TABLE 1).

TABLE 1 *Ticarcillin Serum Levels μg/ml*

Dosage	Route	¼ h	½ h	1 h	2 h	3 h	4 h	6 h
Adults:								
500 mg	IM	—	7.7	8.6	6.0	4.0	—	2.9
1 g	IM	—	31.0	18.7	15.7	9.7	—	3.4
2 g	IM	—	63.6	39.7	32.3	18.9	—	3.4
3 g	IV	190.0	140.0	107.0	52.2	31.3	13.8	4.2
5 g	IV	327.0	280.0	175.0	106.0	63.0	28.5	9.6
3+ g	IV							
		223.0	166.0	123.0	78.0	54.0	35.4	17.1
1 g Probenecid	Oral							
Neonates:								
		½ h	**1 h**	**1½ h**	**2 h**	**4 h**	**8 h**	
50 mg/kg	IM	64.0	70.7	63.7	60.1	33.2	11.6	

As with other penicillins, ticarcillin is eliminated by glomerular filtration and tubular secretion. It is not highly bound to serum protein (approximately 45%) and is excreted unchanged in high concentrations in the urine. After the administration of a 1-2 g IM dose, a urine concentration of 2000-4000 μg/ml may be obtained in patients with normal renal function. The serum half-life of ticarcillin in normal individuals is approximately 70 minutes.

An inverse relationship exists between serum half-life and creatinine clearance, but the dosage of tirarcillin disodium need only be adjusted in cases of severe renal impairment (see DOSAGE AND ADMINISTRATION). The administered ticarcillin may be removed from patients undergoing dialysis; the actual amount removed depends on the duration and type of dialysis.

Ticarcillin can be detected in tissues and interstitial fluid following parenteral administration. Penetration into the cerebrospinal fluid, bile, and pleural fluid has been demonstrated.

MICROBIOLOGY

Ticarcillin is bactericidal and demonstrates substantial *in vitro* activity against both gram-positive and gram-negative organisms. Many strains of the following organisms were found to be susceptible to ticarcillin *in vitro*:

Pseudomonas aeruginosa (and other species); *Escherichia coli; Proteus mirabilis; Morganella morganii* (formerly *Proteus morganii*); *Providencia rettgeri* (formerly *Proteus rettgeri*); *Proteus vulgaris; Enterobacter species; Haemophilus influenzae; Neisseria* species. *Salmonella* species; *Staphylococcus aureus* (non-penicillinase producing); *Staphylococcus epidermidis;* Beta-hemolytic streptococci (Group A); *Streptococcus faecalis* (*Enterococcus*); *Streptococcus pneumoniae. Anaerobic Bacteria, Including: Bacteroides* species including *B. fragilis; Fusobacterium* species; *Veillonella* species; *Clostridium* species; *Eubacterium* species; *Peptococcus* species;*Peptostreptococcus* species.

In vitro synergism between ticarcillin and gentamicin sulfate, tobramycin sulfate or amikacin sulfate against certain strains of *Pseudomonas aeruginosa* has been demonstrated.

T

Some strains of such microorganisms as *Mima-Herellea* (*Acinetobacter*), *Citrobacter* and *Serratia* have shown susceptibility.

Ticarcillin is not stable in the presence of penicillinase.

Some strains of *Pseudomonas* have developed resistance fairly rapidly.

DISK SUSCEPTIBILITY TESTS

Susceptibility Testing

Ticarcillin disks or powders should be used for testing susceptibility to ticarcillin. However, organisms reportedly susceptible to carbenicillin are susceptible to ticarcillin.

Diffusion Techniques

For the disk diffusion method of susceptibility testing a 75 μg tirarcillin disodium disk should be used. The method for this test is the one outlined in NCCLS publication M2-A3[1] with the interpretative criteria found in TABLE 2.

TABLE 2

Culture	Susceptible	Intermediate	Resistant
P. aeruginosa and *Enterobacteriaceae*	≥15 mm	12-14 mm	≤11 mm
The MIC correlates are: Resistant >128 μg/ml; Susceptible ≤64 μg/ml.			

Dilution Techniques

Dilution techniques for determining the MIC (minimum inhibitory concentration) are published by NCCLS for the broth and agar dilution procedures. The MIC data should be interpreted in light of the concentrations present in serum, tissue, and body fluids. Organisms with MIC ≤64 are considered susceptible when they are in tissue but organisms with MIC ≤128 would be susceptible in urine where the tirarcillin disodium concentrations are much greater. At present, only dilution methods can be recommended for testing antibiotic susceptibility of obligate anaerobes.

Susceptibility testing methods require the use of control organisms. The 75 μg ticarcillin disk should give zone diameters between 22 and 28 mm for *P. aeruginosa* ATCC 27853 and 24 and 30 mm for *E. coli* ATCC 25922. Reference strains are available for dilution testing of ticarcillin. 95% of the MIC's should fall within the following MIC ranges and the majority of MIC's should be at values close to the center of the pertinent range. (Reference NCCLS publication M7-A.[2])

S. aureus ATCC 29213, 2.0-8.0 μg/ml; *S. faecalis* ATCC 29212, 16-64 μg/ml; *E. coli* ATCC 25922, 2.0-8.0 μg/ml; *P. aeruginosa* ATCC 27853, 8.0-32 μg/ml.

INDICATIONS AND USAGE

Tirarcillin disodium is indicated for the treatment of the following infections:

Bacterial septicemia.*

Skin and soft-tissue infections.*

Acute and chronic respiratory tract infections.*†

* Caused by susceptible strains of *Pseudomonas aeruginosa, Proteus* species (both indole-positive and indole-negative) and *Escherichia coli.*

† Though clinical improvement has been shown, bacteriological cures cannot be expected in patients with chronic respiratory disease or cystic fibrosis.

Genitourinary tract infections (complicated and uncomplicated) due to susceptible strains of *Pseudomonas aeruginosa, Proteus* species (both indole-positive and indole-negative), *Escherichia coli, Enterobacter* and *Streptococcus faecalis* (enterococcus).

Ticarcillin is also indicated in the treatment of the following infections due to susceptible anaerobic bacteria:

1. Bacterial septicemia.
2. Lower respiratory tract infections such as empyema, anaerobic pneumonitis and lung abscess.
3. Intra-abdominal infections such as peritonitis and intra-abdominal abscess (typically resulting from anaerobic organisms resident in the normal gastrointestinal tract).
4. Infections of the female pelvis and genital tract, such as endometritis, pelvic inflammatory disease, pelvic abscess and salpingitis.
5. Skin and soft-tissue infections.

Although ticarcillin is primarily indicated in gram-negative infections, its *in vitro* activity against gram-positive organisms should be considered in treating infections caused by both gram-negative and gram-positive organisms (see CLINICAL PHARMACOLOGY, Microbiology).

Based on the *in vitro* synergism between ticarcillin and gentamicin sulfate, tobramycin sulfate or amikacin sulfate against certain strains of *Pseudomonas aeruginosa,* combined therapy has been successful, using full therapeutic dosages. (For additional information, see the gentamicin sulfate, tobramycin sulfate, and amikacin sulfate prescribing information.)

Note: Culturing and susceptibility testing should be performed initially and during treatment to monitor the effectiveness of therapy and the susceptibility of the bacteria.

CONTRAINDICATIONS

A history of allergic reaction to any of the penicillins is a contraindication.

WARNINGS

Serious and occasionally fatal hypersensitivity (anaphylactoid) reactions have been reported in patients receiving penicillin. These reactions are more likely to occur in persons with a history of sensitivity to multiple allergens.

There are reports of patients with a history of penicillin hypersensitivity reactions who experience severe hypersensitivity reactions when treated with a cephalosporin. Before therapy with a penicillin, careful inquiry should be made about previous hypersensitivity reactions to penicillins, cephalosporins, and other allergens. If a reaction occurs, the drug should be discontinued unless, in the opinion of the physician, the condition being treated is life-threatening and amenable only to ticarcillin therapy. **Serious anaphylactoid reactions require immediate emergency treatment with epinephrine. Oxygen, intravenous steroids, and airway management, including intubation, should also be administered as indicated.**

Some patients receiving high doses of ticarcillin may develop hemorrhagic manifestations associated with abnormalities of coagulation tests, such as bleeding time and platelet aggregation. On withdrawal of the drug, the bleeding should cease and coagulation abnormalities revert to normal. Other causes of abnormal bleeding should also be considered. Patients with renal impairment, in whom excretion of ticarcillin is delayed, should be observed for bleeding manifestations. Such patients should be dosed strictly according to recommendations (see DOSAGE AND ADMINISTRATION). If bleeding manifestations appear, ticarcillin treatment should be discontinued and appropriate therapy instituted.

Pseudomembranous colitis has been reported with nearly all antibacterial agents, including ticarcillin disodium, and has ranged in severity from mild to life-threatening. Therefore, it is important to consider this diagnosis in patients who present with diarrhea subsequent to the administration of antibacterial agents.

Treatment with antibacterial agents alters the normal flora of the colon and may permit overgrowth of clostridia. Studies indicate that a toxin produced by *Clostridium difficile* is one primary cause of "antibiotic colitis."

Mild cases of pseudomembranous colitis usually respond to drug discontinuation alone. In moderate to severe cases, consideration should be given to management with fluids and electrolytes, protein supplementation and treatment with an antibacterial drug effective against *C. difficile.*

PRECAUTIONS

Although ticarcillin disodium exhibits the characteristic low toxicity of the penicillins, as with any other potent agent, it is advisable to check periodically for organ system dysfunction (including renal, hepatic, and hematopoietic) during prolonged treatment. If overgrowth of resistant organisms occurs, the appropriate therapy should be initiated.

Since the theoretical sodium content is 5.2 mEq (120 mg) per gram of ticarcillin, and the actual vial content can be as high as 6.5 mEq/g, electrolyte and cardiac status should be monitored carefully.

In a few patients receiving intravenous ticarcillin, hypokalemia has been reported. Serum potassium should be measured periodically, and, if necessary, corrective therapy should be implemented.

As with any penicillin, the possibility of an allergic response, including anaphylaxis, exists, particularly in hypersensitive patients.

PREGNANCY

Reproduction studies have been performed in mice and rats and have revealed no evidence of impaired fertility or harm to the fetus due to ticarcillin. There are no well-controlled studies in pregnant women, but investigational experience does not include any positive evidence of adverse effects on the fetus. Although there is no clearly defined risk, such experience cannot exclude the possibility of infrequent or subtle damage to the fetus. Ticarcillin should be used in pregnant women only when clearly needed.

ADVERSE REACTIONS

The following adverse reactions may occur:

Hypersensitivity Reactions: Skin rashes, pruritus, urticaria, drug fever.

Gastrointestinal Disturbances: Nausea and vomiting, pseudomembranous colitis. Onset of pseudomembranous colitis symptoms may occur during or after antibiotic treatment (see WARNINGS).

Hemic and Lymphatic Systems: As with other penicillins, anemia, thrombocytopenia, leukopenia, neutropenia, and eosinophilia.

Abnormalities of Blood, Hepatic, and Renal Laboratory Studies: As with other semisynthetic penicillins, SGOT and SGPT elevations have been reported. To date, clinical manifestations of hepatic or renal disorders have not been observed which could be ascribed solely to ticarcillin.

CNS: Patients, especially those with impaired renal function, may experience convulsions or neuromuscular excitability when very high doses of the drug are administered.

Other: Local reactions such as pain (rarely accompanied by induration) at the site of the injection have been reported. Vein irritation and phlebitis can occur, particularly when undiluted solution is directly injected into the vein.

DOSAGE AND ADMINISTRATION

Clinical experience indicates that in serious urinary tract and systemic infections, intravenous therapy in the higher doses should be used. Intramuscular injections should not exceed 2 g per injection (see TABLE 3 and TABLE 4).

To calculate creatine clearance[3] from a serum creatinine value use the following formula:

Males: $C_{cr} = [(140\text{-Age})(\text{wt in kg})] \div [72 \times S_{cr}\ (\text{mg/100 ml})]$

Females: (Value for males) $\times$ 0.85

Neonates: In the neonate, for severe infections (sepsis) due to susceptible strains of *Pseudomonas, Proteus,* and *E. coli,* the following ticarcillin dosages may be given IM or by 10-20 minutes IV infusion.

Infants under 2000 g body weight: *Aged 0-7 days:* 75 mg/kg/12 hours (150 mg/kg/day); *Aged Over 7 days:* 75 mg/kg/8 hours (225 mg/kg/day).

Infants over 2000 g body weight: *Aged 0-7 days:* 75 mg/kg/8 hours (225 mg/kg/day); *Aged Over 7 days:* 100 mg/kg/8 hours (300 mg/kg/day).

This dosage schedule is intended to produce peak serum concentrations of 125-150 μg/ml 1 hour after a dose of ticarcillin and trough concentrations of 25-50 μg/ml immediately before the next dose.

After reconstitution and prior to administration ticarcillin disodium, as with other parenteral drugs, should be inspected visually for particulate matter and discoloration.

Note: Gentamicin, tobramycin or amikacin may be used concurrently with ticarcillin for initial therapy until results of culture and susceptibility studies are known.

TABLE 3 *Adults*

Bacterial Septicemia	200-300 mg/kg/day by IV infusion in divided doses q4-6h
Respiratory Tract Infections	(The usual dose is 3 g given q4h (18 g/day) or 4 g given q6h (16 g/day) depending on weight and the severity of the infection.)
Skin and Soft-Tissue Infections	
Intra-Abdominal Infections	
Infections of the Female Pelvis and Genital Tract	
Urinary Tract Infections	
Complicated:	150-200 mg/kg/day by IV infusion in divided doses q4-6h (Usual recommended dosage for average [70 kg] adults: 3 g qid)
Uncomplicated:	1 g IM or direct IV q6h
Infections Complicated by Renal Insufficiency:*	Initial loading dose of 3 g IV followed by IV doses, based on creatinine clearance and type of dialysis, as indicated below:
Creatinine Clearance ml/min.:	
over 60	3 g q4h
30-60	2 g q4h
10-30	2 g q8h
less than 10	2 g q12h (or 1 g IM q6h)
less than 10 with hepatic dysfunction	2 g q24h (or 1 g IM q12h)
patients on peritoneal dialysis	3 g q12h
patients on hemodialysis	2 g q12h supplemented with 3 g after each dialysis

* The half-life of ticarcillin in patients with renal failure is approximately 13 hours.

TABLE 4 *Children: Under 40 kg (88 lb)*

The daily dose for children should not exceed the adult dosage.

Bacterial Septicemia	200-300 mg/kg/day by IV infusion in divided doses q4-6h
Respiratory Tract Infections	
Skin and Soft-Tissue	
Intra-Abdominal Infections	
Infections of the Female Pelvis and Genital Tract	
Urinary Tract Infections	
Complicated:	150-200 mg/kg/day by IV infusion in divided doses q4-6h
Uncomplicated:	50-100 mg/kg/day IM or direct IV in divided doses q6-8h
Infections Complicated by Renal Insufficiency:	Clinical data is insufficient to recommend optimum dose.

Children weighing more than 40 kg (88 lb) should receive adult dosages.

Seriously ill patients should receive the higher doses. Tirarcillin disodium has proved to be useful in infections in which protective mechanisms are impaired, such as in acute leukemia and during therapy with immunosuppressive or oncolytic drugs.

DIRECTIONS FOR USE

1 g, 3 g and 6 g Standard Vials

Intramuscular Administration

(Concentration of approximately 385 mg/ml).

For initial reconstitution use sterile water for injection, sodium chloride injection or 1% lidocaine HCl solution* (without epinephrine).

Each gram of ticarcillin should be reconstituted with 2 ml of sterile water for injection, sodium chloride injection or 1% lidocaine HCl solution* (without epinephrine) and used promptly. Each 2.6 ml of the resulting solution will then contain 1 g of ticarcillin.

As with all intramuscular preparations, ticarcillin disodium should be injected well within the body of a relatively large muscle using usual techniques and precautions.

*For more information, refer to the lidocaine HCl prescribing information.

Intravenous Administration

(Concentration of approximately 200 mg/ml).

For initial reconstitution use sodium chloride injection, dextrose injection 5% or lactated Ringer's injection.

Reconstitute each gram of ticarcillin with 4 ml of the appropriate diluent. After the addition of 4 ml of diluent per gram of ticarcillin each 1.0 ml of the resulting solution will have an approximate concentration of 200 mg. Once dissolved, further dilute if desired.

Direct Intravenous Injection: In order to avoid vein irritation, administer solution as slowly as possible.

Intravenous Infusion: Administer by continuous or intermittent intravenous drip. Intermittent infusion should be administered over a 30 minute to 2 hour period in equally divided doses.

3 g Piggyback Bottles

Direct Intravenous Injection

(Concentrations of approximately 29-100 mg/ml).

The 3 g bottle should be reconstituted with a minimum of 30 ml of the desired intravenous solution listed in TABLE 5.

In order to avoid vein irritation, the solution should be administered as slowly as possible. A dilution of approximately 50 mg/ml or more will further reduce the incidence of vein irritation.

Intravenous Infusion

Stability studies in the intravenous solutions (TABLE 6) indicates that ticarcillin disodium will provide sufficient activity at room temperature (70-75°F) within the stated time periods at concentrations between 10 mg/ml and 50 mg/ml.

TABLE 5

Amount of Diluent	Concentration of Solution
100 ml	1 g/34 ml (~29 mg/ml)
60 ml	1 g/20 ml (50 mg/ml)
30 ml	1 g/10 ml (100 mg/ml)

Unused solutions should be discarded after the time periods mentioned above.

After reconstitution and prior to administration ticarcillin disodium as with other parenteral drugs should be inspected visually for particulate matter and discoloration.

TABLE 6 *Stability Period*

Intravenous Solution (concentration of 10-100 mg/ml)	Room Temperature 21-24°C (70-75°F)	Refrigeration 4°C (40°F)
Sodium chloride injection	72 hours	14 days
Dextrose injection 5%	72 hours	14 days
Lactated Ringer's injection	48 hours	14 days

Refrigerated solutions stored longer than 72 hours should not be used for multidose purposes.

After reconstitution and dilution to a concentration of 10-100 mg/ml, this solution can be frozen 18°C (0°F) and stored for up to 30 days. The thawed solution must be used within 24 hours.

Unused solutions should be discarded after the time periods mentioned above.

It is recommended that ticarcillin disodium and gentamicin sulfate, tobramycin sulfate or amikacin sulfate not be mixed together in the same IV solution due to the gradual inactivation of gentamicin sulfate, tobramycin sulfate or amikacin sulfate under these circumstances. The therapeutic effect of ticarcillin disodium and these aminoglycoside drugs remains unimpaired when administered separately.

20 and 30 g Pharmacy Bulk Package

For IV use. RECONSTITUTED STOCK SOLUTION MUST BE TRANSFERRED AND FURTHER DILUTED FOR IV INFUSION.

Not for direct infusion. The pharmacy bulk package is for use in a hospital pharmacy admixture program only under a laminar flow hood. After reconstitution, entry into the vial must be made with a sterile transfer set or other sterile dispensing device, and contents dispensed as aliquots into intravenous solution using aseptic technique. Use of syringe and needle is not recommended as it may cause leakage. After entry with a sterile transfer set or other sterile dispensing device, use entire contents of pharmacy bulk package promptly. Any unused portion must be discarded after 24 hours from time of initial reconstitution. Add 85 ml of sodium chloride injection, dextrose injection 5% or lactated Ringer's injection to the 20 g pharmacy bulk package and shake well. Add 75 ml of sodium chloride injection, dextrose injection 5% or lactated Ringer's injection to the 30 g pharmacy bulk package and shake well. For ease of reconstitution, the amount of diluent may be added in 2 portions. Each 1.0 ml of the resulting concentrated stock solution contains approximately 200 mg of ticarcillin in the 20 g pharmacy bulk package, and 300 mg of ticarcillin in the 30 g pharmacy bulk package.

Intravenous Administration

The desired dosage should be withdrawn from the stock solution and further diluted with sodium chloride injection, dextrose injection 5% or lactated Ringer's injection to a concentration between 10 mg/ml and 100 mg/ml. If the solution is administered as a direct injection, it should be administered as slowly as possible in order to avoid vein irritation. Using a concentration of 50 mg/ml or less will further reduce the incidence of vein irritation. The solutions can be administered by either a continuous or intermittent intravenous infusion should be administered over a 30 minute to 2 hour period in equally divided doses.

Stability/Storage Conditions

The concentrated stock solution must be diluted within 24 hours if stored between 21-24°C (70-75°F) or within 72 hours if kept under refrigeration 4°C (40°F).

Upon further dilution (10-100 mg/ml), the solutions will provide sufficient activity within an additional 24 hours between 21-24°C (70-75°F) or 3 days under refrigeration 4°C (40°F).

If the concentrated stock solution is diluted to concentrations between 10 and 50 mg/ml within 8 hours with diluents listed in TABLE 6, then the following stability periods apply.

Refrigerated solutions stored longer than 72 hours should not be used for multidose purposes.

After reconstitution and dilution to a concentration of 10-100 mg/ml, this solution can be frozen -18°C (0°F) and stored for up to 30 days. The thawed solution must be used within 24 hours.

It is recommended that ticarcillin disodium and gentamicin sulfate, tobramycin sulfate or amikacin sulfate not be mixed together in the same IV solution due to the gradual inactivation of gentamicin sulfate, tobramycin sulfate or amikacin sulfate under these circumstances. The therapeutic effect of ticarcillin disodium and these aminoglycoside drugs remains unimpaired when administered separately.

PRODUCT LISTING - EQUIVALENTS NOT AVAILABLE

Powder For Injection - Injectable - 1 Gm

Pack	Price	Product	NDC
10's	$32.38	TICAR, Glaxosmithkline	00029-6550-22
10's	$127.90	TICAR, Glaxosmithkline	00007-6550-26

Powder For Injection - Injectable - 3 Gm

Pack	Price	Product	NDC
1's	$95.88	TICAR, Glaxosmithkline	00029-6552-40
10's	$114.00	TICAR, Glaxosmithkline	00029-6552-07
10's	$124.09	TICAR, Glaxosmithkline	00029-6552-21
10's	$134.30	TICAR, Glaxosmithkline	00029-6552-26

T

Ticarcillin Disodium; Clavulanate Potassium (000833)

For related information, see the comparative table section in Appendix A.

Categories: Endometritis; Infection, bone; Infection, gynecologic; Infection, intra-abdominal; Infection, joint; Infection, lower respiratory tract; Infection, skin and skin structures; Infection, urinary tract; Peritonitis; Septicemia; Pregnancy Category B; FDA Approved 1985 Apr
Drug Classes: Antibiotics, penicillins
Brand Names: **Timentin**
Foreign Brand Availability: Timenten (Austria; Switzerland); Timentine (Spain)
Cost of Therapy: $6,267.20 (Infection; Timentin Injection; 0.1 g; 3 g; 12.4 g/day; 10 day supply)

DESCRIPTION

Timentin is a sterile injectable antibacterial combination consisting of the semisynthetic antibiotic, ticarcillin disodium, and the β-lactamase inhibitor, clavulanate potassium (the potassium salt of clavulanic acid), for intravenous administration. Ticarcillin is derived from the basic penicillin nucleus, 6-amino-penicillanic acid.

Chemically, it is 4-This-1-azabicyclo[3.2.0]heptane-2-carboxylic acid, 6-[(carboxy-3-thienylacetyl)amino]-3,3-dimethyl-7-oxo-, disodium salt, [2*S*-[2α, 5α, 6β (*S**)]]-.

Clavulanic acid is produced by the fermentation of *Streptomyces clavuligerus.* It is a β-lactam structurally related to the penicillins and possesses the ability to inactivate a wide variety of β-lactamases by blocking the active sites of these enzymes. Clavulanic acid is particularly active against the clinically important plasmid-mediated β-lactamases frequently responsible for transferred drug resistance to penicillins and cephalosporins.

Chemically, clavulanate potassium is potassium 4-Oxa-1-azabicyclo[3.2.0]heptane-2-carboxylic acid, 3-(2-hydroxyethylidene)-7-oxo-, monopotassium salt [2*R*-(2α,3*Z*,5α)]-.

Timentin is supplied as a white to pale yellow powder for reconstitution. Timentin is very soluble in water, its solubility being greater than 600 mg/ml. The reconstituted solution is clear, colorless or pale yellow, having a pH of 5.5-7.5.

For the Timentin 3.1 and 3.2 g dosages, the theoretical sodium content is 4.75 mEq (109 mg) per gram of Timentin. The theoretical potassium content is 0.15 mEq (6 mg) and 0.3 mEq (11.9 mg) per gram of Timentin for the 3.1 and 3.2 g dosages, respectively.

CLINICAL PHARMACOLOGY

After an intravenous infusion (30 min.) of 3.1 or 3.2 g clavulanate potassium; ticarcillin disodium, peak serum concentrations of both ticarcillin and clavulanic acid are attained immediately after completion of infusion. Ticarcillin serum levels are similar to those produced by the administration of equivalent amounts of ticarcillin alone with a mean peak serum level of 330 μg/ml for the 3.1 and 3.2 g formulations. The corresponding mean peak serum levels for clavulanic acid were 8 μg/ml and 16 μg/ml for the 3.1 g and 3.2 g formulations, respectively (see TABLE 1).

TABLE 1 *Serum Levels in Adults After a 30 Minute IV Infusion of Clavulanate Potassium; Ticarcillin Disodium (μg/ml)*

	Ticarcillin serum levels						
Dose	**0**	**15 min**	**30 min**	**1 h**	**1.5 h**	**3.5 h**	**5.5 h**
3.1 g	324 (293-388)	223 (184-293)	176 (135-235)	131 (102-195)	90 (65-119)	27 (19-37)	6 (5-7)
3.2 g	336 (301-386)	214 (180-258)	186 (160-218)	122 (108-136)	78 (33-113)	29 (19-44)	10 (5-15)

TABLE 2 *Clavulanic Acid Serum Levels (μg/ml)*

Dose	0	15 min	30 min	1 h	1.5 h	3.5 h	5.5 h
3.1 g	8.0 (5.3-10.3)	4.6 (3.0-7.6)	2.6 (1.8-3.4)	1.8 (1.6-2.2)	1.2 (0.8-1.6)	0.3 (0.2-0.3)	0
3.2 g	15.8 (11.7-21.0)	8.3 (6.4-10.0)	5.2 (3.5-6.3)	3.4 (1.9-4.0)	2.5 (1.3-3.4)	0.5 (0.2-0.8)	0

The mean area under the serum concentration curves for ticarcillin was 485 μg/h/ml for the clavulanate potassium; ticarcillin disodium 3.1 and 3.2 g formulations. The corresponding areas under the serum concentration curves for clavulanic acid were 8.2 μg/h/ml and 15.6 μg/h/ml for the clavulanate potassium; ticarcillin disodium 3.1 g and 3.2 g formulations, respectively.

The mean serum half-lives of ticarcillin and clavulanic acid in healthy volunteers are 1.1 h and 1.1 h, respectively, following administration of 3.1 g or 3.2 g of clavulanate potassium; ticarcillin disodium.

In pediatric patients receiving approximately 50 mg/kg clavulanate potassium; ticarcillin disodium (30:1 ratio ticarcillin to clavulanate), mean ticarcillin serum half-lives were 4.4 hours in neonates (n=18) and 1.0 hours in infants and children (n=41). The corresponding clavulanate serum half-lives averaged 1.9 hours in neonates (n=14) and 0.9 hours in infants and children (n=40). Area under the serum concentration time curves averaged 339 μg/h/ml in infants and children (n=41), whereas the corresponding mean clavulanate area under the serum concentration time curves was approximately 7 μg/h/ml in the same population (n=40). Approximately 60-70% of ticarcillin and approximately 35-45% of clavulanic acid are excreted unchanged in urine during the first 6 hours after administration of a single dose of clavulanate potassium; ticarcillin disodium to normal volunteers with normal renal function. Two (2) hours after an intravenous injection of 3.1 g or 3.2 g clavulanate potassium; ticarcillin disodium, concentrations of ticarcillin in urine generally exceed 1500 μg/ml. The corresponding concentrations of clavulanic acid in urine generally exceed 40 μg/ml and 70 μg/ml following administration of the 3.1 g and 3.2 g doses, respectively. By 4-6 hours after injection, the urine concentrations of ticarcillin and clavulanic acid usually decline to approximately 190 μg/ml and 2 μg/ml, respectively, for both doses. Neither component of clavulanate potassium; ticarcillin disodium is highly protein bound; ticarcillin has been found to be approximately 45% bound to human serum protein and clavulanic acid approximately 9% bound.

Somewhat higher and more prolonged serum levels of ticarcillin can be achieved with the concurrent administration of probenecid; however, probenecid does not enhance the serum levels of clavulanic acid.

Ticarcillin can be detected in tissues and interstitial fluid following parenteral administration.

Penetration of ticarcillin into bile and pleural fluid has been demonstrated. The results of experiments involving the administration of clavulanic acid to animals suggest that this compound, like ticarcillin, is well distributed in body tissues.

An inverse relationship exists between the serum half-life of ticarcillin and creatinine clearance. The dosage of clavulanate potassium; ticarcillin disodium need only be adjusted in cases of severe renal impairment (see DOSAGE AND ADMINISTRATION).

Ticarcillin may be removed from patients undergoing dialysis; the actual amount removed depends on the duration and type of dialysis.

MICROBIOLOGY

Ticarcillin is a semisynthetic antibiotic with a broad spectrum of bactericidal activity against many gram-positive and gram-negative aerobic and anaerobic bacteria.

Ticarcillin is, however, susceptible to degradation by β-lactamases and, therefore, the spectrum of activity does not normally include organisms which produce these enzymes.

Clavulanic acid is a β-lactam, structurally related to the penicillins, which possesses the ability to inactivate a wide range of β-lactamase enzymes commonly found in microorganisms resistant to penicillins and cephalosporins. In particular, it has good activity against the clinically important plasmid-mediated β-lactamases frequently responsible for transferred drug resistance.

The formulation of ticarcillin with clavulanic acid in clavulanate potassium; ticarcillin disodium protects ticarcillin from degradation by β-lactamase enzymes and effectively extends the antibiotic spectrum of ticarcillin to include many bacteria normally resistant to ticarcillin and other β-lactam antibiotics. Thus clavulanate potassium; ticarcillin disodium possesses the distinctive properties of a broad-spectrum antibiotic and a β-lactamase inhibitor.

While *in vitro* studies have demonstrated the susceptibility of most strains of the following organisms, clinical efficacy for infections other than those included in the INDICATIONS AND USAGE section has not been documented:

Gram-Negative Bacteria: *Pseudomonas aeruginosa* (β-lactamase and non-β-lactamase producing), *Pseudomonas* species including *P. maltophilia* (β-lactamase and non-β-lactamase producing), *Escherichia coli* (β-lactamase and non-β-lactamase producing), *Proteus mirabilis* (β-lactamase and non-β-lactamase producing), *Proteus vulgaris* (β-lactamase and non-β-lactamase producing). *Providencia rettgen* (formerly *Proteus rettgeri*) (β-lactamase and non-β-lactamase producing), *Providencia stuarti* (β-lactamase and non-β-lactamase producing), *Morganella morganii* (formerly *Proteus morganii*) (β-lactamase and non-β-lactamase producing), *Enterobacter* species (Although most strains of Enterobacter species are resistant *in vitro,* clinical efficacy has been demonstrated with clavulanate potassium; ticarcillin disodium in urinary tract infections caused by these organisms.), *Acinetobacter* species (β-lactamase and non-β-lactamase producing), *Hemophilus influenzae* (β-lactamase and non-β-lactamase producing), *Branhamella catarrhalis* (β-lactamase and non-β-lactamase producing), *Serratia* species including *S. marcescens* (β-lactamase and non-β-lactamase producing), *Neissenia gonorrhoeae* (β-lactamase and non-β-lactamase producing), *Neissenia meningitidis**, *Salmonella* species (β-lactamase and non-β-lactamase producing), *Klebsiella* species including *K. pneumoniae* (β-lactamase and non-β-lactamase producing), *Citrobacter* species including *C. freundii, C. diversus* and *C. amalonaticus* (β-lactamase and non-β-lactamase producing).

Gram-Positive Bacteria: *Staphylococcus aureus* (β-lactamase and non-β-lactamase producing), *Staphylococcus saprophyticus, Staphylococcus epidermidis* (coagulase-negative staphylococci) (β-lactamase and non-β-lactamase producing), *Streptococcus pneumoniae** *(D. pneumoniae), Streptococcus bovis**, *Streptococcus agalactiae**(Group B), *Streptococcus faecalis** (Enterococcus), *Streptococcus pyogenes* (Group A, β-hemolytic), Viridans group streptococci*.

Anaerobic Bacteria: Bacteroides species, including *B. fragilis* group *(B. fragilis, B. vulgatus)* (β-lactamase and non-β-lactamase producing), non-*B. fragilis (B. melaninogenicus)* (β-lactamase and non-β-lactamase producing), *B. thetaiotaomicron, B. ovatus, B. distasonis* (β-lactamase and non-β-lactamase producing), *Clostridium* species including *C. perfringens, C. difficile, C. sporogenes, C. ramosum* and *C. bifermentans**, *Eubacterium* species, *Fusobacterium* species including *F. nucleatum* and *F. necrophorum**, *Peptococcus* species*, *Peptostreptococcus* species*, *Veillonella* species.

*These are non β-lactamase-producing strains and therefore are susceptible to ticarcillin alone. Some of the β-lactamase-producing strains are also susceptible to ticarcillin alone.

In vitro synergism between clavulanate potassium; ticarcillin disodium and gentamicin, tobramycin or amikacin against multiresistant strains of *Pseudomonas aeruginosa* has been demonstrated.

SUSCEPTIBILITY TESTING

Diffusion Technique: An 85 μg (75 μg ticarcillin plus 10 μg clavulanic acid) diffusion disk is available for use with the Kirby-Bauer method. Based on the zone sizes given below, a report of "Susceptible" indicates that the infecting organism is likely to respond to clavulanate potassium; ticarcillin disodium therapy, while a report of "Resistant" indicates that the organism is not likely to respond to therapy with this antibiotic. A report of "Intermediate" susceptibility indicates that the organism would be susceptible to clavulanate potassium; ticarcillin disodium at a higher dosage or if the infection is confined to tissues or fluids (*e.g.,* urine) in which high antibiotic levels are attained.

T

Dilution Technique: Broth or agar dilution methods may be used to determine the minimal inhibitory concentration (MIC) values for bacterial isolates to clavulanate potassium; ticarcillin disodium. Tubes should be inoculated with the test culture containing 10^4 to 10^5 CFU/ml or plates spotted with a test solution containing 10^3 to 10^4 CFU/ml.

The recommended dilution pattern utilizes a constant level of clavulanic acid, 2 μg/ml, in all tubes together with varying amounts of ticarcillin. MICs are expressed in terms of the ticarcillin concentration in the presence of 2 μg/ml clavulanic acid.

***TABLE 3** Recommended Ranges for Clavulanate Potassium; Ticarcillin Disodium Susceptibility Testing*

Diffusion Method Disk Zone Size, mm			Dilution Method MIC Correlates*, μg/ml	
Resistant	**Intermediate**	**Susceptible**	**Resistant**	**Susceptible**
≤11	12-14	≥15	≥128	≤64

* Expressed as concentration of ticarcillin in the presence of a constant 2.0 μg/ml concentration of clavulanic acid.

TABLE 4

		Disks	MIC Range (μg/ml)
E. coli	(ATCC 25922)	24-30 mm	2/2-8/2
S. aureus	(ATCC 25923)	32-40 mm	—
Ps. aeruginosa	(ATCC 27853)	20-28 mm	8/2-32/2
E. coli	(ATCC 35218)	21-25 mm	4/2-16/2
S. aureus	(ATCC 29213)	—	0.5/2-2/2

INDICATIONS AND USAGE

Clavulanate potassium; ticarcillin disodium is indicated in the treatment of infections caused by susceptible strains of the designated microorganisms in the conditions listed below:

Septicemia: Including bacteremia, caused by β-lactamase-producing strains of *Klebsiella* spp.*, *E. coli**, *Staphylococcus aureus**, or *Pseudomonas aeruginosa** (or other *Pseudomonas* species*).

Lower Respiratory Infections: Caused by β-lactamase-producing strains of *Staphylococcus aureus, Hemophilus influenzae**, or *Klebsiella* spp.*.

Bone and Joint Infections: Caused by β-lactamase-producing strains of *Staphylococcus aureus.*

Skin and Skin Structure Infections: Caused by β-lactamase-producing strains of *Staphylococcus aureus, Klebsiella* spp.*, or *E. coli**.

Urinary Tract Infections: (Complicated and uncomplicated) caused by β-lactamase-producing strains of *E. coli, Klebsiella* spp., *Pseudomonas aeruginosa** (or other *Pseudomonas* spp.*), *Citrobacter spp.**, *Enterobacter cloacae**, *Serratia marcescens**, or *Staphylococcus aureus**.

Gynecologic Infections: Endometritis caused by β-lactamase-producing strains of *B. melaninogenicus**, *Enterobacter* spp. (including *E. cloacae**), *Escherichia coli, Klebsiella pneumoniae**, *Staphylococcus aureus,* or *Staphylococcus epidermidis.*

Intra-abdominal Infections: Peritonitis caused by β-lactamase-producing strains of *Escherichia coli, Klebsiella pneumoniae,* or *Bacteroides fragilis** group.

* for this organism in this organ system was studied in fewer than 10 infections.

NOTE: For information on use in pediatric patients (≥3 months of age) (see PRECAUTIONS, Pediatric Use). There are insufficient data to support the use of clavulanate potassium; ticarcillin disodium in pediatric patients under 3 months of age or for the treatment of septicemia and/or infections in the pediatric population where the suspected or proven pathogen is *Haemophilus influenzae* type b.

While clavulanate potassium; ticarcillin disodium is indicated only for the conditions listed above, infections caused by ticarcillin-susceptible organisms are also amenable to clavulanate potassium; ticarcillin disodium treatment due to its ticarcillin content. Therefore, mixed infections caused by ticarcillin-susceptible organisms and β-lactamase-producing organisms susceptible to ticarcillin/clavulanic acid should not require the addition of another antibiotic.

Appropriate culture and susceptibility tests should be performed before treatment in order to isolate and identify organisms causing infection and to determine their susceptibility to ticarcillin/clavulanic acid. Because of its broad spectrum of bactericidal activity against gram-positive and gram-negative bacteria. clavulanate potassium; ticarcillin disodium is particularly useful for the treatment of mixed infections and for presumptive therapy prior to the identification of the causative organisms. Clavulanate potassium; ticarcillin disodium has been shown to be effective as single drug therapy in the treatment of some serious infections where normally combination antibiotic therapy might be employed. Therapy with clavulanate potassium; ticarcillin disodium may be initiated before results of such tests are known when there is reason to believe the infection may involve any of the β-lactamase-producing organisms listed above; however, once these results become available, appropriate therapy should be continued.

Based on the *in vitro* synergism between ticarcillin/clavulanic acid and aminoglycosides against certain strains of *Pseudomonas aeruginosa,* combined therapy has been successful, especially in patients with impaired host defenses. Both drugs should be used in full therapeutic doses. As soon as results of culture and susceptibility tests become available, antimicrobial therapy should be adjusted as indicated.

CONTRAINDICATIONS

Clavulanate potassium; ticarcillin disodium is contraindicated in patients with a history of hypersensitivity reactions to any of the penicillins.

WARNINGS

SERIOUS AND OCCASIONALLY FATAL HYPERSENSITIVITY (ANAPHYLACTIC) REACTIONS HAVE BEEN REPORTED IN PATIENTS ON PENICILLIN THERAPY. THESE REACTIONS ARE MORE LIKELY TO OCCUR IN INDIVIDUALS WITH A HISTORY OF PENICILLIN HYPERSENSITIVITY AND/OR A HISTORY OF SENSITIVITY TO MULTIPLE ALLERGENS. THERE HAVE BEEN REPORTS OF INDIVIDUALS WITH A HISTORY OF PENICILLIN HYPERSENSITIVITY WHO HAVE EXPERIENCED SEVERE REACTIONS WHEN TREATED WITH CEPHALOSPORINS. BEFORE INITIATING THERAPY WITH CLAVULANATE POTASSIUM; TICARCILLIN DISODIUM. CAREFUL INQUIRY SHOULD BE MADE CONCERNING PREVIOUS HYPERSENSITIVITY REACTIONS TO PENICILLINS, CEPHALOSPORINS, OR OTHER ALLERGENS. IF AN ALLERGIC REACTION OCCURS, CLAVULANATE POTASSIUM; TICARCILLIN DISODIUM SHOULD BE DISCONTINUED AND THE APPROPRIATE THERAPY INSTITUTED. **SERIOUS ANAPHYLACTIC REACTIONS REQUIRE IMMEDIATE EMERGENCY TREATMENT WITH EPINEPHRINE, OXYGEN, INTRAVENOUS STEROIDS AND AIRWAY MANAGEMENT, INCLUDING INTUBATION, SHOULD ALSO BE PROVIDED AS INDICATED.**

Pseudomembranous colitis has been reported with nearly all antibacterial agents, including clavulanate potassium; ticarcillin disodium, and may range in severity from mild to life-threatening. Therefore, it is important to consider this diagnosis in patients who present with diarrhea subsequent to the administration of antibacterial agents.

Treatment with antibacterial agents alters the normal flora of the colon and may permit overgrowth of clostrida. Studies indicate that a toxin produced by *Clostridium difficile* is one primary cause of "antibiotic-associated colitis."

After the diagnosis of pseudomembranous colitis has been established, therapeutic measures should be initiated. Mild cases of pseudomembranous colitis usually respond to drug discontinuation alone. In moderate to severe cases, consideration should be given to management with fluids and electrolytes, protein supplementation and treatment with an antibacterial drug clinically effective against *C. difficile* colitis.

PRECAUTIONS

GENERAL

While clavulanate potassium; ticarcillin disodium possesses the characteristic low toxicity of the penicillin group of antibiotics, periodic assessment of organ system functions, including renal, hepatic, and hematopoietic function, is advisable during prolonged therapy.

Bleeding manifestations have occurred in some patients receiving β-lactam antibiotics. These reactions have been associated with abnormalities of coagulation tests such as clotting time, platelet aggregation, and prothrombin time and are more likely to occur in patients with renal impairment.

If bleeding manifestations appear, clavulanate potassium; ticarcillin disodium treatment should be discontinued and appropriate therapy instituted.

Clavulanate potassium; ticarcillin disodium has only rarely been reported to cause hypokalemia; however, the possibility of this occurring should be kept in mind particularly when treating patients with fluid and electrolyte imbalance. Periodic monitoring of serum potassium may be advisable in patients receiving prolonged therapy.

The theoretical sodium content is 4.75 mEq (109 mg) per gram of clavulanate potassium; ticarcillin disodium. This should be considered when treating patients requiring restricted salt intake.

As with any penicillin, an allergic reaction, including anaphylaxis, may occur during clavulanate potassium; ticarcillin disodium administration, particularly in a hypersensitive individual.

The possibility of superinfections with mycotic or bacterial pathogens should be kept in mind, particularly during prolonged treatment. If superinfections occur, appropriate measures should be taken.

DRUG/LABORATORY TEST INTERACTIONS

As with other penicillins, the mixing of clavulanate potassium; ticarcillin disodium with an aminoglycoside in solutions for parenteral administration can result in substantial inactivation of the aminoglycoside.

Probenecid interferes with the renal tubular secretion of ticarcillin, thereby increasing serum concentrations and prolonging serum half-life of the antibiotic. High urine concentrations of ticarcillin may produce false-positive protein reactions (pseudoproteinuria) with the following methods: sulfosalicylic acid and boiling test, acetic acid test, biuret reaction and nitric acid test. The bromphenol blue (Multi-stix) reagent strip test has been reported to be reliable.

The presence of clavulanic acid in clavulanate potassium; ticarcillin disodium may cause a nonspecific binding of IgG and albumin by red cell membranes leading to a false-positive Coombs test.

CARCINOGENESIS, MUTAGENESIS, AND IMPAIRMENT OF FERTILITY

Long-term studies in animals have not been performed to evaluate carcinogenic potential. Results of studies performed with clavulanate potassium; ticarcillin disodium *in vitro* and *in vivo* did not indicate a potential for mutagenicity.

PREGNANCY CATEGORY B

Reproduction studies have been performed in rats given doses up to 1050 mg/kg/day and have revealed no evidence of impaired fertility or harm to the fetus due to clavulanate potassium; ticarcillin disodium. There are, however, no adequate and well-controlled studies in pregnant women. Because animal reproduction studies are not always predictive of human response, this drug should be used during pregnancy only if clearly needed.

NURSING MOTHERS

It is not known whether this drug is excreted in human milk. Because many drugs are excreted in human milk, caution should be exercised when clavulanate potassium; ticarcillin disodium is administered to a nursing woman.

PEDIATRIC USE

The safety and effectiveness of clavulanate potassium; ticarcillin disodium have been established in the age group of 3 months to 16 years. Use of clavulanate potassium; ticarcillin disodium in these age groups is supported by evidence from adequate and well-controlled studies of clavulanate potassium; ticarcillin disodium in adults with additional efficacy, safety, and pharmacokinetic data from both comparative and non-comparative studies in pediatric patients. There are insufficient data to support the use of clavulanate potassium; ticarcillin disodium in pediatric patients under 3 months of age or for the treatment of septicemia and/or infections in the pediatric population where the suspected or proven pathogen is *Haemophilus influenzae* type b.

In those patients in whom meningeal seeding from a distant infection site or in whom meningitis is suspected or documented, or in patients who require prophylaxis against central nervous system infection, an alternate agent with demonstrated clinical efficacy in this setting should be used.

ADVERSE REACTIONS

As with other penicillins, the following adverse reactions may occur.

Hypersensitivity Reactions: Skin rash, pruritus, urticaria, arthralgia, myalgia, drug fever, chills, chest discomfort, and anaphylactic reactions.

Central Nervous System: Headache, giddiness, neuromuscular hyperirritability, or convulsive seizures.

Gastrointestinal Disturbances: Disturbances of taste and smell, stomatitis, flatulence, nausea, vomiting and diarrhea, epigastric pain, and pseudomembranous colitis have been reported. Onset of pseudomembranous colitis symptoms may occur during or after antibiotic treatment (see WARNINGS).

Hemic and Lymphatic Systems: Thrombocytopenia, leukopenia, neutropenia, eosinophilia, reduction of hemoglobin or hematocrit, and prolongation of prothrombin time and bleeding time.

Abnormalities of Hepatic and Renal Function Tests: Elevation of serum aspartate aminotransferase (SGOT), serum alanine aminotransferase (SGPT), serum alkaline phosphatase, serum LDH, serum bilirubin. There have been reports of transient hepatitis and cholestatic jaundice—as with some other penicillins and some cephalosporins. Elevation of serum creatinine and/or BUN, hypernatremia, reduction in serum potassium and uric acid.

Local Reactions: Pain, burning, swelling, and induration at the injection site and thrombophlebitis with intravenous administration.

Available safety data for pediatric patients treated with clavulanate potassium; ticarcillin disodium demonstrate a similar adverse event profile to that observed in adult patients.

DOSAGE AND ADMINISTRATION

Clavulanate potassium; ticarcillin disodium should be administered by intravenous infusion (30 min.).

ADULTS

The usual recommended dosage for systemic and urinary tract infections for average (60 kg) adults is 3.1 g clavulanate potassium; ticarcillin disodium (3.1 g vial containing 3 g ticarcillin and 100 mg clavulanic acid) given every 4-6 hours. For gynecologic infections, clavulanate potassium; ticarcillin disodium should be administered as follows: Moderate infections 200 mg/kg/day in divided doses every 6 hours and for severe infections 300 mg/kg/day in divided doses every 4 hours. For patients weighing less than 60 kg, the recommended dosage is 200-300 mg/kg/day, based on ticarcillin content, given in divided doses every 4-6 hours. In urinary tract infections, a dosage of 3.2 g clavulanate potassium; ticarcillin disodium (3.2 g vial containing 3 g ticarcillin and 200 mg clavulanic acid) given every 8 hours is adequate.

PEDIATRIC PATIENTS (≥3 MONTHS)

For Patients <60 kg: In patients <60 kg, clavulanate potassium; ticarcillin disodium is dosed at 50 mg/kg/dose based on the ticarcillin component. clavulanate potassium; ticarcillin disodium should be administered as follows: Mild to moderate infections 200 mg/kg/day in divided doses every 6 hours; for severe infections, 300 mg/kg/day in divided doses every 4 hours.

For Patients ≥60 kg: For mild to moderate infections, 3.1 g (3 g of ticarcillin and 100 mg of clavulanic acid) administered every 6 hours; for severe infections, 3.1 g every 4 hours.

Renal Impairment: For infections complicated by renal insufficiency†, an initial loading dose of 3.1 g should be followed by doses based on creatinine clearance and type of dialysis as indicated in TABLE 5.

TABLE 5

Creatinine Clearance ml/min	Dosage
over 60	3.1 g every 4 h
30-60	2 g every 4 h
10-30	2 g every 8 h
less than 10	2 g every 12 h
less than 10 with hepatic dysfunction	2 g every 24 h
patients on peritoneal dialysis	3.1 g every 12 h
patients on hemodialysis	2 g every 12 h supplemented with 3.1 g after each dialysis

To calculate creatinine clearance* from a serum creatinine value use the following formula.

CCR = [(140-Age)(wt. in kg)] ÷ [72 × SCR (mg/100 ml)]

This is the calculated creatinine clearance for adult males; for females it is 15% less.

* Cockcroft, D.W., *et al.*: Prediction of Creatinine Clearance from Serum Creatinine, Nephron 16.31-41, 1976.

† The half-life of ticarcillin in patients with renal failure is approximately 13 hours.

Dosage for any individual patient must take into consideration the site and severity of infection, the susceptibility of the organisms causing infection, and the status of the patient's host defense mechanisms.

The duration of therapy depends upon the severity of infection. Generally, clavulanate potassium; ticarcillin disodium should be continued for at least 2 days after the signs and symptoms of infection have disappeared. The usual duration is 10-14 days; however, in difficult and complicated infections, more prolonged therapy may be required.

Frequent bacteriologic and clinical appraisals are necessary during therapy of chronic urinary tract infection and may be required for several months after therapy has been completed; persistent infections may require treatment for several weeks, and doses smaller than those indicated above should not be used.

In certain infections, involving abscess formation, appropriate surgical drainage should be performed in conjunction with antimicrobial therapy.

INTRAVENOUS ADMINISTRATION DIRECTIONS FOR USE

3.1 and 3.2 g Vials and Piggyback Bottles: The 3.1 or 3.2 g vial should be reconstituted by adding approximately 13 ml of sterile water for injection or sodium chloride injection and shaking well. When dissolved, the concentration of ticarcillin will be approximately 200 mg/ml with corresponding concentrations of 6.7 mg/ml and 13.4 mg/ml clavulanic acid for the 3.1 and 3.2 g respective doses. Conversely, each 5.0 ml of the 3.1 g dose reconstituted with approximately 13 ml of diluent will contain approximately 1 g of ticarcillin and 33 mg of clavulanic acid. For the 3.2 g dose reconstituted with 13 ml of diluent, each 5.0 ml will contain 1 g of ticarcillin and 66 mg of clavulanic acid.

Intravenous Infusion: The dissolved drug should be further diluted to desired volume using the recommended solution listed in TABLE 6 to a concentration between 10-100 mg/ml. The solution of reconstituted drug may then be administered over a period of 30 minutes by direct infusion or through a Y-type intravenous infusion set. If this method or the "piggyback" method of administration is used, it is advisable to discontinue temporarily the administration of any other solutions during the infusion of clavulanate potassium; ticarcillin disodium.

Stability: For IV solutions, see TABLE 6.

When clavulanate potassium; ticarcillin disodium is given in combination with another antimicrobial, such as an aminoglycoside, each drug should be given separately in accordance with the recommended dosage and routes of administration for each drug.

After reconstitution and prior to administration, clavulanate potassium; ticarcillin disodium, as with other parenteral drugs, should be inspected visually for particulate matter. If this condition is evident, the solution should be discarded.

The color of reconstituted solutions of clavulanate potassium; ticarcillin disodium normally ranges from light to dark yellow depending on concentration, duration and temperature of storage while maintaining label claim characteristics.

COMPATIBILITY AND STABILITY

3.1 Gram and 3.2 Gram Vials and Piggyback Bottles: (Dilutions derived from a stock solution of 200 mg/ml.)

The concentrated stock solution at 200 mg/ml is stable for up to 6 hours at room temperature 21-24°C (70-75°F) or up to 72 hours under refrigeration 4°C (40°F).

If the concentrated stock solution (200 mg/ml) is held for up to 6 hours at room temperature 21-24°C (70-75°F) or up to 72 hours under refrigeration 4°C (40°F) and further diluted to a concentration between 10 mg/ml and 100 mg/ml with any of the diluents listed below, then the following stability periods apply.

TABLE *Stability Period (3.1 and 3.2 g vials and piggyback bottles)*

Intravenous Solution (ticarcillin concentrations of 10-100 mg/ml)	Room Temperature 21-24°C (70-75°F)	Refrigerated 4°C (40°F)
Dextrose injection 5%	24 hours	3 days
Sodium chloride injection	24 hours	7 days
Lactated Ringer's injection	24 hours	7 days

If the concentrated stock solution (200 mg/ml) is stored for up to 6 hours at room temperature and then further diluted to a concentration between 10 mg/ml and 100 mg/ml, solutions of sodium chloride injection and lactated ringer's injection may be stored frozen -18°C (0°F) for up to 30 days. Solutions prepared with Dextrose Injection 5% may be stored frozen -18°C (0°F) for up to 7 days. All thawed solutions should be used within 8 hours or discarded. Once thawed, solutions should not be refrozen.

NOTE: Clavulanate potassium; ticarcillin disodium is incompatible with sodium bicarbonate.

Unused solutions must be discarded after the time periods listed above (see TABLE 6).

HOW SUPPLIED

Clavulanate potassium; ticarcillin disodium vials should be stored at or below 24°C (75°F).

PRODUCT LISTING - EQUIVALENTS NOT AVAILABLE

Powder For Injection - Intravenous - 3 Gm;100 mg/100 ml

10's	$157.00	TIMENTIN, Glaxosmithkline	00029-6571-26
10's	$160.10	TIMENTIN, Glaxosmithkline	00029-6571-40

Powder For Injection - Intravenous - 30 Gm;1 Gm

10's	$1566.80	TIMENTIN, Glaxosmithkline	00029-6579-21

Solution - Intravenous - 3 Gm;100 mg/100 ml

12's	$218.09	TIMENTIN, Glaxosmithkline	00029-6571-31

T

Ticlopidine Hydrochloride *(003063)*

Categories: Stroke, thrombotic, prevention; Thrombosis, stent, prevention; Pregnancy Category B; FDA Approved 1991 Oct
Drug Classes: Platelet inhibitors
Brand Names: Ticlid
Foreign Brand Availability: Agulan (Indonesia); Anagregal (Italy); Antigreg (Singapore); Aplaket (Singapore; Thailand); Cartrilet (Indonesia); Clid (Korea); Declot (China; Taiwan); Desitic (Germany); Licodin (China; Taiwan); Nufaclapide (Indonesia); Panaldine (Japan); Tacron (Singapore); Ticdine (Thailand); Ticlidil (Israel); Ticlodix (Portugal); Ticlodone (Greece; Italy; Korea; Spain); Ticlomed (France); Ticuring (Indonesia); Tikleen (India); Tiklid (Italy; Spain); Tiklyd (Germany); Tilodene (Australia); Tipidin (Singapore); Tipidine (Thailand); Tyklid (India)
Cost of Therapy: $134.64 (Thrombotic Stroke Prevention; Ticlid; 250 mg; 2 tablets/day; 30 day supply)
$111.85 (Thrombotic Stroke Prevention; Generic Tablets; 250 mg; 2 tablets/day; 30 day supply)

WARNING

Ticlopidine HCl can cause life-threatening hematological adverse reactions, including neutropenia/agranulocytosis, thrombotic thrombocytopenic purpura (TTP) and aplastic anemia.

Neutropenia/Agranulocytosis:

Among 2048 patients in clinical trials, there were 50 cases (2.4%) of neutropenia (less than 1200 neutrophils/mm^3), and the neutrophil count was below 450/mm^3 in 17 of these patients (0.8% of the total population).

TTP:

One (1) case of thrombotic thrombocytopenic purpura was reported during clinical trials. Based on postmarketing data, US physicians reported about 100 cases between 1992 and 1997. Based on an estimated patient exposure of 2-4 million, and assuming an event reporting rate of 10% (the true rate is not known), the incidence of ticlopidine associated TTP may be as high as 1 case in every 2000-4000 patients exposed.

Aplastic Anemia:

Aplastic anemia was not seen during clinical trials, but US physicians reported about 50 cases between 1992 and 1998. Based on an estimated patient exposure of 2-4 million, and assuming an event reporting rate of 10% (the true rate is not known), the incidence of ticlopidine-associated aplastic anemia may be as high as 1 case in every 4000-8000 patients exposed.

Monitoring of Clinical and Hematologic Status:

Severe hematological adverse reactions may occur within a few days of the start of therapy. The incidence of TTP peaks after about 3-4 weeks of therapy and neutropenia peaks at approximately 4-6 weeks. The incidence of aplastic anemia peaks after about 4-8 weeks of therapy. The incidence of the hematologic adverse reactions declines thereafter. Only a few cases of neutropenia, TTP, or aplastic anemia have arisen after more than 3 months of therapy.

Hematological adverse reactions cannot be reliably predicted by any identified demographic or clinical characteristics. During the first 3 months of treatment, patients receiving ticlopidine HCl must, therefore, be hematologically and clinically monitored for evidence of neutropenia or TTP. If any such evidence is seen, ticlopidine HCl should be immediately discontinued.

The detection and treatment of ticlopidine-associated hematological adverse reactions are further described under WARNINGS.

DESCRIPTION

Ticlopidine hydrochloride is a platelet aggregation inhibitor. Chemically it is 5-[(2-chlorophenyl)methyl]-4,5,6,7-tetrahydrothieno [3,2-c] pyridine hydrochloride.

Ticlopidine hydrochloride is a white crystalline solid. It is freely soluble in water and self-buffers to a pH of 3.6. It also dissolves freely in methanol, is sparingly soluble in methylene chloride and ethanol, slightly soluble in acetone and insoluble in a buffer solution of pH 6.3. It has a molecular weight of 300.25.

Ticlid tablets for oral administration are provided as white, oval, film-coated, blue-imprinted tablets containing 250 mg of ticlopidine hydrochloride. Each tablet also contains citric acid, magnesium stearate, microcrystalline cellulose, povidone, starch and stearic acid as inactive ingredients. The white film-coating contains hydroxypropylmethyl cellulose, polyethylene glycol and titanium dioxide. Each tablet is printed with blue ink, which includes FD&C blue no. 1 aluminum lake as the colorant. The tablets are identified with "Ticlid" on one side and "250" on the reverse side.

CLINICAL PHARMACOLOGY

MECHANISM OF ACTION

When taken orally, ticlopidine hydrochloride causes a time- and dose-dependent inhibition of both platelet aggregation and release of platelet granule constituents, as well as a prolongation of bleeding time. The intact drug has no significant *in vitro* activity at the concentrations attained *in vivo;* and, although analysis of urine and plasma indicates at least 20 metabolites, no metabolite which accounts for the activity of ticlopidine has been isolated.

Ticlopidine hydrochloride, after oral ingestion, interferes with platelet membrane function by inhibiting ADP-induced platelet-fibrinogen binding and subsequent platelet-platelet interactions. The effect on platelet function is irreversible for the life of the platelet, as shown both by persistent inhibition of fibrinogen binding after washing platelets *ex vivo* and by inhibition of platelet aggregation after resuspension of platelets in buffered medium.

PHARMACOKINETICS AND METABOLISM

After oral administration of a single 250 mg dose, ticlopidine hydrochloride is rapidly absorbed with peak plasma levels occurring at approximately 2 hours after dosing and is extensively metabolized. Absorption is greater than 8004. Administration after meals results in a 20% increase in the AUC of ticlopidine.

Ticlopidine hydrochloride displays nonlinear pharmacokinetics and clearance decreases markedly on repeated dosing. In older volunteers the apparent half-life of ticlopidine after a single 250 mg dose is about 12.6 hours; with repeat dosing at 250 mg bid, the terminal elimination half-life rises to 4-5 days and steady-state levels of ticlopidine hydrochloride in plasma are obtained after approximately 14-21 days.

Ticlopidine hydrochloride binds reversibly (98%) to plasma proteins, mainly to serum albumin and lipoproteins. The binding to albumin and lipoproteins is nonsaturable over a wide concentration range. Ticlopidine also binds to alpha-1 acid glycoprotein. At concentrations attained with the recommended dose, only 15% or less ticlopidine in plasma is bound to this protein. Ticlopidine hydrochloride is metabolized extensively by the liver; only trace amounts of intact drug are detected in the urine. Following an oral dose of radioactive ticlopidine hydrochloride administered in solution, 60% of the radioactivity is recovered in the urine and 23% in the feces. Approximately 1/3 of the dose excreted in the feces is intact ticlopidine hydrochloride, possibly excreted in the bile. Ticlopidine hydrochloride is a minor component in plasma (5%) after a single dose, but at steady-state is the major component (15%). Approximately 40-50% of the radioactive metabolites circulating in plasma are covalently bound to plasma proteins, probably by acylation.Clearance of ticlopidine decreases with age. Steady-state trough values in elderly patients (mean age 70 years) are about twice those in younger volunteer populations.

HEPATICALLY IMPAIRED PATIENTS

The effect of decreased hepatic function on the pharmacokinetics of ticlopidine HCl was studied in 17 patients with advanced cirrhosis. The average plasma concentration of ticlopidine in these subjects was slightly higher than that seen in older subjects in a separate trial (see CONTRAINDICATIONS).

RENALLY IMPAIRED PATIENTS

Patients with mildly (Ccr 50-80 ml/min) or moderately (Ccr 20-50 ml/min) impaired renal function were compared to normal subjects (Ccr 80-150 ml/min) in a study of the pharmacokinetic and platelet pharmacodynamic effects of ticlopidine HCl (250 mg bid) for 11 days. Concentrations of unchanged ticlopidine HCl were measured after a single 250 mg dose and after the final 250 mg dose on Day 11.

AUC values of ticlopidine increased by 28% and 60% in mild and moderately impaired patients, respectively, and plasma clearance decreased by 37% and 52%, respectively, but there were no statistically significant differences in ADP-induced platelet aggregation. In this small study (26 patients), bleeding times showed significant prolongation only in the moderately impaired patients.

PHARMACODYNAMICS

In healthy volunteers over the age of 50, substantial inhibition (over 50%) of ADP-induced platelet aggregation is detected within 4 days after administration of ticlopidine hydrochloride 250 mg bid, and maximum platelet aggregation inhibition (60-70%) is achieved after 8-11 days. Lower doses cause less, and more delayed, platelet aggregation inhibition, while doses above 250 mg bid give little additional effect on platelet aggregation but an increased rate of adverse effects. The dose of 250 mg bid is the only dose that has been evaluated in controlled clinical trials.

After discontinuation of ticlopidine hydrochloride, bleeding time and other platelet function tests return to normal within 2 weeks, in the majority of patients.

At the recommended therapeutic dose (250 mg bid), ticlopidine hydrochloride has no known significant pharmacological actions in man other than inhibition of platelet function and prolongation of the bleeding time.

INDICATIONS AND USAGE

Ticlopidine HCl is indicated:

- To reduce the risk of thrombotic stroke (fatal or nonfatal) in patients who have experienced stroke precursors, and in patients who have had a completed thrombotic stroke. Because ticlopidine HCl is associated with a risk of life-threatening blood dyscrasias including thrombotic thrombocytopenic purpura (TTP), neutropenia/agranulocytosis and aplastic anemia (see BOXED WARNING and WARNINGS), ticlopidine HCl should be reserved for patients who are intolerant or allergic to aspirin therapy or who have failed aspirin therapy.
- As adjunctive therapy with aspirin to reduce the incidence of subacute stent thrombosis in patients undergoing successful coronary stent implantation.

CONTRAINDICATIONS

The use of ticlopidine HCl is contraindicated in the following conditions:

- Hypersensitivity to the drug.
- Presence of hematopoietic disorders such as neutropenia and thrombocytopenia or a past history of either TTP or aplastic anemia.
- Presence of a hemostatic disorder or active pathological bleeding (such as bleeding peptic ulcer or intracranial bleeding).
- Patients with severe liver impairment.

WARNINGS

HEMATOLOGICAL ADVERSE REACTIONS

Neutropenia

Neutropenia may occur suddenly. Bone-marrow examination typically shows a reduction in white blood cell precursors. After withdrawal of ticlopidine, the neutrophil count usually rises to >1200/mm^3 within 1-3 weeks.

Thrombocytopenia

Rarely, thrombocytopenia may occur in isolation or together with neutropenia.

Thrombotic Thrombocytopenic Purpura (TTP)

TTP is characterized by thrombocytopenia, microangiopathic hemolytic anemia (schistocytes [fragmented RBCs] seen on peripheral smear), neurological findings, renal dysfunction, and fever. The signs and symptoms can occur in any order, in particular, clinical symptoms may precede laboratory findings by hours or days. With **prompt** treatment (often including plasmapheresis), 70-80% of patients will survive with minimal or no sequelae. Because platelet transfusions may accelerate thrombosis in patients with TTP on ticlopidine, they should, if possible, be avoided.

T

Aplastic Anemia

Aplastic anemia is characterized by anemia, thrombocytopenia and neutropenia together with a bone marrow examination that shows decreases in the precursor cells for red blood cells, white blood cells, and platelets. Patients may present with signs or symptoms suggestive of infection, in association with low white blood cell and platelet counts. **Prompt** treatment, which may include the use of drugs to stimulate the bone marrow, can minimize the mortality associated with aplastic anemia.

Monitoring for Hematologic Adverse Reactions

Starting just before initiating treatment and continuing through the third month of therapy, patients receiving ticlopidine HCl must be monitored every 2 weeks. Because of ticlopidine's long plasma half-life, patients who discontinue ticlopidine during this 3 month period should continue to be monitored for 2 weeks after discontinuation. More frequent monitoring, and monitoring after the first 3 months of therapy, is necessary only in patients with clinical signs (*e.g.,* signs or symptoms suggestive of infection) or laboratory signs (*e.g.,* neutrophil count less than 70% of the baseline count, decrease in hematocrit or platelet count) that suggest incipient hematological adverse reactions.

Clinically, fever might suggest neutropenia, TTP, or aplastic anemia; TTP might also be suggested by weakness, pallor, petechiae or purpura, dark urine (due to blood, bile pigments, or hemoglobin) or jaundice, or neurological changes. Patients should be told to discontinue ticlopidine HCl and to contact the physician immediately upon the occurrence of any of these findings.

Laboratory monitoring should include a complete blood count, with special attention to the absolute neutrophil count (WBC × % neutrophils), platelet count, and the appearance of the peripheral smear. Ticlopidine is occasionally associated with thrombocytopenia unrelated to TTP or aplastic anemia. Any acute, unexplained reduction in **hemoglobin** or platelet count should prompt further investigation for a diagnosis of TTP, and the appearance of **schistocytes** (fragmented RBCs) on the smear should be treated as presumptive evidence of TTP. A simultaneous decrease in platelet count and WBC count should prompt further investigation for a diagnosis of aplastic anemia. If there are laboratory signs of TTP, or if the neutrophil count is confirmed to be $1200/mm^3$, then ticlopidine HCl should be discontinued immediately.

OTHER HEMATOLOGICAL EFFECTS

Rare cases of agranulocytosis, pancytopenia, or leukemia have been reported in postmarketing experience, some of which have been fatal. All forms of hematological adverse reactions are potentially fatal.

CHOLESTEROL ELEVATION

Ticlopidine HCl therapy causes increased serum cholesterol and triglycerides. Serum total cholesterol levels are increased 8-10% within 1 month of therapy and persist at that level. The ratios of the lipoprotein subfractions are unchanged.

ANTICOAGULANT DRUGS

The tolerance and safety of coadministration of ticlopidine HCl with heparin, oral anticoagulants or fibrinolytic agents have not been established. If a patient is switched from an anticoagulant or fibrinolytic drug to ticlopidine HCl, the former drug should be discontinued prior to ticlopidine HCl administration.

PRECAUTIONS

GENERAL

Ticlopidine HCl should be used with caution in patients who may be at risk of increased bleeding from trauma, surgery or pathological conditions. If it is desired to eliminate the antiplatelet effects of ticlopidine HCl prior to elective surgery, the drug should be discontinued 10-14 days prior to surgery. Several controlled clinical studies have found increased surgical blood loss in patients undergoing surgery during treatment with ticlopidine. In TASS and CATS it was recommended that patients have ticlopidine discontinued prior to elective surgery. Several hundred patients underwent surgery during the trials, and no excessive surgical bleeding was reported.

Prolonged bleeding time is normalized within 2 hours after administration of 20 mg methylprednisolone IV. Platelet transfusions may also be used to reverse the effect of ticlopidine HCl on bleeding. Because platelet transfusions may accelerate thrombosis in patients with TTP on ticlopidine, they should, if possible, be avoided.

GI BLEEDING

Ticlopidine HCl prolongs template bleeding time. The drug should be used with caution in patients who have lesions with a propensity to bleed (such as ulcers). Drugs that might induce such lesions should be used with caution in patients on ticlopidine HCl (see CONTRAINDICATIONS).

USE IN HEPATICALLY IMPAIRED PATIENTS

Since ticlopidine is metabolized by the liver, dosing of ticlopidine HCl or other drugs metabolized in the liver may require adjustment upon starting or stopping concomitant therapy. Because of limited experience in patients with severe hepatic disease, who may have bleeding diatheses, the use of ticlopidine HCl is not recommended in this population (see CLINICAL PHARMACOLOGY and CONTRAINDICATIONS).

USE IN RENALLY IMPAIRED PATIENTS

There is limited experience in patients with renal impairment. Decreased plasma clearance, increased AUC values and prolonged bleeding times can occur in renally impaired patients. In controlled clinical trials no unexpected problems have been encountered in patients having mild renal impairment, and there is no experience with dosage adjustment in patients with greater degrees of renal impairment. Nevertheless, for renally impaired patients, it may be necessary to reduce the dosage of ticlopidine or discontinue it altogether if hemorrhagic or hematopoietic problems are encountered (see CLINICAL PHARMACOLOGY).

INFORMATION FOR THE PATIENT

See the Patient Leaflet which is distributed with the prescription.

Patients should be told that a decrease in the number of white blood cells (neutropenia) or platelets (thrombocytopenia) can occur with ticlopidine HCl, especially during the first 3 months of treatment and that neutropenia, if it is severe, can result in an increased risk of infection. They should be told it is critically important to obtain the scheduled blood tests to detect neutropenia or thrombocytopenia. Patients should also be reminded to contact their physicians if they experience any indication of infection such as fever, chills, or sore throat, any of which might be a consequence of neutropenia. Thrombocytopenia may be part of a syndrome called TTP. Symptoms and signs of TTP, such as fever, weakness, difficulty speaking, seizures, yellowing of skin or eyes, dark or bloody urine, pallor or petechiae (pinpoint hemorrhagic spots on the skin), should be reported immediately.

All patients should be told that it may take them longer than usual to stop bleeding when they take ticlopidine HCl and that they should report any unusual bleeding to their physician. Patients should tell physicians and dentists that they are taking ticlopidine HCl before any surgery is scheduled and before any new drug is prescribed.

Patients should be told to promptly report side effects of ticlopidine HCl such as severe or persistent diarrhea, skin rashes or subcutaneous bleeding or any signs of cholestasis, such as yellow skin or sclera, dark urine, or light-colored stools.

Patients should be told to take ticlopidine HCl with food or just after eating in order to minimize gastrointestinal discomfort.

LABORATORY TESTS

Liver Function

Ticlopidine HCl therapy has been associated with elevations of alkaline phosphatase, bilirubin, and transaminases, which generally occurred within 1-4 months of therapy initiation. In controlled clinical trials the incidence of elevated alkaline phosphatase (greater than 2 times upper limit of normal) was 7.6% in ticlopidine patients, 6% in placebo patients and 2.5% in aspirin patients. The incidence of elevated AST (SGOT) (greater than 2 times upper limit of normal) was 3.1% in ticlopidine patients, 4% in placebo patients and 2.1% in aspirin patients. No progressive increases were observed in closely monitored clinical trials (*e.g.,* no transaminase greater than 10 times the upper limit of normal was seen), but most patients with these abnormalities had therapy discontinued. Occasionally patients had developed minor elevations in bilirubin.

Postmarketing experience includes rare individuals with elevations in their transaminases and bilirubin to >10× above the upper limits of normal. Based on postmarketing and clinical trial experience, liver function testing, including ALT, AST, and GGT, should be considered whenever liver dysfunction is suspected, particularly during the first 4 months of treatment.

FOOD INTERACTION

The oral bioavailability of ticlopidine is increased by 20% when taken after a meal. Administration of ticlopidine HCl with food is recommended to maximize gastrointestinal tolerance. In controlled trials ticlopidine HCl was taken with meals.

CARCINOGENESIS, MUTAGENESIS, AND IMPAIRMENT OF FERTILITY

In a 2 year oral carcinogenicity study in rats, ticlopidine at daily doses of up to 100 mg/kg ($610\ mg/m^2$) was not tumorigenic. For a 70 kg person ($1.73\ m^2$ body surface area) the dose represents 14 times the recommended clinical dose on a mg/kg basis and 2 times the clinical dose on body surface area basis. In a 78 week oral carcinogenicity study in mice, ticlopidine at daily doses up to 275 mg/kg ($1180\ mg/m^2$) was not tumorigenic. The dose represents 40 times the recommended clinical dose on a mg/kg basis and 4 times the clinical dose on body surface area basis.

Ticlopidine was not mutagenic *in vitro* in the Ames test, the rat hepatocyte DNA-repair assay, or the Chinese-hamster fibroblast chromosomal aberration test; or *in vivo* in the mouse spermatozoid morphology test, the Chinese-hamster micronucleus test, or the Chinese-hamster bone-marrow-cell sister-chromatid exchange test. Ticlopidine was found to have no effect on fertility of male and female rats at oral doses up to 400 mg/kg/day.

PREGNANCY, TERATOGENIC EFFECTS, PREGNANCY CATEGORY B

Teratology studies have been conducted in mice (doses up to 200 mg/kg/day), rats (doses up to 400 mg/kg/day) and rabbits (doses up to 200 mg/kg/day). Doses of 400 mg/kg in rats, 200 mg/kg/day in mice and 100 mg/kg in rabbits produced maternal toxicity, as well as fetal toxicity, but there was no evidence of a teratogenic potential of ticlopidine. There are, however, no adequate and well-controlled studies in pregnant women. Because animal reproduction studies are not always predictive of a human response, this drug should be used during pregnancy only if clearly needed.

NURSING MOTHERS

Studies in rats have shown ticlopidine is excreted in the milk. It is not known whether this drug is excreted in human milk. Because many drugs are excreted in human milk and because of the potential for serious adverse reactions in nursing infants from ticlopidine, a decision should be made whether to discontinue nursing or to discontinue the drug, taking into account the importance of the drug to the mother.

PEDIATRIC USE

Safety and effectiveness in pediatric patients have not been established.

GERIATRIC USE

Clearance of ticlopidine is somewhat lower in elderly patients and trough levels are increased. The major clinical trials with ticlopidine HCl were conducted in an elderly population with an average age of 64 years. Of the total number of patients in the therapeutic trials, 45% of patients were over 65 years old and 12% were over 75 years old. No overall differences in effectiveness or safety were observed between these patients and younger patients, and other reported clinical experience has not identified differences in responses between the elderly and younger patients, but greater sensitivity of some older individuals cannot be ruled out.

DRUG INTERACTIONS

Therapeutic doses of ticlopidine HCl caused a 30% increase in the plasma half-life of antipyrine and may cause analogous effects on similarly metabolized drugs. Therefore, the dose of drugs metabolized by hepatic microsomal enzymes with low therapeutic ratios or being given to patients with hepatic impairment may require adjustment to maintain optimal therapeutic blood levels when starting or stopping concomitant therapy with ticlopidine. Studies of specific drug interactions yielded the following results:

Aspirin and Other NSAIDs: Ticlopidine potentiates the effect of aspirin or other NSAIDs on platelet aggregation. The safety of concomitant use of ticlopidine with aspirin or other NSAIDs has not been established. Aspirin did not modify the ticlopidine-mediated inhibition of ADP induced platelet aggregation, but ticlopidine potentiated the effect of aspirin on collagen-induced platelet aggregation. Concomitant use of aspirin and ticlopidine is not recommended (see PRECAUTIONS, General, GI Bleeding).

Antacids: Administration of ticlopidine HCl after antacids resulted in an 18% decrease in plasma levels of ticlopidine.

Cimetidine: Chronic administration of cimetidine reduced the clearance of a single dose of ticlopidine HCl by 50%.

Digoxin: Coadministration of ticlopidine HCl with digoxin resulted in a slight decrease (approximately 15%) in digoxin plasma levels. Little or no change in therapeutic efficacy of digoxin would be expected.

Theophylline: In normal volunteers, concomitant administration of ticlopidine HCl resulted in a significant increase in the theophylline elimination half-life from 8.6 to 12.2 hours and a comparable reduction in total plasma clearance of theophylline.

Phenobarbital: In 6 normal volunteers, the inhibitory effects of ticlopidine HCl on platelet aggregation were not altered by chronic administration of phenobarbital.

Phenytoin: *In vitro* studies demonstrated that ticlopidine does not alter the plasma protein binding of phenytoin. However, the protein binding interactions of ticlopidine and its metabolites have not been studied *in vivo.* Several cases of elevated phenytoin plasma levels with associated somnolence and lethargy have been reported following coadministration with ticlopidine HCl. Caution should be exercised in coadministering this drug with ticlopidine HCl, and it may be useful to remeasure phenytoin blood concentrations.

Propranolol: *In vitro* studies demonstrated that ticlopidine does not alter the plasma protein binding of propranolol. However, the protein binding interactions of ticlopidine and its metabolites have not been studied *in vivo.* Caution should be exercised in coadministering this drug with ticlopidine HCl.

Other Concomitant Therapy: Although specific interaction studies were not performed, in clinical studies ticlopidine HCl was used concomitantly with beta blockers, calcium channel blockers and diuretics without evidence of clinically significant adverse interactions (see PRECAUTIONS).

ADVERSE REACTIONS

Adverse reactions were relatively frequent with over 50% of patients reporting at least one. Most (30-40%) involved the gastrointestinal tract. Most adverse effects are mild, but 21% of patients discontinued therapy because of an adverse event, principally diarrhea, rash, nausea, vomiting, GI pain and neutropenia. Most adverse effects occur early in the course of treatment, but a new onset of adverse effects can occur after several months.

The incidence rates of adverse events listed in TABLE 3 were derived from multicenter, controlled clinical trials described above comparing ticlopidine HCl, placebo and aspirin over study periods of up to 5.8 years. Adverse events considered by the investigator to be probably drug-related that occurred in at least 1% of patients treated with ticlopidine HCl are shown in TABLE 3.

TABLE 3 *Percent of Patients With Adverse Events in Controlled Studies*

	TASS and CATTS		
	Ticlopidine	**Aspirin**	**Placebo**
Event	**(n=2048)**	**(n=1527)**	**(n=536)**
Any events	60.0% (20.9%)	53.2% (14.5%)	34.3% (6.1%)
Diarrhea	12.5% (6.3%)	5.2% (1.8%)	4.5% (1.7%)
Nausea	7.0% (2.6%)	6.2% (1.9%)	1.7% (0.9%)
Dyspepsia	7.0% (1.1%)	9.0% (2.0%)	0.9% (0.2%)
Rash	5.1% (3.4%)	1.5% (0.8%)	0.6% (0.9%)
GI pain	3.7% (1.9%)	5.6% (2.7%)	1.3% (0.4%)
Neutropenia	2.4% (1.3%)	0.8% (0.1%)	1.1% (0.4%)
Purpura	2.2% (0.2%)	1.6% (0.1%)	0.0% (0.0%)
Vomiting	1.9% (1.4%)	1.4% (0.9%)	0.9% (0.4%)
Flatulence	1.5% (0.1%)	1.4% (0.3%)	0.0% (0.0%)
Pruritus	1.3% (0.8%)	0.3% (0.1%)	0.0% (0.0%)
Dizziness	1.1% (0.4%)	0.5% (0.4%)	0.0% (0.0%)
Anorexia	1.0% (0.4%)	0.5% (0.3%)	0.0% (0.0%)
Abnormal liver function test	1.0% (0.7%)	0.3% (0.3%)	0.0% (0.0%)

Incidence of discontinuation, regardless of relationship to therapy, is shown in parentheses.

HEMATOLOGICAL

Neutropenia/thrombocytopenia, TTP, aplastic anemia (see BOXED WARNING and WARNINGS), leukemia, agranulocytosis, eosinophilia, pancytopenia, thrombocytosis and bone-marrow depression have been reported.

GASTROINTESTINAL

Ticlopidine HCl therapy has been associated with a variety of gastrointestinal complaints including diarrhea and nausea. The majority of cases are mild, but about 13% of patients discontinued therapy because of these. They usually occur within 3 months of initiation of therapy and typically are resolved within 1-2 weeks without discontinuation of therapy. If the effect is severe or persistent, therapy should be discontinued. In some cases of severe or bloody diarrhea, colitis was later diagnosed.

HEMORRHAGIC

Ticlopidine HCl has been associated with increased bleeding, spontaneous posttraumatic bleeding and perioperative bleeding including, but not limited to, gastrointestinal bleeding. It has also been associated with a number of bleeding complications such as ecchymosis, epistaxis, hematuria and conjunctival hemorrhage.

Intracerebral bleeding was rare in clinical trials with ticlopidine HCl, with an incidence no greater than that seen with comparator agents (ticlopidine 0.5%, aspirin 0.6%, placebo 0.75%). It has also been reported postmarketing.

RASH

Ticlopidine has been associated with a maculopapular or urticarial rash (often with pruritus). Rash usually occurs within 3 months of initiation of therapy with a mean onset time of 11 days. If drug is discontinued, recovery occurs within several days. Many rashes do not recur on drug rechallenge. There have been rare reports of severe rashes, including Stevens-Johnson syndrome, erythema multiforme and exfoliative dermatitis.

LESS FREQUENT ADVERSE REACTIONS (PROBABLY RELATED)

Clinical adverse experiences occurring in 0.5% to 1% of patients in the controlled trials include:

Digestive System: GI fullness.
Skin and Appendages: Urticaria.
Nervous System: Headache.
Body as a Whole: Asthenia, pain.
Hemostatic System: Epistaxis.
Special Senses: Tinnitus.

In addition, rarer, relatively serious and potentially fatal events associated with the use of ticlopidine HCl have also been reported from postmarketing experience: Hemolytic anemia with reticulocytosis, immune thrombocytopenia, hepatitis, hepatocellular jaundice, cholestatic jaundice, hepatic necrosis, hepatic failure, peptic ulcer, renal failure, nephrotic syndrome, hyponatremia, vasculitis, sepsis, allergic reactions (including angioedema, allergic pneumonitis, and anaphylaxis), systemic lupus (positive ANA), peripheral neuropathy, serum sickness, arthropathy and myositis.

DOSAGE AND ADMINISTRATION

STROKE

The recommended dose of ticlopidine HCl is 250 mg bid taken with food. Other doses have not been studied in controlled trials for these indications.

CORONARY ARTERY STENTING

The recommended dose of ticlopidine HCl is 250 mg bid taken with food together with antiplatelet doses of aspirin for up to 30 days of therapy following successful stent implantation.

HOW SUPPLIED

Ticlid is available in white, oval, film-coated 250 mg tablets, printed in blue with "Ticlid" on one side and "250" on the other.

Storage: Store at 15-30°C (59-86°F).

PRODUCT LISTING - RATED THERAPEUTICALLY EQUIVALENT

Tablet - Oral - 250 mg

30's	$57.63	GENERIC, Geneva Pharmaceuticals	00781-1514-31
30's	$57.69	GENERIC, Eon Labs Manufacturing Inc	00185-0115-30
30's	$57.69	GENERIC, Purepac Pharmaceutical Company	00228-2613-03
30's	$57.69	GENERIC, Major Pharmaceuticals Inc	00904-5378-46
30's	$57.69	GENERIC, Par Pharmaceutical Inc	49884-0599-11
30's	$57.69	GENERIC, Apotex Usa Inc	60505-0027-02
30's	$67.32	TICLID, Allscripts Pharmaceutical Company	54569-4691-00
30's	$69.64	TICLID, Physicians Total Care	54868-3783-00
30's	$69.64	TICLID, Physicians Total Care	54868-3783-01
30's	$76.44	TICLID, Roche Laboratories	00004-0018-23
60's	$90.71	FEDERAL UPPER LIMIT, H.C.F.A. F F P	99999-3063-01
60's	$111.85	GENERIC, Geneva Pharmaceuticals	00781-1514-60
60's	$111.97	GENERIC, Major Pharmaceuticals Inc	00904-5378-52
60's	$111.97	GENERIC, Apotex Usa Inc	60505-0027-04
60's	$111.98	GENERIC, Eon Labs Manufacturing Inc	00185-0115-60
60's	$111.98	GENERIC, Par Pharmaceutical Inc	49884-0599-02
60's	$112.23	GENERIC, Purepac Pharmaceutical Company	00228-2613-06
60's	$134.64	TICLID, Allscripts Pharmaceutical Company	54569-4691-01
60's	$148.34	TICLID, Roche Laboratories	00004-0018-22
100's	$186.00	GENERIC, Teva Pharmaceuticals Usa	00093-0154-01
100's	$186.62	GENERIC, Purepac Pharmaceutical Company	00228-2613-11
100's	$186.62	GENERIC, Par Pharmaceutical Inc	49884-0599-01
100's	$195.79	GENERIC, Major Pharmaceuticals Inc	00904-5378-61

Tiludronate Disodium (003393)

Categories: Paget's disease; FDA Approved 1997 Mar; Pregnancy Category C
Drug Classes: Bisphosphonates
Brand Names: **Skelid**
Cost of Therapy: $1,418.22 (Paget's Disease; Skelid; 200 mg; 2 tablets/day; 84 day supply)

DESCRIPTION

Tiludronate disodium is a bisphosphonate characterized by a (4-chlorophenylthio) group on the carbon atom of the basic P-C-P structure common to all bisphosphonates. Its generic name is tiludronate disodium. Tiludronate disodium is the hydrated hemihydrate form of the disodium salt of tiludronic acid. Its chemical name is [[(4-Chlorophenyl)thio]methylene]bis[phosphoric acid], disodium salt.

The molecular weight of tiludronate disodium is 380.6.

Skelid tablets for oral administration contain 240 mg tiludronate disodium, which is the molar equivalent of 200 mg tiludronic acid. Skelid tablets also contain sodium lauryl sulfate, hydroxypropyl methylcellulose 2910, crospovidone, magnesium stearate, and lactose monohydrate.

CLINICAL PHARMACOLOGY

MECHANISM OF ACTION

In vitro studies indicate that tiludronate disodium acts primarily on bone through a mechanism that involves inhibition of osteoclastic activity with a probable reduction in the enzymatic and transport processes that lead to resorption of the mineralized matrix.

Bone resorption occurs following recruitment, activation, and polarization of osteoclasts. *Tiludronate disodium appears to inhibit osteoclasts through at least two mechanisms:* disruption of the cytoskeletal ring structure, possibly by inhibition of protein-tyrosine-phosphatase, thus leading to detachment of osteoclasts from the bone surface and the inhibition of the osteoclastic proton pump.

PHARMACOKINETICS

ABSORPTION

Relative to an intravenous (IV) reference dose, the mean oral bioavailability of tiludronate disodium in healthy male subjects was 6% after an oral dose equivalent to 400 mg tiludronic acid administered after an overnight fast and 4 hours before a standard breakfast. In single-dose studies, bioavailability was reduced by 90% when an oral dose equivalent to 400 mg tiludronic acid was administered with, or 2 hours after, a standard breakfast compared to the same dose administered after an overnight fast and 4 hours before a standard breakfast. However, in clinical studies, efficacy was seen when tiludronate disodium was dosed at least 2 hours before or after meals.

After administration of a single dose equivalent to 400 mg tiludronic acid to healthy male subjects, tiludronic acid was rapidly absorbed with peak plasma concentrations of approximately 3 mg/L occurring within 2 hours. In pagetic patients, after repeated administration of doses equivalent to 400 mg/day tiludronic acid (2 hours before or 2 hours after a meal) for durations of 12 days to 12 weeks, average plasma concentrations of tiludronic acid occurring between 1 and 2 hours after dosing ranged between 1 and 4.6 mg/L.

DISTRIBUTION

Animal pharmacology studies in rats demonstrate that tiludronic acid is widely distributed to bone and soft tissues. Over a period of days, loss of drug occurs from most tissues with the exception of bone and cartilage. Tiludronate is then slowly released from bone with a half-life in rats of 30 days or longer depending on the status of bone turnover.

After oral administration of doses equivalent to 400 mg/day tiludronic acid to nonpagetic patients with osteoarthrosis, the steady state in bone was not reached after 30 days of dosing.

At plasma concentrations between 1 and 10 mg/L, tiludronic acid was approximately 90% bound to human serum protein (mainly albumin).

METABOLISM

In laboratory animals, tiludronic acid undergoes little if any metabolism. *In vitro,* tiludronic acid is not metabolized in human liver microsomes and hepatocytes.

ELIMINATION

The principal route of elimination of tiludronic acid is in the urine. After IV administration to healthy volunteers, approximately 60% of the dose was excreted in the urine as tiludronic acid within 13 days. Renal clearance is dose independent and is approximately 10 ml/min in healthy subjects. In pagetic patients treated with doses equivalent to 400 mg/day tiludronic acid for 12 days, the mean apparent plasma elimination half-life was approximately 150 hours. The elimination rate from human bone is unknown.

SPECIAL POPULATIONS

Geriatric: No dosage adjustment in elderly patients is necessary. Plasma concentrations of tiludronic acid were higher in elderly pagetic patients (≥65 years of age); however, this difference was not clinically significant.

Pediatric: Tiludronate disodium pharmacokinetics have not been investigated in subjects under the age of 18 years.

Gender: There were no clinically significant differences in plasma concentrations after repeated administration of tiludronate disodium to male and female pagetic patients.

Race: Pharmacokinetic differences due to race have not been studied.

Renal Insufficiency: Tiludronate disodium is not recommended for patients with severe renal failure (creatinine clearance <30 ml/min) due to lack of clinical experience. After a single oral dose equivalent to 400 mg tiludronic acid, subjects with creatinine clearance between 11 and 18 ml/min had C_{max} values (approximately 3 mg/L) in the range of healthy volunteers. However, the plasma elimination half-life was approximately 205 hours, which is longer than that observed in pagetic patients after repeated doses (150 hours) and healthy subjects after single doses (50 hours). These values were obtained in a cross-study comparison between healthy volunteers and pagetic patients.

Hepatic Insufficiency: No dosage adjustment is needed. Since tiludronate undergoes little or no metabolism, no studies were conducted in subjects with hepatic insufficiency.

Drug-Drug Interactions: (See also DRUG INTERACTIONS) The bioavailability of tiludronate disodium is decreased 80% by calcium, when calcium and tiludronate disodium are administered at the same time, and 60% by some aluminum- or magnesium-containing antacids, when administered 1 hour before tiludronate disodium. Aspirin may decrease bioavailability of tiludronate disodium by up to 50% when taken 2 hours after tiludronate disodium. The bioavailability of tiludronate disodium is increased 2-4 fold by indomethacin and is not significantly altered by coadministration of diclofenac. The pharmacokinetic parameters of digoxin are not significantly modified by tiludronate disodium coadministration. *In vitro* studies show that tiludronate disodium does not displace warfarin from its binding site on protein.

TABLE 1 *Summary of Pharmacokinetic Parameters in the Normal Population*

Parameter	Mean (SD)
Absolute bioavailability of two 200-mg tablets taken 4 hrs before standard breakfast	6% (2%)*
Time to peak plasma concentration (taken 4 hrs before first meal of day, n=151)	1.5 (0.9) hr
Maximum plasma concentration after a single 400-mg dose (taken 4 hrs before first meal of day, n=151)	2.66 (1.22) mg/L
Renal clearance after IV administration of 20-mg dose	0.54 (0.14) L/hr

* Bioavailability was reduced by 90% when this oral dose was administered with, or 2 hours after, a standard breakfast.

PHARMACODYNAMICS

Paget's disease of bone is a chronic, focal skeletal disorder characterized by greatly increased and disorderly bone remodeling. Excessive osteoclastic bone resorption is followed by osteoblastic new bone formation, leading to the replacement of the normal bone architecture by disorganized, enlarged, and weakened bone structure.

Clinical manifestations of Paget's disease range from no symptoms to severe bone pain, bone deformity, pathological fractures, and neurological and other complications. Serum alkaline phosphatase, the most frequently used biochemical index of disease activity, provides an objective measure of disease severity and response to therapy.

In pagetic patients treated with tiludronate disodium 400 mg/day for 3 months, changes in urinary hydroxyproline, a biochemical marker of bone resorption, and in serum alkaline phosphatase, a marker of bone formation, indicate a reduction toward normal in the rate of bone turnover. In addition, reduced numbers of osteoclasts by histomorphometric analysis and radiological improvement of lytic lesions indicate that tiludronate disodium can suppress the pagetic disease process.

INDICATIONS AND USAGE

Tiludronate disodium is indicated for treatment of Paget's disease of bone (osteitis deformans).

Treatment is Indicated in Patients with Paget's Disease of Bone:

1. Who have a level of serum alkaline phosphatase (SAP) at least twice the upper limit of normal.
2. Who are symptomatic.
3. Who are at risk for future complications of their disease.

NON-FDA APPROVED INDICATIONS

Bisphosphonates are also used in the treatment of hypercalcemia of malignancy, breast cancer or multiple myeloma associated osteolytic bone disease and in the management of postmenopausal and steroid-induced osteoporosis.

CONTRAINDICATIONS

Tiludronate disodium is contraindicated in individuals with known hypersensitivity to any component of this product.

WARNINGS

Bisphosphonates may cause upper gastrointestinal disorders, such as dysphagia, esophagitis, esophageal ulcer, and gastric ulcer (see ADVERSE REACTIONS).

PRECAUTIONS

GENERAL

Tiludronate disodium is not recommended for patients with severe renal failure, for example, those with creatinine clearance <30 ml/min (see CLINICAL PHARMACOLOGY, Renal Insufficiency).

INFORMATION FOR PATIENTS

Patients Receiving Tiludronate Disodium Should be Instructed To:

1. Take tiludronate disodium with 6 to 8 ounces of plain water.
2. Tiludronate disodium should not be taken within 2 hours of food.
3. Maintain adequate vitamin D and calcium intake.
4. Calcium supplements, aspirin, and indomethacin should not be taken within 2 hours before or 2 hours after tiludronate disodium.
5. Aluminum- or magnesium-containing antacids, if needed, should be taken at least 2 hours after taking tiludronate disodium.

CARCINOGENESIS, MUTAGENESIS, AND IMPAIRMENT OF FERTILITY

Carcinogenicity studies have not yet been completed.

Tiludronate was not genotoxic in the following assays: an *in vitro* microbial mutagenesis assay with and without metabolic activation, a human lymphocyte assay, a yeast cell assay for forward mutation and mitotic crossing over, or the *in vivo* mouse micronucleus test.

Tiludronate had no effect on rat fertility (male or female) at exposures up to two times the 400 mg/day human dose, based on surface area, mg/m^2 (75 mg/kg/day tiludronic acid dose).

PREGNANCY CATEGORY C

In a teratology study in rabbits dosed during days 6-18 of gestation at 42 mg/kg/day and 130 mg/kg/day (2 and 5 times the 400 mg/day human dose based on body surface area), there was dose-related scoliosis likely attributable to the pharmacologic properties of the drug.

Mice receiving 375 mg/kg/day tiludronic acid (7 times the 400 mg/day human dose based on body surface area, mg/m^2) for days 6-15 of gestation showed slight maternal toxicity (decreased body weight gain), increased post-implantation loss, decreased number of fetuses/dam, and decreased fetus body weight. Uncommon malformations of the paw (shortened or missing digits, blood blisters between or in place of digits) were present in six fetuses at 375 mg/kg/day, all from the same litter.

Maternal toxicity (decreased body weight) was also observed in a teratology study in rats dosed during days 6-18 of gestation at 375 mg/kg/day tiludronic acid (10 times the 400 mg/day human dose based on body surface area, mg/m^2). There were reduced percent implantations, increased postimplantation loss, and increased intrauterine deaths in the rats. There were no teratogenic effects on fetuses.

Protracted parturition and maternal death, presumably due to hypocalcemia, occurred at 75 mg/kg/day tiludronic acid (two times the 400 mg/day human dose based on body surface area, mg/m^2) when rats were treated from day 15 of gestation to day 25 postpartum.

There are no adequate and well-controlled studies in pregnant women. Tiludronate disodium should be used during pregnancy only if the potential benefit justifies the potential risk to the fetus.

NURSING MOTHERS

It is not known whether tiludronate is excreted in human milk. Because many drugs are excreted in human milk, caution should be exercised when tiludronate disodium is administered to a nursing woman.

PEDIATRIC USE

Safety and effectiveness of tiludronate disodium in pediatric patients have not been established.

DRUG INTERACTIONS

The bioavailability of tiludronate disodium is decreased 80% by calcium, when calcium and tiludronate disodium are administered at the same time, and 60% by some aluminum- or magnesium-containing antacids, when administered 1 hour before tiludronate disodium. Aspirin may decrease bioavailability of tiludronate disodium by up to 50% when taken 2 hours after tiludronate disodium. The bioavailability of tiludronate disodium is increased 2-4 fold by indomethacin but is not significantly altered by coadministration of diclofenac. The pharmacokinetic parameters of digoxin are not significantly modified by tiludronate disodium coadministration. *In vitro* studies show that tiludronate does not displace warfarin from its binding site on protein.

ADVERSE REACTIONS

The safety of tiludronate disodium has been studied in more than 1100 patients, and the adverse experience profile is similar between controlled and uncontrolled clinical trials. Adverse events occurring in placebo-controlled trials of pagetic patients treated with tiludronate disodium 400 mg/day are presented in TABLE 2.

The most frequently occurring adverse events in patients who received tiludronate disodium 400 mg/day were in the gastrointestinal body system: nausea (9.3%), diarrhea (9.3%), and dyspepsia (5.3%).

Adverse events associated with tiludronate disodium usually have been mild, and generally have not required discontinuation of therapy. In two placebo-controlled trials, 1.3% of patients receiving 400 mg tiludronate disodium and 5.4% of patients receiving placebo discontinued therapy due to any clinical adverse event.

Other adverse events not listed in the table above but reported in $\geq$ 1% of pagetic patients treated with tiludronate disodium in all clinical trials of at least one month duration, regardless of dose and causality assessment, are listed below. The adverse event terms within each body system are listed in the order of decreasing frequency occurring in the population.

Body as a Whole: Asthenia, syncope, fatigue.
Cardiovascular: Hypertension.
Central and Peripheral Nervous Systems: Vertigo, involuntary muscle contractions.
Gastrointestinal: Abdominal pain, constipation, dry mouth, gastritis.
Musculoskeletal: Fracture pathological.
Psychiatric: Anorexia, somnolence, anxiety, nervousness, insomnia.
Respiratory System: Bronchitis.
Skin and Appendages: Pruritus, increased sweating.
Urinary System: Urinary tract infection.
Vascular (extracardiac): Flushing.
Stevens-Johnson type syndrome has been observed rarely; the causality relationship of this to tiludronate disodium has not been established.

TABLE 2 *Adverse Events[a] (%) Reported [b] in > 2% of Pagetic Patients from Placebo-Controlled Studies*

	Tiludronate Disodium 400 mg/day (n=75)	Placebo (n=74)
Body as a Whole		
Pain	21.3	23.0
Back Pain	8.0	8.1
Accidental Injury	4.0	2.7
Influenza-like Symptoms	4.0	5.4
Chest Pain	2.7	0
Peripheral Edema	2.7	1.4
Cardiovascular, General		
Dependent Edema	2.7	0
Central and Peripheral Nervous Systems		
Headache	6.7	12.2
Dizziness	4.0	6.8
Paresthesia	4.0	0
Endocrine		
Hyperparathyroidism	2.7	0
Gastrointestinal		
Diarrhea	9.3	4.1
Nausea	9.3	5.4
Dyspepsia	5.3	8.1
Vomiting	4.0	0
Flatulence	2.7	0
Tooth Disorder	2.7	1.4
Metabolic and Nutritional		
Vitamin D Deficiency	2.7	2.7
Musculoskeletal System		
Arthralgia	2.7	5.4
Arthrosis	2.7	0
Resistance Mechanism		
Infection	2.7	0
Respiratory System		
Rhinitis	5.3	0
Sinusitis	5.3	1.4
Upper Respiratory Tract Infection	5.3	14.9
Coughing	2.7	2.7
Pharyngitis	2.7	1.4
Skin and Appendage		
Rash	2.7	1.4
Skin Disorder	2.7	1.4
Vision		
Cataract	2.7	0
Conjunctivitis	2.7	0
Glaucoma	2.7	0

[a] Reported using WHO terminology
[b] All events reported, irrespective of causality

DOSAGE AND ADMINISTRATION

A single 400-mg daily oral dose of tiludronate disodium, taken with 6 to 8 ounces of plain water only, should be administered for a period of 3 months. Beverages other than plain water (including mineral water), food, and some medications (see DRUG INTERACTIONS) are likely to reduce the absorption of tiludronate disodium (see CLINICAL PHARMACOLOGY, Pharmacokinetics).

Tiludronate disodium should not be taken within 2 hours of food.

Calcium or mineral supplements should be taken at least 2 hours before or two hours after tiludronate disodium. Aluminum- or magnesium-containing antacids, if needed, should be taken at least two hours after taking tiludronate disodium.

Tiludronate disodium should not be taken within 2 hours of indomethacin.

Following therapy, allow an interval of 3 months to assess response. Specific data regarding retreatment are limited, although results from uncontrolled studies indicate favorable biochemical improvement similar to initial tiludronate disodium treatment.

HOW SUPPLIED

Skelid is supplied as white to practically white, biconvex round tablets containing 240 mg tiludronate disodium, which is the molar equivalent of 200 mg tiludronic acid. Skelid tablets are engraved with "S.W" on one side and "200" on the other side .

Storage: Store at 25° C (77°F); excursions permitted to 15° C to 30° C (59° F to 86° F). Tablets should not be removed from the foil strips until they are to be used.

PRODUCT LISTING - EQUIVALENTS NOT AVAILABLE

Tablet - Oral - 200 mg

56's $472.74 SKELID, Sanofi Winthrop Pharmaceuticals 00024-1800-16

T

Timolol *(002353)*

For related information, see the comparative table section in Appendix A.

Categories: Glaucoma, open-angle; Headache, migraine, prophylaxis; Hypertension, essential; Hypertension, ocular; Myocardial infarction, prophylaxis; Pregnancy Category C; FDA Approved 1978 Aug; WHO Formulary

Drug Classes: Antiadrenergics, beta blocking; Ophthalmics

Brand Names: **Betimol**; Blocadren; Dispatim; **Timoptic**; Timoptic-Xe

Foreign Brand Availability: Apo-Timol (Canada); Apo-Timolol (New-Zealand); Apo-Timop (Canada; New-Zealand); Aquanil (Denmark; Finland; Norway; Sweden); Arutinol (Germany); Betim (Denmark; England; Greece; Ireland; Norway); Blocanol (Finland); Cardina (Finland); Chibro-Timoptol (Germany); Cusimolol (Hungary; Spain); Digaol (France); Gen-Timolol (Canada); Glafemak (Greece); Glauco (Thailand); Glauco Oph (Thailand); Glaucopress (Indonesia); Glucomol (India); Hypermol (New-Zealand); Imot Ofteno Al (Costa-Rica; Dominican-Republic; El-Salvador; Guatemala; Honduras; Mexico; Nicaragua; Panama); Isotic Adretor (Indonesia); Molotic Eye Ocupres (India); Noval (Greece); Novo-Timol (Canada); Nylol (Israel); Nyogel (England; Ireland); Nyogel LP (France); Nyolol (Colombia; Mexico; Singapore; Taiwan); Nyolol Gel (Korea); Ocupres (Benin; Burkina-Faso; Ethiopia; Gambia; Ghana; Guinea; India; Ivory-Coast; Kenya; Liberia; Malawi; Mali; Mauritania; Mauritius; Morocco; Niger; Nigeria; Senegal; Seychelles; Sierra-Leone; Sudan; Tanzania; Tunia; Uganda; Zambia; Zimbabwe); Ofal (Argentina); Ofan (Thailand); Oftan Timolol (China); Optimol (Australia; Denmark; Sweden); Proflax (Argentina); Temserin (Germany; Greece); Tenopt (Australia); Tilmat (New-Zealand); Tiloptic (Israel); Timabak (Hong-Kong; Singapore); Timacar (Denmark); Timacor (France); Timoftol (Spain); Timohexal (Germany; Hungary); Timol (Taiwan); Timolo (India); Timolol-POS (Israel); Tim Ophtal (Indonesia); Timoptic (Austria; Bulgaria; Canada; Czech-Republic; Hungary; Japan; Korea; Switzerland); Timoptol (Australia; Belgium; Benin; Burkina-Faso; China; Ecuador; England; Ethiopia; France; Gambia; Germany; Ghana; Guinea; Hong-Kong; Ireland; Italy; Ivory-Coast; Japan; Kenya; Liberia; Malawi; Malaysia; Mali; Mauritania; Mauritius; Mexico; Morocco; Netherlands; New-Zealand; Niger; Nigeria; Philippines; Senegal; Seychelles; Sierra-Leone; South-Africa; Sudan; Taiwan; Tanzania; Thailand; Tunia; Uganda; Zambia; Zimbabwe); Timoptol-XE (China; Hong-Kong; New-Zealand; Peru; Philippines; Singapore); Timozzard (Mexico); Titol (Denmark); Unitimo (Korea); Ximex Opticom (Indonesia); Yesan (Greece)

Cost of Therapy: $39.67 (Hypertension; Blocadren; 10 mg; 2 tablets/day; 30 day supply)
$19.08 (Hypertension; Generic Tablets; 10 mg; 2 tablets/day; 30 day supply)
$18.68 (Glaucoma; Timoptic Ophth. Solution; 0.25%;5 ml; 2 drops/day; variable day supply)
$13.49 (Glaucoma; Generic Ophth. Solution; 0.25%;5 ml; 2 drops/day; variable day supply)

OPHTHALMIC

DESCRIPTION

Note: The trade names have been used throughout this monograph for clarity.

Timolol maleate is a non-selective beta-adrenergic receptor blocking agent. Its chemical name is (-)-1-(*tert*-butylamino)-3-[(4-morpholino-1,2,5-thiadiazol-3-yl)oxy]-2-propanol maleate (1:1) (salt). Timolol maleate possesses an asymmetric carbon atom in its structure and is provided as the levo-isomer.

Its molecular formula is $C_{13}H_{24}N_4O_3S{\cdot}C_4H_4O_4$.

Timolol maleate has a molecular weight of 432.50. It is a white, odorless, crystalline powder which is soluble in water, methanol, and alcohol.

TIMOPTIC OPHTHALMIC SOLUTION

Timoptic ophthalmic solution is stable at room temperature.

Timoptic ophthalmic solution is supplied as a sterile, isotonic, buffered, aqueous solution of timolol maleate in 2 dosage strengths: Each ml of Timoptic 0.25% contains 2.5 mg of timolol (3.4 mg of timolol maleate). Each ml of Timoptic 0.5% contains 5 mg of timolol (6.8 mg of timolol maleate). *Inactive Ingredients:* Monobasic and dibasic sodium phosphate, sodium hydroxide to adjust pH, and water for injection. Benzalkonium chloride 0.01% is added as preservative.

PRESERVATIVE-FREE TIMOPTIC OPHTHALMIC SOLUTION

Preservative-free Timoptic ophthalmic solution is stable at room temperature.

Preservative-free Timoptic ophthalmic solution is supplied in Ocudose, a unit dose container, as a sterile, isotonic, buffered, aqueous solution of timolol maleate in 2 dosage strengths: Each ml of preservative-free Timoptic in Ocudose 0.25% contains 2.5 mg of timolol (3.4 mg of timolol maleate). Each ml of preservative-free Timoptic in Ocudose 0.5% contains 5 mg of timolol (6.8 mg of timolol maleate). *Inactive Ingredients:* Monobasic and dibasic sodium phosphate, sodium hydroxide to adjust pH, and water for injection.

TIMOPTIC-XE STERILE OPHTHALMIC GEL FORMING SOLUTION

Timoptic-XE sterile ophthalmic gel forming solution is supplied as a sterile, isotonic, buffered, aqueous solution of timolol maleate in 2 dosage strengths. Each ml of Timoptic-XE 0.25% contains 2.5 mg of timolol (3.4 mg of timolol maleate). Each ml of Timoptic-XE 0.5% contains 5 mg of timolol (6.8 mg of timolol maleate). *Inactive Ingredients:* Gelrite gellan gum, tromethamine, mannitol, and water for injection. Preservative: benzododecinium bromide 0.012%.

Gelrite is a purified anionic heteropolysaccharide derived from gellan gum. An aqueous solution of Gelrite, in the presence of a cation, has the ability to gel. Upon contact with the precorneal tear film, Timoptic-XE forms a gel that is subsequently removed by the flow of tears.

CLINICAL PHARMACOLOGY

TIMOPTIC OPHTHALMIC SOLUTION AND PRESERVATIVE-FREE OPHTHALMIC SOLUTION

Mechanism of Action

Timolol maleate is a $beta_1$ and $beta_2$ (non-selective) adrenergic receptor blocking agent that does not have significant intrinsic sympathomimetic, direct myocardial depressant, or local anesthetic (membrane-stabilizing) activity.

Beta-adrenergic receptor blockade reduces cardiac output in both healthy subjects and patients with heart disease. In patients with severe impairment of myocardial function, beta-adrenergic receptor blockade may inhibit the stimulatory effect of the sympathetic nervous system necessary to maintain adequate cardiac function.

Beta-adrenergic receptor blockade in the bronchi and bronchioles results in increased airway resistance from unopposed parasympathetic activity. Such an effect in patients with asthma or other bronchospastic conditions is potentially dangerous.

Timoptic ophthalmic solution, when applied topically on the eye, has the action of reducing elevated as well as normal intraocular pressure, whether or not accompanied by glaucoma. Elevated intraocular pressure is a major risk factor in the pathogenesis of glaucomatous visual field loss. The higher the level of intraocular pressure, the greater the likelihood of glaucomatous visual field loss and optic nerve damage.

The onset of reduction in intraocular pressure following administration of timolol maleate can usually be detected within one-half hour after a single dose. The maximum effect usually occurs in 1-2 hours and significant lowering of intraocular pressure can be maintained for periods as long as 24 hours with a single dose. Repeated observations over a period of 1 year indicate that the intraocular pressure-lowering effect of Timoptic is well maintained.

The precise mechanism of the ocular hypotensive action of Timoptic is not clearly established at this time. Tonography and fluorophotometry studies in man suggest that its predominant action may be related to reduced aqueous formation. However, in some studies a slight increase in outflow facility was also observed.

Pharmacokinetics

In a study of plasma drug concentration in 6 subjects, the systemic exposure to timolol was determined following twice daily administration of Timoptic 0.5%. The mean peak plasma concentration following morning dosing was 0.46 ng/ml and following afternoon dosing was 0.35 ng/ml.

TIMOPTIC-XE STERILE OPHTHALMIC GEL FORMING SOLUTION

Mechanism of Action

Timolol maleate is a $beta_1$ and $beta_2$ (non-selective) adrenergic receptor blocking agent that does not have significant intrinsic sympathomimetic, direct myocardial depressant, or local anesthetic (membrane-stabilizing) activity.

Timoptic-XE, when applied topically on the eye, has the action of reducing elevated, as well as normal intraocular pressure, whether or not accompanied by glaucoma. Elevated intraocular pressure is a major risk factor in the pathogenesis of glaucomatous visual field loss and optic nerve damage.

The precise mechanism of the ocular hypotensive action of Timoptic-XE is not clearly established at this time. Tonography and fluorophotometry studies of Timoptic in man suggest that its predominant action may be related to reduced aqueous formation. However, in some studies, a slight increase in outflow facility was also observed.

Beta-adrenergic receptor blockade reduces cardiac output in both healthy subjects and patients with heart disease. In patients with severe impairment of myocardial function, beta-adrenergic receptor blockade may inhibit the stimulatory effect of the sympathetic nervous system necessary to maintain adequate cardiac function.

Beta-adrenergic receptor blockade in the bronchi and bronchioles results in increased airway resistance from unopposed parasympathetic activity. Such an effect in patients with asthma or other bronchospastic conditions is potentially dangerous.

Pharmacokinetics

In a study of plasma drug concentration in 6 subjects, the systemic exposure to timolol was determined following once daily administration of Timoptic-XE 0.5% in the morning. The mean peak plasma concentration following this morning dose was 0.28 ng/ml.

INDICATIONS AND USAGE

Timolol ophthalmic solution is indicated in the treatment of elevated intraocular pressure in patients with ocular hypertension or open-angle glaucoma.

TIMOPTIC PRESERVATIVE-FREE OPHTHALMIC SOLUTION

Preservative-free Timoptic in Ocudose may be used when a patient is sensitive to the preservative in Timoptic ophthalmic solution, benzalkonium chloride, or when use of a preservative-free topical medication is advisable.

CONTRAINDICATIONS

Timolol is contraindicated in patients with:

- Bronchial asthma.
- A history of bronchial asthma.
- Severe chronic obstructive pulmonary disease (see WARNINGS).
- Sinus bradycardia.
- Second or third degree atrioventricular block.
- Overt cardiac failure (see WARNINGS).
- Cardiogenic shock.
- Hypersensitivity to any component of this product.

WARNINGS

As with many topically applied ophthalmic drugs, this drug is absorbed systemically.

The same adverse reactions found with systemic administration of beta-adrenergic blocking agents may occur with topical administration. For example, severe respiratory reactions and cardiac reactions, including death due to bronchospasm in patients with asthma, and rarely death in association with cardiac failure, have been reported following systemic or ophthalmic administration of timolol maleate (see CONTRAINDICATIONS).

CARDIAC FAILURE

Sympathetic stimulation may be essential for support of the circulation in individuals with diminished myocardial contractility, and its inhibition of beta-adrenergic receptor blockade may precipitate more severe failure.

In patients without a history of cardiac failure continued depression of the myocardium with beta-blocking agents over a period of time can, in some cases, lead to cardiac failure. At the first sign or symptom of cardiac failure, timolol should be discontinued.

OBSTRUCTIVE PULMONARY DISEASE

Patients with chronic obstructive pulmonary disease (*e.g.*, chronic bronchitis, emphysema) of mild or moderate severity, bronchospastic disease, or a history of bronchospastic disease [other than bronchial asthma or a history of bronchial asthma, in which timolol is contrain-

T

dicated (see CONTRAINDICATIONS)] should, in general, not receive beta-blockers, including timolol.

MAJOR SURGERY

The necessity or desirability of withdrawal of beta-adrenergic blocking agents prior to major surgery is controversial. Beta-adrenergic receptor blockade impairs the ability of the heart to respond to beta-adrenergically mediated reflex stimuli. This may augment the risk of general anesthesia in surgical procedures. Some patients receiving beta-adrenergic receptor blocking agents have experienced protracted severe hypotension during anesthesia. Difficulty in restarting and maintaining the heartbeat has also been reported. For these reasons, in patients undergoing elective surgery, some authorities recommend gradual withdrawal of beta-adrenergic receptor blocking agents.

The necessity or desirability of withdrawal of beta-adrenergic blocking agents prior to major surgery is controversial. Beta-adrenergic receptor blockade impairs the ability of the heart to respond to beta-adrenergically mediated reflex stimuli. This may augment the risk of general anesthesia in surgical procedures. Some patients receiving beta-adrenergic receptor blocking agents have experienced protracted severe hypotension during anesthesia. Difficulty in restarting and maintaining the heartbeat has also been reported. For these reasons, in patients undergoing elective surgery, some authorities recommend gradual withdrawal of beta-adrenergic receptor blocking agents.

DIABETES MELLITUS

Beta-adrenergic blocking agents should be administered with caution in patients subject to spontaneous hypoglycemia or to diabetic patients (especially those with labile diabetes) who are receiving insulin or oral hypoglycemic agents. Beta-adrenergic receptor blocking agents may mask the signs and symptoms of acute hypoglycemia.

THYROTOXICOSIS

Beta-adrenergic blocking agents may mask certain clinical signs (*e.g.,* tachycardia) of hyperthyroidism. Patients suspected of developing thyrotoxicosis should be managed carefully to avoid abrupt withdrawal of beta-adrenergic blocking agents that might precipitate a thyroid storm.

PRECAUTIONS

GENERAL

Because of potential effects of beta-adrenergic blocking agents on blood pressure and pulse, these agents should be used with caution in patients with cerebrovascular insufficiency. If signs or symptoms suggesting reduced cerebral blood flow develop following initiation of therapy with timolol, alternative therapy should be considered.

There have been reports of bacterial keratitis associated with the use of multiple dose containers of topical ophthalmic products. These containers had been inadvertently contaminated by patients who, in most cases, had a concurrent corneal disease or a disruption of the ocular epithelial surface. (See Information for the Patient.)

Choroidal detachment after filtration procedures has been reported with the administration of aqueous suppressant therapy (*e.g.,* timolol).

Angle-Closure Glaucoma

In patients with angle-closure glaucoma, the immediate objective of treatment is to reopen the angle. This requires constricting the pupil. Timolol maleate has little or no effect on the pupil. Timolol should not be used alone in the treatment of angle-closure glaucoma.

Anaphylaxis

While taking beta-blockers, patients with a history of atopy or a history of severe anaphylactic reactions to a variety of allergens may be more reactive to repeated accidental, diagnostic, or therapeutic challenge with such allergens. Such patients may be unresponsive to the usual doses of epinephrine used to treat anaphylactic reactions.

Muscle Weakness

Beta-adrenergic blockade has been reported to potentiate muscle weakness consistent with certain myasthenic symptoms (*e.g.,* diplopia, ptosis, and generalized weakness). Timolol has been reported rarely to increase muscle weakness in some patients with myasthenia gravis or myasthenic symptoms.

INFORMATION FOR THE PATIENT

Timoptic Ophthalmic Solution

Patients should be instructed to avoid allowing the tip of the dispensing container to contact the eye or surrounding structures.

Patients should also be instructed that ocular solutions, if handled improperly or if the tip of the dispensing container contacts the eye or surrounding structures, can become contaminated by common bacteria known to cause ocular infections. Serious damage to the eye and subsequent loss of vision may result from using contaminated solutions. (See General.)

Patients should also be advised that if they have ocular surgery or develop an intercurrent ocular condition (*e.g.,* trauma or infection), they should immediately seek their physician's advice concerning the continued use of the present multidose container.

Patients with bronchial asthma, a history of bronchial asthma, severe chronic obstructive pulmonary disease, sinus bradycardia, second or third degree atrioventricular block, or cardiac failure should be advised not to take this product. (See CONTRAINDICATIONS.)

Patients should be advised that timolol contains benzalkonium chloride which may be absorbed by soft contact lenses. Contact lenses should be removed prior to administration of the solution. Lenses may be reinserted 15 minutes following timolol administration.

Timoptic Preservative-Free Ophthalmic Solution

Patients should be instructed about the use of preservative-free Timoptic in Ocudose.

Since sterility cannot be maintained after the individual unit is opened, patients should be instructed to use the product immediately after opening, and to discard the individual unit and any remaining contents immediately after use.

Patients with bronchial asthma, a history of bronchial asthma, severe chronic obstructive pulmonary disease, sinus bradycardia, second or third degree atrioventricular block, or cardiac failure should be advised not to take this product. (See CONTRAINDICATIONS.)

Timoptic-XE Sterile Ophthalmic Gel Forming Solution

Patients should be instructed to avoid allowing the tip of the dispensing container to contact the eye or surrounding structures.

Patients should also be instructed that ocular solutions, if handled improperly or if the tip of the dispensing container contacts the eye or surrounding structures, can become contaminated by common bacteria known to cause ocular infections. Serious damage to the eye and subsequent loss of vision may result from using contaminated solutions. (See General.)

Patients should also be advised that if they have ocular surgery or develop an intercurrent ocular condition (*e.g.,* trauma or infection), they should immediately seek their physician's advice concerning the continued use of the present multidose container.

Patients should be instructed to invert the closed container and shake once before each use. It is not necessary to shake the container more than once.

Patients requiring concomitant topical ophthalmic medications should be instructed to administer these at least 10 minutes before instilling Timoptic-XE.

Patients with bronchial asthma, a history of bronchial asthma, severe chronic obstructive pulmonary disease, sinus bradycardia, second or third degree atrioventricular block, or cardiac failure should be advised not to take this product. (See CONTRAINDICATIONS.)

Transient blurred vision, generally lasting from 30 seconds to 5 minutes, following instillation, and potential visual disturbances may impair the ability to perform hazardous tasks such as operating machinery or driving a motor vehicle.

CARCINOGENESIS, MUTAGENESIS, AND IMPAIRMENT OF FERTILITY

In a 2 year study of timolol maleate administered orally to rats, there was a statistically significant increase in the incidence of adrenal pheochromocytomas in male rats administered 300 mg/kg/day (approximately 42,000 times the systemic exposure following the maximum recommended human ophthalmic dose). Similar differences were not observed in rats administered oral doses equivalent to approximately 14,000 times the maximum recommended human ophthalmic dose.

In a lifetime oral study in mice, there were statistically significant increases in the incidence of benign and malignant pulmonary tumors, benign uterine polyps and mammary adenocarcinomas in female mice at 500 mg/kg/day, (approximately 71,000 times the systemic exposure following the maximum recommended human ophthalmic dose), but not at 5 or 50 mg/kg/day (approximately 700 or 7,000, respectively, times the systemic exposure following the maximum recommended human ophthalmic dose). In a subsequent study in female mice, in which post-mortem examinations were limited to the uterus and the lungs, a statistically significant increase in the incidence of pulmonary tumors was again observed at 500 mg/kg/day.

The increased occurrence of mammary adenocarcinomas was associated with elevations in serum prolactin which occurred in female mice administered oral timolol at 500 mg/kg/day, but not at doses of 5 or 50 mg/kg/day. An increased incidence of mammary adenocarcinomas in rodents has been associated with administration of several other therapeutic agents that elevate serum prolactin, but no correlation between serum prolactin levels and mammary tumors has been established in humans. Furthermore, in adult human female subjects who received oral dosages of up to 60 mg of timolol maleate (the maximum recommended human oral dosage), there were no clinically meaningful changes in serum prolactin.

Timolol maleate was devoid of mutagenic potential when tested *in vivo* (mouse) in the micronucleus test and cytogenetic assay (doses up to 800 mg/kg) and *in vitro* in a neoplastic cell transformation assay (up to 100 μg/ml). In Ames tests the highest concentrations of timolol employed, 5,000 or 10,000 μg/plate, were associated with statistically significant elevations of revertants observed with tester strain TA100 (in seven replicate assays), but not in the remaining three strains. In the assays with tester strain TA100, no consistent dose response relationship was observed, and the ratio of test to control revertants did not reach 2. A ratio of 2 is usually considered the criterion for a positive Ames test.

Reproduction and fertility studies in rats demonstrated no adverse effect on male or female fertility at doses up to 21,000 times the systemic exposure following the maximum recommended human ophthalmic dose.

PREGNANCY, TERATOGENIC EFFECTS, PREGNANCY CATEGORY C

Teratogenicity studies with timolol in mice, rats, and rabbits at oral doses up to 50 mg/kg/day (7,000 times the systemic exposure following the maximum recommended human ophthalmic dose) demonstrated no evidence of fetal malformations. Although delayed fetal ossification was observed at this dose in rats, there were no adverse effects on postnatal development of offspring. Doses of 1000 mg/kg/day (142,000 times the systemic exposure following the maximum recommended human ophthalmic dose) were maternotoxic in mice and resulted in an increased number of fetal resorptions. Increased fetal resorptions were also seen in rabbits at doses of 14,000 times the systemic exposure following the maximum recommended human ophthalmic dose, in this case without apparent maternotoxicity.

There are no adequate and well-controlled studies in pregnant women. Timolol should be used during pregnancy only if the potential benefit justifies the potential risk to the fetus.

NURSING MOTHERS

Timolol maleate has been detected in human milk following oral and ophthalmic drug administration. Because of the potential for serious adverse reactions from timolol in nursing infants, a decision should be made whether to discontinue nursing or to discontinue the drug, taking into account the importance of the drug to the mother.

PEDIATRIC USE

Safety and effectiveness in pediatric patients have not been established.

GERIATRIC USE

No overall differences in safety or effectiveness have been observed between elderly and younger patients.

DRUG INTERACTIONS

Although timolol used alone has little or no effect on pupil size, mydriasis resulting from concomitant therapy with timolol and epinephrine has been reported occasionally.

Beta-Adrenergic Blocking Agents: Patients who are receiving a beta-adrenergic blocking agent orally and timolol should be observed for potential additive effects of beta-blockade, both systemic and on intraocular pressure. The concomitant use of two topical beta-adrenergic blocking agents is not recommended.

Calcium Antagonists: Caution should be used in the coadministration of beta-adrenergic blocking agents, such as timolol, and oral or intravenous (IV) calcium antagonists because of possible atrioventricular conduction disturbances, left ventricular failure, and hypotension. In patients with impaired cardiac function, coadministration should be avoided.

Catecholamine-Depleting Drugs: Close observation of the patient is recommended when a beta-blocker is administered to patients receiving catecholamine-depleting drugs such as reserpine, because of possible additive effects and the production of hypotension and/or marked bradycardia, which may result in vertigo, syncope, or postural hypotension.

Digitalis and Calcium Antagonists: The concomitant use of beta-adrenergic blocking agents with digitalis and calcium antagonists may have additive effects in prolonging atrioventricular conduction time.

Quinidine: Potentiated systemic beta-blockade (*e.g.,* decreased heart rate) has been reported during combined treatment with quinidine and timolol, possibly because quinidine inhibits the metabolism of timolol via the P-450 enzyme, CYP2D6.

Clonidine: Oral beta-adrenergic blocking agents may exacerbate the rebound hypertension which can follow the withdrawal of clonidine. There have been no reports of exacerbation of rebound hypertension with ophthalmic timolol maleate.

Injectable Epinephrine: See PRECAUTIONS, General, Anaphylaxis.

ADVERSE REACTIONS

TIMOPTIC OPHTHALMIC SOLUTION AND PRESERVATIVE-FREE OPHTHALMIC SOLUTION

The most frequently reported adverse experiences have been burning and stinging upon instillation (approximately 1 in 8 patients).

The following additional adverse experiences have been reported less frequently with ocular administration of this or other timolol maleate formulations:

Body as a Whole: Headache, asthenia/fatigue, and chest pain.

Cardiovascular: Bradycardia, arrhythmia, hypotension, hypertension, syncope, heart block, cerebral vascular accident, cerebral ischemia, cardiac failure, worsening of angina pectoris, palpitation, cardiac arrest, pulmonary edema, edema, claudication, Raynaud's phenomenon, and cold hands and feet.

Digestive: Nausea, diarrhea, dyspepsia, anorexia, and dry mouth.

Immunologic: Systemic lupus erythematosus.

Nervous System/Psychiatric: Dizziness, increase in signs and symptoms of myasthenia gravis, paresthesia, somnolence, insomnia, nightmares, behavioral changes and psychic disturbances including depression, confusion, hallucinations, anxiety, disorientation, nervousness, and memory loss.

Skin: Alopecia and psoriasiform rash or exacerbation of psoriasis.

Hypersensitivity: Signs and symptoms of systemic allergic reactions, including anaphylaxis, angioedema, urticaria, and localized and generalized rash.

Respiratory: Bronchospasm (predominantly in patients with pre-existing bronchospastic disease), respiratory failure, dyspnea, nasal congestion, cough and upper respiratory infections.

Endocrine: Masked symptoms of hypoglycemia in diabetic patients (see WARNINGS).

Special Senses: Signs and symptoms of ocular irritation including conjunctivitis, blepharitis, keratitis, ocular pain, discharge (*e.g.,* crusting), foreign body sensation, itching and tearing, and dry eyes; ptosis; decreased corneal sensitivity; cystoid macular edema; visual disturbances including refractive changes and diplopia; pseudopemphigoid; choroidal detachment following filtration surgery (see PRECAUTIONS, General); and tinnitus.

Urogenital: Retroperitoneal fibrosis, decreased libido, impotence, and Peyronie's disease.

The following additional adverse effects have been reported in clinical experience with ORAL timolol maleate or other ORAL beta-blocking agents and may be considered potential effects of ophthalmic timolol maleate:

Allergic: Erythematous rash, fever combined with aching and sore throat, laryngospasm with respiratory distress.

Body as a Whole: Extremity pain, decreased exercise tolerance, weight loss.

Cardiovascular: Worsening of arterial insufficiency, vasodilatation.

Digestive: Gastrointestinal pain, hepatomegaly, vomiting, mesenteric arterial thrombosis, ischemic colitis.

Hematologic: Nonthrombocytopenic purpura, thrombocytopenic purpura, agranulocytosis.

Endocrine: Hyperglycemia, hypoglycemia.

Skin: Pruritus, skin irritation, increased pigmentation, sweating.

Musculoskeletal: Arthralgia.

Nervous System/Psychiatric: Vertigo, local weakness, diminished concentration, reversible mental depression progressing to catatonia, an acute reversible syndrome characterized by disorientation for time and place, emotional lability, slightly clouded sensorium, and decreased performance on neuropsychometrics.

Respiratory: Rales, bronchial obstruction.

Urogenital: Urination difficulties.

TIMOPTIC-XE STERILE OPHTHALMIC GEL FORMING SOLUTION

In clinical trials, transient blurred vision upon instillation of the drop was reported in approximately 1 in 3 patients (lasting from 30 seconds to 5 minutes). Less than 1% of patients discontinued from the studies due to blurred vision. The frequency of patients reporting burning and stinging upon instillation was comparable between Timoptic-XE and Timoptic (approximately 1 in 8 patients).

Adverse experiences reported in 1-5% of patients were:

Ocular: Pain, conjunctivitis, discharge (*e.g.,* crusting), foreign body sensation, itching and tearing.

Systemic: Headache, dizziness, and upper respiratory infections.

The following additional adverse experiences have been reported with the ocular administration of this or other timolol maleate formulations:

Body as a Whole: Asthenia/fatigue, and chest pain.

Cardiovascular: Bradycardia, arrhythmia, hypotension, hypertension, syncope, heart block, cerebral vascular accident, cerebral ischemia, cardiac failure, worsening of angina pectoris, palpitation, cardiac arrest, pulmonary edema, edema, claudication, Raynaud's phenomenon, and cold hands and feet.

Digestive: Nausea, diarrhea, dyspepsia, anorexia, and dry mouth.

Immunologic: Systemic lupus erythematosus.

Nervous System/Psychiatric: Increase in signs and symptoms of myasthenia gravis, paresthesia, somnolence, insomnia, nightmares, behavioral changes and psychic disturbances including depression, confusion, hallucinations, anxiety, disorientation, nervousness, and memory loss.

Skin: Alopecia and psoriasiform rash or exacerbation of psoriasis.

Hypersensitivity: Signs and symptoms of systemic allergic reactions including anaphylaxis, angioedema, urticaria, localized and generalized rash.

Respiratory: Bronchospasm (predominantly in patients with pre-existing bronchospastic disease), respiratory failure, dyspnea, nasal congestion, and cough.

Endocrine: Masked symptoms of hypoglycemia in diabetic patients (see WARNINGS).

Special Senses: Signs and symptoms of ocular irritation including blepharitis, keratitis, and dry eyes; ptosis; decreased corneal sensitivity; cystoid macular edema; visual disturbances including refractive changes and diplopia; pseudopemphigoid; choroidal detachment following filtration surgery (see PRECAUTIONSGeneral); and tinnitus.

Urogenital: Retroperitoneal fibrosis, decreased libido, impotence, and Peyronie's disease.

The following additional adverse effects have been reported in clinical experience with ORAL timolol maleate or other ORAL beta-blocking agents and may be considered potential effects of ophthalmic timolol maleate:

Allergic: Erythematous rash, fever combined with aching and sore throat, laryngospasm with respiratory distress.

Body as a Whole: Extremity pain, decreased exercise tolerance, weight loss.

Cardiovascular: Worsening of arterial insufficiency, vasodilatation.

Digestive: Gastrointestinal pain, hepatomegaly, vomiting, mesenteric arterial thrombosis, ischemic colitis.

Hematologic: Nonthrombocytopenic purpura, thrombocytopenic purpura, agranulocytosis.

Endocrine: Hyperglycemia, hypoglycemia.

Skin: Pruritus, skin irritation, increased pigmentation, sweating.

Musculoskeletal: Arthralgia.

Nervous System/Psychiatric: Vertigo, local weakness, diminished concentration, reversible mental depression progressing to catatonia, an acute reversible syndrome characterized by disorientation for time and place, emotional lability, slightly clouded sensorium, and decreased performance on neuropsychometrics.

Respiratory: Rales, bronchial obstruction.

Urogenital: Urination difficulties.

DOSAGE AND ADMINISTRATION

TIMOPTIC OPHTHALMIC SOLUTION

Timoptic ophthalmic solution is available in concentrations of 0.25 and 0.5%. The usual starting dose is 1 drop of 0.25% Timoptic in the affected eye(s) twice a day. If the clinical response is not adequate, the dosage may be changed to 1 drop of 0.5% solution in the affected eye(s) twice a day.

Since in some patients the pressure-lowering response to Timoptic may require a few weeks to stabilize, evaluation should include a determination of intraocular pressure after approximately 4 weeks of treatment with Timoptic.

If the intraocular pressure is maintained at satisfactory levels, the dosage schedule may be changed to 1 drop once a day in the affected eye(s). Because of diurnal variations in intraocular pressure, satisfactory response to the once a day dose is best determined by measuring the intraocular pressure at different times during the day.

Dosages above 1 drop of 0.5% Timoptic twice a day generally have not been shown to produce further reduction in intraocular pressure. If the patient's intraocular pressure is still not at a satisfactory level on this regimen, concomitant therapy with other agent(s) for lowering intraocular pressure can be instituted. The concomitant use of two topical beta-adrenergic blocking agents is not recommended. (See DRUG INTERACTIONS, Beta-Adrenergic Blocking Agents.)

TIMOPTIC PRESERVATIVE-FREE OPHTHALMIC SOLUTION

Preservative-free Timoptic in Ocudose is a sterile solution that does not contain a preservative. The solution from 1 individual unit is to be used immediately after opening for administration to 1 or both eyes. Since sterility cannot be guaranteed after the individual unit is opened, the remaining contents should be discarded immediately after administration.

Preservative-free Timoptic in Ocudose is available in concentrations of 0.25 and 0.5%. The usual starting dose is 1 drop of 0.25% preservative-free Timoptic in Ocudose in the affected eye(s) administered twice a day. Apply enough gentle pressure on the individual container to obtain a single drop of solution. If the clinical response is not adequate, the dosage may be changed to 1 drop of 0.5% solution in the affected eye(s) administered twice a day.

Since in some patients the pressure-lowering response to preservative-free Timoptic in Ocudose may require a few weeks to stabilize, evaluation should include a determination of

T

intraocular pressure after approximately 4 weeks of treatment with preservative-free Timoptic in Ocudose.

If the intraocular pressure is maintained at satisfactory levels, the dosage schedule may be changed to 1 drop once a day in the affected eye(s). Because of diurnal variations in intraocular pressure, satisfactory response to the once a day dose is best determined by measuring the intraocular pressure at different times during the day.

Dosages above 1 drop of 0.5% Timoptic twice a day generally have not been shown to produce further reduction in intraocular pressure. If the patient's intraocular pressure is still not at a satisfactory level on this regimen, concomitant therapy with other agent(s) for lowering intraocular pressure can be instituted taking into consideration that the preparation(s) used concomitantly may contain one or more preservatives. The concomitant use of two topical beta-adrenergic blocking agents is not recommended. (See DRUG INTERACTIONS, Beta-Adrenergic Blocking Agents.)

TIMOPTIC-XE STERILE OPHTHALMIC GEL FORMING SOLUTION

Patients should be instructed to invert the closed container and shake once before each use. It is not necessary to shake the container more than once. Other topically applied ophthalmic medications should be administered at least 10 minutes before Timoptic-XE. (See PRECAUTIONS, Information for the Patient and the Instructions For Use that accompany each prescription.)

Timoptic-XE sterile ophthalmic gel forming solution is available in concentrations of 0.25% and 0.5%. The dose is 1 drop of Timoptic-XE (either 0.25% or 0.5%) in the affected eye(s) once a day.

Because in some patients the pressure-lowering response to Timoptic-XE may require a few weeks to stabilize, evaluation should include a determination of intraocular pressure after approximately 4 weeks of treatment with Timoptic-XE.

Dosages higher than 1 drop of 0.5% Timoptic-XE once a day have not been studied. If the patient's intraocular pressure is still not at a satisfactory level on this regimen, concomitant therapy can be considered. The concomitant use of two topical beta-adrenergic blocking agents is not recommended. (See DRUG INTERACTIONS, Beta-Adrenergic Blocking Agents.)

When patients have been switched from therapy with Timoptic administered twice daily to Timoptic-XE administered once daily, the ocular hypotensive effect has remained consistent.

HOW SUPPLIED

TIMOPTIC OPHTHALMIC SOLUTION

Timoptic sterile ophthalmic solution is a clear, colorless to light yellow solution available in 0.25 and 0.5% concentrations supplied in an Ocmeter Plus container.

Storage

Store at room temperature, 15-30°C (59-86°F). Protect from freezing. Protect from light.

TIMOPTIC PRESERVATIVE-FREE OPHTHALMIC SOLUTION

Preservative-free sterile ophthalmic solution Timoptic in Ocudose is a clear, colorless to light yellow solution available in 0.25 and 0.5% concentrations.

Storage

Store at room temperature, 15-30°C (59-86°F). Protect from freezing. Protect from light.

Because evaporation can occur through the unprotected polyethylene unit dose container and prolonged exposure to direct light can modify the product, the unit dose container should be kept in the protective foil overwrap and used within 1 month after the foil package has been opened.

TIMOPTIC-XE STERILE OPHTHALMIC GEL FORMING SOLUTION

Timoptic-XE sterile ophthalmic gel forming solution is a colorless to nearly colorless, slightly opalescent, and slightly viscous solution available in 0.25 and 0.5% concentrations.

Storage

Store between 15 and 25°C (59 and 77°F). **AVOID FREEZING.** Protect from light.

ORAL

DESCRIPTION

Note: The trade names have been used throughout this monograph for clarity.

Timolol maleate is a non-selective beta-adrenergic receptor blocking agent. The chemical name for timolol maleate is (*S*)-1-[(1,1-dimethylethyl)amino]-3-[[4-(4-morpholinyl)-1,2,5-thiadiazol-3-yl]oxy]-2-propanol(*Z*)-2-butenedioate (1:1) salt. It possesses an asymmetric carbon atom in its structure and is provided as the levo isomer. Its empirical formula is $C_{13}H_{24}N_4O_3S{\cdot}C_4H_4O_4$.

Timolol maleate has a molecular weight of 432.50. It is a white, odorless, crystalline powder which is soluble in water, methanol, and alcohol.

Blocadren is supplied as tablets in three strengths containing 5, 10, or 20 mg timolol maleate for oral administration. Inactive ingredients are cellulose, FD&C blue no. 2, magnesium stearate, and starch.

CLINICAL PHARMACOLOGY

Blocadren is a $beta_1$ and $beta_2$ (non-selective) adrenergic receptor blocking agent that does not have significant intrinsic sympathomimetic, direct myocardial depressant, or local anesthetic activity.

PHARMACODYNAMICS

Clinical pharmacology studies have confirmed the beta-adrenergic blocking activity as shown by (1) changes in resting heart rate and response of heart rate to changes in posture; (2) inhibition of isoproterenol-induced tachycardia; (3) alteration of the response to the Valsalva maneuver and amyl nitrite administration; and (4) reduction of heart rate and blood pressure changes on exercise.

Blocadren decreases the positive chronotropic, positive inotropic, bronchodilator, and vasodilator responses caused by beta-adrenergic receptor agonists. The magnitude of this decreased response is proportional to the existing sympathetic tone and the concentration of Blocadren at receptor sites.

In normal volunteers, the reduction in heart rate response to a standard exercise was dose dependent over the test range of 0.5 to 20 mg, with a peak reduction at 2 hours of approximately 30% at higher doses.

Beta-adrenergic receptor blockade reduces cardiac output in both healthy subjects and patients with heart disease. In patients with severe impairment of myocardial function beta-adrenergic receptor blockade may inhibit the stimulatory effect of the sympathetic nervous system necessary to maintain adequate cardiac function.

Beta-adrenergic receptor blockade in the bronchi and bronchioles results in increased airway resistance from unopposed parasympathetic activity. Such an effect in patients with asthma or other bronchospastic conditions is potentially dangerous.

Clinical studies indicate that Blocadren at a dosage of 20-60 mg/day reduces blood pressure without causing postural hypotension in most patients with essential hypertension. Administration of Blocadren to patients with hypertension results initially in a decrease in cardiac output, little immediate change in blood pressure, and an increase in calculated peripheral resistance. With continued administration of Blocadren, blood pressure decreases within a few days, cardiac output usually remains reduced, and peripheral resistance falls toward pretreatment levels. Plasma volume may decrease or remain unchanged during therapy with Blocadren. In the majority of patients with hypertension Blocadren also decreases plasma renin activity. Dosage adjustment to achieve optimal antihypertensive effect may require a few weeks. When therapy with Blocadren is discontinued, the blood pressure tends to return to pretreatment levels gradually. In most patients the antihypertensive activity of Blocadren is maintained with long-term therapy and is well-tolerated.

The mechanism of the antihypertensive effects of beta-adrenergic receptor blocking agents is not established at this time. Possible mechanisms of action include reduction in cardiac output, reduction in plasma renin activity, and a central nervous system sympatholytic action.

A Norwegian multi-center, double-blind study, which included 20-75 years of age, compared the effects of timolol maleate with placebo in 1884 patients who had survived the acute phase of a myocardial infarction. Patients with systolic blood pressure below 100 mm Hg, sick sinus syndrome and contraindications to beta-blockers, including uncontrolled heart failure, second or third degree AV block and bradycardia (<50 beats/min), were excluded from the multi-center trial. Therapy with Blocadren, begun 7-28 days following infarction, was shown to reduce overall mortality; this was primarily attributable to a reduction in cardiovascular mortality. Blocadren significantly reduced the incidence of sudden deaths (deaths occurring without symptoms or within 24 hours of the onset of symptoms), including those occurring within 1 hour, and particularly instantaneous deaths (those occurring without preceding symptoms). The protective effect of Blocadren was consistent regardless of age, sex or site of infarction. The effect was clearest in patients with a first infarction who were considered at a high risk of dying, defined as those with 1 or more of the following characteristics during the acute phase: transient left ventricular failure, cardiomegaly, newly appearing atrial fibrillation or flutter, systolic hypotension, or SGOT (ASAT) levels greater than 4 times the upper limit of normal. Therapy with Blocadren also reduced the incidence of non-fatal reinfarction. The mechanism of the protective effect of Blocadren is unknown.

Blocadren was studied for the prophylactic treatment of migraine headache in placebo-controlled clinical trials involving 400 patients, mostly women between the ages of 18 and 66 years. Common migraine was the most frequent diagnosis. All patients had at least 2 headaches per month at baseline. Approximately 50% of patients who received Blocadren had a reduction in the frequency of migraine headache of at least 50%, compared to a similar decrease in frequency in 30% of patients receiving placebo. The most common cardiovascular adverse effect was bradycardia (5%).

PHARMACOKINETICS AND METABOLISM

Blocadren is rapidly and nearly completely absorbed (about 90%) following oral ingestion. Detectable plasma levels of timolol occur within one-half hour and peak plasma levels occur in about 1-2 hours. The drug half-life in plasma is approximately 4 hours and this is essentially unchanged in patients with moderate renal insufficiency. Timolol is partially metabolized by the liver and timolol and its metabolites are excreted by the kidney. Timolol is not extensively bound to plasma proteins; *i.e.,* <10% by equilibrium dialysis and approximately 60% by ultrafiltration. An *in vitro* hemodialysis study, using ^{14}C timolol added to human plasma or whole blood, showed that timolol was readily dialyzed from these fluids; however, a study of patients with renal failure showed that timolol did not dialyze readily. Plasma levels following oral administration are about half those following intravenous (IV) administration indicating approximately 50% first pass metabolism. The level of beta sympathetic activity varies widely among individuals, and no simple correlation exists between the dose or plasma level of timolol maleate and its therapeutic activity. Therefore, objective clinical measurements such as reduction of heart rate and/or blood pressure should be used as guides in determining the optimal dosage for each patient.

INDICATIONS AND USAGE

HYPERTENSION

Blocadren is indicated for the treatment of hypertension. It may be used alone or in combination with other antihypertensive agents, especially thiazide-type diuretics.

MYOCARDIAL INFARCTION

Blocadren is indicated in patients who have survived the acute phase of myocardial infarction, and are clinically stable, to reduce cardiovascular mortality and the risk of reinfarction.

MIGRAINE

Blocadren is indicated for the prophylaxis of migraine headache.

CONTRAINDICATIONS

Blocadren is contraindicated in patients with bronchial asthma or with a history of bronchial asthma, or severe chronic obstructive pulmonary disease (see WARNINGS); sinus bradycardia; second and third degree atrioventricular block; overt cardiac failure (see WARNINGS); cardiogenic shock; hypersensitivity to this product.

WARNINGS

CARDIAC FAILURE

Sympathetic stimulation may be essential for support of the circulation in individuals with diminished myocardial contractility, and its inhibition by beta-adrenergic receptor blockade may precipitate more severe failure. Although beta-blockers should be avoided in overt congestive heart failure, they can be used, if necessary, with caution in patients with a history of failure who are well-compensated, usually with digitalis and diuretics. Both digitalis and timolol maleate slow AV conduction. If cardiac failure persists, therapy with Blocadren should be withdrawn.

In patients without a history of cardiac failure continued depression of the myocardium with beta-blocking agents over a period of time can, in some cases, lead to cardiac failure. At the first sign or symptom of cardiac failure, patients receiving Blocadren should be digitalized and/or be given a diuretic, and the response observed closely. If cardiac failure continues, despite adequate digitalization and diuretic therapy, Blocadren should be withdrawn.

Exacerbation of ischemic heart disease following abrupt withdrawal: Hypersensitivity to catecholamines has been observed in patients withdrawn from beta-blocker therapy; exacerbation of angina and, in some cases, myocardial infarction have occurred after *abrupt* discontinuation of such therapy. When discontinuing chronically administered timolol maleate, particularly in patients with ischemic heart disease, the dosage should be gradually reduced over a period of 1-2 weeks and the patient should be carefully monitored. If angina markedly worsens or acute coronary insufficiency develops, timolol maleate administration should be reinstituted promptly, at least temporarily, and other measures appropriate for the management of unstable angina should be taken. Patients should be warned against interruption or discontinuation of therapy without the physician's advice. Because coronary artery disease is common and may be unrecognized, it may be prudent not to discontinue timolol maleate therapy abruptly even in patients treated only for hypertension.

OBSTRUCTIVE PULMONARY DISEASE

PATIENTS WITH CHRONIC OBSTRUCTIVE PULMONARY DISEASE (*e.g.*, CHRONIC BRONCHITIS, EMPHYSEMA) OF MILD OR MODERATE SEVERITY, BRONCHOSPASTIC DISEASE OR A HISTORY OF BRONCHOSPASTIC DISEASE (OTHER THAN BRONCHIAL ASTHMA OR A HISTORY OF BRONCHIAL ASTHMA, IN WHICH 'BLOCADREN' IS CONTRAINDICATED, SEE CONTRAINDICATIONS), SHOULD IN GENERAL NOT RECEIVE BETA-BLOCKERS, INCLUDING 'BLOCADREN'. However, if Blocadren is necessary in such patients, then the drug should be administered with caution since it may block bronchodilation produced by endogenous and exogenous catecholamine stimulation of $beta_2$ receptors.

MAJOR SURGERY

The necessity or desirability of withdrawal of beta-blocking therapy prior to major surgery is controversial. Beta-adrenergic receptor blockade impairs the ability of the heart to respond to beta-adrenergically mediated reflex stimuli. This may augment the risk of general anesthesia in surgical procedures. Some patients receiving beta-adrenergic receptor blocking agents have been subject to protracted severe hypotension during anesthesia. Difficulty in restarting and maintaining the heartbeat has also been reported. For these reasons, in patients undergoing elective surgery, some authorities recommend gradual withdrawal of beta-adrenergic receptor blocking agents.

If necessary during surgery, the effects of beta-adrenergic blocking agents may be reversed by sufficient doses of such agonists as isoproterenol, dopamine, dobutamine or levarterenol.

DIABETES MELLITUS

Blocadren should be administered with caution in patients subject to spontaneous hypoglycemia or to diabetic patients (especially those with labile diabetes) who are receiving insulin or oral hypoglycemic agents. Beta-adrenergic receptor blocking agents may mask the signs and symptoms of acute hypoglycemia.

THYROTOXICOSIS

Beta-adrenergic blockade may mask certain clinical signs (*e.g.*, tachycardia) of hyperthyroidism. Patients suspected of developing thyrotoxicosis should be managed carefully to avoid abrupt withdrawal of beta-blockade which might precipitate a thyroid storm.

PRECAUTIONS

GENERAL

Impaired Hepatic or Renal Function

Since Blocadren is partially metabolized in the liver and excreted mainly by the kidneys, dosage reductions may be necessary when hepatic and/or renal insufficiency is present.

Dosing in the Presence of Marked Renal Failure

Although the pharmacokinetics of Blocadren are not greatly altered by renal impairment, marked hypotensive responses have been seen in patients with marked renal impairment undergoing dialysis after 20 mg doses. Dosing in such patients should therefore be especially cautious.

Muscle Weakness

Beta-adrenergic blockade has been reported to potentiate muscle weakness consistent with certain myasthenic symptoms (*e.g.*, diplopia, ptosis, and generalized weakness). Timolol has been reported rarely to increase muscle weakness in some patients with myasthenia gravis or myasthenic symptoms.

Cerebrovascular Insufficiency

Because of potential effects of beta-adrenergic blocking agents relative to blood pressure and pulse, these agents should be used with caution in patients with cerebrovascular insufficiency. If signs or symptoms suggesting reduced cerebral blood flow are observed, consideration should be given to discontinuing these agents.

CARCINOGENESIS, MUTAGENESIS, AND IMPAIRMENT OF FERTILITY

In a 2 year study of timolol maleate in rats, there was a statistically significant increase in the incidence of adrenal pheochromocytomas in male rats administered 300 mg/kg/day (250 times* the maximum recommended human dose). Similar differences were not observed in rats administered doses equivalent to approximately 20 or 80* times the maximum recommended human dose.

In a lifetime study in mice, there were statistically significant increases in the incidence of benign and malignant pulmonary tumors, benign uterine polyps and mammary adenocarcinoma in female mice at 500 mg/kg/day (approximately 400 times* the maximum recommended human dose), but not at 5 or 50 mg/kg/day. In a subsequent study in female mice, in which post-mortem examinations were limited to uterus and lungs, a statistically significant increase in the incidence of pulmonary tumors was again observed at 500 mg/kg/day.

The increased occurrence of mammary adenocarcinoma was associated with elevations in serum prolactin that occurred in female mice administered timolol at 500 mg/kg/day, but not at doses of 5 or 50 mg/kg/day. An increased incidence of mammary adenocarcinomas in rodents has been associated with administration of several other therapeutic agents which elevate serum prolactin, but no correlation between serum prolactin levels and mammary tumors has been established in man. Furthermore, in adult human female subjects who received oral dosages of up to 60 mg of timolol maleate, the maximum recommended daily human oral dosage, there were no clinically meaningful changes in serum prolactin.

Timolol maleate was devoid of mutagenic potential when evaluated *in vivo* (mouse) in the micronucleus test and cytogenetic assay (doses up to 800 mg/kg) and *in vitro* in a neoplastic cell transformation assay (up to 100 μg/ml). In Ames tests the highest concentrations of timolol employed, 5,000 or 10,000 μg/plate, were associated with statistically significant elevations of revertants observed with tester strain TA100 (in seven replicate assays), but not in three additional strains. In the assays with tester strain TA100, no consistent dose response relationship was observed, nor did the ratio of test to control revertants reach 2. A ratio of 2 is usually considered the criterion for a positive Ames test.

Reproduction and fertility studies in rats showed no adverse effect on male or female fertility at doses up to 125 times* the maximum recommended human dose.

*Based on patient weight of 50 kg.

PREGNANCY CATEGORY C

Teratogenicity studies with timolol in mice, rats and rabbits at doses up to 50 mg/kg/day (approximately 40 times* the maximum recommended daily human dose) showed no evidence of fetal malformations. Although delayed fetal ossification was observed at this dose in rats, there were no adverse effects on postnatal development of offspring. Doses of 1000 mg/kg/day (approximately 830 times* the maximum recommended daily human dose) were maternotoxic in mice and resulted in an increased number of fetal resorptions. Increased fetal resorptions were also seen in rabbits at doses of approximately 40 times* the maximum recommended daily human dose, in this case without apparent maternotoxicity. There are no adequate and well-controlled studies in pregnant women. Blocadren should be used during pregnancy only if the potential benefit justifies the potential risk to the fetus.

*Based on patient weight of 50 kg.

NURSING MOTHERS

Timolol maleate has been detected in human milk.

Because of the potential for serious adverse reactions from timolol in nursing infants, a decision should be made whether to discontinue nursing or to discontinue the drug, taking into account the importance of the drug to the mother.

PEDIATRIC USE

Safety and effectiveness in pediatric patients have not been established.

GERIATRIC USE

Clinical studies of Blocadren for the treatment of hypertension or migraine did not include sufficient numbers of subjects aged 65 and over to determine whether they respond differently from younger subjects.

In a clinical study of Blocadren in patients who had survived the acute phase of a myocardial infarction, approximately 350 patients (37%) were 65-75 years of age. Safety and efficacy were not different between these patients and younger patients (see CLINICAL PHARMACOLOGY, Pharmacodynamics).

Other reported clinical experience has not identified differences in responses between the elderly and younger patients. In general, dose selection for an elderly patient should be cautious, usually starting at the low end of the dosing range, reflecting the greater frequency of decreased hepatic, renal or cardiac function, and of concomitant disease or other drug therapy.

This drug is known to be substantially excreted by the kidney, and the risk of toxic reactions to this drug may be greater in patients with impaired renal function. Because elderly patients are more likely to have decreased renal function, care should be taken in dose selection, and it may be useful to monitor renal function. (See Impaired Hepatic or Renal Function and Dosing in the Presence of Marked Renal Failure.)

DRUG INTERACTIONS

CATECHOLAMINE-DEPLETING DRUGS

Close observation of the patient is recommended when Blocadren is administered to patients receiving catecholamine-depleting drugs such as reserpine, because of possible additive effects and the production of hypotension and/or marked bradycardia, which may produce vertigo, syncope, or postural hypotension.

T

NON-STEROIDAL ANTI-INFLAMMATORY DRUGS

Blunting of the antihypertensive effect of beta-adrenoceptor blocking agents by non-steroidal anti-inflammatory drugs has been reported. When using these agents concomitantly, patients should be observed carefully to confirm that the desired therapeutic effect has been obtained.

CALCIUM ANTAGONISTS

Literature reports suggest that oral calcium antagonists may be used in combination with beta-adrenergic blocking agents when heart function is normal, but should be avoided in patients with impaired cardiac function. Hypotension, AV conduction disturbances, and left ventricular failure have been reported in some patients receiving beta-adrenergic blocking agents when an oral calcium antagonist was added to the treatment regimen. Hypotension was more likely to occur if the calcium antagonist were a dihydropyridine derivative, *e.g.*, nifedipine, while left ventricular failure and AV conduction disturbances were more likely to occur with either verapamil or diltiazem.

Intravenous calcium antagonists should be used with caution in patients receiving beta-adrenergic blocking agents.

DIGITALIS AND EITHER DILTIAZEM OR VERAPAMIL

The concomitant use of beta-adrenergic blocking agents with digitalis and either diltiazem or verapamil may have additive effects in prolonging AV conduction time.

QUINIDINE

Potentiated systemic beta-blockade (*e.g.*, decreased heart rate) has been reported during combined treatment with quinidine and timolol, possibly because quinidine inhibits the metabolism of timolol via the P-450 enzyme, CYP2D6.

CLONIDINE

Beta-adrenergic blocking agents may exacerbate the rebound hypertension which can follow the withdrawal of clonidine. If the two drugs are coadministered, the beta-adrenergic blocking agent should be withdrawn several days before the gradual withdrawal of clonidine. If replacing clonidine by beta-blocker therapy, the introduction of beta-adrenergic blocking agents should be delayed for several days after clonidine administration has stopped.

RISK FROM ANAPHYLACTIC REACTION

While taking beta-blockers, patients with a history of atopy or a history of severe anaphylactic reaction to a variety of allergens may be more reactive to repeated accidental, diagnostic, or therapeutic challenge with such allergens. Such patients may be unresponsive to the usual doses of epinephrine used to treat anaphylactic reactions.

ADVERSE REACTIONS

Blocadren is usually well-tolerated in properly selected patients. Most adverse effects have been mild and transient.

In a multicenter (12 week) clinical trial comparing timolol maleate and placebo in hypertensive patients, the adverse reactions in TABLE 1 were reported spontaneously and considered to be causally related to timolol maleate.

TABLE 1

	Timolol Maleate (n=176)	Placebo (n=168)
Body as a Whole		
Fatigue/tiredness	3.4%	0.6%
Headache	1.7%	1.8%
Chest pain	0.6%	0%
Asthenia	0.6%	0%
Cardiovascular		
Bradycardia	9.1%	0%
Arrhythmia	1.1%	0.6%
Syncope	0.6%	0%
Edema	0.6%	1.2%
Digestive		
Dyspepsia	0.6%	0.6%
Nausea	0.6%	0%
Skin		
Pruritus	1.1%	0%
Nervous System		
Dizziness	2.3%	1.2%
Vertigo	0.6%	0%
Paresthesia	0.6%	0%
Psychiatric		
Decreased libido	0.6%	0%
Respiratory		
Dyspnea	1.7%	0.6%
Bronchial spasm	0.6%	0%
Rales	0.6%	0%
Special Senses		
Eye irritation	1.1%	0.6%
Tinnitus	0.6%	0%

These data are representative of the incidence of adverse effects that may be observed in properly selected patients treated with Blocadren, *i.e.*, excluding patients with bronchospastic disease, congestive heart failure or other contraindications to beta-blocker therapy.

In patients with migraine the incidence of bradycardia was 5%.

In a coronary artery disease population studied in the Norwegian multi-center trial (see CLINICAL PHARMACOLOGY), the frequency of the principal adverse reactions and the frequency with which these resulted in discontinuation of therapy in the timolol and placebo groups are shown in TABLE 2.

TABLE 2

	Adverse Reaction*		Withdrawal†	
	Timolol (n=945)	Placebo (n=939)	Timolol (n=945)	Placebo (n=939)
Asthenia or fatigue	5%	1%	<1%	<1%
Heart rate <40 beats/min	5%	<1%	4%	<1%
Cardiac failure — nonfatal	8%	7%	3%	2%
Hypotension	3%	2%	3%	1%
Pulmonary edema — nonfatal	2%	<1%	<1%	<1%
Claudication	3%	3%	1%	<1%
AV Block — 2nd or 3rd degree	<1%	<1%	<1%	<1%
Sinoatrial block	<1%	<1%	<1%	<1%
Cold hands and feet	8%	<1%	<1%	0%
Nausea or digestive disorders	8%	6%	1%	<1%
Dizziness	6%	4%	1%	0%
Bronchial obstruction	2%	<1%	1%	<1%

* When an adverse reaction recurred in a patient, it is listed only once.
† Only principal reason for withdrawal in each patient is listed. These adverse reactions can also occur in patients treated for hypertension.

The following additional adverse effects have been reported in clinical experience with the drug:

Body as a Whole: Anaphylaxis, extremity pain, decreased exercise tolerance, weight loss, fever.

Cardiovascular: Cardiac arrest, cardiac failure, cerebral vascular accident, worsening of angina pectoris, worsening of arterial insufficiency, Raynaud's phenomenon, palpitations, vasodilatation.

Digestive: Gastrointestinal pain, hepatomegaly, vomiting, diarrhea, dyspepsia.

Hematologic: Nonthrombocytopenic purpura.

Endocrine: Hyperglycemia, hypoglycemia.

Skin: Rash, skin irritation, increased pigmentation, sweating, alopecia.

Musculoskeletal: Arthralgia.

Nervous System: Local weakness, increase in signs and symptoms of myasthenia gravis.

Psychiatric: Depression, nightmares, somnolence, insomnia, nervousness, diminished concentration, hallucinations.

Respiratory: Cough.

Special Senses: Visual disturbances, diplopia, ptosis, dry eyes.

Urogenital: Impotence, urination difficulties.

There have been reports of retroperitoneal fibrosis in patients receiving timolol maleate and in patients receiving other beta-adrenergic blocking agents. A causal relationship between this condition and therapy with beta-adrenergic blocking agents has not been established.

POTENTIAL ADVERSE EFFECTS

In addition, a variety of adverse effects not observed in clinical trials with Blocadren, but reported with other beta-adrenergic blocking agents, should be considered potential adverse effects of Blocadren:

Nervous System: Reversible mental depression progressing to catatonia; an acute reversible syndrome characterized by disorientation for time and place, short-term memory loss, emotional lability, slightly clouded sensorium, and decreased performance on neuropsychometrics.

Cardiovascular: Intensification of AV block (see CONTRAINDICATIONS).

Digestive: Mesenteric arterial thrombosis, ischemic colitis.

Hematologic: Agranulocytosis, thrombocytopenic purpura.

Allergic: Erythematous rash, fever combined with aching and sore throat, laryngospasm with respiratory distress.

Miscellaneous: Peyronie's disease.

There have been reports of a syndrome comprising psoriasiform skin rash, conjunctivitis sicca, otitis, and sclerosing serositis attributed to the beta-adrenergic receptor blocking agent, practolol. This syndrome has not been reported with Blocadren.

CLINICAL LABORATORY TEST FINDINGS

Clinically important changes in standard laboratory parameters were rarely associated with the administration of Blocadren. Slight increases in blood urea nitrogen, serum potassium, uric acid, and triglycerides, and slight decreases in hemoglobin, hematocrit and HDL cholesterol occurred, but were not progressive or associated with clinical manifestations. Increases in liver function tests have been reported.

DOSAGE AND ADMINISTRATION

HYPERTENSION

The usual initial dosage of Blocadren is 10 mg twice a day, whether used alone or added to diuretic therapy. Dosage may be increased or decreased depending on heart rate and blood pressure response. The usual total maintenance dosage is 20-40 mg/day. Increases in dosage to a maximum of 60 mg/day divided into 2 doses may be necessary. There should be an interval of at least 7 days between increases in dosages.

Blocadren may be used with a thiazide diuretic or with other antihypertensive agents. Patients should be observed carefully during initiation of such concomitant therapy.

MYOCARDIAL INFARCTION

The recommended dosage for long-term prophylactic use in patients who have survived the acute phase of a myocardial infarction is 10 mg given twice daily (see CLINICAL PHARMACOLOGY).

MIGRAINE

The usual initial dosage of Blocadren is 10 mg twice a day. During maintenance therapy the 20 mg daily dosage may be administered as a single dose. Total daily dosage may be increased to a maximum of 30 mg, given in divided doses, or decreased to 10 mg once per day, depending on clinical response and tolerability. If a satisfactory response is not obtained after 6-8 weeks use of the maximum daily dosage, therapy with Blocadren should be discontinued.

HOW SUPPLIED

BLOCADREN TABLETS

5 mg: Light blue, round, compressed tablets, with code "MSD 59" on 1 side and "BLOCADREN" on the other.

10 mg: Light blue, round, scored, compressed tablets, with code "MSD 136" on 1 side and "BLOCADREN" on the other.

20 mg: Light blue, capsule shaped, scored, compressed tablets, with code "MSD 437" on 1 side and "BLOCADREN" on the other.

Storage: Store at controlled room temperature, 15-30°C (59-86°F). Keep container tightly closed. Protect from light.

PRODUCT LISTING - RATED THERAPEUTICALLY EQUIVALENT

Gel Forming Solution - Ophthalmic - 0.25%

Size	Price	Product	NDC
2 ml	$16.66	TIMOPTIC-XE, Merck & Company Inc	00006-3557-32
5 ml	$26.16	TIMOPTIC-XE, Allscripts Pharmaceutical Company	54569-4302-00
5 ml	$26.50	GENERIC, Falcon Pharmaceuticals, Ltd.	61314-0224-05
5 ml	$29.03	TIMOPTIC-XE, Physicians Total Care	54868-3263-00
5 ml	$29.44	TIMOPTIC-XE, Merck & Company Inc	00006-3557-03

Gel Forming Solution - Ophthalmic - 0.5%

Size	Price	Product	NDC
2 ml	$19.73	TIMOPTIC-XE, Merck & Company Inc	00006-3558-32
2.50 ml	$17.76	GENERIC, Falcon Pharmaceuticals, Ltd.	61314-0225-25
5 ml	$31.10	TIMOPTIC-XE, Allscripts Pharmaceutical Company	54569-4303-00
5 ml	$31.50	GENERIC, Falcon Pharmaceuticals, Ltd.	61314-0225-05
5 ml	$35.00	TIMOPTIC-XE, Merck & Company Inc	00006-3558-03
5 ml	$35.72	TIMOPTIC-XE, Physicians Total Care	54868-3264-00

Solution - Ophthalmic - 0.25%

Size	Price	Product	NDC
5 ml	$13.49	GENERIC, West Point Pharma	59591-0767-03
5 ml	$13.99	GENERIC, Qualitest Products Inc	00603-7338-37
5 ml	$14.10	GENERIC, Pacific Pharma	60758-0802-05
5 ml	$15.00	GENERIC, Bausch and Lomb	24208-0330-05
5 ml	$18.10	GENERIC, Rexall Group	60814-0720-05
5 ml	$18.68	TIMOPTIC OCUMETER PLUS, Merck & Company Inc	00006-8895-35
10 ml	$6.98	FEDERAL UPPER LIMIT, H.C.F.A. F F P	99999-2353-11
10 ml	$25.72	GENERIC, Fougera	00168-0199-10
10 ml	$26.06	GENERIC, West Point Pharma	59591-0767-10
10 ml	$27.06	GENERIC, Qualitest Products Inc	00603-7338-39
10 ml	$27.20	GENERIC, Pacific Pharma	60758-0802-10
10 ml	$27.75	GENERIC, Apotex Usa Inc	60505-0552-03
10 ml	$27.76	GENERIC, Bausch and Lomb	24208-0330-10
10 ml	$29.50	GENERIC, Rexall Group	60814-0720-10
10 ml	$36.10	TIMOPTIC OCUMETER PLUS, Merck & Company Inc	00006-8895-36
15 ml	$39.00	GENERIC, West Point Pharma	59591-0767-12
15 ml	$39.00	GENERIC, West Point Pharma	59591-3767-03
15 ml	$40.52	GENERIC, Qualitest Products Inc	00603-7338-41
15 ml	$41.55	GENERIC, Pacific Pharma	60758-0802-15
15 ml	$42.02	GENERIC, Apotex Usa Inc	60505-0552-04
15 ml	$42.04	GENERIC, Fougera	00168-0199-15
15 ml	$42.04	GENERIC, Bausch and Lomb	24208-0330-15
15 ml	$44.15	GENERIC, Rexall Group	60814-0720-15

Solution - Ophthalmic - 0.5%

Size	Price	Product	NDC
5 ml	$14.40	GENERIC, Major Pharmaceuticals Inc	00904-5248-05
5 ml	$16.64	GENERIC, Akorn Inc	17478-0288-10
5 ml	$16.70	GENERIC, Pacific Pharma	60758-0801-05
5 ml	$17.00	GENERIC, Bausch and Lomb	24208-0324-05
5 ml	$18.25	GENERIC, Rexall Group	60814-0721-05
10 ml	$27.98	GENERIC, Major Pharmaceuticals Inc	00904-5248-10
10 ml	$32.15	GENERIC, Pacific Pharma	60758-0801-10
10 ml	$32.29	GENERIC, Akorn Inc	17478-0288-11
10 ml	$32.29	GENERIC, Bausch and Lomb	24208-0324-10
10 ml	$32.33	GENERIC, Apotex Usa Inc	60505-0551-03
10 ml	$32.35	GENERIC, Fougera	00168-0200-10
10 ml	$35.10	GENERIC, Rexall Group	60814-0721-10
10 ml	$42.88	TIMOPTIC OCUMETER PLUS, Physicians Total Care	00006-8896-36
15 ml	$13.50	FEDERAL UPPER LIMIT, H.C.F.A. F F P	99999-2353-15
15 ml	$41.78	GENERIC, Major Pharmaceuticals Inc	00904-5248-35
15 ml	$48.32	GENERIC, Akorn Inc	17478-0288-12
15 ml	$48.40	GENERIC, Pacific Pharma	60758-0801-15
15 ml	$48.43	GENERIC, Apotex Usa Inc	60505-0551-04
15 ml	$48.46	GENERIC, Fougera	00168-0200-15
15 ml	$48.75	GENERIC, Bausch and Lomb	24208-0324-15
15 ml	$52.15	GENERIC, Rexall Group	60814-0721-15

Tablet - Oral - 5 mg

Size	Price	Product	NDC
100's	$22.15	GENERIC, Major Pharmaceuticals Inc	00904-3408-60
100's	$23.80	GENERIC, Moore, H.L. Drug Exchange Inc	00839-7584-06
100's	$25.95	GENERIC, Qualitest Products Inc	00603-6071-21
100's	$28.56	GENERIC, Novopharm Usa Inc	55953-0961-40
100's	$28.75	GENERIC, Geneva Pharmaceuticals	00781-1126-01
100's	$28.89	GENERIC, Endo Laboratories Llc	60951-0782-70
100's	$29.25	GENERIC, Mylan Pharmaceuticals Inc	00378-0055-01
100's	$53.45	BLOCADREN, Merck & Company Inc	00006-0059-68

Tablet - Oral - 10 mg

Size	Price	Product	NDC
100's	$31.80	GENERIC, Qualitest Products Inc	00603-6072-21
100's	$33.70	GENERIC, Aligen Independent Laboratories Inc	00405-5020-01
100's	$33.95	GENERIC, West Point Pharma	59591-0194-68
100's	$34.01	GENERIC, Moore, H.L. Drug Exchange Inc	00839-7585-06
100's	$35.25	GENERIC, Major Pharmaceuticals Inc	00904-3409-60
100's	$35.25	GENERIC, Novopharm Usa Inc	55953-0972-40
100's	$35.71	GENERIC, Moore, H.L. Drug Exchange Inc	00839-7936-06
100's	$35.89	GENERIC, Endo Laboratories Llc	60951-0783-70
100's	$36.50	GENERIC, Mylan Pharmaceuticals Inc	00378-0221-01
100's	$66.11	BLOCADREN, Merck & Company Inc	00006-0136-68

Tablet - Oral - 20 mg

Size	Price	Product	NDC
100's	$64.79	GENERIC, Moore, H.L. Drug Exchange Inc	00839-7586-06
100's	$65.00	GENERIC, Novopharm Usa Inc	55953-0984-40
100's	$66.10	GENERIC, Watson/Schein Pharmaceuticals Inc	00364-2359-01
100's	$67.50	GENERIC, Mylan Pharmaceuticals Inc	00378-0715-01
100's	$68.03	GENERIC, Moore, H.L. Drug Exchange Inc	00839-7937-06
100's	$108.26	BLOCADREN, Merck & Company Inc	00006-0437-68

PRODUCT LISTING - EQUIVALENTS NOT AVAILABLE

Solution - Ophthalmic - Hemihydrate 0.25%

Size	Price	Product	NDC
5 ml	$16.50	BETIMOL, Santen Inc	65086-0522-05
10 ml	$32.00	BETIMOL, Santen Inc	65086-0522-10
15 ml	$48.00	BETIMOL, Santen Inc	65086-0522-15

Solution - Ophthalmic - Hemihydrate 0.5%

Size	Price	Product	NDC
5 ml	$19.55	BETIMOL, Santen Inc	65086-0525-05
10 ml	$33.38	BETIMOL, Allscripts Pharmaceutical Company	54569-4306-00
10 ml	$37.90	BETIMOL, Santen Inc	65086-0525-10
15 ml	$50.01	BETIMOL, Allscripts Pharmaceutical Company	54569-4394-00
15 ml	$57.00	BETIMOL, Santen Inc	65086-0525-15

Solution - Ophthalmic - 0.25%

Size	Price	Product	NDC
0.45 ml x 60	$104.68	TIMOPTIC OCUDOSE, Merck & Company Inc	00006-3542-60
0.45 ml x 60	$108.85	TIMOPTIC OCUDOSE, Merck & Company Inc	00006-9689-60
2.50 ml	$9.94	TIMOPTIC OCUMETER, Southwood Pharmaceuticals Inc	58016-1126-01
5 ml	$14.00	GENERIC, Watson/Schein Pharmaceuticals Inc	00364-3077-53
5 ml	$15.00	GENERIC, Falcon Pharmaceuticals, Ltd.	61314-0226-05
5 ml	$20.10	TIMOPTIC OCUMETER, Physicians Total Care	54868-0621-01
10 ml	$9.25	GENERIC, Pharma Pac	54868-3713-00
10 ml	$27.18	GENERIC, Allscripts Pharmaceutical Company	54569-4288-00
10 ml	$27.75	GENERIC, Falcon Pharmaceuticals, Ltd.	61314-0226-10
10 ml	$36.10	TIMOPTIC OCUMETER, Merck & Company Inc	00006-3366-10
10 ml	$38.29	TIMOPTIC OCUMETER, Physicians Total Care	54868-0621-02
15 ml	$40.50	GENERIC, Watson/Schein Pharmaceuticals Inc	00364-3077-72
15 ml	$42.00	GENERIC, Falcon Pharmaceuticals, Ltd.	61314-0226-15
15 ml	$54.04	TIMOPTIC OCUMETER, Merck & Company Inc	00006-3366-12
15 ml	$57.03	TIMOPTIC OCUMETER, Physicians Total Care	54868-0621-00

Solution - Ophthalmic - 0.5%

Size	Price	Product	NDC
0.45 ml x 60	$126.01	TIMOPTIC OCUDOSE, Merck & Company Inc	00006-3543-60
0.45 ml x 60	$131.05	TIMOPTIC OCUDOSE, Merck & Company Inc	00006-9690-60
2 ml	$10.49	TIMOPTIC OCUMETER, Merck & Company Inc	00006-3367-32
2.50 ml	$11.54	TIMOPTIC OCUMETER, Southwood Pharmaceuticals Inc	58016-6331-01
5 ml	$15.96	GENERIC, West Point Pharma	59591-0768-03
5 ml	$15.96	GENERIC, West Point Pharma	59591-3768-01
5 ml	$17.00	GENERIC, Falcon Pharmaceuticals, Ltd.	61314-0227-05
5 ml	$21.25	TIMOPTIC OCUMETER, Allscripts Pharmaceutical Company	54569-1206-00
5 ml	$21.68	TIMOPTIC OCUMETER, Southwood Pharmaceuticals Inc	58016-6216-01
5 ml	$22.10	TIMOPTIC OCUMETER, Merck & Company Inc	00006-3367-03
5 ml	$22.10	TIMOLOL, OPHTHALMIC, Merck & Company Inc	00006-8896-35
5 ml	$23.25	TIMOPTIC OCUMETER, Physicians Total Care	54868-0664-01
5 ml	$39.65	TIMOPTIC OCUMETER, Pharma Pac	52959-0584-03
10 ml	$30.95	GENERIC, West Point Pharma	59591-0768-10
10 ml	$30.95	GENERIC, West Point Pharma	59591-3768-02
10 ml	$32.35	GENERIC, Falcon Pharmaceuticals, Ltd.	61314-0227-10
10 ml	$39.63	TIMOPTIC OCUMETER, Southwood Pharmaceuticals Inc	58016-6069-01

10 ml	$44.58	TIMOPTIC OCUMETER, Physicians Total Care	54868-0664-02
15 ml	$17.08	GENERIC, Physicians Total Care	54868-3714-00
15 ml	$46.31	GENERIC, West Point Pharma	59591-0768-12
15 ml	$46.31	GENERIC, West Point Pharma	59591-3768-03
15 ml	$48.00	GENERIC, Watson/Schein Pharmaceuticals Inc	00364-3078-72
15 ml	$48.75	GENERIC, Falcon Pharmaceuticals, Ltd.	61314-0227-15
15 ml	$66.43	TIMOPTIC OCUMETER, Physicians Total Care	54868-0664-03

Tinzaparin Sodium *(003497)*

For related information, see the comparative table section in Appendix A.

Categories: FDA Approved 2000 Jul; Pregnancy Category C
Drug Classes: Anticoagulants
Brand Names: **Innohep**
Foreign Brand Availability: Logiparin (Austria; Denmark; England; Finland; Greece; Netherlands; Sweden; Switzerland)
Cost of Therapy: $604.80 (Deep Vein Thrombosis; Innohep Injection; 20,000 u/ml; 2 ml; 12,000 units/day; 6 day supply)

WARNING

SPINAL/EPIDURAL HEMATOMAS

When neuraxial anesthesia (epidural/spinal anesthesia) or spinal puncture is employed, patients anticoagulated or scheduled to be anticoagulated with low molecular weight heparins or heparinoids for prevention of thromboembolic complications are at risk of developing an epidural or spinal hematoma which can result in long-term or permanent paralysis.

The risk of these events is increased by the use of indwelling epidural catheters for administration of analgesia or by the concomitant use of drugs affecting hemostasis such as non-steroidal anti-inflammatory drugs (NSAIDs), platelet inhibitors, or other anticoagulants. The risk also appears to be increased by traumatic or repeated epidural or spinal puncture.

Patients should be frequently monitored for signs and symptoms of neurological impairment. If neurological compromise is noted, urgent treatment is necessary.

The physician should consider the potential benefit versus risk before neuraxial intervention in patients anticoagulated or to be anticoagulated for thromboprophylaxis (see WARNINGS, Hemorrhage, and DRUG INTERACTIONS).

DESCRIPTION

Innohep is a sterile solution, containing tinzaparin sodium, a low molecular weight heparin. It is available in a multiple dose 2 ml vial.

Each 2 ml vial contains 20,000 anti-Factor Xa IU (anti-Xa) of tinzaparin sodium per ml, for a total of 40,000 IU, and 3.1 mg/ml sodium metabisulfite as a stabilizer. The vial contains 10 mg/ml benzyl alcohol as a preservative. Sodium hydroxide may be added to achieve a pH range of 5.0-7.5 (seeTABLE 1).

TABLE 1 *Composition of 20,000 Anti-Xa IU/ml Tinzaparin Sodium Injection*

Component	Quantity per ml
Tinzaparin sodium	20,000 anti-Xa IU
Benzyl alcohol	10 mg
Sodium metabisulfite	3.106 mg*
Sodium hydroxide	as necessary
Water for injection	qs to 1 ml

* Corresponding to 3.4 mg/ml sodium bisulfite.

Tinzaparin sodium is the sodium salt of a low molecular weight heparin obtained by controlled enzymatic depolymerization of heparin from porcine intestinal mucosa using heparinase from *Flavobacterium heparinum.* The majority of the components have a 2-O-sulpho-4-enepyranosuronic acid structure at the non-reducing end and a 2-N,6-O-disulpho-D-glucosamine structure at the reducing end of the chain.

Potency is determined by means of a biological assay and interpreted by the first International Low Molecular Weight Heparin Standard as units of anti-factor Xa (anti-Xa) activity per milligram. The mean tinzaparin sodium anti-factor Xa activity is approximately 100 IU per milligram. The average molecular weight ranges between 5500 and 7500 daltons (see TABLE 2).

TABLE 2 *Molecular Weight Distribution*

Molecular Weight	Molecular Weight Distribution
<2000 daltons	<10%
2000-8000 daltons	60%-72%
>8000 daltons	22%-36%

STORAGE

Store at 25°C (77°F); excursions permitted to 15-30°C (59-86°F).

CLINICAL PHARMACOLOGY

Tinzaparin sodium is a low molecular weight heparin with antithrombotic properties. Tinzaparin sodium inhibits reactions that lead to the clotting of blood including the formation of fibrin clots, both *in vitro* and *in vivo.* It acts as a potent co-inhibitor of several activated coagulation factors, especially Factors Xa and IIa (thrombin). The primary inhibitory activity is mediated through the plasma protease inhibitor, antithrombin.

Bleeding time is usually unaffected by tinzaparin sodium. Activated partial thromboplastin time (aPTT) is prolonged by therapeutic doses of tinzaparin sodium used in the treatment of deep vein thrombosis (DVT). Prothrombin time (PT) may be slightly prolonged with tinzaparin sodium treatment but usually remains within the normal range. Neither aPTT nor PT can be used for therapeutic monitoring of tinzaparin sodium.

Neither unfractionated heparin nor tinzaparin sodium have intrinsic fibrinolytic activity; therefore, they do not lyse existing clots. Tinzaparin sodium induces release of tissue factor pathway inhibitor, which may contribute to the antithrombotic effect. Heparin is also known to have a variety of actions that are independent of its anticoagulant effects. These include interactions with endothelial cell growth factors, inhibition of smooth muscle cell proliferation, activation of lipoprotein lipase, suppression of aldosterone secretion, and induction of platelet aggregation.

PHARMACOKINETICS/PHARMACODYNAMICS

Anti-Xa and anti-IIa activities are the primary biomarkers for assessing tinzaparin sodium exposure because plasma concentrations of low molecular weight heparins cannot be measured directly. Because of analytical assay limitations, anti-Xa activity is the more widely used biomarker. The measurements of anti-Xa and anti-IIa activities in plasma serve as surrogates for the concentrations of molecules which contain the high-affinity binding site for antithrombin (anti-Xa and anti-IIa activities). Monitoring patients based on anti-Xa activity is generally not advised. (See TABLE 3.)

Studies with tinzaparin sodium in healthy volunteers and patients have been conducted with both fixed- and weight-adjusted dose administration. Recommended therapy with tinzaparin sodium is based on weight-adjusted dosing. (See DOSAGE AND ADMINISTRATION.)

TABLE 3 *Summary of Pharmacokinetic Parameters (Mean and Standard Deviation) Based on Anti-Xa Activity Following a Single SC Administration of Tinzaparin Sodium to Healthy Volunteers*

	Dose	
Parameter	4500 IU*	175 IU/kg
C_{max} (IU/ml)	0.25 (0.05)	0.87 (0.24)
T_{max} (h)	3.7 (0.9)	4.7 (1.1)
AUC(0-∞) (IU·h/ml)	2.0 (0.5)	9.6 (1.6)
Half-life (h)	3.4 (1.7)	3.9 (0.9)

* Dosing based on fixed dose of 4500 IU. Mean dose administered was 64.3 IU/kg.

Absorption

Plasma levels of anti-Xa activity increase in the first 2-3 hours following SC injection of tinzaparin sodium and reach a maximum within 4-5 hours. Maximum concentrations (C_{max}) of 0.25 and 0.87 IU/ml are achieved following a single SC fixed dose of 4500 IU (approximately 64.3 IU/kg) and weight-adjusted dose of 175 IU/kg of tinzaparin sodium, respectively. Following a single SC injection of tinzaparin sodium, the mean anti-Xa to anti-IIa activity ratio, based on the area under the anti-Xa and anti-IIa time profiles, is 2.8 and is higher than that of unfractionated heparin (approximately 1.2). The absolute bioavailability (following 4500 IU SC and intravenous [IV] administrations) is 86.7% based on anti-Xa activity. Based on the extent of absorption [AUC(0-∞)], a comparison of 4500 IU and 12,250 IU doses indicates that increases in anti-Xa activity are greater than dose proportional relative to the increase in dose.

Distribution

The volume of distribution of tinzaparin sodium ranges from 3.1-5.0 L. These values are similar in magnitude to blood volume, suggesting that the distribution of anti-Xa activity is limited to the central compartment.

Metabolism

Low molecular weight heparins are partially metabolized by desulphation and depolymerization.

Elimination

In healthy volunteers, the elimination half-life following SC administration of 4500 IU or 175 IU/kg tinzaparin sodium is approximately 3-4 hours based on anti-Xa activity. Clearance following IV administration of 4500 IU tinzaparin sodium is approximately 1.7 L/h. The primary route of elimination is renal.

SPECIAL POPULATIONS

Population Pharmacokinetics

Anti-Xa concentrations from approximately 180 patients receiving SC tinzaparin sodium once daily (175 IU/kg body weight) as the treatment of proximal DVT and approximately 240 patients undergoing elective hip replacement surgery receiving SC tinzaparin sodium once daily (∼65 IU/kg body weight) were analyzed by population pharmacokinetic methods. The results indicate that neither age nor gender significantly alter tinzaparin sodium clearance based on anti-Xa activity (see PRECAUTIONS, General). However, a reduction in tinzaparin sodium clearance was observed in patients with impaired renal function (reduced calculated creatinine clearance). Weight is also an important factor for the prediction of tinzaparin sodium clearance, consistent with the recommendation thattinzaparin sodium therapy be based on weight-adjusted dosing (see DOSAGE AND ADMINISTRATION).

Renal Impairment

In 6 patients undergoing hemodialysis for chronic renal failure, the half-life of anti-Xa activity following a single IV dose of 75 IU/kg of tinzaparin sodium was prolonged compared to that for healthy volunteers (5.2 versus 1.6 hours). In patients being treated with tinzaparin sodium (175 IU/kg) for DVT, a population pharmacokinetic (PK) analysis determined that tinzaparin sodium clearance based on anti-Xa activity was related to creatinine clearance calculated by the Cockroft Gault equation. In this PK analysis, a reduction in tinzaparin sodium clearance in moderate (30-50 ml/min) and severe (<30 ml/min) renal impairment was observed. Patients with severe renal impairment exhibited a 24% reduction in tinzaparin sodium clearance relative to the remainder of the patients in the study. Patients with severe renal impairment should be dosed with caution (see PRECAUTIONS).

Hepatic Impairment

No prospective studies have assessed tinzaparin sodium pharmacokinetics or pharmacodynamics in hepatically-impaired patients. However, the hepatic route is not a major route of elimination of low molecular weight heparins (see WARNINGS, Hemorrhage).

Elderly

No prospective studies have assessed tinzaparin sodium pharmacokinetics or pharmacodynamics in healthy elderly volunteers. Since renal function is known to decline with age, elderly patients may show reduced elimination of tinzaparin sodium.

Obesity

No prospective studies have assessed tinzaparin sodium pharmacokinetics or pharmacodynamics in obese subjects. Based on the results of the population PK analysis, dosing should be based on body weight; body weight adjusted exposure is sufficient to explain tinzaparin sodium clearance differences observed in patients of different body mass index (BMI). Clinical trial experience is limited in patients with a BMI >40 kg/m^2.

INDICATIONS AND USAGE

Tinzaparin sodium is indicated for the treatment of acute symptomatic deep vein thrombosis with or without pulmonary embolism when administered in conjunction with warfarin sodium. The safety and effectiveness of tinzaparin sodium were established in hospitalized patients.

CONTRAINDICATIONS

Tinzaparin sodium is contraindicated in patients with active major bleeding, in patients with (or history of) heparin-induced thrombocytopenia, or in patients with hypersensitivity to tinzaparin sodium.

Patients with known hypersensitivity to heparin, sulfites, benzyl alcohol, or pork products should not be treated with tinzaparin sodium.

WARNINGS

Tinzaparin sodium is not intended for intramuscular or intravenous administration.

Tinzaparin sodium cannot be used interchangeably (unit for unit) with heparin or other low molecular weight heparins as they differ in manufacturing process, molecular weight distribution, anti-Xa and anti-IIa activities, units, and dosage. Each of these medications has its own instructions for use.

Tinzaparin sodium should not be used in patients with a history of heparin-induced thrombocytopenia (see CONTRAINDICATIONS).

HEMORRHAGE

Tinzaparin sodium, like other anticoagulants, should be used with extreme caution in conditions with increased risk of hemorrhage, such as bacterial endocarditis; severe uncontrolled hypertension; congenital or acquired bleeding disorders including hepatic failure and amyloidosis; active ulcerative and angiodysplastic gastrointestinal disease; hemorrhagic stroke; shortly after brain, spinal or ophthalmological surgery, or in patients treated concomitantly with platelet inhibitors. Bleeding can occur at any site during therapy with tinzaparin sodium. An unexplained fall in hematocrit, hemoglobin, or blood pressure should lead to serious consideration of a hemorrhagic event. If severe hemorrhage occurs, tinzaparin sodium should be discontinued.

Spinal or epidural hematomas can occur with the associated use of low molecular weight heparins or heparinoids and spinal/epidural anesthesia or spinal puncture which can result in long-term or permanent paralysis. The risk of these events is higher with the use of post-operative indwelling epidural catheters or with the concomitant use of additional drugs affecting hemostasis such as NSAIDs (see BOXED WARNING, and DRUG INTERACTIONS).

THROMBOCYTOPENIA

Thrombocytopenia can occur with the administration of tinzaparin sodium.

In clinical studies, thrombocytopenia (platelet count <100,000/mm^3 if baseline value ≥150,000/mm^3, ≥50% decline if baseline <150,000/mm^3) was identified in 1% of patients given tinzaparin sodium; severe thrombocytopenia (platelet count less than 50,000/mm^3) occurred in 0.13%.

Thrombocytopenia of any degree should be monitored closely. If the platelet count falls below 100,000/mm^3, tinzaparin sodium should be discontinued. Cases of thrombocytopenia with disseminated thrombosis have also been observed in clinical practice with heparins, and low molecular weight heparins, including tinzaparin sodium. Some of these cases were complicated by organ infarction or limb ischemia.

HYPERSENSITIVITY

Tinzaparin sodium contains sodium metabisulfite, a sulfite that may cause allergic-type reactions including anaphylactic symptoms and life-threatening asthmatic episodes in certain susceptible people. The overall prevalence of sulfite sensitivity in the general population is unknown, but is probably low. Sulfite sensitivity is more frequent in asthmatic people than in non-asthmatic people.

PRIAPISM

Priapism has been reported from post-marketing surveillance as a rare occurrence. In some cases surgical intervention was required.

MISCELLANEOUS

Tinzaparin sodium multiple dose vial contains benzyl alcohol as a preservative.The administration of medications containing benzyl alcohol as a preservative to premature neonates has been associated with a fatal "Gasping Syndrome". Because benzyl alcohol may cross the placenta, tinzaparin sodium preserved with benzyl alcohol should be used with caution in pregnant women only if clearly needed (see PRECAUTIONS, Pregnancy).

PRECAUTIONS

GENERAL

Tinzaparin sodium should not be mixed with other injections or infusions.

Tinzaparin sodium should be used with care in patients with a bleeding diathesis, uncontrolled arterial hypertension, or a history of recent gastrointestinal ulceration, diabetic retinopathy, and hemorrhage.

Consistent with expected age-related changes in renal function, elderly patients and patients with renal insufficiency may show reduced elimination of tinzaparin sodium. Tinzaparin sodium should be used with care in these patients (see CLINICAL PHARMACOLOGY, Special Populations).

LABORATORY TESTS

Periodic complete blood counts including platelet count and hematocrit or hemoglobin, and stool tests for occult blood are recommended during treatment with tinzaparin sodium. When administered at the recommended doses, routine anticoagulation tests such as prothrombin time (PT) and activated partial thromboplastin time (aPTT) are relatively insensitive measures of tinzaparin sodium activity and, therefore, are unsuitable for monitoring.

LABORATORY TEST INTERACTIONS

Elevation of Serum Transaminases

Asymptomatic reversible increases in aspartate (AST [SGOT]) and alanine (ALT [SGPT]) aminotransferase levels have occurred in patients during treatment with tinzaparin sodium (see ADVERSE REACTIONS, Elevations of Serum Aminotransferases). Similar increases in transaminase levels have also been observed in patients and volunteers treated with heparin and other low molecular weight heparins.

Since aminotransferase determinations are important in the differential diagnosis of myocardial infarction, liver disease, and pulmonary emboli, elevations that might be caused by drugs like tinzaparin sodium should be interpreted with caution.

CARCINOGENESIS, MUTAGENESIS, AND IMPAIRMENT OF FERTILITY

No long-term studies in animals have been performed to evaluate the carcinogenic potential of tinzaparin sodium.

Tinzaparin sodium displayed no genotoxic potential in an *in vitro* bacterial cell mutation assay (AMES test), *in vitro* Chinese hamster ovary cell forward gene mutation test, *in vitro* human lymphocyte chromosomal aberration assay, and *in vivo* mouse micronucleus assay. Tinzaparin sodium at subcutaneous doses up to 1800 IU/kg/day in rats (about 2 times the maximum recommended human dose based on body surface area) was found to have no effect on fertility and reproductive performance.

PREGNANCY

Teratogenic Effects, Pregnancy Category B

Teratogenicity studies have been performed in rats at subcutaneous doses up to 1800 IU/kg/day (about 2 times the maximum recommended human dose based on body surface area) and in rabbits at subcutaneous doses up to 1900 IU/kg/day (about 4 times the maximum recommended human dose based on body surface area) and have revealed no evidence of impaired fertility or harm to the fetus due to tinzaparin sodium. There are, however, no adequate and well-controlled studies in pregnant women. Because animal reproduction studies are not always predictive of human response, this drug should be used during pregnancy only if clearly needed.

There has been one case each reported of cleft palate, optic nerve hypoplasia, and trisomy 21 (Down's) syndrome in infants of women who received tinzaparin sodium during pregnancy. A cause and effect relationship has not been established.

Nonteratogenic Effects

There have been four reports of fetal death/miscarriage in pregnant women receiving tinzaparin sodium who had high risk pregnancies and/or a prior history of spontaneous abortion. Approximately 6% of pregnancies were complicated by fetal distress. There have been spontaneous reports of one case each of pulmonary hypoplasia or muscular hypotonia in infants of women receiving tinzaparin sodium during pregnancy. A cause and effect relationship for the above observations has not been established.

Approximately 10% of pregnant women receiving tinzaparin sodium experienced significant vaginal bleeding. A cause and effect relationship has not been established.

If tinzaparin sodium is used during pregnancy, or if the patient becomes pregnant while taking this drug, the patient should be apprised of potential hazards to the fetus.

Cases of "Gasping Syndrome" have occurred in premature infants when large amounts of benzyl alcohol have been administered (99-404 mg/kg/day). The 2 ml vial of tinzaparin sodium contains 20 mg of benzyl alcohol (10 mg of benzyl alcohol per ml) (see WARNINGS, Miscellaneous).

NURSING MOTHERS

In studies where tinzaparin sodium was administered subcutaneously to lactating rats, very low levels of tinzaparin sodium were found in breast milk. It is not known whether tinzaparin sodium is excreted in human milk. Because many drugs are excreted in human milk, caution should be exercised when tinzaparin sodium is administered to nursing women.

PEDIATRIC USE

Safety and effectiveness of tinzaparin sodium in pediatric patients have not been established.

GERIATRIC USE

In clinical studies for the treatment of DVT, 58% of patients were 65 or older and 29% were 75 and over. No significant overall differences in safety or effectiveness were observed between these subjects and younger subjects, and other reported clinical experience has not identified differences in responses between the elderly and younger patients, but greater sensitivity to tinzaparin sodium of some older individuals cannot be ruled out.

DRUG INTERACTIONS

Because of increased risk of bleeding, tinzaparin sodium should be used with caution in patients receiving oral anticoagulants, platelet inhibitors (*e.g.,* salicylates, dipyridamole, sulfinpyrazone, dextran, and NSAIDs including ketorolac tromethamine), and thrombolytics. If co-administration is essential, close clinical and laboratory monitoring of these patients is advised (see PRECAUTIONS,Laboratory Tests).

ADVERSE REACTIONS

BLEEDING

Bleeding is the most common adverse event associated with tinzaparin sodium; however, the incidence of major bleeding is low. In clinical trials, the definition of major bleeding included bleeding accompanied by ≥2 g/dl decrease in hemoglobin, requiring transfusion of 2 or more units of blood products, or bleeding which was intracranial, retroperitoneal, or into a major prosthetic joint. (See TABLE 5.)

TABLE 5 *Major Bleeding Events* in Treatment of Acute Deep Vein Thrombosis With or Without Pulmonary Embolism*

Indication	Treatment Group*	
Treatment of Acute DVT With or Without PE	Tinzaparin Sodium (n=519)	Heparin (n=524)
Major bleeding events†	0.8%‡	2.7%‡

* Tinzaparin sodium 175 IU/kg once daily SC. Unfractionated heparin initial IV bolus of 5,000 IU followed by continuous IV infusion adjusted to an aPTT of 1.5-2.5 or initial IV bolus of 50 IU/kg followed by continuous IV infusion adjusted to an aPTT of 2.0-3.0. In all groups treatment continued for approximately 6-8 days, and all patients received oral anticoagulant treatment commencing in the first 2-3 days.
† Bleeding accompanied by ≥2 gram/dl decline in hemoglobin, requiring transfusion of 2 or more units of blood products, or bleeding which was intracranial, retroperitoneal, or into a major prosthetic joint.
‡ The 95% CI on the difference in major bleeding event rates (1.9%) was 0.33%, 3.47%.

THROMBOCYTOPENIA

In clinical studies thrombocytopenia was identified in 1% of patients treated with tinzaparin sodium. Severe thrombocytopenia (platelet count $<50{,}000/mm^3$) occurred in 0.13% (see-WARNINGS, Thrombocytopenia).

ELEVATIONS OF SERUM AMINOTRANSFERASES

Asymptomatic increases in aspartate (AST [SGOT]) and/or alanine (ALT [SGPT]) aminotransferase levels greater than 3 times the upper limit of normal of the laboratory reference range have been reported in up to 8.8% and 13% for AST and ALT, respectively, of patients receiving tinzaparin sodium for the treatment of DVT. Similar increases in aminotransferase levels have also been observed in patients and healthy volunteers treated with heparin and other low molecular weight heparins. Such elevations are reversible and are rarely associated with increases in bilirubin (see PRECAUTIONS, Laboratory Tests).

LOCAL REACTIONS

Mild local irritation, pain, hematoma, and ecchymosis may follow SC injection of tinzaparin sodium. Injection site hematoma has been reported in approximately 16% of tinzaparin sodium treated patients.

HYPERSENSITIVITY

Anaphylactic/anaphylactoid reactions may occur in association with tinzaparin sodium use (see CONTRAINDICATIONS, and WARNINGS).

ADVERSE EVENTS

Adverse events with tinzaparin sodium or heparin, reported at a frequency of ≥1% in clinical trials with patients undergoing treatment for proximal DVT with or without PE are provided inTABLE 6.

OTHER ADVERSE EVENTS IN COMPLETED OR ONGOING TRIALS

Other adverse events reported at a frequency of ≥1% in 4000 patients who received tinzaparin sodium in completed or ongoing clinical trials are listed by body system:

Body as a Whole: Injection site hematoma, reaction unclassified.
Cardiovascular Disorders, General: Hypotension, hypertension.
Central and Peripheral Nervous System Disorders: Dizziness.
Gastrointestinal System Disorders: Flatulence, gastrointestinal disorder (not otherwise specified), dyspepsia.
Heart Rate and Rhythm Disorders: Tachycardia.
Myo-, Endo-, Pericardial and Valve Disorders: Angina pectoris.
Platelet, Bleeding and Clotting Disorders: Hematoma, thrombocytopenia.
Psychiatric Disorders: Insomnia, confusion.
Red Blood Cell Disorders: Anemia.
Resistance Mechanism Disorders: Healing impaired, infection.
Respiratory System Disorders: Pneumonia, respiratory disorder.
Skin and Appendages Disorders: Rash erythematous, pruritus, bullous eruption, skin disorder.
Urinary System Disorders: Urinary retention, dysuria.

TABLE 6 *Adverse Events Occurring in ≥1% in Treatment of Acute Deep Vein Thrombosis With or Without Pulmonary Embolism Studies*

Adverse Event	Treatment Group* Tinzaparin Sodium (n=519)	Heparin (n=524)
Urinary tract infection	19 (3.7%)	18 (3.4%)
Pulmonary embolism	12 (2.3%)	12 (2.3%)
Chest pain	12 (2.3%)	8 (1.5%)
Epistaxis	10 (1.9%)	7 (1.3%)
Headache	9 (1.7%)	9 (1.7%)
Nausea	9 (1.7%)	10 (1.9%)
Hemorrhage (NOS)†	8 (1.5%)	23 (4.4%)
Back pain	8 (1.5%)	2 (0.4%)
Fever	8 (1.5%)	11 (2.1%)
Pain	8 (1.5%)	7 (1.3%)
Constipation	7 (1.3%)	9 (1.7%)
Rash	6 (1.2%)	8 (1.5%)
Dyspnea	6 (1.2%)	9 (1.7%)
Vomiting	5 (1.0%)	8 (1.5%)
Hematuria	5 (1.0%)	6 (1.1%)
Abdominal pain	4 (0.8%)	6 (1.1%)
Diarrhea	3 (0.6%)	7 (1.3%)
Anemia	0	7 (1.3%)

* Tinzaparin sodium 175 IU/kg once daily SC. Unfractionated heparin initial IV bolus of 5000 IU followed by continuous IV infusion adjusted to an aPTT of 1.5-2.5 or initial IV bolus of 50 IU/kg followed by continuous IV infusion adjusted to an aPTT of 2.0-3.0. In all groups treatment continued for approximately 6-8 days, and all patients received oral anticoagulant treatment commencing in the first 2-3 days.
† NOS = Not otherwise specified

Vascular (Extracardiac) Disorders: Thrombophlebitis deep, thrombophlebitis leg deep.

Serious adverse events reported in clinical trials or from post-marketing experience are included in the following tables. (See TABLE 7 and TABLE 8.)

TABLE 7 *Serious Adverse Events Associated With Tinzaparin Sodium in Clinical Trials*

Category	Serious Adverse Event
Bleeding-related	Anorectal bleeding, cerebral/intracranial bleeding, epistaxis, gastrointestinal hemorrhage, hemarthrosis, hematemesis, hematuria, hemorrhage NOS, injection site bleeding, melena, purpura, retroperitoneal/intra-abdominal bleeding, vaginal hemorrhage, wound hematoma
Organ dysfunction	Angina pectoris, cardiac arrythmia, dependent edema, myocardial infarction/coronary thrombosis, thromboembolism
Fetal/neonatal	Congenital anomally, fetal death, fetal distress
Cutaneous	Bullous eruption, erythematous rash, skin necrosis
Hematologic	Granulocytopenia, thrombocytopenia
Allergic reactions	Allergic reaction
Injection site reaction	Cellulitis
Neoplastic	Neoplasm

TABLE 8 *Other Serious Adverse Events Associated With Tinzaparin Sodium From Post-Marketing Surveillance*

Category	Serious Adverse Event
Organ dysfunction	Cholestatic hepatitis, increase in hepatic enzymes, peripheral ischemia, priapism
Bleeding-related	Hemoptysis, ocular hemorrhage, rectal bleeding
Cutaneous reactions	Epidermal necrolysis, ischemic necrosis, urticaria
Hematologic	Agranulocytosis, pancytopenia, thrombocythemia
Injection site reactions	Abscess, necrosis
Allergic reactions	Angioedema
Fetal/neonatal	Neonatal hypotonia
General	Acute febrile reaction

ONGOING SAFETY SURVEILLANCE

When neuraxial anesthesia (epidural/spinal anesthesia) or spinal puncture is employed, patients anticoagulated or scheduled to be anticoagulated with low molecular weight heparins or heparinoids for prevention of thromboembolic complications are at risk of developing an epidural or spinal hematoma which can result in long-term or permanent paralysis (see-BOXED WARNING).

Tinzaparin sodium was first introduced in foreign markets in 1991. There have been no reports of spinal epidural hematoma in association with neuraxial anesthesia or spinal puncture with tinzaparin sodium in clinical trials or in post-marketing surveillance.

There has been one case of spinal epidural hematoma with tinzaparin sodium administered at a therapeutic dose in a patient who had not received neuraxial anesthesia or spinal puncture.

DOSAGE AND ADMINISTRATION

All patients should be evaluated for bleeding disorders before administration of tinzaparin sodium. Since coagulation parameters are unsuitable for monitoring tinzaparin sodium activity, routine monitoring of coagulation parameters is not required (see PRECAUTION-S,Laboratory Tests).

ADULT DOSAGE

The recommended dose of tinzaparin sodium for the treatment of DVT with or without PE is 175 anti-Xa IU/kg of body weight, administered SC once daily for at least 6 days and until the patient is adequately anticoagulated with warfarin (INR at least 2.0 for two consecutive days). Warfarin sodium therapy should be initiated when appropriate (usually within 1-3 days of tinzaparin sodium initiation).

As tinzaparin sodium may theoretically affect the PT/INR, patients receiving both tinsaparin sodium and warfarin should have blood for PT/INR determination drawn just prior to the next scheduled dose of tinzaparin sodium.

TABLE 9 provides tinzaparin sodium doses for the treatment of DVT with or without PE. It is necessary to calculate the appropriate tinzaparin sodium dose for patient weights not displayed in TABLE 9.

An appropriately calibrated syringe should be used to assure withdrawal of the correct volume of drug from tinzaparin sodium vials.

TABLE 9 *Tinzaparin Sodium Weight-Based Dosing for Treatment of Deep Vein Thrombosis With or Without Symptomatic Pulmonary Embolism*

	DVT Treatment 175 IU/kg SC Once Daily 20,000 IU per ml		
Patient Body Weight	**Dose (IU)**	**Amount (ml)**	**Patient Body Weight**
68-80 lb	6,000	0.3	31-36 kg
81-94 lb	7,000	0.35	37-42 kg
95-107 lb	8,000	0.4	43-48 kg
108-118 lb	9,000	0.45	49-53 kg
119-131 lb	10,000	0.5	54-59 kg
132-144 lb	11,000	0.55	60-65 kg
145-155 lb	12,000	0.6	66-70 kg
156-168 lb	13,000	0.65	71-76 kg
169-182 lb	14,000	0.7	77-82 kg
183-195 lb	15,000	0.75	83-88 kg
196-206 lb	16,000	0.8	89-93 kg
207-219 lb	17,000	0.85	94-99 kg
220-232 lb	18,000	0.9	100-105 kg
233-243 lb	19,000	0.95	106-110 kg
244-256 lb	20,000	1	111-116 kg
257-270 lb	21,000	1.05	117-122 kg

To calculate the volume (ml) of an tinzaparin sodium 175 anti-Ca IU per kg subcutaneous dose for treatment of deep vein thrombosis:

Patient weight (kg) × 0.00875 ml/kg = volume to be administered (ml) subcutaneously.

ADMINISTRATION

Tinzaparin sodium is a clear, colorless to slightly yellow solution, and as with other parenteral drug products should be inspected visually for particulate matter and discoloration prior to administration.

Tinzaparin sodium is administered by SC injection. It must not be administered by intramuscular or intravenous injection.

Subcutaneous Injection Technique

Patients should be lying down (supine) or sitting and tinzaparin sodium administered by deep SC injection. Administration should be alternated between the left and right anterolateral and left and right posterolateral abdominal wall. The injection site should be varied daily. The whole length of the needle should be introduced into a skin fold held between the thumb and forefinger; the skin fold should be held throughout the injection. To minimize bruising, do not rub the injection site after completion of the injection.

PRODUCT LISTING - EQUIVALENTS NOT AVAILABLE

Solution - Subcutaneous - 20000 U/ml

2 ml	$168.00	INNOHEP, Dupont Pharmaceuticals	00056-0342-08
2 ml	$168.00	INNOHEP, Pharmion Corporation	54653-0342-08
2 ml	$168.00	INNOHEP, Pharmion Corporation	67211-0342-08
2 ml x 10	$1680.00	INNOHEP, Dupont Pharmaceuticals	00056-0342-53
2 ml x 10	$1680.00	INNOHEP, Pharmion Corporation	54653-0342-53
2 ml x 10	$1680.00	INNOHEP, Pharmion Corporation	67211-0342-53

Tirofiban Hydrochloride (003384)

Categories: Myocardial infarction; FDA Approved 1998 May; Pregnancy Category B
Drug Classes: Platelet inhibitors
Brand Names: Aggrastat
Foreign Brand Availability: Agrastat (Colombia; France); Aggrastet (South-Africa)

DESCRIPTION

Tirofiban hydrochloride, a non-peptide antagonist of the platelet glycoprotein (GP) IIb/IIIa receptor, inhibits platelet aggregation.

Tirofiban hydrochloride monohydrate, a non-peptide molecule, is chemically described as *N*-(butylsulfonyl)-*O*-[4-(4-piperidinyl)butyl]-L-tyrosine monohydrochloride monohydrate.

Its molecular formula is $C_{22}H_{36}N_2O_5S{\cdot}HCl{\cdot}H_2O$.

Tirofiban hydrochloride monohydrate is a white to off-white, non-hygroscopic, free-flowing powder, with a molecular weight of 495.08. It is very slightly soluble in water.

AGGRASTAT INJECTION PREMIXED

Aggrastat injection premixed is supplied as a sterile solution in water for injection, for intravenous (IV) use only, in plastic containers of 100 or 250 ml. Each 100 ml of the premixed, iso-osmotic IV injection contains 5.618 mg tirofiban hydrochloride monohydrate equivalent to 5 mg tirofiban (50 μg/ml) and the following inactive ingredients: 0.9 mg sodium chloride, 54 mg sodium citrate dihydrate, and 3.2 mg citric acid anhydrous. Each 250 ml of the premixed, iso-osmotic IV injection contains 14.045 mg tirofiban hydrochloride monohydrate equivalent to 12.5 mg tirofiban (50 μg/ml) and the following inactive ingredients: 2.25 g sodium chloride, 135 mg sodium citrate dihydrate, and 8 mg citric acid anhydrous.

The pH of the solution ranges from 5.5-6.5 and may have been adjusted with hydrochloric acid and/or sodium hydroxide. The flexible container is manufactured from a specially designed multilayer plastic (PL 2408). Solutions in contact with the plastic container leach out certain chemical components from the plastic in very small amounts; however, biological testing was supportive of the safety of the plastic container materials.

AGGRASTAT INJECTION

Aggrastat injection is a sterile concentrated solution for IV infusion after dilution and is supplied in a 25 or 50 ml vial. Each ml of the solution contains 0.281 mg of tirofiban hydrochloride monohydrate equivalent to 0.25 mg of tirofiban and the following inactive ingredients: 0.16 mg citric acid anhydrous, 2.7 mg sodium citrate dihydrate, 8 mg sodium chloride, and water for injection. The pH ranges from 5.5-6.5 and may have been adjusted with hydrochloric acid and/or sodium hydroxide.

CLINICAL PHARMACOLOGY

MECHANISM OF ACTION

Tirofiban HCl is a reversible antagonist of fibrinogen binding to the GP IIb/IIIa receptor, the major platelet surface receptor involved in platelet aggregation. When administered intravenously, tirofiban HCl inhibits *ex vivo* platelet aggregation in a dose- and concentration-dependent manner. When given according to the recommended regimen, >90% inhibition is attained by the end of the 30 minute infusion. Platelet aggregation inhibition is reversible following cessation of the infusion of tirofiban HCl.

PHARMACOKINETICS

Tirofiban has a half-life of approximately 2 hours. It is cleared from the plasma largely by renal excretion, with about 65% of an administered dose appearing in urine and about 25% in feces, both largely as unchanged tirofiban. Metabolism appears to be limited.

Tirofiban is not highly bound to plasma proteins and protein binding is concentration independent over the range of 0.01 to 25 μg/ml. Unbound fraction in human plasma is 35%. The steady state volume of distribution of tirofiban ranges from 22-42 liters.

In healthy subjects, the plasma clearance of tirofiban ranges from 213-314 ml/min. Renal clearance accounts for 39-69% of plasma clearance. The recommended regimen of a loading infusion followed by a maintenance infusion produces a peak tirofiban plasma concentration that is similar to the steady state concentration during the infusion. In patients with coronary artery disease, the plasma clearance of tirofiban ranges from 152-267 ml/min; renal clearance accounts for 39% of plasma clearance.

SPECIAL POPULATIONS

Gender

Plasma clearance of tirofiban in patients with coronary artery disease is similar in males and females.

Elderly

Plasma clearance of tirofiban is about 19-26% lower in elderly (>65 years) patients with coronary artery disease than in younger (≤65 years) patients.

Race

No difference in plasma clearance was detected in patients of different races.

Hepatic Insufficiency

In patients with mild to moderate hepatic insufficiency, plasma clearance of tirofiban is not significantly different from clearance in healthy subjects.

Renal Insufficiency

Plasma clearance of tirofiban is significantly decreased (>50%) in patients with creatinine clearance <30 ml/min, including patients requiring hemodialysis (see DOSAGE AND ADMINISTRATION, Recommended Dosage). Tirofiban is removed by hemodialysis.

PHARMACODYNAMICS

Tirofiban HCl inhibits platelet function, as demonstrated by its ability to inhibit *ex vivo* adenosine phosphate (ADP)-induced platelet aggregation and prolong bleeding time in healthy subjects and patients with coronary artery disease. The time course of inhibition parallels the plasma concentration profile of the drug. Following discontinuation of an infusion of tirofiban HCl, 0.10 μg/kg/min, *ex vivo* platelet aggregation returns to near baseline in approximately 90% of patients with coronary artery disease in 4-8 hours. The addition of heparin to this regimen does not significantly alter the percentage of subjects with >70% inhibition of platelet aggregation (IPA), but does increase the average bleeding time, as well as the number of patients with bleeding times prolonged to >30 minutes.

In patients with unstable angina, a two-staged IV infusion regimen of tirofiban HCl (loading infusion of 0.4 μg/kg/min for 30 minutes followed by 0.1 μg/kg/min for up to 48 hours in the presence of heparin and aspirin), produces approximately 90% inhibition of *ex vivo* ADP-induced platelet aggregation with a 2.9-fold prolongation of bleeding time during the loading infusion. Inhibition persists over the duration of the maintenance infusion.

INDICATIONS AND USAGE

Tirofiban HCl, in combination with heparin, is indicated for the treatment of acute coronary syndrome, including patients who are to be managed medically and those undergoing PTCA or atherectomy. In this setting, tirofiban HCl has been shown to decrease the rate of a combined endpoint of death, new myocardial infarction or refractory ischemia/repeat cardiac procedure.

Tirofiban HCl has been studied in a setting that included aspirin and heparin.

CONTRAINDICATIONS

Tirofiban HCl is contraindicated in patients with:

- Known hypersensitivity to any component of the product.
- Active internal bleeding or a history of bleeding diathesis within the previous 30 days.
- A history of intracranial hemorrhage, intracranial neoplasm, arteriovenous malformation, or aneurysm.
- A history of thrombocytopenia following prior exposure to tirofiban HCl.
- History of stroke within 30 days or any history of hemorrhagic stroke.
- Major surgical procedure or severe physical trauma within the previous month.
- History, symptoms, or findings suggestive of aortic dissection.
- Severe hypertension (systolic blood pressure >180 mm Hg and/or diastolic blood pressure >110 mm Hg).
- Concomitant use of another parenteral GP IIb/IIIa inhibitor.
- Acute pericarditis.

WARNINGS

Bleeding is the most common complication encountered during therapy with tirofiban HCl. Administration of tirofiban HCl is associated with an increase in bleeding events classified as both major and minor bleeding events by criteria developed by the Thrombolysis in Myocardial Infarction Study group (TIMI).[1] Most major bleeding associated with tirofiban HCl occurs at the arterial access site for cardiac catheterization. Fatal bleedings have been reported (see ADVERSE REACTIONS).

Tirofiban HCl should be used with caution in patients with platelet count <150,000/mm^3, in patients with hemorrhagic retinopathy, and in chronic hemodialysis patients.

Because tirofiban HCl inhibits platelet aggregation, caution should be employed when it is used with other drugs that affect hemostasis. The safety of tirofiban HCl when used in combination with thrombolytic agents has not been established.

During therapy with tirofiban HCl, patients should be monitored for potential bleeding. When bleeding cannot be controlled with pressure, infusion of tirofiban HCl and heparin should be discontinued.

PRECAUTIONS

BLEEDING PRECAUTIONS

Percutaneous Coronary Intervention — Care of the Femoral Artery Access Site

Therapy with tirofiban HCl is associated with increases in bleeding rates particularly at the site of arterial access for femoral sheath placement. Care should be taken when attempting vascular access that only the anterior wall of the femoral artery is punctured. Prior to pulling the sheath, heparin should be discontinued for 3-4 hours and activated clotting time (ACT) <180 seconds or APTT <45 seconds should be documented. Care should be taken to obtain proper hemostasis after removal of the sheaths using standard compressive techniques followed by close observation. While the vascular sheath is in place, patients should be maintained on complete bed rest with the head of the bed elevated 30° and the affected limb restrained in a straight position. Sheath hemostasis should be achieved at least 4 hours before hospital discharge.

Minimize Vascular and Other Trauma

Other arterial and venous punctures, epidural procedures, intramuscular injections, and the use of urinary catheters, nasotracheal intubation and nasogastric tubes should be minimized. When obtaining IV access, non-compressible sites (*e.g.*, subclavian or jugular veins) should be avoided.

Laboratory Monitoring

Platelet counts, and hemoglobin and hematocrit should be monitored prior to treatment, within 6 hours following the loading infusion, and at least daily thereafter during therapy with tirofiban HCl (or more frequently if there is evidence of significant decline). In patients who have previously received GP IIb/IIIa receptor antagonists, consideration should be given to earlier monitoring of platelet count. If the patient experiences a platelet decrease to <90,000/mm^3, additional platelet counts should be performed to exclude pseudothrombocytopenia. If thrombocytopenia is confirmed, tirofiban HCl and heparin should be discontinued and the condition appropriately monitored and treated.

In addition, the activated partial thromboplastin time (APTT) should be determined before treatment and the anticoagulant effects of heparin should be carefully monitored by repeated determinations of APTT and the dose should be adjusted accordingly (see also DOSAGE AND ADMINISTRATION). Potentially life-threatening bleeding may occur especially when heparin is administered with other products affecting hemostasis, such as GP IIb/IIIa receptor antagonists. To monitor unfractionated heparin, APTT should be monitored 6 hours after the start of the heparin infusion; heparin should be adjusted to maintain APTT at approximately 2 times control.

T

SEVERE RENAL INSUFFICIENCY

In clinical studies, patients with severe renal insufficiency (creatinine clearance <30 ml/min) showed decreased plasma clearance of tirofiban HCl. The dosage of tirofiban HCl should be reduced in these patients (see DOSAGE AND ADMINISTRATION).

CARCINOGENESIS, MUTAGENESIS, AND IMPAIRMENT OF FERTILITY

The carcinogenic potential of tirofiban HCl has not been evaluated.

Tirofiban HCl was negative in the *in vitro* microbial mutagenesis and V-79 mammalian cell mutagenesis assays. In addition, there was no evidence of direct genotoxicity in the *in vitro* alkaline elution and *in vitro* chromosomal aberration assays. There was no induction of chromosomal aberrations in bone marrow cells of male mice after the administration of IV doses up to 5 mg tirofiban/kg (about 3 times the maximum recommended daily human dose when compared on a body surface area basis).

Fertility and reproductive performance were not affected in studies with male and female rats given IV doses of tirofiban HCl up to 5 mg/kg/day (about 5 times the maximum recommended daily human dose when compared on a body surface area basis).

PREGNANCY CATEGORY B

Tirofiban has been shown to cross the placenta in pregnant rats and rabbits. Studies with tirofiban HCl at IV doses up to 5 mg/kg/day (about 5 and 13 times the maximum recommended daily human dose for rat and rabbit, respectively, when compared on a body surface area basis) have revealed no harm to the fetus. There are, however, no adequate and well-controlled studies in pregnant women. Because animal reproduction studies are not always predictive of human response, this drug should be used during pregnancy only if clearly needed.

NURSING MOTHERS

It is not known whether tirofiban is excreted in human milk. However, significant levels of tirofiban were shown to be present in rat milk. Because many drugs are excreted in human milk, and because of the potential for adverse effects on the nursing infant, a decision should be made whether to discontinue nursing or discontinue the drug, taking into account the importance of the drug to the mother.

PEDIATRIC USE

Safety and effectiveness of tirofiban HCl in pediatric patients (<18 years old) have not been established.

GERIATRIC USE

Of the total number of patients in controlled clinical studies of tirofiban HCl, 42.8% were 65 years and over, while 11.7% were 75 and over. With respect to efficacy, the effect of tirofiban HCl in the elderly (≥65 years) appeared similar to that seen in younger patients (<65 years). Elderly patients receiving tirofiban HCl with heparin or heparin alone had a higher incidence of bleeding complications than younger patients, but the incremental risk of bleeding in patients treated with tirofiban HCl in combination with heparin compared to the risk in patients treated with heparin alone was similar regardless of age. The overall incidence of non-bleeding adverse events was higher in older patients (compared to younger patients) but this was true both for tirofiban HCl with heparin and heparin alone. No dose adjustment is recommended for the elderly population (see DOSAGE AND ADMINISTRATION, Recommended Dosage).

DRUG INTERACTIONS

Tirofiban HCl has been studied on a background of aspirin and heparin.

The use of tirofiban HCl, in combination with heparin and aspirin, has been associated with an increase in bleeding compared to heparin and aspirin alone (see ADVERSE REACTIONS). Caution should be employed when tirofiban HCl is used with other drugs that affect hemostasis (*e.g.*, warfarin). No information is available about the concomitant use of tirofiban HCl with thrombolytic agents (see PRECAUTIONS, Bleeding Precautions).

In a sub-set of patients (n=762) in the PRISM study, the plasma clearance of tirofiban in patients receiving 1 of the following drugs was compared to that in patients not receiving that drug. There were no clinically significant effects of co-administration of these drugs on the plasma clearance of tirofiban: acebutolol, acetaminophen, alprazolam, amlodipine, aspirin preparations, atenolol, bromazepam, captopril, diazepam, digoxin, diltiazem, docusate sodium, enalapril, furosemide, glyburide, heparin, insulin, isosorbide, lorazepam, lovastatin, metoclopramide, metoprolol, morphine, nifedipine, nitrate preparations, oxazepam, potassium chloride, propranolol, ranitidine, simvastatin, sucralfate and temazepam. Patients who received levothyroxine or omeprazole along with tirofiban HCl had a higher rate of clearance of tirofiban HCl. The clinical significance of this is unknown.

ADVERSE REACTIONS

In clinical trials, 1946 patients received tirofiban HCl in combination with heparin and 2002 patients received tirofiban HCl alone. Duration of exposure was up to 116 hours. Forty-three percent (43%) of the population was >65 years of age and approximately 30% of patients were female.

BLEEDING

The most common drug-related adverse event reported during therapy with tirofiban HCl when used concomitantly with heparin and aspirin, was bleeding (usually reported by the investigators as oozing or mild). The incidences of major and minor bleeding using the TIMI criteria in the PRISM-PLUS and RESTORE studies are shown in TABLE 4.

There were no reports of intracranial bleeding in the PRISM-PLUS study for tirofiban HCl in combination with heparin or in the heparin control group. The incidence of intracranial bleeding in the RESTORE study was 0.1% for tirofiban HCl in combination with heparin and 0.3% for the control group (which received heparin). In the PRISM-PLUS study, the incidences of retroperitoneal bleeding reported for tirofiban HCl in combination with heparin, and for the heparin control group were 0.0% and 0.1%, respectively. In the RESTORE study, the incidences of retroperitoneal bleeding reported for tirofiban HCl in combination with heparin, and the control group were 0.6% and 0.3%, respectively. The incidences of TIMI major gastrointestinal and genitourinary bleeding for tirofiban HCl in combination with heparin in the PRISM-PLUS study were 0.1% and 0.1%, respectively; the incidences in the RESTORE study for tirofiban HCl in combination with heparin were 0.2% and 0.0%, respectively.

The incidence rates of TIMI major bleeding in patients undergoing percutaneous procedures in PRISM-PLUS are shown in TABLE 5.

The incidence rates of TIMI major bleeding (in some cases possibly reflecting hemodilution rather than actual bleeding) in patients undergoing CABG in the PRISM-PLUS and RESTORE studies within 1 day of discontinuation of tirofiban HCl are shown in TABLE 6.

Female and elderly patients receiving tirofiban HCl with heparin or heparin alone had a higher incidence of bleeding complications than male patients or younger patients. The incremental risk of bleeding in patients treated with tirofiban HCl in combination with heparin over the risk in patients treated with heparin alone was comparable regardless of age or gender. No dose adjustment is recommended for these populations (see DOSAGE AND ADMINISTRATION, Recommended Dosage).

TABLE 4

Bleeding	PRISM-PLUS* (UAP/Non-Q-Wave MI Study) Tirofiban HCl † + Heparin‡ (n=773)	Heparin‡ (n=797)	RESTORE* (Angioplasty/Atherectomy Study) Tirofiban HCl§ + Heparin¤ (n=1071)	Heparin¤ (n=1070)
Major bleeding (TIMI criteria)¶	1.4% (11)	0.8% (6)	2.2% (24)	1.6% (17)
Minor bleeding (TIMI criteria)**	10.5% (81)	8.0% (64)	12.0% (129)	6.3% (67)
Transfusions	4.0% (31)	2.8% (22)	4.3% (46)	2.5% (27)

* Patients received aspirin unless contraindicated.
† 0.4 μg/kg/min loading infusion; 0.10 μg/kg/min maintenance infusion.
‡ 5000 U bolus followed by 1000 U/h titrated to maintain an APTT of approximately 2 times control.
§ 10 μg/kg bolus followed by infusion of 0.15 μg/kg/min.
¤ Bolus of 10,000 U or 150 U/kg for patients <70 kg followed by administration as necessary to maintain ACT in approximate range of 300-400 seconds during procedure.
¶ Hemoglobin drop of >50 g/L with or without an identified site, intracranial hemorrhage, or cardiac tamponade.
** Hemoglobin drop of >30 g/L with bleeding from a known site, spontaneous gross hematuria, hematemesis, or hemoptysis.

TABLE 5

	Tirofiban HCl + Heparin		Heparin	
Prior to procedures	2/773	0.3%	1/797	0.1%
Following angiography	9/697	1.3%	5/708	0.7%
Following PTCA	6/239	2.5%	5/236	2.2%

TABLE 6

	Tirofiban HCl + Heparin		Heparin	
PRISM-PLUS	5/29	17.2%	11/31	35.4%
RESTORE	3/12	25.0%	6/16	37.5%

NON-BLEEDING

The incidences of non-bleeding adverse events that occurred at an incidence of >1% and numerically higher than control, regardless of drug relationship, are shown in TABLE 7.

TABLE 7

	Tirofiban HCl + Heparin (n=1953)	Heparin (n=1887)
Body as a Whole		
Edema/swelling	2%	1%
Pain, pelvic	6%	5%
Reaction, vasovagal	2%	1%
Cardiovascular System		
Bradycardia	4%	3%
Dissection, coronary artery	5%	4%
Musculoskeletal System		
Pain, leg	3%	2%
Nervous System/Psychiatric		
Dizziness	3%	2%
Skin and Skin Appendage		
Sweating	2%	1%

Other non-bleeding side effects (considered at least possibly related to treatment) reported at a >1% rate with tirofiban HCl administered concomitantly with heparin were nausea, fever, and headache; these side effects were reported at a similar rate in the heparin group.

In clinical studies, the incidences of adverse events were generally similar among different races, patients with or without hypertension, patients with or without diabetes mellitus, and patients with or without hypercholesteremia.

The overall incidence of non-bleeding adverse events was higher in female patients (compared to male patients) and older patients (compared to younger patients). However, the incidences of non-bleeding adverse events in these patients were comparable between the tirofiban HCl with heparin and the heparin alone groups. (See Bleeding for bleeding adverse events.)

ALLERGIC REACTIONS/READMINISTRATION

Although no patients in the clinical trial database developed anaphylaxis and/or hives requiring discontinuation of the infusion of tirofiban, anaphylaxis has been reported in post-marketing experience (see also Post-Marketing Experience, Hypersensitivity). No information is available regarding the development of antibodies to tirofiban.

LABORATORY FINDINGS

The most frequently observed laboratory adverse events in patients receiving tirofiban HCl concomitantly with heparin were related to bleeding. Decreases in hemoglobin (2.1%) and hematocrit (2.2%) were observed in the group receiving tirofiban HCl compared to 3.1% and 2.6%, respectively, in the heparin group. Increases in the presence of urine and fecal occult blood were also observed (10.7% and 18.3%, respectively) in the group receiving tirofiban HCl compared to 7.8% and 12.2%, respectively, in the heparin group.

Patients treated with tirofiban HCl, with heparin, were more likely to experience decreases in platelet counts than the control group. These decreases were reversible upon discontinuation of tirofiban HCl. The percentage of patients with a decrease of platelets to <90,000/mm^3 was 1.5%, compared with 0.6% in the patients who received heparin alone. The percentage of patients with a decrease of platelets to <50,000/mm^3 was 0.3%, compared with 0.1% of the patients who received heparin alone. Platelet decreases have been observed in patients with no prior history of thrombocytopenia upon readministration of GP IIb/IIIa receptor antagonists.

POST-MARKETING EXPERIENCE

The following additional adverse reactions have been reported in post-marketing experience:

Bleeding: Intracranial bleeding, retroperitoneal bleeding, hemopericardium, pulmonary (alveolar) hemorrhage, and spinal-epidural hematoma. Fatal bleeding events have been reported.

Body as a Whole: Acute and/or severe decreases in platelet counts which may be associated with chills, low-grade fever, or bleeding complications (see Laboratory Findings).

Hypersensitivity: Severe allergic reactions including anaphylactic reactions. The reported cases have occurred during the first day of tirofiban infusion, during initial treatment, and during readministration of tirofiban. Some cases have been associated with severe thrombocytopenia (platelet counts <10,000/mm^3).

DOSAGE AND ADMINISTRATION

Tirofiban HCl injection must first be diluted to the same strength as tirofiban HCl injection premixed, as noted under Directions for Use.

USE WITH ASPIRIN AND HEPARIN

In the clinical studies, patients received aspirin, unless it was contraindicated, and heparin. Tirofiban HCl and heparin can be administered through the same IV catheter.

PRECAUTIONS

Tirofiban HCl is intended for IV delivery using sterile equipment and technique. Do not add other drugs or remove solution directly from the bag with a syringe. Do not use plastic containers in series connections; such use can result in air embolism by drawing air from the first container if it is empty of solution. Any unused solution should be discarded.

DIRECTIONS FOR USE

Prior to use, tirofiban HCl injection (250 μg/ml) must be diluted to the same strength as tyrofiban HCl injection premixed (50 μg/ml). This may be acheived, for example, using 1 of the following 3 methods:

If using a 500 ml bag of sterile 0.9% sodium chloride or 5% dextrose in water, withdraw and discard 100 ml from the bag and replace this volume with 100 ml of tirofiban HCl injection (from four 25 ml vials or two 50 ml vials), **OR**

If using a 250 ml bag of sterile 0.9% sodium chloride or 5% dextrose in water, withdraw and discard 50 ml from the bag and replace this volume with 50 ml of tirofiban HCl injection (from two 25 ml vials or one 50 ml vial), **OR**

If using a 100 ml bag of sterile 0.9% sodium chloride or 5% dextrose in water, add the contents of a 25 ml vial to the bag.

Mix well prior to administration.

Tirofiban HCl injection premixed is supplied as 100 or 250 ml of 0.9% sodium chloride containing 50 μg/ml tirofiban. It is supplied in IntraVia containers. To open the IntraVia container, first tear off its foil overpouch. The plastic may be somewhat opaque because of moisture absorption during sterilization; the opacity will diminish gradually. Check for leaks by squeezing the inner bag firmly; if any leaks are found, the sterility is suspect and the solution should be discarded. Do not use unless the solution is clear and the seal is intact. Suspend the container from its eyelet support, remove the plastic protector from the outlet port, and attach a conventional administration set.

Tirofiban HCl may be administered in the same IV line as dopamine, lidocaine, potassium chloride, and famotidine injection. Tirofiban HCl should not be administered in the same IV line as diazepam.

RECOMMENDED DOSAGE

In most patients, tirofiban HCl should be administered intravenously, at an initial rate of 0.4 μg/kg/min for 30 minutes and then continued at 0.1 μg/kg/min. Patients with severe renal insufficiency (creatinine clearance <30 ml/min) should receive half the usual rate of infusion (see PRECAUTIONS, Severe Renal Insufficiency and CLINICAL PHARMACOLOGY, Special Populations, Renal Insufficiency). TABLE 8 is provided as a guide to dosage adjustment by weight.

Tirofiban HCl injection must first be diluted to the same strength as tirofiban HCl injection premixed, as noted under Directions for Use.

No dosage adjustment is recommended for elderly or female patients (see PRECAUTIONS, Geriatric Use). In PRISM-PLUS, tirofiban HCl was administered in combination with heparin for 48-108 hours. The infusion should be continued through angiography and for 12-24 hours after angioplasty or atherectomy.

HOW SUPPLIED

FOR INTRAVENOUS USE ONLY.

AGGRASTAT INJECTION

Aggrastat injection 6.25 mg per 25 ml (250 μg/ml) and 12.5 mg per 50 ml (250 μg/ml) are non-preserved, clear, colorless concentrated sterile solutions for IV infusion after dilution. **Storage:** Store at 25°C (77°F) with excursions permitted between 15-30°C (59-86°F). Do not freeze. Protect from light during storage.

T

TABLE 8

	Most Patients		Severe Renal Impairment	
Patient Weight	30 Min Loading Infusion Rate	Maintenance Infusion Rate	30 Min Loading Infusion Rate	Maintenance Infusion Rate
30-37 kg	16 ml/h	4 ml/h	8 ml/h	2 ml/h
38-45 kg	20 ml/h	5 ml/h	10 ml/h	3 ml/h
46-54 kg	24 ml/h	6 ml/h	12 ml/h	3 ml/h
55-62 kg	28 ml/h	7 ml/h	14 ml/h	4 ml/h
63-70 kg	32 ml/h	8 ml/h	16 ml/h	4 ml/h
71-79 kg	36 ml/h	9 ml/h	18 ml/h	5 ml/h
80-87 kg	40 ml/h	10 ml/h	20 ml/h	5 ml/h
88-95 kg	44 ml/h	11 ml/h	22 ml/h	6 ml/h
96-104 kg	48 ml/h	12 ml/h	24 ml/h	6 ml/h
105-112 kg	52 ml/h	13 ml/h	26 ml/h	7 ml/h
113-120 kg	56 ml/h	14 ml/h	28 ml/h	7 ml/h
121-128 kg	60 ml/h	15 ml/h	30 ml/h	8 ml/h
129-137 kg	64 ml/h	16 ml/h	32 ml/h	8 ml/h
138-145 kg	68 ml/h	17 ml/h	34 ml/h	9 ml/h
146-153 kg	72 ml/h	18 ml/h	36 ml/h	9 ml/h

AGGRASTAT INJECTION PREMIXED

Aggrastat injection premixed 5 mg tirofiban per 100 ml (50 µg/ml) and 12.5 mg tirofiban per 250 ml (50 µg/ml) are clear, non-preserved, sterile solution premixed in a vehicle made iso-osmotic with sodium chloride.

Storage: Store at 25°C (77°F) with excursions permitted between 15-30°C (59-86°F). Do not freeze. Protect from light during storage.

PRODUCT LISTING - EQUIVALENTS NOT AVAILABLE

Solution - Intravenous - 50 mcg/ml

100 ml	$228.23	AGGRASTAT, Merck & Company Inc	00006-3739-55
250 ml	$496.20	AGGRASTAT, Merck & Company Inc	00006-3739-96

Solution - Intravenous - 250 mcg/ml

25 ml	$243.24	AGGRASTAT, Merck & Company Inc	00006-3713-25
50 ml	$496.20	AGGRASTAT, Merck & Company Inc	00006-3713-50

Tizanidine Hydrochloride *(003321)*

Categories: Spasticity; Pregnancy Category C; FDA Approved 1996 Dec
Drug Classes: Adrenergic agonists; Musculoskeletal agents; Relaxants, skeletal muscle
Brand Names: **Zanaflex**
Foreign Brand Availability: Sirdalud (Austria; Bahamas; Barbados; Belgium; Belize; Benin; Bermuda; Burkina-Faso; Colombia; Curacao; Czech-Republic; Denmark; Ethiopia; Finland; Gambia; Germany; Ghana; Greece; Guinea; Guyana; Hungary; India; Indonesia; Italy; Ivory-Coast; Jamaica; Kenya; Korea; Liberia; Malawi; Mali; Mauritania; Mauritius; Mexico; Morocco; Netherland-Antilles; Netherlands; Niger; Nigeria; Peru; Philippines; Portugal; Senegal; Seychelles; Sierra-Leone; Spain; Sudan; Surinam; Switzerland; Taiwan; Tanzania; Thailand; Trinidad; Tunia; Turkey; Uganda; Zambia; Zimbabwe); Sirdalud MR (Netherlands; Switzerland); Sirdalud Retard (Denmark; Finland); Ternelax (Philippines); Ternelin (Japan)
Cost of Therapy: $244.39 (Muscle Spasticity; Zanaflex; 4 mg; 6 tablets/day; 30 day supply)

DESCRIPTION

Tizanidine hydrochloride is a centrally acting α_2-adrenergic agonist. Tizanidine HCl is a white to off-white, fine crystalline powder, odorless or with a faint characteristic odor. Tizanidine is slightly soluble in water and methanol; solubility in water decreases as the pH increases. Its chemical name is 5-chloro-4-(2-imidazolin-2-ylamino)-2,1,3-benzothiodiazole hydrochloride. Tizanidine's molecular formula is $C_9H_8ClN_5S{\cdot}HCl$, and its molecular weight is 290.2.

Zanaflex is supplied as 2 and 4 mg tablets and 2, 4, and 6 mg capsules for oral administration. Zanaflex tablets are composed of the active ingredient, tizanidine hydrochloride (2.288 mg equivalent to 2 mg tizanidine base and 4.576 mg equivalent to 4 mg tizanidine base), and the inactive ingredients, silicon dioxide colloidal, stearic acid, microcrystalline cellulose and anhydrous lactose.

Zanaflex capsules are composed of the active ingredient, tizanidine hydrochloride (2.29 mg equivalent to 2 mg tizanidine base, 4.58 mg equivalent to 4 mg tizanidine base, and 6.87 mg equivalent to 6 mg tizanidine base), and the inactive ingredients, hydroxypropyl methyl cellulose, silicon dioxide, sugar spheres, titanium dioxide, gelatin, and colorants.

T

CLINICAL PHARMACOLOGY

MECHANISM OF ACTION

Tizanidine is an agonist at α_2-adrenergic receptor sites and presumably reduces spasticity by increasing presynaptic inhibition of motor neurons. In animal models, tizanidine has no direct effect on skeletal muscle fibers or the neuromuscular junction, and no major effect on monosynaptic spinal reflexes. The effects of tizanidine are greatest on polysynaptic pathways. The overall effect of these actions is thought to reduce facilitation of spinal motor neurons.

The imidazoline chemical structure of tizanidine is related to that of the anti-hypertensive drug clonidine and other α_2-adrenergic agonists. Pharmacological studies in animals show similarities between the two compounds, but tizanidine was found to have one-tenth to one-fiftieth (1/50) of the potency of clonidine in lowering blood pressure.

PHARMACOKINETICS

Tizanidine HCl tablets and capsules are bioequivalent to each other under fasted conditions, but not under fed conditions.

A single dose of either two 4 mg tablets or two 4 mg capsules was administered under fed and fasting conditions in an open label, 4 period, randomized crossover study in 96 human volunteers, of whom 81 were eligible for the statistical analysis.

Following oral administration of either the tablet or capsule (in the fasted state), tizanidine has peak plasma concentrations occurring 1.0 hours after dosing with a half-life of approximately 2 hours.

When two 4 mg tablets are administered with food the mean maximal plasma concentration is increased by approximately 30%, and the median time to peak plasma concentration is increased by 25 minutes, to 1 hour and 25 minutes.

In contrast, when two 4 mg capsules are administered with food the mean maximal plasma concentration is decreased by 20%, the median time to peak plasma concentration is increased by 2-3 hours. Consequently, the mean C_{max} for the capsule when administered with food is approximately 2/3 the C_{max} for the tablet when administered with food.

Food also increases the extent of absorption for both the tablets and capsules. The increase with the tablet (~30%) is significantly greater than with the capsule (~10%). Consequently when each is administered with food, the amount absorbed from the capsule is about 80% of the amount absorbed from the tablet.

Administration of the capsule contents sprinkled on applesauce is not bioequivalent to administration of an intact capsule under fasting conditions. Administration of the capsule contents on applesauce results in a 15-20% increase in C_{max} and AUC of tizanidine compared to administration of an intact capsule while fasting, and a 15 minute decrease in the median lag time and time to peak concentration.

SPECIAL POPULATIONS

Age Effects

No specific pharmacokinetic study was conducted to investigate age effects. Cross study comparison of pharmacokinetic data following single dose administration of 6 mg tizanidine showed that younger subjects cleared the drug 4 times faster than the elderly subjects. Tizanidine has not been evaluated in children (see PRECAUTIONS).

Hepatic Impairment

Pharmacokinetic differences due to hepatic impairment have not been studied (see WARNINGS).

Renal Impairment

Tizanidine clearance is reduced by more than 50% in elderly patients with renal insufficiency (creatinine clearance <25 ml/min) compared to healthy elderly subjects; this would be expected to lead to a longer duration of clinical effect. Tizanidine should be used with caution in renally impaired patients (see PRECAUTIONS).

Gender Effects

No specific pharmacokinetic study was conducted to investigate gender effects. Retrospective analysis of pharmacokinetic data, however, following single and multiple dose administration of 4 mg tizanidine showed that gender had no effect on the pharmacokinetics of tizanidine.

Race Effects

Pharmacokinetic differences due to race have not been studied.

Drug Interactions — Oral Contraceptives

No specific pharmacokinetic study was conducted to investigate interaction between oral contraceptives and tizanidine. Retrospective analysis of population pharmacokinetic data following single and multiple dose administration of 4 mg tizanidine, however, showed that women concurrently taking oral contraceptives had 50% lower clearance of tizanidine compared to women not on oral contraceptives (see PRECAUTIONS).

INDICATIONS AND USAGE

Tizanidine is a short-acting drug for the management of spasticity. Because of the short duration of effect, treatment with tizanidine should be reserved for those daily activities and times when relief of spasticity is most important (see DOSAGE AND ADMINISTRATION).

CONTRAINDICATIONS

Tizanidine HCl is contraindicated in patients with know hypersensitivity to tizanidine or its ingredients.

WARNINGS

LIMITED DATA BASE FOR CHRONIC USE OF SINGLE DOSES ABOVE 8 MG AND MULTIPLE DOSES ABOVE 24 MG/DAY

Clinical experience with long-term use of tizanidine at doses of 8-16 mg single doses or total daily doses of 24-36 mg (see DOSAGE AND ADMINISTRATION) is limited. In safety studies, approximately 75 patients have been exposed to individual doses of 12 mg or more for at least 1 year or more and approximately 80 patients have been exposed to total daily doses of 30-36 mg/day for at least 1 year or more. There is essentially no long-term experience with single, daytime doses of 16 mg. Because long-term clinical study experience at high doses is limited, only those adverse events with a relatively high incidence are likely to have been identified (see WARNINGS, PRECAUTIONS, and ADVERSE REACTIONS).

HYPOTENSION

Tizanidine is an α_2-adrenergic agonist (like clonidine) and can produce hypotension. In a single dose study where blood pressure was monitored closely after dosing, two-thirds of patients treated with 8 mg of tizanidine had a 20% reduction in either the diastolic or systolic BP. The reduction was seen within 1 hour after dosing, peaked 2-3 hours after dosing and was associated, at times, with bradycardia, orthostatic hypotension, light-headedness/dizziness and rarely, syncope. The hypotensive effect is dose related and has been measured following single doses of ≥2 mg.

The chance of significant hypotension may possibly be minimized by titration of the dose and by focusing attention on signs and symptoms of hypotension prior to dose advancement.

In addition, patients moving from a supine to a fixed upright position may be at increased risk for hypotension and orthostatic effects.

Caution is advised when tizanidine is to be used in patients receiving concurrent antihypertensive therapy and should not be used with other α_2-adrenergic agonists.

RISK OF LIVER INJURY

Tizanidine occasionally causes liver injury, most often hepatocellular in type. In controlled clinical studies, approximately 5% of patients treated with tizanidine had elevations of liver function tests (ALT/SGPT, AST/SGOT) to greater than 3 times the upper limit of normal (or 2 times if baseline levels were elevated) compared to 0.4% in the control patients. Most cases resolved rapidly upon drug withdrawal with no reported residual problems. In occasional symptomatic cases, nausea, vomiting, anorexia and jaundice have been reported. In postmarketing experience, 3 deaths associated with liver failure have been reported in patients treated with tizanidine. In 1 case, a 49-year-old male developed jaundice and liver enlargement following 2 months of tizanidine treatment, primarily at 6 mg tid. A liver biopsy showed multilobular necrosis without eosinophilic infiltration. Treatment was discontinued and the patient died in hepatic coma 10 days later. There was no evidence of hepatitis B and C in this patient and other therapy included only oxazepam and ranitidine. There was thus no explanation, other than a reaction to tizanidine, to explain the liver injury. In the 2 other cases, patients were taking other drugs with known potential for liver toxicity. One patient, treated with tizanidine at a dose of 4 mg/day, was also on carbamazepine when he developed cholestatic jaundice after 2 months of treatment; this patient died with pneumonia about 20 days later. Another patient, treated with tizanidine for 11 days, was also treated with dantrolene for about 2 weeks prior to developing fatal fulminant hepatic failure.

Monitoring of aminotranferase levels is recommended during the first 6 months of treatment (*e.g.,* baseline, 1, 3, and 6 months) and periodically thereafter, based on clinical status. Because of the potential toxic hepatic effect of tizanidine, the drug should be used only with extreme caution in patients with impaired hepatic function.

SEDATION

In the multiple dose, controlled clinical studies, 48% of patients receiving any dose of tizanidine reported sedation as an adverse event. In 10% of these cases, the sedation was rated as severe compared to <1% in the placebo treated patients. Sedation may interfere with everyday activity.

The effect appears to be dose related. In a single dose study, 92% of the patients receiving 16 mg, when asked, reported that they were drowsy during the 6 hour study. This compares to 76% of the patients on a 8 mg and 35% of the patients on placebo. Patients began noting this effect 30 minutes following dosing. The effect peaked 1.5 hours following dosing. Of the patients who received a single dose of 16 mg, 51% continued to report drowsiness 6 hours following dosing compared to 13% in the patients receiving placebo or 8 mg of tizanidine.

In the multiple dose studies, the prevalence of patients with sedation peaked following the first week of titration and then remained stable for the duration of the maintenance phase of the study.

HALLUCINOSIS/PSYCHOTIC-LIKE SYMPTOMS

Tizanidine use has been associated with hallucinations. Formed, visual hallucinations or delusions have been reported in 5 of 170 patients (3%) in two North American controlled clinical studies. These 5 cases occurred within the first 6 weeks. Most of the patients were aware that the events were unreal. One patient developed psychoses in association with the hallucinations. One patient among these 5 continued to have problems for at least 2 weeks following discontinuation of tizanidine.

PRECAUTIONS

CARDIOVASCULAR

Prolongation of the QT interval and bradycardia were noted in chronic toxicity studies in dogs at doses equal to the maximum human dose on a mg/m^2 basis. ECG evaluation was not performed in the controlled clinical studies. Reduction in pulse rate has been noted in association with decreases in blood pressure in the single dose controlled study (see WARNINGS).

OPHTHALMIC

Dose-related retinal degeneration and corneal opacities have been found in animal studies at doses equivalent to approximately the maximum recommended dose on a mg/m^2 basis. There have been no reports of corneal opacities or retinal degeneration in the clinical studies.

USE IN RENALLY IMPAIRED PATIENTS

Tizanidine should be used with caution in patients with renal insufficiency (creatinine clearance <25 ml/min), as clearance is reduced by more than 50%. In these patients, during titration, the individual doses should be reduced. If higher doses are required, individual doses rather than dosing frequency should be increased. These patients should be monitored closely for the onset or increase in severity of the common adverse events (dry mouth, somnolence, asthenia, and dizziness) as indicators of potential overdose.

USE IN WOMEN TAKING ORAL CONTRACEPTIVES

Tizanidine should be used with caution in women taking oral contraceptives, as clearance of tizanidine is reduced by approximately 50% in such patients. In these patients, during titration, the individual doses should be reduced.

DISCONTINUING THERAPY

If therapy needs to be discontinued, especially in patients who have been receiving high doses for long periods, the dose should be decreased slowly to minimize the risk of withdrawal and rebound hypertension, tachycardia, and hypertonia.

INFORMATION FOR THE PATIENT

Patients should be advised of the limited clinical experience with tizanidine both in regard to duration of use and the higher doses required to reduce muscle tone (see WARNINGS).

Because of the possibility of tizanidine lowering blood pressure, patients should be warned about the risk of clinically significant orthostatic hypotension (see WARNINGS).

Because of the possibility of sedation, patients should be warned about performing activities requiring alertness, such as driving a vehicle or operating machinery (see WARNINGS). Patients should also be instructed that the sedation may be additive when tizanidine is taken in conjunction with drugs (baclofen, benzodiazepines) or substances (*e.g.,* alcohol) that act as CNS depressants.

Patients should be advised of the change in the absorption profile of tizanidine HCl if taken with food and the potential changes in efficacy and adverse effect profiles that may result (see CLINICAL PHARMACOLOGY, Pharmacokinetics).

Patients should be advised not to stop tizanidine suddenly as rebound hypertension and tachycardia may occur (see Discontinuing Therapy).

Tizanidine should be used with caution where spasticity is utilized to sustain posture and balance in locomotion or whenever spasticity is utilized to obtain increased function.

CARCINOGENESIS, MUTAGENESIS, AND IMPAIRMENT OF FERTILITY

No evidence for carcinogenicity was seen in two dietary studies in rodents. Tizanidine was administered to mice for 78 weeks at doses up to 16 mg/kg, which is equivalent to 2 times the maximum recommended human dose on a mg/m^2 basis. Tizanidine was also administered to rats for 104 weeks at doses up to 9 mg/kg, which is equivalent to 2.5 times the maximum recommended human dose on a mg/m^2 basis. There was no statistically significant increase in tumors in either species.

Tizanidine was not mutagenic or clastogenic in the following *in vitro* assays: the bacterial Ames test and the mammalian gene mutation test and chromosomal aberration test in Chinese hamster cells. It was also negative in the following *in vivo* assays: the bone marrow micronucleus test in mice, the bone marrow micronucleus and cytogenecity test in Chinese hamsters, the dominant lethal mutagenicity test in mice, and the unscheduled DNA synthesis (UDS) test in mice.

Tizanidine did not affect fertility in male rats at doses of 10 mg/kg, approximately 2.7 times the maximum recommended human dose on a mg/m^2 basis, and in females at doses of 3 mg/kg, approximately equal to the maximum recommended human dose on a mg/m^2 basis; fertility was reduced in males receiving 30 mg/kg (8 times the maximum recommended human dose on a mg/m^2 basis) and in females receiving 10 mg/kg (2.7 times the maximum recommended human dose on a mg/m^2 basis). At these doses, maternal behavioral effects and clinical signs were observed including marked sedation, weight loss, and ataxia.

PREGNANCY CATEGORY C

Reproduction studies performed in rats at a dose of 3 mg/kg, equal to the maximum recommended human dose on a mg/m^2 basis, and in rabbits at 30 mg/kg, 16 times the recommended human dose on a mg/m^2 basis, did not show evidence of teratogenicity. Tizanidine at doses that are equal to and up to 8 times the maximum recommended human dose on a mg/m^2 basis increased gestation duration in rats. Prenatal and postnatal pup loss was increased and developmental retardation occurred. Postimplantation loss was increased in rabbits at doses of 1 mg/kg or greater, equal to or greater than 0.5 times the maximum recommended human dose on a mg/m^2 basis. Tizanidine has not been studied in pregnant women. Tizanidine should be given to pregnant women only if clearly needed.

LABOR AND DELIVERY

The effect of tizanidine on labor and delivery in humans is unknown.

NURSING MOTHERS

It is not known whether tizanidine is excreted in human milk, although as a lipid soluble drug, it might be expected to pass into breast milk.

GERIATRIC USE

Tizanidine should be used with caution in elderly patients because clearance is decreased 4-fold.

PEDIATRIC USE

There are no adequate and well-controlled studies to document the safety and efficacy of tizanidine in children.

DRUG INTERACTIONS

In vitro studies of cytochrome P450 isoenzymes using human liver microsomes indicate that neither tizanidine nor the major metabolites are likely to affect the metabolism of other drugs metabolized by cytochrome P450 isoenzymes.

Acetaminophen: Tizanidine delayed the T_{max} of acetaminophen by 16 minutes. Acetaminophen did not affect the pharmacokinetics of tizanidine.

Alcohol: Alcohol increased the AUC of tizanidine by approximately 20% while also increasing its C_{max} by approximately 15%. This was associated with an increase in side effects of tizanidine. The CNS depressant effects of tizanidine and alcohol are additive.

Oral Contraceptives: No specific pharmacokinetic study was conducted to investigate interaction between oral contraceptives and tizanidine, but retrospective analysis of population pharmacokinetic data following single and multiple dose administration of 4 mg tizanidine showed that women concurrently taking oral contraceptives had 50% lower clearance of tizanidine than women not on oral contraceptives.

Rofecoxib: Rofecoxib may potentiate the adverse effects of tizanidine. Eight case reports of a potential rofecoxib-tizanidine drug interaction have been identified in postmarketing safety reports. Most of the adverse events reported involved the nervous system (*e.g.,* hallucinations, psychosis, somnolence, hypotonia, etc.) and the cardiovascular system (*e.g.,* hypotension, tachycardia, bradycardia). In all cases, adverse events resolved following discontinuation of tizanidine, rofecoxib, or both.

Rechallenges with both drugs were not performed. The possible mechanism and the potential for a drug interaction between tizanidine and rofecoxib remain unclear.

ADVERSE REACTIONS

In multiple dose, placebo-controlled clinical studies, 264 patients were treated with tizanidine and 261 with placebo. Adverse events, including severe adverse events, were more frequently reported with tizanidine than with placebo.

COMMON ADVERSE EVENTS LEADING TO DISCONTINUATION

Forty-five of 264 (17%) patients receiving tizanidine and 13 of 261 (5%) patients receiving placebo in three multiple dose, placebo-controlled clinical studies, discontinued treatment for adverse events. When patients withdrew from the study, they frequently had more than one reason for discontinuing. The adverse events most frequently leading to withdrawal of tizanidine treated patients in the controlled clinical studies were asthenia (weakness, fatigue and/or tiredness) (3%), somnolence (3%), dry mouth (3%), increased spasm or tone (2%), and dizziness (2%).

MOST FREQUENT ADVERSE CLINICAL EVENTS SEEN IN ASSOCIATION WITH THE USE OF TIZANIDINE

In multiple dose, placebo-controlled clinical studies involving 264 patients with spasticity, the most frequent adverse events were dry mouth, somnolence/sedation, asthenia (weakness, fatigue and/or tiredness), and dizziness. Three-quarters of the patients rated the events as mild to moderate and one-quarter of the patients rated the events as being severe. These events appeared to be dose related.

ADVERSE EVENTS REPORTED IN CONTROLLED STUDIES

The events cited reflect experience gained under closely monitored conditions of clinical studies in a highly selected patient population. In actual clinical practice or in other clinical studies, these frequency estimates may not apply, as the conditions of use, reporting behavior, and the kinds of patients treated may differ. TABLE 1 lists treatment emergent signs and symptoms that were reported in greater than 2% of patients in three multiple dose, placebo-controlled studies who received tizanidine where the frequency in the tizanidine group was at least as common as in the placebo group. These events are not necessarily related to tizanidine treatment. For comparison purposes, the corresponding frequency of the event (per 100 patients) among placebo treated patients is also provided.

TABLE 1 *Multiple Dose, Placebo-Controlled Studies — Frequent (>2%) Adverse Events Reported for Which Tizanidine Incidence Is Greater Than Placebo*

Event	Placebo (n=261)	Tizanidine (n=264)
Dry mouth	10%	49%
Somnolence	10%	48%
Asthenia*	16%	41%
Dizziness	4%	16%
UTI	7%	10%
Infection	5%	6%
Constipation	1%	4%
Liver function tests abnormal	<1%	3%
Vomiting	0%	3%
Speech disorder	0%	3%
Amblyopia (blurred vision)	<1%	3%
Urinary frequency	2%	3%
Flu syndrome	2%	3%
SGPT/ALT increased	<1%	3%
Dyskinesia	0%	3%
Nervousness	<1%	3%
Pharnygitis	1%	3%
Rhinitis	2%	3%

* Weakness, fatigue and/or tiredness.

In the single dose, placebo-controlled study involving 142 patients with spasticity, the patients were specifically asked if they had experienced any of the four most common adverse events: dry mouth, somnolence (drowsiness), asthenia (weakness, fatigue and/or tiredness), and dizziness. In addition, hypotension and bradycardia were observed. The occurrence of the adverse events are summarized in TABLE 2. Other events were, in general, reported at a rate of 2% or less.

TABLE 2 *Single Dose, Placebo-Controlled Study — Common Adverse Events Reported*

Event	Placebo (n=48)	Tizanidine 8 mg (n=45)	Tizanidine 16 mg (n=49)
Somnolence	31%	78%	92%
Dry mouth	35%	76%	88%
Asthenia*	40%	67%	78%
Dizziness	4%	22%	45%
Hypotension	0%	16%	33%
Bradycardia	0%	2%	10%

* Weakness, fatigue and/or tiredness.

OTHER ADVERSE EVENTS OBSERVED DURING THE EVALUATION OF TIZANIDINE

Tizanidine was administered to 1385 patients in additional clinical studies where adverse event information was available. The conditions and duration of exposure varied greatly, and included (in overlapping categories) double-blind and open-label studies, uncontrolled and controlled studies, inpatient and outpatient studies, and titration studies. Untoward events associated with the exposure were recorded by clinical investigators using terminology of their own choosing. Consequently, it is not possible to provide a meaningful estimate of the proportion of individuals experiencing adverse events without first grouping similar types of untoward events into a smaller number of standardized event categories.

In the tabulations that follow, reported adverse events were classified using a standard COSTART-based dictionary terminology. The frequencies presented, therefore, represent the proportion of the 1385 patients exposed to tizanidine who experienced an event of the type cited on at least one occasion while receiving tizanidine. All reported events are included except those already listed in TABLE 1. If the COSTART term for an event was so general as to be uninformative, it was replaced by a more informative term. It is important to emphasize that, although the events reported occurred during treatment with tizanidine, they were not necessarily caused by it.

Events are further categorized by body system and listed in order of decreasing frequency according to the following definitions: *frequent* adverse events are those occurring on one or more occasions in at least 1/100 patients (only those not already listed in the tabulated results from placebo-controlled studies appear in this listing); *infrequent* adverse events are those occurring in 1/100 to 1/1000 patients.

Body as a Whole: *Frequent:* Fever. *Infrequent:* Allergic reaction, moniliasis, malaise, abscess, neck pain, sepsis, cellulitis, death, overdose. *Rare:* Carcinoma, congenital anomaly, suicide attempt.

Cardiovascular System: *Infrequent:* Vasodilatation, postural hypotension, syncope, migraine, arrhythmia. *Rare:* Angina pectoris, coronary artery disorder, heart failure, myocardial infarct, phlebitis, pulmonary embolus, ventricular extrasystoles, ventricular tachycardia.

Digestive System: *Frequent:* Abdomen pain, diarrhea, dyspepsia. *Infrequent:* Dysphagia, cholelithiasis, fecal impaction, flatulence, gastrointestinal hemorrhage, hepatitis, melena. *Rare:* Gastroenteritis, hematemesis, hepatoma, intestinal obstruction, liver damage.

Hemic and Lymphatic System: *Infrequent:* Ecchymosis, hypercholesteremia, anemia, hyperlipemia, leukopenia, leukocytosis, sepsis. *Rare:* Petechia, purpura, thrombocythemia, thrombocytopenia.

Metabolic and Nutritional System: *Infrequent:* Edema, hypothyroidism, weight loss. *Rare:* Adrenal cortex insufficiency, hyperglycemia, hypokalemia, hyponatremia, hypoproteinemia, respiratory acidosis.

Musculoskeletal System: *Frequent:* Myasthenia, back pain. *Infrequent:* Pathological fracture, arthralgia, arthritis, bursitis.

Nervous System: *Frequent:* Depression, anxiety, paresthesia. *Infrequent:* Tremor, emotional lability, convulsion, paralysis, thinking abnormal, vertigo, abnormal dreams, agitation, depersonalization, euphoria, migraine, stupor, dysautonomia, neuralgia. *Rare:* Dementia, hemoplagia, neuropathy.

Respiratory System: *Infrequent:* Sinusitis, pneumonia, bronchitis. *Rare:* Asthma.

Skin and Appendages: *Frequent:* Rash, sweating, skin ulcer. *Infrequent:* Pruritus, dry skin, acne, alopecia, urticaria. *Rare:* Exfoliative dermatitis, herpes simplex, herpes zoster, skin carcinoma.

Special Senses: *Infrequent:* Ear pain, tinnitus, deafness, glaucoma, conjunctivitis, eye pain, optic neuritis, otitis media, retinal hemorrhage, visual field defect. *Rare:* Iritis, keratitis, optic atrophy.

Urogenital System: *Infrequent:* Urinary urgency, cystitis, menorrhagia, pyelonephritis, urinary retention, kidney calculus, uterine fibroids enlarged, vaginal moniliasis, vaginitis. *Rare:* Albuminuria, glycosuria, hematuria, metrorrhagia.

DOSAGE AND ADMINISTRATION

A single dose of 8 mg of tizanidine reduces muscle tone in patients with spasticity for a period of several hours. The effect peaks at approximately 1-2 hours and dissipates between 3-6 hours. Effects are dose-related.

Although single doses of less than 8 mg have not been demonstrated to be effective in controlled clinical studies, the dose-related nature of tizanidine's common adverse events make it prudent to begin treatment with single oral doses of 4 mg. Increase the dose gradually (2-4 mg steps) to optimum effect (satisfactory reduction of muscle tone at a tolerated dose).

The dose can be repeated at 6-8 hour intervals, as needed, to a maximum of 3 doses in 24 hours. The total daily dose should not exceed 36 mg.

Experience with single doses exceeding 8 mg and daily doses exceeding 24 mg is limited. There is essentially no experience with repeated, single, daytime doses greater than 12 mg or total daily doses greater than 36 mg (see WARNINGS).

Food has complex effects on tizanidine pharmacokinetics, which differ with the different formulations. These pharmacokinetic differences may result in clinically significant differences when (1) switching administration of the tablet between the fed or fasted state, (2) switching administration of the capsule between the fed or fasted state, (3) switching between the tablet and capsule in the fed state, or (4) switching between the intact capsule and sprinkling the contents of the capsule on applesauce. These changes may result in increased adverse events or delayed/more rapid onset of activity, depending upon the nature of the switch. For this reason, the prescriber should be thoroughly familiar with the changes in kinetics associated with these different conditions (see CLINICAL PHARMACOLOGY, Pharmacokinetics).

HOW SUPPLIED

ZANAFLEX TABLETS

2 mg: White tablets, with a bisecting score on one side and debossed with "A592" on the other.

4 mg: White tablets, with a quadrisecting score on one side and debossed with "A594" on the other.

Storage: Store at 25°C (77°F); excursions permitted to 15-30°C (59-86°F). Dispense in containers with child resistant closure.

ZANAFLEX CAPSULES

2 mg: Two-piece hard gelatin capsule consisting of a standard blue opaque body with a standard blue opaque cap. The capsules are printed with "2 mg" in white.

T

4 mg: Two-piece hard gelatin capsule consisting of a light blue opaque body with a light blue opaque cap. The capsules are printed with "4 mg" in white.

6 mg: Two-piece hard gelatin capsule consisting of a light blue opaque body with a standard blue opaque cap. The capsules are printed with "6 mg" in white.

Storage: Store at 25°C (77°F); excursions permitted to 15-30°C (59-86°F). Dispense in containers with child resistant closure.

PRODUCT LISTING - RATED THERAPEUTICALLY EQUIVALENT

Tablet - Oral - 2 mg

Qty	Price	Product	NDC
150's	$183.05	GENERIC, Purepac Pharmaceutical Company	00228-2742-15
150's	$183.28	GENERIC, Teva Pharmaceuticals Usa	00093-5163-51

Tablet - Oral - 4 mg

Qty	Price	Product	NDC
150's	$219.76	GENERIC, Teva Pharmaceuticals Usa	00093-5160-51
150's	$219.78	GENERIC, Eon Labs Manufacturing Inc	00185-4400-51

PRODUCT LISTING - EQUIVALENTS NOT AVAILABLE

Tablet - Oral - 2 mg

Qty	Price	Product	NDC
20's	$35.00	GENERIC, Pharma Pac	52959-0691-20
24's	$39.00	GENERIC, Pharma Pac	52959-0691-24
25's	$40.00	GENERIC, Pharma Pac	52959-0691-25
30's	$34.50	ZANAFLEX, Southwood Pharmaceuticals Inc	58016-0521-30
30's	$44.88	GENERIC, Southwood Pharmaceuticals Inc	58016-0737-30
30's	$45.00	GENERIC, Pharma Pac	52959-0691-30
30's	$46.57	ZANAFLEX, Pharma Pac	52959-0636-30
40's	$69.85	ZANAFLEX, Pharma Pac	52959-0636-40
45's	$52.02	GENERIC, Pharma Pac	52959-0691-45
45's	$69.85	ZANAFLEX, Pharma Pac	52959-0636-45
60's	$69.00	ZANAFLEX, Southwood Pharmaceuticals Inc	58016-0521-60
60's	$89.76	GENERIC, Southwood Pharmaceuticals Inc	58016-0737-60
90's	$96.10	GENERIC, Pharma Pac	52959-0691-90
90's	$116.42	ZANAFLEX, Pharma Pac	52959-0636-90
90's	$134.64	GENERIC, Southwood Pharmaceuticals Inc	58016-0737-90
100's	$115.00	ZANAFLEX, Southwood Pharmaceuticals Inc	58016-0521-00
100's	$149.60	GENERIC, Southwood Pharmaceuticals Inc	58016-0737-00
120's	$179.61	GENERIC, Southwood Pharmaceuticals Inc	58016-0737-02
150's	$147.50	GENERIC, Pharma Pac	52959-0691-05
150's	$183.28	GENERIC, Par Pharmaceutical Inc	49884-0782-53
150's	$203.66	ZANAFLEX, Elan Pharmaceuticals	59075-0592-15

Tablet - Oral - 4 mg

Qty	Price	Product	NDC
2's	$2.72	ZANAFLEX, Southwood Pharmaceuticals Inc	58016-0513-02
8's	$10.86	ZANAFLEX, Southwood Pharmaceuticals Inc	58016-0513-08
10's	$13.58	ZANAFLEX, Southwood Pharmaceuticals Inc	58016-0513-10
20's	$27.15	ZANAFLEX, Southwood Pharmaceuticals Inc	58016-0513-20
30's	$40.73	ZANAFLEX, Southwood Pharmaceuticals Inc	58016-0513-30
30's	$45.00	ZANAFLEX, Pharma Pac	52959-0637-30
30's	$64.61	GENERIC, Southwood Pharmaceuticals Inc	58016-0730-30
40's	$54.31	ZANAFLEX, Southwood Pharmaceuticals Inc	58016-0513-40
45's	$61.10	ZANAFLEX, Southwood Pharmaceuticals Inc	58016-0513-45
45's	$69.85	ZANAFLEX, Pharma Pac	52959-0637-45
60's	$68.88	ZANAFLEX, Allscripts Pharmaceutical Company	54569-4975-00
60's	$81.46	ZANAFLEX, Southwood Pharmaceuticals Inc	58016-0513-60
60's	$129.22	GENERIC, Southwood Pharmaceuticals Inc	58016-0730-60
90's	$116.42	ZANAFLEX, Pharma Pac	52959-0637-90
90's	$122.19	ZANAFLEX, Southwood Pharmaceuticals Inc	58016-0513-90
90's	$193.83	GENERIC, Southwood Pharmaceuticals Inc	58016-0730-90
100's	$135.77	ZANAFLEX, Southwood Pharmaceuticals Inc	58016-0513-00
100's	$215.37	GENERIC, Southwood Pharmaceuticals Inc	58016-0730-00
150's	$219.76	GENERIC, Par Pharmaceutical Inc	49884-0783-53
150's	$244.20	ZANAFLEX, Elan Pharmaceuticals	59075-0594-15

Tobramycin *(002355)*

Categories: Conjunctivitis, infectious; Pregnancy Category B; FDA Approval Pre 1982; Orphan Drugs
Drug Classes: Antibiotics, aminoglycosides; Anti-infectives, ophthalmic; Ophthalmics
Brand Names: Aktob; **Tobrex**
Foreign Brand Availability: Artobin (Philippines); Bralifex (Indonesia); Cleo (Taiwan); Eyebrex (Philippines; Taiwan); Ikobel (Greece); Isotic Tobryne (Indonesia); Obry (Mexico); Ocumicin (Colombia); Ocuracin (Korea); Tirselon (Greece); Tobacin (India; Korea); Toberan (Korea); Tobi (England; France; Ireland; Israel); Tobradex (China); Tobramaxin (Germany); Tobrimin (Dominican-Republic); Tobrin (Bahrain; Cyprus; Egypt; Iran; Iraq; Jordan; Kuwait; Lebanon; Libya; Oman; Qatar; Republic-of-Yemen; Saudi-Arabia; Syria; United-Arab-Emirates); Toravin (Korea); Trazil (El-Salvador; Guatemala; Honduras; Nicaragua; Panama); Trazil ofteno (Mexico); Tronamycin (Korea)
Cost of Therapy: $25.60 (Bacterial Conjunctivitis; Tobrex Ophth. Ointment; 0.3%; 3.5 g; 0.5 inch/day; variable day supply)
$22.10 (Bacterial Conjunctivitis; Tobrex Ophthalmic Solution; 0.3%; 5 ml; 6 drops/day; variable day supply)
$4.44 (Bacterial Conjunctivitis; Generic Ophthalmic Solution; 0.3%; 5 ml; 6 drops/day; variable day supply)

OPHTHALMIC

DESCRIPTION

Tobramycin 0.3% is a sterile topical ophthalmic antibiotic formulation prepared specifically for topical therapy of external ophthalmic infections.

Each gram of Tobrex ophthalmic ointment contains: *Active:* Tobramycin 0.3% (3 mg). *Preservative:* Chlorobutanol 0.5%.*Inactives:* Mineral oil, white petrolatum.

Each ml of Tobrex solution contains: *Active:* Tobramycin 0.3% (3 mg). *Preservative:* Benzalkonium Chloride 0.01% (0.1 mg).*Inactives:* Boric acid, sodium sulfate, sodium chloride, tyloxapol, sodium hydroxide and/or sulfuric acid (to adjust pH) and purified water.

Tobramycin is a water-soluble aminoglycoside antibiotic active against a wide variety of gram-negative and gram-positive ophthalmic pathogens.

Chemical Name: O-(3-amino-3-deoxy-α-D-glucopyranosyl-(1→4))-*O*-[2,6-diamino-2,3,6-trideoxy-α-D-*ribo*-hexopyranosyl-(1→6)]-2-deoxystreptamine.

Storage: Store at 8-27°C (46- 80°F).

CLINICAL PHARMACOLOGY

IN VITRO DATA

In vitro studies have demonstrated tobramycin is active against susceptible strains of the following microorganisms: Staphylococci, including *S. aureus* and *S. epidermidis* (coagulase-positive and coagulase-negative), including penicillin-resistant strains.

Streptococci, including some of the Group A-beta-hemolytic species, some nonhemolytic species, and some *Streptococcus pneumoniae.*

Pseudomonas aeruginosa, Escherichia coli, Klebsiella pneumoniae, Enterobacter aerogenes, Proteus mirabilis, Morganella morganii, most *Proteus vulgaris* strains, *Haemophilus influenzae* and *H. aegyptius, Moraxella lacunata, Acinetobacter calcoaceticus* and some *Neisseria* species. Bacterial susceptibility studies demonstrate that in some cases, microorganisms resistant to gentamicin retain susceptibility to tobramycin.

INDICATIONS AND USAGE

Tobramycin is a topical antibiotic indicated in the treatment of external infections of the eye and its adnexa caused by susceptible bacteria. Appropriate monitoring of bacterial response to topical antibiotic therapy should accompany the use of tobramycin. Clinical studies have shown tobramycin to be safe and effective for use in children.

CONTRAINDICATIONS

Tobramycin ophthalmic ointment and ophthalmic solution are contraindicated in patients with known hypersensitivity to any of its components.

WARNINGS

NOT FOR INJECTION INTO THE EYE. Sensitivity to topically applied aminoglycosides may occur in some patients. If a sensitivity reaction to tobramycin occurs, discontinue use. Remove contact lenses before applying ointment or solution.

PRECAUTIONS

GENERAL

As with other antibiotic preparations, prolonged use may result in overgrowth of nonsusceptible organisms, including fungi. If superinfection occurs, appropriate therapy should be initiated. Ophthalmic ointments may retard corneal wound healing.

Cross-sensitivity to other aminoglycoside antibiotics may occur; if hypersensitivity develops with this product, discontinue use and institute appropriate therapy.

INFORMATION FOR THE PATIENT

Ophthalmic Ointment: Do not touch tube tip to any surface, as this may contaminate the ointment.

Ophthalmic Solution: Do not touch dropper tip to any surface, as this may contaminate the solution.

PREGNANCY CATEGORY B

Reproduction studies in 3 types of animals at doses up to 33 times the normal human systemic dose have revealed no evidence of impaired fertility or harm to the fetus due to tobramycin. There are, however, no adequate and well-controlled studies in pregnant women. Because animal studies are not always predictive of human response, this drug should be used during pregnancy only if clearly needed.

NURSING MOTHERS

Because of the potential for adverse reactions in nursing infants from tobramycin, a decision should be made whether to discontinue nursing the infant or discontinue the drug, taking into account the importance of the drug to the mother.

ADVERSE REACTIONS

The most frequent adverse reactions to tobramycin ophthalmic ointment and ophthalmic solution are hypersensitivity and localized ocular toxicity, including lid itching and swelling, and conjunctival erythema. These reactions occur in less than 3 of 100 patients treated with tobramycin. Similar reactions may occur with the topical use of other aminoglycoside antibiotics. Other adverse reactions have not been reported from tobramycin therapy; however, if topical ocular tobramycin is administered concomitantly with systemic aminoglycoside antibiotics, care should be taken to monitor the total serum concentration.

In clinical trials, tobramycin ophthalmic ointment produced significantly fewer adverse reactions (3.7%) than did Garamycin Ophthalmic Ointment (10.6%).

DOSAGE AND ADMINISTRATION

OPHTHALMIC OINTMENT

In mild to moderate disease, apply a half-inch ribbon into the affected eye(s) 2 or 3 times per day. In severe infections, instill a half-inch ribbon into the affected eye(s) every 3-4 hours until improvement, following which treatment should be reduced prior to discontinuation.

How to Apply Tobramycin Ointment:

1. Tilt your head back.
2. Place a finger on your cheek just under your eye and gently pull down until a "V" pocket is formed between your eyeball and your lower lid.
3. Place a small amount (about ½ inch) of tobramycin in the "V" pocket. Do not let the tip of the tube touch your eye.
4. Look downward before closing your eye.

OPHTHALMIC SOLUTION

In mild to moderate disease, instill 1 or 2 drops into the affected eye(s) every 4 hours. In severe infections, instill 2 drops into the eye(s) hourly until improvement, following which treatment should be reduced prior to discontinuation.

INHALATION

DESCRIPTION

Tobramycin is a sterile, clear, slightly yellow, non-pyrogenic, aqueous solution with the pH and salinity adjusted specifically for administration by a compressed air driven reusable nebulizer. The chemical formula for tobramycin is $C_{18}H_{37}N_5O_9$ and the molecular weight is 467.52. Tobramycin is *O*-3-amino-3-deoxy-α-D-glucopyranosyl-(1→4)-*O*-[2,6-diamino-2,3,6-trideoxy-α-D-*ribo*-hexopyranosyl-(1→6)]-2-deoxy-L-streptamine.

Each Tobi single-use 5 ml ampule contains 300 mg tobramycin and 11.25 mg sodium chloride in sterile water for injection. Sulfuric acid and sodium hydroxide are added to adjust the pH to 6.0. Nitrogen is used for sparging. All ingredients meet USP requirements. The formulation contains no preservatives.

CLINICAL PHARMACOLOGY

Tobramycin is specifically formulated for administration by inhalation. When inhaled, tobramycin is concentrated in the airways.

PHARMACOKINETICS

Tobramycin is a cationic polar molecule that does not readily cross epithelial membranes.[1] The bioavailability of tobramycin may vary because of individual differences in nebulizer performance and airway pathology.[2] Following administration, tobramycin remains concentrated primarily in the airways.

Sputum Concentrations

Ten (10) minutes after inhalation of the first 300 mg dose of tobramycin, the average concentration of tobramycin was 1237 μg/g (ranging from 35-7414 μg/g) in sputum. Tobramycin does not accumulate in sputum; after 20 weeks of therapy with the tobramycin regimen, the average concentration of tobramycin at 10 minutes after inhalation was 1154 μg/g (ranging from 39-8085 μg/g) in sputum. High variability of tobramycin concentration in sputum was observed. Two (2) hours after inhalation, sputum concentrations declined to approximately 14% of tobramycin levels at 10 minutes after inhalation.

Serum Concentrations

The average serum concentration of tobramycin 1 hour after inhalation of a single 300 mg dose of tobramycin by cystic fibrosis patients was 0.95 μg/ml. After 20 weeks of therapy on the tobramycin regimen, the average serum concentration 1 hour after dosing was 1.05 μg/ml.

Elimination

The elimination half-life of tobramycin from serum is approximately 2 hours after intravenous (IV) administration. Assuming tobramycin absorbed following inhalation behaves similarly to tobramycin following IV administration, systemically absorbed tobramycin is eliminated principally by glomorular filtration. Unabsorbed tobramycin, following tobramycin administration, is probably eliminated primarily in expectorated sputum.

MICROBIOLOGY

Tobramycin is an aminoglycoside antibiotic produced by *Streptomyces tenebrarius*.[1] It acts primarily by disrupting protein synthesis, leading to altered cell membrane permeability, progressive disruption of the cell envelope, and eventual cell death.[3]

Tobramycin has *in vitro* activity against a wide range of gram-negative organisms including *Pseudomonas aeruginosa*. It is bactericidal at concentrations equal to or slightly greater than inhibitory concentrations.

SUSCEPTIBILITY TESTING

A single sputum sample from a cystic fibrosis patient may contain multiple morphotypes of *Pseudomonas aeruginosa* and each morphotype may have a different level of *in vitro* susceptibility to tobramycin. Treatment for 6 months with tobramycin in two clinical studies did not affect the susceptibility of the majority of *P. aeruginosa* isolates tested; however, increased MICs were noted in some patients. The clinical significance of this information has not been clearly established in the treatment of *P. aeruginosa* in cystic fibrosis patients.

The *in vitro* antimicrobial susceptibility test methods used for parenteral tobramycin therapy can be used to monitor the susceptibility of *P. aeruginosa* isolated from cystic fibrosis patients. If decreased susceptibility is noted, the results should be reported to the clinician.

Susceptibility breakpoints established for parenteral administration of tobramycin do not apply to aerosolized administration of tobramycin. The relationship between *in vitro* susceptibility test results and clinical outcome with tobramycin therapy is not clear.

INDICATIONS AND USAGE

Tobramycin is indicated for the management of cystic fibrosis patients with *P. aeruginosa*.

Safety and efficacy have not been demonstrated in patients under the age of 6 years, patients with FEV_1 <25% or >75% predicted, or patients colonized with *Burkholderia cepacia*.

CONTRAINDICATIONS

Tobramycin is contraindicated in patients with a known hypersensitivity to any aminoglycoside.

WARNINGS

Caution should be exercised when prescribing tobramycin to patients with known or suspected renal, auditory, vestibular, or neuromuscular dysfunction. Patients receiving concomitant parenteral aminoglycoside therapy should be monitored as clinically appropriate.

Aminoglycosides can cause fetal harm when administered to a pregnant woman. Aminoglycosides cross the placenta, and streptomycin has been associated with several reports of total, irreversible, bilateral congenital deafness in pediatric patients exposed *in utero*. Patients who use tobramycin during pregnancy, or become pregnant while taking tobramycin should be apprised of the potential hazard to the fetus.

OTOTOXICITY

Ototoxicity, as measured by complaints of hearing loss or by audiometric evaluations, did not occur with tobramycin therapy during clinical studies. However, transient tinnitus occurred in 8 tobramycin solution-treated patients versus no placebo patients in the clinical studies. Tinnitus is a sentinel symptom of ototoxicity, and therefore the onset of this symptom warrants caution (see ADVERSE REACTIONS). Ototoxicity, manifested as both auditory and vestibular toxicity, has been reported with parenteral aminoglycosides. Vestibular toxicity may be manifested by vertigo, ataxia or dizziness.

NEPHROTOXICITY

Nephrotoxicity was not seen during tobramycin clinical studies but has been associated with aminoglycosides as a class. If nephrotoxicity occurs in a patient receiving tobramycin, tobramycin therapy should be discontinued until serum concentrations fall below 2 μg/ml.

MUSCULAR DISORDERS

Tobramycin should be used cautiously in patients with muscular disorders, such as myasthenia gravis or Parkinson's disease, since aminoglycosides may aggravate muscle weakness because of a potential curare-like effect on neuromuscular function.

BRONCHOSPASM

Bronchospasm can occur with inhalation of tobramycin. In clinical studies of tobramycin, changes in FEV_1 measured after the inhaled dose were similar in the tobramycin and placebo groups. Bronchospasm should be treated as medically appropriate.

PRECAUTIONS

INFORMATION FOR PATIENTS

See the Patient Instructions that are distributed with the prescription.

LABORATORY TESTS

Audiograms

Clinical studies of tobramycin did not identify hearing loss using audiometric tests which evaluated hearing up to 8000 Hz. Tinnitus may be a sentinel symptom of ototoxicity, and therefore the onset of this symptom warrants caution. Physicians should consider an audiogram for patients who show any evidence of auditory dysfunction, or who are at increased risk for auditory dysfunction.

Serum Concentrations

In patients with normal renal function treated with tobramycin, serum tobramycin concentrations are approximately 1 μg/ml 1 hour after dose administration and do not require routine monitoring. Serum concentrations of tobramycin in patients with renal dysfunction or patients treated with concomitant parenteral tobramycin should be monitored at the discretion of the treating physician.

Renal Function

The clinical studies of tobramycin did not reveal any imbalance in the percentage of patients in the tobramycin and placebo groups who experienced at least a 50% rise in serum creatinine from baseline (see ADVERSE REACTIONS). Laboratory tests of urine and renal function should be conducted at the discretion of the treating physician.

CARCINOGENESIS, MUTAGENESIS, AND IMPAIRMENT OF FERTILITY

A 2 year rat inhalation toxicology study to assess carcinogenic potential of tobramycin is in progress.

Tobramycin has been evaluated for genotoxicity in a battery of *in vitro* and *in vivo* tests. The Ames bacterial reversion test, conducted with five tester strains, failed to show a significant increase in revertants with or without metabolic activation in all strains. Tobramycin was negative in the mouse lymphoma forward mutation assay, did not induce chromosomal

T

aberrations in Chinese hamster ovary cells, and was negative in the mouse micronucleus test.

Subcutaneous administration of up to 100 mg/kg of tobramycin did not affect mating behavior or cause impairment of fertility in male or female rats.

PREGNANCY, TERATOGENIC EFFECTS, PREGNANCY CATEGORY D

No reproduction toxicology studies have been conducted with tobramycin. However, subcutaneous administration of tobramycin at doses of 100 or 20 mg/kg/day during organogenesis was not teratogenic in rats or rabbits, respectively. Doses of tobramycin ≥40 mg/kg/day were severely maternally toxic to rabbits and precluded the evaluation of teratogenicity. Aminoglycosides can cause fetal harm (*e.g.*, congenital deafness) when administered to a pregnant woman. Ototoxicity was not evaluated in offspring during nonclinical reproduction toxicity studies with tobramycin. If tobramycin is used during pregnancy, or if the patient becomes pregnant while taking tobramycin, the patient should be apprised of the potential hazard to the fetus. (See WARNINGS).

NURSING MOTHERS

It is not known if tobramycin will reach sufficient concentrations after administration by inhalation to be excreted in human breast milk. Because of the potential for ototoxicity and nephrotoxicity in infants, a decision should be made whether to terminate nursing or discontinue tobramycin.

PEDIATRIC USE

In pediatric patients under 6 years of age, safety and efficacy of tobramycin have not been studied.

DRUG INTERACTIONS

In clinical studies of tobramycin, patients taking tobramycin concomitantly with dornase alfa, β-agonists, inhaled corticosteroids, other anti-pseudomonal antibiotics, or parenteral aminoglycosides demonstrated adverse experience profiles similar to the study population as a whole.

Concurrent and/or sequential use of tobramycin with other drugs with neurotoxic or ototoxic potential should be avoided. Some diuretics can enhance aminoglycoside toxicity by altering antibiotic concentrations in serum and tissue. Tobramycin should not be administered concomitantly with ethacrynic acid, furosemide, urea, or mannitol.

ADVERSE REACTIONS

Tobramycin was generally well tolerated during two clinical studies in 258 cystic fibrosis patients ranging in age from 6-63 years. Patients received tobramycin in alternating periods of 28 days on and 28 days off drug in addition to their standard cystic fibrosis therapy for a total of 24 weeks.

Voice alteration and tinnitus were the only adverse experiences reported by significantly more tobramycin-treated patients. Thirty-three patients (13%) treated with tobramycin complained of voice alteration compared to 17 (7%) placebo patients. Voice alteration was more common in the on-drug periods.

Eight (8) patients from the tobramycin group (3%) reported tinnitus compared to no placebo patients. All episodes were transient, resolved without discontinuation of the tobramycin treatment regimen, and were not associated with loss of hearing in audiograms. Tinnitus is one of the sentinel symptoms of cochlear toxicity, and patients with this symptom should be carefully monitored for high frequency hearing loss. The numbers of patients reporting vestibular adverse experiences such as dizziness were similar in the tobramycin and placebo groups.

Nine (3%) patients in the tobramycin group and 9 (3%) patients in the placebo group had increases in serum creatinine of at least 50% over baseline. In all 9 patients in the tobramycin group, creatinine decreased at the next visit.

TABLE 2 lists the percent of patients with treatment-emergent adverse experiences (spontaneously reported and solicited) that occurred in >5% of tobramycin patients during the two Phase III studies.

DOSAGE AND ADMINISTRATION

The recommended dosage for both adults and pediatric patients 6 years of age and older is 1 single-use ampule (300 mg) administered BID for 28 days. Dosage is not adjusted by weight. All patients should be administered 300 mg BID. The doses should be taken as close to 12 hours apart as possible; they should not be taken less than 6 hours apart.

Tobramycin is inhaled while the patient is sitting or standing upright and breathing normally through the mouthpiece of the nebulizer. Nose clips may help the patient breathe through the mouth.

Tobramycin is administered BID in alternating periods of 28 days. After 28 days of therapy, patients should stop tobramycin therapy for the next 28 days, and then resume therapy for the next 28 day on/28 day off cycle.

Tobramycin is supplied as a single-use ampule and is administered by inhalation, using a hand-held Pari LC Plus reusable nebulizer with a DeVilbiss Pulmo-Aide compressor. Tobramycin is not for subcutaneous, intravenous or Intrathecal administration.

USAGE

Tobramycin is administered by inhalation over a 10-15 minute period, using a hand-held Pari LC Plus reusable nebulizer with a DeVilbiss Pulmo-Aide compressor. Tobramycin should not be diluted or mixed with dornase alfa in the nebulizer.

During clinical studies, patients on multiple therapies were instructed to take them first, followed by tobramycin.

HOW SUPPLIED

Tobi is supplied in single-use, low-density polyethylene plastic 5 ml ampules.

Storage: Tobramycin should be stored under refrigeration at 2-8°C/36-46°F. Upon removal from the refrigerator, or if refrigeration is unavailable, Tobramycin pouches (opened or unopened) may be stored at room temperature (up to 25°C/77°F) for up to 28 days. Tobramycin should not be used beyond the expiration date stamped on the ampule when stored under refrigeration (2-8°C/36-46°F) or beyond 28 days when stored at room temperature (25°C/77°F).

Tobramycin ampules should not be exposed to intense light. The solution in the ampule is slightly yellow, but may darken with age if not stored in the refrigerator; however, the color change does not indicate any change in the quality of the product as long as it is stored within the recommended storage conditions.

***TABLE 2** Percent of Patients With Treatment Emergent Adverse Experiences Occurring in >5% of Tobramycin Patients*

Adverse Event	Tobramycin (n=258)	Placebo (n=262)
Cough increased	46.1%	47.3%
Pharyngitis	38.0%	39.3%
Sputum increased	37.6%	39.7%
Asthenia	35.7%	39.3%
Rhinitis	34.5%	33.6%
Dyspnea	33.7%	38.5%
Fever*	32.9%	43.5%
Lung disorder	31.4%	31.3%
Headache	26.7%	32.1%
Chest pain	26.0%	29.8%
Sputum discoloration	21.3%	19.8%
Hemoptysis	19.4%	23.7%
Anorexia	18.6%	27.9%
Lung function decreased†	16.3%	15.3%
Asthma	15.9%	20.2%
Vomiting	14.0%	22.1%
Abdominal pain	12.8%	23.7%
Voice alteration	12.8%	6.5%
Nausea	11.2%	16.0%
Weight loss	10.1%	15.3%
Pain	8.1%	12.6%
Sinusitis	8.1%	9.2%
Ear pain	7.4%	8.8%
Back pain	7.0%	8.0%
Epistaxis	7.0%	6.5%
Taste perversion	6.6%	6.9%
Diarrhea	6.2%	10.3%
Malaise	6.2%	5.3%
Lower resp. tract infection	5.8%	8.0%
Dizziness	5.8%	7.6%
Hyperventilation	5.4%	9.9%
Rash	5.4%	6.1%

* Includes subjective complaints of fever.
† Includes reported decreases in pulmonary function tests or decreased lung volume on chest radiograph associated with intercurrent illness or study drug administration.

PRODUCT LISTING - RATED THERAPEUTICALLY EQUIVALENT

Solution - Ophthalmic - 0.3%

Size	Price	Product	NDC
5 ml	$5.44	GENERIC, Prescript Pharmaceuticals	00247-0114-05
5 ml	$5.93	FEDERAL UPPER LIMIT, H.C.F.A. F F P	99999-2355-01
5 ml	$7.44	GENERIC, Ocusoft	54799-0513-05
5 ml	$13.38	GENERIC, Aligen Independent Laboratories Inc	00405-6145-05
5 ml	$14.18	GENERIC, Moore, H.L. Drug Exchange Inc	00839-7610-85
5 ml	$14.25	GENERIC, Akorn Inc	17478-0290-10
5 ml	$15.00	GENERIC, Qualitest Products Inc	00603-7345-37
5 ml	$15.00	GENERIC, Bausch and Lomb	24208-0290-05
5 ml	$15.05	GENERIC, Fougera	00168-0254-03
5 ml	$15.50	GENERIC, Ivax Corporation	00182-7044-62
5 ml	$17.19	GENERIC, Major Pharmaceuticals Inc	00904-2970-05
5 ml	$22.10	TOBREX, Southwood Pharmaceuticals Inc	58016-6074-01
5 ml	$22.10	TOBREX, Southwood Pharmaceuticals Inc	58016-6074-05
5 ml	$33.32	TOBREX, Physicians Total Care	54868-0638-00
5 ml	$33.44	TOBREX, Allscripts Pharmaceutical Company	54569-0878-00
5 ml	$43.31	TOBREX, Alcon Laboratories Inc	00065-0643-05
5 ml	$47.76	TOBREX, Pharma Pac	52959-0590-00

PRODUCT LISTING - EQUIVALENTS NOT AVAILABLE

Ointment - Ophthalmic - 0.3%

Size	Price	Product	NDC
3.50 gm	$25.60	TOBREX, Southwood Pharmaceuticals Inc	58016-5013-01
3.50 gm	$25.60	TOBREX, Southwood Pharmaceuticals Inc	58016-5013-03
3.50 gm	$35.63	TOBREX, Allscripts Pharmaceutical Company	54569-1182-00
3.50 gm	$47.50	TOBREX, Alcon Laboratories Inc	00065-0644-35
3.50 gm	$49.06	TOBREX, Pharma Pac	52959-0051-01
3.50 gm	$49.06	TOBREX, Pharma Pac	52959-0051-03
4 gm	$37.50	TOBREX, Physicians Total Care	54868-1682-00

Solution - Ophthalmic - 0.3%

Size	Price	Product	NDC
5 ml	$4.44	GENERIC, Physicians Total Care	54868-3118-00
5 ml	$12.00	GENERIC, Raway Pharmacal Inc	00686-0290-05
5 ml	$14.50	GENERIC, Southwood Pharmaceuticals Inc	58016-6489-00
5 ml	$15.00	GENERIC, Allscripts Pharmaceutical Company	54569-3781-00
5 ml	$15.00	GENERIC, Falcon Pharmaceuticals, Ltd.	61314-0643-05
5 ml	$16.64	GENERIC, Pharma Pac	52959-0108-03
5 ml	$20.05	GENERIC, Alpharma Uspd Makers Of Barre and Nmc	63874-0733-05

Tobramycin Sulfate *(002356)*

Categories: Infection, bone; Infection, central nervous system; Infection, intra-abdominal; Infection, lower respiratory tract; Infection, skin and skin structures; Infection, urinary tract; Meningitis; Peritonitis; Septicemia; Pregnancy Category D; FDA Approved 1975 Jun

Drug Classes: Antibiotics, aminoglycosides

Brand Names: **Nebcin**; Tobradistin; Tobramycin In Sodium Chloride; Tobrasix; Toround

Foreign Brand Availability: Brulamycin (Germany); Dartobcin (Indonesia); Nebcina (Denmark; Finland; Norway; Sweden); Nebcine (France); Nebicina (Italy); Obracin (Belgium; Netherlands; Switzerland); Tobra (Mexico); Tobra-gobens (Spain); Tobraneg (India)

Cost of Therapy: $203.82 (Infection; Nebcin Injection; 80 mg; 210 mg/day; 10 day supply)

HCFA JCODE(S): J3260 up to 80 mg IM, IV

WARNING

Patients treated with tobramycin sulfate injection, and other aminoglycosides should be under close clinical observation, because these drugs have an inherent potential for causing ototoxicity and nephrotoxicity.

Neurotoxicity, manifested as both auditory and vestibular ototoxicity, can occur. The auditory changes are irreversible, are usually bilateral, and may be partial or total. Eighth-nerve impairment and nephrotoxicity may develop, primarily in patients having preexisting renal damage and in those with normal renal function to whom aminoglycosides are administered for longer periods or in higher doses than those recommended. Other manifestations of neurotoxicity may include numbness, skin tingling, muscle twitching, and convulsions. The risk of aminoglycoside-induced hearing loss increases with the degree of exposure to either high peak or high trough serum concentrations. Patients who develop cochlear damage may not have symptoms during therapy to warn them of eighth-nerve toxicity, and partial or total irreversible bilateral deafness may continue to develop after the drug has been discontinued.

Rarely, nephrotoxicity may not become apparent until the first few days after cessation of therapy. Aminoglycoside-induced nephrotoxicity usually is reversible.

Renal and eighth-nerve function should be closely monitored in patients with known or suspected renal impairment and also in those whose renal function is initially normal but who develop signs of renal dysfunction during therapy. Peak and trough serum concentrations of aminoglycosides should be monitored periodically during therapy to assure adequate levels and to avoid potentially toxic levels. Prolonged serum concentrations above 12 µg/ml should be avoided. Rising trough levels (above 2 µg/ml) may indicate tissue accumulation. Such accumulation, excessive peak concentrations, advanced age, and cumulative dose may contribute to ototoxicity and nephrotoxicity (see PRECAUTIONS). Urine should be examined for decreased specific gravity and increased excretion of protein, cells, and casts. Blood urea nitrogen, serum creatinine, and creatinine clearance should be measured periodically. When feasible, it is recommended that serial audiograms be obtained in patients old enough to be tested, particularly high-risk patients. Evidence of impairment of renal, vestibular, or auditory function requires discontinuation of the drug or dosage adjustment.

Tobramycin sulfate injection should be used with caution in premature and neonatal infants because of their renal immaturity and the resulting prolongation of serum half-life of the drug.

Concurrent and sequential use of other neurotoxic and/or nephrotoxic antibiotics, particularly other aminoglycosides (*e.g.,* amikacin, streptomycin, neomycin, kanamycin, gentamicin, and paromomycin), cephaloridine, viomycin, polymyxin B, colistin, cisplatin, and vancomycin, should be avoided. Other factors that may increase patient risk are advanced age and dehydration.

Aminoglycosides should not be given concurrently with potent diuretics, such as ethacrynic acid and furosemide. Some diuretics themselves cause ototoxicity, and intravenously administered diuretics enhance aminoglycoside toxicity by altering antibiotic concentrations in serum and tissue.

Aminoglycosides can cause fetal harm when administered to a pregnant woman (see PRECAUTIONS).

DESCRIPTION

Tobramycin sulfate, a water-soluble antibiotic of the aminoglycoside group, is derived from the actinomycete *Streptomyces tenebrarius.* Tobramycin sulfate injection, is a clear and colorless sterile aqueous solution for parenteral administration.

Tobramycin sulfate is *O*-3-amino-3-deoxy-α-D-glucopyranosyl-(1→4)-*O*-[2,6-diamino-2,3,6-trideoxy-α-D-*ribo*-hexopyranosyl-(1→6)]-2-deoxy-L-streptamine, sulfate (2:5)(salt) and has the chemical formula $(C_{18}H_{37}N_5O_9)_2 \cdot 5\ H_2SO_4$. The molecular weight is 1425.45.

Each ml also contains phenol as a preservative (5 mg, multiple-dose vials; 1.25 mg ADD-Vantage vials), sodium bisulfite (3.2 mg, multiple-dose vials; 1.6 mg, ADD-Vantage vials), 0.1 mg edetate disodium, and water for injection, qs. Sulfuric acid and/or sodium hydroxide may have been added to adjust the pH.

Storage: Store at controlled room temperature 15-30°C (59-86°F).

CLINICAL PHARMACOLOGY

Tobramycin is rapidly absorbed following intramuscular administration. Peak serum concentrations of tobramycin occur between 30 and 90 minutes after intramuscular administration. Following an intramuscular dose of 1 mg/kg of body weight, maximum serum concentrations reach about 4 µg/ml, and measurable levels persist for as long as 8 hours. Therapeutic serum levels are generally considered to range from 4-6 µg/ml. When tobramycin sulfate is administered by intravenous infusion over a 1 hour period, the serum concentrations are similar to those obtained by intramuscular administration. Tobramycin sulfate is poorly absorbed from the gastrointestinal tract.

In patients with normal renal function, except neonates, tobramycin sulfate administered every 8 hours does not accumulate in the serum. However, in those patients with reduced renal function and in neonates, the serum concentration of the antibiotic is usually higher and can be measured for longer periods of time than in normal adults. Dosage for such patients must, therefore, be adjusted accordingly (see DOSAGE AND ADMINISTRATION).

Following parenteral administration, little, if any, metabolic transformation occurs, and tobramycin is eliminated almost exclusively by glomerular filtration. Renal clearance is similar to that of endogenous creatinine. Ultrafiltration studies demonstrate that practically no serum protein binding occurs. In patients with normal renal function, up to 84% of the dose is recoverable from the urine in 8 hours and up to 93% in 24 hours.

Peak urine concentrations ranging from 75-100 µg/ml have been observed following the intramuscular injection of a single dose of 1 mg/kg. After several days of treatment, the amount of tobramycin excreted in the urine approaches the daily dose administered. When renal function is impaired, excretion of tobramycin sulfate is slowed, and accumulation of the drug may cause toxic blood levels.

The serum half-life in normal individuals is 2 hours. An inverse relationship exists between serum half-life and creatinine clearance, and the dosage schedule should be adjusted according to the degree of renal impairment (see DOSAGE AND ADMINISTRATION). In patients undergoing dialysis, 25-70% of the administered dose may be removed, depending on the duration and type of dialysis.

Tobramycin can be detected in tissues and body fluids after parenteral administration. Concentrations in bile and stools ordinarily have been low, which suggests minimum biliary excretion. Tobramycin has appeared in low concentration in the cerebrospinal fluid following parenteral administration, and concentrations are dependent on dose, rate of penetration, and degree of meningeal inflammation. It has also been found in sputum, peritoneal fluid, synovial fluid, and abscess fluids, and it crosses the placental membranes. Concentrations in the renal cortex are several times higher than the usual serum levels.

Probenecid does not affect the renal tubular transport of tobramycin.

MICROBIOLOGY

Tobramycin acts by inhibiting synthesis of protein in bacterial cells.*In vitro* tests demonstrate that tobramycin is bactericidal.

Tobramycin has been shown to be active against most strains of the following organisms both *in vitro* and in clinical infection (see INDICATIONS AND USAGE).

Gram-Positive Aerobes: *Staphylococcus aureus.*

Gram-Negative Aerobes: *Citrobacter* species; *Enterobacter* species; *Escherichia coli; Klebsiella* species; *Morganella morganii; Pseudomonas aeruginosa; Proteus mirabilis; Proteus vulgaris; Providencia* species; *Serratia* species.

Aminoglycosides have a low order of activity against most gram-positive organisms, including *Streptococcus pyogenes, Streptococcus pneumoniae,* and enterococci.

Although most strains of enterococci demonstrate *in vitro* resistance, some strains in this group are susceptible. *In vitro* studies have shown that an aminoglycoside combined with an antibiotic that interferes with cell-wall synthesis affects some enterococcal strains synergistically. The combination of penicillin G and tobramycin results in a synergistic bactericidal effect *in vitro* against certain strains of *Enterococcus faecalis.* However, this combination is not synergistic against other closely related organisms, *e.g., Enterococcus faecium.* Speciation of enterococci alone cannot be used to predict susceptibility. Susceptibility testing and tests for antibiotic synergism are emphasized.

Cross resistance between aminoglycosides may occur.

SUSCEPTIBILITY TESTING

Diffusion Techniques

Quantitative methods that require measurement of zone diameters give the most precise estimates of susceptibility of bacteria to antimicrobial agents. One such procedure is the National Committee for Clinical Laboratory Standards (NCCLS)-approved procedure.[1] This method has been recommended for use with disks to test susceptibility to tobramycin. Interpretation involves correlation of the diameters obtained in the disk test with minimum inhibitory concentrations (MIC) for tobramycin.

Reports from the laboratory giving results of the standard single-disk susceptibility test with a 10 µg tobramycin disk should be interpreted according to the criteria in TABLE 1.

TABLE 1

Zone Diameter (mm)	Interpretation
≥15	(S) Susceptible
13-14	(I) Intermediate
≤12	(R) Resistant

A report of "Susceptible" indicates that the pathogen is likely to be inhibited by generally achievable blood levels. A report of "Intermediate" suggests that the organism would be susceptible if high dosage is used or if the infection is confined to tissues and fluids in which high antimicrobial levels are obtained. A report of "Resistant" indicates that achievable concentrations are unlikely to be inhibitory and other therapy should be selected.

Standardized procedures require the use of laboratory control organisms. The 10 µg tobramycin disk should give the following zone diameters (TABLE 2):

TABLE 2

Organism	Zone Diameter (mm)
E. coli ATCC 25922	18-26
P. aeruginosa ATCC 27853	19-25
S. aureus ATCC 25923	19-29

Dilution Techniques

Broth and agar dilution methods, such as those recommended by the NCCLS,[2] may be used to determine MICs of tobramycin. MIC test results should be interpreted according to TABLE 3:

As with standard diffusion methods, dilution procedures require the use of laboratory control organisms. Standard tobramycin laboratory reagent should give the MIC values shown inTABLE 4.

TABLE 3

MIC (μg/ml)	Interpretation
≤4	(S) Susceptible
8	(I) Intermediate
≥16	(R) Resistant

TABLE 4

Organism	MIC Range (μg/ml)
E. faecalis ATCC 29212	8.0-32.0
E. coli ATCC 25922	0.25-1
P. aeruginosa ATCC 27853	0.12-1
S. aureus ATCC 29213	0.12-1

INDICATIONS AND USAGE

Tobramycin sulfate is indicated for the treatment of serious bacterial infections caused by susceptible strains of the designated microorganisms in the diseases listed below:

- Septicemia in the neonate, child, and adult caused by *P. aeruginosa, E. coli,* and *Klebsiella* spp.
- Lower respiratory tract infections caused by *P. aeruginosa,Klebsiella* spp, *Enterobacter* spp, *Serratia* spp,*E. coli,* and *S. aureus* (penicillinase- and non-penicillinase-producing strains).
- Serious central nervous system infections (meningitis) caused by susceptible organisms.
- Intra-abdominal infections, including peritonitis, caused by *E. coli, Klebsiella* spp, and *Enterobacter* spp.
- Complicated and recurrent urinary tract infections caused by *P. aeruginosa, Proteus* spp (indole-positive and indole-negative),*E. coli, Klebsiella* spp, *Enterobacter* spp,*Serratia* spp, *S. aureus, Providencia* spp, and *Citrobacter* spp.
- Skin, bone, and skin structure infections caused by *P. aeruginosa, Proteus* spp, *E. coli, Klebsiella* spp, *Enterobacter* spp, and *S. aureus.*

Aminoglycosides, including tobramycin sulfate, are not indicated in uncomplicated initial episodes of urinary tract infections unless the causative organisms are not susceptible to antibiotics having less potential toxicity. Tobramycin sulfate may be considered in serious staphylococcal infections when penicillin or other potentially less toxic drugs are contraindicated and when bacterial susceptibility testing and clinical judgment indicate its use.

Bacterial cultures should be obtained prior to and during treatment to isolate and identify etiologic organisms and to test their susceptibility to tobramycin. If susceptibility tests show that the causative organisms are resistant to tobramycin, other appropriate therapy should be instituted. In patients in whom a serious life-threatening gram-negative infection is suspected, including those in whom concurrent therapy with a penicillin or cephalosporin and an aminoglycoside may be indicated, treatment with tobramycin sulfate may be initiated before the results of susceptibility studies are obtained. The decision to continue therapy with tobramycin sulfate should be based on the results of susceptibility studies, the severity of the infection, and the important additional concepts discussed in the BOXED WARNING above.

CONTRAINDICATIONS

A hypersensitivity to any aminoglycoside is a contraindication to the use of tobramycin. A history of hypersensitivity or serious toxic reactions to aminoglycosides may also contraindicate the use of any other aminoglycoside because of the known cross-sensitivity of patients to drugs in this class.

WARNINGS

See BOXED WARNING.

Tobramycin sulfate contains sodium bisulfite, a sulfite that may cause allergic-type reactions, including anaphylactic symptoms and life-threatening or less severe asthmatic episodes, in certain susceptible people. The overall prevalence of sulfite sensitivity in the general population is unknown and probably low. Sulfite sensitivity is seen more frequently in asthmatic than in nonasthmatic people.

Serious allergic reactions including anaphylaxis and dermatologic reactions including exfoliative dermatitis, toxic epidermal necrolysis, erytherma multiforme, and Stevens-Johnson Syndrome have been reported rarely in patients on tobramycin therapy. Although rare, fatalities have been reported. See CONTRAINDICATIONS.

If an allergic reaction occurs, the drug should be discontinued and appropriate therapy instituted.

PRECAUTIONS

Serum and urine specimens for examination should be collected during therapy, as recommended in the BOXED WARNING. Serum calcium, magnesium, and sodium should be monitored.

Peak and trough serum levels should be measured periodically during therapy. Prolonged concentrations above 12 μg/ml should be avoided. Rising trough levels (above 2 μg/ml) may indicate tissue accumulation. Such accumulation, advanced age, and cumulative dosage may contribute to ototoxicity and nephrotoxicity. It is particularly important to monitor serum levels closely in patients with known renal impairment.

A useful guideline would be to perform serum level assays after 2 or 3 doses, so that the dosage could be adjusted if necessary, and at 3-4 day intervals during therapy. In the event of changing renal function, more frequent serum levels should be obtained and the dosage or dosage interval adjusted according to the guidelines provided inDOSAGE AND ADMINISTRATION.

In order to measure the peak level, a serum sample should be drawn about 30 minutes following intravenous infusion or 1 hour after an intramuscular injection. Trough levels are measured by obtaining serum samples at 8 hours or just prior to the next dose of tobramycin sulfate. These suggested time intervals are intended only as guidelines and may vary according to institutional practices. It is important, however, that there be consistency within the individual patient program unless computerized pharmacokinetic dosing programs are available in the institution. These serum-level assays may be especially useful for monitoring the treatment of severely ill patients with changing renal function or of those infected with less susceptible organisms or those receiving maximum dosage.

Neuromuscular blockade and respiratory paralysis have been reported in cats receiving very high doses of tobramycin (40 mg/kg). The possibility of prolonged or secondary apnea should be considered if tobramycin is administered to anesthetized patients who are also receiving neuromuscular blocking agents, such as succinylcholine, tubocurarine, or decamethonium, or to patients receiving massive transfusions of citrated blood. If neuromuscular blockade occurs, it may be reversed by the administration of calcium salts.

Cross-allergenicity among aminoglycosides has been demonstrated.

In patients with extensive burns or cystic fibrosis, altered pharmacokinetics may result in reduced serum concentrations of aminoglycosides. In such patients treated with tobramycin sulfate, measurement of serum concentration is especially important as a basis for determination of appropriate dosage.

Elderly patients may have reduced renal function that may not be evident in the results of routine screening tests, such as BUN or serum creatinine. A creatinine clearance determination may be more useful. Monitoring of renal function during treatment with aminoglycosides is particularly important in such patients.

An increased incidence of nephrotoxicity has been reported following concomitant administration of aminoglycoside antibiotics and cephalosporins.

Aminoglycosides should be used with caution in patients with muscular disorders, such as myasthenia gravis or parkinsonism, since these drugs may aggravate muscle weakness because of their potential curare-like effect on neuromuscular function.

Aminoglycosides may be absorbed in significant quantities from body surfaces after local irrigation or application and may cause neurotoxicity and nephrotoxicity.

Aminoglycosides have not been approved for intraocular and/or subconjunctival use. Physicians are advised that macular necrosis has been reported following administration of aminoglycosides, including tobramycin, by these routes.

See BOXED WARNING regarding concurrent use of potent diuretics and concurrent and sequential use of other neurotoxic or nephrotoxic drugs.

The inactivation of tobramycin and other aminoglycosides by β-lactam-type antibiotics (penicillins or cephalosporins) has been demonstrated *in vitro* and in patients with severe renal impairment. Such inactivation has not been found in patients with normal renal function who have been given the drugs by separate routes of administration.

Therapy with tobramycin may result in overgrowth of nonsusceptible organisms. If overgrowth of nonsusceptible organisms occurs, appropriate therapy should be initiated.

PREGNANCY CATEGORY D

Aminoglycosides can cause fetal harm when administered to a pregnant woman. Aminoglycoside antibiotics cross the placenta, and there have been several reports of total irreversible bilateral congenital deafness in children whose mothers received streptomycin during pregnancy. Serious side effects to mother, fetus, or newborn have not been reported in the treatment of pregnant women with other aminoglycosides. If tobramycin is used during pregnancy or if the patient becomes pregnant while taking tobramycin, she should be apprised of the potential hazard to the fetus.

PEDIATRIC USE

See INDICATIONS AND USAGE and DOSAGE AND ADMINISTRATION.

ADVERSE REACTIONS

NEUROTOXICITY

Adverse effects on both the vestibular and auditory branches of the eighth nerve have been noted, especially in patients receiving high doses or prolonged therapy, in those given previous courses of therapy with an ototoxin, and in cases of dehydration. Symptoms include dizziness, vertigo, tinnitus, roaring in the ears, and hearing loss. Hearing loss is usually irreversible and is manifested initially by diminution of high-tone acuity. Tobramycin and gentamicin sulfates closely parallel each other in regard to ototoxic potential.

NEPHROTOXICITY

Renal function changes, as shown by rising BUN, NPN, and serum creatinine and by oliguria, cylindruria, and increased proteinuria, have been reported, especially in patients with a history of renal impairment who are treated for longer periods or with higher doses than those recommended. Adverse renal effects can occur in patients with initially normal renal function.

Clinical studies and studies in experimental animals have been conducted to compare the nephrotoxic potential of tobramycin and gentamicin. In some of the clinical studies and in the animal studies, tobramycin caused nephrotoxicity significantly less frequently than gentamicin. In some other clinical studies, no significant difference in the incidence of nephrotoxicity between tobramycin and gentamicin was found.

Other reported adverse reactions possibly related to tobramycin sulfate include anemia, granulocytopenia, and thrombocytopenia; and fever, rash, exfoliative dermatitis, itching, urticaria, nausea, vomiting, diarrhea, headache, lethargy, pain at the injection site, mental confusion, and disorientation. Laboratory abnormalities possibly related to tobramycin sulfate include increased serum transaminases (AST [SGOT], ALT [SGPT]); increased serum LDH and bilirubin; decreased serum calcium, magnesium, sodium, and potassium; and leukopenia, leukocytosis, and eosinophilia.

DOSAGE AND ADMINISTRATION

Tobramycin sulfate may be given intramuscularly or intravenously. ADD-Vantage vials are not for intramuscular administration. Recommended dosages are the same for both routes. The patient's pretreatment body weight should be obtained for calculation of correct dosage. It is desirable to measure both peak and trough serum concentrations (see BOXED WARNING and PRECAUTIONS).

T

ADMINISTRATION FOR PATIENTS WITH NORMAL RENAL FUNCTION-ADULTS WITH SERIOUS INFECTIONS

3 mg/kg/day in 3 equal doses every 8 hours (see TABLE 5).

ADULTS WITH LIFE-THREATENING INFECTIONS

Up to 5 mg/kg/day may be administered in 3 or 4 equal doses (see TABLE 5). The dosage should be reduced to 3 mg/kg/day as soon as clinically indicated. To prevent increased toxicity due to excessive blood levels, dosage should not exceed 5 mg/kg/day unless serum levels are monitored (see BOXED WARNING and PRECAUTIONS).

TABLE 5 *Dosage Schedule Guide for Adults With Normal Renal Function (Dosage at 8 Hour Intervals)*

For Patient Weighing		Usual Dose for Serious Infections 1 mg/kg q8h (Total, 3 mg/kg/day)		Maximum Dose for Life-Threatening Infections (Reduce as soon as possible) 1.66 mg/kg q8h (Total, 5 mg/kg/day)	
kg	lb	mg/dose q8h	ml/dose*	mg/dose q8h	ml/dose*
120	264	120 mg	3 ml	200 mg	5 ml
115	253	115 mg	2.9 ml	191 mg	4.75 ml
110	242	110 mg	2.75 ml	183 mg	4.5 ml
105	231	105 mg	2.6 ml	175 mg	4.4 ml
100	220	100 mg	2.5 ml	166 mg	4.2 ml
95	209	95 mg	2.4 ml	158 mg	4 ml
90	198	90 mg	2.25 ml	150 mg	3.75 ml
85	187	85 mg	2.1 ml	141 mg	3.5 ml
80	176	80 mg	2 ml	133 mg	3.3 ml
75	165	75 mg	1.9 ml	125 mg	3.1 ml
70	154	70 mg	1.75 ml	116 mg	2.9 ml
65	143	65 mg	1.6 ml	108 mg	2.7 ml
60	132	60 mg	1.5 ml	100 mg	2.5 ml
55	121	55 mg	1.4 ml	91 mg	2.25 ml
50	110	50 mg	1.25 ml	83 mg	2.1 ml
45	99	45 mg	1.1 ml	75 mg	1.9 ml
40	88	40 mg	1 ml	66 mg	1.6 ml

* Applicable to all product forms except tobramycin sulfate pediatric injection (see HOW SUPPLIED).

PEDIATRIC PATIENTS

Six (6) to 7.5 mg/kg/day in 3 or 4 equally divided doses (2-2.5 mg/kg every 8 hours or 1.5-1.89 mg/kg every 6 hours).

PREMATURE OR FULL-TERM NEONATES 1 WEEK OF AGE OR LESS

Up to 4 mg/kg/day may be administered in 2 equal doses every 12 hours.

It is desirable to limit treatment to a short term. The usual duration of treatment is 7-10 days. A longer course of therapy may be necessary in difficult and complicated infections. In such cases, monitoring of renal, auditory, and vestibular functions is advised, because neurotoxicity is more likely to occur when treatment is extended longer than 10 days.

DOSAGE IN PATIENTS WITH CYSTIC FIBROSIS

In patients with cystic fibrosis, altered pharmacokinetics may result in reduced serum concentrations of aminoglycosides. Measurement of tobramycin serum concentration during treatment is especially important as a basis for determining appropriate dose. In patients with severe cystic fibrosis, an initial dosing regimen of 10 mg/kg/day in 4 equally divided doses is recommended. This dosing regimen is suggested only as a guide. The serum levels of tobramycin should be measured directly during treatment due to wide interpatient variability.

ADMINISTRATION FOR PATIENTS WITH RENAL IMPAIRMENT

Whenever possible, serum tobramycin concentrations should be monitored during therapy.

Following a loading dose of 1 mg/kg, subsequent dosage in these patients must be adjusted, either with reduced doses administered at 8-hour intervals or with normal doses given at prolonged intervals. Both of these methods are suggested as guides to be used when serum levels of tobramycin cannot be measured directly. They are based on either the creatinine clearance level or the serum creatinine level of the patient because these values correlate with the half-life of tobramycin. The dosage schedule derived from either method should be used in conjunction with careful clinical and laboratory observations of the patient and should be modified as necessary. Neither method should be used when dialysis is being performed.

REDUCED DOSAGE AT 8 HOUR INTERVALS

When the creatinine clearance rate is 70 ml or less per minute or when the serum creatinine value is known, the amount of the reduced dose can be determined by multiplying the normal dose from TABLE 5 by the percent of normal dose from the nomogram in the original package insert.

An alternate rough guide for determining reduced dosage at 8 hour intervals (for patients whose steady-state serum creatinine values are known) is to divide the normally recommended dose by the patient's serum creatinine.

NORMAL DOSAGE AT PROLONGED INTERVALS

If the creatinine clearance rate is not available and the patient's condition is stable, a dosage frequency *in hours* for the dosage given in TABLE 5 can be determined by multiplying the patient's serum creatinine by 6.

DOSAGE IN OBESE PATIENTS

The appropriate dose may be calculated by using the patient's estimated lean body weight plus 40% of the excess as the basic weight on which to figure mg/kg.

INTRAMUSCULAR ADMINISTRATION

Tobramycin sulfate may be administered by withdrawing the appropriate dose directly from a vial or by using a prefilled Hyporet. ADD-Vantage vials are not for intramuscular administration.

INTRAVENOUS ADMINISTRATION

For intravenous administration, the usual volume of diluent (0.9% sodium chloride injection or 5% dextrose injection) is 50-100 ml for adult doses. For pediatric patients, the volume of diluent should be proportionately less than that for adults. The diluted solution usually should be infused over a period of 20-60 minutes. Infusion periods of less than 20 minutes are not recommended because peak serum levels may exceed 12 μg/ml (see BOXED WARNING).

USE OF ADD-VANTAGE TOBRAMYCIN SULFATE VIALS

ADD-Vantage tobramycin sulfate vials are not intended for multiple use and should not be used with a syringe in the conventional way. These products are intended for use only with Abbott ADD-Vantage diluent containers and in those instances in which the physician's order specified 60 mg or 80 mg doses. Use within 24 hours after activation.

Tobramycin sulfate should not be physically premixed with other drugs but should be administered separately according to the recommended dose and route.

Prior to administration, parenteral drug products should be inspected visually for particulate matter and discoloration whenever solution and container permit.

PRODUCT LISTING - RATED THERAPEUTICALLY EQUIVALENT

Powder For Injection - Injectable - 1.2 Gm

1's	$338.25	GENERIC, Pharm Tech Packaging Corporation	39822-0412-01
6's	$1919.88	GENERIC, Pharm Tech Packaging Corporation	39822-0412-06

Powder For Injection - Injectable - 60 mg

1's	$6.92	NEBCIN, Lilly, Eli and Company	00002-7293-01

Powder For Injection - Injectable - 80 mg

1's	$7.76	NEBCIN, Lilly, Eli and Company	00002-7294-01

Solution - Injectable - 10 mg/ml

2 ml	$3.65	NEBCIN PEDIATRIC, Lilly, Eli and Company	00002-0501-01
2 ml	$3.65	GENERIC, Lilly, Eli and Company	00002-8988-01
2 ml x 25	$85.54	GENERIC, Geneva Pharmaceuticals	00781-3770-72
2 ml x 25	$93.22	GENERIC, Abbott Pharmaceutical	00074-3577-01
6 ml x 25	$473.25	GENERIC, Abbott Pharmaceutical	00074-3254-03
8 ml x 25	$331.91	GENERIC, Abbott Pharmaceutical	00074-3255-03

Solution - Injectable - 40 mg/ml

1 ml x 25	$252.00	GENERIC, Abbott Pharmaceutical	00074-3582-01
2 ml x 25	$95.50	GENERIC, Bristol-Myers Squibb	00003-2725-10
2 ml x 25	$136.00	GENERIC, Astra-Zeneca Pharmaceuticals	00186-1783-04
2 ml x 25	$153.79	GENERIC, Physicians Total Care	54868-4106-00
2 ml x 25	$155.56	GENERIC, Abbott Pharmaceutical	00074-3578-01
2 ml x 25	$170.53	GENERIC, Geneva Pharmaceuticals	00781-3772-72
2 ml x 25	$182.00	NEBCIN, Lilly, Eli and Company	00002-1499-25
2 ml x 25	$182.00	GENERIC, Lilly, Eli and Company	00002-8989-25
2 ml x 25	$324.25	GENERIC, Abbott Pharmaceutical	00074-3583-01
2 ml x 25	$328.50	GENERIC, Gensia Sicor Pharmaceuticals Inc	00703-9402-04
30 ml	$59.14	GENERIC, Bristol-Myers Squibb	00003-2725-30
30 ml	$70.32	GENERIC, Gensia Sicor Pharmaceuticals Inc	00703-9416-01
30 ml	$92.88	GENERIC, Geneva Pharmaceuticals	00781-3775-90
30 ml x 5	$369.06	GENERIC, Astra-Zeneca Pharmaceuticals	00186-1784-01
50 ml	$73.86	GENERIC, Abbott Pharmaceutical	00074-3590-02
50 ml	$170.75	GENERIC, Vha Supply	00702-2725-11

Solution - Intravenous - 60 mg/50 ml;0.9%

50 ml x 24	$212.04	GENERIC, Abbott Pharmaceutical	00074-3469-13

Solution - Intravenous - 80 mg/100 ml;0.9%

100 ml x 24	$248.64	GENERIC, Abbott Pharmaceutical	00074-3470-23

PRODUCT LISTING - EQUIVALENTS NOT AVAILABLE

Powder For Injection - Injectable - 1.2 Gm

1's	$269.15	NEBCIN, Lilly, Eli and Company	00002-7040-01
6's	$2228.57	NEBCIN, Lilly, Eli and Company	00002-7040-16

Solution - Inhalation - 60 mg/ml

5 ml x 56	$2634.00	TOBI, Pathogenesis	63430-0065-01
5 ml x 56	$3024.56	TOBI, Pathogenesis	53905-0065-01

Solution - Injectable - 40 mg/ml

2 ml	$7.28	NEBCIN, Lilly, Eli and Company	00002-1499-01
2 ml x 25	$182.11	NEBCIN, Lilly, Eli and Company	00002-7381-25
30 ml	$109.26	NEBCIN, Lilly, Eli and Company	00002-7090-01
30 ml x 6	$655.56	NEBCIN, Lilly, Eli and Company	00002-7090-16
30 ml x 6	$655.61	NEBCIN, Lilly, Eli and Company	00002-7382-16

Tocainide Hydrochloride (002357)

For complete prescribing information, refer to the CD-ROM included with the book.

Categories: Arrhythmia, ventricular; Tachycardia, ventricular; Pregnancy Category C; FDA Approved 1984 Nov
Drug Classes: Antiarrhythmics, class IB
Brand Names: Tonocard
Cost of Therapy: $97.45 (Arrhythmia; Tonocard; 400 mg; 3 tablets/day; 30 day supply)

WARNING

Blood Dyscrasias

Agranulocytosis, bone marrow depression, leukopenia, neutropenia, aplastic/hypoplastic anemia, thrombocytopenia and sequelae such as septicemia and septic shock have been reported in patients receiving tocainide HCl. Most of these patients received tocainide HCl within the recommended dosage range. Fatalities have occurred (with approximately 25% mortality in reported agranulocytosis cases). Since most of these events have been noted during the first 12 weeks of therapy, it is recommended that complete blood counts, including white cell, differential and platelet counts be performed, optimally, at weekly intervals for the first 3 months of therapy; and frequently thereafter. Complete blood counts should be performed promptly if the patient develops any signs of infection (such as fever, chills, sore throat, or stomatitis), bruising, or bleeding. If any of these hematologic disorders is identified, tocainide HCl should be discontinued and appropriate treatment should be instituted if necessary. Blood counts usually return to normal within 1 month of discontinuation. Caution should be used in patients with pre-existing marrow failure or cytopenia of any type.

Pulmonary Fibrosis

Pulmonary fibrosis, interstitial pneumonitis, fibrosing alveolitis, pulmonary edema, and pneumonia have been reported in patients receiving tocainide HCl. Many of these events occurred in patients who were seriously ill. Fatalities have been reported. The experiences are usually characterized by bilateral infiltrates on x-ray and are frequently associated with dyspnea and cough. Fever may or may not be present. Patients should be instructed to promptly report the development of any pulmonary symptoms such as exertional dyspnea, cough or wheezing. Chest x-rays are advisable at that time. If these pulmonary disorders develop, tocainide HCl should be discontinued.

DESCRIPTION

Tocainide hydrochloride is a primary amine analog of lidocaine with antiarrhythmic properties useful in the treatment of ventricular arrhythmias. The chemical name for tocainide hydrochloride is 2-amino-*N*-(2,6-dimethylphenyl)propanamide hydrochloride. Its empirical formula is $C_{11}H_{16}N_2O{\cdot}HCl$, with a molecular weight of 228.72.

Tocainide hydrochloride is a white crystalline powder with a bitter taste and is freely soluble in water. It is supplied as 400 and 600 mg tablets for oral administration. Each tablet contains the following inactive ingredients: hydroxypropyl methylcellulose, iron oxide, magnesium stearate, methylcellulose, polyethylene glycol, and titanium dioxide.

INDICATIONS AND USAGE

Tocainide HCl is indicated for the treatment of documented ventricular arrhythmias, such as sustained tachycardia, that, in the judgment of the physician, are life-threatening. Because of the proarrhythmic effects of tocainide HCl, as well as its potential for other serious adverse effects, (see WARNINGS), its use to treat lesser arrhythmias is not recommended. Treatment of patients with asymptomatic ventricular premature contractions should be avoided.

Initiation of treatment with tocainide HCl, as with other antiarrhythmic agents used to treat life-threatening arrhythmias, should be carried out in the hospital. It is essential that each patient given tocainide HCl be evaluated electrocardiographically and clinically prior to, and during, therapy with tocainide HCl to determine whether the response to tocainide HCl supports continued treatment.

Antiarrhythmic drugs have not been shown to enhance survival in patients with ventricular arrhythmias.

CONTRAINDICATIONS

Patients who are hypersensitive to this product or to local anesthetics of the amide type.

Patients with second or third degree atrioventricular block in the absence of an artificial ventricular pacemaker.

WARNINGS

***Mortality*: In the National Heart, Lung and Blood Institute's Cardiac Arrhythmia Suppression Trial (CAST), a long-term, multi-center, randomized, double-blind study in patients with asymptomatic non-life-threatening ventricular arrhythmias who had a myocardial infarction more than 6 days but less than 2 years previously, an excessive mortality or non-fatal cardiac arrest rate (7.7%) was seen in patients treated with encainide or flecainide compared with that seen in patients assigned to matched placebo-treated groups (3.0%). The average duration of treatment with encainide or flecainide in this study was 10 months.**

The applicability of the CAST results to other populations (*e.g.*, those without recent myocardial infarctions) is uncertain. Considering the known proarrhythmic properties of tocainide HCl and the lack of evidence of improved survival for any antiarrhythmic drug in patients without life-threatening arrhythmias, the use of tocainide HCl as well as other antiarrhythmic agents should be reserved for patients with life-threatening ventricular arrhythmias.

ACCELERATION OF VENTRICULAR RATE

Acceleration of ventricular rate occurs infrequently when antiarrhythmics are administered to patients with atrial flutter or fibrillation.

DOSAGE AND ADMINISTRATION

The dosage of tocainide HCl must be individualized on the basis of antiarrhythmic response and tolerance, both of which are dose-related. Clinical and electrocardiographic evaluation (including Holter monitoring if necessary for evaluation) are needed to determine whether the desired antiarrhythmic response has been obtained and to guide titration and dose adjustment. Adverse effects appearing shortly after dosing, for example, suggest a need for dividing the dose further with a shorter dose-interval. Loss of arrhythmia control prior to the next dose suggests use of a shorter dose interval and/or a dose increase. Absence of a clear response suggests reconsideration of therapy.

The recommended initial dosage is 400 mg every 8 hours. The usual adult dosage is between 1200 and 1800 mg/day in a three dose daily divided regimen. Doses beyond 2400 mg/day have been administered infrequently. Patients who tolerate the tid regimen may be tried on a twice daily regimen with careful monitoring.

Some patients, particularly those with renal or hepatic impairment, may be adequately treated with less than 1200 mg/day.

PRODUCT LISTING - EQUIVALENTS NOT AVAILABLE

Tablet - Oral - 400 mg

100's	$88.18	TONOCARD, Astra-Zeneca Pharmaceuticals	61113-0707-28
100's	$93.26	TONOCARD, Astra-Zeneca Pharmaceuticals	00186-0707-28
100's	$108.28	TONOCARD, Astra-Zeneca Pharmaceuticals	00186-0707-68

Tablet - Oral - 600 mg

100's	$106.40	TONOCARD, Astra-Zeneca Pharmaceuticals	61113-0709-68
100's	$111.12	TONOCARD, Astra-Zeneca Pharmaceuticals	61113-0709-28
100's	$121.56	TONOCARD, Astra-Zeneca Pharmaceuticals	00186-0709-68

Tolazamide (002358)

For complete prescribing information, refer to the CD-ROM included with the book.

For related information, see the comparative table section in Appendix A.

Categories: Diabetes mellitus; Pregnancy Category C; FDA Approved 1971 Aug
Drug Classes: Antidiabetic agents; Sulfonylureas, first generation
Brand Names: Diabewas; **Tolinase**; Tolisan
Foreign Brand Availability: Desumide (Taiwan); Norglycin (Germany); Tolanase (England; Ireland)
Cost of Therapy: $33.86 (Diabetes Mellitus; Tolinase; 250 mg; 1 tablet/day; 30 day supply)
$3.94 (Diabetes Mellitus; Generic Tablets; 250 mg; 1 tablet/day; 30 day supply)

DESCRIPTION

Tolinase tablets contain tolazamide, an oral blood glucose lowering drug of the sulfonylurea class. Tolazamide is white or creamy-white powder with a melting point of 165-173°C. The solubility of tolazamide at pH 6.0 (mean urinary pH) is 27.8 mg/100 ml.

The chemical names for tolazamide are (1) Benzenesulfonamide, *N*-[[(hexahydro-1*H*-azepin-1-yl) amino) carbonyl)-4-methyl-; (2) 1- (Hexahydro-1*H*-azepin-1-yl)-3-(*p*-tolylsulfonyl)urea and its molecular weight is 311.40.

Tolinase tablets for oral administration are available as scored, white tablets containing 100, 250 or 500 mg tolazamide. *Inactive Ingredients:* Calcium sulfate, docusate sodium, magnesium stearate, methylcellulose, sodium alginate.

INDICATIONS AND USAGE

Tolazamide tablets are indicated as an adjunct to diet to lower the blood glucose in patients with noninsulin dependent diabetes mellitus (Type II) whose hyperglycemia cannot be satisfactorily controlled by diet alone.

In initiating treatment for noninsulin-dependent diabetes, diet should be emphasized as the primary form of treatment. Caloric restriction and weight loss are essential in the obese diabetic patient. Proper dietary management alone may be effective in controlling the blood glucose and symptoms of hyperglycemia. The importance of regular physical activity should also be stressed and cardiovascular risk factors should be identified and corrective measures taken where possible.

If this treatment program fails to reduce symptoms and/or blood glucose, the use of an oral sulfonylurea or insulin should be considered. Use of tolazamide must be viewed by both the physician and patient as a treatment in addition to diet and not as a substitute for diet or as a convenient mechanism for avoiding dietary restraint. Furthermore, loss of blood glucose control on diet alone may be transient thus requiring only short-term administration of tolazamide.

During maintenance programs, tolazamide should be discontinued if satisfactory lowering of blood glucose is no longer achieved. Judgments should be based on regular clinical and laboratory evaluations.

In considering the use of tolazamide in asymptomatic patients, it should be recognized that controlling the blood glucose in noninsulin-dependent diabetes has not been definitely established to be effective in preventing the long-term cardiovascular or neural complications of diabetes.

CONTRAINDICATIONS

Tolazamide tablets are contraindicated in patients with: 1) known hypersensitivity or allergy to tolazamide; 2) diabetic ketoacidosis, with or without coma. This condition should be treated with insulin; 3) Type I diabetes, as sole therapy.

SPECIAL WARNING ON INCREASED RISK OF CARDIOVASCULAR MORTALITY

The administration of oral hypoglycemic drugs has been reported to be associated with increased cardiovascular mortality as compared to treatment with diet alone or diet

T

plus insulin. This warning is based on the study conducted by the University Group Diabetes Program (UGDP), a long-term prospective clinical trial designed to evaluate the effectiveness of glucose-lowering drugs in preventing or delaying vascular complications in patients with noninsulin-dependent diabetes. The study involved 823 patients who randomly assigned to 1 of 4 treatment groups.[1]

UGDP reported that patients treated for 5-8 years with diet plus a fixed dose of tolbutamide (1.5 g/day) had a rate of cardiovascular mortality approximately 2½ times that of patients with diet alone. A significant increase in total mortality was not observed, but the use of tolbutamide was discontinued based on the increase in cardiovascular mortality, thus limiting the opportunity for the study to show an increase in overall mortality. Despite controversy regarding the interpretation of these results, the findings of the UGDP study provide an adequate basis for this warning. The patient should be informed of the potential risks and advantages of tolazamide and of alternative modes of therapy.

Although only 1 drug in the sulfonylurea class (tolbutamide) was included in this study, it is prudent from a safety standpoint to consider that this warning may also apply to other oral hypoglycemic drugs in this class, in view of their close similarities in mode of action and chemical structure.

DOSAGE AND ADMINISTRATION

There is no fixed dosage regimen for the management of diabetes mellitus with tolazamide tablets or any other hypoglycemic agent. In addition to the usual monitoring of urinary glucose, the patient's blood glucose must also be monitored periodically to determine the minimum effective dose for the patient; to detect primary failure (*i.e.,* inadequate lowering of blood glucose at the maximum recommended dose of medication); and to detect secondary failure (*i.e.,* loss of adequate blood glucose response after an initial period of effectiveness). Glycosylated hemoglobin levels may also be of value in monitoring the patient's response to therapy.

Short-term administration of tolazamide may be sufficient during periods of transient loss of control in patients usually controlled well on diet.

USUAL STARTING DOSE

The usual starting dose of tolazamide tablets for the mild to moderately severe Type II diabetic patient is 100-250 mg daily administered with breakfast or the first main meal. Generally, if the fasting blood glucose is less than 200 mg/dl, the starting dose is 100 mg/day as a single daily dose. If the fasting blood glucose value is greater than 200 mg/dl, the starting dose is 250 mg/day as a single dose. If the patient is malnourished, underweight, elderly, or not eating properly, the initial therapy should be 100 mg once a day. Failure to follow an appropriate dosage regimen may precipitate hypoglycemia. Patients who do not adhere to their prescribed dietary regimen are more prone to exhibit unsatisfactory response to drug therapy.

TRANSFER FROM OTHER HYPOGLYCEMIC THERAPY

Patients Receiving Other Oral Antidiabetic Therapy

Transfer of patients from other oral antidiabetes regimens of tolazamide should be done conservatively. When transferring patients from oral hypoglycemic agents other than chlorpropamide to tolazamide, no transition period or initial or priming dose is necessary. When transferring from chlorpropamide, particular care should be exercised to avoid hypoglycemia.

Tolbutamide

If receiving less than 1 gm/day, begin at 100 mg of tolazamide per day. If receiving 1 gm or more per day, initiate at 250 mg of tolazamide per day as a single dose.

Chlorpropamide

250 mg of chlorpropamide may be considered to provide approximately the same degree of blood glucose control as 250 mg of tolazamide. The patient should be observed carefully for hypoglycemia during the transition period from chlorpropamide to tolazamide (1-2 weeks) due to the prolonged retention of chlorpropamide in the body and the possibility of subsequent overlapping drug effects.

Acetohexamide

100 mg of tolazamide may be considered to provide approximately the same degree of blood glucose control as 250 mg of acetohexamide.

Patients Receiving Insulin

Some Type II diabetic patients who have been treated only with insulin may respond satisfactorily to therapy with tolazamide. If the patient's previous insulin dosage has been less than 20 units, substitution of 100 mg of tolazamide per day as a single daily dose may be tried. If the previous insulin dosage was less than 40 units, but more than 20 units, the patient should be placed directly on 250 mg of tolazamide per day as a single dose. If the previous insulin dosage was greater than 40 units, the insulin dosage should be decreased by 50% and 250 mg of tolazamide per day started. The dosage of tolazamide should be adjusted weekly (or more often in the group previously requiring more than 40 units of insulin). During this conversion period when both insulin and tolazamide are being used, hypoglycemia may rarely occur. During insulin withdrawal, patients should test their urine for glucose and acetone at least 3 times daily and report results to their physician. The appearance of persistent acetonuria with glycosuria indicates that the patients is a Type I diabetic who requires insulin therapy.

MAXIMUM DOSE

Daily doses of greater than 1000 mg are not recommended. Patients will generally have no further response to doses larger than this.

USUAL MAINTENANCE DOSE

The usual maintenance dose is in the range of 100-1000 mg/day with the average maintenance dose being 250-500 mg/day. Following initiation of therapy, dosage adjustment is made in increments of 100-250 mg at weekly intervals based on the patients's blood glucose response.

DOSAGE INTERVAL

Once a day therapy is usually satisfactory. Doses up to 500 mg/day should be given as single dose in the morning. 500 mg once daily is as effective as 250 mg twice daily. When a dose of more than 500 mg/day is required, the dose may be divided and given twice daily.

In elderly patients, debilitated or malnourished patients, and patients with impaired renal or hepatic function, the initial and maintenance dosing should be conservative to avoid hypoglycemic reactions.

PRODUCT LISTING - RATED THERAPEUTICALLY EQUIVALENT

Package	Price	Product	NDC
Tablet - Oral - 100 mg			
25's	$16.73	TOLINASE, Pd-Rx Pharmaceuticals	55289-0289-97
100's	$37.00	GENERIC, Ivax Corporation	00172-2978-60
100's	$50.86	TOLINASE, Pharmacia and Upjohn	00009-0070-02
Tablet - Oral - 250 mg			
90's	$15.84	GENERIC, Pd-Rx Pharmaceuticals	55289-0265-90
100's	$18.64	FEDERAL UPPER LIMIT, H.C.F.A. F F P	99999-2358-05
100's	$19.07	GENERIC, Us Trading Corporation	56126-0103-11
100's	$20.00	GENERIC, Raway Pharmacal Inc	00686-0292-20
100's	$77.00	GENERIC, Ivax Corporation	00172-2979-60
100's	$77.00	GENERIC, Mylan Pharmaceuticals Inc	00378-0217-01
100's	$112.86	TOLINASE, Pharmacia and Upjohn	00009-0114-05
200's	$29.22	GENERIC, Interpharm Inc	53746-0286-02
200's	$92.00	GENERIC, Ivax Corporation	00172-2979-61
200's	$209.69	TOLINASE, Pharmacia and Upjohn	00009-0114-04
Tablet - Oral - 500 mg			
25's	$22.04	GENERIC, Pd-Rx Pharmaceuticals	55289-0187-97
100's	$31.00	GENERIC, Raway Pharmacal Inc	00686-0293-20
100's	$51.50	GENERIC, Martec Pharmaceuticals Inc	52555-0293-01
100's	$67.30	GENERIC, Watson/Schein Pharmaceuticals Inc	00364-0722-90
100's	$67.35	GENERIC, Geneva Pharmaceuticals	00781-1942-13
100's	$138.60	GENERIC, Ivax Corporation	00172-2980-60
100's	$138.60	GENERIC, Mylan Pharmaceuticals Inc	00378-0551-01

PRODUCT LISTING - EQUIVALENTS NOT AVAILABLE

Package	Price	Product	NDC
Tablet - Oral - 100 mg			
100's	$12.50	GENERIC, Cmc-Consolidated Midland Corporation	00223-2081-01
Tablet - Oral - 250 mg			
30's	$9.65	GENERIC, Southwood Pharmaceuticals Inc	58016-0370-30
100's	$13.12	GENERIC, Physicians Total Care	54868-1020-00
100's	$21.00	GENERIC, Cmc-Consolidated Midland Corporation	00223-2082-01
Tablet - Oral - 500 mg			
100's	$35.00	GENERIC, Cmc-Consolidated Midland Corporation	00223-2083-01

Tolbutamide (002360)

For complete prescribing information, refer to the CD-ROM included with the book.

For related information, see the comparative table section in Appendix A.

Categories: Diabetes mellitus; Diagnosis, pancreatic adenoma; Diagnosis, insulinoma; Pregnancy Category C; FDA Approved 1963 Jan; WHO Formulary

Drug Classes: Antidiabetic agents; Sulfonylureas, first generation

Brand Names: Aglicem; Aglycid; Ansulin; Diabecid-R; Dolipol; Fordex; Glucosulfa; Guabeta; Mobenol; Noglucor; Novobutamide; Orabet; **Orinase**; Orinase Diagnostic; Raston; Tolbusal; Tolbutamida Valdecases

Foreign Brand Availability: Abemin (Japan); Arcosal (Denmark); Artosin (Netherlands); Diaben (Japan); Diatol (Hong-Kong; New-Zealand); Glyconon (England); Orsinon (Israel); Rastinon (Australia; Austria; Bahrain; Belgium; Cyprus; Denmark; Egypt; England; Finland; Greece; Iran; Iraq; Italy; Japan; Jordan; Kuwait; Lebanon; Libya; Mexico; Oman; Portugal; Qatar; Republic-of-Yemen; Saudi-Arabia; Spain; Sweden; Switzerland; Syria; United-Arab-Emirates); Tolsiran (Japan)

Cost of Therapy: $16.10 (Diabetes Mellitus; Orinase; 500 mg; 2 tablets/day; 30 day supply)
$5.25 (Diabetes Mellitus; Generic Tablets; 500 mg; 2 tablets/day; 30 day supply)

INTRAVENOUS

DESCRIPTION

Orinase diagnostic sterile powder contains tolbutamide sodium which is a white to off-white, practically odorless, crystalline powder, having a slightly bitter taste. It is freely soluble in water, soluble in alcohol and in chloroform, very slightly soluble in ether.

Each vial contains the equivalent of 1.0 g of free tolbutamide, present as 1.081 g of the sodium salt of 1-Butyl-3-(*p*-tolylsulfonyl)urea. The 81 mg of sodium present should not interdict the diagnostic use of this preparation in patients maintained on salt-poor regimens.

The chemical name for tolbutamide sodium is 1-Butyl-3-(*p*-tolylsulfonyl)urea monosodium salt $C_{12}H_{17}N_2NaO_3S$.

STORAGE

Store unreconstituted product at controlled room temperature 20-25°C (68- 77°F).

Use immediately after reconstitution (within 1 hour) but only if solution is complete and clear.

INDICATIONS AND USAGE

Tolbutamide sodium sterile powder is indicated for use as an aid in the diagnosis of pancreatic islet cell adenoma.

The difficulties of differential diagnosis of spontaneous hypoglycemia have made clear the need for more definitive diagnostic procedures in order to avoid subtotal pancreatic resection in patients in whom surgery is not indicated. Fully 80% of cases of spontaneous hypoglycemia result from one of three causes: functional hyperinsulinism, organic hyperinsulinism, and hepatogenic hypoglycemia. Functional hyperinsulinism is by far the most common form of the disorder, accounting for 70% of all cases. This form of hyperinsulinism is believed to be basically a psychosomatic disorder associated with an imbalance of autonomic nervous system influences on blood glucose control. The management of such patients is dietary, as is that of patients with hepatogenic hypoglycemia. These must be distinguished from organic hyperinsulinism due to pancreatic islet cell adenoma which requires surgery.

Patients with functioning insulinomas exhibit hypoglycemic responses to intravenously administered tolbutamide sodium which are sufficiently distinctive to make this drug a valuable adjunct in the diagnosis of functioning insulinomas.

It will be noted that the administration of 1.0 g of tolbutamide sodium to healthy subjects results in a rapid fall in blood glucose levels for 30-45 minutes, followed by a secondary rise of the blood glucose concentration into the normal range in the ensuing 90-180 minutes. The initial hypoglycemia results from the rapid release of insulin from the pancreatic beta cells, while the secondary rise is due to activation of counter-regulatory factors. In contrast, patients with insulinomas were found to exhibit tolbutamide induced blood glucose decreases of greater magnitude than healthy persons. Of greater significance than the magnitude of blood glucose fall in these patients is the persistence of the hypoglycemia for 3 hours after the administration of tolbutamide sodium sterile powder. It is this phenomenon of persistent tolbutamide induced hypoglycemia for 3 hours rather than degree of blood glucose decrease which is of importance in the diagnosis of pancreatic islet cell adenomas. False positive responses have been observed in a few patients with liver disease, alcohol hypoglycemia, idiopathic hypoglycemia of infancy, severe under nutrition, azotemia, sarcoma, and other extrapancreatic insulin producing tumors.

CONTRAINDICATIONS

Because of the lack of data to establish ideal dosage and the inability to interpret results, use of tolbutamide sodium sterile powder is not recommended in children.

The test should not be performed on persons who have previously shown allergy to tolbutamide or related sulfonylureas.

WARNINGS

Severe and prolonged hypoglycemia following oral administration of tolbutamide has been reported in patients suffering from severe liver disease and severe renal disease.

Severe hypoglycemic symptoms may develop during the test, particularly in patients with fasting blood glucose levels in the hypoglycemic range. If they occur, the test should be terminated immediately by intravenously injecting 12.5-25 g of glucose in a 25-50% solution.

DOSAGE AND ADMINISTRATION

Fajans Test

1. The patient should receive a high carbohydrate diet of from 150-300 g daily for at least 3 days prior to the test.
2. On morning of test, after an overnight fast, withdraw a fasting blood specimen.
3. Inject entire volume (20 ml) of tolbutamide sodium solution intravenously at a constant rate over a 2-3 minute period.
4. Withdraw blood specimens at the following intervals (in minutes) after the midpoint of the injection: 20, 30, 45, 60, 90, 120, 150, and 180. Of greater significance than the magnitude of blood glucose fall in these patients is the persistence of the hypoglycemia for 3 hours after the administration of tolbutamide sodium. The determination of serum insulin levels before, and at 10, 20, and 30 minutes after the intravenous administration of the drug as described below, provides a specific and safer test for insulinoma. It also permits the performance of the test in the presence of moderate fasting hypoglycemia, since interpretation is not based on the decline of the blood glucose.
5. Blood glucose determinations are made by the true glucose procedures. The procedure is terminated with a feeding of readily assimilable carbohydrate or breakfast.

INTERPRETATION OF RESULTS — HEALTHY SUBJECTS

A decrease to a blood glucose of 38-79% of the fasting level may be expected. At 90-120 minutes a level of from 78-100% of initial level may be seen. Similar responses are to be found in patients with functional hyperinsulinism.

INSULINOMA PATIENTS

Minimum blood glucose levels of 17-50% of fasting values are seen. In the 90-180 minute interval, levels are in the range of 40-64%. Some patients with liver disease may show the same type of blood glucose response as to patients with insulinomas. Therefore, appropriate laboratory and clinical tests must be employed to distinguish between these two conditions.

USE WITH SERUM INSULIN DETERMINATION IN INSULINOMA PATIENTS

If a method of assay for serum insulin is available, the test for insulinoma may be made shorter and more specific. Using an immunoassay, serum insulin levels rose to peak values of 160-300 μU/ml in 5 subjects with proven insulinoma (normal range 27-89). In 4 of the subjects the peak was attained in 20-30 minutes, the first determination being performed at 60 minutes in the fifth subject. Excessive increases in plasma insulin of 5 patients with insulinomas (range 118-1055, mean 486 μU/ml) were also found by immunoassay.

The serum insulin response returned to normal after the removal of the insulinoma in 2 other patients.

Accordingly, the determination of serum insulin levels before, and at 10, 20, and 30 minutes after the intravenous administration of the drug described above, provides a specific and safer test for insulinoma, and permits the performance of the test in the presence of moderate fasting hypoglycemia, since interpretation is not based on the decline of the blood glucose. The test may be terminated after the 30 minute specimen by the feeding of carbohydrate as described above.

Preparation of Tolbutamide Sodium Solution:

1. Remove the protective metal cap from the vial and sterilize the top of the rubber stopper with a suitable germicide.
2. Using a 20 ml syringe, inject 20 ml of sterile water for injection into the vial containing tolbutamide sodium sterile powder.
3. Shake thoroughly until solution is complete.

Parenteral drug products should be inspected visually for particulate matter and discoloration prior to administration, whenever solution and container permit.

ORAL

DESCRIPTION

These tablets contain tolbutamide, an oral blood glucose lowering drug of the sulfonylurea category. Tolbutamide is a pure white crystalline compound practically insoluble in water but forming water-soluble salts with alkalies.

The chemical names for tolbutamide are: (1) Benzenesulfonamide,*N*-((butylamino)carbonyl)-4-methyl; (2) 1-Butyl-3-(*p*-tolylsulfonyl)urea and its molecular weight is 270.35.

Each Orinase tablet for oral administration contains 250 or 500 mg tolbutamide. *Inactive Ingredients:* Colloidal silicon dioxide, croscarmellose sodium, magnesium stearate, pregelatinized starch.

Storage: Store at controlled room temperature 15-30°C (59-86°F).

INDICATIONS AND USAGE

Tolbutamide tablets are indicated as an adjunct to diet to lower the blood glucose in patients with noninsulin-dependent diabetes whose hyperglycemia cannot be satisfactorily controlled by diet alone. In initiating treatment for noninsulin dependent diabetes, diet should be emphasized as the primary form of treatment. Caloric restriction and weight loss are essential in the obese diabetic patient. Proper dietary management alone may be effective in controlling the blood glucose and symptoms of hyperglycemia. The importance of regular physical activity should also be stressed and cardiovascular risk factors should be identified and corrective measures taken where possible.

If this treatment program fails to reduce symptoms and/or blood glucose, the use of an oral sulfonylurea or insulin should be considered. Use of tolbutamide must be viewed by both the physician and patient as a treatment in addition to diet, and not as a substitute for diet or as a convenient mechanism for avoiding dietary restraint. Furthermore, loss of blood glucose control on diet alone may be transient, thus requiring only short-term administration of tolbutamide.

During maintenance programs, tolbutamide should be discontinued if satisfactory lowering of blood glucose is no longer achieved. Judgments should be based on regular clinical and laboratory evaluations.

In considering the use of tolbutamide in asymptomatic patients, it should be recognized that controlling the blood glucose in noninsulin-dependent diabetes has not been definitely established to be effective in preventing the long-term cardiovascular or neural complications of diabetes.

CONTRAINDICATIONS

Tolbutamide tablets are contraindicated in patients with: (1) known hypersensitivity or allergy to tolbutamide; (2) diabetic ketoacidosis, with or without coma. This condition should be treated with insulin. (3) Type I diabetes, as sole therapy.

SPECIAL WARNING ON INCREASED RISK OF CARDIOVASCULAR MORTALITY

The administration of oral hypoglycemic drugs has been reported to be associated with increased cardiovascular mortality as compared to treatment with diet alone or diet plus insulin. This warning is based on the study conducted by the University Group Diabetes Program (UGDP), a long-term prospective clinical trial designed to evaluate the effectiveness of glucose-lowering drugs in preventing or delaying vascular complications in patients with noninsulin-dependent diabetes. The study involved 823 patients who were randomly assigned to 1 of 4 treatment groups.[1]

UGDP reported that patients treated for 5-8 years with diet plus a fixed dose of tolbutamide (1.5 g/day) had a rate of cardiovascular mortality approximately 2½ times that of patients with diet alone. A significant increase in total mortality was not observed, but the use of tolbutamide was discontinued based on the increase in cardiovascular mortality, thus limiting the opportunity for the study to show an increase in overall mortality. Despite controversy regarding the interpretation of these results, the findings of the UGDP study provide an adequate basis for this warning. The patient should be informed of the potential risks and advantages of tolbutamide tablets and of alternative modes of therapy.

Although only 1 drug in the sulfonylurea class (tolbutamide) was included in this study, it is prudent from a safety standpoint to consider that this warning may also apply to other oral hypoglycemic drugs in this class, in view of their close similarities in mode of action and chemical structure.

DOSAGE AND ADMINISTRATION

There is no fixed dosage regimen for the management of diabetes mellitus with tolbutamide tablets or any other hypoglycemic agent. In addition to the usual monitoring of urinary glucose, the patient's blood glucose must also be monitored periodically to determine the minimum effective dose for the patient; to detect primary failure, *i.e.,* inadequate lowering of blood glucose at the maximum recommended dose of medication; and to detect secondary failure, *i.e.,* loss of adequate blood glucose response after an initial period of effectiveness. Glycosylated hemoglobin levels may also be of value in monitoring the patient's response to therapy.

Short-term administration of tolbutamide may be sufficient during periods of transient loss of control in patients usually controlled well on diet.

T

USUAL STARTING DOSE

The usual starting dose is 1-2 g daily. This may be increased or decreased depending on individual patient response. Failure to follow an appropriate dosage regimen may precipitate hypoglycemia. Patients who do not adhere to their prescribed dietary regimens are more prone to exhibit unsatisfactory response to drug therapy.

Transfer From Other Hypoglycemic Therapy Patients Receiving Other Antidiabetic Therapy

Transfer of patients from other oral antidiabetes regimens to tolbutamide should be done conservatively. When transferring patients from oral hypoglycemic agents other than chlorpropamide to tolbutamide, no transition period and no initial or priming doses are necessary. When transferring patients from chlorpropamide, however, particular care should be exercised during the first 2 weeks because of the prolonged retention of chlorpropamide in the body and the possibility that subsequent overlapping drug effects might provoke hypoglycemia.

Patients Receiving Insulin

Patients requiring 20 units or less of insulin daily may be placed directly on tolbutamide and insulin abruptly discontinued. Patients whose insulin requirement is between 20 and 40 units daily may be started on therapy with tolbutamide with a concurrent 30-50% reduction in insulin dose, with further daily reduction of the insulin when response to tolbutamide is observed. In patients requiring more than 40 units of insulin daily, therapy with tolbutamide may be initiated in conjunction with a 20% reduction in insulin dose the first day, with further careful reduction of insulin as response is observed. Occasionally, conversion to tolbutamide in the hospital may be advisable in candidates who require more than 40 units of insulin daily. During this conversion period when both insulin and tolbutamide are being used, hypoglycemia may rarely occur. During insulin withdrawal, patients should test their urine for glucose and acetone at least 3 times daily and report results to their physician. The appearance of persistent acetonuria with glycosuria indicates that the patient is a Type I diabetic patient who requires insulin therapy.

MAXIMUM DOSE

Daily doses of greater than 3 grams are not recommended.

USUAL MAINTENANCE DOSE

The maintenance dose is in the range of 0.25 to 3 g daily. Maintenance doses above 2 g are seldom required.

DOSAGE INTERVAL

The total daily dose may be taken either in the morning or in divided doses through the day. While either schedule is usually effective, the divided dose system is preferred by some clinicians from the standpoint of digestive tolerance.

In elderly, debilitated or malnourished patients and patients with impaired renal or hepatic function, the initial and maintenance dosing should be conservative to avoid hypoglycemic reactions.

PRODUCT LISTING - RATED THERAPEUTICALLY EQUIVALENT

Tablet - Oral - 500 mg

100's	$9.77	GENERIC, Major Pharmaceuticals Inc	00904-0223-61
100's	$10.98	GENERIC, Qualitest Products Inc	00603-6121-21
100's	$26.95	GENERIC, Mylan Pharmaceuticals Inc	00378-0215-01
100's	$29.15	GENERIC, Udl Laboratories Inc	51079-0560-20

PRODUCT LISTING - EQUIVALENTS NOT AVAILABLE

Tablet - Oral - 500 mg

100's	$3.65	GENERIC, Alra	51641-0405-01
100's	$8.75	GENERIC, Cmc-Consolidated Midland Corporation	00223-1076-01
100's	$9.15	GENERIC, Physicians Total Care	54868-1361-01

Tolcapone *(003392)*

Categories: Parkinson's disease, adjunct; FDA Approved 1998 Jan; Pregnancy Category C
Drug Classes: Antiparkinson agents; Dopaminergics
Brand Names: Tasmar
Cost of Therapy: $227.71 (Parkinsonism; Tasmar; 100 mg; 3 tablets/day; 30 day supply)
$197.47 (Parkinsonism; Tasmar; 200 mg; 3 tablets/day; 30 day supply)

T

DESCRIPTION

Tolcapone, an inhibitor of catechol-*O*-methyltransferase (COMT), is used in the treatment of Parkinson's disease as an adjunct to levodopa/carbidopa therapy. It is a yellow, odorless, nonhygroscopic, crystalline compound with a relative molecular mass of 273.25. The chemical name of tolcapone is 3,4-dihydroxy-4′-methyl-5-nitrobenzophenone. Its empirical formula is $C_{14}H_{11}NO_5$.

The inactive ingredients in tasmar tablets are: *Core:* Lactose monohydrate, microcrystalline cellulose, dibasic calcium phosphate anhydrous, povidone K-30, sodium starch glycolate, talc and magnesium stearate. *Film Coating:* Hydroxypropyl methyl cellulose, titanium dioxide, talc, ethylcellulose, triacetin and sodium lauryl sulfate, with the following dye systems: *100 mg:* Yellow and red iron oxide. *200 mg:* Red iron oxide.

CLINICAL PHARMACOLOGY

MECHANISM OF ACTION

Tolcapone is a selective and reversible inhibitor of catechol-*O*-methyltransferase (COMT).

In mammals, COMT is distributed throughout various organs. The highest activities are in the liver and kidney. COMT also occurs in the heart, lung, smooth and skeletal muscles, intestinal tract, reproductive organs, various glands, adipose tissue, skin, blood cells and neuronal tissues, especially in glial cells. COMT catalyzes the transfer of the methyl group of S-adenosyl-L-methionine to the phenolic group of substrates that contain a catechol structure. Physiological substrates of COMT include dopa, catecholamines (dopamine, norepinephrine, epinephrine) and their hydroxylated metabolites. The function of COMT is the elimination of biologically active catechols and some other hydroxylated metabolites. In the presence of a decarboxylase inhibitor, COMT becomes the major metabolizing enzyme for levodopa catalyzing the metabolism to 3-methoxy-4-hydroxy-L-phenylalanine (3-OMD) in the brain and periphery.

The precise mechanism of action of tolcapone is unknown, but it is believed to be related to its ability to inhibit COMT and alter the plasma pharmacokinetics of levodopa. When tolcapone is given in conjunction with levodopa and an aromatic amino acid decarboxylase inhibitor, such as carbidopa, plasma levels of levodopa are more sustained than after administration of levodopa and an aromatic amino acid decarboxylase inhibitor alone. It is believed that these sustained plasma levels of levodopa result in more constant dopaminergic stimulation in the brain, leading to greater effects on the signs and symptoms of Parkinson's disease in patients as well as increased levodopa adverse effects, sometimes requiring a decrease in the dose of levodopa. Tolcapone enters the CNS to a minimal extent, but has been shown to inhibit central COMT activity in animals.

PHARMACODYNAMICS

COMT Activity in Erythrocytes

Studies in healthy volunteers have shown that tolcapone reversibly inhibits human erythrocyte catechol-*O*-methyltransferase (COMT) activity after oral administration. The inhibition is closely related to plasma tolcapone concentrations. With a 200 mg single dose of tolcapone, maximum inhibition of erythrocyte COMT activity is on average greater than 80%. During multiple dosing with tolcapone (200 mg tid), erythrocyte COMT inhibition at trough tolcapone blood concentrations is 30% to 45%.

EFFECT ON THE PHARMACOKINETICS OF LEVODOPA AND ITS METABOLITES

When tolcapone is administered together with levodopa/carbidopa, it increases the relative bioavailability (AUC) of levodopa by approximately 2-fold. This is due to a decrease in levodopa clearance resulting in a prolongation of the terminal elimination half-life of levodopa (from approximately 2 hours to 3.5 hours). In general, the average peak levodopa plasma concentration (C_{max}) and the time of its occurrence (T_{max}) are unaffected. The onset of effect occurs after the first administration and is maintained during long-term treatment. Studies in healthy volunteers and Parkinson's disease patients have confirmed that the maximal effect occurs with 100 mg to 200 mg tolcapone. Plasma levels of 3-OMD are markedly and dose-dependently decreased by tolcapone when given with levodopa/carbidopa.

Population pharmacokinetic analyses in patients with Parkinson's disease have shown the same effects of tolcapone on levodopa plasma concentrations that occur in healthy volunteers.

PHARMACOKINETICS OF TOLCAPONE

Tolcapone pharmacokinetics are linear over the dose range of 50-400 mg, independent of levodopa/carbidopa coadministration. The elimination half-life of tolcapone is 2-3 hours and there is no significant accumulation. With tid dosing of 100 mg or 200 mg, C_{max} is approximately 3 μg/ml and 6 μg/ml, respectively.

Absorption

Tolcapone is rapidly absorbed, with a T_{max} of approximately 2 hours. The absolute bioavailability following oral administration is about 65%. Food given within 1 hour before and 2 hours after dosing of tolcapone decreases the relative bioavailability by 10-20% (see DOSAGE AND ADMINISTRATION).

Distribution

The steady-state volume of distribution of tolcapone is small (9 L). Tolcapone does not distribute widely into tissues due to its high plasma protein binding. The plasma protein binding of tolcapone is >99.9% over the concentration range of 0.32 to 210 μg/ml. *In vitro* experiments have shown that tolcapone binds mainly to serum albumin.

Metabolism and Elimination

Tolcapone is almost completely metabolized prior to excretion, with only a very small amount (0.5% of dose) found unchanged in urine. The main metabolic pathway of tolcapone is glucuronidation; the glucuronide conjugate is inactive. In addition, the compound is methylated by COMT to 3-*(O)*-methyl-tolcapone. Tolcapone is metabolized to a primary alcohol (hydroxylation of the methyl group), which is subsequently oxidized to the carboxylic acid. *In vitro* experiments suggest that the oxidation may be catalyzed by cytochrome P450 3A4 and P450 2A6. The reduction to an amine and subsequent *N*-acetylation occur to a minor extent. After oral administration of a ^{14}C-labeled dose of tolcapone, 60% of labeled material is excreted in urine and 40% in feces.

Tolcapone is a low-extraction ratio drug (extraction ratio = 0.15) with a moderate systemic clearance of about 7L/h.

SPECIAL POPULATIONS

Tolcapone pharmacokinetics are independent of sex, age, body weight, and race (Japanese, Black and Caucasian). Polymorphic metabolism is unlikely based on the metabolic pathways involved.

Hepatic Impairment

A study in patients with hepatic impairment has shown that moderate noncirrhotic liver disease had no impact on the pharmacokinetics of tolcapone. In patients with moderate cirrhotic liver disease (Child-Pugh Class B), however, clearance and volume of distribution of unbound tolcapone was reduced by almost 50%. This reduction may increase the average concentration of unbound drug by 2-fold (see DOSAGE AND ADMINISTRATION).

Renal Impairment

The pharmacokinetics of tolcapone have not been investigated in a specific renal impairment study. However, the relationship of renal function and tolcapone pharmacokinetics has been investigated using population pharmacokinetics during clinical trials. The data of more than 400 patients have confirmed that over a wide range of creatinine clearance values (30 ml/min to 130 ml/min) the pharmacokinetics of tolcapone are unaffected by renal function. This could be explained by the fact that only a negligible amount of unchanged tolcapone (0.5%) is excreted in the urine. The glucuronide conjugate of tolcapone is mainly excreted in the urine but is also excreted in the bile. Accumulation of this stable and inactive metabolite should not present a risk in renally impaired patients with creatinine clearance above 25 ml/min (see DOSAGE AND ADMINISTRATION). Given the very high protein binding of tolcapone, no significant removal of the drug by hemodialysis would be expected.

Drug Interactions

See DRUG INTERACTIONS.

INDICATIONS AND USAGE

Tolcapone is indicated as an adjunct to levodopa and carbidopa for the treatment of the signs and symptoms of idiopathic Parkinson's disease.

The effectiveness of tolcapone was demonstrated in randomized controlled trials in patients receiving concomitant levodopa therapy with carbidopa or another aromatic amino acid decarboxylase inhibitor who experienced end of dose wearing-off phenomena as well as in patients who did not experience such phenomena.

CONTRAINDICATIONS

Tolcapone tablets are contraindicated in patients who have demonstrated hypersensitivity to the drug or its ingredients.

WARNINGS

Monoamine oxidase (MAO) and COMT are the two major enzyme systems involved in the metabolism of catecholamines. It is theoretically possible, therefore, that the combination of tolcapone and a non-selective MAO inhibitor (*e.g.*, phenelzine and tranylcypromine) would result in inhibition of the majority of the pathways responsible for normal catecholamine metabolism. For this reason, patients should ordinarily not be treated concomitantly with tolcapone and a non-selective MAO inhibitor.

Tolcapone can be taken concomitantly with a selective MAO-B inhibitor (*e.g.*, selegiline).

PRECAUTIONS

HYPOTENSION/SYNCOPE

Dopaminergic therapy in Parkinson's disease patients has been associated with orthostatic hypotension. Tolcapone enhances levodopa bioavailability and, therefore, may increase the occurrence of orthostatic hypotension. In tolcapone clinical trials, orthostatic hypotension was documented at least once in 8%, 14% and 13% of the patients treated with placebo, 100 mg and 200 mg tolcapone tid, respectively. A total of 2%, 5% and 4% of the patients treated with placebo, 100 mg and 200 mg tolcapone tid, respectively, reported orthostatic symptoms at some time during their treatment and also had at least one episode of orthostatic hypotension documented (however, the episode of orthostatic symptoms itself was invariably not accompanied by vital sign measurements). Patients with orthostasis at baseline were more likely than patients without symptoms to have orthostatic hypotension during the study, irrespective of treatment group. In addition, the effect was greater in tolcapone-treated patients than in placebo-treated patients. Baseline treatment with dopamine agonists or selegiline did not appear to increase the likelihood of experiencing orthostatic hypotension when treated with tolcapone. Approximately 0.7% of the patients treated with tolcapone (5% of patients who were documented to have had at least one episode of orthostatic hypotension) eventually withdrew from treatment due to adverse events presumably related to hypotension.

In controlled Phase 3 trials, approximately 5%, 4% and 3% of tolcapone 200 mg tid, 100 mg tid and placebo patients, respectively, reported at least one episode of syncope. Reports of syncope were generally more frequent in patients in all three treatment groups who had an episode of documented hypotension (although the episodes of syncope, obtained by history, were themselves not documented with vital sign measurement) compared to patients who did not have any episodes of documented hypotension.

DIARRHEA

In clinical trials, diarrhea developed in approximately 8%, 16% and 18% of patients treated with placebo, 100 mg and 200 mg tolcapone tid, respectively. While diarrhea was generally regarded as mild to moderate in severity, approximately 3% to 4% of patients on tolcapone had diarrhea which was regarded as severe. Diarrhea was the adverse event which most commonly led to discontinuation, with approximately 1%, 5% and 6% of patients treated with placebo, 100 mg and 200 mg tolcapone tid, respectively, withdrawing from the trials prematurely. Discontinuing tolcapone for diarrhea was related to the severity of the symptom. Diarrhea resulted in withdrawal in approximately 8%, 40% and 70% of patients with mild, moderate and severe diarrhea, respectively. Although diarrhea generally resolved after discontinuation of tolcapone, it led to hospitalization in 0.3%, 0.7% and 1.7% of patients in the placebo, 100 mg and 200 mg tolcapone tid groups.

Typically, diarrhea presents 6 to 12 weeks after tolcapone is started, but it may appear as early as 2 weeks and as late as many months after the initiation of treatment. Clinical trial data suggested that diarrhea associated with tolcapone use may sometimes be associated with anorexia (decreased appetite).

No consistent description of tolcapone-induced diarrhea has been derived from clinical trial data, and the mechanism of action is currently unknown.

It is recommended that all cases of persistent diarrhea should be followed up with an appropriate work-up (including occult blood samples).

HALLUCINATIONS

In clinical trials, hallucinations developed in approximately 5%, 8% and 10% of patients treated with placebo, 100 mg and 200 mg tolcapone tid, respectively. Hallucinations led to drug discontinuation and premature withdrawal from clinical trials in 0.3%, 1.4% and 1.0% of patients treated with placebo, 100 mg and 200 mg tolcapone tid, respectively. Hallucinations led to hospitalization in 0.0%, 1.7% and 0.0% of patients in the placebo, 100 mg and 200 mg tolcapone tid groups, respectively.

In general, hallucinations present shortly after the initiation of therapy with tolcapone (typically within the first 2 weeks). Clinical trial data suggest that hallucinations associated with tolcapone use may be responsive to levodopa dose reduction. Patients whose hallucinations resolved had a mean levodopa dose reduction of 175 mg to 200 mg (20% to 25%) after the onset of the hallucinations. Hallucinations were commonly accompanied by confusion and to a lesser extent sleep disorder (insomnia) and excessive dreaming.

DYSKINESIA

Tolcapone may potentiate the dopaminergic side effects of levodopa and may cause and/or exacerbate preexisting dyskinesia. Although decreasing the dose of levodopa may ameliorate this side effect, many patients in controlled trials continued to experience frequent dyskinesias despite a reduction in their dose of levodopa. The rates of withdrawal for dyskinesia were 0.0%, 0.3% and 1.0% for placebo, 100 mg and 200 mg tolcapone tid, respectively.

RENAL AND HEPATIC

Renal Impairment

No dosage adjustment is needed in patients with mild to moderate renal impairment, however, patients with severe renal impairment should be treated with caution (see CLINICAL PHARMACOLOGY, Pharmacokinetics of Tolcapone and DOSAGE AND ADMINISTRATION).

Renal Toxicity

When rats were dosed daily for 1 or 2 years (exposures 6 times the human exposure or greater) there was a high incidence of proximal tubule cell damage consisting of degeneration, single cell necrosis, hyperplasia, karyocytomegaly and atypical nuclei. These effects were not associated with changes in clinical chemistry parameters, and there is no established method for monitoring for the possible occurrence of these lesions in humans. Although it has been speculated that these toxicities may occur as the result of a species-specific mechanism, experiments which would confirm that theory have not been conducted.

Hepatic Impairment

Patients with moderate non-cirrhotic liver disease need no adjustment of dose. Patients with moderate cirrhotic liver disease have reduced clearance of unbound tolcapone by almost 50%, increasing the average concentration of unbound drug by about 2-fold. Dosage should be reduced in such patients (see CLINICAL PHARMACOLOGY, Pharmacokinetics of Tolcapone and DOSAGE AND ADMINISTRATION). Patients with severe liver impairment should be treated with caution.

Hepatic Enzyme Abnormalities

In Phase 3 controlled trials, increases to more than 3 times the upper limit of normal in ALT or AST occurred in approximately 1% of patients at 100 mg tid and 3% of patients at 200 mg tid. Females were more likely than males to have an increase in hepatic enzymes (approximately 5% vs 2%). Approximately one-third of patients with elevated enzymes had diarrhea. Increases to more than 8 times the upper limit of normal in hepatic enzymes occurred in 0.3% at 100 mg tid and 0.7% at 200 mg tid. Elevated enzymes led to discontinuation in 0.3% and 1.7% of patients treated with 100 mg tid and 200 mg tid, respectively. Elevations usually occurred within 6 weeks to 6 months of starting treatment. In about half the cases with elevated hepatic enzymes, enzyme levels returned to baseline values within 1 to 3 months while patients continued tolcapone treatment. When treatment was discontinued, enzymes generally declined within 2 to 3 weeks but in some cases took as long as 1 to 2 months to return to normal.

One patient, a 55-year-old woman who had received treatment with tolcapone 200 mg tid for 53 days, had the onset of diarrhea followed 4 days later by yellowing of the skin and eyes. She died 7 days after the onset of the diarrhea. No liver function tests were performed after the onset of symptoms.

It is recommended that liver enzymes be monitored monthly during the first 3 months of tolcapone treatment, and every 6 weeks for the next 3 months of treatment. Tolcapone should be discontinued for enzyme elevations greater than or equal to 5 times the upper limit of normal or at the appearance of jaundice (see PRECAUTIONS, Laboratory Tests).

Hematuria

The rates of hematuria in placebo-controlled trials were approximately 2%, 4% and 5% in placebo, 100 mg and 200 mg tolcapone tid, (respectively. The etiology of the increase with tolcapone has not always been explained (for example, by urinary tract infection or coumadin therapy). In placebo-controlled trials in the US (n=593) rates of microscopically confirmed hematuria were approximately 3%, 2% and 2% in placebo, 100 mg and 200 mg tolcapone tid, respectively.

EVENTS REPORTED WITH DOPAMINERGIC THERAPY

The events listed below are known to be associated with the use of drugs that increase dopaminergic activity, although they are most often associated with the use of direct dopamine agonists. While cases of Withdrawal Emergent Hyperpyrexia and Confusion have been reported in association with tolcapone withdrawal, the expected incidence of fibrotic complications is so low that even if tolcapone caused these complications at rates similar to those attributable to other dopaminergic therapies, it is unlikely that even a single example would have been detected in a cohort of the size exposed to tolcapone.

Withdrawal Emergent Hyperpyrexia and Confusion

Four cases of a symptom complex resembling the neuroleptic malignant syndrome (characterized by elevated temperature, muscular rigidity, and altered consciousness), similar to

T

that reported in association with the rapid dose reduction or withdrawal of other dopaminergic drugs, have been reported in association with the abrupt withdrawal or lowering of the dose of tolcapone. In 3 of these cases, CPK was elevated as well. One patient died, and the other 3 patients recovered over periods of approximately 2, 4 and 6 weeks.

FIBROTIC COMPLICATIONS

Cases of retroperitoneal fibrosis, pulmonary infiltrates, pleural effusion, and pleural thickening have been reported in some patients treated with ergot derived dopaminergic agents. While these complications may resolve when the drug is discontinued, complete resolution does not always occur. Although these adverse events are believed to be related to the ergoline structure of these compounds, whether other, nonergot derived drugs (*e.g.*, tolcapone) that increase dopaminergic activity can cause them is unknown.

Three cases of pleural effusion, one with pulmonary fibrosis, occurred during clinical trials. These patients were also on concomitant dopamine agonists (pergolide or bromocriptine) and had a prior history of cardiac disease or pulmonary pathology (nonmalignant lung lesion).

INFORMATION FOR THE PATIENT

Patients should be instructed to take tolcapone only as prescribed.

Patients should be informed that hallucinations can occur.

Patients should be advised that they may develop postural (orthostatic) hypotension with or without symptoms such as dizziness, nausea, syncope, and sometimes sweating. Hypotension may occur more frequently during initial therapy. Accordingly, patients should be cautioned against rising rapidly after sitting or lying down, especially if they have been doing so for prolonged periods, and especially at the initiation of treatment with tolcapone.

Patients should be advised that they should neither drive a car nor operate other complex machinery until they have gained sufficient experience on tolcapone to gauge whether or not it affects their mental and/or motor performance adversely. Because of the possible additive sedative effects, caution should be used when patients are taking other CNS depressants in combination with tolcapone.

Patients should be informed that nausea may occur, especially at the initiation of treatment with tolcapone.

Patients should be advised of the possibility of an increase in dyskinesia and/or dystonia.

Although tolcapone has not been shown to be teratogenic in animals, it is always given in conjunction with levodopa/carbidopa, which is known to cause visceral and skeletal malformations in the rabbit. Accordingly, patients should be advised to notify their physicians if they become pregnant or intend to become pregnant during therapy (see Pregnancy Category C).

Tolcapone is excreted into maternal milk in rats. Because of the possibility that tolcapone may be excreted into human maternal milk, patients should be advised to notify their physicians if they intend to breastfeed or are breastfeeding an infant.

LABORATORY TESTS

It is recommended that transaminases be monitored monthly for the first 3 months of treatment with tolcapone, after which LFTs should be monitored every 6 weeks for the next 3 months. If elevations occur, and a decision is made to continue to treat the patient, more frequent monitoring of complete liver function is recommended. Treatment should be discontinued if ALT exceeds 5 × ULN or if jaundice develops.

SPECIAL POPULATIONS

Parkinson's disease patients with moderate to severe liver impairment or severe renal impairment should be treated with caution (see DOSAGE AND ADMINISTRATION).

CARCINOGENESIS, MUTAGENESIS, AND IMPAIRMENT OF FERTILITY

Carcinogenesis

Carcinogenicity studies in which tolcapone was administered in the diet were conducted in mice and rats. Mice were treated for 80 (female) or 95 (male) weeks with doses of 100, 300 and 800 mg/kg/day, equivalent to 0.8, 1.6 and 4 times human exposure (AUC = 80 μg·h/ml) at the recommended daily clinical dose of 600 mg. Rats were treated for 104 weeks with doses of 50, 250 and 450 mg/kg/day. Tolcapone exposures were 1, 6.3 and 13 times the human exposure in male rats and 1.7, 11.8 and 26.4 times the human exposure in female rats. There was an increased incidence of uterine adenocarcinomas in female rats at exposure equivalent to 26.4 times the human exposure. There was evidence of renal tubular injury and renal tubular tumor formation in rats. A low incidence of renal tubular cell adenomas occurred in middle- and high-dose female rats; tubular cell carcinomas occurred in middle- and high-dose male and high-dose female rats, with a statistically significant increase in high-dose males. Exposures were equivalent to 6.3 (males) or 11.8 (females) times the human exposure or greater; no renal tumors were observed at exposures of 1 (males) or 1.7 (females) times the human exposure. Minimal-to-marked damage to the renal tubules, consisting of proximal tubule cell degeneration, singe cell necrosis, hyperplasia and karyocytomegaly, occurred at the doses associated with renal tumors. Renal tubule damage, characterized by proximal tubule cell degeneration and the presence of atypical nuclei, as well as one adenocarcinoma in a high-dose male, were observed in a 1-year study in rats receiving doses of tolcapone of 150 and 450 mg/kg/day. These histopathological changes suggest the possibility that renal tumor formation might be secondary to chronic cell damage and sustained repair, but this relationship has not been established, and the relevance of these findings to humans is not known. There was no evidence of carcinogenic effects in the long-term mouse study. The carcinogenic potential of tolcapone in combination with levodopa/carbidopa has not been examined.

T

Mutagenesis

Tolcapone was clastogenic in the *in vitro* mouse lymphoma/thymidine kinase assay in the presence of metabolic activation. Tolcapone was not mutagenic in the Ames test, the *in vitro* V79/HPRT gene mutation assay, or the unscheduled DNA synthesis assay. It was not clastogenic in an *in vitro* chromosomal aberration assay in cultured human lymphocytes, or an *in vivo* micronucleus assay in mice.

Impairment of Fertility

Tolcapone did not affect fertility and general reproductive performance in rats at doses up to 300 mg/kg/day (5.7 times the human dose on a mg/m^2 basis).

PREGNANCY CATEGORY C

Tolcapone, when administered alone during organogenesis, was not teratogenic at doses of up to 300 mg/kg/day in rats or up to 400 mg/kg/day in rabbits (5.7 times and 15 times the recommended daily clinical dose of 600 mg, on a mg/m^2 basis, respectively). In rabbits, however, an increased rate of abortion occurred at a dose of 100 mg/kg/day (3.7 times the daily clinical dose on a mg/m^2 basis) or greater. Evidence of maternal toxicity (decreased weight gain, death) was observed at 300 mg/kg in rats and 400 mg/kg in rabbits. When tolcapone was administered to female rats during the last part of gestation and throughout lactation, decreased litter size and impaired growth and learning performance in female pups were observed at a dose of 250/150 mg/kg/day (dose reduced from 250 to 150 mg/kg/day during late gestation due to high rate of maternal mortality; equivalent to 4.8/2.9 times the clinical dose on a mg/m^2 basis).

Tolcapone is always given concomitantly with levodopa/carbidopa, which is known to cause visceral and skeletal malformations in rabbits. The combination of tolcapone (100 mg/kg/day) with levodopa/carbidopa (80/20 mg/kg/day) produced an increased incidence of fetal malformations (primarily external and skeletal digit defects) compared to levodopa/carbidopa alone when pregnant rabbits were treated throughout organogenesis. Plasma exposures to tolcapone (based on AUC) were 0.5 times the expected human exposure, and plasma exposures to levodopa were 6 times higher than those in humans under therapeutic conditions. In a combination embryo-fetal development study in rats, fetal body weights were reduced by the combination of tolcapone (10, 30 and 50 mg/kg/day) and levodopa/carbidopa (120/30 mg/kg/day) and by levodopa/carbidopa alone. Tolcapone exposures were 0.5 times expected human exposure or greater; levodopa exposures were 21 times expected human exposure or greater. The high dose of 50 mg/kg/day of tolcapone given alone was not associated with reduced fetal body weight (plasma exposures of 1.4 times the expected human exposure).

There is no experience from clinical studies regarding the use of tolcapone in pregnant women. Therefore, tolcapone should be used during pregnancy only if the potential benefit justifies the potential risk to the fetus.

NURSING MOTHERS

In animal studies, tolcapone was excreted into maternal rat milk.

It is not known whether tolcapone is excreted in human milk. Because many drugs are excreted in human milk, caution should be exercised when tolcapone is administered to a nursing woman.

PEDIATRIC USE

There is no identified potential use of tolcapone in pediatric patients.

DRUG INTERACTIONS

PROTEIN BINDING

Although tolcapone is highly protein bound, *in vitro* studies have shown that tolcapone at a concentration of 50 μg/ml did not displace other highly protein-bound drugs from their binding sites at therapeutic concentrations. The experiments included warfarin (0.5 to 7.2 μg/ml), phenytoin (4.0 to 38.7 μg/ml), tolbutamide (24.5 to 96.1 μg/ml) and digitoxin (9.0 to 27.0 μg/ml).

DRUGS METABOLIZED BY CATECHOL-O-METHYLTRANSFERASE (COMT)

Tolcapone may influence the pharmacokinetics of drugs metabolized by COMT. However, no effects were seen on the pharmacokinetics of the COMT substrate carbidopa. The effect of tolcapone on the pharmacokinetics of other drugs of this class such as α-methyldopa, dobutamine, apomorphine, and isoproterenol has not been evaluated. A dose reduction of such compounds should be considered when they are coadministered with tolcapone.

EFFECT OF TOLCAPONE ON THE METABOLISM OF OTHER DRUGS

In vitro experiments have been performed to assess the potential of tolcapone to interact with isoenzymes of cytochrome P450 (CYP). No relevant interactions with substrates for CYP 2A6 (coumadin), CYP 1A2 (caffeine), CYP 3A4 (midazolam, terfenadine, cyclosporine), CYP 2C19 (S-mephenytoin) and CYP 2D6 (desipramine) were observed *in vitro*. The absence of an interaction with desipramine, a drug metabolized by cytochrome P450 2D6, was also confirmed in an *in vivo* study where tolcapone did not change the pharmacokinetics of desipramine.

Due to its affinity to cytochrome P450 2C9 *in vitro*, tolcapone may interfere with drugs, whose clearance is dependent on this metabolic pathway, such as tolbutamide and warfarin. However, in an *in vivo* interaction study, tolcapone did not change the pharmacokinetics of tolbutamide.

Therefore, clinically relevant interactions involving cytochrome P450 2C9 appear unlikely. Similarly, tolcapone did not affect the pharmacokinetics of desipramine, a drug metabolized by cytochrome P450 2D6, indicating that interactions with drugs metabolized by that enzyme are unlikely. Since clinical information is limited regarding the combination of warfarin and tolcapone, coagulation parameters should be monitored when these two drugs are coadministered.

DRUGS THAT INCREASE CATECHOLAMINES

Tolcapone did not influence the effect of ephedrine, an indirect sympathomimetic, on hemodynamic parameters or plasma catecholamine levels, either at rest or during exercise. Since tolcapone did not alter the tolerability of ephedrine, these drugs can be coadministered.

When tolcapone was given together with levodopa/carbidopa and desipramine, there was no significant change in blood pressure, pulse rate and plasma concentrations of desipramine. Overall, the frequency of adverse events increased slightly. These adverse events were predictable based on the known adverse reactions to each of the three drugs individually. Therefore, caution should be exercised when desipramine is administered to Parkinson's disease patients being treated with tolcapone and levodopa/carbidopa.

In clinical trials, patients receiving tolcapone/levodopa preparations reported a similar adverse event profile independent of whether or not they were also concomitantly administered selegiline (a selective MAO-B inhibitor).

ADVERSE REACTIONS

During the pre-marketing development of tolcapone, two distinct patient populations were studied, patients with end-of-dose wearing-off phenomena and patients with stable responses to levodopa therapy. All patients received concomitant treatment with levodopa preparations, however, and were similar in other clinical aspects. Adverse events are, therefore, shown for these two populations combined.

The most commonly observed adverse events (>5%) in the double-blind, placebo-controlled trials (n=892) associated with the use of tolcapone not seen at an equivalent frequency among the placebo-treated patients were dyskinesia, nausea, sleep disorder, dystonia, dreaming excessive, anorexia, cramps muscle, orthostatic complaints, somnolence, diarrhea, confusion, dizziness, headache, hallucination, vomiting, constipation, fatigue, upper respiratory tract infection, falling, sweating increased, urinary tract infection, xerostomia, abdominal pain, urine discoloration.

Approximately 16% of the 592 patients who participated in the double-blind, placebo-controlled trials discontinued treatment due to adverse events compared to 10% of the 298 patients who received placebo. Diarrhea was by far the most frequent cause of discontinuation (approximately 6% in tolcapone patients vs 1% on placebo).

ADVERSE EVENT INCIDENCE IN CONTROLLED CLINICAL STUDIES

TABLE 4 lists treatment emergent adverse events that occurred in at least 1% of patients treated with tolcapone participating in the double-blind, placebo-controlled studies and were numerically more common in at least one of the tolcapone groups. In these studies, either tolcapone or placebo were added to levodopa/carbidopa (or benserazide).

The prescriber should be aware that these figures cannot be used to predict the incidence of adverse events in the course of usual medical practice where patient characteristics and other factors differ from those that prevailed in the clinical studies. Similarly, the cited frequencies cannot be compared with figures obtained from other clinical investigations involving different treatments, uses, and investigators. However, the cited figures do provide the prescriber with some basis for estimating the relative contribution of drug and nondrug factors to the adverse events incidence rate in the population studied.

Other events reported by 1% or more of patients treated with tolcapone but that were equally or more frequent in the placebo group were arthralgia, pain limbs, anxiety, micturition frequency, fractures, vision blurred, pneumonia, paresis, lethargy, asthenia, edema peripheral, gait abnormal, taste alteration, weight decrease and sinusitis.

Effects of gender and age on adverse reactions: Experience in clinical trials have suggested that patients greater than 75 years of age may be more likely to develop hallucinations than patients less than 75 years of age, while patients over 75 may be less likely to develop dystonia. Females may be more likely to develop somnolence than males.

OTHER ADVERSE EVENTS OBSERVED DURING ALL TRIALS IN PATIENTS WITH PARKINSON'S DISEASE

Tolcapone has been administered in 1536 patients with Parkinson's disease in clinical trials. During these trials, all adverse events were recorded by the clinical investigators using terminology of their own choosing. To provide a meaningful estimate of the proportion of individuals having adverse events, similar types of adverse events were grouped into a smaller number of standardized categories using COSTART dictionary terminology. These categories are used in the listing below.

All reported events that occurred at least twice (or once for serious or potentially serious events), except those already listed above, trivial events and terms too vague to be meaningful are included, without regard to determination of a causal relationship to tolcapone.

Events are further classified within body system categories and enumerated in order of decreasing frequency using the following definitions: *frequent* adverse events are defined as those occurring in at least 1/100 patients; *infrequent* adverse events are defined as those occurring in between 1/100 and 1/1000 patients; and *rare* adverse events are defined as those occurring in fewer than 1/1000 patients.

Nervous System: *Frequent:* Depression, hypesthesia, tremor, speech disorder, vertigo, emotional lability; *Infrequent:* Neuralgia, amnesia, extrapyramidal syndrome, hostility, libido increased, manic reaction, nervousness, paranoid reaction, cerebral ischemia, cerebrovascular accident, delusions, libido decreased, neuropathy, apathy, choreoathetosis, myoclonus, psychosis, thinking abnormal, twitching; *Rare:* Antisocial reaction, delirium, encephalopathy, hemiplegia, meningitis.

Digestive System: *Frequent:* Tooth disorder; *Infrequent:* Dysphagia, gastrointestinal hemorrhage, gastroenteritis, mouth ulceration, increased salivation, abnormal stools, esophagitis, cholelithiasis, colitis, tongue disorder, rectal disorder; *Rare:* Cholecystitis, duodenal ulcer, gastrointestinal carcinoma, stomach atony.

Body as a Whole: *Frequent:* Flank pain, accidental injury, abdominal pain, infection; *Infrequent:* Hernia, pain, allergic reaction, cellulitis, infection fungal, viral infection, carcinoma, chills, infection bacterial, neoplasm, abscess, face edema; *Rare:* Death.

Cardiovascular System: *Frequent:* Palpitation; *Infrequent:* Hypertension, vasodilation, angina pectoris, heart failure, atrial fibrillation, tachycardia, migraine, aortic stenosis, arrythmia, arteriospasm, bradycardia, cerebral hemorrhage, coronary artery disorder, heart arrest, myocardial infarct, myocardial ischemia, pulmonary embolus; *Rare:* Arteriosclerosis, cardiovascular disorder, pericardial effusion, thrombosis.

Musculoskeletal System: *Frequent:* Myalgia; *Infrequent:* Tenosynovitis, arthrosis, joint disorder.

Urogenital System: *Frequent:* Urinary incontinence, impotence; *Infrequent:* Prostatic disorder, dysuria, nocturia, polyuria, urinary retention, urinary tract disorder, hematuria, kidney calculus, prostatic carcinoma, breast neoplasm, oliguria, uterine atony, uterine disorder, vaginitis; *Rare:* Bladder calculus, ovarian carcinoma, uterine hemorrhage.

TABLE 4 *Summary of Patients With Adverse Events After Start of Trial Drug Administration (At Least 1% in Tolcapone Group and at Least One Tolcapone Dose Group > Placebo)*

		Tolcapone tid	
Adverse Events	**Placebo (n=298)**	**Placebo (n=296)**	**200 mg (n=298)**
Dyskinesia	20%	42%	51%
Nausea	18%	30%	35%
Sleep disorder	18%	24%	25%
Dystonia	17%	19%	22%
Dreaming excessive	17%	21%	16%
Anorexia	13%	19%	23%
Cramps muscle	17%	17%	18%
Orthostatic complaints	14%	17%	17%
Somnolence	13%	18%	14%
Diarrhea	8%	16%	18%
Confusion	9%	11%	10%
Dizziness	10%	13%	6%
Headache	7%	10%	11%
Hallucination	5%	8%	10%
Vomiting	4%	8%	10%
Constipation	5%	6%	8%
Fatigue	6%	7%	3%
Upper respiratory tract infection	3%	5%	7%
Falling	4%	4%	6%
Sweating increased	2%	4%	7%
Urinary tract infection	4%	5%	5%
Xerostomia	2%	5%	6%
Abdominal pain	3%	5%	6%
Syncope	3%	4%	5%
Urine discoloration	1%	2%	7%
Dyspepsia	2%	4%	3%
Influenza	2%	3%	4%
Dyspnea	2%	3%	3%
Balance loss	2%	3%	2%
Flatulence	2%	2%	4%
Hyperkinesia	1%	3%	2%
Chest pain	1%	3%	1%
Hypotension	1%	2%	2%
Paresthesia	2%	3%	1%
Stiffness	1%	2%	2%
Arthritis	1%	2%	1%
Chest discomfort	1%	1%	2%
Hypokinesia	1%	1%	3%
Micturition disorder	1%	2%	1%
Pain neck	1%	2%	2%
Burning	0%	2%	1%
Sinus congestion	0%	2%	1%
Agitation	0%	1%	1%
Bleeding dermal	0%	1%	1%
Irritability	0%	1%	1%
Mental deficiency	0%	1%	1%
Hyperactivity	0%	1%	1%
Malaise	0%	1%	0%
Panic reaction	0%	1%	0%
Tumor skin	0%	1%	0%
Cataract	0%	1%	0%
Euphoria	0%	1%	0%
Fever	0%	0%	1%
Alopecia	0%	1%	0%
Eye inflamed	0%	1%	0%
Hypertonia	0%	0%	1%
Tumor uterus	0%	1%	0%

Respiratory System: *Frequent:* Bronchitis, pharyngitis; *Infrequent:* Cough increased, rhinitis, asthma, epistaxis, hyperventilation, laryngitis, hiccup; *Rare:* Apnea, hypoxia, lung edema.

Skin and Appendages: *Frequent:* Rash; *Infrequent:* Herpes zoster, pruritus, seborrhea, skin discoloration, eczema, erythema multiforme, skin disorder, furunculosis, herpes simplex, urticaria.

Special Senses: *Frequent:* Tinnitus; *Infrequent:* Diplopia, ear pain, eye hemorrhage, eye pain, lacrimation disorder, otitis media, parosmia; *Rare:* Glaucoma.

Metabolic and Nutritional: *Infrequent:* Edema, hypercholesteremia, thirst, dehydration.

Hemic and Lymphatic System: *Infrequent:* Anemia; *Rare:* Leukemia, thrombocytopenia.

Endocrine System: *Infrequent:* Diabetes mellitus.

Unclassified: *Infrequent:* Surgical procedure.

DOSAGE AND ADMINISTRATION

Therapy with tolcapone may be initiated with 100 mg or 200 mg tid, always as an adjunct to levodopa/carbidopa therapy. Although clinical trial data suggest that initial treatment with 200 mg tid (a daily dose of 600 mg) is reasonably well tolerated, the prescriber may wish to begin treatment with 100 mg tid because of the potential for increased dopaminergic side effects (*e.g.,* dyskinesias) and the possible necessary adjustment of the concomitant levodopa/carbidopa dose. In clinical trials, the first dose of the day of tolcapone was always taken together with the first dose of the day of levodopa/carbidopa, and the subsequent doses of tolcapone were given approximately 6 and 12 hours later.

In clinical trials, the majority of patients required a decrease in their daily levodopa dose if their daily dose of levodopa was >600 mg or if patients had moderate or severe dyskinesias before beginning treatment.

The maximum recommended dose of tolcapone is 600 mg a day, given as tid dosing. To optimize an individual patient's response, reductions in daily levodopa dose may be necessary. In clinical trials, the average reduction in daily levodopa dose was about 30% in

T

those patients requiring a levodopa dose reduction. (Greater than 70% of patients with levodopa doses above 600 mg daily required such a reduction.)

The safety and effectiveness of daily doses greater than 600 mg, or of single doses greater than 200 mg, have not been systematically evaluated.

Tolcapone can be combined with both the immediate and sustained release formulations of levodopa/carbidopa.

Tolcapone may be taken with or without food (see CLINICAL PHARMACOLOGY).

PATIENTS WITH IMPAIRED RENAL OR HEPATIC FUNCTION

Patients with moderate to severe cirrhosis of the liver should not be escalated to 200 mg tolcapone tid (see CLINICAL PHARMACOLOGY).

No dose adjustment of tolcapone is recommended for patients with mild to moderate renal impairment. The safety of tolcapone has not been examined in subjects who had creatinine clearance less than 25 ml/min (see CLINICAL PHARMACOLOGY).

HOW SUPPLIED

Tasmar is supplied as film-coated tablets containing 100 or 200 mg tolcapone. The 100 mg beige tablet and the 200 mg reddish-brown tablet are hexagonal and biconvex. Imprinted with black ink on one side of the tablet is "TASMAR" and the tablet strength (100 or 200), on the other side is "ROCHE".

Storage: Store at controlled room temperature 20-25°C (68-77°F) in tight containers.

PRODUCT LISTING - EQUIVALENTS NOT AVAILABLE

Tablet - Oral - 100 mg			
90's	$227.71	TASMAR, Roche Laboratories	00004-5920-01
Tablet - Oral - 200 mg			
90's	$244.41	TASMAR, Roche Laboratories	00004-5921-01

Tolmetin Sodium *(002361)*

For complete prescribing information, refer to the CD-ROM included with the book.

For related information, see the comparative table section in Appendix A.

Categories: Arthritis, osteoarthritis; Arthritis, rheumatoid; Pregnancy Category C; FDA Approved 1979 Oct
Drug Classes: Analgesics, non-narcotic; Nonsteroidal anti-inflammatory drugs
Brand Names: Donison; Midocil; Reutol; Safitex; **Tolectin**
Cost of Therapy: $148.93 (Osteoarthritis; Tolectin DS; 400 mg; 3 capsules/day; 30 day supply)
$62.06 (Osteoarthritis; Generic Capsules; 400 mg; 3 capsules/day; 30 day supply)

DESCRIPTION

Tolmetin Sodium 200 mg tablets for oral administration contain tolmetin sodium as the dihydrate in an amount equivalent to 200 mg of tolmetin (scored for 100 mg). Each tablet contains 18 mg (0.784 mEq) of sodium and the following inactive ingredients: cellulose, magnesium stearate, silicon dioxide, corn starch and talc.

Tolmetin Sodium capsules for oral administration contain tolmetin sodium as the dihydrate in an amount equivalent to 400 mg of tolmetin. Each capsule contains 36 mg (1.568 mEq) of sodium and the following inactive ingredients: gelatin, magnesium stearate, corn starch, talc, FD&C Red No. 3, FD&C Yellow No. 6 and titanium dioxide.

Tolmetin Sodium 600 mg tablets for oral administration contain tolmetin sodium as the dihydrate in an amount equivalent to 600 mg of tolmetin. Each tablet contains 54 mg (2.35 mEq) of sodium and the following inactive ingredients: cellulose, silicon dioxide, crospovidone, hydroxypropyl methyl cellulose, magnesium stearate, polyethylene glycol, corn starch, titanium dioxide, FD&C Yellow No. 6 and D&C Yellow No. 10.

The pKa of tolmetin is 3.5 and tolmetin sodium is freely soluble in water.

Tolmetin sodium is a nonsteroidal anti-inflammatory agent.

INDICATIONS AND USAGE

Tolmetin Sodium is indicated for the relief of signs and symptoms of rheumatoid arthritis and osteoarthritis. Tolmetin Sodium is indicated in the treatment of acute flares and the long-term management of the chronic disease.

Tolmetin Sodium is also indicated for treatment of juvenile rheumatoid arthritis. The safety and effectiveness of tolmetin sodium have not been established in children under 2 years of age see DOSAGE AND ADMINISTRATION.

NON-FDA APPROVED INDICATIONS

While not FDA approved conditions, tolmetin has also been used in the management of pain as well as acute gout.

CONTRAINDICATIONS

Anaphylactoid reactions have been reported with tolmetin sodium as with other nonsteroidal anti-inflammatory drugs. Because of the possibility of cross-sensitivity to other nonsteroidal anti-inflammatory drugs, particularly zomepirac sodium, anaphylactoid reactions may be more likely to occur in patients who have exhibited allergic reactions to these compounds. For this reason, tolmetin sodium should not be given to patients in whom aspirin and other nonsteroidal anti-inflammatory drugs induce symptoms of asthma, rhinitis, urticaria or other symptoms of allergic or anaphylactoid reactions. Patients experiencing anaphylactoid reactions on tolmetin sodium should be treated with conventional therapy, such as epinephrine, antihistamines and/or steroids.

WARNINGS

RISK OF GI ULCERATION, BLEEDING AND PERFORATION WITH NSAID THERAPY

Serious gastrointestinal toxicity such as bleeding, ulceration, and perforation, can occur at any time, with or without warning symptoms, in patients treated chronically with NSAID (Nonsteroidal Anti-Inflammatory Drug) therapy. Although minor upper gastrointestinal problems, such as dyspepsia, are common, usually developing early in therapy, physicians should remain alert for ulceration and bleeding in patients treated chronically with NSAID's even in the absence of previous GI tract symptoms. In patients observed in clinical trials of several months to two years duration, symptomatic upper GI ulcers, gross bleeding or perforation appear to occur in approximately 1% of patients treated for 3-6 months, and in about 2-4% of patients treated for one year. Physicians should inform patients about the signs and/or symptoms of serious GI toxicity and what steps to take if they occur.

Studies to date have not identified any subset of patients not at risk of developing peptic ulceration and bleeding. Except for a prior history of serious GI events and other risk factors known to be associated with peptic ulcer disease, such as alcoholism, smoking, etc., no risk factors (*e.g.*, age, sex) have been associated with increased risk. Elderly or debilitated patients seem to tolerate ulceration or bleeding less well than other individuals and most spontaneous reports of fatal GI events are in this population. Studies to date are inconclusive concerning the relative risk of various NSAID's in causing such reactions. High doses of any NSAID probably carry a greater risk of these reactions, although controlled clinical trials showing this do not exist in most cases. In considering the use of relatively large doses (within the recommended dosage range), sufficient benefit should be anticipated to offset the potential increased risk of GI toxicity.

DOSAGE AND ADMINISTRATION

In adults with rheumatoid arthritis or osteoarthritis, the recommended starting dose is 400 mg three times daily (1200 mg daily), preferably including a dose on arising and a dose at bedtime. To achieve optimal therapeutic effect the dose should be adjusted according to the patient's response after one to two weeks. Control is usually achieved at doses of 600-1800 mg daily in divided doses (generally t.i.d.). Doses larger than 1800 mg/day have not been studied and are not recommended.

The recommended starting dose for children (2 years and older) is 20 mg/kg/day in divided doses (t.i.d. or q.i.d.). When control has been achieved, the usual dose ranges from 15 to 30 mg/kg/day. Doses higher than 30 mg/kg/day have not been studied and, therefore, are not recommended.

A therapeutic response to tolmetin sodium can be expected in a few days to a week. Progressive improvement can be anticipated during succeeding weeks of therapy. If gastrointestinal symptoms occur, tolmetin sodium can be administered with antacids other than sodium bicarbonate. Tolmetin Sodium bioavailability and pharmacokinetics are not significantly affected by acute or chronic administration of magnesium and aluminum hydroxides; however, bioavailability is affected by food or milk.

Store at controlled room temperature (15-30°C, 59-86°F). Protect from light.

PRODUCT LISTING - RATED THERAPEUTICALLY EQUIVALENT

Capsule - Oral - 400 mg			
14's	$11.48	GENERIC, Allscripts Pharmaceutical Company	54569-3730-01
21's	$28.63	TOLECTIN DS, Allscripts Pharmaceutical Company	54569-1467-07
24's	$19.24	GENERIC, Pharmaceutical Corporation Of America	51655-0562-30
30's	$23.25	GENERIC, Allscripts Pharmaceutical Company	54569-3730-00
30's	$24.17	GENERIC, Heartland Healthcare Services	61392-0573-30
30's	$24.17	GENERIC, Heartland Healthcare Services	61392-0573-39
30's	$26.70	GENERIC, Medirex Inc	57480-0360-06
30's	$40.89	TOLECTIN DS, Allscripts Pharmaceutical Company	54569-1467-01
31's	$24.97	GENERIC, Heartland Healthcare Services	61392-0573-31
32's	$25.78	GENERIC, Heartland Healthcare Services	61392-0573-32
45's	$36.25	GENERIC, Heartland Healthcare Services	61392-0573-45
60's	$48.33	GENERIC, Heartland Healthcare Services	61392-0573-60
90's	$72.50	GENERIC, Heartland Healthcare Services	61392-0573-90
100's	$68.95	GENERIC, Baker Norton Pharmaceuticals	50732-0900-01
100's	$74.50	GENERIC, Geneva Pharmaceuticals	00781-2182-01
100's	$80.00	GENERIC, Aligen Independent Laboratories Inc	00405-5035-01
100's	$81.50	GENERIC, Ivax Corporation	00172-3627-60
100's	$81.50	GENERIC, Ivax Corporation	00182-1931-01
100's	$82.00	GENERIC, Novopharm Usa Inc	55953-0815-01
100's	$85.04	GENERIC, Moore, H.L. Drug Exchange Inc	00839-7671-06
100's	$89.50	GENERIC, Ivax Corporation	00182-1931-89
100's	$106.15	GENERIC, Major Pharmaceuticals Inc	00904-7653-60
100's	$112.40	GENERIC, Mylan Pharmaceuticals Inc	00378-5200-01
100's	$112.44	GENERIC, Novopharm Usa Inc	55953-0815-40
100's	$118.25	GENERIC, Teva Pharmaceuticals Usa	00093-8815-01
100's	$118.25	GENERIC, Purepac Pharmaceutical Company	00228-2520-10
100's	$165.48	TOLECTIN DS, Janssen Pharmaceuticals	00045-0414-60
Tablet - Oral - 200 mg			
100's	$52.37	GENERIC, Aligen Independent Laboratories Inc	00405-5033-01
100's	$60.74	GENERIC, Moore, H.L. Drug Exchange Inc	00839-7729-06
100's	$65.00	GENERIC, Mutual/United Research Laboratories	00677-1425-01
100's	$65.00	GENERIC, Mutual Pharmaceutical Co Inc	53489-0506-01
Tablet - Oral - 600 mg			
100's	$85.92	GENERIC, Aligen Independent Laboratories Inc	00405-5034-01
100's	$89.89	GENERIC, Mutual/United Research Laboratories	00677-1447-01
100's	$94.90	GENERIC, Geneva Pharmaceuticals	00781-1428-01

100's	\$95.03	GENERIC, Moore, H.L. Drug Exchange Inc	00839-7690-06
100's	\$95.06	GENERIC, Qualitest Products Inc	00603-6131-21
100's	\$95.25	GENERIC, Major Pharmaceuticals Inc	00904-7694-60
100's	\$99.00	GENERIC, Parmed Pharmaceuticals Inc	00349-8964-01
100's	\$105.95	GENERIC, Ivax Corporation	00182-1932-01
100's	\$110.00	GENERIC, Vangard Labs	00615-3564-13
100's	\$123.25	GENERIC, Mylan Pharmaceuticals Inc	00378-0313-01
100's	\$129.65	GENERIC, Purepac Pharmaceutical Company	00228-2480-10

PRODUCT LISTING - EQUIVALENTS NOT AVAILABLE

Capsule - Oral - 400 mg

30's	\$26.75	GENERIC, Pharma Pac	52959-0342-30
30's	\$42.00	GENERIC, Southwood Pharmaceuticals Inc	58016-0614-30
60's	\$84.00	GENERIC, Southwood Pharmaceuticals Inc	58016-0614-60
90's	\$126.00	GENERIC, Southwood Pharmaceuticals Inc	58016-0614-90
100's	\$140.00	GENERIC, Southwood Pharmaceuticals Inc	58016-0614-00

Tablet - Oral - 600 mg

30's	\$53.14	GENERIC, Physicians Total Care	54868-2421-01
100's	\$132.03	GENERIC, Physicians Total Care	54868-2421-00
100's	\$200.78	TOLECTIN 600, Janssen Pharmaceuticals	00045-0416-60

Tolterodine Tartrate *(003309)*

Categories: Bladder, overactive; Incontinence, urinary, urge; Urinary frequency; Urinary urgency; FDA Approved 1998 Mar; Pregnancy Category C

Drug Classes: Anticholinergics; Relaxants, urinary tract

Brand Names: **Detrol**

Foreign Brand Availability: Detrusitol (Bahrain; Colombia; Cyprus; Egypt; England; France; Germany; Hong-Kong; Indonesia; Iran; Iraq; Ireland; Israel; Jordan; Korea; Kuwait; Lebanon; Libya; Mexico; Oman; Peru; Philippines; Qatar; Republic-of-Yemen; Saudi-Arabia; Singapore; South-Africa; Sweden; Syria; Taiwan; Thailand; United-Arab-Emirates)

Cost of Therapy: \$112.22 (Overactive Bladder; Detrol; 2 mg; 2 tablets/day; 30 day supply)
\$92.33 (Overactive Bladder; Detrol LA; 4 mg; 1 tablet/day; 30 day supply)

DESCRIPTION

Note: The trade names have been used throughout this monograph for clarity.

DETROL

Detrol tablets contain tolterodine tartrate. The active moiety, tolterodine, is a muscarinic receptor antagonist. The chemical name of tolterodine tartrate is (R)-2-[3-[bis(1-methylethyl)-amino]-1-phenylpropyl]-4-methylphenol [R-(R*,R*)]-2,3- dihydroxybutanedioate (1:1) (salt). The empirical formula of tolterodine tartrate is $C_{26}H_{37}NO_7$, and its molecular weight is 475.6.

Tolterodine tartrate is a white, crystalline powder. The pKa value is 9.87 and the solubility in water is 12 mg/ml. It is soluble in methanol, slightly soluble in ethanol, and practically insoluble in toluene. The partition coefficient (Log D) between n-octanol and water is 1.83 at pH 7.3.

Detrol tablets for oral administration contain 1 or 2 mg of tolterodine tartrate. The inactive ingredients are colloidal anhydrous silica, calcium hydrogen phosphate dihydrate, cellulose microcrystalline, hydroxypropyl methylcellulose, magnesium stearate, sodium starch glycolate (pH 3.0-5.0), stearic acid, and titanium dioxide.

DETROL LA

Detrol LA capsules contain tolterodine tartrate. The active moiety, tolterodine, is a muscarinic receptor antagonist. The chemical name of tolterodine tartrate is (R)-N,N-diisopropyl-3-(2-hydroxy-5-methylphenyl)- 3-phenylpropanamine L-hydrogen tartrate. The empirical formula of tolterodine tartrate is $C_{26}H_{37}NO_7$, and its molecular weight is 475.6.

Tolterodine tartrate is a white, crystalline powder. The pKa value is 9.87 and the solubility in water is 12 mg/ml. It is soluble in methanol, slightly soluble in ethanol, and practically insoluble in toluene. The partition coefficient (Log D) between n-octanol and water is 1.83 at pH 7.3.

Detrol LA for oral administration contains 2 or 4 mg of tolterodine tartrate. Inactive ingredients are sucrose, starch, hydroxypropyl methylcellulose, ethylcellulose, medium chain triglycerides, oleic acid, gelatin, and FD&C blue no. 2. The 2 mg capsules also contain yellow iron oxide. Both capsule strengths are imprinted with a pharmaceutical grade printing ink that contains shellac glaze, titanium dioxide, propylene glycol, and simethicone.

CLINICAL PHARMACOLOGY

DETROL

Tolterodine is a competitive muscarinic receptor antagonist. Both urinary bladder contraction and salivation are mediated via cholinergic muscarinic receptors.

After oral administration, tolterodine is metabolized in the liver, resulting in the formation of the 5-hydroxymethyl derivative, a major pharmacologically active metabolite. The 5-hydroxymethyl metabolite, which exhibits an antimuscarinic activity similar to that of tolterodine, contributes significantly to the therapeutic effect. Both tolterodine and the 5-hydroxymethyl metabolite exhibit a high specificity for muscarinic receptors, since both show negligible activity or affinity for other neurotransmitter receptors and other potential cellular targets, such as calcium channels.

Tolterodine has a pronounced effect on bladder function. Effects on urodynamic parameters before and 1 and 5 hours after a single 6.4 mg dose of tolterodine immediate release were determined in healthy volunteers. The main effects of tolterodine at 1 and 5 hours were an increase in residual urine, reflecting an incomplete emptying of the bladder, and a decrease in detrusor pressure. These findings are consistent with an antimuscarinic action on the lower urinary tract.

Pharmacokinetics

Absorption

In a study with ^{14}C-tolterodine solution in healthy volunteers who received a 5 mg oral dose, at least 77% of the radiolabeled dose was absorbed. Tolterodine immediate release is rapidly absorbed, and maximum serum concentrations (C_{max}) typically occur within 1-2 hours after dose administration. C_{max} and area under the concentration-time curve (AUC) determined after dosage of tolterodine immediate release are dose-proportional over the range of 1-4 mg.

Effect of Food

Food intake increases the bioavailability of tolterodine (average increase 53%), but does not affect the levels of the 5-hydroxymethyl metabolite in extensive metabolizers. This change is not expected to be a safety concern and adjustment of dose is not needed.

Distribution

Tolterodine is highly bound to plasma proteins, primarily α_1-acid glycoprotein. Unbound concentrations of tolterodine average 3.7% ± 0.13% over the concentration range achieved in clinical studies. The 5-hydroxymethyl metabolite is not extensively protein bound, with unbound fraction concentrations averaging 36% ± 4.0%. The blood to serum ratio of tolterodine and the 5-hydroxymethyl metabolite averages 0.6 and 0.8, respectively, indicating that these compounds do not distribute extensively into erythrocytes. The volume of distribution of tolterodine following administration of a 1.28 mg intravenous dose is 113 ± 26.7 liters.

Metabolism

Tolterodine is extensively metabolized by the liver following oral dosing. The primary metabolic route involves the oxidation of the 5-methyl group and is mediated by the cytochrome P450 2D6 (CYP2D6) and leads to the formation of a pharmacologically active 5-hydroxymethyl metabolite. Further metabolism leads to formation of the 5-carboxylic acid and *N*-dealkylated 5-carboxylic acid metabolites, which account for 51% ± 14% and 29% ± 6.3% of the metabolites recovered in the urine, respectively.

Variability in Metabolism

A subset (about 7%) of the population is devoid of CYP2D6, the enzyme responsible for the formation of the 5-hydroxymethyl metabolite of tolterodine. The identified pathway of metabolism for these individuals ("poor metabolizers") is dealkylation via cytochrome P450 3A4 (CYP3A4) to *N*-dealkylated tolterodine. The remainder of the population is referred to as "extensive metabolizers". Pharmacokinetic studies revealed that tolterodine is metabolized at a slower rate in poor metabolizers than in extensive metabolizers; this results in significantly higher serum concentrations of tolterodine and in negligible concentrations of the 5-hydroxymethyl metabolite.

Excretion

Following administration of a 5 mg oral dose of ^{14}C-tolterodine solution to healthy volunteers, 77% of radioactivity was recovered in urine and 17% was recovered in feces in 7 days. Less than 1% (<2.5% in poor metabolizers) of the dose was recovered as intact tolterodine, and 5-14% (<1% in poor metabolizers) was recovered as the active 5-hydroxymethyl metabolite.

A summary of mean (± standard deviation) pharmacokinetic parameters of tolterodine immediate release and the 5-hydroxymethyl metabolite in extensive (EM) and poor (PM) metabolizers is provided in TABLE 1. These data were obtained following single- and multipledoses of tolterodine 4 mg administered twice daily to 16 healthy male volunteers (8 EM, 8 PM).

***TABLE 1** Summary of Mean (±SD) Pharmacokinetic Parameters of Tolterodine and its Active Metabolite (5-Hydroxymethyl Metabolite) in Healthy Volunteers*

	Single-Dose		Multiple-Dose	
Phenotype (CYP 2D6)	**EM**	**PM**	**EM**	**PM**
Tolterodine				
T_{max} (h)	1.6 ± 1.5	1.4 ± 0.5	1.2 ± 0.5	1.9 ± 1.0
C_{max}* (μg/L)	1.6 ± 1.2	10 ± 4.9	2.6 ± 2.8	19 ± 7.5
C_{avg}* (μg/L)	0.50 ± 0.35	8.3 ± 4.3	0.58 ± 0.54	12 ± 5.1
T½ (h)	2.0 ± 0.7	6.5 ± 1.6	2.2 ± 0.4	9.6 ± 1.5
CL/F (L/h)	534 ± 697	17 ± 7.3	415 ± 377	11 ± 4.2
5-Hydroxymethyl Metabolite				
T_{max} (h)	1.8 ± 1.4	—†	1.2 ± 0.5	—
C_{max}* (μg/L)	1.8 ± 0.7	—	2.4 ± 1.3	—
C_{avg}* (μg/L)	0.62 ± 0.26	—	0.92 ± 0.46	—
T½ (h)	3.1 ± 0.7	—	2.9 ± 0.4	—

* Parameter was dose-normalized from 4 mg to 2 mg.
† Not applicable.
C_{max} = Maximum plasma concentration; T_{max} = Time of occurence of C_{max}; C_{avg} = Average plasma concentration; T½ = Terminal elimination half-life; CL/F = Apparent oral clearance.

Pharmacokinetics in Special Populations

Age

In Phase 1, multiple-dose studies in which tolterodine immediate release 4 mg (2 mg bid) was administered, serum concentrations of tolterodine and of the 5-hydroxymethyl metabolite were similar in healthy elderly volunteers (aged 64 through 80 years) and healthy young volunteers (aged less than 40 years). In another Phase 1 study, elderly volunteers (aged 71 through 81 years) were given tolterodine immediate release 2 or 4 mg (1 or 2 mg bid). Mean serum concentrations of tolterodine and the 5-hydroxymethyl metabolite in these elderly volunteers were approximately 20% and 50% higher, respectively, than reported in young healthy volunteers. However, no overall differences were observed in safety between older and younger patients on tolterodine in Phase 3, 12 week, controlled clinical studies; therefore, no tolterodine dosage adjustment for elderly patients is recommended (see PRECAUTIONS, Detrol, Geriatric Use).

T

Pediatric

The pharmacokinetics of tolterodine have not been established in pediatric patients.

Gender

The pharmacokinetics of tolterodine immediate release and the 5-hydroxymethyl metabolite are not influenced by gender. Mean C_{max} of tolterodine (1.6 mg/L in males versus 2.2 mg/L in females) and the active 5-hydroxymethyl metabolite (2.2 mg/L in males versus 2.5 mg/L in females) are similar in males and females who were administered tolterodine immediate release 2 mg. Mean AUC values of tolterodine (6.7 µg·h/L in males versus 7.8 µg·h/L in females) and the 5-hydroxymethyl metabolite (10 µg·h/L in males versus 11 µg·h/L in females) are also similar. The elimination half-life of tolterodine for both males and females is 2.4 hours, and the half-life of the 5-hydroxymethyl metabolite is 3.0 hours in females and 3.3 hours in males.

Race

Pharmacokinetic differences due to race have not been established.

Renal Insufficiency

Renal impairment can significantly alter the disposition of tolterodine immediate release and its metabolites. In a study conducted in patients with creatinine clearance between 10 and 30 ml/min, tolterodine immediate release and the 5-hydroxymethyl metabolite levels were approximately 2- to 3-fold higher in patients with renal impairment than in healthy volunteers. Exposure levels of other metabolites of tolterodine (*e.g.*, tolterodine acid, *N*-dealkylated tolterodine acid, *N*-dealkylated tolterodine, and *N*-dealkylated hydroxylated tolterodine) were significantly higher (10- to 30-fold) in renally impaired patients as compared to the healthy volunteers. The recommended dosage for patients with significantly reduced renal function is Detrol 1 mg twice daily (see PRECAUTIONS, Detrol, General).

Hepatic Insufficiency

Liver impairment can significantly alter the disposition of tolterodine immediate release. In a study conducted in cirrhotic patients, the elimination half-life of tolterodine immediate release was longer in cirrhotic patients (mean, 8.7 hours) than in healthy, young and elderly volunteers (mean, 2-4 hours). The clearance of orally administered tolterodine was substantially lower in cirrhotic patients (1.1 ± 1.7 L/h/kg) than in the healthy volunteers (5.7 ± 3.8 L/h/kg). The recommended dose for patients with significantly reduced hepatic function is Detrol 1 mg twice daily (see PRECAUTIONS, Detrol, General).

Drug-Drug Interactions

Fluoxetine

Fluoxetine is a selective serotonin reuptake inhibitor and a potent inhibitor of CYP2D6 activity. In a study to assess the effect of fluoxetine on the pharmacokinetics of tolterodine immediate release and its metabolites, it was observed that fluoxetine significantly inhibited the metabolism of tolterodine immediate release in extensive metabolizers, resulting in a 4.8-fold increase in tolterodine AUC. There was a 52% decrease in C_{max} and a 20% decrease in AUC of the 5-hydroxymethyl metabolite. Fluoxetine thus alters the pharmacokinetics in patients who would otherwise be extensive metabolizers of tolterodine immediate release to resemble the pharmacokinetic profile in poor metabolizers. The sums of unbound serum concentrations of tolterodine immediate release and the 5-hydroxy-methyl metabolite are only 25% higher during the interaction. No dose adjustment is required when Detrol and fluoxetine are coadministered.

Other Drugs Metabolized by Cytochrome P450 Isoenzymes

Tolterodine immediate release does not cause clinically significant interactions with other drugs metabolized by the major drug metabolizing CYP enzymes. *In vivo* drug-interaction data show that tolterodine immediate release does not result in clinically relevant inhibition of CYPIA2, 2D6, 2C9, 2C19, or 3A4 as evidenced by lack of influence on the marker drugs caffeine, debrisoquine, S-warfarin, and omeprazole. *In vitro* data show that tolterodine immediate release is a competitive inhibitor of CYP2D6 at high concentrations (Ki 1.05 µM), while tolterodine immediate release as well as the 5-hydroxymethyl metabolite are devoid of any significant inhibitory potential regarding the other isoenzymes.

CYP3A4 Inhibitors

The effect of 200 mg daily dose of ketoconazole on the pharmacokinetics of tolterodine immediate release was studied in 8 healthy volunteers, all of whom were poor metabolizers (see Pharmacokinetics, Metabolism, Variability in Metabolism for discussion of poor metabolizers). In the presence of ketoconazole, the mean C_{max} and AUC of tolterodine increased by 2- and 2.5-fold, respectively. Based on these findings, other potent CYP3A inhibitors such as other azole antifungals (*e.g.*, itraconazole, miconazole) or macrolide antibiotics (*e.g.*, erythromycin, clarithromycin) or cyclosporine or vinblastine may also lead to increases of tolterodine plasma concentrations (see PRECAUTIONS, Detrol and DOSAGE AND ADMINISTRATION, Detrol).

Warfarin

In healthy volunteers, coadministration of tolterodine immediate release 4 mg (2 mg bid) for 7 days and a single dose of warfarin 25 mg on day 4 had no effect on prothrombin time, Factor VII suppression, or on the pharmacokinetics of warfarin.

Oral Contraceptives

Tolterodine immediate release 4 mg (2 mg bid) had no effect on the pharmacokinetics of an oral contraceptive (ethinyl estradiol 30 mg/levonorgestrel 150 mg) as evidenced by the monitoring of ethinyl estradiol and levonorgestrel over a 2 month cycle in healthy female volunteers.

Diuretics

Coadministration of tolterodine immediate release up to 8 mg (4 mg bid) for up to 12 weeks with diuretic agents, such as indapamide, hydrochlorothiazide, triamterene, bendroflumethiazide, chlorothiazide, methylchlorothiazide, or furosemide, did not cause any adverse electrocardiographic (ECG) effects.

DETROL LA

Tolterodine is a competitive muscarinic receptor antagonist. Both urinary bladder contraction and salivation are mediated via cholinergic muscarinic receptors.

After oral administration, tolterodine is metabolized in the liver, resulting in the formation of the 5-hydroxymethyl derivative, a major pharmacologically active metabolite. The 5-hydroxymethyl metabolite, which exhibits an antimuscarinic activity similar to that of tolterodine, contributes significantly to the therapeutic effect. Both tolterodine and the 5-hydroxymethyl metabolite exhibit a high specificity for muscarinic receptors, since both show negligible activity or affinity for other neurotransmitter receptors and other potential cellular targets, such as calcium channels.

Tolterodine has a pronounced effect on bladder function. Effects on urodynamic parameters before and 1 and 5 hours after a single 6.4 mg dose of tolterodine immediate release were determined in healthy volunteers. The main effects of tolterodine at 1 and 5 hours were an increase in residual urine, reflecting an incomplete emptying of the bladder, and a decrease in detrusor pressure. These findings are consistent with an antimuscarinic action on the lower urinary tract.

Pharmacokinetics

Absorption

In a study with ^{14}C-tolterodine solution in healthy volunteers who received a 5 mg oral dose, at least 77% of the radiolabeled dose was absorbed. C_{max} and area under the concentration-time curve (AUC) determined after dosage of tolterodine immediate release are dose-proportional over the range of 1-4 mg. Based on the sum of unbound serum concentrations of tolterodine and the 5-hydroxymethyl metabolite ("active moiety"), the AUC of tolterodine extended release 4 mg daily is equivalent to tolterodine immediate release 4 mg (2 mg bid). C_{max} and C_{min} levels of tolterodine extended release are about 75% and 150% of tolterodine immediate release, respectively. Maximum serum concentrations of tolterodine extended release are observed 2-6 hours after dose administration.

Effect of Food

There is no effect of food on the pharmacokinetics of tolterodine extended release.

Distribution

Tolterodine is highly bound to plasma proteins, primarily α_1-acid glycoprotein. Unbound concentrations of tolterodine average 3.7% ± 0.13% over the concentration range achieved in clinical studies. The 5-hydroxymethyl metabolite is not extensively protein bound, with unbound fraction concentrations averaging 36% ± 4.0%. The blood to serum ratio of tolterodine and the 5-hydroxymethyl metabolite averages 0.6 and 0.8, respectively, indicating that these compounds do not distribute extensively into erythrocytes. The volume of distribution of tolterodine following administration of a 1.28 mg intravenous dose is 113 ± 26.7 liters.

Metabolism

Tolterodine is extensively metabolized by the liver following oral dosing. The primary metabolic route involves the oxidation of the 5-methyl group and is mediated by the cytochrome P450 2D6 (CYP2D6) and leads to the formation of a pharmacologically active 5-hydroxymethyl metabolite. Further metabolism leads to formation of the 5-carboxylic acid and *N*-dealkylated 5-carboxylic acid metabolites, which account for 51% ± 14% and 29% ± 6.3% of the metabolites recovered in the urine, respectively.

Variability in Metabolism

A subset (about 7%) of the Caucasian population is devoid of CYP2D6, the enzyme responsible for the formation of the 5-hydroxymethyl metabolite of tolterodine. The identified pathway of metabolism for these individuals ("poor metabolizers") is dealkylation via cytochrome P450 3A4 (CYP3A4) to *N*-dealkylated tolterodine. The remainder of the population is referred to as "extensive metabolizers". Pharmacokinetic studies revealed that tolterodine is metabolized at a slower rate in poor metabolizers than in extensive metabolizers; this results in significantly higher serum concentrations of tolterodine and in negligible concentrations of the 5-hydroxymethyl metabolite.

Excretion

Following administration of a 5 mg oral dose of ^{14}C-tolterodine solution to healthy volunteers, 77% of radioactivity was recovered in urine and 17% was recovered in feces in 7 days. Less than 1% (<2.5% in poor metabolizers) of the dose was recovered as intact tolterodine, and 5-14% (<1% in poor metabolizers) was recovered as the active 5-hydroxymethyl metabolite.

A summary of mean (± standard deviation) pharmacokinetic parameters of tolterodine extended release and the 5-hydroxymethyl metabolite in extensive (EM) and poor (PM) metabolizers is provided in TABLE 2. These data were obtained following single and multiple doses of tolterodine extended release administered daily to 17 healthy male volunteers (13 EM, 4 PM).

Pharmacokinetics in Special Populations

Age

In Phase 1, multiple-dose studies in which tolterodine immediate release 4 mg (2 mg bid) was administered, serum concentrations of tolterodine and of the 5-hydroxymethyl metabolite were similar in healthy elderly volunteers (aged 64 through 80 years) and healthy young volunteers (aged less than 40 years). In another Phase 1 study, elderly volunteers (aged 71 through 81 years) were given tolterodine immediate release 2 or 4 mg (1 or 2 mg bid). Mean serum concentrations of tolterodine and the 5-hydroxymethyl metabolite in these elderly volunteers were approximately 20% and 50% higher, respectively, than reported in young healthy volunteers. However, no overall differences were observed in safety between older and younger patients on tolterodine in the Phase 3, 12 week, controlled clinical studies; therefore, no tolterodine dosage adjustment for elderly patients is recommended (see PRECAUTIONS, Detrol LA, Geriatric Use).

Pediatric

The pharmacokinetics of tolterodine has not been established in pediatric patients.

T

TABLE 2 *Summary of Mean (±SD) Pharmacokinetic Parameters of Tolterodine Extended Release and its Active Metabolite (5-Hydroxymethyl Metabolite) in Healthy Volunteers*

	Single Dose (4 mg)*	Multiple Dose (4 mg)	
	EM	EM	PM
Tolterodine			
T_{max}† (h)	4 (2-6)	4 (2-6)	4 (3-6)
C_{max} (μg/L)	1.3 (0.8)	3.4 (4.9)	19 (16)
C_{avg} (μg/L)	0.8 (0.57)	1.7 (2.8)	13 (11)
T½ (h)	8.4 (3.2)	6.9 (3.5)	18 (16)
5-Hydroxymethyl Metabolite			
T_{max}† (h)	4 (3-6)	4 (2-6)	—‡
C_{max} (μg/L)	1.6 (0.5)	2.7 (0.90)	—
C_{avg} (μg/L)	1.0 (0.32)	1.4 (0.6)	—
T½ (h)	8.8 (5.9)	9.9 (4.0)	—

* Parameter dose-normalized from 8 to 4 mg for the single-dose data.
† Data presented as median (range).
‡ Not applicable.
C_{max} = Maximum serum concentration; T_{max} = Time of occurrence of C_{max}; C_{avg} = Average serum concentration; T½ = Terminal elimination half-life.

Gender

The pharmacokinetics of tolterodine immediate release and the 5-hydroxymethyl metabolite are not influenced by gender. Mean C_{max} of tolterodine immediate release (1.6 μg/L in males versus 2.2 μg/L in females) and the active 5-hydroxymethyl metabolite (2.2 μg/L in males versus 2.5 μg/L in females) are similar in males and females who were administered tolterodine immediate release 2 mg. Mean AUC values of tolterodine (6.7 μg·h/L in males versus 7.8 μg·h/L in females) and the 5-hydroxymethyl metabolite (10 μg·h/L in males versus 11 μg·h/L in females) are also similar. The elimination half-life of tolterodine immediate release for both males and females is 2.4 hours, and the half-life of the 5-hydroxymethyl metabolite is 3.0 hours in females and 3.3 hours in males.

Race

Pharmacokinetic differences due to race have not been established.

Renal Insufficiency

Renal impairment can significantly alter the disposition of tolterodine immediate release and its metabolites. In a study conducted in patients with creatinine clearance between 10 and 30 ml/min, tolterodine immediate release and the 5-hydroxymethyl metabolite levels were approximately 2-3 fold higher in patients with renal impairment than in healthy volunteers. Exposure levels of other metabolites of tolterodine (*e.g.,* tolterodine acid, *N*-dealkylated tolterodine acid, *N*-dealkylated tolterodine and *N*-dealkylated hydroxy tolterodine) were significantly higher (10- to 30-fold) in renally impaired patients as compared to the healthy volunteers. The recommended dose for patients with significantly reduced renal function is tolterodine 2 mg daily (see PRECAUTIONS, Detrol LA, General).

Hepatic Insufficiency

Liver impairment can significantly alter the disposition of tolterodine immediate release. In a study of tolterodine immediate release conducted in cirrhotic patients, the elimination half-life of tolterodine immediate release was longer in cirrhotic patients (mean, 7.8 hours) than in healthy, young and elderly volunteers (mean, 2-4 hours). The clearance of orally administered tolterodine immediate release was substantially lower in cirrhotic patients (1.0 ± 1.7 L/h/kg) than in the healthy volunteers (5.7 ± 3.8 L/h/kg). The recommended dose for patients with significantly reduced hepatic function is tolterodine 2 mg daily (see PRECAUTIONS, Detrol LA, General).

Drug-Drug Interactions

Fluoxetine

Fluoxetine is a selective serotonin reuptake inhibitor and a potent inhibitor of CYP2D6 activity. In a study to assess the effect of fluoxetine on the pharmacokinetics of tolterodine immediate release and its metabolites, it was observed that fluoxetine significantly inhibited the metabolism of tolterodine immediate release in extensive metabolizers, resulting in a 4.8-fold increase in tolterodine AUC. There was a 52% decrease in C_{max} and a 20% decrease in AUC of the 5-hydroxymethyl metabolite. Fluoxetine thus alters the pharmacokinetics in patients who would otherwise be extensive metabolizers of tolterodine immediate release to resemble the pharmacokinetic profile in poor metabolizers. The sums of unbound serum concentrations of tolterodine immediate release and the 5-hydroxymethyl metabolite are only 25% higher during the interaction. No dose adjustment is required when tolterodine and fluoxetine are coadministered.

Other Drugs Metabolized by Cytochrome P450 Isoenzymes

Tolterodine immediate release does not cause clinically significant interactions with other drugs metabolized by the major drug metabolizing CYP enzymes. *In vivo* drug-interaction data show that tolterodine immediate release does not result in clinically relevant inhibition of CYP1A2, 2D6, 2C9, 2C19, or 3A4 as evidenced by lack of influence on the marker drugs caffeine, debrisoquine, S-warfarin, and omeprazole. *In vitro* data show that tolterodine immediate release is a competitive inhibitor of CYP2D6 at high concentrations (Ki 1.05 μM), while tolterodine immediate release as well as the 5-hydroxymethyl metabolite are devoid of any significant inhibitory potential regarding the other isoenzymes.

CYP3A4 Inhibitors

The effect of 200 mg daily dose of ketoconazole on the pharmacokinetics of tolterodine immediate release was studied in 8 healthy volunteers, all of whom were poor metabolizers (see Pharmacokinetics, Metabolism, Variability in Metabolism for discussion of poor metabolizers). In the presence of ketoconazole, the mean C_{max} and AUC of tolterodine increased by 2- and 2.5-fold, respectively. Based on these findings, other potent CYP3A4 inhibitors such as other azole antifungals (*e.g.,* itraconazole, miconazole) or macrolide antibiotics (*e.g.,* erythromycin, clarithromycin) or cyclosporine or vinblastine may also lead to increases of tolterodine plasma concentrations (see PRECAUTIONS, Detrol LA and DOSAGE AND ADMINISTRATION, Detrol LA).

Warfarin

In healthy volunteers, coadministration of tolterodine immediate release 4 mg (2 mg bid) for 7 days and a single dose of warfarin 25 mg on day 4 had no effect on prothrombin time, Factor VII suppression, or on the pharmacokinetics of warfarin.

Oral Contraceptives

Tolterodine immediate release 4 mg (2 mg bid) had no effect on the pharmacokinetics of an oral contraceptive (ethinyl estradiol 30 μg/levo-norgestrel 150 μg) as evidenced by the monitoring of ethinyl estradiol and levo-norgestrel over a 2 month period in healthy female volunteers.

Diuretics

Coadministration of tolterodine immediate release up to 8 mg (4 mg bid) for up to 12 weeks with diuretic agents, such as indapamide, hydrochlorothiazide, triamterene, bendroflumethiazide, chlorothiazide, methylchlorothiazide, or furosemide, did not cause any adverse electrocardiographic (ECG) effects.

INDICATIONS AND USAGE

DETROL

Detrol tablets are indicated for the treatment of overactive bladder with symptoms of urge urinary incontinence, urgency, and frequency.

DETROL LA

Detrol LA capsules are once daily extended release capsules indicated for the treatment of overactive bladder with symptoms of urge urinary incontinence, urgency, and frequency.

CONTRAINDICATIONS

DETROL

Detrol tablets are contraindicated in patients with urinary retention, gastric retention, or uncontrolled narrow-angle glaucoma. Detrol is also contraindicated in patients who have demonstrated hypersensitivity to the drug or its ingredients.

DETROL LA

Detrol LA capsules are contraindicated in patients with urinary retention, gastric retention, or uncontrolled narrow-angle glaucoma. Detrol LA is also contraindicated in patients who have demonstrated hypersensitivity to the drug or its ingredients.

PRECAUTIONS

DETROL

General

Risk of Urinary Retention and Gastric Retention

Detrol tablets should be administered with caution to patients with clinically significant bladder outflow obstruction because of the risk of urinary retention and to patients with gastrointestinal obstructive disorders, such as pyloric stenosis, because of the risk of gastric retention (see CONTRAINDICATIONS, Detrol).

Controlled Narrow-Angle Glaucoma

Detrol should be used with caution in patients being treated for narrow-angle glaucoma.

Reduced Hepatic and Renal Function

For patients with significantly reduced hepatic function or renal function, the recommended dose of Detrol is 1 mg twice daily (see CLINICAL PHARMACOLOGY, Detrol, Pharmacokinetics in Special Populations).

Information for the Patient

Patients should be informed that antimuscarinic agents such as Detrol may produce the following effects: blurred vision, dizziness, or drowsiness.

Drug/Laboratory Test Interactions

Interactions between tolterodine and laboratory tests have not been studied.

Carcinogenesis, Mutagenesis, and Impairment of Fertility

Carcinogenicity studies with tolterodine were conducted in mice and rats. At the maximum tolerated dose in mice (30 mg/kg/day), female rats (20 mg/kg/day), and male rats (30 mg/kg/day), AUC values obtained for tolterodine were 355, 291, and 462 mg·h/L, respectively. In comparison, the human AUC value for a 2 mg dose administered twice daily is estimated at 34 mg·h/L. Thus, tolterodine exposure in the carcinogenicity studies was 9- to 14-fold higher than expected in humans. No increase in tumors was found in either mice or rats.

No mutagenic effects of tolterodine were detected in a battery of *in vitro* tests, including bacterial mutation assays (Ames test) in four strains of *Salmonella typhimurium* and in two strains of *Escherichia coli,* a gene mutation assay in L5178Y mouse lymphoma cells, and chromosomal aberration tests in human lymphocytes. Tolterodine was also negative *in vivo* in the bone marrow micronucleus test in the mouse.

In female mice treated for 2 weeks before mating and during gestation with 20 mg/kg/day (corresponding to AUC value of about 500 mg·h/L), neither effects on reproductive performance or fertility were seen. Based on AUC values, the systemic exposure was about 15-fold higher in animals than in humans. In male mice, a dose of 30 mg/kg/day did not induce any adverse effects on fertility.

Pregnancy Category C

At oral doses of 20 mg/kg/day (approximately 14 times the human exposure), no anomalies or malformations were observed in mice. When given at doses of 30-40 mg/kg/day, tolterodine has been shown to be embryolethal, reduce fetal weight, and increase the incidence of fetal abnormalities (cleft palate, digital abnormalities, intra-abdominal hemorrhage, and various skeletal abnormalities, primarily reduced ossification) in mice. At these doses, the AUC values were about 20- to 25-fold higher than in humans. Rabbits treated subcutaneously at a dose of 0.8 mg/kg/day achieved an AUC of 100 mg·h/L, which is about 3-fold higher than that resulting from the human dose. This dose did not result in any embryotoxicity or teratogenicity. There are no studies of tolterodine in pregnant women. Therefore, Detrol should be used during pregnancy only if the potential benefit for the mother justifies the potential risk to the fetus.

Nursing Mothers

Tolterodine is excreted into the milk in mice. Offspring of female mice treated with tolterodine 20 mg/kg/day during the lactation period had slightly reduced body-weight gain. The offspring regained the weight during the maturation phase. It is not known whether tolterodine is excreted in human milk; therefore, Detrol should not be administered during nursing. A decision should be made whether to discontinue nursing or to discontinue Detrol in nursing mothers.

Pediatric Use

The safety and effectiveness of Detrol in pediatric patients have not been established.

Geriatric Use

Of the 1120 patients who were treated in the four Phase 3, 12 week clinical studies of Detrol, 474 (42%) were 65-91 years of age. No overall differences in safety were observed between the older and younger patients (see CLINICAL PHARMACOLOGY, Detrol, Pharmacokinetics in Special Populations).

DETROL LA

General

Risk of Urinary Retention and Gastric Retention

Detrol LA capsules should be administered with caution to patients with clinically significant bladder outflow obstruction because of the risk of urinary retention and to patients with gastrointestinal obstructive disorders, such as pyloric stenosis, because of the risk of gastric retention (see CONTRAINDICATIONS, Detrol LA).

Controlled Narrow-Angle Glaucoma

Detrol LA should be used with caution in patients being treated for narrow-angle glaucoma.

Reduced Hepatic and Renal Function

For patients with significantly reduced hepatic function or renal function, the recommended dose for Detrol LA is 2 mg daily (see CLINICAL PHARMACOLOGY, Detrol LA, Pharmacokinetics in Special Populations).

Information for the Patient

Patients should be informed that antimuscarinic agents such as Detrol LA may produce the following effects: blurred vision, dizziness, or drowsiness.

Drug/Laboratory Test Interactions

Interactions between tolterodine and laboratory tests have not been studied.

Carcinogenesis, Mutagenesis, and Impairment of Fertility

Carcinogenicity studies with tolterodine immediate release were conducted in mice and rats. At the maximum tolerated dose in mice (30 mg/kg/day), female rats (20 mg/kg/day), and male rats (30 mg/kg/day), AUC values obtained for tolterodine were 355, 291, and 462 μg·h/L, respectively. In comparison, the human AUC value for a 2 mg dose administered twice daily is estimated at 34 μg·h/L. Thus, tolterodine exposure in the carcinogenicity studies was 9- to 14-fold higher than expected in humans. No increase in tumors was found in either mice or rats.

No mutagenic effects of tolterodine were detected in a battery of *in vitro* tests, including bacterial mutation assays (Ames test) in four strains of *Salmonella typhimurium* and in two strains of *Escherichia coli*, a gene mutation assay in L5178Y mouse lymphoma cells, and chromosomal aberration tests in human lymphocytes. Tolterodine was also negative *in vivo* in the bone marrow micronucleus test in the mouse.

In female mice treated for 2 weeks before mating and during gestation with 20 mg/kg/day (corresponding to AUC value of about 500 μg·h/L), neither effects on reproductive performance or fertility were seen. Based on AUC values, the systemic exposure was about 15-fold higher in animals than in humans. In male mice, a dose of 30 mg/kg/day did not induce any adverse effects on fertility.

T

Pregnancy Category C

At oral doses of 20 mg/kg/day (approximately 14 times the human exposure), no anomalies or malformations were observed in mice. When given at doses of 30-40 mg/kg/day, tolterodine has been shown to be embryolethal and reduce fetal weight, and increase the incidence of fetal abnormalities (cleft palate, digital abnormalities, intra-abdominal hemorrhage, and various skeletal abnormalities, primarily reduced ossification) in mice. At these doses, the AUC values were about 20- to 25-fold higher than in humans. Rabbits treated subcutaneously at a dose of 0.8 mg/kg/day achieved an AUC of 100 μg·h/L, which is about 3-fold higher than that resulting from the human dose. This dose did not result in any embryotoxicity or teratogenicity. There are no studies of tolterodine in pregnant women. Therefore, Detrol LA should be used during pregnancy only if the potential benefit for the mother justifies the potential risk to the fetus.

Nursing Mothers

Tolterodine immediate release is excreted into the milk in mice. Offspring of female mice treated with tolterodine 20 mg/kg/day during the lactation period had slightly reduced body-weight gain. The offspring regained the weight during the maturation phase. It is not known whether tolterodine is excreted in human milk; therefore, Detrol LA should not be administered during nursing. A decision should be made whether to discontinue nursing or to discontinue Detrol LA in nursing mothers.

Pediatric Use

The safety and effectiveness of tolterodine in pediatric patients has not been established.

Geriatric Use

No overall differences in safety were observed between the older and younger patients treated with tolterodine (see CLINICAL PHARMACOLOGY, Detrol LA, Pharmacokinetics in Special Populations).

DRUG INTERACTIONS

DETROL

CYP3A4 Inhibitors

Ketoconazole, an inhibitor of the drug metabolizing enzyme CYP3A4, significantly increased plasma concentrations of tolterodine when coadministered to subjects who were poor metabolizers (see CLINICAL PHARMACOLOGY, Detrol, Pharmacokinetics, Metabolism, Variability in Metabolism and CLINICAL PHARMACOLOGY, Drug-Drug Interactions). For patients receiving ketoconazole or other potent CYP3A4 inhibitors such as other azole anitfungals (*e.g.*, itraconazole, miconazole) or macrolide antibiotics (*e.g.*, erythromycin, clarithromycin) or cyclosporine or vinblastin, the recommended dose of Detrol is 1 mg twice daily.

DETROL LA

CYP3A4 Inhibitors

Ketoconazole, an inhibitor of the drug metabolizing enzyme CYP3A4, significantly increased plasma concentrations of tolterodine when coadministered to subjects who were poor metabolizers (see CLINICAL PHARMACOLOGY, Detrol LA, Pharmacokinetics, Metabolism, Variability in Metabolism and CLINICAL PHARMACOLOGY, Drug-Drug Interactions). For patients receiving ketoconazole or other potent CYP3A4 inhibitors such as other azole antifungals (*e.g.*, itraconazole, miconazole) or macrolide antibiotics (*e.g.*, erythromycin, clarithromycin) or cyclosporine or vinblastine, the recommended dose of Detrol LA is 2 mg daily.

ADVERSE REACTIONS

DETROL

The Phase 2 and 3 clinical trial program for Detrol tablets included 3071 patients who were treated with Detrol (n=2133) or placebo (n=938). The patients were treated with 1, 2, 4, or 8 mg/day for up to 12 months. No differences in the safety profile of tolterodine were identified based on age, gender, race, or metabolism.

The data described below reflect exposure to Detrol 2 mg bid in 986 patients and to placebo in 683 patients exposed for 12 weeks in five Phase 3, controlled clinical studies. Because clinical trials are conducted under widely varying conditions, adverse reaction rates observed in the clinical trials of a drug cannot be directly compared to rates in the clinical trials of another drug and may not reflect the rates observed in practice. The adverse reaction information from clinical trials does, however, provide a basis for identifying the adverse events that appear to be related to drug use and approximating rates.

Sixty-six percent (66%) of patients receiving Detrol 2 mg bid reported adverse events versus 56% of placebo patients. The most common adverse events reported by patients receiving Detrol were dry mouth, headache, constipation, vertigo/ dizziness, and abdominal pain. Dry mouth, constipation, abnormal vision (accommodation abnormalities), urinary retention, and xerophthalmia are expected side effects of antimuscarinic agents.

Dry mouth was the most frequently reported adverse event for patients treated with Detrol 2 mg bid in the Phase 3 clinical studies, occurring in 34.8% of patients treated with Detrol and 9.8% of placebo-treated patients. One percent (1%) of patients treated with Detrol discontinued treatment due to dry mouth.

The frequency of discontinuation due to adverse events was highest during the first 4 weeks of treatment. Seven percent (7%) of patients treated with Detrol 2 mg bid discontinued treatment due to adverse events versus 6% of placebo patients. The most common adverse events leading to discontinuation of Detrol were dizziness and headache.

Three percent (3%) of patients treated with Detrol 2 mg bid reported a serious adverse event versus 4% of placebo patients. Significant ECG changes in QT and QTc have not been demonstrated in clinical-study patients treated with Detrol 2 mg bid. TABLE 6 lists the adverse events reported in 1% or more of the patients treated with Detrol 2 mg bid in the 12 week studies. The adverse events are reported regardless of causality.

Postmarketing Surveillance

The following events have been reported in association with tolterodine use in clinical practice: Anaphylactoid reactions, tachycardia, and peripheral edema. Because these spontaneously reported events are from the worldwide postmarketing experience, the frequency of events and the role of tolterodine in their causation cannot be reliably determined.

DETROL LA

The Phase 2 and 3 clinical trial program for Detrol LA capsules included 1073 patients who were treated with Detrol LA (n=537) or placebo (n=536). The patients were treated with 2, 4, 6, or 8 mg/day for up to 15 months. Because clinical trials are conducted under widely varying conditions, adverse reaction rates observed in the clinical trials of a drug cannot be directly compared to rates in the clinical trials of another drug and may not reflect the rates observed in practice. The adverse reaction information from clinical trials does, however, provide a basis for identifying the adverse events that appear to be related to drug use and for approximating rates. The data described below reflect exposure to Detrol LA 4 mg once daily every morning in 505 patients and to placebo in 507 patients exposed for 12 weeks in the Phase 3, controlled clinical study.

Adverse events were reported in 52% (n=263) of patients receiving Detrol LA and in 49% (n=247) of patients receiving placebo. The most common adverse events reported by patients receiving Detrol LA were dry mouth, headache, constipation, and abdominal pain. Dry mouth was the most frequently reported adverse event for patients treated with Detrol

TABLE 6 *Incidence* (%) of Adverse Events Exceeding Placebo Rate and Reported in ≥1% of Patients Treated With Detrol Tablets (2 mg bid) in 12 Week, Phase 3 Clinical Studies*

Body System / Adverse Event	Detrol (n=986)	Placebo (n=683)
Autonomic Nervous		
Accommodation abnormal	2%	1%
Dry mouth	35%	10%
General		
Chest pain	2%	1%
Fatigue	4%	3%
Headache	7%	5%
Influenza-like symptoms	3%	2%
Central/Peripheral Nervous		
Vertigo/dizziness	5%	3%
Gastrointestinal		
Abdominal pain	5%	3%
Constipation	7%	4%
Diarrhea	4%	3%
Dyspepsia	4%	1%
Urinary		
Dysuria	2%	1%
Skin/Appendages		
Dry skin	1%	0%
Musculoskeletal		
Arthralgia	2%	1%
Vision		
Xerophthalmia	3%	2%
Psychiatric		
Somnolence	3%	2%
Metabolic/Nutritional		
Weight gain	1%	0%
Resistance Mechanism		
Infection	1%	0%

* In nearest integer.

LA occurring in 23.4% of patients treated with Detrol LA and 7.7% of placebo-treated patients. Dry mouth, constipation, abnormal vision (accommodation abnormalities), urinary retention, and dry eyes are expected side effects of antimuscarinic agents. A serious adverse event was reported by 1.4% (n=7) of patients receiving Detrol LA and by 3.6% (n=18) of patients receiving placebo.

The frequency of discontinuation due to adverse events was highest during the first 4 weeks of treatment. Similar percentages of patients treated with Detrol LA or placebo discontinued treatment due to adverse events. Treatment was discontinued due to adverse events and dry mouth was reported as an adverse event in 2.4% (n=12) of patients treated with Detrol LA and in 1.2% (n=6) of patients treated with placebo.

TABLE 7 lists the adverse events reported in 1% or more of patients treated with Detrol LA 4 mg once daily in the 12 week study. The adverse events were reported regardless of causality.

TABLE 7 *Incidence* (%) of Adverse Events Exceeding Placebo Rate and Reported in ≥1% of Patients Treated With Detrol LA (4 mg daily) in a 12 Week, Phase 3 Clinical Trial*

Body System / Adverse Event	Detrol LA n=505	Placebo n=507
Autonomic Nervous		
Dry mouth	23%	8%
General		
Headache	6%	4%
Fatigue	2%	1%
Central/Peripheral Nervous		
Dizziness	2%	1%
Gastrointestinal		
Consitpation	6%	4%
Abdominal pain	4%	2%
Dyspepsia	3%	1%
Vision		
Xerophthalmia	3%	2%
Vision abnormal	1%	0%
Psychiatric		
Somnolence	3%	2%
Anxiety	1%	0%
Respiratory		
Sinusitis	2%	1%
Urinary		
Dysuria	1%	0%

* In nearest integer.

Postmarketing Surveillance

The following events have been reported in association with tolterodine use in clinical practice: Anaphylactoid reactions, tachycardia, and peripheral edema. Because these spontaneously reported events are from the worldwide postmarketing experience, the frequency of events and the role of tolterodine in their causation cannot be reliably determined.

DOSAGE AND ADMINISTRATION

DETROL

The initial recommended dose of Detrol tablets is 2 mg twice daily. The dose may be lowered to 1 mg twice daily based on individual response and tolerability. For patients with significantly reduced hepatic or renal function or who are currently taking drugs that are potent inhibitors of CYP3A4, the recommended dose of Detrol is 1 mg twice daily (see PRECAUTIONS, Detrol, General and DRUG INTERACTIONS, Detrol).

DETROL LA

The recommended dose of Detrol LA capsules are 4 mg daily. Detrol LA should be taken once daily with liquids and swallowed whole. The dose may be lowered to 2 mg daily based on individual response and tolerability, however, limited efficacy data is available for Detrol LA 2 mg.

For patients with significantly reduced hepatic or renal function or who are currently taking drugs that are potent inhibitors of CYP3A4, the recommended dose of Detrol LA is 2 mg daily (see CLINICAL PHARMACOLOGY, Detrol LA and DRUG INTERACTIONS, Detrol LA).

HOW SUPPLIED

DETROL

Detrol tablets are available in:

1 mg: White, round, biconvex, film-coated tablets engraved with arcs above and below the letters "TO".

2 mg: White, round, biconvex, film-coated tablets engraved with arcs above and below the letters "DT".

Storage: Store at 25°C (77°F); excursions permitted to 15-30°C (59-86°F).

DETROL LA

Detrol LA capsules are available in:

2 mg: Blue-green with symbol and "2" printed in white ink.

4 mg: Blue with symbol and "4" printed in white ink.

Storage: Store at 25°C (77°F); excursions permitted to 15-30°C (59-86°F). Protect from light.

PRODUCT LISTING - EQUIVALENTS NOT AVAILABLE

Capsule, Extended Release - Oral - 2 mg

30's	$89.96	DETROL LA, Pharmacia and Upjohn	00009-5190-01
90's	$269.88	DETROL LA, Pharmacia and Upjohn	00009-5190-02
100's	$275.36	DETROL LA, Pharmacia and Upjohn	00009-5190-04

Capsule, Extended Release - Oral - 4 mg

30's	$92.33	DETROL LA, Pharmacia and Upjohn	00009-5191-01
90's	$276.98	DETROL LA, Pharmacia and Upjohn	00009-5191-02
100's	$282.60	DETROL LA, Pharmacia and Upjohn	00009-5191-04

Tablet - Oral - 1 mg

60's	$108.25	DETROL, Pharmacia and Upjohn	00009-4541-02
140's	$255.25	DETROL, Pharmacia and Upjohn	00009-4541-01

Tablet - Oral - 2 mg

30's	$38.79	DETROL, Allscripts Pharmaceutical Company	54569-4590-00
60's	$111.10	DETROL, Pharmacia and Upjohn	00009-4544-02
140's	$261.84	DETROL, Pharmacia and Upjohn	00009-4544-01

Topiramate *(003312)*

Categories: Lennox-Gastaut syndrome; Seizures, generalized tonic-clonic; Seizures, partial; FDA Approved 1996 Dec; Pregnancy Category C; Orphan Drugs
Drug Classes: Anticonvulsants
Brand Names: **Topamax**
Foreign Brand Availability: Epitomax (Finland); Topamax Sprinkle (Hong-Kong; Israel; Korea; New-Zealand)
Cost of Therapy: $265.41 (Epilepsy; Topamax; 200 mg; 2 tablets/day; 30 day supply)

DESCRIPTION

Topiramate is a sulfamate-substituted monosaccharide that is intended for use as an anti-epileptic drug. Topamax tablets are available as 25, 100, and 200 mg round tablets for oral administration. Topamax sprinkle capsules are available as 15 and 25 mg sprinkle capsules for oral administration as whole capsules or opened and sprinkled onto soft food.

Topiramate is a white crystalline powder with a bitter taste. Topiramate is most soluble in alkaline solutions containing sodium hydroxide or sodium phosphate and having a pH of 9-10. It is freely soluble in acetone, chloroform, dimethylsulfoxide, and ethanol. The solubility in water is 9.8 mg/ml. Its saturated solution has a pH of 6.3. Topiramate has the molecular formula $C_{12}H_{21}NO_8S$ and a molecular weight of 339.37. Topiramate is designated chemically as 2,3:4,5-Di-*O*-isopropylidene-β-D-fructopyranose sulfamate.

Topamax tablets contain the following inactive ingredients: lactose monohydrate, pregelatinized starch, microcrystalline cellulose, sodium starch glycolate, magnesium stearate, purified water, carnauba wax, hydroxypropyl methylcellulose, titanium dioxide, polyethylene glycol, synthetic iron oxide (100 and 200 mg tablets), and polysorbate 80.

Topamax sprinkle capsules contain topirimate coated beads in a hard gelatin capsule. The inactive ingredients are: sugar spheres (sucrose and starch), povidone, cellulose acetate, gelatin, silicone dioxide, sodium lauryl sulfate, titanium dioxide, and black pharmaceutical ink.

CLINICAL PHARMACOLOGY

MECHANISM OF ACTION

The precise mechanism by which topiramate exerts its antiseizure effect is unknown; however, electrophysiological and biochemical studies of the effects of topiramate on cultured neurons have revealed three properties that may contribute to topiramate's antiepileptic efficacy. First, action potentials elicited repetitively by a sustained depolarization of the neurons are blocked by topiramate in a time-dependent manner, suggestive of a state-dependent sodium channel blocking action. Second, topiramate increases the frequency at which γ-aminobutyrate (GABA) activates $GABA_A$ receptors, and enhances the ability of GABA to induce a flux of chloride ions into neurons, suggesting that topiramate potentiates the activity of this inhibitory neurotransmitter. This effect was not blocked by flumazenil, a

T

benzodiazepine antagonist, nor did topiramate increase the duration of the channel open time, differentiating topiramate from barbiturates that modulate $GABA_A$ receptors. Third, topiramate antagonizes the ability of kainate to activate the kainate/AMPA (α-amino-3-hydroxy-5-methylisoxazole-4-propionic acid; non-NMDA) subtype of excitatory amino acid (glutamate) receptor, but has no apparent effect on the activity of N-methyl-D-aspartate (NMDA) at the NMDA receptor subtype. These effects of topiramate are concentration-dependent within the range of 1-200 μM.

Topiramate also inhibits some isoenzymes of carbonic anhydrase (CA-II and CA-IV). This pharmacologic effect is generally weaker than that of acetazolamide, a known carbonic anhydrase inhibitor, and is not thought to be a major contributing factor to topiramate's antiepileptic activity.

PHARMACODYNAMICS

Topiramate has anticonvulsant activity in rat and mouse maximal electroshock seizure (MES) tests. Topiramate is only weakly effective in blocking clonic seizures induced by the $GABA_A$ receptor antagonist, pentylenetetrazole. Topiramate is also effective in rodent models of epilepsy, which include tonic and absence-like seizures in the spontaneous epileptic rat (SER) and tonic and clonic seizures induced in rats by kindling of the amygdala or by global ischemia.

PHARMACOKINETICS

The sprinkle formulation is bioequivalent to the immediate release tablet formulation and, therefore, may be substituted as a therapeutic equivalent.

Absorption of topiramate is rapid, with peak plasma concentrations occurring at approximately 2 hours following a 400 mg oral dose. The relative bioavailability of topiramate from the tablet formulation is about 80% compared to a solution. The bioavailability of topiramate is not affected by food.

The pharmacokinetics of topiramate are linear with dose proportional increases in plasma concentration over the dose range studied (200-800 mg/day). The mean plasma elimination half-life is 21 hours after single or multiple doses. Steady-state is thus reached in about 4 days in patients with normal renal function. Topiramate is 13-17% bound to human plasma proteins over the concentration range of 1-250 μg/ml.

METABOLISM AND EXCRETION

Topiramate is not extensively metabolized and is primarily eliminated unchanged in the urine (approximately 70% of an administered dose). Six metabolites have been identified in humans, none of which constitutes more than 5% of an administered dose. The metabolites are formed via hydroxylation, hydrolysis, and glucuronidation. There is evidence of renal tubular reabsorption of topiramate. In rats, given probenecid to inhibit tubular reabsorption, along with topiramate, a significant increase in renal clearance of topiramate was observed. This interaction has not been evaluated in humans. Overall, oral plasma clearance (CL/F) is approximately 20-30 ml/min in humans following oral administration.

PHARMACOKINETIC INTERACTIONS

See also DRUG INTERACTIONS.

Antiepileptic Drugs

Potential interactions between topiramate and standard AEDs were assessed in controlled clinical pharmacokinetic studies in patients with epilepsy. The effect of these interactions on mean plasma AUCs are summarized in PRECAUTIONS and TABLE 3.

SPECIAL POPULATIONS

Renal Impairment

The clearance of topiramate was reduced by 42% in moderately renally impaired (creatinine clearance 30-69 ml/min/1.73 m^2) and by 54% in severely renally impaired subjects (creatinine clearance <30 ml/min/1.73 m^2) compared to normal renal function subjects (creatinine clearance >70 ml/min/1.73 m^2). Since topiramate is presumed to undergo significant tubular reabsorption, it is uncertain whether this experience can be generalized to all situations of renal impairment. It is conceivable that some forms of renal disease could differentially affect glomerular filtration rate and tubular reabsorption resulting in a clearance of topiramate not predicted by creatinine clearance. In general, however, use of one-half the usual dose is recommended in patients with moderate or severe renal impairment.

Hemodialysis

Topiramate is cleared by hemodialysis. Using a high efficiency, counterflow, single pass-dialysate hemodialysis procedure, topiramate dialysis clearance was 120 ml/min with blood flow through the dialyzer at 400 ml/min. This high clearance (compared to 20-30 ml/min total oral clearance in healthy adults) will remove a clinically significant amount of topiramate from the patient over the hemodialysis treatment period. Therefore, a supplemental dose may be required (see DOSAGE AND ADMINISTRATION).

Hepatic Impairment

In hepatically impaired subjects, the clearance of topiramate may be decreased; the mechanism underlying the decrease is not well understood.

Age, Gender, and Race

Clearance of topiramate was not affected by age (18-67 years), gender, or race.

Pediatric Pharmacokinetics

Pharmacokinetics of topiramate were evaluated in patients ages 4-17 years receiving 1 or 2 other antiepileptic drugs. Pharmacokinetic profiles were obtained after 1 week at doses of 1, 3, and 9 mg/kg/day. Clearance was independent of dose.

Pediatric patients have a 50% higher clearance and consequently shorter elimination half-life than adults. Consequently, the plasma concentration for the same mg/kg dose may be lower in pediatric patients compared to adults. As in adults, hepatic enzyme-inducing antiepileptic drugs decrease the steady-state plasma concentrations of topiramate.

INDICATIONS AND USAGE

Topiramate tablets and sprinkle capsules are indicated as adjunctive therapy for adults and pediatric patients ages 2-16 years with partial onset seizures, or primary generalized tonic-clonic seizures, and in paitents 2 years of age and older with seizures associated with Lennox-Gastaut syndrome.

NON-FDA APPROVED INDICATIONS

Topiramate has also shown efficacy as monotherapy in patients with refractory partial and generalized seizures. However, use of this drug as monotherapy has not been approved by the FDA. In one small study (n=11), an antimanic response has been reported to be reproducibly linked to the addition of topiramate. Use of topiramate as an antimanic agent has also not been approved by the FDA.

CONTRAINDICATIONS

Topiramate is contraindicated in patients with a history of hypersensitivity to any component of this product.

WARNINGS

ACUTE MYOPIA AND SECONDARY ANGLE CLOSURE GLAUCOMA

A syndrome consisting of acute myopia associated with secondary angle closure glaucoma has been reported in patients recieving topiramate. Symptoms include acute onset of decreased visual acuity and/or ocular pain. Opthalmologic findings can include myopia, anterior chamber shallowing, ocular hyperemia (redness) and increased intracoular pressure. Mydriasis may or may not be present. This syndrome may be associated with supraciliary effusion resulting in anterior displacement of the lens and iris, with secondary angle closure glaucoma. Symptoms typically occur within 1 month of initiating topiramate therapy. In contrast to primary narrow angle glaucoma, which is rare under 40 years of age, secondary angle closure glaucoma associated with topiramate has been reported in pediatric patients as well as adults. The primary treatment to reverse symptoms is discontinution of topiramate as rapidly as possible, according to the judgement of the treating physician. Other measures, in conjunction with discontinuation of topiramate, may be helpful.

Elevated intracular pressure of any etiology, if left untreated, can lead to serious sequelae including permanent vision loss.

WITHDRAWAL OF AEDS

Antiepileptic drugs, including topiramate, should be withdrawn gradually to minimize the potential of increased seizure frequency.

COGNITIVE/NEUROPSYCHIATRIC ADVERSE EVENTS

Adults

Adverse events most often associated with the use of topiramate were central nervous system related. In adults, the most significant of these can be classified into two general categories: (1) psychomotor slowing, difficulty with concentration, and speech or language problems, in particular, word-finding difficulties and (2) somnolence or fatigue. Additional nonspecific CNS effects occasionally observed with topiramate as add-on therapy include dizziness or imbalance, confusion, memory problems, and exacerbation of mood disturbances (*e.g.*, irritability and depression).

Reports of psychomotor slowing, speech and language problems, and difficulty with concentration and attention were common in adults. Although in some cases these events were mild to moderate, they at times led to withdrawal from treatment. The incidence of psychomotor slowing is only marginally dose-related, but both language problems and difficulty with concentration or attention clearly increased in frequency with increasing dosage in the five double-blind trials (see TABLE 5).

Somnolence and fatigue were the most frequently reported adverse events during clinical trials with topiramate. These events were generally mild to moderate and occurred early in therapy. While the incidence of somnolence does not appear to be dose-related, that of fatigue increases at dosages above 400 mg/day.

Pediatric Patients

In double-blind clinical studies, the incidences of cognitive/neuropsychiatric adverse events in pediatric patients were generally lower than previously observed in adults. These events included psychomotor slowing, difficutly with concentration/attention, speech disorders/related speech problems and language problems. The most frequently reported neuropsychiatric events in this population were somnolence and fatigue. No patients discontinued treatment due to adverse events in double-blind trials.

SUDDEN UNEXPLAINED DEATH IN EPILEPSY (SUDEP)

During the course of premarketing development of topiramate tablets, 10 sudden and unexplained deaths were recorded among a cohort of treated patients (2796 subject years of exposure). This represents an incidence of 0.0035 deaths per patient year. Although this rate exceeds that expected in a healthy population matched for age and sex, it is within the range of estimates for the incidence of sudden unexplained deaths in patients with epilepsy not receiving topiramate (ranging from 0.0005 for the general population of patients with epilepsy, to 0.003 for a clinical trial population similar to that in the topiramate program, to 0.005 for patients with refractory epilepsy).

PRECAUTIONS

GENERAL

Kidney Stones

A total of 32/2086 (1.5%) of adults exposed to topiramate during its development reported the occurrence of kidney stones, an incidence about 2-4 times than expected in a similar, untreated population. As in the general population, the incidence of stone formation among topiramate treated patients was higher in men. Kidney stones have also been reported in pediatric patients.

An explanation for the association of topiramate and kidney stones may lie in the fact that topiramate is a weak carbonic anhydrase inhibitor. Carbonic anhydrase inhibitors, *e.g.*, acetazolamide or dichlorphenamide, promote stone formation by reducing urinary citrate excretion and by increasing urinary pH. The concomitant use of topiramate with other carbonic anhydrase inhibitors or potentially in patients on a ketogenic diet may create a physiological environment that increases the risk of kidney stone formation, and should therefore be avoided.

Increased fluid intake increases the urinary output, lowering the concentration of substances involved in stone formation. Hydration is recommended to reduce new stone formation.

Paresthesia

Paresthesia, an effect associated with the use of other carbonic anhydrase inhibitors, appears to be a common effect of topiramate.

Adjustment of Dose in Renal Failure

The major route of elimination of unchanged topiramate and its metabolites is via the kidney. Dosage adjustment may be required (see DOSAGE AND ADMINISTRATION).

Decreased Hepatic Function

In hepatically impaired patients, topiramate should be administered with caution as the clearance of topiramate may be decreased.

INFORMATION FOR THE PATIENT

Patients taking topiramate should be told to seek immediate medical attention if they experience blurred vision or periorbital pain.

Patients, particularly those with predisposing factors, should be instructed to maintain an adequate fluid intake in order to minimize the risk of renal stone formation (see General, for support regarding hydration as a preventative measure).

Patients should be warned about the potential for somnolence, dizziness, confusion, and difficulty concentrating and advised not to drive or operate machinery until they have gained sufficient experience on topiramate to gauge whether it adversely affects their mental and/or motor performance.

Additional food intake may be considered if the patient is losing weight while on this medication.

Please refer to the important information included with the prescription on how to take topiramate sprinkle capsules.

LABORATORY TESTS

There are no known interactions of topiramate with commonly used laboratory tests.

CARCINOGENESIS, MUTAGENESIS, AND IMPAIRMENT OF FERTILITY

An increase in urinary bladder tumors was observed in mice given topiramate (20, 75, and 300 mg/kg) in the diet for 21 months. The elevated bladder tumor incidence, which was statistically significant in males and females receiving 300 mg/kg, was primarily due to the increased occurrence of a smooth muscle tumor considered histomorphologically unique to mice. Plasma exposures in mice receiving 300 mg/kg were approximately 0.5-1 times steady-state exposures measured in patients receiving topiramate monotherapy at the recommended human dose (RHD) of 400 mg, and 1.5-2 times steady-state topiramate exposures in patients receiving 400 mg of topiramate plus phenytoin. The relevance of this finding to human carcinogenic risk is uncertain. No evidence of carcinogenicity was seen in rats following oral administration of topiramate for 2 years at doses up to 120 mg/kg (approximately 3 times the RHD on a mg/m^2 basis).

Topiramate did not demonstrate genotoxic potential when tested in a battery of *in vitro* and *in vivo* assays. Topiramate was not mutagenic in the Ames test or the *in vitro* mouse lymphoma assay; it did not increase unscheduled DNA synthesis in rat hepatocytes *in vitro;* and it did not increase chromosomal aberrations in human lymphocytes *in vitro* or in rat bone marrow *in vivo.*

No adverse effects on male or female fertility were observed in rats at doses up to 100 mg/kg (2.5 times the RHD on a mg/m^2 basis).

PREGNANCY CATEGORY C

Topiramate has demonstrated selective developmental toxicity, including teratogenicity, in experimental animal studies. When oral doses of 20, 100, or 500 mg/kg were administered to pregnant mice during the period of organogenesis, the incidence of fetal malformations (primarily craniofacial defects) was increased at all doses. The low dose is approximately 0.2 times the recommended human dose (RHD = 400 mg/day) on a mg/m^2 basis. Fetal body weights and skeletal ossification were reduced at 500 mg/kg in conjunction with decreased maternal body weight gain.

In rat studies (oral doses of 20, 100, and 500 mg/kg or 0.2, 2.5, 30, and 400 mg/kg), the frequency of limb malformations (ectrodactyly, micromelia, and amelia) was increased among the offspring of dams treated with 400 mg/kg (10 times the RHD on a mg/m^2 basis) or greater during the organogenesis period of pregnancy. Embryotoxicity (reduced fetal body weights, increased incidence of structural variations) was observed at doses as low as 20 mg/kg (0.5 times the RHD on a mg/m^2 basis). Clinical signs of maternal toxicity were seen at 400 mg/kg and above, and maternal body weight gain was reduced during treatment with 100 mg/kg or greater.

In rabbit studies (20, 60, and 180 mg/kg or 10, 35, and 120 mg/kg orally during organogenesis), embryo/fetal mortality was increased at 35 mg/kg (2 times the RHD on a mg/m^2 basis) or greater, and teratogenic effects (primarily rib and vertebral malformations) were observed at 120 mg/kg (6 times the RHD on a mg/m^2 basis). Evidence of maternal toxicity (decreased body weight gain, clinical signs, and/or mortality) was seen at 35 mg/kg and above.

When female rats were treated during the latter part of gestation and throughout lactation (0.2, 4, 20, and 100 mg/kg or 2, 20, and 200 mg/kg), offspring exhibited decreased viability and delayed physical development at 200 mg/kg (5 times the RHD on a mg/m^2 basis) and reductions in pre- and/or postweaning body weight gain at 2 mg/kg (0.05 times the RHD on a mg/m^2 basis) and above. Maternal toxicity (decreased body weight gain, clinical signs) was evident at 100 mg/kg or greater.

In a rat embryo/fetal development study with a postnatal component (0.2, 2.5, 30 or 400 mg/kg during organogenesis; noted above), pups exhibited delayed physical development at 400 mg/kg (10 times the RHD on a mg/m^2 basis) and persistent reductions in body weight gain at 30 mg/kg (1 times the RHD on a mg/m^2 basis) and higher.

There are no studies using topiramate in pregnant women. Topiramate should be used during pregnancy only if the potential benefit outweighs the potential risk to the fetus.

In postmarketing experience, cases of hypospadias have been reported in male infants exposed *in utero* to topiramate, with or without other anticonvulsants; however, a causal relationship with topiramate has not been established.

LABOR AND DELIVERY

In studies of rats where dams were allowed to deliver pups naturally, no drug-related effects on gestation length or parturition were observed at dosage levels up to 200 mg/kg/day.

The effect of topiramate on labor and delivery in humans is unknown.

NURSING MOTHERS

Topiramate is excreted in the milk of lactating rats. It is not known if topiramate is excreted in human milk. Since many drugs are excreted in human milk, and because the potential for serious adverse reactions in nursing infants to topiramate is unknown, the potential benefit to the mother should be weighed against the potential risk to the infant when considering recommendations regarding nursing.

PEDIATRIC USE

Safety and effectiveness in patients below the age of 2 years have not been established.

GERIATRIC USE

In clinical trials, 2% of patients were over 60. No age related difference in effectiveness or adverse effects were seen. There were no pharmacokinetic differences related to age alone, although the possibility of age-associated renal functional abnormalities should be considered.

RACE AND GENDER EFFECTS

Evaluation of effectiveness and safety in clinical trials has shown no race or gender related effects.

DRUG INTERACTIONS

ANTIEPILEPTIC DRUGS

Potential interactions between topiramate and standard AEDs were assessed in controlled clinical pharmacokinetic studies in patients with epilepsy. The effects of these interactions on mean plasma AUCs are summarized in TABLE 3.

In TABLE 3, the second column (AED Concentration) describes what happens to the concentration of the AED listed in the first column when topiramate is added.

The third column (Topiramate Concentration) describes how the coadministration of a drug listed in the first column modifies the concentration of topiramate in experimental settings when topiramate was given alone.

TABLE 3 *Summary of AED Interactions With Topiramate*

AED Coadministered	AED Concentration	Topiramate Concentration
Phenytoin	NC or 25% increase*	48% decrease
Carbamazepine (CBZ)	NC	40% decrease
CBZ epoxide †	NC	NE
Valproic acid	11% decrease	14% decrease
Phenobarbital	NC	NE
Primidone	NC	NE

* Plasma concentration increased 25% in some patients, generally those on a bid dosing regimen of phenytoin.
† Is not administered but is an active metabolite of carbamazepine.
NC Less than 10% change in plasma concentration.
AED Antiepileptic drug.
NE Not Evaluated.

OTHER DRUG INTERACTIONS

Digoxin: In a single-dose study, serum digoxin AUC was decreased by 12% with concomitant topiramate administration. The clinical relevance of this observation has not been established.

CNS Depressants: Concomitant administration of topiramate and alcohol or other CNS depressant drugs has not been evaluated in clinical studies. Because of the potential of topiramate to cause CNS depression, as well as other cognitive and/or neuropsychiatric adverse events, topiramate should be used with extreme caution if used in combination with alcohol and other CNS depressants.

Oral Contraceptives: In a pharmacokinetic interaction study with oral contraceptives using a combination product containing norethindrone and ethinyl estradiol, topiramate did not significantly affect the clearance of norethindrone. The mean oral clearance of ethinyl estradiol at 800 mg/day dose was increased by 47% (range: 13-107%). The mean total exposure to the estrogenic component decreased by 18%, 21%, and 30% at daily doses of 200, 400, and 800 mg/day, respectively. Therefore, efficacy of oral contraceptives may be compromised by topiramate. Patients taking oral contraceptives should be asked to report any change in their bleeding patterns. The effect of oral contraceptives on the pharmacokinetics of topiramate is not known.

Metformin: A drug-drug interaction study conducted in healthy volunteers evaluated the steady-state pharmacokinetics of metformin and topiramate in plasma when metformin was given alone and when metformin and topiramate were given simultaneously. The results of this study indicated that metformin mean C_{max} and mean AUC(0-12h) increased by 18% and 25%, respectively, while mean CL/F decreased 20% when metformin was coadministered with topiramate. Topiramate did not affect metformin T_{max}. The clinical significance of the effect of topiramate on metformin pharmacokinetics is unclear. Oral plasma clearance of topiramate appears to be reduced when administered with metformin. The extent of change in the clearance is unknown. The clinical significance of the effect of metformin on topiramate pharmacokinetics is unclear. When topiramate is added or withdrawn in patients on metformin therapy, careful attention should be given to the routine monitoring for adequate control of their diabetic disease state.

Others: Concomitant use of topiramate, a weak carbonic anhydrase inhibitor, with other carbonic anhydrase inhibitors, *e.g.*, acetazolamide or dichlorphenamide, may create a physiological environment that increases the risk of renal stone formation, and should therefore be avoided.

ADVERSE REACTIONS

The data described in the following section were obtained using topiramate tablets.

The most commonly observed adverse events associated with the use of topiramate at dosages of 200-400 mg/day in controlled trials in adults with partial onset seizures, primary generalized tonic-clonic seizures, or Lennox-Gastaut syndrome, that were seen at greater frequency in topiramate-treated patients and did not appear to be dose-related were: somnolence, dizziness, ataxia, speech disorders and related speech problems, psychomotor slowing, abnormal vision, difficulty with memory, paresthesia and diplopia (see TABLE 4). The most common dose-related adverse events at dosages of 200-1000 mg/day were: fatigue, nervousness, difficulty with concentration or attention, confusion, depression, anorexia, language problems, anxiety, mood problems, and weight decreased (see TABLE 5).

Adverse events associated with the use of topiramate at dosages of 5-9 mg/kg/day in controlled trials in pediatric patients with partial onset seizures, primary generalized tonic-clonic seizures, or Lennox-Gastaut syndrome, that were seen at greater frequency in topiramate-treated patients were: fatigue, somnolence, anorexia, nervousness, difficulty with concentration/attention, difficulty with memory, aggressive reaction, and weight decrease (see TABLE 6).

In controlled clinical trials in adults, 11% of patients receiving topiramate 200-400 mg/day as adjunctive therapy discontinued due to adverse events. This rate appeared to increase at dosages above 400 mg/day. Adverse events associated with discontinuing therapy included somnolence, dizziness, anxiety, difficulty with concentration or attention, fatigue, and paresthesia and increased at dosages above 400 mg/day. None of the pediatric patients who received topiramate adjunctive therapy at 5-9 mg/kg/day in controlled clinical trials discontinued due to adverse events.

Approximately 28% of the 1757 adults with epilepsy who received topiramate at dosages of 200-1600 mg/day in clinical studies discontinued treatment because of adverse events; an individual patient could have reported more than one adverse event. These adverse events were: psychomotor slowing (4.0%), difficulty with memory (3.2%), fatigue (3.2%), confusion (3.1%), somnolence (3.2%), difficulty with concentration/attention (2.9%), anorexia (2.7%), depression (2.6%), dizziness (2.5%), weight decrease (2.5%), nervousness (2.3%), ataxia (2.1%), and paresthesia (2.0%). Approximately 11% of the 310 pediatric patients who received topiramate at dosages up to 30 mg/kg/day discontinued due to adverse events. Adverse events associated with discontinuing therapy included aggravated convulsions (2.3%), difficulty with concentration/attention (1.6%), language problems (1.3%), personality disorder (1.3%), and somnolence (1.3%).

INCIDENCE IN CONTROLLED CLINICAL TRIALS — ADD-ON THERAPY

TABLE 4 lists treatment-emergent adverse events that occurred in at least 1% of adults treated with 200-400 mg/day topiramate in controlled trials that were numerically more common at this dose than in the patients treated with placebo. In general, most patients who experienced adverse events during the first 8 weeks of these trials no longer experienced them by their last visit. TABLE 6 lists treatment-emergent adverse events that occurred in at least 1% of pediatric patients treated with 5-9 mg/kg topiramate in controlled trials that were numerically more common than in patients treated with placebo.

The prescriber should be aware that these data were obtained when topiramate was added to concurrent antiepileptic drug therapy and cannot be used to predict the frequency of adverse events in the course of usual medical practice where patient characteristics and other factors may differ from those prevailing during clinical studies. Similarly, the cited frequencies cannot be directly compared with data obtained from other clinical investigations involving different treatments, uses, or investigators. Inspection of these frequencies, however, does provide the prescribing physician with a basis to estimate the relative contribution of drug and non-drug factors to the adverse event incidences in the population studied.

OTHER ADVERSE EVENTS OBSERVED

Other events that occurred in more than 1% of adults treated with 200-400 mg of topiramate in placebo-controlled trials but with equal or greater frequency in the placebo group were: headache, injury, anxiety, rash, pain, convulsions aggravated, coughing, fever, diarrhea, vomiting, muscle weakness, insomnia, personality disorder, dysmenorrhea, upper respiratory tract infection, and eye pain.

OTHER ADVERSE EVENTS OBSERVED DURING ALL CLINICAL TRIALS

Topiramate, initiated as adjunctive therapy, has been administered to 1757 adults and 310 pediatric patients with epilepsy during all clinical studies. During these studies, all adverse events were recorded by the clinical investigators using terminology of their own choosing. To provide a meaningful estimate of the proportion of individuals having adverse events, similar types of events were grouped into a smaller number of standardized categories using modified WHOART dictionary terminology. The frequencies presented represent the proportion of patients who experienced an event of the type cited on at least one occasion while receiving topiramate. Reported events are included except those already listed in the previous table or text, those too general to be informative, and those not reasonably associated with the use of the drug.

Events are classified within body system categories and enumerated in order of decreasing frequency using the following definitions: *frequent* occurring in at least 1/100 patients; *infrequent* occurring in 1/100 to 1/1000 patients; *rare* occurring in fewer than 1/1000 patients.

Autonomic Nervous System Disorders: *Infrequent:* Vasodilation.

Body as a Whole: *Frequent:* Fever. *Infrequent:* Syncope, abdomen enlarged. *Rare:* Alcohol intolerance.

Cardiovascular Disorders, General: *Infrequent:* Hypotension, postural hypotension.

T

TABLE 4 *Incidence of Treatment-Emergent Adverse Events in Placebo-Controlled, Add-On Trials in Adults*† Where Rate Was >1% in Either Topiramate Group and Greater Than the Rate in Placebo-Treated Patients*

Body System		Topiramate Dosage (mg/day)	
	Placebo	200-400	600-1000
Adverse Event‡	(n=291)	(n=183)	(n=414)
Body as a Whole — General Disorders			
Fatigue	13%	15%	30%
Asthenia	1%	6%	3%
Back pain	4%	5%	3%
Chest pain	3%	4%	2%
Influenza-like symptoms	2%	3%	4%
Leg pain	2%	2%	4%
Hot flushes	1%	2%	1%
Allergy	1%	2%	3%
Edema	1%	2%	1%
Body odor	0%	1%	0%
Rigors	0%	1%	<1%
Central and Peripheral Nervous System Disorders			
Dizziness	15%	25%	32%
Ataxia	7%	16%	14%
Speech disorders/related speech problems	2%	13%	11%
Paresthesia	4%	11%	19%
Nystagmus	7%	10%	11%
Tremor	6%	9%	9%
Language problems	1%	6%	10%
Coordination abnormal	2%	4%	4%
Hypoaesthesia	1%	2%	1%
Gait abnormal	1%	3%	2%
Muscle contractions involuntary	1%	2%	2%
Stupor	0%	2%	1%
Vertigo	1%	1%	2%
Gastrointestinal System Disorders			
Nausea	8%	10%	12%
Dyspepsia	6%	7%	6%
Abdominal pain	4%	6%	7%
Constipation	2%	4%	3%
Gastroenteritis	1%	2%	1%
Dry mouth	1%	2%	4%
Gingivitis	<1%	1%	1%
GI disorder	<1%	1%	0%
Hearing and Vestibular Disorders			
Hearing decreased	1%	2%	1%
Metabolic and Nutritional Disorders			
Weight decrease	3%	9%	13%
Musculoskeletal System Disorders			
Myalgia	1%	2%	2%
Skeletal pain	0%	1%	0%
Platelet, Bleeding and Clotting Disorders			
Epistaxis	1%	2%	1%
Psychiatric Disorders			
Somnolence	12%	29%	28%
Nervousness	6%	16%	19%
Psychomotor slowing	2%	13%	21%
Difficulty with memory	3%	12%	14%
Anorexia	4%	10%	12%
Confusion	5%	11%	14%
Depression	5%	5%	13%
Difficulty with concentration/attention	2%	6%	14%
Mood problems	2%	4%	9%
Agitation	2%	3%	3%
Aggressive reaction	2%	3%	3%
Emotional lability	1%	3%	3%
Cognitive problems	1%	3%	3%
Libido decreased	1%	2%	<1%
Apathy	1%	1%	3%
Depersonalization	1%	1%	2%
Reproductive Disorders, Female			
Breast pain	2%	4%	0%
Amenorrhea	1%	2%	2%
Menorrhagia	0%	2%	1%
Menstrual disorder	1%	2%	1%
Reproductive Disorders, Male			
Prostatic disorder	<1%	2%	0%
Resistance Mechanism Disorders			
Infection	1%	2%	1%
Infection viral	1%	2%	<1%
Moniliasis	<1%	1%	0%
Respiratory System Disorders			
Pharyngitis	2%	6%	3%
Rhinitis	6%	7%	6%
Sinusitis	4%	5%	6%
Dyspnea	1%	1%	2%

(Table continued in next column)

Central and Peripheral Nervous System Disorders: *Frequent:* Hypertonia. *Infrequent:* Neuropathy, apraxia, hyperaesthesia, dyskinesia, dysphonia, scotoma, ptosis, dystonia, visual field defect, encephalopathy, upper motor neuron lesion, EEG abnormal. *Rare:* Cerebellar syndrome, tongue paralysis.

Gastrointestinal System Disorders: *Frequent:* Diarrhea, vomiting, hemorrhoids. *Infrequent:* Stomatitis, melena, gastritis, tongue edema, esophagitis.

Hearing and Vestibular Disorders: *Frequent:* Tinnitus.

Heart Rate and Rhythm Disorders: *Infrequent:* AV block, bradycardia.

Liver and Biliary System Disorders: *Infrequent:* SGPT increased, SGOT increased, gamma-GT increased.

Metabolic and Nutritional Disorders: *Frequent:* Dehydration. *Infrequent:* Hypokalemia, alkaline phosphatase increased, hypocalcemia, hyperlipemia, acidosis, hyper-

TABLE 4 (cont.) *Incidence of Treatment-Emergent Adverse Events in Placebo-Controlled, Add-On Trials in Adults*† Where Rate Was >1% in Either Topiramate Group and Greater Than the Rate in Placebo-Treated Patients*

Body System		Topiramate Dosage (mg/day)	
Adverse Event‡	Placebo (n=291)	200-400 (n=183)	600-1000 (n=414)
Skin and Appendages Disorders			
Skin disorder	<1%	2%	1%
Sweating increased	<1%	1%	<1%
Rash erythematous	<1%	1%	<1%
Special Senses Other, Disorders			
Taste perversion	0%	2%	4%
Urinary System Disorders			
Hematuria	1%	2%	<1%
Urinary tract infection	1%	2%	3%
Micturition frequency	1%	1%	2%
Urinary incontinence	<1%	2%	1%
Urine abnormal	0%	1%	<1%
Vision Disorders			
Vision abnormal	2%	13%	10%
Diplopia	5%	10%	10%
White Cell and RES Disorders			
Leukopenia	1%	2%	1%

* Patients in these add-on trials were receiving 1-2 concomitant antiepileptic drugs in addition to topiramate or placebo.
† Values represent the percentage of patients reporting a given adverse event. Patients may have reported more than one adverse event during the study and can be included in more than one adverse event category.
‡ Adverse events reported by at least 1% of patients in the topiramate 200-400 mg/day group and more common than in the placebo group are listed in this table.

TABLE 5 *Incidence (%) of Dose-Related Adverse Events From Placebo-Controlled, Add-On Trials in Adults With Partial Onset Seizures**

		Topiramate Dosage (mg/day)		
Adverse Event	Placebo (n=216)	200 (n=45)	400 (n=68)	600-1000 (n=414)
Fatigue	13%	11%	12%	30%
Nervousness	7%	13%	18%	19%
Difficulty with concentration/ attention	1%	7%	9%	14%
Confusion	4%	9%	10%	14%
Depression	6%	9%	7%	13%
Anorexia	4%	4%	6%	12%
Language problems	<1%	2%	9%	10%
Anxiety	6%	2%	3%	10%
Mood problems	2%	0%	6%	9%
Weight decrease	3%	4%	9%	13%

* Dose-response studies were not conducted for other adult indications or for pediatric indications.

glycemia, hyperchloremia, xerophthalmia. *Rare:* Diabetes mellitus, hypernatremia, hyponatremia, hypocholesterolemia, hypophosphatemia, creatinine increased.

Musculoskeletal System Disorders: *Frequent:* Arthralgia, muscle weakness. *Infrequent:* Arthrosis.

Myo-, Endo-, Pericardial and Valve Disorders: *Infrequent:* Angina pectoris.

Neoplasms: *Infrequent:* Thrombocythemia. *Rare:* Polycythemia.

Platelet, Bleeding, and Clotting Disorders: *Infrequent:* Gingival bleeding, pulmonary embolism.

Psychiatric Disorders: *Frequent:* Impotence, hallucination, euphoria, psychosis. *Infrequent:* Paranoid reaction, delusion, paranoia, delirium, abnormal dreaming, neurosis, libido increased, manic reaction, suicide attempt.

Red Blood Cell Disorders: *Frequent:* Anemia. *Rare:* Marrow depression, pancytopenia.

Reproductive Disorders, Male: *Infrequent:* Ejaculation disorder, breast discharge.

Skin and Appendages Disorders: *Frequent:* Acne, urticaria. *Infrequent:* Photosensitivity reaction, sweating decreased, abnormal hair texture. *Rare:* Chloasma.

Special Senses Other, Disorders: *Infrequent:* Taste loss, parosmia.

Urinary System Disorders: *Frequent:* Dysuria, renal calculus. *Infrequent:* Urinary retention, face edema, renal pain, albuminuria, polyuria, oliguria.

Vascular (extracardiac) Disorders: *Infrequent:* Flushing, deep vein thrombosis, phlebitis. *Rare:* Vasospasm.

Vision Disorders: *Frequent:* Conjunctivitis. *Infrequent:* Abnormal accommodation, photophobia, strabismus, mydriasis. *Rare:* Iritis.

White Cell and Reticuloendothelial System Disorders: *Infrequent:* Lymphadenopathy, eosinophilia, lymphopenia, granulocytopenia, lymphocytosis.

TABLE 6 *Incidence (%) of Treatment-Emergent Adverse Events in Placebo-Controlled, Add-On Trials in Pediatric Patients Ages 2-16 Years*†‡*

Body System Adverse Event	Placebo (n=101)	Topiramate (n=98)
Body as a Whole — General Disorders		
Fatigue	5%	16%
Injury	13%	14%
Allergic reaction	1%	2%
Back pain	0%	1%
Pallor	0%	1%
Cardiovascular Disorders, General		
Hypertension	0%	1%
Central and Peripheral Nervous System Disorders		
Gait abnormal	5%	8%
Ataxia	2%	6%
Hyperkinesia	4%	5%
Dizziness	2%	4%
Speech disorders/related speech problems	2%	4%
Hyporeflexia	0%	2%
Convulsions grand mal	0%	1%
Fecal incontinence	0%	1%
Paresthesia	0%	1%
Gastrointestinal System Disorders		
Nausea	5%	6%
Saliva increased	4%	6%
Constipation	4%	5%
Gastroenteritis	2%	3%
Dysphagia	0%	1%
Flatulence	0%	1%
Gastroesophageal reflux	0%	1%
Glossitis	0%	1%
Gum hyperplasia	0%	1%
Heart Rate and Rhythm Disorders		
Bradycardia	0%	1%
Metabolic and Nutritional Disorders		
Weight decrease	1%	9%
Thirst	1%	2%
Hypoglycemia	0%	1%
Weight increase	0%	1%
Platelet, Bleeding, and Clotting Disorders		
Purpura	4%	8%
Epistaxis	1%	4%
Hematoma	0%	1%
Prothrombin increased	0%	1%
Thrombocytopenia	0%	1%
Psychiatric Disorders		
Somnolence	16%	26%
Anorexia	15%	24%
Nervousness	7%	14%
Personality disorder (behavior problems)	9%	11%
Difficulty with concentration/attention	2%	10%
Aggressive reaction	4%	9%
Insomnia	7%	8%
Difficulty with memory NOS	0%	5%
Confusion	3%	4%
Psychomotor slowing	2%	3%
Appetite increased	0%	1%
Neurosis	0%	1%
Reproductive Disorders, Female		
Leukorrhoea	0%	2%
Resistance Mechanism Disorders		
Infection viral	3%	7%
Respiratory System Disorders		
Pneumonia	1%	5%
Respiratory disorder	0%	1%
Skin and Appendages Disorders		
Skin disorder	2%	3%
Alopecia	1%	2%
Dermatitis	0%	2%
Hypertrichosis	1%	2%
Rash erythematous	0%	2%
Eczema	0%	1%
Seborrhoea	0%	1%
Skin discoloration	0%	1%
Urinary System Disorders		
Urinary incontinence	2%	4%
Nocturia	0%	1%
Vision Disorders		
Eye abnormality	1%	2%
Vision abnormal	1%	2%
Diplopia	0%	1%
Lacrimation abnormal	0%	1%
Myopia	0%	1%
White Cell and RES Disorders		
Leukopenia	0%	2%

* Events that occurred in at least 1% of topiramate-treated patients and occurred more frequently in topiramate-treated than placebo-treated patients.
† Patients in these add-on trials were receiving 1-2 concomitant antiepileptic drugs in addition to topiramate or placebo.
‡ Values represent the percentage of patients reporting a given adverse event. Patients may have reported more than one adverse event during the study and can be included in more than one adverse event category.

POSTMARKETING AND OTHER EXPERIENCE

In addition to the adverse experiences reported during clinical testing of topiramate, the following adverse experiences have been reported worldwide in patients receiving topiramate post-approval. These adverse experiences have not been listed above and data are insufficient to support an estimate of their incidence or to establish causation. The listing is alphabetized: hepatic failure, (including fatalities), hepatitis, pancreatitis, and renal tubular acidosis.

DOSAGE AND ADMINISTRATION

Topiramate has been shown to be effective in adults and pediatric patients ages 2-16 years with partial onset seizures or primary generalized tonic-clonic seizures, and in patients 2 years of age and older with seizures associated with Lennox-Gastaut syndrome. In the controlled add-on trials, no correlation has been demonstrated between trough plasma concentrations of topiramate and clinical efficacy. No evidence of tolerance has been demonstrated

T

in humans. Doses above 400 mg/day (600, 800, or 1000 mg/day) have not been shown to improve responses in dose-response studies in adults with partial onset seizures.

It is not necessary to monitor topiramate plasma concentrations to optimize topiramate therapy. On occasion, the addition of topiramate to phenytoin may require an adjustment of the dose of phenytoin to achieve optimal clinical outcome. Addition or withdrawal of phenytoin and/or carbamazepine during adjunctive therapy with topiramate may require adjustment of the dose of topiramate. Because of the bitter taste, tablets should not be broken.

Topiramate can be taken without regard to meals.

ADULTS (17 YEARS OF AGE AND OVER)

The recommended total daily dose of topiramate as adjunctive therapy is 400 mg/day in two divided doses. In studies of adults with partial onset seizures, a daily dose of 200 mg/day has inconsistent effects and is less effective than 400 mg/day. It is recommended that therapy be initiated at 25-50 mg/day followed by titration to an effective dose in increments of 25-50 mg/week. Titrating in increments of 25 mg/week may delay the time to reach an effective dose. Daily doses above 1600 mg have not been studied.

In the study of primary generalized tonic-clonic seizures the initial titration rate was slower than in previous studies; the assigned dose was reached at the end of 8 weeks.

PEDIATRIC PATIENTS (AGES 2-16 YEARS) — PARTIAL SEIZURES, PRIMARY GENERALIZED TONIC-CLONIC SEIZURES, OR LENNOX-GASTAUT SYNDROME

The recommended total daily dose of topiramate as adjunctive therapy for patients with partial seizures, primary generalized tonic-clonic seizures, or seizures associated with Lennox-Gastaut syndrome is approximately 5-9 mg/kg/day in two divided doses. Titration should begin at 25 mg (or less, based on a range of 1-3 mg/kg/day) nightly for the first week. The dosage should then be increased at 1 or 2 week intervals by increments of 1-3 mg/kg/day (administered in two divided doses), to achieve optimal clinical response. Dose titration should be guided by clinical outcome.

In the study of primary generalized tonic-clonic seizures the initial titration rate was slower than in previous studies; the assigned dose of 6 mg/kg/day was reached at the end of 8 weeks.

ADMINISTRATION OF TOPIRAMATE SPRINKLE CAPSULES

Topiramate sprinkle capsules may be swallowed whole or may be administered by carefully opening the capsule and sprinkling the entire contents on a small amount (teaspoon) of soft food. This drug/food mixture should be swallowed immediately and not chewed. It should not be stored for future use.

PATIENTS WITH RENAL IMPAIRMENT

In renally impaired subjects (creatinine clearance less than 70 ml/min/1.73 m^2), one-half of the usual adult dose is recommended. Such patients will require a longer time to reach steady-state at each dose.

PATIENTS UNDERGOING HEMODIALYSIS

Topiramate is cleared by hemodialysis at a rate that is 4-6 times greater than a normal individual. Accordingly, a prolonged period of dialysis may cause topiramate concentration to fall below that required to maintain an anti-seizure effect. To avoid rapid drops in topiramate plasma concentration during hemodialysis, a supplemental dose of topiramate may be required. The actual adjustment should take into account (1) the duration of dialysis period, (2) the clearance rate of the dialysis system being used, and (3) the effective renal clearance of topiramate in the patient being dialyzed.

PATIENTS WITH HEPATIC DISEASE

In hepatically impaired patients topiramate plasma concentrations may be increased. The mechanism is not well understood.

HOW SUPPLIED

TOPAMAX TABLETS

Topamax is available as debossed, coated, round tablets in the following strengths and colors:

25 mg: White and coded with "TOP" on one side; "25" on the other.
100 mg: Yellow and coded with "TOPAMAX" on one side; "100" on the other.
200 mg: Salmon and coded with "TOPAMAX" on one side; "200" on the other.

Storage: Topamax tablets should be stored in tightly-closed containers at controlled room temperature, 15-30°C (59-86°F). Protect from moisture.

TOPAMAX SPRINKLE CAPSULES

Topamax sprinkle capsules contain small, white to off-white spheres. The gelatin capsules are white and clear. They are marked as follows:

15 mg: With "TOP" and "15 mg" on the side.
25 mg: With "TOP" and "25 mg" on the side.

Storage: Topamax sprinkle capsules should be stored in tightly-closed containers at or below 25°C (77°F). Protect from moisture.

PRODUCT LISTING - EQUIVALENTS NOT AVAILABLE

Capsule - Oral - 15 mg

60's	$91.46	TOPAMAX SPRINKLE, Janssen Pharmaceuticals	00045-0647-65

Capsule - Oral - 25 mg

60's	$110.55	TOPAMAX SPRINKLE, Janssen Pharmaceuticals	00045-0645-65

Tablet - Oral - 25 mg

10's	$17.40	TOPAMAX, Southwood Pharmaceuticals Inc	58016-0478-10
20's	$28.80	TOPAMAX, Southwood Pharmaceuticals Inc	58016-0478-20
30's	$52.20	TOPAMAX, Southwood Pharmaceuticals Inc	58016-0478-30
40's	$69.59	TOPAMAX, Southwood Pharmaceuticals Inc	58016-0478-40
60's	$79.28	TOPAMAX, Allscripts Pharmaceutical Company	54569-4831-00
60's	$96.70	TOPAMAX, Janssen Pharmaceuticals	00045-0639-65
60's	$104.39	TOPAMAX, Southwood Pharmaceuticals Inc	58016-0478-60
90's	$156.59	TOPAMAX, Southwood Pharmaceuticals Inc	58016-0478-90
100's	$173.98	TOPAMAX, Southwood Pharmaceuticals Inc	58016-0478-00

Tablet - Oral - 100 mg

60's	$226.70	TOPAMAX, Janssen Pharmaceuticals	00045-0641-65

Tablet - Oral - 200 mg

60's	$265.41	TOPAMAX, Janssen Pharmaceuticals	00045-0642-65

Topotecan Hydrochloride *(003288)*

Categories: Carcinoma, lung; Carcinoma, ovarian; Pregnancy Category D; FDA Approved 1996 May
Drug Classes: Antineoplastics, topoisomerase inhibitors
Brand Names: Hycamtin
Foreign Brand Availability: Oncotecan (Colombia); Topotel (India)
HCFA JCODE(S): J9350 4 mg IV

WARNING

Topotecan HCl for injection should be administered under the supervision of a physician experienced in the use of cancer chemotherapeutic agents. Appropriate management of complications is possible only when adequate diagnostic and treatment facilities are readily available.

Therapy with topotecan HCl should not be given to patients with baseline neutrophil counts of less than 1500 cells/mm^3. In order to monitor the occurrence of bone marrow suppression, primarily neutropenia, which may be severe and result in infection and death, frequent peripheral blood cell counts should be performed on all patients receiving topotecan HCl.

DESCRIPTION

Topotecan hydrochloride is a semisynthetic derivative of camptothecin and is an anti-tumor drug with topoisomerase I-inhibitory activity.

Hycamtin for injection is supplied as a sterile lyophilized, buffered, light yellow to greenish powder available in single-dose vials. Each vial contains topotecan HCl equivalent to 4 mg of topotecan as free base. The reconstituted solution ranges in color from yellow to yellow-green and is intended for administration by intravenous infusion.

Inactive ingredients are mannitol, 48 mg, and tartaric acid, 20 mg. Hydrochloric acid and sodium hydroxide may be used to adjust the pH. The solution pH ranges from 2.5-3.5.

The chemical name for topotecan HCl is (*S*)-10-[(dimethylamino)methyl]-4-ethyl-4,9-dihydroxy-1*H*-pyrano[3',4':6,7] indolizino [1,2-*b*]quinoline-3,14-(4*H*,12*H*)-dione monohydrochloride. It has the molecular formula $C_{23}H_{23}N_3O_5$·HCl and a molecular weight of 457.9.

It is soluble in water and melts with decomposition at 213-218°C.

CLINICAL PHARMACOLOGY

MECHANISM OF ACTION

Topoisomerase I relieves torsional strain in DNA by inducing reversible single strand breaks. Topotecan binds to the topoisomerase I-DNA complex and prevents religation of these single strand breaks. The cytotoxicity of topotecan is thought to be due to double strand DNA damage produced during DNA synthesis when replication enzymes interact with the ternary complex formed by topotecan, topoisomerase I and DNA. Mammalian cells cannot efficiently repair these double strand breaks.

PHARMACOKINETICS

The pharmacokinetics of topotecan have been evaluated in cancer patients following doses of 0.5-1.5 mg/m^2 administered as a 30 minute infusion. Topotecan exhibits multiexponential pharmacokinetics with a terminal half-life of 2-3 hours. Total exposure (AUC) is approximately dose-proportional. Binding of topotecan to plasma proteins is about 35%.

Metabolism and Elimination

Topotecan undergoes a reversible pH dependent hydrolysis of its lactone moiety; it is the lactone form that is pharmacologically active. At pH ≤4 the lactone is exclusively present whereas the ring-opened hydroxy-acid form predominates at physiologic pH. *In vitro* studies in human liver microsomes indicate that metabolism of topotecan to a N-demethylated metabolite represents a minor metabolic pathway.

In humans, about 30% of the dose is excreted in the urine and renal clearance is an important determinant of topotecan elimination (see Special Populations).

SPECIAL POPULATIONS

Gender

The overall mean topotecan plasma clearance in male patients was approximately 24% higher than in female patients, largely reflecting difference in body size.

Geriatrics

Topotecan pharmacokinetics have not been specifically studied in an elderly population, but population pharmacokinetic analysis in female patients did not identify age as a significant factor. Decreased renal clearance, common in the elderly, is a more important determinant of topotecan clearance.

Race
The effect of race on topotecan pharmacokinetics has not been studied.

Renal Impairment
In patients with mild renal impairment (creatinine clearance of 40-60 ml/min), topotecan plasma clearance was decreased to about 67% of the value in patients with normal renal function. In patients with moderate renal impairment (CLCR of 20-39 ml/min), topotecan plasma clearance was reduced to about 34% of the value in control patients, with an increase in half-life. Mean half-life, estimated in 3 renally impaired patients, was about 5.0 hours. Dosage adjustment is recommended for these patients (see DOSAGE AND ADMINISTRATION).

Hepatic Impairment
Plasma clearance in patients with hepatic impairment (serum bilirubin levels between 1.7 and 15.0 mg/dl) was decreased to about 67% of the value in patients without hepatic impairment. Topotecan half-life increased slightly, from 2.0-2.5 hours, but these hepatically impaired patients tolerated the usual recommended topotecan dosage regimen (see DOSAGE AND ADMINISTRATION).

Drug Interactions
Pharmacokinetic studies of the interaction of topotecan with concomitantly administered medications have not been formally investigated. *In vitro* inhibition studies using marker substrates known to be metabolized by human P450 CYP1A2, CYP2A6, CYP2C8/9, CYP2C19, CYP2D6, CYP2E, CYP3A, or CYP4A or dihydropyrimidine dehydrogenase indicate that the activities of these enzymes were not altered by topotecan. Enzyme inhibition by topotecan has not been evaluated *in vivo*.

PHARMACODYNAMICS
The dose-limiting toxicity of topotecan is leukopenia. White blood cell count decreases with increasing topotecan dose or topotecan AUC. When topotecan is administered at a dose of 1.5 mg/m^2/day for 5 days, an 80-90% decrease in white blood cell count at nadir is typically observed after the first cycle of therapy.

INDICATIONS AND USAGE

Topotecan HCl is indicated for the treatment of:

Metastatic carcinoma of the ovary after failure of initial or subsequent chemotherapy.

Small cell lung cancer sensitive disease after failure of first-line chemotherapy. In clinical studies submitted to support approval, sensitive disease was defined as disease responding to chemotherapy but subsequently progressing at least 60 days (in the Phase 3 study) or at least 90 days (in the Phase 2 studies) after chemotherapy.

NON-FDA APPROVED INDICATIONS
While not approved by the FDA, activity has been demonstrated in breast cancer, non-small cell lung cancer, soft tissue sarcoma, and acute leukemias (including the lymphocytic, lymphoblastic, and myeloid forms). Limited activity has been demonstrated in colorectal cancer. Topotecan has been shown to have significant effectiveness in the treatment of myelodysplastic syndrome and chronic myelomonocytic leukemia.

CONTRAINDICATIONS

Topotecan HCl is contraindicated in patients who have a history of hypersensitivity reactions to topotecan or to any of its ingredients. Topotecan HCl should not be used in patients who are pregnant or breast-feeding, or those with severe bone marrow depression.

WARNINGS

Bone marrow suppression (primarily neutropenia) is the dose-limiting toxicity of topotecan. Neutropenia is not cumulative over time. The following data on myelosuppression with topotecan is based on the combined experience of 879 patients with metastatic ovarian cancer or small cell lung cancer.

NEUTROPENIA
Grade 4 neutropenia (<500 cells/mm^3) was most common during course 1 of treatment (60% of patients) and occurred in 39% of all courses, with a median duration of 7 days. The nadir neutrophil count occurred at a median of 12 days. Therapy-related sepsis or febrile neutropenia occurred in 23% of patients and sepsis was fatal in 1%.

THROMBOCYTOPENIA
Grade 4 thrombocytopenia (<25,000/mm^3) occurred in 27% of patients and in 9% of courses, with a median duration of 5 days and platelet nadir at a median of 15 days. Platelet transfusions were given to 15% of patients in 4% of courses.

ANEMIA
Grade 3/4 anemia (<8 g/dl) occurred in 37% of patients and in 14% of courses. Median nadir was at day 15. Transfusions were needed in 52% of patients in 22% of courses.

In ovarian cancer, the overall treatment-related death rate was 1%. In the comparative study in small cell lung cancer, however, the treatment-related death rates were 5% for topotecan HCl and 4% for CAV.

MONITORING OF BONE MARROW FUNCTION
Topotecan HCl should only be administered in patients with adequate bone marrow reserves, including baseline neutrophil count of at least 1500 cells/mm^3 and platelet count at least 100,000/mm^3. Frequent monitoring of peripheral blood cell counts should be instituted during treatment with topotecan HCl. Patients should not be treated with subsequent course of topotecan HCl until neutrophils recover to >1000 cells/mm^3, platelets recover to >100,000 cells/mm^3 and hemoglobin levels recover to 9.0 g/dl (with transfusion if necessary). Severe myelotoxicity has been reported when topotecan HCl is used in combination with cisplatin (see DRUG INTERACTIONS).

PREGNANCY
Topotecan HCl may cause fetal harm when administered to a pregnant woman. The effects of topotecan on pregnant women have not been studied. If topotecan is used during a patient's pregnancy, or if a patient becomes pregnant while taking topotecan, she should be warned of the potential hazard to the fetus. Fecund women should be warned to avoid becoming pregnant. In rabbits, a dose of 0.10 mg/kg/day (about equal to the clinical dose on a mg/m^2 basis) given on days 6 through 20 of gestation caused maternal toxicity, embryolethality, and reduced fetal body weight. In the rat, a dose of 0.23 mg/kg/day (about equal to the clinical dose on a mg/m^2 basis) given for 14 days before mating through gestation day 6 caused fetal resorption, microphthalmia, pre-implant loss, and mild maternal toxicity. A dose of 0.10 mg/kg/day (about half the clinical dose on a mg/m^2 basis) given to rats on days 6 through 17 of gestation caused an increase in post-implantation mortality. This dose also caused an increase in total fetal malformations. The most frequent malformations were of the eye (microphthalmia, anophthalmia, rosette formation of the retina, coloboma of the retina, ectopic orbit), brain (dilated lateral and third ventricles), skull and vertebrae.

PRECAUTIONS

GENERAL
Inadvertent extravasation with topotecan HCl has been associated only with mild local reactions such as erythema and bruising.

INFORMATION FOR THE PATIENT
As with other chemotherapeutic agents, topotecan HCl may cause asthenia or fatigue; if these symptoms occur, caution should be observed when driving or operating machinery.

HEMATOLOGY
Monitoring of bone marrow function is essential (see WARNINGS and DOSAGE AND ADMINISTRATION).

CARCINOGENESIS, MUTAGENESIS, AND IMPAIRMENT OF FERTILITY
Carcinogenicity testing of topotecan has not been performed. Topotecan, however, is known to be genotoxic to mammalian cells and is a probable carcinogen. Topotecan was mutagenic to L5178Y mouse lymphoma cells and clastogenic to cultured human lymphocytes with and without metabolic activation. It was also clastogenic to mouse bone marrow. Topotecan did not cause mutations in bacterial cells.

PREGNANCY CATEGORY D
See WARNINGS.

NURSING MOTHERS
It is not known whether the drug is excreted in human milk. Breast-feeding should be discontinued when women are receiving topotecan HCl (see CONTRAINDICATIONS).

PEDIATRIC USE
Safety and effectiveness in pediatric patients have not been established.

DRUG INTERACTIONS

Concomitant administration of G-CSF can prolong the duration of neutropenia, so if G-CSF is to be used, it should not be initiated until day 6 of the course of therapy, 24 hours after completion of treatment with topotecan HCl.[1]

Myelosuppression was more severe when topotecan HCl was given in combination with cisplatin in Phase 1 studies. In a reported study on concomitant administration of cisplatin 50 mg/m^2 and topotecan HCl at a dose of 1.25 mg/m^2/day × 5 days, 1 of 3 patients had severe neutropenia for 12 days and a second patient died with neutropenic sepsis. There are no adequate data to define a safe and effective regimen for topotecan HCl and cisplatin in combination.

ADVERSE REACTIONS

Data in the following section are based on the combined experience of 453 patients with metastatic ovarian carcinoma, and 426 patients with small cell lung cancer treated with topotecan HCl. TABLE 4 lists the principal hematologic toxicities and TABLE 5A and TABLE 5B list non-hematologic toxicities occurring in at least 15% of patients.

TABLE 4 *Summary of Hematologic Adverse Events in Patients Receiving Topotecan HCl*

Hematologic Adverse Events	Patients (n=879) Incidence	Courses (n=4124) Incidence
Neutropenia		
<1500 cells/mm^3	97%	81%
<500 cells/mm^3	78%	39%
Leukopenia		
<3000 cells/mm^3	97%	80%
<1000 cells/mm^3	32%	11%
Thrombocytopenia		
<75,000/mm^3	69%	42%
<25,000/mm^3	27%	9%
Anemia		
<10 g/dl	89%	71%
<8 g/dl	37%	14%
Sepsis or fever/infection with Grade 4 neutropenia	23%	7%
Platelet transfusions	15%	4%
RBC transfusions	52%	22%

T

TABLE 5A *Summary of Non-Hematologic Adverse Events in Patients Receiving Topotecan HCl*

Non-Hematologic Adverse Events	All Grades Incidence	
	n=879	n=4124
	Patients	Courses
Gastrointestinal		
Nausea	64%	42%
Vomiting	45%	22%
Diarrhea	32%	14%
Constipation	29%	15%
Abdominal pain	22%	10%
Stomatitis	18%	8%
Anorexia	19%	9%
Body as a Whole		
Fatigue	29%	22%
Fever	28%	11%
Pain*	23%	11%
Asthenia	25%	13%
Skin/Appendages		
Alopecia	49%	54%
Rash†	16%	6%
Respiratory System		
Dyspnea	22%	11%
Coughing	15%	7%
CNS/Peripheral Nervous System		
Headache	18%	7%

* Pain includes body pain, back pain and skeletal pain.
† Rash also includes pruritus, rash erythematous, urticaria, dermatitis, bullous eruption and rash maculopapular.

TABLE 5B *Summary of Non-Hematologic Adverse Events in Patients Receiving Topotecan HCl*

Non-Hematologic Adverse Events	Grade 3 Incidence		Grade 4 Incidence	
	n=879	n=4124	n=879	n=4124
	Patients	Courses	Patients	Courses
Gastrointestinal				
Nausea	7%	2%	1%	<1%
Vomiting	4%	1%	1%	<1%
Diarrhea	3%	1%	1%	<1%
Constipation	2%	1%	1%	<1%
Abdominal pain	2%	1%	2%	<1%
Stomatitis	1%	<1%	<1%	<1%
Anorexia	2%	1%	<1%	<1%
Body as a Whole				
Fatigue	5%	2%	0%	0%
Fever	1%	<1%	<1%	<1%
Pain*	2%	1%	1%	<1%
Asthenia	4%	1%	2%	<1%
Skin/Appendages				
Alopecia	NA	NA	NA	NA
Rash†	1%	<1%	0%	0%
Respiratory System				
Dyspnea	5%	2%	3%	1%
Coughing	1%	<1%	0%	0%
CNS/Peripheral Nervous System				
Headache	1%	<1%	<1%	0%

* Pain includes body pain, back pain and skeletal pain.
† Rash also includes pruritus, rash erythematous, urticaria, dermatitis, bullous eruption and rash maculopapular.

Premedications were not routinely used in these clinical studies.

Hematologic: See WARNINGS.

Gastrointestinal: The incidence of nausea was 64% (8% Grade 3/4) and vomiting occurred in 45% (6% Grade 3/4) of patients (see TABLE 5A and TABLE 5B). The prophylactic use of antiemetics was not routine in patients treated with topotecan HCl. Thirty-two percent (32%) of patients had diarrhea (4% Grade 3/4), 29% constipation (2% Grade 3/4) and 22% had abdominal pain (4% Grade 3/4). Grade 3/4 abdominal pain was 6% in ovarian cancer patients and 2% in small cell lung cancer patients.

Skin/Appendages: Total alopecia (Grade 2) occurred in 31% of patients.

Central and Peripheral Nervous System: Headache (18% of patients) was the most frequently reported neurologic toxicity. Paresthesia occurred in 7% of patients but was generally Grade 1.

Liver/Biliary: Grade 1 transient elevations in hepatic enzymes occurred in 8% of patients. Greater elevations, Grade 3/4, occurred in 4%. Grade 3/4 elevated bilirubin occurred in <2% of patients.

Respiratory: The incidence of Grade 3/4 dyspnea was 4% in ovarian cancer patients and 12% in small cell lung cancer patients.

TABLE 6 shows the Grade 3/4 hematologic and major non-hematologic adverse events in the topotecan/paclitaxel comparator trial in ovarian cancer.

Premedications were not routinely used in patients randomized to topotecan HCl, while patients receiving paclitaxel received routine pretreatment with corticosteroids, diphenhydramine, and histamine receptor type 2 blockers.

TABLE 7 shows the Grade 3/4 hematologic and major non-hematologic adverse events in the topotecan/CAV comparator trial in small cell lung cancer.

TABLE 6 *Comparative Toxicity Profiles for Ovarian Cancer Patients Randomized to Receive Topotecan HCl or Paclitaxel*

Adverse Event	Topotecan HCl		Paclitaxel	
	Pts	Courses	Pts	Courses
	n=112	n=597	n=114	n=589
Hematologic Grade 3/4				
Grade 4 neutropenia (<500 cells/ml)	80%	36%	21%	9%
Grade 3/4 anemia (Hgb <8 g/dl)	41%	16%	6%	2%
Grad 4 thrombocytopenia (<25,000 plts/ml)	27%	10%	3%	<1%
Fever/Grade 4 neutropenia	23%	6%	4%	1%
Documented sepsis	5%	1%	2%	<1%
Death related to sepsis	2%	NA	0%	NA
Non-Hematologic Grade 3/4				
Gastrointestinal				
Abdominal pain	5%	1%	4%	1%
Constipation	5%	1%	0%	0%
Diarrhea	6%	2%	1%	<1%
Intestinal obstruction	5%	1%	4%	1%
Nausea	10%	3%	2%	<1%
Stomatitis	1%	<1%	1%	<1%
Vomiting	10%	2%	3%	<1%
Constitutional				
Anorexia	4%	1%	0%	0%
Dyspnea	6%	2%	5%	1%
Fatigue	7%	2%	6%	2%
Malaise	2%	<1%	2%	<1%
Neuromuscular				
Arthralgia	1%	<1%	3%	<1%
Asthenia	5%	2%	3%	1%
Chest pain	2%	<1%	1%	<1%
Headache	1%	<1%	2%	1%
Myalgia	0%	0%	3%	2%
Pain*	5%	1%	7%	2%
Skin/Appendages				
Rash†	0%	0%	1%	<1%
Liver/Biliary				
Increased hepatic enzymes‡	1%	<1%	1%	<1%

* Pain includes body pain, skeletal pain and back pain.
† Rash also includes pruritus, rash erythematous, urticaria, dermatitis, bullous eruption and rash maculopapular.
‡ Increased hepatic enzymes includes increased SGOT/AST, increased SGPT/ALT and increased hepatic enzymes.

TABLE 7 *Comparative Toxicity Profiles for Small Cell Lung Cancer Patients Randomized to Receive Topotecan HCl or CAV*

Adverse Event	Topotecan HCl		CAV	
	Pts	Courses	Pts	Courses
	n=107	n=446	n=104	n=359
Hematologic Grade 3/4				
Grade 4 neutropenia (<500 cells/ml)	70%	38%	72%	51%
Grade 3/4 anemia (Hgb <8 g/dl)	42%	18%	20%	7%
Grade 4 thrombocytopenia (<25,000 plts/ml)	29%	10%	5%	1%
Fever/Grade 4 neutropenia	28%	9%	26%	13%
Documented sepsis	5%	1%	5%	1%
Death related to sepsis	3%	NA	1%	NA
Non-Hematologic Grade 3/4				
Gastrointestinal				
Abdominal pain	6%	1%	4%	2%
Constipation	1%	<1%	0%	0%
Diarrhea	1%	<1%	0%	0%
Nausea	8%	2%	6%	2%
Stomatitis	2%	<1%	1%	<1%
Vomiting	3%	<1%	3%	1%
Constitutional				
Anorexia	3%	1%	4%	2%
Dyspnea	9%	5%	14%	7%
Fatigue	6%	4%	10%	3%
Neuromuscular				
Asthenia	9%	4%	7%	2%
Headache	0%	0%	2%	<1%
Pain*	5%	2%	7%	4%
Respiratory System				
Coughing	2%	1%	0%	0%
Pneumonia	8%	2%	6%	2%
Skin/Appendages				
Rash†	1%	<1%	1%	<1%
Liver/Biliary				
Increased hepatic enzymes‡	1%	<1%	0%	0%

* Pain includes body pain, skeletal pain and back pain.
† Rash also includes pruritus, rash erythematous, urticaria, dermatitis, bullous eruption and rash maculopapular.
‡ Increased hepatic enzymes includes increased SGOT/AST, increased SGPT/ALT and increased hepatic enzymes.

Premedications were not routinely used in patients randomized to topotecan HCl, while patients receiving CAV received routine pretreatment with corticosteroids, diphenhydramine, and histamine receptor type 2 blockers.

POSTMARKETING REPORTS OF ADVERSE EVENTS

Reports of adverse events in patients taking topotecan HCl received after market introduction, which are not listed above, include the following:

Hematologic: *Rare:* Severe bleeding (in association with thrombocytopenia).

Skin/Appendages: *Rare:* Severe dermatitis, severe pruritus.

Body as a Whole: *Infrequent:* Allergic manifestations; *Rare:* Anaphylactoid reactions, angioedema.

DOSAGE AND ADMINISTRATION

Prior to administration of the first course of topotecan HCl, patients must have a baseline neutrophil count of >1500 cells/mm^3 and a platelet count of >100,000 cells/mm^3. The recommended dose of topotecan HCl is 1.5 mg/m^2 by intravenous infusion over 30 minutes daily for 5 consecutive days, starting on day 1 of a 21 day course. In the absence of tumor progression, a minimum of four courses is recommended because tumor response may be delayed. The median time to response in three ovarian clinical trials was 9-12 weeks and median time to response in four small cell lung cancer trials was 5-7 weeks. In the event of severe neutropenia during any course, the dose should be reduced by 0.25 mg/m^2 for subsequent courses. Dose should be similarly reduced if the platelet count falls below 25,000 cells/mm^3. Alternatively, in the event of severe neutropenia, G-CSF may be administered following the subsequent course (before resorting to dose reduction) starting from day 6 of the course (24 hours after completion of topotecan administration).

DOSE ADJUSTMENT IN SPECIAL POPULATIONS

Hepatic Impairment: No dosage adjustment appears to be required for treating patients with impaired hepatic function (plasma bilirubin >1.5 to <10 mg/dl).

Renal Functional Impairment: No dosage adjustment appears to be required for treating patients with mild renal impairment (CLCR 40-60 ml/min). Dosage adjustment to 0.75 mg/m^2 is recommended for patients with moderate renal impairment (20-39 ml/min). Insufficient data are available in patients with severe renal impairment to provide a dosage recommendation.

Elderly Patients: No dosage adjustment appears to be needed in the elderly, other than adjustments related to renal function.

PREPARATION FOR ADMINISTRATION

Precautions

Topotecan HCl is a cytotoxic anticancer drug. As with other potentially toxic compounds, topotecan HCl should be prepared under a vertical laminar flow hood while wearing gloves and protective clothing. If topotecan HCl solution contacts the skin, wash the skin immediately and thoroughly with soap and water. If topotecan HCl contacts mucous membranes, flush thoroughly with water.

Preparation for Intravenous Administration

Each topotecan HCl 4 mg vial is reconstituted with 4 ml sterile water for injection. Then the appropriate volume of the reconstituted solution is diluted in either 0.9% sodium chloride intravenous infusion or 5% dextrose intravenous infusion prior to administration.

Because the lyophilized dosage form contains no antibacterial preservative, the reconstituted product should be used immediately.

STABILITY

Unopened vials of topotecan HCl are stable until the date indicated on the package when stored between 20-25°C (68-77°F) and protected from light in the original package. Because the vials contain no preservative, contents should be used immediately after reconstitution.

Reconstituted vials of topotecan HCl diluted for infusion are stable at approximately 20-25°C (68-77°F) and ambient lighting conditions for 24 hours.

HOW SUPPLIED

Hycamtin for injection is supplied in 4 mg (free base) single-dose vials.

Storage: Store the vials protected from light in the original cartons at controlled room temperature between 20 and 25°C (68-77°F).

Handling and Disposal: Procedures for proper handling and disposal of anticancer drugs should be used. Several guidelines on this subject have been published.[1-7] There is no general agreement that all of the procedures recommended in the guidelines are necessary or appropriate.

PRODUCT LISTING - EQUIVALENTS NOT AVAILABLE

Powder For Injection - Intravenous - 4 mg

1's	$875.71	HYCAMTIN, Glaxosmithkline	00007-4201-01
5's	$4378.55	HYCAMTIN, Glaxosmithkline	00007-4201-05

Toremifene Citrate (003273)

Categories: Carcinoma, breast; FDA Approved 1997 May; Pregnancy Category D; Orphan Drugs
Drug Classes: Antineoplastics, antiestrogens; Estrogen receptor modulators, selective; Hormones/hormone modifiers
Brand Names: **Fareston**
Cost of Therapy: $122.40 (Breast Cancer; Fareston; 60 mg; 1 tablet/day; 30 day supply)

DESCRIPTION

Fareston tablets for oral administration each contain 88.5 mg of toremifene citrate, which is equivalent to 60 mg toremifene.

Toremifene citrate is a nonsteroidal antiestrogen. The chemical name of toremifene is 2-(p-[(Z)-4-chloro-1,2-diphenyl-1-butenyl]phenoxy)-N,N-dimethylethylamine citrate (1:1) and the molecular formula is $C_{26}H_{28}ClNO \cdot C_6H_8O_7$. The molecular weight of toremifene citrate is 598.10. The pKa is 8.0. Water solubility at 37°C is 0.63 mg/ml and in 0.02 N HCl at 37°C is 0.38 mg/ml.

Toremifene citrate is available only as tablets for oral administration. Inactive ingredients: starch, lactose, povidone, sodium starch glycolate, magnesium stearate, microcrystalline cellulose, and colloidal silicon dioxide.

CLINICAL PHARMACOLOGY

MECHANISM OF ACTION

Toremifene is a nonsteroidal triphenylethylene derivative. Toremifene binds to estrogen receptors and may exert estrogenic, antiestrogenic, or both activities, depending upon the duration of treatment, animal species, gender, target organ, or endpoint selected. In general, however, nonsteroidal triphenylethylene derivatives are predominantly antiestrogenic in rats and humans and estrogenic in mice. In rats, toremifene causes regression of established dimethylbenzanthracene (DMBA)-induced mammary tumors. The antitumor effect of toremifene in breast cancer is believed to be mainly due to its antiestrogenic effects, *i.e.*, its ability to compete with estrogen for binding sites in the cancer, blocking the growth-stimulating effects of estrogen in the tumor.

Toremifene causes a decrease in the estradiol-induced vaginal cornification index in some postmenopausal women, indicative of its antiestrogenic activity. Toremifene also has estrogenic activity as shown by decreases in serum gonadotropin concentrations (FSH and LH).

PHARMACOKINETICS

The plasma concentration time profile of toremifene declines biexponentially after absorption with a mean distribution half-life of about 4 hours and an elimination half-life of about 5 days. Elimination half-lives of major metabolites, N-demethyltoremifene and (deamino-hydroxy) toremifene were 6 and 4 days, respectively. Mean total clearance of toremifene was approximately 5 L/h.

Absorption and Distribution

Toremifene is well absorbed after oral administration and absorption is not influenced by food. Peak plasma concentrations are obtained within 3 hours. Toremifene displays linear pharmacokinetics after single oral doses of 10 to 680 mg. After multiple dosing, dose proportionality was observed for doses of 10-400 mg. Steady-state concentrations were reached in about 4-6 weeks. Toremifene has an apparent volume of distribution of 580 L and binds extensively (>99.5%) to serum proteins, mainly to albumin.

Metabolism and Excretion

Toremifene is extensively metabolized, principally by CYP3A4 to N-demethyltoremifene, which is also antiestrogenic but with weak *in vivo* antitumor potency. Serum concentrations of N-demethyltoremifene are 2-4 times higher than toremifene at steady state. Toremifene is eliminated as metabolites predominantly in the feces, with about 10% excreted in the urine during a 1 week period. Elimination of toremifene is slow, in part because of enterohepatic circulation.

SPECIAL POPULATIONS

Renal Insufficiency

The pharmacokinetics of toremifene and N-demethyltoremifene were similar in normals and in patients with impaired kidney function.

Hepatic Insufficiency

The mean elimination half-life of toremifene was increased by less than 2-fold in 10 patients with hepatic impairment (cirrhosis or fibrosis) compared to subjects with normal hepatic function. The pharmacokinetics of N-demethyltoremifene were unchanged in these patients. Ten (10) patients on anticonvulsants (phenobarbital, clonazepam, phenytoin, and carbamazepine) showed a 2-fold increase in clearance and a decrease in the elimination half-life of toremifene.

Geriatric Patients

The pharmacokinetics of toremifene were studied in 10 healthy young males and 10 elderly females following a single 120 mg dose under fasting conditions. Increases in the elimination half-life (4.2 vs 7.2 days) and the volume of distribution (457 vs 627 L) of toremifene were seen in the elderly females without any change in clearance or AUC.

Race

The pharmacokinetics of toremifene in patients of different races has not been studied.

INDICATIONS AND USAGE

Toremifene citrate is indicated for the treatment of metastatic breast cancer in postmenopausal women with estrogen-receptor positive or unknown tumors.

CONTRAINDICATIONS

Toremifene citrate is contraindicated in patients with known hypersensitivity to the drug.

WARNINGS

HYPERCALCEMIA AND TUMOR FLARE

As with other antiestrogens, hypercalcemia and tumor flare have been reported in some breast cancer patients with bone metastases during the first weeks of treatment with toremifene citrate. Tumor flare is a syndrome of diffuse musculoskeletal pain and erythema with increased size of tumor lesions that later regress. It is often accompanied by hypercalcemia. Tumor flare does not imply failure of treatment or represent tumor progression. If hypercalcemia occurs, appropriate measures should be instituted and if hypercalcemia is severe, toremifene citrate treatment should be discontinued.

TUMORIGENICITY

Since most toremifene trials have been conducted in patients with metastatic disease, adequate data on the potential endometrial tumorigenicity of long-term treatment with toremifene citrate are not available. Endometrial hyperplasia has been reported. Some patients treated with toremifene citrate have developed endometrial cancer, but circumstances (short duration of treatment or prior antiestrogen treatment or premalignant conditions) make it difficult to establish the role of toremifene citrate.

Endometrial hyperplasia of the uterus was observed in monkeys following 52 weeks of treatment at $\geq$1 mg/kg and in dogs following 16 weeks of treatment at $\geq$3 mg/kg with toremifene (about ¼ and 1.4 times, respectively, the daily maximum recommended human dose on a mg/m^2 basis).

PREGNANCY

Toremifene citrate may cause fetal harm when administered to pregnant women. Studies in rats at doses $\geq$1.0 mg/kg/day (about ¼ the daily maximum recommended human dose on a mg/m^2 basis) administered during the period of organogenesis, have shown that toremifene is embryotoxic and fetotoxic, as indicated by intrauterine mortality, increased resorption, reduced fetal weight, and fetal anomalies; including malformation of limbs, incomplete ossification, misshapen bones, ribs/spine anomalies, hydroureter, hydronephrosis, testicular displacement, and subcutaneous edema. Fetal anomalies may have been a consequence of maternal toxicity. Toremifene has been shown to cross the placenta and accumulate in the rodent fetus.

In rodent models of fetal reproductive tract development, toremifene produced inhibition of uterine development in female pups similar to diethylstilbestrol (DES) and tamoxifen. The clinical relevance of these changes is not known.

Embryotoxicity and fetotoxicity were observed in rabbits at doses $\geq$1.25 mg/kg/day and 2.5 mg/kg/day, respectively (about ⅓ and ⅔ the daily maximum recommended human dose on a mg/m^2 basis); fetal anomalies included incomplete ossification and anencephaly.

There are no studies in pregnant women. If toremifene citrate is used during pregnancy, or if the patient becomes pregnant while receiving this drug, the patient should be apprised of the potential hazard to the fetus or potential risk for loss of the pregnancy.

PRECAUTIONS

GENERAL

Patients with a history of thromboembolic diseases should generally not be treated with toremifene citrate. In general, patients with preexisting endometrial hyperplasia should not be given long-term toremifene citrate treatment. Patients with bone metastases should be monitored closely for hypercalcemia during the first weeks of treatment (see WARNINGS). Leukopenia and thrombocytopenia have been reported rarely; leukocyte and platelet counts should be monitored when using toremifene citrate in patients with leukopenia or thrombocytopenia.

INFORMATION FOR THE PATIENT

Vaginal bleeding has been reported in patients using toremifene citrate. Patients should be informed about this and instructed to contact their physician if such bleeding occurs.

Patients with bone metastases should be informed about the typical signs and symptoms of hypercalcemia and instructed to contact their physician for further assessment if such signs or symptoms occur.

LABORATORY TESTS

Periodic complete blood counts, calcium levels, and liver function tests should be obtained.

CARCINOGENESIS, MUTAGENESIS, AND IMPAIRMENT OF FERTILITY

Conventional carcinogenesis studies in rats at doses of 0.12 to 12 mg/kg/day (about 1/100 to 1.5 times daily maximum recommended human dose on a mg/m^2 basis) for up to 2 years did not show evidence of carcinogenicity. Studies in mice at doses of 1.0-30.0 mg/kg/day (about 1/15 to 2 times the daily maximum recommended human dose on a mg/m^2 basis) for up to 2 years revealed increased incidence of ovarian and testicular tumors, and increased incidence of osteoma and osteosarcoma. The significance of the mouse findings is uncertain because of the different role of estrogens in mice and the estrogenic effect of toremifene in mice. An increased incidence of ovarian and testicular tumors in mice has also been observed with other human antiestrogenic agents that have primarily estrogenic activity in mice.

Toremifene has not been shown to be mutagenic in *in vitro* tests (Ames and *E. coli* bacterial tests). Toremifene is clastogenic *in vitro* (chromosomal aberrations and micronuclei formation in human lymphoblastoid MCL-5 cells) and *in vivo* (chromosomal aberrations in rat hepatocytes). No significant adduct formation could be detected using ^{32}P post-labeling in liver DNA from rats administered toremifene when compared to tamoxifen at similar doses. A study in cultured human lymphocytes indicated that adducting activity of toremifene, detected by ^{32}P post-labeling, was about one-sixth that of tamoxifen at approximately equipotent concentrations. In addition, the DNA adducting activity of toremifene in salmon sperm, using ^{32}P post-labeling, was one-sixth and one-fourth that observed with tamoxifen at equivalent concentrations following activation by rat and human microsomal systems, respectively. However, toremifene exposure is 4-fold the exposure of tamoxifen based on human AUC in serum at recommended clinical doses.

Toremifene produced impairment of fertility and conception in male and female rats at doses $\geq$25.0 and 0.14 mg/kg/day, respectively (about 3.5 times and 1/50 the daily maximum recommended human dose on a mg/m^2 basis). At these doses, sperm counts, fertility index, and conception rate were reduced in males with atrophy of seminal vesicles and prostate. In females, fertility and reproductive indices were markedly reduced with increased pre- and post-implantation loss. In addition, offspring of treated rats exhibited depressed reproductive indices. Toremifene produced ovarian atrophy in dogs administered doses $\geq$3 mg/kg/day (about 1.5 times the daily maximum recommended human dose on a mg/m^2 basis) for 16 weeks. Cystic ovaries and reduction in endometrial stromal cellularity were observed in monkeys at doses $\geq$1 mg/kg/day (about ¼ the daily maximum recommended human dose on a mg/m^2 basis) for 52 weeks.

PREGNANCY CATEGORY D

See WARNINGS.

NURSING MOTHERS

Toremifene has been shown to be excreted in the milk of lactating rats. It is not known if this drug is excreted in human milk. (See WARNINGS and PRECAUTIONS.)

PEDIATRIC USE

There is no indication for use of toremifene citrate in pediatric patients.

GERIATRIC USE

The median ages in the three controlled studies ranged from 60-66 years. No significant age-related differences in toremifene citrate effectiveness or safety were noted.

RACE

Fourteen percent (14%) of patients in the North American Study were non-Caucasian. No significant race-related differences in toremifene citrate effectiveness or safety were noted.

DRUG INTERACTIONS

No formal drug-drug interaction studies with toremifene have been performed.

Drugs that decrease renal calcium excretion, *e.g.*, thiazide diuretics may increase the risk of hypercalcemia in patients receiving toremifene citrate. There is a known interaction between antiestrogenic compounds of the triphenylethylene derivative class and coumarin-type anticoagulants (*e.g.*, warfarin), leading to an increased prothrombin time. When concomitant use of anticoagulants with toremifene citrate is necessary, careful monitoring of the prothrombin time is recommended.

Cytochrome P450 3A4 enzyme inducers, such as phenobarbital, phenytoin, and carbamazepine increase the rate of toremifene metabolism, lowering the steady-state concentration in serum. Metabolism of toremifene may be inhibited by drugs known to inhibit the CYP3A4-6 enzymes. Examples of such drugs are ketoconazole and similar antimycotics as well as erythromycin and similar macrolides. This interaction has not been studied and its clinical relevance is uncertain.

ADVERSE REACTIONS

Adverse drug reactions are principally due to the antiestrogenic hormonal actions of toremifene citrate and typically occur at the beginning of treatment.

The incidences of the following eight clinical toxicities were prospectively assessed in the North American Study (TABLE 2). The incidence reflects the toxicities that were considered by the investigator to be drug related or possibly drug related.

Approximately 1% of patients receiving toremifene citrate (n=592) in the three controlled studies discontinued treatment as a result of adverse events (nausea and vomiting, fatigue,

TABLE 2 *North American Study*

	FAR60 (n=221)	TAM20 (n=215)
Hot flashes	35%	30%
Sweating	20%	17%
Nausea	14%	15%
Vaginal discharge	13%	16%
Dizziness	9%	7%
Edema	5%	5%
Vomiting	4%	2%
Vaginal bleeding	2%	4%

TABLE 3

	North American		Eastern European		Nordic	
	FAR60	TAM20	FAR60	TAM40	FAR60	TAM40
Adverse Events	n=221	n=215	n=157	n=149	n=214	n=201
Cardiac						
Cardiac failure	2 (1%)	1 (<1%)	—	1 (<1%)	2 (1%)	3 (1.5%)
Myocardial infarction	2 (1%)	3 (1.5%)	1 (<1%)	2 (1%)	—	1 (<1%)
Arrhythmia	—	—	—	—	3 (1.5%)	1 (<1%)
Angina pectoris	—	—	1 (<1%)	—	1 (<1%)	2 (1%)
Ocular*						
Cataracts	22 (10%)	16 (7.5%)	—	—	—	5 (3%)
Dry eyes	20 (9%)	16 (7.5%)	—	—	—	—
Abnormal visual fields	8 (4%)	10 (5%)	—	—	—	1 (<1%)
Corneal keratopathy	4 (2%)	2 (1%)	—	—	—	—
Glaucoma	3 (1.5%)	2 (1%)	1 (<1%)	—	—	1 (<1%)
Abnormal vision/ diplopia	—	—	—	—	3 (1.5%)	—
Thromboembolic						
Pulmonary embolism	4 (2%)	2 (1%)	1 (<1%)	—	—	1 (<1%)
Thrombophlebitis	—	2 (1%)	1 (<1%)	1 (<1%)	4 (2%)	3 (1.5%)
Thrombosis	—	1 (<1%)	1 (<1%)	—	3 (1.5%)	4 (2%)
CVA/TIA	1 (<1%)	—	—	1 (<1%)	4 (2%)	4 (2%)
Elevated Liver Tests†						
SGOT	11 (5%)	4 (2%)	30 (19%)	22 (15%)	32 (15%)	35 (17%)
Alkaline phosphatase	41 (19%)	24 (11%)	16 (10%)	13 (9%)	18 (8%)	31 (15%)
Bilirubin	3 (1.5%)	4 (2%)	2 (1%)	1 (<1%)	2 (1%)	3 (1.5%)
Hypercalcemia	6 (3%)	6 (3%)	1 (<1%)	—	—	—

* Most of the ocular abnormalities were observed in the North American Study in which on-study and biannual ophthalmic examinations were performed. No cases of retinopathy were observed in any arm.

† Elevated defined as follows: North American Study: SGOT >100 IU/L; alkaline phosphatase >200 IU/L; bilirubin >2 mg/dL. Eastern European and Nordic studies: SGOT, alkaline phosphatase, and bilirubin — WHO Grade 1 (1.25 times the upper limit of normal).

thrombophlebitis, depression, lethargy, anorexia, ischemic attack, arthritis, pulmonary embolism, and myocardial infarction).

Serious adverse events occurring in patients receiving toremifene citrate in the three major trials are listed in TABLE 3.

Other adverse events of unclear causal relationship to toremifene citrate included leukopenia and thrombocytopenia, skin discoloration or dermatitis, constipation, dyspnea, paresis, tremor, vertigo, pruritus, anorexia, reversible corneal opacity (corneal verticulata), asthenia, alopecia, depression, jaundice, and rigors.

In the 200 and 240 mg toremifene citrate dose arms, the incidence of SGOT elevation and nausea was higher. Approximately 4% of patients were withdrawn for toxicity from the high-dose toremifene citrate treatment arms. Reasons for withdrawal included hypercalcemia, abnormal liver function tests, and one case each of toxic hepatitis, depression, dizziness, incoordination, ataxia, blurry vision, diffuse dermatitis, and a constellation of symptoms consisting of nausea, sweating, and tremor.

DOSAGE AND ADMINISTRATION

The dosage of toremifene citrate is 60 mg, once daily, orally. Treatment is generally continued until disease progression is observed.

HOW SUPPLIED

Fareston tablets, containing toremifene citrate in an amount equivalent to 60 mg of toremifene, are round, convex, unscored, uncoated, and white, or almost white. Fareston tablets are identified with "TO 60" embossed on one side.

Storage: Store at 25°C (77°F). Protect from heat and light.

PRODUCT LISTING - EQUIVALENTS NOT AVAILABLE

Tablet - Oral - 60 mg

30's	$122.39	FARESTON, Shire Richwood Pharmaceutical Company Inc	54092-0170-30
100's	$408.01	FARESTON, Shire Richwood Pharmaceutical Company Inc	54092-0170-01

Torsemide *(003179)*

Categories: Edema; Hypertension, essential; FDA Approved 1993 Aug; Pregnancy Category B
Drug Classes: Diuretics, loop
Brand Names: **Demadex**; Presaril
Foreign Brand Availability: Toral (Indonesia); Torem (England; Germany; Korea; Sweden; Switzerland); Unat (Germany; Hong-Kong; Indonesia; Portugal; South-Africa)
Cost of Therapy: $23.69 (Edema; Demadex; 10 mg; 1 tablet/day; 30 day supply)
$21.08 (Edema; Generic Tablets; 10 mg; 1 tablet/day; 30 day supply)
$27.67 (Edema; Demadex; 20 mg; 1 tablet/day; 30 day supply)
$24.62 (Edema; Generic Tablets; 20 mg; 1 tablet/day; 30 day supply)
HCFA JCODE(S): J3265 10 mg/ml IV

DESCRIPTION

Torsemide is a diuretic of the pyridine-sulfonylurea class. Its chemical name is 1-isopropyl-3-[(4-*m*-toluidino-3-pyridyl)sulfonyl]urea.

Its empirical formula is $C_{16}H_{20}N_4O_3S$, its pKa is 7.1, and its molecular weight is 348.43.

Demadex is a white to off-white crystalline powder. The tablets for oral administration also contain lactose, crospovidone, povidone, microcrystalline cellulose, and magnesium stearate. Demadex ampuls for intravenous injection contain a sterile solution of torsemide (10 mg/ml), polyethylene glycol-400, tromethamine, and sodium hydroxide (as needed to adjust pH) in water for injection.

CLINICAL PHARMACOLOGY

MECHANISM OF ACTION

Micropuncture studies in animals have shown that torsemide acts from within the lumen of the thick ascending portion of the loop of Henle, where it inhibits the $Na^+/K^+/2Cl^-$ carrier system. Clinical pharmacology studies have confirmed this site of action in humans, and effects in other segments of the nephron have not been demonstrated. Diuretic activity thus correlates better with the rate of drug excretion in the urine than with the concentration in the blood.

Torsemide increases the urinary excretion of sodium, chloride, and water, but it does not significantly alter glomerular filtration rate, renal plasma flow, or acid-base balance.

PHARMACOKINETICS AND METABOLISM

Bioavailability

The bioavailability of torsemide tablets is approximately 80%, with little intersubject variation; the 90% confidence interval is 75-89%. The drug is absorbed with little first-pass metabolism, and the serum concentration reaches its peak (C_{max}) within 1 hour after oral administration. C_{max} and area under the serum concentration-time curve (AUC) after oral administration are proportional to dose over the range of 2.5 to 200 mg. Simultaneous food intake delays the time to C_{max} by about 30 minutes, but overall bioavailability (AUC) and diuretic activity are unchanged. Absorption is essentially unaffected by renal or hepatic dysfunction.

Volume of Distribution

The volume of distribution of torsemide is 12-15 L in normal adults or in patients with mild to moderate renal failure or congestive heart failure. In patients with hepatic cirrhosis, the volume of distribution is approximately doubled.

Elimination Half-Life

In normal subjects the elimination half-life of torsemide is approximately 3.5 hours. Torsemide is cleared from the circulation by both hepatic metabolism (approximately 80% of total clearance) and excretion into the urine (approximately 20% of total clearance in patients with normal renal function). The major metabolite in humans is the carboxylic acid derivative, which is biologically inactive. Two of the lesser metabolites possess some diuretic activity, but for practical purposes metabolism terminates the action of the drug.

Because torsemide is extensively bound to plasma protein (>99%), very little enters tubular urine via glomerular filtration. Most renal clearance of torsemide occurs via active secretion of the drug by the proximal tubules into tubular urine.

In patients with decompensated congestive heart failure, hepatic and renal clearance are both reduced, probably because of hepatic congestion and decreased renal plasma flow, respectively. The total clearance of torsemide is approximately 50% of that seen in healthy volunteers, and the plasma half-life and AUC are correspondingly increased. Because of reduced renal clearance, a smaller fraction of any given dose is delivered to the intraluminal site of action, so at any given dose there is less natriuresis in patients with congestive heart failure than in normal subjects.

In patients with renal failure, renal clearance of torsemide is markedly decreased but total plasma clearance is not significantly altered. A smaller fraction of the administered dose is delivered to the intraluminal site of action, and the natriuretic action of any given dose of diuretic is reduced. A diuretic response in renal failure may still be achieved if patients are given higher doses. The total plasma clearance and elimination half-life of torsemide remain normal under the conditions of impaired renal function because metabolic elimination by the liver remains intact.

In patients with hepatic cirrhosis, the volume of distribution, plasma half-life, and renal clearance are all increased, but total clearance in unchanged.

The pharmacokinetic profile of torsemide in healthy elderly subjects is similar to that in young subjects except for a decrease in renal clearance related to the decline in renal function that commonly occurs with aging. However, total plasma clearance and elimination half-life remain unchanged.

CLINICAL EFFECTS

The diuretic effects of torsemide begin within 10 minutes of intravenous dosing and peak within the first hour. With oral dosing, the onset of diuresis occurs within 1 hour and the peak effect occurs during the first or second hour. Independent of the route of administration, diuresis lasts about 6-8 hours. In healthy subjects given doses, the dose-response relationship for sodium excretion is linear over the dose range of 2.5 to 20 mg. The increase in potassium excretion is negligible after a single dose of up to 10 mg and only slight (5-15 mEq) after a single dose of 20 mg.

Congestive Heart Failure

Torsemide has been studied in controlled rials in patients with New York Heart Association Class II to Class IV congestive heart failure. Patients who received 10-20 mg of daily torsemide in these studies achieved significantly greater reductions in weight and edema than did patients who received placebo.

Nonanuric Renal Failure

In single-dose studies in patients with nonanuric renal failure, high doses of torsemide (20-200 mg) caused marked increases in water and sodium excretion. In patients with nonanuric renal failure severe enough to require hemodialysis, chronic treatment with up to 200 mg of daily torsemide has not been shown to change steady-state fluid retention. When patients in a study of acute renal failure received total daily doses of 520-1200 mg of torsemide, 19% experienced seizures. 96 total patients were treated in this study; 6/32 treated with torsemide experienced seizures, 6/32 treated with comparably high doses of furosemide experienced seizures, and 1/32 treated with placebo experienced a seizure.

Hepatic Cirrhosis

When given with aldosterone antagonists, torsemide also caused increases in sodium and fluid excretion in patients with edema or ascites due to hepatic cirrhosis. Urinary sodium excretion rate relative to the urinary excretion rate of torsemide is less in cirrhotic patients than in healthy subjects (possibly because of the hyperaldosteronism and resultant sodium retention that are characteristic of portal hypertension and ascites). However, because of the increased renal clearance of torsemide in patients with hepatic cirrhosis, these factors tend to balance each other, and the result is an overall natriuretic response that is similar to that seen in healthy subjects. Chronic use of any diuretic in hepatic disease has not been studied in adequate and well-controlled trials.

Essential Hypertension

In patients with essential hypertension, torsemide has been shown in controlled studies to lower blood pressure when administered once a day at doses of 5-10 mg. The antihypertensive effect is near maximal after 4-6 weeks of treatment, but it may continue to increase for up to 12 weeks. Systolic and diastolic supine and standing blood pressures are all reduced. There is no significant orthostatic effect, and there is only a minimal peak-trough difference in blood pressure reduction.

The antihypertensive effects of torsemide are, like those of other diuretics, on the average greater in black patients (a low-renin population) than in non-black patients.

When torsemide is first administered, daily urinary sodium excretion increases for at least a week. With chronic administration, however, daily sodium loss comes into balance with dietary sodium intake. If the administration of torsemide is suddenly stopped, blood pressure returns to pretreatment levels over several days, without overshoot.

Torsemide has been administered together with β-adrenergic blocking agents, ACE inhibitors, and calcium-channel blockers. Adverse drug interactions have not been observed, and special dosage adjustment has not been necessary.

INDICATIONS AND USAGE

Torsemide is indicated for the treatment of edema associated with congestive heart failure, renal disease, or hepatic disease. Use of torsemide has been found to be effective in the treatment of edema associated with chronic renal failure. Chronic use of any diuretic in renal or hepatic disease has not been studied in adequate and well-controlled trials.

Torsemide intravenous injection is indicated when a rapid onset of diuresis is desired or when oral administration is impractical.

T

Torsemide is indicated for the treatment of hypertension alone or in combination with other antihypertensive agents.

CONTRAINDICATIONS

Torsemide is contraindicated in patients with known hypersensitivity to torsemide or to sulfonylureas.

Torsemide is contraindicated in patients who are anuric.

WARNINGS

HEPATIC DISEASE WITH CIRRHOSIS AND ASCITES

Torsemide should be used with caution in patients with hepatic disease with cirrhosis and ascites, since sudden alterations of fluid and electrolyte balance may precipitate hepatic coma. In these patients, diuresis with torsemide (or any other diuretic) is best initiated in the hospital. To prevent hypokalemia and metabolic alkalosis, an aldosterone antagonist or potassium-sparing drug should be used concomitantly with torsemide.

OTOTOXICITY

Tinnitus and hearing loss (usually reversible) have been observed after rapid intravenous injection of other loop diuretics and have also been observed after oral torsemide. It is not certain that these events were attributable to torsemide. Ototoxicity has also been seen in animal studies when very high plasma levels of torsemide were induced. Administered intravenously, torsemide should be injected slowly over 2 minutes, and single doses should not exceed 200 mg.

VOLUME AND ELECTROLYTE DEPLETION

Patients receiving diuretics should be observed for clinical evidence of electrolyte imbalance, hypovolemia, or perenal azotemia. Symptoms of these disturbances may include one or more of the following: dryness of the mouth, thirst, weakness, lethargy, drowsiness, restlessness, muscle pains or cramps, muscular fatigue, hypotension, oliguria, tachycardia, nausea, and vomiting. Excessive diuresis may cause dehydration, blood-volume reduction, and possibly thrombosis and embolism, especially in elderly patients. In patients who develop fluid and electrolyte imbalances, hypovolemia, or perenal azotemia, the observed laboratory changes may include hyper- or hyponatremia, hyper- or hypochloremia, hyper- or hypokalemia, acid-base abnormalities, and increased blood urea nitrogen. If any of these occur, torsemide should be discontinued until the situation is corrected; torsemide may be restarted at a lower dose.

In controlled studies in the US, torsemide was administered to hypertensive patients at doses of 5 or 10 mg daily. After 6weeks at these doses, the mean decrease in serum potassium was approximately 0.1 mEq/L. The percentage of patients who had a serum potassium level below 3.5 mEq/L at any time during the studies was essentially the same in patients who received torsemide (1.5%) as in those who received placebo (3%). In patients followed for 1 year, there was no further change in mean serum potassium levels. In patients with congestive heart failure, hepatic cirrhosis, or renal disease treated with torsemide at doses higher than those studied in US antihypertensive trials, hypokalemia was observed with greater frequency, in a dose-related manner.

In patients with cardiovascular disease, especially those receiving digitalis glycosides, diuretic-induced hypokalemia may be a risk factor for the development of arrhythmias. The risk of hypokalemia is greatest in patients with cirrhosis of the liver, in patients experiencing a brisk diuresis, in patients who are receiving inadequate oral intake of electrolytes, and in patients receiving concomitant therapy with corticosteroids or ACTH.

Periodic monitoring of serum potassium and other electrolytes is advised in patients treated with torsemide.

PRECAUTIONS

LABORATORY VALUES

Potassium

See statement in WARNINGS.

Calcium

Single doses of torsemide increased the urinary excretion of calcium by normal subjects, but serum calcium levels were slightly increased in 4-6 week hypertension trials. In a long-term study of patients with congestive heart failure, the average 1 year change in serum calcium was a decrease of 0.10 mg/dl (0.02 mmol/L). Among 426 patients treated with torsemide for an average of 11 months, hypocalcemia was not reported as an adverse event.

T

Magnesium

Single doses of torsemide caused healthy volunteers to increase the urinary excretion of magnesium, but serum magnesium levels were slightly increased in 4-6 week hypertension trials. In long-term hypertension studies, the average 1 year change in serum magnesium was an increase of 0.03 mg/dl (0.01 mmol/L). Among 426 patients treated with torsemide for an average of 11 months, one case of hypomagnesemia (1.3 mg/dl (0.53 mmol/L)) was reported as an adverse event.

In a long-term clinical study of torsemide in patients with congestive heart failure, the estimated annual change in serum magnesium was an increase of 0.2 mg/dl (0.08 mmol/L), but these data are confounded by the fact that many of these patients received magnesium supplements. In a 4 week study in which magnesium supplementation was not given, the rate of occurrence of serum magnesium levels below 1.7 mg/dl (0.70 mmol/L was 6% and 9% in the groups receiving 5 and 10 mg of torsemide, respectively.

Blood Urea Nitrogen (Bun), Creatinine, and Uric Acid

Torsemide produces small dose-related increases in each of these laboratory values. In hypertensive patients who received 10 mg of torsemide daily for 6 weeks, the mean increase in blood urea nitrogen was 1.8 mg/dl (0.6 mmol/L), the mean increase in serum creatinine was 0.05 mg/dl (4 μmol/L), and the mean increase in serum uric acid was 1.2 mg/dl (70 μmol/L). Little further change occurred with long-term treatment, and all changes reversed when treatment was discontinued.

Symptomatic gout has been reported in patients receiving torsemide, but its incidence has been similar to that seen in patients receiving placebo.

Glucose

Hypertensive patients who received 10 mg of daily torsemide experienced a mean increase in serum glucose concentration of 5.5 mg/dl (0.3 mmol/L) after 6 weeks of therapy, with a further increase of 1.8 mg/dl (0.1 mmol/L) during the subsequent year. In long-term studies in diabetics, mean fasting glucose values were not significantly changed from baseline. Cases of hyperglycemia have been reported but are uncommon.

Serum Lipids

In the controlled short-term hypertension studies in the US, daily doses of 5,10, and 20 mg of torsemide were associated with increases in total plasma cholesterol of 4, 4, and 8 mg/dl (0.10 to 0.20 mmol/L), respectively. The changes subsided during chronic therapy.

In the same short-term hypertension studies, daily doses of 5, 10, and 20 mg of torsemide were associated with mean increases in plasma triglycerides of 16, 13, and 71 mg/dl (0.15 to 0.80 mmmol/L), respectively.

In long-term studies of 5-20 mg of torsemide daily, no clinically significant differences from baseline lipid values were observed after 1 year of therapy.

Other

In long-term studies in hypertensive patients, torsemide has been associated with small mean decreases in hemoglobin, hematocrit, and erythrocyte count and small mean increases in white blood cell count, platelet count, and serum alkaline phosphatase. Although statistically significant, all of these changes were medically inconsequential. No significant trends have been observed in any liver enzyme tests other than alkaline phosphatase.

CARCINOGENESIS, MUTAGENESIS, AND IMPAIRMENT OF FERTILITY

No overall increase in tumor incidence was found when torsemide was given to rats and mice throughout their lives at dose up to 9 mg/kg/day (rats) and 32 mg/kg/day (mice). On a body-weight basis, these doses are 27-96 times a human dose of 20 mg; on a body-surface-area basis, they are 5-8 times this dose. In the rat study, the high-dose female group demonstrated renal tubular injury, interstitial inflammation, and a statistically significant increase in renal adenomas and carcinomas. The tumor incidence in this group was, however, not much higher than the incidence sometimes seen in historical controls. Similar signs of chronic non-neoplastic renal injury have been reported in high- dose animal studies of other diuretics such as furosemide and hydrochlorothiazide.

No mutagenic activity was detected in any of a variety of *in vivo* and *in vitro* tests of torsemide and its major human metabolite. The tests included the Ames test in bacteria (with and without metabolic activation), tests for chromosome aberrations and sister-chromatid exchanges in human lymphocytes, tests for various nuclear anomalies in cells found in hamster and murine bone marrow, tests for unscheduled DNA synthesis in mice and rats, and others.

In doses up to 25 mg/kg/day (75 times a human dose of 20 mg on a body-weight basis; 13 times this dose on a body-surface-area basis), torsemide had no adverse effect on the reproductive performance of male or female rats.

PREGNANCY CATEGORY B

There was no fetotoxicity or teratogenicity in rats treated with up to 5 mg/kg/day of torsemide (on a mg/kg basis, this is 15 times a human dose of 20 mg/day; on a mg/m^2 basis, the animal dose is 10 times the human dose) or in rabbits, treated with 1.6 mg/kg/day (on an mg/kg basis, 5 times the human dose of 20 mg/kg/day; on a mg/m basis 1.7 times this dose). Fetal and maternal toxicity (decrease in average body weight, increase in fetal resorption, and delayed fetal ossification) occurred in rabbits and rats given doses 4 (rabbits) and 5 (rats) times larger. Adequate and well-controlled studies have not been carried out in pregnant women. Because animal reproduction studies are not always predictive of human response, this drug should be used during pregnancy only if clearly needed.

LABOR AND DELIVERY

The effect of torsemide on labor and delivery is unknown.

NURSING MOTHERS

It is not known whether torsemide is excreted in human milk. Because many drugs are excreted in human milk, caution should be exercised when torsemide is administered to a nursing woman.

GERIATRIC USE

Of the total number of patients who received torsemide in US clinical studies, 24% were 65 or older while about 4% were 75 or older. No specific age-related differences in effectiveness or safety were observed between younger patients and elderly patients.

PEDIATRIC USE

Safety and effectiveness in children have not been established.

Administration of another loop diuretic to severely premature infants with edema due to patent ductus arteriosus and hyaline membrane disease has occasionally been associated with renal calcifications, sometimes barely visible on x-ray but sometimes in staghorn form, filling the renal pelves. Some of these calculi have been dissolved, and hypercalciuria has been reported to have decreased, when chlorothiazide has been coadministered along with the loop diuretic. In other premature neonates with hyaline membrane disease, another loop diuretic has been reported to increase the risk of persistent patent ductus arteriosus, possibly through a prostaglandin-E-mediated process. The use of torsemide in such patients has not been studied.

DRUG INTERACTIONS

In patients with essential hypertension, torsemide has been administered together with β-blockers, ACE inhibitors, and calcium-channel blockers. In patients with congestive heart failure, torsemide has been administered together with digitalis glycosides, ACE inhibitors, and organic nitrates. None of these combined uses was associated with new or unexpected adverse events.

Torsemide does not affect the protein binding of **glyburide** or of **warfarin,** the anticoagulant effect of **phenprocoumon** (a related coumarin derivative), or the pharmacokinetics of **digoxin** or **carvedilol** (a vasodilator/β-blocker). In healthy subjects, coadministration of torsemide was associated with significant reduction in the renal clearance of **spironolactone,** with corresponding increases in the AUC. However, clinical experience indicates that dosage adjustment of either agent is not required.

Because torsemide and salicylates compete for secretion by renal tubules, patients receiving high doses of **salicylates** may experience salicylate toxicity when torsemide is concomitantly administered. Also, although possible interactions between torsemide and **nonsteroidal anti-inflammatory agents (including aspirin)** have not been studied, coadministration of these agents with another loop diuretic (furosemide) has occasionally been associated with renal dysfunction.

The natriuretic effect of torsemide (like that of many other diuretics) is partially inhibited by the concomitant administration of **indomethacin.** This effect has been demonstrated for torsemide under conditions of dietary sodium restriction (50 mEq/day) but not in the presence of normal sodium intake (150 mEq/day).

The pharmacokinetic profile and diuretic activity of torsemide are not altered by **cimetidine** or **spironolactone.** Coadministration of **digoxin** is reported to increase the area under the curve for torsemide by 50%, but dose adjustment of torsemide is not necessary.

Concomitant use of torsemide and cholestyramine has not been studied in humans but, in a study of animals, coadministration of cholestyramine decreased the absorption of orally administered torsemide. If torsemide and cholestyramine are used concomitantly, simultaneous administration is not recommended.

Coadministration of **probenecid** reduces secretion of torsemide into the proximal tubule and thereby decreases the diuretic activity of torsemide.

Other diuretics are known to reduce the renal clearance of **lithium,** inducing a high risk of lithium toxicity, so coadministration of lithium and diuretics should be undertaken with great caution, if at all. Coadministration of lithium and torsemide has not been studied.

Other diuretics have been reported to increase the ototoxic potential of **aminoglycoside antibiotics** and of **ethacrynic acid,** especially in the presence of impaired renal function. These potential interactions with torsemide have not been studied.

ADVERSE REACTIONS

At the time of approval, torsemide had been evaluated for safety in approximately 4000 subjects: over 800 of these subjects received torsemide for at least 6 months, and over 380 were treated for more than 1 year. Among these subjects were 564 who received torsemide during US-based trials in which 274 other subjects received placebo.

The reported side effects of torsemide were generally transient, and there was no relationship between side effects and age, sex, race, or duration of therapy. Discontinuation of therapy due to side effects occurred in 3.5% of US patients treated with torsemide and in 4.4% of patients treated with placebo. In studies conducted in the US and Europe, discontinuation rates due to side effects were 3.0% (38/1250) with torsemide and 3.4% (13/380) with furosemide in patients with congestive heart failure, 2.0% (8/409) with torsemide and 4.8% (11/230) with furosemide in patients with renal insufficiency, and 7.6% (13/170) with torsemide and 0% (0/33) with furosemide in patients with cirrhosis.

The most common reasons for discontinuation of therapy with torsemide were (in descending order of frequency) dizziness, headache, nausea, weakness, vomiting, hyperglycemia, excessive urination, hyperuricemia, hypokalemia, excessive thirst, hypovolemia, impotence, esophageal hemorrhage, and dyspepsia. Dropout rates for these adverse events ranged from 0.1-0.5%.

The side effects considered possibly or probably related to study drug that occurred in US placebo-controlled trials in more than 1% of patients treated with torsemide are shown in TABLE 1.

***TABLE 1** Reactions Possibly or Probably Drug-Related US Placebo-Controlled Studies Incidence (Percentages of Patients)*

	Torsemide (n=564)	Placebo (n=274)
Headache	7.3%	9.1%
Excessive urination	6.7%	2.2%
Dizziness	3.2%	4.0%
Rhinitis	2.8%	2.2%
Asthenia	2.0%	1.5%
Diarrhea	2.0%	1.1%
ECG abnormality	2.0%	0.4%
Cough increase	2.0%	1.5%
Constipation	1.8%	0.7%
Nausea	1.8%	0.4%
Arthralgia	1.8%	0.7%
Dyspepsia	1.6%	0.7%
Sore throat	1.6%	0.7%
Myalgia	1.6%	1.5%
Chest pain	1.2%	0.4%
Insomnia	1.2%	1.8%
Edema	1.1%	1.1%
Nervousness	1.1%	0.4%

The daily doses of torsemide used in these trials ranged from 1.25 to 20 mg, with most patients receiving 5-10 mg; the duration of treatment ranged from 1 to 52 days, with a median of 41 days. Of the side effects listed in the table, only "excessive urination" occurred significantly more frequently in patients treated with torsemide than in patients treated with placebo. In the placebo-controlled hypertension studies whose design allowed side-effect rates to be attributed to dose, excessive urination was reported by 1% of the patients receiving placebo, 4% of those treated with 5 mg of daily torsemide, and 15% of those treated with 10 mg. The complaint of excessive urination was generally not reported as an adverse event among patients who received torsemide for cardiac, renal, or hepatic failure.

Serious adverse events reported in the clinical studies for which a drug relationship could not be excluded were atrial fibrillation, chest pain, diarrhea, digitalis intoxication, gastrointestinal hemorrhage, hyperglycemia, hyperuricemia, hypokalemia, hypotension, hypovolemia, shunt thrombosis, rash, rectal bleeding, syncope, and ventricular tachycardia.

Angioedema has been reported in a patient exposed to torsemide who was later found to be allergic to sulfa drugs.

Of the adverse reactions during placebo-controlled trials listed without taking into account assessment of relatedness to drug therapy, arthritis and various other nonspecific musculoskeletal problems were more frequently reported in association with torsemide than with placebo, even though gout was somewhat more frequently associated with placebo. These reactions did not increase in frequency or severity with the dose of torsemide. One patient in the group treated with torsemide withdrew due to myalgia, and one in the placebo group withdrew due to gout.

HYPOKALEMIA

See statement in WARNINGS.

DOSAGE AND ADMINISTRATION

GENERAL

Torsemide tablets may be given at any time in relation to a meal, as convenient. Special dosage adjustment in the elderly is not necessary.

Because of the high bioavailability of torsemide, oral and intravenous doses are therapeutically equivalent, so patients may be switched to and from the intravenous form with no change in dose. Torsemide intravenous injection should be administered slowly over a period of 2 minutes.

If torsemide is administered through an IV line, itis recommended that, as with other IV injections, the IV line be flushed with normal saline (sodium chloride injection) before and after administration. Torsemide injection is formulated above pH 8.3. Flushing the line is recommended to avoid the potential for incompatabilities caused by differences in pH which could be indicated by color change, haziness or the formulation of a precipitate in the solution.

Before administration, the solution of torsemide should be visually inspected for discoloration and particulate matter. If either is found, the ampul should not be used.

CONGESTIVE HEART FAILURE

The usual initial dose is 10 or 20 mg of once-daily oral or intravenous torsemide. If the diuretic response is inadequate, the dose should be titrated upward by approximately doubling until the desired diuretic response is obtained. Single doses higher than 200 mg have not been adequately studied.

CHRONIC RENAL FAILURE

The usual initial dose of torsemide is 20 mg of once-daily oral or intravenous torsemide. If the diuretic response is inadequate, the dose should be titrated upward by approximately doubling until the desired diuretic response is obtained. Single doses higher than 200 mg have not been adequately studied.

HEPATIC CIRRHOSIS

The usual initial dose is 5-10 mg of once-daily oral or intravenous torsemide, administered together with an aldosterone antagonist or a potassium-sparing diuretic. If the diuretic response is inadequate, the dose should be titrated upward by approximately doubling until the desired diuretic response is obtained. Single doses higher than 40 mg have not been adequately studied.

Chronic use of any diuretic in hepatic disease has not been studied in adequate and well-controlled trials.

HYPERTENSION

The usual initial dose is 5 mg once daily. If the 5 mg dose does not provide adequate reduction in blood pressure within 4-6 weeks, the dose may be increased to 10 mg once daily. If the response to 10 mg is insufficient, an additional antihypertensive agent should be added to the treatment regimen.

HOW SUPPLIED

Torsemide for oral administration is available as white, scored tablets containing 5, 10, 20, or 100 mg of torsemide. The 5, 10 and 20 mg tablets are oval. The 100 mg tablet is capsule shaped.

Each tablet is debossed on the scored side with the Boehringer Mannheim logo and a portion (102, 103, 104, or 105) of the National Drug Code. On the opposite side, the tablet is debossed with 5, 10, 20, or 100 to indicate the dose.

Torsemide for intravenous injection is supplied in clear ampuls containing 2 ml (20 mg,) or 5 ml (50 mg) of a 10 mg/ml sterile solution.

Storage: Store all dosage forms at controlled room temperature, 15-30°C (59-86°F). Do not freeze.

T

PRODUCT LISTING - RATED THERAPEUTICALLY EQUIVALENT

Tablet - Oral - 5 mg

100's	$63.41	GENERIC, Teva Pharmaceuticals Usa	00093-7127-01

Tablet - Oral - 10 mg

100's	$70.27	GENERIC, Teva Pharmaceuticals Usa	00093-7128-01

Tablet - Oral - 20 mg

100's	$82.08	GENERIC, Teva Pharmaceuticals Usa	00093-7129-01

Tablet - Oral - 100 mg

100's	$304.10	GENERIC, Teva Pharmaceuticals Usa	00093-7130-01

PRODUCT LISTING - EQUIVALENTS NOT AVAILABLE

Solution - Injectable - 10 mg/ml

2 ml x 10	$55.40	DEMADEX I.V., Roche Laboratories	00004-0267-06
5 ml x 10	$77.60	DEMADEX I.V., Roche Laboratories	00004-0268-06

Tablet - Oral - 5 mg			
100's	$71.25	DEMADEX, Roche Laboratories	00004-0262-01
100's	$71.25	DEMADEX, Roche Laboratories	00004-0262-49
Tablet - Oral - 10 mg			
30's	$16.14	DEMADEX, Allscripts Pharmaceutical Company	54569-4439-00
100's	$61.31	DEMADEX, Roche Laboratories	00004-0263-49
100's	$78.95	DEMADEX, Roche Laboratories	00004-0263-01
Tablet - Oral - 20 mg			
100's	$65.06	DEMADEX, Boehringer Mannheim	53169-0104-60
100's	$92.23	DEMADEX, Roche Laboratories	00004-0264-01
100's	$92.23	DEMADEX, Roche Laboratories	00004-0264-49
Tablet - Oral - 100 mg			
100's	$241.20	DEMADEX, Boehringer Mannheim	53169-0105-60
100's	$265.36	DEMADEX, Roche Laboratories	00004-0265-49
100's	$341.69	DEMADEX, Roche Laboratories	00004-0265-01

Tramadol Hydrochloride *(003255)*

For related information, see the comparative table section in Appendix A.

Categories: Pain, moderate to moderately severe; FDA Approved 1995 Mar; Pregnancy Category C
Drug Classes: Analgesics, narcotic-like
Brand Names: **Ultram**
Foreign Brand Availability: Adamon (Costa-Rica; Dominican-Republic; El-Salvador; Guatemala; Honduras; Nicaragua; Panama); Analab (Thailand); Analdol (Bahrain; Cyprus; Egypt; Iran; Iraq; Jordan; Kuwait; Lebanon; Libya; Oman; Qatar; Republic-of-Yemen; Saudi-Arabia; Syria; United-Arab-Emirates); Andalpha (Indonesia); Bellatram (Indonesia); Biodalgic (France); Contramal (France; India); Contramal LP (France); Dolana (Indonesia); Dolotral (Philippines); Dromadol (England); Exopen (Korea); Katrasic (Indonesia); Mabron (Bahrain; China; Cyprus; Egypt; Iran; Iraq; Jordan; Kuwait; Lebanon; Libya; Oman; Qatar; Republic-of-Yemen; Saudi-Arabia; Syria; Thailand; United-Arab-Emirates); Mosepan (Philippines); Omnidol (Colombia); O.P. Pain (Korea); Nonalges (Indonesia); Pengesic (Singapore); Penimadol (Korea); Prontofort (Mexico); Radol (Indonesia); Sefmal (Hong-Kong; Singapore); Takadol (France); Tamolan (Thailand); Tandol (Korea); Tarol (Bahrain; Cyprus; Egypt; Iran; Iraq; Jordan; Kuwait; Lebanon; Libya; Oman; Qatar; Republic-of-Yemen; Saudi-Arabia; Syria; United-Arab-Emirates); Topalgic (France); Trabar (Israel); Trabilin (Bahamas; Barbados; Belize; Bermuda; Curacao; Guyana; Jamaica; Netherland-Antilles; Puerto-Rico; Surinam; Trinidad); Tradol (Mexico); Tradol-Puren (Germany); Tradonal (Philippines); Tralic (Mexico); Tramadex (Israel); Tramagetic (Germany); Tramagit (Germany); Tramahexal (South-Africa); Tramake (England; Ireland); Tramal (Australia; Austria; Bahrain; Benin; Bulgaria; Burkina-Faso; China; Colombia; Cyprus; Ecuador; Egypt; Ethiopia; Gambia; Germany; Ghana; Guinea; Hong-Kong; Iran; Iraq; Ivory-Coast; Jordan; Kenya; Kuwait; Lebanon; Liberia; Libya; Malawi; Malaysia; Mali; Mauritania; Mauritius; Morocco; Netherlands; New-Zealand; Niger; Nigeria; Oman; Peru; Philippines; Qatar; Republic-of-Yemen; Saudi-Arabia; Senegal; Seychelles; Sierra-Leone; South-Africa; Sudan; Switzerland; Syria; Taiwan; Tanzania; Thailand; Tunia; Uganda; United-Arab-Emirates; Zambia; Zimbabwe); Tramal SR (Australia); Tramazac (Benin; Burkina-Faso; Ethiopia; Gambia; Ghana; Guinea; India; Ivory-Coast; Kenya; Liberia; Malawi; Mali; Mauritania; Mauritius; Morocco; Niger; Nigeria; Senegal; Seychelles; Sierra-Leone; Sudan; Tanzania; Tunia; Uganda; Zambia; Zimbabwe); Tramed (Taiwan); Tramol (Poland); Trasedal (France); Trasik (Indonesia); TRD-Contin (India); Trexol (Mexico); Tridol (Korea); Unitral (Philippines); Urgendol (India); Zamadol (England); Zamudol (France); Zodol (Peru); Zumatran (Indonesia); Zydol (England; Ireland); Zytram BD (New-Zealand); Zytram XL SR (Korea)
Cost of Therapy: $45.51 (Pain; Ultram; 50 mg; 4 tablets/day; 14 day supply)
$44.07 (Pain; Generic Tablets; 50 mg; 4 tablets/day; 14 day supply)

DESCRIPTION

Tramadol hydrochloride is a centrally acting analgesic. The chemical name for tramadol hydrochloride is (±)*cis*-2-[(dimethylamino)methyl]-1-(3-methoxyphenyl) cyclohexanol hydrochloride. The molecular weight of tramadol hydrochloride is 299.8.

Tramadol hydrochloride is a white, bitter, crystalline and odorless powder. It is readily soluble in water and ethanol and has a pKa of 9.41. The water/n-octanol partition coefficient is 1.35 at pH 7.

Ultram tablets contain 50 mg of tramadol hydrochloride and are white in color. Inactive ingredients in the tablet are corn starch, hydroxypropyl methylcellulose, lactose, magnesium stearate, microcrystalline cellulose, polyethylene glycol, polysorbate 80, sodium starch glycolate, titanium dioxide and wax.

CLINICAL PHARMACOLOGY

PHARMACODYNAMICS

Tramadol is a centrally acting synthetic analgesic compound. Although its mode of action is not completely understood, from animal tests, at least two complementary mechanisms appear applicable: binding of parent and M1 metabolite to μ-opioid receptors and weak inhibition of reuptake of norepinephrine and serotonin. Opioid activity is due to both low affinity binding of the parent compound and higher affinity binding of the O-demethylated metabolite M1 to μ-opioid receptors. In animal models, M1 is up to 6 times more potent than tramadol in producing analgesia and 200 times more potent in μ-opioid binding. Tramadol-induced analgesia is only partially antagonized by the opiate antagonist naloxone in several animal tests. The relative contribution of both tramadol and M1 to human analgesia is dependent upon the plasma concentrations of each compound (see Pharmacokinetics).

Tramadol has been shown to inhibit reuptake of norepinephrine and serotonin *in vitro*, as have some other opioid analgesics. These mechanisms may contribute independently to the overall analgesic profile of tramadol HCl. Analgesia in humans begins approximately within 1 hour after administration and reaches a peak in approximately 2-3 hours.

Apart from analgesia, tramadol administration may produce a constellation of symptoms (including dizziness, somnolence, nausea, constipation, sweating and pruritus) similar to that of an opioid. However, tramadol causes less respiratory depression than morphine at recommended doses. In contrast to morphine, tramadol has not been shown to cause histamine release. At therapeutic doses, tramadol has no effect on heart rate, left-ventricular function or cardiac index. Orthostatic hypotension has been observed.

PHARMACOKINETICS

The analgesic activity of tramadol HCl is due to both parent drug and the M1 metabolite (see Pharmacodynamics). Tramadol is administered as a racemate and both the [-] and [+] forms of both tramadol and M1 are detected in the circulation. Tramadol is well absorbed orally with an absolute bioavailability of 75%. Tramadol has a volume of distribution of approximately 2.7 L/kg and is only 20% bound to plasma proteins. Tramadol is extensively metabolized by a number of pathways, including CYP2D6 and CYP3A4, as well as by conjugation of parent and metabolites. One metabolite, M1, is pharmacologically active in animal models. The formation of M1 is dependent upon Cytochrome P-450(2D6) and as such is subject to both metabolic induction and inhibition which may affect the therapeutic response (see DRUG INTERACTIONS). Tramadol and its metabolites are excreted primarily in the urine with observed plasma half-lives of 6.3 and 7.4 hours for tramadol and M1, respectively. Linear pharmacokinetics have been observed following multiple doses of 50 and 100 mg to steady-state.

Absorption

Racemic tramadol is rapidly and almost completely absorbed after oral administration. The mean absolute bioavailability of a 100 mg oral dose is approximately 75%. The mean peak plasma concentration of racemic tramadol and M1 occurs at 2 and 3 hours, respectively, after administration in healthy adults. In general, both enantiomers of tramadol and M1 follow a parallel time course in the body following single and multiple doses although small differences (~10%) exist in the absolute amount of each enantiomer present.

Steady-state plasma concentrations of both tramadol and M1 are achieved within 2 days with qid dosing. There is no evidence of self-induction (see TABLE 1).

TABLE 1 *Mean (%CV) Pharmacokinetic Parameters for Racemic Tramadol and M1 Metabolite*

	Peak Conc. (ng/ml)	Time to Peak (hours)	Clearance/F* (ml/min/kg)	T½ (hours)
Healthy Adults, 100 mg qid, Multiple Dose po				
Tramadol	592 (30)	2.3 (61)	5.90 (25)	6.7 (15)
M1	110 (29)	2.4 (46)	NA	7.0 (14)
Healthy Adults, 100 mg Single Dose po				
Tramadol	308 (25)	1.6 (63)	8.50 (31)	5.6 (20)
M1	55.0 (36)	3.0 (51)	NA	6.7 (16)
Geriatric, (>75 years) 50 mg Single Dose po				
Tramadol	208 (31)	2.1 (19)	6.89 (25)	7.0 (23)
M1	NM	NM	NA	NM
Hepatic Impaired, 50 mg Single Dose po				
Tramadol	217 (11)	1.9 (16)	4.23 (56)	13.3 (11)
M1	19.4 (12)	9.8 (20)	NA	18.5 (15)
Renal Impaired, CLCR 10-30 ml/min 100 mg Single Dose IV				
Tramadol	NA	NA	4.23 (54)	10.6 (31)
M1	NA	NA	NA	11.5 (40)
Renal Impaired, CLCR <5 ml/min 100 mg Single Dose IV				
Tramadol	NA	NA	3.73 (17)	11.0 (29)
M1	NA	NA	NA	16.9 (18)

* F represents the oral bioavailability of tramadol
NA Not applicable
NM Not measured

Food Effect on Absorption

Oral administration of tramadol HCl with food does not significantly affect its rate or extent of absorption, therefore, tramadol HCl can be administered without regard to food.

Distribution

The volume of distribution of tramadol was 2.6 and 2.9 L/kg in male and female subjects, respectively following a 100 mg intravenous dose. The binding of tramadol to human plasma proteins is approximately 20% and binding also appears to be independent of concentration up to 10 μg/ml. Saturation of plasma protein binding occurs only at concentrations outside the clinically relevant range. Although not confirmed in humans, tramadol has been shown in rats to cross the blood-brain barrier.

Metabolism

Tramadol is extensively metabolized after oral administration. Approximately 30% of the dose is excreted in the urine as unchanged drug, whereas 60% of the dose is excreted as metabolites. The remainder is excreted either as unidentified or as unextractable metabolites. The major metabolic pathways appear to be *N*- and *O*-demethylation and glucuronidation or sulfation in the liver. One metabolite (*O*-desmethyltramadol, denoted M1) is pharmacologically active in animal models. Production of M1 is dependent on the CYP2D6 isoenzyme of cytochrome P-450 and as such is subject to both metabolic induction and inhibition which may affect the therapeutic response (see DRUG INTERACTIONS).

Approximately 7% of the population has reduced activity of the CYP2D6 isoenzyme of cytochrome P-450. These individuals are "poor metabolizers" of debrisoquine, dextromethorphan, tricyclic antidepressants, among other drugs. After a single oral dose of tramadol, concentrations of tramadol were only slightly higher in "poor metabolizers" versus "extensive metabolizers", while M1 concentrations were lower. Concomitant therapy with inhibitors of CYP2D6 such as fluoxetine, paroxetine, and quinidine could result in significant drug interactions. *In vitro* drug interaction studies in human liver microsomes indicate that inhibitors of CYP2D6 such as fluoxetine and its metabolite norfluoxetine, amitriptyline and quinidine inhibit the metabolism of tramadol to various degrees, suggesting that concomitant administration of these compounds could result in increases in tramadol concentrations and decreased concentrations of M1. The pharmacological impact of these alterations in terms of either efficacy or safety is unknown.

Elimination

The mean terminal plasma elimination half-lives of racemic tramadol and racemic M1 are 6.3 ± 1.4 and 7.4 ± 1.4 hours, respectively. The plasma elimination half-life of racemic tramadol increased from approximately 6-7 hours upon multiple dosing.

SPECIAL POPULATIONS

Renal

Impaired renal function results in a decreased rate and extent of excretion of tramadol and its active metabolite, M1. In patients with creatinine clearances of less than 30 ml/min,

T

adjustment of the dosing regimen is recommended (see DOSAGE AND ADMINISTRATION). The total amount of tramadol and M1 removed during a 4 hour dialysis period is less than 7% of the administered dose.

Hepatic

Metabolism of tramadol and M1 is reduced in patients with advanced cirrhosis of the liver, resulting in both a larger area under the concentration time curve for tramadol and longer tramadol and M1 elimination half-lives (13 hours for tramadol and 19 hours for M1). In cirrhotic patients adjustment of the dosing regimen is recommended (see DOSAGE AND ADMINISTRATION).

Age

Healthy elderly subjects aged 65-75 years have plasma tramadol concentrations and elimination half-lives comparable to those observed in healthy subjects less than 65 years of age. In subjects over 75 years, maximum serum concentrations are slightly elevated (208 vs 162 ng/ml) and the elimination half-life is slightly prolonged (7 vs 6 hours) compared to subjects 65-75 years of age. Adjustment of the daily dose is recommended for patients older than 75 years (see DOSAGE AND ADMINISTRATION).

Gender

The absolute bioavailability of tramadol was 73% in males and 79% in females. The plasma clearance was 6.4 ml/min/kg in males and 5.7 ml/min/kg in females following a 100 mg IV dose of tramadol. Following a single oral dose, and after adjusting for body weight, females had a 12% higher peak tramadol concentration and a 35% higher area under the concentration-time curve compared to males. The clinical significance of this difference is unknown.

INDICATIONS AND USAGE

Tramadol is indicated for the management of moderate to moderately severe pain.

NON-FDA APPROVED INDICATIONS

Tramadol has also been reported to have shown efficacy in the treatment of diabetic neuropathy and restless legs syndrome. However, these uses have not been approved by the FDA.

CONTRAINDICATIONS

Tramadol should not be administered to patients who have previously demonstrated hypersensitivity to tramadol, any other component of this product or opioids. It is also contraindicated in cases of acute intoxication with alcohol, hypnotics, centrally acting analgesics, opioids or psychotropic drugs.

WARNINGS

SEIZURE RISK

Seizures have been reported in patients receiving tramadol HCl within the recommended dosage range. Spontaneous post-marketing reports indicate that seizure risk is increased with doses of tramadol HCl above the recommended range. Concomitant use of tramadol HCl increases the seizure risk in patients taking:

- **Selective serotonin reuptake inhibitors (SSRI antidepressants or anoretics).**
- **Tricyclic antidepressants (TCAs), and other tricyclic compounds (*e.g.,* cyclobenzaprine, promethazine, etc.).**
- **Opioids.**

Administration of tramadol HCl may enhance the seizure risk in patients taking:

MAO inhibitors (see also WARNINGS, Use With MAO Inhibitors).

Neuroleptics.

Other drugs that reduce the seizure threshold.

Risk of convulsions may also increase in patients with epilepsy, those with a history of seizures, or in patients with a recognized risk for seizure (such as head trauma, metabolic disorders, alcohol and drug withdrawal, CNS infections). In tramadol HCl overdose, naloxone administration may increase the risk of seizure.

ANAPHYLACTOID REACTIONS

Serious and rarely fatal anaphylactoid reactions have been reported in patients receiving therapy with tramadol HCl. These reactions often occur following the first dose. Other reported reactions include pruritus, hives, bronchospasm, and angioedema. Patients with a history of anaphylactoid reactions to codeine and other opioids may be at increased risk and therefore should not receive tramadol HCl (see CONTRAINDICATIONS).

USE IN OPIOID-DEPENDENT PATIENTS

Tramadol HCl should not be used in opioid-dependent patients. Tramadol HCl has been shown to reinitiate physical dependence in some patients that have been previously dependent on other opioids. Consequently, in patients with a tendency to opioid abuse or opioid dependence, treatment with tramadol HCl is not recommended.

USE WITH CNS DEPRESSANTS

Tramadol should be used with caution and in reduced dosages when administered to patients receiving CNS depressants such as alcohol, opioids, anesthetic agents, phenothiazines, tranquilizers or sedative hypnotics.

USE WITH MAO INHIBITORS

Tramadol should be used with great caution in patients taking monoamine oxidase inhibitors, because animal studies have shown increased deaths with combined administration.

PRECAUTIONS

RESPIRATORY DEPRESSION

Administer tramadol HCl cautiously in patients at risk for respiratory depression. When large doses of tramadol HCl are administered with anesthetic medications or alcohol, respiratory depression may result. Treat such cases as an overdose. If naloxone is to be administered, use cautiously because it may precipitate seizures (see WARNINGS, Seizure Risk).

INCREASED INTRACRANIAL PRESSURE OR HEAD TRAUMA

Tramadol should be used with caution in patients with increased intracranial pressure or head injury. Pupillary changes (miosis) from tramadol may obscure the existence, extent, or course of intracranial pathology. Clinicians should also maintain a high index of suspicion for adverse drug reaction when evaluating altered mental status in these patients if they are receiving tramadol.

ACUTE ABDOMINAL CONDITIONS

The administration of tramadol may complicate the clinical assessment of patients with acute abdominal conditions.

WITHDRAWAL

Withdrawal symptoms may occur if tramadol HCl is discontinued abruptly. These symptoms may include: anxiety, sweating, insomnia, rigors, pain, nausea, tremors, diarrhoea, upper respiratory symptoms, piloerection, and rarely hallucinations. Clinical experience suggests that withdrawal symptoms may be relieved by tapering the medication.

PATIENTS PHYSICALLY DEPENDENT ON OPIOIDS

Tramadol is not recommended for patients who are dependent on opioids. Patients who have recently taken substantial amounts of opioids may experience withdrawal symptoms. Because of the difficulty in assessing dependence in patients who have previously received substantial amounts of opioid medication, administer tramadol cautiously to such patients.

USE IN RENAL AND HEPATIC DISEASE

Impaired renal function results in a decreased rate and extent of excretion of tramadol and its active metabolite, M1. In patients with creatinine clearances of less than 30 ml/min, dosing reduction is recommended (see DOSAGE AND ADMINISTRATION).

Metabolism of tramadol and M1 is reduced in patients with advanced cirrhosis of the liver. In cirrhotic patients, dosing reduction is recommended (see DOSAGE AND ADMINISTRATION).

With the prolonged half-life in these conditions, achievement of steady state is delayed, so that it may take several days for elevated plasma concentrations to develop.

INFORMATION FOR THE PATIENT

- Tramadol HCl may impair mental or physical abilities required for the performance of potentially hazardous tasks such as driving a car or operating machinery.
- Tramadol HCl should not be taken with alcohol containing beverages.
- Tramadol HCl should be used with caution when taking medications such as tranquilizers, hypnotics or other opiate containing analgesics.
- Patients should be instructed to inform the physician if they are pregnant, think they might become pregnant, or are trying to become pregnant (see Labor and Delivery).
- The patient should understand the single-dose and 24 hour dose limit and the time interval between doses, since exceeding these recommendations can result in respiratory depression and seizures.

CARCINOGENESIS, MUTAGENESIS, AND IMPAIRMENT OF FERTILITY

Tramadol was not mutagenic in the following assays: Ames *Salmonella* microsomal activation test, CHO/HPRT mammalian cell assay, mouse lymphoma assay (in the absence of metabolic activation), dominant lethal mutation tests in mice, chromosome aberration test in Chinese hamsters, and bone marrow micronucleus tests in mice and Chinese hamsters. Weakly mutagenic results occurred in the presence of metabolic activation in the mouse lymphoma assay and micronucleus test in rats. Overall, the weight of evidence from these tests indicates that tramadol does not pose a genotoxic risk to humans.

A slight, but statistically significant, increase in 2 common murine tumors, pulmonary and hepatic, was observed in a mouse carcinogenicity study, particularly in aged mice (dosing orally up to 30 mg/kg for approximately 2 years, although the study was not done with the Maximum Tolerated Dose). This finding is not believed to suggest risk in humans. No such finding occurred in a rat carcinogenicity study.

No effects on fertility were observed for tramadol at oral dose levels up to 50 mg/kg in male rats and 75 mg/kg in female rats.

PREGNANCY, TERATOGENIC EFFECTS, PREGNANCY CATEGORY C

There are no adequate and well-controlled studies in pregnant women. Tramadol should be used during pregnancy only if the potential benefit justifies the potential risk to the fetus.

Tramadol has been shown to be embryotoxic and fetotoxic in mice, rats and rabbits at maternally toxic doses 3-15 times the maximum human dose or higher (120 mg/kg in mice, 25 mg/kg or higher in rats and 75 mg/kg or higher in rabbits), but was not teratogenic at these dose levels. No harm to the fetus due to tramadol was seen at doses that were not maternally toxic.

No drug-related teratogenic effects were observed in progeny of mice, rats or rabbits treated with tramadol by various routes (up to 140 mg/kg for mice, 80 mg/kg for rats or 300 mg/kg for rabbits). Embryo and fetal toxicity consisted primarily of decreased fetal weights, skeletal ossification and increased supernumerary ribs at maternally toxic dose levels. Transient delays in developmental or behavioral parameters were also seen in pups from rat dams allowed to deliver. Embryo and fetal lethality were reported only in one rabbit study at 300 mg/kg, a dose that would cause extreme maternal toxicity in the rabbit.

In peri- and post-natal studies in rats, progeny of dams receiving oral (gavage) dose levels of 50 mg/kg or greater had decreased weights, and pup survival was decreased early in lactation at 80 mg/kg (6-10 times the maximum human dose). No toxicity was observed for progeny of dams receiving 8, 10, 20, 25 or 40 mg/kg. Maternal toxicity was observed at all dose levels, but effects on progeny were evident only at higher dose levels where maternal toxicity was more severe.

LABOR AND DELIVERY

Tramadol should not be used in pregnant women prior to or during labor unless the potential benefits outweigh the risks. Safe use in pregnancy has not been established. Chronic use during pregnancy may lead to physical dependance and post-partum withdrawl symptoms in the newborn. Tramadol has been shown to cross the placenta. The mean ratio of serum tramadol in the umbilical veins compared to maternal veins was 0.83 for 40 women given tramadol during labor.

The effect of tramadol, if any, on the later growth, development, and functional maturation of the child is unknown.

NURSING MOTHERS

Tramadol is not recommended for obstetrical preoperative medication or for post-delivery analgesia in nursing mothers because its safety in infants and newborns has not been studied. Following a single IV 100 mg dose of tramadol, the cumulative excretion in breast milk within 16 hours postdose was 100 μg of tramadol (0.1% of the maternal dose) and 27 μg of M1.

PEDIATRIC USE

The pediatric use of tramadol is not recommended because safety and efficacy in patients under 16 years of age have not been established.

GERIATRIC USE

In subjects over the age of 75 years, serum concentrations are slightly elevated and the elimination half-life is slightly prolonged. The aged also can be expected to vary more widely in their ability to tolerate adverse drug effects. Daily doses in excess of 300 mg are not recommended in patients over 75 (see DOSAGE AND ADMINISTRATION).

DRUG INTERACTIONS

Tramadol does not appear to induce its own metabolism in humans, since observed maximal plasma concentrations after multiple oral doses are higher than expected based on single-dose data. Tramadol is a mild inducer of selected drug metabolism pathways measured in animals.

Use With Carbamazepine: Concomitant administration of tramadol hydrochloride with **carbamazepine** causes a significant increase in tramadol metabolism, presumably through metabolic induction by carbamazepine. Patients receiving chronic carbamazepine doses of up to 800 mg daily may require up to twice the recommended dose of tramadol.

Use With Quinidine: Tramadol is metabolized to M1 by the CYP2D6 P-450 isoenzyme. **Quinidine** is a selective inhibitor of that isoenzyme; so that concomitant administration of quinidine and tramadol results in increased concentrations of tramadol and reduced concentrations of M1. The clinical consequences of this effect have not been fully investigated, and the effect on quinidine concentrations is unknown. *In vitro* drug interaction studies in human liver microsomes indicate that tramadol has no effect on quinidine metabolism.

Use With Inhibitors of CYP2D6: *In vitro* drug interaction studies in human liver microsomes indicate that concomitant administration with inhibitors of CYP2D6 such as fluoxetine, paroxetine, and amitriptyline could result in some inhibition of the metabolism of tramadol.

Use With Cimetidine: Concomitant administration of tramadol with **cimetidine** does not result in clinically significant changes in tramadol pharmacokinetics. Therefore, no alteration of the tramadol dosage regimen is recommended.

Use With MAO Inhibitors: Interactions with **MAO Inhibitors** due to interference with detoxification mechanisms, have been reported for some centrally acting drugs (see WARNINGS, Use With MAO Inhibitors)).

Use With Digoxin and Warfarin: Post-marketing surveillance has revealed rare reports of digoxin toxicity and alteration of warfarin effect, including elevation of prothrombin times.

ADVERSE REACTIONS

Tramadol hydrochloride was administered to 550 patients during the double-blind or open-label extension periods in US studies of chronic nonmalignant pain. Of these patients, 375 were 65 years old or older. TABLE 2 reports the cumulative incidence rate of adverse reactions by 7, 30 and 90 days for the most frequent reactions (5% or more by 7 days). The most frequently reported events were in the central nervous system and gastrointestinal system. Although the reactions listed in the table are felt to be probably related to tramadol administration, the reported rates also include some events that may have been due to underlying disease or concomitant medication. The overall incidence rates of adverse experiences in these trials were similar for tramadol and the active control groups, acetaminophen 300 mg with codeine phosphate 30 mg, and aspirin 325 mg with codeine phosphate 30 mg. (TABLE 2)

INCIDENCE 1% TO LESS THAN 5%, POSSIBLY CASUALLY RELATED

The following lists adverse reactions that occurred with an incidence of 1% to less than 5% in clinical trials, and for which the possibility of a casual relationship with tramadol exists.

Body as a Whole: Malaise.

Cardiovascular: Vasodilation.

Central Nervous System: Anxiety, confusion, coordination disturbance, euphoria, nervousness, sleep disorder.

Gastrointestinal: Abdominal pain, anorexia, flatulence.

Musculoskeletal: Hypertonia.

Skin: Rash.

Special Senses: Visual disturbance.

Urogenital: Urinary retention, urinary frequency, menopausal symptoms.

INCIDENCE LESS THAN 1%, POSSIBLE CAUSALLY RELATED

The following lists adverse reactions that occurred with an incidence of less than 1% in clinical trials and/or reported in post-marketing experience.

Body as a Whole: Allergic reaction, accidental injury, weight loss, anaphylaxis.

TABLE 2 *Cumulative Incidence of Adverse Reactions for Tramadol HCl In Chronic Trials of Nonmalignant Pain (n=427)*

	Up to 7 Days	Up to 30 Days	Up to 90 Days
Dizziness/vertigo	26%	31%	33%
Nausea	24%	34%	40%
Constipation	24%	38%	46%
Headache	18%	26%	32%
Somnolence	16%	23%	25%
Vomiting	9%	13%	17%
Pruritus	8%	10%	11%
CNS stimulation*	7%	11%	14%
Asthenia	6%	11%	12%
Sweating	6%	7%	9%
Dyspepsia	5%	9%	13%
Dry mouth	5%	9%	10%
Diarrhea	5%	6%	10%

* CNS Stimulation is a composite of nervousness, anxiety, agitation, tremor, spasticity, euphoria, emotional lability and hallucinations.

Cardiovascular: Syncope, orthostatic hypotension, tachycardia.

Central Nervous System: Seizure (see WARNINGS), paresthesia, cognitive dysfunction, hallucinations, tremor, amnesia, difficulty in concentration, abnormal gait, depression.

Respiratory: Dyspnea.

Skin: Urticaria, vesicles, Stevens-Johnson syndrome/toxic epidermal necrolysis.

Special Senses: Dysgeusia.

Urogenital: Dysuria, menstrual disorder.

OTHER ADVERSE EXPERIENCES, CAUSAL RELATIONSHIP UNKNOWN

A variety of other adverse events were reported infrequently in patients taking tramadol during clinical trials and/or reported in post-marketing experience. A causal relationship between tramadol and these events has not been determined. However, the most significant events are listed below as alerting information to the physician.

Body as a Whole: Suicidal tendency.

Cardiovascular: Abnormal ECG, hypertension, hypotension, myocardial ischemia, palpitations.

Central Nervous System: Migraine, speech disorders.

Gastrointestinal: Gastrointestinal bleeding, hepatitis, stomatitis.

Laboratory Abnormalities: Creatinine increase, elevated liver enzymes, hemoglobin decrease, proteinuria.

Sensory: Cataracts, deafness, tinnitus.

Skin: Pruritus.

DOSAGE AND ADMINISTRATION

For the treatment of painful conditions tramadol 50-100 mg can be administered as needed for relief every 4-6 hours, **not to exceed 400 mg/day.** For moderate pain tramadol 50 mg may be adequate as the initial dose, and for more severe pain, tramadol 100 mg is usually more effective as the initial dose.

INDIVIDUALIZATION OF DOSE

Available data do not suggest that a dosage adjustment is necessary in elderly patients 65-75 years of age unless they also have renal or hepatic impairment. For elderly patients **over 75 years old,** not more than 300 mg/day in divided doses as above is recommended. In all patients with **creatine clearance less than 30 ml/min,** it is recommended that the dosing interval of tramadol HCl be increased to 12 hours with a maximum daily dose of 200 mg. Since only 7% of an administered dose is removed by hemodialysis, **dialysis patients** can receive their regular dose on the day of dialysis. The recommended dose for patients with **cirrhosis** is 50 mg every 12 hours. Patients receiving chronic **carbamazepine** doses up to 800 mg daily may require up to twice the recommended dose of tramadol HCl.

HOW SUPPLIED

Ultram 50 mg (white, film-coated capsule-shaped tablet) is engraved "McNeil" on one side and "659" on the other side.

Storage: Dispense in a tight container. Store at controlled room temperature (up to 25°C [77°F]).

PRODUCT LISTING - RATED THERAPEUTICALLY EQUIVALENT

Tablet - Oral - 50 mg

100's	$78.69	GENERIC, Mallinckrodt Medical Inc	00406-7171-01
100's	$79.58	GENERIC, Mutual/United Research Laboratories	53489-0499-01
100's	$79.60	GENERIC, Udl Laboratories Inc	51079-0991-20
100's	$82.90	GENERIC, Teva Pharmaceuticals Usa	00093-0058-01
100's	$83.37	GENERIC, Sidmak Laboratories Inc	50111-0616-01
100's	$83.40	GENERIC, Dixon-Shane Inc	17236-0363-01
100's	$83.70	GENERIC, Purepac Pharmaceutical Company	00228-2714-11
100's	$83.81	GENERIC, Caraco Pharmaceutical Laboratories	57664-0377-08
100's	$83.84	GENERIC, Eon Labs Manufacturing Inc	00185-0311-01

PRODUCT LISTING - EQUIVALENTS NOT AVAILABLE

Tablet - Oral - 50 mg

2's	$1.70	ULTRAM, Allscripts Pharmaceutical Company	54569-4089-07
6's	$5.11	ULTRAM, Allscripts Pharmaceutical Company	54569-4089-08
7's	$5.69	ULTRAM, Southwood Pharmaceuticals Inc	58016-0387-07

T

7's	$6.51	GENERIC, Southwood Pharmaceuticals Inc	58016-0708-07
10's	$8.13	ULTRAM, Southwood Pharmaceuticals Inc	58016-0387-10
10's	$8.52	ULTRAM, Allscripts Pharmaceutical Company	54569-4089-04
10's	$9.30	GENERIC, Southwood Pharmaceuticals Inc	58016-0708-10
10's	$20.01	GENERIC, Pharma Pac	52959-0688-10
10's	$22.23	ULTRAM, Pharma Pac	52959-0414-10
14's	$16.82	ULTRAM, Dhs Inc	55887-0897-14
15's	$12.19	ULTRAM, Southwood Pharmaceuticals Inc	58016-0387-15
15's	$12.78	ULTRAM, Allscripts Pharmaceutical Company	54569-4089-05
15's	$13.94	GENERIC, Southwood Pharmaceuticals Inc	58016-0708-15
15's	$14.85	ULTRAM, Physicians Total Care	54868-3605-03
15's	$19.65	ULTRAM, Pd-Rx Pharmaceuticals	55289-0650-15
15's	$27.28	GENERIC, Pharma Pac	52959-0688-15
15's	$30.31	ULTRAM, Pharma Pac	52959-0414-15
20's	$16.25	ULTRAM, Southwood Pharmaceuticals Inc	58016-0387-20
20's	$17.88	ULTRAM, Allscripts Pharmaceutical Company	54569-4089-00
20's	$18.59	GENERIC, Southwood Pharmaceuticals Inc	58016-0708-20
20's	$19.40	ULTRAM, Physicians Total Care	54868-3605-00
20's	$22.72	ULTRAM, St. Mary'S Mpp	60760-0659-20
20's	$24.06	ULTRAM, Dhs Inc	55887-0897-20
20's	$24.86	ULTRAM, Pd-Rx Pharmaceuticals	55289-0650-20
20's	$34.78	GENERIC, Pharma Pac	52959-0688-20
20's	$38.64	ULTRAM, Pharma Pac	52959-0414-20
21's	$17.07	ULTRAM, Southwood Pharmaceuticals Inc	58016-0387-21
21's	$19.52	GENERIC, Southwood Pharmaceuticals Inc	58016-0708-21
21's	$36.51	GENERIC, Pharma Pac	52959-0688-21
24's	$32.81	ULTRAM, Pd-Rx Pharmaceuticals	55289-0650-24
24's	$40.22	GENERIC, Pharma Pac	52959-0688-24
24's	$44.69	ULTRAM, Pharma Pac	52959-0414-24
25's	$20.32	ULTRAM, Southwood Pharmaceuticals Inc	58016-0387-25
25's	$23.24	GENERIC, Southwood Pharmaceuticals Inc	58016-0708-25
28's	$22.75	ULTRAM, Southwood Pharmaceuticals Inc	58016-0387-28
28's	$26.03	GENERIC, Southwood Pharmaceuticals Inc	58016-0708-28
28's	$45.16	GENERIC, Pharma Pac	52959-0688-28
28's	$50.18	ULTRAM, Pharma Pac	52959-0414-28
30's	$24.38	ULTRAM, Southwood Pharmaceuticals Inc	58016-0387-30
30's	$25.56	ULTRAM, Allscripts Pharmaceutical Company	54569-4089-01
30's	$27.89	GENERIC, Southwood Pharmaceuticals Inc	58016-0708-30
30's	$28.52	ULTRAM, Physicians Total Care	54868-3605-02
30's	$34.08	ULTRAM, St. Mary'S Mpp	60760-0659-30
30's	$37.21	ULTRAM, Dhs Inc	55887-0897-30
30's	$37.64	ULTRAM, Pd-Rx Pharmaceuticals	55289-0650-30
30's	$47.63	GENERIC, Pharma Pac	52959-0688-30
30's	$52.92	ULTRAM, Pharma Pac	52959-0414-30
40's	$32.51	ULTRAM, Southwood Pharmaceuticals Inc	58016-0387-40
40's	$37.18	GENERIC, Southwood Pharmaceuticals Inc	58016-0708-40
40's	$57.46	GENERIC, Pharma Pac	52959-0688-40
40's	$63.84	ULTRAM, Pharma Pac	52959-0414-40
42's	$34.13	ULTRAM, Southwood Pharmaceuticals Inc	58016-0387-42
42's	$39.04	GENERIC, Southwood Pharmaceuticals Inc	58016-0708-42
50's	$40.63	ULTRAM, Southwood Pharmaceuticals Inc	58016-0387-50
50's	$42.61	ULTRAM, Allscripts Pharmaceutical Company	54569-4089-02
50's	$46.48	GENERIC, Southwood Pharmaceuticals Inc	58016-0708-50
60's	$48.76	ULTRAM, Southwood Pharmaceuticals Inc	58016-0387-60
60's	$55.77	GENERIC, Southwood Pharmaceuticals Inc	58016-0708-60
60's	$55.86	ULTRAM, Physicians Total Care	54868-3605-05
60's	$68.16	ULTRAM, St. Mary'S Mpp	60760-0659-60
60's	$91.09	GENERIC, Pharma Pac	52959-0688-60
60's	$101.21	ULTRAM, Pharma Pac	52959-0414-60
90's	$73.14	ULTRAM, Southwood Pharmaceuticals Inc	58016-0387-90
90's	$83.66	GENERIC, Southwood Pharmaceuticals Inc	58016-0708-90
100's	$81.27	ULTRAM, Southwood Pharmaceuticals Inc	58016-0387-00
100's	$83.37	GENERIC, Watson Laboratories Inc	00591-0466-01
100's	$83.75	GENERIC, Par Pharmaceutical Inc	49884-0742-01
100's	$85.21	ULTRAM, Allscripts Pharmaceutical Company	54569-4089-03
100's	$88.22	ULTRAM, Physicians Total Care	54868-3605-04
100's	$92.95	GENERIC, Southwood Pharmaceuticals Inc	58016-0708-00
100's	$106.48	ULTRAM, Janssen Pharmaceuticals	00045-0659-60
100's	$117.11	ULTRAM, Janssen Pharmaceuticals	00045-0659-10
100's	$126.00	GENERIC, Pharma Pac	52959-0688-00
100's	$135.10	ULTRAM, Pharma Pac	52959-0414-00
120's	$111.54	GENERIC, Southwood Pharmaceuticals Inc	58016-0708-02
120's	$143.64	GENERIC, Pharma Pac	52959-0688-02
140's	$130.13	GENERIC, Southwood Pharmaceuticals Inc	58016-0708-81
150's	$139.43	GENERIC, Southwood Pharmaceuticals Inc	58016-0708-03
200's	$170.42	ULTRAM, Allscripts Pharmaceutical Company	54569-4089-06
200's	$185.90	GENERIC, Southwood Pharmaceuticals Inc	58016-0708-89

Trandolapril (003286)

For related information, see the comparative table section in Appendix A.

Categories: Hypertension, essential; Pregnancy Category C, 1st Trimester; Pregnancy Category D, 2nd & 3rd Trimesters; FDA Approved 1996 Apr
Drug Classes: Angiotensin converting enzyme inhibitors
Brand Names: **Mavik**
Foreign Brand Availability: Gopten (Australia; Colombia; Czech-Republic; Denmark; England; Finland; France; Germany; Italy; Mexico; Netherlands; New-Zealand; Portugal; South-Africa; Spain; Switzerland; Turkey); Odace (Philippines); Odrik (Australia; Denmark; England; Finland; France; Greece; Italy; New-Zealand; Peru; Portugal; Spain); Udrik (Germany)
Cost of Therapy: $28.83 (Hypertension; Mavik; 2 mg; 1 tablet/day; 30 day supply)

WARNING

Use in Pregnancy

When used in pregnancy during the second and third trimesters, ACE inhibitors can cause injury and even death to the developing fetus. When pregnancy is detected, trandolapril should be discontinued as soon as possible. (See WARNINGS, Mortality.)

DESCRIPTION

Trandolapril is the ethyl ester prodrug of a nonsulfhydryl angiotensin converting enzyme (ACE) inhibitor, trandolaprilat. Trandolapril is chemically described as (2S, 3aR, 7aS)-1-[(S)-N-[(S)-1-Carboxy-3-phenylpropyl]alanyl] hexahydro-2-indolinecarboxylic acid, 1-ethyl ester. Its empirical formula is $C_{24}H_{34}N_2O_5$. It has a molecular weight of 430.54 and a melting point of 125°C.

Trandolapril is a colorless, crystalline substance that is soluble (>100 mg/ml) in chloroform, dichloromethane, and methanol. Mavik tablets contain 1, 2, or 4 mg of trandolapril for oral administration. Each tablet also contains corn starch , croscarmellose sodium, hydroxypropyl methylcellulose, iron oxide, lactose, povidone, sodium stearyl fumarate.

CLINICAL PHARMACOLOGY

MECHANISM OF ACTION

Trandolapril is deesterified to the diacid metabolite, trandolaprilat, which is approximately 8 times more active as an inhibitor of ACE activity. ACE is a peptidyl dipeptidase that catalyzes the conversion of angiotensin I to the vasoconstrictor, angiotensin II. Angiotensin II is a potent peripheral vasoconstrictor that also stimulates secretion of aldosterone by the adrenal cortex and provides negative feedback for renin secretion. The effect of trandolapril in hypertension appears to result primarily from the inhibition of circulating and tissue ACE activity thereby reducing angiotensin II formation, decreasing vasoconstriction, decreasing aldosterone secretion, and increasing plasma renin. Decreased aldosterone secretion leads to diuresis, natriuresis, and a small increase of serum potassium. In controlled clinical trials, treatment with trandolapril alone resulted in mean increases in potassium of 0.1 mEq/L. (See PRECAUTIONS.)

ACE is identical to kininase II, an enzyme that degrades bradykinin, a potent peptide vasodilator; whether increased levels of bradykinin play a role in the therapeutic effect of trandolapril remains to be elucidated.

While the principal mechanism of antihypertensive effect is thought to be through the renin-angiotensin-aldosterone system, trandolapril exerts antihypertensive actions even in patients with low-renin hypertension. Trandolapril was an effective antihypertensive in all races studied. Both black patients (usually a predominantly low-renin group) and non-black patients responded to 2-4 mg of trandolapril.

PHARMACOKINETICS AND METABOLISM

Pharmacokinetics

Trandolapril's ACE-inhibiting activity is primarily due to its diacid metabolite, trandolaprilat. Cleavage of the ester group of trandolapril, primarily in the liver, is responsible for conversion. Absolute bioavailability after oral administration of trandolapril is about 10% as trandolapril and 70% as trandolaprilat. After oral trandolapril under fasting conditions, peak trandolapril levels occur at about 1 hour and peak trandolaprilat levels occur between 4 and 10 hours. The elimination half lives of trandolapril and trandolaprilat are about 6 and 10 hours, respectively, but, like all ACE inhibitors, trandolaprilat also has a prolonged terminal elimination phase, involving a small fraction of administered drug, probably representing binding to plasma and tissue ACE. During multiple dosing of trandolapril, there is no significant accumulation of trandolaprilat. Food slows absorption of trandolapril, but does not effect AUC or C_{max} of trandolaprilat or C_{max} of trandolapril.

Metabolism and Excretion

After oral administration of trandolapril, about 33% of parent drug and metabolites are recovered in urine, mostly as trandolaprilat, with about 66% in feces. The extent of the absorbed dose which is biliary excreted has not been determined. Plasma concentrations (C_{max} and AUC of trandolapril and C_{max} of trandolaprilat) are dose proportional over the 1-4 mg range, but the AUC of trandolaprilat is somewhat less than dose proportional. In addition to trandolaprilat, at least 7 other metabolites have been found, principally glucuronides or deesterification products.

Serum protein binding of trandolapril is about 80%, and is independent of concentration. Binding of trandolaprilat is concentration-dependent, varying from 65% at 1000 ng/ml to 94% at 0.1 ng/ml, indicating saturation of binding with increasing concentration.

The volume of distribution of trandolapril is about 18 L. Total plasma clearances of trandolapril and trandolaprilat after approximately 2 mg IV doses are about 52 L/hour and 7L/hour respectively. Renal clearance of trandolaprilat varies from 1-4 L/hour, depending on dose.

T

SPECIAL POPULATIONS

Pediatric

Trandolapril pharmacokinetics have not been evaluated in patients <18 years of age.

Geriatric and Gender

Trandolapril pharmacokinetics have been investigated in the elderly (>65 years) and in both genders. The plasma concentration of trandolapril is increased in elderly hypertensive patients, but the plasma concentration of trandolaprilat and inhibition of ACE activity are similar in elderly and young hypertensive patients. The pharmacokinetics of trandolapril and trandolaprilat and inhibition of ACE activity are similar in male and female elderly hypertensive patients.

Race

Pharmacokinetic differences have not been evaluated in different races.

Renal Insufficiency

Compared to normal subjects, the plasma concentrations of trandolapril and trandolaprilat are approximately 2-fold greater and renal clearance is reduced by about 85% in patients with creatinine clearance below 30 ml/min and in patients on hemodialysis. Dosage adjustment is recommended in renally impaired patients. (See DOSAGE AND ADMINISTRATION.)

Hepatic Insufficiency

Following oral administration in patients with mild to moderate alcoholic cirrhosis, plasma concentrations of trandolapril and trandolaprilat were, respectively, 9- and 2-fold greater than in normal subjects, but inhibition of ACE activity was not affected. Lower doses should be considered in patients with hepatic insufficiency. (See DOSAGE AND ADMINISTRATION.)

PHARMACODYNAMICS AND CLINICAL EFFECTS

A single 2-mg dose of trandolapril produces 70-85% inhibition of plasma ACE activity at 4 hours with about 10% decline at 24 hours and about half the effect manifest at 8 days. Maximum ACE inhibition is achieved with a plasma trandolaprilat concentration of 2 ng/ml. ACE inhibition is a function of trandolaprilat concentration, not trandolapril concentration. The effect of trandolapril on exogenous angiotensin I was not measured.

HYPERTENSION

Four placebo-controlled dose response studies were conducted using once-daily oral dosing of trandolapril in doses from 0.25-16 mg/day in 827 black and non-black patients with mild to moderate hypertension. The minimal effective once-daily dose was 1 mg in non-black patients and 2 mg in black patients. Further decreases in trough supine diastolic blood pressure were obtained in non-black patients with higher doses, and no further response was seen with doses above 4 mg (up to 16 mg). The antihypertensive effect diminished somewhat at the end of the dosing interval, but trough/peak ratios are well above 50% for all effective doses. There was a slightly greater effect on the diastolic pressure, but no difference on systolic pressure with bid dosing. During chronic therapy, the maximum reduction in blood pressure with any dose is achieved within 1 week. Following 6 weeks of monotherapy in placebo-controlled trials in patients with mild to moderate hypertension, once-daily doses of 2-4 mg lowered supine or standing systolic/diastolic blood pressure 24 hours after dosing by an average 7-10/4-5 mm Hg below placebo responses in non-black patients. Once-daily doses of 2-4 mg lowered blood pressure 4-6/3-4 mm Hg in black patients. Trough to peak ratios for effective doses ranged from 0.5-0.9. There were no differences in response between men and women, but responses were somewhat greater in patients under 60 than in patients over 60 years old. Abrupt withdrawal of trandolapril has not been associated with a rapid increase in blood pressure.

Administration of trandolapril to patients with mild to moderate hypertension results in a reduction of supine, sitting and standing blood pressure to about the same extent without compensatory tachycardia.

Symptomatic hypotension is infrequent, although it can occur in patients who are salt-and/or volume-depleted. (See WARNINGS.) Use of trandolapril in combination with thiazide diuretics gives a blood pressure lowering effect greater than that seen with either agent alone, and the additional effect of trandolapril is similar to the effect of monotherapy.

Heart Failure Post Myocardial Infarction or Left-Ventricular Dysfunction Post Myocardial Infarction

The Trandolapril Cardiac Evaluation (TRACE) Trial was a Danish, 27-center, double-blind, placebo controlled, parallel-group study of the effect of trandolapril on all-cause mortality in stable patients with echocardiographic evidence of left-ventricular dysfunction 3-7 days after a myocardial infarction. Subjects with residual ischemia or overt heart failure were included. Patients tolerant of a test dose of 1 mg trandolapril were randomized to placebo (n=873) or trandolapril (n=876) and followed for 24 months. Among patients randomized to trandolapril, who began treatment on 1 mg, 62% were successfully titrated to a target dose of 4 mg once daily over a period of weeks. The use of trandolapril was associated with a 16% reduction in the risk of all-cause mortality (p=0.042), largely cardiovascular mortality. Trandolapril was also associated with a 20% reduction in the risk of progression of heart failure (p=0.047), defined by a time-to-first-event analysis of death attributed to heart failure, hospitalization for heart failure, or requirement for open-label ACE inhibitor for the treatment of heart failure. There was no significant effect of treatment on other end-points: subsequent hospitalization, incidence of recurrent myocardial infarction, exercise tolerance, ventricular function, ventricular dimensions, or NYHA class.

The population in TRACE was entirely Caucasian and had less usage than would be typical in a US population of other post-infarction interventions: 42% thrombolysis, 16% beta-adrenergic blockade, and 6.7% PTCA or CABG during the entire period of follow-up. Blood pressure control, especially in the placebo group, was poor: 47-53% of patients randomized to placebo and 32-40% of patients randomized to trandolapril had blood pressures >140/95 at 90 day follow-up visits.

INDICATIONS AND USAGE

HYPERTENSION

Trandolapril is indicated for the treatment of hypertension. It may be used alone or in combination with other antihypertensive medication such as hydrochlorothiazide.

In considering the use of trandolapril, it should be noted that in controlled trials ACE inhibitors (for which adequate data are available) cause a higher rate of angioedema in black than in non-black patients. (See WARNINGS, Anaphylactoid and Possibly Related Reactions, Angioedema.)

When using trandolapril, consideration should be given to the fact that another angiotensin converting enzyme inhibitor, captopril, has caused agranulocytosis, particularly in patients with renal impairment or collagen-vascular disease. Available data are insufficient to show that trandolapril does not have a similar risk. (See WARNINGS.)

HEART FAILURE POST MYOCARDIAL INFARCTION OR LEFT-VENTRICULAR DYSFUNCTION POST MYOCARDIAL INFARCTION

Trandolapril is indicated in stable patients who have evidence of left-ventricular systolic dysfunction (identified by wall motion abnormalities) or who are symptomatic from congestive heart failure within the first few days after sustaining acute myocardial infarction. Administration of trandolapril to Caucasian patients has been shown to decrease the risk of death (principally cardiovascular death) and to decrease the risk of heart failure-related hospitalization. (See CLINICAL PHARMACOLOGY, Hypertension, Heart Failure Post Myocardial Infarction or Left-Ventricular Dysfunction Post Myocardial Infarction for details of the survival trial.)

NON-FDA APPROVED INDICATIONS

ACE inhibitors have also been used for the treatment of diabetic nephropathy (proteinuria greater than 500 mg/day) in patients with diabetes mellitus and retinopathy.

CONTRAINDICATIONS

Trandolapril is contraindicated in patients who are hypersensitive to this product and in patients with a history of angioedema related to previous treatment with an ACE inhibitor.

WARNINGS

ANAPHYLACTOID AND POSSIBLY RELATED REACTIONS

Presumably because angiotensin converting enzyme inhibitors affect the metabolism of eicosanoids and polypeptides, including endogenous bradykinin, patients receiving ACE inhibitors, including trandolapril, may be subject to a variety of adverse reactions, some of them serious.

Angioedema

Angioedema of the face, extremities, lips, tongue, glottis, and larynx has been reported in patients treated with ACE inhibitors including trandolapril. Symptoms suggestive of angioedema or facial edema occurred in 0.13% of trandolapril-treated patients. Two (2) of the 4 cases were life-threatening and resolved without treatment or with medication (corticosteroids). Angioedema associated with laryngeal edema can be fatal. If laryngeal stridor or angioedema of the face, tongue or glottis occurs, treatment with trandolapril should be discontinued immediately, the patient treated in accordance with accepted medical care and carefully observed until the swelling disappears. In instances where swelling is confined to the face and lips, the condition generally resolves without treatment; antihistamines may be useful in relieving symptoms. **Where there is involvement of the tongue, glottis, or larynx, likely to cause airway obstruction, emergency therapy, including but not limited to subcutaneous epinephrine solution 1:1000 (0.3-0.5 ml) should be promptly administered.** (See PRECAUTIONS, Information for the Patient and ADVERSE REACTIONS.)

Anaphylactoid Reactions During Desensitization

Two (2) patients undergoing desensitizing treatment with hymenoptera venom while receiving ACE inhibitors sustained life-threatening anaphylactoid reactions. In the same patients, these reactions did not occur when ACE inhibitors were temporarily withheld, but they reappeared when the ACE inhibitors were inadvertently readministered.

Anaphylactoid Reactions During Membrane Exposure:

Anaphylactoid reactions have been reported in patients dialyzed with high-flux membranes and treated concomitantly with an ACE inhibitor. Anaphylactoid reactions have also been reported in patients undergoing low-density lipoprotein apheresis with dextran sulfate absorption.

HYPOTENSION

Trandolapril can cause symptomatic hypotension. Like other ACE inhibitors, trandolapril has only rarely been associated with symptomatic hypotension in uncomplicated hypertensive patients. Symptomatic hypotension is most likely to occur in patients who have been salt- or volume-depleted as a result of prolonged treatment with diuretics, dietary salt restriction, dialysis, diarrhea, or vomiting. Volume and/or salt depletion should be corrected before initiating treatment with trandolapril. (See DRUG INTERACTIONS and ADVERSE REACTIONS.) In controlled and uncontrolled studies, hypotension was reported as an adverse event in 0.6% of patients and led to discontinuations in 0.1% of patients.

In patients with concomitant congestive heart failure, with or without associated renal insufficiency, ACE inhibitor therapy may cause excessive hypotension, which may be associated with oliguria or azotemia, and rarely, with acute renal failure and death. In such patients, trandolapril therapy should be started at the recommended dose under close medical supervision. These patients should be followed closely during the first 2 weeks of treatment and, thereafter, whenever the dosage of trandolapril or diuretic is increased. (See DOSAGE AND ADMINISTRATION.) Care in avoiding hypotension should also be taken in patients with ischemic heart disease, aortic stenosis, or cerebrovascular disease.

If symptomatic hypotension occurs, the patient should be placed in the supine position and, if necessary, normal saline may be administered intravenously. A transient hypotensive response is not a contraindication to further doses; however, lower doses of trandolapril or reduced concomitant diuretic therapy should be considered.

NEUTROPENIA/AGRANULOCYTOSIS

Another ACE inhibitor, captopril, has been shown to cause agranulocytosis and bone marrow depression rarely in patients with uncomplicated hypertension, but more frequently in patients with renal impairment, especially if they also have a collagen-vascular disease such as systemic lupus erythematosus or scleroderma. Available data from clinical trials of trandolapril are insufficient to show that trandolapril does not cause agranulocytosis at similar rates. As with other ACE inhibitors, periodic monitoring of white blood cell counts in patients with collagen-vascular disease and/or renal disease should be considered.

HEPATIC FAILURE

ACE inhibitors rarely have been associated with a syndrome of cholestatic jaundice, fulminant hepatic necrosis, and death. The mechanism of this syndrome is not understood. Patients receiving ACE inhibitors who develop jaundice should discontinue the ACE inhibitor and receive appropriate medical follow-up.

FETAL/NEONATAL MORBIDITY AND MORTALITY

ACE inhibitors can cause fetal and neonatal morbidity and death when administered to pregnant women. Several dozen cases have been reported in the world literature. When pregnancy is detected, ACE inhibitors should be discontinued as soon as possible.

The use of ACE inhibitors during the second and third trimesters of pregnancy has been associated with fetal and neonatal injury, including hypotension, neonatal skull hypoplasia, anuria, reversible or irreversible renal failure, and death. Oligohydramnios has also been reported, presumably resulting from decreased fetal renal function; oligohydramnios in this setting has been associated with fetal limb contractures, craniofacial deformation, and hypoplastic lung development. Prematurity, intrauterine growth retardation, and patent ductus arteriosus have also been reported, although it is not clear whether these occurrences were due to the ACE inhibitor exposure.

These adverse effects do not appear to have resulted from intrauterine ACE-inhibitor exposure that has been limited to the first trimester. Mothers whose embryos and fetuses are exposed to ACE inhibitors only during the first trimester should be so informed. Nonetheless, when patients become pregnant, physicians should make every effort to discontinue the use of trandolapril as soon as possible.

Rarely (probably less often than once in every thousand pregnancies), no alternative to ACE inhibitors will be found. In these rare cases, the mothers should be apprised of the potential hazards to their fetuses, and serial ultrasound examinations should be performed to assess the intra-amniotic environment.

If oligohydramnios is observed, trandolapril should be discontinued unless it is considered life-saving for the mother. Contraction stress testing (CST), a non-stress test (NST), or biophysical profiling (BPP) may be appropriate, depending upon the week of pregnancy.

Patients and physicians should be aware, however, that oligohydramnios may not appear until after the fetus has sustained irreversible injury.

Infants with histories of *in utero* exposure to ACE inhibitors should be closely observed for hypotension, oliguria, and hyperkalemia. If oliguria occurs, attention should be directed toward support of blood pressure and renal perfusion. Exchange transfusions or dialysis may be required as a means of reversing hypotension and/or substituting for disordered renal function.

Doses of 0.8 mg/kg/day (9.4 mg/m^2/day) in rabbits, 1000 mg/kg/day (7000 mg/m^2/day) in rats, and 25 mg/kg/day (295 mg/m^2/day) in cynomolgus monkeys did not produce teratogenic effects. These doses represent 10 and 3 times (rabbits), 1250 and 2564 times (rats), and 312 and 108 times (monkeys) the maximum projected human dose of 4 mg based on body-weight and body-surface-area, respectively assuming a 50 kg woman.

PRECAUTIONS

GENERAL

Impaired Renal Function

As a consequence of inhibiting the renin-angiotensin-aldosterone system, changes in renal function may be anticipated in susceptible individuals. In patients with severe heart failure whose renal function may depend on the activity of the renin-angiotensin-aldosterone system, treatment with ACE inhibitors, including trandolapril, may be associated with oliguria and/or progressive azotemia and rarely with acute renal failure and/or death.

In hypertensive patients with unilateral or bilateral renal artery stenosis, increases in blood urea nitrogen and serum creatinine have been observed in some patients following ACE inhibitor therapy. These increases were almost always reversible upon discontinuation of the ACE inhibitor and/or diuretic therapy. In such patients, renal function should be monitored during the first few weeks of therapy.

Some hypertensive patients with no apparent preexisting renal vascular disease have developed increases in blood urea and serum creatinine, usually minor and transient, especially when ACE inhibitors have been given concomitantly with a diuretic. This is more likely to occur in patients with preexisting renal impairment. Dosage reduction and/or discontinuation of any diuretic and/or the ACE inhibitor may be required.

Evaluation of hypertensive patients should always include assessment of renal function. (See DOSAGE AND ADMINISTRATION.)

Hyperkalemia and Potassium-Sparing Diuretics

In clinical trials, hyperkalemia (serum potassium >6.00 mEq/L) occurred in approximately 0.4% of hypertensive patients receiving trandolapril. In most cases, elevated serum potassium levels were isolated values, which resolved despite continued therapy. None of these patients were discontinued from the trials because of hyperkalemia. Risk factors for the development of hyperkalemia include renal insufficiency, diabetes mellitus, and the concomitant use of potassium-sparing diuretics, potassium supplements, and/or potassium-containing salt substitutes, which should be used cautiously, if at all, with trandolapril. (See DRUG INTERACTIONS.)

Cough

Presumably due to the inhibition of the degradation of endogenous bradykinin, persistent nonproductive cough has been reported with all ACE inhibitors, always resolving after discontinuation of therapy. ACE inhibitor-induced cough should be considered in the differential diagnosis of cough. In controlled trials of trandolapril, cough was present in 2% of trandolapril patients and 0% of patients given placebo. There was no evidence of a relationship to dose.

Surgery/Anesthesia

In patients undergoing major surgery or during anesthesia with agents that produce hypotension, trandolapril will block angiotensin II formation secondary to compensatory renin release. If hypotension occurs and is considered to be due to this mechanism, it can be corrected by volume expansion.

INFORMATION FOR THE PATIENT

Angioedema

Angioedema, including laryngeal edema, may occur at any time during treatment with ACE inhibitors, including trandolapril. Patients should be so advised and told to report immediately any signs or symptoms suggesting angioedema (swelling of face, extremities, eyes, lips, tongue, difficulty in swallowing or breathing) and to stop taking the drug until they have consulted with their physician. (See WARNINGS and ADVERSE REACTIONS.)

Symptomatic Hypotension

Patients should be cautioned that light-headedness can occur, especially during the first days of trandolapril therapy, and should be reported to a physician. If actual syncope occurs, patients should be told to stop taking the drug until they have consulted with their physician. (See WARNINGS.)

All patients should be cautioned that inadequate fluid intake, excessive perspiration, diarrhea, or vomiting, resulting in reduced fluid volume, may precipitate an excessive fall in blood pressure with the same consequences of light-headedness and possible syncope.

Patients planning to undergo any surgery and/or anesthesia should be told to inform their physician that they are taking an ACE inhibitor that has a long duration of action.

Hyperkalemia

Patients should be told not to use potassium supplements or salt substitutes containing potassium without consulting their physician. (See PRECAUTIONS.)

Neutropenia

Patients should be told to report promptly any indication of infection (*e.g.,* sore throat, fever) which could be a sign of neutropenia.

Pregnancy

Female patients of childbearing age should be told about the consequences of second- and third-trimester exposure to ACE inhibitors, and they should also be told that these consequences do not appear to have resulted from intrauterine ACE-inhibitor exposure that has been limited to the first trimester. These patients should be asked to report pregnancies to their physicians as soon as possible.

Note: As with many other drugs, certain advice to patients being treated with trandolapril is warranted. This information is intended to aid in the safe and effective use of this medication. It is not a disclosure of all possible adverse or intended effects.

CARCINOGENESIS, MUTAGENESIS, AND IMPAIRMENT OF FERTILITY

Long-term studies were conducted with oral trandolapril administered by gavage to mice (78 weeks) and rats (104 and 106 weeks). No evidence of carcinogenic potential was seen in mice dosed up to 25 mg/kg/day (85 mg/m^2/day) or rats dosed up to 8 mg/kg/day (60 mg/m^2/day). These doses are 313 and 32 times (mice), and 100 and 23 times (rats) the maximum recommended human daily dose (MRHDD) of 4 mg based on body-weight and body-surface-area, respectively assuming a 50 kg individual. The genotoxic potential of trandolapril was evaluated in the microbial mutagenicity (Ames) test, the point mutation and chromosome aberration assays in Chinese hamster V79 cells, and the micronucleus test in mice. There was no evidence of mutagenic or clastogenic potential in these *in vitro* and *in vivo* assays.

Reproduction studies in rats did not show any impairment of fertility at doses up to 100 mg/kg/day (710 mg/m^2/day) of trandolapril, or 1250 and 260 times the MRHDD on the basis of body-weight and body-surface-area, respectively.

PREGNANCY CATEGORY C (FIRST TRIMESTER) AND PREGNANCY CATEGORY D (SECOND AND THIRD TRIMESTERS)

See WARNINGS, Fetal/Neonatal Morbidity and Mortality.

NURSING MOTHERS

Radiolabeled trandolapril or its metabolites are secreted in rat milk. Trandolapril should not be administered to nursing mothers.

GERIATRIC USE

In placebo-controlled studies of trandolapril, 31.1% of patients were 60 years and older, 20.1% were 65 years and older, and 2.3% were 75 years and older. No overall differences in effectiveness or safety were observed between these patients and younger patients. (Greater sensitivity of some older individual patients cannot be ruled out.)

PEDIATRIC USE

The safety and effectiveness of trandolapril in pediatric patients have not been established.

DRUG INTERACTIONS

Trandolapril did not affect the plasma concentration (pre-dose and 2 hours post-dose) of oral digoxin (0.25 mg). Coadministration of trandolapril and cimetidine led to an increase of about 44% in C_{max} for trandolapril, but no difference in the pharmacokinetics of trandolaprilat or in ACE inhibition. Coadministration of trandolapril and furosemide led to an increase of about 25% in the renal clearance of trandolaprilat, but no effect was seen on the pharmacokinetics of furosemide or trandolaprilat or on ACE inhibition.

CONCOMITANT DIURETIC THERAPY

As with other ACE inhibitors, patients on diuretics, especially those on recently instituted diuretic therapy, may experience an excessive reduction of blood pressure after initiation of therapy with trandolapril. The possibility of exacerbation of hypotensive effects with trandolapril may be minimized by either discontinuing the diuretic or cautiously increasing salt intake prior to initiation of treatment with trandolapril. If it is not possible to discontinue the diuretic, the starting dose of trandolapril should be reduced. (See DOSAGE AND ADMINISTRATION.)

AGENTS INCREASING SERUM POTASSIUM

Trandolapril can attenuate potassium loss caused by thiazide diuretics and increase serum potassium when used alone. Use of potassium-sparing diuretics (spironolactone, triamterene, or amiloride), potassium supplements, or potassium-containing salt substitutes concomitantly with ACE inhibitors can increase the risk of hyperkalemia. If concomitant use of such agents is indicated, they should be used with caution and with appropriate monitoring of serum potassium. (See PRECAUTIONS.)

LITHIUM

Increased serum lithium levels and symptoms of lithium toxicity have been reported in patients receiving concomitant lithium and ACE inhibitor therapy. These drugs should be coadministered with caution, and frequent monitoring of serum lithium levels is recommended. If a diuretic is also used, the risk of lithium toxicity may be increased.

OTHER

No clinically significant interaction has been found between trandolaprilat and food, cimetidine, digoxin, or furosemide. The anticoagulant effect of warfarin was not significantly changed by trandolapril.

ADVERSE REACTIONS

The safety experience in US placebo-controlled trials included 1067 hypertensive patients, of whom 831 received trandolapril. Nearly 200 hypertensive patients received trandolapril for over 1 year in open-label trials. In controlled trials, withdrawals for adverse events were 2.1% on placebo and 1.4% on trandolapril. Adverse events considered at least possibly related to treatment occurring in 1% of trandolapril-treated patients and more common on trandolapril than placebo, pooled for all doses, are shown in TABLE 1, together with the frequency of discontinuation of treatment because of these events.

TABLE 1 *Adverse Events in Placebo-Controlled Hypertension Trials*

	Occurring at 1% or Greater	
	Trandolapril (n=832)	Placebo (n=237)
Adverse Event	% Incidence (% Discontinuance)	% Incidence (% Discontinuance)
Cough	1.9% (0.1%)	0.4% (0.4%)
Dizziness	1.3% (0.2%)	0.4% (0.4%)
Diarrhea	1.0% (0.0%)	0.4% (0.0%)

Headache and fatigue were all seen in more than 1% of trandolapril-treated patients but were more frequently seen on placebo. Adverse events were not usually persistent or difficult to manage.

LEFT-VENTRICULAR DYSFUNCTION POST MYOCARDIAL INFARCTION

Adverse reactions related to trandolapril, occurring at a rate greater than that observed in placebo-treated patients with left-ventricular dysfunction, are shown in TABLE 2. The incidences represent the experiences from the TRACE study. The follow-up time was between 24 and 50 months for this study.

TABLE 2 *Percentage of Patients With Adverse Events Greater Than Placebo*

	Placebo-Controlled (TRACE) Mortality Study	
Adverse Event	Trandolapril (n=876)	Placebo (n=873)
Cough	35%	22%
Dizziness	23%	17%
Hypotension	11%	6.8%
Elevated serum uric acid	15%	13%
Elevated BUN	9.0%	7.6%
PICA or CABG	7.3%	6.1%
Dyspepsia	6.4%	6.0%
Syncope	5.9%	3.3%
Hyperkalemia	5.3%	2.8%
Bradycardia	4.7%	4.4%
Hypocalcemia	4.7%	3.9%
Myalgia	4.7%	3.1%
Elevated creatinine	4.7%	2.4%
Gastritis	4.2%	3.6%
Cardiogenic shock	3.8%	<2%
Intermittent claudication	3.8%	<2%
Stroke	3.3%	3.2%
Asthenia	3.3%	2.6%

Clinical adverse experiences possibly or probably related or of uncertain relationship to therapy occurring in 0.3-1.0% (except as noted) of the patients treated with trandolapril (with or without concomitant calcium ion antagonist or diuretic) in controlled or uncontrolled trials (n=1134) and less frequent, clinically significant events seen in clinical trials or post-marketing experience (the rarer events are in italics) include (listed by body system):

General Body Function: Chest pain.

Cardiovascular: AV first degree block, bradycardia, edema, flushing, hypotension, palpitations.

Central Nervous System: Drowsiness, insomnia, paresthesia, vertigo.

Dermatologic: Pruritus, rash, pemphigus.

Eye, Ear, Nose, Throat: Epistaxis, throat inflammation, upper respiratory tract infection.

Emotional, Mental, Sexual States: Anxiety, impotence, decreased libido.

Gastrointestinal: Abdominal distention, abdominal pain/cramps, constipation, dyspepsia, diarrhea, vomiting, *pancreatitis.*

Hemopoietic: *Decreased leukocytes, decreased neutrophils.*

Metabolism and Endocrine: *Increased creatinine, increased potassium,* increased SGPT (ALT).

Musculoskeletal System: Extremity pain, muscle cramps, gout.

Pulmonary: Dyspnea.

Angioedema: Angioedema has been reported in 4 (0.13%) patients receiving trandolapril in US and foreign studies. Angioedema associated with laryngeal edema may be fatal. If angioedema of the face, extremities, lips, tongue, glottis, and/or larynx occurs, treatment with trandolapril should be discontinued and appropriate therapy instituted immediately. (See WARNINGS.)

Hypotension: In hypertensive patients, symptomatic hypotension occurred in 0.6% and near syncope occurred in 0.2%. Hypotension or syncope was a cause for discontinuation of therapy in 0.1% of hypertensive patients.

Fetal/Neonatal Morbidity and Mortality: See WARNINGS, Fetal/Neonatal Morbidity and Mortality.

Cough: See PRECAUTIONS, General, Cough.

Clinical Laboratory Test Findings

Hematologic: (See WARNINGS.) Low white blood cells, low neutrophils, low lymphocytes, thrombocytopenia.

Serum Electrolytes: Hyperkalemia (see PRECAUTIONS), hyponatremia.

Creatinine and Blood Urea Nitrogen: Increases in creatinine levels occurred in 1.1% of patients receiving trandolapril alone and 7.3% of patients treated with trandolapril, a calcium ion antagonist and a diuretic. Increases in blood urea nitrogen levels occurred in 0.6% of patients receiving trandolapril alone and 1.4% of patients receiving trandolapril, a calcium ion antagonist, and a diuretic. None of these increases required discontinuation of treatment. Increases in these laboratory values are more likely to occur in patients with renal insufficiency or those pretreated with a diuretic and, based on experience with other ACE inhibitors, would be expected to be especially likely in patients with renal artery stenosis. (See PRECAUTIONS and WARNINGS.)

Liver Function Tests: Occasional elevation of transaminases at the rate of 3x upper normals occurred in 0.8% of patients and persistent increase in bilirubin occurred in 0.2% of patients. Discontinuation for elevated liver enzymes occurred in 0.2% of patients.

DOSAGE AND ADMINISTRATION

HYPERTENSION

The recommended initial dosage of trandolapril for patients not receiving a diuretic is 1 mg once daily in non-black patients and 2 mg in black patients. Dosage should be adjusted according to the blood pressure response. Generally, dosage adjustments should be made at intervals of at least 1 week. Most patients have required dosages of 2-4 mg once daily. There is little clinical experience with doses above 8 mg.

Patients inadequately treated with once-daily dosing at 4 mg may be treated with twice-daily dosing. If blood pressure is not adequately controlled with trandolapril monotherapy, a diuretic may be added.

In patients who are currently being treated with a diuretic, symptomatic hypotension occasionally can occur following the initial dose of trandolapril. To reduce the likelihood of hypotension, the diuretic should, if possible, be discontinued 2-3 days prior to beginning therapy with trandolapril. (See WARNINGS.) Then, if blood pressure is not controlled with trandolapril alone, diuretic therapy should be resumed. If the diuretic cannot be discontinued, an initial dose of 0.5 mg trandolapril should be used with careful medical supervision for several hours until blood pressure has stabilized. The dosage should subsequently be titrated (as described above)-the optimal response. (See WARNINGS, PRECAUTIONS, and DRUG INTERACTIONS.)

Concomitant administration of trandolapril with potassium supplements, potassium salt substitutes, or potassium-sparing diuretics can lead-increases of serum potassium. (See PRECAUTIONS.)

HEART FAILURE POST MYOCARDIAL INFARCTION OR LEFT-VENTRICULAR DYSFUNCTION POST MYOCARDIAL INFARCTION

The recommended starting dose is 1 mg, once daily. Following the initial dose, all patients should be titrated (as tolerated) toward a target dose of 4 mg, once daily. If a 4 mg dose is not tolerated, patients can continue therapy with the greatest tolerated dose.

DOSE ADJUSTMENT IN RENAL IMPAIRMENT OR HEPATIC CIRRHOSIS

For patients with creatinine clearance <30 ml/min or with hepatic cirrhosis, the recommended starting dose, based on clinical and pharmacokinetic data, is 0.5 mg daily. Patients should subsequently have their dosage titrated (as described above) — the optimal response.

HOW SUPPLIED

Mavik tablets are available as follows:

1 mg: The Mavik 1 mg tablets are salmon colored, round shaped, scored and compressed with code "KNOLL 1" on one side.

2 mg: The Mavik 2 mg tablets are yellow colored, round shaped and compressed with code "KNOLL 2" on one side.

4 mg: The Mavik 4 mg tablets are rose colored, round shaped and compressed with code "KNOLL 4" on one side.

Storage: Store at controlled room temperature: 20-25°C (68-77°F).

T

PRODUCT LISTING - EQUIVALENTS NOT AVAILABLE

Tablet - Oral - 1 mg

100's	$60.00	MAVIK, Knoll Pharmaceutical Company	00048-5805-41
100's	$96.11	MAVIK, Knoll Pharmaceutical Company	00048-5805-01
100's	$98.51	MAVIK, Abbott Pharmaceutical	00074-2278-13

Tablet - Oral - 2 mg

100's	$84.49	MAVIK, Knoll Pharmaceutical Company	00048-5806-41
100's	$96.11	MAVIK, Knoll Pharmaceutical Company	00048-5806-01
100's	$98.51	MAVIK, Abbott Pharmaceutical	00074-2279-13

Tablet - Oral - 4 mg

100's	$60.00	MAVIK, Knoll Pharmaceutical Company	00048-5807-41
100's	$96.11	MAVIK, Knoll Pharmaceutical Company	00048-5807-01
100's	$98.51	MAVIK, Abbott Pharmaceutical	00074-2280-13

Tranylcypromine Sulfate *(002366)*

For related information, see the comparative table section in Appendix A.

Categories: Depression; FDA Approved 1985 Aug; Pregnancy Category C
Drug Classes: Antidepressants, monoamine oxidase inhibitors
Brand Names: Parnate
Cost of Therapy: $61.45 (Depression; Parnate; 10 mg; 3 tablets/day; 30 day supply)

DESCRIPTION

Before prescribing, the physician should be familiar with the entire contents of this prescribing information.

Chemically, tranylcypromine sulfate is (±)-*trans*-2-phenylcyclopropylamine sulfate (2:1).

Each round, rose-red, film-coated tablet is imprinted with the product name "PARNATE" and "SKF" and contains tranylcypromine sulfate equivalent to 10 mg of tranylcypromine. Inactive ingredients consist of cellulose, citric acid, croscarmellose sodium, D&C red no. 7, FD&C blue no. 2, FD&C red no. 40, FD&C yellow no. 6, gelatin, iron oxide, lactose, magnesium stearate, talc, titanium dioxide and trace amounts of other inactive ingredients. **NOTE:** Parnate tablets have been changed from rose-red sugar-coated tablets to rose-red film-coated tablets. The film-coated tablets differ in size from the sugar-coated tablets, but the drug content remains unchanged.

CLINICAL PHARMACOLOGY

ACTION

Tranylcypromine is a non-hydrazine monoamine oxidase inhibitor with a rapid onset of activity. It increases the concentration of epinephrine, norepinephrine and serotonin in storage sites throughout the nervous system and, in theory, this increased concentration of monoamines in the brain stem is the basis for its antidepressant activity. When tranylcypromine is withdrawn, monoamine oxidase activity is recovered in 3-5 days, although the drug is excreted in 24 hours.

INDICATIONS AND USAGE

For the treatment of major depressive episode without melancholia.

Tranylcypromine sulfate should be used in adult patients who can be closely supervised. It should rarely be the first antidepressant drug given. Rather, the drug is suited for patients who have failed to respond to the drugs more commonly administered for depression.

The effectiveness of tranylcypromine sulfate has been established in adult outpatients, most of whom had a depressive illness which would correspond to a diagnosis of major depressive episode without melancholia. As described in the American Psychiatric Association's Diagnostic and Statistical Manual, third edition (DSM III). major depressive episode implies a prominent and relatively persistent (nearly every day for at least 2 weeks) depressed or dysphoric mood that usually interferes with daily functioning and includes at least 4 of the following 8 symptoms: change in appetite, change in sleep, psychomotor agitation or retardation, loss of interest in usual activities or decrease in sexual drive, increased fatigability, feelings of guilt or worthlessness, slowed thinking or impaired concentration and suicidal ideation or attempts.

The effectiveness of tranylcypromine sulfate in patients who meet the criteria for major depressive episode with melancholia (endogenous features) has not been established.

SUMMARY OF CONTRAINDICATIONS

Tranylcypromine sulfate should not be administered in combination with any of the following: MAO inhibitors or dibenzazepine derivatives; sympathomimetics (including amphetamines); some central nervous system depressants (including narcotics and alcohol); antihypertensive, diuretic, antihistaminic, sedative or anesthetic drugs; bupropion HCl; buspirone HCl; dextromethorphan; cheese or other foods with a high tyramine content; or excessive quantities of caffeine.

Tranylcypromine sulfate should not be administered to any patient with a confirmed or suspected cerebrovascular defect or to any patient with cardiovascular disease, hypertension or history of headache.

(For a complete discussion, see CONTRAINDICATIONS and WARNINGS.)

CONTRAINDICATIONS

Tranylcypromine sulfate is contraindicated:

In patients with cerebrovascular defects or cardiovascular disorders: Tranylcypromine sulfate should not be administered to any patient with a confirmed or suspected cerebrovascular defect or to any patient with cardiovascular disease or hypertension.

In the presence of pheochromocytoma: Tranylcypromine sulfate should not be used in the presence of pheochromocytoma since such tumors secrete pressor substances.

In combination with MAO inhibitors or with dibenzazepine-related entities: Tranylcypromine sulfate should not be administered together or in rapid succession with other MAO inhibitors or with dibenzazepine-related entities. Hypertensive crises or severe convulsive seizures may occur in patients receiving such combinations.

In patients being transferred to tranylcypromine sulfate from another MAO inhibitor or from a dibenzazepine-related entity, allow a medication-free interval of at least a week, then initiate tranylcypromine sulfate using half the normal starting dosage for at least the first week of therapy. Similarly, at least a week should elapse between the discontinuance of tranylcypromine sulfate and the administration of another MAO inhibitor or a dibenzazepine-related entity, or the readministration of tranylcypromine sulfate.

The following list includes some other MAO inhibitors, dibenzazepine-related entities and tricyclic antidepressants.

Other MAO inhibitors:

Furazolidone, isocarboxazid, pargyline HCl, pargyline HCl and methyclothiazide, phenelzine sulfate, procarbazine HCl.

Dibenzazepine-related and other tricyclics:

Amitriptyline HCl, perphenazine and amitriptyline HCl, clomipramine HCl, desipramine HCl, imipramine HCl, nortriptyline HCl, protriptyline HCl, doxepin HCl, carbamazepine, cyclobenzaprine HCl, amoxapine, maprotiline HCl, trimipramine maleate.

In combination with bupropion: The concurrent administration of a MAO inhibitor and bupropion HCl is contraindicated. At least 14 days should elapse between discontinuation of a MAO inhibitor and initiation of treatment with bupropion HCl.

In combination with dexfenfluramine HCl: Because dexfenfluramine HCl is a serotonin releaser and reuptake inhibitor, it should not be used concomitantly with tranylcypromine sulfate.

In combination with selective serotonin reuptake inhibitors (SSRIs): As a general rule, tranylcypromine sulfate should not be administered in combination with any SSRI. There have been reports of serious, sometimes fatal, reactions (including hyperthermia, rigidity, myoclonus, autonomic instability with possible rapid fluctuations of vital signs, and mental status changes that include extreme agitation progressing to delirium and coma) in patients receiving fluoxetine in combination with a monoamine oxidase inhibitor (MAOI), and in patients who have recently discontinued fluoxetine and are then started on a MAOI. Some cases presented with features resembling neuroleptic malignant syndrome. Therefore, fluoxetine and other SSRIs should not be used in combination with a MAOI, or within 14 days of discontinuing therapy with a MAOI. Since fluoxetine and its major metabolite have very long elimination half-lives, at least 5 weeks should be allowed after stopping fluoxetine before starting a MAOI.

At least 2 weeks should be allowed after stopping sertraline or paroxetine before starting a MAOI.

In combination with buspirone: Tranylcypromine sulfate should not be used in combination with buspirone HCl, since several cases of elevated blood pressure have been reported in patients taking MAO inhibitors who were then given buspirone HCl. At least 10 days should elapse between the discontinuation of tranylcypromine sulfate and the institution of buspirone HCl.

In combination with sympathomimetics: Tranylcypromine sulfate should not be administered in combination with sympathomimetics, including amphetamines, and over-the-counter drugs such as cold, hay fever or weight-reducing preparations that contain vasoconstrictors.

During tranylcypromine sulfate therapy, it appears that certain patients are particularly vulnerable to the effects of sympathomimetics when the activity of certain enzymes is inhibited. Use of sympathomimetics and compounds such as guanethidine, methyldopa, reserpine, dopamine, levodopa and tryptophan with tranylcypromine sulfate may precipitate hypertension, headache and related symptoms. In addition, use with tryptophan may precipitate disorientation, memory impairment and other neurologic and behavioral signs.

In combination with meperidine: Do not use meperidine concomitantly with MAO inhibitors or within 2 or 3 weeks following MAOI therapy. Serious reactions have been precipitated with concomitant use, including coma, severe hypertension or hypotension, severe respiratory depression, convulsions, malignant hyperpyrexia, excitation, peripheral vascular collapse and death. It is thought that these reactions may be mediated by accumulation of 5-HT (serotonin) consequent to MAO inhibition.

In combination with dextromethorphan: The combination of MAO inhibitors and dextromethorphan has been reported to cause brief episodes of psychosis or bizarre behavior.

In combination with cheese or other foods with a high tyramine content: Hypertensive crises have sometimes occurred during tranylcypromine sulfate therapy after ingestion of foods with a high tyramine content. In general, the patient should avoid protein foods in which aging or protein breakdown is used to increase flavor. In particular, patients should be instructed not to take foods such as cheese (particularly strong or aged varieties), sour cream, Chianti wine, sherry, beer (including nonalcoholic beer), liqueurs, pickled herring, anchovies, caviar, liver, canned figs, dried fruit (raisins, prunes, etc.), bananas, raspberries, avocados, overripe fruit, chocolate, soy sauce, sauerkraut, the pods of broad beans (fava beans), yeast extracts, yogurt, meat extracts or meat prepared with tenderizers.

In patients undergoing elective surgery: Patients taking tranylcypromine sulfate should not undergo elective surgery requiring general anesthesia. Also, they should not be given cocaine or local anesthesia containing sympathomimetic vasoconstrictors. The possible combined hypotensive effects of tranylcypromine sulfate and spinal anesthesia should be kept in mind. Tranylcypromine sulfate should be discontinued at least 10 days prior to elective surgery.

ADDITIONAL CONTRAINDICATIONS

In general, the physician should bear in mind the possibility of a lowered margin of safety when tranylcypromine sulfate is administered in combination with potent drugs.

Tranylcypromine sulfate should not be used in combination with some central nervous system depressants such as narcotics and alcohol, or with hypotensive agents. A marked potentiating effect on these classes of drugs has been reported.

T

Anti-parkinsonism drugs should be used with caution in patients receiving tranylcypromine sulfate since severe reactions have been reported.

Tranylcypromine sulfate should not be used in patients with a history of liver disease or in those with abnormal liver function tests.

Excessive use of caffeine in any form should be avoided in patients receiving tranylcypromine sulfate.

WARNINGS

WARNING TO PHYSICIANS

Tranylcypromine sulfate is a potent agent with the capability of producing serious side effects. Tranylcypromine sulfate is not recommended in those depressive reactions where other antidepressant drugs may be effective. **It should be reserved for patients who can be closely supervised and who have not responded satisfactorily to the drugs more commonly administered for depression.**

Before prescribing, the physician should be completely familiar with the full material on dosage, side effects and contraindications on these pages, with the principles of MAO inhibitor therapy and the side effects of this class of drugs. Also, the physician should be familiar with the symptomatology of mental depressions and alternate methods of treatment to aid in the careful selection of patients for tranylcypromine sulfate therapy. In depressed patients, the possibility of suicide should always be considered and adequate precautions taken.

PREGNANCY WARNING

Use of any drug in pregnancy, during lactation or in women of childbearing age requires that the potential benefits of the drug be weighed against its possible hazards to mother and child.

Animal reproductive studies show that tranylcypromine sulfate passes through the placental barrier into the fetus of the rat, and into the milk of the lactating dog. The absence of a harmful action of tranylcypromine sulfate on fertility or on postnatal development by either prenatal treatment or from the milk of treated animals has not been demonstrated. Tranylcypromine is excreted in human milk.

WARNING TO THE PATIENT

Patients should be instructed to report promptly the occurrence of headache or other unusual symptoms, *i.e.*, palpitation and/or tachycardia, a sense of constriction in the throat or chest, sweating, dizziness, neck stiffness, nausea or vomiting.

Patients should be warned against eating the foods listed in CONTRAINDICATIONS while on tranylcypromine sulfate therapy. Also, they should be told not to drink alcoholic beverages. The patient should also be warned about the possibility of hypotension and faintness, as well as drowsiness sufficient to impair performance of potentially hazardous tasks such as driving a car or operating machinery.

Patients should also be cautioned not to take concomitant medications, whether prescription or over-the-counter drugs such as cold, hay fever or weight-reducing preparations, without the advice of a physician. They should be advised not to consume excessive amounts of caffeine in any form. Likewise, they should inform other physicians, and their dentist, about their use of tranylcypromine sulfate.

HYPERTENSIVE CRISES

The most important reaction associated with tranylcypromine sulfate is the occurrence of hypertensive crises which have sometimes been fatal.

These crises are characterized by some or all of the following symptoms: occipital headache which may radiate frontally, palpitation, neck stiffness or soreness, nausea or vomiting, sweating (sometimes with fever and sometimes with cold, clammy skin) and photophobia. Either tachycardia or bradycardia may be present, and associated constricting chest pain and dilated pupils may occur. **Intracranial bleeding, sometimes fatal in outcome, has been reported in association with the paradoxical increase in blood pressure.**

In all patients taking tranylcypromine sulfate blood pressure should be followed closely to detect evidence of any pressor response. It is emphasized that full reliance should not be placed on blood pressure readings, but that the patient should also be observed frequently.

Therapy should be discontinued immediately upon the occurrence of palpitation or frequent headaches during tranylcypromine sulfate therapy. These signs may be prodromal of a hypertensive crisis.

Important — Recommended Treatment in Hypertensive Crises

If a hypertensive crisis occurs, tranylcypromine sulfate should be discontinued and therapy to lower blood pressure should be instituted immediately. Headache tends to abate as blood pressure is lowered. On the basis of present evidence, phentolamine is recommended. (The dosage reported for phentolamine is 5 mg IV.) Care should be taken to administer this drug slowly in order to avoid producing an excessive hypotensive effect. Fever should be managed by means of external cooling. Other symptomatic and supportive measures may be desirable in particular cases. Do not use parenteral reserpine.

PRECAUTIONS

HYPOTENSION

Hypotension has been observed during tranylcypromine sulfate therapy. Symptoms of postural hypotension are seen most commonly but not exclusively in patients with pre-existent hypertension; blood pressure usually returns rapidly to pretreatment levels upon discontinuation of the drug. At doses above 30 mg daily, postural hypotension is a major side effect and may result in syncope. Dosage increases should be made more gradually in patients showing a tendency toward hypotension at the beginning of therapy. Postural hypotension may be relieved by having the patient lie down until blood pressure returns to normal.

Also, when tranylcypromine sulfate is combined with those phenothiazine derivatives or other compounds known to cause hypotension, the possibility of additive hypotensive effects should be considered.

OTHER PRECAUTIONS

There have been reports of drug dependency in patients using doses of tranylcypromine significantly in excess of the therapeutic range. Some of these patients had a history of previous substance abuse. The following withdrawal symptoms have been reported: restlessness, anxiety, depression, confusion, hallucinations, headache, weakness and diarrhea.

Drugs which lower the seizure threshold, including MAO inhibitors, should not be used with metrizamide. As with other MAO inhibitors, tranylcypromine sulfate should be discontinued at least 48 hours before myelography and should not be resumed for at least 24 hours postprocedure.

In depressed patients, the possibility of suicide should always be considered and adequate precautions taken. Exclusive reliance on drug therapy to prevent suicidal attempts is unwarranted as there may be a delay in the onset of therapeutic effect or an increase in anxiety and agitation. Also, some patients fail to respond to drug therapy or may respond only temporarily.

MAO inhibitors may have the capacity to suppress anginal pain that would otherwise serve as a warning of myocardial ischemia.

The usual precautions should be observed in patients with impaired renal function since there is a possibility of cumulative effects in such patients.

Older patients may suffer more morbidity than younger patients during and following an episode of hypertension or malignant hyperthermia. Older patients have less compensatory reserve to cope with any serious adverse reaction. Therefore, tranylcypromine sulfate should be used with caution in the elderly population.

Although excretion of tranylcypromine sulfate is rapid, inhibition of MAO may persist up to 10 days following discontinuation.

Because the influence of tranylcypromine sulfate on the convulsive threshold is variable in animal experiments, suitable precautions should be taken if epileptic patients are treated.

Some MAO inhibitors have contributed to hypoglycemic episodes in diabetic patients receiving insulin or oral hypoglycemic agents. Therefore, tranylcypromine sulfate should be used with caution in diabetics using these drugs.

Tranylcypromine sulfate may aggravate coexisting symptoms in depression, such as anxiety and agitation.

Use tranylcypromine sulfate with caution in hyperthyroid patients because of their increased sensitivity to pressor amines.

Tranylcypromine sulfate should be administered with caution to patients receiving disulfiram. In a single study, rats given high intraperitoneal doses of *d* or *l* isomers of tranylcypromine sulfate plus disulfiram experienced severe toxicity including convulsions and death. Additional studies in rats given high oral doses of racemic tranylcypromine sulfate and disulfiram produced no adverse interaction.

ADVERSE REACTIONS

Overstimulation which may include increased anxiety, agitation and manic symptoms is usually evidence of excessive therapeutic action. Dosage should be reduced, or a phenothiazine tranquilizer should be administered concomitantly.

Patients may experience restlessness or insomnia; may notice some weakness, drowsiness, episodes of dizziness or dry mouth; or may report nausea, diarrhea, abdominal pain or constipation. Most of these effects can be relieved by lowering the dosage or by giving suitable concomitant medication.

Tachycardia, significant anorexia, edema, palpitation, blurred vision, chills and impotence have each been reported.

Headaches without blood pressure elevation have occurred.

Rare instances of hepatitis, skin rash, and alopeica have been reported.

Impaired water excretion compatible with the syndrome of inappropriate secretion of antidiuretic hormone (SIADH) has been reported.

Tinnitus, muscle spasm, tremors, myoclonic jerks, numbness, paresthesia, urinary retention and retarded ejaculation have been reported.

Hematologic disorders including anemia, leukopenia, agranulocytosis and thrombocytopenia have been reported.

POST-INTRODUCTION REPORTS

The following are spontaneously reported adverse events temporally associated with tranylcypromine sulfate therapy. No clear relationship between tranylcypromine sulfate and these events has been established. Localized scleroderma, flare-up of cystic acne, ataxia, confusion, disorientation, memory loss, urinary frequency, urinary incontinence, urticaria, fissuring in corner of mouth, akinesia.

DOSAGE AND ADMINISTRATION

Dosage should be adjusted to the requirements of the individual patient. Improvement should be seen within 48 hours to 3 weeks after starting therapy.

The usual effective dosage is 30 mg/day, usually given in divided doses. If there are no signs of improvement after a reasonable period (up to 2 weeks), then the dosage may be increased in 10 mg/day increments at intervals of 1-3 weeks; the dosage range may be extended to a maximum of 60 mg/day from the usual 30 mg/day.

HOW SUPPLIED

Parnate is supplied as round, rose-red, film-coated tablets imprinted with the product name "PARNATE" and "SB" and contains tranylcypromine sulfate equivalent to 10 mg of tranylcypromine.

Storage: Store between 15 and 30°C (59 and 86°F).

PRODUCT LISTING - EQUIVALENTS NOT AVAILABLE

Tablet - Oral - 10 mg

100's	$68.28	PARNATE, Glaxosmithkline	00007-4471-20

Trastuzumab (003419)

Categories: Carcinoma, breast; FDA Approved 1998 Sep; Pregnancy Category B
Drug Classes: Antineoplastics, monoclonal antibodies; Monoclonal antibodies
Brand Names: Herceptin

WARNING

Cardiomyopathy

Trastuzumab administration can result in the development of ventricular dysfunction and congestive heart failure. Left ventricular function should be evaluated in all patients prior to and during treatment with trastuzumab. Discontinuation of trastuzumab treatment should be strongly considered in patients who develop a clinically significant decrease in left ventricular function. The incidence and severity of cardiac dysfunction was particularly high in patients who received trastuzumab in combination with anthracyclines and cyclophosphamide. (See WARNINGS.)

DESCRIPTION

Herceptin is a recombinant DNA-derived humanized monoclonal antibody that selectively binds with high affinity in a cell-based assay (Kd = 5 nM) to the extracellular domain of the human epidermal growth factor receptor 2 protein, HER2.[1,2] The antibody is an IgG_1 kappa that contains human framework regions with the complementarity-determining regions of a murine antibody (4D5) that binds to HER2.

The humanized antibody against HER2 is produced by a mammalian cell (Chinese Hamster Ovary) [CHO] suspension culture in a nutrient medium containing the antibiotic gentamicin. Gentamicin is not detectable in the final product.

Herceptin is a sterile, white to pale yellow, preservative-free lyophilized powder for intravenous (IV) administration. Each vial of Herceptin contains 440 mg trastuzumab, 9.9 mg L-histidine HCl, 6.4 mg L-histidine, 400 mgα,α-trehalose dihydrate, and 1.8 mg polysorbate 20. Reconstitution with 20 ml of the supplied bacteriostatic water for injection, (BWFI), containing 1.1% benzyl alcohol as a preservative, yields 21 ml of a multi-dose solution containing 21 mg/ml trastuzumab, at a pH of approximately 6.

CLINICAL PHARMACOLOGY

GENERAL

The HER2 (or c-erbB2) proto-oncogene encodes a transmembrane receptor protein of 185 kDa, which is structurally related to the epidermal growth factor receptor.[1] HER2 protein overexpression is observed in 25-30% of primary breast cancers. HER2 protein overexpression can be determined using an immunohistochemistry-based assessment of fixed tumor blocks.[3]

Trastuzumab has been shown, in both *in vitro* assays and in animals, to inhibit the proliferation of human tumorcells that overexpress HER2.[4-6]

Trastuzumab is a mediator of antibody-dependent cellular cytotoxicity (ADCC).[7,8] *In vitro*, trastuzumab-mediated ADCC has been shown to be preferentially exerted on HER2 overexpressing cancer cells compared with cancer cells that do not overexpress HER2.

PHARMACOKINETICS

The pharmacokinetics of trastuzumab were studied in breast cancer patients with metastatic disease. Short duration intravenous infusions of 10-500 mg once weekly demonstrated dose-dependent pharmacokinetics. Mean half-life increased and clearance decreased with increasing dose level. The half-life averaged 1.7 and 12 days at the 10 and 500 mg dose levels, respectively. Trastuzumab's volume of distribution was approximately that of serum volume (44 ml/kg). At the highest weekly dose studied (500 mg), mean peak serum concentrations were 377 μg/ml.

In studies using a loading dose of 4 mg/kg followed by a weekly maintenance dose of 2 mg/kg, a mean half-life of 5.8 days (range = 1-32 days) was observed. Between weeks 16 and 32, trastuzumab serum concentrations reached a steady-state with a mean trough and peak concentrations of approximately 79 μg/ml and 123 μg/ml, respectively.

Detectable concentrations of the circulating extracellular domain of the HER2 receptor (shed antigen) are found in the serum of some patients with HER2 overexpressing tumors. Determination of shed antigen in baseline serum samples revealed that 64% (286/447) of patients had detectable shed antigen, which ranged as high as 1880 ng/ml (median=11 ng/ml). Patients with higher baseline shed antigen levels were more likely to have lower serum trough concentrations. However, with weekly dosing, most patients with elevated shed antigen levels achieved target serum concentrations of trastuzumab by week 6.

Data suggest that the disposition of trastuzumab is not altered based on age or serum creatinine (up to 2.0 mg/dl). No formal interaction studies have been performed.

Mean serum trough concentrations of trastuzumab, when administered in combination with paclitaxel, were consistently elevated approximately 1.5-fold as compared with serum concentrations of trastuzumab used in combination with anthracycline plus cyclophosphamide. In primate studies, administration of trastuzumab with paclitaxel resulted in a reduction in trastuzumab clearance. Serum levels of trastuzumab in combination with cisplatin, doxorubicin or epirubicin plus cyclophosphamide did not suggest any interactions; no formal drug interaction studies were performed.

INDICATIONS AND USAGE

Trastuzumab as a single agent is indicated for the treatment of patients with metastatic breast cancer whose tumors overexpress the HER2 protein and who have received one or more chemotherapy regimens for their metastatic disease. Trastuzumab in combination with paclitaxel is indicated for treatment of patients with metastatic breast cancer whose tumors overexpress the HER2 protein and who have not received chemotherapy for their metastatic disease. Trastuzumab should only be used in patients whose tumors have HER2 protein overexpression.

CONTRAINDICATIONS

None known.

WARNINGS

See BOXED WARNING.

CARDIOTOXICITY

Signs and symptoms of cardiac dysfunction, such as dyspnea, increased cough, paroxysmal nocturnal dyspnea, peripheral edema, S_3 gallop, or reduced ejection fraction, have been observed in patients treated with trastuzumab. Congestive heart failure associated with trastuzumab therapy may be severe and has been associated with disabling cardiac failure, death, and mural thrombosis leading to stroke. The clinical status of patients in the trials who developed congestive heart failure were classified for severity using the New York Heart Association classification system (I-IV, where IV is the most severe level of cardiac failure). (See TABLE 3.)

TABLE 3 *Incidence and Severity of Cardiac Dysfunction*

	TRZ* alone	TRZ + PAC†	PAC	TRZ + AC†	AC†
	n=213	n=91	n=95	n=143	n=135
Any cardiac dysfunction	7%	11%	1%	28%	7%
Class III-IV	5%	4%	1%	19%	3%

* Open-label, single-agent Phase 2 study (94% received prior anthracyclines).
† Randomized Phase 3 study comparing chemotherapy plus trastuzumab to chemotherapy alone, where chemotherapy is either anthracycline/cyclophosphamide or paclitaxel.
TRZ Trastuzumab.
PAC Paclitaxel.
AC = Anthracycline (doxorubicin or epirubicin) and cyclophosphamide.

Candidates for treatment with trastuzumab should undergo thorough baseline cardiac assessment including history and physical exam and one or more of the following: EKG, echocardiogram, and MUGA scan. There are no data regarding the most appropriate method of evaluation for the identification of patients at risk for developing cardiotoxicity. Monitoring may not identify all patients who will develop cardiac dysfunction.

Extreme caution should be exercised in treating patients with pre-existing cardiac dysfunction.

Patients receiving trastuzumab should undergo frequent monitoring for deteriorating cardiac function.

The probability of cardiac dysfunction was highest in patients who received trastuzumab concurrently with anthracyclines. The data suggest that advanced age may increase the probability of cardiac dysfunction.

Pre-existing cardiac disease or prior cardiotoxic therapy (*e.g.*, anthracycline or radiation therapy to the chest) may decrease the ability to tolerate trastuzumab therapy; however, the data are not adequate to evaluate the correlation between trastuzumab-induced cardiotoxicity and these factors.

Discontinuation of trastuzumab therapy should be strongly considered in patients who develop clinically significant congestive heart failure. In the clinical trials, most patients with cardiac dysfunction responded to appropriate medical therapy often including discontinuation of trastuzumab. The safety of continuation or resumption of trastuzumab in patients who have previously experienced cardiac toxicity has not been studied. There are insufficient data regarding discontinuation of trastuzumab therapy in patients with asymptomatic decreases in ejection fraction; such patients should be closely monitored for evidence of clinical deterioration.

PRECAUTIONS

GENERAL

Trastuzumab therapy should be used with caution in patients with known hypersensitivity to trastuzumab, Chinese Hamster Ovary cell proteins, or any component of this product.

BENZYL ALCOHOL

For patients with a known hypersensitivity to benzyl alcohol (the preservative in bacteriostatic water for injection) reconstitute trastuzumab with sterile water for injection (SWFI). DISCARD THE SWFI-RECONSTITUTED TRASTUZUMAB VIAL FOLLOWING A SINGLE USE.

IMMUNOGENICITY

Of 903 patients that have been evaluated, human anti-human antibody (HAHA) to trastuzumab was detected in 1 patient, who had no allergic manifestations.

CARCINOGENESIS, MUTAGENESIS, AND IMPAIRMENT OF FERTILITY

Carcinogenesis

Trastuzumab has not been tested for its carcinogenic potential.

Mutagenesis

No evidence of mutagenic activity was observed in Ames tests using six different test strains of bacteria, with and without metabolic activation, at concentrations of up to 5000 g/ml trastuzumab. Human peripheral blood lymphocytes treated *in vitro* at concentrations of up to 5000 g/plate trastuzumab, with and without metabolic activation, revealed no evidence of mutagenic potential. In an *in vivo* mutagenic assay (the micronucleus assay), no evidence of chromosomal damage to mouse bone marrow cells was observed following bolus intravenous doses of up to 118 mg/kg trastuzumab.

T

Impairment of Fertility

A fertility study has been conducted in female cynomolgus monkeys at doses up to 25 times the weekly human maintenance dose of 2 mg/kg trastuzumab and has revealed no evidence of impaired fertility.

PREGNANCY CATEGORY B

Reproduction studies have been conducted in cynomolgus monkeys at doses up to 25 times the weekly human maintenance dose of 2 mg/kg trastuzumab and have revealed no evidence of impaired fertility or harm to the fetus. However, HER2 protein expression is high in many embryonic tissues including cardiac and neural tissues; in mutant mice lacking HER2, embryos died in early gestation.[9] Placental transfer of trastuzumab during the early (days 20-50 of gestation) and late (Days 120-150 of gestation) fetal development period was observed. There are, however, no adequate and well-controlled studies in pregnant women. Because animal reproduction studies are not always predictive of human response, this drug should be used during pregnancy only if clearly needed.

NURSING MOTHERS

A study conducted in lactating cynomolgus monkeys at doses 25 times the weekly human maintenance dose of 2 mg/kg trastuzumab demonstrated that trastuzumab is secreted in the milk. The presence of trastuzumab in the serum of infant monkeys was not associated with any adverse effects on their growth or development from birth to 3 months of age. It is not known whether trastuzumab is excreted in human milk. Because human IgG is excreted in human milk, and the potential for absorption and harm to the infant is unknown, women should be advised to discontinue nursing during trastuzumab therapy and for 6 months after the last dose of trastuzumab.

PEDIATRIC USE

The safety and effectiveness of trastuzumab in pediatric patients have not been established.

GERIATRIC USE

Trastuzumab has been administered to 133 patients who were 65 years of age or over. The risk of cardiac dysfunction may be increased in geriatric patients. The reported clinical experience is not adequate to determine whether older patients respond differently from younger patients.

DRUG INTERACTIONS

There have been no formal drug interaction studies performed with trastuzumab in humans. Administration of paclitaxel in combination with trastuzumab resulted in a 2-fold decrease in trastuzumab clearance in a non-human primate study and in a 1.5-fold increase in trastuzumab serum levels in clinical studies (see CLINICAL PHARMACOLOGY, Pharmacokinetics).

ADVERSE REACTIONS

A total of 958 patients have received trastuzumab alone or in combination with chemotherapy. Data in TABLE 4 are based on the experience with the recommended dosing regimen for trastuzumab in the randomized controlled clinical trial in 234 patients who received trastuzumab in combination with chemotherapy and four open-label studies of trastuzumab as a single agent in 352 patients at doses of 10-500 mg administered weekly.

Cardiac Failure/Dysfunction: For a description of cardiac toxicities, see WARNINGS.

Anemia and Leukopenia: An increased incidence of anemia and leukopenia was observed in the treatment group receiving trastuzumab and chemotherapy, especially in the trastuzumab and AC subgroup, compared with the treatment group receiving chemotherapy alone. The majority of these cytopenic events were mild or moderate in intensity, reversible, and none resulted in discontinuation of therapy with trastuzumab.

Hematologic toxicity is infrequent following the administration of trastuzumab as a single agent, with an incidence of Grade III toxicities for WBC, platelets, hemoglobin all 1%. No Grade IV toxicities were observed.

Diarrhea: Of patients treated with trastuzumab as a single agent, 25% experienced diarrhea. An increased incidence of diarrhea, primarily mild to moderate in severity, was observed in patients receiving trastuzumab in combination with chemotherapy.

Infection: An increased incidence of infections, primarily mild upper respiratory infections of minor clinical significance or catheter infections, was observed in patients receiving trastuzumab in combination with chemotherapy.

Infusion-Associated Symptoms: During the first infusion with trastuzumab, a symptom complex most commonly consisting of chills and/or fever was observed in about 40% of patients. The symptoms were usually mild to moderate in severity and were treated with acetaminophen, diphenhydramine, and meperidine (with or without reduction in the rate of trastuzumab infusion). Trastuzumab discontinuation was infrequent. Other signs and/or symptoms may include nausea, vomiting, pain (in some cases at tumor sites), rigors, headache, dizziness, dyspnea, hypotension, rash, and asthenia. The symptoms occurred infrequently with subsequent trastuzumab infusions.

OTHER SERIOUS ADVERSE EVENTS

The following other serious adverse events occurred in at least 1 of the 958 patients treated with trastuzumab:

Body as a Whole: Cellulitis, anaphylactoid reaction, ascites, hydrocephalus, radiation injury, deafness, amblyopia.

Cardiovascular: Vascular thrombosis, pericardial effusion, heart arrest, hypotension, syncope, hemorrhage, shock arrhythmia.

Digestive: Hepatic failure, gastroenteritis, hematemesis, ileus, intestinal obstruction, colitis, esophageal ulcer, stomatitis, pancreatitis, hepatitis.

Endocrine: Hypothyroidism.

Hematological: Pancytopenia, acute leukemia, coagulation disorder, lymphangitis.

Metabolic: Hypercalcemia, hypomagnesemia, hyponatremia, hypoglycemia, growth retardation, weight loss.

Musculoskeletal: Pathological fractures, bone necrosis, myopathy.

TABLE 4 *Adverse Events Occurring in ≥5% of Patients or at Increased Incidence in the Trastuzumab Arm of the Randomized Study*

	Single Agent n=352	TRZ + PAC n=91	PAC Alone n=95	TRZ + AC n=143	AC Alone n=135
Body as a Whole					
Pain	47%	61%	62%	57%	42%
Asthenia	42%	62%	57%	54%	55%
Fever	36%	49%	23%	56%	34%
Chills	32%	41%	4%	35%	11%
Headache	26%	36%	28%	44%	31%
Abdominal pain	22%	34%	22%	23%	18%
Back pain	22%	34%	30%	27%	15%
Infection	20%	47%	27%	47%	31%
Flu syndrome	10%	12%	5%	12%	6%
Accidental injury	6%	13%	3%	9%	4%
Allergic Reaction	3%	8%	2%	4%	2%
Cardiovascular					
Tachycardia	5%	12%	4%	10%	5%
Congestive heart failure	7%	11%	1%	28%	7%
Digestive					
Nausea	33%	51%	9%	76%	77%
Diarrhea	25%	45%	29%	45%	26%
Vomiting	23%	37%	28%	53%	49%
Nausea and vomiting	8%	14%	11%	18%	9%
Anorexia	14%	24%	16%	31%	26%
Hematic & Lymphatic					
Anemia	4%	14%	9%	36%	26%
Leukopenia	3%	24%	17%	52%	34%
Metabolic					
Peripheral edema	10%	22%	20%	20%	17%
Edema	8%	10%	8%	11%	5%
Musculoskeletal					
Bone pain	7%	24%	18%	7%	7%
Arthralgia	6%	37%	21%	8%	9%
Nervous					
Insomnia	14%	25%	13%	29%	15%
Dizziness	13%	22%	24%	24%	18%
Paresthesia	9%	48%	39%	17%	11%
Depression	6%	12%	13%	20%	12%
Peripheral neuritis	2%	23%	16%	2%	2%
Neuropathy	1%	13%	5%	4%	4%
Respiratory					
Cough increased	26%	41%	22%	43%	29%
Dyspnea	22%	27%	26%	42%	25%
Rhinitis	14%	22%	5%	22%	16%
Pharyngitis	12%	22%	14%	30%	18%
Sinusitis	9%	21%	7%	13%	6%
Skin					
Rash	18%	38%	18%	27%	17%
Herpes simplex	2%	12%	3%	7%	9%
Acne	2%	11%	3%	3%	<1%
Urogenital					
Urinary tract infection	5%	18%	14%	13%	7%

Nervous: Convulsion, ataxia, confusion, manic reaction.

Respiratory: Apnea, pneumothorax, asthma, hypoxia, laryngitis.

Skin: Herpes zoster, skin ulceration.

Urogenital: Hydronephrosis, kidney failure, cervical cancer, hematuria, hemorrhagic cystitis, pyelonephritis.

DOSAGE AND ADMINISTRATION

USUAL DOSE

The recommended initial loading dose is 4 mg/kg trastuzumab administered as a 90-minute infusion. The recommended weekly maintenance dose is 2 mg/kg trastuzumab and can be administered as a 30-minute infusion if the initial loading dose was well tolerated. Trastuzumab may be administered in an outpatient setting. **DO NOT ADMINISTER AS AN IV PUSH OR BOLUS** (see Administration).

PREPARATION FOR ADMINISTRATION

Use appropriate aseptic technique. Each vial of trastuzumab should be reconstituted with 20 ml of BWFI, 1.1% benzyl alcohol preserved, as supplied, to yield a multi-dose solution containing 21 mg/ml trastuzumab. Immediately upon reconstitution with BWFI, the vial of trastuzumab must be labeled in the area marked "Do not use after:" with the future date that is 28 days from the date of reconstitution.

If the patient has known hypersensitivity to benzyl alcohol, trastuzumab must be reconstituted with sterile water for injection (see PRECAUTIONS). TRASTUZUMAB WHICH HAS BEEN RECONSTITUTED WITH SWFI MUST BE USED IMMEDIATELY AND ANY UNUSED PORTION DISCARDED. USE OF OTHER RECONSTITUTION DILUENTS SHOULD BE AVOIDED.

Determine the number in mg of trastuzumab needed, based on a loading dose of 4 mg trastuzumab/kg body weight or a maintenance dose of 2 mg trastuzumab/kg body weight. Calculate the volume of 21 mg/ml trastuzumab solution and withdraw this amount from the vial and add it to an infusion bag containing 250 ml of 0.9% sodium chloride. **DEXTROSE (5%) SOLUTION SHOULD NOT BE USED.** Gently invert the bag to mix the solution. The reconstituted preparation results in a colorless to pale yellow transparent solution. Parenteral drug products should be inspected visually for particulates and discoloration prior to administration.

No incompatibilities between trastuzumab and polyvinylchloride or polyethylene bags have been observed.

ADMINISTRATION

Treatment may be administered in an outpatient setting by administration of a 4 mg/kg trastuzumab loading dose by intravenous (IV) infusion over 90 minutes. **DO NOT ADMINISTER AS AN IV PUSH OR BOLUS.** Patients should be observed for fever and chills or other infusion-associated symptoms (see ADVERSE REACTIONS). If prior infusions are well tolerated, subsequent weekly doses of 2 mg/kg trastuzumab may be administered over 30 minutes. Trastuzumab should not be mixed or diluted with other drugs. Trastuzumab infusions should not be administered or mixed with dextrose solutions.

HOW SUPPLIED

Herceptin is supplied as a lyophilized, sterile powder containing 440 mg trastuzumab per vial under vacuum.

STABILITY AND STORAGE

Vials of trastuzumab are stable at 2-8°C (36-46°F) prior to reconstitution. Do not use beyond the expiration date stamped on the vial. A vial of trastuzumab reconstituted with BWFI, as supplied, is stable for 28 days after reconstitution when stored refrigerated at 2-8°C (36-46°F), and the solution is preserved for multiple use. Discard any remaining multi-dose reconstituted solution after 28 days. If unpreserved SWFI (not supplied) is used, the reconstituted trastuzumab solution should be used immediately and any unused portion must be discarded. DO NOT FREEZE TRASTUZUMAB THAT HAS BEEN RECONSTITUTED.

Storage

Solution of trastuzumab for infusion diluted in polyvinylchloride or polyethylene bags containing 0.9% sodium chloride for injection, may be stored at 2-8°C (36-46°F) for up to 24 hours prior to use. Diluted trastuzumab has been shown to be stable for up to 24 hours at room temperature (2-25°C). However, since diluted trastuzumab contains no effective preservative, the reconstituted and diluted solution should be stored refrigerated (2-8°C).

PRODUCT LISTING - EQUIVALENTS NOT AVAILABLE

Kit - Intravenous - 440 mg

1's $2692.38 HERCEPTIN, Genentech 50242-0134-60

Travoprost *(003263)*

Categories: Glaucoma, open-angle; Hypertension, ocular; FDA Approved 2001 Mar; Pregnancy Category C

Drug Classes: Ophthalmics; Prostaglandins

Brand Names: **Betimol**

Foreign Brand Availability: Apo-Timop (Canada; New-Zealand); Aquanil (Denmark; Finland; Norway; Sweden); Arutinol (Germany); Blocadren (Norway; Sweden); Blocanol (Finland); Chibro-Timoptol (Germany); Cusimolol (Hong-Kong; Hungary; Spain); Digaol (France); Gen-Timolol (Canada); Glafemak (Greece); Glauco (Thailand); Glauco Oph (Hong-Kong; Thailand); Glaucopress (Indonesia); Glucomol (India); Imot Ofteno Al (Costa-Rica; Dominican-Republic; El-Salvador; Guatemala; Honduras; Mexico; Nicaragua; Panama); Isotic Adretor (Indonesia); Molotic Eye Ocupres (India); Noval (Greece); Nylol (Israel); Nyolol (Colombia; Mexico; Taiwan); Nyolol Gel (Korea); Ocupres (Benin; Burkina-Faso; Ethiopia; Gambia; Ghana; Guinea; India; Ivory-Coast; Kenya; Liberia; Malawi; Mali; Mauritania; Mauritius; Morocco; Niger; Nigeria; Senegal; Seychelles; Sierra-Leone; Sudan; Tanzania; Tunia; Uganda; Zambia; Zimbabwe); Ofal (Argentina); Ofan (Thailand); Optimol (Australia; Colombia; Denmark; Sweden); Temserin (Greece); Tenopt (Australia); Tiloptic (Israel); Timacar (Denmark); Timoftol (Spain); Timohexal (Germany; Hungary); Timol (Taiwan); Timolol-POS (Israel); Tim Ophtal (Indonesia); Timoptic (Austria; Bulgaria; Canada; Czech-Republic; Hungary; Japan; Korea; Switzerland); Timoptic XE (Bahamas; Barbados; Belize; Bermuda; Curacao; Guyana; Jamaica; Netherland-Antilles; Surinam; Trinidad); Timoptol (Australia; Belgium; Benin; Burkina-Faso; Colombia; Ecuador; England; Ethiopia; France; Gambia; Germany; Ghana; Guinea; Hong-Kong; Italy; Ivory-Coast; Japan; Kenya; Liberia; Malawi; Malaysia; Mali; Mauritania; Mauritius; Mexico; Morocco; Netherlands; New-Zealand; Niger; Nigeria; Philippines; Senegal; Seychelles; Sierra-Leone; South-Africa; Sudan; Taiwan; Tanzania; Thailand; Tunia; Uganda; Zambia; Zimbabwe); Timoptol-XE (Hong-Kong; New-Zealand; Peru; Philippines); Timozzard (Mexico); Titol (Denmark); Ximex Opticom (Indonesia); Yesan (Greece)

Cost of Therapy: $55.75 (Glaucoma; Travatan Ophth. Solution; 0.004%; 2.5 ml; 1 drop/day; variable day supply)

DESCRIPTION

Travoprost is a synthetic prostaglandin $F_{2\alpha}$ analogue. Its chemical name is isopropyl (Z)-7-[(1*R*,2*R*,3*R*,5S)-3,5-dihydroxy-2-[(1*E*,3*R*)-3-hydroxy-4-[(α,α,α-trifluoro-*m*-tolyl)oxy]-1-butenyl]cyclopentyl]-5-heptenoate. It has a molecular formula of $C_{26}H_{35}F_3O_6$ and a molecular weight of 500.56.

Travoprost is a clear, colorless to slightly yellow oil that is very soluble in acetonitrile, methanol, octanol, and chloroform. It is practically insoluble in water.

Travatan ophthalmic solution 0.004% is supplied as sterile, buffered aqueous solution of travoprost with a pH of approximately 6.0 and an osmolality of approximately 290 mOsmol/kg.

Each ml of travatan 0.004% contains 40 μg travoprost. Benzalkonium chloride 0.015% is added as a preservative. Inactive ingredients are: polyoxyl 40 hydrogenated castor oil, tromethamine, boric acid, mannitol, edetate disodium, sodium hydroxide and/or hydrochloric acid (to adjust pH) and purified water.

CLINICAL PHARMACOLOGY

MECHANISM OF ACTION

Travoprost free acid is a selective FP prostanoid receptor agonist which is believed to reduce intraocular pressure by increasing uveoscleral outflow. The exact mechanism of action is unknown at this time.

PHARMACOKINETICS/PHARMACODYNAMICS

Absorption

Travoprost is absorbed through the cornea. In humans, peak plasma concentrations of travoprost free acid (25 pg/ml or less) were reached within 30 minutes following topical ocular administration and was rapidly eliminated.

Metabolism

Travoprost, an isopropyl ester prodrug, is hydrolyzed by esterases in the cornea to its biologically active free acid. Systemically, travoprost free acid is metabolized to inactive metabolites via beta-oxidation of the α(carboxylic acid) chain to give the 1,2-dinor and 1,2,3,4-tetranor analogs, via oxidation of the 15-hydroxyl moiety, as well as via reduction of the 13,14 double bond.

Excretion

Elimination of travoprost free acid from human plasma is rapid. Plasma levels are below the limit of quantitation (<10 pg/ml) within 1 hour following ocular instillation.

INDICATIONS AND USAGE

Travoprost ophthalmic solution is indicated for the reduction of elevated intraocular pressure in patients with open-angle glaucoma or ocular hypertension who are intolerant of other intraocular pressure lowering medications or insufficiently responsive (failed to achieve target IOP determined after multiple measurements over time) to another intraocular pressure lowering medication.

CONTRAINDICATIONS

Known hypersensitivity to travoprost, benzalkonium chloride or any other ingredients in this product. Travoprost may interfere with the maintenance of pregnancy and should not be used by women during pregnancy or by women attempting to become pregnant.

WARNINGS

Travoprost has been reported to cause changes to pigmented tissues. The most frequently reported changes have been increased pigmentation of the iris and periorbital tissue (eyelid) and increased pigmentation and growth of eyelashes. These changes may be permanent.

Travoprost may gradually change eye color, increasing the amount of brown pigmentation in the iris by increasing the number of melanosomes (pigment granules) in melanocytes. The long term effects on the melanocytes and the consequences of potential injury to the melanocytes and/or deposition of pigment granules to other areas of the eye are currently unknown. The change in iris color occurs slowly and may not be noticeable for months to years. Patients should be informed of the possibility of iris color change.

Eyelid skin darkening has been reported in association with the use of travoprost.

Travoprost may gradually change eyelashes in the treated eye; these changes include increased length, thickness, pigmentation, and/or number of lashes.

Patients who are expected to receive treatment in only 1 eye should be informed about the potential for increased brown pigmentation of the iris, periorbital and/or eyelid tissue, and eyelashes in the treated eye and thus heterochromia between the eyes. They should also be advised of the potential for a disparity between the eyes in length, thickness, and/or number of eyelashes.

PRECAUTIONS

GENERAL

There have been reports of bacterial keratitis associated with the use of multiple-dose containers of topical ophthalmic products. These containers had been inadvertently contaminated by patients who, in most cases, had a concurrent corneal disease or a disruption of the epithelial surface (see Information for the Patient).

Patients may slowly develop increased brown pigmentation of the iris. This change may not be noticeable for months to years (see WARNINGS). Iris pigmentation changes may be more noticeable in patients with mixed colored irides, *i.e.*, blue-brown, grey-brown, yellow-brown, and green-brown; however, it has also been observed in patients with brown eyes. The color change is believed to be due to increased melanin content in the stromal melanocytes of the iris. The exact mechanism of action is unknown at this time. Typically the brown pigmentation around the pupil spreads concentrically towards the periphery in affected eyes, but the entire iris or parts of it may become more brownish. Until more information about increased brown pigmentation is available, patients should be examined regularly and, depending on the situation, treatment may be stopped if increased pigmentation ensues.

Travoprost should be used with caution in patients with active intraocular inflammation (iritis/uveitis).

Macular edema, including cystoid macular edema, has been reported during treatment with prostaglandin $F_{2\alpha}$ analogues. These reports have mainly occurred in aphakic patients, pseudophakic patients with a torn posterior lens capsule, or in patients with known risk factors for macular edema. Travoprost should be used with caution in these patients.

Travoprost has not been evaluated for the treatment of angle closure, inflammatory or neovascular glaucoma.

Travoprost has not been studied in patients with renal or hepatic impairment and should be used with caution in such patients.

Travoprost should not be administered while wearing contact lenses.

Patients should be advised that travoprost contains benzalkonium chloride which may be adsorbed by contact lenses. Contact lenses should be removed prior to the administration of the solution. Lenses may be reinserted 15 minutes following administration of travoprost.

Since prostaglandins are biologically active and may be absorbed through the skin, women who are pregnant or attempting to become pregnant should exercise appropriate precautions to avoid direct exposure to the contents of the bottle. In case of accidental contact with the contents of the bottle, thoroughly cleanse the exposed area with soap and water immediately.

INFORMATION FOR THE PATIENT

Patients should be advised concerning all the information contained in WARNINGS and PRECAUTIONS.

Patients should also be instructed to avoid allowing the tip of the dispensing container to contact the eye or surrounding structures because this could cause the tip to become contaminated by common bacteria known to cause ocular infections. Serious damage to the eye and subsequent loss of vision may result from using contaminated solutions.

Patients also should be advised that if they develop an intercurrent ocular condition (*e.g.*, trauma, or infection) or have ocular surgery, they should immediately seek their physician's advice concerning the continued use of the multi-dose container.

T

Patients should be advised that if they develop any ocular reactions, particularly conjunctivitis and lid reactions, they should immediately seek their physician's advice.

If more than one topical ophthalmic drug is being used, the drugs should be administered at least 5 minutes apart.

CARCINOGENESIS, MUTAGENESIS, AND IMPAIRMENT OF FERTILITY

Travoprost was not mutagenic in the Ames test, mouse micronucleus test and rat chromosome aberration assay. A slight increase in the mutant frequency was observed in 1 of 2 mouse lymphoma assays in the presence of rat S-9 activation enzymes.

Travoprost did not affect mating or fertility indices in male or female rats at subcutaneous doses up to 10 μg/kg/day [250 times the maximum recommended human ocular dose of 0.04 μg/kg/day on a μg/kg basis (MRHOD)]. At 10 μg/kg/day, the mean number of corpora lutea was reduced, and the post-implantation losses were increased. These effects were not observed at 3 μg/kg/day (75 times the MRHOD).

PREGNANCY, TERATOGENIC EFFECTS, PREGNANCY CATEGORY C

Travoprost was teratogenic in rats, at an intravenous (IV) dose up to 10 μg/kg/day (250 times the MRHOD), evidenced by an increase in the incidence of skeletal malformations as well as external and visceral malformations, such as fused sternebrae, domed head and hydrocephaly. Travoprost was not teratogenic in rats at IV doses up to 3 μg/kg/day (75 times the MRHOD), and in mice at subcutaneous doses up to 1.0 μg/kg/day (25 times the MRHOD). Travoprost produced an increase in post-implantation losses and a decrease in fetal viability in rats at IV doses >3 μg/kg/day (75 times the MRHOD) and in mice at subcutaneous doses >0.3 μg/kg/day (7.5 times the MRHOD).

In the offspring of female rats that received travoprost subcutaneously from Day 7 of pregnancy to lactation Day 21 at the doses of ≥0.12 μg/kg/day (3 times the MRHOD), the incidence of postnatal mortality was increased, and neonatal body weight gain was decreased. Neonatal development was also affected, evidenced by delayed eye opening, pinna detachment and preputial separation, and by decreased motor activity.

No adequate and well-controlled studies have been performed in pregnant women. Travoprost may interfere with the maintenance of pregnancy and should not be used by women during pregnancy or by women attempting to become pregnant.

NURSING MOTHERS

A study in lactating rats demonstrated that radiolabeled travoprost and/or its metabolites were excreted in milk. It is not known whether this drug or its metabolites are excreted in human milk. Because many drugs are excreted in human milk, caution should be exercised when travoprost is administered to a nursing woman.

PEDIATRIC USE

Safety and effectiveness in pediatric patients have not been established.

GERIATRIC USE

No overall differences in safety or effectiveness have been observed between elderly and other adult patients.

ADVERSE REACTIONS

The most common ocular adverse event observed in controlled clinical studies with travoprost 0.004% was ocular hyperemia which was reported in 35-50% of patients. Approximately 3% of patients discontinued therapy due to conjunctival hyperemia.

Ocular adverse events reported at an incidence of 5-10% included decreased visual acuity, eye discomfort, foreign body sensation, pain, and pruritus.

Ocular adverse events reported at an incidence of 1-4% included, abnormal vision, blepharitis, blurred vision, cataract, cells, conjunctivitis, dry eye, eye disorder, flare, iris discoloration, keratitis, lid margin crusting, photophobia, subconjunctival hemorrhage, and tearing.

Nonocular adverse events reported at a rate of of 1-5% were accidental injury, angina pectoris, anxiety, arthritis, back pain, bradycardia, bronchitis, chest pain, cold syndrome, depression, dyspepsia, gastrointestinal disorder, headache, hypercholesterolemia, hypertension, hypotension, infection, pain, prostate disorder, sinusitis, urinary incontinence, and urinary tract infection.

DOSAGE AND ADMINISTRATION

The recommended dosage is 1 drop in the affected eye(s) once-daily in the evening. The dosage of travoprost should not exceed once-daily since it has been shown that more frequent administration may decrease the intraocular pressure lowering effect.

Reduction of intraocular pressure starts approximately 2 hours after administration, and the maximum effect is reached after 12 hours.

Travoprost may be used concomitantly with other topical ophthalmic drug products to lower intraocular pressure. If more than one topical ophthalmic drug is being used, the drugs should be administered at least 5 minutes apart.

HOW SUPPLIED

Travatan (travoprost ophthalmic solution) 0.004% is a sterile, isotonic, buffered, preserved, aqueous solution of travoprost (0.04 mg/ml) supplied in Alcon's oval Drop-Tainer package system inside a sealed foil pouch.

Travatan is supplied as a 2.5 ml solution in a 3.5 ml natural polypropylene dispenser bottle with a natural polypropylene dropper tip and a turquoise polypropylene overcap. Tamper evidence is provided with a shrink band around the closure and neck area of the package. **Storage:** Store between 2-25°C (36-77°F). Discard the container within 6 weeks of removing it from the sealed pouch.

PRODUCT LISTING - EQUIVALENTS NOT AVAILABLE

Solution - Ophthalmic - 0.004%

2.50 ml	$55.75	TRAVATAN, Alcon Laboratories Inc	00065-0266-25
2.50 ml x 2	$111.50	TRAVATAN, Alcon Laboratories Inc	00065-0266-17

T

Trazodone Hydrochloride *(002367)*

For related information, see the comparative table section in Appendix A.

Categories: Depression; Pregnancy Category C; FDA Approved 1981 Dec
Drug Classes: Antidepressants, miscellaneous
Brand Names: **Desyrel**; Sideril; Trazalon; Trazonil
Foreign Brand Availability: Azonz (Finland); Beneficat (Argentina); Bimaran (Argentina); Deprax (Spain); Depresil (Philippines); Depyrel (Israel); Desirel (Thailand); Manegan (Argentina); Molipaxin (England; Ireland; South-Africa); Pragmarel (France); Reslin (Japan); Taxagon (Argentina); Thombran (Germany); Trazodil (Israel); Trazolan (Belgium; India; Netherlands); Trazone (Indonesia; Portugal; Taiwan); Trittico (Austria; Colombia; Greece; Hong-Kong; Italy; Peru; Switzerland)
Cost of Therapy: $120.11 (Depression; Desyrel; 50 mg; 3 tablets/day; 30 day supply)
$8.89 (Depression; Generic Tablets; 50 mg; 3 tablets/day; 30 day supply)

DESCRIPTION

Trazodone HCl, is an antidepressant chemically unrelated to tricyclic, tetracyclic, or other known antidepressant agents. It is a triazolopyridine derivative designated as 2-[3-{4 -(*m*-Chlorophenyl)-1-piperazinyl} propyl]s-triazolo[4,3-*a*]-pyridin-3(2*H*)-one monohydrochloride. Trazodone HCl is a white to off-white crystalline powder which is sparingly soluble in chloroform and water. Its molecular weight is 408.3. The empirical formula is $C_{19}H_{22}ClN_5O{\cdot}HCl$.

Trazodone HCl is supplied for oral administration in 50 mg, 100 mg, 150 mg, and 300 mg tablets.

Trazodone HCl tablets, 50 mg, contain the following inactive ingredients: dibasic calcium phosphate, castor oil, microcrystalline cellulose, ethylcellulose, FD&C yellow no. 6 (aluminum lake), lactose, magnesium stearate, povidone, sodium starch glycolate, and starch (corn).

Trazodone HCl tablets, 100 mg, contain the following inactive ingredients: dibasic calcium phosphate, castor oil, microcrystalline cellulose, ethylcellulose, lactose, magnesium stearate, povidone, sodium starch glycolate, and starch (corn).

Trazodone HCl tablets, 150 mg, contain the following in active ingredients: microcrystalline cellulose, FD&C yellow no. 6 (aluminum lake), magnesium stearate, pre-gelatinized starch, and stearic acid.

Trazodone HCl tablets, 300 mg, contain the following inactive ingredients: microcrystalline cellulose, yellow ferric oxide, magnesium stearate, sodium starch glycolate, pregelatinized starch, and stearic acid.

STORAGE

Store at controlled room temperature 15-30°C (59-86°F).

Dispense in tight, light-resistant container with a child-resistant closure.

CLINICAL PHARMACOLOGY

The mechanism of trazodone HCl's antidepressant action in man is not fully understood. In animals, trazodone HCl selectively inhibits serotonin uptake by brain synaptosomes and potentiates the behavioral changes induced by the serotonin precursor, 5-hydroxytryptophan. Cardiac conduction effects of trazodone HCl in the anesthetized dog are qualitatively dissimilar and quantitatively less pronounced than those seen with tricyclic antidepressants. Trazodone HCl is not a monoamine oxidase inhibitor and, unlike amphetamine-type drugs, does not stimulate the central nervous system.

In man, trazodone HCl is well absorbed after oral administration without selective localization in any tissue. When trazodone HCl is taken shortly after ingestion of food, there may be an increase in the amount of drug absorbed, a decrease in maximum concentration and a lengthening in the time to maximum concentration. Peak plasma levels occur approximately 1 hour after dosing when trazodone HCl tablets are taken on an empty stomach or 2 hours after dosing when taken with food. Elimination of trazodone HCl is biphasic, consisting of an initial phase (half-life 3-6 hours) followed by a slower phase (half-life 5-9 hours), and is unaffected by the presence or absence of food. Since the clearance of trazodone HCl from the body is sufficiently variable, is some patients trazodone HCl may accumulate in the plasma.

For those patients who responded to trazodone HCl, one-third of the inpatients and one-half of the outpatients had a significant therapeutic response by the end of the first week of treatment. Three-fourths of all responders demonstrated a significant therapeutic effect by the end of the second week. One-fourth of responders required 2-4 weeks for a significant therapeutic response.

INDICATIONS AND USAGE

Trazodone HCl is indicated for the treatment of depression. The efficacy of trazodone HCl has been demonstrated in both inpatient and outpatient settings and for depressed patients with and without prominent anxiety. The depressive illness of patients studied corresponds to the Major Depressive Episode criteria of the American Psychiatric Association's Diagnostic and Statistical Manual, III.[1]

Major Depressive Episode implies a prominent and relatively persistent (nearly every day for at least 2 weeks) depressed or dysphoric mood that usually interferes with daily functioning, and includes at least four of the following eight symptoms: change in appetite, change in sleep, psychomotor agitation or retardation, loss of interest in usual activities or decrease in sexual drive, increased fatigability, feelings of guilt or worthlessness, slowed thinking or impaired concentration, and suicidal ideation or attempts.

NON-FDA APPROVED INDICATIONS

Preliminary data suggest trazodone may also be effective in reducing the three primary clusters of symptoms of posttraumatic stress disorder. However, this use is not approved by the FDA and further clinical testing is needed.

CONTRAINDICATIONS

Trazodone HCl is contraindicated in patients hypersensitive to the drug substance.

WARNINGS

TRAZODONE HAS BEEN ASSOCIATED WITH THE OCCURRENCE OF PRIAPISM. IN APPROXIMATELY 1/3 OF THE CASES REPORTED, SURGICAL INTERVENTION WAS REQUIRED AND, IN A PORTION OF THESE CASES, PERMANENT IMPAIRMENT OF ERECTILE FUNCTION OR IMPOTENCE RESULTED. MALE PATIENTS WITH PROLONGED OR INAPPROPRIATE ERECTIONS SHOULD IMMEDIATELY DISCONTINUE THE DRUG AND CONSULT THEIR PHYSICIAN.

The detumescence of priapism and drug-induced penile erections by the intracavernosal injection of alpha-adrenergic stimulants such as epinephrine and metaraminol has been reported.[2-7] For one case of priapism (of some 12-24 hours' duration) in a trazodone HCl treated patient in whom the intracavernosal injection of epinephrine was accomplished, prompt detumescence occurred with return of normal erectile activity.

This procedure should be performed under the supervision of a urologist or a physician familiar with the procedure and should not be initiated without urologic consultation if the priapism has persisted for more than 24 hours.

Trazodone HCl is not recommended for use during the initial recovery phase of myocardial infarction.

Caution should be used when administering trazodone HCl to patients with cardiac disease, and such patients should be closely monitored, since antidepressant drugs (including trazodone HCl) have been associated with the occurrence of cardiac arrhythmias. Recent clinical studies in patients with pre-existing cardiac disease indicate that trazodone HCl may be arrhythmogenic in some patients in that population. Arrhythmias identified include isolated PVCs, ventricular couplets, and in 2 patients short episodes (3-4 beats) of ventricular tachycardia.

PRECAUTIONS

GENERAL

The possibility of suicide in seriously depressed patients is inherent in the illness and may persist until significant remission occurs. Therefore, prescriptions should be written for the smallest number of tablets consistent with good patient management.

Hypotension, including orthostatic hypotension and syncope, has been reported to occur in patients receiving trazodone HCl. Concomitant administration of antihypertensive therapy with trazodone HCl may require a reduction in the dose of the antihypertensive drug.

Little is known about the interaction between trazodone HCl and general anesthetics; therefore, prior to elective surgery, trazodone HCl should be discontinued for as long as clinically feasible.

As with all antidepressants, the use of trazodone HCl should be given on the consideration of the physician that the expected benefits of therapy outweigh potential risk factors.

INFORMATION FOR THE PATIENT

Because priapism has been reported to occur in patients receiving trazodone HCl, patients with prolonged or inappropriate penile erection should immediately discontinue the drug and consult with the physician (see WARNINGS).

Antidepressants may impair the mental and/or physical ability required for the performance of potentially hazardous tasks, such as operating an automobile or machinery; the patient should be cautioned accordingly.

Trazodone HCl may enhance the response to alcohol, barbiturates, and other CNS depressants.

Trazodone HCl should be given shortly after a meal or light snack. Within any individual patient, total drug absorption may be up to 20% higher when the drug is taken with food rather than on an empty stomach. The risk of dizziness/lightheadedness may increase under fasting conditions.

LABORATORY TESTS

Occasional low white blood cell and neutrophil counts have been noted in patients receiving trazodone HCl. These were not considered clinically significant and did not necessitate discontinuation of the drug; however, the drug should be discontinued in any patient whose white blood cell count or absolute neutrophil count falls below normal levels. White blood cell and differential counts are recommended for patients who develop fever and sore throat (or other signs of infection) during therapy.

THERAPEUTIC INTERACTIONS

Concurrent administration with electroshock therapy should be avoided because of the absence of experience in this area.

There have been reports of increased and decreased prothrombin time occurring in patients taking warfarin and trazodone HCl.

CARCINOGENESIS, MUTAGENESIS, AND IMPAIRMENT OF FERTILITY

No drug- or dose-related occurrence of carcinogenesis was evident in rats receiving trazodone HCl in daily oral doses up to 300 mg/kg for 18 months.

PREGNANCY CATEGORY C

Trazodone HCl has been shown to cause increased fetal resorption and other adverse effects on the fetus in two studies using the rat when given at dose levels approximately 30-50 times the proposed maximum human dose. There was also an increase in congenital anomalies in one of three rabbit studies at approximately 15-50 times the maximum human dose. There are no adequate and well-controlled studies in pregnant women. Trazodone HCl should be used during pregnancy only if the potential benefit justifies the potential risk to the fetus.

NURSING MOTHERS

Trazodone HCl and/or its metabolites have been found in the milk of lactating rats, suggesting that the drug may be secreted in human milk. Caution should be exercised when trazodone HCl is administered to a nursing woman.

PEDIATRIC USE

Safety and effectiveness in children below the age of 18 have not been established.

DRUG INTERACTIONS

Increased serum digoxin or phenytoin levels have been reported to occur in patients receiving trazodone HCl concurrently with either of those 2 drugs.

It is not known whether interactions will occur between monoamine oxidase (MAO) inhibitors and trazodone HCl. Due to the absence of clinical experience, if MAO inhibitors are discontinued shortly before or are to be given concomitantly with trazodone HCl, therapy should be initiated cautiously with gradual increase in dosage until optimum response is achieved.

ADVERSE REACTIONS

Because the frequency of adverse drug effects is affected by diverse factors (*e.g.,* drug dose, methods of detection, physician judgment, disease under treatment, etc.) a single meaningful estimate of adverse event incidence is difficult to obtain. This problem is illustrated by the variation in adverse event incidence observed and reported from the inpatients and outpatients treated with trazodone HCl. It is impossible to determine precisely what accounts for the differences observed.

CLINICAL TRIAL REPORTS

TABLE 1 is presented solely to indicate the relative frequency of adverse events reported in representative controlled clinical studies conducted to evaluate the safety and efficacy of trazodone HCl.

The figures cited cannot be used to predict precisely the incidence of untoward events in the course of usual medical practice where patient characteristics and other factors often differ from those which prevailed in the clinical trials. These incidence figures, also, cannot be compared with those obtained from other clinical studies involving related drug products and placebo, as each group of drug trials is conducted under a different set of conditions.

TABLE 1

	Treatment-Emergent Symptom Incidence			
	Inpatients		Outpatients	
	Trazodone HCl	Placebo	Trazodone HCl	Placebo
Number of Patients	142	95	157	158
% of Patients Reporting				
Allergic				
Skin condition/edema	2.8	1.1	7.0	1.3
Autonomic				
Blurred vision	6.3	4.2	14.7	3.8
Constipation	7.0	4.2	7.6	5.7
Dry mouth	14.8	8.4	33.8	20.3
Cardiovascular				
Hypertension	2.1	1.1	1.3	*
Hypotension	7.0	1.1	3.8	0.0
Shortness of breath	*	1.1	1.3	0.0
Syncope	2.8	2.1	4.5	1.3
Tachycardia/palpitations	0.0	0.0	7.0	7.0
CNS				
Anger/Hostility	3.5	6.3	1.3	2.5
Confusion	4.9	0.0	5.7	7.6
Decreased concentration	2.8	2.1	1.3	0.0
Disorientation	2.1	0.0	*	0.0
Dizziness/lightheadedness	19.7	5.3	28.0	15.2
Drowsiness	23.9	6.3	40.8	19.6
Excitement	1.4	1.1	5.1	5.7
Fatigue	11.3	4.2	5.7	2.5
Headache	9.9	5.3	19.8	15.8
Insomnia	9.9	10.5	6.4	12.0
Impaired memory	1.4	0.0	*	*
Nervousness	14.8	10.5	6.4	8.2
Gastrointestinal				
Abdominal/gastric disorder	3.5	4.2	5.7	4.4
Bad taste in mouth	1.4	0.0	0.0	0.0
Diarrhea	0.0	1.1	4.5	1.9
Nausea/vomiting	9.9	1.1	12.7	9.5
Musculoskeletal				
Musculoskeletal Aches/Pains	5.6	3.2	5.1	2.5
Neurological				
Incoordination	4.9	0.0	1.9	0.0
Paresthesia	1.4	0.0	0.0	*
Tremors	2.8	1.1	5.1	3.8
Sexual Function				
Decreased libido	*	1.1	1.3	*
Other				
Decreased appetite	3.5	5.3	0.0	*
Eyes red/Tired/Itching	2.8	0.0	0.0	0.0
Head full-heavy	2.8	0.0	0.0	0.0
Malaise	2.8	0.0	0.0	0.0
Nasal/Sinal congestion	2.8	0.0	5.7	3.2
Nightmares/Vivid dreams	*	1.1	5.1	5.7
Sweating/Clamminess	1.4	1.1	*	*
Tinnitus	1.4	0.0	0.0	*
Weight gain	1.4	0.0	4.5	1.9
Weight loss	*	3.2	5.7	2.5

* Incidence less than 1%.

Occasional sinus bradycardia has occurred in long-term studies.

In addition to the relatively common (*i.e.,* greater than 1%) untoward events enumerated above, the following adverse events have been reported to occur in association with the use of trazodone HCl in the controlled clinical studies: akathisia, allergic reaction, anemia, chest pain, delayed urine flow, early menses, flatulence, hallucinations/delusions, hematuria, hypersalivation, hypomania, impaired speech, impotence, increased appetite, increased libido, increased urinary frequency, missed periods, muscle twitches, numbness, and retrograde ejaculation.

POSTINTRODUCTION REPORTS

Although the following adverse reactions have been reported in trazodone HCl users, the causal association has neither been confirmed nor refuted.

Voluntary Reports Received Since Market Introduction Include the Following

Agitation, alopecia, apnea, ataxia, breast enlargement or engorgement, diplopia, edema, extrapyramidal symptoms, grand mal seizures, hallucinations, hemolytic anemia, hyperbilirubinemia, leukonychia, jaundice, lactation, liver enzyme alterations, methemoglobinemia, nausea/vomiting (most frequently), paresthesia, priapism (See WARNINGS and PRECAUTIONS, Information for the Patient; some patients may require surgical intervention), pruritus, psychosis, rash, stupor, inappropriate ADH syndrome, tardive dyskinesia, unexplained death, urinary incontinence, urinary retention, urticaria, vasodilation, vertigo, and weakness.

Cardiovascular System Effects Which Have Been Reported Include the Following

Conduction block, orthostatic hypotension and syncope, palpitations, bradycardia, atrial fibrillation, myocardial infarction, cardiac arrest, arrhythmia, and ventricular ectopic activity, including ventricular tachycardia (see WARNINGS).

DOSAGE AND ADMINISTRATION

The dosage should be initiated at a low level and increased gradually, noting the clinical response and any evidence of intolerance. Occurrence of drowsiness may require the administration of a major portion of the daily dose at bedtime or a reduction of dosage. Trazodone HCl should be taken shortly after a meal or light snack. Symptomatic relief may be seen during the first week, with optimal antidepressant effects typically evident within 2 weeks. Twenty-five percent (25%) of those who respond to trazodone HCl require more than 2 weeks (up to 4 weeks) of drug administration.

USUAL ADULT DOSAGE

An initial dose of 150 mg/day in divided doses is suggested. The dose may be increased by 50 mg/day every 3-4 days. The maximum dose for outpatients usually should not exceed 400 mg/day in divided doses. Inpatients (*i.e.*, more severely depressed patients) may be given up to but not in excess of 600 mg/day in divided doses.

MAINTENANCE

Dosage during prolonged maintenance therapy should be kept at the lowest effective level. Once an adequate response has been achieved, dosage may be gradually reduced, with subsequent adjustment depending on therapeutic response.

Although there has been no systematic evaluation of the efficacy of trazodone HCl beyond 6 weeks, it is generally recommended that a course of antidepressant drug treatment should be continued for several months.

PRODUCT LISTING - RATED THERAPEUTICALLY EQUIVALENT

Tablet - Oral - 50 mg

Size	Price	Product	NDC
7's	$5.03	GENERIC, Pd-Rx Pharmaceuticals	55289-0064-07
14's	$7.43	GENERIC, Pd-Rx Pharmaceuticals	55289-0064-14
20's	$42.66	DESYREL, Pharma Pac	52959-0350-20
25's	$3.72	GENERIC, Udl Laboratories Inc	51079-0427-19
30 x 25	$310.43	GENERIC, Sky Pharmaceuticals Packaging, Inc	63739-0245-01
30 x 25	$310.43	GENERIC, Sky Pharmaceuticals Packaging, Inc	63739-0245-03
30's	$8.10	GENERIC, Pd-Rx Pharmaceuticals	55289-0064-30
30's	$9.97	GENERIC, Golden State Medical	60429-0187-30
30's	$12.15	GENERIC, Heartland Healthcare Services	61392-0487-30
30's	$12.15	GENERIC, Heartland Healthcare Services	61392-0487-39
30's	$60.39	DESYREL, Pharma Pac	52959-0350-30
31 x 10	$139.93	GENERIC, Vangard Labs	00615-2578-53
31 x 10	$139.93	GENERIC, Vangard Labs	00615-2578-63
31's	$12.56	GENERIC, Heartland Healthcare Services	61392-0487-31
32's	$12.96	GENERIC, Heartland Healthcare Services	61392-0487-32
45's	$18.23	GENERIC, Heartland Healthcare Services	61392-0487-45
60's	$19.35	GENERIC, Golden State Medical	60429-0187-60
60's	$24.30	GENERIC, Heartland Healthcare Services	61392-0487-60
90's	$28.74	GENERIC, Golden State Medical	60429-0187-90
90's	$36.45	GENERIC, Heartland Healthcare Services	61392-0487-90
100's	$6.84	FEDERAL UPPER LIMIT, H.C.F.A. F F P	99999-2367-01
100's	$11.72	GENERIC, Us Trading Corporation	56126-0368-11
100's	$12.00	GENERIC, Raway Pharmacal Inc	00686-0472-20
100's	$14.93	GENERIC, Interstate Drug Exchange Inc	00814-7980-14
100's	$24.07	GENERIC, Qualitest Products Inc	00603-6144-21
100's	$25.20	GENERIC, Major Pharmaceuticals Inc	00904-3990-60
100's	$28.40	GENERIC, Martec Pharmaceuticals Inc	52555-0260-01
100's	$28.65	GENERIC, Major Pharmaceuticals Inc	00904-5219-60
100's	$28.75	GENERIC, Warner Chilcott Laboratories	00047-0577-24
100's	$30.71	GENERIC, Moore, H.L. Drug Exchange Inc	00839-7251-06
100's	$41.73	GENERIC, Parmed Pharmaceuticals Inc	00349-8906-01
100's	$41.73	GENERIC, Watson/Rugby Laboratories Inc	00536-4715-01
100's	$41.73	GENERIC, Barr Laboratories Inc	00555-0489-02
100's	$42.42	GENERIC, Ivax Corporation	00182-1259-89
100's	$42.42	GENERIC, Udl Laboratories Inc	51079-0427-20
100's	$43.51	GENERIC, Major Pharmaceuticals Inc	00904-3990-61
100's	$56.50	GENERIC, Teva Pharmaceuticals Usa	00093-0637-01
100's	$56.52	GENERIC, Sidmak Laboratories Inc	50111-0433-01
100's	$56.54	GENERIC, Watson/Schein Pharmaceuticals Inc	00364-2109-01
100's	$56.54	GENERIC, Mutual/United Research Laboratories	00677-1133-01
100's	$56.54	GENERIC, Geneva Pharmaceuticals	00781-1807-01
100's	$56.54	GENERIC, Martec Pharmaceuticals Inc	52555-0727-01
100's	$56.54	GENERIC, Mutual Pharmaceutical Co Inc	53489-0510-01
100's	$56.79	GENERIC, Purepac Pharmaceutical Company	00228-2439-10
100's	$133.45	DESYREL, Pharma Pac	52959-0350-00
100's	$217.28	DESYREL, Bristol-Myers Squibb	00087-0775-41

Tablet - Oral - 100 mg

Size	Price	Product	NDC
15's	$10.22	GENERIC, Heartland Healthcare Services	61392-0490-15
25 x 30	$549.23	GENERIC, Sky Pharmaceuticals Packaging, Inc	63739-0246-03
25's	$4.77	GENERIC, Udl Laboratories Inc	51079-0428-19
30's	$8.69	GENERIC, Pd-Rx Pharmaceuticals	55289-0223-30
30's	$16.27	GENERIC, Golden State Medical	60429-0188-30
30's	$20.43	GENERIC, Heartland Healthcare Services	61392-0490-30
30's	$20.43	GENERIC, Heartland Healthcare Services	61392-0490-39
31 x 10	$238.47	GENERIC, Vangard Labs	00615-2579-53
31 x 10	$238.47	GENERIC, Vangard Labs	00615-2579-63
31's	$21.11	GENERIC, Heartland Healthcare Services	61392-0490-31
32's	$21.79	GENERIC, Heartland Healthcare Services	61392-0490-32
45's	$30.65	GENERIC, Heartland Healthcare Services	61392-0490-45
60's	$31.97	GENERIC, Golden State Medical	60429-0188-60
60's	$40.86	GENERIC, Heartland Healthcare Services	61392-0490-60
90's	$61.29	GENERIC, Heartland Healthcare Services	61392-0490-90
100's	$9.52	FEDERAL UPPER LIMIT, H.C.F.A. F F P	99999-2367-05
100's	$18.00	GENERIC, Raway Pharmacal Inc	00686-0428-20
100's	$23.90	GENERIC, Us Trading Corporation	56126-0369-11
100's	$23.93	GENERIC, Interstate Drug Exchange Inc	00814-7982-14
100's	$39.75	GENERIC, Major Pharmaceuticals Inc	00904-3991-60
100's	$41.00	GENERIC, Qualitest Products Inc	00603-6145-21
100's	$41.78	GENERIC, Moore, H.L. Drug Exchange Inc	00839-7252-06
100's	$46.40	GENERIC, Martec Pharmaceuticals Inc	52555-0261-01
100's	$47.45	GENERIC, Major Pharmaceuticals Inc	00904-5220-60
100's	$70.18	GENERIC, Barr Laboratories Inc	00555-0490-02
100's	$73.20	GENERIC, Teva Pharmaceuticals Usa	00093-0638-01
100's	$73.25	GENERIC, Sidmak Laboratories Inc	50111-0434-01
100's	$73.26	GENERIC, Watson/Schein Pharmaceuticals Inc	00364-2110-01
100's	$73.26	GENERIC, Watson/Schein Pharmaceuticals Inc	00591-5599-01
100's	$73.26	GENERIC, Mutual/United Research Laboratories	00677-1134-01
100's	$73.26	GENERIC, Geneva Pharmaceuticals	00781-1808-01
100's	$73.26	GENERIC, Martec Pharmaceuticals Inc	52555-0728-01
100's	$73.26	GENERIC, Mutual Pharmaceutical Co Inc	53489-0511-01
100's	$73.51	GENERIC, Purepac Pharmaceutical Company	00228-2441-10
100's	$73.59	GENERIC, Ivax Corporation	00182-1260-89
100's	$73.59	GENERIC, Udl Laboratories Inc	51079-0428-20
100's	$76.94	GENERIC, Geneva Pharmaceuticals	00781-1808-13
100's	$78.43	GENERIC, Major Pharmaceuticals Inc	00904-3991-61
100's	$295.68	DESYREL, Bristol-Myers Squibb	00087-0776-42
100's	$379.69	DESYREL, Bristol-Myers Squibb	00087-0776-41
250's	$116.15	GENERIC, Parmed Pharmaceuticals Inc	00349-8907-25

Tablet - Oral - 150 mg

Size	Price	Product	NDC
14's	$14.25	GENERIC, Pd-Rx Pharmaceuticals	55289-0060-14
15's	$53.22	DESYREL DIVIDOSE, Physicians Total Care	54868-2549-00
30's	$25.70	DESYREL DIVIDOSE, Pharmaceutical Corporation Of America	51655-0277-24
30's	$31.14	GENERIC, Heartland Healthcare Services	61392-0491-30
30's	$31.14	GENERIC, Heartland Healthcare Services	61392-0491-39
30's	$44.98	GENERIC, Mutual/United Research Laboratories	00677-1302-07
30's	$97.92	DESYREL DIVIDOSE, Pd-Rx Pharmaceuticals	55289-0489-30
31's	$32.17	GENERIC, Heartland Healthcare Services	61392-0491-31
32's	$33.21	GENERIC, Heartland Healthcare Services	61392-0491-32
45's	$46.70	GENERIC, Heartland Healthcare Services	61392-0491-45
60's	$62.27	GENERIC, Heartland Healthcare Services	61392-0491-60
90's	$93.41	GENERIC, Heartland Healthcare Services	61392-0491-90
100's	$31.13	FEDERAL UPPER LIMIT, H.C.F.A. F F P	99999-2367-09
100's	$70.35	GENERIC, Major Pharmaceuticals Inc	00904-3992-60
100's	$77.20	GENERIC, Qualitest Products Inc	00603-6146-21
100's	$88.50	GENERIC, Ivax Corporation	00182-1298-01
100's	$89.90	GENERIC, Martec Pharmaceuticals Inc	52555-0132-01
100's	$94.49	GENERIC, Moore, H.L. Drug Exchange Inc	00839-7507-06
100's	$96.88	GENERIC, Watson/Rugby Laboratories Inc	00536-4691-01
100's	$146.91	GENERIC, Sidmak Laboratories Inc	50111-0441-01
100's	$146.92	GENERIC, Watson/Schein Pharmaceuticals Inc	00364-2300-01
100's	$146.92	GENERIC, Barr Laboratories Inc	00555-0732-02
100's	$146.92	GENERIC, Watson/Schein Pharmaceuticals Inc	00591-2300-01
100's	$146.92	GENERIC, Mutual/United Research Laboratories	00677-1302-01
100's	$146.92	GENERIC, Martec Pharmaceuticals Inc	52555-0729-01
100's	$146.92	GENERIC, Mutual Pharmaceutical Co Inc	53489-0517-01
100's	$327.09	DESYREL DIVIDOSE, Bristol-Myers Squibb	00087-0778-43
250's	$149.00	GENERIC, Major Pharmaceuticals Inc	00904-3392-70
250's	$184.90	GENERIC, Major Pharmaceuticals Inc	00904-3992-70
250's	$189.95	GENERIC, Parmed Pharmaceuticals Inc	00349-8824-25

Tablet - Oral - 300 mg

100's	$426.52	GENERIC, Barr Laboratories Inc	00555-0733-02
100's	$582.18	DESYREL DIVIDOSE, Bristol-Myers Squibb	00087-0796-41

PRODUCT LISTING - EQUIVALENTS NOT AVAILABLE

Tablet - Oral - 50 mg

10's	$15.10	GENERIC, Southwood Pharmaceuticals Inc	58016-0263-10
12's	$18.96	TRAZODONE HYDROCHLORIDE, Southwood Pharmaceuticals Inc	58016-0263-12
15's	$23.70	TRAZODONE HYDROCHLORIDE, Southwood Pharmaceuticals Inc	58016-0263-15
20's	$10.79	GENERIC, Pharma Pac	52959-0378-20
28's	$44.24	TRAZODONE HYDROCHLORIDE, Southwood Pharmaceuticals Inc	58016-0263-28
30's	$4.38	GENERIC, Physicians Total Care	54868-0122-02
30's	$13.39	GENERIC, Pharmaceutical Corporation Of America	51655-0634-24
30's	$13.54	GENERIC, Allscripts Pharmaceutical Company	54569-1470-00
30's	$16.63	GENERIC, Pharma Pac	52959-0378-30
30's	$47.40	TRAZODONE HYDROCHLORIDE, Southwood Pharmaceuticals Inc	58016-0263-30
60's	$33.92	GENERIC, Allscripts Pharmaceutical Company	54569-1470-06
60's	$94.80	GENERIC, Southwood Pharmaceuticals Inc	58016-0263-60
90's	$142.20	GENERIC, Southwood Pharmaceuticals Inc	58016-0263-90
100's	$9.88	GENERIC, Physicians Total Care	54868-0122-00
100's	$45.14	GENERIC, Allscripts Pharmaceutical Company	54569-1470-01
100's	$158.00	TRAZODONE HYDROCHLORIDE, Southwood Pharmaceuticals Inc	58016-0263-00
120's	$189.60	GENERIC, Southwood Pharmaceuticals Inc	58016-0263-02

Tablet - Oral - 100 mg

12's	$27.37	GENERIC, Southwood Pharmaceuticals Inc	58016-0862-12
15's	$34.21	GENERIC, Southwood Pharmaceuticals Inc	58016-0862-15
20's	$45.61	GENERIC, Southwood Pharmaceuticals Inc	58016-0862-20
30's	$5.57	GENERIC, Physicians Total Care	54868-1223-01
30's	$18.31	GENERIC, Pharmaceutical Corporation Of America	51655-0666-24
30's	$60.50	GENERIC, Pharma Pac	52959-0140-30
30's	$68.42	GENERIC, Southwood Pharmaceuticals Inc	58016-0862-30
50's	$114.00	GENERIC, Southwood Pharmaceuticals Inc	58016-0862-50
60's	$43.96	GENERIC, Allscripts Pharmaceutical Company	54569-1999-02
100's	$15.44	GENERIC, Physicians Total Care	54868-1223-00
100's	$73.26	GENERIC, Allscripts Pharmaceutical Company	54569-1999-01
100's	$228.06	GENERIC, Southwood Pharmaceuticals Inc	58016-0862-00

Tablet - Oral - 150 mg

6's	$8.82	GENERIC, Allscripts Pharmaceutical Company	54569-3732-01
12's	$23.58	GENERIC, Southwood Pharmaceuticals Inc	58016-0880-12
15's	$7.57	GENERIC, Physicians Total Care	54868-1959-02
15's	$29.47	GENERIC, Southwood Pharmaceuticals Inc	58016-0880-15
20's	$39.30	GENERIC, Southwood Pharmaceuticals Inc	58016-0880-20
30's	$13.81	GENERIC, Physicians Total Care	54868-1959-01
30's	$44.08	GENERIC, Allscripts Pharmaceutical Company	54569-3732-02
30's	$58.94	GENERIC, Southwood Pharmaceuticals Inc	58016-0880-30
100's	$146.90	GENERIC, Apothecon Inc	59772-3171-01
100's	$196.48	GENERIC, Southwood Pharmaceuticals Inc	58016-0880-00

Tablet - Oral - 300 mg

12's	$68.44	GENERIC, Southwood Pharmaceuticals Inc	58016-0701-12
15's	$85.55	GENERIC, Southwood Pharmaceuticals Inc	58016-0701-15
20's	$114.07	GENERIC, Southwood Pharmaceuticals Inc	58016-0701-20
30's	$171.10	GENERIC, Southwood Pharmaceuticals Inc	58016-0701-30
50's	$285.17	GENERIC, Southwood Pharmaceuticals Inc	58016-0701-50
60's	$342.20	GENERIC, Southwood Pharmaceuticals Inc	58016-0701-60
90's	$513.30	GENERIC, Southwood Pharmaceuticals Inc	58016-0701-90
100's	$570.33	GENERIC, Southwood Pharmaceuticals Inc	58016-0701-00

Treprostinil Sodium *(003560)*

Categories: Hypertension, pulmonary; FDA Approved 2002 May; Pregnancy Category B; Orphan Drugs
Drug Classes: Platelet inhibitors; Prostaglandins; Vasodilators
Brand Names: Remodulin

DESCRIPTION

Remodulin (treprostinil sodium) Injection is a sterile sodium salt formulated for subcutaneous administration. Remodulin is supplied in 20 ml multi-use vials in four strengths, containing 1.0, 2.5, 5.0 or 10.0 mg/ml of treprostinil. Each ml also contains 5.3 mg sodium chloride (except for the 10.0 mg/ml strength which contains 4.0 mg sodium chloride), 3.0 mg metacresol, 6.3 mg sodium citrate, and water for injection. Sodium hydroxide and hydrochloric acid may be added to adjust pH between 6.0 and 7.2.

Treprostinil is chemically stable at room temperature and neutral pH.

Treprostinil sodium is (1R,2R,3aS,9aS)-[[2,3,3a,4,9,9a-Hexahydro-2-hydroxy-1-[(3S)-3-hydroxyoctyl]-1H-benz[f]inden-5-yl]oxy]acetic acid monosodium salt. Treprostinil sodium has a molecular weight of 412.49 and a molecular formula of $C_{23}H_{33}NaO_5$.

CLINICAL PHARMACOLOGY

GENERAL

The major pharmacological actions of treprostinil are direct vasodilation of pulmonary and systemic arterial vascular beds and inhibition of platelet aggregation. In animals, the vasodilatory effects reduce right and left ventricular afterload and increase cardiac output and stroke volume. Other studies have shown that treprostinil causes a dose-related negative inotropic and lusitropic effect. No major effects on cardiac conduction have been observed.

PHARMACOKINETICS

The pharmacokinetics of continuous subcutaneous treprostinil sodium are linear over the dose range of 1.25 to 22.5 ng/kg/min (corresponding to plasma concentrations of about 0.03 to 8 μg/L) and can be described by a two-compartment model. Dose proportionality at infusion rates greater than 22.5 ng/kg/min has not been studied.

Absorption

Treprostinil sodium is relatively rapidly and completely absorbed after subcutaneous infusion, with an absolute bioavailability approximating 100%. Steady-state concentrations occurred in approximately 10 hours. Concentrations in patients treated with an average dose of 9.3 ng/kg/min were approximately 2 μg/L.

Distribution

The volume of distribution of the drug in the central compartment is approximately 14 L/70 kg ideal body weight. Treprostinil sodium at *in vitro* concentrations ranging from 330-10,000 μg/L was 91% bound to human plasma protein.

Metabolism

Treprostinil sodium is substantially metabolized by the liver, but the precise enzymes responsible are unknown. Five metabolites have been described (HU1 through HU5). The biological activity and metabolic fate of these metabolites are unknown. The chemical structure of HU1 is unknown. HU5 is the glucuronide conjugate of treprostinil. The other metabolites are formed by oxidation of the 3-hydroxyoctyl side chain (HU2) and subsequent additional oxidation (HU3) or dehydration (HU4). Based on the results of *in vitro* human hepatic cytochrome P450 studies, treprostinil sodium does not inhibit CYP-1A2, 2C9, 2C19, 2D6, 2E1, or 3A. Whether treprostinil sodium induces these enzymes has not been studied.

Excretion

The elimination of treprostinil sodium is biphasic, with a terminal half-life of approximately 2-4 hours. Approximately 79% of an administered dose is excreted in the urine as unchanged drug (4%) and as the identified metabolites (64%). Approximately 13% of a dose is excreted in the feces. Systemic clearance is approximately 30 L/h for a 70 kg ideal body weight person.

SPECIAL POPULATIONS

Hepatic Insufficiency

In patients with portopulmonary hypertension and mild (n=4) or moderate (n=5) hepatic insufficiency, treprostinil sodium at a subcutaneous dose of 10 ng/kg/min for 150 minutes had a C_{max} that was increased 2-fold and 4-fold, respectively, and AUC(0-∞) was increased 3-fold and 5-fold, respectively, compared to healthy subjects. Clearance in patients with hepatic insufficiency was reduced by up to 80% compared to healthy adults.

In patients with mild or moderate hepatic insufficiency, the initial dose of treprostinil sodium should be decreased to 0.625 ng/kg/min ideal body weight and should be increased cautiously. Treprostinil sodium has not been studied in patients with severe hepatic insufficiency.

Renal Insufficiency

No studies have been performed in patients with renal insufficiency, so no specific advice about dosing in such patients can be given. Although only 4% of the administered dose is excreted unchanged in the urine, the five identified metabolites are all excreted in the urine.

Effect of Other Drugs on Treprostinil Sodium

In vitro studies: Treprostinil sodium did not significantly affect the plasma protein binding of normally observed concentrations of digoxin or warfarin.

In vivo studies: *Acetaminophen*— Analgesic doses of acetaminophen, 1000 mg every 6 hours for seven doses, did not affect the pharmacokinetics of treprostinil sodium, at a subcutaneous infusion rate of 15 ng/kg/min.

INDICATIONS AND USAGE

Treprostinil sodium is indicated as a continuous subcutaneous infusion for the treatment of pulmonary arterial hypertension in patients with NYHA Class II-IV symptoms to diminish symptoms associated with exercise.

CONTRAINDICATIONS

Treprostinil sodium is contraindicated in patients with known hypersensitivity to the drug or to structurally related compounds.

WARNINGS

Treprostinil sodium is indicated for subcutaneous use only.

PRECAUTIONS

GENERAL

Treprostinil sodium should be used only by clinicians experienced in the diagnosis and treatment of PAH.

Treprostinil sodium is a potent pulmonary and systemic vasodilator. Initiation of treprostinil sodium must be performed in a setting with adequate personnel and equipment for physiological monitoring and emergency care. Subcutaneous therapy with treprostinil sodium may be used for prolonged periods, and the patient's ability to administer treprostinil sodium and care for an infusion system should be carefully considered.

Dose should be increased for lack of improvement in, or worsening of, symptoms and it should be decreased for excessive pharmacological effects or for unacceptable infusion site symptoms (see DOSAGE AND ADMINISTRATION).

Abrupt withdrawal or sudden large reductions in dosage of treprostinil sodium may result in worsening of PAH symptoms and should be avoided.

INFORMATION FOR THE PATIENT

Patients receiving treprostinil sodium should be given the following information: Treprostinil sodium is infused continuously through a subcutaneous catheter, via an infusion pump. Therapy with treprostinil sodium will be needed for prolonged periods, possibly years, and the patient's ability to accept, place, and care for a subcutaneous catheter and to use an infusion pump should be carefully considered. Additionally, patients should be aware that subsequent disease management may require the initiation of an intravenous therapy.

HEPATIC AND RENAL IMPAIRMENT

Caution should be used in patients with hepatic or renal impairment (see CLINICAL PHARMACOLOGY, Special Populations).

CARCINOGENESIS, MUTAGENESIS, AND IMPAIRMENT OF FERTILITY

Long-term studies have not been performed to evaluate the carcinogenic potential of treprostinil. *In vitro* and *in vivo* mutagenicity studies did not demonstrate any mutagenic or clastogenic effects of treprostinil. Treprostinil sodium did not affect fertility or mating performance of male or female rats given continuous subcutaneous infusion at rates of up to 450 ng treprostinil/kg/min [about 59 times the recommended starting human rate of infusion (1.25 ng/kg/min) and about 8 times the average rate (9.3 ng/kg/min) achieved in clinical trials, on a ng/m^2 basis]. In this study, males were dosed from 10 weeks prior to mating and through the 2 week mating period. Females were dosed from 2 weeks prior to mating until gestational day 6.

PREGNANCY CATEGORY B

In pregnant rats, continuous subcutaneous infusion of treprostinil sodium during the period of organogenesis and late gestational development, at rates as high as 900 ng treprostinil/kg/min (about 117 times the starting human rate of infusion, on a ng/m^2 basis and about 16 times the average rate achieved in clinical trials), resulted in no evidence of harm to the fetus. In pregnant rabbits, effects of continuous subcutaneous infusion of treprostinil during organogenesis were limited to an increased incidence of fetal skeletal variations (bilateral full rib or right rudimentary rib on lumbar 1) associated with maternal toxicity (reduction in body weight and food consumption) at an infusion rate of 150 ng treprostinil/kg/min (about 41 times the starting human rate of infusion, on a ng/m^2 basis, and 5 times the average rate used in clinical trials). In rats, continuous subcutaneous infusion of treprostinil from implantation to the end of lactation, at rates of up to 450 ng treprostinil/kg/min, did not affect the growth and development of offspring. Because animal reproduction studies are not always predictive of human response, treprostinil sodium should be used during pregnancy only if clearly needed.

LABOR AND DELIVERY

No treprostinil sodium treatment-related effects on labor and delivery were seen in animal studies. The effect of treprostinil sodium on labor and delivery in humans is unknown.

NURSING MOTHERS

It is not known whether treprostinil is excreted in human milk or absorbed systemically after ingestion. Because many drugs are excreted in human milk, caution should be exercised when treprostinil sodium is administered to nursing women.

PEDIATRIC USE

Safety and effectiveness in pediatric patients have not been established. Clinical studies of treprostinil sodium did not include sufficient numbers of patients aged ≤16 years to determine whether they respond differently from older patients. In general, dose selection should be cautious.

GERIATRIC USE

Clinical studies of treprostinil sodium did not include sufficient numbers of patients aged 65 and over to determine whether they respond differently from younger patients. In general, dose selection for an elderly patient should be cautious, reflecting the greater frequency of decreased hepatic, renal, or cardiac function, and of concomitant disease or other drug therapy.

DRUG INTERACTIONS

Reduction in blood pressure caused by treprostinil sodium may be exacerbated by drugs that by themselves alter blood pressure, such as diuretics, antihypertensive agents, or vasodilators. Since treprostinil sodium inhibits platelet aggregation, there is also a potential for increased risk of bleeding, particularly among patients maintained on anticoagulants. During clinical trials, treprostinil sodium was used concurrently with anticoagulants, diuretics, cardiac glycosides, calcium channel blockers, analgesics, antipyretics, nonsteroidal anti-inflammatories, opioids, corticosteroids, and other medications.

EFFECT OF OTHER DRUGS ON TREPROSTINIL SODIUM

In vitro studies: Treprostinil sodium did not significantly affect the plasma protein binding of normally observed concentrations of digoxin or warfarin.

In vivo studies: *Acetaminophen*— Analgesic doses of acetaminophen, 1000 mg every 6 hours for seven doses, did not affect the pharmacokinetics of treprostinil sodium, at a subcutaneous infusion rate of 15 ng/kg/min.

Treprostinil sodium has not been studied in conjunction with Flolan (epoprostenol sodium) or Tracleer (bosentan).

EFFECT OF TREPROSTINIL SODIUM ON OTHER DRUGS

In vivo studies: *Warfarin*— Treprostinil sodium does not affect the pharmacokinetics or pharmacodymamics of warfarin. The pharmacokinetics of R- and S-warfarin and the INR in healthy subjects given a single 25 mg dose of warfarin were unaffected by continuous subcutaneous treprostinil sodium at an infusion rate of 10 ng/kg/min.

ADVERSE REACTIONS

Patients receiving treprostinil sodium reported a wide range of adverse events, many potentially related to the underlying disease (dyspnea, fatigue, chest pain, right ventricular heart failure, and pallor). During clinical trials infusion site pain and reaction were the most common adverse events among those treated with treprostinil sodium. Infusion site reaction was defined as any local adverse event other than pain or bleeding/bruising at the infusion site and included symptoms such as erythema, induration or rash. Infusion site reactions were sometimes severe and could lead to discontinuation of treatment.

TABLE 2 *Percentages of Subjects Reporting Infusion Site Adverse Events*

	Reaction		Pain	
	Placebo	Treprostinil Sodium	Placebo	Treprostinil Sodium
Severe	1%	38%	2%	39%
Requiring narcotics*	NA†	NA†	1%	32%
Leading to discontinuation	0	3%	0	7%

* Based on prescriptions for narcotics, not actual use.
† Medications used to treat infusion site pain were not distinguished from those used to treat site reactions.

Other adverse events included diarrhea, jaw pain, edema, vasodilatation and nausea.

ADVERSE EVENTS DURING CHRONIC DOSING

TABLE 3 lists adverse events that occurred at a rate of at least 3% and were more frequent in patients treated with treprostinil sodium than with placebo in controlled trials in PAH.

TABLE 3 *Adverse Events in Controlled Studies of Patients With PAH, Occurring With at Least 3% Incidence and More Common on Treprostinil Sodium Than on Placebo*

Adverse Event	Treprostinil Sodium (n=236)	Placebo (n=233)
Infusion site pain	85%	27%
Infusion site reaction	83%	27%
Headache	27%	23%
Diarrhea	25%	16%
Nausea	22%	18%
Rash	14%	11%
Jaw pain	13%	5%
Vasodilatation	11%	5%
Dizziness	9%	8%
Edema	9%	3%
Pruritus	8%	6%
Hypotension	4%	2%

Reported adverse events (at least 3%) are included except those too general to be informative, and those not plausibly attributable to the use of the drug, because they were associated with the condition being treated or are very common in the treated population.

ADVERSE EVENTS ATTRIBUTABLE TO THE DRUG DELIVERY SYSTEM IN PAH CONTROLLED TRIALS

There were no reports of infection related to the drug delivery system. There were 187 infusion system complications reported in 28% of patients (23% treprostinil sodium, 33% placebo); 173 (93%) were pump related and 14 (7%) related to the infusion set. Most delivery system complications were easily managed (*e.g.*, replace syringe or battery, reprogram pump, straighten crimped infusion line). Eight of these patients (4 treprostinil sodium, 4 placebo) reported non-serious adverse events resulting from infusion system complications. Adverse events resulting from problems with the delivery systems were typically related to either symptoms of excess treprostinil sodium (*e.g.*, nausea) or return of PAH symptoms (*e.g.*, dyspnea). These events were generally resolved by correcting the delivery system pump or infusion set problem. Adverse events resulting from problems with the delivery system did not lead to clinical instability or rapid deterioration.

DOSAGE AND ADMINISTRATION

Treprostinil sodium is supplied in 20 ml vials in concentrations of 1.0, 2.5, 5.0 and 10.0 mg/ml. Treprostinil sodium is meant to be administered without further dilution.

INITIAL DOSE

Treprostinil sodium is administered by continuous subcutaneous infusion. The infusion rate is initiated at 1.25 ng/kg/min. If this initial dose cannot be tolerated, the infusion rate should be reduced to 0.625 ng/kg/min.

DOSAGE ADJUSTMENTS

The goal of chronic dosage adjustments is to establish a dose at which PAH symptoms are improved, while minimizing excessive pharmacological effects of treprostinil sodium (headache, nausea, emesis, restlessness, anxiety and infusion site pain or reaction).

The infusion rate should be increased in increments of no more than 1.25 ng/kg/min/week for the first 4 weeks and then no more than 2.5 ng/kg/min/week for the remaining duration of infusion, depending on clinical response. There is little experience with doses >40 ng/kg/min. Abrupt cessation of infusion should be avoided (see PRECAUTIONS).

T

ADMINISTRATION

Treprostinil sodium is administered by continuous subcutaneous infusion, via a self-inserted subcutaneous catheter, using an infusion pump designed for subcutaneous drug delivery. To avoid potential interruptions in drug delivery, the patient must have immediate access to a backup infusion pump and subcutaneous infusion sets. The ambulatory infusion pump used to administer treprostinil sodium should: (1) be small and lightweight, (2) be adjustable to approximately 0.002 ml/h, (3) have occlusion/no delivery, low battery, programming error and motor malfunction alarms, (4) have delivery accuracy of ±6% or better and (5) be positive pressure driven. The reservoir should be made of polyvinyl chloride, polypropylene or glass.

Infusion rates are calculated using the following formula:

Infusion Rate (ml/h) = Dose (ng/kg/min) × Weight (kg) × [0.00006/Remodulin dosage strength concentration (mg/ml)]

HOW SUPPLIED

Remodulin is supplied in 20 ml multi-use vials at concentrations of 1.0, 2.5, 5.0, and 10.0 mg/ml treprostinil, as sterile solutions in water for injection, individually packaged in a carton. Each ml contains treprostinil sodium equivalent to 1.0, 2.5, 5.0, or 10.0 mg/ml treprostinil. Unopened vials of Remodulin are stable until the date indicated when stored at 15-25°C (59-77°F). Store at 25°C (77°F), with excursions permitted to15-30°C (59-86°F).

During use, a single reservoir (syringe) of Remodulin can be administered up to 72 hours at 37°C. A single vial of Remodulin should be used for no more than 14 days after the initial introduction into the vial.

Parenteral drug products should be inspected visually for particulate matter and discoloration prior to administration whenever solution and container permit. If either particulate matter or discoloration is noted, Remodulin should not be administered.

Tretinoin *(002368)*

Categories: Acne vulgaris; Hyperpigmentation, facial; Leukemia, acute promyelocytic; Wrinkles, facial; Pregnancy Category C; FDA Approval Pre 1982; Patent Expiration 2005 Oct; Orphan Drugs

Drug Classes: Antineoplastics, retinoids; Dermatologics; Keratolytics; Retinoids

Brand Names: Avita; Renova; **Retin-A**; Retinoic Acid; **Vesanoid**

Foreign Brand Availability: Aberel (France); Aberela (Sweden); A-Acido (Argentina); Acid A Vit (Belgium; Netherlands); Acne Free (Bahrain; Cyprus; Egypt; Iran; Iraq; Jordan; Kuwait; Lebanon; Libya; Oman; Qatar; Republic-of-Yemen; Saudi-Arabia; Syria; United-Arab-Emirates); Acta (Hong-Kong); Airol (Argentina; Czech-Republic; Greece; Italy; Malaysia; Mexico; Norway; Switzerland; Taiwan); Alquingel (Colombia); Avitcid (Finland); Derm A (Philippines); Dermairol (Sweden); Dermik A (China); Effederm (France); Eudyna (Hong-Kong; India; Indonesia; Malaysia; Taiwan); Facenol (Indonesia); Ilotycin-A (South-Africa); Locacid (Israel); Reacel-A (Mexico); Retacnyl (Costa-Rica; Dominican-Republic; El-Salvador; Guatemala; Honduras; Nicaragua; Panama; Peru; Philippines; Singapore; South-Africa); Retavit (Israel); Retiderma (Spain); Retin A (Austria; Bulgaria; Czech-Republic; France; Greece; Hungary; Israel; Portugal); Retinova (New-Zealand; Singapore); Retrieve Cream (Australia); Stieva-A (Australia; Colombia; Costa-Rica; Dominican-Republic; El-Salvador; Guatemala; Honduras; Korea; Malaysia; Mexico; Nicaragua; Panama; Thailand); Stieva A (Canada); Trentin (Indonesia); Vitamin A Acid (Canada)

Cost of Therapy: $36.76 (Acne; Retin-A Micro Gel; 0.1%; 20 g; 1 application/day; variable day supply)
$41.19 (Acne; Retin-A Cream; 0.1%; 20 g; 1 application/day; variable day supply)
$38.17 (Acne; Generic Cream; 0.1%; 20 g; 1 application/day; variable day supply)
$4,289.83 (Acute Promyelocytic Leukemia; Vesanoid; 10 mg; 8 capsules/day; 30 day supply)

ORAL

WARNING

Experienced Physician and Institution: Patients with acute promyelocytic leukemia (APL) are at high risk in general and can have severe adverse reactions to tretinoin. Tretinoin should therefore be administered under the supervision of a physician who is experienced in the management of patients with acute leukemia and in a facility with laboratory and supportive services sufficient to monitor drug tolerance and protect and maintain a patient compromised by drug toxicity, including respiratory compromise. Use of tretinoin requires that the physician concludes that the possible benefit to the patient outweighs the following known adverse effects of the therapy.

Retinoic Acid-APL Syndrome: About 25% of patients with APL treated with tretinoin have experienced a syndrome called the retinoic-acid-APL (RA-APL) syndrome characterized by fever, dyspnea, weight gain, radiographic pulmonary infiltrates and pleural or pericardial effusions. This syndrome has occasionally been accompanied by impaired myocardial contractility and episodic hypotension. It has been observed with or without concomitant leukocytosis. Endotracheal intubation and mechanical ventilation have been required in some cases due to progressive hypoxemia, and several patients have expired with multiorgan failure. The syndrome generally occurs during the first month of treatment, with some cases reported following the first dose of tretinoin.

The management of the syndrome has not been defined rigorously, but high-dose steroids given at the first suspicion of the RA-APL syndrome appear to reduce morbidity and mortality. At the first signs suggestive of the syndrome (unexplained fever, dyspnea and/or weight gain, abnormal chest auscultatory findings or radiographic abnormalities), high-dose steroids (dexamethasone 10 mg intravenously administered every 12 hours for 3 days or until the resolution of symptoms) should be immediately initiated, irrespective of the leukocyte count. The majority of patients do not require termination of tretinoin therapy during treatment of the RA-APL syndrome.

Leukocytosis at Presentation and Rapidly Evolving Leukocytosis During Tretinoin Treatment: During tretinoin treatment about 40% of patients will develop rapidly evolving leukocytosis. Patients who present with high WBC at diagnosis (>5 × 10^9/L) have an increased risk of a further rapid increase in WBC counts. Rapidly evolving leukocytosis is associated with a higher risk of life-threatening complications.

If signs and symptoms of the RA-APL syndrome are present together with leukocytosis, treatment with high-dose steroids should be initiated immediately. Some investigators routinely add chemotherapy to tretinoin treatment in the case of patients presenting with a WBC count of >5 × 10^9/L or in the case of a rapid increase in WBC count for patients leukopenic at start of treatment, and have

WARNING — Cont'd

reported a lower incidence of the RA-APL syndrome. Consideration could be given to adding full-dose chemotherapy (including an anthracycline if not contraindicated) to the tretinoin therapy on day 1 or 2 for patients presenting with a WBC count of >5 × 10^9/L, or immediately, for patients presenting with a WBC count of <5 × 10^9/L, if the WBC count reaches ≥6 × 10^9/L by day 5, or ≥10 × 10^9/L by day 10, or ≥15 × 10^9/L by day 28.

Teratogenic Effects, Pregnancy Category D: See WARNINGS. There is a high risk that a severely deformed infant will result if tretinoin is administered during pregnancy. If, nonetheless, it is determined that tretinoin represents the best available treatment for a pregnant woman or a woman of childbearing potential, it must be assured that the patient has received full information and warnings of the risk to the fetus if she were to be pregnant and of the risk of possible contraception failure and has been instructed in the need to use 2 reliable forms of contraception simultaneously during therapy and for 1 month following discontinuation of therapy, and has acknowledged her understanding of the need for using dual contraception, unless abstinence is the chosen method.

Within 1 week prior to the institution of tretinoin therapy, the patient should have blood or urine collected for a serum or urine pregnancy test with a sensitivity of at least 50 mIU/L. When possible, tretinoin therapy should be delayed until a negative result from this test is obtained. When a delay is not possible the patient should be placed on two reliable forms of contraception. Pregnancy testing and contraception counseling should be repeated monthly throughout the period of tretinoin treatment.

DESCRIPTION

Vesanoid (tretinoin) is a retinoid that induces maturation of acute promyelocytic leukemia (APL) cells in culture. It is available in a 10 mg soft gelatin capsule for oral administration. Each capsule also contains beeswax, butylated hydroxyanisole, edetate disodium, hydrogenated soybean oil flakes, hydrogenated vegetable oils and soybean oil. The gelatin capsule shell contains glycerin, yellow iron oxide, red iron oxide, titanium dioxide, methylparaben, and propylparaben. Chemically, tretinoin is all-*trans* retinoic acid and is related to retinol (vitamin A). It is a yellow to light orange crystalline powder with a molecular weight of 300.44.

CLINICAL PHARMACOLOGY

MECHANISM OF ACTION

Tretinoin is not a cytolytic agent but instead induces cytodifferentiation and decreased proliferation of APL cells in culture and *in vivo*. In APL patients, tretinoin treatment produces an initial maturation of the primitive promyelocytes derived from the leukemic clone, followed by a repopulation of the bone marrow and peripheral blood by normal, polyclonal hematopoietic cells in patients achieving complete remission (CR). The exact mechanism of action of tretinoin in APL is unknown.

PHARMACOKINETICS

Tretinoin activity is primarily due to the parent drug. In human pharmacokinetics studies, orally administered drug was well absorbed into the systemic circulation, with approximately two-thirds of the administered radiolabel recovered in the urine. The terminal elimination half-life of tretinoin following initial dosing is 0.5 to 2 hours in patients with APL. There is evidence that tretinoin induces its own metabolism. Plasma tretinoin concentrations decrease on average to one-third of their day 1 values during 1 week of continuous therapy. Mean ±SD peak tretinoin concentrations decreased from 394 ± 89 to 138 ± 139 ng/ml, while area under the curve (AUC) values decreased from 537 ± 191 ng·h/ml to 249 ± 185 ng·h/ml during 45 mg/m^2 daily dosing in 7 APL patients. Increasing the dose to "correct" for this change has not increased response.

Absorption

A single 45 mg/m^2 (~80 mg) oral dose to APL patients resulted in a mean ±SD peak tretinoin concentration of 347 ± 266 ng/ml. Time to reach peak concentration was between 1 and 2 hours.

Distribution

The apparent volume of distribution of tretinoin has not been determined. Tretinoin is greater than 95% bound in plasma, predominately to albumin. Plasma protein binding remains constant over the concentration range of 10-500 ng/ml.

Metabolism

Tretinoin metabolites have been identified in plasma and urine. Cytochrome P450 enzymes have been implicated in the oxidative metabolism of tretinoin. Metabolites include 13-*cis* retinoic acid, 4-oxo *trans* retinoic acid, 4-oxo *cis* retinoic acid, and 4-oxo *trans* retinoic acid glucuronide. In APL patients, daily administration of a 45 mg/m^2 dose of tretinoin resulted in an approximately 10-fold increase in the urinary excretion of 4-oxo *trans* retinoic acid glucuronide after 2-6 weeks of continuous dosing, when compared to baseline values.

Excretion

Studies with radiolabeled drug have demonstrated that after the oral administration of 2.75 and 50 mg doses of tretinoin, greater than 90% of the radioactivity was recovered in the urine and feces. Based upon data from 3 subjects, approximately 63% of radioactivity was recovered in the urine within 72 hours and 31% appeared in the feces within 6 days.

Special Populations

The pharmacokinetics of tretinoin have not been separately evaluated in women, in members of different ethnic groups, or in individuals with renal or hepatic insufficiency.

Drug-Drug Interactions

In 13 patients who had received daily doses of tretinoin for 4 consecutive weeks, administration of ketoconazole 400-1200 mg oral dose 1 hour prior to the administration of the tretinoin dose on day 29 led to a 72% increase (218 ± 224 vs 375 ± 285 ng·h/ml) in tretinoin mean plasma AUC. The precise cytochrome P450 enzymes involved in these in-

T

teractions have not been specified; *CYP*, 3A4, 2C8, and 2E have been implicated in various preliminary reports.

INDICATIONS AND USAGE

Tretinoin capsules are indicated for the induction of remission in patients with acute promyelocytic leukemia (APL), French-American-British (FAB) classification M3 (including the M3 variant), characterized by the presence of the t(15;17) translocation and/or the presence of the PML/RARα gene who are refractory to, or who have relapsed from, anthracycline chemotherapy, or for whom anthracycline-based chemotherapy is contraindicated. Tretinoin is for the induction of remission only. The optimal consolidation or maintenance regimens have not been defined, but all patients should receive an accepted form of remission consolidation and/or maintenance therapy for APL after completion of induction therapy with tretinoin.

CONTRAINDICATIONS

Tretinoin is contraindicated in patients with a known hypersensitivity to retinoids. Tretinoin should not be given to patients who are sensitive to parabens, which are used as preservatives in the gelatin capsule.

WARNINGS

PREGNANCY CATEGORY D

See BOXED WARNING.

Tretinoin has teratogenic and embryotoxic effects in mice, rats, hamsters, rabbits and pigtail monkeys, and may be expected to cause fetal harm when administered to a pregnant woman. Tretinoin causes fetal resorptions and a decrease in live fetuses in all animals studied. Gross external, soft tissue, and skeletal alterations occurred at doses higher than 0.7 mg/kg/day in mice, 2 mg/kg/day in rats, 7 mg/kg/day in hamsters, and at a dose of 10 mg/kg/day, the only dose tested, in pigtail monkeys (about 1/20, 1/4, and 1/2 and 4 times the human dose, respectively, on a mg/m^2 basis).

There are no adequate and well-controlled studies in pregnant women. Although experience with humans administered tretinoin is extremely limited, increased spontaneous abortions and major human fetal abnormalities related to the use of other retinoids have been documented in humans. Reported defects include abnormalities of the CNS, musculoskeletal system, external ear, eye, thymus, and great vessels; and facial dysmorphia, cleft palate, and parathyroid hormone deficiency. Some of these abnormalities were fatal. Cases of IQ scores less than 85, with or without obvious CNS abnormalities, have also been reported. All fetuses exposed during pregnancy can be affected and at the present time there is no antepartum means of determining which fetuses are and are not affected.

Effective contraception must be used by all females during tretinoin therapy and for 1 month following discontinuation of therapy. Contraception must be used even when there is a history of infertility or menopause, unless a hysterectomy has been performed. Whenever contraception is required, it is recommended that 2 reliable forms of contraception be used simultaneously, unless abstinence is the chosen method. If pregnancy does occur during treatment, the physician and patient should discuss the desirability of continuing or terminating the pregnancy.

PATIENTS WITHOUT THE T(15;17) TRANSLOCATION

Initiation of therapy with tretinoin may be based on the morphological diagnosis of acute promyelocytic leukemia. Confirmation of the diagnosis of APL should be sought by detection of the t(15;17) genetic marker by cytogenetic studies. If these are negative, PML/RARα fusion should be sought using molecular diagnostic techniques. The response rate of other AML subtypes to tretinoin has not been demonstrated; therefore, patients who lack the genetic marker should be considered for alternative treatment.

RETINOIC ACID-APL (RA-APL) SYNDROME

In up to 25% of patients with APL treated with tretinoin, a syndrome occurs which can be fatal (see BOXED WARNING and ADVERSE REACTIONS).

LEUKOCYTOSIS AT PRESENTATION AND RAPIDLY EVOLVING LEUKOCYTOSIS DURING TRETINOIN TREATMENT

See BOXED WARNING.

PSEUDOTUMOR CEREBRI

Retinoids, including tretinoin, have been associated with pseudotumor cerebri (benign intracranial hypertension), especially in pediatric patients. Early signs and symptoms of pseudotumor cerebri include papilledema, headache, nausea and vomiting, and visual disturbances. Patients with these symptoms should be evaluated for pseudotumor cerebri, and, if present, appropriate care should be instituted in concert with neurological assessment.

LIPIDS

Up to 60% of patients experienced hypercholesterolemia and/or hypertriglyceridemia, which were reversible upon completion of treatment. The clinical consequences of temporary elevation of triglycerides and cholesterol are unknown, but venous thrombosis and myocardial infarction have been reported in patients who ordinarily are at low risk for such complications.

ELEVATED LIVER FUNCTION TEST RESULTS

Elevated liver function test results occur in 50-60% of patients during treatment. Liver function test results should be carefully monitored during treatment and consideration be given to a temporary withdrawal of tretinoin if test results reach >5 times the upper limit of normal values. However, the majority of these abnormalities resolve without interruption of tretinoin or after completion of treatment.

PRECAUTIONS

GENERAL

Tretinoin has potentially significant toxic side effects in APL patients. Patients undergoing therapy should be closely observed for signs of respiratory compromise and/or leukocytosis (see BOXED WARNING). Supportive care appropriate for APL patients; *e.g.*, prophylaxis for bleeding, prompt therapy for infection, should be maintained during therapy with tretinoin.

LABORATORY TESTS

The patient's hematologic profile, coagulation profile, liver function test results, and triglyceride and cholesterol levels should be monitored frequently.

EFFECT OF FOOD

No data on the effect of food on the absorption of tretinoin are available. The absorption of retinoids as a class has been shown to be enhanced when taken together with food.

CARCINOGENESIS, MUTAGENESIS, AND IMPAIRMENT OF FERTILITY

No long-term carcinogenicity studies with tretinoin have been conducted. In short-term carcinogenicity studies, tretinoin at a dose of 30 mg/kg/day (about 2 times the human dose on a mg/m^2 basis) was shown to increase the rate of diethylnitrosamine (DEN)-induced mouse liver adenomas and carcinomas. Tretinoin was negative when tested in the Ames and Chinese hamster V79 cell HGPRT assays for mutagenicity. A 2-fold increase in the sister chromatid exchange (SCE) has been demonstrated in human diploid fibroblasts, but other chromosome aberration assays, including an *in vitro* assay in human peripheral lymphocytes and an *in vivo* mouse micronucleus assay, did not show a clastogenic or aneuploidogenic effect. Adverse effects on fertility and reproductive performance were not observed in studies conducted in rats at doses of up to 5 mg/kg/day (about 2/3 the human dose on a mg/m^2 basis). In a 6 week toxicology study in dogs, minimal to marked testicular degeneration, with increased numbers of immature spermatozoa, were observed at 10 mg/kg/day (about 4 times the equivalent human dose in mg/m^2).

NURSING MOTHERS

It is not known whether this drug is excreted in human milk. Because many drugs are excreted in human milk, and because of the potential for serious adverse reactions from tretinoin in nursing infants, mothers should discontinue nursing prior to taking this drug.

PEDIATRIC USE

There are limited clinical data on the pediatric use of tretinoin. Of 15 pediatric patients (age range: 1-16 years) treated with tretinoin, the incidence of complete remission was 67%. Safety and effectiveness in pediatric patients below the age of 1 year have not been established. Some pediatric patients experience severe headache and pseudotumor cerebri, requiring analgesic treatment and lumbar puncture for relief. Increased caution is recommended in the treatment of pediatric patients. Dose reduction may be considered for pediatric patients experiencing serious and/or intolerable toxicity; however, the efficacy and safety of tretinoin at doses lower than 45 mg/m^2/day have not been evaluated in the pediatric population.

GERIATRIC USE

Of the total number of subjects in clinical studies of tretinoin, 21.4% were 60 and over. No overall differences in safety and effectiveness were observed between these subjects and younger subjects, and other reported clinical experience has not identified differences in responses between the elderly and younger patients, but greater sensitivity of some older individuals cannot be ruled out.

DRUG INTERACTIONS

Limited clinical data on potential drug interactions are available. As tretinoin is metabolized by the hepatic P450 system, there is a potential for alteration of pharmacokinetics parameters in patients administered concomitant medications that are also inducers or inhibitors of this system. Medications that generally induce hepatic P450 enzymes include rifampicin, glucocorticoids, phenobarbital, and pentobarbital. Medications that generally inhibit hepatic P450 enzymes include ketoconazole, cimetidine, erythromycin, verapamil, diltiazem, and cyclosporin. To date there are no data to suggest that co-use with these medications increases or decreases either efficacy or toxicity of tretinoin.

ADVERSE REACTIONS

Virtually all patients experience some drug-related toxicity, especially headache, fever, weakness, and fatigue. These adverse effects are seldom permanent or irreversible nor do they usually require interruption of therapy. Some of the adverse events are common in patients with APL, including hemorrhage, infections, gastrointestinal hemorrhage, disseminated intravascular coagulation, pneumonia, septicemia, and cerebral hemorrhage.

The following describes the adverse events, regardless of drug relationship, that were observed in patients treated with tretinoin:

Typical retinoid toxicity: The most frequently reported adverse events were similar to those described in patients taking high doses of vitamin A and included headache (86%), fever (83%), skin/mucous membrane dryness (77%), bone pain (77%), nausea/vomiting (57%), rash (54%), mucositis (26%), pruritus (20%), increased sweating (20%), visual disturbances (17%), ocular disorders (17%), alopecia (14%), skin changes (14%), changed visual acuity (6%), bone inflammation (3%), visual field defects (3%).

RA-APL syndrome: APL patients treated with tretinoin have experienced a syndrome characterized by fever, dyspnea, weight gain, radiographic pulmonary infiltrates, and pleural or pericardial effusions. This syndrome has occasionally been accompanied by impaired myocardial contractility and episodic hypotension and has been observed with or without concomitant leukocytosis. Some patients have expired due to progressive hypoxemia and multiorgan failure. The syndrome generally occurs during the first month of treatment, with some cases reported following the first dose of tretinoin. The management of the syndrome has not been defined rigorously, but high-dose steroids given at the first signs of the syndrome appear to reduce morbidity and mortality. Treatment with dexamethasone, 10 mg intravenously administered every 12 hours for 3 days or until resolution of symptoms, should be initiated without delay at the first suspicion of symptoms (1 or more of the following: fever, dyspnea, weight gain, abnormal chest auscultatory findings, or radiographic abnormalities). Sixty percent (60%) or more of patients treated with tretinoin may require high-dose steroids because of these symptoms. The majority of patients do not require termination of tretinoin therapy during treatment of the syndrome.

Body as a whole: General disorders related to tretinoin administration and/or associated with APL included malaise (66%), shivering (63%), hemorrhage (60%), infections (58%), peripheral edema (52%), pain (37%), chest discomfort (32%), edema (29%), disseminated intravascular coagulation (26%), weight increase (23%), injection site reactions (17%), anorexia (17%), weight decrease (17%), myalgia (14%), flank pain (9%), cellulitis (8%), face edema (6%), fluid imbalance (6%), pallor (6%), lymph disorders (6%), acidosis (3%), hypothermia (3%), ascites (3%).

Respiratory system disorders: Respiratory system disorders were commonly reported in APL patients administered tretinoin. The majority of these events are symptoms of the RA-APL syndrome (see BOXED WARNING). Respiratory system adverse events included upper respiratory tract disorders (63%), dyspnea (60%), respiratory insufficiency (26%), pleural effusion (20%), pneumonia (14%), rales (14%), expiratory wheezing (14%), lower respiratory tract disorders (9%), pulmonary infiltration (6%), bronchial asthma (3%), pulmonary edema (3%), larynx edema (3%), unspecified pulmonary disease (3%).

Ear disorders: Ear disorders were consistently reported, with earache or feeling of fullness in the ears reported by 23% of the patients. Hearing loss and other unspecified auricular disorders were observed in 6% of patients, with infrequent (<1%) reports of irreversible hearing loss.

Gastrointestinal disorders: GI disorders included GI hemorrhage (34%), abdominal pain (31%), other gastrointestinal disorders (26%), diarrhea (23%), constipation (17%), dyspepsia (14%), abdominal distention (11%), hepatosplenomegaly (9%), hepatitis (3%), ulcer (3%), unspecified liver disorder (3%).

Cardiovascular and heart rate and rhythm disorders: Arrhythmias (23%), flushing (23%), hypotension (14%), hypertension (11%), phlebitis (11%), cardiac failure (6%) and for 3% of patients: cardiac arrest, myocardial infarction, enlarged heart, heart murmur, ischemia, stroke, myocarditis, pericarditis, pulmonary hypertension, secondary cardiomyopathy.

Central and peripheral nervous system disorders and psychiatric: Dizziness (20%), paresthesias (17%), anxiety (17%), insomnia (14%), depression (14%), confusion (11%), cerebral hemorrhage (9%), intracranial hypertension (9%), agitation (9%), hallucination (6%) and for 3% of patients: abnormal gait, agnosia, aphasia, asterixis, cerebellar edema, cerebellar disorders, convulsions, coma, CNS depression, dysarthria, encephalopathy, facial paralysis, hemiplegia, hyporeflexia, hypotaxia, no light reflex, neurologic reaction, spinal cord disorder, tremor, leg weakness, unconsciousness, dementia, forgetfulness, somnolence, slow speech.

Urinary system disorders: Renal insufficiency (11%), dysuria (9%), acute renal failure (3%), micturition frequency (3%), renal tubular necrosis (3%), enlarged prostate (3%).

Miscellaneous adverse events: Isolated cases of erythema nodosum, basophilia and hyperhistaminemia, Sweet's syndrome, organomegaly, hypercalcemia, pancreatitis, and myositis have been reported.

DOSAGE AND ADMINISTRATION

The recommended dose is 45 mg/m^2/day administered as 2 evenly divided doses until complete remission is documented. Therapy should be discontinued 30 days after achievement of complete remission or after 90 days of treatment, whichever occurs first.

If after initiation of treatment of tretinoin the presence of the t(15;17) translocation is not confirmed by cytogenetics and/or by polymerase chain reaction studies and the patient has not responded to tretinoin, alternative therapy appropriate for acute myelogenous leukemia should be considered.

Tretinoin is for the induction of remission only. Optimal consolidation or maintenance regimens have not been determined. All patients should, therefore, receive a standard consolidation and/or maintenance chemotherapy regimen for APL after induction therapy with tretinoin, unless otherwise contraindicated.

HOW SUPPLIED

Vesanoid is supplied as 10 mg capsules, 2-tone (lengthwise), orange-yellow and reddish-brown and imprinted "VESANOID 10 ROCHE".

Storage: Store at 15-30°C (59-86°F). Protect from light.

TOPICAL

DESCRIPTION

Note: The trade names were used throughout this monograph for clarity.

RETIN-A

FOR TOPICAL USE ONLY. NOT FOR OPHTHALMIC, ORAL, OR INTRAVAGINAL USE.

Chemically, tretinoin is all-*trans*-retinoic acid, also known as (all-*E*)-3,7-dimethyl-9-(2,6,6-trimethyl-1-cyclohexen-1-yl)-2,4,6,8-nonatetraenoic acid. It is a member of the retinoid family of compounds, and a metabolite of naturally occurring vitamin A. Tretinoin has a molecular weight of 300.44.

Retin-A Micro Microsphere, 0.1% and 0.04%

Retin-A Micro microsphere, 0.1% and 0.04%, is a formulation containing 0.1 or 0.04%, by weight, tretinoin for topical treatment of acne vulgaris. This formulation uses patented methyl methacrylate/glycol dimethacrylate crosspolymer porous microspheres (Microsponge System) to enable inclusion of the active ingredient, tretinoin, in an aqueous gel. Other components of this formulation are purified water, carbomer 974P (0.04% formulation), carbomer 934P (0.1% formulation), glycerin, disodium EDTA, propylene glycol, sorbic acid, PPG-20 methyl glucose ether distearate, cyclomethicone and dimethicone copolyol, benzyl alcohol, trolamine, and butylated hydroxytoluene.

Retin-A Cream, Gel and Liquid

Retin-A gel, cream and liquid, containing tretinoin are used for the topical treatment of acne vulgaris. Retin-A gel contains tretinoin (retinoic acid, vitamin A acid) in either of two strengths, 0.025% or 0.01% by weight, in a gel vehicle of butylated hydroxytoluene, hydroxypropyl cellulose and alcohol (denatured with *tert*-butyl alcohol and brucine sulfate) 90% w/w. Retin-A cream contains tretinoin in either of three strengths, 0.1, 0.05, or 0.025% by weight, in a hydrophilic cream vehicle of stearic acid, isopropyl myristate, polyoxyl 40 stearate, stearyl alcohol, xanthan gum, sorbic acid, butylated hydroxytoluene, and purified water. Retin-A liquid contains tretinoin 0.05% by weight, polyethylene glycol 400, butylated hydroxytoluene and alcohol (denatured with *tert*-butyl alcohol and brucine sulfate) 55%.

RENOVA

FOR TOPICAL USE ON THE FACE. NOT FOR OPHTHALMIC, ORAL, OR INTRAVAGINAL USE.

Renova contains the active ingredient tretinoin in a cream base. Tretinoin is a yellow- to light-orange crystalline powder having a characteristic floral odor. Tretinoin is soluble in dimethylsulfoxide, slightly soluble in polyethylene glycol 400, octanol, and 100% ethanol. It is practically insoluble in water and mineral oil, and it is insoluble in glycerin. The chemical name for tretinoin is (all-*E*)-3,7-dimethyl-9-(2,6,6-trimethyl-1-cyclohexen-1-yl)-2,4,6,8-nonatetraenoic acid. Tretinoin is also referred to as all-*trans*-retinoic acid and has a molecular weight of 300.44.

Renova 0.02%

Tretinoin is available as Renova at a concentration of 0.02% w/w in an oil-in-water emulsion formulation consisting of benzyl alcohol, butylated hydroxytoluene, caprylic/capric triglyceride, cetyl alcohol, edetate disodium, fragrance, methylparaben, propylparaben, purified water, stearic acid, stearyl alcohol, steareth 2, steareth 20, and xanthan gum.

Renova 0.05%

Tretinoin is available as Renova at a concentration of 0.05% w/w in a water-in-oil emulsion formulation consisting of butylated hydroxytoluene, citric acid monohydrate, dimethicone 50 cs, edetate disodium, fragrance, hydroxyoctacosanyl hydroxystearate, light mineral oil, methoxy PEG-22/dodecyl glycol copolymer, methylparaben, PEG-45/dodecyl glycol copolymer, purified water, quaternium-15, stearoxytrimethylsilane and stearyl alcohol, and sorbitol solution.

CLINICAL PHARMACOLOGY

RETIN-A

Tretinoin is a retinoid metabolite of vitamin A that binds to intracellular receptors in the cytosol and nucleus, but cutaneous levels of tretinoin in excess of physiologic concentrations occur following application of a tretinoin-containing topical drug product.

Although tretinoin activates three members of the retinoid acid (RAR) nuclear receptors (RARα, RARβ, and RARγ) which may act to modify gene expression, subsequent protein synthesis, and epithelial cell growth and differentiation, it has not been established whether the clinical effects of tretinoin are mediated through activation of retinoic acid receptors, other mechanisms, or both.

Mode of Action

Although the exact mode of action of tretinoin is unknown, current evidence suggests that the effectiveness of tretinoin in acne is due primarily to its ability to modify abnormal follicular keratinization. Comedones form in follicles with an excess of keratinized epithelial cells. Tretinoin promotes detachment of cornified cells and the enhanced shedding of corneocytes from the follicle. By increasing the mitotic activity of follicular epithelia, tretinoin also increases the turnover rate of thin, loosely-adherent corneocytes. Through these actions, the comedo contents are extruded and the formation of the microcomedo, the precursor lesion of acne vulgaris, is reduced.

Additionally, tretinoin acts by modulating the proliferation and differentiation of epidermal cells. These effects are mediated by tretinoin's interaction with a family of nuclear retinoic acid receptors. Activation of these nuclear receptors causes changes in gene expression. The exact mechanisms whereby tretinoin-induced changes in gene expression regulate skin function are not understood.

Pharmacokinetics

Tretinoin is a metabolite of vitamin A metabolism in man. Percutaneous absorption, as determined by the cumulative excretion of radiolabeled drug into urine and feces, was assessed in 44 healthy men and women. Estimates of *in vivo* bioavailability, mean (SD)%, following both single and multiple daily applications, for a period of 28 days with the 0.1% gel, were 0.82 (0.11)% and 1.41 (0.54)%, respectively. The plasma concentrations of tretinoin and its metabolites, 13-*cis*-retinoic acid, all-trans-4-oxo-retinoic acid, and 13-*cis*-4-oxo-retinoic acid, generally ranged from 1-3 ng/ml and were essentially unaltered after either single or multiple daily applications of Retin-A Micro microsphere, 0.1%, relative to baseline levels. Clinical pharmacokinetic studies have not been performed with Retin-A Micro microsphere, 0.04%.

RENOVA

Tretinoin is an endogenous retinoid metabolite of vitamin A that binds to intracellular receptors in the cytosol and nucleus, but cutaneous levels of tretinoin in excess of physiologic concentrations occur following application of a tretinoin-containing topical drug product. Although tretinoin activates three members of the retinoic acid (RAR) nuclear receptors (RARα, RARβ, and RARγ) which may act to modify gene expression, subsequent protein synthesis, and epithelial cell growth and differentiation, it has not been established whether the clinical effects of tretinoin are mediated through activation of retinoic acid receptors, other mechanisms such as irritation, or both.

The effect of tretinoin on skin with chronic photodamage has not been evaluated in animal studies. When hairless albino mice were treated topically with tretinoin shortly after a period of UVB irradiation, new collagen formation was demonstrated only in photodamaged skin. However, in human skin treated topically, adequate data have not been provided to demonstrate any increase in desmosine, hydroxyproline, or elastin mRNA. Application of 0.1% tretinoin cream to photodamaged human forearm skin was associated with an increase in antibody staining for procollagen I propeptide. No correlation was made between procollagen I propeptide staining with collagen I levels or with observed clinical effects. Thus, the relationships between the increased collagen in rodents, increased procollagen I propeptide in humans, and the clinical effects of tretinoin have not yet been clearly defined.

Tretinoin was shown to enhance UV-stimulated melanogenesis in pigmented mice. Generalized amyloid deposition in the basal layer of tretinoin-treated skin was noted in a 2 year mouse study. In a different study, hyalinization at tretinoin-treated skin sites was noted at doses beginning at 0.25 mg/kg in CD-1 mice.

The transdermal absorption of tretinoin from various topical formulations ranged from 1-31% of applied dose, depending on whether it was applied to healthy skin or dermatitic skin. No percutaneous absorption study was conducted with Renova 0.02% in human volunteers. When percutaneous absorption of the oil-in-water emulsion formulation at 0.05% concentration was assessed in healthy male subjects with radiolabeled cream after a single application (n=7), as well as after repeated daily applications (n=7) for 28 days, the absorption of tretinoin was less than 2% and the extent of bioavailability was less after repeated application. No significant difference in endogenous concentrations of tretinoin was observed between single and repeated daily applications.

INDICATIONS AND USAGE

RETIN-A

Retin-A and Retin-A Micro microsphere, 0.1% and 0.04%, is indicated for topical application in the treatment of acne vulgaris. The safety and efficacy of the use of this product in the treatment of other disorders have not been established.

RENOVA

(To understand fully the indication for this product, please read the entire INDICATIONS AND USAGE section of the labeling.)

Renova 0.02%

Renova 0.02% is indicated as an adjunctive agent (see second bullet point below) for use in the mitigation (palliation) of fine facial wrinkles in patients who use comprehensive skin care and sunlight avoidance programs. **RENOVA DOES NOT ELIMINATE WRINKLES, REPAIR SUN-DAMAGED SKIN, REVERSE PHOTOAGING, or RESTORE MORE YOUTHFUL or YOUNGER SKIN.** In double-blinded, vehicle-controlled clinical studies, many patients in the vehicle group achieved desired palliative effects on fine wrinkling of facial skin with the use of comprehensive skin care and sunlight avoidance programs including sunscreens, protective clothing, and non-prescription emollient creams.

- Renova 0.02% has NOT DEMONSTRATED A MITIGATING EFFECT on significant signs of chronic sunlight exposure such as coarse or deep wrinkling, tactile roughness, mottled hyperpigmentation, lentigines, telangiectasia, skin laxity, keratinocytic atypia, melanocytic atypia, or dermal elastosis.
- Renova 0.02% should be used under medical supervision as an adjunct to a comprehensive skin care and sunlight avoidance program that includes the use of effective sunscreens (minimum SPF of 15) and protective clothing.
- Patients with visible actinic keratoses and patients with a history of skin cancer were excluded from clinical trials of Renova 0.02%. Thus the effectiveness and safety of Renova 0.02% in these populations are not known at this time.
- Neither the safety nor the effectiveness of Renova for the prevention or treatment of actinic keratoses or skin neoplasms has been established.
- Neither the safety nor the efficacy of using Renova 0.02% daily for greater than 52 weeks has been established, and daily use beyond 52 weeks has not been systematically and histologically investigated in adequate and well-controlled trials. (See WARNINGS.)

Renova 0.05%

Renova 0.05% is indicated as an adjunctive agent (see second bullet point below) for use in the mitigation (palliation) of fine wrinkles, mottled hyperpigmentation, and tactile roughness of facial skin in patients who use comprehensive skin care and sunlight avoidance programs (see bullet point 3 for populations in which effectiveness has not been established). **RENOVA DOES NOT ELIMINATE WRINKLES, REPAIR SUN DAMAGED SKIN, REVERSE PHOTOAGING, or RESTORE MORE YOUTHFUL or YOUNGER SKIN.** In double-blinded, vehicle-controlled clinical studies, many patients in the vehicle group achieved desired palliative effects on fine wrinkling, mottled hyperpigmentation, and tactile roughness of facial skin with the use of comprehensive skin care and sunlight avoidance programs including sunscreens, protective clothing, and non-prescription emollient creams.

- Renova 0.05% has NOT DEMONSTRATED A MITIGATING EFFECT on significant signs of chronic sun exposure such as coarse or deep wrinkling, skin yellowing, lentigines, telangiectasia, skin laxity, keratinocytic atypia, melanocytic atypia, or dermal elastosis.
- Renova 0.05% should be used under medical supervision as an adjunct to a comprehensive skin care and sunlight avoidance program that includes the use of effective sunscreens (minimum SPF of 15) and protective clothing when desired results on fine wrinkles, mottled hyperpigmentation, and roughness of facial skin have not been achieved with a comprehensive skin care and sunlight avoidance program alone.
- The effectiveness of Renova 0.05% in the mitigation of fine wrinkles, mottled hyperpigmentation, and tactile roughness of facial skin has not been established in people greater than 50 years of age OR in people with moderately to heavily pigmented skin. In addition, patients with visible actinic keratoses and patients with a history of skin cancer were excluded from clinical trials of Renova 0.05%. Thus the effectiveness and safety of Renova 0.05% in these populations are not known at this time.
- Neither the safety nor the effectiveness of Renova 0.05% for the prevention or treatment of actinic keratoses or skin neoplasms has been established.
- Neither the safety nor the efficacy of using Renova 0.05% daily for greater than 48 weeks has been established, and daily use beyond 48 weeks has not been systematically and histologically investigated in adequate and well-controlled trials. (See WARNINGS.)

CONTRAINDICATIONS

RETIN-A

This drug is contraindicated in individuals with a history of sensitivity reactions to any of its components. It should be discontinued if hypersensitivity to any of its ingredients is noted.

RENOVA

This drug is contraindicated in individuals with a history of sensitivity reactions to any of its components. It should be discontinued if hypersensitivity to any of its ingredients is noted.

WARNINGS

RENOVA

- Renova 0.02% is a dermal irritant, and the results of continued irritation of the skin for greater than 52 weeks in chronic use with Renova are not known. There is evidence of atypical changes in melanocytes and keratinocytes and of increased dermal elastosis in some patients treated with Renova 0.05% for longer than 48 weeks. The significance of these findings and their relevance for Renova 0.02% are unknown.
- Safety and effectiveness of Renova 0.05% in individuals with moderately or heavily pigmented skin have not been established.
- Renova should not be administered if the patient is also taking drugs known to be photosensitizers (*e.g.,* thiazides, tetracyclines, fluoroquinolones, phenothiazines, sulfonamides) because of the possibility of augmented phototoxicity.

Exposure to sunlight (including sunlamps) should be avoided or minimized during use of Renova because of heightened sunburn susceptibility. Patients should be warned to use sunscreens (minimum SPF of 15) and protective clothing when using Renova. Patients with sunburn should be advised not to use Renova until fully recovered. Patients who may have considerable sun exposure, *e.g.,* due to their occupation, and those patients with inherent sensitivity to sunlight should exercise caution when using Renova and follow the precautions outlined in the Patient Package Insert.

Renova should be kept out of the eyes, mouth, angles of the nose, and mucous membranes. Topical use may cause severe local erythema, pruritus, burning, stinging, and peeling at the site of application. If the degree of local irritation warrants, patients should be directed to use less medication, decrease the frequency of application, discontinue use temporarily, or discontinue use altogether and consider additional appropriate therapy.

Tretinoin has been reported to cause severe irritation on eczematous skin and should be used only with caution in patients with this condition.

Application of larger amounts of medication than recommended has not been shown to lead to more rapid or better results, and marked redness, peeling, or discomfort may occur.

PRECAUTIONS

RETIN-A

General

The skin of certain individuals may become excessively dry, red, swollen, or blistered. If the degree of irritation warrants, patients should be directed to temporarily reduce the amount or frequency of application of the medication, discontinue use temporarily, or discontinue use all together. Efficacy at reduced frequencies of application has not been established. If a reaction suggesting sensitivity occurs, use of the medication should be discontinued. Excessive skin dryness may also be experienced; if so, use of an appropriate emollient during the day may be helpful.

Unprotected exposure to sunlight, including sunlamps, should be minimized during the use of Retin-A and Retin-A Micro microsphere, 0.1% and 0.04%, and patients with sunburn should be advised not to use the product until fully recovered because of heightened susceptibility to sunlight as a result of the use of tretinoin. Patients who may be required to have considerable sun exposure due to occupation and those with inherent sensitivity to the sun should exercise particular caution. Use of sunscreen products (SPF 15) and protective clothing over treated areas are recommended when exposure cannot be avoided.

Weather extremes, such as wind or cold, also may be irritating to patients under treatment with tretinoin.

Retin-A and Retin-A Micro microsphere, 0.1% and 0.04%, should be kept away from the eyes, the mouth, paranasal creases of the nose, and mucous membranes.

Tretinoin has been reported to cause severe irritation on eczematous skin and should be used with utmost caution in patients with this condition.

GELS ARE FLAMMABLE. *Note:* Keep away from heat and flame. Keep tube tightly closed.

Information for the Patient

See Patient Information leaflet.

Carcinogenesis, Mutagenesis, and Impairment of Fertility

In a 91 week dermal study in which CD-1 mice were administered 0.017% and 0.035% formulations of tretinoin, cutaneous squamous cell carcinomas and papillomas in the treatment area were observed in some female mice. These concentrations are near the tretinoin concentration of these clinical formulations (0.04% and 0.1%). A dose-related incidence of liver tumors in male mice was observed at those same doses. The maximum systemic doses associated with the administered 0.017% and 0.035% formulations are 0.5 and 1.0 mg/kg/day, respectively. These doses are 2 and 4 times the maximum human systemic dose applied topically, when normalized for total body surface area. The biological significance of these findings is not clear because they occurred at doses that exceeded the dermal maximally tolerated dose (MTD) of tretinoin and because they were within the background natural occurrence rate for these tumors in this strain of mice. There was no evidence of carcinogenic potential when 0.025 mg/kg/day of tretinoin was administered topically to mice (0.1 times the maximum human systemic dose, normalized for total body surface area). For purposes of comparisons of the animal exposure to systemic human exposure, the maximum human systemic dose applied topically is defined as 1 g of Retin-A Micro microsphere, 0.1% applied daily to a 50 kg person (0.02 mg tretinoin/kg body weight).

Dermal carcinogenicity testing has not been performed with Retin-A Micro microsphere, 0.04% or 0.1%.

Studies in hairless albino mice suggest that concurrent exposure to tretinoin may enhance the tumorigenic potential of carcinogenic doses of UVB and UVA light from a solar simulator. This effect has been confirmed in a later study in pigmented mice, and dark pigmentation did not overcome the enhancement of photocarcinogenesis by 0.05% tretinoin. Although the significance of these studies to humans is not clear, patients should minimize exposure to sunlight or artificial ultraviolet irradiation sources.

The mutagenic potential of tretinoin was evaluated in the Ames assay and in the *in vivo* mouse micronucleus assay, both of which were negative.

The components of the microspheres have shown potential for genetic toxicity and teratogenesis. EGDMA, a component of the excipient acrylates copolymer, was positive for induction of structural chromosomal aberrations in the *in vitro* chromosomal aberration assay in mammalian cells in the absence of metabolic activation, and negative for genetic toxicity in the Ames assay, the HGPRT forward mutation assay, and the mouse micronucleus assay.

In dermal Segment I fertility studies of another tretinoin formulation in rats, slight (not statistically significant) decreases in sperm count and motility were seen at 0.5 mg/kg/day (4 times the maximum human systemic dose applied topically, and normalized for total body surface area), and slight (not statistically significant) increases in the number and percent of nonviable embryos in females treated with 0.25 mg/kg/day (2 times the maximum human systemic dose applied topically and normalized for total body surface area) and above were observed. In oral Segment I and Segment III studies in rats with tretinoin, decreased survival of neonates and growth retardation were observed at doses in excess of 2 mg/kg/day (17 times the human topical dose normalized for total body surface area).

Dermal fertility and perinatal development studies with Retin-A Micro microsphere, 0.1% or 0.04%, have not been performed in any species.

Pregnancy, Teratogenic Effects, Pregnancy Category C

In a study of pregnant rats treated with topical application of Retin-A Micro microsphere, 0.1%, at doses of 0.5 to 1 mg/kg/day on gestation days 6-15 (4-8 times the maximum human systemic dose of tretinoin normalized for total body surface area after topical administration of Retin-A Micro microsphere, 0.1%) some alterations were seen in vertebrae and ribs of offspring. In another study, pregnant New Zealand white rabbits were treated with Retin-A Micro microsphere, 0.1%, at doses of 0.2, 0.5, and 1.0 mg/kg/day, administered topically for 24 hours a day while wearing Elizabethan collars to prevent ingestion of the drug. There appeared to be increased incidences of certain alterations, including domed head and hydrocephaly, typical of retinoid-induced fetal malformations in this species, at 0.5 and 1.0 mg/kg/day. Similar malformations were not observed at 0.2 mg/kg/day, 3 times the maximum human systemic dose of tretinoin after topical administration of Retin-A Micro microsphere, 0.1%, normalized for total body surface area. In a repeat study of the highest topical dose (1.0 mg/kg/day) in pregnant rabbits, these effects were not seen, but a few alterations that may be associated with tretinoin exposure were seen. Other pregnant rabbits exposed topically for 6 hours to 0.5 or 0.1 mg/kg/day tretinoin while restrained in stocks to prevent ingestion, did not show any teratogenic effects at doses up to 17 times (1.0 mg/kg/day) the maximum human systemic dose after topical administration of Retin-A Micro microsphere, 0.1%, adjusted for total body surface area, but fetal resorptions were increased at 0.5 mg/kg. In addition, topical tretinoin in non Retin-A Micro microsphere formulations was not teratogenic in rats and rabbits when given in doses of 42 and 27 times the maximum human systemic dose after topical administration of Retin-A Micro microsphere, 0.1%, normalized for total body surface area, respectively, (assuming a 50 kg adult applied a daily dose of 1.0 g of 0.1% gel topically.) At these topical doses, however, delayed ossification of several bones occurred in rabbits. In rats, a dose-dependent increase of supernumerary ribs was observed.

Oral tretinoin has been shown to be teratogenic in rats, mice, rabbits, hamsters, and subhuman primates. Tretinoin was teratogenic in Wistar rats when given orally or topically in doses greater than 1 mg/kg/day (8 times the maximum human systemic dose normalized for total body surface area). However, variations in teratogenic doses among various strains of rats have been reported. In the cynomolgus monkey, which metabolically is more similar to humans than other species in its handling of tretinoin, fetal malformations were reported for doses of 10 mg/kg/day or greater, but none were observed at 5 mg/kg/day (83 times the maximum human systemic dose normalized for total body surface area), although increased skeletal variations were observed at all doses. Dose-related increases in embryolethality and abortion also were reported. Similar results have also been reported in pigtail macaques.

Topical tretinoin in animal teratogenicity tests has generated equivocal results. There is evidence for teratogenicity (shortened or kinked tail) of topical tretinoin in Wistar rats at doses greater than 1 mg/kg/day (8 times the maximum human systemic dose normalized for total body surface area). Anomalies (humerus: short 13%, bent 6%, os parietal incompletely ossified 14%) have also been reported when 10 mg/kg/day was topically applied. Supernumerary ribs have been a consistent finding in rats when dams were treated topically or orally with retinoids.

There are no adequate and well-controlled studies in pregnant women. Retin-A Micro should be used during pregnancy only if the potential benefit justifies the potential risk to the fetus.

With widespread use of any drug, a small number of birth defect reports associated temporally with the administration of the drug would be expected by chance alone. Thirty (30) human cases of temporally associated congenital malformations have been reported during 2 decades of clinical use of Retin-A. Although no definite pattern of teratogenicity and no causal association has been established from these cases, 5 of the reports describe the rare birth defect category holoprosencephaly (defects associated with incomplete midline development of the forebrain). The significance of these spontaneous reports in terms of risk to the fetus is not known.

Nonteratogenic Effects

Topical tretinoin has been shown to be fetotoxic in rabbits when administered 0.5 mg/kg/day (8 times the maximum human systemic dose applied topically and normalized for total body surface area), resulting in fetal resorptions and variations in ossification. Oral tretinoin has been shown to be fetotoxic, resulting in skeletal variations and increased intrauterine death in rats when administered 2.5 mg/kg/day (21 times the maximum human systemic dose applied topically and normalized for total body surface area).

There are, however, no adequate and well-controlled studies in pregnant women.

Nursing Mothers

It is not known whether this drug is excreted in human milk. Because many drugs are excreted in human milk, caution should be exercised when Retin-A and Retin-A Micro microsphere, 0.1% or 0.04%, is administered to a nursing woman.

Pediatric Use

Safety and effectiveness in children below the age of 12 have not been established.

Geriatric Use

Safety and effectiveness in a geriatric population have not been established. Clinical studies of Retin-A Micro did not include sufficient numbers of subjects aged 65 and over to determine whether they respond differently from younger subjects.

RENOVA

General

Renova should be used only as an adjunct to a comprehensive skin care and sunlight avoidance program. (See INDICATIONS AND USAGE, Renova.)

If a drug sensitivity, chemical irritation, or a systemic adverse reaction develops, use of Renova should be discontinued.

Weather extremes, such as wind or cold, may be more irritating to patients using tretinoin-containing products.

Information for the Patient

Renova is to be used as described below unless otherwise directed by your physician:

- It is for use on the face.
- Avoid contact with the eyes, ears, nostrils, angles of the nose, and mouth. Renova may cause severe redness, itching, burning, stinging, and peeling if used on these areas.
- In the evening, gently wash your face with a mild soap. Pat skin dry and wait 20-30 minutes before applying Renova. Apply only a small pearl-sized (about ¼ inch or 5 millimeter diameter) amount of Renova to your face at one time. This should be enough to cover the entire affected area lightly.
- Do not wash your face for at least 1 hour after applying Renova.
- For best results, you are advised not to apply another skin care product or cosmetic for at least 1 hour after applying Renova.
- In the morning, apply a moisturizing sunscreen, SPF 15 or greater.
- Renova is a serious medication. Do not use Renova if you are pregnant or attempting to become pregnant. If you become pregnant while using Renova, please contact your physician immediately.
- Avoid sunlight and other medicines that may increase your sensitivity to sunlight.
- Renova does not remove wrinkles or repair sun-damaged skin.

Please refer to the Patient Package Insert for additional patient information.

Carcinogenesis, Mutagenesis, and Impairment of Fertility

In a 91 week dermal study in which CD-1 mice were administered 0.017% and 0.035% formulations of tretinoin, cutaneous squamous cell carcinomas and papillomas in the treatment area were observed in some female mice. These concentrations are near the tretinoin concentration of this clinical formulation (0.02%). A dose-related incidence of liver tumors in male mice was observed at those same doses. The maximum systemic doses associated with the 0.017% and 0.035% formulations are 0.5 and 1.0 mg/kg/day. These doses are 10 and 20 times the maximum human systemic dose, when adjusted for total body surface area. The biological significance of these findings is not clear because they occurred at doses that exceeded the dermal maximally tolerated dose (MTD) of tretinoin and because they were within the background natural occurrence rate for these tumors in this strain of mice. There was no evidence of carcinogenic potential when 0.025 mg/kg/day of tretinoin was administered topically to mice (0.5 times the maximum human systemic dose, adjusted for total body surface area). For purposes of comparisons of the animal exposure to systemic human exposure, the maximum human systemic dose is defined as 1 g of 0.02% Renova applied daily to a 50 kg person (0.004 mg tretinoin/kg body weight).

Studies in hairless albino mice suggest that concurrent exposure to tretinoin may enhance the tumorigenic potential of carcinogenic doses of UVB and UVA light from a solar simulator. This effect has been confirmed in a later study in pigmented mice, and dark pigmentation did not overcome the enhancement of photocarcinogenesis by 0.05% tretinoin. Although the significance of these studies to humans is not clear, patients should minimize exposure to sunlight or artificial ultraviolet irradiation sources.

The mutagenic potential of tretinoin was evaluated in the Ames assay and in the *in vivo* mouse micronucleus assay, both of which were negative.

In dermal Segment I fertility studies in rats, slight (not statistically significant) decreases in sperm count and motility were seen at 0.5 mg/kg/day (20 times the maximum human systemic dose adjusted for total body surface area), and slight (not statistically significant) increases in the number and percent of nonviable embryos in females treated with 0.25 mg/kg/day (10 times the maximum human systemic dose adjusted for total body surface area) and above were observed. A dermal Segment III study with Renova has not been performed in any species. In oral Segment I and Segment III studies in rats with tretinoin, decreased survival of neonates and growth retardation were observed at doses in excess of 2 mg/kg/day (83 times the human topical dose adjusted for total body surface area).

T

Pregnancy Category C

Teratogenic Effects

ORAL tretinoin has been shown to be teratogenic in rats, mice, rabbits, hamsters, and subhuman primates. It was teratogenic and fetotoxic in Wistar rats when given orally or topically in doses greater than 1 mg/kg/day (42 times the maximum human systemic dose normalized for total body surface area). However, variations in teratogenic doses among various strains of rats have been reported. In the cynomolgus monkey, which, metabolically, is closer to humans for tretinoin than the other species examined, fetal malformations were reported at doses of 10 mg/kg/day or greater, but none were observed at 5 mg/kg/day (417 times the maximum human systemic dose adjusted for total body surface area), although increased skeletal variations were observed at all doses. A dose-related increase in embryolethality and abortion was reported. Similar results have also been reported in pigtail macaques.

TOPICAL tretinoin in animal teratogenicity tests has generated equivocal results. There is evidence for teratogenicity (shortened or kinked tail) of topical tretinoin in Wistar rats at doses greater than 1 mg/kg/day (42 times the maximum human systemic dose adjusted for total body surface area). Anomalies (humerus: short 13%, bent 6%, os parietal incompletely ossified 14%) have also been reported when 10 mg/kg/day was dermally applied.

There are other reports in New Zealand White rabbits administered doses of greater than 0.2 mg/kg/day (17 times the maximum human systemic dose adjusted for total body surface area) of an increased incidence of domed head and hydrocephaly, typical of retinoid-induced fetal malformations in this species.

In contrast, several well-controlled animal studies have shown that dermally applied tretinoin may be fetotoxic, but not overtly teratogenic, in rats and rabbits at doses of 1.0 and 0.5 mg/kg/day, respectively (42 times the maximum human systemic dose adjusted for total body surface area in both species).

With widespread use of any drug, a small number of birth defect reports associated temporally with the administration of the drug would be expected by chance alone. Thirty (30) human cases of temporally-associated congenital malformations have been reported during 2 decades of clinical use of another formulation of topical tretinoin (Retin-A). Although no definite pattern of teratogenicity and no causal association has been established from these cases, 5 of the reports describe the rare birth defect category holoprosencephaly (defects associated with incomplete midline development of the forebrain). The significance of these spontaneous reports in terms of risk to the fetus is not known.

Nonteratogenic Effects

Dermal tretinoin has been shown to be fetotoxic in rabbits when administered 0.5 mg/kg/day (42 times the maximum human systemic dose normalized for total body surface area). Oral tretinoin has been shown to be fetotoxic, resulting in skeletal variations and increased intrauterine death, in rats when administered 2.5 mg/kg/day (104 times the maximum human systemic dose adjusted for total body surface area).

There are, however, no adequate and well-controlled studies in pregnant women. Renova should not be used during pregnancy.

Nursing Mothers

It is not known whether this drug is excreted in human milk. Since many drugs are excreted in human milk, mitigation of fine wrinkles, mottled hyperpigmentation, and tactile roughness on the face with Renova may be postponed in nursing mothers until after completion of the nursing period.

Pediatric Use

Safety and effectiveness in patients less than 18 years of age have not been established.

Geriatric Use

In clinical studies with Renova 0.02%, patients aged 65-71 did not demonstrate a significant difference for improvement in fine wrinkling when compared to patients under the age of 65. Patients aged 65 and over may demonstrate slightly more irritation, although the differences were not statistically significant in the clinical studies for Renova 0.02%. Safety and effectiveness of Renova 0.02% in individuals older than 71 years of age have not been established.

Clinical studies of Renova 0.05% did not include sufficient number of subjects aged 65 and over to determine whether they respond differently from younger subjects. Other reported clinical experience has not identified differences in responses between elderly and younger patients.

DRUG INTERACTIONS

RETIN-A

Concomitant topical medication, medicated or abrasive soaps and cleansers, products that have a strong drying effect, products with high concentrations of alcohol, astringents, or spices should be used with caution because of possible interaction with tretinoin. Avoid contact with the peel of limes. Particular caution should be exercised with the concomitant use of topical over-the-counter acne preparations containing benzoyl peroxide, sulfur, resorcinol, or salicylic acid with Retin-A and Retin-A Micro microsphere, 0.1% and 0.04%. It also is advisable to allow the effects of such preparations to subside before use of Retin-A and Retin-A Micro microsphere, 0.1% and 0.04%, is begun.

RENOVA

Concomitant topical medications, medicated or abrasive soaps, shampoos, cleansers, cosmetics with a strong drying effect, products with high concentrations of alcohol, astringents, spices or lime, permanent wave solutions, electrolysis, hair depilatories or waxes, and products that may irritate the skin should be used with caution in patients being treated with Renova because they may increase irritation with Renova.

Renova should not be administered if the patient is also taking drugs known to be photosensitizers (*e.g.*, thiazides, tetracyclines, fluoroquinolones, phenothiazines, sulfonamides) because of the possibility of augmented phototoxicity.

ADVERSE REACTIONS

RETIN-A

Irritation Potential

Acne Clinical Trial Results

In separate clinical trials for each concentration, acne patients treated with Retin-A Micro microsphere 0.1% or 0.04%, analysis over the 12 week period showed that cutaneous irritation scores for erythema, peeling, dryness, burning/stinging, or itching peaked during the initial 2 weeks of therapy, decreasing thereafter.

Approximately half of the patients treated with Retin-A Micro 0.04% had cutaneous irritation at week 2. Of those patients who did experience cutaneous side effects, most had signs or symptoms that were mild in severity (Severity was ranked on a 4-point ordinal scale: 0=none, 1=mild, 2=moderate, and 3=severe). Less than 10% of patients experienced moderate cutaneous irritation and there was no severe irritation at week 2.

In studies on Retin-A Micro microsphere 0.04%, throughout the treatment period the majority of patients experienced some degree of irritation (mild, moderate, or severe) with 1% (2/225) of patients having scores indicative of a severe irritation rating; and 1.3% (3/225) of patients treated with Retin-A Micro microsphere, 0.04%, discontinued treatment due to irritation, which included dryness in 1 patient and peeling and urticaria in another.

In studies on Retin-A Micro microsphere 0.1%, no more than 3% of patients had cutaneous irritation scores indicative of a severe irritation rating; although, 6% (14/224) of patients treated with Retin-A Micro microsphere 0.1% discontinued treatment due to irritation. Of these 14 patients, 4 had severe irritation after 3-5 days of treatment, with blistering in 1 patient.

Results in Studies of Subjects Without Acne

In a half-face comparison trial conducted for up to 14 days in women with sensitive skin, but without acne, Retin-A Micro microsphere, 0.1% was statistically less irritating than tretinoin cream, 0.1%. In addition, a cumulative 21 day irritation evaluation in subjects with normal skin showed that Retin-A Micro microsphere, 0.1%, had a lower irritation profile than tretinoin cream, 0.1%. The clinical significance of these irritation studies for patients with acne is not established. Comparable effectiveness of Retin-A Micro microsphere, 0.1% and tretinoin cream, 0.1%, has not been established. The lower irritancy of Retin-A Micro microsphere, 0.1% in subjects without acne may be attributable to the properties of its vehicle. The contribution to decreased irritancy by the Microsponge System has not been established. No irritation studies have been performed to compare Retin-A Micro microsphere, 0.04%, with either Retin-A Micro microsphere, 0.1%, or tretinoin cream, 0.1%.

The skin of certain sensitive individuals may become excessively red, edematous, blistered, or crusted. If these effects occur, the medication should either be discontinued until the integrity of the skin is restored, or the medication should be adjusted to a level the patient can tolerate. However, efficacy has not been established for lower dosing frequencies (see DOSAGE AND ADMINISTRATION).

True contact allergy to topical tretinoin is rarely encountered. Temporary hyper- or hypopigmentation has been reported with repeated application of tretinoin. Some individuals have been reported to have heightened susceptibility to sunlight while under treatment with tretinoin.

RENOVA

See WARNINGS, Renova and PRECAUTIONS, Renova.

In double-blind, vehicle-controlled studies involving 339 patients who applied Renova 0.02% to their faces, adverse reactions associated with the use of Renova were limited primarily to the skin. Almost all patients reported 1 or more local reactions such as peeling, dry skin, burning, stinging, erythema, and pruritus. In 24% of all study patients, skin irritation was reported that was either severe (about 7%), led to temporary discontinuation of Renova 0.02% (about 20%), or led to use of a mild topical corticosteroid. About 5% of patients using Renova 0.02%, compared to less than 1% of the control patients, had sufficiently severe local irritation to warrant short-term use of mild topical corticosteroids to alleviate local irritation. About 4% of patients had to discontinue use of Renova because of adverse reactions.

In double-blind, vehicle-controlled studies involving 179 patients who applied Renova 0.05% to their face, adverse reactions associated with the use of Renova 0.05% were limited primarily to the skin. During these trials, 4% of patients had to discontinue use of Renova 0.05% because of adverse reactions. These discontinuations were due to skin irritation or related cutaneous adverse reactions.

Local reactions such as peeling, dry skin, burning, stinging, erythema, and pruritus were reported by almost all subjects during therapy with Renova 0.05%. These signs and symptoms were usually of mild to moderate severity and generally occurred early in therapy. In most patients the dryness, peeling, and redness recurred after an initial (24 week) decline.

Approximately 2% of spontaneous post-marketing adverse event reporting for Renova 0.05% were for skin hypo- or hyperpigmentation. Other spontaneously reported adverse events for Renova 0.05% predominantly appear to be local reactions similar to those seen in clinical trials.

DOSAGE AND ADMINISTRATION

RETIN-A

Retin-A Micro Microsphere, 0.1% and 0.04%

Retin-A Micro microsphere, 0.1% and 0.04%, should be applied once a day, in the evening, to the skin where acne lesions appear, using enough to cover the entire affected area lightly. Application of excessive amounts of gel may result in "caking" of the gel, and will not provide incremental efficacy.

A transitory feeling of warmth or slight stinging may be noted on application. In cases where it has been necessary to temporarily discontinue therapy or to reduce the frequency of application, therapy may be resumed or the frequency of application increased as the patient becomes able to tolerate the treatment. Frequency of application should be closely monitored by careful observation of the clinical therapeutic response and skin tolerance. Efficacy has not been established for less than once daily dosing frequencies.

During the early weeks of therapy, an apparent exacerbation of inflammatory lesions may occur. If tolerated, this should not be considered a reason to discontinue therapy.

Therapeutic results may be noticed after 2 weeks, but more than 7 weeks of therapy are required before consistent beneficial effects are observed.

Patients treated with Retin-A Micro microsphere, 0.1% and 0.04%, may use cosmetics, but the areas to be treated should be cleansed thoroughly before the medication is applied.

Retin-A Cream, Gel or Liquid

Retin-A gel, cream or liquid should be applied once a day, before retiring, to the skin where acne lesions appear, using enough to cover the entire affected area lightly. *Liquid:* The liquid may be applied using a fingertip, gauze pad, or cotton swab. If gauze or cotton is employed, care should be taken not to oversaturate it to the extent that the liquid would run into areas where treatment is not intended. *Gel:* Excessive application results in "pilling" of the gel, which minimizes the likelihood of over application by the patient.

Alterations of vehicle, drug concentration, or dose frequency should be closely monitored by careful observation of the clinical therapeutic response and skin tolerance.

Therapeutic results should be noticed after 2-3 weeks but more than 6 weeks of therapy may be required before definite beneficial effects are seen.

Once the acne lesions have responded satisfactorily, it may be possible to maintain the improvement with less frequent applications, or other dosage forms.

RENOVA

- Do NOT use Renova if the patient is pregnant or is attempting to become pregnant or is at high risk of pregnancy.
- Do NOT use Renova if the patient is sunburned or if the patient has eczema or other chronic skin conditions of the face.
- Do NOT use Renova if the patient is inherently sensitive to sunlight.
- Do NOT use Renova if the patient is also taking drug(s) known to be photosensitizers (*e.g.*, thiazides, tetracyclines, fluoroquinolones, phenothiazines, sulfonamides) because of the possibility of augmented phototoxicity.

Patients require detailed instruction to obtain maximal benefits and to understand all the precautions necessary to use this product with greatest safety. The physician should review the Patient Package Insert.

Renova should be applied to the face once a day in the evening, using only enough to cover the entire affected area lightly. Patients should gently wash their faces with a mild soap, pat the skin dry, and wait 20-30 minutes before applying Renova. The patient should apply a small pearl-sized (about ¼ inch or 5 mm diameter) amount of cream to cover the entire affected area lightly. Caution should be taken when applying the cream to avoid the eyes, ears, nostrils, and mouth.

Application of Renova may cause a transitory feeling of warmth or slight stinging.

Mitigation (palliation) of fine facial wrinkling may occur gradually over the course of therapy. Up to 6 months of therapy may be required before the effects are seen.

Mitigation (palliation) of facial fine wrinkling, mottled hyperpigmentation and tactile roughness may occur gradually over the course of therapy. Up to 6 months of therapy may be required before the effects are seen. Most of the improvement noted with Renova 0.05% is seen during the first 24 weeks of therapy. Thereafter, therapy primarily maintains the improvement realized during the first 24 weeks.

With discontinuation of Renova therapy, some patients may lose the mitigating effects of Renova on fine facial wrinkles. **The safety and effectiveness of using Renova 0.02% daily for greater than 52 weeks have not been established.**

With discontinuation of Renova 0.05% therapy, a majority of patients will lose most mitigating effects of Renova 0.05% on fine wrinkles, mottled hyperpigmentation, and tactile roughness of facial skin; **however, the safety and effectiveness of using Renova 0.05% daily for greater than 48 weeks have not been established.**

Application of larger amounts of medication than recommended may not lead to more rapid or better results, and marked redness, peeling, or discomfort may occur.

Patients treated with Renova may use cosmetics but the areas to be treated should be cleansed before the medication is applied. (See PRECAUTIONS, Renova.)

ANIMAL PHARMACOLOGY

RETIN-A

In male mice treated topically with Retin-A Micro microsphere 0.1%, at 0.5, 2.0, or 5.0 mg/kg/day tretinoin (2, 8, or 21 times the maximum human systemic dose after topical administration of Retin-A Micro microsphere, 0.1%, normalized for total body surface area) for 90 days, a reduction in testicular weight, but with no pathological changes were observed at the 2 highest doses. Similarly, in female mice there was a reduction in ovarian weights, but without any underlying pathological changes, at 5.0 mg/kg/day (21 times the maximum human dose). In this study there was a dose-related increase in the plasma concentration of tretinoin 4 hours after the first dose. A separate toxicokinetic study in mice indicates that systemic exposure is greater after topical application to unrestrained animals than to restrained animals, suggesting that the systemic toxicity observed is probably related to ingestion. Male and female dogs treated with Retin-A Micro microsphere, 0.1%, at 0.2, 0.5, or 1.0 mg/kg/day tretinoin (5, 12, or 25 times the maximum human systemic dose after topical administration of Retin-A Micro microsphere, 0.1%, normalized for total body surface area, respectively) for 90 days showed no evidence of reduced testicular or ovarian weights or pathological changes.

HOW SUPPLIED

RETIN-A

Retin-A Micro

Retin-A Micro microsphere, 0.1% and 0.04%, is supplied in 20 and 45 g tubes.

Storage Conditions: Store at 15-25°C (59-77°F).

Retin-A Cream, Gel or Liquid

Retin-A cream, gel or liquid is supplied in the following strengths:

Retin-A Cream

0.025%: 20 and 45 g

0.05%: 20 and 45 g

0.1%: 20 and 45 g

Retin-A Gel

0.01%: 15 and 45 g

0.025%: 15 and 45 g

Retin-A Liquid

0.05%: 28 ml

Storage Conditions: *Retin-A liquid, 0.05%, and Retin-A gel, 0.025% and 0.01%:* Store below 86°F. *Retin-A cream, 0.1%, 0.05%, and 0.025%:* Store below 80°F.

RENOVA

Renova 0.02%

Renova 0.02% is available in tubes containing 40 g.

Storage: Store at 25°C (77°F), excursions permitted to 15-30°C (59-86°F).

Renova 0.05%

Renova 0.05% is available in 20, 40, and 60 g tubes.

Storage: Store at 25°C (77°F), excursions permitted to 15-30°C (59-86°F). DO NOT FREEZE.

PRODUCT LISTING - RATED THERAPEUTICALLY EQUIVALENT

Size	Price	Product	NDC
Cream - Topical - 0.025%			
20 gm	$29.16	GENERIC, Geneva Pharmaceuticals	00781-7045-22
20 gm	$31.85	RETIN-A, Southwood Pharmaceuticals Inc	58016-3072-01
20 gm	$32.08	GENERIC, Upsher-Smith Laboratories Inc	00245-9045-22
20 gm	$33.90	RETIN-A, Allscripts Pharmaceutical Company	54569-2276-00
20 gm	$34.59	RETIN-A, Pharma Pac	52959-0571-01
20 gm	$38.28	RETIN-A, Physicians Total Care	54868-1760-01
20 gm	$38.91	GENERIC, Spear Pharmaceuticals	66530-0243-20
20 gm	$39.34	GENERIC, Alpharma Uspd Makers Of Barre and Nmc	00472-0117-20
20 gm	$42.49	AVITA, Bertek Pharmaceuticals Inc	62794-0141-02
20 gm	$43.76	RETIN-A, Janssen Pharmaceuticals	00062-0165-01
20 gm	$57.94	RETIN-A, Southwood Pharmaceuticals Inc	58016-3299-01
45 gm	$55.20	GENERIC, Geneva Pharmaceuticals	00781-7045-19
45 gm	$60.74	GENERIC, Upsher-Smith Laboratories Inc	00245-9045-19
45 gm	$64.18	RETIN-A, Allscripts Pharmaceutical Company	54569-2277-00
45 gm	$71.95	RETIN-A, Physicians Total Care	54868-1760-02
45 gm	$73.65	GENERIC, Spear Pharmaceuticals	66530-0243-45
45 gm	$74.48	GENERIC, Alpharma Uspd Makers Of Barre and Nmc	00472-0117-45
45 gm	$80.08	AVITA, Bertek Pharmaceuticals Inc	62794-0141-03
45 gm	$82.85	RETIN-A, Janssen Pharmaceuticals	00062-0165-02
Cream - Topical - 0.05%			
20 gm	$32.71	GENERIC, Geneva Pharmaceuticals	00781-7047-22
20 gm	$34.73	RETIN-A, Southwood Pharmaceuticals Inc	58016-3073-01
20 gm	$35.98	GENERIC, Upsher-Smith Laboratories Inc	00245-9047-22
20 gm	$38.03	RETIN-A, Allscripts Pharmaceutical	54569-1152-00
20 gm	$43.64	GENERIC, Spear Pharmaceuticals	66530-0242-20
20 gm	$43.91	RETIN-A, Physicians Total Care	54868-0267-01
20 gm	$49.09	RETIN-A, Janssen Pharmaceuticals	00062-0175-12
45 gm	$59.56	RETIN-A, Southwood Pharmaceuticals Inc	58016-3142-01
45 gm	$61.32	GENERIC, Geneva Pharmaceuticals	00781-7047-19
45 gm	$67.46	GENERIC, Upsher-Smith Laboratories Inc	00245-9047-19
45 gm	$71.29	RETIN-A, Allscripts Pharmaceutical Company	54569-1145-00
45 gm	$77.27	RETIN-A, Physicians Total Care	54868-0267-02
45 gm	$81.81	GENERIC, Spear Pharmaceuticals	66530-0242-45
45 gm	$92.03	RETIN-A, Janssen Pharmaceuticals	00062-0175-13
Cream - Topical - 0.1%			
20 gm	$38.17	GENERIC, Geneva Pharmaceuticals	00781-7049-22
20 gm	$41.99	GENERIC, Upsher-Smith Laboratories Inc	00245-9049-22
20 gm	$44.38	RETIN-A, Allscripts Pharmaceutical Company	54569-1147-00
20 gm	$50.93	GENERIC, Spear Pharmaceuticals	66530-0241-20
20 gm	$51.13	RETIN-A, Physicians Total Care	54868-0268-01
20 gm	$57.29	RETIN-A, Janssen Pharmaceuticals	00062-0275-23
45 gm	$68.44	RETIN-A, Southwood Pharmaceuticals Inc	58016-9039-01
45 gm	$71.47	GENERIC, Geneva Pharmaceuticals	00781-7049-19
45 gm	$78.64	GENERIC, Upsher-Smith Laboratories Inc	00245-9049-19
45 gm	$87.35	RETIN-A, Physicians Total Care	54868-0268-02
45 gm	$95.37	GENERIC, Spear Pharmaceuticals	66530-0241-45
45 gm	$107.28	RETIN-A, Janssen Pharmaceuticals	00062-0275-01
Gel - Topical - 0.01%			
15 gm	$30.89	GENERIC, Spear Pharmaceuticals	66530-0245-15
45 gm	$72.92	GENERIC, Spear Pharmaceuticals	66530-0245-45
Gel - Topical - 0.025%			
15 gm	$25.35	TRETINOIN TOPICAL, Geneva Pharmaceuticals	00781-7061-27
15 gm	$25.69	RETIN-A, Southwood Pharmaceuticals Inc	58016-3076-01
15 gm	$26.71	RETIN-A, Pharma Pac	52959-0570-00
15 gm	$29.83	RETIN-A, Allscripts Pharmaceutical Company	54569-1090-00
15 gm	$31.16	GENERIC, Spear Pharmaceuticals	66530-0244-15
15 gm	$35.05	RETIN-A, Janssen Pharmaceuticals	00062-0475-42
45 gm	$59.33	TRETINOIN TOPICAL, Geneva Pharmaceuticals	00781-7061-19
45 gm	$61.16	RETIN-A, Southwood Pharmaceuticals Inc	58016-3173-01
45 gm	$63.60	RETIN-A, Pharma Pac	52959-0570-01
45 gm	$73.52	GENERIC, Spear Pharmaceuticals	66530-0244-45
45 gm	$74.05	RETIN-A, Physicians Total Care	54868-0270-01
45 gm	$82.70	RETIN-A, Janssen Pharmaceuticals	00062-0475-45
Liquid - Topical - 0.05%			
28 ml	$49.46	GENERIC, Geneva Pharmaceuticals	00781-6031-82
28 ml	$50.47	GENERIC, Teva Pharmaceuticals Usa	00093-9655-31

T

30 ml	$45.40	GENERIC, Morton Grove Pharmaceuticals Inc	60432-0151-30

PRODUCT LISTING - RATED NOT THERAPEUTICALLY EQUIVALENT

Cream - Topical - 0.1%

20 gm	$41.19	RETIN-A, Southwood Pharmaceuticals Inc	58016-3074-01

Gel - Topical - 0.025%

20 gm	$33.38	AVITA, Allscripts Pharmaceutical Company	54569-4811-00
20 gm	$38.61	AVITA, Bertek Pharmaceuticals Inc	62794-0140-02
45 gm	$83.70	AVITA, Bertek Pharmaceuticals Inc	62794-0140-03

PRODUCT LISTING - EQUIVALENTS NOT AVAILABLE

Capsule - Oral - 10 mg

100's	$1787.43	VESANOID, Roche Laboratories	00004-0250-01

Cream - Topical - 0.02%

40 gm	$73.50	RENOVA, Janssen Pharmaceuticals	00062-0187-02

Cream - Topical - 0.025%

20 gm	$28.71	GENERIC, Allscripts Pharmaceutical Company	54569-4808-00
20 gm	$35.50	GENERIC, Southwood Pharmaceuticals Inc	58016-5569-01
45 gm	$54.57	GENERIC, Allscripts Pharmaceutical Company	54569-4809-00

Cream - Topical - 0.05%

20 gm	$30.20	RENOVA, Allscripts Pharmaceutical Company	54569-4632-00
20 gm	$39.50	GENERIC, Southwood Pharmaceuticals Inc	58016-5568-01
40 gm	$60.16	RENOVA, Allscripts Pharmaceutical Company	54569-4261-00
40 gm	$68.63	RENOVA, Physicians Total Care	54868-3710-00
40 gm	$73.50	RENOVA, Janssen Pharmaceuticals	00062-0185-05
60 gm	$76.75	RENOVA, Allscripts Pharmaceutical Company	54569-4262-00
60 gm	$82.59	RENOVA, Physicians Total Care	54868-3710-01
60 gm	$93.76	RENOVA, Janssen Pharmaceuticals	00062-0185-03

Gel - Topical - 0.01%

15 gm	$25.73	RETIN-A, Southwood Pharmaceuticals Inc	58016-3075-01
15 gm	$29.42	RETIN-A, Prescript Pharmaceuticals	00247-0255-15
15 gm	$29.58	RETIN-A, Allscripts Pharmaceutical Company	54569-1079-00
15 gm	$31.47	RETIN-A, Physicians Total Care	54868-0269-02
15 gm	$34.75	RETIN-A, Janssen Pharmaceuticals	00062-0575-44
45 gm	$82.03	RETIN-A, Janssen Pharmaceuticals	00062-0575-46

Gel - Topical - 0.04%

20 gm	$43.45	RETIN A MICRO GEL, Janssen Pharmaceuticals	00062-0204-02
45 gm	$82.16	RETIN A MICRO GEL, Janssen Pharmaceuticals	00062-0204-03

Gel - Topical - 0.1%

20 gm	$36.76	RETIN A MICRO GEL, Allscripts Pharmaceutical Company	54569-4506-00
20 gm	$43.45	RETIN A MICRO GEL, Janssen Pharmaceuticals	00062-0190-02
45 gm	$82.16	RETIN A MICRO GEL, Janssen Pharmaceuticals	00062-0190-03

Liquid - Topical - 0.05%

28 ml	$41.58	RETIN-A, Southwood Pharmaceuticals Inc	58016-3277-01
28 ml	$73.51	RETIN-A, Janssen Pharmaceuticals	00062-0075-07

Triamcinolone *(002370)*

For related information, see the comparative table section in Appendix A.

Categories: Anemia, acquired hemolytic; Anemia, congenital hypoplastic; Ankylosing spondylitis; Arthritis, gouty; Arthritis, post-traumatic; Arthritis, psoriatic; Arthritis, rheumatoid; Asthma; Berylliosis; Bursitis; Carditis, rheumatic; Chorioretinitis; Choroiditis; Colitis, ulcerative; Conjunctivitis, allergic; Crohn's disease; Dermatitis herpetiformis; Dermatitis, atopic; Dermatitis, contact; Dermatitis, exfoliative; Dermatitis, seborrheic; Epicondylitis; Erythema multiforme; Erythroblastopenia; Herpes zoster ophthalmicus; Hypercalcemia, secondary to cancer; Hyperplasia, adrenal; Hypersensitivity reactions; Iridocyclitis; Iritis; Keratitis; Leukemia; Loffler's syndrome; Lupus erythematosus, systemic; Lymphoma; Meningitis, tuberculous; Multiple sclerosis; Mycosis fungoides; Nephrotic syndrome; Neuritis, optic; Ophthalmia, sympathetic; Pemphigus; Pneumonitis, aspiration; Psoriasis; Rhinitis, allergic; Sarcoidosis; Serum sickness; Stevens-Johnson syndrome; Synovitis, secondary to osteoarthritis; Tenosynovitis; Thrombocytopenia, secondary; Thrombocytopenic purpura, idiopathic; Thyroiditis, nonsuppurative; Trichinosis; Tuberculosis, disseminated; Tuberculosis, fulminating; Ulcer, allergic corneal marginal; Uveitis; FDA Approved 1964 Sep; Pregnancy Category C

Drug Classes: Corticosteroids

Brand Names: Aristo-Pak; **Aristocort**; Kenacort

Foreign Brand Availability: Adcortyl (England; Ireland); Azmacor (South-Africa); Azmacort (Peru); Delphicort (Austria; Germany; Hungary); Korticoid (Germany); Ledercort (Belgium; Denmark; Ecuador; England; Finland; India; Italy; Japan; Korea; Netherlands; Norway; Spain; Sweden; Switzerland); Sterocort (Israel); Triamsicort (Mexico); Volon (Austria; Germany)

Cost of Therapy: $88.70 (Asthma; Aristocort; 4 mg; 2 tablet/day; 30 day supply)
$3.30 (Asthma; Generic Tablets; 4 mg; 2 tablet/day; 30 day supply)

T

DESCRIPTION

Triamcinolone is a synthetic adrenocorticosteroid. Aristocort tablets contain triamcinolone, 9-Fluoro-11β, 16α, 17,21-tetrahydroxypregna-1,4-diene-3,20-dione.

Aristocort Tablets contain 1, 2, 4, or 8 mg triamcinolone.

Inactive Ingredients: Corn starch dibasic calcium phosphate, docusate sodium, lactose, magnesium stearate, microcrystalline cellulose, red 30, sodium benzoate, sodium starch glycolate and yellow 10.

Storage: Store at controlled room temperature 15-30°C (59-86°F).

CLINICAL PHARMACOLOGY

Triamcinolone is primarily glucocorticoid in action and has potent anti-inflammatory, hormonal and metabolic effects common to cortisone-like drugs. It is essentially devoid of mineralocorticoid activity when administered in therapeutic doses, causing little or no sodium retention, with potassium excretion minimal or absent. The body's immune responses to diverse stimuli are also modified by its action.

INDICATIONS AND USAGE

Endocrine Disorders:

Primary or secondary adrenocortical insufficiency (hydrocortisone or cortisone is the first choice; synthetic analogs may be used in conjunction with mineralocorticoids where applicable; in infancy mineralocorticoid supplementation is of particular importance).

Congenital adrenal hyperplasia

Nonsuppurative thyroiditis

Hypercalcemia associated with cancer

Rheumatic Disorders:

As adjunctive therapy for short-term administration (to tide the patient over an acute episode or exacerbation) in:

Psoriatic arthritis

Rheumatoid arthritis, including juvenile rheumatoid arthritis (selected cases may require low-dose maintenance therapy)

Ankylosing spondylitis

Acute and subacute bursitis

Acute nonspecific tenosynovitis

Acute gouty arthritis

Posttraumatic osteoarthritis

Synovitis of osteoarthritis

Epicondylitis

Collagen Diseases:

During an exacerbation or as maintenance therapy in selected cases of:

Systemic lupus erythematosus

Acute rheumatic carditis

Dermatologic Diseases:

Pemphigus

Bullous dermatitis herpetiformis

Severe erythema multiforme (Stevens-Johnson syndrome)

Exfoliative dermatitis

Mycosis fungoides

Severe psoriasis

Severe seborrheic dermatitis

Allergic States:

Control of severe or incapacitating allergic conditions intractable to adequate trials of conventional treatment:

Seasonal or perennial allergic rhinitis

Bronchial asthma

Contact dermatitis

Atopic dermatitis

Serum sickness

Drug hypersensitivity reactions

Ophthalmic Diseases:

Severe acute and chronic allergic and inflammatory processes involving the eye and its adnexa such as:

Allergic conjunctivitis

Keratitis

Allergic corneal marginal ulcers

Herpes zoster ophthalmicus

Iritis and iridocyclitis

Chorioretinitis

Anterior segment inflammation

Diffuse posterior uveitis and choroiditis

Optic neuritis

Sympathetic ophthalmia

Respiratory Disease:

Symptomatic sarcoidosis

Loeffler's syndrome not manageable by other means

Berylliosis

Fulminating or disseminated pulmonary tuberculosis when used concurrently with appropriate antituberculous chemotherapy

Aspiration pneumonitis

Hematologic Disorders:

Idiopathic thrombocytopenic purpura in adults

Secondary thrombocytopenia in adults

Acquired (autoimmune) hemolytic anemia

Erythroblastopenia (RBC anemia)

Congenital (erythroid) hypoplastic anemia

Neoplastic Diseases:

For palliative management of:

Leukemias and lymphomas in adults

Acute leukemia of childhood

Edematous States:

To induce a diuresis or remission of proteinuria in the nephrotic syndrome, without uremia, of the idiopathic type or that due to lupus erythematosus

Gastrointestinal Diseases:

To tide the patient over a critical period of the disease in:

Ulcerative colitis

Regional enteritis

Nervous System:
Acute exacerbations of multiple sclerosis
Miscellaneous:
Tuberculous meningitis with subarachnoid block or impending block when used concurrently with appropriate antituberculous chemotherapy
Trichinosis with neurologic or myocardial involvement

CONTRAINDICATIONS

Systemic fungal infections.
Sensitivity to the drug or any of its components.

WARNINGS

In patients on corticosteroid therapy subjected to unusual stress, increased dosage of rapidly acting corticosteroids before, during, and after the stressful situation is indicated.

Corticosteroids may mask some signs of infection, and new infections may appear during their use. There may be decreased resistance and inability to localize infection when corticosteroids are used.

Prolonged use of corticosteroids may produce posterior subcapsular cataracts, glaucoma with possible damage to the optic nerves, and may enhance the establishment of secondary ocular infections due to fungi or viruses.

USE IN PREGNANCY

Since adequate human reproduction studies have not been done with corticosteroids the use of these drugs in pregnancy, nursing mothers or women of childbearing potential requires that the possible benefit of the drug be weighed against the potential hazards to the mother and embryo or fetus. Infants born of mothers who have received substantial doses of corticosteroids during pregnancy should be carefully observed for signs of hypoadrenalism.

Average and large doses of hydrocortisone or cortisone can cause elevation of blood pressure, salt and water retention, and increased excretion of potassium. These effects are less likely to occur with triamcinolone except when used in large doses. Dietary salt restriction and potassium supplementation may be necessary. All corticosteroids increase calcium excretion.

While on Corticosteroid Therapy, Patients Should NOT Be Vaccinated Against Smallpox. Other immunization procedures should not be undertaken in patients who are on corticosteroids, especially on high doses, because of possible hazards of neurological complications and lack of antibody response.

The use of triamcinolone in active tuberculosis should be restricted to those cases of fulminating or disseminated tuberculosis in which the corticosteroid is used for the management of the disease in conjunction with appropriate antituberculous regimen.

If corticosteroids are indicated in patients with latent tuberculosis or tuberculin reactivity, close observation is necessary as reactivation of the disease may occur. During prolonged corticosteroid therapy, these patients should receive chemoprophylaxis.

Children who are on immunosuppressant drugs are more susceptible to infections than healthy children. Chickenpox and measles, for example, can have a more serious or even fatal course in children on immunosuppressant corticosteroids. In such children, or in adults who have not had these diseases, particular care should be taken to avoid exposure. If exposed, therapy with varicella zoster immune globulin (VZIG) or pooled intravenous immunoglobulin (IVIG), as appropriate, may be indicated. If chickenpox develops, treatment with antiviral agents may be considered.

PRECAUTIONS

Drug-induced secondary adrenocortical insufficiency may be minimized by gradual reduction of dosage. This type of relative insufficiency may persist for months after discontinuation of therapy; therefore, in any situation of stress occurring during that period, hormone therapy should be reinstituted. Since mineralocorticoid secretion may be impaired, salt and/or a mineralocorticoid should be administered concurrently.

There is an enhanced effect of corticosteroids on patients with hypothyroidism and in those with cirrhosis.

Corticosteroids should be used cautiously in patients with ocular herpes simplex because of possible corneal perforation.

The lowest possible dose of corticosteroids should be used to control the condition under treatment, and when reduction in dosage is possible, the reduction should be gradual.

Psychic derangements may appear when corticosteroids are used, ranging from euphoria, insomnia, mood swings, personality changes and severe depression to frank psychotic manifestations. Also, existing emotional instability or psychotic tendencies may be aggravated by corticosteroids.

Aspirin should be used cautiously in conjunction with corticosteroids in hypoprothrombinemia.

Steroids should be used with caution in nonspecific ulcerative colitis if there is a probability of impending perforation, abscess or other pyogenic infection, diverticulitis, fresh intestinal anastomoses, active or latent peptic ulcer, renal insufficiency, hypertension, osteoporosis, and myasthenia gravis.

Growth and development of infants and children on prolonged corticosteroid therapy should be carefully observed.

Although controlled clinical trials have shown corticosteroids to be effective in speeding the resolution of acute exacerbations of multiple sclerosis they do not show that they affect the ultimate outcome or natural history of the disease. The studies do show that relatively high doses of corticosteroids are necessary to demonstrate a significant effect. (See DOSAGE AND ADMINISTRATION.)

Since complications of treatment with glucocorticoid are dependent on the size of the dose and the duration of treatment a risk/benefit decision must be made in each individual case as to dose and duration of treatment and as to whether daily or intermittent therapy should be used.

Information for the Patient: Patients who are on immunosuppressant doses of corticosteroids should be warned to avoid exposure to chickenpox or measles and, if exposed, to obtain medical advice.

ADVERSE REACTIONS

Fluid and Electrolyte Disturbances: Sodium retention, fluid retention, congestive heart failure in susceptible patients, potassium loss, hypokalemic alkalosis, hypertension.
Musculoskeletal: Muscle weakness, steroid myopathy, loss of muscle mass, osteoporosis, vertebral compression fractures, aseptic necrosis of femoral and humeral heads, pathologic fracture of long bones.
Gastrointestinal: Peptic ulcer with possible subsequent perforation and hemorrhage, pancreatitis, abdominal distention, ulcerative esophagitis.
Dermatologic: Impaired wound healing, thin fragile skin, petechiae and ecchymoses, facial erythema, increased sweating, may suppress reactions to skin tests.
Neurological: Convulsions, increased intracranial pressure with papilledema (pseudotumor cerebri) usually after treatment, vertigo, headache.
Endocrine: Menstrual irregularities, development of cushingoid state, suppression of growth in children, secondary adrenocortical and pituitary unresponsiveness, particularly in times of stress, as in trauma, surgery or illness, decreased carbohydrate tolerance, manifestations of latent diabetes mellitus, increased requirements for insulin or oral hypoglycemic agents in diabetics.
Ophthalmic: Posterior subcapsular cataracts, increased intraocular pressure, glaucoma, exophthalmos.
Metabolic: Negative nitrogen balance due to protein catabolism.
Hypersensitivity Reactions: Anaphylactoid reactions have been reported rarely with products of this class.

DOSAGE AND ADMINISTRATION

GENERAL PRINCIPLES

1. The initial dosage of triamcinolone may vary from 4-48 mg/day depending on the specific disease entity being treated. In situations of less severity lower doses will generally suffice while in selected patients higher initial doses may be required. The initial dosage should be maintained or adjusted until a satisfactory response is noted. If after a reasonable period of time there is a lack of satisfactory clinical response, the drug should be discontinued and the patient transferred to other appropriate therapy. **IT SHOULD BE EMPHASIZED THAT DOSAGE REQUIREMENTS ARE VARIABLE AND MUST BE INDIVIDUALIZED ON THE BASIS OF THE DISEASE UNDER TREATMENT AND THE RESPONSE ON THE PATIENT.** After a favorable response is noted, the proper maintenance dosage should be determined by decreasing the initial drug dosage in small increments at appropriate time intervals until the lowest dosage is reached which will maintain an adequate clinical response. It should be kept in mind that constant monitoring is needed in regard to drug dosage. Included in the situation which may make dosage adjustment necessary are changes in clinical status secondary to remissions or exacerbations in the disease process, the patient's individual drug responsiveness, and the effect of patient exposure to stressful situations not directly related to the disease entity under treatment; in this latter situation it may be necessary to increase the dosage of triamcinolone for a period of time consistent with the patient's condition. It after long-term therapy the drug is to be stopped, it is recommended that it be withdrawn gradually rather than abruptly.
2. Dosage should be individualized according to the severity of the disease and the response of the patient. For infants and children, the recommended dosage should be governed by the same considerations rather than by strict adherence to the ratio indicated by age or body weight.
3. Hormone therapy is an adjunct to, and not a replacement for, conventional therapy.
4. The severity, prognosis and expected duration of the disease and the reaction of the patient to medication are primary factors in determining dosage.
5. If a period of spontaneous remission occurs in a chronic condition, treatment should be discontinued.
6. Blood pressure, body weight, routine laboratory studies, including 2 hour postprandial blood glucose and serum potassium, and a chest X-ray should be obtained at regular intervals during prolonged therapy. Upper GI X-rays are desirable in patients with known or suspected peptic ulcer disease.
7. Suppression of autogenous pituitary function, a common effect of exogenous corticosteroids administration, may be reduced, modified or minimized by revision of dose schedules. The time of maximum corticoid effect is from midnight to 8 AM and minimal during the intervening hours. Use of a single daily dose at or about 8 AM will be effective in most conditions, will lower corticoid overload and will cause the least interference with the diurnal system of endogenous secretion and hypothalamopituitary-adrenal function; alternate-day dosage in some conditions in certain severe disorders requiring long-term and/or high dose maintenance levels have proven both clinically effective and less likely to produce adverse reactions.
8. ***Alternate-Day Therapy:*** After the conventional dose has been established, some patients may be maintained on alternate-day therapy. It has been shown that the activity of the adrenal cortex varies throughout the day, being greatest from about midnight to 8:00 AM. Exogenous corticoid suppresses this activity least when given at the time of maximum activity. A 48 hour interval appears to be necessary since shorter intervals are accompanied by adrenal suppression similar to that of conventional daily divided doses. Therefore, with the alternate-day dose plan, a total 48 hour requirement is given every other day at 8:00 AM. As with other regimens, the minimum effective dose level should be sought.

The maximum daily morning dose not associated with lasting adrenocorticoid suppression is 8 mg.

SPECIFIC DOSAGE RECOMMENDATIONS

Endocrine Disorders

Wide variation in dosage requirements for the endocrine disorders such as *congenital adrenal hyperplasia, non-suppurative thyroiditis,* and *hypercalcemia* associated with cancer precludes specific recommendation except for*adrenocortical insufficiency* where the dose is usually 4-12 mg daily in addition to mineralocorticoid therapy.

Rheumatic Disorders
Rheumatoid arthritis; acute gouty arthritis; ankylosing spondylitis; and *selected cases* of *psoriatic arthritis;* in *acute* and *subacute bursitis;* and in*acute nonspecific tenosynovitis.* The initial suppressive dose of triamcinolone in these conditions ranges from 8-16 mg/day, although the occasional patient may require higher doses.

Patients may show an early or a delayed effect, characterized by a reduction in the inflammatory reaction and in joint swelling, together with alleviation of pain and stiffness, resulting in an increased range of motion of the affected joints or tissues. Maintenance doses are adjusted to keep symptoms at a level tolerable to the patient. Rapid reduction of the steroid or its abrupt discontinuance may result in recurrence or even exacerbation of signs and symptoms. Short-term administration is desirable as a rule. Triamcinolone is ordinarily administered as a single morning dose, daily or on alternate days depending on the need of the patient. Occasional patients may secure more effective relief on divided daily doses, either 2-4 times daily.

Collagen Diseases
Systemic Lupus Erythematosus
The initial dose is usually 20-32 mg daily continued until the desired response is obtained, when reduced maintenance levels are sought. Patients with more severe symptoms may require higher initial doses, 48 mg or more daily, and higher maintenance doses. Although some patients with systemic lupus erythematosus appear to have spontaneous remissions or to tolerate the disorder in its milder forms for prolonged periods of time, adjustment of dosage scheduling to reduce adverse suppression of the pituitary-adrenal axis may be useful.

Acute Rheumatic Carditis
In severely ill patients with carditis, pericardial effusion and/or congestive heart failure, corticosteroid therapy is effective in the control of the acute and severe inflammatory changes and may be lifesaving. Initial dose of triamcinolone may be from 20-60 mg daily, and clinical response is usually rapid and the drug can then be reduced. Maintenance therapy should be continued for at least 6-8 weeks and is seldom required beyond a period of 3 months. Corticosteroid therapy does not preclude conventional treatment, including antibiotics and salicylization.

Dermatological Disorders
Pemphigus; bullous dermatitis herpetiformis; severe erythema multiforme (Stevens-Johnson syndrome); *exfoliative dermatitis;* and *mycosis fungoides*. The initial dose is 8-16 mg daily. In these conditions, as well as in certain allergic dermatoses, *alternate-day* administration has been found effective and apparently less likely to produce adverse side effects.

Severe Psoriasis
Triamcinolone may produce reduction or remission of the disabling skin manifestations following initial doses of 8-16 mg daily. The period of maintenance is dependent on the clinical response. Corticosteroid reduction or discontinuation of therapy should be attempted with caution since relapse may occur and may appear in more aggravated form, the so-called "rebound phenomenon."

Allergic States
Triamcinolone is administered is doses of 8-12 mg daily in acute seasonal or perennial *allergic rhinitis*. Intractable cases may require high initial and maintenance doses. In*bronchial asthma*, 8-16 mg daily are usually effective. The usual therapeutic measures for control of bronchial asthma should be carried out in addition to triamcinolone therapy. In both allergic rhinitis and bronchial asthma, therapy is directed at alleviation of acute distress and chronic long-term use of corticosteroids is neither desirable nor often essential. Some patients may be maintained on alternate-day therapy. In such conditions as *contact dermatitis* and atopic dermatitis, topical therapy may be supplemented with short courses of triamcinolone by mouth in doses of 8-16 mg daily. In severely ill patients with *serum sickness*, epinephrine may be the drug of choice for immediate therapy, often supplemented by antihistamines.

Triamcinolone is frequently useful as adjunctive treatment in such cases, with the dosage determined by the severity of the disorder, the speed with which therapeutic response is desired and the response of the patient to initial therapy.

Ophthalmological Diseases
Allergic conjunctivitis; keratitis; iridocyclitis; chorioretinitis; anterior segment inflammation; diffuse posterior uveitis and choroiditis, optic neuritis and sympathetic ophthalmia. Initial doses range from 12-40 mg daily depending on the severity of the condition, the nature and degree of involvement of ocular structure, but response is usually rapid and therapy of short-term duration.

Respiratory Diseases
Symptomatic sarcoidosis; Loeffler's syndrome' berylliosis; and in certain cases of fulminating or disseminated pulmonary tuberculosis when concurrently accompanied by appropriate antituberculous chemotherapy. Initial doses are usually in the range of 16-48 mg daily.

Hematologic Disorders
Idiopathic and secondary thrombocytopenia in adults, acquired (autoimmune) hemolytic anemia; erythroblastopenia (RBC anemia;) congenital (erythroid) hypoplastic anemia. Triamcinolone is used to produce a remission of symptoms and may, in some instances, produce an apparent regression of abnormal cellular blood elements to normal states, temporary or permanent. The recommended dose varies between 16-60 mg daily, with reduction after adequate clinical response.

Neoplastic Diseases
Acute leukemia in childhood. The usual dose of triamcinolone is 1 mg/kg of body weight daily, although as much as 2 mg/kg may be necessary. Initial response is usually seen within 6-21 days and therapy continued from 4-6 weeks.

Acute Leukemia and Lymphoma in Adults
The usual dose of triamcinolone is 16-40 mg daily, although it may be necessary to give as much as 100 mg daily in leukemia. Triamcinolone therapy in these neoplasias is only palliative and not curative. Other therapeutic and supportive measures must be used when appropriate.

Edematous States
Nephrotic Syndrome
Triamcinolone may be used to induce a diuresis or remission of proteinuria in the nephrotic syndrome, without uremia, of the idiopathic type or that due to lupus erythematosus. The average dose is 16-20 mg (up to 48 mg) daily until diuresis occurs. The diuresis may be massive and usually occurs by the 14th day, but occasionally may be delayed. After diuresis begins it is advisable to continue treatment until maximal or complete chemical and clinical remission occurs, at which time the dosage should be reduced gradually and then discontinued. In less severe cases maintenance dosages of as little as 4 mg daily may be adequate. Alternatively and when maintenance therapy may be prolonged, triamcinolone may be administered on alternate-day dose schedules.

Miscellaneous
Tuberculous Meningitis
Triamcinolone may be useful when accompanied by appropriate antituberculous therapy when there is subarachnoid block or impending block. The average dosage is 32-48 mg daily in either single or divided doses (TABLE 1).

TABLE 1

	Anti-inflammatory Relative Potency		Frequently Used Tablet Strength (mg)		Tablet X Potency Equivalent Value
Hydrocortisone	1	X	20	=	20
Prednisolone	4	X	5	=	20
Triamcinolone	5	X	4	=	20
Dexamethasone	25	X	0.75	=	18.75

PRODUCT LISTING - RATED NOT THERAPEUTICALLY EQUIVALENT

Tablet - Oral - 4 mg

16's	$9.12	GENERIC, Vangard Labs	00615-0527-26
16's	$9.72	GENERIC, Qualitest Products Inc	00603-6170-14
16's	$12.02	GENERIC, Major Pharmaceuticals Inc	00904-0884-44
30's	$43.16	ARISTOCORT, Fujisawa	57317-0600-30
30's	$46.67	ARISTOCORT, Fujisawa	00469-5124-30
100's	$5.50	GENERIC, Global Pharmaceutical Corporation	00115-4840-01
100's	$6.75	GENERIC, Moore, H.L. Drug Exchange Inc	00839-5009-06
100's	$7.90	GENERIC, Major Pharmaceuticals Inc	00904-0884-60
100's	$8.07	GENERIC, Aligen Independent Laboratories Inc	00405-5042-01
100's	$10.75	GENERIC, Cmc-Consolidated Midland Corporation	00223-2110-01
100's	$14.25	GENERIC, Interstate Drug Exchange Inc	00814-8000-14
100's	$147.84	ARISTOCORT, Fujisawa	00469-5124-71

Tablet - Oral - 8 mg

50's	$107.57	ARISTOCORT, Fujisawa	57317-0603-50

T

Triamcinolone Acetonide *(002371)*

For related information, see the comparative table section in Appendix A.

Categories: Alopecia areata; Anemia, acquired hemolytic; Ankylosing spondylitis; Arthritis, gouty; Arthritis, post-traumatic; Arthritis, rheumatoid; Asthma; Berylliosis; Bursitis; Carditis, rheumatic; Chorioretinitis; Choroiditis; Colitis, ulcerative; Crohn's disease; Dermatitis herpetiformis; Dermatitis, atopic; Dermatitis, contact; Dermatitis, exfoliative; Dermatitis, seborrheic; Dermatosis, corticosteroid responsive; Epicondylitis; Erythema multiforme; Granuloma annulare; Herpes zoster ophthalmicus; Iridocyclitis; Iritis; Keloid; Leukemia, palliation; Lichen planus; Lichen simplex chronicus; Lupus erythematosus, discoid; Lupus erythematosus, systemic; Lymphoma, palliation; Necrobiosis lipoidica diabeticorum; Nephrotic syndrome; Neuritis, optic; Ophthalmia, sympathetic; Pemphigus; Pneumonitis, aspiration; Psoriasis; Rhinitis, allergic; Sarcoidosis; Synovitis, secondary to osteoarthritis; Tenosynovitis; Thyroiditis, nonsuppurative; Ulcer, aphthous; Uveitis; Pregnancy Category C; FDA Approved 1958 Oct

Drug Classes: Corticosteroids; Corticosteroids, inhalation; Corticosteroids, topical; Dermatologics

Brand Names: Acetocot; Aricin; Aristocort Topical; Aristogel; Azmacort; Cenocort A-40; Cinalog; Cinolar; Cinonide 40; Delta-Tritex; Flutex; Kena-Plex 40; Kenac; Kenaject-40; **Kenalog**; Kenonel; Nasacort; Oracort; Oralone; Sholog K; Tac; Tramacort 40; Tri-Kort; Triacet; Triacort; Triam-A; Triamcinair; Triamcot; Triamonide 40; Trianide; Triatex; Triderm; Trilog; Trylone A; Trymex

Foreign Brand Availability: Adcortyl (England; Israel); Adcortyl in Orabase (England; Ireland); Aftab (Germany); Ahbina (Korea); Albicort (Belgium); Aristocort (Bahamas; Barbados; Belize; Bermuda; Curacao; Guyana; Jamaica; Netherland-Antilles; Surinam; Trinidad); Aristocort A (Hong-Kong; Malaysia; Thailand); Delphi Creme (Netherlands); Delphicort (Austria; Germany); Denkacort Forte (Hong-Kong); Dermacort (Hong-Kong; Malaysia); Facort (Thailand); Ftorocort (Bahamas; Barbados; Belize; Bermuda; Curacao; Guyana; Jamaica; Netherland-Antilles; Surinam; Trinidad); Gemicort (Korea); Generlog (Thailand); Invert Plaster (Korea); Kemzid (Hong-Kong); Kenacort (India); Kenacort A (Belgium; China; Colombia; Netherlands; Philippines; Switzerland); Kenacort A I.A.-I.D. (Costa-Rica; Ecuador; El-Salvador; Guatemala; Honduras; Nicaragua; Panama); Kenacort A I.M. (Bahrain; Costa-Rica; Ecuador; El-Salvador; Guatemala; Honduras; Indonesia; Iraq; Jordan; Kuwait; Lebanon; Libya; Malaysia; Nicaragua; Oman; Panama; Qatar; Republic-of-Yemen; Saudi-Arabia; Syria; United-Arab-Emirates); Kenacort A in Orabase (Switzerland); Kenacort-A (Australia; Bahrain; Egypt; Hong-Kong; Indonesia; Kenya; Malaysia; New-Zealand; Peru; Taiwan; Tanzania; Uganda); Kenacort-A IM (Hong-Kong; Taiwan; Thailand); Kenacort-A in Orabase (Netherlands); Kenacort-A Intra-articular Intra-dermal (Philippines); Kenacort-A IA ID (Hong-Kong; Indonesia; Taiwan; Thailand); Kenacort A IA ID (Bahrain; Jordan; Malaysia); Kenacort E (Peru); Kenacort IM (Colombia; Mexico); Kenacort Retard (France); Kenacort T (Finland; Norway); Kenacort T Munnsalve (Norway); Kenalog-40 (Canada); Kenalog Dental (Mexico); Kenalog in Orabase (Australia; Benin; Burkina-Faso; Canada; Ethiopia; Gambia; Ghana; Guinea; Indonesia; Ivory-Coast; Kenya; Liberia; Malawi; Malaysia; Mali; Mauritania; Mauritius; Morocco; New-Zealand; Niger; Nigeria; Senegal; Seychelles; Sierra-Leone; South-Africa; Sudan; Tanzania; Thailand; Tunia; Uganda; Zambia; Zimbabwe); Laver (Thailand); Ledercort (Bahrain; Cyprus; Egypt; England; India; Iran; Iraq; Jordan; Kuwait; Lebanon; Libya; Oman; Qatar; Republic-of-Yemen; Saudi-Arabia; South-Africa; Syria; United-Arab-Emirates); Ledercort A (Philippines); Manolone (Thailand); Metoral (Thailand); Nasocor AQ (Benin; Burkina-Faso; Ethiopia; Gambia; Ghana; Guinea; Ivory-Coast; Kenya; Liberia; Malawi; Mali; Mauritania; Mauritius; Morocco; Niger; Nigeria; Senegal; Seychelles; Sierra-Leone; Sudan; Tanzania; Tunia; Uganda; Zambia; Zimbabwe); Nasacort AQ (Canada; Colombia; Hong-Kong; Mexico; Peru); Nincort (China; Taiwan); Oramedy (Korea; Singapore); Shincort (Malaysia; Thailand); Steronase AQ (Israel); Tess (India); Triaderm (Canada); Tricort (Finland); Tricot (Korea); Trigon (Spain); Trinolone (Singapore); Unif (Thailand); Volon A (Austria); Volon A Antibiotikafrei (Austria; Germany); Volon A 10 (Germany); Volon A 40 (Germany); Volon A Spray (Austria)

Cost of Therapy: $55.40 (Asthma; Azmacort Aerosol; 100 μg/inh; 20 g; 6 inhalations/day; 40 day supply)
$43.64 (Nasacort Spray; Allergic Rhinitis; 55 μg/inh; 10 g; 4 sprays/day; 25 day supply)
$42.34 (Allergic Rhinitis; Nasacort AQ Spray; 55 μg/inh; 10 g; 4 sprays/day; 30 day supply)

HCFA JCODE(S): J3301 per 10 mg IM

DENTAL

DESCRIPTION

Kenalog in Orabase contains the corticosteroid triamcinolone acetonide in an adhesive vehicle suitable for application to oral tissues. Triamcinolone acetonide is designated chemically as 9-fluoro-11β,16α,17,21-tetrahydroxypregna-1,4-diene-3,20-dione cyclic 16,17-acetal with acetone. The structural formula of triamcinolone acetonide is $C_{24}H_{31}FO_6$ and the molecular weight is 434.50.

Each gram of Kenalog in Orabase contains 1 mg triamcinolone acetonide in a dental paste containing gelatin, pectin, and carboxymethylcellulose sodium in plastibase (plasticized hydrocarbon gel), a polyethylene and mineral oil gel base.

CLINICAL PHARMACOLOGY

Like other topical corticosteroids, triamcinolone acetonide has anti-inflammatory, antipruritic, and vasoconstrictive properties. The mechanism of the anti-inflammatory activity of the topical steroids, in general, is unclear. However, corticosteroids are thought to act by the induction of phospholipase A_2 inhibitory proteins, collectively called lipocortins. It is postulated that these proteins control the biosynthesis of potent mediators of inflammation such as prostaglandins and leukotrienes by inhibiting the release of their common precursor, arachidonic acid. Arachidonic acid is released from membrane phospholipids by phospholipase A_2.

PHARMACOKINETICS

The extent of absorption through the oral mucosa is determined by multiple factors including the vehicle, the integrity of the mucosal barrier, the duration of therapy, and the presence of inflammation and/or other disease processes. Once absorbed through the mucous membranes, the disposition of corticosteroids is similar to that of systemically administered corticosteroids. Corticosteroids are bound to the plasma proteins in varying degrees. Corticosteroids are metabolized primarily in the liver and are then excreted by the kidneys; some corticosteroids and their metabolites are also excreted into the bile.

INDICATIONS AND USAGE

Triamcinolone acetonide dental paste 0.1% is indicated for adjunctive treatment and for the temporary relief of symptoms associated with oral inflammatory lesions and ulcerative lesions resulting from trauma.

CONTRAINDICATIONS

Triamcinolone acetonide dental paste 0.1% is contraindicated in those patients with a history of hypersensitivity to any of the components of the preparations; it is also contraindicated in the presence of fungal, viral, or bacterial infections of the mouth or throat.

PRECAUTIONS

GENERAL

Triamcinolone acetonide dental paste 0.1% may cause local adverse reactions. If irritation develops, triamcinolone acetonide dental paste 0.1% should be discontinued and appropriate therapy instituted. Allergic contact sensitization with corticosteroids is usually diagnosed by observing failure to heal rather than noting a clinical exacerbation as with most topical products not containing corticosteroids. Such an observation should be corroborated with appropriate diagnostic patch testing.

If concomitant mucosal infections are present or develop, an appropriate antifungal or antibacterial agent should be used. If a favorable response does not occur promptly, use of triamcinolone acetonide dental paste 0.1% should be discontinued until the infection has been adequately controlled.

If significant regeneration or repair of oral tissues has not occurred in 7 days, additional investigation into the etiology of the oral lesion is advised.

Systemic absorption of topical corticosteroids has produced reversible hypothalamic-pituitary-adrenal (HPA) axis suppression, manifestations of Cushing's syndrome, hyperglycemia, glucosuria, and other adverse effects known to occur with parenterally-administered steroid preparations; therefore, it may be advisable to periodically evaluate patients on prolonged therapy with corticosteroid-containing dental pastes for evidence of HPA axis suppression (see PRECAUTIONS, Laboratory Tests). If HPA axis suppression is noted, an attempt should be made to withdraw the drug or to reduce the frequency of application. Recovery of HPA axis function is generally prompt and complete upon discontinuation of therapy.

INFORMATION FOR THE PATIENT

Patients using topical corticosteroids should receive the following information and instructions:

This medication is to be used as directed by the physician or dentist. It is for oral use only; it is not intended for ophthalmic or dermatological use.

Patients should be advised not to use this medication for any disorder other than for which it was prescribed.

Patients should report any signs of adverse reactions.

As with other corticosteroids, therapy should be discontinued when control is achieved. If no improvement is seen within 2 weeks, contact the physician or dentist.

LABORATORY TESTS

A urinary free cortisol test and ACTH stimulation test may be helpful in evaluating HPA axis suppression.

CARCINOGENESIS, MUTAGENESIS, AND IMPAIRMENT OF FERTILITY

Animal studies have not been performed to evaluate triamcinolone acetonide for potential to induce carcinogenesis, mutagenesis, or impairment of fertility.

PREGNANCY, TERATOGENIC EFFECTS, PREGNANCY CATEGORY C

Triamcinolone acetonide has been shown to induce teratogenic effects in several species. In mice and rabbits, triamcinolone acetonide induced an increased incidence of cleft palate at dosages of approximately 120 μg/kg/day and 24 μg/kg/day, respectively (approximately 12 times and 10 times the amount in a typical daily human dose of triamcinolone acetonide dental paste 0.1% when compared following normalization of the data on the basis of body surface area estimates, respectively). In monkeys, triamcinolone acetonide induced cranial skeletal malformations at the lowest dosage studied (500 μg/kg/day), which was approximately 200 times the amount in a typical daily human dose of triamcinolone acetonide dental paste 0.1% when compared following normalization of the data on the basis of body surface area estimates. There are no adequate and well-controlled studies in pregnant women. However, a retrospective analysis of birth defects among children born to mothers that used drugs of the same class as triamcinolone acetonide dental paste 0.1% (corticosteroids) during pregnancy found an approximately 3 times increased incidence of cleft palate. Triamcinolone acetonide dental paste 0.1% should be used during pregnancy only if the potential benefit justifies the potential risk to the fetus.

NURSING MOTHERS

It is not known whether oral application of corticosteroids could result in sufficient systemic absorption to produce detectable quantities in breast milk. Caution should be exercised when corticosteroid-containing dental pastes are prescribed for a nursing woman.

PEDIATRIC USE

The safety and efficacy of triamcinolone acetonide dental paste 0.1% in children is unknown. Pediatric patients may demonstrate greater susceptibility to topical corticosteroid-induced HPA axis suppression and Cushing's Syndrome than mature patients because of a larger skin surface area to body weight ratio. Administration of corticosteroid-containing dental pastes to children should be limited to the least amount compatible with an effective therapeutic regimen. Chronic corticosteroid therapy may interfere with the growth and development of children.

GERIATRIC USE

Clinical studies of triamcinolone acetonide dental paste 0.1% did not include sufficient numbers of subjects age 65 and older to determine whether they respond differently from younger subjects. Other reported clinical experience has not identified differences in responses between the elderly and younger patients.

ADVERSE REACTIONS

The following local adverse reactions may occur with corticosteroid-containing dental pastes: burning, itching, irritation, dryness, blistering or peeling not present prior to therapy, perioral dermatitis, allergic contact dermatitis, maceration of the oral mucosa, secondary infection, and atrophy of the oral mucosa.

Also, see PRECAUTIONS for potential effects of systemic absorption.

DOSAGE AND ADMINISTRATION

Press a small dab (about ¼ inch) to the lesion until a thin film develops. A larger quantity may be required for coverage of some lesions. For optimal results use only enough to coat the lesion with a thin film. Do not rub in. Attempting to spread this preparation may result in granular, gritty sensation and cause it to crumble. After application, however, a smooth, slippery film develops.

The preparation should be applied at bedtime to permit steroid contact with the lesion throughout the night. Depending on the severity of symptoms, it may be necessary to apply the preparation 2 or 3 times a day, preferably after meals. If significant repair or regeneration has not occurred in 7 days, further investigation is advisable.

HOW SUPPLIED

Kenalog in Orabase (triamcinolone acetonide dental paste), 0.1% tube contains 5 g of dental paste.

Storage: Keep tightly closed. Store at controlled room temperature, 15-25°C (59-77°F).

INHALATION

DESCRIPTION

Triamcinolone acetonide, the active ingredient in Azmacort inhalation aerosol, is a corticosteroid with a molecular weight of 434.5 and with the chemical designation 9-Fluoro-11β,16α,17,21-tetrahydroxypregna-1,4-diene-3,20-dione cyclic 16,17-acetal with acetone ($C_{24}H_{31}FO_6$).

Azmacort inhalation aerosol is a metered-dose aerosol unit containing a microcrystalline suspension of triamcinolone acetonide in the propellant dichlorodifluoromethane and dehydrated alcohol 1% w/w. Each canister contains 60 mg triamcinolone acetonide. The canister must be primed prior to the first use. After an initial priming of 2 actuations, each actuation delivers 200 μg triamcinolone acetonide from the valve and 100 μg from the spacer-mouthpiece under defined *in vitro* test conditions. The canister will remain primed for 3 days. If the canister is not used for more than 3 days, then it should be reprimed with 2 actuations. There are at least 240 actuations in 1 Azmacort inhalation aerosol canister. **After 240 actuations, the amount delivered per actuation may not be consistent and the unit should be discarded.**

CLINICAL PHARMACOLOGY

Triamcinolone acetonide is a more potent derivative of triamcinolone. Although triamcinolone itself is approximately 1-2 times as potent as prednisone in animal models of inflammation, triamcinolone acetonide is approximately 8 times more potent than prednisone.

The precise mechanism of the action of glucocorticoids in asthma is unknown. However, the inhaled route makes it possible to provide effective local anti-inflammatory activity with reduced systemic corticosteroid effects. Though highly effective for asthma, glucocorticoids do not affect asthma symptoms immediately. While improvement in asthma may occur as soon as 1 week after initiation of triamcinolone acetonide inhalation aerosol therapy, maximum improvement may not be achieved for 2 weeks or longer.

Based upon intravenous (IV) dosing of triamcinolone acetonide phosphate ester, the half-life of triamcinolone acetonide was reported to be 88 minutes. The volume of distribution (Vd) reported was 99.5 L (SD ± 27.5) and clearance was 45.2 L/h (SD ± 9.1) for triamcinolone acetonide. The plasma half-life of glucocorticoids does not correlate well with the biologic half-life.

The pharmacokinetics of radiolabeled triamcinolone acetonide [^{14}C] were evaluated following a single oral dose of 800 μg to healthy male volunteers. Radiolabeled triamcinolone acetonide was found to undergo relatively rapid absorption following oral administration with maximum plasma triamcinolone acetonide and [^{14}C]-derived radioactivity occurring between 1.5 and 2 hours. Plasma protein binding of triamcinolone acetonide appears to be relatively low and consistent over a wide plasma triamcinolone acetonide concentration range as a function of time. The overall mean percent fraction bound was approximately 68%.

The metabolism and excretion of triamcinolone acetonide were both rapid and extensive with no parent compound being detected in the plasma after 24 hours post-dose and a low ratio (10.6%) of parent compound AUC(0-∞) to total [^{14}C] radioactivity AUC(0-∞). Greater than 90% of the oral [^{14}C]-radioactive dose was recovered within 5 days after administration in 5 out of the 6 subjects in the study. Of the recovered [^{14}C]-radioactivity, approximately 40% and 60% were found in the urine and feces, respectively.

Three metabolites of triamcinolone acetonide have been identified. They are 6β-hydroxytriamcinolone acetonide, 21-carboxytriamcinolone acetonide and 21-carboxy-6β-hydroxytriamcinolone acetonide. All 3 metabolites are expected to be substantially less active than the parent compound due to (a) the dependence of anti-inflammatory activity on the presence of a 21-hydroxyl group, (b) the decreased activity observed upon 6-hydroxylation, and (c) the markedly increased water solubility favoring rapid elimination. There appeared to be some quantitative differences in the metabolites among species. No differences were detected in metabolic pattern as a function of route of administration.

INDICATIONS AND USAGE

Triamcinolone acetonide inhalation aerosol is indicated in the maintenance treatment of asthma as prophylactic therapy. Triamcinolone acetonide inhalation aerosol is also indicated for asthma patients who require systemic corticosteroid administration, where adding triamcinolone acetonide may reduce or eliminate the need for the systemic corticosteroids.

Triamcinolone acetonide inhalation aerosol is NOT indicated for the relief of acute bronchospasm.

CONTRAINDICATIONS

Triamcinolone acetonide inhalation aerosol is contraindicated in the primary treatment of status asthmaticus or other acute episodes of asthma where intensive measures are required.

Hypersensitivity to triamcinolone acetonide or any of the other ingredients in this preparation contraindicates its use.

WARNINGS

Particular care is needed in patients who are transferred from systemically active corticosteroids to triamcinolone acetonide inhalation aerosol because deaths due to adrenal insufficiency have occurred in asthmatic patients during and after transfer from systemic corticosteroids to aerosolized steroids in recommended doses. After withdrawal from systemic corticosteroids, a number of months is usually required for recovery of hypothalamic-pituitary-adrenal (HPA) function. For some patients who have received large doses of oral steroids for long periods of time before therapy with triamcinolone acetonide inhalation aerosol is initiated, recovery may be delayed for 1 year or longer. During this period of HPA suppression, patients may exhibit signs and symptoms of adrenal insufficiency when exposed to trauma, surgery, or infections, particularly gastroenteritis or other conditions with acute electrolyte loss. Although triamcinolone acetonide inhalation aerosol may provide control of asthmatic symptoms during these episodes, in recommended doses it supplies only normal physiological amounts of corticosteroid systemically and does NOT provide the increased systemic steroid which is necessary for coping with these emergencies. During periods of stress or a severe asthmatic attack, patients who have been recently withdrawn from systemic corticosteroids should be instructed to resume systemic steroids (in large doses) immediately and to contact their physician for further instruction. These patients should also be instructed to carry a warning card indicating that they may need supplementary systemic steroids during periods of stress or a severe asthma attack.

Localized infections with *Candida albicans* have occurred infrequently in the mouth and pharynx. These areas should be examined by the treating physician at each patient visit. The percentage of positive mouth and throat cultures for *Candida albicans* did not change during a year of continuous therapy. The incidence of clinically apparent infection is low (2.5%). These infections may disappear spontaneously or may require treatment with appropriate antifungal therapy or discontinuance of treatment with triamcinolone acetonide inhalation aerosol.

Children who are on immunosuppressant drugs are more susceptible to infections than healthy children. Chickenpox and measles, for example, can have a more serious or even fatal course in children on immunosuppressant doses of corticosteroids. In such children, or in adults who have not had these diseases, particular care should be taken to avoid exposure. If exposed, therapy with varicella zoster immune globulin (VZIG) or pooled IV immunoglobulin (IVIG), as appropriate, may be indicated. If chickenpox develops, treatment with antiviral agents may be considered.

Triamcinolone acetonide inhalation aerosol is not to be regarded as a bronchodilator and is not indicated for rapid relief of bronchospasm.

As with other inhaled asthma medications, bronchospasm may occur with an immediate increase in wheezing following dosing. If bronchospasm occurs following use of triamcinolone acetonide inhalation aerosol, it should be treated immediately with a fast-acting inhaled bronchodilator. Treatment with triamcinolone acetonide inhalation aerosol should be discontinued and alternative treatment should be instituted.

Patients should be instructed to contact their physician immediately when episodes of asthma which are not responsive to bronchodilators occur during the course of treatment with triamcinolone acetonide inhalation aerosol. During such episodes, patients may require therapy with systemic corticosteroids.

The use of triamcinolone acetonide inhalation aerosol with systemic prednisone, dosed either daily or on alternate days, could increase the likelihood of HPA suppression compared to a therapeutic dose of either one alone. Therefore, triamcinolone acetonide inhalation aerosol should be used with caution in patients already receiving prednisone treatment for any disease.

Transfer of patients from systemic steroid therapy to triamcinolone acetonide inhalation aerosol may unmask allergic conditions previously suppressed by the systemic steroid therapy, *e.g.*, rhinitis, conjunctivitis, and eczema.

PRECAUTIONS

During withdrawal from oral steroids, some patients may experience symptoms of systemically active steroid withdrawal, *e.g.*, joint and/or muscular pain, lassitude, and depression, despite maintenance or even improvement of respiratory function. (See DOSAGE AND ADMINISTRATION.) Although steroid withdrawal effects are usually transient and not severe, severe and even fatal exacerbation of asthma can occur if the previous daily oral corticosteroid requirement had significantly exceeded 10 mg/day of prednisone or equivalent.

In responsive patients, inhaled corticosteroids will often permit control of asthmatic symptoms with less suppression of HPA function than therapeutically equivalent oral doses of prednisone. Since triamcinolone acetonide is absorbed into the circulation and can be systemically active, the beneficial effects of triamcinolone acetonide inhalation aerosol in minimizing or preventing HPA dysfunction may be expected only when recommended dosages are not exceeded.

Suppression of HPA function has been reported in volunteers who received 4000 μg daily of triamcinolone acetonide by oral inhalation. In addition, suppression of HPA function has been reported in some patients who have received recommended doses for as little as 6-12 weeks. Since the response of HPA function to inhaled corticosteroids is highly individualized, the physician should consider this information when treating patients.

When used at excessive doses or at recommended doses in a small number of susceptible individuals, systemic corticosteroid effects such as hypercorticoidism and adrenal suppression may appear. If such changes occur, triamcinolone acetonide inhalation aerosol should be discontinued slowly, consistent with accepted procedures for reducing systemic steroid therapy and for management of asthma symptoms.

Triamcinolone acetonide inhalation aerosol should be used with caution, if at all, in patients with active or quiescent tuberculosis infection of the respiratory tract; untreated systemic fungal, bacterial, parasitic, or viral infections; or ocular herpes simplex.

The long-term local and systemic effects of triamcinolone acetonide inhalation aerosol in human subjects are still not fully known. While there has been no clinical evidence of adverse experiences, the effects resulting from chronic use of triamcinolone acetonide inhalation aerosol on developmental or immunologic processes in the mouth, pharynx, trachea, and lung are unknown.

Because of the possibility of systemic absorption of inhaled corticosteroids, patients treated with these drugs should be observed carefully for any evidence of systemic corticosteroid effects including suppression of growth in children. Particular care should be taken in observing patients postoperatively or during periods of stress for evidence of a decrease in adrenal function.

INFORMATION FOR THE PATIENT

Patients being treated with triamcinolone acetonide inhalation aerosol should receive the following information and instructions. This information is intended to aid them in the safe and effective use of this medication. It is not a complete disclosure of all possible adverse or intended effects.

Patients should use triamcinolone acetonide inhalation aerosol at regular intervals as directed. Results of clinical trials indicate that significant improvement in asthma may occur by 1 week, but maximum benefit may not be achieved for 2 weeks or more. The patient should not increase the prescribed dosage but should contact the physician if symptoms do not improve or if the condition worsens.

In clinical studies and post-marketing experience with triamcinolone acetonide inhalation aerosol, local infections of the oropharynx with *Candida albicans* have occurred. When such an infection develops, it should be treated with appropriate local or systemic (*i.e.*, oral antifungal) therapy while remaining on treatment with triamcinolone acetonide inhalation aerosol. However, at times therapy with triamcinolone acetonide inhalation aerosol may need to be interrupted.

Patients should be instructed to track their use of triamcinolone acetonide inhalation aerosol and to dispose of the canister after 240 actuations since reliable dose delivery cannot be assured after 240 doses.

Patients who are on immunosuppressant doses of corticosteroids should be warned to avoid exposure to chickenpox or measles and, if exposed, to obtain medical advice.

CARCINOGENESIS, MUTAGENESIS, AND IMPAIRMENT OF FERTILITY

No evidence of treatment-related carcinogenicity was demonstrated after 2 years of once daily gavage of triamcinolone acetonide at doses of 0.05, 0.2, and 1.0 μg/kg (approximately 0.02, 0.07, and 0.4% of the maximum recommended human daily inhalation dose on a μg/m^2 basis) in the rat and 0.1, 0.6, and 3.0 μg/kg (approximately 0.02, 0.1, and 0.6% of the maximum recommended human daily inhalation dose on a μg/m^2 basis) in a mouse.

Mutagenesis studies with triamcinolone acetonide have not been carried out.

No evidence of impaired fertility was manifested when oral doses of up to 15.0 μg/kg (8% of the maximum recommended human daily inhalation dose on a μg/m^2 basis) were administered to female and male rats. However, triamcinolone acetonide at oral doses of 8 μg/kg (approximately 4% of the maximum recommended human daily inhalation dose on a μg/m^2 basis) caused dystocia and prolonged delivery and at oral doses of 5.0 μg/kg (approximately 2.5% of the maximum recommended human daily inhalation dose on a μg/m^2 basis) and above caused increases in fetal resorptions and stillbirths and decreases in pup body weight and survival. At a lower dose of 1.0 μg/kg (approximately 0.5% of the maximum recommended human daily inhalation dose on a μg/m^2 basis) it did not induce the above mentioned effects.

PREGNANCY CATEGORY C

Triamcinolone acetonide has been shown to be teratogenic at inhalational doses of 20, 40, and 80 μg/kg in rats (approximately 0.1, 0.2, and 0.4 times the maximum recommended human daily inhalation dose on a μg/m^2 basis, respectively), in rabbits at the same doses (approximately 0.2, 0.4, and 0.8 times the maximum recommended human daily inhalation dose on a μg/m^2 basis, respectively) and in monkeys, at an inhalational dose of 500 μg/kg (approximately 5 times the maximum recommended human daily inhalation dose on a μg/m^2 basis). Dose related teratogenic effects in rats and rabbits included cleft palate and/or internal hydrocephaly and axial skeletal defects whereas the teratogenic effects observed in the monkey were CNS and/or cranial malformations. There are no adequate and well controlled studies in pregnant women. Triamcinolone acetonide should be used during pregnancy only if the potential benefit justifies the potential risk to the fetus.

Experience with oral glucocorticoids since their introduction in pharmacologic as opposed to physiologic doses suggests that rodents are more prone to teratogenic effects from glucocorticoids than humans. In addition, because there is a natural increase in glucocorticoid production during pregnancy, most women will require a lower exogenous steroid dose and many will not need glucocorticoid treatment during pregnancy.

Nonteratogenic Effects: Hypoadrenalism may occur in infants born of mothers receiving corticosteroids during pregnancy. Such infants should be carefully observed.

NURSING MOTHERS

It is not known whether triamcinolone acetonide is excreted in human milk. Because other corticosteroids are excreted in human milk, caution should be exercised when triamcinolone acetonide inhalation aerosol is administered to nursing women.

PEDIATRIC USE

Safety and effectiveness have not been established in pediatric patients below the age of 6. Oral corticosteroids have been shown to cause growth suppression in children and teenagers, particularly with higher doses over extended periods. If a child or teenager on any corticosteroid appears to have growth suppression, the possibility that they are particularly sensitive to this effect of steroids should be considered.

ADVERSE REACTIONS

TABLE 2 describes the incidence of common adverse experiences based upon three placebo-controlled, multicenter US clinical trials of 507 patients [297 female and 210 male adults (age range 18-64)]. These trials included asthma patients who had previously received inhaled beta$_2$-agonists alone, as well as those who previously required inhaled corticosteroid therapy for the control of their asthma. The patients were treated with triamcinolone acetonide inhalation aerosol (including doses ranging from 200-800 μg twice daily for 6 weeks) or placebo.

Adverse events that occurred at an incidence of 1-3% in the overall triamcinolone acetonide inhalation aerosol treatment group and greater than placebo included:

Body as a Whole: Facial edema, pain, abdominal pain, photosensitivity.
Digestive System: Diarrhea, oral monilia, toothache, vomiting.
Metabolic and Nutrition: Weight gain.

TABLE 2 *Adverse Events Occurring at an Incidence of Greater Than 3% and Greater Than Placebo*

	Triamcinolone Acetonide Dose			
Adverse Event	200 μg bid (n=57)	400 μg bid (n=170)	800 μg bid (n=57)	Placebo (n=167)
Sinusitis	5 (9%)	7 (4%)	1 (2%)	6 (4%)
Pharyngitis	4 (7%)	42 (25%)	10 (18%)	19 (11%)
Headache	4 (7%)	35 (21%)	7 (12%)	24 (14%)
Flu syndrome	2 (4%)	8 (5%)	1 (2%)	5 (3%)
Back pain	2 (4%)	3 (2%)	2 (4%)	3 (2%)

Musculoskeletal System: Bursitis, myalgia, tenosynovitis.
Nervous System: Dry mouth.
Organs of Special Sense: Rash.
Respiratory System: Chest congestion, voice alteration.
Urogenital System: Cystitis, urinary tract infection, vaginal monilia.

In older controlled clinical trials of steroid dependent asthmatics, urticaria was reported rarely. Anaphylaxis was not reported in these controlled trials. Typical steroid withdrawal effects including muscle aches, joint aches, and fatigue were noted in clinical trials when patients were transferred from oral steroid therapy to triamcinolone acetonide inhalation aerosol. Easy bruisability was also noted in these trials.

Hoarseness, dry throat, irritated throat, dry mouth, facial edema, increased wheezing, and cough have been reported. These adverse effects have generally been mild and transient. Cases of oral candidiasis occurring with clinical use have been reported. (See WARNINGS.) Anaphylaxis has also been reported from post-marketing surveillance.

DOSAGE AND ADMINISTRATION

ADULTS

The usual recommended dosage is 2 inhalations (200 μg) given 3-4 times a day or 4 inhalations (400 μg) given twice daily. The maximal daily intake should not exceed 16 inhalations (1600 μg) in adults. Higher initial doses (12-16 inhalations/day) may be considered in patients with more severe asthma.

CHILDREN 6-12 YEARS OF AGE

The usual recommended dosage is 1 or 2 inhalations (100-200 μg) given 3-4 times a day or 2-4 inhalations (200-400 μg) given twice daily. The maximal daily intake should not exceed 12 inhalations (1200 μg) in children 6-12 years of age. Insufficient clinical data exist with respect to the safety and efficacy of the administration of triamcinolone acetonide inhalation aerosol to children below the age of 6. The long-term effects of inhaled steroids, including triamcinolone acetonide inhalation aerosol, on growth are still not fully known. Rinsing the mouth after inhalation is advised.

Different considerations must be given to the following groups of patients in order to obtain the full therapeutic benefit of triamcinolone acetonide inhalation aerosol:

Note: In all patients, it is desirable to titrate to the lowest effective dose once asthma stability has been achieved.

Patients Not Receiving Systemic Corticosteroids: Patients who require maintenance therapy of their asthma may benefit from treatment with triamcinolone acetonide inhalation aerosol at the doses recommended above. In patients who respond to triamcinolone acetonide inhalation aerosol, improvement in pulmonary function is usually apparent within 1-2 weeks after the initiation of therapy.

Patients Maintained on Systemic Corticosteroids: Clinical studies have shown that triamcinolone acetonide inhalation aerosol may be effective in the management of asthmatics dependent or maintained on systemic corticosteroids and may permit replacement or significant reduction in the dosage of systemic corticosteroids.

The patient's asthma should be reasonably stable before treatment with triamcinolone acetonide inhalation aerosol is started. Initially, triamcinolone acetonide inhalation aerosol should be used concurrently with the patient's usual maintenance dose of systemic corticosteroid. After approximately 1 week, gradual withdrawal of the systemic corticosteroid is started by reducing the daily or alternate daily dose. Reductions may be made after an interval of 1 or 2 weeks, depending on the response of the patient. A slow rate of withdrawal is strongly recommended. Generally, these decrements should not exceed 2.5 mg of prednisone or its equivalent. During withdrawal, some patients may experience symptoms of systemic corticosteroid withdrawal, *e.g.*, joint and/or muscular pain, lassitude, and depression, despite maintenance or even improvement in pulmonary function. Such patients should be encouraged to continue with the inhaler but should be monitored for objective signs of adrenal insufficiency. If evidence of adrenal insufficiency occurs, the systemic corticosteroid doses should be increased temporarily and thereafter withdrawal should continue more slowly. Inhaled corticosteroids should be used with caution when used chronically in patients receiving prednisone regimens, either daily or alternate day. (See WARNINGS.)

During periods of stress or a severe asthma attack, transfer patients may require supplementary treatment with systemic corticosteroids.

Directions for Use: An illustrated leaflet of patient instructions for proper use accompanies each package of triamcinolone acetonide inhalation aerosol.

HOW SUPPLIED

Azmacort inhalation aerosol contains 60 mg triamcinolone acetonide in a 20 g package which delivers at least 240 actuations. It is supplied with a white plastic actuator, a white plastic spacer-mouthpiece and patient's leaflet of instructions: box of 1. Each actuation delivers 200 μg triamcinolone acetonide from the valve and 100 μg from the spacer-mouthpiece under defined *in vitro* test conditions.

Avoid spraying in eyes.

For best results, the canister should be at room temperature before use.

Shake well before using.

CONTENTS UNDER PRESSURE. Do not puncture. Do not use or store near heat or open flame. Exposure to temperatures above 120°F may cause bursting. Never throw canister into fire or incinerator. Keep out of reach of children unless otherwise prescribed. Store at controlled room temperature 20-25°C (68-77°F).

Note: The indented statement below is required by the Federal government's Clean Air Act for all products containing or manufactured with chlorofluorocarbons (CFCs):

WARNING: Contains CFC-12, a substance which harms public health and the environment by destroying ozone in the upper atmosphere.

A notice similar to the above warning has been placed in the Patient Information that is distributed with the prescription under the Environmental Protection Agency's (EPA's) regulations. The patient's warning states that the patient should consult his or her physician if there are questions about alternatives.

INTRANASAL

DESCRIPTION

NASAL INHALER

For Intranasal Use Only.

Shake Well Before Using.

Triamcinolone acetonide, the active ingredient in Nasacort nasal inhaler, is a glucocorticosteroid with a molecular weight of 434.5 and with the chemical designation 9-Fluoro-11β,16α,17,21-tetrahydroxypregna-1,4-diene-3,20-dione cyclic 16,17-acetal with acetone ($C_{24}H_{31}FO_6$).

Nasacort nasal inhaler is a metered-dose aerosol unit containing a microcrystalline suspension of triamcinolone acetonide in dichlorodifluoromethane and dehydrated alcohol 0.7% w/w. Each canister contains 15 mg triamcinolone acetonide. Each actuation delivers 55 μg triamcinolone acetonide from the nasal actuator to the patient (estimated from *in vitro* testing). There are at least 100 actuations in 1 Nasacort nasal inhaler canister. **After 100 actuations, the amount delivered per actuation may not be consistent and the unit should be discarded.** Patients are provided with a check-off card to track usage as part of the Information for Patients tear-off sheet.

NASAL SPRAY

For Intranasal Use Only.

Shake Well Before Using.

Triamcinolone acetonide, the active ingredient in Nasacort AQ nasal spray, is a corticosteroid with a molecular weight of 434.51 and with the chemical designation 9-Fluoro-11β,16α,17,21-tetrahydroxypregna-1,4-diene-3,20-dione cyclic 16,17-acetal with acetone ($C_{24}H_{31}FO_6$).

Nasacort AQ nasal spray is an unscented, thixotropic, water-based metered-dose pump spray formulation unit containing a microcrystalline suspension of triamcinolone acetonide in an aqueous medium. Microcrystalline cellulose, carboxymethylcellulose sodium, polysorbate 80, dextrose, benzalkonium chloride, and edetate disodium are contained in this aqueous medium; hydrochloric acid or sodium hydroxide may be added to adjust the pH to a target of 5.0 within a range of 4.5 and 6.0.

Each actuation delivers 55 μg triamcinolone acetonide from the nasal actuator after an initial priming of 5 sprays. It will remain adequately primed for 2 weeks. If the product is not used for more than 2 weeks, then it can be adequately reprimed with 1 spray. The contents of one 6.5 g sample bottle provide 30 actuations, and the contents of one 16.5 g bottle provide 120 actuations. **After either 30 actuations or 120 actuations, the amount of triamcinolone acetonide delivered per actuation may not be consistent and the unit should be discarded.** Each 30 actuation sample bottle contains 3.575 mg of triamcinolone acetonide and each 120 actuation bottle contains 9.075 mg of triamcinolone acetonide.

In the Information for Patients tear-off sheet, patients are provided with a check-off form to track usage.

CLINICAL PHARMACOLOGY

Triamcinolone acetonide is a more potent derivative of triamcinolone. Although triamcinolone itself is approximately 1-2 times as potent as prednisone in animal models of inflammation, triamcinolone acetonide is approximately 8 times more potent than prednisone.

NASAL INHALER

Although the precise mechanism of corticosteroid antiallergic action is unknown, corticosteroids are very effective. However, they do not have an immediate effect on allergic signs and symptoms. When allergic symptoms are very severe, local treatment with recommended doses (microgram) of any available topical corticosteroids are not as effective as treatment with larger doses (milligram) of oral or parenteral formulations. When corticosteroids are prematurely discontinued, symptoms may not recur for several days.

Based upon intravenous (IV) dosing of triamcinolone acetonide phosphate ester, the half-life of triamcinolone acetonide was reported to be 88 minutes. The volume of distribution (Vd) reported was 99.5 L (SD ± 27.5) and clearance was 45.2 L/h (SD ± 9.1) for triamcinolone acetonide. The plasma half-life of corticosteroids does not correlate well with the biologic half-life.

When administered intranasally to man at 440 μg/day dose, the peak plasma concentration was <1 ng/ml and occurred on average at 3.4 hours (range 0.5-8.0 hours) postdosing. The apparent half-life was 4.0 hours (range 1.0-7.0 hours); however, this value probably reflects lingering absorption. Intranasal doses below 440 μg/day gave sparse data and did not allow for the calculation of meaningful pharmacokinetic parameters.

In animal studies using rats and dogs, three metabolites of triamcinolone acetonide have been identified. They are 6β-hydroxytriamcinolone acetonide, 21-carboxytriamcinolone acetonide and 21-carboxy-6β-hydroxytriamcinolone acetonide. All three metabolites are expected to be substantially less active than the parent compound due to (a) the dependence of anti-inflammatory activity on the presence of a 21-hydroxyl group, (b) the decreased activity observed upon 6-hydroxylation, and (c) the markedly increased water solubility favoring rapid elimination. There appeared to be some quantitative differences in the metabolites among species. No differences were detected in metabolic pattern as a function of route of administration.

NASAL SPRAY

Although the precise mechanism of corticosteroid antiallergic action is unknown, corticosteroids are very effective. However, when allergic symptoms are very severe, local treatment with recommended doses (microgram) of any available topical corticosteroid are not as effective as treatment with larger doses (milligram) of oral or parenteral formulations. Based upon IV dosing of triamcinolone acetonide phosphate ester in adults, the half-life of triamcinolone acetonide was reported to be 88 minutes. The volume of distribution (Vd) reported was 99.5 L (SD ± 27.5) and clearance was 45.2 L/h (SD ± 9.1) for triamcinolone acetonide. The plasma half-life of corticosteroids does not correlate well with the biologic half-life.

Pharmacokinetic characterization of the triamcinolone acetonide nasal spray formulation was determined in both normal adult subjects and patients with allergic rhinitis. Single dose intranasal administration of 220 μg of triamcinolone acetonide nasal spray in normal adult subjects and patients demonstrated minimal absorption of triamcinolone acetonide. The mean peak plasma concentration was approximately 0.5 ng/ml (range: 0.1-1.0 ng/ml) and occurred at 1.5 hours post dose. The mean plasma drug concentration was less than 0.06 ng/ml at 12 hours, and below the assay detection limit at 24 hours. The average terminal half-life was 3.1 hours. The range of mean AUC(0-∞) values was 1.4-4.7 ng·h/ml between doses of 110-440 μg in both patients and healthy volunteers. Dose proportionality was demonstrated in both normal adult subjects and in allergic rhinitis patients following single intranasal doses of 110 or 220 μg triamcinolone acetonide nasal spray. The C_{max} and AUC of the 440 μg dose increased less than proportionally when compared to 110 and 220 μg doses. Following multiple doses in pediatric patients receiving 440 μg/day, plasma drug concentrations, AUC, C_{max} and T_{max} were similar to those values observed in adult patients.

In animal studies using rats and dogs, three metabolites of triamcinolone acetonide have been identified. They are 6β-hydroxytriamcinolone acetonide, 21-carboxytriamcinolone acetonide and 21-carboxy-6β-hydroxytriamcinolone acetonide. All three metabolites are expected to be substantially less active than the parent compound due to (a) the dependence of anti-inflammatory activity on the presence of a 21-hydroxyl group, (b) the decreased activity observed upon 6-hydroxylation, and (c) the markedly increased water solubility favoring rapid elimination. There appeared to be some quantitative differences in the metabolites among species. No differences were detected in metabolic pattern as a function of route of administration.

In order to determine if systemic absorption plays a role in triamcinolone acetonide nasal spray's treatment of allergic rhinitis symptoms, a 2 week double-blind, placebo-controlled clinical study was conducted comparing triamcinolone acetonide nasal spray, orally ingested triamcinolone acetonide, and placebo in 297 adult patients with seasonal allergic rhinitis. The study demonstrated that the therapeutic efficacy of triamcinolone acetonide nasal spray can be attributed to the topical effects of triamcinolone acetonide.

In order to evaluate the effects of systemic absorption on the Hypothalamic-Pituitary-Adrenal (HPA) axis, a clinical study was performed in adults comparing 220 or 440 μg triamcinolone acetonide nasal spray per day, or 10 mg prednisone per day with placebo for 42 days. Adrenal response to a 6 hour cosyntropin stimulation test showed that triamcinolone acetonide nasal spray administered at doses of 220 and 440 μg had no statistically significant effect on HPA activity versus placebo. Conversely, oral prednisone at 10 mg/day significantly reduced the response to ACTH.

A study evaluating plasma cortisol response 30 and 60 minutes after cosyntropin stimulation in 80 pediatric patients who received 220 or 440 μg (twice the maximum recommended daily dose) daily for 6 weeks was conducted. No abnormal response to cosyntropin infusion (peak serum cortisol <18 μg/dl) was observed in any pediatric patient after 6 weeks of dosing with triamcinolone acetonide nasal spray at 440 μg/day.

INDICATIONS AND USAGE

Triamcinolone acetonide nasal inhaler or nasal spray is indicated for the nasal treatment of seasonal and perennial allergic rhinitis symptoms in adults and children 6 years of age and older.

CONTRAINDICATIONS

Hypersensitivity to any of the ingredients of this preparation contraindicates its use.

WARNINGS

The replacement of a systemic corticosteroid with a topical corticoid can be accompanied by signs of adrenal insufficiency and, in addition, some patients may experience symptoms of withdrawal, *e.g.*, joint and/or muscular pain, lassitude and depression. Patients previously treated for prolonged periods with systemic corticosteroids and transferred to topical corticoids should be carefully monitored for acute adrenal insufficiency in response to stress. In those patients who have asthma or other clinical conditions requiring long-term systemic corticosteroid treatment, too rapid a decrease in systemic corticosteroids may cause a severe exacerbation of their symptoms.

Children who are on immunosuppressant drugs are more susceptible to infections than healthy children. Chickenpox and measles, for example, can have a more serious or even fatal course in children on immunosuppressant doses of corticosteroids. In such children, or in adults who have not had these diseases, particular care should be taken to avoid exposure. If exposed, therapy with varicella-zoster immune globulin (VZIG) or pooled IV immunoglobulin (IVIG), as appropriate, may be indicated. If chickenpox develops, treatment with antiviral agents may be considered.

NASAL INHALER

The use of triamcinolone acetonide nasal inhaler with alternate-day systemic prednisone could increase the likelihood of hypothalamic-pituitaryadrenal (HPA) suppression compared to a therapeutic dose of either one alone. Therefore, triamcinolone acetonide nasal inhaler should be used with caution in patients already receiving alternate-day prednisone treatment for any disease.

PRECAUTIONS

NASAL INHALER

General

In clinical studies with triamcinolone acetonide administered intranasally, the development of localized infections of the nose and pharynx with *Candida albicans* has rarely occurred. When such an infection develops, it may require treatment with appropriate local therapy and discontinuance of treatment with triamcinolone acetonide nasal inhaler.

Triamcinolone acetonide administered intranasally has been shown to be absorbed into the systemic circulation in humans.

Patients with active rhinitis showed absorption similar to that found in normal volunteers. Triamcinolone acetonide nasal inhaler at 440 μg/day for 42 days did not measurably affect adrenal response to a 6 hour cosyntropin test. In the same study, prednisone 10 mg/day significantly reduced adrenal response to ACTH over the same period.

Triamcinolone acetonide nasal inhaler should be used with caution, if at all, in patients with active or quiescent tuberculous infections of the respiratory tract or in patients with untreated fungal, bacterial, or systemic viral infections or ocular herpes simplex.

Because of the inhibitory effect of corticosteroids on wound healing in patients who have experienced recent nasal septal ulcers, nasal surgery or trauma, a corticosteroid should be used with caution until healing has occurred. As with other nasally inhaled corticosteroids, nasal septal perforations have been reported in rare instances.

When used at excessive doses, systemic corticosteroid effects such as hypercorticism and adrenal suppression may appear. If such changes occur, triamcinolone acetonide nasal inhaler should be discontinued slowly, consistent with accepted procedures for discontinuing oral steroid therapy.

Information for the Patient

Patients being treated with triamcinolone acetonide nasal inhaler should receive the following information and instructions.

Patients who are on immunosuppressant doses of corticosteroids should be warned to avoid exposure to chickenpox or measles and, if exposed, to obtain medical advice.

Patients should use triamcinolone acetonide nasal inhaler at regular intervals since its effectiveness depends on its regular use. A decrease in symptoms may occur as soon as 12 hours after starting steroid therapy and generally can be expected to occur within a few days of initiating therapy in allergic rhinitis. The patient should take the medication as directed and should not exceed the prescribed dosage. The patient should contact the physician if symptoms do not improve after 3 weeks, or if the condition worsens. Nasal irritation and/or burning or stinging after use of the spray occur only rarely with this product. The patient should contact the physician if they occur.

For the proper use of this unit and to attain maximum improvement, the patient should read and follow the accompanying patient instructions carefully. Spraying triamcinolone acetonide directly onto the nasal septum should be avoided. Because the amount dispensed per puff may not be consistent, it is important to shake the canister well. Also, the canister should be discarded after 100 actuations.

Carcinogenesis, Mutagenesis

No evidence of treatment-related carcinogenicity was demonstrated after 2 years of once daily gavage administration of triamcinolone acetonide at doses of 0.05, 0.2 and 1.0 μg/kg (approximately 0.1, 0.4 and 1.8% of the recommended clinical dose on a μg/m^2 basis) in the rat and 0.1, 0.6 and 3.0 μg/kg (approximately 0.1, 0.6 and 3.0% of the recommended clinical dose on a μg/m^2 basis) in the mouse.

Mutagenesis studies with triamcinolone acetonide have not been conducted.

Impairment of Fertility

No evidence of impaired fertility was demonstrated when oral doses up to 15 μg/kg (approximately 28% of the recommended clinical dose on a μg/m^2 basis) were administered to female and male rats. However, triamcinolone acetonide at oral doses of 8.0 μg/kg (approximately 15.0% of the recommended clinical dose on a μg/m^2 basis) caused dystocia and prolonged delivery and at oral doses of 5.0 μg/kg (approximately 9.0% of the recommended clinical dose on a μg/m^2 basis) and above produced increases in fetal resorptions and stillbirths as well as decreases in pup body weight and survival. At an oral dose of 1.0 μg/kg (approximately 2.0% of the recommended clinical dose on a μg/m^2 basis), it did not manifest the above mentioned effects.

Pregnancy Category C

Triamcinolone acetonide was teratogenic at inhalational doses of 20, 40 and 80 μg/kg in rats (approximately 0.4, 0.75 and 1.5 times the recommended clinical dose on a μg/m^2 basis, respectively) and rabbits (approximately 0.75, 1.5 and 3.0 times the recommended dose on a μg/m^2 basis, respectively). Triamcinolone acetonide was also teratogenic at an inhalational dose of 500 μg/kg in monkeys (approximately 18 times the recommended clinical dose on a μg/m^2 basis). Dose-related teratogenic effects in rats and rabbits included cleft palate, internal hydrocephaly, and axial skeletal defects. Teratogenic effects observed in the monkey were CNS and cranial malformations. There are no adequate and well-controlled studies in pregnant women. Triamcinolone acetonide should be used during pregnancy only if the potential benefits justify the potential risk to the fetus.

Experience with oral corticoids since their introduction in pharmacologic as opposed to physiologic doses suggests that rodents are more prone to teratogenic effects from corticoids than humans. In addition, because there is a natural increase in glucocorticoid production during pregnancy, most women will require a lower exogenous steroid dose and many will not need corticoid treatment during pregnancy.

Nonteratogenic Effects: Hypoadrenalism may occur in infants born of mothers receiving corticosteroids during pregnancy. Such infants should be carefully observed.

Nursing Mothers

It is not known whether triamcinolone acetonide is excreted in human milk. Because other corticosteroids are excreted in human milk, caution should be exercised when triamcinolone acetonide nasal inhaler is administered to nursing women.

Pediatric Use

Safety and effectiveness in pediatric patients below the age of 6 have not been established. Oral corticosteroids have been shown to cause growth suppression in children and teenagers, particularly with higher doses over extended periods. If a child or teenager on any corticosteroid appears to have growth suppression, the possibility that they are particularly sensitive to this effect of steroids should be considered.

NASAL SPRAY

General

In clinical studies with triamcinolone acetonide nasal spray, the development of localized infections of the nose and pharynx with *Candida albicans* has rarely occurred. When such an infection develops it may require treatment with appropriate local or systemic therapy and discontinuance of treatment with triamcinolone acetonide nasal spray.

Triamcinolone acetonide nasal spray should be used with caution, if at all, in patients with active or quiescent tuberculous infection of the respiratory tract or in patients with untreated fungal, bacterial, or systemic viral infections or ocular herpes simplex.

Because of the inhibitory effect of corticosteroids, in patients who have experienced recent nasal septal ulcers, nasal surgery, or trauma, a corticosteroid should be used with caution until healing has occurred. As with other nasally inhaled corticosteroids, nasal septal perforations have been reported in rare instances.

When used at excessive doses, systemic corticosteroid effects such as hypercorticism and adrenal suppression may appear. If such changes occur, triamcinolone acetonide nasal spray should be discontinued slowly, consistent with accepted procedures for discontinuing oral steroid therapy.

Information for the Patient

Patients being treated with triamcinolone acetonide nasal spray should receive the following information and instructions. Patients who are on immunosuppressant doses of corticosteroids should be warned to avoid exposure to chickenpox or measles and, if exposed, to obtain medical advice.

Patients should use triamcinolone acetonide nasal spray at regular intervals since its effectiveness depends on its regular use. (See DOSAGE AND ADMINISTRATION, Nasal Spray.)

An improvement in some patient symptoms may be seen within the first day of treatment, and generally, it takes 1 week of treatment to reach maximum benefit. Initial assessment for response should be made during this time frame and periodically until the patient's symptoms are stabilized.

The patient should take the medication as directed and should not exceed the prescribed dosage. The patient should contact the physician if symptoms do not improve after 3 weeks, or if the condition worsens. Patients who experience recurrent episodes of epistaxis (nose bleeds) or nasal septum discomfort while taking this medication should contact their physician. For the proper use of this unit and to attain maximum improvement, the patient should read and follow the accompanying patient instructions carefully.

It is important to shake the bottle well before each use. **Also, the bottle should be discarded after 120 actuations since the amount of triamcinolone acetonide delivered thereafter per actuation may be substantially less than 55 μg of drug.** Do not transfer any remaining suspension to another bottle.

Carcinogenesis, Mutagenesis, and Impairment of Fertility

In a 2 year study in rats, triamcinolone acetonide caused no treatment-related carcinogenicity at oral doses up to 1.0 μg/kg (approximately 1/30 and 1/50 of the maximum recommended daily intranasal dose in adults and children on a μg/m^2 basis, respectively). In a 2 year study in mice, triamcinolone acetonide caused no treatment-related carcinogenicity at oral doses up to 3.0 μg/kg (approximately 1/12 and 1/30 of the maximum recommended daily intranasal dose in adults and children on a μg/m^2 basis, respectively).

No mutagenicity studies with triamcinolone acetonide have been performed.

In male and female rats, triamcinolone acetonide caused no change in pregnancy rate at oral doses up to 15.0 μg/kg (approximately 1/2 of the maximum recommended daily intranasal dose in adults on a μg/m^2 basis). Triamcinolone acetonide caused increased fetal resorptions and stillbirths and decreases in pup weight and survival at doses of 5.0 μg/kg and above (approximately 1/5 of the maximum recommended daily intranasal dose in adults on a μg/m^2 basis). At 1.0 μg/kg (approximately 1/30 of the maximum recommended daily intranasal dose in adults on a μg/m^2 basis), it did not induce the above mentioned effects.

Pregnancy Category C

Teratogenic Effects

Triamcinolone acetonide was teratogenic in rats, rabbits, and monkeys. In rats, triamcinolone acetonide was teratogenic at inhalation doses of 20 μg/kg and above (approximately 7/10 of the maximum recommended daily intranasal dose in adults on a μg/m^2 basis). In rabbits, triamcinolone acetonide was teratogenic at inhalation doses of 20 μg/kg and above (approximately 2 times the maximum recommended daily intranasal dose in adults on a μg/m^2 basis). In monkeys, triamcinolone acetonide was teratogenic at an inhalation dose of 500 μg/kg (approximately 37 times the maximum recommended daily intranasal dose in adults on a μg/m^2 basis). Dose-related teratogenic effects in rats and rabbits included cleft palate and/or internal hydrocephaly and axial skeletal defects, whereas the effects observed in the monkey were cranial malformations.

There are no adequate and well-controlled studies in pregnant women. Therefore, triamcinolone acetonide should be used in pregnancy only if the potential benefit justifies the potential risk to the fetus. Since their introduction, experience with oral corticosteroids in pharmacologic as opposed to physiologic doses suggests that rodents are more prone to teratogenic effects from corticosteroids than humans. In addition, because there is a natural increase in glucocorticoid production during pregnancy, most women will require a lower exogenous corticosteroid dose and many will not need corticosteroid treatment during pregnancy.

Nonteratogenic Effects

Hypoadrenalism may occur in infants born of mothers receiving corticosteroids during pregnancy. Such infants should be carefully observed.

Nursing Mothers

It is not known whether triamcinolone acetonide is excreted in human milk. Because other corticosteroids are excreted in human milk, caution should be exercised when triamcinolone acetonide nasal spray is administered to nursing women.

Pediatric Use

Safety and effectiveness in pediatric patients below the age of 6 years have not been established.

Corticosteroids have been shown to cause growth suppression in children and teenagers, particularly with higher doses over extended periods. If a child or teenager on any corticosteroid appears to have growth suppression, the possibility that they are particularly sensitive to this effect of corticosteroids should be considered.

ADVERSE REACTIONS

NASAL INHALER

Adults and Children 12 Years of Age and Older

In controlled and uncontrolled studies, 1257 adult and adolescent patients received treatment with intranasal triamcinolone acetonide. Adverse reactions are based on the 567 patients who received a product similar to the marketed triamcinolone acetonide nasal inhaler canister.

These patients were treated for an average of 48 days (range 1-117 days). The 145 patients enrolled in uncontrolled studies received treatment from 1-820 days (average 332 days). The most prevalent adverse experience was headache, being reported by approximately 18% of the patients who received triamcinolone acetonide nasal inhaler. Nasal irritation was reported by 2.8% of the patients receiving triamcinolone acetonide nasal inhaler.

Other nasopharyngeal side effects were reported by fewer than 5% of the patients who received triamcinolone acetonide nasal inhaler and included: dry mucous membranes, naso-sinus congestion, throat discomfort, sneezing, and epistaxis. The complaints do not usually interfere with treatment and in the controlled and uncontrolled studies approximately 1% of patients have discontinued because of these nasal adverse effects. In the event of accidental overdose, an increased potential for these adverse experiences may be expected, but systemic adverse experiences are unlikely.

Children 6-11 Years of Age

Adverse event data in children 6-11 years of age are derived from two controlled clinical trials of 2 and 4 weeks duration. In these trials, 127 patients received fixed doses of 220 µg/day of triamcinolone acetonide for an average of 22 days (range 8-33 days).

Adverse events occurring at an incidence of 3% or greater and more common among children treated with 220 µg triamcinolone acetonide daily than vehicle placebo are shown in TABLE 3.

TABLE 3

Adverse Events	220 µg of Triamcinolone Acetonide Daily (n=127)	Vehicle Placebo (n=322)
Epistaxis	11.0%	9.3%
Cough	9.4%	9.3%
Fever	7.9%	5.6%
Nausea	6.3%	3.1%
Throat discomfort	5.5%	5.3%
Otitis	4.7%	3.7%
Dyspepsia	4.7%	2.2%

Adverse events occurring at a rate of 3% or greater that were more common in the placebo group were upper respiratory tract infection, headache and concurrent infection.

Only 1.6% of patients discontinued due to adverse experiences. No patient discontinued due to a serious adverse event related to triamcinolone acetonide nasal inhaler therapy.

Though not observed in controlled clinical trials of triamcinolone acetonide nasal inhaler in children, cases of nasal septum perforation among pediatric users have been reported in post-marketing surveillance of this product.

NASAL SPRAY

In placebo-controlled, double-blind, and open-label clinical studies, 1483 adults and children 12 years and older received treatment with triamcinolone acetonide aqueous nasal spray. These patients were treated for an average duration of 51 days. In the controlled trials (2-5 weeks duration) from which the following adverse reaction data are derived, 1394 patients were treated with triamcinolone acetonide nasal spray for an average of 19 days. In a long-term, open-label study, 172 patients received treatment for an average duration of 286 days.

Adverse events occurring at an incidence of 2% or greater and more common among triamcinolone acetonide nasal spray-treated patients than placebo-treated patients in controlled adult clinical trials are shown in TABLE 4.

TABLE 4

Adverse Events	Patients Treated With 220 µg Triamcinolone Acetonide (n=857)	Vehicle Placebo (n=962)
Pharyngitis	5.1%	3.6%
Epistaxis	2.7%	0.8%
Increase in cough	2.1%	1.5%

A total of 602 children 6-12 years of age were studied in three double-blind, placebo-controlled clinical trials. Of these, 172 received 110 µg/day and 207 received 220 µg/day of triamcinolone acetonide nasal spray for 2, 6, or 12 weeks. The longest average durations of treatment for patients receiving 110 µg/day and 220 µg/day were 76 days and 80 days, respectively. Only 1% of those patients treated with triamcinolone acetonide nasal spray were discontinued due to adverse experiences. No patient receiving 110 µg/day discontinued due to a serious adverse event and 1 patient receiving 220 µg/day discontinued due to a serious event that was considered not drug related. Overall, these studies found the adverse experience profile for triamcinolone acetonide nasal spray to be similar to placebo. A similar adverse event profile was observed in pediatric patients 6-12 years of age as compared to older children and adults with the exception of epistaxis which occurred in less than 2% of the pediatric patients studied.

Adverse events occurring at an incidence of 2% or greater and more common among adult patients treated with placebo than triamcinolone acetonide nasal spray were: headache, and rhinitis. In children aged 6-12 years these events included: asthma, epistaxis, headache, infection, otitis media, sinusitis, and vomiting.

In clinical trials, nasal septum perforation was reported in 1 adult patient although relationship to triamcinolone acetonide nasal spray has not been established.

In the event of accidental overdose, an increased potential for these adverse experiences may be expected, but acute systemic adverse experiences are unlikely.

DOSAGE AND ADMINISTRATION

NASAL INHALER

A decrease in symptoms may occur as soon as 12 hours after starting steroid therapy and generally can be expected to occur within a few days of initiating therapy in allergic rhinitis.

If improvement is not evident after 2-3 weeks, the patient should be re-evaluated.

Adults and Children 12 Years of Age and Older

The recommended starting dose of triamcinolone acetonide nasal inhaler is 220 µg/day given as 2 sprays (55 µg/spray) in each nostril once-a-day. If needed, the dose may be increased to 440 µg/day (55 µg/spray) either as once-a-day dosage or divided up to 4 times a day, *i.e.,* twice a day (2 sprays/nostril), or 4 times a day (1 spray/nostril). After the desired effect is obtained, some patients may be maintained on a dose of as little as 1 spray (55 µg) in each nostril once-a-day (total daily dose 110 µg/day).

Children 6-11 Years of Age

The recommended starting dose of triamcinolone acetonide nasal inhaler is 220 µg/day given as 2 sprays (55 µg/spray) in each nostril once-a-day. Once the maximal effect has been achieved, it is always desirable to titrate the patient to the minimum effective dose.

Triamcinolone acetonide nasal inhaler is not recommended for children below 6 years of age since adequate numbers of patients have not been studied in this age group.

Directions for Use: Illustrated Patient's Instructions for use accompany each package of triamcinolone acetonide nasal inhaler.

NASAL SPRAY

Recommended Doses

Adults and Children 12 Years of Age and Older

The recommended starting and maximum dose is 220 µg/day as 2 sprays in each nostril once daily.

Children 6-12 Years of Age

The recommended starting dose is 110 µg/day given as 1 spray in each nostril once daily. The maximum recommended dose is 220 µg/day as 2 sprays/nostril once daily.

Triamcinolone acetonide nasal spray is not recommended for children under 6 years of age since adequate numbers of patients have not been studied in this age group.

Individualization Of Dosage

It is always desirable to titrate an individual patient to the minimum effective dose to reduce the possibility of side effects. In adults, when the maximum benefit has been achieved and symptoms have been controlled, reducing the dose to 110 µg /day (1 spray in each nostril once-a-day) has been shown to be effective in maintaining control of the allergic rhinitis symptoms in patients who were initially controlled at 220 µg/day.

In children 6-12 years of age, the recommended starting dose is 110 µg/day given as 1 spray in each nostril once daily. The maximum recommended daily dose in children 6-12 years of age is 220 µg/day (2 sprays in each nostril once daily). Some patients who do not achieve maximum symptom control at a dose of 110 µg/day may benefit from a dose of 220 µg given as 2 sprays in each nostril once daily. The minimum effective dose should be used to ensure continued control of symptoms. Once symptoms are controlled, pediatric patients may be able to be maintained on 110 µg/day (1 spray in each nostril once daily).

An improvement in some patient symptoms may be seen within the first day of treatment, and generally, it takes 1 week of treatment to reach maximum benefit. Initial assessment for response should be made during this time frame and periodically until the patient's symptoms are stabilized. If adequate relief of symptoms has not been obtained after 3 weeks of treatment, triamcinolone acetonide nasal spray should be discontinued. (See WARNINGS; PRECAUTIONS, Nasal Spray, Information for the Patient; and ADVERSE REACTIONS, Nasal Spray.)

Directions For Use: Illustrated Patient's Instructions for use accompany each package of triamcinolone acetonide nasal spray.

HOW SUPPLIED

NASAL INHALER

Nasacort nasal inhaler is supplied as an aerosol canister which will provide 100 metered dose actuations. Each actuation delivers 55 µg triamcinolone acetonide through the nasal actuator. The Nasacort nasal inhaler canister and accompanying nasal actuator are designed to be used together. The Nasacort nasal inhaler canister should not be used with other nasal actuators and the supplied nasal actuator should not be used with other products' canisters. Nasacort nasal inhaler is supplied with a white plastic nasal actuator and patient instructions. Net weight of the canister contents is 10 g.

CONTENTS UNDER PRESSURE.

Avoid spraying in eyes.

Storage: Do not puncture. Do not use or store near heat or open flame. Exposure to temperatures above 120°F may cause bursting. Never throw container into fire or incinerator. Keep out of reach of children. Store at controlled room temperature 20-25°C (68-77°F).

Note: The indented statement below is required by the Federal government's Clean Air Act for all products containing or manufactured with chlorofluorocarbons (CFCs):

> ***WARNING:*** Contains CFC-12, a substance which harms public health and the environment by destroying ozone in the upper atmosphere.

A notice similar to the above warning has been placed in the Patient Information that is distributed with the prescription under the Environmental Protection Agency's (EPA's) regulations. The patient's warning states that the patient should consult his or her physician if there are questions about alternatives.

NASAL SPRAY

Nasacort AQ nasal spray is a nonchlorofluorocarbon (non-CFC) containing metered-dose pump spray. The contents of one 6.5 g sample bottle provide 30 actuations, and the contents of one 16.5 g bottle provide 120 actuations. The bottle should be discarded when the labeled number of actuations have been reached even though the bottle is not completely empty.

It is supplied in a white high-density polyethylene container with a metered-dose pump unit, white nasal adapter, and patient instructions.

Keep out of reach of children.

Storage: Store at controlled room temperature, 20-25°C (68-77°F).

TOPICAL

DESCRIPTION

The topical corticosteroids constitute a class of primarily synthetic steroids used as anti-inflammatory and antipruritic agents. The steroids in this class include triamcinolone acetonide. Triamcinolone acetonide is designated chemically as 9-Fluoro-11β,16α,17,21-tetrahydroxypregna-1,4-diene-3,20-dione cyclic 16,17-acetal with acetone. The empirical formula is $C_{24}H_{31}FO_6$ and the molecular weight is 434.50.

CREAM

Each gram of 0.025%, 0.1% and 0.5% Kenalog cream (triamcinolone acetonide cream) provides 0.25 mg, 1 mg or 5 mg triamcinolone acetonide, respectively, in a vanishing cream base containing propylene glycol, cetearyl monostearate, polyethylene glycol monostearate, simethicone, sorbic acid, and purified water.

LOTION

Each gram of 0.025%, 0.1% and 0.5% Kenalog lotion (triamcinolone acetonide lotion) provides 0.25 mg and 1 mg triamcinolone acetonide, respectively, in a lotion base containing propylene glycol, cetyl alcohol, stearyl alcohol, sorbitan monopalmitate, polysorbate 20, simethicone, and purified water.

OINTMENT

Each gram of 0.025%, 0.1% and 0.5% Kenalog ointment (triamcinolone acetonide ointment) provides 0.25 mg, 1 mg or 5 mg triamcinolone acetonide, respectively, in Plastibase (plasticized hydrocarbon gel), a polyethylene and mineral oil gel base.

AEROSOL SPRAY

A 2 second application, which covers an area approximately the size of the hand, delivers an amount of triamcinolone acetonide not exceeding 0.2 mg. After spraying, the nonvolatile remaining on the skin contains approximately 0.2% triamcinolone acetonide. Each gram of spray provides 0.147 mg triamcinolone acetonide in a vehicle of isopropyl palmitate, dehydrated alcohol (10.3%), and isobutane propellant.

CLINICAL PHARMACOLOGY

Topical corticosteroids share anti-inflammatory, antipruritic and vasoconstrictive actions.

The mechanism of anti-inflammatory activity of the topical corticosteroids is unclear. Various laboratory methods, including vasoconstrictor assays are used to compare and predict potencies and/or clinical efficacies of the topical corticosteroids. There is some evidence to suggest that a recognizable correlation exists between vasoconstrictor potency and therapeutic efficacy in man.

PHARMACOKINETICS

The extent of percutaneous absorption of topical corticosteroids is determined by many factors including the vehicle, the integrity of the epidermal barrier, and the use of occlusive dressings.

Topical corticosteroids can be absorbed from normal intact skin. Inflammation and/or other disease processes in the skin increase percutaneous absorption. Occlusive dressings substantially increase the percutaneous absorption of topical corticosteroids. Thus, occlusive dressings may be a valuable therapeutic adjunct for treatment of resistant dermatoses (see DOSAGE AND ADMINISTRATION).

Once absorbed through the skin, topical corticosteroids are handled through pharmacokinetic pathways similar to systemically administered corticosteroids. Corticosteroids are bound to plasma proteins in varying degrees. Corticosteroids are metabolized primarily in the liver and are then excreted by the kidneys. Some of the topical corticosteroids and their metabolites are also excreted into the bile.

INDICATIONS AND USAGE

Topical triamcinolone acetonide is indicated for the relief of the inflammatory and pruritic manifestations of corticosteroid-responsive dermatoses.

CONTRAINDICATIONS

Topical corticosteroids are contraindicated in those patients with a history of hypersensitivity to any of the components of the preparations.

PRECAUTIONS

GENERAL

Systemic absorption of topical corticosteroids has produced reversible hypothalamic-pituitary-adrenal (HPA) axis suppression, manifestations of Cushing's syndrome, hyperglycemia, and glucosuria in some patients.

Conditions which augment systemic absorption include the application of the more potent steroids, use over large surface areas, prolonged use, and the addition of occlusive dressings.

Therefore, patients receiving a large dose of any potent topical steroid applied to a large surface area or under an occlusive dressing should be evaluated periodically for evidence of HPA axis suppression by using the urinary free cortisol and ACTH stimulation tests, and for impairment of thermal homeostasis. If HPA axis suppression or elevation of the body temperature occurs, an attempt should be made to withdraw the drug, to reduce the frequency of application, substitute a less potent steroid, or use a sequential approach when utilizing the occlusive technique.

Recovery of HPA axis function and thermal homeostasis are generally prompt and complete upon discontinuation of the drug. Infrequently, signs and symptoms of steroid withdrawal may occur, requiring supplemental systemic corticosteroids. Occasionally, a patient may develop a sensitivity reaction to a particular occlusive dressing material or adhesive and a substitute material may be necessary.

Children may absorb proportionally larger amounts of topical corticosteroids and thus be more susceptible to systemic toxicity (see Pediatric Use).

If irritation develops, topical corticosteroids should be discontinued and appropriate therapy instituted.

In the presence of dermatological infections, the use of an appropriate antifungal or antibacterial agent should be instituted. If a favorable response does not occur promptly, the corticosteroid should be discontinued until the infection has been adequately controlled.

These preparations are not for ophthalmic use.

INFORMATION FOR THE PATIENT

Patients using topical corticosteroids should receive the following information and instructions:

This medication is to be used as directed by the physician. It is for dermatologic use only. Avoid contact with the eyes.

Patients should be advised not to use this medication for any disorder *other than for which it was prescribed.*

The treated skin area should not be bandaged or otherwise covered or wrapped as to be occlusive unless directed by the physician.

Patients should report any signs of local adverse reactions especially under occlusive dressing.

Parents of pediatric patients should be advised not to use tight-fitting diapers or plastic pants on a child being treated in the diaper area, as these garments may constitute occlusive dressings.

LABORATORY TESTS

A urinary free cortisol test and ACTH stimulation test may be helpful in evaluating HPA axis suppression.

CARCINOGENESIS, MUTAGENESIS, AND IMPAIRMENT OF FERTILITY

Long-term animal studies have not been performed to evaluate the carcinogenic potential or the effect on fertility of topical corticosteroids.

Studies to determine mutagenicity with prednisolone and hydrocortisone showed negative results.

PREGNANCY, TERATOGENIC EFFECTS, PREGNANCY CATEGORY C

Corticosteroids are generally teratogenic in laboratory animals when administered systemically at relatively low dosage levels. The more potent corticosteroids have been shown to be teratogenic after dermal application in laboratory animals. There are no adequate and well-controlled studies in pregnant women on teratogenic effects from topically applied corticosteroids. Therefore, topical corticosteroids should be used during pregnancy only if the potential benefit justifies the potential risk to the fetus. Drugs of this class should not be used extensively on pregnant patients, in large amounts, or for prolonged periods of time.

NURSING MOTHERS

It is not known whether topical administration of corticosteroids could result in sufficient systemic absorption to produce detectable quantities in breast milk. Systemically administered corticosteroids are secreted into breast milk in quantities **not** likely to have a deleterious effect on the infant. Nevertheless, caution should be exercised when topical corticosteroids are administered to a nursing woman.

PEDIATRIC USE

Pediatric patients may demonstrate greater susceptibility to topical corticosteroid-induced HPA axis suppression and Cushing's syndrome than mature patients because of a larger skin surface area to body weight ratio.

HPA axis suppression, Cushing's syndrome, and intracranial hypertension have been reported in children receiving topical corticosteroids. Manifestations of adrenal suppression in children include linear growth retardation, delayed weight gain, low plasma cortisol levels, and absence of response to ACTH stimulation. Manifestation of intracranial hypertension include bulging fontanelles, headaches, and bilateral papilledema.

Administration of topical corticosteroids to children should be limited to the least amount compatible with an effective therapeutic regimen. Chronic corticosteroid therapy may interfere with the growth and development of children.

ADVERSE REACTIONS

The following local adverse reactions are reported infrequently with topical corticosteroids, but may occur more frequently with the use of occlusive dressings (reactions are listed in an approximate decreasing order of occurrence): burning, itching, irritation, dryness, folliculitis, hypertrichosis, acneiform eruptions, hypopigmentation, perioral dermatitis, allergic contact dermatitis, maceration of the skin, secondary infection, skin atrophy, striae, and miliaria.

DOSAGE AND ADMINISTRATION

CREAM

Apply triamcinolone acetonide cream 0.025% to the affected area 2-4 times daily. Rub in gently.

Apply the 0.1% or the 0.5% triamcinolone acetonide cream, as appropriate, to the affected area 2-3 times daily. Rub in gently.

Occlusive Dressing Technique

Occlusive dressings may be used for the management of psoriasis or other recalcitrant conditions. Gently rub a small amount of cream into the lesion until it disappears. Reapply the preparation leaving a thin coating on the lesion, cover with pliable nonporous film, and seal the edges. If needed, additional moisture may be provided by covering the lesion with a dampened clean cotton cloth before the nonporous film is applied or by briefly wetting the affected area with water immediately prior to applying the medication. The frequency of changing dressings is best determined on an individual basis. It may be convenient to apply triamcinolone acetonide cream under an occlusive dressing in the evening and to remove the dressing in the morning (*i.e.,* 12 hour occlusion). When utilizing the 12 hour occlusion regimen, additional cream should be applied, without occlusion, during the day. Reapplication is essential at each dressing change.

If an infection develops, the use of occlusive dressings should be discontinued and appropriate antimicrobial therapy instituted.

LOTION

Apply the 0.025% triamcinolone acetonide lotion to the affected area 2-4 times daily. Rub in gently.

Apply the 0.1% or the 0.5% triamcinolone acetonide lotion to the affected area 2-3 times daily. Rub in gently.

Occlusive Dressing Technique

Occlusive dressings may be used for the management of psoriasis or other recalcitrant conditions. Gently rub a small amount of lotion into the lesion until it disappears. Reapply the preparation leaving a thin coating on the lesion, cover with pliable nonporous film, and seal the edges. If needed, additional moisture may be provided by covering the lesion with a dampened clean cotton cloth before the nonporous film is applied or by briefly wetting the affected area with water immediately prior to applying the medication. The frequency of changing dressings is best determined on an individual basis. It may be convenient to apply triamcinolone acetonide lotion under an occlusive dressing in the evening and to remove the dressing in the morning (*i.e.,* 12 hour occlusion). When utilizing the 12 hour occlusion regimen, additional lotion should be applied, without occlusion, during the day. Reapplication is essential at each dressing change.

If an infection develops, the use of occlusive dressings should be discontinued and appropriate antimicrobial therapy instituted.

OINTMENT

Apply a thin film of triamcinolone acetonide ointment 0.025% to the affected area 2-4 times daily.

Apply a thin film of the 0.1% or the 0.5% triamcinolone acetonide ointment, as appropriate, to the affected area 2-3 times daily. Rub in gently.

Occlusive Dressing Technique

Occlusive dressings may be used for the management of psoriasis or other recalcitrant conditions. Apply a thin film of ointment to the lesion, cover with pliable nonporous film, and seal the edges. If needed, additional moisture may be provided by covering the lesion with a dampened clean cotton cloth before the nonporous film is applied or by briefly wetting the affected area with water immediately prior to applying the medication. The frequency of changing dressings is best determined on an individual basis. It may be convenient to apply triamcinolone acetonide ointment under an occlusive dressing in the evening and to remove the dressing in the morning (*i.e.,* 12 hour occlusion). When utilizing the 12 hour occlusion regimen, additional ointment should be applied, without occlusion, during the day. Reapplication is essential at each dressing change.

If an infection develops, the use of occlusive dressings should be discontinued and appropriate antimicrobial therapy instituted.

T

AEROSOL SPRAY

Directions for use of the spray can are provided on the label. The preparation may be applied to any area of the body, but when it is sprayed about the face, care should be taken to see that the eyes are covered, and that inhalation of the spray is avoided.

Three (3) or 4 applications daily of triamcinolone acetonide spray are generally adequate.

Occlusive Dressing Technique

Occlusive dressings may be used for the management of psoriasis or other recalcitrant conditions. Spray a small amount of preparation onto the lesion, cover with a pliable nonporous film, and seal the edges. If needed, additional moisture may be provided by covering the lesion with a dampened clean cotton cloth before the nonporous film is applied or by briefly wetting the affected area with water immediately prior to applying the medication. The frequency of changing dressings is best determined on an individual basis. It may be convenient to apply the spray under an occlusive dressing in the evening and to remove the dressing in the morning (*i.e.,* 12 hour occlusion). When utilizing the 12 hour occlusion regimen, additional spray should be applied, without occlusion, during the day.

If an infection develops, the use of occlusive dressings should be discontinued.

HOW SUPPLIED

KENALOG CREAMS

Kenalog cream is available in 0.025%, 0.1% and 0.5% dosage strengths.

Storage: Store at room temperature; avoid freezing.

KENALOG LOTION

Kenalog lotion is available in 0.025% and 0.1% dosage strengths.

Storage: Store at room temperature; avoid freezing.

KENALOG OINTMENT

Kenalog ointment is available in 0.025%, 0.1% and 0.5% dosage strengths.

Storage: Store at room temperature.

KENALOG SPRAY

Kenalog spray is supplied in 23 g and 63 g aerosol cans.

Storage: Store a room temperature; avoid excessive heat.

PRODUCT LISTING - RATED THERAPEUTICALLY EQUIVALENT

Size	Price	Product, Manufacturer	NDC
Cream - Topical - 0.025%			
15 gm	$0.96	GENERIC, Syosset Laboratories Company	47854-0575-17
15 gm	$1.00	GENERIC, Raway Pharmacal Inc	00686-0063-35
15 gm	$1.20	GENERIC, Thames Pharmacal Company Inc	49158-0139-20
15 gm	$1.28	GENERIC, Moore, H.L. Drug Exchange Inc	00839-6127-47
15 gm	$1.40	GENERIC, Taro Pharmaceuticals U.S.A. Inc	51672-1283-01
15 gm	$1.40	GENERIC, Taro Pharmaceuticals U.S.A. Inc	51672-1285-01
15 gm	$1.41	GENERIC, Qualitest Products Inc	00603-7850-74
15 gm	$1.50	GENERIC, Clay-Park Laboratories Inc	45802-0063-35
15 gm	$1.55	GENERIC, Major Pharmaceuticals Inc	00904-2740-36
15 gm	$1.60	GENERIC, Ivax Corporation	00182-1216-51
15 gm	$1.65	GENERIC, Interstate Drug Exchange Inc	00814-0850-93
15 gm	$1.74	GENERIC, Watson/Schein Pharmaceuticals Inc	00591-7211-86
15 gm	$1.79	GENERIC, Major Pharmaceuticals Inc	00904-2738-36
15 gm	$1.82	GENERIC, Fougera	00168-0003-15
15 gm	$10.00	ARISTOCORT A, Fujisawa	00469-5101-15
29 gm	$3.00	GENERIC, Syosset Laboratories Company	47854-0575-05
60 gm	$24.64	ARISTOCORT A, Fujisawa	00469-5101-60
80 gm	$2.55	GENERIC, Moore, H.L. Drug Exchange Inc	00839-6392-46
80 gm	$2.64	GENERIC, Syosset Laboratories Company	47854-0575-28
80 gm	$2.80	GENERIC, Raway Pharmacal Inc	00686-0063-36
80 gm	$2.91	FEDERAL UPPER LIMIT, H.C.F.A. F F P	99999-2371-08
80 gm	$3.27	GENERIC, Qualitest Products Inc	00603-7850-90
80 gm	$3.31	GENERIC, Moore, H.L. Drug Exchange Inc	00839-6127-46
80 gm	$3.50	GENERIC, Clay-Park Laboratories Inc	00414-0063-36
80 gm	$3.50	GENERIC, Alpharma Uspd Makers Of Barre and Nmc	00472-0300-80
80 gm	$3.50	GENERIC, Major Pharmaceuticals Inc	00904-2738-11
80 gm	$3.50	GENERIC, Clay-Park Laboratories Inc	45802-0063-36
80 gm	$3.60	GENERIC, Interstate Drug Exchange Inc	00814-0850-97
80 gm	$4.16	GENERIC, Taro Pharmaceuticals U.S.A. Inc	51672-1283-08
80 gm	$4.16	GENERIC, Taro Pharmaceuticals U.S.A. Inc	51672-1285-08
80 gm	$4.26	GENERIC, Fougera	00168-0003-80
80 gm	$4.32	GENERIC, Watson/Schein Pharmaceuticals Inc	00364-7211-60
80 gm	$6.12	GENERIC, Thames Pharmacal Company Inc	49158-0139-21
80 gm	$6.25	GENERIC, G and W Laboratories Inc	00713-0226-80
100 gm	$1.85	GENERIC, Cmc-Consolidated Midland Corporation	00223-4447-15
100 gm	$1.90	GENERIC, Cmc-Consolidated Midland Corporation	00223-4449-15
454 gm	$6.25	GENERIC, Raway Pharmacal Inc	00686-0063-05
454 gm	$7.35	GENERIC, Syosset Laboratories Company	47854-0575-13
454 gm	$8.86	GENERIC, Clay-Park Laboratories Inc	00414-0063-05
454 gm	$8.86	GENERIC, Clay-Park Laboratories Inc	45802-0063-05
454 gm	$8.99	GENERIC, Major Pharmaceuticals Inc	00904-2738-27
454 gm	$9.18	GENERIC, Alpharma Uspd Makers Of Barre and Nmc	00472-0300-16
454 gm	$9.35	GENERIC, Ivax Corporation	00182-1216-45
480 gm	$8.59	GENERIC, Thames Pharmacal Company Inc	49158-0139-16
2270 gm	$20.64	GENERIC, Moore, H.L. Drug Exchange Inc	00839-6127-48
2270 gm	$32.40	GENERIC, Clay-Park Laboratories Inc	45802-0063-29
Cream - Topical - 0.1%			
15 gm	$1.30	GENERIC, Thames Pharmacal Company Inc	49158-0140-20
15 gm	$1.65	GENERIC, Interstate Drug Exchange Inc	00814-0851-93
15 gm	$1.80	GENERIC, Clay-Park Laboratories Inc	45802-0064-35
15 gm	$2.00	GENERIC, Physicians Total Care	54868-0843-01
15 gm	$2.01	GENERIC, Qualitest Products Inc	00603-7851-74
15 gm	$2.03	GENERIC, Watson/Rugby Laboratories Inc	00536-5225-20
15 gm	$2.05	GENERIC, Ivax Corporation	00182-1217-51
15 gm	$2.05	GENERIC, Major Pharmaceuticals Inc	00904-2741-36
15 gm	$2.08	GENERIC, Taro Pharmaceuticals U.S.A. Inc	51672-1284-01

Size	Price	Product	NDC
15 gm	$2.64	GENERIC, G and W Laboratories Inc	00713-0225-15
15 gm	$2.70	GENERIC, Fougera	00168-0004-15
15 gm	$4.25	GENERIC, Alpharma Uspd Makers Of Barre and Nmc	00472-0301-15
15 gm	$8.48	ARISTOCORT TOPICAL, Allscripts Pharmaceutical Company	54569-2799-00
15 gm	$13.22	ARISTOCORT A, Physicians Total Care	54868-0966-01
15 gm	$13.35	ARISTOCORT A, Fujisawa	00469-5102-15
15 gm	$15.77	KENALOG, Bristol-Myers Squibb	00003-0506-20
29 gm	$2.60	GENERIC, Syosset Laboratories Company	47854-0576-05
30 gm	$2.33	GENERIC, Interstate Drug Exchange Inc	00814-0851-72
30 gm	$2.50	GENERIC, Watson/Schein Pharmaceuticals Inc	00364-7212-56
30 gm	$2.50	GENERIC, Watson Laboratories Inc	00591-7212-30
30 gm	$2.50	GENERIC, Watson/Schein Pharmaceuticals Inc	00591-7346-30
30 gm	$3.45	GENERIC, Physicians Total Care	54868-0843-00
30 gm	$4.20	GENERIC, Thames Pharmacal Company Inc	49158-0140-08
30 gm	$4.28	GENERIC, Dermol Pharmaceuticals Inc	50744-0105-05
30 gm	$4.28	GENERIC, Dermol Pharmaceuticals Inc	50744-0576-05
30 gm	$7.46	GENERIC, Del Ray Laboratories Inc	00316-0170-01
57 gm	$7.95	GENERIC, Syosset Laboratories Company	47854-0576-07
60 gm	$34.13	ARISTOCORT A, Fujisawa	00469-5102-60
60 gm	$38.49	KENALOG, Bristol-Myers Squibb	00003-0506-46
80 gm	$3.58	FEDERAL UPPER LIMIT, H.C.F.A. F F P	99999-2371-11
80 gm	$3.80	GENERIC, Thames Pharmacal Company Inc	49158-0140-21
80 gm	$4.02	GENERIC, Syosset Laboratories Company	47854-0576-28
80 gm	$4.37	GENERIC, Physicians Total Care	54868-0843-02
80 gm	$4.64	GENERIC, Qualitest Products Inc	00603-7851-90
80 gm	$4.80	GENERIC, Watson/Schein Pharmaceuticals Inc	00364-7212-60
80 gm	$4.80	GENERIC, Watson Laboratories Inc	00591-7212-84
80 gm	$4.88	GENERIC, Interstate Drug Exchange Inc	00814-0851-97
80 gm	$5.10	GENERIC, Suppositoria Laboratories Inc	00414-0064-36
80 gm	$5.10	GENERIC, Watson/Rugby Laboratories Inc	00536-5225-30
80 gm	$5.10	GENERIC, Clay-Park Laboratories Inc	45802-0064-36
80 gm	$5.10	GENERIC, Taro Pharmaceuticals U.S.A. Inc	51672-1284-08
80 gm	$5.39	GENERIC, Ivax Corporation	00182-1217-53
80 gm	$5.72	GENERIC, Fougera	00168-0004-80
80 gm	$5.75	GENERIC, Alpharma Uspd Makers Of Barre and Nmc	00472-0301-80
80 gm	$6.43	GENERIC, Mutual/United Research Laboratories	00677-0747-46
80 gm	$6.44	GENERIC, G and W Laboratories Inc	00713-0225-80
80 gm	$6.53	GENERIC, Major Pharmaceuticals Inc	00904-2741-11
80 gm	$8.08	GENERIC, Dermol Pharmaceuticals Inc	50744-0576-80
80 gm	$46.52	KENALOG, Bristol-Myers Squibb	00003-0506-49
90 gm	$11.05	GENERIC, Del Ray Laboratories Inc	00316-0170-03
100 gm	$1.95	GENERIC, Cmc-Consolidated Midland Corporation	00223-4446-15
100 gm	$2.25	GENERIC, Cmc-Consolidated Midland Corporation	00223-4448-15
454 gm	$15.98	GENERIC, Thames Pharmacal Company Inc	49158-0140-16
454 gm	$16.98	GENERIC, Syosset Laboratories Company	47854-0576-13
454 gm	$18.11	GENERIC, Physicians Total Care	54868-0843-03
454 gm	$18.53	GENERIC, Major Pharmaceuticals Inc	00904-2741-27
454 gm	$19.50	GENERIC, Ivax Corporation	00182-1217-45
454 gm	$19.90	GENERIC, Suppositoria Laboratories Inc	00414-0055-05
454 gm	$19.90	GENERIC, Clay-Park Laboratories Inc	45802-0064-05
454 gm	$21.50	GENERIC, Fougera	00168-0004-16
454 gm	$22.14	GENERIC, Alpharma Uspd Makers Of Barre and Nmc	00472-0301-16
454 gm	$26.39	GENERIC, Mutual/United Research Laboratories	00677-0747-44
480 gm	$19.90	GENERIC, Suppositoria Laboratories Inc	00414-0064-05
2270 gm	$48.75	GENERIC, Clay-Park Laboratories Inc	45802-0064-29
2270 gm	$60.24	GENERIC, Moore, H.L. Drug Exchange Inc	00839-6126-48
2270 gm	$66.48	GENERIC, Major Pharmaceuticals Inc	00904-2741-33
2270 gm	$74.88	GENERIC, Thames Pharmacal Company Inc	49158-0140-22
2270 gm	$77.48	GENERIC, Alpharma Uspd Makers Of Barre and Nmc	00472-0301-05
2270 gm	$77.50	GENERIC, Mutual/United Research Laboratories	00677-0747-47
2270 gm	$79.58	GENERIC, Clay-Park Laboratories Inc	00414-0064-29

Cream - Topical - 0.5%

Size	Price	Product	NDC
15 gm	$2.83	FEDERAL UPPER LIMIT, H.C.F.A. F F P	99999-2371-11
15 gm	$2.96	GENERIC, Moore, H.L. Drug Exchange Inc	00839-6128-47
15 gm	$3.90	GENERIC, Interstate Drug Exchange Inc	00814-0852-93
15 gm	$3.95	GENERIC, Qualitest Products Inc	00603-7852-74
15 gm	$4.00	GENERIC, Major Pharmaceuticals Inc	00904-2744-36
15 gm	$4.27	GENERIC, Mutual/United Research Laboratories	00677-0751-40
15 gm	$4.28	GENERIC, Watson/Schein Pharmaceuticals Inc	00364-7213-72
15 gm	$4.28	GENERIC, Watson/Rugby Laboratories Inc	00536-5200-20
15 gm	$4.28	GENERIC, Watson/Rugby Laboratories Inc	00591-7213-86
15 gm	$4.55	GENERIC, Ivax Corporation	00182-1218-51
15 gm	$4.61	GENERIC, Fougera	00168-0002-15
15 gm	$4.95	GENERIC, Geneva Pharmaceuticals	00781-7046-27
15 gm	$4.99	GENERIC, Clay-Park Laboratories Inc	45802-0065-35
15 gm	$6.32	GENERIC, Thames Pharmacal Company Inc	49158-0141-20
15 gm	$36.62	ARISTOCORT A, Fujisawa	00469-5104-15
20 gm	$45.74	KENALOG, Westwood Squibb Pharmaceutical Corporation	00003-1483-20
29 gm	$10.95	GENERIC, Syosset Laboratories Company	47854-0577-05
100 gm	$5.00	GENERIC, Cmc-Consolidated Midland Corporation	00223-4443-20
100 gm	$5.00	GENERIC, Cmc-Consolidated Midland Corporation	00223-4444-20
227 gm	$26.20	GENERIC, Syosset Laboratories Company	47854-0577-11

Lotion - Topical - 0.025%

Size	Price	Product	NDC
60 ml	$7.50	GENERIC, Raway Pharmacal Inc	00686-1248-02
60 ml	$37.79	GENERIC, Morton Grove Pharmaceuticals Inc	60432-0560-60
60 ml	$44.22	KENALOG, Bristol-Myers Squibb	00003-0173-60

Lotion - Topical - 0.1%

Size	Price	Product	NDC
60 ml	$7.29	FEDERAL UPPER LIMIT, H.C.F.A. F F P	99999-2371-23
60 ml	$8.28	GENERIC, Qualitest Products Inc	00603-7855-49
60 ml	$8.76	GENERIC, Moore, H.L. Drug Exchange Inc	00839-6726-50
60 ml	$8.78	GENERIC, Watson/Schein Pharmaceuticals Inc	00364-7346-58
60 ml	$8.78	GENERIC, Watson/Schein Pharmaceuticals Inc	00364-7346-60
60 ml	$8.78	GENERIC, Watson/Rugby Laboratories Inc	00591-7346-60
60 ml	$10.22	GENERIC, Ivax Corporation	00182-1777-68
60 ml	$42.42	GENERIC, Morton Grove Pharmaceuticals Inc	60432-0561-60
60 ml	$49.65	KENALOG, Bristol-Myers Squibb	00003-0502-70

Ointment - Topical - 0.025%

Size	Price	Product	NDC
15 gm	$1.07	GENERIC, Moore, H.L. Drug Exchange Inc	00839-6392-47
15 gm	$1.34	GENERIC, Qualitest Products Inc	00603-7858-74
15 gm	$1.50	GENERIC, Clay-Park Laboratories Inc	45802-0054-35
15 gm	$2.75	GENERIC, Raway Pharmacal Inc	00686-0054-35
60 gm	$8.20	GENERIC, Major Pharmaceuticals Inc	00904-2739-03
80 gm	$2.80	GENERIC, Raway Pharmacal Inc	00686-0054-36
80 gm	$3.50	GENERIC, Clay-Park Laboratories Inc	45802-0054-36
80 gm	$4.25	GENERIC, Ivax Corporation	00182-1394-53
80 gm	$4.50	GENERIC, Clay-Park Laboratories Inc	00414-0054-36
80 gm	$4.92	GENERIC, Fougera	00168-0005-80
100 gm	$8.95	GENERIC, Cmc-Consolidated Midland Corporation	00223-6635-60
454 gm	$6.25	GENERIC, Raway Pharmacal Inc	00686-0054-05
454 gm	$8.86	GENERIC, Clay-Park Laboratories Inc	00414-0054-05
454 gm	$8.86	GENERIC, Clay-Park Laboratories Inc	45802-0054-05
454 gm	$9.36	GENERIC, Ivax Corporation	00182-1394-45
2270 gm	$32.40	GENERIC, Clay-Park Laboratories Inc	45802-0054-29

Ointment - Topical - 0.1%

Size	Price	Product	NDC
15 gm	$1.55	GENERIC, Moore, H.L. Drug Exchange Inc	00839-6391-47
15 gm	$1.80	GENERIC, Clay-Park Laboratories Inc	45802-0055-35
15 gm	$2.01	GENERIC, Qualitest Products Inc	00603-7859-74
15 gm	$2.03	GENERIC, Watson/Rugby Laboratories Inc	00536-5180-20
15 gm	$2.05	GENERIC, Ivax Corporation	00182-1395-51
15 gm	$2.05	GENERIC, Watson/Schein Pharmaceuticals Inc	00364-7360-72
15 gm	$2.05	GENERIC, Watson Laboratories Inc	00591-7360-86
15 gm	$2.25	GENERIC, Major Pharmaceuticals Inc	00904-2743-36
15 gm	$2.70	GENERIC, Fougera	00168-0006-15
15 gm	$2.75	GENERIC, Alpharma Uspd Makers Of Barre and Nmc	00472-0306-15
15 gm	$3.60	GENERIC, Thames Pharmacal Company Inc	49158-0160-20
15 gm	$11.75	ARISTOCORT A, Fujisawa	00469-5105-15
15 gm	$15.13	KENALOG, Allscripts Pharmaceutical Company	54569-0766-00
15 gm	$15.76	KENALOG, Bristol-Myers Squibb	00003-0508-20
30 gm	$4.20	GENERIC, Thames Pharmacal Company Inc	49158-0160-08
30 gm	$7.16	GENERIC, Del Ray Laboratories Inc	00316-0175-01
60 gm	$9.00	GENERIC, Major Pharmaceuticals Inc	00904-2742-03
60 gm	$10.95	GENERIC, Geneva Pharmaceuticals	00781-7048-61
60 gm	$30.06	ARISTOCORT A, Fujisawa	00469-5105-60
60 gm	$38.09	KENALOG, Bristol-Myers Squibb	00003-0508-56
80 gm	$4.02	FEDERAL UPPER LIMIT, H.C.F.A. F F P	99999-2371-28
80 gm	$4.88	GENERIC, Interstate Drug Exchange Inc	00814-0854-97
80 gm	$5.10	GENERIC, Clay-Park Laboratories Inc	00414-0055-36
80 gm	$5.10	GENERIC, Watson/Rugby Laboratories Inc	00536-5180-30
80 gm	$5.10	GENERIC, Major Pharmaceuticals Inc	00904-2743-11
80 gm	$5.10	GENERIC, Clay-Park Laboratories Inc	45802-0055-36
80 gm	$5.72	GENERIC, Fougera	00168-0006-80
80 gm	$5.75	GENERIC, Alpharma Uspd Makers Of Barre and Nmc	00472-0306-80
80 gm	$6.60	GENERIC, Thames Pharmacal Company Inc	49158-0160-21
90 gm	$10.51	GENERIC, Del Ray Laboratories Inc	00316-0175-03
100 gm	$9.95	GENERIC, Cmc-Consolidated Midland Corporation	00223-6636-60
454 gm	$19.90	GENERIC, Clay-Park Laboratories Inc	45802-0055-05
454 gm	$20.50	GENERIC, Major Pharmaceuticals Inc	00904-2743-27
454 gm	$26.40	GENERIC, Ivax Corporation	00182-1395-45
454 gm	$26.40	GENERIC, Thames Pharmacal Company Inc	49158-0160-16

Size	Price	Product	NDC
2270 gm	$77.76	GENERIC, Clay-Park Laboratories Inc	45802-0055-29
Ointment - Topical - 0.5%			
15 gm	$4.99	GENERIC, Clay-Park Laboratories Inc	45802-0049-35
15 gm	$5.88	GENERIC, Ivax Corporation	00182-5068-51
Paste - Dental - 0.1%			
5 gm	$4.14	FEDERAL UPPER LIMIT, H.C.F.A. F F P	99999-2371-37
Paste - Mucous Membrane - 0.1%			
5 gm	$4.44	GENERIC, Moore, H.L. Drug Exchange Inc	00839-7403-41
5 gm	$4.65	GENERIC, Qualitest Products Inc	00603-7870-69
5 gm	$6.40	GENERIC, Ivax Corporation	00182-5047-49
5 gm	$8.89	GENERIC, Watson/Schein Pharmaceuticals Inc	00364-2218-53
5 gm	$9.80	GENERIC, Major Pharmaceuticals Inc	00904-3643-68
5 gm	$9.89	GENERIC, Geneva Pharmaceuticals	00781-7039-39
5 gm	$9.90	GENERIC, Taro Pharmaceuticals U.S.A. Inc	51672-1267-05
5 gm	$14.13	GENERIC, Allscripts Pharmaceutical Company	54569-3473-00
5 gm	$16.99	KENALOG, Allscripts Pharmaceutical Company	54569-1091-00
5 gm	$17.70	KENALOG, Bristol-Myers Squibb	00003-0496-20

PRODUCT LISTING - RATED NOT THERAPEUTICALLY EQUIVALENT

Size	Price	Product	NDC
Suspension - Injectable - acetonide 40 mg/ml			
1 ml	$4.66	GENERIC, Moore, H.L. Drug Exchange Inc	00839-6287-82
1 ml	$6.20	KENALOG-40, Southwood Pharmaceuticals Inc	58016-9799-01
1 ml	$6.79	KENALOG-40, Bristol-Myers Squibb	00003-0293-05
1 ml	$8.07	KENALOG-40, Physicians Total Care	54868-0235-00
5 ml	$6.95	GENERIC, Roberts/Hauck Pharmaceutical Corporation	43797-0002-11
5 ml	$7.00	GENERIC, Med Tek Pharmaceuticals Inc	52349-0112-05
5 ml	$8.49	KEN-JEC 40, Hauser, A.F. Inc	52637-0040-05
5 ml	$9.25	GENERIC, Roberts/Hauck Pharmaceutical Corporation	43797-0114-11
5 ml	$10.00	GENERIC, Bolan Pharmaceutical Inc	44437-0182-75
5 ml	$10.33	GENERIC, Forest Pharmaceuticals	00785-8047-05
5 ml	$11.00	GENERIC, Keene Pharmaceuticals Inc	00588-5373-75
5 ml	$11.25	GENERIC, Interstate Drug Exchange Inc	00814-8007-38
5 ml	$11.35	GENERIC, Hyrex Pharmaceuticals	00314-3400-75
5 ml	$14.93	GENERIC, General Injectables and Vaccines Inc	52584-0204-05
5 ml	$17.50	GENERIC, Forest Pharmaceuticals	00456-0781-05
5 ml	$17.60	GENERIC, Major Pharmaceuticals Inc	00904-0886-05
5 ml	$17.96	GENERIC, Moore, H.L. Drug Exchange Inc	00839-6287-25
5 ml	$19.25	GENERIC, Geneva Pharmaceuticals	00781-3116-75
5 ml	$19.80	GENERIC, Interstate Drug Exchange Inc	00814-8008-38
5 ml	$31.48	KENALOG-40, Allscripts Pharmaceutical Company	54569-1398-00
5 ml	$34.43	KENALOG-40, Bristol-Myers Squibb	00003-0293-20
5 ml	$38.52	KENALOG-40, Physicians Total Care	54868-0235-01
10 ml	$51.43	KENALOG-40, Bristol-Myers Squibb	00003-0293-28
25 ml	$81.25	GENERIC, Cmc-Consolidated Midland Corporation	00223-8691-25
100 ml	$6.50	GENERIC, Cmc-Consolidated Midland Corporation	00223-8691-05
100 ml	$8.00	GENERIC, Cmc-Consolidated Midland Corporation	00223-8690-05

PRODUCT LISTING - EQUIVALENTS NOT AVAILABLE

Size	Price	Product	NDC
Aerosol - Nasal - 55 mcg/Inh			
10 gm	$43.64	NASACORT, Allscripts Pharmaceutical Company	54569-3557-00
10 gm	$49.88	NASACORT, Physicians Total Care	54868-2163-01
10 gm	$59.85	NASACORT, Aventis Pharmaceuticals	00075-1505-43
Aerosol with Adapter - Inhalation - 100 mcg/Inh			
20 gm	$55.40	AZMACORT, Allscripts Pharmaceutical Company	54569-0053-00
20 gm	$63.12	AZMACORT, Pharma Pac	52959-0286-03
20 gm	$63.16	AZMACORT, Physicians Total Care	54868-1268-01
20 gm	$72.69	AZMACORT, Aventis Pharmaceuticals	00075-0060-37
20 gm	$75.96	AZMACORT, Prescript Pharmaceuticals	00247-0190-20
Cream - Topical - 0.025%			
15 gm	$1.79	GENERIC, Physicians Total Care	54868-1060-01
15 gm	$1.88	GENERIC, Allscripts Pharmaceutical Company	54569-1121-00
15 gm	$4.12	GENERIC, Prescript Pharmaceuticals	00247-0018-15
15 gm	$4.88	GENERIC, Southwood Pharmaceuticals Inc	58016-3034-01
15 gm	$9.95	GENERIC, Pharma Pac	52959-0199-03
30 gm	$4.89	GENERIC, Prescript Pharmaceuticals	00247-0018-30
60 gm	$6.42	GENERIC, Prescript Pharmaceuticals	00247-0018-60
80 gm	$3.75	GENERIC, Physicians Total Care	54868-1060-00
80 gm	$4.25	GENERIC, Allscripts Pharmaceutical Company	54569-1774-01
80 gm	$7.45	GENERIC, Prescript Pharmaceuticals	00247-0018-80
80 gm	$12.75	GENERIC, Pharma Pac	52959-0199-01
Cream - Topical - 0.1%			
15 gm	$2.33	GENERIC, Allscripts Pharmaceutical Company	54569-1084-00
15 gm	$3.12	GENERIC, Alpharma Uspd Makers Of Barre and Nmc	63874-0820-15
15 gm	$4.12	GENERIC, Prescript Pharmaceuticals	00247-0017-15
15 gm	$10.98	GENERIC, Southwood Pharmaceuticals Inc	58016-3035-01
15 gm	$12.15	GENERIC, Pharma Pac	52959-0096-00
28 gm	$4.80	GENERIC, Prescript Pharmaceuticals	00247-0017-29
30 gm	$4.89	GENERIC, Prescript Pharmaceuticals	00247-0017-30
30 gm	$13.91	GENERIC, Pharma Pac	52959-0096-30
45 gm	$5.66	GENERIC, Prescript Pharmaceuticals	00247-0017-45
45 gm	$15.23	GENERIC, Pharma Pac	52959-0096-45
60 gm	$6.42	GENERIC, Prescript Pharmaceuticals	00247-0017-60
80 gm	$4.90	GENERIC, Allscripts Pharmaceutical Company	54569-0765-00
80 gm	$7.28	GENERIC, Alpharma Uspd Makers Of Barre and Nmc	63874-0820-80
80 gm	$7.45	GENERIC, Prescript Pharmaceuticals	00247-0017-80
80 gm	$8.37	GENERIC, Southwood Pharmaceuticals Inc	58016-3108-01
80 gm	$16.34	GENERIC, Pharma Pac	52959-0096-01
454 gm	$19.44	GENERIC, Allscripts Pharmaceutical Company	54569-4781-00
Cream - Topical - 0.5%			
15 gm	$4.43	GENERIC, Physicians Total Care	54868-0844-01
15 gm	$5.13	GENERIC, Allscripts Pharmaceutical Company	54569-2025-00
15 gm	$6.83	GENERIC, Southwood Pharmaceuticals Inc	58016-3127-01
15 gm	$8.24	GENERIC, Pharma Pac	52959-0136-00
15 gm	$8.28	CINALOG, Economed Pharmaceuticals Inc	38130-0047-15
Lotion - Topical - 0.1%			
60 ml	$8.50	GENERIC, Raway Pharmacal Inc	00686-1250-02
60 ml	$11.58	GENERIC, Physicians Total Care	54868-3097-00
60 ml	$13.64	GENERIC, Thames Pharmacal Company Inc	49158-0211-32
Ointment - Topical - 0.025%			
15 gm	$1.82	GENERIC, Allscripts Pharmaceutical Company	54569-2452-00
15 gm	$2.24	GENERIC, Physicians Total Care	54868-1590-01
30 gm	$5.13	GENERIC, Southwood Pharmaceuticals Inc	58016-3161-01
80 gm	$3.53	GENERIC, Physicians Total Care	54868-1590-02
Ointment - Topical - 0.1%			
15 gm	$1.00	CINOLAR, Ocumed Inc	51944-2255-02
15 gm	$2.28	GENERIC, Allscripts Pharmaceutical Company	54569-1124-00
15 gm	$3.20	GENERIC, Southwood Pharmaceuticals Inc	58016-3208-01
15 gm	$10.05	GENERIC, Pharma Pac	52959-0156-00
80 gm	$4.59	GENERIC, Physicians Total Care	54868-1591-02
80 gm	$5.38	GENERIC, Allscripts Pharmaceutical Company	54569-0767-00
80 gm	$8.37	GENERIC, Southwood Pharmaceuticals Inc	58016-3253-01
80 gm	$13.35	GENERIC, Pharma Pac	52959-0156-02
454 gm	$18.88	GENERIC, Physicians Total Care	54868-1591-03
Paste - Mucous Membrane - 0.1%			
5 gm	$5.00	GENERIC, Thames Pharmacal Company Inc	49158-0231-03
Spray - Nasal - 50 mcg/Inh			
15 ml	$42.98	TRI-NASAL, Muro Pharmaceuticals Inc	00451-5050-15
Spray - Nasal - 55 mcg/Inh			
16.50 gm	$42.34	NASACORT AQ, Allscripts Pharmaceutical Company	54569-4476-00
16.50 gm	$66.21	NASACORT AQ, Aventis Pharmaceuticals	00075-1506-16
Spray - Topical - 0.147 mg/Gm			
63 gm	$32.98	KENALOG, Physicians Total Care	54868-3255-00
63 gm	$33.53	KENALOG, Allscripts Pharmaceutical Company	54569-2153-00
63 gm	$34.92	KENALOG, Bristol-Myers Squibb	00003-0501-62
Suspension - Injectable - acetonide 40 mg/ml			
5 ml	$8.40	GENERIC, C.O. Truxton Inc	00463-1091-05
5 ml	$8.49	GENERIC, Hauser, A.F. Inc	52637-0540-05
5 ml	$12.00	GENERIC, Primedics Laboratories	00684-0199-05
5 ml	$16.20	GENERIC, C.O. Truxton Inc	00463-1100-05
5 ml	$23.75	CLINALOG, Clint Pharmaceutical Inc	55553-0204-05
5 ml	$25.86	GENERIC, Physicians Total Care	54868-0284-00
Suspension - Injectable - 3 mg/ml			
5 ml	$10.43	TAC 3, Parnell Pharmaceuticals Inc	50930-0218-05
5 ml	$10.54	TAC 3, Allergan Inc	00023-0218-05
Suspension - Injectable - 10 mg/ml			
5 ml	$8.02	KENALOG-10, Allscripts Pharmaceutical Company	54569-1827-01
5 ml	$8.76	KENALOG-10, Bristol-Myers Squibb	00003-0494-20
5 ml	$10.26	KENALOG-10, Physicians Total Care	54868-0234-00

T

Triamcinolone Diacetate *(002372)*

For complete prescribing information, refer to the CD-ROM included with the book.

For related information, see the comparative table section in Appendix A.

Categories: Anemia, acquired hemolytic; Anemia, congenital hypoplastic; Ankylosing spondylitis; Arthritis, gouty; Arthritis, posttraumatic; Arthritis, psoriatic; Arthritis, rheumatoid; Asthma; Beryliiosis; Bursitis; Carditis, rheumatic; Chorioretinitis; Choroiditis; Colitis, ulcerative; Conjunctivitis, allergic; Crohn's disease; Dermatitis herpetiformis; Dermatitis, atopic; Dermatitis, contact; Dermatitis, exfoliative; Dermatitis, seborrheic; Epicondylitis; Erythema multiforme; Erythroblastopenia; Herpes zoster ophthalmicus; Hypercalcemia, secondary to neoplasia; Hyperplasia, congenital adrenal; Hypersensitivity reactions; Iridocyclitis; Iritis; Keratitis; Leukemia; Loffler's syndrome; Lupus erythematosus, systemic; Lymphoma; Meningitis, tuberculous; Multiple sclerosis; Mycosis fungoides; Nephrotic syndrome; Neuritis, optic; Ophthalmia, sympathetic; Pemphigus; Pneumonitis, aspiration; Psoriasis; Rhinitis, perennial allergic; Rhinitis, seasonal allergic; Sarcoidosis; Serum sickness; Stevens-Johnson syndrome; Synovitis, secondary to osteoarthritis; Tenosynovitis; Thrombocytopenia, secondary; Thyroiditis, nonsuppurative; Trichinosis; Tuberculosis, disseminated; Tuberculosis, fulminating; Ulcer, allergic corneal marginal; Uveitis; FDA Approved 1959 Mar; Pregnancy Category C

Drug Classes: Corticosteroids

Brand Names: Amcort; **Aristocort Forte**; Aristocort Suspension; Articulose-L.A.; Cenocort Forte; Kenacort; Sholog A; Tramacort-D; Tri-Med; Triam-Forte; Triamcot; Triamolone 40; Trilone; Tristo-Plex; Tristoject; Trylone D; U-Tri-Lone

HCFA JCODE(S): J3302 per 5 mg IM

DESCRIPTION

25 mg/ml Aristocort Intralesional: Aristocort possesses glucocorticoid properties while being essentially devoid of mineralocorticoid activity thus causing little or no sodium retention. Aristocort is supplied as a sterile suspension of 25 mg/ml micronized triamcinolone diacetate in the vehicle listed below.

40 mg/ml Aristocort Forte Parenteral: A sterile suspension of 40 mg/ml of triamcinolone diacetate (micronized). Aristocort Forte is suspended in a vehicle consisting of the ingredients listed below.

Vehicle ingredients for both the 25 mg/ml and 40 mg/ml Aristocort formulations:

Polysorbate 80: 0.20%
Polyethylene glycol 3350: 3%
Sodium chloride: 0.85%
Benzyl alcohol (preservative): 0.90%
Water for injection: 100%

Hydrochloric acid and/or sodium hydroxide may be used during manufacture to adjust pH of suspension to approximately 6.

Irreversible clumping occurs when product is frozen.

Chemically triamcinolone diacetate is 9-Fluoro-11β, 16α, 17, 21-tetrahydroxypregna-1,4-diene-3,20-dione 16,21-diacetate.

The molecular weight is 478.51.

Additional Information for 40 mg/ml Parenteral Formulation: This preparation is a slightly soluble suspension suitable for parenteral administration through a 24-gauge needle (or larger), but NOT suitable for intravenous use. It may be administered by the intramuscular, intra-articular, or intrasynovial routes, depending upon the situation. The response to each glucocorticoid varies considerably with each type of disease indication and each corticosteroid prescribed.

INDICATIONS AND USAGE

25 MG/ML INTRALESIONAL

Triamcinolone diacetate intralesional is indicated by the intralesional route for:

- Keloids.
- Localized hypertrophic, infiltrated, inflammatory lesion of:
  - Lichen planus, psoriatic plaques, granuloma annulare, and lichen simplex chronicus (neurodermatitis).
  - Discoid lupus erythematosus.
  - Necrobiosis lipoidica diabeticorum.
  - Alopecia areata.

It may also be useful in cystic tumors of an aponeurosis or tendon (ganglia).

When used intra-articularly it is also indicated for:

- Adjunctive therapy for short-term administration (to tide the patient over an acute episode or exacerbation) in:
  - Synovitis of osteoarthritis.
  - Rheumatoid arthritis.
  - Acute and subacute bursitis.
  - Acute gouty arthritis.
  - Epicondylitis.
  - Acute nonspecific tenosynovitis.
  - Posttraumatic osteoarthritis.

40 MG/ML PARENTERAL

Where oral therapy is not feasible or temporarily desirable in the judgement of the physician, sterile triamcinolone diacetate suspension, 40 mg/ml, is indicated for intramuscular use as follows:

1. Endocrine disorders.
Primary or secondary adrenocortical insufficiency (hydrocortisone or cortisone is the drug of choice; synthetic analogs may be used in conjunction with mineralocorticoids where applicable; in infancy, mineralocorticoid supplementation is of particular importance).
Preoperatively and in the event of serious trauma or illness, in patients with known adrenal insufficiency or when adrenocortical reserve is doubtful.
Congenital adrenal hyperplasia.
Nonsuppurative thyroiditis.
Hypercalcemia associated with cancer.

2. Rheumatic disorders. As adjunctive therapy for short-term administration (to tide the patient over an acute episode or exacerbation) in:
Posttraumatic osteoarthritis.
Synovitis of osteoarthritis.
Rheumatoid arthritis, including juvenile rheumatoid arthritis (selected cases may require low-dose maintenance therapy).
Acute and subacute bursitis.
Epicondylitis.
Acute nonspecific tenosynovitis.
Acute gouty arthritis.
Psoriatic arthritis.
Ankylosing spondylitis.

3. Collagen diseases. During an exacerbation or as maintenance therapy in selected cases of:
Systemic lupus erythematosus.
Acute rheumatic carditis.

4. Dermatologic diseases. Pemphigus.
Severe erythema multiforme (Stevens-Johnson syndrome).
Exfoliative dermatitis.
Bullous dermatitis herpetiformis.
Severe seborrheic dermatitis.
Severe psoriasis.
Mycosis fungoides.

5. Allergic states. Control of severe or incapacitating allergic conditions intractable to adequate trials of conventional treatment in:
Bronchial asthma.
Contact dermatitis.
Atopic dermatitis.
Serum sickness.
Seasonal or perennial allergic rhinitis.
Drug hypersensitivity reactions.
Urticarial transfusion reactions.
Acute noninfectious laryngeal edema (epinephrine is the drug of first choice).

6. Ophthalmic diseases. Severe acute and chronic allergic and inflammatory processes involving the eye, such as:
Herpes zoster ophthalmicus.
Iritis, iridocyclitis.
Chorioretinitis.
Diffuse posterior uveitis and choroiditis.
Optic neuritis.
Sympathetic ophthalmia.
Allergic conjunctivitis.
Allergic corneal marginal ulcers.
Keratitis.

7. Gastrointestinal disease. To tide the patient over a critical period of disease in:
Ulcerative colitis—(Systemic therapy).
Regional enteritis—(Systemic therapy).

8. Respiratory diseases.
Symptomatic sarcoidosis.
Berylliosis.
Fulminating or disseminated pulmonary tuberculosis when used concurrently with appropriate antituberculous chemotherapy.
Loeffler's syndrome not manageable by other means.
Aspiration pneumonitis.

9. Hematologic disorders.
Acquired (autoimmune) hemolytic anemia.
Secondary thrombocytopenia in adults.
Erythroblastopenia (RBC anemia).
Congenital (erythroid) hypoplastic anemia.

10. Neoplastic diseases. For palliative management of:
Leukemias and lymphomas in adults.
Acute leukemia of childhood.

11. Edematous state. To induce diuresis or remission of proteinuria in the nephrotic syndrome, without uremia, of the idiopathic type or that due to lupus erythematosus.

12. Nervous system, acute exacerbations of multiple sclerosis.

13. Miscellaneous. Tuberculous meningitis with subarachnoid block or impending block when used concurrently with appropriate antituberculous chemotherapy. Trichinosis with neurologic or myocardial involvement.

Triamcinolone diacetate 40 mg/ml is indicated for intra-articular or soft tissue use as follows:

As adjunctive therapy for short-term administration (to tide the patient over an acute episode or exacerbation) in:
Synovitis of osteoarthritis.
Rheumatoid arthritis.
Acute and subacute bursitis.
Acute gouty arthritis.
Epicondylitis.
Acute nonspecific tenosynovitis.
Posttraumatic osteoarthritis.

Triamcinolone diacetate is indicated for intralesional use as follows:

Keloids.
Localized hypertrophic, infiltrated, inflammatory lesion of: Lichen planus, psoriatic plaques, granuloma annulare and lichen simplex chronicus (neurodermatitis).
Discoid lupus erythematosus.
Necrobiosis lipoidica diabeticorum.
Alopecia areata.

It may also be useful in cystic tumors of an aponeurosis or tendon (ganglia).

CONTRAINDICATIONS

Systemic fungal infections.

WARNINGS

In patients on corticosteroid therapy subjected to any unusual stress, increased dosage of rapidly acting corticosteroids before, during, and after the stressful situation is indicated.

Corticosteroids may mask some signs of infection, and new infections may appear during their use. There may be decreased resistance and inability to localize infection when corticosteroids are used.

Prolonged use of corticosteroids may produce posterior subcapsular cataracts, glaucoma with possible damage to the optic nerves and may enhance the establishment of secondary ocular infections due to fungi or viruses.

Use in Pregnancy: Since adequate human reproduction studies have not been done with corticosteroids, the use of these drugs in pregnancy, nursing mothers, or women of childbearing potential requires that the possible benefits of the drug be weighed against the potential hazards to the mother and embryo or fetus. Infants born of mothers who have received substantial doses of corticosteroids during pregnancy should be carefully observed for signs of hypoadrenalism.

Average and large doses of cortisone or hydrocortisone can cause elevation of blood pressure, salt and water retention, and increased excretion of potassium. These effects are less likely to occur with the synthetic derivatives except when used in large doses. Dietary salt restriction and potassium supplementation may be necessary. All corticosteroids increase calcium excretion.

While on corticosteroid therapy patients should not be vaccinated against smallpox. Other immunization procedures should not be undertaken in patients who are on corticosteroids, especially in high doses, because of possible hazards of neurological complications and lack of antibody response.

The use of triamcinolone diacetate in active tuberculosis should be restricted to those cases of fulminating or disseminated tuberculosis in which the corticosteroid is used for the management of the disease in conjunction with appropriate antituberculous regimen.

If corticosteroids are indicated in patients with latent tuberculosis or tuberculin reactivity, close observation is necessary as reactivation of the disease may occur. During prolonged corticosteroid therapy, these patients should receive chemoprophylaxis.

Because rare instances of anaphylactoid reactions have occurred in patients receiving parenteral corticosteroid therapy, appropriate precautionary measures should be taken prior to administration, especially when the patient has a history of allergy to any drug.

Postinjection flare (following intra-articular use) and Charcot-like arthropathy have been associated with parenteral corticosteroid therapy.

Persons who are on drugs which suppress the immune system are more susceptible to infections than healthy individuals. Chickenpox and measles, for example, can have a more serious or even fatal course in nonimmune children or adults on corticosteroids. In such children or adults who have not had these diseases, particular care should be taken to avoid exposure. How the dose, route and duration of corticosteroid administration affects the risk of developing a disseminated infection is not known. The contribution of the underlying disease and/or prior corticosteroid treatment to the risk is also not known. If exposed to chickenpox, prophylaxis with varicella zoster immune globulin (VZIG) may be indicated. If exposed to measles, prophylaxis with pooled intramuscular immunoglobulin (IG) may be indicated. (See the respective package inserts for complete VZIG and IG prescribing information.) If chickenpox develops, treatment with antiviral agents may be considered.

Additional Information for 25 mg/ml Intralesional Formulation: Intralesional or sublesional injection of excessive dosage whether by single or multiple injection into any given area may cause cutaneous or subcutaneous atrophy.

DOSAGE AND ADMINISTRATION

GENERAL

The initial intralesional or intramuscular dosage of sterile triamcinolone diacetate may vary from 3 to 48 mg per day depending on the specific disease entity being treated. In situations of less severity, lower doses will generally suffice while in selected patients higher initial doses may be required. Usually the parenteral dosage ranges are one-third to one-half the oral dose given every 12 hours. However, in certain overwhelming, acute, life-threatening situations, administration in dosages exceeding the usual dosages may be justified and may be in multiples of the oral dosages.

The initial dosage should be maintained or adjusted until a satisfactory response is noted. If after a reasonable period of time there is a lack of satisfactory clinical response triamcinolone diacetate should be discontinued and the patient transferred to other appropriate therapy. **It should be emphasized that dosage requirements are variable and must be individualized on the basis of the disease under treatment and the response of the patient.** After a favorable response is noted, the proper maintenance dosage should be determined by decreasing the initial drug dosage in small increments at appropriate time intervals until the lowest dosage which will maintain an adequate clinical response is reached. It should be kept in mind that constant monitoring is needed in regard to drug dosage. Included in the situations which may make dosage adjustments necessary are changes in clinical status secondary to remissions or exacerbations in the disease process, the patient's individual drug responsiveness, and the effect of patient exposure to stressful situations not directly related to the disease entity under treatment; in this latter situation it may be necessary to increase the dosage of triamcinolone diacetate for a period of time consistent with the patient's condition. If after long-term therapy the drug is to be stopped, it is recommended that it be withdrawn gradually rather than abruptly.

Additional Information for 25 mg/ml Intralesional Formulation: For intra-articular, intralesional and soft tissue use, a lesser initial dosage range of triamcinolone diacetate may produce the desired effect when the drug is administered to provide a localized concentration. The site of the injection and the volume of the injection should be carefully considered when triamcinolone diacetate is administered for this purpose.

SPECIFIC

25 mg/ml Intralesional

When triamcinolone diacetate intralesional is administered by injection, strict aseptic technique is mandatory. Full strength suspensions may be employed, or if preferred, the suspension may be diluted, either to a 1:1 or 1:10 concentration, thus obtaining a working concentration of 12.5 mg/ml or approximately 2.5 mg/ml respectively. Normal (isotonic) saline solution alone or equal parts of normal (isotonic) saline solution and 1% procaine or other local anesthetics may be used as diluents. These dilutions usually retain full potency for at least one week. Topical ethyl chloride spray may be used as a local anesthetic. The use of diluents containing preservatives such as methylparaben, propylparaben, phenol, etc., must be avoided as these preparations tend to cause flocculations of the steroid.

Since this product has been designed for ease of administration, a small bore needle (not smaller than 24 gauge) may be used.

Intralesional or Sublesional

For small lesions, injection is usually well tolerated and a local anesthetic is not necessary. The location and type of lesion will determine the route of injection: intralesional, sublesional, intradermal, subdermal, intracutaneous, or subcutaneous. The size of the lesion will determine: the total amount of drug needed, the concentration used, and the number and pattern of injection sites utilized (*e.g.,* from a total of 5 mg triamcinolone diacetate intralesional in a 2 ml volume divided over several locations in small lesions, ranging up to 48 mg total triamcinolone diacetate intralesional for large psoriatic plaques). Avoid injecting too superficially. In general, no more than 12.5 mg per injection site should be used. An average of 25 mg is the usual limit for any one lesion. Large areas require multiple injections with smaller doses per injection.

For a majority of conditions, sublesional injection directly through the lesion into the deep dermal tissue is suggested. In cases where it is difficult to inject intradermally, the suspension may be introduced subcutaneously, as superficially as possible.

Two or three injections at one to two week intervals may suffice as an average course of treatment for many conditions. Within 5 to 7 days after initial injection involution of the lesion can usually be seen, with pronounced clearing towards normal tissue after 12 to 14 days. Multiple injections of small amounts of equal strength may be convenient in alopecia areata and in psoriasis where there are large or confluent lesions. This is best accomplished by a series of fan-like injections ½ to 1 inch apart.

Alopecia areata and totalis require an average dose of 25 mg to 30 mg in a concentration of 10 mg/ml subcutaneously 1 to 2 times a week, to stimulate hair regrowth. Results may be expected in 3 to 6 weeks on this dosage, and hair growth may last 3 to 6 months after initial injection. No more than 0.5 ml should be given in any one site, because excessive deposition may produce local skin atrophy. Continued periodic local injections may be necessary to maintain response and continued hair growth. Use of more dilute solutions diminish the incidence and degree of local atrophy in the injection site.

In keloids and similar dense scars injections are usually made directly into the lesion.

Injections may be repeated as required, but probably a total of no more than 75 mg of triamcinolone diacetate a week should be given to any one patient. The need for repeated injections is best determined by clinical response. Remissions may be expected to last from a few weeks up to eleven months.

Intra-articular or Intrasynovial

Strict surgical asepsis is mandatory. The physician should be familiar with anatomical relationships as described in standard textbooks. A recent paper details the anatomy and the technical approach in arthrocentesis.

It is usually recommended that infiltration by local anesthetic of the soft tissue precede intra-articular injection. A 22-gauge or larger needle on a dry syringe should be inserted into the joint and excess fluid if present should be aspirated. The specific dose depends primarily on the size of the joint. The usual dose varies from 5 mg to 40 mg with the average for the knee being 25 mg. Smaller joints as in the fingers require 2 mg to 5 mg. The duration of effect varies from one week to two months. However, acutely inflamed joints may require more frequent injections. Accidental injection into soft tissue is usually not harmful but decreases the local effectiveness. Injection into subcutaneous lipoid tissue may produce "pseudoatrophy" with a persistent depression of the overlying dermis, lasting several weeks or months.

Administration and dosage of triamcinolone diacetate intralesional must be individualized according to the nature, severity and chronicity of the disease or disorder treated, and should be undertaken with a view of the patient's entire clinical condition. Corticosteroid therapy is considered an adjunct to and not usually a replacement for conventional therapy. Therapy with triamcinolone diacetate intralesional, as with all steroids, is of the suppressive type, related to its anti-inflammatory effect. The dose should be regulated during therapy according to the degree of therapeutic response, and should be reduced gradually to maintenance levels, whereby the patient obtains adequate or acceptable control of symptoms. When such control occurs, consideration should be given to gradual decrease in dosage and eventual cessation of therapy. Remission of symptoms may be due to therapy or may be spontaneous and a therapeutic test of gradual withdrawal of steroid treatment is usually indicated.

Parenteral drug products should be inspected visually for particulate matter and discoloration prior to administration, whenever solution and container permit.

40 mg/ml Parenteral Formulation

Sterile triamcinolone diacetate (40 mg/ml) is suspended in a suitable vehicle. The full-strength suspension may be employed. If preferred, the suspension may be diluted with normal saline or water. The diluent may also be prepared by mixing equal parts of normal saline and 1% procaine hydrochloride or other similar local anesthetics. The use of diluents containing preservatives such as methylparaben, propylparaben, phenol, etc. must be avoided as these preparations tend to cause flocculation of the steroid. These dilutions retain full potency for at least one week. Topical ethyl chloride spray may be used locally prior to injection.

Since this product has been designed for ease of administration, a small bore needle (not smaller than 24 gauge) may be used.

Intramuscular

Although triamcinolone diacetate Parenteral may be administered intramuscularly for initial therapy, most physicians prefer to adjust the dose orally until adequate control is attained. Intramuscular administration provides a sustained or depot action which can be used to supplement or replace initial oral therapy. With intramuscular therapy, greater supervision of the amount of steroid used is made possible in the patient who is inconsistent in following

T

an oral dosage schedule. In maintenance therapy, the patient-to-patient response is not uniform and, therefore, the dose must be individualized for optimal control.

Although triamcinolone diacetate may possess greater anti-inflammatory potency than many glucocorticoids, this is only dose-related since side effects, such as osteoporosis, peptic ulcer, etc. related to glucocorticoid activity, have not been diminished.

The average dose is 40 mg (1 ml) administered intramuscularly once a week for conditions in which anti-inflammatory action is desired.

In general, a single parenteral dose 4 to 7 times the oral daily dose may be expected to control the patient from 4 to 7 days up to 3 to 4 weeks. Dosage should be adjusted to the point where adequate but not necessarily complete relief of symptoms is obtained.

Intra-Articular and Intrasynovial

The usual dose varies from 5 to 40 mg. The average for the knee, for example, is 25 mg. The duration of effect varies from one week to 2 months. However, acutely inflamed joints may require more frequent injections.

A lesser initial dosage range of sterile triamcinolone diacetate may produce the desired effect when the drug is administered to provide a localized concentration. The site of the injection and the volume of the injection should be carefully considered when triamcinolone diacetate is administered for this purpose.

A specific dose depends largely on the size of the joint.

Strict surgical asepsis is mandatory. The physician should be familiar with anatomical relationships as described in standard textbooks. Triamcinolone diacetate parenteral may be used in any accessible joint except the intervertebrals. In general, intrasynovial therapy is suggested under the following circumstances:

1. When systemic steroid therapy is contraindicated because of side effects such as peptic ulcer.
2. When it is desirable to secure relief in one or two specific joints.
3. When good systemic maintenance fails to control flare-ups in a few joints and it is desirable to secure relief without increasing oral therapy.

Such treatment should not be considered to constitute a cure; for although this method will ameliorate the joint symptoms, it does not preclude the need for the conventional measures usually employed.

It is suggested that infiltration of the soft tissue by local anesthetic precede intra-articular injection. A 24-gauge or larger needle on a dry syringe may be inserted into the joint and excess fluid aspirated. For the first few hours following injection, there may be local discomfort in the joint but this is usually followed rapidly by effective relief of pain and improvement in local function.

TABLE 1

	Anti-Inflammatory Relative Potency		Frequently Used Tablet Strength (mg)		Tablet × Potency Equivalent Value
Hydrocortisone	1	×	20	=	20
Prednisolone	4	×	5	=	20
Triamcinolone	5	×	4	=	20
Dexamethasone	25	×	0.75	=	18.75

Parenteral drug products should be inspected visually for particulate matter and discoloration prior to administration, whenever solution and container permit.

PRODUCT LISTING - RATED NOT THERAPEUTICALLY EQUIVALENT

Suspension - Injectable - Diacetate 40 mg/ml

1 ml	$7.21	ARISTOCORT FORTE, Fujisawa	00469-5116-01
1 ml	$21.01	ARISTOCORT FORTE, Physicians Total Care	54868-3344-00
5 ml	$8.98	GENERIC, General Injectables and Vaccines Inc	52584-0042-05
5 ml	$10.38	GENERIC, Moore, H.L. Drug Exchange Inc	00839-5057-25
5 ml	$11.48	GENERIC, Hyrex Pharmaceuticals	00314-0775-75
5 ml	$12.50	GENERIC, Forest Pharmaceuticals	00456-1060-05
5 ml	$12.75	GENERIC, Major Pharmaceuticals Inc	00904-0885-05
5 ml	$13.81	GENERIC, Steris Laboratories Inc	00402-0042-05
5 ml	$14.38	ARISTOCORT FORTE, Fujisawa	00469-5116-05
5 ml	$17.23	ARISTOCORT FORTE, Physicians Total Care	54868-0926-00
5 ml	$27.13	ARISTOCORT FORTE, Allscripts Pharmaceutical Company	54569-2184-00

PRODUCT LISTING - EQUIVALENTS NOT AVAILABLE

Suspension - Injectable - Diacetate 40 mg/ml

5 ml	$14.00	CLINACORT, Clint Pharmaceutical Inc	55553-0042-05

Suspension - Injectable - 25 mg/ml

5 ml	$23.30	ARISTOCORT, Fujisawa	00469-5117-05

Triamterene *(002374)*

Categories: Edema; Pregnancy Category B; FDA Approved 1974 Dec
Drug Classes: Diuretics, potassium sparing
Brand Names: **Dyrenium**
Cost of Therapy: $107.42 (Edema; Dyrenium; 100 mg; 2 capsules/day; 30 day supply)

WARNING

Abnormal elevation of serum potassium levels (greater than or equal to 5.5 mEq/L) can occur with all potassium-sparing agents, including triamterene. Hyperkalemia is more likely to occur in patients with renal impairment, and diabetes (even without evidence of renal impairment), elderly or severely ill patients. Since uncorrected hyperkalemia may be fatal, serum potassium levels must be monitored at frequent intervals especially in patients receiving triamterene, when dosages are changed or with any illness that may influence renal function.

DESCRIPTION

Dyrenium (triamterene) is a potassium-conserving diuretic.

Triamterene is 2,4,7-triamino-6-phenylpteridine. Its molecular weight is 253.27. At 50°C, triamterene is slightly soluble in water. It is soluble in dilute ammonia, dilute aqueous sodium hydroxide and dimethylformamide. It is sparingly soluble in methanol.

Each capsule for oral administration, with opaque red cap and body, contains triamterene, 50 or 100 mg, and is imprinted with the product name Dyrenium, strength (50 or 100), and WPC 002 (50mg) or WPC 003 (100mg). Inactive ingredients consist of benzyl alcohol, cetylpyridinium chloride, D&C red no. 33, FD&C yellow no. 6, gelatin, lactose, magnesium stearate, povidone, sodium lauryl sulfate, titanium dioxide and trace amounts of other inactive ingredients.

CLINICAL PHARMACOLOGY

Triamterene has a unique mode of action; it inhibits the reabsorption of sodium ions in exchange for potassium and hydrogen ions at that segment of the distal tubule under the control of adrenal mineralocorticoids (especially aldosterone). This activity is not directly related to aldosterone secretion or antagonism; it is a result of a direct effect on the renal tubule.

The fraction of filtered sodium reaching this distal tubular exchange site is relatively small, and the amount which is exchanged depends on the level of mineralocorticoid activity. Thus, the degree of natriuresis and diuresis produced by inhibition of the exchange mechanism is necessarily limited. Increasing the amount of available sodium and the level of mineralocorticoid activity by the use of more proximally acting diuretics will increase the degree of diuresis and potassium conservation.

Triamterene occasionally causes increases in serum potassium which can result in hyperkalemia. It does not produce alkalosis because it does not cause excessive excretion of titratable acid and ammonium.

Triamterene has been shown to cross the placental barrier and appear in the cord blood of animals.

PHARMACOKINETICS

Onset of action is 2-4 hours after ingestion. In normal volunteers the mean peak serum levels were 30 ng/ml at 3 hours. The average percent of drug recovered in the urine (0-48 hours) was 21%. Triamterene is primarily metabolized to the sulfate conjugate of hydroxytriamterene. Both the plasma and urine levels of this metabolite greatly exceed triamterene levels. Triamterene is rapidly absorbed, with somewhat less than 50% of the oral dose reaching the urine. Most patients will respond to triamterene during the first day of treatment. Maximum therapeutic effect, however, may not be seen for several days. Duration of diuresis depends on several factors, especially renal function, but it generally tapers off 7-9 hours after administration.

INDICATIONS AND USAGE

Triamterene is indicated in the treatment of edema associated with congestive heart failure, cirrhosis of the liver, and the nephrotic syndrome; also in steroid-induced edema, idiopathic edema, and edema due to secondary hyperaldosteronism.

Triamterene may be used alone or with other diuretics either for its added diuretic effect or its potassium-conserving potential. It also promotes increased diuresis when patients prove resistant or only partially responsive to thiazides or other diuretics because of secondary hyperaldosteronism.

USAGE IN PREGNANCY

The routine use of diuretics in an otherwise healthy woman is inappropriate and exposes mother and fetus to unnecessary hazard. Diuretics do not prevent development of toxemia of pregnancy, and there is no satisfactory evidence that they are useful in the treatment of developed toxemia.

Edema during pregnancy may arise from pathological causes or from the physiologic and mechanical consequences of pregnancy. Diuretics are indicated in pregnancy when edema is due to pathologic causes, just as they are in the absence of pregnancy (see PRECAUTIONS). Dependent edema in pregnancy, resulting from restriction of venous return by the expanded uterus, is properly treated through elevation of the lower extremities and use of support hose; use of diuretics to lower intravascular volume in this case is illogical and unnecessary. There is hypervolemia during normal pregnancy which is harmful to neither the fetus nor the mother (in the absence of cardiovascular disease), but which is associated with edema, including generalized edema, in the majority of pregnant women. If this edema produces discomfort, increased recumbency will often provide relief. In rare instances, this edema may cause extreme discomfort which is not relieved by rest. In these cases, a short course of diuretics may provide relief and may be appropriate.

CONTRAINDICATIONS

Anuria. Severe or progressive kidney disease or dysfunction with the possible exception of nephrosis. Severe hepatic disease. Hypersensitivity to the drug.

Triamterene should not be used in patients with preexisting elevated serum potassium, as is sometimes seen in patients with impaired renal function or azotemia, or in patients who develop hyperkalemia while on the drug. Patients should not be placed on dietary potassium supplements, potassium salts, or potassium-containing salt substitutes in conjunction with triamterene.

Triamterene should not be given to patients receiving other potassium-sparing agents such as spironolactone, amiloride hydrochloride, or other formulations containing triamterene. Two deaths have been reported in patients receiving concomitant spironolactone and triamterene or Dyazide. Although dosage recommendations were exceeded in one case and in the other serum electrolytes were not properly monitored, these 2 drugs should not be given concomitantly.

WARNINGS

There have been isolated reports of hypersensitivity reactions; therefore, patients should be observed regularly for the possible occurrence of blood dyscrasias, liver damage, or other idiosyncratic reactions.

Periodic BUN and serum potassium determinations should be made to check kidney function, especially in patients with suspected or confirmed renal insufficiency. It is particularly important to make serum potassium determinations in elderly or diabetic patients receiving the drug; these patients should be observed carefully for possible serum potassium increases.

If hyperkalemia is present or suspected, an electrocardiogram should be obtained. If the ECG shows no widening of the QRS or arrhythmia in the presence of hyperkalemia, it is usually sufficient to discontinue triamterene and any potassium supplementation and substitute a thiazide alone. Sodium polystyrene sulfonate (Kayexalate, Winthrop) may be administered to enhance the excretion of excess potassium. **The presence of a widened QRS complex or arrhythmia in association with hyperkalemia requires prompt additional therapy.** For tachyarrhythmia, infuse 44 mEq of sodium bicarbonate or 10 ml of 10% calcium gluconate or calcium chloride over several minutes. For asystole, bradycardia, or A-V block transvenous pacing is also recommended.

The effect of calcium and sodium bicarbonate is transient and repeated administration may be required. When indicated by the clinical situation, excess K^+ may be removed by dialysis or oral or rectal administration of Kayexalate. Infusion of glucose and insulin has also been used to treat hyperkalemia.

PRECAUTIONS

GENERAL

Triamterene tends to conserve potassium rather than to promote the excretion as do many diuretics and, occasionally, can cause increases in serum potassium which, in some instances, can result in hyperkalemia. In rare instances, hyperkalemia has been associated with cardiac irregularities.

Electrolyte imbalance often encountered in such diseases as congestive heart failure, renal disease, or cirrhosis may be aggravated or caused independently by any effective diuretic agent including triamterene. The use of full doses of a diuretic when salt intake is restricted can result in a low-salt syndrome.

Triamterene can cause mild nitrogen retention which is reversible upon withdrawal of the drug and is seldom observed with intermittent (every-other-day) therapy.

Triamterene may cause a decreasing alkali reserve with the possibility of metabolic acidosis.

By the very nature of their illness, cirrhotics with splenomegaly sometimes have marked variations in their blood pictures. Since triamterene is a weak folic acid antagonist, it may contribute to the appearance of megaloblastosis in cases where folic acid stores have been depleted. Therefore, periodic blood studies in these patients are recommended. They should also be observed for exacerbations of underlying liver disease.

Triamterene has elevated uric acid, especially in persons predisposed to gouty arthritis.

Triamterene has been reported in renal stones in association with other calculus components. Triamterene should be used with caution in patients with histories of renal stones.

INFORMATION FOR THE PATIENT

To help avoid stomach upset, it is recommended that the drug be taken after meals.

If a single daily dose is prescribed, it may be preferable to take it in the morning to minimize the effect of increased frequency of urination on nighttime sleep.

If a dose is missed, the patient should not take more than the prescribed dose at the next dosing interval.

LABORATORY TESTS

Hyperkalemia will rarely occur in patients with adequate urinary output, but it is a possibility if large doses are used for considerable periods of time. If hyperkalemia is observed, Triamterene should be withdrawn. The normal adult range of serum potassium is 3.5-5.0 mEq/L with 4.5 mEq often being used for a reference point. Potassium levels persistently above 6 mEq/L require careful observation and treatment. Normal potassium levels tend to be higher in neonates (7.7 mEq/L) than in adults.

Serum potassium levels do not necessarily indicate true body potassium concentration. A rise in plasma pH may cause a decrease in plasma potassium concentration and an increase in the intracellular potassium concentration. Because triamterene conserves potassium, it has been theorized that in patients who have received intensive therapy or been given the drug for prolonged periods, a rebound kaliuresis could occur upon abrupt withdrawal. In such patients withdrawal of triamterene should be gradual.

DRUG/LABORATORY TEST INTERACTIONS

Triamterene and quinidine have similar fluorescence spectra; thus, triamterene will interfere with the fluorescent measurement of quinidine.

CARCINOGENESIS, MUTAGENESIS, AND IMPAIRMENT OF FERTILITY

Long-term studies to determine the carcinogenic potential of triamterene are not available. Studies to determine the mutagenic potential of triamterene are not available. Reproductive studies have been performed in rats at doses up to 30 times the human dose and have revealed no evidence of impaired fertility.

PREGNANCY CATEGORY B

Teratogenic Effects

Reproduction studies have been performed in rats at doses up to 30 times the human dose and have revealed no evidence of impaired fertility or harm to the fetus due to triamterene. There are, however, no adequate and well-controlled studies in pregnant women. Because animal reproductive studies are not always predictive of human response, this drug should be used during pregnancy only if clearly needed.

Nonteratogenic Effects

Triamterene has been shown to cross the placental barrier and appear in the cord blood of animals; this may occur in humans. The use of triamterene in pregnant women requires that the anticipated benefit be weighed against possible hazards to the fetus. These possible hazards include adverse reactions which have occurred in the adult.

NURSING MOTHERS

Triamterene appears in animal milk; this may occur in humans. If use of the drug is deemed essential, the patient should stop nursing.

PEDIATRIC USE

Safety and effectiveness in children have not been established.

DRUG INTERACTIONS

Caution should be used when lithium and diuretics are used concomitantly because diuretic-induced sodium loss may reduce the renal clearance of lithium and increase serum lithium levels with risk of lithium toxicity. Patients receiving such combined therapy should have serum lithium levels monitored closely and the lithium dosage adjusted if necessary.

A possible interaction resulting in acute renal failure has been reported in a few subjects when indomethacin, a nonsteroidal anti-inflammatory agent, was given with triamterene. Caution is advised in administering nonsteroidal anti-inflammatory agents with triamterene.

The effects of the following drugs may be potentiated when given together with triamterene: antihypertensive medication, other diuretics, preanesthetic and anesthetic agents, skeletal muscle relaxants (nondepolarizing).

Potassium-sparing agents should be used with caution in conjunction with angiotensin-converting enzyme (ACE) inhibitors due to an increased risk of hyperkalemia.

The following agents, given together with triamterene, may promote serum potassium accumulation and possibly result in hyperkalemia because of the potassium-sparing nature of triamterene, especially in patients with renal insufficiency: blood from blood bank (may contain up to 30 mEq of potassium per L of plasma or up to 65 mEq/L of whole blood when stored for more than 10 days); low-salt milk (may contain up to 60 mEq of potassium per L); potassium-containing medications (such as parenteral penicillin G potassium); salt substitutes (most contain substantial amounts of potassium).

Triamterene may raise blood glucose levels; for adult-onset diabetes, dosage adjustments of hypoglycemic agents may be necessary during and after therapy; concurrent use with chlorpropamide may increase the risk of severe hyponatremia.

ADVERSE REACTIONS

Adverse effects are listed in decreasing order of frequency; however, the most serious adverse effects are listed first regardless of frequency. All adverse effects occur rarely (that is, 1 in 1000, or less).

Hypersensitivity: anaphylaxis, rash, photosensitivity.

Metabolic: hyperkalemia, hypokalemia.

Renal: azotemia, elevated BUN and creatinine, renal stones, acute interstitial nephritis (rare), acute renal failure (one case of irreversible renal failure has been reported).

Gastrointestinal: jaundice and/or liver enzyme abnormalities, nausea and vomiting, diarrhea.

Hematologic: thrombocytopenia, megaloblastic anemia.

Central Nervous System: weakness, fatigue, dizziness, headache, dry mouth.

DOSAGE AND ADMINISTRATION

ADULT DOSAGE

Dosage should be titrated to the needs of the individual patient. When used alone, the usual starting dose is 100 mg twice daily after meals. When combined with another diuretic or antihypertensive agent, the total daily dosage of each agent should usually be lowered initially and then adjusted to the patient's needs. The total daily dosage should not exceed 300 mg. Please refer to PRECAUTIONS, General.

When triamterene is added to other diuretic therapy or when patients are switched to triamterene from other diuretics, all potassium supplementation should be discontinued.

HOW SUPPLIED

Capsules: 50 mg and 100 mg.

Storage: Store at controlled room temperature (59-86° F). Protect from light.

PRODUCT LISTING - EQUIVALENTS NOT AVAILABLE

Capsule - Oral - 50 mg

100's	$98.46	DYRENIUM, Wellspring Pharmaceutical Corporation	65197-0002-01

Capsule - Oral - 100 mg

100's	$179.03	DYRENIUM, Wellspring Pharmaceutical Corporation	65197-0003-01

Triazolam (002375)

Categories: Insomnia; Pregnancy Category X; DEA Class CIV; FDA Approved 1982 Nov
Drug Classes: Benzodiazepines; Sedatives/hypnotics
Brand Names: **Halcion**; Somniton; Tialam; Trizam
Foreign Brand Availability: Apo-Triazo (Canada); Arring (Taiwan); Dumozolam (Sweden); Hypam (New-Zealand); Novidorm (Argentina); Novodorm (Spain); Nuctane (Argentina); Rilamir (Denmark; Finland); Somese (Colombia; Ecuador; Malaysia; Peru); Songar (Italy); Trialam (Taiwan); Trycam (New-Zealand; Thailand); Zolmin (Korea)
Cost of Therapy: $14.04 (Insomnia; Halcion; 0.25 mg; 1 tablet/day; 10 day supply)
$6.47 (Insomnia; Generic Tablets; 0.25 mg; 1 tablet/day; 10 day supply)

DESCRIPTION

Halcion tablets contain triazolam, a triazolobenzodiazepine hypnotic agent.

Triazolam is a white crystalline powder, soluble in alcohol and poorly soluble in water. It has a molecular weight of 343.21.

The chemical name for triazolam is 8-chloro-6-(o-chlorophenyl)-1-methyl -4H-s-triazolo-[4,3-α][1,4] benzodiazepine.

Each halcion tablet, for oral administration, contains 0.125 mg or 0.25 mg of triazolam. **Inactive Ingredients:** *0.125 mg:* Cellulose, corn starch, docusate sodium, lactose, magnesium stearate, silicon dioxide, sodium benzoate; *0.25 mg:* Cellulose, corn starch, docusate sodium, FD&C blue no. 2, lactose, magnesium stearate, silicon dioxide, sodium benzoate.

CLINICAL PHARMACOLOGY

CLINICAL STUDIES

Triazolam is a hypnotic with a short mean plasma half-life reported to be in the range of 1.5-5.5 hours. In normal subjects treated for 7 days with 4 times the recommended dosage, there was no evidence of altered systemic bioavailability, rate of elimination, or accumulation. Peak plasma levels are reached within 2 hours following oral administration. Following recommended doses of triazolam, triazolam peak plasma levels in the range of 1-6 ng/ml are seen. The plasma levels achieved are proportional to the dose given.

Triazolam and its metabolites, principally as conjugated glucuronides, which are presumably inactive, are excreted primarily in the urine. Only small amounts of unmetabolized triazolam appear in the urine. The 2 primary metabolites accounted for 79.9% of urinary excretion. Urinary excretion appeared to be biphasic in its time course.

Triazolam tablets 0.5 mg, in 2 separate studies, did not affect the prothrombin times or plasma warfarin levels in male volunteers administered sodium warfarin orally.

Extremely high concentrations of triazolam do not displace bilirubin bound to human serum albumin *in vitro*.

Triazolam ^{14}C was administered orally to pregnant mice. Drug-related material appeared uniformly distributed in the fetus with ^{14}C concentrations approximately the same as in the brain of the mother.

In sleep laboratory studies, triazolam tablets significantly decreased sleep latency, increased the duration of sleep, and decreased the number of nocturnal awakenings. After 2 weeks of consecutive nightly administration, the drug's effect on total wake time is decreased, and the values recorded in the last third of the night approach baseline levels. On the first and/or second night after drug discontinuance (first or second post-drug night), total time asleep, percentage of time spent sleeping, and rapidity of falling asleep frequently were significantly less than on baseline (predrug) nights. This effect is often called "rebound" insomnia.

PHARMACOKINETICS AND PHARMACODYNAMICS

The type and duration of hypnotic effects and the profile of unwanted effects during administration of benzodiazepine drugs may be influenced by the biologic half-life of administered drug and any active metabolites formed. When half-lives are long, the drug or metabolites may accumulate during periods of nightly administration and be associated with impairments of cognitive and motor performance during waking hours; the possibility of interaction with other psychoactive drugs or alcohol will be enhanced. In contrast, if half-lives are short, the drug and metabolites will be cleared before the next dose is ingested, and carry-over effects related to excessive sedation or CNS depression should be minimal or absent. However, during nightly use for an extended period pharmacodynamic tolerance or adaptation to some effects of benzodiazepine hypnotics may develop. If the drug has a short half-life of elimination, it is possible that a relative deficiency of the drug or its active metabolites (*i.e.*, in relationship to the receptor site) may occur at some point in the interval between each night's use. This sequence of events may account for 2 clinical findings reported to occur after several weeks of nightly use of rapidly eliminated benzodiazepine hypnotics: (1) increased wakefulness during the last third of the night and (2) the appearance of increased daytime anxiety after 10 days of continuous treatment.

INDICATIONS AND USAGE

Triazolam is indicated for the short-term treatment of insomnia (generally 7-10 days). Use for more than 2-3 weeks requires complete reevaluation of the patient (see WARNINGS).

Prescriptions for triazolam should be written for short-term use (7-10 days) and it should not be prescribed in quantities exceeding a 1 month supply.

CONTRAINDICATIONS

Triazolam tablets are contraindicated in patients with known hypersensitivity to this drug or other benzodiazepines.

Triazolam is contraindicated in pregnant women. If there is a likelihood of the patient becoming pregnant while receiving triazolam, she should be warned of the potential risk to the fetus. Patients should be instructed to discontinue the drug prior to becoming pregnant. The possibility that a woman of childbearing potential may be pregnant at the time of institution of therapy should be considered.

Triazolam is contraindicated with ketoconazole, itraconazole, and nefazodone, medications that significantly impair the oxidative metabolism mediated by cytochrome P450 3A (CYP 3A) (see WARNINGS and DRUG INTERACTIONS).

PREGNANCY

Benzodiazepines may cause fetal damage when administered during pregnancy. An increased risk of congenital malformations associated with the use of diazepam and chlordiazepoxide during the first trimester of pregnancy has been suggested in several studies. Transplacental distribution has resulted in neonatal CNS depression following the ingestion of therapeutic doses of a benzodiazepine hypnotic during the last weeks of pregnancy.

WARNINGS

Sleep disturbance may be the presenting manifestation of a physical and/or psychiatric disorder. Consequently, a decision to initiate symptomatic treatment of insomnia should only be made after the patient has been carefully evaluated.

The failure of insomnia to remit after 7-10 days of treatment may indicate the presence of a primary psychiatric and/or medical illness.

Worsening of insomnia or the emergence of new abnormalities of thinking or behavior may be the consequence of an unrecognized psychiatric or physical disorder. These have also been reported to occur in association with the use of triazolam.

Because some of the adverse effects of triazolam appear to be dose related (see PRECAUTIONS and DOSAGE AND ADMINISTRATION), it is important to use the smallest possible effective dose. Elderly patients are especially susceptible to dose related adverse effects.

An increase in daytime anxiety has been reported for triazolam after as few as 10 days of continuous use. In some patients this may be a manifestation of interdose withdrawal (see CLINICAL PHARMACOLOGY). If increased daytime anxiety is observed during treatment, discontinuation of treatment may be advisable.

IDIOSYNCRATIC REACTIONS

A variety of abnormal thinking and behavior changes have been reported to occur in association with the use of benzodiazepine hypnotics including triazolam. Some of these changes may be characterized by decreased inhibition (*e.g.*, aggressiveness and extroversion that seem excessive), similar to that seen with alcohol and other CNS depressants (*e.g.*, sedative/hypnotics). Other kinds of behavioral changes have also been reported, for example, bizarre behavior, agitation, hallucinations, depersonalization. In primarily depressed patients, the worsening of depression, including suicidal thinking, has been reported in association with the use of benzodiazepines.

It can rarely be determined with certainty whether a particular instance of the abnormal behaviors listed above is drug induced, spontaneous in origin, or a result of an underlying psychiatric or physical disorder. Nonetheless, the emergence of any new behavioral sign or symptom of concern requires careful and immediate evaluation.

Because of its depressant CNS effects, patients receiving triazolam should be cautioned against engaging in hazardous occupations requiring complete mental alertness such as operating machinery or driving a motor vehicle. For the same reason, patients should be cautioned about the concomitant ingestion of alcohol and other CNS depressant drugs during treatment with triazolam tablets.

As with some, but not all benzodiazepines, anterograde amnesia of varying severity and paradoxical reactions have been reported following therapeutic doses of triazolam. Data from several sources suggest that anterograde amnesia may occur at a higher rate with triazolam than with other benzodiazepine hypnotics.

TRIAZOLAM INTERACTION WITH DRUGS THAT INHIBIT METABOLISM VIA CYTOCHROME P450 3A

The initial stop in triazolam metabolism is hydroxylation catalyzed by cytochrome P450 3A (CYP 3A). Drugs that inhibit this metabolic pathway may have a profound effect on the clearance of triazolam. Consequently, triazolam should be avoided in patients receiving very potent inhibitors of CYP 3A. With drugs inhibiting CYP 3A to a lesser but still significant degree, triazolam should be used only with caution and consideration of appropriate dosage reduction. For some drugs, an interaction with triazolam has been quantified with clinical data; for other drugs, interactions are predicted from *in vitro* data and/or experience with similar drugs in the same pharmacologic class.

The following are examples of drugs known to inhibit the metabolism of triazolam and/or related benzodiazepines, presumably through inhibition of CYP 3A.

Potent CYP 3A Inhibitors

Potent inhibitors of CYP 3A that should not be used concomitantly with triazolam include ketoconazole, itraconazole, and nefazodone. Although data concerning the effects of azole-type antifungal agents other than ketoconazole and itraconazole on triazolam metabolism are not available, they should be considered potent CYP 3A inhibitors, and their coadministration with triazolam is not recommended (see CONTRAINDICATIONS).

Drugs Demonstrated To Be CYP 3A Inhibitors on the Basis of Clinical Studies Involving Triazolam

Caution and consideration of dose reduction are recommended during coadministration with triazolam.

Macrolide Antibiotics

Coadministration of erythromycin increased the maximum plasma concentration of triazolam by 46%, decreased clearance by 53%, and increased half-life by 35%; caution and consideration of appropriate triazolam dose reductions are recommended. Similar caution should be observed during coadministration with clarithromycin and other macrolide antibiotics.

Cimetidine

Coadministration of cimetidine increased the maximum plasma concentration of triazolam by 51%, decreased clearance by 55%, and increased half-life by 68%; caution and consideration of appropriate triazolam dose reduction are recommended.

Other Drugs Possibly Affecting Triazolam Metabolism

Other drugs possibly affecting triazolam metabolism by inhibition of CYP 3A are discussed in DRUG INTERACTIONS.

T

PRECAUTIONS

GENERAL

In elderly and/or debilitated patients it is recommended that treatment with triazolam tablets be initiated at 0.125 mg to decrease the possibility of development of oversedation, dizziness, or impaired coordination.

Some side effects reported in association with the use of triazolam appear to be dose related. These include drowsiness, dizziness, light-headedness, and amnesia.

The relationship between dose and what may be more serious behavioral phenomena is less certain. Specifically, some evidence, based on spontaneous marketing reports, suggests that confusion, bizarre or abnormal behavior, agitation, and hallucinations may also be dose related, but this evidence is inconclusive. In accordance with good medical practice it is recommended that therapy be initiated at the lowest effective dose (see DOSAGE AND ADMINISTRATION).

Cases of "traveler's amnesia" have been reported by individuals who have taken triazolam to induce sleep while traveling, such as during an airplane flight. In some of these cases, insufficient time was allowed for the sleep period prior to awakening and before beginning activity. Also, the concomitant use of alcohol may have been a factor in some cases.

Caution should be exercised if triazolam is prescribed to patients with signs or symptoms of depression that could be intensified by hypnotic drugs. Suicidal tendencies may be present in such patients and protective measures may be required. Intentional overdosage is more common in these patients, and the least amount of drug that is feasible should be available to the patient at any one time.

The usual precautions should be observed in patients with impaired renal or hepatic function, chronic pulmonary insufficiency, and sleep apnea. In patients with compromised respiratory function, respiratory depression and apnea have been reported infrequently.

INFORMATION FOR THE PATIENT

See the Patient Instructions that are distributed with the prescription. To assure safe and effective use of triazolam, the information and instructions provided in the Patient Instructions should be discussed with patients.

LABORATORY TESTS

Laboratory tests are not ordinarily required in otherwise healthy patients.

CARCINOGENESIS, MUTAGENESIS, AND IMPAIRMENT OF FERTILITY

No evidence of carcinogenic potential was observed in mice during a 24 month study with triazolam in doses up to 4000 times the human dose.

PREGNANCY, TERATOGENIC EFFECTS, PREGNANCY CATEGORY X

See CONTRAINDICATIONS.

NONTERATOGENIC EFFECTS

It is to be considered that the child born of a mother who is on benzodiazepines may be at some risk for withdrawal symptoms from the drug, during the postnatal period. Also, neonatal flaccidity has been reported in an infant born of a mother who had been receiving benzodiazepines.

NURSING MOTHERS

Human studies have not been performed; however, studies in rats have indicated that triazolam and its metabolites are secreted in milk. Therefore, administration of triazolam to nursing mothers is not recommended.

PEDIATRIC USE

Safety and effectiveness of triazolam in individuals below 18 years of age have not been established.

DRUG INTERACTIONS

Both pharmacodynamic and pharmacokinetic interactions have been reported with benzodiazepines. In particular, triazolam produces additive CNS depressant effects when coadministered with other psychotropic medications, anticonvulsants, antihistamines, ethanol, and other drugs which themselves produce CNS depression.

DRUGS THAT INHIBIT TRIAZOLAM METABOLISM VIA CYTOCHROME P450 3A

The initial step in triazolam metabolism is hydroxylation catalyzed by cytochrome P450 3A (CYP 3A). Drugs which inhibit this metabolic pathway may have a profound effect on the clearance of triazolam (CONTRAINDICATIONS and WARNINGS for additional drugs of this type).

T

DRUGS AND OTHER SUBSTANCES DEMONSTRATED TO BE CYP 3A INHIBITORS OF POSSIBLE CLINICAL SIGNIFICANCE ON THE BASIS OF CLINICAL STUDIES INVOLVING TRIAZOLAM

Caution is recommended during coadministration with triazolam.

Isoniazid: Coadministration of isoniazid increased the maximum plasma concentration of triazolam by 20%, decreased clearance by 42%, and increased half-life by 31%.

Oral Contraceptives: Coadministration of oral contraceptives increased maximum plasma concentration by 6%, decreased clearance by 32%, and increased half-life by 16%.

Grapefruit Juice: Coadministration of grapefruit juice increased the maximum plasma concentration of triazolam by 25%, increased the area under the concentration curve by 48%, and increased half-life by 18%.

DRUGS DEMONSTRATED TO BE CYP 3A INHIBITORS ON THE BASIS OF CLINICAL STUDIES INVOLVING BENZODIAZEPINES METABOLIZED SIMILARLY TO TRIAZOLAM OR ON THE BASIS OF IN VITRO STUDIES WITH TRIAZOLAM OR OTHER BENZODIAZEPINES

Caution is recommended during coadministration with triazolam.

Available data from clinical studies of benzodiazepines other than triazolam suggest a possible drug interaction with triazolam for the following: fluvoxamine, diltiazem, and verapamil. Data from *in vitro* studies of triazolam suggest a possible drug interaction with triazolam for the following: sertraline and paroxetine. Data from *in vitro* studies of benzodiazepines other than triazolam suggest a possible drug interaction with triazolam for the following: ergotamine, cyclosporine, amiodarone, nicardipine, and nifedipine. Caution is recommended during coadministration of any of these drugs with triazolam (see WARNINGS).

DRUGS THAT AFFECT TRIAZOLAM PHARMACOKINETICS BY OTHER MECHANISMS

Ranitidine: Coadministration of ranitidine increased the maximum plasma concentration of triazolam by 30%, increased the area under the concentration curve by 27%, and increased half-life by 3.3%. Caution is recommended during coadministration with triazolam.

ADVERSE REACTIONS

During placebo-controlled clinical studies in which 1003 patients received triazolam tablets, the most troublesome side effects were extensions of the pharmacologic activity of triazolam (*e.g.*, drowsiness, dizziness, or light-headedness).

The figures cited in TABLE 1 are estimates of untoward clinical event incidence among subjects who participated in the relatively short duration (*i.e.*, 1-42 days) placebo-controlled clinical trials of triazolam. The figures cannot be used to predict precisely the incidence of untoward events in the course of usual medical practice where patient characteristics and other factors often differ from those in clinical trials. These figures cannot be compared with those obtained from other clinical studies involving related drug products and placebo, as each group of drug trials is conducted under a different set of conditions.

Comparison of the cited figures, however, can provide the prescriber with some basis for estimating the relative contributions of drug and nondrug factors to the untoward event incidence rate in the population studied. Even this use must be approached cautiously, as a drug may relieve a symptom in one patient while inducing it in others. (For example, an anticholinergic, anxiolytic drug may relieve dry mouth [a sign of anxiety] in some subjects but induce it [an untoward event] in others.) (See TABLE 1.)

TABLE 1

Number of Patients	Triazolam	Placebo
% Patients Reporting	1003	997
Central Nervous System		
Drowsiness	14.0%	6.4%
Headache	9.7%	8.4%
Dizziness	7.8%	3.1%
Nervousness	5.2%	4.5%
Light-headedness	4.9%	0.9%
Coordination disorders/ataxia	4.6%	0.8%
Gastrointestinal		
Nausea/vomiting	4.6%	3.7%

In addition to the relatively common (*i.e.*, 1% or greater) untoward events enumerated above, the following adverse events have been reported less frequently (*i.e.*, 0.9-0.5%): euphoria, tachycardia, tiredness, confusional states/memory impairment, cramps/pain, depression, visual disturbances.

Rare (*i.e.*, less than 0.5%) adverse reactions included constipation, taste alterations, diarrhea, dry mouth, dermatitis/allergy, dreaming/nightmares, insomnia, paresthesia, tinnitus, dysesthesia, weakness, congestion, death from hepatic failure in a patient also receiving diuretic drugs.

In addition to these untoward events for which estimates of incidence are available, the following adverse events have been reported in association with the use of triazolam and other benzodiazepines: amnestic symptoms (anterograde amnesia with appropriate or inappropriate behavior), confusional states (disorientation, derealization, depersonalization, and/or clouding of consciousness), dystonia, anorexia, fatigue, sedation, slurred speech, jaundice, pruritus, dysarthria, changes in libido, menstrual irregularities, incontinence, and urinary retention. Other factors may contribute to some of these reactions (*e.g.*, concomitant intake of alcohol or other drugs, sleep deprivation, an abnormal premorbid state, etc.).

Other events reported include: Paradoxical reactions such as stimulation, mania, an agitational state (restlessness, irritability, and excitation), increased muscle spasticity, sleep disturbances, hallucinations, delusions, aggressiveness, falling, somnambulism, syncope,

TABLE 2

Number of Patients	Triazolam 380		Placebo 361	
% of Patients Reporting	Low	High	Low	High
Hematology				
Hematocrit	*	*	*	*
Hemoglobin	*	*	*	*
Total WBC count	1.7%	2.1%	*	1.3%
Neutrophil count	1.5%	1.5%	3.3%	1.0%
Lymphocyte count	2.3%	4.0%	3.1%	3.8%
Monocyte count	3.6%	*	4.4%	1.5%
Eosinophil count	10.2%	3.2%	9.8%	3.4%
Basophil count	1.7%	2.1%	*	1.8%
Urinalysis				
Albumin	—	1.1%	—	*
Sugar	—	*	—	*
RBC/HPF	—	2.9%	—	2.9%
WBC/HPF	—	11.7%	—	7.9%
Blood Chemistry				
Creatinine	2.4%	1.9%	3.6%	1.5%
Bilirubin	*	1.5%	1.0%	*
SGOT	*	5.3%	*	4.5%
Alkaline phosphatase	*	2.2%	*	2.6%

* Less than 1%

inappropriate behavior and other adverse behavioral effects. Should these occur, use of the drug should be discontinued.

The following events have also been reported: Chest pain, burning tongue/glossitis/stomatitis.

Laboratory analyses were performed on all patients participating in the clinical program for triazolam. The following incidences of abnormalities were observed in patients receiving triazolam and the corresponding placebo group. None of these changes were considered to be of physiological significance (see TABLE 2).

When treatment with triazolam is protracted, periodic blood counts, urinalysis, and blood chemistry analyses are advisable.

Minor changes in EEG patterns, usually low-voltage fast activity, have been observed in patients during therapy with triazolam and are of no known significance.

DOSAGE AND ADMINISTRATION

It is important to individualize the dosage of triazolam tablets for maximum beneficial effect and to help avoid significant adverse effects.

The recommended dose for most adults is 0.25 mg before retiring. A dose of 0.125 mg may be found to be sufficient for some patients (*e.g.*, low body weight). A dose of 0.5 mg should be used only for exceptional patients who do not respond adequately to a trial of a lower dose since the risk of several adverse reactions increases with the size of the dose administered. A dose of 0.5 mg should not be exceeded.

In geriatric and/or debilitated patients the recommended dosage range is 0.125-0.25 mg. Therapy should be initiated at 0.125 mg in this group and the 0.25 mg dose should be used only for exceptional patients who do not respond to a trial of the lower dose. A dose of 0.25 mg should not be exceeded in these patients.

As with all medications, the lowest effective dose should be used.

HOW SUPPLIED

Halicon 0.125 mg Tablets: White, elliptical, imprinted "HALCION 0.125".
Halicon 0.25 mg Tablets: Powder blue, elliptical, scored, imprinted "HALCION 0.25".
Storage: Store at controlled room temperature 20-25°C (68-77°F).

PRODUCT LISTING - RATED THERAPEUTICALLY EQUIVALENT

Tablet - Oral - 0.125 mg

10 x 10	$60.22	GENERIC, Watson/Schein Pharmaceuticals Inc	00364-2598-33
10 x 10	$61.00	GENERIC, Par Pharmaceutical Inc	49884-0453-01
10 x 10	$67.30	GENERIC, Par Pharmaceutical Inc	49884-0453-12
10 x 10	$128.30	HALCION, Pharmacia Corporation	00009-0010-38
10's	$4.04	FEDERAL UPPER LIMIT, H.C.F.A. F F P	99999-2375-06
10's	$61.63	GENERIC, Par Pharmaceutical Inc	49884-0453-62
10's	$64.90	GENERIC, Roxane Laboratories Inc	00054-4858-06
10's	$67.30	GENERIC, Greenstone Limited	59762-3717-04
100's	$59.68	GENERIC, Greenstone Limited	59762-3717-01
100's	$61.63	GENERIC, Ivax Corporation	00182-0175-13
100's	$64.00	GENERIC, Roxane Laboratories Inc	00054-8858-25
100's	$64.87	GENERIC, Aligen Independent Laboratories Inc	00405-0192-10
100's	$128.30	HALCION, Pharmacia Corporation	00009-0010-32

Tablet - Oral - 0.25 mg

10 x 10	$72.30	GENERIC, Par Pharmaceutical Inc	49884-0454-12
10's	$63.10	GENERIC, Roxane Laboratories Inc	00054-4859-06
10's	$66.68	GENERIC, Par Pharmaceutical Inc	49884-0454-01
10's	$72.30	GENERIC, Greenstone Limited	59762-3718-04
100's	$64.73	GENERIC, Watson/Schein Pharmaceuticals Inc	00364-2599-33
100's	$66.68	GENERIC, Geneva Pharmaceuticals	00781-1442-83
100's	$67.17	GENERIC, Ivax Corporation	00182-0176-13
100's	$67.17	GENERIC, Par Pharmaceutical Inc	49884-0454-62
100's	$67.22	GENERIC, Geneva Pharmaceuticals	00781-1442-13
100's	$69.00	GENERIC, Roxane Laboratories Inc	00054-8859-25
100's	$70.70	GENERIC, Aligen Independent Laboratories Inc	00405-0193-10

PRODUCT LISTING - EQUIVALENTS NOT AVAILABLE

Tablet - Oral - 0.125 mg

12's	$8.89	GENERIC, Southwood Pharmaceuticals Inc	58016-0338-12
15's	$10.17	GENERIC, Southwood Pharmaceuticals Inc	58016-0338-15
20's	$13.56	GENERIC, Southwood Pharmaceuticals Inc	58016-0338-20
30's	$20.33	GENERIC, Southwood Pharmaceuticals Inc	58016-0338-30

Tablet - Oral - 0.25 mg

5's	$4.76	GENERIC, Southwood Pharmaceuticals Inc	58016-0757-05
10's	$9.52	GENERIC, Southwood Pharmaceuticals Inc	58016-0757-10
12's	$11.41	GENERIC, Southwood Pharmaceuticals Inc	58016-0757-12
15's	$14.27	GENERIC, Southwood Pharmaceuticals Inc	58016-0757-15
20's	$19.02	GENERIC, Southwood Pharmaceuticals Inc	58016-0757-20
30's	$28.53	GENERIC, Southwood Pharmaceuticals Inc	58016-0757-30
60's	$57.06	GENERIC, Southwood Pharmaceuticals Inc	58016-0757-60
100's	$95.10	GENERIC, Southwood Pharmaceuticals Inc	58016-0757-00
100's	$140.25	HALCION, Pharmacia and Upjohn	00009-0017-55
100's	$140.40	HALCION, Pharmacia and Upjohn	00009-0017-59

Trifluoperazine Hydrochloride *(002382)*

Categories: Anxiety disorder, generalized; Schizophrenia; FDA Approved 1958 Oct; Pregnancy Category C
Drug Classes: Antipsychotics; Phenothiazines
Brand Names: **Stelazine**; Suprazine; Tfp
Foreign Brand Availability: Eskazine (Spain); Espazine (India); Flurazin (Taiwan); Iremo-pierol (Greece); Jatroneural (Germany); Jatroneural Retard (Austria); Modalina (Italy); Modiur (Colombia); Nerolet (Argentina); Nylipton (Greece); Operzine (Korea); Oxyperazine (Greece); Psyrazine (Thailand); Sporalon (Greece); Terfluzine (Hungary; Netherlands); Triflumed (Thailand); Trinicalm (India)
Cost of Therapy: $76.13 (Schizophrenia; Stelazine; 5 mg; 2 tablets/day; 30 day supply)
$24.29 (Schizophrenia; Generic Tablets; 5 mg; 2 tablets/day; 30 day supply)

DESCRIPTION

STELAZINE TABLETS

Each stelazine tablet contains trifluoperazine hydrochloride equivalent to trifluoperazine in 1, 2, 5, or 10 mg. Inactive ingredients consist of cellulose, croscarmellose sodium, FD&C blue no. 2, FD&C yellow no. 6, FD&C red no. 40, gelatin, iron oxide, lactose, magnesium stearate, talc, titanium dioxide and trace amounts of other inactive ingredients.

STELAZINE MULTI-DOSE VIALS

Stelazine multi-dose vials are available in 10 ml (2 mg/ml) vials. Each ml contains, in aqueous solution, trifluoperazine, 2 mg, as the hydrochloride; sodium tartrate, 4.75 mg; sodium biphosphate, 11.6 mg; sodium saccharin, 0.3 mg; benzyl alcohol, 0.75%, as preservative.

STELAZINE CONCENTRATE

Each ml of clear, yellow, banana-vanilla-flavored liquid contains 10 mg of trifluoperazine as the hydrochloride. Inactive ingredients consist of D&C yellow no. 10, FD&C yellow no. 6, flavor, sodium benzoate, sodium bisulfite, sucrose, and water.

N.B.: The concentrate is for use in schizophrenia when oral medication is preferred and other oral forms are considered impractical.

INDICATIONS AND USAGE

For the management of schizophrenia.

Trifluoperazine HCl is effective for the short-term treatment of generalized non-psychotic anxiety. However, trifluoperazine HCl is not the first drug to be used in therapy for most patients with non-psychotic anxiety because certain risks associated with its use are not shared by common alternative treatments (*i.e.*, benzodiazepines).

When used in the treatment of non-psychotic anxiety, trifluoperazine HCl should not be administered at doses of more than 6 mg/day or for longer than 12 weeks because the use of trifluoperazine HCl at higher doses or for longer intervals may cause persistent tardive dyskinesia that may prove irreversible (see WARNINGS).

The effectiveness of trifluoperazine HCl as a treatment for non-psychotic anxiety was established in a 4 week clinical multicenter study of outpatients with generalized anxiety disorder (DSM-III). This evidence does not predict that trifluoperazine HCl will be useful in patients with other non-psychotic conditions in which anxiety, or signs that mimic anxiety, are found (*i.e.*, physical illness, organic mental conditions, agitated depression, character pathologies, etc.).

Trifluoperazine HCl has not been shown effective in the management of behavioral complications in patients with mental retardation.

CONTRAINDICATIONS

A known hypersensitivity to phenothiazines, comatose or greatly depressed states due to central nervous system (CNS) depressants and, in cases of existing blood dyscrasias, bone marrow depression and pre-existing liver damage.

WARNINGS

TARDIVE DYSKINESIA

Tardive dyskinesia, a syndrome consisting of potentially irreversible, involuntary, dyskinetic movements, may develop in patients treated with antipsychotic drugs. Although the prevalence of the syndrome appears to be highest among the elderly, especially elderly women, it is impossible to rely upon prevalence estimates to predict, at the inception of antipsychotic treatment, which patients are likely to develop the syndrome. Whether antipsychotic drug products differ in their potential to cause tardive dyskinesia is unknown.

Both the risk of developing the syndrome and the likelihood that it will become irreversible are believed to increase as the duration of treatment and the total cumulative dose of antipsychotic drugs administered to the patient increase. However, the syndrome can develop, although much less commonly, after relatively brief treatment periods at low doses.

There is no known treatment for established cases of tardive dyskinesia, although the syndrome may remit, partially or completely, if antipsychotic treatment is withdrawn. Antipsychotic treatment itself, however, may suppress (or partially suppress) the signs and symptoms of the syndrome and thereby may possibly mask the underlying disease process. The effect that symptomatic suppression has upon the long-term course of the syndrome is unknown.

Given these considerations, antipsychotics should be prescribed in a manner that is most likely to minimize the occurrence of tardive dyskinesia. Chronic antipsychotic treatment should generally be reserved for patients who suffer from a chronic illness that (1) is known to respond to antipsychotic drugs, and, (2) for whom alternative, equally effective, but potentially less harmful treatments are *not* available or appropriate. In patients who do require chronic treatment, the smallest dose and the shortest duration of treatment producing a satisfactory clinical response should be sought. The need for continued treatment should be reassessed periodically.

If signs and symptoms of tardive dyskinesia appear in a patient on antipsychotics, drug discontinuation should be considered. However, some patients may require treatment despite the presence of the syndrome.

For further information about the description of tardive dyskinesia and its clinical detection, please refer to PRECAUTIONS and ADVERSE REACTIONS.

NEUROLEPTIC MALIGNANT SYNDROME (NMS)

A potentially fatal symptom complex sometimes referred to as Neuroleptic Malignant Syndrome (NMS) has been reported in association with antipsychotic drugs. Clinical manifestations of NMS are hyperpyrexia, muscle rigidity, altered mental status and evidence of autonomic instability (irregular pulse or blood pressure, tachycardia, diaphoresis, and cardiac dysrhythmias).

The diagnostic evaluation of patients with this syndrome is complicated. In arriving at a diagnosis, it is important to identify cases where the clinical presentation includes both serious medical illness (*e.g.*, pneumonia, systemic infection, etc.) and untreated or inadequately treated extrapyramidal signs and symptoms (EPS). Other important considerations in the differential diagnosis include central anticholinergic toxicity, heat stroke, drug fever, and primary central nervous system (CNS) pathology.

The management of NMS should include (1) immediate discontinuation of antipsychotic drugs and other drugs not essential to concurrent therapy, (2) intensive symptomatic treatment and medical monitoring, and (3) treatment of any concomitant serious medical problems for which specific treatments are available. There is no general agreement about specific pharmacological treatment regimens for uncomplicated NMS.

If a patient requires antipsychotic drug treatment after recovery from NMS, the potential reintroduction of drug therapy should be carefully considered. The patient should be carefully monitored, since recurrences of NMS have been reported.

An encephalopathic syndrome (characterized by weakness, lethargy, fever, tremulousness and confusion, extrapyramidal symptoms, leukocytosis, elevated serum enzymes, BUN and FBS) has occurred in a few patients treated with lithium plus an antipsychotic. In some instances, the syndrome was followed by irreversible brain damage. Because of a possible causal relationship between these events and the concomitant administration of lithium and antipsychotics, patients receiving such combined therapy should be monitored closely for early evidence of neurologic toxicity and treatment discontinued promptly if such signs appear. This encephalopathic syndrome may be similar to or the same as NMS.

Patients who have demonstrated a hypersensitivity reaction (*e.g.*, blood dyscrasias, jaundice) with a phenothiazine should not be re-exposed to any phenothiazine, including trifluoperazine HCl, unless in the judgment of the physician the potential benefits of treatment outweigh the possible hazard.

Trifluoperazine HCl concentrate contains sodium bisulfite, a sulfite that may cause allergic-type reactions including anaphylactic symptoms and life-threatening or less severe asthmatic episodes in certain susceptible people. The overall prevalence of sulfite sensitivity in the general population is unknown and probably low. Sulfite sensitivity is seen more frequently in asthmatic than in non-asthmatic people.

Trifluoperazine HCl may impair mental and/or physical abilities, especially during the first few days of therapy. Therefore, caution patients about activities requiring alertness (*e.g.*, operating vehicles or machinery).

If agents such as sedatives, narcotics, anesthetics, tranquilizers or alcohol are used either simultaneously or successively with the drug, the possibility of an undesirable additive depressant effect should be considered.

USE IN PREGNANCY

Safety for the use of trifluoperazine HCl during pregnancy has not been established. Therefore, it is not recommended that the drug be given to pregnant patients except when, in the judgment of the physician, it is essential. The potential benefits should clearly outweigh possible hazards. There are reported instances of prolonged jaundice, extrapyramidal signs, hyperreflexia or hyporeflexia in newborn infants whose mothers received phenothiazines.

Reproductive studies in rats given over 600 times the human dose showed an increased incidence of malformations above controls and reduced litter size and weight linked to maternal toxicity. These effects were not observed at half this dosage. No adverse effect on fetal development was observed in rabbits given 700 times the human dose nor in monkeys given 25 times the human dose.

NURSING MOTHERS

There is evidence that phenothiazines are excreted in the breast milk of nursing mothers. Because of the potential for serious adverse reactions in nursing infants from trifluoperazine, a decision should be made whether to discontinue nursing or to discontinue the drug, taking into account the importance of the drug to the mother.

PRECAUTIONS

GENERAL

Given the likelihood that some patients exposed chronically to antipsychotics will develop tardive dyskinesia, it is advised that all patients in whom chronic use is contemplated be given, if possible, full information about this risk. The decision to inform patients and/or their guardians must obviously take into account the clinical circumstances and the competency of the patient to understand the information provided.

Thrombocytopenia and anemia have been reported in patients receiving the drug. Agranulocytosis and pancytopenia have also been reported — warn patients to report the sudden appearance of sore throat or other signs of infection. If white blood cell and differential counts indicate cellular depression, stop treatment and start antibiotic and other suitable therapy.

Jaundice of the cholestatic type of hepatitis or liver damage has been reported. If fever with grippe-like symptoms occurs, appropriate liver studies should be conducted. If tests indicate an abnormality, stop treatment.

One result of therapy may be an increase in mental and physical activity. For example, a few patients with angina pectoris have complained of increased pain while taking the drug. Therefore, angina patients should be observed carefully and, if an unfavorable response is noted, the drug should be withdrawn.

Because hypotension has occurred, large doses and parenteral administration should be avoided in patients with impaired cardiovascular systems. To minimize the occurrence of hypotension after injection, keep patient lying down and observe for at least ½ hour. If hypotension occurs from parenteral or oral dosing, place patient in head-low position with legs raised. If a vasoconstrictor is required, norepinephrine bitartrate and phenylephrine HCl are suitable. Other pressor agents, including epinephrine, should not be used as they may cause a paradoxical further lowering of blood pressure.

Since certain phenothiazines have been reported to produce retinopathy, the drug should be discontinued if ophthalmoscopic examination or visual field studies should demonstrate retinal changes.

An antiemetic action of trifluoperazine HCl may mask the signs and symptoms of toxicity or overdosage of other drugs and may obscure the diagnosis and treatment of other conditions such as intestinal obstruction, brain tumor and Reye's syndrome.

With prolonged administration at high dosages, the possibility of cumulative effects, with sudden onset of severe CNS or vasomotor symptoms, should be kept in mind.

Antipsychotic drugs elevate prolactin levels; the elevation persists during chronic administration. Tissue culture experiments indicate that approximately 1/3 of human breast cancers are prolactin-dependent *in vitro*, a factor of potential importance if the prescribing of these drugs is contemplated in a patient with a previously detected breast cancer. Although disturbances such as galactorrhea, amenorrhea, gynecomastia and impotence have been reported, the clinical significance of elevated serum prolactin levels is unknown for most patients. An increase in mammary neoplasms has been found in rodents after chronic administration of antipsychotic drugs. Neither clinical nor epidemiologic studies conducted to date, however, have shown an association between chronic administration of these drugs and mammary tumorigenesis; the available evidence is considered too limited to be conclusive at this time.

Chromosomal aberrations in spermatocytes and abnormal sperm have been demonstrated in rodents treated with certain antipsychotics.

Because phenothiazines may interfere with thermoregulatory mechanisms, use with caution in persons who will be exposed to extreme heat.

As with all drugs which exert an anticholinergic effect, and/or cause mydriasis, trifluoperazine should be used with caution in patients with glaucoma.

Phenothiazines may diminish the effect of oral anticoagulants.

Phenothiazines can produce alpha-adrenergic blockade.

Concomitant administration of propranolol with phenothiazines results in increased plasma levels of both drugs.

Antihypertensive effects of guanethidine and related compounds may be counteracted when phenothiazines are used concurrently.

Thiazide diuretics may accentuate the orthostatic hypotension that may occur with phenothiazines.

Phenothiazines may lower the convulsive threshold; dosage adjustments of anticonvulsants may be necessary. Potentiation of anticonvulsant effects does not occur. However, it has been reported that phenothiazines may interfere with the metabolism of phenytoin sodium and thus precipitate phenytoin sodium toxicity.

Drugs which lower the seizure threshold, including phenothiazine derivatives, should not be used with metrizamide. As with other phenothiazine derivatives, trifluoperazine HCl should be discontinued at least 48 hours before myelography, should not be resumed for at least 24 hours postprocedure and should not be used for the control of nausea and vomiting occurring either prior to myelography or postprocedure with metrizamide.

The presence of phenothiazines may produce false-positive phenylketonuria (PKU) test results.

Long-Term Therapy

To lessen the likelihood of adverse reactions related to cumulative drug effect, patients with a history of long-term therapy with trifluoperazine HCl and/or other antipsychotics should be evaluated periodically to decide whether the maintenance dosage could be lowered or drug therapy discontinued.

ADVERSE REACTIONS

Drowsiness, dizziness, skin reactions, rash, dry mouth, insomnia, amenorrhea, fatigue, muscular weakness, anorexia, lactation, blurred vision, and neuromuscular (extrapyramidal) reactions.

NEUROMUSCULAR (EXTRAPYRAMIDAL) REACTIONS

These symptoms are seen in a significant number of hospitalized mental patients. They may be characterized by motor restlessness, be of the dystonic type, or they may resemble parkinsonism.

Depending on the severity of symptoms, dosage should be reduced or discontinued. If therapy is reinstituted, it should be at a lower dosage. Should these symptoms occur in children or pregnant patients, the drug should be stopped and not reinstituted. In most cases barbiturates by suitable route of administration will suffice. (Or, injectable diphenhydramine HCl may be useful.) In more severe cases, the administration of an anti-parkinsonism agent, except levodopa, usually produces rapid reversal of symptoms. Suitable supportive measures such as maintaining a clear airway and adequate hydration should be employed.

Motor Restlessness

Symptoms may include agitation or jitteriness and sometimes insomnia. These symptoms often disappear spontaneously. At times these symptoms may be similar to the original neurotic or psychotic symptoms. Dosage should not be increased until these side effects have subsided.

If this phase becomes too troublesome, the symptoms can usually be controlled by a reduction of dosage or change of drug. Treatment with anti-parkinsonism agents, benzodiazepines or propranolol may be helpful.

Dystonias

Symptoms May Include: Spasm of the neck muscles, sometimes progressing to torticollis; extensor rigidity of back muscles, sometimes progressing to opisthotonos; carpopedal spasm, trismus, swallowing difficulty, oculogyric crisis, and protrusion of the tongue.

These usually subside within a few hours, and almost always within 24-48 hours, after the drug has been discontinued.

In mild cases, reassurance or a barbiturate is often sufficient.*In moderate cases,* barbiturates will usually bring rapid relief.*In more severe adult cases,* the administration of an anti-parkinsonism agent, except levodopa, usually produces rapid reversal of symptoms. Also, IV caffeine with sodium benzoate seems to be effective. *In children,* reassurance and barbiturates will usually control symptoms. (Or, injectable diphenhydramine HCl may be useful.) *Note:* See diphenhydramine HCl prescribing information for appropriate children's dosage. If appropriate treatment with anti-parkinsonism agents or diphenhydramine HCl fails to reverse the signs and symptoms, the diagnosis should be reevaluated.

Pseudo-Parkinsonism

Symptoms May Include: Mask-like facies; drooling; tremors; pill-rolling motion; cog-wheel rigidity; and shuffling gait. Reassurance and sedation are important. In most cases these symptoms are readily controlled when an anti-parkinsonism agent is administered concomitantly. Anti-parkinsonism agents should be used only when required. Generally, therapy of a few weeks to 2-3 months will suffice. After this time patients should be evaluated to determine their need for continued treatment. (*Note:* Levodopa has not been found effective in pseudo-parkinsonism.) Occasionally it is necessary to lower the dosage of trifluoperazine HCl or to discontinue the drug.

Tardive Dyskinesia

As with all antipsychotic agents, tardive dyskinesia may appear in some patients on long-term therapy or may appear after drug therapy has been discontinued. The syndrome can also develop, although much less frequently, after relatively brief treatment periods at low doses. This syndrome appears in all age groups. Although its prevalence appears to be highest among elderly patients, especially elderly women, it is impossible to rely upon prevalence estimates to predict at the inception of antipsychotic treatment which patients are likely to develop the syndrome. The symptoms are persistent and in some patients appear to be irreversible. The syndrome is characterized by rhythmical involuntary movements of the tongue, face, mouth or jaw (*e.g.,* protrusion of tongue, puffing of cheeks, puckering of mouth, chewing movements). Sometimes these may be accompanied by involuntary movements of extremities. In rare instances, these involuntary movements of the extremities are the only manifestations of tardive dyskinesia. A variant of tardive dyskinesia, tardive dystonia, has also been described.

There is no known effective treatment for tardive dyskinesia; anti-parkinsonism agents do not alleviate the symptoms of this syndrome. If clinically feasible, it is suggested that all antipsychotic agents be discontinued if these symptoms appear. Should it be necessary to reinstitute treatment, or increase the dosage of the agent, or switch to a different antipsychotic agent, the syndrome may be masked.

It has been reported that fine vermicular movements of the tongue may be an early sign of the syndrome and if the medication is stopped at that time the syndrome may not develop.

Adverse Reactions Reported With Trifluoperazine HCl or Other Phenothiazine Derivatives

Adverse effects with different phenothiazines vary in type, frequency, and mechanism of occurrence, *i.e.,* some are dose-related, while others involve individual patient sensitivity. Some adverse effects may be more likely to occur, or occur with greater intensity, in patients with special medical problems, *e.g.,* patients with mitral insufficiency or pheochromocytoma have experienced severe hypotension following recommended doses of certain phenothiazines.

Neuroleptic Malignant Syndrome (NMS) has been reported in association with antipsychotic drugs. (See WARNINGS.)

Not all of the following adverse reactions have been observed with every phenothiazine derivative, but they have been reported with 1 or more and should be borne in mind when drugs of this class are administered: extrapyramidal symptoms (opisthotonos, oculogyric crisis, hyperreflexia, dystonia, akathisia, dyskinesia, parkinsonism) some of which have lasted months and even years — particularly in elderly patients with previous brain damage; grand mal and petit mal convulsions, particularly in patients with EEG abnormalities or history of such disorders; altered cerebrospinal fluid proteins; cerebral edema; intensification and prolongation of the action of CNS depressants (opiates, analgesics, antihistamines, barbiturates, alcohol), atropine, heat, organophosphorus insecticides; autonomic reactions (dryness of mouth, nasal congestion, headache, nausea, constipation, obstipation, adynamic ileus, ejaculatory disorders/impotence, priapism, atonic colon, urinary retention, miosis and mydriasis); reactivation of psychotic processes, catatonic-like states; hypotension (sometimes fatal); cardiac arrest; blood dyscrasias (pancytopenia, thrombocytopenic purpura, leukopenia, agranulocytosis, eosinophilia, hemolytic anemia, aplastic anemia); liver damage (jaundice, biliary stasis); endocrine disturbances (hyperglycemia, hypoglycemia, glycosuria, lactation, galactorrhea, gynecomastia, menstrual irregularities, false-positive pregnancy tests); skin disorders (photosensitivity, itching, erythema, urticaria, eczema up to exfoliative dermatitis); other allergic reactions (asthma, laryngeal edema, angioneurotic edema, anaphylactoid reactions); peripheral edema; reversed epinephrine effect; hyperpyrexia; mild fever after large IM doses; increased appetite; increased weight; a systemic lupus erythematosus-like syndrome; pigmentary retinopathy; with prolonged administration of substantial doses, skin pigmentation, epithelial keratopathy, and lenticular and corneal deposits.

EKG changes — particularly nonspecific, usually reversible Q and T wave distortions — have been observed in some patients receiving phenothiazine antipsychotics. Although phenothiazines cause neither psychic nor physical dependence, sudden discontinuance in long-term psychiatric patients may cause temporary symptoms, *e.g.,* nausea and vomiting, dizziness, tremulousness.

Note: There have been occasional reports of sudden death in patients receiving phenothiazines. In some cases, the cause appeared to be cardiac arrest or asphyxia due to failure of the cough reflex.

DOSAGE AND ADMINISTRATION

ADULTS

Dosage should be adjusted to the needs of the individual. The lowest effective dosage should always be used. Dosage should be increased more gradually in debilitated or emaciated patients. When maximum response is achieved, dosage may be reduced gradually to a maintenance level. Because of the inherent long action of the drug, patients may be controlled on convenient bid administration; some patients may be maintained on once-a-day administration.

When trifluoperazine HCl is administered by IM injection, equivalent oral dosage may be substituted once symptoms have been controlled.

Note: Although there is little likelihood of contact dermatitis due to the drug, persons with known sensitivity to phenothiazine drugs should avoid direct contact.

Elderly Patients

In general, dosages in the lower range are sufficient for most elderly patients. Since they appear to be more susceptible to hypotension and neuromuscular reactions, such patients should be observed closely. Dosage should be tailored to the individual, response carefully monitored, and dosage adjusted accordingly. Dosage should be increased more gradually in elderly patients.

Non-Psychotic Anxiety

Usual dosage is 1 or 2 mg twice daily. Do not administer at doses of more than 6 mg/day or for longer than 12 weeks.

Shizophrenia

Oral

Usual starting dosage is 2-5 mg bid. (Small or emaciated patients should always be started on the lower dosage.)

Most patients will show optimum response on 15 or 20 mg daily, although a few may require 40 mg/day or more. Optimum therapeutic dosage levels should be reached within 2 or 3 weeks.

When the concentrate dosage form is to be used, it should be added to 60 ml (2 fl oz) or more of diluent *just prior to administration* to insure palatability and stability. Vehicles suggested for dilution are: tomato or fruit juice, milk, simple syrup, orange syrup, carbonated beverages, coffee, tea, or water. Semisolid foods (soup, puddings, etc.) may also be used.

Intramuscular (for prompt control of severe symptoms)

Usual dosage is 1-2 mg (½ to 1 ml) by deep IM injection q4-6h, prn. More than 6 mg within 24 hours is rarely necessary.

Only in very exceptional cases should IM dosage exceed 10 mg within 24 hours. Injections should not be given at intervals of less than 4 hours because of a possible cumulative effect.

Note: Trifluoperazine HCl injection has been usually well tolerated and there is little, if any, pain and irritation at the site of injection.

This solution should be protected from light. This is a clear, colorless to pale yellow solution; a slight yellowish discoloration will not alter potency. If markedly discolored, solution should be discarded.

SHIZOPHRENIA IN CHILDREN

Dosage should be adjusted to the weight of the child and severity of the symptoms. These dosages are for children, ages 6-12, who are hospitalized or under close supervision.

Oral

The starting dosage is 1 mg administered once a day or bid. Dosage may be increased gradually until symptoms are controlled or until side effects become troublesome.

While it is usually not necessary to exceed dosages of 15 mg daily, some older children with severe symptoms may require higher dosages.

Intramuscular

There has been little experience with the use of trifluoperazine HCl injection in children. However, if it is necessary to achieve rapid control of severe symptoms, 1 mg (½ ml) of the drug may be administered intramuscularly once or twice a day.

HOW SUPPLIED

Stelazine Tablets: Each round, blue, film-coated tablet contains trifluoperazine hydrochloride equivalent to trifluoperazine as follows:

1 mg: Imprinted "SKF" and "S03".
2 mg: Imprinted "SKF" and "S04".
5 mg: Imprinted "SKF" and "S06".
10 mg: Imprinted "SKF" and "S07".

Stelazine Multi-Dose Vials: Available in 10 ml (2 mg/ml) vials.

Stelazine Concentrate (for institutional use): Available as 10 mg/ml in 2 fl oz bottles. The concentrate form is light-sensitive. For this reason, it should be protected from light and dispensed in amber bottles. *Refrigeration is not required.*

Storage: Store all Stelazine formulations between 15 and 30°C (59 and 86°F).

PRODUCT LISTING - RATED THERAPEUTICALLY EQUIVALENT

Solution - Intramuscular - 2 mg/ml			
10 ml	$67.79	STELAZINE, Glaxosmithkline	00108-4902-01
Tablet - Oral - 1 mg			
10 x 10	$60.05	GENERIC, Udl Laboratories Inc	51079-0572-20
100's	$24.33	FEDERAL UPPER LIMIT, H.C.F.A. F F P	99999-2382-08
100's	$54.40	GENERIC, Geneva Pharmaceuticals	00781-1030-01
100's	$55.50	GENERIC, Dixon-Shane Inc	17236-0379-01
100's	$56.64	GENERIC, Apothecon Inc	62269-0278-24
100's	$58.30	GENERIC, Mylan Pharmaceuticals Inc	00378-2401-01
100's	$67.97	GENERIC, Geneva Pharmaceuticals	00781-1030-13
Tablet - Oral - 2 mg			
30's	$20.77	GENERIC, Pd-Rx Pharmaceuticals	61392-0152-30
30's	$20.77	GENERIC, Pd-Rx Pharmaceuticals	61392-0152-39
31 x 10	$259.92	GENERIC, Vangard Labs	00615-3598-53
31's	$21.46	GENERIC, Pd-Rx Pharmaceuticals	61392-0152-31
32's	$22.15	GENERIC, Pd-Rx Pharmaceuticals	61392-0152-32
45's	$31.15	GENERIC, Pd-Rx Pharmaceuticals	61392-0152-45

T

60's	$41.53	GENERIC, Pd-Rx Pharmaceuticals	61392-0152-60
90's	$62.30	GENERIC, Pd-Rx Pharmaceuticals	61392-0152-90
100's	$35.52	FEDERAL UPPER LIMIT, H.C.F.A. F F P	99999-2382-11
100's	$40.30	GENERIC, Major Pharmaceuticals Inc	00904-0561-60
100's	$80.24	GENERIC, Apothecon Inc	62269-0279-24
100's	$81.85	GENERIC, Dixon-Shane Inc	17236-0293-01
100's	$83.54	GENERIC, Geneva Pharmaceuticals	00781-1032-01
100's	$83.85	GENERIC, Geneva Pharmaceuticals	00781-1032-13
100's	$85.90	GENERIC, Mylan Pharmaceuticals Inc	00378-2402-01
100's	$88.48	GENERIC, Udl Laboratories Inc	51079-0573-20
100's	$122.90	STELAZINE, Glaxosmithkline	00108-4904-20
200 x 5	$835.45	GENERIC, Vangard Labs	00615-3598-43
Tablet - Oral - 5 mg			
30's	$26.14	GENERIC, Pd-Rx Pharmaceuticals	61392-0154-30
30's	$26.14	GENERIC, Pd-Rx Pharmaceuticals	61392-0154-39
31's	$27.01	GENERIC, Pd-Rx Pharmaceuticals	61392-0154-31
32's	$27.88	GENERIC, Pd-Rx Pharmaceuticals	61392-0154-32
45's	$39.21	GENERIC, Pd-Rx Pharmaceuticals	61392-0154-45
60's	$52.28	GENERIC, Pd-Rx Pharmaceuticals	61392-0154-60
90's	$78.42	GENERIC, Pd-Rx Pharmaceuticals	61392-0154-90
100's	$14.33	GENERIC, Us Trading Corporation	56126-0315-11
100's	$42.71	FEDERAL UPPER LIMIT, H.C.F.A. F F P	99999-2382-13
100's	$47.50	GENERIC, Major Pharmaceuticals Inc	00904-0562-60
100's	$100.98	GENERIC, Apothecon Inc	62269-0280-24
100's	$103.00	GENERIC, Mylan Pharmaceuticals Inc	00378-2405-01
100's	$103.00	GENERIC, Dixon-Shane Inc	17236-0296-01
100's	$105.14	GENERIC, Geneva Pharmaceuticals	00781-1034-01
100's	$111.45	GENERIC, Udl Laboratories Inc	51079-0574-20
100's	$126.89	STELAZINE, Southwood Pharmaceuticals Inc	58016-0684-00
100's	$154.70	STELAZINE, Glaxosmithkline	00108-4906-20
Tablet - Oral - 10 mg			
30's	$39.40	GENERIC, Heartland Healthcare Services	61392-0151-30
30's	$39.40	GENERIC, Heartland Healthcare Services	61392-0151-39
31 x 10	$492.99	GENERIC, Vangard Labs	00615-1503-53
31 x 10	$492.99	GENERIC, Vangard Labs	00615-1503-63
31's	$40.71	GENERIC, Heartland Healthcare Services	61392-0151-31
32's	$42.02	GENERIC, Heartland Healthcare Services	61392-0151-32
45's	$59.09	GENERIC, Heartland Healthcare Services	61392-0151-45
60's	$78.79	GENERIC, Heartland Healthcare Services	61392-0151-60
90's	$118.19	GENERIC, Heartland Healthcare Services	61392-0151-90
100's	$14.85	GENERIC, Us Trading Corporation	56126-0316-11
100's	$54.03	FEDERAL UPPER LIMIT, H.C.F.A. F F P	99999-2382-09
100's	$60.00	GENERIC, Major Pharmaceuticals Inc	00904-0563-60
100's	$137.45	GENERIC, Vangard Labs	00615-1503-29
100's	$152.24	GENERIC, Apothecon Inc	62269-0281-24
100's	$155.30	GENERIC, Mylan Pharmaceuticals Inc	00378-2410-01
100's	$155.30	GENERIC, Dixon-Shane Inc	17236-0334-01
100's	$158.47	GENERIC, Geneva Pharmaceuticals	00781-1036-01
100's	$167.99	GENERIC, Udl Laboratories Inc	51079-0575-20
100's	$190.16	GENERIC, Geneva Pharmaceuticals	00781-1036-13
100's	$217.32	STELAZINE, Glaxosmithkline	00108-4907-20
200 x 5	$1590.29	GENERIC, Vangard Labs	00615-1503-43

PRODUCT LISTING - EQUIVALENTS NOT AVAILABLE

Tablet - Oral - 5 mg			
100's	$40.48	GENERIC, Physicians Total Care	54868-1352-00
Tablet - Oral - 10 mg			
100's	$66.78	GENERIC, Physicians Total Care	54868-2356-01

Trihexyphenidyl Hydrochloride *(002385)*

Categories: Extrapyramidal disorder, drug-induced; Parkinson's disease; FDA Approved 1949 May; Pregnancy Category C
Drug Classes: Anticholinergics; Antiparkinson agents
Brand Names: Aparkane; **Artane**; Tremin; Trihexane; Trihexidyl; Trihexy; Tritane
Foreign Brand Availability: Acamed (Thailand); Apo-Trihex (Canada; Malaysia); Arkine (Indonesia); Beahexol (Singapore); Hipokinon (Mexico); Pacitane (India); Pargitan (Sweden); Parkinane LP (France); Parkines (Japan); Parkisonal (Japan); Parkopan (Germany); Partane (Israel); Stobrun (Japan); Tridyl (Thailand); Trihexin (Japan)
Cost of Therapy: $8.18 (Parkinsonism; Generic Tablets; 2 mg; 3 tablets/day; 30 day supply)

T

DESCRIPTION

Trihexyphenidyl HCl is a synthetic antispasmodic drug.

Trihexyphenidyl HCl is a white or slightly off-white, crystalline powder, having not more than a very faint odor.

Trihexyphenidyl HCl is the substituted piperidine salt, (±)-α-Cyclohexyl-α-phenyl-1-piperidine-propanol hydrochloride. Its molecular formula is $C_{20}H_{31}NO{\cdot}HCl$.

Storage: Store at controlled room temperature 15-30°C (59-86°F). DO NOT FREEZE THE ELIXIR.

CLINICAL PHARMACOLOGY

Trihexyphenidyl HCl exerts a direct inhibitory effect upon the parasympathetic nervous system. It also has a relaxing effect on smooth musculature; exerted both directly upon the muscle tissue itself and indirectly through an inhibitory effect upon the parasympathetic nervous system. Its therapeutic properties are similar to those of atropine although undesirable side effects are ordinarily less frequent and severe than with the latter.

INDICATIONS AND USAGE

Trihexyphenidyl HCl is indicated as an adjunct in the treatment of all forms of parkinsonism (postencephalitic, arteriosclerotic, and idiopathic). It is often useful as adjuvant therapy when treating these forms of parkinsonism with levodopa. Additionally, it is indicated for the control of extrapyramidal disorders caused by central nervous system drugs such as the dibenzoxazepines, phenothiazines, thioxanthenes, and butyrophenones.

Sequels: For maintenance therapy after patients have been stabilized on trihexyphenidyl HCl in conventional dosage forms (tablets or elixir).

NON-FDA APPROVED INDICATIONS

Trihexyphenidyl has also been used in the treatment of primary dystonia of different etiologies, although this use is not approved by the FDA.

WARNINGS

Patients to be treated with trihexyphenidyl HCl should have a gonioscope evaluation and close monitoring of intraocular pressures at regular periodic intervals.

PRECAUTIONS

Although trihexyphenidyl HCl is not contraindicated for patients with cardiac, liver, or kidney disorders, or with hypertension, such patients should be maintained under close observation. Since the use of trihexyphenidyl HCl may in some cases continue indefinitely and since it has atropine-like properties, patients should be subjected to constant and careful long-term observation to avoid allergic and other untoward reactions. Inasmuch as trihexyphenidyl HCl possesses some parasympatholytic activity, it should be used with caution in patients with glaucoma, obstructive disease of the gastrointestinal or genitourinary tracts, and in elderly males with possible prostatic hypertrophy. Geriatric patients, particularly over the age of 60, frequently develop increased sensitivity to the actions of drugs of this type, and hence, require strict dosage regulation. Incipient glaucoma may be precipitated by parasympatholytic drugs such as trihexyphenidyl HCl.

Tardive dyskinesia may appear in some patients on long-term therapy with antipsychotic drugs or may occur after therapy with these drugs has been discontinued. Antiparkinsonism agents do not alleviate the symptoms of tardive dyskinesia, and in some instances may aggravate them. However, parkinsonism and tardive dyskinesia often coexist in patients receiving chronic neuroleptic treatment, and anticholinergic therapy with trihexyphenidyl HCl may relieve some of these parkinsonism symptoms.

ADVERSE REACTIONS

Minor side effects, such as dryness of the mouth, blurring of vision, dizziness, mild nausea, or nervousness, will be experienced by 30-50% of all patients. These sensations, however, are much less troublesome with trihexyphenidyl HCl than with belladonna alkaloids and are usually less disturbing than unalleviated parkinsonism. Such reactions tend to become less pronounced, and even to disappear, as treatment continues. Even before these reactions have remitted spontaneously, they may often be controlled by careful adjustment of dosage form, amount of drug, or interval between doses.

Isolated instances of suppurative parotitis secondary to excessive dryness of the mouth, skin rashes, dilatation of the colon, paralytic ileus, and certain psychiatric manifestations such as delusions and hallucinations, plus one doubtful case of paranoia all of which may occur with any of the atropine-like drugs, have been reported rarely with trihexyphenidyl HCl.

Patients with arteriosclerosis or with a history of idiosyncrasy to other drugs may exhibit reactions of mental confusion, agitation, disturbed behavior, or nausea and vomiting. Such patients should be allowed to develop a tolerance through the initial administration of a small dose and gradual increase in dose until an effective level is reached. If a severe reaction should occur, administration of the drug should be discontinued for a few days and then resumed at a lower dosage. Psychiatric disturbances can result from indiscriminate use (leading to overdosage) to sustain continued euphoria.

Potential side effects associated with the use of any atropine-like drugs include constipation, drowsiness, urinary hesitancy or retention, tachycardia, dilation of the pupil, increased intraocular tension, weakness, vomiting, and headache.

The occurrence of angle-closure glaucoma due to long-term treatment with trihexyphenidyl HCl has been reported.

DOSAGE AND ADMINISTRATION

Dosage should be individualized. The initial dose should be low and then increased gradually, especially in patients over 60 years of age. Whether trihexyphenidyl HCl may best be given before or after meals should be determined by the way the patient reacts. Postencephalitic patients, who are usually more prone to excessive salivation, may prefer to take it after meals and may, in addition, require small amounts of atropine which, under such circumstances, is sometimes an effective adjuvant. If trihexyphenidyl HCl tends to dry the mouth excessively, it may be better to take it before meals, unless it causes nausea. If taken after meals, the thirst sometimes induced can be allayed by mint candies, chewing gum, or water.

TRIHEXYPHENIDYL HCl IN IDIOPATHIC PARKINSONISM

As initial therapy for parkinsonism, 1 mg of trihexyphenidyl HCl in tablet or elixir form may be administered the first day. The dose may then be increased by 2 mg increments at intervals of 3-5 days, until a total of 6-10 mg is given daily. The total daily dose will depend upon what is found to be the optimal level. Many patients derive maximum benefit from this daily total of 6-10 mg, but some patients, chiefly those in the postencephalitic group, may require a total daily dose of 12-15 mg.

TRIHEXYPHENIDYL HCl IN DRUG-INDUCED PARKINSONISM

The size and frequency of dose of trihexyphenidyl HCl needed to control extrapyramidal reactions to commonly employed tranquilizers, notably the phenothiazines, thioxanthenes, and butyrophenones, must be determined empirically. The total daily dosage usually ranges between 5 and 15 mg although, in some cases, these reactions have been satisfactorily controlled on as little as 1 mg daily. It may be advisable to commence therapy with a single 1 mg dose. If the extrapyramidal manifestations are not controlled in a few hours, the subsequent doses may be progressively increased until satisfactory control is achieved. Satisfactory control may sometimes be more rapidly achieved by temporarily reducing the dosage of the tranquilizer on instituting trihexyphenidyl HCl therapy and then adjusting dosage of both drugs until the desired ataractic effect is retained without onset of extrapyramidal reactions.

It is sometimes possible to maintain the patient on a reduced trihexyphenidyl HCl dosage after the reactions have remained under control for several days. Instances have been reported in which these reactions have remained in remission for long periods after trihexyphenidyl HCl therapy was discontinued.

CONCOMITANT USE OF TRIHEXYPHENIDYL HCl WITH LEVODOPA

When trihexyphenidyl HCl is used concomitantly with levodopa, the usual dose of each may need to be reduced. Careful adjustment is necessary, depending on side effects and degree of symptom control. Trihexyphenidyl HCl dosage of 3-6 mg daily, in divided doses, is usually adequate.

CONCOMITANT USE OF TRIHEXYPHENIDYL HCl WITH OTHER PARASYMPATHETIC INHIBITORS

Trihexyphenidyl HCl may be substituted, in whole or in part, for other parasympathetic inhibitors. The usual technique is partial substitution initially, with progressive reduction in the other medication as the dose of trihexyphenidyl HCl is increased.

TRIHEXYPHENIDYL HCl TABLETS AND ELIXIR

The total daily intake of trihexyphenidyl HCl tablets or elixir is tolerated best if divided into 3 doses and taken at mealtimes. High doses (>10 mg daily) may be divided unto 4 parts, with 3 doses administered at mealtimes and the fourth at bedtime.

TRIHEXYPHENIDYL HCl SEQUELS

Because of the relatively high dosage in each controlled-release capsule, this dosage form should not be used for initial therapy. After patients are stabilized on trihexyphenidyl HCl in conventional dosage forms (tablet or elixir), for convenience of administration they may be switched to the controlled-release capsules on a milligram per milligram total daily dose basis, as a single dose after breakfast or in 2 divided doses 12 hours apart. Most patients will be adequately maintained on the controlled-release form, but some may develop an exacerbation of parkinsonism and have to be returned to the conventional form.

PRODUCT LISTING - RATED THERAPEUTICALLY EQUIVALENT

Elixir - Oral - 2 mg/5 ml

5 ml x 40	$48.00	GENERIC, Pharmaceutical Assoc Inc Div Beach Products	00121-0658-05
10 ml x 40	$96.00	GENERIC, Pharmaceutical Assoc Inc Div Beach Products	00121-0658-10
12.50 ml x 40	$120.00	GENERIC, Pharmaceutical Assoc Inc Div Beach Products	00121-0658-12
473 ml	$30.00	GENERIC, Pharmaceutical Assoc Inc Div Beach Products	00121-0658-16
480 ml	$20.00	GENERIC, Liquipharm Inc	54198-0107-16
480 ml	$30.99	GENERIC, Cypress Pharmaceutical Inc	60258-0081-16
480 ml	$42.84	ARTANE, Lederle Laboratories	00005-4440-65

Tablet - Oral - 2 mg

25 x 30	$127.58	GENERIC, Sky Pharmaceuticals Packaging, Inc	63739-0249-03
31 x 10	$58.44	GENERIC, Vangard Labs	00615-0675-53
31 x 10	$58.44	GENERIC, Vangard Labs	00615-0675-63
100's	$9.09	GENERIC, Richmond Pharmaceuticals	54738-0554-01
100's	$9.50	GENERIC, Raway Pharmacal Inc	00686-0115-20
100's	$12.36	GENERIC, Aligen Independent Laboratories Inc	00405-5061-01
100's	$12.75	FEDERAL UPPER LIMIT, H.C.F.A. F F P	99999-2385-02
100's	$12.81	GENERIC, Moore, H.L. Drug Exchange Inc	00839-1699-06
100's	$14.25	GENERIC, Major Pharmaceuticals Inc	00904-2041-60
100's	$14.75	GENERIC, Ivax Corporation	00182-0627-01
100's	$15.00	GENERIC, Cmc-Consolidated Midland Corporation	00223-2126-01
100's	$15.43	GENERIC, Vangard Labs	00615-0675-29
100's	$16.10	GENERIC, Major Pharmaceuticals Inc	00904-2041-61
100's	$17.65	GENERIC, Medirex Inc	57480-0368-01
100's	$18.28	GENERIC, West Ward Pharmaceutical Corporation	00143-1764-01
100's	$18.28	GENERIC, Vintage Pharmaceuticals Inc	00254-5971-28
100's	$18.28	GENERIC, Mutual/United Research Laboratories	00677-1751-01
100's	$18.29	GENERIC, Watson/Schein Pharmaceuticals Inc	00364-0408-01
100's	$18.29	GENERIC, Watson/Schein Pharmaceuticals Inc	00591-5335-01
100's	$18.29	GENERIC, Watson/Rugby Laboratories Inc	52544-0575-01
100's	$21.30	ARTANE, Lederle Laboratories	00005-4434-23
200 x 5	$188.52	GENERIC, Vangard Labs	00615-0675-43

Tablet - Oral - 5 mg

60's	$3.52	GENERIC, Circle Pharmaceuticals Inc	00659-0402-60
100's	$6.54	GENERIC, Us Trading Corporation	56126-0318-11
100's	$10.00	GENERIC, Raway Pharmacal Inc	00686-0124-20
100's	$18.30	GENERIC, Richmond Pharmaceuticals	54738-0555-01
100's	$25.50	GENERIC, Major Pharmaceuticals Inc	00904-2050-60
100's	$25.80	FEDERAL UPPER LIMIT, H.C.F.A. F F P	99999-2385-01
100's	$27.50	GENERIC, Cmc-Consolidated Midland Corporation	00223-2127-01
100's	$27.87	GENERIC, Major Pharmaceuticals Inc	00904-2050-61
100's	$28.22	GENERIC, Ivax Corporation	00182-0628-01
100's	$29.28	GENERIC, Moore, H.L. Drug Exchange Inc	00839-1698-06
100's	$31.06	GENERIC, Aligen Independent Laboratories Inc	00405-5062-01
100's	$35.47	GENERIC, Watson/Rugby Laboratories Inc	52544-0576-01
100's	$36.37	GENERIC, West Ward Pharmaceutical Corporation	00143-1763-01
100's	$36.37	GENERIC, Vintage Pharmaceuticals Inc	00254-5972-28
100's	$36.37	GENERIC, Mutual/United Research Laboratories	00677-1752-01
100's	$36.38	GENERIC, Watson/Schein Pharmaceuticals Inc	00364-0409-01
100's	$39.43	ARTANE, Lederle Laboratories	00005-4436-60

PRODUCT LISTING - EQUIVALENTS NOT AVAILABLE

Elixir - Oral - 2 mg/5 ml

480 ml	$30.60	GENERIC, Versapharm Inc	61748-0054-16

Tablet - Oral - 2 mg

30's	$6.93	GENERIC, Physicians Total Care	54868-2340-02
60's	$12.53	GENERIC, Physicians Total Care	54868-2340-03

Trimethobenzamide Hydrochloride (002390)

Categories: Nausea; Vomiting; FDA Approved 1974 Jul; Pregnancy Category C
Drug Classes: Anticholinergics; Antiemetics/antivertigo
Brand Names: Anaus; Arrestin; Benzacot; Bio-Gan; Ibikin; Navogan; Stemetic; T-Gen; Tebamide; Tegamide; Ti-Plex; Ticon; **Tigan**; Tiject-20; Triban; Tribenzagan; Trimazide
Cost of Therapy: $46.31 (Nausea; Tigan; 250 mg; 3 capsules/day; 30 day supply)
$24.30 (Nausea; Generic Capsules; 250 mg; 3 capsules/day; 30 day supply)
HCFA JCODE(S): J3250 up to 200 mg IM

DESCRIPTION

Chemically, trimethobenzamide HCl is N-[p-[2-(dimethylamino)-ethoxy]benzyl]-3,4,5-trimethoxybenzamide hydrochloride. It has a molecular weight of 424.93.

CAPSULES

Each 100 mg Tigan capsule for oral use contains trimethobenzamide hydrochloride equivalent to 100 mg. The capsule has an opaque blue cap marked "Tigan" and an opaque white body marked "ROBERTS" "186". Each 250 mg Tigan capsule for oral use contains trimethobenzamide hydrochloride equivalent to 250 mg. The capsule has an opaque blue cap marked "Tigan" and an opaque blue body marked "ROBERTS" "187".
Inactive Ingredients: FD&C blue no. 1, FD&C red no. 3, lactose, magnesium stearate, starch and titanium dioxide.

SUPPOSITORIES (200 MG)

Each suppository contains 200 mg trimethobenzamide hydrochloride and 2% benzocaine in a base compounded with polysorbate 80, white beeswax and propylene glycol monostearate.

SUPPOSITORIES, PEDIATRIC (100 MG)

Each suppository contains 100 mg trimethobenzamide hydrochloride and 2% benzocaine in a base compounded with polysorbate 80, white beeswax and propylene glycol monostearate.

AMPULS

Each 2 ml ampul contains 200 mg trimethobenzamide hydrochloride compounded with 0.2% parabens (methyl and propyl) as preservatives, 1 mg sodium citrate and 0.4 mg citric acid as buffers and pH adjusted to approximately 5.0 with sodium hydroxide.

MULTI-DOSE VIALS

Each ml contains 100 mg trimethobenzamide hydrochloride compounded with 0.45% phenol as preservative, 0.5 mg sodium citrate and 0.2 mg citric acid as buffers and pH adjusted to approximately 5.0 with sodium hydroxide.

THERA-JECT (DISPOSABLE SYRINGES)

Each 2 ml contains 200 mg trimethobenzamide hydrochloride compounded with 0.45% phenol as preservative, 1 mg sodium citrate and 0.4 mg citric acid as buffers, 0.2 mg disodium edetate as stabilizer and pH adjusted to approximately 5.0 with sodium hydroxide.

STORAGE

Store Tigan from 15-30°C (59-86°F).

CLINICAL PHARMACOLOGY

The mechanism of action of trimethobenzamide HCl as determined in animals is obscure, but may be the chemoreceptor trigger zone (CTZ), an area in the medulla oblongata through which emetic impulses are conveyed to the vomiting center; direct impulses to the vomiting center apparently are not similarly inhibited. In dogs pretreated with trimethobenzamide HCl, the emetic response to apomorphine is inhibited, while little or no protection is afforded against emesis induced by intragastric copper sulfate.

INDICATIONS AND USAGE

Trimethobenzamide HCl is indicated for the control of nausea and vomiting.

CONTRAINDICATIONS

The injectable form of trimethobenzamide HCl in children, the suppositories in premature or newborn infants, and use in patients with known hypersensitivity to trimethobenzamide

T

are contraindicated. Since the suppositories contain benzocaine they should not be used in patients known to be sensitive to this or similar local anesthetics.

WARNINGS

Caution should be exercised when administering trimethobenzamide HCl to children for the treatment of vomiting. Antiemetics are not recommended for treatment of uncomplicated vomiting in children and their use should be limited to prolonged vomiting of known etiology. There are three principal reasons for caution:

There has been some suspicion that centrally acting antiemetics may contribute, in combination with viral illnesses (a possible cause of vomiting in children), to development of Reye's syndrome, a potentially fatal acute childhood encephalopathy with visceral fatty degeneration, especially involving the liver. Although there is no confirmation of this suspicion, caution is nevertheless recommended.

The extrapyramidal symptoms which can occur secondary to trimethobenzamide HCl may be confused with the central nervous system signs of an undiagnosed primary disease responsible for the vomiting, *e.g.,* Reye's syndrome or other encephalopathy.

It has been suspected that drugs with hepatotoxic potential, such as trimethobenzamide HCl, may unfavorably alter the course of Reye's syndrome. Such drugs should therefore be avoided in children whose signs and symptoms (vomiting) could represent Reye's syndrome. It should also be noted that salicylates and acetaminophen are hepatotoxic at large doses. Although it is not known that at usual doses they would represent a hazard in patients with the underlying hepatic disorder of Reye's syndrome, these drugs, too, should be avoided in children whose signs and symptoms could represent Reye's syndrome, unless alternative methods of controlling fever are not successful.

Trimethobenzamide HCl may produce drowsiness. Patients should not operate motor vehicles or other dangerous machinery until their individual responses have been determined. Reye's syndrome has been associated with the use of trimethobenzamide HCl and other drugs, including antiemetics, although their contribution, if any, to the cause and course of the disease has not been established. This syndrome is characterized by an abrupt onset shortly following a non-specific febrile illness, with persistent, severe vomiting, lethargy, irrational behavior, progressive encephalopathy leading to coma, convulsions and death.

USAGE IN PREGNANCY

Trimethobenzamide HCl was studied in reproduction experiments in rats and rabbits and no teratogenicity was suggested. The only effects observed were an increased percentage of embryonic resorptions or stillborn pups in rats administered 20 mg and 100 mg/kg and increased resorptions in rabbits receiving 100 mg/kg. In each study these adverse effects were attributed to 1 or 2 dams. The relevance to humans is not known. Since there is no adequate experience in pregnant or lactating women who have received this drug, safety in pregnancy or in nursing mothers has not been established.

USAGE WITH ALCOHOL

Concomitant use of alcohol with trimethobenzamide HCl may result in an adverse drug interaction.

PRECAUTIONS

During the course of acute febrile illness, encephalitides, gastroenteritis, dehydration and electrolyte imbalance, especially in children and the elderly or debilitated, CNS reactions such as opisthotonos, convulsions, coma and extrapyramidal symptoms have been reported with and without use of trimethobenzamide hydrochloride or other antiemetic agents. In such disorders caution should be exercised in administering trimethobenzamide HCl, particularly to patients who have recently received other CNS-acting agents (phenothiazines, barbiturates, belladonna derivatives). It is recommended that severe emesis should not be treated with an antiemetic drug alone; where possible the cause of vomiting should be established. Primary emphasis should be directed toward the restoration of body fluids and electrolyte balance, the relief of fever and relief of the causative disease process. Overhydration should be avoided since it may result in cerebral edema.

The antiemetic effects of trimethobenzamide HCl may render diagnosis more difficult in such conditions as appendicitis and obscure signs of toxicity due to overdosage of other drugs.

ADVERSE REACTIONS

There have been reports of hypersensitivity reactions and Parkinson-like symptoms. There have been instances of hypotension reported following parenteral administration to surgical patients. There have been reports of blood dyscrasias, blurring of vision, coma, convulsions, depression of mood, diarrhea, disorientation, dizziness, drowsiness, headache, jaundice, muscle cramps and opisthotonos. If these occur, the administration of the drug should be discontinued. Allergic-type skin reactions have been observed; therefore, the drug should be discontinued at the first sign of sensitization. While these symptoms will usually disappear spontaneously, symptomatic treatment may be indicated in some cases.

T

DOSAGE AND ADMINISTRATION

See WARNINGS and PRECAUTIONS.

Dosage should be adjusted according to the indication for therapy, severity of symptoms and the response of the patient.

Capsules, 250 mg and 100 mg

Usual Adult Dosage: One 250 mg capsule tid or qid.

Usual Children's Dosage: 30-90 lb: One or two 100 mg capsules tid or qid.

Suppositories, 200 mg (not to be used in premature or newborn infants)

Usual Adult Dosage: One suppository (200 mg) tid or qid.

Usual Children's Dosage:

Under 30 lb: One-half suppository (100 mg) tid or qid.

30-90 lb: One-half to one suppository (100-200 mg) tid or qid.

Suppositories, Pediatric, 100 mg (not to be used in premature or newborn infants)

Usual Children's Dosage:

Under 30 lb: One suppository (100 mg) tid or qid.

30-90 lb: One to two suppositories (100-200 mg) tid or qid.

Injectable, 100 mg/ml (not for use in children)

Usual Adult Dosage: 2 ml (200 mg) tid or qid intramuscularly.

Note: The injectable form is intended for intramuscular administration only; it is not recommended for intravenous use.

Intramuscular administration may cause pain, stinging, burning, redness and swelling at the site of injection. Such effects may be minimized by deep injection into the upper outer quadrant of the gluteal region, and by avoiding the escape of solution along the route.

PRODUCT LISTING - RATED THERAPEUTICALLY EQUIVALENT

Solution - Intramuscular - 100 mg/ml

2 ml x 10	$28.38	GENERIC, Abbott Pharmaceutical	00074-1252-02
2 ml x 10	$28.50	GENERIC, Abbott Pharmaceutical	00074-1952-02
2 ml x 10	$58.10	TIGAN, Monarch Pharmaceuticals Inc	61570-0540-02
20 ml	$8.68	GENERIC, Moore, H.L. Drug Exchange Inc	00839-6676-33
20 ml	$9.95	GENERIC, Roberts/Hauck Pharmaceutical Corporation	43797-0143-26
20 ml	$10.00	GENERIC, Cmc-Consolidated Midland Corporation	00223-8700-20
20 ml	$12.75	GENERIC, Interstate Drug Exchange Inc	00814-8064-44
20 ml	$32.18	TIGAN, Physicians Total Care	54868-0756-00
20 ml	$45.26	TIGAN, Allscripts Pharmaceutical Company	54569-1796-01
20 ml	$48.88	TIGAN, Roberts Pharmaceutical Corporation	54092-0541-20
20 ml	$51.81	TIGAN, Monarch Pharmaceuticals Inc	61570-0541-20

Suppository - Rectal - 2%;200 mg

10's	$31.16	TIGAN ADULT, Monarch Pharmaceuticals Inc	61570-0504-10
50's	$140.98	TIGAN ADULT, Monarch Pharmaceuticals Inc	61570-0504-50

PRODUCT LISTING - EQUIVALENTS NOT AVAILABLE

Capsule - Oral - 100 mg

15's	$9.58	TIGAN, Physicians Total Care	54868-1485-01
100's	$42.68	TIGAN, Roberts Pharmaceutical Corporation	00029-4082-30
100's	$59.67	TIGAN, Roberts Pharmaceutical Corporation	54092-0186-01
100's	$64.44	TIGAN, Monarch Pharmaceuticals Inc	61570-0186-01

Capsule - Oral - 250 mg

4's	$2.88	TIGAN, Allscripts Pharmaceutical Company	54569-0363-03
4's	$4.05	GENERIC, Prescript Pharmaceuticals	00247-0267-04
5's	$4.21	GENERIC, Prescript Pharmaceuticals	00247-0267-05
6's	$4.39	GENERIC, Prescript Pharmaceuticals	00247-0267-06
8's	$3.78	GENERIC, Southwood Pharmaceuticals Inc	58016-0973-08
8's	$4.73	GENERIC, Prescript Pharmaceuticals	00247-0267-08
8's	$5.76	TIGAN, Allscripts Pharmaceutical Company	54569-0363-04
10's	$3.26	GENERIC, Pharmaceutical Corporation Of America	51655-0523-53
10's	$4.72	GENERIC, Southwood Pharmaceuticals Inc	58016-0973-10
10's	$5.07	GENERIC, Prescript Pharmaceuticals	00247-0267-10
10's	$7.20	TIGAN, Allscripts Pharmaceutical Company	54569-0363-05
10's	$7.44	TIGAN, Southwood Pharmaceuticals Inc	58016-0721-10
10's	$8.40	TIGAN, Pharma Pac	52959-0226-10
10's	$10.37	GENERIC, Pharma Pac	52959-0479-10
10's	$10.44	TIGAN, Pd-Rx Pharmaceuticals	55289-0428-10
12's	$4.39	GENERIC, Allscripts Pharmaceutical Company	54569-3407-00
12's	$5.42	GENERIC, Prescript Pharmaceuticals	00247-0267-12
12's	$5.66	GENERIC, Southwood Pharmaceuticals Inc	58016-0973-12
12's	$9.96	TIGAN, Pharma Pac	52959-0226-12
12's	$12.59	GENERIC, Pharma Pac	52959-0479-12
15's	$5.66	GENERIC, Physicians Total Care	54868-2973-00
15's	$5.93	GENERIC, Prescript Pharmaceuticals	00247-0267-15
15's	$7.08	GENERIC, Southwood Pharmaceuticals Inc	58016-0973-15
15's	$9.88	TIGAN, Southwood Pharmaceuticals Inc	58016-0721-15
20's	$6.80	GENERIC, Prescript Pharmaceuticals	00247-0267-20
20's	$9.44	GENERIC, Southwood Pharmaceuticals Inc	58016-0973-20
20's	$10.89	GENERIC, Dhs Inc	55887-0741-20
20's	$11.12	GENERIC, Pd-Rx Pharmaceuticals	55289-0219-20
20's	$16.16	GENERIC, Pharma Pac	52959-0479-20
24's	$11.33	GENERIC, Southwood Pharmaceuticals Inc	58016-0973-24
30's	$9.99	GENERIC, Physicians Total Care	54868-2973-03
30's	$14.16	GENERIC, Southwood Pharmaceuticals Inc	58016-0973-30
30's	$22.89	GENERIC, Pharma Pac	52959-0479-30
40's	$10.24	GENERIC, Prescript Pharmaceuticals	00247-0267-40
50's	$23.60	GENERIC, Southwood Pharmaceuticals Inc	58016-0973-50
100's	$27.00	GENERIC, Concord Laboratories	20254-0018-01
100's	$29.51	GENERIC, Physicians Total Care	54868-2973-02
100's	$34.55	GENERIC, Ivax Corporation	00182-1396-01
100's	$34.55	GENERIC, Qualitest Products Inc	00603-6256-21
100's	$36.48	GENERIC, Watson/Rugby Laboratories Inc	00536-4727-01
100's	$36.95	GENERIC, Mutual/United Research Laboratories	53489-0293-01
100's	$37.80	GENERIC, Aligen Independent Laboratories Inc	00405-5066-01
100's	$37.80	GENERIC, Breckenridge Inc	51991-0625-01
100's	$38.59	GENERIC, Liquipharm Inc	57779-0144-04
100's	$38.95	GENERIC, Iomed Laboratories Inc	61646-0308-01
100's	$39.95	GENERIC, Pecos Pharmaceutical	59879-0115-01

100's	$45.71	GENERIC, Major Pharmaceuticals Inc	00904-3291-60
100's	$45.75	GENERIC, Amide Pharmaceutical Inc	52152-0166-02
100's	$47.20	GENERIC, Southwood Pharmaceuticals Inc	58016-0973-00
100's	$51.45	TIGAN, Roberts Pharmaceutical Corporation	00029-4083-30
100's	$64.75	GENERIC, Ethex Corporation	58177-0037-04
100's	$71.95	TIGAN, Roberts Pharmaceutical Corporation	54092-0187-01
100's	$77.70	TIGAN, Monarch Pharmaceuticals Inc	61570-0187-01
100's	$88.17	TIGAN, Pd-Rx Pharmaceuticals	55289-0428-17
Capsule - Oral - 300 mg			
100's	$112.63	TIGAN, Monarch Pharmaceuticals Inc	61570-0079-01
Solution - Intramuscular - 100 mg/ml			
2 ml x 25	$32.60	GENERIC, Physicians Total Care	54868-0608-00
20 ml	$14.40	BENZACOT, C.O. Truxton Inc	00463-1108-20
Suppository - Rectal - 2%;100 mg			
4's	$3.08	TEBAMIDE, Pharma Pac	52959-0290-04
4's	$9.18	TIGAN PEDIATRIC, Allscripts Pharmaceutical Company	54569-0364-01
5's	$3.80	TEBAMIDE, Pharma Pac	52959-0290-05
5's	$5.93	TEBAMIDE PEDIATRIC, Pd-Rx Pharmaceuticals	55289-0529-05
5's	$6.58	TEBAMIDE, Allscripts Pharmaceutical Company	54569-1897-01
5's	$13.02	TIGAN PEDIATRIC, Physicians Total Care	54868-0340-01
10's	$4.31	TEBAMIDE, Moore, H.L. Drug Exchange Inc	00839-6540-95
10's	$5.55	GENERIC, Paddock Laboratories Inc	00574-7220-10
10's	$5.75	GENERIC, Watson/Schein Pharmaceuticals Inc	00364-7347-10
10's	$5.75	GENERIC, Qualitest Products Inc	00603-8150-10
10's	$5.80	GENERIC, Ivax Corporation	00182-1428-23
10's	$5.97	TEBAMIDE, G and W Laboratories Inc	00713-0107-09
10's	$6.15	GENERIC, Major Pharmaceuticals Inc	00904-2735-15
10's	$6.58	TEBAMIDE, Allscripts Pharmaceutical Company	54569-1897-00
10's	$6.75	GENERIC, Bio Pharm Inc	59741-0305-09
10's	$7.34	TEBAMIDE, Pharma Pac	52959-0290-10
10's	$8.99	GENERIC, Clay-Park Laboratories Inc	45802-0723-90
10's	$9.50	GENERIC, Cmc-Consolidated Midland Corporation	00223-5904-10
10's	$10.07	NAVOGAN, International Ethical Laboratories Inc	11584-0421-01
10's	$10.75	GENERIC, Elge Inc	58298-0140-10
10's	$15.90	GENERIC, Southwood Pharmaceuticals Inc	58016-3091-01
10's	$16.40	TIGAN PEDIATRIC, Roberts Pharmaceutical Corporation	00029-4088-38
10's	$22.94	TIGAN PEDIATRIC, Roberts Pharmaceutical Corporation	54092-0503-10
10's	$24.23	TIGAN PEDIATRIC, Physicians Total Care	54868-0340-00
10's	$26.26	TIGAN PEDIATRIC, Monarch Pharmaceuticals Inc	61570-0503-10
50's	$22.60	GENERIC, Clay-Park Laboratories Inc	45802-0723-32
50's	$29.35	GENERIC, Bio Pharm Inc	59741-0305-50
100's	$27.10	GENERIC, Bio Pharm Inc	59741-0305-49
Suppository - Rectal - 2%;200 mg			
2's	$1.74	GENERIC, Allscripts Pharmaceutical Company	54569-1896-03
3's	$2.87	GENERIC, Physicians Total Care	54868-3487-00
4's	$2.98	GENERIC, Allscripts Pharmaceutical Company	54569-1896-02
5's	$3.73	GENERIC, Allscripts Pharmaceutical Company	54569-1896-01
5's	$3.89	GENERIC, Physicians Total Care	54868-3487-01
5's	$13.61	TIGAN ADULT, Allscripts Pharmaceutical Company	54569-0365-01
10's	$4.85	TEBAMIDE, Moore, H.L. Drug Exchange Inc	00839-6541-95
10's	$5.37	GENERIC, Cheshire Drugs	55175-1201-01
10's	$6.00	GENERIC, Ivax Corporation	00182-1427-23
10's	$6.14	GENERIC, Qualitest Products Inc	00603-8151-10
10's	$6.39	TEBAMIDE, G and W Laboratories Inc	00713-0108-09
10's	$6.47	GENERIC, Physicians Total Care	54868-3487-02
10's	$6.95	GENERIC, Paddock Laboratories Inc	00574-7222-10
10's	$7.25	GENERIC, Cmc-Consolidated Midland Corporation	00223-5905-10
10's	$7.43	GENERIC, Watson/Schein Pharmaceuticals Inc	00364-7348-10
10's	$7.45	GENERIC, Allscripts Pharmaceutical Company	54569-1896-00
10's	$9.26	GENERIC, Major Pharmaceuticals Inc	00904-2736-15
10's	$9.98	GENERIC, Clay-Park Laboratories Inc	45802-0724-90
10's	$12.54	GENERIC, Elge Inc	58298-0145-10
10's	$13.95	GENERIC, Bio Pharm Inc	59741-0304-09
10's	$14.60	TEBAMIDE, Pharma Pac	52959-0573-01
10's	$17.85	GENERIC, Southwood Pharmaceuticals Inc	58016-3092-10
10's	$20.10	GENERIC, Southwood Pharmaceuticals Inc	58016-3092-01
10's	$29.40	TIGAN PEDIATRIC, Monarch Pharmaceuticals Inc	54092-0504-10
15's	$8.94	TEBAMIDE, Pharma Pac	52959-0573-05
50's	$21.25	GENERIC, Bio Pharm Inc	59741-0304-49
50's	$24.10	GENERIC, Paddock Laboratories Inc	00574-7222-50
50's	$26.10	GENERIC, Ivax Corporation	00182-1427-19
50's	$26.88	GENERIC, Clay-Park Laboratories Inc	45802-0724-32
50's	$30.62	TEBAMIDE, G and W Laboratories Inc	00713-0108-50
50's	$34.50	GENERIC, Cmc-Consolidated Midland Corporation	00223-5905-50
50's	$49.10	GENERIC, Elge Inc	58298-0145-50
100's	$48.45	GENERIC, Bio Pharm Inc	59741-0304-50

Trimetrexate Glucuronate *(003189)*

Categories: Pneumonia, pneumocystis; FDA Approved 1993 Dec; Pregnancy Category D; Orphan Drugs
Drug Classes: Antibiotics, folate antagonists; Antiprotozoals
Brand Names: **Neutrexin**
HCFA JCODE(S): J3305 per 25 mg IV

WARNING

TRIMETREXATE GLUCURONATE FOR INJECTION MUST BE USED WITH CONCURRENT LEUCOVORIN (LEUCOVORIN PROTECTION) TO AVOID POTENTIALLY SERIOUS OR LIFE-THREATENING TOXICITIES (SEE PRECAUTIONS AND DOSAGE AND ADMINISTRATION).

DESCRIPTION

Neutrexin is the brand name for trimetrexate glucuronate. Trimetrexate, a 2,4-diaminoquinazoline, nonclassical folate antagonist, is a synthetic inhibitor of the enzyme dihydrofolate reductase (DHFR). Neutrexin is available as a sterile lyophilized powder, containing trimetrexate glucuronate equivalent to either 200 mg or 25 mg of trimetrexate without any preservatives or excipients. The powder is reconstituted prior to intravenous infusion (see DOSAGE AND ADMINISTRATION, Reconstitution and Dilution).

Trimetrexate glucuronate is chemically known as 2,4-diamino-5-methyl-6-[(3,4,5-trimethoxyanilino)methyl] quinazoline mono-D-glucuronate.

The empirical formula for trimetrexate glucuronate is $C_{19}H_{23}N_5O_3 \cdot C_6H_{10}O_7$ with a molecular weight of 563.56. The active ingredient, trimetrexate free base, has an empirical formula of $C_{19}H_{23}N_5O_3$ with a molecular weight of 369.42. Trimetrexate glucuronate for injection is a pale greenish-yellow powder or cake. Trimetrexate glucuronate is soluble in water (>50 mg/ml), whereas trimetrexate free base is practically insoluble in water (<0.1 mg/ml). The pKa of trimetrexate free base in 50% methanol/water is 8.0. The logarithm_{10} of the partition coefficient of trimetrexate free base between octanol and water is 1.63.

CLINICAL PHARMACOLOGY

MECHANISM OF ACTION

In vitro studies have shown that trimetrexate is a competitive inhibitor of dihydrofolate reductase (DHFR) from bacterial, protozoan, and mammalian sources. DHFR catalyzes the reduction of intracellular dihydrofolate to the active coenzyme tetrahydrofolate. Inhibition of DHFR results in the depletion of this coenzyme, leading directly to interference with thymidylate biosynthesis, as well as inhibition of folate-dependent formyltransferases, and indirectly to inhibition of purine biosynthesis. The end result is disruption of DNA, RNA, and protein synthesis, with consequent cell death. Leucovorin (folinic acid) is readily transported into mammalian cells by an active, carrier-mediated process and can be assimilated into cellular folate pools following its metabolism. *In vitro* studies have shown that leucovorin provides a source of reduced folates necessary for normal cellular biosynthetic processes. Because the *Pneumocystis carinii* organism lacks the reduced folate carrier-mediated transport system, leucovorin is prevented from entering the organism. Therefore, at concentrations achieved with therapeutic doses of trimetrexate plus leucovorin, the selective transport of trimetrexate, but not leucovorin, into the *Pneumocystis carinii* organism allows the concurrent administration of leucovorin to protect normal host cells from the cytotoxicity of trimetrexate without inhibiting the antifolate's inhibition of *Pneumocystis carinii*. It is not known if considerably higher doses of leucovorin would affect trimetrexate's effect on *Pneumocystis carinii*.

MICROBIOLOGY

Trimetrexate inhibits, in a dose-related manner, *in vitro* growth of the trophozoite stage of rat *Pneumocystis carinii* cultured on human embryonic lung fibroblast cells. Trimetrexate concentrations between 3 and 54.1 μM were shown to inhibit the growth of trophozoites. Leucovorin alone at a concentration of 10 μM did not alter either the growth of the trophozoites or the anti-pneumocystis activity of trimetrexate. Resistance to trimetrexate's antimicrobial activity against *Pneumocystis carinii* has not been studied.

PHARMACOKINETICS

Trimetrexate pharmacokinetics were assessed in 6 patients with acquired immunodeficiency syndrome (AIDS) who had *Pneumocystis carinii* pneumonia (4 patients) or toxoplasmosis (2 patients). Trimetrexate was administered intravenously as a bolus injection at a dose of 30 mg/m^2/day along with leucovorin 20 mg/m^2 every 6 hours for 21 days. Trimetrexate clearance (mean ±SD) was 38 ± 15 $ml/min/m^2$ and volume of distribution at steady state (Vdss) was 20 ± 8 L/m^2. The plasma concentration time profile declined in a biphasic manner over 24 hours with a terminal half-life of 11 ± 4 hours.

The pharmacokinetics of trimetrexate without the concomitant administration of leucovorin have been evaluated in cancer patients with advanced solid tumors using various dosage regimens. The decline in plasma concentrations over time has been described by either biexponential or triexponential equations. Following the single-dose administration of 10-130 mg/m^2 to 37 patients, plasma concentrations were obtained for 72 hours. Nine plasma concentration time profiles were described as biexponential. The alpha phase half-life was 57 ± 28 minutes, followed by a terminal phase with a half-life of 16 ± 3 hours. The plasma concentrations in the remaining patients exhibited a triphasic decline with half-lives of 8.6 ± 6.5 minutes, 2.4 ± 1.3 hours, and 17.8 ± 8.2 hours.

T

Trimetrexate clearance in cancer patients has been reported as 53 ± 41 ml/min (14 patients) and 32 ± 18 ml/min/m^2 (23 patients) following single-dose administration. After a 5 day infusion of trimetrexate to 16 patients, plasma clearance was 30 ± 8 ml/min/m^2.

Renal clearance of trimetrexate in cancer patients has varied from about 4 ± 2 ml/min/m^2 to 10 ± 6 ml/min/m^2. Ten percent (10%) to 30% of the administered dose is excreted unchanged in the urine. Considering the free fraction of trimetrexate, active tubular secretion may possibly contribute to the renal clearance of trimetrexate. Renal clearance has been associated with urine flow, suggesting the possibility of tubular reabsorption as well.

The Vdss of trimetrexate in cancer patients after single-dose administration and for whom plasma concentrations were obtained for 72 hours was 36.9 ± 17.6 L/m^2 (n=23) and 0.62 ± 0.24 L/kg (n=14). Following a constant infusion of trimetrexate for 5 days, Vdss was 32.8 ± 16.6 L/m^2. The volume of the central compartment has been estimated as 0.17 ± 0.08 L/kg and 4.0 ± 2.9 L/m^2.

There have been inconsistencies in the reporting of trimetrexate protein binding. The *in vitro* plasma protein binding of trimetrexate using ultrafiltration is approximately 95% over the concentration range of 18.75 to 1000 ng/ml. There is a suggestion of capacity limited binding (saturable binding) at concentrations greater than about 1000 ng/ml, with free fraction progressively increasing to about 9.3% as concentration is increased to 15 μg/ml. Other reports have declared trimetrexate to be greater than 98% bound at concentrations of 0.1 to 10 μg/ml; however, specific free fractions were not stated. The free fraction of trimetrexate also has been reported to be about 15-16% at a concentration of 60 ng/ml, increasing to about 20% at a trimetrexate concentration of 6 μg/ml.

Trimetrexate metabolism in man has not been characterized. Preclinical data strongly suggest that the major metabolic pathway is oxidative O-demethylation, followed by conjugation to either glucuronide or the sulfate. N-demethylation and oxidation is a related minor pathway. Preliminary findings in humans indicate the presence of a glucuronide conjugate with DHFR inhibition and a demethylated metabolite in urine.

The presence of metabolite(s) in human plasma following the administration of trimetrexate is suggested by the differences seen in trimetrexate plasma concentrations when measured by HPLC and a nonspecific DHFR inhibition assay. The profiles are similar initially, but diverge with time; concentrations determined by DHFR being higher than those determined by HPLC. This suggests the presence of 1 or more metabolites with DHFR inhibition activity. After intravenous administration of trimetrexate to humans, urinary recovery averaged about 40%, using a DHFR assay, in comparison to 10% urinary recovery as determined by HPLC, suggesting the presence of 1 or more metabolites that retain inhibitory activity against DHFR. Fecal recovery of trimetrexate over 48 hours after intravenous administration ranged from 0.09-7.6% of the dose as determined by DHFR inhibition and 0.02-5.2% of the dose as determined by HPLC.

The pharmacokinetics of trimetrexate have not been determined in patients with renal insufficiency or hepatic dysfunction.

INDICATIONS AND USAGE

Trimetrexate glucuronate for injection with concurrent leucovorin administration (leucovorin protection) is indicated as an alternative therapy for the treatment of moderate-to-severe *Pneumocystis carinii* pneumonia (PCP) in immunocompromised patients, including patients with the acquired immunodeficiency syndrome (AIDS), who are intolerant of, or are refractory to, trimethoprim-sulfamethoxazole therapy or for whom trimethoprim-sulfamethoxazole is contraindicated.

This indication is based on the results of a randomized, controlled double-blind trial comparing trimetrexate glucuronate with concurrent leucovorin protection (TMTX/LV) to trimethoprim-sulfamethoxazole (TMP/SMX) in patients with moderate-to-severe *Pneumocystis carinii* pneumonia, as well as results of a Treatment IND.

NON-FDA APPROVED INDICATIONS

Trimetrexate is being evaluated for the treatment of non-small cell lung cancer, prostate cancer, and colorectal cancer.

CONTRAINDICATIONS

Trimetrexate glucuronate for injection is contraindicated in patients with clinically significant sensitivity to trimetrexate, leucovorin, or methotrexate.

WARNINGS

Trimetrexate glucuronate for injection must be used with concurrent leucovorin to avoid potentially serious or life-threatening complications including bone marrow suppression, oral and gastrointestinal mucosal ulceration, and renal and hepatic dysfunction. Leucovorin therapy must extend for 72 hours past the last dose of trimetrexate glucuronate. Patients should be informed that failure to take the recommended dose and duration of leucovorin can lead to fatal toxicity. Patients should be closely monitored for the development of serious hematologic adverse reactions (see PRECAUTIONS and DOSAGE AND ADMINISTRATION).

Trimetrexate glucuronate can cause fetal harm when administered to a pregnant woman. Trimetrexate has been shown to be fetotoxic and teratogenic in rats and rabbits. Rats administered 1.5 and 2.5 mg/kg/day intravenously on gestational days 6-15 showed substantial postimplantation loss and severe inhibition of maternal weight gain. Trimetrexate administered intravenously to rats at 0.5 and 1.0 mg/kg/day on gestational days 6-15 retarded normal fetal development and was teratogenic. Rabbits administered trimetrexate intravenously at daily doses of 2.5 and 5.0 mg/kg/day on gestational days 6-18 resulted in significant maternal and fetal toxicity. In rabbits, trimetrexate at 0.1 mg/kg/day was teratogenic in the absence of significant maternal toxicity. These effects were observed using doses 1/20-1/2 the equivalent human therapeutic dose based on a mg/m^2 basis. Teratogenic effects included skeletal, visceral, ocular, and cardiovascular abnormalities. If trimetrexate glucuronate is used during pregnancy, or if the patient becomes pregnant while taking this drug, the patient should be apprised of the potential hazard to the fetus. Women of childbearing potential should be advised to avoid becoming pregnant.

PRECAUTIONS

GENERAL

Patients receiving trimetrexate glucuronate for injection may experience severe hematologic, hepatic, renal, and gastrointestinal toxicities. Caution should be used in treating patients with impaired hematologic, renal, or hepatic function. Patients who require concomitant therapy with nephrotoxic, myelosuppressive, or hepatotoxic drugs should be treated with trimetrexate glucuronate at the discretion of the physician and monitored carefully. To allow for full therapeutic doses of trimetrexate glucuronate, treatment with zidovudine should be discontinued during trimetrexate glucuronate therapy.

Trimetrexate glucuronate-associated myelosuppression, stomatitis, and gastrointestinal toxicities generally can be ameliorated by adjusting the dose of leucovorin. Mild elevations in transaminases and alkaline phosphatase have been observed with trimetrexate glucuronate administration and are usually not cause for modification of trimetrexate glucuronate therapy (see DOSAGE AND ADMINISTRATION). Seizures have been reported rarely (<1%) in AIDS patients receiving trimetrexate glucuronate; however, a causal relationship has not been established. Trimetrexate is a known inhibitor of histamine metabolism. Hypersensitivity/allergic type reactions including but not limited to rash, chills/rigors, fever, diaphoresis and dypsnea have occurred with trimetrexate primarily when it is administered as a bolus infusion or at doses higher than those recommended for PCP, and most frequently in combination with 5FU and leucovorin. In rare cases, anaphylactoid reactions, including acute hypotension and loss of consciousness have occurred.

Trimetrexate glucuronate has not been evaluated clinically for the treatment of concurrent pulmonary conditions such as bacterial, viral, or fungal pneumonia or mycobacterial diseases. *In vitro* activity has been observed against *Toxoplasma gondii, Mycobacterium avium* complex, gram positive cocci, and gram negative rods. If clinical deterioration is observed in patients, they should be carefully evaluated for other possible causes of pulmonary disease and treated with additional agents as appropriate.

LABORATORY TESTS

Patients receiving trimetrexate glucuronate with leucovorin protection should be seen frequently by a physician. Blood tests to assess the following parameters should be performed at least twice a week during therapy: hematology (absolute neutrophil counts [ANC], platelets), renal function (serum creatinine, BUN), and hepatic function (AST, ALT, alkaline phosphatase).

CARCINOGENESIS, MUTAGENESIS, AND IMPAIRMENT OF FERTILITY

Carcinogenesis

Long term studies in animals to evaluate the carcinogenic potential of trimetrexate have not been performed.

Mutagenesis

Trimetrexate was not mutagenic when tested using the standard Ames *Salmonella* mutagenicity assay with and without metabolic activation. Trimetrexate did not induce mutations in Chinese hamster lung cells or sister-chromatid exchange in Chinese hamster ovary cells. Trimetrexate did induce an increase in the chromosomal aberration frequency of cultured Chinese hamster lung cells; however, trimetrexate showed no clastogenic activity in a mouse micronucleus assay.

Impairment of Fertility

No studies have been conducted to evaluate the potential of trimetrexate to impair fertility. However, during standard toxicity studies conducted in mice and rats, degeneration of the testes and spermatocytes including the arrest of spermatogenesis was observed.

PREGNANCY, TERATOGENIC EFFECTS, PREGNANCY CATEGORY D

See WARNINGS.

NURSING MOTHERS

It is not known if trimetrexate is excreted in human milk. Because many drugs are excreted in human milk and because of the potential for serious adverse reactions in nursing infants from trimetrexate, it is recommended that breast feeding be discontinued if the mother is treated with trimetrexate glucuronate.

PEDIATRIC USE

The safety and effectiveness of trimetrexate glucuronate for the treatment of histologically confirmed PCP has not been established for patients under 18 years of age. Two children, ages 15 and 9 months, were treated with trimetrexate and leucovorin using a dose of 45 mg/m^2 of trimetrexate per day for 21 days and 20 mg/m^2 of leucovorin every 6 hours for 24 days. There were no serious or unexpected adverse effects.

DRUG INTERACTIONS

Since trimetrexate is metabolized by a P450 enzyme system, drugs that induce or inhibit this drug metabolizing enzyme system may elicit important drug-drug interactions that may alter trimetrexate plasma concentrations. Agents that might be coadministered with trimetrexate in AIDS patients for other indications that could elicit this activity include erythromycin, rifampin, rifabutin, ketoconazole, and fluconazole. *In vitro* perfusion of isolated rat liver has shown that cimetidine caused a significant reduction in trimetrexate metabolism and that acetaminophen altered the relative concentration of trimetrexate metabolites possibly by competing for sulfate metabolites. Based on an *in vitro* rat liver model, nitrogen substituted imidazole drugs (clotrimazole, ketoconazole, miconazole) were potent, non-competitive inhibitors of trimetrexate metabolism. Patients medicated with these drugs and trimetrexate should be carefully monitored.

ADVERSE REACTIONS

Because many patients who participated in clinical trials of trimetrexate glucuronate for injection had complications of advanced HIV disease, it is difficult to distinguish adverse events caused by trimetrexate glucuronate from those resulting from underlying medical conditions.

TABLE 3 lists the adverse events that occurred in ≥1% of the patients who participated in the Comparative Study of trimetrexate glucuronate plus leucovorin versus TMP/SMX.

TABLE 3 *Trimetrexate Glucuronate Comparative Trial — Comparison of Adverse Events Reported for ≥1% of Patients*

Adverse Events	TMTX/LV (n=109)	TMP/SMX (n=111)
Non-Laboratory Adverse Events		
Fever	9 (8.3%)	14 (12.6%)
Rash/pruritus	6 (5.5%)	14 (12.6%)
Nausea/vomiting	5 (4.6%)*	15 (13.5%)*
Confusion	3 (2.8%)	3 (2.7%)
Fatigue	2 (1.8%)	0 (0.0%)
Hematologic Toxicity		
Neutropenia (≤1000/mm^3)	33 (30.3%)	37 (33.3%)
Thrombocytopenia (≤75,000/mm^3)	11 (10.1%)	17 (15.3%)
Anemia (Hgb <8 g/dl)	8 (7.3%)	10 (9.0%)
Hepatotoxicity		
Increased AST (>5 × ULN)	15 (13.8%)	10 (9.0%)
Increased ALT (>5 × ULN)	12 (11.0%)	13 (11.7%)
Increased alkaline phosphatase (>5 × ULN)	5 (4.6%)	3 (2.7%)
Increased bilirubin (2.5 × ULN)	2 (1.8%)	1 (0.9%)
Renal		
Increased serum creatinine (>3 × ULN)	1 (0.9%)	2 (1.8%)
Electrolyte Imbalance		
Hyponatremia	5 (4.6%)	10 (9.0%)
Hypocalcemia	2 (1.8%)	0 (0.0%)
No. of patients with at least 1 adverse event†	**58 (53.2%)**	**60 (54.1%)**

* Statistically significant difference between treatment groups (Chi-square: p=0.022).
† Patients could have reported more than 1 adverse event; therefore the sum of adverse events exceeds the number of patients.
ULN = Upper limit of normal range.

Laboratory toxicities were generally manageable with dose modification of trimetrexate/leucovorin (see DOSAGE AND ADMINISTRATION).

TABLE 4 lists the adverse events resulting in discontinuation of study therapy in the Trimetrexate Glucuronate Comparative Study with TMP/SMX. Twenty-nine percent (29%) of the patients on the TMP/SMX arm discontinued therapy due to adverse events compared to 10% of the patients treated with TMTX/LV (p <0.001).

TABLE 4 *Trimetrexate Glucuronate Comparative Trial — Adverse Events Resulting in Discontinuation of Therapy**

Adverse Events	TMTX/LV (n=109)	TMP/SMX (n=111)
Non-Laboratory Adverse Events		
Rash/pruritus	3 (2.8%)	5 (4.5%)
Fever	2 (1.8%)	4 (3.6%)
Nausea/vomiting	1 (0.9%)	8 (7.2%)
Neurologic toxicity	1 (0.9%)†	2 (1.8%)
Hematologic Toxicity		
Neutropenia (≤1000/mm^3)	4 (3.7%)	6 (5.4%)
Thrombocytopenia (≤75,000/mm^3)	0 (0.0%)	4 (3.6%)
Anemia (Hgb <8 g/dl)	0 (0.0%)	4 (3.6%)
Hepatotoxicity		
Increased AST (>5 × ULN)	3 (2.8%)	9 (8.1%)
Increased ALT (>5 × ULN)	1 (0.9%)	4 (3.6%)
Increased alkaline phosphatase (>5 × ULN)	0 (0.0%)	1 (0.9%)
Electrolyte Imbalance		
Hyponatremia	0 (0.0%)	3 (2.7%)
No. of patients discontinuing therapy due to an adverse event*	**11 (10.1%)‡**	**32 (28.8%)‡**

ULN = Upper limit of normal range.
* Patients could discontinue therapy due to more than 1 toxicity; therefore the sum exceeds number of patients who discontinued due to toxicity.
† Patient discontinued TMTX/LV due to seizure, though causal relationship could not be established.
‡ Statistically significant difference between treatment groups (Chi-square: p <0.001).

Hematologic toxicity was the principal dose-limiting side effect.

DOSAGE AND ADMINISTRATION

Caution: Trimetrexate glucuronate for injection must be administered with concurrent leucovorin (leucovorin protection) to avoid potentially serious or life-threatening toxicities. Leucovorin therapy must extend for 72 hours past the last dose of trimetrexate glucuronate.

Trimetrexate glucuronate for injection is administered at a dose of 45 mg/m^2 once daily by intravenous infusion over 60 minutes. Leucovorin must be administered daily during treatment with trimetrexate glucuronate and for 72 hours past the last dose of trimetrexate glucuronate. Leucovorin may be administered intravenously at a dose of 20 mg/m^2 over 5-10 minutes every 6 hours for a total daily dose of 80 mg/m^2, or orally as 4 doses of 20 mg/m^2 spaced equally throughout the day. The oral dose should be rounded up to the next higher 25 mg increment. The recommended course of therapy is 21 days of trimetrexate glucuronate and 24 days of leucovorin.

Trimetrexate glucuronate and leucovorin may alternatively be dosed on a mg/kg basis, depending on the patient's body weight, using the conversion factors shown in TABLE 5.

TABLE 5

Body Weight	Trimetrexate Glucuronate Dose	Leucovorin
<50 kg	1.5 mg/kg/day	0.6 mg/kg/qid
50-80 kg	1.2 mg/kg/day	0.5 mg/kg/qid
>80 kg	1.0 mg/kg/day	0.5 mg/kg/qid

DOSAGE MODIFICATIONS

Hepatic Toxicity

Transient elevations of transaminases and alkaline phosphatase have been observed in patients treated with trimetrexate glucuronate. Interruption of treatment is advisable if transaminase levels or alkaline phosphatase levels increase to >5 times the upper limit of normal range.

Renal Toxicity

Interruption of trimetrexate glucuronate is advisable if serum creatinine levels increase to >2.5 mg/dl and the elevation is considered to be secondary to trimetrexate glucuronate.

Other Toxicities

Interruption of treatment is advisable in patients who experience severe mucosal toxicity that interferes with oral intake. Treatment should be discontinued for fever (oral temperature ≥105°F/40.5°C) that cannot be controlled with antipyretics.

Leucovorin therapy must extend for 72 hours past the last dose of trimetrexate glucuronate.

Hematologic Toxicity

Trimetrexate glucuronate for injection and leucovorin doses should be modified based on the worst hematologic toxicity according to TABLE 6A and TABLE 6B. If leucovorin is given orally, doses should be rounded up to the next higher 25 mg increment.

TABLE 6A *Dose Modifications for Hematologic Toxicity*

Toxicity Grade	Neutrophils (Polys and Bands)	Platelets	Recommended Dosage of Trimetrexate Glucuronate
1	>1000/mm^3	>75,000/mm^3	45 mg/m^2 once daily
2	750-1000/mm^3	50,000-75,000/mm^3	45 mg/m^2 once daily
3	500-749/mm^3	25,000-49,999/mm^3	22 mg/m^2 once daily
4	<500/mm^3	<25,000/mm^3	Day 1-9 discontinue
4	<500/mm^3	<25,000/mm^3	Day 10-21 interrupt up to 96 h*

* If Grade 4 hematologic toxicity occurs prior to Day 10, trimetrexate glucuronate should be discontinued. Leucovorin (40 mg/m^2, q6h) should be administered for an additional 72 hours. If Grade 4 hematologic toxicity occurs at Day 10 or later, trimetrexate glucuronate may be held up to 96 hours to allow counts to recover. If counts recover to Grade 3 within 96 hours, trimetrexate glucuronate should be administered at a dose of 22 mg/m^2 and leucovorin maintained at 40 mg/m^2, q6h. When counts recover to Grade 2 toxicity, trimetrexate glucuronate dose may be increased to 45 mg/m^2, but the leucovorin dose should be maintained at 40 mg/m^2 for the duration of treatment. If counts do not improve to ≤Grade 3 toxicity within 96 hours, trimetrexate glucuronate should be discontinued. Leucovorin at a dose of 40 mg/m^2,q6h should be administered for 72 hours following the last dose of trimetrexate glucuronate.

TABLE 6B *Dose Modifications for Hematologic Toxicity*

Toxicity Grade	Neutrophils (Polys and Bands)	Platelets	Recommended Dosage of Leucovorin
1	>1000/mm^3	>75,000/mm^3	20 mg/m^2 every 6 h
2	750-1000/mm^3	50,000-75,000/mm^3	40 mg/m^2 every 6 h
3	500-749/mm^3	25,000-49,999/mm^3	40 mg/m^2 every 6 h
4	<500/mm^3	>25,000/mm^3	40 mg/m^2 every 6 h

RECONSTITUTION AND DILUTION

Each vial of trimetrexate glucuronate for injection should be reconstituted in accordance with labeled instructions with either 5% dextrose injection, or sterile water for injection, to yield a concentration of 12.5 mg of trimetrexate per ml (complete dissolution should occur within 30 seconds). The reconstituted product will appear as a pale greenish-yellow solution and must be inspected visually prior to dilution. **Do not use if cloudiness or precipitate is observed.** Trimetrexate glucuronate should not be reconstituted with solutions containing either chloride ion or leucovorin, since precipitation occurs instantly. After reconstitution, the solution should be used immediately; however, the solution is stable for 6 hours at room temperature (20-25°C), or 24 hours under refrigeration (2-8°C).

Prior to administration, the reconstituted solution should be further diluted with 5% dextrose injection, to yield a final concentration of 0.25 to 2 mg of trimetrexate per ml. The diluted solution should be administered by intravenous infusion over 60 minutes. Trimetrexate glucuronate should not be mixed with solutions containing either chloride ion or leucovorin, since precipitation occurs instantly. The diluted solution is stable under refrigeration or at room temperature for up to 24 hours. Do not freeze. Discard any unused portion after 24 hours. The intravenous line must be flushed thoroughly with at least 10 ml of 5% dextrose injection, before and after administering trimetrexate glucuronate.

Leucovorin protection may be administered prior to or following trimetrexate glucuronate. In either case, the intravenous line must be flushed thoroughly with at least 10 ml of 5% dextrose injection. Leucovorin calcium for injection should be diluted according to the instructions in the leucovorin package insert, and administered over 5-10 minutes every 6 hours.

Caution: Parenteral products should be inspected visually for particulate matter and discoloration prior to administration, whenever solution and container permit. Trimetrexate glucuronate forms a precipitate instantly upon contact with chloride ion or leucovorin, therefore it should not be added to solutions containing sodium chloride or other anions. Trimetrexate glucuronate and leucovorin solutions must be administered separately. Intravenous lines should be flushed with at least 10 ml of 5% dextrose injection, between trimetrexate glucuronate and leucovorin infusions.

HANDLING AND DISPOSAL

If trimetrexate glucuronate for injection contacts the skin or mucosa, immediately wash thoroughly with soap and water. Procedures for proper disposal of cytotoxic drugs should be considered. Several guidelines on this subject have been published.[1-5]

HOW SUPPLIED

Neutrexin (trimetrexate glucuronate for injection) is supplied as a sterile lyophilized powder in either 5 ml or 30 ml vials. Each 5 ml vial contains trimetrexate glucuronate equivalent to 25 mg of trimetrexate. Each 30 ml vial contains trimetrexate glucuronate equivalent to 200 mg of trimetrexate.

Storage: Store at controlled room temperature 20-25°C (68-77°F). **Protect from exposure to light.**

PRODUCT LISTING - EQUIVALENTS NOT AVAILABLE

Powder For Injection - Intravenous - 25 mg

10's	$700.00	NEUTREXIN, Us Bioscience	58178-0020-10
50's	$6250.00	NEUTREXIN, Us Bioscience	58178-0020-50

Trimipramine Maleate *(002392)*

For related information, see the comparative table section in Appendix A.

Categories: Depression; Pregnancy Category C; FDA Approved 1982 Sep
Drug Classes: Antidepressants, tricyclic
Brand Names: **Surmontil**
Foreign Brand Availability: Rhotrimine (Canada); Stangyl (Germany); Sapilent (China); Sumontil (Japan); Tripress (New-Zealand)
Cost of Therapy: $84.01 (Depression; Surmontil; 50 mg; 2 capsules/day; 30 day supply)

DESCRIPTION

Trimipramine maleate is 5-(3-dimethylamino-2-methylpropyl)-10,11-dihydro-5H-dibenz (b,f) azepine acid maleate (racemic form).

Trimipramine maleate capsules contain trimipramine maleate equivalent to 25 mg, 50 mg, or 100 mg of trimipramine as the base. The inactive ingredients present are FD&C blue 1, gelatin, lactose, magnesium stearate, and titanium dioxide. The 25 mg dosage strength also contains D&C yellow 10 and FD&C yellow 6; the 50 mg dosage strength also contains D&C red 28, FD&C red 40, and FD&C yellow 6.

Trimipramine maleate is prepared as a racemic mixture which can be resolved into levorotatory and dextrorotatory isomers. The asymmetric center responsible for optical isomerism is marked in the formula by an asterisk. Trimipramine maleate is an almost odorless, white or slightly cream-colored, crystalline substance, melting at 140-144°C. It is very slightly soluble in ether and water, is slightly soluble in ethyl alcohol and acetone, and freely soluble in chloroform and methanol at 20°C.

STORAGE

Keep bottles tightly closed.

Dispense in a tight container.

Protect capsules packaged in blister strips from moisture.

CLINICAL PHARMACOLOGY

Trimipramine maleate is an antidepressant with an anxiety-reducing sedative component to its action. The mode of action of trimipramine maleate on the central nervous system is not known. However, unlike amphetamine-type compounds it does not act primarily by stimulation of the central nervous system. It does not act by inhibition of the monoamine oxidase system.

INDICATIONS AND USAGE

Trimipramine maleate is indicated for the relief of symptoms of depression. Endogenous depression is more likely to be alleviated than other depressive states. In studies with neurotic outpatients, the drug appeared to be equivalent to amitriptyline in the less-depressed patients but somewhat less effective than amitriptyline in the more severely depressed patients. In hospitalized depressed patients, trimipramine and imipramine were equally effective in relieving depression.

CONTRAINDICATIONS

Trimipramine maleate is contraindicated in cases of known hypersensitivity to the drug. The possibility of cross-sensitivity to other dibenzazepine compounds should be kept in mind. Trimipramine maleate should not be given in conjunction with drugs of the monoamine oxidase inhibitor class (*e.g.,* tranylcypromine, isocarboxazid or phenelzine sulfate). The concomitant use of monoamine oxidase inhibitors (MAOI) and tricyclic compounds similar to trimipramine maleate has caused severe hyperpyretic reactions, convulsive crises, and death in some patients. At least 2 weeks should elapse after cessation of therapy with MAOI before instituting therapy with trimipramine maleate. Initial dosage should be low and increased gradually with caution and careful observation of the patient. The drug is contraindicated during the acute recovery period after a myocardial infarction.

WARNINGS

USE IN CHILDREN

This drug is not recommended for use in children, since safety and effectiveness in the pediatric age group have not been established.

GENERAL

Extreme caution should be used when this drug is given to patients with any evidence of cardiovascular disease because of the possibility of conduction defects, arrhythmias, myocardial infarction, strokes, and tachycardia.

Caution is advised in patients with increased intraocular pressure, history of urinary retention, or history of narrow-angle glaucoma because of the drug's anticholinergic properties; hyperthyroid patients or those on thyroid medication because of the possibility of cardiovascular toxicity; patients with a history of seizure disorder, because this drug has been shown to lower the seizure threshold; patients receiving guanethidine or similar agents, since trimipramine maleate may block the pharmacologic effects of these drugs.

Since the drug may impair the mental and/or physical abilities required for the performance of potentially hazardous tasks, such as operating an automobile or machinery, the patient should be cautioned accordingly.

PRECAUTIONS

The possibility of suicide is inherent in any severely depressed patient and persists until a significant remission occurs. When a patient with a serious suicidal potential is not hospitalized, the prescription should be for the smallest amount feasible.

In schizophrenic patients activation of the psychosis may occur and require reduction of dosage or the addition of a major tranquilizer to the therapeutic regime.

Manic or hypomanic episodes may occur in some patients, in particular those with cyclic-type disorders. In some cases therapy with trimipramine maleate must be discontinued until the episode is relieved, after which therapy may be reinstituted at lower dosages if still required.

Concurrent administration of trimipramine maleate and electroshock therapy may increase the hazards of therapy. Such treatment should be limited to those patients for whom it is essential. When possible, discontinue the drug for several days prior to elective surgery.

There is evidence that cimetidine inhibits the elimination of tricyclic antidepressants. Downward adjustment of trimipramine maleate dosage may be required if cimetidine therapy is initiated; upward adjustment if cimetidine therapy is discontinued.

Patients should be warned that the concomitant use of alcoholic beverages may be associated with exaggerated effects.

It has been reported that tricyclic antidepressants can potentiate the effects of catecholamines. Similarly, atropinelike effects may be more pronounced in patients receiving anticholinergic therapy.

Therefore, particular care should be exercised when it is necessary to administer tricyclic antidepressants with sympathomimetic amines, local decongestants, local anesthetics containing epinephrine, atropine or drugs with an anticholinergic effect. In resistant cases of depression in adults, a dose of 2.5 mg/kg/day may have to be exceeded. If a higher dose is needed, ECG monitoring should be maintained during the initiation of therapy and at appropriate intervals during stabilization of dose.

PREGNANCY CATEGORY C

Trimipramine maleate has shown evidence of embryo-toxicity and/or increased incidence of major anomalies in rats or rabbits at doses 20 times the human dose. There are no adequate and well-controlled studies in pregnant women. Trimipramine maleate should be used during pregnancy only if the potential benefit justifies the potential risk to the fetus.

Semen studies in man (4 schizophrenics and 9 normal volunteers) revealed no significant changes in sperm morphology. It is recognized that drugs having a parasympathetic effect, including tricyclic antidepressants, may alter the ejaculatory response.

Chronic animal studies showed occasional evidence of degeneration of seminiferous tubules at the highest dose of 60 mg/kg/day.

Trimipramine maleate should be used with caution in patients with impaired liver function.

Chronic animal studies showed occasional occurrence of hepatic congestion, fatty infiltration, or increased serum liver enzymes at the highest dose of 60 mg/kg/day.

Both elevation and lowering of blood sugar have been reported with tricyclic antidepressants.

ADVERSE REACTIONS

Note: The pharmacological similarities among the tricyclic antidepressants require that each of the reactions be considered when trimipramine maleate is administered. Some of the adverse reactions included in this listing have not in fact been reported with trimipramine maleate.

Cardiovascular: Hypotension, hypertension, tachycardia, palpitation, myocardial infarction, arrhythmias, heart block, stroke.

Psychiatric: Confusional states (especially the elderly) with hallucinations, disorientation, delusions; anxiety, restlessness, agitation; insomnia and nightmares; hypomania; exacerbation of psychosis.

Neurological: Numbness, tingling, paresthesias of extremities; incoordination, ataxia, tremors; peripheral neuropathy; extrapyramidal symptoms; seizures, alterations in EEG patterns; tinnitus; syndrome of inappropriate ADH (antidiuretic hormone) secretion.

Anticholinergic: Dry mouth and, rarely, associated sublingual adenitis; blurred vision, disturbances of accommodation, mydriasis, constipation, paralytic ileus; urinary retention, delayed micturition, dilation of the urinary tract.

Allergic: Skin rash, petechiae, urticaria, itching, photosensitization, edema of face and tongue.

Hematologic: Bone-marrow depression including agranulocytosis, eosinophilia; purpura; thrombocytopenia. Leukocyte and differential counts should be performed in any patient who develops fever and sore throat during therapy; the drug should be discontinued if there is evidence of pathological neutrophil depression.

Gastrointestinal: Nausea and vomiting, anorexia, epigastric distress, diarrhea, peculiar taste, stomatitis, abdominal cramps, black tongue.

Endocrine: Gynecomastia in the male; breast enlargement and galactorrhea in the female; increased or decreased libido, impotence; testicular swelling; elevation or depression of blood-sugar levels.

Other: Jaundice (simulating obstructive); altered liver function; weight gain or loss; perspiration; flushing; urinary frequency; drowsiness, dizziness, weakness, and fatigue; headache; parotid swelling; alopecia.

Withdrawal Symptoms: Though not indicative of addiction, abrupt cessation of treatment after prolonged therapy may produce nausea, headache, and malaise.

DOSAGE AND ADMINISTRATION

Dosage should be initiated at a low level and increased gradually, noting carefully the clinical response and any evidence of intolerance.

Lower dosages are recommended for elderly patients and adolescents. Lower dosages are also recommended for outpatients as compared to hospitalized patients who will be under close supervision. It is not possible to prescribe a single dosage schedule of trimipramine maleate that will be therapeutically effective in all patients. The physical psychodynamic factors contributing to depressive symptomatology are very complex; spontaneous remissions or exacerbations of depressive symptoms may occur with or without drug therapy. Consequently, the recommended dosage regimens are furnished as a guide which may be modified by factors such as the age of the patient, chronicity and severity of the disease, medical condition of the patient, and degree of psychotherapeutic support.

Most antidepressant drugs have a lag period of 10 days to 4 weeks before a therapeutic response is noted. Increasing the dose will not shorten this period but rather increase the incidence of adverse reactions.

USUAL ADULT DOSE

Outpatients and Office Patients

Initially, 75 mg/day in divided doses, increased to 150 mg/day. Dosages over 200 mg/day are not recommended. Maintenance therapy is in the range of 50-150 mg/day. For convenient therapy and to facilitate patient compliance, the total dosage requirement may be given at bedtime.

Hospitalized Patients

Initially, 100 mg/day in divided doses. This may be increased gradually in a few days to 200 mg/day, depending upon individual response and tolerance. If improvement does not occur in 2-3 weeks, the dose may be increased to the maximum recommended dose of 250-300 mg/day.

Adolescent and Geriatric Patients

Initially, a dose of 50 mg/day is recommended, with gradual increments up to 100 mg/day, depending upon patient response and tolerance.

Maintenance

Following remission, maintenance medication may be required for a longer period of time, at the lowest dose that will maintain remission. Maintenance therapy is preferably administered as a single dose at bedtime. To minimize relapse, maintenance therapy should be continued for about 3 months.

PRODUCT LISTING - RATED THERAPEUTICALLY EQUIVALENT

Capsule - Oral - 25 mg

100's	$85.58	SURMONTIL, Wyeth-Ayerst Laboratories	00008-4132-01
100's	$108.26	SURMONTIL, Odyssey Pharmaceutical	65473-0718-01

Capsule - Oral - 50 mg

100's	$140.01	SURMONTIL, Wyeth-Ayerst Laboratories	00008-4133-01
100's	$177.11	SURMONTIL, Odyssey Pharmaceutical	65473-0719-01

Capsule - Oral - 100 mg

100's	$203.54	SURMONTIL, Wyeth-Ayerst Laboratories	00008-4158-01
100's	$257.48	SURMONTIL, Odyssey Pharmaceutical	65473-0720-01

Triptorelin Pamoate *(003495)*

Categories: Carcinoma, prostate; FDA Approved 2000 Jun; Pregnancy Category X
Drug Classes: Antineoplastics, hormones/hormone modifiers; Hormones/hormone modifiers
Brand Names: Trelstar Depot
Foreign Brand Availability: Arvekap (Greece); Decapeptyl (Bahrain; Belgium; Bulgaria; China; Colombia; Cyprus; Egypt; England; France; Germany; Hong-Kong; Hungary; Iran; Iraq; Ireland; Italy; Jordan; Kuwait; Lebanon; Libya; Netherlands; Oman; Peru; Portugal; Qatar; Republic-of-Yemen; Saudi-Arabia; Spain; Syria; United-Arab-Emirates); Decapeptyl CR (Bahrain; Cyprus; Egypt; Iran; Iraq; Jordan; Korea; Kuwait; Lebanon; Libya; Malaysia; Oman; Qatar; Republic-of-Yemen; Saudi-Arabia; Syria; Taiwan; Thailand; United-Arab-Emirates); Decapeptyl Depot (Austria; Denmark; Finland; Germany; Korea; Sweden); Decapeptyl L (South-Africa); Decapeptyl LP (France); Decapeptyl Retard (Switzerland); Diphereline (China); Diphereline PR (Hong-Kong; Taiwan); Diphereline SR (Israel); Trelstar (Mexico)

DESCRIPTION

Note: The trade names have been used throughout this monograph for clarity.

TRELSTAR DEPOT

Trelstar Depot contains a pamoate salt of triptorelin, and triptorelin is a synthetic decapeptide agonist analog of luteinizing hormone releasing hormone (LHRH or GnRH) with greater potency than the naturally occurring LHRH. The chemical name of triptorelin pamoate is 5-oxo-L-prolyl-L-histidyl-L-tryptophyl-L-seryl-L-tyrosyl-D-tryptophyl-L-leucyl-L-arginyl-L-prolylglycine amide (pamoate salt); the empirical formula is $C_{64}H_{82}N_{18}O_{13}{\cdot}C_{23}H_{16}O_6$ and the molecular weight is 1699.9.

Trelstar Depot is a sterile, lyophilized biodegradable microgranule formulation supplied as a single-dose vial containing triptorelin pamoate (3.75 mg as the peptide base), 170 mg poly-*d,l*-lactide-co-glycolide, 85 mg mannitol, 30 mg carboxymethylcellulose sodium, 2 mg polysorbate 80. When 2 ml sterile water for injection is added to the vial containing Trelstar Depot and mixed, a suspension is formed which is intended as a monthly intramuscular injection.

TRELSTAR LA

Trelstar LA contains a pamoate salt of triptorelin, and triptorelin is a synthetic decapeptide agonist analog of luteinizing hormone releasing hormone (LHRH or GnRH) with greater potency than the naturally occurring LHRH. The chemical name of triptorelin pamoate is 5-oxo-L-prolyl-L-histidyl-L-tryptophyl-L-seryl-L-tyrosyl-D-tryptophyl-L-leucyl-L-arginyl-L-prolylglycine amide (pamoate salt); the empirical formula is $C_{64}H_{82}N_{18}O_{13}{\cdot}C_{23}H_{16}O_6$ and the molecular weight is 1699.9.

Trelstar LA is a sterile, lyophilized biodegradable microgranule formulation supplied as a single-dose vial containing triptorelin pamoate (11.25 mg as the peptide base), 145 mg poly-*d,l*-lactide-coglycolide, 85 mg mannitol, 30 mg carboxymethylcellulose sodium, 2 mg polysorbate 80. When 2 ml sterile water for injection is added to the vial containing Trelstar LA and mixed, a suspension is formed which is intended as an intramuscular injection to be administered every 84 days (*i.e.*, every 12 weeks). Trelstar LA is available in 2 packaging configurations: (a) Trelstar LA vial alone or (b) Trelstar LA vial plus a separate pre-filled syringe that contains 2 ml of sterile water for injection (Debioclip).

CLINICAL PHARMACOLOGY

TRELSTAR DEPOT

Mechanism of Action

Triptorelin is a potent inhibitor of gonadotropin secretion when given continuously and in therapeutic doses. Following the first administration, there is a transient surge in circulating levels of luteinizing hormone (LH), follicle-stimulating hormone (FSH), testosterone, and estradiol (see ADVERSE REACTIONS, Trelstar Depot). After chronic and continuous administration, usually 2-4 weeks after initiation of therapy, a sustained decrease in LH and FSH secretion and marked reduction of testicular and ovarian steroidogenesis is observed. In men, a reduction of serum testosterone concentration to a level typically seen in surgically castrated men is obtained. Consequently, the result is that tissues and functions that depend on these hormones for maintenance become quiescent. These effects are usually reversible after cessation of therapy.

Following a single intramuscular (IM) injection of Trelstar Depot to healthy male volunteers, serum testosterone levels first increased, peaking on day 4, and declined thereafter to low levels by week 4. Similar testosterone profiles were observed in patients with advanced prostate cancer, when injected with Trelstar Depot. In healthy volunteers, testosterone serum levels returned to near baseline by week 8.

Pharmacokinetics

Results of pharmacokinetic investigations conducted in healthy men indicate that after intravenous (IV) bolus administration, triptorelin is distributed and eliminated according to a 3-compartment model and corresponding half-lives are approximately 6 minutes, 45 minutes, and 3 hours.

Absorption

Triptorelin pamoate is not active when given orally. Intramuscular injection of the depot formulation provides plasma concentrations of triptorelin over a period of 1 month. The pharmacokinetic parameters following a single IM injection of 3.75 mg of Trelstar Depot to 20 healthy male volunteers are listed in TABLE 1. The plasma concentrations declined to 0.084 ng/ml at 4 weeks.

TABLE 1 *Pharmacokinetic Parameters Following Intramuscular Administration of Trelstar Depot to Healthy Male Volunteers*

Dose (n=20)	C_{max} (ng/ml)	T_{max} (hours)	AUC(0-28 d) (h·ng/ml)	F* (%)
3.75 mg	28.43 ± 7.31†	1.0 (1.0-3.0)‡	223.15 ± 46.96†	83 (28 days)

* Mean ±SD.
† Median (range).
‡ Computed as the mean AUC of the study divided by the mean AUC of healthy volunteers corrected for dose where AUC=36.1 h·ng/ml and 500 μg IV bolus dose of triptorelin was administered.

Distribution

The volume of distribution following an IV bolus dose of 0.5 mg of triptorelin peptide was 30-33 L in healthy male volunteers. There is no evidence that triptorelin, at clinically relevant concentrations, binds to plasma proteins.

Metabolism

The metabolism of triptorelin in humans is unknown, but is unlikely to involve hepatic microsomal enzymes (cytochrome P-450). However, the effect of triptorelin on the activity of other drug metabolizing enzymes is unknown. Thus far, no metabolites of triptorelin have been identified. Pharmacokinetic data suggest that C-terminal fragments produced by tissue degradation are either completely degraded in the tissues, or rapidly degraded in plasma, or cleared by the kidneys.

Excretion

Triptorelin is eliminated by both the liver and the kidneys. Following IV administration of 0.5 mg triptorelin peptide to 6 healthy male volunteers with a creatinine clearance of 149.9 ml/min, 41.7% of the dose was excreted in urine as intact peptide with a total triptorelin clearance of 211.9 ml/min. This percentage increased to 62.3% in patients with liver disease who have a lower creatinine clearance (89.9 ml/min). It has also been observed that the non-renal clearance of triptorelin (patient anuric, Cl_{creat}=0) was 76.2 ml/min, thus indicating that the nonrenal elimination of triptorelin is mainly dependent on the liver (see Special Populations).

Special Populations

Renal and Hepatic Impairment

After an IV injection of 0.5 mg triptorelin peptide, the two distribution half-lives were unaffected by renal and hepatic impairment, but renal insufficiency led to a decrease in total triptorelin clearance proportional to the decrease in creatinine clearance as well as an increase in volume of distribution and consequently an increase in elimination half-life (TABLE 2). The decrease in triptorelin clearance was more pronounced in subjects with liver insufficiency, but the half-life was prolonged similarly in subjects with renal insufficiency, since the volume of distribution was only minimally increased.

T

TABLE 2 *Pharmacokinetic Parameters (Mean ±SD) in Healthy Volunteers and Special Populations*

	6 Healthy Male Volunteers	6 Males With Moderate Renal Impairment	6 Males With Severe Renal Impairment	6 Males With Liver Disease
C_{max} (ng/ml)	48.2 ± 11.8	45.6 ± 20.5	46.5 ± 14.0	54.1 ± 5.3
AUC(∞) (h·ng/ml)	36.1 ± 5.8	69.9 ± 24.6	88.0 ± 18.4	131.9 ± 18.1
CL_p (ml/min)	211.9 ± 31.6	120.0 ± 45.0	88.6 ± 19.7	57.8 ± 8.0
Cl_{renal} (ml/min)	90.6 ± 35.3	23.3 ± 17.6	4.3 ± 2.9	35.9 ± 5.0
T½ (hours)	2.81 ± 1.21	6.56 ± 1.25	7.65 ± 1.25	7.58 ± 1.17
Cl_{creat} (ml/min)	149.9 ± 7.3	39.7 ± 22.5	8.9 ± 6.0	89.9 ± 15.1

Age and Race

The effects of age and race on triptorelin pharmacokinetics have not been systematically studied. However, pharmacokinetic data obtained in young healthy male volunteers aged 20-22 years with an elevated creatinine clearance (approximately 150 ml/min) indicates that triptorelin was eliminated twice as fast in this young population (see Special Populations, Renal and Hepatic Impairment) as compared to patients with moderate renal insufficiency. This is related to the fact that triptorelin clearance is partly correlated to total creatinine clearance, which is well known to decrease with age.

Pharmacokinetic Drug-Drug Interactions

No pharmacokinetic drug-drug interaction studies have been conducted with triptorelin (see DRUG INTERACTIONS, Trelstar Depot).

TRELSTAR LA

Mechanism of Action

Triptorelin is a potent inhibitor of gonadotropin secretion when given continuously and in therapeutic doses. Following the first administration, there is a transient surge in circulating levels of luteinizing hormone (LH), follicle-stimulating hormone (FSH), testosterone, and estradiol (see ADVERSE REACTIONS, Trelstar LA). After chronic and continuous administration, usually 2-4 weeks after initiation of therapy, a sustained decrease in LH and FSH secretion and marked reduction of testicular and ovarian steroidogenesis is observed. In men, a reduction of serum testosterone concentration to a level typically seen in surgically castrated men is obtained. Consequently, the result is that tissues and functions that depend on these hormones for maintenance become quiescent. These effects are usually reversible after cessation of therapy.

Following a single intramuscular (IM) injection of Trelstar LA to men with advanced prostate cancer, serum testosterone levels first increased, peaking on days 2-3, and declined thereafter to low levels by weeks 3-4.

Pharmacokinetics

Results of pharmacokinetic investigations conducted in healthy men indicate that after intravenous (IV) bolus administration, triptorelin is distributed and eliminated according to a 3-compartment model and corresponding half-lives are approximately 6 minutes, 45 minutes, and 3 hours.

Absorption

Triptorelin pamoate is not active when given orally. The pharmacokinetic parameters following a single IM injection of 11.25 mg of Trelstar LA to 13 patients with prostate cancer are listed in TABLE 3. Triptorelin did not accumulate over 9 months of treatment.

TABLE 3 *Pharmacokinetic Parameters (Mean ±SD) Following Intramuscular Administration of Trelstar LA to Patients With Prostate Cancer*

Dose (n=13)	$C_{max\ (0\text{-}85\ d)}$ (ng/ml)	$T_{max\ (0\text{-}85\ d)}$ (hours)	AUC(1-85 d) (h·ng/ml)
11.25 mg	38.5 ± 10.5	2.9 ± 1.3	2268.0 ± 444.6

Distribution

The volume of distribution following a single IV bolus dose of 0.5 mg of triptorelin peptide was 30-33 L in healthy male volunteers. There is no evidence that triptorelin, at clinically relevant concentrations, binds to plasma proteins.

Metabolism

The metabolism of triptorelin in humans is unknown, but is unlikely to involve hepatic microsomal enzymes (cytochrome P-450). However, the effect of triptorelin on the activity of other drug metabolizing enzymes is unknown. Thus far, no metabolites of triptorelin have been identified. Pharmacokinetic data suggest that C-terminal fragments produced by tissue degradation are either completely degraded in the tissues, or rapidly degraded in plasma, or cleared by the kidneys.

Excretion

Triptorelin is eliminated by both the liver and the kidneys. Following IV administration of 0.5 mg triptorelin peptide to 6 healthy male volunteers with a creatinine clearance of 149.9 ml/min, 41.7% of the dose was excreted in urine as intact peptide with a total triptorelin clearance of 211.9 ml/min. This percentage increased to 62.3% in patients with liver disease who have a lower creatinine clearance (89.9 ml/min). It has also been observed that the nonrenal clearance of triptorelin (patient anuric, Cl_{creat}=0) was 76.2 ml/min, thus indicating that the nonrenal elimination of triptorelin is mainly dependent on the liver (see Special Populations).

Special Populations

Renal and Hepatic Impairment

After an IV bolus injection of 0.5 mg triptorelin peptide, the two distribution half-lives were unaffected by renal and hepatic impairment, but renal insufficiency led to a decrease in total triptorelin clearance proportional to the decrease in creatinine clearance as well as an increase in volume of distribution and consequently an increase in elimination half-life (TABLE 2). The decrease in triptorelin clearance was more pronounced in subjects with liver insufficiency, but the half-life was prolonged similarly in subjects with renal insufficiency, since the volume of distribution was only minimally increased. Patients with renal or hepatic impairment had 2- to 4-fold higher exposure (AUC values) than young healthy males.

Age and Race

The effects of age and race on triptorelin pharmacokinetics have not been systematically studied. However, pharmacokinetic data obtained in young healthy male volunteers aged 20-22 years with an elevated creatinine clearance (approximately 150 ml/min) indicates that triptorelin was eliminated twice as fast in this young population (see Special Populations, Renal and Hepatic Impairment) as compared to patients with moderate renal insufficiency. This is related to the fact that triptorelin clearance is partly correlated to total creatinine clearance, which is well known to decrease with age.

Pharmacokinetic Drug-Drug Interactions

No pharmacokinetic drug-drug interaction studies have been conducted with triptorelin (See DRUG INTERACTIONS, Trelstar LA).

INDICATIONS AND USAGE

TRELSTAR DEPOT

Trelstar Depot is indicated in the palliative treatment of advanced prostate cancer. It offers an alternative treatment for prostate cancer when orchiectomy or estrogen administration are either not indicated or unacceptable to the patient.

TRELSTAR LA

Trelstar LA is indicated in the palliative treatment of advanced prostate cancer. It offers an alternative treatment for prostate cancer when orchiectomy or estrogen administration are either not indicated or unacceptable to the patient.

NON-FDA APPROVED INDICATIONS

The drug has also been shown to have efficacy in the treatment of endometriosis. However, further studies are needed and this use has not been approved by the FDA.

CONTRAINDICATIONS

TRELSTAR DEPOT

Trelstar Depot is contraindicated in individuals with a known hypersensitivity to triptorelin or any other component of the product, other LHRH agonists or LHRH. Three (3) postmarketing reports of anaphylactic shock and 7 postmarketing reports of angioedema related to triptorelin administration have been reported since 1986 (see WARNINGS, Trelstar Depot).

Trelstar Depot may cause fetal harm when administered to a pregnant woman.

TRELSTAR LA

Trelstar LA is contraindicated in individuals with a known hypersensitivity to triptorelin or any other component of the product, other LHRH agonists or LHRH.

Trelstar LA is contraindicated in women who are or may become pregnant while receiving the drug. Trelstar LA may cause fetal harm when administered to a pregnant woman.

WARNINGS

TRELSTAR DEPOT

Initially, triptorelin, like other LHRH agonists, causes a transient increase in serum testosterone levels. As a result, isolated cases of worsening of signs and symptoms of prostate cancer during the first weeks of treatment have been reported with LHRH agonists. Patients may experience worsening of symptoms or onset of new symptoms, including bone pain, neuropathy, hematuria, or urethral or bladder outlet obstruction. Cases of spinal cord compression, which may contribute to paralysis with or without fatal complications, have been reported with LHRH agonists.

If spinal cord compression or renal impairment develops, standard treatment of these complications should be instituted, and in extreme cases an immediate orchiectomy considered.

Trelstar Depot should not be administered to individuals who are hypersensitive to triptorelin, other LHRH agonists, or LHRH. In the event of a hypersensitivity reaction, therapy with Trelstar Depot should be discontinued immediately and the appropriate supportive and symptomatic care should be administered.

TRELSTAR LA

Rare reports of anaphylactic shock and angioedema related to triptorelin administration have been reported. In the event of a reaction, therapy with Trelstar LA should be discontinued immediately and the appropriate supportive and symptomatic care should be administered.

Initially, triptorelin, like other LHRH agonists, causes a transient increase in serum testosterone levels. As a result, isolated cases of worsening of signs and symptoms of prostate cancer during the first weeks of treatment have been reported with LHRH agonists. Patients may experience worsening of symptoms or onset of new symptoms, including bone pain, neuropathy, hematuria, or urethral or bladder outlet obstruction. Cases of spinal cord compression, which may contribute to paralysis with or without fatal complications, have been reported with LHRH agonists.

If spinal cord compression or renal impairment develops, standard treatment of these complications should be instituted, and in extreme cases an immediate orchiectomy considered.

PRECAUTIONS

TRELSTAR DEPOT

General

Patients with metastatic vertebral lesions and/or with upper or lower urinary tract obstruction should be closely observed during the first few weeks of therapy (see WARNINGS, Trelstar Depot). Hypersensitivity and anaphylactic reactions have been reported with triptorelin as with other LHRH agonists (see CONTRAINDICATIONS, Trelstar Depot and WARNINGS, Trelstar Depot).

Laboratory Tests

Response to Trelstar Depot should be monitored by measuring serum levels of testosterone and prostate-specific antigen.

Drug/Laboratory Test Interactions

Chronic or continuous administration of triptorelin in therapeutic doses results in suppression of the pituitary-gonadal axis. Diagnostic tests of the pituitary-gonadal function conducted during treatment and after cessation of therapy may therefore be misleading.

Pregnancy, Teratogenic Effects, Pregnancy Category X

See CONTRAINDICATIONS, Trelstar Depot.

Trelstar Depot is contraindicated in women who are or may become pregnant while receiving the drug. Studies in pregnant rats administered triptorelin at doses of 2, 10, and 100 µg/kg/day (approximately equivalent to 0.2, 0.8, and 8 times the recommended human therapeutic dose based on body surface area) during the period of organogenesis displayed maternal toxicity and embryotoxicity, but no fetotoxicity or teratogenicity. Similarly, no teratogenic effects were observed when mice were administered doses of 2, 20, and 200 µg/kg/day (approximately equivalent to 0.1, 0.7, and 7 times the recommended human therapeutic dose based on body surface area). If this drug is used during pregnancy or if the patient becomes pregnant while taking this drug, she should be apprised of the potential hazard to the fetus.

Carcinogenesis, Mutagenesis, and Impairment of Fertility

In rats, doses of 120, 600, and 3000 µg/kg given every 28 days (approximately 0.3, 2.0, and 8 times the recommended human therapeutic dose based on body surface area) resulted in increased mortality with a drug treatment period of 13-19 months. The incidence of benign and malignant pituitary tumors and histiosarcomas were increased in a dose related manner. No oncogenic effect was observed in mice administered triptorelin for 18 months at doses up to 6000 µg/kg every 28 days (approximately 8 times the human therapeutic dose based on body surface area).

Mutagenicity studies performed with triptorelin using bacterial and mammalian systems (*in vitro* Ames test and chromosomal aberration test in CHO cells and an *in vivo* mouse micronucleus test) provided no evidence of mutagenic potential.

After 60 days of treatment followed by a minimum of four estrus cycles prior to mating, triptorelin, at doses of 2, 20, and 200 µg/kg/day in saline (approximately 0.2, 2.0, and 16 times the recommended human therapeutic dose based on body surface area) or 20 µg/kg/day in slow release microspheres, had no effect on the fertility or general reproductive performance of female rats. Treatment did not elicit embryotoxicity, teratogenicity, or any effects on the development of the offspring (F_1 generation) or their reproductive performance.

No studies were conducted to assess the effect of triptorelin on male fertility.

Geriatric Use

Prostate cancer occurs primarily in an older patient population. Clinical studies with Trelstar Depot have been conducted primarily in patients ≥65 years.

Nursing Mothers

It is not known whether Trelstar Depot is excreted in human milk. Because many drugs are excreted in human milk, and because the effects of Trelstar Depot on lactation and/or the breastfed child have not been determined, Trelstar Depot should not be used by nursing mothers.

Pediatric Use

Trelstar Depot has not been studied in pediatric patients.

TRELSTAR LA

General

Patients with metastatic vertebral lesions and/or with upper or lower urinary tract obstruction should be closely observed during the first few weeks of therapy (see WARNINGS, Trelstar LA). Hypersensitivity and anaphylactic reactions have been reported with triptorelin as with other LHRH agonists (see CONTRAINDICATIONS, Trelstar LA and WARNINGS, Trelstar LA).

Laboratory Tests

Response to Trelstar LA should be monitored by measuring serum levels of testosterone and prostate-specific antigen. Testosterone levels should be measured immediately prior to or immediately after dosing.

Drug/Laboratory Test Interactions

Chronic or continuous administration of triptorelin in therapeutic doses results in suppression of the pituitary-gonadal axis. Diagnostic tests of the pituitary-gonadal function conducted during treatment and after cessation of therapy may therefore be misleading.

Pregnancy, Teratogenic Effects, Pregnancy Category X

See CONTRAINDICATIONS, Trelstar LA.

Trelstar LA is contraindicated in women who are or may become pregnant while receiving the drug. Studies in pregnant rats administered triptorelin at doses of 2, 10, and 100 µg/kg/day (approximately equivalent to 0.2, 0.8, and 8 times the recommended human therapeutic dose based on body surface area) during the period of organogenesis displayed maternal toxicity and embryotoxicity, but no fetotoxicity or teratogenicity. Similarly, no teratogenic effects were observed when mice were administered doses of 2, 20, and 200 µg/kg/day (approximately equivalent to 0.1, 0.7, and 7 times the recommended human therapeutic dose based on body surface area). If this drug is used during pregnancy or if the patient becomes pregnant while taking this drug, she should be apprised of the potential hazard to the fetus (see PRECAUTIONS, Trelstar LA).

Carcinogenesis, Mutagenesis, and Impairment of Fertility

In rats, doses of 120, 600, and 3000 µg/kg given every 28 days (approximately 0.3, 2, and 8 times the recommended human therapeutic dose based on body surface area) resulted in increased mortality with a drug treatment period of 13-19 months. The incidence of benign and malignant pituitary tumors and histiosarcomas were increased in a dose related manner. No oncogenic effect was observed in mice administered triptorelin for 18 months at doses up to 6000 µg/kg every 28 days (approximately 8 times the human therapeutic dose based on body surface area).

Mutagenicity studies performed with triptorelin using bacterial and mammalian systems (*in vitro* Ames test and chromosomal aberration test in CHO cells and an *in vivo* mouse micronucleus test) provided no evidence of mutagenic potential.

After 60 days of treatment followed by a minimum of four estrus cycles prior to mating, triptorelin, at doses of 2, 20, and 200 µg/kg/day in saline (approximately 0.2, 2.0, and 16 times the recommended human therapeutic dose based on body surface area) or 20 µg/kg/day in slow release microspheres, had no effect on the fertility or general reproductive performance of female rats. Treatment did not elicit embryotoxicity, teratogenicity, or any effects on the development of the offspring (F_1 generation) or their reproductive performance.

No studies were conducted to assess the effect of triptorelin on male fertility.

Geriatric Use

Prostate cancer occurs primarily in an older patient population. Clinical studies with Trelstar LA have been conducted primarily in patients ≥65 years old.

Use in Women

Trelstar LA has not been studied in women and is not indicated for use in women.

Nursing Mothers

It is not known whether Trelstar LA is excreted in human milk. Because many drugs are excreted in human milk and because the effects of Trelstar LA on lactation and/or the breastfed child have not been determined, Trelstar LA should not be used by nursing mothers.

Pediatric Use

Trelstar LA has not been studied in pediatric patients and is not indicated for use in pediatric patients.

DRUG INTERACTIONS

TRELSTAR DEPOT

No drug-drug interaction studies involving triptorelin have been conducted. In the absence of relevant data and as a precaution, hyperprolactinemic drugs should not be prescribed concomitantly with Trelstar Depot since hyperprolactinemia reduces the number of pituitary GnRH receptors.

TRELSTAR LA

No drug-drug interaction studies involving triptorelin have been conducted. In the absence of relevant data and as a precaution, hyperprolactinemic drugs should not be prescribed concomitantly with Trelstar LA since hyperprolactinemia reduces the number of pituitary GnRH receptors.

ADVERSE REACTIONS

TRELSTAR DEPOT

In the majority of patients, testosterone levels increased above baseline during the first week following the initial injection, declining thereafter to baseline levels or below by the end of the second week of treatment. The transient increase in testosterone levels may be associated with temporary worsening of disease signs and symptoms, including bone pain, hematuria, and bladder outlet obstruction. Isolated cases of spinal cord compression with weakness or paralysis of the lower extremities have occurred (see WARNINGS, Trelstar Depot).

In a controlled, comparative clinical trial, the following adverse reactions were reported to have a possible or probable relationship to therapy as ascribed by the treating physician in 1% or more of the patients receiving triptorelin (TABLE 4). Often, causality is difficult to assess in patients with metastatic prostate cancer. Reactions considered not drug-related are excluded.

Changes in Laboratory Values During Treatment

There were no clinically meaningful changes in laboratory values during or following therapy with Trelstar Depot.

TRELSTAR LA

In the majority of patients, testosterone levels increased above baseline during the first week following the initial injection, declining thereafter to baseline levels or below by the end of the second week of treatment. The transient increase in testosterone levels may be associated with temporary worsening of disease signs and symptoms, including bone pain, hematuria, and bladder outlet obstruction. Isolated cases of spinal cord compression with weakness or paralysis of the lower extremities have occurred (see WARNINGS, Trelstar LA).

In a controlled, comparative clinical trial, the following adverse reactions were reported to have a possible or probable relationship to therapy as ascribed by the treating physician in 1% or more of the patients receiving triptorelin (TABLE 5). Often, causality is difficult

T

TABLE 4 *Related Adverse Events Reported by 1% or More of Patients During Treatment With Trelstar Depot (n=140)*

Adverse Event	n (%)
Application Site Disorders	
Injection site pain	5 (3.6%)
Body as a Whole	
Hot flushes*	82 (58.6%)
Pain	3 (2.1%)
Leg pain	3 (2.1%)
Fatigue	3 (2.1%)
Cardiovascular	
Hypertension	5 (3.6%)
Central and Peripheral Nervous System Disorders	
Headache	7 (5.0%)
Dizziness	2 (1.4%)
Gastrointestinal Disorders	
Diarrhea	2 (1.4%)
Vomiting	3 (2.1%)
Musculokeletal System Disorders	
Skeletal pain	17 (12.1%)
Psychiatric	
Insomnia	3 (2.1%)
Impotence*	10 (7.1%)
Emotional lability	2 (1.4%)
Red Blood Cell Disorders	
Anemia	2 (1.4%)
Skin and Appendages Disorders	
Pruritus	2 (1.4%)
Urinary System	
Urinary retention	2 (1.4%)
Urinary tract infection	2 (1.4%)

* Expected pharmacologic consequences of testosterone suppression.

to assess in patients with metastatic prostate cancer. Reactions considered not drug-related or unlikely to be related are excluded.

TABLE 5 *Treatment-Related Adverse Events Reported by 1% or More of Patients During Treatment With Trelstar LA (n=174)*

Adverse Event	n (%)
Application Site	
Injection site pain	7 (4.0%)
Body as a Whole	
Hot flushes*	127 (73.0%)
Leg pain	9 (5.2%)
Pain	6 (3.4%)
Back pain	5 (2.9%)
Fatigue	4 (2.3%)
Chest pain	3 (1.7%)
Asthenia	2 (1.1%)
Peripheral edema	2 (1.1%)
Cardiovascular	
Hypertension	7 (4.0%)
Dependent edema	4 (2.3%)
Central and Peripheral Nervous System	
Headache	12 (6.9%)
Dizziness	5 (2.9%)
Leg cramps	3 (1.7%)
Endocrine	
Breast pain	4 (2.3%)
Gynecomastia	3 (1.7%)
Gastrointestinal	
Nausea	5 (2.9%)
Consitpation	3 (1.7%)
Dyspepsia	3 (1.7%)
Diarrhea	2 (1.1%)
Abdominal pain	2 (1.1%)
Liver and Bilary System	
Abnormal hepatic function	2 (1.1%)
Metabolic and Nutritional	
Edema in legs	11 (6.3%)
Increased alkaline phosphatase	3 (1.7%)
Musculoskeletal System	
Skeletal pain	23 (13.2%)
Arthralgia	4 (2.3%)
Myalgia	2 (1.1%)
Psychiatric	
Decreased libido*	4 (2.3%)
Impotence*	4 (2.3%)
Insomnia	3 (1.7%)
Anorexia	3 (1.7%)
Respiratory System	
Coughing	3 (1.7%)
Dyspnea	2 (1.1%)
Pharyngitis	2 (1.1%)
Skin and Appendages	
Rash	3 (1.7%)
Urinary System	
Dysuria	8 (4.6%)
Urinary retention	2 (1.1%)
Vision Disorders	
Eye pain	2 (1.1%)
Conjuctivitis	2 (1.1%)

* Expected pharmacologic consequences of testosterone suppression.

Changes in Laboratory Values During Treatment

The following abnormalities in laboratory values not present at baseline were observed in 10% or more of patients at the Day 253 visit: decreased hemoglobin and RBC count and increased glucose, BUN, SGOT, SGPT, and alkaline phosphatase. The relationship of these changes to drug treatment is difficult to assess in this population.

DOSAGE AND ADMINISTRATION

TRELSTAR DEPOT

Trelstar Depot Must Be Administered Under the Supervision of a Physician.

The recommended dose of Trelstar Depot is 3.75 mg incorporated in a depot formulation and is administered monthly as a single intramuscular injection. The lyophilized microgranules are to be reconstituted **in sterile water. No other diluent should be used.**

The suspension should be discarded if not used immediately after reconstitution.

As with other drugs administered by intramuscular injection, the injection site should be altered periodically.

Dosage Adjustments

Patients with renal or hepatic impairment showed 2- to 4-fold higher exposure than young healthy males. The clinical consequences of this increase, as well as the potential need for dose adjustment, is unknown.

TRELSTAR LA

Trelstar LA Must Be Administered Under the Supervision of a Physician.

The recommended dose of Trelstar LA is 11.25 mg incorporated in a long acting formulation administered every 84 days as a single intramuscular injection administered in either buttock. The lyophilized microgranules are to be reconstituted **in sterile water. No other diluent should be used.**

The suspension should be discarded if not used immediately after reconstitution.

As with other drugs administered by intramuscular injection, the injection site should be altered periodically.

HOW SUPPLIED

TRELSTAR DEPOT

Trelstar Depot is supplied in a single-dose vial with a flip-off seal containing sterile lyophilized triptorelin pamoate microgranules equivalent to 3.75 mg triptorelin peptide base, incorporated in a biodegradable copolymer of lactic and glycolic acids. A single dose vial of Trelstar Depot contains triptorelin pamoate (3.75 mg as peptide base units), poly-*d,l*-lactide-co-glycolide (170 mg), mannitol (85 mg), carboxymethylcellulose sodium (30 mg), and polysorbate 80 (2 mg).

Trelstar Depot is also supplied in the Trelstar Depot Debioclip single-dose delivery system consisting of a vial with a flip-off seal containing sterile lyophilized triptorelin pamoate microgranules equivalent to 3.75 mg of triptorelin peptide base, incorporated in a biodegradable copolymer of lactic and glycolic acids, and a pre-filled syringe containing 2 ml sterile water for injection.

When mixed with sterile water for injection, Trelstar Depot is administered every 28 days as a single intramuscular injection.

Storage: Store at 25°C (77°F); excursions permitted to 15-30°C (59-86°F).

TRELSTAR LA

Trelstar LA is supplied in a single-dose vial with a flip-off seal containing sterile lyophilized triptorelin pamoate microgranules equivalent to 11.25 mg triptorelin peptide base, incorporated in a biodegradable copolymer of lactic and glycolic acids.

A single dose vial of Trelstar LA contains triptorelin pamoate (11.25 mg as peptide base units), poly-*d,l*-lactide-co-glycolide (145 mg), mannitol (85 mg), carboxymethylcellulose sodium (30 mg), and polysorbate 80 (2 mg).

Trelstar LA is also supplied in the Trelstar LA Debioclip single-dose delivery system consisting of a vial with a flip-off seal containing sterile lyophilized triptorelin pamoate microgranules equivalent to 11.25 mg of triptorelin peptide base, incorporated in a biodegradable copolymer of lactic and glycolic acids, and a pre-filled syringe containing 2 ml sterile water for injection.

When mixed with sterile water for injection, Trelstar LA is administered every 84 days as a single intramuscular injection.

Storage: Store at 20-25°C (68-77°F); excursions permitted to 15-30°C (59-86°F). Do not freeze.

PRODUCT LISTING - EQUIVALENTS NOT AVAILABLE

Powder For Injection - Intramuscular - 3.75 mg

1's	$437.09	TRELSTAR DEPOT, Pharmacia Corporation	00009-5219-01
1's	$437.09	TRELSTAR DEPOT, Pharmacia Corporation	00009-7664-01

T

Trovafloxacin Mesylate (003379)

For complete prescribing information, refer to the CD-ROM included with the book.

For related information, see the comparative table section in Appendix A.

Categories: Abortion, septic; Bronchitis, chronic, acute exacerbation; Endomyometritis; Gonorrhea; Infection, gynecologic; Infection, intra-abdominal; Infection, lower respiratory tract; Infection, post-partum; Infection, skin and skin structures; Infection, upper respiratory tract; Infection, urinary tract; Infection, postoperative; Parametritis; Pelvic inflammatory disease; Pneumonia, community-acquired; Pneumonia, nosocomial; Prophylaxis, perioperative; Prostatitis; Sinusitis; Pregnancy Category C; FDA Approved 1997 Dec

Drug Classes: Antibiotics, quinolones

Brand Names: Trovan

WARNING

TROVAFLOXACIN MESYLATE HAS BEEN ASSOCIATED WITH SERIOUS LIVER INJURY LEADING TO LIVER TRANSPLANTATION AND/OR DEATH. TROVAFLOXACIN MESYLATE-ASSOCIATED LIVER INJURY HAS BEEN REPORTED WITH BOTH SHORT-TERM AND LONG-TERM DRUG EXPOSURE. TROVAFLOXACIN MESYLATE USE EXCEEDING 2 WEEKS IN DURATION IS ASSOCIATED WITH A SIGNIFICANTLY INCREASED RISK OF SERIOUS LIVER INJURY. LIVER INJURY HAS ALSO BEEN REPORTED FOLLOWING TROVAFLOXACIN MESYLATE RE-EXPOSURE. TROVAFLOXACIN MESYLATE SHOULD BE RESERVED FOR USE IN PATIENTS WITH SERIOUS, LIFE- OR LIMB-THREATENING INFECTIONS WHO RECEIVE THEIR INITIAL THERAPY IN AN IN-PATIENT HEALTH CARE FACILITY (*I.E.,* HOSPITAL OR LONG-TERM NURSING CARE FACILITY). TROVAFLOXACIN MESYLATE SHOULD NOT BE USED WHEN SAFER, ALTERNATIVE ANTIMICROBIAL THERAPY WILL BE EFFECTIVE. (SEE WARNINGS.)

DESCRIPTION

TROVAN TABLETS

Trovafloxacin mesylate is a synthetic broad-spectrum antibacterial agent for oral administration. Chemically, trovafloxacin mesylate, a fluoronaphthyridone related to the fluoroquinolone antibacterials, is (1α,5α,6α)-7-(6-amino-3-azabicyclo[3.1.0]hex-3-yl)-1-(2,4-difluorophenyl)-6-fluoro-1,4-dihydro-4-oxo-1,8-naphthyridine-3-carboxylic acid, monomethanesulfonate. Trovafloxacin mesylate differs from other quinolone derivatives by having a 1,8-naphthyridine nucleus.

Its empirical formula is $C_{20}H_{15}F_3N_4O_3 \cdot CH_3SO_3H$ and its molecular weight is 512.46.

Trovafloxacin mesylate is a white to off-white powder.

Trovan tablets are available in 100 and 200 mg (trovafloxacin equivalent) blue, film-coated tablets. Trovan tablets contain microcrystalline cellulose, cross-linked sodium carboxymethylcellulose and magnesium stearate. The tablet coating is a mixture of hydroxypropylcellulose, hydroxypropylmethylcellulose, titanium dioxide, polyethylene glycol, and FD&C blue no. 2 aluminum lake.

TROVAN IV

Trovan IV contains alatrofloxacin mesylate, the L-alanyl-L-alanyl prodrug of trovafloxacin mesylate. Chemically, alatrofloxacin mesylate is (1α,5α,6α)-L-alanyl-*N*-[3-[6-carboxy-8-(2,4-difluorophenyl)-3-fluoro-5,8-dihydro-5-oxo-1,8-naphthyridine-2-yl]-3-azabicyclo[3.1.0]hex-6-yl]-L-alaninamide, monomethanesulfonate. It is intended for administration by intravenous infusion.

Following intravenous administration, the alanine substituents in alatrofloxacin are rapidly hydrolyzed *in vivo* to yield trovafloxacin.

Its empirical formula is $C_{26}H_{25}F_3N_6O_5 \cdot CH_3SO_3H$ and its molecular weight is 654.62.

Alatrofloxacin mesylate is a white to light yellow powder.

Trovan IV is available in 40 and 60 ml single use vials as a sterile, preservative-free aqueous concentrate of 5 mg trovafloxacin/ml as alatrofloxacin mesylate intended for dilution prior to intravenous administration of doses of 200 or 300 mg of trovafloxacin, respectively.

The formulation contains water for injection, and may contain sodium hydroxide or hydrochloric acid for pH adjustment. The pH range for the 5 mg/ml aqueous concentrate is 3.5-4.3.

INDICATIONS AND USAGE

Trovafloxacin mesylate is indicated for the treatment of patients initiating therapy in in-patient health care facilities (*i.e.,* hospitals and long term nursing care facilities) with serious, life- or limb-threatening infections caused by susceptible strains of the designated microorganisms in the conditions listed below. (See DOSAGE AND ADMINISTRATION.)

Nosocomial pneumonia caused by *Escherichia coli, Pseudomonas aeruginosa, Haemophilus influenzae,* or *Staphylococcus aureus.* As with other antimicrobials, where *Pseudomonas aeruginosa* is a documented or presumptive pathogen, combination therapy with either an aminoglycoside or aztreonam may be clinically indicated.

Community acquired pneumonia caused by *Streptococcus pneumoniae, Haemophilus influenzae, Klebsiella pneumoniae, Staphylococcus aureus, Mycoplasma pneumoniae, Moraxella catarrhalis, Legionella pneumophila,* or *Chlamydia pneumoniae.*

Complicated intra-abdominal infections, including post-surgical infections caused by *Escherichia coli, Bacteroides fragilis,* viridans group streptococci, *Pseudomonas aeruginosa, Klebsiella pneumoniae, Peptostreptococcus species,* or *Prevotella* species.

Gynecologic and pelvic infections including endomyometritis, parametritis, septic abortion and post-partum infections caused by *Escherichia coli, Bacteroides fragilis,* viridans group streptococci, *Enterococcus faecalis, Streptococcus agalactiae, Peptostreptococcus* species, *Prevotella* species, or *Gardnerella vaginalis.*

Complicated skin and skin structure infections, including diabetic foot infections, caused by *Staphylococcus aureus, Streptococcus agalactiae, Pseudomonas aeruginosa, Enterococcus faecalis, Escherichia coli,* or *Proteus mirabilis. Note:* Trovafloxacin mesylate has not been studied in the treatment of osteomyelitis. (See WARNINGS.)

CONTRAINDICATIONS

Trovafloxacin mesylate is contraindicated in persons with a history of hypersensitivity to trovafloxacin, alatrofloxacin, quinolone antimicrobial agents or any other components of these products.

WARNINGS

(SEE BOXED WARNING.) TROVAFLOXACIN MESYLATE-ASSOCIATED LIVER ENZYME ABNORMALITIES, SYMPTOMATIC HEPATITIS, JAUNDICE, AND LIVER FAILURE (INCLUDING RARE REPORTS OF ACUTE HEPATIC NECROSIS WITH EOSINOPHILIC INFILTRATION, LIVER TRANSPLANTATION AND/OR DEATH) HAVE BEEN REPORTED WITH BOTH SHORT-TERM AND LONG-TERM DRUG EXPOSURE IN MEN AND WOMEN. TROVAFLOXACIN MESYLATE USE EXCEEDING 2 WEEKS IN DURATION IS ASSOCIATED WITH A SIGNIFICANTLY INCREASED RISK OF SERIOUS LIVER INJURY. LIVER INJURY HAS ALSO BEEN REPORTED FOLLOWING TROVAFLOXACIN MESYLATE RE-EXPOSURE. CLINICIANS SHOULD MONITOR LIVER FUNCTION TESTS (*E.G.,* AST, ALT, BILIRUBIN) IN TROVAFLOXACIN MESYLATE RECIPIENTS WHO DEVELOP SIGNS OR SYMPTOMS CONSISTENT WITH HEPATITIS. CLINICIANS SHOULD CONSIDER DISCONTINUING TROVAFLOXACIN MESYLATE IN THOSE PATIENTS WHO DEVELOP LIVER FUNCTION TEST ABNORMALITIES.

THE SAFETY AND EFFECTIVENESS OF TROVAFLOXACIN IN PEDIATRIC POPULATIONS LESS THAN 18 YEARS OF AGE, PREGNANT WOMEN, AND NURSING WOMEN HAVE NOT BEEN ESTABLISHED.

As with other members of the quinolone class, trovafloxacin has caused arthropathy and/or chondrodysplasia in immature rats and dogs. The significance of these findings to humans is unknown.

Convulsions, increased intracranial pressure, and psychosis have been reported in patients receiving quinolones. Quinolones may also cause central nervous system stimulation which may lead to tremors, restlessness, lightheadedness, confusion, hallucinations, paranoia, depression, nightmares, and insomnia. These reactions may occur following the first dose. If these reactions occur in patients receiving trovafloxacin or alatrofloxacin, the drug should be discontinued and appropriate measures instituted.

As with other quinolones, trovafloxacin mesylate should be used with caution in patients with known or suspected CNS disorders, such as severe cerebral atherosclerosis, epilepsy, and other factors that predispose to seizures.

Serious and occasionally fatal hypersensitivity and/or anaphylactic reactions have been reported in patients receiving therapy with quinolones. These reactions may occur following the first dose. Some reactions have been accompanied by cardiovascular collapse, hypotension/shock, seizure, loss of consciousness, tingling, angioedema (including tongue, laryngeal, throat or facial edema/swelling), airway obstruction (including bronchospasm, shortness of breath, and acute respiratory distress), dyspnea, urticaria, itching, and other serious skin reactions.

Trovafloxacin mesylate should be discontinued at the first appearance of a skin rash or any other sign of hypersensitivity. Serious acute hypersensitivity reactions may require treatment with epinephrine and other resuscitative measures, including oxygen, intravenous fluids, antihistamines, corticosteroids, pressor amines and airway management, as clinically indicated.

Serious and sometimes fatal events, some due to hypersensitivity and some due to uncertain etiology, have been reported in patients receiving therapy with all antibiotics. These events may be severe and generally occur following the administration of multiple doses. Clinical manifestations may include 1 or more of the following: fever, rash or severe dermatologic reactions (*e.g.,* toxic epidermal necrolysis, Stevens-Johnson Syndrome); vasculitis, arthralgia, myalgia, serum sickness; allergic pneumonitis, interstitial nephritis; acute renal insufficiency or failure; hepatitis, jaundice, acute hepatic necrosis or failure; anemia, including hemolytic and aplastic; thrombocytopenia, including thrombotic thrombocytopenic purpura; leukopenia; agranulocytosis; pancytopenia; and/or other hematologic abnormalities.

Pseudomembranous colitis has been reported with nearly all antibacterial agents, including trovafloxacin mesylate, and may range in severity from mild to life-threatening. Therefore, it is important to consider this diagnosis in patients who present with diarrhea subsequent to the administration of any antibacterial agent.

Treatment with antibacterial agents alters the flora of the colon and may permit overgrowth of clostridia. Studies indicate that a toxin produced by *Clostridium difficile* is the primary cause of "antibiotic-associated colitis."

After the diagnosis of pseudomembranous colitis has been established, therapeutic measures should be initiated. Mild cases of pseudomembranous colitis usually respond to drug discontinuation alone. In moderate to severe cases, consideration should be given to management with fluids and electrolytes, protein supplementation, and treatment with an antibacterial drug clinically effective against *C. difficile* colitis.

Although not seen in trovafloxacin mesylate clinical trials, ruptures of the shoulder, hand, and Achilles tendons that required surgical repair or resulted in prolonged disability have been reported in patients receiving quinolones. Trovafloxacin mesylate should be discontinued if the patient experiences pain, inflammation or rupture of a tendon. Patients should rest and refrain from exercise until the diagnosis of tendinitis or tendon rupture has been confidently excluded. Tendon rupture can occur during or after therapy with quinolones.

Trovafloxacin has not been shown to be effective in the treatment of syphilis. Antimicrobial agents used in high doses for short periods of time to treat gonorrhea may mask or delay the symptoms of incubating syphilis. All patients with gonorrhea should have a serologic test for syphilis at the time of diagnosis.

DOSAGE AND ADMINISTRATION

The recommended dosage for trovafloxacin mesylate for the treatment of serious, life- or limb-threatening infections is described in TABLE 17. Doses of trovafloxacin mesylate are administered once every 24 hours. Trovafloxacin mesylate should not usually be administered for more than 2 weeks. It should only be administered for longer than 2 weeks if the treating physician believes the benefits to the individual patients clearly outweigh the risks of such longer-term treatment. (See BOXED WARNING.)

Oral doses should be administered at least 2 hours before or 2 hours after antacids containing magnesium or aluminum, as well as sucralfate, citric acid buffered with sodium citrate (*e.g.,* Bicitra) and metal cations (*e.g.,* ferrous sulfate) and didanosine (Videx), chewable/buffered tablets or the pediatric powder for oral solution.

Intravenous morphine should be administered at least 2 hours after oral trovafloxacin mesylate dosing in the fasted state and at least 4 hours after oral trovafloxacin mesylate is taken with food.

Patients whose therapy is started with alatrofloxacin mesylate IV may be switch to trovafloxin mesylate tablets to complete the course of therapy, if deemed appropriate by the treating physician. In certain patients with serious and life- or limb-threatening infections as described in INDICATIONS AND USAGE, trovafloxin mesylate tablets may be considered appropriate initial therapy, when the treating physician believes that the benefit of the product for the patient outweighs the potential risk.

Alatrofloxacin mesylate IV should only be administered by INTRAVENOUS infusion. It is not for intramuscular, intrathecal, intraperitoneal, or subcutaneous administration.

Single-use vials require dilution prior to administration. (See Preparation of Alatrofloxacin Mesylate Injection For Administration.)

TABLE 17 *Dosage Guidelines*

Infection*/Location and Type	Daily Unit Dose and Route of Administration	Total Duration‡
Nosocomial Pneumonia§	300 mg IV† followed by 200 mg oral	10-14 days
Community Acquired Pneumonia	200 mg oral or 200 mg IV followed by 200 mg oral	7-14 days
Complicated Intra-Abdominal Infections, including post-surgical infections	300 mg IV† followed by 200 mg oral	7-14 days
Gynecologic and Pelvic Infections	300 mg IV† followed by 200 mg oral	7-14 days
Skin and Skin Structure Infections, Complicated, including diabetic foot infections	200 mg oral or 200 mg IV followed by 200 mg oral	10-14 days

* Due to the designated pathogens. (See INDICATIONS AND USAGE.)
† Where the 300 mg alatrofloxacin mesylate IV dose is indicated, therapy should be decreased to the 200 mg dose as soon as clinically indicated.
‡ See WARNINGS
§ As with other antimicrobials, where *Pseudomonas aeruginosa* is a documented or presumptive pathogen, combination therapy with either an aminoglycoside or aztreonam may be clinically indicated.

IMPAIRED RENAL FUNCTION

No adjustment in the dosage of trovafloxacin mesylate is necessary in patients with impaired renal function. Trovafloxacin is eliminated primarily by biliary excretion. Trovafloxacin is not efficiently removed from the body by hemodialysis.

CHRONIC HEPATIC DISEASE (CIRRHOSIS)

TABLE 18 provides dosing guidelines for patients with mild or moderate cirrhosis (Child-Pugh Class A and B) There are no data in patients with severe cirrhosis (Child-Pugh Class C).

TABLE 18

Indicated Dose (Normal Hepatic Function)	Chronic Hepatic Disease Dose
300 mg IV	200 mg IV
200 mg IV or oral	100 mg IV or oral

INTRAVENOUS ADMINISTRATION

AFTER DILUTION WITH AN APPROPRIATE DILUENT, ALATROFLOXACIN MESYLATE IV SHOULD BE ADMINISTERED BY INTRAVENOUS INFUSION OVER A PERIOD OF 60 MINUTES. *CAUTION:* RAPID OR BOLUS INTRAVENOUS INFUSION SHOULD BE AVOIDED.

Trovan IV is supplied in single-use vials containing a concentrated solution of alatrofloxacin mesylate in water for injection (equivalent of 200 mg or 300 mg as trovafloxacin). Each ml contains alatrofloxacin mesylate equivalent to 5 mg trovafloxacin. THESE ALATROFLOXACIN MESYLATE IV SINGLE-USE VIALS MUST BE FURTHER DILUTED WITH AN APPROPRIATE SOLUTION PRIOR TO INTRAVENOUS ADMINISTRATION. This parenteral drug product should be inspected visually for discoloration and particulate matter prior to dilution and administration. Since no preservative or bacteriostatic agent is present in this product, aseptic technique must be used in preparation of the final parenteral solution.

Preparation of Alatrofloxacin Mesylate Injection For Administration

The intravenous dose should be prepared by aseptically withdrawing the appropriate volume of concentrate from the vials of alatrofloxacin mesylate IV. This should be diluted with a suitable intravenous solution to a final concentration of 1-2 mg/ml. (See Compatible Intravenous Solutions.) The resulting solution should be infused over a period of 60 minutes by direct infusion or through a Y-type intravenous infusion set which may already be in place.

Since the vials are for single use only, any unused portion should be discarded.

Since only limited data are available on the compatibility of alatrofloxacin intravenous injection with other intravenous substances, additives or other medications should not be added to alatrofloxacin mesylate IV in single-use vials or infused simultaneously through the same intravenous line.

If the same intravenous line is used for sequential infusion of several different drugs, the line should be flushed before and after infusion of alatrofloxacin mesylate IV with an infusion solution compatible with alatrofloxacin mesylate IV and with any other drug(s) administered via this common line.

If alatrofloxacin mesylate IV is to be given concomitantly with another drug, each drug should be given separately in accordance with the recommended dosage and route of administration for each drug.

The desired dosage of alatrofloxacin mesylate IV may be prepared according to TABLE 19.

TABLE 19

Dosage Strength*	Volume to Withdraw (ml)	Diluent Volume (ml)	Total Volume (ml)	Infusion Conc. (mg/ml)
100 mg	20	30	50	2
100 mg	20	80	100	1
200 mg	40	60	100	2
200 mg	40	160	200	1
300 mg	60	90	150	2
300 mg	60	240	300	1

* Trovafloxacin equivalent.

For example, to prepare a 200 mg dose at an infusion concentration of 2 mg/ml (as trovafloxacin), 40 ml of alatrofloxacin mesylate IV is withdrawn from a vial and diluted with 60 ml of a compatible intravenous fluid to produce a total infusion solution volume of 100 ml.

Compatible intravenous solutions:

5% dextrose injection
0.45% sodium chloride injection
5% dextrose and 0.45% sodium chloride injection
5% dextrose and 0.2% sodium chloride injection
Lactated Ringer's and 5% dextrose injection.

Alatrofloxacin mesylate IV should not be diluted with 0.9% sodium chloride injection (normal saline), alone or in combination with other diluents. A precipitate may form under these conditions. In addition, alatrofloxacin mesylate IV should not be diluted with lactated Ringer's.

Normal saline, 0.9% sodium chloride injection, can be used for flushing IV lines prior to or after administration of alatrofloxacin mesylate IV.

Stability of alatrofloxacin mesylate IV as supplied: When stored under recommended conditions, alatrofloxacin mesylate IV, as supplied in 40 ml or 60 ml vials, is stable through the expiration date printed on the label.

Stability of alatrofloxacin mesylate IV following dilution: Alatrofloxacin mesylate IV, when diluted with the compatible intravenous solutions to concentrations of 0.5-2.0 mg/ml (as trovafloxacin), is physically and chemically stable for up to 7 days when refrigerated or up to 3 days at room temperature stored in glass bottles or plastic (PVC type) intravenous containers.

PRODUCT LISTING - EQUIVALENTS NOT AVAILABLE

Solution - Intravenous - 5 mg/ml

40 ml	$40.08	TROVAN, Pfizer U.S. Pharmaceuticals	00049-3890-28
60 ml	$60.45	TROVAN, Pfizer U.S. Pharmaceuticals	00049-3900-28

Tablet - Oral - 100 mg

30's	$193.60	TROVAN, Pfizer U.S. Pharmaceuticals	00049-3780-30

Tablet - Oral - 200 mg

30's	$234.35	TROVAN, Pfizer U.S. Pharmaceuticals	00049-3790-30

Unoprostone Isopropyl (003502)

Categories: Glaucoma, open-angle; Glaucoma, secondary; FDA Approved 2000 Aug; Pregnancy Category C
Drug Classes: Ophthalmics; Prostaglandins
Brand Names: Rescula
Cost of Therapy: $51.50 (Glaucoma; Rescula Ophth. Solution; 0.15%; 5 ml; 2 drops/day; variable day supply)

DESCRIPTION

Unoprostone isopropyl is a docosanoid, a structural analogue of an inactive biosynthetic cyclic derivative of arachidonic acid, 13, 14-dihydro-15-keto-prostaglandin $F_{2\alpha}$. Its chemical name is isopropyl (+)-(*Z*)-7-[(1*R*,2*R*,3*R*,5*S*)-3,5-dihydroxy-2-(3-oxodecyl) cyclopentyl]-5-heptenoate. Its molecular formula is $C_{25}H_{44}O_5$.

Unoprostone isopropyl is a clear, colorless viscous liquid that is very soluble in acetonitrile, ethanol, ethyl acetate, isopropanol, dioxane, ether, and hexane. It is practically insoluble in water. Rescula (unoprostone isopropyl ophthalmic solution) 0.15% is supplied as a sterile, isotonic, buffered aqueous solution of unoprostone isopropyl with a pH of 5.0-6.5 and an osmolality of 235-300 mOsmol/kg.

Each ml of Rescula contains 1.5 mg of unoprostone isopropyl. Benzalkonium chloride 0.015% is added as a preservative. Inactive ingredients are: mannitol, polysorbate 80, edetate disodium, sodium hydroxide or hydrochloric acid (to adjust pH), and water for injection.

CLINICAL PHARMACOLOGY

MECHANISM OF ACTION

When instilled in the eye, unoprostone isopropyl ophthalmic solution is believed to reduce elevated intraocular pressure (IOP), by increasing the outflow of aqueous humor, but the exact mechanism is unknown at this time.

PHARMACOKINETICS AND PHARMACODYNAMICS

Absorption

After application to the eye, unoprostone isopropyl is absorbed through the cornea and conjuctival epithelium where it is hydrolyzed by esterases to unoprostone free acid.

A study conducted with 18 healthy volunteers dosed bilaterally with unoprostone isopropyl ophthalmic solution twice daily for 14 days demonstrated little systemic absorption of unoprostone isopropyl. The systemic exposure of its metabolite unoprostone free acid was minimal following the ocular administration. Mean peak unoprostone free acid concentration was less than 1.5 ng/ml. Little or no accumulation of unoprostone free acid was observed.

Elimination

Elimination of unoprostone free acid from human plasma is rapid, with a half-life of 14 minutes. Plasma levels of unoprostone free acid dropped below the lower limit of quantitation (<0.25 ng/ml) 1 hour following ocular instillation. The metabolites are excreted predominately in urine.

INDICATIONS AND USAGE

Unoprostone isopropyl ophthalmic solution 0.15% is indicated for the lowering of intraocular pressure in patients with open-angle glaucoma or ocular hypertension who are intolerant of other intraocular pressure lowering medications or insufficiently responsive (failed to achieve target IOP determined after multiple measurements over time) to another intraocular pressure lowering medication.

CONTRAINDICATIONS

Known hypersensitivity to unoprostone isopropyl, benzalkonium chloride or any other ingredients in this product.

WARNINGS

Unoprostone isopropyl ophthalmic solution has been reported to cause changes to pigmented tissue. These changes may be permanent.

Unoprostone isopropyl ophthalmic solution may gradually change eye color, increasing the amount of brown pigment in the iris. The long-term effects and the consequences of potential injury to the eye are currently unknown. The change in iris color occurs slowly and may not be noticeable for months to several years. Patients should be informed of the possibility of iris color change.

PRECAUTIONS

GENERAL

There have been reports of bacterial keratitis associated with the use of multiple-dose containers of topical ophthalmic products. These containers had been inadvertently contaminated by patients who, in most cases, had a concurrent corneal disease or a disruption of the ocular epithelial surface (see Information for the Patient).

Unoprostone isopropyl ophthalmic solution should be used with caution in patients with active intraocular inflammation (*e.g.*, uveitis).

Unoprostone isopropyl ophthalmic solution has not been evaluated for the treatment of angle closure, inflammatory or neovascular glaucoma.

Unoprostone isopropyl ophthalmic solution has not been studied in patients with renal or hepatic impairment and should be used with caution in such patients.

Unoprostone isopropyl ophthalmic solution should not be administered while wearing contact lenses.

Patients should also be advised that unoprostone isopropyl ophthalmic solution contains benzalkonium chloride which may be adsorbed by contact lenses. Contact lenses should be removed prior to administration of the solution. Lenses may be reinserted 15 minutes following administration of unoprostone isopropyl ophthalmic solution.

INFORMATION FOR THE PATIENT

Patients should be instructed to avoid allowing the tip of the dispensing container to contact the eye or surrounding structures because this could cause the tip to become contaminated by common bacteria known to cause ocular infections. Serious damage to the eye and subsequent loss of vision may result from using contaminated solutions.

Patients should also be advised that if they develop an intercurrent ocular condition (*e.g.*, trauma or infection) or have ocular surgery, they should immediately seek their physician's advice concerning the continued use of the multidose container.

Patients should be advised that if they develop any ocular reactions, particularly conjunctivitis and eyelid reactions, they should immediately seek their physician's advice.

If more than one topical ophthalmic drug is being used the drugs should be administered at least 5 minutes apart.

CARCINOGENESIS, MUTAGENESIS, AND IMPAIRMENT OF FERTILITY

Unoprostone isopropyl ophthalmic solution was not carcinogenic in rats administered oral doses up to 12 mg/kg/day for up to 2 years (approximately 580- and 240-fold the recommended human dose of 0.005 mg/kg/day based on AUC(0-24 h) in male and female rats, respectively).

Under the conditions tested, unoprostone isopropyl and unoprostone free acid were neither mutagenic in an Ames assay nor clastogenic in a chromosome aberration assay in Chinese hamster lung-derived fibroblast cells. Under the conditions tested, unoprostone isopropyl was not genotoxic in a mouse lymphoma mutation assay or clastogenic in an *in vivo* chromosomal aberration test in mouse bone marrow.

Unoprostone isopropyl did not impair male or female fertility in rats at subcutaneous doses up to 50 mg/kg (approximately 10,000-fold the recommended human dose of 0.005 mg/kg/day).

PREGNANCY, TERATOGENIC EFFECTS, PREGNANCY CATEGORY C

There were no teratogenic effects observed in rats and rabbits up to 5 and 0.3 mg/kg/day (approximately 1000- and 60-fold the recommended human dose of 0.005 mg/kg/day in the rat and rabbit, respectively). There was an increase in the incidence of miscarriages and a decrease in live birth index in rats administered unoprostone isopropyl during organogenesis at subcutaneous doses of 5 mg/kg. There was an increase in incidence of miscarriages and resorptions and a decrease in the number of live fetuses in rabbits administered unoprostone isopropyl during organogenesis at subcutaneous doses of 0.3 mg/kg. The no observable adverse effect level (NOAEL) for embryofetal toxicity in rats and rabbits was 2.0 and 0.1 mg/kg (approximately 400- and 20-fold the recommended human dose of 0.005 mg/kg/day in the rat and rabbit, respectively).

There was an increase in incidence of premature delivery, a decrease in live birth index, and a decrease in weight at birth and through postpartum Day 7 in rats administered unoprostone isopropyl during late gestation through postpartum Day 21 at subcutaneous doses of 1.25 mg/kg. In addition, pups from rats administered 1.25 mg/kg subcutaneously exhibited delayed growth and development characterized by delayed incisor eruption and eye opening. There was an increase in the number of stillborn pups and a decrease in perinatal survival in rats administered unoprostone isopropyl during late gestation through weaning at subcutaneous doses of ≥0.5 mg/kg. The NOAEL for pre and postnatal toxicity in rats was 0.2 mg/kg (approximately 40-fold the recommended human dose of 0.005 mg/kg/day).

There are no adequate and well-controlled studies in pregnant women. Because animal studies are not always predictive of human response, unoprostone isopropyl ophthalmic solution should be used during pregnancy only if the potential benefit justifies the potential risk to the fetus.

NURSING MOTHERS

Unoprostone isopropyl has been identified in breast milk in rats following intravenous administration. It is not known whether topical ocular administration could result in sufficient systemic absorption to produce detectable quantities in breast milk. Nevertheless, caution should be exercised when unoprostone isopropyl ophthalmic solution is administered to a nursing mother.

PEDIATRIC USE

Pediatric Use: Safety and effectiveness in pediatric patients have not been established.

GERIATRIC USE

No overall differences in safety or effectiveness have been observed between elderly and other adult patients.

ADVERSE REACTIONS

In clinical studies, the most common ocular adverse events were burning/stinging, burning/stinging upon drug instillation, dry eyes, itching, increased length of eyelashes and injection. These were reported in approximately 10-25% of patients. Approximately 10-14% of patients were observed to have an increase in the length of eyelashes (≥1 mm) at 12 months, while 7% of patients were observed to have a decrease in the length of eyelashes.

Ocular adverse events occurring in approximately 5-10% of patients were abnormal vision, eyelid disorder, foreign body sensation, and lacrimation disorder.

Ocular adverse events occurring in approximately 1-5% of patients were blepharitis, cataract, conjunctivitis, corneal lesion, discharge from the eye, eye hemorrhage, eye pain, keratitis, irritation, photophobia, and vitreous disorder.

Other ocular adverse events reported in less than 1% of patients were acute elevated intraocular pressure, color blindness, corneal deposits, corneal edema, corneal opacity, diplopia, hyperpigmentation of the eyelid, increased number of eyelashes, iris hyperpigmentation, iritis, optic atrophy, ptosis, retinal hemorrhage, and visual field defect.

The most frequently reported nonocular adverse event associated with the use of unoprostone isopropyl ophthalmic solution in the clinical trials was flu syndrome that was observed in approximately 6% of patients. Nonocular adverse events reported in the 1-5% of patients were accidental injury, allergic reaction, back pain, bronchitis, cough increased, diabetes mellitus, dizziness, headache, hypertension, insomnia, pharyngitis, pain, rhinitis, and sinusitis.

DOSAGE AND ADMINISTRATION

The recommended dosage is 1 drop in the affected eye(s) twice daily. Unoprostone isopropyl ophthalmic solution may be used concomitantly with other topical ophthalmic drug products to lower intraocular pressure. If 2 drugs are used, they should be administered at least 5 minutes apart.

ANIMAL PHARMACOLOGY

In cynomolgus monkeys administered unoprostone isopropyl ophthalmic solution for twelve months at 150 μg/eye/day (equal to the human dose), 1 of 10 animals exhibited increased pigmentation of the iris. The incidence did not change when the administered dose was increased to 300 μg/eye/day (twice the human dose) for an additional 6 months.

HOW SUPPLIED

Rescula (unoprostone isopropyl ophthalmic solution) 0.15% is a clear, isotonic, buffered, preserved colorless solution of unoprostone isopropyl 0.15% (1.5 mg/ml). Rescula 0.15% is supplied as 5 ml solution in a 7.5 ml natural polypropylene bottle with a natural polypropylene dropper tip, a turquoise polypropylene closure and a clear tamper-evident shrink-band.

Storage: Store between 2-25°C (36-77°F).

PRODUCT LISTING - EQUIVALENTS NOT AVAILABLE

Solution - Ophthalmic - 0.15%

5 ml $51.50 RESCULA, Ciba Vision Ophthalmics 58768-0961-05

Uracil Mustard (002410)

Categories: Leukemia, chronic lymphocytic; Leukemia, chronic myelogenous; Lymphoma, non-Hodgkin's; Mycosis fungoides; Polycythemia vera; FDA Approval Pre 1982

Drug Classes: Antineoplastics, alkylating agents

Cost of Therapy: $51.83 (CLL; Generic Tablets; 1 mg; 10 tablets/week; 28 day supply)

DESCRIPTION

Uracil Mustard Capsules, USP contain uracil mustard. Uracil mustard, 5-(bis (2-chloroethyl) amino) uracil.

Uracil mustard is an off-white, odorless crystalline compound which is slightly soluble in methanol and in acetone. It is unstable in the presence of water and reacts with many organic substances, including the carbonyl and amino groups of proteins including, in all probability, the nucleoproteins of the cell nucleus.

Uracil Mustard Capsules, USP, for oral administration contain 1 mg of uracil mustard. Uracil Mustard Capsules also contain the following inactive ingredients: erythrosine sodium, FD&C Blue No. 1, FD&C Yellow No. 5, FD&C Yellow No. 6, gelatin, lactose, mineral oil, talc, and titanium dioxide.

CLINICAL PHARMACOLOGY

Uracil mustard is an orally active alkylating agent belonging to the class of substances known as nitrogen mustards. Clinically uracil mustard, like other nitrogen mustards, has been found to be of value in the palliative treatment of certain neoplasms affecting the reticuloendothelial system.

INDICATIONS AND USAGE

Chronic lymphocytic leukemia: Uracil mustard is usually effective in the palliative treatment of symptomatic chronic lymphocytic leukemia.

Non-Hodgkin's lymphomas: Uracil mustard is effective for palliative treatment of lymphomas of the histiocytic or lymphocytic type.

Chronic myelogenous leukemia: Uracil mustard may be effective in the palliative treatment of patients with chronic myelogenous leukemia. It is not effective in the acute blastic crisis or in patients with acute leukemia.

Other conditions: Uracil mustard may be effective in the palliative treatment of early stages of polycythemia vera before the development of leukemia or myelofibrosis. It may also be beneficial as palliative therapy in mycosis fungoides.

CONTRAINDICATIONS

Uracil mustard should not be given to any patient with severe leukopenia or thrombocytopenia.

WARNINGS

USE IN PREGNANCY

Drugs of the nitrogen mustard group have been shown to produce fetal abnormalities in experimental animals when given during pregnancy. Uracil mustard should not be used during pregnancy unless in the opinion of the physician the potential benefits outweigh the possible hazards.

Alkylating agents are carcinogenic in animals and suspect as carcinogens in humans. Their possible effect on fertility should be considered; amenorrhea and impaired spermatogenesis have been reported following therapy with alkylating compounds.

Uracil mustard has a cumulative toxic effect against the hematopoietic system. Blood counts including platelet counts should be done once or twice weekly.

PRECAUTIONS

Patients receiving uracil mustard must be followed carefully to avoid the possibility of irreversible damage to the bone marrow. Therapy with this agent should be discontinued if severe depression of the bone marrow occurs, as indicated by sharp diminution in any of the formed blood elements.

While therapy with uracil mustard need not be discontinued following initial depression of blood counts, it should be realized that maximum depression of bone marrow function may not occur until 2 to 4 weeks after discontinuance of the drug, and that as the total accumulated doses approach 1 mg/kg there is real danger of producing irreversible damage to the bone marrow.

While there is no specific therapy for severe depression of the bone marrow, frequent blood and blood component transfusions, with antibiotics to combat secondary infection, may sustain the patient until recovery has occurred.

This preparation contains FD&C Yellow No. 5 (tartrazine) which may cause allergic-type reactions (including bronchial asthma) in certain susceptible individuals. Although the overall incidence of FD&C Yellow No. 5 (tartrazine) sensitivity in the general population is low, it is frequently seen in patients who also have aspirin hypersensitivity.

ADVERSE REACTIONS

In addition to its toxic effects on the hematopoietic system (see PRECAUTIONS and CONTRAINDICATIONS) evidence of toxicity may be manifested by nausea, vomiting or diarrhea of varying degrees of severity. These are related to the size of the dose, i.e. the greater the dose, the more severe the symptoms. Other side reactions, some of which may not be related to administration of the drug, include nervousness, irritability or depression and various skin reactions such as pruritus, dermatitis and some loss of hair. Frank alopecia has not been reported to date.

DOSAGE AND ADMINISTRATION

Uracil mustard should not be administered until about 2 or 3 weeks after the maximum effect of any previous X-ray or cytotoxic drug therapy upon the bone marrow has been obtained. An increasing white blood cell count is probably the best criterion for determining that such maximum effect has subsided. Some investigators prefer to wait until the blood count has returned to normal before beginning a new course of therapy. In the presence of pronounced leukopenia, thrombocytopenia, or aplastic anemia, uracil mustard should not be administered. In the presence of bone marrow infiltrated with malignant cells, hematopoietic toxicity may be increased and judicious care must be used during administration.

The following are suggested dosage schedules:

Adults: A single weekly dose of 0.15 mg/kg of body weight should be given for 4 weeks to provide an adequate trial.

Children: A single weekly dose of 0.30 mg/kg of body weight should be given for 4 weeks to provide an adequate trial.

If response occurs, the same dose may be continued weekly until relapse. These dosages must be carefully individualized and the dose reduced or discontinued in accordance with the severity of depression of bone marrow function.

Procedures for proper handling and disposal of anticancer drugs should be considered. Several guidelines on this subject have been published.[1-6] There is no general agreement that all of the procedures recommended in the guidelines are necessary or appropriate.

ANIMAL PHARMACOLOGY

Pharmacologic studies have shown that uracil mustard is readily absorbed following oral administration, the orally effective dose in certain rat tumors being almost the same as the parenteral dose. In rats the LD_{50}'s are 7.5 mg/kg orally, 6.2 mg/kg subcutaneously and 3.7 mg/kg intraperitoneally. Thus, the oral and subcutaneous toxicities appear to be about one-half the intraperitoneal toxicity.

Subacute and chronic oral toxicity studies in animals indicate that uracil mustard produces toxic effects characteristic of nitrogen mustards. These effects include depression of the hematopoietic system as indicated initially by severe thrombocytopenia, granulocytic and lymphocytic leukopenia and later by depression of the erythrocyte count and hemoglobin values. Other evidence of toxicity in laboratory animals included anorexia, weight loss, bleeding from the gastrointestinal tract, muscular weakness and moribund states.

Experimental studies have shown that uracil mustard is a highly potent inducer of malignant lung tumors in A-strain mice.

PRODUCT LISTING - EQUIVALENTS NOT AVAILABLE

Capsule - Oral - 1 mg

50's $64.79 GENERIC, Roberts Pharmaceutical Corporation 54092-0039-50

Urokinase (002417)

Categories: Embolism, pulmonary; Infarction, myocardial; Occlusion, intravenous catheter; Thrombosis, coronary artery; Pregnancy Category B; FDA Pre 1938 Drugs

Drug Classes: Thrombolytics

Brand Names: Abbokinase

Foreign Brand Availability: Actosolv (Austria; Germany; Italy); Alphakinase (Germany); Medacinase (Netherlands); Persolv (Italy); Ukidan (Austria; Bahrain; Bangladesh; Cyprus; Czech-Republic; Egypt; England; Germany; Greece; Hong-Kong; Hungary; India; Indonesia; Iran; Iraq; Italy; Jordan; Kuwait; Lebanon; Libya; Malaysia; Oman; Pakistan; Peru; Portugal; Qatar; Republic-of-Yemen; Saudi-Arabia; Sweden; Switzerland; Syria; United-Arab-Emirates); Urokine (Korea)

HCFA JCODE(S): J3364 5,000 IU vial IV; J3365 250,000 IU vial IV

DESCRIPTION

INJECTION AND OPEN-CATH

Urokinase is an enzyme (protein) produced by the kidney, and found in the urine. There are two forms of urokinase differing in molecular weight but having similar clinical effects. Abbokinase (urokinase for injection) is a thrombolytic agent obtained from human kidney cells by tissue culture techniques and is primarily the low molecular weight form. It is supplied as a sterile lyophilized white powder containing mannitol (25 mg/vial), Albumin (Human) (250 mg/vial), and sodium chloride (50 mg/vial).

INJECTION

Urokinase should be used in hospitals where the recommended diagnostic and monitoring techniques are available. Thrombolytic therapy should be considered in all situations where the benefits to be achieved outweigh the risk of potentially serious hemorrhage. When internal bleeding does occur, it may be more difficult to manage than that which occurs with conventional anticoagulant therapy.

Urokinase treatment should be instituted as soon as possible after onset of pulmonary embolism, preferably no later than seven days after onset. Any delay in instituting lytic therapy to evaluate the effect of heparin decreases the potential for optimal efficacy.[1]

When urokinase is used for treatment of coronary artery thrombosis associated with evolving transmural myocardial infarction, therapy should be instituted within 6 hours of symptom onset.

Thin translucent filaments may occasionally occur in reconstituted urokinase vials, but do not indicate any decrease in potency of this product. No clinical problems have been associated with these filaments. See DOSAGE AND ADMINISTRATION .

Following reconstitution with 5 ml of sterile water for injection, it is a clear, slightly straw-colored solution; each ml contains 50,000 IU of urokinase activity, 0.5% mannitol, 5% Albumin (Human), and 1% sodium chloride. The pH is adjusted with sodium hydroxide and/or hydrochloric acid prior to lyophilization.

Urokinase is for intravenous and intracoronary infusion only.

U

IV CATHETER CLEARANCE

Each ml of reconstituted Abbokinase Open-Cath solution contains 5000 IU of urokinase activity, 5 mg gelatin, 15 mg mannitol, 1.7 mg sodium chloride and 4.6 mg monobasic sodium phosphate anhydrous. The pH is adjusted with sodium hydroxide and/or hydrochloric acid prior to lyophilization.

Storage: Store powder below 25°C (77°F). Avoid freezing. *For Injection:* Store powder at 2-8°C.

CLINICAL PHARMACOLOGY

Urokinase acts on the endogenous fibrinolytic system. It is converts plasminogen to the enzyme plasmin. Plasmin degrades fibrin clots as well as fibrinogen and other plasma proteins.

Intravenous infusion of urokinase in doses recommended for lysis of pulmonary embolism is followed by increased fibrinolytic activity. This effect disappears within a few hours after discontinuation, but a decrease in plasma levels of fibrinogen and plasminogen and an increase in the amount of circulating fibrin (ogen) degradation products may persist for 12-24 hours.[2,3] There is a lack of correlation between embolus resolution and changes in coagulation and fibrinolytic assay results.

Information is incomplete about the pharmacokinetic properties in man. Urokinase administered by intravenous infusion is cleared rapidly by the liver. The serum half-life in man is 20 minutes or less. Patients with impaired liver function (*e.g.,* cirrhosis) would be expected to show a prolongation in half-life. Small fractions of an administered dose are excreted in bile and urine.

IV Catheter Clearance: When used as directed for IV catheter clearance, only small amounts of urokinase may reach the circulation; therefore, therapeutic serum levels are not expected to be achieved. Nevertheless, one should be aware of the clinical pharmacology of urokinase.

INDICATIONS AND USAGE

PULMONARY EMBOLISM

Urokinase is indicated in adults:

- For the lysis of acute massive pulmonary emboli, defined as obstruction of blood flow to a lobe or multiple segments.
- For the lysis of pulmonary emboli accompanied by unstable hemodynamics, *i.e.* failure to maintain blood pressure without supportive measures.

The diagnosis should be confirmed by objective means, such as pulmonary angiography via an upper extremity vein, or non-invasive procedures such as lung scanning.

Angiographic and hemodynamic measurements demonstrate a more rapid improvement with lytic therapy than with heparin therapy.[4-8]

CORONARY ARTERY THROMBOSIS

Urokinase has been reported to lyse acute thrombi obstructing coronary arteries, associated with evolving transmural myocardial infarction.[9] The majority of patients who received urokinase by intracoronary infusion within 6 hours following onset of symptoms showed recanalization of the involved vessel.

IT HAS BEEN ESTABLISHED THAT INTRACORONARY ADMINISTRATION OF UROKINASE DURING EVOLVING TRANSMURAL MYOCARDIAL INFARCTION RESULTS IN SALVAGE OF MYOCARDIAL TISSUE, NOR THAT IT REDUCES MORTALITY. THE PATIENTS WHO MIGHT BENEFIT FROM THIS THERAPY CANNOT BE DEFINED.

IV CATHETER CLEARANCE

Urokinase is indicated for the restoration of patency to intravenous catheters, including central venous catheters, obstructed by clotted blood or fibrin.[10,11]

NON-FDA APPROVED INDICATIONS

Urokinase is also used without FDA approval for selected patients with deep vein thrombosis and to restore patency to clotted hemodialysis fistulae.

CONTRAINDICATIONS

Injection and IV Catheter Clearance: Because thrombolytic therapy increases the risk of bleeding, urokinase is contraindicated in the following situations: (See WARNINGS.)

- Active internal bleeding.
- History of cerebrovascular accident.
- Recent (within two months) intracranial or intraspinal surgery.
- Recent trauma including cardiopulmonary resuscitation.
- Intracranial neoplasm, arteriovenous malformation, or aneurysm.
- Known bleeding diathesis.
- Severe uncontrolled arterial hypertension.

IV Catheter Clearance: There have been no reports, however, which would suggest a contraindication for the use of urokinase for IV catheter clearance.

WARNINGS

INJECTION

Bleeding: The aim of urokinase is the production of sufficient amounts of plasmin for lysis of intravascular deposits of fibrin; however, fibrin deposits which provide hemostasis, for example, at sites of needle puncture, will also lyse, and bleeding from such sites may occur.

Intramuscular injections and nonessential handling of the patient must be avoided during treatment with urokinase. Venipunctures should be performed carefully and as infrequently as possible.

Should an arterial puncture be necessary (except for intracoronary administration), upper extremity vessels are preferable. Pressure should be applied for at least 30 minutes, a pressure dressing applied, and the puncture site checked frequently for evidence of bleeding.

In the following conditions, the risks of therapy may be increased and should be weighed against the anticipated benefits:

- Recent (within 10 days) major surgery, obstetrical delivery, organ biopsy, previous puncture of non-compressible vessels.
- Recent (within 10 days) serious gastrointestinal bleeding.
- High likelihood of a left heart thrombus, *e.g.,* mitral stenosis with atrial fibrillation.
- Subacute bacterial endocarditis.
- Hemostatic defects including those secondary to severe hepatic or renal disease.
- Pregnancy.
- Cerebrovascular disease.
- Diabetic hemorrhagic retinopathy.
- Any other condition in which bleeding might constitute a significant hazard or be particularly difficult to manage because of its location.

Should serious spontaneous bleeding (not controlled by local pressure) occur, the infusion of urokinase should be terminated immediately, and treatment instituted as described under ADVERSE REACTIONS.

USE OF ANTICOAGULANTS

Concurrent use of anticoagulants with intravenous administration of urokinase is not recommended. However, concurrent use of heparin may be required during intracoronary administration of urokinase. A clinical study[9] with concurrent use of heparin and urokinase during intracoronary administration has demonstrated no tendency toward increased bleeding that would not be attributable to the procedure or urokinase alone. Nevertheless, careful monitoring for excessive bleeding is advised.

ARRHYTHMIAS

Rapid lysis of coronary thrombi has been reported occasionally to cause atrial or ventricular dysrhythmias as a result of reperfusion requiring immediate treatment. Careful monitoring for arrhythmias should be maintained during and immediately following intracoronary administration of urokinase.

IV CATHETER CLEARANCE

Excessive pressure should be avoided when urokinase solution is injected into the catheter. Such force could cause rupture of the catheter or expulsion of the clot into the circulation. During attempts to determine catheter occlusion, vigorous suction should not be applied due to possible damage to the vascular wall or collapse of soft-wall catheters.

Catheters may be occluded by substances other than fibrin clots such as drug precipitates. Urokinase solution is not effective in such cases and there is the possibility that the substances may be forced into the vascular system.

PRECAUTIONS

LABORATORY TESTS

Injection

Before commencing thrombolytic therapy, obtain a hematocrit, platelet count, and a thrombin time (TT), activated partial thromboplastin time (APTT), or prothrombin time (PT). If heparin has been given, it should be discontinued unless it is to be used in conjunction with urokinase for intracoronary administration. TT or APTT should be less than twice the normal control value before thrombolytic therapy is started.

During the infusion, coagulation tests and/or measures of fibrinolytic activity may be performed if desired. Results do not, however, reliably predict either efficacy or a risk of bleeding. The clinical response should be observed frequently, and vital signs, *i.e.,* pulse, temperature, respiratory rate and blood pressure, should be checked at least every 4 hours. The blood pressure should not be taken in the lower extremities to avoid dislodgment of possible deep vein thrombi.

Following the intravenous infusion *before (re) instituting heparin,* the TT or APTT should be less than twice the upper limits of normal. Following intracoronary infusion of urokinase, blood coagulation parameters should be determined and heparin therapy continued as appropriate.

CARCINOGENICITY

Injection and IV Catheter Clearance: Adequate data are not available on the long-term potential for carcinogenicity in animals or humans.

PREGNANCY CATEGORY B

Reproduction studies have been performed in mice and rats at doses up to 1000 times the human dose and have revealed no evidence of impaired fertility or harm to the fetus due to urokinase. There are, however, no adequate and well-controlled studies in pregnant women. Because animal reproduction studies are not always predictive of human response, this drug should be used during pregnancy only if clearly needed.

NURSING MOTHERS

It is known whether this drug is excreted in human milk. Because many drugs are excreted in human milk, caution should be exercised when urokinase is administered to a nursing woman.

PEDIATRIC USE

Safety and effectiveness in children have not been established.

DRUG INTERACTIONS

INJECTION

The interaction of urokinase with other drugs has not been studied. Drugs that alter platelet function should not be used. Common examples are: aspirin, indomethacin and phenylbutazone.

Although a bolus dose of heparin is recommended prior to intracoronary use of urokinase, oral anticoagulants or heparin should not be given concurrently with large doses of urokinase such as those used for pulmonary embolism. Concomitant use of intravenous urokinase and oral anticoagulants or heparin may increase the risk of hemorrhage. (See WARNINGS.)

ADVERSE REACTIONS

THE FOLLOWING ADVERSE REACTIONS HAVE BEEN ASSOCIATED WITH INTRAVENOUS THERAPY BUT MAY ALSO OCCUR WITH INTRACORONARY ARTERY INFUSION.

Bleeding

Injection and IV Catheter Clearance: The type of bleeding associated with thrombolytic therapy can be placed into two broad categories:

- Superficial or surface bleeding, observed mainly at invaded or disturbed sites (*e.g.*, venous cutdowns, arterial punctures, sites of recent surgical intervention, etc.).
- Internal bleeding, involving, *e.g.*, the gastrointestinal tract, genitourinary tract, vagina, or intramuscular, retroperitoneal, or intracranial sites.

Several fatalities due to intracranial or retroperitoneal hemorrhage have occurred during thrombolytic therapy.

Should serious bleeding occur, urokinase infusion should be discontinued and, if necessary, blood loss and reversal of the bleeding tendency can be effectively managed with whole blood (fresh blood preferable), packed red blood cells and cryoprecipitate or fresh frozen plasma. Dextran should not be used. Although the use of aminocaproic acid (ACA, AMICAR) in humans as an antidote for urokinase has not been documented, it may be considered in an emergency situation.

Allergic Reactions

In vitro tests with urokinase, as well as intradermal tests in humans, gave no evidence of induced antibody formation. Relatively mild allergic type reactions, *e.g.*, bronchospasm and skin rash, have been reported. When such reactions occur, they usually respond to conventional therapy. In addition, rare cases of anaphylaxis have been reported.

Miscellaneous

Fever and chills, including shaking chills (rigors), nausea and/or vomiting, transient hypotension or hypertension, dyspnea, tachycardia, cyanosis, back pain, hypoxemia, and acidosis have been reported together and separately. Rare cases of myocardial infarction have also been reported. A cause and effect relationship has not been established.

Aspirin is not recommended for treatment of fever.

DOSAGE AND ADMINISTRATION

UROKINASE IS INTENDED FOR INTRAVENOUS AND INTRACORONARY INFUSION ONLY.

PULMONARY EMBOLISM: PREPARATION

Injection

Reconstitute urokinase by aseptically adding 5 ml of sterile water for injection to the vial. (It is important that urokinase be reconstituted *only* with sterile water for injection *without* preservatives. Bacteriostatic water for injection should *not* be used.) Each vial should be visually inspected for discoloration (slightly straw-colored solution) and for the presence of particulate material. Highly colored solutions should not be used. Because urokinase contains no preservatives, it should not be reconstituted until immediately before using. Any unused portion of the reconstituted material should be discarded.

To minimize formation of filaments, avoid shaking the vial during reconstitution. Roll and tilt the vial to enhance reconstitution. The solution may be terminally filtered, *e.g.* through a 0.45 micron or smaller cellulose membrane filter. No other medication should be added to this solution.

Reconstituted urokinase is diluted with 0.9% sodium chloride injection or 5% dextrose injection prior to intravenous infusion. See TABLE 1, Dose Preparation, Pulmonary Embolism.

Administration

Administer urokinase by means of a constant infusion pump that is capable of delivering a total volume of 195 ml. The following table may be used as an aid in the preparation of urokinase for administration.

TABLE 1 *Dose Preparation-Pulmonary Embolism*

Weight (lbs)	Total Dose* Urokinase (IU)	Number Vials Abbokinase (urokinase for injection)	Volume of Abbokinase After Reconstitution (ml)† +	Volume of Diluent (ml) =	Final Volume (ml)
81-90	2,250,000	9	45	150	195
91-100	2,500,000	10	50	145	195
101-110	2,750,000	11	55	140	195
111-120	3,000,000	12	60	135	195
121-130	3,250,000	13	65	130	195
131-140	3,500,000	14	70	125	195
141-150	3,750,000	15	75	120	195
151-160	4,000,000	16	80	115	195
161-170	4,250,000	17	85	110	195
171-180	4,500,000	18	90	105	195
181-190	4,750,000	19	95	100	195
191-200	5,000,000	20	100	95	195
201-210	5,250,000	21	105	90	195
211-220	5,500,000	22	110	85	195
221-230	5,750,000	23	115	80	195
231-240	6,000,000	24	120	75	195
241-250	6,250,000	25	125	70	195
Infusion Rate:	Priming Dose: 15 ml/10 min‡		Dose for 12-Hour Period: 15 ml/hr for 12 hrs		

* Priming dose + dose administered during 12-hour period.
† After addition of 5 ml of sterile water for injection, per vial. (See Preparation.)
‡ Pump rate = 90 ml/hr

A priming dose of 2000 IU/lb (4400 IU/kg) of urokinase is given as the urokinase-0.9% sodium chloride injection or 5% dextrose injection admixture at a rate of 90 ml/hour over a period of 10 minutes. This is followed by a continuous infusion of 2000 IU/lb/hr (4400 IU/kg/hr) of urokinase at a rate of 15 ml/hour for 12 hours. Since some urokinase admixture will remain in the tubing at the end of an infusion pump delivery cycle, the following flush procedure should be performed to insure that the total dose of urokinase is administered. A solution of 0.9% sodium chloride injection or 5% dextrose injection approximately equal in amount to the volume of the tubing in the infusion set should be administered via the pump to flush the urokinase admixture from the entire length of the infusion set. The pump should be set to administer the flush solution at the continuous infusion rate of 15 ml/hour.

Anticoagulation After Terminating Urokinase Treatment

At the end of urokinase therapy, treatment with heparin by continuous intravenous infusion is recommended to prevent recurrent thrombosis. Heparin treatment without a loading dose, should not begin until the thrombin time has decreased to *less than twice* the normal control value (approximately 3-4 hours after completion of the infusion). See manufacturer's prescribing information for proper use of heparin. This should then be followed by oral anticoagulants in the conventional manner.

LYSIS OF CORONARY ARTERY THROMBI[9]

Preparation

Reconstitute three 250,000 IU vials of urokinase by aseptically adding 5 ml of sterile water for injection to each vial. (It is important that urokinase be reconstituted *only* with sterile water for injection *without* preservatives. Bacteriostatic water for injection should *not* be used.) Each vial should be visually inspected for discoloration (slightly straw-colored solution) and for the presence of particulate material. Highly colored solutions should not be used. Because urokinase contains no preservatives, it should not be reconstituted until immediately before using. Any unused portion of the reconstituted material should be discarded.

To minimize formation of filaments, avoid shaking the vial during reconstitution. Roll and tilt the vial to enhance reconstitution. The solution may be terminally filtered, *e.g.* through a 0.45 micron or smaller cellulose membrane filter.

Add the contents of the three reconstituted urokinase vials to 500 ml of 5% dextrose injection. The following solution admixture will have a concentration of approximately 1500 IU/ml. No other medication should be added to the solution.

The admixture should be administered immediately as described under Administration. Any solution remaining after administration should be discarded.

Note: Adsorption of drug from dilute protein solution to various materials has been reported in the literature. Therefore, the directions for Preparation and Administration must be followed to assure that significant drug loss does not occur.

Administration

Prior to the infusion of urokinase, a bolus dose of heparin ranging from 2500-10,000 units should be administered intravenously. Prior heparin administration should be considered when calculating the heparin dose for this procedure. Following the bolus dose of heparin, the prepared urokinase solution should be infused into the occluded artery at a rate of 4 ml/minute (6000 IU/minute) for periods up to 2 hours. In a clinical study the average total dose of urokinase utilized for lysis of coronary artery thrombi was 500,000 IU.[9]

To determine response to urokinase therapy, periodic angiography during the infusion is recommended. It is suggested that the angiography be repeated at approximately 15 minute intervals. urokinase therapy should be continued until the artery is maximally opened, usually 15-30 minutes after the initial opening. Following the infusion, coagulation parameters should be determined. It is advisable to continue heparin therapy after the artery is opened by urokinase.

When urokinase was administered selectively into thrombosed coronary arteries via coronary catheter within 6 hours following onset of symptoms of acute transmural myocardial infarction, 60% of the occlusions were opened.[9]

IV CATHETER CLEARANCE

BECAUSE UROKINASE OPEN-CATH POWDER CONTAINS NO PRESERVATIVE, RECONSTITUTED SOLUTION SHOULD BE USED IMMEDIATELY AFTER RECONSTITUTION. DISCARD ANY UNUSED PORTION.

Preparation of Solution

Univial:

1. Remove protective cap. Turn plunger-stopper a quarter turn and press to force diluent into lower chamber.
2. Roll and tilt to effect solution. Use only a clear, essentially colorless solution.
3. Sterilize top of stopper with a suitable germicide.
4. Insert needle through the center of stopper until tip is barely visible. Withdraw dose.

It is recommended that vigorous shaking be avoided during reconstitution; roll and tilt to enhance reconstitution.

Parenteral drug products should be inspected visually for particulate matter and discoloration prior to administration, whenever solution and container permit.

Administration

When the following procedure is used to clear a central venous catheter, the patient should be instructed to exhale and hold his breath any time the catheter is not connected to IV tubing or a syringe. This is to prevent air from entering the open catheter.

Aseptically disconnect the IV tubing connection at the catheter hub and attach a 10 ml syringe. Determine occlusion of the catheter by *gently* attempting to aspirate blood from the catheter with the 10 ml syringe. If aspiration is not possible, remove the 10 ml syringe and attach a 1 ml tuberculin syringe filled with prepared urokinase to the catheter. Slowly and gently inject an amount of urokinase equal to the volume of the catheter. Aseptically remove the tuberculin syringe and connect a 5 ml syringe to the catheter. Wait at least 5 minutes before attempting to aspirate the drug and residual clot with the 5 ml syringe. Repeat aspiration attempts every 5 minutes. If the catheter is not open within 30 minutes, the catheter may be capped allowing urokinase to remain in the catheter for 30-60 minutes before again attempting to aspirate. A second injection of urokinase may be necessary in resistant cases.

When patency is restored, aspirate 4-5 ml of blood to assure removal of all drug and clot residual. Remove the blood-filled syringe and replace it with a 10 ml syringe filled with 0.9% sodium chloride injection. The catheter should then be gently irrigated with this solution to assure patency of the catheter. After the catheter has been irrigated, remove the 10 ml syringe and aseptically reconnect sterile IV tubing to the catheter hub.

PRODUCT LISTING - EQUIVALENTS NOT AVAILABLE

Powder For Injection - Injectable - 5000 IU

1's $56.61 ABBOKINASE OPEN-CATH, Abbott Pharmaceutical 00074-6111-01

Powder For Injection - Injectable - 9000 IU

1's $98.72 ABBOKINASE OPEN-CATH, Abbott Pharmaceutical 00074-6145-02

Powder For Injection - Injectable - 250000 IU

1's $539.78 ABBOKINASE, Abbott Pharmaceutical 00074-6109-05

Ursodiol *(002418)*

Categories: Calculus, biliary; Pregnancy Category B; FDA Approved 1987 Dec; Orphan Drugs
Drug Classes: Gallstone solubilizers
Brand Names: Actigall
Foreign Brand Availability: Cholacid (Germany); Dehychol (Taiwan); Deursil (Italy); Estazor (Indonesia); Pramur (Indonesia); Urdafalk (Indonesia); Ursacol (Italy); Ursochol (Netherlands; Switzerland); Ursodamor (Italy); Ursofalk (Canada; Colombia; Germany; Hong-Kong; Korea; Malaysia; Mexico; Peru; Philippines; Thailand); Ursolin (Thailand); Ursolit (Israel); Ursolvan (France); Urso-Ratiopharm (Germany)
Cost of Therapy: $209.90 (Gall Stones; Actigall; 300 mg; 2 capsules/day; 30 day supply)
$154.62 (Gall Stones; Generic Capsules; 300 mg; 2 capsules/day; 30 day supply)

DESCRIPTION

SPECIAL NOTE: Gallbladder stone dissolution with ursodiol treatment requires months of therapy. Complete dissolution does not occur in all patients and recurrence of stones within 5 years has been observed in up to 50% of patients who do dissolve their stones on bile acid therapy. Patients should be carefully selected for therapy with ursodiol, and alternative therapies should be considered.

Ursodiol is a bile acid available as 300 mg capsules suitable for oral administration.

Actigall is ursodiol (ursodeoxycholic acid), a naturally occurring bile acid found in small quantities in normal human bile and in large quantities in the biles of certain species of bears. It is a bitter-tasting, white powder freely soluble in ethanol, methanol, and in glacial acetic acid; slightly soluble in chloroform; sparingly soluble in ether; and insoluble in water. The chemical name for ursodiol is 3α,7β-dihydroxy-5β-cholan-24-oic acid ($C_{24}H_{40}O_4$). Ursodiol has a molecular weight of 392.58.

Inactive Ingredients: Colloidal silicon dioxide, ferric oxide, gelatin, magnesium stearate, starch (corn), and titanium dioxide.

CLINICAL PHARMACOLOGY

About 90% of a therapeutic dose of ursodiol is absorbed in the small bowel after oral administration. After absorption, ursodiol enters the portal vein and undergoes efficient extraction from portal blood by the liver (*i.e.*, there is a large "first-pass" effect) where it is conjugated with either glycine or taurine and is then secreted into the hepatic bile ducts. Ursodiol in bile is concentrated in the gallbladder and expelled into the duodenum in gallbladder bile via the cystic and common ducts by gallbladder contractions provoked by physiologic responses to eating. Only small quantities of ursodiol appear in the systemic circulation and very small amounts are excreted into urine. The sites of the drug's therapeutic actions are in the liver, bile and gut lumen.

Beyond conjugation, ursodiol is not altered or catabolized appreciably by the liver or intestinal mucosa. A small proportion of orally administered drug undergoes bacterial degradation with each cycle of enterohepatic circulation. Ursodiol can be both oxidized and reduced at the 7-carbon, yielding either 7-keto-lithocholic acid or lithocholic acid, respectively. Further, there is some bacterially catalyzed deconjugation of glyco- and tauro-ursodeoxycholic acid in the small bowel. Free ursodiol, 7-keto-lithocholic acid, and lithocholic acid are relatively insoluble in aqueous media and larger proportions of these compounds are lost from the distal gut into the feces. Reabsorbed free ursodiol is reconjugated by the liver. Eighty percent (80%) of lithocholic acid formed in the small bowel is excreted in the feces, but the 20% that is absorbed is sulfated at the 3-hydroxyl group in the liver to relatively insoluble lithocholyl conjugates which are excreted into bile and lost in feces. Absorbed 7-keto-lithocholic acid is stereospecifically reduced in the liver to chenodiol.

Lithocholic acid causes cholestatic liver injury and can cause death from liver failure in certain species unable to form sulfate conjugates. Lithocholic acid is formed by 7-dehydroxylation of the dihydroxy bile acids (ursodiol and chenodiol) in the gut lumen. The 7-dehydroxylation reaction appears to be alpha-specific, *i.e.*, chenodiol is more efficiently 7-dehydroxylated than ursodiol and, for equimolar doses of ursodiol and chenodiol, levels of lithocholic acid appearing in bile are lower with the former. Man has the capacity to sulfate lithocholic acid. Although liver injury has not been associated with ursodiol therapy, a reduced capacity to sulfate may exist in some individuals, but such a deficiency has not yet been clearly demonstrated.

PHARMACODYNAMICS

Ursodiol suppresses hepatic synthesis and secretion of cholesterol, and also inhibits intestinal absorption of cholesterol. It appears to have little inhibitory effect on synthesis and secretion into bile of endogenous bile acids, and does not appear to affect secretion of phospholipids into bile.

With repeated dosing, bile ursodeoxycholic acid concentrations reach a steady state in about 3 weeks. Although insoluble in aqueous media, cholesterol can be solubilized in at least two different ways in the presence of dihydroxy bile acids. In addition to solubilizing cholesterol in micelles, ursodiol acts by an apparently unique mechanism to cause dispersion of cholesterol as liquid crystals in aqueous media. Thus, even though administration of high doses (*e.g.*, 15-18 mg/kg/day) does not result in a concentration of ursodiol higher than 60% of the total bile acid pool, ursodiol-rich bile effectively solubilizes cholesterol. The overall effect of ursodiol is to increase the concentration level at which saturation of cholesterol occurs.

The various actions of ursodiol combine to change the bile of patients with gallstones from cholesterol-precipitating to cholesterol-solubilizing, thus resulting in bile conducive to cholesterol stone dissolution.

After ursodiol dosing is stopped, the concentration of the bile acid in bile falls exponentially, declining to about 5-10% of its steady-state level in about 1 week.

INDICATIONS AND USAGE

Ursodiol is indicated for patients with radiolucent, noncalcified gallbladder stones <20 mm in greatest diameter in whom elective cholecystectomy would be undertaken except for the presence of increased surgical risk due to systemic disease, advanced age, idiosyncratic reaction to general anesthesia, or for those patients who refuse surgery. Safety of use of ursodiol beyond 24 months is not established.

Ursodiol is indicated for the prevention of gallstone formation in obese patients experiencing rapid weight loss.

NON-FDA APPROVED INDICATIONS

Although not approved by the FDA, ursodiol has been used in combination with chenodeoxycholic acid and in conjunction with extracorporeal shock-wave lithotripsy for the dissolution of gallstones.

CONTRAINDICATIONS

- Ursodiol will not dissolve calcified cholesterol stones, radiopaque stones, or radiolucent bile pigment stones. Hence, patients with such stones are not candidates for ursodiol therapy.
- Patients with compelling reasons for cholecystectomy including unremitting acute cholecystitis, cholangitis, biliary obstruction, gallstone pancreatitis or biliary-gastrointestinal fistula are not candidates for ursodiol therapy.
- Allergy to bile acids.

PRECAUTIONS

LIVER TESTS

Ursodiol therapy has not been associated with liver damage. Lithocholic acid, a naturally occurring bile acid, is known to be a liver-toxic metabolite. This bile acid is formed in the gut from ursodiol less efficiently and in smaller amounts than that seen from chenodiol. Lithocholic acid is detoxified in the liver by sulfation and although man appears to be an efficient sulfater, it is possible that some patients may have a congenital or acquired deficiency in sulfation, thereby predisposing them to lithocholate-induced liver damage.

Abnormalities in liver enzymes have not been associated with ursodiol therapy and, in fact, ursodiol has been shown to decrease liver enzyme levels in liver disease. However, patients given ursodiol should have SGOT (AST) and SGPT (ALT) measured at the initiation of therapy and thereafter as indicated by the particular clinical circumstances.

CARCINOGENESIS, MUTAGENESIS, AND IMPAIRMENT OF FERTILITY

Ursodeoxycholic acid was tested in 2 year oral carcinogenicity studies in CD-1 mice and Sprague-Dawley rats at daily doses of 50, 250, and 1000 mg/kg/day. It was not tumorigenic in mice. In the rat study, it produced statistically significant dose-related increased incidences of pheochromocytomas of adrenal medulla in males (p=0.014, Peto trend test) and females (p=0.004, Peto trend test). A 78 week rat study employing intrarectal instillation of lithocholic acid and tauro-deoxycholic acid, metabolites of ursodiol and chenodiol, has been conducted. These bile acids alone did not produce any tumors. A tumor-promoting effect of both metabolites was observed when they were co-administered with a carcinogenic agent. Results of epidemiologic studies suggest that bile acids might be involved in the pathogenesis of human colon cancer in patients who had undergone a cholecystectomy, but direct evidence is lacking. Ursodiol is not mutagenic in the Ames test. Dietary administration of lithocholic acid to chickens is reported to cause hepatic adenomatous hyperplasia.

PREGNANCY CATEGORY B

Reproduction studies have been performed in rats and rabbits with ursodiol doses up to 200-fold the therapeutic dose and have revealed no evidence of impaired fertility or harm to the fetus at doses of 20- to 100-fold the human dose in rats and at 5-fold the human dose (highest dose tested) in rabbits. Studies employing 100- to 200-fold the human dose in rats have shown some reduction in fertility rate and litter size. There have been no adequate and well-controlled studies of the use of ursodiol in pregnant women, but inadvertent exposure of 4 women to therapeutic doses of the drug in the first trimester of pregnancy during the ursodiol trials led to no evidence of effects on the fetus or newborn baby. Although it seems unlikely, the possibility that ursodiol can cause fetal harm cannot be ruled out; hence, the drug is not recommended for use during pregnancy.

NURSING MOTHERS

It is not known whether ursodiol is excreted in human milk. Because many drugs are excreted in human milk, caution should be exercised when ursodiol is administered to a nursing mother.

PEDIATRIC USE

The safety and effectiveness of ursodiol in pediatric patients have not been established.

DRUG INTERACTIONS

Bile acid sequestering agents such as cholestyramine and colestipol may interfere with the action of ursodiol by reducing its absorption. Aluminum-based antacids have been shown to adsorb bile acids *in vitro* and may be expected to interfere with ursodiol in the same manner as the bile acid sequestering agents. Estrogens, oral contraceptives and clofibrate (and perhaps other lipid-lowering drugs) increase hepatic cholesterol secretion, and encourage cholesterol gallstone formation and hence may counteract the effectiveness of ursodiol.

ADVERSE REACTIONS

The nature and frequency of adverse experiences were similar across all groups.

TABLE 2 and TABLE 3 provide comprehensive listings of the adverse experiences reported that occurred with a 5% incidence level.

TABLE 2 *Gallstone Dissolution*

	Ursodiol 8-10 mg/kg/day (n=155)	Placebo (n=159)
Body as a Whole		
Allergy	8 (5.2%)	7 (4.4%)
Chest pain	5 (3.2%)	10 (6.3%)
Fatigue	7 (4.5%)	8 (5.0%)
Infection viral	30 (19.4%)	41 (25.8%)
Digestive System		
Abdominal pain	67 (43.2%)	70 (44.0%)
Cholecystitis	8 (5.2%)	7 (4.4%)
Constipation	15 (9.7%)	14 (8.8%)
Diarrhea	42 (27.1%)	34 (21.4%)
Dyspepsia	26 (16.8%)	18 (11.3%)
Flatulence	12 (7.7%)	12 (7.5%)
Gastrointestinal disorder	6 (3.9%)	8 (5.0%)
Nausea	22 (14.2%)	27 (17.0%)
Vomiting	15 (9.7%)	11 (6.9%)
Musculoskeletal System		
Arthralgia	12 (7.7%)	24 (15.1%)
Arthritis	9 (5.8%)	4 (2.5%)
Back pain	11 (7.1%)	18 (11.3%)
Myalgia	9 (5.8%)	9 (5.7%)
Nervous System		
Headache	28 (18.1%)	34 (21.4%)
Insomnia	3 (1.9%)	8 (5.0%)
Respiratory System		
Bronchitis	10 (6.5%)	6 (3.8%)
Coughing	11 (7.1%)	7 (4.4%)
Pharyngitis	13 (8.4%)	5 (3.1%)
Rhinitis	8 (5.2%)	11 (6.9%)
Sinusitis	17 (11.0%)	18 (11.3%)
Upper respiratory tract infection	24 (15.5%)	21 (13.2%)
Urogenital System		
Urinary tract infection	10 (6.5%)	7 (4.4%)

TABLE 3 *Gallstone Prevention*

	Ursodiol 600 mg (n=322)	Placebo (n=325)
Body as a Whole		
Fatigue	25 (7.8%)	33 (10.2%)
Infection viral	29 (9.0%)	29 (8.9%)
Influenza-like symptoms	21 (6.5%)	19 (5.8%)
Digestive System		
Abdominal pain	20 (6.2%)	39 (12.0%)
Constipation	85 (26.4%)	72 (22.2%)
Diarrhea	81 (25.2%)	68 (20.9%)
Flatulence	15 (4.7%)	24 (7.4%)
Nausea	56 (17.4%)	43 (13.2%)
Vomiting	44 (13.7%)	44 (13.5%)
Muscoloskeletal System		
Back pain	38 (11.8%)	21 (6.5%)
Musculoskeletal pain	19 (5.9%)	15 (4.6%)
Nervous System		
Dizziness	53 (16.5%)	42 (12.9%)
Headache	80 (24.8%)	78 (24.0%)
Respiratory System		
Pharyngitis	10 (3.1%)	19 (5.8%)
Sinusitis	17 (5.3%)	18 (5.5%)
Upper respiratory tract infection	40 (12.4%)	35 (10.8%)
Skin and Appendages		
Alopecia	17 (5.3%)	8 (2.5%)
Urogenital System		
Dysmenorrhea	18 (5.6%)	19 (5.8%)

DOSAGE AND ADMINISTRATION

GALLSTONE DISSOLUTION

The recommended dose for ursodiol treatment of radiolucent gallbladder stones is 8-10 mg/kg/day given in 2 or 3 divided doses.

Ultrasound images of the gallbladder should be obtained at 6 month intervals for the first year of ursodiol therapy to monitor gallstone response. If gallstones appear to have dissolved, ursodiol therapy should be continued and dissolution confirmed on a repeat ultrasound examination within 1-3 months. Most patients who eventually achieve complete stone dissolution will show partial or complete dissolution at the first on-treatment reevaluation. If partial stone dissolution is not seen by 12 months of ursodiol therapy, the likelihood of success is greatly reduced.

GALLSTONE PREVENTION

The recommended dosage of ursodiol for gallstone prevention in patients undergoing rapid weight loss is 600 mg/day (300 mg bid).

HOW SUPPLIED

Actigall Capsules

300 mg: Opaque, white, pink (imprinted "Actigall 300 mg").

STORAGE

Store at 25°C (77°F); excursions permitted to 15-30°C (59-86°F).

Dispense in tight container.

PRODUCT LISTING - RATED THERAPEUTICALLY EQUIVALENT

Capsule - Oral - 300 mg

100's	$257.70	GENERIC, Udl Laboratories Inc	51079-0970-20
100's	$257.75	GENERIC, Teva Pharmaceuticals Usa	00093-9380-01
100's	$282.25	GENERIC, Amide Pharmaceutical Inc	52152-0060-02

PRODUCT LISTING - EQUIVALENTS NOT AVAILABLE

Capsule - Oral - 300 mg

100's	$349.84	ACTIGALL, Novartis Pharmaceuticals	00078-0319-05
100's	$349.84	ACTIGALL, Watson Laboratories Inc	52544-0930-01

Tablet - Oral - 250 mg

100's	$220.73	URSO, Scandipharm Inc	58914-0785-10

Valacyclovir Hydrochloride *(003265)*

Categories: Herpes genitalis; Herpes labialis; Herpes zoster; Infection, herpes simplex virus; Infection, varicella-zoster virus; Pregnancy Category B; FDA Approved 1995 Jun

Drug Classes: Antivirals

Brand Names: **Valtrex**

Foreign Brand Availability: Rapivir (Mexico); Valcyclor (Colombia); Zelitrex (France; South-Africa)

Cost of Therapy: $148.09 (Genital Herpes; Valtrex; 1 g; 2 tablets/day; 10 day supply)
$155.49 (Herpes Zoster; Valtrex; 1 g; 3 tablets/day; 7 day supply)

DESCRIPTION

Valacyclovir hydrochloride is the hydrochloride salt of *L*-valyl ester of the antiviral drug acyclovir.

Valtrex caplets are for oral administration. Each caplet contains valacyclovir hydrochloride equivalent to 500 mg or 1 g valacyclovir and the inactive ingredients carnauba wax, colloidal silicon dioxide, crospovidone, FD&C blue no. 2 lake, hypromellose, magnesium stearate, microcrystalline cellulose, polyethylene glycol, polysorbate 80, povidone, and titanium dioxide. The blue, film-coated caplets are printed with edible white ink.

The chemical name of valacyclovir hydrochloride is *L*-valine, 2-[(2-amino-1,6-dihydro-6-oxo-9*H*-purin-9-yl)methoxy]ethyl ester, monohydrochloride.

Valacyclovir hydrochloride is a white to off-white powder with a molecular formula $C_{13}H_{20}N_6O_4 \cdot HCl$ and a molecular weight of 360.80. The maximum solubility in water at 25°C is 174 mg/ml. The pKa's for valacyclovir hydrochloride are 1.90, 7.47, and 9.43.

CLINICAL PHARMACOLOGY

MICROBIOLOGY

Mechanism of Antiviral Action

Valacyclovir HCl is rapidly converted to acyclovir which has demonstrated antiviral activity against herpes simplex virus types 1 (HSV-1) and 2 (HSV-2) and varicella-zoster virus (VZV) both *in vitro* and *in vivo*.

The inhibitory activity of acyclovir is highly selective due to its affinity for the enzyme thymidine kinase (TK) encoded by HSV and VZV. This viral enzyme converts acyclovir into acyclovir monophosphate, a nucleotide analogue. The monophosphate is further converted into diphosphate by cellular guanylate kinase and into triphosphate by a number of cellular enzymes. *In vitro*, acyclovir triphosphate stops replication of herpes viral DNA. This is accomplished in 3 ways: (1) competitive inhibition of viral DNA polymerase, (2) incorporation and termination of the growing viral DNA chain, and (3) inactivation of the viral DNA polymerase. The greater antiviral activity of acyclovir against HSV compared to VZV is due to its more efficient phosphorylation by the viral TK.

Antiviral Activities

The quantitative relationship between the *in vitro* susceptibility of herpes viruses to antivirals and the clinical response to therapy has not been established in humans, and virus sensitivity testing has not been standardized. Sensitivity testing results, expressed as the concentration of drug required to inhibit by 50% the growth of virus in cell culture (IC_{50}), vary greatly depending upon a number of factors. Using plaque-reduction assays, the IC_{50} against herpes simplex virus isolates ranges from 0.02-13.5 μg/ml for HSV-1 and from 0.01-9.9 μg/ml for HSV-2. The IC_{50} for acyclovir against most laboratory strains and clinical isolates of VZV ranges from 0.12-10.8 μg/ml. Acyclovir also demonstrates activity against the Oka vaccine strain of VZV with a mean IC_{50} of 1.35 μg/ml.

Drug Resistance

Resistance of HSV and VZV to acyclovir can result from qualitative and quantitative changes in the viral TK and/or DNA polymerase. Clinical isolates of VZV with reduced susceptibility to acyclovir have been recovered from patients with AIDS. In these cases, TK-deficient mutants of VZV have been recovered.

Resistance of HSV and VZV to acyclovir occurs by the same mechanisms. While most of the acyclovir-resistant mutants isolated thus far from immunocompromised patients have been found to be TK-deficient mutants, other mutants involving the viral TK gene (TK partial and TK altered) and DNA polymerase have also been isolated. TK-negative mutants may cause severe disease in immunocompromised patients. The possibility of viral resistance to valacyclovir (and therefore, to acyclovir) should be considered in patients who show poor clinical response during therapy.

After oral administration, valacyclovir HCl is rapidly absorbed from the gastrointestinal tract and nearly completely converted to acyclovir and *L*-valine by first-pass intestinal and/or hepatic metabolism.

PHARMACOKINETICS

The pharmacokinetics of valacyclovir and acyclovir after oral administration of valacyclovir HCl have been investigated in 14 volunteer studies involving 283 adults.

Absorption and Bioavailability

The absolute bioavailability of acyclovir after administration of valacyclovir HCl is 54.5 ± 9.1% as determined following a 1 g oral dose of valacyclovir HCl and a 350 mg intravenous acyclovir dose to 12 healthy volunteers. Acyclovir bioavailability from the administration of valacyclovir HCl is not altered by administration with food (30 minutes after an 873 Kcal breakfast, which included 51 g of fat).

There was a lack of dose proportionality in acyclovir maximum concentration (C_{max}) and area under the acyclovir concentration-time curve (AUC) after single-dose administration of 100 mg, 250 mg, 500 mg, 750 mg, and 1 g of valacyclovir HCl to 8 healthy volunteers. The mean C_{max} (±SD) was 0.83 (±0.14), 2.15 (±0.50), 3.28 (±0.83), 4.17 (±1.14), and 5.65 (±2.37) μg/ml, respectively; and the mean AUC (±SD) was 2.28 (±0.40), 5.76 (±0.60), 11.59 (±1.79), 14.11 (±3.54), and 19.52 (±6.04) h·μg/ml, respectively.

There was also a lack of dose proportionality in acyclovir C_{max} and AUC after the multiple-dose administration of 250 mg, 500 mg, and 1 g of valacyclovir HCl administered 4 times daily for 11 days in parallel groups of 8 healthy volunteers. The mean C_{max} (±SD) was 2.11 (±0.33), 3.69 (±0.87), and 4.96 (±0.64) μg/ml, respectively, and the mean AUC (±SD) was 5.66 (±1.09), 9.88 (±2.01), and 15.70 (±2.27) h·μg/ml, respectively.

There is no accumulation of acyclovir after the administration of valacyclovir at the recommended dosage regimens in healthy volunteers with normal renal function.

Distribution

The binding of valacyclovir to human plasma proteins ranged from 13.5-17.9%.

Metabolism

After oral administration, valacyclovir HCl is rapidly absorbed from the gastrointestinal tract. Valacyclovir is converted to acyclovir and *L*-valine by first-pass intestinal and/or hepatic metabolism. Acyclovir is converted to a small extent to inactive metabolites by aldehyde oxidase and by alcohol and aldehyde dehydrogenase. Neither valacyclovir nor acyclovir is metabolized by cytochrome P450 enzymes. Plasma concentrations of unconverted valacyclovir are low and transient, generally becoming non-quantifiable by 3 hours after administration. Peak plasma valacyclovir concentrations are generally less than 0.5 μg/ml at all doses. After single-dose administration of 1 g of valacyclovir HCl, average plasma valacyclovir concentrations observed were 0.5, 0.4, and 0.8 μg/ml in patients with hepatic dysfunction, renal insufficiency, and in healthy volunteers who received concomitant cimetidine and probenecid, respectively.

Elimination

The pharmacokinetic disposition of acyclovir delivered by valacyclovir is consistent with previous experience from intravenous and oral acyclovir. Following the oral administration of a single 1 g dose of radiolabeled valacyclovir to 4 healthy subjects, 45.60% and 47.12% of administered radioactivity was recovered in urine and feces over 96 hours, respectively. Acyclovir accounted for 88.60% of the radioactivity excreted in the urine. Renal clearance of acyclovir following the administration of a single 1 g dose of valacyclovir HCl to 12 healthy volunteers was approximately 255 ± 86 ml/min which represents 41.9% of total acyclovir apparent plasma clearance.

The plasma elimination half-life of acyclovir typically averaged 2.5-3.3 hours in all studies of valacyclovir HCl in volunteers with normal renal function.

End-Stage Renal Disease (ESRD)

Following administration of valacyclovir HCl to volunteers with ESRD, the average acyclovir half-life is approximately 14 hours. During hemodialysis, the acyclovir half-life is approximately 4 hours. Approximately one-third of acyclovir in the body is removed by dialysis during a 4 hour hemodialysis session. Apparent plasma clearance of acyclovir in dialysis patients was 86.3 ± 21.3 ml/min/1.73 m^2, compared to 679.16 ± 162.76 ml/min/1.73 m^2 in healthy volunteers.

Reduction in dosage is recommended in patients with renal impairment (see DOSAGE AND ADMINISTRATION).

Geriatrics

After single-dose administration of 1 g of valacyclovir HCl in healthy geriatric volunteers, the half-life of acyclovir was 3.11 ± 0.51 hours, compared to 2.91 ± 0.63 hours in healthy volunteers. The pharmacokinetics of acyclovir following single- and multiple-dose oral administration of valacyclovir HCl in geriatric volunteers varied with renal function. Dose reduction may be required in geriatric patients, depending on the underlying renal status of the patient (see PRECAUTIONS and DOSAGE AND ADMINISTRATION).

Pediatrics

Valacyclovir pharmacokinetics have not been evaluated in pediatric patients.

Liver Disease

Administration of valacyclovir HCl to patients with moderate (biopsy-proven cirrhosis) or severe (with and without ascites and biopsy-proven cirrhosis) liver disease indicated that the rate but not the extent of conversion of valacyclovir to acyclovir is reduced, and the acyclovir half-life is not affected. Dosage modification is not recommended for patients with cirrhosis.

HIV Disease

In 9 patients with HIV disease and CD4 cell counts <150 cells/mm^3 who received valacyclovir HCl at a dosage of 1 g four times daily for 30 days, the pharmacokinetics of valacyclovir and acyclovir were not different from that observed in healthy volunteers (see WARNINGS).

Drug Interactions

The pharmacokinetics of digoxin was not affected by coadministration of valacyclovir HCl 1 g three times daily, and the pharmacokinetics of acyclovir after a single dose of valacyclovir HCl (1 g) was unchanged by coadministration of digoxin (2 doses of 0.75 mg), single doses of antacids (Al^{3+} or Mg^{++}), or multiple doses of thiazide diuretics. Acyclovir C_{max} and AUC following a single dose of valacyclovir HCl (1 g) increased by 8% and 32%, respectively, after a single dose of cimetidine (800 mg), or by 22% and 49%, respectively, after probenecid (1 g), or by 30% and 78%, respectively, after a combination of cimetidine and probenecid, primarily due to a reduction in renal clearance of acyclovir. These effects are not considered to be of clinical significance in subjects with normal renal function. Therefore, no dosage adjustment is recommended when valacyclovir HCl is coadministered with digoxin, antacids, thiazide diuretics, cimetidine, or probenecid in subjects with normal renal function.

INDICATIONS AND USAGE

Herpes Zoster: Valacyclovir HCl is indicated for the treatment of herpes zoster (shingles).

Genital Herpes: Valacyclovir HCl is indicated for the treatment or suppression of genital herpes in immunocompetent individuals and for the suppression of recurrent genital herpes in HIV-infected individuals.

Cold Sores (herpes labialis): Valacyclovir HCl is indicated for the treatment of cold sores (herpes labialis).

CONTRAINDICATIONS

Valacyclovir HCl is contraindicated in patients with a known hypersensitivity or intolerance to valacyclovir, acyclovir, or any component of the formulation.

WARNINGS

Thrombotic thrombocytopenic purpura/hemolytic uremic syndrome (TTP/HUS), in some cases resulting in death, has occurred in patients with advanced HIV disease and also in allogenic bone marrow transplant and renal transplant recipients participating in clinical trials of valacyclovir HCl at doses of 8 g/day.

PRECAUTIONS

Dosage reduction is recommended when administering valacyclovir HCl to patients with renal impairment (see DOSAGE AND ADMINISTRATION). Acute renal failure and central nervous system symptoms have been reported in patients with underlying renal disease who have received inappropriately high doses of valacyclovir HCl for their level of renal function. Similar caution should be exercised when administering valacyclovir HCl to geriatric patients (see Geriatric Use) and patients receiving potentially nephrotoxic agents.

Given the dosage recommendations for treatment of cold sores, special attention should be paid when prescribing valacyclovir HCl for cold sores in patients who are elderly or who have impaired renal function (see DOSAGE AND ADMINISTRATION and Geriatric Use). Treatment should not exceed 1 day (2 doses of 2 g in 24 hours). Therapy beyond 1 day does not provide additional clinical benefit.

Precipitation of acyclovir in renal tubules may occur when the solubility (2.5 mg/ml) is exceeded in the intratubular fluid. In the event of acute renal failure and anuria, the patient may benefit from hemodialysis until renal function is restored (see DOSAGE AND ADMINISTRATION).

The safety and efficacy of valacyclovir HCl have not been established in immunocompromised patients other than for the suppression of genital herpes in HIV-infected patients. The safety and efficacy of valacyclovir HCl for suppression of recurrent genital herpes in patients with advanced HIV disease (CD4 cell count <100 cells/mm^3) have not been established. The efficacy of valacyclovir HCl for the treatment of genital herpes in HIV-infected patients has not been established. The safety and efficacy of valacyclovir HCl have not been established for the treatment of disseminated herpes zoster.

INFORMATION FOR THE PATIENT

Herpes Zoster

There are no data on treatment initiated more than 72 hours after onset of the zoster rash. Patients should be advised to initiate treatment as soon as possible after a diagnosis of herpes zoster.

Genital Herpes

Patients should be informed that valacyclovir HCl is not a cure for genital herpes. There are no data evaluating whether valacyclovir HCl will prevent transmission of infection to others. Because genital herpes is a sexually transmitted disease, patients should avoid contact with lesions or intercourse when lesions and/or symptoms are present to avoid infecting partners. Genital herpes can also be transmitted in the absence of symptoms through asymptomatic viral shedding. If medical management of a genital herpes recurrence is indicated, patients should be advised to initiate therapy at the first sign or symptom of an episode.

There are no data on the effectiveness of treatment initiated more than 72 hours after the onset of signs and symptoms of a first episode of genital herpes or more than 24 hours of the onset of signs and symptoms of a recurrent episode.

There are no data on the safety or effectiveness of chronic suppressive therapy of more than 1 year's duration in otherwise healthy patients. There are no data on the safety or effectiveness of chronic suppressive therapy of more than 6 months' duration in HIV-infected patients.

Cold Sores (herpes labialis)

Patients should be advised to initiate treatment at the earliest symptom of a cold sore (*e.g.*, tingling, itching, or burning). There are no data on the effectiveness of treatment initiated after the development of clinical signs of a cold sore (*e.g.*, papule, vesicle, or ulcer). Patients should be instructed that treatment for cold sores should not exceed 1 day (2 doses) and that

V

their doses should be taken about 12 hours apart. Patients should be informed that valacyclovir HCl is not a cure for cold sores (herpes labialis).

CARCINOGENESIS, MUTAGENESIS, AND IMPAIRMENT OF FERTILITY

The data presented below include references to the steady-state acyclovir AUC observed in humans treated with 1 g valacyclovir HCl given orally 3 times a day to treat herpes zoster. Plasma drug concentrations in animal studies are expressed as multiples of human exposure to acyclovir (see CLINICAL PHARMACOLOGY, Pharmacokinetics).

Valacyclovir was noncarcinogenic in lifetime carcinogenicity bioassays at single daily doses (gavage) of up to 120 mg/kg/day for mice and 100 mg/kg/day for rats. There was no significant difference in the incidence of tumors between treated and control animals, nor did valacyclovir shorten the latency of tumors. Plasma concentrations of acyclovir were equivalent to human levels in the mouse bioassay and 1.4-2.3 times human levels in the rat bioassay.

Valacyclovir was tested in 5 genetic toxicity assays. An Ames assay was negative in the absence or presence of metabolic activation. Also negative were an *in vitro* cytogenetic study with human lymphocytes and a rat cytogenetic study at a single oral dose of 3000 mg/kg (8-9 times human plasma levels).

In the mouse lymphoma assay, valacyclovir was not mutagenic in the absence of metabolic activation. In the presence of metabolic activation (76-88% conversion to acyclovir), valacyclovir was mutagenic.

Valacyclovir was not mutagenic in a mouse micronucleus assay at 250 mg/kg but positive at 500 mg/kg (acyclovir concentrations 26-51 times human plasma levels).

Valacyclovir did not impair fertility or reproduction in rats at 200 mg/kg/day (6 times human plasma levels).

PREGNANCY, TERATOGENIC EFFECTS, PREGNANCY CATEGORY B

Valacyclovir was not teratogenic in rats or rabbits given 400 mg/kg (which results in exposures of 10 and 7 times human plasma levels, respectively) during the period of major organogenesis.

There are no adequate and well-controlled studies of valacyclovir HCl or acyclovir in pregnant women. A prospective epidemiologic registry of acyclovir use during pregnancy was established in 1984 and completed in April 1999. There were 749 pregnancies followed in women exposed to systemic acyclovir during the first trimester of pregnancy resulting in 756 outcomes. The occurrence rate of birth defects approximates that found in the general population. However, the small size of the registry is insufficient to evaluate the risk for less common defects or to permit reliable or definitive conclusions regarding the safety of acyclovir in pregnant women and their developing fetuses. Valacyclovir HCl should be used during pregnancy only if the potential benefit justifies the potential risk to the fetus.

NURSING MOTHERS

There is no experience with valacyclovir HCl. However, acyclovir concentrations have been documented in breast milk in 2 women following oral administration of acyclovir and ranged from 0.6-4.1 times corresponding plasma levels. These concentrations would potentially expose the nursing infant to a dose of acyclovir as high as 0.3 mg/kg/day. Valacyclovir HCl should be administered to a nursing mother with caution and only when indicated.

PEDIATRIC USE

Safety and effectiveness of valacyclovir HCl in pre-pubertal pediatric patients have not been established.

GERIATRIC USE

Of the total number of subjects in clinical studies of valacyclovir HCl, 889 were 65 and over, and 350 were 75 and over. In a clinical study of herpes zoster, the duration of pain after healing (post-herpetic neuralgia) was longer in patients 65 and older compared with younger adults. Elderly patients are more likely to have reduced renal function and require dose reduction. Elderly patients are also more likely to have renal or CNS adverse events. With respect to CNS adverse events observed during clinical practice, agitation, hallucinations, confusion, delirium, and encephalopathy were reported more frequently in elderly patients (see CLINICAL PHARMACOLOGY; ADVERSE REACTIONS, Observed During Clinical Practice; and DOSAGE AND ADMINISTRATION).

DRUG INTERACTIONS

See CLINICAL PHARMACOLOGY, Pharmacokinetics.

ADVERSE REACTIONS

Frequently reported adverse events in clinical trials of valacyclovir HCl in healthy patients are listed in TABLE 3, TABLE 4A and TABLE 4B.

TABLE 3 *Incidence of Adverse Events in Herpes Zoster Study Populations*

Adverse Event	Valacyclovir HCl (1 g tid) (n=967)	Placebo (n=195)
Nausea	15%	8%
Headache	14%	12%
Vomiting	6%	3%
Dizziness	3%	2%
Abdominal pain	3%	2%

Laboratory abnormalities reported in clinical trials of valacyclovir HCl in otherwise healthy patients are listed in TABLE 5A, TABLE 5B, and TABLE 5C.

SUPPRESSION OF GENITAL HERPES IN HIV-INFECTED PATIENTS

In HIV-infected patients, frequently reported adverse events for valacyclovir HCl (500 mg twice daily; n=194, median days on therapy = 172) and placebo (n=99, median days on therapy = 59), respectively, included headache (13% vs 8%), fatigue (8% vs 5%), and rash (8% vs 1%). Post-randomization laboratory abnormalities that were reported more frequently in valacyclovir subjects versus placebo included elevated alkaline phosphatase (4% vs 2%), elevated ALT (14% vs 10%), elevated AST (16% vs 11%), decreased neutrophil counts (18% vs 10%), and decreased platelet counts (3% vs 0%).

TABLE 4A *Incidence of Adverse Events in Genital Herpes Treatment Study Populations*

Adverse Event	Valacyclovir HCl 1 g bid (n=1194)	Valacyclovir HCl 500 mg bid (n=1159)	Placebo (n=439)
Nausea	6%	5%	8%
Headache	16%	15%	14%
Vomiting	1%	<1%	<1%
Dizziness	3%	2%	3%
Abdominal pain	2%	1%	3%
Dysmenorrhea	<1%	<1%	1%
Arthralgia	<1%	<1%	<1%
Depression	1%	0%	<1%

TABLE 4B *Incidence of Adverse Events in Genital Herpes Suppression Study Populations*

Adverse Event	Valacyclovir HCl 1 g qd (n=269)	Valacyclovir HCl 500 mg qd (n=266)	Placebo (n=134)
Nausea	11%	11%	8%
Headache	35%	38%	34%
Vomiting	3%	3%	2%
Dizziness	4%	2%	1%
Abdominal pain	11%	9%	6%
Dysmenorrhea	8%	5%	4%
Arthralgia	6%	5%	4%
Depression	7%	5%	5%

TABLE 5A *Incidence of Laboratory Abnormalities in Herpes Zoster Study Populations*

Laboratory Abnormality	Valacyclovir HCl (1 g tid)	Placebo
Hemoglobin (<0.8 × LLN)	0.8%	0%
White blood cells (<0.75 × LLN)	1.3%	0.6%
Platelet count (<100,000/mm³)	1.0%	1.2%
AST (SGOT) (>2 × ULN)	1.0%	0%
Serum creatinine (>1.5 × ULN)	0.2%	0%

LLN = Lower limit of normal.
ULN = Upper limit of normal.

TABLE 5B *Incidence of Laboratory Abnormalities in Genital Herpes Treatment Study Populations*

Laboratory Abnormality	Valacyclovir HCl 1 g bid	Valacyclovir HCl 500 mg bid	Placebo
Hemoglobin (<0.8 × LLN)	0.3%	0.2%	0%
White blood cells (<0.75 × LLN)	0.7%	0.6%	0.2%
Platelet count (<100,000/mm³)	0.3%	0.1%	0.7%
AST (SGOT) (>2 × ULN)	1.0%	*	0.5%
Serum creatinine (>1.5 × ULN)	0.7%	0%	0%

* Data were not collected prospectively.
LLN = Lower limit of normal.
ULN = Upper limit of normal.

TABLE 5C *Incidence of Laboratory Abnormalities in Genital Herpes Suppression Study Populations*

Laboratory Abnormality	Valacyclovir HCl 1 g qd	Valacyclovir HCl 500 mg qd	Placebo
Hemoglobin (<0.8 × LLN)	0%	0.8%	0.8%
White blood cells (<0.75 × LLN)	0.7%	0.8%	1.5%
Platelet count (<100,000/mm³)	0.4%	1.1%	1.5%
AST (SGOT) (>2 × ULN)	4.1%	3.8%	3.0%
Serum creatinine (>1.5 × ULN)	0%	0%	0%

LLN = Lower limit of normal.
ULN = Upper limit of normal.

COLD SORES (HERPES LABIALIS)

In clinical studies for the treatment of cold sores, the adverse events reported by patients receiving valacyclovir HCl (n=609) or placebo (n=609) included headache (valacyclovir HCl 14%, placebo 10%) and dizziness (valacyclovir HCl 2%, placebo 1%). The frequencies of abnormal ALT (>2 × ULN) were 1.8% for patients receiving valacyclovir HCl compared with 0.8% for placebo. Other laboratory abnormalities (hemoglobin, white blood cells, alkaline phosphatase, and serum creatinine) occurred with similar frequencies in the 2 groups.

OBSERVED DURING CLINICAL PRACTICE

The following events have been identified during post-approval use of valacyclovir HCl in clinical practice. Because they are reported voluntarily from a population of unknown size, estimates of frequency cannot be made. These events have been chosen for inclusion due to either their seriousness, frequency of reporting, causal connection to valacyclovir HCl, or a combination of these factors.

General: Facial edema, hypertension, tachycardia.

Allergic: Acute hypersensitivity reactions including anaphylaxis, angioedema, dyspnea, pruritus, rash, and urticaria.

CNS Symptoms: Aggressive behavior; agitation; ataxia; coma; confusion; decreased consciousness; dysarthria; encephalopathy; mania; and psychosis, including auditory and visual hallucinations; seizures; tremors (see PRECAUTIONS).

Eye: Visual abnormalities.

Gastrointestinal: Diarrhea.

Hepatobiliary Tract and Pancreas: Liver enzyme abnormalities, hepatitis.

Renal: Elevated creatinine, renal failure.

Hematologic: Thrombocytopenia, aplastic anemia, leukocytoclastic vasculitis, TTP/HUS.

Skin: Erythema multiforme, rashes including photosensitivity, alopecia.

RENAL IMPAIRMENT

Renal failure and CNS symptoms have been reported in patients with renal impairment who received valacyclovir HCl or acyclovir at greater than the recommended dose. **Dose reduction is recommended in this patient population (see DOSAGE AND ADMINISTRATION).**

DOSAGE AND ADMINISTRATION

Valacyclovir HCl caplets may be given without regard to meals.

HERPES ZOSTER

The recommended dosage of valacyclovir HCl for the treatment of herpes zoster is 1 g orally 3 times daily for 7 days. Therapy should be initiated at the earliest sign or symptom of herpes zoster and is most effective when started within 48 hours of the onset of zoster rash. No data are available on efficacy of treatment started greater than 72 hours after rash onset.

GENITAL HERPES

Initial Episodes

The recommended dosage of valacyclovir HCl for treatment of initial genital herpes is 1 g twice daily for 10 days.

There are no data on the effectiveness of treatment with valacyclovir HCl when initiated more than 72 hours after the onset of signs and symptoms. Therapy was most effective when administered within 48 hours of the onset of signs and symptoms.

Recurrent Episodes

The recommended dosages of valacyclovir HCl for the treatment of recurrent genital herpes is 500 mg twice daily for 3 days.

If medical management of a genital herpes recurrence is indicated, patients should be advised to initiate therapy at the first sign or symptom of an episode. There are no data on the effectiveness of treatment with valacyclovir HCl when initiated more than 24 hours after the onset of signs or symptoms.

Suppressive Therapy

The recommended dosage of valacyclovir HCl for chronic suppressive therapy of recurrent genital herpes is 1 g once daily in patients with normal immune function. In patients with a history of 9 or fewer recurrences/year, an alternative dose is 500 mg once daily. The safety and efficacy of therapy with valacyclovir HCl beyond 1 year have not been established.

In HIV-infected patients with CD4 cell count ≥100 cells/mm^3, the recommended dosage of valacyclovir HCl for chronic suppressive therapy of recurrent genital herpes is 500 mg twice daily. The safety and efficacy of therapy with valacyclovir HCl beyond 6 months in patients with HIV infection have not been established.

Cold Sores (herpes labialis)

The recommended dosage of valacyclovir HCl for the treatment of cold sores is 2 g twice daily for 1 day taken about 12 hours apart. Therapy should be initiated at the earliest symptom of a cold sore (*e.g.*, tingling, itching, or burning). There are no data on the effectiveness of treatment initiated after the development of clinical signs of a cold sore (*e.g.*, papule, vesicle, or ulcer).

PATIENTS WITH ACUTE OR CHRONIC RENAL IMPAIRMENT

In patients with reduced renal function, reduction in dosage is recommended (see TABLE 6).

HEMODIALYSIS

During hemodialysis, the half-life of acyclovir after administration of valacyclovir HCl is approximately 4 hours. About one-third of acyclovir in the body is removed by dialysis during a 4 hour hemodialysis session. Patients requiring hemodialysis should receive the recommended dose of valacyclovir HCl after hemodialysis.

PERITONEAL DIALYSIS

There is no information specific to administration of valacyclovir HCl in patients receiving peritoneal dialysis. The effect of chronic ambulatory peritoneal dialysis (CAPD) and continuous arteriovenous hemofiltration/dialysis (CAVHD) on acyclovir pharmacokinetics has been studied. The removal of acyclovir after CAPD and CAVHD is less pronounced than with hemodialysis, and the pharmacokinetic parameters closely resemble those observed in patients with ESRD not receiving hemodialysis. Therefore, supplemental doses of valacyclovir HCl should not be required following CAPD or CAVHD.

TABLE 6 *Dosages for Patients With Renal Impairment*

Indications	Normal Dosage Regimen (Creatinine Clearance ≥50)	Creatinine Clearance (ml/min)		
		30-49	10-29	<10
Herpes Zoster	1 g q8h	1 g q12h	1 g q24h	500 mg q24h
Genital Herpes				
Initial treatment	1 g q12h	no reduction	1 g q24h	500 mg q24h
Recurrent episodes	500 mg q12h	no reduction	500 mg q24h	500 mg q24h
Suppressive therapy	1 g q24h	no reduction	500 mg q24h	500 mg q24h
Suppressive therapy	500 mg q24h	no reduction	500 mg q48h	500 mg q48h
Suppressive therapy in HIV-infected patients	500 mg q12h	no reduction	500 mg q24h	500 mg q24h
Herpes Labialis (Cold Sores)*	Two 2 g doses†	Two 1 g doses†	Two 500 mg doses†	500 mg single dose

*** Do not exceed 1 day of treatment.**
† Taken about 12 hours apart.

HOW SUPPLIED

Valtrex Caplets

500 mg: Blue, film-coated, capsule-shaped tablets containing valacyclovir HCl equivalent to 500 mg valacyclovir and printed with "VALTREX 500 mg".

1 g: Blue, film-coated, capsule-shaped tablets containing valacyclovir HCl equivalent to 1 g valacyclovir and printed with "VALTREX 1 gram".

Storage: Store at 15-25°C (59-77°F).

PRODUCT LISTING - EQUIVALENTS NOT AVAILABLE

Tablet - Oral - 1 Gm

Qty	Price	Product	NDC
20's	$112.98	VALTREX, Glaxo Wellcome	00173-0565-00
21's	$155.49	VALTREX, Glaxosmithkline	00173-0565-02

Tablet - Oral - 500 mg

Qty	Price	Product	NDC
7's	$31.28	VALTREX, Pd-Rx Pharmaceuticals	55289-0926-07
10's	$33.83	VALTREX, Allscripts Pharmaceutical Company	54569-4280-00
10's	$35.20	VALTREX, Physicians Total Care	54868-3804-00
10's	$50.15	VALTREX, Pd-Rx Pharmaceuticals	55289-0926-10
10's	$52.25	VALTREX, Pharma Pac	52959-0641-10
14's	$47.36	VALTREX, Allscripts Pharmaceutical Company	54569-4280-01
14's	$71.68	VALTREX, Pharma Pac	52959-0641-14
14's	$115.92	VALTREX, Pd-Rx Pharmaceuticals	55289-0926-14
30's	$130.50	VALTREX, Glaxosmithkline	00173-0933-08
30's	$148.80	VALTREX, Pharma Pac	52959-0641-30
42's	$142.09	VALTREX, Allscripts Pharmaceutical Company	54569-4280-02
42's	$155.11	VALTREX, Physicians Total Care	54868-3804-01
42's	$169.26	VALTREX, Glaxosmithkline	00173-0933-03
42's	$186.56	VALTREX, Pharma Pac	52959-0641-42
100's	$444.70	VALTREX, Glaxosmithkline	00173-0933-56

Valdecoxib *(003541)*

For related information, see the comparative table section in Appendix A.

Categories: Arthritis, osteoarthritis; Arthritis, rheumatoid; Dysmenorrhea; FDA Approved 2001 Nov; Pregnancy Category C
Drug Classes: Analgesics, non-narcotic; COX-2 inhibitors; Nonsteroidal anti-inflammatory drugs
Brand Names: **Bextra**
Foreign Brand Availability: Valus (India)
Cost of Therapy: $91.47 (Arthritis; Bextra; 10 mg; 1 tablet/day; 30 day supply)
$182.95 (Dysmenorrhea; Bextra; 20 mg; 2 tablets/day; 30 day supply)

DESCRIPTION

Valdecoxib is chemically designated as 4-(5-methyl-3-phenyl-4-isoxazolyl)benzenesulfonamide and is a diaryl substituted isoxazole.

The empirical formula for valdecoxib is $C_{16}H_{14}N_2O_3S$, and the molecular weight is 314.36. Valdecoxib is a white crystalline powder that is relatively insoluble in water (10 µg/ml) at 25°C and pH 7.0, soluble in methanol and ethanol, and freely soluble in organic solvents and alkaline (pH=12) aqueous solutions.

Bextra tablets for oral administration contain either 10 or 20 mg of valdecoxib. Inactive ingredients include lactose monohydrate, microcrystalline cellulose, pregelatinized starch, croscarmellose sodium, magnesium stearate, hydroxypropyl methylcellulose, polyethylene glycol, polysorbate 80, and titanium dioxide.

CLINICAL PHARMACOLOGY

MECHANISM OF ACTION

Valdecoxib is a nonsteroidal anti-inflammatory drug (NSAID) that exhibits anti-inflammatory, analgesic and antipyretic properties in animal models. The mechanism of action is believed to be due to inhibition of prostaglandin synthesis primarily through inhibition of cyclooxygenase-2 (COX-2). At therapeutic plasma concentrations in humans valdecoxib does not inhibit cyclooxygenase-1 (COX-1).

V

PHARMACOKINETICS

Absorption

Valdecoxib achieves maximal plasma concentrations in approximately 3 hours. The absolute bioavailability of valdecoxib is 83% following oral administration of valdecoxib compared to IV infusion of valdecoxib.

Dose proportionality was demonstrated after single doses (1-400 mg) of valdecoxib. With multiple doses (up to 100 mg/day for 14 days), valdecoxib exposure as measured by the AUC, increases in a more than proportional manner at doses above 10 mg bid. Steady state plasma concentrations of valdecoxib are achieved by Day 4.

The steady state pharmacokinetic parameters of valdecoxib in healthy male subjects are shown in TABLE 1.

***TABLE 1** Mean (SD) Steady State Pharmacokinetic Parameters After Valdecoxib 10 mg Once Daily for 14 Days*

Pharmacokinetic Parameter	Healthy Male Subjects (n=8, 20-42 years)
AUC(0-24h) (h·ng/ml)	1479.0 (291.9)
C_{max} (ng/ml)	161.1 (48.1)
T_{max} (h)	2.25 (0.71)
C_{min} (ng/ml)	21.9 (7.68)
Elimination half-life (h)	8.11 (1.32)

No clinically significant age or gender differences were seen in pharmacokinetic parameters that would require dosage adjustments.

Effect of Food and Antacid

Valdecoxib can be taken with or without food. Food had no significant effect on either the peak plasma concentration (C_{max}) or extent of absorption (AUC) of valdecoxib when valdecoxib was taken with a high fat meal. The time to peak plasma concentration (T_{max}), however, was delayed by 1-2 hours. Administration of valdecoxib with antacid (aluminum/magnesium hydroxide) had no significant effect on either the rate or extent of absorption of valdecoxib.

Distribution

Plasma protein binding for valdecoxib is about 98% over the concentration range (21-2384 ng/ml). Steady state apparent volume of distribution (Vss/F) of valdecoxib is approximately 86 L after oral administration. Valdecoxib and its active metabolite preferentially partition into erythrocytes with a blood to plasma concentration ratio of about 2.5:1. This ratio remains approximately constant with time and therapeutic blood concentrations.

Metabolism

In humans, valdecoxib undergoes extensive hepatic metabolism involving both P450 isoenzymes (3A4 and 2C9) and non-P450 dependent pathways (*i.e.,* glucuronidation). Concomitant administration of valdecoxib with known CYP 3A4 and 2C9 inhibitors (*e.g.,* fluconazole and ketoconazole) can result in increased plasma exposure of valdecoxib (see DRUG INTERACTIONS).

One active metabolite of valdecoxib has been identified in human plasma at approximately 10% the concentration of valdecoxib. This metabolite, which is a less potent COX-2 specific inhibitor than the parent, also undergoes extensive metabolism and constitutes less than 2% of the valdecoxib dose excreted in the urine and feces. Due to its low concentration in the systemic circulation, it is not likely to contribute significantly to the efficacy profile of valdecoxib.

Excretion

Valdecoxib is eliminated predominantly via hepatic metabolism with less than 5% of the dose excreted unchanged in the urine and feces. About 70% of the dose is excreted in the urine as metabolites, and about 20% as valdecoxib N-glucuronide. The apparent oral clearance (CL/F) of valdecoxib is about 6 L/h. The elimination half-life ($T_{½}$) ranges from 8-11 hours and increases with age.

SPECIAL POPULATIONS

Geriatric

In elderly subjects (>65 years), weight-adjusted steady state plasma concentrations [AUC(0-12h)] are about 30% higher than in young subjects. No dose adjustment is needed based on age.

Pediatric

Valdecoxib has not been investigated in pediatric patients below 18 years of age.

Race

Pharmacokinetic differences due to race have not been identified in clinical and pharmacokinetic studies conducted to date.

Hepatic Insufficiency

Valdecoxib plasma concentrations are significantly increased (130%) in patients with moderate (Child-Pugh Class B) hepatic impairment. In clinical trials, doses of valdecoxib above those recommended have been associated with fluid retention. Hence, treatment with valdecoxib should be initiated with caution in patients with mild to moderate hepatic impairment and fluid retention. The use of valdecoxib in patients with severe hepatic impairment (Child-Pugh Class C) is not recommended.

Renal Insufficiency

The pharmacokinetics of valdecoxib have been studied in patients with varying degrees of renal impairment. Because renal elimination of valdecoxib is not important to its disposition, no clinically significant changes in valdecoxib clearance were found even in patients with severe renal impairment or in patients undergoing renal dialysis. In patients undergoing hemodialysis the plasma clearance (CL/F) of valdecoxib was similar to the CL/F found in healthy elderly subjects (CL/F about 6-7 L/h) with normal renal function (based on creatinine clearance).

NSAIDs have been associated with worsening renal function and use in advanced renal disease is not recommended (see PRECAUTIONS, Renal Effects).

DRUG INTERACTIONS

Also see DRUG INTERACTIONS.

General

Valdecoxib undergoes both P450 (CYP) dependent and non-P450 dependent (glucuronidation) metabolism. *In vitro* studies indicate that valdecoxib is not a significant inhibitor of CYP 1A2, 3A4, or 2D6 and is only a weak inhibitor of CYP 2C9 and 2C19 at therapeutic concentrations. The P450-mediated metabolic pathway of valdecoxib predominantly involves the 3A4 and 2C9 isozymes. Using prototype inhibitors and substrates of these isozymes, the following results were obtained. Coadministration of a known inhibitor of CYP 2C9/3A4 (fluconazole) and a CYP 3A4 (ketoconazole) inhibitor enhanced the total plasma exposure (AUC) of valdecoxib. Coadministration of valdecoxib with warfarin caused a small, but statistically significant increase in plasma exposures of R-warfarin and S-warfarin, and also in the pharmacodynamic effects (International Normalized Ratio-INR) of warfarin. (See DRUG INTERACTIONS.)

Coadministration of valdecoxib, or its injectable prodrug, with substrates of CYP 2C9 (propofol) and CYP 3A4 (midazolam, alfentanil, fentanyl) did not inhibit the metabolism of either substrate.

Coadministration of valdecoxib with a CYP 3A4 substrate (glyburide) or a CYP 2D6 substrate (dextromethorphan) did not result in clinically important inhibition in the metabolism of these agents.

INDICATIONS AND USAGE

Valdecoxib tablets are indicated:

For relief of the signs and symptoms of osteoarthritis and adult rheumatoid arthritis.

For the treatment of primary dysmenorrhea.

CONTRAINDICATIONS

Valdecoxib should not be given to patients who have demonstrated allergic-type reactions to sulfonamides. Valdecoxib tablets are contraindicated in patients with known hypersensitivity to valdecoxib. Valdecoxib should not be given to patients who have experienced asthma, urticaria, or allergic-type reactions after taking aspirin or NSAIDs. Severe, rarely fatal, anaphylactic-like reactions to NSAIDs are possible in such patients (see WARNINGS, Anaphylactoid Reactions; and PRECAUTIONS, Preexisting Asthma).

WARNINGS

GASTROINTESTINAL (GI) EFFECTS — RISK OF GI ULCERATION, BLEEDING, AND PERFORATION

Serious gastrointestinal toxicity such as bleeding, ulceration and perforation of the stomach, small intestine or large intestine can occur at any time with or without warning symptoms in patients treated with nonsteroidal anti-inflammatory drugs (NSAIDs). Minor gastrointestinal problems such as dyspepsia are common and may also occur at any time during NSAID therapy. Therefore, physicians and patients should remain alert for ulceration and bleeding even in the absence of previous GI tract symptoms. Patients should be informed about the signs and symptoms of serious GI toxicity and the steps to take if they occur. The utility of periodic laboratory monitoring has not been demonstrated, nor has it been adequately assessed. Only 1 in 5 patients who develop a serious upper GI adverse event on NSAID therapy is symptomatic. It has been demonstrated that upper GI ulcers, gross bleeding or perforation caused by NSAIDs appear to occur in approximately 1% of patients treated for 3-6 months and 2-4% of patients treated for 1 year. These trends continue, thus increasing the likelihood of developing a serious GI event at some time during the course of therapy. However, even short-term therapy is not without risk.

NSAIDs should be prescribed with extreme caution in patients with a prior history of ulcer disease or gastrointestinal bleeding. Most spontaneous reports of fatal GI events are in elderly or debilitated patients and therefore special care should be taken in treating this population. For high risk patients, alternate therapies that do not involve NSAIDs should be considered.

Studies have shown that patients with a *prior history of peptic ulcer disease and/or gastrointestinal bleeding* and who use NSAIDs, have a greater than 10-fold higher risk for developing a GI bleed than patients with neither of these risk factors. In addition to a past history of ulcer disease, pharmacoepidemiological studies have identified several other co-therapies or co-morbid conditions that may increase the risk for GI bleeding such as: treatment with oral corticosteroids, treatment with anticoagulants, longer duration of NSAID therapy, smoking, alcoholism, older age, and poor general health status.

SERIOUS SKIN REACTIONS

Serious skin reactions, including exfoliative dermatitis, Stevens-Johnson syndrome, and toxic epidermal necrolysis, have been reported through postmarketing surveillance in patients receiving valdecoxib (see ADVERSE REACTIONS, Postmarketing Experience). As these reactions can be life-threatening, valdecoxib should be discontinued at the first appearance of skin rash or any other sign of hypersensitivity.

ANAPHYLACTOID REACTIONS

In postmarketing experience, cases of hypersensitivity reactions (anaphylactic reactions and angioedema) have been reported in patients receiving valdecoxib (see ADVERSE REACTIONS, Postmarketing Experience). These cases have occurred in patients with and without a history of allergic-type reactions to sulfonamides (see CONTRAINDICATIONS). Valdecoxib should not be given to patients with the aspirin triad. This symptom complex typically occurs in asthmatic patients who experience rhinitis with or without nasal polyps, or who exhibit severe, potentially fatal bronchospasm after taking aspirin or other NSAIDs (see CONTRAINDICATIONS and PRECAUTIONS, Preexisting Asthma). Emergency help should be sought in cases where an anaphylactoid reaction occurs.

ADVANCED RENAL DISEASE

No information is available regarding the safe use of valdecoxib tablets in patients with advanced kidney disease. Therefore, treatment with valdecoxib is not recommended in these patients. If therapy with valdecoxib must be initiated, close monitoring of the patient's kidney function is advisable (see PRECAUTIONS, Renal Effects).

PREGNANCY

In late pregnancy, valdecoxib should be avoided because it may cause premature closure of the ductus arteriosus.

PRECAUTIONS

GENERAL

Valdecoxib tablets cannot be expected to substitute for corticosteroids or to treat corticosteroid insufficiency. Abrupt discontinuation of corticosteroids may lead to exacerbation of corticosteroid-responsive illness. Patients on prolonged corticosteroid therapy should have their therapy tapered slowly if a decision is made to discontinue corticosteroids.

The pharmacological activity of valdecoxib in reducing fever and inflammation may diminish the utility of these diagnostic signs in detecting complications of presumed noninfectious, painful conditions.

HEPATIC EFFECTS

Borderline elevations of 1 or more liver tests may occur in up to 15% of patients taking NSAIDs. Notable elevations of ALT or AST (approximately 3 or more times the upper limit of normal) have been reported in approximately 1% of patients in clinical trials with NSAIDs. These laboratory abnormalities may progress, may remain unchanged, or may remain transient with continuing therapy. Rare cases of severe hepatic reactions, including jaundice and fatal fulminant hepatitis, liver necrosis and hepatic failure (some with fatal outcome) have been reported with NSAIDs. In controlled clinical trials of valdecoxib, the incidence of borderline (defined as 1.2- to 3.0-fold) elevations of liver tests was 8.0% for valdecoxib and 8.4% for placebo, while approximately 0.3% of patients taking valdecoxib, and 0.2% of patients taking placebo, had notable (defined as greater than 3-fold) elevations of ALT or AST.

A patient with symptoms and/or signs suggesting liver dysfunction, or in whom an abnormal liver test has occurred, should be monitored carefully for evidence of the development of a more severe hepatic reaction while on therapy with valdecoxib. If clinical signs and symptoms consistent with liver disease develop, or if systemic manifestations occur (*e.g.*, eosinophilia, rash), valdecoxib should be discontinued.

RENAL EFFECTS

Long-term administration of NSAIDs has resulted in renal papillary necrosis and other renal injury. Renal toxicity has also been seen in patients in whom renal prostaglandins have a compensatory role in the maintenance of renal perfusion. In these patients, administration of a nonsteroidal anti-inflammatory drug may cause a dose-dependent reduction in prostaglandin formation and, secondarily, in renal blood flow, which may precipitate overt renal decompensation. Patients at greatest risk of this reaction are those with impaired renal function, heart failure, liver dysfunction, those taking diuretics and Angiotensin Converting Enzyme (ACE) inhibitors, and the elderly. Discontinuation of NSAID therapy is usually followed by recovery to the pretreatment state.

Caution should be used when initiating treatment with valdecoxib in patients with considerable dehydration. It is advisable to rehydrate patients first and then start therapy with valdecoxib. Caution is also recommended in patients with preexisting kidney disease. (See WARNINGS, Advanced Renal Disease.)

HEMATOLOGICAL EFFECTS

Anemia is sometimes seen in patients receiving valdecoxib. Patients on long-term treatment with valdecoxib should have their hemoglobin or hematocrit checked if they exhibit any signs or symptoms of anemia.

Valdecoxib does not generally affect platelet counts, prothrombin time (PT), or activated partial thromboplastin (APTT), and does not appear to inhibit platelet aggregation at indicated dosages.

FLUID RETENTION AND EDEMA

Fluid retention and edema have been observed in some patients taking valdecoxib (see ADVERSE REACTIONS). Therefore, valdecoxib should be used with caution in patients with fluid retention, hypertension, or heart failure.

PREEXISTING ASTHMA

Patients with asthma may have aspirin-sensitive asthma. The use of aspirin in patients with aspirin-sensitive asthma has been associated with severe bronchospasm, which can be fatal. Since cross reactivity, including bronchospasm, between aspirin and other nonsteroidal anti-inflammatory drugs has been reported in such aspirin-sensitive patients, valdecoxib should not be administered to patients with this form of aspirin sensitivity and should be used with caution in patients with preexisting asthma.

INFORMATION FOR THE PATIENT

Valdecoxib can cause GI discomfort and, rarely, more serious GI side effects, which may result in hospitalization and even fatal outcomes. Although serious GI tract ulcerations and bleeding can occur without warning symptoms, patients should be alert for the signs and symptoms of ulcerations and bleeding, and should ask for medical advice when observing any indicative sign or symptoms.

Patients should be apprised of the importance of this follow-up (see WARNINGS, Gastrointestinal (GI) Effects — Risk of GI Ulceration, Bleeding, and Perforation).

Patients should report to their physicians, signs or symptoms of gastrointestinal ulceration or bleeding, skin rash, weight gain, or edema.

Patients should be informed of the warning signs and symptoms of hepatotoxicity (*e.g.*, nausea, fatigue, lethargy, pruritus, jaundice, right upper quadrant tenderness, and flu-like symptoms). If these occur, patients should be instructed to stop therapy and seek immediate medical attention.

Patients should also be instructed to seek immediate emergency help in the case of an anaphylactoid reaction (see WARNINGS, Anaphylactoid Reactions).

In late pregnancy, valdecoxib should be avoided because it may cause premature closure of the ductus arteriosus.

LABORATORY TESTS

Because serious GI tract ulcerations and bleeding can occur without warning symptoms, physicians should monitor for signs and symptoms of GI bleeding.

CARCINOGENESIS, MUTAGENESIS, AND IMPAIRMENT OF FERTILITY

Valdecoxib was not carcinogenic in rats given oral doses up to 7.5 mg/kg/day for males and 1.5 mg/kg/day for females [equivalent to approximately 2- to 6-fold human exposure at 20 mg qd as measured by the AUC(0-24h)] or in mice given oral doses up to 25 mg/kg/day for males and 50 mg/kg/day for females [equivalent to approximately 0.6- to 2.4-fold human exposure at 20 mg qd as measured by the AUC(0-24h)] for 2 years.

Valdecoxib was not mutagenic in an Ames test or a mutation assay in Chinese hamster ovary (CHO) cells, nor was it clastogenic in a chromosome aberration assay in CHO cells or in an *in vivo* micronucleus test in rat bone marrow.

Valdecoxib did not impair male rat fertility at oral doses up to 9.0 mg/kg/day [equivalent to approximately 3- to 6-fold human exposure at 20 mg qd as measured by the AUC(0-24h)]. In female rats, a decrease in ovulation with increased pre- and post-implantation loss resulted in decreased live embryos/fetuses at doses ≥2 mg/kg/day [equivalent to approximately 2-fold human exposure at 20 mg qd as measured by the AUC(0-24h) for valdecoxib]. The effects on female fertility were reversible. This effect is expected with inhibition of prostaglandin synthesis and is not the result of irreversible alteration of female reproductive function.

PREGNANCY

Teratogenic Effects: Pregnancy Category C

The incidence of fetuses with skeletal anomalies such as semi-bipartite thoracic vertebra centra and fused sternebrae was slightly higher in rabbits at an oral dose of 40 mg/kg/day [equivalent to approximately 72-fold human exposures at 20 mg qd as measured by the AUC(0-24h)] throughout organogenesis. Valdecoxib was not teratogenic in rabbits up to an oral dose of 10 mg/kg/day [equivalent to approximately 8-fold human exposures at 20 mg qd as measured by the AUC(0-24h)].

Valdecoxib was not teratogenic in rats up to an oral dose of 10 mg/kg/day [equivalent to approximately 19-fold human exposure at 20 mg qd as measured by the AUC(0-24h)]. There are no studies in pregnant women. However, valdecoxib crosses the placenta in rats and rabbits. Valdecoxib should be used during pregnancy only if the potential benefit justifies the potential risk to the fetus.

Nonteratogenic Effects

Valdecoxib caused increased pre-and post-implantation loss with reduced live fetuses at oral doses ≥10 mg/kg/day [equivalent to approximately 19-fold human exposure at 20 mg qd as measured by the AUC(0-24h)] in rats and an oral dose of 40 mg/kg/day [equivalent to approximately 72-fold human exposure at 20 mg qd as measured by the AUC(0-24h)] in rabbits throughout organogenesis. In addition, reduced neonatal survival and decreased neonatal body weight when rats were treated with valdecoxib at oral doses ≥6 mg/kg/day [equivalent to approximately 7-fold human exposure at 20 mg qd as measured by the AUC(0-24h)] throughout organogenesis and lactation period. No studies have been conducted to evaluate the effect of valdecoxib on the closure of the ductus arteriosus in humans. Therefore, as with other drugs known to inhibit prostaglandin synthesis, use of valdecoxib during the third trimester of pregnancy should be avoided.

LABOR AND DELIVERY

Valdecoxib produced no evidence of delayed labor or parturition at oral doses up to 10 mg/kg/day in rats [equivalent to approximately 19-fold human exposure at 20 mg qd as measured by the AUC(0-24h)]. The effects of valdecoxib on labor and delivery in pregnant women are unknown.

NURSING MOTHERS

Valdecoxib and its active metabolite are excreted in the milk of lactating rats. It is not known whether this drug is excreted in human milk. Because many drugs are excreted in human milk, and because of the potential for adverse reactions in nursing infants from valdecoxib, a decision should be made whether to discontinue nursing or to discontinue the drug, taking into account the importance of the drug to the mother and the importance of nursing to the infant.

PEDIATRIC USE

Safety and effectiveness of valdecoxib in pediatric patients below the age of 18 years have not been evaluated.

GERIATRIC USE

Of the patients who received valdecoxib in arthritis clinical trials of 3 months duration, or greater, approximately 2100 were 65 years of age or older, including 570 patients who were 75 years or older. No overall differences in effectiveness were observed between these patients and younger patients.

DRUG INTERACTIONS

The drug interaction studies with valdecoxib were performed both with valdecoxib and a rapidly hydrolyzed IV prodrug form. The results from trials using the IV prodrug are reported in this section as they relate to the role of valdecoxib in drug interactions.

General: In humans, valdecoxib metabolism is predominantly mediated via CYP 3A4 and 2C9 with glucuronidation being a further (20%) route of metabolism. *In vitro* studies indicate that valdecoxib is a moderate inhibitor of CYP 2C19 (IC_{50} = 6 µg/ml), and a weak inhibitor of both 3A4 (IC_{50} = 44 µg/ml) and 2C9 (IC_{50} = 13 µg/ml). In view of the limitations of *in vitro* studies and the high valdecoxib IC_{50} values, the

V

potential for such metabolic inhibitory effects *in vivo* at therapeutic doses of valdecoxib is low.

Aspirin: Concomitant administration of aspirin with valdecoxib may result in an increased risk of GI ulceration and complications compared to valdecoxib alone. Because of its lack of anti-platelet effect valdecoxib is not a substitute for aspirin for cardiovascular prophylaxis.

In a parallel group drug interaction study comparing the IV prodrug form of valdecoxib at 40 mg bid (n=10) vs placebo (n=9), valdecoxib had no effect on *in vitro* aspirin-mediated inhibition of arachidonate- or collagen-stimulated platelet aggregation.

Methotrexate: Valdecoxib 10 mg bid did not show a significant effect on the plasma exposure or renal clearance of methotrexate.

ACE-Inhibitors: Reports suggest that NSAIDs may diminish the antihypertensive effect of ACE-inhibitors. This interaction should be given consideration in patients taking valdecoxib concomitantly with ACE-inhibitors.

Furosemide: Clinical studies, as well as post-marketing observations, have shown that NSAIDs can reduce the natriuretic effect of furosemide and thiazides in some patients. This response has been attributed to inhibition of renal prostaglandin synthesis.

Anticonvulsants: Anticonvulsant drug interaction studies with valdecoxib have not been conducted. As with other drugs, routine monitoring should be performed when therapy with valdecoxib is either initiated or discontinued in patients on anticonvulsant therapy.

Dextromethorphan: Dextromethorphan is primarily metabolized by CYP 2D6 and to a lesser extent by 3A4. Coadministration with valdecoxib (40 mg bid for 7 days) resulted in a significant increase in dextromethorphan plasma levels suggesting that, at these doses, valdecoxib is a weak inhibitor of 2D6. Dextromethorphan plasma concentrations in the presence of high doses of valdecoxib were almost 5-fold lower than those seen in CYP 2D6 poor metabolizers.

Lithium: Valdecoxib 40 mg bid for 7 days produced significant decreases in lithium serum clearance (25%) and renal clearance (30%) with a 34% higher serum exposure compared to lithium alone. Lithium serum concentrations should be monitored closely when initiating or changing therapy with valdecoxib in patients receiving lithium. Lithium carbonate (450 mg bid for 7 days) had no effect on valdecoxib pharmacokinetics.

Warfarin: The effect of valdecoxib on the anticoagulant effect of warfarin (1-8 mg/day) was studied in healthy subjects by coadministration of valdecoxib 40 mg bid for 7 days. Valdecoxib caused a statistically significant increase in plasma exposures of R-warfarin and S-warfarin (12% and 15%, respectively), and in the pharmacodynamic effects (prothrombin time, measured as INR) of warfarin. While mean INR values were only slightly increased with coadministration of valdecoxib, the day-to-day variability in individual INR values was increased. Anticoagulant therapy should be monitored, particularly during the first few weeks, after initiating therapy with valdecoxib in patients receiving warfarin or similar agents.

Fluconazole and Ketoconazole: Ketoconazole and fluconazole are predominantly CYP 3A4 and 2C9 inhibitors, respectively. Concomitant single dose administration of valdecoxib 20 mg with multiple doses of ketoconazole and fluconazole produced a significant increase in exposure of valdecoxib. Plasma exposure (AUC) to valdecoxib was increased 62% when coadministered with fluconazole and 38% when coadministered with ketoconazole.

Glyburide: Glyburide is a CYP 3A4 substrate. Coadministration of valdecoxib (10 mg bid for 7 days) with glyburide (5 mg qd or 10 mg bid) did not affect the pharmacokinetics (exposure) of glyburide.

ADVERSE REACTIONS

Of the patients treated with valdecoxib tablets in controlled arthritis trials, 2665 were patients with OA, and 2684 were patients with RA. More than 4000 patients have received a chronic total daily dose of valdecoxib 10 mg or more. More than 2800 patients have received valdecoxib 10 mg/day, or more, for at least 6 months and 988 of these have received valdecoxib for at least 1 year.

OSTEOARTHRITIS AND RHEUMATOID ARTHRITIS

TABLE 4 lists all adverse events, regardless of causality, that occurred in ≥2.0% of patients receiving valdecoxib 10 and 20 mg/day in studies of 3 months or longer from 7 controlled studies conducted in patients with OA or RA that included a placebo and/or a positive control group.

In these placebo- and active-controlled clinical trials, the discontinuation rate due to adverse events was 7.5% for arthritis patients receiving valdecoxib 10 mg daily, 7.9% for arthritis patients receiving valdecoxib 20 mg daily and 6.0% for patients receiving placebo.

In the 7 controlled OA and RA studies, the following adverse events occurred in 0.1-1.9% of patients treated with valdecoxib 10-20 mg daily, regardless of causality.

Application Site Disorders: Cellulitis, dermatitis contact.

Cardiovascular: Aggravated hypertension, aneurysm, angina pectoris, arrhythmia, cardiomyopathy, congestive heart failure, coronary artery disorder, heart murmur, hypotension.

Central, Peripheral Nervous System: Cerebrovascular disorder, hypertonia, hypoesthesia, migraine, neuralgia, neuropathy, paresthesia, tremor, twitching, vertigo.

Endocrine: Goiter.

Female Reproductive: Amenorrhea, dysmenorrhea, leukorrhea, mastitis, menstrual disorder, menorrhagia, menstrual bloating, vaginal hemorrhage.

Gastrointestinal: Abnormal stools, constipation, diverticulosis, dry mouth, duodenal ulcer, duodenitis, eructation, esophagitis, fecal incontinence, gastric ulcer, gastritis, gastroenteritis, gastroesophageal reflux, hematemesis, hematochezia, hemorrhoids, hemorrhoids bleeding, hiatal hernia, melena, stomatitis, stool frequency increased, tenesmus, tooth disorder, vomiting.

General: Allergy aggravated, allergic reaction, asthenia, chest pain, chills, cyst NOS, edema generalized, face edema, fatigue, fever, hot flushes, halitosis, malaise, pain, periorbital swelling, peripheral pain.

Hearing and Vestibular: Ear abnormality, earache, tinnitus.

TABLE 4 *Adverse Events With Incidence ≥2.0% in Valdecoxib Treatment Groups: Controlled Arthritis Trials of 3 Months or Longer*

Adverse Event	Placebo n=973	Valdecoxib* 10 mg n=1214	Valdecoxib* 20 mg n=1358	Diclofenac* 150 mg n=711	Ibuprofen* 2400 mg n=207	Naproxen* 1000 mg n=766
Autonomic Nervous System Disorders						
Hypertension	0.6%	1.6%	2.1%	2.5%	2.4%	1.7%
Body as a Whole						
Back pain	1.6%	1.6%	2.7%	2.8%	1.4%	1.0%
Edema peripheral	0.7%	2.4%	3.0%	3.2%	2.9%	2.1%
Influenza-like symptoms	2.2%	2.0%	2.2%	3.1%	2.9%	2.0%
Injury accident	2.8%	4.0%	3.7%	3.9%	3.9%	3.0%
Central and Peripheral Nervous System Disorders						
Dizziness	2.1%	2.6%	2.7%	4.2%	3.4%	2.7%
Headache	7.1%	4.8%	8.5%	6.6%	4.3%	5.5%
Gastrointestinal System Disorders						
Abdominal fullness	2.0%	2.1%	1.9%	3.0%	2.9%	2.5%
Abdominal pain	6.3%	7.0%	8.2%	17.0%	8.2%	10.1%
Diarrhea	4.2%	5.4%	6.0%	10.8%	3.9%	4.7%
Dyspepsia	6.3%	7.9%	8.7%	13.4%	15.0%	12.9%
Flatulence	4.1%	2.9%	3.5%	3.1%	7.7%	5.4%
Nausea	5.9%	7.0%	6.3%	8.4%	7.7%	8.7%
Musculoskeletal System Disorders						
Myalgia	1.6%	2.0%	1.9%	2.4%	2.4%	1.4%
Respiratory System Disorders						
Sinusitis	2.2%	2.6%	1.8%	1.1%	3.4%	3.4%
Upper respiratory track infection	6.0%	6.7%	5.7%	6.3%	4.3%	6.4%
Skin and Appendages Disorders						
Rash	1.0%	1.4%	2.1%	1.5%	0.5%	1.4%

* Total daily dose.

Heart Rate and Rhythm: Bradycardia, palpitation, tachycardia.

Hemic: Anemia.

Liver and Biliary System: Hepatic function abnormal, hepatitis, ALT increased, AST increased.

Male Reproductive: Impotence, prostatic disorder.

Metabolic and Nutritional: Alkaline phosphatase increased, BUN increased, CPK increased, creatinine increased, diabetes mellitus, glycosuria, gout, hypercholesterolemia, hyperglycemia, hyperkalemia, hyperlipemia, hyperuricemia, hypocalcemia, hypokalemia, LDH increased, thirst increased, weight decrease, weight increase, xerophthalmia.

Musculoskeletal: Arthralgia, fracture accidental, neck stiffness, osteoporosis, synovitis, tendonitis.

Neoplasm: Breast neoplasm, lipoma, malignant ovarian cyst.

Platelets (bleeding or clotting): Ecchymosis, epistaxis, hematoma NOS, thrombocytopenia.

Psychiatric: Anorexia, anxiety, appetite increased, confusion, depression, depression aggravated, insomnia, nervousness, morbid dreaming, somnolence.

Resistance Mechanism Disorders: Herpes simplex, herpes zoster, infection fungal, infection soft tissue, infection viral, moniliasis, moniliasis genital, otitis media.

Respiratory: Abnormal breath sounds, bronchitis, bronchospasm, coughing, dyspnea, emphysema, laryngitis, pneumonia, pharyngitis, pleurisy, rhinitis.

Skin and Appendages: Acne, alopecia, dermatitis, dermatitis fungal, eczema, photosensitivity allergic reaction, pruritus, rash erythematous, rash maculopapular, rash psoriaform, skin dry, skin hypertrophy, skin ulceration, sweating increased, urticaria.

Special Senses: Taste perversion.

Urinary System: Albuminuria, cystitis, dysuria, hematuria, micturition frequency increased, pyuria, urinary incontinence, urinary tract infection.

Vascular: Claudication intermittent, hemangioma acquired, varicose vein.

Vision: Blurred vision, cataract, conjunctival hemorrhage, conjunctivitis, eye pain, keratitis, vision abnormal.

White Cell and RES Disorders: Eosinophilia, leukopenia, leukocytosis, lymphadenopathy, lymphangitis, lymphopenia.

Other serious adverse events that were reported rarely (estimated <0.1%) in clinical trials, regardless of causality, in patients taking valdecoxib:

Autonomic Nervous System Disorders: Hypertensive encephalopathy, vasospasm.

Cardiovascular: Abnormal ECG, aortic stenosis, atrial fibrillation, carotid stenosis, coronary thrombosis, heart block, heart valve disorders, mitral insufficiency, myocardial infarction, myocardial ischemia, pericarditis, syncope, thrombophlebitis, unstable angina, ventricular fibrillation.

Central, Peripheral Nervous System: Convulsions.

Endocrine: Hyperparathyroidism.

Female Reproductive: Cervical dysplasia.

Gastrointestinal: Appendicitis, colitis with bleeding, dysphagia, esophageal perforation, gastrointestinal bleeding, ileus, intestinal obstruction, peritonitis.

Hemic: Lymphoma-like disorder, pancytopenia.

Liver and Biliary System: Cholelithiasis.

Metabolic: Dehydration.
Musculoskeletal: Pathological fracture, osteomyelitis.
Neoplasm: Benign brain neoplasm, bladder carcinoma, carcinoma, gastric carcinoma, prostate carcinoma, pulmonary carcinoma.
Platelets (bleeding or clotting): Embolism, pulmonary embolism, thrombosis.
Psychiatric: Manic reaction, psychosis.
Renal: Acute renal failure.
Resistance Mechanism Disorders: Sepsis.
Respiratory: Apnea, pleural effusion, pulmonary edema, pulmonary fibrosis, pulmonary infarction, pulmonary hemorrhage, respiratory insufficiency.
Skin: Basal cell carcinoma, malignant melanoma.
Urinary System: Pyelonephritis, renal calculus.
Vision: Retinal detachment.

POSTMARKETING EXPERIENCE

The following reactions have been identified during postmarketing use of valdecoxib. These reactions have been chosen for inclusion either due to their seriousness, reporting frequency, possible causal relationship to valdecoxib, or a combination of these factors. Because these reactions were reported voluntarily from a population of uncertain size, it is not possible to reliably estimate their frequency or establish a causal relationship to drug exposure.
General: Hypersensitivity reactions (including anaphylactic reactions and angioedema).
Skin and appendages: Erythema multiforme, exfoliative dermatitis, Stevens-Johnson syndrome, toxic epidermal necrolysis.

DOSAGE AND ADMINISTRATION

OSTEOARTHRITIS AND ADULT RHEUMATOID ARTHRITIS

The recommended dose of valdecoxib tablets for the relief of the signs and symptoms of arthritis is 10 mg once daily.

PRIMARY DYSMENORRHEA

The recommended dose of valdecoxib tablets for treatment of primary dysmenorrhea is 20 mg twice daily, as needed.

HOW SUPPLIED

Bextra tablets are available in:

10 mg: White, film-coated, and capsule-shaped, debossed "10" on one side with a 4 pointed star shape on the other.

20 mg: White, film-coated, and capsule-shaped, debossed "20" on one side with a 4 pointed star shape on the other.

Storage: Store at 25°C (77°F); excursions permitted to 15-30°C (59-86°F).

PRODUCT LISTING - EQUIVALENTS NOT AVAILABLE

Tablet - Oral - 10 mg

10's	$51.13	BEXTRA, Pharma Pac	52959-0667-10
14's	$68.65	BEXTRA, Pharma Pac	52959-0667-14
15's	$72.96	BEXTRA, Pharma Pac	52959-0667-15
20's	$58.20	BEXTRA, Southwood Pharmaceuticals Inc	58016-0670-20
20's	$89.66	BEXTRA, Pharma Pac	52959-0667-20
25's	$72.75	BEXTRA, Southwood Pharmaceuticals Inc	58016-0670-25
30's	$87.30	BEXTRA, Southwood Pharmaceuticals Inc	58016-0670-30
30's	$118.88	BEXTRA, Pharma Pac	52959-0667-30
52's	$186.63	BEXTRA, Pharma Pac	52959-0667-52
55's	$190.82	BEXTRA, Pharma Pac	52959-0667-55
60's	$195.74	BEXTRA, Pharma Pac	52959-0667-60
100's	$304.91	BEXTRA, Pharmacia Corporation	00025-1975-31
100's	$309.49	BEXTRA, Pharmacia Corporation	00025-1975-34

Tablet - Oral - 20 mg

10's	$51.13	BEXTRA, Pharma Pac	52959-0683-10
14's	$68.65	BEXTRA, Pharma Pac	52959-0683-14
15's	$72.96	BEXTRA, Pharma Pac	52959-0683-15
20's	$58.20	BEXTRA, Southwood Pharmaceuticals Inc	58016-0665-20
20's	$89.66	BEXTRA, Pharma Pac	52959-0683-20
21's	$92.01	BEXTRA, Pharma Pac	52959-0683-21
25's	$72.75	BEXTRA, Southwood Pharmaceuticals Inc	58016-0665-25
28's	$127.01	BEXTRA, Pharma Pac	52959-0683-28
30's	$87.30	BEXTRA, Southwood Pharmaceuticals Inc	58016-0665-30
30's	$129.15	BEXTRA, Pharma Pac	52959-0683-30
40's	$140.30	BEXTRA, Pharma Pac	52959-0683-40
52's	$163.85	BEXTRA, Pharma Pac	52959-0683-52
55's	$172.94	BEXTRA, Pharma Pac	52959-0683-55
60's	$197.34	BEXTRA, Pharma Pac	52959-0683-60
100's	$304.91	BEXTRA, Pharmacia Corporation	00025-1980-31
100's	$309.49	BEXTRA, Pharmacia Corporation	00025-1980-34

Valganciclovir Hydrochloride *(001640)*

Categories: Infection, cytomegalovirus; FDA Approved 2001 Mar; Pregnancy Category C
Drug Classes: Antivirals
Brand Names: Valcyte
Foreign Brand Availability: Valixa (Colombia)
Cost of Therapy: $2,517.90 (CMV Retinitis Induction; Valcyte; 450 mg; 4 tablets/day; 21 day supply)
$1,798.50 (CMV Retinitis Maintenance; Valcyte; 450 mg; 2 tablets/day; 30 day supply)

WARNING

THE CLINICAL TOXICITY OF VALGANCICLOVIR HCl, WHICH IS METABOLIZED TO GANCICLOVIR, INCLUDES GRANULOCYTOPENIA, ANEMIA AND THROMBOCYTOPENIA. IN ANIMAL STUDIES GANCICLOVIR WAS CARCINOGENIC, TERATOGENIC AND CAUSED ASPERMATOGENESIS.

DESCRIPTION

Valcyte contains valganciclovir hydrochloride (valganciclovir HCl), a hydrochloride salt of the L-valyl ester of ganciclovir that exists as a mixture of two diastereomers. Ganciclovir is a synthetic guanine derivative active against cytomegalovirus (CMV).

Valcyte is available as a 450 mg tablet for oral administration. Each tablet contains 496.3 mg of valganciclovir HCl (corresponding to 450 mg of valganciclovir), and the inactive ingredients microcrystalline cellulose, povidone K-30, crospovidone, and stearic acid. The film-coat applied to the tablets contains Opadry Pink.

Valganciclovir HCl is a white to off-white crystalline powder with a molecular formula of $C_{14}H_{22}N_6O_5 \cdot HCl$ and a molecular weight of 390.83. The chemical name for valganciclovir HCl is L-Valine, 2-[(2-amino-1,6-dihydro-6-oxo-9H-purin-9-yl)methoxy]-3-hydroxypropyl ester, monohydrochloride. Valganciclovir HCl is a polar hydrophilic compound with a solubility of 70 mg/ml in water at 25°C at a pH of 7.0 and an n-octanol/water partition coefficient of 0.0095 at pH 7.0. The pKa for valganciclovir is 7.6.

All doses in this insert are specified in terms of valganciclovir.

CLINICAL PHARMACOLOGY

MECHANISM OF ACTION

Valganciclovir is an L-valyl ester (prodrug) of ganciclovir that exists as a mixture of two diastereomers. After oral administration, both diastereomers are rapidly converted to ganciclovir by intestinal and hepatic esterases. Ganciclovir is a synthetic analogue of 2′-deoxyguanosine, which inhibits replication of human cytomegalovirus *in vitro* and *in vivo*.

In CMV-infected cells ganciclovir is initially phosphorylated to ganciclovir monophosphate by the viral protein kinase, pUL97. Further phosphorylation occurs by cellular kinases to produce ganciclovir triphosphate, which is then slowly metabolized intracellularly (half-life 18 hours). As the phosphorylation is largely dependent on the viral kinase, phosphorylation of ganciclovir occurs preferentially in virus-infected cells. The virustatic activity of ganciclovir is due to inhibition of viral DNA synthesis by ganciclovir triphosphate.

Antiviral Activity

The quantitative relationship between the *in vitro* susceptibility of human herpesviruses to antivirals and clinical response to antiviral therapy has not been established, and virus sensitivity testing has not been standardized. Sensitivity test results, expressed as the concentration of drug required to inhibit the growth of virus in cell culture by 50% (IC_{50}), vary greatly depending upon a number of factors. Thus the IC_{50} of ganciclovir that inhibits human CMV replication *in vitro* (laboratory and clinical isolates) has ranged from 0.02-5.75 μg/ml (0.08-22.94 μM). Ganciclovir inhibits mammalian cell proliferation (CIC_{50}) *in vitro* at higher concentrations ranging from 10.21 to >250 μg/ml (40 to >1000 μM). Bone marrow-derived colony-forming cells are more sensitive (CIC_{50} = 0.69-3.06 μg/ml: 2.7 to 12 μM).

Viral Resistance

Viruses resistant to ganciclovir can arise after prolonged treatment with valganciclovir by selection of mutations in either the viral protein kinase gene (UL97) responsible for ganciclovir monophosphorylation and/or in the viral polymerase gene (UL54). Virus with mutations in the UL97 gene is resistant to ganciclovir alone, whereas virus with mutations in the UL54 gene may show cross-resistance to other antivirals with a similar mechanism of action.

The current working definition of CMV resistance to ganciclovir in *in vitro* assays is IC_{50} ≥1.5 μg/ml ≥6.0 μM). CMV resistance to ganciclovir has been observed in individuals with AIDS and CMV retinitis who have never received ganciclovir therapy. Viral resistance has also been observed in patients receiving prolonged treatment for CMV retinitis with ganciclovir. The possibility of viral resistance should be considered in patients who show poor clinical response or experience persistent viral excretion during therapy.

PHARMACOKINETICS

BECAUSE THE MAJOR ELIMINATION PATHWAY FOR GANCICLOVIR IS RENAL, DOSAGE REDUCTIONS ACCORDING TO CREATININE CLEARANCE ARE REQUIRED FOR VALGANCICLOVIR HCl TABLETS. FOR DOSING INSTRUCTIONS IN PATIENTS WITH RENAL IMPAIRMENT, REFER TO DOSAGE AND ADMINISTRATION.

The ganciclovir pharmacokinetic measures following administration of 900 mg valganciclovir and 5 mg/kg intravenous ganciclovir and 1000 mg three times daily oral ganciclovir are summarized in TABLE 1.

The area under the plasma concentration-time curve (AUC) for ganciclovir administered as valganciclovir HCl tablets is comparable to the ganciclovir AUC for intravenous ganciclovir. Ganciclovir C_{max} following valganciclovir administration is 40% lower than following intravenous ganciclovir administration.

During maintenance dosing, ganciclovir AUC(0-24h) and C_{max} following oral ganciclovir administration (1000 mg three times daily) are lower relative to valganciclovir and intravenous ganciclovir. The ganciclovir C_{min} following intravenous ganciclovir and valganciclovir administration are less than the ganciclovir C_{min} following oral ganciclovir administration. The clinical significance of the differences in ganciclovir pharmacokinetics for these three ganciclovir delivery systems is unknown.

Absorption

Valganciclovir, a prodrug of ganciclovir, is well absorbed from the gastrointestinal tract and rapidly metabolized in the intestinal wall and liver to ganciclovir. The absolute bioavailability of ganciclovir from valganciclovir HCl tablets following administration with food was approximately 60% (3 studies, n=18; n=16; n=28). Ganciclovir median T_{max} following administration of 450-2625 mg valganciclovir tablets ranged from 1-3 hours. Dose proportionality with respect to ganciclovir AUC following administration of valganciclovir tablets was demonstrated only under fed conditions. Systemic exposure to the prodrug, valganciclovir, is transient and low, and the AUC(24) and C_{max} values are approximately 1% and 3% of those of ganciclovir, respectively.

TABLE 1 *Mean Ganciclovir Pharmacokinetic* Measures in Healthy Volunteers and HIV-Positive/CMV-Positive Adults at Maintenance Dosage Formulation*

	Formulation		
	Valganciclovir HCl Tablets	Cytovene -IV	Cytovene
Dosage	900 mg once daily with food	5 mg/kg once daily	1000 mg three times daily with food
AUC(0-24h) (μg·h/ml)	29.1 ± 9.7 (3 studies, n=57)	26.5 ± 5.9 (4 studies, n=68)	Range of means 12.3-19.2 (6 studies, n=94)
C_{max} (μg/ml)	5.61 ± 1.52 (3 studies, n=58)	9.46 ± 2.02 (4 studies, n=68)	Range of means 0.955-1.40 (6 studies, n=94)
Absolute oral bioavailability (%)	59.4 ± 6.1 (2 studies, n=32)	Not Applicable	Range of means 6.22 ± 1.29-8.53 ± 1.53(2 studies, n=32)
Elimination half-life (h)	4.08 ± 0.76 (4 studies, n=73)	3.81 ± 0.71 (4 studies, n=69)	Range of means 3.86-5.03 (4 studies, n=61)
Renal clearance (ml/min/kg)	3.21 ± 0.75 (1 study, n=20)	2.99 ± 0.67 (1 study, n=16)	Range of means 2.67-3.98 (3 studies, n=30)

* Data were obtained from single and multiple dose studies in healthy volunteers, HIV-positive patients, and HIV-positive/CMV-positive patients with and without retinitis. Patients with CMV retinitis tended to have higher ganciclovir plasma concentrations than patients without CMV retinitis.

Food Effects

When valganciclovir tablets were administered with a high fat meal containing approximately 600 total calories (31.1 g fat, 51.6 g carbohydrates, and 22.2 g protein) at a dose of 875 mg once daily to 16 HIV-positive subjects, the steady-state ganciclovir AUC increased by 30% (95% CI 12-51%), and the C_{max} increased by 14% (95% CI -5-36%), without any prolongation in time to peak plasma concentrations (T_{max}). Valganciclovir HCl tablets should be administered with food (see DOSAGE AND ADMINISTRATION).

Distribution

Due to the rapid conversion of valganciclovir to ganciclovir, plasma protein binding of valganciclovir was not determined. Plasma protein binding of ganciclovir is 1-2% over concentrations of 0.5 and 51 μg/ml. When ganciclovir was administered intravenously, the steady state volume of distribution of ganciclovir was 0.703 ± 0.134 L/kg (n=69).

After administration of valganciclovir tablets, no correlation was observed between ganciclovir AUC and reciprocal weight; oral dosing of valganciclovir tablets according to weight is not required.

Metabolism

Valganciclovir is rapidly hydrolyzed to ganciclovir; no other metabolites have been detected. No metabolite of orally-administered radiolabeled ganciclovir (1000 mg single dose) accounted for more than 1-2% of the radioactivity recovered in the feces or urine.

Elimination

The major route of elimination of valganciclovir is by renal excretion as ganciclovir through glomerular filtration and active tubular secretion. Systemic clearance of intravenously administered ganciclovir was 3.07 ± 0.64 ml/min/kg (n=68) while renal clearance was 2.99 ± 0.67 ml/min/kg (n=16).

The terminal half-life ($T_{1/2}$) of ganciclovir following oral administration of valganciclovir tablets to either healthy or HIV-positive/CMV-positive subjects was 4.08 ± 0.76 hours (n=73), and that following administration of intravenous ganciclovir was 3.81 ± 0.71 hours (n=69).

Special Populations

Renal Impairment

The pharmacokinetics of ganciclovir from a single oral dose of 900 mg valganciclovir HCl tablets were evaluated in 24 otherwise healthy individuals with renal impairment.

TABLE 2 *Pharmacokinetics of Ganciclovir From a Single Oral Dose of 900 mg Valganciclovir HCl Tablets*

Estimated Creatinine Clearance (ml/min)	n	Apparent Clearnace (ml/min) Mean ± SD	AUC(last) (μg·h/ml) Mean ± SD	Half-Life (hours) Mean ± SD
51-70	6	249 ± 99	49.5 ± 22.4	4.85 ± 1.4
21-50	6	136 ± 64	91.9 ± 43.9	10.2 ± 4.4
11-20	6	45 ± 11	223 ± 46	21.8 ± 5.2
≤10	6	12.8 ± 8	366 ± 66	67.5 ± 34

Decreased renal function results in decreased clearance of ganciclovir from valganciclovir, and a corresponding increase in terminal half-life. Therefore, dosage adjustment is required for patients with impaired renal function (see PRECAUTIONS, General).

Hemodialysis

Hemodialysis reduces plasma concentrations of ganciclovir by about 50% following valganciclovir administration. Patients receiving hemodialysis (CRCL <10 ml/min) cannot use valganciclovir HCl tablets because the daily dose of valganciclovir HCl tablets required for these patients is less than 450 mg (see PRECAUTIONS, General and DOSAGE AND ADMINISTRATION, Hemodialysis Patients).

Liver Transplant Patients

In liver transplant patients, the ganciclovir AUC(0-24h) achieved with 900 mg valganciclovir was 41.7 ± 9.9 μg·h/ml (n=28) and the AUC(0-24h) achieved with the approved dosage of 5 mg/kg intravenous ganciclovir was 48.2 ± 17.3 μg/ml (n=27).

Race/Ethnicity and Gender

Insufficient data are available to demonstrate any effect of race or gender on the pharmacokinetics of valganciclovir.

Pediatrics

Valganciclovir HCl tablets have not been studied in pediatric patients; the pharmacokinetic characteristics of valganciclovir HCl tablets in these patients have not been established (see PRECAUTIONS, Pediatric Use).

Geriatrics

No studies of valganciclovir HCl tablets have been conducted in adults older than 65 years of age (see PRECAUTIONS, Geriatric Use).

INDICATIONS AND USAGE

Valganciclovir HCl tablets are indicated for the treatment of cytomegalovirus (CMV) retinitis in patients with acquired immunodeficiency syndrome (AIDS).

CONTRAINDICATIONS

Valganciclovir HCl tablets are contraindicated in patients with hypersensitivity to valganciclovir or ganciclovir.

WARNINGS

THE CLINICAL TOXICITY OF VALGANCICLOVIR HCl, WHICH IS METABOLIZED TO GANCICLOVIR, INCLUDES GRANULOCYTOPENIA, ANEMIA AND THROMBOCYTOPENIA. IN ANIMAL STUDIES GANCICLOVIR WAS CARCINOGENIC, TERATOGENIC AND CAUSED ASPERMATOGENESIS.

HEMATOLOGIC

Valganciclovir HCl tablets should not be administered if the absolute neutrophil count is less than 500 cells/μl, the platelet count is less than 25,000/μl, or the hemoglobin is less than 8 g/dl.

Severe leukopenia, neutropenia, anemia, thrombocytopenia, pancytopenia, bone marrow depression and aplastic anemia have been observed in patients treated with valganciclovir HCl tablets (and ganciclovir) (see PRECAUTIONS, Laboratory Testing and ADVERSE REACTIONS).

Valganciclovir HCl tablets should, therefore, be used with caution in patients with preexisting cytopenias, or who have received or who are receiving myelosuppressive drugs or irradiation. Cytopenia may occur at any time during treatment and may increase with continued dosing. Cell counts usually begin to recover within 3-7 days of discontinuing drug.

IMPAIRMENT OF FERTILITY

Animal data indicate that administration of ganciclovir causes inhibition of spermatogenesis and subsequent infertility. These effects were reversible at lower doses and irreversible at higher doses (see PRECAUTIONS, Carcinogenesis, Mutagenesis, and Impairment of Fertility). It is considered probable that in humans, valganciclovir at the recommended doses may cause temporary or permanent inhibition of spermatogenesis. Animal data also indicate that suppression of fertility in females may occur.

TERATOGENESIS, CARCINOGENESIS AND MUTAGENESIS

Because of the mutagenic and teratogenic potential of ganciclovir, women of childbearing potential should be advised to use effective contraception during treatment. Similarly, men should be advised to practice barrier contraception during, and for at least 90 days following, treatment with valganciclovir HCl tablets (see PRECAUTIONS: Carcinogenesis, Mutagenesis, and Impairment of Fertility and Pregnancy Category C).

In animal studies, ganciclovir was found to be mutagenic and carcinogenic. Valganciclovir should, therefore, be considered a potential teratogen and carcinogen in humans with the potential to cause birth defects and cancers (see DOSAGE AND ADMINISTRATION, Handling and Disposal).

PRECAUTIONS

GENERAL

Strict adherence to dosage recommendations is essential to avoid overdose.

The bioavailability of ganciclovir from valganciclovir HCl tablets is significantly higher than from ganciclovir capsules. Patients switching from ganciclovir capsules should be advised of the risk of overdosage if they take more than the prescribed number of valganciclovir HCl tablets. **Valganciclovir HCl tablets cannot be substituted for Cytovene capsules on a one-to-one basis** (see DOSAGE AND ADMINISTRATION).

Since ganciclovir is excreted by the kidneys, normal clearance depends on adequate renal function. **IF RENAL FUNCTION IS IMPAIRED, DOSAGE ADJUSTMENTS ARE REQUIRED FOR VALGANCICLOVIR HCl TABLETS.** Such adjustments should be based on measured or estimated creatinine clearance values (see DOSAGE AND ADMINISTRATION, Renal Impairment).

For patients on hemodialysis (CRCL <10 ml/min) it is recommended that ganciclovir be used (in accordance with the dose-reduction algorithm cited in the Cytovene-IV and Cytovene prescribing information, DOSAGE AND ADMINISTRATION, Renal Impairment) rather than valganciclovir HCl tablets (see DOSAGE AND ADMINISTRATION, Hemodialysis and CLINICAL PHARMACOLOGY, Pharmacokinetics, Special Populations, Hemodialysis).

INFORMATION FOR THE PATIENT

See the Patient Instructions that are distributed with the prescription.

Valganciclovir HCl tablets cannot be substituted for ganciclovir capsules on a one-to-one basis. Patients switching from ganciclovir capsules should be advised of the risk of overdosage if they take more than the prescribed number of valganciclovir HCl tablets (see DOSAGE AND ADMINISTRATION).

Valganciclovir HCl is changed to ganciclovir once it is absorbed into the body. All patients should be informed that the major toxicities of ganciclovir include granulocytopenia (neutropenia), anemia and thrombocytopenia and that dose modifications may be required, including discontinuation. The importance of close monitoring of blood counts while on therapy should be emphasized. Patients should be informed that ganciclovir has been associated with elevations in serum creatinine.

Patients should be instructed to take valganciclovir HCl tablets with food to maximize bioavailability.

Patients should be advised that ganciclovir has caused decreased sperm production in animals and may cause decreased fertility in humans. Women of childbearing potential should be advised that ganciclovir causes birth defects in animals and should not be used during pregnancy. Because of the potential for serious adverse events in nursing infants, mothers should be instructed not to breastfeed if they are receiving valganciclovir HCl tablets. Women of childbearing potential should be advised to use effective contraception during treatment with valganciclovir HCl tablets. Similarly, men should be advised to practice barrier contraception during and for at least 90 days following treatment with valganciclovir HCl tablets.

Although there is no information from human studies, patients should be advised that ganciclovir should be considered a potential carcinogen.

Convulsions, sedation, dizziness, ataxia and/or confusion have been reported with the use of valganciclovir HCl tablets and/or ganciclovir. If they occur, such effects may affect tasks requiring alertness including the patient's ability to drive and operate machinery.

Patients should be told that ganciclovir is not a cure for CMV retinitis, and that they may continue to experience progression of retinitis during or following treatment. Patients should be advised to have ophthalmologic follow-up examinations at a minimum of every 4-6 weeks while being treated with valganciclovir HCl tablets. Some patients will require more frequent follow-up.

LABORATORY TESTING

Due to the frequency of neutropenia, anemia and thrombocytopenia in patients receiving valganciclovir HCl tablets (see ADVERSE REACTIONS), it is recommended that complete blood counts and platelet counts be performed frequently, especially in patients in whom ganciclovir or other nucleoside analogues have previously resulted in leukopenia, or in whom neutrophil counts are less than 1000 cells/μl at the beginning of treatment. Increased monitoring for cytopenias may be warranted if therapy with oral ganciclovir is changed to oral valganciclovir, because of increased plasma concentrations of ganciclovir after valganciclovir administration (see CLINICAL PHARMACOLOGY).

Increased serum creatinine levels have been observed in trials evaluating valganciclovir HCl tablets. Patients should have serum creatinine or creatinine clearance values monitored carefully to allow for dosage adjustments in renally impaired patients (see DOSAGE AND ADMINISTRATION, Renal Impairment). The mechanism of impairment of renal function is not known.

*CARCINOGENESIS, MUTAGENESIS, AND IMPAIRMENT OF FERTILITY**

No long-term carcinogenicity studies have been conducted with valganciclovir. However, upon oral administration, valganciclovir is rapidly and extensively converted to ganciclovir. Therefore, like ganciclovir, valganciclovir is a potential carcinogen.

Ganciclovir was carcinogenic in the mouse at oral doses of 20 and 1000 mg/kg/day (approximately 0.1× and 1.4×, respectively, the mean drug exposure in humans following the recommended intravenous dose of 5 mg/kg, based on area under the plasma concentration curve [AUC] comparisons). At the dose of 1000 mg/kg/day there was a significant increase in the incidence of tumors of the preputial gland in males, forestomach (nonglandular mucosa) in males and females, and reproductive tissues (ovaries, uterus, mammary gland, clitoral gland and vagina) and liver in females. At the dose of 20 mg/kg/day, a slightly increased incidence of tumors was noted in the preputial and harderian glands in males, forestomach in males and females, and liver in females. No carcinogenic effect was observed in mice administered ganciclovir at 1 mg/kg/day (estimated as 0.01× the human dose based on AUC comparison). Ganciclovir should be considered a potential carcinogen in humans.

Valganciclovir increases mutations in mouse lymphoma cells. In the mouse micronucleus assay, valganciclovir was clastogenic at a dose of 1500 mg/kg (60× human mean exposure for ganciclovir based upon AUC). Valganciclovir was not mutagenic in the Ames *Salmonella* assay. Ganciclovir increased mutations in mouse lymphoma cells and DNA damage in human lymphocytes *in vitro*. In the mouse micronucleus assay, ganciclovir was clastogenic at doses of 150 and 500 mg/kg (IV) (2.8 to 10× human exposure based on AUC) but not 50 mg/kg (exposure approximately comparable to the human based on AUC). Ganciclovir was not mutagenic in the Ames *Salmonella* assay.

Valganciclovir is converted to ganciclovir and therefore is expected to have similar reproductive toxicity effects as ganciclovir (see WARNINGS, Impairment of Fertility). Ganciclovir caused decreased mating behavior, decreased fertility, and an increased incidence of embryolethality in female mice following intravenous doses of 90 mg/kg/day (approximately 1.7× the mean drug exposure in humans following the dose of 5 mg/kg, based on AUC comparisons). Ganciclovir caused decreased fertility in male mice and hypospermatogenesis in mice and dogs following daily oral or intravenous administration of doses ranging from 0.2 to 10 mg/kg. Systemic drug exposure (AUC) at the lowest dose showing toxicity in each species ranged from 0.03 to 0.1× the AUC of the recommended human intravenous dose. Valganciclovir caused similar effects on spermatogenesis in mice, rats, and dogs. It is considered likely that ganciclovir (and valganciclovir) could cause inhibition of human spermatogenesis.

*PREGNANCY CATEGORY C**

Valganciclovir is converted to ganciclovir and therefore is expected to have reproductive toxicity effects similar to ganciclovir. Ganciclovir has been shown to be embryotoxic in rabbits and mice following intravenous administration, and teratogenic in rabbits. Fetal resorptions were present in at least 85% of rabbits and mice administered 60 mg/kg/day and 108 mg/kg/day (2× the human exposure based on AUC comparisons), respectively. Effects observed in rabbits included: fetal growth retardation, embryolethality, teratogenicity and/or maternal toxicity. Teratogenic changes included cleft palate, anophthalmia/microphthalmia, aplastic organs (kidney and pancreas), hydrocephaly and brachygnathia. In mice, effects observed were maternal/fetal toxicity and embryolethality.

Daily intravenous doses of 90 mg/kg administered to female mice prior to mating, during gestation, and during lactation caused hypoplasia of the testes and seminal vesicles in the month-old male offspring, as well as pathologic changes in the nonglandular region of the stomach (see WARNINGS, Teratogenesis, Carcinogenesis and Mutagenesis). The drug exposure in mice as estimated by the AUC was approximately 1.7× the human AUC.

Data obtained using an *ex vivo* human placental model show that ganciclovir crosses the placenta and that simple diffusion is the most likely mechanism of transfer. The transfer was not saturable over a concentration range of 1-10 mg/ml and occurred by passive diffusion.

Valganciclovir may be teratogenic or embryotoxic at dose levels recommended for human use. There are no adequate and well-controlled studies in pregnant women. Valganciclovir HCl tablets should be used during pregnancy only if the potential benefit justifies the potential risk to the fetus.

***Footnote:** All dose comparisons presented in the Carcinogenesis, Mutagenesis, Impairment of Fertility, and Pregnancy subsections are based on the human AUC following administration of a single 5 mg/kg infusion of intravenous ganciclovir.

NURSING MOTHERS

It is not known whether ganciclovir or valganciclovir is excreted in human milk. Because valganciclovir caused granulocytopenia, anemia and thrombocytopenia in clinical trials and ganciclovir was mutagenic and carcinogenic in animal studies, the possibility of serious adverse events from ganciclovir in nursing infants is possible (see WARNINGS). Because of potential for serious adverse events in nursing infants, **mothers should be instructed not to breastfeed if they are receiving valganciclovir HCl tablets.** In addition, the Centers for Disease Control and Prevention recommend that HIV-infected mothers not breastfeed their infants to avoid risking postnatal transmission of HIV.

PEDIATRIC USE

Safety and effectiveness of valganciclovir HCl tablets in pediatric patients have not been established.

GERIATRIC USE

The pharmacokinetic characteristics of valganciclovir HCl in elderly patients have not been established. Since elderly individuals frequently have a reduced glomerular filtration rate, particular attention should be paid to assessing renal function before and during administration of valganciclovir HCl (see DOSAGE AND ADMINISTRATION).

Clinical studies of valganciclovir HCl did not include sufficient numbers of subjects aged 65 and over to determine whether they respond differently from younger subjects. In general, dose selection for an elderly patient should be cautious, reflecting the greater frequency of decreased hepatic, renal, or cardiac function, and of concomitant disease or other drug therapy. Valganciclovir HCl is known to be substantially excreted by the kidney, and the risk of toxic reactions to this drug may be greater in patients with impaired renal function. Because elderly patients are more likely to have decreased renal function, care should be taken in dose selection. In addition, renal function should be monitored and dosage adjustments should be made accordingly (see PRECAUTIONS, General, CLINICAL PHARMACOLOGY, Pharmacokinetics, Special Populations, Renal Impairment, and DOSAGE AND ADMINISTRATION, Renal Impairment).

DRUG INTERACTIONS

DRUG INTERACTION STUDIES CONDUCTED WITH VALGANCICLOVIR

No *in vivo* drug-drug interaction studies were conducted with valganciclovir. However, because valganciclovir is rapidly and extensively converted to ganciclovir, interactions associated with ganciclovir will be expected for valganciclovir HCl tablets.

DRUG INTERACTION STUDIES CONDUCTED WITH GANCICLOVIR

Binding of ganciclovir to plasma proteins is only about 1-2%, and drug interactions involving binding site displacement are not anticipated.

Drug-drug interaction studies were conducted in patients with normal renal function. Patients with impaired renal function may have increased concentrations of ganciclovir and the coadministered drug following concomitant administration of valganciclovir HCl tablets and drugs excreted by the same pathway as ganciclovir. Therefore, these patients should be closely monitored for toxicity of ganciclovir and the coadministered drug.

ADVERSE REACTIONS

EXPERIENCE WITH VALGANCICLOVIR HCl TABLETS

Valganciclovir, a prodrug of ganciclovir, is rapidly converted to ganciclovir after oral administration. Adverse events known to be associated with ganciclovir usage can therefore be expected to occur with valganciclovir HCl tablets.

As shown in TABLE 6, the safety profiles of valganciclovir HCl tablets and intravenous ganciclovir during 28 days of randomized therapy (21 days induction dose and 7 days maintenance dose) in 158 patients were comparable, with the exception of catheter-related infection, which occurred with greater frequency in patients randomized to receive IV ganciclovir (see TABLE 6).

TABLE 7 and TABLE 8 show the pooled adverse event data and abnormal laboratory values from two single arm, open-label clinical trials, WV15376 (after the initial 4 weeks of randomized therapy) and WV15705). A total of 370 patients received maintenance therapy with valganciclovir tablets 900 mg q day. Approximately 252 (68%) of these patients received valganciclovir HCl tablets for more than 9 months (maximum duration was 36 months).

Serious adverse events reported from these two clinical trials (n=370) with a frequency of less than 5% and which are not mentioned in the two tables above, are listed below:

***TABLE 4** Results of Drug Interaction Studies With Ganciclovir — Effects of Co-Administered Drug on Ganciclovir Plasma AUC and C_{max} Values*

Co-Administered Drug	Ganciclovir Dosage	n	Ganciclovir Pharmacokinetic (PK) Parameter	Clinical Comment
Zidovudine 100 mg every 4 h	1000 mg every 8 h dose	12	AUC dec 17 ± 25% (range: -52% to 23%)	Zidovudine and valganciclovir HCl each have the potential to cause neutropenia and anemia. Some patients may not tolerate concomitant therapy at full dosage.
Didanosine 200 mg every 12 h administered 2 h before ganciclovir	1000 mg every 8 h dose	12	AUC dec 21 ± 17% (range: -44% to 5%)	Effect not likely to be clinically significant.
Didanosine 200 mg every 12 h simultaneously administered with ganciclovir	1000 mg every 8 h dose (n=12); IV ganciclovir 5 mg/kg twice daily (n=11); IV ganciclovir 5 mg/kg once daily (n=11)		No effect on ganciclovir PK parameters observed	No effect expected.
Probenecid 500 mg every 6 h	1000 mg every 8 h	10	AUC inc 53 ± 91% (range: -14% to 299%) Ganciclovir renal clearance dec 22 ± 20% (Range: -54% to -4%)	Patients taking probenecid and valganciclovir HCl should be monitored for evidence of ganciclovir toxicity.
Zalcitabine 0.75 mg every 8 h administered 2 h before ganciclovir	1000 mg every 8 h	10	AUC inc 13%	Effect not likely to be clinically significant.
Trimethoprim 200 mg once daily	1000 mg every 8 h	12	Ganciclovir renal clearance dec 16.3% Half-life inc 15%	Effect not likely to be clinically significant.
Mycophenolate mofetil 1.5 g single dose	IV ganciclovir 5 mg/kg single dose	12	No effect on ganciclovir PK parameters observed (patients with normal renal function)	Patients with renal impairment should be monitored carefully as levels of metabolites of both drugs may increase.

***TABLE 5** Results of Drug Interaction Studies With Ganciclovir — Effects of Ganciclovir on Plasma AUC and C_{max} Values of Co-Administered Drug*

Co-Administered Drug	Ganciclovir Dosage	n	Co-Administered Drug Pharmacokinetic (PK) Parameter	Clinical Comment
Zidovudine 100 mg every 4 h	1000 mg every 8 h dose	12	AUC(0-4) inc 19 ± 27% (range: -11% to 74%)	Zidovudine and valganciclovir HCl each have the potential to cause neutropenia and anemia. Some patients may not tolerate concomitant therapy at full dosage.
Didanosine 200 mg every 12 h when administered 2 h prior to or concurrent with ganciclovir	1000 mg every 8 h dose	12	AUC(0-12) inc 111 ± 114% (range 10% to 493%)	Patients should be closely monitored for didanosine toxicity.
Didanosine 200 mg every 12 h	IV ganciclovir 5 mg/kg twice daily	11	AUC(0-12) inc 70 ± 40% (range 3% to 121%) C_{max} inc 49 ± 48% (range -28% to 125%)	Patients should be closely monitored for didanosine toxicity.
Didanosine 200 mg every 12 h	IV ganciclovir 5 mg/kg once daily	11	AUC(0-12) inc 50 ± 26% (range 22% to 110%) C_{max} inc 36 ± 36% (range -27% to 94%)	Patients should be closely monitored for didanosine toxicity.
Zalcitabine 0.75 mg every 8 h administered 2 hours before ganciclovir	1000 mg every 8 h	10	No clinically relevant PK parameter changes	No effect expected.
Trimethoprim 200 mg once daily	1000 mg every 8 h	12	Increase in C_{min}	Effect not likely to be clinically significant.
Mycophenolate mofetil 1.5 g single dose	IV ganciclovir 5 mg/kg single dose	12	No PK interaction observed (patients with normal renal function)	Patients with renal impairment should be monitored carefully as levels of metabolites of both drugs may increase.

***TABLE 6** Percentage of Selected Adverse Events Occurring During the Randomized Phase of Study WV15376*

Adverse Event	Valganciclovir Arm n=79	IV Ganciclovir Arm n=79
Diarrhea	16%	10%
Neutropenia	11%	13%
Nausea	8%	14%
Headache	9%	5%
Anemia	8%	8%
Catheter-related infection	3%	11%

***TABLE 7** Pooled Selected Adverse Events Reported in ≥5% of Patients in Two Clinical Studies*

Adverse Events According to Body System	% Patients n=370
Gastrointestinal System	
Diarrhea	41%
Nausea	30%
Vomiting	21%
Abdominal pain	15%
Body as a Whole	
Pyrexia	31%
Headache	22%
Hemic and Lymphatic System	
Neutropenia	27%
Anemia	26%
Thrombocytopenia	6%
Central and Peripheral Nervous System	
Insomnia	16%
Peripheral neuropathy	9%
Paresthesia	8%
Special Senses	
Retinal detachment	15%

Hemic and Lymphatic System: Pancytopenia, bone marrow depression, aplastic anemia.

Urogenital System: Decreased creatinine clearance.

Infections: Local and systemic infections and sepsis.

Bleeding Complications: Potentially life-threatening bleeding associated with thrombocytopenia.

Central and Peripheral Nervous System: Convulsion, psychosis, hallucinations, confusion, agitation.

Body as a Whole: Valganciclovir hypersensitivity.

Laboratory abnormalities reported with valganciclovir HCl tablets are listed in TABLE 8.

***TABLE 8** Pooled Laboratory Abnormalities Reported in Two Clinical Studies*

Laboratory Abnormalities	n=370
Neutropenia: ANC /µl	
<500	19%
500 to <750	17%
750 to <1000	17%
Anemia: Hemoglobin g/dl	
<6.5	7%
6.5 to <8.0	13%
8.0 to <9.5	16%
Thrombocytopenia: Platelets /µl	
<25,000	4%
25,000 to <50,000	6%
50,000 to <100,000	22%
Serum Creatinine: mg/dl	
>2.5	3%
>1.5 to 2.5	12%

EXPERIENCE WITH GANCICLOVIR

Valganciclovir is rapidly converted to ganciclovir upon oral administration. Adverse events reported with valganciclovir HCl in general were similar to those reported with ganciclovir (Cytovene). Please refer to the Cytovene label for more information on post-marketing adverse events associated with ganciclovir.

DOSAGE AND ADMINISTRATION

Strict adherence to dosage recommendations is essential to avoid overdose. Valganciclovir HCl tablets cannot be substituted for Cytovene capsules on a one-to-one basis.

Valganciclovir HCl tablets are administered orally, and should be taken with food (see CLINICAL PHARMACOLOGY, Pharmacokinetics, Absorption). After oral administration, valganciclovir is rapidly and extensively converted into ganciclovir. The bioavailability of ganciclovir from valganciclovir HCl tablets is significantly higher than from ganciclovir capsules. Therefore the dosage and administration of valganciclovir HCl tablets as described below should be closely followed (see PRECAUTIONS, General).

FOR THE TREATMENT OF CMV RETINITIS IN PATIENTS WITH NORMAL RENAL FUNCTION

Induction: For patients with active CMV retinitis, the recommended dosage is 900 mg (two 450 mg tablets) twice a day for 21 days with food.

Maintenance: Following induction treatment, or in patients with inactive CMV retinitis, the recommended dosage is 900 mg (two 450 mg tablets) once daily with food.

V

RENAL IMPAIRMENT

Serum creatinine or creatinine clearance levels should be monitored carefully. Dosage adjustment is required according to creatinine clearance as shown in TABLE 9 (see PRECAUTIONS, General and CLINICAL PHARMACOLOGY, Pharmacokinetics, Special Populations, Renal Impairment). Increased monitoring for cytopenias may be warranted in patients with renal impairment (see PRECAUTIONS, Laboratory Testing).

TABLE 9 *Dose Modifications for Patients With Impaired Renal Function*

CRCL* (ml/min)	Induction Dose	Maintenance Dose
≥60	900 mg twice daily	900 mg once daily
40-59	450 mg twice daily	450 mg once daily
25-39	450 mg once daily	450 mg every 2 days
10-24	450 mg every 2 days	450 mg twice weekly

* An estimated creatinine clearance can be related to serum creatinine by the following formulas: **For males** = {(140 - age [years]) × (body weight [kg])} ÷ {(72) × (serum creatinine [mg/dl])}; **For females** = 0.85 × male value

HEMODIALYSIS PATIENTS

Valganciclovir HCl should not be prescribed to patients receiving hemodialysis (see CLINICAL PHARMACOLOGY, Pharmacokinetics, Special Populations, Hemodialysis and PRECAUTIONS, General).

HANDLING AND DISPOSAL

Caution should be exercised in the handling of valganciclovir HCl tablets. Tablets should not be broken or crushed. Since valganciclovir is considered a potential teratogen and carcinogen in humans, caution should be observed in handling broken tablets (see WARNINGS, Teratogenesis, Carcinogenesis and Mutagenesis). Avoid direct contact of broken or crushed tablets with skin or mucous membranes. If such contact occurs, wash thoroughly with soap and water, and rinse eyes thoroughly with plain water.

Because ganciclovir shares some of the properties of antitumor agents (*i.e.*, carcinogenicity and mutagenicity), consideration should be given to handling and disposal according to guidelines issued for antineoplastic drugs. Several guidelines on this subject have been published (see REFERENCES).

There is no general agreement that all of the procedures recommended in the guidelines are necessary or appropriate.

HOW SUPPLIED

Valcyte (valganciclovir HCl tablets) is available as 450 mg pink convex oval tablets with "VGC" on one side and "450" on the other side. Each tablet contains valganciclovir HCl equivalent to 450 mg valganciclovir.

Storage: Store at 25°C (77°F); excursions permitted to 15-30°C (59-86°F).

PRODUCT LISTING - EQUIVALENTS NOT AVAILABLE

Tablet - Oral - 450 mg

60's $1798.50 VALCYTE, Roche Laboratories 00004-0038-22

Valproate Sodium *(003326)*

Categories: Seizures, absence; Seizures, complex partial; Pregnancy Category D; FDA Approved 1997 Jan

Drug Classes: Anticonvulsants

Brand Names: **Depacon**

Foreign Brand Availability: Convulex (Germany); Depakene (Japan); Depakin (Bulgaria; Turkey); Depakine (Austria; Bahrain; Belgium; Cyprus; Egypt; France; Greece; Hungary; Iran; Iraq; Jordan; Korea; Kuwait; Lebanon; Libya; Netherlands; Oman; Portugal; Qatar; Republic-of-Yemen; Saudi-Arabia; Spain; Switzerland; Syria; Thailand; United-Arab-Emirates); Depakine Chrono (Belgium; Hungary; Poland; Portugal; Taiwan; Thailand); Depakine Druppels (Netherlands); Depakote (France); Depalept (Israel); Depalept Chrono (Israel); Epilam (Korea); Epilex (Turkey); Epilim (Australia; Bahamas; Barbados; Belize; Benin; Bermuda; Burkina-Faso; China; Curacao; England; Ethiopia; Gambia; Ghana; Guinea; Guyana; Hong-Kong; Ireland; Ivory-Coast; Jamaica; Kenya; Liberia; Malawi; Malaysia; Mali; Mauritania; Mauritius; Morocco; Netherland-Antilles; New-Zealand; Niger; Nigeria; Senegal; Seychelles; Sierra-Leone; South-Africa; Sudan; Surinam; Tanzania; Trinidad; Tunia; Uganda; Zambia; Zimbabwe); Epilim Chrono (Malaysia); Epival (Bahrain; Costa-Rica; Cyprus; Dominican-Republic; Egypt; El-Salvador; Guatemala; Honduras; Iran; Iraq; Jordan; Kuwait; Lebanon; Libya; Nicaragua; Oman; Panama; Qatar; Republic-of-Yemen; Saudi-Arabia; Syria; United-Arab-Emirates); Leptilan (Bahamas; Barbados; Belize; Benin; Bermuda; Burkina-Faso; Curacao; Ecuador; Ethiopia; Gambia; Ghana; Guinea; Guyana; Indonesia; Ivory-Coast; Jamaica; Kenya; Liberia; Malawi; Malaysia; Mali; Mauritania; Mauritius; Mexico; Morocco; Netherland-Antilles; Niger; Nigeria; Senegal; Seychelles; Sierra-Leone; Sudan; Surinam; Taiwan; Tanzania; Trinidad; Tunia; Uganda; Zambia; Zimbabwe); Orfil (Korea); Orfiril (Hong-Kong; Israel; Peru); Orfiril Retard (Singapore); Petilin (Bahamas; Bahrain; Barbados; Belize; Benin; Bermuda; Burkina-Faso; Curacao; Cyprus; Egypt; Ethiopia; Gambia; Ghana; Guinea; Guyana; Iran; Iraq; Ivory-Coast; Jamaica; Jordan; Kenya; Kuwait; Lebanon; Liberia; Libya; Malawi; Mali; Mauritania; Mauritius; Morocco; Netherland-Antilles; Niger; Nigeria; Oman; Qatar; Republic-of-Yemen; Saudi-Arabia; Senegal; Seychelles; Sierra-Leone; Sudan; Surinam; Syria; Tanzania; Trinidad; Tunia; Uganda; United-Arab-Emirates; Zambia; Zimbabwe); Valcote (Ecuador); Valeptol (Korea); Valoin (Korea); Valpakine (Costa-Rica; Dominican-Republic; Ecuador; El-Salvador; Guatemala; Honduras; Peru); Valparin (Thailand); Valporal (Israel); Valprax (Peru); Valpro (Australia; Hong-Kong); Valsup (Colombia)

WARNING

HEPATOTOXICITY:

HEPATIC FAILURE RESULTING IN FATALITIES HAS OCCURRED IN PATIENTS RECEIVING VALPROIC ACID AND ITS DERIVATIVES. EXPERIENCE HAS INDICATED THAT CHILDREN UNDER THE AGE OF 2 YEARS ARE AT A CONSIDERABLY INCREASED RISK OF DEVELOPING FATAL HEPATOTOXICITY, ESPECIALLY THOSE ON MULTIPLE ANTICONVULSANTS, THOSE WITH CONGENITAL METABOLIC DISORDERS, THOSE WITH SEVERE SEIZURE DISORDERS ACCOMPANIED BY MENTAL RETARDATION, AND THOSE WITH ORGANIC BRAIN DISEASE. WHEN VALPROATE SODIUM FOR INJECTION IS USED IN THIS PATIENT GROUP, IT SHOULD BE USED WITH EXTREME CAUTION AND AS A SOLE AGENT. THE BENEFITS OF THERAPY SHOULD BE WEIGHED AGAINST THE RISKS. ABOVE THIS AGE GROUP, EXPERIENCE IN EPILEPSY HAS INDICATED THAT THE INCIDENCE OF FATAL HEPATOTOXICITY DECREASES CONSIDERABLY IN PROGRESSIVELY OLDER PATIENT GROUPS.

WARNING — Cont'd

THESE INCIDENTS USUALLY HAVE OCCURRED DURING THE FIRST 6 MONTHS OF TREATMENT. SERIOUS OR FATAL HEPATOTOXICITY MAY BE PRECEDED BY NON-SPECIFIC SYMPTOMS SUCH AS MALAISE, WEAKNESS, LETHARGY, FACIAL EDEMA, ANOREXIA, AND VOMITING. IN PATIENTS WITH EPILEPSY, A LOSS OF SEIZURE CONTROL MAY ALSO OCCUR. PATIENTS SHOULD BE MONITORED CLOSELY FOR APPEARANCE OF THESE SYMPTOMS. LIVER FUNCTION TESTS SHOULD BE PERFORMED PRIOR TO THERAPY AND AT FREQUENT INTERVALS THEREAFTER, ESPECIALLY DURING THE FIRST 6 MONTHS.

TERATOGENICITY:

VALPROATE CAN PRODUCE TERATOGENIC EFFECTS SUCH AS NEURAL TUBE DEFECTS (*e.g.*, SPINA BIFIDA), ACCORDINGLY, THE USE OF VALPROATE PRODUCTS IN WOMEN OF CHILDBEARING POTENTIAL REQUIRES THAT THE BENEFITS OF ITS USE BE WEIGHED AGAINST THE RISK OF INJURY TO THE FETUS.

PANCREATITIS:

CASES OF LIFE-THREATENING PANCREATITIS HAVE BEEN REPORTED IN BOTH CHILDREN AND ADULTS RECEIVING VALPROATE. SOME OF THE CASES HAVE BEEN DESCRIBED AS HEMORRHAGIC WITH A RAPID PROGRESSION FROM INITIAL SYMPTOMS TO DEATH. CASES HAVE BEEN REPORTED SHORTLY AFTER INITIAL USE AS WELL AS AFTER SEVERAL YEARS OF USE. PATIENTS AND GUARDIANS SHOULD BE WARNED THAT ABDOMINAL PAIN, NAUSEA, VOMITING, AND/OR ANOREXIA CAN BE SYMPTOMS OF PANCREATITIS THAT REQUIRE PROMPT MEDICAL EVALUATION. IF PANCREATITIS IS DIAGNOSED, VALPROATE SHOULD ORDINARILY BE DISCONTINUED. ALTERNATIVE TREATMENT FOR THE UNDERLYING MEDICAL CONDITION SHOULD BE INITIATED AS CLINICALLY INDICATED. (SEE WARNINGS AND PRECAUTIONS.)

DESCRIPTION

Valproate sodium is the sodium salt of valproic acid designated as sodium 2-propylpentanoate. Valproate sodium has a molecular weight of 166.2. It occurs as an essentially white and odorless, crystalline, deliquescent powder.

Depacon solution is available in 5 ml single-dose vials for intravenous injection. Each ml contains valproate sodium equivalent to 100 mg valproic acid, edetate disodium 0.40 mg, and water for injection to volume. The pH is adjusted to 7.6 with sodium hydroxide and/or hydrochloric acid. The solution is clear and colorless.

CLINICAL PHARMACOLOGY

Valproate sodium exists as the valproate ion in the blood. The mechanisms by which valproate exerts its therapeutic effects have not been established. It has been suggested that its activity in epilepsy is related to increased brain concentrations of gamma-aminobutyric acid (GABA).

PHARMACOKINETICS

Bioavailability

Equivalent doses of intravenous (IV) valproate and oral valproate products are expected to result in equivalent C_{max}, C_{min}, and total systemic exposure to the valproate ion. However, the rate of valproate ion absorption may vary with the formulation used. These differences should be of minor clinical importance under the steady state conditions achieved in chronic use in the treatment of epilepsy.

Administration of divalproex sodium tablets and IV valproate (given as a 1 hour infusion), 250 mg every 6 hours for 4 days to 18 healthy male volunteers resulted in equivalent AUC, C_{max}, C_{min} as steady state, as well as after the first dose. The T_{max} after IV valproate sodium occurs at the end of the 1 hour infusion, while the T_{max} after oral dosing with divalproex sodium occurs at approximately 4 hours. Because the kinetics of unbound valproate are linear, bioequivalence between valproate sodium and divalproex sodium up to the maximum recommended dose of 60 mg/kg/day can be assumed. The AUC and C_{max} resulting from administration of IV valproate 500 mg as a single 1 hour infusion and a single 500 mg dose of valproic acid syrup to 17 healthy male volunteers were also equivalent.

Patients maintained on valproic acid doses of 750 mg to 4250 mg daily (given in divided doses every 6 hours) as oral divalproex sodium alone (n=24) or with another stabilized antiepileptic drug [carbamazepine (n=15), phenytoin (n=11), or phenobarbital (n=1)], showed comparable plasma levels for valproic acid when switching from oral divalproex sodium to IV valproate (1-hour infusion).

Distribution

Protein Binding

The plasma protein binding of valproate is concentration dependent and the free fraction increases from approximately 10% at 40 μg/ml to 18.5% at 130 μg/ml. Protein binding of valproate is reduced in the elderly, in patients with chronic hepatic diseases, in patients with renal impairment, and in the presence of other drugs (*e.g.*, aspirin). Conversely, valproate may displace certain protein-bound drugs (*e.g.*, phenytoin, carbamazepine, warfarin, and tolbutamide). (See DRUG INTERACTIONS for more detailed information on the pharmacokinetic interactions of valproate with other drugs.)

CNS Distribution

Valproate concentration in cerebrospinal fluid (CSF) approximate unbound concentrations in plasma (about 10% of total concentration).

Metabolism

Valproate is metabolized almost entirely by the liver. In adult patients on monotherapy, 30-50% of an administered dose appears in urine as a glucuronide conjugate. Mitochondrial β-oxidation is the other major metabolic pathway, typically accounting for over 40% of the dose. Usually, less than 15-20% of the dose is eliminated by other oxidative mechanisms. Less than 3% of an administered dose is excreted unchanged in urine.

The relationship between dose and total valproate concentration is nonlinear; concentration does not increase proportionally with the dose, but rather, increases to a lesser extent due to saturable plasma protein binding. The kinetics of unbound drug are linear.

Elimination

Mean plasma clearance and volume of distribution for total valproate are 0.56 L/h/1.73 m^2 and 11 L/1.73 m^2, respectively. Mean terminal half-life for valproate monotherapy after a 60 minute intravenous infusion of 1000 mg was 16 ± 3.0 hours.

The estimates cited apply primarily to patients who are not taking drugs that affect hepatic metabolizing enzyme systems. For example, patients taking enzyme-inducing antepileptic drugs (carbamazepine, phenytoin, and phenobarbital) will clear valproate more rapidly. Because of these changes in valproate clearance, monitoring of antiepileptic concentrations should be intensified whenever concomitant antiepileptics are introduced or withdrawn.

Special Populations

Effects of Age

Neonates: Children within the first 2 months of life have a markedly decreased ability to eliminate valproate compared to older children and adults. This is a result of reduced clearance (perhaps due to delay in development of glucuronosyltransferase and other enzyme systems involved in valproate elimination) as well as increased volume of distribution (in part due to decreased plasma protein binding). For example, in one study, the half-life in children under 10 days ranged from 10-67 hours compared to a range of 7-13 hours in children greater than 2 months.

Children: Pediatric patients (*i.e.,* between 3 months and 10 years) have 50% higher clearances expressed on weight (*i.e.,* ml/min/kg) than do adults. Over the age of 10 years, children have pharmacokinetic parameters that approximate those of adults.

Elderly: The capacity of elderly patients (age range: 68-89 years) to eliminate valproate has been shown to be reduced compared to younger adults (age range: 22-26 years). Intrinsic clearance is reduced by 39%; the free fraction is increased by 44%. Accordingly, the initial dosage should be reduced in the elderly. (See DOSAGE AND ADMINISTRATION.)

Effects of Gender

There are no differences in the body surface area adjusted unbound clearance between males and females (4.8 ± 0.17 and 4.7 ± 0.07 L/h/1.73 m^2, respectively).

Effects of Race

The effects of race on the kinetics of valproate have not been studied.

Effects of Disease

Liver Disease: (See BOXED WARNING, CONTRAINDICATIONS, WARNINGS.) Liver disease impairs the capacity to eliminate valproate. In one study, the clearance of free valproate was decreased by 50% in 7 patients with cirrhosis and by 16% in 4 patients with acute hepatitis, compared with 6 healthy subjects. In that study, the half-life of valproate was increased from 12-18 hours. Liver disease is also associated with decreased albumin concentrations and larger unbound fractions (2- to 2.6-fold increase) of valproate. Accordingly, monitoring of total concentrations may be misleading since free concentrations may be substantially elevated in patients with hepatic disease whereas total concentrations may appear to be normal.

Renal Disease: A slight reduction (27%) in the unbound clearance of valproate has been reported in patients with renal failure (creatinine clearance <10 ml/minute); however, hemodialysis typically reduces valproate concentrations by about 20%. Therefore, no dosage adjustment appears to be necessary in patients with renal failure. Protein binding in these patients is substantially reduced; thus, monitoring total concentrations may be misleading.

PLASMA LEVELS AND CLINICAL EFFECT

The relationship between plasma concentration and clinical response is not well documented. One contributing factor is the nonlinear, concentration dependent protein binding of valproate which affects the clearance of the drug. Thus, monitoring of total serum valproate cannot provide a reliable index of the bioactive valproate species.

For example, because the plasma protein binding of valproate is concentration dependent, the free fraction increases from approximately 10% at 40 µg/ml to 18.5% at 130 µg/ml. Higher than expected free fractions occur in the elderly, in hyperlipidemic patients, and in patients with hepatic and renal diseases.

Epilepsy: The therapeutic range in epilepsy is commonly considered to be 50-100 µg/ml of total valproate, although some patients may be controlled with lower or higher plasma concentrations.

Equivalent doses of valproate sodium and divalproex sodium yield equivalent plasma levels of the valproate ion (see Pharmacokinetics).

V

INDICATIONS AND USAGE

Valproate sodium injection is indicated as an intravenous alternative in patients for whom oral administration of valproate products is temporarily not feasible in the following conditions:

Valproate sodium is indicated as monotherapy and adjunctive therapy in the treatment of patients with complex partial seizures that occur either in isolation or in association with other types of seizures.

Valproate sodium is also indicated for use as sole and adjunctive therapy in the treatment of patients with simple and complex absence seizures, and adjunctively in patients with multiple seizure types that include absence seizures.

Simple absence is defined as very brief clouding of the sensorium or loss of consciousness accompanied by certain generalized epileptic discharges without other detectable clinical signs. Complex absence is the term used when other signs are also present. (SEE WARNINGS FOR STATEMENT REGARDING FATAL HEPATIC DYSFUNCTION.)

CONTRAINDICATIONS

VALPROATE SODIUM INJECTION SHOULD NOT BE ADMINISTERED TO PATIENTS WITH HEPATIC DISEASE OR SIGNIFICANT HEPATIC DYSFUNCTION.

Valproate sodium injection is contraindicated in patients with known hypersensitivity to the drug.

WARNINGS

HEPATOTOXICITY

Hepatic failure resulting in fatalities has occurred in patients receiving valproic acid. These incidents usually have occurred during the first 6 months of treatment. Serious or fatal hepatotoxicity may be preceded by non-specific symptoms such as malaise, weakness, lethargy, facial edema, anorexia, and vomiting. In patients with epilepsy, a loss of seizure control may also occur. Patients should be monitored closely for appearance of these symptoms. Liver function tests should be performed prior to therapy and at frequent intervals thereafter, especially during the first 6 months of valproate therapy. However, physicans should not rely totally on serum biochemistry since these tests may not be abnormal in all instances, but should also consider the result of careful interim medical history and physical examination.

Caution should be observed when administering valproate products to patients with a prior history of hepatic disease. Patients on multiple anticonvulsants, children, those with congenital metabolic disorders, those with severe seizure disorders accompanied by mental retardation, and those with organic brain disease may be at particular risk. Experience has indicated that children under the age of 2 years are at a considerably increased risk of developing fatal hepatotoxicity, especially those with the aforementioned conditions. When valproate sodium is used in this patient group, it should be used with extreme caution and as a sole agent. The benefits of therapy should be weighed against the risks. Use of valproate sodium has not been studied in children below the age of 2 years. Above this age group, experience with valproate products in epilepsy has indicated that the incidence of fatal hepatotoxicity decreases considerably in progressively older patient groups.

The drug should be discontinued immediately in the presence of significant hepatic dysfunction, suspected or apparent. In some cases, hepatic dysfunction has progressed in spite of discontinuation of drug.

PANCREATITIS

Cases of life-threatening pancreatitis have been reported in both children and adults receiving valproate. Some of the cases have been described as hemorrhagic with a rapid progression from initial symptoms to death. Some cases have occurred shortly after initial use as well as after several years of use. The rate based upon the reported case exceeds that expected in the general population and there have been cases in which pancreatitis recurred after rechallenge with valproate. In clinical trials, there were 2 cases of pancreatitis without alternative etiology in 2416 patients, representing 1044 patient-years experience. Patients and guardians should be warned that abdominal pain, nausea, vomiting, and/or anorexia can be symptoms of pancreatitis that require prompt medical evaluation. If pancreatitis is diagnosed, valproate should ordinarily be discontinued. Alternative treatment for the underlying medical condition should be initiated as clinically indicated (see BOXED WARNING).

SOMNOLENCE IN THE ELDERLY

In a double-blind, multicenter trial of valproate in elderly patients with dementia (mean age = 83 years), doses were increased by 125 mg/day to a target dose of 20 mg/kg/day. A significantly higher proportion of valproate patients had somnolence compared to placebo, and although not statistically significant, there was a higher proportion of patients with dehydration. Discontinuations for somnolence were also significantly higher than with placebo. In some patients with somnolence (approximately one-half), there was associated reduced nutritional intake and weight loss. There was a trend for the patients who experienced these events to have a lower baseline albumin concentration, lower valproate clearance, and a higher BUN. In elderly patients, dosage should be increased more slowly and with regular monitoring for fluid and nutritional intake, dehydration, somnolence, and other adverse events. Dose reductions or discontinuation of valproate should be considered in patients with decreased food or fluid intake and in patients with excessive somnolence (see DOSAGE AND ADMINISTRATION).

THROMBOCYTOPENIA

The frequency of adverse effects (particularly elevated liver enzymes and thrombocytopenia [see PRECAUTIONS]) may be dose-related. In a clinical trial of divalproex sodium as monotherapy in patients with epilepsy, 34/126 patients (27%) receiving approximately 50 mg/kg/day on average, had at least one value of platelets $\leq 75 \times 10^9$/L. Approximately half of these patients had treatment discontinued, with return of platelet counts to normal. In the remaining patients, platelet counts normalized with continued treatment. In this study, the probability of thrombocytopenia appeared to increase significantly at total valproate concentrations of ≥110 µg/ml (females) or ≥135 µg/ml (males). The therapeutic benefit which may accompany the higher doses should therefore be weighed against the possibility of a greater incidence of adverse effects.

POST-TRAUMATIC SEIZURES

A study was conducted to evaluate the effect of IV valproate in the prevention of post-traumatic seizures in patients with acute head injuries. Patients were randomly assigned to receive either IV valproate given for 1 week (followed by oral valproate products for either 1 or 6 months per random treatment assignment) or IV phenytoin given for 1 week (followed by placebo). In this study, the incidence of death was found to be higher in the two groups assigned to valproate treatment compared to the rate in those assigned to the IV phenytoin treatment group (13% vs 8.5%, respectively). Many of these patients were critically ill with multiple and/or severe injuries, and evaluation of the causes of death did not suggest any specific drug-related causation. Further, in the absence of a concurrent placebo control during the initial week of intravenous therapy, it is impossible to determine if the mortality rate in the patients treated with valproate was greater or less than that expected in a similar group not treated with valproate, or whether the rate seen in the IV phenytoin treated patients was lower than would be expected. Nonetheless, until further information is available, it seems prudent not to use valproate sodium in patients with acute head trauma for the prophylaxis of post-traumatic seizures.

USE IN PREGNANCY

ACCORDING TO PUBLISHED AND UNPUBLISHED REPORTS, VALPROIC ACID MAY PRODUCE TERATOGENIC EFFECTS IN THE OFFSPRING OF HUMAN FEMALES RECEIVING THE DRUG DURING PREGNANCY.

THERE ARE MULTIPLE REPORTS IN THE CLINICAL LITERATURE WHICH INDICATE THAT THE USE OF ANTIEPILEPSY DRUGS DURING PREGNANCY RESULT IN AN INCREASED INCIDENCE OF BIRTH DEFECTS IN THE OFFSPRING. ALTHOUGH DATA ARE MORE EXTENSIVE WITH RESPECT TO TRIMETHADIONE, PARAMETHADIONE, PHENYTOIN, AND PHENOBARBITAL, REPORTS INDICATE A POSSIBLE SIMILAR ASSOCIATION WITH THE USE OF OTHER ANTIEPILEPSY DRUGS. THEREFORE, ANTIEPILEPSY DRUGS SHOULD BE ADMINISTERED TO WOMEN OF CHILDBEARING POTENTIAL ONLY IF THEY ARE CLEARLY SHOWN TO BE ESSENTIAL IN THE MANAGEMENT OF THEIR SEIZURES.

THE INCIDENCE OF NEURAL TUBE DEFECTS IN THE FETUS MAY BE INCREASED IN MOTHERS RECEIVING VALPROATE DURING THE FIRST TRIMESTER OF PREGNANCY. THE CENTERS FOR DISEASE CONTROL (CDC) HAS ESTIMATED THE RISK OF VALPROIC ACID EXPOSED WOMEN HAVING CHILDREN WITH SPINA BIFIDA TO BE APPROXIMATELY 1-2%.

OTHER CONGENITAL ANOMALIES (*e.g.,* CRANIOFACIAL DEFECTS, CARDIOVASCULAR MALFORMATIONS, AND ANOMALIES INVOLVING VARIOUS BODY SYSTEMS), COMPATIBLE AND INCOMPATIBLE WITH LIFE, HAVE BEEN REPORTED. SUFFICIENT DATA TO DETERMINE THE INCIDENCE OF THESE CONGENITAL ANOMALIES IS NOT AVAILABLE.

THE HIGHER INCIDENCE OF CONGENITAL ANOMALIES IN ANTIEPILEPSY DRUG-TREATED WOMEN WITH SEIZURE DISORDERS CANNOT BE REGARDED AS A CAUSE AND EFFECT RELATIONSHIP. THERE ARE INTRINSIC METHODOLOGIC PROBLEMS IN OBTAINING ADEQUATE DATA ON DRUG TERATOGENICITY IN HUMANS; GENETIC FACTORS OR THE EPILEPTIC CONDITION ITSELF, MAY BE MORE IMPORTANT THAN DRUG THERAPY IN CONTRIBUTING TO CONGENITAL ANOMALIES.

PATIENTS TAKING VALPROATE MAY DEVELOP CLOTTING ABNORMALITIES. A PATIENT WHO HAD LOW FIBRINOGEN WHEN TAKING MULTIPLE ANTICONVULSANTS INCLUDING VALPROATE GAVE BIRTH TO AN INFANT WITH AFIBRINOGENEMIA WHO SUBSEQUENTLY DIED OF HEMORRHAGE. IF VALPROATE IS USED IN PREGNANCY THE CLOTTING PARAMETERS SHOULD BE MONITORED CAREFULLY.

HEPATIC FAILURE, RESULTING IN THE DEATH OF A NEWBORN AND OF AN INFANT, HAS BEEN REPORTED FOLLOWING THE USE OF VALPROATE DURING PREGNANCY.

Animal studies have demonstrated valproate-induced teratogenicity. Increased frequencies of malformations, as well as intrauterine growth retardation and death, have been observed in mice, rats, rabbits, and monkeys following prenatal exposure to valproate. Malformations of the skeletal system are the most common structural abnormalities produced in experimental animals, but neural tube closure defects have been seen in mice exposed to maternal plasma valproate concentrations exceeding 230 μg/ml (2.3 times the upper limit of the human therapeutic range) during susceptible periods of embryonic development. Administration of an oral dose of 200 mg/kg/day or greater (50% of the maximum human daily dose or greater on a mg/m^2 basis) to pregnant rats during organogenesis produced malformations (skeletal, cardiac, and urogenital) and growth retardation in the offspring. These doses resulted the peak maternal plasma valproate levels of approximately 340 μg/ml or greater (3.4 times the upper limit of the human therapeutic range or greater). Behavioral deficits have been reported in the offspring of rats given a dose of 200 mg/kg/day throughout most of pregnancy. An oral dose of 350 mg/kg/day (2 times the maximum human daily dose on a mg/m^2 basis) produced skeletal and visceral malformations in rabbits exposed during organogenesis. Skeletal malformations, growth retardation, and death were observed in rhesus monkeys following administration of an oral dose of 200 mg/kg/day (equal to the maximum human daily dose on a mg/m^2 basis) during organogenesis. This dose resulted in peak maternal plasma valproate levels of approximately 280 μg/ml (2.8 times the upper limit of the human therapeutic range).

The prescribing physician will wish to weigh the benefits of therapy against the risks in treating or counseling women of childbearing potential. If this drug is used during pregnancy, or if the patient becomes pregnant while taking this drug, the patient should be apprised of the potential hazard to the fetus.

Antiepilepsy drugs should not be discontinued abruptly in patients in whom the drug is administered to prevent major seizures because of the strong possibility of precipitating status epilepticus with attendant hypoxia and threat to life. In individual cases where the severity and frequency of the seizure disorder are such that the removal of medication does not pose a serious threat to the patient, discontinuation of the drug may be considered prior to and during pregnancy, although it cannot be said with any confidence that even minor seizures do not pose some hazard to the developing embryo or fetus.

Tests to detect neural tube and other defects using current accepted procedures should be considered a part of routine prenatal care in childbearing women receiving valproate.

PRECAUTIONS

HEPATIC DYSFUNCTION

See BOXED WARNING, CONTRAINDICATIONS and WARNINGS.

PANCREATITIS

See BOXED WARNING and WARNINGS.

GENERAL

Because of reports of thrombocytopenia (see WARNINGS), inhibition of the secondary phase of platelet aggregation, and abnormal coagulation parameters, (*e.g.,* low fibrinogen), platelet counts and coagulation tests are recommended before initiating therapy and at periodic intervals. It is recommended that patients receiving valproate sodium be monitored for platelet count and coagulation parameters prior to planned surgery. In a clinical trial of divalproex sodium as monotherapy in patients with epilepsy, 34/126 patients (27%) receiving approximately 50 mg/kg/day on average, had at least one value of platelets $\leq 75 \times 10^9$/L. Approximately half of these patients had treatment discontinued, with return of platelet counts to normal. In the remainng patients, platelet counts normalized with continued treatment. In this study, the probability of thrombocytopenia appeared to increase significantly at total valproate concentrations of $\geq$110 μg/ml (females) or $\geq$135 μg/ml (males). Evidence of hemorrhage, bruising, or a disorder of hemostasis/coagulation is an indication for reduction of the dosage or withdrawal of therapy.

Hyperammonemia with or without lethargy or coma has been reported and may be present in the absence of abnormal liver function tests. Asymptomatic elevations of ammonia are more common and when present require more frequent monitoring. If clinically significant symptoms occur, valproate sodium therapy should be modified or discontinued.

Since valproate sodium may interact with concurrently administered drugs which are capable of enzyme induction, periodic plasma concentration determinations of valproate and concomitant drugs are recommended during the early course of therapy. (See DRUG INTERACTIONS.)

Valproate is partially eliminated in the urine as a keto-metabolite which may lead to false interpretation of the urine ketone test.

There have been reports of altered thyroid function tests associated with valproate. The clinical significance of these is unknown.

There are *in vitro* studies that suggest valproate stimulates the replication of the HIV and CMV viruses under certain experimental conditions. The clinical consequence, if any, is not known. Additionally, the relevance of these *in vitro* findings is uncertain for patients receiving maximally suppressive antiretroviral therapy. Nevertheless, these data should be borne in mind when interpreting the results from regular monitoring of the viral load in HIV infected patients receiving valproate or when following CMV infected patients clinically.

INFORMATION FOR THE PATIENT

Patients and guardians should be warned that abdominal pain, nausea, vomiting, and/or anorexia can be symptoms of pancreatitis and, therefore, require further medical evaluation promptly.

Since valproate sodium may produce CNS depression, especially when combined with another CNS depressant (*e.g.,* alcohol) patients should be advised not to engage in hazardous activities, such as driving an automobile or operating dangerous machinery, until it is known that they do not become drowsy from the drug.

CARCINOGENESIS, MUTAGENESIS, AND IMPAIRMENT OF FERTILITY

Carcinogenesis

Valproic acid was administered orally to Sprague Dawley rats and ICR (HA/ICR) mice at doses of 80 and 170 mg/kg/day (approximately 10-50% of the maximum human daily dose on a mg/m^2 basis) for 2 years. A variety of neoplasms were observed in both species. The chief findings were a statistically significant increase in the incidence of subcutaneous fibrosarcomas in high dose male rats receiving valproic acid and a statistically significant dose-related trend for benign pulmonary adenomas in male mice receiving valproic acid. The significance of these findings for humans is unknown.

Mutagenesis

Valproate was not mutagenic in an *in vitro* bacterial assay (Ames test), did not produce dominant lethal effects in mice, and did not increase chromosome aberration frequency in an *in vivo* cytogenetic study in rats. Increased frequencies of sister chromatid exchange (SCE) have been reported in a study of epileptic children taking valproate, but this association was not observed in another study conducted in adults. There is some evidence that increased SCE frequencies may be associated with epilepsy. The biological significance of an increase in SCE frequency is not known.

Fertility

Chronic toxicity studies in juvenile and adult rats and dogs demonstrated reduced spermatogenesis and testicular atrophy at oral doses of 400 mg/kg/day or greater in rats (approximately equivalent to or greater than the maximum human daily dose on a mg/m^2 basis) and 150 mg/kg/day or greater in dogs (approximately 1.4 times the maximum human daily dose or greater on a mg/m^2 basis). Segment I fertility studies in rats have shown oral doses up to 350 mg/kg/day (approximately equal to the maximum human daily dose on a mg/m^2 basis) for 60 days to have no effect on fertility. THE EFFECT OF VALPROATE ON TESTICULAR DEVELOPMENT AND ON SPERM PRODUCTION AND FERTILITY IN HUMANS IS UNKNOWN.

PREGNANCY CATEGORY D

See WARNINGS.

NURSING MOTHERS

Valproate is excreted in breast milk. Concentrations in breast milk have been reported to be 1-10% of serum concentrations. It is not known what effect this would have on a nursing infant. Consideration should be given to discontinuing nursing when valproate is administered to a nursing woman.

PEDIATRIC USE

Experience with oral valproate has indicated that pediatric patients under the age of 2 years are at a considerably increased risk of developing fatal hepatotoxicity, especially those with the aforementioned conditions (see BOXED WARNING). The safety of valproate sodium has not been studied in individuals below the age of 2 years. If a decision is made to use valproate sodium in this age group, it should be used with extreme caution and as a sole agent. The benefits of therapy should be weighed against the risks. Above the age of 2 years, experience in epilepsy has indicated that the incidence of fatal hepatotoxicity decreases considerably in progressively older patient groups.

Younger children, especially those receiving enzyme-inducing drugs, will require larger maintenance doses to attain targeted total and unbound valproic acid concentrations.

The variability in free fraction limits the clinical usefulness of monitoring total serum valproic acid concentrations. Interpretation of valproic acid concentrations in children should include consideration of factors that affect hepatic metabolism and protein binding.

No unique safety concerns were identified in the 24 patients age 2-17 years who received valproate sodium in clinical trials.

The basic toxicology and pathologic manifestations of valproate sodium in neonatal (4 day old) and juvenile (14 day old) rats are similar to those seen in young adult rats. However, additional findings, including renal alterations in juvenile rats and renal alterations and retinal dysplasia in neonatal rats, have been reported. These findings occurred at 240 mg/kg/day, a dosage approximately equivalent to the human maximum recommended daily dose on a mg/m^2 basis. They were not seen at 90 mg/kg, or 40% of the maximum human daily dose on a mg/m^2 basis.

GERIATRIC USE

No patients above the age of 65 years were enrolled in double-blind prospective clinical trials of mania associated with bipolar illness. In a case review study of 583 patients, 72 patients (12%) were greater than 65 years of age. A higher percentage of patients above 65 years of age reported accidental injury, infection, pain, somnolence, and tremor. Discontinuation of valproate was occasionally associated with the latter 2 events. It is not clear whether these events indicate additional risk or whether they result from preexisting medical illness and concomitant medication use among these patients.

A study of elderly patients with dementia revealed drug related somnolence and discontinuation for somnolence (see WARNINGS, Somnolence in the Elderly). The starting dose should be reduced in these patients, and dosage reductions or discontinuation should be considered in patients with excessive somnolence (see DOSAGE AND ADMINISTRATION).

No unique safety concerns were identified in the 19 patients >65 years of age receiving valproate sodium in clinical trials.

DRUG INTERACTIONS

EFFECTS OF CO-ADMINISTERED DRUGS ON VALPROATE CLEARANCE

Drugs that affect the level of expression of hepatic enzymes, particularly those that elevate levels of glucuronosyltransferases, may increase the clearance of valproate. For example, phenytoin, carbamazepine, and phenobarbital (or primidone) can double the clearance of valproate. Thus, patients on monotherapy will generally have longer half-lives and higher concentrations than patients receiving polytherapy with antiepilepsy drugs.

In contrast, drugs that are inhibitors of cytochrome P450 isozymes, (*e.g.*, antidepressants), may be expected to have little effect on valproate clearance because cytochrome P450 microsomal mediated oxidation is a relatively minor secondary metabolic pathway compared to glucuronidation and beta-oxidation.

Because of these changes in valproate clearance, monitoring of valproate and concomitant drug concentrations should be increased whenever enzyme inducing drugs are introduced or withdrawn.

The following list provides information about the potential for an influence of several commonly prescribed medications on valproate pharmacokinetics. The list is not exhaustive nor could it be, since new interactions are continuously being reported.

DRUGS FOR WHICH A POTENTIALLY IMPORTANT INTERACTION HAS BEEN OBSERVED

Aspirin: A study involving the co-administration of aspirin at antipyretic doses (11-16 mg/kg) with valproate to pediatric patients (n=6) revealed a decrease in protein binding and an inhibition of metabolism of valproate. Valproate free fraction was increased 4-fold in the presence of aspirin compared to valproate alone. The β-oxidation pathway consisting of 2-E-valproic acid, 3-OH-valproic acid, and 3-keto valproic acid was decreased from 25% of total metabolites excreted on valproate alone to 8.3% in the presence of aspirin. Caution should be observed if valproate and aspirin are to be co-administered.

Felbamate: A study involving the co-administration of 1200 mg/day of felbamate with valproate to patients with epilepsy (n=10) revealed an increase in mean valproate peak concentration by 35% (from 86-115 μg/ml) compared to valproate alone. Increasing the felbamate dose to 2400 mg/day increased the mean valproate peak concentration to 133 μg/ml (another 16% increase). A decrease in valproate dosage may be necessary when felbamate therapy is initiated.

Rifampin: A study involving the administration of a single dose of valproate (7 mg/kg) 36 hours after 5 nights of daily dosing with rifampin (600 mg) revealed a 40% increase in the oral clearance of valproate. Valproate dosage adjustment may be necessary when it is co-administered with rifampin.

DRUGS FOR WHICH EITHER NO INTERACTION OR A LIKELY CLINICALLY UNIMPORTANT INTERACTION HAS BEEN OBSERVED

Antacids: A study involving the co-administration of valproate 500 mg with commonly administered antacids (Maalox, Trisogel, and Titralac - 160 mEq doses) did not reveal any effect on the extent of absorption of valproate.

Chlorpromazine: A study involving the administration of 100-300 mg/day of chlorpromazine to schizophrenic patients already receiving valproate (200 mg bid) revealed a 15% increase in trough plasma levels of valproate.

Haloperidol: A study involving the administration of 6-10 mg/day of haloperidol to schizophrenic patients already receiving valproate (200 mg bid) revealed no significant changes in valproate trough plasma levels.

Cimetidine and Ranitidine: Cimetidine and ranitidine do not affect the clearance of valproate.

EFFECTS OF VALPROATE ON OTHER DRUGS

Valproate has been found to be a weak inhibitor of some P450 isozymes, epoxide hydrase, and glucuronyltransferases.

The following list provides information about the potential for an influence of valproate co-administration on the pharmacokinetics or pharmacodynamics of several commonly prescribed medications. The list is not exhaustive, since new interactions are continuously being reported.

DRUGS FOR WHICH A POTENTIALLY IMPORTANT VALPROATE INTERACTION HAS BEEN OBSERVED

Amitriptyline/Nortriptyline: Administration of a single oral 50 mg dose of amitriptyline to 15 normal volunteers (10 males and 5 females) who received valproate (500 mg bid) resulted in a 21% decrease in plasma clearance of amitriptyline and a 34% decrease in the net clearance of nortriptyline. Rare postmarketing reports of concurrent use of valproate and amitriptyline resulting in an increased amitriptyline level have been received. Concurrent use of valproate and amitriptyline has rarely been associated with toxicity. Monitoring of amitriptyline levels should be considered for patients taking valproate concomitantly with amitriptyline. Consideration should be given to lowering the dose of amitriptyline/nortriptyline in the presence of valproate.

Carbamazepine/Carbamazepine-10,11-Epoxide: Serum levels of carbamazepine (CBZ) decreased 17% while that of carbamazepine-10, 11-epoxide (CBZ-E) increased by 45% upon co-administration of valproate and CBZ to epileptic patients.

Clonazepam: The concomitant use of valproic acid and clonazepam may induce absence status in patients with a history of absence type seizures.

Diazepam: Valproate displaces diazepam from its plasma albumin binding sites and inhibits its metabolism. Co-administration of valproate (1500 mg daily) increased the free fraction of diazepam (10 mg) by 90% in healthy volunteers (n=6). Plasma clearance and volume of distribution for free diazepam were reduced by 25% and 20%, respectively, in the presence of valproate. The elimination half-life of diazepam remained unchanged upon addition of valproate.

Ethosuximide: Valproate inhibits the metabolism of ethosuximide. Administration of a single ethosuximide dose of 500 mg with valproate (800-1600 mg/day) to healthy volunteers (n=6) was accompanied by a 25% increase in elimination half-life of ethosuximide and a 15% decrease in its total clearance as compared to ethosuximide alone. Patients receiving valproate and ethosuximide, especially along with other anticonvulsants, should be monitored for alterations in serum concentrations of both drugs.

Lamotrigine: In a steady-state study involving 10 healthy volunteers, the elimination half-life of lamotrigine increased from 26-70 hours with valproate co-administration (a 165% increase). The dose of lamotrigine should be reduced when co-administered with valproate.

Phenobarbital: Valproate was found to inhibit the metabolism of phenobarbital. Co-administration of valproate (250 mg bid for 14 days) with phenobarbital to normal subjects (n=6) resulted in a 50% increase in half-life and a 30% decrease in plasma clearance of phenobarbital (60 mg single-dose). The fraction of phenobarbital dose excreted unchanged increased by 50% in presence of valproate.

There is evidence for severe CNS depression, with or without significant elevations of barbiturate or valproate serum concentrations. All patients receiving concomitant barbiturate therapy should be closely monitored for neurological toxicity. Serum barbiturate concentrations should be obtained, if possible, and the barbiturate dosage decreased, if appropriate.

Primidone, which is metabolized to a barbiturate, may be involved in a similar interaction with valproate.

Phenytoin: Valproate displaces phenytoin from its plasma albumin binding sites and inhibits its hepatic metabolism. Co-administration of valproate (400 mg tid) with phenytoin (250 mg) in normal volunteers (n=7) was associated with a 60% increase in the free fraction of phenytoin. Total plasma clearance and apparent volume of distribution of phenytoin increased 30% in the presence of valproate. Both the clearance and appparent volume of distribution of free phenytoin were reduced by 25%.

In patients with epilepsy, there have been reports of breakthrough seizures occurring with the combination of valproate and phenytoin. The dosage of phenytoin should be adjusted as required by the clinical situation.

Tolbutamide: From *in vitro* experiments, the unbound fraction of tolbutamide was increased from 20-50% when added to plasma sample taken from patients treated with valproate. The clinical relevance of this displacement is unknown.

Warfarin: In an *in vitro* study, valproate increased the unbound fraction of warfarin by up to 32.6%. The therapeutic relevance of this is unknown; however, coagulation tests should be monitored if valproate therapy is instituted in patients taking anticoagulants.

Zidovudine: In 6 patients who were seropositive for HIV, the clearance of zidovudine (100 mg q8h) was decreased by 38% after administration of valproate (250 or 500 mg q8h); the half-life of zidovudine was unaffected.

DRUGS FOR WHICH EITHER NO INTERACTION OR A LIKELY CLINICALLY UNIMPORTANT INTERACTION HAS BEEN OBSERVED

Acetaminophen: Valproate had no effect on any of the pharmacokinetic parameters of acetaminophen when it was concurrently administered to 3 epileptic patients.

Clozapine: In psychotic patients (n=11), no interaction was observed when valproate was co-administered with clozapine.

Lithium: Co-administration of valproate (500 mg bid) and lithium carbonate (300 mg tid) to normal male volunteers (n=16) had no effect on the steady-state kinetics of lithium.

Lorazepam: Concomitant administration of valproate (500 mg bid) and lorazepam (1 mg bid) in normal male volunteers (n=9) was accompanied by a 17% decrease in the plasma clearance of lorazepam.

Oral Contraceptive Steroids: Administration of a single-dose of ethinyloestradiol (50 µg)/levonorgestrel (250 µg) to 6 women on valproate (200 mg bid) therapy for 2 months did not reveal any pharmacokinetic interaction.

ADVERSE REACTIONS

The adverse events that can result from valproate sodium use include all of those associated with oral forms or valproate. The following describes experience specifically with valproate sodium. Valproate sodium has been generally well tolerated in clinical trials involving 111 healthy adult male volunteers and 352 patients with epilepsy, given at doses of 125-6000 mg (total daily dose). A total of 2% of patients discontinued treatment with valproate sodium due to adverse events. The most common adverse events leading to discontinuation were 2 cases each of nausea/vomiting and elevated amylase. Other adverse events leading to discontinuation were hallucinations, pneumonia, headache, injection site reaction, and abnormal gait. Dizziness and injection site pain were observed more frequently at a 100 mg/ml infusion rate than at rates up to 33 mg/min. At a 200 mg/min rate, dizziness and taste perversion occurred more frequently than at a 100 mg/min rate. The maximum rate of infusion studied was 200 mg/min.

Adverse events reported by at least 0.5% of all subjects/patients in clinical trials of valproate sodium are summarized in TABLE 3.

TABLE 3 *Adverse Events Reported During Studies of Valproate Sodium*

Body System/Event	n=463
Body as a Whole	
Chest pain	1.7%
Headache	4.3%
Injection site inflammation	0.6%
Injection site pain	2.6%
Injection site reaction	2.4%
Pain (unspecified)	1.3%
Cardiovascular	
Vasodilation	0.9%
Dermatologic	
Sweating	0.9%
Digestive System	
Abdominal pain	1.1%
Diarrhea	0.9%
Nausea	3.2%
Vomiting	1.3%
Nervous System	
Dizziness	5.2%
Euphoria	0.9%
Hypesthesia	0.6%
Nervousness	0.9%
Paresthesia	0.9%
Somnolence	1.7%
Tremor	0.6%
Respiratory	
Pharyngitis	0.6%
Special Senses	
Taste perversion	1.9%

EPILEPSY

Based on placebo-controlled trial of adjunctive therapy for treatment of complex partial seizures, divalproex sodium was generally well tolerated with most adverse events rated as mild to moderate in severity. Intolerance was the primary reason for discontinuation in the divalproex sodium-treated patients (6%), compared to 1% of placebo-treated patients.

TABLE 4 lists treatment-emergent adverse events which were reported by ≥5% of divalproex sodium-treated patients and for which the incidence was greater than in the placebo group, in the placebo-controlled trial of adjunctive therapy for treatment of complex partial seizures. Since patients were also treated with other antiepilepsy drugs, it is not possible, in most cases, to determine whether the adverse events listed in TABLE 4 can be ascribed to divalproex sodium alone, or the combination of divalproex sodium and other antiepilepsy drugs.

TABLE 5 lists treatment-emergent adverse events which were reported by ≥5% of patients in the high dose divalproex sodium group, and for which the incidence was greater than in the low dose group, in a controlled trial of divalproex sodium monotherapy treatment of complex partial seizures. Since patients were being titrated off another antiepilepsy drug during the first portion of the trial, it is not possible, in many cases, to determine whether the following adverse events can be ascribed to divalproex sodium alone, or the combination of divalproex sodium and other antiepilepsy drugs.

The following additional adverse events were reported by greater than 1% but less than 5% of the 358 patients treated with divalproex sodium in the controlled trials of complex partial seizures:

Body as a Whole: Back pain, chest pain, malaise.
Cardiovascular System: Tachycardia, hypertension, palpitation.
Digestive System: Increased appetite, flatulence, hematemesis, eructation, pancreatitis, periodontal abscess.
Hemic and Lymphatic System: Petechia.
Metabolic and Nutritional Disorders: SGOT increased, SGPT increased.
Musculoskeletal System: Myalgia, twitching, arthralgia, leg cramps, myasthenia.
Nervous System: Anxiety, confusion, abnormal gait, paresthesia, hypertonia, incoordination, abnormal dreams, personality disorder.
Respiratory System: Sinusitis, cough increased, pneumonia, epistaxis.
Skin and Appendages: Rash, pruritus, dry skin.
Special Senses: Taste perversion, abnormal vision, deafness, otitis media.
Urogenital System: Urinary incontinence, vaginitis, dysmenorrhea, amenorrhea, urinary frequency.

OTHER PATIENT POPULATIONS

Adverse events that have been reported with all dosage forms of valproate from epilepsy trials, spontaneous reports, and other sources are listed below by body system.

TABLE 4 *Adverse Events Reported by ≥5% of Patients Treated with Divalproex Sodium During Placebo-Controlled Trial of Adjunctive Therapy for Complex Partial Seizures*

Body System Event	Divalproex Sodium (n=77)	Placebo (n=70)
Body as a Whole		
Headache	31%	21%
Asthenia	27%	7%
Fever	6%	4%
Gastrointestinal System		
Nausea	48%	14%
Vomiting	27%	7%
Abdominal pain	23%	6%
Diarrhea	13%	6%
Anorexia	12%	0%
Dyspepsia	8%	4%
Constipation	5%	1%
Nervous System		
Somnolence	27%	11%
Tremor	25%	6%
Dizziness	25%	13%
Diplopia	16%	9%
Amblyopia/blurred vision	12%	9%
Ataxia	8%	1%
Nystagmus	8%	1%
Emotional lability	6%	4%
Thinking abnormal	6%	0%
Amnesia	5%	1%
Respiratory System		
Flu syndrome	12%	9%
Infection	12%	6%
Bronchitis	5%	1%
Rhinitis	5%	4%
Other		
Alopecia	6%	1%
Weight loss	6%	0%

TABLE 5 *Adverse Events Reported by ≥5% of Patients in the High Dose Group in the Controlled Trial of Divalproex Sodium Monotherapy for Complex Partial Seizures**

Body System Event	High Dose (n=131)	Low Dose (n=134)
Body as a Whole		
Asthenia	21%	10%
Digestive System		
Nausea	34%	26%
Diarrhea	23%	19%
Vomiting	23%	15%
Abdominal pain	12%	9%
Anorexia	11%	4%
Dyspepsia	11%	10%
Hemic/Lymphatic System		
Thrombocytopenia	24%	1%
Ecchymosis	5%	4%
Metabolic /Nutritional		
Weight gain	9%	4%
Peripheral edema	8%	3%
Nervous System		
Tremor	57%	19%
Somnolence	30%	18%
Dizziness	18%	13%
Insomnia	15%	9%
Nervousness	11%	7%
Amnesia	7%	4%
Nystagmus	7%	1%
Depression	5%	4%
Respiratory System		
Infection	20%	13%
Pharyngitis	8%	2%
Dyspnea	5%	1%
Skin Appendages		
Alopecia	24%	13%
Special Senses		
Amblyopia/blurred vision	8%	4%
Tinnitus	7%	1%

* Headache was the only adverse event that occurred in ≥5% of patients in the high dose group and at an equal or greater incidence in the low dose group.

Gastrointestinal: The most commonly reported side effects at the initiation of therapy are nausea, vomiting, and indigestion. These effects are usually transient and rarely require discontinuation of therapy. Diarrhea, abdominal cramps, and constipation have been reported. Both anorexia with some weight loss and increased appetite with weight gain have also been reported. The administration of delayed-release divalproex sodium may result in reduction of gastrointestinal side effects in some patients using oral therapy.

CNS Effects: Sedative effects have occurred in patients receiving valproate alone but occur most often in patients receiving combination therapy. Sedation usually abates upon reduction of the other antiepileptic medication. Tremor (may be dose-related), hallucinations, ataxia, headache, nystagmus, diplopia, asterixis, "spots before eyes", dysarthria, dizziness, confusion, hypesthesia, vertigo, incoordination and parkinsonism. Rare cases of coma, have occurred in patients receiving valproate alone or in conjunction with phenobarbital. In rare instances encephalophathy, with fever has developed shortly after the introduction of valproate monotherapy without evidence of hepatic dysfunction or inappropriate plasma levels; all patients recovered after the drug was withdrawn. Several reports have noted reversible cerebral atrophy and dementia in association with valproate therapy.

Dermatologic: Transient hair loss, skin rash, photosensitivity, generalized pruritus, erythema multiforme, and Stevens-Johnson syndrome. Rare cases of toxic epidermal necrolysis have been reported including a fatal case in a 6 month old infant taking valproate and several other concomitant medications. An additional case of toxic epidermal necrosis resulting in death was reported in a 35 year old patient with AIDS taking several concomitant medications and with a history of multiple cutaneous drug reactions.

Psychiatric: Emotional upset, depression, psychosis, aggression, hyperactivity, hostility, and behavioral deterioration.

Musculoskeletal: Weakness.

Hematologic: Thrombocytopenia and inhibition of the secondary phase of platelet aggregation may be reflected in altered bleeding time, petechiae, bruising, hematoma formation, epistaxis, and frank hemorrhage (see PRECAUTIONS, General and DRUG INTERACTIONS). Relative lymphocytosis, macrocytosis, hypofibrinogenemia, leukopenia, eosinophilia, anemia including macrocytic with or without folate deficiency, bone marrow suppression, pancytopenia, aplastic anemia, and acute intermittent porphyria.

Hepatic: Minor elevations of transaminases (*e.g.*, SGOT and SGPT) and LDH are frequent and appear to be dose-related. Occasionally, laboratory test results include increases in serum bilrubin and abnormal changes in other liver function tests. These results may reflect potentially serious hepatotoxicity (see WARNINGS).

Endocrine: Irregular menses, secondary amenorrhea, breast enlargement, galactorrhea, and parotid gland swelling. Abnormal thyroid function tests (see PRECAUTIONS). There have been rare spontaneous reports of polycystic ovary disease. A cause and effect relationship has not been established.

Pancreatic: Acute pancreatitis including fatalitites (see WARNINGS).

Metabolic: Hyperammonemia, (see PRECAUTIONS), hyponatremia, and inappropriate ADH secretion. There have been rare reports of Fanconi's syndrome occurring chiefly in children. Decreased carnitine concentrations have been reported although the clinical relevance is undetermined. Hyperglycinemia has occurred and was associated with a fatal outcome in a patient with preexistent nonketotic hyperglycinemia.

Genitourinary: Enuresis and urinary tract infection.

Special Senses: Hearing loss, either, reversible or irreversible, has been reported; however, a cause and effect relationship has not been established. Ear pain has also been reported.

Other: Anaphylaxis, edema of the extremities, lupus erythematosus, bone pain, cough increased, pneumonia, otitis media, bradycardia, cutaneous vasculitis, and fever.

MANIA

Although valproate sodium has not been evaluated for safety and efficacy in the treatment of manic episodes associated with bipolar disorder, the following adverse events not listed above were reported by 1% or more of patients from two placebo-controlled clinical trials of divalproex sodium tablets.

Body as a Whole: Chills, neck pain, neck rigidity.
Cardiovascular System: Hypotension, postural hypotension, vasodilation.
Digestive System: Fecal incontinence, gastroenteritis, glossitis.
Musculoskeletal System: Arthrosis.
Nervous System: Agitation, catatonic reaction, hypokinesia, reflexes increased, tardive dyskinesia, vertigo.
Skin and Appendages: Furunculosis, maculopapular rash, seborrhea.
Special Senses: Conjunctivitis, dry eyes, eye pain.
Urogenital System: Dysuria.

MIGRAINE

Although valproate sodium has not been evaluated for safety and efficacy in the prophylactic treatment of migraine headaches, the following adverse events not listed above were reported by 1% or more of patients from two placebo-controlled clinical trials of divalproex sodium tablets.

Body as a Whole: Face edema.
Digestive System: Dry mouth, stomatitis.
Urogenital System: Cystitis, metrorrhagia, and vaginal hemorrhage.

DOSAGE AND ADMINISTRATION

VALPROATE SODIUM FOR INTRAVENOUS USE ONLY.

Use of valproate sodium for periods of more than 14 days has not been studied. Patients should be switched to oral valproate products as soon as it is clinically feasible.

Valproate sodium should be administered as a 60 minute infusion (but not more than 20 mg/min) with the same frequency as the oral products, although plasma concentration monitoring and dosage adjustments may be necessary.

V

INITIAL EXPOSURE TO VALPROATE

The following dosage recommendations were obtained from studies utilizing oral divalproex sodium products.

Complex Partial Seizures: For adults and children 10 years of age or older.

Monotherapy (Initial Therapy)

Valproate sodium has not been systematically studied as initial therapy. Patients should initiate therapy at 10-15 mg/kg/day. The dosage should be increased by 5-10 mg/kg/week to achieve optimal clinical response. Ordinarily, optimal clinical response is acieved at daily doses below 60 mg/kg/day. If satisfactory clinical response has not been achieved, plasma levels should be measured to determine whether or not they are in the usually accepted therapeutic range (50-100 µg/ml). No recommendation regarding the safety of valproate for use at doses above 60 mg/kg/day can be made.

The probability of thrombocytopenia increases significantly at total trough valproate plasma concentrations above 110 µg/ml in females and 135 µg/ml in males. The benefit of improved seizure control with higher doses should be weighed against the possibility of a greater incidence of adverse reactions.

Conversion to Monotherapy

Patients should initiate therapy at 10-15 mg/kg/day. The dosage should be increased by 5-10 mg/kg/week to achieve optimal clinical response. Ordinarily, optimal clinical response is achieved at daily doses below 60 mg/kg/day. If satisfactory clinical response has not been achieved, plasma levels should be measured to determine whether or not they are in the usually accepted therapeutic range (50-100 µg/ml). No recommendation regarding the safety of valproate for use at doses above 60 mg/kg/day can be made. Concomitant antiepilepsy drug (AED) dosage can ordinarily be reduced by approximately 25% every 2 weeks. This reduction may be started at initiation of valproate sodium therapy, or delayed by 1-2 weeks if there is a concern that seizures are likely to occur with a reduction. The speed and duration of withdrawal of the concomitant AED can be highly variable, and patients should be monitored closely during this period for increased seizure frequency.

Adjunctive Therapy

Valproate sodium may be added to the patient's regimen at a dosage of 10-15 mg/kg/day. The dosage may be increased by 5-10 mg/kg/week to achieve optimal clinical response. Ordinarily, optimal clinical response is achieved at daily doses below 60 mg/kg/day. If satisfactory clinical response has not been achieved, plasma levels should be measured to determine whether or not they are in the usually accepted therapeutic range (50-100 µg/ml). No recommendation regarding the safety of valproate for use at doses above 60 mg/kg/day can be made. If the total daily dose exceeds 250 mg, it should be given in divided doses.

In a study of adjunctive therapy for complex partial seizures in which patients were receiving either carbamazepine or phenytoin in addition to divalproex sodium, no adjustment of carbamazepine or phenytoin dosage was needed. However, since valproate may interact with these or other concurrently administered AEDs as well as other drugs (see DRUG INTERACTIONS), periodic plasma concentration determinations of concomitant AEDs are recommended during the early course of therapy (see DRUG INTERACTIONS).

Simple and Complex Absence Seizures

The recommended intial dose is 15 mg/kg/day, increasing at 1 week intervals by 5-10 mg/kg/day until seizures are controlled or side effects preclude further increases. The maximum recommended dosage is 60 mg/kg/day. If the total daily dose exceeds 250 mg, it should be given in divided doses.

A good correlation has not been established between daily dose, serum concentrations, and therapeutic effect. However, therapeutic valproate serum concentrations for most patients with absence seizures is considered to range from 50-100 µg/ml. Some patients may be controlled with lower or higher serum concentrations (see CLINICAL PHARMACOLOGY).

As the valproate sodium dosage is titrated upward, blood concentrations of phenobarbital and/or phenytoin may be affected (see PRECAUTIONS).

Antiepilepsy drugs should not be abruptly discontinued in patients in whom the drug is administered to prevent major seizures because of the strong possibility of precipitating status epilepticus with attendant hypoxia and threat to life.

REPLACEMENT THERAPY

When switching from oral valproate products, the total daily dose of valproate sodium should be equivalent to the total daily dose of the oral valproate product (see CLINICAL PHARMACOLOGY), and should be administered as a 60 minute infusion (but not more that 20 mg/min) with the same frequency as the oral products, although plasma concentration monitoring and dosage adjustments may be necessary. Patients receiving doses near the maximum recommended daily dose of 60 mg/kg/day, particularly those not receiving enzyme-inducing drugs, should be monitored more closely. If the total daily dose exceeds 250 mg, it should be given in a divided regimen. However, the equivalence shown between valproate sodium and oral valproate products (divalproex sodium) at steady state was only evaluated in an every 6 hour regimen. Whether, when valproate sodium is given less frequently (*i.e.*, 2 or 3 times a day), trough levels fall below those that result from an oral dosage form given via the same regimen is unknown. For this reason, when valproate sodium is given twice or three times a day, close monitoring of trough plasma levels may be needed.

GENERAL DOSING ADVICE

Dosing in Elderly Patients

Due to a decrease in unbound clearance of valproate and possibly a greater sensitivity to somnolence in the elderly, the starting dose should be reduced in these patients. Dosage should be increased more slowly and with regular monitoring for fluid and nutritional intake, dehydration, somnolence, and other adverse events. Dose reductions or discontinuation of valproate should be considered in patients with decreased food or fluid intake and in patients with excessive somnolence. The ultimate therapeutic dose should be achieved on the basis of both tolerability and clinical response (see WARNINGS).

Dose-Related Adverse Events

The frequency of adverse effects (particularly elevated liver enzymes and thrombocytopenia) may be dose-related. The probability of thrombocytopenia appears to increase significantly at total valproate concentrations of ≥110 µg/ml (females) or ≥135 µg/ml (males) (see PRECAUTIONS). The benefit of improved therapeutic effect with higher doses should be weighed against the possibility of a greater incidence of adverse reactions.

ADMINISTRATION

Rapid infusion of valproate sodium has been associated with an increase in adverse events. Infusion times of less than 60 minutes or rates of infusion >20 mg/min have not been studied in patients with epilepsy (see ADVERSE REACTIONS).

Valproate sodium should be administered intravenously as a 60 minute infusion, as noted above. It should be diluted with at least 50 ml of a compatible diluent. Any unused portion of the vial contents should be discarded.

Parenteral drug products should be inspected visually for particulate matter and discoloration prior to administration whenever solution and container permit.

COMPATIBILITY AND STABILITY

Valproate was found to be physically compatible and chemically stable in the following parenteral solutions for at least 24 hours when stored in glass or polyvinyl chloride (PVC) bags at controlled room temperature 15-30°C (59-86°F): dextrose (5%) injection, sodium chloride (0.9%) injection and lactated Ringer's injection.

HOW SUPPLIED

Depacon (valproate sodium injection), equivalent to 100 mg of valproic acid per ml, is a clear, colorless solution in 5 ml single-dose vials.
Storage: Store vials at controlled room temperature 15-30°C (59-86°F). No preservatives have been added. Unused portion of container should be discarded.

Valproic Acid *(002419)*

Categories: Seizures, absence; Pregnancy Category D; FDA Approved 1978 Feb; WHO Formulary
Drug Classes: Anticonvulsants
Brand Names: **Depakene**; Myproic Acid
Foreign Brand Availability: Convulex (Belgium; South-Africa; Taiwan); Depakin (Italy); Depakine (Taiwan); Epilim (Malaysia); Leptilan (Portugal); Orfiril (Germany); Valporal (Israel); Valprosid (Mexico)
Cost of Therapy: $239.52 (Epilepsy; Depakene; 250 mg; 4 capsules/day; 30 day supply)
$26.40 (Epilepsy; Generic Capsules; 250 mg; 4 capsules/day; 30 day supply)

WARNING

HEPATIC FAILURE RESULTING IN FATALITIES HAS OCCURRED IN PATIENTS RECEIVING VALPROIC ACID. EXPERIENCE HAS INDICATED THAT CHILDREN UNDER THE AGE OF 2 YEARS ARE AT A CONSIDERABLY INCREASED RISK OF DEVELOPING FATAL HEPATOTOXICITY, ESPECIALLY THOSE ON MULTIPLE ANTICONVULSANTS, THOSE WITH CONGENITAL METABOLIC DISORDERS, THOSE WITH SEVERE SEIZURE DISORDERS ACCOMPANIED BY MENTAL RETARDATION, AND THOSE WITH ORGANIC BRAIN DISEASE. WHEN VALPROIC ACID PRODUCTS ARE USED IN THIS PATIENT GROUP, THEY SHOULD BE USED WITH EXTREME CAUTION AND AS A SOLE AGENT. THE BENEFITS OF SEIZURE CONTROL SHOULD BE WEIGHED AGAINST THE RISKS. ABOVE THIS AGE GROUP, EXPERIENCE HAS INDICATED THAT THE INCIDENCE OF FATAL HEPATOTOXICITY DECREASES CONSIDERABLY IN PROGRESSIVELY OLDER PATIENT GROUPS.

THESE INCIDENTS USUALLY HAVE OCCURRED DURING THE FIRST 6 MONTHS OF TREATMENT. SERIOUS OR FATAL HEPATOTOXICITY MAY BE PRECEDED BY NON-SPECIFIC SYMPTOMS SUCH AS LOSS OF SEIZURE CONTROL, MALAISE, WEAKNESS, LETHARGY, FACIAL EDEMA, ANOREXIA AND VOMITING. PATIENTS SHOULD BE MONITORED CLOSELY FOR APPEARANCE OF THESE SYMPTOMS. LIVER FUNCTION TESTS SHOULD BE PERFORMED PRIOR TO THERAPY AND AT FREQUENT INTERVALS THEREAFTER, ESPECIALLY DURING THE FIRST 6 MONTHS.

DESCRIPTION

Valproic acid is a carboxylic acid designated as 2-propyl-pentanoic acid. It is also known as dipropylacetic acid.

Valproic acid (pKa 4.8) has a molecular weight of 144 and occurs as a colorless liquid with a characteristic odor. It is slightly soluble in water (1.3 mg/ml) and very soluble in organic solvents.

Valproic acid capsules and syrup are antiepileptics for oral administration. Each soft elastic capsule contains 250 mg valproic acid. The syrup contains the equivalent of 250 mg valproic acid per 5 ml as the sodium salt.
Storage: Store capsules at 15-25°C (59-77°F). Store syrup below 30°C (86°F).

CLINICAL PHARMACOLOGY

Valproic acid is an antiepileptic agent which dissociates to the valproate ion in the gastrointestinal tract. The mechanism by which valproate exerts its antiepileptic effects has not yet been established. It has been suggested that its activity is related to increased brain levels of gamma-aminobutyric acid (GABA).

Valproic acid is rapidly absorbed after oral administration. Peak plasma concentrations of valproate ion are observed 1-4 hours after a single dose of valproic acid. A slight delay in absorption occurs when the drug is administered with meals but this does not affect the total absorption.

Accordingly, administration of oral valproate products with food, and substitution among the various valproic acid and divalproex sodium products should be without consequence. Nonetheless, any changes in dosage administration or the addition or discontinuance of concomitant drugs, should ordinarily be accompanied by close monitoring of clinical status and valproate plasma concentrations.

The plasma half-life of valproate is typically in the range of 6-16 hours. Half-lives in the lower part of the range are usually found in patients taking other antiepileptic drugs capable of enzyme induction.

Valproate is primarily metabolized in the liver. The major metabolic routes are glucuronidation, mitochondrial beta oxidation, and microsomal oxidation. The major metabolites formed are the glucuronide conjugate, 2-propyl-3-keto-pentanoic acid, and 2-propylhydroxypentanoic acids. Other unsaturated metabolites have been reported. The major route of elimination of these metabolites is in the urine.

Patients on monotherapy will generally have longer half-lives and higher concentrations of valproate at a given dosage than patients receiving polytherapy. This is primarily due to enzyme induction caused by other antiepileptics, which results in enhanced clearance of valproate by glucuronidation and microsomal oxidation. Because of these changes in valproate clearance, monitoring of antiepileptic concentrations should be intensified whenever concomitant antiepileptics are introduced or withdrawn.

The therapeutic range is commonly considered to be 50-100 µg/ml of total valproate, although some patients may be controlled with lower or higher plasma concentrations.[4] Valproate is highly bound (90%) to plasma proteins in the therapeutic range; however, protein binding is concentration-dependent and decreases at high valproate concentrations. The binding is variable among patients, and may be affected by fatty acids or by highly bound drugs such as salicylate. Some clinicians favor monitoring free valproate concentrations, which may more accurately reflect CNS penetration of valproate. As yet, a consensus on the therapeutic range of free concentrations has not been established; however; monitoring total and free valproate may be informative when there are changes in clinical status, concomitant medication or valproate dosage.

INDICATIONS AND USAGE

Valproic acid is indicated for use as sole and adjunctive therapy in the treatment of simple and complex absence seizures, and adjunctively in patients with multiple seizure types which include absence seizures.

Simple absence is defined as very brief clouding of the sensorium or loss of consciousness, accompanied by certain generalized epileptic discharges without other detractable clinical signs. Complex absence is the term used when other signs are also present.

SEE WARNINGS FOR STATEMENT REGARDING FATAL HEPATIC DYSFUNCTION.

NON-FDA APPROVED INDICATIONS

Valproic acid has been used in the treatment of bipolar disorder in patients who fail to respond to other treatments or who do not tolerate other medications. While this use is not explicitly approved, the FDA has approved divalproex sodium tablets for the treatment of manic episodes associated with bipolar disorder. In addition, valproic acid may have utility in the prophylaxis of migraine headaches and possibly even in acute migraine attacks. While these uses are not explicitly approved, the FDA has also approved divalproex sodium for the prophylaxis of migraine.

CONTRAINDICATIONS

VALPROIC ACID SHOULD NOT BE ADMINISTERED TO PATIENTS WITH HEPATIC DISEASE OR SIGNIFICANT DYSFUNCTION.

Valproic acid is contraindicated in patients with known hypersensitivity to the drug.

WARNINGS

Hepatic failure resulting in fatalities has occurred in patients receiving valproic acid. These incidents usually have occurred during the first 6 months of treatment. Serious or fatal hepatotoxicity may be preceded by non-specific symptoms such as loss of seizure control, malaise, weakness, lethargy, facial edema, anorexia and vomiting. Patients should be monitored closely for the appearance of these symptoms. Liver function tests should be performed prior to therapy and at frequent intervals thereafter, especially during the first 6 months. However, physicians should not rely totally on serum biochemistry since these tests may not be abnormal in all instances, but should also consider the results of careful interim medical history and physical examination. Caution should be observed when administering valproic acid to patients with a prior history of hepatic disease. Patients on multiple anticonvulsants, children, those with congenital metabolic disorders, those with severe seizure disorders accompanied by mental retardation, and those with organic brain disease may be at particular risk. Experience has indicated that children under the age of 2 years are at a considerably increased risk of developing fatal hepatotoxicity, especially those with the aforementioned conditions. When valproic acid products are used in this patient group, it should be with extreme caution and as a sole agent. The benefits of seizure control should be weighed against the risks. Above this age group, experience has indicated that the incidence of fatal hepatotoxicity decreases considerably in progressively older patient groups.

The drug should be discontinued immediately in the presence of significant hepatic dysfunction, suspected or apparent. In some cases, hepatic dysfunction has progressed in spite of discontinuation of drug.

The frequency of adverse effects (particularly elevated liver enzymes) may be dose-related. The benefit of improved seizure control which may be accompanied at higher doses should therefore be weighed against the possibility of a greater incidence of adverse effects.

USAGE IN PREGNANCY

ACCORDING TO PUBLISHED AND UNPUBLISHED REPORTS, VALPROIC ACID MAY PRODUCE TERATOGENIC EFFECTS IN THE OFFSPRING OF HUMAN FEMALES RECEIVING THE DRUG DURING PREGNANCY.

THERE ARE MULTIPLE REPORTS IN THE CLINICAL LITERATURE WHICH MAY INDICATE THAT THE USE OF ANTIEPILEPTIC DRUGS DURING PREGNANCY RESULTS IN AN INCREASED INCIDENCE OF BIRTH DEFECTS IN THE OFFSPRING. ALTHOUGH DATA ARE MORE EXTENSIVE WITH RESPECT TO TRIMETHADIONE, PARAMETHADIONE, PHENYTOIN, AND PHENOBARBITAL, REPORTS INDICATE A POSSIBLE SIMILAR ASSOCIATION WITH THE USE OF OTHER ANTIEPILEPTIC DRUGS. THEREFORE, ANTIEPILEPTIC DRUGS SHOULD BE ADMINISTERED TO WOMEN OF CHILDBEARING POTENTIAL ONLY IF THEY ARE CLEARLY SHOWN TO BE ESSENTIAL IN THE MANAGEMENT OF SEIZURES.

THE INCIDENCE OF NEURAL TUBE DEFECTS IN THE FETUS MAY BE INCREASED IN MOTHERS RECEIVING VALPROATE DURING THE FIRST TRIMESTER OF PREGNANCY. THE CENTERS FOR DISEASE CONTROL (CDC) HAS ESTIMATED THE RISK OF VALPROIC ACID EXPOSED TO WOMEN HAVING CHILDREN WITH SPINA BIFIDA TO BE APPROXIMATELY 1-2%.[1] THIS RISK IS SIMILAR TO THAT FOR NONEPILEPTIC WOMEN WHO HAVE HAD CHILDREN WITH NEURAL TUBE DEFECTS (ANENCEPHALY AND SPINA BIFIDA).

OTHER CONGENITAL ANOMALIES (*e.g.,* CRANIOFACIAL DEFECTS, CARDIOVASCULAR MALFORMATIONS AND ANOMALIES INVOLVING VARIOUS BODY SYSTEMS), COMPATIBLE AND INCOMPATIBLE WITH LIFE, HAVE BEEN RE-

PORTED. SUFFICIENT DATA TO DETERMINE THIS INCIDENCE OF THESE CONGENITAL ANOMALIES IS NOT AVAILABLE.

THE HIGHER INCIDENCE OF CONGENITAL ANOMALIES IN ANTIEPILEPTIC DRUG-TREATED WOMEN WITH SEIZURE DISORDERS CANNOT BE REGARDED AS A CAUSE AND EFFECT RELATIONSHIP. THERE ARE INTRINSIC METHODOLOGIC PROBLEMS IN ATTAINING ADEQUATE DATA ON DRUG TERATOGENICITY IN HUMANS; GENETIC FACTORS OR THE EPILEPTIC CONDITION ITSELF, MAY BE MORE IMPORTANT THAN DRUG THERAPY IN CONTRIBUTING TO CONGENITAL ANOMALIES.

PATIENTS TAKING VALPROATE MAY DEVELOP CLOTTING ABNORMALITIES. A PATIENT WHO HAD LOW FIBROGEN WHEN TAKING MULTIPLE ANTICONVULSANTS INCLUDING VALPROATE GAVE BIRTH TO AN INFANT WHO SUBSEQUENTLY DIED OF HEMORRHAGE. IF VALPROATE IS USED IN PREGNANCY, THE CLOTTING PARAMETERS SHOULD BE MONITORED CAREFULLY.

HEPATIC FAILURE RESULTING IN THE DEATH OF A NEWBORN AND OF AN INFANT, HAVE BEEN REPORTED FOLLOWING THE USE OF VALPROATE DURING PREGNANCY.

ANIMAL STUDIES HAVE ALSO DEMONSTRATED VALPROATE INDUCED TERATOGENICITY. Studies in rats and human females demonstrated placental transfer of the drug. Doses greater than 65 mg/kg/day given to pregnant rats and mice produced skeletal abnormalities in the offspring, primarily involving ribs and vertebrae; doses greater than 150 mg/kg/day given to pregnant rabbits produced fetal resorptions and (primarily) soft-tissue abnormalities in the offspring. In rats a dose-related delay in the onset of parturition was noted. Potential growth and survival of the progeny were adversely affected, particularly when the drug administration spanned the entire gestation and early lactation period.

Antiepileptic drugs should not be discontinued in patients in whom the drug is administered to prevent seizures because of the strong possibility of precipitating status epilepticus with attendant hypoxia and threat to life. In individual cases where the severity and frequency of the seizure disorder are such that the removal of medication does not pose a serious threat to the patient, discontinuation of the drug may be considered prior to and during pregnancy, although it cannot be said with any confidence that even minor seizures do not pose some hazard to the developing embryo or fetus.

The prescribing physicians will wish to weigh these considerations in treating or counseling epileptic women of childbearing potential.

Tests to detect neural tube and other defects using current accepted procedures should be considered a part of routine prenatal care in childbearing women receiving valproate.

PRECAUTIONS

HEPATIC DYSFUNCTION

See BOXED WARNING, CONTRAINDICATIONS, AND WARNINGS.

GENERAL

Because of reports of thrombocytopenia, inhibition of the secondary phase of platelet aggregation, and abnormal coagulation parameters, (*e.g.*, low fibrinogen), platelet counts and coagulation tests are recommended before initiating therapy and at periodic intervals. It is recommended that patients receiving valproic acid be monitored for platelet count and coagulation parameters prior to planned surgery. Evidence of hemorrhage, bruising or a disorder of hemostasis/coagulation is an indication for reduction of the dosage or withdrawal of therapy.

Hyperammonemia with or without lethargy or coma has been reported and may be present in the absence of abnormal liver function tests. Asymptomatic elevations of ammonia are more common and when present require more frequent monitoring. If clinically significant symptoms occur, valproic acid therapy should be modified or discontinued.

Since valproate may interact with concurrently administered antiepileptic drugs, periodic plasma concentrations of concomitant antiepileptic drugs are recommended during the early course of therapy (see DRUG INTERACTIONS).

Valproate is partially eliminated in the urine as a keto-metabolite which may lead to a false interpretation of the urine ketone test.

There have also been reports of altered thyroid function tests associated with valproate. The clinical significance of these is unknown.

INFORMATION FOR THE PATIENT

Since valproic acid products may produce CNS depression, especially when combined with another CNS depressant (*e.g.*, alcohol), patients should be advised not to operate an automobile or dangerous machinery until it is known that they do not become drowsy from the drug.

CARCINOGENESIS

Valproic acid was administered to Sprague Dawley rats and ICR (HA/ICR) mice at doses of 0, 80, and 170 mg/kg/day for 2 years. A variety of neoplasms were observed in both species. The chief findings were a statistically significant increase in the incidence of subcutaneous fibrosarcomas in high dose male rats receiving valproic acid and a statistically significant dose-related trend for benign pulmonary adenomas in male mice receiving valproic acid. The significance of these findings for man is unknown.

MUTAGENESIS

Studies on valproate have been performed using bacterial and mammalian systems. These studies have provided no evidence of a mutagenic potential for valproate.

FERTILITY

Chronic toxicity studies in juvenile and adult rats and dogs demonstrated reduced spermatogenesis and testicular atrophy at doses greater than 200 mg/kg/day in rats and greater than 90 mg/kg/day in dogs. Segment I fertility studies in rats have shown doses up to 350 mg/kg/day for 60 days to have no effect on fertility. THE EFFECT OF VALPROATE ON TESTICULAR DEVELOPMENT AND ON SPERM PRODUCTION AND FERTILITY IN HUMANS IS UNKNOWN.

PREGNANCY CATEGORY D

See WARNINGS.

NURSING MOTHERS

Valproate is excreted in breast milk. Concentrations in breast milk have been reported to be 1-10% of serum concentrations. It is not known what effect this would have on a nursing infant. Caution should be exercised when valproic acid is administered to a nursing woman.

DRUG INTERACTIONS

Valproate may potentiate the CNS depressants (*i.e.,* alcohol., benzodiazepines, etc.).

The concomitant administration of valproate with drugs that exhibit extensive protein binding (*e.g.,* aspirin, carbamazepine, dicumarol, and phenytoin) may result in alteration of serum drug concentrations.

THERE IS EVIDENCE THAT VALPROATE CAN CAUSE AN INCREASE IN SERUM PHENOBARBITAL CONCENTRATIONS BY IMPAIRMENT OF NON-RENAL CLEARANCE. THIS PHENOMENON CAN RESULT IN SEVERE CNS DEPRESSION. THE COMBINATION OF VALPROATE AND PHENOBARBITAL HAS ALSO BEEN REPORTED TO PRODUCE CNS DEPRESSION WITHOUT SIGNIFICANT ELEVATIONS OF BARBITURATE OR VALPROATE SERUM CONCENTRATIONS. ALL PATIENTS RECEIVING CONCOMITANT BARBITURATE THERAPY SHOULD BE CLOSELY MONITORED FOR NEUROLOGICAL TOXICITY, SERUM BARBITURATE CONCENTRATIONS SHOULD BE OBTAINED, IF POSSIBLE AND THE BARBITURATE DOSAGE DECREASED, IF APPROPRIATE.

Primidone is metabolized into a barbiturate and, therefore, may also be involved in a similar or identical interaction.

THERE HAVE ALSO BEEN REPORTS OF BREAKTHROUGH SEIZURES OCCURRING WITH THE COMBINATION OF VALPROATE AND PHENYTOIN. MOST REPORTS HAVE NOTED A DECREASE IN TOTAL PLASMA PHENYTOIN CONCENTRATION. HOWEVER, INCREASES IN TOTAL PHENYTOIN SERUM CONCENTRATIONS HAVE BEEN REPORTED. AN INITIAL FALL WITH SUBSEQUENT INCREASE IN TOTAL PHENYTOIN CONCENTRATIONS HAS ALSO BEEN REPORTED. IN ADDITION, A DECREASE IN TOTAL SERUM PHENYTOIN WITH AN INCREASE IN THE FREE VS PROTEIN BOUND PHENYTOIN CONCENTRATIONS HAS BEEN REPORTED. THE DOSAGE OF PHENYTOIN SHOULD BE ADJUSTED AS REQUIRED BY THE CLINICAL SITUATION.

THE CONCOMITANT USE OF VALPROIC ACID AND CLONAZEPAM MAY PRODUCE ABSENCE STATUS IN PATIENTS WITH A HISTORY OF ABSENCE TYPE SEIZURES.

There is inconclusive evidence regarding the effects of valproate on serum ethosuximide concentrations. Patients receiving valproate and ethosuximide, especially along with other anticonvulsants, should be monitored for alterations in serum concentrations of both drugs.

Caution is recommended when valproate is used with drugs affecting coagulation (*e.g.,* aspirin, warfarin). See ADVERSE REACTIONS.

Evidence suggests that there is an association between the use of certain antiepileptics and failure of oral contraceptives. One explanation for this interaction is that enzyme-inducing antiepileptics effectively lower plasma concentrations of the relevant steroid hormones, resulting in unimpaired ovulation. However, other mechanisms, not related to enzyme induction may contribute to the failure of oral contraceptives. While valproate is not a significant enzyme inducer, and, therefore, would not be expected to decrease concentrations of steroid hormones, clinical data about the interaction of valproate with oral contraceptives is minimal.[2]

ADVERSE REACTIONS

Since valproic acid has usually been used with other antiepileptic drugs, it is not possible, in most cases, to determine whether the following adverse reactions can be ascribed to valproic acid alone, or the combination of drugs.

Gastrointestinal: The most commonly reported side effects at the initiation of therapy are nausea, vomiting, and indigestion. These effects are usually transient and rarely require discontinuation of therapy. Diarrhea, abdominal cramps and constipation have been reported. Both anorexia with some weight loss and increased appetite with weight gain have also been reported. Some patients experiencing gastrointestinal side effects may benefit by converting therapy from valproic acid to divalproex sodium.[3]

CNS Effects: Sedative effects have occurred in patients receiving valproate alone but occur most often in patients receiving combination therapy. Sedation usually abates upon reduction of other antiepileptic medication. Tremor has been reported in patients receiving valproate and may be dose-related. Ataxia, headache, nystagmus, diplopia, asterixis, "spots before eyes", dysarthria, dizziness, and incoordination have rarely been noted. Rare cases of coma have been noted in patients receiving valproic acid alone or in conjunction with phenobarbital. In rare instances encephalopathy with fever has developed shortly after the introduction of valproate monotherapy without evidence of hepatic dysfunction or inappropriate plasma levels; all patients recovered after the drug was withdrawn.

Dermatologic: Transient hair loss, skin rash, photosensitivity, generalized pruritus, erythema multiforme, and Stevens-Johnson syndrome. A case of fatal epidermal necrolysis has been reported in a 6 month old infant taking valproate and several other concomitant medications.

Psychiatric: Emotional upset, depression, psychosis, aggression, hyperactivity and behavioral deterioration.

Musculoskeletal: Weakness.

Hematologic: Thrombocytopenia and inhibition of the secondary phase of platelet aggregation may be reflected in altered bleeding time, petechiae, bruising, hematoma formation and frank hemorrhage. (SeeDRUG INTERACTIONS.) Relative lymphocytosis, macrocytosis, hypofibrinogenemia, leukopenia, eosinophilia, anemia, bone marrow suppression, and acute intermittent porphyria.

Hepatic: Minor elevations of transaminases (*e.g.,*SGOT and SGPT) and LDH are frequent and appear to be dose related. Occasionally, laboratory test results include

V

increases in serum bilirubin and abnormal changes in other liver function tests. These results may reflect potentially serious hepatotoxicity. (See WARNINGS.)

Endocrine: Irregular menses, secondary amenorrhea, breast enlargement, galactorrhea, and parotid gland swelling. Abnormal thyroid function tests (see PRECAUTIONS).

Pancreatic: Acute pancreatitis, including fatalities.

Metabolic: Hyperammonemia (see PRECAUTIONS), hyponatremia, and inappropriate ADH secretion.

There have been rare reports of Fanconi's syndrome occurring chiefly in children.

Decreased carnitine concentrations have been reported although the clinical relevance is undetermined.

Hyperglycinemia has occurred and was associated with a fatal outcome in a patient with pre-existing nonketotic hyperglycinemia.

Other: Edema of the extremities.

DOSAGE AND ADMINISTRATION

Valproic acid is administered orally. The recommended initial dose is 15 mg/kg/day, increasing at 1 week intervals by 5-10 mg/kg/day, until seizures are controlled or side effects preclude further increases. The maximum recommended dosage is 60 mg/kg/day. If the total daily dose exceeds 250 mg, it should be given in a divided regimen.

TABLE 1 is a guide for the initial daily dose of valproic acid (15 mg/kg/day).

TABLE 1

Weight		Total Daily Dose	Number of Capsules or Teaspoonfuls of Syrup		
			Dose 1	Dose 2	Dose 3
10-24.9 kg	22-54.9 lb	250 mg	0	0	1
25-39.9 kg	55-87.9 lb	500 mg	1	0	1
40-59.9 kg	88-131.9 lb	750 mg	1	1	1
60-74.9 kg	132-164.9 lb	1000 mg	1	1	2
75-89.9 kg	165-197.9 lb	1250 mg	2	1	2

The frequency of adverse effects (particularly elevated liver enzymes) may be dose related. The benefits of improved seizure control with higher doses should be weighed against the possibility of a greater incidence of adverse reactions.

A good correlation has not been established between daily dose, serum concentration and therapeutic effect. However, therapeutic valproate serum concentrations for most patients will range from 50-100 µg/ml. Some patients may be controlled with lower or higher serum concentrations (see CLINICAL PHARMACOLOGY).

As the valproic acid dosage is titrated upward, blood concentrations of phenobarbital and/or phenytoin may be affected. (See PRECAUTIONS.)

Patients who experience GI irritation may benefit from administration of the drug with food or by slowly building up the dose from an initial low level.

THE CAPSULES SHOULD BE SWALLOWED WITHOUT CHEWING TO AVOID LOCAL IRRITATION OF THE MOUTH AND THROAT.

PRODUCT LISTING - RATED THERAPEUTICALLY EQUIVALENT

Capsule - Oral - 250 mg

Package	Price	Product	NDC
25 x 30	$209.70	GENERIC, Sky Pharmaceuticals Packaging, Inc	63739-0251-03
30's	$10.97	GENERIC, Heartland Healthcare Services	61392-0157-30
30's	$10.97	GENERIC, Heartland Healthcare Services	61392-0157-39
31 x 10	$188.36	GENERIC, Vangard Labs	00615-1325-53
31 x 10	$188.36	GENERIC, Vangard Labs	00615-1325-63
31's	$11.34	GENERIC, Heartland Healthcare Services	61392-0157-31
32's	$11.70	GENERIC, Heartland Healthcare Services	61392-0157-32
45's	$16.46	GENERIC, Heartland Healthcare Services	61392-0157-45
60's	$21.94	GENERIC, Heartland Healthcare Services	61392-0157-60
90's	$32.91	GENERIC, Heartland Healthcare Services	61392-0157-90
100's	$16.40	GENERIC, Us Trading Corporation	56126-0106-11
100's	$18.82	FEDERAL UPPER LIMIT, H.C.F.A. F F P	99999-2419-01
100's	$22.00	GENERIC, Chase Laboratories Inc	54429-3194-01
100's	$27.00	GENERIC, Interstate Drug Exchange Inc	00814-8240-14
100's	$34.44	GENERIC, Martec Pharmaceuticals Inc	52555-0325-01
100's	$36.10	GENERIC, Aligen Independent Laboratories Inc	00405-5094-01
100's	$42.51	GENERIC, Moore, H.L. Drug Exchange Inc	00839-7180-06
100's	$47.10	GENERIC, Major Pharmaceuticals Inc	00904-2101-60
100's	$47.10	GENERIC, Major Pharmaceuticals Inc	00904-7765-60
100's	$58.45	GENERIC, Ivax Corporation	00182-1754-01
100's	$59.00	GENERIC, Martec Pharmaceuticals Inc	52555-0688-01
100's	$64.49	GENERIC, Qualitest Products Inc	00603-6334-21
100's	$79.40	GENERIC, Watson/Schein Pharmaceuticals Inc	00364-0822-01
100's	$79.40	GENERIC, Udl Laboratories Inc	51079-0298-20
100's	$82.15	GENERIC, Rosemont Pharmaceutical Corporation	00832-1007-00
100's	$82.51	GENERIC, Upsher-Smith Laboratories Inc	00832-1008-00
100's	$88.22	GENERIC, Sidmak Laboratories Inc	50111-0852-01
100's	$199.60	DEPAKENE, Abbott Pharmaceutical	00074-5681-13
200 x 5	$607.62	GENERIC, Vangard Labs	00615-1325-43

Syrup - Oral - 250 mg/5 ml

Package	Price	Product	NDC
5 ml x 40	$31.20	GENERIC, Pharmaceutical Assoc Inc Div Beach Products	00121-0675-05
5 ml x 100	$194.02	GENERIC, Xactdose Inc	50962-0226-61
473 ml	$50.02	GENERIC, Hi-Tech Pharmacal Company Inc	50383-0792-16
480 ml	$28.51	FEDERAL UPPER LIMIT, H.C.F.A. F F P	99999-2419-02
480 ml	$32.22	GENERIC, Physicians Total Care	54868-4285-00
480 ml	$46.75	GENERIC, Ivax Corporation	00182-6115-40
480 ml	$46.75	GENERIC, Qualitest Products Inc	00603-1840-58
480 ml	$46.80	GENERIC, Aligen Independent Laboratories Inc	00405-3890-16
480 ml	$49.01	GENERIC, Moore, H.L. Drug Exchange Inc	00839-7195-69
480 ml	$56.00	GENERIC, Major Pharmaceuticals Inc	00904-2103-16
480 ml	$62.50	GENERIC, Pharmaceutical Assoc Inc Div Beach Products	00121-0675-16
480 ml	$69.17	GENERIC, Geneva Pharmaceuticals	00781-6701-16
480 ml	$72.75	GENERIC, Teva Pharmaceuticals Usa	00093-9633-16
480 ml	$72.75	GENERIC, Morton Grove Pharmaceuticals Inc	60432-0621-16
480 ml	$204.01	DEPAKENE, Abbott Pharmaceutical	00074-5682-16

PRODUCT LISTING - EQUIVALENTS NOT AVAILABLE

Capsule - Oral - 250 mg

Package	Price	Product	NDC
100's	$22.15	GENERIC, Physicians Total Care	54868-1689-01

Solution - Injectable - 100 mg/ml

Package	Price	Product	NDC
5 ml x 10	$124.10	GENERIC, Bedford Laboratories	55390-0007-10
5 ml x 10	$129.00	DEPACON, Abbott Pharmaceutical	00074-1564-10

Syrup - Oral - 250 mg/5 ml

Package	Price	Product	NDC
480 ml	$29.00	GENERIC, Raway Pharmacal Inc	00686-0792-16
480 ml	$72.75	GENERIC, Alpharma Uspd Makers Of Barre and Nmc	00472-0210-16

Valrubicin (003401)

Categories: FDA Approved 1997 Jun; Pregnancy Category C; Orphan Drugs
Drug Classes: Antineoplastics, antibiotics
Brand Names: Valstar

DESCRIPTION

Valrubicin (N-trifluoroacetyladriamycin-14-valerate), a semisynthetic analog of the anthracycline doxorubicin, is a cytotoxic agent with the chemical name, (2*S*-*cis*)-2-[1,2,3,4,6,11-hexahydro-2,5,12-trihydroxy-7-methoxy-6,11-dioxo-4-[[2,3,6-trideoxy-3-[(trifluoroacetyl)amino]-α-L-*lyxo*-hexopyranosyl]oxyl]-2-naphthacenyl]-2-oxoethyl pentanoate. Valrubicin is an orange or orange-red powder that is highly lipophilic, soluble in methylene chloride, ethanol, methanol and acetone and relatively insoluble in water. Its chemical formula is $C_{34}H_{36}F_3NO_{13}$ and its molecular weight is 723.65.

Valstar sterile solution for intravesical instillation is intended for intravesical administration in the urinary bladder. It is supplied as a nonaqueous solution that should be diluted before intravesical administration. Each vial of Valstar contains valrubicin at a concentration of 40 mg/ml in 50% cremophor EL (polyoxyethyleneglycol triricinoleate)/50% dehydrated alcohol, without preservatives or other additives. The solution is sterile and nonpyrogenic.

CLINICAL PHARMACOLOGY

MECHANISM OF ACTION

Valrubicin is an anthracycline that affects a variety of inter-related biological functions, most of which involve nucleic acid metabolism. It readily penetrates into cells, where it inhibits the incorporation of nucleosides into nucleic acids, causes extensive chromosomal damage, and arrests cell cycle in G_2. Although valrubicin does not bind strongly to DNA, a principal mechanism of its action, mediated by valrubicin metabolites, is interference with the normal DNA breaking-resealing action of DNA topoisomerase II.

PHARMACOKINETICS AFTER INTRAVESICAL ADMINISTRATION OF VALRUBICIN

When 800 mg valrubicin was administered intravesically to patients with carcinoma *in situ*, valrubicin penetrated into the bladder wall. The mean total anthracycline concentration measured in bladder tissue exceeded the levels causing 90% cytoxicity to human bladder cells cultured *in vitro*. During the 2 hour dose-retention period, the metabolism of valrubicin to its major metabolites N-trifluoroacetyladriamycin and N-trifluoroacetyladriamycinol was neglible. After retention, the drug was almost completely excreted by voiding the instillate. Mean percent recovery of valrubicin, N-trifluoroacetyladriamycin, and total anthracyclines in 14 urine samples from 6 patients was 98.6%, 0.4%, and 99.0% of the total administered drug, respectively. During the 2 hour dose-retention period, only nanogram quantities of valrubicin were absorbed into the plasma. Valrubicin metabolites N-trifluoroacetyladriamycin and N-trifluoroacetyladriamycinol were measured in blood.

Total systemic exposure to anthracyclines during and after intravesical administration of valrubicin is dependent upon the condition of the bladder wall. The mean AUC(0-6h) (total anthracyclines exposure) for an intravesical dose of 900 mg of valrubicin administered 2 weeks after transurethral resection of bladder tumors (n=6) was 78 nmol/L·h. In patients receiving 800 mg of valrubicin 5-51 minutes after typical (n=8) and extensive (n=5) transurethral resection of bladder tumors (TURBs), the mean AUC(0-6h) values for total anthracyclines were 409 and 788 nmol/L·h, respectively. The AUC(0-6h) total exposure to anthracyclines was 18,382 nmol/L·h in 1 patient who experienced a perforated bladder following a transurethral resection that occurred 5 minutes before administration of an intravesical dose of 800 mg of valrubicin. Administration of a comparable intravenous dose of valrubicin (600 mg/m^2; n=2) as a 24 hour infusion resulted in an AUC(0-6h) for total anthracyclines of 11,975 nmol/L·h.

The patient with a perforated bladder who received 800 mg of valrubicin intravesically developed severe leukopenia and neutropenia approximately 2 weeks after drug administration. Systemic hematologic toxicity from valrubicin was not seen after an intravesical dose of 800 mg of valrubicin unless perforation of the urinary bladder occurred.

V

INDICATIONS AND USAGE

Valrubicin is indicated for intravesical therapy of BCG-refractory carcinoma *in situ* (CIS) of the urinary bladder in patients for whom immediate cystectomy would be associated with unacceptable morbidity or mortality.

CONTRAINDICATIONS

Valrubicin is contraindicated in patients with known hypersensitivity to anthracyclines or cremophor EL (polyoxyethyleneglycol triricinoleate).

Patients with concurrent urinary tract infections should not receive valrubicin.

Valrubicin should not be administered to a patient with a small bladder capacity, *i.e.*, unable to tolerate a 75 ml instillation.

WARNINGS

Patients should be informed that valrubicin has been shown to induce complete response in only about 1 in 5 patients with BCG—refractory CIS, and that delaying cystectomy could lead to development of metastatic bladder cancer, which is lethal. The exact risk of developing metastatic bladder cancer from such a delay may be difficult to assess but increases the longer cystectomy is delayed in the presence of persisting CIS. **If there is not a complete response of CIS to treatment after 3 months or if CIS recurs, cystectomy must be reconsidered.**

Valrubicin should not be administered to patients with a perforated bladder or to those in whom the integrity of the bladder mucosa has been compromised (see PRECAUTIONS and CLINICAL PHARMACOLOGY).

In order to avoid possible dangerous systemic exposure to valrubicin for the patients undergoing transurethral resection of the bladder, the status of the bladder should be evaluated before the intravesical instillation of drug. In case of bladder perforation, the administration of valrubicin should be delayed until bladder integrity has been restored.

Valrubicin should be administered under the supervision of a physician experienced in the use of intravesical cancer chemotherapeutic agents.

PRECAUTIONS

GENERAL

Aseptic techniques must be used during administration of intravesical valrubicin to avoid introducing contaminants into the urinary tract or traumatizing unduly the urinary mucosa.

INFORMATION FOR PATIENTS

Patients should be informed that valrubicin has been shown to induce complete responses in only about 1 in 5 patients, and that delaying cystectomy could lead to development of metastatic bladder cancer, which is lethal. They should discuss with their physician the relative risk of cystectomy versus the risk of metastatic bladder cancer and be aware that the risk increases the longer cystectomy is delayed in the presence of persisting CIS.

Patients should be informed that the major acute toxicities from valrubicin are related to irritable bladder symptoms that may occur during instillation and retention of valrubicin and for a limited period following voiding. For the first 24 hours following administration, red-tinged urine is typical. Patients should report prolonged irritable bladder symptoms or prolonged passage of red-colored urine immediately to their physician.

Women of child-bearing potential should be advised not to become pregnant during treatment. Men should be advised to refrain from engaging in procreative activities while receiving therapy with valrubicin. All patients of reproductive age should be advised to use an effective contraception method during the treatment period.

IRRITABLE BLADDER SYMPTOMS

Valrubicin should be used with caution in patients with severe irritable bladder symptoms. Bladder spasm and spontaneous discharge of the intravesical instillate may occur; clamping of the urinary catheter is not advised and, if performed, should be executed under medical supervision and with caution.

CARCINOGENESIS, MUTAGENESIS, AND IMPAIRMENT OF FERTILITY

The carcinogenic potential of valrubicin has not been evaluated, but the drug does cause damage to DNA *in vitro*. Valrubicin was mutagenic in *in vitro* assays in *Salmonella typhimurium* and *Escherichia coli*. Valrubicin was clastogenic in the chromosomal aberration assay in CHO cells. Studies of the effects of valrubicin on male or female fertility have not been done.

PREGNANCY CATEGORY C

Valrubicin can cause fetal harm if a pregnant woman is exposed to the drug systemically. Such exposure could occur after perforation of the urinary bladder during valrubicin therapy. Daily intravenous doses of 12 mg/kg (about one-sixth of the recommended human intravesical dose on a mg/m^2 basis) given to rats during fetal development caused fetal malformations. A dose of 24 mg/kg (about one-third the recommended human intravesical dose on a mg/m^2 basis) caused numerous, severe alterations in the skull and skeleton of the developing fetuses. This dose also caused an increase in fetal resorptions and a decrease in viable fetuses. Thus, valrubicin is embryotoxic and teratogenic. There are no preclinical studies of the effects of intravesical valrubicin on fetal development and no adequate and well controlled studies of valrubicin in pregnant women. If valrubicin is used during pregnancy, or if the patient becomes pregnant while receiving this drug, the patient should be apprized of the potential hazard to the fetus. It should be used during pregnancy only if the potential benefit justifies the potential risk to the fetus. Women who might become pregnant should be advised to avoid doing so during therapy with valrubicin.

NURSING MOTHERS

It is not known whether valrubicin is excreted in human milk. Nevertheless, the drug is highly lipophilic and any exposure of infants to valrubicin could pose serious health risks. Women should discontinue nursing before the initiation of valrubicin therapy.

PEDIATRIC USE

Safety and effectiveness in pediatric patients have not been established.

GERIATRIC USE

Because carcinoma *in situ* of the bladder generally occurs in older individuals, 85% of the patients enrolled in the clinical studies of valrubicin were more than 60 years of age (49% of the patients were more than 70 years of age). In the primary efficacy studies, the mean age of the population was 69.5 years. There are no specific precautions regarding use of valrubicin product in geriatric patients who are otherwise in good health.

DRUG INTERACTIONS

Because systemic exposure to valrubicin is negligible following intravesical administration, the potential for drug interactions is low. No drug interaction studies were conducted.

ADVERSE REACTIONS

Approximately 84% of patients who received intravesical valrubicin in clinical studies experienced local adverse events, but approximately half of the patients reported irritable bladder symptoms prior to treatment. The local adverse reactions associated with valrubicin usually occur during or shortly after instillation and resolve within 1-7 days after the instillate is removed from the bladder.

TABLE 1 displays the frequency of the local adverse experiences at baseline and during treatment among 170 patients who received 800 mg doses of valrubicin in a multiple-cycle treatment regimen. Only 7 of 143 patients who were scheduled to receive six doses failed to receive all of the planned doses because of the occurrence of local bladder symptoms.

TABLE 1 *Occurrence of Local Adverse Reactions Before and After Intravesical Administration of Valrubicin — Patients Who Received Multiple-Cycle Treatment Regimen at 800 mg/dose (n=170)*

Reaction	Before Treatment	During Treatment
Any local bladder symptom	45%	88%
Urinary frequency	30%	61%
Dysuria	11%	56%
Urinary urgency	27%	57%
Bladder spasm	3%	31%
Hematuria	11%	29%
Bladder pain	6%	28%
Urinary incontinence	7%	22%
Cystitis	4%	15%
Nocturia	2%	7%
Local burning symptoms - procedure related	0%	5%
Urethral pain	0%	3%
Pelvic pain	1%	1%
Hematuria (gross)	0%	1%

Most systemic adverse events associated with use of valrubicin have been mild in nature and self-limited, resolving within 24 hours after drug administration. TABLE 2 displays the adverse events other than local bladder symptoms that occurred in 1% or more of the 230 patients who received at least one dose of valrubicin (200 to 900 mg) in a clinical trial. It can not be determined whether these events are drug-related.

TABLE 2 *Most Commonly Reported Systemic Adverse Reactions Following Intravesical Administration of Valrubicin*

Body System Preferred Term	(n=230)
Body as a Whole	
Abdominal pain	5%
Asthenia	4%
Back pain	3%
Chest pain	3%
Fever	2%
Headache	4%
Malaise	4%
Cardiovascular	
Vasodilation	2%
Digestive	
Diarrhea	3%
Flatulence	1%
Nausea	5%
Vomiting	2%
Hemic and Lymphatic	
Anemia	2%
Metabolic and Nutritional	
Hyperglycemia	1%
Peripheral edema	1%
Musculoskeletal	
Myalgia	1%
Nervous	
Dizziness	3%
Respiratory	
Pneumonia	1%
Skin and Appendages	
Rash	3%
Urogenital	
Hematuria (microscopic)	3%
Urinary retention	4%
Urinary tract infection	15%

Adverse reactions other than local reactions that occurred in less than 1% of the patients who received valrubicin intravesically in clinical trials are listed below. This list includes only adverse reactions that were suspected of being related to treatment.

Digestive System: Tenesmus.
Metabolic and Nutritional: Nonprotein nitrogen increased.
Skin and Appendages: Pruritus.
Special Senses: Taste loss.
Urogenital System: Local skin irritation, poor urine flow, and urethritis.

V

Inadvertent paravenous extravasation of valrubicin was not associated with skin ulceration or necrosis.

DOSAGE AND ADMINISTRATION

Valrubicin is recommended at a dose of 800 mg administered intravesically once a week for 6 weeks. Administration should be delayed at least 2 weeks after transurethral resection and/or fulguration. For each instillation, four 5 ml vials (200 mg valrubicin/5 ml per vial) should be allowed to warm slowly to room temperature, but should not be heated. Twenty milliliters (20 ml) of valrubicin should then be withdrawn from the four vials and diluted with 55 ml 0.9% sodium chloride injection, providing 75 ml of a diluted valrubicin solution. A urethral catheter should then be inserted into the patient's bladder under aseptic conditions, the bladder drained, and the diluted 75 ml valrubicin solution instilled slowly via gravity flow over a period of several minutes. The catheter should then be withdrawn. The patient should retain the drug for 2 hours before voiding. At the end of 2 hours, all patients should void. (Some patients will be unable to retain the drug for the full 2 hours.) Patients should be instructed to maintain adequate hydration following treatment.

Patients receiving valrubicin for refractory carcinoma *in situ* must be monitored closely for disease recurrence or progression. Recommended evaluations include cystoscopy, biopsy, and urine cytology every 3 months.

ADMINISTRATION PRECAUTIONS

As recommended with other cytotoxic agents, caution should be exercised in handling and preparing the solution of valrubicin. Contact toxicity, common and severe with other anthracyclines, is not typical with valrubicin and, when observed, has been mild. Skin reactions may occur with accidental exposure, and the use of gloves during dose preparation and administration is recommended. Irritation of the eye has also been reported with accidental exposure. If this happens, the eye should be flushed with water immediately and thoroughly.

Valstar sterile solution contains cremophor EL, which has been known to cause leaching of di(2-ethylhexyl)phthalate(DEHP) a hepatotoxic plasticizer, from polyvinyl chloride (PVC) bags and intravenous tubing. Valstar solutions should be prepared and stored in glass, polypropylene, or polyolefin containers and tubing. It is recommended that non-DEHP containing administration sets, such as those that are polyethylene-lined, be used.

Procedures for proper handling and disposal of anticancer drugs should be used. Spills should be cleaned up with undiluted chlorine bleach.

PREPARATION FOR ADMINISTRATION

Valrubicin sterile solution for intravesical instillation is a clear red solution. It should be visually inspected for particulate matter and discoloration prior to administration. At temperatures below 4°C, cremophor EL may begin to form a waxy precipitate. If this happens, the vial should be warmed in the hand until the solution is clear. If particulate matter is still seen, valrubicin should not be administered.

STABILITY

Unopened vials of valrubicin are stable until the date indicated on the package when stored under refrigerated conditions at 2-8°C (36-46°F). Vials should not be heated. Valrubicin diluted in 0.9% sodium chloride injection, for administration is stable for 12 hours at temperatures up to 25°C (77°F). Since compatibility data are not available, valrubicin should not be mixed with other drugs.

HOW SUPPLIED

Valstar sterile solution for intravesical instillation is a clear red solution in cremophor EL/dehydrated alcohol, containing 40 mg valrubicin per ml.

Storage: Store vials under refrigeration at 2-8°C (36-46°F) in the carton. DO NOT FREEZE.

PRODUCT LISTING - EQUIVALENTS NOT AVAILABLE

Solution - Irrigation - 40 mg/ml

5 ml x 4	$1782.00	VALSTAR, Celltech Pharmacueticals Inc	53014-0216-70
5 ml x 4	$2217.60	VALSTAR, Celltech Pharmacueticals Inc	53014-0216-04
5 ml x 24	$13305.60	VALSTAR, Celltech Pharmacueticals Inc	53014-0216-24

Valsartan (003320)

For related information, see the comparative table section in Appendix A.

Categories: Heart failure, congestive; Hypertension, essential; Pregnancy Category C, 1st Trimester; Pregnancy Category D, 2nd & 3rd Trimesters; FDA Approved 1996 Feb; Patent Expiration 2012 Mar
Drug Classes: Angiotensin II receptor antagonists
Brand Names: Diovan
Foreign Brand Availability: Nisis (France); Provas (Germany); Tareg (France)
Cost of Therapy: $41.93 (Hypertension; Diovan; 80 mg; 1 capsule/day; 30 day supply)

WARNING

USE IN PREGNANCY

When used in pregnancy during the second and third trimesters, drugs that act directly on the renin-angiotensin system can cause injury and even death to the developing fetus. When pregnancy is detected, valsartan should be discontinued as soon as possible. See WARNINGS, Fetal/Neonatal Morbidity and Mortality.

DESCRIPTION

Diovan (valsartan) is a nonpeptide, orally active, and specific angiotensin II antagonist acting on the AT_1 receptor subtype.

Valsartan is chemically described as *N*-(1-oxopentyl)-N-[[2′-(1*H*-tetrazol-5-yl)[1,1′-biphenyl]-4-yl]methyl]-L-valine. Its empirical formula is $C_{24}H_{29}N_5O_3$, its molecular weight is 435.5.

Valsartan is a white to practically white fine powder. It is soluble in ethanol and methanol and slightly soluble in water.

CAPSULES

Diovan is available as capsules for oral administration, containing either 80 or 160 mg of valsartan. The inactive ingredients of the capsules are cellulose compounds, crospovidone, gelatin, iron oxides, magnesium stearate, povidone, sodium lauryl sulfate, and titanium dioxide.

TABLETS

Diovan is available as tablets for oral administration, containing 40, 80, 160 or 320 mg of valsartan. The inactive ingredients of the tablets are colloidal silicon dioxide, crospovidone, hydroxypropyl methylcellulose, iron oxides (yellow, black and/or red), magnesium stearate, microcrystalline cellulose, polyethylene glycol 8000, and titanium dioxide.

CLINICAL PHARMACOLOGY

MECHANISM OF ACTION

Angiotensin II is formed from angiotensin I in a reaction catalyzed by angiotensin-converting enzyme (ACE, kininase II). Angiotensin II is the principal pressor agent of the renin-angiotensin system, with effects that include vasoconstriction, stimulation of synthesis and release of aldosterone, cardiac stimulation, and renal reabsorption of sodium. Valsartan blocks the vasoconstrictor and aldosterone-secreting effects of angiotensin II by selectively blocking the binding of angiotensin II to the AT_1 receptor in many tissues, such as vascular smooth muscle and the adrenal gland. Its action is therefore independent of the pathways for angiotensin II synthesis.

There is also an AT_2 receptor found in many tissues, but AT_2 is not known to be associated with cardiovascular homeostasis. Valsartan has much greater affinity (about 20,000-fold) for the AT_1 receptor than for the AT_2 receptor. The increased plasma levels of angiotensin II following AT_1 receptor blockade with valsartan may stimulate the unblocked AT_2 receptor. The primary metabolite of valsartan is essentially inactive with an affinity for the AT_1 receptor about one 200th that of valsartan itself.

Blockade of the renin-angiotensin system with ACE inhibitors, which inhibit the biosynthesis of angiotensin II from angiotensin I, is widely used in the treatment of hypertension. ACE inhibitors also inhibit the degradation of bradykinin, a reaction also catalyzed by ACE. Because valsartan does not inhibit ACE (kininase II), it does not affect the response to bradykinin. Whether this difference has clinical relevance is not yet known. Valsartan does not bind to or block other hormone receptors or ion channels known to be important in cardiovascular regulation.

Blockade of the angiotensin II receptor inhibits the negative regulatory feedback of angiotensin II on renin secretion, but the resulting increased plasma renin activity and angiotensin II circulating levels do not overcome the effect of valsartan on blood pressure.

PHARMACOKINETICS

Valsartan peak plasma concentration is reached 2-4 hours after dosing. Valsartan shows bi-exponential decay kinetics following intravenous (IV) administration, with an average elimination half-life of about 6 hours. Absolute bioavailability for valsartan is about 25% (range 10-35%). Food decreases the exposure (as measured by AUC) to valsartan by about 40% and peak plasma concentration (C_{max}) by about 50%. AUC and C_{max} values of valsartan increase approximately linearly with increasing dose over the clinical dosing range. Valsartan does not accumulate appreciably in plasma following repeated administration.

METABOLISM AND ELIMINATION

Valsartan, when administered as an oral solution, is primarily recovered in feces (about 83% of dose) and urine (about 13% of dose). The recovery is mainly as unchanged drug, with only about 20% of dose recovered as metabolites. The primary metabolite, accounting for about 9% of dose, is valeryl 4-hydroxy valsartan. The enzyme(s) responsible for valsartan metabolism have not been identified but do not seem to be CYP 450 isozymes.

Following IV administration, plasma clearance of valsartan is about 2 L/h and its renal clearance is 0.62 L/h (about 30% of total clearance).

DISTRIBUTION

The steady state volume of distribution of valsartan after IV administration is small (17 L), indicating that valsartan does not distribute into tissues extensively. Valsartan is highly bound to serum proteins (95%), mainly serum albumin.

SPECIAL POPULATIONS

Pediatric

The pharmacokinetics of valsartan have not been investigated in patients <18 years of age.

Geriatric

Exposure (measured by AUC) to valsartan is higher by 70% and the half-life is longer by 35% in the elderly than in the young. No dosage adjustment is necessary (see DOSAGE AND ADMINISTRATION).

Gender

Pharmacokinetics of valsartan does not differ significantly between males and females.

Heart Failure

The average time to peak concentration and elimination half-life of valsartan in heart failure patients are similar to that observed in healthy volunteers. AUC and C_{max} values of valsartan increase linearly and are almost proportional with increasing dose over the clinical dosing range (40-160 mg twice a day). The average accumulation factor is about 1.7. The apparent clearance of valsartan following oral administration is approximately 4.5 L/h. Age does not affect the apparent clearance in heart failure patients.

Renal Insufficiency

There is no apparent correlation between renal function (measured by creatinine clearance) and exposure (measured by AUC) to valsartan in patients with different degrees of renal impairment. Consequently, dose adjustment is not required in patients with mild-to-moderate renal dysfunction. No studies have been performed in patients with severe impairment of renal function (creatinine clearance <10 ml/min). Valsartan is not removed from the plasma by hemodialysis. In the case of severe renal disease, exercise care with dosing of valsartan (see DOSAGE AND ADMINISTRATION).

Hepatic Insufficiency

On average, patients with mild-to-moderate chronic liver disease have twice the exposure (measured by AUC values) to valsartan of healthy volunteers (matched by age, sex and weight). In general, no dosage adjustment is needed in patients with mild-to-moderate liver disease. Care should be exercised in patients with liver disease (see DOSAGE AND ADMINISTRATION).

PHARMACODYNAMICS AND CLINICAL EFFECTS

Hypertension

Valsartan inhibits the pressor effect of angiotensin II infusions. An oral dose of 80 mg inhibits the pressor effect by about 80% at peak with approximately 30% inhibition persisting for 24 hours. No information on the effect of larger doses is available.

Removal of the negative feedback of angiotensin II causes a 2- to 3-fold rise in plasma renin and consequent rise in angiotensin II plasma concentration in hypertensive patients. Minimal decreases in plasma aldosterone were observed after administration of valsartan; very little effect on serum potassium was observed.

In multiple-dose studies in hypertensive patients with stable renal insufficiency and patients with renovascular hypertension, valsartan had no clinically significant effects on glomerular filtration rate, filtration fraction, creatinine clearance, or renal plasma flow.

In multiple-dose studies in hypertensive patients, valsartan had no notable effects on total cholesterol, fasting triglycerides, fasting serum glucose, or uric acid.

The antihypertensive effects of valsartan were demonstrated principally in 7 placebo-controlled, 4-12 week trials (one in patients over 65) of dosages from 10-320 mg/day in patients with baseline diastolic blood pressures of 95-115. The studies allowed comparison of once-daily and twice-daily regimens of 160 mg/day; comparison of peak and trough effects; comparison (in pooled data) of response by gender, age, and race; and evaluation of incremental effects of hydrochlorothiazide.

Administration of valsartan to patients with essential hypertension results in a significant reduction of sitting, supine, and standing systolic and diastolic blood pressure, usually with little or no orthostatic change.

In most patients, after administration of a single oral dose, onset of antihypertensive activity occurs at approximately 2 hours, and maximum reduction of blood pressure is achieved within 6 hours. The antihypertensive effect persists for 24 hours after dosing, but there is a decrease from peak effect at lower doses (40 mg) presumably reflecting loss of inhibition of angiotensin II. At higher doses, however (160 mg), there is little difference in peak and trough effect. During repeated dosing, the reduction in blood pressure with any dose is substantially present within 2 weeks, and maximal reduction is generally attained after 4 weeks. In long-term follow-up studies (without placebo control), the effect of valsartan appeared to be maintained for up to 2 years. The antihypertensive effect is independent of age, gender or race. The latter finding regarding race is based on pooled data and should be viewed with caution, because antihypertensive drugs that affect the renin-angiotensin system (that is, ACE inhibitors and angiotensin-II blockers) have generally been found to be less effective in low-renin hypertensives (frequently blacks) than in high-renin hypertensives (frequently whites). In pooled, randomized, controlled trials of valsartan that included a total of 140 blacks and 830 whites, valsartan and an ACE-inhibitor control were generally at least as effective in blacks as whites. The explanation for this difference from previous findings is unclear.

Abrupt withdrawal of valsartan has not been associated with a rapid increase in blood pressure.

The blood pressure lowering effect of valsartan and thiazide-type diuretics are approximately additive.

The 7 studies of valsartan monotherapy included over 2000 patients randomized to various doses of valsartan and about 800 patients randomized to placebo. Doses below 80 mg were not consistently distinguished from those of placebo at trough, but doses of 80, 160 and 320 mg produced dose-related decreases in systolic and diastolic blood pressure, with the difference from placebo of approximately 6-9/3-5 mm Hg at 80-160 mg and 9/6 mm Hg at 320 mg. In a controlled trial the addition of HCTZ to valsartan 80 mg resulted in additional lowering of systolic and diastolic blood pressure by approximately 6/3 and 12/5 mm Hg for 12.5 and 25 mg of HCTZ, respectively, compared to valsartan 80 mg alone.

Patients with an inadequate response to 80 mg once daily were titrated to either 160 mg once daily or 80 mg twice daily, which resulted in a comparable response in both groups.

In controlled trials, the antihypertensive effect of once-daily valsartan 80 mg was similar to that of once-daily enalapril 20 mg or once-daily lisinopril 10 mg.

There was essentially no change in heart rate in valsartan-treated patients in controlled trials.

Heart Failure

The Valsartan Heart Failure Trial (Val-HeFT) was a multinational, double-blind study in which 5010 patients with NYHA class II (62%) to IV (2%) heart failure and LVEF <40%, on baseline therapy chosen by their physicians, were randomized to placebo or valsartan (titrated from 40 mg twice daily to the highest tolerated dose or 160 mg twice daily) and followed for a mean of about 2 years. Although Val-HeFT's primary goal was to examine the effect of valsartan when added to an ACE inhibitor, about 7% were not receiving an ACE inhibitor. Other background therapy included diuretics (86%), digoxin (67%), and beta-blockers (36%). The population studied was 80% male, 46% 65 years or older and 89% Caucasian. At the end of the trial, patients in the valsartan group had a blood pressure that was 4 mm Hg systolic and 2 mm Hg diastolic lower than the placebo group. There were 2 primary end points, both assessed as time to first event: all-cause mortality and heart failure morbidity, the latter defined as all-cause mortality, sudden death with resuscitation, hospitalization for heart failure, and the need for IV inotropic or vasodilatory drugs for at least 4 hours. These results are summarized in TABLE 1.

TABLE 1

	Placebo n=2499	Valsartan n=2511	Hazard Ratio (95% CI*)	Nominal p-value
All-cause mortality	484 (19.4%)	495 (19.7%)	1.02 (0.90-1.15)	0.80
HF morbidity	801 (32.1%)	723 (28.8%)	0.87 (0.79-0.97)	0.009

* CI = Confidence Interval.

Although the overall morbidity result favored valsartan, this result was largely driven by the 7% of patients not receiving an ACE inhibitor, as shown in TABLE 2.

TABLE 2

	Without ACE Inhibitor		With ACE Inhibitor	
	Placebo (n=181)	Valsartan (n=185)	Placebo (n=2318)	Valsartan (n=2326)
Events (%)	77 (42.5%)	46 (24.9%)	724 (31.2%)	677 (29.1%)
Hazard ratio (95% CI)	0.51 (0.35, 0.73)		0.92 (0.82, 1.02)	
p-value	0.0002		0.0965	

The modest favorable trend in the group receiving an ACE inhibitor was largely driven by the patients receiving less than the recommended dose of ACE inhibitor. Thus, there is little evidence of further clinical benefit when valsartan is added to an adequate dose of ACE inhibitor.

Secondary end points in the subgroup not receiving ACE inhibitors are shown in TABLE 3.

TABLE 3

	Placebo n=181	Valsartan n=185	Hazard Ratio (95% CI)
Components of HF Morbidity			
All-cause mortality	499 (27.1%)	32 (17.3%)	0.59 (0.37, 0.91)
Sudden death with resuscitation	2 (1.1%)	1 (0.5%)	0.47 (0.04, 5.20)
CHF therapy	1 (0.6%)	0 (0.0%)	—
CHF hospitalization	48 (26.5%)	24 (13.0%)	0.43 (0.27, 0.71)
Cardiovascular Mortality	40 (22.1%)	29 (15.7%)	0.65 (0.40, 1.05)
Non-Fatal Morbidity	49 (27.1%)	24 (13.0%)	0.42 (0.26, 0.69)

In patients not receiving an ACE inhibitor, valsartan-treated patients had an increase in ejection fraction and reduction in left ventricular internal diastolic diameter (LVIDD).

Concomitant use of an ACE inhibitor, a beta-blocker, and valsartan was associated with a worse outcome for heart failure morbidity, as shown in TABLE 4.

TABLE 4

	Placebo (n=816)	Valsartan (n=794)	Hazard Ratio (95% CI)
Heart failure morbidity	179 (21.9%)	202 (25.4%)	1.18 (0.97, 1.45)
All-cause mortality	97 (11.9%)	129 (16.2%)	1.42 (1.09, 1.85)

It is not known if this is a reproducible effect or a chance occurrence. The use of a beta-blocker did not appear to influence the effect of valsartan in patients not receiving an ACE inhibitor.

Effects were generally consistent across subgroups defined by age and gender for the population of patients not receiving an ACE inhibitor. The number of black patients was small and does not permit a meaningful assessment in this subset of patients.

INDICATIONS AND USAGE

HYPERTENSION

Valsartan is indicated for the treatment of hypertension. It may be used alone or in combination with other antihypertensive agents.

HEART FAILURE

Valsartan is indicated for the treatment of heart failure (NYHA class II-IV) in patients who are intolerant of angiotensin converting enzyme inhibitors. In a controlled clinical trial, valsartan significantly reduced hospitalizations for heart failure. There is no evidence that valsartan provides added benefits when it is used with an adequate dose of an ACE inhibitor. (See CLINICAL PHARMACOLOGY, Pharmacodynamics and Clinical Effects, Heart Failure.)

CONTRAINDICATIONS

Valsartan is contraindicated in patients who are hypersensitive to any component of this product.

WARNINGS

FETAL/NEONATAL MORBIDITY AND MORTALITY

Drugs that act directly on the renin-angiotensin system can cause fetal and neonatal morbidity and death when administered to pregnant women. Several dozen cases have been reported in the world literature in patients who were taking angiotensin-converting enzyme inhibitors. When pregnancy is detected, valsartan should be discontinued as soon as possible.

The use of drugs that act directly on the renin-angiotensin system during the second and third trimesters of pregnancy has been associated with fetal and neonatal injury, including hypotension, neonatal skull hypoplasia, anuria, reversible or irreversible renal failure, and death. Oligohydramnios has also been reported, presumably resulting from decreased fetal renal function; oligohydramnios in this setting has been associated with fetal limb contractures, craniofacial deformation, and hypoplastic lung development. Prematurity, intrauterine growth retardation, and patent ductus arteriosus have also been reported, although it is not clear whether these occurrences were due to exposure to the drug.

These adverse effects do not appear to have resulted from intrauterine drug exposure that has been limited to the first trimester. Mothers whose embryos and fetuses are exposed to an angiotensin II receptor antagonist only during the first trimester should be so informed. Nonetheless, when patients become pregnant, physicians should advise the patient to discontinue the use of valsartan as soon as possible.

Rarely (probably less often than once in every 1000 pregnancies), no alternative to a drug acting on the renin-angiotensin system will be found. In these rare cases, the mothers should be apprised of the potential hazards to their fetuses, and serial ultrasound examinations should be performed to assess the intra-amniotic environment.

If oligohydramnios is observed, valsartan should be discontinued unless it is considered life-saving for the mother. Contraction stress testing (CST), a nonstress test (NST), or biophysical profiling (BPP) may be appropriate, depending upon the week of pregnancy. Patients and physicians should be aware, however, that oligohydramnios may not appear until after the fetus has sustained irreversible injury.

Infants with histories of *in utero* exposure to an angiotensin II receptor antagonist should be closely observed for hypotension, oliguria, and hyperkalemia. If oliguria occurs, attention should be directed toward support of blood pressure and renal perfusion. Exchange transfusion or dialysis may be required as means of reversing hypotension and/or substituting for disordered renal function.

No teratogenic effects were observed when valsartan was administered to pregnant mice and rats at oral doses up to 600 mg/kg/day and to pregnant rabbits at oral doses up to 10 mg/kg/day. However, significant decreases in fetal weight, pup birth weight, pup survival rate, and slight delays in developmental milestones were observed in studies in which parental rats were treated with valsartan at oral, maternally toxic (reduction in body weight gain and food consumption) doses of 600 mg/kg/day during organogenesis or late gestation and lactation. In rabbits, fetotoxicity (*i.e.*, resorptions, litter loss, abortions, and low body weight) associated with maternal toxicity (mortality) was observed at doses of 5 and 10 mg/kg/day. The no observed adverse effect doses of 600, 200 and 2 mg/kg/day in mice, rats and rabbits represent 9, 6, and 0.1 times, respectively, the maximum recommended human dose on a mg/m^2 basis. (Calculations assume an oral dose of 320 mg/day and a 60 kg patient.)

HYPOTENSION

Excessive hypotension was rarely seen (0.1%) in patients with uncomplicated hypertension treated with valsartan alone. In patients with an activated renin-angiotensin system, such as volume- and/or salt-depleted patients receiving high doses of diuretics, symptomatic hypotension may occur. This condition should be corrected prior to administration of valsartan, or the treatment should start under close medical supervision.

If excessive hypotension occurs, the patient should be placed in the supine position and, if necessary, given an IV infusion of normal saline. A transient hypotensive response is not a contraindication to further treatment, which usually can be continued without difficulty once the blood pressure has stabilized.

HYPOTENSION IN HEART FAILURE PATIENTS

Caution should be observed when initiating therapy in patients with heart failure. Patients with heart failure given valsartan commonly have some reduction in blood pressure, but discontinuation of therapy because of continuing symptomatic hypotension usually is not necessary when dosing instructions are followed. In controlled trials, the incidence of hypotension in valsartan-treated patients was 5.5% compared to 1.8% in placebo-treated patients.

PRECAUTIONS

GENERAL

Impaired Hepatic Function

As the majority of valsartan is eliminated in the bile, patients with mild-to-moderate hepatic impairment, including patients with biliary obstructive disorders, showed lower valsartan clearance (higher AUCs). Care should be exercised in administering valsartan to these patients.

Impaired Renal Function

Hypertension

In studies of ACE inhibitors in hypertensive patients with unilateral or bilateral renal artery stenosis, increases in serum creatinine or blood urea nitrogen have been reported. In a 4 day trial of valsartan in 12 hypertensive patients with unilateral renal artery stenosis, no significant increases in serum creatinine or blood urea nitrogen were observed. There has been no long-term use of valsartan in patients with unilateral or bilateral renal artery stenosis, but an effect similar to that seen with ACE inhibitors should be anticipated.

Heart Failure

As a consequence of inhibiting the renin-angiotensin-aldosterone system, changes in renal function may be anticipated in susceptible individuals. In patients with severe heart failure whose renal function may depend on the activity of the renin-angiotensin-aldosterone system, treatment with angiotensin-converting enzyme inhibitors and angiotensin receptor antagonists has been associated with oliguria and/or progressive azotemia and (rarely) with acute renal failure and/or death. Similar outcomes have been reported with valsartan.

Some patients with heart failure have developed increases in blood urea nitrogen, serum creatinine, and potassium. These effects are usually minor and transient, and they are more likely to occur in patients with pre-existing renal impairment. Dosage reduction and/or discontinuation of the diuretic and/or valsartan may be required. In the Valsartan Heart Failure Trial, in which 93% of patients were on concomitant ACE inhibitors, treatment was discontinued for elevations in creatinine or potassium (total of 1.0% on valsartan versus 0.2% on placebo). Evaluation of patients with heart failure should always include assessment of renal function.

Concomitant Therapy in Patients With Heart Failure

In patients with heart failure, concomitant use of valsartan, an ACE inhibitor, and a beta blocker is not recommended. In the Valsartan Heart Failure Trial, this triple combination was associated with an unfavorable heart failure outcome (see CLINICAL PHARMACOLOGY, Pharmacodynamics and Clinical Effects, Heart Failure).

INFORMATION FOR THE PATIENT

Pregnancy

Female patients of childbearing age should be told about the consequences of second- and third-trimester exposure to drugs that act on the renin-angiotensin system, and they should also be told that these consequences do not appear to have resulted from intrauterine drug exposure that has been limited to the first trimester. These patients should be asked to report pregnancies to their physicians as soon as possible.

CARCINOGENESIS, MUTAGENESIS, AND IMPAIRMENT OF FERTILITY

There was no evidence of carcinogenicity when valsartan was administered in the diet to mice and rats for up to 2 years at doses up to 160 and 200 mg/kg/day, respectively. These doses in mice and rats are about 2.6 and 6 times, respectively, the maximum recommended human dose on a mg/m^2 basis. (Calculations assume an oral dose of 320 mg/day and a 60 kg patient.)

Mutagenicity assays did not reveal any valsartan-related effects at either the gene or chromosome level. These assays included bacterial mutagenicity tests with *Salmonella* (Ames) and *E. coli;* a gene mutation test with Chinese hamster V79 cells; a cytogenetic test with Chinese hamster ovary cells; and a rat micronucleus test.

Valsartan had no adverse effects on the reproductive performance of male or female rats at oral doses up to 200 mg/kg/day. This dose is 6 times the maximum recommended human dose on a mg/m^2 basis. (Calculations assume an oral dose of 320 mg/day and a 60 kg patient.)

PREGNANCY CATEGORY C (FIRST TRIMESTER) AND PREGNANCY CATEGORY D (SECOND AND THIRD TRIMESTERS)

See WARNINGS, Fetal/Neonatal Morbidity and Mortality.

NURSING MOTHERS

It is not known whether valsartan is excreted in human milk, but valsartan was excreted in the milk of lactating rats. Because of the potential for adverse effects on the nursing infant, a decision should be made whether to discontinue nursing or discontinue the drug, taking into account the importance of the drug to the mother.

PEDIATRIC USE

Safety and effectiveness in pediatric patients have not been established.

GERIATRIC USE

In the controlled clinical trials of valsartan, 1214 (36.2%) of hypertensive patients treated with valsartan were ≥65 years and 265 (7.9%) were ≥75 years. No overall difference in the efficacy or safety of valsartan was observed in this patient population, but greater sensitivity of some older individuals cannot be ruled out.

Of the 2511 patients with heart failure randomized to valsartan in the Valsartan Heart Failure Trial, 45% (1141) were 65 years of age or older. There were no notable differences in efficacy or safety between older and younger patients.

DRUG INTERACTIONS

No clinically significant pharmacokinetic interactions were observed when valsartan was coadministered with amlodipine, atenolol, cimetidine, digoxin, furosemide, glyburide, hydrochlorothiazide, or indomethacin. The valsartan-atenolol combination was more antihypertensive than either component, but it did not lower the heart rate more than atenolol alone.

Coadministration of valsartan and warfarin did not change the pharmacokinetics of valsartan or the time-course of the anticoagulant properties of warfarin.

CYP 450 Interactions: The enzyme(s) responsible for valsartan metabolism have not been identified but do not seem to be CYP 450 isozymes. The inhibitory or induction potential of valsartan on CYP 450 is also unknown.

As with other drugs that block angiotensin II or its effects, concomitant use of potassium sparing diuretics (*e.g.*, spironolactone, triamterene, amiloride), potassium supplements, or salt substitutes containing potassium may lead to increases in serum potassium and in heart failure patients to increases in serum creatinine.

ADVERSE REACTIONS

HYPERTENSION

Valsartan has been evaluated for safety in more than 4000 patients, including over 400 treated for over 6 months, and more than 160 for over 1 year. Adverse experiences have generally been mild and transient in nature and have only infrequently required discontinuation of therapy. The overall incidence of adverse experiences with valsartan was similar to placebo.

The overall frequency of adverse experiences was neither dose-related nor related to gender, age, race, or regimen. Discontinuation of therapy due to side effects was required in 2.3% of valsartan patients and 2.0% of placebo patients. The most common reasons for discontinuation of therapy with valsartan were headache and dizziness.

The adverse experiences that occurred in placebo-controlled clinical trials in at least 1% of patients treated with valsartan and at a higher incidence in valsartan (n=2316) than placebo (n=888) patients included viral infection (3% vs 2%), fatigue (2% vs 1%), and abdominal pain (2% vs 1%).

Headache, dizziness, upper respiratory infection, cough, diarrhea, rhinitis, sinusitis, nausea, pharyngitis, edema, and arthralgia occurred at a more than 1% rate but at about the same incidence in placebo and valsartan patients.

In trials in which valsartan was compared to an ACE inhibitor with or without placebo, the incidence of dry cough was significantly greater in the ACE-inhibitor group (7.9%) than in the groups who received valsartan (2.6%) or placebo (1.5%). In a 129 patient trial limited to patients who had had dry cough when they had previously received ACE inhibitors, the incidences of cough in patients who received valsartan, HCTZ, or lisinopril were 20%, 19%, and 69% respectively ($p < 0.001$).

Dose-related orthostatic effects were seen in less than 1% of patients. An increase in the incidence of dizziness was observed in patients treated with valsartan 320 mg (8%) compared to 10-160 mg (2-4%).

Valsartan has been used concomitantly with hydrochlorothiazide without evidence of clinically important adverse interactions.

Other adverse experiences that occurred in controlled clinical trials of patients treated with valsartan (>0.2% of valsartan patients) are listed below. It cannot be determined whether these events were causally related to valsartan.

Body as a Whole: Allergic reaction and asthenia.
Cardiovascular: Palpitations.
Dermatologic: Pruritus and rash.
Digestive: Constipation, dry mouth, dyspepsia, and flatulence.
Musculoskeletal: Back pain, muscle cramps, and myalgia.
Neurologic and Psychiatric: Anxiety, insomnia, paresthesia, and somnolence.
Respiratory: Dyspnea.
Special Senses: Vertigo.
Urogenital: Impotence.

Other reported events seen less frequently in clinical trials included chest pain, syncope, anorexia, vomiting, and angioedema.

HEART FAILURE

The adverse experience profile of valsartan in heart failure patients was consistent with the pharmacology of the drug and the health status of the patients. In the Valsartan Heart Failure Trial, comparing valsartan in total daily doses up to 320 mg (n=2506) to placebo (n=2494), 10% of valsartan patients discontinued for adverse events versus 7% of placebo patients.

TABLE 5 shows adverse events in double-blind short-term heart failure trials, including the first 4 months of the Valsartan Heart Failure Trial, with an incidence of at least 2% that were more frequent in valsartan-treated patients than in placebo-treated patients. All patients received standard drug therapy for heart failure, frequently as multiple medications, which could include diuretics, digitalis, beta-blockers, or ACE inhibitors.

TABLE 5

	Valsartan (n=3282)	Placebo (n=2740)
Dizziness	17%	9%
Hypotension	7%	2%
Diarrhea	5%	4%
Arthralgia	3%	2%
Fatigue	3%	2%
Back pain	3%	2%
Dizziness, postural	2%	1%
Hyperkalemia	2%	1%
Hypotension, postural	2%	1%

Other adverse events with an incidence greater than 1% and greater than placebo included headache NOS, nausea, renal impairment NOS, syncope, blurred vision, upper abdominal pain and vertigo.

(NOS = not otherwise specified.)

From the long term data in the Valsartan Heart Failure Trial, there did not appear to be any significant adverse events not previously identified.

POST-MARKETING EXPERIENCE

The following additional adverse reactions have been reported in post-marketing experience:

Hypersensitivity: There are rare reports of angioedema.
Digestive: Elevated liver enzymes and very rare reports of hepatitis.
Renal: Impaired renal function.
Clinical Laboratory Tests: Hyperkalemia.
Dermatologic: Alopecia.

CLINICAL LABORATORY TEST FINDINGS

In controlled clinical trials, clinically important changes in standard laboratory parameters were rarely associated with administration of valsartan.

Creatinine: Minor elevations in creatinine occurred in 0.8% of patients taking valsartan and 0.6% given placebo in controlled clinical trials of hypertensive patients. In heart failure trials, greater than 50% increases in creatinine were observed in 3.9% of valsartan-treated patients compared to 0.9% of placebo-treated patients.

Hemoglobin and Hematocrit: Greater than 20% decreases in hemoglobin and hematocrit were observed in 0.4% and 0.8%, respectively, of valsartan patients, compared with 0.1% and 0.1% in placebo-treated patients. One valsartan patient discontinued treatment for microcytic anemia.

Liver Function Tests: Occasional elevations (greater than 150%) of liver chemistries occurred in valsartan-treated patients. Three patients (<0.1%) treated with valsartan discontinued treatment for elevated liver chemistries.

Neutropenia: Neutropenia was observed in 1.9% of patients treated with valsartan and 0.8% of patients treated with placebo.

Serum Potassium: In hypertensive patients, greater than 20% increases in serum potassium were observed in 4.4% of valsartan-treated patients compared to 2.9% of placebo-treated patients. In heart failure patients, greater than 20% increases in serum potassium were observed in 10.0% of valsartan-treated patients compared to 5.1% of placebo-treated patients.

Blood Urea Nitrogen (BUN): In heart failure trials, greater than 50% increases in BUN were observed in 16.6% of valsartan-treated patients compared to 6.3% of placebo-treated patients.

DOSAGE AND ADMINISTRATION

HYPERTENSION

The recommended starting dose of valsartan is 80 or 160 mg once daily when used as monotherapy in patients who are not volume-depleted. Patients requiring greater reductions may be started at the higher dose. Valsartan may be used over a dose range of 80-320 mg daily, administered once-a-day.

The antihypertensive effect is substantially present within 2 weeks and maximal reduction is generally attained after 4 weeks. If additional antihypertensive effect is required over the starting dose range, the dose may be increased to a maximum of 320 mg or a diuretic may be added. Addition of a diuretic has a greater effect than dose increases beyond 80 mg.

No initial dosage adjustment is required for elderly patients, for patients with mild or moderate renal impairment, or for patients with mild or moderate liver insufficiency. Care should be exercised with dosing of valsartan in patients with hepatic or severe renal impairment.

Valsartan may be administered with other antihypertensive agents.

Valsartan may be administered with or without food.

HEART FAILURE

The recommended starting dose of valsartan is 40 mg twice daily. Uptitration to 80 and 160 mg twice daily should be done to the highest dose, as tolerated by the patient. Consideration should be given to reducing the dose of concomitant diuretics. The maximum daily dose administered in clinical trials is 320 mg in divided doses.

Concomitant use with an ACE inhibitor and a beta blocker is not recommended.

HOW SUPPLIED

CAPSULES

Diovan is available as opaque capsules containing valsartan 80 or 160 mg. Capsules are imprinted as follows:

80 mg: Light grey, imprinted "CG FZF".
160 mg: Dark grey, imprinted "CG GOG".

Storage: Store at 25°C (77°F); excursions permitted to 15-30°C (59-86°F). Protect from moisture. Dispense in tight container.

TABLETS

Diovan is available as tablets containing valsartan 40, 80, 160 or 320 mg. All tablets are unscored and debossed as follows:

40 mg: Yellow, round and slightly convex with bevelled edges, debossed with "DO" on 1 side and "NVR" on the other.
80 mg: Pale red, almond-shaped with beveled edges, debossed with "DV" on 1 side and "NVR" on the other.
160 mg: Grey-orange, almond-shaped with beveled edges, debossed with "DX" on 1 side and "NVR" on the other.
320 mg: Dark grey-violet, almond-shaped with beveled edges, debossed with "DXL" on 1 side and "NVR" on the other.

Storage: Store at 25°C (77°F); excursions permitted to 15-30°C (59-86°F). Protect from moisture. Dispense in tight container.

PRODUCT LISTING - EQUIVALENTS NOT AVAILABLE

Tablet - Oral - 40 mg

30's	$39.00	DIOVAN, Novartis Pharmaceuticals	00078-0376-15
100's	$130.00	DIOVAN, Novartis Pharmaceuticals	00078-0376-06

Tablet - Oral - 80 mg

30's	$38.81	DIOVAN, Allscripts Pharmaceutical Company	54569-4697-00
100's	$139.75	DIOVAN, Novartis Pharmaceuticals	00083-4000-01
100's	$139.75	DIOVAN, Novartis Pharmaceuticals	00083-4000-61
100's	$155.39	DIOVAN, Novartis Pharmaceuticals	00078-0358-05
100's	$155.39	DIOVAN, Novartis Pharmaceuticals	00078-0358-06

Tablet - Oral - 160 mg

30's	$42.09	DIOVAN, Allscripts Pharmaceutical Company	54569-4698-00
100's	$151.70	DIOVAN, Novartis Pharmaceuticals	00083-4001-01
100's	$151.70	DIOVAN, Novartis Pharmaceuticals	00083-4001-61
100's	$167.08	DIOVAN, Novartis Pharmaceuticals	00078-0359-05
100's	$167.08	DIOVAN, Novartis Pharmaceuticals	00078-0359-06

Tablet - Oral - 320 mg

100's	$203.25	DIOVAN, Novartis Pharmaceuticals	00078-0360-06
100's	$211.38	DIOVAN, Novartis Pharmaceuticals	00078-0360-05

Vancomycin Hydrochloride (002420)

Categories: Colitis, pseudomembranous; Endocarditis; Enterocolitis; Infection, bone; Infection, lower respiratory tract; Infection, skin and skin structures; Septicemia; Pregnancy Category C; FDA Approved 1964 Nov; WHO Formulary
Drug Classes: Antibiotics, glycopeptides
Brand Names: Lyphocin; **Vancocin**; Vancoled; Vancor
Foreign Brand Availability: Balcorin (Mexico); Diatracin (Spain); Edicin (Thailand); Ifavac (Mexico); Vanauras (Mexico); Vancam (Mexico); Vanccostacin (Korea); Vanco (Germany); Vancocin CP (Australia; Bulgaria; China; Czech-Republic; Hong-Kong; Hungary; Malaysia; Mexico; New-Zealand; South-Africa; Taiwan; Thailand); Vancocina (Italy; Peru); Vancocine (France); Vanco-Teva (Israel); Vancox (Mexico); Vanmicina (Mexico); Voncon (Greece)
Cost of Therapy: $121.26 (Infection; Generic Injection; 1 g; 2 g/day; 10 day supply)
HCFA JCODE(S): J3370 up to 500 mg IV, IM

ORAL

WARNING

Note: The trade name has been used throughout this monograph for clarity.

Vancocin HCl Pulvules

This preparation for the treatment of colitis is for oral use only and is not systemically absorbed. Vancocin HCl must be given orally for treatment of staphylococcal enterocolitis and antibiotic-associated pseudomembranous colitis caused by *Clostridium difficile*. Orally administered Vancocin HCl is *not* effective for other types of infection.

Parenteral administration of Vancocin HCl is not effective for treatment of staphylococcal enterocolitis and antibiotic-associated pseudomembranous colitis caused by *C. difficile*. If parenteral vancomycin therapy is desired, use Vancocin HCl (sterile vancomycin hydrochloride), IntraVenous, and consult package insert accompanying that preparation.

Vancocin HCl Oral Solution

This preparation for the treatment of colitis is for oral use only and is not systemically absorbed. Vancocin HCl must be given orally for treatment of staphylococcal enterocolitis and antibiotic-associated pseudomembranous colitis caused by *Clostridium difficile*. Orally administered Vancocin HCl is *not* effective for other types of infection.

Parenteral administration of Vancocin HCl is not effective for treatment of staphylococcal enterocolitis and antibiotic-associated pseudomembranous colitis caused by *C. difficile*. If parenteral vancomycin therapy is desired, use Vancocin HCl (sterile vancomycin hydrochloride), IntraVenous, and consult package insert accompanying that preparation.

DESCRIPTION

VANCOCIN HCl PULVULES

Pulvules Vancocin HCl (vancomycin hydrochloride capsules) contain chromatographically purified vancomycin hydrochloride, a tricyclic glycopeptide antibiotic derived from *Amycolatopsis orientalis* (formerly *Nocardia orientalis*), which has the chemical formula $C_{66}H_{75}Cl_2N_9O_{24}$·HCl. The molecular weight of vancomycin hydrochloride is 1485.73; 500 mg of the base is equivalent to 0.34 mmol.

The pulvules contain vancomycin hydrochloride equivalent to 125 mg (0.08 mmol) or 250 mg (0.17 mmol) vancomycin. The pulvules also contain FD&C blue no. 2, gelatin, iron oxide, polyethylene glycol, titanium dioxide, and other inactive ingredients.

VANCOCIN HCl ORAL SOLUTION

Vancocin HCl for oral solution (vancomycin hydrochloride for oral solution) contains chromatographically purified vancomycin hydrochloride, a tricyclic glycopeptide antibiotic derived from *Amycolatopsis orientalis* (formerly *Nocardia orientalis*), which has the chemical formula $C_{66}H_{75}Cl_2N_9O_{24}$·HCl. The molecular weight of vancomycin hydrochloride is 1485.73; 500 mg of the base is equivalent to 0.34 mmol.

Vancocin HCl for oral solution contains vancomycin hydrochloride equivalent to 10 g (6.7 mmol) or 1 g (0.67 mmol) vancomycin. Calcium disodium edetate, equivalent to 0.2 mg edetate per gram of vancomycin, is added at the time of manufacture. The 10 g bottle may contain up to 40 mg of ethanol per gram of vancomycin.

CLINICAL PHARMACOLOGY

VANCOCIN HCl PULVULES

Vancomycin is poorly absorbed after oral administration. During multiple dosing of 250 mg every 8 hours for 7 doses, fecal concentrations of vancomycin in volunteers exceeded 100 mg/kg in the majority of samples. No blood concentrations were detected and urinary recovery did not exceed 0.76%. Additional data using the oral solution dosage form follow. In anephric patients with no inflammatory bowel disease, blood concentrations of vancomycin were barely measurable (0.66 µg/ml) in 2 of 5 subjects who received 2 g of Vancocin HCl for oral solution daily for 16 days. No measurable blood concentrations were attained in the other 3 patients. With doses of 2 g daily, very high concentrations of drug can be found in the feces (>3100 mg/kg) and very low concentrations (<1 µg/ml) can be found in the serum of patients with normal renal function who have pseudomembranous colitis. Orally administered vancomycin does not usually enter the systemic circulation even when inflammatory lesions are present. After multiple-dose oral administration of vancomycin, measurable serum concentrations may infrequently occur in patients with active *C. difficile*-induced pseudomembranous colitis, and, in the presence of renal impairment, the possibility of accumulation exists.

Microbiology

The bactericidal action of vancomycin results primarily from inhibition of cell-wall biosynthesis. In addition, vancomycin alters bacterial-cell-membrane permeability and RNA synthesis.

There is no cross-resistance between vancomycin and other antibiotics.

NOTE: The oral form of vancomycin is effective only for the infections noted in INDICATIONS AND USAGE. The oral form is ***not*** effective for any other type of infection.

Vancomycin has been shown to be active against most strains of the following microorganisms in clinical infections as described in INDICATIONS AND USAGE:

Aerobic Gram-Positive Microorganisms: *Staphylococcus aureus* (gram-positive microorganisms including methicillin-resistant strains) associated with enterocolitis.

Anaerobic Gram-Positive Microorganisms: *Clostridium difficile* antibiotic-associated pseudomembranous colitis.

VANCOCIN HCl ORAL SOLUTION

Vancomycin is poorly absorbed after oral administration. During multiple dosing of 250 mg every 8 hours for 7 doses, fecal concentrations of vancomycin in volunteers exceeded 100 mg/kg in the majority of samples. No blood concentrations were detected and urinary recovery did not exceed 0.76%. In anephric patients with no inflammatory bowel disease, blood concentrations of vancomycin were barely measurable (0.66 µg/ml) in 2 of 5 subjects who received 2 g of Vancocin HCl for oral solution daily for 16 days. No measurable blood concentrations were attained in the other 3 patients. With doses of 2 g daily, very high concentrations of drug can be found in the feces (>3100 mg/kg) and very low concentrations (<1 µg/ml) can be found in the serum of patients with normal renal function who have pseudomembranous colitis. Orally administered vancomycin does not usually enter the systemic circulation even when inflammatory lesions are present. After multiple-dose oral administration of vancomycin, measurable serum concentrations may infrequently occur in patients with active *C. difficile*-induced pseudomembranous colitis, and, in the presence of renal impairment, the possibility of accumulation exists.

Microbiology

The bactericidal action of vancomycin results primarily from inhibition of cell-wall biosynthesis. In addition, vancomycin alters bacterial-cell-membrane permeability and RNA synthesis. There is no cross-resistance between vancomycin and other antibiotics. Vancomycin is active against *C. difficile* (*e.g.*, toxigenic strains implicated in pseudomembranous enterocolitis). It is also active against staphylococci, including *Staphylococcus aureus*.

For further information, see prescribing information for Vancocin HCl, intravenous.

Vancomycin is not active *in vitro* against gram-negative bacilli, mycobacteria, or fungi.

Disk Susceptibility Tests

The standardized disk and/or dilution methods described by the National Committee for Clinical Laboratory Standards have been recommended to test susceptibility to vancomycin.

INDICATIONS AND USAGE

VANCOCIN HCl PULVULES

Vancocin HCl pulvules may be administered orally for treatment of enterocolitis caused by *Staphylococcus aureus* (including methicillin-resistant strains) and antibiotic-associated pseudomembranous colitis caused by *C. difficile*. Parenteral administration of Vancocin HCl is not effective for the above indications; therefore, Vancocin HCl must be given orally for these indications. **Orally administered Vancocin HCl is not effective for other types of infection.**

VANCOCIN HCl ORAL SOLUTION

Vancocin HCl for oral solution is administered orally for treatment of staphylococcal enterocolitis and antibiotic-associated pseudomembranous colitis caused by *C. difficile*. Parenteral administration of Vancocin HCl is not effective for the above indications; therefore, Vancocin HCl must be given orally for these indications. **Orally administered Vancocin HCl is not effective for other types of infection.**

CONTRAINDICATIONS

VANCOCIN HCl PULVULES AND ORAL SOLUTION

Vancocin HCl is contraindicated in patients with known hypersensitivity to this antibiotic.

PRECAUTIONS

VANCOCIN HCl PULVULES

General

Clinically significant serum concentrations have been reported in some patients who have taken multiple oral doses of vancomycin for active *C. difficile*-induced pseudomembranous colitis; therefore, monitoring of serum concentrations may be appropriate in some instances, *e.g.*, in patients with renal insufficiency and/or colitis.

Some patients with inflammatory disorders of the intestinal mucosa may have significant systemic absorption of vancomycin and, therefore, may be at risk for the development of adverse reactions associated with the parenteral administration of vancomycin. (See full prescribing information accompanying the intravenous preparation.) The risk is greater if renal impairment is present. It should be noted that the total systemic and renal clearances of vancomycin are reduced in the elderly.

Ototoxicity has occurred in patients receiving Vancocin HCl. It may be transient or permanent. It has been reported mostly in patients who have been given excessive intravenous doses, who have an underlying hearing loss, or who are receiving concomitant therapy with another ototoxic agent, such as an aminoglycoside. Serial tests of auditory function may be helpful in order to minimize the risk of ototoxicity.

When patients with underlying renal dysfunction or those receiving concomitant therapy with an aminoglycoside are being treated, serial monitoring of renal function should be performed.

Carcinogenesis, Mutagenesis, and Impairment of Fertility

No long-term carcinogenesis studies in animals have been conducted.

At concentrations up to 1000 µg/ml, vancomycin had no mutagenic effect *in vitro* in the mouse lymphoma forward mutation assay or the primary rat hepatocyte unscheduled DNA synthesis assay. The concentrations tested *in vitro* were above the peak plasma vancomycin concentrations of 20-40 µg/ml usually achieved in humans after slow infusion of the maximum recommended dose of 1 g. Vancomycin had no mutagenic effect *in vivo* in the Chinese hamster sister chromatid exchange assay (400 mg/kg IP) or the mouse micronucleus assay (800 mg/kg IP).

No definitive fertility studies have been conducted.

Pregnancy, Teratogenic Effects, Pregnancy Category B

The highest doses of vancomycin tested were not teratogenic in rats given up to 200 mg/kg/day IV (1180 mg/m^2 or 1 times the recommended maximum human dose based on a mg/m^2 basis) or in rabbits given up to 120 mg/kg/day IV (1320 mg/m^2 or 1.1 times the recommended maximum human dose based on a mg/m^2 basis). No effects on fetal weight or development were seen in rats at the highest dose tested or in rabbits given 80 mg/kg/day (880 mg/m^2 or 0.74 times the recommended maximum human dose based on mg/m^2).

In a controlled clinical study, the potential ototoxic and nephrotoxic effects of Vancocin HCl on infants were evaluated when the drug was administered intravenously to pregnant women for serious staphylococcal infections complicating intravenous drug abuse. Vancocin HCl was found in cord blood. No sensorineural hearing loss or nephrotoxicity attributable to Vancocin HCl was noted. One (1) infant whose mother received Vancocin HCl in the third trimester experienced conductive hearing loss that was not attributed to the administration of Vancocin HCl. Because the number of patients treated in this study was limited and Vancocin HCl was administered only in the second and third trimesters, it is not known whether Vancocin HCl causes fetal harm. Because animal reproduction studies are not always predictive of human response, Vancocin HCl should be given to a pregnant woman only if clearly needed.

Nursing Mothers

Vancocin HCl is excreted in human milk based on information obtained with the intravenous administration of Vancocin HCl. However, systemic absorption of vancomycin is very low following oral administration of Vancocin HCl pulvules (see CLINICAL PHARMACOLOGY). It is not known whether oral vancomycin is excreted in human milk, as no studies of vancomycin concentration in human milk after oral administration have been done. Caution should be exercised when Vancocin HCl is administered to a nursing woman. Because of the potential for adverse events, a decision should be made whether to discontinue nursing or discontinue the drug, taking into account the importance of the drug to the mother.

Pediatric Use

Safety and effectiveness in pediatric patients have not been established.

VANCOCIN HCl ORAL SOLUTION

General

Clinically significant serum concentrations have been reported in some patients who have taken multiple oral doses of vancomycin for active *C. difficile*-induced pseudomembranous colitis; therefore, monitoring of serum concentrations may be appropriate.

Some patients with inflammatory disorders of the intestinal mucosa may have significant systemic absorption of vancomycin and, therefore, may be at risk for the development of adverse reactions associated with the parenteral administration of vancomycin. (See prescribing information accompanying the intravenous preparation.) The risk is greater if renal impairment is present. It should be noted that the total systemic and renal clearances of vancomycin are reduced in the elderly.

Ototoxicity has occurred in patients receiving Vancocin HCl. It may be transient or permanent. It has been reported mostly in patients who have been given excessive intravenous doses, who have an underlying hearing loss, or who are receiving concomitant therapy with another ototoxic agent, such as an aminoglycoside. Serial tests of auditory function may be helpful in order to minimize the risk of ototoxicity.

When patients with underlying renal dysfunction or those receiving concomitant therapy with an aminoglycoside are being treated, serial monitoring of renal function should be performed.

Pregnancy Category C

Animal reproduction studies have not been conducted with Vancocin HCl. It is not known whether Vancocin HCl can affect reproduction capacity. In a controlled clinical study, the potential ototoxic and nephrotoxic effects of Vancocin HCl on infants were evaluated when the drug was administered intravenously to pregnant women for serious staphylococcal infections complicating intravenous drug abuse. Vancocin HCl was found in cord blood. No sensorineural hearing loss or nephrotoxicity attributable to Vancocin HCl was noted. One (1) infant whose mother received Vancocin HCl in the third trimester experienced conductive hearing loss that was not attributed to the administration of Vancocin HCl. Because the number of patients treated in this study was limited and Vancocin HCl was administered only in the second and third trimesters, it is not known whether Vancocin HCl causes fetal harm. Vancocin HCl should be given to a pregnant woman only if clearly needed.

Nursing Mothers

Vancocin HCl is excreted in human milk based on information obtained with the intravenous administration of Vancocin HCl. Blood concentrations achieved with oral administration are very low (*see* CLINICAL PHARMACOLOGY). Caution should be exercised when Vancocin HCl is administered to a nursing woman. Because of the potential for adverse events, a decision should be made whether to discontinue nursing or discontinue the drug, taking into account the importance of the drug to the mother.

ADVERSE REACTIONS

VANCOCIN HCl PULVULES

Nephrotoxicity

Rarely, renal failure, principally manifested by increased serum creatinine or BUN concentrations, especially in patients given large doses of intravenously administered Vancocin HCl has been reported. Rare cases of interstitial nephritis have been reported. Most of these have occurred in patients who were given aminoglycosides concomitantly or who had preexisting kidney dysfunction. When Vancocin HCl was discontinued, azotemia resolved in most patients.

Ototoxicity

A few dozen cases of hearing loss associated with intravenously administered Vancocin HCl have been reported. Most of these patients had kidney dysfunction or a preexisting hearing loss or were receiving concomitant treatment with an ototoxic drug. Vertigo, dizziness, and tinnitus have been reported rarely.

Hematopoietic

Reversible neutropenia, usually starting 1 week or more after onset of intravenous therapy with Vancocin HCl or after a total dose of more than 25 g, has been reported for several dozen patients. Neutropenia appears to be promptly reversible when Vancocin HCl is discontinued. Thrombocytopenia has rarely been reported.

Miscellaneous

Infrequently, patients have been reported to have had anaphylaxis, drug fever, chills, nausea, eosinophilia, rashes (including exfoliative dermatitis), Stevens-Johnson syndrome, toxic epidermal necrolysis, and rare cases of vasculitis in association with the administration of Vancocin HCl.

A condition has been reported that is similar to the IV-induced syndrome with symptoms consistent with anaphylactoid reactions, including hypotension, wheezing, dyspnea, urticaria, pruritus, flushing of the upper body ("Red Man Syndrome"), pain and muscle spasm of the chest and back. These reactions usually resolve within 20 minutes but may persist for several hours.

VANCOCIN HCl ORAL SOLUTION

Nephrotoxicity

Rarely, renal failure, principally manifested by increased serum creatinine or BUN concentrations, especially in patients given large doses of intravenously administered Vancocin HCl, has been reported. Rare cases of interstitial nephritis have been reported. Most of these have occurred in patients who were given aminoglycosides concomitantly or who had preexisting kidney dysfunction. When Vancocin HCl was discontinued, azotemia resolved in most patients.

Ototoxicity

A few dozen cases of hearing loss associated with intravenously administered Vancocin HCl have been reported. Most of these patients had kidney dysfunction or a preexisting hearing loss or were receiving concomitant treatment with an ototoxic drug. Vertigo, dizziness, and tinnitus have been reported rarely.

Hematopoietic

Reversible neutropenia, usually starting 1 week or more after onset of intravenous therapy with Vancocin HCl or after a total dosage of more than 25 g, has been reported for several dozen patients. Neutropenia appears to be promptly reversible when Vancocin HCl is discontinued. Thrombocytopenia has rarely been reported.

Miscellaneous

Infrequently, patients have been reported to have had anaphylaxis, drug fever, chills, nausea, eosinophilia, rashes (including exfoliative dermatitis), Stevens-Johnson syndrome, toxic epidermal necrolysis, and rare cases of vasculitis in association with the administration of Vancocin HCl.

A condition has been reported that is similar to the IV-induced syndrome with symptoms consistent with anaphylactoid reactions, including hypotension, wheezing, dyspnea, urticaria, pruritus, flushing of the upper body ("Red Man Syndrome"), pain and muscle spasm of the chest and back. These reactions usually resolve within 20 minutes but may persist for several hours.

DOSAGE AND ADMINISTRATION

VANCOCIN HCl PULVULES

Adults

Oral Vancocin HCl is used in treating antibiotic-associated pseudomembranous colitis caused by *C. difficile* and staphylococcal enterocolitis. Vancocin HCl is not effective by the oral route for other types of infections. The usual adult total daily dosage is 500 mg to 2 g administered orally in 3 or 4 divided doses for 7-10 days.

Pediatric Patients

The usual daily dosage is 40 mg/kg in 3 or 4 divided doses for 7-10 days. The total daily dosage should not exceed 2 g.

VANCOCIN HCl ORAL SOLUTION

Adults

Oral Vancocin HCl is used in treating antibiotic-associated pseudomembranous colitis caused by *C. difficile* and staphylococcal enterocolitis. Vancocin HCl is not effective by the oral route for other types of infections. The usual adult total daily dosage is 500 mg to 2 g administered orally in 3 or 4 divided doses for 7-10 days.

Pediatric Patients

The usual daily dosage is 40 mg/kg in 3 or 4 divided doses for 7-10 days. The total daily dosage should not exceed 2 g.

Preparation and Stability

The contents of the 10 g bottle may be mixed with distilled or deionized water (115 ml) for oral administration. When mixed with 115 ml of water, each 6 ml provides approximately 500 mg of vancomycin. The contents of the 1 g bottle may be mixed with distilled or deionized water (20 ml). When reconstituted with 20 ml, each 5 ml contains approximately 250 mg of vancomycin. Mix thoroughly to dissolve. These mixtures may be kept for 2 weeks in a refrigerator without significant loss of potency.

The appropriate oral solution dose may be diluted in 1 oz of water and given to the patient to drink. Common flavoring syrups may be added to the solution to improve the taste for oral administration. The diluted material may be administered via nasogastric tube.

HOW SUPPLIED

VANCOCIN HCl PULVULES

Vancocin HCl Pulvules (or vancomycin hydrochloride capsules) are available in:

125 mg: The 125 mg (equivalent to vancomycin) pulvules have an opaque blue cap and opaque brown body imprinted with "3125" on the cap and "VANCOCIN HCl 125 MG" on the body in white ink.

250 mg: The 250 mg (equivalent to vancomycin) pulvules have an opaque blue cap and opaque lavender body imprinted with "3126" on the cap and "VANCOCIN HCl 250 MG" on the body in white ink.

Storage: Store at controlled room temperature, 15-30°C (59-86°F).

VANCOCIN HCl ORAL SOLUTION

Vancocin HCl for oral solution (or vancomycin hydrochloride for oral solution) is available in 10 g and 1 g bottles.

Storage: Prior to reconstitution, store at controlled room temperature, 15-30°C (59-86°F).

INTRAVENOUS

DESCRIPTION

Note: The trade name has been used throughout this monograph for clarity.

Vancocin HCl (sterile vancomycin hydrochloride), IntraVenous, is a chromatographically purified, tricyclic glycopeptide antibiotic derived from *Amycolatopsis orientalis* (formerly *Nocardia orientalis*) and has the chemical formula $C_{66}H_{75}Cl_2H_9O_{24}$·HCl. The molecular weight is 1485.73; 500 mg of the base is equivalent to 0.34 mmol.

The vials contain sterile vancomycin hydrochloride equivalent to either 500 mg or 1 g vancomycin activity. Vancomycin hydrochloride is an off-white lyophilized plug. When reconstituted in water, it forms a clear solution with a pH range of 2.5-4.5. This produce is oxygen sensitive.

CLINICAL PHARMACOLOGY

Vancomycin is poorly absorbed after oral administration; it is given intravenously for therapy of systemic infections. Intramuscular injection is painful.

In subjects with normal kidney function, multiple intravenous dosing of 1 g of vancomycin (15 mg/kg) infused over 60 minutes produces mean plasma concentrations of approximately 63 μg/ml immediately after the completion of infusion, mean plasma concentrations of approximately 23 μg/ml 2 hours after infusion, and mean plasma concentrations of approximately 8 μg/ml 11 hours after the end of the infusion. Multiple dosing of 500 mg infused over 30 minutes produces mean plasma concentrations of about 49 μg/ml at the completion of infusion, mean plasma concentrations of about 19 μg/ml 2 hours after infusion, and mean plasma concentrations of about 10 μg/ml 6 hours after infusion. The plasma concentrations during multiple dosing are similar to those after a single dose.

The mean elimination half-life of vancomycin from plasma is 4-6 hours in subjects with normal renal function. In the first 24 hours, about 75% of an administered dose of vancomycin is excreted in urine by glomerular filtration. Mean plasma clearance is about 0.058 L/kg/h, and mean renal clearance is about 0.048 L/kg/h. Renal dysfunction slows excretion of vancomycin. In anephric patients, the average half-life of elimination is 7.5 days. The distribution coefficient is from 0.3-0.43 L/kg. There is no apparent metabolism of the drug. About 60% of an intraperitoneal dose of vancomycin administered during peritoneal dialysis is absorbed systemically in 6 hours. Serum concentrations of about 10 μg/ml are achieved by intraperitoneal injection of 30 mg/kg of vancomycin. Although vancomycin is not effectively removed by either hemodialysis or peritoneal dialysis, there have been reports of increased vancomycin clearance with hemoperfusion and hemofiltration.

Total systemic and renal clearance of vancomycin may be reduced in the elderly.

Vancomycin is approximately 55% serum protein bound as measured by ultrafiltration at vancomycin serum concentrations of 10-100 μg/ml. After IV administration of Vancocin HCl, inhibitory concentrations are present in pleural, pericardial, ascitic, and synovial fluids; in urine; in peritoneal dialysis fluid; and in atrial appendage tissue. Vancocin HCl does not readily diffuse across normal meninges into the spinal fluid; but, when the meninges are inflamed, penetration into the spinal fluid occurs.

MICROBIOLOGY

The bactericidal action of vancomycin results primarily from inhibition of cell-wall biosynthesis. In addition, vancomycin alters bacterial-cell-membrane permeability and RNA synthesis. There is no cross-resistance between vancomycin and other antibiotics. Vancomycin is active against staphylococci, including *Staphylococcus aureus* and *Staphylococcus epidermidis* (including heterogeneous methicillin-resistant strains); streptococci, including *Streptococcus pyogenes, Streptococcus pneumoniae* (including penicillin-resistant strains), *Streptococcus agalactiae,* the viridans group, *Streptococcus bovis,* and enterococci (*e.g., Enterococcus faecalis* [formerly *Streptococcus faecalis*]); *Clostridium difficile* (*e.g.,* toxigenic strains implicated in pseudomembranous enterocolitis); and diphtheroids. Other organisms that are susceptible to vancomycin *in vitro* include *Listeria monocytogenes, Lactobacillus* species, *Actinomyces* species, *Clostridium* species, and *Bacillus* species. Vancomycin is not active *in vitro* against gram-negative bacilli, mycobacteria, or fungi.

SYNERGY

The combination of vancomycin and an aminoglycoside acts synergistically *in vitro* against many strains of *S. aureus,* nonenterococcal group D streptococci, enterococci, and *Streptococcus* species (viridans group).

DISK SUSCEPTIBILITY TESTS

The standardized disk method described by the National Committee for Clinical Laboratory Standards has been recommended to test susceptibility to vancomycin. Results of standard susceptibility tests with a 30 μg vancomycin hydrochloride disk should be interpreted according to the following criteria: Susceptible organisms produce zones greater than or equal to 12 mm, indicating that the test organism is likely to respond to therapy. Organisms that produce zones of 10 or 11 mm are considered to be of intermediate susceptibility. Organisms in this category are likely to respond if the infection is confined to tissues or fluids in which high antibiotic concentrations are attained. Resistant organisms produce zones of 9 mm or less, indicating that other therapy should be selected.

Using a standardized dilution method, a bacterial isolate may be considered susceptible if the MIC value for vancomycin is 4 μg/ml or less. Organisms are considered resistant to vancomycin if the MIC is greater than or equal to 16 μg/ml. Organisms having an MIC value of less than 16 μg/ml but greater than 4 μg/ml are considered to be of intermediate susceptibility.[1-2]

Standardized procedures require the use of laboratory control organisms. The 30 μg vancomycin disk should give zone diameters between 15 and 19 mm for *S. aureus* ATCC 25923. As with the standard diffusion methods, dilution procedures require the use of laboratory control organisms. Standard vancomycin powder should give MIC values in the range of 0.5-2.0 μg/ml for *S. aureus* ATCC 29213. For *E. faecalis* ATCC 29212, the MIC range should be 1.0-4.0 μg/ml.

INDICATIONS AND USAGE

Vancocin HCl is indicated for the treatment of serious or severe infections caused by susceptible strains of methicillin-resistant (beta-lactam-resistant) staphylococci. It is indicated for penicillin-allergic patients, for patients who cannot receive or who have failed to respond to other drugs, including the penicillins or cephalosporins, and for infections caused by vancomycin-susceptible organisms that are resistant to other antimicrobial drugs. Vancocin HCl is indicated for initial therapy when methicillin-resistant staphylococci are suspected, but after susceptibility data are available, therapy should be adjusted accordingly.

Vancocin HCl is effective in the treatment of staphylococcal endocarditis. Its effectiveness has been documented in other infections due to staphylococci, including septicemia, bone infections, lower respiratory tract infections, and skin and skin structure infections. When staphylococcal infections are localized and purulent, antibiotics are used as adjuncts to appropriate surgical measures.

Vancocin HCl has been reported to be effective alone or in combination with an aminoglycoside for endocarditis caused by *Streptococcus viridans* or *S. bovis.* For endocarditis caused by enterococci (*e.g., E. faecalis*), Vancocin HCl has been reported to be effective only in combination with an aminoglycoside.

Vancocin HCl has been reported to be effective for the treatment of diphtheroid endocarditis. Vancocin HCl has been used successfully in combination with either rifampin, an aminoglycoside, or both in early-onset prosthetic valve endocarditis caused by *S. epidermidis* or diphtheroids.

Specimens for bacteriologic cultures should be obtained in order to isolate and identify causative organisms and to determine their susceptibilities to Vancocin HCl.

The parenteral form of Vancocin HCl may be administered orally for treatment of antibiotic-associated pseudomembranous colitis caused by *C. difficile* and for staphylococcal enterocolitis. Parenteral administration of Vancocin HCl alone is of unproven benefit for these indications. **Vancocin HCl is not effective by the oral route for other types of infection.** Although no controlled clinical efficacy studies have been conducted, intravenous vancomycin has been suggested by the American Heart Association and the American Dental Association as prophylaxis against bacterial endocarditis in penicillin-allergic patients who have congenital heart disease or rheumatic or other acquired valvular heart disease when these patients undergo dental procedures or surgical procedures of the upper respiratory tract.

Note: When selecting antibiotics for the prevention of bacterial endocarditis, the physician or dentist should read the full joint statement of the American Heart Association and the American Dental Association.[3]

CONTRAINDICATIONS

Vancocin HCl is contraindicated in patients with known hypersensitivity to this antibiotic.

WARNINGS

Rapid bolus administration (*e.g.,* over several minutes) may be associated with exaggerated hypotension, and, rarely, cardiac arrest.

Vancocin HCl should be administered in a dilute solution over a period of not less than 60 minutes to avoid rapid-infusion-related reactions. Stopping the infusion usually results in prompt cessation of these reactions.

Ototoxicity has occurred in patients receiving Vancocin HCl. It may be transient or permanent. It has been reported mostly in patients who have been given excessive doses, who have an underlying hearing loss, or who are receiving concomitant therapy with another ototoxic agent, such as an aminoglycoside. Vancomycin should be used with caution in patients with renal insufficiency because the risk of toxicity is appreciably increased by high, prolonged blood concentrations.

Dosage of Vancocin HCl must be adjusted for patients with renal dysfunction (*see* PRECAUTIONS and DOSAGE AND ADMINISTRATION).

Psuedomembranous colitis has been reported with nearly all antibacterial agents, including vancomycin, and may range in severity from mild to life-threatening. Therefore, it is important to consider this diagnosis in patients who present with diarrhea subsequent to the administration of antibacterial agents.

Treatment with antibacterial agents alters the normal flora of the colon and may permit overgrowth of clostridia. Studies indicate that a toxin produced by *Clostridium difficile* is a primary cause of "antibiotic-associated colitis." After the diagnosis of pseudomembranous colitis has been established, therapeutic measures should be initiated. Mild cases of pseudomembranous colitis usually respond to drug discontamination alone. In moderate to severe cases, consideration should be given to management with fluids and electrolytes, protein supplementation, and treatment with an antibacterial drug clinically effective against *C. difficile* colitis.

PRECAUTIONS

GENERAL

Clinically significant serum concentrations have been reported in some patients who have taken multiple oral doses of vancomycin for active *C. difficile*-induced pseudomembranous colitis.

Prolonged use of Vancocin HCl may result in the overgrowth of nonsusceptible organisms. Careful observation of the patient is essential. If superinfection occurs during therapy, appropriate measures should be taken.

In order to minimize the risk of nephrotoxicity when treating patients with underlying renal dysfunction or patients receiving concomitant therapy with an aminoglycoside, serial monitoring of renal function should be performed and particular care should be taken in following appropriate dosing schedules (*see* DOSAGE AND ADMINISTRATION). Serial tests of auditory function may be helpful in order to minimize the risk of ototoxicity.

Reversible neutropenia has been reported in patients receiving Vancocin HCl (*see* ADVERSE REACTIONS). Patients who will undergo prolonged therapy with Vancocin HCl or those who are receiving concomitant drugs that may cause neutropenia should have periodic monitoring of the leukocyte count.

Vancocin HCl is irritating to tissue and must be given by a secure intravenous route of administration. Pain, tenderness, and necrosis occur with intramuscular injection of Vancocin HCl or with inadvertent extravasation. Thrombophlebitis may occur, the frequency and severity of which can be minimized by administering the drug slowly as a dilute solution (2.5-5 g/L) and by rotating the sites of infusion. There have been reports that the frequency of infusion-related events (including hypotension, flushing, erythema, urticaria, and pruritus) increases with the concomitant administration of anesthetic agents. Infusion-related events may be minimized by the administration of Vancocin HCl as a 60 minute infusion prior to anesthetic induction.

The safety and efficacy of vancomycin administration by the intrathecal (intralumbar or intraventricular) routes have not been assessed.

Reports have revealed that administration of sterile vancomycin HCl by the intraperitoneal route during continuous ambulatory peritoneal dialysis (CAPD) has resulted in a syndrome of chemical peritonitis. To date, this syndrome has ranged from a cloudy dialysate alone to a cloudy dialysate accompanied by variable degrees of abdominal pain and fever. This syndrome appears to be short-lived after discontinuation of intraperitoneal vancomycin.

PREGNANCY CATEGORY C

Animal reproduction studies have not been conducted with Vancocin HCl. It is not known whether Vancocin HCl can affect reproduction capacity. In a controlled clinical study, the potential ototoxic and nephrotoxic effects of Vancocin HCl on infants were evaluated when the drug was administered to pregnant women for serious staphylococcal infections complicating intravenous drug abuse. Vancocin HCl was found in cord blood. No sensorineural hearing loss or nephrotoxicity attributable to Vancocin HCl was noted. One (1) infant whose mother received Vancocin HCl in the third trimester experienced conductive hearing loss that was not attributed to the administration of Vancocin HCl. Because the number of patients treated in this study was limited and Vancocin HCl was administered only in the second and third trimesters, it is not known whether Vancocin HCl causes fetal harm. Vancocin HCl should be given to a pregnant woman only if clearly needed.

NURSING MOTHERS

Vancocin HCl is excreted in human milk. Caution should be exercised when Vancocin HCl is administered to a nursing woman. Because of the potential for adverse events, a decision should be made whether to discontinue nursing or to discontinue the drug, taking into account the importance of the drug to the mother.

PEDIATRIC USE

In premature neonates and young infants, it may be appropriate to confirm desired vancomycin serum concentrations. Concomitant administration of vancomycin and anesthetic agents has been associated with erythema and histamine-like flushing in children (*see* ADVERSE REACTIONS).

GERIATRIC USE

The natural decrement of glomerular filtration with increasing age may lead to elevated vancomycin serum concentrations if dosage is not adjusted. Vancomycin dosage schedules should be adjusted in elderly patients (*see* DOSAGE AND ADMINISTRATION).

DRUG INTERACTIONS

Concomitant administration of vancomycin and anesthetic agents has been associated with erythema and histamine-like flushing (*see* PRECAUTIONS, Pediatric Use) and anaphylactoid reactions (*see* ADVERSE REACTIONS).

Concurrent and/or sequential systemic or topical use of other potentially neurotoxic and/or nephrotoxic drugs, such as amphotericin B, aminoglycosides, bacitracin; polymyxin B, colistin, viomycin, or cisplatin, when indicated, requires careful monitoring.

V

ADVERSE REACTIONS

INFUSION-RELATED EVENTS

During or soon after rapid infusion of Vancocin HCl, patients may develop anaphylactoid reactions, including hypotension (*see* ANIMAL PHARMACOLOGY), wheezing, dyspnea, urticaria, or pruritus. Rapid infusion may also cause flushing of the upper body ("Red Man Syndrome") or pain and muscle spasm of the chest and back. These reactions usually resolve within 20 minutes or may persist for several hours. Such events are infrequent. Vancocin HCl is given by a slow infusion over 60 minutes. In studies of normal volunteers, infusion-related events did not occur when Vancocin HCl was administered at a rate of 10 mg/min or less.

NEPHROTOXICITY

Rarely, renal failure, principally manifested by increased serum creatinine or BUN concentrations, especially in patients given large doses of Vancocin HCl, has been reported. Rare cases of interstitial nephritis have been reported. Most of these have occurred in patients who were given aminoglycosides concomitantly or who had preexisting kidney dysfunction. When Vancocin HCl was discontinued, azotemia resolved in most patients.

GASTROINTESTINAL

Onset of pseudomembranous colitis symptoms may occur during or after antibiotic treatment (*see* WARNINGS).

OTOTOXICITY

A few dozen cases of hearing loss associated with Vancocin HCl have been reported. Most of these patients had kidney dysfunction or a preexisting hearing loss or were receiving concomitant treatment with an ototoxic drug. Vertigo, dizziness, and tinnitus have been reported rarely.

HEMATOPOIETIC

Reversible neutropenia, usually starting 1 week or more after onset of therapy with Vancocin HCl or after a total dosage of more than 25 g, has been reported for several dozen patients. Neutropenia appears to be promptly reversible when Vancocin HCl is discontinued. Thrombocytopenia has rarely been reported.

Although a causal relationship has not been established, reversible agranulocytosis (granulocytes $<500/mm^3$) has been reported rarely.

PHLEBITIS

Inflammation at the injection site has been reported.

MISCELLANEOUS

Infrequently, patients have been reported to have had anaphylaxis, drug fever, nausea, chills, eosinophilia, rashes (including exfoliative dermatitis), Stevens-Johnson syndrome, toxic epidermal necrolysis, and rare cases of vasculitis in association with administration of Vancocin HCl.

Chemical peritonitis has been reported following intraperitoneal administration of vancomycin (*see* PRECAUTIONS).

DOSAGE AND ADMINISTRATION

Infusion-related events are related to both concentration and rate of administration of vancomycin. Concentrations of no more than 5 mg/ml and rates of no more than 10 mg/min are recommended in adults (see also age-specific recommendations). In selected patients in need of fluid restriction, a concentration up to 10 mg/ml may be used; use of such higher concentrations may increase the risk of infusion-related events. Infusion-related events may occur, however, at any rate or concentration.

PATIENTS WITH NORMAL RENAL FUNCTION

Adults

The usual daily intravenous dose is 2 g divided either as 500 mg every 6 hours or 1 g every 12 hours. Each dose should be administered at no more than 10 mg/min or over a period of at least 60 minutes, whichever is longer. Other patient factors, such as age or obesity, may call for modification of the usual intravenous daily dose.

Children

The usual intravenous dosage of Vancocin HCl is 10 mg/kg per dose given every 6 hours. Each dose should be administered over a period of at least 60 minutes.

Infants and Neonates

In neonates and young infants, the total daily intravenous dosage may be lower. In both neonates and infants, an initial dose of 15 mg/kg is suggested, followed by 10 mg/kg every 12 hours for neonates in the 1st week of life and every 8 hours thereafter up to the age of 1 month. Each dose should be administered over 60 minutes. Close monitoring of serum concentrations of vancomycin may be warranted in these patients.

PATIENTS WITH IMPAIRED RENAL FUNCTION AND ELDERLY PATIENTS

Dosage adjustment must be made in patients with impaired renal function. In premature infants and the elderly, greater dosage reductions than expected may be necessary because of decreased renal function. Measurement of vancomycin serum concentrations can be helpful in optimizing therapy, especially in seriously ill patients with changing renal function. Vancomycin serum concentrations can be determined by use of microbiologic assay, radioimmunoassay, fluorescence polarization immunoassay, fluorescence immunoassay, or high-pressure liquid chromatography.

If creatinine clearance can be measured or estimated accurately, the dosage for most patients with renal impairment can be calculated using TABLE 1. The dosage of Vancocin HCl per day in mg is about 15 times the glomerular filtration rate in ml/min:

TABLE 1 *Dosage Table for Vancomycin in Patients With Impaired Renal Function — (Adapted From Moellering, et al.)*[4]

Creatinine Clearance	Vancomycin Dose
100 ml/min	1545 mg/24 h
90 ml/min	1390 mg/24 h
80 ml/min	1235 mg/24 h
70 ml/min	1080 mg/24 h
60 ml/min	925 mg/24 h
50 ml/min	770 mg/24 h
40 ml/min	620 mg/24 h
30 ml/min	465 mg/24 h
20 ml/min	310 mg/24 h
10 ml/min	155 mg/24 h

The initial dose should be no less than 15 mg/kg, even in patients with mild to moderate renal insufficiency.

TABLE 1 is not valid for functionally anephric patients. For such patients, an initial dose of 15 mg/kg of body weight should be given to achieve prompt therapeutic serum concentrations. The dose required to maintain stable concentrations is 1.9 mg/kg/24 h. In patients with marked renal impairment, it may be more convenient to give maintenance doses of 250-1000 mg once every several days rather than administering the drug on a daily basis. In anuria, a dose of 1000 mg every 7-10 days has been recommended.

When only the serum creatinine concentration is known, the following formula (based on sex, weight, and age of the patient) may be used to calculate creatinine clearance. Calculated creatinine clearances (ml/min) are only estimates. The creatinine clearance should be measured promptly.

Men: Weight (kg) × (140 − age in years) ÷ 72 × serum creatinine concentration (mg/dl)

Women: 0.85 × above value

The serum creatinine must represent a steady state of renal function. Otherwise, the estimated value for creatinine clearance is not valid. Such a calculated clearance is an overestimate of actual clearance in patients with conditions: (1) characterized by decreasing renal function, such as shock, severe heart failure, or oliguria; (2) in which a normal relationship between muscle mass and total body weight is not present, such as obese patients or those with liver disease, edema, or ascites; and (3) accompanied by debilitation, malnutrition, or inactivity.

The safety and efficacy of vancomycin administration by the intrathecal (intralumbar or intraventricular) routes have not been assessed.

Intermittent infusion is the recommended method of administration.

PREPARATION AND STABILITY

At the time of use, reconstitute by adding either 10 ml of sterile water for injection to the 500 mg vial or 20 ml of sterile water for injection to the 1 g vial of dry, sterile vancomycin powder. Vials reconstituted in this manner will give a solution of 50 mg/ml. FURTHER DILUTION IS REQUIRED.

After reconstitution with sterile water for injection, 5% dextrose injection, of 0.9% sodium chloride for injection, the vials may be stored in a refrigerator for 14 days without significant loss of potency. Reconstituted solutions containing 500 mg of vancomycin must be diluted with at least 100 ml of diluent. Reconstituted solutions containing 1 g of vancomycin must be diluted with at least 200 ml of diluent. The desired dose, diluted in this manner, should be administered by intermittent intravenous infusion over a period of at least 60 minutes.

Compatibility With Intravenous Fluids

Solutions that are diluted with 5% dextrose injection or 0.9% sodium chloride injection may be stored in a refrigerator for 14 days without significant loss of potency.

Solutions that are diluted with the following infusion fluids may be stored in a refrigerator for 96 hours:

- 5% dextrose injection and 0.9% sodium chloride injection
- Lactated Ringer's injection
- Lactated Ringer's and 5% dextrose injection
- Normosol-M and 5% dextrose
- Isolyte E
- Acetated Ringer's injection

Vancomycin solution has a low pH and may cause chemical or physical instability when it is mixed with other compounds.

Prior to administration, parenteral drug products should be inspected visually for particulate matter and discoloration whenever solution or container permits.

For Oral Administration

Oral Vancocin HCl is used in treating antibiotic-associated pseudomembranous colitis caused by *C. difficile* and for staphylococcal enterocolitis. Vancocin HCl is not effective by the oral route for other types of infections. The usual adult total daily dosage is 500 mg to 2 g given in 3 or 4 divided doses for 7-10 days. The total daily dosage in children is 40 mg/kg of body weight in 3 or 4 divided doses for 7-10 days. The total daily dosage should not exceed 2 g. The appropriate dose may be diluted in 1 oz of water and given to the patient to drink. Common flavoring syrups may be added to the solution to improve the taste for oral administration. The diluted solution may be administered via a nasogastric tube.

ANIMAL PHARMACOLOGY

In animal studies, hypotension and bradycardia occurred in dogs receiving an intravenous infusion of vancomycin hydrochloride, 25 mg/kg, at a concentration of 25 mg/ml and an infusion rate of 13.3 ml/min.

HOW SUPPLIED

VANCOCIN HCl VIALS

Vancocin HCl vials (or sterile vancomycin hydrochloride) are available in:

The 500 mg (equivalent to vancomycin), 10 ml vials.

The 1 g (equivalent to vancomycin), 20 ml vials.

Storage: Prior to reconstitution, the vials may be stored at room temperature, 15-30°C (59-86°F).

VANCOCIN HCl ADD-VANTAGE VIALS

Vancocin HCl ADD-Vantage vials (or sterile vancomycin hydrochloride) are available in:

The 500 mg (equivalent to vancomycin), 15 ml vials.

The 1 g (equivalent to vancomycin), 15 ml vials.

Storage: Prior to reconstitution, the vials may be stored at room temperature, 15-30°C (59-86°F).

VANCOCIN HCl PHARMACY BULK PACKAGE

Vancocin HCl pharmacy bulk package (or vancomycin hydrochloride for injection) are available in the 10 g (equivalent to vancomycin), 100 ml vials.

Storage: Prior to reconstitution, the vials may be stored at room temperature, 15-30°C (59-86°F).

PRODUCT LISTING - RATED THERAPEUTICALLY EQUIVALENT

Package	Price	Product, Manufacturer	NDC
Powder For Injection - Injectable - 1 Gm			
1's	$16.08	VANCOCIN HCL, Lilly, Eli and Company	00002-7298-01
10's	$60.63	GENERIC, Abbott Pharmaceutical	00074-6533-01
10's	$90.13	GENERIC, Abbott Pharmaceutical	00074-6535-01
10's	$109.39	VANCOLED, Lederle Laboratories	00205-3154-15
10's	$140.25	GENERIC, Vha Supply	00074-6535-49
10's	$162.50	GENERIC, American Pharmaceutical Partners	63323-0284-20
10's	$167.50	VANCOCIN HCL, Lilly, Eli and Company	00002-7298-10
10's	$177.25	GENERIC, Vha Supply	00074-6533-49
10's	$245.39	VANCOLED, Allscripts Pharmaceutical Company	54569-4669-00
Powder For Injection - Injectable - 5 Gm			
1's	$38.26	GENERIC, Abbott Pharmaceutical	00074-6509-01
1's	$54.33	GENERIC, Vha Supply	00074-6509-49
1's	$89.38	GENERIC, American Pharmaceutical Partners	63323-0295-61
Powder For Injection - Injectable - 10 Gm			
1's	$178.75	GENERIC, American Pharmaceutical Partners	63323-0314-61
Powder For Injection - Injectable - 500 mg			
1's	$8.28	VANCOCIN HCL, Lilly, Eli and Company	00002-7297-01
10's	$41.90	GENERIC, Abbott Pharmaceutical	00074-6534-01
10's	$73.38	GENERIC, Abbott Pharmaceutical	00074-6534-49
10's	$82.80	VANCOCIN HCL, Lilly, Eli and Company	00002-7297-10
10's	$86.57	GENERIC, Abbott Pharmaceutical	00074-4332-01
10's	$89.25	GENERIC, Vha Supply	00074-4332-49
25's	$218.75	GENERIC, American Pharmaceutical Partners	63323-0221-10
Powder For Reconstitution - Oral - 250 mg/5 ml			
10 ml x 6	$183.96	GENERIC, Esi Lederle Generics	59911-5875-02
Solution - Intravenous - 5%;1 Gm/200 ml			
200 ml x 6	$216.00	VANCOCIN HCL, Baxter Healthcare Corporation	00338-3552-48
Solution - Intravenous - 5%;500 mg/100 ml			
100 ml	$123.75	VANCOMYCIN HCL, Baxter Healthcare Corporation	00338-3551-48

PRODUCT LISTING - EQUIVALENTS NOT AVAILABLE

Package	Price	Product, Manufacturer	NDC
Capsule - Oral - 125 mg			
20's	$141.25	VANCOCIN HCL PULVULES, Lilly, Eli and Company	00002-3125-42
Capsule - Oral - 250 mg			
20's	$282.50	VANCOCIN HCL PULVULES, Lilly, Eli and Company	00002-3126-42
Powder For Reconstitution - Oral - 250 mg/5 ml			
10 ml	$37.08	VANCOCIN HCL, Lilly, Eli and Company	00002-5105-01
20 ml x 6	$231.36	VANCOCIN HCL, Lilly, Eli and Company	00002-5105-16
Powder For Reconstitution - Oral - 500 mg/6 ml			
120 ml	$326.95	VANCOCIN HCL, Lilly, Eli and Company	00002-2372-37

Varicella Vaccine *(003195)*

For complete prescribing information, refer to the CD-ROM included with the book.

Categories: Immunization, varicella; FDA Approved 1995 Mar; Pregnancy Category C
Drug Classes: Vaccines
Brand Names: Varivax
Foreign Brand Availability: Okavax (Hong-Kong); Suduvax (Korea); Varilrix (Australia; Bahamas; Barbados; Belize; Bermuda; Costa-Rica; Curacao; Dominican-Republic; El-Salvador; Guatemala; Guyana; Honduras; Hong-Kong; India; Indonesia; Israel; Jamaica; Korea; Netherland-Antilles; New-Zealand; Nicaragua; Panama; Peru; Philippines; Puerto-Rico; Surinam; Taiwan; Thailand; Trinidad); Varivax II (Australia); V-Z Vax (Philippines)

DESCRIPTION

Varivax (varicella vaccine) is a preparation of the Oka/Merck strain of live attenuated varicella virus. The virus was initially obtained from a child with natural varicella, then introduced into human embryonic lung cell cultures, adapted to and propagated in embryonic guinea pig cell cultures and finally propagated in human diploid cell cultures (WI-38). Further passage of the virus for varicella vaccine was performed at Merck Research Laboratories (MRL) in human diploid cell cultures (MRC-5) that were free of adventitious agents. This live, attenuated varicella vaccine is a lyophilized preparation containing sucrose, phosphate, glutamate, and processed gelatin as stabilizers.

Varicella vaccine, when reconstituted as directed, is a sterile preparation for subcutaneous administration. Each 0.5 ml dose contains the following: a minimum of 1350 PFU (plaque forming units) of Oka/Merck varicella virus when reconstituted and stored at room temperature for 30 minutes, approximately 25 mg of sucrose, 12.5 mg hydrolyzed gelatin, 3.2 mg sodium chloride, 0.5 mg monosodium L-glutamate, 0.45 mg of sodium phosphate dibasic, 0.08 mg of potassium phosphate monobasic, 0.08 mg of potassium chloride; residual components of MRC-5 cells including DNA and protein; and trace quantities of sodium phosphate monobasic, EDTA, neomycin, and fetal bovine serum. The product contains no preservative.

To maintain potency, the lyophilized vaccine must be kept frozen at an average temperature of -15°C (+5°F) or colder and must be used before the expiration date.

V

STABILITY AND STORAGE

Varivax retains a potency level of 1500 PFU or higher per dose for at least 18 months in a frost-free freezer with an average temperature of -15°C (+5°F) or colder.

Varivax has a minimum potency level approximately 1350 PFU 30 minutes after reconstitution at room temperature (20-25°C, 68-77°F).

For information regarding stability at temperatures other than those recommended for storage call 1-800-9-Varivax.

During shipment, to ensure that there is no loss of potency, the vaccine must be maintained at a temperature of -20°C (-4°F) or colder.

Before reconstitution, store the lyophilized vaccine in a freezer at an average temperature of -15°C (+5°F) or colder. Storage in a frost-free freezer with an average temperature of -15°C (+5°F) or colder is acceptable.

Before reconstitution, protect from light.

The diluent should be stores separately at room temperature, or in the refrigerator.

INDICATIONS AND USAGE

Varicella vaccine is indicated for vaccination against varicella in individuals 12 months of age and older.

REVACCINATION

The duration of protection of varicella vaccine is unknown at present and the need for booster doses is not defined. However, a boost in antibody levels has been observed in vaccinees following exposure to natural varicella as well as following a booster dose of varicella vaccine administered 4-6 years postvaccination.[5]

In a highly vaccinated population, immunity for some individuals may wane due to lack of exposure to natural varicella as a result of shifting epidemiology. Post-marketing surveillance studies are ongoing to evaluate the need and timing for booster vaccination.

Vaccination with varicella vaccine may not result in protection of all healthy, susceptible children, adolescents, and adults.

CONTRAINDICATIONS

A history of hypersensitivity to any component of the vaccine, including gelatin.

A history of anaphylactoid reaction to neomycin (each dose of reconstituted vaccine contains trace quantities of neomycin).

Individuals with blood dyscrasias, leukemia, lymphomas of any type, or other malignant neoplasms affecting the bone marrow or lymphatic systems.

Individuals receiving immunosuppressive therapy. Individuals who are on immunosuppressant drugs are more susceptible to infections than healthy individuals. Vaccination with live attenuated varicella vaccine can result in a more extensive vaccine-associated rash or disseminated disease in individuals on immunosuppressant doses of corticosteroids.

Individuals with primary and acquired immunodeficiency states, including those who are immunosuppressed in association with AIDS or other clinical manifestations of infection with human immunodeficiency virus;[23] cellular immune deficiencies; and hypogammaglobulinemic and dysgammaglobulinemic states.

A family history of congenital or hereditary immunodeficiency, unless the immune competence of the potential vaccine recipient is demonstrated.

Active untreated tuberculosis.

Any febrile respiratory illness or other active febrile infection.

Pregnancy; the possible effects of the vaccine on fetal development are unknown at this time. However, natural varicella is known to sometimes cause fetal harm. If vaccination of postpubertal females is undertaken, pregnancy should be avoided for 3 months following vaccination.

WARNINGS

Children and adolescents with acute lymphoblastic leukemia (ALL) in remission can receive the vaccine under an investigational protocol. More information is available by contacting the varicella vaccine coordinating center, Bio-Pharm Clinical Services, Inc., 4 Valley Square, Blue Bell, PA 19422 (215) 283-0897.

DOSAGE AND ADMINISTRATION

FOR SUBCUTANEOUS ADMINISTRATION. Do not inject intravenously.

Children 12 month to 12 years of age should receive a single 0.5 ml dose administered subcutaneously.

Adolescents and adults 13 years of age and older should receive a 0.5 ml dose administered subcutaneously at elected date and a second 0.5 ml dose 4-8 weeks later.

Varicella vaccine is for subcutaneous administration. The outer aspect of the upper arm (deltoid) is the preferred site of injection.

Varicella vaccine **MUST BE STORED FROZEN** at an average temperature of -15°C (+5°F) or colder is acceptable. The diluent should be stored separately at room temperature or in the refrigerator. To reconstitute the vaccine, first withdraw 0.7 ml of diluent into the syringe to be used for reconstitution. Inject all the diluent in the syringe into the vial of lyophilized vaccine and gently agitate to mix thoroughly. Withdraw the entire contents into a syringe, change the needle, and inject the total volume (about 0.5 ml) of reconstituted vaccine subcutaneously, preferably into the outer aspect of the upper arm (deltoid) or the anterolateral thigh. **IT IS RECOMMENDED THAT THE VACCINE BE ADMINISTERED IMMEDIATELY AFTER RECONSTITUTION, TO MINIMIZE LOSS OF POTENCY. DISCARD IF RECONSTITUTED VACCINE IS NOT USED WITHIN 30 MINUTES.**

CAUTION

A sterile syringe free of preservatives, antiseptics, and detergents should be used for each injection and/or reconstitution of varicella vaccine because these substances may inactivate the vaccine virus.

It is important to use a separate sterile syringe and needle for each patient to prevent transmission of infectious agents from one individual to another.

To reconstitute the vaccine, use only the diluent supplied, since it is free of preservatives or other anti-viral substances which might inactivate the vaccine virus.

Do not freeze reconstituted vaccine.

Do not give immune globulin including Varicella Zoster Immune Globulin concurrently with varicella vaccine.

Parenteral drug products should be inspected visually for particulate matter and discoloration prior to administration, whenever solution and container permit. Varicella vaccine when reconstituted is a clear, colorless to pale yellow liquid.

PRODUCT LISTING - EQUIVALENTS NOT AVAILABLE

Powder For Injection - Subcutaneous - Strength n/a

1's	$62.63	VARIVAX, Allscripts Pharmaceutical Company	54569-4055-00
1's	$76.18	VARIVAX, Merck & Company Inc	00006-4826-00
10's	$597.06	VARIVAX, Allscripts Pharmaceutical Company	54569-4056-00
10's	$726.33	VARIVAX, Merck & Company Inc	00006-4827-00

Varicella-Zoster Immune Globulin (Human) *(003337)*

For complete prescribing information, refer to the CD-ROM included with the book.

Categories: Immunization, varicella; Pregnancy Category C
Drug Classes: Immune globulins
Brand Names: VZIG
Foreign Brand Availability: Varitect (Hong-Kong; Taiwan; Thailand)

DESCRIPTION

Varicella-Zoster Immune Globulin (Human) (VZIG) is a sterile 10.0-18.0% solution of the globulin fraction of human plasma, primarily immunoglobulin G (IgG) in 0.3 M glycine.[1] VZIG contains no preservative. VZIG is derived from adult human plasma selected for high titers of varicella-zoster antibodies.[2] Plasma pools are fractionated by ethanol precipitation of the proteins according to Methods 6 and 9 of Cohn. A widely utilized solvent-detergent viral inactivation process is also used.[3] Each milliliter contains 100-180 mg of protein, principally IgG, and trace amounts of IgA and IgM. The product is to be administered by intramuscular injection. The recommended dose is based on body weight.

INDICATIONS AND USAGE

VZIG is intended for the passive immunization of exposed, susceptible individuals who are at greater risk of complications from varicella than healthy children. High-risk groups include immunocompromised children, newborns of mothers with varicella shortly before or after delivery, premature infants, immunocompromised adults and normal susceptible adults[8] and may also include susceptible high risk infants less than a year of age.

IMMUNOCOMPROMISED CHILDREN

VZIG is recommended for passive immunization of susceptible, immunocompromised children after significant exposure to chickenpox or zoster. These children include those with primary cellular immune deficiency disorders or neoplastlc diseases and those currently receiving immunosuppressive treatments. Although VZIG administration has been shown to reduce the severity of disease and decrease the rate of complications, severe varicella and death may still occur in exposed immunocompromised children despite VZIG administration. Antiviral chemotherapy should be considered if significant clinical varicella develops after VZIG administration.

NEWBORNS OF MOTHERS WITH VARICELLA SHORTLY BEFORE OR AFTER DELIVERY

VZIG is indicated for newborns of mothers who develop chickenpox within 5 days before or within 48 hours after delivery.[9-11] Despite VZIG administration some of these neonates may still develop varicella[10-15] which can be severe or fatal.[8] Antiviral chemotherapy should be considered in neonates who develop clinical varicella following VZIG administration.

PREMATURE INFANTS

Although the risk of post-natally acquired varicella in the premature infant is unknown, it has been judged prudent to administer VZIG to exposed premature infants of 28 weeks gestation or more if their mothers have a negative or uncertain history of varicella.[8] Premature infants of less than 28 weeks gestation or birth weight of less than 1000 g should be considered for VZIG regardless of maternal history since they may not yet have acquired transplacental maternal antibody.

FULL TERM INFANTS LESS THAN 1 YEAR OF AGE

Mortality from varicella in the first year of life is 4 times higher than that in older children, but lower than mortality in immunocompromised children or normal adults.[16,17] The decision to administer VZIG to infants less than 1 year of age should be evaluated on an individual basis. After careful evaluation of the type of exposure, susceptibility to varicella including maternal history of varicella and zoster, and presence of underlying disease, VZIG may be administered to selected infants.

IMMUNOCOMPROMISED ADULTS

The complication rate for immunocompromised adults who contract varicella is likely to be substantially greater than for normal adults. Approximately 90% of immunocompromised adults with negative or unknown histories of prior varicella are likely to be immune. After a careful evaluation, which might include the measurement of antibody to Varicella-Zoster virus by a reliable and sensitive assay such as Fluorescent Antibody to Membrane Antigen (FAMA), adults who are believed susceptible should receive VZIG.

HEALTHY ADULTS

Chickenpox can be severe in normal adults. The decision to administer VZIG to an adult should be evaluated on an individual basis. Approximately 90% of adults with negative or uncertain histories of varicella will be immune. The objective is to modify rather than prevent illness in hopes of inducing lifelong immunity. The clinician should consider the patient's health status, type of exposure, and likelihood of previous unrecognized varicella infection in deciding whether to administer VZIG. Adults who are older siblings of large families and adults whose children have had varicella are more likely to be immune. If reliable and sensitive tests for varicella antibody are available, they might be used to determine susceptibility, if time permits. If, after careful evaluation, a normal adult with significant exposure to varicella is believed susceptible, VZIG may be administered.

PREGNANT WOMEN

Pregnant women may be at higher risk of complications of chickenpox than healthy adults.[18] They should be evaluated the same way as other adults. There is no evidence that administration of VZIG to a susceptible, pregnant woman will prevent viremia, fetal infection or congenital varicella syndrome. Therefore the primary indication for VZIG in pregnant women is to prevent complications of varicella in a susceptible adult patient rather than to prevent intrauterine infection. Pregnant women should be evaluated for type of exposure and history of previous infection as described for healthy adults.

TIMING OF VZIG AFTER VARICELLA OR ZOSTER EXPOSURE

Greatest effectiveness of treatment is to be expected when it is begun within 96 hours after exposure; treatment after 96 hours is of uncertain value. There is no evidence that established infections with Varicella-Zoster virus can be modified by VZIG. There is no indication for the prophylactic use of VZIG in immunodeficient children or adults when there is a past history of varicella, unless the patient has undergone bone marrow transplantation.

MULTIPLE EXPOSURES

The duration of protection from a single dose of VZIG is not known. Therefore a second dose of VZIG should be considered when high risk patients have second exposures to Varicella-Zoster.

CONTRAINDICATIONS

A history of prior severe reaction associated with the administration of human immune globulin, or severe thrombocytopenia.

WARNINGS

The parenteral administration of any biologic should be surrounded by every precaution for the prevention and arrest of allergic and other untoward reactions.

Persons with immunoglobulin A deficiency have the potential for developing antibodies to immunoglobulin A and could have anaphylactic reactions to subsequent administration of blood products that contain immunoglobulin A. Therefore VZIG should be given to such persons only if the expected benefits outweigh the potential risks.

DOSAGE AND ADMINISTRATION

Administer the product by deep intramuscular injection in the gluteal muscle, or in a physician-directed site if there are contraindications to the gluteal site. NEVER ADMINISTER THIS MATERIAL INTRAVENOUSLY. The recommended dose of VZIG is based on body weight according to the schedule in TABLE 1.

TABLE 1 *Dosing Schedule for VZIG*

Weight of Patients		Dose Units	Dose Number of Vials
0-10 kg	0-22 lb	125	1 125 units
10.1-20 kg	22.1-44 lb	250	2 125 units
20.1-30 kg	44.1-66 lb	375	3 125 units
30.1-40 kg	66.1-88 lb	500	4 125 units
Over 40 kg	Over 88 lb	625	1 625 units or 5 125 units

Since VZIG does not contain a preservative administer the entire contents of each vial. Each 125 unit vial contains 125 units of antibody to varicella-zoster virus in a volume of approximately 1.25 ml and each 625 unit vial contains 625 units of antibody in a volume of approximately 6.25 ml. For patients weighing 10 kg or less, 125 units (1.25 ml) may be given in a single injection site. For patients weighing more than 10 kg, we recommend that no more than 2.5 ml be given in a single injection site, however some clinicians elect to give larger or smaller volumes.

The number of units required to prevent pneumonia and death and to reduce the number of pox is unknown. The proposed dosage regimen was found to be effective in significantly modifying the expected severity of chickenpox and reducing the observed frequency of death, pneumonia and encephalitis to less than 25% of the expected rate without treatment.

Parenteral drug products should be inspected visually for particulate matter and discoloration prior to administration whenever solution and container permit.

To prevent the transmission of hepatitis viruses or other infectious agents from one person to another, a separate sterile disposable syringe and needle should be used for each individual patient.

PRODUCT LISTING - EQUIVALENTS NOT AVAILABLE

Solution - Intramuscular - 125 U

1.25 ml	$118.80	VARICELLA ZOSTER IMMUNE GLOBULIN, American Red Cross Blood Services	52769-0574-11
1.25 ml	$125.00	VARICELLA ZOSTER IMMUNE GLOBULIN, American Red Cross Blood Services	52769-0118-02
2 ml	$93.75	VARICELLA ZOSTER IMMUNE GLOBULIN, American Red Cross Blood Services	14362-0118-02

Solution - Intramuscular - 625 U

2 ml	$448.20	VARICELLA ZOSTER IMMUNE GLOBULIN, American Red Cross Blood Services	14362-0118-10
6.25 ml	$118.80	VARICELLA ZOSTER IMMUNE GLOBULIN, American Red Cross Blood Services	52769-0574-66
6.25 ml	$562.50	VARICELLA ZOSTER IMMUNE GLOBULIN, American Red Cross Blood Services	52769-0118-10

Vasopressin *(002422)*

Categories: Diabetes insipidus; Distention, abdominal, postoperative; Imaging, abdominal, adjunct; Pregnancy Category C; FDA Pre 1938 Drugs
Drug Classes: Antidiuretics; Hormones/hormone modifiers
Brand Names: **Pitressin**
Foreign Brand Availability: Pressyn (Canada)

DESCRIPTION

Vasopressin injection synthetic is a sterile, aqueous solution of synthetic vasopressin (8-Arginine vasopressin) of the posterior pituitary gland.

It is substantially free from the oxytocic principle and is standardized to contain 20 pressor units/ml. The solution contains 0.5% Chloretone (chlorobutanol) (chloroform derivative) as a preservative. The acidity of the solution is adjusted with acetic acid.

Storage: Store between 15-25°C (59-77°F).

CLINICAL PHARMACOLOGY

The antidiuretic action of vasopressin is ascribed to increasing reabsorption of water by the renal tubules.

Vasopressin can cause contraction of smooth muscle of the gastrointestinal tract and of all parts of the vascular bed, especially the capillaries, small arterioles and venules with less effect on the smooth musculature of the large veins. The direct effect on the contractile elements is neither antagonized by adrenergic blocking agents nor prevented by vascular denervation.

Following subcutaneous or intramuscular administration of vasopressin injection, the duration of antidiuretic activity is variable but effects are usually maintained for 2-8 hours.

The majority of a dose of vasopressin is metabolized and rapidly destroyed in the liver and kidneys. Vasopressin has a plasma half-life of about 10-20 minutes. Approximately 5% of a subcutaneous dose of vasopressin is excreted in urine unchanged after four hours.

INDICATIONS AND USAGE

Vasopressin injection is indicated for prevention and treatment of postoperative abdominal distention, in abdominal roentgenography to dispel interfering gas shadows, and in diabetes insipidus.

NON-FDA APPROVED INDICATIONS

Unapproved uses include management of bleeding esophageal varices and von Willebrand's disease (the polypeptide appears to increase factor VIII activity).

CONTRAINDICATIONS

Anaphylaxis or hypersensitivity to the drug or its components.

WARNINGS

This drug should not be used in patients with vascular disease, especially disease of the coronary arteries, except with extreme caution. In such patients, even small doses may precipitate anginal pain, and with larger doses, the possibility of myocardial infarction should be considered.

Vasopressin may produce water intoxication. The early signs of drowsiness, listlessness, and headaches should be recognized to prevent terminal coma and convulsions.

PRECAUTIONS

GENERAL

Vasopressin should be used cautiously in the presence of epilepsy, migraine, asthma, heart failure or any state in which a rapid addition to extracellular water may produce hazard for an already overburdened system.

Chronic nephritis with nitrogen retention contraindicates the use of vasopressin until reasonable nitrogen blood levels have been attained.

INFORMATION FOR THE PATIENT

Side effects such as blanching of skin, abdominal cramps, and nausea may be reduced by taking 1 or 2 glasses of water at the time of vasopressin administration. These side effects are usually not serious and probably will disappear within a few minutes.

LABORATORY TESTS

Electrocardiograms (ECG) and fluid and electrolyte status determinations are recommended at periodic intervals during therapy.

PREGNANCY CATEGORY C

Animal reproduction studies have not been conducted with vasopressin injection. It is also not known whether Vasopressin injection can cause fetal harm when administered to a pregnant woman or can affect reproduction capacity. Vasopressin injection should be given to a pregnant woman only if clearly needed.

LABOR AND DELIVERY

Doses of vasopressin sufficient for an antidiuretic effect are not likely to produce tonic uterine contractions that could be deleterious to the fetus or threaten the continuation of the pregnancy.

NURSING MOTHERS

Caution should be exercised when vasopressin injection is administered to a nursing woman.

DRUG INTERACTIONS

1) The following drugs may potentiate the antidiuretic effect of vasopressin when used concurrently: carbamazepine; chlorpropamide; clofibrate; urea; fludrocortisone; tricyclic antidepressants. 2) The following drugs may decrease the antidiuretic effect of vasopressin when used concurrently: demeclocycline; norepinephrine; lithium; heparin; alcohol. 3) Ganglionic blocking agents may produce a marked increase in sensitivity to the pressor effects of vasopressin.

ADVERSE REACTIONS

Local or systemic allergic reactions may occur in hypersensitive individuals.

The following side effects have been reported following the administration of vasopressin:

Body as a Whole: Anaphylaxis (cardiac arrest and/or shock) has been observed shortly after injection of vasopressin.

Cardiovascular: Cardiac arrest, circumoral pallor, arrhythmias, decreased cardiac output, angina, myocardial ischemia, peripheral vasoconstriction and gangrene.

Gastrointestinal: Abdominal cramps, nausea, vomiting, passage of gas.

Nervous System: Tremor, vertigo, "pounding" in head.

Respiratory: Bronchial constriction.

Skin and Appendages: Sweating, urticaria, cutaneous gangrene.

DOSAGE AND ADMINISTRATION

Vasopressin injection may be administered subcutaneously or intramuscularly.

Ten units of vasopressin injection (0.5 ml) will usually elicit full physiologic response in adult patients; 5 units will be adequate in many cases. Vasopressin injection should be given intramuscularly at three- or four-hour intervals as needed. The dosage should be proportionately reduced for children. (For an additional discussion of dosage, consult the sections below.)

When determining the dose of vasopressin injection for a given case, the following should be kept in mind.

It is particularly desirable to give a dose not much larger than is just sufficient to elicit the desired physiologic response. Excessive doses may cause undesirable side effects—blanching of the skin, abdominal cramps, nausea—which, though not serious, may be alarming to the patient. Spontaneous recovery from such side effects occurs in a few minutes. It has been found that one or two glasses of water given at the time vasopressin injection is administered reduce such symptoms.

ABDOMINAL DISTENTION

In the average postoperative adult patient, give 5 units (0.25 ml) initially, increase to 10 units (0.5 ml) at subsequent injections if necessary. It is recommended that vasopressin injection be given intramuscularly and that injections be repeated at three-or four-hour intervals as required. Dosage to be reduced proportionately for children.

Vasopressin injection used in this manner will frequently prevent or relieve postoperative distension. These recommendations apply also to distention complicating pneumonia or other acute toxemias.

ABDOMINAL ROENTGENOGRAPHY

For the average case, two injections of 10 units each (0.5 ml) are suggested. These should be given two hours and one-half hour, respectively, before films are exposed. Many roentgenologists advise giving an enema prior to the first dose of vasopressin injection.

DIABETES INSIPIDUS

Vasopressin injection may be given by injection or administered intranasally on cotton pledgets, by nasal spray, or by dropper. The dose by injection is 5-10 units (0.25-0.5 ml) repeated two or three times daily as needed. When vasopressin injection is administered intranasally by spray or on pledgets, the dosage and interval between treatments must be determined for each patient.

PRODUCT LISTING - EQUIVALENTS NOT AVAILABLE

Solution - Injectable - 20 U/ml

0.50 ml x 25	$75.00	GENERIC, American Regent Laboratories Inc	00517-0510-25
1 ml x 10	$90.70	PITRESSIN, Monarch Pharmaceuticals Inc	61570-0420-01
1 ml x 25	$135.00	GENERIC, American Regent Laboratories Inc	00517-1020-25
1 ml x 25	$181.25	GENERIC, American Pharmaceutical Partners	63323-0302-01
1 ml x 25	$209.88	PITRESSIN, Monarch Pharmaceuticals Inc	61570-0420-03
10 ml x 10	$193.80	GENERIC, American Regent Laboratories Inc	00517-0410-10

Venlafaxine Hydrochloride *(003166)*

For related information, see the comparative table section in Appendix A.

Categories: Anxiety disorder, generalized; Depression; FDA Approved 1993 Dec; Pregnancy Category C

Drug Classes: Antidepressants, miscellaneous

Brand Names: **Effexor**

Foreign Brand Availability: Efexor (Australia; Austria; Bahrain; Canada; Colombia; Cyprus; Denmark; Egypt; England; Greece; Hong-Kong; Iran; Iraq; Israel; Jordan; Korea; Kuwait; Lebanon; Libya; Mexico; Netherlands; New-Zealand; Oman; Peru; Philippines; Qatar; Republic-of-Yemen; Saudi-Arabia; South-Africa; Sweden; Switzerland; Syria; Thailand; United-Arab-Emirates); Efexor XR (Australia; Canada; Colombia; Israel; New-Zealand; Philippines; Singapore; Thailand); Efexor-XR SR (Korea); Trevilor (Germany; Switzerland); Trewilor (Austria); Vaxor (Bahrain; Cyprus; Egypt; Iran; Iraq; Jordan; Kuwait; Lebanon; Libya; Oman; Qatar; Republic-of-Yemen; Saudi-Arabia; Syria; United-Arab-Emirates); Venix-XR (India)

Cost of Therapy: $94.98 (Depression; Effexor; 75 mg; 2 tablets/day; 30 day supply)
$81.15 (Depression; Effexor XR; 75 mg; 1 tablet/day; 30 day supply)

DESCRIPTION

Effexor XR is an extended-release capsule for oral administration that contains venlafaxine hydrochloride, a structurally novel antidepressant. Venlafaxine hydrochloride is chemically unrelated to tricyclic, tetracyclic, and other available antidepressants and to other agents used to treat Generalized Anxiety Disorder. It is designated (R/S)-1-[2-(dimethylamino)-1-(4-methoxyphenyl)ethyl] cyclohexanol hydrochloride or (±)-1-[α-[(dimethylamino)methyl]-p-methoxybenzyl] cyclohexanol hydrochloride and has the empirical formula of $C_{17}H_{27}NO_2$ hydrochloride. Its molecular weight is 313.87.

Venlafaxine hydrochloride is a white to off-white crystalline solid with a solubility of 572 mg/ml in water (adjusted to ionic strength of 0.2 M with sodium chloride). Its octanol:water (0.2 M sodium chloride) partition coefficient is 0.43.

Effexor XR is formulated as an extended-release capsule for once-a-day oral administration. Drug release is controlled by diffusion through the coating membrane on the spheroids and is not pH dependent. Capsules contain venlafaxine hydrochloride equivalent to 37.5, 75, or 150 mg venlafaxine. Inactive ingredients consist of cellulose, ethylcellulose, gelatin, hypromellose, iron oxide, and titanium dioxide. The 37.5 mg capsule also contains D&C red no. 28, D&C yellow no. 10, and FD&C blue no. 1.

CLINICAL PHARMACOLOGY

PHARMACODYNAMICS

The mechanism of the antidepressant action of venlafaxine in humans is believed to be associated with its potentiation of neurotransmitter activity in the CNS. Preclinical studies have shown that venlafaxine and its active metabolite, O-desmethylvenlafaxine (ODV), are potent inhibitors of neuronal serotonin and norepinephrine reuptake and weak inhibitors of dopamine reuptake. Venlafaxine and ODV have no significant affinity for muscarinic cholinergic, H_1-histaminergic, or α_1-adrenergic receptors *in vitro*. Pharmacologic activity at these receptors is hypothesized to be associated with the various anticholinergic, sedative, and cardiovascular effects seen with other psychotropic drugs. Venlafaxine and ODV do not possess monoamine oxidase (MAO) inhibitory activity.

PHARMACOKINETICS

Steady-state concentrations of venlafaxine and ODV in plasma are attained within 3 days of oral multiple dose therapy. Venlafaxine and ODV exhibited linear kinetics over the dose range of 75-450 mg/day. Mean ± SD steady-state plasma clearance of venlafaxine and ODV is 1.3 ± 0.6 and 0.4 ± 0.2 L/h/kg, respectively; apparent elimination half-life is 5 ± 2 and 11 ± 2 hours, respectively; and apparent (steady-state) volume of distribution is 7.5 ± 3.7 and 5.7 ± 1.8 L/kg, respectively. Venlafaxine and ODV are minimally bound at therapeutic concentrations to plasma proteins (27% and 30%, respectively).

Absorption

Venlafaxine is well absorbed and extensively metabolized in the liver. ODV is the only major active metabolite. On the basis of mass balance studies, at least 92% of a single oral dose of venlafaxine is absorbed. The absolute bioavailability of venlafaxine is about 45%.

Administration of venlafaxine HCl extended-release (150 mg q24h) generally resulted in lower C_{max} (150 ng/ml for venlafaxine and 260 ng/ml for ODV) and later T_{max} (5.5 hours for venlafaxine and 9 hours for ODV) than for immediate-release venlafaxine tablets (C_{max}'s for immediate-release 75 mg q12h were 225 ng/ml for venlafaxine and 290 ng/ml for ODV; T_{max}'s were 2 hours for venlafaxine and 3 hours for ODV). When equal daily doses of venlafaxine were administered as either an immediate-release tablet or the extended-release capsule, the exposure to both venlafaxine and ODV was similar for the two treatments, and the fluctuation in plasma concentrations was slightly lower with the venlafaxine HCl extended-release capsule. Venlafaxine HCl extended-release, therefore, provides a slower rate of absorption, but the same extent of absorption compared with the immediate-release tablet.

Food did not affect the bioavailability of venlafaxine or its active metabolite, ODV. Time of administration (AM vs PM) did not affect the pharmacokinetics of venlafaxine and ODV from the 75 mg venlafaxine HCl extended-release capsule.

Metabolism and Excretion

Following absorption, venlafaxine undergoes extensive presystemic metabolism in the liver, primarily to ODV, but also to N-desmethylvenlafaxine, N,O-didesmethylvenlafaxine, and other minor metabolites. *In vitro* studies indicate that the formation of ODV is catalyzed by CYP2D6; this has been confirmed in a clinical study showing that patients with low CYP2D6 levels ("poor metabolizers") had increased levels of venlafaxine and reduced levels of ODV compared to people with normal CYP2D6 ("extensive metabolizers"). The differences between the CYP2D6 poor and extensive metabolizers, however, are not expected to be clinically important because the sum of venlafaxine and ODV is similar in the 2 groups and venlafaxine and ODV are pharmacologically approximately equiactive and equipotent.

Approximately 87% of a venlafaxine dose is recovered in the urine within 48 hours as unchanged venlafaxine (5%), unconjugated ODV (29%), conjugated ODV (26%), or other

PREGNANCY CATEGORY C

Teratogenic Effects

Venlafaxine did not cause malformations in offspring of rats or rabbits given doses up to 2.5 times (rat) or 4 times (rabbit) the maximum recommended human daily dose on a mg/m^2 basis. However, in rats, there was a decrease in pup weight, an increase in stillborn pups, and an increase in pup deaths during the first 5 days of lactation, when dosing began during pregnancy and continued until weaning. The cause of these deaths is not known. These effects occurred at 2.5 times (mg/m^2) the maximum human daily dose. The no effect dose for rat pup mortality was 0.25 times the human dose on a mg/m^2 basis. There are no adequate and well-controlled studies in pregnant women. Because animal reproduction studies are not always predictive of human response, this drug should be used during pregnancy only if clearly needed.

Nonteratogenic Effects

If venlafaxine is used until or shortly before birth, discontinuation effects in the newborn should be considered.

LABOR AND DELIVERY

The effect of venlafaxine on labor and delivery in humans is unknown.

NURSING MOTHERS

Venlafaxine and ODV have been reported to be excreted in human milk. Because of the potential for serious adverse reactions in nursing infants from venlafaxine HCl extended-release, a decision should be made whether to discontinue nursing or to discontinue the drug, taking into account the importance of the drug to the mother.

PEDIATRIC USE

Safety and effectiveness in pediatric patients have not been established.

GERIATRIC USE

Approximately 4% (14/357) and 6% (77/1381) of venlafaxine HCl extended-release-treated patients in placebo-controlled premarketing depression and GAD trials, respectively, were 65 years of age or over. Of 2897 venlafaxine HCl immediate-release-treated patients in premarketing phase depression studies, 12% (357) were 65 years of age or over. No overall differences in effectiveness or safety were observed between geriatric patients and younger patients, and other reported clinical experience generally has not identified differences in response between the elderly and younger patients. However, greater sensitivity of some older individuals cannot be ruled out. As with other antidepressants, several cases of hyponatremia and syndrome of inappropriate antidiuretic hormone secretion (SIADH) have been reported, usually in the elderly.

The pharmacokinetics of venlafaxine and ODV are not substantially altered in the elderly (see CLINICAL PHARMACOLOGY). No dose adjustment is recommended for the elderly on the basis of age alone, although other clinical circumstances, some of which may be more common in the elderly, such as renal or hepatic impairment, may warrant a dose reduction (see DOSAGE AND ADMINISTRATION).

DRUG INTERACTIONS

As with all drugs, the potential for interaction by a variety of mechanisms is a possibility.

ALCOHOL

A single dose of ethanol (0.5 g/kg) had no effect on the pharmacokinetics of venlafaxine or ODV when venlafaxine was administered at 150 mg/day in 15 healthy male subjects. Additionally, administration of venlafaxine in a stable regimen did not exaggerate the psychomotor and psychometric effects induced by ethanol in these same subjects when they were not receiving venlafaxine.

CIMETIDINE

Concomitant administration of cimetidine and venlafaxine in a steady-state study for both drugs resulted in inhibition of first-pass metabolism of venlafaxine in 18 healthy subjects. The oral clearance of venlafaxine was reduced by about 43%, and the exposure (AUC) and maximum concentration (C_{max}) of the drug were increased by about 60%. However, coadministration of cimetidine had no apparent effect on the pharmacokinetics of ODV, which is present in much greater quantity in the circulation than venlafaxine. The overall pharmacological activity of venlafaxine plus ODV is expected to increase only slightly, and no dosage adjustment should be necessary for most normal adults. However, for patients with pre-existing hypertension, and for elderly patients or patients with hepatic dysfunction, the interaction associated with the concomitant use of venlafaxine and cimetidine is not known and potentially could be more pronounced. Therefore, caution is advised with such patients.

DIAZEPAM

Under steady-state conditions for venlafaxine administered at 150 mg/day, a single 10 mg dose of diazepam did not appear to affect the pharmacokinetics of either venlafaxine or ODV in 18 healthy male subjects. Venlafaxine also did not have any effect on the pharmacokinetics of diazepam or its active metabolite, desmethyldiazepam, or affect the psychomotor and psychometric effects induced by diazepam.

HALOPERIDOL

Venlafaxine administered under steady-state conditions at 150 mg/day in 24 healthy subjects decreased total oral-dose clearance (Cl/F) of a single 2 mg dose of haloperidol by 42%, which resulted in a 70% increase in haloperidol AUC. In addition, the haloperidol C_{max} increased 88% when coadministered with venlafaxine, but the haloperidol elimination half-life ($T_{1/2}$) was unchanged. The mechanism explaining this finding is unknown.

LITHIUM

The steady-state pharmacokinetics of venlafaxine administered at 150 mg/day were not affected when a single 600 mg oral dose of lithium was administered to 12 healthy male subjects. ODV also was unaffected. Venlafaxine had no effect on the pharmacokinetics of lithium.

DRUGS HIGHLY BOUND TO PLASMA PROTEINS

Venlafaxine is not highly bound to plasma proteins; therefore, administration of venlafaxine HCl extended-release to a patient taking another drug that is highly protein bound should not cause increased free concentrations of the other drug.

DRUGS THAT INHIBIT CYTOCHROME P450 ISOENZYMES

CYP2D6 Inhibitors

In vitro and *in vivo* studies indicate that venlafaxine is metabolized to its active metabolite, ODV, by CYP2D6, the isoenzyme that is responsible for the genetic polymorphism seen in the metabolism of many antidepressants. Therefore, the potential exists for a drug interaction between drugs that inhibit CYP2D6-mediated metabolism of venlafaxine, reducing the metabolism of venlafaxine to ODV, resulting in increased plasma concentrations of venlafaxine and decreased concentrations of the active metabolite. CYP2D6 inhibitors such as quinidine would be expected to do this, but the effect would be similar to what is seen in patients who are genetically CYP2D6 poor metabolizers (see CLINICAL PHARMACOLOGY, Metabolism and Excretion). Therefore, no dosage adjustment is required when venlafaxine is coadministered with a CYP2D6 inhibitor.

The concomitant use of venlafaxine with a drug treatment(s) that potentially inhibits both CYP2D6 and CYP3A4, the primary metabolizing enzymes for venlafaxine, has not been studied.

Therefore, caution is advised should a patient's therapy include venlafaxine and any agent(s) that produce simultaneous inhibition of these two enzyme systems.

DRUGS METABOLIZED BY CYTOCHROME P450 ISOENZYMES

CYP2D6

In vitro studies indicate that venlafaxine is a relatively weak inhibitor of CYP2D6. These findings have been confirmed in a clinical drug interaction study comparing the effect of venlafaxine with that of fluoxetine on the CYP2D6-mediated metabolism of dextromethorphan to dextrorphan.

Imipramine

Venlafaxine did not affect the pharmacokinetics of imipramine and 2-OH-imipramine. However, desipramine AUC, C_{max}, and C_{min} increased by about 35% in the presence of venlafaxine. The 2-OH-desipramine AUCs increased by at least 2.5-fold (with venlafaxine 37.5 mg q12h) and by 4.5-fold (with venlafaxine 75 mg q12h). Imipramine did not affect the pharmacokinetics of venlafaxine and ODV. The clinical significance of elevated 2-OH-desipramine levels is unknown.

Risperidone

Venlafaxine administered under steady-state conditions at 150 mg/day slightly inhibited the CYP2D6-mediated metabolism of risperidone (administered as a single 1 mg oral dose) to its active metabolite, 9-hydroxyrisperidone, resulting in an approximate 32% increase in risperidone AUC. However, venlafaxine coadministration did not significantly alter the pharmacokinetic profile of the total active moiety (risperidone plus 9-hydroxyrisperidone).

CYP3A4

Venlafaxine did not inhibit CYP3A4 *in vitro*. This finding was confirmed *in vivo* by clinical drug interaction studies in which venlafaxine did not inhibit the metabolism of several CYP3A4 substrates, including alprazolam, diazepam, and terfenadine.

Indinavir

In a study of 9 healthy volunteers, venlafaxine administered under steady-state conditions at 150 mg/day resulted in a 28% decrease in the AUC of a single 800 mg oral dose of indinavir and a 36% decrease in indinavir C_{max}. Indinavir did not affect the pharmacokinetics of venlafaxine and ODV. The clinical significance of this finding is unknown.

CYP1A2

Venlafaxine did not inhibit CYP1A2 *in vitro*. This finding was confirmed *in vivo* by a clinical drug interaction study in which venlafaxine did not inhibit the metabolism of caffeine, a CYP1A2 substrate.

CYP2C9

Venlafaxine did not inhibit CYP2C9 *in vitro*. The clinical significance of this finding is unknown.

CYP2C19

Venlafaxine did not inhibit the metabolism of diazepam, which is partially metabolized by CYP2C19 (see Diazepam).

MONOAMINE OXIDASE INHIBITORS

See CONTRAINDICATIONS and WARNINGS.

CNS-ACTIVE DRUGS

The risk of using venlafaxine in combination with other CNS-active drugs has not been systematically evaluated (except in the case of those CNS-active drugs noted above). Consequently, caution is advised if the concomitant administration of venlafaxine and such drugs is required.

ELECTROCONVULSIVE THERAPY

There are no clinical data establishing the benefit of electroconvulsive therapy combined with venlafaxine HCl extended-release capsules treatment.

POSTMARKETING SPONTANEOUS DRUG INTERACTION REPORTS

See ADVERSE REACTIONS, Postmarketing Reports.

ADVERSE REACTIONS

The information included in Adverse Findings Observed in Short-Term, Placebo-Controlled Studies with Venlafaxine HCl Extended-Release is based on data from a pool of three 8 and

12 week controlled clinical trials in depression (includes two U.S. trials and one European trial) and on data up to 8 weeks from a pool of five controlled clinical trials in GAD with venlafaxine HCl extended-release. Information on additional adverse events associated with venlafaxine HCl extended-release in the entire development program for the formulation and with venlafaxine HCl (the immediate release formulation of venlafaxine) is included in the Other Adverse Events Observed During the Premarketing Evaluation of Venlafaxine HCl Immediate-Release and Extended-Release (see also WARNINGS and PRECAUTIONS).

ADVERSE FINDINGS OBSERVED IN SHORT-TERM, PLACEBO-CONTROLLED STUDIES WITH VENLAFAXINE HCl EXTENDED-RELEASE

Adverse Events Associated With Discontinuation of Treatment

Approximately 11% of the 357 patients who received venlafaxine HCl extended-release capsules in placebo-controlled clinical trials for depression discontinued treatment due to an adverse experience, compared to 6% of the 285 placebo-treated patients in those studies. Approximately 18% of the 1381 patients who received venlafaxine HCl extended-release capsules in placebo-controlled clinical trials for GAD discontinued treatment due to an adverse experience, compared with 12% of the 555 placebo-treated patients in those studies. The most common events leading to discontinuation and considered to be drug-related (*i.e.*, leading to discontinuation in at least 1% of the venlafaxine HCl extended-release-treated patients at a rate at least twice that of placebo for either indication) are shown in TABLE 2.

Adverse Events Occurring at an Incidence of 2% or More Among Venlafaxine HCl

TABLE 2 *Common Adverse Events Leading to Discontinuation of Treatment in Placebo-Controlled Trials**

	% of Patients Discontinuing Due to Adverse Event			
	Depression Indication†		GAD Indication‡§	
Adverse Event	Venlafaxine HCl Extended-Release (n=357)	Placebo (n=285)	Venlafaxine HCl Extended-Release (n=1381)	Placebo (n=555)
Body as a Whole				
Asthenia	-	-	3%	<1%
Digestive System				
Nausea	4%	<1%	8%	<1%
Anorexia	1%	<1%	-	-
Dry mouth	1%	0%	2%	<1%
Vomiting	-	-	1%	<1%
Nervous System				
Dizziness	2%	1%	-	-
Insomnia	1%	<1%	3%	<1%
Somnolence	2%	<1%	3%	<1%
Nervousness	—	—	2%	<1%
Tremor	—	—	1%	0%
Skin				
Sweating	-	-	2%	<1%

* Two of the depression studies were flexible dose and one was fixed dose. Four of the GAD studies were fixed dose and one was flexible dose.

† In US placebo-controlled trials for depression, the following were also common events leading to discontinuation and were considered to be drug-related for venlafaxine HCl extended-release-treated patients (% venlafaxine HCl extended-release [n=192], % Placebo [n=202]): hypertension (1%, <1%); diarrhea (1%, 0%); paresthesia (1%, 0%); tremor (1%, 0%); abnormal vision, mostly blurred vision (1%, 0%); and abnormal, mostly delayed, ejaculation (1%, 0%).

‡ In two short-term U.S. placebo-controlled trials for GAD, the following were also common events leading to discontinuation and were considered to be drug-related for venlafaxine HCl extended-release-treated patients (% venlafaxine HCl extended-release [n= 476]), % Placebo [n=201]: headache (4%, <1%); vasodilatation (1%, 0%); anorexia (2%, <1%); dizziness (4%, 1%); thinking abnormal (1%, 0%); and abnormal vision (1%, 0%).

§ In long-term placebo-controlled trials for GAD, the following was also a common event leading to discontinuation and was considered to be drug-related for venlafaxine HCl extended-release-treated patients (% venlafaxine HCl extended-release [n=535], % Placebo [n=257]): decreased libido (1%, 0%).

Extended-Release-Treated Patients

TABLE 3 and TABLE 4 enumerate the incidence, rounded to the nearest percent, of treatment-emergent adverse events that occurred during acute therapy of depression (up to 12 weeks; dose range of 75-225 mg/day) and of GAD (up to 8 weeks; dose range of 37.5-225 mg/day), respectively, in 2% or more of patients treated with venlafaxine HCl extended-release where the incidence in patients treated with venlafaxine HCl extended-release was greater than the incidence for the respective placebo-treated patients. TABLE 3 and TABLE 4 show the percentage of patients in each group who had at least 1 episode of an event at some time during their treatment. Reported adverse events were classified using a standard COSTART-based Dictionary terminology.

The prescriber should be aware that these figures cannot be used to predict the incidence of side effects in the course of usual medical practice where patient characteristics and other factors differ from those which prevailed in the clinical trials. Similarly, the cited frequencies cannot be compared with figures obtained from other clinical investigations involving different treatments, uses and investigators. The cited figures, however, do provide the prescribing physician with some basis for estimating the relative contribution of drug and non-drug factors to side effect incidence in the population studied.

Commonly Observed Adverse Events From TABLE 3 and TABLE 4

Depression

Note in particular the following adverse events that occurred in at least 5% of venlafaxine HCl extended-release patients and at a rate at least twice that of the placebo group for all placebo-controlled trials for the depression indication (see TABLE 3): abnormal ejaculation, gastrointestinal complaints (nausea, dry mouth, and anorexia), CNS complaints (dizziness, somnolence, and abnormal dreams), and sweating. In the two US placebo-controlled trials, the following additional events occurred in at least 5% of venlafaxine HCl extended-release-treated patients (n=192) and at a rate at least twice that of the placebo group: abnormalities of sexual function (impotence in men, anorgasmia in women, and libido decreased), gastrointestinal complaints (constipation and flatulence), CNS complaints (insomnia, nervousness, and tremor), problems of special senses (abnormal vision), cardiovascular effects (hypertension and vasodilatation), and yawning.

TABLE 3 *Treatment-Emergent Adverse Event Incidence in Short-Term Placebo-Controlled Venlafaxine HCl Extended-Release Clinical Trials in Depressed Patients*†*

Body System / Preferred Term	Venlafaxine HCl Extended-Release (n=357)	Placebo (n=285)
Body as a Whole		
Asthenia	8%	7%
Cardiovascular System		
Vasodilatation‡	4%	2%
Hypertension	4%	1%
Digestive System		
Nausea	31%	12%
Constipation	8%	5%
Anorexia	8%	4%
Vomiting	4%	2%
Flatulence	4%	3%
Metabolic/Nutritional		
Weight loss	3%	0%
Nervous System		
Dizziness	20%	9%
Somnolence	17%	8%
Insomnia	17%	11%
Dry mouth	12%	6%
Nervousness	10%	5%
Abnormal dreams§	7%	2%
Tremor	5%	2%
Depression	3%	<1%
Paresthesia	3%	1%
Libido decreased	3%	<1%
Agitation	3%	1%
Respiratory System		
Pharyngitis	7%	6%
Yawn	3%	0%
Skin		
Sweating	14%	3%
Special Senses		
Abnormal vision¤	4%	<1%
Urogenital System		
Abnormal ejaculation (male)¶**	16%	<1%
Impotence**	4%	<1%
Anorgasmia (female)††‡‡	3%	<1%

* Incidence, rounded to the nearest %, for events reported by at least 2% of patients treated with venlafaxine HCl extended-release, except the following events which had an incidence equal to or less than placebo: abdominal pain, accidental injury, anxiety, back pain, bronchitis, diarrhea, dysmenorrhea, dyspepsia, flu syndrome, headache, infection, pain, palpitation, rhinitis, and sinusitis.

† <1% indicates an incidence greater than zero but less than 1%.

‡ Mostly "hot flashes."

§ Mostly "vivid dreams," "nightmares," and "increased dreaming."

¤ Mostly "blurred vision" and "difficulty focusing eyes."

¶ Mostly "delayed ejaculation."

** Incidence is based on the number of male patients.

†† Mostly "delayed orgasm" or "anorgasmia."

‡‡ Incidence is based on the number of female patients.

Generalized Anxiety Disorder

Note in particular the following adverse events that occurred in at least 5% of the venlafaxine HCl extended-release patients and at a rate at least twice that of the placebo group for all placebo-controlled trials for the GAD indication (see TABLE 4): abnormalities of sexual function (abnormal ejaculation and impotence), gastrointestinal complaints (nausea, dry mouth, anorexia, and constipation), problems of special senses (abnormal vision), and sweating.

Vital Sign Changes

Venlafaxine HCl extended-release capsules treatment for up to 12 weeks in premarketing placebo-controlled depression trials was associated with a mean final on-therapy increase in pulse rate of approximately 2 beats/min, compared with 1 beat/min for placebo. Venlafaxine HCl extended-release treatment for up to 8 weeks in premarketing placebo-controlled GAD trials was associated with a mean final on-therapy increase in pulse rate of approximately 2 beats/min, compared with less than 1 beat/min for placebo. (See WARNINGS, Sustained Hypertension for effects on blood pressure.)

In a flexible-dose study, with venlafaxine HCl immediate-release doses in the range of 200-375 mg/day and mean dose greater than 300 mg/day, the mean pulse was increased by about 2 beats/min compared with a decrease of about 1 beat/min for placebo.

Laboratory Changes

Venlafaxine HCl extended-release capsules treatment for up to 12 weeks in premarketing placebo-controlled trials for major depressive disorder was associated with a mean final on-therapy increase in serum cholesterol concentration of approximately 1.5 mg/dl compared with a mean final decrease of 7.4 mg/dl for placebo. Venlafaxine HCl extended-release treatment for up to 8 weeks and up to 6 months in premarketing placebo-controlled GAD trials was associated with mean final on-therapy increases in serum cholesterol con-

TABLE 4 *Treatment-Emergent Adverse Event Incidence in Short-Term Placebo-Controlled Venlafaxine HCl Extended-Release Clinical Trials in GAD Patients*†*

Body System Preferred Term	Venlafexine HCl Extended-Release (n=1381)	Placebo (n=555)
Body as a Whole		
Asthenia	12%	8%
Cardiovascular System		
Vasodilatation‡	4%	2%
Digestive System		
Nausea	35%	12%
Constipation	10%	4%
Anorexia	8%	2%
Vomiting	5%	3%
Nervous System		
Dizziness	16%	11%
Dry mouth	16%	6%
Insomnia	15%	10%
Somnolence	14%	8%
Nervousness	6%	4%
Libido decreased	4%	2%
Tremor	4%	<1%
Abnormal Dreams§	3%	2%
Hypertonia	3%	2%
Paresthesia	2%	1%
Respiratory System		
Yawn	3%	<1%
Skin		
Sweating	10%	3%
Special Senses		
Abnormal vision¤	5%	<1%
Urogenital System		
Abnormal ejaculation (male)¶**	11%	<1%
Impotence**	5%	<1%
Orgasmic dysfunction (female)††‡‡	2%	0%

* Adverse events for which the venlafaxine HCl extended-release reporting rate was less than or equal to the placebo rate are not included. These events are: abdominal pain, accidental injury, anxiety, back pain, diarrhea, dysmenorrhea, dyspepsia, flu syndrome, headache, infection, myalgia, pain, palpitation, pharyngitis, rhinitis, tinnitus, and urinary frequency.
† <1% means greater than zero but less than 1%.
‡ Mostly "hot flashes."
§ Mostly "vivid dreams," "nightmares," and "increased dreaming."
¤ Mostly "blurred vision" and "difficulty focusing eyes."
¶ Includes "delayed ejaculation" and "anorgasmia."
** Percentage based on the number of males (venlafaxine HCl extended-release=525, placebo=220).
†† Includes "delayed orgasm," "abnormal orgasm," and "anorgasmia."
‡‡ Percentage based on the number of females (venlafaxine HCl extended-release=856, placebo=335).

centration of approximately 1.0 mg/dl and 2.3 mg/dl, respectively while placebo subjects experienced mean final decreases of 4.9 mg/dl and 7.7 mg/dl, respectively.

Patients treated with venlafaxine HCl tablets (the immediate-release form of venlafaxine) for at least 3 months in placebo-controlled 12 month extension trials had a mean final on-therapy increase in total cholesterol of 9.1 mg/dl compared with a decrease of 7.1 mg/dl among placebo-treated patients. This increase was duration dependent over the study period and tended to be greater with higher doses. Clinically relevant increases in serum cholesterol, defined as (1) a final on-therapy increase in serum cholesterol ≥50 mg/dl from baseline and to a value ≥261 mg/dl, or (2) an average on-therapy increase in serum cholesterol ≥50 mg/dl from baseline and to a value ≥261 mg/dl, were recorded in 5.3% of venlafaxine-treated patients and 0.0% of placebo-treated patients (see PRECAUTIONS, General, Serum Cholesterol Elevation).

ECG Changes

In a flexible-dose study, with venlafaxine HCl immediate-release doses in the range of 200-375 mg/day and mean dose greater than 300 mg/day, the mean change in heart rate was 8.5 beats/min compared with 1.7 beats/min for placebo.

See PRECAUTIONS, Use in Patients With Concomitant Illnesses.

OTHER ADVERSE EVENTS OBSERVED DURING THE PREMARKETING EVALUATION OF VENLAFAXINE HCl IMMEDIATE-RELEASE AND EXTENDED-RELEASE

During its premarketing assessment, multiple doses of venlafaxine HCl extended-release were administered to 705 patients in Phase 3 depression studies and venlafaxine HCl immediate-release was administered to 96 patients. During its premarketing assessment, multiple doses of venlafaxine HCl extended-release were administered to 1381 patients in Phase 3 GAD studies. In addition, in premarketing assessment of venlafaxine HCl immediate-release, multiple doses were administered to 2897 patients in Phase 2 and 3 depression studies. The conditions and duration of exposure to venlafaxine in both development programs varied greatly, and included (in overlapping categories) open and double-blind studies, uncontrolled and controlled studies, inpatient (venlafaxine HCl immediate-release only) and outpatient studies, fixed-dose, and titration studies. Untoward events associated with this exposure were recorded by clinical investigators using terminology of their own choosing. Consequently, it is not possible to provide a meaningful estimate of the proportion of individuals experiencing adverse events without first grouping similar types of untoward events into a smaller number of standardized event categories.

In the tabulations that follow, reported adverse events were classified using a standard COSTART-based Dictionary terminology. The frequencies presented, therefore, represent the proportion of the 5079 patients exposed to multiple doses of either formulation of venlafaxine who experienced an event of the type cited on at least 1 occasion while receiving venlafaxine. All reported events are included except those already listed in TABLE 3 and TABLE 4 and those events for which a drug cause was remote. If the COSTART term for an event was so general as to be uninformative, it was replaced with a more informative term. It is important to emphasize that, although the events reported occurred during treatment with venlafaxine, they were not necessarily caused by it.

Events are further categorized by body system and listed in order of decreasing frequency using the following definitions: *Frequent:* Adverse events are defined as those occurring on one or more occasions in at least 1/100 patients; *Infrequent:* Adverse events are those occurring in 1/100 to 1/1000 patients; *Rare:* Events are those occurring in fewer than 1/1000 patients.

Body as a Whole: *Frequent:* Chest pain substernal, chills, fever, neck pain; *Infrequent:* Face edema, intentional injury, malaise, moniliasis, neck rigidity, pelvic pain, photosensitivity reaction, suicide attempt, withdrawal syndrome; *Rare:* Appendicitis, bacteremia, carcinoma, cellulitis.

Cardiovascular System: *Frequent:* Migraine, postural hypotension, tachycardia; *Infrequent:* Angina pectoris, arrhythmia, extrasystoles, hypotension, peripheral vascular disorder (mainly cold feet and/or cold hands), syncope, thrombophlebitis; *Rare:* Aortic aneurysm, arteritis, first-degree atrioventricular block, bigeminy, bradycardia, bundle branch block, capillary fragility, cerebral ischemia, coronary artery disease, congestive heart failure, heart arrest, cardiovascular disorder (mitral valve and circulatory disturbance), mucocutaneous hemorrhage, myocardial infarct, pallor.

Digestive System: *Frequent:* Eructation, increased appetite;*Infrequent:* Bruxism, colitis, dysphagia, tongue edema, esophagitis, gastritis, gastroenteritis, gastrointestinal ulcer, gingivitis, glossitis, rectal hemorrhage, hemorrhoids, melena, oral moniliasis, stomatitis, mouth ulceration; *Rare:* Cheilitis, cholecystitis, cholelithiasis, esophageal spasms, duodenitis, hematemesis, gastrointestinal hemorrhage, gum hemorrhage, hepatitis, ileitis, jaundice, intestinal obstruction, parotitis, proctitis, increased salivation, soft stools, tongue discoloration.

Endocrine System: *Rare:* Goiter, hyperthyroidism, hypothyroidism, thyroid nodule, thyroiditis.

Hemic and Lymphatic System: *Frequent:* Ecchymosis; *Infrequent:* Anemia, leukocytosis, leukopenia, lymphadenopathy, thrombocythemia, thrombocytopenia; *Rare:* Basophilia, bleeding time increased, cyanosis, eosinophilia, lymphocytosis, multiple myeloma, purpura.

Metabolic and Nutritional: *Frequent:* Edema, weight gain; *Infrequent:* Alkaline phosphatase increased, dehydration, hypercholesteremia, hyperglycemia, hyperlipemia, hypokalemia, SGOT increased, SGPT increased, thirst; *Rare:* Alcohol intolerance, bilirubinemia, BUN increased, creatinine increased, diabetes mellitus, glycosuria, gout, healing abnormal, hemochromatosis, hypercalcinuria, hyperkalemia, hyperphosphatemia, hyperuricemia, hypocholesteremia, hypoglycemia, hyponatremia, hypophosphatemia, hypoproteinemia, uremia.

Musculoskeletal System: *Frequent:* Arthralgia; *Infrequent:* Arthritis, arthrosis, bone pain, bone spurs, bursitis, leg cramps, myasthenia, tenosynovitis; *Rare:* Pathological fracture, myopathy, osteoporosis, osteosclerosis, rheumatoid arthritis, tendon rupture.

Nervous System: *Frequent:* Amnesia, confusion, depersonalization, emotional lability, hypesthesia, thinking abnormal, trismus, vertigo; *Infrequent:* Apathy, ataxia, circumoral paresthesia, CNS stimulation, euphoria, hallucinations, hostility, hyperesthesia, hyperkinesia, hypotonia, incoordination, manic reaction, myoclonus, neuralgia, neuropathy, psychosis, seizure, abnormal speech, stupor, twitching; *Rare:* Akathisia, akinesia, alcohol abuse, aphasia, bradykinesia, buccoglossal syndrome, cerebrovascular accident, loss of consciousness, delusions, dementia, dystonia, facial paralysis, abnormal gait, Guillain-Barre Syndrome, hyperchlorhydria, hypokinesia, impulse control difficulties, libido increased, neuritis, nystagmus, paranoid reaction, paresis, psychotic depression, reflexes decreased, reflexes increased, suicidal ideation, torticollis.

Respiratory System: *Frequent:* Cough increased, dyspnea; *Infrequent:* Asthma, chest congestion, epistaxis, hyperventilation, laryngismus, laryngitis, pneumonia, voice alteration; *Rare:* Atelectasis, hemoptysis, hypoventilation, hypoxia, larynx edema, pleurisy, pulmonary embolus, sleep apnea.

Skin and Appendages: *Frequent:* Rash, pruritus; *Infrequent:* Acne, alopecia, brittle nails, contact dermatitis, dry skin, eczema, skin hypertrophy, maculopapular rash, psoriasis, urticaria; *Rare:* Erythema nodosum, exfoliative dermatitis, lichenoid dermatitis, hair discoloration, skin discoloration, furunculosis, hirsutism, leukoderma, petechial rash, pustular rash, vesiculobullous rash, seborrhea, skin atrophy, skin striae.

Special Senses: *Frequent:* Abnormality of accommodation, mydriasis, taste perversion; *Infrequent:* Cataract, conjunctivitis, corneal lesion, diplopia, dry eyes, eye pain, hyperacusis, otitis media, parosmia, photophobia, taste loss, visual field defect; *Rare:* Blepharitis, chromatopsia, conjunctival edema, deafness, exophthalmos, glaucoma, retinal hemorrhage, subconjunctival hemorrhage, keratitis, labyrinthitis, miosis, papilledema, decreased pupillary reflex, otitis externa, scleritis, uveitis.

Urogenital System: *Frequent:* Dysuria, metrorrhagia,* prostatic disorder (prostatitis and enlarged prostate),* urination impaired, vaginitis;* *Infrequent:* Albuminuria, amenorrhea,* cystitis, hematuria, leukorrhea,* menorrhagia,* nocturia, bladder pain, breast pain, polyuria, pyuria, urinary incontinence, urinary retention, urinary urgency, vaginal hemorrhage;* *Rare:* Abortion,* anuria, breast discharge, breast engorgement, balanitis,* breast enlargement, endometriosis,* female lactation,* fibrocystic breast, calcium crystalluria, cervicitis,* orchitis,* ovarian cyst,* prolonged erection,* gynecomastia (male),* hypomenorrhea,* kidney calculus, kidney pain, kidney function abnormal, mastitis, menopause,* pyelonephritis, oliguria, salpingitis,* urolithiasis, uterine hemorrhage,* uterine spasm.*

* Based on the number of men and women as appropriate.

POSTMARKETING REPORTS

Voluntary reports of other adverse events temporally associated with the use of venlafaxine that have been received since market introduction and that may have no causal relationship with the use of venlafaxine include the following: agranulocytosis, anaphylaxis, aplastic

V

anemia, catatonia, congenital anomalies, CPK increased, deep vein thrombophlebitis, delirium, EKG abnormalities such as QT prolongation; cardiac arrhythmias including atrial fibrillation, supraventricular tachycardia, ventricular extrasystoles, and rare reports of ventricular fibrillation and ventricular tachycardia, including torsade de pointes; epidermal necrosis/Stevens-Johnson Syndrome, erythema multiforme, extrapyramidal symptoms (including tardive dyskinesia), hemorrhage (including eye and gastrointestinal bleeding), hepatic events (including GGT elevation; abnormalities of unspecified liver function tests; liver damage, necrosis, or failure; and fatty liver), involuntary movements, LDH increased, neuroleptic malignant syndrome-like events (including a case of a 10-year-old who may have been taking methylphenidate, was treated and recovered), neutropenia, night sweats, pancreatitis, pancytopenia, panic, prolactin increased, pulmonary eosinophilia, renal failure, serotonin syndrome, shock-like electrical sensations (in some cases, subsequent to the discontinuation of venlafaxine or tapering of dose), and syndrome of inappropriate antidiuretic hormone secretion (usually in the elderly).

There have been reports of elevated clozapine levels that were temporally associated with adverse events, including seizures, following the addition of venlafaxine. There have been reports of increases in prothrombin time, partial thromboplastin time, or INR when venlafaxine was given to patients receiving warfarin therapy.

DOSAGE AND ADMINISTRATION

Venlafaxine HCl extended-release should be administered in a single dose with food either in the morning or in the evening at approximately the same time each day. Each capsule should be swallowed whole with fluid and not divided, crushed, chewed, or placed in water, or it may be administered by carefully opening the capsule and sprinkling the entire contents on a spoonful of applesauce. This drug/food mixture should be swallowed immediately without chewing and followed with a glass of water to ensure complete swallowing of the pellets.

INITIAL TREATMENT

Depression

For most patients, the recommended starting dose for venlafaxine HCl extended-release is 75 mg/day, administered in a single dose. In the clinical trials establishing the efficacy of venlafaxine HCl extended-release in moderately depressed outpatients, the initial dose of venlafaxine was 75 mg/day. For some patients, it may be desirable to start at 37.5 mg/day for 4-7 days, to allow new patients to adjust to the medication before increasing to 75 mg/day. While the relationship between dose and antidepressant response for venlafaxine HCl extended-release has not been adequately explored, patients not responding to the initial 75 mg/day dose may benefit from dose increases to a maximum of approximately 225 mg/day. Dose increases should be in increments of up to 75 mg/day, as needed, and should be made at intervals of not less than 4 days, since steady-state plasma levels of venlafaxine and its major metabolites are achieved in most patients by Day 4. In the clinical trials establishing efficacy, upward titration was permitted at intervals of 2 weeks or more; the average doses were about 140-180 mg/day.

It should be noted that, while the maximum recommended dose for moderately depressed outpatients is also 225 mg/day for venlafaxine HCl (the immediate-release form of venlafaxine), more severely depressed inpatients in one study of the development program for that product responded to a mean dose of 350 mg/day (range of 150-375 mg/day). Whether or not higher doses of venlafaxine HCl extended-release are needed for more severely depressed patients is unknown; however, the experience with venlafaxine HCl extended-release doses higher than 225 mg/day is very limited (see PRECAUTIONS, General, Use in Patients With Concomitant Illness).

Generalized Anxiety Disorder (GAD)

For most patients, the recommended starting dose for venlafaxine HCl extended-release is 75 mg/day, administered in a single dose. In clinical trials establishing the efficacy of venlafaxine HCl extended-release in outpatients with GAD, the initial dose of venlafaxine was 75 mg/day. For some patients, it may be desirable to start at 37.5 mg/day for 4-7 days, to allow new patients to adjust to the medication before increasing to 75 mg/day. Although a dose-response relationship for effectiveness in GAD was not clearly established in fixed-dose studies, certain patients not responding to the initial 75 mg/day dose may benefit from dose increases to a maximum of approximately 225 mg/day. Dose increases should be in increments of up to 75 mg/day, as needed, and should be made at intervals of not less than 4 days (see PRECAUTIONS, General, Use in Patients With Concomitant Illness).

SWITCHING PATIENTS FROM VENLAFAXINE HCl IMMEDIATE-RELEASE TABLETS

Depressed patients who are currently being treated at a therapeutic dose with venlafaxine HCl immediate-release may be switched to venlafaxine HCl extended-release at the nearest equivalent dose (mg/day), *e.g.,* 37.5 mg venlafaxine two-times-a-day to 75 mg venlafaxine HCl extended-release once daily. However, individual dosage adjustments may be necessary.

PATIENTS WITH HEPATIC IMPAIRMENT

Given the decrease in clearance and increase in elimination half-life for both venlafaxine and ODV that is observed in patients with hepatic cirrhosis compared with normal subjects (see CLINICAL PHARMACOLOGY), it is recommended that the starting dose be reduced by 50% in patients with moderate hepatic impairment. Because there was much individual variability in clearance between patients with cirrhosis, individualization of dosage may be desirable in some patients.

PATIENTS WITH RENAL IMPAIRMENT

Given the decrease in clearance for venlafaxine and the increase in elimination half-life for both venlafaxine and ODV that is observed in patients with renal impairment (GFR = 10-70 ml/min) compared with normal subjects (see CLINICAL PHARMACOLOGY), it is recommended that the total daily dose be reduced by 25-50%. In patients undergoing hemodialysis, it is recommended that the total daily dose be reduced by 50% and that the dose be withheld until the dialysis treatment is completed (4 h). Because there was much individual variability in clearance between patients with renal impairment, individualization of dosage may be desirable in some patients.

ELDERLY PATIENTS

No dose adjustment is recommended for elderly patients solely on the basis of age. As with any drug for the treatment of depression or generalized anxiety disorder, however, caution should be exercised in treating the elderly. When individualizing the dosage, extra care should be taken when increasing the dose.

MAINTENANCE TREATMENT

There is no body of evidence available from controlled trials to indicate how long patients with depression or GAD should be treated with venlafaxine HCl extended-release.

It is generally agreed that acute episodes of depression require several months or longer of sustained pharmacological therapy beyond response to the acute episode. In one study, in which patients responding during 8 weeks of acute treatment with venlafaxine HCl extended-release were assigned randomly to placebo or to the same dose of venlafaxine HCl extended-release (75, 150, or 225 mg/day, qAM) during 26 weeks of maintenance treatment as they had received during the acute stabilization phase, longer-term efficacy was demonstrated. A second longer-term study has demonstrated the efficacy of venlafaxine HCl immediate-release in maintaining an antidepressant response in patients with recurrent depression who had responded and continued to be improved during an initial 26 weeks of treatment and were then randomly assigned to placebo or venlafaxine HCl immediate-release for periods of up to 52 weeks on the same dose (100-200 mg/day, on a bid schedule) (see CLINICAL STUDIES). Based on these limited data, it is not known whether or not the dose of venlafaxine HCl immediate or extended-release needed for maintenance treatment is identical to the dose needed to achieve an initial response. Patients should be periodically reassessed to determine the need for maintenance treatment and the appropriate dose for such treatment.

In patients with GAD, venlafaxine HCl extended-release has been shown to be effective in 6 month clinical trials. The need for continuing medication in patients with GAD who improve with venlafaxine HCl extended-release treatment should be periodically reassessed.

DISCONTINUING VENLAFAXINE HCl EXTENDED-RELEASE

When discontinuing venlafaxine HCl extended-release after more than 1 week of therapy, it is generally recommended that the dose be tapered to minimize the risk of discontinuation symptoms. Patients who have received venlafaxine HCl extended-release for 6 weeks or more should have their dose tapered over at least a 2 week period. In clinical trials with venlafaxine HCl extended-release, tapering was achieved by reducing the daily dose by 75 mg at 1 week intervals. Individualization of tapering may be necessary.

Discontinuation symptoms have been systematically evaluated in patients taking venlafaxine, to include prospective analyses of clinical trials in GAD and retrospective surveys of trials in depression. Abrupt discontinuation or dose reduction of venlafaxine at various doses has been found to be associated with the appearance of new symptoms, the frequency of which increased with increased dose level and with longer duration of treatment. Reported symptoms include agitation, anorexia, anxiety, confusion, coordination impaired, diarrhea, dizziness, dry mouth, dysphoric mood, fasciculation, fatigue, headaches, hypomania, insomnia, nausea, nervousness, nightmares, sensory disturbances (including shock-like electrical sensations), somnolence, sweating, tremor, vertigo, and vomiting. It is therefore recommended that the dosage of venlafaxine HCl extended-release be tapered gradually and the patient monitored. The period required for tapering may depend on the dose, duration of therapy and the individual patient. Discontinuation effects are well known to occur with antidepressants.

SWITCHING PATIENTS TO OR FROM A MONOAMINE OXIDASE INHIBITOR

At least 14 days should elapse between discontinuation of an MAOI and initiation of therapy with venlafaxine HCl extended-release. In addition, at least 7 days should be allowed after stopping venlafaxine HCl extended-release before starting an MAOI (see CONTRAINDICATIONS and WARNINGS).

HOW SUPPLIED

Effexor XR capsules are available as follows:

37.5 mg: Gray cap/peach body with "W" and "Effexor XR" on the cap and "37.5" on the body.

75 mg: Peach cap and body with "W" and "Effexor XR" on the cap and "75" on the body.

150 mg: Dark orange cap and body with "W" and "Effexor XR" on the cap and "150" on the body.

Storage: Store at controlled room temperature, 20-25°C (68-77°F). Protect from light.

PRODUCT LISTING - EQUIVALENTS NOT AVAILABLE

Capsule, Extended Release - Oral - 37.5 mg

7's	$15.81	EFFEXOR XR, Allscripts Pharmaceutical Company	54569-5265-00
100's	$254.54	EFFEXOR XR, Wyeth-Ayerst Laboratories	00008-0837-01
100's	$254.54	EFFEXOR XR, Wyeth-Ayerst Laboratories	00008-0837-03

Capsule, Extended Release - Oral - 75 mg

30's	$79.83	EFFEXOR XR, Pharma Pac	52959-0550-30
30's	$81.15	EFFEXOR XR, Southwood Pharmaceuticals Inc	58016-0615-30
60's	$162.30	EFFEXOR XR, Southwood Pharmaceuticals Inc	58016-0615-60
100's	$270.50	EFFEXOR XR, Southwood Pharmaceuticals Inc	58016-0615-00
100's	$285.14	EFFEXOR XR, Wyeth-Ayerst Laboratories	00008-0833-01
100's	$285.14	EFFEXOR XR, Wyeth-Ayerst Laboratories	00008-0833-03

Capsule, Extended Release - Oral - 150 mg

10's	$33.08	EFFEXOR XR, Physicians Total Care	54868-4252-01
30's	$78.44	EFFEXOR XR, Allscripts Pharmaceutical Company	54569-5231-00
30's	$80.25	EFFEXOR XR, Pharma Pac	52959-0388-30

30's	$82.68	EFFEXOR XR, Southwood Pharmaceuticals Inc	58016-0616-30
30's	$96.83	EFFEXOR XR, Physicians Total Care	54868-4252-00
60's	$165.36	EFFEXOR XR, Southwood Pharmaceuticals Inc	58016-0616-60
100's	$275.60	EFFEXOR XR, Southwood Pharmaceuticals Inc	58016-0616-00
100's	$310.60	EFFEXOR XR, Wyeth-Ayerst Laboratories	00008-0836-01
100's	$310.60	EFFEXOR XR, Wyeth-Ayerst Laboratories	00008-0836-03
Tablet - Oral - 25 mg			
10's	$14.53	EFFEXOR, Southwood Pharmaceuticals Inc	58016-0350-10
14's	$20.34	EFFEXOR, Southwood Pharmaceuticals Inc	58016-0350-14
15's	$21.80	EFFEXOR, Southwood Pharmaceuticals Inc	58016-0350-15
20's	$29.06	EFFEXOR, Southwood Pharmaceuticals Inc	58016-0350-20
21's	$30.51	EFFEXOR, Southwood Pharmaceuticals Inc	58016-0350-21
28's	$40.68	EFFEXOR, Southwood Pharmaceuticals Inc	58016-0350-28
30's	$43.59	EFFEXOR, Southwood Pharmaceuticals Inc	58016-0350-30
40's	$58.12	EFFEXOR, Southwood Pharmaceuticals Inc	58016-0350-40
50's	$72.65	EFFEXOR, Southwood Pharmaceuticals Inc	58016-0350-50
60's	$87.18	EFFEXOR, Southwood Pharmaceuticals Inc	58016-0350-60
90's	$130.77	EFFEXOR, Southwood Pharmaceuticals Inc	58016-0350-90
100's	$145.30	EFFEXOR, Southwood Pharmaceuticals Inc	58016-0350-00
100's	$150.26	EFFEXOR, Wyeth-Ayerst Laboratories	00008-0701-01
100's	$150.26	EFFEXOR, Wyeth-Ayerst Laboratories	00008-0701-02
Tablet - Oral - 37.5 mg			
4's	$12.13	EFFEXOR, Prescript Pharmaceuticals	00247-0853-04
6's	$16.52	EFFEXOR, Prescript Pharmaceuticals	00247-0853-06
8's	$20.91	EFFEXOR, Prescript Pharmaceuticals	00247-0853-08
10's	$14.95	EFFEXOR, Southwood Pharmaceuticals Inc	58016-0349-10
14's	$20.93	EFFEXOR, Southwood Pharmaceuticals Inc	58016-0349-14
15's	$22.43	EFFEXOR, Southwood Pharmaceuticals Inc	58016-0349-15
20's	$29.91	EFFEXOR, Southwood Pharmaceuticals Inc	58016-0349-20
20's	$34.05	EFFEXOR, Physicians Total Care	54868-3414-02
21's	$31.40	EFFEXOR, Southwood Pharmaceuticals Inc	58016-0349-21
30's	$37.63	EFFEXOR, Allscripts Pharmaceutical Company	54569-4131-01
30's	$44.73	EFFEXOR, Physicians Total Care	54868-3414-00
30's	$44.86	EFFEXOR, Southwood Pharmaceuticals Inc	58016-0349-30
30's	$69.19	EFFEXOR, Prescript Pharmaceuticals	00247-0853-30
40's	$59.81	EFFEXOR, Southwood Pharmaceuticals Inc	58016-0349-40
50's	$74.77	EFFEXOR, Southwood Pharmaceuticals Inc	58016-0349-50
60's	$89.72	EFFEXOR, Southwood Pharmaceuticals Inc	58016-0349-60
60's	$135.04	EFFEXOR, Prescript Pharmaceuticals	00247-0853-60
90's	$134.58	EFFEXOR, Southwood Pharmaceuticals Inc	58016-0349-90
90's	$200.87	EFFEXOR, Prescript Pharmaceuticals	00247-0853-90
100's	$138.23	EFFEXOR, Physicians Total Care	54868-3414-01
100's	$149.53	EFFEXOR, Southwood Pharmaceuticals Inc	58016-0349-00
100's	$154.75	EFFEXOR, Wyeth-Ayerst Laboratories	00008-0781-01
100's	$154.75	EFFEXOR, Wyeth-Ayerst Laboratories	00008-0781-02
Tablet - Oral - 50 mg			
10's	$15.41	EFFEXOR, Southwood Pharmaceuticals Inc	58016-0351-10
14's	$21.57	EFFEXOR, Southwood Pharmaceuticals Inc	58016-0351-14
15's	$23.12	EFFEXOR, Southwood Pharmaceuticals Inc	58016-0351-15
20's	$30.82	EFFEXOR, Southwood Pharmaceuticals Inc	58016-0351-20
21's	$32.36	EFFEXOR, Southwood Pharmaceuticals Inc	58016-0351-21
28's	$43.15	EFFEXOR, Southwood Pharmaceuticals Inc	58016-0351-28
30's	$46.23	EFFEXOR, Southwood Pharmaceuticals Inc	58016-0351-30
40's	$61.64	EFFEXOR, Southwood Pharmaceuticals Inc	58016-0351-40
50's	$77.05	EFFEXOR, Southwood Pharmaceuticals Inc	58016-0351-50
60's	$92.46	EFFEXOR, Southwood Pharmaceuticals Inc	58016-0351-60
90's	$138.69	EFFEXOR, Southwood Pharmaceuticals Inc	58016-0351-90
100's	$154.10	EFFEXOR, Southwood Pharmaceuticals Inc	58016-0351-00
100's	$159.36	EFFEXOR, Wyeth-Ayerst Laboratories	00008-0703-01
100's	$159.36	EFFEXOR, Wyeth-Ayerst Laboratories	00008-0703-02
Tablet - Oral - 75 mg			
10's	$16.34	EFFEXOR, Southwood Pharmaceuticals Inc	58016-0323-10
14's	$22.88	EFFEXOR, Southwood Pharmaceuticals Inc	58016-0323-14
15's	$24.51	EFFEXOR, Southwood Pharmaceuticals Inc	58016-0323-15
20's	$32.68	EFFEXOR, Southwood Pharmaceuticals Inc	58016-0323-20
21's	$34.31	EFFEXOR, Southwood Pharmaceuticals Inc	58016-0323-21
28's	$45.75	EFFEXOR, Southwood Pharmaceuticals Inc	58016-0323-28
30's	$41.09	EFFEXOR, Allscripts Pharmaceutical Company	54569-4132-01
30's	$49.02	EFFEXOR, Southwood Pharmaceuticals Inc	58016-0323-30
30's	$51.30	EFFEXOR, Physicians Total Care	54868-3523-01
40's	$65.36	EFFEXOR, Southwood Pharmaceuticals Inc	58016-0323-40
50's	$81.70	EFFEXOR, Southwood Pharmaceuticals Inc	58016-0323-50
60's	$74.04	EFFEXOR, Prescript Pharmaceuticals	00247-1035-60
60's	$98.04	EFFEXOR, Southwood Pharmaceuticals Inc	58016-0323-60
60's	$101.39	EFFEXOR, Physicians Total Care	54868-3523-00
90's	$109.36	EFFEXOR, Prescript Pharmaceuticals	00247-1035-90
90's	$147.06	EFFEXOR, Southwood Pharmaceuticals Inc	58016-0323-90
100's	$158.30	EFFEXOR, Physicians Total Care	54868-3523-02
100's	$163.40	EFFEXOR, Southwood Pharmaceuticals Inc	58016-0323-00
100's	$168.99	EFFEXOR, Wyeth-Ayerst Laboratories	00008-0704-01
100's	$168.99	EFFEXOR, Wyeth-Ayerst Laboratories	00008-0704-02
Tablet - Oral - 100 mg			
10's	$17.32	EFFEXOR, Southwood Pharmaceuticals Inc	58016-0352-10
14's	$24.25	EFFEXOR, Southwood Pharmaceuticals Inc	58016-0352-14
15's	$25.98	EFFEXOR, Southwood Pharmaceuticals Inc	58016-0352-15
20's	$34.64	EFFEXOR, Southwood Pharmaceuticals Inc	58016-0352-20
21's	$36.37	EFFEXOR, Southwood Pharmaceuticals Inc	58016-0352-21
28's	$48.50	EFFEXOR, Southwood Pharmaceuticals Inc	58016-0352-28
30's	$51.96	EFFEXOR, Southwood Pharmaceuticals Inc	58016-0352-30
40's	$69.28	EFFEXOR, Southwood Pharmaceuticals Inc	58016-0352-40
50's	$86.60	EFFEXOR, Southwood Pharmaceuticals Inc	58016-0352-50
60's	$103.92	EFFEXOR, Southwood Pharmaceuticals Inc	58016-0352-60
90's	$155.88	EFFEXOR, Southwood Pharmaceuticals Inc	58016-0352-90
100's	$173.20	EFFEXOR, Southwood Pharmaceuticals Inc	58016-0352-00
100's	$179.09	EFFEXOR, Wyeth-Ayerst Laboratories	00008-0705-01
100's	$179.09	EFFEXOR, Wyeth-Ayerst Laboratories	00008-0705-02

Verapamil Hydrochloride *(002425)*

For related information, see the comparative table section in Appendix A.

Categories: Angina pectoris; Angina, chronic stable; Angina, variant; Arrhythmia, atrial fibrillation; Arrhythmia, atrial flutter; Arrhythmia, paroxysmal supraventricular tachycardia; Arrhythmia, ventricular; Hypertension, essential; Pregnancy Category C; FDA Approved 1981 Aug; WHO Formulary

Drug Classes: Antiarrhythmics, class IV; Calcium channel blockers

Brand Names: **Calan**; Calan SR; Covera-Hs; Isoptin; Isoptin SR; Verelan

Foreign Brand Availability: Akilen (Hong-Kong); Anpec (Australia; Taiwan); Apoacor (Israel); Apo-Verap (Canada); Azupamil (Germany); Berkatens (England; Ireland); Calaptin (India); Calaptin 240 SR (India); Cardiover (Indonesia); Caveril (Bahamas; Bahrain; Barbados; Belize; Bermuda; Curacao; Cyprus; Egypt; Ethiopia; Ghana; Guyana; Iran; Iraq; Israel; Jamaica; Jordan; Kenya; Kuwait; Lebanon; Libya; Mauritius; Netherland-Antilles; Oman; Qatar; Republic-of-Yemen; Saudi-Arabia; Surinam; Syria; Tanzania; Trinidad; United-Arab-Emirates); Civicor (Thailand); Coraver (Sweden); Cordilox (England); Cordilox SR (Australia); Corpamil (Indonesia); Dilacoran (Mexico); Dilacoran HTA (Mexico); Flamon (Bahamas; Barbados; Belize; Bermuda; Curacao; Guyana; Jamaica; Malaysia; Netherland-Antilles; Surinam; Switzerland; Trinidad); Geangin (Denmark; England; Netherlands; Norway); Hexasoptin (Denmark; Finland); Hexasoptin Retard (Denmark); Ikacor (Israel); Ikapress (Israel); Iso-Card SR (South-Africa); Isoptin Retard (Austria; Costa-Rica; Denmark; Dominican-Republic; Ecuador; El-Salvador; Finland; Germany; Greece; Guatemala; Honduras; Italy; Nicaragua; Panama; Peru; Portugal; Sweden; Switzerland); Isoptine (Belgium; France); Isoptino (Argentina); Manidon (Spain); Manidon Retard (Spain); Novopressan (China); Novo-Veramil (Canada); Quasar (Italy); Ravamil SR (South-Africa); Securon (England); Vasolan (Japan); Vasomil (South-Africa); Vasopten (India; Thailand); Veracaps SR (Australia); Veracor (Israel); Verahexal (Australia; Germany); Veraloc (Denmark; Sweden; Switzerland); Veramex (Germany); Veramil (India); Verapin (Thailand); Verapress 240 SR (Israel); Veratad (Colombia); Verdilac (Mexico); Verpamil (Bahrain; Cyprus; Egypt; Iran; Iraq; Israel; Jordan; Kuwait; Lebanon; Libya; Oman; Qatar; Republic-of-Yemen; Saudi-Arabia; Syria; United-Arab-Emirates); Vetrimil (Taiwan); Zolvera (England)

Cost of Therapy: $68.72 (Angina; Calan; 80 mg; 3 tablets/day; 30 day supply)
$8.42 (Angina; Generic Tablets; 80 mg; 3 tablets/day; 30 day supply)
$42.63 (Hypertension; Calan SR; 180 mg; 1 tablet/day; 30 day supply)
$57.38 (Hypertension; Verelen PM; 200 mg; 1 tablet/day; 30 day supply)
$12.44 (Hypertension; Covera HS; 180 mg; 1 tablet/day; 30 day supply)
$14.36 (Hypertension; Generic Extended Release Tablets; 180 mg; 1 tablet/day; 30 day supply)

DESCRIPTION

Verapamil HCl is a calcium ion influx inhibitor (slow channel blocker or calcium ion antagonist). Verapamil is administered as a racemic mixture of the R and S enantiomers. Verapamil HCl is an almost white, crystalline powder, practically free of odor, with a bitter taste. It is soluble in water, chloroform, and methanol. Verapamil HCl is not chemically related to other cardioactive drugs.

$C_{27}H_{38}N_2O_4 \cdot HCl$.

The molecular weight of verapamil HCl is 491.08.

Chemical Name: Benzeneacetonitrile, α-[3-[[2-(3,4-dimethoxyphenyl)ethyl]methylamino] propyl]-3,4-dimethoxy-α-(1- methylethyl)monohydrochloride.

VERAPAMIL HCl IS AVAILABLE IN THE FOLLOWING FORMS

Tablets

Calan is available for oral administration in film-coated tablets containing 40, 80, or 120 mg of verapamil HCl. *Inactive Ingredients:* Microcrystalline cellulose, corn starch, gelatin, hydroxypropyl cellulose, hydroxypropyl methylcellulose, iron oxide colorant, lactose, magnesium stearate, polyethylene glycol, talc, and titanium dioxide.

Capsules

Verapamil HCl is available for oral administration as a 240 mg hard gelatin capsule (dark blue cap/yellow body), a 180 mg hard gelatin capsule (light gray cap/yellow body), and a 120 mg hard gelatin capsule (yellow cap/yellow body). These pellet filled capsules provide a sustained-release of the drug in the gastrointestinal tract.

Sustained-Release/Extended-Release Tablets

The tablets are designed for sustained release of the drug in the gastrointestinal tract; sustained-release characteristics are not altered when the tablet is divided in half.

Sustained-Release Caplets

Calan SR is available for oral administration as light green, capsule-shaped, scored, film-coated tablets (caplets) containing 240 mg of verapamil HCl; as light pink, oval, scored, film-coated tablets (caplets) containing 180 mg of verapamil HCl; and as light violet, oval, film-coated tablets (caplets) containing 120 mg of verapamil HCl. The caplets are designed for sustained release of the drug in the gastrointestinal tract; sustained release characteristics are not altered when the caplet is divided in half. *Inactive Ingredients:* Alginate, carnauba wax, hydroxypropyl methylcellulose, magnesium stearate, microcrystalline cellulose, polyethylene glycol, polyvinyl pyrcolidone, talc, titanium dioxide, and coloring agents; *240 mg:* D&C yellow no. 10 lake and FD&C blue no. 2 lake; *120 and 180 mg:* Iron oxide.

Extended-Release Capsules, Controlled-Onset

Verelan PM is available for oral administration as a 100 mg hard gelatin capsule (white opaque cap/amethyst body), a 200 mg hard gelatin capsule (amethyst opaque cap/amethyst body), and as a 300 mg hard gelatin capsule (lavender opaque cap/amethyst body). *Inactive Ingredients:* D&C red no. 28, FD&C blue no. 1, FD&C red no. 40, fumaric acid, gelatin, povidone, shellac, silicon dioxide, sodium lauryl sulfate, starch, sugar spheres, talc, and titanium dioxide.

CLINICAL PHARMACOLOGY

Verapamil HCl is a calcium ion influx inhibitor (slow-channel blocker or calcium ion antagonist) that exerts its pharmacologic effects by modulating the influx of ionic calcium across the cell membrane of the arterial smooth muscle as well as in conductile and contractile myocardial cells without altering serum calcium concentrations.

ADDITIONAL INFORMATION FOR VERAPAMIL EXTENDED-RELEASE, CONTROLLED-ONSET CAPSULES ONLY

System Components and Performance

Verapamil HCl, extended-release, controlled-onset capsules uses the proprietary CODAS (Chronotherapeutic Oral Drug Absorption System) technology, which is designed for bedtime dosing, incorporating a 4-5 hour delay in drug delivery. The controlled-onset delivery system results in a maximum plasma concentration (C_{max}) of verapamil in the morning hours. These pellet filled capsules provide for extended-release of the drug in the gastrointestinal tract. The verapamil HCl, extended-release, controlled-onset capsules formulation has been designed to initiate the release of verapamil 4-5 hours after ingestion. This delay is introduced by the level of non-enteric release-controlling polymer applied to drug loaded beads. The release-controlling polymer is a combination of water soluble and water insoluble polymers. As water from the gastrointestinal tract comes into contact with the polymer coated beads, the water soluble polymer slowly dissolves and the drug diffuses through the resulting pores in the coating. The water insoluble polymer continues to act as a barrier, maintaining the controlled release of the drug. The rate of release is essentially independent of pH, posture, and food. Multiparticulate systems such as verapamil HCl, extended-release, controlled-onset capsules have been shown to be independent of gastrointestinal motility.

MECHANISM OF ACTION

Angina

The precise mechanism of action of verapamil HCl as an antianginal agent remains to be fully determined, but includes the following two mechanisms:

1. ***Relaxation and Prevention of Coronary Artery Spasm:*** Verapamil HCl dilates the main coronary arteries and coronary arterioles, both in normal and ischemic regions, and is a potent inhibitor of coronary artery spasm, whether spontaneous or ergonovine-induced. This property increases myocardial oxygen delivery in patients with coronary artery spasm and is responsible for the effectiveness of verapamil HCl in vasospastic (Prinzmetal's or variant) as well as unstable angina at rest. Whether this effect plays any role in classical effort angina is not clear, but studies of exercise tolerance have not shown an increase in the maximum exercise rate-pressure product, a widely accepted measure of oxygen utilization. This suggests that, in general, relief of spasm or dilation of coronary arteries is not an important factor in classical angina.
2. ***Reduction of Oxygen Utilization:*** Verapamil HCl regularly reduces the total peripheral resistance (afterload) against which the heart works both at rest and at a given level of exercise by dilating peripheral arterioles. This unloading of the heart reduces myocardial energy consumption and oxygen requirements and probably accounts for the effectiveness of verapamil HCl in chronic stable effort angina.

Arrhythmia

Electrical activity through the AV node depends, to a significant degree, upon calcium influx through the slow channel. By decreasing the influx of calcium, verapamil HCl prolongs the effective refractory period within the AV node and slows AV conduction in a rate-related manner. This property accounts for the ability of verapamil HCl to slow the ventricular rate in patients with chronic atrial flutter or atrial fibrillation.

Normal sinus rhythm is usually not affected, but in patients with sick sinus syndrome, verapamil HCl may interfere with sinus-node impulse generation and may induce sinus arrest or sinoatrial block. Atrioventricular block can occur in patients without preexisting conduction defects (see WARNINGS). Verapamil HCl decreases the frequency of episodes of paroxysmal supraventricular tachycardia.

Verapamil HCl does not alter the normal atrial action potential or intraventricular conduction time, but in depressed atrial fibers it decreases amplitude, velocity of depolarization, and conduction velocity. Verapamil HCl may shorten the antegrade effective refractory period of the accessory bypass tract. Acceleration of ventricular rate and/or ventricular fibrillation has been reported in patients with atrial flutter or atrial fibrillation and a coexisting accessory AV pathway following administration of verapamil HCl (see WARNINGS).

Verapamil HCl has a local anesthetic action that is 1.6 times that of procaine on an equimolar basis. It is not known whether this action is important at the doses used in man.

In Vitro: Verapamil binding is voltage-dependent with affinity increasing as the vascular smooth muscle membrane potential is reduced. In addition, verapamil binding is frequency dependent and apparent affinity increases with increased frequency of depolarizing stimulus.

The L-type calcium channel is an oligomeric structure consisting of five putative subunits designated alpha-1, alpha-2, beta, tau, and epsilon. Biochemical evidence points to separate binding sites for 1,4-dihydropyridines, phenylalkylamines, and the benzothiazepines (all located on the alpha-1 subunit). Although they share a similar mechanism of action, calcium channel blockers represent three heterogeneous categories of drugs with differing vascular-cardiac selectivity ratios.

V

Essential Hypertension

Verapamil HCl exerts antihypertensive effects by decreasing systemic vascular resistance, usually without orthostatic decreases in blood pressure or reflex tachycardia; bradycardia (rate less than 50 beats/min) is uncommon (1.4%). During isometric or dynamic exercise verapamil HCl does not alter systolic cardiac function in patients with normal ventricular function.

Verapamil regularly reduces the total systemic resistance (afterload) against which the heart works both at rest and at a given level of exercise by dilating peripheral arterioles.

Verapamil HCl does not alter total serum calcium levels. However, one report suggested that calcium levels above the normal range may alter the therapeutic effect of verapamil HCl.

PHARMACOKINETICS AND METABOLISM

Immediate-Release Tablets and Sustained-Release Caplets

With the immediate-release formulation, more than 90% of the orally administered dose of verapamil HCl is absorbed. Because of rapid biotransformation of verapamil during its first pass through the portal circulation, bioavailability ranges from 20-35%. Peak plasma concentrations are reached between 1 and 2 hours after oral administration. Chronic oral administration of 120 mg of verapamil HCl every 6 hours resulted in plasma levels of verapamil ranging from 125-400 ng/ml, with higher values reported occasionally. A nonlinear correlation between the verapamil dose administered and verapamil plasma levels does exist. In early dose titration with verapamil a relationship exists between verapamil plasma concentration and prolongation of the PR interval. However, during chronic administration this relationship may disappear. The mean elimination half-life in single-doses studies ranged from 2.8-7.4 hours. In these same studies, after repetitive dosing, the half-life increased to a range from 4.5-12.0 hours (after less than 10 consecutive doses given 6 hours apart). Half-life of verapamil may increase during titration. No relationship has been established between the plasma concentration of verapamil and a reduction in blood pressure.

In a randomized, single-dose, crossover study using healthy volunteers, administration of 240 mg verapamil HCl sustained-release with food produced peak plasma verapamil concentrations of 79 ng/ml; time to peak plasma verapamil concentration of 7.71 hours; and AUC (0-24 h) of 841 ng·h/ml. When verapamil HCl, sustained-release caplets were administered to fasting subjects, peak plasma verapamil concentration was 164 ng/ml; time to peak plasma verapamil concentration was 5.21 hours; and AUC (0-24 h) was 1478 ng·h/ml. Similar results were demonstrated for plasma norverapamil. Food thus produces decreased bioavailability (AUC) but a narrower peak-to-trough ration. Good correlation of dose and response is not available, but controlled studies of verapamil HCl sustained-release caplets have shown effectiveness of doses similar to the effective doses of verapamil HCl (immediate release).

In healthy men, orally administered verapamil HCl undergoes extensive metabolism in the liver. Twelve metabolites have been identified in plasma; all except norverapamil are present in trace amounts only. Norverapamil can reach steady-state plasma concentrations approximately equal to those of verapamil itself. The cardiovascular activity of norverapamil appears to be approximately 20% that of verapamil. Approximately 70% of an administered dose is excreted as metabolites in the urine and 16% or more in the feces within 5 days. About 3-4% is excreted in the urine as unchanged drug. Approximately 90% is bound to plasma proteins. In patients with hepatic insufficiency, metabolism of immediate-release verapamil is delayed and elimination half—life prolonged up to 14-16 hours (see PRECAUTIONS); the volume of distribution is increased and plasma clearance reduced to about 30% of normal. Verapamil clearance values suggest that patients with liver dysfunction may attain therapeutic verapamil plasma concentrations with one-third of the oral daily dose required for patients with normal liver function.

In randomized, single dose, crossover studies using healthy volunteers, administration of verapamil extended-release tablets with food produced lower peak concentrations, delayed time to peak, and lesser total absorption (AUC), than when the product was administered to fasting subjects. Similar results were demonstrated for plasma norverapamil. Food thus produces decreased bioavailability (AUC) but a narrower peak to trough ratio. Good correlation of dose and response is not available, but controlled studies of extended-release verapamil have shown effectiveness of doses similar to the effective doses of immediate-release verapamil.

In 10 healthy males, administration of oral verapamil (80 mg every 8 hours for 6 days) and a single oral dose of ethanol (0.8 g/kg) resulted in a 17% increase in mean peak ethanol concentrations (106.45 $\pm$ 21.40 to 124.23 $\pm$ 24.74 mg·h/dl) compared to placebo. The area under the blood ethanol concentration versus time curve (AUC over 12 hours) increased by 30% (365.67 $\pm$ 93.52 to 475.07 $\pm$ 97.24 mg·h/dl). Verapamil AUCs were positively correlated (r=0.71) to increased ethanol blood AUC values (see DRUG INTERACTIONS).

Aging may affect the pharmacokinetics of verapamil. In general, bioavailability of verapamil is higher and half life longer in older (>65 yrs) subjects. Lean body weight also affects its pharmacokinetics inversely. In multiple-dose studies under fasting conditions, the bioavailability, measured by AUC, of verapamil HCl sustained-release was similar to verapamil HCl (immediate release); rates of absorption were, of course, different.

It was not possible to observe a gender difference in the clinical trials of verapamil HCl, extended-release, controlled-onset capsules due to the small sample size. However, there are conflicting data in the literature suggesting that verapamil clearance decreased with age in women to a greater degree than in men.

After 4 weeks of oral dosing (120 mg qid), verapamil and norverapamil levels were noted in the cerebrospinal fluid with estimated partition coefficient of 0.06 for verapamil and 0.04 for norverapamil.

Sustained-Release, Controlled-Onset Capsules

Note: See Pharmacokinetics and Metabolism, Immediate-Release Tablets and Sustained-Release Caplets for additional information.

Verapamil is administered as a racemic mixture of the R and S enantiomers. The systemic concentrations of R and S enantiomers, as well as overall bioavailability, are dependent upon the route of administration and the rate and extent of release from the dosage forms. Upon oral administration, there is rapid stereoselective biotransformation during the first pass of verapamil through the portal circulation. In a study in 5 subjects with oral immediate-release verapamil, the systemic bioavailability was from 33-65% for the R enantiomer and from 13-34% for the S enantiomer. Following oral administration of an immediately releasing formulation every 8 hours in 24 subjects, the relative systemic availability of the S enantiomer compared to the R enantiomer was approximately 13% following a single day's administration and approximately 18% following administration to steady-state. The degree of stereoselectivity of metabolism for verapamil HCl, extended-release, controlled-onset capsules capsules was similar to that for the immediately releasing formulation. The R and S enantiomers have differing levels of pharmacologic activity. In studies in animals and humans, the S enantiomer has 8-20 times the activity of the R enantiomer in slowing AV conduction. In animal studies, the S enantiomer has 15-50 times the activity of the R enantiomer in reducing myocardial contractility in isolated blood-perfused dog papillary muscle, respectively, and twice the effect in reducing peripheral resistance. In isolated septal strip preparations from 5 patients, the S enantiomer was 8 times more potent than the

R in reducing myocardial contractility. Dose escalation study data indicate that verapamil concentrations increase disproportionally to dose as measured by relative peak plasma concentrations (C_{max}) or areas under the plasma concentration vs time curves (AUC).

Although some evidence of lack of dose linearity was observed for verapamil HCl, extended-release, controlled-onset capsules, this non-linearity was enantiomer specific, with the R enantiomer showing the greatest degree of non-linearity.

TABLE 1 *Pharmacokinetic Characteristics of Verapamil Enantiomers After Administration of Escalating Doses of Verapamil HCl, Extended-Release, Controlled-Onset Capsules*

	Isomer	200	300	400
Dose Ratio		1	1.5	2
Relative C_{max}	R	1	1.89	2.34
	S	1	1.88	2.5
Relative AUC	R	1	1.67	2.34
	S	1	1.35	2.20

Racemic verapamil is released from verapamil HCl, extended-release, controlled-onset capsules by diffusion following the gradual solubilization of the water soluble polymer. The rate of solubilization of the water soluble polymer produces a lag period in drug release for approximately 4-5 hours. The drug release phase is prolonged with the peak plasma concentration (C_{max}) occurring approximately 11 hours after administration. Trough concentrations occur approximately 4 hours after bedtime dosing while the patient is sleeping. Steady-state pharmacokinetics were determined in healthy volunteers. Steady-state concentration is achieved by day 5 of dosing.

In healthy volunteers, following administration of verapamil HCl, extended-release, controlled-onset capsules (200 mg/day), steady-state pharmacokinetics of the R and S enantiomers of verapamil is as follows: Mean C_{max} of the R isomer was 77.8 ng/ml and 16.8 ng/ml for the S isomer; AUC (0-24h) of the R isomer was 1037 ng·h/ml and 195 ng·h/ml for the S isomer.

Consumption of a high fat meal just prior to dosing in the morning had no effect on the extent of absorption and a modest effect on the rate of absorption from verapamil HCl, extended-release, controlled-onset capsules. The rate of absorption was not affected by whether the volunteers were supine 2 hours after night-time dosing or non-supine for 4 hours following morning dosing. Administering verapamil HCl, extended-release, controlled-onset capsules in the morning increased the extent of absorption of verapamil and/or decreased the metabolism to norverapamil.

Orally administered verapamil undergoes extensive metabolism in the liver. Verapamil is metabolized by O-demethylation (25%) and N-dealkylation (40%), and is subject to presystemic hepatic metabolism with elimination of up to 80% of the dose. The metabolism is mediated by hepatic cytochrome P_{450}, and animal studies have implied that the monooxygenase is the specific isoenzyme of the P_{450} family. Thirteen metabolites have been identified in urine. Norverapamil enantiomers can reach steady-state plasma concentrations approximately equal to those of the enantiomers of the parent drug. For verapamil HCl, extended-release, controlled-onset capsules, the norverapamil R enantiomer reached steady-state plasma concentrations similar to the verapamil R enantiomer, but the norverapamil S enantiomer concentrations were approximately twice that of the verapamil S enantiomer concentrations. The cardiovascular activity of norverapamil appears to be approximately 20% that of verapamil. Approximately 70% of an administered dose is excreted as metabolites in the urine and 16% or more in the feces within 5 days. About 3-4% is excreted in the urine as unchanged drug.

R verapamil is 94% bound to plasma albumin, while S verapamil is 88% bound. In addition, R verapamil is 92% and S verapamil 86% bound to alpha-1 acid glycoprotein. In patients with hepatic insufficiency, metabolism of immediate-release verapamil is delayed and elimination half-life prolonged up to 14-16 hours because of the extensive hepatic metabolism (see PRECAUTIONS). In addition, in these patients there is a reduced first pass effect, and verapamil is more bioavailable. Verapamil clearance values suggest that patients with liver dysfunction may attain therapeutic verapamil plasma concentrations with one-third of the oral daily dose required for patients with normal liver function.

HEMODYNAMICS AND MYOCARDIAL METABOLISM

Verapamil HCl reduces afterload and myocardial contractility. During isometric or dynamic exercise, verapamil does not alter systolic cardiac funcion in patients with normal ventricular function. Improved left ventricular diastolic function in patients with IHSS and those with coronary heart disease has also been observed with verapamil HCl therapy. In most patients, including those with organic cardiac disease, the negative inotropic action of verapamil HCl is countered by reduction of afterload, and cardiac index is usually not reduced. However, in patients with severe left ventricular dysfunction (*e.g.,* pulmonary wedge pressure above 20 mm Hg or ejection fraction less than 30%), or in patients taking beta-adrenergic blocking agents or other cardiodepressant drugs, deterioration of ventricular function may occur (see DRUG INTERACTIONS).

PULMONARY FUNCTION

Verapamil HCl does not induce bronchoconstriction and, hence, does not impair ventilatory function. Verapamil has been shown to have either a neutral or relaxant effect on bronchial smooth muscle.

INDICATIONS AND USAGE

VERAPAMIL HCl IMMEDIATE-RELEASE TABLETS ARE INDICATED FOR THE TREATMENT OF THE FOLLOWING

Angina:

1. Angina at rest including vasospastic (Prinzmetal's variant) angina; Unstable (crescendo, pre-infarction) angina.
2. Chronic stable angina (classic effort-associated angina).

Arrhythmias:

1. In association with digitalis for the control of ventricular rate at rest and during stress in patients with chronic atrial flutter and/or atrial fibrillation (see WARNINGS, Accessory Bypass Tract).
2. Prophylaxis of repetitive paroxysmal supraventricular tachycardia.

VERAPAMIL HCl IS INDICATED FOR THE TREATMENT OF THE FOLLOWING

Essential Hypertension

NON-FDA APPROVED INDICATIONS

Unapproved uses include treatment of bipolar disorder, cluster headaches, hypertrophic cardiomyopathy, and as prophylaxis against migraine headaches.

CONTRAINDICATIONS

Verapamil HCl is Contraindicated in:

1. Severe left ventricular dysfunction (see WARNINGS).
2. Hypotension (systolic pressure less than 90 mm Hg) or cardiogenic shock.
3. Sick sinus syndrome (except in patients with a functioning artificial ventricular pacemaker).
4. Second- or third-degree AV block (except in patients with a functioning artificial ventricular pacemaker).
5. Patients with atrial flutter or atrial fibrillation and an accessory bypass tract (*e.g.,* Wolff-Parkinson-White, Lown-Ganong-Levine syndromes). (See WARNINGS.)
6. Patients with known hypersensitivity to verapamil HCl.

WARNINGS

HEART FAILURE

Verapamil has a negative inotropic effect, which in most patients is compensated by its afterload reduction (decreased systemic vascular resistance) properties without a net impairment of ventricular performance. In clinical experience with 4954 patients (primarily with immediate-release verapamil), 87 (1.8%) developed congestive heart failure or pulmonary edema. Verapamil should be avoided in patients with severe left ventricular dysfunction (*e.g.,* ejection fraction less than 30%) or moderate to severe symptoms of cardiac failure and in patients with any degree of ventricular dysfunction if they are receiving a beta-adrenergic blocker (see DRUG INTERACTIONS). Patients with milder ventricular dysfunction should, if possible, be controlled with optimum doses of digitalis and/or diuretics before verapamil treatment. **(Note interactions with digoxin under DRUG INTERACTIONS; Digitalis.)**

HYPOTENSION

Occasionally, the pharmacologic action of verapamil may produce a decrease in blood pressure below normal levels, which may result in dizziness or symptomatic hypotension. The incidence of hypotension observed in 4954 patients enrolled in clinical trials was 2.5%. In hypertensive patients, decreases in blood pressure below normal are unusual. Tilt-table testing (60 degrees) was not able to induce orthostatic hypotension. In clinical studies of Verelan PM, 1.7% of the patients developed significant hypotension.

ELEVATED LIVER ENZYMES

Elevations of transaminases with and without concomitant elevations in alkaline phosphatase and bilirubin have been reported. Such elevations have sometimes been transient and may disappear even with continued verapamil treatment. Several cases of hepatocellular injury related to verapamil have been proven by rechallenge; half of these had clinical symptoms (malaise, fever, and/or right upper quadrant pain), in addition to elevation of SGOT, SGPT, and alkaline phosphatase. Periodic monitoring of liver function in patients receiving verapamil is therefore prudent.

ACCESSORY BYPASS TRACT (WOLFF-PARKINSON-WHITE OR LOWN-GANONG-LEVINE)

Some patients with paroxysmal and/or chronic atrial fibrillation or atrial flutter and a coexisting accessory AV pathway have developed increased antegrade conduction across the accessory pathway bypassing the AV node, producing a very rapid ventricular response or ventricular fibrillation after receiving intravenous verapamil (or digitalis). Although a risk of this occurring with oral verapamil has not been established, such patients receiving oral verapamil may be at risk and its use in these patients is contraindicated (see CONTRAINDICATIONS). Treatment is usually DC-cardioversion. Cardioversion has been used safety and effectively after oral verapamil HCl.

ATRIOVENTRICULAR BLOCK

The effect of verapamil on AV conduction and the SA node may cause asymptomatic first-degree AV block and transient bradycardia, sometimes accompanied by nodal escape rhythms. PR-interval prolongation is correlated with verapamil plasma concentrations especially during the early titration phase of therapy. Higher degrees of AV block, however, were infrequently (0.8%) observed. Marked first-degree block or progressive development to second- or third-degree AV block requires a reduction in dosage, or, in rare instances, discontinuation of verapamil HCl and institution of appropriate therapy, depending on the clinical situation.

PATIENTS WITH HYPERTROPHIC CARDIOMYOPATHY (IHSS)

In 120 patients with hypertrophic cardiomyopathy (most of them refractory or intolerant to propranolol) who received therapy with verapamil at doses up to 720 mg/day, a variety of serious adverse effects were seen. Three (3) patients died in pulmonary edema; all had severe left ventricular outflow obstruction and a past history of left ventricular dysfunction. Eight (8) other patients had pulmonary edema and/or severe hypotension; abnormally high (greater than 20 mm Hg) pulmonary wedge pressure and a marked left ventricular outflow obstruction were present in most of these patients. Concomitant administration of quinidine (see DRUG INTERACTIONS) preceded the severe hypotension in 3 of the 8 patients (2 of whom developed pulmonary edema). Sinus bradycardia occurred in 11% of the patients, second-degree AV block in 4%, and sinus arrest in 2%. It must be appreciated that this group of patients had a serious disease with a high mortality rate. Most adverse effects responded well to dose reduction, and only rarely did verapamil use have to be discontinued.

PRECAUTIONS

THE CONTENTS OF THE VERAPAMIL HCL, EXTENDED-RELEASE, CONTROLLED-ONSET CAPSULE SHOULD NOT BE CRUSHED OR CHEWED.

GENERAL

Use in Patients With Impaired Hepatic Function

Since verapamil is highly metabolized by the liver, it should be administered cautiously to patients with impaired hepatic function. Severe liver dysfunction prolongs the elimination half-life of verapamil to about 14-16 hours; hence, approximately 30% of the dose given to patients with normal liver function should be administered to these patients. Careful monitoring for abnormal prolongation of the PR interval or other signs of excessive pharmacologic effects should be carried out.

Use in Patients With Attenuated (Decreased) Neuromuscular Transmission

It has been reported that verapamil decreases neuromuscular transmission in patients with Duchenne's muscular dystrophy, and that verapamil prolongs recovery from the neuromuscular blocking agent vecuronium. It may be necessary to decrease the dosage of verapamil when it is administered to patients with attenuated neuromuscular transmission.

Use in Patients With Impaired Renal Function

About 70% of an administered dose of verapamil is excreted as metabolites in the urine. Verapamil is not removed by hemodialysis. Until further data are available, verapamil should be administered cautiously to patients with impaired renal function. These patients should be carefully monitored for abnormal prolongation of the PR interval or other signs of overdosage.

CARCINOGENESIS, MUTAGENESIS, AND IMPAIRMENT OF FERTILITY

An 18-month toxicity study in rats, at a low multiple (6-fold) of the maximum recommended human dose, and not the maximum tolerated dose, did not suggest a tumorigenic potential. There was no evidence of a carcinogenic potential of verapamil administered in the diet of rats for 2 years at doses of 10, 35, and 120 mg/kg/day or approximately 1, 3.5, and 12 times, respectively, the maximum recommended human daily dose (480 mg/day or 9.6 mg/kg/day). Likewise, no evidence of a carcinogenic potential was found for verapamil capsules administered in the diet of rats for 2 years at doses of 10, 35, and 120 mg/kg/day or approximately 1.2, 4.4, and 15 times the maximum recommended human daily dose (400 mg/day or 8 mg/kg/day).

Verapamil was not mutagenic in the Ames test in 5 test strains at 3 mg/plate, with or without metabolic activation.

Studies in female rats at daily dietary doses up to 5.5 times (55 mg/kg/day) the maximum recommended human dose (6.9 times (55 mg/kg/day) for capsules) did not show impaired fertility. Effects on male fertility have not been determined.

PREGNANCY CATEGORY C

Reproduction studies have been performed in rabbits and rats at oral doses up to 1.5 (15 mg/kg/day) and 6 (60 mg/kg/day) times the human oral daily dose (1.9 and 7.5 times the human daily dose for capsules), respectively, have revealed no evidence of teratogenicity. In the rat, however, this multiple of the human dose was embryocidal and retarded fetal growth and development, probably because of adverse maternal effects reflected in reduced weight gains of the dams. This oral dose has also been shown to cause hypotension in rats. There are no adequate and well-controlled studies in pregnant women. Because animal reproduction studies are not always predictive of human response, this drug should be used during pregnancy only if clearly needed. Verapamil crosses the placental barrier and can be detected in umbilical blood at delivery.

LABOR AND DELIVERY

It is not known whether the use of verapamil during labor or delivery has immediate or delayed adverse effects on the fetus, or whether it prolongs the duration of labor or increases the need for forceps delivery or other obstetric intervention. Such adverse experiences have not been reported in the literature, despite a long history of use of verapamil in Europe in the treatment of cardiac side effects of beta-adrenergic agonist agents used to treat premature labor.

NURSING MOTHERS

Verapamil is excreted in human milk. Because of the potential for adverse reactions in nursing infants from verapamil, nursing should be discontinued while verapamil is administered.

PEDIATRIC USE

Safety and efficacy of verapamil HCl in pediatric patients below the age of 18 years have not been established.

GERIATRIC USE

Clinical studies of verapamil HCl, extended-release, controlled-onset capsules were not adequate to determine if subjects aged 65 or over respond differently from younger patients. Other reported clinical experience has not identified differences in response between the elderly and younger patients; however, greater sensitivity to verapamil HCl, extended-release, controlled-onset capsules by some older individuals cannot be ruled out.

Aging may affect the pharmacokinetics of verapamil. Elimination half-life may be prolonged in the elderly (see CLINICAL PHARMACOLOGY, Pharmacokinetics and Metabolism).

Verapamil is highly metabolized by the liver, and about 70% of the administered dose is excreted as metabolites in the urine. Clinical circumstances, some of which may be more common in the elderly, such as hepatic or renal impairment, should be considered (See General). In general, lower initial doses of verapamil HCl, extended-release, controlled-onset capsules may be warranted in the elderly (see DOSAGE AND ADMINISTRATION, Essential Hypertension).

DRUG INTERACTIONS

Verapamil undergoes biotransformation by predominantly CYP3A4, however CYP1A2 and members of the CYP2C subfamily are involved in its metabolism. Coadministration of verapamil with other drugs metabolized by the above-mentioned enzymes may alter the bioavailability of either verapmail and/or the other drugs. Therefore, coadministration of narrow therapeutic index drugs with similar metabolic pathwyas as verapamil should be carefully monitored. Similarly, verapamil plasma levels in patients with hepatic cysfuction whould be carefully monitored, due to decreased clearanc of verapmil in these patients.

ALCOHOL

Verapamil has been found to inhibit ethanol elimination significantly, resulting in elevated blood ethanol concentrations that may prolong the intoxicating effects of alcohol (see Pharmacokinetics and Metabolism).

ANTINEOPLASTIC AGENTS

Verapamil can increase the efficacy of doxorubicin both in tissue culture systems and in patients. It raises the serum doxorubicin levels. The absorption of verapamil can be reduced by the cyclophosphamide, oncovin, procarbazine, prednisone (COPP) and the vindesine, adriamycin, cisplatin (VAC) cytotoxic drug regimens. Concomitant administration of R verapamil can decrease the clearance of paclitaxel.

ASPIRIN

In a few reported cases, coadministration of verapamil with aspirin has led to increased bleeding times greater than observed with aspirin alone.

BETA-BLOCKERS

Controlled studies in small numbers of patients suggest that the concomitant use of verapamil and oral beta-adrenergic blocking agents may be beneficial in certain patients with chronic stable angina or hypertension, but available information is not sufficient to predict with confidence the effects of concurrent treatment in patients with left ventricular dysfunction or cardiac conduction abnormalities. Concomitant therapy with beta-adrenergic blockers and verapamil may result in additive negative effects on hear rate, atrioventricular conduction and/or cardiac contractility.

The combination of sustained-release verapamil and beta-adrenergic blocking agents has not been studied. However, there have been reports of excessive bradycardia and AV block, including complete heart block, when the combination has been used for the treatment of hypertension. For hypertensive patients, the risks of combined therapy may outweigh the potential benefits. The combination should be used only with caution and close monitoring.

In one study involving 15 patients treated with high doses of propranolol (median dose, 480 mg/day; range 160-1280 mg/day) for severe angina, with preserved left ventricular function (ejection fraction greater than 35%), the hemodynamic effects of additional therapy with verapamil HCl were assessed using invasive methods. The addition of verapamil to high-dose beta-blockers induced modest negative inotropic and chronotropic effects that were not severe enough to limit short-term (48 hours) combination therapy in this study. These modest cardiodepressant effects persisted for greater than 6 but less than 30 hours after abrupt withdrawal of beta-blockers and were closely related to plasma levels of propranolol. The primary verapamil/beta-blocker interaction in this study appeared to be hemodynamic rather than electrophysiologic.

In other studies verapamil did not generally induce significant negative inotropic, chronotropic, or dromotropic effects in patients with preserved left ventricular function receiving low or moderate doses of propranolol (less than or equal to 320 mg/day); in some patients, however, combined therapy did produce such effects. Therefore, if combined therapy is used, close surveillance of clinical status should be carried out. Combined therapy should usually be avoided in patients with atrio-ventricular conduction abnormalities and those with depressed left ventricular function.

Asymptomatic bradycardia (36 beats/min) with a wandering atrial pacemaker has been observed in a patient receiving concomitant timolol (a beta-adrenergic blocker) eyedrops and oral verapamil.

A decrease in metoprolol and propranolol clearance has been observed when either drug is administered concomitantly with verapamil. A variable effect has been seen when verapamil and atenolol were given together.

DIGITALIS

Clinical use of verapamil in digitalized patients has shown the combination to be well tolerated if digoxin doses are properly adjusted. However, chronic verapamil treatment can increase serum digoxin levels by 50-75% during the first week of therapy, and this can result in digitalis toxicity. In patients with hepatic cirrhosis, the influence of verapamil on digoxin kinetics is magnified. Verapamil may reduce total body clearance and extrarenal clearance of digitoxin by 27% and 29%, respectively. Maintenance and digitalization doses should be reduced when verapamil is administered, and the patient should be reassessed to avoid over- or underdigitalization. Whenever overdigitalization is suspected, the daily dose of digitalis should be reduced or temporarily discontinued. On discontinuation of verapamil HCl use, the patient should be reassessed to avoid underdigitalization. In previous clinical trials with other verapamil formulations related to the control of ventricular response in digitalized patients who had atrial fibrillation or atrial flutter, ventricular rates below 50/min at rest occurred in 15% of patients, and asymptomatic hypotension occurred in 5% of patients.

ANTIHYPERTENSIVE AGENTS

Verapamil administered concomitantly with oral antihypertensive agents (*e.g.*, vasodilators, angiotensin-converting enzyme inhibitors, diuretics, beta-blockers) will usually have an additive effect on lowering blood pressure. Patients receiving these combinations should be appropriately monitored. Concomitant use of agents that attenuate alpha-adrenergic function with verapamil may result in a reduction in blood pressure that is excessive in some patients. Such an effect was observed in one study following the concomitant administration of verapamil and prazosin.

ANTIARRHYTHMIC AGENTS

Disopyramide: Until data on possible interactions between verapamil and disopyramide are obtained, disopyramide should not be administered within 48 hours before or 24 hours after verapamil administration.

Flecainide: A study in healthy volunteers showed that the concomitant administration of flecainide and verapamil may have additive effects on myocardial contractility, AV conduction, and repolarization. Concomitant therapy with flecainide and verapamil may result in additive negative inotropic effect and prolongation of atrioventricular conduction.

Quinidine: In a small number of patients with hypertrophic cardiomyopathy (IHSS), concomitant use of verapamil and quinidine resulted in significant hypotension. Until further data are obtained, combined therapy of verapamil and quinidine in patients with hypertrophic cardiomyopathy should probably be avoided.

The electrophysiologic effects of quinidine and verapamil on AV conduction were studied in 8 patients. Verapamil significantly counteracted the effects of quinidine on AV conduction. There has been a report of increased quinidine levels during verapamil therapy.

OTHER

Nitrates: Verapamil has been given concomitantly with short- and long-acting nitrates without any undesirable drug interactions. The pharmacologic profile of both drugs and the clinical experience suggest beneficial interactions.

Cimetidine: The interaction between cimetidine and chronically administered verapamil has not been studied. Variable results on clearance have been obtained in acute studies of healthy volunteers; clearance of verapamil was either reduced or unchanged.

Lithium: Increased sensitivity to the effects of lithium (neurotoxicity) has been reported during concomitant verapamil-lithium therapy; lithium levels have been observed sometimes to increase, sometimes to decrease, and sometimes to be unchanged. Patients receiving both drugs must be monitored carefully.

Carbamazepine: Verapamil therapy may increase carbamazepine concentrations during combined therapy. This may produce carbamazepine side effects such as diplopia, headache, ataxia, or dizziness.

Rifampin: Therapy with rifampin may markedly reduce oral verapamil bioavailability.

Phenobarbital: Phenobarbital therapy may increase verapamil clearance.

Cyclosporin: Verapamil therapy may increase serum levels of cyclosporin.

Theophylline: Verapamil may inhibit the clearance and increase the plasma levels of theophylline.

Inhalation Anesthetics: Animal experiments have shown that inhalation anesthetics depress cardiovascular activity by decreasing the inward movement of calcium ions. When used concomitantly, inhalation anesthetics and calcium antagonists, such as verapamil, should each be titrated carefully to avoid excessive cardiovascular depression.

Neuromuscular Blocking Agents: Clinical data and animal studies suggest that verapamil may potentiate the activity of neuromuscular blocking agents (curare-like and depolarizing). It may be necessary to decrease the dose of verapamil and/or the dose of the neuromuscular blocking agent when the drugs are used concomitantly.

ADVERSE REACTIONS

Serious adverse reactions are uncommon when verapamil HCl therapy is initiated with upward dose titration within the recommended single and total daily dose. See WARNINGS for discussion of heart failure, hypotension, elevated liver enzymes, AV block, and rapid ventricular response. Reversible (upon discontinuation of verapamil) non-obstructive, paralytic ileus has been infrequently reported in association with the use of verapamil. Reactions to orally administered verapamil occurred at rates greater than 1.0% or occurred at lower rates but appeared clearly drug-related in clinical trials in 4954 patients are shown below.

TABLE 2

Constipation	7.3%
Dizziness	3.3%
Nausea	2.7%
Hypotension	2.5%
Headache	2.2%
Edema	1.9%
CHF, pulmonary edema	1.8%
Fatigue	1.7%
Dyspnea	1.4%
Bradycardia (HR <50/min)	1.4%
AV block total (1°, 2°,3 °)	1.2%
2° and 3°	0.8%
Rash	1.2%
Flushing	0.6%

For information concerning elevated liver enzymes see WARNINGS.

In clinical trials related to the control of ventricular response in digitalized patients who had atrial fibrillation or flutter, ventricular rates below 50/min at rest occurred in 15% of patients and asymptomatic hypotension occurred in 5% of patients.

ADDITIONAL INFORMATION FOR VERAPAMIL HCl, SUSTAINED-RELEASE, CONTROLLED-RELEASE

The following reactions, reported in 2.0% or less of patients, occurred under conditions (open trials, marketing experience) where a causal relationship is uncertain; they are listed to alert the physician to a possible relationship.

Cardiovascular: Angina pectoris, atrioventricular dissociation, chest pain, claudication, myocardial infarction, palpitations, purpura (vasculitis), syncope.

Digestive System: Diarrhea, dry mouth, gastrointestinal distress, gingival hyperplasia.

Hemic and Lymphatic: Ecchymosis or bruising.

Nervous System: Cerebrovascular accident, confusion, equilibrium disorders, insomnia, muscle cramps, paresthesia, psychotic symptoms, shakiness, somnolence.

Respiratory: Dypnea.

Skin: Arthralgia and rash, exanthema, hair loss, hyperkeratosis, macules, sweating urticaria, Stevens-Johnson syndrome, erythema multiforme.

Special Senses: Blurred vision, tinnitus.

Urogenital: Gynecomastia, galactorrhea/hyperprolactinemia, increased urination, spotty menstruation, impotence.

Other: Allergy aggravated.

TREATMENT OF ACUTE CARDIOVASCULAR ADVERSE REACTIONS

The frequency of cardiovascular adverse reactions that require therapy is rare; hence, experience with their treatment is limited. Whenever severe hypotension or complete AV block occurs following oral administration of verapamil, the appropriate emergency measures should be applied immediately; *e.g.,* intravenously administered norepinephrine bitartrate, atropine sulfate, isoproterenol HCl (all in the usual doses), or calcium gluconate (10% solution). In patients with hypertrophic cardiomyopathy (IHSS), alpha-adrenergic agents (phenylephrine HCl, metaraminol bitartrate, or methoxamine HCl) should be used to maintain blood pressure, and isoproterenol and norepinephrine should be avoided. If further support is necessary, dopamine HCl or dobutamine HCl may be administered. Actual treatment and dosage should depend on the severity of the clinical situation and the judgment and experience of the treating physician.

SUSTAINED-RELEASE, CONTROLLED-ONSET CAPSULES

The following reactions to orally administered verapamil HCl, extended-release, controlled-onset capsules shown in TABLE 3 occurred at rates of 2.0% or greater or occurred at lower rates but appeared to be drug-related in clinical trials in hypertension.

TABLE 3

	Placebo n=116	All Doses Studied n=297
Headache	11.2%	12.1%
Infection	6.9%	12.1%*
Constipation	0.9%	8.8%*
Flu syndrome	2.6%	3.7%
Peripheral edema	0.9%	3.7%
Dizziness	0.9%	3.0%
Pharyngitis	2.6%	3.0%
Sinusitis	2.6%	3.0%
Dyspepsia	1.7%	2.7%
Rhinitis	2.6%	2.7%
Diarrhea	1.7%	2.4%
Pain	1.7%	2.4%
Rash	2.6%	2.4%
Asthenia	3.4%	2.0%
ECG abnormal	3.4%	2.0%
Hypertension	2.0%	1.7%
Edema	0.0%	1.7%
Nausea	0.0%	1.7%
Accidental injury	0.0%	1.5%

* Infection, primarily upper respiratory infection (URI) and unrelated to study medication. Constipation was typically mild and easily manageable. At the usual once-daily dose of 200 mg, the observed incidence of constipation was 3.9%.

DOSAGE AND ADMINISTRATION

IMMEDIATE-RELEASE TABLETS

The dose of verapamil must be individualized by titration. The usefulness and safety of dosages exceeding 480 mg/day have not been established; therefore, this daily dosage should not be exceeded. Since the half-life of verapamil increases during chronic dosing, maximum response may be delayed.

Angina

Clinical trials show that the usual dose is 80-120 mg three times a day. However, 40 mg three times a day may be warranted in patients who may have an increased response to verapamil (*e.g.,* decreased hepatic function, elderly, etc). Upward titration should be based on therapeutic efficacy and safety evaluated approximately 8 hours after dosing. Dosage may be increased at daily (*e.g.,* patients with unstable angina) or weekly intervals until optimum clinical response is obtained.

Arrhythmias

The dosage in digitalized patients with chronic atrial fibrillation (see PRECAUTIONS) ranges from 240-320 mg/day in divided (tid or qid) doses. The dosage for prophylaxis of PSVT (non-digitalized patients) ranges from 240-480 mg/day in divided (tid or qid) doses. In general, maximum effects for any given dosage will be apparent during the first 48 hours of therapy.

Essential Hypertension

Dose should be individualized by titration. The usual initial monotherapy dose in clinical trials was 80 mg three times a day (240 mg/day). Daily dosages of 360 and 480 mg have been used but there is no evidence that dosages beyond 360 mg provided added effect. Consideration should be given to beginning titration at 40 mg three times per day in patients who might respond to lower doses, such as the elderly or people of small stature. The antihypertensive effects of verapamil HCl are evident within the first week of therapy. Upward titration should be based on therapeutic efficacy, assessed at the end of the dosing interval.

SUSTAINED-RELEASE CAPLETS

Essential Hypertension

The dose of verapamil HCl should be individualized by titration and should be administered with food. Initiate therapy with 180 mg of sustained-release verapamil HCl given in the morning. Lower initial doses of 120 mg a day may be warranted in patients who may have an increased response to verapamil HCl (*e.g.,* the elderly or small people). Upward titration should be based on therapeutic efficacy and safety evaluated weekly and approximately 24 hours after the previous dose. The antihypertensive effects of verapamil HCl sustained release are evident within the first week of therapy.

If adequate response is not obtained with 180 mg of verapamil HCl sustained-release, the dose may be titrated upward in the following manner:

(a) 240 mg each morning.
(b) 180 mg each morning plus 180 mg each evening; or 240 mg each morning plus 120 mg each evening.
(c) 240 mg every 12 hours.

When switching from immediate-release to sustained-release verapamil HCl the total daily dose in milligrams may remain the same.

SUSTAINED-RELEASE CAPSULES

Essential Hypertension

The dose of verapamil HCl should be individualized by titration. The usual daily dose of sustained-release verapamil, in clinical trials has been 240 mg given by mouth once daily in the morning. However, initial doses of 120 mg a day may be warranted in patients who may have an increased response to verapamil (*e.g.*, elderly, small people, etc.). Upward titration should be based on therapeutic efficacy and safety evaluated approximately 24 hours after dosing. The antihypertensive effects of verapamil HCl are evident within the first week of therapy.

If adequate response is not obtained with 120 of verapamil HCl, the dose may be titrated upward in the following manner:

(a) 180 mg in the morning.
(b) 240 mg in the morning.
(c) 360 mg in the morning.
(d) 480 mg in the morning.

Verapamil HCl sustained-release capsules are for once-a-day administration. When switching from immediate-release verapamil to verapamil HCl capsules, the same total daily dose of verapamil HCl can be used.

As with immediate-release verapamil, dosages of verapamil HCl capsules should be individualized and titration may be needed in some patients.

SUSTAINED-RELEASE, CONTROLLED-ONSET CAPSULES

Essential Hypertension

Verapamil HCl, extended-release, controlled-onset should be administered once daily at bedtime. Clinical trials studied doses of 100, 200, 300, and 400 mg. The usual daily dose of verapamil HCl, extended-release, controlled-onset capsules in clinical trials has been 200 mg given by mouth once daily at bedtime. In rare instances, initial doses of 100 mg a day may be warranted in patients who have an increased response to verapamil [*e.g.*, patients with impaired renal function (see PRECAUTIONS), impaired hepatic function, elderly, small people, etc.]. Upward titration should be based on therapeutic efficacy and safety evaluated approximately 24 hours after dosing. The antihypertensive effects of verapamil HCl, extended-release, controlled-onset capsules are evident within the first week of therapy.

If an adequate response is not obtained with 200 mg of verapamil HCl, extended-release, controlled-onset capsules, the dose may be titrated upward in the following manner:

(a) 300 mg each evening.
(b) 400 mg each evening (2×200 mg).

When verapamil HCl, extended-release, controlled-onset capsules is administered at bedtime, office evaluation of blood pressure during morning and early afternoon hours is essentially a measure of peak effect. The usual evaluation of trough effect, which sometimes might be needed to evaluate the appropriateness of any given dose of verapamil HCl, extended-release, controlled-onset capsules would be just prior to bedtime.

As with immediate-release and sustained-release verapamil, dosages of verapamil HCl, extended-release, controlled-onset capsules should be individualized and titration may be needed in some patients.

ANIMAL PHARMACOLOGY

In chronic animal toxicology studies verapamil caused lenticular and/or suture line changes at 30 mg/kg/day or greater, and frank cataracts at 62.5 mg/kg/day or greater in the beagle dog, but not in the rat. Development of cataracts due to verapamil has not been reported in man.

HOW SUPPLIED

CALAN

40 mg Tablets: Round, pink, film coated, with "CALAN" debossed on one side and "40" on the other.

80 mg Tablets: Oval, peach colored, scored, film coated, with "CALAN" debossed on one side and "80" on the other.

120 mg Tablets: Oval, brown, scored, film coated, with "CALAN 120" debossed on one side.

CALAN SR

240 mg Caplets: Light green, capsule shaped, scored, film coated, with "CALAN' debossed on one side and "SR 240' on the other.

180 mg Caplets: Light pink, oval, scored, film coated, with "CALAN" debossed on one side and "SR 180" on the other.

120 mg Caplets: Light violet, oval, film coated, with "CALAN" debossed on one side and "SR 120" on the other.

VERELAN PM PELLET FILLED CAPSULES ARE SUPPLIED IN THREE DOSAGE STRENGTHS

100 mg: Two piece size 2 hard gelatin capsule, white opaque cap imprinted "SCHWARZ/4085" and amethyst body imprinted with "100 mg".

200 mg: Two piece size 0 hard gelatin capsule, amethyst opaque cap imprinted "SCHWARZ/4086" and amethyst body imprinted with "200 mg".

300 mg: Two piece size 00 hard gelatin capsule, lavender opaque cap imprinted "SCHWARZ/4087" and amethyst body imprinted "300 mg".

STORAGE

Store at controlled room temperature 15-30°C (59-86°F), protected from moisture.

Dispense in a tight, light-resistant container.

PRODUCT LISTING - RATED THERAPEUTICALLY EQUIVALENT

Capsule, Extended Release - Oral - 120 mg			
100's	$82.50	FEDERAL UPPER LIMIT, H.C.F.A. F F P	99999-2425-17
100's	$93.73	GENERIC, Udl Laboratories Inc	51079-0894-20
100's	$130.25	GENERIC, Udl Laboratories Inc	51079-0917-20
100's	$130.50	GENERIC, Teva Pharmaceuticals Usa	00093-5151-01
100's	$130.55	GENERIC, Mylan Pharmaceuticals Inc	00378-6320-01
100's	$203.98	VERELAN, Schwarz Pharma	00091-2490-23
Capsule, Extended Release - Oral - 180 mg			
100's	$87.00	FEDERAL UPPER LIMIT, H.C.F.A. F F P	99999-2425-18
100's	$136.67	GENERIC, Teva Pharmaceuticals Usa	00093-5152-01
100's	$137.00	GENERIC, Mylan Pharmaceuticals Inc	00378-6380-01
100's	$148.22	GENERIC, Udl Laboratories Inc	51079-0918-20
100's	$213.60	VERELAN, Schwarz Pharma	00091-2489-23
Capsule, Extended Release - Oral - 240 mg			
80's	$167.68	GENERIC, Udl Laboratories Inc	51079-0919-08
100's	$99.00	FEDERAL UPPER LIMIT, H.C.F.A. F F P	99999-2425-19
100's	$154.25	GENERIC, Teva Pharmaceuticals Usa	00093-5153-01
100's	$155.00	GENERIC, Mylan Pharmaceuticals Inc	00378-6440-01
100's	$241.08	VERELAN, Schwarz Pharma	00091-2491-23
Solution - Intravenous - 2.5 mg/ml			
2 ml	$12.99	ISOPTIN I.V., Knoll Pharmaceutical Company	00044-1816-21
2 ml x 5	$4.51	GENERIC, Abbott Pharmaceutical	00074-4011-01
2 ml x 5	$6.06	GENERIC, Abbott Pharmaceutical	00074-1144-01
2 ml x 5	$9.38	GENERIC, American Regent Laboratories Inc	00517-0501-72
2 ml x 5	$12.20	GENERIC, American Regent Laboratories Inc	00517-5402-05
2 ml x 10	$29.52	GENERIC, Sanofi Winthrop Pharmaceuticals	00024-2110-41
2 ml x 10	$32.89	GENERIC, Abbott Pharmaceutical	00074-1982-22
2 ml x 25	$107.75	GENERIC, Abbott Pharmaceutical	00074-4000-01
4 ml x 5	$6.65	GENERIC, Abbott Pharmaceutical	00074-1144-02
4 ml x 5	$13.45	GENERIC, American Regent Laboratories Inc	00517-5404-05
4 ml x 10	$48.93	GENERIC, Abbott Pharmaceutical	00074-9633-05
4 ml x 10	$63.40	GENERIC, Abbott Pharmaceutical	00074-1143-15
Tablet - Oral - 40 mg			
30's	$9.59	GENERIC, Heartland Healthcare Services	61392-0158-30
30's	$9.59	GENERIC, Heartland Healthcare Services	61392-0158-39
31's	$9.91	GENERIC, Heartland Healthcare Services	61392-0158-31
32's	$10.23	GENERIC, Heartland Healthcare Services	61392-0158-32
45's	$14.39	GENERIC, Heartland Healthcare Services	61392-0158-45
60's	$19.18	GENERIC, Heartland Healthcare Services	61392-0158-60
90's	$28.77	GENERIC, Heartland Healthcare Services	61392-0158-90
100's	$19.63	FEDERAL UPPER LIMIT, H.C.F.A. F F P	99999-2425-06
100's	$26.15	GENERIC, Qualitest Products Inc	00603-6356-21
100's	$26.75	GENERIC, Creighton Products Corporation	50752-0305-05
100's	$27.25	GENERIC, Major Pharmaceuticals Inc	00904-7799-60
100's	$27.31	GENERIC, Caremark Inc	00339-5857-12
100's	$27.47	GENERIC, Moore, H.L. Drug Exchange Inc	00839-7921-06
100's	$27.66	GENERIC, Watson/Rugby Laboratories Inc	00591-0404-01
100's	$27.66	GENERIC, Geneva Pharmaceuticals	00781-1014-01
100's	$27.66	GENERIC, Watson Laboratories Inc	52544-0404-01
100's	$28.75	GENERIC, Ivax Corporation	00182-1601-01
100's	$30.74	ISOPTIN, Knoll Pharmaceutical Company	00044-1821-02
100's	$53.09	CALAN, Searle	00025-1771-31
Tablet - Oral - 80 mg			
8's	$1.92	GENERIC, Pd-Rx Pharmaceuticals	55289-0896-08
25's	$5.66	GENERIC, Pd-Rx Pharmaceuticals	55289-0896-97
25's	$8.07	GENERIC, Udl Laboratories Inc	51079-0682-19
30's	$11.36	GENERIC, Heartland Healthcare Services	61392-0493-30
30's	$11.36	GENERIC, Heartland Healthcare Services	61392-0493-39
31's	$11.74	GENERIC, Heartland Healthcare Services	61392-0493-31
32's	$12.12	GENERIC, Heartland Healthcare Services	61392-0493-32
45's	$17.05	GENERIC, Heartland Healthcare Services	61392-0493-45
50's	$14.95	GENERIC, Mutual Pharmaceutical Co Inc	53489-0154-02
60's	$22.73	GENERIC, Heartland Healthcare Services	61392-0493-60
90's	$22.29	GENERIC, Golden State Medical	60429-0196-90
90's	$34.09	GENERIC, Heartland Healthcare Services	61392-0493-90
100's	$6.23	FEDERAL UPPER LIMIT, H.C.F.A. F F P	99999-2425-08
100's	$10.43	GENERIC, Interstate Drug Exchange Inc	00814-8280-14
100's	$10.71	GENERIC, Us Trading Corporation	56126-0360-11
100's	$21.18	GENERIC, Moore, H.L. Drug Exchange Inc	00839-7253-06
100's	$21.18	GENERIC, Moore, H.L. Drug Exchange Inc	00839-7267-06
100's	$22.05	GENERIC, Major Pharmaceuticals Inc	00904-2920-60
100's	$23.10	GENERIC, Martec Pharmaceuticals Inc	52555-0179-01
100's	$23.55	GENERIC, Caremark Inc	00339-5621-12
100's	$23.90	GENERIC, Creighton Products Corporation	50752-0306-05
100's	$25.92	GENERIC, Aligen Independent Laboratories Inc	00405-5099-01
100's	$26.80	GENERIC, Mutual Pharmaceutical Co Inc	53489-0154-01
100's	$27.65	GENERIC, Geneva Pharmaceuticals	00781-1016-01
100's	$27.70	GENERIC, Ivax Corporation	00182-1300-01
100's	$29.00	GENERIC, Mylan Pharmaceuticals Inc	00378-0512-01

Qty	Price	Product	NDC
100's	$30.75	GENERIC, Purepac Pharmaceutical Company	00228-2473-10
100's	$36.70	GENERIC, Auro Pharmaceutical	55829-0561-10
100's	$42.09	GENERIC, Geneva Pharmaceuticals	00781-1016-13
100's	$42.09	GENERIC, Udl Laboratories Inc	51079-0682-20
100's	$44.19	GENERIC, Ivax Corporation	00182-1300-89
100's	$46.77	ISOPTIN, Knoll Pharmaceutical Company	00044-1822-10
100's	$53.38	GENERIC, Watson Laboratories Inc	00591-0343-01
100's	$53.38	GENERIC, Watson Laboratories Inc	00591-0344-01
100's	$53.38	GENERIC, Watson Laboratories Inc	52544-0343-01
100's	$53.38	GENERIC, Watson Laboratories Inc	52544-0344-01
100's	$57.00	GENERIC, Major Pharmaceuticals Inc	00904-2920-61
100's	$76.36	CALAN, Searle	00025-1851-31

Tablet - Oral - 120 mg

Qty	Price	Product	NDC
30's	$15.17	GENERIC, Heartland Healthcare Services	61392-0496-30
30's	$15.17	GENERIC, Heartland Healthcare Services	61392-0496-39
30's	$29.63	CALAN, Physicians Total Care	54868-0933-00
30's	$337.00	GENERIC, Medirex Inc	57480-0375-06
31's	$15.67	GENERIC, Heartland Healthcare Services	61392-0496-31
32's	$16.18	GENERIC, Heartland Healthcare Services	61392-0496-32
45's	$22.75	GENERIC, Heartland Healthcare Services	61392-0496-45
60's	$9.86	GENERIC, Pd-Rx Pharmaceuticals	55289-0481-60
60's	$27.35	GENERIC, Golden State Medical	60429-0197-60
60's	$30.33	GENERIC, Heartland Healthcare Services	61392-0496-60
90's	$45.50	GENERIC, Heartland Healthcare Services	61392-0496-90
100's	$8.61	FEDERAL UPPER LIMIT, H.C.F.A. F F P	99999-2425-12
100's	$9.66	GENERIC, Us Trading Corporation	56126-0361-11
100's	$12.30	GENERIC, Pd-Rx Pharmaceuticals	55289-0481-01
100's	$14.93	GENERIC, Interstate Drug Exchange Inc	00814-8281-14
100's	$27.90	GENERIC, Qualitest Products Inc	00603-6358-21
100's	$28.27	GENERIC, Moore, H.L. Drug Exchange Inc	00839-7254-06
100's	$28.27	GENERIC, Moore, H.L. Drug Exchange Inc	00839-7268-06
100's	$29.20	GENERIC, Major Pharmaceuticals Inc	00904-2924-60
100's	$29.75	GENERIC, Creighton Products Corporation	50752-0307-05
100's	$30.83	GENERIC, Caremark Inc	00339-5622-12
100's	$30.85	GENERIC, Martec Pharmaceuticals Inc	52555-0180-01
100's	$34.25	GENERIC, Mutual Pharmaceutical Co Inc	53489-0155-01
100's	$34.65	GENERIC, Aligen Independent Laboratories Inc	00405-5100-01
100's	$35.45	GENERIC, Warner Chilcott Laboratories	00047-0329-24
100's	$35.45	GENERIC, Geneva Pharmaceuticals	00781-1017-01
100's	$37.20	GENERIC, Mylan Pharmaceuticals Inc	00378-0772-01
100's	$40.15	GENERIC, Purepac Pharmaceutical Company	00228-2475-10
100's	$48.40	GENERIC, Auro Pharmaceutical	55829-0562-10
100's	$56.16	GENERIC, Geneva Pharmaceuticals	00781-1017-13
100's	$56.16	GENERIC, Udl Laboratories Inc	51079-0683-20
100's	$57.85	GENERIC, Ivax Corporation	00182-1301-89
100's	$59.80	ISOPTIN, Knoll Pharmaceutical Company	00044-1823-02
100's	$62.40	ISOPTIN, Knoll Pharmaceutical Company	00044-1823-10
100's	$68.43	GENERIC, Watson Laboratories Inc	00591-0345-01
100's	$68.43	GENERIC, Watson Laboratories Inc	00591-0346-01
100's	$68.43	GENERIC, Watson Laboratories Inc	52544-0345-01
100's	$68.43	GENERIC, Watson Laboratories Inc	52544-0346-01
100's	$75.00	GENERIC, Major Pharmaceuticals Inc	00904-2924-61
100's	$103.28	CALAN, Searle	00025-1861-31

Tablet, Extended Release - Oral - 120 mg

Qty	Price	Product	NDC
30's	$40.76	CALAN SR, Physicians Total Care	54868-2147-02
100's	$86.79	GENERIC, Duramed Pharmaceuticals Inc	51285-0480-02
100's	$107.29	GENERIC, Ivax Corporation	00172-4285-60
100's	$107.29	GENERIC, Mylan Pharmaceuticals Inc	00378-1120-01
100's	$135.55	ISOPTIN SR, Abbott Pharmaceutical	00074-1149-14
100's	$141.60	CALAN SR, Pharmacia Corporation	00025-1901-34
100's	$143.63	CALAN SR, Pharmacia Corporation	00025-1901-31

Tablet, Extended Release - Oral - 180 mg

Qty	Price	Product	NDC
30's	$2.70	GENERIC, Heartland Healthcare Services	61392-0345-30
30's	$2.70	GENERIC, Heartland Healthcare Services	61392-0345-39
30's	$47.86	CALAN SR, Allscripts Pharmaceutical Company	54569-3802-00
31's	$2.79	GENERIC, Heartland Healthcare Services	61392-0345-31
32's	$2.88	GENERIC, Heartland Healthcare Services	61392-0345-32
45's	$4.05	GENERIC, Heartland Healthcare Services	61392-0345-45
60's	$5.40	GENERIC, Heartland Healthcare Services	61392-0345-60
90's	$8.10	GENERIC, Heartland Healthcare Services	61392-0345-90
100's	$43.50	FEDERAL UPPER LIMIT, H.C.F.A. F F P	99999-2425-01
100's	$97.75	GENERIC, Qualitest Products Inc	00603-6359-21
100's	$97.80	GENERIC, Geneva Pharmaceuticals	00781-1239-01
100's	$97.80	GENERIC, Major Pharmaceuticals Inc	00904-7871-60
100's	$97.80	GENERIC, Major Pharmaceuticals Inc	00904-7931-60
100's	$98.50	GENERIC, West Point Pharma	59591-0286-68
100's	$99.27	GENERIC, Caremark Inc	00339-5811-12
100's	$101.57	GENERIC, Baker Norton Pharmaceuticals	50732-0915-01
100's	$102.95	GENERIC, Aligen Independent Laboratories Inc	00405-5101-01
100's	$103.60	GENERIC, Martec Pharmaceuticals Inc	52555-0536-01
100's	$105.50	GENERIC, Watson/Rugby Laboratories Inc	00536-5630-01
100's	$107.20	GENERIC, Moore, H.L. Drug Exchange Inc	00839-7878-06
100's	$111.00	GENERIC, Mylan Pharmaceuticals Inc	00378-1180-01
100's	$120.10	GENERIC, Udl Laboratories Inc	51079-0899-20
100's	$143.96	GENERIC, Ivax Corporation	00172-4286-60
100's	$158.50	CALAN SR, Physicians Total Care	54868-1550-03
100's	$182.03	CALAN SR, Pharmacia Corporation	00025-1911-31
100's	$191.11	CALAN SR, Pharmacia Corporation	00025-1911-34

Tablet, Extended Release - Oral - 240 mg

Qty	Price	Product	NDC
25's	$30.48	GENERIC, Udl Laboratories Inc	51079-0869-19
30's	$3.00	GENERIC, Heartland Healthcare Services	61392-0500-30
30's	$3.00	GENERIC, Heartland Healthcare Services	61392-0500-39
30's	$18.32	GENERIC, Pd-Rx Pharmaceuticals	55289-0723-30
30's	$68.99	ISOPTIN SR, Pd-Rx Pharmaceuticals	55289-0078-30
31's	$3.10	GENERIC, Heartland Healthcare Services	61392-0500-31
32's	$3.20	GENERIC, Heartland Healthcare Services	61392-0500-32
45's	$4.50	GENERIC, Heartland Healthcare Services	61392-0500-45
60's	$6.00	GENERIC, Heartland Healthcare Services	61392-0500-60
90's	$9.00	GENERIC, Heartland Healthcare Services	61392-0500-90
90's	$115.72	GENERIC, Golden State Medical	60429-0198-90
90's	$116.21	ISOPTIN SR, Allscripts Pharmaceutical Company	54569-8012-00
100's	$35.93	FEDERAL UPPER LIMIT, H.C.F.A. F F P	99999-2425-03
100's	$103.75	GENERIC, West Point Pharma	59591-0280-68
100's	$107.45	GENERIC, Qualitest Products Inc	00603-6360-21
100's	$111.91	GENERIC, Geneva Pharmaceuticals	00781-1018-01
100's	$112.79	GENERIC, Caremark Inc	00339-5809-12
100's	$115.44	GENERIC, Moore, H.L. Drug Exchange Inc	00839-7670-06
100's	$116.20	GENERIC, Baker Norton Pharmaceuticals	50732-0901-01
100's	$118.00	GENERIC, Sidmak Laboratories Inc	50111-0488-01
100's	$118.00	GENERIC, Martec Pharmaceuticals Inc	52555-0537-01
100's	$120.95	GENERIC, Mylan Pharmaceuticals Inc	00378-0411-01
100's	$126.80	GENERIC, Major Pharmaceuticals Inc	00904-7723-60
100's	$163.55	GENERIC, Ivax Corporation	00172-4280-60
100's	$196.54	ISOPTIN SR, Abbott Pharmaceutical	00074-1625-14
100's	$208.25	CALAN SR, Searle	00025-1891-31

PRODUCT LISTING - RATED NOT THERAPEUTICALLY EQUIVALENT

Capsule, Extended Release - Oral - 180 mg

Qty	Price	Product	NDC
100's	$135.16	GENERIC, Watson Laboratories Inc	00591-2882-01

Tablet, Extended Release - Oral - 180 mg/24 Hours

Qty	Price	Product	NDC
30's	$41.48	COVERA-HS, Allscripts Pharmaceutical Company	54569-4498-00
100's	$146.41	COVERA-HS, Searle	00025-2011-34
100's	$153.81	COVERA-HS, Searle	00025-2011-31

Tablet, Extended Release - Oral - 240 mg

Qty	Price	Product	NDC
30's	$36.29	GENERIC, Allscripts Pharmaceutical Company	54569-3691-00

Tablet, Extended Release - Oral - 240 mg/24 Hours

Qty	Price	Product	NDC
30's	$56.86	COVERA-HS, Allscripts Pharmaceutical Company	54569-4499-00
100's	$170.93	COVERA-HS, Searle	00025-2021-34
100's	$216.03	COVERA-HS, Searle	00025-2021-31

PRODUCT LISTING - EQUIVALENTS NOT AVAILABLE

Capsule, Extended Release - Oral - 100 mg/24 Hours

Qty	Price	Product	NDC
100's	$148.50	VERELAN PM, Schwarz Pharma	00091-4085-01

Capsule, Extended Release - Oral - 120 mg

Qty	Price	Product	NDC
100's	$129.05	GENERIC, Mylan Pharmaceuticals Inc	00364-2880-01

Capsule, Extended Release - Oral - 180 mg

Qty	Price	Product	NDC
100's	$135.16	GENERIC, Watson/Schein Pharmaceuticals Inc	00364-2882-01

Capsule, Extended Release - Oral - 200 mg/24 Hours

Qty	Price	Product	NDC
100's	$191.26	VERELAN PM, Schwarz Pharma	00091-4086-01

Capsule, Extended Release - Oral - 240 mg

Qty	Price	Product	NDC
100's	$152.54	GENERIC, Watson/Schein Pharmaceuticals Inc	00364-2884-01

Capsule, Extended Release - Oral - 300 mg/24 Hours

Qty	Price	Product	NDC
100's	$278.06	VERELAN PM, Schwarz Pharma	00091-4087-01

Capsule, Extended Release - Oral - 360 mg

Qty	Price	Product	NDC
100's	$209.94	GENERIC, Watson/Schein Pharmaceuticals Inc	00364-2886-01
100's	$209.94	GENERIC, Watson Laboratories Inc	00591-2886-01
100's	$354.36	VERELAN, Schwarz Pharma	00091-2495-23

Solution - Intravenous - 2.5 mg/ml

Qty	Price	Product	NDC
2 ml	$1.65	GENERIC, Physicians Total Care	54868-3809-00
2 ml	$3.35	GENERIC, Allscripts Pharmaceutical Company	54569-3744-01
2 ml x 5	$16.75	GENERIC, Allscripts Pharmaceutical Company	54569-3744-00

Tablet - Oral - 40 mg

Qty	Price	Product	NDC
30's	$8.05	GENERIC, Physicians Total Care	54868-2885-00

Tablet - Oral - 80 mg

Qty	Price	Product	NDC
8's	$4.49	GENERIC, Southwood Pharmaceuticals Inc	58016-0511-08
30's	$3.97	GENERIC, Physicians Total Care	54868-0120-03
30's	$9.15	GENERIC, Allscripts Pharmaceutical Company	54569-0639-01
30's	$16.85	GENERIC, Southwood Pharmaceuticals Inc	58016-0511-30
60's	$6.28	GENERIC, Physicians Total Care	54868-0120-00
60's	$18.30	GENERIC, Allscripts Pharmaceutical Company	54569-0639-02
100's	$9.36	GENERIC, Physicians Total Care	54868-0120-01
100's	$22.50	GENERIC, Cmc-Consolidated Midland Corporation	00223-1735-01
100's	$30.50	GENERIC, Allscripts Pharmaceutical Company	54569-0639-00
100's	$56.15	GENERIC, Southwood Pharmaceuticals Inc	58016-0511-00

Tablet - Oral - 120 mg

Qty	Price	Product	NDC
12's	$12.78	GENERIC, Southwood Pharmaceuticals Inc	58016-0509-12
15's	$15.98	GENERIC, Southwood Pharmaceuticals Inc	58016-0509-15
20's	$21.30	GENERIC, Southwood Pharmaceuticals Inc	58016-0509-20
30's	$4.97	GENERIC, Physicians Total Care	54868-0121-06

30's	$11.73	GENERIC, Allscripts Pharmaceutical Company	54569-0646-02
30's	$31.95	GENERIC, Southwood Pharmaceuticals Inc	58016-0509-30
60's	$8.27	GENERIC, Physicians Total Care	54868-0121-05
60's	$23.46	GENERIC, Allscripts Pharmaceutical Company	54569-0646-01
100's	$12.67	GENERIC, Physicians Total Care	54868-0121-01
100's	$22.50	GENERIC, Cmc-Consolidated Midland Corporation	00223-1736-01
100's	$39.10	GENERIC, Allscripts Pharmaceutical Company	54569-0646-00
100's	$106.50	GENERIC, Southwood Pharmaceuticals Inc	58016-0509-00
120's	$37.20	GENERIC, Pharmaceutical Corporation Of America	51655-0586-82
Tablet, Extended Release - Oral - 120 mg			
60's	$63.90	GENERIC, Southwood Pharmaceuticals Inc	58016-0509-60
100's	$135.55	ISOPTIN SR, Knoll Pharmaceutical Company	00044-1827-02
Tablet, Extended Release - Oral - 180 mg			
7's	$7.77	GENERIC, Allscripts Pharmaceutical Company	54569-4447-00
30's	$8.21	GENERIC, Physicians Total Care	54868-3300-02
90's	$99.90	GENERIC, Allscripts Pharmaceutical Company	54569-4447-01
100's	$22.93	GENERIC, Physicians Total Care	54868-3300-01
100's	$171.79	ISOPTIN SR, Knoll Pharmaceutical Company	00044-1825-02
Tablet, Extended Release - Oral - 240 mg			
12's	$18.58	GENERIC, Southwood Pharmaceuticals Inc	58016-0860-12
15's	$23.22	GENERIC, Southwood Pharmaceuticals Inc	58016-0860-15
20's	$30.96	GENERIC, Southwood Pharmaceuticals Inc	58016-0860-20
30's	$7.93	GENERIC, Physicians Total Care	54868-2207-02
30's	$46.44	GENERIC, Southwood Pharmaceuticals Inc	58016-0860-30
30's	$56.06	GENERIC, Pharma Pac	52959-0050-30
30's	$56.06	GENERIC, Southwood Pharmaceuticals Inc	58016-0374-30
60's	$12.84	GENERIC, Physicians Total Care	54868-2207-00
100's	$27.74	GENERIC, Physicians Total Care	54868-2207-03
100's	$120.85	GENERIC, Warner Chilcott Laboratories	00047-0474-24
100's	$121.87	GENERIC, Udl Laboratories Inc	51079-0869-20
100's	$154.80	GENERIC, Southwood Pharmaceuticals Inc	58016-0860-00
100's	$196.54	ISOPTIN SR, Knoll Pharmaceutical Company	00044-1826-02
100's	$205.33	CALAN SR, Searle	00025-1891-34

Verteporfin *(003481)*

For complete prescribing information, refer to the CD-ROM included with the book.

Categories: Choroidal neovascularization; Histoplasmosis, ocular; Macular degeneration; Myopia, pathologic; FDA Approved 2000 Apr; Pregnancy Category C

Drug Classes: Ophthalmics

Foreign Brand Availability: Visudyne (Australia; Austria; Belgium; Bulgaria; Canada; Colombia; Czech-Republic; Denmark; England; Finland; France; Germany; Greece; Hong-Kong; Hungary; Ireland; Israel; Italy; Korea; Netherlands; Norway; Philippines; Poland; Portugal; Singapore; Slovenia; Spain; Sweden; Switzerland; Thailand; Turkey)

DESCRIPTION

Visudyne (verteporfin for injection) is a light activated drug used in photodynamic therapy. The finished drug product is a lyophilized dark green cake. Verteporfin is a 1:1 mixture of two regioisomers (I and II).

The chemical names for the verteporfin regioisomers are: 9-methyl (I) and 13-methyl (II) *trans*-(±)-18-ethenyl-4,4a-dihydro-3,4-bis(methoxycarbonyl)-4a,8,14,19-tetramethyl-23*H*,25*H*-benzo[*b*]porphine-9,13-dipropanoate.

The molecular formula is $C_{41}H_{42}N_4O_8$ with a molecular weight of approximately 718.8.

Each ml of reconstituted Visudyne contains: *Active:* Verteporfin, 2 mg; *Inactives:* Lactose, egg phosphatidylglycerol, dimyristoyl phosphatidylcholine, ascorbyl palmitate and butylated hydroxytoluene.

INDICATIONS AND USAGE

Verteporfin therapy is indicated for the treatment of patients with predominantly classic subfoveal choroidal neovascularization due to age-related macular degeneration, pathologic myopia or presumed ocular histoplasmosis.

There is insufficient evidence to indicate verteporfin for the treatment of predominantly occult subfoveal choroidal neovascularization.

NON-FDA APPROVED INDICATIONS

Although not approved by the FDA, case reports have described the use of photodynamic therapy with verteporfin in the treatment of circumscribed choroidal hemangioma.

CONTRAINDICATIONS

Verteporfin is contraindicated for patients with porphyria or a known hypersensitivity to any component of this preparation.

WARNINGS

Following injection with verteporfin, care should be taken to avoid exposure of skin or eyes to direct sunlight or bright indoor light for 5 days. In the event of extravasation during infusion, the extravasation area must be thoroughly protected from direct light until the swelling and discoloration have faded in order to prevent the occurrence of a local burn which could be severe. If emergency surgery is necessary within 48 hours after treatment, as much of the internal tissue as possible should be protected from intense light.

Patients who experience severe decrease of vision of 4 lines or more within 1 week after treatment should not be retreated, at least until their vision completely recovers to pretreatment levels and the potential benefits and risks of subsequent treatment are carefully considered by the treating physician.

Use of incompatible lasers that do not provide the required characteristics of light for the photoactivation of verteporfin could result in incomplete treatment due to partial photoactivation of verteporfin, overtreatment due to overactivation of verteporfin, or damage to surrounding normal tissue.

DOSAGE AND ADMINISTRATION

A course of verteporfin therapy is a two-step process requiring administration of both drug and light.

The first step is the intravenous infusion of verteporfin. The second step is the activation of verteporfin with light from a nonthermal diode laser.

The physician should re-evaluate the patient every 3 months and if choroidal neovascular leakage is detected on fluorescein angiography, therapy should be repeated.

LESION SIZE DETERMINATION

The greatest linear dimension (GLD) of the lesion is estimated by fluorescein angiography and color fundus photography. All classic and occult CNV, blood and/or blocked fluorescence, and any serous detachments of the retinal pigment epithelium should be included for this measurement. Fundus cameras with magnification within the range of 2.4-2.6× are recommended. The GLD of the lesion on the fluorescein angiogram must be corrected for the magnification of the fundus camera to obtain the GLD of the lesion on the retina.

SPOT SIZE DETERMINATION

The treatment spot size should be 1000 microns larger than the GLD of the lesion on the retina to allow a 500 micron border, ensuring full coverage of the lesion. The maximum spot size used in the clinical trials was 6400 microns.

The nasal edge of the treatment spot must be positioned at least 200 microns from the temporal edge of the optic disc, even if this will result in lack of photoactivation of CNV within 200 microns of the optic nerve.

VERTEPORFIN ADMINISTRATION

Reconstitute each vial of verteporfin with 7 ml of sterile water for injection to provide 7.5 ml containing 2 mg/ml. Reconstituted verteporfin must be protected from light and used within 4 hours. It is recommended that reconstituted verteporfin be inspected visually for particulate matter and discoloration prior to administration. Reconstituted verteporfin is an opaque dark green solution.

The volume of reconstituted verteporfin required to achieve the desired dose of 6 mg/m^2 body surface area is withdrawn from the vial and diluted with 5% dextrose for injection to a total infusion volume of 30 ml. The full infusion volume is administered intravenously over 10 minutes at a rate of 3 ml/min, using an appropriate syringe pump and in-line filter. The clinical studies were conducted using a standard infusion line filter of 1.2 microns.

Precautions should be taken to prevent extravasation at the injection site. If extravasation occurs, protect the site from light.

LIGHT ADMINISTRATION

Initiate 689 nm wavelength laser light delivery to the patient 15 minutes after the start of the 10 minute infusion with verteporfin.

Photoactivation of verteporfin is controlled by the total light dose delivered. In the treatment of choroidal neovascularization, the recommended light dose is 50 J/cm^2 of neovascular lesion administered at an intensity of 600 mW/cm^2. This dose is administered over 83 seconds.

Light dose, light intensity, ophthalmic lens magnification factor and zoom lens setting are important parameters for the appropriate delivery of light to the predetermined treatment spot. Follow the laser system manuals for procedure set up and operation.

The laser system must deliver a stable power output at a wavelength of 689 ± 3 nm. Light is delivered to the retina as a single circular spot via a fiber optic and a slit lamp, using a suitable ophthalmic magnification lens.

The following laser systems have been tested for compatibility with verteporfin and are approved for delivery of a stable power output at a wavelength of 689 ± 3 nm:

Coherent Opal Photoactivator laser console and modified Coherent LaserLink adapter, manufactured by Lumenus, Inc., Santa Clara, CA.

Zeiss VISULAS 690s laser and VISULINK PDT/U adapter, manufactured by Carl Zeiss Inc., Thornwood, NY.

CONCURRENT BILATERAL TREATMENT

The controlled trials only allowed treatment of 1 eye per patient. In patients who present with eligible lesions in both eyes, physicians should evaluate the potential benefits and risks of treating both eyes concurrently. If the patient has already received previous verteporfin therapy in 1 eye with an acceptable safety profile, both eyes can be treated concurrently after a single administration of verteporfin. The more aggressive lesion should be treated first, at 15 minutes after the start of infusion. Immediately at the end of light application to the first eye, the laser settings should be adjusted to introduce the treatment parameters for the second eye, with the same light dose and intensity as for the first eye, starting no later than 20 minutes from the start of infusion.

In patients who present for the first time with eligible lesions in both eyes without prior verteporfin therapy, it is prudent to treat only 1 eye (the most aggressive lesion) at the first course. One week after the first course, if no significant safety issues are identified, the second eye can be treated using the same treatment regimen after a second verteporfin infusion. Approximately 3 months later, both eyes can be evaluated and concurrent treatment following a new verteporfin infusion can be started if both lesions still show evidence of leakage.

PRODUCT LISTING - EQUIVALENTS NOT AVAILABLE

Powder For Injection - Intravenous - 15 mg
1's $1535.00 VISUDYNE, Ciba Vision Ophthalmics 58768-0150-15

Vidarabine (002426)

Categories: Encephalitis; Keratitis; Keratoconjunctivitis; Pregnancy Category C; FDA Approved 1976 Nov
Drug Classes: Anti-infectives, ophthalmic; Antivirals; Ophthalmics
Brand Names: Vira-A
Foreign Brand Availability: Adena A ungena (Mexico); Arasena-A (Japan)

DESCRIPTION

Vira-A is the trade name for vidarabine (also known as adenine arabinoside and Ara-A), an antiviral drug for the treatment of epithelial keratitis caused by Herpes simplex virus. Vidarabine is a purine nucleoside obtained from fermentation cultures of *Streptomyces antibioticus*.

INFUSION

Each ml of sterile suspension contains 200 mg of vidarabine monohydrate equivalent to 187.4 mg of vidarabine. Each ml contains 0.1 mg Phemerol (benzethonium chloride) as a preservative; sodium phosphate, 1.8 mg, and sodium biphosphate, 4.8 mg as buffering agents. Hydrochloric acid may have been added to adjust pH. Vidarabine is a white, crystalline solid with this empirical formula: $C_{10}H_{13}N_5O_4 \cdot H_2O$. The molecular weight is 285.2; the solubility is 0.45 mg/ml at 25°C; and the melting point ranges from 260-270°C. The chemical name is 9-β-D-arabinofuranosyladenine monohydrate.

OPHTHALMIC OINTMENT

The chemical name of vidarabine ophthalmic ointment is 9H-Purin-6-amine, 9-β-D-arabinofuranosyl-, monohydrate. Each gram of the ophthalmic ointment contains 30 mg of vidarabine monohydrate equivalent to 28.11 mg of vidarabine in a sterile, inert, petrolatum base. The empirical formula is $C_{10}H_{13}N_5O_4 \cdot H_2O$. The molecular weight is 285.26.

CLINICAL PHARMACOLOGY

INFUSION

Following intravenous administration, vidarabine is rapidly deaminated into arabinosylhypoxanthine (Ara-Hx), the principal metabolite, which is promptly distributed into the tissues. Peak Ara-Hx and Ara-A plasma levels ranging from 3-6 μg/ml and 0.2-0.4 μg/ml, respectively, are attained after slow intravenous infusion of vidarabine doses of 10 mg/kg of body weight. These levels reflect the rate of infusion and show no accumulation across time. The mean half-life of Ara-Hx is 3.3 hours. Ara-Hx penetrates into the cerebrospinal fluid (CSF) to give a CSF/plasma ratio of approximately 1:3.

Excretion of vidarabine is principally via the kidneys. Urinary excretion is constant over 24 hours. Forty-one (41) to 53% of the daily dose is recovered in the urine as Ara-Hx with 1-3% appearing as the parent compound. There is no evidence of fecal excretion of drug or metabolites. In patients with impaired renal function Ara-Hx may accumulate in the plasma and reach levels several-fold higher than those described above.

Vidarabine possesses *in vitro* and *in vivo* antiviral activity against *Herpes virus* simplex (Herpes simplex virus) types 1 and 2.

The antiviral mechanism of action has not yet been established. The drug is converted into nucleotides which appear to be involved with the inhibition of viral replication. In KB cells infected with Herpes simplex virus type 1, vidarabine inhibits viral DNA synthesis. Vidarabine is rapidly deaminated to Ara-Hx, the principal metabolite, in cell cultures, laboratory animals, and humans.

Ara-Hx also possesses *in vitro* antiviral activity but this activity is significantly less than the activity of vidarabine.

OPHTHALMIC OINTMENT

Vidarabine is rapidly deaminated to arabinosylhypoxanthine (Ara-Hx), the principal metabolite. Ara-Hx also possesses *in vitro* antiviral activity but this activity is less than that of vidarabine. Because of the low solubility of vidarabine, trace amounts of both vidarabine and Ara-Hx can be detected in the aqueous humor only if there is an epithelial defect in the cornea. If the cornea is normal, only trace amounts of Ara-Hx can be recovered from the aqueous humor.

Systemic absorption of vidarabine should not be expected to occur following ocular administration and swallowing lacrimal secretions. In laboratory animals, vidarabine is rapidly deaminated in the gastrointestinal tract to Ara-Hx.

In contrast to topical idoxuridine, vidarabine demonstrated less cellular toxicity in the regenerating corneal epithelium of the rabbit.

In controlled and uncontrolled clinical trials, an average of 7 and 9 days of continuous vidarabine therapy was required to achieve corneal re-epithelialization. In the controlled trials, 70 of 81 subjects (86%) re-epithelialized at the end of 3 weeks of therapy. In the uncontrolled trials, 101 of 142 subjects (71%) re-epithelialized at the end of 3 weeks. Seventy-five percent (75%) of the subjects in these uncontrolled trials had either not healed previously or had developed hypersensitivity to topical idoxuridine therapy.

Microbiology

Vidarabine is a purine nucleoside obtained from fermentation cultures of *Streptomyces antibioticus*. The antiviral mechanism of action has not been established. Vidarabine appears to interfere with the early steps of viral DNA synthesis.

Vidarabine has been shown to possess antiviral activity against the following viruses *in vitro*:

Herpes simplex types 1 and 2.
Vaccinia.
Varicella-Zoster.

Except for Rhabdovirus and Oncornavirus, vidarabine does not display *in vitro* antiviral activity against other RNA or DNA viruses, including Adenovirus.

Susceptibility Testing

No universal, standardized, quantitative *in vitro* procedures have as yet been developed to estimate the susceptibility of viruses to antiviral agents.

INDICATIONS AND USAGE

INFUSION

Vidarabine is indicated in the treatment of Herpes simplex virus encephalitis. Controlled studies indicated that vidarabine therapy will reduce the mortality caused by Herpes simplex virus encephalitis from 70-28% 30 days following onset. In a larger uncontrolled study of 75 patients with biopsy-proven herpes simplex encephalitis, the mortality 6 months from onset was 39%, similar to 44% in the initial controlled study at 6 months.

Morbidity from both studies 1 year after onset was: normal 53%, moderately debilitated 29%, and severely damaged 18%. Vidarabine does not appear to alter morbidity and resulting serious neurological sequelae in the comatose patient. Therefore early diagnosis and treatment are essential.

Herpes simplex virus encephalitis should be suspected in patients with a history of an acute febrile encephalopathy associated with disordered mentation, altered level of consciousness and focal cerebral signs.

Studies which may support the suspected diagnosis include examination of cerebrospinal fluid and localization of an intra-cerebral lesion by brain scan, electroencephalography or computerized axial tomography (CAT).

Brain biopsy is required in order to confirm the etiological diagnosis by means of viral isolation in cell cultures.

Detection of Herpes simplex virus in the biopsied brain tissue can also be reliably done by specific fluorescent antibody techniques. Detection of Herpes virus-like particles by electron microscopy or detection of intranuclear inclusions by histopathologic techniques only provides a presumptive diagnosis.

OPHTHALMIC OINTMENT

Vidarabine is indicated for the treatment of acute keratoconjunctivitis and recurrent epithelial keratitis due to Herpes simplex virus types 1 and 2. The clinical diagnosis of keratitis caused by Herpes simplex virus is usually established by the presence of typical dendritic or geographic lesions on slit-lamp examination. It is also effective in superficial keratitis caused by Herpes simplex virus which has not responded to topical idoxuridine or when toxic or hypersensitivity reactions due to idoxuridine have occurred. The effectiveness of vidarabine against stromal keratitis and uveitis due to Herpes simplex virus has not been established.

CONTRAINDICATIONS

Vidarabine is contraindicated in patients who develop hypersensitivity reactions to it.

WARNINGS

INFUSION

Vidarabine should not be administered by the intramuscular or subcutaneous route because of its low solubility and poor absorption.

There are no reports available to indicate that vidarabine for infusion is effective in the management of encephalitis due to varicella-zoster or vaccinia viruses. Vidarabine is not effective against infections caused by adenovirus or RNA viruses. It is also not effective against bacterial or fungal infections. There are no data to support efficacy of vidarabine against cytomegalovirus, vaccinia virus, or smallpox virus.

OPHTHALMIC OINTMENT

Normally, corticosteroids alone are contraindicated in Herpes simplex virus infections of the eye. If vidarabine is administered concurrently with topical corticosteroid therapy, corticosteroid-induced ocular side effects must be considered. These include corticosteroid-induced glaucoma or cataract formation and progression of a bacterial or viral infection.

Vidarabine is not effective against RNA virus or adenoviral ocular infections. It is also not effective against bacterial, fungal, or chlamydial infections of the cornea or nonviral trophic ulcers.

Although viral resistance to vidarabine has not been observed, this possibility may exist.

PRECAUTIONS

GENERAL

Infusion

Treatment should be discontinued in the patient with a brain biopsy negative for Herpes simplex virus in cell culture.

Special care should be exercised when administering vidarabine to patients susceptible to fluid overloading or cerebral edema. Examples are patients with CNS infections and impaired renal function.

Patients with impaired renal function, such as post-operative renal transplant recipients, may have a slower rate of renal excretion of Ara-Hx. Therefore, the dose of vidarabine may need to be adjusted according to the severity of impairment. These patients should be carefully monitored.

Patients with impaired liver function should also be observed for possible adverse effects.

Although clear evidence of adverse experience in humans from simultaneous vidarabine and allopurinol administration has not been reported, laboratory studies indicate that allopurinol may interfere with vidarabine metabolism. Therefore, caution is recommended when administering vidarabine to patients receiving allopurinol.

Ophthalmic Ointment

The diagnosis of keratoconjunctivitis due to Herpes simplex virus should be established clinically prior to prescribing vidarabine.

Patients should be forewarned that vidarabine like any ophthalmic ointment, may produce a temporary visual haze.

LABORATORY TESTS

Infusion

Appropriate hematologic tests are recommended during vidarabine administration since hemoglobin, hematocrit, white blood cells, and platelets may be depressed during therapy.

Some degree of immunocompetence must be present in order for vidarabine to achieve clinical response.

CARCINOGENESIS, MUTAGENESIS, AND IMPAIRMENT OF FERTILITY

Carcinogenesis

Chronic parenteral (IM) studies of vidarabine have been conducted in mice and rats.

In the mouse study, there was a statistically significant increase in liver tumor incidence among the vidarabine-treated females. In the same study, some vidarabine-treated male mice developed kidney neoplasia. No renal tumors were found in the vehicle-treated control mice or the vidarabine-treated female mice.

In the rat study, intestinal, testicular, and thyroid neoplasia occurred with greater frequency among the vidarabine-treated animals than in the vehicle-treated controls. The increases in thyroid adenoma incidence in the high-dose (50 mg/kg) males and the low-dose (30 mg/kg) females were statistically significant.

Hepatic megalocytosis, associated with vidarabine treatment, has been found in short- and long-term rodent (rat and mouse) studies. It is not clear whether or not this represents a preneoplastic change.

The recommended frequency and duration of administration should not be exceeded (see DOSAGE AND ADMINISTRATION).

Mutagenesis

Results of *in vitro* experiments indicate that vidarabine can be incorporated into mammalian DNA and can induce mutation in mammalian cells (mouse L5178Y cell line). Thus far, *in vivo* studies have not been as conclusive, but there is some evidence (dominant lethal assay in mice) that vidarabine may be capable of producing mutagenic effects in male germ cells.

It has also been reported that vidarabine causes chromosome breaks and gaps when added to human leukocytes *in vitro*. While the significance of these effects in terms of mutagenicity is not fully understood, there is a well-known correlation between the ability of various agents to produce such effects and their ability to produce heritable genetic damage.

PREGNANCY CATEGORY C

Infusion

Vidarabine given parenterally is teratogenic in rats and rabbits. Doses of 5 mg/kg or higher given intramuscularly to pregnant rabbits during organogenesis induced fetal abnormalities. Doses of 3 mg/kg or less did not induce teratogenic changes in pregnant rabbits. Vidarabine doses ranging from 30-250 mg/kg were given intramuscularly to pregnant rats during organogenesis; signs of maternal toxicity were induced at doses of 100 mg/kg or higher and frank fetal anomalies were found at doses of 150-250 mg/kg.

A safe dose for the human embryo or fetus has not been established.

There are no adequate and well controlled studies in pregnant women, vidarabine should be used during pregnancy only if the potential benefit justifies the potential risk to the fetus.

Ophthalmic Ointment

Vidarabine parenterally is teratogenic in rats and rabbits. Ten percent (10%) vidarabine ointment applied to 10% of the body surface during organogenesis induced fetal abnormalities in rabbits. When 10% vidarabine ointment was applied to 2-3% of the body surface of rabbits, no fetal abnormalities were found. This dose greatly exceeds the total recommended ophthalmic dose in humans. The possibility of embryonic or fetal damage in pregnant women receiving vidarabine is remote. The topical ophthalmic dose is small, and the drug relatively insoluble. Its ocular penetration is very low. However, a safe dose for a human embryo or fetus has not been established. There are no adequate and well-controlled studies in pregnant women. Vidarabine should be used during pregnancy only of the potential benefit justifies the potential risk to the fetus.

NURSING MOTHERS

It is not known whether vidarabine is secreted in human milk. Because many drugs are excreted in human milk and because of the potential tumorigenicity shown for vidarabine in animal studies, a decision should be made whether to discontinue nursing or to discontinue the drug, taking into account the importance of the drug to the mother.

Ophthalmic Ointment Only: However, breast milk excretion is unlikely because vidarabine is rapidly deaminated in the gastrointestinal tract.

PEDIATRIC USE

Ophthalmic Ointment Only: The safety and effectiveness in pediatric patients below the age of 2 years have not been established.

ADVERSE REACTIONS

INFUSION

The principal adverse reactions involve the gastrointestinal tract and are anorexia, nausea, vomiting, and diarrhea. These reactions are mild to moderate, and seldom require termination of vidarabine therapy.

CNS disturbances have been reported at therapeutic doses. These are tremor, dizziness, hallucinations, confusion, psychosis, and ataxia.

Hematologic clinical laboratory changes noted in controlled and uncontrolled studies were a decrease in hemoglobin or hematocrit, white blood cell count, and platelet count. SGOT elevations were also observed. Other changes occasionally observed were decreases in reticulocyte count and elevated total bilirubin.

Other symptoms which have been reported are weight loss, malaise, pruritus, rash, hematemesis, and pain at the injection site.

OPHTHALMIC OINTMENT

Lacrimation, foreign body sensation, conjunctival injection, burning, irritation, superficial punctate keratitis, pain, photophobia, punctal occlusion, and sensitivity have been reported with vidarabine. The following have also been reported but appear disease-related: uveitis, stromal edema, secondary glaucoma, trophic defects, corneal vascularization, and hyphema.

DOSAGE AND ADMINISTRATION

INFUSION

CAUTION — THE CONTENTS OF THE VIAL MUST BE DILUTED IN AN APPROPRIATE INTRAVENOUS SOLUTION PRIOR TO ADMINISTRATION. RAPID OR BOLUS INJECTION MUST BE AVOIDED.

Dosage: Herpes simplex virus encephalitis — 15 mg/kg/day for 10 days.

Method of Preparation: Each 5 ml vial contains 1 gram of vidarabine (200 mg/ml of suspension). The solubility of vidarabine in intravenous infusion fluids is limited. Each 1 mg of vidarabine requires 2.22 ml of intravenous infusion fluid for complete solubilization. Therefore, each 1 L of intravenous infusion fluid will solubilize a maximum of 450 mg of vidarabine.

Any appropriate intravenous solution is suitable for use as a diluent*EXCEPT* biologic or colloidal fluids (*e.g.*, blood products, protein solutions, etc.).

Shake the vidarabine vial well to obtain a homogeneous suspension before measuring and transferring.

Prepare the vidarabine solution for intravenous administration by aseptically transferring the proper dose of vidarabine into an appropriate intravenous infusion fluid. The intravenous infusion fluid used to prepare the vidarabine solution should be prewarmed to 35-40°C (95-100°F) to facilitate solution of the drug following its transference. Depending on the dose to be given, more than 1 L of intravenous infusion fluid may be required. Thoroughly agitate the prepared admixture until*completely* clear. Complete solubilization of the drug, as indicated by a completely clear solution, is ascertained by careful visual inspection. Final filtration with an in-line membrane filter (0.45 μ pore size or smaller) is necessary.

Dilution should be made just prior to administration and used at least within 48 hours. Subsequent agitation, shaking, or inversion of the bottle is unnecessary once the drug is completely in solution. DO NOT REFRIGERATE THE DILUTION.

Administration: Using aseptic technique, slowly infuse the total daily dose by intravenous infusion (prepared as discussed above) at a constant rate over a 12-24 hour period.

OPHTHALMIC OINTMENT

Administer approximately one-half inch of vidarabine into the lower conjunctival sac 5 times daily at 3 hour intervals.

If there are no signs of improvement after 7 days, or complete re-epithelialization has not occurred by 21 days, other forms of therapy should be considered. Some severe cases may require longer treatment.

Too frequent administration should be avoided.

After re-epithelialization has occurred, treatment for an additional 7 days at a reduced dosage (such as twice daily) is recommended in order to prevent recurrence.

The following topical antibiotics: gentamicin, erythromycin, chloramphenicol; or topical steroids: prednisolone or dexamethasone have been administered concurrently with vidarabine.

ANIMAL PHARMACOLOGY

INFUSION

Acute Toxicity

The Intraperitoneal LD_{50} for vidarabine ranged from 3890-4500 mg/kg in mice, and from 2239-2512 mg/kg in rats, suggesting a low order of toxicity to a single parenteral dose. Hepatic megalocytosis was observed in rats after single, intraperitoneal injections at doses near and exceeding the LD_{50} value. The hepatic megalocytosis appeared to regress completely over several months. Acute intravenous LD_{50} values could not be obtained because of the limited solubility of vidarabine.

Subacute Toxicity

Rats, dogs, and monkeys have been given daily intramuscular injections of vidarabine as a 20% suspension for 28 days. These animal species showed dose related decreases in hemoglobin, hematocrit, and lymphocytes. Bone marrow depression was also observed in monkeys. Except for localized, injection-site injury and weight gain inhibition or loss, rats tolerated daily doses up to 150 mg/kg, and dogs tolerated daily doses up to 50 mg/kg. Megalocytosis was not seen in the rats dosed by the intramuscular route for 28 days. Rhesus monkeys were particularly sensitive to vidarabine. Daily intramuscular doses of 15 mg/kg were tolerable, but doses of 25 mg/kg or higher induced progressively severe clinical signs of CNS toxicity. Three (3) monkeys given slow intravenous infusions of vidarabine in solution at a dose of 15 mg/kg daily for 28 days had no significant adverse reactions.

HOW SUPPLIED

OPHTHALMIC OINTMENT

The Vira-A Ophthalmic Ointment base isa 60:40 mixture of solid and liquid petrolatum.

Storage: Store at room temperature 15-30°C (59-86°F).

PRODUCT LISTING - EQUIVALENTS NOT AVAILABLE

Ointment - Ophthalmic - 3%

3.50 gm $27.05 VIRA-A, Monarch Pharmaceuticals Inc 61570-0367-71

Vinblastine Sulfate *(002427)*

Categories: Carcinoma, breast; Carcinoma, embryonal cell; Carcinoma, testicular; Choriocarcinoma; Histiocytosis X; Lymphoma, histiocytic; Lymphoma, Hodgkin's; Lymphoma, lymphocytic; Mycosis fungoides; Sarcoma, Kaposi's; Teratocarcinoma; Pregnancy Category D; FDA Approved 1961 Mar; WHO Formulary
Drug Classes: Antineoplastics, antimitotics
Brand Names: **Velban**; Velsar
Foreign Brand Availability: Blastovin (Israel); Cytoblastin (India); Lemblastine (Mexico); Velbe (Australia; Austria; Belgium; Benin; Bulgaria; Burkina-Faso; Canada; China; Czech-Republic; Denmark; England; Ethiopia; Finland; France; Gambia; Germany; Ghana; Greece; Guinea; Ireland; Italy; Ivory-Coast; Kenya; Liberia; Malawi; Malaysia; Mali; Mauritania; Mauritius; Morocco; Netherlands; Niger; Nigeria; Norway; Peru; Poland; Portugal; Senegal; Seychelles; Sierra-Leone; Slovenia; Sudan; Sweden; Switzerland; Tanzania; Tunia; Uganda; Zambia; Zimbabwe)
HCFA JCODE(S): J9360 1 mg IV

WARNING

Caution: This preparation should be administered by individuals experienced in the administration of vinblastine sulfate. It is extremely important that the intravenous needle or catheter be properly positioned before any vinblastine sulfate is injected. Leakage into surrounding tissue during intravenous administration of vinblastine sulfate may cause considerable irritation. If extravasation occurs, the injection should be discontinued immediately, and any remaining portion of the dose should then be introduced into another vein. Local injection of hyaluronidase and the application of moderate heat to the area of leakage help disperse the drug and are thought to minimize discomfort and the possibility of cellulitis.

FATAL IF GIVEN INTRATHECALLY. FOR INTRAVENOUS USE ONLY.

See WARNINGS for the treatment of patients given intrathecal vinblastine sulfate.

DESCRIPTION

Velban (vinblastine sulfate for injection) is vincaleukoblastine, sulfate (1:1) (salt). It is the salt of an alkaloid extracted from *Vinca rosea* Linn, a common flowering herb known as the periwinkle (more properly known as *Catharanthus roseus* G. Don). Previously, the generic name was vincaleukoblastine, abbreviated VLB. It is a stathmokinetic oncolytic agent. When treated *in vitro* with this preparation, growing cells are arrested in metaphase.

Chemical and physical evidence indicate that vinblastine sulfate has the empirical formula $C_{46}H_{58}N_4O_9 \cdot H_2SO_4$ and that it is a dimeric alkaloid containing both indole and dihydroindole moieties. It has a molecular weight of 909.07.

Vinblastine sulfate is a white to off-white powder. It is freely soluble in water, soluble in methanol, and slightly soluble in ethanol. It is insoluble in benzene, ether, and naphtha. The clinical formulation is supplied in a sterile form for intravenous use only. Vials of Velban contain 10 mg (0.011 mmol) of vinblastine sulfate, in the form of a white, amorphous, solid lyophilized plug, without excipients. After reconstitution with sodium chloride solution, the pH of the resulting solution lies in the range of 3.5 to 5.

CLINICAL PHARMACOLOGY

Experimental data indicate that the action of vinblastine sulfate is different from that of other recognized antineoplastic agents. Tissue-culture studies suggest an interference with metabolic pathways of amino acids leading from glutamic acid to the citric acid cycle and to urea. *In vivo* experiments tend to confirm the *in vitro* results. A number of studies *in vitro* and *in vivo* have demonstrated that vinblastine sulfate produces a stathmokinetic effect and various atypical mitotic figures. The therapeutic responses, however, are not fully explained, by the cytologic changes, since these changes are sometimes observed clinically and experimentally in the absence of any oncolytic effects.

Reversal of the antitumor effect of vinblastine sulfate by glutamic acid or tryptophan has been observed. In addition, glutamic acid and aspartic acid have protected mice from lethal doses of vinblastine sulfate. Aspartic acid was relatively ineffective in reversing the antitumor effect.

Other studies indicate that vinblastine sulfate has an effect on cell-energy production required for mitosis and interferes with nucleic acid synthesis. The mechanism of action of vinblastine sulfate has been related to the inhibition of microtubule formation in the mitotic spindle, resulting in an arrest of dividing cells at the metaphase stage.

Pharmacokinetic studies in patients with cancer have shown a triphasic serum decay pattern following rapid intravenous injection. The initial, middle, and terminal half-lives are 3.7 minutes, 1.6 hours, and 24.8 hours respectively. The volume of the central compartment is 70% of body weight, probably reflecting very rapid tissue binding to formed elements of the blood. Extensive reversible tissue binding occurs. Low body stores are present at 48 and 72 hours after injection. Since the major route of excretion may be through the biliary system, toxicity from this drug may be increased when there is hepatic excretory insufficiency. The metabolism of vinca alkaloids has been shown to be mediated by hepatic cytochrome P450 isoenzymes in the CYP 3A subfamily. This metabolic pathway may be impaired in patients with hepatic dysfunction or who are taking concomitant potent inhibitors of these isoenzymes such as erythromycin. Enhanced toxicity has been reported in patients receiving concomitant erythromycin (see PRECAUTIONS). Following injection of tritiated vinblastine in the human cancer patient, 10% of the radioactivity was found in the feces and 14% in the urine; the remaining activity was not accounted for. Similar studies in dogs demonstrated that, over 9 days, 30-36% of radioactivity was found in the bile and 12-17% in the urine. A similar study in the rat demonstrated that the highest concentrations of radioactivity were found in the lung, liver, spleen, and kidney 2 hours after injection.

HEMATOLOGIC EFFECTS

Clinically, leukopenia is an expected effect of vinblastine sulfate, and the level of the leukocyte count is an important guide to therapy with this drug. In general, the larger the dose employed, the more profound and longer lasting the leukopenia will be. The fact that the white-blood-cell count returns to normal levels after drug-induced leukopenia is an indication that the white-cell-producing mechanism is not permanently depressed. Usually, the white count has completely returned to normal after the virtual disappearance of white cells from the peripheral blood.

Following therapy with vinblastine sulfate, the nadir in white-blood-cell count may be expected to occur 5-10 days after the last day of drug administration. Recovery of the white blood count is fairly rapid thereafter and is usually complete within another 7-14 days. With the smaller doses employed for maintenance therapy, leukopenia may not be a problem.

Although the thrombocyte count ordinarily is not significantly lowered by therapy with vinblastine sulfate, patients whose bone marrow has been recently impaired by prior therapy with radiation or with other oncolytic drugs may show thrombocytopenia (less than 200,000 platelets/mm^3). When other chemotherapy or radiation has not been employed previously, thrombocyte reduction below the level of 200,000/mm^3 is rarely encountered, even when vinblastine sulfate may be causing significant leukopenia. Rapid recovery from thrombocytopenia within a few days is the rule.

The effect of vinblastine sulfate upon the red-cell count and hemoglobin is usually insignificant when other therapy does not complicate the picture. It should be remembered, however, that patients with malignant disease may exhibit anemia even in the absence of any therapy.

INDICATIONS AND USAGE

Vinblastine sulfate is indicated in the palliative treatment of the following:

1. ***Frequently Responsive Malignancies:***
   - Generalized Hodgkin's disease (Stages III and IV, Ann Arbor modification of Rye staging system).
   - Lymphocytic lymphoma (nodular and diffuse, poorly and well differentiated).
   - Histiocytic lymphoma.
   - Mycosis fungoides (advanced stages).
   - Advanced carcinoma of the testis.
   - Kaposi's sarcoma.
   - Letterer-Siwe disease (histiocytosis X).
2. ***Less Frequently Responsive Malignancies:***
   - Choriocarcinoma resistant to other chemotherapeutic agents.
   - Carcinoma of the breast, unresponsive to appropriate endocrine surgery and hormonal therapy.

Current principles of chemotherapy for many types of cancer include the concurrent administration of several antineoplastic agents. For enhanced therapeutic effect without additive toxicity, agents with different dose-limiting clinical toxicities and different mechanisms of action are generally selected. Therefore, although vinblastine sulfate is effective as a single agent in the aforementioned indications, it is usually administered in combination with other antineoplastic drugs. Such combination therapy produces a greater percentage of response than does a single-agent regimen. These principles have been applied, for example, in the chemotherapy of Hodgkin's disease.

HODGKIN'S DISEASE

Vinblastine sulfate has been shown to be one of the most effective single agents for the treatment of Hodgkin's disease. Advanced Hodgkin's disease has also been successfully treated with several multiple-drug regimens that included vinblastine sulfate. Patients who had relapses after treatment with the MOPP program — mechiorethamine hydrochloride (nitrogen mustard), vincristine sulfate (Oncovin), prednisone, and procarbazine — have likewise responded to combination-drug therapy that included vinblastine sulfate. A protocol using cyclophosphamide in place of nitrogen mustard and vinblastine sulfate instead of vincristine sulfate is an alternative therapy for previously untreated patients with advanced Hodgkin's disease.

Advanced testicular germinal-cell cancers (embryonal carcinoma, teratocarcinoma, and choriocarcinoma) are sensitive to vinblastine sulfate alone, but better clinical results are achieved when vinblastine sulfate is administered concomitantly with other antineoplastic agents. The effect of bleomycin is significantly enhanced if vinblastine sulfate is administered 6-8 hours prior to the administration of bleomycin; this schedule permits more cells to be arrested during metaphase, the stage of the cell cycle in which bleomycin is active.

NON-FDA APPROVED INDICATIONS

The drug has also been used without FDA approval in the treatment of bladder cancer, melanoma, cervical cancer, non-small cell lung cancer and head and neck cancer.

CONTRAINDICATIONS

Vinblastine sulfate is contraindicated in patients who have significant granulocytopenia unless this is a result of the disease being treated. It should not be used in the presence of bacterial infections. Such infections must be brought under control prior to the initiation of therapy with vinblastine sulfate.

WARNINGS

This preparation is for intravenous use only. It should be administered by individuals experienced in the administration of vinblastine sulfate. The intrathecal administration of vinblastine sulfate usually results in death. Syringes containing this product should be labeled, using the auxiliary sticker provided, to state "FATAL IF GIVEN INTRATHECALLY. FOR INTRAVENOUS USE ONLY."

Extemporaneously prepared syringes containing this product must be packaged in an overwrap which is labeled 'DO NOT REMOVE COVERING UNTIL MOMENT OF INJECTION. FATAL IF GIVEN INTRATHECALLY. FOR INTRAVENOUS USE ONLY.'

After inadvertent intrathecal administration of vinca alkaloids, immediate neurosurgical intervention is required in order to prevent ascending paralysis leading to death. In a very small number of patients, life-threatening paralysis and subsequent death was averted but resulted in devastating neurological sequelae, with limited recovery afterwards.

There are no published cases of survival following intrathecal administration of vinblastine sulfate to base treatment on. However, based on the published management of survival cases involving the related vinca alkaloid vincristine sulfate,1-3 if vinblastine sulfate is mistakenly given by the intrathecal route, the following treatment should be initiated immediately after the injection:

1. Removal of as much CSF as is safely possible through the lumbar access.

V

Cont'd

2. **Insertion of an epidural catheter into the subarachnoid space via the intervertebral space above initial lumbar access and CSF irrigation with lactated Ringer's solution. Fresh frozen plasma should be requested and, when available, 25 ml should be added to every 1 liter of lactated Ringer's solution.**
3. **Insertion of an intraventricular drain or catheter by a neurosurgeon and continuation of CSF irrigation with fluid removal through the lumbar access connected to a closed drainage system. Lactated Ringer's solution should be given by continuous infusion at 150 ml/h, or at a rate of 75 ml/h when fresh frozen plasma has been added as above.The rate of infusion should be adjusted to maintain a spinal fluid protein level of 150 mg/dl.The following measures have also been used in addition but may not be essential: Glutamic acid, 10 g, has been given intravenously over 24 hours, followed by 500 mg three times daily by mouth for 1 month. Folinic acid has been administered intravenously as a 100 mg bolus and then infused at a rate of 25 mg/h for 24 hours, then bolus doses of 25 mg every 6 hours for 1 week. Pyridoxine has been given at a dose of 50 mg every 8 hours by intravenous infusion over 30 minutes. Their roles in the reduction of neurotoxicity are unclear.**

PREGNANCY CATEGORY D

Caution is necessary with the administration of all oncolytic drugs during pregnancy. Information on the use of vinblastine sulfate during human pregnancy is very limited. Animal studies with vinblastine sulfate suggest that teratogenic effects may occur. Vinblastine sulfate can cause fetal harm when administered to a pregnant woman. Laboratory animals given this drug early in pregnancy suffer resorption of the conceptus: surviving fetuses demonstrate gross deformities. There are no adequate and well-controlled studies in pregnant women. If this drug is used during pregnancy, or if the patient becomes pregnant while receiving this drug, she should be apprised of the potential hazard to the fetus. Women of childbearing potential should be advised to avoid becoming pregnant.

Aspermia has been reported in man. Animal studies show metaphase arrest and degenerative changes in germ cells.

Leukopenia (granulocytopenia) may reach dangerously low levels following administration of the higher recommended doses. It is therefore important to follow the dosage technique recommended in DOSAGE AND ADMINISTRATION. Stomatitis and neurologic toxicity, although not common or permanent, can be disabling.

PRECAUTIONS

GENERAL

Toxicity may be enhanced in the presence of hepatic insufficiency.

If leukopenia with less than 2000 white blood cells/mm^3 occurs following a dose of vinblastine sulfate, the patient should be watched carefully for evidence of infection until the white-blood-cell count has returned to a safe level.

When cachexia or ulcerated areas of the skin surface are present, there may be a more profound leukopenic response to the drug; therefore, its use should be avoided in older persons suffering from either of these conditions.

In patients with malignant-cell infiltration of the bone marrow, the leukocyte and platelet counts have sometimes fallen precipitously after moderate doses of vinblastine sulfate. Further use of the drug in such patients is inadvisable.

Acute shortness of breath and severe bronchospasm have been reported following the administration of vinca alkaloids. These reactions have been encountered most frequently when the vinca alkaloid was used in combination with mitomycin C and may require aggressive treatment, particularly when there is pre-existing pulmonary dysfunction. The onset may be within minutes or several hours after the vinca is injected and may occur up to 2 weeks following a dose of mitomycin. Progressive dyspnea requiring chronic therapy may occur. Vinblastine sulfate should not be readministered.

The use of small amounts of vinblastine sulfate daily for long periods is not advised, even though the resulting total weekly dosage may be similar to that recommended. Little or no added therapeutic effect has been demonstrated when such regimens have been used. *Strict adherence to the recommended dosage schedule is very important.* When amounts equal to several times the recommended weekly dosage were given in 7 daily installments for long periods, convulsions, severe and permanent central-nervous-system damage, and even death occurred.

Care must be taken to avoid contamination of the eye with concentrations of vinblastine sulfate used clinically. If accidental contamination occurs, severe irritation (or, if the drug was delivered under pressure, even corneal ulceration) may result. The eye should be washed with water immediately and thoroughly.

It is not necessary to use preservative-containing solvents if unused portions of the remaining solutions are discarded immediately. Unused preservative-containing solutions should be refrigerated for future use.

INFORMATION FOR THE PATIENT

The patient should be warned to report immediately the appearance of sore throat, fever, chills, or sore mouth. Advice should be given to avoid constipation, and the patient should be made aware that alopecia may occur and that jaw pain and pain in the organs containing tumor tissue may occur. The latter is thought possibly to result from swelling of tumor tissue during its response to treatment. Scalp hair will regrow to its pretreatment extent even with continued treatment with vinblastine sulfate. Nausea and vomiting, although not common, may occur. Any other serious medical event should be reported to the physician.

LABORATORY TESTS

Since dose-limiting clinical toxicity is the result of depression of the white-blood-cell count, it is imperative that this count be obtained just before the planned dose of vinblastine sulfate. Following administration of vinblastine sulfate, a fall in the white-blood-cell count may occur. The nadir of this fall is observed from 5-10 days following a dose. Recovery to pretreatment levels is usually observed from 7-14 days after treatment. These effects will be exaggerated when preexisting bone marrow damage is present and also with the higher recommended doses (see DOSAGE AND ADMINISTRATION). The presence of this drug or its metabolites in blood or body tissues is not known to interfere with clinical laboratory tests.

V

CARCINOGENESIS, MUTAGENESIS, AND IMPAIRMENT OF FERTILITY

Aspermia has been reported in man. Animal studies suggest that teratogenic effects may occur. See WARNINGS regarding impaired fertility. Animal studies have shown metaphase arrest and degenerative changes in germ cells. Amenorrhea has occurred in some patients treated with the combination consisting of an alkylating agent, procarbazine, prednisone, and vinblastine sulfate. Its occurrence was related to the total dose of these 4 agents used. Recovery of menses was frequent. The same combination of drugs given to male patients produced azoospermia; if spermatogenesis did return, it was not likely to do so with less than 2 years of unmaintained remission.

Mutagenicity

Tests in *Salmonella typhimurium* and with the dominant lethal assay in mice failed to demonstrate mutagenicity. Sperm abnormalities have been noted in mice. Vinblastine sulfate has produced an increase in micronuclei formation in bone marrow cells of mice; however, since vinblastine sulfate inhibits mitotic spindle formation, it cannot be concluded that this is evidence of mutagenicity. Additional studies in mice demonstrated no reduction in fertility of males. Chromosomal translocations did occur in male mice. First-generation male offspring of these mice were not heterozygous translocation carriers.

In vitro tests using hamster lung cells in culture have produced chromosomal changes, including chromatid breaks and exchanges, whereas tests using another type of hamster cell failed to demonstrate mutation. Breaks and aberrations were not observed on chromosome analysis of marrow cells from patients being treated with this drug.

It is not clear from the literature how this drug affects synthesis of DNA and RNA. Some believe that there is no interference. Others believe that vinblastine interferes with nucleic acid metabolism but may not do so by direct effect but possibly as the result of biochemical disturbance in some other part of the molecular organization of the cell. No inhibition of RNA synthesis occurred in rat hepatoma cells exposed in culture to noncytotoxic levels of vinblastine. Conflicting results have been noted by others regarding interference with DNA synthesis.

Carcinogenesis

There is no currently available evidence to indicate that vinblastine sulfate itself has been carcinogenic in humans since the inception of its clinical use in the late 1950s. Patients treated for Hodgkin's disease have developed leukemia following radiation therapy and administration of vinblastine sulfate in combination with other chemotherapy including agents known to intercalate with DNA. It is not known to what extent vinblastine sulfate may have contributed to the appearance of leukemia. Available data in rats and mice have failed to demonstrate clearly evidence of carcinogenesis when the animals were treated with the maximum tolerated dose and with one half that dose for 6 months. This testing system demonstrated that other agents were clearly carcinogenic, whereas vinblastine sulfate was in the group of drugs causing slightly increased or the same tumor incidence as controls in one study and 1.5- to 2-fold increase in tumor incidence over controls in another study.

USAGE IN PREGNANCY — PREGNANCY CATEGORY D

See WARNINGS.

Vinblastine sulfate should be given to a pregnant woman only if clearly needed. Animal studies suggest that teratogenic effects may occur.

PEDIATRIC USE

The dosage schedule for pediatric patients is indicated under DOSAGE AND ADMINISTRATION.

NURSING MOTHERS

It is not known whether this drug is excreted in human milk. Because many drugs are excreted in human milk and because of the potential for serious adverse reactions from vinblastine sulfate in nursing infants, a decision should be made whether to discontinue nursing or the drug, taking into account the importance of the drug to the mother.

DRUG INTERACTIONS

Solutions should be made with normal saline (with or without preservative) and should not be combined in the same container with any other chemical. Unused portions of the remaining solutions that do not contain preservatives should be discarded immediately.

The simultaneous oral or intravenous administration of phenytoin and antineoplastic chemotherapy combinations that included vinblastine sulfate has been reported to have reduced blood levels of the anticonvulsant and to have increased seizure activity. Dosage adjustment should be based on serial blood level monitoring. The contribution of vinblastine sulfate to this interaction is not certain. The interaction may result from either reduced absorption of phenytoin or an increase in the rate of its metabolism and elimination.

Caution should be exercised in patients concurrently taking drugs known to inhibit drug metabolism by hepatic cytochrome P450 isoenzymes in the CYP 3A subfamily, or in patients with hepatic dysfunction. Concurrent administration of vinblastine sulfate with an inhibitor of this metabolic pathway may cause an earlier onset and/or an increased severity of side effects. Enhanced toxicity has been reported in patients receiving concomitant erythromycin (see ADVERSE REACTIONS).

ADVERSE REACTIONS

Prior to the use of the drug, patients should be advised of the possibility of untoward symptoms.

In general, the incidence of adverse reactions attending the use of vinblastine sulfate appears to be related to the size of the dose employed. With the exception of epilation, leukopenia, and neurologic side effects, adverse reactions generally have not persisted for longer than 24 hours. Neurologic side effects are not common; but when they do occur, they often last for more than 24 hours. Leukopenia, the most common adverse reaction, is usually the dose-limiting factor.

The following are manifestations that have been reported as adverse reactions, in decreasing order of frequency. The most common adverse reactions are underlined:

Hematologic: Leukopenia (granulocytopenia), anemia, thrombocytopenia (myelosuppression).

Dermatologic: Alopecia is common. A single case of light sensitivity associated with this product has been reported.

Gastrointestinal: Constipation, anorexia, nausea, vomiting, abdominal pain, ileus, vesiculation of the mouth, pharyngitis, diarrhea, hemorrhagic enterocolitis, bleeding from an old peptic ulcer, rectal bleeding.

Neurologic: Numbness of digits (paresthesias), loss of deep tendon reflexes, peripheral neuritis, mental depression, headache, convulsions.

Treatment with vinca alkaloids has resulted rarely in both vestibular and auditory damage to the eighth cranial nerve. Manifestations include partial or total deafness which may be temporary or permanent, and difficulties with balance including dizziness, nystagmus, and vertigo. Particular caution is warranted when vinblastine sulfate is used in combination with other agents known to be ototoxic such as the platinum-containing oncolytics.

Cardiovascular: Hypertension. Cases of unexpected myocardial infarction and cerebrovascular accidents have occurred in patients undergoing combination chemotherapy with vinblastine, bleomycin, and cisplatin. Raynaud's phenomenon has also been reported with this combination.

Pulmonary: See PRECAUTIONS.

Miscellaneous: Malaise, bone pain, weakness, pain in tumor-containing tissue, dizziness, jaw pain, skin vesiculation, hypertension, Raynaud's phenomenon when patients are being treated with vinblastine sulfate in combination with bleomycin and cis-platinum for testicular cancer. The syndrome of inappropriate secretion of antidiuretic hormone has occurred with higher than recommended doses.

Nausea and vomiting usually may be controlled with ease by antiemetic agents. When epilation develops, it frequently is not total; and, in some cases, hair regrows while maintenance therapy continues.

Extravasation during intravenous injection may lead to cellulitis and phlebitis. If the amount of extravasation is great, sloughing may occur.

DOSAGE AND ADMINISTRATION

This preparation is for intravenous use only (see WARNINGS).

SPECIAL DISPENSING INFORMATION

WHEN DISPENSING VELBAN IN OTHER THAN THE ORIGINAL CONTAINER, IT IS IMPERATIVE THAT IT BE PACKAGED IN AN OVERWRAP BEARING THE STATEMENT: "DO NOT REMOVE COVERING UNTIL MOMENT OF INJECTION. FATAL IF GIVEN INTRATHECALLY. FOR INTRAVENOUS USE ONLY" (see WARNINGS).

A syringe containing a specific dose must be labeled, using fhe auxiliary sticker provided, to state "FATAL IF GIVEN INTRATHECALLY. FOR INTRAVENOUS USE ONLY."

Caution: *It is extremely important that the needle be properly positioned in the vein before this product is injected. If leakage into surrounding tissue should occur during intravenous administration of vinblastine sulfate, it may cause considerable irritation. The injection should be discontinued immediately, and any remaining portion of the dose should then be introduced into another vein. Local injection of hyaluronidase and the application of moderate heat to the area of leakage help disperse the drug and are thought to minimize discomfort and the possibility of cellulitis.*

There are variations in the depth of the leukopenic response that follows therapy with vinblastine sulfate. For this reason, it is recommended that the drug be given no more frequently than once every 7 days.

ADULT PATIENTS

It is wise to initiate therapy for adults by administering a single intravenous dose of 3.7 mg/m^2 of body surface area (bsa). Thereafter, white-blood-cell counts should be made to determine the patient's sensitivity to vinblastine sulfate.

A simplified and conservative incremental approach to dosage at *weekly intervals* for adults may be outlined as follows (see TABLE 1).

TABLE 1

First dose	3.7 mg/m^2 bsa
Second dose	5.5 mg/m^2 bsa
Third dose	7.4 mg/m^2 bsa
Fourth dose	9.25 mg/m^2 bsa
Fifth dose	11.1 mg/m^2 bsa

The above mentioned increases may be used until a maximum dose not exceeding 18.5 mg/m^2 bsa for adults is reached. The dose should not be increased after that dose which reduces the white-cell count to approximately 3000 cells/mm^3. In some adults, 3.7 mg/m^2 bsa may produce this leukopenia; other adults may require more than 11.1 mg/m^2 bsa; and, very rarely, as much as 18.5 mg/m^2 bsa may be necessary. For most adult patients, however, the weekly dose will prove to be 5.5-7.4 mg/m^2 bsa.

When the dose of vinblastine sulfate which will produce the above degree of leukopenia has been established, a dose of *1 increment smaller* than this should be administered at weekly intervals for maintenance. Thus, the patient is receiving the maximum dose that does not cause leukopenia. *It should be emphasized that, even though 7 days have elapsed, the next dose of vinblastine sulfate should not be given until the white-cell count has returned to at least 4000/mm^3.* In some cases, oncolytic activity may be encountered before leukopenic effect. When this occurs, there is no need to increase the size of subsequent doses (see PRECAUTIONS).

PEDIATRIC PATIENTS

A review of published literature from 1993-1995 showed that initial doses of vinblastine sulfate in pediatric patients varied depending on the schedule used and whether vinblastine sulfate was administered as a single agent or incorporated within a particular chemotherapeutic regimen. As a single agent for Letterer-Siwe disease (histiocytosis X), the initial dose of vinblastine sulfate was reported as 6.5 mg/m^2. When vinblastine sulfate was used in combination with other chemotherapeutic agents for the treatment of Hodgkin's disease, the initial dose was reported as 6 mg/m^2. For testicular germ cell carcinomas, the initial dose of vinblastine sulfate was reported as 3 mg/m^2 in a combination regimen. Dose modifications should be guided by hematologic tolerance.

PATIENTS WITH RENAL OR HEPATIC IMPAIRMENT

A reduction of 50% in the dose of vinblastine sulfate is recommended for patients having a direct serum bilirubin value above 3 mg/100 ml. Since metabolism and excretion are primarily hepatic, no modification is recommended for patients with impaired renal function.

The duration of maintenance therapy varies according to the disease being treated and the combination of antineoplastic agents being used. There are differences of opinion regarding the duration of maintenance therapy with the same protocol for a particular disease; for example, various durations have been used with the MOPP program in treating Hodgkin's disease. Prolonged chemotherapy for maintaining remissions involves several risks, among which are life-threatening infectious diseases, sterility, and possibly the appearance of other cancers through suppression of immune surveillance.

In some disorders, survival following complete remission may not be as prolonged as that achieved with shorter periods of maintenance therapy. On the other hand, failure to provide maintenance therapy in some patients may lead to unnecessary relapse; complete remissions in patients with testicular cancer, unless maintained for at least 2 years, often result in early relapse.

To prepare a solution containing 1 mg of vinblastine sulfate/ml, add 10 ml of bacteriostatic sodium chloride injection (preserved with benzyl alcohol) or 10 ml of sodium chloride injection (unpreserved) to the 10 mg of vinblastine sulfate in the sterile vial. Do not use other solutions. The drug dissolves instantly to give a clear solution.

Parenteral drug products should be inspected visually for particulate matter and discoloration prior to administration, whenever solution and container permit.

Unused portions of the remaining solutions made with normal saline that do not contain preservatives should be discarded immediately. Unused preservative-containing solutions made with normal saline may be stored in a refrigerator for future use for a maximum of 28 days.

The dose of vinblastine sulfate (calculated to provide the desired amount) may be injected either into the tubing of a running intravenous infusion or directly into a vein. The latter procedure is readily adaptable to outpatient therapy. In either case, the injection may be completed in about 1 minute. If care is taken to insure that the needle is securely within the vein and that no solution containing vinblastine sulfate is spilled extravascularly, cellulitis and/or phlebitis will not occur. To minimize further the possibility of extravascular spillage, it is suggested that the syringe and needle be rinsed with venous blood before withdrawal of the needle. The dose should not be diluted in large volumes of diluent (*i.e.,* 100-250 ml) or given intravenously for prolonged periods (ranging from 30-60 minutes or more), since this frequently results in irritation of the vein and increases the chance of extravasation.

Because of the enhanced possibility of thrombosis, it is considered inadvisable to inject a solution of vinblastine sulfate into an extremity in which the circulation is impaired or potentially impaired by such conditions as compressing or invading neoplasm, phlebitis, or varicosity.

Procedures for proper handling and disposal of anticancer drugs should be considered. Several guidelines on this subject have been published.1-7 There is no general agreement that all of the procedures recommended in the guidelines are necessary or appropriate.

SPECIAL DISPENSING INFORMATION

When dispensing vinblastine sulfate in other than the original container, *e.g.,* a syringe containing a specific dose, it is imperative that it be packaged in an overwrap bearing the statement: "DO NOT REMOVE COVERING UNTIL MOMENT OF INJECTION. FATAL IF GIVEN INTRATHECALLY. FOR INTRAVENOUS USE ONLY" (see WARNINGS).

HOW SUPPLIED

Vials of Velban contain 10 mg (0.011 mmol) of vinblastine sulfate, in the form of a white, amorphous, solid lyophilized plug, without excipients.

Storage: The vials should be stored in a refrigerator (2-8°C, or 36-46°F) to assure extended stability.

PRODUCT LISTING - RATED THERAPEUTICALLY EQUIVALENT

Powder For Injection - Intravenous - 10 mg

1's	$37.50	GENERIC, Faulding Pharmaceutical Company	61703-0310-18
1's	$40.54	VELBAN, Lilly, Eli and Company	00002-1452-01
10's	$120.00	GENERIC, Bedford Laboratories	55390-0091-10
25's	$33.13	GENERIC, American Pharmaceutical Partners	63323-0278-10

Vincristine Sulfate (002428)

V

Categories: Leukemia, acute; Lymphoma, Hodgkin's; Lymphoma, non-Hodgkin's; Neuroblastoma; Rhabdomyosarcoma; Wilms' tumor; Pregnancy Category D; FDA Approved 1984 Mar; WHO Formulary

Drug Classes: Antineoplastics, antimitotics

Brand Names: **Oncovin**; Vincasar Pfs; Vincrex

Foreign Brand Availability: Citomid (Mexico); Cytocristin (India); Farmistin CS (Germany); Krebin (Indonesia); Neocristin (India); Vincrisul (Spain); Vintec (Mexico)

HCFA JCODE(S): J9370 1 mg IV; J9375 2 mg IV; J9380 5 mg IV

WARNING

Caution - This preparation should be administered by individuals experienced in the administration of vincristine sulfate. It is extremely important that the intravenous needle or catheter be properly positioned before any vincristine is injected. Leakage into surrounding tissue during intravenous administration of vincristine sulfate may cause considerable irritation. If extravasation occurs, the injection

WARNING — Cont'd

should be discontinued immediately, and any remaining portion of the dose should then be introduced into another vein. Local injection of hyaluronidase and the application of moderate heat to the area of leakage help disperse the drug and are thought to minimize discomfort and the possibility of cellulitis.

FATAL IF GIVEN INTRATHECALLY. FOR INTRAVENOUS USE ONLY.

See WARNINGS for the treatment of patients given intrathecal vincristine sulfate.

DESCRIPTION

Vincristine sulfate is the salt of an alkaloid obtained from a common flowering herb, the periwinkle plant *(Vinca rosea Linn)*. Originally known as leurocristine, it has also been referred to as LCR and VCR. The empirical formula for vincristine sulfate is: $C_{46}H_{56}N_4O_{10} \cdot H_2SO_4$.

It has a molecular weight of 923.04.

Vincristine sulfate is a white to off-white powder. It is soluble in methanol, freely soluble in water, but only slightly soluble in 95% ethanol. In 98% ethanol, vincristine sulfate has an ultraviolet spectrum with maxima at 221 nm (8 + 47,100).

Each ml contains vincristine sulfate, 1 mg (1.08 μmol); mannitol, 100 mg; methylparaben, 1.3 mg; propylparaben, 0.2 mg; and water for injection, qs. Acetic acid and sodium acetate have been added for pH control. The pH of oncovin solution ranges from 3.5-5.5. This product is a sterile solution for cancer/oncolytic use.

Storage: This product should be refrigerated.

CLINICAL PHARMACOLOGY

The mechanisms of action of vincristine sulfate remain under investigation.[1] The mechanism of action of vincristine sulfate has been related to the inhibition of microtubule formation in the mitotic spindle, resulting in an arrest of dividing cells at the metaphase stage.

Central-nervous-system leukemia has been reported in patients undergoing otherwise successful therapy with vincristine sulfate. This suggests that vincristine sulfate does not penetrate well into the cerebrospinal fluid.

Pharmacokinetic studies in patients with cancer have shown a triphasic serum decay pattern following rapid intravenous injection. The initial, middle, and terminal half-lives are 5 minutes, 2.3 hours, and 85 hours respectively; however, the range of the terminal half-life in humans is from 19-155 hours. The liver is the major excretory organ in humans and animals; about 80% of an injected dose of vincristine sulfate appears in the feces and 10-20% can be found in the urine. Within 15-30 minutes after injection, over 90% of the drug is distributed from the blood into tissue, where it remains tightly, but not irreversibly, bound.[2]

Current principles of cancer chemotherapy involve the simultaneous use of several agents. Generally, each agent used has a unique toxicity and mechanism of action so that therapeutic enhancement occurs without additive toxicity. It is rarely possible to achieve equally good results with single-agent methods of treatment. Thus, vincristine sulfate is often chosen as part of polychemotherapy because of lack of significant bone-marrow suppression (at recommended doses) and of unique clinical toxicity (neuropathy). See DOSAGE AND ADMINISTRATION for possible increased toxicity when used in combination therapy.

INDICATIONS AND USAGE

Vincristine sulfate is indicated in acute leukemia.

Vincristine sulfate has also been shown to be useful in combination with other oncolytic agents in Hodgkin's disease,[3] non-Hodgkin's malignant lymphomas[4-6] (lymphocytic, mixed-cell, histiocytic, undifferentiated, nodular, and diffuse types), rhabdomyosarcoma,[7] neuroblastoma,[8] and Wilms' tumor.[9]

NON-FDA APPROVED INDICATIONS

The drug has been used without FDA approval in the treatment of thrombotic thrombocytopenic purpura.

CONTRAINDICATIONS

Patients with the demyelinating form of Charcot-Marie-Tooth syndrome should not be given vincristine sulfate. Careful attention should be given to those conditions listed under WARNINGS and PRECAUTIONS.

WARNINGS

This preparation is for intravenous use only. It should be administered by individuals experienced in the administration of vincristine sulfate. The intrathecal administration of vincristine sulfate usually results in death. Syringes containing this product should be labeled "WARNING—FOR IV USE ONLY."

Extemporaneously prepared syringes containing this product must be packaged in an overwrap which is labeled "DO NOT REMOVE COVERING UNTIL MOMENT OF INJECTION. FATAL IF GIVEN INTRATHECALLY. FOR INTRAVENOUS USE ONLY."

Treatment of patients following intrathecal administration of vincristine sulfate has included immediate removal of spinal fluid and flushing with Lactated Ringer's, as well as other solutions and has not prevented ascending paralysis and death. In one case, progressive paralysis in an adult was arrested by the following treatment initiated immediately after the intrathecal injection:

1. **As much spinal fluid was removed as could be safely done through lumbar access.**
2. **The subarachnoid space was flushed with Lactated Ringer's solution infused continuously through a catheter in a cerebral lateral ventricle at the rate of 150 ml/h. The fluid was removed through a lumbar access.**
3. **As soon as fresh frozen plasma became available, the fresh frozen plasma, 25 ml, diluted in 1 L of Lactated Ringer's solution was infused through the cerebral ventricular catheter at the rate 75 ml/h with removal through the lumbar access. The rate of infusion was adjusted to maintain a protein level in the spinal fluid of 150 mg/dl.**
4. **Glutamic acid, 10 g, was given intravenously over 24 hours followed by 500 mg 3 times daily by mouth for 1 month or until neurological dysfunction stabilized. The role of glutamic acid in this treatment is not certain and may not be essential.**

PREGNANCY CATEGORY D

Vincristine sulfate can cause fetal harm when administered to a pregnant woman. When pregnant mice and hamsters were given doses of vincristine sulfate that caused the resorption of 23-85% of fetuses, fetal malformations were produced in those that survived. Five monkeys were given since doses of vincristine sulfate between days 27 and 34 of their pregnancies; 3 of the fetuses were normal at term, and 2 viable fetuses had grossly evident malformations at term.[10] In several animal species, vincristine sulfate can induce teratogenesis as well as embryo death at doses that are nontoxic to the pregnant animal. There are no adequate and well-controlled studies in pregnant women. If this drug is used during pregnancy or if the patient becomes pregnant while receiving this drug, she should be apprised of the potential hazard to the fetus. Women of childbearing potential should be advised to avoid becoming pregnant.

PRECAUTIONS

GENERAL

Acute uric acid nephropathy, which may occur after the administration of oncolytic agents, has also been reported with vincristine sulfate. In the presence of leukopenia or a complicating infection, administration of the next dose of vincristine sulfate warrants careful consideration.

If central-nervous-system leukemia is diagnosed, additional agents may be required because vincristine sulfate does not appear to cross the blood-brain barrier in adequate amounts.

Particular attention should be given to dosage and neurologic side effects if vincristine sulfate is administered to patients with preexisting neuromuscular disease and when other drugs with neurotoxic potential are also being used.

Acute shortness of breath and severe bronchospasm have been reported following the administration of vinca alkaloids. These reactions have been encountered most frequently when the vinca alkaloid was used in combination with mitomycin-C and may require aggressive treatment, particularly when there is preexisting pulmonary, dysfunction. The onset of these reactions may occur minutes to several hours after the vinca alkaloid is injected and may occur up to 2 weeks following the dose of mitomycin. Progressive dyspnea requiring chronic therapy may occur. Vincristine sulfate should not be read ministered.

Care must be taken to avoid contamination of the eye with concentrations of vincristine sulfate used clinically. If accidental contamination occurs, severe irritation (or, if the drug was delivered under pressure, even corneal ulceration) may result. The eye should be washed immediately and thoroughly.

LABORATORY TESTS

Because dose-limiting clinical toxicity is manifested as neurotoxicity, clinical evaluation (*e.g.*, history, physical examination) is necessary to detect the need for dosage modification. Following administration of vincristine sulfate, some individuals may have a fall in the white-blood-cell count or platelet count, particularly when previous therapy or the disease itself has reduced bone-marrow function. Therefore, a complete blood count should be done before administration of each dose. Acute elevation of serum uric acid may also occur during induction of remission in acute leukemia; thus, such levels should be determined frequently during the first 3-4 weeks of treatment or appropriate measures taken to prevent uric acid nephropathy. The laboratory performing these tests should be consulted for its range of normal values.

CARCINOGENESIS, MUTAGENESIS, AND IMPAIRMENT OF FERTILITY

Neither in vivo nor in vitro laboratory tests have conclusively demonstrated the mutagenicity of this product.[10] Fertility following treatment with vincristine sulfate alone for malignant disease has not been studied in humans. Clinical reports of both male and female patients who received multiple-agent chemotherapy that included vincristine sulfate indicate that azoospermia and amenorrhea can occur in postpubertal patients. Recovery occurred many months after completion of chemotherapy in some but not all patients. When the same treatment is administered to prepubertal patients, permanent azoospermia and amenorrhea are much less likely.[12-18]

Patients who received chemotherapy with vincristine sulfate in combination with anticancer drugs known to be carcinogenic have developed second malignancies. The contributing role of vincristine sulfate in this development has not been determined. No evidence of carcinogenicity was found following intraperitoneal administration of vincristine sulfate in rats and mice, although this study was limited.[10]

PREGNANCY CATEGORY D

See WARNINGS.

NURSING MOTHERS

It is not known whether this drug is excreted in human milk. Because many drugs are excreted in human milk and because of the potential for serious adverse reactions due to vincristine sulfate in nursing infants a decision should be made either to discontinue nursing or the drug, taking into account the importance of the drug to the mother.

DRUG INTERACTIONS

The simultaneous oral or intravenous administration of phenytoin and antineoplastic chemotherapy combinations that included vincristine sulfate has been reported to reduce blood levels of the anticonvulsant and to increase seizure activity.[11] Dosage adjustment should be based on serial blood level monitoring. The contribution of vincristine sulfate to this interaction is not certain. The interaction may result from reduced absorption of phenytoin and an increase in the rate of its metabolism and elimination.

Vincristine sulfate should not be diluted in solutions that raise or lower the pH outside the range of 3.5-5.5. It should not be mixed with anything other than normal saline or glucose in water.

Whenever solution and container permit, parenteral drug products should be inspected visually for particulate matter and discoloration prior to administration.

V

Procedures for proper handling and disposal of anticancer drugs should be considered. Several guidelines on this subject have been published.[20-25] There is no general agreement that all of the procedures recommended in the guidelines are necessary or appropriate.

ADVERSE REACTIONS

Prior to the use of this drug, patients and/or their parents/guardian should be advised of the possibility of untoward symptoms.

In general, adverse reactions are reversible and are related to dosage. The most common adverse reaction is hair loss; the most troublesome adverse reactions are neuromuscular in origin.

When single, weekly doses of the drug are employed, the adverse reactions of leukopenia, neuritic pain, and constipation occur but are usually of short duration (*i.e.*, less than 7 days). When the dosage is reduced, these reactions may lessen or disappear. The severity of such reactions seems to increase when the calculated amount of drug is given in divided doses. Other adverse reactions, such as hair loss, sensory loss, paresthesia, difficulty in walking, slapping gait, loss of deep-tendon reflexes, and muscle wasting, may persist for at least as long as therapy is continued. Generalized sensorimotor dysfunction may become progressively more severe with continued treatment, some neuromuscular difficulties may persist for prolonged periods in some patients. Regrowth of hair may occur while maintenance therapy continues.

The following adverse reactions have been reported:

Hypersensitivity: Rare cases of allergic-type reactions, such as anaphylaxis, rash, and edema, that are temporally related to vincristine therapy have been reported in patients receiving vincristine as a part of multidrug chemotherapy regimens.

Gastrointestinal: Constipation, abdominal cramps, weight loss, nausea, vomiting, oral ulceration, diarrhea, paralytic ileus, intestinal necrosis and/or perforation, and anorexia have occurred. Constipation may take the form of upper-colon impaction, and, on physical examination, the rectum may be empty. Colicky abdominal pain coupled with an empty rectum may mislead the physician. A flat film of the abdomen is useful in demonstrating this condition. All cases have responded to high enemas and laxatives. A routine prophylactic regimen against constipation is recommended for all patients receiving vincristine sulfate. Paralytic ileus (which mimics the "surgical abdomen") may occur, particularly in young children. The ileus will reverse itself with temporary discontinuance of vincristine sulfate and with symptomatic care.

Genitourinary: Polyuria, dysuria, and urinary retention due to bladder atony have occurred. Other drugs known to cause urinary retention (particularly in the elderly) should, if possible, be discontinued for the first few days following administration of vincristine sulfate.

Cardiovascular: Hypertension and hypotension have occurred. Chemotherapy combinations that have included vincristine sulfate, when given to patients previously treated with mediastinal radiation, have been associated with coronary artery disease and myocardial infarction. Causality has not been established.

Neurologic: Frequently, there is a sequence to the development of neuromuscular side effects. Initially, only sensory impairment and paresthesia may be encountered. With continued treatment, neuritic pain and, later, motor difficulties may occur. There have been no reports of any agent that can reverse the neuromuscular manifestations that may accompany therapy with vincristine sulfate. Loss of deep-tendon reflexes, foot drop, ataxia, and paralysis have been reported with continued administration. Cranial nerve manifestations, including isolated paresis and/or paralysis of muscles controlled by cranial motor nerves, may occur in the absence of motor impairment elsewhere; extraocular and laryngeal muscles are those most commonly involved. aw pain, pharyngeal pain, parotid gland pain, bone pain, back pain, limb pain, and myalgias have been reported; pain in these areas may be severe. Convulsions, frequently with hypertension, have been reported in a few patients receiving vincristine sulfate. Several instances of convulsions followed by coma have been reported in children. Transient cortical blindness and optic atrophy with blindness have been reported.

Pulmonary: See PRECAUTIONS.

Endocrine: Rare occurrences of a syndrome attributable to inappropriate antidiuretic hormone secretion have been observed in patients treated with vincristine sulfate. This syndrome is characterized by high urinary sodium excretion in the presence of hyponatremia; renal or adrenal disease, hypotension, dehydration, azotemia, and clinical edema are absent. With fluid deprivation, improvement occurs in the hyponatremia and in the renal loss of sodium.

Hematologic: Vincristine sulfate does not appear to have any constant or significant effect on platelets or red blood cells. Serious bone-marrow depression is usually not a major dose-limiting event. However, anemia, leukopenia, and thrombocytopenia have been reported. Thrombocytopenia, if present when therapy with vincristine sulfate is begun, may actually improve before the appearance of marrow remission.

Skin: Alopecia and rash have been reported.

Other: Fever and headache have occurred.

DOSAGE AND ADMINISTRATION

This preparation is for intravenous use only (see WARNINGS).

Neurotoxicity appears to be dose related. Extreme care must be used in calculating and administering the dose of vincristine sulfate since overdosage may have a very serious or fatal outcome.

The concentration of vincristine contained in all vials and Hyporets of vincristine sulfate is 1 mg/ml. Do not add extra fluid to the vial prior to removal of the dose. Withdraw the solution of vincristine sulfate into an accurate dry syringe, measuring the dose carefully. Do not add extra fluid to the vial in an attempt to empty it completely.

Caution — It is extremely important that the intravenous needle or catheter be properly positioned before any vincristine is injected. Leakage into surrounding tissue during intravenous administration of vincristine sulfate may cause considerable irritation. If extravasation occurs, the injection should be discontinued immediately and any remaining portion of the dose should then be introduced into another vein. Local injection of hyaluronidase and the application of moderate heat to the area of leakage will help disperse the drug and may minimize discomfort and the possibility of cellulitis.

Vincristine sulfate must be administered via an intact, free-flowing intravenous needle or catheter. Care should be taken that there is no leakage or swelling occurring during administration (see BOXED WARNING).

The solution may be injected either directly into a vein or into the tubing of a running intravenous infusion (see DRUG INTERACTIONS). Injection of vincristine sulfate should be accomplished within 1 minute.

The drug is administered intravenously *at weekly intervals.*

The usual dose of vincristine sulfate for children is 2 mg/m^2. For children weighing 10 kg or less, the starting dose should be 0.05 mg/kg, administered once a week. The usual dose of vincristine sulfate for adults is 1.4 mg/m^2. A 50% reduction in the dose of Vincristine sulfate is recommended for patients having a direct serum bilirubin value above 3 mg/100 ml.[19]

Vincristine sulfate should not be given to patients while they are receiving radiation therapy through ports that include the liver. When vincristine sulfate is used in combination with L-asparaginase, vincristine sulfate should be given 12-24 hours before administration of the enzyme in order to minimize toxicity; administering L-asparaginase before vincristine sulfate may reduce hepatic clearance of vincristine sulfate.

SPECIAL DISPENSING INFORMATION

When dispensing vincristine sulfate in other than the original container, (*e.g.*, a syringe containing a specific dose), it is imperative that it be packaged in an overwrap bearing the statement: "DO NOT REMOVE COVERING UNTIL MOMENT OF INJECTION. FATAL IF GIVEN INTRATHECALLY. FOR INTRAVENOUS USE ONLY" (see WARNINGS).

PRODUCT LISTING - RATED THERAPEUTICALLY EQUIVALENT

Solution - Intravenous - 1 mg/ml

Size	Price	Product	NDC
1 ml	$18.81	GENERIC, Gensia Sicor Pharmaceuticals Inc	00703-4402-11
1 ml	$31.75	GENERIC, Faulding Pharmaceutical Company	61703-0309-06
1 ml	$36.06	ONCOVIN, Lilly, Eli and Company	00002-7198-01
1 ml	$43.23	VINCASAR PFS, Pharmacia and Upjohn	00013-7456-86
2 ml	$37.63	GENERIC, Gensia Sicor Pharmaceuticals Inc	00703-4412-11
2 ml	$38.25	GENERIC, Faulding Pharmaceutical Company	61703-0309-16
2 ml	$86.46	VINCASAR PFS, Pharmacia and Upjohn	00013-7466-86

Vinorelbine Tartrate *(003190)*

Categories: Carcinoma, lung; FDA Approved 1994 Dec; Pregnancy Category D
Drug Classes: Antineoplastics, antimitotics
Brand Names: **Navelbine**
Foreign Brand Availability: Navelbin (Bulgaria; Hungary)
HCFA JCODE(S): *J9390 per 10 mg IV*

WARNING

Vinorelbine tartrate injection should be administered under the supervision of a physician experienced in the use of cancer chemotherapeutic agents. This product is for intravenous (IV) use only. Intrathecal administration of other vinca alkaloids has resulted in death. Syringes containing this product should be labeled "*WARNING:* FOR IV USE ONLY. FATAL if given intrathecally."

Severe granulocytopenia resulting in increased susceptibility to infection may occur. Granulocyte counts should be $\geq$1000 cells/mm^3 prior to the administration of vinorelbine tartrate. The dosage should be adjusted according to complete blood counts with differentials obtained on the day of treatment.

Caution: It is extremely important that the intravenous (IV) needle or catheter be properly positioned before vinorelbine tartrate is injected. Administration of vinorelbine tartrate may result in extravasation causing local tissue necrosis and/or thrombophlebitis (see DOSAGE AND ADMINISTRATION, Administration Precautions).

DESCRIPTION

Navelbine (vinorelbine tartrate) injection is for intravenous administration. Each vial contains vinorelbine tartrate equivalent to 10 mg (1 ml vial) or 50 mg (5 ml vial) vinorelbine in water for injection. No preservatives or other additives are present. The aqueous solution is sterile and nonpyrogenic.

Vinorelbine tartrate is a semi-synthetic vinca alkaloid with antitumor activity. The chemical name is 3′,4′-didehydro-4′-deoxy-*C*′-norvincaleukoblastine [*R*-(*R**,*R**)-2,3- dihydroxybutanedioate (1:2)(salt)].

Vinorelbine tartrate is a white to yellow or light brown amorphous powder with the molecular formula $C_{45}H_{54}N_4O_8 \cdot 2C_4H_6O_6$ and molecular weight of 1079.12. The aqueous solubility is >1000 mg/ml in distilled water. The pH of vinorelbine tartrate injection is approximately 3.5.

CLINICAL PHARMACOLOGY

Vinorelbine is a vinca alkaloid that interferes with microtubule assembly. The vinca alkaloids are structurally similar compounds comprised of 2 multiringed units, vindoline and catharanthine. Unlike other vinca alkaloids, the catharanthine unit is the site of structural modification for vinorelbine. The antitumor activity of vinorelbine is thought to be due primarily to inhibition of mitosis at metaphase through its interaction with tubulin. Like other vinca alkaloids, vinorelbine may also interfere with: (1) amino acid, cyclic AMP, and

V

glutathione metabolism; (2) calmodulin-dependent Ca^{++}-transport ATPase activity; (3) cellular respiration; and (4) nucleic acid and lipid biosynthesis. In intact tectal plates from mouse embryos, vinorelbine, vincristine, and vinblastine inhibited mitotic microtubule formation at the same concentration (2 μM), inducing a blockade of cells at metaphase. Vincristine produced depolymerization of axonal microtubules at 5 μM, but vinblastine and vinorelbine did not have this effect until concentrations of 30 μM and 40 μM, respectively. These data suggest relative selectivity of vinorelbine for mitotic microtubules.

PHARMACOKINETICS

The pharmacokinetics of vinorelbine were studied in 49 patients who received doses of 30 mg/m^2 in 4 clinical trials. Doses were administered by 15-20 minute constant-rate infusions. Following IV administration, vinorelbine concentration in plasma decays in a triphasic manner. The initial rapid decline primarily represents distribution of drug to peripheral compartments followed by metabolism and excretion of the drug during subsequent phases. The prolonged terminal phase is due to relatively slow efflux of vinorelbine from peripheral compartments. The terminal phase half-life averages 27.7-43.6 hours and the mean plasma clearance ranges from 0.97-1.26 L/h/kg. Steady-state volume of distribution (Vss) values range from 25.4-40.1 L/kg.

Vinorelbine demonstrated high binding to human platelets and lymphocytes. The free fraction was approximately 0.11 in pooled human plasma over a concentration range of 234-1169 ng/ml. The binding to plasma constituents in cancer patients ranged from 79.6-91.2%. Vinorelbine binding was not altered in the presence of cisplatin, 5-fluorouracil, or doxorubicin.

Vinorelbine undergoes substantial hepatic elimination in humans, with large amounts recovered in feces after IV administration to humans. Two metabolites of vinorelbine have been identified in human blood, plasma, and urine; vinorelbine N-oxide and deacetylvinorelbine. Deacetylvinorelbine has been demonstrated to be the primary metabolite of vinorelbine in humans, and has been shown to possess antitumor activity similar to vinorelbine. Therapeutic doses of vinorelbine tartrate (30 mg/m^2) yield very small, if any, quantifiable levels of either metabolite in blood or urine. The metabolism of vinca alkaloids has been shown to be mediated by hepatic cytochrome P450 isoenzymes in the CYP3A subfamily. This metabolic pathway may be impaired in patients with hepatic dysfunction or who are taking concomitant potent inhibitors of these isoenzymes (see PRECAUTIONS). The effects of renal or hepatic dysfunction on the disposition of vinorelbine have not been assessed, but based on experience with other anticancer vinca alkaloids, dose adjustments are recommended for patients with impaired hepatic function (see DOSAGE AND ADMINISTRATION).

The disposition of radiolabeled vinorelbine given intravenously was studied in a limited number of patients. Approximately 18% and 46% of the administered dose was recovered in the urine and in the feces, respectively. Incomplete recovery in humans is consistent with results in animals where recovery is incomplete, even after prolonged sampling times. A separate study of the urinary excretion of vinorelbine using specific chromatographic analytical methodology showed that 10.9% ± 0.7% of a 30 mg/m^2 IV dose was excreted unchanged in the urine.

The influence of age on the pharmacokinetics of vinorelbine was examined using data from 44 cancer patients (average age, 56.7 ± 7.8 years; range, 41-74 years; with 12 patients ≥60 years and 6 patients ≥65 years) in 3 studies. CL (the mean plasma clearance), $T_{½}$ (the terminal phase half-life), and Vz (the volume of distribution during terminal phase) were independent of age. A separate pharmacokinetic study was conducted in 10 elderly patients with metastatic breast cancer (age range, 66-81 years; 3 patients >75 years; normal liver function tests) receiving vinorelbine 30 mg/m^2 intravenously. CL, Vss, and $T_{½}$ were similar to those reported for younger adult patients in previous studies. No relationship between age, systemic exposure [AUC(0-∞)] and hematological toxicity was observed.

The pharmacokinetics of vinorelbine are not influenced by the concurrent administration of cisplatin with vinorelbine tartrate (see DRUG INTERACTIONS).

INDICATIONS AND USAGE

Vinorelbine tartrate is indicated as a single agent or in combination with cisplatin for the first-line treatment of ambulatory patients with unresectable, advanced nonsmall cell lung cancer (NSCLC). In patients with Stage 4 NSCLC, vinorelbine tartrate is indicated as a single agent or in combination with cisplatin. In Stage 3 NSCLC, vinorelbine tartrate is indicated in combination with cisplatin.

NON-FDA APPROVED INDICATIONS

Vinorelbine has also been reported to have efficacy in the treatment of patients with metastatic breast cancer and advanced AIDS related Kaposi's sarcoma which has been previously treated with one or more chemotherapy regimens. One study has reported that the drug shows promise in the palliation of patients with malignant pleural mesothelioma. However, these uses have not been approved by the FDA and further clinical trials are needed.

CONTRAINDICATIONS

Administration of vinorelbine tartrate is contraindicated in patients with pretreatment granulocyte counts <1000 $cells/mm^3$ (see WARNINGS).

WARNINGS

Vinorelbine tartrate should be administered in carefully adjusted doses by or under the supervision of a physician experienced in the use of cancer chemotherapeutic agents.

Patients treated with vinorelbine tartrate should be frequently monitored for myelosuppression both during and after therapy. Granulocytopenia is dose-limiting. Granulocyte nadirs occur between 7 and 10 days after dosing with granulocyte count recovery usually within the following 7-14 days. Complete blood counts with differentials should be performed and results reviewed prior to administering each dose of vinorelbine tartrate. Vinorelbine tartrate should not be administered to patients with granulocyte counts <1000 $cells/mm^3$. Patients developing severe granulocytopenia should be monitored carefully for evidence of infection and/or fever. See DOSAGE AND ADMINISTRATION for recommended dose adjustments for granulocytopenia.

Acute shortness of breath and severe bronchospasm have been reported infrequently, following the administration of vinorelbine tartrate and other vinca alkaloids, most commonly when the vinca alkaloid was used in combination with mitomycin. These adverse events may require treatment with supplemental oxygen, bronchodilators, and/or corticosteroids, particularly when there is pre-existing pulmonary dysfunction.

Reported cases of interstitial pulmonary changes and acute respiratory distress syndrome (ARDS), most of which were fatal, occurred in patients treated with single-agent vinorelbine tartrate. The mean time to onset of these symptoms after vinorelbine administration was 1 week (range 3-8 days). Patients with alterations in their baseline pulmonary symptoms or with new onset of dyspnea, cough, hypoxia, or other symptoms should be evaluated promptly.

Vinorelbine tartrate has been reported to cause severe constipation (*e.g.*, Grade 3-4), paralytic ileus, intestinal obstruction, necrosis, and/or perforation. Some events have been fatal.

PREGNANCY CATEGORY D

Vinorelbine tartrate may cause fetal harm if administered to a pregnant woman. A single dose of vinorelbine has been shown to be embryo- and/or fetotoxic in mice and rabbits at doses of 9 mg/m^2 and 5.5 mg/m^2, respectively (one-third and one-sixth the human dose). At nonmaternotoxic doses, fetal weight was reduced and ossification was delayed. There are no studies in pregnant women. If vinorelbine tartrate is used during pregnancy, or if the patient becomes pregnant while receiving this drug, the patient should be apprised of the potential hazard to the fetus. Women of childbearing potential should be advised to avoid becoming pregnant during therapy with vinorelbine tartrate.

PRECAUTIONS

GENERAL

Most drug-related adverse events of vinorelbine tartrate are reversible. If severe adverse events occur, vinorelbine tartrate should be reduced in dosage or discontinued and appropriate corrective measures taken. Reinstitution of therapy with vinorelbine tartrate should be carried out with caution and alertness as to possible recurrence of toxicity.

Vinorelbine tartrate should be used with extreme caution in patients whose bone marrow reserve may have been compromised by prior irradiation or chemotherapy, or whose marrow function is recovering from the effects of previous chemotherapy (see DOSAGE AND ADMINISTRATION).

Administration of vinorelbine tartrate to patients with prior radiation therapy may result in radiation recall reactions (see ADVERSE REACTIONS and DRUG INTERACTIONS).

Patients with a prior history or pre-existing neuropathy, regardless of etiology, should be monitored for new or worsening signs and symptoms of neuropathy while receiving vinorelbine tartrate.

Care must be taken to avoid contamination of the eye with concentrations of vinorelbine tartrate used clinically. Severe irritation of the eye has been reported with accidental exposure to another vinca alkaloid. If exposure occurs, the eye should immediately be thoroughly flushed with water.

INFORMATION FOR THE PATIENT

Patients should be informed that the major acute toxicities of vinorelbine tartrate are related to bone marrow toxicity, specifically granulocytopenia with increased susceptibility to infection. They should be advised to report fever or chills immediately. Women of childbearing potential should be advised to avoid becoming pregnant during treatment. Patients should be advised to contact their physician if they experience increased shortness of breath, cough, or other new pulmonary symptoms, or if they experience symptoms of abdominal pain or constipation.

LABORATORY TESTS

Since dose-limiting clinical toxicity is the result of depression of the white blood cell count, it is imperative that complete blood counts with differentials be obtained and reviewed on the day of treatment prior to each dose of vinorelbine tartrate (see ADVERSE REACTIONS, Hematologic).

HEPATIC

There is no evidence that the toxicity of vinorelbine tartrate is enhanced in patients with elevated liver enzymes. No data are available for patients with severe baseline cholestasis, but the liver plays an important role in the metabolism of vinorelbine tartrate. Because clinical experience in patients with severe liver disease is limited, caution should be exercised when administering vinorelbine tartrate to patients with severe hepatic injury or impairment (see DOSAGE AND ADMINISTRATION).

CARCINOGENESIS, MUTAGENESIS, AND IMPAIRMENT OF FERTILITY

The carcinogenic potential of vinorelbine tartrate has not been studied. Vinorelbine has been shown to affect chromosome number and possibly structure *in vivo* (polyploidy in bone marrow cells from Chinese hamsters and a positive micronucleus test in mice). It was not mutagenic in the Ames test and gave inconclusive results in the mouse lymphoma TK Locus assay. The significance of these or other short-term test results for human risk is unknown. Vinorelbine did not affect fertility to a statistically significant extent when administered to rats on either a once-weekly (9 mg/m^2, approximately one-third the human dose) or alternate-day schedule (4.2 mg/m^2, approximately one-seventh the human dose) prior to and during mating. However, biweekly administration for 13 or 26 weeks in the rat at 2.1 and 7.2 mg/m^2 (approximately one-fifteenth and one-fourth the human dose) resulted in decreased spermatogenesis and prostate/seminal vesicle secretion.

PREGNANCY CATEGORY D

See WARNINGS.

NURSING MOTHERS

It is not known whether the drug is excreted in human milk. Because many drugs are excreted in human milk and because of the potential for serious adverse reactions in nursing infants from vinorelbine tartrate, it is recommended that nursing be discontinued in women who are receiving therapy with vinorelbine tartrate.

PEDIATRIC USE

Safety and effectiveness in pediatric patients have not been established.

GERIATRIC USE

Of the total number of patients in North American clinical studies of IV vinorelbine tartrate, approximately one-third were 65 years of age or greater. No overall differences in effectiveness or safety were observed between these patients and younger adult patients. Other reported clinical experience has not identified differences in responses between the elderly and younger adult patients, but greater sensitivity of some older individuals cannot be ruled out.

The pharmacokinetics of vinorelbine in elderly and younger adult patients are similar (see CLINICAL PHARMACOLOGY).

DRUG INTERACTIONS

Acute pulmonary reactions have been reported with vinorelbine tartrate and other anticancer vinca alkaloids used in conjunction with mitomycin. Although the pharmacokinetics of vinorelbine are not influenced by the concurrent administration of cisplatin, the incidence of granulocytopenia with vinorelbine tartrate used in combination with cisplatin is significantly higher than with single-agent vinorelbine tartrate. Patients who receive vinorelbine tartrate and paclitaxel, either concomitantly or sequentially, should be monitored for signs and symptoms of neuropathy. Administration of vinorelbine tartrate to patients with prior or concomitant radiation therapy may result in radiosensitizing effects.

Caution should be exercised in patients concurrently taking drugs known to inhibit drug metabolism by hepatic cytochrome P450 isoenzymes in the CYP3A subfamily, or in patients with hepatic dysfunction. Concurrent administration of vinorelbine tartrate with an inhibitor of this metabolic pathway may cause an earlier onset and/or an increased severity of side effects.

ADVERSE REACTIONS

The pattern of adverse reactions is similar whether vinorelbine tartrate injection is used as a single agent or in combination. Adverse reactions from studies with single-agent and combination use of vinorelbine tartrate injection are summarized in TABLE 2, TABLE 3A, TABLE 3B, TABLE 4A, TABLE 4B, TABLE 5A, TABLE 5B, and TABLE 5C.

SINGLE-AGENT VINORELBINE TARTRATE INJECTION

Data in TABLE 2, TABLE 3A, and TABLE 3B are based on the experience of 365 patients (143 patients with NSCLC; 222 patients with advanced breast cancer) treated with IV vinorelbine tartrate as a single agent in 3 clinical studies. The dosing schedule in each study was 30 mg/m^2 vinorelbine tartrate on a weekly basis.

TABLE 2 *Summary of Adverse Events in 365 Patients Receiving Single-Agent Vinorelbine Tartrate*†*

Adverse Event (Bone Marrow)	All Patients (n=365)	NSCLC (n=143)
Granulocytopenia		
<2000 cells/mm^3	90%	80%
<500 cells/mm^3	36%	29%
Leukopenia		
<4000 cells/mm^3	92%	81%
<1000 cells/mm^3	15%	12%
Thrombocytopenia		
<100,000 cells/mm^3	5%	4%
<50,000 cells/mm^3	1%	1%
Anemia		
<11 g/dl	83%	77%
<8 g/dl	9%	1%
Hospitalizations due to granulocytopenic complications	9%	8%

* None of the reported toxicities were influenced by age. Grade based on modified criteria from the National Cancer Institute.
† Patients with NSCLC had not received prior chemotherapy. The majority of the remaining patients had received prior chemotherapy.

TABLE 3A *Summary of Adverse Events in 365 Patients Receiving Single-Agent Vinorelbine Tartrate*†*

Adverse Event (All Grades)	All Patients	NSCLC
Clinical Chemistry Elevations		
Total bilirubin (n=351)	13%	9%
SGOT (n=346)	67%	54%
General		
Asthenia	36%	27%
Injection site reactions	28%	38%
Injection site pain	16%	13%
Phlebitis	7%	10%
Digestive		
Nausea	44%	34%
Vomiting	20%	15%
Constipation	35%	29%
Diarrhea	17%	13%
Peripheral Neuropathy‡	25%	20%
Dyspnea	7%	3%
Alopecia	12%	12%

* None of the reported toxicities were influenced by age. Grade based on modified criteria from the National Cancer Institute.
† Patients with NSCLC had not received prior chemotherapy. The majority of the remaining patients had received prior chemotherapy.
‡ Incidence of paresthesia + hypesthesia.

TABLE 3B *Summary of Adverse Events in 365 Patients Receiving Single-Agent Vinorelbine Tartrate*†*

	Grade 3		Grade 4	
Adverse Event	All Patients	NSCLC	All Patients	NSCLC
Clinical Chemistry Elevations				
Total bilirubin (n=351)	4%	3%	3%	2%
SGOT (n=346)	5%	2%	1%	1%
General				
Asthenia	7%	5%	0%	0%
Injection site reactions	2%	5%	0%	0%
Injection site pain	2%	1%	0%	0%
Phlebitis	<1%	1%	0%	0%
Digestive				
Nausea	2%	1%	0%	0%
Vomiting	2%	1%	0%	0%
Constipation	3%	2%	0%	0%
Diarrhea	1%	1%	0%	0%
Peripheral Neuropathy‡	1%	1%	<1%	0%
Dyspnea	2%	2%	1%	0%
Alopecia	≤1%	1%	0%	0%

* None of the reported toxicities were influenced by age. Grade based on modified criteria from the National Cancer Institute.
† Patients with NSCLC had not received prior chemotherapy. The majority of the remaining patients had received prior chemotherapy.
‡ Incidence of paresthesia + hypesthesia.

HEMATOLOGIC

Granulocytopenia is the major dose-limiting toxicity with vinorelbine tartrate. Dose adjustments are required for hematologic toxicity and hepatic insufficiency (see DOSAGE AND ADMINISTRATION). Granulocytopenia was generally reversible and not cumulative over time. Granulocyte nadirs occurred 7-10 days after the dose, with granulocyte recovery usually within the following 7-14 days. Granulocytopenia resulted in hospitalizations for fever and/or sepsis in 8% of patients. Septic deaths occurred in approximately 1% of patients. Prophylactic hematologic growth factors have not been routinely used with vinorelbine tartrate. If medically necessary, growth factors may be administered at recommended doses no earlier than 24 hours after the administration of cytotoxic chemotherapy. Growth factors should not be administered in the period 24 hours before the administration of chemotherapy.

Whole blood and/or packed red blood cells were administered to 18% of patients who received vinorelbine tartrate.

NEUROLOGIC

Loss of deep tendon reflexes occurred in less than 5% of patients. The development of severe peripheral neuropathy was infrequent (1%) and generally reversible.

SKIN

Like other anticancer vinca alkaloids, vinorelbine tartrate is a moderate vesicant. Injection site reactions, including erythema, pain at injection site, and vein discoloration, occurred in approximately one-third of patients; 5% were severe. Chemical phlebitis along the vein proximal to the site of injection was reported in 10% of patients.

GASTROINTESTINAL

Prophylactic administration of antiemetics was not routine in patients treated with single-agent vinorelbine tartrate. Due to the low incidence of severe nausea and vomiting with single-agent vinorelbine tartrate, the use of serotonin antagonists is generally not required.

HEPATIC

Transient elevations of liver enzymes were reported without clinical symptoms.

CARDIOVASCULAR

Chest pain was reported in 5% of patients. Most reports of chest pain were in patients who had either a history of cardiovascular disease or tumor within the chest. There have been rare reports of myocardial infarction.

PULMONARY

Shortness of breath was reported in 3% of patients; it was severe in 2% (see WARNINGS). Interstitial pulmonary changes were documented.

OTHER

Fatigue occurred in 27% of patients. It was usually mild or moderate but tended to increase with cumulative dosing.

Other toxicities that have been reported in less than 5% of patients include jaw pain, myalgia, arthralgia, and rash. Hemorrhagic cystitis and the syndrome of inappropriate ADH secretion were each reported in <1% of patients.

COMBINATION USE

Adverse events for combination use are summarized in TABLE 4A, TABLE 4B, TABLE 5A, TABLE 5B, and TABLE 5C .

Vinorelbine Tartrate Injection in Combination With Cisplatin

Vinorelbine Tartrate Injection + Cisplatin versus Single-Agent Cisplatin

See TABLE 4A and TABLE 4B.

Myelosuppression was the predominant toxicity in patients receiving combination therapy, Grade 3 and 4 granulocytopenia of 82% compared to 5% in the single-agent cisplatin arm. Fever and/or sepsis related to granulocytopenia occurred in 11% of patients on vinorelbine tartrate injection and cisplatin compared to 0% on the cisplatin arm.

Four patients on the combination died of granulocytopenia-related sepsis. During this study, the use of granulocyte colony-stimulating factor ([G-CSF] filgrastim) was permitted, but not mandated, after the first course of treatment for patients who experienced Grade 3 or 4 granulocytopenia ($\leq$1000 cells/mm^3) or in those who developed neutropenic fever between cycles of chemotherapy. Beginning 24 hours after completion of chemotherapy, G-CSF was started at a dose of 5 μg/kg/day and continued until the total granulocyte count was >1000 cells/mm^3 on 2 successive determinations. G-CSF was not administered on the day of treatment.

Grade 3 and 4 anemia occurred more frequently in the combination arm compared to control, 24% vs 8%, respectively. Thrombocytopenia occurred in 6% of patients treated with vinorelbine tartrate injection + cisplatin compared to 2% of patients treated with cisplatin.

The incidence of severe non-hematologic toxicity was similar among the patients in both treatment groups. Patients receiving vinorelbine tartrate injection + cisplatin compared to single-agent cisplatin experienced more Grade 3 and/or 4 peripheral numbness (2% vs <1%), phlebitis/thrombosis/embolism (3% vs <1%), and infection (6% vs <1%). Grade 3-4 constipation and/or ileus occurred in 3% of patients treated with combination therapy and in 1% of patients treated with cisplatin.

Seven (7) deaths were reported on the combination arm; 2 were related to cardiac ischemia, 1 massive cerebrovascular accident, 1 multisystem failure due to an overdose of vinorelbine tartrate injection, and 3 from febrile neutropenia. One death, secondary to respiratory infection unrelated to granulocytopenia, occurred with single-agent cisplatin.

Vinorelbine Tartrate Injection + Cisplatin versus Vindesine + Cisplatin versus Single-Agent Vinorelbine Tartrate Injection

See TABLE 5A, TABLE 5B, and TABLE 5C.

Myelosuppression, specifically Grade 3 and 4 granulocytopenia, was significantly greater with the combination of vinorelbine tartrate injection + cisplatin (79%) than with either single-agent vinorelbine tartrate injection (53%) or vindesine + cisplatin (48%), P <0.0001. Hospitalization due to documented sepsis occurred in 4.4% of patients treated with vinorelbine tartrate injection + cisplatin; 2% of patients treated with vindesine and cisplatin, and 4% of patients treated with single-agent vinorelbine tartrate injection. Grade 3 and 4 thrombocytopenia was infrequent in patients receiving combination chemotherapy and no events were reported with single-agent vinorelbine tartrate injection.

The incidence of Grade 3 and/or 4 nausea and vomiting, alopecia, and renal toxicity were reported more frequently in the cisplatin-containing combinations compared to single-agent vinorelbine tartrate injection. Severe local reactions occurred in 2% of patients treated with combinations containing vinorelbine tartrate injection; none were observed in the vindesine + cisplatin arm. Grade 3 and 4 neurotoxicity was significantly more frequent in patients receiving vindesine + cisplatin (17%) compared to vinorelbine tartrate injection + cisplatin (7%) and single-agent vinorelbine tartrate injection (9%) (P <0.005). Cisplatin did not appear to increase the incidence of neurotoxicity observed with single-agent vinorelbine tartrate injection.

TABLE 4A *Selected Adverse Events From a Comparative Trial of Vinorelbine Tartrate Injection + Cisplatin versus Single-Agent Cisplatin**

	Vinorelbine Tartrate Injection 25 mg/m^2 + Cisplatin 100 mg/m^2 (n=212)		
Adverse Event	**All Grades**	**Grade 3**	**Grade 4**
Bone Marrow			
Granulocytopenia	89%	22%	60%
Anemia	88%	21%	3%
Leukopenia	88%	39%	19%
Thrombocytopenia	29%	4%	1%
Febrile Neutropenia	NA	NA	11%
Hepatic			
Elevated transaminase	1%	0%	0%
Renal			
Elevated creatinine	37%	2%	2%
Non-Laboratory			
Malaise/fatigue/lethargy	67%	12%	0%
Vomiting	60%	7%	6%
Nausea	58%	14%	0%
Anorexia	46%	0%	0%
Constipation	35%	3%	0%
Alopecia	34%	0%	0%
Weight loss	34%	1%	0%
Fever without infection	20%	2%	0%
Hearing	18%	4%	0%
Local (injection site reactions)	17%	<1%	0%
Diarrhea	17%	2%	<1%
Paresthesias	17%	<1%	0%
Taste alterations	17%	0%	0%
Peripheral numbness	11%	2%	0%
Myalgia/arthralgia	12%	<1%	0%
Phlebitis/thrombosis/embolism	10%	3%	0%
Weakness	12%	2%	<1%
Dizziness/vertigo	9%	<1%	0%
Infection	11%	5%	<1%
Respiratory infection	10%	4%	<1%

* Graded according to the standard SWOG criteria.

OBSERVED DURING CLINICAL PRACTICE

In addition to the adverse events reported from clinical trials, the following events have been identified during post-approval use of vinorelbine tartrate. Because they are reported voluntarily from a population of unknown size, estimates of frequency cannot be made. These events have been chosen for inclusion due to a combination of their seriousness, frequency of reporting, or potential causal connection to vinorelbine tartrate.

Body as a Whole: Systemic allergic reactions reported as anaphylaxis, pruritus, urticaria, and angioedema; flushing; and radiation recall events such as dermatitis and esophagitis (see PRECAUTIONS) have been reported.

Hematologic: Thromboembolic events, including pulmonary embolus and deep venous thrombosis, have been reported primarily in seriously ill and debilitated patients with known predisposing risk factors for these events.

Neurologic: Peripheral neurotoxicities such as, but not limited to, muscle weakness and disturbance of gait, have been observed in patients with and without prior symptoms. There may be increased potential for neurotoxicity in patients with pre-existing neuropathy, regardless of etiology, who receive vinorelbine tartrate. Vestibular and auditory deficits have been observed with vinorelbine tartrate, usually when used in combination with cisplatin.

Skin: Injection site reactions, including localized rash and urticaria, blister formation, and skin sloughing have been observed in clinical practice. Some of these reactions may be delayed in appearance.

Gastrointestinal: Dysphagia, mucositis, and pancreatitis have been reported.

Cardiovascular: Hypertension, hypotension, vasodilation, tachycardia, and pulmonary edema have been reported.

Pulmonary: Pneumonia has been reported.

TABLE 4B *Selected Adverse Events From a Comparative Trial of Vinorelbine Tartrate Injection + Cisplatin versus Single-Agent Cisplatin**

	Vinorelbine Tartrate Injection 25 mg/m^3 + Cisplatin 100 mg/m^2 (n=212)		
Adverse Event	**All Grades**	**Grade 3**	**Grade 4**
Bone Marrow			
Granulocytopenia	26%	4%	1%
Anemia	72%	7%	<1%
Leukopenia	31%	<1%	0%
Thrombocytopenia	21%	1%	<1%
Febrile Neutropenia	NA	NA	0%
Hepatic			
Elevated transaminase	<1%	<1%	0%
Renal			
Elevated creatinine	28%	4%	<1%
Non-Laboratory			
Malaise/fatigue/lethargy	49%	8%	0%
Vomiting	60%	10%	4%
Nausea	57%	12%	0%
Anorexia	37%	0%	0%
Constipation	16%	1%	0%
Alopecia	14%	0%	0%
Weight loss	21%	<1%	0%
Fever without infection	4%	0%	0%
Hearing	18%	3%	<1%
Local (injection site reactions)	1%	0%	0%
Diarrhea	11%	1%	<1%
Paresthesias	10%	<1%	0%
Taste alterations	15%	0%	0%
Peripheral numbness	7%	<1%	0%
Myalgia/arthralgia	3%	<1%	0%
Phlebitis/thrombosis/embolism	<1%	0%	<1%
Weakness	7%	2%	0%
Dizziness/vertigo	3%	<1%	0%
Infection	<1%	<1%	0%
Respiratory infection	3%	3%	0%

* Graded according to the standard SWOG criteria.

TABLE 5A *Selected Adverse Events From a Comparative Trial of Vinorelbine Tartrate Injection + Cisplatin versus Vindesine + Cisplatin versus Single-Agent Vinorelbine Tartrate Injection**

	Vinorelbine Tartrate Injection/Cisplatin†		
Adverse Event	**All Grades**	**Grade 3**	**Grade 4**
Bone Marrow			
Neutropenia	95%	20%	58%
Leukopenia	94%	40%	17%
Thrombocytopenia	15%	3%	1%
Febrile Neutropenia	NA	NA	4%
Hepatic			
Elevated bilirubin‡	6%	NA	NA
Renal			
Elevated creatinine‡	46%	NA	NA
Non-Laboratory			
Nausea/vomiting	74%	27%	3%
Alopecia	51%	7%	0.5%
Ototoxicity	10%	1%	1%
Local reactions	17%	2%	0.5%
Diarrhea	25%	1.5%	0%
Neurotoxicity§	44%	7%	0%

* Grade based on criteria from the World Health Organization (WHO).
† n=194-207; all patients receiving vinorelbine tartrate injection/cisplatin with laboratory and non-laboratory data.
‡ Categorical toxicity grade not specified.
§ Neurotoxicity includes peripheral neuropathy and constipation.

TABLE 5B *Selected Adverse Events From a Comparative Trial of Vinorelbine Tartrate Injection + Cisplatin versus Vindesine + Cisplatin versus Single-Agent Vinorelbine Tartrate Injection**

Adverse Event	Vindesine/Cisplatin† All Grades	Grade 3	Grade 4
Bone Marrow			
Neutropenia	79%	26%	22%
Leukopenia	82%	24%	3%
Thrombocytopenia	10%	3%	0.5%
Febrile Neutropenia	NA	NA	2%
Hepatic			
Elevated bilirubin‡	5%	NA	NA
Renal			
Elevated creatinine‡	37%	NA	NA
Non-Laboratory			
Nausea/vomiting	72%	24%	1%
Alopecia	56%	14%	0%
Ototoxicity	14%	1%	0%
Local reactions	7%	0%	0%
Diarrhea	24%	1%	0%
Neurotoxicity§	58%	16%	1%

* Grade based on criteria from the World Health Organization (WHO).
† n=173-192; all patients receiving vindesine/cisplatin with laboratory and non-laboratory data.
‡ Categorical toxicity grade not specified.
§ Neurotoxicity includes peripheral neuropathy and constipation.

TABLE 5C *Selected Adverse Events From a Comparative Trial of Vinorelbine Tartrate Injection + Cisplatin versus Vindesine + Cisplatin versus Single-Agent Vinorelbine Tartrate Injection**

Adverse Event	Vinorelbine Tartrate Injection† All Grades	Grade 3	Grade 4
Bone Marrow			
Neutropenia	85%	25%	28%
Leukopenia	83%	26%	6%
Thrombocytopenia	3%	0%	0%
Febrile Neutropenia	NA	NA	4%
Hepatic			
Elevated bilirubin‡	5%	NA	NA
Renal			
Elevated creatinine‡	13%	NA	NA
Non-Laboratory			
Nausea/vomiting	31%	1%	1%
Alopecia	30%	2%	0%
Ototoxicity	1%	0%	0%
Local reactions	22%	2%	0%
Diarrhea	12%	0%	0.5%
Neurotoxicity§	44%	8%	0.5%

* Grade based on criteria from the World Health Organization (WHO).
† n=165-201; all patients receiving vinorelbine tartrate injection with laboratory and non-laboratory data.
‡ Categorical toxicity grade not specified.
§ Neurotoxicity includes peripheral neuropathy and constipation.

Musculoskeletal: Headache has been reported, with and without other musculoskeletal aches and pains.

Other: Pain in tumor-containing tissue, back pain, and abdominal pain have been reported. Electrolyte abnormalities, including hyponatremia with or without the syndrome of inappropriate ADH secretion, have been reported in seriously ill and debilitated patients.

Combination Use

Patients with prior exposure to paclitaxel and who have demonstrated neuropathy should be monitored closely for new or worsening neuropathy. Patients who have experienced neuropathy with previous drug regimens should be monitored for symptoms of neuropathy while receiving vinorelbine tartrate. Vinorelbine tartrate may result in radiosensitizing effects with prior or concomitant radiation therapy (see PRECAUTIONS).

DOSAGE AND ADMINISTRATION

SINGLE-AGENT VINORELBINE TARTRATE INJECTION

The usual initial dose of single-agent vinorelbine tartrate injection is 30 mg/m^2 administered weekly. The recommended method of administration is an IV injection over 6-10 minutes. In controlled trials, single-agent vinorelbine tartrate injection was given weekly until progression or dose-limiting toxicity.

VINORELBINE TARTRATE INJECTION IN COMBINATION WITH CISPLATIN

Vinorelbine tartrate injection may be administered weekly at a dose of 25 mg/m^2 in combination with cisplatin given every 4 weeks at a dose of 100 mg/m^2.

Blood counts should be checked weekly to determine whether dose reductions of vinorelbine tartrate injection and/or cisplatin are necessary. In the SWOG study, most patients required a 50% dose reduction of vinorelbine tartrate injection at day 15 of each cycle and a 50% dose reduction of cisplatin by cycle 3.

Vinorelbine tartrate injection may also be administered weekly at a dose of 30 mg/m^2 in combination with cisplatin, given on days 1 and 29, then every 6 weeks at a dose of 120 mg/m^2.

DOSE MODIFICATIONS FOR VINORELBINE TARTRATE INJECTION

The dosage should be adjusted according to hematologic toxicity or hepatic insufficiency, whichever results in the lower dose for the corresponding starting dose of vinorelbine tartrate injection (see TABLE 6).

Dose Modification for Hematologic Toxicity

Granulocyte counts should be ≥1000 cells/mm^3 prior to the administration of vinorelbine tartrate. Adjustments in the dosage of vinorelbine tartrate should be based on granulocyte counts obtained on the day of treatment according to TABLE 6.

TABLE 6 *Dose Adjustments Based on Granulocyte Counts*

Granulocytes on Days of Treatment	Percentage of Starting Dose of Vinorelbine Tartrate
≥1500 cells/mm^3	100%
1000-1499 cells/mm^3	50%
<1000 cells/mm^3	Do not administer. Repeat granulocyte count in 1 week. If 3 consecutive weekly doses are held because granulocyte count is <1000 cells/mm^3, discontinue vinorelbine tartrate.
Note: For patients who, during treatment with vinorelbine tartrate experienced fever and/or sepsis while granulocytopenic or had 2 consecutive weekly doses held due to granulocytopenia, subsequent doses of vinorelbine tartrate should be:	
≥1500 cells/mm^3	75%
1000-1499 cells/mm^3	37.5%
<1000 cells/mm^3	See above.

Dose Modification for Hepatic Insufficiency

Vinorelbine tartrate should be administered with caution to patients with hepatic insufficiency. In patients who develop hyperbilirubinemia during treatment with vinorelbine tartrate, the dose should be adjusted for total bilirubin according to TABLE 7.

TABLE 7 *Dose Modification Based on Total Bilirubin*

Total Bilirubin	Percentage of Starting Dose of Vinorelbine Tartrate
≤2.0 mg/dl	100%
2.1-3.0 mg/dl	50%
>3.0 mg/dl	25%

Dose Modification for Concurrent Hematologic Toxicity and Hepatic Insufficiency

In patients with both hematologic toxicity and hepatic insufficiency, the lower of the doses based on the corresponding starting dose of vinorelbine tartrate injection determined from TABLE 6 and TABLE 7 should be administered.

Dose Modifications for Renal Insufficiency

No dose adjustments for vinorelbine tartrate injection are required for renal insufficiency. Appropriate dose reductions for cisplatin should be made when vinorelbine tartrate injection is used in combination.

Dose Modifications for Neurotoxicity

If Grade ≥2 neurotoxicity develops, vinorelbine tartrate injection should be discontinued.

ADMINISTRATION PRECAUTIONS

Caution: Vinorelbine tartrate must be administered intravenously. It is extremely important that the IV needle or catheter be properly positioned before any vinorelbine tartrate is injected. Leakage into surrounding tissue during intravenous administration of vinorelbine tartrate may cause considerable irritation, local tissue necrosis, and/or thrombophlebitis. If extravasation occurs, the injection should be discontinued immediately, and any remaining portion of the dose should then be introduced into another vein. Since there are no established guidelines for the treatment of extravasation injuries with vinorelbine tartrate, institutional guidelines may be used. The *ONS Chemotherapy Guidelines* provide additional recommendations for the prevention of extravasation injuries.[1]

As with other toxic compounds, caution should be exercised in handling and preparing the solution of vinorelbine tartrate. Skin reactions may occur with accidental exposure. The use of gloves is recommended. If the solution of vinorelbine tartrate contacts the skin or mucosa, immediately wash the skin or mucosa thoroughly with soap and water. Severe irritation of the eye has been reported with accidental contamination of the eye with another vinca alkaloid. If this happens with vinorelbine tartrate, the eye should be flushed with water immediately and thoroughly.

Procedures for proper handling and disposal of anticancer drugs should be used. Several guidelines on this subject have been published.[2-8] There is no general agreement that all of the procedures recommended in the guidelines are necessary or appropriate.

Vinorelbine tartrate injection is a clear, colorless to pale yellow solution. Parenteral drug products should be visually inspected for particulate matter and discoloration prior to administration whenever solution and container permit. If particulate matter is seen, vinorelbine tartrate should not be administered.

V

PREPARATION FOR ADMINISTRATION

Vinorelbine tartrate injection must be diluted in either a syringe or IV bag using one of the recommended solutions. The diluted vinorelbine tartrate should be administered over 6-10 minutes into the side port of a free-flowing IV **closest to the IV bag** followed by flushing with at least 75-125 ml of one of the solutions. Diluted vinorelbine tartrate may be used for up to 24 hours under normal room light when stored in polypropylene syringes or polyvinyl chloride bags at 5-30°C (41-86°F).

Syringe

The calculated dose of vinorelbine tartrate should be diluted to a concentration between 1.5 and 3.0 mg/ml.

The following solutions may be used for dilution:
5% Dextrose injection
0.9% Sodium chloride injection

IV Bag

The calculated dose of vinorelbine tartrate should be diluted to a concentration between 0.5 and 2 mg/ml.

The following solutions may be used for dilution:
5% Dextrose injection
0.9% Sodium chloride injection
0.45% Sodium chloride injection
5% Dextrose and 0.45% sodium chloride injection
Ringer's injection
Lactated Ringer's injection

Stability

Unopened vials of vinorelbine tartrate are stable until the date indicated on the package when stored under refrigeration at 2-8°C (36-46°F) and protected from light in the carton. Unopened vials of vinorelbine tartrate are stable at temperatures up to 25°C (77°F) for up to 72 hours. This product should not be frozen.

HOW SUPPLIED

Navelbine injection is a clear, colorless to pale yellow solution in water for injection, containing 10 mg vinorelbine per milliliter. Navelbine injection is available in single-use, clear glass vials with elastomeric stoppers and royal blue caps.

Storage: Store the vials under refrigeration at 2-8°C (36-46°F) in the carton. Protect from light. DO NOT FREEZE.

PRODUCT LISTING - EQUIVALENTS NOT AVAILABLE

Solution - Intravenous - 10 mg/ml

1 ml	$119.53	NAVELBINE, Glaxosmithkline	00173-0656-01
5 ml	$597.64	NAVELBINE, Glaxosmithkline	00173-0656-44

Vitamin E (002438)

Categories: Deficiency, vitamin and mineral; FDA Pre 1938 Drugs
Drug Classes: Vitamins/minerals
Brand Names: Lactinol-E; Tocopherol
Foreign Brand Availability: Aquasol E (Colombia); Dermorelle (France); Detulin (Germany); E Perle (Italy); E Recordati (Costa-Rica; Dominican-Republic; El-Salvador; Guatemala; Honduras; Mexico; Panama); Ephynal (Austria; Belgium; England; France; Greece; Hungary; Ireland; Italy; Portugal; Spain; Sweden; Switzerland); Evion (India); Livingpherol (Korea)

CLINICAL PHARMACOLOGY

Involved in digestion and metabolism of polyunsaturated fats, decreases platelet aggregation, decreases blood clot formation, promotes normal growth and development of muscle tissue, prostaglandin synthesis.

PHARMACOKINETICS

Vitamin E is metabolized in the liver and excreted in bile.

INDICATIONS AND USAGE

Vitamin E deficiency.

PRECAUTIONS

PREGNANCY

Pregnancy Category A if doses do not exceed the recommended daily allowance of 15 IU. Pregnancy Category C if doses exceed the recommended daily allowance.

NURSING MOTHERS

Vitamin E is excreted in breast milk which is 5 times richer in vitamin E than cow's milk. The recommended daily allowance in lactating mothers is 16 IU.

DRUG INTERACTIONS

Iron: Impaired hematological response to iron in children with iron-deficiency anemia.
Oral Anticoagulant: Vitamin E increases hypoprothombinemic response to oral anticoagulants, especially in doses >400 IU/day.

ADVERSE REACTIONS

Central Nervous System: Fatigue, headache.
Special Senses: Blurred vision.
Gastrointestinal: Cramps, diarrhea, nausea.
Genitourinary: Gonadal dysfunction.
Metabolic: Altered metabolism of thyroid, pituitary, and adrenal hormones.
Musculoskeletal: Weakness.
Skin: Contact dermatitis, sterile abscess.

DOSAGE AND ADMINISTRATION

Adults: 60-75 IU per day, not to exceed 300 IU/day.
Pediatric Patients: 1 IU/kg/day.

PRODUCT LISTING - EQUIVALENTS NOT AVAILABLE

Capsule - Oral - 200 IU

100's	$7.99	VITAMIN E, Cypress Pharmaceutical Inc	60258-0109-01

Voriconazole (003556)

For related information, see the comparative table section in Appendix A.

Categories: Aspergillosis; Infection, fungal, systemic; Pregnancy Category D; FDA Approved 2002 May
Drug Classes: Antifungals
Brand Names: Vfend
Cost of Therapy: $1,8775.00 (Fungal Infections; Vfend; 200 mg; 2 tablets/day; 30 day supply)

DESCRIPTION

Vfend (voriconazole), a triazole antifungal agent, is available as film-coated tablets for oral administration, and as a lyophilized powder for solution for intravenous infusion.

Voriconazole is designated chemically as (2R, 3S)-2-(2,4-difluorophenyl)-3-(5-fluoro-4-pyrimidinyl)-1-(1*H*-1,2,4-triazol-1-yl)-2-butanol with an empirical formula of $C_{16}H_{14}F_3N_5O$ and a molecular weight of 349.3.

Voriconazole drug substance is a white to light-colored powder.

Vfend Tablets contain 50 or 200 mg of voriconazole. The inactive ingredients include lactose monohydrate, pregelatinized starch, croscarmellose sodium, povidone, magnesium stearate and a coating containing hydroxypropyl methylcellulose, titanium dioxide, lactose monohydrate and triacetin.

Vfend IV is a white lyophilized powder containing nominally 200 mg voriconazole and 3200 mg sulfobutyl ether beta-cyclodextrin sodium in a 30 ml Type I clear glass vial.

Vfend IV is intended for administration by intravenous infusion. It is a single dose, unpreserved product. Vials containing 200 mg lyophilized voriconazole are intended for reconstitution with water for injection to produce a solution containing 10 mg/ml voriconazole and 160 mg/ml of sulfobutyl ether beta-cyclodextrin sodium. The resultant solution is further diluted prior to administration as an intravenous infusion (see DOSAGE AND ADMINISTRATION).

CLINICAL PHARMACOLOGY

PHARMACOKINETICS

General Pharmacokinetic Characteristics

The pharmacokinetics of voriconazole have been characterized in healthy subjects, special populations and patients.

The pharmacokinetics of voriconazole are non-linear due to saturation of its metabolism. The interindividual variability of voriconazole pharmacokinetics is high. Greater than proportional increase in exposure is observed with increasing dose. It is estimated that, on average, increasing the oral dose in healthy subjects from 200 mg q12h to 300 mg q12h leads to a 2.5-fold increase in exposure (AUCτ) while increasing the intravenous dose from 3 mg/kg q12h to 4 mg/kg q12h produces a 2.3-fold increase in exposure (TABLE 1).

TABLE 1 *Population Pharmacokinetic Parameters of Voriconazole in Volunteers*

	200 mg Oral q12h	300 mg Oral q12h	3 mg/kg IV q12h	4 mg/kg IV q12h
AUCτ* (μg·h/ml)	19.86	50.32	21.81	50.40
(CV%)	(94%)	(74%)	(100%)	(83%)

* Mean AUCτ are predicted values from population pharmacokinetic analysis of data from 236 volunteers.

During oral administration of 200 or 300 mg twice daily for 14 days in patients at risk of aspergillosis (mainly patients with malignant neoplasms of lymphatic or hematopoietic tissue), the observed pharmacokinetic characteristics were similar to those observed in healthy subjects (TABLE 2).

TABLE 2 *Pharmacokinetic Parameters of Voriconazole in Patients at Risk for Aspergillosis*

	200 mg Oral q12h (n=9)	300 mg Oral q12h (n=9)
AUCτ* (μg·h/ml)	20.31	36.51
(CV%)	(69%)	(45%)
C_{max}* (μg/ml)	3.00	4.66
(CV%)	(51%)	(35%)

* Geometric mean values on Day 14 of multiple dosing in 2 cohorts of patients.

Sparse plasma sampling for pharmacokinetics was conducted in the therapeutic studies in patients aged 12-18 years. In 11 adolescent patients who received a mean voriconazole maintenance dose of 4 mg/kg IV, the median of the calculated mean plasma concentrations was 1.60 μg/ml (inter-quartile range 0.28-2.73 μg/ml). In 17 adolescent patients for whom mean plasma concentrations were calculated following a mean oral maintenance dose of 200 mg q12h, the median of the calculated mean plasma concentrations was 1.16 μg/ml (inter-quartile range 0.85-2.14 μg/ml).

When the recommended intravenous or oral loading dose regimens are administered to healthy subjects, peak plasma concentrations close to steady state are achieved within the first 24 hours of dosing. Without the loading dose, accumulation occurs during twice-daily multiple dosing with steady-state peak plasma voriconazole concentrations being achieved by day 6 in the majority of subjects (TABLE 3).

Steady state trough plasma concentrations with voriconazole are achieved after approximately 5 days of oral or intravenous dosing without a loading dose regimen. However, when an intravenous loading dose regimen is used, steady state trough plasma concentrations are achieved within 1 day.

TABLE 3 *Pharmacokinetic Parameters of Voriconazole From Loading Dose and Maintenance Dose Regimens (Individual Studies in Volunteers)*

	400 mg q12h on Day 1, 200 mg q12h on Days 2-10 (n=17)		6 mg/kg IV† q12h on Day 1, 3 mg/kg IV q12h on Days 2-10 (n=9)	
	Day 1, 1st dose	Day 10	Day 1, 1st dose	Day 10
AUCτ* (μg·h/ml)	9.31	11.13	13.22	13.25
(CV%)	(38%)	(103%)	(22%)	(58%)
C_{max}* (μg/ml)	2.30	2.08	4.70	3.06
(CV%)	(19%)	(62%)	(22%)	(31%)

Pharmacokinetic parameters for loading and maintenance doses summarized for same cohort of volunteers.
* AUCτ values are calculated over dosing interval of 12 hours.
† IV infusion over 60 minutes.

Absorption
The pharmacokinetic properties of voriconazole are similar following administration by the intravenous and oral routes. Based on a population pharmacokinetic analysis of pooled data in healthy subjects (n=207), the oral bioavailability of voriconazole is estimated to be 96% (CV 13%).

Maximum plasma concentrations (C_{max}) are achieved 1-2 hours after dosing. When multiple doses of voriconazole are administered with high fat meals, the mean C_{max} and AUCτ are reduced by 34% and 24%, respectively (see DOSAGE AND ADMINISTRATION).

In healthy subjects, the absorption of voriconazole is not affected by coadministration of oral ranitidine, cimetidine, or omeprazole, drugs that are known to increase gastric pH.

Distribution
The volume of distribution at steady state for voriconazole is estimated to be 4.6 L/kg, suggesting extensive distribution into tissues. Plasma protein binding is estimated to be 58% and was shown to be independent of plasma concentrations achieved following single and multiple oral doses of 200 or 300 mg (approximate range: 0.9-15 μg/ml). Varying degrees of hepatic and renal insufficiency do not affect the protein binding of voriconazole.

Metabolism
In vitro studies showed that voriconazole is metabolized by the human hepatic cytochrome P450 enzymes, CYP2C19, CYP2C9 and CYP3A4 (see CLINICAL PHARMACOLOGY, Drug Interactions).

In vivo studies indicated that CYP2C19 is significantly involved in the metabolism of voriconazole. This enzyme exhibits genetic polymorphism. For example, 15-20% of Asian populations may be expected to be poor metabolizers. For Caucasians and Blacks, the prevalence of poor metabolizers is 3-5%. Studies conducted in Caucasian and Japanese healthy subjects have shown that poor metabolizers have, on average, 4-fold higher voriconazole exposure (AUCτ) than their homozygous extensive metabolizer counterparts. Subjects who are heterozygous extensive metabolizers have, on average, 2-fold higher voriconazole exposure than their homozygous extensive metabolizer counterparts.

The major metabolite of voriconazole is the N-oxide, which accounts for 72% of the circulating radiolabelled metabolites in plasma. Since this metabolite has minimal antifungal activity, it does not contribute to the overall efficacy of voriconazole.

Excretion
Voriconazole is eliminated via hepatic metabolism with less than 2% of the dose excreted unchanged in the urine. After administration of a single radiolabelled dose of either oral or IV voriconazole, preceded by multiple oral or IV dosing, approximately 80-83% of the radioactivity is recovered in the urine. The majority (>94%) of the total radioactivity is excreted in the first 96 hours after both oral and intravenous dosing.

As a result of non-linear pharmacokinetics, the terminal half-life of voriconazole is dose dependent and therefore not useful in predicting the accumulation or elimination of voriconazole.

Pharmacokinetic-Pharmacodynamic Relationships
In ten clinical trials, the median values for the average and maximum voriconazole plasma concentrations in individual patients across these studies (n=1121) was 2.51 μg/ml (inter-quartile range 1.21-4.44 μg/ml) and 3.79 μg/ml (inter-quartile range 2.06-6.31 μg/ml), respectively. A pharmacokinetic-pharmacodynamic analysis of patient data from 6 of these 10 clinical trials (n=280) could not detect a positive association between mean, maximum or minimum plasma voriconazole concentration and efficacy. However, PK/PD analyses of the data from all 10 clinical trials identified positive associations between plasma voriconazole concentrations and rate of both liver function test abnormalities and visual disturbances (see ADVERSE REACTIONS).

Pharmacokinetics in Special Populations

Gender
In a multiple oral dose study, the mean C_{max} and AUCτ for healthy young females were 83% and 113% higher, respectively, than in healthy young males (18-45 years). In the same study, no significant differences in the mean C_{max} and AUCτ were observed between healthy elderly males and healthy elderly females (≥65 years).

In the clinical program, no dosage adjustment was made on the basis of gender. The safety profile and plasma concentrations observed in male and female subjects were similar. Therefore, no dosage adjustment based on gender is necessary.

Geriatric
In an oral multiple dose study the mean C_{max} and AUCτ in healthy elderly males (≥65 years) were 61% and 86% higher, respectively, than in young males (18-45 years). No significant differences in the mean C_{max} and AUCτ were observed between healthy elderly females (≥65 years) and healthy young females (18-45 years).

In the clinical program, no dosage adjustment was made on the basis of age. An analysis of pharmacokinetic data obtained from 552 patients from 10 voriconazole clinical trials showed that the median voriconazole plasma concentrations in the elderly patients (>65 years) were approximately 80-90% higher than those in the younger patients (≤65 years) after either IV or oral administration. However, the safety profile of voriconazole in young and elderly subjects was similar and, therefore, no dosage adjustment is necessary for the elderly.

Pediatric
A population pharmacokinetic analysis was conducted on pooled data from 35 immunocompromised pediatric patients aged 2 to <12 years old who were included in two pharmacokinetic studies of intravenous voriconazole (single dose and multiple dose). Twenty-four (24) of these patients received multiple intravenous maintenance doses of 3 and 4 mg/kg. A comparison of the pediatric and adult population pharmacokinetic data revealed that the predicted average steady state plasma concentrations were similar at the maintenance dose of 4 mg/kg every 12 hours in children and 3 mg/kg every 12 hours in adults (medians of 1.19 μg/ml and 1.16 μg/ml in children and adults, respectively). (See PRECAUTIONS, Pediatric Use.)

Hepatic Insufficiency
After a single oral dose (200 mg) of voriconazole in 8 patients with mild (Child-Pugh Class A) and 4 patients with moderate (Child-Pugh Class B) hepatic insufficiency, the mean systemic exposure (AUC) was 3.2-fold higher than in age and weight matched controls with normal hepatic function. There was no difference in mean peak plasma concentrations (C_{max}) between the groups. When only the patients with mild (Child-Pugh Class A) hepatic insufficiency were compared to controls, there was still a 2.3-fold increase in the mean AUC in the group with hepatic insufficiency compared to controls.

In an oral multiple dose study, AUCτ was similar in 6 subjects with moderate hepatic impairment (Child-Pugh Class B) given a lower maintenance dose of 100 mg twice daily compared to 6 subjects with normal hepatic function given the standard 200 mg twice daily maintenance dose. The mean peak plasma concentrations (C_{max}) were 20% lower in the hepatically impaired group.

It is recommended that the standard loading dose regimens be used but that the maintenance dose be halved in patients with mild to moderate hepatic cirrhosis (Child-Pugh Class A and B) receiving voriconazole. No pharmacokinetic data are available for patients with severe hepatic cirrhosis (Child-Pugh Class C) (see DOSAGE AND ADMINISTRATION).

Renal Insufficiency
In a single oral dose (200 mg) study in 24 subjects with normal renal function and mild to severe renal impairment, systemic exposure (AUC) and peak plasma concentration (C_{max}) of voriconazole were not significantly affected by renal impairment. Therefore, no adjustment is necessary for oral dosing in patients with mild to severe renal impairment.

In a multiple dose study of IV voriconazole (6 mg/kg IV loading dose × 2, then 3 mg/kg IV × 5.5 days) in 7 patients with moderate renal dysfunction (creatinine clearance 30-50 ml/min), the systemic exposure (AUC) and peak plasma concentrations (C_{max}) were not significantly different from those in 6 volunteers with normal renal function.

However, in patients with moderate renal dysfunction (creatinine clearance 30-50 ml/min), accumulation of the intravenous vehicle, SBECD, occurs. The mean systemic exposure (AUC) and peak plasma concentrations (C_{max}) of SBECD were increased by 4-fold and almost 50%, respectively, in the moderately impaired group compared to the normal control group.

Intravenous voriconazole should be avoided in patients with moderate or severe renal impairment (creatinine clearance <50 ml/min), unless an assessment of the benefit/risk to the patient justifies the use of intravenous voriconazole (see DOSAGE AND ADMINISTRATION, Dose Adjustment).

A pharmacokinetic study in subjects with renal failure undergoing hemodialysis showed that voriconazole is dialyzed with clearance of 121 ml/min. The intravenous vehicle, SBECD, is hemodialyzed with clearance of 55 ml/min. A 4 hour hemodialysis session does not remove a sufficient amount of voriconazole to warrant dose adjustment.

DRUG INTERACTIONS

Effects of Other Drugs on Voriconazole
Voriconazole is metabolized by the human hepatic cytochrome P450 enzymes CYP2C19, CYP2C9, and CYP3A4. Results of *in vitro* metabolism studies indicate that the affinity of voriconazole is highest for CYP2C19, followed by CYP2C9, and is appreciably lower for CYP3A4. Inhibitors or inducers of these three enzymes may increase or decrease voriconazole systemic exposure (plasma concentrations), respectively.

The systemic exposure to voriconazole is significantly reduced or is expected to be reduced by the concomitant administration of the following agents and their use is contraindicated:

Rifampin (potent CYP450 inducer): Rifampin (600 mg once daily) decreased the steady state C_{max} and AUCτ of voriconazole (200 mg q12h × 7 days) by an average of 93% and 96%, respectively, in healthy subjects. Doubling the dose of voriconazole to 400 mg q12h does not restore adequate exposure to voriconazole during coadministration with rifampin. **Coadministration of voriconazole and rifampin is contraindicated** (see CONTRAINDICATIONS and DRUG INTERACTIONS).

Carbamazepine and long acting barbiturates (potent CYP450 inducers): Although not studied *in vitro* or *in vivo*, carbamazepine and long acting barbiturates (*e.g.*, phenobarbital, mephobarbital) are likely to significantly decrease plasma voriconazole concentrations. **Coadministration of voriconazole with carbamazepine or long acting barbiturates is contraindicated** (see CONTRAINDICATIONS and DRUG INTERACTIONS).

V

Minor or no significant pharmacokinetic interactions that do not require dosage adjustment:

Cimetidine (non-specific CYP450 inhibitor and increases gastric pH): Cimetidine (400 mg q12h × 8 days) increased voriconazole steady state C_{max} and AUCτ by an average of 18% (90% CI: 6%, 32%) and 23% (90% CI: 13%, 33%), respectively, following oral doses of 200 mg q12h × 7 days to healthy subjects.

Ranitidine (increases gastric pH): Ranitidine (150 mg q12h) had no significant effect on voriconazole C_{max} and AUCτ following oral doses of 200 mg q12h × 7 days to healthy subjects.

Macrolide antibiotics: Coadministration of **erythromycin** (CYP3A4 inhibitor; 1g q12h for 7 days) or **azithromycin** (500 mg qd for 3 days) with voriconazole 200 mg q12h for 14 days had no significant effect on voriconazole steady state C_{max} and AUCτ in healthy subjects. The effects of voriconazole on the pharmacokinetics of either erythromycin or azithromycin are not known.

Effects of Voriconazole on Other Drugs

In vitro studies with human hepatic microsomes show that voriconazole inhibits the metabolic activity of the cytochrome P450 enzymes CYP2C19, CYP2C9, and CYP3A4. In these studies, the inhibition potency of voriconazole for CYP3A4 metabolic activity was significantly less than that of two other azoles, ketoconazole and itraconazole. *In vitro* studies also show that the major metabolite of voriconazole, voriconazole N-oxide, inhibits the metabolic activity of CYP2C9 and CYP3A4 to a greater extent than that of CYP2C19. Therefore, there is potential for voriconazole and its major metabolite to increase the sytemic exposure (plasma concentrations) of other drugs metabolized by these CYP450 enzymes.

The systemic exposure of the following drugs is significantly increased or is expected to be significantly increased by coadministration of voriconazole and their use is contraindicated:

Sirolimus (CYP3A4 substrate): Repeat dose administration of oral voriconazole (400 mg q12h for 1 day, then 200 mg q12h for 8 days) increased the C_{max} and AUC of sirolimus (2 mg single dose) an average of 7-fold (90% CI: 5.7, 7.5) and 11-fold (90% CI: 9.9, 12.6), respectively, in healthy subjects. **Coadministration of voriconazole and sirolimus is contraindicated** (see CONTRAINDICATIONS and DRUG INTERACTIONS).

Terfenadine, astemizole, cisapride, pimozide and quinidine (CYP3A4 substrates): Although not studied *in vitro* or *in vivo,* concomitant administration of voriconazole with terfenadine, astemizole, cisapride, pimozide or quinidine may result in inhibition of the metabolism of these drugs. Increased plasma concentrations of these drugs can lead to QT prolongation and rare occurrences of *torsade de pointes.* **Coadministration of voriconazole and terfenidine, astemizole, cisapride, pimozide and quinidine is contraindicated** (see CONTRAINDICATIONS and DRUG INTERACTIONS).

Ergot alkaloids: Although not studied *in vitro* or *in vivo,* voriconazole may increase the plasma concentration of ergot alkaloids (ergotamine and dihydroergotamine) and lead to ergotism. **Coadministration of voriconazole with ergot alkaloids is contraindicated** (see CONTRAINDICATIONS and DRUG INTERACTIONS).

Coadministration of voriconazole with the following agents results in increased exposure or is expected to result in increased exposure to these drugs. Therefore, careful monitoring and/or dosage adjustment of these drugs is needed:

Cyclosporine (CYP3A4 substrate): In stable renal transplant recipients receiving chronic cyclosporine therapy, concomitant administration of oral voriconazole (200 mg q12h for 8 days) increased cyclosporine C_{max} and AUCτ an average of 1.1 times (90% CI: 0.9, 1.41) and 1.7 times (90% CI: 1.5, 2.0), respectively, as compared to when cyclosporine was administered without voriconazole. When initiating therapy with voriconazole in patients already receiving cyclosporine, it is recommended that the cyclosporine dose be reduced to one-half of the original dose and followed with frequent monitoring of the cyclosporine blood levels. Increased cyclosporine levels have been associated with nephrotoxicity. When voriconazole is discontinued, cyclosporine levels should be frequently monitored and the dose increased as necessary (see DRUG INTERACTIONS).

Tacrolimus (CYP3A4 substrate): Repeat oral dose administration of voriconazole (400 mg q12h × 1 day then 200 mg q12h × 6 days) increased tacrolimus (0.1 mg/kg single dose) C_{max} and AUCτ [in healthy subjects by an average of 2-fold (90% CI: 1.9, 2.5] and 3-fold (90% CI: 2.7, 3.8), respectively. When initiating therapy with voriconazole in patients already receiving tacrolimus, it is recommended that the tacrolimus dose be reduced to one-third of the original dose and followed with frequent monitoring of the tacrolimus blood levels. Increased tacrolimus levels have been associated with nephrotoxicity. When voriconazole is discontinued, tacrolimus levels should be carefully monitored and the dose increased as necessary (see DRUG INTERACTIONS).

Warfarin (CYP2C9 substrate): Coadministration of voriconazole (300 mg q12h × 12 days) with warfarin (30 mg single dose) significantly increased maximum prothrombin time by approximately 2 times that of placebo in healthy subjects. Close monitoring of prothrombin time or other suitable anti-coagulation tests is recommended if warfarin and voriconazole are coadministered and the warfarin dose adjusted accordingly (see DRUG INTERACTIONS).

Oral Coumarin Anticoagulants (CYP2C9, CYP3A4 substrates): Although not studied *in vitro* or *in vivo,* voriconazole may increase the plasma concentrations of coumarin anticoagulants and therefore may cause an increase in prothrombin time. If patients receiving coumarin preparations are treated simultaneously with voriconazole, the prothrombin time or other suitable anti-coagulation tests should be monitored at close intervals and the dosage of anticoagulants adjusted accordingly (see DRUG INTERACTIONS).

Statins (CYP3A4 substrates): Although not studied clinically, voriconazole has been shown to inhibit lovastatin metabolism *in vitro* (human liver microsomes). Therefore, voriconazole is likely to increase the plasma concentrations of statins that are metabolized by CYP3A4. It is recommended that dose adjustment of the statin be considered during coadministration. Increased statin concentrations in plasma have been associated with rhabdomyolysis (see DRUG INTERACTIONS).

Benzodiazepines (CYP3A4 substrates): Although not studied clinically, voriconazole has been shown to inhibit midazolam metabolism *in vitro* (human liver microsomes). Therefore, voriconazole is likely to increase the plasma concentrations of benzodiazepines that are metabolized by CYP3A4 (*e.g.,* midazolam, triazolam, and alprazolam) and lead to a prolonged sedative effect. It is recommended that dose adjustment of the benzodiazepine be considered during coadministration (see DRUG INTERACTIONS).

Calcium Channel Blockers (CYP3A4 substrates): Although not studied clinically, voriconazole has been shown to inhibit felodipine metabolism *in vitro* (human liver microsomes). Therefore, voriconazole may increase the plasma concentrations of calcium channel blockers that are metabolized by CYP3A4. Frequent monitoring for adverse events and toxicity related to calcium channel blockers is recommended during coadministration. Dose adjustment of the calcium channel blocker may be needed (see DRUG INTERACTIONS).

Sulfonylureas (CYP2C9 substrates): Although not studied *in vitro* or *in vivo,* voriconazole may increase plasma concentrations of sulfonylureas (*e.g.,* tolbutamide, glipizide, and glyburide) and therefore cause hypoglycemia. Frequent monitoring of blood glucose and appropriate adjustment (*i.e.,* reduction) of the sulfonylurea dosage is recommended during coadministration (see DRUG INTERACTIONS).

Vinca Alkaloids (CYP3A4 substrates): Although not studied *in vitro* or *in vivo,* voriconazole may increase the plasma concentrations of the vinca alkaloids (*e.g.,* vincristine and vinblastine) and lead to neurotoxicity. Therefore, it is recommended that dose adjustment of the vinca alkaloid be considered.

No significant pharmacokinetic interactions were observed when voriconazole was coadministered with the following agents. Therefore, no dosage adjustment for these agents is recommended.

Prednisolone (CYP3A4 substrate): Voriconazole (200 mg q12h × 30 days) increased C_{max} and AUC of prednisolone (60 mg single dose) by an average of 11% and 34%, respectively in healthy subjects.

Digoxin (P-glycoprotein mediated transport): Voriconazole (200 mg q12h × 12 days) had no significant effect on steady state C_{max} and AUCτ of digoxin (0.25 mg once daily for 10 days) in healthy subjects.

Mycophenolic Acid (UDP-glucuronyl transferase substrate): Voriconazole (200 mg q12h × 5 days) had no significant effect on the C_{max} and AUCτ of mycophenolic acid and its major metabolite, mycophenolic acid glucuronide after administration of a 1 g single oral dose of mycophenolate mofetil.

Two-Way Interactions

Concomitant use of the following agent with voriconazole is contraindicated:

Rifabutin (potent CYP450 inducer): Rifabutin (300 mg once daily) decreased the C_{max} and AUCτ of voriconazole at 200 mg twice daily by an average of 67% (90% CI: 58%, 73%) and 79% (90% CI: 71%, 84%), respectively, in healthy subjects. During coadministration with rifabutin (300 mg once daily), the steady state C_{max} and AUCτ of voriconazole following an increased dose of 400 mg twice daily were on average approximately 2 times higher, compared with voriconazole alone at 200 mg twice daily. Coadministration of voriconazole at 400 mg twice daily with rifabutin 300 mg twice daily increased the C_{max} and AUCτ of rifabutin by an average of 3 times (90% CI: 2.2, 4.0) and 4 times (90% CI: 3.5, 5.4), respectively, compared to rifabutin given alone. **Coadministration of voriconazole and rifabutin is contraindicated.**

Significant drug interactions that may require dosage adjustment, frequent monitoring of drug levels and/or frequent monitoring of drug-related adverse events/toxicity:

Phenytoin (CYP2C9 substrate and potent CYP450 inducer): Repeat dose administration of phenytoin (300 mg once daily) decreased the steady state C_{max} and AUCτ of orally administered voriconazole (200 mg q12h × 14 days) by an average of 50% and 70%, respectively, in healthy subjects. Administration of a higher voriconazole dose (400 mg q12h × 7 days) with phenytoin (300 mg once daily) resulted in comparable steady state voriconazole C_{max} and AUCτ estimates as compared to when voriconazole was given at 200 mg q12h without phenytoin.

Phenytoin may be coadministered with voriconazole if the maintenance dose of voriconazole is increased from 4-5 mg/kg intravenously every 12 hours or from 200-400 mg orally, every 12 hours (100-200 mg orally, every 12 hours in patients less than 40 kg) (see DOSAGE AND ADMINISTRATION).

Repeat dose administration of voriconazole (400 mg q12h × 10 days) increased the steady state C_{max} and AUCτ of phenytoin (300 mg once daily) by an average of 70% and 80%, respectively, in healthy subjects. The increase in phenytoin C_{max} and AUC when coadministered with voriconazole may be expected to be as high as 2 times the C_{max} and AUC estimates when phenytoin is given without voriconazole. Therefore, frequent monitoring of plasma phenytoin concentrations and phenytoin-related adverse effects is recommended when phenytoin is coadministered with voriconazole (see DRUG INTERACTIONS).

Omeprazole (CYP2C19 inhibitor; CYP2C19 and CYP3A4 substrate): Coadminstration of omeprazole (40 mg once daily × 10 days) with oral voriconazole (400 mg q12h × 1 day, then 200 mg q12h × 9 days) increased the steady state C_{max} and AUCτ of voriconazole by an average of 15% (90% CI: 5%, 25%) and 40% (90% CI: 29%, 55%), respectively in healthy subjects. No dosage adjustment of voriconazole is recommended.

Coadministration of voriconazole (400 mg q12h × 1 day, then 200 mg × 6 days) with omeprazole (40 mg once daily × 7 days) to healthy subjects significantly increased the steady state C_{max} and AUCτ of omeprazole an average of 2 times (90% CI: 1.8, 2.6) and 4 times (90% CI: 3.3, 4.4), respectively, as compared to when omeprazole is given without voriconazole. When initiating voriconazole in patients already receiving omeprazole doses of 40 mg or greater, it is recommended that the omeprazole dose be reduced by one-half (see DRUG INTERACTIONS).

The metabolism of other proton pump inhibitors that are CYP2C19 substrates may also be inhibited by voriconazole and may result in increased plasma concentrations of these drugs.

No significant pharmacokinetic interaction was seen and no dosage adjustment of these drugs is recommended:

Indinavir (CYP3A4 inhibitor and substrate): Repeat dose administration of indinavir (800 mg tid for 10 days) had no significant effect on voriconazole C_{max} and AUC following repeat dose administration (200 mg q12h for 17 days) in healthy subjects.

Repeat dose administration of voriconazole (200 mg q12h for 7 days) did not have a significant effect on steady state C_{max} and AUCτ of indinavir following repeat dose administration (800 mg tid for 7 days) in healthy subjects.

Other two-way interactions expected to be significant based on *in vitro* findings:

Other HIV Protease Inhibitors (CYP3A4 substrates and inhibitors): *In vitro* studies (human liver microsomes) suggest that voriconazole may inhibit the metabolism of HIV protease inhibitors (*e.g.,* saquinavir, amprenavir and nelfenavir). *In vitro* studies (human liver microsomes) also show that the metabolism of voriconazole may be inhibited by HIV protease inhibitors (*e.g.,* ritonavir, saquinavir, and amprenavir). Patients should be frequently monitored for drug toxicity during the coadministration of voriconazole and HIV protease inhibitors (see DRUG INTERACTIONS).

Non-Nucleoside Reverse Transcriptase Inhibitors (NNRTI) (CYP3A4 substrates, inhibitors or CYP450 inducers): *In vitro* studies (human liver microsomes) show that the metabolism of voriconazole may be inhibited by an NNRTI (*e.g.,* delavirdine and efavirenz). Although not studied *in vitro* or *in vivo,* the metabolism of voriconazole may be induced by an NNRTI, such as efavirenz or nevirapine. *In vitro* studies (human liver microsomes) show that voriconazole may also inhibit the metabolism of an NNRTI (*e.g.,* delavirdine). Patients should be frequently monitored for drug toxicity during the coadministration of voriconazole and an NNRTI (see DRUG INTERACTIONS).

MICROBIOLOGY

Mechanism of Action

Voriconazole is a triazole antifungal agent. The primary mode of action of voriconazole is the inhibition of fungal cytochrome P-450-mediated 14 alpha-lanosterol demethylation, an essential step in fungal ergosterol biosynthesis. The accumulation of 14 alpha-methyl sterols correlates with the subsequent loss of ergosterol in the fungal cell wall and may be responsible for the antifungal activity of voriconazole. Voriconazole has been shown to be more selective for fungal cytochrome P-450 enzymes than for various mammalian cytochrome P-450 enzyme systems.

Activity In Vitro and In Vivo

Voriconazole has demonstrated *in vitro* activity against *Aspergillus fumigatus* isolates as well as *A. flavus, A. niger* and *A. terreus.* Variable *in vitro* activity against *Scedosporium apiospermum* and *Fusarium* spp., including *Fusarium solani,* has been seen. Most of the speciated isolates from clinical studies were *Aspergillus fumigatus* but clinical efficacy was also seen in a small number of species other than *A. fumigatus* (see INDICATIONS AND USAGE).

In vitro susceptibility testing was performed according to the National Committee for Clinical Laboratory Standards (NCCLS) proposed method (M38-P). Voriconazole breakpoints have not been established for any fungi. The relationship between clinical outcome and *in vitro* susceptibility results remains to be elucidated.

Voriconazole has demonstrated *in vivo* activity in normal and immunocompromised guinea pigs with established systemic *A. fumigatus* infections in which the endpoints were prolonged survival of infected animals and reduction of mycological burden from target organs. Activity has also been shown in immunocompromised guinea pigs with pulmonary *A. fumigatus* infections. Voriconazole demonstrated activity in immunocompromised guinea pigs with systemic infections produced by an *A. fumigatus* isolate with reduced susceptibility to itraconazole (itraconazole MIC 3.1 μg/ml). The exact mechanism of resistance was not identified for that particular isolate. In one experiment, voriconazole exhibited activity against *Scedosporium apiospermum* infections in immune competent guinea pigs.

Drug Resistance

Voriconazole drug resistance development has not been adequately studied *in vitro* against the filamentous fungi, including *Aspergillus, Scedosporium* and *Fusarium* species. The frequency of drug resistance development for the various fungi for which this drug is indicated is not known.

Fungal isolates exhibiting reduced susceptibility to fluconazole or itraconazole may also show reduced susceptibility to voriconazole, suggesting cross-resistance can occur among these azoles. The relevance of cross-resistance and clinical outcome has not been fully characterized. Clinical cases where azole cross-resistance is demonstrated may require alternative antifungal therapy.

INDICATIONS AND USAGE

Voriconazole is indicated for use in the treatment of the following fungal infections:

Treatment of invasive aspergillosis. In clinical trials, the majority of isolates recovered were *Aspergillus fumigatus.* There was a small number of cases of culture-proven disease due to species of *Aspergillus* other than *A. fumigatus* (see CLINICAL PHARMACOLOGY, Microbiology).

Treatment of serious fungal infections caused by *Scedosporium apiospermum* (asexual form of *Pseudallescheria boydii*) and *Fusarium* spp. including *Fusarium solani,* in patients intolerant of, or refractory to, other therapy.

Specimens for fungal culture and other relevant laboratory studies (including histopathology) should be obtained prior to therapy to isolate and identify causative organism(s). Therapy may be instituted before the results of the cultures and other laboratory studies are known. However, once these results become available, antifungal therapy should be adjusted accordingly.

CONTRAINDICATIONS

Voriconazole is contraindicated in patients with known hypersensitivity to voriconazole or its excipients. There is no information regarding cross-sensitivity between voriconazole and other azole antifungal agents. Caution should be used when prescribing voriconazole to patients with hypersensitivity to other azoles.

Coadministration of the CYP3A4 substrates, terfenadine, astemizole, cisapride, pimozide or quinidine with voriconazole are contraindicated since increased plasma concentrations of these drugs can lead to QT prolongation and rare occurrences of *torsade de pointes* (see CLINICAL PHARMACOLOGY, Drug Interactions; DRUG INTERACTIONS).

Coadministration of voriconazole with sirolimus is contraindicated because voriconazole significantly increases sirolimus concentrations in healthy subjects (see CLINICAL PHARMACOLOGY, Drug Interactions; DRUG INTERACTIONS).

Coadministration of voriconazole with rifampin, carbamazepine and long-acting barbiturates is contraindicated since these drugs are likely to decrease plasma voriconazole concentrations significantly (see CLINICAL PHARMACOLOGY, Drug Interactions; DRUG INTERACTIONS).

Coadministration of voriconazole with rifabutin is contraindicated since voriconazole significantly increases rifabutin plasma concentrations and rifabutin also significantly decreases voriconazole plasma concentrations (see CLINICAL PHARMACOLOGY, Drug Interactions; DRUG INTERACTIONS).

Coadministration of voriconazole with ergot alkaloids (ergotamine and dihydroergotamine) is contraindicated because voriconazole may increase the plasma concentration of ergot alkaloids, which may lead to ergotism.

WARNINGS

VISUAL DISTURBANCES

The effect of voriconazole on visual function is not known if treatment continues beyond 28 days. If treatment continues beyond 28 days, visual function including visual acuity, visual field and color perception should be monitored (see PRECAUTIONS, Information for the Patient and ADVERSE REACTIONS, Visual Disturbances).

HEPATIC TOXICITY

In clinical trials, there have been uncommon cases of serious hepatic reactions during treatment with voriconazole (including clinical hepatitis, cholestasis and fulminant hepatic failure, including fatalities). Instances of hepatic reactions were noted to occur primarily in patients with serious underlying medical conditions (predominantly hematological malignancy). Hepatic reactions, including hepatitis and jaundice, have occurred among patients with no other identifiable risk factors. Liver dysfunction has usually been reversible on discontinuation of therapy (see PRECAUTIONS, Laboratory Tests and ADVERSE REACTIONS, Clinical Laboratory Values).

MONITORING OF HEPATIC FUNCTION

Liver function tests should be evaluated at the start of and during the course of voriconazole therapy. Patients who develop abnormal liver function tests during voriconazole therapy should be monitored for the development of more severe hepatic injury. Patient management should include laboratory evaluation of hepatic function (particularly liver function tests and bilirubin). Discontinuation of voriconazole must be considered if clinical signs and symptoms consistent with liver disease develop that may be attributable to voriconazole (see PRECAUTIONS, Laboratory Tests; DOSAGE AND ADMINISTRATION, Dose Adjustment; ADVERSE REACTIONS, Clinical Laboratory Values).

PREGNANCY CATEGORY D

Voriconazole can cause fetal harm when administered to a pregnant woman.

Voriconazole was teratogenic in rats (cleft palates, hydronephrosis/hydroureter) from 10 mg/kg (0.3 times the recommended maintenance dose (RMD) on a mg/m^2 basis) and embryotoxic in rabbits at 100 mg/kg (6 times the RMD). Other effects in rats included reduced ossification of sacral and caudal vertebrae, skull, pubic and hyoid bone, super numerary ribs, anomalies of the sternebrae and dilatation of the ureter/renal pelvis. Plasma estradiol in pregnant rats was reduced at all dose levels. Voriconazole treatment in rats produced increased gestational length and dystocia, which were associated with increased perinatal pup mortality at the 10 mg/kg dose. The effects seen in rabbits were an increased embryomortality, reduced fetal weight and increased incidences of skeletal variations, cervical ribs and extra sternebral ossification sites.

If this drug is used during pregnancy, or if the patient becomes pregnant while taking this drug, the patient should be apprised of the potential hazard to the fetus.

GALACTOSE INTOLERANCE

Voriconazole tablets contain lactose and should not be given to patients with rare hereditary problems of galactose intolerance, Lapp lactase deficiency or glucose-galactose malabsorption.

PRECAUTIONS

GENERAL

See WARNINGS; DOSAGE AND ADMINISTRATION.

Some azoles, including voriconazole, have been associated with prolongation of the QT interval on the electrocardiogram. During clinical development and post-marketing surveillance, there have been rare cases of torsade de pointes in patients taking voriconazole. These reports involved seriously ill patients with multiple confounding risk factors, such as history of cardiotoxic chemotherapy, cardiomyopathy, hypokalemia and concomitant medications that may have been contributory.

Voriconazole should be administered with caution to patients with these potentially proarrhythmic conditions.

Rigorous attempts to correct potassium, magnesium and calcium should be made before starting voriconazole.

INFUSION RELATED REACTIONS

During infusion of the intravenous formulation of voriconazole in healthy subjects, anaphylactoid-type reactions, including flushing, fever, sweating, tachycardia, chest tightness, dyspnea, faintness, nausea, pruritus and rash, have occurred uncommonly. Symptoms

V

appeared immediately upon initiating the infusion. Consideration should be given to stopping the infusion should these reactions occur.

INFORMATION FOR THE PATIENT

Patients Should Be Advised:

That voriconazole tablets should be taken at least 1 hour before, or 1 hour following, a meal.

That they should not drive at night while taking voriconazole. Voriconazole may cause changes to vision, including blurring and/or photophobia.

That they should avoid potentially hazardous tasks, such as driving or operating machinery if they perceive any change in vision.

That strong, direct sunlight should be avoided during voriconazole therapy.

LABORATORY TESTS

Electrolyte disturbances such as hypokalemia, hypomagnesemia and hypocalcemia should be corrected prior to initiation of voriconazole therapy.

Patient management should include laboratory evaluation of renal (particularly serum creatinine) and hepatic function (particularly liver function tests and bilirubin).

PATIENTS WITH HEPATIC INSUFFICIENCY

It is recommended that the standard loading dose regimens be used but that the maintenance dose be halved in patients with mild to moderate hepatic cirrhosis (Child-Pugh Class A and B) receiving voriconazole (see CLINICAL PHARMACOLOGY, Pharmacokinetics, Pharmacokinetics in Special Populations, Hepatic Insufficiency; DOSAGE AND ADMINISTRATION, Use In Patients With Hepatic Insufficiency).

Voriconazole has not been studied in patients with severe cirrhosis (Child-Pugh Class C). Voriconazole has been associated with elevations in liver function tests and clinical signs of liver damage, such as jaundice, and should only be used in patients with severe hepatic insufficiency if the benefit outweighs the potential risk. Patients with hepatic insufficiency must be carefully monitored for drug toxicity.

PATIENTS WITH RENAL INSUFFICIENCY

In patients with moderate to severe renal dysfunction (creatinine clearance <50 ml/min), accumulation of the intravenous vehicle, SBECD, occurs. Oral voriconazole should be administered to these patients, unless an assessment of the benefit/risk to the patient justifies the use of intravenous voriconazole. Serum creatinine levels should be closely monitored in these patients, and if increases occur, consideration should be given to changing to oral voriconazole therapy (see CLINICAL PHARMACOLOGY, Pharmacokinetics, Pharmacokinetics in Special Populations, Renal Insufficiency; DOSAGE AND ADMINISTRATION, Use in Patients With Renal Insufficiency).

Renal Adverse Events

Acute renal failure has been observed in severely ill patients undergoing treatment with voriconazole. Patients being treated with voriconazole are likely to be treated concomitantly with nephrotoxic medications and have concurrent conditions that may result in decreased renal function.

Monitoring of Renal Function

Patients should be monitored for the development of abnormal renal function. This should include laboratory evaluation, particularly serum creatinine.

DERMATOLOGICAL REACTIONS

Patients have rarely developed serious cutaneous reactions, such as Stevens-Johnson syndrome, during treatment with voriconazole. If patients develop a rash, they should be monitored closely and consideration given to discontinuation of voriconazole. Voriconazole has been infrequently associated with photosensitivity skin reaction, especially during long-term therapy. It is recommended that patients avoid strong, direct sunlight during voriconazole therapy.

CARCINOGENESIS, MUTAGENESIS, AND IMPAIRMENT OF FERTILITY

Two year carcinogenicity studies were conducted in rats and mice. Rats were given oral doses of 6, 18 or 50 mg/kg voriconazole, or 0.2, 0.6, or 1.6 times the recommended maintenance dose (RMD) on a mg/m^2 basis. Hepatocellular adenomas were detected in females at 50 mg/kg and hepatocellular carcinomas were found in males at 6 and 50 mg/kg. Mice were given oral doses of 10, 30 or 100 mg/kg voriconazole, or 0.1, 0.4, or 1.4 times the RMD on a mg/m^2 basis. In mice, hepatocellular adenomas were detected in males and females and hepatocellular carcinomas were detected in males at 1.4 times the RMD of voriconazole.

Voriconazole demonstrated clastogenic activity (mostly chromosome breaks) in human lymphocyte cultures *in vitro.* Voriconazole was not genotoxic in the Ames assay, CHO assay, the mouse micronucleus assay or the DNA repair test (Unscheduled DNA Synthesis assay).

Voriconazole produced a reduction in the pregnancy rates of rats dosed at 50 mg/kg, or 1.6 times the RMD. This was statistically significant only in the preliminary study and not in a larger fertility study.

PREGNANCY, TERATOGENIC EFFECTS, PREGNANCY CATEGORY D

See WARNINGS.

WOMEN OF CHILD-BEARING POTENTIAL

Women of childbearing potential should use effective contraception during treatment.

NURSING MOTHERS

The excretion of voriconazole in breast milk has not been investigated. Voriconazole should not be used by nursing mothers unless the benefit clearly outweighs the risk.

PEDIATRIC USE

Safety and effectiveness in pediatric patients below the age of 12 years have not been established.

A total of 22 patients aged 12-18 years with invasive aspergillosis were included in the therapeutic studies. Twelve out of 22 (55%) patients had successful response after treatment with a maintenance dose of voriconazole 4 mg/kg q12h.

Sparse plasma sampling for pharmacokinetics in adolescents was conducted in the therapeutic studies (see CLINICAL PHARMACOLOGY, Pharmacokinetics, General Pharmacokinetic Characteristics).

GERIATRIC USE

In multiple dose therapeutic trials of voriconazole, 9.2% of patients were ≥65 years of age and 1.8% of patients were ≥75 years of age. In a study in healthy volunteers, the systemic exposure (AUC) and peak plasma concentrations (C_{max}) were increased in elderly males compared to young males. Pharmacokinetic data obtained from 552 patients from 10 voriconazole therapeutic trials showed that voriconazole plasma concentrations in the elderly patients were approximately 80-90% higher than those in younger patients after either IV or oral administration. However, the overall safety profile of the elderly patients was similar to that of the young so no dosage adjustment is recommended (see CLINICAL PHARMACOLOGY, Pharmacokinetics, Pharmacokinetics in Special Populations).

DRUG INTERACTIONS

TABLE 6 and TABLE 7 provide a summary of significant drug interactions with voriconazole that either have been studied *in vivo* (clinically) or that may be expected to occur based on results of *in vitro* metabolism studies with human liver microsomes. For more details, see CLINICAL PHARMACOLOGY, Drug Interactions.

TABLE 6 *Effect of Other Drugs on Voriconazole Pharmacokinetics*

Drug/Drug Class (Mechanism of Interaction by the Drug)	Voriconazole Plasma Exposure (C_{max} and AUCτ After 200 mg q12h)
Rifampin* and rifabutin* (CYP450 induction)	Significantly reduced; ***Recommendation:* Contraindicated.**
Carbamazepine (CYP450 induction)	Not studied *in vivo* or *in vitro,* but likely to result in significant reduction; ***Recommendation:* Contraindicated.**
Long acting barbiturates (CYP450 induction)	Not studied *in vivo* or *in vitro,* but likely to result in significant reduction; ***Recommendation:* Contraindicated.**
Phenytoin* (CYP450 induction)	Significantly reduced; ***Recommendation:*** Increase voriconazole maintenance dose from 4 to 5 mg/kg IV q12h or from 200 to 400 mg orally q12h (100-200 mg orally q12h in patients weighing less than 40 kg).
HIV protease inhibitors (CYP3A4 inhibition)	*In vivo* studies showed no significant effects of indinavir on voriconazole exposure; ***Recommendation:*** No dosage adjustment in the voriconazole dosage needed when coadministered with indinavir.
	In vitro studies demonstrate potential for inhibition of voriconazole metabolism (increased plasma exposure); ***Recommendation:*** Frequent monitoring for adverse events and toxicity related to voriconazole when coadministered with other HIV protease inhibitors.
NNRTI† (CYP3A4 inhibition or CYP450 induction)	*In vitro* studies demonstrate potential for inhibition of voriconazole metabolism (increased plasma exposure); ***Recommendation:*** Frequent monitoring for adverse events and toxicity related to voriconazole.
	Not studied *in vitro* or *in vivo,* but metabolism of voriconazole may also be induced (decreased plasma exposure); ***Recommendation:*** Careful assessment of voriconazole effectiveness.

* Results based on *in vivo* clinical studies generally following repeat oral dosing with 200 mg q12h voriconazole to healthy subjects.
† Non-nucleoside reverse transcriptase inhibitors.

ADVERSE REACTIONS

OVERVIEW

The most frequently reported adverse events (all causalities) in the therapeutic trials were visual disturbances, fever, rash, vomiting, nausea, diarrhea, headache, sepsis, peripheral edema, abdominal pain, and respiratory disorder. The treatment-related adverse events which most often led to discontinuation of voriconazole therapy were elevated liver function tests, rash, and visual disturbances (see WARNINGS, Hepatic Toxicity and ADVERSE REACTIONS: Clinical Laboratory Values, Dermatologic Reactions and Visual Disturbances).

DISCUSSION OF ADVERSE REACTIONS

The data described in TABLE 8A and TABLE 8B reflect exposure to voriconazole in 1493 patients in the therapeutic studies. This represents a heterogeneous population, including immunocompromised patients, *e.g.,* patients with hematological malignancy or HIV and non-neutropenic patients. This subgroup does not include healthy volunteers and patients treated in the compassionate use and non-therapeutic studies. This patient population was 62% male, had a mean age of 45.1 years (range 12-90, including 49 patients aged 12-18 years), and was 81% white and 9% black. Five hundred sixty-one (561) patients had a duration of voriconazole therapy of greater than 12 weeks, with 136 patients receiving voriconazole for over 6 months. TABLE 8A and TABLE 8B include all adverse events which were reported in therapeutic studies at an incidence of ≥1% as well as events of concern which occurred at an incidence of <1% during voriconazole therapy.

In study 307/602, 381 patients (196 on voriconazole, 185 on amphotericin B) were treated to compare voriconazole to amphotericin B followed by other licensed antifungal therapy in the primary treatment of patients with acute invasive aspergillosis. Study 305 evaluated the effects of oral voriconazole (200 patients) and oral fluconazole (191 patients) for another indication in immunocompromised (primarily HIV) patients. Laboratory test abnormalities for these studies are discussed under Clinical Laboratory Values.

V

TABLE 7 *Effect of Voriconazole on Pharmacokinetics of Other Drugs*

Drug/Drug Class (Mechanism of Interaction by Voriconazole)	Drug Plasma Exposure (C_{max} and AUCτ)
Sirolimus* (CYP3A4 inhibition)	Significantly increased; ***Recommendation:*** **Contraindicated.**
Rifabutin* (CYP3A4 inhibition)	Significantly increased; ***Recommendation:*** **Contraindicated.**
Terfenadine, astemizole, cisapride, pimozide, quinidine (CYP3A4 inhibition)	Not studied *in vivo* or *in vitro,* but drug plasma exposure likely to be increased; ***Recommendation:*** **Contraindicated** because of potential for QT prolongation and rare occurrence of *torsade de pointes.*
Ergot alkaloids (CYP450 inhibition)	Not studied *in vivo* or *in vitro,* but drug plasma exposure likely to be increased; ***Recommendation:*** **Contraindicated.**
Cyclosporine* (CYP3A4 inhibition)	AUCτ significantly increased; no significant effect on C_{max}; ***Recommendation:*** When initiating therapy with voriconazole in patients already receiving cyclosporine, reduce the cyclosporine dose to one-half of the starting dose and follow with frequent monitoring of cyclosporine blood levels. Increased cyclosporine levels have been associated with nephrotoxicity. When voriconazole is discontinued, cyclosporine concentrations must be frequently monitored and the dose increased as necessary.
Tacrolimus* (CYP3A4 inhibition)	Significantly increased; ***Recommendation:*** When initiating therapy with voriconazole in patients already receiving tacrolimus, reduce the tacrolimus dose to one-third of the starting dose and follow with frequent monitoring of tacrolimus blood levels. Increased tacrolimus levels have been associated with nephrotoxicity. When voriconazole is discontinued, tacrolimus concentrations must be frequently monitored and the dose increased as necessary.
Phenytoin* (CYP2C9 inhibition)	Significantly increased; ***Recommendation:*** Frequent monitoring of phenytoin plasma concentrations and frequent monitoring of adverse effects related to phenytoin.
Warfarin* (CYP2C9 inhibition)	Prothrombin time significantly increased; ***Recommendation:*** Monitor PT or other suitable anticoagulation tests. Adjustment of warfarin dosage may be needed.
Omeprazole* (CYP2C19/3A4 inhibition)	Significantly increased; ***Recommendation:*** When initiating therapy with voriconazole in patients already receiving omeprazole doses of 40 mg or greater, reduce the omeprazole dose by one-half. The metabolism of other proton pump inhibitors that are CYP2C19 substrates may also be inhibited by voriconazole and may result in increased plasma concentrations of other proton pump inhibitors.
HIV protease inhibitors (CYP3A4 inhibition)	*In vivo* studies showed no significant effects on indinavir exposure; ***Recommendation:*** No dosage adjustment for indinavir when coadministered with voriconazole. *In vitro* studies demonstrate potential for voriconazole to inhibit metabolism (increased plasma exposure); ***Recommendation:*** Frequent monitoring for adverse events and toxicity related to other HIV protease inhibitors
NNRTI† (CYP3A4 inhibition)	*In vitro* studies demonstrate potential for voriconazole to inhibit metabolism (increased plasma exposure); ***Recommendation:*** Frequent monitoring for adverse events and toxicity related to NNRTI.
Benzodiazepines (CYP3A4 inhibition)	*In vitro* studies demonstrate potential for voriconazole to inhibit metabolism (increased plasma exposure); ***Recommendation:*** Frequent monitoring for adverse events and toxicity (*i.e.,* prolonged sedation) related to benzodiazepines metabolized by CYP3A4 (*e.g.,* midazolam, triazolam, alprazolam). Adjustment of benzodiazepine dosage may be needed.
HMG-CoA reductase inhibitors (statins) (CYP3A4 inhibition)	*In vitro* studies demonstrate potential for voriconazole to inhibit metabolism (increased plasma exposure); ***Recommendation:*** Frequent monitoring for adverse events and toxicity related to statins. Increased statin concentrations in plasma have been associated with rhabdomyolysis. Adjustment of the statin dosage may be needed.
Dihydropyridine calcium channel blockers (CYP3A4 inhibition)	*In vitro* studies demonstrate potential for voriconazole to inhibit metabolism (increased plasma exposure); ***Recommendation:*** Frequent monitoring for adverse events and toxicity related to calcium channel blockers. Adjustment of calcium channel blocker dosage may be needed.
Sulfonylurea oral hypoglycemics (CYP2C9 inhibition)	Not studied *in vivo* or *in vitro,* but drug plasma exposure likely to be increased; ***Recommendation:*** Frequent monitoring of blood glucose and for signs and symptoms of hypoglycemia. Adjustment of oral hypoglycemic drug dosage may be needed.
Vinca alkaloids (CYP3A4 inhibition)	Not studied *in vivo* or *in vitro,* but drug plasma exposure likely to be increased; ***Recommendation:*** Frequent monitoring for adverse events and toxicity (*i.e.,* neurotoxicity) related to vinca alkaloids. Adjustment of vinca alkaloid dosage may be needed.

* Results based on *in vivo* clinical studies generally following repeat oral dosing with 200 mg bid voriconazole to healthy subjects.
† Non-nucleoside reverse transcriptase inhibitors.

TABLE 8A *Treatment-Emergent Adverse Events: Rate ≥1% or Adverse Events of Concern in All Therapeutic Studies Possibly Related to Therapy or Causality Unknown*

	Voriconazole n=1493
Special Senses*	
Abnormal vision	307 (20.6%)
Photophobia	36 (2.4%)
Chromatopsia	20 (1.3%)
Eye hemorrhage	3 (0.2%)
Body as a Whole	
Fever	93 (6.2%)
Chills	61 (4.1%)
Headache	48 (3.2%)
Abdominal pain	25 (1.7%)
Chest pain	13 (0.9%)
Cardiovascular System	
Tachycardia	37 (2.5%)
Hypertension	29 (1.9%)
Hypotension	26 (1.7%)
Vasodilatation	23 (1.5%)
Digestive System	
Nausea	88 (5.9%)
Vomiting	71 (4.8%)
Liver function tests abnormal	41 (2.7%)
Diarrhea	16 (1.1%)
Cholestatic jaundice	16 (1.1%)
Dry mouth	15 (1.0%)
Jaundice	3 (0.2%)
Hemic and Lymphatic System	
Thrombocytopenia	7 (0.5%)
Anemia	2 (0.1%)
Leukopenia	4 (0.3%)
Pancytopenia	1 (0.1%)
Metabolic and Nutritional Systems	
Alkaline phosphatase increased	54 (3.6%)
Hepatic enzymes increased	28 (1.9%)
SGOT increased	28 (1.9%)
SGPT increased	27 (1.8%)
Hypokalemia	24 (1.6%)
Peripheral edema	16 (1.1%)
Hypomagnesemia	16 (1.1%)
Bilirubinemia	12 (0.8%)
Creatinine increased	4 (0.3%)
Nervous System	
Hallucinations	37 (2.5%)
Dizziness	20 (1.3%)
Skin and Appendages	
Rash	86 (5.8%)
Pruritus	16 (1.1%)
Maculopapular rash	17 (1.1%)
Urogenital	
Kidney function abnormal	8 (0.5%)
Acute kidney failure	7 (0.5%)

* See WARNINGS, Visual Disturbances; PRECAUTIONS, Information for the Patient.

VISUAL DISTURBANCES

Voriconazole treatment-related visual disturbances are common. In clinical trials, approximately 30% of patients experienced altered/enhanced visual perception, blurred vision, color vision change and/or photophobia. The visual disturbances were generally mild and rarely resulted in discontinuation. Visual disturbances may be associated with higher plasma concentrations and/or doses.

The mechanism of action of the visual disturbance is unknown, although the site of action is most likely to be within the retina. In a study in healthy volunteers investigating the effect of 28 day treatment with voriconazole on retinal function, voriconazole caused a decrease in the electroretinogram (ERG) waveform amplitude, a decrease in the visual field, and an alteration in color perception. The ERG measures electrical currents in the retina. The effects were noted early in administration of voriconazole and continued through the course of study drug dosing.

Fourteen (14) days after end of dosing, ERG, visual fields and color perception returned to normal (see WARNINGS; PRECAUTIONS, Information for the Patient).

DERMATOLOGIC REACTIONS

Dermatological reactions were common in the patients treated with voriconazole. The mechanism underlying these dermatologic adverse events remains unknown. In clinical trials, rashes considered related to therapy were reported by 6% (86/1493) of voriconazole-treated patients. The majority of rashes were of mild to moderate severity. Cases of photosensitivity reactions appear to be more likely to occur with long-term treatment. Patients have rarely developed serious cutaneous reactions, including Stevens-Johnson syndrome, toxic epidermal necrolysis and erythema multiforme during treatment with voriconazole. If patients develop a rash, they should be monitored closely and consideration given to discontinuation of voriconazole. It is recommended that patients avoid strong, direct sunlight during voriconazole therapy.

LESS COMMON ADVERSE EVENTS

The following adverse events occurred in <1% of all voriconazole-treated patients, including healthy volunteers and patients treated under compassionate use protocols (total n=2090). This listing includes events where a causal relationship to voriconazole cannot be ruled out or those which may help the physician in managing the risks to the patients. The list does not include events included in TABLE 8A and TABLE 8B and does not include every event reported in the voriconazole clinical program.

TABLE 8B *Treatment-Emergent Adverse Events: Rate ≥1% or Adverse Events of Concern in Protocol 305 and Protocol 307/602 Possibly Related to Therapy or Causality Unknown*

	Protocol 305		Protocol 307/602	
	Oral Therapy		IV/Oral Therapy	
	Voriconazole	Fluconazole	Voriconazole	Ampho B†
	n=200	n=191	n=196	n=185
Special Senses*				
Abnormal vision	31 (15.5%)	8 (4.2%)	55 (28.1%)	1 (0.5%)
Photophobia	5 (2.5%)	2 (1.0%)	7 (3.6%)	0
Chromatopsia	2 (1.0%)	0	2 (1.0%)	0
Eye hemorrhage	0	0	0	0
Body as a Whole				
Fever	0	0	7 (3.6%)	25 (13.5%)
Chills	1 (0.5%)	0	0	36 (19.5%)
Headache	0	1 (0.5%)	7 (3.6%)	8 (4.3%)
Abdominal pain	0	0	5 (2.6%)	6 (3.2%)
Chest pain	0	0	4 (2.0%)	2 (1.1%)
Cardiovascular System				
Tachycardia	0	0	5 (2.6%)	5 (2.7%)
Hypertension	0	0	1 (0.5%)	2 (1.1%)
Hypotension	1 (0.5%)	0	1 (0.5%)	3 (1.6%)
Vasodilatation	0	0	2 (1.0%)	2 (1.1%)
Digestive System				
Nausea	2 (1.0%)	3 (1.6%)	14 (7.1%)	29 (15.7%)
Vomiting	2 (1.0%)	1 (0.5%)	11 (5.6%)	18 (9.7%)
Liver function tests abnormal	6 (3.0%)	2 (1.0%)	9 (4.6%)	4 (2.2%)
Diarrhea	0	0	3 (1.5%)	6 (3.2%)
Cholestatic jaundice	3 (1.5%)	0	4 (2.0%)	0
Dry mouth	0	1 (0.5%)	3 (1.5%)	0
Jaundice	1 (0.5%)	0	0	0
Hemic and Lymphatic System				
Thrombocytopenia	0	1 (0.5%)	2 (1.0%)	2 (1.1%)
Anemia	0	0	0	5 (2.7%)
Leukopenia	0	0	1 (0.5%)	0
Pancytopenia	0	0	0	0
Metabolic and Nutritional Systems				
Alkaline phosphatase increased	10 (5.0%)	3 (1.6%)	6 (3.1%)	4 (2.2%)
Hepatic enzymes increased	3 (1.5%)	0	7 (3.6%)	5 (2.7%)
SGOT increased	8 (4.0%)	2 (1.0%)	1 (0.5%)	0
SGPT increased	6 (3.0%)	2 (1.0%)	3 (1.5%)	1 (0.5%)
Hypokalemia	0	0	1 (0.5%)	36 (19.5%)
Peripheral edema	1 (0.5%)	0	7 (3.6%)	9 (4.9%)
Hypomagnesemia	0	0	2 (1.0%)	10 (5.4%)
Bilirubinemia	1 (0.5%)	0	1 (0.5%)	3 (1.6%)
Creatinine increased	1 (0.5%)	0	0	59 (31.9%)
Nervous System				
Hallucinations	0	0	10 (5.1%)	1 (0.5%)
Dizziness	0	2 (1.0%)	5 (2.6%)	0
Skin and Appendages				
Rash	3 (1.5%)	1 (0.5%)	13 (6.6%)	7 (3.8%)
Pruritus	0	0	2 (1.0%)	2 (1.1%)
Maculopapular rash	3 (1.5%)	0	1 (0.5%)	0
Urogenital				
Kidney function abnormal	1 (0.5%)	1 (0.5%)	4 (2.0%)	40 (21.6%)
Acute kidney failure	0	0	0	11 (5.9%)

* See WARNINGS, Visual Disturbances; PRECAUTIONS, Information for the Patient.
† Amphotericin B followed by other licensed antifungal therapy.

Body as a Whole: Abdomen enlarged, allergic reaction, anaphylactoid reaction (see PRECAUTIONS), ascites, asthenia, back pain, cellulitis, edema, face edema, flank pain, flu syndrome, graft versus host reaction, granuloma, infection, bacterial infection, fungal infection, injection site pain, injection site infection/inflammation, mucous membrane disorder, multi-organ failure, pain, pelvic pain, peritonitis, sepsis, substernal chest pain.

Cardiovascular: Atrial arrhythmia, atrial fibrillation, AV block complete, bigeminy, bradycardia, bundle branch block, cardiomegaly, cardiomyopathy, cerebral hemorrhage, cerebral ischemia, cerebrovascular accident, congestive heart failure, deep thrombophlebitis, endocarditis, extrasystoles, heart arrest, myocardial infarction, nodal arrhythmia, palpitation, phlebitis, postural hypotension, pulmonary embolus, QT interval prolonged, supraventricular tachycardia, syncope, thrombophlebitis, vasodilatation, ventricular arrhythmia, ventricular fibrillation, ventricular tachycardia (including possible *torsade de pointes*).

Digestive: Anorexia, cheilitis, cholecystitis, cholelithiasis, constipation, duodenal ulcer perforation, duodenitis, dyspepsia, dysphagia, esophageal ulcer, esophagitis, flatulence, gastroenteritis, gastrointestinal hemorrhage, GGT/LDH elevated, gingivitis, glossitis, gum hemorrhage, gum hyperplasia, hematemesis, hepatic coma, hepatic failure, hepatitis, intestinal perforation, intestinal ulcer, enlarged liver, melena, mouth ulceration, pancreatitis, parotid gland enlargement, periodontitis, proctitis, pseudomembranous colitis, rectal disorder, rectal hemorrhage, stomach ulcer, stomatitis, tongue edema.

Endocrine: Adrenal cortex insufficiency, diabetes insipidus, hyperthyroidism, hypothyroidism.

Hemic and Lymphatic: Agranulocytosis, anemia (macrocytic, megaloblastic, microcytic, normocytic), aplastic anemia, hemolytic anemia, bleeding time increased, cyanosis, DIC, ecchymosis, eosinophilia, hypervolemia, lymphadenopathy, lymphangitis, marrow depression, petechia, purpura, enlarged spleen, thrombotic thrombocytopenic purpura.

Metabolic and Nutritional: Albuminuria, BUN increased, creatine phosphokinase increased, edema, glucose tolerance decreased, hypercalcemia, hypercholesteremia, hyperglycemia, hyperkalemia, hypermagnesemia, hypernatremia, hyperuricemia, hypocalcemia, hypoglycemia, hyponatremia, hypophosphatemia, uremia.

Musculoskeletal: Arthralgia, arthritis, bone necrosis, bone pain, leg cramps, myalgia, myasthenia, myopathy, osteomalacia, osteoporosis.

Nervous System: Abnormal dreams, acute brain syndrome, agitation, akathisia, amnesia, anxiety, ataxia, brain edema, coma, confusion, convulsion, delirium, dementia, depersonalization, depression, diplopia, encephalitis, encephalopathy, euphoria, extrapyramidal syndrome, grand mal convulsion, Guillain-Barré syndrome, hypertonia, hypesthesia, insomnia, intracranial hypertension, libido decreased, neuralgia, neuropathy, nystagmus, oculogyric crisis, paresthesia, psychosis, somnolence, suicidal ideation, tremor, vertigo.

Respiratory System: Cough increased, dyspnea, epistaxis, hemoptysis, hypoxia, lung edema, pharyngitis, pleural effusion, pneumonia, respiratory disorder, respiratory distress syndrome, respiratory tract infection, rhinitis, sinusitis, voice alteration.

Skin and Appendages: Alopecia, angioedema, contact dermatitis, discoid lupus erythematosis, eczema, erythema multiforme, exfoliative dermatitis, fixed drug eruption, furunculosis, herpes simplex, melanosis, photosensitivity skin reaction, psoriasis, skin discoloration, skin disorder, skin dry, Stevens-Johnson syndrome, sweating, toxic epidermal necrolysis, urticaria.

Special Senses: Abnormality of accommodation, blepharitis, color blindness, conjunctivitis, corneal opacity, deafness, ear pain, eye pain, dry eyes, keratitis, keratoconjunctivitis, mydriasis, night blindness, optic atrophy, optic neuritis, otitis externa, papilledema, retinal hemorrhage, retinitis, scleritis, taste loss, taste perversion, tinnitus, uveitis, visual field defect.

Urogenital: Anuria, blighted ovum, creatinine clearance decreased, dysmenorrhea, dysuria, epididymitis, glycosuria, hemorrhagic cystitis, hematuria, hydronephrosis, impotence, kidney pain, kidney tubular necrosis, metrorrhagia, nephritis, nephrosis, oliguria, scrotal edema, urinary incontinence, urinary retention, urinary tract infection, uterine hemorrhage, vaginal hemorrhage.

CLINICAL LABORATORY VALUES

The overall incidence of clinically significant transaminase abnormalities in the voriconazole clinical program was 13.4% (200/1493) of patients treated with voriconazole. Increased incidence of liver function test abnormalities may be associated with higher plasma concentrations and/or doses. The majority of abnormal liver function tests either resolved during treatment without dose adjustment or following dose adjustment, including discontinuation of therapy.

Voriconazole has been infrequently associated with cases of serious hepatic toxicity including cases of jaundice and rare cases of hepatitis and hepatic failure leading to death. Most of these patients had other serious underlying conditions.

Liver function tests should be evaluated at the start of and during the course of voriconazole therapy. Patients who develop abnormal liver function tests during voriconazole therapy should be monitored for the development of more severe hepatic injury. Patient management should include laboratory evaluation of hepatic function (particularly liver function tests and bilirubin). Discontinuation of voriconazole must be considered if clinical signs and symptoms consistent with liver disease develop that may be attributable to voriconazole (see WARNINGS and PRECAUTIONS, Laboratory Tests).

Acute renal failure has been observed in severely ill patients undergoing treatment with voriconazole. Patients being treated with voriconazole are likely to be treated concomitantly with nephrotoxic medications and have concurrent conditions that may result in decreased renal function. It is recommended that patients are monitored for the development of abnormal renal function. This should include laboratory evaluation, particularly serum creatinine.

TABLE 9 and TABLE 10 show the number of patients with hypokalemia and clinically significant changes in renal and liver function tests in two randomized, comparative multicenter studies. In Study 305, patients were randomized to either oral voriconazole or oral fluconazole to evaluate an indication other than invasive aspergillosis in immunocompromised patients. In Study 307/602, patients with definite or probable invasive aspergillosis were randomized to either voriconazole or amphotericin B therapy.

TABLE 9 *Protocol 305: Clinically Significant Laboratory Test Abnormalities*

	Criteria*	Voriconazole n/N (%)	Fluconazole n/N (%)
T. Bilirubin	>1.5 × ULN	8/185 (4.3%)	7/186 (3.8%)
AST	>3.0 × ULN	38/187 (20.3%)	15/186 (8.1%)
ALT	>3.0 × ULN	20/187 (10.7%)	12/186 (6.5%)
Alk phos	>3.0 × ULN	19/187 (10.2%)	14/186 (7.5%)

* Without regard to baseline value.
n =Number of patients with a clinically significant abnormality while on study therapy.
N =Total number of patients with at least one observation of the given lab test while on study therapy.
ULN =Upper limit of normal.

DOSAGE AND ADMINISTRATION

ADMINISTRATION

Voriconazole tablets should be taken at least 1 hour before, or 1 hour following, a meal.

Voriconazole IV for injection requires reconstitution to 10 mg/ml and subsequent dilution to 5 mg/ml or less prior to administration as an infusion, at a maximum rate of 3 mg/kg/h over 1-2 hours (see Intravenous Administration).

NOT FOR IV BOLUS INJECTION.

V

TABLE 10 *Protocol 307/602: Clinically Significant Laboratory Test Abnormalities*

	Criteria*	Voriconazole n/N (%)	Amphotericin B† n/N (%)
T. Bilirubin	>1.5 × ULN	35/180 (19.4%)	46/173 (26.6%)
AST	>3.0 × ULN	21/180 (11.7%)	18/174 (10.3%)
ALT	>3.0 × ULN	34/180 (18.9%)	40/173 (23.1%)
Alk phos	>3.0 × ULN	29/181 (16.0%)	38/173 (22.0%)
Creatinine	>1.3 × ULN	39/182 (21.4%)	102/177 (57.6%)
Potassium	<0.9 × LLN	30/181 (16.6%)	70/178 (39.3%)

* Without regard to baseline value.
† Amphotericin B followed by other licensed antifungal therapy.
n =Number of patients with a clinically significant abnormality while on study therapy.
N =Total number of patients with at least one observation of the given lab test while on study therapy.
ULN =Upper limit of normal.
LLN =Lower limit of normal.

Electrolyte disturbances such as hypokalemia, hypomagnesemia and hypocalcemia should be corrected prior to initiation of voriconazole therapy (see PRECAUTIONS).

Use in Adults

Therapy must be initiated with the specified loading dose regimen of intravenous voriconazole to achieve plasma concentrations on Day 1 that are close to steady state. On the basis of high oral bioavailability, switching between intravenous and oral administration is appropriate when clinically indicated (see CLINICAL PHARMACOLOGY).

For the treatment of adults with invasive aspergillosis and infections due to *Fusarium* spp. and *Scedosporium apiospermum,* the recommended dosing regimen of voriconazole is as follows:

Loading dose of 6 mg/kg voriconazole IV every 12 hours for 2 doses, followed by a maintenance dose of 4 mg/kg voriconazole IV every 12 hours.

Once the patient can tolerate medication given by mouth, the oral tablet form of voriconazole may be utilized. Patients who weigh more than 40 kg should receive an oral maintenance dose of 200 mg voriconazole tablet every 12 hours. Adult patients who weigh less than 40 kg should receive an oral maintenance dose of 100 mg every 12 hours.

DOSE ADJUSTMENT

If patient response is inadequate, the oral maintenance dose may be increased from 200 mg every 12 hours to 300 mg every 12 hours. For adult patients weighing less than 40 kg, the oral maintenance dose may be increased from 100 mg every 12 hours to 150 mg every 12 hours.

If patients are unable to tolerate treatment, reduce the intravenous maintenance dose to 3 mg/kg every 12 hours and the oral maintenance dose by 50 mg steps to a minimum of 200 mg every 12 hours (or to 100 mg every 12 hours for adult patients weighing less than 40 kg).

Phenytoin may be coadministered with voriconazole if the maintenance dose of voriconazole is increased to 5 mg/kg IV every 12 hours, or from 200 mg to 400 mg every 12 hours orally (100-200 mg every 12 hours orally in adult patients weighing less than 40 kg) (see CLINICAL PHARMACOLOGY; DRUG INTERACTIONS).

Duration of therapy should be based on the severity of the patient's underlying disease, recovery from immunosuppression, and clinical response.

USE IN GERIATRIC PATIENTS

No dose adjustment is necessary for geriatric patients.

USE IN PATIENTS WITH HEPATIC INSUFFICIENCY

In the clinical program, patients were included who had baseline liver function tests (ALT, AST) up to 5 times the upper limit of normal. No dose adjustment is necessary in patients with this degree of abnormal liver function, but continued monitoring of liver function tests for further elevations is recommended (see WARNINGS).

It is recommended that the standard loading dose regimens be used but that the maintenance dose be halved in patients with mild to moderate hepatic cirrhosis (Child-Pugh Class A and B).

Voriconazole has not been studied in patients with severe hepatic cirrhosis (Child-Pugh Class C) or in patients with chronic hepatitis B or chronic hepatitis C disease. Voriconazole has been associated with elevations in liver function tests and clinical signs of liver damage, such as jaundice, and should only be used in patients with severe hepatic insufficiency if the benefit outweighs the potential risk. Patients with hepatic insufficiency must be carefully monitored for drug toxicity.

USE IN PATIENTS WITH RENAL INSUFFICIENCY

The pharmacokinetics of orally administered voriconazole are not significantly affected by renal insufficiency. Therefore, no adjustment is necessary for oral dosing in patients with mild to severe renal impairment (see CLINICAL PHARMACOLOGY, Pharmacokinetics, Pharmacokinetics in Special Populations).

In patients with moderate or severe renal insufficiency (creatinine clearance <50 ml/min), accumulation of the intravenous vehicle, SBECD, occurs. Oral voriconazole should be administered to these patients, unless an assessment of the benefit/risk to the patient justifies the use of intravenous voriconazole. Serum creatinine levels should be closely monitored in these patients, and, if increases occur, consideration should be given to changing to oral voriconazole therapy (see DOSAGE AND ADMINISTRATION).

Voriconazole is hemodialyzed with clearance of 121 ml/min. The intravenous vehicle, SBECD, is hemodialyzed with clearance of 55 ml/min. A 4 hour hemodialysis session does not remove a sufficient amount of voriconazole to warrant dose adjustment.

INTRAVENOUS ADMINISTRATION

Voriconazole IV for Injection

Reconstitution

The powder is reconstituted with 19 ml of water for injection to obtain an extractable volume of 20 ml of clear concentrate containing 10 mg/ml of voriconazole. It is recommended that a standard 20 ml (non-automated) syringe be used to ensure that the exact amount (19.0 ml) of water for injection is dispensed. Discard the vial if a vacuum does not pull the diluent into the vial. Shake the vial until all the powder is dissolved.

Dilution

Voriconazole must be infused over 1-2 hours, at a concentration of 5 mg/ml or less. Therefore, the required volume of the 10 mg/ml voriconazole concentrate should be further diluted as follows (appropriate diluents listed below):

Calculate the volume of 10 mg/ml voriconazole concentrate required based on the patient's weight (see TABLE 11).

In order to allow the required volume of voriconazole concentrate to be added, withdraw and discard at least an equal volume of diluent from the infusion bag or bottle to be used. The volume of diluent remaining in the bag or bottle should be such that when the 10 mg/ml voriconazole concentrate is added, the final concentration is not less than 0.5 mg/ml nor greater than 5 mg/ml.

Using a suitable size syringe and aseptic technique, withdraw the required volume of voriconazole concentrate from the appropriate number of vials and add to the infusion bag or bottle. DISCARD PARTIALLY USED VIALS.

The final voriconazole solution must be infused over 1-2 hours at a maximum rate of 3 mg/kg/h.

TABLE 11 *Required Volumes of 10 mg/ml Voriconazole Concentrate*

	Volume of Voriconazole Concentrate (10 mg/ml) Required for:		
Body Weight	3 mg/kg Dose (No. of Vials)	4 mg/kg Dose (No. of Vials)	6 mg/kg Dose (No. of Vials)
30 kg	9.0 ml (1)	12 ml (1)	18 ml (1)
35 kg	10.5 ml (1)	14 ml (1)	21 ml (2)
40 kg	12.0 ml (1)	16 ml (1)	24 ml (2)
45 kg	13.5 ml (1)	18 ml (1)	27 ml (2)
50 kg	15.0 ml (1)	20 ml (1)	30 ml (2)
55 kg	16.5 ml (1)	22 ml (2)	33 ml (2)
60 kg	18.0 ml (1)	24 ml (2)	36 ml (2)
65 kg	19.5 ml (1)	26 ml (2)	39 ml (2)
70 kg	21.0 ml (2)	28 ml (2)	42 ml (3)
75 kg	22.5 ml (2)	30 ml (2)	45 ml (3)
80 kg	24.0 ml (2)	32 ml (2)	48 ml (3)
85 kg	25.5 ml (2)	34 ml (2)	51 ml (3)
90 kg	27.0 ml (2)	36 ml (2)	54 ml (3)
95 kg	28.5 ml (2)	38 ml (2)	57 ml (3)
100 kg	30.0 ml (2)	40 ml (2)	60 ml (3)

Voriconazole is a single dose unpreserved sterile lyophile. Therefore, from a microbiological point of view, once reconstituted, the product should be used immediately. If not used immediately, in-use storage times and conditions prior to use are the responsibility of the user and should not be longer than 24 hours at 2-8°C (37-46°F). This medicinal product is for single use only and any unused solution should be discarded. Only clear solutions without particles should be used.

The reconstituted solution can be diluted with:

9 mg/ml (0.9%) sodium chloride
Lactated Ringers
5% Dextrose and lactated Ringers
5% Dextrose and 0.45% sodium chloride
5% Dextrose
5% Dextrose and 20 mEq potassium chloride
0.45% Sodium chloride
5% Dextrose and 0.9% sodium chloride

The compatibility of voriconazole IV with diluents other than those described above is unknown (see Incompatibilities).

Parenteral drug products should be inspected visually for particulate matter and discoloration prior to administration, whenever solution and container permit.

Incompatibilities

Voriconazole IV must not be infused into the same line or cannula concomitantly with other drug infusions, including parenteral nutrition, *e.g.,* Aminofusin 10% Plus. Aminofusin 10% Plus is physically incompatible, with an increase in subvisible particulate matter after 24 hours storage at 4°C.

Infusions of blood products not occur simultaneously with voriconazole IV.

Infusions of total parenteral nutrition can occur simultaneously with voriconazole IV.

Voriconazole IV must not be diluted with 4.2% sodium bicarbonate infusion. The mildly alkaline nature of this diluent caused slight degradation of voriconazole after 24 hours storage at room temperature. Although refrigerated storage is recommended following reconstitution, use of this diluent is not recommended as a precautionary measure. Compatibility with other concentrations is unknown.

STABILITY

Voriconazole Tablets: Store at controlled room temperature 15-30°C (59-86°F).
Voriconazole IV for Injection: Store at controlled room temperature 15-30°C (59-86°F).

HOW SUPPLIED

VFEND TABLETS

50 mg: White, film-coated, round, debossed with "Pfizer" on one side and "VOR50" on the reverse.

200 mg: White, film-coated, capsule shaped, debossed with "Pfizer" on one side and "VOR200" on the reverse.

Storage and Stability

Vfend Tablets should be stored at controlled room temperature 15-30°C (59-86°F).

POWDER FOR SOLUTION FOR INJECTION

Vfend IV for injection is supplied in a single use vial as a sterile lyophilized powder equivalent to 200 mg Vfend and 3200 mg sulfobutyl ether betacyclodextrin sodium (SBECD).

Storage and Stability

Unreconstituted vials should be stored at controlled room temperature 15-30°C (59-86°F). Vfend is a single dose unpreserved sterile lyophile. From a microbiological point of view, following reconstitution of the lyophile with water for injection, the reconstituted solution should be used immediately. If not used immediately, in-use storage times and conditions prior to use are the responsibility of the user and should not be longer than 24 hours at 2-8°C (37-46°F). Chemical and physical in-use stability has been demonstrated for 24 hours at 2-8°C (37-46°F). This medicinal product is for single use only and any unused solution should be discarded. Only clear solutions without particles should be used (see DOSAGE AND ADMINISTRATION, Intravenous Administration).

PRODUCT LISTING - EQUIVALENTS NOT AVAILABLE

Powder For Injection - Intravenous - 200 mg
1's $106.25 VFEND, Pfizer U.S. Pharmaceuticals 00049-3190-28
Tablet - Oral - 50 mg
30's $234.38 VFEND, Pfizer U.S. Pharmaceuticals 00049-3170-30
Tablet - Oral - 200 mg
30's $937.50 VFEND, Pfizer U.S. Pharmaceuticals 00049-3180-30

Warfarin Sodium *(002444)*

Categories: Arrhythmias, atrial fibrillation, with embolism; Embolism, pulmonary; Embolism, pulmonary, prophylaxis; Myocardial infarction, prophylaxis; Stroke, prophylaxis; Thrombosis, venous; Thrombosis, venous, prophylaxis; Pregnancy Category X; FDA Approved 1955 Nov; WHO Formulary

Drug Classes: Anticoagulants

Brand Names: Coumadin

Foreign Brand Availability: Aldocumar (Spain); Coumadan Sodico (Argentina); Coumadine (France); Farin (Thailand); Marevan (Australia; Belgium; Denmark; England; Finland; New-Zealand; Norway); Orfarin (Malaysia; Thailand); Panwarfin (Greece); Simarc-2 (Indonesia); UniWarfin (India); Waran (Sweden); Warfar (Colombia); Warfil 5 (Dominican-Republic); Warfilone (Canada)

Cost of Therapy: $20.78 (Thromboembolism; Coumadin; 5 mg; 1 tablet/day; 30 day supply)
$17.46 (Thromboembolism; Generic Tablets; 5 mg; 1 tablet/day; 30 day supply)

DESCRIPTION

Crystalline warfarin sodium is an anticoagulant which acts by inhibiting vitamin K-dependent coagulation factors. Chemically, it is 3-(α-acetonylbenzyl)-4-hydroxycoumarin and is a racemic mixture of the R- and S-enantiomers. Crystalline warfarin sodium is an isopropanol clathrate. The crystallization of warfarin sodium virtually eliminates trace impurities present in amorphous warfarin. Its empirical formula is $C_{19}H_{15}NaO_4$.

Crystalline warfarin sodium occurs as a white, odorless, crystalline powder, is discolored by light and is very soluble in water; freely soluble in alcohol; very slightly soluble in chloroform and in ether.

COUMADIN TABLETS

Coumadin tablets for oral use also contain: *All Strengths:* Lactose, starch and magnesium stearate; *1 mg:* D&C red no. 6 barium lake; *2 mg:* FD&C blue no. 2 aluminum lake and FD&C red no. 40 aluminum lake; *2½ mg:* D&C yellow no. 10 aluminum lake and FD&C blue no. 1 aluminum lake; *3 mg:* FD&C yellow no. 6 aluminum lake, FD&C blue no. 2 aluminum lake and FD&C red no. 40 aluminum lake; *4 mg:* FD&C blue no. 1 aluminum lake; *5 mg:* FD&C yellow no. 6 aluminum lake; *6 mg:* FD&C yellow no. 6 aluminum lake and FD&C blue no. 1 aluminum lake; *7½ mg:* D&C yellow no. 10 aluminum lake and FD&C yellow no. 6 aluminum lake; *10 mg:* Dye free.

COUMADIN FOR INJECTION

Coumadin for injection is supplied as a sterile, lyophilized powder, which, after reconstitution with 2.7 ml sterile water for injection, contains: *Warfarin Sodium:* 2 mg/ml; *Sodium Phosphate, Dibasic, Heptahydrate:* 4.98 mg/ml; *Sodium Phosphate, Monobasic, Monohydrate:* 0.194 mg/ml; *Sodium Chloride:* 0.1 mg/ml; *Mannitol:* 38.0 mg/ml; *Sodium Hydroxide, as needed for pH adjustment to:* 8.1-8.3.

CLINICAL PHARMACOLOGY

Warfarin sodium and other coumarin anticoagulants act by inhibiting the synthesis of vitamin K dependent clotting factors, which include Factors II, VII, IX and X, and the anticoagulant proteins C and S. Half-lives of these clotting factors are as follows: Factor II — 60 hours, VII — 4-6 hours, IX — 24 hours, and X — 48-72 hours. The half-lives of proteins C and S are approximately 8 hours and 30 hours, respectively. The resultant *in vivo* effect is a sequential depression of Factors VII, IX, X and II activities. Vitamin K is an essential cofactor for the post ribosomal synthesis of the vitamin K dependent clotting factors. The vitamin promotes the biosynthesis of α-carboxyglutamic acid residues in the proteins which are essential for biological activity. Warfarin is thought to interfere with clotting factor synthesis by inhibition of the regeneration of vitamin K_1 epoxide. The degree of depression is dependent upon the dosage administered. Therapeutic doses of warfarin decrease the total amount of the active form of each vitamin K dependent clotting factor made by the liver by approximately 30-50%.

An anticoagulation effect generally occurs within 24 hours after drug administration. However, peak anticoagulant effect may be delayed 72-96 hours. The duration of action of a single dose of racemic warfarin is 2-5 days. The effects of warfarin sodium may become more pronounced as effects of daily maintenance doses overlap. Anticoagulants have no direct effect on an established thrombus, nor do they reverse ischemic tissue damage. However, once a thrombus has occurred, the goal of anticoagulant treatment is to prevent further extension of the formed clot and prevent secondary thromboembolic complications which may result in serious and possibly fatal sequelae.

PHARMACOKINETICS

Warfarin sodium is a racemic mixture of the R- and S-enantiomers. The S-enantiomer exhibits 2-5 times more anticoagulant activity than the R-enantiomer in humans, but generally has a more rapid clearance.

Absorption

Warfarin sodium is essentially completely absorbed after oral administration with peak concentration generally attained within the first 4 hours.

Distribution

There are no differences in the apparent volumes of distribution after IV and oral administration of single doses of warfarin solution. Warfarin distributes into a relatively small apparent volume of distribution of about 0.14 L/kg. A distribution phase lasting 6-12 hours is distinguishable after rapid IV or oral administration of an aqueous solution. Using a one compartment model, and assuming complete bioavailability, estimates of the volumes of distribution of R- and S-warfarin are similar to each other and to that of the racemate. Concentrations in fetal plasma approach the maternal values, but warfarin has not been found in human milk (see WARNINGS, Lactation). Approximately 99% of the drug is bound to plasma proteins.

Metabolism

The elimination of warfarin is almost entirely by metabolism. Warfarin sodium is stereoselectively metabolized by hepatic microsomal enzymes (cytochrome P-450) to inactive hydroxylated metabolites (predominant route) and by reductases to reduced metabolites (warfarin alcohols). The warfarin alcohols have minimal anticoagulant activity. The metabolites are principally excreted into the urine; and to a lesser extent into the bile. The metabolites of warfarin that have been identified include dehydrowarfarin, two diastereoisomer alcohols, 4'-, 6-, 7-, 8- and 10-hydroxywarfarin. The cytochrome P-450 isozymes involved in the metabolism of warfarin include 2C9, 2C19, 2C8, 2C18, 1A2, and 3A4. 2C9 is likely to be the principal form of human liver P-450 which modulates the *in vivo* anticoagulant activity of warfarin.

Excretion

The terminal half-life of warfarin after a single dose is approximately 1 week; however, the effective half-life ranges from 20-60 hours, with a mean of about 40 hours. The clearance of R-warfarin is generally half that of S-warfarin, thus as the volumes of distribution are similar, the half-life of R-warfarin is longer than that of S-warfarin. The half-life of R-warfarin ranges from 37-89 hours, while that of S-warfarin sodium ranges from 21-43 hours. Studies with radiolabeled drug have demonstrated that up to 92% of the orally administered dose is recovered in urine. Very little warfarin is excreted unchanged in urine. Urinary excretion is in the form of metabolites.

Elderly

Patients 60 years or older appear to exhibit greater than expected prothombin time (PT)/ International Normalized Ratio (INR) response to the anticoagulant effects of warfarin. The cause of the increased sensitivity to the anticoagulant effects of warfarin in this age group is unknown. This increased anticoagulant effect from warfarin may be due to a combination of pharmacokinetic and pharmacodynamic factors. Racemic warfarin clearance may be unchanged or reduced with increasing age. Limited information suggests there is no difference in the clearance of S-warfarin in the elderly versus young subjects. However, there may be a slight decrease in the clearance of R-warfarin in the elderly as compared to the young. Therefore, as patient age increases, a lower dose of warfarin is usually required to produce a therapeutic level of anticoagulation.

Asians

Asian patients may require lower initiation and maintenance doses of warfarin. One non-controlled study conducted in 151 Chinese outpatients reported a mean daily warfarin requirement of 3.3 ± 1.4 mg to achieve an INR of 2 to 2.5. These patients were stabilized on warfarin for various indications. Patient age was the most important determinant of warfarin requirement in Chinese patients with a progressively lower warfarin requirement with increasing age.

Renal Dysfunction

Renal clearance is considered to be a minor determinant of anticoagulant response to warfarin. No dosage adjustment is necessary for patients with renal failure.

Hepatic Dysfunction

Hepatic dysfunction can potentiate the response to warfarin through impaired synthesis of clotting factors and decreased metabolism of warfarin.

The administration of warfarin sodium via the intravenous (IV) route should provide the patient with the same concentration of an equal oral dose, but maximum plasma concentration will be reached earlier. However, the full anticoagulant effect of a dose of warfarin sodium may not be achieved until 72-96 hours after dosing, indicating that the administration of IV warfarin sodium should not provide any increased biological effect or earlier onset of action.

INDICATIONS AND USAGE

Warfarin sodium is indicated for the prophylaxis and/or treatment of venous thrombosis and its extension, and pulmonary embolism.

Warfarin sodium is indicated for the prophylaxis and/or treatment of the thromboembolic complications associated with atrial fibrillation and/or cardiac valve replacement.

Warfarin sodium is indicated to reduce the risk of death, recurrent myocardial infarction, and thromboembolic events such as stroke or systemic embolization after myocardial infarction.

NON-FDA APPROVED INDICATIONS

Warfarin has been used without FDA approval for the treatment of heart failure. In general, routine anticoagulation for patients with heart failure is controversial. Most experts believe that heart failure in patients with (1) a history of pulmonary or systemic thromboemboli, (2) atrial fibrillation, or (3) left ventricular thrombi should definitely be treated with warfarin therapy unless strong contraindications exist.

CONTRAINDICATIONS

Anticoagulation is contraindicated in any localized or general physical condition or personal circumstance in which the hazard of hemorrhage might be greater than the potential clinical benefits of anticoagulation, such as:

Pregnancy: Warfarin sodium is contraindicated in women who are or may become pregnant because the drug passes through the placental barrier and may cause fatal hemorrhage to the fetus *in utero*. Furthermore, there have been reports of birth malformations in children born to mothers who have been treated with warfarin during pregnancy.

Embryopathy characterized by nasal hypoplasia with or without stippled epiphyses (chondrodysplasia punctata) has been reported in pregnant women exposed to warfarin during the first trimester. Central nervous system abnormalities also have been reported, including dorsal midline dysplasia characterized by agenesis of the corpus callosum, Dandy-Walker malformation, and midline cerebellar atrophy. Ventral midline dysplasia, characterized by optic atrophy, and eye abnormalities have been observed. Mental retardation, blindness, and other central nervous system abnormalities have been reported in association with second and third trimester exposure. Although rare, teratogenic reports following *in utero* exposure to warfarin include urinary tract anomalies such as single kidney, asplenia, anencephaly, spina bifida, cranial nerve palsy, hydrocephalus, cardiac defects and congenital heart disease, polydactyly, deformities of toes, diaphragmatic hernia, corneal leukoma, cleft palate, cleft lip, schizencephaly, and microcephaly.

Spontaneous abortion and still birth are known to occur and a higher risk of fetal mortality is associated with the use of warfarin. Low birth weight and growth retardation have also been reported.

Women of childbearing potential who are candidates for anticoagulant therapy should be carefully evaluated and the indications critically reviewed with the patient. If the patient becomes pregnant while taking this drug, she should be apprised of the potential risks to the fetus, and the possibility of termination of the pregnancy should be discussed in light of those risks.

Hemorrhagic tendencies or blood dyscrasias.

Recent or contemplated surgery of: (1) central nervous system; (2) eye; (3) traumatic surgery resulting in large open surfaces.

Bleeding tendencies associated with active ulceration or overt bleeding of: (1) gastrointestinal, genitourinary or respiratory tracts; (2) cerebrovascular hemorrhage; (3) aneurysms-cerebral, dissecting aorta; (4) pericarditis and pericardial effusions; (5) bacterial endocarditis.

Threatened abortion, eclampsia, and preeclampsia.

Inadequate laboratory facilities.

Unsupervised patients with senility, alcoholism, psychosis, or other lack of patient cooperation.

Spinal puncture and other diagnostic or therapeutic procedures with potential for uncontrollable bleeding.

Miscellaneous: Major regional, lumbar block anesthesia, malignant hypertension and known hypersensitivity to warfarin or to any other components of this product.

WARNINGS

The most serious risks associated with anticoagulant therapy with warfarin sodium are hemorrhage in any tissue or organ and, less frequently (<0.1%), necrosis and/or gangrene of skin and other tissues. The risk of hemorrhage is related to the level of intensity and the duration of anticoagulant therapy. Hemorrhage and necrosis have in some cases been reported to result in death or permanent disability. Necrosis appears to be associated with local thrombosis and usually appears within a few days of the start of anticoagulant therapy. In severe cases of necrosis, treatment through debridement or amputation of the affected tissue, limb, breast or penis has been reported. Careful diagnosis is required to determine whether necrosis is caused by an underlying disease. Warfarin therapy should be discontinued when warfarin is suspected to be the cause of developing necrosis and heparin therapy may be considered for anticoagulation. Although various treatments have been attempted, no treatment for necrosis has been considered uniformly effective. See below for information on predisposing conditions. These and other risks associated with anticoagulant therapy must be weighed against the risk of thrombosis or embolization in untreated cases.

It cannot be emphasized too strongly that treatment of each patient is a highly individualized matter. Warfarin sodium, a narrow therapeutic range (index) drug, may be affected by factors such as other drugs and dietary vitamin K. Dosage should be controlled by periodic determinations of PT/INR or other suitable coagulation tests. Determinations of whole blood clotting and bleeding times are not effective measures for control of therapy. Heparin prolongs the one-stage PT. When heparin and warfarin sodium are administered concomitantly, refer to DOSAGE AND ADMINISTRATION, Conversion From Heparin Therapy for recommendations.

Caution should be observed when warfarin sodium is administered in any situation or in the presence of any predisposing condition where added risk of hemorrhage, necrosis, and/or gangrene is present.

Anticoagulation therapy with warfarin sodium may enhance the release of atheromatous plaque emboli, thereby increasing the risk of complications from systemic cholesterol microembolization, including the "purple toes syndrome". Discontinuation of warfarin sodium therapy is recommended when such phenomena are observed.

Systemic atheroemboli and cholesterol microemboli can present with a variety of signs and symptoms including purple toes syndrome, livedo reticularis, rash, gangrene, abrupt and intense pain in the leg, foot, or toes, foot ulcers, myalgia, penile gangrene, abdominal pain, flank or back pain, hematuria, renal insufficiency, hypertension, cerebral ischemia, spinal cord infarction, pancreatitis, symptoms stimulating polyarteritis, or any other sequelae of vascular compromise due to embolic occlusion. The most commonly involved visceral organs are the kidneys followed by the pancreas, spleen, and liver. Some cases have progressed to necrosis or death.

Purple toes syndrome is a complication of oral anticoagulation characterized by a dark, purplish or mottled color of the toes, usually occurring between 3-10 weeks, or later, after the initiation of therapy with warfarin or related compounds. Major features of this syndrome include purple color of plantar surfaces and sides of the toes that blanches on moderate pressure and fades with elevation of the legs; pain and tenderness of the toes; waxing and waning of the color over time. While the purple toes syndrome is reported to be reversible, some cases progress to gangrene or necrosis which may require debridement of the affected area, or may lead to amputation.

Heparin-Induced Thrombocytopenia: Warfarin sodium should be used with caution in patients with heparin-induced thrombocytopenia and deep venous thrombosis. Cases of venous limb ischemia, necrosis, and gangrene have occurred in patients with heparin-induced thrombocytopenia and deep venous thrombosis when heparin treatment was discontinued and warfarin therapy was started or continued. In some patients sequelae have included amputation of the involved area and/or death (Warkentin *et al.,* 1997).

A severe elevation (>50 seconds) in activated partial thromboplastin time (aPTT) with a PT/INR in the desired range has been identified as an indication of increased risk of postoperative hemorrhage.

The decision to administer anticoagulants in the following conditions must be based upon clinical judgment in which the risks of anticoagulant therapy are weighed against the benefits:

Lactation: Based on very limited published data, warfarin has not been detected in the breast milk of mothers treated with warfarin. The same limited published data reports that breast-fed infants, whose mothers were treated with warfarin, had neither detectable warfarin in their plasma, nor clinically significant changes in coagulation tests. Although warfarin was not detected in the plasma of the breast-fed infants, the possibility of an anticoagulant effect by warfarin cannot be excluded. It is prudent to perform coagulation tests on infants at risk for bleeding tendencies before advising women taking warfarin to breast-feed. Effects in premature infants have not been evaluated.

Severe to moderate hepatic or renal insufficiency.

Infectious diseases or disturbances of intestinal flora: Sprue, antibiotic therapy.

Trauma which may result in internal bleeding.

Surgery or trauma resulting in large exposed raw surfaces.

Indwelling catheters.

Severe to moderate hypertension.

Known or suspected deficiency in protein C mediated anticoagulant response: Hereditary or acquired deficiencies of protein C or its cofactor, protein S, have been associated with tissue necrosis following warfarin administration. Not all patients with these conditions develop necrosis, and tissue necrosis occurs in patients without these deficiencies. Inherited resistance to activated protein C has been described in many patients with venous thromboembolic disorders but has not yet been evaluated as a risk factor for tissue necrosis. The risk associated with these conditions, both for recurrent thrombosis and for adverse reaction, is difficult to evaluate since it does not appear to be the same for everyone. Decisions about testing and therapy must be made on an individual basis. It has been reported that concomitant anticoagulation therapy with heparin for 5-7 days during initiation of therapy with warfarin sodium may minimize the incidence of tissue necrosis. Warfarin therapy should be discontinued when warfarin is suspected to be the cause of developing necrosis and heparin therapy may be considered for anticoagulation.

Miscellaneous: Polycythemia vera, vasculitis, and severe diabetes.

Minor and severe allergic/hypersensitivity reactions and anaphylactic reactions have been reported.

In patients with acquired or inherited warfarin resistance, decreased therapeutic responses to warfarin sodium have been reported. Exaggerated therapeutic responses have been reported in other patients.

Patients with congestive heart failure may exhibit greater than expected PT/INR response to warfarin sodium, thereby requiring more frequent laboratory monitoring, and reduced doses of warfarin sodium.

Concomitant use of anticoagulants with streptokinase or urokinase is not recommended and may be hazardous. (Please note recommendations accompanying these preparations.)

PRECAUTIONS

Periodic determination of PT/INR or other suitable coagulation test is essential.

Numerous factors, alone or in combination, including travel, changes in diet, environment, physical state and medication, including botanicals, may influence response of the patient to anticoagulants. It is generally good practice to monitor the patient's response with additional PT/INR determinations in the period immediately after discharge from the hospital, and whenever other medications, including botanicals, are initiated, discontinued or taken irregularly. The following factors are listed for reference; however, other factors may also affect the anticoagulant response. (See DRUG INTERACTIONS.)

Drugs may interact with warfarin sodium through pharmacodynamic or pharmacokinetic mechanisms. Pharmacodynamic mechanisms for drug interactions with warfarin sodium are synergism (impaired hemostasis, reduced clotting factor synthesis), competitive antagonism (vitamin K), and altered physiologic control loop for vitamin K metabolism (hereditary resistance). Pharmacokinetic mechanisms for drug interactions with warfarin sodium are mainly enzyme induction, enzyme inhibition, and reduced plasma protein binding. It is important to note that some drugs may interact by more than one mechanism. (See DRUG INTERACTIONS.)

W

INFORMATION FOR THE PATIENT

The objective of anticoagulant therapy is to decrease the clotting ability of the blood so that thrombosis is prevented, while avoiding spontaneous bleeding. Effective therapeutic levels with minimal complications are in part dependent upon cooperative and well-instructed patients who communicate effectively with their physician. Patients should be advised: strict adherence to prescribed dosage schedule is necessary. Do not take or discontinue any other medication, including salicylates (*e.g.,* aspirin and topical analgesics), other over-the-counter medications, and botanical (herbal) products (*e.g.,* bromelains, coenzyme Q_{10}, danshen, dong quai, garlic, Ginkgo biloba, and St. John's wort) except on advice of the physician. Avoid alcohol consumption. Do not take warfarin sodium during pregnancy and do not become pregnant while taking it (see CONTRAINDICATIONS). Avoid any activity or sport that may result in traumatic injury. Prothrombin time tests and regular visits to the physician or clinic are needed to monitor therapy. Carry identification stating that warfarin sodium is being taken. If the prescribed dose of warfarin sodium is forgotten, notify the physician immediately. Take the dose as soon as possible on the same day but do not take a double dose of warfarin sodium the next day to make up for the missed doses. The amount of vitamin K in food may affect therapy with warfarin sodium. Eat a normal, balanced diet maintaining a consistent amount of vitamin K. Avoid drastic changes in dietary habits, such as eating large amounts of green leafy vegetables. Contact physician to report any illness, such as diarrhea, infection or fever. Notify physician immediately if any unusual bleeding or symptoms occur. Signs and symptoms of bleeding include: pain, swelling or discomfort, prolonged bleeding from cuts, increased menstrual flow or vaginal bleeding, nosebleeds, bleeding of gums from brushing, unusual bleeding or bruising, red or dark brown urine, red or tar black stools, headache, dizziness, or weakness. If therapy with warfarin sodium is discontinued, patients should be cautioned that the anticoagulant effects of warfarin sodium may persist for about 2-5 days. **Patients should be informed that all warfarin sodium products represent the same medication, and should not be taken concomitantly, as overdosage may result.**

CARCINOGENESIS, MUTAGENESIS, AND IMPAIRMENT OF FERTILITY

Carcinogenicity and mutagenicity studies have not been performed with warfarin sodium. The reproductive effects of warfarin sodium have not been evaluated.

PREGNANCY CATEGORY X

See CONTRAINDICATIONS.

PEDIATRIC USE

Safety and effectiveness in pediatric patients below the age of 18 have not been established in randomized, controlled clinical trials. However, the use of warfarin sodium in pediatric patients is well-documented for the prevention and treatment of thromboembolic events. Difficulty achieving and maintaining therapeutic PT/INR ranges in the pediatric patient has been reported. More frequent PT/INR determinations are recommended because of possible changing warfarin requirements.

GERIATRIC USE

Patients 60 years or older appear to exhibit greater than expected PT/INR response to the anticoagulant effects of warfarin (see CLINICAL PHARMACOLOGY). Warfarin sodium is contraindicated in any unsupervised patient with senility. Caution should be observed with administration of warfarin sodium to elderly patients in any situation or physical condition where added risk of hemorrhage is present. Low initiation and maintenance doses of warfarin sodium are recommended for elderly patients (see DOSAGE AND ADMINISTRATION).

DRUG INTERACTIONS

The following factors, alone or in combination, may be responsible for INCREASED PT/INR response:

Endogenous Factors: Cancer, collagen vascular disease, congestive heart failure, diarrhea, elevated temperature, hyperthyroidism, poor nutritional state, steatorrhea and vitamin K deficiency. *Hepatic Disorders:* Infectious hepatitis and jaundice. *Blood Dyscrasias:* See CONTRAINDICATIONS.

Exogenous Factors: Potential drug interactions with warfarin sodium are listed below by drug class and by specific drugs.

Classes of Drugs:

5-lipoxygenase inhibitor, adrenergic stimulants (central), alcohol abuse reduction preparations, analgesics, anesthetics (inhalation), antiandrogen, antiarrhythmics§*, anticoagulants, anticonvulsants*, antidepressants*, antimalarial agents, antineoplastics*, antiparasitic/antimicrobials, antiplatelet drugs/effects, antithyroid drugs*, beta-adrenergic blockers, cholelitholytic agents, diabetes agents (oral), diuretics*, fungal medications (systemic)*, gastric acidity and peptic ulcer agents*, gastrointestinal (prokinetic agents and ulcerative colitis agents), gout treatment agents, hemorrheologic agents, hepatotoxic drugs, hyperglycemic agents, hypertensive emergency agents, hypnotics*, leukotriene receptor antagonist, monoamine oxidase inhibitors, narcotics (prolonged), nonsteroidal anti-inflammatory agents, psychostimulants, pyrazolones, salicylates, selective serotonin reuptake inhibitors, steroids (adrenocortical)*, steroids [anabolic (17-alkyl testosterone derivatives)], thrombolytics, thyroid drugs, tuberculosis agents*, uricosuric agents, vaccines, vitamins.* *Antibiotics:** Aminoglycosides (oral), cephalosporins (parenteral), macrolides, miscellaneous, penicillins (intravenous, high dose), quinolones (fluoroquinolones), sulfonamides (long acting), and tetracyclines. *Hypolipidemics:** Bile acid-binding resins*, fibric acid derivatives, HMG-CoA reductase inhibitors*.

Specific Drugs Reported:

Acetaminophen, alcohol*, allopurinol, aminosalicylic acid, amiodarone HCl, aspirin, azithromycin, capecitabine, cefamandole, cefazolin, cefoperazone, cefotetan, cefoxitin, ceftriaxone, celecoxib, cerivastatin, chenodiol, chloramphenicol, chloral hydrate*, chlorpropamide, cholestyramine*, cimetidine, ciprofloxacin, cisapride, clarithromycin, clofibrate, warfarin sodium overdose, cyclophosphamide*, danazol, dextran, dextrothyroxine, diazoxide, diclofenac, dicumarol, diflunisal, disulfiram, doxycycline, erythromycin, ethacrynic acid, fenofibrate, fenoprofen, fluconazole, fluorouracil, fluoxetine, flutamide, fluvastatin, fluvoxamine, gemfibrozil, glucagon, halothane, heparin, ibuprofen, ifosamide, indomethacin, influenza virus vaccine, itraconazole, ketoprofen, ketorolac, levamisole, levofloxacin, levothyroxine, liothyronine, lovastatin, mefenamic acid, methimazole*, methyldopa, methylphenidate, methylsalicylate ointment (topical), metronidazole, miconazole, moricizine HCl*, nalidixic acid, naproxen, neomycin, norfloxacin, ofloxacin, olsalazine, omeprazole, oxaprozin, oxymetholone, paroxetine, penicillin G (intravenous), pentoxifylline, phenylbutazone, phenytoin*, piperacillin, piroxicam, prednisone*, propafenone, propoxyphene, propranolol, propylthiouracil*, quinidine, quinine, ranitidine*, rofecoxib, sertraline, simvastatin, stanozolol, streptokinase, sulfamethizole, sulfamethoxazole, sulfinpyrazone, sulfisoxazole, sulindac, tamoxifen, tetracycline, thyroid, ticarcillin, ticlopidine, tissue plasminogen activator (t-PA), tolbutamide, tramadol, trimethoprim/sulfamethoxazole, urokinase, valproate, vitamin E, zafirlukast, zileuton.

Also: Other medications affecting blood elements which may modify hemostasis; dietary deficiencies, prolonged hot weather and unreliable PT/INR determinations.

* Increased and decreased PT/INR responses have been reported.

The following factors, alone or in combination, may be responsible for DECREASED PT/INR response:

Endogenous Factors: Edema, hereditary warfarin sodium resistance, hyperlipemia, hypothyroidism, and nephrotic syndrome.

Exogenous Factors: Potential drug interactions with warfarin sodium are listed below by drug class and by specific drugs.

Classes of Drugs:

Adrenal cortical steroid inhibitors, antacids, antianxiety agents, antiarrhythmics†, antibiotics†, anticonvulsants†, antidepressants†, antihistamines, antineoplastics†, antipsychotic medications, antithyroid drugs†, barbiturates, diuretics†, enteral nutritional supplements, fungal medications (systemic)†, gastric acidity and peptic ulcer agents†, hypnotics†, immunosuppressives, oral contraceptives (estrogen containing), selective estrogen receptor modulators, steroids (adrenocortical)†, tuberculosis agents†, vitamins†. *Hypolipidemics:*† Bile acid-binding resins† and HMG-CoA reductase inhibitors†.

Specific Drugs Reported:

Alcohol†, aminoglutethimide, amobarbital, atorvastatin, azathioprine, butabarbital, butalbital, carbamazepine, chloral hydrate†, chlordiazepoxide, chlorthalidone, cholestyramine†, clozapine, corticotropin, cortisone, warfarin sodium underdosage, cyclophosphamide†, dicloxacillin, ethchlorvynol, glutethimide, griseofulvin, haloperidol, meprobamate, 6-mercaptopurine, methimazole†, moricizine HCl†, nafcillin, paraldehyde, pentobarbital, phenobarbital, phenytoin†, prednisone†, primidone, propylthiouracil†, raloxifene, ranitidine†, rifampin, secobarbital, spironolactone, sucralfate, trazodone, vitamin C (high dose), and vitamin K.

Also: Diet high in vitamin K and unreliable PT/INR determinations.

† Increased and decreased PT/INR responses have been reported.

Because a patient may be exposed to a combination of the above factors, the net effect of warfarin sodium on PT/INR response may be unpredictable. More frequent PT/INR monitoring is therefore advisable. Medications of unknown interaction with coumarins are best regarded with caution. When these medications are started or stopped, more frequent PT/INR monitoring is advisable.

It has been reported that concomitant administration of warfarin sodium and ticlopidine may be associated with cholestatic hepatitis.

BOTANICAL (HERBAL) MEDICINES

Caution should be exercised when botanical medicines (botanicals) are taken concomitantly with warfarin sodium. Few adequate, well-controlled studies exist evaluating the potential for metabolic and/or pharmacologic interactions between botanicals and warfarin sodium. Due to a lack of manufacturing standardization with botanical medicinal preparations, the amount of active ingredients may vary. This could further confound the ability to assess potential interactions and effects on anticoagulation. It is good practice to monitor the patient's response with additional PT/INR determinations when initiating or discontinuing botanicals.

Specific botanicals reported to affect warfarin sodium therapy include the following:

- Bromelains, danshen, dong quai *(Angelica sinensis),* garlic, and Ginkgo biloba are associated most often with an INCREASE in the effects of warfarin sodium.
- Coenzyme Q_{10} (ubidecarenone) and St. John's wort are associated most often with a DECREASE in the effects of warfarin sodium.

Some botanicals may cause bleeding events when taken alone (*e.g.,* garlic and Ginkgo biloba) and may have anticoagulant, antiplatelet, and/or fibrinolytic properties. These effects would be expected to be additive to the anticoagulant effects of warfarin sodium. Conversely, other botanicals may have coagulant properties when taken alone or may decrease the effects of warfarin sodium.

Some botanicals that may affect coagulation are listed below for reference; however, this list should not be considered all-inclusive. Many botanicals have several common names and scientific names. The most widely recognized common botanical names are listed.

Botanicals that contain coumarins with potential anticoagulant effects: Alfalfa, angelica (dong quai), aniseed, arnica, asa foetida, bogbean‡, boldo, buchu, capsicum§, cassia¤, celery, chamomile (German and Roman), dandelion¤, fenugreek, horse chestnut, horseradish, licorice¤, meadowsweet‡, nettle, parsley, passion flower, prickly ash (Northern), quassia, red clover, sweet clover, sweet woodruff, tonka beans, wild carrot, wild lettuce.

Miscellaneous botanicals with anticoagulant properties: Bladder wrack *(Fucus)* and pau d'arco.

Botanicals that contain salicylate and/or have antiplatelet properties: Agrimony¶, aloe gel, aspen, black cohosh, black haw, bogbean‡, cassia¤, clove, dandelion¤, feverfew, garlic**, German sarsaparilla, ginger, Ginkgo biloba, ginseng *(Panax)***,

W

licorice¤, meadowsweet‡, onion**, policosanol, poplar, senega, tamarind, willow, wintergreen.

Botanicals with fibrinolytic properties: Bromelains, capsicum§, garlic**, ginseng *(Panax)***, inositol nicotinate, onion**.

Botanicals with coagulant properties: Agrimony¶, goldenseal, mistletoe, yarrow.

‡ Contains coumarins and salicylate.
§ Contains coumarins and has fibrinolytic properties.
¤ Contains coumarins and has antiplatelet properties.
¶ Contains salicylate and has coagulant properties.
** Has antiplatelet and fibrinolytic properties.

EFFECT ON OTHER DRUGS

Coumarins may also affect the action of other drugs. Hypoglycemic agents (chlorpropamide and tolbutamide) and anticonvulsants (phenytoin and phenobarbital) may accumulate in the body as a result of interference with either their metabolism or excretion.

SPECIAL RISK PATIENTS

Warfarin sodium is a narrow therapeutic range (index) drug, and caution should be observed when warfarin sodium is administered to certain patients such as the elderly or debilitated or when administered in any situation or physical condition where added risk of hemorrhage is present.

Intramuscular (IM) injections of concomitant medications should be confined to the upper extremities which permits easy access for manual compression, inspections for bleeding and use of pressure bandages.

Caution should be observed when warfarin sodium is administered concomitantly with nonsteroidal anti-inflammatory drugs (NSAIDs), including aspirin, to be certain that no change in anticoagulation dosage is required. In addition to specific drug interactions that might affect PT/INR, NSAIDS, including aspirin, can inhibit platelet aggregation, and can cause gastrointestinal bleeding, peptic ulceration and/or perforation.

Acquired or inherited warfarin resistance should be suspected if large daily doses of warfarin sodium are required to maintain a patient's PT/INR within a normal therapeutic range.

ADVERSE REACTIONS

POTENTIAL ADVERSE REACTIONS TO WARFARIN SODIUM MAY INCLUDE

- ***Fatal or nonfatal hemorrhage from any tissue or organ:*** This is a consequence of the anticoagulant effect. The signs, symptoms, and severity will vary according to the location and degree or extent of the bleeding. Hemorrhagic complications may present as paralysis; paresthesia; headache, chest, abdomen, joint, muscle, or other pain; dizziness; shortness of breath, difficult breathing or swallowing; unexplained swelling; weakness; hypotension; or unexplained shock. Therefore, the possibility of hemorrhage should be considered in evaluating the condition of any anticoagulated patient with complaints which do not indicate an obvious diagnosis. Bleeding during anticoagulant therapy does not always correlate with PT/INR.
- **Bleeding** which occurs when the PT/INR is within the therapeutic range warrants diagnostic investigation since it may unmask a previously unsuspected lesion, *e.g.,* tumor, ulcer, etc.
- ***Necrosis of skin and other tissues:*** See WARNINGS.
- ***Adverse reactions reported infrequently include:*** Hypersensitivity/allergic reactions, systemic cholesterol microembolization, purple toes syndrome, hepatitis, cholestatic hepatic injury, jaundice, elevated liver enzymes, vasculitis, edema, fever, rash, dermatitis, including bullous eruptions, urticaria, abdominal pain including cramping, flatulence/bloating, fatigue, lethargy, malaise, asthenia, nausea, vomiting, diarrhea, pain, headache, dizziness, taste perversion, pruritus, alopecia, cold intolerance, and paresthesia including feeling cold and chills.

Rare events of tracheal or tracheobronchial calcification have been reported in association with long-term warfarin sodium therapy. The clinical significance of this event is unknown.

Priapism has been associated with anticoagulant administration, however, a causal relationship has not been established.

DOSAGE AND ADMINISTRATION

The dosage and administration of warfarin sodium must be individualized for each patient according to the particular patient's PT/INR response to the drug. The dosage should be adjusted based upon the patient's PT/INR. (See Laboratory Control for full discussion on INR.)

VENOUS THROMBOEMBOLISM (INCLUDING PULMONARY EMBOLISM)

Available clinical evidence indicates that an INR of 2.0-3.0 is sufficient for prophylaxis and treatment of venous thromboembolism and minimizes the risk of hemorrhage associated with higher INRs. In patients with risk factors for recurrent venous thromboembolism including venous insufficiency, inherited thrombophilia, idiopathic venous thromboembolism, and a history of thrombotic events, consideration should be given to longer term therapy (Schulman *et al.,* 1995 and Schulman *et al.,* 1997).

ATRIAL FIBRILLATION

Five recent clinical trials evaluated the effects of warfarin in patients with non-valvular atrial fibrillation (AF). Meta-analysis findings of these studies revealed that the effects of warfarin in reducing thromboembolic events including stroke were similar at either moderately high INR (2.0-4.5) or low INR (1.4-3.0). There was a significant reduction in minor bleeds at the low INR. Similar data from clinical studies in valvular atrial fibrillation patients are not available. The trials in non-valvular atrial fibrillation support the American College of Chest Physicians' (ACCP) recommendation that an INR of 2.0-3.0 be used for long term warfarin therapy in appropriate AF patients.

POST-MYOCARDIAL INFARCTION

In post-myocardial infarction patients, warfarin sodium therapy should be initiated early (2-4 weeks post-infarction) and dosage should be adjusted to maintain an INR of 2.5-3.5 long-term. The recommendation is based on the results of the WARIS study in which treatment was initiated 2-4 weeks after the infarction. In patients thought to be at an increased risk of bleeding complications or on aspirin therapy, maintenance of warfarin sodium therapy at the lower end of this INR range is recommended.

MECHANICAL AND BIOPROSTHETIC HEART VALVES

In patients with mechanical heart valve(s), long term prophylaxis with warfarin to an INR of 2.5-3.5 is recommended. In patients with bioprosthetic heart valve(s), based on limited data, the American College of Chest Physicians recommends warfarin therapy to an INR of 2.0-3.0 for 12 weeks after valve insertion. In patients with additional risk factors such as atrial fibrillation or prior thromboembolism, consideration should be given for longer term therapy.

RECURRENT SYSTEMIC EMBOLISM

In cases where the risk of thromboembolism is great, such as in patients with recurrent systemic embolism, a higher INR may be required.

An INR of greater than 4.0 appears to provide no additional therapeutic benefit in most patients and is associated with a higher risk of bleeding.

INITIAL DOSAGE

The dosing of warfarin sodium must be individualized according to patient's sensitivity to the drug as indicated by the PT/INR. Use of a large loading dose may increase the incidence of hemorrhagic and other complications, does not offer more rapid protection against thrombi formation, and is not recommended. Lower initiation and maintenance doses are recommended for elderly and/or debilitated patients and patients with potential to exhibit greater than expected PT/INR response to warfarin sodium (see PRECAUTIONS). Based on limited data, Asian patients may also require lower initiation and maintenance doses of warfarin sodium (see CLINICAL PHARMACOLOGY). It is recommended that warfarin sodium therapy be initiated with a dose of 2-5 mg/day with dosage adjustments based on the results of PT/INR determinations.

MAINTENANCE

Most patients are satisfactorily maintained at a dose of 2-10 mg daily. Flexibility of dosage is provided by breaking scored tablets in half. The individual dose and interval should be gauged by the patient's prothrombin response.

DURATION OF THERAPY

The duration of therapy in each patient should be individualized. In general, anticoagulant therapy should be continued until the danger of thrombosis and embolism has passed.

MISSED DOSE

The anticoagulant effect of warfarin sodium persists beyond 24 hours. If the patient forgets to take the prescribed dose of warfarin sodium at the scheduled time, the dose should be taken as soon as possible on the same day. The patient should not take the missed dose by doubling the daily dose to make up for missed doses, but should refer back to his or her physician.

INTRAVENOUS ROUTE OF ADMINISTRATION

Warfarin sodium for injection provides an alternate administration route for patients who cannot receive oral drugs. The IV dosages would be the same as those that would be used orally if the patient could take the drug by the oral route. Warfarin sodium for injection should be administered as a slow bolus injection over 1-2 minutes into a peripheral vein. It is not recommended for intramuscular administration. The vial should be reconstituted with 2.7 ml of sterile water for injection and inspected for particulate matter and discoloration immediately prior to use. Do not use if either particulate matter and/or discoloration is noted. After reconstitution, warfarin sodium for injection is chemically and physically stable for 4 hours at room temperature. It does not contain any antimicrobial preservative and, thus, care must be taken to assure the sterility of the prepared solution. The vial is not recommended for multiple use and unused solution should be discarded.

LABORATORY CONTROL

The PT reflects the depression of vitamin K dependent Factors VII, X, and II. There are several modifications of the one-stage PT and the physician should become familiar with the specific method used in his laboratory. The degree of anticoagulation indicated by any range of PTs may be altered by the type of thromboplastin used; the appropriate therapeutic range must be based on the experience of each laboratory. The PT should be determined daily after the administration of the initial dose until PT/INR results stabilize in the therapeutic range. Intervals between subsequent PT/INR determinations should be based upon the physician's judgement of the patient's reliability and response to warfarin sodium in order to maintain the individual within the therapeutic range. Acceptable intervals for PT/INR determinations are normally within the range of 1-4 weeks after a stable dosage has been determined. To ensure adequate control, it is recommended that additional PT tests are done when other warfarin products are interchanged with warfarin sodium tablets as well as whenever other medications are initiated, discontinued, or taken irregularly (see PRECAUTIONS).

Different thromboplastin reagents vary substantially in their sensitivity to sodium warfarin-induced effects on PT. To define the appropriate therapeutic regimen it is important to be familiar with the sensitivity of the thromboplastin reagent used in the laboratory and its relationship to the International Reference Preparation (IRP), a sensitive thromboplastin reagent prepared from human brain.

A system of standardizing the PT in oral anticoagulant control was introduced by the World Health Organization in 1983. It is based upon the determination of an International Normalized Ratio (INR) which provides a common basis for communication of PT results and interpretations of therapeutic ranges. The INR system of reporting is based on a logarithmic relationship between the PT ratios of the test and reference preparation. The INR is the PT ratio that would be obtained if the International Reference Preparation (IRP), which has an ISI of 1.0, were used to perform the test. Early clinical studies of oral anticoagulants, which formed the basis for recommended therapeutic ranges of 1.5-2.5 times control mean normal PT, used sensitive human brain thromboplastin. When using the less sensitive rabbit brain thromboplastins commonly employed in PT assays today, adjustments must be made to the targeted PT range that reflect this decrease in sensitivity.

The INR can be calculated as:

$INR = (\text{observed PT ratio})^{ISI}$

where the ISI (International Sensitivity Index) is the correction factor in the equation that relates the PT ratio of the local reagent to the reference preparation and is a measure of the sensitivity of a given thromboplastin to reduction of vitamin K-dependent coagulation factors; the lower the ISI, the more "sensitive" the reagent and the closer the derived INR will be to the observed PT ratio.[1]

The proceedings and recommendations of the 1992 National Conference on Antithrombotic Therapy[2-4] review and evaluate issues related to oral anticoagulant therapy and the sensitivity of thromboplastin reagents and provide additional guidelines for defining the appropriate therapeutic regimen.

The conversion of the INR to PT ratios for the less-intense (INR 2.0-3.0) and more intense (INR 2.5-3.5) therapeutic range recommended by the ACCP for thromboplastins over a range of ISI values shown in TABLE 3.[5]

TABLE 3 *Relationship Between INR and PT Ratios for Thromboplastins With Different ISI Values (sensitivities)*

	PT Ratios				
	ISI 1.0	ISI 1.4	ISI 1.8	ISI 2.3	ISI 2.8
INR = 2.0-3.0	2.0-3.0	1.6-2.2	1.5-1.8	1.4-1.6	1.3-1.5
INR = 2.5-3.5	2.5-3.5	1.9-2.4	1.7-2.0	1.5-1.7	1.4-1.6

TREATMENT DURING DENTISTRY AND SURGERY

The management of patients who undergo dental and surgical procedures requires close liaison between attending physicians, surgeons and dentists. PT/INR determination is recommended just prior to any dental or surgical procedure. In patients undergoing minimal invasive procedures who must be anticoagulated prior to, during, or immediately following these procedures, adjusting the dosage of warfarin sodium to maintain the PT/INR at the low end of the therapeutic range may safely allow for continued anticoagulation. The operative site should be sufficiently limited and accessible to permit the effective use of local procedures for hemostasis. Under these conditions, dental and minor surgical procedures may be performed without undue risk of hemorrhage. Some dental or surgical procedures may necessitate the interruption of warfarin sodium therapy. When discontinuing warfarin sodium even for a short period of time, the benefits and risks should be strongly considered.

CONVERSION FROM HEPARIN THERAPY

Since the anticoagulant effect of warfarin sodium is delayed, heparin is preferred initially for rapid anticoagulation. Conversion to warfarin sodium may begin concomitantly with heparin therapy or may be delayed 3-6 days. To ensure continuous anticoagulation, it is advisable to continue full dose heparin therapy and the warfarin sodium therapy be overlapped with heparin for 4-5 days, until warfarin sodium has produced the desired therapeutic response as determined by PT/INR. When warfarin sodium has produced the desired PT/INR or prothombin activity, heparin may be discontinued.

Warfarin sodium may increase the aPTT test, even in the absence of heparin. During initial therapy with warfarin sodium, the interference with heparin anticoagulation is of minimal clinical significance.

As heparin may affect the PT/INR, patients receiving both heparin and warfarin sodium should have blood for PT/INR determination drawn at least:

- 5 hours after the last IV bolus dose of heparin, or
- 4 hours after cessation of a continuous IV infusion of heparin, or
- 24 hours after the last subcutaneous heparin injection.

HOW SUPPLIED

COUMADIN TABLETS

For oral use, single scored with one face imprinted numerically with 1, 2, 2½, 3, 4, 5, 6, 7½ or 10 superimposed and inscribed with "COUMADIN" and with the opposite face plain.

The 1 mg tablet is pink.
The 2 mg tablet is lavender.
The 2½ mg tablet is green.
The 3 mg tablet is tan.
The 4 mg tablet is blue.
The 5 mg tablet is peach.
The 6 mg tablet is teal.
The 7½ mg tablet is yellow.
The 10 mg tablet is white (dye free).

Storage: Protect from light. Store at controlled room temperature (15-30°C, 59-86°F). Dispense in a tight, light-resistant container.

COUMADIN INJECTION

Available for intravenous use only. Not recommended for intramuscular administration. Reconstitute with 2.7 ml of sterile water for injection to yield 2 mg/ml. Net contents 5.4 mg lyophilized powder. Maximum yield 2.5 ml.

Storage: Protect from light. Keep vial in box until used. Store at controlled room temperature (15-30°C, 59-86°F).

After reconstitution, store at controlled room temperature (15-30°C, 59-86°F) and use within 4 hours. Do not refrigerate. Discard any unused solution.

PRODUCT LISTING - RATED THERAPEUTICALLY EQUIVALENT

Tablet - Oral - 1 mg

30's	$19.06	COUMADIN, Allscripts Pharmaceutical Company	54569-4443-00
90's	$55.14	GENERIC, Apothecon Inc	59772-0352-04
100's	$53.35	GENERIC, Bristol-Myers Squibb	59772-0352-07
100's	$53.35	GENERIC, Bristol-Myers Squibb	59772-0352-70
100's	$56.02	GENERIC, Barr Laboratories Inc	00555-0831-02
100's	$58.34	GENERIC, Ivax Corporation	00182-2671-01
100's	$58.34	GENERIC, Ivax Corporation	00182-2671-89
100's	$58.34	GENERIC, Caremark Inc	00339-6537-12
100's	$58.35	GENERIC, Taro Pharmaceuticals U.S.A. Inc	51672-4027-01
100's	$61.26	GENERIC, Geneva Pharmaceuticals	00781-0352-07
100's	$75.11	COUMADIN, Bristol-Myers Squibb	00056-0169-70
100's	$75.11	COUMADIN, Bristol-Myers Squibb	00056-0169-75

Tablet - Oral - 2 mg

25's	$23.69	COUMADIN, Pd-Rx Pharmaceuticals	55289-0143-97
30's	$19.89	COUMADIN, Allscripts Pharmaceutical Company	54569-0158-00
90's	$57.54	GENERIC, Apothecon Inc	59772-0363-04
100's	$55.67	GENERIC, Bristol-Myers Squibb	59772-0363-70
100's	$55.68	GENERIC, Bristol-Myers Squibb	59772-0363-07
100's	$58.46	GENERIC, Barr Laboratories Inc	00555-0869-02
100's	$60.89	GENERIC, Ivax Corporation	00182-2672-01
100's	$60.89	GENERIC, Ivax Corporation	00182-2672-89
100's	$60.89	GENERIC, Caremark Inc	00339-6538-12
100's	$60.89	GENERIC, Taro Pharmaceuticals U.S.A. Inc	51672-4028-01
100's	$63.93	GENERIC, Geneva Pharmaceuticals	00781-0363-07
100's	$66.28	COUMADIN, Allscripts Pharmaceutical Company	54569-0158-01
100's	$78.38	COUMADIN, Bristol-Myers Squibb	00056-0170-70
100's	$78.38	COUMADIN, Bristol-Myers Squibb	00056-0170-75

Tablet - Oral - 2.5 mg

30's	$20.51	COUMADIN, Allscripts Pharmaceutical Company	54569-0212-01
90's	$59.39	GENERIC, Apothecon Inc	59772-0364-04
100's	$57.45	GENERIC, Apothecon Inc	59772-0364-07
100's	$57.46	GENERIC, Apothecon Inc	59772-0364-70
100's	$60.33	GENERIC, Barr Laboratories Inc	00555-0832-02
100's	$62.84	GENERIC, Ivax Corporation	00182-2673-01
100's	$62.84	GENERIC, Ivax Corporation	00182-2673-89
100's	$62.84	GENERIC, Caremark Inc	00339-6539-12
100's	$62.85	GENERIC, Taro Pharmaceuticals U.S.A. Inc	51672-4029-01
100's	$65.98	GENERIC, Geneva Pharmaceuticals	00781-0364-07
100's	$80.88	COUMADIN, Bristol-Myers Squibb	00056-0176-70
100's	$80.88	COUMADIN, Bristol-Myers Squibb	00056-0176-75

Tablet - Oral - 3 mg

100's	$60.55	GENERIC, Barr Laboratories Inc	00555-0925-02
100's	$62.23	GENERIC, Caremark Inc	00339-6540-12
100's	$63.07	GENERIC, Ivax Corporation	00182-2674-01
100's	$63.07	GENERIC, Ivax Corporation	00182-2674-89
100's	$63.07	GENERIC, Taro Pharmaceuticals U.S.A. Inc	51672-4030-01
100's	$63.07	GENERIC, Geneva Pharmaceuticals	59772-0366-07
100's	$66.22	GENERIC, Geneva Pharmaceuticals	00781-0366-07
100's	$81.19	COUMADIN, Bristol-Myers Squibb	00056-0188-70
100's	$81.19	COUMADIN, Bristol-Myers Squibb	00056-0188-75

Tablet - Oral - 4 mg

100's	$57.83	GENERIC, Bristol-Myers Squibb	59772-0369-70
100's	$57.84	GENERIC, Bristol-Myers Squibb	59772-0369-07
100's	$60.73	GENERIC, Barr Laboratories Inc	00555-0874-02
100's	$63.25	GENERIC, Ivax Corporation	00182-2675-01
100's	$63.25	GENERIC, Ivax Corporation	00182-2675-89
100's	$63.25	GENERIC, Caremark Inc	00339-6541-12
100's	$63.25	GENERIC, Taro Pharmaceuticals U.S.A. Inc	51672-4031-01
100's	$66.41	GENERIC, Geneva Pharmaceuticals	00781-0369-07
100's	$81.40	COUMADIN, Bristol-Myers Squibb	00056-0168-70
100's	$81.40	COUMADIN, Bristol-Myers Squibb	00056-0168-75

Tablet - Oral - 5 mg

25's	$24.72	COUMADIN, Pd-Rx Pharmaceuticals	55289-0286-97
30's	$20.78	COUMADIN, Allscripts Pharmaceutical Company	54569-0159-00
30's	$31.43	COUMADIN, Pd-Rx Pharmaceuticals	55289-0286-30
50's	$51.51	COUMADIN, Pd-Rx Pharmaceuticals	55289-0286-50
90's	$51.41	COUMADIN, Allscripts Pharmaceutical Company	54569-8542-00
90's	$60.18	GENERIC, Apothecon Inc	59772-0377-04
100's	$58.21	GENERIC, Bristol-Myers Squibb	59772-0377-07
100's	$58.21	GENERIC, Bristol-Myers Squibb	59772-0377-70
100's	$61.13	GENERIC, Barr Laboratories Inc	00555-0833-02
100's	$63.68	GENERIC, Ivax Corporation	00182-2676-01
100's	$63.68	GENERIC, Ivax Corporation	00182-2676-89
100's	$63.68	GENERIC, Caremark Inc	00339-6542-12
100's	$63.68	GENERIC, Taro Pharmaceuticals U.S.A. Inc	51672-4032-01
100's	$66.86	GENERIC, Geneva Pharmaceuticals	00781-0377-07
100's	$69.28	COUMADIN, Allscripts Pharmaceutical Company	54569-0159-01
100's	$84.29	COUMADIN, Bristol-Myers Squibb	00056-0172-70
100's	$84.29	COUMADIN, Bristol-Myers Squibb	00056-0172-75

Tablet - Oral - 6 mg

100's	$86.69	GENERIC, Barr Laboratories Inc	00555-0926-02
100's	$89.10	GENERIC, Caremark Inc	00339-6543-12
100's	$90.30	GENERIC, Ivax Corporation	00182-2677-01
100's	$90.30	GENERIC, Ivax Corporation	00182-2677-89
100's	$90.30	GENERIC, Geneva Pharmaceuticals	00781-0381-07
100's	$90.30	GENERIC, Taro Pharmaceuticals U.S.A. Inc	51672-4033-01
100's	$90.30	GENERIC, Geneva Pharmaceuticals	59772-0381-07

100's $108.59 COUMADIN, Bristol-Myers Squibb 00056-0189-70
100's $108.59 COUMADIN, Bristol-Myers Squibb 00056-0189-75

Tablet - Oral - 7.5 mg
100's $85.43 GENERIC, Bristol-Myers Squibb 59772-0386-07
100's $85.43 GENERIC, Bristol-Myers Squibb 59772-0386-70
100's $89.70 GENERIC, Barr Laboratories Inc 00555-0834-02
100's $93.44 GENERIC, Ivax Corporation 00182-2678-01
100's $93.44 GENERIC, Ivax Corporation 00182-2678-89
100's $93.44 GENERIC, Caremark Inc 00339-6544-12
100's $93.44 GENERIC, Taro Pharmaceuticals U.S.A. Inc 51672-4034-01
100's $98.11 GENERIC, Geneva Pharmaceuticals 00781-0386-07
100's $112.35 COUMADIN, Bristol-Myers Squibb 00056-0173-70
100's $112.35 COUMADIN, Bristol-Myers Squibb 00056-0173-75

Tablet - Oral - 10 mg
100's $88.61 GENERIC, Bristol-Myers Squibb 59772-0387-07
100's $88.61 GENERIC, Bristol-Myers Squibb 59772-0387-70
100's $93.04 GENERIC, Barr Laboratories Inc 00555-0835-02
100's $96.91 GENERIC, Ivax Corporation 00182-2679-01
100's $96.91 GENERIC, Ivax Corporation 00182-2679-89
100's $96.91 GENERIC, Caremark Inc 00339-6545-12
100's $96.91 GENERIC, Taro Pharmaceuticals U.S.A. Inc 51672-4035-01
100's $101.76 GENERIC, Geneva Pharmaceuticals 00781-0387-07
100's $116.54 COUMADIN, Bristol-Myers Squibb 00056-0174-70
100's $116.54 COUMADIN, Bristol-Myers Squibb 00056-0174-75

PRODUCT LISTING - EQUIVALENTS NOT AVAILABLE

Powder For Injection - Intravenous - 5 mg
6's $135.47 COUMADIN, Bristol-Myers Squibb 00059-0324-35
6's $135.47 COUMADIN, Dupont Pharmaceuticals 00590-0324-35

Tablet - Oral - 1 mg
30's $28.72 GENERIC, Physicians Total Care 54868-4349-00
100's $58.34 GENERIC, Vangard Labs 00615-4547-29

Tablet - Oral - 2 mg
30's $24.30 GENERIC, Physicians Total Care 54868-4422-00
100's $60.89 GENERIC, Vangard Labs 00615-1509-29

Tablet - Oral - 2.5 mg
30's $24.88 GENERIC, Physicians Total Care 54868-4400-00
100's $62.84 GENERIC, Vangard Labs 00615-1510-29

Tablet - Oral - 3 mg
100's $63.07 GENERIC, Vangard Labs 00615-4548-29

Tablet - Oral - 4 mg
30's $26.09 GENERIC, Physicians Total Care 54868-4402-00
100's $63.25 GENERIC, Vangard Labs 00615-4549-29

Tablet - Oral - 5 mg
30's $19.10 GENERIC, Allscripts Pharmaceutical Company 54569-4934-00
30's $32.04 GENERIC, Physicians Total Care 54868-4286-00
100's $63.68 GENERIC, Vangard Labs 00615-1512-29

Tablet - Oral - 6 mg
100's $90.30 GENERIC, Vangard Labs 00615-4550-29

Tablet - Oral - 7.5 mg
100's $93.44 GENERIC, Vangard Labs 00615-4551-29

Zafirlukast *(003303)*

Categories: Asthma; Pregnancy Category B; FDA Approved 1996 Aug
Drug Classes: Leucotriene antagonists/inhibitors
Brand Names: Accolate
Foreign Brand Availability: Zuvair (India)
Cost of Therapy: $75.59 (Asthma; Accolate; 20 mg; 2 tablets/day; 30 day supply)

DESCRIPTION

Zafirlukast is a synthetic, selective peptide leukotriene receptor antagonist (LTRA), with the chemical name 4-(5-cyclopentyloxy-carbonylamino-1-methyl-indol-3-ylmethyl)-3-methoxy-N-o-tolylsulfonylbenzamide. The molecular weight of zafirlukast is 575.7.
The Empirical Formula is: $C_{31}H_{33}N_3O_6S$.
Zafirlukast, a fine white to pale yellow amorphous powder, is practically insoluble in water. It is slightly soluble in methanol and freely soluble in tetrahydrofuran, dimethylsulfoxide, and acetone.

Accolate is supplied as 10 and 20 mg tablets for oral administration.
Inactive Ingredients: Film-coated tablets containing croscarmellose sodium, lactose, magnesium stearate, microcrystalline cellulose, povidone, hydroxypropylmethylcellulose, and titanium dioxide.

CLINICAL PHARMACOLOGY

MECHANISM OF ACTION

Zafirlukast is a selective and competitive receptor antagonist of leukotriene D_4 and E_4 (LTD_4 and LTE_4), components of slow-reacting substance of anaphylaxis (SRSA). Cysteinyl leukotriene production and receptor occupation have been correlated with the pathophysiology of asthma, including airway edema, smooth muscle constriction, and altered cellular activity associated with the inflammatory process, which contribute to the signs and symptoms of asthma. Patients with asthma were found in one study to be 25-100 times more sensitive to the bronchoconstricting activity of inhaled LTD_4 than nonasthmatic subjects.

In vitro studies demonstrated that zafirlukast antagonized the contractile activity of three leukotrienes (LTC_4, LTD_4, and LTE_4) in conducting airway smooth muscle from laboratory animals and humans. Zafirlukast prevented intradermal LTD_4-induced increases in cutaneous vascular permeability and inhibited inhaled LTD_4-induced influx of eosinophils into animal lungs. Inhalational challenge studies in sensitized sheep showed that zafirlukast suppressed the airway responses to antigen; this included both the early- and late-phase response and the nonspecific hyperresponsiveness.

In humans, zafirlukast inhibited bronchoconstriction caused by several kinds of inhalational challenges. Pretreatment with single oral doses of zafirlukast inhibited the bronchoconstriction caused by sulfur dioxide and cold air in patients with asthma. Pretreatment with single doses of zafirlukast attenuated the early- and late-phase reaction caused by inhalation of various antigens such as grass, cat dander, ragweed, and mixed antigens in patients with asthma. Zafirlukast also attenuated the increase in bronchial hyperresponsiveness to inhaled histamine that followed inhaled allergen challenge.

CLINICAL PHARMACOKINETICS AND BIOAVAILABILITY

Absorption

Zafirlukast is rapidly absorbed following oral administration. Peak plasma concentrations are generally achieved 3 hours after oral administration. The absolute bioavailability of zafirlukast is unknown. In two separate studies, one using a high fat and the other a high protein meal, administration of zafirlukast with food reduced the mean bioavailability by approximately 40%.

Distribution

Zafirlukast is more than 99% bound to plasma proteins, predominantly albumin. The degree of binding was independent of concentration in the clinically relevant range. The apparent steady-state volume of distribution (Vss/F) is approximately 70 L, suggesting moderate distribution into tissues. Studies in rats using radiolabeled zafirlukast indicate minimal distribution across the blood-brain barrier.

Metabolism

Zafirlukast is extensively metabolized. The most common metabolic products are hydroxylated metabolites which are excreted in the feces. The metabolites of zafirlukast identified in plasma are at least 90 times less potent as LTD_4 receptor antagonists than zafirlukast in a standard *in vitro* test of activity. *In vitro* studies using human liver microsomes showed that the hydroxylated metabolites of zafirlukast excreted in the feces are formed through the cytochrome P450 2C9 (CYP2C9) pathway. Additional *in vitro* studies utilizing human liver microsomes show that zafirlukast inhibits the cytochrome P450 CYP3A4 and CYP2C9 isoenzymes at concentrations close to the clinically achieved total plasma concentrations. (See Drug Interactions.)

Excretion

The apparent oral clearance (CL/f) of zafirlukast is approximately 20 L/h. Studies in the rat and dog suggest that biliary excretion is the primary route of excretion. Following oral administration of radiolabeled zafirlukast to volunteers, urinary excretion accounts for approximately 10% of the dose and the remainder is excreted in feces. Zafirlukast is not detected in urine.

In the pivotal bioequivalence study, the mean terminal half-life of zafirlukast is approximately 10 hours in both normal adult subjects and patients with asthma. In other studies, the mean plasma half-life of zafirlukast ranged from approximately 8-16 hours in both normal subjects and patients with asthma. The pharmacokinetics of zafirlukast are approximately linear over the range from 5-80 mg. Steady-state plasma concentrations of zafirlukast are proportional to the dose and predictable from single-dose pharmacokinetic data. Accumulation of zafirlukast in the plasma following twice daily dosing is approximately 45%.

The pharmacokinetic parameters of zafirlukast 20 mg administered as a single dose to 36 male volunteers are shown in TABLE 1.

TABLE 1 *Mean (% coefficient of variation) Pharmacokinetic Parameters of Zafirlukast Following Single 20 mg Oral Dose Administration to Male Volunteers (n=36)*

C_{max} (ng/ml)	T_{max}* (h)	AUC (ng·h/ml)	$T_{½}$ (h)	CL/f (L/h)
326 (31.0)	2 (0.5-5.0)	1137 (34)	13.3 (75.6)	19.4 (32)

* Median and range.

Special Populations

Gender

The pharmacokinetics of zafirlukast are similar in males and females. Weight-adjusted apparent oral clearance does not differ due to gender.

Race

No differences in the pharmacokinetics of zafirlukast due to race have been observed.

Elderly

The apparent oral clearance of zafirlukast decreases with age. In patients above 65 years of age, there is an approximately 2- to 3-fold greater C_{max} and AUC compared to young adult patients.

Children

Following administration of a single 20 mg dose of zafirlukast to 20 boys and girls between 7 and 11 years of age, and in a second study, to 29 boys and girls between 5 and 6 years of age, the following pharmacokinetic parameters were obtained (see TABLE 2).

Weight unadjusted apparent clearance was 11.4 L/h (42%) in the 7-11 year old children, which resulted in greater systemic drug exposure than that obtained in adults for an identical dose. To maintain similar exposure levels in children compared to adults, a dose of 10 mg bid is recommended in children 5-11 years of age (see DOSAGE AND ADMINISTRATION).

Zafirlukast disposition was unchanged after multiple dosing (20 mg bid) in children and the degree of accumulation in plasma was similar to that observed in adults.

TABLE 2

Parameter	Children age 5-6 years Mean (% coefficient of variation)	Children age 7-11 years Mean (% coefficient of variation)
C_{max} (ng/ml)	756 (39%)	601 (45%)
AUC (ng·h/ml)	2458 (34%)	2027 (38%)
T_{max} (h)	2.1 (61%)	2.5 (55%)
CL/F (L/h)	9.2 (37%)	11.4 (42%)

Hepatic Insufficiency

In a study of patients with hepatic impairment (biopsy-proven cirrhosis), there was a reduced clearance of zafirlukast resulting in a 50-60% greater C_{max} and AUC compared to normal subjects.

Renal Insufficiency

Based on a cross-study comparison, there are no apparent differences in the pharmacokinetics of zafirlukast between renally-impaired patients and normal subjects.

Drug Interactions

The following drug interaction studies have been conducted with zafirlukast. (See DRUG INTERACTIONS.)

- Coadministration of multiple doses of zafirlukast (160 mg/day) to steady-state with a single 25 mg dose of warfarin (a substrate of CYP2C9) resulted in a significant increase in the mean AUC (+63%) and half-life (+36%) of S-warfarin. The mean prothrombin time increased by approximately 35%. The pharmacokinetics of zafirlukast were unaffected by coadministration with warfarin.
- Coadministration of zafirlukast (80 mg/day) at steady-state with a single dose of a liquid theophylline preparation (6 mg/kg) in 13 asthmatic patients, 18-44 years of age, resulted in decreased mean plasma concentrations of zafirlukast by approximately 30%, but no effect on plasma theophylline concentrations was observed.
- Coadministration of zafirlukast (20 mg/day) or placebo at steady-state with a single dose of sustained release theophylline preparation (16 mg/kg) in 16 healthy boys and girls (6-11 years of age) resulted in no significant differences in the pharmacokinetic parameters of theophylline.
- Coadministration of zafirlukast dosed at 40 mg bid in a single-blind, parallel-group, 3 week study in 39 healthy female subjects taking oral contraceptives, resulted in no significant effect on ethinyl estradiol plasma concentrations or contraceptive efficacy.
- Coadministration of zafirlukast (40 mg/day) with aspirin (650 mg four times daily) resulted in mean increased plasma concentrations of zafirlukast by approximately 45%.
- Coadministration of a single dose of zafirlukast (40 mg) with erythromycin (500 mg three times daily for 5 days) to steady-state in 11 asthmatic patients, resulted in decreased mean plasma concentrations of zafirlukast by approximately 40% due to a decrease in zafirlukast bioavailability.

INDICATIONS AND USAGE

Zafirlukast is indicated for the prophylaxis and chronic treatment of asthma in adults and children 5 years of age and older.

CONTRAINDICATIONS

Zafirlukast is contraindicated in patients who are hypersensitive to zafirlukast or any of its inactive ingredients.

WARNINGS

Zafirlukast is not indicated for use in the reversal of bronchospasm in acute asthma attacks, including status asthmaticus. Therapy with zafirlukast can be continued during acute exacerbations of asthma.

Coadministration of zafirlukast with warfarin results in a clinically significant increase in prothrombin time (PT). Patients on oral warfarin anticoagulant therapy and zafirlukast should have their prothrombin times monitored closely and anticoagulant dose adjusted accordingly (see DRUG INTERACTIONS).

PRECAUTIONS

INFORMATION FOR THE PATIENT

Zafirlukast is indicated for the chronic treatment of asthma and should be taken regularly as prescribed, even during symptom-free periods. Zafirlukast is not a bronchodilator and should not be used to treat acute episodes of asthma. Patients receiving zafirlukast should be instructed not to decrease the dose or stop taking any other antiasthma medications unless instructed by a physician. Women who are breast-feeding should be instructed not to take zafirlukast (see Nursing Mothers). Alternative antiasthma medication should be considered in such patients.

The bioavailability of zafirlukast may be decreased when taken with food. Patients should be instructed to take zafirlukast at least 1 hour before or 2 hours after meals.

Patients should be told that a rare side effect of zafirlukast is hepatic dysfunction, and to contact their physician immediately if they experience symptons of hepatic dysfunction (*e.g.*, right upper quadrant abdominal pain, nausea, fatigue, lethargy, pruritus, jaundice, flu-like symptoms, and anorexia).

HEPATIC

Rarely, elevations of one or more liver enzymes have occurred in patients receiving zafirlukast in controlled clinical trials. In clinical trials, most of these have been observed at doses 4 times higer than the recommended dose. The following hepatic events (which have occurred predominantly in females) have been reported from postmarketing adverse event surveillance of patients who have received the recommended dose of zafirlukast (40 mg/day): cases of symptomatic hepatitus (with or without hyperbilirubinemia) without other attributable cause; and rarely, hyperbilirubinemia without other elevated liver function tests. In most, but not all, postmarketing reports, the patient's symptoms abated and the liver enzymes returned to normal or near normal after stopping zafirlukast. In rare cases, patients have progressed to hepatic failure.

If liver dysfunction is suspected based upon clinical signs or symptoms (*e.g.*, right upper quadrant abdominal pain, nausea, fatigue, lethargy, pruritus, jaundice, flu-like symptoms, anorexia, and enlarged liver) zafirlukast should be discontinued. Liver function tests, in particular serum ALT, should be measured immediately and the patient managed accordingly. If liver function tests are consistent with hepatic dysfunction, zafirlukast therapy should not be resumed. Patients in whom zafirlukast was withdrawn because of hepatic dysfunction where no other attributable cause is identified should not be re-exposed to zafirlukast (see Information for the Patient and ADVERSE REACTIONS).

EOSINOPHILIC CONDITIONS

In rare cases, patients on zafirlukast therapy may present with systemic eosinophilia, sometimes presenting with clinical features of vasculitis consistent with Churg-Strauss syndrome, a condition which is often treated with systemic steroid therapy. These events usually, but not always, have been associated with the reduction of oral steroid therapy. Physicians should be alert to eosinophilia, vasculitic rash, worsening pulmonary symptoms, cardiac complications, and/or neuropathy presenting in their patients. A causal association between zafirlukast and these underlying conditions has not been established (see ADVERSE REACTIONS).

CARCINOGENESIS, MUTAGENESIS, AND IMPAIRMENT OF FERTILITY

In 2 year carcinogenicity studies, zafirlukast was administered at dietary doses of 10, 100, and 300 mg/kg to mice and 40, 400, and 2000 mg/kg to rats. Male mice given 300 mg/kg/day (approximately 30 times the maximum recommended daily oral dose in adults and children based on a mg/m^2 showed an increased incidence of hepatocellular adenomas; female mice at this dose showed a greater incidence of whole body histocytic sarcomas. Male and female rats given an oral dose of 2000 mg/kg/day (resulting in approximately 160 times the exposure to drug plus metabolites from the maximum recommended daily oral dose in adults and children based on a comparison of the plasma area-under the curve [AUC] values) of zafirlukast showed an increased incidence of urinary bladder transitional cells. Zafirlukast was not tumorigenic at oral doses up to 100 mg/kg (approximately 10 times the maximum recommended daily oral dose in adults and children on a mg/m^2 basis) in mice and at oral doses up to 400 mg/kg (resulting in approximately 140 times the exposure of drug plus metabolites from the maximum recommended daily oral dose in adults and children based on a comparison of the AUCs) in rats. The clinical significance of these findings for the long-term use of zafirlukast is unknown.

Zafirlukast showed no evidence of mutagenic potential in the reverse microbial assay, in 2 forward point mutation (CHO-HGPRT and mouse lymphoma) assays or in two assays for chromosomal aberrations (the *in vitro* human peripheral blood lymphocyte clastogenic assay and the *in vitro* rat bone marrow micronucleus assay).

No evidence of impairment of fertility and reproduction was seen in male and female rats treated with zafirlukast at oral doses up to 2000 mg/kg (approximately 410 times the maximum recommended daily oral dose in adults on a mg/m^2 basis).

PREGNANCY CATEGORY B

No teratogenicity was observed at oral doses up to 1600 mg/kg/day in mice (approximately 160 times the maximum recommended human oral daily dose on a mg/m^2 basis), 2000 mg/kg/day in rats (approximately 410 times the maximum recommended daily oral dose in adults on a mg/m^2 basis) and 2000 mg/kg/day in cynomolgus monkeys (approximately 20 times the exposure to drug plus metabolites compared to that from the maximum recommended daily oral dose in adults based on comparison of the AUCs values). At an oral dose of 2000 mg/kg/day in rats, maternal toxicity and deaths were seen with increased incidence of early fetal resorption. Spontaneous abortions occurred in cynomolgus monkeys at the maternally toxic dose of 2000 mg/kg/day. There are no adequate and well-controlled trials in pregnant women. Because animal reproduction studies are not always predictive of human response, zafirlukast should be used during pregnancy only if clearly needed.

NURSING MOTHERS

Zafirlukast is excreted in breast milk. Following repeated 40 mg twice-a-day dosing in healthy women, average steady-state concentrations of zafirlukast in breast milk were 50 ng/ml compared to 255 ng/ml in plasma. Because of the potential for tumorigenicity shown for zafirlukast in mouse and rat studies and the enhanced sensitivity of neonatal rats and dogs to the adverse effects of zafirlukast, zafirlukast should not be administered to mothers who are breast-feeding.

PEDIATRIC USE

The safety of zafirlukast at doses of 10 mg bid has been demonstrated in 205 pediatric patients 5-11 years of age in placebo-controlled trials lasting up to 6 weeks and with 179 patients in this age range participating in 52 weeks of treatment in an open label extension.

The effectiveness of zafirlukast for the prophylaxis and chronic treatment of asthma in pediatric patients 5-11 years of age is based on an extrapolation of the demonstrated efficacy of zafirlukast in adults with asthma and the likelihood that the disease course, and pathophysiology and the drug's effect are substantially similar between the two populations. The recommended dose for the patients 5-11 years of age is based upon a cross-study comparison of the pharmacokinetics of zafirlukast in adults and pediatric subjects, and on the safety profile of zafirlukast in both adult and pediatric patients at doses equal to or higher than the recommended dose.

The safety and effectiveness of zafirlukast for pediatric patients less than 5 years of age has not been established.

GERIATRIC USE

Based on cross study comparison, the clearance of zafirlukast is reduced in patients 65 years of age and older such that C_{max} and AUC are approximately 2- to 3-fold greater than those of younger patients (see DOSAGE AND ADMINISTRATION and CLINICAL PHARMACOLOGY).

A total of 8094 patients were exposed to zafirlukast in North American and European short-term placebo-controlled clinical trials. Of these, 243 patients were elderly (age 65 years and older). No overall difference in adverse events was seen in the elderly patients, except for an increase in the frequency of infection among zafirlukast-treated elderly patients compared to placebo treated elderly patients (7.0% vs 2.9%). The infections were not severe, occurred mostly in the lower respiratory tract, and did not necessitate withdrawal of therapy.

An open-label, uncontrolled, 4 week trial of 3759 asthma patients compared the safety and efficacy of zafirlukast 20 mg given twice daily in 3 patient age groups, adolescents (12-17 years), adults (18-65 years), and elderly (greater than 65 years). A higher percentage of elderly patients (n=384) reported adverse events when compared to adults and adolescents. These elderly patients showed less improvement in efficacy measures. In the elderly patients, adverse events occurring in greater than 1% of the population included headache (4.7%), diarrhea and nausea (1.8%), and pharyngitis (1.3%). The elderly reported the lowest percentage of infections of all 3 age groups in this study.

DRUG INTERACTIONS

In a drug interaction study in 16 healthy male volunteers, coadministration of multiple doses of zafirlukast (160 mg/day) to steady-state with a single 25 mg dose of warfarin resulted in a significant increase in the mean AUC (+63%) and half-life (+36%) of S-warfarin. The mean prothrombin time (PT) increased by approximately 35%. This interaction is probably due to an inhibition by zafirlukast of the cytochrome P450 2C9 isoenzyme system. Patients on oral warfarin anticoagulant therapy and zafirlukast should have their prothrombin times monitored closely and anticoagulant dose adjusted accordingly (see WARNINGS). No formal drug-drug interaction studies with zafirlukast and other drugs known to be metabolized by the cytochrome P450 2C9 isoenzyme (*e.g.*, tolbutamide, phenytoin, carbamazepine) have been conducted; however, care should be exercised when zafirlukast is coadministered with these drugs.

In a drug interaction study in 11 asthmatic patients, coadministration of a single dose of zafirlukast (40 mg) with erythromycin (500 mg three times daily for 5 days) to steady-state resulted in decreased mean plasma levels of zafirlukast by approximately 40% due to a decrease in zafirlukast bioavailability.

Coadministration of zafirlukast (20 mg/day) or placebo at steady-state with a single dose of sustained release theophylline preparation (16 mg/kg) in 16 healthy boys and girls (6-11 years of age) resulted in no significant differences in the pharmacokinetic parameters of theophylline.

Coadministration of zafirlukast (80 mg/day) at steady-state with a single dose of a liquid theophylline preparation (6 mg/kg) in 13 asthmatic patients, 18-44 years of age, resulted in decreased mean plasma levels of zafirlukast by approximately 30%, but no effect on plasma theophylline levels was observed.

Rare cases of patients experiencing increased theophylline levels with or without clinical signs or symptoms of theophylline toxicity after the addition of zafirlukast to an existing theophylline regimen have been reported. The mechanism of the interaction between zafirlukast and theophylline in these patients is unknown (see ADVERSE REACTIONS).

Coadministration of zafirlukast (40 mg/day) with aspirin (650 mg four times daily) resulted in mean increased plasma levels of zafirlukast by approximately 45%.

In a single-blind, parallel-group, 3 week study in 39 healthy female subjects taking oral contraceptives, 40 mg bid of zafirlukast had no significant effect on ethinyl estradiol plasma concentrations or contraceptive efficacy.

No formal drug-drug interaction studies between zafirlukast and marketed drugs known to be metabolized by the P450 3A4 (CYP 3A4) isoenzyme (*e.g.*, dihydropyridine calcium-channel blockers, cyclosporin, cisapride) have been conducted. As zafirlukast is known to be an inhibitor of CYP 3A4 *in vitro*, it is reasonable to employ appropriate clinical monitoring when these drugs are coadministered with zafirlukast.

ADVERSE REACTIONS

ADULTS AND CHILDREN 12 YEARS OF AGE AND OLDER

The safety database for zafirlukast consists of more than 4000 healthy volunteers and patients who received zafirlukast, of which 1723 were asthmatics enrolled in trials of 13 weeks duration or longer. A total of 671 patients received zafirlukast for 1 year or longer. The majority of the patients were 18 years of age or older; however, 222 patients between the age of 12 and 18 years received zafirlukast.

A comparison of adverse events reported by ≥1% of zafirlukast-treated patients, and at rates numerically greater than in placebo-treated patients, is shown for all trials in TABLE 4.

TABLE 4

Adverse Event	Zafirlukast n=4058	Placebo n=2032
Headache	12.9%	11.7%
Infection	3.5%	3.4%
Nausea	3.1%	2.0%
Diarrhea	2.8%	2.1%
Pain (generalized)	1.9%	1.7%
Asthenia	1.8%	1.6%
Abdominal pain	1.8%	1.1%
Accidental injury	1.6%	1.5%
Dizziness	1.6%	1.5%
Myalgia	1.6%	1.5%
Fever	1.6%	1.1%
Back pain	1.5%	1.2%
Vomiting	1.5%	1.1%
SGPT elevation	1.5%	1.1%
Dyspepsia	1.3%	1.2%

The frequency of less common adverse events was comparable between zafirlukast and placebo.

Rarely, elevations of one or more liver enzymes have occurred in patients receiving zafirlukast in controlled clinical trials. In clinical trials, most of these have been observed at doses 4 times higher than the recommended dose. The following hepatic events (which have occurred predominantly in females) have been reported from postmarketing adverse event surveillance of patients who have received the recommended dose of zafirlukast (40 mg/day): cases of symptomatic hepatitis (with or without hyperbilirubinemia) without other attributable cause; and rarely, hyperbilirubinemia without other elevated liver function tests. In most, but not all, postmarketing reports, the patient's symptoms abated and the liver enzymes returned to normal or near normal after stopping zafirlukast. In rare cases, patients have progressed to hepatic failure.

In clinical trials, an increased proportion of zafirlukast patients over the age of 55 years reported infections as compared to placebo-treated patients. A similar finding was not observed in other age groups studied. These infections were mostly mild or moderate in intensity and predominantly affected the respiratory tract. Infections occurred equally in both sexes, were dose-proportional to total milligrams of zafirlukast exposure, and were associated with coadministration of inhaled corticosteroids. The clinical significance of this finding is unknown.

In rare cases, patients on zafirlukast therapy may present with systemic eosinophilia, sometimes presenting with clinical features of vasculitis consistent with Churg-Strauss syndrome, a condition which is often treated with systemic steroid therapy. These events usually, but not always, have been associated with the reduction of oral steroid therapy. Physicians should be alert to eosinophilia, vasculitic rash, worsening pulmonary symptoms, cardiac complications, and/or neuropathy presenting in their patients. A causal association between zafirlukast and these underlying conditions has not been established. (See PRECAUTIONS, Eosinophilic Conditions.)

Hypersensitivity reactions, including urticaria, angioedema, and rashes, with or without blistering, have been reported in association with zafirlukast therapy. Additionally, there have been reports of patients experiencing agranulocytosis, bleeding, bruising, or edema, arthralgia and myalgia in association with zafirlukast therapy.

Rare cases of patients experiencing increased theophylline levels with or without clinical signs or symptoms of theophylline toxicity after the addition of zafirlukast to an existing theophylline regimen have been reported. The mechanism of the interaction between zafirlukast and theophylline in these patients is unknown and not predicted by available *in vitro* metabolism data and the results of two clinical drug interaction studies (see CLINICAL PHARMACOLOGY and DRUG INTERACTIONS).

PEDIATRIC PATIENTS 5-11 YEARS OF AGE

Zafirlukast has been evaluated for safety in 788 pediatric patients 5-11 years of age. Cumulatively, 313 pediatric patients were treated with zafirlukast 10 mg bid or higher for at least 6 months, and 113 of them were treated for 1 year or longer in clinical trials. The safety profile of zafirlukast 10 mg bid versus placebo in the 4 and 6 week double-blind trials was generally similar to that observed in the adult clinical trials with zafirlukast 20 mg bid.

In pediatric patients receiving zafirlukast in multidose clinical trials, the following events occurred with a frequency of ≥2% and more frequently than in pediatric patients who received placebo, regardless of causality assessment: Headache (4.5 vs 4.2%) and abdominal pain (2.8 vs 2.3%).

DOSAGE AND ADMINISTRATION

Because food can reduce the bioavailability of zafirlukast, zafirlukast should be taken at least 1 hour before or 2 hours after meals.

Adults and Children 12 Years of Age and Older: The recommended dose of zafirlukast in adults and children 12 years and older is 20 mg bid.

Pediatric Patients 5-11 Years of Age: The recommended dose of zafirlukast in children 5-11 years of age is 10 mg bid.

Elderly Patients: Based on cross-study comparisons, the clearance of zafirlukast is reduced in elderly patients (65 years of age and older), such that C_{max} and AUC are approximately twice those of younger adults. In clinical trials, a dose of 20 mg bid was not associated with an increase in the overall incidence of adverse events or withdrawals because of adverse events in elderly patients.

Patients With Hepatic Impairment: The clearance of zafirlukast is reduced in patients with stable alcoholic cirrhosis such that the C_{max} and AUC are approximately 50-60% greater than those of normal adults. Zafirlukast has not been evaluated in patients with hepatitis or in long-term studies of patients with cirrhosis.

Patients With Renal Impairment: Dosage adjustment is not required for patients with renal impairment.

HOW SUPPLIED

Accolate 10 mg Tablets: White, unflavored, round, biconvex, film-coated, mini-tablets identified with "ZENECA" debossed on one side and "ACCOLATE 10" debossed on the other side.

Accolate 20 mg Tablets: White, round, biconvex, coated tablets identified with "ZENECA" debossed on one side and "ACCOLATE 20" debossed on the other side.

Storage: Store at controlled room temperature, 20-25°C (68-77°F). Protect from light and moisture. Dispense in the original air-tight container.

PRODUCT LISTING - EQUIVALENTS NOT AVAILABLE

Tablet - Oral - 10 mg

60's	$75.59	ACCOLATE, Astra-Zeneca Pharmaceuticals	00310-0401-60
100's	$112.58	ACCOLATE, Astra-Zeneca Pharmaceuticals	00310-0401-39

Tablet - Oral - 20 mg

60's	$75.59	ACCOLATE, Astra-Zeneca Pharmaceuticals	00310-0402-60
100's	$125.98	ACCOLATE, Astra-Zeneca Pharmaceuticals	00310-0402-39

Zalcitabine (003076)

For related information, see the comparative table section in Appendix A.

Categories: Infection, human immunodeficiency virus; Pregnancy Category C; FDA Approved 1992 Jun; Orphan Drugs
Drug Classes: Antivirals; Nucleoside reverse transcriptase inhibitors
Brand Names: D.D.C.; ddC; Dideoxycytidine; **HIVID**
Cost of Therapy: $206.93 (HIV; Hivid; 0.75 mg; 3 tablets/day; 30 day supply)

WARNING

THE USE OF ZALCITABINE HAS BEEN ASSOCIATED WITH SIGNIFICANT CLINICAL ADVERSE REACTIONS, SOME OF WHICH ARE POTENTIALLY FATAL. ZALCITABINE CAN CAUSE SEVERE PERIPHERAL NEUROPATHY AND BECAUSE OF THIS SHOULD BE USED WITH EXTREME CAUTION IN PATIENTS WITH PREEXISTING NEUROPATHY. ZALCITABINE MAY ALSO RARELY CAUSE PANCREATITIS AND PATIENTS WHO DEVELOP ANY SYMPTOMS SUGGESTIVE OF PANCREATITIS WHILE USING ZALCITABINE SHOULD HAVE THERAPY SUSPENDED IMMEDIATELY UNTIL THIS DIAGNOSIS IS EXCLUDED.

LACTIC ACIDOSIS AND SEVERE HEPATOMEGALY WITH STEATOSIS, INCLUDING FATAL CASES, HAVE BEEN REPORTED WITH THE USE OF ANTIRETROVIRAL NUCLEOSIDE ANALOGUES ALONE OR IN COMBINATION, INCLUDING ZALCITABINE (SEE WARNINGS).

IN ADDITION, RARE CASES OF HEPATIC FAILURE AND DEATH CONSIDERED POSSIBLY RELATED TO UNDERLYING HEPATITIS B AND ZALCITABINE HAVE BEEN REPORTED (SEE WARNINGS AND PRECAUTIONS).

DESCRIPTION

Hivid is the Hoffmann-La Roche brand of zalcitabine [formerly called 2′,3′-dideoxycytidine (ddC)], a synthetic pyrimidine nucleoside analogue active against the human immunodeficiency virus (HIV). Hivid is available as film-coated tablets for oral administration in strengths of 0.375 and 0.750 mg. Each tablet also contains the inactive ingredients lactose, microcrystalline cellulose, croscarmellose sodium, magnesium stearate, hydroxypropyl methylcellulose, polyethylene glycol, and polysorbate 80 along with the following colorant system: 0.375 mg tablet — synthetic brown, black, red and yellow iron oxides, and titanium dioxide; 0.750 mg tablet — synthetic black iron oxide and titanium dioxide. The chemical name for zalcitabine is 4-amino-1-beta-D-2′,3′-dideoxyribofuranosyl-2-(1H)-pyrimidone or 2′,3′-dideoxycytidine with the molecular formula $C_9H_{13}N_3O_3$ and a molecular weight of 211.22.

Zalcitabine is a white to off-white crystalline powder with an aqueous solubility of 76.4 mg/ml at 25°C.

CLINICAL PHARMACOLOGY

MICROBIOLOGY

Mechanism of Action

Zalcitabine is a synthetic nucleoside analogue of the naturally occurring nucleoside deoxycytidine, in which the 3′-hydroxyl group is replaced by hydrogen. Within cells, zalcitabine is converted to the active metabolite, dideoxycytidine 5′-triphosphate (ddCTP), by the sequential action of cellular enzymes. Dideoxycytidine 5′-triphosphate inhibits the activity of the HIV-reverse transcriptase both by competing for utilization of the natural substrate, deoxycytidine 5′-triphosphate (dCTP), and by its incorporation into viral DNA. The lack of a 3′-OH group in the incorporated nucleoside analogue prevents the formation of the 5′ to 3′ phosphodiester linkage essential for DNA chain elongation and, therefore, the viral DNA growth is terminated. The active metabolite, ddCTP, is also an inhibitor of cellular DNA polymerase-beta and mitochondrial DNA polymerase-gamma and has been reported to be incorporated into the DNA of cells in culture.

In Vitro HIV Susceptibility

The *in vitro* anti-HIV activity of zalcitabine was assessed by infecting cell lines of lymphoblastic and monocytic origin and peripheral blood lymphocytes with laboratory and clinical isolates of HIV. The IC_{50} and IC_{95} values (50% and 95% inhibitory concentration) were in the range of 30-500 nM and 100-1000 nM, respectively (1 nM = 0.21 ng/ml). Zalcitabine showed antiviral activity in all acute infections; however, activity was substantially less in chronically infected cells. In drug combination studies with zidovudine (ZDV) or saquinavir, zalcitabine showed additive to synergistic activity in cell culture. The relationship between the *in vitro* susceptibility of HIV to reverse-transcriptase inhibitors and the inhibition of HIV replication in humans has not been established.

Drug Resistance

HIV isolates with a reduction in sensitivity to zalcitabine (ddC) have been isolated from a small number of patients treated with zalcitabine by 1 year of therapy. Genetic analysis of these isolates showed point mutations (Lys 65 Arg or Asn, Thr 69 Asp, Leu 74 Val, Val 75 Thr or Ala, Met 184 Val or Tyr 215 Cys) in the pol gene that encodes for the reverse transcriptase. Combination therapy with zalcitabine and ZDV does not appear to prevent the emergence of zidovudine-resistant isolates.

Cross-Resistance

The potential for cross-resistance between HIV-reverse transcriptase inhibitors and HIV-protease inhibitors is low because of the different enzyme targets involved. The point mutation at position 69 appears to be specific to ddC in its selection and effect. Additionally, the point mutations at positions 65, 74, 75, and 184 are associated with resistance to didanosine (ddI), that at position 75 with resistance to stavudine (d4T), and those at positions 65 (Lys to Arg), and 184 (Met to Val) with resistance to lamivudine (3TC). HIV isolates with multidrug resistance to ZDV, ddI, ddC, d4T, and 3TC were recovered from a small number of patients treated for 1 year with the combination of ZDV, ddI or ddC. The pattern of resistance mutations in the combination therapy was different (Ala 62 Val, Val 75 Ile, Phe 77 Leu, Phe 116 Tyr and Gln 151 Met) from monotherapy with mutation 151 being most significant for multidrug resistance.

PHARMACOKINETICS

The pharmacokinetics of zalcitabine has been evaluated in studies in HIV-infected patients following 0.01 mg/kg, 0.03 mg/kg, and 1.5 mg oral doses, and a 1.5 mg intravenous dose administered as a 1 hour infusion.

Absorption and Bioavailability in Adults

Following oral administration to HIV-infected patients, the mean absolute bioavailability of zalcitabine was >80% (30% CV, range 23-124%, n=19). The absorption rate of a 1.5 mg oral dose of zalcitabine (n=20) was reduced when administered with food. This resulted in a 39% decrease in mean maximum plasma concentrations (C_{max}) from 25.2 ng/ml (35% CV, range 11.6-37.5 ng/ml) to 15.5 ng/ml (24% CV, range 9.1-23.7 ng/ml), and a 2-fold increase in time to achieve maximum plasma concentrations from a mean of 0.8 hours under fasting conditions to 1.6 hours when the drug was given with food. The extent of absorption (as reflected by AUC) was decreased by 14%, from 72 ng·h/ml (28% CV, range 43-119 ng·h/ml) to 62 ng·h/ml (23% CV, range 42-91 ng·h/ml). The clinical relevance of these decreases is unknown. Absorption of zalcitabine does not appear to be reduced in patients with diarrhea not caused by an identified pathogen.

Distribution in Adults

The steady-state volume of distribution following intravenous administration of a 1.5 mg dose of zalcitabine averaged 0.534 (±0.127) L/kg (24% CV, range 0.304-0.734 L/kg, n=20). Cerebrospinal fluid obtained from 9 patients at 2 to 3.5 hours following 0.06 or 0.09 mg/kg intravenous infusion showed measurable concentrations of zalcitabine. The CSF plasma concentration ratio ranged from 9-37% (mean 20%), demonstrating penetration of the drug through the blood-brain barrier. The clinical relevance of these ratios has not been evaluated.

Metabolism and Elimination in Adults

Zalcitabine is phosphorylated intracellularly to zalcitabine triphosphate, the active substrate for HIV-reverse transcriptase. Concentrations of zalcitabine triphosphate are too low for quantitation following administration of therapeutic doses to humans.

Zalcitabine does not undergo a significant degree of metabolism by the liver. The primary metabolite of zalcitabine that has been identified is dideoxyuridine (ddU), which accounts for less than 15% of an oral dose in both urine and feces (n=4). Approximately 10% of an orally administered radiolabeled dose of zalcitabine appears in the feces (n=10), comprised primarily of unchanged drug and ddU. Renal excretion of unchanged drug appears to be the primary route of elimination, accounting for approximately 80% of an intravenous dose and 60% of an orally administered dose within 24 hours after dosing (n=19). The mean elimination half-life is 2 hours and generally ranges from 1-3 hours in individual patients. Total clearance following an intravenous dose averaged 285 ml/min (29% CV, range 165-447 ml/min, n=20). Renal clearance averaged approximately 235 ml/min or about 80% of total clearance (30% CV, range 129-348 ml/min, n=20). Renal clearance exceeds glomerular filtration rate suggesting renal tubular secretion contributes to the elimination of zalcitabine by the kidneys.

In patients with impaired kidney function, prolonged elimination of zalcitabine may be expected. Preliminary results from 7 patients with renal impairment (estimated creatinine clearance <55 ml/min) indicate that the half-life was prolonged (up to 8.5 hours) in these patients compared to those with normal renal function. Maximum plasma concentrations were higher in some patients after a single dose (see PRECAUTIONS).

In patients with normal renal function, the pharmacokinetics of zalcitabine was not altered during 3 times daily multiple dosing (n=9). Accumulation of drug in plasma during this regimen was negligible. The drug was <4% bound to plasma proteins, indicating that drug interactions involving binding-site displacement are unlikely (see DRUG INTERACTIONS).

Drug Interactions

Zidovudine: There was no significant pharmacokinetic interaction between zidovudine and zalcitabine when single doses of zalcitabine (1.5 mg) and zidovudine (200 mg) were coadministered to 12 HIV-positive patients.

Probenecid: Following administration of a single oral 1.5 mg dose of zalcitabine alone during probenecid treatment (500 mg at 8 and 2 hours before and 4 hours after zalcitabine dosing) to 12 HIV-positive patients, mean renal clearance decreased from 310 ml/min (28% CV) to 180 ml/min (22% CV) and AUC increased from 59 ng·h/ml (27% CV) to 91 ng·h/ml (22% CV), indicating an increase in exposure of approximately 50% to zalcitabine. Mean half-life of zalcitabine increased from 1.7 to 2.5 hours (see PRECAUTIONS).

Cimetidine: Administration of a single dose of 1.5 mg zalcitabine with a single dose of 800 mg cimetidine to 12 HIV-positive patients resulted in a decrease in renal clearance from 224 ml/min (27% CV) to 171 ml/min (39% CV) and an increase in AUC from 75 ng·h/ml (29% CV) to 102 ng·h/ml (35% CV) (see PRECAUTIONS) indicating an increase in exposure of approximately 36% to zalcitabine.

Maalox: Concomitant administration of Maalox TC (30 ml) with single dose of 1.5 mg zalcitabine to 12 HIV-positive patients resulted in a decrease in mean C_{max} from 25.2 ng/ml (28% CV) to 18.4 ng/ml (34% CV) and AUC from 75 ng·h/ml (29% CV, n=10) to 58 ng·h/ml (36% CV, n=10) indicating a decrease in bioavailability of approximately 25% to zalcitabine (see PRECAUTIONS).

Metoclopramide: Administration of a single dose of 1.5 mg zalcitabine with 20 mg metoclopramide (10 mg 1 hour before and 10 mg 4 hours after zalcitabine dose) to 12 HIV-positive patients resulted in a decrease in AUC from 69 ng·h/ml (16% CV) to 62 ng·h/ml (21% CV) indicating a decrease in bioavailability of approximately 10% (see PRECAUTIONS).

Loperamide: Administration of a single dose of 1.5 mg zalcitabine during loperamide treatment (4 mg 16 hours before zalcitabine, 2 mg at 10 hours and 4 hours before zalcitabine, and 2 mg 2 hours after the zalcitabine dose) to 12 HIV-positive patients with diarrhea resulted in no significant pharmacokinetic interaction between zalcitabine and loperamide.

Pharmacokinetics in Pediatric Patients

For pharmacokinetic properties in pediatric patients, see PRECAUTIONS, Pediatric Use. Limited pharmacokinetic data have been reported for 5 HIV-positive pediatric patients using doses of 0.03 and 0.04 mg/kg zalcitabine administered orally every 6 hours.[1] The mean bioavailability of zalcitabine in these pediatric patients was 54% and mean apparent systemic clearance was 150 ml/min/m^2. Due to the small number of subjects and different analytical techniques, it is difficult to make comparisons between pediatric and adult data.

INDICATIONS AND USAGE

Zalcitabine is indicated in combination with antiretroviral agents for the treatment of HIV infection. This indication is based on study results showing a reduction in the rate of disease progression (AIDS-defining events or death) in patients with limited prior antiretroviral therapy who were treated with the combination of zalcitabine and zidovudine. This indication is also based on a study showing a reduction in both mortality and AIDS-defining clinical events for patients who received saquinavir mesylate in combination with zalcitabine compared to patients who received either zalcitabine or saquinavir mesylate alone.

CONTRAINDICATIONS

Zalcitabine is contraindicated in patients with clinically significant hypersensitivity to zalcitabine or to any of the excipients contained in the tablets.

WARNINGS

SIGNIFICANT CLINICAL ADVERSE REACTIONS, SOME OF WHICH ARE POTENTIALLY FATAL, HAVE BEEN REPORTED WITH ZALCITABINE. PATIENTS WITH DECREASED CD4 CELL COUNTS APPEAR TO HAVE AN INCREASED INCIDENCE OF ADVERSE EVENTS.

PERIPHERAL NEUROPATHY

THE MAJOR CLINICAL TOXICITY OF ZALCITABINE IS PERIPHERAL NEUROPATHY, WHICH MAY OCCUR IN UP TO 1/3 OF PATIENTS WITH ADVANCED DISEASE TREATED WITH ZALCITABINE. The incidence in patients with less-advanced disease is lower.

Zalcitabine-related peripheral neuropathy is a sensorimotor neuropathy characterized initially by numbness and burning dysesthesia involving the distal extremities. These symptoms may be followed by sharp shooting pains or severe continuous burning pain if the drug is not withdrawn. The neuropathy may progress to severe pain requiring narcotic analgesics and is potentially irreversible. In some patients, symptoms of neuropathy may initially progress despite discontinuation of zalcitabine. With prompt discontinuation of zalcitabine, the neuropathy is usually slowly reversible.

There are no data regarding the use of zalcitabine in patients with preexisting peripheral neuropathy since these patients were excluded from clinical trials; therefore, zalcitabine should be used with extreme caution in these patients. Individuals with moderate or severe peripheral neuropathy, as evidenced by symptoms accompanied by objective findings, are advised to avoid zalcitabine.

Zalcitabine should be used with caution in patients with a risk of developing peripheral neuropathy: patients with low CD4 cell counts (CD4 <50 cells/mm^3), diabetes, weight loss and/or patients receiving zalcitabine concomitantly with drugs that have the potential to cause peripheral neuropathy (see DRUG INTERACTIONS). Careful monitoring is strongly recommended for these individuals.

Zalcitabine should be stopped promptly if signs or symptoms of peripheral neuropathy occurs, such as when moderate discomfort from numbness, tingling, burning or pain of the extremities progresses, or any related symptoms occur that are accompanied by an objective finding (see DOSAGE AND ADMINISTRATION).

PANCREATITIS

PANCREATITIS, WHICH HAS BEEN FATAL IN SOME CASES, HAS BEEN OBSERVED WITH THE ADMINISTRATION OF ZALCITABINE. Pancreatitis is an uncommon complication of zalcitabine occurring in up to 1.1% of patients.

Patients with a history of pancreatitis or known risk factors for the development of pancreatitis should be followed more closely while on zalcitabine therapy. Of 528 zalcitabine-treated patients enrolled in an expanded-access safety study (N3544), who had a history of prior pancreatitis or increased amylase, 28 (5.3%) developed pancreatitis and an additional 23 (4.4%) developed asymptomatic elevated serum amylase.

Treatment with zalcitabine should be stopped immediately if clinical signs or symptoms (nausea, vomiting, abdominal pain) or if abnormalities in laboratory values (hyperamylasemia associated with dysglycemia, rising triglyceride level, decreasing serum calcium) suggestive of pancreatitis should occur. If clinical pancreatitis develops during zalcitabine administration, it is recommended that zalcitabine be permanently discontinued. Treatment with zalcitabine should also be interrupted if treatment with another drug known to cause pancreatitis (*e.g.,* intravenous pentamidine) is required (see DRUG INTERACTIONS).

LACTIC ACIDOSIS/SEVERE HEPATOMEGALY WITH STEATOSIS AND HEPATIC TOXICITY

Lactic acidosis and severe hepatomegaly with steatosis, including fatal cases, have been reported with the use of nucleoside analogues alone or in combination, including zalcitabine and other antiretrovirals.[5,6] A majority of these cases have been in women. Obesity and prolonged nucleoside exposure may be risk factors. Particular caution should be exercised when administering zalcitabine to any patient with known risk factors for liver disease; however, cases have also been reported in patients with no known risk factors. Treatment with zalcitabine should be suspended in any patient who develops clinical or laboratory findings suggestive of lactic acidosis or pronounced hepatotoxicity (which may include hepatomegaly and steatosis even in the absence of marked transaminase elevations).

IN ADDITION, RARE CASES OF HEPATIC FAILURE AND DEATH CONSIDERED POSSIBLY RELATED TO UNDERLYING HEPATITIS B AND ZALCITABINE HAVE BEEN REPORTED. Treatment with zalcitabine in patients with preexisting liver disease, liver enzyme abnormalities, a history of ethanol abuse or hepatitis should be approached with caution. Treatment with zalcitabine should be suspended in any patient who develops clinical or laboratory findings suggestive of pronounced hepatotoxicity. In clinical trials, drug interruption was recommended if liver function tests exceeded >5 times the upper limit of normal.

OTHER SERIOUS TOXICITIES

Oral Ulcers: Severe oral ulcers occurred in up to 3% of patients receiving zalcitabine in CPCRA 002 and ACTG 175; less severe oral ulcerations have occurred at higher frequencies in other clinical trials.

Esophageal Ulcers: Infrequent cases of esophageal ulcers have also been attributed to zalcitabine therapy. Interruption of zalcitabine should be considered in patients who develop esophageal ulcers that do not respond to specific treatment for opportunistic pathogens in order to assess a possible relationship to zalcitabine.

Cardiomyopathy/Congestive Heart Failure: Cardiomyopathy and congestive heart failure in patients with AIDS have been associated with the use of nucleoside analogues. Infrequent cases have been reported in patients receiving zalcitabine. Treatment with zalcitabine in patients with baseline cardiomyopathy or history of congestive heart failure should be approached with caution.

Anaphylactoid Reaction: An anaphylactoid reaction was reported in a patient receiving both zalcitabine and zidovudine. In addition, there have been several reports of hypersensitivity reactions (including anaphylactic reaction or urticaria without other signs of anaphylaxis).

PRECAUTIONS

GENERAL

Renal Impairment

Patients with renal impairment (estimated creatinine clearance <55 ml/min) may be at a greater risk of toxicity from zalcitabine due to decreased drug clearance. Dosage adjustment is recommended in these patients (see DOSAGE AND ADMINISTRATION).

Lymphoma

High doses of zalcitabine, administered for 3 months to $B_6C_3F_1$ mice (resulting in plasma concentrations over 1000 times those seen in patients taking the recommended doses of zalcitabine) induced an increased incidence of thymic lymphoma.[7] Although the pathogenesis of the effect is uncertain, a predisposition to chemically induced thymic lymphoma and high rates of spontaneous lymphoreticular neoplasms have previously been noted in this strain of mice.[8]

The incidence of lymphomas was reviewed in 13 comparative studies conducted by Roche, the NIAID and the NCI, as well as 7 Roche expanded-access studies that included zalcitabine. In one study, ACTG 155, a statistically significant increased rate of lymphomas was seen in patients receiving zalcitabine or combination zalcitabine and zidovudine compared to zidovudine alone (rates of 0, 1.3, and 2.3 per 100 person years for zidovudine, zalcitabine, and combination zalcitabine and zidovudine, respectively; log rank p-value = 0.01, pooling zalcitabine, and combination zalcitabine and zidovudine vs zidovudine, p-value = 0.003). Based on review of the literature, the incidence of lymphomas in HIV-infected patients with advanced disease on zidovudine monotherapy would be expected to be approximately 1-2 per 100 person years of follow-up.

None of the other comparative studies evaluated showed a statistically significant difference in rates of lymphomas in patients receiving zalcitabine. In a large, controlled clinical trial (ACTG 175) zalcitabine in combination with zidovudine was not associated with an increase in the incidence of lymphoma over that seen with zidovudine monotherapy (6 of 615 and 9 of 619, respectively).

Lymphoma has been identified as a consequence of HIV infection. This most likely represents a consequence of prolonged immunosuppression; however, an association between the occurrence of lymphoma and antiviral therapy can not be excluded.

Fat Redistribution

Redistribution/accumulation of body fat including central obesity, dorsocervical fat enlargement (buffalo hump), peripheral wasting, facial wasting, breast enlargement, and "cushingoid appearance" have been observed in patients receiving antiretroviral therapy. The mechanism and long-term consequences of these events are currently unknown. A causal relationship has not been established.

Patients receiving zalcitabine or any other antiretroviral therapy may continue to develop opportunistic infections and other complications of HIV infections, and therefore should remain under close clinical observation by physicians experienced in the treatment of patients with associated HIV diseases.

The duration of clinical benefit from antiretroviral therapy may be limited. Alterations in antiretroviral therapy should be considered in cases of disease progression, either clinical or as demonstrated by viral rebound (increase in HIV RNA after initial decline).

INFORMATION FOR THE PATIENT

Patients should be informed that zalcitabine is not a cure for HIV infection and that they may continue to acquire illnesses associated with advanced HIV infection, including opportunistic infections.

Patients should be told that there is currently no data demonstrating that zalcitabine therapy can reduce the risk of transmitting HIV to others through sexual contact or blood contamination.

Patients should be advised to take zalcitabine every day as prescribed. Patients should not alter the dose or discontinue therapy without consulting with their physician. If a dose is missed, patients should take the dose as soon as possible and then return to their normal schedule. However, if a dose is skipped, the patient should not double the next dose.

Patients should be instructed that the major toxicity of zalcitabine is peripheral neuropathy. Pancreatitis and hepatic toxicity are other serious potentially life-threatening toxicities that have been reported in patients treated with zalcitabine. Patients should be advised of the early symptoms of these conditions and instructed to promptly report them to their physician. Since the development of peripheral neuropathy appears to be dose-related to zalcitabine, patients should be advised to follow their physicians' instructions regarding the prescribed dose.

Patients should be informed that redistribution or accumulation of body fat may occur in patients receiving antiretroviral therapy and that the cause and long-term health effects of these conditions are not known at this time.

LABORATORY TESTS

Complete blood counts and clinical chemistry tests should be performed prior to initiating zalcitabine therapy and at appropriate intervals thereafter. Baseline testing of serum amylase and triglyceride levels should be performed in individuals with a prior history of pancreatitis, increased amylase, those on parenteral nutrition or with a history of ethanol abuse.

CARCINOGENESIS, MUTAGENESIS, AND IMPAIRMENT OF FERTILITY

Carcinogenesis

Zalcitabine was administered orally by dietary admixture to CRL:CD-1 (ICR) Br mice at dosages of 3, 83, or 250 mg/kg/day for 2 years. Plasma exposures (as measured by AUC) at these doses were 6- to 704-fold greater than the systemic exposure in humans with the therapeutic dose. Zalcitabine was administered orally by dietary admixture to CDF (F-344)/CrlBR/CdBR rats at dosages of 3, 28, 83, or 250 mg/kg/day. At the highest dose tested, the systemic exposure to zalcitabine was 833 times the systemic exposure in humans with the therapeutic dose.

A significant increase in thymic lymphoma in all zalcitabine dose groups and Harderian gland (a gland of the eye of rodents) adenoma in the two highest dose groups was observed in female CD1 mice after 2 years of dosing. No increase in tumor incidence was observed in rats or male mice treated with zalcitabine. In an independent study, administration of zalcitabine to $B_6C_3F_1$ mice at a dose of 1000 mg/kg/day for 3 months induced an increased incidence of thymic lymphoma. A high rate of spontaneous lymphoreticular neoplasms have previously been noted in this strain of mice.

Mutagenesis

Zalcitabine was positive in a cell transformation assay and induced chromosomal aberrations *in vitro* in human peripheral blood lymphocytes. Oral doses of zalcitabine at 2500 and 4500 mg/kg were clastogenic in the mouse micronucleus assay. Zalcitabine showed no evidence of mutagenicity in Ames tests, Chinese hamster lung cell assays and the mouse lymphoma assay. An unscheduled DNA synthesis assay in rat hepatocytes showed that zalcitabine had no effect on DNA repair.

Impairment of Fertility

Fertility and reproductive performance were assessed in rats at plasma concentrations up to 2142 times those achieved with the maximum recommended human dose (MRHD) based on AUC measurements. No adverse effects on rate of conception or general reproductive performance were observed. The highest dose was associated with embryolethality and evidence of teratogenicity. The next lower dose studied (plasma concentrations equivalent to 485 times the MRHD) was associated with a lower frequency of embryotoxicity but no teratogenicity. The fertility of F_1 males was significantly reduced at a calculated dose of 2142 (but not 485) times the MRHD (based on AUC measurements) in a teratology study in which rat mothers were dosed on gestation days 7-15. No adverse effects were observed on the fertility of parents or F_1 generation in the study of fertility and general reproductive performance or in the perinatal and postnatal reproduction study.

PREGNANCY

Teratogenic Effects, Pregnancy Category C

Zalcitabine has been shown to be teratogenic in mice at calculated exposure levels of 1365 and 2730 times that of the MRHD (based on AUC measurements). In rats, zalcitabine was teratogenic at a calculated exposure level of 2142 times the MRHD but not at an exposure level of 485 times the MRHD. In a perinatal and postnatal study in the rat, a high incidence of hydrocephalus was observed in the F_1 offspring derived from litters of dams treated with 1071 (but not 485) times the MRHD (based on AUC measurements). There are no adequate and well-controlled studies of zalcitabine in pregnant women. Zalcitabine should be used during pregnancy only if the potential benefit justifies the potential risk to the fetus. Fertile women should not receive zalcitabine unless they are using effective contraception during therapy. If pregnancy occurs, physicians are encouraged to report such cases by calling (800) 526-6367.

Nonteratogenic Effects

Increased embryolethality was observed in pregnant mice at doses 2730 times the MRHD and in pregnant rats above 485 (but not 98) times the MRHD (based on AUC measurements). Average fetal body weight was significantly decreased in mice at doses of 1365 times the MRHD and in rats at 2142 times the MRHD (based on AUC measurements). In a perinatal and postnatal study, the learning and memory of a significant number of F_1 offspring were impaired, and they tended to stay hyperactive for a longer period of time. These effects, observed at a calculated exposure level of 1071 (but not 485) times the MRHD (based on AUC measurements), were considered to result from extensive damage to or gross underdevelopment of the brain of these F_1 offspring consistent with the finding of hydrocephalus.

Antiretroviral Pregnancy Registry

To monitor maternal-fetal outcomes of pregnant women exposed to antiretroviral medications, including zalcitabine, an Antiretroviral Pregnancy Registry has been established. Physicians are encouraged to register patients by calling 1-800-258-4263.

NURSING MOTHERS

The Centers for Disease Control and Prevention recommend HIV-infected mothers not breast-feed their infants to avoid risking postnatal transmission of HIV. It is not known whether zalcitabine is excreted in human milk. Because of both the potential for HIV transmission and the potential for serious adverse reactions in nursing infants, **mothers should be instructed not to breast-feed if they are receiving antiretroviral medications, including zalcitabine.**

PEDIATRIC USE

Pharmacokinetics in Pediatric Patients

Limited pharmacokinetic data have been reported for 5 HIV-positive pediatric patients using doses of 0.03 and 0.04 mg/kg zalcitabine administered orally every 6 hours.[1] The mean bioavailability of zalcitabine in these pediatric patients was 54% and mean apparent systemic clearance was 150 ml/min/m^2. Due to the small number of subjects and different analytical techniques, it is difficult to make comparisons between pediatric and adult data.

Safety and effectiveness of zalcitabine in HIV-infected pediatric patients younger than 13 years of age have not been established.

GERIATRIC USE

Clinical studies of zalcitabine did not include sufficient numbers of subjects aged 65 and over to determine whether they respond differently from younger subjects. In general, dose selection for an elderly patient should be cautious, reflecting the greater frequency of decreased hepatic, renal, or cardiac function, and of concomitant disease or other drug therapy. Zalcitabine is known to be substantially excreted by the kidney, and the risk of toxic reactions to this drug may be greater in patients with impaired renal function. Because elderly patients are more likely to have decreased renal function, care should be taken in dose selection. In addition, renal function should be monitored and dosage adjustments should be made accordingly (see PRECAUTIONS, General, Renal Impairment and DOSAGE AND ADMINISTRATION).

DRUG INTERACTIONS

ZIDOVUDINE

There is no significant pharmacokinetic interaction between ZDV and zalcitabine which has been confirmed clinically. Zalcitabine also has no significant effect on the intracellular phosphorylation of ZDV, as shown *in vitro* in peripheral blood mononuclear cells or in 2 other cell lines (U937 and Molt-4). In the same study it was shown that didanosine and stavudine had no significant effect on the intracellular phosphorylation of zalcitabine in peripheral blood mononuclear cells[1].

LAMIVUDINE

In vitro studies[2, 3, 4] in peripheral blood mononuclear cells, U937 and Molt-4 cells revealed that lamivudine significantly inhibited zalcitabine phosphorylation in a dose dependent manner. Effects were already seen with doses corresponding to relevant plasma levels in humans, and the intracellular phosphorylation of zalcitabine to its 3 metabolites (including the active zalcitabine triphosphate metabolite) was significantly inhibited. Zalcitabine inhibited lamivudine phosphorylation at high concentration ratios (10 and 100); however, it is considered to be unlikely that this decrease of phosphorylated lamivudine concentration is of clinical significance, as lamivudine is a more efficient substrate for deoxycytidine kinase than zalcitabine. These *in vitro* studies suggest that concomitant administration of zalcitabine and lamivudine in humans may result in sub-therapeutic concentrations of active phosphorylated zalcitabine, which may lead to a decreased antiretroviral effect of zalcitabine. It is unknown how the effect seen in these *in vitro* studies translates into clinical consequences. **Concomitant use of zalcitabine and lamivudine is not recommended.**

SAQUINAVIR

The combination of zalcitabine, saquinavir, and ZDV has been studied (as triple combination) in adults. Pharmacokinetic data suggest that absorption, metabolism, and elimination of each of these drugs are unchanged when they are used together.

DRUGS ASSOCIATED WITH PERIPHERAL NEUROPATHY

The concomitant use of zalcitabine with drugs that have the potential to cause peripheral neuropathy should be avoided where possible. Drugs that have been associated with peripheral neuropathy include antiretroviral nucleoside analogues, chloramphenicol, cisplatin, dapsone, disulfiram, ethionamide, glutethimide, gold, hydralazine, iodoquinol, isoniazid, metronidazole, nitrofurantoin, phenytoin, ribavirin, and vincristine. Concomitant use of zalcitabine with didanosine is not recommended.

INTRAVENOUS PENTAMIDINE

Treatment with zalcitabine should be interrupted when the use of a drug that has the potential to cause pancreatitis is required. Death due to fulminant pancreatitis possibly related to intravenous pentamidine and zalcitabine has been reported. If intravenous pentamidine is required to treat *Pneumocystis carinii* pneumonia, treatment with zalcitabine should be interrupted (see WARNINGS).

AMPHOTERICIN, FOSCARNET, AND AMINOGLYCOSIDES

Drugs such as amphotericin, foscarnet, and aminoglycosides may increase the risk of developing peripheral neuropathy (see WARNINGS, Peripheral Neuropathy) or other zalcitabine-associated adverse events by interfering with the renal clearance of zalcitabine (thereby raising systemic exposure). Patients who require the use of one of these drugs with zalcitabine should have frequent clinical and laboratory monitoring with dosage adjustment for any significant change in renal function.

PROBENECID OR CIMETIDINE

Concomitant administration of probenecid or cimetidine decreases the elimination of zalcitabine, most likely by inhibition of renal tubular secretion of zalcitabine. Patients receiving these drugs in combination with zalcitabine should be monitored for signs of toxicity and the dose of zalcitabine reduced if warranted.

MAGNESIUM/ALUMINUM-CONTAINING ANTACID PRODUCTS

Absorption of zalcitabine is moderately reduced (approximately 25%) when coadministered with magnesium/aluminum-containing antacid products. The clinical significance of this reduction is not known, hence zalcitabine is not recommended to be ingested simultaneously with magnesium/aluminum-containing antacids.

METOCLOPRAMIDE

Bioavailability is mildly reduced (approximately 10%) when zalcitabine and metoclopramide are coadministered (see CLINICAL PHARMACOLOGY, Pharmacokinetics, Drug Interactions).

DOXORUBICIN

Doxorubicin caused a decrease in zalcitabine phosphorylation (>50% inhibition of total phosphate formation) in U937/Molt 4 cells. Although there may be decreased zalcitabine activity because of lessened active metabolite formation, the clinical relevance of these *in vitro* results are not known.

ADVERSE REACTIONS

See WARNINGS.

TABLE 2 and TABLE 3 summarize the clinical adverse events and laboratory abnormalities, respectively, that occurred in ≥1% of patients in the comparative monotherapy trial (CPCRA 002) of zalcitabine (ddC) versus didanosine (ddI), and the comparative combination trial (ACTG 175) of zidovudine (ZDV) monotherapy versus zalcitabine and zidovudine combination therapy, respectively. Other studies have found a higher or lower incidence of adverse experiences depending upon disease status, generally being lower in patients with less advanced disease.

TABLE 2 *Percentage of Patients With Clinical Adverse Experience ≥Grade 3*† in ≥1% of Patients Receiving Zalcitabine*

	CPCRA 002*		ACTG 175‡	
	ZDV Intolerant or Failure		ZDV Naive/Experienced	
	ddC	ddI	ZDV	ddC + ZDV
	0.750 mg	250 mg	200 mg	0.750 mg + 200 mg
Body System	q8h	q12h	q8h	q8h
Adverse Event	n=237	n=230	n=619	n=615
Systemic				
Fatigue	3.8%	2.6%	2.7%	2.3%
Headache	2.1%	1.3%	2.4%	2.6%
Fever	1.7%	0.4%	2.7%	2.9%
Gastrointestinal				
Abdominal pain	3.0%	7.0%	2.3%	1.8%
Oral lesions/stomatitis§	3.0%	0.0%	0.6%	1.5%
Vomiting/nausea§	3.4%	7.0%	4.9%	2.1%
Diarrhea/constipation§	2.5%	17.4%	2.9%	1.0%
Hepatic				
Abnormal hepatic function	8.9%	7.0%	¤	¤
Neurological				
Convulsions	1.3%	2.2%		
Peripheral neuropathy¶	28.3%	13.0%	3.1%	3.3%
Skin				
Rash/pruritus/urticaria	3.4%	3.9%	1.8%	1.6%
Metabolic and Nutrition				
Pancreatitis	0.0%	1.7%	0.2%	0.5%
Psychological				
Depression	0.4%	0.0%	1.1%	1.8%
Musculoskeletal				
Painful/swollen joints	0.4%	0.0%	0.3%	1.0%

* Grade 2 adverse events possibly or probably related to treatment or unassessable were included if study drug dosage was changed or interrupted.
† *Grade 3 Severity:* Event causing marked limitation in activity, requiring medical care and possible hospitalization. *Grade 4 Severity:* Completely disabling, unable to care for self, requiring active medical intervention, probable hospitalization or hospice care.
‡ All relationships.
§ Adverse experiences were combined to form this category.
¤ See TABLE 3.
¶ CPCRA 002 included patients who were dose-adjusted for Grade 2 events; ACTG 175 required dose adjustment for Grade 2 peripheral neuropathy but recorded only Grade 3 events.

TABLE 3 *Percentage of Patients With Laboratory Abnormalities Protocol Grade 3/4*

	CPCRA 002*		ACTG 175	
	ZDV Intolerant or Failure		ZDV Naive/Experienced	
	ddC	ddI	ZDV	ddC + ZDV
	0.750 mg	250 mg	200 mg	0.750 mg + 200 mg
	q8h	q12h	q8h	q8h
Laboratory Abnormality	n=237	n=230	n=619	n=615
Anemia (<7.5 g/dl)	8.4%	7.4%	1.8%	3.1%
Leukopenia (<1500 cells/mm^3)	13.1%	9.6%	N/A	N/A
Eosinophilia (>1000 cells/mm^3 or 25%)	2.5%	1.7%	N/A	N/A
Neutropenia (<750 cells/mm^3)	16.9%	11.7%	1.9%	4.2%
Thrombocytopenia (<50,000 cells/mm^3)	1.3%	4.8%	1.1%	1.8%
CPK elevation* (>4 × ULN)	0.8%	0.0%	5.8%	5.7%
ALT (SGPT) (>5 × ULN)	N/A	N/A	3.6%	5.0%
AST (SGOT) (>5 × ULN)	7.6%	5.7%	2.9%	4.1%
Bilirubin (>2.5 × ULN)	0.8%	0.9%	0.5%	1.0%
GGT (>5 × ULN)	N/A	N/A	0.5%	1.0%
Amylase (>2 × ULN)	5.1%	3.9%	1.0%	1.5%
Hyperglycemia* (>250 mg/dl)	0.0%	1.7%	0.8%	2.0%

* Grade 3 or higher reported for CPCRA 002.
N/A Not available.

Additional clinical adverse experiences associated with zalcitabine that occurred in <1% of patients in CPCRA 002 (at least possibly related, Grade 3 or higher), ACTG 175 (any relationship, Grade 3/4) or in other clinical studies are listed below by body system. Several of these events occurred in slightly higher rates in other studies. The incidence of adverse experiences varied in different studies, generally being lower in patients with less-advanced disease.

Body as a Whole: Abnormal weight loss, asthenia, cachexia, chest tightness or pain, chills, cutaneous/allergic reaction, debilitation, difficulty moving, dry eyes/mouth, edema, facial pain or swelling, flank pain, flushing, increased sweating, lymphadenopathy, hypersensitivity reactions (see WARNINGS), malaise, night sweats, pain, pelvic/groin pain, rigors, redistribution/accumulation of body fat (see PRECAUTIONS, Fat Redistribution).

Cardiovascular: Abnormal cardiac movement, arrhythmia, atrial fibrillation, cardiac failure, cardiac dysrhythmias, cardiomyopathy, heart racing, hypertension, palpitation, subarachnoid hemorrhage, syncope, tachycardia, ventricular ectopy.

Endocrine/Metabolic: Abnormal triglycerides, abnormal lipase, altered serum glucose, decreased bicarbonate, diabetes mellitus, glycosuria, gout, hot flushes, hypercalcemia, hyperkalemia, hyperlipemia, hypernatremia, hyperuricemia, hypocalcemia, hypoglycemia, hypokalemia, hypomagnesemia, hyponatremia, hypophosphatemia, increased nonprotein nitrogen, lactic acidosis.

Gastrointestinal: Abdominal bloating or cramps, acute pancreatitis, anal/rectal pain, anorexia, bleeding gums, bloody or black stools, colitis, dental abscess, dry mouth, dyspepsia, dysphagia, enlarged abdomen, epigastric pain, eructation, esophageal pain, esophageal ulcers, esophagitis, flatulence, gagging with pills, gastritis, gastrointestinal hemorrhage, gingivitis, glossitis, gum disorder, heartburn, hemorrhagic pancreatitis, hemorrhoids, increased saliva, left quadrant pain, melena, mouth lesion, odynophagia, painful sore gums, painful swallowing, pancreatitis, rectal hemorrhage, rectal mass, rectal ulcers, salivary gland enlargement, sore tongue, sore throat, tongue disorder, tongue ulcer, toothache, unformed/loose stools, vomiting.

Hematologic: Absolute neutrophil count alteration, anemia, epistaxis, decreased hematocrit, granulocytosis, hemoglobinemia, leukopenia, neutrophilia, platelet alteration, purpura, thrombus, unspecified hematologic toxicity, white blood cell alteration.

Hepatic: Abnormal lactate dehydrogenase, bilirubinemia, cholecystitis, decreased alkaline phosphatase, hepatitis, hepatocellular damage, hepatomegaly, increased alkaline phosphatase, jaundice.

Musculoskeletal: Arthralgia, arthritis, arthropathy, arthrosis, back pain, backache, bone pains/aches, bursitis, cold extremities, extremity pain, joint inflammation, leg cramps, muscle aches, muscle weakness, muscle disorder, muscle stiffness, muscle cramps, myalgia, myopathy, myositis, neck pain, rib pain, stiff neck.

Neurological: Abnormal coordination, aphasia, ataxia, Bell's palsy, confusion, decreased concentration, decreased neurological function, disequilibrium, dizziness, dysphonia, facial nerve palsy, focal motor seizures, grand mal seizure, hyperkinesia, hypertonia, hypokinesia, memory loss, migraine, neuralgia, neuritis, paralysis, seizures, speech disorder, status epilepticus, stupor, tremor, twitch, vertigo.

Psychological: Acute psychotic disorder, acute stress reaction, agitation, amnesia, anxiety, confusion, decreased motivation, decreased sexual desire, depersonalization, emotional lability, euphoria, hallucination, impaired concentration, insomnia, manic reaction, mood swings, nervousness, paranoid state, somnolence, suicide attempt, dementia.

Respiratory: Acute nasopharyngitis, chest congestion, coughing, cyanosis, difficulty breathing, dry nasal mucosa, dyspnea, flu-like symptoms, hemoptysis, nasal discharge, pharyngitis, rales/rhonchi, respiratory distress, sinus congestion, sinus pain, sinusitis, wheezing.

Skin: Acne, alopecia, bullous eruptions, carbuncle/furuncle, cellulitis, cold sore, dermatitis, dry skin, dry rash desquamation, erythematous rash, exfoliative dermatitis, finger inflammation, follicular rash, impetigo, infection, itchy rash, lip blisters/lesions, macular/papular rash, maculopapular rash, moniliasis, mucocutaneous/skin disorder, nail disorder, photosensitivity reaction, pruritic disorder, pruritus, skin disorder, skin lesions, skin fissure, skin ulcer, urticaria.

Special Senses: Abnormal vision, blurred vision, burning eyes, decreased taste, decreased vision, ear pain/problem, ear blockage, eye abnormality, eye inflammation, eye itching, eye pain, eye irritation, eye redness, eye hemorrhage, fluid in ears, hearing loss, increased tears, loss of taste, mucopurulent conjunctivitis, parosmia, photophobia, smell dysfunction, taste perversion, tinnitus, unequal-sized pupils, xerophthalmia, yellow sclera.

Urogenital: Abnormal renal function, acute renal failure, albuminuria, bladder pain, dysuria, frequent urination, genital lesion/ulcer, increased blood urea nitrogen, increased creatinine, micturition frequency, nocturia, painful penis sore, pain on urination, penile edema, polyuria, renal cyst, renal calculus, testicular swelling, toxic nephropathy, urinary retention, vaginal itch, vaginal ulcer, vaginal pain, vaginal/cervix disorder, vaginal discharge.

DOSAGE AND ADMINISTRATION

Patients should be advised that zalcitabine is recommended for use in combination with active antiretroviral therapy. Greater activity has been observed when new antiretroviral therapies are begun at the same time as zalcitabine. Concomitant therapy should be based on a patient's prior drug exposure. The recommended regimen is one 0.750 mg tablet of zalcitabine orally every 8 hours (2.25 mg zalcitabine total daily dose) in combination with other antiretroviral agents. Please refer to the complete product information for each of the other antiretroviral agents for the recommended doses of these agents. Based on preliminary data, the recommended zalcitabine dosage reduction for patients with impaired renal function is: creatinine clearance 10-40 ml/min: 0.750 mg of zalcitabine every 12 hours; creatinine clearance <10 ml/min: 0.750 mg of zalcitabine every 24 hours.

MONITORING OF PATIENTS

Complete blood counts and clinical chemistry tests should be performed prior to initiating zalcitabine therapy and at appropriate intervals thereafter. For comprehensive patient monitoring recommendations for other antiretroviral therapies, physicians should refer to the complete product information for these drugs. Serum amylase levels should be monitored in those individuals who have a history of elevated amylase, pancreatitis, ethanol abuse, who are on parenteral nutrition or who are otherwise at high risk of pancreatitis. Careful monitoring for signs or symptoms suggestive of peripheral neuropathy is recommended, particularly in individuals with a low CD4 cell count or who are at a greater risk of developing peripheral neuropathy while on therapy (see WARNINGS).

DOSE ADJUSTMENT FOR ZALCITABINE

For toxicities that are likely to be associated with zalcitabine (*e.g.,* peripheral neuropathy, severe oral ulcers, pancreatitis, elevated liver function tests especially in patients with chronic Hepatitis B), zalcitabine should be interrupted or dose reduced. FOR SEVERE TOXICITIES OR THOSE PERSISTING AFTER DOSE REDUCTION, ZALCITABINE SHOULD BE INTERRUPTED. For recipients of combination therapy with zalcitabine and other antiretroviral agents, dose adjustments or interruption for each drug should be based on the known toxicity profile of the individual drugs. SEE INFORMATION FOR EACH DRUG USED IN COMBINATION FOR A DESCRIPTION OF KNOWN DRUG-ASSOCIATED ADVERSE REACTIONS.

Patients developing moderate discomfort with signs or symptoms of peripheral neuropathy should stop zalcitabine. Zalcitabine-associated peripheral neuropathy may continue to worsen despite interruption of zalcitabine. Zalcitabine should be reintroduced at 50% dose — 0.375 mg every 8 hours only if all findings related to peripheral neuropathy have improved to mild symptoms. Zalcitabine should be permanently discontinued if patients experience severe discomfort related to peripheral neuropathy or moderate discomfort that progresses. If other moderate to severe clinical adverse reactions or laboratory abnormalities (such as increased liver function tests) occur, then zalcitabine and/or the other potential causative agent(s) should be interrupted until the adverse reaction abates. Zalcitabine and/or the other potential causative agent(s) should then be carefully reintroduced at lower doses if appropriate. If adverse reactions recur at the reduced dose, therapy should be discontinued. The minimum effective dose of zalcitabine in combination with zidovudine for the treatment of adult patients with advanced HIV infection has not been established.

In patients with poor bone marrow reserve, particularly those patients with advanced symptomatic HIV disease, frequent monitoring of hematologic indices is recommended to detect serious anemia or granulocytopenia. Significant toxicities, such as anemia (hemoglobin of <7.5 g/dl or reduction of >25% of baseline) and/or granulocytopenia (granulocyte count of <750 cells/mm^3 or reduction of >50% from baseline), may require a treatment interruption of zalcitabine and zidovudine until evidence of marrow recovery is observed. For less severe anemia or granulocytopenia, a reduction in daily dose of zidovudine in those patients receiving combination therapy may be adequate. In patients who experience hematologic toxicity, reduction in hemoglobin may occur as early as 2-4 weeks after initiation of therapy, and granulocytopenia usually occurs after 6-8 weeks of therapy. In patients who develop significant anemia, dose modification does not necessarily eliminate the need for transfusion. If marrow recovery occurs following dose modification, gradual increases in dose may be appropriate depending on hematologic indices and patient tolerance. For more details, refer to the complete product information for zidovudine.

HOW SUPPLIED

Hivid tablets are supplied as:

0.375 mg: Oval, beige, film-coated tablets with "HIVID 0.375" imprinted on one side and "ROCHE" on the other side.

0.750 mg: Oval, gray, film-coated tablets with "HIVID 0.750" imprinted on one side and "ROCHE" on the other side.

Storage: The tablets should be stored in tightly closed bottles at 15-30°C (59-86°F).

PRODUCT LISTING - EQUIVALENTS NOT AVAILABLE

Tablet - Oral - 0.375 mg

100's	$204.98	HIVID, Physicians Total Care	54868-2499-01
100's	$226.93	HIVID, Roche Laboratories	00004-0220-01

Tablet - Oral - 0.75 mg

15's	$41.75	HIVID, Physicians Total Care	54868-2500-02
90's	$225.03	HIVID, Allscripts Pharmaceutical Company	54569-3877-01
100's	$229.92	HIVID, Allscripts Pharmaceutical Company	54569-3877-00
100's	$256.05	HIVID, Physicians Total Care	54868-2500-01
100's	$284.43	HIVID, Roche Laboratories	00004-0221-01

Zaleplon *(003449)*

Categories: Insomnia; FDA Approved 1999 Aug; Pregnancy Category C
Drug Classes: Sedatives/hypnotics
Foreign Brand Availability: Sonata (Austria; Belgium; Bulgaria; Czech-Republic; Denmark; England; Finland; France; Germany; Greece; Hungary; Ireland; Italy; Mexico; Netherlands; Norway; Poland; Portugal; Slovenia; Spain; Sweden; Switzerland; Turkey); Starnoc (Canada); Zaplon (India); Zerene (Austria; Belgium; Bulgaria; Czech-Republic; Denmark; England; Finland; France; Germany; Greece; Hungary; Ireland; Italy; Netherlands; Norway; Poland; Portugal; Slovenia; Spain; Sweden; Switzerland; Turkey)
Cost of Therapy: $25.71 (Insomnia; Sonata; 10 mg; 1 tablet/day; 10 day supply)

DESCRIPTION

Zaleplon is a nonbenzodiazepine hypnotic from the pyrazolopyrimidine class. The chemical name of zaleplon is N-[3-(3-cyanopyrazolo[1,5-a]pyrimidin-7-yl)phenyl]-N-ethylacetamide. Its empirical formula is $C_{17}H_{15}N^5O$, and its molecular weight is 305.34.

Zaleplon is a white to off-white powder that is practically insoluble in water and sparingly soluble in alcohol or propylene glycol. Its partition coefficient in octanol/water is constant (log PC = 1.23) over the pH range of 1-7.

Sonata capsules contain zaleplon as the active ingredient. Inactive ingredients consist of microcrystalline cellulose, pregelatinized starch, silicon dioxide, sodium lauryl sulfate, magnesium stearate, lactose, gelatin, titanium dioxide, D&C yellow no. 10, FD&C blue no. 1, FD&C green no. 3, and FD&C yellow no. 5.

CLINICAL PHARMACOLOGY

PHARMACODYNAMICS AND MECHANISM OF ACTION

While zaleplon is a hypnotic agent with a chemical structure unrelated to benzodiazepines, barbiturates, or other drugs with known hypnotic properties, it interacts with the gamma-aminobutyric acid-benzodiazepine (GABA-BZ) receptor complex. Subunit modulation of the GABA-BZ receptor chloride channel macromolecular complex is hypothesized to be responsible for some of the pharmacological properties of benzodiazepines, which include sedative, anxiolytic, muscle relaxant, and anticonvulsive effects in animal models.

Other nonclinical studies have also shown that zaleplon binds selectively to the brain omega-1 receptor situated on the alpha subunit of the $GABA_A$/chloride ion channel receptor complex and potentiates t-butyl-bicyclophosphorothionate (TBPS) binding. Studies of binding of zaleplon to recombinant $GABA_A$ receptors ($\alpha_1\beta_1\gamma_2$ [omega-1] and $\alpha_2\beta_1\gamma_2$ [omega-2]) have shown that zaleplon has a low affinity for these receptors, with preferential binding to the omega-1 receptor.

PHARMACOKINETICS

The pharmacokinetics of zaleplon have been investigated in more than 500 healthy subjects (young and elderly), nursing mothers, and patients with hepatic disease or renal disease. In healthy subjects, the pharmacokinetic profile has been examined after single doses of up to 60 mg and once-daily administration at 15 and 30 mg for 10 days. Zaleplon was rapidly absorbed with a time to peak concentration (T_{max}) of approximately 1 hour and a terminal-phase elimination half-life ($T_{1/2}$) of approximately 1 hour. Zaleplon does not accumulate with once-daily administration and its pharmacokinetics are dose proportional in the therapeutic range.

Absorption

Zaleplon is rapidly and almost completely absorbed following oral administration. Peak plasma concentrations are attained within approximately 1 hour after oral administration. Although zaleplon is well absorbed, its absolute bioavailability is approximately 30% because it undergoes significant presystemic metabolism.

Distribution

Zaleplon is a lipophilic compound with a volume of distribution of approximately 1.4 L/kg following intravenous (IV) administration, indicating substantial distribution into extravascular tissues. The *in vitro* plasma protein binding is approximately 60 ± 15% and is independent of zaleplon concentration over the range of 10-1000 ng/ml. This suggests that zaleplon disposition should not be sensitive to alterations in protein binding. The blood to plasma ratio for zaleplon is approximately 1, indicating that zaleplon is uniformly distributed throughout the blood with no extensive distribution into red blood cells.

Metabolism

After oral administration, zaleplon is extensively metabolized, with less than 1% of the dose excreted unchanged in urine. Zaleplon is primarily metabolized by aldehyde oxidase to form 5-oxo-zaleplon. Zaleplon is metabolized to a lesser extent by cytochrome P450 (CYP)3A4 to form desethylzaleplon, which is quickly converted, presumably by aldehyde oxidase, to 5-oxo-desethylzaleplon. These oxidative metabolites are then converted to glucuronides and eliminated in urine. All of zaleplon's metabolites are pharmacologically inactive.

Elimination

After either oral or IV administration, zaleplon is rapidly eliminated with a mean $T_{1/2}$ of approximately 1 hour. The oral-dose plasma clearance of zaleplon is about 3 L/h/kg and the IV zaleplon plasma clearance is approximately 1 L/h/kg. Assuming normal hepatic blood flow and negligible renal clearance of zaleplon, the estimated hepatic extraction ratio of zaleplon is approximately 0.7, indicating that zaleplon is subject to high first-pass metabolism.

After administration of a radiolabeled dose of zaleplon, 70% of the administered dose is recovered in urine within 48 hours (71% recovered within 6 days), almost all as zaleplon metabolites and their glucuronides. An additional 17% is recovered in feces within 6 days, most as 5-oxo-zaleplon.

Effect of Food

In healthy adults a high-fat/heavy meal prolonged the absorption of zaleplon compared to the fasted state, delaying T_{max} by approximately 2 hours and reducing C_{max} by approximately 35%. Zaleplon AUC and elimination half-life were not significantly affected. These results suggest that the effects of zaleplon on sleep onset may be reduced if it is taken with or immediately after a high-fat, heavy meal.

SPECIAL POPULATIONS

Age

The pharmacokinetics of zaleplon have been investigated in three studies with elderly men and women ranging in age from 65-85 years. The pharmacokinetics of zaleplon in elderly subjects, including those over 75 years of age, are not significantly different from those in young healthy subjects.

Gender

There is no significant difference in the pharmacokinetics of zaleplon in men and women.

Race

The pharmacokinetics of zaleplon have been studied in Japanese subjects as representative of Asian populations. For this group, C_{max} and AUC were increased 37% and 64%, respectively. This finding can likely be attributed to differences in body weight, or alternatively, may represent differences in enzyme activities resulting from differences in diet, environment, or other factors. The effects of race on pharmacokinetic characteristics in other ethnic groups have not been well characterized.

Hepatic Impairment

Zaleplon is metabolized primarily by the liver and undergoes significant presystemic metabolism. Consequently, the oral clearance of zaleplon was reduced by 70% and 87% in compensated and decompensated cirrhotic patients, respectively, leading to marked increases in mean C_{max} and AUC (up to 4-fold and 7-fold in compensated and decompensated patients, respectively), in comparison with healthy subjects. The dose of zaleplon should therefore be reduced in patients with mild to moderate hepatic impairment (see DOSAGE AND ADMINISTRATION). Zaleplon is not recommended for use in patients with severe hepatic impairment.

Renal Impairment

Because renal excretion of unchanged zaleplon accounts for less than 1% of the administered dose, the pharmacokinetics of zaleplon are not altered in patients with renal insufficiency. No dose adjustment is necessary in patients with mild to moderate renal impairment. Zaleplon has not been adequately studied in patients with severe renal impairment.

DRUG-DRUG INTERACTIONS

Because zaleplon is primarily metabolized by aldehyde oxidase, and to a lesser extent by CYP3A4, inhibitors of these enzymes might be expected to decrease zaleplon's clearance and inducers of these enzymes might be expected to increase its clearance. Zaleplon has been shown to have minimal effects on the kinetics of warfarin (both R- and S-forms), imipramine, ethanol, ibuprofen, diphenhydramine, thioridazine, and digoxin. However, the effects of zaleplon on inhibition of enzymes involved in the metabolism of other drugs have not been studied. (See DRUG INTERACTIONS.)

INDICATIONS AND USAGE

Zaleplon is indicated for the short-term treatment of insomnia. Zaleplon has been shown to decrease the time to sleep onset for up to 30 days in controlled clinical studies. It has not been shown to increase total sleep time or decrease the number of awakenings.

Hypnotics should generally be limited to 7-10 days of use, and reevaluation of the patient is recommended if they are to be taken for more than 2-3 weeks. Zaleplon should not be prescribed in quantities exceeding a 1 month supply (see WARNINGS).

CONTRAINDICATIONS

Hypersensitivity to zaleplon or any excipients in the formulation (see also PRECAUTIONS).

WARNINGS

Because sleep disturbances may be the presenting manifestation of a physical and/or psychiatric disorder, symptomatic treatment of insomnia should be initiated only after a careful evaluation of the patient. The failure of insomnia to remit after 7-10 days of treatment may indicate the presence of a primary psychiatric and/or medical illness that should be evaluated. Worsening of insomnia or the emergence of new thinking or behavior abnormalities may be the consequence of an unrecognized psychiatric or physical disorder. Such findings have emerged during the course of treatment with sedative/hypnotic drugs, including zaleplon. Because some of the important adverse effects of zaleplon appear to be dose-related, it is important to use the lowest possible effective dose, especially in the elderly (see DOSAGE AND ADMINISTRATION).

A variety of abnormal thinking and behavior changes have been reported to occur in association with the use of sedative/hypnotics. Some of these changes may be characterized by decreased inhibition (*e.g.,* aggressiveness and extroversion that seem out of character), similar to effects produced by alcohol and other CNS depressants. Other reported behavioral changes have included bizarre behavior, agitation, hallucinations, and depersonalization. Amnesia and other neuropsychiatric symptoms may occur unpredictably. In primarily depressed patients, worsening of depression, including suicidal thinking, has been reported in association with the use of sedative/hypnotics.

It can rarely be determined with certainty whether a particular instance of the abnormal behaviors listed above are drug induced, spontaneous in origin, or a result of an underlying psychiatric or physical disorder. Nonetheless, the emergence of any new behavioral sign or symptom of concern requires careful and immediate evaluation.

Following rapid dose decrease or abrupt discontinuation of the use of sedative/hypnotics, there have been reports of signs and symptoms similar to those associated with withdrawal from other CNS-depressant drugs.

Zaleplon, like other hypnotics, has CNS-depressant effects. Because of the rapid onset of action, zaleplon should only be ingested immediately prior to going to bed or after the patient has gone to bed and has experienced difficulty falling asleep. Patients receiving zaleplon should be cautioned against engaging in hazardous occupations requiring complete mental alertness or motor coordination (*e.g.,* operating machinery or driving a motor vehicle) after ingesting the drug, including potential impairment of the performance of such activities that may occur the day following ingestion of zaleplon. Zaleplon, as well as other hypnotics, may produce additive CNS-depressant effects when coadministered with other psychotropic medications, anticonvulsants, antihistamines, narcotic analgesics, anesthetics, ethanol, and other drugs that themselves produce CNS depression. Zaleplon should not be taken with alcohol. Dosage adjustment may be necessary when zaleplon is administered with other CNS-depressant agents because of the potentially additive effects.

PRECAUTIONS

GENERAL

Timing of Drug Administration

Zaleplon should be taken immediately before bedtime or after the patient has gone to bed and has experienced difficulty falling asleep. As with all sedative/hypnotics, taking zaleplon while still up and about may result in short-term memory impairment, hallucinations, impaired coordination, dizziness, and lightheadedness.

Use in the Elderly and/or Debilitated Patients

Impaired motor and/or cognitive performance after repeated exposure or unusual sensitivity to sedative/hypnotic drugs is a concern in the treatment of elderly and/or debilitated patients. A dose of 5 mg is recommended for elderly patients to decrease the possibility of side effects (see DOSAGE AND ADMINISTRATION). Elderly and/or debilitated patients should be monitored closely.

Use in Patients With Concomitant Illness

Clinical experience with zaleplon in patients with concomitant systemic illness is limited. Zaleplon should be used with caution in patients with diseases or conditions that could affect metabolism or hemodynamic responses.

Although preliminary studies did not reveal respiratory depressant effects at hypnotic doses of zaleplon in normal subjects, caution should be observed if zaleplon is prescribed to patients with compromised respiratory function, because sedative/hypnotics have the capacity to depress respiratory drive. Controlled trials of acute administration of zaleplon 10 mg in patients with mild to moderate chronic obstructive pulmonary disease or moderate obstructive sleep apnea showed no evidence of alterations in blood gases or apnea/hypopnea index, respectively. However, patients with compromised respiration due to preexisting illness should be monitored carefully.

The dose of zaleplon should be reduced to 5 mg in patients with mild to moderate hepatic impairment (see DOSAGE AND ADMINISTRATION). It is not recommended for use in patients with severe hepatic impairment.

No dose adjustment is necessary in patients with mild to moderate renal impairment. Zaleplon has not been adequately studied in patients with severe renal impairment.

Use in Patients With Depression

As with other sedative/hypnotic drugs, zaleplon should be administered with caution to patients exhibiting signs or symptoms of depression. Suicidal tendencies may be present in such patients and protective measures may be required. Intentional overdosage is more common in this group of patients; therefore, the least amount of drug that is feasible should be prescribed for the patient at any one time.

This product contains FD&C yellow no. 5 (tartrazine) which may cause allergic-type reactions (including bronchial asthma) in certain susceptible persons. Although the overall incidence of FD&C yellow no. 5 (tartrazine) sensitivity in the general population is low, it is frequently seen in patients who also have aspirin hypersensitivity.

INFORMATION FOR THE PATIENT

Patient information is printed at the end of the insert supplied with the prescription. To assure safe and effective use of zaleplon, the information and instructions provided in the patient information section should be discussed with patients.

LABORATORY TESTS

There are no specific laboratory tests recommended.

CARCINOGENESIS, MUTAGENESIS, AND IMPAIRMENT OF FERTILITY

Carcinogenesis

Lifetime carcinogenicity studies of zaleplon were conducted in mice and rats. Mice received doses of 25, 50, 100, and 200 mg/kg/day in the diet for 2 years. These doses are equivalent to 6-49 times the maximum recommended human dose (MRHD) of 20 mg on a mg/m^2 basis. There was a significant increase in the incidence of hepatocellular adenomas in female mice in the high dose group. Rats received doses of 1, 10, and 20 mg/kg/day in the diet for 2 years. These doses are equivalent to 0.5-10 times the maximum recommended human dose (MRHD) of 20 mg on a mg/m^2 basis. Zaleplon was not carcinogenic in rats.

Mutagenesis

Zaleplon was clastogenic, both in the presence and absence of metabolic activation, causing structural and numerical aberrations (polyploidy and endoreduplication), when tested for chromosomal aberrations in the *in vitro* Chinese hamster ovary cell assay. In the *in vitro* human lymphocyte assay, zaleplon caused numerical, but not structural, aberrations only in the presence of metabolic activation at the highest concentrations tested. In other *in vitro* assays, zaleplon was not mutagenic in the Ames bacterial gene mutation assay or the Chinese hamster ovary HGPRT gene mutation assay. Zaleplon was not clastogenic in 2 *in vivo* assays, the mouse bone marrow micronucleus assay and the rat bone marrow chromosomal aberration assay, and did not cause DNA damage in the rat hepatocyte unscheduled DNA synthesis assay.

Impairment of Fertility

In a fertility and reproductive performance study in rats, mortality and decreased fertility were associated with administration of an oral dose of zaleplon of 100 mg/kg/day to males and females prior to and during mating. This dose is equivalent to 49 times the maximum recommended human dose (MRHD) of 20 mg on a mg/m^2 basis. Follow-up studies indicated that impaired fertility was due to an effect on the female.

PREGNANCY CATEGORY C

In embryofetal development studies in rats and rabbits, oral administration of up to 100 and 50 mg/kg/day, respectively, to pregnant animals throughout organogenesis produced no evidence of teratogenicity. These doses are equivalent to 49 (rat) and 48 (rabbit) times the maximum recommended human dose (MRHD) of 20 mg on a mg/m^2 basis. In rats, pre- and postnatal growth was reduced in the offspring of dams receiving 100 mg/kg/day. This dose was also maternally toxic, as evidenced by clinical signs and decreased maternal body weight gain during gestation. The no-effect dose for rat offspring growth reduction was 10 mg/kg (a dose equivalent to 5 times the MRHD of 20 mg on a mg/m^2 basis). No adverse effects on embryofetal development were observed in rabbits at the doses examined.

In a pre- and postnatal development study in rats, increased stillbirth and postnatal mortality, and decreased growth and physical development, were observed in the offspring of females treated with doses of 7 mg/kg/day or greater during the latter part of gestation and throughout lactation. There was no evidence of maternal toxicity at this dose. The no-effect dose for offspring development was 1 mg/kg/day (a dose equivalent to 0.5 times the MRHD of 20 mg on a mg/m^2 basis). When the adverse effects on offspring viability and growth were examined in a cross-fostering study, they appeared to result from both *in utero* and lactational exposure to the drug.

There are no studies of zaleplon in pregnant women; therefore, zaleplon is not recommended for use in women during pregnancy.

LABOR AND DELIVERY

Zaleplon has no established use in labor and delivery.

NURSING MOTHERS

A study in lactating mothers indicated that the clearance and half-life of zaleplon is similar to that in young normal subjects. A small amount of zaleplon is excreted in breast milk, with the highest excreted amount occurring during a feeding at approximately 1 hour after zaleplon administration. Since the small amount of the drug from breast milk may result in potentially important concentrations in infants, and because the effects of zaleplon on a nursing infant are not known, it is recommended that nursing mothers not take zaleplon.

PEDIATRIC USE

The safety and effectiveness of zaleplon in pediatric patients have not been established.

GERIATRIC USE

A total of 628 patients in double-blind, placebo-controlled, parallel-group clinical trials who received zaleplon were at least 65 years of age; of these, 311 received 5 mg and 317 received 10 mg. In both sleep laboratory and outpatient studies, elderly patients with insomnia responded to a 5 mg dose with a reduced sleep latency, and thus 5 mg is the recommended dose in this population. During short-term treatment (14 night studies) of elderly patients with zaleplon, no adverse event with a frequency of at least 1% occurred at a significantly higher rate with either 5 or 10 mg zaleplon than with placebo.

DRUG INTERACTIONS

As with all drugs, the potential exists for interaction with other drugs by a variety of mechanisms.

CNS-ACTIVE DRUGS

Ethanol

Zaleplon 10 mg potentiated the CNS-impairing effects of ethanol 0.75 g/kg on balance testing and reaction time for 1 hour after ethanol administration and on the digit symbol substitution test (DSST), symbol copying test, and the variability component of the divided attention test for 2.5 hours after ethanol administration. The potentiation resulted from a CNS pharmacodynamic interaction; zaleplon did not affect the pharmacokinetics of ethanol.

Imipramine

Coadministration of single doses of zaleplon 20 mg and imipramine 75 mg produced additive effects on decreased alertness and impaired psychomotor performance for 2-4 hours after administration. The interaction was pharmacodynamic with no alteration of the pharmacokinetics of either drug.

Paroxetine

Coadministration of a single dose of zaleplon 20 mg and paroxetine 20 mg daily for 7 days did not produce any interaction on psychomotor performance. Additionally, paroxetine did not alter the pharmacokinetics of zaleplon, reflecting the absence of a role of CYP2D6 in zaleplon's metabolism.

Thioridazine

Coadministration of single doses of zaleplon 20 mg and thioridazine 50 mg produced additive effects on decreased alertness and impaired psychomotor performance for 2-4 hours after administration. The interaction was pharmacodynamic with no alteration of the pharmacokinetics of either drug.

Venlafaxine

Coadministration of multiple doses of zaleplon 10 mg and venlafaxine ER (extended release) 75 or 150 mg did not produce any interaction on psychomotor performance. Additionally, there was no pharmacokinetic interaction between zaleplon and venlafaxine ER.

Promethazine

There was no pharmacokinetic interaction between zaleplon and promethazine following the administration of a single dose (10 and 25 mg, respectively) of each drug.

DRUGS THAT INDUCE CYP3A4

Rifampin

CYP3A4 is ordinarily a minor metabolizing enzyme of zaleplon. Multiple-dose administration of the potent CYP3A4 inducer rifampin (600 mg q24h for 14 days), however, reduced zaleplon C_{max} and AUC by approximately 80%. The coadministration of a potent CYP3A4 enzyme inducer, although not posing a safety concern, thus could lead to ineffectiveness of zaleplon. An alternative non-CYP3A4 substrate hypnotic agent may be considered in patients taking CYP3A4 inducers such as rifampin, phenytoin, carbamazepine and phenobarbital.

DRUGS THAT INHIBIT CYP3A4

CYP3A4 is a minor metabolic pathway for the elimination of zaleplon because the sum of desethylzaleplon (formed via CYP3A4 *in vitro*) and its metabolites, 5-oxo-desethylzaleplon and 5-oxo-desethylzaleplon glucuronide, account for only 9% of the urinary recovery of a zaleplon dose. Coadministration of zaleplon with erythromycin, a strong, selective CYP3A4 inhibitor, produced a 34% increase in zaleplon's plasma concentrations. Similar increases would be expected with other stong, selective CYP3A4 inhibitors, such as ketaconazole. A routine dosage adjustment of zaleplon is not considered necessary.

DRUGS THAT INHIBIT ALDEHYDE OXIDASE

The aldehyde oxidase enzyme system is less well studied than the cytochrome P450 enzyme system.

Diphenhydramine

Diphenhydramine is reported to be a weak inhibitor of aldehyde oxidase in rat liver, but its inhibitory effects in human liver are not known. There is no pharmacokinetic interaction between zaleplon and diphenhydramine following the administration of a single dose (10 mg and 50 mg, respectively) of each drug. However, because both of these compounds have CNS effects, an additive pharmacodynamic effect is possible.

DRUGS THAT INHIBIT BOTH ALDEHYDE OXIDASE AND CYP3A4

Cimetidine

Cimetidine inhibits both aldehyde oxidase (*in vitro*) and CYP3A4 (*in vitro* and *in vivo*), the primary and secondary enzymes, respectively, responsible for zaleplon metabolism. Concomitant administration of zaleplon (10 mg) and cimetidine (800 mg) produced an 85% increase in the mean C_{max} and AUC of zaleplon. An initial dose of 5 mg should be given to patients who are concomitantly being treated with cimetidine (see DOSAGE AND ADMINISTRATION).

DRUGS HIGHLY BOUND TO PLASMA PROTEIN

Zaleplon is not highly bound to plasma proteins (fraction bound 60 ± 15%); therefore, the disposition of zaleplon is not expected to be sensitive to alterations in protein binding. In addition, administration of zaleplon to a patient taking another drug that is highly protein bound should not cause transient increase in free concentrations of the other drug.

DRUGS WITH A NARROW THERAPEUTIC INDEX

Digoxin

Zaleplon (10 mg) did not affect the pharmacokinetic or pharmacodynamic profile of digoxin (0.375 mg q24h for 8 days).

Warfarin

Multiple oral doses of zaleplon (20 mg q24h for 13 days) did not affect the pharmacokinetics of warfarin (R+)- or (S-)-enantiomers or the pharmacodynamics (prothrombin time) following a single 25 mg oral dose of warfarin.

DRUGS THAT ALTER RENAL EXCRETION

Ibuprofen

Ibuprofen is known to affect renal function and, consequently, alter the renal excretion of other drugs. There was no apparent pharmacokinetic interaction between zaleplon and ibuprofen following single dose administration (10 mg and 600 mg, respectively) of each drug. This was expected because zaleplon is primarily metabolized, and renal excretion of unchanged zaleplon accounts for less than 1% of the administered dose.

ADVERSE REACTIONS

The premarketing development program for zaleplon included zaleplon exposures in patients and/or normal subjects from 2 different groups of studies: approximately 900 normal subjects in clinical pharmacology/pharmacokinetic studies; and approximately 2900 exposures from patients in placebo-controlled clinical effectiveness studies, corresponding to approximately 450 patient exposure years. The conditions and duration of treatment with zaleplon varied greatly and included (in overlapping categories) open-label and double-blind phases of studies, inpatients and outpatients, and short-term or longer-term exposure. Adverse reactions were assessed by collecting adverse events, results of physical examinations, vital signs, weights, laboratory analyses, and ECGs.

Adverse events during exposure were obtained primarily by general inquiry and recorded by clinical investigators using terminology of their own choosing. Consequently, it is not possible to provide a meaningful estimate of the proportion of individuals experiencing adverse events without first grouping similar types of events into a smaller number of standardized event categories. In the tables and tabulations that follow, COSTART terminology has been used to classify reported adverse events.

The stated frequencies of adverse events represent the proportion of individuals who experienced, at least once, a treatment-emergent adverse event of the type listed. An event was considered treatment emergent if it occurred for the first time or worsened while receiving therapy following baseline evaluation.

ADVERSE FINDINGS OBSERVED IN SHORT-TERM, PLACEBO-CONTROLLED TRIALS

Adverse Events Associated With Discontinuation of Treatment

In premarketing placebo-controlled, parallel-group Phase 2 and Phase 3 clinical trials, 3.1% of 744 patients who received placebo and 3.7% of 2149 patients who received zaleplon discontinued treatment because of an adverse clinical event. This difference was not statistically significant. No event that resulted in discontinuation occurred at a rate of ≥1%.

Adverse Events Occurring at an Incidence of 1% or More Among Zaleplon 20 mg-Treated Patients

TABLE 1 enumerates the incidence of treatment-emergent adverse events for a pool of three 28 hight and one 35 night placebo-controlled studies of zaleplon at doses of 5 or 10 mg and 20 mg. The table includes only those events that occurred in 1% or more of patients treated with zaleplon 20 mg and that had a higher incidence in patients treated with zaleplon 20 mg than in placebo-treated patients.

The prescriber should be aware that these figures cannot be used to predict the incidence of adverse events in the course of usual medical practice where patient characteristics and other factors differ from those which prevailed in the clinical trials. Similarly, the cited frequencies cannot be compared with figures obtained from other clinical investigations involving different treatments, uses, and investigators. The cited figures, however, do provide the prescribing physician with some basis for estimating the relative contribution of drug and non-drug factors to the adverse event incidence rate in the population studied.

TABLE 1 *Incidence (%) of Treatment-Emergent Adverse Events in Long-Term (28 and 35 nights) Placebo-Controlled Clinical Trials of Zaleplon**

Body System		Zaleplon	
Preferred Term	Placebo (n=344)	5 or 10 mg (n=569)	20 mg (n=297)
Body as a Whole			
Abdominal pain	3%	6%	6%
Asthenia	5%	5%	7%
Headache	35%	30%	42%
Malaise	<1%	<1%	2%
Photosensitivity reaction	<1%	<1%	1%
Digestive System			
Anorexia	<1%	<1%	2%
Colitis	0%	0%	1%
Nausea	7%	6%	8%
Metabolic and Nutritional			
Peripheral edema	<1%	<1%	1%
Nervous System			
Amnesia	1%	2%	4%
Confusion	<1%	<1%	1%
Depersonalization	<1%	<1%	2%
Dizziness	7%	7%	9%
Hallucinations	<1%	<1%	1%
Hypertonia	<1%	1%	1%
Hypesthesia	<1%	<1%	2%
Paresthesia	1%	3%	3%
Somnolence	4%	5%	6%
Tremor	1%	2%	2%
Vertigo	<1%	<1%	1%
Respiratory System			
Epistaxis	<1%	<1%	1%
Special Senses			
Abnormal vision	<1%	<1%	2%
Ear pain	0%	<1%	1%
Eye pain	2%	4%	3%
Hyperacusis	<1%	1%	2%
Parosmia	<1%	<1%	2%
Urogenital System			
Dysmenorrhea	2%	3%	4%

* Events for which the incidence for zaleplon 20 mg-treated patients was at least 1% and greater than the incidence among placebo-treated patients. Incidence greater than 1% has been rounded to the nearest whole number.

OTHER ADVERSE EVENTS OBSERVED DURING THE PREMARKETING EVALUATION OF ZALEPLON

Listed below are COSTART terms that reflect treatment-emergent adverse events as defined in the introduction to ADVERSE REACTIONS. These events were reported by patients treated with zaleplon at doses in a range of 5-20 mg/day during premarketing Phase 2 and 3 clinical trials throughout the US, Canada, and Europe including approximately 2900 patients. All reported events are included except those already listed in TABLE 1 or elsewhere in labeling, those events for which a drug cause was remote, and those event terms that were so general as to be uninformative. It is important to emphasize that although the events reported occurred during treatment with zaleplon, they were not necessarily caused by it.

Events are further categorized by body system and listed in order of decreasing frequency according to the following definitions: *Frequent:* Adverse events are those occurring on 1 or more occasions in at least 1/100 patients; *Infrequent:* Adverse events are those occurring in less than 1/100 patients but at least 1/1000 patients; *Rare:* Events are those occurring in fewer than 1/1000 patients.

Body as a Whole: *Frequent:* Back pain, chest pain, fever; *Infrequent:* Chest pain substernal, chills, face edema, generalized edema, hangover effect, neck rigidity.

Cardiovascular System: *Frequent:* Migraine; *Infrequent:* Angina pectoris, bundle branch block, hypertension, hypotension, palpitation, syncope, tachycardia, vasodilatation, ventricular extrasystoles; *Rare:* Bigeminy, cerebral ischemia, cyanosis, pericardial effusion, postural hypotension, pulmonary embolus, sinus bradycardia, thrombophlebitis, ventricular tachycardia.

Digestive System: *Frequent:* Constipation, dry mouth, dyspepsia; *Infrequent:* Eructation, esophagitis, flatulence, gastritis, gastroenteritis, gingivitis, glossitis, increased appetite, melena, mouth ulceration, rectal hemorrhage, stomatitis; *Rare:* Aphthous stomatitis, biliary pain, bruxism, cardiospasm, cheilitis, cholelithiasis, duodenal ulcer, dysphagia, enteritis, gum hemorrhage, increased salivation, intestinal obstruction, abnormal liver function tests, peptic ulcer, tongue discoloration, tongue edema, ulcerative stomatitis.

Endocrine System: *Rare:* Diabetes mellitus, goiter, hypothyroidism.

Hemic and Lymphatic System: *Infrequent:* Anemia, ecchymosis, lymphadenopathy; *Rare:* Eosinophilia, leukocytosis, lymphocytosis, purpura.

Metabolic and Nutritional: *Infrequent:* Edema, gout, hypercholesteremia, thirst, weight gain; *Rare:* Bilirubinemia, hyperglycemia, hyperuricemia, hypoglycemia, hypoglycemic reaction, ketosis, lactose intolerance, AST (SGOT) increased, ALT (SGPT) increased, weight loss.

Musculoskeletal System: *Frequent:* Arthralgia, arthritis, myalgia; *Infrequent:* Arthrosis, bursitis, joint disorder (mainly swelling, stiffness, and pain), myasthenia, tenosynovitis; *Rare:* Myositis, osteoporosis.

Nervous System: *Frequent:* Anxiety, depression, nervousness, thinking abnormal (mainly difficulty concentrating); *Infrequent:* Abnormal gait, agitation, apathy, ataxia, circumoral paresthesia, emotional lability, euphoria, hyperesthesia, hyperkinesia, hypotonia, incoordination, insomnia, libido decreased, neuralgia, nystagmus; *Rare:* CNS stimulation, delusions, dysarthria, dystonia, facial paralysis, hostility, hypokinesia, myoclonus, neuropathy, psychomotor retardation, ptosis, reflexes decreased, reflexes increased, sleep talking, sleep walking, slurred speech, stupor, trismus.

Respiratory System: *Frequent:* Bronchitis; *Infrequent:* Asthma, dyspnea, laryngitis, pneumonia, snoring, voice alteration; *Rare:* Apnea, hiccup, hyperventilation, pleural effusion, sputum increased.

Skin and Appendages: *Frequent:* Pruritus, rash; *Infrequent:* Acne, alopecia, contact dermatitis, dry skin, eczema, maculopapular rash, skin hypertrophy, sweating, urticaria, vesiculobullous rash; *Rare:* Melanosis, psoriasis, pustular rash, skin discoloration.

Special Senses: *Frequent:* Conjunctivitis, taste perversion; *Infrequent:* Diplopia, dry eyes, photophobia, tinnitus, watery eyes; *Rare:* Abnormality of accommodation, blepharitis, cataract specified, corneal erosion, deafness, eye hemorrhage, glaucoma, labyrinthitis, retinal detachment, taste loss, visual field defect.

Urogenital System: *Infrequent:* Bladder pain, breast pain, cystitis, decreased urine stream, dysuria, hematuria, impotence, kidney calculus, kidney pain, menorrhagia, metrorrhagia, urinary frequency, urinary incontinence, urinary urgency, vaginitis; *Rare:* Albuminuria, delayed menstrual period, leukorrhea, menopause, urethritis, urinary retention, vaginal hemorrhage.

DOSAGE AND ADMINISTRATION

The dose of zaleplon should be individualized. The recommended dose of zaleplon for most nonelderly adults is 10 mg. For certain low weight individuals, 5 mg may be a sufficient dose. Although the risk of certain adverse events associated with the use of zaleplon appears to be dose dependent, the 20 mg dose has been shown to be adequately tolerated and may be considered for the occasional patient who does not benefit from a trial of a lower dose. Doses above 20 mg have not been adequately evaluated and are not recommended.

Zaleplon should be taken immediately before bedtime or after the patient has gone to bed and has experienced difficulty falling asleep (see PRECAUTIONS). Taking zaleplon with or immediately after a heavy, high-fat meal results in slower absorption and would be expected to reduce the effect of zaleplon on sleep latency (see CLINICAL PHARMACOLOGY,Pharmacokinetics).

SPECIAL POPULATIONS

Elderly patients and debilitated patients appear to be more sensitive to the effects of hypnotics, and respond to 5 mg of zaleplon. The recommended dose for these patients is therefore 5 mg. Doses over 10 mg are not recommended.

Hepatic Insufficiency: Patients with mild to moderate hepatic impairment should be treated with zaleplon 5 mg because clearance is reduced in this population. Zaleplon is not recommended for use in patients with severe hepatic impairment.

Renal Insufficiency: No dose adjustment is necessary in patients with mild to moderate renal impairment. Zaleplon has not been adequately studied in patients with severe renal impairment.

An initial dose of 5 mg should be given to patients concomitantly taking cimetidine because zaleplon clearance is reduced in this population (see DRUG INTERACTIONS).

HOW SUPPLIED

Sonata capsules are available in the following dosage strengths:

5 mg: Opaque green cap and opaque pale green body with "5 mg" on the cap and "SONATA" on the body.

10 mg: Opaque green cap and opaque light green body with "10 mg" on the cap and "SONATA" on the body.

Storage: Store at controlled room temperature, 20-25°C (68-77°F). Dispense in a light-resistant container.

PRODUCT LISTING - EQUIVALENTS NOT AVAILABLE

Capsule - Oral - 5 mg

100's	$208.99	SONATA, Wyeth-Ayerst Laboratories	00008-0925-81

Capsule - Oral - 10 mg

100's	$257.05	SONATA, Wyeth-Ayerst Laboratories	00008-0926-81

Zanamivir (003439)

Categories: Influenza; FDA Approved 1999 Jul; Pregnancy Category B
Drug Classes: Antivirals
Brand Names: Relenza
Cost of Therapy: $46.18 (Influenza; Relenza; 5 mg/inhalation; 4 inhalations/day; 5 day supply)

DESCRIPTION

For Oral Inhalation Only.

For Use With the Diskhaler Inhalation Device.

The active component of Relenza is zanamivir. The chemical name of zanamivir is 5-(acetylamino)-4-[(aminoiminomethyl)-amino]-2,6-anhydro-3,4,5-trideoxy-D-glycero-D-galacto-non-2-enonic acid. It has a molecular formula of $C_{12}H_{20}N_4O_7$ and a molecular weight of 332.3.

Zanamivir is a white to off-white powder with a solubility of approximately 18 mg/ml in water at 20°C.

Relenza is for administration to the respiratory tract by oral inhalation only. Each Relenza Rotadisk contains 4 regularly spaced double-foil blisters with each blister containing a powder mixture of 5 mg of zanamivir and 20 mg of lactose. The contents of each blister are inhaled using a specially designed breath-activated plastic device for inhaling powder called the Diskhaler. After a Relenza Rotadisk is loaded into the Diskhaler, a blister that contains medication is pierced and the zanamivir is dispersed into the air stream created when the patient inhales through the mouthpiece. The amount of drug delivered to the respiratory tract will depend on patient factors such as inspiratory flow. Under standardized *in vitro* testing, Relenza Rotadisk delivers 4 mg of zanamivir from the Diskhaler device when tested at a pressure drop of 3 kPa (corresponding to a flow rate of about 62-65 L/min) for 3 seconds. In a study of 5 adult and 5 adolescent patients with obstructive airway diseases, the combined peak inspiratory flow rates (PIFR) ranged from 66-140 L/min. In a separate study of 16 pediatric patients, PIFR results were more variable; 4 did not achieve measurable flow rates, and PIFR for measurable inhalations by 12 children ranged from 30.5-122.4 L/min. Only 1 of 4 children under age 8 had a measurable flow rate (see CLINICAL PHARMACOLOGY, Pediatric Patients and PRECAUTIONS,Pediatric Use).

CLINICAL PHARMACOLOGY

MICROBIOLOGY

Mechanism of Action

The proposed mechanism of action of zanamivir is via inhibition of influenza virus neuraminidase with the possibility of alteration of virus particle aggregation and release.

Antiviral Activity In Vitro

The antiviral activity of zanamivir against laboratory and clinical isolates of influenza virus was determined in cell culture assays. The concentrations of zanamivir required for inhibition of influenza virus were highly variable depending on the assay method used and virus isolate tested. The 50% and 90% inhibitory concentrations (IC_{50} and IC_{90}) of zanamivir were in the range of 0.005 to 16.0 µm and 0.05 to >100 µm, respectively (1 µm = 0.33 µg/ml). The relationship between the *in vitro* inhibition of influenza virus by zanamivir and the inhibition of influenza virus replication in humans has not been established.

Drug Resistance

Influenza viruses with reduced susceptibility to zanamivir have been recovered *in vitro* by passage of the virus in the presence of increasing concentrations of the drug. Genetic analysis of these viruses showed that the reduced susceptibility *in vitro* to zanamivir is associated with mutations that result in amino acid changes in the viral neuraminidase or viral hemagglutinin or both.

In an immunocompromised patient infected with influenza B virus, a variant virus emerged after treatment with an investigational nebulized solution of zanamivir for 2 weeks. Analysis of this variant showed a hemagglutinin mutation (Thr 198 IIe) which resulted in a reduced affinity for human cell receptors, and a mutation in the neuraminidase active site (Arg 152 Lys) which reduced the enzyme's activity to zanamivir by 1000-fold.

Insufficient information is available to characterize the risk of emergence of zanamivir resistance in clinical use.

Cross-Resistance

Cross-resistance has been observed between zanamivir-resistant and oseltamivir-resistant influenza virus mutants generated *in vitro*. No studies have been performed to assess risk of emergence of cross-resistance during clinical use.

Influenza Vaccine Interaction Study

An interaction study (n=138) was conducted to evaluate the effects of zanamivir (10 mg once daily) on the serological response to a single dose of trivalent inactivated influenza vaccine, as measured by hemagglutination inhibition titers. There was no clear difference in hemagglutination inhibition antibody titers at 2 and 4 weeks after vaccine administration between zanamivir and placebo recipients.

Influenza Challenge Studies

Antiviral activity of zanamivir was supported for influenza A, and to a more limited extent for influenza B, by Phase 1 studies in volunteers who received intranasal inoculations of challenge strains of influenza virus, and received an intranasal formulation of zanamivir or placebo starting before or shortly after viral inoculation.

PHARMACOKINETICS

Absorption and Bioavailability

Pharmacokinetic studies of orally inhaled zanamivir indicate that approximately 4-17% of the inhaled dose is systemically absorbed. The peak serum concentrations ranged from 17-142 ng/ml within 1-2 hours following a 10 mg dose. The area under the serum concentration versus time curve [AUC(∞)] ranged from 111-1364 ng·h/ml.

Distribution

Zanamivir has limited plasma protein binding (<10%).

Metabolism

Zanamivir is renally excreted as unchanged drug. No metabolites have been detected in humans.

Elimination

The serum half-life of zanamivir following administration by oral inhalation ranges from 2.5-5.1 hours. It is excreted unchanged in the urine with excretion of a single dose completed within 24 hours. Total clearance ranges from 2.5-10.9 L/h. Unabsorbed drug is excreted in the feces.

Special Populations

Impaired Hepatic Function

The pharmacokinetics of zanamivir have not been studied in patients with impaired hepatic function.

Impaired Renal Function

Systemic exposure is limited after inhalation (see Absorption and Bioavailability). After a single intravenous dose of 4 or 2 mg of zanamivir in volunteers with mild/moderate or severe renal impairment, respectively, significant decreases in renal clearance (and hence total clearance: normals 5.3 L/h, mild/moderate 2.7 L/h, and severe 0.8 L/h; median values) and significant increases in half-life (normals 3.1 h, mild/moderate 4.7 h, and severe 18.5 h; median values) and systemic exposure were observed. Safety and efficacy have not been documented in the presence of severe renal insufficiency.

Pediatric Patients

The pharmacokinetics of zanamivir were evaluated in pediatric patients with signs and symptoms of respiratory illness. Sixteen (16) patients, 6-12 years of age, received a single dose of 10 mg zanamivir dry powder via inhalation device. Five (5) patients had either undetectable zanamivir serum concentrations or had low drug concentrations (8.32-10.38 ng/ml) that were not detectable after 1.5 hours. Eleven (11) patients had C_{max} median values of 43 ng/ml (range 15-74) and AUC(∞) median values of 167 ng·h/ml (range 58-279). Low or undetectable serum concentrations were related to lack of measurable PIFR in individual patients (see DESCRIPTION and PRECAUTIONS, Pediatric Use).

Geriatric Patients

The pharmacokinetics of zanamivir have not been studied in patients over 65 years of age (see PRECAUTIONS, Geriatric Use).

Gender, Race, and Weight

In a population pharmacokinetic analysis in patient studies, no clinically significant differences in serum concentrations and/or pharmacokinetic parameters (V/F, CL/F, Ka, AUC(0-3), C_{max}, T_{max}, CLR, and percent excreted in urine) were observed when demographic variables (gender, age, race, and weight) and indices of infection (laboratory evidence of infection, overall symptoms, symptoms of upper respiratory illness, and viral titers) were considered. There were no significant correlations between measures of systemic exposure and safety parameters.

Drug Interactions

No clinically significant pharmacokinetic drug interactions are predicted based on data from *in vitro* studies.

Zanamivir is not a substrate nor does it affect cytochrome P450 (CYP) isoenzymes (CYP1A1/2, 2A6, 2C9, 2C18, 2D6, 2E1, and 3A4) in human liver microsomes.

INDICATIONS AND USAGE

Zanamivir is indicated for treatment of uncomplicated acute illness due to influenza A and B virus in adults and pediatric patients 7 years and older who have been symptomatic for no more than 2 days (see PRECAUTIONS).

CONTRAINDICATIONS

Zanamivir is contraindicated in patients with a known hypersensitivity to any component of the formulation.

WARNINGS

BRONCHOSPASM AND DECLINE IN LUNG FUNCTION HAVE BEEN REPORTED IN SOME PATIENTS RECEIVING ZANAMIVIR. MANY BUT NOT ALL OF THESE PATIENTS HAD UNDERLYING AIRWAYS DISEASE SUCH AS ASTHMA OR CHRONIC OBSTRUCTIVE PULMONARY DISEASE. BECAUSE OF THE RISK OF SERIOUS ADVERSE EVENTS AND BECAUSE EFFICACY HAS NOT BEEN DEMONSTRATED IN THIS POPULATION, ZANAMIVIR IS NOT GENERALLY RECOMMENDED FOR TREATMENT OF PATIENTS WITH UNDERLYING AIRWAYS DISEASE (SEE PRECAUTIONS). Some patients with serious adverse events during treatment with zanamivir have had fatal outcomes, although causality was difficult to assess.

ZANAMIVIR SHOULD BE DISCONTINUED IN ANY PATIENT WHO DEVELOPS BRONCHOSPASM OR DECLINE IN RESPIRATORY FUNCTION; immediate treatment and hospitalization may be required. Some patients without prior pulmonary disease may also have respiratory abnormalities from acute respiratory infection that could resemble adverse drug reactions or increase patient vulnerability to adverse drug reactions.

PRECAUTIONS

GENERAL

Patients should be instructed in the use of the delivery system. Instructions should include a demonstration whenever possible. Patients should read and follow carefully the Patient Instructions for Use accompanying the product. Effective and safe use of zanamivir requires proper use of the inhalation device to inhale the drug.

There is no evidence for efficacy of zanamivir in any illness caused by agents other than influenza virus A and B.

No data are available to support safety or efficacy in patients who begin treatment after 48 hours of symptoms.

Safety and efficacy of repeated treatment courses have not been studied.

PATIENTS WITH RESPIRATORY DISEASE

SAFETY AND EFFICACY OF ZANAMIVIR HAVE NOT BEEN DEMONSTRATED IN PATIENTS WITH UNDERLYING CHRONIC PULMONARY DISEASE (SEE WARNINGS). IN PARTICULAR, ZANAMIVIR HAS NOT BEEN SHOWN TO BE EFFECTIVE IN PATIENTS WITH SEVERE OR DECOMPENSATED CHRONIC OBSTRUCTIVE PULMONARY DISEASE OR ASTHMA, AND SERIOUS ADVERSE EVENTS HAVE BEEN REPORTED IN SUCH PATIENTS. THEREFORE, ZANAMIVIR IS NOT GENERALLY RECOMMENDED FOR TREATMENT OF PATIENTS WITH UNDERLYING AIRWAYS DISEASE SUCH AS ASTHMA OR CHRONIC OBSTRUCTIVE PULMONARY DISEASE (SEE WARNINGS).

Bronchospasm was documented following administration of zanamivir in 1 of 13 patients with mild or moderate asthma (but without acute influenza-like illness) in a Phase 1 study. In interim results from an ongoing treatment study in patients with acute influenza-like illness superimposed on underlying asthma or chronic obstructive pulmonary disease, more patients on zanamivir than on placebo experienced greater than 20% decline in FEV_1 or peak expiratory flow rate.

If treatment with zanamivir is considered for a patient with underlying airways disease, the potential risks and benefits should be carefully weighed. If a decision is made to prescribe zanamivir for such a patient, this should be done only under conditions of careful

Z

monitoring of respiratory function, close observation, and appropriate supportive care including availability of fast-acting bronchodilators.

ALLERGIC REACTIONS

Allergic-like reactions, including oropharyngeal edema and serious skin rashes, have been reported in post-marketing experience with zanamivir. Zanamivir should be stopped and appropriate treatment instituted if an allergic reaction occurs or is suspected.

BACTERIAL INFECTIONS

Serious bacterial infections may begin with influenza-like symptoms or may coexist with or occur as complications during the course of influenza. Zanamivir has not been shown to prevent such complications.

PREVENTION OF INFLUENZA

Use of zanamivir should not affect the evaluation of individuals for annual influenza vaccination in accordance with guidelines of the Centers for Disease Control and Prevention Advisory Committee on Immunization Practices. Safety and efficacy of zanamivir have not been established for prophylactic use of zanamivir to prevent influenza.

LIMITATIONS OF POPULATIONS STUDIED

Safety and efficacy have not been demonstrated in patients with high-risk underlying medical conditions (see WARNINGS). No information is available regarding treatment of influenza in patients with any medical condition sufficiently severe or unstable to be considered at imminent risk of requiring inpatient management.

INFORMATION FOR THE PATIENT

Patients should be instructed in use of the delivery system. Instructions should include a demonstration whenever possible.

For the proper use of zanamivir, the patient should read and follow carefully the accompanying Patient Instructions for Use.

Patients should be advised that the use of zanamivir for treatment of influenza has not been shown to reduce the risk of transmission of influenza to others.

Patients should be advised of the risk of bronchospasm, especially in the setting of underlying airways disease, and should stop zanamivir and contact their physician if they experience increased respiratory symptoms during treatment such as worsening wheezing, shortness of breath, or other signs or symptoms of bronchospasm (see WARNINGS). If a decision is made to prescribe zanamivir for a patient with asthma or chronic obstructive pulmonary disease, the patient should be made aware of the risks and should have a fast-acting bronchodilator available. Patients scheduled to take inhaled bronchodilators at the same time as zanamivir should be advised to use their bronchodilators before taking zanamivir.

CARCINOGENESIS, MUTAGENESIS, AND IMPAIRMENT OF FERTILITY

Carcinogenesis

In 2 year carcinogenicity studies conducted in rats and mice using a powder formulation administered through inhalation, zanamivir induced no statistically significant increases in tumors over controls. The maximum daily exposures in rats and mice were approximately 23-25 and 20-22 times, respectively, greater than those in humans at the proposed clinical dose based on AUC comparisons.

Mutagenesis

Zanamivir was not mutagenic in *in vitro* and *in vivo* genotoxicity assays which included bacterial mutation assays in *S. typhimurium* and *E. coli,* mammalian mutation assays in mouse lymphoma, chromosomal aberration assays in human peripheral blood lymphocytes, and the *in vivo* mouse bone marrow micronucleus assay.

Impairment of Fertility

The effects of zanamivir on fertility and general reproductive performance were investigated in male (dosed for 10 weeks prior to mating, and throughout mating, gestation/lactation, and shortly after weaning) and female rats (dosed for 3 weeks prior to mating through day 19 of pregnancy, or day 21 post partum) at IV doses 1, 9, and 90 mg/kg/day. Zanamivir did not impair mating or fertility of male or female rats, and did not affect the sperm of treated male rats. The reproductive performance of the F1 generation born to female rats given zanamivir was not affected. Based on a subchronic study in rats at a 90 mg/kg/day IV dose, AUC values ranged between 142 and 199 μg·h/ml (>300 times the human exposure at the proposed clinical dose).

PREGNANCY CATEGORY C

Embryo/fetal development studies were conducted in rats (dosed from days 6-15 of pregnancy) and rabbits (dosed from days 7-19 of pregnancy) using the same IV doses. Pre- and post-natal developmental studies were performed in rats (dosed from day 16 of pregnancy until litter day 21 to 23). In all studies, intravenous (1, 9, and 90 mg/kg/day) instead of the inhalational route of drug administration was used. No malformations, maternal toxicity, or embryotoxicity were observed in pregnant rats or rabbits and their fetuses. Because of insufficient blood sampling timepoints in both rat and rabbit reproductive toxicity studies, AUC values were not available. However, in a subchronic study in rats at the 90 mg/kg/day IV dose, the AUC values were greater than 300 times the human exposure at the proposed clinical dose.

An additional embryo/fetal study, in a different strain of rat, was conducted using subcutaneous administration of zanamivir, 3 times daily, at doses of 1, 9, or 80 mg/kg during days 7-17 of pregnancy. There was an increase in the incidence rates of a variety of minor skeleton alterations and variants in the exposed offspring in this study. Based on AUC measurements, the high dose in the study produced an exposure greater than 1000 times the human exposure at the proposed clinical dose. However, the individual incidence rate of each skeletal alteration or variant, in most instances, remained within the background rates of the historical occurrence in the strain studied.

Zanamivir has been shown to cross the placenta in rats and rabbits. In these animals, fetal blood concentrations of zanamivir were significantly lower than zanamivir concentrations in the maternal blood.

There are no adequate and well-controlled studies of zanamivir in pregnant women. Zanamivir should be used during pregnancy only if the potential benefit justifies the potential risk to the fetus.

NURSING MOTHERS

Studies in rats have demonstrated that zanamivir is excreted in milk. However, nursing mothers should be instructed that it is not known whether zanamivir is excreted in human milk. Because many drugs are excreted in human milk, caution should be exercised when zanamivir is administered to a nursing mother.

PEDIATRIC USE

Safety and effectiveness of zanamivir have not been established in pediatric patients under 7 years of age.

The safety and effectiveness of zanamivir have been studied in a Phase 3 treatment study in pediatric patients, where 471 children 5-12 years of age received zanamivir or placebo (see ADVERSE REACTIONS and DOSAGE AND ADMINISTRATION). In a Phase 1 study of 16 children ages 6-12 years with signs and symptoms of respiratory disease, 4 did not produce a measurable peak inspiratory flow rate (PIFR) through the inhalation device (3 with no adequate inhalation on request, 1 with missing data), 9 had measurable PIFR on each of 2 inhalations, and 3 achieved measurable PIFR on only 1 of 2 inhalations. Neither of the two 6-year-olds and one of two 7-year-olds produced measurable PIFR. Overall, 8 of the 16 children (including all those under 8 years old) either did not produce measurable inspiratory flow through the inhalation device or produced peak inspiratory flow rates below the 60 L/min considered optimal for the device under standardized *in vitro* testing; lack of measurable flow rate was related to low or undetectable serum concentrations (see DESCRIPTION and CLINICAL PHARMACOLOGY, Pediatric Patients). Prescribers should carefully evaluate the ability of young children to use the delivery system if prescription of zanamivir is considered. When zanamivir is prescribed for children, it should be used only under adult supervision and with attention to proper use of the delivery system.

Adolescents were included in the 3 principal Phase 3 adult treatment studies. In these studies, 67 patients were 12-16 years of age. No definite differences in safety and efficacy were observed between these adolescent patients and young adults.

GERIATRIC USE

Of the total number of patients in 6 clinical treatment studies of zanamivir, 59 were 65 and over, while 24 were 75 and over. No overall differences in safety or effectiveness were observed between these subjects and younger patients, and other reported clinical experience has not identified differences in responses between the elderly and younger patients, but greater sensitivity of some older individuals cannot be ruled out.

DRUG INTERACTIONS

No clinically significant pharmacokinetic drug interactions are predicted based on data from *in vitro* studies.

ADVERSE REACTIONS

See WARNINGS and PRECAUTIONS for information about risk of serious adverse events such as bronchospasm and allergic-like reactions, and for safety information in patients with underlying respiratory disease.

CLINICAL TRIALS IN ADULTS AND ADOLESCENTS

Adverse events that occurred with an incidence ≥1.5% in treatment studies are listed in TABLE 1. This table shows adverse events occurring in patients ≥12 years of age receiving zanamivir 10 mg inhaled twice daily, zanamivir in all inhalation regimens, and placebo inhaled twice daily (where placebo consisted of the same lactose vehicle used in zanamivir).

TABLE 1 *Summary of Adverse Events ≥1.5% Incidence During Treatment in Adults and Adolescents*

	Zanamivir		
	10 mg bid Inhaled	All Dosing Regimens*	Placebo (Lactose Vehicle†)
Adverse Event	(n=1132)	(n=2289)	(n=1520)
Body as a Whole			
Headaches	2%	2%	3%
Digestive			
Diarrhea	3%	3%	4%
Nausea	3%	3%	3%
Vomiting	1%	1%	2%
Respiratory			
Nasal signs and symptoms	2%	3%	3%
Bronchitis	2%	2%	3%
Cough	2%	2%	3%
Sinusitis	3%	2%	2%
Ear, nose, & throat infections	2%	1%	2%
Nervous System			
Dizziness	2%	1%	<1%

* Includes studies where zanamivir was administered intranasally (6.4 mg 2-4 times per day in addition to inhaled preparation) and/or inhaled more frequently (qid) than the currently recommended dose.

† Because the placebo consisted of inhaled lactose powder, which is also the vehicle for the active drug, some adverse events occurring at similar frequencies in different treatment groups could be related to lactose vehicle inhalation.

Additional adverse reactions occurring in less than 1.5% of patients receiving zanamivir included malaise, fatigue, fever, abdominal pain, myalgia, arthralgia, and urticaria.

The most frequent laboratory abnormalities in Phase 3 treatment studies included elevations of liver enzymes and CPK, lymphopenia, and neutropenia. These were reported in similar proportions of zanamivir and lactose vehicle placebo recipients with acute influenza-like illness.

CLINICAL TRIALS IN PEDIATRIC PATIENTS

Adverse events that occurred with an incidence of ≥1.5% in children receiving treatment doses of zanamivir in two Phase 3 studies are listed in TABLE 2. This table shows adverse events occurring in pediatric patients 5-12 years old receiving zanamivir 10 mg inhaled twice daily, and placebo inhaled twice daily (where placebo consisted of the same lactose vehicle used in zanamivir).

TABLE 2 *Summary of Adverse Events ≥ 1.5% Incidence During Treatment in Pediatric Patients**

Adverse Event	Zanamivir 10 mg bid Inhaled (n=291)	Placebo (Lactose Vehicle†) (n=318)
Respiratory		
Ear, nose, & throat infections	5%	5%
Ear, nose, & throat hemorrhage	<1%	2%
Asthma	<1%	2%
Cough	<1%	2%
Digestive		
Vomiting	2%	3%
Diarrhea	2%	2%
Nausea	<1%	2%

* Includes a subset of patients receiving zanamivir for treatment of influenza in a prophylaxis study.

† Because the placebo consisted of inhaled lactose powder, which is also the vehicle for the active drug, some adverse events occurring at similar frequencies in different treatment groups could be related to lactose vehicle inhalation.

In 1 of the 2 studies described in TABLE 2, some additional information is available from children (5-12 years old) without acute influenza-like illness who received an investigational prophylaxis regimen of zanamivir; 132 children received zanamivir and 145 children received placebo. Among these children, nasal signs and symptoms (zanamivir 20%, placebo 9%), cough (zanamivir 16%, placebo 8%), and throat/tonsil discomfort and pain (zanamivir 11%, placebo 6%) were reported more frequently with zanamivir than placebo. In a subset with chronic respiratory disease, lower respiratory adverse events (described as asthma, cough, or viral respiratory infections which could include influenza-like symptoms) were reported in 7 of 7 zanamivir recipients and 5 of 12 placebo recipients.

OBSERVED DURING CLINICAL PRACTICE

In addition to adverse events reported from clinical trials, the following events have been identified during post-marketing use of zanamivir. Because they are reported voluntarily from a population of unknown size, estimates of frequency cannot be made. These events have been chosen for inclusion due to a combination of their seriousness, frequency of reporting, or potential causal connection to zanamivir.

General: Allergic or allergic-like reaction, including oropharyngeal edema (see PRECAUTIONS).

Cardiac: Arrhythmias, syncope.

Neurologic: Seizures.

Respiratory: Bronchospasm, dyspnea (see WARNINGS and PRECAUTIONS).

Skin: Facial edema; rash, including serious cutaneous reactions (see PRECAUTIONS).

DOSAGE AND ADMINISTRATION

Zanamivir is for administration to the respiratory tract by oral inhalation only, using the inhalation device provided. **Patients should be instructed in the use of the delivery system. Instructions should include a demonstration whenever possible. If zanamivir is prescribed for children, it should be used only under adult supervision and instruction, and the supervising adult should first be instructed by a healthcare professional (see PRECAUTIONS).**

The recommended dose of zanamivir for treatment of influenza in adult and pediatric patients ages 7 years and older is 2 inhalations (one 5 mg blister per inhalation for a total dose of 10 mg) twice daily (approximately 12 hours apart) for 5 days. Two doses should be taken on the first day of treatment whenever possible provided there is at least 2 hours between doses. On subsequent days, doses should be about 12 hours apart (*e.g.,* morning and evening) at approximately the same time each day. There are no data on the effectiveness of treatment with zanamivir when initiated more than 2 days after the onset of signs or symptoms.

Patients scheduled to use an inhaled bronchodilator at the same time as zanamivir should use their bronchodilator before taking zanamivir. (See WARNINGS and PRECAUTIONS regarding patients with chronic respiratory disease and other medical conditions.)

HOW SUPPLIED

Relenza is supplied in a circular double-foil pack (a Rotadisk) containing 4 blisters of the drug. Five Rotadisks are packaged in a white polypropylene tube. The tube is packaged in a carton with 1 blue and gray Diskhaler inhalation device.

Storage: Store at 25°C (77°F); excursions permitted to 15-30°C (59-86°F). Keep out of reach of children. Do not puncture any Relenza Rotadisk blister until taking a dose using the Diskhaler.

PRODUCT LISTING - EQUIVALENTS NOT AVAILABLE

Powder - Inhalation - 5 mg

4 x 5	$52.53	RELENZA, Glaxosmithkline	00173-0681-01
20's	$46.18	RELENZA, Allscripts Pharmaceutical Company	54569-4830-00

Zidovudine (002451)

Categories: Infection, human immunodeficiency virus; Maternal-fetal HIV transmission prevention; Pregnancy Category C; FDA Approved 1987 Mar; Orphan Drugs; WHO Formulary

Drug Classes: Antivirals; Nucleoside reverse transcriptase inhibitors

Brand Names: AZT; Retrovir

Foreign Brand Availability: Adovi (Indonesia); Apo-Zidovudine (Canada); Aviral (Colombia); Avirzid (Indonesia); Novo-AZT (Canada); Pranadox (Mexico); Retrocar (Peru); Retrovir-AZT (Mexico; Peru); T-Za (Thailand); Zidis (Thailand); Zidovir (India); Zydowin (Benin; Burkina-Faso; Ethiopia; Gambia; Ghana; Guinea; Ivory-Coast; Kenya; Liberia; Malawi; Mali; Mauritania; Mauritius; Morocco; Niger; Nigeria; Senegal; Seychelles; Sierra-Leone; Sudan; Tanzania; Tunia; Uganda; Zambia; Zimbabwe)

Cost of Therapy: $318.52 (HIV; Retrovir; 300 mg; 2 tablets/day; 30 day supply)
$307.73 (HIV; Retrovir; 100 mg; 5 capsules/day; 30 day supply)

INTRAVENOUS

WARNING

FOR INTRAVENOUS INFUSION ONLY

ZIDOVUDINE HAS BEEN ASSOCIATED WITH HEMATOLOGIC TOXICITY, INCLUDING NEUTROPENIA AND SEVERE ANEMIA, PARTICULARLY IN PATIENTS WITH ADVANCED HIV DISEASE (SEE WARNINGS). PROLONGED USE OF ZIDOVUDINE HAS BEEN ASSOCIATED WITH SYMPTOMATIC MYOPATHY.

LACTIC ACIDOSIS AND SEVERE HEPATOMEGALY WITH STEATOSIS, INCLUDING FATAL CASES, HAVE BEEN REPORTED WITH THE USE OF NUCLEOSIDE ANALOGUES ALONE OR IN COMBINATION, INCLUDING ZIDOVUDINE AND OTHER ANTIRETROVIRALS (SEE WARNINGS).

DESCRIPTION

Retrovir is the brand name for zidovudine (formerly called azidothymidine [AZT]), a pyrimidine nucleoside analogue active against human immunodeficiency virus (HIV). Retrovir IV infusion is a sterile solution for intravenous (IV) infusion only. Each ml contains 10 mg zidovudine in water for injection. Hydrochloric acid and/or sodium hydroxide may have been added to adjust the pH to approximately 5.5. Retrovir IV infusion contains no preservatives.

The chemical name of zidovudine is 3′-azido-3′-deoxythymidine.

Zidovudine is a white to beige, odorless, crystalline solid with a molecular weight of 267.24 and a solubility of 20.1 mg/ml in water at 25°C. The molecular formula is $C_{10}H_{13}N_5O_4$.

CLINICAL PHARMACOLOGY

MICROBIOLOGY

Mechanism of Action

Zidovudine is a synthetic nucleoside analogue of the naturally occurring nucleoside, thymidine, in which the 3′-hydroxy (-OH) group is replaced by an azido (-N_3) group. Within cells, zidovudine is converted to the active metabolite, zidovudine 5′-triphosphate (AztTP), by the sequential action of the cellular enzymes. Zidovudine 5′-triphosphate inhibits the activity of the HIV reverse transcriptase both by competing for utilization with the natural substrate, deoxythymidine 5′-triphosphate (dTTP), and by its incorporation into viral DNA. The lack of a 3′-OH group in the incorporated nucleoside analogue prevents the formation of the 5′ to 3′ phosphodiester linkage essential for DNA chain elongation and, therefore, the viral DNA growth is terminated. The active metabolite AztTP is also a weak inhibitor of the cellular DNA polymerase-alpha and mitochondrial polymerase-gamma and has been reported to be incorporated into the DNA of cells in culture.

In Vitro HIV Susceptibility

The *in vitro* anti-HIV activity of zidovudine was assessed by infecting cell lines of lymphoblastic and monocytic origin and peripheral blood lymphocytes with laboratory and clinical isolates of HIV. The IC_{50} and IC_{90} values (50% and 90% inhibitory concentrations) were 0.003-0.013 and 0.03-0.13 μg/ml, respectively (1 nM = 0.27 ng/ml). The IC_{50} and IC_{90} values of HIV isolates recovered from 18 untreated AIDS/ARC patients were in the range of 0.003-0.013 μg/ml and 0.03 to 0.3 μg/ml, respectively. Zidovudine showed antiviral activity in all acutely infected cell lines; however, activity was substantially less in chronically infected cell lines. In drug combination studies with zalcitabine, didanosine, lamivudine, saquinavir, indinavir, ritonavir, nevirapine, delavirdine, or interferon-alpha, zidovudine showed additive to synergistic activity in cell culture. The relationship between the *in vitro* susceptibility of HIV to reverse transcriptase inhibitors and the inhibition of HIV replication in humans has not been established.

Drug Resistance

HIV isolates with reduced sensitivity to zidovudine have been selected *in vitro* and were also recovered from patients treated with zidovudine. Genetic analysis of the isolates showed mutations that result in 5 amino acid substitutions (Met41→Leu, A67→Asn, Lys70→Arg, Thr215→Tyr or Phe, and Lys219→Gln) in the viral reverse transcriptase. In general, higher levels of resistance were associated with greater number of mutations, with 215 mutation being the most significant.

Cross-Resistance

The potential for cross-resistance between HIV reverse transcriptase inhibitors and protease inhibitors is low because of the different enzyme targets involved. Combination therapy with zidovudine plus zalcitabine or didanosine does not appear to prevent the emergence of zidovudine-resistant isolates. Combination therapy with zidovudine plus lamivudine delayed the emergence of mutations conferring resistance to zidovudine. In some patients harboring zidovudine-resistant virus, combination therapy with zidovudine plus lamivudine restored phenotypic sensitivity to zidovudine by 12 weeks of treatment. HIV isolates with multidrug resistance to zidovudine, didanosine, zalcitabine, stavudine, and lamivudine were recovered from a small number of patients treated for ≥1 year with the combination of zidovudine and didanosine or zalcitabine. The pattern of resistant mutations in the combination therapy was different (Ala62→Val, Val75→Ile, Phe77→116Tyr, and Gln→151Met) from monotherapy, with mutation 151 being most significant for multidrug resistance. Site-directed mutagenesis studies showed that these mutations could also result in resistance to zalcitabine, lamivudine, and stavudine.

PHARMACOKINETICS

Adults

The pharmacokinetics of zidovudine have been evaluated in 22 adult HIV-infected patients in a Phase 1 dose-escalation study. Following IV dosing, dose-independent kinetics was observed over the range of 1-5 mg/kg. the major metabolite of zidovudine is 3′-azido-3′-deoxy-5′-*O*-β-*D*—glucopyranuronosylthymidine (GZDV). GZDV area under the curve (AUC) is about 3-fold greater than the zidovudine AUC. Urinary recvoer of zidovudine and GZDV accounts for 18% and 60%, respectively, following IV dosing. A second metabolite, 3′-amino-3′-deoxythymidine (AMT), has been identified in the plasma following single-dose IV administration of zidovudine. The AMT AUC was one-fifth of the zidovudine AUC.

The mean steady-state peak and trough concentrations of zidovudine at 2.5 mg/kg every 4 hours were 1.06 and 0.12 μg/ml, respectively.

The zidovudine cerebrospinal fluid (CSF)/plasma concentration ratio was determined in 39 patients receiving chronic therapy with zidovudine. The median ratio measured in 50 paired samples drawn 1-8 hours after the last dose of zidovudine was 0.6.

TABLE 1 *Zidovudine Pharmacokinetic Parameters Following Intravenous Administration in HIV-Infected Patients*

Parameter	n	Mean ±SD (except where noted)
Apparent volume of distribution (L/kg)	11	1.6 ± 0.6
Plasma proetin binding (%)		<38
CSF:plasma ratio*	39	0.6 [0.04-2.62]
Systemic clearance (L/h/kg)	18	1.6 (0.8-2.7)
Renal clearance (L/h/kg)	16	0.34 ± 0.05
Elimination half-life (h)†	19	1.1 (0.5-2.9)

* Median [range].
† Approximate range.

Adults With Impaired Renal Function

Zidovudine clearance was decreased resulting in increased zidovudine and GZDV half-life and AUC in patients with impaired renal function (n=14) following a single 200 mg oral dose (TABLE 2). Plasma concentrations of AMT were not determined. A dose adjustment should not be necessary for patients with creatinine clearance (CRCL) ≥15 ml/min.

TABLE 2 *Zidovudine Pharmacokinetic Parameters in Patients With Severe Renal Impairment**

Parameter	Control Subjects† (n=6)	Patients With Renal Impairment (n=14)
CRCL (ml/min)	120 ± 8	18 ± 2
Zidovudine AUC (ng·h/ml)	1400 ± 200	3100 ± 300
Zidovudine half-life (h)	1.0 ± 0.2	1.4 ± 0.1

* Data are expressed as mean ± standard deviation.
† Normal renal function.

The pharmacokinetics and tolerance of oral zidovudine were evaluated in a multiple-dose study in patients undergoing hemodialysis (n=5) or peritoneal dialysis (n=6) recieving escalating doses up to 200 mg 5 times daily for 8 weeks. Daily doses of 500 mg or less were well tolerated despite significantly elevated GZDV plasma concentrations. Apparent zidovudine oral clearance was approximately 50% of that reported in patients with normal renal function. Hemodialysis and peritoneal dialysis appear to have a negligible effect on the removal of zidovudine, whereas GZDV elimination is enhanced. A dosage adjustment is recommended for patients undergoing hemodialysis or peritoneal dialysis (see DOSAGE AND ADMINISTRATION, Dose Adjustment).

Adults With Impaired Hepatic Function

Data describing the effect of hepatic impairment on the pharmacokinetics of zidovudine are limited. However, because zidovudine is eliminated primarily by hepatic metabolism, it is expected that zidovudine clearance would be decreased and plasma concentrations would be increased following administration of the recommended adult doses to patients with hepatic impairment (see DOSAGE AND ADMINISTRATION, Dose Adjustment).

Pediatrics

Zidovudine pharmacokinetics have been evaluated in HIV-infected pediatric patients (TABLE 3).

Patients From 3 Months to 12 Years of Age

Overall, zidovudine pharmacokinetics in pediatric patients >3 months of age are similar to those in adult patients. Proportional increases in plasma zidovudine concentrations were observed following administration of oral solution from 90-240 mg/m^2 every 6 hours. Oral bioavailability, terminal half-life, and oral clearance were comparable to adult values. As in adult patients, the major route of elimination was by metabolism to GZDV. After IV dosing, about 29% of the dose was excreted in the urine unchanged and about 45% of the dose was excreted as GZDV (see DOSAGE AND ADMINISTRATION).

Patients Younger Than 3 Months of Age

Zidovudine pharmacokinetics have been evaluated in pediatric patients from birth to 3 months of life. Zidovudine elimination was determined immediately following birth in 8 neonates who were exposed to zidovudine *in utero*. The half-life was 13.0 ± 5.8 hours. In neonates ≤14 days old, bioavailability was greater, total body clearance was slower, and half-life was longer than in pediatric patients >14 days old. For dose recommendations for neonates, see DOSAGE AND ADMINISTRATION, Neonatal Dosing.

TABLE 3 *Zidovudine Pharmacokinetic Parameters in Pediatric Patients**

Parameter	Birth to 14 Days of Age	14 Days to 3 Months of Age	3 Months to 12 Years of Age
Oral bioavailability (%)	89 ± 19 n=15	61 ± 19 n=17	65 ± 24 n=18
CSF:plasma ratio	no data	no data	0.26 ± 0.17† n=28
CL (L/h/kg)	0.65 ± 0.29 n=18	1.14 ± 0.24 n=16	1.85 ± 0.47 n=20
Elimination half-life (h)	3.1 ± 1.2 n=21	1.9 ± 0.7 n=18	1.5 ± 0.7 n=21

* Data presented as mean ± standard deviation except where noted.
† CSF ratio determined at steady-state on constant IV infusion.

Pregnancy

Zidovudine pharmacokinetics have been studied in a Phase 1 study of 8 women during the last trimester of pregnancy. As pregnancy progressed, there was no evidence of drug accumulation. Zidovudine pharmacokinetics were similar to that of nonpregnant adults. Consistent with passive transmission of the drug across the placenta, zidovudine concentrations in neonatal plasma at birth were essentially equal to those in maternal plasma at delivery. Although data are limited, methadone maintenance therapy in 5 pregnant women did not appear to alter zidovudine pharmacokinetics. However, in another patient population, a potential for interaction has been identified (see PRECAUTIONS).

Nursing Mothers

The Centers for Disease Control and Prevention recommend that HIV-infected mothers not breastfeed their infants to avoid risking postnatal transmission of HIV. After administration of a single dose of 200 mg zidovudine to 13 HIV-infected women, the mean concentration of zidovudine was similar in human milk and serum (see PRECAUTIONS, Nursing Mothers).

Geriatric Patients

Zidovudine pharmacokinetics have not been studied in patients over 65 years of age.

Gender

A pharmacokinetic study in healthy male (n=12) and female (n=12) subjects showed no differences in zidovudine exposure (AUC) when a single dose of zidovudine was administered as the 300 mg zidovudine tblet.

DRUG INTERACTIONS

See TABLE 4 and DRUG INTERACTIONS.

Zidovudine Plus Lamivudine

No clinically significant alterations in lamivudine or zidovudine pharmacokinetics were observed in 12 asymptomatic HIV-infected adult patients given a single oral dose of zidovudine (200 mg) in combination with multiple oral doses of lamivudine (300 mg every 12 hours).

INDICATIONS AND USAGE

Zidovudine IV infusion in combination with other antiretroviral agents is indicated for the treatment of HIV infection.

MATERNAL-FETAL HIV TRANSMISSION

Zidovudine is also indicated for the prevention of maternal-fetal HIV transmission as part of a regimen that includes oral zidovudine beginning between 14 and 34 weeks of gestation, IV zidovudine during labor, and administration of zidovudine syrup to the neonate after birth. The efficacy of this regimen for preventing HIV transmission in women who have received zidovudine for a prolonged period before pregnancy has not been evaluated. The safety of zidovudine for the mother or fetus during the first trimester of pregnancy has not been assessed.

NON-FDA APPROVED INDICATIONS

In addition, zidovudine may be given prophylactically to health care workers to reduce the risk of seroconversion following inadvertent exposure to HIV, although this use is not approved by the FDA.

CONTRAINDICATIONS

Zidovudine IV infusion is contraindicated for patients who have potentially life-threatening allergic reactions to any of the components of the formulation.

TABLE 4 *Effect of Coadministered Drugs on Zidovudine AUC**

Coadministered Drug and Dose	Zidovudine Oral Dose	n	Zidovudine Concentrations AUC	Variability	Concentration of Coadministered Drug
Atovaquone 750 mg q12h with food	200 mg q8h	14	Inc 31%	Range 23-78%†	NS
Fluconazole 400 mg daily	200 mg q8h	12	Inc 74%	95% CI: 54-98%	Not reported
Methadone 30-90 mg daily	200 mg q4h	9	Inc 43%	Range 16-64%†	NS
Nelfinavir 750 mg q8h × 7-10 days	Single 200 mg	11	Dec 35%	Range 28-41%	NS
Probenecid 500 mg q6h × 2 days	2 mg/kg q8h × 3 days	3	Inc 106%	Range 100-170%†	Not assessed
Ritonavir 300 mg q6h × 4 days	200 mg q8h × 4 days	9	Dec 25%	95% CI: 15-34%	NS
Valproic acid 250 or 500 mg q8h × 4 days	100 mg q8h × 4 days	6	Inc 80%	Range 64-130%†	Not assessed

Note: ROUTINE DOSE MODIFICATION OF ZIDOVUDINE IS NOT WARRANTED WITH COADMINISTRATION OF THE DRUGS LISTED IN THIS TABLE.
* This table is not all inclusive.
† Estimated range of percent difference.
I Increase.
D Decrease.
NS No significant change.

WARNINGS

Combivir and Trizivir are combination product tablets that contain zidovudine as one of their components. Retrovir should not be administered concomitantly with Combivir or Trizivir .

The incidence of adverse reactions appears to increase with disease progression; patients should be monitored carefully, especially as disease progression occurs.

BONE MARROW SUPPRESSION

Zidovudine should be used with caution in patients who have bone marrow compromise evidenced by granulocyte count <1000 cells/mm^3 or hemoglobin <9.5 g/dl. In patients with advanced symptomatic HIV disease, anemia and neutropenia were the most significant adverse events observed. There have been reports of pancytopenia associated with the use of zidovudine, which was reversible in most instances, after discontinuance of the drug. However, significant anemia, in many cases requiring dose adjustment, discontinuation of zidovudine, and/or blood transfusions, has occurred during treatment with zidovudine alone or in combination with other antiretrovirals.

Frequent blood counts are strongly recommended in patients with advanced HIV disease who are treated with zidovudine. For HIV-infected individuals and patients with asymptomatic or early HIV disease, periodic blood counts are recommended. If anemia or neutropenia develops, dosage adjustments may be necessary (see DOSAGE AND ADMINISTRATION).

MYOPATHY

Myopathy and myositis with pathological changes, similar to that produced by HIV disease, have been associated with prolonged use of zidovudine.

LACTIC ACIDOSIS/SEVERE HEPATOMEGALY WITH STEATOSIS

Lactic acidosis and severe hepatomegaly with steatosis, including fatal cases, have been reported with the use of nucleoside analogues alone or in combination, including zidovudine and other antiretrovirals. A majority of these cases have been in women. Obesity and prolonged exposure to antiretroviral nucleoside analogues may be risk factors. Particular caution should be exercised when administering zidovudine to any patient with known risk factors for liver disease; however, cases have also been reported in patients with no known risk factors. Treatment with zidovudine should be suspended in any patient who develops clinical or laboratory findings suggestive of lactic acidosis or pronounced hepatotoxicity (which may include hepatomegaly and steatosis even in the absence of marked transaminase elevations).

PRECAUTIONS

GENERAL

Zidovudine is eliminated from the body primarily by renal excretion following metabolism in the liver (glucuronidation). In patients with severely impaired renal function (CRCL <15 ml/min), dosage reduction is recommended. Although the data are limited, zidovudine concentrations appear to be increased in patients with severely impaired hepatic function which may increase the risk of hematologic toxicity (see CLINICAL PHARMACOLOGY, Pharmacokinetics and DOSAGE AND ADMINISTRATION).

INFORMATION FOR THE PATIENT

Zidovudine is not a cure for HIV infection, and patients may continue to acquire illnesses associated with HIV infection, including opportunistic infections. Therefore, patients should be advised to seek medical care for any significant change in their health status.

The safety and efficacy of zidovudine in treating women, intravenous drug users, and racial minorities is not significantly different than that observed in white males.

Patients should be informed that the major toxicities of zidovudine are neutropenia and/or anemia. The frequency and severity of these toxicities are greater in patients with more advanced disease and in those who initiate therapy later in the course of their infection. They should be told that if toxicity develops, they may require transfusions or drug discontinuation. They should be told of the extreme importance of having their blood counts followed closely while on therapy, especially for patients with advanced symptomatic HIV disease. They should be cautioned about the use of other medications, including ganciclovir and interferon-alpha, which may exacerbate the toxicity of zidovudine (see DRUG INTERACTIONS). Patients should be informed that other adverse effects of zidovudine include nausea and vomiting. Patients should also be encouraged to contact their physician if they experience muscle weakness, shortness of breath, symptoms of hepatitis or pancreatitis, or any other unexpected adverse events while being treated with zidovudine.

Pregnant women considering the use of zidovudine during pregnancy for prevention of HIV transmission to their infants should be advised that transmission may still occur in some cases despite therapy. The long-term consequences of *in utero* and neonatal exposure to zidovudine are unknown, including the possible risk of cancer.

HIV-infected pregnant women should be advised not to breastfeed to avoid postnatal transmission of HIV to a child who may not yet be infected.

Patients should be advised that therapy with zidovudine has not been shown to reduce the risk of transmission of HIV to others through sexual contact or blood contamination.

CARCINOGENESIS, MUTAGENESIS, AND IMPAIRMENT OF FERTILITY

Zidovudine was administered orally at 3 dosage levels to separate groups of mice and rats (60 females and 60 males in each group). Initial single daily doses were 30, 60, and 120 mg/kg/day in mice and 80, 220, and 600 mg/kg/day in rats. The doses in mice were reduced to 20, 30, and 40 mg/kg/day after day 90 because of treatment-related anemia, whereas in rats only the high dose was reduced to 450 mg/kg/day on day 91, and then to 300 mg/kg/day on day 279.

In mice, 7 late-appearing (after 19 months) vaginal neoplasms (5 nonmetastasizing squamous cell carcinomas, 1 squamous cell papilloma, and 1 squamous polyp) occurred in animals given the highest dose. One late-appearing squamous cell papilloma occurred in the vagina of a middle-dose animal. No vaginal tumors were found at the lowest dose.

In rats, 2 late-appearing (after 20 months), nonmetastasizing vaginal squamous cell carcinomas occurred in animals given the highest dose. No vaginal tumors occurred at the low or middle dose in rats. No other drug-related tumors were observed in either sex of either species.

At doses that produced tumors in mice and rats, the estimated drug exposure (as measured by AUC) was approximately 3 times (mouse) and 24 times (rat) the estimated human exposure at the recommended therapeutic dose of 100 mg every 4 hours.

Two transplacental carcinogenicity studies were conducted in mice. One study administered zidovudine at doses of 20 or 40 mg/kg/day from gestation day 10 through parturition and lactation with dosing continuing in offspring for 24 months postnatally. The doses of zidovudine employed in this study produced zidovudine exposures approximately 3 times the estimated human exposure at recommended doses. After 24 months, an increase in incidence of vaginal tumors was noted with no increase in tumors in the liver or lung or any other organ in either gender. These findings are consistent with results of the standard oral carcinogenicity study in mice, as described earlier. A second study administered zidovudine at maximum tolerated doses of 12.5 or 25 mg/day (~1000 mg/kg nonpregnant body weight or ~450 mg/kg of term body weight) to pregnant mice from days 12-18 of gestation. There was an increase in the number of tumors in the lung, liver, and female reproductive tracts in the offspring of mice receiving the higher dose level of zidovudine. It is not known how predictive the results of rodent carcinogenicity studies may be for humans.

Zidovudine was mutagenic in a 5178Y/TK$^{+/-}$ mouse lymphoma assay, positive in an *in vitro* cell transformation assay, clastogenic in a cytogenetic assay using cultured human lymphocytes, and positive in mouse and rat micronucleus tests after repeated doses. It was negative in a cytogenetic study in rats given a single dose.

Zidovudine, administered to male and female rats at doses up to 7 times the usual adult dose based on body surface area considerations, had no effect on fertility judged by conception rates.

PREGNANCY CATEGORY C

Oral teratology studies in the rat and in the rabbit at doses up to 500 mg/kg/day revealed no evidence of teratogenicity with zidovudine. Zidovudine treatment resulted in embryo/fetal toxicity as evidenced by an increase in the incidence of fetal resorptions in rats given 150 or 450 mg/kg/day and rabbits given 500 mg/kg/day. The doses used in the teratology studies resulted in peak zidovudine plasma concentrations (after one-half of the daily dose) in rats 66-226 times, and in rabbits 12-87 times, mean steady-state peak human plasma concentrations (after one-sixth of the daily dose) achieved with the recommended daily dose (100 mg every 4 hours). In an *in vitro* experiment with fertilized mouse oocytes, zidovudine exposure resulted in a dose-dependent reduction in blastocyst formation. In an additional teratology study in rats, a dose of 3000 mg/kg/day (very near the oral median lethal dose in rats of 3683 mg/kg) caused marked maternal toxicity and an increase in the incidence of fetal malformations. This dose resulted in peak zidovudine plasma concentrations 350 times peak human plasma concentrations. (Estimated area-under-the-curve [AUC] in rats at this dose level was 300 times the daily AUC in humans given 600 mg/day.) No evidence of teratogenicity was seen in this experiment at doses of 600 mg/kg/day or less.

Two rodent transplacental carcinogenicity studies were conducted (see Carcinogenesis, Mutagenesis, and Impairment of Fertility).

A randomized, double-blind, placebo-controlled trial was conducted in HIV-infected pregnant women to determine the utility of zidovudine for the prevention of maternal-fetal HIV transmission. Congenital abnormalities occurred with similar frequency between neonates born to mothers who received zidovudine and neonates born to mothers who received placebo. Abnormalities were either problems in embryogenesis (prior to 14 weeks) or were recognized on ultrasound before or immediately after initiation of study drug.

Antiretroviral Pregnancy Registry: To monitor maternal-fetal outcomes of pregnant women exposed to zidovudine, an Antiretroviral Pregnancy Registry has been established. Physicians are encouraged to register patients by calling 1-800-258-4263.

NURSING MOTHERS

The Centers for Disease Control and Prevention recommend that HIV-infected women not breastfeed their infants to avoid risking postnatal transmission of HIV.

Zidovudine is excreted in human milk (see CLINICAL PHARMACOLOGY, Pharmacokinetics, Nursing Mothers). Because of both the potential for HIV transmission and the potential for serious adverse reactions in nursing infants, **mothers should be instructed not to breastfeed if they are receiving zidovudine** (see Pediatric Use and INDICATIONS AND USAGE, Maternal-Fetal HIV Transmission).

PEDIATRIC USE

Zidovudine has been studied in HIV-infected pediatric patients over 3 months of age who have HIV-related symptoms or who are asymptomatic with abnormal laboratory values indicating significant HIV-related immunosuppression. Zidovudine has also been studied in neonates perinatally exposed to HIV (see ADVERSE REACTIONS; DOSAGE AND ADMINISTRATION; and CLINICAL PHARMACOLOGY, Pharmacokinetics).

GERIATRIC USE

Clinical studies of zidovudine did not include sufficient numbers of subjects aged 65 and over to determine whether they respond differently from younger subjects. Other reported clinical experience has not identified differences in responses between the elderly and younger patients. In general, dose selection for an elderly patient should be cautious, reflecting the greater frequency of decreased hepatic, renal, or cardiac function, and of concomitant disease or other drug therapy.

DRUG INTERACTIONS

See TABLE 4 for information on zidovudine concentrations when coadministered with other drugs. For patients experiencing pronounced anemia or other severe zidovudine-associated events while receiving chronic administration of zidovudine and some of the drugs (*e.g.*, fluconazole, valproic acid) listed in TABLE 4, zidovudine dose reduction may be considered.

ANTIRETROVIRAL AGENTS

Concomitant use of zidovudine with stavudine should be avoided since an antagonistic relationship has been demonstrated *in vitro*.

Some nucleoside analogues affecting DNA replication, such as ribavirin, antagonize the *in vitro* antiviral activity of zidovudine against HIV; concomitant use of such drugs should be avoided.

DOXORUBICIN

Concomitant use of zidovudine with doxorubicin should be avoided since an antagonistic relationship has been demonstrated *in vitro* (see CLINICAL PHARMACOLOGY for additional drug interactions).

PHENYTOIN

Phenytoin plasma levels have been reported to be low in some patients receiving zidovudine, while in 1 case a high level was documented. However, in a pharmacokinetic interaction study in which 12 HIV-positive volunteers received a single 300 mg phenytoin dose alone and during steady-state zidovudine conditions (200 mg every 4 hours), no change in phenytoin kinetics was observed. Although not designed to optimally assess the effect of phenytoin on zidovudine kinetics, a 30% decrease in oral zidovudine clearance was observed with phenytoin.

OVERLAPPING TOXICITIES

Coadministration of ganciclovir, interferon-alpha, and other bone marrow suppressive or cytotoxic agents may increase the hematologic toxicity of zidovudine.

ADVERSE REACTIONS

The adverse events reported during IV administration of zidovudine IV infusion are similar to those reported with oral administration; neutropenia and anemia were reported most frequently. Long-term IV administration beyond 2-4 weeks has not been studied in adults and may enhance hematologic adverse events. Local reaction, pain, and slight irritation during IV administration occur infrequently.

ADULTS

The frequency and severity of adverse events associated with the use of oral zidovudine are greater in patients with more advanced infection at the time of initiation of therapy.

TABLE 5summarizes events reported at a statistically significantly greater incidence for patients receiving zidovudine orally in a monotherapy study.

***TABLE 5** Percentage (%) of Patients With Adverse Events* in Asymptomatic HIV Infection (ACTG 019)*

Adverse Event	Zidovudine 500 mg/day (n=453)	Placebo (n=428)
Body as a Whole		
Asthenia	8.6%	5.8%
Headache	62.5%	52.6%
Malaise	53.2%	44.9%
Gastrointestinal		
Anorexia	20.1%	10.5%
Constipation	6.4%†	3.5%
Nausea	51.4%	29.9%
Vomiting	17.2%	9.8%

* Reported in ≥5% of study population.
† Not statistically significant versus placebo.

In addition to the adverse events listed in TABLE 5, other adverse events observed in clinical studies were abdominal cramps, abdominal pain, arthralgia, chills, dyspepsia, fatigue, hyperbilirubinemia, insomnia, musculoskeletal pain, myalgia, and neuropathy.

Selected laboratory abnormalities observed during a clinical study of monotherapy with oral zidovudine are shown in TABLE 6.

***TABLE 6** Frequencies of Selected (Grade 3/4) Laboratory Abnormalities in Patients With Asymptomatic HIV Infection (ACTG 019)*

Adverse Event	Zidovudine 500 mg/day (n=453)	Placebo (n=428)
Anemia (Hgb <8 g/dl)	1.1%	0.2%
Granulocytopenia (<750 cells/mm^3)	1.8%	1.6%
Thrombocytopenia (platelets <50,000/mm^3)	0%	0.5%
ALT (>5 × ULN)	3.1%	2.6%
AST (>5 × ULN)	0.9%	1.6%
Alkaline phosphatase (>5 × ULN)	0%	0%

ULN = Upper limit of normal.

PEDIATRICS

Study ACTG300

Selected clinical adverse events and physical findings with a ≥5% frequency during therapy with lamivudine 4 mg/kg twice daily plus zidovudine 160 mg/m^2 orally 3 times daily compared with didanosine in therapy-naive (≤56 days of antiretroviral therapy) pediatric patients are listed in TABLE 7.

***TABLE 7** Selected Clinical Adverse Events and Physical Findings (≥5% Frequency) in Pediatric Patients in Study ACTG300*

Adverse Events	Lamivudine plus Zidovudine (n=236)	Didanosine (n=235)
Body as a Whole		
Fever	25%	32%
Digestive		
Hepatomegaly	11%	11%
Nausea & vomiting	8%	7%
Diarrhea	8%	6%
Stomatitis	6%	12%
Splenomegaly	5%	8%
Respiratory		
Cough	15%	18%
Abnormal breath sounds/wheezing	7%	9%
Ear, Nose, and Throat		
Signs or symptoms of ears*	7%	6%
Nasal discharge or congestion	8%	11%
Other		
Skin rashes	12%	14%
Lymphadenopathy	9%	11%

* Includes pain, discharge, erythema, or swelling of an ear.

Selected laboratory abnormalities experienced by therapy-naive (≤56 days of antiretroviral therapy) pediatric patients are listed in TABLE 8.

***TABLE 8** Frequencies of Selected (Grade 3/4) Laboratory Abnormalities in Pediatric Patients in Study ACTG300*

Test (Abnormal Level)	Lamivudine plus Zidovudine	Didanosine
Neutropenia (ANC <400 cells/mm^3)	8%	3%
Anemia (Hgb <7.0 g/dl)	4%	2%
Thrombocytopenia (platelets <50,000/mm^3	1%	3%
ALT (>10 × ULN)	1%	3%
AST (>10 × ULN)	2%	4%
Lipase (>2.5 × ULN)	3%	3%
Total amylase (>2.5 × ULN)	3%	3%

ULN = Upper limit of normal.
ANC = Absolute neutrophil count.

Additional adverse events reported in open-label studies in pediatric patients receiving zidovudine 180 mg/m^2 every 6 hours were congestive heart failure, decreased reflexes, ECG abnormality, edema, hematuria, left ventricular dilation, macrocytosis, nervousness/irritability, and weight loss.

The clinical adverse events reported among adult recipients of zidovudine may also occur in pediatric patients.

USE FOR THE PREVENTION OF MATERNAL-FETAL TRANSMISSION OF HIV

In a randomized, double-blind, placebo-controlled trial in HIV-infected women and their neonates conducted to determine the utility of zidovudine for the prevention of maternal-fetal HIV transmission, zidovudine syrup at 2 mg/kg was administered every 6 hours for 6 weeks to neonates beginning within 12 hours after birth. The most commonly reported adverse experiences were anemia (hemoglobin <9.0 g/dl) and neutropenia (<1000 cells/mm^3). Anemia occurred in 22% of the neonates who received zidovudine and in 12% of the neonates who received placebo. The mean difference in hemoglobin values was less than 1.0 g/dl for neonates receiving zidovudine compared to neonates receiving placebo. No neonates with anemia required transfusion, and all hemoglobin values spontaneously returned to normal within 6 weeks after completion of therapy with zidovudine. Neutropenia was reported with similar frequency in the group that received zidovudine (21%) and in the

Z

group that received placebo (27%). The long-term consequences of *in utero* and neonatal exposure to zidovudine are unknown.

OBSERVED DURING CLINICAL PRACTICE

In addition to adverse events reported from clinical trials, the following events have been identified during use of zidovudine in clinical practice. Because they are reported voluntarily from a population of unknown size, estimates of frequency cannot be made. These events have been chosen for inclusion due to either their seriousness, frequency of reporting, potential causal connection to zidovudine, or a combination of these factors.

Body as a Whole: Back pain, chest pain, flu-like syndrome, generalized pain.

Cardiovascular: Cardiomyopathy, syncope.

Endocrine: Gynecomastia.

Eye: Macular edema.

Gastrointestinal: Constipation, dysphagia, flatulence, oral mucosal pigmentation, mouth ulcer.

General: Sensitization reactions including anaphylaxis and angioedema, vasculitis.

Hemic and Lymphatic: Aplastic anemia, hemolytic anemia, leukopenia, lymphadenopathy, pancytopenia with marrow hypoplasia, pure red cell aplasia.

Hepatobiliary Tract and Pancreas: Hepatitis, hepatomegaly with steatosis, jaundice, lactic acidosis, pancreatitis.

Musculoskeletal: Increased CPK, increased LDH, muscle spasm, myopathy and myositis with pathological changes (similar to that produced by HIV disease), rhabdomyolysis, tremor.

Nervous: Anxiety, confusion, depression, dizziness, loss of mental acuity, mania, paresthesia, seizures, somnolence, vertigo.

Respiratory: Cough, dyspnea, rhinitis, sinusitis.

Skin: Changes in skin and nail pigmentation, pruritus, rash, Stevens-Johnson syndrome, toxic epidemal necrolysis, sweat, urticaria.

Special Senses: Amblyopia, hearing loss, photophobia, taste perversion.

Urogenital: Urinary frequency, urinary hesitancy.

DOSAGE AND ADMINISTRATION

ADULTS

The recommended IV dose is 1 mg/kg infused over 1 hour. This dose should be administered 5-6 times daily (5-6 mg/kg daily). The effectiveness of this dose compared to higher dosing regimens in improving the neurologic dysfunction associated with HIV disease is unknown. A small randomized study found a greater effect of higher doses of zidovudine on improvement of neurological symptoms in patients with pre-existing neurological disease.

Patients should receive zidovudine IV infusion only until oral therapy can be administered. The IV dosing regimen equivalent to the oral administration of 100 mg every 4 hours is approximately 1 mg/kg intravenously every 4 hours.

MATERNAL-FETAL HIV TRANSMISSION

The recommended dosing regimen for administration to pregnant women (>14 weeks of pregnancy) and their neonates is:

Maternal Dosing: 100 mg orally 5 times per day until the start of labor. During labor and delivery, IV zidovudine should be administered at 2 mg/kg (total body weight) over 1 hour followed by a continuous IV infusion of 1 mg/kg/h (total body weight) until clamping of the umbilical cord.

Neonatal Dosing 2 mg/kg orally every 6 hours starting within 12 hours after birth and continuing through 6 weeks of age. Neonates unable to receive oral dosing may be administered zidovudine intravenously at 1.5 mg/kg, infused over 30 minutes, every 6 hours. (See PRECAUTIONS if hepatic disease or renal insufficiency is present.)

MONITORING OF PATIENTS

Hematologic toxicities appear to be related to pretreatment bone marrow reserve and to dose and duration of therapy. In patients with poor bone marrow reserve, particularly in patients with advanced symptomatic HIV disease, frequent monitoring of hematologic indices is recommended to detect serious anemia or neutropenia (see WARNINGS). In patients who experience hematologic toxicity, reduction in hemoglobin may occur as early as 2-4 weeks, and neutropenia usually occurs after 6-8 weeks.

DOSE ADJUSTMENT

Anemia

Significant anemia (hemoglobin of <7.5 g/dl or reduction of >25% of baseline) and/or significant neutropenia (granulocyte count of <750 cells/mm^3 or reduction of >50% from baseline) may require a dose interruption until evidence of marrow recovery is observed (see WARNINGS). In patients who develop significant anemia, dose interruption does not necessarily eliminate the need for transfusion. If marrow recovery occurs following dose interruption, resumption in dose may be appropriate using adjunctive measures such as epoetin alfa at recommended doses, depending on hematologic indices such as serum erythropoetin level and patient tolerance.

For patients experiencing pronounced anemia while receiving chronic coadministration of zidovudine and some of the drugs (*e.g.*, fluconazole, valproic acid) listed in TABLE 4, zidovudine dose reduction may be considered.

End-Stage Renal Disease

In patients maintained on hemodialysis or peritoneal dialysis (CRCL <15 ml/min), recommended dosing is 1 mg/kg every 6-8 hours (see CLINICAL PHARMACOLOGY, Pharmacokinetics).

Hepatic Impairment

There are insufficient data to recommend dose adjustment of zidovudine in patients with mild to moderate impaired hepatic function or liver cirrhosis. Since zidovudine is primarily eliminated by hepatic metabolism, a reduction in the daily dose may be necessary in these patients. Frequent monitoring of hematologic toxicities is advised (see CLINICAL PHARMACOLOGY, Pharmacokinetics and PRECAUTIONS, General).

METHOD OF PREPARATION

Zidovudine IV infusion must be diluted prior to administration. The calculated dose should be removed from the 20 ml vial and added to 5% dextrose injection solution to achieve a concentration no greater than 4 mg/ml. Admixture in biologic or colloidal fluids (*e.g.*, blood products, protein solutions, etc.) is not recommended.

After dilution, the solution is physically and chemically stable for 24 hours at room temperature and 48 hours if refrigerated at 2-8°C (36-46°F). Care should be taken during admixture to prevent inadvertent contamination. As an additional precaution, the diluted solution should be administered within 8 hours if stored at 25°C (77°F) or 24 hours if refrigerated at 2-8°C to minimize potential administration of a microbially contaminated solution.

Parenteral drug products should be inspected visually for particulate matter and discoloration prior to administration whenever solution and container permit. Should either be observed, the solution should be discarded and fresh solution prepared.

ADMINISTRATION

Zidovudine IV infusion is administered intravenously at a constant rate over 1 hour. Rapid infusion or bolus injection should be avoided. Zidovudine IV infusion should not be given intramuscularly.

HOW SUPPLIED

Retrovir IV infusion, 10 mg zidovudine in each ml in a 20 ml single-use vial.
Storage: Store vials at 15-25°C (59-77°F) and protect from light.

ORAL

WARNING

ZIDOVUDINE HAS BEEN ASSOCIATED WITH HEMATOLOGIC TOXICITY INCLUDING NEUTROPENIA AND SEVERE ANEMIA PARTICULARLY IN PATIENTS WITH ADVANCED HIV DISEASE (SEE WARNINGS). PROLONGED USE OF ZIDOVUDINE HAS BEEN ASSOCIATED WITH SYMPTOMATIC MYOPATHY.

LACTIC ACIDOSIS AND SEVERE HEPATOMEGALY WITH STEATOSIS, INCLUDING FATAL CASES, HAVE BEEN REPORTED WITH THE USE OF NUCLEOSIDE ANALOGUES ALONE OR IN COMBINATION, INCLUDING ZIDOVUDINE AND OTHER ANTIRETROVIRALS (SEE WARNINGS).

DESCRIPTION

Retrovir is the brand name for zidovudine (formerly called azidothymidine [AZT]), a pyrimidine nucleoside analogue active against human immunodeficiency virus (HIV).

TABLETS

Retrovir tablets are for oral administration. Each film-coated tablet contains 300 mg of zidovudine and the inactive ingredients hydroxypropyl methylcellulose, magnesium stearate, microcrystalline cellulose, polyethylene glycol, sodium starch glycolate, and titanium dioxide.

CAPSULES

Retrovir capsules are for oral administration. Each capsule contains 100 mg of zidovudine and the inactive ingredients corn starch, magnesium stearate, microcrystalline cellulose, and sodium starch glycolate. The 100 mg empty hard gelatin capsule, printed with edible black ink, consists of black iron oxide, dimethylpolysiloxane, gelatin, pharmaceutical shellac, soya lecithin, and titanium dioxide. The blue band around the capsule consists of gelatin and FD&C blue no. 2.

SYRUP

Retrovir syrup is for oral administration. Each teaspoonful (5 ml) of Retrovir syrup contains 50 mg of zidovudine and the inactive ingredients sodium benzoate 0.2% (added as a preservative), citric acid, flavors, glycerin, and liquid sucrose. Sodium hydroxide may be added to adjust pH.

The chemical name of zidovudine is 3′-azido-3′-deoxythymidine.

Zidovudine is a white to beige, odorless, crystalline solid with a molecular weight of 267.24 and a solubility of 20.1 mg/ml in water at 25°C. The molecular formula is $C_{10}H_{13}N_5O_4$.

CLINICAL PHARMACOLOGY

MICROBIOLOGY

Mechanism of Action

Zidovudine is a synthetic nucleoside analogue of the naturally occurring nucleoside, thymidine, in which the 3′-hydroxy (-OH) group is replaced by an azido ($-N_3$) group. Within cells, zidovudine is converted to the active metabolite, zidovudine 5′-triphosphate (AztTP), by the sequential action of the cellular enzymes. Zidovudine 5′-triphosphate inhibits the activity of the HIV reverse transcriptase both by competing for utilization with the natural substrate, deoxythymidine 5′-triphosphate (dTTP), and by its incorporation into viral DNA. The lack of a 3′-OH group in the incorporated nucleoside analogue prevents the formation of the 5′ to 3′ phosphodiester linkage essential for DNA chain elongation and, therefore, the viral DNA growth is terminated. The active metabolite AztTP is also a weak inhibitor of the cellular DNA polymerase-alpha and mitochondrial polymerase-gamma and has been reported to be incorporated into the DNA of cells in culture.

In Vitro HIV Susceptibility

The *in vitro* anti-HIV activity of zidovudine was assessed by infecting cell lines of lymphoblastic and monocytic origin and peripheral blood lymphocytes with laboratory and clinical isolates of HIV. The IC_{50} and IC_{90} values (50% and 90% inhibitory concentrations) were 0.003-0.013 and 0.03-0.13 μg/ml, respectively (1 nM = 0.27 ng/ml).The IC_{50} and IC_{90} values of HIV isolates recovered from 18 untreated AIDS/ARC patients were in the range of 0.003-0.013 μg/ml and 0.03 to 0.3 μg/ml, respectively. Zidovudine showed antiviral activity in all acutely infected cell lines; however, activity was substantially less in chronically infected cell lines. In drug combination studies with zalcitabine, didanosine, lamivudine, saquinavir, indinavir, ritonavir, nevirapine, delavirdine, or interferon-alpha, zidovudine showed additive to synergistic activity in cell culture. The relationship between the *in vitro* susceptibility of HIV to reverse transcriptase inhibitors and the inhibition of HIV replication in humans has not been established.

Drug Resistance

HIV isolates with reduced sensitivity to zidovudine have been selected *in vitro* and were also recovered from patients treated with zidovudine. Genetic analysis of the isolates showed mutations that result in 5 amino acid substitutions (Met41→Leu, A67→Asn, Lys70→Arg, Thr215→Tyr or Phe, and Lys219→Gln) in the viral reverse transcriptase. In general, higher levels of resistance were associated with greater number of mutations with 215 mutation being the most significant.

Cross-Resistance

The potential for cross-resistance between HIV reverse transcriptase inhibitors and protease inhibitors is low because of the different enzyme targets involved. Combination therapy with zidovudine plus zalcitabine or didanosine does not appear to prevent the emergence of zidovudine-resistant isolates. Combination therapy with zidovudine plus lamivudine delayed the emergence of mutations conferring resistance to zidovudine. In some patients harboring zidovudine-resistant virus, combination therapy with zidovudine plus lamivudine restored phenotypic sensitivity to zidovudine by 12 weeks of treatment. HIV isolates with multidrug resistance to zidovudine, didanosine, zalcitabine, stavudine, and lamivudine were recovered from a small number of patients treated for ≥1 year with the combination of zidovudine and didanosine or zalcitabine. The pattern of resistant mutations in the combination therapy was different (Ala62→Val, Val75→Ile, Phe77→116Tyr, and Gln→151Met) from monotherapy, with mutation 151 being most significant for multidrug resistance. Site-directed mutagenesis studies showed that these mutations could also result in resistance to zalcitabine, lamivudine, and stavudine.

PHARMACOKINETICS

Adults

The pharmacokinetic properties of zidovudine in fasting patients are summarized in TABLE 9. Following oral administration, zidovudine is rapidly absorbed and extensively distributed, with peak serum concentrations occurring within 0.5-1.5 hours. Binding to plasma protein is low. Zidovudine is primarily eliminated by hepatic metabolism. The major metabolite of zidovudine is 3′-azido-3′-deoxy-5′-*O*-β-*D*-glucopyranuronosylthymidine (GZDV). GZDV area under the curve (AUC) is about 3-fold greater than the zidovudine AUC. Urinary recovery of zidovudine and GZDV accounts for 14% and 74%, respectively, of the dose following oral administration. A second metabolite, 3′-amino-3′-deoxythymidine (AMT), has been identified in the plasma following single-dose intravenous (IV) administration of zidovudine. The AMT AUC was one-fifth of the zidovudine AUC. Pharmacokinetics of zidovudine were dose independent at oral dosing regimens ranging from 2 mg/kg every 8 hours to 10 mg/kg every 4 hours.

The extent of absorption (AUC) was equivalent when zidovudine was administered as zidovudine tablets or syrup compared to zidovudine capsules.

TABLE 9 *Zidovudine Pharmacokinetic Parameters in Fasting Adult Patients*

Parameter	Mean ±SD (except where noted)
Oral bioavailability (%)	64 ± 10 (n=5)
Aparent volume of distribution (L/kg)	1.6 ± 0.6 (n=8)
Plama protein binding (%)	<38
CSF:Plasma ratio*	0.6 [0.04-2.62] (n=39)
Systemic clearance (L/h/kg)	1.6 ± 0.6 (n=6)
Renal clearance (L/h/kg)	0.34 ± 0.05 (n=9)
Elimination half-life (h)†	0.5 to 3 (n=19)

* Median [range].
† Approximate range.

Adults With Impaired Renal Function

Zidovudine clearance was decreased resulting in increased zidovudine and GZDV half-life and AUC in patients with impaired renal function (n=14) following a single 200 mg oral dose (TABLE 10). Plasma concentrations of AMT were not determined. A dose adjustment should not be necessary for patients with creatinine clearance (CRCL) ≥15 ml/min.

TABLE 10 *Zidovudine Pharmacokinetic Parameters in Patients With Severe Renal Impairment**

Parameter	Control Subjects (Normal Renal Function) (n=6)	Patients With Renal Impairment (n=14)
CRCL (ml/min)	120 ± 8	18 ± 2
Zidovudine AUC (ng·h/ml)	1400 ± 200	3100 ± 300
Zidovudine half-life (h)	1.0 ± 0.2	1.4 ± 0.1

* Data are expressed as mean ± standard deviation.

The pharmacokinetics and tolerance of zidovudine were evaluated in a multiple-dose study in patients undergoing hemodialysis (n=5) or peritoneal dialysis (n=6) receiving escalating doses up to 200 mg 5 times daily for 8 weeks. Daily doses of 500 mg or less were well tolerated despite significantly elevated GZDV plasma concentrations. Apparent zidovudine oral clearance was approximately 50% of that reported in patients with normal renal function. Hemodialysis and peritoneal dialysis appeared to have a negligible effect on the removal of zidovudine, whereas GZDV elimination was enhanced. A dosage adjustment is recommended for patients undergoing hemodialysis or peritoneal dialysis (see DOSAGE AND ADMINISTRATION, Dose Adjustment).

Adults With Impaired Hepatic Function

Data describing the effect of hepatic impairment on the pharmacokinetics of zidovudine are limited. However, because zidovudine is eliminated primarily by hepatic metabolism, it is expected that zidovudine clearance would be decreased and plasma concentrations would be increased following administration of the recommended adult doses to patients with hepatic impairment (see DOSAGE AND ADMINISTRATION, Dose Adjustment).

Pediatrics

Zidovudine pharmacokinetics have been evaluated in HIV-infected pediatric patients (TABLE 11).

Patients From 3 Months to 12 Years of Age

Overall, zidovudine pharmacokinetics in pediatric patients greater than 3 months of age are similar to those in adult patients. Proportional increases in plasma zidovudine concentrations were observed following administration of oral solution from 90-240 mg/m^2 every 6 hours. Oral bioavailability, terminal half-life, and oral clearance were comparable to adult values. As in adult patients, the major route of elimination was by metabolism to GZDV. After IV dosing, about 29% of the dose was excreted in the urine unchanged, and about 45% of the dose was excreted as GZDV (see DOSAGE AND ADMINISTRATION, Pediatrics).

Patients Younger Than 3 Months of Age

Zidovudine pharmacokinetics have been evaluated in pediatric patients from birth to 3 months of life. Zidovudine elimination was determined immediately following birth in 8 neonates who were exposed to zidovudine *in utero*. The half-life was 13.0 ± 5.8 hours. In neonates ≤14 days old, bioavailability was greater, total body clearance was slower, and half-life was longer than in pediatric patients >14 days old. For dose recommendations for neonates, see DOSAGE AND ADMINISTRATION, Neonatal Dosing.

TABLE 11 *Zidovudine Pharmacokinetic Parameters in Pediatric Patients**

Parameter	Birth to 14 Days of Age	14 Days to 3 Months of Age	3 Months to 12 Years of Age
Oral bioavailability (%)	89 ± 19 (n=15)	61 ± 19 (n=17)	65 ± 24 (n=18)
CSF:Plasma ratio	no data	no data	0.68 (0.03-3.25)† (n=38)
CL (L/h/kg)	0.65 ± 0.29 (n=18)	1.14 ± 0.24 (n=16)	1.85 ± 0.47 (n=20)
Elimination half-life (h)	3.1 ± 1.2 (n=21)	1.9 ± 0.7 (n=18)	1.5 ± 0.7 (n=21)

* Data presented as mean ± standard deviation except where noted.
† Median [range].

Pregnancy

Zidovudine pharmacokinetics have been studied in a Phase 1 study of 8 women during the last trimester of pregnancy. As pregnancy progressed, there was no evidence of drug accumulation. Zidovudine pharmacokinetics were similar to that of nonpregnant adults. Consistent with passive transmission of the drug across the placenta, zidovudine concentrations in neonatal plasma at birth were essentially equal to those in maternal plasma at delivery. Although data are limited, methadone maintenance therapy in 5 pregnant women did not appear to alter zidovudine pharmacokinetics. However, in another patient population, a potential for interaction has been identified (see PRECAUTIONS).

Nursing Mothers

The Centers for Disease Control and Prevention recommend that HIV-infected mothers not breastfeed their infants to avoid risking postnatal transmission of HIV. After administration of a single dose of 200 mg zidovudine to 13 HIV-infected women, the mean concentration of zidovudine was similar in human milk and serum (see PRECAUTIONS, Nursing Mothers).

Geriatric Patients

Zidovudine pharmacokinetics have not been studied in patients over 65 years of age.

Gender

A pharmacokinetic study in healthy male (n=12) and female (n=12) subjects showed no differences in zidovudine exposure (AUC) when a single dose of zidovudine was administered as the 300 mg zidovudine tablet.

Effect of Food on Absorption

Zidovudine may be administered with or without food. The extent of zidovudine absorption (AUC) was similar when a single dose of zidovudine was administered with food.

Drug Interactions

See TABLE 12 and DRUG INTERACTIONS.

Zidovudine Plus Lamivudine

No clinically significant alterations in lamivudine or zidovudine pharmacokinetics were observed in 12 asymptomatic HIV-infected adult patients given a single dose of zidovudine (200 mg) in combination with multiple doses of lamivudine (300 mg every 12 hours).

INDICATIONS AND USAGE

Zidovudine in combination with other antiretroviral agents is indicated for the treatment of HIV infection.

TABLE 12 *Effect of Coadministered Drugs on Zidovudine AUC*†*

Coadministered Drug and Dose	Zidovudine Dose	n	Zidovudine Conc. AUC	Variability	Conc. of Coadministered Drug
Atovaquone 750 mg q12h with food	200 mg q8h	14	inc AUC 31%	Range: 23-78%‡	NS
Fluconazole 400 mg daily	200 mg q8h	12	inc AUC 74%	95% CI: 54-98%	Not reported
Methadone 30-90 mg daily	200 mg q4h	9	inc AUC 43%	Range: 16-64%‡	NS
Nelfinavir 750 mg q8h × 7-10 days	single 200 mg	11	dec AUC 35%	Range: 28-41%	NS
Probenecid 500 mg q6h × 2 days	2 mg/kg q8h × 3 days	3	inc AUC 106%	Range: 100-170%‡	Not assessed
Rifampin 600 mg daily × 14 days	200 mg q8h × 14 days	8	dec AUC 47%	90% CI: 41-53%	Not assessed
Ritonavir 300 mg q6h × 4 days	200 mg q8h × 4 days	9	dec AUC 25%	95% CI: 15-34%	NS
Valproic acid 250 or 500 mg q8h × 4 days	100 mg q8h × 4 days	6	inc AUC 80%	Range: 64-130%‡	Not assessed

inc = Increase; dec = Decrease; NS = no significant change; AUC = area under the concentration versus time curve; CI = confidence interval.
* This table is not all inclusive.
† **Note:** Routine dose modification of zidovudine is not warranted with coadministration of the drugs listed in this table.
‡ Estimated range of percent difference.

MATERNAL-FETAL HIV TRANSMISSION

Zidovudine is also indicated for the prevention of maternal-fetal HIV transmission as part of a regimen that includes oral zidovudine beginning between 14 and 34 weeks of gestation, IV zidovudine during labor, and administration of zidovudine syrup to the neonate after birth. The efficacy of this regimen for preventing HIV transmission in women who have received zidovudine for a prolonged period before pregnancy has not been evaluated. The safety of zidovudine for the mother or fetus during the first trimester of pregnancy has not been assessed.

CONTRAINDICATIONS

Zidovudine tablets, capsules, and syrup are contraindicated for patients who have potentially life-threatening allergic reactions to any of the components of the formulations.

WARNINGS

Combivir and trizivir are combination product tablets that contain zidovudine as one of their components. Zidovudine should not be administered concomitantly with Combivir or Trizivir.

The incidence of adverse reactions appears to increase with disease progression; patients should be monitored carefully, especially as disease progression occurs.

BONE MARROW SUPPRESSION

Zidovudine should be used with caution in patients who have bone marrow compromise evidenced by granulocyte count <1000 cells/mm^3 or hemoglobin <9.5 g/dl. In patients with advanced symptomatic HIV disease, anemia and neutropenia were the most significant adverse events observed. There have been reports of pancytopenia associated with the use of zidovudine, which was reversible in most instances after discontinuance of the drug. However, significant anemia, in many cases requiring dose adjustment, discontinuation of zidovudine, and/or blood transfusions, has occurred during treatment with zidovudine alone or in combination with other antiretrovirals.

Frequent blood counts are strongly recommended in patients with advanced HIV disease who are treated with zidovudine. For HIV-infected individuals and patients with asymptomatic or early HIV disease, periodic blood counts are recommended. If anemia or neutropenia develops, dosage adjustments may be necessary (see DOSAGE AND ADMINISTRATION).

MYOPATHY

Myopathy and myositis with pathological changes, similar to that produced by HIV disease, have been associated with prolonged use of zidovudine.

LACTIC ACIDOSIS/SEVERE HEPATOMEGALY WITH STEATOSIS

Lactic acidosis and severe hepatomegaly with steatosis, including fatal cases, have been reported with the use of nucleoside analogues alone or in combination, including zidovudine and other antiretrovirals. A majority of these cases have been in women. Obesity and prolonged exposure to antiretroviral nucleoside analogues may be risk factors. Particular caution should be exercised when administering zidovudine to any patient with known risk factors for liver disease; however, cases have also been reported in patients with no known risk factors. Treatment with zidovudine should be suspended in any patient who develops clinical or laboratory findings suggestive of lactic acidosis or pronounced hepatotoxicity (which may include hepatomegaly and steatosis even in the absence of marked transaminase elevations).

PRECAUTIONS

GENERAL

Zidovudine is eliminated from the body primarily by renal excretion following metabolism in the liver (glucuronidation). In patients with severely impaired renal function (CRCL <15 ml/min), dosage reduction is recommended. Although the data are limited, zidovudine concentrations appear to be increased in patients with severely impaired hepatic function which may increase the risk of hematologic toxicity (see CLINICAL PHARMACOLOGY, Pharmacokinetics and DOSAGE AND ADMINISTRATION).

INFORMATION FOR THE PATIENT

Zidovudine is not a cure for HIV infection, and patients may continue to acquire illnesses associated with HIV infection, including opportunistic infections. Therefore, patients should be advised to seek medical care for any significant change in their health status.

The safety and efficacy of zidovudine in women, IV drug users, and racial minorities is not significantly different than that observed in white males.

Patients should be informed that the major toxicities of zidovudine are neutropenia and/or anemia. The frequency and severity of these toxicities are greater in patients with more advanced disease and in those who initiate therapy later in the course of their infection. They should be told that if toxicity develops, they may require transfusions or drug discontinuation. They should be told of the extreme importance of having their blood counts followed closely while on therapy, especially for patients with advanced symptomatic HIV disease. They should be cautioned about the use of other medications, including ganciclovir and interferon-alpha, that may exacerbate the toxicity of zidovudine (see DRUG INTERACTIONS). Patients should be informed that other adverse effects of zidovudine include nausea and vomiting. Patients should also be encouraged to contact their physician if they experience muscle weakness, shortness of breath, symptoms of hepatitis or pancreatitis, or any other unexpected adverse events while being treated with zidovudine.

Zidovudine tablets, capsules, and syrup are for oral ingestion only. Patients should be told of the importance of taking zidovudine exactly as prescribed. They should be told not to share medication and not to exceed the recommended dose. Patients should be told that the long-term effects of zidovudine are unknown at this time.

Pregnant women considering the use of zidovudine during pregnancy for prevention of HIV-transmission to their infants should be advised that transmission may still occur in some cases despite therapy. The long-term consequences of *in utero* and infant exposure to zidovudine are unknown, including the possible risk of cancer.

HIV-infected pregnant women should be advised not to breastfeed to avoid postnatal transmission of HIV to a child who may not yet be infected.

Patients should be advised that therapy with zidovudine has not been shown to reduce the risk of transmission of HIV to others through sexual contact or blood contamination.

CARCINOGENESIS, MUTAGENESIS, AND IMPAIRMENT OF FERTILITY

Zidovudine was administered orally at 3 dosage levels to separate groups of mice and rats (60 females and 60 males in each group). Initial single daily doses were 30, 60, and 120 mg/kg/day in mice and 80, 220, and 600 mg/kg/day in rats. The doses in mice were reduced to 20, 30, and 40 mg/kg/day after day 90 because of treatment-related anemia, whereas in rats only the high dose was reduced to 450 mg/kg/day on day 91 and then to 300 mg/kg/day on day 279.

In mice, 7 late-appearing (after 19 months) vaginal neoplasms (5 nonmetastasizing squamous cell carcinomas, 1 squamous cell papilloma, and 1 squamous polyp) occurred in animals given the highest dose. One late-appearing squamous cell papilloma occurred in the vagina of a middle-dose animal. No vaginal tumors were found at the lowest dose.

In rats, 2 late-appearing (after 20 months), nonmetastasizing vaginal squamous cell carcinomas occurred in animals given the highest dose. No vaginal tumors occurred at the low or middle dose in rats. No other drug-related tumors were observed in either sex of either species.

At doses that produced tumors in mice and rats, the estimated drug exposure (as measured by AUC) was approximately 3 times (mouse) and 24 times (rat) the estimated human exposure at the recommended therapeutic dose of 100 mg every 4 hours.

Two transplacental carcinogenicity studies were conducted in mice. One study administered zidovudine at doses of 20 or 40 mg/kg/day from gestation day 10 through parturition and lactation with dosing continuing in offspring for 24 months postnatally. The doses of zidovudine employed in this study produced zidovudine exposures approximately 3 times the estimated human exposure at recommended doses. After 24 months, an increase in incidence of vaginal tumors was noted with no increase in tumors in the liver or lung or any other organ in either gender. These findings are consistent with results of the standard oral carcinogenicity study in mice, as described earlier. A second study administered zidovudine at maximum tolerated doses of 12.5 or 25 mg/day (~1000 mg/kg nonpregnant body weight or ~450 mg/kg of term body weight) to pregnant mice from days 12-18 of gestation. There was an increase in the number of tumors in the lung, liver, and female reproductive tracts in the offspring of mice receiving the higher dose level of zidovudine.

It is not known how predictive the results of rodent carcinogenicity studies may be for humans.

Zidovudine was mutagenic in a 5178Y/TK$^{+/-}$ mouse lymphoma assay, positive in an *in vitro* cell transformation assay, clastogenic in a cytogenetic assay using cultured human lymphocytes, and positive in mouse and rat micronucleus tests after repeated doses. It was negative in a cytogenetic study in rats given a single dose.

Zidovudine, administered to male and female rats at doses up to 7 times the usual adult dose based on body surface area considerations, had no effect on fertility judged by conception rates.

PREGNANCY CATEGORY C

Oral teratology studies in the rat and in the rabbit at doses up to 500 mg/kg/day revealed no evidence of teratogenicity with zidovudine. Zidovudine treatment resulted in embryo/fetal toxicity as evidenced by an increase in the incidence of fetal resorptions in rats given 150 or 450 mg/kg/day and rabbits given 500 mg/kg/day. The doses used in the teratology studies resulted in peak zidovudine plasma concentrations (after one-half of the daily dose) in rats 66-226 times, and in rabbits 12-87 times, mean steady-state peak human plasma concentrations (after one-sixth of the daily dose) achieved with the recommended daily dose (100 mg every 4 hours). In an *in vitro* experiment with fertilized mouse oocytes, zidovudine exposure resulted in a dose-dependent reduction in blastocyst formation. In an additional teratology study in rats, a dose of 3000 mg/kg/day (very near the oral median lethal dose in rats of 3683 mg/kg) caused marked maternal toxicity and an increase in the incidence of fetal malformations. This dose resulted in peak zidovudine plasma concentrations 350 times peak human plasma concentrations. (Estimated area-under-the-curve [AUC] in rats at this dose level was 300 times the daily AUC in humans given 600 mg/day.) No evidence of teratogenicity was seen in this experiment at doses of 600 mg/kg/day or less.

Two rodent transplacental carcinogenicity studies were conducted (see Carcinogenesis, Mutagenesis, and Impairment of Fertility).

A randomized, double-blind, placebo-controlled trial was conducted in HIV-infected pregnant women to determine the utility of zidovudine for the prevention of maternal-fetal HIV-transmission. Congenital abnormalities occurred with similar frequency between neonates born to mothers who received zidovudine and neonates born to mothers who received placebo. Abnormalities were either problems in embryogenesis (prior to 14 weeks) or were recognized on ultrasound before or immediately after initiation of study drug.

Antiretroviral Pregnancy Registry: To monitor maternal-fetal outcomes of pregnant women exposed to zidovudine, an Antiretroviral Pregnancy Registry has been established. Physicians are encouraged to register patients by calling 1-800-258-4263.

NURSING MOTHERS

The Centers for Disease Control and Prevention recommend that HIV-infected mothers not breastfeed their infants to avoid risking postnatal transmission of HIV. Zidovudine is excreted in human milk (see CLINICAL PHARMACOLOGY, Pharmacokinetics, Nursing Mothers). Because of both the potential for HIV transmission and the potential for serious adverse reactions in nursing infants, **mothers should be instructed not to breastfeed if they are receiving zidovudine** (see Pediatric Use and INDICATIONS AND USAGE, Maternal-Fetal HIV Transmission).

PEDIATRIC USE

Zidovudine has been studied in HIV-infected pediatric patients over 3 months of age who had HIV-related symptoms or who were asymptomatic with abnormal laboratory values indicating significant HIV-related immunosuppression. Zidovudine has also been studied in neonates perinatally exposed to HIV (see ADVERSE REACTIONS; DOSAGE AND ADMINISTRATION; and CLINICAL PHARMACOLOGY, Pharmacokinetics).

GERIATRIC USE

Clinical studies of zidovudine did not include sufficient numbers of subjects aged 65 and over to determine whether they respond differently from younger subjects. Other reported clinical experience has not identified differences in responses between the elderly and younger patients. In general, dose selection for an elderly patient should be cautious, reflecting the greater frequency of decreased hepatic, renal, or cardiac function, and of concomitant disease or other drug therapy.

DRUG INTERACTIONS

See TABLE 11 for information on zidovudine concentrations when coadministered with other drugs. For patients experiencing pronounced anemia or other severe zidovudine-associated events while receiving chronic administration of zidovudine and some of the drugs (*e.g.*, fluconazole, valproic acid) listed in TABLE 11, zidovudine dose reduction may be considered.

ANTIRETROVIRAL AGENTS

Concomitant use of zidovudine with stavudine should be avoided since an antagonistic relationship has been demonstrated *in vitro*.

Some nucleoside analogues affecting DNA replication, such as ribavirin, antagonize the *in vitro* antiviral activity of zidovudine against HIV; concomitant use of such drugs should be avoided.

DOXORUBICIN

Concomitant use of zidovudine with doxorubicin should be avoided since an antagonistic relationship has been demonstrated *in vitro* (see CLINICAL PHARMACOLOGY for additional drug interactions).

PHENYTOIN

Phenytoin plasma levels have been reported to be low in some patients receiving zidovudine, while in one case a high level was documented. However, in a pharmacokinetic interaction study in which 12 HIV-positive volunteers received a single 300 mg phenytoin dose alone and during steady-state zidovudine conditions (200 mg every 4 hours), no change in phenytoin kinetics was observed. Although not designed to optimally assess the effect of phenytoin on zidovudine kinetics, a 30% decrease in oral zidovudine clearance was observed with phenytoin.

OVERLAPPING TOXICITIES

Coadministration of ganciclovir, interferon-alpha, and other bone marrow suppressive or cytotoxic agents may increase the hematologic toxicity of zidovudine.

ADVERSE REACTIONS

ADULTS

The frequency and severity of adverse events associated with the use of zidovudine are greater in patients with more advanced infection at the time of initiation of therapy.

TABLE 14 summarizes events reported at a statistically significant greater incidence for patients receiving zidovudine in a monotherapy study.

In addition to the adverse events listed in TABLE 14, other adverse events observed in clinical studies were abdominal cramps, abdominal pain, arthralgia, chills, dyspepsia, fatigue, hyperbilirubinemia, insomnia, musculoskeletal pain, myalgia, and neuropathy.

Selected laboratory abnormalities observed during a clinical study of monotherapy with zidovudine are shown in TABLE 15.

TABLE 14 *Percentage (%) of Patients With Adverse Events* in Asympotmatic HIV Infection (ACTG 019)*

Adverse Event	Zidovudine 500 mg/day (n=453)	Placebo (n=428)
Body as a Whole		
Asthenia	8.6%†	5.8%
Headache	62.5%	52.6%
Malaise	53.2%	44.9%
Gastrointestinal		
Anorexia	20.1%	10.5%
Constipation	6.4%†	3.5%
Nausea	51.4%	29.9%
Vomiting	17.2%	9.8%

* Reported in ≥5% of study population.
† Not statistically significant versus placebo.

TABLE 15 *Frequencies of Selected (Grade 3/4) Laboratory Abnormalities in Patients With Asymptomatic HIV Infection (ACTG 019)*

Adverse Event	Zidovudine 500 mg/day (n=453)	Placebo (n=428)
Anemia (Hgb <8 g/dl)	1.1%	0.2%
Granulocytopenia (<750 cells/mm^3)	1.8%	1.6%
Thrombocytopenia (platelets <50,000/mm^3)	0%	0.5%
ALT (>5 × ULN)	3.1%	2.6%
AST (>5 × ULN)	0.9%	1.6%
Alkaline phosphatase (>5 × ULN)	0%	0%

ULN = Upper limit of normal.

PEDIATRICS

Study ACTG300

Selected clinical adverse events and physical findings with a ≥5% frequency during therapy with lamivudine 4 mg/kg twice daily plus zidovudine 160 mg/m^2 three times daily compared with didanosine in therapy-naive (≤56 days of antiretroviral therapy) pediatric patients are listed in TABLE 16.

TABLE 16 *Selected Clinical Adverse Events and Physical Findings (≥5% Frequency) in Pediatric Patients in Study ACTG300*

Adverse Event	Lamivudine + Zidovudine (n=236)	Didanosine (n=235)
Body as a Whole		
Fever	25%	32%
Digestive		
Hepatomegaly	11%	11%
Nausea & vomiting	8%	7%
Diarrhea	8%	6%
Stomatitis	6%	12%
Splenomegaly	5%	8%
Respiratory		
Cough	15%	18%
Abnormal breath sounds/wheezing	7%	9%
Ear, Nose, and Throat		
Signs or symptoms of ears*	7%	6%
Nasal discharge or congestion	8%	11%
Other		
Skin rashes	12%	14%
Lymphadenopathy	9%	11%

* Includes pain, discharge, erythema, or swelling of an ear.

Selected laboratory abnormalities experienced by therapy-naive (≤56 days of antiretroviral therapy) pediatric patients are listed in TABLE 17.

TABLE 17 *Frequencies of Selected (Grade 3/4) Laboratory Abnormalities in Pediatric Patients in Study ACTG300*

Test (abnormal level)	Lamivudine + Zidovudine	Didanosine
Neutropenia (ANC <400 cells/mm^3)	8%	3%
Anemia (Hgb <7.0 g/dl)	4%	2%
Thrombocytopenia (platelets <50,000/mm^3)	1%	3%
ALT (>10 × ULN)	1%	3%
AST (>10 × ULN)	2%	4%
Lipase (>2.5 × ULN)	3%	3%
Total amylase (>2.5 × ULN)	3%	3%

ULN = Upper limit of normal.
ANC = Absolute neutrophil count.

Additional adverse events reported an open-label studies in pediatric patients receiving zidovudine 180 mg/m^2 every 6 hours were congestive heart failure, decreased reflexes, ECG abnormality, edema, hematuria, left ventricular dilation, macrocytosis, nervousness/irritability, and weight loss.

The clinical adverse events reported among adult recipients of zidovudine may also occur in pediatric patients.

USE FOR THE PREVENTION OF MATERNAL-FETAL TRANSMISSION OF HIV

In a randomized, double-blind, placebo-controlled trial in HIV-infected women and their neonates conducted to determine the utility of zidovudine for the prevention of maternal-fetal HIV transmission, zidovudine syrup at 2 mg/kg was administered every 6 hours for 6 weeks to neonates beginning within 12 hours following birth. The most commonly reported adverse experiences were anemia (hemoglobin <9.0 g/dl) and neutropenia (<1000 cells/mm^3). Anemia occurred in 22% of the neonates who received zidovudine and in 12% of the neonates who received placebo. The mean difference in hemoglobin values was less than 1.0 g/dl for neonates receiving zidovudine compared to neonates receiving placebo. No neonates with anemia required transfusion and all hemoglobin values spontaneously returned to normal within 6 weeks after completion of therapy with zidovudine. Neutropenia was reported with similar frequency in the group that received zidovudine (21%) and in the group that received placebo (27%). The long-term consequences of *in utero* and infant exposure to zidovudine are unknown.

OBSERVED DURING CLINICAL PRACTICE

In addition to adverse events reported from clinical trials, the following events have been identified during use of zidovudine in clinical practice. Because they are reported voluntarily from a population of unknown size, estimates of frequency cannot be made. These events have been chosen for inclusion due to either their seriousness, frequency of reporting, potential causal connection to zidovudine, or a combination of these factors.

Body as a Whole: Back pain, chest pain, flu-like syndrome, generalized pain.
Cardiovascular: Cardiomyopathy, syncope.
Eye: Macular edema.
Endocrine: Gynecomastia.
Gastrointestinal: Constipation, dysphagia, flatulence, mouth ulcer.
General: Sensitization reactions including anaphylaxis and angioedema, vasculitis.
Hemic and Lymphatic: Aplastic anemia, hemolytic anemia, leukopenia, lymphadenopathy, pancytopenia with marrow hypoplasia, pure red cell aplasia.
Hepatobiliary Tract and Pancreas: Hepatitis, hepatomegaly with steatosis, jaundice, lactic acidosis, pancreatitis.
Musculoskeletal: Increased CPK, increased LDH, muscle spasm, myopathy and myositis with pathological changes (similar to that produced by HIV disease), rhabdomyolysis, tremor.
Nervous: Anxiety, confusion, depression, dizziness, loss of mental acuity, mania, paresthesia, seizures, somnolence, vertigo.
Respiratory: Cough, dyspnea, rhinitis, sinusitis.
Skin: Changes in skin and nail pigmentation, pruritus, rash, Stevens-Johnson syndrome, toxic epidermal necrolysis, sweat, urticaria.
Special Senses: Amblyopia, hearing loss, photophobia, taste perversion.
Urogenital: Urinary frequency, urinary hesitancy.

DOSAGE AND ADMINISTRATION

ADULTS

The recommended oral dose of zidovudine is 600 mg/day in divided doses in combination with other antiretroviral agents.

PEDIATRICS

The recommended dose in pediatric patients 6 weeks to 12 years of age is 160 mg/m^2 every 8 hours (480 mg/m^2/day up to a maximum of 200 mg every 8 hours) in combination with other antiretroviral agents.

MATERNAL-FETAL HIV TRANSMISSION

The recommended dosing regimen for administration to pregnant women (>14 weeks of pregnancy) and their neonates is:

Maternal Dosing: 100 mg orally 5 times per day until the start of labor. During labor and delivery, IV zidovudine should be administered at 2 mg/kg (total body weight) over 1 hour followed by a continuous IV infusion of 1 mg/kg/h (total body weight) until clamping of the umbilical cord.

Neonatal Dosing: 2 mg/kg orally every 6 hours starting within 12 hours after birth and continuing through 6 weeks of age. Neonates unable to receive oral dosing may be administered zidovudine intravenously at 1.5 mg/kg, infused over 30 minutes, every 6 hours. (See PRECAUTIONS if hepatic disease or renal insufficiency is present.)

MONITORING OF PATIENTS

Hematologic toxicities appear to be related to pretreatment bone marrow reserve and to dose and duration of therapy. In patients with poor bone marrow reserve, particularly in patients with advanced symptomatic HIV disease, frequent monitoring of hematologic indices is recommended to detect serious anemia or neutropenia (see WARNINGS). In patients who experience hematologic toxicity, reduction in hemoglobin may occur as early as 2-4 weeks, and neutropenia usually occurs after 6-8 weeks.

DOSE ADJUSTMENT

Anemia

Significant anemia (hemoglobin of <7.5 g/dl or reduction of >25% of baseline) and/or significant neutropenia (granulocyte count of <750 cells/mm^3 or reduction of >50% from baseline) may require a dose interruption until evidence of marrow recovery is observed (see WARNINGS). In patients who develop significant anemia, dose interruption does not necessarily eliminate the need for transfusion. If marrow recovery occurs following dose interruption, resumption in dose may be appropriate using adjunctive measures such as epoetin alfa at recommended doses, depending on hematologic indices such as serum erythropoetin level and patient tolerance.

For patients experiencing pronounced anemia while receiving chronic coadministration of zidovudine and some of the drugs (*e.g.,* fluconazole, valproic acid) listed in TABLE 10, zidovudine dose reduction may be considered.

End-Stage Renal Disease

In patients maintained on hemodialysis or peritoneal dialysis, recommended dosing is 100 mg every 6-8 hours (see CLINICAL PHARMACOLOGY, Pharmacokinetics).

Hepatic Impairment

There are insufficient data to recommend dose adjustment of zidovudine in patients with mild to moderate impaired hepatic function or liver cirrhosis. Since zidovudine is primarily eliminated by hepatic metabolism, a reduction in the daily dose may be necessary in these patients. Frequent monitoring for hematologic toxicities is advised (see CLINICAL PHARMACOLOGY, Pharmacokinetics and PRECAUTIONS, General).

HOW SUPPLIED

RETROVIR TABLETS

Retrovir tablets 300 mg (biconvex, white, round, film-coated) containing 300 mg zidovudine, one side engraved "GX CW3" and "300" on the other side.
Storage: Store at 15-25°C (59-77°F).

RETROVIR CAPSULES

Retrovir capsules 100 mg (white, opaque cap and body with a dark blue band) containing 100 mg zidovudine and printed with "Wellcome" and unicorn logo on cap and "Y9C" and "100" on body.
Storage: Store at 15-25°C (59-77°F) and protect from moisture.

RETROVIR SYRUP

Retrovir syrup (colorless to pale yellow, strawberry-flavored) containing 50 mg zidovudine in each teaspoonful (5 ml).
Storage: Store at 15-25°C (59- 77°F).

PRODUCT LISTING - EQUIVALENTS NOT AVAILABLE

Capsule - Oral - 100 mg			
6's	$13.43	RETROVIR, Pharma Pac	52959-0509-06
10's	$19.92	RETROVIR, Physicians Total Care	54868-1974-02
12's	$26.37	RETROVIR, Pharma Pac	52959-0509-12
15's	$29.29	RETROVIR, Physicians Total Care	54868-1974-00
18's	$26.87	RETROVIR, Allscripts Pharmaceutical Company	54569-1772-03
18's	$33.44	RETROVIR, Southwood Pharmaceuticals Inc	58016-0690-18
18's	$36.78	RETROVIR, Quality Care Pharmaceuticals Inc	60346-1015-01
18's	$39.35	RETROVIR, Pharma Pac	52959-0509-18
20's	$30.96	RETROVIR, Allscripts Pharmaceutical Company	54569-1772-02
20's	$35.35	RETROVIR, Compumed Pharmaceuticals	00403-4049-20
20's	$35.97	RETROVIR, Pharma Pac	52959-0509-20
24's	$47.17	RETROVIR, Pharma Pac	52959-0509-24
24's	$56.22	RETROVIR, Quality Care Pharmaceuticals Inc	60346-1015-02
28's	$54.47	RETROVIR, Pharma Pac	52959-0509-28
30's	$57.76	RETROVIR, Pharma Pac	52959-0509-30
42's	$74.32	RETROVIR, Allscripts Pharmaceutical Company	54569-1772-05
100's	$148.25	RETROVIR, Compumed Pharmaceuticals	00403-4049-01
100's	$159.29	RETROVIR, Glaxosmithkline	00081-0108-56
100's	$159.29	RETROVIR, Allscripts Pharmaceutical Company	54569-1772-00
100's	$177.57	RETROVIR, Physicians Total Care	54868-1974-03
100's	$205.15	RETROVIR, Glaxosmithkline	00173-0108-55
100's	$205.15	RETROVIR, Glaxosmithkline	00173-0108-56
180's	$318.51	RETROVIR, Allscripts Pharmaceutical Company	54569-1772-04
240's	$183.18	RETROVIR, Cheshire Drugs	55175-4494-01
Solution - Intravenous - 10 mg/ml			
20 ml x 10	$221.90	RETROVIR, Glaxosmithkline	00173-0107-93
Syrup - Oral - 50 mg/5 ml			
240 ml	$42.47	RETROVIR, Allscripts Pharmaceutical Company	54569-4334-00
240 ml	$49.24	RETROVIR, Glaxosmithkline	00173-0113-18
Tablet - Oral - 300 mg			
60's	$318.52	RETROVIR, Allscripts Pharmaceutical Company	54569-4538-00
60's	$369.27	RETROVIR, Glaxosmithkline	00173-0501-00

Zileuton *(003257)*

Categories: Asthma; FDA Approved 1996 Dec; Pregnancy Category C
Drug Classes: Leucotriene antagonists/inhibitors
Brand Names: Zyflo
Cost of Therapy: $105.14 (Asthma; Zyflo; 600 mg; 4 tablets/day; 30 day supply)

DESCRIPTION

Zileuton is an orally active inhibitor of 5-lipoxygenase, the enzyme that catalyzes the formation of leukotrienes from arachidonic acid. Zileuton has the chemical name (±)-1-(1-Benzo[b] thien-2-ylethyl)-1 -hydroxyurea. Zileuton has the molecular formula $C_{11}H_{12}N_2O_2S$ and molecular weight of 236.29. It is a racemic mixture (50:50) of R(+) and S(-) enantiomers. Zileuton is a practically odorless, white, crystalline powder that is soluble in methanol and ethanol, slightly soluble in acetonitrile and practically insoluble in water and hexane. The melting point ranges from 144.2-145.2°C. Zyflo tablets for oral administration is supplied in one dosage strength containing 600 mg of zileuton.

Zyflo Inactive Ingredients: Crospovidone, hydroxypropyl cellulose, hydroxypropyl methylcellulose, magnesium stearate, microcrystalline cellulose, pregelatinized starch, propylene glycol, sodium starch glycolate, talc, and titanium dioxide.

CLINICAL PHARMACOLOGY

MECHANISM OF ACTION

Zileuton is a specific inhibitor of 5-lipoxygenase and thus inhibits leukotriene (LTB_4, LTC_4, LTD_4 and LTE_4) formation. Both the R(+) and S(-) enantiomers are pharmacologically active as 5-lipoxygenase inhibitors in *in vitro* systems. Leukotrienes are substances that induce numerous biological effects including augmentation of neutrophil and eosinophil migration, neutrophil and monocyte aggregation, leukocyte adhesion, increased capillary permeability, and smooth muscle contraction. These effects contribute to inflammation, edema, mucous secretion, and bronchoconstriction in the airways of asthmatic patients. Sulfido-peptide leukotrienes (LTC_4, LTD_4, LTE_4, also known as the slow-releasing substances of anaphylaxis) and LTB_4, a chemoattractant for neutrophils and eosinophils, can be measured in a number of biological fluids including bronchoalveolar lavage fluid (BALF) from asthmatic patients.

Zileuton is an orally active inhibitor of *ex vivo* LTB_4 formation in several species, including dogs, monkeys, rats, sheep, and rabbits. Zileuton inhibits arachidonic acid-induced ear edema in mice, neutrophil migration in mice in response to polyacrylamide gel, and eosinophil migration into the lungs of antigen-challenged sheep.

Zileuton inhibits leukotriene-dependent smooth muscle contractions *in vitro* in guinea pig and human airways. The compound inhibits leukotriene-dependent bronchospasm in antigen and arachidonic acid-challenged guinea pigs. In antigen-challenged sheep, zileuton inhibits late-phase bronchoconstriction and airway hyperactivity. In humans, pretreatment with zileuton attenuated bronchoconstriction caused by cold air challenge in patients with asthma.

PHARMACOKINETICS

Zileuton is rapidly absorbed upon oral administration with a mean time to peak plasma concentration (T_{max}) of 1.7 hours and a mean peak level (C_{max}) of 4.98 µg/ml. The absolute bioavailability of zileuton is unknown. Systemic exposure (mean AUC) following 600 mg zileuton administration is 19.2 µg/hr/ml. Plasma concentrations of zileuton are proportional to dose, and steady-state levels are predictable from single-dose pharmacokinetic data. Administration of zileuton with food resulted in a small but statistically significant increase (27%) in zileuton C_{max} without significant changes in the extent of absorption (AUC) or T_{max}. Therefore, zileuton can be administered with or without food (see DOSAGE AND ADMINISTRATION).

The apparent volume of distribution (V/F) of zileuton is approximately 1.2 L/kg. Zileuton is 93% bound to plasma proteins, primarily to albumin, with minor binding to α1-acid glycoprotein.

Elimination of zileuton is predominantly via metabolism with a mean terminal half-life of 2.5 hours. Apparent oral clearance of zileuton is 7.0 ml/min/kg. Zileuton activity is primarily due to the parent drug. Studies with radiolabeled drug demonstrated that orally administered zileuton is well absorbed into the systemic circulation with 94.5% and 2.2% of the radiolabeled dose recovered in urine and feces, respectively. Several zileuton metabolites have been identified in human plasma and urine. These include two diastereomeric O-glucuronide conjugates (major metabolites) and an N-dehydroxylated metabolite of zileuton. The urinary excretion of the inactivated N-dehydroxylated metabolite and unchanged zileuton each accounted for less than 0.5% of the dose. *In vitro* studies utilizing human liver microsomes have shown that zileuton and its N-dehydroxylated metabolite can be oxidatively metabolized by the cytochrome P450 isoenzymes 1A2, 2C9 and 3A4 (CYP1A2, CYP2C9 and CYP3A4).

SPECIAL POPULATIONS

Effect of Age

Zileuton pharmacokinetics were similar in healthy elderly subjects (>65 years) compared to healthy younger adults (18-40 years).

Effect of Gender

Across several studies, no significant gender effects were observed on the pharmacokinetics of zileuton.

Renal Insufficiency

The pharmacokinetics of zileuton were similar in healthy subjects and in subjects with mild, moderate, and severe renal insufficiency. In subjects with renal failure requiring hemodialysis, zileuton pharmacokinetics were not altered by hemodialysis and a very small percentage of the administered zileuton dose (<0.5%) was removed by hemodialysis. Hence, dosing adjustment in patients with renal dysfunction or undergoing hemodialysis is not necessary.

Hepatic Insufficiency

Zileuton is contraindicated in patients with active liver disease (see CONTRAINDICATIONS and PRECAUTIONS, Hepatic) .

INDICATIONS AND USAGE

Zileuton is indicated for the prophylaxis and chronic treatment of asthma in adults and children 12 years of age and older.

CONTRAINDICATIONS

Zileuton tablets are contraindicated in patients with:

- Active liver disease or transaminase elevations greater than or equal to 3 times the upper limit of normal (≥3 × ULN) (see PRECAUTIONS, Hepatic).
- Hypersensitivity to zileuton or any of its inactive ingredients.

WARNINGS

Zileuton is not indicated for use in the reversal of bronchospasm in acute asthma attacks, including status astmaticus. Therapy with zileuton can be continued during acute exacerbations of asthma.

PRECAUTIONS

HEPATIC

Elevations of one or more liver function tests may occur during zileuton therapy. These laboratory abnormalities may progress, remain unchanged, or resolve with continued therapy. In a few cases, initial transaminase elevations were first noted after discontinuing treatment, usually within 2 weeks. The ALT (SGPT) test is considered the most sensitive indicator of liver injury. In placebo-controlled clinical trials, the frequency of ALT elevations greater than or equal to 3 times the upper limits of normal (3 x ULN) was 1.9% for zileuton treated patients, compared with 0.2% for placebo-treated patients.

In a long-term safety surveillance study, 2458 patients received zileuton in addition to their usual asthma care and 489 received their usual asthma care. In patients treated for up to 12 months with zileuton in addition to their usual asthma care, 4.6% developed an ALT of at least 3 × ULN, compared with 1.1% of patients receiving only their usual asthma care. Sixty-one percent (61%) of these elevations occurred during the first 2 months of zileuton therapy. After 2 months of treatment, the rate of new ALT elevations ≥3 × ULN stabilized at a mean of 0.30% per month for patients receiving zileuton-plus usual-asthma care compared with 0.11% per month for patients receiving usual asthma care alone. Of the 61 zileuton plus usual asthma care patients with ALT elevations between 3 to 5 × ULN, 32 patients (52%) had ALT values decrease to below 2 × ULN while continuing zileuton therapy. Twenty-one of the 61 patients (34%) had further increases in ALT levels to ≥5 × ULN and were withdrawn from the study in accordance with the study protocol. In patients who discontinued zileuton, elevated ALT levels returned to <2 × ULN in an average of 32 days (range 1-111 days).

In controlled and uncontrolled clinical trials involving more than 5000 patients treated with zileuton, the overall rate of ALT elevation ≥3 × ULN was 3.2%. In these trials, 1 patient developed symptomatic hepatitis with jaundice, which resolved upon discontinuation of therapy. An additional 3 patients with transaminase elevations developed mild hyperbilirubinemia that was less than 3 times the upper limit of normal. There was no evidence of hypersensitivity or other alternative etiologies for these findings. In subsequent analyses, females over the age of 65 appeared to be at an increased risk for ALT elevations. Patients with pre-existing transaminase elevations may also be at an increased risk for ALT elevations (see CONTRAINDICATIONS).

It is recommended that hepatic transaminases be evaluated at initiation of, and during therapy with, zileuton. Serum ALT should be monitored before treatment begins, once-a-month for the first 3 months, every 2-3 months for the remainder of the first year, and periodically thereafter for patients receiving long-term zileuton therapy. If clinical signs and/or symptoms of liver dysfunction (*e.g*, right upper quadrant pain, nausea, fatigue, lethargy, pruritus, jaundice, or "flu-like" symptoms) develop or transaminase elevations greater than 5 times the ULN occur, zileuton should be discontinued and transaminase levels followed until normal.

Since treatment with zileuton may result in increased hepatic transaminases, zileuton should be used with caution in patients who consume substantial quantities of alcohol and/or have a past history of liver disease.

INFORMATION FOR THE PATIENT

Patients should be told that:

- Zileuton is indicated for the chronic treatment of asthma and should be taken regularly as prescribed, even during symptom-free periods.
- Zileuton is not a bronchodilator and should not be used to treat acute episodes of asthma.
- When taking zileuton, they should not decrease the dose or stop taking any other anti-asthma medications unless instructed by a physician.
- While using zileuton, medical attention should be sought if short-acting bronchodilators are needed more often than usual, or if more than the maximum number of inhalations of short-acting bronchodilator treatment prescribed for a 24 hour period are needed.
- The most serious side effect of zileuton is elevation of liver enzyme tests and that, while taking zileuton, they must return for liver enzyme test monitoring on a regular basis.
- If they experience signs and/or symptoms of liver dysfunction (*e.g.*, right upper quadrant pain, nausea, fatigue, lethargy, pruritus, jaundice, or "flu-like" symptoms), they should contact their physician immediately.
- Zileuton can interact with other drugs and that, while taking zileuton, they should consult their doctor before starting or stopping any prescription or non-prescription medicines.

CARCINOGENESIS, MUTAGENESIS, AND IMPAIRMENT OF FERTILITY

In 2 year carcinogenicity studies, increases in the incidence of liver, kidney, and vascular tumors in female mice and a trend towards an increase in the incidence of liver tumors in male mice were observed at 450 mg/kg/day (providing approximately 4 times [females] or 7 times [males] the systemic exposure [AUC] achieved at the maximum recommended human daily oral dose). No increase in the incidence of tumors was observed at 150 mg/kg/day (providing approximately 2 times the systemic exposure [AUC] achieved at the maximum recommended human daily oral dose). In rats, an increase in the incidence of kidney tumors was observed in both sexes at 170 mg/kg/day (providing approximately 6 times [males] or 14 times [females] the systemic exposure [AUC] achieved at the maximum recommended human daily oral dose). No increased incidence of kidney tumors was seen at 80 mg/kg/day (providing approximately 4 times [males] or 6 times [females] the systemic exposure [AUC] achieved at the maximum recommended human daily oral dose). Although a dose-related increased incidence of benign Leydig cell tumors was observed, Leydig cell tumorogenesis was prevented by supplementing male rats with testosterone.

Zileuton was negative in genotoxicity studies including bacterial reverse mutation (Ames) using *S. typhimurium* and *E. coli*, chromosome aberration in human lymphocytes, *in vitro* unscheduled DNA synthesis (UDS), in rat hepatocytes with or without zileuton pretreatment and in mouse and rat kidney cells with zileuton pretreatment, and mouse micronucleus assays. However, a dose-related increase in DNA adduct formation was reported in kidneys and livers of female mice treated with zileuton. Although some evidence of DNA damage was observed in a UDS assay in hepatocytes isolated from Aroclor-1254 treated rats, no such finding was noticed in hepatocytes isolated from monkeys, where the metabolic profile of zileuton is more similar to that of humans.

In reproductive performance/fertility studies, zileuton produced no effects on fertility in rats at oral doses up to 300 mg/kg/day (providing approximately 8 times [male rats] and 18 times [female rats] the systemic exposure [AUC] achieved at the maximum recommended human daily oral dose). Comparative systemic exposure (AUC) is based on measurements in male rats or nonpregnant female rats at similar dosages. However, reduction in fetal implants was observed at oral doses of 150 mg/kg/day and higher (providing approximately 9 times the systemic exposure [AUC] achieved at the maximum recommended human daily oral dose). Increases in gestation length, prolongation of estrous cycle, and increases in stillbirths were observed at oral doses of 70 mg/kg/day and higher (providing approximately 4 times the systemic exposure (AUC) achieved at the maximum recommended human daily oral dose). In a perinatal/postnatal study in rats, reduced pup survival and growth were noted at an oral dose of 300 mg/kg/day (providing approximately 18 times the systemic exposure [AUC] achieved at the maximum recommended human daily oral dose).

PREGNANCY, TERATOGENIC EFFECTS, PREGNANCY CATEGORY C

Developmental studies indicated adverse effects (reduced body weight and increased skeletal variations) in rats at an oral dose of 300 mg/kg/day (providing approximately 18 times the systemic exposure [AUC] achieved at the maximum recommended human daily oral dose). Comparative systemic exposure [AUC] is based on measurements in nonpregnant female rats at a similar dosage. Zileuton and/or its metabolites cross the placental barrier of rats. Three of 118 (2.5%) rabbit fetuses had cleft palates at an oral dose of 150 mg/kg/day (equivalent to the maximum recommended human daily oral dose on a mg/m^2 basis). There are no adequate and well-controlled studies in pregnant women. Zileuton should be used during pregnancy only if the potential benefit justifies the potential risk to the fetus.

NURSING MOTHERS

Zileuton and/or its metabolites are excreted in rat milk. It is not known if zileuton is excreted in human milk. Because many drugs are excreted in human milk, and because of the potential for tumorogenicity shown for zileuton in animal studies, a decision should be made whether to discontinue nursing or to discontinue the drug, taking into account the importance of the drug to the mother.

PEDIATRIC USE

The safely and effectiveness of zileuton in pediatric patients under 12 years of age have not been established.

DRUG INTERACTIONS

In a drug-interaction study in 16 healthy volunteers, co-administration of multiple doses of zileuton (800 mg every 12 hours) and theophylline (200 mg every 6 hours) for 5 days resulted in a significant decrease (approximately 50%) in steady-state clearance of theophylline, an approximate doubling of theophylline AUC, and an increase in theophylline C_{max} by 73%). The elimination half-life of theophylline was increased by 24%. Also, during co-administration, theophylline-related adverse events were observed more frequently than after theophylline alone. Upon initiation of zileuton in patients receiving theophylline, the theophylline dosage should be reduced by approximately one-half and plasma theophylline concentrations monitored. Similarly, when initiating therapy with theophylline in a patient receiving zileuton, the maintenance dose and/or dosing interval of theophylline should be adjusted accordingly and guided by serum theophylline determinations (see WARNINGS).

Concomitant administration of multiple doses of zileuton (600 mg every 6 hours) and warfarin (fixed daily dose obtained by titration in each subject) to 30 healthy male volunteers resulted in a 15% decrease in R-warfarin clearance and an increase in AUC of 22%. The pharmacokinetics of S-warfarin were not affected. These pharmacokinetic changes were accompanied by a clinically significant increase in prothrombin times. Monitoring of prothrombin time, or other suitable coagulation tests, with the appropriate dose titration of warfarin is recommended in patients receiving concomitant zileuton and warfarin therapy (see WARNINGS).

Co-administration of zileuton and propranolol results in a significant increase in propranolol concentrations. Administration of a single 80 mg dose of propranolol in 16 healthy male volunteers who received zileuton 600 mg every 6 hours for 5 days resulted in a 42% decrease in propranolol clearance. This resulted in an increase in propranolol C_{max}, AUC, and elimination half-life by 52%, 104%, and 25%, respectively. There was an increase in β-blockade and decrease in heart rate associated with the co-administration of these drugs. Patients on zileuton and propranolol should be closely monitored and the dose of propranolol reduced as necessary (see WARNINGS). No formal drug-drug interaction studies between zileuton and other beta-adrenergic blocking agents (*i.e.,* β-blockers) have been conducted. It is reasonable to employ appropriate clinical monitoring when these drugs are co-administered with zileuton.

In a drug interaction study in 16 healthy volunteers, co-administration of multiple doses of terfenadine (600 mg every 12 hours) and zileuton (600 mg every 6 hours) for 7 days resulted in a decrease in clearance of terfenadine by 22% leading to a statistically significant increase in mean AUC and C_{max} of terfenadine of approximately 35%. This increase in terfenadine plasma concentration in the presence of zileuton was not associated with a significant prolongation of the QTc interval. Although there was no cardiac effect in this small number of healthy volunteers, given the high inter-individual pharmacokinetic variability of terfenadine, co-administration of zileuton and terfenadine is not recommended.

Drug-drug interaction studies conducted in healthy volunteers between zileuton and prednisone and ethinyl estradiol (oral contraceptive), drugs known to be metabolized by the P450 3A4 (CYP3A4) isoenzyme, have shown no significant interaction. However, no formal drug-drug interaction studies between zileuton and dihydropyridine, calcium channel blockers, cyclosporine, cisapride, and astemizole, also metabolized by CYP3A4 have been conducted. It is reasonable to employ appropriate clinical monitoring when these drugs are co-administered with zileuton.

Drug-drug interaction studies in healthy volunteers have been conducted with zileuton and digoxin, phenytoin, sulfasalazine, and naproxen. There was no significant interaction between zileuton and any of these drugs.

Co-administration of zileuton and theophylline results in, on average, an approximate doubling of serum theophylline concentrations. Theophylline dosage in these patients should be reduced and serum theophylline concentrations monitored closely (see DRUG INTERACTIONS).

ADVERSE REACTIONS

In clinical studies a total of 5542 patients have been exposed to zileuton in clinical trials, 2252 of them for greater than 6 months and 742 for greater than 1 year.

Adverse events most frequently occurring (frequency ≥3%) in zileuton-treated patients and at a frequency greater than placebo-treated patients are summarized in TABLE 2.

TABLE 2 *Proportion of Patients Experiencing Adverse Events in Placebo-Controlled Studies in Asthma*

Body System Event	Zileuton 600 mg 4× Daily (n=475)	Placebo (n=491)
Body as a Whole		
Headache	24.6%	24.0%
Pain (unspecified)	7.8%	5.3%
Abdominal pain	4.6%	2.4%
Asthenia	3.8%	2.4%
Accidental injury	3.4%	2.0%
Digestive System		
Dyspepsia	8.2%*	2.9%
Nausea	5.5%	3.7%
Musculoskeletal		
Myalgia	3.2%	2.9%

* p ≤0.05 vs placebo

Less common adverse events occurring at a frequency of greater than 1% and more commonly in zileuton-treated patients included: arthralgia, chest pain, conjunctivitis constipation, dizziness, fever, flatulence, hypertonia, insomnia, lymphadenopathy, malaise, neck pain/rigidity, nervousness, pruritus, somnolence, urinary tract infection, vaginitis, and vomiting.

The frequency of discontinuation from the asthma clinical studies due to any adverse event was comparable between zileuton (9.7%) and placebo-treated (8. 4%) groups.

In placebo-controlled clinical trials, the frequency of ALT elevations ≥3 × ULN was 1.9% for zileuton-treated patients, compared with 0.2% for placebo-treated patients. In controlled and uncontrolled trials, 1 patient developed symptomatic hepatitis with jaundice, which resolved upon discontinuation of therapy. An additional 3 patients with transaminase elevations developed mild hyperbilirubinemia that was less than 3 times the upper limit of normal. There was no evidence of hypersensitivity or other alternative etiologies for these findings. Zileuton is contraindicated in patients with active liver disease or transaminase elevations greater than or equal to 3 × ULN (see CONTRAINDICATIONS). It is recommended that hepatic transaminases be evaluated at initiation of and during therapy with zileuton (see PRECAUTIONS, Hepatic).

Occurrences of low white blood cell count ≤2.8 × 10^9/L) were observed in 1.0% of 1673 patients taking zileuton and 0.6% of 1056 patients taking placebo in placebo-controlled studies. These findings were transient and the majority of cases returned toward normal or baseline with continued zileuton dosing. All remaining cases returned toward normal or baseline after discontinuation of zileuton. Similar findings were also noted in a long-term safety surveillance study of 2458 patients treated with zileuton plus usual asthma care versus 489 patients treated only with usual asthma care for up to 1 year. The clinical significance of these observations is not known.

In the long-term safety surveillance trial of zileuton plus usual asthma care versus usual asthma care alone, a similar adverse event profile was seen as in other clinical trials.

DOSAGE AND ADMINISTRATION

The recommended dosage of zileuton for the symptomatic treatment of patients with asthma is one 600 mg tablet 4 times a day for a total daily dose of 2400 mg. For ease of administration, zileuton may be taken with meals and at bedtime. Hepatic transaminases should be evaluated prior to initiation of zileuton and periodically during treatment (see PRECAUTIONS, Hepatic).

HOW SUPPLIED

Zyflo Filmtab Tablets are available as 1 dosage strength: 600 mg white ovaloid tablets with single bisect, debossed on bisect side with Abbott logo and "ZL (Abbo-Code)", and "600" on the opposite side.

Storage: Store tablets at controlled room temperature between 20-25°C (68-77°F). Protect from light.

PRODUCT LISTING - EQUIVALENTS NOT AVAILABLE

Tablet - Oral - 600 mg

120's	$105.14	ZYFLO, Abbott Pharmaceutical	00074-8036-22

Zinc Sulfate *(002459)*

Categories: Deficiency, vitamin and mineral; FDA Approved 1987 May
Drug Classes: Vitamins/minerals
Brand Names: Z Span; Zinc-220; Zinca-Pak; Zincate; Zincomed

DESCRIPTION

Each opaque blue and pink capsule contains zinc sulfate 220 mg delivering 55 mg of elemental zinc. Zinc-220 capsules do not contain dextrose or glucose.

INDICATIONS AND USAGE

Zinc sulfate capsules are indicated as a dietary supplement. Normal growth and tissue repair are directly dependent upon an adequate supply of zinc in the diet. Zinc functions as an integral part of a number of enzymes important to protein and carbohydrate metabolism.

Zinc sulfate capsules are recommended for deficiencies or the prevention of deficiencies of zinc.

WARNINGS

Zinc sulfate capsules if administered in stat dosages of 2 g (9 capsules) will cause an emetic effect. This product should not be used by pregnant or lactating women.

PRECAUTIONS

It is recommended that zinc sulfate capsules be taken with meals or milk to avoid gastric distress.

DOSAGE AND ADMINISTRATION

One (1) capsule daily with milk or meals. One (1) capsule daily provides approximately 5.3 times the recommended adult requirement of zinc.

PRODUCT LISTING - EQUIVALENTS NOT AVAILABLE

Solution - Intravenous - 1 mg/ml

10 ml	$1.89	GENERIC, Mcguff Company	49072-0993-10
10 ml x 25	$40.00	GENERIC, Raway Pharmacal Inc	00686-6110-25
10 ml x 25	$62.25	GENERIC, American Regent Laboratories Inc	00517-6110-25

Solution - Intravenous - 5 mg/ml

5 ml x 25	$60.00	GENERIC, Raway Pharmacal Inc	00686-8105-25
5 ml x 25	$124.75	GENERIC, American Regent Laboratories Inc	00517-8105-25

Ziprasidone *(001900)*

Categories: Agitation, psychomotor; Schizophrenia; FDA Approved 2001 Feb; Pregnancy Category C
Drug Classes: Antipsychotics
Brand Names: **Geodon**
Foreign Brand Availability: Zeldox (Hong-Kong; Philippines)
Cost of Therapy: $268.21 (Schizophrenia; Geodon; 20 mg; 2 capsules/day; 30 day supply)

DESCRIPTION

Geodon is available as Geodon capsules (ziprasidone hydrochloride) for oral administration and as Geodon for Injection (ziprasidone mesylate) for intramuscular (IM) injection. Ziprasidone is an antipsychotic agent that is chemically unrelated to phenothiazine or butyrophenone antipsychotic agents. It has a molecular weight of 412.94 (free base), with the following chemical name: 5-[2-[4-(1,2-benzisothiazol-3-yl)-1-piperazinyl]ethyl]-6-chloro-1,3-dihydro-2*H*-indol-2-one. The empirical formula is $C_{21}H_{21}ClN_4OS$ (free base of ziprasidone).

CAPSULES

Geodon capsules contain a monohydrochloride, monohydrate salt of ziprasidone. Chemically, ziprasidone hydrochloride monohydrate is 5-[2-[4-(1,2-benzisothiazol-3-yl)-1-piperazinyl]ethyl]-6-chloro-1,3-dihydro-2*H*-indol-2-one, monohydrochloride, monohydrate. The empirical formula is $C_{21}H_{21}ClN_4OS{\cdot}HCl{\cdot}H_2O$ and its molecular weight is 467.42. Ziprasidone hydrochloride monohydrate is a white to slightly pink powder.

Geodon capsules are supplied for oral administration in 20 mg (blue/white), 40 mg (blue/blue), 60 mg (white/white), and 80 mg (blue/white) capsules. Geodon capsules contain ziprasidone hydrochloride monohydrate, lactose, pregelatinized starch, and magnesium stearate.

INJECTION

FOR IM USE ONLY.

Geodon for Injection contains a lyophilized form of ziprasidone mesylate trihydrate. Chemically, ziprasidone mesylate trihydrate is 5-[2-[4-(1,2-benzisothiazol-3-yl)-1-piperazinyl]ethyl]-6-chloro-1,3-dihydro-2H-indol-2-one, methanesulfonate, trihydrate. The empirical formula is $C_{21}H_{21}ClN_4OS{\cdot}CH_3SO_3H{\cdot}3H_2O$ and its molecular weight is 563.09.

Geodon for Injection is available in a single dose vial as ziprasidone mesylate (20 mg ziprasidone/ml when reconstituted according to label instructions — see DOSAGE AND ADMINISTRATION, Preparation for Administration) for IM administration. Each ml of ziprasidone mesylate for injection (when reconstituted) contains 20 mg of ziprasidone and 4.7 mg of methanesulfonic acid solubilized by 294 mg of sulfobutylether β-cyclodextrin sodium (SBECD).

CLINICAL PHARMACOLOGY

PHARMACODYNAMICS

Ziprasidone exhibited high *in vitro* binding affinity for the dopamine D_2 and D_3, the serotonin $5HT_{2A}$, $5HT_{2C}$, $5HT_{1A}$, $5HT_{1D}$ and α_1-adrenergic receptors (Ki's of 4.8, 7.2, 0.4, 1.3, 3.4, 2, and 10 nM, respectively) and moderate affinity for the histamine H_1 receptor (Ki = 47 nM). Ziprasidone functioned as an antagonist at the D_2, $5HT_{2A}$, and $5HT_{1D}$ receptors, and as an agonist at the $5HT_{1A}$ receptor. Ziprasidone inhibited synaptic reuptake of serotonin and norepinephrine. No appreciable affinity was exhibited for other receptor/binding sites tested, including the cholinergic muscarinic receptor (IC_{50} >1 μM).

The mechanism of action of ziprasidone, as with other drugs having efficacy in schizophrenia, is unknown. However, it has been proposed that this drug's efficacy in schizophrenia is mediated through a combination of dopamine Type 2 (D_2) and serotonin Type 2 ($5HT_2$) antagonism. Antagonism at receptors other than dopamine and $5HT_2$ with similar receptor affinities may explain some of the other therapeutic and side effects of ziprasidone.

Ziprasidone's antagonism of histamine H_1 receptors may explain the somnolence observed with this drug.

Ziprasidone's antagonism of α_1-adrenergic receptors may explain the orthostatic hypotension observed with this drug.

ORAL PHARMACOKINETICS

Ziprasidone's activity is primarily due to the parent drug. The multiple-dose pharmacokinetics of ziprasidone are dose-proportional within the proposed clinical dose range, and ziprasidone accumulation is predictable with multiple dosing. Elimination of ziprasidone is mainly via hepatic metabolism with a mean terminal half-life of about 7 hours within the proposed clinical dose range. Steady-state concentrations are achieved within 1-3 days of dosing. The mean apparent systemic clearance is 7.5 ml/min/kg. Ziprasidone is unlikely to interfere with the metabolism of drugs metabolized by cytochrome P450 enzymes.

Absorption

Ziprasidone is well absorbed after oral administration, reaching peak plasma concentrations in 6-8 hours. The absolute bioavailability of a 20 mg dose under fed conditions is approximately 60%. The absorption of ziprasidone is increased up to 2-fold in the presence of food.

Distribution

Ziprasidone has a mean apparent volume of distribution of 1.5 L/kg. It is greater than 99% bound to plasma proteins, binding primarily to albumin and α_1-acid glycoprotein. The *in vitro* plasma protein binding of ziprasidone was not altered by warfarin or propranolol, two highly protein-bound drugs, nor did ziprasidone alter the binding of these drugs in human plasma. Thus, the potential for drug interactions with ziprasidone due to displacement is minimal.

Metabolism and Elimination

Ziprasidone is extensively metabolized after oral administration with only a small amount excreted in the urine (<1%) or feces (<4%) as unchanged drug. Ziprasidone is primarily cleared via three metabolic routes to yield four major circulating metabolites, benzisothiazole (BITP) sulphoxide, BITP sulphone, ziprasidone sulphoxide, and S-methyl-dihydroziprasidone. Approximately 20% of the dose is excreted in the urine, with approximately 66% being eliminated in the feces. Unchanged ziprasidone represents about 44% of total drug-related material in serum. *In vitro* studies using human liver subcellular fractions indicate that S-methyl-dihydroziprasidone is generated in 2 steps. The data indicate that the reduction reaction is mediated by aldehyde oxidase and the subsequent methylation is mediated by thiol methyltransferase. *In vitro* studies using human liver microsomes and recombinant enzymes indicate that CYP3A4 is the major CYP contributing to the oxidative metabolism of ziprasidone. CYP1A2 may contribute to a much lesser extent. Based on *in vivo* abundance of excretory metabolites, less than one-third of ziprasidone metabolic clearance is mediated by cytochrome P450 catalyzed oxidation and approximately two-thirds via reduction by aldehyde oxidase. There are no known clinically relevant inhibitors or inducers of aldehyde oxidase.

INTRAMUSCULAR PHARMACOKINETICS

Systemic Bioavailability

The bioavailability of ziprasidone administered intramuscularly is 100%. After IM administration of single doses, peak serum concentrations typically occur at approximately 60 minutes post-dose or earlier and the mean half-life ($T_{1/2}$) ranges from 2-5 hours. Exposure increases in a dose-related manner and following 3 days of IM dosing, little accumulation is observed.

Metabolism and Elimination

Although the metabolism and elimination of IM ziprasidone have not been systematically evaluated, the IM route of administration would not be expected to alter the metabolic pathways.

SPECIAL POPULATIONS

Age and Gender Effects

In a multiple-dose (8 days of treatment) study involving 32 subjects, there was no difference in the pharmacokinetics of ziprasidone between men and women or between elderly (>65 years) and young (18-45 years) subjects. Additionally, population pharmacokinetic evaluation of patients in controlled trials has revealed no evidence of clinically significant age or gender-related differences in the pharmacokinetics of ziprasidone. Dosage modifications for age or gender are, therefore, not recommended.

Ziprasidone IM has not been systematically evaluated in elderly patients (65 years and over).

Race

No specific pharmacokinetic study was conducted to investigate the effects of race. Population pharmacokinetic evaluation has revealed no evidence of clinically significant race-related differences in the pharmacokinetics of ziprasidone. Dosage modifications for race are, therefore, not recommended.

Smoking

Based on *in vitro* studies utilizing human liver enzymes, ziprasidone is not a substrate for CYP1A2; smoking should therefore not have an effect on the pharmacokinetics of ziprasidone. Consistent with these *in vitro* results, population pharmacokinetic evaluation has not revealed any significant pharmacokinetic differences between smokers and nonsmokers.

Renal Impairment

Because ziprasidone is highly metabolized, with less than 1% of the drug excreted unchanged, renal impairment alone is unlikely to have a major impact on the pharmacokinetics of ziprasidone. The pharmacokinetics of ziprasidone following 8 days of 20 mg bid dosing were similar among subjects with varying degrees of renal impairment (n=27), and subjects with normal renal function, indicating that dosage adjustment based upon the degree of renal impairment is not required. Ziprasidone is not removed by hemodialysis.

Hepatic Impairment

As ziprasidone is cleared substantially by the liver, the presence of hepatic impairment would be expected to increase the AUC of ziprasidone; a multiple-dose study at 20 mg bid for 5 days in subjects (n=13) with clinically significant (Childs-Pugh Class A and B) cirrhosis revealed an increase in AUC(0-12) of 13% and 34% in Childs-Pugh Class A and B, respectively, compared to a matched control group (n=14). A half-life of 7.1 hours was observed in subjects with cirrhosis compared to 4.8 hours in the control group.

Intramuscular ziprasidone has not been systematically evaluated in elderly patients or in patients with hepatic or renal impairment. As the cyclodextrin excipient is cleared by renal filtration, ziprasidone IM should be administered with caution to patients with impaired renal function.

DRUG-DRUG INTERACTIONS

An *in vitro* enzyme inhibition study utilizing human liver microsomes showed that ziprasidone had little inhibitory effect on CYP1A2, CYP2C9, CYP2C19, CYP2D6 and CYP3A4, and thus would not likely interfere with the metabolism of drugs primarily metabolized by these enzymes. *In vivo* studies have revealed no effect of ziprasidone on the pharmacokinetics of dextromethorphan, estrogen, progesterone, or lithium (see DRUG INTERACTIONS).

In vivo studies have revealed an approximately 35% decrease in ziprasidone AUC by concomitantly administered carbamazepine, an approximately 35-40% increase in ziprasidone AUC by concomitantly administered ketoconazole, but no effect on ziprasidone's pharmacokinetics by cimetidine or antacid (see DRUG INTERACTIONS).

INDICATIONS AND USAGE

Ziprasidone is indicated for the treatment of schizophrenia. When deciding among the alternative treatments available for this condition, the prescriber should consider the finding of ziprasidone's greater capacity to prolong the QT/QTc interval compared to several other antipsychotic drugs (see WARNINGS). Prolongation of the QTc interval is associated in some other drugs with the ability to cause torsade de pointes-type arrhythmia, a potentially fatal polymorphic ventricular tachycardia, and sudden death. In many cases this would lead to the conclusion that other drugs should be tried first. Whether ziprasidone will cause torsade de pointes or increase the rate of sudden death is not yet known (see WARNINGS).

The efficacy of oral ziprasidone was established in short-term (4 and 6 week) controlled trials of schizophrenic inpatients (see CLINICAL PHARMACOLOGY).

In a placebo-controlled trial involving the follow-up for up to 52 weeks of stable schizophrenic inpatients, ziprasidone was demonstrated to delay the time to and rate of relapse. The physician who elects to use ziprasidone for extended periods should periodically reevaluate the long-term usefulness of the drug for the individual patient.

Ziprasidone IM is indicated for the treatment of acute agitation in schizophrenic patients for whom treatment with ziprasidone is appropriate and who need IM antipsychotic medication for rapid control of the agitation. "Psychomotor agitation" is defined in DSM-IV as "excessive motor activity associated with a feeling of inner tension." Schizophrenic patients experiencing agitation often manifest behaviors that interfere with their diagnosis and care, *e.g.*, threatening behaviors, escalating or urgently distressing behavior, or self-exhausting behavior, leading clinicians to the use of IM antipsychotic medications to achieve immediate control of the agitation. The efficacy of IM ziprasidone for acute agitation in schizophrenia was established in single-day controlled trials of schizophrenic inpatients (see CLINICAL PHARMACOLOGY). Since there is no experience regarding the safety of administering ziprasidone IM to schizophrenic patients already taking oral ziprasidone, the practice of co-administration is not recommended.

NON-FDA APPROVED INDICATIONS

Initial data have reported ziprasidone to be effective and well tolerated in the treatment of Tourette's syndrome. However, additional studies are needed and this use has not been approved by the FDA.

CONTRAINDICATIONS

QT PROLONGATION

Because of ziprasidone's dose-related prolongation of the QT interval and the known association of fatal arrhythmias with QT prolongation by some other drugs, ziprasidone is contraindicated in patients with a known history of QT prolongation (including congenital long QT syndrome), with recent acute myocardial infarction, or with uncompensated heart failure (see WARNINGS).

Pharmacokinetic/pharmacodynamic studies between ziprasidone and other drugs that prolong the QT interval have not been performed. An additive effect of ziprasidone and other drugs that prolong the QT interval cannot be excluded. Therefore, ziprasidone should not be given with dofetilide, sotalol, quinidine, other Class Ia and III anti-arrhythmics, mesoridazine, thioridazine, chlorpromazine, droperidol, pimozide, sparfloxacin, gatifloxacin, moxifloxacin, halofantrine, mefloquine, pentamidine, arsenic trioxide, levomethadyl acetate, dolasetron mesylate, probucol or tacrolimus. Ziprasidone is also contraindicated with drugs that have demonstrated QT prolongation as one of their pharmacodynamic effects and have this effect described in the full prescribing information as a contraindication or a boxed or bolded warning (see WARNINGS).

HYPERSENSITIVITY

Ziprasidone is contraindicated in individuals with a known hypersensitivity to the product.

WARNINGS

QT PROLONGATION AND RISK OF SUDDEN DEATH

Ziprasidone use should be avoided in combination with other drugs that are known to prolong the QTc interval (see CONTRAINDICATIONS, and DRUG INTERACTIONS). Additionally, clinicians should be alert to the identification of other drugs that have been consistently observed to prolong the QTc interval. Such drugs should not be prescribed with ziprasidone. Ziprasidone should also be avoided in patients with congenital long QT syndrome and in patients with a history of cardiac arrhythmias (see CONTRAINDICATIONS).

A study directly comparing the QT/QTc prolonging effect of oral ziprasidone with several other drugs effective in the treatment of schizophrenia was conducted in patient volunteers. In the first phase of the trial, ECGs were obtained at the time of maximum plasma concentration when the drug was administered alone. In the second phase of the trial, ECGs were obtained at the time of maximum plasma concentration while the drug was coadministered with an inhibitor of the CYP4503A4 metabolism of the drug.

In the first phase of the study, the mean change in QTc from baseline was calculated for each drug, using a sample-based correction that removes the effect of heart rate on the QT interval. The mean increase in QTc from baseline for ziprasidone ranged from approximately 9-14 milliseconds greater than for four of the comparator drugs (risperidone, olanzapine, quetiapine, and haloperidol), but was approximately 14 milliseconds less than the prolongation observed for thioridazine.

In the second phase of the study, the effect of ziprasidone on QTc length was not augmented by the presence of a metabolic inhibitor (ketoconazole 200 mg bid).

In placebo-controlled trials, oral ziprasidone increased the QTc interval compared to placebo by approximately 10 milliseconds at the highest recommended daily dose of 160 mg. In clinical trials with oral ziprasidone, the electrocardiograms of 2/2988 (0.06%) patients who received ziprasidone and 1/440 (0.23%) patients who received placebo revealed QTc intervals exceeding the potentially clinically relevant threshold of 500 milliseconds. In the ziprasidone-treated patients, neither case suggested a role of ziprasidone. One patient had a history of prolonged QTc and a screening measurement of 489 milliseconds; QTc was 503 milliseconds during ziprasidone treatment. The other patient had a QTc of 391 milliseconds at the end of treatment with ziprasidone and upon switching to thioridazine experienced QTc measurements of 518 and 593 milliseconds.

Some drugs that prolong the QT/QTc interval have been associated with the occurrence of torsade de pointes and with sudden unexplained death. The relationship of QT prolongation to torsade de pointes is clearest for larger increases (20 milliseconds and greater) but it is possible that smaller QT/QTc prolongations may also increase risk, or increase it in susceptible individuals, such as those with hypokalemia, hypomagnesemia, or genetic predisposition. Torsade de pointes has not been observed in association with the use of ziprasidone at recommended doses in premarketing studies.

A study evaluating the QT/QTc prolonging effect of IM ziprasidone, with IM haloperidol as a control, was conducted in patient volunteers. In the trial, ECGs were obtained at the time of maximum plasma concentration following 2 injections of ziprasidone (20 mg then 30 mg) or haloperidol (7.5 mg then 10 mg) given 4 hours apart. Note that a 30 mg dose of IM ziprasidone is 50% higher than the recommended therapeutic dose. The mean change in QTc from baseline was calculated for each drug, using a sample based correction that removes the effect of heart rate on the QT interval. The mean increase in QTc from baseline for ziprasidone was 4.6 milliseconds following the first injection and 12.8 milliseconds following the second injection. The mean increase in QTc from baseline for haloperidol was 6.0 milliseconds following the first injection and 14.7 milliseconds following the second injection. In this study, no patients had a QTc interval exceeding 500 milliseconds.

As with other antipsychotic drugs and placebo, sudden unexplained deaths have been reported in patients taking ziprasidone at recommended doses. The premarketing experience for ziprasidone did not reveal an excess risk of mortality for ziprasidone compared to other antipsychotic drugs or placebo, but the extent of exposure was limited, especially for the drugs used as active controls and placebo. Nevertheless, ziprasidone's larger prolongation of QTc length compared to several other antipsychotic drugs raises the possibility that the risk of sudden death may be greater for ziprasidone than for other available drugs for treating schizophrenia. This possibility needs to be considered in deciding among alternative drug products (see INDICATIONS AND USAGE).

Certain circumstances may increase the risk of the occurrence of torsade de pointes and/or sudden death in association with the use of drugs that prolong the QTc interval, including (1) bradycardia; (2) hypokalemia or hypomagnesemia; (3) concomitant use of other drugs that prolong the QTc interval; and (4) presence of congenital prolongation of the QT interval.

It is recommended that patients being considered for ziprasidone treatment who are at risk for significant electrolyte disturbances, hypokalemia in particular, have baseline serum potassium and magnesium measurements. Hypokalemia (and/or hypomagnesemia) may increase the risk of QT prolongation and arrhythmia. Hypokalemia may result from diuretic therapy, diarrhea, and other causes. Patients with low serum potassium and/or magnesium should be repleted with those electrolytes before proceeding with treatment. It is essential to periodically monitor serum electrolytes in patients for whom diuretic therapy is introduced during ziprasidone treatment. Persistently prolonged QTc intervals may also increase the risk of further prolongation and arrhythmia, but it is not clear that routine screening ECG measures are effective in detecting such patients. Rather, ziprasidone should be avoided in patients with histories of significant cardiovascular illness, *e.g.*, QT prolongation, recent acute myocardial infarction, uncompensated heart failure, or cardiac arrhythmia. Ziprasidone should be discontinued in patients who are found to have persistent QTc measurements >500 milliseconds.

For patients taking ziprasidone who experience symptoms that could indicate the occurrence of torsade de pointes, *e.g.*, dizziness, palpitations, or syncope, the prescriber should initiate further evaluation, *e.g.*, Holter monitoring may be useful.

NEUROLEPTIC MALIGNANT SYNDROME (NMS)

A potentially fatal symptom complex sometimes referred to as Neuroleptic Malignant Syndrome (NMS) has been reported in association with administration of antipsychotic drugs. Clinical manifestations of NMS are hyperpyrexia, muscle rigidity, altered mental status and evidence of autonomic instability (irregular pulse or blood pressure, tachycardia, diaphoresis and cardiac dysrhythmia). Additional signs may include elevated creatinine phosphokinase, myoglobinuria (rhabdomyolysis), and acute renal failure.

The diagnostic evaluation of patients with this syndrome is complicated. In arriving at a diagnosis, it is important to exclude cases where the clinical presentation includes both serious medical illness (*e.g.*, pneumonia, systemic infection, etc.) and untreated or inadequately treated extrapyramidal signs and symptoms (EPS). Other important considerations in the differential diagnosis include central anticholinergic toxicity, heat stroke, drug fever, and primary central nervous system (CNS) pathology.

The management of NMS should include: (1) Immediate discontinuation of antipsychotic drugs and other drugs not essential to concurrent therapy; (2) intensive symptomatic treatment and medical monitoring; and (3) treatment of any concomitant serious medical problems for which specific treatments are available. There is no general agreement about specific pharmacological treatment regimens for NMS.
If a patient requires antipsychotic drug treatment after recovery from NMS, the potential reintroduction of drug therapy should be carefully considered. The patient should be carefully monitored, since recurrences of NMS have been reported.

TARDIVE DYSKINESIA

A syndrome of potentially irreversible, involuntary, dyskinetic movements may develop in patients undergoing treatment with antipsychotic drugs. Although the prevalence of the syndrome appears to be highest among the elderly, especially elderly women, it is impossible to rely upon prevalence estimates to predict, at the inception of antipsychotic treatment, which patients are likely to develop the syndrome. Whether antipsychotic drug products differ in their potential to cause tardive dyskinesia is unknown.

The risk of developing tardive dyskinesia and the likelihood that it will become irreversible are believed to increase as the duration of treatment and the total cumulative dose of antipsychotic drugs administered to the patient increase. However, the syndrome can develop, although much less commonly, after relatively brief treatment periods at low doses.

There is no known treatment for established cases of tardive dyskinesia, although the syndrome may remit, partially or completely, if antipsychotic treatment is withdrawn. Antipsychotic treatment, itself, however, may suppress (or partially suppress) the signs and symptoms of the syndrome and thereby may possibly mask the underlying process. The effect that symptomatic suppression has upon the long-term course of the syndrome is unknown.

Given these considerations, ziprasidone should be prescribed in a manner that is most likely to minimize the occurrence of tardive dyskinesia. Chronic antipsychotic treatment should generally be reserved for patients who suffer from a chronic illness that (1) is known to respond to antipsychotic drugs and (2) for whom alternative, equally effective, but potentially less harmful treatments are not available or appropriate. In patients who do require chronic treatment, the smallest dose and the shortest duration of treatment producing a satisfactory clinical response should be sought. The need for continued treatment should be reassessed periodically.

If signs and symptoms of tardive dyskinesia appear in a patient on ziprasidone, drug discontinuation should be considered. However, some patients may require treatment with ziprasidone despite the presence of the syndrome.

PRECAUTIONS

GENERAL

Rash

In premarketing trials with ziprasidone, about 5% of patients developed rash and/or urticaria, with discontinuation of treatment in about one-sixth of these cases. The occurrence of rash was related to dose of ziprasidone, although the finding might also be explained by the longer exposure time in the higher dose patients. Several patients with rash had signs and symptoms of associated systemic illness, *e.g.,* elevated WBCs. Most patients improved promptly with adjunctive treatment with antihistamines or steroids and/or upon discontinuation of ziprasidone, and all patients experiencing these events were reported to recover completely. Upon appearance of rash for which an alternative etiology cannot be identified, ziprasidone should be discontinued.

Orthostatic Hypotension

Ziprasidone may induce orthostatic hypotension associated with dizziness, tachycardia and, in some patients, syncope, especially during the initial dose-titration period, probably reflecting its α_1-adrenergic antagonist properties. Syncope was reported in 0.6% of the patients treated with ziprasidone.

Ziprasidone should be used with particular caution in patients with known cardiovascular disease (history of myocardial infarction or ischemic heart disease, heart failure or conduction abnormalities), cerebrovascular disease or conditions that would predispose patients to hypotension (dehydration, hypovolemia, and treatment with antihypertensive medications).

Seizures

During clinical trials, seizures occurred in 0.4% of patients treated with ziprasidone. There were confounding factors that may have contributed to the occurrence of seizures in many of these cases. As with other antipsychotic drugs, ziprasidone should be used cautiously in patients with a history of seizures or with conditions that potentially lower the seizure threshold, *e.g.,* Alzheimer's dementia. Conditions that lower the seizure threshold may be more prevalent in a population of 65 years or older.

Hyperprolactinemia

As with other drugs that antagonize dopamine D_2 receptors, ziprasidone elevates prolactin levels in humans. Increased prolactin levels were also observed in animal studies with this compound, and were associated with an increase in mammary gland neoplasia in mice; a similar effect was not observed in rats (see PRECAUTIONS, Carcinogenesis, Mutagenesis, and Impairment of Fertility, Carcinogenesis). Tissue culture experiments indicate that approximately one-third of human breast cancers are prolactin-dependent *in vitro,* a factor of potential importance if the prescription of these drugs is contemplated in a patient with previously detected breast cancer. Although disturbances such as galactorrhea, amenorrhea, gynecomastia, and impotence have been reported with prolactin-elevating compounds, the clinical significance of elevated serum prolactin levels is unknown for most patients. Neither clinical studies nor epidemiologic studies conducted to date have shown an association between chronic administration of this class of drugs and tumorigenesis in humans; the available evidence is considered too limited to be conclusive at this time.

Potential for Cognitive and Motor Impairment

Somnolence was a commonly reported adverse event in patients treated with ziprasidone. In the 4 and 6 week placebo-controlled trials, somnolence was reported in 14% of patients on ziprasidone compared to 7% of placebo patients. Somnolence led to discontinuation in 0.3% of patients in short-term clinical trials. Since ziprasidone has the potential to impair judgment, thinking, or motor skills, patients should be cautioned about performing activities requiring mental alertness, such as operating a motor vehicle (including automobiles) or operating hazardous machinery until they are reasonably certain that ziprasidone therapy does not affect them adversely.

Priapism

One case of priapism was reported in the premarketing database. While the relationship of the event to ziprasidone use has not been established, other drugs with alpha-adrenergic blocking effects have been reported to induce priapism, and it is possible that ziprasidone may share this capacity. Severe priapism may require surgical intervention.

Body Temperature Regulation

Although not reported with ziprasidone in premarketing trials, disruption of the body's ability to reduce core body temperature has been attributed to antipsychotic agents. Appropriate care is advised when prescribing ziprasidone for patients who will be experiencing conditions which may contribute to an elevation in core body temperature, *e.g.,* exercising strenuously, exposure to extreme heat, receiving concomitant medication with anticholinergic activity, or being subject to dehydration.

Dysphagia

Esophageal dysmotility and aspiration have been associated with antipsychotic drug use. Aspiration pneumonia is a common cause of morbidity and mortality in elderly patients, in particular those with advanced Alzheimer's dementia. Ziprasidone and other antipsychotic drugs should be used cautiously in patients at risk for aspiration pneumonia.

Suicide

The possibility of a suicide attempt is inherent in psychotic illness and close supervision of high-risk patients should accompany drug therapy. Prescriptions for ziprasidone should be written for the smallest quantity of capsules consistent with good patient management in order to reduce the risk of overdose.

Use in Patients With Concomitant Illness

Clinical experience with ziprasidone in patients with certain concomitant systemic illnesses (see CLINICAL PHARMACOLOGY, Special Populations: Renal Impairment and Hepatic Impairment) is limited.

Ziprasidone has not been evaluated or used to any appreciable extent in patients with a recent history of myocardial infarction or unstable heart disease. Patients with these diagnoses were excluded from premarketing clinical studies. Because of the risk of QTc prolongation and orthostatic hypotension with ziprasidone, caution should be observed in cardiac patients (see WARNINGS, QT Prolongation, and PRECAUTIONS, General, Orthostatic Hypotension).

INFORMATION FOR THE PATIENT

Please refer to the patient package insert that is distributed with the prescription for complete instructions. To assure safe and effective use of ziprasidone, the information and instructions provided in the patient information should be discussed with patients.

LABORATORY TESTS

Patients being considered for ziprasidone treatment that are at risk of significant electrolyte disturbances should have baseline serum potassium and magnesium measurements. Low serum potassium and magnesium should be repleted before proceeding with treatment. Patients who are started on diuretics during ziprasidone therapy need periodic monitoring of serum potassium and magnesium. Ziprasidone should be discontinued in patients who are found to have persistent QTc measurements >500 milliseconds. (See WARNINGS.)

CARCINOGENESIS, MUTAGENESIS, AND IMPAIRMENT OF FERTILITY

Carcinogenesis

Lifetime carcinogenicity studies were conducted with ziprasidone in Long Evans rats and CD-1 mice. Ziprasidone was administered for 24 months in the diet at doses of 2, 6, or 12 mg/kg/day to rats, and 50, 100, or 200 mg/kg/day to mice (0.1-0.6 and 1-5 times the maximum recommended human dose [MRHD] of 200 mg/day on a mg/m^2 basis, respectively]. In the rat study, there was no evidence of an increased incidence of tumors compared to controls. In male mice, there was no increase in incidence of tumors relative to controls. In female mice, there were dose-related increases in the incidences of pituitary gland adenoma and carcinoma, and mammary gland adenocarcinoma at all doses tested (50-200 mg/kg/day or 1-5 times the MRHD on a mg/m^2 basis). Proliferative changes in the pituitary and mammary glands of rodents have been observed following chronic administration of other antipsychotic agents and are considered to be prolactin-mediated. Increases in serum prolactin were observed in a 1 month dietary study in female, but not male, mice at 100 and 200 mg/kg/day (or 2.5 and 5 times the MRHD on a mg/m^2 basis). Ziprasidone had no effect on serum prolactin in rats in a 5 week dietary study at the doses that were used in the carcinogenicity study. The relevance for human risk of the findings of prolactin-mediated endocrine tumors in rodents is unknown (see PRECAUTIONS, General, Hyperprolactinemia).

Mutagenesis

Ziprasidone was tested in the Ames bacterial mutation assay, the *in vitro* mammalian cell gene mutation mouse lymphoma assay, the *in vitro* chromosomal aberration assay in human lymphocytes, and the *in vivo* chromosomal aberration assay in mouse bone marrow. There was a reproducible mutagenic response in the Ames assay in one strain of *S. typhimurium* in the absence of metabolic activation. Positive results were obtained in both the *in vitro* mammalian cell gene mutation assay and the *in vitro* chromosomal aberration assay in human lymphocytes.

Impairment of Fertility

Ziprasidone was shown to increase time to copulation in Sprague-Dawley rats in two fertility and early embryonic development studies at doses of 10-160 mg/kg/day (0.5 to 8 times

Z

the MRHD of 200 mg/day on a mg/m^2 basis). Fertility rate was reduced at 160 mg/kg/day (8 times the MRHD on a mg/m^2 basis). There was no effect on fertility at 40 mg/kg/day (2 times the MRHD on a mg/m^2 basis). The effect on fertility appeared to be in the female since fertility was not impaired when males given 160 mg/kg/day (8 times the MRHD on a mg/m^2 basis) were mated with untreated females. In a 6 month study in male rats given 200 mg/kg/day (10 times the MRHD on a mg/m^2 basis) there were no treatment-related findings observed in the testes.

PREGNANCY CATEGORY C

In animal studies ziprasidone demonstrated developmental toxicity, including possible teratogenic effects at doses similar to human therapeutic doses. When ziprasidone was administered to pregnant rabbits during the period of organogenesis, an increased incidence of fetal structural abnormalities (ventricular septal defects and other cardiovascular malformations and kidney alterations) was observed at a dose of 30 mg/kg/day (3 times the MRHD of 200 mg/day on a mg/m^2 basis). There was no evidence to suggest that these developmental effects were secondary to maternal toxicity. The developmental no-effect dose was 10 mg/kg/day (equivalent to the MRHD on a mg/m^2 basis). In rats, embryofetal toxicity (decreased fetal weights, delayed skeletal ossification) was observed following administration of 10-160 mg/kg/day (0.5 to 8 times the MRHD on a mg/m^2 basis) during organogenesis or throughout gestation, but there was no evidence of teratogenicity. Doses of 40 and 160 mg/kg/day (2 and 8 times the MRHD on a mg/m^2 basis) were associated with maternal toxicity. The developmental no-effect dose was 5 mg/kg/day (0.2 times the MRHD on a mg/m^2 basis).

There was an increase in the number of pups born dead and a decrease in postnatal survival through the first 4 days of lactation among the offspring of female rats treated during gestation and lactation with doses of 10 mg/kg/day (0.5 times the MRHD on a mg/m^2 basis) or greater. Offspring developmental delays and neurobehavioral functional impairment were observed at doses of 5 mg/kg/day (0.2 times the MRHD on a mg/m^2 basis) or greater. A no-effect level was not established for these effects.

There are no adequate and well-controlled studies in pregnant women. Ziprasidone should be used during pregnancy only if the potential benefit justifies the potential risk to the fetus.

LABOR AND DELIVERY

The effect of ziprasidone on labor and delivery in humans is unknown.

NURSING MOTHERS

It is not known whether, and if so in what amount, ziprasidone or its metabolites are excreted in human milk. It is recommended that women receiving ziprasidone should not breast feed.

PEDIATRIC USE

The safety and effectiveness of ziprasidone in pediatric patients have not been established.

GERIATRIC USE

Of the approximately 4500 patients treated with ziprasidone in clinical studies, 2.4% (109) were 65 years of age or over. In general, there was no indication of any different tolerability of ziprasidone or for reduced clearance of ziprasidone in the elderly compared to younger adults. Nevertheless, the presence of multiple factors that might increase the pharmacodynamic response to ziprasidone, or cause poorer tolerance or orthostasis, should lead to consideration of a lower starting dose, slower titration, and careful monitoring during the initial dosing period for some elderly patients.

DRUG INTERACTIONS

Drug-drug interactions can be pharmacodynamic (combined pharmacologic effects) or pharmacokinetic (alteration of plasma levels). The risks of using ziprasidone in combination with other drugs have been evaluated as described below. All interaction studies have been conducted with oral ziprasidone. Based upon the pharmacodynamic and pharmacokinetic profile of ziprasidone, possible interactions could be anticipated:

PHARMACODYNAMIC INTERACTIONS

Ziprasidone should not be used with any drug that prolongs the QT interval (see CONTRAINDICATIONS).

Given the primary CNS effects of ziprasidone, caution should be used when it is taken in combination with other centrally acting drugs.

Because of its potential for inducing hypotension, ziprasidone may enhance the effects of certain antihypertensive agents.

Ziprasidone may antagonize the effects of levodopa and dopamine agonists.

PHARMACOKINETIC INTERACTIONS

The Effect of Other Drugs on Ziprasidone

Carbamazepine: Carbamazepine is an inducer of CYP3A4; administration of 200 mg bid for 21 days, resulted in a decrease of approximately 35% in the AUC of ziprasidone. This effect may be greater when higher doses of carbamazepine are administered.

Ketoconazole: Ketoconazole, a potent inhibitor of CYP3A4, at a dose of 400 mg qd for 5 days, increased the AUC and C_{max} of ziprasidone by about 35-40%. Other inhibitors of CYP3A4 would be expected to have similar effects.

Cimetidine: Cimetidine at a dose of 800 mg qd for 2 days did not affect ziprasidone pharmacokinetics.

Antacid: The coadministration of 30 ml of Maalox with ziprasidone did not affect the pharmacokinetics of ziprasidone.

In addition, population pharmacokinetic analysis of schizophrenic patients enrolled in controlled clinical trials has not revealed evidence of any clinically significant pharmacokinetic interactions with benztropine, propranolol, or lorazepam.

Effect of Ziprasidone on Other Drugs

In vitro studies revealed little potential for ziprasidone to interfere with the metabolism of drugs cleared primarily by CYP1A2, CYP2C9, CYP2C19, CYP2D6, and CYP3A4, and little potential for drug interactions with ziprasidone due to displacement (see CLINICAL PHARMACOLOGY, Pharmacokinetics).

Lithium: Ziprasidone at a dose of 40 mg bid administered concomitantly with lithium at a dose of 450 mg bid for 7 days did not affect the steady-state level or renal clearance of lithium.

Oral Contraceptives: Ziprasidone at a dose of 20 mg bid did not affect the pharmacokinetics of concomitantly administered oral contraceptives, ethinylestradiol (0.03 mg) and levonorgestrel (0.15 mg).

Dextromethorphan: Consistent with *in vitro* results, a study in normal healthy volunteers showed that ziprasidone did not alter the metabolism of dextromethorphan, a CYP2D6 model substrate, to its major metabolite, dextrorphan. There was no statistically significant change in the urinary dextromethorphan/dextrorphan ratio.

ADVERSE REACTIONS

The premarketing development program for oral ziprasidone included over 5400 patients and/or normal subjects exposed to one or more doses of ziprasidone. Of these 5400 subjects, over 4500 were patients who participated in multiple-dose effectiveness trials, and their experience corresponded to approximately 1733 patient years. The conditions and duration of treatment with ziprasidone included open-label and double-blind studies, inpatient and outpatient studies, and short-term and longer-term exposure. The premarketing development program for IM ziprasidone included 570 patients and/or normal subjects who received 1 or more injections of ziprasidone. Over 325 of these subjects participated in trials involving the administration of multiple doses.

Adverse events during exposure were obtained by collecting voluntarily reported adverse experiences, as well as results of physical examinations, vital signs, weights, laboratory analyses, ECGs, and results of ophthalmologic examinations. Adverse experiences were recorded by clinical investigators using terminology of their own choosing. Consequently, it is not possible to provide a meaningful estimate of the proportion of individuals experiencing adverse events without first grouping similar types of events into a smaller number of standardized event categories. In the tables and tabulations that follow, standard COSTART dictionary terminology has been used to classify reported adverse events.

The stated frequencies of adverse events represent the proportion of individuals who experienced, at least once, a treatment-emergent adverse event of the type listed. An event was considered treatment emergent if it occurred for the first time or worsened while receiving therapy following baseline evaluation.

ADVERSE FINDINGS OBSERVED IN SHORT-TERM, PLACEBO-CONTROLLED TRIALS WITH ORAL ZIPRASIDONE

The following findings are based on a pool of two 6 week, and two 4 week placebo-controlled trials in which ziprasidone was administered in doses ranging from 10-200 mg/day.

Adverse Events Associated With Discontinuation of Treatment in Short-Term, Placebo-Controlled Trials of Oral Ziprasidone

Approximately 4.1% (29/702) of ziprasidone-treated patients in short-term, placebo-controlled studies discontinued treatment due to an adverse event, compared with about 2.2% (6/273) on placebo. The most common event associated with dropout was rash, including 7 dropouts for rash among ziprasidone patients (1%) compared to no placebo patients (see PRECAUTIONS).

Adverse Events Occurring at an Incidence of 1% or More Among Ziprasidone-Treated Patients in Short-Term, Oral, Placebo-Controlled Trials

TABLE 1 enumerates the incidence, rounded to the nearest percent, of treatment-emergent adverse events that occurred during acute therapy (up to 6 weeks) in predominantly schizophrenic patients, including only those events that occurred in 1% or more of patients treated with ziprasidone and for which the incidence in patients treated with ziprasidone was greater than the incidence in placebo-treated patients.

The prescriber should be aware that these figures cannot be used to predict the incidence of side effects in the course of usual medical practice where patient characteristics and other factors differ from those which prevailed in the clinical trials. Similarly, the cited frequencies cannot be compared with figures obtained from other clinical investigations involving different treatments, uses, and investigators. The cited figures, however, do provide the prescribing physician with some basis for estimating the relative contribution of drug and non-drug factors to the side effect incidence rate in the population studied.

In these studies, the most commonly observed adverse events associated with the use of ziprasidone (incidence of 5% or greater) and observed at a rate on ziprasidone at least twice that of placebo were somnolence (14%), extrapyramidal syndrome (5%), and respiratory disorder (8%).

Explorations for interactions on the basis of gender did not reveal any clinically meaningful differences in the adverse event occurrence on the basis of this demographic factor.

Dose Dependency of Adverse Events in Short-Term, Placebo-Controlled Trials

An analysis for dose response in this 4-study pool revealed an apparent relation of adverse event to dose for the following events: Asthenia, postural hypotension, anorexia, dry mouth, increased salivation, arthralgia, anxiety, dizziness, dystonia, hypertonia, somnolence, tremor, rhinitis, rash, and abnormal vision.

Extrapyramidal Symptoms (EPS)

The incidence of reported EPS for ziprasidone-treated patients in the short-term, placebo-controlled trials was 5% vs 1% for placebo. Objectively collected data from those trials on the Simpson Angus Rating Scale (for EPS) and the Barnes Akathisia Scale (for akathisia) did not generally show a difference between ziprasidone and placebo.

Vital Sign Changes

Ziprasidone is associated with orthostatic hypotension (see PRECAUTIONS).

TABLE 1 *Treatment-Emergent Adverse Event Incidence in Short-Term Oral Placebo-Controlled Trials*

Body System Adverse Event	Ziprasidone (n=702)	Placebo (n=273)
Body as a Whole		
Asthenia	5%	3%
Accidental injury	4%	2%
Cardiovascular		
Tachycardia	2%	1%
Postural hypotension	1%	0%
Digestive		
Nausea	10%	7%
Constipation	9%	8%
Dyspepsia	8%	7%
Diarrhea	5%	4%
Dry mouth	4%	2%
Anorexia	2%	1%
Musculoskeletal		
Myalgia	1%	0%
Nervous		
Somnolence	14%	7%
Akathisia	8%	7%
Dizziness	8%	6%
Extrapyramidal syndrome	5%	1%
Dystonia	4%	2%
Hypertonia	3%	2%
Respiratory		
Respiratory disorder*	8%	3%
Rhinitis	4%	2%
Cough increased	3%	1%
Skin and Appendages		
Rash	4%	3%
Fungal dermatitis	2%	1%
Special Senses		
Abnormal vision	3%	2%

* Cold symptoms and upper respiratory infection account for >90% of investigator terms pointing to "respiratory disorder".

Weight Gain

The proportions of patients meeting a weight gain criterion of ≥7% of body weight were compared in a pool of four 4 and 6 week placebo-controlled clinical trials, revealing a statistically significantly greater incidence of weight gain for ziprasidone (10%) compared to placebo (4%). A median weight gain of 0.5 kg was observed in ziprasidone patients compared to no median weight change in placebo patients. In this set of clinical trials, weight gain was reported as an adverse event in 0.4% and 0.4% of ziprasidone and placebo patients, respectively. During long-term therapy with ziprasidone, a categorization of patients at baseline on the basis of body mass index (BMI) revealed the greatest mean weight gain and highest incidence of clinically significant weight gain (>7% of body weight) in patients with low BMI (<23) compared to normal (23-27) or overweight patients (>27). There was a mean weight gain of 1.4 kg for those patients with a "low" baseline BMI, no mean change for patients with a "normal" BMI, and a 1.3 kg mean weight loss for patients who entered the program with a "high" BMI.

ECG Changes

Ziprasidone is associated with an increase in the QTc interval (see WARNINGS). Ziprasidone was associated with a mean increase in heart rate of 1.4 beats per minute compared to a 0.2 beats per minute decrease among placebo patients.

OTHER ADVERSE EVENTS OBSERVED DURING THE PREMARKETING EVALUATION OF ORAL ZIPRASIDONE

Following is a list of COSTART terms that reflect treatment-emergent adverse events as defined in the introduction to ADVERSE REACTIONS reported by patients treated with ziprasidone at multiple doses >4 mg/day within the database of 3834 patients. All reported events are included except those already listed in TABLE 1 or elsewhere in labeling, those event terms that were so general as to be uninformative, events reported only once and that did not have a substantial probability of being acutely life-threatening, events that are part of the illness being treated or are otherwise common as background events, and events considered unlikely to be drug-related. It is important to emphasize that, although the events reported occurred during treatment with ziprasidone, they were not necessarily caused by it.

Events are further categorized by body system and listed in order of decreasing frequency according to the following definitions: *Frequent* adverse events are those occurring in at least 1/100 patients (only those not already listed in the tabulated results from placebo-controlled trials appear in this listing); *infrequent* adverse events are those occurring in 1/100 to 1/1000 patients; *rare* events are those occurring in fewer than 1/1000 patients.

Body as a Whole: *Frequent:* Abdominal pain, flu syndrome, fever, accidental fall, face edema, chills, photosensitivity reaction, flank pain, hypothermia, motor vehicle accident.

Cardiovascular System: *Frequent:* Hypertension; *Infrequent:* Bradycardia, angina pectoris, atrial fibrillation; *Rare:* First degree AV block, bundle branch block, phlebitis, pulmonary embolus, cardiomegaly, cerebral infarct, cerebrovascular accident, deep thrombophlebitis, myocarditis, thrombophlebitis.

Digestive System: *Frequent:* Vomiting; *Infrequent:* Rectal hemorrhage, dysphagia, tongue edema; *Rare:* Gum hemorrhage, jaundice, fecal impaction, gamma glutamyl transpeptidase increased, hematemesis, cholestatic jaundice, hepatitis, hepatomegaly, leukoplakia of mouth, fatty liver deposit, melena.

Endocrine: *Rare:* Hypothyroidism, hyperthyroidism, thyroditis.

Hemic and Lymphatic System: *Infrequent:* Anemia, ecchymosis, leukocytosis, leukopenia, eosinophilia, lymphadenopathy; *Rare:* Thrombocytopenia, hypochromic anemia, lymphocytosis, monocytosis, basophilia, lymphedema, polycythemia, thrombocythemia.

Metabolic and Nutritional Disorders: *Infrequent:* Thirst, transaminase increased, peripheral edema, hyperglycemia, creatine phosphokinase increased, alkaline phosphatase increased, hypercholesteremia, dehydration, lactic dehydrogenase increased, albuminuria, hypokalemia; *Rare:* BUN increased, creatinine increased, hyperlipemia, hypocholesteremia, hyperkalemia, hypochloremia, hypoglycemia, hyponatremia, hypoproteinemia, glucose tolerance decreased, gout, hyperchloremia, hyperuricemia, hypocalcemia, hypoglycemic reaction, hypomagnesemia, ketosis, respiratory alkalosis.

Musculoskeletal System: *Infrequent:* Tenosynovitis; *Rare:* Myopathy.

Nervous System: *Frequent:* Agitation, tremor, dyskinesia, hostility, parathesia, confusion, vertigo, hypokinesia, hyperkinesia, abnormal gait, oculogyric crisis, hypesthesia, ataxia, amnesia, cogwheel rigidity, delerium, hypotonia, akinesia, dysarthria, withdrawal syndrome, buccoglossal syndrome, choreoathetosis, diplopia, incoordination, neuropathy; *Rare:* Myoclonus, nystagmus, torticollis, circumoral paresthesia, opisthotonos, reflexes increased, trismus.

Respiratory System: *Frequent:* Dyspnea; *Infrequent:* Pneumonia, epistaxis; *Rare:* Hemoptysis, laryngismus.

Skin and Appendages: *Infrequent:* Maculopapular rash, urticaria, alopecia, eczema, exfoliative dermatitis, contact dermatitis, vesiculobullous rash.

Special Senses: *Infrequent:* Conjunctivitis, dry eyes, tinnitus, blepharitis, cataract, photophobia; *Rare:* Eye hemorrhage, visual field defect, keratitis, keratoconjunctivitis.

Urogenital System: *Infrequent:* Impotence, abnormal ejaculation, amenorrhea, hematuria, menorrhagia, female lactation, polyuria, urinary retention, metrorrhagia, male sexual dysfunction, anorgasmia, glycosuria; *Rare:* Gynecomastia, vaginal hemorrhage, nocturia, oliguria, female sexual dysfunction, uterine hemorrhage.

ADVERSE FINDINGS OBSERVED IN TRIALS OF IM ZIPRASIDONE

Adverse Events Occurring at an Incidence of 1% or More Among Ziprasidone-Treated Patients in Short-Term Trials of IM Ziprasidone

TABLE 2 enumerates the incidence, rounded to the nearest percent, of treatment-emergent adverse events that occurred during acute therapy with IM ziprasidone in 1% or more of patients.

In these studies, the most commonly observed adverse events associated with the use of IM ziprasidone (incidence of 5% or greater) and observed at a rate on IM ziprasidone (in the higher dose groups) at least twice that of the lowest IM ziprasidone group were headache (13%), nausea (12%), and somnolence (20%).

TABLE 2 *Treatment-Emergent Adverse Event Incidence in Short-Term Fixed-Dose Intramuscular Trials*

	Ziprasidone		
Body System Adverse Event	2 mg (n=92)	10 mg (n=63)	20 mg (n=41)
Body as a Whole			
Headache	3%	13%	5%
Injection site pain	9%	8%	7%
Asthenia	2%	0%	0%
Abdominal pain	0%	2%	0%
Flu syndrome	1%	0%	0%
Back pain	1%	0%	0%
Cardiovascular			
Postural hypotension	0%	0%	5%
Hypertension	2%	0%	0%
Bradycardia	0%	0%	2%
Vasodilation	1%	0%	0%
Digestive			
Nausea	4%	8%	12%
Rectal hemorrhage	0%	0%	2%
Diarrhea	3%	3%	0%
Vomiting	0%	3%	0%
Dyspepsia	1%	3%	2%
Anorexia	0%	2%	0%
Constipation	0%	0%	2%
Tooth disorder	1%	0%	0%
Dry mouth	1%	0%	0%
Nervous			
Dizziness	3%	3%	10%
Anxiety	2%	0%	0%
Insomnia	3%	0%	0%
Somnolence	8%	8%	20%
Akathisia	0%	2%	0%
Agitation	2%	2%	0%
Extrapyramidal syndrome	2%	0%	0%
Hypertonia	1%	0%	0%
Cogwheel rigidity	1%	0%	0%
Paresthesia	0%	2%	0%
Personality disorder	0%	2%	0%
Psychosis	1%	0%	0%
Speech disorder	0%	2%	0%
Respiratory			
Rhinitis	1%	0%	0%
Skin and Appendages			
Furunculosis	0%	2%	0%
Sweating	0%	0%	2%
Urogenital			
Dysmenorrhea	0%	2%	0%
Priapism	1%	0%	0%

DOSAGE AND ADMINISTRATION

When deciding among the alternative treatments available for schizophrenia, the prescriber should consider the finding of ziprasidone's greater capacity to prolong the QT/QTc interval compared to several other antipsychotic drugs (see WARNINGS).

INITIAL TREATMENT

Ziprasidone capsules should be administered at an initial daily dose of 20 mg bid with food. In some patients daily dosage may subsequently be adjusted on the basis of individual clinical status up to 80 mg bid. Dosage adjustments, if indicated, should generally occur at intervals of not less than 2 days, as steady-state is achieved within 1-3 days. In order to ensure use of the lowest effective dose, ordinarily patients should be observed for improvement for several weeks before upward dosage adjustment.

Efficacy in schizophrenia was demonstrated in a dose range of 20-100 mg bid in short-term, placebo-controlled clinical trials. There were trends toward dose response within the range of 20-80 mg bid, but results were not consistent. An increase to a dose greater than 80 mg bid is not generally recommended. The safety of doses above 100 mg bid has not been systematically evaluated in clinical trials.

MAINTENANCE TREATMENT

While there is no body of evidence available to answer the question of how long a patient treated with ziprasidone should remain on it, systematic evaluation of ziprasidone has shown that its efficacy in schizophrenia is maintained for periods of up to 52 weeks at a dose of 20-80 mg bid (see CLINICAL PHARMACOLOGY). No additional benefit was demonstrated for doses above 20 mg bid. Patients should be periodically reassessed to determine the need for maintenance treatment.

INTRAMUSCULAR ADMINISTRATION

The recommended dose is 10-20 mg administered as required up to a maximum dose of 40 mg/day. Doses of 10 mg may be administered every 2 hours; doses of 20 mg may be administered every 4 hours up to a maximum of 40 mg/day. Intramuscular administration of ziprasidone for more than 3 consecutive days has not been studied.

If long-term therapy is indicated, oral ziprasidone hydrochloride capsules should replace the IM administration as soon as possible.

Since there is no experience regarding the safety of administering ziprasidone IM to schizophrenic patients already taking oral ziprasidone, the practice of co-administration is not recommended.

DOSING IN SPECIAL POPULATIONS

Oral

Dosage adjustments are generally not required on the basis of age, gender, race, or renal or hepatic impairment.

Intramuscular

Ziprasidone IM has not been systematically evaluated in elderly patients or in patients with hepatic or renal impairment. As the cyclodextrin excipient is cleared by renal filtration, ziprasidone IM should be administered with caution to patients with impaired renal function. Dosing adjustments are not required on the basis of gender or race.

PREPARATION FOR ADMINISTRATION

Ziprasidone for injection should only be administered by intramuscular injection. Single-dose vials require reconstitution prior to administration; any unused portion should be discarded.

Add 1.2 ml of sterile water for injection to the vial and shake vigorously until all the drug is dissolved. Each ml of reconstituted solution contains 20 mg ziprasidone. Since no preservative or bacteriostatic agent is present in this product, aseptic technique must be used in preparation of the final solution. This medicinal product must not be mixed with other medicinal products or solvents other than sterile water for injection.

Parenteral drug products should be inspected visually for particulate matter and discoloration prior to administration, whenever solution and container permit.

HOW SUPPLIED

CAPSULES

Geodon capsules are available in the following dosage strengths:

20 mg: Blue/white capsules imprinted in black ink with "Pfizer" and"396".
40 mg: Blue/blue capsules imprinted in black ink with "Pfizer" and"397".
60 mg: White/white capsules imprinted in black ink with "Pfizer" and"398".
80 mg: Blue/white capsules imprinted in black ink with "Pfizer" and"399".

Storage and Handling

Geodon capsules should be stored at controlled room temperature, 15-30°C (59-86°F).

INJECTION

Geodon for Injection is available in a single dose vial as ziprasidone mesylate (20 mg ziprasidone/ml when reconstituted according to label instructions — see DOSAGE AND ADMINISTRATION, Preparation for Administration) for IM administration. Each ml of ziprasidone mesylate for injection (when reconstituted) affords a colorless to pale pink solution that contains 20 mg of ziprasidone and 4.7 mg of methanesulfonic acid solubilized by 294 mg of sulfobutylether β-cyclodextrin sodium (SBECD).

Storage and Handling

Geodon for Injection should be stored at controlled room temperature, 15-30°C (59-86°F) in dry form. Protect from light. Following reconstitution, Geodon for Injection can be stored, when protected from light, for up to 24 hours at 15-30°C (59-86°F) or up to 7 days refrigerated, 2-8°C (36-46°F).

PRODUCT LISTING - EQUIVALENTS NOT AVAILABLE

Capsule - Oral - 20 mg

60's	$268.21	GEODON, Pfizer U.S. Pharmaceuticals	00049-3960-60
80's	$357.61	GEODON, Pfizer U.S. Pharmaceuticals	00049-3960-41

Capsule - Oral - 40 mg

60's	$268.21	GEODON, Pfizer U.S. Pharmaceuticals	00049-3970-60
80's	$357.61	GEODON, Pfizer U.S. Pharmaceuticals	00049-3970-41

Capsule - Oral - 60 mg

60's	$268.21	GEODON, Pfizer U.S. Pharmaceuticals	00049-3980-60
80's	$357.61	GEODON, Pfizer U.S. Pharmaceuticals	00049-3980-41

Capsule - Oral - 80 mg

60's	$268.21	GEODON, Pfizer U.S. Pharmaceuticals	00049-3990-60
80's	$357.61	GEODON, Pfizer U.S. Pharmaceuticals	00049-3990-41

Powder For Injection - Intramuscular - 20 mg

1's	$437.50	GEODON, Roerig Division	00049-3920-83

Zolmitriptan *(003375)*

For related information, see the comparative table section in Appendix A.

Categories: Headache, migraine; FDA Approved 1997 Nov; Pregnancy Category C
Drug Classes: Serotonin receptor agonists
Brand Names: **Zomig**; Zomig ZMT
Foreign Brand Availability: Ascotop (Germany); Myslee (Japan); Zomig Rapimelt (Israel); Zomigoro (France)
Cost of Therapy: $15.94 (Migraine Headache; Zomig; 2.5 mg; 1 tablet/day; 6 day supply)
$15.94 (Migraine Headache; Zomig-ZMT; 2.5 mg; 1 tablet/day; 6 day supply)

DESCRIPTION

Zomig tablets and orally disintegrating tablets contain zolmitriptan, which is a selective 5-hydroxytryptamine $_{1B/1D}$ ($5\text{-}HT_{1B/1D}$) receptor agonist. Zolmitriptan is chemically designated as (S)-4-[[3-[2-(Dimethylamino)ethyl]-1H-indol-5-yl]methyl]-2-oxazolidinone.

The empirical formula is $C_{16}H_{21}N_3O_2$, representing a molecular weight of 287.36. Zolmitriptan is a white to almost white powder that is readily soluble in water.

ZOMIG TABLETS

Zomig tablets are available as 2.5 mg (yellow) and 5 mg (pink) film coated tablets for oral administration. The film coated tablets contain anhydrous lactose, microcrystalline cellulose, sodium starch glycolate, magnesium stearate, hydroxypropyl methylcellulose, titanium dioxide, polyethylene glycol 400, yellow iron oxide (2.5 mg tablet), red iron oxide (5 mg tablet), and polyethylene glycol 8000.

ZOMIG-ZMT ORALLY DISINTEGRATING TABLETS

Zomig-ZMT orally disintegrating tablets are available as 2.5 and 5.0 mg white uncoated tablets for oral administration. The orally disintegrating tablets contain mannitol, microcrystalline cellulose, crospovidone, aspartame, sodium bicarbonate, citric acid anhydrous, colloidal silicon dioxide, magnesium stearate and orange flavor SN 027512.

CLINICAL PHARMACOLOGY

MECHANISM OF ACTION

Zolmitriptan binds with high affinity to human recombinant $5\text{-}HT_{1D}$ and $5\text{-}HT_{1B}$ receptors. Zolmitriptan exhibits modest affinity for $5\text{-}HT_{1A}$ receptors, but has no significant affinity (as measured by radioligand binding assays) or pharmacological activity at $5\text{-}HT_2$, $5\text{-}HT_3$, $5\text{-}HT_4$, alpha$_1$-, alpha$_2$- or beta$_1$-adrenergic; H_1, H_2, histaminic; muscarinic; dopamine$_1$, or dopamine$_2$ receptors. The N-desmethyl metabolite also has high affinity for $5\text{-}HT_{1B/1D}$ and modest affinity for $5\text{-}HT_{1A}$ receptors.

Current theories proposed to explain the etiology of migraine headache suggest that symptoms are due to local cranial vasodilatation and/or to the release of sensory neuropeptides (vasoactive intestinal peptide, substance P and calcitonin gene-related peptide) through nerve endings in the trigeminal system. The therapeutic activity of zolmitriptan for the treatment of migraine headache can most likely be attributed to the agonist effects at the $5\text{-}HT_{1B/1D}$ receptors on intracranial blood vessels (including the arterio-venous anastomoses) and sensory nerves of the trigeminal system which result in cranial vessel constriction and inhibition of pro-inflammatory neuropeptide release.

CLINICAL PHARMACOKINETICS AND BIOAVAILABILITY

Absorption

Zolmitriptan is well absorbed after oral administration for both the conventional tablets and the orally disintegrating tablets. Zolmitriptan displays linear kinetics over the dose range of 2.5 to 50 mg.

The AUC and C_{max} of zolmitriptan are similar following administration of zolmitriptan tablets and orally disintegrating tablets, but the T_{max} is somewhat later with zolmitriptan orally disintegrating tablets, with a median T_{max} of 3 hours for the orally disintegrating tablet compared with 1.5 hours for the conventional tablet. The AUC, C_{max}, and T_{max} for the active N-desmethyl metabolite are similar for the 2 formulations.

During a moderate to severe migraine attack, mean AUC(0-4) and C_{max} for zolmitriptan, dosed as a conventional tablet, were decreased by 40% and 25%, respectively, and mean T_{max} was delayed by one-half hour compared to the same patients during a migraine free period.

Food has no significant effect on the bioavailiability of zolmitriptan. No accumulation occurred on multiple dosing.

Distribution

Mean absolute bioavailability is approximately 40%. The mean apparent volume of distribution is 7.0 L/kg. Plasma protein binding of zolmitriptan is 25% over the concentration range of 10-1000 ng/ml.

Metabolism

Zolmitriptan is converted to an active N-desmethyl metabolite such that the metabolite concentrations are about two-thirds that of zolmitriptan. Because the $5\text{-}HT_{1B/1D}$ potency of the metabolite is 2-6 times that of the parent, the metabolite may contribute a substantial portion of the overall effect after zolmitriptan administration.

Elimination

Total radioactivity recovered in urine and feces was 65% and 30% of the administered dose, respectively. About 8% of the dose was recovered in the urine as unchanged zolmitriptan. Indole acetic acid metabolite accounted for 31% of the dose, followed by N-oxide (7%) and N-desmethyl (4%) metabolites. The indole acetic acid and N-oxide metabolites are inactive.

Mean total plasma clearance is 31.5 ml/min/kg, of which one-sixth is renal clearance. The renal clearance is greater than the glomerular filtration rate suggesting renal tubular secretion.

Special Populations

Age

Zolmitriptan pharmacokinetics in healthy elderly non-migraineur volunteers (age 65-76 years) were similar to those in younger non-migraineur volunteers (age 18-39 years).

Gender

Mean plasma concentrations of zolmitriptan were up to 1.5-fold higher in females than males.

Renal Impairment

Clearance of zolmitriptan was reduced by 25% in patients with severe renal impairment (CLCR ≥5 ≤25 ml/min) compared to the normal group (CLCR ≥70 ml/min); no significant change in clearance was observed in the moderately renally impaired group (CLCR ≥26 ≤50 ml/min).

Hepatic Impairment

In severely hepatically impaired patients, the mean C_{max}, T_{max}, and AUC(0-∞) of zolmitriptan were increased 1.5, 2 (2 vs 4 hr), and 3-fold, respectively, compared to normals. Seven (7) out of 27 patients experienced 20-80 mm Hg elevations in systolic and/or diastolic blood pressure after a 10 mg dose. Zolmitriptan should be administered with caution in subjects with liver disease, generally using doses less than 2.5 mg (see WARNINGS and PRECAUTIONS).

Hypertensive Patients

No differences in the pharmacokinetics of zolmitriptan or its effects on blood pressure were seen in mild to moderate hypertensive volunteers compared to normotensive controls.

Race

Retrospective analysis of pharmacokinetic data between Japanese and Caucasians revealed no significant differences.

Drug Interactions

All drug interaction studies were performed in healthy volunteers using a single 10 mg dose of zolmitriptan and a single dose of the other drug except where otherwise noted.

Fluoxetine

The pharmacokinetics of zolmitriptan as well as its effect on blood pressure were unaffected by 4 weeks of pretreatment with oral fluoxetine (20 mg/day).

MAO Inhibitors

Following 1 week of administration of 150 mg bid moclobemide, a specific MAO-A inhibitor, there was an increase of about 25% in both C_{max} and AUC for zolmitriptan and a 3-fold increase in the C_{max} and AUC of the active N-desmethyl metabolite of zolmitriptan (see CONTRAINDICATIONS and PRECAUTIONS).

Selegiline, a selective MAO-B inhibitor, at a dose of 10 mg/day for 1 week, had no effect on the pharmacokinetics of zolmitriptan and its metabolite.

Propranolol

C_{max} and AUC of zolmitriptan increased 1.5-fold after 1 week of dosing with propranolol (160 mg/day). C_{max} and AUC of the N-desmethyl metabolite were reduced by 30% and 15%, respectively. There were no interactive effects on blood pressure or pulse rate following administration of propranolol with zolmitriptan.

Acetaminophen

A single 1 g dose of acetaminophen does not alter the pharmacokinetics of zolmitriptan and its N-desmethyl metabolite. However, zolmitriptan delayed the T_{max} of acetaminophen by 1 hour.

Metoclopramide

A single 10 mg dose of metoclopramide had no effect on the pharmacokinetics of zolmitriptan or its metabolites.

Oral Contraceptives

Retrospective analysis of pharmacokinetic data across studies indicated that mean plasma concentrations of zolmitriptan were generally higher in females taking oral contraceptives compared to those not taking oral contraceptives. Mean C_{max} and AUC of zolmitriptan were found to be higher by 30% and 50%, respectively, and T_{max} was delayed by one-half hour in females taking oral contraceptives. The effect of zolmitriptan on the pharmacokinetics of oral contraceptives has not been studied.

Cimetidine

Following the administration of cimetidine, the half-life and AUC of a 5 mg dose of zolmitriptan and its active metabolite were approximately doubled (see PRECAUTIONS).

INDICATIONS AND USAGE

Zolmitriptan is indicated for the acute treatment of migraine with or without aura in adults.

Zolmitriptan is not intended for the prophylactic therapy of migraine or for use in the management of hemiplegic or basilar migraine (see CONTRAINDICATIONS). Safety and effectiveness of zolmitriptan have not been established for cluster headache, which is present in an older, predominantly male population.

CONTRAINDICATIONS

Zolmitriptan should not be given to patients with ischemic heart disease (angina pectoris, history of myocardial infarction, or documented silent ischemia) or to patients who have symptoms or findings consistent with ischemic heart disease, coronary artery vasospasm, including Prinzmetal's variant angina, or other significant underlying cardiovascular disease (see WARNINGS).

Because zolmitriptan may increase blood pressure, it should not be given to patients with uncontrolled hypertension (see WARNINGS).

Zolmitriptan should not be used within 24 hours of treatment with another 5-HT_1 agonist, or an ergotamine-containing or ergot-type medication like dihydroergotamine or methysergide.

Zolmitriptan should not be administered to patients with hemiplegic or basilar migraine.

Concurrent administration of MAO-A inhibitors or use of zolmitriptan within 2 weeks of discontinuation of MAO-A inhibitor therapy is contraindicated (see CLINICAL PHARMACOLOGY, Drug Interactions and DRUG INTERACTIONS).

Zolmitriptan is contraindicated in patients who are hypersensitive to zolmitriptan or any of its inactive ingredients.

WARNINGS

Zolmitriptan should only be used where a clear diagnosis of migraine has been established.

RISK OF MYOCARDIAL ISCHEMIA AND/OR INFARCTION AND OTHER ADVERSE CARDIAC EVENTS

Zolmitriptan should not be given to patients with documented ischemic or vasospastic coronary artery disease (see CONTRAINDICATIONS). It is strongly recommended that zolmitriptan not be given to patients in whom unrecognized coronary artery disease (CAD) is predicted by the presence of risk factors (*e.g.,* hypertension, hypercholesterolemia, smoker, obesity, diabetes, strong family history of CAD, female with surgical or physiological menopause, or male over 40 years of age) unless a cardiovascular evaluation provides satisfactory clinical evidence that the patient is reasonably free of coronary artery and ischemic myocardial disease or other significant underlying cardiovascular disease. The sensitivity of cardiac diagnostic procedures to detect cardiovascular disease or predisposition to coronary artery vasospasm is modest, at best. If, during the cardiovascular evaluation, the patient's medical history, electrocardiographic or other investigations reveal findings indicative of, or consistent with, coronary artery vasospasm or myocardial ischemia, zolmitriptan should not be administered (see CONTRAINDICATIONS). For patients with risk factors predictive of CAD, who are determined to have a satisfactory cardiovascular evaluation, it is strongly recommended that administration of the first dose of zolmitriptan take place in the setting of a physician's office or similar medically staffed and equipped facility unless the patient has previously received zolmitriptan. Because cardiac ischemia can occur in the absence of clinical symptoms, consideration should be given to obtaining on the first occasion of use an electrocardiogram (ECG) during the interval immediately following zolmitriptan, in these patients with risk factors.

It is recommended that patients who are intermittent long-term users of zolmitriptan and who have or acquire risk factors predictive of CAD, as described above, undergo periodic interval cardiovascular evaluation as they continue to use zolmitriptan.

The systematic approach described above is intended to reduce the likelihood that patients with unrecognized cardiovascular disease will be inadvertently exposed to zolmitriptan.

CARDIAC EVENTS AND FATALITIES

Serious adverse cardiac events, including acute myocardial infarction, have been reported within a few hours following the administration of zolmitriptan. Life-threatening disturbances of cardiac rhythm, and death have been reported within a few hours following the administration of other 5-HT_1 agonists. Considering the extent of use of 5-HT_1 agonists in patients with migraine, the incidence of these events is extremely low.

Zolmitriptan can cause coronary vasospasm; at least 1 of these events occurred in a patient with no cardiac disease history and with documented absence of coronary artery disease. Because of the close proximity of the events to zolmitriptan use, a causal relationship cannot be excluded. In the cases where there has been known underlying coronary artery disease, the relationship is uncertain.

Patients with symptomatic Wolff-Parkinson-White syndrome or arrhythmias associated with other cardiac accessory conduction pathway disorders should not receive zolmitriptan.

Premarketing Experience With Zolmitriptan

Among the more than 2500 patients with migraine who participated in premarketing controlled clinical trials of zolmitriptan tablets, no deaths or serious cardiac events were reported.

Postmarketing Experience With Zolmitriptan

Serious cardiovascular events have been reporterd in association with the use of zolmitriptan. The uncontrolled nature of postmarketing surveillance, however, makes it impossible to determine definitively the proportion of the reported cases that were actually caused by zolmitriptan or to reliably assess causation in individual cases.

CEREBROVASCULAR EVENTS AND FATALITIES WITH 5-HT_1 AGONISTS

Cerebral hemorrhage, subarachnoid hemorrhage, stroke, and other cerebrovascular events have been reported in patients treated with 5-HT_1 agonists; and some have resulted in fatalities. In a number of cases, it appears possible that the cerebrovascular events were primary, the agonist having been administered in the incorrect belief that the symptoms experienced were a consequence of migraine, when they were not. It should be noted that patients with migraine may be at increased risk of certain cerebrovascular events (*e.g.*, stroke, hemorrhage, transient ischemic attack).

OTHER VASOSPASM-RELATED EVENTS

5-HT_1 agonists may cause vasospastic reactions other than coronary artery vasospasm. Both peripheral vascular ischemia and colonic ischemia with abdominal pain and bloody diarrhea have been reported with 5-HT_1 agonists.

INCREASE IN BLOOD PRESSURE

Significant elevations in systemic blood pressure have been reported on rare occasions in patients with and without a history of hypertension treated with 5-HT_1 agonists. Zolmitriptan is contraindicated in patients with uncontrolled hypertension. In volunteers, an increase of 1 and 5 mm Hg in the systolic and diastolic blood pressure, respectively, was seen at 5 mg. In the headache trials, vital signs were measured only in the small inpatient study and no effect on blood pressure was seen. In a study of patients with moderate to severe liver disease, 7 of 27 experienced 20-80 mm Hg elevations in systolic and/or diastolic blood pressure after a dose of 10 mg of zolmitriptan (see CONTRAINDICATIONS).

An 18% increase in mean pulmonary artery pressure was seen following dosing with another 5-HT_1 agonist in a study evaluating subjects undergoing cardiac catheterization.

PRECAUTIONS

GENERAL

As with other 5-$HT_{1B/1D}$ agonists, sensations of tightness, pain, pressure, and heaviness have been reported after treatment with zolmitriptan tablets in the precordium, throat, neck and jaw. Because zolmitriptan may cause coronary artery vasospasm, patients who experience signs or symptoms suggestive of angina following dosing should be evaluated for the presence of CAD or a predisposition to Prinzmetal's variant angina before receiving additional doses of medication, and should be monitored electrocardiographically if dosing is resumed and similar symptoms recur. Similarly, patients who experience other symptoms or signs suggestive of decreased arterial flow, such as ischemic bowel syndrome or Raynaud's syndrome following the use of any 5-HT agonist are candidates for further evaluation (see WARNINGS).

Zolmitriptan should also be administered with caution to patients with diseases that may alter the absorption, metabolism, or excretion of drugs, such as impaired hepatic function (see CLINICAL PHARMACOLOGY).

For a given attack, if a patient does not respond to the first dose of zolmitriptan, the diagnosis of migraine headache should be reconsidered before administration of a second dose.

BINDING TO MELANIN-CONTAINING TISSUES

When pigmented rats were given a single oral dose of 10 mg/kg of radiolabeled zolmitriptan, the radioactivity in the eye after 7 days, the latest time point examined, was still 75% of the value measured after 4 hours. This suggests that zolmitriptan and/or its metabolites may bind to the melanin of the eye. Because there could be accumulation in melanin rich tissues over time, this raises the possibility that zolmitriptan could cause toxicity in these tissues after extended use. However, no effects on the retina related to treatment with zolmitriptan were noted in any of the toxicity studies. Although no systematic monitoring of ophthalmologic function was undertaken in clinical trials, and no specific recommendations for ophthalmologic monitoring are offered, prescribers should be aware of the possibility of long-term ophthalmologic effects.

PHENYLKETONURICS

Phenylketonuric patients should be informed that zolmitriptan orally disintegrating tablets contain phenylalanine (a component of aspartame). Each 2.5 mg orally disintegrating tablet contains 2.81 mg phenylalanine. Each 5 mg orally disintegrating tablet contains 5.62 mg phenylalanine.

INFORMATION FOR THE PATIENT

Refer to the Patient Instructions that are distributed with the prescription.

Zolmitriptan Orally Disintegrating Tablets

The orally disintegrating tablet is packaged in a blister. Patients should be instructed not to remove the tablet from the blister until just prior to dosing. The blister pack should then be peeled open, and the orally disintegrating tablet placed on the tongue, where it will dissolve and be swallowed with the saliva.

LABORATORY TESTS

No monitoring of specific laboratory tests is recommended.

DRUG/LABORATORY TEST INTERACTIONS

Zolmitriptan is not known to interfere with commonly employed clinical laboratory tests.

CARCINOGENESIS, MUTAGENESIS, AND IMPAIRMENT OF FERTILITY

Carcinogenesis

Carcinogenicity studies by oral gavage were carried out in mice and rats at doses up to 400 mg/kg/day. Mice were dosed for 85 weeks (males) and 92 weeks (females). The exposure (plasma AUC of parent drug) at the highest dose level was approximately 800 times that seen in humans after a single 10 mg dose (the maximum recommended total daily dose). There was no effect of zolmitriptan on tumor incidence. Control, low dose and middle dose rats were dosed for 104-105 weeks; the high dose group was sacrificed after 101 weeks (males) and 86 weeks (females) due to excess mortality. Aside from an increase in the incidence of thyroid follicular cell hyperplasia and thyroid follicular cell adenomas seen in male rats receiving 400 mg/kg/day, an exposure approximately 3000 times that seen in humans after dosing with 10 mg, no tumors were noted.

Mutagenesis

Zolmitriptan was mutagenic in an Ames test, in 2 of 5 strains of *S. typhimurium* tested, in the presence of, but not in the absence of, metabolic activation. It was not mutagenic in an *in vitro* mammalian gene cell mutation (CHO/HGPRT) assay. Zolmitriptan was clastogenic in an *in vitro* human lymphocyte assay both in the absence of and the presence of metabolic activation; it was not clastogenic in an *in vivo* mouse micronucleus assay. It was also not genotoxic in an unscheduled DNA synthesis study.

Impairment of Fertility

Studies of male and female rats administered zolmitriptan prior to and during mating and up to implantation have shown no impairment of fertility at doses up to 400 mg/kg/day. Exposure at this dose was approximately 3000 times exposure at the maximum recommended human dose of 10 mg/day.

PREGNANCY CATEGORY C

There are no adequate and well controlled studies in pregnant women; therefore, zolmitriptan should be used during pregnancy only if the potential benefit justifies the potential risk to the fetus.

In reproductive toxicity studies in rats and rabbits, oral administration of zolmitriptan to pregnant animals was associated with embryolethality and fetal abnormalities. When pregnant rats were administered oral zolmitriptan during the period of organogenesis at doses of 100, 400 and 1200 mg/kg/day, there was a dose-related increase in embryolethality which became statistically significant at the high dose. The maternal plasma exposures at these doses were approximately 280, 1100 and 5000 times the exposure in humans receiving the maximum recommended total daily dose of 10 mg. The high dose was maternally toxic, as evidenced by a decreased maternal body weight gain during gestation. In a similar study in rabbits, embryolethality was increased at the maternally toxic doses of 10 and 30 mg/kg/day (maternal plasma exposures equivalent to 11 and 42 times exposure in humans receiving the maximum recommended total daily dose of 10 mg), and increased incidences of fetal malformations (fused sternebrae, rib anomalies) and variations (major blood vessel variations, irregular ossification pattern of ribs) were observed at 30 mg/kg/day. Three mg/kg/day was a no effect dose (equivalent to human exposure at a dose of 10 mg). When female rats were given zolmitriptan during gestation, parturition, and lactation, an increased incidence of hydronephrosis was found in the offspring at the maternally toxic dose of 400 mg/kg/day (1100 times human exposure).

NURSING MOTHERS

It is not known whether zolmitriptan is excreted in human milk. Because many drugs are excreted in human milk, caution should be exercised when zolmitriptan is administered to a nursing woman. Lactating rats dosed with zolmitriptan had milk levels equivalent to maternal plasma levels at 1 hour and 4 times higher than plasma levels at 4 hours.

PEDIATRIC USE

Safety and effectiveness of zolmitriptan in pediatric patients have not been established; therefore, zolmitriptan is not recommended for the use in patients under 18 years of age.

Postmarketing experience with other triptans includes a limited number of reports that describe pediatric patients who have experienced clinically serious adverse events that are similar in nature to those reported rarely in adults.

USE IN THE ELDERLY

Although the pharmacokinetic disposition of the drug in the elderly is similar to that seen in younger adults, there is no information about the safety and effectiveness of zolmitriptan in this population because patients over age 65 were excluded from the controlled clinical trials (see CLINICAL PHARMACOLOGY, Pharmacokinetics and Bioavailability, Special Populations).

DRUG INTERACTIONS

Ergot-containing drugs have been reported to cause prolonged vasospastic reactions. Because there is a theoretical basis that these effects may be additive, use of ergotamine-containing or ergot-type medications (like dihydroergotamine or methysergide) and zolmitriptan within 24 hours of each other should be avoided (see CONTRAINDICATIONS).

MAO-A inhibitors increase the systemic exposure of zolmitriptan. Therefore, the use of zolmitriptan in patients receiving MAO-A inhibitors is contraindicated (see CLINICAL PHARMACOLOGY and CONTRAINDICATIONS).

Concomitant use of other 5-$HT_{1B/1D}$ agonists within 24 hours of zolmitriptan treatment is not recommended (see CONTRAINDICATIONS).

Following administration of cimetidine, the half-life and AUC of zolmitriptan and its active metabolites were approximately doubled (see CLINICAL PHARMACOLOGY).

Selective serotonin reuptake inhibitors (SSRIs) (*e.g.*, fluoxetine, fluvoxamine, paroxetine, sertraline) have been reported, rarely, to cause weakness, hyperreflexia, and incoordination when coadministered with 5-HT_1 agonists. If concomitant treatment with zolmitriptan and an SSRI is clinically warranted, appropriate observation of the patient is advised.

ADVERSE REACTIONS

Serious cardiac events, including myocardial infarction, have occurred following the use of zolmitriptan tablets. These events are extremely rare and most have been reported in patients with risk factors predictive of CAD. Events reported, in association with drugs of this class, have included coronary artery vasospasm, transient myocardial ischemia, myocardial infarction, ventricular tachycardia, and ventricular fibrillation (see CONTRAINDICATIONS, WARNINGS, and PRECAUTIONS).

INCIDENCE IN CONTROLLED CLINICAL TRIALS

Among 2633 patients treated with zolmitriptan tablets in the active and placebo controlled trials, no patients withdrew for reasons related to adverse events, but as patients treated a single headache in these trials, the opportunity for discontinuation was limited. In a long-term, open label study where patients were allowed to treat multiple migraine attacks for up to 1 year, 8% (167 out of 2058) withdrew from the trial because of adverse experience. The most common events were paresthesia, asthenia, nausea, dizziness, pain, chest or neck tightness or heaviness, somnolence and warm sensation.

TABLE 2 lists the adverse events that occurred in ≥2% of the 2074 patients in any one of the zolmitriptan 1, 2.5 or 5 mg tablets dose groups of the controlled clinical trials. Only events that were more frequent in a zolmitriptan group compared to the placebo groups are included. The events cited reflect experience gained under closely monitored conditions of clinical trials in a highly selected patient population. In actual clinical practice or in other clinical trials, these frequency estimates may not apply, as the conditions of use, reporting behavior, and the kinds of patients treated may differ.

Several of the adverse events appear dose related, notably paresthesia, sensation of heaviness or tightness in chest, neck, jaw, and throat, dizziness, somnolence, and possibly asthenia and nausea.

***TABLE 2** Adverse Experience Incidence in Five Placebo-Controlled Migraine Clinical Trials — Events Reported by ≥2% Patients Treated With Zolmitriptan Tablets*

		Zolmitriptan		
Adverse Event Type	**Placebo (n=401)**	**1 mg (n=163)**	**2.5 mg (n=498)**	**5 mg (n=1012)**
Atypical Sensations	**6%**	**12%**	**12%**	**18%**
Hypesthesia	1%	1%	1%	2%
Paresthesia (all types)	2%	5%	7%	9%
Sensation warm/cold	4%	6%	5%	7%
Pain and Pressure Sensations	**7%**	**13%**	**14%**	**22%**
Chest — pain/tightness/ pressure and/or heaviness	1%	2%	3%	4%
Neck/throat/jaw — pain/ tightness/pressure	3%	4%	7%	10%
Heaviness other than chest or neck	1%	1%	2%	5%
Pain — location specified	1%	2%	2%	3%
Other — pressure/ tightness/heaviness	0%	2%	2%	2%
Digestive	**8%**	**11%**	**16%**	**14%**
Dry mouth	2%	5%	3%	3%
Dyspepsia	1%	3%	2%	1%
Dysphagia	0%	0%	0%	2%
Nausea	4%	4%	9%	6%
Neurological	**10%**	**11%**	**17%**	**21%**
Dizziness	4%	6%	8%	10%
Somnolence	3%	5%	6%	8%
Vertigo	0%	0%	0%	2%
Other				
Asthenia	3%	5%	3%	9%
Palpitations	1%	0%	<1%	2%
Myalgia	<1%	1%	1%	2%
Myasthenia	<1%	0%	1%	2%
Sweating	1%	0%	2%	3%

Zolmitriptan is generally well tolerated. Across all doses, most adverse reactions were mild and transient and did not lead to long-lasting effects. The incidence of adverse events in controlled clinical trials was not affected by gender, weight, or age of the patients; use of prophylactic medications; or presence of aura. There were insufficient data to assess the impact of race on the incidence of adverse events.

Other Events

In the paragraphs that follow, the frequencies of less commonly reported adverse clinical events are presented. Because the reports include events observed in open and uncontrolled studies, the role of zolmitriptan in their causation cannot be reliably determined. Furthermore, variability associated with adverse event reporting, the terminology used to describe adverse events, etc., limit the value of the quantitative frequency estimates provided. Event frequencies are calculated as the number of patients who used zolmitriptan tablets (n=4027) and reported an event divided by the total number of patients exposed to zolmitriptan tablets. All reported events are included except those already listed in the previous table, those too general to be informative, and those not reasonably associated with the use of the drug.

Events are further classified within body system categories and enumerated in order of decreasing frequency using the following definitions: *infrequent* adverse events are those occurring in 1/100 to 1/1000 patients and *rare* adverse events are those occurring in fewer than 1/1000 patients.

Atypical Sensation: *Infrequent:* Hyperesthesia.

General: *Infrequent:* Allergy reaction, chills, facial edema, fever, malaise and photosensitivity.

Cardiovascular: *Infrequent:* Arrhythmias, hypertension and syncope. *Rare:* Bradycardia, extrasystoles, postural hypotension, QT prolongation, tachycardia and thrombophlebitis.

Digestive: *Infrequent:* Increased appetite, tongue edema, esophagitis, gastroenteritis, liver function abnormality and thirst. *Rare:* Anorexia, constipation, gastritis, hematemesis, pancreatitis, melena and ulcer.

Hemic: *Infrequent:* Ecchymosis. *Rare:* Cyanosis, thrombocytopenia, eosinophilia and leukopenia.

Metabolic: *Infrequent:* Edema. *Rare:* Hyperglycemia and alkaline phosphatase increased.

Musculoskeletal: *Infrequent:* Back pain, leg cramps and tenosynovitis. *Rare:* Arthritis, asthenia, tetany and twitching.

Neurological: *Infrequent:* Agitation, anxiety, depression, emotional lability and insomnia. *Rare:* Akathesia, amnesia, apathy, ataxia, dystonia, euphoria, hallucinations, cerebral ischemia, hyperkinesia, hypotonia, hypertonia and irritability.

Respiratory: *Infrequent:* Bronchitis, bronchospasm, epistaxis, hiccup, laryngitis and yawn. *Rare:* Apnea and voice alteration.

Skin: *Infrequent:* Pruritus, rash and urticaria.

Special Senses: *Infrequent:* Dry eye, eye pain, hyperacusis, ear pain, parosmia, and tinnitus. *Rare:* Diplopia and lacrimation.

Urogenital: *Infrequent:* Hematuria, cystitis, polyuria, urinary frequency, urinary urgency. *Rare:* Miscarriage and dysmenorrhea.

The adverse experiences profile seen with zolmitriptan orally disintegrating tablets was similar to that seen with the zolmitriptan tablets.

POSTMARKETING EXPERIENCE

The following section enumerates potentially important adverse events that have occurred in clinical practice and which have been reported spontaneously to various surveillance systems. The events enumerated represent reports arising from both domestic and nondomestic use of zolmitriptan. The events enumerated include all except those already listed above or those too general to be informative. Because the reports cite events reported spontaneously from worldwide postmarketing experience, frequency of events and the role of zolmitriptan in their causation cannot be reliably determined.

Cardiovascular: Coronary artery vasospasm; transient myocardial ischemia, angina pectoris, and myocardial infarction.

General: As with other 5-$HT_{1B/1D}$ agonists, there have been very rare reports of anaphylaxis or anaphylactoid reactions in patients receiving zolmitriptan.

DOSAGE AND ADMINISTRATION

ZOLMITRIPTAN TABLETS

In controlled clinical trials, single doses of 1, 2.5 and 5 mg of zolmitriptan tablets were effective for the acute treatment of migraines in adults. A greater proportion of patients had headache response following a 2.5 or 5 mg dose than following a 1 mg dose. In the only direct comparison of 2.5 and 5 mg, there was little added benefit from the larger dose but side effects are generally increased at 5 mg (see TABLE 2). Patients should, therefore, be started on 2.5 mg or lower. A dose lower than 2.5 mg can be achieved by manually breaking the scored 2.5 mg tablet in half.

If the headache returns, the dose may be repeated after 2 hours, not to exceed 10 mg within a 24 hour period. Controlled trials have not adequately established the effectiveness of a second dose if the initial dose is ineffective.

The safety of treating an average of more than 3 headaches in a 30 day period has not been established.

ZOLMITRIPTAN ORALLY DISINTEGRATING TABLETS

In a controlled clincial trial, a single dose of 2.5 mg of zolmitriptan orally disintegrating tablets was effective for the acute treatment of migraines in adults.

If the headache returns, the dose may be repeated after 2 hours, not to exceed 10 mg within a 24 hour period. Controlled trials have not adequately established the effectiveness of a second dose if the initial dose is ineffective.

The safety of treating an average of more than 3 headaches in a 30 day period has not been established.

Administration with liquid is not necessary. The orally disintegrating tablet is packaged in a blister. Patients should be instructed not to remove the tablet from the blister until just prior to dosing. The blister pack should then be peeled open, and the orally disintegrating tablet placed on the tongue, where it will dissolve and be swallowed with the saliva. It is not recommended to break the orally disintegrating tablet.

HEPATIC IMPAIRMENT

Patients with moderate to severe hepatic impairment have decreased clearance of zolmitriptan and significant elevation in blood pressure was observed in some patients. Use of a low dose with blood pressure monitoring is recommended (see CLINICAL PHARMACOLOGY and WARNINGS).

HOW SUPPLIED

ZOMIG TABLETS

2.5 mg: Yellow, biconvex, round, film-coated, scored tablets contain 2.5 mg of zolmitriptan identified with "ZOMIG" and "2.5" debossed on one side.

5 mg: Pink, biconvex, film-coated tablets contain 5 mg of zolmitriptan identified with "ZOMIG" and "5" debossed on one side.

ZOMIG-ZMT

2.5 mg: White, flat faced, uncoated, bevelled tablet containing 2.5 mg of zolmitriptan identified with a debossed "Z" on one side.

5 mg: White, flat faced, round, uncoated, bevelled tablet containing 5.0 mg of zolmitriptan identified with a debossed "Z" and "5" on one side.

STORAGE

Store both Zomig tablets and Zomig-ZMT tablets at controlled room temperature, 20-25°C (68-77°F). Protect from light and moisture.

PRODUCT LISTING - EQUIVALENTS NOT AVAILABLE

Tablet - Oral - 2.5 mg

6's	$95.63	ZOMIG, Astra-Zeneca Pharmaceuticals	00310-0210-20

Tablet - Oral - 5 mg

3's	$54.38	ZOMIG, Astra-Zeneca Pharmaceuticals	00310-0211-25

Tablet, Disintegrating - Oral - 2.5 mg

6's	$95.63	ZOMIG-ZMT, Astra-Zeneca Pharmaceuticals	00310-0209-20

Tablet, Disintegrating - Oral - 5 mg

3's	$54.38	ZOMIG-ZMT, Astra-Zeneca Pharmaceuticals	00310-0213-21

Zolpidem Tartrate *(003145)*

Categories: Insomnia; DEA Class CIV; FDA Approved 1992 Dec; Pregnancy Category B
Drug Classes: Sedatives/hypnotics
Brand Names: Ambien
Foreign Brand Availability: Niotal (Italy); Nitrest (India); Somnil (Colombia); Somno (Peru); Stilnoct (Belgium; Denmark); Stilnox (Australia; Belgium; Benin; Burkina-Faso; Colombia; Czech-Republic; Ethiopia; France; Gambia; Germany; Ghana; Greece; Guinea; Hong-Kong; Hungary; Israel; Italy; Ivory-Coast; Kenya; Liberia; Malawi; Malaysia; Mali; Mauritania; Mauritius; Mexico; Morocco; Niger; Nigeria; Peru; Philippines; Senegal; Seychelles; Sierra-Leone; South-Africa; Spain; Sudan; Switzerland; Taiwan; Tanzania; Thailand; Tunia; Uganda; Zambia; Zimbabwe); Supedal (Peru)
Cost of Therapy: $28.06 (Insomnia; Ambien ; 10 mg; 1 tablet/day; 10 day supply)

DESCRIPTION

Zolpidem tartrate, is a non-benzodiazepine hypnotic of the imidazopyridine class and is available in 5 mg and 10 mg strength tablets for oral administration.

Chemically, zolpidem is N,N,6-trimethyl-2-p-toyl-imidazo(1,2,-a)pyridine-3-acetamide L-(+)-tartrate (2:1).

Zolpidem tartrate is a white to off-white crystalline powder that is sparingly soluble in water, alcohol, and propylene glycol. It has a molecular weight of 764.88.

Each Ambien tablet includes the following inactive ingredients: hydroxypropyl methylcellulose, lactose, magnesium stearate, microcrystalline cellulose, polyethylene glycol, sodium starch glycolate, titanium dioxide; the 5 mg tablet also contains FD&C red no. 40, iron oxide colorant, and polysorbate 80.

CLINICAL PHARMACOLOGY

PHARMACODYNAMICS

Subunit modulation of the $GABA_a$ receptor chloride channel macromolecular complex is hypothesized to be responsible for sedative, anticonvulsant, anxiolytic, and myorelaxant drug properties. The major modulatory site of the $GABA_a$ receptor complex is located on its alpha (α) subunit and is referred to as the benzodiazepine (BZ) or Ω receptor. At least three subtypes of the Ω receptor have been identified.

While zolpidem is a hypnotic agent with a chemical structure unrelated to benzodiazepines, barbiturates, or other drugs with known hypnotic properties, it interacts with a GABA-BZ receptor complex and shares some of the pharmacological properties of the benzodiazepines. In contrast to the benzodiazepines, which non-selectively bind to and activate all three omega receptor subtypes, zolpidem *in vitro* binds the (ω_1) receptor preferentially. The Ω_1) receptor is found primarily on the Lamina IV of the sensorimotor cortical regions, substantia nigra (pars reticulata), cerebellum molecular layer, olfactory bulb, ventral thalamic complex, pons, inferior colliculus, and globus pallidus. This selective binding of zolpidem on the Ω_1) receptor is not absolute, but it may explain the relative absence of myorelaxant and anticonvulsant effects in animal studies as well as the preservation of deep sleep (stages 3 and 4) in human studies of zolpidem at hypnotic doses.

PHARMACOKINETICS

The pharmacokinetic profile of zolpidem tartrate is characterized by rapid absorption from the GI tract and a short elimination half-life ($T_{1/2}$) in healthy subjects. In a single- dose crossover study in 45 healthy subjects administered 5 and 10 mg zolpidem tartrate tablets, the mean peak concentrations (C_{max}) were 59 (range: 29-113) and 121 (range: 58-272) ng/ml, respectively, occurring at a mean time (T_{max}) of 1.6 hours for both. The mean zolpidem tartrate elimination half-life was 2.6 (range: 1.4-4.5) and 2.5 (range: 1.4-3.8) hours, for the 5 and 10 mg tablets, respectively. Zolpidem tartrate is converted to inactive metabolites that are eliminated primarily by renal excretion. Zolpidem tartrate demonstrated linear kinetics in the dose range of 5-20 mg. Total protein binding was found to be 92.5 ± 0.1% and remained constant, independent of concentration between 40 and 790 ng/ml. Zolpidem did not accumulate in young adults following nightly dosing with 20 mg zolpidem tartrate tablets for 2 weeks.

A food-effect study in 30 healthy male volunteers compared the pharmacokinetics of zolpidem tartrate 10 mg when administered while fasting or 20 minutes after a meal. Results demonstrated that with food, mean AUC and C_{max}were decreased by 15% and 25% respectively, while mean $T_{max}$was prolonged by 60% (from 1.4-2.2 h). The half-life remained unchanged. These results suggest that, for faster sleep onset, zolpidem tartrate should not be administered with or immediately after a meal.

In the elderly, the dose for zolpidem tartrate should be 5 mg (see PRECAUTIONS and DOSAGE AND ADMINISTRATION). This recommendation is based on several studies in which the mean C_{max}, $T_{1/2}$, and AUC were significantly increased when compared to results in young adults. In one study of 8 elderly subjects (> 70 years), the means for C_{max}, $T_{1/2}$, and AUC significantly increased by 50% (255 vs 284 ng/ml), 32% (2.2 vs 2.9 h), and 64% (955 vs 1562 ng·h/ml), respectively, as compared to younger adults (20-40 years) following a single 20 mg oral zolpidem dose. Zolpidem tartrate did not accumulate in elderly subjects following nightly oral dosing of 10 mg for 1 week.

The pharmacokinetics of zolpidem tartrate in 8 patients with chronic hepatic insufficiency were compared to results in healthy subjects. Following a single 20 mg oral zolpidem dose, mean C_{max} and AUC were found to be 2 times (250 vs 499 ng/ml) and 5 times (788 vs 4,203 ng·h/ml) higher, respectively, in hepatically compromised patients. T_{max} did not change. The mean half-life in cirrhotic patients of 9.9 h (range: 4.1-25.8 h) was greater than that observed in normals of 2.2 h (range: 1.6-2.4 h). Dosing should be modified accordingly in patients with hepatic insufficiency (see PRECAUTIONS and DOSAGE AND ADMINISTRATION).

The pharmacokinetics of zolpidem tartrate were studied in 11 patients with end-stage renal failure (mean Cl_{cr}= 6.5 ± 1.5 ml/min) undergoing hemodialysis 3 times a week, who were dosed with zolpidem 10 mg orally each day for 14-21 days. No statistically significant differences were observed for C_{max}, T_{max}, half-life, and AUC between the first and last days of drug administration when baseline concentration adjustments were made. On day 1, C_{max} was 172 ± 29 ng/ml (range: 46-344 ng/ml). After repeated dosing for 14 or 21 days, C_{max} was 203 ± 32 ng/ml (range 28-316 ng/ml). On day 1, T_{max} was 1.7 ± 0.3 h (range 0.5-3.0 h); after repeated dosing T_{max} 0.8 ± 0.2 h (range 0.5-2.0 h). This variation is accounted for by noting that last-day serum sampling began 10 hours after the previous dose, rather than after 24 hours. This resulted in residual drug concentration and a shorter period to reach maximal serum concentration. On day 1, $T_{1/2}$ was 2.4 ± 0.4 h (range 0.4-5.1 h). After repeated dosing, $T_{1/2}$ was 2.5 ± 0.4 h (range: 0.7-4.2 h). AUC was 796 ± 159 ng · h/ml after the first dose and 818 ± 170 ng · h/ml after repeated dosing. Zolpidem was not hemodialyzable. No accumulation of unchanged drug appeared after 14 or 21 days. Zolpidem tartrate pharmacokinetics were not significantly different in renally impaired patients. No dosage adjustment is necessary in patients with compromised renal function. As a general precaution, these patients should be closely monitored.

POSTULATED RELATIONSHIP BETWEEN ELIMINATION RATE OF HYPNOTICS AND THEIR PROFILE OF COMMON UNTOWARD EFFECTS

The type and duration of hypnotic effects and the profile of unwanted effects during administration of hypnotic drugs may be influenced by the biologic half- life of administered drug and any active metabolites formed. When half-lives are long, drug or metabolites may accumulate during periods of nightly administration and may be associated with impairment of cognitive and/or motor performance during waking hours; the possibility of interaction with other psychoactive drugs or alcohol will be enhanced. In contrast, if half-lives, including half-lives of active metabolites, are short, drug and metabolites will be cleared before the next dose is ingested, and carryover effects related to excessive sedation or CNS depression should be minimal or absent. Zolpidem tartrate has a short half-life and no active metabolites. During nightly use for an extended period, pharmacodynamic tolerance or adaptation to some effects of hypnotics may develop. If the drug has a short elimination half-life, it is possible that a relative deficiency of the drug or its active metabolites (*i.e.,* in relationship to the receptor site) may occur at some point in the interval between each night's use. This sequence of events may account for two clinical findings reported to occur after several weeks of nightly use of other rapidly eliminated hypnotics, namely, increased wakefulness during the last third of the night, and the appearance of increased signs of daytime anxiety. Increased wakefulness during the last third of the night as measured by polysomnography has not been observed in clinical trials with zolpidem tartrate.

CONTROLLED TRIALS SUPPORTING SAFETY AND EFFICACY

Transient Insomnia

Normal adults experiencing transient insomnia (n=462) during the first night in a sleep laboratory were evaluated in a double blind, parallel group, single-night trial comparing 2 doses of zolpidem (7.5 and 10 mg) and placebo. Both zolpidem doses were superior to placebo on objective (polysomnographic) measures of sleep latency, sleep duration, and number of awakenings.

Chronic Insomnia

Adult outpatients, with chronic insomnia (n=75) were evaluated in a double-blind, parallel group, 5-week trial comparing 2 doses of zolpidem tartrate (10 and 15 mg) and placebo. On objective (polysomnographic) measures of sleep latency and sleep efficiency, zolpidem 15 mg was superior to placebo for all 5 weeks; zolpidem 10 mg was superior to placebo on sleep latency for the first 4 weeks and on sleep efficiency for weeks 2 and 4. Zolpidem was comparable to placebo on number of awakenings at both doses studied.

Adult outpatients (n=141) with chronic insomnia were evaluated in a double-blind, parallel group, 4-week trial comparing 2 doses of zolpidem (10 and 15 mg) and placebo. Zolpidem 10 mg was superior to placebo on a subjective measure of sleep latency for all 4 weeks, and on subjective measures of total sleep time, number of awakenings, and sleep quality for the first treatment week. Zolpidem 15 mg was superior to placebo on a subjective measure of sleep latency for the first 3 weeks, on a subjective measure of total sleep time for the first week, and on number of awakenings and sleep quality for the first 2 weeks.

Next-Day Residual Effects

There was no evidence of residual next-day effects seen with zolpidem tartrate in several studies utilizing the Multiple Sleep latency Test (MSLT), the Digit Symbol Substitution Test (DSST), and patient ratings of alertness. In one study involving elderly patients, there was a small but statistically significant decrease in one measure of performance, the DSST, but no impairment was seen in the MSLT study.

Rebound Effects

There was no objective (polysomnographic) evidence of rebound insomnia at recommended doses seen in studies evaluating sleep on the nights following discontinuation of zolpidem tartrate. There was subjective evidence of impaired sleep in the elderly on the first post-treatment night at doses above the recommended elderly dose of 5 mg.

Memory Impairment

Two small studies (n=6 and n=9) utilizing objective measures of memory yielded little evidence for memory impairment following the administration of zolpidem tartrate. There was subjective evidence from adverse event data for anterograde amnesia occurring in association with the administration zolpidem tartrate, predominantly at doses above 10 mg.

Effects on Sleep Stages

In studies that measured the percentage of sleep time spent in each sleep stage, zolpidem tartrate has generally been shown to preserve sleep stages. Sleep time spent in stages 3 and 4 (deep sleep) was found comparable to placebo with only inconsistent, minor changes in REM (paradoxical) sleep at the recommended dose.

INDICATIONS AND USAGE

Zolpidem tartrate is indicated for the short-term treatment of insomnia. Hypnotics should generally be limited to 7-10 days of use; and reevaluation of the patient is recommended if they are to be taken for more than 2-3 weeks.

Zolpidem tartrate should not be prescribed in quantities exceeding a 1 month supply (see WARNINGS).

Zolpidem tartrate has been shown to decrease sleep latency and increase the duration of sleep for up to 5 weeks in controlled clinical studies (see CLINICAL PHARMACOLOGY).

CONTRAINDICATIONS

None known.

WARNINGS

Since sleep disturbances may be the presenting manifestation of a physical and/or psychiatric disorder, symptomatic treatment of the insomnia should be initiated only after a careful evaluation of the patient. The failure of insomnia to remit after 7-10 days of treatment may indicate the presence of a primary psychiatric and/or medical illness which should be evaluated. Worsening of insomnia or the emergence of new thinking or behavior abnormalities may be the consequence of an unrecognized psychiatric or physical disorder. Such findings have emerged during the course of treatment with sedative/hypnotic drugs, including zolpidem tartrate. Because some of the important adverse effects of zolpidem tartrate appear to be dose related (see PRECAUTIONS and DOSAGE AND ADMINISTRATION), it is important to use the smallest possible effective dose, especially in the elderly.

A variety of abnormal thinking and behavior changes have been reported to occur in association with the use of sedative/hypnotics. Some of these changes may be characterized by decreased inhibition (*e.g.*, aggressiveness and extroversion that seemed out of character), similar to effects produced by alcohol and other CNS depressants. Other reported behavioral changes have included bizarre behavior, agitation, hallucinations, and depersonalization. Amnesia and other neuropsychiatric symptoms may occur unpredictably. In primarily depressed patients, worsening of depression, including suicidal thinking, has been reported in association with the use of sedative/hypnotics.

It can rarely be determined with certainty whether a particular instance of the abnormal behaviors listed above are drug induced, spontaneous in origin, or a result of an underlying psychiatric or physical disorder. Nonetheless, the emergence of any new behavioral sign or symptom of concern requires careful and immediate evaluation.

Following the rapid dose decrease or abrupt discontinuation of sedative/hypnotics, there have been reports of signs and symptoms similar to those associated with withdrawal from other CNS-depressant drugs.

Zolpidem tartrate, like other sedative/hypnotic drugs, has CNS-depressant effects. Due to the rapid onset of action, zolpidem tartrate should only be ingested immediately prior to going to bed. Patients should be cautioned against engaging in hazardous occupations requiring complete mental alertness or motor coordination such as operating machinery or driving a motor vehicle after ingesting the drug, including potential impairment of the performance of such activities that may occur the day following ingestion of zolpidem tartrate. Zolpidem tartrate showed additive effects when combined with alcohol and should not be taken with alcohol. Patients should also be cautioned about possible combined effects with other CNS-depressant drugs. Dosage adjustments may be necessary when zolpidem tartrate is administered with such agents because of the potentially additive effects.

PRECAUTIONS

GENERAL

Use in the Elderly and/or Debilitated Patients

Impaired motor and/or cognitive performance after repeated exposure or unusual sensitivity to sedative/hypnotic drugs is a concern in the treatment of elderly and/or debilitated patients. Therefore, the recommended zolpidem tartrate dosage is 5 mg in such patients (see DOSAGE AND ADMINISTRATION) to decrease the possibility of side effects. These patients should be closely monitored.

Use in Patients With Concomitant Illness

Clinical experience with zolpidem tartrate in patients with concomitant systemic illness is limited. Caution is advisable in using zolpidem tartrate in patients with diseases or conditions that could affect metabolism or hemodynamic responses. Although preliminary studies did not reveal respiratory depressant effects at hypnotic doses of zolpidem tartrate in normals, precautions should be observed if zolpidem tartrate is prescribed to patients with compromised respiratory function, since sedative/hypnotics have the capacity to depress respiratory drive. Post-marketing reports or respiratory insufficiency, most of which involved patients with pre-existing respiratory impairment, have been received. Data in end-stage renal failure patients repeatedly treated with zolpidem tartrate did not demonstrate drug accumulation or alterations in pharmacokinetic parameters. No dosage adjustment in renally impaired patients is required; however, these patients should be closely monitored (see CLINICAL PHARMACOLOGY, Pharmacokinetics). A study in subjects with hepatic impairment did reveal prolonged elimination in this group; therefore, treatment should be initiated with 5 mg in patients with hepatic compromise, and they should be closely monitored.

Use in Depression

As with other sedative/hypnotic drugs, zolpidem tartrate should be administered with caution to patients exhibiting signs or symptoms of depression. Suicidal tendencies may be present in such patients and protective measures may be required. Intentional overdosage is more common in this group of patients; therefore, the least amount of drug that is feasible should be prescribed for the patient at any one time.

INFORMATION FOR THE PATIENT

Patient information is provided with the prescription. To assure safe and effective use of zolpidem tartrate, this information and instructions provided in the patient information should be discussed with patients.

LABORATORY TESTS

There are no specific laboratory tests recommended.

DRUG/LABORATORY TEST INTERACTIONS

Zolpidem is not known to interfere with commonly employed clinical laboratory tests.

CARCINOGENESIS, MUTAGENESIS, AND IMPAIRMENT OF FERTILITY

Carcinogenesis

Zolpidem was administered to rats and mice for 2 years at dietary dosages of 4, 18, and 80 mg/kg/day. In mice, these doses are 26-520 times or 2-35 times the maximum 10 mg human dose on a mg/kg or mg/m^2 basis, respectively. In rats these doses are 43-876 times or 6-115 times the maximum 10 mg human dose on a mg/kg or mg/m^2 basis, respectively. No evidence of carcinogenic potential was observed in mice. Renal lipocarcinomas were seen in 4/100 rats (3 males, 1 female) receiving 80 mg/kg/day and a renal lipoma was observed in 1 male rat at the 18 mg/kg/day dose. Incidence rates of lipoma and liposarcoma for zolpidem were comparable to those seen in historical controls and the tumor findings are thought be a spontaneous occurrence.

Mutagenesis

Zolpidem did not have mutagenic activity in several tests including the Ames test, genotoxicity in mouse lymphoma cells *in vitro*, chromosomal aberration in cultured human lymphocytes, unscheduled DNA synthesis in rat hepatocytes *in vitro*, and the micronucleus test in mice.

Impairment of Fertility

In a rat reproduction study, the high dose (100 mg/base/kg) of zolpidem resulted in irregular estrus cycles and prolonged precoital intervals, but there was no effect on male or female fertility after daily oral doses of 4-100 mg base/mg or 5-130 times the recommended human dose in mg/m^2. No effects on any other fertility parameters were noted.

PREGNANCY CATEGORY B

Teratogenic Effects

Studies to assess the effects of zolpidem on human reproduction and development have not been conducted.

Teratology studies were conducted in rats and rabbits.

In rats, adverse maternal and fetal effects occurred at 20 and 100 mg base/kg and included dose-related maternal lethargy and ataxia and a dose-related trend to incomplete ossification of fetal skull bones. Under-ossification of various fetal bone indicated a delay in maturation and is often seen in rats treated with sedative/hypnotic drugs. There were no teratogenic effects after zolpidem administration. The no-effect dose for maternal or fetal toxicity was 4 mg base/kg or 5 times the maximum human dose on a mg/m^2 basis.

In rabbits, dose-related maternal sedation and decreased weight gain occurred at all doses tested. At the high dose, 16 mg base/kg, there was an increase in postimplantation fetal loss and underossification of sternebrae in viable fetuses. These fetal findings in rabbits are often secondary to reductions in maternal weight gain. There were no frank teratogenic effects. The no-effect dose for fetal toxicity was 4 mg base/kg or 7 times the maximum human dose on a mg/m^2 basis.

Because animal reproduction studies are not always predictive of human response, this drug should be used during pregnancy only if clearly needed.

Nonteratogenic Effects

Studies to assess the effects on children whose mother took zolpidem during pregnancy have not been conducted. However, children born of mothers taking sedative/hypnotic drugs may be at some risk for withdrawal symptoms from the drug during the postnatal period. In addition, neonatal flaccidity has been reported in infants born of mothers who received sedative/hypnotic drugs during pregnancy.

LABOR AND DELIVERY

Zolpidem tartrate has no established use in labor and delivery.

NURSING MOTHERS

Studies in lactating mothers indicate that the half-life of zolpidem is similar to that in young normal volunteers (2.6 ± 0.3 h). Between 0.004 and 0.019% of the total administered dose is excreted into milk, but the effect of zolpidem on the infant is unknown.

In addition, in a rat study, zolpidem inhibited the secretion of milk. The no-effect dose was 4 mg base/kg or 6 times the recommended human dose in mg/m^2.

The use of zolpidem tartrate in nursing mothers is not recommended.

PEDIATRIC USE

Safety and effectiveness in children below the age of 18 have not been established.

DRUG INTERACTIONS

CNS-ACTIVE DRUGS

Zolpidem tartrate was evaluated in healthy volunteers in single-dose interaction studies for several CNS drugs. A study involving haloperidol and zolpidem revealed no effect of haloperidol on the pharmacokinetics or pharmacodynamics of zolpidem. Imipramine in combination with zolpidem produced no pharmacokinetic interaction other a 20% decrease in peak levels of imipramine, but there was an additive effect of decreased alertness. Similarly, chlorpromazine in combination with zolpidem produced no pharmacokinetic interaction, but there was an additive effect of decreased alertness and psychomotor performance. The lack of a drug interaction following single-dose administration does not predict a lack following chronic administration.

An additive effect on psychomotor performance between alcohol and zolpidem was demonstrated.

Since the systemic evaluation of zolpidem tartrate in combination with other CNS-active drugs have been limited, careful consideration should be given to the pharmacology of any CNS-active drug to be used with zolpidem. Any drug with CNS-depressant effects could potentially enhance the CNS- depressant effects of zolpidem.

OTHER DRUGS

A study involving cimetidine/zolpidem and ranitidine/zolpidem combinations revealed no effect of either drug on the pharmacokinetics or pharmacodynamics of zolpidem. Zolpidem had no effect on digoxin kinetics and did not effect prothrombin time when given with warfarin in normal subjects. Zolpidem's sedative/hypnotic effect was reversed by flumazenil; however, no significant alterations in zolpidem pharmacokinetics were found.

ADVERSE REACTIONS

ASSOCIATED WITH DISCONTINUATION OF TREATMENT

Approximately 4% of 1,701 patients who received zolpidem at all doses (1.25 to 90 mg) in US pre-marketing clinical trial discontinued treatment because of an adverse clinical event. Events most commonly associated with discontinuation from US trials were daytime drowsiness (0.5%), dizziness (0.4%), headache (0.5%), nausea (0.6%), and vomiting (0.5%).

Approximately 6% of 1320 patients who received zolpidem at all doses (5-50 mg) in similar foreign trials discontinued treatment because of an adverse event. Events most commonly associated with discontinuation from these trials were daytime drowsiness (1.6%), amnesia (0.6%), dizziness (0.6%), headache (0.6%), nausea (0.6%).

INCIDENCE IN CONTROLLED CLINICAL TRIALS

Most Commonly Observed Adverse Events in Controlled Trials

During short-term treatment (up to 10 nights) with zolpidem tartrate at doses up to 10 mg, the most commonly observed adverse events associated with the use of zolpidem and seen at statistically significant differences from placebo-treated patients were drowsiness (reported by 2% of zolpidem patients), dizziness (1%), and diarrhea(1%). During longer- term treatment (28-35 nights) with zolpidem at doses up to 10 mg, the most commonly observed adverse events associated with the use of zolpidem and seen at statistically significant differences from placebo-treated patients were dizziness (5%) and drugged feelings (3%).

Adverse Events Observed at an Incidence of ≥1% in Controlled Trials

TABLE 1 and TABLE 2 enumerate treatment-emergent adverse event frequencies that were observed at an incidence equal to 1% or greater among patients with insomnia who received zolpidem tartrate in US placebo-controlled trials. Events reported by investigators were classified utilizing a modified World Health Organization (WHO) dictionary of preferred terms for the purpose of establishing event frequencies. The prescriber should be aware that these figures cannot be used to predict the incidence of side effects in the course of usual medical practice, in which patient characteristics and other factors differ from those that prevailed in these clinical trials. Similarly, the cited frequencies cannot be compared with figure obtained from other clinical investigators involving related drug products and uses, since each group of drug trials is conducted under a different set of conditions. However, the cited figures provide the physician with a basis for estimating the relative contribution of drug and nondrug factors to the incidence of side effects in the population studied.

TABLE 1 was derived from a pool of 11 placebo-controlled short-term US efficacy trials involving zolpidem in doses ranging from 1.25 to 20 mg. The table is limited to data from doses up to and including 10 mg, the highest dose recommended for use.

TABLE 1 *Incidence of Treatment-Emergent Adverse Experiences in Short-Term Placebo-Controlled Clinical Trials (percentage of patients reporting)*

Body System/ Adverse Event*	Zolpidem (≤10 mg) (n=685)	Placebo (n=473)
Central and Peripheral Nervous System		
Headache	7%	6%
Drowsiness	2%	—
Dizziness	1%	—
Gastrointestinal System		
Nausea	2%	3%
Diarrhea	1%	—
Musculoskeletal System		
Myalgia	1%	2%

* Events reported by at least 1% of Ambien patients are included.

TABLE 2 was derived from a pool of three placebo-controlled long-term efficacy trials involving zolpidem tartrate. These trials involved patients with chronic insomnia who were treated for 28-35 nights with zolpidem at doses of 5, 10, or 15 mg. TABLE 2 is limited to data from doses up to and including 10 mg, the highest dose recommended for use. TABLE 2 includes only adverse events occurring at an incidence of at least 1% for zolpidem patients.

Dose Relationship for Adverse Events

There is evidence from dose comparison trials suggesting a dose relationship for many of the adverse events associated with zolpidem use, particularly for certain CNS and gastrointestinal adverse events.

ADVERSE EVENT INCIDENCE ACROSS THE ENTIRE PRE-APPROVAL DATABASE

Zolpidem tartrate was administered to 3021 subjects in clinical trials throughout the US, Canada, and Europe. Treatment-emergent adverse events associated with clinical trial participation were recorded by clinical investigators using terminology of their own choosing. To provide a meaningful estimate of the proportion of individuals experiencing treatment-emergent adverse events, similar types of untoward events were grouped into a smaller number of standardized event categories and classified utilizing a modified World Health Organization (WHO) dictionary of preferred terms. The frequencies presented, therefore, represent the proportions of the 3021 individuals exposed to zolpidem, at all doses, who experienced an event of the type cited on at least one occasion while receiving zolpidem. All reported treatment-emergent adverse events are included, except those already listed in the table above of adverse events in placebo-controlled studies, those coding terms that are so general as to be uninformative, and those events where a drug cause was remote. It is important to emphasize that, although the events reported did occur during treatment with zolpidem tartrate, they were not necessarily caused by it.

TABLE 2 *Incidence of Treatment-Emergent Adverse Experiences in Long-term Placebo-Controlled Clinical Trials (percentage of patients reporting)*

Body System/ Adverse Event*	Zolpidem (≤10 mg) (n=152)	Placebo (n=161)
Autonomic Nervous System		
Dry mouth	3%	1%
Body as a Whole		
Allergy	4%	1%
Back pain	3%	2%
Influenza-like symptoms	2%	—
Chest pain	1%	—
Fatigue	1%	2%
Cardiovascular System		
Palpitation	2%	—
Central and Peripheral Nervous System		
Headache	19%	22%
Drowsiness	8%	5%
Dizziness	5%	1%
Lethargy	3%	1%
Drugged feeling	3%	—
Lightheadedness	2%	1%
Depression	2%	1%
Abnormal dreams	1%	—
Amnesia	1%	—
Anxiety	1%	1%
Nervousness	1%	3%
Sleep disorder	1%	—
Gastrointestinal System		
Nausea	6%	6%
Dyspepsia	5%	6%
Diarrhea	3%	2%
Abdominal pain	2%	2%
Constipation	2%	1%
Anorexia	1%	1%
Vomiting	1%	1%
Immunologic system infection	1%	1%
Musculoskeletal System		
Myalgia	7%	7%
Arthralgia	4%	4%
Respiratory System		
Upper respiratory infection	5%	6%
Sinusitis	4%	2%
Pharyngitis	3%	1%
Rhinitis	1%	3%
Skin and Appendages		
Rash	2%	1%
Urogenital System		
Urinary tract infection	2%	2%

* Events reported by at least 1% of patients treated with Ambien.

Adverse events are further classified within body system categories and enumerated in order of decreasing frequency using the following definitions: *frequent* adverse events are defined as those occurring in greater than 1/100 subjects; *infrequent* adverse events are those occurring in 1/100 to 1/1000 patients; *rare* events are those occurring in less than 1/1,000 patients.

Autonomic Nervous System: *Infrequent:* Increased sweating, pallor, postural hypotension. *Rare:* Altered saliva, flushing, glaucoma, hypotension, impotence, syncope, tenesmus.

Body as a Whole: *Infrequent:* Asthenia, edema, falling, fever, malaise, trauma. *Rare:* Allergic reaction, allergy aggravated, abdominal body sensation, anaphylactic shock, face edema, hot flashes, increased ESR, pain, restless legs, rigors, tolerance increased, weight decrease.

Cardiovascular System: *Infrequent:* Cerebrovascular disorder, hypertension, tachycardia. *Rare:* Arrhythmia, arteritis, circulatory failure, extrasystoles, hypertension aggravated, myocardial infarction, phlebitis, pulmonary embolism, pulmonary edema, varicose veins, ventricular tachycardia.

Central and Peripheral Nervous System: *Frequent:* Ataxia, confusion, euphoria, insomnia, vertigo. *Infrequent:* Agitation, decreased cognition, detached, difficulty concentrating, dysarthria, emotional lability, hallucination, hypoesthesia, migraine, paresthesia, sleeping (after daytime dosing), stupor, tremor. *Rare:* Abnormal thinking, aggressive reaction, appetite increased, decreased libido, delusion, dementia, depersonalization, dysphasia, feeling strange, hypotonia, hysteria, illusion, intoxicated feeling, leg cramps, manic reaction, neuralgia, neuritis, neuropathy, neurosis, panic attacks, paresis, personality disorder, somnambulism, suicide attempts, tetany, yawning.

Gastrointestinal System: *Infrequent:* Constipation, dysphagia, flatulence, gastroenteritis, hiccup. *Rare:* Enteritis, eructation, esophagospasm, gastritis, hemorrhoids, intestinal obstruction, rectal hemorrhage, tooth caries.

Hematologic and Lymphatic System: *Rare:* Anemia, hyperhemoglobinemia, leukopenia, lymphadenopathy, macrocytic anemia, purpura.

Immunologic System: *Rare:* Abscess, herpes simplex, herpes zoster, otitis externa, otitis media.

Liver and Biliary System: *Infrequent:* Increased SGPT. *Rare:* Abnormal hepatic function, bilirubinemia, increased SGOT.

Metabolic and Nutritional: *Infrequent:* Hyperglycemia. *Rare:* Gout, hypercholesteremia, hyperlipidemia, increased BUN, periorbital edema, thirst, weight decrease.

Musculoskeletal System: *Infrequent:* Arthritis. *Rare:* Arthrosis, muscle weakness, sciatica, tendinitis.

Reproductive System: *Infrequent:* Menstrual disorder, vaginitis. *Rare:* Breast fibroadenosis, breast neoplasm, breast pain.

Respiratory System: *Infrequent:* Bronchitis, coughing, dyspnea. *Rare:* Bronchospasm, epistaxis, hypoxia, laryngitis, pneumonia.

Skin and Appendages: *Rare:* Acne, bullous eruption, dermatitis, furunculosis, injection-site inflammation, photosensitivity reaction, urticaria.

Special Senses: *Frequent:* Diplopia, vision abnormal. *Infrequent:* Eye irritation, scleritis, taste perversion, tinnitus. *Rare:* Corneal ulceration, eye pain, lacrimation abnormal, photopsia.

Urogenital System: *Infrequent:* Cystitis, urinary incontinence. *Rare:* Acute renal failure, dysuria, micturition frequency, polyuria, pyelonephritis, renal pain, urinary retention.

DOSAGE AND ADMINISTRATION

The dose of zolpidem tartrate should be individualized.

The recommended dose for adults is 10 mg immediately before bedtime.

Downward dosage adjustment may be necessary when zolpidem is administered with agents having known CNS-depressant effects because of the potentially additive effects.

Elderly or debilitated patients may be especially sensitive to the effects of zolpidem tartrate. Patients with hepatic insufficiency do not clear the drug as rapidly as normals. An initial 5 mg dose is recommended in these patients (see PRECAUTIONS).

The total zolpidem tartrate dose should not exceed 10 mg.

HOW SUPPLIED

Ambien 5 mg Tablets: Capsule-shaped, pink, film coated, identified with markings of "AMB 5" on one side and "5401" on the other side.

Ambien 10 mg Tablets: Capsule-shaped, white, film coated, identified with markings of "AMB 10" on one side and "5421" on the other.

Storage: Store below 30°C (86°F).

PRODUCT LISTING - EQUIVALENTS NOT AVAILABLE

Tablet - Oral - 5 mg

10's	$20.75	AMBIEN, Southwood Pharmaceuticals Inc	58016-0342-10
15's	$41.76	AMBIEN, Pharma Pac	52959-0362-15
20's	$41.51	AMBIEN, Southwood Pharmaceuticals Inc	58016-0342-20
20's	$54.46	AMBIEN, Pharma Pac	52959-0362-20
30's	$62.26	AMBIEN, Southwood Pharmaceuticals Inc	58016-0342-30
30's	$75.75	AMBIEN, Pharma Pac	52959-0362-30
40's	$83.01	AMBIEN, Southwood Pharmaceuticals Inc	58016-0342-40
60's	$124.52	AMBIEN, Southwood Pharmaceuticals Inc	58016-0342-60
60's	$139.21	AMBIEN, Pharma Pac	52959-0362-60
90's	$186.78	AMBIEN, Southwood Pharmaceuticals Inc	58016-0342-90
100's	$207.56	AMBIEN, Searle	00025-5401-31
100's	$217.93	AMBIEN, Searle	00025-5401-34
100's	$228.10	AMBIEN, Sanofi Winthrop Pharmaceuticals	00024-5401-31
100's	$239.50	AMBIEN, Sanofi Winthrop Pharmaceuticals	00024-5401-34

Tablet - Oral - 10 mg

10's	$25.53	AMBIEN, Southwood Pharmaceuticals Inc	58016-0341-10
10's	$41.50	AMBIEN, Pharma Pac	52959-0363-10
15's	$60.20	AMBIEN, Pharma Pac	52959-0363-15
20's	$51.06	AMBIEN, Southwood Pharmaceuticals Inc	58016-0341-20
20's	$79.14	AMBIEN, Pharma Pac	52959-0363-20
30's	$76.59	AMBIEN, Southwood Pharmaceuticals Inc	58016-0341-30
30's	$100.66	AMBIEN, Pharma Pac	52959-0363-30
40's	$102.12	AMBIEN, Southwood Pharmaceuticals Inc	58016-0341-40
60's	$153.18	AMBIEN, Southwood Pharmaceuticals Inc	58016-0341-60
60's	$195.75	AMBIEN, Pharma Pac	52959-0363-60
90's	$229.77	AMBIEN, Southwood Pharmaceuticals Inc	58016-0341-90
100's	$255.30	AMBIEN, Searle	00025-5421-31
100's	$268.09	AMBIEN, Searle	00025-5421-34
100's	$280.56	AMBIEN, Sanofi Winthrop Pharmaceuticals	00024-5421-31
100's	$294.63	AMBIEN, Sanofi Winthrop Pharmaceuticals	00024-5421-34

Zonisamide (003473)

Categories: Seizures, partial; Pregnancy Category C; FDA Approved 2000 Mar
Drug Classes: Anticonvulsants
Brand Names: Zonegran
Cost of Therapy: $65.10 (Epilepsy; Zonegran; 100 mg; 1 tablet/day; 30 day supply)

DESCRIPTION

Zonegran (zonisamide) is an antiseizure drug chemically classified as a sulfonamide and unrelated to other antiseizure agents. The active ingredient is zonisamide, 1,2-benzisoxazole-3-methanesulfonamide. The empirical formula is $C_8H_8N_2O_3S$ with a molecular weight of 212.23. Zonisamide is a white powder, pKa = 10.2, and is moderately soluble in water (0.80 mg/ml) and 0.1 N HCl (0.50 mg/ml).

Zonegran is supplied for oral administration as capsules containing 100 mg zonisamide. Each capsule contains the labeled amount of zonisamide plus the following inactive ingredients: microcrystalline cellulose, hydrogenated vegetable oil, sodium laurel sulfate, gelatin, and colorants.

CLINICAL PHARMACOLOGY

MECHANISM OF ACTION

The precise mechanism(s) by which zonisamide exerts its antiseizure effect is unknown. Zonisamide demonstrated anticonvulsant activity in several experimental models. In animals, zonisamide was effective against tonic extension seizures induced by maximal electroshock but ineffective against clonic seizures induced by subcutaneous pentylenetetrazol. Zonisamide raised the threshold for generalized seizures in the kindled rat model and reduced the duration of cortical focal seizures induced by electrical stimulation of the visual cortex in cats. Furthermore, zonisamide suppressed both interictal spikes and the secondarily generalized seizures produced by cortical application of tungstic acid gel in rats or by cortical freezing in cats. The relevance of these models to human epilepsy is unknown.

Zonisamide may produce these effects through action at sodium and calcium channels. *In vitro* pharmacological studies suggest that zonisamide blocks sodium channels and reduces voltage-dependent, transient inward currents (T-type Ca^{2+} currents), consequently stabilizing neuronal membranes and suppressing neuronal hypersynchronization. *In vitro* binding studies have demonstrated that zonisamide binds to the GABA/benzodiazepine receptor ionophore complex in an allosteric fashion which does not produce changes in chloride flux. Other *in vitro* studies have demonstrated that zonisamide (10-30 μg/ml) suppresses synaptically-driven electrical activity without affecting postsynaptic GABA or glutamate responses (cultured mouse spinal cord neurons) or neuronal or glial uptake of [^{3}H]-GABA (rat hippocampal slices). Thus, zonisamide does not appear to potentiate the synaptic activity of GABA. *In vivo* microdialysis studies demonstrated that zonisamide facilitates both dopaminergic and serotonergic neurotransmission. Zonisamide also has weak carbonic anhydrase inhibiting activity, but this pharmacologic effect is not thought to be a major contributing factor in the antiseizure activity of zonisamide.

PHARMACOKINETICS

Following a 200-400 mg oral zonisamide dose, peak plasma concentrations (range: 2-5 μg/ml) in normal volunteers occur within 2-6 hours. In the presence of food, the time to maximum concentration is delayed, occurring at 4-6 hours, but food has no effect on the bioavailability of zonisamide. Zonisamide extensively binds to erythrocytes, resulting in an 8-fold higher concentration of zonisamide in red blood cells (RBC) than in plasma. The pharmacokinetics of zonisamide are dose proportional in the range of 200-400 mg, but the C_{max} and AUC increase disproportionately at 800 mg, perhaps due to saturable binding of zonisamide to RBC. Once a stable dose is reached, steady state is achieved within 14 days. The elimination half-life of zonisamide in plasma is about 63 hours. The elimination half-life of zonisamide in RBC is approximately 105 hours.

The apparent volume of distribution (V/F) of zonisamide is about 1.45 L/kg following a 400 mg oral dose. Zonisamide, at concentrations of 1.0-7.0 μg/ml, is approximately 40% bound to human plasma proteins. Protein binding of zonisamide is unaffected in the presence of therapeutic concentrations of phenytoin, phenobarbital or carbamazepine.

METABOLISM AND EXCRETION

Following oral administration of ^{14}C-zonisamide to healthy volunteers, only zonisamide was detected in plasma. Zonisamide is excreted primarily in urine as parent drug and as the glucuronide of a metabolite. Following multiple dosing, 62% of the ^{14}C dose was recovered in the urine, with 3% in the feces by Day 10. Zonisamide undergoes acetylation to form N-acetyl zonisamide and reduction to form the open ring metabolite, 2-sulfamoylacetyl phenol (SMAP). Of the excreted dose, 35% was recovered as zonisamide, 15% as N-acetyl zonisamide, and 50% as the glucuronide of SMAP. Reduction of zonisamide to SMAP is mediated by cytochrome P450 isozyme 3A4 (CYP3A4). Zonisamide does not induce its own metabolism. Plasma clearance of zonisamide is approximately 0.30-0.35 ml/min/kg in patients not receiving enzyme-inducing antiepilepsy drugs (AEDs). The clearance of zonisamide is increased to 0.5 ml/min/kg in patients concurrently on enzyme-inducing AEDs.

Renal clearance is about 3.5 ml/min. The clearance of an oral dose of zonisamide from RBC is 2 ml/min.

SPECIAL POPULATIONS

Renal Insufficiency

Single 300 mg zonisamide doses were administered to 3 groups of volunteers. Group 1 was a healthy group with a creatinine clearance ranging from 70-152 ml/min. Group 2 and Group 3 had creatinine clearances ranging from 14.5-59 ml/min and 10-20 ml/min, respectively. Zonisamide renal clearance decreased with decreasing renal function (3.42, 2.50, 2.23 ml/min, respectively). Marked renal impairment (creatinine clearance <20 ml/min) was associated with an increase in zonisamide AUC of 35% (see DOSAGE AND ADMINISTRATION).

Hepatic Disease

The pharmacokinetics of zonisamide in patients with impaired liver function have not been studied (see DOSAGE AND ADMINISTRATION).

Age

The pharmacokinetics of a 300 mg single dose of zonisamide was similar in young (mean age 28 years) and elderly subjects (mean age 69 years).

Gender and Race

Information on the effect of gender and race on the pharmacokinetics of zonisamide is not available.

Interactions of Zonisamide With Other Antiepilepsy Drugs (AEDs)

Concurrent medication with drugs that either induce or inhibit CYP3A4 may alter serum concentrations of zonisamide. Concomitant administration of phenytoin and carbamazepine increases zonisamide plasma clearance from 0.30-0.35 ml/min/kg to 0.35-0.5 ml/min/kg. The half-life of zonisamide is decreased to 27 hours by phenytoin, to 38 hours by phenobarbital and carbamazepine, and to 46 hours by valproate. Plasma protein binding of phenytoin and carbamazepine was not affected by zonisamide administration (see DRUG INTERACTIONS).

INDICATIONS AND USAGE

Zonisamide is indicated as adjunctive therapy in the treatment of partial seizures in adults with epilepsy.

CONTRAINDICATIONS

Zonisamide is contraindicated in patients who have demonstrated hypersensitivity to sulfonamides or zonisamide.

WARNINGS

POTENTIALLY FATAL REACTIONS TO SULFONAMIDES

Fatalities have occurred, although rarely, as a result of severe reactions to sulfonamides (zonisamide is a sulfonamide) including Stevens-Johnson syndrome, toxic epidermal necrolysis, fulminant hepatic necrosis, agranulocytosis, aplastic anemia, and other blood dyscrasias. Such reactions may occur when a sulfonamide is readministered irrespective of the route of administration. If signs of hypersensitivity or other serious reactions occur, discontinue zonisamide immediately. Specific experience with sulfonamide-type adverse reaction to zonisamide is described below.

SERIOUS SKIN REACTIONS

Consideration should be given to discontinuing zonisamide in patients who develop an otherwise unexplained rash. If the drug is not discontinued, patients should be observed frequently. Seven deaths from severe rash [*i.e.*, Stevens Johnson Syndrome (SJS) and toxic epidermal necrolysis (TEN)] were reported in the first 11 years of marketing in Japan. All of the patients were receiving other drugs in addition to zonisamide. In post-marketing experience from Japan, a total of 49 cases of SJS or TEN have been reported, a reporting rate of 46/million patient-years of exposure. Although this rate is greater than background, it is probably an underestimate of the true incidence because of under-reporting. There were no confirmed cases of SJS or TEN in the US, European, or Japanese development programs.

In the US and European randomized controlled trials, 6 of 269 (2.2%) zonisamide patients discontinued treatment because of rash compared to none on placebo. Across all trials during the US and European development, rash that led to discontinuation of zonisamide was reported in 1.4% of patients (12.0 events/1000 patient-years of exposure). During Japanese development, serious rash or rash that led to study drug discontinuation was reported in 2.0% of patients (27.8 events/1000 patient-years). Rash usually occurred early in treatment, with 85% reported within 16 weeks in the US and European studies and 90% reported within 2 weeks in the Japanese studies. There was no apparent relationship of dose to the occurrence of rash.

SERIOUS HEMATOLOGIC EVENTS

Two confirmed cases of aplastic anemia and 1 confirmed case of agranulocytosis were reported in the first 11 years of marketing in Japan, rates greater than generally accepted background rates. There were no cases of aplastic anemia and 2 confirmed cases of agranulocytosis in the US, European, or Japanese development programs. There is inadequate information to assess the relationship, if any, between dose and duration of treatment and these events.

OLIGOHYDROSIS AND HYPERTHERMIA IN PEDIATRIC PATIENTS

Oligohydrosis, sometimes resulting in heat stroke and hospitalization, is seen in association with zonisamide in pediatric patients.

During the pre-approval development program in Japan, 1 case of oligohydrosis was reported in 403 pediatric patients, an incidence of 1 case/285 patient-years of exposure. While there were no cases reported in the US or European development programs, fewer than 100 pediatric patients participated in these trials.

In the first 11 years of marketing in Japan, 38 cases were reported, an estimated reporting rate of about 1 case/10,000 patient-years of exposure. In the first year of marketing in the US, 2 cases were reported, an estimated reporting rate of about 12 cases/10,000 patient-years of exposure. These rates are underestimates of the true incidence because of under-reporting. There has also been 1 report of heat stroke in an 18-year-old patient in the US.

Decreased sweating and an elevation in body temperature above normal characterized these cases. Many cases were reported after exposure to elevated environmental temperatures. Heat stroke, requiring hospitalization, was diagnosed in some cases. There have been no reported deaths.

Pediatric patients appear to be at an increased risk for zonisamide-associated oligohydrosis and hyperthermia. Patients, especially pediatric patients, treated with zonisamide should be monitored closely for evidence of decreased sweating and increased body temperature, especially in warm or hot weather. Caution should be used when zonisamide is prescribed with other drugs that predispose patients to heat-related disorders; these drugs include, but are not limited to, carbonic anhydrase inhibitors and drugs with anticholinergic activity.

The practitioner should be aware that the safety and effectiveness of zonisamide in pediatric patients have not been established, and that zonisamide is not approved for use in pediatric patients.

SEIZURES ON WITHDRAWAL

As with other AEDs, abrupt withdrawal of zonisamide in patients with epilepsy may precipitate increased seizure frequency or status epilepticus. Dose reduction or discontinuation of zonisamide should be done gradually.

TERATOGENICITY

Women of child bearing potential who are given zonisamide should be advised to use effective contraception. Zonisamide was teratogenic in mice, rats, and dogs and embryolethal in monkeys when administered during the period of organogenesis. A variety of fetal abnormalities, including cardiovascular defects, and embryo-fetal deaths occurred at maternal plasma levels similar to or lower than therapeutic levels in humans. These findings suggest that the use of zonisamide during pregnancy in humans may present a significant risk to the fetus (see PRECAUTIONS, Pregnancy Category C). It cannot be said with any confidence, however, that even mild seizures do not pose some hazards to the developing fetus. Zonisamide should be used during pregnancy only if the potential benefit justifies the potential risk to the fetus.

COGNITIVE/NEUROPSYCHIATRIC ADVERSE EVENTS

Use of zonisamide was frequently associated with central nervous system-related adverse events. The most significant of these can be classified into 3 general categories: (1) psychiatric symptoms, including depression and psychosis, (2) psychomotor slowing, difficulty with concentration, and speech or language problems, in particular, word-finding difficulties, and (3) somnolence or fatigue.

In placebo-controlled trials, 2.2% of patients discontinued zonisamide or were hospitalized for depression compared to 0.4% of placebo patients, while 1.1% of zonisamide and 0.4% of placebo patients attempted suicide. Among all epilepsy patients treated with zonisamide, 1.4% were discontinued and 1.0% were hospitalized because of reported depression or suicide attempts. In placebo-controlled trials, 2.2% of patients discontinued zonisamide or were hospitalized due to psychosis or psychosis-related symptoms compared to none of the placebo patients. Among all epilepsy patients treated with zonisamide, 0.9% were discontinued and 1.4% were hospitalized because of reported psychosis or related symptoms.

Psychomotor slowing and difficulty with concentration occurred in the first month of treatment and were associated with doses above 300 mg/day. Speech and language problems tended to occur after 6-10 weeks of treatment and at doses above 300 mg/day. Although in most cases these events were of mild to moderate severity, they at times led to withdrawal from treatment.

Somnolence and fatigue were frequently reported CNS adverse events during clinical trials with zonisamide. Although in most cases these events were of mild to moderate severity, they led to withdrawal from treatment in 0.2% of the patients enrolled in controlled trials. Somnolence and fatigue tended to occur within the first month of treatment. Somnolence and fatigue occurred most frequently at doses of 300-500 mg/day. **Patients should be cautioned about this possibility and special care should be taken by patients if they drive, operate machinery, or perform any hazardous task.**

PRECAUTIONS

GENERAL

Somnolence is commonly reported, especially at higher doses of zonisamide (see WARNINGS, Cognitive/Neuropsychiatric Adverse Events). Zonisamide is metabolized by the liver and eliminated by the kidneys; caution should therefore be exercised when administering zonisamide to patients with hepatic and renal dysfunction (see CLINICAL PHARMACOLOGY, Special Populations).

KIDNEY STONES

Among the 991 patients treated during the development of zonisamide, 40 patients (4.0%) with epilepsy receiving zonisamide developed clinically possible or confirmed kidney stones (*e.g.*, clinical symptomatology, sonography, etc.), a rate of 34/1000 patient-years of exposure (40 patients with 1168 years of exposure). Of these, 12 were symptomatic, and 28 were described as possible kidney stones based on sonographic detection. In 9 patients, the diagnosis was confirmed by a passage of a stone or by a definitive sonographic finding. The rate of occurrence of kidney stones was 28.7/1000 patient-years of exposure in the first 6 months, 62.6/1000 patient-years of exposure between 6 and 12 months, and 24.3/1000 patient-years of exposure after 12 months of use. There are no normative sonographic data available for either the general population or patients with epilepsy. The clinical significance of the sonographic finding is unknown. The analyzed stones were composed of calcium or urate salts. In general, increasing fluid intake and urine output can help reduce the risk of stone formation, particularly in those with predisposing risk factors. It is unknown, however, whether these measures will reduce the risk of stone formation in patients treated with zonisamide.

EFFECT ON RENAL FUNCTION

In several clinical studies, zonisamide was associated with a statistically significant 8% mean increase from baseline of serum creatinine and blood urea nitrogen (BUN) compared to essentially no change in the placebo patients. The increase appeared to persist over time but was not progressive; this has been interpreted as an effect on glomerular filtration rate (GFR). There were no episodes of unexplained acute renal failure in clinical development in the US, Europe, or Japan. The decrease in GFR appeared within the first 4 weeks of treatment. In a 30 day study, the GFR returned to baseline within 2-3 weeks of drug discontinuation. There is no information about reversibility, after drug discontinuation, of the effects on GFR after long-term use. Zonisamide should be discontinued in patients who develop acute renal failure or a clinically significant sustained increase in the creatinine/BUN concentration. Zonisamide should not be used in patients with renal failure (estimated GFR <50 ml/min) as there has been insufficient experience concerning drug dosing and toxicity.

SUDDEN UNEXPLAINED DEATH IN EPILEPSY

During the development of zonisamide, 9 sudden unexplained deaths occurred among 991 patients with epilepsy receiving zonisamide for whom accurate exposure data are available. This represents an incidence of 7.7 deaths/1000 patient-years. Although this rate exceeds that expected in a healthy population, it is within the range of estimates for the incidence of sudden unexplained deaths in patients with refractory epilepsy not receiving zonisamide (ranging from 0.5/1000 patient-years for the general population of patients with epilepsy, to 2-5/1000 patient-years for patients with refractory epilepsy; higher incidences range from 9-15/1000 patient-years among surgical candidates and surgical failures). Some of the deaths could represent seizure-related deaths in which the seizure was not observed.

STATUS EPILEPTICUS

Estimates of the incidence of treatment emergent status epilepticus in zonisamide-treated patients are difficult because a standard definition was not employed. Nonetheless, in controlled trials, 1.1% of patients treated with zonisamide had an event labeled as status epilepticus compared to none of the patients treated with placebo. Among patients treated with zonisamide across all epilepsy studies (controlled and uncontrolled), 1.0% of patients had an event reported as status epilepticus.

INFORMATION FOR THE PATIENT

Patients should be advised as follows:

Zonisamide may produce drowsiness, especially at higher doses. Patients should be advised not to drive a car or operate other complex machinery until they have gained experience on zonisamide sufficient to determine whether it affects their performance.

Patients should contact their physician immediately if a skin rash develops or seizures worsen.

Patients should contact their physician immediately if they develop signs or symptoms, such as sudden back pain, abdominal pain, and/or blood in the urine, that could indicate a kidney stone. Increasing fluid intake and urine output may reduce the risk of stone formation, particularly in those with predisposing risk factors for stones.

Patients should contact their physician immediately if a child has been taking zonisamide and is not sweating as usual with or without a fever.

Because zonisamide can cause hematological complications, patients should contact their physician immediately if they develop a fever, sore throat, oral ulcers, or easy bruising.

As with other AEDs, patients should contact their physician if they intend to become pregnant or are pregnant during zonisamide therapy. Patients should notify their physician if they intend to breast-feed or are breast-feeding an infant.

LABORATORY TESTS

In several clinical studies, zonisamide was associated with a mean increase in the concentration of serum creatinine and blood urea nitrogen (BUN) of approximately 8% over the baseline measurement. Consideration should be given to monitoring renal function periodically (see Effect on Renal Function).

Zonisamide was associated with an increase in serum alkaline phosphatase. In the randomized, controlled trials, a mean increase of approximately 7% over baseline was associated with zonisamide compared to a 3% mean increase in placebo-treated patients. These changes were not statistically significant. The clinical relevance of these changes is unknown.

CARCINOGENESIS, MUTAGENESIS, AND IMPAIRMENT OF FERTILITY

No evidence of carcinogenicity was found in mice or rats following dietary administration of zonisamide for 2 years at doses of up to 80 mg/kg/day. In mice, this dose is approximately equivalent to the maximum recommended human dose (MRHD) of 400 mg/day on a mg/m^2 basis. In rats, this dose is 1-2 times the MRHD on a mg/m^2 basis.

Zonisamide increased mutation frequency in Chinese hamster lung cells in the absence of metabolic activation. Zonisamide was not mutagenic or clastogenic in the Ames test, mouse lymphoma assay, sister chromatid exchange test, and human lymphocyte cytogenetics assay *in vitro,* and the rat bone marrow cytogenetics assay *in vivo.*

Rats treated with zonisamide (20, 60, or 200 mg/kg) before mating and during the initial gestation phase showed signs of reproductive toxicity (decreased corpora lutea, implantations, and live fetuses) at all doses. The low dose in this study is approximately 0.5 times the maximum recommended human dose (MRHD) on a mg/m^2 basis. The effect of zonisamide on human fertility is unknown.

PREGNANCY CATEGORY C

See WARNINGS, Teratogenicity.

Zonisamide was teratogenic in mice, rats, and dogs and embryolethal in monkeys when administered during the period of organogenesis. Fetal abnormalities or embryo-fetal deaths occurred in these species at zonisamide dosage and maternal plasma levels similar to or lower than therapeutic levels in humans, indicating that use of this drug in pregnancy entails a significant risk to the fetus. A variety of external, visceral, and skeletal malformations was produced in animals by prenatal exposure to zonisamide. Cardiovascular defects were prominent in both rats and dogs.

Following administration of zonisamide (10, 30, or 60 mg/kg/day) to pregnant dogs during organogenesis, increased incidences of fetal cardiovascular malformations (ventricular septal defects, cardiomegaly, various valvular and arterial anomalies) were found at doses of 30 mg/kg/day or greater. The low effect dose for malformations produced peak maternal plasma zonisamide levels (25 μg/ml) about 0.5 times the highest plasma levels measured in patients receiving the maximum recommended human dose (MRHD) of 400 mg/day. In dogs, cardiovascular malformations were found in approximately 50% of all fetuses exposed to the high dose, which was associated with maternal plasma levels (44 μg/ml) approximately equal to the highest levels measured in humans receiving the MRHD. Incidences of skeletal malformations were also increased at the high dose, and fetal growth retardation and increased frequencies of skeletal variations were seen at all doses in this study. The low dose produced maternal plasma levels (12 μg/ml) about 0.25 times the highest human levels.

In cynomolgus monkeys, administration of zonisamide (10 or 20 mg/kg/day) to pregnant animals during organogenesis resulted in embryo-fetal deaths at both doses. The possibility that these deaths were due to malformations cannot be ruled out. The lowest embryolethal dose in monkeys was associated with peak maternal plasma zonisamide levels (5 μg/ml) approximately 0.1 times the highest levels measured in patients at the MRHD.

In a mouse embryo-fetal development study, treatment of pregnant animals with zonisamide (125, 250, or 500 mg/kg/day) during the period of organogenesis resulted in increased incidences of fetal malformations (skeletal and/or craniofacial defects) at all doses tested. The low dose in this study is approximately 1.5 times the MRHD on a mg/m^2 basis. In rats, increased frequencies of malformations (cardiovascular defects) and variations (persistent cords of thymic tissue, decreased skeletal ossification) were observed among the offspring of dams treated with zonisamide (20, 60, or 200 mg/kg/day) throughout organogenesis at all doses. The low effect dose is approximately 0.5 times the MRHD on a mg/m^2 basis.

Perinatal death was increased among the offspring of rats treated with zonisamide (10, 30, or 60 mg/kg/day) from the latter part of gestation up to weaning at the high dose, or approximately 1.4 times the MRHD on a mg/m^2 basis. The no effect level of 30 mg/kg/day is approximately 0.7 times the MRHD on a mg/m^2 basis.

There are no adequate and well-controlled studies in pregnant women. Zonisamide should be used during pregnancy only if the potential benefit justifies the potential risk to the fetus.

LABOR AND DELIVERY

The effect of zonisamide on labor and delivery in humans is not known.

NURSING MOTHERS

It is not known whether zonisamide is excreted in human milk. Because many drugs are excreted in human milk and because of the potential for serious adverse reactions in nursing infants from zonisamide, a decision should be made whether to discontinue nursing or to discontinue drug, taking into account the importance of the drug to the mother. Zonisamide should be used in nursing mothers only if the benefits outweigh the risks.

PEDIATRIC USE

The safety and effectiveness of zonisamide in children under age 16 have not been established. Cases of oligohydrosis and hyperpyrexia have been reported (see WARNINGS, Oligohydrosis and Hyperthermia in Pediatric Patients).

GERIATRIC USE

Single dose pharmacokinetic parameters are similar in elderly and young healthy volunteers (see CLINICAL PHARMACOLOGY, Special Populations). Clinical studies of zonisamide did not include sufficient numbers of subjects aged 65 and over to determine whether they respond differently from younger subjects. Other reported clinical experience has not identified differences in responses between the elderly and younger patients. In general, dose selection for an elderly patient should be cautious, usually starting at the low end of the dosing range, reflecting the greater frequency of decreased hepatic, renal, or cardiac function, and of concomitant disease or other drug therapy.

DRUG INTERACTIONS

EFFECTS OF ZONISAMIDE ON THE PHARMACOKINETICS OF OTHER ANTIEPILEPSY DRUGS (AEDS)

Zonisamide had no appreciable effect on the steady state plasma concentrations of phenytoin, carbamazepine, or valproate during clinical trials. Zonisamide did not inhibit mixed-function liver oxidase enzymes (cytochrome P450), as measured in human liver microsomal preparations, *in vitro.* Zonisamide is not expected to interfere with the metabolism of other drugs that are metabolized by cytochrome P450 isozymes.

EFFECTS OF OTHER DRUGS ON ZONISAMIDE PHARMACOKINETICS

Drugs that induce liver enzymes increase the metabolism and clearance of zonisamide and decrease its half-life. The half-life of zonisamide following a 400 mg dose in patients concurrently on enzyme-inducing AEDs such as phenytoin, carbamazepine, or phenobarbital was between 27-38 hours; the half-life of zonisamide in patients concurrently on the non-enzyme inducing AED, valproate, was 46 hours. Concurrent medication with drugs that either induce or inhibit CYP3A4 would be expected to alter serum concentrations of zonisamide.

INTERACTION WITH CIMETIDINE

Zonisamide single dose pharmacokinetic parameters were not affected by cimetidine (300 mg four times/day for 12 days).

ADVERSE REACTIONS

The most commonly observed adverse events associated with the use of zonisamide in controlled clinical trials that were not seen at an equivalent frequency among placebo-treated patients were somnolence, anorexia, dizziness, headache, nausea, and agitation/irritability.

In controlled clinical trials, 12% of patients receiving zonisamide as adjunctive therapy discontinued due to an adverse event compared to 6% receiving placebo. Approximately 21% of the 1336 patients with epilepsy who received zonisamide in clinical studies discontinued treatment because of an adverse event. The adverse events most commonly associated with discontinuation were somnolence, fatigue and/or ataxia (6%), anorexia (3%), difficulty concentrating (2%), difficulty with memory, mental slowing, nausea/vomiting (2%), and weight loss (1%). Many of these adverse events were dose-related (see WARNINGS and PRECAUTIONS).

ADVERSE EVENT INCIDENCE IN CONTROLLED CLINICAL TRIALS

TABLE 3 lists treatment-emergent adverse events that occurred in at least 2% of patients treated with zonisamide in controlled clinical trials that were numerically more common in the zonisamide group. In these studies, either zonisamide or placebo was added to the patient's current AED therapy. Adverse events were usually mild or moderate in intensity.

The prescriber should be aware that these figures, obtained when zonisamide was added to concurrent AED therapy, cannot be used to predict the frequency of adverse events in the course of usual medical practice when patient characteristics and other factors may differ from those prevailing during clinical studies. Similarly, the cited frequencies cannot be directly compared with figures obtained from other clinical investigations involving different treatments, uses, or investigators. An inspection of these frequencies, however, does provide the prescriber with 1 basis by which to estimate the relative contribution of drug and non-drug factors to the adverse event incidences in the population studied.

OTHER ADVERSE EVENTS OBSERVED DURING CLINICAL TRIALS

Zonisamide has been administered to 1598 individuals during all clinical trials, only some of which were placebo-controlled. During these trials, all events were recorded by the investigators using their own terms. To provide a useful estimate of the proportion of individuals having adverse events, similar events have been grouped into a smaller number of standardized categories using a modified COSTART dictionary. The frequencies represent the proportion of the 1598 individuals exposed to zonisamide who experienced an event on at least 1 occasion. All events are included except those already listed in TABLE 3 or discussed in WARNINGS or PRECAUTIONS, trivial events, those too general to be informative, and those not reasonably associated with zonisamide.

Events are further classified within each category and listed in order of decreasing frequency as follows: *frequent* occurring in at least 1:100 patient; *infrequent* occurring in 1:100 to 1:1000 patients; *rare* occurring in fewer than 1:1000 patients.

Body as a Whole: *Frequent:* Accidental injury, asthenia. *Infrequent:* Chest pain, flank pain, malaise, allergic reaction, face edema, neck rigidity. *Rare:* Lupus erythematosus.

Z

TABLE 3 *Incidence (%) of Treatment-Emergent Adverse Events in Placebo-Controlled, Add-On Trials (Events That Occurred in at Least 2% of Zonisamide-Treated Patients and Occured More Frequently in Zonisamide-Treated Than Placebo-Treated Patients)*

Body System/Preferred Term	Zonisamide (n=269)	Placebo (n=230)
Body as a Whole		
Headache	10%	8%
Abdominal pain	6%	3%
Flu syndrome	4%	3%
Digestive		
Anorexia	13%	6%
Nausea	9%	6%
Diarrhea	5%	2%
Dyspepsia	3%	1%
Constipation	2%	1%
Dry mouth	2%	1%
Hematologic and Lymphatic		
Ecchymosis	2%	1%
Metabolic and Nutritional		
Weight loss	3%	2%
Nervous System		
Dizziness	13%	7%
Ataxia	6%	1%
Nystagmus	4%	2%
Paresthesia	4%	1%
Neuropsychiatric and Cognitive Dysfunction — Altered Cognitive Function		
Confusion	6%	3%
Difficulty concentrating	6%	2%
Difficulty with memory	6%	2%
Mental slowing	4%	2%
Neuropsychiatric and Cognitive Dysfunction — Behavioral Abnormalities (non-psychosis-related)		
Agitation/irritability	9%	4%
Depression	6%	3%
Insomnia	6%	3%
Anxiety	3%	2%
Nervousness	2%	1%
Neuropsychiatric and Cognitive Dysfunction — Behavioral Abnormalities (psychosis-related)		
Schizophrenic/schizophreniform behavior	2%	0%
Neuropsychiatric and Cognitive Dysfunction — CNS Depression		
Somnolence	17%	7%
Fatigue	8%	6%
Tiredness	7%	5%
Neuropsychiatric and Cognitive Dysfunction — Speech and Language Abnormalities		
Speech abnormalities	5%	2%
Difficulties in verbal expression	2%	<1%
Respiratory		
Rhinitis	2%	1%
Skin and Appendages		
Rash	3%	2%
Special Senses		
Diplopia	6%	3%
Taste perversion	2%	0%

Cardiovascular: *Infrequent:* Palpitation, tachycardia, vascular insufficiency, hypotension, hypertension, thrombophlebitis, syncope, bradycardia. *Rare:* Atrial fibrillation, heart failure, pulmonary embolus, ventricular extrasystoles.

Digestive: *Frequent:* Vomiting. *Infrequent:* Flatulence, gingivitis, gum hyperplasia, gastritis, gastroenteritis, stomatitis, cholelithiasis, glossitis, melena, rectal hemorrhage, ulcerative stomatitis, gastro-duodenal ulcer, dysphagia, gum hemorrhage. *Rare:* Cholangitis, hematemesis, cholecystitis, cholestatic jaundice, colitis, duodenitis, esophagitis, fecal incontinence, mouth ulceration.

Hematologic and Lymphatic: *Infrequent:* Leukopenia, anemia, immunodeficiency, lymphadenopathy. *Rare:* Thrombocytopenia, microcytic anemia, petechia.

Metabolic and Nutritional: *Infrequent:* Peripheral edema, weight gain, edema, thirst, dehydration. *Rare:* Hypoglycemia, hyponatremia, lactic dehydrogenase increased, SGOT increased, SGPT increased.

Musculoskeletal: *Infrequent:* Leg cramps, myalgia, myasthenia, arthralgia, arthritis.

Nervous System: *Frequent:* Tremor, convulsion, abnormal gait, hyperesthesia, incoordination. *Infrequent:* Hypertonia, twitching, abnormal dreams, vertigo, libido decreased, neuropathy, hyperkinesia, movement disorder, dysarthria, cerebrovascular accident, hypotonia, peripheral neuritis, parathesia, reflexes increased. *Rare:* Circumoral paresthesia, dyskinesia, dystonia, encephalopathy, facial paralysis, hypokinesia, hyperesthesia, myoclonus, oculogyric crisis.

Behavioral Abnormalities — Non-Psychosis-Related: *Infrequent:* Euphoria.

Respiratory: *Frequent:* Pharyngitis, cough increased. *Infrequent:* Dyspnea. *Rare:* Apnea, hemoptysis.

Skin and Appendages: *Frequent:* Pruritus. *Infrequent:* Maculopapular rash, acne, alopecia, dry skin, sweating, eczema, urticaria, hirsutism, pustular rash, vesiculobullous rash.

Special Senses: *Frequent:* Amblyopia, tinnitus. *Infrequent:* Conjunctivitis, parosmia, deafness, visual field defect, glaucoma. *Rare:* Photophobia, iritis.

Urogenital: *Infrequent:* Urinary frequency, dysuria, urinary incontinence, hematuria, impotence, urinary retention, urinary urgency, amenorrhea, polyuria, nocturia. *Rare:* Albuminuria, enuresis, bladder pain, bladder calculus, gynocomastia, mastitis, menorrhagia.

DOSAGE AND ADMINISTRATION

Zonisamide is recommended as adjunctive therapy for the treatment of partial seizures in adults. Safety and efficacy in pediatric patients below the age of 16 have not been established. Zonisamide should be administered once or twice daily, except for the daily dose of 100 mg at the initiation of therapy. Zonisamide is given orally and can be taken with or without food. Capsules should be swallowed whole.

ADULTS OVER AGE 16

The prescriber should be aware that, because of the long half-life of zonisamide, up to 2 weeks may be required to achieve steady state levels upon reaching a stable dose or following dosage adjustment. Although the regimen described below is one that has been shown to be tolerated, the prescriber may wish to prolong the duration of treatment at the lower doses in order to fully assess the effects of zonisamide at steady state, noting that many of the side effects of zonisamide are more frequent at doses of 300 mg/day and above. Although there is some evidence of greater response at doses above 100-200 mg/day, the increase appears small and formal dose-response studies have not been conducted.

The initial dose should be 100 mg daily. After 2 weeks, the dose may be increased to 200 mg/day for at least 2 weeks. It can be increased to 300 mg/day and 400 mg/day, with the dose stable for at least 2 weeks to achieve steady state at each level. Evidence from controlled trials suggests that zonisamide doses of 100-600 mg/day are effective, but there is no suggestion of increasing response above 400 mg/day. There is little experience with doses greater than 600 mg/day.

PATIENTS WITH RENAL OR HEPATIC DISEASE

Because zonisamide is metabolized in the liver and excreted by the kidneys, patients with renal or hepatic disease should be treated with caution, and might require slower titration and more frequent monitoring (see CLINICAL PHARMACOLOGY and PRECAUTIONS).

ANIMAL PHARMACOLOGY

In dogs treated with zonisamide (10, 30, or 75 mg/kg/day) for 1 year, dark brown discoloration of the liver and concentric lamellar bodies in the cytoplasm of hepatocytes were observed in association with clinical chemistry changes indicative of liver damage (elevated alkaline phosphatase, gamma glutamyl transferase, and alanine amino transferase; decreased albumin) and altered drug metabolism at the highest dose, which is approximately 6 times the maximum recommended human dose (MRHD) of 400 mg/day on a mg/m^2 basis. Gross liver changes not clearly accompanied by biochemical evidence of hepatotoxicity were noted at 30 mg/kg/day, or approximately 2.4 times the MRHD on mg/m^2 basis. The no effect dose of 10 mg/kg/day is slightly less than the MRHD on mg/m^2 basis. The significance of these finding for humans is not known.

HOW SUPPLIED

Zonegran is available as a 100 mg two-piece hard gelatin capsule consisting of a white opaque body with a red opaque cap. The capsules are printed with a company logo and "ZONEGRAN 100" in black.

Storage: Store at 25°C (77°F), excursions permitted to 15-30°C (59-86°F), in a dry place and protected from light.

PRODUCT LISTING - EQUIVALENTS NOT AVAILABLE

Capsule - Oral - 100 mg

100's $217.00 ZONEGRAN, Elan Pharmaceuticals 59075-0680-10

Z

HERBAL AND SUPPLEMENT INFORMATION

Comprehensive information for the 50 most commonly used herbs and supplements is provided in this section. The monographs are arranged in alphabetical order by common name allowing for quick access to the information. In addition, the subsections of each herbal and supplement monograph are listed in a logical order that is analogous to the drug information monographs.

- Each monograph contains the following sections: brand names of clinically tested products, description, pharmacology, clinical studies, proposed indications and usage, warnings, precautions, drug interactions, adverse reactions, overdosage, proposed dosage and administration, patient information, and references.

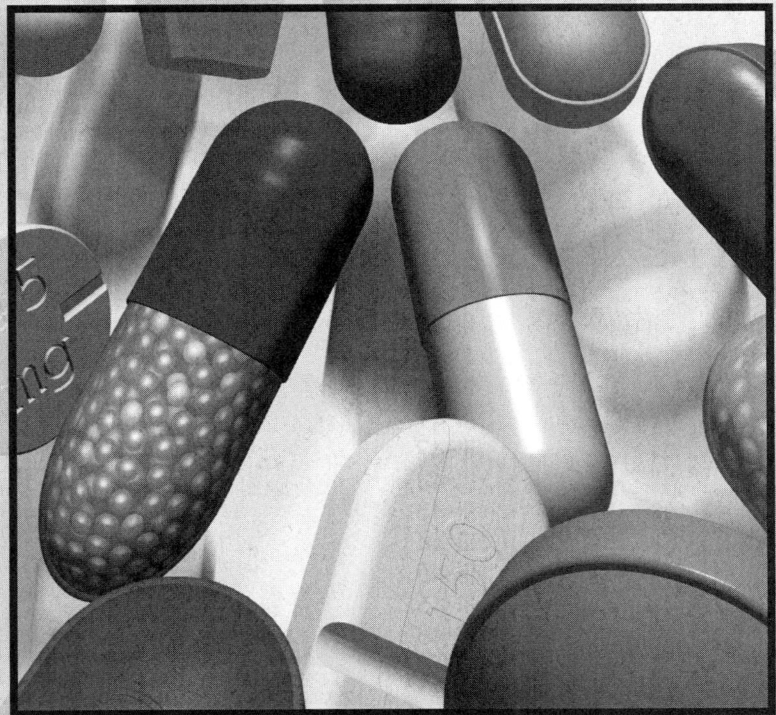

Contents

Aloe Vera Gel

Aloe Vera

U.S. BRAND NAMES OF CLINICALLY TESTED PRODUCTS

None.

DESCRIPTION

The gel found in the leaves of the aloe plant has a long traditional use as a topical treatment for burns, wound infections, and other skin conditions. Currently popular uses of topical aloe gel remain similar, along with speculative oral usage in diabetes, HIV, and numerous other conditions. However, there is little evidence that aloe is effective for any of these purposes.

PHARMACOLOGY

Aloe gel contains mono- and polysaccharides, tannins, sterols, saponins, cyclooxygenase, and various nutrients. The mannan polysaccharide acemannan derived from aloe has immunomodulatory and antiviral actions. It is an FDA-approved treatment for fibrosarcoma in cats and dogs, and is also used against feline leukemia virus and feline immunodeficiency virus.

CLINICAL STUDIES

Research into topical or oral aloe to date is limited to preliminary and often poorly designed trials.

GENITAL HERPES (TOPICAL ALOE)

A 2-week double-blind placebo-controlled trial enrolled 60 men with active genital herpes.[1] Use of aloe cream resulted in a reduced mean time to healing and increased total number of healed patients by the end of the trial. A previous double-blind placebo-controlled study by the same researchers enrolled 120 men with genital herpes and compared aloe cream and aloe gel against placebo.[2] Aloe cream proved more effective than gel and superior to placebo.

PSORIASIS (TOPICAL ALOE)

A double-blind placebo-controlled study of 60 patients with mild to moderate psoriasis compared the effects of topical *Aloe vera* extract (0.5%) to placebo cream, applied 3 times daily for 4 weeks.[3] Significant comparative improvement was seen in both groups.

SEBORRHEA (TOPICAL ALOE)

A double-blind placebo-controlled study of 44 individuals reported that 4 to 6 weeks of treatment with aloe ointment significantly reduced symptoms of seborrhea.[4]

OTHER SKIN CONDITIONS (TOPICAL AND ORAL ALOE)

Aloe gel may offer adjuvant benefits when combined with hydrocortisone acetate cream.[5]

Although several animal studies suggest that oral administration as well as topical aloe gel application may improve healing of various forms of wounds,[6,7,8] a study of secondary intention post-surgical wound healing in 21 women showed a significant *delay* in wound healing in the group receiving standard wound care and aloe gel compared to the group receiving standard wound care alone.[9]

Similarly, despite its popularity for sunburn, topical aloe appears to be ineffective for this condition, and may actually be detrimental to the healing of second-degree burns.[10,11]

Topical aloe has also been found ineffective for protecting the skin during radiation therapy.[12]

DIABETES (ORAL ALOE)

A poorly reported single-blind placebo-controlled trial evaluated the effects of aloe gel in an unspecified number of individuals with diabetes, and indicated that significant reductions in fasting glucose levels were seen.[13] In addition, a 6-week single-blind placebo-controlled trial evaluated the effects of aloe gel in nonresponders to glibenclamide and also reported improvements.[14]

PROPOSED DOSAGE AND ADMINISTRATION

Topical aloe gel preparations are typically applied 3 to 4 times daily. Studies of aloe for diabetes treatment have used *Aloe vera* gel at a dose of 1 tablespoon twice daily.

PROPOSED INDICATIONS AND USAGE

Despite an almost complete lack of evidence of effectiveness, topical aloe is widely marketed for the treatment of a great variety of skin conditions, and is included in numerous cosmetic products. Oral aloe is additionally popular for HIV and general "immune weakness," based primarily on the immunomodulatory effects of acemannan. Lay use of oral *Aloe vera* for diabetes is growing based on results of recent preliminary trials.

WARNINGS

Drug aloe ("aloes"), a potent anthraquinone laxative produced from the aloe leaf rather than the gel, can cause hypokalemia and other effects secondary to diarrhea.[15] Oral aloe gel does not present the same risks.

PRECAUTIONS

Maximum safe dosages for pregnant or lactating women, young children, or individuals with severe hepatic or renal disease are not known.

DRUG INTERACTIONS

None known. However, it is conceivable that the known immunomodulatory effects of acemannan could interfere with the action of immune-suppressant drugs. If aloe gel does indeed possess significant hypoglycemic effects, interactions with oral hypoglycemic agents or insulin might be a possibility.

ADVERSE REACTIONS

Other than occasional hypersensitivity reactions, no serious adverse effects have been reported with topical or oral aloe gel. However, comprehensive safety studies are lacking.

PATIENT INFORMATION

Aloe gel is a popular treatment for burns and wounds. However, there is no real evidence that it works. In addition, aloe might actually make severe wounds heal more slowly.

Internal use of aloe gel has no proven benefits. However, there is some evidence that oral aloe might reduce blood sugar levels in people with diabetes. If you have diabetes, consult with your physician before taking this herb (or any other supplement). Keep in mind that if it does reduce blood sugar, a hypoglycemic reaction is possible. Reduction of drug dosage could be necessary.

The maximum safe dosage of aloe for pregnant or nursing women or young children has not been established. Individuals with severe liver or kidney disease, or those taking a drug that suppresses the immune system, should consult a physician before using this (or any other) supplement.

REFERENCES

1. Syed TA, Afzal M, Ashfaq Ahmad S, et al. Management of genital herpes in men with 0.5% Aloe vera extract in a hydrophilic cream: a placebo-controlled double-blind study. *J Dermatol Treat.* 1997;8:99-102. **2.** Syed TA, Cheema KM, Ashfaq A, et al. Aloe vera extract 0.5% in a hydrophilic cream versus Aloe vera gel for the management of genital herpes in males. A placebo-controlled, double-blind, comparative study [letter]. *J Eur Acad Dermatol Venereol.* 1996;7:294-295. **3.** Syed TA, Ahmad SA, Holt AH, et al. Management of psoriasis with Aloe vera extract in a hydrophilic cream: a placebo-controlled, double-blind study. *Trop Med Int Health.* 1996;1:505-509. **4.** Vardy DA, Cohen AD, Tchetov T, et al. A double blind, placebo-controlled trial of an Aloe vera (A. barbadensis) emulsion in the treatment of seborrheic dermatitis. *J Dermatol Treat.* 1999;10:7-11. **5.** Davis RH, Parker WL, Murdoch DP. Aloe vera as a biologically active vehicle for hydrocortisone acetate. *J Am Podiatr Assoc.* 1991;81:1-9. **6.** Chithra P, Sajithlal GB, Chandrakasan G. Influence of Aloe vera on collagen characteristics in healing dermal wounds in rats. *Mol Cell Biochem.* 1998;181:71-76. **7.** Fulton JE Jr. The stimulation of post-dermabrasion wound healing with stabilized aloe vera gel-polyethylene oxide dressing. *J Dermatol Surg Oncol.* 1990;16:460-467. **8.** Davis RH, Leitner MG, Russo JM, et al. Wound healing. Oral and topical activity of Aloe vera. *J Am Podiatr Med Assoc.* 1989;79:559-562. **9.** Schmidt JM, Greenspoon JS. Aloe vera dermal wound gel is associated with a delay in wound healing. *Obstet Gynecol.* 1991;78:115-117. **10.** Kaufman T, Kalderon N, Ullmann Y, et al. Aloe vera gel hindered wound healing of experimental second-degree burns: a quantitative controlled study. *J Burn Care Rehabil.* 1988;9:156-159. **11.** Crowell J, Penneys N. The effect of Aloe vera on cutaneus erythema and blood-flow following ultraviolet-B (UVB) exposure [abstract]. *Clin Res.* 1987;35:A676. **12.** Williams MS, Burk M, Loprinzi CL, et al. Phase III double-blind evaluation of an aloe vera gel as a prophylactic agent for radiation-induced skin toxicity. *Int J Radiat Oncol Biol Phys.* 1996;36:345-349. **13.** Yongchaiyudha S, Rungpitarangsi V, Bunyapraphatsara N, et al. Antidiabetic activity of Aloe vera L. juice. I. Clinical trial in new cases of diabetes mellitus. *Phytomedicine.* 1996;3:241-243. **14.** Bunyapraphatsara N, Yongchaiyudha S, Rungpitarangsi V, et al. Antidiabetic activity of Aloe vera L. juice II. Clinical trial in diabetes mellitus patients in combination with glibenclamide. *Phytomedicine.* 1996;3:245-248. **15.** Shah AH, Qureshi S, Tariq M, et al. Toxicity studies on six plants used in the traditional Arab system of medicine. *Phytother Res.* 1989;3:25-29.

Bilberry Fruit

Vaccinium Myrtillus

U.S. BRAND NAMES OF CLINICALLY TESTED PRODUCTS

None.

DESCRIPTION

The genus *Vaccinium* comprises many well-known berries, including cranberry, huckleberry, and blueberry. Bilberry is traditionally used in the preparation of jams, pies, cobblers, and cakes. It also has a long medicinal history, with traditional uses for conditions as diverse as typhoid fever, bladder stones, liver disorders, coughs, lung diseases, intestinal disorders, gout, urinary tract infections, hemorrhoids, and infections of the mouth and skin. Current popular usage focuses on eye-related conditions: most prominently, enhancing night vision. However, there is no meaningful clinical evidence that bilberry has beneficial effects in any condition.

PHARMACOLOGY

Raw bilberry fruit contains 5% to 10% catechins, 30% invertose, and relatively small amounts of anthocyanosides and flavone glycosides.[1] The pharmacokinetics of bilberry anthocyanosides are known only from animal studies. In male rats, plasma anthocyanosides achieve peak levels of 2 to 3 mcg/ml at 15 minutes and decline rapidly within 2 hours, with an absolute bioavailability of only 1.2% of the administered dose.[2,3]

Anthocyanosides have received the most attention, and commercial bilberry products are standardized to anthocyanoside content. Some evidence suggests that anthocyanosides may increase cross-linkage of collagen fibers, normalize capillary permeability, inhibit collagen degradation, promote collagen biosynthesis, reduce inflammatory activity, and scavenge free radicals.[4-10] Bilberry anthocyanosides have numerous effects in the retina, including enhancing recovery of rhodopsin and altering a variety of enzymatic reactions, although the clinical significance of these findings remains unclear.[11,12,13]

Like other flavonoids, at very high doses anthocyanosides inhibit platelet aggregation in vitro and in vivo.[14-17]

Bilberry leaves, as opposed to the much more commonly used fruit, have entirely different constituents and have been investigated for hypoglycemic and hypolipidemic effects.[18]

CLINICAL STUDIES

VISION-RELATED CONDITIONS

There is no reliable evidence that bilberry has any medicinal effect in vision-related conditions.

Two small controlled studies of bilberry from the 1960s found short-term improvements in visual acuity in semidarkness as well as shortened time to dark adaptation and improved recovery from glare as compared to placebo.[19,20] Short-term benefits were also seen in a double-blind placebo-controlled study of 40 healthy subjects, which found that a single dose of bilberry extract improved pupillary photomotor response for 2 hours.[21]

However, more recent trials have failed to find improvements in night vision through the use of bilberry. For example, a 3-week double-blind crossover trial of 15 individuals found no immediate or delayed improvement in night vision attributable to bilberry extract (25% anthocyanosides) taken at a dose of 160 mg twice daily.[22] Negative results were seen in a similar double-blind placebo-controlled crossover trial of 18 subjects,[23] and another of 16 subjects.[24]

A double-blind placebo-controlled trial of bilberry extract in 14 patients with diabetic and/or hypertensive retinopathy reported improvements as shown by ophthalmoscopic and angiographic examination.[25] Animal studies suggest that bilberry can help prevent macular degeneration.[26] According to one double-blind placebo-controlled trial of 50 individuals with mild cataracts (involving 62 eyes), a combination of vitamin E and bilberry slowed lens opacity progression.[27]

CHRONIC VENOUS INSUFFICIENCY

In a single-blind placebo-controlled study of 60 patients with venous insufficiency, use of bilberry extract resulted in a significant decrease in signs and symptoms over a period of 30 days.[28]

PROPOSED INDICATIONS AND USAGE

Despite the absence of evidence showing efficacy, oral bilberry fruit is widely marketed for oral use in the prevention and treatment of eye disorders of all types, including poor night vision, macular degeneration, glaucoma, diabetic retinopathy, and cataracts.

Bilberry is also often added to herb and supplement combinations intended for the treatment of chronic venous insufficiency/varicose veins. However, the evidence for other natural products such as horse chestnut, diosmin/hesperidin, oxerutins, and butcher's broom is considerably stronger.

WARNINGS

Bilberry leaf may have hypoglycemic effects and should not be confused with bilberry fruit.

PRECAUTIONS

Because bilberry anthocyanosides mildly inhibit platelet aggregation, it is possible that bilberry could have adverse effects in individuals with impaired hemostasis.

Safety in young children, pregnant or lactating women, or in individuals with severe hepatic or renal dysfunction has not been established. However, there are no known or suspected problems with such uses, and pregnant women have been given bilberry in clinical trials without apparent adverse effects.[29]

There are no known risks with overdosage of bilberry fruit; bilberry leaf, however, has been associated with toxicity.

DRUG INTERACTIONS

Based on known anti-platelet effects, potentiation of anticoagulant and antiplatelet agents is possible.

ADVERSE REACTIONS

Bilberry fruit is a food and as such would appear to have a high safety threshold. However, it must be kept in mind that bilberry herbal extracts sold as medicinal products may contain artificially high levels of anthocyanosides. Nonetheless, very high doses have been administered to rats without toxic effects.[30,2] One drug-monitoring study of 2,295 patients showed no serious side effects and only a 4% incidence of mild reactions such as gastrointestinal distress, skin rashes, and drowsiness.[31]

PROPOSED DOSAGE AND ADMINISTRATION

The typical dose of bilberry is 160 mg twice a day of a fruit extract standardized to contain 25% bilberry anthocyanosides.

PATIENT INFORMATION

Extracts of bilberry fruit are widely marketed for improving night vision and helping the eyes in other ways. However, there is no real evidence that it works, and recent studies have found no effect.

Warning: Do not confuse bilberry leaf with bilberry fruit. The leaf can be toxic.

The safety of bilberry fruit in pregnant or nursing women or young children has not been established. Individuals with severe liver or kidney disease should consult a physician before using this (or any other) supplement.

REFERENCES

1. Schulz V, Hansel R, Tyler VE. *Rational Phytotherapy: A Physicians' Guide to Herbal Medicine.* 3rd ed. Berlin, Germany: Springer-Verlag; 1998. **2.** Lietti A, Forni G. Studies on vaccinium myrtillus anthocyanosides. II. Aspects of anthocyanins pharmacokinetics in the rat. *Arzneimittelforschung.* 1976;26:832-835. **3.** Morazzoni P, Livio S, Scilingo A, et al. Vaccinium myrtillus anthocyanosides pharmacokinetics in rats. *Arzneimittelforschung.* 1991;41:128-131. **4.** Gabor M. Pharmacologic effects of flavonoids on blood vessels. *Angiologica.* 1972;9:355-374 **5.** Havsteen B. Flavonoids, a class of natural products of high pharmacological potency. *Biochem Pharmacol.* 1983;32:1141-1148. **6.** Mian E, Curri SB, Lietti A, et al. Anthocyanosides and microvessels wall: new findings on the mechanism of action of their protective effect in syndromes due to abnormal capillary fragility [in Italian]. *Minerva Med.* 1977;68:3565-3581. **7.** Monboisse JC, Braquet P, Randoux A, et al. Non-enzymatic degradation of acid-soluble calf skin collagen by superoxide ion: protective effect of flavonoids. *Biochem Pharmacol.* 1983;32:53-58. **8.** Morazzoni P, Bombardelli E. Vaccinium myrtillus L. *Fitoterapia.* 1996;67:3-29. **9.** Pulliero G, Montin S, Bettini R, et al. Ex vivo study of the inhibitory effects of Vaccinium myrtillus anthocyanosides on human platelet aggregation. *Fitoterapia.* 1989;60:69-75. **10.** Berta V, Zucchi C. *Fitoterapia.* 1988;59(suppl 1):27. Cited by: Bone K. Bilberry-The vision herb. *Mediherb Professional Rev.* 1997;59(3):1-4. **11.** Cluzel C, Bastide P, Wegman R, et al. Enzymatic activities in the retina and anthocyanosides extracted from Vaccinium myrtillus [translated from French]. *Biochem Pharmacol.* 1970;19:2295-2302. **12.** Wegmann R, et al. Effects of anthocyanosides on photo receptors. Cyto-enzymatic aspects [translated from French]. *Ann Histochim.* 1969;14:237-256. **13.** Bertuglia S, Malandrino S, Colantuoni A. Effect of Vaccinium myrtillus anthocyanosides on ischaemia reperfusion injury in hamster cheek pouch microcirculation. *Pharmacol Res.* 1995;31:183-187. **14.** Bottecchia D, Bettini V, Martino R, et al. Preliminary report on the inhibitory effect of Vaccinium myrtillus anthocyanosides on platelet aggregation and clot retraction. *Fitoterapia.* 1987;58:3-8. **15.** Morazzoni P, Magistretti MJ. Effects of Vaccinium myrtillus anthocyanosides on prostacyclin-like activity in rat arterial tissue. *Fitoterapia.* 1986;57:11-14. **16.** Morazzoni P, Magistretti MJ. Activity of Myrtocyan(r), an anthocyanoside complex from Vaccinium myrtillus (VMA), on platelet aggregation and adhesiveness. *Fitoterapia.* 1990;61:13-19. **17.** Zaragoza F, Iglesias I, Benedi J. Comparative study of the anti-aggregation effects of anthocyanosides and other agents [in Spanish]. *Arch Farmacol Toxicol.* 1985;11:183-188. **18.** Cignarella A, Nastasi M, Cavalli E, et al. Novel lipid-lowering properties of Vaccinium myrtillus L. leaves, a traditional antidiabetic treatment, in several models of rat dyslipidaemia: a comparison with ciprofibrate. *Thromb Res.* 1996;84:311-322. **19.** Jayle GE, Aubert L. Action of anthocyan glucosides on the scotopic and mesopic vision of the normal subject [in French; English abstract]. *Therapie.* 1964;19:171-185. **20.** Jayle GE, Aubry M, Gavini H, et al. Study concerning the action of anthocyanoside extracts of Vaccinium Myrtillus on night vision [in French]. *Ann Ocul (Paris).* 1965;198:556-562. **21.** Vannini L, Samually R, Coffano M, et al. Pupillographic study after administration of anthocyanosides [in Italian]. *Boll Ocul.* 1986;65:569-577. **22.** Muth ER, Laurent JM, Jasper P. The effect of bilberry nutritional supplementation on night visual acuity and contrast sensitivity. *Altern Med Rev.* 2000;5:164-173. **23.** Zadok D, Levy Y, Glovinsky Y. The effect of anthocyanosides in a multiple oral dose on night vision. *Eye.* 1999;13:734-736. **24.** Levy Y, Glovinsky Y. The effect of anthocyanosides on night vision. *Eye.* 1998;12:967-969. **25.** Perossini M, Guidi G, Chiellini S, et al. Diabetic and hypertensive retinopathy therapy with Vaccinium Myrtillus anthocyanosides (tegens): double blind placebo-controlled clinical trial [in Italian; English abstract]. *Ann Ottalmol Clin Ocul.* 1987;12:1174-1190. **26.** Pautler EL, Ennis SR. The effect of diet on inherited retinal dystrophy in the rat. *Curr Eye Res.* 1984;3:1221-1224. **27.** Bravetti G, Fraboni E, Maccolini E. Preventive medical treatment of senile cataract with vitamin E and Vaccinium myrtillus anthocianosides: clinical evaluation [in Italian; English abstract]. *Ann Ottalmol Clin Ocul.* 1989;115:109-116. **28.** Gatta L, et al. *Fitoterapia.* 1988;59(suppl 1):19. Cited by: Bone K. Bilberry-The vision herb. *Mediherb Professional Rev.* 1997;59(3):1-4. **29.** Grismondi GL. Angiology: The treatment of venous disease caused by stasis during pregnancy [translated from Italian]. *Minerva Ginecol.* 1981;33:221-230. **30.** Lietti A, Cristoni A, Picci M. Studies on vaccinium myrtillus anthocyanosides I. Vasoprotective and antiinflammatory activity. *Arzneimittelforschung.* 1976;26:829-832. **31.** Eandi M. Unpublished results. Cited in Morazzoni P, et al. (1996). *Vaccinium myrtillus. Fitoterapia.* 1996;67:3-29.

Black Cohosh

Cimicifuga Racemosa

U.S. BRAND NAMES OF CLINICALLY TESTED PRODUCTS

Remifemin (PhytoPharmica/Enzymatic Therapy) =
Remifemin (Schaper and Brummer) in Europe

DESCRIPTION

The black cohosh plant is native to eastern North America, where it grows as a tall perennial. Its root is used medicinally. Native Americans introduced the use of this herb to European colonists.

Early studies suggested that extracts of black cohosh could stimulate menstruation. Research escalated in the 1980s with a focus on estrogen-like benefits in menopause. Soon thereafter, Germany's Commission E approved standardized extracts of black cohosh for use in menopause, dysmenorrhea, and premenstrual discomfort.

However, supportive evidence is weak. Although some human studies found indications that black cohosh produces estrogenic effects, the preponderance of current evidence suggests that black cohosh is not significantly estrogenic.

PHARMACOLOGY

Black cohosh contains a variety of triterpene glycosides including actein, deoxyactein, cimigoside, cimicifugoside, and racemoside, as well as phytosterins, isoflavones, isoferulic acid, and miscellaneous volatile oils. Black cohosh extracts are usually standardized to deoxyactein content.

Much of the apparent vasomotor and/or endocrine effect of black cohosh is believed to reside in the triterpene glycoside constituents, although the phytosterin and flavone derivatives have also been investigated.[1,2,3] Black cohosh has been found in animal studies to inhibit pituitary LH production without affecting FSH or prolactin release.[1,2] Similar results were seen in an open study of 110 female patients over the course of 2 months, which found suppression of LH in the black cohosh group as compared to the placebo group, but no significant FSH changes.[4] This LH-specific effect was not consistent with a purely estrogenic action. Fractionation studies have identified three classes of active compounds in black cohosh: (1) those that bind to estrogen receptors and inhibit LH release, (2) those that bind to estrogen receptors but do not inhibit LH release, and (3) constituents that do not bind to estrogen receptors but nonetheless inhibit LH release.[4]

More recent human and animal studies have found no effect on LH or FSH, nor any estrogenic effects.[5,6,7] Some preliminary evidence suggests that black cohosh may have selective action on estrogen receptors outside of the uterine area, making it a type of phyto-SERM.[8,9,10]

Animal studies have found that actein in high doses exerts a hypotensive effect in rabbits and cats, but not reliably in dogs.[11] Similar effects were not seen in humans.

CLINICAL STUDIES

The case for black cohosh as a treatment for menopausal syndrome has grown weaker in recent years.

Numerous open studies, some large, reported benefit; however, menopausal symptoms have been found to improve dramatically in the placebo arm of numerous placebo-controlled trials, making such results meaningless.[12]

There has been only one double-blind placebo-controlled trial of black cohosh for menopausal syndrome, and its results were challenged by subsequent findings. This randomized study of 80 patients at one gynecological practice compared the benefits of black cohosh, conjugated estrogens (0.625 mg), and placebo over a period of 12 weeks.[13] Black cohosh produced significantly greater improvements than placebo in the Kupperman Index, the Hamilton Anxiety Scale, and the degree of proliferation of the vaginal epithelium. Surprisingly, estrogen failed to prove more effective than placebo.

However, these results were cast in doubt by a subsequent double-blind comparative study of 152 patients with at least a moderate degree of menopausal symptoms on the Kupperman Index.[14] One group was given Remifemin at the usual dose of 2 tablets twice daily, while the other received half this dose. No changes were seen in vaginal cytology or levels of LH, FSH, prolactin, estradiol, or sex hormone-binding globulin. Equivalent and statistically significant clinical improvement was seen in both groups, but because the study lacked placebo control it is possible that the clinical improvements seen were due entirely to nonspecific effects.

Based on this study as well as other evidence indicating that black cohosh is not estrogenic (see Pharmacology), a 2-month double-blind placebo-controlled trial evaluated the use of black cohosh in 85 breast cancer survivors with menopause-like symptoms.[15] No benefits were seen.

PROPOSED INDICATIONS AND USAGE

Despite the paucity of evidence, black cohosh is widely marketed for the treatment of some menopausal symptoms, as well as for other women's conditions such as PMS and dysmenorrhea.

WARNINGS

Traditional herbology contraindicates the use of black cohosh during pregnancy, due to supposed increased risk of spontaneous abortion.

PRECAUTIONS

The possibility of estrogenic effects outside the uterus suggests that black cohosh should be used with caution in conditions where estrogen levels or activity are an issue.

Studies in rats showed no significant toxicity when black cohosh was given at 90 times the therapeutic dose for a period of 6 months.[16] This length of time in rat trials is generally regarded as corresponding to an unlimited treatment period in humans. Ames tests have shown no evidence of mutagenicity.[5]

Studies of breast cancer cells have found that black cohosh, unlike estradiol, does not exhibit any stimulatory effect in vitro, a finding that is not surprising in view of the absence of estrogenic effects,[17,18,19] and black cohosh has been used in a trial of breast cancer survivors without apparent adverse effects.[15] Nonetheless, it should be emphasized that black cohosh has not yet been subjected to large-scale, retrospective epidemiology studies similar to those conducted for estrogens. For this reason, safety for individuals with previous breast cancer is not known.

In addition, because of its apparent effects on LH as well as traditional warnings, black cohosh is not recommended for adolescents or pregnant or lactating females, except in a research setting. Safety in young children or in individuals with severe hepatic or renal dysfunction has not been established.

DRUG INTERACTIONS

None are known. However, formal drug interaction studies have not been performed, and interactions with estrogen and related hormones are possible. There are weak indications of potential interactions with antihypertensive medications.[7,20]

ADVERSE REACTIONS

Generally, black cohosh is well tolerated, producing only occasional mild gastrointestinal distress. Other occasionally reported side effects of unclear causal connection include headaches, weight gain, and breast tenderness.

PROPOSED DOSAGE AND ADMINISTRATION

The usual dosage of black cohosh is 1 or 2 tablets twice a day of a standardized extract such as Remifemin, which is manufactured to contain 1 mg of 27-deoxyactein per tablet. Germany's Commission E recommends the use of black cohosh for no more than 6 months due to the lack of long-term safety data in humans.

PATIENT INFORMATION

Black cohosh is widely marketed as a treatment for menopause. However, there is very little evidence that it really works. Black cohosh is often described as a "natural estrogen"; however, recent studies indicate that black cohosh does not have any estrogen-like effects. In particular, there is no indication that black cohosh can help prevent osteoporosis.

Warning: Black cohosh should not be confused with the toxic herb blue cohosh.

The safety of black cohosh in pregnant or nursing women, or women with a history of breast cancer has not been established. Individuals with severe liver or kidney disease should consult a physician before using this (or any other) supplement.

REFERENCES

1. Jarry H, Harnischfeger G. Studies on the endocrine effects of the contents of Cimicifuga racemosa: 1. Influence on the serum concentrations of pituitary hormones in ovariectomized rats [translated from German]. *Planta Med.* 1985;51:46-49. **2.** Jarry H, Harnischfeger G, Duker E. The endocrine effects of constituents of Cimicifuga racemosa. 2. In vitro binding of constituents to estrogen receptors [translated from German]. *Planta Med.* 1985;51:316-319. **3.** Schulz V, Hansel R, Tyler VE. *Rational Phytotherapy: A Physicians' Guide to Herbal Medicine.* 3rd ed. Berlin, Germany: Springer-Verlag; 1998. **4.** Duker EM, Kopanski L, Jarry H, et al. Effects of extracts from Cimicifuga racemosa on gonadotropin release in menopausal women and ovariectomized rats. *Planta Med.* 1991;57:420-424. **5.** Liske, E. Therapeutic efficacy and safety of *Cimicifuga racemosa* for gynecological disorders. *Adv Ther.* 1998;15:45-53. **6.** Nesselhut T, Liske E. Pharmacological measures in postmenopausal women with an isopropanolic aqueous extract of Cimicifugae racemosae rhizoma [abstract]. *Menopause.* 1999;6:99.012. **7.** Einer-Jensen N, Zhao J, Andersen KP, Kristoffersen K. Cimicifuga and Melbrosia lack oestrogenic effects in mice and rats. *Maturitas.* 1996;25:149-153. **8.** Seidlova-Wuttke D, Wuttke W. Selective estrogen receptor modulator activity of Cimicifuga racemosa extract: clinical data [abstract]. *Phytomedicine.* 2000;7(suppl 2):11. **9.** Seidlova-Wuttke D, Jarry H, Heiden I, et al. Effects of Cimicifuga racemosa on estrogen-dependent tissues [abstract]. *Phytomedicine.* 2000;7(suppl 2):11-12. **10.** Wuttke W, Jarry H, Heiden I, et al. Selective estrogen receptor modulator (SERM) activity of the Cimicifuga racemosa extract BNO 1055: pharmacology and mechanisms of action [abstract]. *Phytomedicine.* 2000;7(suppl 2):12. **11.** Genazzani E, Sorrentino L. Vascular action of acteina: active constituent of Actaea racemosa L. *Nature.* 1962;194:544-545. **12.** MacLennan A, Lester S, Moore V. Oral estrogen replacement therapy versus placebo for hot flushes: a systematic review. *Climacteric.* 2001;4:58-74. **13.** Stoll W. Phythopharmacon influences atrophic vaginal epithelium. Double-blind study: Cimicifuga vs. estrogenic substances [translated from German]. *Therapeutikon.* 1987;1:23-26, 28, 30-31. **14.** Liske E, and Wüstenberg P. Therapy of climacteric complaints with *Cimicifuga racemosa:* herbal medicine with clinically proven evidence [abstract]. *Menopause.* 1998;5:250. **15.** Jacobson JS, Troxel AB, Evans J, et al. Randomized trial of black cohosh for the treatment of hot flashes among women with a history of breast cancer. *J Clin Oncol.* 2001;19:2739-2745. **16.** Korn, WD. Six month oral toxicity study with Remifemin-granulate in rats followed by an 8-week recovery period. Hannover, Germany: International Bioresearch;1991. **17.** Nesselhut T, Schellhase C, Dietrich R, et al. Investigations into the growth-inhibitive efficiacy of phytopharmacopia with estrogen-like influences on mammary gland carcinoma cells [translated from German]. *Arch Gynecol Obstet.* 1993;254:817-818. **18.** Zava DT, Dollbaum CM, Blen M. Estrogen and progestin bioactivity of foods, herbs, and spices. *Proc Soc Exp Biol Med.* 1998;217:369-378. **19.** Freudenstein J, Dasenbrock C, Nisslein T. Lack of promotion of estrogen dependent mammary gland tumors in vivo by an isopropanolic black cohosh extract [abstract]. *Phytomedicine.* 2000;7(suppl 2):13. **20.** Lehmann-Willenbrock VE, Riedel H-H. Clinical and endocrinologic examinations about therapy of climacteric symptoms following hysterectomy with remaining ovaries [in German; English abstract]. *Zentralbl Gynakol.* 1988;110:611-618.

Blue Cohosh

Caulophyllum Thalictroides

Alternate/Related Names: Beechdrops, Blue or Yellow Ginseng, Blueberry Root, Papoose Root, Squawroot

U.S. BRAND NAMES OF CLINICALLY TESTED PRODUCTS

None.

DESCRIPTION

Blue cohosh is a flowering herb native to North America, which grows in forested areas from the southeastern United States to Canada. Sometimes known as squaw root or papoose root, this toxic plant may have been used medicinally by Native Americans, although this is controversial. Other common names for the herb include yellow ginseng and blue ginseng. Blue cohosh should not be confused with the similarly named (but unrelated and safer herb) black cohosh.

PHARMACOLOGY

Blue cohosh contains numerous potentially toxic chemicals, including alkaloids in the quinolizidine and isoquinoline families, cardioactive saponins, and N-methylcytisine (similar to nicotine).[1] Animal and in vitro studies of saponin glycoside extracts of blue cohosh have documented smooth muscle stimulation in the uterus, small intestines, and heart, leading to significant constriction of coronary vessels and negative inotropic effects.[2]

CLINICAL STUDIES

None.

PROPOSED INDICATIONS AND USAGE

Despite known toxic risks, blue cohosh is widely prescribed by herbalists and midwives today. According to a survey, 64% of certified nurse-midwives who prescribe herbal medicines use blue cohosh to induce labor.[1] It is also sometimes tried as an abortifacient.

WARNINGS

Due to serious safety concerns, blue cohosh should be avoided entirely.

PRECAUTIONS

The use of blue cohosh in pregnant or lactating women is strongly contraindicated. One case report documents profound congestive heart failure in a newborn whose mother used blue cohosh to induce labor.[1] Multiple severe neonatal complications were seen in another case as well.[3]

Blue cohosh's constituents anagyrine, N-methylcytisine, and taspine can reportedly cause severe birth defects in cattle and laboratory rats.[1] Antifertility effects in rats have also been reported.[4]

DRUG INTERACTIONS

None known, although interactions with cardioactive agents are probable.

ADVERSE REACTIONS

Use of blue cohosh has been associated with severe neonatal complications including congestive heart failure, congenital defects, and spontaneous abortions. Hypertension and gastrointestinal distress due to the nicotinic effects of N-methylcytisine have also been reported.

PROPOSED DOSAGE AND ADMINISTRATION

Blue cohosh is usually used as a tincture. Typical dosages range from 5 to 10 drops taken every 2 to 4 hours.

PATIENT INFORMATION

Blue cohosh is a toxic herb that should be strictly avoided, especially by pregnant women.

REFERENCES

1. Jones TK, Lawson BM. Profound neonatal congestive heart failure caused by maternal consumption of blue cohosh herbal medication. *J Pediatr.* 1998;132(3 pt 1): 550-552. **2.** Ferguson HC, Edwards LD. A pharmacological study of a crystallin glycoside of caulophyllum thalictroides. *J Am Pharm Assoc.* 1954;43:16-21. **3.** Gunn TR, Wright IM. The use of black and blue cohosh in labour. *N Z Med J.* 1996;109:410-411. **4.** Chaudresekkhar K. Studies on the effect of Caulophyllum on implantation in rats. *J Reprod Fertil.* 1974;38:245-246.

Boldo

Peumus Boldus

U.S. BRAND NAMES OF CLINICALLY TESTED PRODUCTS

None.

DESCRIPTION

Boldo is an evergreen shrub native to South America. The leaves of the boldo plant have traditionally been used as a treatment for liver and bladder disorders, various forms of arthritis, and a wide variety of other ailments, including headache, earache, congestion, menstrual pain, and syphilis.

PHARMACOLOGY

Some evidence suggests that boldo may possess choleretic actions.[1,2,3] The isoquinoline alkaloid boldine, an apomorphine-like substance with antioxidant properties, is thought to be one of the active ingredients.[3,4,5] Other constituents include volatile oils and flavonoids.

CLINICAL STUDIES

In Europe, nonulcer dyspepsia is commonly attributed to inadequate bile production. Based on its apparent choleretic properties, boldo is a common ingredient in combination digestive therapies. Boldo taken alone has not been clinically evaluated as a treatment for dyspepsia; however, in a double-blind trial, 60 individuals were given either a boldo-artichoke leaf-celandine combination or placebo.[6] The results showed statistically significant comparative improvements in dyspepsia symptoms after 14 days of treatment.

NOTE: There are indications that celandine may have hepatotoxic properties.[7,8,9]

PROPOSED INDICATIONS AND USAGE

Germany's Commission E has approved boldo for "spastic gastrointestinal complaints and dyspepsia." Boldo is also sometimes recommended as a hepatoprotectant, laxative, and anti-inflammatory agent.

WARNINGS

Boldo should be avoided by pregnant or lactating women, and by individuals with hepatic, renal, or gallbladder disease.

PRECAUTIONS

In rats, hydro-alcohol extract of boldo as well as isolated boldine exhibited abortive and teratogenic actions, and also caused changes in bilirubin, cholesterol, glucose, alanine aminotransferase, aspartate aminotransferase, and urea.[10] Over a period of 90-day usage, histological transformations were not seen. In addition, the plant's essential oils can cause kidney damage if taken alone or if large amounts of the leaf are ingested.

These findings contraindicate boldo for pregnant or lactating women as well as individuals with hepatic or renal disease. In addition, because of its apparent choleretic properties, boldo use in individuals with gallbladder disease should be approached with caution.

DRUG INTERACTIONS

None reported. However, concomitant use with hepatotoxic drugs should be avoided.

PROPOSED DOSAGE AND ADMINISTRATION

Germany's Commission E recommends 3 g of the dried leaf or its equivalent per day for digestive complaints.

ADVERSE REACTIONS

Due to the lack of clinical trials, an accurate estimate of the side-effect rate of boldo is not known.

PATIENT INFORMATION

Boldo is marketed as a treatment for nonspecific indigestion, sometimes called dyspepsia. However, there is no meaningful evidence that it works, and it may have toxic effects.

The safety of boldo in pregnant or nursing women or young children has not been established. Individuals with severe liver or kidney disease should consult a physician before using this (or any other) supplement.

REFERENCES

1. Magistretti MJ. Remarks on the pharmacological examination of plant extracts. *Fitoterapia.* 1980;51:67-79. **2.** Lanhers MC, Joyeux M, Soulimani R, et al. Hepatoprotective and anti-inflammatory effects of a traditional medicinal plant of Chile, Peumus boldus. *Planta Med.* 1991;57:110-115. **3.** Speisky H, Cassels BK. Boldo and boldine: an emerging case of natural drug development. *Pharmacol Res.* 1994;29:1-12. **4.** Jimenez I, Speisky H. Biological disposition of boldine: in vitro and in vivo studies. *Phytother Res.* 2000;14:254-260. **5.** Jimenez I, Garrido A, Bannach R, et al. Protective effects of boldine against free radical-induced erythrocyte lysis. *Phytother Res.* 2000;15:339-343. **6.** Kupke D, von Sanden H, Trinczek-Gartner H, et al. An evaluation of the choleretic activity of a plant-based cholagogue [translated from German]. *Z Allgemeinmed.* 1991;67:1046-1058. **7.** Greving I, Meister V, Monnerjahn C, et al. Chelidonium majus: a rare reason for severe hepatotoxic reaction. *Pharmacoepidemiol Drug Safety.* 1998;7:S66-S69. **8.** Benninger J, Schneider HT, Schuppan, et al. Acute hepatitis induced by greater celandine (Chelidonium majus). *Gastroenterology.* 1999;117:1234-1237. **9.** Strahl S, Ehret V, Dahm HH, et al. Necrotizing hepatitis after taking herbal remedies [translated from German]. *Dtsch Med Wochenschr.* 1998;123:1410-1414. **10.** Almeida ER, Melo AM, Xavier H. Toxicological evaluation of the hydro-alcohol extract of the dry leaves of Peumus boldus and boldine in rats. *Phytother Res.* 2000;14:99-102.

Butterbur

Petasites spp, including Petasites Hybridus, P. Albus, P. Vulgaris

U.S. BRAND NAMES OF CLINICALLY TESTED PRODUCTS

Petadolex (Weber & Weber) = Petadolex (Weber & Weber) in Europe

DESCRIPTION

A large-leaved, unpleasant-smelling herb in the Asteraceae family, butterbur has a long history of medicinal uses for conditions including stomach cramps, whooping cough, and asthma.

PHARMACOLOGY

The active ingredients of butterbur are thought to be angelic acid esters of sesquiterpine alcohols, including petasin, isopetasin, and furanopetasin.[1] Petasin is unstable and spontaneously shifts into isopetasin. In vitro studies suggest that these substances may possess anti-inflammatory, antispasmodic, antihistaminic, and antidopaminergic effects.[1-5] Butterbur extracts appear to affect peptido-leukotrienes but not prostaglandins; the net effect may be gastric cytoprotection rather than gastric irritation.[6,7] Furanopetasin extracts containing furanoeremophilanes have shown cytotoxic properties.[3] Other constituents of butterbur include flavonoids, volatile oils, and potentially hepatotoxic and carcinogenic pyrrolizidine alkaloids.

The pharmacokinetics of butterbur have not been explored.

CLINICAL STUDIES

A double-blind placebo-controlled study of 60 individuals with a history of at least 3 migraines per month evaluated the effectiveness of butterbur as a migraine prophylactic.[8] After a 4-week washout period, participants were given either 50 mg of butterbur extract or placebo twice daily for 3 months. Both the number of migraine attacks and the total number of days of migraine pain were significantly reduced in the treatment group as compared to the placebo group. Three out of four individuals taking butterbur reported improvement, as compared to only one out of four in the placebo group.

PROPOSED INDICATIONS AND USAGE

One small double-blind trial supports the use of butterbur in migraine prophylaxis.

Based on pharmacological evidence suggesting that butterbur has spasmolytic and analgesic effects, butterbur has also been marketed for use in asthma, abdominal pain, tension headaches, back pain, bladder spasms, and gallbladder pain.

WARNINGS

Raw butterbur may contain hepatotoxic and possibly carcinogenic pyrrolizidine alkaloids.

PRECAUTIONS

Unprocessed butterbur contains potentially hepatotoxic and carcinogenic pyrrolizidine alkaloids.[9] These must be removed during the manufacturing process to create a safe product.[10]

Safety in pregnant or lactating women, young children, or individuals with severe hepatic or renal disease is not known.

DRUG INTERACTIONS

None reported.

ADVERSE REACTIONS

No significant side effects were reported in the one published clinical trial of butterbur (n=60).[8]

PROPOSED DOSAGE AND ADMINISTRATION

The usual dosage of butterbur as a migraine preventive is 50 mg twice daily of an extract that has been processed to remove pyrrolizidine alkaloids.

PATIENT INFORMATION

One study suggests that butterbur may help prevent migraine headaches. It is also marketed for other conditions such as asthma, tension headaches, and back pain, but there is no real evidence that it works for these conditions.

Raw butterbur may contain liver toxic ingredients. These must be removed in a special manufacturing process to create a safe product.

The safety of butterbur in pregnant or nursing women or young children has not been established. Individuals with severe liver or kidney disease should consult a physician before using this (or any other) supplement.

REFERENCES

1. Carle R. Plant-based antiphlogistics and spasmolytics [translated from German]. *Z Phytother.* 1988;9:67-76. **2.** Grossman W. Migraine prophylaxis with a phytopharmaceutical remedy: the results of a randomized, placebo-controlled, double-blind clinical study with Petadolex(tm). *Der Freie Arzt.* 1996;(3):1-7. **3.** Scheidegger C, Dahinden C, Wiesmann U. Effects of extracts and of individual components from Petasites on prostaglandin synthesis in cultured skin fibroblasts and on leucotriene synthesis in isolated human peripheral leucocytes. *Pharm Acta Helv.* 1998;72:376-378. **4.** Reglin F. Butterbur root—a pain reliever with wide range application possibilities. *Praxis-Telegram.* 1998;1:13-14. **5.** Berger D, Burkard W, Schaffner W. Influence of Petasites hybridus on dopamine-D2 and histamine-H1 receptors. *Pharm Acta Helv.* 1998;72:373-375. **6.** Brune K, Bickel D, Peskar BA. Gastro-protective effects by extracts of Petasites hybridus: the role of inhibition of peptido-leukotriene synthesis. *Planta Med.* 1993;59:494-496. **7.** Bickel D, Roder T, Bestmann HJ, et al. Identification and characterization of inhibitors of peptido-leukotriene-synthesis from Petasites hybridus. *Planta Med.* 1994;60:318-322. **8.** Grossmann M, Schmidramsl H. An extract of Petasites hybridus is effective in the prophylaxis of migraine. *Int J Clin Pharmacol Ther.* 2000;38:430-435. **9.** Luthy J, Zweifel U, Schmid P, et al. Pyrrolizidine alkaloids in Petasites hybridus L. and P. albus L. [in German; English abstract]. *Pharm Acta Helv.* 1983;58:98-100. **10.** Mauz C, Candrian U, Luthy J, et al. Method for the reduction of pyrrolizidine alkaloids from medicinal plant extracts [in German; English abstract]. *Pharm Acta Helv.* 1985;60:256-259.

Carnitine

Alternate/Related Names: L-Carnitine, L-Acetyl-Carnitine (LAC), Propionyl L-Carnitine (PLC), Acetyl-L-Carnitine (ALC)

U.S. BRAND NAMES OF CLINICALLY TESTED PRODUCTS

Not applicable.

DESCRIPTION

When it was first identified, carnitine was briefly known as vitamin B_T. However, because the body can synthesize carnitine from lysine, this substance has subsequently been classified as a nonessential nutrient. In Europe, physicians have used various forms of carnitine for the adjunctive treatment of angina, intermittent claudication, congestive heart failure, post-myocardial-infarction cardioprotection, dementia, and dysthymia. Recently, supplemental carnitine has also been suggested as a treatment to correct the carnitine depletion possibly caused by various antiseizure drugs as well as to counter the cardiotoxic effects of zidovudine (AZT).

Oral L-carnitine is generally well tolerated.

PHARMACOLOGY

Carnitine synthesis depends on the presence of vitamin B_6, vitamin C, niacin, and iron and is primarily performed in the liver, kidney, and brain. However, infants (especially preterm ones) cannot synthesize carnitine well and must rely on breast milk as an exogenous source. For this reason, formula should be fortified with carnitine.

Orally administered L-carnitine reaches peak plasma concentrations in 3.5 to 5 hours, with a half-life of 2 to 15 hours.[1] Tracer studies in humans suggest that exogenous carnitine is rapidly taken up and retained by the myocardium.[2]

Carnitine is an essential factor for the transport of long-chain fatty acids into the mitochondria. Necropsy has shown decreased L-carnitine concentrations in the infarct area of patients who have suffered fatal MIs.[3] This is attributed to diffusion of L-carnitine away from ischemic tissue.[4]

Free fatty acids and acetylene-CoA in long chains accumulate under ischemic conditions. These substances degrade cellular membranes and also inhibit adenine nucleotide translocase, which catalyses the movement of ADP from cytoplasm to mitochondria and of ATP in the reverse direction. Repletion with L-carnitine may protect the failing heart by stimulating oxidative metabolism of fatty acids and acetylene-CoA.[1,4-6]

In patients with acute MI, controlled studies have shown that oral or intravenous administration of carnitine reduced the levels of the MB fraction of creatine kinase.[7] Furthermore, intravenous administration of L-carnitine in patients with moderately impaired left-ventricular function produced a positive inotropic effect.[1] In healthy individuals, infusion of propionyl-L-carnitine (PLC) increased heart rate and the effective and functional refractory period of the AV node.[8]

The apparent benefits of carnitine in intermittent claudication are presumed to be due to improved muscle function rather than to normalized circulation.[9,10]

Some evidence suggests that L-carnitine may inhibit thyroid hormone entry into cells, suggesting potential usage in hyperthyroidism.[11]

Acetyl-L-carnitine (ALC) has been postulated to mimic some of the CNS effects of acetylcholine.[12-18] It may also exert a neuroprotective effect.[19]

In certain congenital metabolic diseases, such as systemic carnitine deficiency, a failure of carnitine synthesis leads to progressive weakness, hepatic encephalopathy, and early death. Decreased levels of serum carnitine also appear to be associated with the use of various antiseizure medications or their combinations, including phenobarbital, valproic acid, phenytoin, and carbamazepine.[20-23] Most of the interest has focused on children taking valproic acid, supported by evidence of defects of fat metabolism consistent with a meaningful carnitine deficiency.[24,25] However, the one double-blind clinical study on carnitine supplementation during therapy with valproic acid found no benefit (see Clinical Studies).

CLINICAL STUDIES

The best evidence for carnitine can be found in its use as adjunctive therapy in post-MI cardioprotection and intermittent claudication. The carnitine derivative ALC does not appear to be effective for the treatment of dementia.

POST-MI CARDIOPROTECTION (L-CARNITINE)

Two double-blind placebo-controlled studies that followed a total of 632 individuals post-MI found that over a 1-year period adjunctive use of L-carnitine caused significant decreases in ventricular hypertrophy,[26] anginal attacks, and mortality,[27] as well as improvement in some hemodynamic parameters.[27] The dosage in the larger of the two studies was 9 g daily intravenously for 5 days followed by 6 g daily orally; the other used 4 g daily orally.

Another double-blind placebo-controlled study that followed 101 postinfarct patients for 1 month found that use of L-carnitine reduced mean infarct size and other postinfarct complications.[28]

INTERMITTENT CLAUDICATION (L-CARNITINE AND PROPIONYL-L-CARNITINE)

A 12-month double-blind placebo-controlled trial of 485 patients with intermittent claudication found that PLC at a dose of 1 g twice daily produced a significant (44%) improvement in maximal walking distance in those with initial maximal walking distance less than or equal to 250 m; however, no response was seen in those with milder disease.[29] Benefits were seen in most but not all other studies using L-carnitine or PLC.[9,30-39]

ANGINA (L-CARNITINE AND PROPIONYL-L-CARNITINE)

A controlled (but not blinded) study of 200 patients taking conventional medical therapy for exercise-induced angina found significant reduction of ST-segment depression during maximal effort and improvement of hemodynamic parameters in the group receiving L-carnitine supplementation over 6 months, compared to the placebo group.[4] In addition, patient needs for primary medications were reduced, as were plasma cholesterol and triglyceride levels. Other studies using L-carnitine or PLC also found positive effects.[40-44]

CONGESTIVE HEART FAILURE (L-CARNITINE AND PROPIONYL-L-CARNITINE)

Acute infusion of PLC improves myocardial contractility and relaxation and cardiac pump function in patients with ventricular dysfunction.[45,46,47]

A double-blind placebo-controlled trial that followed 50 patients with NYHA class II CHF for a period of 6 months reported that use of PLC increased exercise duration and improved hemodynamic parameters.[48] Similar results were seen in other studies.[4,49,50]

DEMENTIA (ACETYL-L-CARNITINE)

Numerous double- or single-blind studies involving a total of over 1,400 patients have evaluated ALC in the treatment of Alzheimer's disease and other forms of dementia.[13-17,19,51-55] Though some have reported positive results in some measures of mental function, on balance the evidence is negative. For example, a 1-year double-blind placebo-controlled study followed 431 patients with mild to moderate dementia (thought most likely to be Alzheimer's disease).[18] The results showed no significant improvement with supplemental carnitine as compared to placebo. Based on benefits noted in subgroup analysis, the same researcher performed a subsequent study to evaluate whether ALC was useful in early-onset Alzheimer's.[38] This 1-year double-blind placebo-controlled trial followed 229 patients, and found no benefits.

PROPOSED INDICATIONS AND USAGE

Promising but far from definitive evidence suggests that L-carnitine and PLC may be of use as adjunctive treatment for post-MI cardioprotection, intermittent claudication, angina, and congestive heart failure.

ALC is widely marketed as a treatment for dementia, but overall the evidence is more negative than positive. Similarly, although L-carnitine is widely marketed as an ergogenic aid, studies have yielded contradictory results at best.[56-64]

Mixed evidence suggests that intravenous L-carnitine, in various forms, may offer cardioprotective effects in cardiac surgery and improve heart function in cardiogenic shock.[45,65-68]

Other potential uses of carnitine with weak or mixed supporting evidence include reducing bone breakdown in hyperthyroidism,[69] decreasing incidence and mortality of myocarditis in childhood diphtheria,[70] reducing zidovudine toxicity,[71,72] enhancing immune function in HIV-infected individuals,[73,74,75] improving coordination and muscle tone in cerebellar ataxia,[76] increasing exercise tolerance in individuals with COPD (presumably by improving muscular efficiency in the lungs and other muscles),[77,78,79] preventing diabetic cardiac autonomic neuropathy,[80] treating dysthymia,[81] and reducing levels of Lp(a).[82]

Despite evidence that antiseizure drugs may reduce serum carnitine levels and cause carnitine-dependent metabolic dysfunction,[21,83-87] a double-blind crossover study of 47 children taking anticonvulsants found no measurable benefit with carnitine supplementation.[88]

WARNINGS

None.

PRECAUTIONS

A single report suggests that patients undergoing hemodialysis might require reduced doses of carnitine.[89] However, a more recent study suggests that hemodialysis causes a transient carnitine deficiency.[90]

In contrast to L-carnitine, D-carnitine is known to cause numerous problems by competitively inhibiting the L-form.[63] DL-carnitine has caused a myasthenia gravis-like syndrome in hemodialysis patients.[1]

Maximum safe dosage for young children, pregnant or lactating women, or people with severe hepatic or renal disease has not been established.

DRUG INTERACTIONS

None are known. However, formal drug interaction studies have not been performed.

ADVERSE REACTIONS

L-carnitine in its three forms appears to be safe. In a 12-month drug-monitoring study involving more than 4,000 patients with cardiovascular disease, the most common adverse effects were stomach discomfort (6%), nausea (4%), and diarrhea (2%).[1]

PROPOSED DOSAGE AND ADMINISTRATION

Carnitine is used in its L-form, as L-carnitine, propionyl-L-carnitine (PLC), and acetyl-L-carnitine (ALC). The D- and DL-forms of carnitine should not be used. Generally, L-carnitine or PLC are most often recommended in heart-related conditions, whereas ALC is used in Alzheimer's and other CNS conditions. The daily dosage usually ranges from 1,500 to 3,000 mg for all forms, given in 3 divided doses.

PATIENT INFORMATION

There is some evidence that L-carnitine might be helpful in certain heart conditions, not as a replacement for standard medications, but as a supplement to them. However, due to the serious nature of heart disease, it is not advisable for individuals with heart-related conditions to take carnitine (or any other supplement) except under the supervision of a physician.

One form of carnitine, acetyl-L-carnitine is marketed as a treatment for Alzheimer's disease and related conditions. However, on balance, the evidence suggests that it does not work.

The maximum safe dosage of carnitine for pregnant or nursing women or young children has not been established. Individuals with severe liver or kidney disease should consult a physician before using this (or any other) supplement.

REFERENCES

1. Goa KL, Brogden RN. L-carnitine: a preliminary review of its pharmacokinetics, and its therapeutic use in ischaemic cardiac disease and primary and secondary carnitine deficiencies in relationship to its role in fatty acid metabolism. *Drugs.* 1987;34:1-24. **2.** Cunningham VJ, Rosen SD, Boyd H, et al. Uptake of [N-methyl-11C] propionyl-L-carnitine (PLC) in human myocardium. *J Pharmacol Exp Ther.* 1996;277:511-517. **3.** Spagnoli LG, Corsi M, Villaschi S, et al. Myocardial carnitine deficiency in acute myocardial infarction. *Lancet.* 1982;1:1419-1420. **4.** Cacciatore L, Cerio R, Ciarimboli M, et al. The therapeutic effect of L-carnitine in patients with exercise-induced stable angina: a controlled study. *Drugs Exp Clin Res.* 1991;17:225-235. **5.** Opie LH. Role of carnitine in fatty acid metabolism of normal and ischemic myocardium. *Am Heart J.* 1979;97:375-388. **6.** Ferrari R, Cucchini F, Di Lisa F, et al. The effect of L-carnitine (carnitene) on myocardial metabolism of patients with coronary artery disease. *Clin Trials J.* 1984;21:40-50. **7.** Rebuzzi AG, Schiavoni G, Amico CM, et al. Beneficial effects of L-carnitine in the reduction of the necrotic area in acute myocardial infarction. *Drugs Exp Clin Res.* 1984;10:219-223. **8.** Di Biase M, Tritto M, Pitzalis MV, et al. Electrophysiologic evaluation of intravenous L-propionylcarnitine in man. *Int J Cardiol.* 1991;30:329-333. **9.** Brevetti G, Perna S, Sabba C, et al. Propionyl-L-carnitine in intermittent claudication: double-blind, placebo-controlled, dose titration, multicenter study. *J Am Coll Cardiol.* 1995;26:1411-1416. **10.** Brevetti G, Perna S, Sabba C, et al. Effect of propionyl-L-carnitine on quality of life in intermittent claudication. *Am J Cardiol.* 1997;79:777-780. **11.** Benvenga S, Lakshmanan M, Trimarchi F. Carnitine is a naturally occurring inhibitor of thyroid hormone nuclear uptake. *Thyroid.* 2000;10:1043-1050. **12.** Carta A, Calvani M, Bravi D, et al. Acetyl-L-carnitine and Alzheimer's disease: pharmacological considerations beyond the cholinergic sphere. *Ann N Y Acad Sci.* 1993;695:324-326. **13.** Cipolli C, Chiari G. Effects of L-acetylcarnitine on mental deterioration in the aged: initial results [in Italian; English abstract]. *Clin Ter.* 1990;132(6 suppl):479-510. **14.** Garzya G, Corallo D, Fiore A, et al. Evaluation of the effects of L-acetylcarnitine on senile patients suffering from depression. *Drugs Exp Clin Res.* 1990;16:101-106. **15.** Passeri M, Cucinotta D, Bonati PA, et al. Acetyl-L-carnitine in the treatment of mildly demented elderly patients. *Int J Clin Pharmacol Res.* 1990;10:75-79. **16.** Salvioli G, Neri M. L-acetylcarnitine treatment of mental decline in the elderly. *Drugs Exp Clin Res.* 1994;20:169-176. **17.** Spagnoli A, Lucca U, Menasce G, et al. Long-term acetyl-L-carnitine treatment in Alzheimer's disease. *Neurology.* 1991;41:1726-1732. **18.** Thal LJ, Carta A, Clarke WR, et al. A 1-year multicenter placebo-controlled study of acetyl-L-carnitine in patients with Alzheimer's disease. *Neurology.* 1996;47:705-711. **19.** Calvani M, Carta A, Caruso G, et al. Action of acetyl-L-carnitine in neurodegeneration and Alzheimer's disease. *Ann N Y Acad Sci.* 1992;663:483-486. **20.** Hiraoka A, Arato T, Tominaga I. Reduction in blood free carnitine levels in association with changes in sodium valproate (VPA) disposition in epileptic patients treated with VPA and other anti-epileptic drugs. *Biol Pharm Bull.* 1997;20:91-93. **21.** Hug C, McGraw CA, Bates SR, et al. Reduction of serum carnitine concentrations during anticonvulsant therapy with phenobarbital, valproic acid, phenytoin, and carbamazepine in children. *J Pediatr.* 1991;119:799-802. **22.** Opala G, Winter S, Vance C, et al. The effect of valproic acid on plasma carnitine levels. *Am J Dis Child.* 1991;145:999-1001. **23.** Van Wouwe JP. Carnitine deficiency during valproic acid treatment. *Int J Vitam Nutr Res.* 1995;65:211-214. **24.** Melegh B, Pap M, Morava E, et al. Carnitine-dependent changes of metabolic fuel consumption during long-term treatment with valproic acid. *J Pediatr.* 1994;125:317-321. **25.** Melegh B, Trombitas K. Valproate treatment induces lipid globule accumulation with ultrastructural abnormalities of mitochondria in skeletal muscle. *Neuropediatrics.* 1997;28:257-261. **26.** Iliceto S, Scrutinio D, Bruzzi P, et al. Effects of L-carnitine administration on left ventricular remodeling after acute anterior myocardial infarction: the L-Carnitine Ecocardiografia Digitalizzata Infarto Miocardico (CEDIM) Trial. *J Am Coll Cardiol.* 1995;26:380-387. **27.** Davini P, Bigalli A, Lamanna F, et al. Controlled study on L-carnitine therapeutic efficacy in post-infarction. *Drugs Exp Clin Res.* 1992;18:355-365. **28.** Singh RB, Niaz MA, Agarwal P, et al. A randomised, double-blind, placebo-controlled trial of L-carnitine in suspected acute myocardial infarction. *Postgrad Med J.* 1996;72:45-50. **29.** Brevetti G, Diehm C, Lambert D. European multicenter study on propionyl-L-carnitine in intermittent claudication. *J Am Coll Cardiol.* 1999;34:1618-1624. **30.** Bolognesi M, Amodio P, Merkel C, et al. Effect of 8-day therapy with propionyl-L-carnitine on muscular and subcutaneous blood flow of the lower limbs in patients with peripheral arterial disease. *Clin Physiol.* 1995;15:417-423. **31.** Brevetti G, Perna S, Sabba C, et al. Superiority of L-propionylcarnitine vs L-carnitine in improving walking capacity in patients with peripheral vascular disease: an acute, intravenous, double-blind, cross-over study. *Eur Heart J.* 1992;13:251-255. **32.** Greco AV, Mingrone G, Bianchi M, et al. Effect of propionyl-L-carnitine in the treatment of diabetic angiopathy: controlled double blind trial versus placebo. *Drugs Exp Clin Res.* 1992;18:69-80. **33.** Brevetti G, Chiariello M, Ferulano G, et al. Increases in walking distance in patients with peripheral vascular disease treated with L-carnitine: a double-blind, cross-over study.*Circulation.* 1988;77:767-773. **34.** Deckert J. Propionyl-L-carnitine for intermittent claudication. *J Fam Pract.* 1997;44:533-534. **35.** Sabba C, Berardi E, Antonica G, et al. Comparison between the effect of L-propionylcarnitine, L-acetylcarnitine and nitroglycerin in chronic peripheral arterial disease: a haemodynamic double blind echo-Doppler study. *Eur Heart J.* 1994;15:1348-1352. **36.** Pepine CJ. The therapeutic potential of carnitine in cardiovascular disorders. *Clin Ther.* 1991;13:2-21. **37.** Brevetti G, Attisano T, Perna S, et al. Effect of L-carnitine on the reactive hyperemia in patients affected by peripheral vascular disease: a double-blind, crossover study. *Angiology.* 1989;40:857-862. **38.** Thal LJ, Calvani M, Amato A, et al. A 1-year controlled trial of acetyl-l-carnitine in early-onset AD. *Neurology.* 2000;55:805-810. **39.** Hiatt WR, Regensteiner JG, Creager MA, et al. Propionyl-L-carnitine improves exercise performance and functional status in patients with claudication. *Am J Med.* 2001;110:616-622. **40.** Bartels GL, Remme WJ, Pillay M, et al. Effects of L-propionylcarnitine on ischemia-induced myocardial dysfunction in men with angina pectoris. *Am J Cardiol.* 1994;74:125-130. **41.** Bartels GL, Remme WJ, den Hartog FR, et al. Additional antiischemic effects of long-term L-Propionylcarnitine in anginal patients treated with conventional antianginal therapy. *Cardiovasc Drugs Ther.* 1995;9:749-753. **42.** Bartels GL, Remme WJ, Holwerda KJ, et al. Anti-ischaemic efficacy of L-propionylcarnitine—a promising novel metabolic approach to ischaemia? *Eur Heart J.* 1996;17:414-420. **43.** Cherchi A, Lai C, Angelino F, et al. Effects of L-carnitine on exercise tolerance in chronic stable angina: a multicenter, double-blind, randomized, placebo controlled crossover study. *Int J Clin Pharmacol Ther Toxicol.* 1985;23:569-572. **44.** Lagioia R, Scrutinio D, Mangini SG, et al. Propionil-L-carnitine: a new compound in the metabolic approach to the treatment of effort angina. *Int J Cardiol.* 1992;34:167-172. **45.** Bartels GL, Remme WJ, Pillay M, et al. Acute improvement of cardiac function with intravenous L-propionylcarnitine in humans. *J Cardiovasc Pharmacol.* 1992;20:157-164. **46.** Chiddo A, Gaglione A, Musci S, et al. Hemodynamic study of intravenous propionyl-L-carnitine in patients with ischemic heart disease and normal left ventricular function. *Cardiovasc Drugs Ther.* 1991;5(suppl 1):107-111. **47.** Anand I, Chandrashekhan Y, De Giuli F, et al. Acute and chronic effects of propionyl-L-carnitine on the hemodynamics, exercise capacity, and hormones in patients with congestive heart failure. *Cardiovasc Drugs Ther.* 1998;12:291-299. **48.** Caponnetto S, Canale C, Masperone MA, et al. Efficacy of L-propionylcarnitine treatment in patients with left ventricular dysfunction. *Eur Heart J.* 1994;15:1267-1273. **49.** Mancini M, Rengo F, Lingetti M, et al. Controlled study on the therapeutic efficacy of propionyl-L-carnitine in patients with congestive heart failure. *Arzneimittelforschung.* 1992;42:1101-1104. **50.** Pucciarelli G, Mastursi M, Latte S, et al. The clinical and hemodynamic effects of propionyl-L-carnitine in patients with congestive heart failure [in Italian; English abstract]. *Clin Ter.* 1992;141:379-384. **51.** Bonavita E. Study of the efficacy and tolerability of L-acetylcarnitine therapy in the senile brain. *Int J Clin Pharmacol Ther Toxicol.* 1986;24:511-516. **52.** Campi N, Todeschini GP, Scarzella L. Selegiline versus L-acetylcarnitine in the treatment of Alzheimer-type dementia. *Clin Ther.* 1990;12:306-314. **53.** Rai G, Wright G, Scott L, et al. Double-blind, placebo controlled study of acetyl-l-carnitine in patients with Alzheimer's dementia. *Curr Med Res Opin.* 1990;11:638-647. **54.** Sano M, Bell K, Cote L, et al. Double-blind parallel design pilot study of acetyl levocarnitine in patients with Alzheimer's disease. *Arch Neurol.* 1992;49:1137-1141. **55.** Vecchi GP, Chiari G, Cipolli C, et al. Acetyl-l-carnitine treatment of mental impairment in the elderly: evidence from a multicentre study. *Arch Gerontol Geriatr.* 1991;(suppl 2):159-168. **56.** Decombaz J, Deriaz O, Acheson K, et al. Effect of L-carnitine on submaximal exercise metabolism after depletion of muscle glycogen. *Med Sci Sports Exerc.* 1993;25:733-740. **57.** Dragan AM, Vasilic D, Eremia NMD. Studies concerning some acute biological changes after endovenous administration of 1 g L-carnitine in elite athletes. *Physiologie.* 1987;24:231-234. **58.** Dragan GI, Wagner W, Ploesteanu E. Studies concerning the ergogenic value of protein supply and L-carnitine in elite junior cyclists. *Physiologie.* 1988;25:129-132. **59.** Greig C, Finch KM, Jones DA, et al. The effect of oral supplementation with L-carnitine on maximum and submaximum exercise capacity. *Eur J Appl Physiol Occup Physiol.* 1987;56:457-460. **60.** Marconi C, Sassi G, Carpinelli A, Cerretelli P. Effects of L-carnitine loading on the aerobic and anaerobic performance of endurance athletes. *Eur J Appl Physiol.* 1985;54:131-135. **61.** Soop M, Bjorkman O, Cederblad G, et al. Influence of carnitine supplementation on muscle substrate and carnitine metabolism during exercise. *J Appl Physiol.* 1988;88:2394-2399. **62.** Vecchiet L, Di Lisa F, Pieralisi G, et al. Influence of L-carnitine administration on maximal physical exercise. *Eur J Appl Physiol.* 1990;61:486-490. **63.** Watanabe S, Ajisaka R, Masuoka T, et al. Effects of L- and DL-carnitine on patients with impaired exercise tolerance. *Jpn Heart J.* 1995;36:319-331. **64.** Heinonen OJ. Carnitine and physical exercise. *Sports Med.* 1996;22:109-132. **65.** Golba KS, Wos S, Deja MA, et al. Cardioplegia supplementation with L-carnitine enhances myocardial protection in patients with low ejection fraction. *Kardiol Pol.* 2000;51:181-184. **66.** Pastoris O, Dossena M, Foppa P, et al. Effect of L-carnitine on myocardial metabolism: results of a balanced, placebo-controlled, double-blind study in patients undergoing open heart surgery. *Pharmacol Res.* 1998;37:115-122. **67.** Corbucci GG, Loche F. L-carnitine in cardiogenic shock therapy: pharmacodynamic aspects and clinical data. *Int J Clin Pharmacol Res.* 1993;13:87-91. **68.** Gasparetto A, Corbucci GG, De Blasi RA, et al. Influence of acetyl-L-carnitine infusion on haemodynamic parameters and survival of circulatory-shock patients. *Int J Clin Pharmacol Res.* 1991;11:83-92. **69.** Benvenga S, Ruggeri RM, Russo A, et al. Usefulness of l-carnitine, a naturally occurring peripheral antagonist of thyroid hormone action, in iatrogenic hyperthyroidism: a randomized, double-blind, placebo-controlled clinical trial. *J Clin Endocrinol Metab.* 2001;86:3579-3594. **70.** Ramos AC, Barrucand L, Elias PR, et al. Carnitine supplementation in diphtheria. *Indian Pediatr.* 1992;29(12):1501-1505. **71.** Dalakas MC, Leon-Monzon ME, Bernardini I, et al. Zidovudine-induced mitochondrial myopathy is associated with muscle carnitine deficiency and lipid storage. *Ann Neurol.* 1994;35:482-487. **72.** Semino-Mora MC, Leon-Monzon ME, Dalakas MC. Effect of L-carnitine on the zidovudine-induced destruction of human myotubes. Part I: L-carnitine prevents the myotoxicity of AZT in vitro. *Lab Invest.* 1994;71:102-112. **73.** Moretti S, Alesse E, Di Marzio L, et al. Effect of L-carnitine on human immunodeficiency virus-1 infection-associated apoptosis: a pilot study. *Blood.* 1998;91:3817-3824. **74.** De Simone C, Cifone MG, Alesse E, et al. Cell-associated ceramide in HIV-1-infected subjects. *AIDS.* 1996;10:675-676. **75.** Kroemer G, Zamzami N, Susin SA. Mitochondrial control of apoptosis. *Immunol Today.* 1997;18:44-51. **76.** Sorbi S, Forleo P, Fani C, et al. Double-blind, crossover, placebo-controlled clinical trial with L-acetylcarnitine in patients with degenerative cerebellar ataxia. *Clin Neuropharmacol.* 2000;23:114-118. **77.** Dal Negro R, Pomari G, Zoccatelli O, et al. L-carnitine and rehabilitative respiratory physiokinesitherapy: metabolic and ventilatory response in chronic respiratory insufficiency. *Int J Clin Pharmacol Ther Toxicol.* 1986;24:453-456. **78.** Dal Negro R, Turco P, Pomari C, et al. Effects of L-carnitine on physical performance in chronic respiratory insufficiency. *Int J Clin Pharmacol Ther Toxicol.* 1988;26:269-272. **79.** Dal Negro R, Zoccatelli D, Pomari C, et al. L-carnitine and physiokinesiotherapy in chronic respiratory insufficiency. Preliminary results. *Clin Trials J.* 1985;22:353-360. **80.** Turpeinen AK, Kuikka JT, Vanninen E, et al. Long-term effect of acetyl-L-carnitine on myocardial 123I-MIBG uptake in patients with diabetes. *Clin Auton Res.* 2000;10:13-16. **81.** Bella R, Biondi R, Raffaele R, et al. Effect of acetyl-L-carnitine on geriatric patients suffering from dysthymic disorders. *Int J Clin Pharmacol Res.* 1990;10:355-360. **82.** Sirtori CR, Calabresi L, Ferrara S, et al. L-carnitine reduces plasma lipoprotein(a) levels in patients with hyper Lp(a). *Nutr Metab Cardiovasc Dis.* 2000;10:247-251. **83.** Matsuda I, Ohtani Y. Carnitine status in Reye and Reye-like syndromes. *Pediatr Neurol.* 1986;2:90-94. **84.** Camina MF, Rozas I, Gomez M, et al. Short-term effects of administration of anticonvulsant drugs on free carnitine and acylcarnitine in mouse serum and tissues. *Br J Pharmacol.* 1991;103:1179-1183. **85.** De Vivo DC, Bohan TP, Coulter DL, et al. L-Carnitine supplementation in childhood epilepsy: current perspectives. *Epilepsia.* 1998;39:1216-1225. **86.** Zelnik N, Fridkis I, Gruener N. Reduced carnitine and antiepileptic drugs: cause relationship or co-existence? *Acta Paediatr.* 1995;84:93-95. **87.** Rodriguez-Segade S, de la Pena CA, Tutor JC, et al. Carnitine deficiency associated with anticonvulsant therapy. *Clin Chim Acta.* 1989;181:175-181. **88.** Freeman JM, Vining EP, Cost S, et al. Does carnitine administration improve the symptoms attributed to anticonvulsant medications?: A double-blinded, crossover study. *Pediatrics.* 1994;93(6 Pt 1):893-895. **89.** Weschler A, Aviram M, Levin M. High dose of L-carnitine increases platelet aggregation and plasma triglyceride levels in uremic patients on hemodialysis. *Nephron.* 1984;38:120-124. **90.** Jackson, JM, Lee HA. L-Carnitine and acetyl-L-carnitine status during hemodialysis with acetate in humans: a kinetic analysis. *Am J Clin Nutr.* 1996;64:922-927.

Chasteberry

Vitex Agnus-Castus

Alternate/Related Names: Chaste Tree

U.S. BRAND NAMES OF CLINICALLY TESTED PRODUCTS

Femaprin (Nature's Way) = Agnolyt (Madaus) in Europe

DESCRIPTION

Chasteberry is a shrub in the verbena family, commonly found on river banks and nearby foothills in central Asia and around the Mediterranean Sea. For medicinal purposes, this fruit is harvested ripe and then dried. It was traditionally used to suppress libido, as well as a digestive aid and as a reducer of uterine bleeding.

PHARMACOLOGY

Chasteberry fruit contains 5% volatile oil as well as the iridoid glycosides agnoside and aucubin. Pharmacokinetic and pharmacodynamic data are lacking, as are meaningful studies on the species-specific constituents of chasteberry.

In vitro, animal, and preliminary human trials in women suggest that chasteberry extracts inhibit prolactin release, apparently through dopaminergic stimulation of D2-type receptor cells in the pituitary.[1-8] However, a double-blind study of 20 normal men showed no clear dose-dependent change in prolactin profile produced by vitex extract.[9]

CLINICAL STUDIES

Many studies of chasteberry used Mastodynon, a product containing chasteberry plus other herbs in homeopathic dilutions; others used chasteberry extract alone.

CYCLIC MASTALGIA

A double-blind placebo-controlled trial of 97 women with symptoms of cyclic mastalgia found that treatment with chasteberry extract (as Mastodynon) significantly reduced pain intensity at the end of the first and the second menstrual cycle as compared to placebo.[10] However, in the third cycle, benefits of chasteberry treatment plateaued, while improvements continued in the placebo group. This effect reduced the still-existing difference between the groups to a point where it was no longer statistically significant.

Benefits were also seen in a double-blind trial that enrolled 160 women with cyclic mastodynia. Patients were given either chasteberry (as Mastodynon), a progestin (lynestrenol), or placebo, and followed for at least 4 menstrual cycles.[11] The results in evaluable patients (38 placebo, 28 progestin, and 55 chasteberry) showed that both chasteberry and progestin were superior to placebo.

Another double-blind trial included 104 patients in an intention-to-treat analysis, comparing placebo against two forms of chasteberry (liquid and tablet) for at least 3 menstrual cycles.[1] The results showed statistically significant and comparable improvements in the treated groups as compared to the placebo group.

PREMENSTRUAL SYNDROME

A double-blind placebo-controlled study of 178 women found that treatment with chasteberry over 3 menstrual cycles significantly reduced PMS symptoms.[12] The dose used was 1 tablet 3 times daily of the chasteberry dry extract ZE 440. Women in the treatment group experienced significant improvements in symptoms, including irritability, depression, headache, and breast tenderness.

Another double-blind study followed 175 women with PMS for 3 months; half received a standard chasteberry preparation (Agnolyt), and the others received 200 mg of pyridoxine (vitamin B_6) daily.[13] Over the 3-month study period, chasteberry use was associated with slightly better results than the vitamin. However, the effectiveness of B_6 in PMS is controversial and modest at best.[14]

LUTEAL PHASE DEFECT

A double-blind trial followed 52 women with luteal phase defect due to latent hyperprolactinemia.[6] After 3 months, reduction in prolactin release, normalization of luteal phase length, and improvements in secondary progesterone synthesis occurred in the treated group but not in the control group. No other hormonal parameters changed except 17 beta-estradiol, which increased during the luteal phase.

PROPOSED INDICATIONS AND USAGE

Preliminary evidence suggests that chasteberry may have utility for cyclic mastalgia and general PMS symptoms.

Based on its antiprolactin effects, chasteberry has also been tried as a fertility drug.[15] However, the two double-blind trials designed to evaluate this use were too small for the results to achieve statistical significance on primary endpoints.[16,17] Chasteberry has also been tried as a treatment for secondary amenorrhea.[18]

In addition, chasteberry is marketed as a treatment for menopause, but there is no supporting evidence for this use.

WARNINGS

None.

PRECAUTIONS

A clinical pharmacology study using high doses of chasteberry extract produced no more than mild nonspecific side effects, such as gastrointestinal disturbances.[9] A fertility clinic has reported a single case of mild ovarian hyperstimulation in a woman who self-prescribed.[19] However, there was no solid evidence of a cause-and-effect relationship in this report.

Chasteberry is definitely not recommended for use in pregnancy and lactation because of its effects on prolactin. Safety in young children and individuals with severe hepatic or renal disease has not been established.

DRUG INTERACTIONS

Based on its mechanism of action, chasteberry might interact with bromocriptine or other agents with endocrine or pituitary activity.

ADVERSE REACTIONS

Widespread use of chasteberry in Germany has not led to any reports of significant adverse effects.[20] In drug-monitoring studies enrolling a total of over 3,000 participants, the rate of minor side effects was less than 2.5%, primarily nausea, headaches, and allergy.[21,22]

PROPOSED DOSAGE AND ADMINISTRATION

Chasteberry dosages depend on the specific formulation. Label instructions should be followed.

PATIENT INFORMATION

Chasteberry is marketed as a treatment for a variety of conditions affecting women. Preliminary evidence suggests that it might offer benefit for cyclic breast discomfort and general PMS symptoms. However, there is no real evidence that it is helpful for any other conditions.

Note: Do not use chasteberry for amenorrhea (lack of menstruation) or irregular menstruation without first seeing a physician to rule out potentially dangerous causes of these conditions.

Chasteberry should not be used by pregnant or nursing women. Safety for individuals with severe liver or kidney disease has not been established. Do not use chasteberry if you are taking other medications that affect your hormones.

REFERENCES

1. Wuttke W, Splitt G, Gorkow C, et al. Treatment of cyclical mastalgia: results of a randomised, placebo-controlled, double-blind study [translated from German]. *Geburtsh Frauenheilk.* 1997;57:569-574. **2.** Meier B, Berger D, Hoberg E, et al. Pharmacological activities of Vitex agnus-castus extracts in vitro. *Phytomedicine.* 2000;7:373-381. **3.** Jarry H, Leonhardt S, Wuttke W, et al. Agnus castus as a dopaminergic active principle in Mastodynon(r) N [in German; English abstract]. *Z Phytother.* 1991;12:77-82. **4.** Jarry H, Leonhardt S, Gorkow C, et al. In vitro prolactin but not LH and FSH release is inhibited by compounds in extracts of Agnus castus: direct evidence for a dopaminergic principle by the dopamine receptor assay. *Exp Clin Endocrinol.* 1994;102:448-454. **5.** Winterhoff H. Medicinal plants witwh endocrine efficacy. Effects on thyroid and ovary function [translated from German]. *Z Phytother.* 1993;14:83-94. **6.** Milewicz A, Gejdel E, Sworen H, et al. Vitex agnus castus extract in the treatment of luteal phase defects due to latent hyperprolactinemia. Results of a randomized placebo-controlled double-blind study [translated from German]. *Arzneimittelforschung.* 1993;43:752-756. **7.** Amann W. Elimination of obstipation with Agnolyt(r) [in German]. *Ther Gegw.* 1965;104:1263-1265. **8.** Weiss RF. *Herbal medicine. Ab arcanum.* Gothenburg, Sweden; 1988:317-318. **9.** Merz PG, Gorkow C, Schrodter A, et al. The effects of a special Agnus castus extract (BP1095E1) on prolactin secretion in healthy male subjects. Exp Clin Endocrinol Diabetes. 1996;104:447-453. **10.** Halaska M, Beles P, Gorkow C, et al. Treatment of cyclical mastalgia with a solution containing a Vitex agnus castus extract: results of a placebo-controlled double-blind study. *Breast.* 1999;8:175-181. **11.** Kubista E, Muller G, Spona J. Treatment of mastopathy associated with cyclic mastodynia: clinical results and hormone profiles [translated from German]. *Gynakol Rundsch.* 1986;26:65-79. **12.** Schellenberg R. Treatment for the premenstrual syndrome with agnus castus fruit extract: prospective, randomised, placebo controlled study. *BMJ.* 2001;322:134-137. **13.** Lauritzen C, Reuter HD, Repges R, et al. Treatment of premenstrual tension syndrome with Vitex agnus castus. Controlled, double-blind study versus pyridoxine. *Phytomedicine.* 1997;4:183-189. **14.** Kleijnen J, Ter Riet G, Knipschild P. Vitamin B6 in the treatment of the premenstrual syndrome—a review. *Br J Obstet Gynaecol.* 1990;97:847-852. **15.** Propping D, Katzorke T, Belkien L. Diagnosis and therapy of corpus luteum deficiency in general practice [translated from German]. *Therapiewoche.* 1988;38:2992-3001. **16.** Bergmann J, Luft B, Boehmann S, et al. The effectiveness of the complex agent, Phyto-Hypophyson(r) L, in female sterility of hormonal origin [translated from German]. *Forsch Komplementarmed Klass Naturheilkd.* 2000;7:190-199. **17.** Gerhard I, Patek A, Monga B, et al. Mastodynon(r) for female infertility [in German; English abstract]. *Forsch Komplementarmed.* 1998;5:272-278. **18.** Loch E-G, Kaiser E. Diagnosis and treatment of amenorrhea in practice [in German]. *Gynakol Praxis.* 1990;14:489-495. **19.** Cahill DJ, Fox R, Wardle PG, et al. Multiple follicular development associated with herbal medicine. *Hum Reprod.* 1994;9:1469-1470. **20.** Schulz V, Hansel R, Tyler VE. *Rational Phytotherapy: A Physicians' Guide to Herbal Medicine.* 3rd ed. Berlin, Germany: Springer-Verlag; 1998:278. **21.** Dittmar FW, Bohnert KJ, Peeters M, et al. Premenstrual syndrome: treatment with a phytopharmaceutical [translated from German]. *Ther Gynakol.* 1992;5:60-68. **22.** Propping D, Bohnert KJ, Peeters M, et al. Agnus-castus: treatment of gynaecological syndromes [translated from German]. *Therapeutikon.* 1991;5:581-585.

Chitosan

Alternate/Related Names: Chitin

U.S. BRAND NAMES OF CLINICALLY TESTED PRODUCTS

Liposan Ultra (Vanson, Inc.) (U.S. product only)

DESCRIPTION

Chitosan is a form of poorly soluble fiber chemically derived from crustaceans or squid. Like other forms of fiber, chitosan may impair fat absorption. For this reason, it has been tried for weight loss and hyperlipidemia.

PHARMACOLOGY

Chitosan is a cationic polysaccharide containing polyglucosamine polymer chains with nonacetylated amines. Similarly to other forms of fiber, chitosan is thought to bind bile acids and dietary lipids. The solubility and activity of chitosan may be altered by the molecular weight of the particular product used.

CLINICAL STUDIES

Only weak and inconsistent evidence supports the use of chitosan for any condition.

WEIGHT LOSS

An 8-week, double-blind placebo-controlled trial of 59 overweight individuals evaluated the effects of 1.5 g of chitosan taken prior to each of the two largest meals of the day.[1] Over the course of the study, participants in the placebo group gained a mean of 1.5 kg, while those in the chitosan group lost 1.0 kg, a statistically significant difference.

However, a 4-week double-blind placebo-controlled trial of 30 overweight individuals given chitosan at the lower dose of 1 g twice daily failed to find any weight-loss effects.[2] Differences in dosing, duration, and the form of chitosan used may explain the negative results.

HYPERLIPIDEMIA

Despite evidence from preclinical trials suggesting that chitosan possesses hypolipidemic properties,[3-10] a 4-month double-blind placebo-controlled trial of 88 individuals found no benefit.[11]

PROPOSED INDICATIONS AND USAGE

Chitosan products are widely marketed as weight-loss aids, although clinical evidence for its effectiveness is limited to the one positive trial described above. Chitosan is also frequently included in supplement mixtures claimed to normalize cholesterol levels, again despite the lack of success in clinical trials.

Other potential uses are based on very weak evidence. One open trial suggests that chitosan might offer benefits in renal failure by binding toxins in the intestinal lumen.[12] Studies in dogs suggest that topically applied chitosan might aid wound healing.[13] Oral chitosan has also been proposed as an antihypertensive, an immune stimulant, and a cancer treatment.

WARNINGS

Use of chitosan may further impair nutrition in malnourished individuals.

PRECAUTIONS

There is significant evidence that long-term, high-dose chitosan supplementation can result in malabsorption of some crucial nutrients, including calcium, magnesium, selenium, and vitamins A, D, E, and K.[8,13] In turn, this may create risk of osteoporosis in adults and growth retardation in children. For this reason, individuals using chitosan require general multinutrient supplementation.

Chitosan may alter intestinal flora, potentially allowing overgrowth of pathogenic bacteria.[13]

Due to its antinutrient effects, chitosan should not be used by pregnant or lactating women or young children. Safety in individuals with severe hepatic or renal disease has not been established.

DRUG INTERACTIONS

None known.

ADVERSE REACTIONS

Gastrointestinal side effects such as discomfort, flatulence, increased stool bulkiness, bloating, and mild nausea may occur with use of chitosan.[1] Increased water consumption may reduce these symptoms.

PROPOSED DOSAGE AND ADMINISTRATION

The usual dosage of chitosan is 3 to 6 g per day, taken in divided doses prior to meals.

PATIENT INFORMATION

Chitosan is a form of fiber extracted from crustaceans. It is widely marketed as a weight loss aid. However, the evidence that it works is limited to one small study. Chitosan is also said to reduce cholesterol levels, but it does not appear to be effective for this purpose. Other proposed uses of chitosan have no evidence at all behind them.

Use of chitosan can cause digestive discomfort. In addition, chitosan can cause depletion of various nutrients. This may lead to a risk of osteoporosis in adults and growth retardation in children. Taking a multivitamin and mineral supplement might help prevent these side effects.

Chitosan should not be used by pregnant or nursing women or young children. Individuals with severe liver or kidney disease should consult a physician before using this (or any other) supplement.

REFERENCES

1. Schiller RN, Barrager E, Schauss AG, et al. A randomized, double-blind, placebo-controlled study examining the effects of a rapidly soluble chitosan dietary supplement on weight loss and body composition in overweight and mildly obese individuals. *J Am Nutraceutical Assoc.* 2001;4:42-49. **2.** Pittler MH, Abbot NC, Harkness EF, et al. Randomized, double-blind trial of chitosan for body weight reduction. *Eur J Clin Nutr.* 1999;53:379-381. **3.** Maezaki Y, Tsuji K, Nakagawa Y, et al. Hypocholesterolemic effect of chitosan in adult males. *Biosci Biotechnol Biochem.* 1993;57:1439-1444. **4.** Jing SB, Li L, Ji D, et al. Effect of chitosan on renal function in patients with chronic renal failure. *J Pharm Pharmacol.* 1997;49:721-723. **5.** Ormrod D, Holmes CC, Miller TE. Dietary chitosan inhibits hypercholesterolaemia and atherogenesis in the apolipoprotein E-deficient mouse model of atherosclerosis. *Atherosclerosis.* 1998;138:329-334. **6.** Deuchi K, Kanauchi O, Imasato Y, et al. Decreasing effect of chitosan on the apparent fat digestibility by rats fed on a high-fat diet. *Biosci Biotechnol Biochem.* 1994;58:1613-1616. **7.** Deuchi K, Kanauchi O, Imasato Y, et al. Effect of the viscosity or deacetylation degree of chitosan on fecal fat excreted from rats fed on a high-fat diet. *Biosci Biotechnol Biochem.* 1995;59:781-785. **8.** Deuchi K, Kanauchi O, Shizukuishi M, et al. Continuous and massive intake of chitosan affects mineral and fat-soluble vitamin status in rats fed on a high-fat diet. *Biosci Biotechnol Biochem.* 1995;59:1211-1216. **9.** Kanauchi O, Deuchi K, Imasato Y, et al. Increasing effect of a chitosan and ascorbic acid mixture on fecal dietary fat excretion. *Biosci Biotechnol Biochem.* 1994;58:1617-1620. **10.** Kobayashi T, Otsuka S, Yugari Y. Effect of chitosan on serum and liver cholesterol levels in cholesterol-fed rats. *Nutr Rep Int.* 1979;19:327-334. **11.** Ho SC, Tai ES, Eng PH, et al. In the absence of dietary surveillance, chitosan does not reduce plasma lipids or obesity in hypercholesterolaemic obese Asian subjects. *Singapore Med J.* 2001;42:6-10. **12.** Jing SB, Li L, Ji D, et al. Effect of chitosan on renal function in patients with chronic renal failure. *J Pharm Pharmacol.* 1997;49:721-723. **13.** Koide SS. Chitin-chitosan: properties, benefits and risks. *Nutr Res.* 1998;18:1091-1101.

Chondroitin Sulfate

Alternate/Related Names: Chondroitin

U.S. BRAND NAMES OF CLINICALLY TESTED PRODUCTS

Cosamin DS (Nutramax Laboratories) (U.S. product only.)

DESCRIPTION

Chondroitin sulfate is a major natural component of the proteoglycans found in articular cartilage. Early studies on chondroitin concentrated on its use in the form of an intra-articular injection into osteoarthritic joints, but oral uses have come to predominate.

PHARMACOLOGY

Chondroitin sulfate is a hydrophilic sulfated glycosaminoglycan, composed of a long, unbranched polydisaccharide chain with alternating units of N-acetylgalactosamine and glucuronic acid. The N-acetylgalactosamine components are primarily mono-sulfated, usually in the 4- or 6-position, although some are unsulfated or disulfated.

It was once assumed that chondroitin could not be absorbed orally due to the size of the molecule. However, more recent animal studies using radiolabeled chondroitin sulfate have found that more than 70% of the radioactive material is absorbed after oral administration.[1] Not all of this radioactivity represents intact chondroitin; perhaps 5% to 15% of the total chondroitin intake is absorbed whole. Other studies suggest that absorption depends on molecular weight, with lower-molecular weight chondroitin products more readily absorbed.[2] In human volunteers, orally administered chondroitin was found to reach maximum plasma concentration in 5 hours, with a half-life of 10 hours and a time to steady-state concentration of 2 to 3 days.

Chondroitin may help retard osteoarthritic damage in several ways: by blocking the action of proteolytic enzymes (e.g., collagenase, elastase, proteoglycanase), enhancing repair mechanisms by stimulating proteoglycan synthesis, and by increasing levels of protective hyaluronic acid.[3,4,5] Furthermore, chondroitin may exert a mild, direct anti-inflammatory effect.[5]

CLINICAL STUDIES

Evidence from several studies suggests that chondroitin relieves symptoms of osteoarthritis more effectively than placebo, and that the results endure for at least 1 year. Weaker evidence suggests that chondroitin can alter the natural history of osteoarthritis by slowing progressive joint damage.

OSTEOARTHRITIS: SYMPTOMATIC IMPROVEMENT

Three recent double-blind placebo-controlled studies involving a total of about 250 participants have found that chondroitin can relieve symptoms of osteoarthritis.

One enrolled 85 people with osteoarthritis of the knee and followed them for 6 months.[6] Participants received either 400 mg of chondroitin sulfate twice daily or placebo, and evaluated the intensity of spontaneous daily joint pain using a Visual Analogue Scale (VAS). Other measurements included locomotor capacity, global efficacy and tolerability as judged by patients and physicians, and Lequesne's Index. Acetaminophen use as rescue medication was allowed but measured. Statistically significant differences between the treatment and control group were seen in most measures.

Comparable results were found in a 3-month double-blind placebo-controlled study of 127 individuals.[7] A third double-blind placebo-controlled study involved only 42 participants; however, it followed them for a full year.[8] Chondroitin took 3 months to reach its full effect, but eventually relieved symptoms more successfully than placebo.

Another double-blind study enrolled 146 individuals and compared the effects of chondroitin against diclofenac sodium.[9] The results showed that chondroitin acted less rapidly, but its results lingered for at least 3 months after cessation of treatment.

Generally positive results were also seen in other studies.[10-13]

OSTEOARTHRITIS: DISEASE-MODIFYING ACTIONS

Two studies in humans and one in animals provide suggestive evidence that chondroitin can slow the progression of osteoarthritis.

The 1-year trial of 42 individuals described above followed radiological and biochemical evidence of joint damage in addition to symptoms.[8] At month 12, the medial femorotibial joint space had decreased significantly in the placebo group but not in the chondroitin sulfate group. Biochemical markers of bone turnover also suggested a relative decrease in degradation.

Additional evidence comes from another double-blind placebo-controlled trial radiographically examining the progression of finger-joint osteoarthritis in 119 individuals for a full 3 years.[14] Over the study period, only 9% of the chondroitin group developed severely damaged joints, compared with almost 30% of the placebo group. Unfortunately, the researchers failed to report whether this difference was statistically significant.

Finally, the effects of both oral and injected chondroitin were assessed in rabbits with damaged cartilage in the knee.[15] After 84 days of treatment, the rabbits given chondroitin had significantly more healthy cartilage remaining in the damaged knee than the untreated animals. Oral chondroitin proved as effective as injection.

PROPOSED INDICATIONS AND USAGE

Meaningful but not definitive evidence suggests that low molecular weight chondroitin might offer symptomatic benefits in osteoarthritis. Weaker evidence suggests a possible disease-modifying effect.

Based on highly preliminary evidence, chondroitin has been proposed as a treatment for other conditions such as atherosclerosis, high cholesterol, and kidney stones.[16,17,18]

WARNINGS

None.

PRECAUTIONS

In clinical trials of chondroitin, hematological, renal, and hepatic assessments have showed no significant difference between treatment and placebo groups.[4,6-8]

Intake of about 1.5 g/kg has caused no mortality in rats or mice, and subacute and chronic administration of 100 mg/kg was not associated with any significant toxicity.[4] Mutagenicity studies and tests for alteration of blood coagulation also were negative.

Teratogenesis studies in rats and rabbits found no malformation of fetuses. However, the newborn of chondroitin sulfate-treated pregnant animals did weigh approximately 10% to 20% less than those of untreated controls. For this reason, chondroitin cannot be recommended for pregnant women at this time. Safety for young children, lactating women, or people with severe hepatic or renal disease has also not been established.

DRUG INTERACTIONS

None are known. However, formal drug interaction studies have not been performed.

ADVERSE REACTIONS

Other than occasional mild digestive disturbances and allergic reactions, orally administered chondroitin sulfate has not been associated with any significant side effects in clinical trials.[4,6-8]

PROPOSED DOSAGE AND ADMINISTRATION

The usual dosage of chondroitin is 400 mg taken 3 times daily, although 1,200 mg once per day has also been tried.[7] Studies suggest that a minimum treatment period of 3 months is necessary for full effect.

There are large differences between chondroitin products based on molecular weight and sulfation, leading to differences in absorption and hence effectiveness. The products most commonly used in double-blind trials are proprietary. It is not clear which competing products are equally effective, although it appears that low molecular weight chondroitin (less than 16,900 daltons) is better absorbed orally than products of higher molecular weight.[2]

For retail sale, chondroitin is often combined with glucosamine. Although there is evidence from human and veterinary trials that such combination products are effective,[19-23] there is only weak evidence that this more expensive combination therapy is superior to either treatment alone.[24,25]

PATIENT INFORMATION

Chondroitin is marketed as a treatment for osteoarthritis, and there is some evidence that it may be effective. Chondroitin appears to be a generally safe supplement. However, the safety of chondroitin sulfate for pregnant or nursing women or young children has not been established. In addition, individuals with severe liver or kidney disease should consult a physician before using this (or any other) supplement.

REFERENCES

1. Conte A, Volpi N, Palmieri L, et al. Biochemical and pharmacokinetic aspects of oral treatment with chondroitin sulfate. *Arzneimittelforschung.* 1995;45:918-925. **2.** Adebowale AO, Cox DS, Liang Z, et al. Analysis of glucosamine and chondroitin sulfate content in marketed products and the Caco-2 permeability of chondroitin sulfate raw materials. *J Am Nutraceutical Assoc.* 2000;3:37-44. **3.** Hungerford DS. Treating osteoarthritis with chondroprotective agents. *Orthop Spec Ed.* 1998;4:39-42. **4.** Paroli E, Antonilli L, Biffoni M. A pharmacological approach to glycosaminoglycans. *Drugs Exp Clin Res.* 1991;17:9-20. **5.** Ronca F, Palmieri L, Panicucci P, et al. Anti-inflammatory activity of chondroitin sulfate. *Osteoarthritis Cartilage.* 1998;6:14-21. **6.** Bucsi L, Poor G. Efficacy and tolerability of oral chondroitin sulfate as a symptomatic slow-acting drug for osteoarthritis (SYSADOA) in the treatment of knee osteoarthritis. *Osteoarthritis Cartilage.* 1998;6 Suppl A:31-36. **7.** Bourgeois P, Chales G, Dehais J, et al. Efficacy and tolerability of chondroitin sulfate 1200 mg/day vs chondroitin sulfate 3 × 400 mg/day vs placebo. *Osteoarthritis Cartilage.* 1998;6 Suppl A:25-30. **8.** Uebelhart D, Thonar EJ, Delmas PD, et al. Effects of oral chondroitin sulfate on the progression of knee osteoarthritis: a pilot study. *Osteoarthritis Cartilage.* 1998;6 Suppl A:39-46. **9.** Morreale P, Manopulo R, Galati M, et al. Comparison of the antiinflammatory efficacy of chondroitin sulfate and diclofenac sodium in patients with knee osteoarthritis. *J Rheumatol.* 1996;23:1385-1391. **10.** Conrozier T. Anti-arthrosis treatments: efficacy and tolerance of chondroitin sulfates (CS 4&6) [translated from French]. *Presse Med.* 1998;27:1862-1865. **11.** L'Hirondel JL. Double-blind clinical study with oral administration of chondroitin sulphate versus placebo in tibiofemoral gonarthrosis (125 patients) [in German]. *Litera Rheumatol.* 1992;14:77-84. **12.** Mazieres B, Loyau G, Menkes CJ, et al. Chondroitin sulfate in the treatment of gonarthrosis and coxarthrosis. 5-months result of a multicenter double-blind controlled prospective study using placebo [in French; English abstract]. *Rev Rhum Mal Osteoartic.* 1992;59:466-472. **13.** Mazieres B, Combe B, Phan Van A, et al. Chondroitin sulfate in osteoarthritis of the knee: a prospective, double blind, placebo controlled multicenter clinical study. *J Rheumatol.* 2001;28:173-181. **14.** Verbruggen G, Goemaere S, Veys EM. Chondroitin sulfate: S/DMOAD (structure/disease modifying anti-osteoarthritis drug) in the treatment of finger joint OA. *Osteoarthritis Cartilage.* 1998;6 Suppl A:37-38. **15.** Uebelhart D, Thonar EJ, Zhang J, et al. Protective effect of exogenous chondroitin 4,6-sulfate in the acute degradation of articular cartilage in the rabbit. *Osteoarthritis Cartilage.* 1998;6 Suppl A:6-13. **16.** Baggio B, Gambaro G, Marchini F, et al. Correction of erythrocyte abnormalities in idiopathic calcium-oxalate nephrolithiasis and reduction of urinary oxalate by oral glycosaminoglycans. *Lancet.* 1991;338:403-405. **17.** Nakazawa K. Effect of chondroitin sulfates on atherosclerosis. I. Long term oral administration of chondroitin sulfates to atherosclerotic subjects [in Japanese]. *Nippon Naika Gakkai Zasshi.* 1970;59:1084-1092. **18.** Nakazawa K, Murata K. Comparative study of the effects of chondroitin sulfate isomers on atherosclerotic subjects. *ZFA.* 1979;34:153-159. **19.** Leffler CT, Philippi AF, Leffler SG, et al. Glucosamine, chondroitin, and manganese ascorbate for degenerative joint disease of the knee or low back: a randomized, double-blind, placebo-controlled pilot study. *Mil Med.* 1999;164:85-91. **20.** Canapp SO Jr, McLaughlin RM Jr, Hoskinson JJ, et al. Scintigraphic evaluation of dogs with acute synovitis after treatment with glucosamine hydrochloride and chondroitin sulfate. *Am J Vet Res.* 1999;60:1552-1557. **21.** Hanson RR, Brawner WR, Hammad TA. The clinical profile of a glucosamine-chondroitin sulfate compound in a double-blinded, placebo-controlled, randomized trial as a selective symptom modifying nutraceutical for navicular syndrome: current data and perspectives. *Veterinary Orthopedic Society.* 1998;Feb:63. **22.** McNamara PS, Johnston SA, Todhunter RJ. Slow-acting, disease modifying osteoarthritis agents. *Vet Clin North Am Small Anim Pract.* 1997;27:863-881. **23.** Moore MG. Promising responses to a new oral treatment for degenerative joint disorders. *Canine Practice.* 1996;21:7-11. **24.** Lippiello L, Woodward J, Karpman R, et al. In vivo chondroprotection and metabolic synergy of glucosamine and chondroitin sulfate. *Clin Orthop.* 2000;381:229-240. **25.** Lippiello L, Karpman RR, Hammad T. Synergistic effect of glucosamine HCL and chondroitin sulfate on in vitro proteoglycan synthesis by bovine chondrocytes. Presented at: American Academy of Orthopaedic Surgeons 67th Annual Meeting; March 15-19, 2000; Orlando, Fla.

Chromium Picolinate

Alternate/Related Names: Chromium Picolinate, Chromium Polynicotinate, Chromium Chloride, High-Chromium Brewer's Yeast

U.S. BRAND NAMES OF CLINICALLY TESTED PRODUCTS

Not applicable.

DESCRIPTION

Chromium is believed to function physiologically as a low molecular weight Cr-nicotinic acid complex named glucose tolerance factor (GTF). It is believed essential to the action of insulin, potentiating and perhaps even permitting its effect.[1,2] Chromium picolinate is the most widely marketed form of chromium; chromium chloride and chromium polynicotinate are also available.

PHARMACOLOGY

Evidence from animal trials and three reports of patients on total peripheral nutrition (TPN) without chromium added has shown that chromium deficiency results in impaired glucose tolerance, elevated levels of serum insulin, weight loss, peripheral neuropathy, CNS disturbances, and elevated serum lipids.[2,3] These signs and symptoms are refractory to insulin but reversible with chromium administration. Chromium levels have been shown to fall when insulin concentrations rise, in both the short term and the long term.[4] This is believed to be related to chromium uptake by insulin-sensitive tissues.[5]

The low tissue concentrations of chromium involved and the potential contamination from sources such as tubing have made the task of isolating, identifying, and crystallizing GTF surprisingly difficult. One study has clouded the issue by finding that the GTF activity of yeast is not dependent on chromium concentrations.[6] The study authors suggest that GTF might not be a single substance. Other researchers have even suggested that GTF is based on cobalt rather than chromium.[2] It has been suggested that chromium can act as a membrane phosphotyrosine phosphatase activator.[7]

The effects and prevalence of mild chromium deficiency are unclear, partially due to the lack of an adequate protocol for determining chromium nutriture.[2] However, reports based on dietary analysis as well as other experimental techniques suggest that chromium is commonly marginally deficient in the American diet, especially in pregnant women and the elderly.[1,3,8-12] Marginal chromium deficiency may be a cause of subclinical impaired glucose tolerance and insulin resistance. Steroid-induced diabetes mellitus may also be partially related to chromium deficiency.[13]

CLINICAL STUDIES

SUBCLINICAL IMPAIRED GLUCOSE INTOLERANCE

A randomized double-blind study of fasting insulin levels in healthy young adults (n=26) found that 90 days of chromium (III)-nicotinate containing 220 mcg of chromium produced a significant decrease in immunoreactive insulin in those patients with initial fasting levels greater than 35 pmol/L.[14] Improvements in insulin sensitivity were seen in another small double-blind trial.[15]

A double-blind crossover study of 76 healthy individuals found that, among individuals with impaired glucose tolerance, chromium normalized glucose responses.[16] This occurred whether the abnormality was elevated or depressed serum glucose. Chromium had no effect on participants with normal glucose tolerance. However, a study of 26 elderly subjects with impaired glucose tolerance randomly treated with either chromium-rich yeast (160 mcg CR/day) or placebo showed no effect on glucose tolerance.[17]

DIABETES

A 4-month study reported in 1997 followed 180 Chinese men and women with type 2 diabetes, comparing the effects of 1,000 mcg chromium, 200 mcg chromium, and placebo. HbA_{1c} values improved significantly after 2 months in the group receiving 1,000 mcg, and in both chromium groups after 4 months. Fasting glucose was also lower in the higher-dose chromium group at 2 and 4 months, but not in the moderate-dose chromium group. Serum insulin levels decreased significantly in both groups at 2 and 4 months.[18]

Another double-blind trial compared placebo against chromium from Brewer's yeast (23.3 mcg chromium daily) and chromium chloride (200 mcg chromium daily) in 78 type 2 diabetics.[19] This rather complex crossover study consisted of four 8-week intervals of treatment in random order. The results in the 67 completers showed that both active treatments significantly improved glycemic control.

A study of 243 type 1 and type 2 diabetics found that chromium supplementation decreased insulin or oral hypoglycemic medication requirements in a significant percentage of cases.[20] However, only 10 participants were enrolled in a double-blind protocol; the remainder of the study was open label.

A double-blind study of 30 pregnant women with gestational diabetes found that supplementation with chromium at a dose of 4 or 8 mcg/kg chromium picolinate significantly improved blood sugar control as determined by HbA_{1c} measurement, as well as by measures of serum glucose and insulin.[21] The lower dose follows a common recommendation for pregnant women; the higher dose did not prove more effective.

Some small studies have found no effect on glucose tolerance.[22,23]

HYPERLIPIDEMIA

Studies of chromium's effects on serum lipids have shown a modest effect. In one double-blind trial, 76 patients with atherosclerotic disease were given either 250 mcg/day of chromium or placebo and were followed for an average of 11 months.[24] HDL cholesterol levels rose from 0.94 to 1.14 in the chromium-treated group but did not change significantly in the control group. Serum triglycerides at the end of the trial were lower in the treated group than in the control group (1.68 nmol/L vs. 2.10 nmol/L). No significant changes in total serum cholesterol were observed.

A double-blind crossover study followed 28 volunteers given either 200 mcg of chromium picolinate or placebo for 42 days and then switched after a 14-day period off treatments.[25] The results showed a modest but statistically significant drop in total cholesterol, LDL, and apolipoprotein B during chromium treatment and an increase in apolipoprotein A-I. Triglycerides did not change.

A study of 72 men taking beta-blockers, primarily for hypertension, showed a clinically useful increase in HDL cholesterol (>0.04 mmol/L) but no change in total cholesterol, triglycerides, or body weight.[26]

Another study found modest improvements in triglyceride levels in diabetics.[27] However, in other trials, no change in lipid levels was observed at all.[16,28] Furthermore, elevated lipids were not seen in three cases of TPN-induced severe chromium deficiency.[2]

WEIGHT LOSS AND BODYBUILDING

In a double-blind trial, 154 individuals were given either placebo or 200 or 400 mcg of chromium picolinate daily.[29] Over a period of 72 days, individuals taking chromium demonstrated increase in lean body mass and loss of fat mass, resulting in a net overall weight loss versus the placebo group. However, in a similar double-blind study by the same team, no statistically significant differences were seen.[30] The researchers resorted to additional statistical analysis in an attempt to show benefit.

A 16-week double-blind placebo-controlled study of 95 Navy personnel found no change in lean body mass with 400 mcg of chromium daily.[31] Smaller studies have produced generally negative results as well.[32-37]

HEART DISEASE PREVENTION

Insulin resistance and mildly impaired glucose tolerance have been strongly associated with increased risk of cardiovascular disease.[38-45] Based on chromium's influence on insulin resistance, as well as its potential effects on weight and lipid variables, chromium status has been evaluated for possible association with heart disease risk.

An observational trial using measurements of toenail chromium found associations between higher chromium intake and reduced risk of myocardial infarction.[46]

PROPOSED INDICATIONS AND USAGE

Based on current evidence, a trial of chromium supplementation at nutritional doses may be warranted in patients with impaired glucose tolerance or hyperlipidemia.

In diabetes, supranutritional doses of chromium might improve glucose control, but such treatment could cause symptoms of heavy metal toxicity in some patients (see Adverse Reactions).

Chromium is extensively marketed as a weight-loss aid, but the balance of the evidence is more negative than positive. Chromium has not been shown effective as an ergogenic aid.

WARNINGS

Chromium is a heavy metal, and in some cases tissue accumulation has apparently occurred at dosage only several times higher than the estimated safe and adequate intake. Exanthematous pustulosis has also been reported. There are also theoretical concerns that picolinate might alter levels of neurotransmitters or cause adverse effects on DNA.

PRECAUTIONS

Chromium supplementation above nutritional requirements is not recommended for individuals with renal or hepatic disease (see Adverse Reactions).

Concerns have also been raised over the use of the picolinate form of chromium in individuals suffering from affective or psychotic disorders, because picolinic acids can change levels of neurotransmitters.[47] There are also theoretical concerns that chromium picolinate could cause adverse effects on DNA.[48]

Several toxicological studies have shown that hexavalent chromium can present health risks.[2] However, this is not the form used nutritionally.

Maximum safe dosage for young children, pregnant or lactating women, or individuals with severe hepatic or renal disease has not been established. Because of the theoretical possibility of DNA damage, forms of chromium other than chromium picolinate may be preferable in pregnancy.

DRUG INTERACTIONS

If chromium therapy proves successful, reduction in dosages of hypoglycemic agents may be necessary.

Beta-blockers may reduce HDL cholesterol levels. According to a double-blind placebo-controlled trial of 72 men, chromium supplementation may correct this side effect, raising HDL levels in individuals.[26]

Simultaneous intake of calcium carbonate may impair chromium absorption.[49]

ADVERSE REACTIONS

Trivalent chromium, the form taken in OTC supplements, is generally well tolerated and dosages within the nutritional recommendations given above are believed to be safe. Studies sponsored by the U.S. Department of Agriculture have shown no toxicity in rats even at a 100 mg/kg dose of chromium chloride or chromium tripicolinate over a period of 24 weeks.[50] However, supranutritional doses of chromium may at times idiosyncratically produce symptoms of heavy-metal toxicity. One case report has been published of anemia, thrombocytopenia, hemolysis, weight loss, and hepatic and renal toxicity in a woman taking 1,200 to 2,400 mcg of chromium picolinate daily for 4 to 5 months,[51] and another found acute interstitial nephritis in a woman taking only 600 mcg of chromium daily for 6 weeks.[52]

In addition, there has been one report of acute generalized exanthematous pustulosis caused by chromium picolinate at a dose of 1,000 mcg daily.[53]

PROPOSED DOSAGE AND ADMINISTRATION

Estimated safe and adequate daily intakes of chromium are as follows: under 6 months, 10 to 40 mcg; 6 months to 1 year, 20 to 60 mcg; 1 to 3 years, 20 to 80 mcg; 4 to 6 years, 30 to 120 mcg; and over 7 years, 50 to 200 mcg. For pregnant women, a dose of 4 mcg/kg has been proposed.

In studies of chromium for diabetes, a dose of 1,000 mcg daily has been used. However, case reports suggest the possibility of idiosyncratic toxic reactions at this dose (see Adverse Reactions).

PATIENT INFORMATION

Chromium is a mineral that is essential for good nutrition. Some evidence suggests that making sure to get enough chromium might improve blood sugar control and cholesterol levels. However, taking excessive doses of chromium could be dangerous. In addition, if you have diabetes, do not use chromium (or any other supplement) without consulting a physician.

Chromium is widely marketed as a weight loss aid. However, most studies have found it ineffective for this purpose. There is no evidence that chromium improves sports performance.

Pregnant or nursing women and individuals with liver or kidney disease should consult a physician before taking chromium.

REFERENCES

1. Anderson RA. Chromium, glucose tolerance, and diabetes. *Biol Trace Elem Res.* 1992;32:19-24. **2.** Mertz W. Chromium in human nutrition: a review. *J Nutr.* 1993;123:626-633. **3.** Anderson RA. Chromium and parenteral nutrition. *Nutrition.* 1995;11:83-86. **4.** Morris BW, Blumsohn A, Mac Neil S, et al. The trace element chromium—a role in glucose homeostasis. *Am J Clin Nutr.* 1992;55:989-991. **5.** Morris BW, Gray TA, Macneil S. Glucose-dependent uptake of chromium in human and rat insulin-sensitive tissues. *Clin Sci.* 1993;84:477-482. **6.** Simonoff M, Shapcott D, Alameddine S, et al. The isolation of glucose tolerance factors from brewer's yeast and their relation to chromium. *Biol Trace Elem Res.* 1992;32:25-38. **7.** Davis CM, Sumrall KH, Vincent JB. A biologically active form of chromium may activate a membrane phosphotyrosine phosphatase (PTP). *Biochemistry.* 1996;35:12963-12969. **8.** Anderson RA. Recent advances in the clinical and biochemical effects of chromium deficiency. *Prog Clin Biol Res.* 1993;380:221-234. **9.** Anderson RA, Kozlovsky AS. Chromium intake, absorption and excretion of subjects consuming self-selected diets. *Am J Clin Nutr.* 1985;41:1177-1183. **10.** Davies S, McLaren Howard J, Hunnisett A, et al. Age-related decreases in chromium levels in 51,665 hair, sweat, and serum samples from 40,872 patients—implications for the prevention of cardiovascular disease and type II diabetes mellitus. *Metabolism.* 1997;46:469-473. **11.** Schroeder HA. The role of chromium in mammalian nutrition. *Am J Clin Nutr.* 1968;21:230-244. **12.** Mossop RT. Trivalent chromium, in atherosclerosis and diabetes. *Cent Afr J Med.* 1991;37:369-374. **13.** Ravina A, Slezak L, Mirsky N, et al. Control of steriod-induced diabetes with supplemental chromium. *J Trace Elem Exp Med.* 1999;12:375-378. **14.** Wilson BE, Gondy A. Effects of chromium supplementation on fasting insulin levels and lipid parameters in healthy, non-obese young subjects. *Diabetes Res Clin Pract.* 1995;28:179-184. **15.** Cefalu WT, Bell-Farrow AD, Stegner J, et al. Effect of chromium picolinate on insulin sensitivity in vivo. *J Trace Elem Exp Med.* 1999;12:71-83. **16.** Anderson RA, Polansky MM, Bryden NA, et al. Chromium supplementation of human subjects: effects on glucose, insulin, and lipid variables. *Metabolism.* 1983;32:894-899. **17.** Uusitupa MI, Mykkanen L, Siitonen O, et al. Chromium supplementation in impaired glucose tolerance of elderly: effects on blood glucose, plasma insulin, C-peptide and lipid levels. *Br J Nutr.* 1992;68:209-216. **18.** Anderson RA, Cheng N, Bryden NA, et al. Elevated intakes of supplemental chromium improve glucose and insulin variables in individuals with type 2 diabetes. *Diabetes.* 1997;46:1786-1791. **19.** Bahijiri SM, Mira SA, Mufti AM, et al. The effects of inorganic chromium and brewer's yeast supplementation on glucose tolerance, serum lipids and drug dosage in individuals with type 2 diabetes. *Saudi Med J.* 2000;21:831-837. **20.** Ravina A, Slezack L. Chromium in the treatment of clinical diabetes mellitus [translated from Hebrew]. *Harefuah.* 1993;125:142-145. **21.** Jovanovic L, Gutierrez M, Peterson CM. Chromium supplementation for women with gestational diabetes mellitus. *J Trace Elem Exp Med.* 1999;12;91-97. **22.** Rabinowitz MB, Gonick HC, Levin SR, et al. Effects of chromium and yeast supplements on carbohydrate and lipid metabolism in diabetic men. *Diabetes Care.* 1983;6:319-327. **23.** Trow LG, Lewis J, Greenwood RH, et al. Lack of effect of dietary chromium supplementation on glucose tolerance, plasma insulin and lipoprotein levels in patients with type 2 diabetes. *Int J Vitam Nutr Res.* 2000;70:14-18. **24.** Abraham AS, Brooks BA, Eylath U. The effects of chromium supplementation on serum glucose and lipids in patients with and without non-insulin-dependent diabetes. *Metabolism.* 1992;41:768-771. **25.** Press RI, Geller J, Evans GW. The effect of chromium picolinate on serum cholesterol and apolipoprotein fractions in human subjects. *West J Med.* 1990;152:41-45. **26.** Roeback JR Jr, Hla KM, Chambless LE, et al. Effects of chromium supplementation on serum high-density lipoprotein cholesterol levels in men taking beta-blockers. A randomized, controlled trial. *Ann Intern Med.* 1991;115:917-924. **27.** Lee NA, Reasner CA. Beneficial effect of chromium supplementation on serum triglyceride levels in NIDDM. *Diabetes Care.* 1994;17:1449-1452. **28.** Offenbacher EG, Rinko CJ, Pi-Sunyer FX. The effects of inorganic chromium and brewer's yeast on glucose tolerance, plasma lipids, and plasma chromium in elderly subjects. *Am J Clin Nutr.* 1985;42:454-461. **29.** Kaats GR, Blum K, Fisher JA, et al. Effects of chromium picolinate supplementation on body composition: a randomized, double-masked, placebo-controlled study. *Curr Ther Res.* 1996;57:747-765. **30.** Kaats GR, Blum K, Pullin D, et al. A randomized, double-masked, placebo-controlled study of the effects of chromium picolinate supplementation on body composition: a replication and extension of a previous study. *Curr Ther Res.* 1998;59:379-388. **31.** Trent LK, Thieding-Cancel D. Effects of chromium picolinate on body composition. *J Sports Med Phys Fitness.* 1995;35:273-280. **32.** Clancy SP, Clarkson PM, DeCheke ME, et al. Effects of chromium picolinate supplementation on body composition, strength, and urinary chromium loss in football players. *Int J Sport Nutr.* 1994;4:142-153. **33.** Amato P, Morales AJ, Yen SS. Effects of chromium picolinate supplementation on insulin sensitivity, serum lipids, and body composition in healthy, nonobese, older men and women. *J Gerontol A Biol Sci Med Sci.* 2000;55:M260-M263. **34.** Lukaski HC, Bolonchuk WW, Siders WA, et al. Chromium supplementation and resistance training: effects on body composition, strength, and trace element status of men. *Am J Clin Nutr.* 1996;63:954-964. **35.** Hallmark MA, Reynolds TH, DeSouza CA, et al. Effects of chromium and resistive training on muscle strength and body composition. *Med Sci Sports Exerc.* 1996;28:139-144. **36.** Volpe SL, Huang HW, Larpadisorn K, et al. Effect of chromium supplementation and exercise on body composition, resting metabolic rate and selected biochemical parameters in moderately obese women following an exercise program. *J Am Coll Nutr.* 2001;20:293-306. **37.** Grant KE, Chandler RM, Castle AL, et al. Chromium and exercise training: effect on obese women. *Med Sci Sports Exerc.* 1997;29:992-998. **38.** Laws A, King AC, Haskell WL, et al. Relation of fasting plasma insulin concentration to high density lipoprotein cholesterol and triglyceride concentrations in men. *Arterioscler Thromb.* 1991;11:1636-1642. **39.** Job FP, Wolfertz J, Meyer R, et al. Hyperinsulinism in patients with coronary artery disease. *Coron Artery Dis.* 1994;5:487-492. **40.** Fontbonne A, Tchobroutsky G, Eschwege E, et al. Coronary heart disease mortality risk: plasma insulin level is a more sensitive marker than hypertension or abnormal glucose tolerance in overweight males. The Paris Prospective Study. *Int J Obes.* 1988;12:557-565. **41.** Despres JP, Lamarche B, Mauriege P, et al. Hyperinsulinemia as an independent risk factor for ischemic heart disease. *N Engl J Med.* 1996;334:952-957. **42.** Pyorala K, Savolainen E, Kaukola S, et al. Plasma insulin as coronary heart disease risk factor: relationship to other risk factors and predictive value during 9 1/2-year follow-up of the Helsinki Policemen Study population. *Acta Med Scand Suppl.* 1985;701:38-52. **43.** Lamarche B, Tchernof A, Mauriege P, et al. Fasting insulin and apolipoprotein B levels and low-density lipoprotein particle size as risk factors for ischemic heart disease. *JAMA.* 1998;279:1955-1961. **44.** Saydah SH, Eberhardt MS, Loria CM, et al. Subclinical states of glucose intolerance and the risk of death in the United States [abstract]. *Diabetes.* 1999;48(suppl 1):A#068. **45.** Haffner SM. The importance of hyperglycemia in the nonfasting state to the development of cardiovascular disease. *Endocr Rev.* 1998;19:583-592. **46.** Guallar E, Jimenez J, van t' Veer P, et al. The association of chromium with the risk of a first myocardial infaction in men. The EURAMIC Study [abstract]. *Circulation.* 2001;103:1366. **47.** Reading SAJ, Wecker L. Chromium picolinate. *J Fla Med Assoc.* 1996;83;29-31. **48.** Speetjens JK, Collins RA, Vincent JB, et al. The nutritional supplement chromium (III) tris(picolinate) cleaves DNA. *Chem Res Toxicol.* 1999;12:483-487. **49.** Seaborn CD, Stoecker BJ. Effects of antacid or ascorbic acid on tissue accumulation and urinary excretion of 51-chromium. *Nutr Res.* 1990;10:1401-1407. **50.** Anderson RA, Bryden NA, Polansky MM. Lack of toxicity of chromium chloride and chromium picolinate in rats. *J Am Coll Nutr.* 1997;16:273-279. **51.** Cerulli J, Grabe DW, Gauthier I, et al. Chromium picolinate toxicity. *Ann Pharmacother.* 1998;32:428-431. **52.** Wasser WG, Feldman NS, D'Agati VD. Chronic renal failure after ingestion of over-the-counter chromium picolinate [letter]. *Ann Intern Med.* 1997;126:410. **53.** Young PC, Turiansky GW, Bonner MW, et al. Acute generalized exanthematous pustulosis induced by chromium picolinate. *J Am Acad Dermatol.* 1999;41:820-823.

Coenzyme Q_{10}

Alternate/Related Names: CoQ_{10}

U.S. BRAND NAMES OF CLINICALLY TESTED PRODUCTS

None.

DESCRIPTION

Coenzyme Q_{10} (CoQ_{10}) is widely utilized in Europe, Israel, and Japan as an approved adjunctive treatment for a variety of cardiovascular conditions. Its use is based on the theory that local CoQ_{10} deficiency is a central process in congestive heart failure (CHF) and other cardiovascular diseases. In addition, numerous pharmaceuticals used in cardiovascular conditions, such as statins and many antihypertensives and diuretics, appear to reduce production or impair activity of endogenous CoQ_{10}; therefore, supplemental CoQ_{10} might correct potential harm caused by the use of these agents. However, the evidence base for using CoQ_{10} as adjunctive therapy for any condition remains incomplete.

PHARMACOLOGY

CoQ_{10} serves as a major redox component in the coupled mitochondrial mechanisms of electron transfer and oxidative phosphorylation. Certain illnesses such as CHF have been associated with reduced tissue levels of CoQ_{10}.[1,2] It has been suggested that mitochondrial dysfunction and consequent energy starvation due to this relative deficiency as well as other factors may be a primary physiological disturbance in CHF and cardiomyopathies.[2,3,4] Proponents of this view believe that CoQ_{10} supplementation may be a metabolically appropriate treatment for these conditions, improving myocardial aerobic energy production and hence cardiac function.

In reperfusion after ischemia, CoQ_{10} may function by preventing oxidative damage to creatine kinase and other substances.[5] Other authors have concluded that CoQ_{10} does not scavenge the free radicals produced in reperfusion, but rather enhances the recovery of high-energy phosphates, thereby preventing Ca^{2+} overload.[6]

Bioavailability tests using low doses of oral CoQ_{10} (30 mg) show peak plasma levels of about 1 mg/L.[7] Dietary CoQ_{10} appears to function like vitamin E in preventing lipid peroxidation[8,9] and can exert a vitamin E-sparing effect.[10]

CLINICAL STUDIES

CONGESTIVE HEART FAILURE

A double-blind multicenter study followed 641 patients with NYHA class III or IV failure for 1 year.[3] Half were given 2 mg/kg of CoQ_{10} orally, and the rest placebo. Conventional therapy was continued. The results showed a progressive and statistically significant reduction in CHF class as well as a reduced need for hospitalizations over the course of the study in the treated group as compared to the placebo group.

Benefits were seen in other studies involving a total of about 300 individuals.[11,12,13] However, a 6-month double-blind study of 45 individuals with CHF found no benefit.[14]

CARDIOMYOPATHY

The evidence base for the use of CoQ_{10} for cardiomyopathy consists primarily of low-quality trials. Most were not blinded.[15,16,17] One double-blind trial followed 80 patients with various cardiomyopathies over a period of 3 years, and found some evidence of benefit with CoQ_{10} at 100 mg daily.[18] However, the involvement of participants with mixed diagnoses detracts from the meaningfulness of the results. In addition, a double-blind placebo-controlled crossover study that followed 25 patients with idiopathic dilated cardiomyopathy for a total period of 8 months found no benefit with CoQ_{10} at a dose of 100 mg/day.[19]

CARDIOPROTECTION IN CARDIAC SURGERY

Animal studies of CoQ_{10} for reducing reperfusion injury have yielded contradictory results.[6,20-22] The results of small human trials using CoQ_{10} pretreatment in cardiac surgery are similarly mixed.[5,23-25]

HYPERTENSION

An 8-week double-blind placebo-controlled study of 59 hypertensive men receiving conventional treatment found that 120 mg CoQ_{10} daily reduced average systolic blood pressure by 10% and diastolic blood pressure by about 9%, while insignificant changes were seen in the placebo group.[26] Significant improvements in systolic and diastolic blood pressure were seen in a small ($n=18$) double-blind crossover study of CoQ_{10} with 10-week treatment periods.[27]

CORRECTION OF DRUG-INDUCED RELATIVE DEPLETION

Some evidence suggests that a variety of pharmaceuticals might cause depletion of CoQ_{10} or interfere with its action. It has been suggested that CoQ_{10} deficiency or inhibition may play a role in the known side effects of these pharmaceuticals, and that concomitant CoQ_{10} supplementation may be beneficial. However, there is little direct evidence for either of these assertions.

The best evidence for pharmaceutical-induced depletion of or interference with endogenous CoQ_{10} involves agents in the statin family. HMG-CoA reductase is necessary for the synthesis of both cholesterol and CoQ_{10}; for this reason, statin drugs would be expected to reduce CoQ_{10} levels. Double-blind placebo-controlled trials have found that lovastatin, pravastatin, and simvastatin significantly reduce plasma CoQ_{10} levels[28]; one of these studies found that CoQ_{10} supplementation can prevent both plasma and platelet CoQ_{10} reduction without affecting the therapeutic effect of simvastatin.[29] Highly preliminary evidence suggests that statin-induced reductions in endogenous CoQ_{10} may be clinically significant.[30]

The evidence for drug-induced depletion of or interference with CoQ_{10} is more indirect for several other categories of drugs, including sulfonylureas (acetohexamide, glyburide, phenformin, and tolazamide; tolbutamide, glipizide, and chlorpropamide may be relatively noninhibitory), beta-blockers (propranolol, metoprolol, and alprenolol; timolol was relatively noninhibitory), phenothiazines, tricyclic antidepressants (supplemental CoQ_{10} may be protective against cardiac side effects), diazoxide, methyldopa, hydrochlorothiazide, clonidine, and hydralazine.[31-35]

CARDIOPROTECTIVE EFFECT IN DOXORUBICIN CHEMOTHERAPY

Animal and preliminary human trials suggest that CoQ_{10} might protect against doxorubicin cardiotoxicity.[16,36,37]

EXERCISE PERFORMANCE

Many small studies have evaluated CoQ_{10} as a potential ergogenic aid, but most have failed to find evidence of benefit.[38-44]

PERIODONTAL DISEASE

Although several studies purport to find that CoQ_{10} can help periodontal disease,[45,46] the meaningfulness of these poorly designed and inadequately reported studies has been sharply criticized.[47]

PROPOSED INDICATIONS AND USAGE

CoQ_{10} may be useful adjunctive treatment in CHF, possibly improving functional capacity and decreasing the incidence of hospitalization. Other potential uses include cardioprotection during cardiac surgery, and the treatment of cardiomyopathy and hypertension, but the evidence is weak at best.

CoQ_{10} may be a useful repletion therapy in patients taking drugs that reduce endogenous CoQ_{10} levels, such as HMG-CoA reductase inhibitors, but this has not been proven.[29] Similarly, CoQ_{10} might help prevent cardiac toxicity caused by doxorubicin, but more research is needed to establish this.

Pilot trials suggest that CoQ_{10} might be useful in Duchenne, Becker, and the limb-girdle muscular dystrophies as well as in myotonic dystrophy, Charcot-Marie-Tooth disease, and Kugelberg-Welander disease disease.[48]

CoQ_{10} is widely marketed for preventing heart disease and cancer, improving energy, aiding in weight loss, and enhancing sports performance, despite the lack of any meaningful evidence that it is effective for these purposes.

WARNINGS

There have been anecdotal reports of a CoQ_{10}-withdrawal syndrome in CHF, leading to temporarily worsening failure.

PRECAUTIONS

A study of hypertensive men unexpectedly found reduction of fasting glucose levels in the group treated with CoQ_{10}.[26] However, another trial in diabetics found no effect on glycemic control.[49] Nonetheless, serum glucose monitoring appears appropriate if diabetics begin using CoQ_{10} (to offset the potential CoQ_{10} depletion apparently caused by some oral hypoglycemic agents, for example).

Abrupt discontinuation of CoQ_{10} during treatment of CHF should be avoided.

Maximum safe dosage in young children, pregnant or lactating women, or individuals with severe hepatic or renal disease has not been established.

DRUG INTERACTIONS

One animal study suggests that CoQ_{10} can prolong the effects of antihypertensives without increasing their maximum hypotensive effect.[50]

CoQ_{10} was found to reduce fasting glucose levels in a recent study of individuals with hypertension.[26] This has led to the suggestion that a reduction in oral hypoglycemic dose may be necessary in individuals using CoQ_{10} for repletion therapy (or during concomitant use for any reason). However, another trial in diabetics found no effect on glycemic control.[49]

ADVERSE REACTIONS

CoQ_{10} is generally well tolerated. In large double-blind and open studies lasting up to 1 year, no serious side effects or drug interactions were noted, and the incidence of minor side effects was generally less than 1.5%.[3,51] A 6-year study of 143 patients showed no toxicity or intolerance.[15]

PROPOSED DOSAGE AND ADMINISTRATION

The typical dose of CoQ_{10} ranges from 30 to 150 mg/day, given in 2 or 3 divided doses at the higher levels. This fat-soluble substance is better absorbed when taken in oil-based soft-gel form.[52]

PATIENT INFORMATION

CoQ_{10} is a substance that occurs naturally in the body. It plays an important role in the process by which cells produce energy.

There is some evidence that supplemental CoQ_{10} may be useful in congestive heart failure (CHF). However, because CHF is a dangerous illness, medical supervision is strongly advised before self-treatment with CoQ_{10} or any other supplement. Additionally, keep in mind that CoQ_{10} has only been investigated as an addition to standard treatment, not a substitute for it. Furthermore, discontinuation of CoQ_{10} by individuals with CHF may be dangerous.

A wide variety of medications are believed to reduce CoQ_{10} levels, or impair its action in the body. For this reason, supplemental CoQ_{10} has been advocated for people taking these medications. However, there is no real evidence as yet that taking extra CoQ_{10} will actually provide any noticeable benefit.

CoQ_{10} has been suggested for other heart-related conditions, such as high blood pressure, but the there is little evidence that it is effective. Other proposed uses of CoQ_{10}, such as preventing heart disease and cancer, improving energy, aiding in weight loss, and enhancing sports performance, have no evidence behind them.

The maximum safe dosage of CoQ_{10} for pregnant or nursing women or young children has not been established. Individuals with severe liver or kidney disease should consult a physician before using this (or any other) supplement.

REFERENCES

1. Kitamura N, et al. Myocardial tissue level of coenzyme Q_{10} in patients with cardiac failure. In Folkers K and Y Yamamura, eds. *Biomedical and clinical aspects of Coenzyme Q*, Vol 4. Amsterdam: Elsevier Science Publishers;1994. **2.** Mortensen SA, Vadhanavikit S, Muratsu K, et al. Coenzyme Q10: clinical benefits with biochemical correlates suggesting a scientific breakthrough in the management of chronic heart failure. *Int J Tissue React.* 1990;12:155-162. **3.** Morisco C, Trimarco B, Condorelli M. Effect of coenzyme Q10 therapy in patients with congestive heart failure: a long-term multicenter randomized study. *Clin Investig.* 1993;71:s134-s136. **4.** Folkers K. Heart failure is a dominant deficiency of coenzyme Q10 and challenges for future clinical research on CoQ10. *Clin Investig.* 1993;71(suppl 8):S51-S54. **5.** Chello M, Mastroroberto P, Romano R, et al. Protection by coenzyme Q10 from myocardial reperfusion injury during coronary artery bypass grafting. *Ann Thorac Surg.* 1994;58:1427-1432. **6.** Hano O, Thompson-Gorman S, Zweifer J, et al. Coenzyme Q10 enhances cardiac functional and metabolic recovery and reduces Ca2+ overload during postischemic reperfusion. *Am J Physiol.* 1994;266:H2174-H2181. **7.** Weber C, Bysted A, Holmer G. Intestinal absorption of coenzyme Q10 administered in a meal or as capsules to healthy subjects. *Nutr Res.* 1997;17:941-945. **8.** Weber C, Jakobsen TS, Mortensen SA, et al. Effect of dietary coenzyme Q10 as an antioxidant in human plasma. *Mol Aspects Med.* 1994;15(Suppl):S97-S102. **9.** Weber C, Sejersgard Jakobsen T, Mortensen SA, et al. Antioxidative effect of dietary coenzyme Q10 in human blood plasma. *Int J Vitam Nutr Res.* 1994;64:311-315. **10.** Alleva R, Tomasetti M, Battino M, et al. The roles of coenzyme Q10 and vitamin E on the peroxidation of human low density lipoprotein subfractions. *Proc Natl Acad Sci U S A.* 1995;92:9388-9391. **11.** Hashiba K, Kuramoto K, Ishimi Z, et al. Coenzyme-Q10 [in Japanese]. *Heart (Japanese).* 1972;4:1579-1589. **12.** Hofman-Bang C, Rehnquist N, Swedberg K, et al. Coenzyme Q10 as an adjunctive in treatment of congestive heart failure. *J Am Coll Cardiol.* 1992;19:216A. **13.** Munkholm H, Hansen HH, Rasmussen K. Coenzyme Q10 treatment in serious heart failure. *Biofactors.* 1999;9:285-289. **14.** Khatta M, Alexander BS, Krichten CM, et al. Long-term efficacy of coenzyme Q10 therapy for congestive heart failure. Presented at: 72nd Scientific Sessions of the American Heart Association; November 7-10, 1999; Atlanta, Ga. **15.** Langsjoen PH, Langsjoen PH, Foilkers K. A six-year clinical study of therapy of cardiomyopathy with coenzyme Q10. *Int J Tissue React.* 1990;12:169-171. **16.** Judy WV, Hall JH, Dugan W, et al. Coenzyme Q10 reduction of Adriamycin cardiotoxicity. *Biomed Clin Aspects Coenzyme Q.* 1984;4:231-241. **17.** Manzoli U, Rossi E, Littarru GP, et al. Coenzyme Q10 in dilated cardiomyopathy. *Int J Tissue React.* 1990;12:173-178. **18.** Langsjoen PH, Vadhhanavikit S, Folkers K. Response of patients in classes III and IV of cardiomyopathy to therapy in a blind and crossover trial with coenzyme Q10. *Proc Natl Acad Sci.* 1985;82:4240-4244. **19.** Permanetter B, Rossy W, Klein G, et al. Ubiquinone (coenzyme Q10) in the long-term treatment of idiopathic dilated cardiomyopathy.*Eur Heart J.* 1992;13:1528-1533. **20.** Birnbaum Y, Hale SL, Kloner RA. The effect of coenzyme Q10 on infarct size in a rabbit model of ischemia/reperfusion. *Cardiovasc Res.* 1996;32:861-868. **21.** Matsushima T, Sueda T, Matsuura Y, et al. Protection by coenzyme Q10 of canine myocardial reperfusion injury after preservation. *J Thorac Cardiovasc Surg.* 1992;103:945-951. **22.** Rosenfeldt FL, Pepe S, Ou R, et al. Coenzyme Q10 improves the tolerance of the senescent myocardium to aerobic and ischemic stress: studies in rats and in human atrial tissue. *Biofactors.* 1999;9:291-299. **23.** Taggart DP, Jenkins M, Hooper J, et al. Effects of short-term supplementation with coenzyme Q10 on myocardial protection during cardiac operations. *Ann Thorac Surg.* 1996;61:829-833. **24.** Judy WV, Stogsdill WW, Folkers K. Myocardial preservation by therapy with coenzyme Q10 during heart surgery. *Clin Investig.* 1993;71(8 Suppl):S155 - S161. **25.** Chen YF, Lin YT, We SC, et al. Effectiveness of coenzyme Q10 on myocardial preservation during hypothermic cardioplegic arrest. *J Thorac Cardiovasc Surg.* 1994;107:242-247. **26.** Singh R, Niaz M, Rastogi S, et al. Effect of hydrosoluble coenzyme Q10 on blood pressures and insulin resistance in hypertensive patients with coronary artery disease. *J Hum Hypertens.* 1999;13:203-208. **27.** Digiesi V, Cantini F, Brodbeck B. Effect of coenzyme Q10 on essential arterial hypertension. *Curr Ther Res.* 1990;47:841-845. **28.** Ghirlanda G, Oradei A, Manto A, et al. Evidence of plasma CoQ10-lowering effect by HMG-CoA reductase inhibitors: a double-blind, placebo-controlled study. *J Clin Pharmacol.* 1993;33:226-229. **29.** Bargossi AM, Battino M, Gaddi A, et al. Exogenous CoQ10 preserves plasma ubiquinone levels in patients treated with 3-hydroxy-3-methylglutaryl coenzyme A reductase inhibitors. *Int J Clin Lab Res.* 1994;24:171-176. **30.** Folkers K, Langsjoen P, Willis R, et al. Lovastatin decreases coenzyme Q levels in humans. *Proc Natl Acad Sci U S A.* 1990;87:8931-8934. **31.** Kishi T, Kishi H, Watanabe T, Folkers K. Bioenergetics in clinical medicine. XI. Studies on coenzyme Q and diabetes mellitus. *J Med.* 1976;7:307-321. **32.** Kishi T, Watanabe T, Folkers K. Bioenergetics in clinical medicine XV. Inhibition of coenzyme Q10-enzymes by clinically used adrenergic blockers of beta-receptors. *Res Commun Chem Pathol Pharmacol.* 1977;17:157-164. **33.** Kishi T, Makino K, Okamoto T, et al. Inhibition of myocardial respiration by psychotherapeutic drugs and prevention by coenzyme Q. *Biomed Clin Aspects Coenzyme Q.* 1980;2:139-157. **34.** Kishi H, Kishi T, Folkers K. Bioenergetics in clinical medicine. III. Inhibition of coenzyme Q10-enzymes by clinically used anti-hypertensive drugs. *Res Commun Chem Pathol Pharmacol.* 1975;12:533-540. **35.** Folkers K. Basic chemical research on coenzyme Q10 and integrated clinical research on therapy of diseases. *Biomed Clin Aspects Coenzyme Q.* 1985;5:457-478. **36.** Combs AB, Choe JY, Truong DH, et al. Reduction by coenzyme Q10 of the acute toxicity of adriamycin in mice. *Res Commun Chem Pathol Pharmacol.* 1977;18:565-568. **37.** Sugiyama S, Yamada K, Hayakawa M, et al. Approaches that mitigate doxorubicin-induced delayed adverse effects on mitochondrial functions in rat hearts; Liposome-encapsulated doxorubican or combination therapy with antioxidant. *Biochem Mol Biol Int.* 1995;36:1001-1007. **38.** Braun B, Clarkson M, Freedson PS, et al. Effects of coenzyme Q10 supplementation on exercise performance, VO2 max and lipid peroxidation in trained cyclists. *Int J Sport Nutr.* 1991;1:353-365. **39.** Snider IP, Bazarre TL, Murdoch SD, et al. Effects of coenzyme athletic performance system as an ergogenic aid on endurance performances to exhaustion. *Int J Sport Nutr.* 1992;2:272-286. **40.** Porter DA, Costill DL, Zachwieja JJ, et al. The effect of oral coenzyme Q10 on the exercise tolerance of middle-aged, untrained men. *Int J Sports Med.* 1995;16:421-427. **41.** Malm C, Svensson M, Ekblom B, et al. Effects of ubiquinone-10 supplementation and high intensity training on physical performance in humans. *Acta Physiol Scand.* 1997;161:379-984. **42.** Weston SB, Zhou S, Weatherby RP, et al. Does exogenous coenzyme Q10 affect aerobic capacity in endurance athletes? *Int J Sport Nutr.* 1997;7:197-206. **43.** Zuliani U, Bonetti A, Campana M, et al. The influence of ubiquinone (Co Q10) on the metabolic response to work. *J Sports Med Phys Fitness.* 1989;29:57-62. **44.** Ylikoski T, et al. The effect of coenzyme Q10 on the exercise performance of cross-country skiers. *Mol Aspects Med.* 1997;18:S283-S290. **45.** Folkers K, Watanabe T. Bioenergetics in clinical medicine-X. Survey of the adjunctive use of coenzyme Q with oral therapy in treating periodontal disease. *J Med.* 1977;8:333-348. **46.** Iwamoto Y, Watanabe T, Okamoto H, et al. Clinical effect of coenzyme Q10 on periodontal disease. *Biomed Clin Aspects Coenzyme Q.* 1981;3:109-119. **47.** Watts TL. Coenzyme Q10 and periodontal treatment: is there any beneficial effect? *Br Dent J.* 1995;178:209-213. **48.** Folkers K, Simonsen R. Two successful double-blind trials with coenzyme Q10 (vitamin Q10) on muscular dystrophies and neurogenic atrophies. *Biochim Biophys Acta.* 1995;1271:281-286. **49.** Eriksson JG, Forsen TJ, Mortensen SA, et al. The effect of coenzyme Q10 administration on metabolic control in patients with type 2 diabetes mellitus. *Biofactors.* 1999;9:315-318. **50.** Danysz A, Oledzka K, Bukowska-Kiliszek M. Influence of coenzyme Q-10 on the hypotensive effects of enalapril and nitrendipine in spontaneously hypertensive rats. *Pol J Pharmacol.* 1994;46:457-461. **51.** Baggio E, Gandini R, Plancher AC, et al. Italian multicenter study on the safety and efficacy of coenzyme Q10 as adjunctive therapy in heart failure. CoQ10 Drug Surveillance Investigators. *Mol Aspects Med.* 1994;15:s287-s294. **52.** Weis M, Mortensen SA, Rassing MR, et al. Bioavailability of four oral coenzyme Q10 formulations in healthy volunteers. *Mol Aspects Med.* 1994;15:S273-S280.

Cranberry

Vaccinium Macrocarpon

U.S. BRAND NAMES OF CLINICALLY TESTED PRODUCTS

None identified.

DESCRIPTION

Cranberry was used medically to treat urinary tract infections (UTIs) before antibiotics were developed, under the erroneous assumption that cranberry inhibits bacterial growth by acidifying the urine. More recent investigations suggest that cranberry might act by impairing bacterial adherence to epithelial cells of the urinary tract.

Cranberry is most widely used by women with recurrent UTIs for prophylaxis of acute infection. It has also been tried for chronic bacteriuria/pyuria. However, the evidence base for any of these uses is weak. In addition, there is no evidence that cranberry juice is an effective treatment for acute cystitis.

PHARMACOLOGY

The primary mechanism of action of cranberry juice is believed to be the reduction of adherence of bacteria to the epithelial cells of the bladder by interference with the activity of adhesins that attach to oligo- or monosaccharide receptors.[1-6] These adhesins are produced by fimbriae, proteinaceous fibers on the bacterial cell wall. Proanthocyanidins in cranberry at a concentration of 10 to 50 mcg/ml inhibit the attachment of p-fimbriated *E. coli.*[1] Inhibition has also been documented in *Proteus, Klebsiella, Enterobacter,* and *Pseudomonas.* Some evidence suggests that, in women who experience recurrent bladder infections, bacterial adherence occurs to a greater-than-normal extent.[7]

Cranberry also causes a decrease in urinary pH and an increase in urinary hippuric acid. However, these effects do not appear to be clinically relevant.[4]

CLINICAL STUDIES

PROPHYLAXIS OF ACUTE CYSTITIS

An unpublished trial presented at the June 2001 meeting of the American Urological Association provides the only real evidence for the use of cranberry as prophylaxis for acute UTIs. This 1-year double-blind placebo-controlled study of 150 sexually active women compared placebo against both cranberry juice and cranberry tablets (dosage not stated in abstract).[8] Both forms of cranberry significantly reduced the number of episodes of symptomatic UTI; however, cranberry tablets were more cost-effective.

A widely reported yearlong open trial of women with recurrent UTIs found cranberry to exert superior prophylaxis as compared to probiotics or no treatment; but given the reputation of cranberry, placebo effect and observer bias cannot be excluded from the results.[9]

CHRONIC BACTERIURIA/PYURIA

A double-blind placebo-controlled study designed to examine the effects of cranberry on bacteriuria/pyuria followed 153 women with a mean age of 78.5 years for a period of 6 months.[10] Half were given a standard commercial cranberry drink and the other half placebo (prepared to look and taste the same). Despite the weak preparation of cranberry used, the results for the treated group showed a 58% decrease in bacteriuria/pyuria compared to the control group. Furthermore, in women who were initially bacteriuric/pyuric, their chance of remaining so was 73% less in the treated group than in the control group. However, subsequent responses to this report called it into question on statistical and methodological grounds.[11,12]

A double-blind placebo-controlled crossover study of 15 children with neurogenic bladder reported no reduction in bacteriuria attributable to the cranberry concentrate used.[13]

PROPOSED INDICATIONS AND USAGE

Despite cranberry's widespread use for prophylaxis and treatment of acute UTIs, the evidence base for the former is weak and for the latter is nonexistent. Similarly, the evidence regarding cranberry for chronic bacteriuria/pyuria is highly preliminary at best.

Based on observations that cranberry acts against oral flora, cranberry has been proposed as a prophylactic treatment for periodontal disease.[14] However, the sweetening agents that are typically added to cranberry to make it palatable would be expected to exert a harmful effect in this regard.

WARNINGS

Cranberry may be contraindicated in individuals with a history of urolithiasis.

PRECAUTIONS

Regular use of cranberry concentrates has been found to increase excretion of oxalate, calcium, phosphate, sodium, magnesium, and potassium.[15] Because some of these ions are lithogenic and others antilithogenic, the overall effect is not clear. Nonetheless, caution is warranted.

There are no known risks or side effects of cranberry in adults, children, and pregnant or lactating women. Maximum safe doses in severe hepatic or renal disease have not been determined.

DRUG INTERACTIONS

Urine acidification by excessive use of cranberry juice can increase the excretion and thus reduce blood levels of some drugs, including certain antidepressants, antipsychotics, and morphine-based analgesics. Use of cranberry juice has been suggested as an antidote in phencyclidine (PCP) overdose.[16]

ADVERSE REACTIONS

None known.

PROPOSED DOSAGE AND ADMINISTRATION

Optimum doses of cranberry have not been determined. The typical dose of dry cranberry juice extract is 300 to 400 mg twice daily; the juice is taken at a dose of 1/2 to 1 cup twice daily. Cranberry juice "cocktail" contains very little cranberry juice; however, the pure juice is extremely bitter.

PATIENT INFORMATION

Cranberry juice has a reputation for helping to treat and prevent bladder infections. One study does suggest that regular use of cranberry may help prevent bladder infections. However, there is no evidence at all that cranberry can cure an acute bladder infection once it has started. If you have symptoms such as urgency to urinate, frequent urination, burning discomfort during urination, and pain in the abdomen or lower back, seek medical attention.

Note: Cranberry does not appear to be effective for preventing bladder infections in individuals at special risk, such as those with an indwelling catheter or neurogenic bladder.

The maximum safe dose of cranberry in pregnant or nursing women or young children has not been established. Individuals with severe liver or kidney disease should consult a physician before using this (or any other) supplement.

REFERENCES

1. Howell AB, Vorsa N, Der Marderosian A, et al. Inhibition of the adherence of P-fimbriated Escherichia coli to uroepithelial-cell surfaces by proanthocyanidin extracts from cranberries [letter]. *N Engl J Med.* 1998;339:1085-1086. **2.** Ofek I, Goldhar J, Zafriri D, et al. Anti-Escherichia coli adhesin activity of cranberry and blueberry juices [letter]. *N Engl J Med.* 1991;324:1599. **3.** Schmidt DR, Sobota AE. An examination of the anti-adherence activity of cranberry juice on urinary and nonurinary bacterial isolates. *Microbios.* 1988;55:173-181. **4.** Sobota AE. Inhibition of bacterial adherence by cranberry juice: potential use for the treatment of urinary tract infections. *J Urol.* 1984;131:1013-1016. **5.** Zafriri D, Ofek I, Adar R, et al. Inhibitory activity of cranberry juice on adherence of type 1 and type P fimbriated Escherichia coli to eucaryotic cells. *Antimicrob Agents Chemother.* 1989;33:92-98. **6.** Habash MB, Van der Mei HC, Busscher HJ, et al. The effect of water, ascorbic acid, and cranberry derived supplementation on human urine and uropathogen adhesion to silicone rubber. *Can J Microbiol.* 1999;45:691-694. **7.** Schaeffer AJ. Recurrent urinary tract infections in the female patient. *Urology.* 1988;32(Suppl):12-15. **8.** Stothers L. A randomized placebo controlled trial to evaluate naturopathic cranberry products as prophylaxis against urinary tract infection in women. Presented at: American Urological Association 2001 Annual Meeting; June 2-7, 2001; Anaheim, Calif. **9.** Kontiokari T, Sundqvist K, Nuutinen M, et al. Randomised trial of cranberry-lingonberry juice and Lactobacillus GG drink for the prevention of urinary tract infections in women. *BMJ.* 2001;322:1-5. **10.** Avorn J, Monane M, Gurwitz JH, et al. Reduction of bacteriuria and pyuria after ingestion of cranberry juice. *JAMA.* 1994;271:751-754. **11.** Hopkins WJ, Heisey DM, Jonler M, et al. Reduction of bacteriuria and pyuria using cranberry juice [letter]. *JAMA.* 1994;272:588-589. **12.** Katz LM. Reduction of bacteriuria and pyuria using cranberry juice [letter]. *JAMA.* 1994;272:589. **13.** Schlager TA, Anderson S, Trudell J, et al. Effect of cranberry juice on bacteriuria in children with neurogenic bladder receiving intermittent catheterization. *J Pediatr.* 1999;135:698-702. **14.** Weiss EI, Lev-Dor R, Kashamn Y, et al. Inhibiting interspecies coaggregation of plaque bacteria with a cranberry juice constituent. *JADA.* 1998;129:1719-1723. **15.** Terris MK, Issa MM, Tacker JR. Dietary supplementation with cranberry concentrate tablets may increase the risk of nephrolithiasis. *Urology.* 2001;57:26-29. **16.** Simpson GM, Khajawall AM. Urinary acidifiers in phencyclidine detoxification. *Hillside J Clin Psychiatry.* 1983;5:161-168.

Creatine

Alternate/Related Names: Creatine Monohydrate

U.S. BRAND NAMES OF CLINICALLY TESTED PRODUCTS

None.

DESCRIPTION

Creatine plays a physiological role in the generation of energy in skeletal muscle. Creatine is also found in cardiac muscle, the brain, spermatozoa, and retina. In its phosphorylated form, creatine serves as a reserve of phosphorus that can be transferred to ADP to produce ATP. The muscle's supply of phosphorylated creatine can be depleted rapidly during exercise and is a limiting factor in anaerobic energy production. Using creatine supplements to increase the amount of creatine and phosphocreatine in muscle has been proposed as a technique for improving athletic performance.

PHARMACOLOGY

Creatine is a nitrogenous amine that is synthesized in the liver, kidneys, and pancreas from the amino acids glycine, arginine, and methionine. Both endogenous and exogenous creatine are catabolized in the body to sarcosine and urea, and thence to methylamine and glyoxalate.[1] Excess creatine is also excreted in the urine. The normal requirement of about 2 g/day can be supplied by endogenous synthesis and by a diet that includes animal products. Vegetarians have lower levels of creatine in the serum and decreased output in the urine.[2]

An average 70-kg male has about 120 g of creatine in his body, of which 95% to 98% is found in skeletal muscle. The normal concentration of creatine in the muscle ranges from 100 to 140 mmol/kg dry mass. Phosphocreatine accounts for about 60% of the total while free creatine equals about 40%.

The phosphorylated form of creatine participates in energy generation via creatine kinase, contributing a phosphate group in the conversion of ADP to ATP. This reaction is rapid and reversible; however, stores of both ATP and phosphocreatine can be exhausted within 10 seconds during high-intensity exercise. During periods of recovery, phosphocreatine is resynthesized. Creatine supplementation is thought to increase muscle reserves of phosphocreatine, and aid resynthesis during rests between bouts of high-intensity exercise.[2-9]

Studies using muscle biopsy suggest that a dose of 20 to 30 g creatine monohydrate/day for 5 to 6 days can result in about a 20% increase in the concentration of intramuscular total creatine with approximately 30% of that increase attributable to phosphocreatine.[2,6,9,10] These results have been confirmed by NMR measurements of phosphocreatine.[7] In the initial 2 days of creatine supplementation, approximately 30% of the administered dose was retained. Renal excretion of creatine increased from 40% of the creatine dose on day 1 to 61% on day 2 and 68% on day 3.

A single 20 to 30 g dose of creatine monohydrate has been found to raise plasma creatine concentrations to levels of 690 to 1,000 μmol/L within 1 hour.[2] The half-life of creatine in the plasma is 1 to 1.5 hours. A dose of 2 g/day after a loading dose of 20 g/day for 6 days was sufficient to keep the concentration of total creatine in the muscle at levels >140 mmol/kg dry weight. Creatine doses of 3 g/day for 28 days resulted in the equivalent concentration of intramuscular total creatine as 20 g/day for 6 days.[9] A 28-day washout period has been found sufficient to return creatine muscle stores to baseline levels.[10]

The potential mechanism of action of creatine in treatment of muscular disorders is not well elucidated. Diminished levels of creatine in muscle may be due to disturbances in ion homeostasis that result in decreased creatine transport into the cells.[11] Diminished intramuscular creatine and phosphocreatine results in increased concentrations of lactic acid and hydrogen ions that may directly affect the contractile apparatus of the muscle. Acidosis also results in more rapid depletion of phosphocreatine and inhibits the enzymes of glycolysis.[4]

Impairment of energy production due to mitochondrial defects may result in lower concentrations of phosphorylated creatine and ATP, leading ultimately to cell death. Phosphorylated creatine produced in the mitochondria from ATP is transported to sites of energy consumption such as the brain or muscles. Supplemental creatine may stabilize mitochondrial creatine kinase and inhibit the opening of the mitochondrial transition pore.

Increasing creatine concentrations may increase the cerebral energy reserve and offer neuroprotection in conditions such as Huntington's disease.[12]

In addition, phosphocreatine serves as an energy source for glutamate uptake into synaptic vesicles; impaired glutamate uptake has been implicated in the pathogenesis of ALS.

CLINICAL STUDIES

Hundreds of small studies have attempted to evaluate creatine as an ergogenic aid, with highly mixed results. Other proposed uses of creatine have preliminary documentation.

HIGH-INTENSITY REPETITIVE BURST EXERCISE WITH SHORT REST PERIODS

Based on the mechanism of action of creatine (increased muscle ability to regenerate phosphocreatine and hence replenish ATP), performance of repeated short bursts of high-intensity exercise (less than 10 seconds) separated by short rest periods (e.g., 30 seconds) might be expected to respond to creatine supplementation. Many but not all studies support this view.[3,5,13-16]

For example, one trial studied 16 male physical education students.[15] The protocol was 10 6-second bouts of high-intensity cycling separated by 30-second rest periods between bouts. Performance in the 2- to 4-second interval of bouts 1 to 6 was similar for both the creatine and placebo groups, but the creatine group showed much less fatigue in the 4- to 6-second interval of bouts 7 to 10.

OTHER POTENTIAL ERGOGENIC USES

In studies of exercise with longer rest periods, the results of creatine supplementation have been uniformly unimpressive, presumably due to the relative lack of stress on the rephosphorylation mechanism.[5,10,17,18] Similarly negative results have been seen in studies involving longer-term exercise (in which rapid phosphorylation of ATP is less significant).[5] However, some studies of resistance training have found potential benefit.[5,19-21]

CONGESTIVE HEART FAILURE

Because patients with congestive heart failure (CHF) suffer from muscle fatigue due to loss of skeletal muscle mass and strength, altered fiber composition, decreased oxidative capacity, and other abnormalities of muscle metabolism, creatine supplementation has been suggested as a means to improve these parameters. A double-blind study examined 17 male subjects with CHF who were given 20 g creatine daily for 10 days.[22] Performance in one-legged and two-legged exercise capacity and muscle strength increased significantly in the creatine-treated group. No marked change was seen in ejection fraction at rest or during exercise.

Similarly, muscle endurance during handgrip exercises improved in a double-blind placebo-controlled crossover study of 20 males with CHF.[23] Compared to baseline values, the number of contractions until exhaustion increased after treatment with 20 g creatine for 5 days. No improvement was seen in the placebo group.

NEUROMUSCULAR DISORDERS

Because Duchenne muscular dystrophy involves muscular atrophy with lowered muscular levels of creatine and phosphocreatine, creatine supplementation could theoretically alleviate some of the clinical symptoms.[11] Studies in cell culture with *mdx* skeletal muscle cells demonstrated that creatine supplementation (20 mmol/L) resulted in increased cellular phosphocreatine levels, myotube formation, and cell survival.[24] A double-blind placebo-controlled trial of creatine in 36 individuals with various types of muscular dystrophy found evidence of benefit in muscle strength and daily life activities.[25]

In a single-blind placebo-controlled trial of 21 individuals with various neuromuscular disorders (such as dermatomyositis and myotonic dystrophy), creatine monohydrate (10 g for 5 days followed by 5 g for 5 to 7 days) produced improvements in handgrip, dorsiflexion, and knee extensor strength.[26] Improved exercise performance was also seen in a small controlled trial of individuals with McArdle's disease.[27]

DEFECTS OF ENERGY PRODUCTION BY THE MITOCHONDRIA

In mitochondrial cytopathies, defects in the mitochondria result in energy failures that lead to increased reliance upon glycolytic and phosphocreatine pathways for energy generation. Consequently, patients with these conditions have reduced levels of resting phosphocreatine and delayed post-exercise recovery of phosphocreatine in skeletal muscle. Theoretically, supplementation with creatine could increase phosphocreatine levels, regenerate ATP, buffer H+ accumulation, and allow maximal activation of glycolysis and glycogenolysis.

Results of preliminary trials of creatine for mitochondrial defects have been somewhat promising. In a randomized double-blind crossover study, 5 g creatine monohydrate or glucose placebo was given to seven patients twice daily for 2 weeks followed by 2 g twice daily for 1 week.[28] Following a 5-week washout period, the treatments were reversed. The authors reported a 19% increase in isometric grip strength at 10 and 40 seconds with creatine treatment but observed no effect on aerobic cycle ergometry or body composition.

PROPOSED INDICATIONS AND USAGE

Despite the lack of consistent evidence, creatine is widely marketed as a sports supplement. Based on highly preliminary evidence, creatine has also been tried for congestive heart failure; Duchenne muscular dystrophy, McArdle's disease, and other neuromuscular disorders; congenital defects in creatine synthesis; mitochondrial disorders; progressive neurological disorders; and hyperlipidemia.

WARNINGS

Use of high-dose creatine is contraindicated in individuals with renal failure.

PRECAUTIONS

The preponderance of data documenting side effects is taken from short-term studies involving healthy and/or athletic subjects; large, systematic, long-term safety studies have not been performed.[29] A long-term placebo-controlled study of 100 football players found no increase in injury or cramping during 1 year of creatine supplementation.[30] Creatine does not appear to adversely affect the body's ability to exercise under hot conditions.[31]

Concerns have been expressed regarding creatine and renal function. One case report indicates that creatine may impair renal function in individuals with existing renal disease[32]; plasma creatinine and creatinine clearance levels in this individual returned to normal 1 month after stopping creatine. Studies have not found any adverse effects upon renal function among individuals with healthy kidneys.[33,34] Nevertheless, there is one report of impaired renal functioning apparently attributable to creatine use in a healthy individual.[35] This 20-year-old man complained of nausea, vomiting, and flank pain about 4 weeks after starting a creatine supplementation regimen of 20 g per day. Serum creatinine and urinary protein were elevated. A renal biopsy revealed interstitial nephritis and focal tubular injury. He recovered after discontinuing the creatine supplement. These effects may have been due to consumption of creatine exceeding the normal recommended loading dose of 20 g/day for only 5 to 7 days.

Safety in pregnant or lactating women, young children, or individuals with severe hepatic disease has not been established.

DRUG INTERACTIONS

No drug interactions with creatine have been reported, although most of the studies have prohibited concurrent use of other drugs, supplements, or steroids.

ADVERSE REACTIONS

The most common side effect of creatine supplementation is weight gain due to an increase in water content or in the diameter of fast-twitch (type II) glycolytic muscle fibers.[5,9,15,36,37] Other side effects of creatine may include muscle cramping, dehydration, and gastrointestinal distress.[5,38]

PROPOSED DOSAGE AND ADMINISTRATION

The most common proposed dosage schedule for creatine begins with a loading dose of 20 to 30 g creatine monohydrate (equivalent to 17.6 to 26.4 g creatine) for 5 to 7 days, usually ingested daily in 4 divided doses of 5 to 6 g. This is followed by doses of 2 g/day to maintain elevated creatine concentrations in the muscle.[9] An alternative schedule avoids a loading dose and simply employs 3 g/day for 28 days. Combining carbohydrates with creatine may be helpful,[39] perhaps due to insulin-augmented creatine accumulation[40] or enhanced muscle glycogen supercompensation.[41]

PATIENT INFORMATION

Creatine is widely marketed as a sports supplement. There is some evidence that it may be useful in high-intensity, repetitive burst exercise, (such as repeated 10-second bursts of high-intensity exercise separated by 30-second rest periods); however, many studies have found no benefit. Creatine does not appear to be at all helpful for other forms of exercise.

Creatine is also sometimes advocated for treatment of numerous conditions involving fatigue or muscle weakness, but there is no real evidence as yet that it is actually helpful.

Creatine should not be used by individuals with kidney problems. The safety of creatine for pregnant or nursing women or young children, or individuals with severe liver disease has not been established.

REFERENCES

1. Yu PH, Deng Y. Potential cytotoxic effect of chronic administration of creatine, a nutrition supplement to augment athletic performance. *Med Hypotheses.* 2000;54:726-728. **2.** Harris RC, Soderlund K, Hultman E. Elevation of creatine in resting and exercised muscle of normal subjects by creatine supplementation. *Clin Sci (Lond).* 1992;83:367-374. **3.** Mujika I, Padilla S. Creatine supplementation as an ergogenic acid for sports performance in highly trained athletes: a critical review. *Int J Sports Med.* 1997;18:491-496. **4.** Volek JS, Kraemer WJ. Creatine supplementation: its effect on human muscular performance and body composition. *J Strength Cond Res.* 1996;10:200-210. **5.** Williams MH, Branch JD. Creatine supplementation and exercise performance: an update. *J Am Coll Nutr.* 1998;17:216-234. **6.** Casey A, Constantin-Teodosiu D, Howell S, et al. Creatine ingestion favorably affects performance and muscle metabolism during maximal exercise in humans. *Am J Physiol.* 1996;271(1 Pt 1):E31-E37. **7.** Francaux M, Demeure R, Goudemant JF. Effect of exogenous creatine supplementation on muscle PCr metabolism. *Int J Sport Med.* 2000;21:139-145. **8.** Greenhaff PL, Bodin K, Soderlund K, et al. Effect of oral creatine supplementation on skeletal muscle phosphocreatine resynthesis. *Am J Physiol.* 1994;266(5 Pt 1):E725-730. **9.** Hultman E, Soderlund K, Timmons JA, et al. Muscle creatine loading in men. *J Appl Physiol.* 1996;81:232-237. **10.** Febbraio MA, Flanagan TR, Snow RJ, et al. Effect of creatine supplementation on intramuscular TCr, metabolism and performance during intermittent, supramaximal exercise in humans. *Acta Physiol Scand.* 1995;155:387-395. **11.** Wyss M, Felber S, Skladal D, et al. The therapeutic potential of oral creatine supplementation in muscle disease. *Med Hypotheses.* 1998;51:333-336. **12.** Matthews RT, Yang L, Jenkins BG, et al. Neuroprotective effects of creatine and cyclocreatine in animal models of Huntington's disease. *J Neurosci.* 1998;18:156-163. **13.** Mujika I, Padilla S, Ibanez J, et al. Creatine supplementation and sprint performance in soccer players. *Med Sci Sports Exerc.* 2000;32:518-525. **14.** Gilliam JD, Hohzorn C, Martin D, et al. Effect of oral creatine supplementation on isokinetic torque production. *Med Sci Sports Exerc.* 2000;32:993-996. **15.** Balsom PD, Ekblom B, Soderlund K, et al. Creatine supplementation and dynamic high-intensity intermittent exercise. *Scand J Med Sci Sport.* 1993;3:143-149. **16.** Finn JP, Ebert TR, Withers RT, et al. Effect of creatine supplementation on metabolism and performance in humans during intermittent sprint cycling. *Eur J Appl Physiol.* 2001;84:238-243. **17.** Burke LM, Pyne DB, Telford RD. Effect of oral creatine supplementation on single-effort sprint performance in elite swimmers. *Int J Sport Nutr.* 1996;6:222-233. **18.** Mujika I, Chatard JC, Lacoste L, et al. Creatine supplementation does not improve sprint performance in competitive swimmers. *Med Sci Sports Exerc.* 1996;28:1435-1441. **19.** Kraemer WJ, Volek JS. Creatine supplementation. Its role in human performance. *Clin Sports Med.* 1999;1:651-666. **20.** Kreider RB, Ferreira M, Wilson P, et al. Effects of creatine supplementation on body composition, strength and sprint performance. *Med Sci Sports Exerc.* 1998;30:73-82. **21.** Volek JS, Kraemer WJ, Bush JA, et al. Creatine supplementation enhances muscular performance during high-intensity resistance exercise. *J Am Diet Assoc.* 1997;97:765-770. **22.** Gordon A, Hultman E, Kaijser L, et al. Creatine supplementation in chronic heart failure increases skeletal muscle creatine phosphate and muscle performance. *Cardiovasc Res.* 1995;30:413-418. **23.** Andrews R, Greenhaff P, Curtis S, et al. The effect of dietary creatine supplementation on skeletal muscle metabolism in congestive heart failure. *Eur Heart J.* 1998;19:617-622. **24.** Pulido SM, Passaquin AC, Leijendekker WJ, et al. Creatine supplementation improves intracellular Ca2+ handling and survival in mdx skeletal muscle cells. *FEBS Lett.* 1998;439:357-362. **25.** Walter MC, Lochmuller H, Reilich P, et al. Creatine monohydrate in muscular dystrophies: a double-blind, placebo-controlled clinical study. *Neurology.* 2000;54:1848-1850. **26.** Tarnopolsky MA, Martin J. Creatine monohydrate increases strength in patients with neuromuscular disease. *Neurology.* 1999;52:854-857. **27.** Vorgerd M, Grehl T, Jager M, et al. Creatine therapy in myophosphorylase deficiency (McArdle disease): a placebo-controlled crossover trial. *Arch Neurol.* 2000;57:956-963. **28.** Tarnopolsky MA, Roy BD, MacDonald JR. A randomized, controlled trial of creatine monohydrate in patients with mitochondrial cytopathies. *Muscle Nerve.* 1997;20:1502-1509. **29.** Juhn MS, Tarnopolsky M. Potential side effects of oral creatine supplementation: a critical review. *Clin J Sport Med.* 1998;8:298-304. **30.** Kreider R, Rasmeussen C, Melton C, et al. Long-tem creatine supplementation does not adversely affect clinical markers of health. Presented at: American College of Sports Medicine 2000 Annual Scientific Meeting; May 31-June 3, 2000; Indianapolis, Indiana. **31.** Volek JS, Mazzetti SA, Farquhar WB, et al. Physiological responses to short-term exercise in the heat after creatine loading. *Med Sci Sports Exerc.* 2001;33:1101-1108. **32.** Pritchard NR, Kalra PA. Renal dysfunction accompanying oral creatine supplements. *Lancet.* 1998;351:1252-1253. **33.** Mihic S, MacDonald JR, McKenzie S, et al. Acute creatine loading increases fat-free mass, but does not affect blood pressure, plasma creatinine, or CK activity in men and women. *Med Sci Sports Exerc.* 2000;32:291-296. **34.** Poortmans JR, Francaux M. Long-term oral creatine supplementation does not impair renal function in healthy athletes. *Med Sci Sports Exerc.* 1999;31:1108-1110. **35.** Koshy KM, Griswold E, Schneeberger EE. Interstitial nephritis in a patient taking creatine. *N Engl J Med.* 1999;340:814-815. **36.** Sipila I, Rapola J, Simell O, et al. Supplementary creatine as a treatment for gyrate atrophy of the choroid and retina. *N Engl J Med.* 1981;304:867-870. **37.** Earnest CP, Snell PG, Rodriguez R, et al. The effect of creatine monohydrate ingestion on anaerobic power indices, muscular strength and body composition. *Acta Physiol Scand.* 1995;153:207-209. **38.** Graham AS, Hatton RC. Creatine: A review of efficacy and safety. *J Am Pharm Assoc.* 1999;39:803-810. **39.** Green AL, Hultman E, Macdonald IA, et al. Carbohydrate ingestion augments skeletal muscle creatine accumulation during creatine supplementation in humans. *Am J Physiol.* 1996;271(5 Pt 1):E821-826. **40.** Steenge GR, Lambourne J, Casey A, et al. Stimulatory effect of insulin on creatine accumulation in human skeletal muscle. *Am J Physiol.* 1998;275:E974-E979. **41.** Nelson AG, Arnall DA, Kokkonen J, et al. Muscle glycogen supercompensation is enhanced by prior creatine supplementation. *Med Sci Sports Exerc.* 2001;33:1096-1100.

Dong Quai

Angelica Sinensis

Alternate/Related Names: Dang Quai, Tang Quai, Dang Kwai, Dong Kwai

U.S. BRAND NAMES OF CLINICALLY TESTED PRODUCTS

None.

DESCRIPTION

Dong quai (also transliterated as dang quai, dang gui, tang kuei, and tang quai) is a staple herb in the repertoire of Chinese herbology. It has become quite popular as a "women's herb" in the United States. However, there is no scientific evidence that dong quai is effective for treating any condition.

PHARMACOLOGY

Dong quai root contains numerous potentially active substances, including butylidene phthalide, ferulic acid, and beta-sitosterol. Nutritionally, it is a source of nicotinic acid, uracil, adenine, folinic acid, vitamin E, carotene, and a subnutritional amount of vitamin B12. Dong quai does not appear to have estrogenic actions.[1,2]

In vitro and animal studies suggest that dong quai can cause both uterine contractions and uterine relaxation, as well as suppress heart dysrhythmias, inhibit platelet aggregation, and lower blood pressure.[3,4,5] However, the clinical relevance of these findings is not known.

CLINICAL STUDIES

MENOPAUSAL SYMPTOMS

A 12-week study compared the effects of dong quai against placebo in 71 postmenopausal women.[2] The results showed no statistically significant differences between groups in endometrial thickness, vaginal maturation index score, number of vasomotor flushes, or Kupperman Index score.

PROPOSED INDICATIONS AND USAGE

Dong quai is widely sold as an ingredient in herbal mixtures said to be helpful for a variety of conditions, including menopausal syndrome, dysmenorrhea, amenorrhea, fibrocystic breast disease, and PMS. However, there is no evidence that it is effective for any of these purposes, and some evidence that it is *ineffective* for menopausal syndrome.

WARNINGS

Dong quai may interact with warfarin (see Drug Interactions).

Chinese patent medicines containing dong quai are widely marketed; however, such products have been found in the past to contain unlisted, potentially dangerous pharmaceuticals and other contaminants.[6]

PRECAUTIONS

The furanocoumarin constituents of dong quai have been associated with photosensitivity.

Safety for young children, pregnant or lactating women, or individuals with severe hepatic or renal disease has not been established. One case report suggests that maternal dong quai usage caused hypertension in both mother and child.[7]

DRUG INTERACTIONS

Dong quai may interact with warfarin. In one case report, concurrent administration of dong quai at a dose of 565 mg once to twice daily with warfarin 5 mg daily resulted in a 2.5-fold increase in PT and INR in a previously stabilized patient.[8] This could be attributed to dong quai's coumarin content as well as to a direct antithrombotic effect.

Because of its furanocoumarin content, dong quai might potentiate photosensitivity reactions if combined with photosensitizing drugs.

ADVERSE REACTIONS

Dong quai possesses a low order of toxicity. In rats, the LD50 of 4:1-concentrated dong quai extract is approximately 100 g/kg.[5] Reported side effects are rare and consist primarily of mild gastrointestinal distress and occasional allergic reactions. There is one report suggesting that maternal dong quai usage caused hypertension in both mother and child.[7]

In addition, a man using a patent herb product containing dong quai developed gynecomastia.[9] However, such products are known to be contaminated at times with pharmaceuticals not listed on the label[6,10]; as noted above, there is no evidence that dong quai possesses estrogenic effects.

PROPOSED DOSAGE AND ADMINISTRATION

Typical recommended dosages of dong quai vary widely.

PATIENT INFORMATION

Dong quai is a Chinese herb advocated as a treatment for various "women's conditions," such as menopause. However, there is no evidence that the herb is effective for any condition. Contrary to some reports, dong quai does not act as a "natural estrogen." Be cautious about using prepackaged dong quai formulas manufactured in Asia, as there are reports of contamination with unlabelled prescription drugs, heavy metals, and other toxic substances.

The safety of dong quai in pregnant or nursing women or young children has not been established. Individuals with severe liver or kidney disease should consult a physician before using this (or any other) supplement.

REFERENCES

1. Zava DT, Dollbaum CM, Blen M. Estrogen and progestin bioactivity of foods, herbs, and spices. *Proc Soc Exp Biol Med.* 1998;217:369-378. **2.** Hirata JD, Swiersz LM, Zell B, et al. Does dong quai have estrogenic effects in postmenopausal women? A double-blind, placebo controlled trial. *Fertil Steril.* 1997;68:981-986. **3.** Bensky D, Gamble A. *Chinese herbal medicine: Materia medica.* Seattle, WA: Eastland Press; 1986:474-476. **4.** Hsu HY, et al. *Oriental Materia Medica: A concise guide.* Long Beach, CA: Oriental Healing Arts Institute; 1986:540-542. **5.** Zhu D. Dong quai. *Am J Chin Med.* 1987;15:117-125. **6.** American Association of Oriental Medicine Boycott. Available at: http://www.acupuncturetcm.com/aaom.htm. Accessed August 27, 2001. **7.** Nambiar S, Schwartz RH, Constantino A. Hypertension in mother and baby linked to ingestion of Chinese herbal medicine [letter]. *West J Med.* 1999;171:152. **8.** Page RL II, Lawrence JD. Potentiation of warfarin by dong quai. *Pharmacotherapy.* 1999;19:870-876. **9.** Goh SY, Loh KC. Gynaecomastia and the herbal tonic "Dong Quai". *Singapore Med J.* 2001;42:115-116. **10.** Nortier JL, Martinez MC, Schmeiser HH, et al. Urothelial Carcinoma Associated with the Use of a Chinese Herb (Aristolochia fangchi). *N Engl J Med.* 2000;342:1686-1692.

Echinacea

Echinacea Purpurea

Alternate/Related Names: Purple Coneflower, *E. angustifolia, E. pallida*

U.S. BRAND NAMES OF CLINICALLY TESTED PRODUCTS

EchinaGuard (Nature's Way) = Echinacin (Madaus) in Europe
Echinoforce (Bioforce AG) = Echinoforce (Bioforce AG) in Europe

DESCRIPTION

Echinacea purpurea is known colloquially as purple coneflower. Its near relatives *E. angustifolia* and *E. pallida* are also used medicinally. Preparations variously consist of the above-ground portion of echinacea, the root, or the whole plant.

PHARMACOLOGY

The above-ground portion of *E. purpurea* contains numerous high and middle molecular weight polysaccharides, including arabinogalactans, as well as cichoric acid, inulin, flavonoids, and caffeic acids. The root is also rich in caffeic acids, including one known as echinacoside, as well as polyacetylenes, alkylamides (including isobutylamide), alkaloids, and volatile oils.[1,2,3] *Echinacea pallida* and *E. angustifolia* contain similar constituents.

In vitro and animal studies using injectable echinacea extracts have found numerous immunomodulatory effects, including increases in antibody production, elevation of white blood cell count, stimulation of T-cells and natural killer cells, increases in macrocyte phagocytosis and IgG response to antigens, antitumor activity, and activation of the alternative complement pathway.[1,4-11] The effect on neutrophils and macrophages appears to be greater than the effect on lymphocytes, except in in vitro studies involving very high concentrations of echinacea extract.[12] Isobutylamide also inhibits cyclo-oxygenase and lipoxygenase in vitro.[13] Studies in humans have found that oral doses of an alcoholic tincture of echinacea enhance carbon particle phagocytosis as compared to placebo.[1] However, the clinical relevance of these findings is unclear.

The active constituents of echinacea have not been identified. It has been proposed that the polysaccharide constituents of echinacea stimulate immune activity by virtue of their similarities to bacterial wall polysaccharides.[1,4,6,9-11] However, other than the arabinogalactans, these polysaccharides are present in low to negligible amounts in most oral preparations of echinacea. Cichoric acid and the alkylamide isobutylamide also have been found to exert immunomodulatory actions, and they are present in typical oral preparations.

CLINICAL STUDIES

Numerous studies support the use of echinacea for reducing the severity and duration of URI symptoms. However, echinacea has failed to prove effective for prophylaxis of URIs or genital herpes.

REDUCING SEVERITY AND DURATION OF RESPIRATORY INFECTIONS

Double-blind trials involving a total of more than 750 participants support the use of echinacea for reducing the severity and duration of respiratory infections. Trials have involved many different preparations of echinacea, including all three species and differing mixtures of root and herb, without any consistent pattern of optimum efficacy.

For example, in a double-blind placebo-controlled trial, 246 individuals with recent onset of a respiratory infection were given either placebo or one of three *E. purpurea* preparations: two concentrations of a 95%-herb (consisting of leaves, stems, and flowers) and 5%-root combination, and one made only from the roots of the plant.[14] The primary outcome measure was reduction in symptoms on day 7. An intention-to-treat analysis showed significant reduction of illness severity and duration with the two above-ground preparations, but not with the root-only formula.

However, in another double-blind study of 180 individuals with flu symptoms, use of a root-only extract produced statistically significant improvements in the severity and duration of symptoms, beginning at about day 3 and continuing to the end of the 10-day study.[15]

In other double-blind placebo-controlled trials, benefits were seen with *E. pallida* root[16]; a beverage tea containing above-ground portions of *E. purpurea* and *E. angustifolia* as well as an extract of *E. purpurea*[17]; and juice extracted from the above-ground parts of *E. purpurea* harvested during the flowering stage.[18,19] Earlier studies also found benefits; however, they used a mixed formulation that included other herbs as well as homeopathic preparations.[20]

PROPHYLAXIS OF RESPIRATORY INFECTIONS

Studies testing echinacea as a prophylactic treatment for URIs have not found evidence of benefit, and one unpublished study actually found a slight increase in infection rate.

A double-blind placebo-controlled study compared *E. purpurea, E. angustifolia,* and placebo for a 12-week period in 302 volunteers.[21] The results failed to show a significant reduction in number of infections in either treatment group as compared to the placebo group. Similar lack of benefit was seen in two other trials enrolling a total of over 200 individuals.[22,23] Furthermore, in an unpublished double-blind placebo-controlled study of 200 individuals, prophylactic use of echinacea was associated with a 20% higher rate of URI.[24]

One study widely quoted as evidence of prophylactic benefit found positive results only in a subgroup analysis. This double-blind placebo-controlled study followed 609 university students, half of whom were treated with a prophylactic dose of a combination product (Resistan) containing echinacea for at least 8 weeks.[25] Among a subgroup rated as more infection prone on the basis of frequency of colds in the previous year, there was a statistically significant reduction of URI incidence. However, in the treatment group as a whole, no significant effect was seen.

PROPHYLAXIS OF GENITAL HERPES

In a 1-year double-blind placebo-controlled crossover trial of 50 individuals with frequently recurrent genital herpes, treatment with *E. purpurea* extract (Echinaforce, 800 mg b.i.d.) failed to impact disease recurrence.[26]

PROPOSED INDICATIONS AND USAGE

Meaningful evidence suggests that various forms of echinacea can significantly reduce the severity and duration of URIs. However, echinacea has failed to prove effective for prophylaxis of URIs.

Echinacea has been tried as a prophylactic treatment for other viral infections, such as genital herpes, but effectiveness has not been shown. Echinacea is also sometimes marketed as a treatment for candidal vaginitis, but the only supporting study lacked blinding and placebo control.[27]

WARNINGS

Based on echinacea's apparent immunomodulatory actions, individuals with autoimmune illnesses as well as those on immunosuppressant agents should avoid use of echinacea.

PRECAUTIONS

Germany's Commission E warns against using echinacea in autoimmune disorders such as multiple sclerosis, lupus, and rheumatoid arthritis, as well as tuberculosis and leukocytosis of any origin. These are theoretical warnings based on concerns over possible immune activation rather than actual case reports of adverse effects.

Commission E also recommends against using echinacea for more than 8 weeks, based on evidence that parenteral echinacea reversibly depresses immune parameters.[28] However, in studies where echinacea was taken orally for up to 6 months, no changes in immune parameters were detected.[12,26,27]

Safety of echinacea for pregnant or lactating women, or individuals with severe hepatic or renal disease, has not been established. Safety of oral echinacea for children has also not been established; however, over 1,000 children with either whooping cough or tuberculosis have been given parenteral echinacea extract in German studies without evidence of harm.[12]

DRUG INTERACTIONS

None are known. However, weak evidence suggests that *E. angustifolia* might inhibit CYP 3A4.[29]

Based on echinacea's immunomodulatory actions, interactions with immunosuppressants are possible.

ADVERSE REACTIONS

Echinacea is generally well tolerated. In clinical trials, oral echinacea has been associated only with minor, nonspecific side effects.[12] In rats, echinacea extracts have not been found to cause either acute or chronic toxicity, even when taken in very high doses.[30]

PROPOSED DOSAGE AND ADMINISTRATION

Echinacea dosages vary with the specific product and should be taken according to label instructions. Treatment is usually begun at the first sign of a cold and continued for 7 to 14 days.

Echinacea products frequently contain the herb goldenseal as well. However, there is no evidence that oral goldenseal is helpful in colds, nor did traditional herbalists use it for that purpose.[31]

PATIENT INFORMATION

The herb echinacea is widely marketed as an "immune stimulant." There is some evidence that short-term use of echinacea may be useful for those with colds or other minor respiratory infections. However, long-term use of echinacea does not appear to help prevent colds or any other infections.

Individuals with autoimmune diseases, or taking drugs that suppress the immune system, should not use echinacea.

Safety of echinacea for pregnant or nursing women or young children has not been established. Individuals with severe liver or kidney disease should consult a physician before using this (or any other) supplement.

REFERENCES

1. Bauer R, Wagner H. Echinacea species as potential immunostimulatory drugs. *Econ Med Plant Res.* 1991;5:253-321. **2.** Heinzer F, et al. *Echinacea pallida* and *Echinacea purpurea:* follow-up of weight development and chemical composition for the first two culture years. [36th Annual Congress - Freiburg, Germany]. *Soc Medicinal Plant Res.* 1988. **3.** Hobbs C. *The Echinacea handbook.* Portland, OR: Eclectic Medical Publications; 1989: 118. **4.** Luettig B, Steinmuller C, Gifford GE, et al. Macrophage activation by the polysaccharide arabinogalactan isolated from plant cell cultures of Echinacea purpurea. *J Natl Cancer Inst.* 1989;81:669-675. **5.** Melchart D, Linde K, Worku F, et al. Results of five randomized studies on the immunomodulatory activity of preparations of Echinacea. *J Altern Complement Med.* 1995;1:145-160. **6.** Mose JR. The effect of echinacin on phagocytosis and natural killer cells [in German; English abstract]. *Med Welt.* 1983;34:1463-1467. **7.** Rehman J, Dillow JM, Carter SM, et al. Increased production of antigen-specific immunoglobulins G and M following in vivo treatment with the medicinal plants Echinacea angustifolia and Hydrastis canadensis. *Immunol Lett.* 1999;68:391-395. **8.** See DM, Broumand N, Sahl L, et al. In vitro effects of echinacea and ginseng on natural killer cells and antibody-dependent cell cytoxicity in healthy subjects and chronic fatigue syndrome or acquired immunodeficiency patients. *Immunopharmacology.* 1997;35:229-235. **9.** Stimple M, Proksch A, Wagner H, et al. Macrophage activation and induction of macrophage cytotoxicity by purified polysaccharide fractions from the plant Echinacea purpurea. *Infect Immun.* 1984;46:845-849. **10.** Vomel T. The effect of a nonspecific immunostimulant on the phagocytosis of erythrocytes and ink by the reticulohistiocyte system in the isolated, perfused liver of rats of various ages [in German; English abstract]. *Arzneimittelforschung.* 1984;34:691-695. **11.** Wagner VH, Proksch A, Riess-Maurer I, et al. Immunostimulating polysaccharides (heteroglycans) of higher plants [translated from German]. *Arzneimittelforschung.* 1985;35:1069-1075. **12.** Parnham MJ. Benefit-risk assessment of the squeezed sap of the purple coneflower (Echinacea purpurea) for long-term oral immunostimulation. *Phytomedicine.* 1996;3:95-102. **13.** Muller-Jakic B, Breu W, Probstle A, et al. In vitro inhibition of cyclooxygenase and 5-lipoxygenase by alkamides from Echinacea and Achillea species. *Planta Med.* 1994;60:37-40. **14.** Brinkeborn RM, Shah DV, Degenring FH. Echinaforce and other Echinacea fresh plant preparations in the treatment of the common cold. A randomized, placebo controlled, double-blind clinical trial. *Phytomedicine.* 1999;6:1-5. **15.** Braunig B, Dorn M, Limburg, et al. Echinacea purpureae radix for strengthening the immune response in flu-like infections [translated from German]. *Z Phytother.* 1992;13:7-13. **16.** Dorn M, Knick E, Lewith G. Placebo-controlled double-blind study of Echinacea pallidae radix in upper respiratory tract infections. *Complement Ther Med.* 1997;5:40-42. **17.** Lindenmuth GF, Lindenmuth EB. The efficacy of echinacea compound herbal tea preparation on the severity and duration of upper respiratory and flu symptoms: a randomized, double-blind placebo-controlled study. *J Altern Complement Med.* 2000;6:327-334. **18.** Hoheisel O, Sandberg M, Bertram S, et al. Echinagard(r) treatment shortens the course of the common cold: a double-blind placebo-controlled clinical trial. *Eur J Clin Res.* 1997;9:261-268. **19.** Schulten B, Bulitta M, Ballering-Bruhl B, et al. Efficacy of Echinacea purpurea in patients with a common cold. A placebo-controlled, randomised, double-blind clinical trial. *Arzneimittelforschung.* 2001;51:563-568. **20.** Melchart MD, Linde K, Worku F, et al. Immunomodulation with echinacea: A systemic review of controlled clinical trials. *Phytomedicine.* 1994;1:245-254. **21.** Melchart D, Walther E, Linde K, et al. Echinacea Root Extracts for the Prevention of Upper Respiratory Tract Infections. *Arch Fam Med.* 1998;7:541-545. **22.** Grimm W, Muller HH. A randomized controlled trial of the effect of fluid extract of echinacea purpurea on the incidence and severity of colds and respiratory infections. *Am J Med.* 1999;106:138-143. **23.** Turner RB, Riker DK, Gangemi JD. Ineffectiveness of echinacea for prevention of experimental rhinovirus colds. *Antimicrob Agents Chemother.* 2000;44:1708-1709. **24.** Chamberlain C. Take echinacea? Bless you. ABC News. 1999. Available at: http://www.abcnews.go.com/sections/living/DailyNews/echinacea990427.html. Accessed July 15, 2000. **25.** Schmidt U, Albrecht M, Schenk N. Immunostimulator decreases the frequency of influenza-like syndromes. Double-blind placebo-controlled trial on 646 students of the University of Cologne [in German; English abstract]. *Natur und Ganzheitsmedizin.* 1990;3:277-281. **26.** Vonau B, Chard S, Mandalia S, et al. Does the extract of the plant Echinacea purpurea influence the clinical course of recurrent genital herpes? *Int J STD AIDS.* 2001;12:154-158. **27.** Coeugniet E, Kuhnast R. Recurrent candidiasis: adjuvant immunotherapy with different formulations of Echinacin(r) [translated from German]. *Therapiewoche.* 1986;36:3352-3358. **28.** Bergner P. *The healing power of Echinacea and Goldenseal.* Rocklin, CA: Prima Publishing; 1997:91, 118. **29.** Budzinski JW, Foster BC, Vandenhoek S, et al. An in vitro evaluation of human cytochrome P450 3A4 inhibition by selected commercial herbal extracts and tinctures. *Phytomedicine.* 2000;7:273-282. **30.** Mengs U, Clare CB, Poiley JA. Toxicity of echinacea purpurea. Acute, subacute and genotoxicity studies. *Arzneimittelforschung.* 1991;41:1076-1081. **31.** Bergner P. Goldenseal and the common cold: the antibiotic myth. *Med Herbalism.* 1996/1997;8(4):1,4-6.

Eleutherococcus

Eleutherococcus Senticosus

Alternate/Related names: Russian Ginseng, Siberian Ginsing, Eleutheroginseng

U.S. BRAND NAMES OF CLINICALLY TESTED PRODUCTS

Elagen (Eladon) = Elagen (Eladon) in Europe

DESCRIPTION

Eleutherococcus senticosus (commonly but incorrectly known as Siberian or Russian ginseng) is only distantly related to the true ginseng species *(Panax ginseng)*. Its popularity stems from the work of Russian scientist I.I. Brekhman, who considered eleutherococcus to be functionally identical to *P. ginseng* and wrote extensively on its properties. Eleutherococcus' major advantage over true ginseng was its far lower cost.

Brekhman believed that *E. senticosus* is an adaptogen, a hypothetical substance that helps the body adapt to stresses of various kinds, minimizing the damaging effects of heat, cold, exertion, trauma, sleep deprivation, toxic exposure, radiation, infection, and psychological stress. Furthermore, a proposed adaptogen must also satisfy the following three criteria: (1) It causes few to no side effects or overt physiological changes, (2) it has a nonspecific action that functions in many circumstances, and (3) it has a normalizing action that tends to return an organism toward homeostasis regardless of the direction in which it is out of balance.

The treatment that comes closest to satisfying the definition of an adaptogen is a healthful lifestyle (except, of course, that this is not a substance). There is no convincing evidence that eleutherococcus (or any other substance) possesses adaptogenic properties.

PHARMACOLOGY

Eleutherococcus contains sterols, coumarins, phenylpropanoids, oleanolic acids, lignans, triterpenes, and phenylpropanoid derivatives, collectively called eleutherosides A-M.[1] This nomenclature was deliberately designed in imitation of the ginsenosides found in *P. ginseng;* however, the eleutherosides are not chemically related to the ginsenosides nor to each other.

Numerous human and animal studies performed in the former Soviet Union suggest that eleutherococcus and its constituents have adaptogenic effects[1]; however, few of these trials were conducted at modern standards of scientific rigor. A German study suggests that eleutherococcus may have immunomodulatory effects.[2] In this 4-week placebo-controlled human trial, eleutherococcus increased the absolute number of immunocompetent cells, especially T-lymphocytes of the helper/inducer type.

CLINICAL STUDIES

GENITAL HERPES

A 6-month double-blind placebo-controlled trial of 93 men and women with recurrent herpes infections found that treatment with eleutherococcus (2 g daily) reduced the frequency of infections by approximately 50%.[3]

SPORTS PERFORMANCE ENHANCEMENT

A double-blind placebo-controlled study of 20 athletes over an 8-week period found no improvement in physical performance.[4] In addition, a small double-blind crossover trial found eleutherococcus ineffective for improving performance in endurance exercise.[5]

ADAPTOGEN

Soviet-era studies enrolling more than 4,300 healthy and nonhealthy individuals report that eleutherococcus may have adaptogenic effects.[1] However, the meaningfulness of these clinical trials is limited by poor design.

PROPOSED INDICATIONS AND USAGE

Eleutherococcus is widely marketed as a sports supplement, despite the absence of meaningful evidence that it is effective. Other purported effects include enhancing energy and strengthening immunity. Based on the one clinical trial reported above, eleutherococcus has recently been marketed as a treatment for genital herpes.

WARNINGS

None.

PRECAUTIONS

Soviet-era animal studies finding eleutherococcus nonteratogenic are not entirely reassuring. Safety in pregnant or lactating women, young children, or individuals with hepatic or renal disease has not been established, although there are no known risks in those populations.

DRUG INTERACTIONS

None reported.

There has been one report of otherwise unexplained elevated digoxin levels in a patient taking digoxin and eleutherococcus.[6] This appears to have been a case of interference with a diagnostic test, rather than actual elevation of digoxin levels.

ADVERSE REACTIONS

Eleutherococcus is generally well tolerated. Human clinical trials have not reported any significant side effects. According to studies performed primarily in the former Soviet Union, eleutherococcus appears to present a low order of toxicity in both the short and long term.[1] The LD_{50} of *E. senticosus* root in mice has been determined to be 31.0 g/kg. In rats, administration of a 33% ethanol extract at a dose of 5 ml/kg for 320 days produced no toxic manifestations. Studies of rats, mink, lamb, and rabbits have found no evidence of teratogenicity.

PROPOSED DOSAGE AND ADMINISTRATION

The usual daily dose of *E. senticosus* is 2 to 3 g of whole herb or 300 to 400 mg of extract.

PATIENT INFORMATION

Eleutherococcus (often incorrectly called Russian or Siberian ginseng) is an herb widely stated to improve the body's ability to respond to stress. However, it has not been proven effective for this, or any other purposes, including improving sports performance.

If you take the drug digoxin, eleutherococcus might interfere with lab tests designed to measure the levels of digoxin in your body.

The safety of eleutherococcus for pregnant or nursing women or young children has not been established. Individuals with severe liver or kidney disease should consult a physician before using this (or any other) supplement.

REFERENCES

1. Farnsworth NR, Kinghorn AD, Soejarto DD, et al. Siberian ginseng *(Eleutherococcus senticosus):* current status as an adaptogen. *Econ Med Plant Res.* 1985;1:156-215. **2.** Bohn B, Nebe CT, Birr C. Flowcytometric studies with *Eleutherococcus senticosus* extract as an immunomodulatory agent. *Arzneimittelforschung.* 1987;37:1193-1196. **3.** Williams M. Immuno-protection against herpes simplex type II infection by eleutherococcus root extract. *Int J Alt Complement Med.* 1995;13:9-12. **4.** Dowling EA, Redondo DR, Branch JD, et al. Effect of *Eleutherococcus senticosus* on submaximal and maximal exercise performance. *Med Sci Sports Exerc.* 1996;28:482-489. **5.** Eschbach LF, Webster MJ, Boyd JC, et al. The effect of Siberian ginseng *(Eleutherococcus senticosus)* on substrate utilization and performance. *Int J Sport Nutr Exerc Metab.* 2000;10:444-451. **6.** McRae S. Elevated serum digoxin levels in a patient taking digoxin and Siberian ginseng. *CMAJ.* 1996;155:293-295.

Fenugreek

Trigonella Foenumgraecum

U.S. BRAND NAMES OF CLINICALLY TESTED PRODUCTS

None.

DESCRIPTION

For millennia, fenugreek seed has been used both as a medicine and as a food spice in Egypt, India, and the Middle East. It was traditionally recommended for the treatment of wounds, bronchitis, digestive problems, arthritis, kidney problems, and male reproductive conditions.

PHARMACOLOGY

Defatted fenugreek seed contains about 50% dietary fiber (much of which is pectin) and 28% protein.[1] Constituents present in small amounts include steroid saponins, steroid saponin-peptide esters, flavonoids, sterols, and volatile oils. Although the mechanism of action of fenugreek is not fully understood, animal studies suggest that the seed's fiber may impair glucose absorption in the intestines, among other potential mechanisms.[2,3]

CLINICAL STUDIES

The evidence base for fenugreek is weak. Animal studies, open trials, and one small single-blind controlled study have reported improvements in overall blood sugar control, blood sugar elevations in response to a meal, and cholesterol levels.[1,2,4]

PROPOSED INDICATIONS AND USAGE

Scant preliminary evidence suggests that fenugreek seed may have hypoglycemic properties. Additional proposed uses parallel those of other high-fiber foods, such as preventing heart disease and cancer and aiding weight loss.

WARNINGS

None.

PRECAUTIONS

As a commonly eaten food, fenugreek seed is generally regarded as safe. The only common side effect is mild gastrointestinal distress when it is taken in high doses.

Extracts of fenugreek seed have been shown to stimulate uterine contractions in guinea pigs.[5] For this reason, pregnant women should not take fenugreek in dosages higher than are commonly used as a spice (perhaps 5 g daily).

Maximum safe dosages for young children, lactating women, and those with hepatic or renal disease have not been established.

DRUG INTERACTIONS

Fenugreek seed could conceivably cause hypoglycemia in diabetic patients who use insulin or other hypoglycemic drugs.

ADVERSE REACTIONS

None reported other than mild, self-limited gastrointestinal distress.

PROPOSED DOSAGE AND ADMINISTRATION

The typical dosage is 5 to 33 g of defatted fenugreek seeds taken 3 times a day with meals. Because the seeds are somewhat bitter, they are often taken in capsule form or added to foods.

PATIENT INFORMATION

Fenugreek seed is a food spice that has been marketed as a treatment for diabetes. However, there has been little scientific study of this herb. Individuals with diabetes who use fenugreek should closely monitor blood sugar levels to avoid possible hypoglycemic reactions.

Pregnant women should not take fenugreek in doses higher than common food uses (5 g daily).

The maximum safe dosage of fenugreek for nursing women, young children, or individuals with severe liver or kidney disease has not been established.

REFERENCES

1. Sharma RD, Raghuram TC, Rao NS. Effect of fenugreek seeds on blood glucose and serum lipids in type I diabetes. *Eur J Clin Nutr.* 1990;44:301-306. **2.** Madar Z, Abel R, Samish S, et al. Glucose-lowering effect of fenugreek in non-insulin dependent diabetics. *Eur J Clin Nutr.* 1988;42:51-54. **3.** Madar Z. New sources of dietary fibre. *Int J Obes.* 1987;11(Suppl):57-65. **4.** Sharma RD, Sarkar A, Hazra DK, et al. Use of fenugreek seed powder in the management of non-insulin dependent diabetes mellitus. *Nutr Res.* 1996;16:1331-1339. **5.** Leung A, et al. *Encyclopedia of common natural ingredients used in food, drugs, and cosmetics.* New York: John Wiley and Sons; 1996: 243-244.

Feverfew

Tanacetum Parthenium

U.S. BRAND NAMES OF CLINICALLY TESTED PRODUCTS

None.

DESCRIPTION

Feverfew's feathery and aromatic leaves have long been used medicinally to assist in childbirth, promote menstruation, induce abortions, relieve rheumatic pain, and treat severe headaches. Its most common current use is to prevent migraine headaches.

PHARMACOLOGY

Feverfew contains many sesquiterpene lactones with an alpha-methylenebutyrolactone structure, of which the germacranolide parthenolide is the primary constituent.[1] It also contains camphor, terpenes, and pyrethrin (used as an insecticide). The relative preponderance of these various constituents vary widely, depending on the variety of feverfew used and the conditions in which it was grown.

In vitro studies suggest that feverfew extract can suppress prostaglandin production without an effect on cyclo-oxygenase.[2] Furthermore, lactones (parthenolide and epoxyartemorin) isolated from feverfew have been found to have inhibitory effects, with IC50 values ranging from approximately 1 to 5 μg/ml, irreversibly inhibiting eicosanoid generation.[3]

Although parthenolide has long been considered the active ingredient in feverfew, this hypothesis was recently called into question by negative results with an extract standardized to its parthenolide concentration.[4] Tanetin, a lipophilic avonol (6-hydroxykaempferol 3,7,4'-trimethyl ether), has also been identified as a feverfew constituent that inhibits generation of pro-inflammatory eicosanoids.[5]

CLINICAL STUDIES

MIGRAINE HEADACHES

Three small double-blind studies using whole feverfew leaf for migraine prophylaxis returned positive results; two trials of feverfew extract found either no benefit or benefit only on subgroup analysis, respectively.

One trial used feverfew leaf from British sources with a parthenolide content of 0.66%.[6] In this 8-month crossover study of 59 patients, treatment with 82 mg feverfew daily was associated with a 24% reduction in the number of migraines, a significant decrease in nausea and vomiting during attacks, and a trend toward reduced severity of headache pain.

In the second study, all 57 migraine patients were initially treated with 50 mg twice daily of an Israeli whole feverfew leaf containing 0.2% parthenolide for 2 months, followed by a 2-month double-blind crossover trial.[7] The results showed significant improvement in intensity of headache pain, nausea, vomiting, and photophobia, and light sensitivity. Unfortunately, the study did not report whether there was an effect on migraine frequency.

Benefits were also seen in a poorly designed double-blind placebo-controlled trial of 17 individuals.[8]

In contrast to these positive results, a randomized double-blind placebo-controlled trial of 50 individuals given an alcohol extract of feverfew standardized to its parthenolide content found no benefit.[4] This negative outcome, in conjunction with the positive results of the low-parthenolide study mentioned above, suggests that the identification of parthenolide as the active principle was premature.

In addition, an unpublished double-blind placebo-controlled study of 147 individuals found equivocal evidence at best for a proprietary CO_2 feverfew extract called Mig-99.[9] The primary outcome measure was reduction of migraine incidence during the final 4-week period of the 12-week treatment phase as compared to migraine incidence during a 4-week baseline interval. Three doses of feverfew extract were compared to placebo. No statistically significant differences were seen in the feverfew group as a whole as compared to the placebo group. However, in a predefined subgroup of 47 individuals with four or more migraines during the baseline interval, the two higher doses of feverfew significantly reduced the number of migraine attacks.

RHEUMATOID ARTHRITIS

A double-blind placebo-controlled study followed 41 symptomatic rheumatoid arthritis patients over 6 weeks, and reported no benefit with feverfew treatment.[10]

PROPOSED INDICATIONS AND USAGE

Feverfew is widely used in the United Kingdom for prophylaxis of chronic migraine headaches, and has become popular in the United States as well. It is also marketed as "herbal aspirin" for fever, joint pain, etc.; however, feverfew, despite its name, does not appear to reduce fevers.

WARNINGS

None.

PRECAUTIONS

Chewing whole feverfew leaf can cause mouth sores.

Safety has definitely not been established in pregnancy, since feverfew has a folk history as an abortifacient. Safety for lactating women, young children or individuals with severe hepatic or renal disease has also not been established.

DRUG INTERACTIONS

Because parthenolide affects platelet activity, it has been suggested that caution should be exercised with the concomitant use of feverfew and anticoagulants or antiplatelet agents. One study comparing platelet aggregation in a group of 10 patients who had taken feverfew over a period of 3.5 to 8 years against a control group that had discontinued feverfew for 6 months or more found no significant difference.[11] However, it is possible that drug combinations could amplify otherwise marginal effects.

ADVERSE REACTIONS

Feverfew is generally well tolerated. Animal studies have shown no adverse effects at 100 times the human daily dose; an LD_{50} has not been determined.[12] A study of 30 feverfew users and matched case controls found no chromosomal changes in circulating lymphocytes among chronic users of feverfew.[13] In the 8-month Nottingham clinical trial of 72 patients (59 completed the study), no significant differences in side effects between feverfew-treated patients and the control group were observed.[6] There were also no changes in standard chem panels, blood counts, and urinalysis.

In a 300-patient survey, 11.3% reported mouth ulcerations from chewing feverfew leaf, occasionally accompanied by general inflammation of tissues in the mouth, and 6.5% reported mild gastrointestinal distress.[8] However, in the Nottingham study, which used capsulated feverfew, this did not occur.

One report described a "postfeverfew syndrome" that consisted of withdrawal symptoms such as headache, insomnia, nervousness, and joint discomfort,[8] but this pattern was not seen in another study.[6] Feverfew was used for a longer time in the former case.

PROPOSED DOSAGE AND ADMINISTRATION

The daily dosage of feverfew used in the Nottingham study was 82 mg of dried leaf, containing 0.66% parthenolide. Subsequent dosage recommendations tended to concentrate on reproducing the same daily quantity of parthenolide. However, now that the primacy of parthenolide has been challenged, it is no longer clear which forms of feverfew are effective or precisely at which dose they should be taken.

PATIENT INFORMATION

Feverfew is an herb marketed for preventing migraine headaches. However, the evidence that it works is very weak.

Chewing whole feverfew can cause mouthsores. Individuals taking drugs that impair blood clotting should avoid feverfew. These drugs include Coumadin (warfarin), heparin, and aspirin.

Pregnant women should not use feverfew.

Safety for nursing women, young children, or individuals with severe liver or kidney disease has not been established.

REFERENCES

1. European Scientific Cooperative on Phytotherapy. *Tanaceti parthenii* herba/folium (feverfew). Exeter, UK: ESCOP; 1996-1997. Monographs on the Medicinal Uses of Plant Drugs, Fascicule 2:1. **2.** Collier HO, Butt NM, McDonald-Gibson WJ, et al. Extract of feverfew inhibits prostaglandin biosynthesis [letter]. *Lancet.* 1980;2:922-923. **3.** Sumner H, Salan U, Knight DW, et al. Inhibition of 5-lipoxygenase and cyclo-oxygenase in leukocytes by feverfew. Involvement of sesquiterpene lactones and other components. *Biochem Pharmacol.* 1992;43:2313-2320. **4.** De Weerdt CJ, Bootsma HPR, Hendriks H. Herbal medicines in migraine prevention. Randomized double-blind placebo-controlled crossover trial of a feverfew preparation. *Phytomedicine.* 1996;3:225-230. **5.** Williams CA, Hoult JRS, Harborne JB, et al. A biologically active lipophilic flavonol from Tanacetum parthenium. *Phytochemistry.* 1995;38:267-270. **6.** Murphy JJ, Heptinstall S, Mitchell JRA. Randomised double-blind placebo-controlled trial of feverfew in migraine prevention. *Lancet.* 1988;23:189-192. **7.** Palevitch DG, Earon G, Carasso R. Feverfew (Tanacetum parthenium) as a prophylactic treatment for migraine: a double-blind placebo-controlled study. *Phytother Res.* 1997;11:508-511. **8.** Johnson ES, Kadam NP, Hylands DM, et al. Efficacy of feverfew as prophylactic treatment of migraine. *Br Med J (Clin Res Ed).* 1985;291:569-573. **9.** Pfaffenrath V, Fischer M, Friede M, et al. Clinical dose-response study for the investigation of efficacy and tolerability of Tanacetum parthenium in migraine prophylaxis. Presented at: Deutscher Schmerzkongress; October 20-24, 1999; Munich, Germany. **10.** Pattrick M, Heptinstall S, Doherty M. Feverfew in rheumatoid arthritis: a double blind, placebo controlled study. *Ann Rheum Dis.* 1989;48:547-549. **11.** Groenewegen WA, Knight DW, Heptinstall S. Progress in the medicinal chemistry of the herb feverfew. *Prog Med Chem.* 1992;29:217-238. **12.** Baldwin CA, Anderson LA, Philipson JD. What pharmacists should know about feverfew. *Pharm J.* 1987;239:237-238. **13.** Johnson ES, Kadam NP, Anderson D, et al. Investigation of possible genetoxic effects of feverfew in migraine patients. *Hum Toxicol.* 1987;6:533-534.

Garlic

Allium Sativum

Alternate/Related Names: ***Allium spp.***

U.S. BRAND NAMES OF CLINICALLY TESTED PRODUCTS

Kwai (Lichtwer Pharma) = Kwai (Lichtwer Pharma) in Europe
Kyolic (Wakanuga) = Kyolic (Wakanuga) in Europe

DESCRIPTION

Garlic has been used as a food and medicine since ancient times, and throughout most of the world. In the early twentieth century, it was most commonly used as a topical antibiotic, and internally for the treatment of hypertension and atherosclerosis.

PHARMACOLOGY

Fresh garlic contains 0.35% sulfur by weight, bound to cysteine and its derivatives. Some of the most investigated bioactive constituents or breakdown products include alliin, allicin, ajoene, allylpropyl sulfide, diallyl disulfide, diallyl trisulfide, s-allylcysteine, and vinyldithiins.

Little to no allicin exists in an intact garlic bulb. However, when garlic is crushed or cut, the enzyme allinase is brought in contact with alliin, yielding allicin. Allicin breaks down rapidly and non-enzymatically into vinyldithiins, diallyl disulfide, and ajoene. At room temperature, the half-life of allicin is 3 hours, and 20 minutes of cooking suffices to degrade it entirely. Garlic oil and aged garlic possess neither alliin nor allicin, and therefore are presumed to differ significantly in medical properties from fresh intact garlic and from garlic powder manufactured to contain alliin.

Pharmacokinetic studies in rats have found that alliin is absorbed well orally, reaching maximum serum concentrations within 10 minutes, and urinary measurements suggest a minimum absorption rate of 65% for allicin and 73% for vinyldithiins.[1] Studies of isolated rat liver found that allicin administered at 400 mcg/minute was 95% metabolized on first pass into diallyl sulfide, allyl mercaptan, and other breakdown products.[2] Oral s-allylcysteine was well absorbed in rats, mice, and dogs.[3]

In vitro experiments on animal hepatocytes have found that allicin and (to a lesser extent) ajoene, s-allylcysteine, and related chemicals reduce cholesterol biosynthesis by inhibiting HMG-CoA reductase as well as 14-alpha-demethylase.[4-9] Garlic's apparent antihypertensive, fibrinolytic, and antiplatelet effects may be mediated through activation of nitric oxide synthetase.[10] Garlic concentrates selenium in a readily absorbable form, which may partially explain its observed antioxidant and chemopreventive properties.[11] In addition, the sulfuric components of garlic may also directly bind and inactivate reactive genotoxic metabolites.[12]

Animal studies support the assertion that garlic can favorably alter lipid profiles.[13,14] Garlic preparations including both fresh garlic and garlic oil have also been found to retard or reverse atherosclerosis in rats, rabbits, and humans, reducing the size of atheromatous lesions by nearly 50%.[15-19] This anti-atheromatous effect appears to reside primarily in the lipophilic, sulfur-containing fractions of whole garlic.

Garlic extracts have been found to reduce blood pressure in dogs and rats.[19] Fibrinolytic and antiplatelet activity has also been demonstrated in human, animal, and in vitro studies of various forms of garlic.[20-25] Both garlic powder and aged garlic have been found to produce antithrombotic effects, perhaps indicating a wide spectrum of active components. Ajoene, alliin, allicin, vinyldithiins, and diallyl disulfide all appear to inhibit platelet aggregation.[26,27]

Antioxidant properties have been found with whole garlic.[28,29,30] However, another study with powdered garlic found no reduction in the oxidation of lipids.[31] Various garlic extracts have also been shown in animals to suppress the DNA-damaging activity of several well-known toxins.[12] Tumor-inhibiting properties have been seen in several animal studies.[24]

Several animal and in vitro studies have demonstrated that garlic (and specifically allicin) possesses broad-spectrum antibiotic, antifungal, and antihelminthic actions, although systemic effectiveness has not been shown.[20,32] Garlic extracts also increase certain measures of immunological activity,[14,33,34] although these effects have not been proven clinically meaningful.

Despite early studies showing that garlic stimulates insulin production, therapeutic studies have found no such effect.[19,35]

CLINICAL STUDIES

Highly imperfect evidence suggests that garlic possesses anti-atherosclerotic effects, mediated through numerous separate actions.

ATHEROSCLEROSIS

In a 4-year double-blind placebo-controlled study that enrolled 280 individuals, standardized garlic powder at a dose of 900 mg/day significantly slowed the development of atherosclerosis as quantified by ultrasound measurement of intimal-medial thickness.[36] However, a high drop-out rate makes the results unreliable.

Evidence from an observational cross-section case-control study suggests that garlic has an overall atherosclerosis-retarding effect.[37] Finally, one placebo-controlled (but not blinded) study of 432 patients who had suffered myocardial infarction showed significant reductions in reinfarction rate (35%) and mortality (45%) with the use of garlic-oil extract over a period of 3 years.[38]

HYPERLIPIDEMIA

Despite extensive German literature finding garlic effective for hypercholesterolemia,[39-42] most recent trials have found no effect.[43-48] The explanation may lie in garlic's apparently modest benefit. A meta-analysis that accepted 13 trials found evidence of cholesterol reduction in the range of 5% compared to placebo.[49] Reported negative trials lacked statistical power to identify a benefit this small.

HYPERTENSION

According to two small double-blind placebo-controlled trials of hypertensive individuals, garlic may reduce blood pressure mildly, in the average range of 10 mm Hg for systolic blood pressure and 5 mm Hg for diastolic blood pressure, as compared to placebo.[50,51] Blood pressure reduction with garlic has also been seen in normotensive individuals.[50]

ANTITHROMBOTIC EFFECTS

In a 4-week double-blind controlled trial, 64 individuals with consistently increased spontaneous platelet aggregation were treated with either placebo or 900 mg of standardized garlic powder daily.[22] A significant decrease in spontaneous platelet aggregation was seen in the treated group. Similar effects were seen in a smaller trial using aged garlic at a dose of 7.2 g daily.[52]

Garlic has also been found in human trials to increase fibrinolytic activity, either when taken in a single dose or over an extended period of time.[27]

CHEMOPREVENTION

Several retrospective and prospective epidemiological studies have shown that individuals whose diet includes relatively large amounts of garlic tend to develop cancer of various types less frequently.[14,20,33,34,53,54]

ANTIMICROBIAL EFFECTS

Raw garlic extracts kill a wide variety of microorganisms in vitro, including fungi, bacteria, viruses, and protozoa.[20,32,55,56] However, there are no clinical trials on this potential use of garlic. Topical effects could also theoretically make garlic useful for treating intestinal infections[57,58] as well as protecting against *Helicobacter pylori*.[59] However, in vivo studies of garlic for *H. pylori* infection have not been promising.[60,61] There is no real evidence that garlic functions as a systemic antibiotic.

PROPOSED INDICATIONS AND USAGE

Garlic may possess antithrombotic, antihypertensive, antihyperlipidemic, and antioxidant actions, potentially leading to an overall anti-atherosclerotic effect. However, the evidence base for these claims is highly imperfect.

Epidemiological evidence suggests that regular use of dietary garlic may decrease the incidence of cancer. Raw garlic possesses topical antimicrobial activity, although there is essentially no clinical evidence of benefit. Folklore suggesting that garlic ingestion can ward off insect bites may have some truth to it.[62]

Oral garlic is widely promoted as a systemic antibiotic, antiviral, antifungal, and immunostimulant agent, and as a treatment for colds. Garlic has additionally been proposed for blood glucose regulation in diabetes and "hypoglycemia," asthma, allergies, fungal infections including tinea pedis and vaginitis, congestive heart failure, intermittent claudication, Raynaud's disease, parasites, arthritis, and traveler's diarrhea. There is no clinical evidence, however, to justify any of these claims.

WARNINGS

Garlic may possess significant antithrombotic and fibrinolytic actions, making its use risky in individuals with altered coagulation hemostasis, during pregnancy and labor and delivery, and within the perisurgical period.

PRECAUTIONS

Based on reports of increased bleeding following surgery, as well as other evidence of potential bleeding complications (see Pharmacology, Drug Interactions, and Adverse Reactions sections), the European Scientific Cooperative on Phytotherapy recommends against using garlic before, during, or immediately after surgical procedures.[2,63,64] For the same reason, it appears wise to caution against garlic use in the period before and after labor and delivery.

Topical garlic can cause skin irritation, blistering, and even third-degree burns.[65]

Based on theoretical reasons rather than case reports, garlic is not recommended for patients with brittle diabetes (possible hypoglycemic effect), pemphigus (activation by sulfur-containing compounds), organ transplants (possible activation of immune rejection), or acute rheumatoid arthritis (possible increase in autoimmunity).

Cooked garlic in dietary doses is presumed to be safe in pregnancy and lactation, based on its extensive food use. However, there are few toxicity studies on the most commonly used garlic extracts, and no studies on teratogenicity or embryotoxicity for any form of garlic.[2] For this reason, use of standardized garlic extracts should be avoided during pregnancy, as well as in young children and individuals with severe hepatic or renal disease.

DRUG INTERACTIONS

There are case reports of increased bleeding time in two patients combining warfarin and garlic supplements.[66] Based on this, as well as evidence discussed earlier, patients taking anticoagulants or antiplatelet agents should avoid using garlic extracts. It is also conceivable that garlic could interact with other natural substances possessing anticoagulant or antithrombotic effects, such as ginkgo, policosanol, and high-dose vitamin E.

Garlic has been found to reduce plasma concentrations of saquinavir.[67] In addition, two individuals with HIV experienced severe gastrointestinal toxicity from ritonavir after taking garlic supplements.[68]

ADVERSE REACTIONS

Based on its food use, garlic is on the FDA's GRAS (generally recognized as safe) list. However, garlic in the diet is usually cooked. Typical standardized garlic products contain substances (such as alliin) not found in cooked garlic, making them more similar to raw garlic. There are few toxicity studies on these products. Only aged garlic has been well studied, and it lacks many active and potentially toxic components found in standardized garlic powder (as well as in raw garlic). Rats fed up to 2,000 mg/kg of aged garlic extract for 6 months showed no significant toxicity.[69] Genotoxicity and mutagenicity studies have been negative for both aged and fresh garlic.[70,71]

One case report associated garlic supplement use with a spontaneous spinal epidural hematoma.[72] However, in extensive clinical trials, standardized garlic extract as well as aged garlic powder have not been associated with serious side effects.[73] The most common problem with garlic is the odor. The use of so-called "odorless" products can alleviate, though not entirely eliminate, this problem.[19]

PROPOSED DOSAGE AND ADMINISTRATION

In most of the studies evaluating the proposed hypolipidemic effects of garlic, researchers used a dried form that supplies a daily dose of at least 10 mg of alliin, or a total allicin potential of 4 to 5 mg. However, not all manufacturers agree that allicin or alliin are at all relevant to garlic's activity. The widely available deodorized form of garlic called Kyolic lacks allicin and many other constituents of garlic. Nonetheless, such products have provided positive results in studies and appear to have fewer gastric side effects.[41,52]

Garlic is also sometimes sold as an oil extract. Such products contain no allicin or alliin but high levels of ajoene, dithiins, and other breakdown products.[74]

PATIENT INFORMATION

Garlic is widely marketed as an herb for lowering cholesterol and preventing cardiovascular disease. However, evidence suggests that garlic is only minimally effective, if at all, for high cholesterol. It may help protect the heart in other ways, but the evidence isn't strong.

Garlic is also said to enhance the immune system and also act as a natural antibiotic. However, there is no scientific evidence for these claims.

Garlic interferes with the ability of the blood to clot. For this reason, individuals taking anticoagulant drugs should not use garlic. These drugs include Coumadin (warfarin), aspirin, heparin, Plavix (clopidogrel), and Trental (pentoxifylline). It is possible that garlic could also interact with other natural substances that interfere with blood clotting, such as ginkgo, policosanol, and high-dose vitamin E. Furthermore, garlic should be avoided in other circumstances where excessive bleeding is a risk, such as surgery and labor and delivery. Hemophiliacs should also avoid garlic.

Individuals with HIV should not use garlic, as it might interfere with the actions of anti-HIV medications or increase their side effects.

The maximum safe dosage of garlic for pregnant or nursing women or young children has not been established. Individuals with severe liver or kidney disease should consult a physician before using this (or any other) herb.

REFERENCES

1. Lachmann G, Lorenz D, Radeck W, et al. The pharmacokinetics of the S35 labeled garlic constituents alliin, allicin and vinyldithiine [in German; English abstract]. *Arzneimittelforschung.* 1994;44:734-743. **2.** European Scientific Cooperative on Phytotherapy. *Allii sativi bulbus* (garlic). Exeter, UK: ESCOP; 1996-1997. Monographs on the Medicinal Uses of Plant Drugs, Fascicule 3: 1, 4-5. **3.** Nagae S, Ushijima M, Hatono S, et al. Pharmacokinetics of the garlic compound S-allylcysteine. *Planta Med.* 1994;60:214-217. **4.** Gebhardt R. Multiple inhibitory effects of garlic extracts on cholesterol biosynthesis in hepatocytes. *Lipids.* 1993;28:613-619. **5.** Gebhardt R, Beck H, Wagner KG. Inhibition of cholesterol biosynthesis by allicin and ajoene in rat hepatocytes and HepG2 cells. *Biochim Biophys Acta.* 1994;1213:57-62. **6.** Gebhardt R, Beck H. Differential inhibitory effects of garlic-derived organosulfur compounds on cholesterol biosynthesis in primary rat hepatocyte cultures. *Lipids.* 1996;31:1269-1276. **7.** Qureshi AA, Abuirmeileh N, Din ZZ, et al. Inhibition of cholesterol and fatty acid biosynthesis in liver enzymes and chicken hepatocytes by polar fractions of garlic. *Lipids.* 1983;18:343-348. **8.** Yeh YY, Yeh SM. Garlic reduces plasma lipids by inhibiting hepatic cholesterol and triacylglycerol synthesis. *Lipids.* 1994;29:189-193. **9.** Yeh YY, Liu L. Cholesterol-lowering effect of garlic extracts and organosulfur compounds: human and animal studies. *J Nutr.* 2001;131:989S-993S. **10.** Das I, Khan NS, Sooranna SR. Potent activation of nitric oxide synthase by garlic: a basis for its therapeutic applications. *Curr Med Res Opin.* 1995;13:257-263. **11.** Ip C; Lisk DJ. Efficacy of cancer prevention by high-selenium garlic is primarily dependent on the action of selenium. *Carcinogenesis.*

1995;16:2649-2652. **12.** Das T, Roychoudhury A, Sharma A, et al. Modification of clastogenicity of three known clastogens by garlic extract in mice in vivo. *Environ Mol Mutagen.* 1993;21:383-388. **13.** Kamanna VS, Chandrasekhara N. Effect of garlic (Allium sativum linn) on serum lipoproteins and lipoprotein cholesterol levels in albino rats rendered hypercholesteremic by feeding cholesterol. *Lipids.* 1982;17:483-488. **14.** Lau BH, Tadi PP, Tosk JM. Allium sativum (garlic) and cancer prevention. *Nutr Res.* 1990;10:937-948. **15.** Bordia A, Verma SK, Srivastava KC. Effect of ginger (*Zingiber officinale* rosc.) and fenugreek (*Trigonella foenumgraecum* L.) on blood lipids, blood sugar and platelet aggregation in patients with coronary artery disease. *Prostaglandins Leukot Essent Fatty Acids.* 1997;56:379-384. **16.** Efendy JL, Simmons DL, Campbell GR, et al. The effect of the aged garlic extract, "kyolic," on the development of experimental atherosclerosis. *Atherosclerosis.* 1997;132:37-42. **17.** Heinle H, Betz E. Effects of dietary garlic supplementation in a rat model of atherosclerosis. *Arzneimittelforschung.* 1994;44:614-617. **18.** Jain RC, Konar DB. Effect of garlic oil in experimental cholesterol atherosclerosis. *Atherosclerosis.* 1978;29:125-129. **19.** Schulz V, Hansel R, Tyler VE. *Rational Phytotherapy: A Physicians' Guide to Herbal Medicine.* 3rd ed. Berlin, Germany: Springer-Verlag; 1998:112, 115, 121. **20.** Agarwal KC. Therapeutic actions of garlic constituents. *Med Res Rev.* 1996;16:111-124. **21.** Chutani SK, Bordia A. The effect of fried versus raw garlic on fibrinolytic activity in man. *Atherosclerosis.* 1981;38:417-421. **22.** Kiesewetter H, Jung F, Pindur G, et al. Effect of garlic on thrombocyte aggregation, microcirculation, and other risk factors. *Int J Clin Pharmacol Ther Toxicol.* 1991;29:151-155. **23.** Legnani C, Grascaro M, Guazzaloca G, et al. Effects of dried garlic preparation on fibrinolysis and platelet aggregation in healthy subjects. *Arzneimittelforschung.* 1993;43:119-122. **24.** Reuter HD, Sendl A. Allium sativum and Allium ursinum: chemistry, pharmacology and medical applications. *Econ Med Plant Res.* 1994;6:55-113. **25.** Steiner M, Lin RS. Changes in platelet function and susceptibility of lipoproteins to oxidation associated with administration of aged garlic extract. *J Cardiovasc Pharmacol.* 1998;31:904-908. **26.** Kleijnen J, Knipschild P, ter Riet G. Garlic, onions and cardiovascular risk factors. A review of the evidence from human experiments with emphasis on commercially available preparations. *Br J Clin Pharmacol.* 1989;28:535-544. **27.** Reuter HD. Allium sativum and Allium ursinum: part 2 pharmacology and medicinal application. *Phytomedicine.* 1995;2:73-91. **28.** Popov I, Blumstein A, Lewin G. Antioxidant effects of aqueous garlic extract: 1st communication: direct detection using photochemoluminescence. *Arzneimittelforschung.* 1994;44:602-604. **29.** Prasad K, Laxdal VA, Yu M, et al. Antioxidant activity of allicin, an active principle in garlic. *Mol Cell Biochem.* 1995;148:183-189. **30.** Torok B, Belagyi J, Rietz B, et al. Effectiveness of garlic on radical activity in radical generating systems. *Arzneimittelforschung.* 1994;44:608-611. **31.** Byrne DJ, Neil HAW, Vallance DT, et al. A pilot study of garlic consumption shows no significant effect on markers of oxidation or sub-fraction composition of low-density lipoprotein including lipoprotein(a) after allowance for non-compliance and the placebo effect. *Clin Chim Acta.* 1999;285:21-33. **32.** Hughes BG, Lawson LD. Antimicrobial effects of Allium sativum L. (garlic), Allium ampeloprasum L. (elephant garlic), and Allium cepa L. (onion), garlic compounds and commercial garlic supplement products. *Phytother Res.* 1991;5:154-158. **33.** Dausch JG, Nixon DW. Garlic: a review of its relationship to malignant disease. *Prev Med.* 1990;19:346-361. **34.** Dorant E, van den Brandt PA, Goldbohm RA, et al. Garlic and its significance for the prevention of cancer in humans: a critical view. *Br J Cancer.* 1993;67:424-429. **35.** Bever BO, Zahnd GR. Plants with oral hypoglycaemic action. *Q J Crude Drug Res.* 1979;17:139-196. **36.** Koscielny J, Klussendorf D, Latza R, et al. The antiatherosclerotic effect of Allium sativum. *Atherosclerosis.* 1999;144:237-249. **37.** Breithaupt-Grogler K, Ling M, Boudoulas H, et al. Protective effect of chronic garlic intake on elastic properties of aorta in the elderly. *Circulation.* 1997;96:2649-2655. **38.** Bordia A. Garlic and coronary heart disease. The effects of garlic extract therapy over three years on the reinfarction and mortality rate [translated from German]. *Dtsch Apoth Ztg.* 1989;129(suppl 15):16-17. **39.** Warshafsky S, Kamer RS, Sivak SL. Effect of garlic on total serum cholesterol. A meta-analysis. *Ann Intern Med.* 1993;119:599-605.] **40.** Mader FH. Treatment of hyperlipidaemia with garlic-powder tablets. Evidence from the German Association of General Practitioners' multicentric placebo-controlled double-blind study. *Arzneimittelforschung.* 1990;40:1111-1116. **41.** Steiner M, Khan AH, Holbert D, et al. A double-blind crossover study in moderately hypercholesterolemic men that compared the effect of aged garlic extract and placebo administration on blood lipids. *Am J Clin Nutr.* 1996;64:866-870. **42.** Holzgartner H, Schmidt U, Kuhn U. Comparison of the efficacy and tolerance of a garlic preparation vs. bezafibrate. *Arzneimittelforschung.* 1992;42:1473-1477. **43.** Neil HA, Silagy CA, Lancaster T, et al. Garlic powder in the treatment of moderate hyperlipidaemia: a controlled trial and meta-analysis. *J R Coll Physicians Lond.* 1996;30:329-334. **44.** Simons LA, Balasubramaniam S, von Konigsmark M, et al. On the effect of garlic on plasma lipids and lipoproteins in mild hypercholesterolaemia. *Atherosclerosis.* 1995;113:219-225. **45.** Superko HR, Krauss RM. Garlic powder, effect on plasma lipids, postprandial lipemia, low-density lipoprotein particle size, high-density lipoprotein subclass distribution and lipoprotein (a).*J Am Coll Cardiol.* 2000;35:321-326. **46.** Isaacsohn JL, Moser M, Stein EA, et al. Garlic powder and plasma lipids and lipoproteins: a multicenter, randomized, placebo-controlled trial. *Arch Intern Med.* 1998;158:1189-1194. **47.** Gardner CD, Chatterjee LM, Carlson JJ. The effect of a garlic preparation on plasma lipid levels in moderately hypercholesterolemic adults. *Atherosclerosis.* 2001;154:213-220. **48.** Kannar D, Wattanapenpaiboon N, Savige GS, et al. Hypocholesterolemic effect of an enteric-coated garlic supplement. *J Am Coll Nutr.* 2001;20:225-231. **49.** Stevinson C, Pittler MH, Ernst E. Garlic for treating hypercholesterolemia. A meta-analysis of randomized clinical trials. *Ann Intern Med.* 2000;133:420-429. **50.** Silagy CA, Neil HA. A meta-analysis of the effect of garlic on blood pressure. *J Hypertens.* 1994;12:463-468. **51.** Auer W, Eiber A, Hertkorn E, et al. Hypertension and hyperlipidaemia: garlic helps in mild cases. *Br J Clin Pract Suppl.* 1990;69:3-6. **52.** Steiner M, Lin RS. Changes in platelet function and susceptibility of lipoproteins to oxidation associated with administration of aged garlic extract. *J Cardiovasc Pharmacol.* 1998;31:904-908. **53.** Steinmetz KA, Kushi LH, Bostick RM, et al. Vegetables, fruit and colon cancer in the Iowa women's health study. *Am J Epidemiol.* 1994;139:1-13. **54.** You WC, Blot WJ, Chang YS, et al. Allium vegetables and reduced risk of stomach cancer. *J Natl Cancer Inst.* 1989;81:162-164. **55.** Ghannoum MA. Studies on the anticandidal mode of action of Allium sativum (garlic). *J Gen Microbiol.* 1988;134:2917-2924. **56.** Sandhu DK, Warraich MK, Singh S. Sensitivity of yeasts isolated from cases of vaginitis to aqueous extracts of garlic. *Mykosen.* 1980;23:691-698. **57.** Chowdhury AKA, Ahsan M, Islam SN, et al. Efficacy of aqueous extract of garlic & allicin in experimental shigellosis in rabbits. *Indian J Med Res.* 1991;93:33-36. **58.** Sharma VD, Sethi MS, Kumar A, et al. Antibacterial property of Allium sativum Linn.: in vivo & in vitro studies. *Indian J Exp Biol.* 1977;15:466-468. **59.** Sivam GP. Protection against Helicobacter pylori and other bacterial infections by garlic. *J Nutr.* 2001;131(3 suppl):1106S-1108S. **60.** Graham DY, Anderson SY, Lang T. Garlic or jalapeno peppers for treatment of *Helicobacter pylori* infection. *Am J Gastroenterol.* 1999;94:1200-1202. **61.** Aydin A, Ersoz G, Tekesin O, et al. Garlic oil and *Helicobacter pylori* infection [letter]. *Am J Gastroenterol.* 2000;95:563-564. **62.** Stjernberg L, Berglund J. Garlic as an insect repellent [letter]. *JAMA.* 2000;284:831. **63.** Burnham BE.Garlic as a possible risk for postoperative bleeding [letter]. *Plast Reconstr Surg.* 1995;95:213. **64.** German K, Kumar U, Blackford HN. Garlic and the risk of TURP bleeding. *Br J Urol.* 1995;76:518. **65.** Garty BZ. Garlic burns. *Pediatrics.* 1993;91:658-659. **66.** Sunter W. Warfarin and garlic (letter). *Pharm J.* 1991;246:722. **67.** Piscitelli SC, Burstein AH, Welden N, et al. Garlic supplements decrease saquinavir plasma concentrations. Presented at: 8th Conference on Retroviruses and Opportunistic Infections; February 4-8, 2001; Chicago, Ill. **68.** Piscitelli SC. Use of complementary medicines by patients with HIV: full sail into uncharted waters. *Medscape HIV/AIDS.* 2000:6(3). **69.** Sumiyoshi H, Kanezawa A, Masamoto K, et al. Chronic toxicity test of garlic extract in rats [in Japanese; English abstract]. *J Toxicol Sci.* 1984;9:61-75. **70.** Abraham SK, Kesavan PC. Genotoxicity of garlic, turmeric and asafoetida in mice. *Mutat Res.* 1984;136:85-88. **71.** Yoshida S, Hirao Y, Nakagawa S. Mutagenicity and cytotoxicity tests of garlic [in Japanese; English abstract]. *J Toxicol Sci.* 1984;9:77-86. **72.** Rose KD, Croissant PD, Parliament CF, et al. Spontaneous spinal epidural hematoma with associated platelet dysfunction from excessive garlic ingestion: a case report. *Neurosurgery.* 1990;26:880-882. **73.** Beck E, Grunwald J. Allium sativum in der Stufentherapie der Hyperlipidamie. Studie mit 1997 Patienten belegt Wirksamkeit und Vertraglichkeit [English abstract]. *Med Welt.* 1993;44:516-520. **74.** Lawson LD, Wang ZJ, Hughes BG. Identification and HPLC quantitation of the sulfides and dialk(en)yl thiosulfinates in commercial garlic products. *Planta Med.* 1991;57:363-370.

Ginger

Zingiber Officinale

U.S. BRAND NAMES OF CLINICALLY TESTED PRODUCTS

Zintona (Pharmaton) = Zintona (Dalidar Pharma) in Europe

DESCRIPTION

Ginger root consists of the rhizome (underground stem) of the plant with its bark-like outer covering scraped off. Ginger has a long history as both a food and medicinal herb. Chinese medical texts of the fourth century B.C. suggest that ginger is effective in nausea, diarrhea, stomachache, cholera, toothache, bleeding, and rheumatism. Later, ginger was also used in a variety of respiratory conditions, including coughs and the early stages of a cold.

PHARMACOLOGY

Ginger rhizome contains approximately 50% starches, 9% proteins, 6% to 8% lipids, and 1% to 3% volatile oils. The pungent substances in ginger include gingerols, shogaols, and related phenolic ketone derivatives.[1] Other constituents include essential oil, diarylheptenones, 6-gingesulfonic acids, and monoacyldigalactosylglycerols.

In cannulated rats, a 3 mg/kg IV bolus of 6-gingerol found a terminal half-life of 7.23 minutes and a total body clearance of 16.8 ml/min/kg.[2]

In vitro studies have found that ginger constituents inhibit prostaglandin and leukotriene synthesis, reduce platelet thromboxane production, and inhibit platelet aggregation.[3-7] However, many of these effects may not occur when whole ginger is taken orally.[8,9,10]

The mechanism of action of ginger in nausea is not known. Studies suggest that ginger does not influence the inner ear or oculomotor system,[11] and rather acts on the stomach alone, perhaps overriding central nervous system stimuli. Ginger appears to increase gastrointestinal motility without affecting gastric emptying.[12,13,14] Acetone extracts of ginger (150 mg/kg) protected against emesis in shrews when administered orally 1 hour before cyclophosphamide. 6-Gingerol (50 mg/kg orally) provided equivalent protection.[15]

Shogaols may exert a capsaicin-like effect on substance P.[16]

CLINICAL STUDIES

MOTION SICKNESS

The preponderance of the evidence suggests that ginger exerts a modest anti-motion sickness effect.

A double-blind placebo-controlled study of 79 Swedish naval cadets found that 1 g ginger could decrease vomiting and cold sweating but without significantly decreasing nausea and vertigo.[17] Benefits were also seen in a smaller double-blind trial controlled with placebo and dimenhydrinate.[18]

A double-blind comparative study that followed 1,489 individuals aboard ship found ginger equally effective as cinnarizine, cinnarizine with domperidone, cyclizine, dimenhydrinate with caffeine, meclozine with caffeine, and scopolamine.[5] Benefits were seen in other comparative trials as well.[19,20]

However, a double-blind placebo-controlled trial of 28 volunteers found no benefit with ginger compared to scopolamine or placebo.[21] Lack of comparative benefit was seen in two other small comparative studies that used strong nausea stimuli.[22,23]

NAUSEA AND VOMITING OF PREGNANCY

A double-blind placebo-controlled trial of 70 pregnant women evaluated the effectiveness of ginger for morning sickness.[24] Participants received either placebo or 250 mg of freshly prepared powdered ginger 3 times daily for a period of 4 days. The results indicated that ginger significantly reduced nausea and number of vomiting episodes. Benefits were also seen in a double-blind crossover trial of 27 women.[25]

POSTSURGICAL NAUSEA

The evidence regarding ginger's effectiveness in postsurgical nausea is almost perfectly mixed. It is possible that discrepancies may be due to the form of ginger used.

A double-blind British study (n=60) compared the effects of 1 g ginger, placebo, and metoclopramide in the treatment of nausea following gynecological surgery.[26] The results showed that both treatments produced a similar and statistically significant benefit compared to placebo. Similar results were seen in a study of comparable design that followed 120 women receiving elective laparoscopic gynecological surgery.[27] However, two other studies of similar size and design found no benefit.[28,29]

CHEMOTHERAPY-INDUCED NAUSEA

A small open trial suggests that ginger may reduce nausea caused by 8-MOP.[30]

OSTEOARTHRITIS

A double-blind placebo-controlled crossover trial compared ginger extract, ibuprofen, and placebo in 56 individuals with osteoarthritis of the hip or knee.[31] Ginger failed to prove more effective at reducing symptoms than placebo.

PROPOSED INDICATIONS AND USAGE

There is some evidence that ginger might offer modest benefits for motion sickness and the nausea and vomiting of pregnancy. Evidence regarding its use for other forms of nausea is inconclusive.

Ginger is sometimes marketed for the treatment of various forms of joint pain, but there is some evidence that it is not effective for this purpose.

Without any clinical supporting evidence, ginger has also been suggested as treatment for headaches, rheumatoid arthritis, hypercholesterolemia, burns, ulcers, depression, impotence, upper respiratory infections, and hepatotoxicity.

WARNINGS

None.

PRECAUTIONS

Ginger is on the FDA's GRAS (generally recognized as safe) list.

Germany's Commission E mentions gallstones as a relative contraindication for reasons that are not evident.

Isolated 6-gingerol appears to be a potent mutagen, but the addition of whole ginger juice counteracts this effect.[32] Opposing effects have also been seen in other models of mutagenicity.[33] Ginger was found to possess antimutagenic activity in *Salmonella* TA98 using tryptophan pyrolysate as mutagen and S9 liver homogenate as activator.[34] Ginger has not been systematically tested in mammalian cell cultures.[1]

Like onions and garlic, extracts of ginger inhibit platelet aggregation and thromboxane synthesis in vitro. This has led to a concern that ginger might prolong bleeding time.

However, European studies with oral ginger in normal quantities have not found any significant anticoagulant effects in vivo.[8,9,10]

Safety in young children, pregnant or lactating women, or individuals with severe renal or hepatic disease has not been established. However, pregnant women have been enrolled in studies of ginger without apparent adverse effect.

DRUG INTERACTIONS

Due to its possible antiplatelet action, ginger use may be inadvisable in patients taking other antiplatelet or anticoagulant agents.

ADVERSE REACTIONS

Ginger is generally well tolerated. The acute oral LD_{50} of ginger in rats exceeded 5 g of ginger oil/kg.[23] In mice, an 80% ethanolic ginger extract was well tolerated at 2.5 mg/kg by gastric gavage.[35]

PROPOSED DOSAGE AND ADMINISTRATION

The typical dose of powdered ginger is 1 to 4 g daily taken in 2 to 4 divided doses.

PATIENT INFORMATION

Ginger is a common food spice that might offer some benefits in mild cases of nausea. In cases of severe nausea, or nausea associated with pregnancy or surgery, seek medical advice before self-treating with ginger. Individuals taking medications that impair blood clotting should avoid ginger. These include Coumadin (warfarin), heparin, and aspirin.

The safety of ginger for pregnant or nursing women or young children has not been established. Individuals with severe liver or kidney disease should consult a physician before using this (or any other) supplement.

REFERENCES

1. European Scientific Cooperative on Phytotherapy. *Zingiberis rhizoma.* Exeter, UK: ESCOP; 1996-1997. Monographs on the Medicinal Uses of Plant Drugs, Fascicule 1:5. **2.** Ding GH, Naora K, Hayashibara M, et al. Pharmacokinetics of [6]-gingerol after intravenous administration in rats. *Chem Pharm Bull (Tokyo).* 1991;39:1612-1614. **3.** Kiuchi F, et al. Inhibitors of Prostaglandin Biosynthesis from Ginger. *Chem Pharm Bull (Tokyo).* 1982;30:754-757. **4.** Kiuchi F, et al. Inhibition of Prostaglandin and Leukotriene Biosynthesis by Gingerols and Diarylheptanoids. *Chem Pharm Bull (Tokyo).* 1992;40:387-391. **5.** Srivastava KC. Effects of aqueous extracts of onion, garlic and ginger on platelet aggregation and metabolism of arachidonic acid in the blood vascular system: in vitro study. *Prostaglandins Leukot Med.* 1984;13:227-235. **6.** Srivastava KC. Isolation and effects of some ginger components on platelet aggregation and eicosanoid biosynthesis. *Prostaglandins Leukot Med.* 1986;25:187-198. **7.** Srivastava KC. Effect of onion and ginger consumption on platelet thromboxane production in humans. *Prostaglandins Leukot Essent Fatty Acids.* 1989;35:183-185. **8.** Bordia A, Verma SK, Srivastava KC. Effect of ginger (Zingiber officinale rosc.) and fenugreek (Trigonella foenumgraecum L.) on blood lipids, blood sugar and platelet aggregation in patients with coronary artery disease. *Prostaglandins Leukot Essent Fatty Acids.* 1997;56:379-384. **9.** Janssen PLTMK, Meyboom S, van Staveren WA, et al. Consumption of ginger (Zingiber officinale roscoe) does not affect ex vivo platelet thromboxane production in humans. *Eur J Clin Nutr.* 1996;50:772-774. **10.** Lumb AB. Effect of dried ginger on human platelet function. *Thromb Haemost.* 1994;71:110-111. **11.** Holtmann S, Clarke AH, Scherer H, et al. The anti-motion sickness mechanism of ginger. A comparative study with placebo and dimenhydrinate. *Acta Otolaryngol.* 1989;108:168-174. **12.** Micklefield G, Redeker Y, Meister V, et al. Effects of ginger on gastroduodenal motility. *Int J Clin Pharmacol Ther.* 1999;37:341-346. **13.** Phillips S, Hutchinson S, Ruggier R. Zingiber officinale does not affect gastric emptying rate. A randomised, placebo-controlled, crossover trial. *Anaesthesia.* 1993;48:393-395. **14.** Yamahara J, Huang Q, Li Y, et a. Gastrointestinal motility enhancing effect of ginger and its active constituents. *Chem Pharm Bull (Tokyo).* 1990;38:430-431. **15.** Yamahara J, Rong HQ, Naitoh Y, et al. Inhibition of cytotoxic drug-induced vomiting in suncus by a ginger constituent. *J Ethnopharmacol.* 1989;27:353-355. **16.** Onogi T, Minami M, Kuraishi Y, et al. Capsaicin-like effect of (6)-shogaol on substance P-containing primary afferents of rats: a possible mechanism of its analgesic action. *Neuropharmacology.* 1992;31:1165-1169. **17.** Grontved A, Brask T, Kambskard J, et al. Ginger root against seasickness: a controlled trial on the open sea. *Acta Otolaryngol (Stockh).* 1988;105:45-49. **18.** Mowrey DB, Clayson DE. Motion sickness, ginger, and psychophysics. *Lancet.* 1982;Mar:655-657. **19.** Riebenfeld D, Borzone L. Randomized double-blind study comparing ginger (Zintona(r)) and dimenhydrinate in motion sickness. *Healthnotes Rev.* 1999;6:98-101. **20.** Careddu P. Motion sickness in children: results of a double-blind study with ginger (Zintona(r)) and dimenhydrinate. *Healthnotes Rev.* 1999;6:102-107. **21.** Stewart JJ, Wood MJ, Wood CD, et al. Effects of ginger on motion sickness susceptibility and gastric function. *Pharmacology.* 1991;42:111-120. **22.** Stott JR, Hubble MP, Spencer MB. A double-blind comparative trial of powdered ginger root, hyosine hydrobromide, and cinnarizine in the prophylaxis of motion sickness induced by cross coupled stimulation. *AGARD Conf Proc.* 1985;(372):1-6. **23.** Wood CD, Manno JE, Wood MJ, et al. Comparison of efficacy of ginger with various antimotion sickness drugs. *Clin Res Pract Drug Regul Aff.* 1988;6:129-136. **24.** Vutyavanich T, Kraisarin T, Ruangsri R. Ginger for nausea and vomiting in pregnancy: randomized, double-masked, placebo-controlled trial. *Obstet Gynecol.* 2001;97:577-582. **25.** Fischer-Rasmussen W, Kjaer SK, Dahl C, et al. Ginger treatment of hyperemesis gravidarum. *Eur J Obstet Gynecol Reprod Biol.* 1991;38:19-24. **26.** Bone ME, Wilkinson DJ, Young JR, et al. Ginger root: a new antiemetic. The effect of ginger root on postoperative nausea and vomiting after major gynaecological sugery. *Anaesthesia.* 1990;45:669-671. **27.** Phillips S, Ruggier R, Hutchinson SE, et al. Zingiber officinale (ginger): an antiemetic for day case surgery. *Anaesthesia.* 1993;48:715-717. **28.** Arfeen Z, Owen H, Plummer JL, et al. A double-blind randomized controlled trial of ginger for the prevention of postoperative nausea and vomiting. *Anaesth Intensive Care.* 1995;23:449-452. **29.** Visalyaputra S, Petchpaisit N, Somcharoen K, et al. The efficacy of ginger root in the prevention of postoperative nausea and vomiting after outpatient gynaecological laparoscopy. *Anaesthesia.* 1998;53:486-510. **30.** Meyer K, Schwartz J, Crater D, et al. Zingiber officinale (ginger) used to prevent 8-Mop associated nausea. *Dermatol Nurs.* 1995;7:242-244. **31.** Bliddal H, Rosetzsky A, Schlichting P, et al. A randomized, placebo-controlled, cross-over study of ginger extracts and ibruprofen in osteoarthritis. *Osteoarthritis Cartilage.* 2000;8:9-12. **32.** Nakamura H, Yamamoto T. Mutagen and anti-mutagen in ginger, Zingiber officinale. *Mutat Res.* 1982;103:119-126. **33.** Nagabhushan M, Amonkar AJ, Bhide SV. Mutagenicity of gingerol and shogaol and antimutagenicity of zingerone in Salmonella/microsome assay. *Cancer Lett.* 1987;36:221-233. **34.** Kada T, Morita K, Inoue T. Anti-mutagenic action of vegetable factor(s) on the mutagenic principle of tryptophan pyrolysate. *Mutat Res.* 1978;53:351-353. **35.** Mascolo N, Jain R, Jain SC, et al. Ethnopharmacologic investigation of ginger (Zingiber officinale). *J Ethnopharmacol.* 1989;27:129-140.

Ginkgo

Ginkgo Biloba

U.S. BRAND NAMES OF CLINICALLY TESTED PRODUCTS

Ginkoba (Pharmaton), Ginkgold (Nature's Way) = EGb 761 (Schwabe) in Europe
Ginkai (Lichtwer Pharma) = LI 1370 (Lichtwer Pharma) in Europe

DESCRIPTION

The seeds of the ginkgo tree have a long history of medicinal use in China. However, current ginkgo products are highly processed extracts manufactured from ginkgo leaf, and bear no resemblance to the traditional herb.

PHARMACOLOGY

Numerous biochemically active flavonoids known as ginkgo-flavonol glycosides are found in ginkgo leaf, as are several terpene lactones named ginkgolides A, B, and C, and bilobalide. Potentially toxic alkylphenols (ginkgolic acids, cardanols, and dardols) are also present in raw ginkgo, but are removed from commercial products.

Pharmacokinetic studies of ginkgo extracts show 98% to 100% bioavailability for ginkgolide A, 79% to 93% for ginkgolide B, and 70% for bilobalide. Maximal plasma flavonoid levels are seen at 2 to 3 hours.[1]

In vitro and animal studies have found some evidence that ginkgo extracts increase tolerance to cerebral hypoxia; reduce stroke infarct volume and capillary fragility; inhibit post-traumatic and toxin-induced brain edema, nitric oxide production by macrophages under proinflammatory conditions, and PAF; scavenge free radicals; retard age-related decline of muscarinic choline receptors and alpha2-adrenergic receptors; and promote choline uptake in the hippocampus.[2,3,4] Animal and preliminary human evidence suggests that ginkgo extracts improve capillary microcirculation through a variety of mechanisms, including decreased blood viscosity, antagonism of PAF, and prolonged half-life of endothelium-derived relaxing factor.[5-11]

When dementia was attributed largely to impaired cerebral circulation (the so-called "cerebral insufficiency syndrome"), ginkgo's mechanism of action in dementia was assumed to involve improved capillary microcirculation. However, the more modern view is that ginkgo (and other nootropic drugs) stimulate nerve cell activity or protect nerve cell populations from further injury.[3,12] Isolated ginkgolides and bilobalide have exhibited neuroprotective properties and inhibition of PAF.[3,8] One study suggests that ginkgo extract can competitively inhibit monoamine oxidase A and B at therapeutic levels,[13] although no MAO-inhibitor-like reactions have been reported in the wide European usage of ginkgo. This in vitro finding is echoed by an earlier demonstration in mice of protection by ginkgo against neurotoxicity from MPTP, a neurotoxin that requires metabolic activation by MAO to exert its toxic effects.[14]

Ginkgo's apparent benefits in intermittent claudication are attributed to improved circulation.[5-8]

CLINICAL STUDIES

ALZHEIMER'S AND NON-ALZHEIMER'S DEMENTIA

A well-regarded double-blind placebo-controlled study of *Ginkgo biloba* in dementia (primarily Alzheimer's), involving 309 patients in a 52-week parallel-group multicenter trial, found significant improvement in a performance-based test of memory and language (the cognitive subscale of the Alzheimer's Disease Assessment Scale, or ADAS-Cog) and a caregivers' evaluation (the Geriatric Evaluation by Relative's Rating Instrument, or GERRI).[15]

Other recent European studies have evaluated the effectiveness of ginkgo in Alzheimer's and non-Alzheimer's dementia and also found benefit.[16,17] Additionally over 40 earlier double-blind controlled trials had evaluated the benefits of ginkgo in "cerebral insufficiency" prior to 1992.[10] Of these, eight were rated of good quality, involving a total of about 1,000 patients, and results were positive in all but one study.

However, a 24-week double-blind placebo-controlled study of 214 participants found no benefit with ginkgo extract at a dose of 160 or 240 mg daily.[18] This study enrolled both individuals with mild to moderate dementia as well as those with ordinary age-associated memory loss.

AGE-ASSOCIATED MEMORY IMPAIRMENT (AAMI)

The results of six double-blind studies suggest that ginkgo might be useful for Age-Associated Memory Impairment (AAMI) and other forms of fairly mild memory loss, although a seventh study found no benefit.[18-24]

For example, in a double-blind placebo-controlled trial, 241 seniors complaining of mildly impaired memory were given either placebo or low-dose or high-dose ginkgo for 24 weeks.[19] The results showed modest improvements in certain types of memory, especially in the low-dose ginkgo group (120 mg daily).

IMPROVING MEMORY AND MENTAL FUNCTION IN YOUNGER ADULTS

In a double-blind placebo-controlled crossover trial, 20 healthy individuals aged 19 to 24 received a one-time dose of ginkgo at 120, 240, or 360 mg, or placebo.[25] The results showed improvement in some measures of mental performance, most markedly in one that measured ability to perform attention-related tasks rapidly. However, a double-blind placebo-controlled study of 30 healthy males found no significant improvement in memory after 5 days treatment with ginkgo at a dose of 120 mg daily.[26] Inconsistent results were seen in two smaller double-blind placebo-controlled crossover trials.[27,28]

INTERMITTENT CLAUDICATION

A 2000 meta-analysis of studies of ginkgo for intermittent claudication evaluated eight double-blind placebo-controlled trials.[29] In aggregate, the results found a modest but statistically significant improvement in pain-free walking distance. For example, a 24-week double-blind placebo-controlled study that enrolled 111 patients found a significant improvement with ginkgo compared to placebo.[30]

A 4-week multicenter double-blind placebo-controlled dose-comparison study of 74 individuals with intermittent claudication reported that ginkgo at a dose of 120 mg twice daily was more effective than 60 mg twice daily.[31]

TINNITUS

Three double-blind placebo-controlled trials enrolling a total of about 220 individuals have evaluated oral *Ginkgo biloba* extract as a treatment for tinnitus, with generally positive results.[32-35] However, a more recent and much larger study found no benefit.

In this double-blind trial, 1,121 individuals with tinnitus were given 12 weeks' treatment either with placebo or standardized ginkgo at a dose of 50 mg 3 times daily.[36] The results showed no difference between the treated and placebo groups.

PROPOSED INDICATIONS AND USAGE

Significant evidence supports the use of *Ginkgo biloba* extract for the treatment of dementia of the Alzheimer's and non-Alzheimer's varieties. Weaker evidence supports its use in ordinary age-associate memory impairment. Its popular use as a "brain stimulator" in younger adults has little substantiation.

Some evidence suggests that ginkgo extract may be useful in intermittent claudication; however, ginkgo's effects on coagulation hemostasis make combination therapy with standard treatments questionable (see Drug Interactions).

Pilot trials suggest that ginkgo might be helpful for PMS,[37] altitude sickness,[38] vertiginous syndromes,[39] and depression.[40,41] Despite wide marketing of ginkgo as a treatment for tinnitus, the preponderance of current evidence suggests that it is not effective for this purpose.

Case reports and highly preliminary studies suggest that ginkgo might help reduce the sexual side effects of SSRIs, including impotence in men and inability to achieve orgasm in women.[42-46] Because sexual dysfunction is a major deterrent to patient compliance with the SSRI antidepressants, this potential effect of ginkgo is being investigated more thoroughly.

Weak and in some cases contradictory evidence suggests that ginkgo extract might be helpful for macular degeneration, diabetic microvascular disease, cochlear deafness, pancreatic cancer, schizophrenia, and allergies.[5,11,47,48]

WARNINGS

Do not combine ginkgo extract with anticoagulant or antiplatelet drugs.

Ginkgo should not be self-harvested from ginkgo trees; the extract used in clinical trials has been processed to remove toxins.

PRECAUTIONS

There have been two case reports of subdural hematoma and hyphema associated with ginkgo use.[49,50] In the former case, the patient was also taking 325 mg aspirin daily. Due to this potential risk, it might be advisable to avoid ginkgo during the perioperative period.

The ginkgo extracts approved for use in Germany are processed to remove alkylphenols, including ginkgolic acids, which have been found to be cytoxic.[51] The same ginkgo extracts are available in the United States. However, other ginkgo extracts and whole ginkgo leaf might contain appreciable levels of these dangerous constituents.

Another toxin, 4'-O-methylpyridoxine (ginkgotoxin), is a neurotoxic anti-vitamin B_6 found primarily in ginkgo seeds rather than leaves. However, very low (and probably harmless) levels have been found in the leaves as well.[52]

One study found evidence that prolonged ginkgo administration increases insulin secretion in response to an oral glucose load[53]; the researchers expressed concern that this effect might potentially lead to insulin resistance.

In vitro evidence suggests that ginkgo might function as an MAO inhibitor,[13] although this has not been correlated by any reports of MAO-like reactions in humans.

Use of ginkgo during pregnancy and lactation, or by young children, is not recommended. Maximum safe dosages in individuals with severe hepatic or renal disease are not known.

DRUG INTERACTIONS

A limited human trial has shown that 400 mg/day of ginkgo extract does not alter hepatic microsomal enzyme activity as indicated by antipyrine clearance.[54]

One case report suggests a possible interaction between ginkgo and aspirin.[49] This would not be surprising, as ginkgo is known to inhibit platelet activation factor. For this reason, it is advisable to use caution when combining ginkgo with warfarin, heparin, aspirin, or any other drugs with anticoagulant effects. In most of the double-blind studies of ginkgo, patients who used such drugs were excluded, so the true magnitude of this risk is not known. It is also conceivable that ginkgo could interact with garlic, phosphatidylserine, policosanol, high-dose vitamin E, and other natural products with relatively mild anticoagulant or antiplatelet effects.

ADVERSE REACTIONS

In pooled clinical trials involving a total of almost 10,000 patients, the incidence of side effects produced by ginkgo extract was extremely small. There were 21 cases of gastrointestinal discomfort and even fewer cases of headache, dizziness, and allergic skin reactions.[5] However, these trials excluded individuals with known risk factors for altered hemostasis.

Contact with live ginkgo plants can cause severe allergic reactions, and ginkgo seeds are toxic.

No evidence of mutagenicity or carcinogenicity has been reported to date. Animal studies of the long-term effects of continued ingestion of ginkgo extract report no evidence of organ damage, impairment of reproductive, renal, or hepatic function, or damage to health of offspring.

PROPOSED DOSAGE AND ADMINISTRATION

The standard dose of ginkgo extract is 120 to 240 mg daily given in 3 divided doses. Studied extracts consist of a 50:1 acetone/water extract standardized to contain 24% ginkgo-flavone glycosides and 6% terpenoids (2.8% to 3.4% ginkgolides A, B, and C, and 2.6% to 3.2% bilobalide).[55] Ginkgolic acid content is kept under 5 ppm.

PATIENT INFORMATION

Ginkgo is an herbal extract widely marketed for improving memory and mental function. There is some meaningful evidence that it might offer modest benefits for individuals with Alzheimer's disease or other forms of serious declining mental function. Weaker evidence suggests that it might be helpful for individuals with ordinary age-related memory loss. There is no evidence that ginkgo can "boost memory" in young adults or children.

NOTE: Symptoms of Alzheimer's disease require a full medical work-up to rule out brain tumors and other treatable conditions.

Commercially available ginkgo extract is a highly processed product. Raw gingko leaves will not be effective and could be toxic.

Ginkgo is a "blood thinner." For this reason, individuals with bleeding disorders such as hemophilia should avoid ginkgo. It should also be avoided around the time of surgery or labor and delivery. Additionally, individuals taking medications that impair blood clotting, such as Coumadin (warfarin), heparin, and aspirin, should avoid gingko. Combination treatment might cause internal bleeding. Natural products that "thin" the blood might also be dangerous if combined with ginkgo. These include garlic, policosanol, and high-dose vitamin E.

Use of ginkgo during pregnancy or nursing, or by young children, is not recommended. Individuals with severe liver or kidney disease should consult a physician before using this (or any other) supplement.

REFERENCES

1. Nieder M. Pharmakokinetics of Ginkgo flavonoles in plasma [in German]. *MMW Munch Med Wochenschr.* 1991;133 (suppl 1):61-62. **2.** Clark WM, Rinker LG, Lessov NS, et al.Therapeutic efficacy of *Ginkgo biloba* in transient focal ischemia. Poster presented at: 52nd annual meeting of the American Academy of Neurology, May 2, 2000; San Diego, Calif. **3.** Schulz V, Hansel R, Tyler VE. *Rational Phytotherapy: A Physicians' Guide to Herbal Medicine.* 3rd ed. Berlin, Germany: Springer-Verlag; 1998:40, 43, 46, 47, 126. **4.** Kobuchi H, et al. *Ginkgo biloba* Extract (Egb 761): inhibitory effect on nitric oxide production in the macrophage cell line RAW 264.7. *Biochem Pharmacol.* 1997;53:897-903. **5.** De Feudis FV. *Ginkgo biloba extract (EGb 761): Pharmacological activities and clinical applications.* Paris: Elsevier; 1991:143-146. **6.** Funfgeld EW. *Rokan* (Ginkgo biloba): *Recent results in pharmacology and clinic.* New York: Springer-Verlag; 1988. **7.** Kleijnen J, Knipschild P. Ginkgo Biloba. *Lancet.* 1992;340:1136-1139. **8.** Klein J, Chatterjee SS, Loffelholz K. Phospholipid breakdown and choline release under hypoxic conditions: inhibition by bilobalide, a constituent of *Ginkgo biloba. Brain Res.* 1997;755:347-350. **9.** Jung F, Mrowietz C, Kiesewetter H, et al. Effect of *Ginkgo biloba* on fluidity of blood and peripheral microcirculation in volunteers. *Arzneimittelforschung.* 1990;40:589-593. **10.** Kleijnen J, Knipschild P. *Ginkgo biloba* for cerebral insufficiency. *Br J Clin Pharmacol.* 1992;34:352-358. **11.** Sikora R, Sohn M, Deutz FJ, et al. *Ginkgo biloba* extract in the therapy of erectile dysfunction. *J Urol.* 1989;142:188A. **12.** Rapin JR, Zaibi M, Drieu K. In vitro and in vivo effects of an extract of *Ginkgo biloba* (EGb 761), ginkgolide B, and bilobalide on apoptosis in primary cultures of rat hippocampal neurons. *Drug Res.* 1998;45:23-29. **13.** White HL, Scates PW, Cooper BR. Extracts of *Ginkgo biloba* leaves inhibit monoamine oxidase. *Life Sci.* 1996;58:1315-1321. **14.** Ramassamy C, Clostre F, Christen Y, et al. Prevention by a *Ginkgo biloba* extract (GBE 761) of the dopaminergic neurotoxicity of MPTP. *J Pharm Pharmacol.* 1990;42:785-789. **15.** Le Bars PL, Katz MM, Berman N, et al. A placebo-controlled, double-blind, randomized trial of an extract of *Ginkgo biloba* for dementia. North American EGb Study Group. *JAMA.* 1997;278:1327-1332. **16.** Hofferberth B. The efficacy of EGb 761 in patients with senile dementia of the Alzheimer type, a double-blind, placebo-controlled study on different levels of investigation. *Hum Psychopharmacol.* 1994;9:215-222. **17.** Kanowski S, Herrmann WM, Stephan K, et al. Proof of efficacy of the *Ginkgo biloba* special extract Egb 761 in outpatients suffering from mild to moderate primary degenerative dementia of the Alzheimer type or multi-infarct dementia. *Pharmacopsychiatry.* 1996;29:47-56. **18.** van Dongen MC, van Rossum E, Kessels AG, et al. The efficacy of ginkgo for elderly people with dementia and age-associated memory impairment: new results of a randomized clinical trial. *J Am Geriatr Soc.* 2000;48:1183-1194. **19.** Brautigam MR, Blommaert FA, Verleye G, et al. Treatment of age-related memory complaints with *Ginkgo biloba* extract: a randomized double blind placebo-controlled study. *Phytomedicine.* 1998;5:425-434. **20.** Mix JA, Crews WD Jr. An examination of the efficacy of *Ginkgo biloba* extract EGb 761 on the neuropsychologic functioning of cognitively intact older adults. *J Altern Complement Med.* 2000;6:219-229. **21.** Winther K, Randlov C, Rein E, et al. Effects of *Ginkgo biloba* extract on cognitive function and blood pressure in elderly subjects. *Curr Ther Res.* 1998;59:881-888. **22.** Rai GS, Shovlin C, Wesnes KA. A double-blind, placebo controlled study of *Ginkgo biloba* extract ('Tanakan(tm)') in elderly outpatients with mild to moderate memory impairment. *Curr Med Res Opin.* 1991;12:350-355. **23.** Rigney U, Kimber S, Hindmarch I. The effects of acute doses of standardized *Ginkgo biloba* extract on memory and psychomotor performance in volunteers. *Phytotherapy Res.* 1999;13:408-415. **24.** Allain H, Raoul P, Lieury A, et al. Effect of two doses of *Ginkgo biloba* extract (EGb 761) on the dual-coding test in elderly subjects. *Clin Ther.* 1993;15:549-558. **25.** Kennedy DO, Scholey AB, Wesnes KA. The dose-dependent cognitive effects of acute administration of Ginkgo biloba to healthy young volunteers. *Psychopharmacology (Berl).* 2000;151:416-423. **26.** Moulton PL, Boyko LN, Fitzpatrick JL, et al. The effect of Ginkgo biloba on memory in healthy male volunteers. *Physiol Behav.* 2001;73:659-665. **27.** Hindmarch I.Activity of Ginkgo biloba extract on short term memory [in French; English abstract]. *Presse Med.* 1986;15:1592-1594. **28.** Warot D, Lacomblez L, Danjou P, et al. Comparative effects of Ginkgo biloba extracts on psychomotor performances and memory in healthy subjects [in French; English abstract]. *Therapie.* 1991;46:33-36. **29.** Pittler MH, Ernst E. *Ginkgo biloba* extract for the treatment of intermittent claudication: a meta-analysis of randomized trials. *Am J Med.* 2000;108:276-281. **30.** Peters H, Kieser M, Holscher U. Demonstration of the efficacy of *Ginkgo biloba* special extract EGb 761 on intermittent claudication-a placebo-controlled, double-blind multicenter trial. *Vasa.* 1998;27:106-110. **31.** Schweizer J, Hautmann C. Comparison of two dosages of ginkgo biloba extract EGb 761 in patients with peripheral arterial occlusive disease Fontaine's stage IIb. A randomised, double-blind, multicentric clinical trial. *Arzneimittelforschung.* 1999;49:900-904. **32.** Ernst E, Stevinson C. *Ginkgo biloba* for tinnitus: a review. *Clin Otolaryngol.* 1999;24:164-167. **33.** Holgers KM, Axelsson A, Pringle I. *Ginkgo biloba* extract for the treatment of tinnitus. *Audiology.* 1994;33:85-92. **34.** Meyer B. Multicenter randomized double-blind drug vs. placebo study of the treatment of tinnitus with *Ginkgo biloba* extract [translated from French]. *Presse Med.* 1986;15:1562-1564. **35.** Morgenstern C, Biermann E. Long-term tinnitus therapy with ginkgo special extract EGb 761 [translated from German]. *Fortschr Med.* 1997;115(29):57-58. **36.** Drew S, Davies E. Effectiveness of *Ginkgo biloba* in treating tinnitus: double blind, placebo controlled trial. *BMJ.* 2001;322:73-75. **37.** Tamborini A, Taurell R. Value of standardized *Ginkgo biloba* extract (Egb 761) in the management of congestive symptoms of premenstrual syndrome [translated from French]. *Rev Fr Gynecol Obstet.* 1993;88:447-457. **38.** Roncin JP, Schwartz F, D'Arbigny P. EGb 761 in control of acute mountain sickness and vascular reactivity to cold exposure. *Aviat Space Environ Med.* 1996;67:445-452. **39.** Haguenauer JP, Cantenot F, Koskas H, et al. Treatment of equilibrium disorders with *Ginkgo biloba* extract. A multicenter double-blind drug vs. placebo study [translated from French]. *Presse Med.* 1986;15:1569-1572. **40.** Schubert H, Halama P. Depressive episode primarily unresponsive to therapy in elderly patients: efficacy of *Ginkgo biloba* extract EGb 761 in combination with antidepressants [translated from German]. *Geriatr Forsch.* 1993;3:45-53. **41.** Eckmann F. Cerebral insufficiency-treatment with *Ginkgo-biloba* extract. Time of onset of effect in a double-blind study with 60 inpatients [translated from German] *Fortschr Med.* 1990;108:557-560. **42.** Cohen A. Treatment of antidepressant-induced sexual dysfunction with Ginkgo biloba extract. Presented at: 149th Annual Meeting of the American Psychiatric Association; May 5-8, 1996. Abstract #716. **43.** Cohen A. Long term safety and efficacy of *Ginkgo biloba* extract in the treatment of antidepressant-induced sexual dysfunction (1997). Priory Lodge Education web site. Available at: http://www.priory.com/pharmol/gingko.htm. Accessed: July 1, 1997. **44.** Cohen AJ, Bartlik B. *Ginkgo biloba* for antidepressant-induced sexual dysfunction. *J Sex Marital Ther.* 1998;24:139-143. **45.** Cohen A, Bartlik B. Treatment of sexual dysfunction with Ginkgo biloba extract [scientific reports]. Presented at: 150th Annual Meeting of the American Psychiatric Association; May 18-21, 1997; San Diego, Calif. **46.** McCann B. Botanical could improve sex life of patients on SSRIs. *Drug Topics.* 1997;141:33. **47.** Hauns B, Haring B, Kohler S, et al. Phase II study with 5-fluorouracil and ginkgo biloba extract (GBE 761 ONC) in patients with pancreatic cancer. *Arzneimittelforschung.* 1999;49:1030-1034. **48.** Liu P, Luo H-C, Shen Y-C, et al. Combined use of ginkgo biloba extracts on the efficacy and adverse reactions of various antipsychotics [translated from Chinese]. *Chin J Clin Pharmacol.* 1997;13:193-198. **49.** Rosenblatt M, Mindel J. Spontaneous hyphema associated with ingestion of *Ginkgo biloba* extract. *N Engl J Med.* 1997;336:1108. **50.** Rowen J, Lewis SL. Spontaneous bilateral subdural hematomas associated with chronic *Ginkgo biloba* ingestion. *Neurology.* 1996;46:1775-1776. **51.** Siegers CP. Cytotoxicity of alkylphenols from *Ginkgo biloba*. *Phytomedicine.* 1999;6:281-283. **52.** Arenz A, Klein M, Fiehe K, et al. Occurrence of neurotoxic 4'-O-methylpyridoxine in *Ginkgo biloba* leaves, ginkgo medications and Japanese ginkgo food. *Planta Med.* 1996;62:548-551. **53.** Kudolo GB. The effect of 3-month ingestion of *Ginkgo biloba* extract on pancreatic beta-cell function in response to glucose loading in normal glucose tolerant individuals. *J Clin Pharmacol.* 2000;40:647-654. **54.** Duche JC, Barre J, Guinot P, et al. Effect of *Ginkgo biloba* extract on microsomal enzyme induction. *Int J Clin Pharmacol Res.* 1989;9:165-168. **55.** Blumenthal M, et al., eds. *The Complete German Commission E Monographs.* Boston: Integrative Medicine Communications; 1998:136.

Ginseng

Panax Ginseng

Alternate/Related Names: True Ginseng, Asian Ginseng, Chinese Ginseng, Korean Ginseng; American Ginseng *(P. quinquefolius)*

U.S. BRAND NAMES OF CLINICALLY TESTED PRODUCTS

Ginsana (Pharmaton) = G115 (Pharmaton) in Europe

DESCRIPTION

Panax ginseng species are perennial herbs with a taproot reminiscent of the human form. Dried, unprocessed ginseng root is called white ginseng, whereas a steamed, heat-dried root is called red ginseng. Asian or Korean ginseng *(P. ginseng)* and American ginseng *(P. quinquefolius)* are closely related. So-called Siberian or Russian ginseng *(Eleutherococcus senticosus)* is only distantly related to *Panax* species and possesses altogether distinct constituents.

Panax ginseng has long been an important herb in both academic Chinese herbal medicine and Asian folk medicine. Emperors believed that it would make them live (and stay potent) forever. Prior to World War II, Russian scientists developed the concept of an *adaptogen,* and concluded that *P. ginseng* was a prime example. By definition, an adaptogen helps the body adapt to stresses of various kinds, minimizing the damaging effects of heat, cold, exertion, trauma, sleep deprivation, toxic exposure, radiation, infection, and psychological stress. An adaptogen must also satisfy the following three criteria: (1) It causes few to no side effects or overt physiological changes, (2) it has a nonspecific action that functions in many circumstances, and (3) it has a normalizing action that tends to return an organism toward homeostasis regardless of the direction in which it is out of balance. The treatment that comes closest to satisfying the definition of an adaptogen is a healthful lifestyle (except, of course, that this is not a substance). There is no convincing evidence that ginseng (or any other substance) possesses adaptogenic properties.

PHARMACOLOGY

Panax ginseng contains 2% to 3% triterpenoid saponins named ginsenosides, of which 18 have been identified.[1] Pharmacokinetic data on ginseng bioavailability are scarce. Aglycone metabolites of ginsenosides have been detected in the urine of human subjects taking ginseng orally, but only about 1.2% of the dose could be recovered over a 5-day period.[2,3]

A large body of in vitro and animal studies of ginsenosides and whole ginseng extracts exists, reporting a wide variety of effects, including prolonged swimming time; CNS stimulation; protective effects against radiation, infections, and toxins; reduction of biological changes produced by physical exhaustion and psychological stress; alterations of glucose and lipid metabolism; increases in RNA and protein synthesis; and activation of white blood cells.[4-15] However, many of these studies involved intraperitoneal injection rather than oral use and few reached modern standards of scientific rigor. In humans, some evidence suggests that ginseng can improve glycogen utilization, alcohol clearance, serum lipid levels, and other metabolic parameters, which is taken by proponents as evidence of a pro-homeostasis, adaptogenic effect.[9,16]

In cells infected with herpes virus, *P. ginseng* extract was found to enhance antibody-dependent cellular cytotoxicity and NK-cell activity.[17] A study in humans found that *P. ginseng* increased PMN phagocytosis, T-helper to T-suppressor cell ratio, and NK activity.[18] However, another human trial found no effect on total or differential peripheral blood leukocytes, or on lymphocyte subsets (T-cells, B-cells, T-helper cells, T-suppressor cells, interleukin-2-receptor cells, or helper/suppressor ratio).[19] An in vitro trial found that an extract of American ginseng decreased cell proliferation in breast cancer cell lines, and augmented the effect of most breast cancer therapeutics tested.[20]

One study weakly suggests that ginsenosides may be the active hypoglycemic constituents in American ginseng,[21] although the lack of dose dependency seen in another trial by the same researcher tends to discount this conclusion.[22]

CLINICAL STUDIES

Only trials of ginseng conducted since the late 1980s are described here.

ADJUVANT USE WITH INFLUENZA VACCINE

A double-blind placebo-controlled study of 227 participants evaluated the potential immune-stimulating effects of *P. ginseng.*[23] After 4 weeks of treatment with 100 mg daily of Ginsana or placebo, all participants received influenza vaccine. The results showed a statistically significant decline in the frequency of colds and flus in the treated group compared to the placebo group from week 4 to 12. Antibody titers and measures of NK-cell activity were also higher in the treated group.

IMPROVING MENTAL ACUITY

Several studies have found that ginseng can improve mental function, but the effects reported are inconsistent between trials and show no general trend.[24-29]

For example, in a 22-month double-blind placebo-controlled study, 112 healthy, middle-aged adults were given either ginseng or placebo.[24] The results showed that ginseng improved abstract thinking ability. However, there was no significant difference in reaction time, memory, concentration, or overall subjective experience between the two groups. In contrast, a double-blind placebo-controlled study of 120 individuals found that ginseng gradually improved reaction time over a 12-week treatment period among those 40 to 60 years old.[25]

DIABETES

A double-blind placebo-controlled study evaluated the effects of *P. ginseng* (100 or 200 mg daily) on 36 newly diagnosed type 2 diabetics over an 8-week period.[30] The results showed reduction in fasting serum glucose levels and improved glycosylated hemoglobin and physical capacity in the ginseng group.

A double-blind placebo-controlled crossover study of nine subjects with type 2 diabetes found that a single 3-g dose of *P. quinquefolius* significantly reduced postprandial glycemia whether given simultaneously with the glucose challenge or 40 minutes before.[31] Hypoglycemic effects were seen with ginseng in other small trials as well.[32] Dose dependency was evaluated in one of these trials, but was not found within a range of 1 to 3 g.[22]

ATHLETIC PERFORMANCE ENHANCEMENT

Small trials testing *P. ginseng* as an ergogenic aid have yielded conflicting results.[33-42]

"WELL-BEING"

Three double-blind placebo-controlled studies of *P. ginseng* attempted to evaluate general sense of "well-being," an ill-defined parameter possibly related to adaptogenic effects. One followed 625 individuals (average age just under 40) for 12 weeks and found that treatment with ginseng improved in results on a standardized questionnaire.[43] Another followed 120 individuals and found that *P. ginseng* improved well-being scores among women aged 30 to 60 and men aged 40 to 60, but not among men aged 30 to 39.[25] However, a 60-day double-blind placebo-controlled trial of 83 adults in their mid-20s found no benefit with ginseng treatment in measurements of affect and mood.[44]

MENOPAUSAL SYNDROME

A double-blind placebo-controlled study of 384 postmenopausal women found no significant benefits for menopausal symptoms, and no evidence of hormonal effects.[45]

PROPOSED INDICATIONS AND USAGE

Ginseng is widely marketed in the United States as a stimulant, despite lack of any evidence that it exerts stimulant properties. In Europe, the adaptogen concept is prevalent, and ginseng is frequently recommended as a treatment for stress, mostly for older men. However, there is little clinical evidence documenting that ginseng actually possesses adaptogenic properties.

Ginseng is also marketed for enhancing physical performance, prolonging life, and increasing sexual potency. However, the evidence base for these uses is weak to nonexistent. Ginseng is sometimes recommended for symptomatic relief in postmenopausal women, but a large trial found it ineffective.

Some evidence supports using ginseng as adjuvant therapy for diabetes and influenza vaccination.

WARNINGS

Contamination of ginseng products with caffeine, other stimulants, eleutherococcus, or toxic substances such as germanium may be widespread.

PRECAUTIONS

Overstimulation and insomnia have also been reported with ginseng, and anecdotal evidence suggests that excessive doses may mildly elevate blood pressure. In addition, there has been one report of cerebral arteritis associated with ginseng use.[46] However, because there have been numerous reports of adulteration of ginseng with other herbs, with germanium (a nephrotoxic substance), and with caffeine and other stimulants, it is not clear if these reported side effects are actually due to ginseng itself.[47,48]

Reports in 1979 of a ginseng-abuse syndrome involving addiction, marked blood pressure elevation, agitation, severe sleeplessness, and hypersexuality have been discredited.[12,49]

Safety in pregnant or lactating women, young children, or individuals with severe hepatic or renal disease is not known.

DRUG INTERACTIONS

One case report suggests that ginseng may inhibit CYP 3A4.[50] According to another case report, *P. ginseng* may reduce the effectiveness of warfarin.[51] However, a study in rats found no pharmacokinetic or pharmacodynamic interaction between warfarin and ginseng.[52]

There have been reports of apparent interaction between ginseng and phenelzine, resulting in headache, tremulousness, and manic-like symptoms.[53] Whether this generalizes into a drug interaction with other MAO inhibitors or drugs with MAOI potential at high doses, such as selegiline, is not known. It is possible the ginseng involved in these case reports may have been contaminated with caffeine.

One report indicates otherwise unexplained elevated digoxin levels in a patient taking digoxin and eleutherococcus.[54] (Because eleutherococcus is sometimes substituted for *P. ginseng*, this finding is mentioned here.) However, this appears to have been a case of interference with a diagnostic test, rather than an actual elevation of digoxin.

Based on results of clinical trials of ginseng for diabetes, it is possible that concomitant use of ginseng might require a reduction in insulin or oral hypoglycemic dose.

Finally, if ginseng does have immunomodulatory actions as purported, interactions with immunosuppressive drugs are possible.

ADVERSE REACTIONS

Ginseng appears to present a low order of toxicity in both short-term and long-term use, according to the results of studies in mice, rats, dogs, chickens, mink, deer, lambs, and dwarf pigs. Ginseng also does not appear to be teratogenic or carcinogenic.[9,47,55,56] Studies of individual ginsenosides have shown little toxicity.

Side effects from whole ginseng taken at appropriate doses are rare. Occasionally, women taking ginseng report menstrual abnormalities and breast tenderness.[57-60] However, this side effect has not been formally documented, and large double-blind placebo-controlled trials have found no effects on sex hormones or gonadotropins.[25,45]

PROPOSED DOSAGE AND ADMINISTRATION

The usual recommended daily dose of *P. ginseng* is 1 g crude herb or 200 g extract standardized to contain 4% to 7% ginsenosides, taken in 2 divided doses. In one study of American ginseng for diabetes, the dose used was 3 g.

PATIENT INFORMATION

Ginseng is an herb widely marketed as an "energy booster." However, there is no evidence that ginseng has any stimulant properties. Some proponents of ginseng claim that it helps the body adapt to stress (making it an "adaptogen"), but there is little evidence for this concept.

Ginseng itself appears to be relatively safe. However, commercial ginseng products may at times be contaminated with unlisted stimulants or other hazardous substances.

The safety of ginseng for pregnant or nursing women or young children has not been established. Individuals with severe liver or kidney disease should consult a physician before using this (or any other) supplement.

REFERENCES

1. Sonnenborn U, Proppert Y. Ginseng (Panax ginseng CA Meyer) [in German]. *Z Phytother.* 1990;11:35-49, 272. **2.** Cui JF, Garle M, Bjorkhem I, et al. Determination of aglycones of ginsenosides in ginseng preparations sold in Sweden and in urine samples from Swedish athletes consuming ginseng. *Scand J Clin Lab Invest.* 1996;56:151-160. **3.** Cui J-F, Bjorkhem I, Eneroth P. Gas chromatographic-mass spectrometric determination of 20(S)-protopanaxadiol and 20(S)-protopanaxatriol for study on human urinary excretion of ginsenosides after ingestion of ginseng preparations. *J Chromatogr.* 1997;689:349-355. **4.** Bittles AH, Fulder SJ, Grant EC, et al. The effect of ginseng on the lifespan and stress responses in mice. *Gerontology.* 1979;25:125-131. **5.** Brekhman II, Dardymov IV. Pharmacological investigation of glycosides from Ginseng and Eleutherococcus. *Lloydia.* 1969;32:46-51. **6.** Dua PR, Shanker G, Srimal RC, et al. Adaptogenic activity of Indian Panax pseudoginseng. *Indian J Exp Biol.* 1989;27:631-634. **7.** Grandhi A, Mujumdar AM, Patwardhan B. A comparative pharmacological investigation of Ashwagandha and Ginseng. *J Ethnopharmacol.* 1994;44:131-135. **8.** Hiai S, Yokoyaa H, Oura H. Features of ginseng saponin induced corticosterone secretion. *Endocrinol Jpn.* 1979;26:737-740. **9.** Newall C, et al. *Herbal medicines: A guide for health-care professionals.* London: The Pharmaceutical Press; 1996:141-143; 146-148. **10.** Oura HS, Hiai S, Nabetani S, et al. Effect of ginseng extract on endoplasmic reticulum and ribosome. *Planta Med.* 1975;28:76-88. **11.** Ramachandran U, Divekar HM, Grover SK, et al. New experimental model for the evaluation of adaptogenic products. *J Ethnopharmacol.* 1990;29:275-281. **12.** Schulz V, Hansel R, Tyler VE. *Rational Phytotherapy: A Physicians' Guide to Herbal Medicine.* 3rd ed. Berlin, Germany: Springer-Verlag; 1998: 271-278. **13.** Singh VK, George CX, Singh N. Combined treatment of mice with Panax ginseng extract and interferon inducer. Amplification of host resistance to Semliki forest virus. *Planta Med.* 1983;47:234-236. **14.** Singh VK, Agarwal SS, Gupta BM. Immunomodulatory activity of Panax ginseng extract. *Planta Med.* 1984;50:462-465. **15.** Song ZJ, Moser C, Wu H, et al. Ginseng Treatment Induces a Th1 Cytokine Response in a Mouse Model of Pseudomonas aeruginosa Lung Infection. Poster presented at: 100th General Meeting American Society for Microbiology, Los Angeles, California; May 21-25, 2000. **16.** Avakian EV, Evonuk E. Effect of Panax ginseng extract on tissue glycogen and adrenal cholesterol depletion during prolonged exercise. *Planta Med.* 1979;36:43-48. **17.** See DM, Broumand N, Sahl L, et al. In vitro effects of echinacea and ginseng on natural killer cells and antibody-dependent cell cytoxicity in healthy subjects and chronic fatigue syndrome or acquired immunodeficiency patients. *Immunopharmacology.* 1997;35:229-235. **18.** Scaglione F, Ferrara F, Dugnani S, et al. Immunomodulatory effects of two extracts of Panax ginseng C.A. Meyer. *Drugs Exp Clin Res.* 1990;16:537-542. **19.** Srisurapanon S, Rungroeng K, Apibal S, et al. The effect of standardized ginseng extract on peripheral blood leukocytes and lymphocyte subsets: a preliminary study in young healthy adults. *J Med Assoc Thai.* 1997;80 (suppl 1):S81-85. **20.** Duda RB. American ginseng and breast cancer therapeutic agents synergistically inhit MCF-7 breast cancer cell growth. *J Surg Oncol.* 1999;72:230-239. **21.** Sievenpiper JL, Stavro MP, Leiter LA, et al. Variable effects of ginseng: American Ginseng (Panax Quinquefolius L.) with a low ginsenoside content does not affect postprandial glycemia in normal subjects [abstract]. *Diabetes.* 2001;50(suppl 2):Abst #1771-PO. **22.** Vuksan V, Sievenpiper JL, Wong J, et al. American ginseng (*Panax quinquefolius* L.) attenuates postprandial glycemia in a time-dependent but not dose-dependent manner in healthy individuals. *Am J Clin Nutr.* 2001;73:753-758. **23.** Scaglione F, Cattaneo G, Alessandria M, et al. Efficacy and safety of the standardised Ginseng extract G115 for potentiating vaccination against the influenza syndrome and protection against the common cold. *Drugs Exp Clin Res.* 1996;22:65-72. **24.** Sorenson H, Sonne J. A double-masked study of the effects of ginseng on cognitive functions. *Curr Ther Res.* 1996;57:959-968. **25.** Forgo I, Kayasseh L, Staub JJ. Effect of a standardized ginseng extract on general well-being, reaction time, lung function and gonadal hormones [translated from German]. *Med Welt.* 1981;32:751-756. **26.** Siegl C, Siegl HJ. The possible revision of impaired mental abilities in old age: a double-blind study with Panax ginseng [translated from German]. *Therapiewoche.* 1979;29:4206, 4209-4216. **27.** Sandberg F, Dencker L. Experimental and clinical tests on ginseng. *Z Phytother.* 1994;15:38-42. **28.** D'Angelo L, Grimaldi R, Caravaggi M, et al. A double-blind, placebo-controlled clinical study on the effect of a standardized ginseng extract on psychomotor performance in healthy volunteers. *J Ethnopharmacol.* 1986;16:15-22. **29.** Wesnes KA, Faleni RA, Hefting NR, et al. The cognitive, subjective, and physical effects of a Ginkgo biloba/Panax ginseng combination in healthy volunteers with neurasthenic complaints. *Psychopharmacol Bull.* 1997;33:677-683. **30.** Sotaniemi EA, Haapakoski E, Rautio A. Ginseng therapy in non-insulin-dependent diabetic patients. *Diabetes Care.* 1995;18:1373-1375. **31.** Vuksan V, Sievenpiper JL, Koo VY, et al. American ginseng (*Panax quinquefolius* L) reduces postprandial glycemia in nondiabetic subjects and subjects with type 2 diabetes mellitus. *Arch Intern Med.* 2000;160:1009-1013. **32.** Vuksan V, Xu Z, Jenkins AL, et al. American ginseng (*Panax quinquefolium* L.) improves long term glycemic control in type 2 diabetes. Presented at: 60th Scientific Sessions of the American Diabetes Association; June 9-13, 2000; San Antonio, Tex. **33.** Cherdrungsi P, Rungroeng K. Effects of standardized ginseng extract and exercise training on aerobic and anaerobic capacities in humans. *Korean J Ginseng Sci.* 1995;19:93-100. **34.** Forgo I. Effect of drugs on physical exertion and the hormonal system of athletes. 2 [translated from German]. *MMW Munch Med Wochenschr.* 1983;125:822-824. **35.** McNaughton LG, Egan G, Caelli G. A comparison of Chinese and Russian ginseng as ergogenic aids to improve various facets of physical fitness. *Int J Clin Nutr Rev.* 1989;9:32-35. **36.** Engels HJ, Wirth JC. No ergogenic effects of ginseng (Panax ginseng C.A. Meyer) during graded maximal aerobic exercise. *J Am Diet Assoc.* 1997;97:1110-1115. **37.** Allen JD, McLung J, Nelson AG, et al. Ginseng supplementation does not enhance healthy young adults' peak aerobic exercise performance. *J Am Coll Nutr.* 1998;17:462-466. **38.** Engels HJ, Said JM, Wirth JC. Failure of chronic ginseng supplementation to affect work performance and energy metabolism in healthy adult females. *Nutr Res.* 1996;16:1295-1306. **39.** Kolokouri I, Englels H-J, Cieslak T, et al. Effect of chronic ginseng supplementation on short duration, supramaximal exercise test performance [abstract]. *Med Sci Sports Exerc.* 1999;31(5 suppl):S117. **40.** Lifton B, Otto RM, Wygand J. The effect of ginseng on acute maximal aerobic exercise [abstract]. *Med Sci Sports Exerc.* 1997;29(5 suppl):S249. **41.** Morris AC, Jacobs I, McLellan TM, et al. No ergogenic effect of ginseng ingestion. *Int J Sport Nutr.* 1996;6:263-271. **42.** Teves MA, Wright JE, Welch MJ, et al. Effects of ginseng on repeated bouts of exhaustive exercise [abstract]. *Med Sci Sports Exerc.* 1983;15:162. **43.** Caso Marasco A, Vargas Ruiz R, Salas Villagomez A, et al. Double-blind study of a multivitamin complex supplemented with ginseng extract. *Drugs Exp Clin Res.* 1996;22:323-329. **44.** Cardinal BJ, Engels HJ. Ginseng does not enhance psychological well-being in healthy, young adults: results of a double-blind placebo-controlled, randomized clinical trial. *J Am Diet Assoc.* 2001;101:655-660. **45.** Wiklund IK, Mattsson LA, Lindgren R, et al. Effects of a standardized ginseng extract on quality of life and physiological parameters in symptomatic postmenopausal women: a double-blind, placebo-controlled trial. *Int J Clin Pharmacol Res.* 1999;19:89-99. **46.** Ryu SJ, Chien YY. Ginseng-associated cerebral arteritis. *Neurology.* 1995;45:829-830. **47.** Baldwin CA, Anderson LA, Phillipson JD. What pharmacists should know about ginseng. *Pharm J.* 1986;237:583-586. **48.** Cui J, Garle M, Eneroth P, et al. What do commercial ginseng preparations contain? [letter]. *Lancet.* 1994;344:134. **49.** Tyler VE. *Herbs of Choice.* New York, NY: Pharmaceutical Products Press; 1994:172. **50.** Kroll D. University of Colorado School of Pharmacy (unpublished communication) 1998. **51.** Janetzky K, Morreale AP. Probable interaction between warfarin and ginseng. *Am J Health Syst Pharm.* 1997;54:692-693. **52.** Zhu M, Chan W, Ng S, et al. Possible influences of ginseng on the pharmacokinetics and pharmacodynamics of warfarin in rats. *J Pharm Pharmacol.* 1999;51:175-180. **53.** Jones BD, Runikis AM. Interaction of ginseng with phenelzine [letter]. *J Clin Psychopharmacol.* 1987;7:201-202. **54.** McRae S. Elevated serum digoxin levels in a patient taking digoxin and Siberian ginseng. *CMAJ.* 1996;155:293-295. **55.** Hess FG, Parent RA, Cox GE, et al. Reproduction study in rats of ginseng extract G115. *Food Chem Toxicol.* 1982;20:189-192. **56.** Sonnenborn U, Proppert Y. Ginseng (Panax ginseng C.A. Meyer). *Br J Phytother.* 1991;2:3-14. **57.** Greenspan EM. Ginseng and vaginal bleeding[letter]. *JAMA.* 1983;249:2018. **58.** Hammond TG, Whitworth JA. Adverse reactions to ginseng[letter]. *Med J Aust.* 1981;1:492. **59.** Palmer BV, Montgomery AC, Monteiro JC. Gin Seng and mastalgia[letter]. *Br Med J.* 1978;1:1284. **60.** Punnonen R, Lukola A. Oestrogen-like effect of ginseng. *Br Med J.* 1980;281:1110.

Gamma-Linolenic Acid (GLA)

Alternate/Related Names: Omega-6 Oil(s), Omega-6 Fatty Acids, Sources of GLA include Black Currant Seed Oil, Borage Oil, Evening Primrose Oil

U.S. BRAND NAMES OF CLINICALLY TESTED PRODUCTS

Efamol (Efamol Nutraceuticals) = Efamol (Efamol Ltd.) in Europe

DESCRIPTION

Gamma-linolenic acid (GLA) is an omega-6 fatty acid, one of the essential fatty acids (EFAs). Sources of GLA include evening primrose oil (EPO), black currant oil, and borage oil.

PHARMACOLOGY

The evening primrose has been artificially bred to produce plants whose seeds reliably yield 7% to 10% GLA. Other EPO constituents include saturated fats (10%), oleic acid (9%), and linoleic acid (72%). Because of the confounding effects of these other constituents, artificially purified GLA has been used in some studies. Borage and black currant oil are also used to supply GLA; based on their fatty acid composition, it has been proposed that EPO is superior; these claims may not be entirely disinterested.[1,2]

Omega-6 fatty acids are essential nutrients whose exact daily requirement is not known. The body primarily utilizes dietary linoleic acid as a precursor, converting it to GLA in a rate-limiting step involving delta-6 desaturase. An elongase enzyme then creates dihomo-GLA, which can be converted to subscript 1-series prostaglandins and subscript 3-series leukotrienes. Additionally, delta-5 desaturase converts dihomo-GLA to arachidonic acid, with its subsequent "unfavorable" prostaglandin and leukotriene metabolites.

The rate-limiting delta-6 desaturase conversion of dietary linoleic acid into GLA may be impaired by numerous conditions, including advanced age, diabetes, high alcohol intake, eczema, cyclic mastitis, viral infections, excessive saturated fat intake, elevated cholesterol levels, excessive dietary intake of trans and positional isomers of linoleic acid, and deficiencies of pyridoxine, zinc, magnesium, biotin, or calcium.[1-6] In these conditions, GLA may be useful as a "downstream" supplement, one that skips the rate-limiting delta-6 desaturase step.

GLA is susceptible to oxidative stress, leading to the formation of potentially toxic peroxides and hydroperoxides. Vitamin E, ascorbate, selenium, superoxide dismutase, and glutathione peroxidase act to inhibit this transformation.[2]

CLINICAL STUDIES

DIABETIC NEUROPATHY

One randomized double-blind placebo-controlled study of 111 patients with mild diabetic neuropathy given 6 g EPO daily for 1 year demonstrated improvement in neuropathy symptoms without change in serum glucose levels.[7] A small double-blind placebo-controlled trial demonstrated improvement in symptoms, motor conduction velocity, muscle action potential amplitudes, nerve action potential amplitudes, and ankle heat and cold thresholds after 6 months of GLA therapy.[8]

RHEUMATOID ARTHRITIS

In a double-blind study of 56 patients with RA, 16 of the 21 treated with GLA for 1 year significantly improved as compared to the placebo group.[9] This study utilized very high doses of purified GLA (2.8 g/day, equivalent to about 30 g EPO daily). Benefits were also seen in other small trials.[2,10-13]

CYCLIC MASTALGIA (AND PMS)

EPO has been used for a variety of breast disorders, but supporting evidence has been reported regarding symptomatic relief in mastalgia only when significant cysts or fibroadenomas are not present.

In a randomized double-blind placebo-controlled crossover study, 73 patients with cyclic or noncyclic mastalgia (with or without palpable nodularity) experienced significantly less discomfort during the 3-month treatment period with 3 g/day EPO.[14] However, according to a 1-year double-blind study of 200 women with cysts large enough to be aspirated, EPO was not more effective than placebo.[15,16] Lack of benefit was also seen in a small 6-month placebo-controlled study of 23 women with fibroadenomas.[17]

Although several small studies suggest that EPO is helpful in reducing general PMS symptoms, all suffer from serious flaws.[18]

ECZEMA

Despite its widespread use in Europe, evidence on the use of EPO for eczema is more negative than positive. Studies with negative results include three double-blind placebo-controlled trials: a 24-week study of 160 adults given GLA from borage oil,[19] a 16-week trial of EPO in 58 children,[20] and a 16-week study of EPO or EPO and fish oil in 102 patients.[21]

A 1989 review of the literature found significant benefit in nine double-blind controlled studies performed to that date, with the greatest benefit in pruritus.[22] However, that review has been criticized for including poorly designed and unpublished studies and for possibly misinterpreting study results.[21]

One recent double-blind trial of 51 children did find overall therapeutic benefit with EPO.[23]

OBESITY

A 12-week double-blind study that enrolled 100 significantly overweight women compared the effectiveness of EPO to placebo.[24] No difference was seen between the groups.

Another double-blind trial ($n=47$) tested the unusual hypothesis that EPO might prove effective only in individuals with a family history of obesity.[25] Use of EPO produced a small but significant weight loss, especially in participants with both parents obese.

CHRONIC FATIGUE SYNDROME

While one 3-month double-blind placebo-controlled study of 63 people with chronic fatigue syndrome found that a combination of EFAs containing EPO and fish oil resulted in significant improvements,[26] a more precisely structured replication of this study in 1999 found no benefit.[27]

PROPOSED INDICATIONS AND USAGE

Based on weak and/or inconsistent evidence, EPO is widely used in Europe for the treatment of diabetic neuropathy, cyclic mastitis, and eczema.

Based on still weaker evidence, GLA or EPO have also been advocated as treatments for obesity, chronic fatigue syndrome, rheumatoid arthritis, general PMS symptoms, Raynaud's phenomenon, Sjogren's disease, endometriosis, osteoporosis, and prostate disease.

WARNINGS

None.

PRECAUTIONS

It has been suggested that supplemental GLA might raise levels of arachidonic acid, with potential adverse consequences.

Maximum safe dosage for young children, pregnant or lactating women, or individuals with severe renal or hepatic disease has not been established.

DRUG INTERACTIONS

None are known.

ADVERSE REACTIONS

Over 4,000 patients have participated in trials of GLA, primarily in the form of EPO. No adverse effects or significant differences in rate of side effects between the treated group and placebo group have been attributed to this treatment.[2] In animal studies, EPO has been found to be nontoxic and noncarcinogenic.

Early reports suggested the possibility of exacerbation of temporal lobe epilepsy and mania by EPO ingestion, but further evidence has not been reported.[28]

PROPOSED DOSAGE AND ADMINISTRATION

Because EPO is the most common form of GLA, dosages will be given in those terms.

For cyclic mastitis, the standard dosage of EPO is 3 g daily in 2 or 3 divided doses. RA has been treated with 5 to 10 g daily, although one study used concentrated GLA equivalent to 30 g of EPO. Diabetic neuropathy is typically treated with 4 to 6 g daily. There may be value in combining lipoic acid with EPO when treating this condition.[29,30] Children with eczema have been given 2 to 4 g daily. For all these conditions, the proposed minimum duration of treatment is several months.

PATIENT INFORMATION

Evening primrose oil is a source of gamma-linolenic acid (GLA), an essential fatty acid. Other sources of GLA include black currant oil and borage oil.

Evening primrose oil and GLA are widely marketed for the treatment for eczema, diabetic neuropathy, cyclic breast pain, and many other conditions. However, the evidence that they work is very weak.

The maximum safe dosage of GLA for pregnant or nursing women or young children has not been established. Individuals with severe liver or kidney disease should consult a physician before using this (or any other) supplement.

REFERENCES

1. Barre DE, Holub BJ, Chapkin RS. The effect of borage oil supplementation on human platelet aggregation, thromboxane B2, prostaglandin E1, and E2 formation. *Nutr Res.* 1993;13:739-751. **2.** Horrobin DF. Nutritional and medical importance of gamma-linolenic acid. *Prog Lipid Res.* 1992;31:163-194. **3.** Horrobin DF. The use of gamma-linolenic acid in diabetic neuropathy. *Agents Actions Suppl.* 1992;37:120-144. **4.** Horrobin DF. Gamma linolenic acid: an intermediate in essential fatty acid metabolism with potential as an ethical pharmaceutical and as a food. *Rev Contemp Pharmacother.* 1990;1:1-41. **5.** Horrobin DF, Manku M, Brush M, et al. Abnormalities in plasma essential fatty acid levels in women with premenstrual syndrome and with nonmalignant breast disease. *J Nutr Med.* 1991;2:259-264. **6.** Manku MS, Horrobin DF, Morse NL, et al. Essential fatty acids in the plasma phospholipids of patients with atopic eczema. *Br J Dermatol.* 1984;110:643-648. **7.** Keen H, Payan J, Allawi J, et al. Treatment of diabetic neuropathy with gamma-linolenic acid: the gamma-linolenic acid multicenter trial group. *Diabetes Care.* 1993;16:8-15. **8.** Jamal GA, Carmichael H. The effect of gamma-linolenic acid on human diabetic peripheral neuropathy: a double-blind placebo-controlled trial. *Diabetic Medicine.* 1990;7:319-323. **9.** Zurier RB, Rossetti RG, Jacobson EW, et al. Gamma-Linolenic acid treatment of rheumatoid arthritis. A randomized, placebo-controlled trial. *Arthritis Rheum.* 1996;39:1808-1817. **10.** Leventhal LJ, Boyce EG, Zurier RB. Treatment of rheumatoid arthritis with gammalinolenic acid. *Ann Intern Med.* 1993;119:867-873. **11.** Leventhal LJ, Boyce EG, Zurier RB. Treatment of rheumatoid arthritis with blackcurrant seed oil. *Br J Rheumatol.* 1994;33:847-852. **12.** Rothman D, DeLuca P, Zurier RB. Botanical lipids: effects on inflammation, immune responses, and rheumatoid arthritis. *Semin Arthritis Rheum.* 1995;25:87-96. **13.** Belch JJ, Ansell D, Madhok R, et al. Effects of altering dietary essential fatty acids on requirements for non-steroidal anti-inflammatory drugs in patients with rheumatoid arthritis: a double blind placebo controlled study. *Ann Rheum Dis.* 1988;47:96-104. **14.** Pashby NL, Mansel RE, Hughes LE, et al. A clinical trial of evening primrose oil in mastalgia [abstract]. *Br J Surg.* 1981;68:801. **15.** Mansel RE, Gateley CA, Harrison BJ, et al. Effects and tolerability of n-6 essential fatty acid supplementation in patients with recurrent breast cysts: a randomized double-blind placebo-controlled trial. *J Nutr Med.* 1990;1:195-200. **16.** Mansel RE, Harrison BJ, Melhuish J, et al. A randomized trial of dietary intervention with essential fatty acids in patients with categorized cysts. *Ann N Y Acad Sci.* 1990;586:288-294. **17.** Kollias J, Macmillan RD, Sibbering DM, et al. Effect of evening primrose oil on clinically diagnosed fibroadenomas. *Breast.* 2000;9:35-36. **18.** Budeiri D, Li Wan Po A, Dornan JC. Is evening primrose oil of value in the treatment of premenstrual syndrome? *Control Clin Trials.* 1996;17:60-68. **19.** Henz BM, Jablonska S, van de Kerkhof PC, et al. Double-blind, multicentre analysis of the efficacy of borage oil in patients with atopic eczema. *Br J Dermatol.* 1999;140:685-688. **20.** Hederos CA, Berg A. Epogam evening primrose oil treatment in atopic dermatitis and asthma. *Arch Dis Child.* 1996;75:494-497. **21.** Berth-Jones J, Graham-Brown RAC. Placebo-controlled trial of essential fatty acid supplementation in atopic dermatitis. *Lancet.* 1993;341:1557-1560. **22.** Morse PF, Horrobin DF, Manku MS, et al. Meta-analysis of placebo-controlled studies of the efficacy of Epogam in the treatment of atopic eczema. Relationship between plasma essential fatty acid changes and clinical response. *Br J Dermatol.* 1989;121:75-90. **23.** Biagi PL, Bordoni A, Hrelia S, et al. The effect of gamma-linolenic acid on clinical status, red cell fatty acid composition and membrane microviscosity in infants with atopic dermatitis. *Drugs Exp Clin Res.* 1994;20:77-84. **24.** Haslett C, Douglas JG, Chalmers SR, et al. A double-blind evaluation of evening primrose oil as an antiobesity agent. *Int J Obes.* 1983;7:549-553. **25.** Garcia CM, Carter J, Chou A. Gamma linolenic acid causes weight loss and lower blood pressure in overweight patients with family history of obesity. *Swed J Biol Med.* 1986;4:8-11. **26.** Behan PO, Behan WM, Horrobin D. Effect of high doses of essential fatty acids on the postviral fatigue syndrome. *Acta Neurol Scand.* 1990;82:209-216. **27.** Warren G, McKendrick M, Peet M. The role of essential fatty acids in chronic fatigue syndrome. A case-controlled study of red-cell membrane essential fatty acids (EFA) and a placebo-controlled treatment study with high dose of EFA. *Acta Neurol Scand.* 1999;99:112-116. **28.** Vaddadi KS. The use of gamma-linolenic acid and linoleic acid to differentiate between temporal lobe epilepsy and schizophrenia. *Prostaglandins Med.* 1981;6:375-379. **29.** Cameron NE, Cotter MA, Horrobin DH, et al. Effects of alpha-lipoic acid on neurovascular function in diabetic rats: interaction with essential fatty acids. *Diabetologia.* 1998;41:390-399. **30.** Hounsom L, Horrobin DF, Tritschler H, et al. A lipoic acid-gamma linolenic acid conjugate is effective against multiple indices of experimental diabetic neuropathy. *Diabetologia.* 1998;41:839-843.

Glucosamine

Alternate/Related Names: Glucosamine Sulfate, Glucosamine Hydrochloride, N-Acetyl Glucosamine, Glucosamine Chloride

U.S. BRAND NAMES OF CLINICALLY TESTED PRODUCTS

Not applicable.

DESCRIPTION

Glucosamine is a constituent of cartilage and other connective tissues. Exogenous glucosamine (virtually always as glucosamine sulfate) has been used since the early 1980s as a treatment for osteoarthritis.

PHARMACOLOGY

Glucosamine is a simple molecule formed of glucose and an amine moiety. It plays a significant role in the manufacture of proteoglycans, both as raw material and as a possible stimulant of chondrocyte activity.[1,2,3]

Pharmacokinetic studies show that glucosamine sulfate, when taken orally, is absorbed at a rate approaching 90% and is ultimately taken up by articular cartilage and other tissues.[4,5]

Although the pathogenesis of osteoarthritis is not fully understood, it appears that the initial stages involve damage to collagen structure and subsequent leakage of proteoglycans, followed by a compensatory rise in the manufacture of proteoglycans. Eventually, proteoglycan levels cannot be maintained, and when they drop, end-stage osteoarthritis develops. Supplemental glucosamine may slow this process by stimulating the synthesis of proteoglycans and collagen by cartilage cells, reducing phospholipase A2 activity, and inhibiting enzymatic degradation of collagen.[6-12]

Glucosamine is also believed to exert a weak anti-inflammatory effect unrelated to prostaglandins, but it does not produce direct analgesia.[2,6,13-15]

CLINICAL STUDIES

OSTEOARTHRITIS: SYMPTOM REDUCTION

A double-blind placebo-controlled study compared the effectiveness of glucosamine sulfate and placebo in 252 patients with radiologic stage I-III osteoarthritis of the knee.[16] The participants were treated with oral glucosamine sulfate (500 mg 3 times daily, the dose used in virtually all studies) or placebo. At the end of the 4-week study period, ratings on Lequesne's index (a measure of osteoarthritic severity) significantly improved in the treated group as compared to the placebo group. Smaller double-blind studies performed in the early 1980s reported similar results.[6,17,18] However, there have been negative results as well.[19,20]

Comparison trials have also been reported. One double-blind study followed 200 subjects with osteoarthritis of the knee, half of whom received 1,200 mg/day ibuprofen and the other half glucosamine sulfate.[2] Although ibuprofen reduced symptoms more rapidly, both groups experienced comparable relief at the end of 4 weeks. A similar trial of 178 patients with knee osteoarthritis yielded essentially the same results.[10] In addition, a 3-month double-blind trial of 45 individuals with temporomandibular joint osteoarthritis found that glucosamine sulfate was at least as effective as ibuprofen (again, 1200 mg daily).[21]

Another double-blind study (published in abstract form only) followed 329 patients given piroxicam (20 mg daily), glucosamine sulfate, placebo, or glucosamine sulfate plus piroxicam for 3 months.[14] It found piroxicam and glucosamine sulfate to be equally effective, and combination treatment to be without significant additional benefit.

OSTEOARTHRITIS: DISEASE-MODIFYING EFFECTS

A double-blind placebo-controlled study of 212 participants over 3 years found radiologic evidence of reduced cartilage loss in the group treated with glucosamine sulfate, suggesting that the supplement is a disease-modifying agent in osteoarthritis.[22]

PROPOSED INDICATIONS AND USAGE

A moderate level of evidence suggests that glucosamine sulfate is an effective treatment for osteoarthritis.[23] Compared to NSAIDs, it appears to act more slowly but ultimately achieves the same level of efficacy. Additionally, glucosamine sulfate may alter the natural history of osteoarthritis by slowing progressive joint damage. However, the research record is far from definitive at this time.

Sports teams frequently use glucosamine sulfate as a prophylactic against muscle and tendon injury; however, there is no evidence that it is effective for this purpose.

WARNINGS

Some evidence suggests that diabetics should not use glucosamine (see Precautions).

PRECAUTIONS

There are concerns that supplemental glucosamine might affect glucose metabolism through the hexosamine pathway because of the chemical similarity between glucosamine-6-phosphate and glucose-6-phosphate. Evidence from animal studies suggests that glucosamine may increase insulin resistance in diabetics.[24-28] While decreased insulin sensitivity has not been seen in human trials,[29] it has been found to increase plasma fasting glucose levels.[30] Glucosamine might increase the rate of glycosylation of tissues such as the lens, thereby increasing risk of long-term diabetic side effects.[31]

Maximum safe dosages for pregnant or lactating women, young children, or individuals with severe hepatic or renal disease are not known.

DRUG INTERACTIONS

None known.

ADVERSE REACTIONS

Glucosamine sulfate appears to be essentially nontoxic.[4,5,11,12] A large open study of 1,502 patients showed a 12% incidence of side effects, mainly consisting of mild to moderate gastrointestinal distress.[32] Double-blind studies have found an incidence of side effects comparable to that of placebo.[2,14]

PROPOSED DOSAGE AND ADMINISTRATION

Glucosamine is typically taken in the sulfate form at a dose of 500 mg 3 times daily. Full benefits appear to require 4 to 6 weeks to develop.

The relative efficacy of other glucosamine compounds such as glucosamine hydrochloride and N-acetyl-glucosamine (NAG) remains unclear.

Glucosamine sulfate is often sold in combination with chondroitin sulfate; however, the evidence for a synergistic effect is limited to preliminary animal studies.[33,34]

PATIENT INFORMATION

Meaningful although not definitive evidence suggests that glucosamine sulfate is an effective treatment for osteoarthritis. It is a slow acting treatment that may require months to reach its full effect.

There are concerns that individuals with diabetes should not use glucosamine sulfate.

The maximum safe dosage of glucosamine sulfate for pregnant or nursing women or young children has not been established. Individuals with severe liver or kidney disease should consult a physician before using this (or any other) supplement.

REFERENCES

1. Karzel K, Domenjoz R. Effects of hexosamine derivatives and uronic acid derivatives on glycosaminoglycane metabolism of fibroblast cultures. *Pharmacology.* 1971;5:337-345. **2.** Muller-Fassbender H, Bach GL, Haase W, et al. Glucosamine sulfate compared to ibuprofen in osteoarthritis of the knee. *Osteoarthritis Cartilage.* 1994;2:61-69. **3.** Vidal y Plana RR, Bizzarri D, Rovati AL. Articular cartilage pharmacology: I. In vitro studies on glucosamine and non steroidal antiinflammatory drugs. *Pharmacol Res Commun.* 1978;10:557-569. **4.** Setnikar I, Giacchetti C, Zanolo G. Pharmacokinetics of glucosamine in the dog and in man. *Arzneimittelforschung.* 1986;36:729-735. **5.** Setnikar I, Palumbo R, Canali S, et al. Pharmacokinetics of glucosamine in man. *Arzneimittelforschung.* 1993;43:1109-1113. **6.** Crolle G, D'Este E. Glucosamine sulphate for the management of arthrosis: a controlled clinical investigation. *Curr Med Res Opin.* 1980;7:104-109. **7.** Hellio MP. The effects of glucosamine on human osteoarthritic chondrocytes. Presented at: The Ninth EULAR Symposium; October 7-10, 1996; Madrid, Spain. **8.** Jimenez SA. The effects of glucosamine on human chondrocyte gene expression. Presented at: The Ninth EULAR Symposium; October 7-10, 1996; Madrid, Spain. **9.** Piperno M, Reboul P, Hellio Le Graverand MP, et al. Glucosamine sulfate modulates dysregulated activities of human osteoarthritic chondrocytes in vitro. *Osteoarthritis Cartilage.* 2000;8:207-212. **10.** Qiu GX, Gao SN, Giacovelli G, et al. Efficacy and safety of glucosamine sulfate versus ibuprofen in patients with knee osteoarthritis. *Arzneimittelforschung.* 1998;48:469-474. **11.** Setnikar I, Pacini MA, Revel L. Antiarthritic effects of glucosamine sulfate studied in animal models. *Arzneimittelforschung.* 1991;41:542-545. **12.** Setnikar I. Antireactive properties of "chondroprotective" drugs. *Int J Tissue React.* 1992;14:253-261. **13.** Reichelt A, Forster KK, Fischer M, et al. Efficacy and safety of intramuscular glucosamine sulfate in osteoarthritis of the knee. A randomised, placebo-controlled, double-blind study. *Arzneimittelforschung.* 1994;44:75-80. **14.** Rovati LC, Giacovelli G, Annefeld M, et al. A large, randomized, placebo controlled, double-blind study of glucosamine sulfate vs. piroxicam and vs. their association, on the kinetics of the symptomatic effect in knee osteoarthritis [abstract]. *Osteoarthritis Cartilage.* 1994;2(suppl 1):56. **15.** Lopes Vaz A. Double-blind clinical evaluation of the relative efficacy of ibuprofen and glucosamine sulphate in the management of osteoarthrosis of the knee in out-patients. *Curr Med Res Opin.* 1982;8:145-149. **16.** Noack W, Fischer M, Forster KK, et al. Glucosamine sulfate in osteoarthritis of the knee. *Osteoarthritis Cartilage.* 1994;2:51-59. **17.** D'Ambrosio E, Casa B, Bompani R, et al. Glucosamine sulphate: a controlled clinical investigation in arthrosis. *Pharmatherapeutica.* 1981;2:504-508. **18.** Drovanti A, Bignamini AA, Rovati AL. Therapeutic activity of oral glucosamine sulfate in osteoarthrosis: a placebo-controlled double-blind investigation. *Clin Ther.* 1980;3:260-272. **19.** Rindone JP, Hiller D, Collacott E, et al. Randomized, controlled trial of glucosamine for treating osteoarthritis of the knee. *West J Med.* 2000;172:91-94. **20.** Houpt JB, McMillian R, Wein C, et al. Effect of glucosamine hydrochloride in the treatment of pain and osteoarthritis of the knee. *J Rheumatol.* 1999;26:2423-2430. **21.** Thie NM, Prasad NG, Major PW. Evaluation of glucosamine sulfate compared to ibuprofen for the treatment of temporomandibular joint osteoarthritis: a randomized double blind controlled 3 month clinical trial. *J Rheumatol.* 2001;28:1347-1355. **22.** Reginster JY, Deroisy R, Rovati L, et al. Long-term effects of glucosamine sulphate on osteoarthritis progression: a randomised, placebo-controlled clinical trial. *Lancet* 2001;357:251-256. **23.** McAlindon TE, LaValley MP, Felson DT. Efficacy of glucosamine and chondroitin for treatment of osteoarthritis. *JAMA.* 2000;284:1241. **24.** Almada AL, et al. Effect of chronic oral glucosamine sulfate upon fasting insulin resistance index (FIRI) in nondiabetic individuals. Poster presented at: Experimental Biology 2000; April 15-18, 2000; San Diego, CA; Program number 521.15. **25.** Head K. Personal communication of case reports. 1999. **26.** Patti ME, Virkamaki A, Landaker EJ, et al. Activation of the hexosamine pathway by glucosamine in vivo induces insulin resistance of early postreceptor insulin signaling events in skelatal muscle. *Diabetes.* 1999;48:1562-1571. **27.** Shankar RR, Zhu JS, Baron AD. Glucosamine infusion in rats mimics the beta-cell dysfunction of non- insulin-dependant diabetes mellitus. *Metabolism.* 1998;47:573-577. **28.** Virkamaki A, Yki-Jarvinen H. Allosteric regulation of glycogen synthase and hexokinase by glucosamine-6-phosphate during glucosamine-induced insulin resistance in skeletal muscle and heart. *Diabetes.* 1999;48:1101-1107. **29.** Pouwels MJ, Jacobs JR, Span PN, et al. Short-term glucosamine infusion does not affect insulin sensitivity in humans. *J Clin Endocrinol Metab.* 2001;86:2099-2103. **30.** Monauni T, Zenti MG, Cretti A, et al. Effects of glucosamine infusion on insulin secretion and insulin action in humans. *Diabetes.* 2000;49:926-935. **31.** Ajiboye R, Harding JJ. The non-enzymic glycosylation of bovine lens proteins by glucosamine and its inhibition by aspirin, ibuprofen and glutathione. *Exp Eye Res.* 1989;49:31-41. **32.** Tapadinhas MJ, Rivera IC, Bignamini AA. Oral glucosamine sulphate in the management of arthrosis: report on a multi-centre open investigation in Portugal. *Pharmatherapeutica.* 1982;3:157-168. **33.** Lippiello L, Woodward J, Karpman R, et al. In vivo chondroprotection and metabolic synergy of glucosamine and chondroitin sulfate. *Clin Orthop.* 2000;381:229-240. **34.** Lippiello L, Karpman RR, Hammad T. Synergistic effect of glucosamine HCL and chondroitin sulfate on in vitro proteoglycan synthesis by bovine chondrocytes. Presented at: American Academy of Orthopaedic Surgeons 67th Annual Meeting; March 15-19, 2000; Orlando, Fla.

Goldenseal

Hydrastis Canadensis

Alternate/Related Names: Yellow Root, Indian Dye, Indian Paint

U.S. BRAND NAMES OF CLINICALLY TESTED PRODUCTS

None.

DESCRIPTION

Goldenseal is a low-lying perennial that is native to the forests of the eastern United States. Its root was widely used by Native Americans both as a dye plant and as a treatment for skin disorders, digestive problems, liver disease, diarrhea, and eye irritations. European settlers learned of the herb from the Iroquois and other tribes and quickly adopted goldenseal as a part of early colonial medical care. In the early 1800s, an herbalist named Samuel Thompson created a simplistic but highly popular system of medicine in which goldenseal was regarded as a virtual cure-all.

Goldenseal remains a best-selling herb today, despite a complete absence of evidence that it is effective for any medical condition.

PHARMACOLOGY

The biologically active ingredients in goldenseal are believed to be hydrastine (2% to 4% total weight) and berberine (2% to 3% total weight). Most of the scientific investigation relevant to goldenseal has focused on berberine.

Berberine possesses antimicrobial activity against a wide variety of bacteria and fungi and may inhibit the growth of several intestinal parasites.[1,2,3] Berberine does not appear to directly influence bacterial cell growth; however, it may inhibit bacterial adhesion to epithelial tissues.[4]

Berberine also appears to possess choleretic[5,6] and possible chemopreventive actions.[7,8,9] Animal studies have found that berberine increases blood flow to the spleen, and an in vitro study found macrophage activity enhancement.[7,10] One study in rats found that goldenseal caused an increase in IgM response to the antigen keyhole limpet hemocyanin (KLH).[11]

In animal studies, berberine and hydrastine have also exhibited hypotensive and hypertensive effects; potentiation of barbiturate activity; antipyretic, antimuscarinic, and antihistaminic actions; and uterine stimulation.[12] However, the clinical relevance of these and other documented effects of goldenseal constituents is unknown.

CLINICAL STUDIES

Whole goldenseal root has not been the subject of clinical trials. Although there is some evidence from low-quality trials that purified berberine may offer benefits in intestinal infections such as cholera and *Giardia,*[13-16] an impossibly high dosage of goldenseal would be necessary to deliver the same amount of berberine.

PROPOSED INDICATIONS AND USAGE

Goldenseal has no evidence-based uses. It is widely sold in combination with echinacea for use at the onset of cold symptoms, but there is no scientific evidence that goldenseal offers any benefits when used in this way. Furthermore, traditional herbalists did not consider it effective for this purpose.

Goldenseal creams are sold as topical antibiotics, but these products have not been evaluated clinically. Goldenseal tea is sometimes used as a douche for vaginal candidiasis, but again there is no clinical evidence of efficacy.

Goldenseal is also widely used in the false belief that it can produce a negative result on urine drug tests.

WARNINGS

Goldenseal should not be used during pregnancy or by individuals with hepatic disease.

PRECAUTIONS

Berberine displaces bilirubin from albumin, raising bilirubin levels, and has also been reported to cause uterine contractions in animals.[17,18] For these reasons, goldenseal is not recommended for use during pregnancy or lactation, or by young children or individuals with hepatic disease. Maximum safe doses in renal disease are not known.

If goldenseal is used as a topical treatment for skin wounds, the wound should be cleaned at least once a day to prevent goldenseal particles from becoming trapped in the healing tissues.

DRUG INTERACTIONS

None reported. However, evidence suggests that goldenseal might inhibit CYP 3A4.[19]

ADVERSE REACTIONS

The toxicology of whole goldenseal root is not known. The LD_{50} for berberine in mice is 300 mg/kg,[18] which translates to a dose of 10,000 mg/kg whole goldenseal root. Side effects of oral goldenseal appear to be uncommon, although there have been anecdotal reports of gastrointestinal distress and increased nervousness in patients who take very high doses.

PROPOSED DOSAGE AND ADMINISTRATION

For systemic use, a typical dose of powdered goldenseal is 250 to 500 mg 3 times daily.

PATIENT INFORMATION

Goldenseal is an expensive herb with no proven medical uses. It is widely combined with echinacea in products advertised for the treatment of the common cold. However, unlike echinacea, goldenseal is not believed to offer any benefits for colds. Additionally, goldenseal is popularly supposed to help produce a "clean" urine drug test, but it does not work.

Goldenseal should not be used by pregnant or nursing women, young children, or individuals with severe liver or kidney disease.

REFERENCES

1. Amin AH, Subbaiah TV, Abbasi KM. Berberine sulfate: antimicrobial activity, bioassay, and mode of action. *Can J Microbiol.* 1969;15:1067-1076. **2.** Hahn FE, Ciak J. Berberine. *Antibiotics.* 1976;3:577-584. **3.** Kaneda Y, Torii M, Tanaka T, et al. In vitro effects of berberine sulphate on the growth and structure of Entamoeba histolytica, Giardia lamblia and Trichomonas vaginalis. *Ann Trop Med Parasitol.* 1991;85:417-425. **4.** Sun D, Abraham SN, Beachey EH. Influence of berberine sulfate on synthesis and expression of Pap fimbrial adhesin in uropathogenic Escherichia coli. *Antimicrob Agents Chemother.* 1988;32:1274-1277. **5.** Chan MY. The effect of berberine on bilirubin excretion in the rat. *Comp Med East West.* 1977;5:161-168. **6.** Preininger V. The pharmacology and toxicology of the Papaveracae alkaloids. *Alkaloids.* 1975;15:207-261. **7.** Kumazawa Y, Itagaki A, Fukumoto M, Fujisawa H, et al. Activation of peritoneal macrophages by berberine-type alkaloids in terms of induction of cytostatic activity. *Int J Immunopharmacol.* 1984;6:587-592. **8.** Kuo CL, Chou CC, Yung BY. Berberine complexes with DNA in the berberine-induced apoptosis in human leukemic HL-60 cells. *Cancer Lett.* 1995;93:193-200. **9.** Nishino H, Kitagawa K, Fujiki H, et al. Berberine sulfate inhibits tumor-promoting activity of teleocidin in two-stage carcinogenesis on mouse skin. *Oncology.* 1986;43:131-134. **10.** Sabir M, Bhide NK. Study of some pharmacological actions of berberine. *Indian J Physiol Pharmacol.* 1971;15:111-132. **11.** Rehman J, Dillow JM, Carter SM, et al. Increased production of antigen-specific immunoglobulins G and M following in vivo treatment with the medicinal plants Echinacea angustifolia and Hydrastis canadensis. *Immunol Lett.* 1999;68:391-395. **12.** Newall C, et al. *Herbal medicines: a guide for healthcare professionals.* London: The Pharmaceutical Press; 1996:151. **13.** Rabbani GH, Butler T, Knight J, et al. Randomized controlled trial of berberine sulfate therapy for diarrhea due to enterotoxigenic Escherichia coli and Vibrio cholerae. *J Infect Dis.* 1987;155:979-984. **14.** Khin-Maung-U, Myo-Khin, Nyunt-Nyunt-Wai, et al. Clinical trial of berberine in acute watery diarrhoea. *Br Med J (Clin Res Ed).* 1985;291:1601-1605. **15.** Choudhry VP, Sabir M, Bhide VN. Berberine in giardiasis. *Indian Pediatr.* 1972;9:143-146. **16.** Gupte S. Use of berberine in treatment of giardiasis. *Am J Dis Child.* 1975;129:866. **17.** Chan E. Displacement of bilirubin from albumin by berberine. *Biol Neonat.* 1993;63:201-208. **18.** DeSmet PAGM, et al., eds. *Adverse effects of herbal drugs.* Vol. I. Berlin: Springer-Verlag; 1992:97-104. **19.** Budzinski JW, Foster BC, Vandenhoek S, et al. An in vitro evaluation of human cytochrome P450 3A4 inhibition by selected commercial herbal extracts and tinctures. *Phytomedicine.* 2000;7;273-282.

Gotu Kola

Centella Asiatica

Alternate/Related Names: Indian Ginseng

U.S. BRAND NAMES OF CLINICALLY TESTED PRODUCTS

None.

DESCRIPTION

Gotu kola is a creeping plant native to subtropical and tropical climates. Commonly confused with the dried seed leaf of the common kola nut, gotu kola is an unrelated herb and contains no caffeine.

Like ginseng, gotu kola has been associated historically with an unusually large array of health claims, ranging from long life to increased sexual potency. However, there is little evidence that gotu kola is effective for any condition other than, possibly, venous insufficiency.

PHARMACOLOGY

Subspecies of gotu kola from various parts of Asia contain different proportions of known ingredients. In general, gotu kola leaf consists of volatile terpene oils, flavonoids, alkaloids, and 1.1% to 8% triterpene saponins. The latter group of substances has been investigated the most for medicinal effects. In the Madagascar species of gotu kola, these triterpenes consist of asiaticoside (40%), asiatic acid (29% to 30%), madecassic acid (29% to 30%), and madecassoside (1% to 2%).[1]

Weak evidence suggests that asiaticoside extracted from gotu kola can stimulate hair and nail growth; speed wound healing; promote blood vessel development; increase the formation of hyaluronic acid, collagen, fibronectin, and chondroitin sulfate; dissolve the protective coating of *Mycobacterium leprae;* and increase the keratinization of the epidermis.[2-10]

CLINICAL STUDIES

VENOUS INSUFFICIENCY

A double-blind study of 94 patients with venous insufficiency of the lower limbs evaluated the comparative benefits of *C. asiatica* extract at 120 and 60 mg/day versus placebo.[11] The results showed a significant dose-related improvement in the treated groups in symptoms such as subjective heaviness, discomfort, and edema.

In a double-blind study of 87 patients with chronic venous hypertensive microangiopathy, patients were divided into three groups, one receiving placebo and the others 30 mg twice daily or 60 mg twice daily of standardized *C. asiatica* extract.[12] The results showed a dose-related improvement in perimalleolar skin flux at rest and in transcutaneous PO_2 and PCO_2.

Benefits with gotu kola were also seen in smaller studies of venous insufficiency.[13-18]

PROPOSED INDICATIONS AND USAGE

Preliminary evidence suggests that gotu kola might offer benefits in chronic venous insufficiency.[18] Gotu kola has been suggested for hemorrhoids on the reasoning that they represent a form of varicose veins but this application has not been studied.

Based on weak to nonexistent evidence, oral or topical gotu kola has also been proposed as a treatment for numerous skin conditions, including scleroderma, psoriasis, burns, wounds, keloids (both prevention and treatment), mycosis fungoides, and anal fissures; other proposed uses of gotu kola with similarly weak substantiation include anxiety, bladder ulcers, dermatitis, fibrocystic breast disease, leprosy, liver cirrhosis, lupus erythematosus, memory loss, peptic ulcer, periodontal disease, retinal detachment, and tuberculosis.[5,19,20]

WARNINGS

None.

PRECAUTIONS

Safety in young children, pregnant or lactating women, or individuals with severe renal or hepatic disease has not been established.

However, rabbit studies suggest that gotu kola extracts are not teratogenic,[21] and gotu kola has been used as a treatment for venous insufficiency during pregnancy.[22]

DRUG INTERACTIONS

None known.

ADVERSE REACTIONS

Gotu kola is generally well tolerated, the only reported side effect being rare allergic skin rash. Toxicology studies suggest that oral asiaticoside at a dose of 1 g/kg, and whole fresh gotu kola leaves at 16 g/kg are safe.[5,20] Asiaticoside has been found to possess weak tumor-promotion properties in hairless mouse epidermis and dermis.[23]

PROPOSED DOSAGE AND ADMINISTRATION

The usual dose of gotu kola is 20 to 40 mg 3 times daily of a triterpenic extract standardized to contain 40% asiaticoside, 29% to 30% asiatic acid, 29% to 30% madecassic acid, and 1% to 2% madecassoside.

PATIENT INFORMATION

Gotu kola is marketed as a treatment for numerous skin problems, including keloid scars, scleroderma, psoriasis, burns, wounds, and anal fissures. However, there is little evidence that it is effective for any of these conditions.

The safety of gotu kola for pregnant or nursing women or young children has not been established. Individuals with severe liver or kidney disease should consult a physician before using this (or any other) supplement.

REFERENCES

1. Castellani C, Marai A, Vacchi P. The Centella asiatica [in Italian]. *Boll Chim Farm.* 1981;120:570-605. **2.** Abou-Chaar Cl. Few drugs from higher plants recently introduced into therapeutics. *Leban Pharm J.* 1963;8:14-37. **3.** Boiteau P, Nigeon-Dureuil M, Ratsimamanga AR. Action of asiaticoside on reticuloendothelial tissue [in French]. *C R Acad Sci Hebd Seances Acad Sci D.* 1951;232:760-762. **4.** Boiteau P, Ratsimamanga AR. Asiaticoside extracted from Centella asiatica, its therepautic uses in the healing of experimental or refractory wounds, leprosy, skin tuberculosis, and lupus [in French]. *Therapie.* 1956;11:125-149. **5.** Kartnig T. Clinical applications of Centella asiatica (L.). *Herbs Spices Med Plants.* 1988;3:146-173. **6.** Lawrence JC. The morphological and pharmacological effects of asiaticoside upon skin in vitro and in vivo. *Eur J Pharmacol.* 1967;1:414-424. **7.** Lawrence JC. The effect of asiaticoside on guinea pig skin. *J Invest Dermatol.* 1967;49:95-96. **8.** May A. The effect of asiaticoside on pig skin in organ culture. *Eur J Pharmacol.* 1968;4:331-339. **9.** Shukla A, Rasik AM, Jain GK, et al. In vitro and in vivo wound healing activity of asiaticoside isolated from Centella asiatica. *J Ethnopharmacol.* 1999;65:1-11. **10.** Tenni R, Zanaboni G, de Agostini MP, et al. Effect of the triterpenoid fraction of Centella asiatica on macromolecules of the connective matrix in human skin fibroblast cultures. *Ital J Biochem.* 1988;37:69-77. **11.** Pointel JP, Boccalon H, Cloarec M, et al. Titrated extract of Centella asiatica (TECA) in the treatment of venous insufficiency of the lower limbs. *Angiology.* 1987;38:46-50. **12.** Cesarone MR, Laurora G, De Sactis MT, et al. The microcirculatory activity of centella asiatica in venous insufficiency. A double-blind study [translated from Italian]. *Minerva Cardioangiol.* 1994;42:299-304. **13.** Belcaro GV, Rulo A, Grimaldi R. Capillary filtration and ankle edema in patients with venous hypertension treated with TTFCA. *Angiology.* 1990;41:12-18. **14.** Allegra C, Pollari G, Criscuolo A, et al. Centella asiatica extract in venous disorders of the lower limbs. Comparative clinico-instrumental studies with a placebo [in Italian; English abstract]. *Clin Ter.* 1981;99:507-513. **15.** Barletta S, Borgioli A, Corsi C, et al. Results with Centella asiatica in chronic venous insufficiency [in Italian; English abstract]. *Gazz Med Ital.* 1981;140:33-35. **16.** Cospite M, Ferrara F, Milio G, et al. Study about pharmacologic and clinical activity of Centella asiatica titrated extract in the chronic venous deficiency of the lower limbs: valuation with strain gauge plethismography [in Italian; English abstract]. *Gazz Ital Angiol.* 1984;4:200-205. **17.** Frausini G, Rotatori P, Oliva S, et al. Controlled trial on clinical-dynamic effects of three treatments in chronic venous insufficiency [in Italian; English abstract]. *Gazz Ital Angiol.* 1985;5:147-151. **18.** Cesarone MR, Laurora G, De Sanctis MT, et al. Activity of Centella asiatica in venous insufficiency [in Italian; English abstract]. *Minerva Cardioangiol.* 1992;40:137-143. **19.** Bradwejn J, Zhou Y, Koszycki D, et al. A double-blind, placebo-controlled study on the effects of Gotu Kola (Centella asiatica) on acoustic startle response in healthy subjects. *J Clin Psychopharmacol.* 2000;20:680-684. **20.** Nalini K, Aroor AR, Karanth KS, et al. Effects of Centella asiatica fresh leaf aqueous extract on learning and memory and biogenic amine turnover in albino rats. *Fitoterapia.* 1992;63:232-237. **21.** Bosse JP, Papillon J, Frenette G, et al. Clinical study of a new antikeloid agent. *Ann Plast Surg.* 1979;3:13-21. **22.** Basellini A, Agus GB, Antonucci E, et al. Varices in pregnancy (an up-date). *Ann Ostet Ginecol Med Perinat.* 1985;106:337-341. **23.** Laerum OD, Iversen OH. Reticuloses and epidermal tumors in hairless mice after topical skin applications of cantharidin and asiaticoside. *Cancer Res.* 1972;32:1463-1469.

Grass Pollen

Alternate/Related Names: Rye Pollen Extract, Timothy Pollen Extract

U.S. BRAND NAMES OF CLINICALLY TESTED PRODUCTS

Cernilton Pollen Extract (Cerniton), Cernitin (Graminex) =
Cernilton Pollen Extract (Cerniton) in Europe

DESCRIPTION

Like the more famous saw palmetto, grass pollen extract is used to treat benign prostatic hyperplasia (BPH). The grasses used for this preparation are 92% rye, 5% timothy, and 3% corn, processed to remove allergenic components.

PHARMACOLOGY

The pharmacology of grass pollen has not been fully elucidated. Active constituents are believed to include a water soluble fraction called T-60, and an acetone soluble fraction called GBX, which contains 3-beta-sterols.[1,2] GBX and the combination of GBX and T-60 have been found to inhibit noradrenaline-induced contraction of mouse urethral strips, although only GBX alone was effective on pig urethral muscle strips. GBX also appears to inhibit 5-alpha reductase, and T-60 has been found to inhibit prostate carcinoma cell lines. No effects on LH, FSH, testosterone, or DHT have been seen in human clinical trials. Animal studies have found evidence of reduction in the weight of prostate ventral and dorsal lobes. Anti-inflammatory effects have been seen in studies of rye pollen extract.[3]

CLINICAL STUDIES

Two double-blind placebo-controlled studies found that grass pollen extract improved symptoms of BPH. The first enrolled 103 men with BPH for 12 weeks.[4] The results showed significant improvements in signs and symptoms. The second trial followed 57 men for 6 months, and demonstrated a similar outcome and significant decrease in prostate size.[1]

PROPOSED INDICATIONS AND USAGE

Preliminary evidence from double-blind trials suggests that grass pollen extract might be effective for BPH.

Highly preliminary evidence suggests that grass pollen might be useful for prostatitis,[5,6,7] prostate cancer,[8,9,10] and hypercholesterolemia.[11]

WARNINGS

None.

PRECAUTIONS

Although many people are allergic to grass pollen, the grass pollen products discussed in this article are processed to remove allergenic proteins.[1] It is therefore unlikely that grass-allergic individuals will have an allergic reaction to a properly prepared product. However, due to the lack of government supervision of dietary supplements, it is possible that some products on the market are not properly prepared.

Maximum safe dosages in individuals with severe hepatic or renal disease are not known.

Grass pollen extract has no proposed clinical use for pregnant or lactating women, or young children.

DRUG INTERACTIONS

None reported, although interaction studies have not been performed.

ADVERSE REACTIONS

No adverse reactions were observed in any of the clinical trials discussed above, although one review author mentioned rare reports of stomach upset and skin rash.[12]

PROPOSED DOSAGE AND ADMINISTRATION

The usual dosage for grass pollen extract in tablet form is 80 to 120 mg/day.[12]

PATIENT INFORMATION

Special grass pollen extracts are used in Europe for the treatment of prostate enlargement (benign prostatic hyperplasia). However, the herb saw palmetto has been much better studied.

The maximum safe dosage of grass pollen for pregnant or nursing women or young children has not been established. Individuals with severe liver or kidney disease should consult a physician before using this (or any other) supplement.

REFERENCES

1. Buck AC, Cox R, Rees RWM, et al. Treatment of outflow tract obstruction due to benign prostatic hyperplasia with the pollen extract, Cernilton: A double-blind, placebo-controlled study. *Br J Urol.* 1990;66:398-404. **2.** Buck AC. Phytotherapy for the prostate. *Br J Urol.* 1996;78:325-336. **3.** Loschen G, Ebeling L. Inhibition of the arachidonate metabolism by an extract of rye pollen [in German; English abstract]. *Arzneimittelforschung.* 1991;41:162-167. **4.** Becker H, Ebeling L. Conservative therapy of benign prostate hyperplasia (BPH) with Cernilton(r)N. Results of a placebo-controlled double-blind study. *Urologe [B].* 1988;28:301-306. **5.** Rugendorff EW, Weidner W, Ebeling L, et al. Results of treatment with pollen extract (Cernilton N) in chronic prostatitis and prostatodynia. *Br J Urol.* 1993;71:433-438. **6.** Buck AC, Rees RWM, Ebeling L. Treatment of chronic prostatitis and prostatodynia with pollen extract. *Br J Urol.* 1989;64:496-499. **7.** Suzuki T, Kurokawa K, Mashimo T, et al. Clinical effect of Cernilton in chronic prostatitis [in Japanese; English abstract]. *Hinyokika Kiyo.* 1992;38:489-494. **8.** Habib FK, Ross M, Buck AC, et al. In vitro evaluation of the pollen extract, cernitin T-60, in the regulation of prostate cell growth. *Br J Urol.* 1990;66:393-397. **9.** Roberts KP, Iyer RA, Prasad G, et al. Cyclic hydroxamic acid inhibitors of prostate cancer cell growth: selectivity and structure activity relationships. *Prostate.* 1998;34:92-99. **10.** Zhang X, Habib FK, Ross M, et al. Isolation and characterization of a cyclic hydroxamic acid from a pollen extract, which inhibits cancerous cell growth in vitro. *J Med Chem.* 1995;38:735-738. **11.** Wojcicki J, Samochowiec L, Bartlomowicz B, et al. Effect of pollen extract on the development of experimental atherosclerosis in rabbits. *Atherosclerosis.* 1986;62:39-45. **12.** Schulz V, Hansel R, Tyler VE. *Rational Phytotherapy: A Physicians' Guide to Herbal Medicine.* 3rd ed. Berlin, Germany: Springer-Verlag; 1998: 230-231.

Guggul

Commiphora Mukul

Alternate/Related Names: Mukul Myrrh, False Myrrh, Gum Guggulu, Gum Guggul, Gugulipid

U.S. BRAND NAMES OF CLINICALLY TESTED PRODUCTS

None.

DESCRIPTION

Guggul, the sticky gum resin from the mukul myrrh tree, plays a major role in the traditional herbal medicine of India. Guggul was traditionally combined with other herbs for the treatment of arthritis, skin diseases, pains in the nervous system, obesity, digestive problems, infections in the mouth, and menstrual problems.

PHARMACOLOGY

Guggul contains a family of ketonic steroid compounds called guggulsterones. Most studies have used a standardized ethyl acetate extract of the resin, containing 4.09% total of two compounds known as Z- and E-guggulsterone. Its mechanism of action is not known.

CLINICAL STUDIES

HYPERLIPIDEMIA

A double-blind placebo-controlled study enrolled 61 hyperlipidemic individuals and followed them for 24 weeks.[1] After 24 weeks of treatment, the treated group experienced an 11.7% decrease in total cholesterol, a 12.7% decrease in LDL, a 12% decrease in triglycerides, and an 11.1% decrease in the total cholesterol/HDL ratio. These improvements were significantly greater than those seen in the placebo group.

Similar results were seen in a double-blind placebo-controlled trial of 40 individuals.[2] In a double-blind comparative trial, equivalent hypolipidemic effects were seen in 228 individuals given either guggul or clofibrate.[3]

WEIGHT LOSS

A small double-blind placebo-controlled trial found no weight loss benefits.[4]

PROPOSED INDICATIONS AND USAGE

Preliminary evidence suggests that guggul might have hypolipidemic effects.

Based on extremely weak evidence that guggul has thyroid-stimulating properties, guggul has been marketed as a weight loss agent. However, there is no evidence that it is effective, and one trial (noted above) found it ineffective.

Very weak evidence has been used to justify marketing guggul for acne and diabetes.[5,6]

WARNINGS

None.

PRECAUTIONS

Safety for pregnant or lactating women, young children, or individuals with hepatic or renal disease is not known.

DRUG INTERACTIONS

None reported.

ADVERSE REACTIONS

In clinical trials of standardized guggul extract, no significant side effects other than occasional mild gastrointestinal distress have been seen.[1,3,7] Laboratory tests conducted in the course of these trials did not reveal any alterations in hepatic or renal function, hematologic parameters, cardiac function, or blood chemistry. Animal studies reportedly found no evidence of toxicity.[3]

PROPOSED DOSAGE AND ADMINISTRATION

Guggul is manufactured in a standardized form that provides a fixed amount of guggulsterones. The typical daily dose should provide 100 mg of guggulsterones.

PATIENT INFORMATION

Guggul is an extract of the mukul myrrh tree that is widely sold as a treatment for high cholesterol. However, there is much better evidence for the safety and effectiveness of other natural substances, including policosanol, soy protein, and stanol esters.

Guggul is also marketed as a weight loss treatment, but there is no evidence that it works, and one study found it ineffective.

The safety of guggul for pregnant or nursing women or young children has not been established. Individuals with severe liver or kidney disease should consult a physician before using this (or any other) supplement.

REFERENCES

1. Singh RB, Niaz MA, Ghosh S. Hypolipidemic and antioxidant effects of *Commiphora mukul* as an adjunct to dietary therapy in patients with hypercholesterolemia. *Cardiovasc Drugs Ther.* 1994;8:659-664. **2.** Verma SK, Bordia A. Effect of *Commiphora mukul* (gum guggulu) in patients of hyperlipidemia with special reference to HDL-cholesterol. *Indian J Med Res.* 1988;87:356-360. **3.** Nityanand S, Srivastava JS, Asthana OP. Clinical trials with gugulipid. A new hypolipidaemic agent. *J Assoc Physicians India.* 1989;37:323-328. **4.** Antonio J, Colker CM, Torina GC, et al. Effects of a standardized guggulsterone phosphate supplement on body composition in overweight adults: a pilot study. *Curr Ther Res.* 1999;60:220-227. **5.** Thappa DM, Dogra J. Nodulocystic acne: oral gugulipid versus tetracycline. *J Dermatol.* 1994;21:729-731. **6.** Subramaniam A, Stocker C, Sennitt MV, et al. Guggul lipid reduces insulin resistance and body weight gain in C57B1/6 lep/lep mice [abstract]. *Int J Obes Relat Metab Disord.* 2001;25(suppl 2):S24. **7.** Agarwal RC, Singh SP, Saran RK, et al. Clinical trial of gugulipid-a new hyperlipidemic agent of plant origin in primary hyperlipidemia. *Indian J Med Res.* 1986;84:626-634.

Gymnema

Gymnema Sylvestre

U.S. BRAND NAMES OF CLINICALLY TESTED PRODUCTS

None.

DESCRIPTION

Native to the forests of India, gymnema has a long tradition of use in diabetes.

PHARMACOLOGY

An ethanolic extract of gymnema leaves called GS4 is thought to contain the active constituents of the herb. In human and animal studies, GS4 administration has resulted in reduced blood glucose levels.[1] Histopathologic examination of pancreatic tissue in one study found evidence of an increase in the number of beta cells after GS4 supplementation.

CLINICAL STUDIES

Two controlled studies (blinding not stated) examined the effects of a gymnema extract on diabetics.[1,2] Both insulin-dependent and noninsulin-dependent individuals showed reductions in blood glucose, glycosylated hemoglobin, and glycosylated plasma proteins, as well as decreased pharmaceutical requirements. In addition, endogenous insulin secretion appeared to be enhanced.

PROPOSED INDICATIONS AND USAGE

Poorly reported pilot studies provide weak evidence that gymnema may be an effective hypoglycemic agent.

WARNINGS

None.

PRECAUTIONS

Although gymnema has not been proven effective, if it were to reduce serum glucose, hypoglycemic reactions could occur. Monitoring of serum glucose is therefore recommended.

Safety in pregnant or lactating women, young children, or individuals with severe hepatic or renal disease has not been established.

DRUG INTERACTIONS

Gymnema could theoretically potentiate the action of insulin or other hypoglycemic medications.

ADVERSE REACTIONS

Gymnema appears to be well tolerated, although comprehensive safety testing has not been undertaken.

PROPOSED DOSAGE AND ADMINISTRATION

Gymnema extract is usually taken at a dosage of 400 to 600 mg daily. Some products are standardized to contain 24% gymnemic acid.

PATIENT INFORMATION

Gymnema is an herb sold as a treatment for diabetes. However, it has not been proven effective.

NOTE: Do not substitute gymnema for standard diabetes therapy. In addition, keep in mind that if gymnema is added to standard therapy, it could conceivably cause a hypoglycemic reaction.

The safety of gymnema for pregnant or nursing women or young children has not been established. Individuals with severe liver or kidney disease should consult a physician before using this (or any other) supplement.

REFERENCES

1. Shanmugasundaram ER, Rajeswari G, Baskaran K, et al. Use of Gymnema sylvestre leaf extract in the control of blood glucose in insulin-dependent diabetes mellitus. *J Ethnopharmacol.* 1990;30:281-294. **2.** Baskaran K, Kizar Ahamath B, Radha Shanmugasundaram K, et al. Antidiabetic effect of a leaf extract from Gymnema sylvestre in non-insulin-dependent diabetes mellitus patients. *J Ethnopharmacol.* 1990;30;295-305.

Hawthorn

Crataegus Laevigata, C. Monogyna, C. Oxyacantha, C. Pentagyna

U.S. BRAND NAMES OF CLINICALLY TESTED PRODUCTS

HeartCare (Nature's Way) = Crataegutt forte, WS 1442 (Schwabe) in Europe

DESCRIPTION

This spiny shrub tree is widely used as a hedge plant in Europe, its original name being hedgethorn, from which hawthorn is a corruption. Dioscorides mentioned hawthorn as a heart drug in the first century A.D., but most early literature focuses on the symbolic use of hawthorn for religious rites and political ceremonies. During the Middle Ages, hawthorn was occasionally used for the treatment of dropsy, an outdated term for congestive heart failure.

PHARMACOLOGY

The primary constituents of hawthorn include flavonoids (including quercetin and vitexin), oligomeric procyanidins (OPCs, such as found in grape seed), catechins, purine derivatives, amines, triterpenoids, and aromatic carboxylic acids.[1]

Animal studies suggest that hawthorn extracts simultaneously increase the force, amplitude, and volume of cardiac contraction while lengthening the cardiac refractory period.[2,3,4] This combination of effects may give hawthorn a particular safety factor when used in heart disease. Protection from myocardial reperfusion injury has also been seen in animal studies.[5,6]

The mechanism of action of hawthorn remains unknown. Recent evidence suggests that hawthorn blocks repolarizing potassium currents in ventricular myocytes, giving the herb a functional similarity to class III antiarrhythmic drugs.[7] Other proposed explanations include activation of potassium channels, inhibition of cyclic AMP phosphodiesterase, and inhibition of angiotensin-converting enzyme.[8-11] Some evidence suggests that inotropic effect of hawthorn is cAMP independent.[12]

Some of hawthorn's effects in reperfusion may be mediated through coronary artery dilation.[13,14,15] However, one animal study suggests that hawthorn extract may aid reperfusion recovery of the myocardium through some mechanism other than increased blood flow.[16] An antioxidant mechanism has been proposed.[8,17]

CLINICAL STUDIES

CHF

Since 1981, at least 14 controlled clinical studies (the majority of them double-blind) have been published on the therapeutic efficacy of hawthorn (WS 1442) in CHF.[4,18-21] Most of the approximately 800 patients participating in these studies had NYHA class II CHF. Significant improvement was generally (but not uniformly) noted in exercise tolerance, anaerobic threshold, ejection fraction, and subjective complaints. The doses of hawthorn used in these studies ranged from 180 to 900 mg/day taken for a period of 21 to 84 days (most studies lasted 42 or 56 days).

There is no evidence that hawthorn reduces CHF morbidity or mortality.

ANGINA

In a double-blind study of 60 patients with angina, treatment for 3 weeks with 180 mg/day of hawthorn extract increased exercise tolerance.[22]

PROPOSED INDICATIONS AND USAGE

There is some evidence that hawthorn may be effective for the treatment of NYHA class II congestive heart failure. However, while the long-term benefits of ACE inhibitors have been established in numerous studies, there is no evidence that hawthorn reduces the morbidity or mortality of CHF. Hawthorn might offer safety advantages over digoxin in early CHF, including apparent lack of arrhythmogenic potential, a large therapeutic window, no contraindication in renal impairment, and no contraindication to coadministration with diuretics and laxatives.[4]

Weaker evidence supports the use of hawthorn in angina. Based on animal trials, hawthorn could also be useful in the prevention of arrhythmias following myocardial infarction. However, clinical trials in humans are lacking.

Hawthorn is often added to dietary products marketed for hypertension. However, there is no evidence that hawthorn has any significant effect on blood pressure.

Hawthorn is sometimes recommended by herbalists as a treatment for minor, benign arrhythmias, but there is no scientific basis for this usage.

WARNINGS

None.

PRECAUTIONS

Germany's Commission E lists no known risks or contraindications with hawthorn. However, safety in young children, pregnant or lactating women, or individuals with severe renal or hepatic disease has not been established.

DRUG INTERACTIONS

Because hawthorn appears to possess cardioactive properties the possibility of interaction with or potentiation of other cardiovascular drugs is not unlikely.

ADVERSE REACTIONS

In clinical trials, hawthorn has been connected only with nonspecific side effects such as mild gastrointestinal distress and allergic reactions. Toxicity studies in animals suggest that the LD_{50} of hawthorn is about 500 to 1,000 times the usual therapeutic dose in humans.[23] Studies in rats and dogs have shown no toxicity after administration of 300 mg/kg for 26 weeks.[4]

A water and alcohol extract of hawthorn has been shown to be nonmutagenic.[4] Other hawthorn extracts have shown mutagenicity in *Salmonella* cultures. This is presumed due to the presence of quercetin. However, because the quercetin content of typical hawthorn products is low compared to the amount of quercetin normally ingested with food, it has been suggested that use of hawthorn is unlikely to add significant additional risk.[4]

PROPOSED DOSAGE AND ADMINISTRATION

The standard dose of hawthorn is 100 to 300 mg 3 times daily of an extract standardized to contain about 2% to 3% flavonoids or 18% to 20% procyanidins. The effectiveness of hawthorn appears to require a 4- to 8-week course.

PATIENT INFORMATION

The herb hawthorn is marketed as a treatment for various heart conditions. There is some evidence that it may be helpful for congestive heart failure (CHF); however, CHF is a dangerous condition that should not be self-treated. Furthermore, while standard treatments have been shown to prevent serious complications of CHF, hawthorn has not been shown to provide the same benefit.

Hawthorn has not been shown to reduce blood pressure or provide any other specific benefits for the heart. Do not combine hawthorn with standard heart drugs except on the advice of a physician.

The safety of hawthorn for pregnant or nursing women or young children has not been established. Individuals with severe liver or kidney disease should consult a physician before using this (or any other) supplement.

REFERENCES

1. Wagner H, et al. *Plant drug analysis.* New York: Springer-Verlag; 1984:166, 178, 179. **2.** Joseph G, Zhao Y, Klaus W. Pharmacologic profile of crataegus extract compared to epinephrine, amrinone, milrinone and digoxin in isolated guinea pig hearts [in German; English abstract]. *Arzneimittelforschung.* 1995;45:1261-1265. **3.** Popping S, Rose H, Ionescu I, et al. Effect of a hawthorn extract on contraction and energy turnover of isolated rat cardiomyocytes. *Arzneimittelforschung.* 1995;45;1157-1161. **4.** Schulz V, Hansel R, Tyler VE. *Rational Phytotherapy: A Physicians' Guide to Herbal Medicine.* 3rd ed. Berlin, Germany: Springer-Verlag; 1998:93-98. **5.** Al Makdessi S, Sweidan H, Dietz K, et al. Protective effect of Crataegus oxyacantha against reperfusion arrhythmias after global no-flow ischemia in the rat heart [published correction appears in *Basic Res Cardiol.* 1999;94:294]. *Basic Res Cardiol.* 1999;94:71-77. **6.** Kurcok A. Ischemia and reperfusion-induced cardiac injury: effects of two flavonoid containing plant extracts possessing radical scavenging properties [abstract]. *Naunyn Schmiedebergs Arch Pharmacol.* 1992;345(suppl 1):R81. **7.** Muller A, Linke W, Klaus W. Crataegus extract blocks potassium currents in guinea pig ventricular cardiac myocytes. *Planta Med.* 1999;65:335-339. **8.** Bahorun T, Trotin F, Pommery J, et al. Antioxidant activities of Crataegus monogyna extracts. *Planta Med.* 1994;60:323-328. **9.** Petkov E, Nikolov N, Uzunov P. Inhibitory effect of some flavonoids and falvonoid mixtures on cyclic AMP phosphodiesterase activity of rat heart. *Planta Med.* 1981;43:183-186. **10.** Siegel G, Casper U, Schnalke F. Molecular physiological effector mechanisms of hawthorn extract in cardiac papillary muscle and coronary vascular smooth muscle. *Phytother Res.* 1996;10:S195-S198. **11.** Uchida S, Ikari N, Ohta H, et al. Inhibitory effects of condensed tannins on angiotensin converting enzyme. *Jpn J Pharmacol.* 1987;43:242-246. **12.** Schwinger RH, Pietsch M, Frank K, et al. Crataegus special extract WS 1442 increases force of contraction in human myocardium cAMP-independently. *J Cardiovasc Pharmacol.* 2000;35:700-707. **13.** Siegel G, Casper U, Walter A, et al. Concentration-response study with the Crataegus extract LI 132 on membrane potential and tone of human coronary arteries and canine papillary muscle [in German; English abstract]. *MMW Munch Med Wochenschr.* 1994;136(suppl 1):S47-S56. **14.** Siegel G, Casper U. Crataegi folium cum flore. In: Loew D, Rietbrock N, eds. Phytopharmaka in Forschung und klinischer Anwendung. Darmstadt, Germany: Steinkopff Verlage; 1995:1-14. Cited by: Schulz V, Hansel R, Tyler VE. *Rational Phytotherapy: A Physicians' Guide to Herbal Medicine.* 3rd ed. Berlin, Germany: Springer-Verlag; 1998. **15.** Mavers VWH, Hensel H. Changes in local myocardial blood flow following oral administration of a crataegus extract to non-anesthetized dogs [in German]. *Arzneimittelforschung.* 1974;24:783-785. **16.** Nasa Y, Hashizume H, Hoque AN, et al. Protective effect of crataegus extract on the cardiac mechanical dysfunction in isolated perfused working rat heart. *Arzneimittelforschung.* 1993;43:945-949. **17.** Bahorun T, Gressier B, Trotin F, et al. Oxygen species scavenging activity of phenolic extracts from hawthorn fresh plant organs and pharmaceutical preparations. *Arzneimittelforschung.* 1996;46:1086-1089. **18.** Leuchtgens VH. Crataegus Special Extract WS 1442 in NYHA II heart failure. A placebo controlled randomized double-blind study [in German]. *Fortschr Med.* 1993;111:36-38. **19.** Schmidt U, Kuhn U, Ploch M, et al. Efficacy of the Hawthorn (Crataegus) preparation L1 132 in 78 patients with chronic congestive heart failure defined as NYHA functional class II. Phytomedicine. 1994;1:17-24. **20.** Tauchert M, Siegel G, Schulz V. Hawthorn extract as plant medication for the heart; a new evaluation of its therapeutic effectiveness [translated from German]. *MMW Munch Med Wochenschr.* 1994;136(suppl 1):S3-S5. **21.** Zapfe jun G. Clinical efficacy of crataegus extract WS 1442 in congestive heart failure NYHA class II. *Phytomedicine.* 2001;8:262-266. **22.** Hanak T, Bruckel MH. The treatment of mild stable forms of angina pectoris using Crategutt(r) novo [in German; English abstract]. *Therapiewoche.* 1983;33:4331-4333. **23.** Ammon HPT, Handel M. Crataegus, toxicology and pharmacology Part I: Toxicity [translated from German]. *Planta Med.* 1981;43:105-120.

Horse Chestnut

Aesculus hippocastanum L.

Alternate/Related Names: Buckeye, Spanish Chestnut

U.S. BRAND NAMES OF CLINICALLY TESTED PRODUCTS

None.

DESCRIPTION

The horse chestnut tree, grows to 25 meters and is native to northern Greece, Iran, the Caucasus, and northern India. The tree was introduced to Europe in the sixteenth century and is naturalized throughout Europe and the central and eastern temperate zones of North America. The leaves, bark, and seeds have been used medicinally. Horse chestnut extract (HCSE) is prepared from the dried seeds.

Horse chestnuts have traditionally been considered to possess analgesic, anticoagulant, antipyretic, astringent, expectorant, tonic, and vasoconstricting properties. Preparations have been used to treat topical ulcers, hemorrhoids, phlebitis, nocturnal leg cramps, whooping cough, and diarrhea.[1]

PHARMACOLOGY

Horse chestnut seeds contain coumarins, flavonoids, saponins, tannins, and other constituents, including allantoin and a number of amino acids. Escin, a heterogeneous mixture of triterpenoid saponin glycosides, is considered to be the most important active constituent; the German-pharmacopoeia-standardized HCSE is specified to contain 16% to 20% triterpenoid glycosides calculated as escin.[2] Horse chestnut also contains esculin, a toxic coumarin glucoside, which is removed during the preparation of many European products.

Escin is comprised of β-escin and α-escin fractions. The bioavailability of escin is about 10% to 15%, with a half-life of 10 to 19 hours.[3] Maximum plasma level after a single capsule of delayed release HCSE is 20 to 30 ng/ml after 2 to 3 hours.[4] In a study of the bioavailability of β-escin in a delayed release formulation versus a normal release preparation (Noricaven mono), both standardized to 50 mg escin, area under the curve for the normal release product was reported to be 30% higher and time to maximum concentration greater.[3] Because there are no findings regarding the effective concentration of a marker compound at the target (vein wall), the clinical relevance of this finding is unclear. No adverse effects were observed for either preparation.

The mechanism underlying the anti-exudative actions of HCSE has been proposed to be related to reduced capillary permeability, a tonic effect on veins, inhibition of lysosomal glycosaminoglycan hydrolases involved in collagen breakdown, anti-inflammatory activity, and increased activity of prostaglandins involved in venous contraction.[5-8] In an in vitro study, escin (250 ng/ml) was shown to strongly inhibit the adherence of neutrophil-like HL60 cells to hypoxic venous endothelium but not to normoxic venous endothelium.[9] Adherence of activated neutrophils may lead to alterations in the venous wall similar to those in chronic venous insufficiency. The clinical significance of these findings and those of other in vitro and animal studies is, of course, difficult to ascertain.

CLINICAL STUDIES

Although the research record is not complete, the balance of existing evidence indicates that HCSE, either alone or in combination with leg compression stockings, is a useful treatment at least for the beginning stages of venous insufficiency.

Four reasonably well designed studies were published in 1986.[10-13] In general, subjective complaints of pain, itching, leg fatigue, and feelings of tension in the legs improved significantly with HCSE treatment in these studies. For example, one double-blind placebo-controlled study of 40 patients found a significant reduction in extravascular volume after a 14-day treatment with 1 capsule twice daily of delayed-release HCSE versus placebo; however, no significant difference in venous capacity was noted.[12] Another study using venous plethysmography to measure the transcapillary filtration coefficient and intravascular volume of the lower leg 3 hours after a single dose of 600 mg HCSE standardized to 100 mg escin found that the filtration coefficient was significantly reduced in the verum group.[10] Both sets of authors concluded that HCSE does not exert a significant tonic effect on veins, but that its contribution to reduced capillary permeability is probably of therapeutic significance.

Subsequent studies involving a total of 321 individuals also found HCSE to be significantly better than placebo for reducing leg volume and/or relieving subjective complaints.[14,15,16]

In addition, a partially blinded study of 240 patients treated for 12 weeks with placebo, compression stockings (unblinded), or HCSE (1 capsule of delayed-release horse chestnut twice daily) found the two therapies to be statistically equivalent and superior to placebo.[5]

PROPOSED INDICATIONS AND USAGE

Meaningful but not definitive evidence suggests that oral horse chestnut preparations may be effective for the treatment of chronic venous insufficiency. There is as yet no evidence that horse chestnut improves existing visible varicosities, although some practitioners believe that regular use of the herb can help prevent new ones from developing.

Based on the supposition that horse chestnut functions by reducing capillary leakage, horse chestnut or escin alone is sometimes used for reduction of edema following injuries such as sprains or surgery, and there is some evidence that they may be effective.[17]

In Europe, horse chestnut is sometimes administered along with standard therapy for phlebitis. Additionally, because hemorrhoids are a form of varicose veins, horse chestnut has been proposed for that condition as well. However, there is little or no corroborating data for these proposed indications.

WARNINGS

Due to the presence of toxic ingredients, whole horse chestnut should not be used.

PRECAUTIONS

Whole horse chestnut is classified as an unsafe herb by the FDA. Poisoning by ingestion of the nuts or a tea made from the leaves and twigs is characterized by nausea, vomiting, diarrhea, salivation, headache, hemolysis, convulsions, and circulatory and respiratory failure possibly leading to death.[1] However, typical European standardized extract formulations remove the most toxic constituents (i.e., esculin) and standardize the quantity of escin.

Use of oral HCSE in patients with renal or hepatic dysfunction should be approached with caution, as renal toxicity after high-dose oral escin has been reported.[18] In addition, acute renal failure has occurred in patients receiving intravenous escin at doses greater than 20 mg to prevent and treat post-surgical edema.[19] Drugs that displace escin from plasma-protein-binding sites may also increase its nephrotoxic potential.[20] Hepatotoxicity as well as shock was reported in a patient receiving an intramuscular injection of an HCSE product,[21] but there are no reports of such events involving oral HCSE products.

Two trials reported use of HCSE in pregnancy-related varicose veins, with good tolerability.[13,22] In addition, animal studies to date have not shown embryotoxicity or teratogenicity.[23] However, it is prudent to use compression stockings rather than HCSE in pregnant women.

Safety in lactating women or young children has not been established.

DRUG INTERACTIONS

Since horse chestnut contains coumarins, interference with anticoagulant therapy is a possibility.

Escin is known to bind to plasma proteins and thus may compete with or displace drugs that are highly protein-bound. Drugs that displace escin from plasma-protein binding sites may also increase escin's nephrotoxic potential.[20]

ADVERSE REACTIONS

The saponins in horse chestnut extract are irritating to the gastrointestinal tract. This is the rationale for the use of controlled release products, which reduce incidence of irritation to below 1%, even at higher doses.[5] Calf cramps and pruritis are occasionally reported.

Acute oral toxicity of HCSE and escin has been studied in several animal species.[23] The no-effect dose is approximately 8 times higher than the recommended human dose. Mutagenic and carcinogenic studies have not been published.

PROPOSED DOSAGE AND ADMINISTRATION

The most common dosage of HCSE in reported clinical trials is 300 mg standardized to 50 mg escin given twice daily in a delayed release formulation. HCSE preparations should certify that esculin has been removed. The delayed release formulation prevents the gastrointestinal upset typically caused by normal release products.

PATIENT INFORMATION

Horse chestnut extract is an herbal product marketed for venous insufficiency, a condition related to varicose veins. There is some evidence horse chestnut extract may reduce symptoms such as tenderness and swelling. However, there is no evidence that horse chestnut treatment will cause visible varicose veins to disappear.

Note: Until it is specially processed, horse chestnut is toxic.

Individuals taking blood-thinning drugs such as aspirin, Plavix (clopidogrel), Trental (pentoxifylline), Coumadin (warfarin), or heparin should avoid horse chestnut.

The safety of horse chestnut for pregnant or nursing women or young children has not been established. Individuals with severe liver or kidney disease should not use horse chestnut.

REFERENCES

1. Chandler RF. Horse chestnut. *Can Pharm J.* 1993;126:297-300, 306. **2.** Blumenthal M, et al., ed. *Horse chestnut seed. The Complete German Commission E Monographs.* Boston: Integrative Medicine Communications; 1998:560. **3.** Schrader E, Schwankl W, Sieder C, et al. Comparison of the bioavailability of beta-aescin after single oral administration of two different drug formulations containing an extract of horse-chestnut seeds. *Pharmazie.* 1995;50:623-627. **4.** Schulz V, Hansel R, Tyler VE. *Rational Phytotherapy: A Physicians' Guide to Herbal Medicine.* 3rd ed. Berlin, Germany: Springer-Verlag; 1998:130. **5.** Diehm C. The role of oedema protective drugs in the treatment of chronic venous insufficiency: A review of evidence based on placebo-controlled clinical trials with regard to efficacy and tolerance. *Phlebology.* 1996;11:23-29. **6.** Hitzenberger G. The therapeutic effect of horse chestnut seed extract (translated from German). *Wien Med Wschr.* 1989;139:385-389. **7.** Kreysel HW, Nissen HP, Enghofer E. A possible role of lysosomal enzymes in the pathogenesis of varicosis and the reduction in their serum activity by Venostasin(r). *Vasa.* 1983;12:377-382. **8.** Newall CA, et al. *Herbal Medicine: A Guide for Health-care Professionals.* London: The Pharmaceutical Press; 1996:166-167. **9.** Bougelet C, Roland IH, Ninane N, et al. Effect of aescine on hypoxia-induced neutrophil adherence to umbilical vein endothelium. *Eur J Pharmacol.* 1998;345:89-95. **10.** Bisler H, Pfeifer R, Kluken N, et al. Effect of horse chestnut seed extract on transcapillary filtration in chronic venous insufficiency [translated from German]. *Dtsch Med Wschr.* 1986;111: 1321-1329. **11.** Lohr E, Garanin G, Jesau P, Fischer H. Antiedemic therapy in chronic venous insufficciency with tendency to formation of edema [translated from German]. *MMW Munch Med Wochenschr.* 1986;128:579-581. **12.** Rudofsky G, Neiss A, Otto K, Seibel K. Antiedematous effects and clinical effectiveness of horse chestnut seed extract in double blind studies [translated from German]. *Phlebol Proktol.* 1986;15:47-54. **13.** Steiner M, Hillemanns HG. Investigation of the anti-edemic efficacy of Venostatin [translated from German]. *Munch Med Wschr.* 1986;128:551-552. **14.** Diehm C, Vollbrecht D, Amendt K, et al. Medical edema protection-clinical benefit in patients with chronic deep vein incompetence. *Vasa.* 1992;21:188-192. **15.** Friederich HC, Vogelsberg H, Neiss A. A contribution to the evaluation of vein medications that work internally [translated from German]. *Z Hautkr.* 1978;53:369-374. **16.** Neiss A, Bohm C. Proof of the efficacy of horse chestnut seed extract in the treatment of varicose syndrome [translated from German]. *Munch Med Wschr.* 1976;118:213-216. **17.** Wilhelm K, Feldmeier C. Thermometric investigations about the efficacy of beta-escin to reduce postoperative edema. *Med Klin.* 1977;72:128-134. **18.** Grasso A, Corvaglia E. Two cases of suspected toxic tubulonephrosis due to escine. *Gass Med Ital.* 1976;135:581-584. **19.** Reynolds JEF, ed. *Martindale, The Extra Pharmacopeia.* London: The Pharmaceutical Press; 1989:1539-1540. **20.** Rothkopf M, Vogel G, Lang W, et al. Animal experiments on the question of the renal toleration of the horse chestnut saponin aescin. *Arzneimittelforschung.* 1977;27:598-605. **21.** Takegoshi K, Tohyama T, Okuda K, et al. A case of Venoplant-induced hepatic injury. *Gastroenterol Jpn.* 1986;21:62-65. **22.** Alter H. Medication therapy for varicosis [translated from German]. *Z Allgemeinmed.* 1973;49:1301-1304. **23.** Hansel R, et al. *Hagers Handbuch der Pharmazeutischen Praxis,* 5th Ed. Berlin: Springer Verlag; 1992:108-122.

Ipriflavone

7-Isopropoxyisoflavone

U.S. BRAND NAMES OF CLINICALLY TESTED PRODUCTS

Not applicable.

DESCRIPTION

Ipriflavone, or 7-isopropoxyisoflavone, is chemically related to the isoflavone daidzein, a naturally occurring phytoestrogen found in soy and other plant products. Ipriflavone was first synthesized in 1969 in an attempt to develop isoflavones with selective estrogen-like properties. In vitro screening of ipriflavone revealed calcium-retaining effects, a discovery that led to investigations of its usefulness in treating bone loss. Testing of ipriflavone began on animals in 1974 and on humans in 1981. By 1989, ipriflavone was approved for the treatment of osteoporosis in 21 countries.

PHARMACOLOGY

Ipriflavone (7-isopropoxy-3-phenyl-4H-1-benzopyran-4-one) is metabolized in the liver and excreted in the urine.[1,2] Ipriflavone is rapidly absorbed through the small intestine and absorption is enhanced if it is taken with food. In humans, there are four major active metabolites. The most abundant in plasma is the unconjugated metabolite MV, followed by the conjugated metabolites MI, MII, and MIII. MII is daidzein, a phytoestrogen found in soy that possesses weak estrogenic activity. Following the administration of 200 mg ipriflavone 3 times daily, steady states are achieved within 3 days for ipriflavone and the metabolites MI, MII, and MIII, and 7 days for MV. After a single 200-mg dose, the mean excretion half-life of ipriflavone was 9.8 hours and the half-life of its metabolites ranged from 2.7 hours for MIII to 16.1 hours for MV.

Although a derivative of isoflavone, ipriflavone has not shown any estrogenic effects in vitro or in vivo.[3,4] Ipriflavone binding sites were not found in the MCF7 breast cancer cell line. A study of the affinity of various phytoestrogens for the estrogen receptors ER-alpha and ER-beta showed that ipriflavone had a 10,000-fold lower affinity than 17-beta-estradiol.[5] In addition, ipriflavone and its metabolites MI, MIII, and MV were not able to displace 17-beta-estradiol from the numerous estrogen receptors in the human preosteoclastic cell line FLG 29.1; however, preincubation with ipriflavone and its metabolites increased 17-beta-estradiol binding in those cells, suggesting that ipriflavone and its metabolites may act synergistically? with estrogen.[6]

The mechanism of action of ipriflavone in osteoporosis has been suggested to be primarily antiresorptive, although osteoblastic stimulatory effects may occur as well.[7-13] An animal study using normal and ovariectomized rats demonstrated that ipriflavone administered at 400 mg/kg daily significantly reduced bone resorption when given for 7 days before or 7 days after surgery. A study of bone strength and mineral composition in male rats showed that a 1-month treatment with 400 mg/kg ipriflavone resulted in a 1.5-fold increase in the amount of energy required to produce a fracture of the femur.[14] A 12-week study of crystal formation at the same dose of ipriflavone, however, did not show significant modifications of bone crystallinity using x-ray diffraction analysis.[14]

CLINICAL STUDIES

OSTEOPOROSIS

In most double-blind placebo-controlled studies of ipriflavone, involving a total of over 1,700 enrolled subjects, results demonstrated either a significant bone-sparing effect or improvement in bone mineral density measured at the radius, whole body, or vertebrae.[12,15-26]

These studies ranged in length from 6 months to 2 years and involved postmenopausal women (naturally, surgically, or GnRh-induced) and women with senile osteoporosis. In those studies that found improvement of bone mineral density in the ipriflavone groups, increases ranged from 0.7% to 7.1% over the course of the study. By comparison, placebo groups had losses as high as 5.0%.

One 2-year multicenter double-blind study evaluated ipriflavone's benefit in a group of 453 postmenopausal women (aged 50 to 65) with vertebral or radial mineral density 1 SD below age-matched controls.[26] They received 200 mg ipriflavone 3 times daily plus 1 g supplemental calcium, or placebo plus calcium. Bone mass was maintained in the ipriflavone group, but the control group exhibited a significant loss in bone density. After 2 years, the results (calculated as a bone-sparing effect) were +1.6% at the lumbar spine ($p<.05$) and +3.5% at the radius ($p<.05$) compared with placebo.

However, the most recent double-blind placebo-controlled study of ipriflavone for osteoporosis found no benefits.[27] In this 3-year trial, 474 postmenopausal women took 500 mg calcium plus either 600 mg ipriflavone or placebo daily. No intergroup differences were seen in spine, hip, or forearm density. The explanation for these negative results may lie in the calcium dosage: virtually all other studies of ipriflavone used 1 g calcium daily.

Evidence also suggests that ipriflavone can reduce the number of bone fractures. A 2-year multicenter randomized double-blind study involving 100 women over 65 years of age found that patients treated with ipriflavone had a significant reduction in new fractures (along with an increase in bone mineral density).[20] A smaller study found a 50% reduction in the rate of new vertebral fractures in the first year of ipriflavone treatment.[21]

Other studies suggest that adjunctive use of ipriflavone may allow reduction of estrogen dosage while achieving an equivalent bone-sparing effect.[28-35] (See Drug Interactions for potential interaction between estrogens and ipriflavone.)

Several studies of osteoporosis have noted pain reduction during treatment with ipriflavone.[20,36,37]

Ipriflavone may also protect bone in hyperparathyroidism and during corticosteroid treatment.[38,39]

PAGET'S DISEASE

Weak evidence from a small randomized controlled crossover trial suggests that ipriflavone treatment at 1,200 mg/day followed by 600 mg/day may reduce biochemical parameters of disease activity and bone pain in patients with Paget's disease.[40]

PROPOSED INDICATIONS AND USAGE

Considerable evidence suggests that ipriflavone may have significant bone-sparing effects. However, concerns about iatrogenic lymphopenia need to be taken into account when considering this treatment approach (see Precautions). Combination treatment with low-dose hormone-replacement therapy may also be worth considering.

Much weaker evidence suggests that ipriflavone might be helpful for Paget's disease. Ipriflavone is also marketed as a sports supplement, although there is no evidence that it is effective for this purpose.

WARNINGS

Use of ipriflavone has been associated with a reduction in serum lymphocyte levels.

PRECAUTIONS

In a 3-year study of 474 postmenopausal women, ipriflavone decreased average serum lymphocyte levels and caused asymptomatic lymphopenia in 29 participants.[27] Similar effects were seen in a previous, much smaller study.[12] The clinical significance of this unexpected finding is not clear; however, at present it appears prudent to recommend that lymphopenic or immunosuppressed individuals avoid ipriflavone, and that healthy individuals taking ipriflavone should have routine blood counts performed.

In addition, some ipriflavone study subjects have exhibited altered hepatic and renal function test results as well as glucose and lipid metabolism changes.[41] None of these changes were permanent or resulted in disease states. However, this data cannot be used to rule out serious but rare adverse effects or those due to ipriflavone treatment beyond the average 2- to 3-year study period.

Use of ipriflavone has been associated with mild gastrointestinal upset. In addition, a published case reported the reoccurrence of a gastric ulcer in a patient administered ipriflavone after surgery for a femoral fracture.[42] As studies of ipriflavone have excluded subjects with possible gastrointestinal diseases, risk for increased gastrointestinal symptoms or increased severity due to treatment with ipriflavone in this population is unknown.

Current research suggests that ipriflavone does not increase the risk of breast cancer or other forms of cancer that are sensitive to estrogen receptor activity.[5-7,43] However, caution should be exercised in persons who have already had an occurrence of breast or reproductive cancer (see also Drug Interactions).

One study found a need for ipriflavone dosage adjustment in individuals with moderate to severe renal disease.[2] Maximum safe dosages in individuals with severe hepatic disease are not known.

Similarly, safety in pregnant or lactating women, or young children, has not been established.

DRUG INTERACTIONS

Ipriflavone may interact with numerous CYP enzymes, including CYP3A, CYP1A2, and CYP2C9.[44,45,46] These interactions may lead to increased serum levels of theophylline, caffeine, theobromine, other polycyclic aromatic compounds, tolbutamide, phenytoin, and warfarin. Both warfarin and phenytoin contribute to osteoporosis, and warfarin is frequently prescribed for the elderly; the use of ipriflavone to treat iatrogenic osteoporosis caused by these pharmaceuticals could result in elevated serum levels of the drugs and potentially serious consequences.

Although ipriflavone by itself appears to have no effect on estrogen-sensitive tissues other than one, it may potentiate the effects of estrogen on reproductive tissue, specifically the uterus.[4,6,47] For this reason, HRT is preferable to ERT when ipriflavone-hormone combination treatment is considered. The finding that such potentiation is possible also suggests that there might be an increased risk of estrogen-dependent breast malignancies with such combination therapy, but thus far this potential risk has not been evaluated.

Because of ipriflavone's apparent ability to cause lymphopenia, potential interactions with immunosupressant drugs should be considered.

ADVERSE REACTIONS

Although ipriflavone is generally well tolerated, mild gastrointestinal distress has been reported. It has been postulated that, in studies, the usual coadministration of 1 g calcium/day with ipriflavone may be the source of gastrointestinal disturbances.[22] Atypical reactions reported for ipriflavone include rash, itching, erythema, headache, drowsiness, depression, asthenia, fatigue, and tachycardia.

PROPOSED DOSAGE AND ADMINISTRATION

The usual dosage of ipriflavone is 200-mg tablets taken 3 times daily with meals, along with 1 g calcium daily. A 300-mg ipriflavone capsule introduced for twice-daily dosing has produced excellent compliance without increased risk of adverse effects.[22] Studies of ipriflavone for Paget's disease and hyperparathyroidism have used 1,200 mg/day dosing.[38,40]

PATIENT INFORMATION

Ipriflavone is sold as an over-the-counter nutritional supplement for the treatment of osteoporosis. Although some evidence suggests that it may be effective, ipriflavone may reduce the amount of immune cells in your blood, with potentially dangerous consequences. Individuals with immune deficiency syndromes such as AIDS, or taking drugs that suppress the immune system, should definitely avoid ipriflavone. Ipriflavone can interact harmfully with numerous other drugs as well, including warfarin (Coumadin), phenytoin (Dilantin), and theophylline. Finally, there may be risks in combining ipriflavone and estrogen.

The safety of ipriflavone for pregnant or nursing women or young children has not been established. Individuals with severe liver or kidney disease should consult a physician before using this (or any other) supplement.

REFERENCES

1. Reginster JY. Ipriflavone: pharmacological properties and usefulness in postmenopausal osteoporosis. *Bone Miner.* 1993;23:223-232. **2.** Rondelli I, Acerbi D, Ventura P. Steady-state pharmacokinetics of ipriflavone and its metabolites in patients with renal failure. *Int J Clin Pharmacol Res.* 1991;11:183-192. **3.** Melis GB, Paoletti AM, Cagnacci A, et al. Lack of any estrogenic effect of ipriflavone in postmenopausal women. *J Endocrinol Invest.* 1992;15:755-761. **4.** Cecchini MG, Fleisch H, Muhibauer RC. Ipriflavone inhibits bone resorption in intact and ovariectomized rats. *Calcif Tissue Int.* 1997;61(suppl 1):S9-S11. **5.** Kuiper GG, Lemmen JG, Carlsson B, et al. Interaction of estrogenic chemicals and phytoestrogens with estrogen receptor beta. *Endocrinology.* 1998;139:4252-4263. **6.** Petilli M, Fiorelli G, Benvenuti S, et al. Interactions between ipriflavone and the estrogen receptor. *Calcif Tissue Int.* 1995;56:160-165. **7.** Benvenuti S, Petilli M, Frediani U, et al. Binding and bioeffects of Ipriflavone on a human preosteoclastic cell line. *Biochem Biophys Res Commun.* 1994;201:1084-1089. **8.** Bonucci E, Silvestrini G, Ballanti P, et al. Cytological and ultrastructural investigation on osteoblastic and preosteoclastic cells grown in vitro in the presence of ipriflavone: preliminary results. *Bone Miner.* 1992;19(suppl):S15-25. **9.** Brandi ML. Ipriflavone influences the osteoblastic phenotype in vitro. *Osteoporos Int.* 1993;3(suppl 1):226-229. **10.** Cheng SL, Zhang SF, Nelson TL, et al. Stimulation of human osteoblast differentiation and function by ipriflavone and its metabolites. *Calcif Tissue Int.* 1994;55:356-362. **11.** Shibano K, Watanabe J, Iwamoto M, et al. Culture of stromal cells derived from medullary cavity of human long bone in the presence of 1,25-dihydroxyvitamin D3, recombinant human bone morphogenetic protein-2, or ipriflavone. *Bone.* 1998;22:251-258. **12.** Agnusdei D, Bufalino L. Efficacy of ipriflavone in established osteoporosis and long-term safety. *Calcif Tissue Int.* 1997;61(suppl 1):S23-S27. **13.** Kakai Y, Kawase T, Nakano T, et al. Effect of ipriflavone and estrogen on the differentiation and proliferation of osteogenic cells. *Calcif Tissue Int.* 1992;51(suppl 1):S11-S15. **14.** Civitelli R. In vitro and in vivo effects of ipriflavone on bone formation and bone biomechanics. *Calcif Tissue Int.* 1997;61(suppl 1):S12-S14. **15.** Agnusdei D, Zacchei F, Bigazzi S, et al. Metabolic and clinical effects of ipriflavone in established post-menopausal osteoporosis. *Drugs Exp Clin Res.* 1989;15:97-104. **16.** Agnusdei D, Adami S, Cervetti R, et al. Effects of ipriflavone on bone mass and calcium metabolism in postmenopausal osteoporosis. *Bone Miner.* 1992;19(suppl 1):S43-S48. **17.** Gambacciani M, Spinetti A, Piaggesi L, et al. Ipriflavone prevents the bone mass reduction in premenopausal women treated with gonadotropin hormone-releasing hormone agonists. *Bone Miner.* 1994;26:19-26. **18.** Gambacciani M, Cappagli B, Piaggesi L, et al. Ipriflavone prevents the loss of bone mass in pharmacological menopause induced by GnRH-agonists. *Calcif Tissue Int.* 1997;61(Suppl 1):S15-18. **19.** Kovacs AB. Efficacy of ipriflavone in the prevention and treatment of postmenopausal osteoporosis. *Agents Actions.* 1994;41:86-87. **20.** Maugeri D, Panebianco P, Russo MS, et al. Ipriflavone-treatment of senile osteoporosis: results of a multicenter, double-blind clinical trial of 2 years. *Arch Gerontol Geriatr.* 1994;19:253-263. **21.** Passeri M, Biondi M, Costi D, et al. Effects of 2-year therapy with ipriflavone in elderly women with established osteoporosis. *Ital J Miner Electrolyte Metab.* 1995;9:137-144. **22.** Valente M, Bufalino L, Castiglione GN, et al. Effects of 1-year treatment with ipriflavone on bone in postmenopausal women with low bone mass. *Calcif Tissue Int.* 1994;54:377-380. **23.** Alexandersen P, Toussaint A, Reginster J, et al. Ipriflavone has no effect on bone metabolism and causes lymphopenia in osteopenic women [abstract]. *J Bone Miner Res.* 2000;15(suppl 1):S198. **24.** Melis GB, Paoletti AM, Cagnacci A. Ipriflavone prevents bone loss in postmenopausal women. *Menopause.* 1996;3:27-32. **25.** Gennari C. Ipriflavone: background. *Calcif Tissue Int.* 1997;61:S3-S4. **26.** Gennari C, Adami S, Agnusdei D, et al. Effect of chronic treatment with ipriflavone in postmenopausal women with low bone mass. *Calcif Tissue Int.* 1997;61:s19-s22. **27.** Alexandersen P, Toussaint A, Christiansen C, et al. Ipriflavone in the treatment of postmenopausal osteoporosis: a randomized controlled trial. *JAMA.* 2001;285:1482-1488. **28.** Agnusdei D, Gennari C, Bufalino L. Prevention of early postmenopausal bone loss using low doses of conjugated estrogens and the non-hormonal, bone-active drug ipriflavone. *Osteoporos Int.* 1995;5:462-466. **29.** Choi YK, Han IK, Yoon HK. Ipriflavone for the treatment of osteoporosis. *Osteoporos Int.* 1997;7(suppl 3):S174-S178. **30.** de Aloysio D, Gambacciani M, Altieri P, de Aloysio D, et al. Bone density changes in postmenopausal women with the administration of ipriflavone alone or in association with low-dose ERT. *Gynecol Endocrinol.* 1997;11:289-293. **31.** Gambacciani M, Ciaponi M, Cappagli B, et al. Effects of combined low dose of the isoflavone derivative ipriflavone and estrogen replacement on bone mineral density and metabolism in postmenopausal women. *Maturitas.* 1997;28:75-81. **32.** Melis GB, Paoletti AM, Bartolini R, et al. Ipriflavone and low doses of estrogens in the prevention of bone mineral loss in climacterium. *Bone Miner.* 1992;19(suppl 1):S49-S56. **33.** Nozaki M, Hashimoto K, Inoue Y, et al. Treatment of bone loss in oophorectomized women with a combination of ipriflavone and conjugated equine estrogen. *Int J Gynaecol Obstet.* 1998;62:69-75. **34.** Hanabayashi T, Imai A, Tamaya T. Effects of ipriflavone and estriol on postmenopausal osteoporotic changes. *Int J Gynaecol Obstet.* 1995;51:63-64. **35.** Ushiroyama T, Okamura S, Ikeda A, et al. Efficacy of ipriflavone and 1 alpha vitamin D therapy for the cessation of vertebral bone loss. *Int J Gynaecol Obstet.* 1995;48:283-288. **36.** Moscarini M, Patacchiola F, Spacca G, et al. New perspectives in the treatment of postmenopausal osteoporosis: ipriflavone. *Gynecol Endocrinol.* 1994;8:203-207. **37.** Scali G, Mansanti P, Zurlo A, et al. Analgesic effect of ipriflavone versus Calcitonin in the treatment of osteoporotic vertebral pain. *Curr Ther Res.* 1991;49:1004-1010. **38.** Mazzuoli G, Romagnoli E, Carnevale V, et al. Effects of ipriflavone on bone remodeling in primary hyperparathyroidism. *Bone Miner.* 1992;19(suppl 1):S27-S33. **39.** Yamazaki I, Shino A, Shimizu Y, et al. Effect of ipriflavone on glucocorticoid-induced osteoporosis in rats. *Life Sci.* 1986;38:951-958. **40.** Agnusdei D, Camporeale A, Gonnelli S, et al. Short-term treatment of Paget's disease of bone with ipriflavone. *Bone Miner.* 1992;19(suppl 1):S35-S42. **41.** Agnusdei D, Crepaldi G, Isaia G, et al. A double blind, placebo-controlled trial of ipriflavone for prevention of postmenopausal spinal bone loss. *Calcif Tissue Int.* 1997;61:142-147. **42.** Matsuoka M, Yoshida Y, Hayakawa K, et al. Gastrojejunal fistula caused by gastric ulcer. *J Gastroenterol.* 1998;33:267-271. **43.** Ferrandina G, Almadori G, Maggiano N, et al. Growth-inhibitory effect of tamoxifen and quercetin and presence of type II estrogen binding sites in human laryngeal cancer cell lines and primary laryngeal tumors. *Int J Cancer.* 1998;77:747-754. **44.** Monostory K, Vereczkey L. Interaction of theophylline and ipriflavone at the cytochrome P450 level. *Eur J Drug Metab Pharmacokinet.* 1995;20:43-47. **45.** Takahashi J, Kawakatsu K, Wakayama T, et al. Elevation of serum theophylline levels by ipriflavone in a patient with chronic obstructive pulmonary disease. *Eur J Clin Pharmacol.* 1992;43:207-208. **46.** Monostory K, Vereczkey L, Levai F, et al. Ipriflavone as an inhibitor of human cytochrome P450 enzymes. *Br J Pharmacol.* 1998;123:605-610. **47.** Yamazaki I. Effect of ipriflavone on the response of uterus and thyroid to estrogen. *Life Sci.* 1986;38:757-764.

Kava

Piper Methysticum

Alternate/Related Names: Ava, Ava Pepper, Intoxicating Pepper, Kava-Kava, Kawa

U.S. BRAND NAMES OF CLINICALLY TESTED PRODUCTS

Kavatrol (Natrol) = Kavatrol (Natrol) in Europe

DESCRIPTION

Kava is a member of the pepper family, which has long been cultivated by Pacific Islanders for use as a relaxing drink in social and ceremonial settings. Dependent entirely on human intervention for propagation, the kava plant is a slow-growing shrub that can reach 9 feet in height. The pithy root and rootstock are used for medicinal purposes.

PHARMACOLOGY

The active constituents of kava are fat-soluble lactones (kavalactones) that make up 5.5% to 8.3% of the root. The kavalactones include dihydrokavain, kavain, methysticin, and dihydromethysticin. The water-soluble ingredients of kava produce little to no effect.[1]

Kavalactones are well absorbed by the digestive tract and have been shown to readily cross the blood-brain barrier in mice.[2] Their plasma half-life ranges from 90 minutes to several hours.

Dihydrokavain has been found to produce a sedative, anticonvulsant, and analgesic effect.[3-6] Mixed kavalactones have been found to cause a mephenesin-like relaxation of skeletal muscles and at very high doses can cause ataxia and paralysis without loss of consciousness.[6,7,8] Peripherally, nonhydrated kavalactones (kavain and methysticin) and to a lesser extent hydrated kavalactones (dihydrokavain and dihydromethysticin) produce local anesthesia similar to that of cocaine.[9] Methysticin and dihydromethysticin exhibit neuroprotective properties in rodents, similar to memantine (a glutamate antagonist at NMDA-glutamate receptors, not marketed in the United States). In double-blind placebo-controlled and comparison studies, DL-kavain has been found to produce anti-anxiety effects similar to those of benzodiazepines.[2]

The analgesia of kava is not reversed by opioid antagonists.[4] Initial reports suggested that kavalactones do not significantly interact with GABA receptors.[10] This led to further investigations of excitatory neuronal mechanisms. Two recent reports suggest that kavain, methysticin, or both can inhibit voltage-dependent sodium channels and suppress the release of the excitatory amino acid neurotransmitter glutamate.[11,12] However, later research suggests that the effects of kavalactones may indeed involve GABA receptors, by increasing their prevalence, especially in the hippocampus and amygdala.[13] EEG studies also suggest that kavalactones act preferentially on the amygdalar complex of the limbic system.[14] Earlier investigations may have erred by examining areas of the brain where kava is not believed to be active, specifically the frontal cortex and cerebellum. It appears that kavalactones interact with some other site on GABA-A receptors besides the benzodiazepine binding site.[15] One study found a direct interaction at nanomolar concentrations between a kavain derivative and cortical neurons, suggesting a ligand-receptor interaction.[16]

CLINICAL STUDIES

ANXIETY

Altogether, over 400 patients with various anxiety syndromes have participated in double-blind controlled studies of kava.[17-21]

The largest of these was a 6-month double-blind placebo-controlled trial that tested 300 mg/day of a 70% kavalactone extract in 101 outpatients with anxiety-related disorders meeting DSM-III-R criteria.[17] Participants were evaluated using the Hamilton Anxiety Scale (HAM-A; quantifying restlessness, nervousness, heart palpitations, stomach discomfort, dizziness, and chest pain) and the Clinical Global Impressions scale (CGI) as well as self-rating scales. The study found that HAM-A scores in the treated group showed clinically and statistically significant reduction compared to the placebo group beginning at 8 weeks, and that this relative improvement increased throughout the duration of the study. At 12 weeks, the CGI scale also showed statistically significant improvement in treated patients compared to the placebo group. Self-rating scales showed similar changes. This study, however, has been criticized for its heterogeneous treatment group (patients had more than one anxiety-related diagnosis) and significant differences in average HAM-A scores between centers.

While this large study found a delayed anxiolytic effect with kava, other studies have found anxiolysis within one week.[2,18]

A 1993 double-blind comparative study followed 174 patients with anxiety symptoms, for a period of 6 weeks. Patients received 300 mg/day of a 70% kavalactone extract, 15 mg/day of oxazepam (a subtherapeutic dose), or 9 mg/day of bromazepam (a full therapeutic dose).[21] A similar improvement in HAM-A scores was seen in all groups, but no intergroup statistical analysis was reported.

Other double-blind placebo-controlled studies have found anxiolytic effects with the single kavalactone kavain.[2,22,23] Furthermore, isolated kavain has been found to produce effects comparable to those of benzodiazepines.[2] However, the results of small controlled trials suggest that kava or kavalactones may impair mental function to a lesser extent than benzodiazepines.[24-27]

WITHDRAWAL FROM BENZODIAZEPINES

A double-blind placebo controlled crossover trial of 40 individuals with various anxiety disorders found that use of kava facilitated withdrawal from benzodiazepine therapy, reducing withdrawal symptoms and maintaining control of anxiety.[28]

PROPOSED INDICATIONS AND USAGE

Some evidence supports the use of kava for the treatment of anxiety disorders, as well as for facilitation of benzodiazepine withdrawal.

Kava is also widely marketed as a component of natural products said to induce sleep; however, there is no clinical evidence that it is effective for this purpose.

WARNINGS

There have been reports of idiopathic hepatotoxicity associated with use of kava products. Individuals with Parkinson's disease or risk factors for dystonic reactions should avoid use of kava.

Kava should not be combined with other sedatives.

PRECAUTIONS

Although kava has not been shown to possess hepatotoxic effects, a 50-year-old man who had been taking an appropriate dose of a well-regarded kava product for 2 months experienced fulminant hepatic failure requiring transplantation,[29] for which causality appears likely. Another case report found a temporal association between use of a kava product and acute hepatitis with confluence necrosis in a 39-year-old woman.[30] However, because the product was not analyzed, it isn't clear whether kava itself or a contaminant in the kava preparation was responsible; the authors also could not rule out acute viral hepatitis or autoimmune hepatitis. Nonetheless, these reports suggest that individuals with hepatic disease or those taking potentially hepatotoxic medications should avoid use of kava.

When taken in typical doses, kava or synthetic kavain does not appear to impair reaction time or mental function.[2,24-27,31,32] However, high doses are known to cause inebriation. Driving while taking kava may be unsafe.

Individuals with Parkinson's disease or risk factors for dystonic reactions should avoid use of kava (see Adverse Reactions).

Safety for pregnant or lactating women, young children, or individuals with renal disease is not known.

DRUG INTERACTIONS

There has been a case report of delirium apparently resulting from the concomitant use of kava extract and the benzodiazepine alprazolam (Xanax).[33] In addition, high doses of alcohol potentiate the effects and toxicity of kava in mice.[4] However, in humans, kava tends to counter some of the safety-related adverse effects of mild alcohol consumption.[34] Nonetheless, based on current evidence, kava should not be combined with other sedatives.

Kava might increase risk of dystonic reactions in individuals on phenothiazines, and could additionally counteract the effectiveness of L-dopa.[35]

ADVERSE REACTIONS

Kava is usually well tolerated. A 4-week drug-monitoring study of 3,029 patients given 800 mg/day of a 30% kavalactone extract yielded a 2.3% incidence of side effects, including mild headache, gastrointestinal distress, and allergic rashes. Another study of 4,049 patients who took a much lower dose found side effects in 1.5% of cases, also limited mainly to mild gastrointestinal complaints or allergic rashes.[2]

Long-term kava use (months to years) in excess of 400 mg kavalactones per day can create a characteristic generalized dry, scaly dermopathy that appears primarily on the palms, soles, forearms, shins, and back.[36] The rash promptly disappears on cessation of kava.

The LD_{50} of kavalactones is about 300 to 400 mg/kg in test animals.[7] Dogs and rats tolerate daily doses of 24 mg/kg and 20 mg/kg, respectively, of 70% kava extract with no adverse effects.[2,7] Up to 320 mg/kg of this extract in rats caused only mild histopathological changes. No evidence of mutagenicity was observed.

Three case reports appear to represent kava-induced dystonic reactions.[35] In one, a 28-year-old man exhibited abnormal ocular movements and neck spasms approximately 90 minutes after ingesting 100 mg of kava extract. This episode lasted about 40 minutes. Similar reactions were seen in two women, aged 22 and 63. In a fourth case, kava increased symptoms of Parkinson's disease. These reports suggest an antidopaminergic effect, indicating that kava should not be used by individuals with Parkinson's disease or those who have had dystonic reactions to antipsychotic medications.

Addiction has not been observed in European patients taking kava extracts, and animal studies suggest that typical kava products do not cause physiological tolerance or dependence.[2,37]

PROPOSED DOSAGE AND ADMINISTRATION

For use as an antianxiety agent, the typical dose of kava extract supplies 60 to 210 mg of kavalactones per day, given in two or three divided doses. The total dose of kavalactones should not exceed 300 mg/day.[2] Germany's Commission E recommends a maximum treatment duration of 3 months.

PATIENT INFORMATION

Kava is an herb marketed for the treatment of anxiety and insomnia. Some research suggests that it may be helpful for anxiety; however, the evidence is not strong. No evidence supports using kava for insomnia.

NOTE: Do not suddenly discontinue benzodiazepine medications and switch to kava.

Individuals taking kava should not drive or operate heavy machinery, and the herb should not be taken concurrently with alcohol or other sedatives. Individuals with liver disease or who are taking medications that can inflame the liver should avoid kava. Individuals with Parkinson's disease or those who have had dystonic reactions to antipsychotic medications should also avoid kava.

The safety of kava for pregnant or nursing women or young children has not been established. Individuals with severe kidney disease should consult a physician before using this (or any other) supplement.

REFERENCES

1. Jamieson DD, Duffield PH, Cheng D, et al. Comparison of the central nervous system activity of the aqueous and lipid extract of kava (Piper methysticum). *Arch Int Pharmacodyn Ther.* 1989;301:66-80. **2.** Schulz V, Hansel R, Tyler VE. *Rational Phytotherapy: A Physicians' Guide to Herbal Medicine.* 3rd ed. Berlin, Germany: Springer-Verlag; 1998:67-68, 70-72. **3.** Bruggemann VF, Meyer HJ. Studies on the analagesic efficacy of the kava constituents dihydrokavain (DHK) and dihydromethysticin (DHM) [in German; English abstract]. *Arzneimittelforschung.* 1963;13:407-409. **4.** Jamieson DD, Duffield PH. Positive interaction of ethanol and kava resin in mice. *Clin Exp Pharmacol Physiol.* 1990;17:509-514. **5.** Klohs MW, Keller F, Williams RE, et al. A chemical and pharmacological investigation of Piper methysticum Forst. *J Med Pharm Chem.* 1959;1:95-103. **6.** Meyer HJ, Kretzschmar R. Kava pyrones—a new substance class of central muscle relaxants of the mephenesin type [translated from German]. *Klin Wochenschr.* 1966;44:902-903. **7.** Meyer HJ. Pharmacology of the active compounds of the kava rhizomel (Piper methysticum Forst) [translated from German]. *Arch Int Pharmacodyn Ther.* 1962;138:505-536. **8.** Singh YN. Effects of kava on neuromuscular transmission and muscle contractility. *J Ethnopharmacol.* 1983;7:267-276. **9.** Meyer HJ, May HU. Local anaesthetic properties of natural Kava pyrones [translated from German]. *Klin Wochenschr.* 1964;42:407. **10.** Davies LP, Drew CA, Duffield P, et al. Kava pyrones and resin: studies on GABAA, GABAB and benzodiazepine binding sites in rodent brain. *Pharmacol Toxicol.* 1992;71:120-126. **11.** Gleitz J, Friese J, Beile A, et al. Anticonvulsive action of (±)-kavain estimated from its properties on stimulated synaptosomes and Na+ channel receptor sites. *Eur J Pharmacol.* 1996;315:89-97. **12.** Magura EI, Kopanitsa MV, Gleitz J, et al. Kava extract ingredients, (+)-methysticin and (±)-kavain inhibit voltage-operated Na(+)-channels in rat CA1 hippocampal neurons. *Neuroscience.* 1997;81:345-351. **13.** Jussofie A, Schmiz A, Hiemke C. Kavapyrone enriched extract from Piper methysticum as modulator of the GABA binding site in different regions of rat brain. *Psychopharmacology (Berl).* 1994;116:469-474. **14.** Holm E, Staedt U, Heep J, et al. The action profile of D,L-kavain. Cerebral sites and sleep-wakefulness-rhythm in animals [in German]. *Arzneimittelforschung.* 1991;41:673-683. **15.** Boonen G, Haberlein H. Influence of genuine kavapyrone enantiomers on the GABA-A binding site. *Planta Med.* 1998;64:504-506. **16.** Boonen G, Pramanik A, Rigler R, et al. Evidence for specific interactions between kavain and human cortical neurons monitored by fluorescence correlation spectroscopy. *Planta Med.* 2000;66:7-10. **17.** Volz HP, Kieser M. Kava-kava extract WS 1490 versus placebo in anxiety disorders-a randomized placebo-controlled 25-week outpatient trial. *Pharmacopsychiatry.* 1997;30:1-5. **18.** Warnecke G. Psychosomatic disorders in the female climacterium, clinical efficacy and tolerance of kava extract WS 1490 [translated from German]. *Fortschr Med.* 1991;109:119-122. **19.** Warnecke G, Pfaender H, Gerster G, et al. Efficacy of an extract of kava root in patients with climacteric syndrome. A double blind study with a new mono-preparation [translated from German]. *Z Phytother.* 1990;11:81-86. **20.** Kinzler E, Kromer J, Lehmann E. Effect of a special kava extract in patients with anxiety-, tension-, and excitation states of non-psychotic genesis. Double blind study with placebos over 4 weeks [translated from German]. *Arzneimittelforschung.* 1991;41:584-588. **21.** Woelk H, Kapoula O, Lehrl S, et al. The treatment of patients with anxiety. A double-blind study: kava extract WS 1490 versus benzodiazepine [translated from German]. *Z Allgemeinmed.* 1993;69:271-277. **22.** Lindenberg D, Pitule-Schodel H. D, L-Kavain in comparison with oxazepam in anxiety disorders. A double-blind study of clinical effectiveness [translated from German]. *Fortschr Med.* 1990;108:48-54. **23.** Scholing WE, Clausen HD. On the effect of D,L-kavain: experience with Neuronika(r) [in German]. *Med Klin.* 1977;72:1301-1306. **24.** Munte TF, Heinze HJ, Matzke M, et al. Effects of oxazepam and an extract of kava roots (Piper methysticum) on event-related potentials in a word recognition task. *Neuropsychobiology.* 1993;27:46-53. **25.** Heinze HJ, Munthe TF, Steitz J, et al. Pharmacopsychological effects of oxazepam and kava-extract in a visual search paradigm assessed with event-related potentials. *Pharmacopsychiatry.* 1994;27:224-230. **26.** Gessner B, Cnota P. Extract of the kava-kava rhizome in comparison with diazepam and placebo [in German; English abstract]. *Z Phytother.* 1994;15:30-37. **27.** Saletu B, Grunberger J, Linzmayer L, et al. EEG-brain mapping, psychometric and psychophysiological studies on central effects of Kavain-a kava plant derivative. *Hum Psychopharmacol.* 1989;4:169-190. **28.** Malsch U, Klement S. Randomized placebo-controlled double-blind clinical trial of a special extract of kava roots (WS 1490) in patients with anxiety disorders of non-psychotic origin [abstract]. Eur Phytojournal [serial online]. 2000; Issue 1. Available at: http://www.escop.com/issue_1.htm. Accessed May 10, 2001. **29.** Escher M, Desmeules J, Giostra E, et al. Hepatitis associated with Kava, a herbal remedy for anxiety. *BMJ.* 2001;322:139. **30.** Strahl S, Ehret V, Dahm H, et al. Necrotizing hepatitis after taking herbal remedies [translated from German]. *Dtsch Med Wochenschr.* 1998;123:1410-1414. **31.** Prescott J, Jamieson D, Emdur N, et al. Acute effects of kava on measures of cognitive performance, physiological function and mood. *Drug Alcohol Rev.* 1993;12:49-57. **32.** Russell PN, Bakker D, Singh NN. The effects of kava on alerting and speed of access of information from long-term memory. *Bull Psychonomic Soc.* 1987;25:236-237. **33.** Almeida JC, Grimsley EW. Coma from the health food store: interaction between kava and alprazolam [letter]. *Ann Intern Med.* 1996;125:940-941. **34.** Herberg K-W. Driving capability after intake of Kava special extract WS 1490 [in German]. *Z Allgemeinmed.* 1991;67:842-846. **35.** Schelosky L, Raffauf C, Jendroska K, et al. Kava and dopamine antagonism [letter]. *J Neurol Neurosurg Psychiatry.* 1995;58:639-640. **36.** Norton SA, Ruze P. Kava dermopathy. *J Am Acad Dermatol.* 1994;31:89-97. **37.** Duffield PH, Jamieson D. Development of tolerance to kava in mice. *Clin Exp Pharmacol Physiol.* 1991;18:571-578.

Lemon Balm

Melissa Officinalis

Alternate/Related Names: Cure-All, Dropsy Plant, Honey Plant, Melissa, Sweet Mary, Balm Mint

U.S. BRAND NAMES OF CLINICALLY TESTED PRODUCTS

Herpalieve (PhytoPharmica), Herpilyn (Enzymatic Therapy) = Lomaherpan (Lomapharm) in Europe

DESCRIPTION

Lemon balm is a native of southern Europe, widely planted in gardens for the purpose of attracting bees. Its leaves give off a delicate lemon odor when bruised.

Authorities as far back as Pliny and Dioscorides mention topical lemon balm as a treatment for wounds. Later applications focused on oral uses for influenza, insomnia, anxiety, depression, and nervous stomach.

PHARMACOLOGY

The major constituents of lemon balm are volatile oils, consisting primarily of citral a and b, as well as flavonoids, polyphenolics, and triterpenic acids.

Numerous in vitro studies have found antiviral properties in lemon balm extracts used topically, and commercial products are standardized by bioassay.[1,2,3] The antiviral mechanism of action of *M. officinalis* is not known. However, the leading theory is that the herb blocks virus receptors on host cells.[3] In addition, lemon balm extract also has the ability to inhibit protein synthesis at the level of elongation factor eEF-2.[4]

In an animal study, lyophilised hydroethanolic extracts of lemon balm were found to produce dose-dependent sedation and potentiation of pentobarbital.[5]

CLINICAL STUDIES

ORAL AND GENITAL HERPES (TOPICAL USE)

A double-blind trial evaluated 116 patients with genital or oral herpes given either lemon balm cream or placebo for a period of 5 days.[3] The largest intergroup differences were seen at day 2 of treatment, showing statistically significant improvements in favor of the treated group. In addition, the total number of patients who were completely recovered on day 5 was significantly higher in the treated group than in the placebo group. Physician and patient evaluation of the course of the outbreak was also strongly in favor of the treated group.

Another double-blind placebo-controlled study followed 66 individuals who were just beginning to develop oral herpes.[6] Treatment with lemon balm cream produced significant benefits on day 2, reducing intensity of discomfort, number of blisters, and the size of the lesions. Long-term but somewhat informal follow-up by the same researchers suggested that the lemon balm application also delayed the next herpes flare-up.

INSOMNIA (ORAL USE)

No clinical studies of oral lemon balm alone have been reported. However, a double-blind placebo-controlled crossover study of 20 insomnia patients compared the effectiveness of a lemon balm and valerian combination against triazolam.[7] The results showed comparable benefit in the two treatment groups and a significant difference from placebo.

PROPOSED INDICATIONS AND USAGE

Weak evidence suggests that lemon balm cream may be modestly effective in the treatment of genital and oral herpes if used at the onset of symptoms.

Oral lemon balm is often added to herbal combinations for insomnia, but there is no meaningful clinical evidence that it is effective for this purpose.

Lemon balm is often used as an ingredient in cosmetics to improve skin and hair.

Lemon balm is also sometimes used for fevers, flus, menstrual problems, muscle spasms, anxiety, nausea, nervous stomach and nervous headaches; again, without evidence of effectiveness.

WARNINGS

Oral lemon balm might potentiate the action of sedatives.

PRECAUTIONS

None.

DRUG INTERACTIONS

One animal study suggests that lemon balm might potentiate the action of sedatives.[5]

ADVERSE REACTIONS

Topical lemon balm has not been associated with any significant side effects, although allergic reactions are always possible. Oral lemon balm is on the FDA's GRAS (Generally Recognized As Safe) list. The Ames test (with and without metabolic activation) has been found negative with oral lemon balm tincture.[8]

PROPOSED DOSAGE AND ADMINISTRATION

For treatment of an active flare-up of herpes, the proper dose is 4 thick daily applications of a standard lemon balm 70:1 extract cream. This can be reduced to twice daily for preventive purposes.

The most studied product in Europe is Lomaherpan, a lemon balm extract standardized by bioassay. Human or animal cell lines are grown in a petri dish and then infected with herpes virus. Standard paper disks infiltrated with lemon balm extract are then inserted. The commercial extract is standardized so that a dose of 200 μg/disc forms a 20 to 30 mm zone of inhibition of viral cellular lysis.[3]

When taken orally, the standard dose of lemon balm is 1.5 to 4.5 g/day of dried herb.

PATIENT INFORMATION

Creams containing the herb lemon balm are marketed for the treatment of herpes flare-ups, and some evidence suggests these products may be helpful. However, lemon balm cream should not be regarded as effective for preventing spread of genital herpes to newborns or sexual partners.

Oral lemon balm is often included in herbal combinations for promoting sleep or relaxation, but the herb has not been proven effective for this purpose.

The maximum safe dosage of lemon balm for pregnant or nursing women or young children has not been established. Individuals with severe liver or kidney disease should consult a physician before using this (or any other) supplement. Lemon balm should not be taken at the same time as sedative medications.

REFERENCES

1. Dimitrova Z, Dimov B, Manolova N, et al. Antiherpes effect of Melissa officinalis L. extracts. *Acta Microbiol Bulg.* 1993;29:65-72. **2.** May VG, Willuhn G. Antiviral activity of aqueous extracts from medicinal plants in tissue cultures [in German]. *Arzneimittelforschung.* 1978;28:1-7. **3.** Wolbling RH, Leonhardt K. Local therapy of herpes simplex with dried extract from Melissa officinalis. *Phytomedicine.* 1994;1:25-31. **4.** Chlabicz J, Galasinski W. The components of Melissa officinalis L. that influence protein biosynthesis in-vitro. *J Pharm Pharmacol.* 1986;38:791-794. **5.** Soulimani R, Fleurentin J, Mortier F, et al. Neurotropic action of the hydroalcoholic extract of Melissa officinalis in the mouse. *Planta Med.* 1991;57:105-109. **6.** Koytchev R, Alken RG, Dundarov S. Balm mint extract (Lo-701) for topical treatment of recurring herpes labialis. *Phytomedicine.* 1999;6:225-230. **7.** Dressing H, Riemann D, Low H, Schredl M, et al. Insomnia: are valerian/balm combinations of equal value to benzodiazepines? [translated from German]. *Therapiewoche.* 1992;42:726-736. **8.** Schimmer O, Kruger A, Paulini H, et al. An evaluation of 55 commercial plant extracts in the Ames mutagenicity test. *Pharmazie.* 1994;49:448-451.

Licorice

Glycyrrhiza Glabra

Alternate/Related Names: Deglycyrrhizinated Licorice, DGL, Sweet Root; *Glycyrrhiza glanulifera, G. pallida, G. tyica, G. violocea*

U.S. BRAND NAMES OF CLINICALLY TESTED PRODUCTS

None.

DESCRIPTION

A member of the pea family, licorice root has been used since ancient times both as food and as medicine.

PHARMACOLOGY

Licorice contains coumarins, flavonoids, terpenoids, and volatile oils. The most studied ingredients are the terpenoids, glycyrrhizin glycoside (glycyrrhizinic acid), and its hydrolysis product glycyrrhetinic acid. These terpenoids exert significant mineralocorticoid effects, suppressing aldosterone secretion and plasma renin activity, and increasing blood pressure in a linear dose-responsive manner.[1-4] Glycyrrhizin glycoside and glycyrrhetinic acid bind to mineralocorticoid and glucocorticoid receptors. However, because mineralocorticoid actions are not seen in adrenalectomized animals, other mechanisms of action have been proposed.[5] These include inhibition of 11-Beta-OHSD, an enzyme that catalyzes the conversion of cortisol to inactive cortisone,[5] as well as displacement of cortisol from transcortin.[6] In order to avoid these undesired actions, glycyrrhizin is removed during the preparation of some licorice products, which are sold as deglycyrrhizinated licorice (DGL).

Glycyrrhetinic acid may possess anti-inflammatory, antiviral, estrogenic, and hepatoprotective actions.[7-19]

An ester derivative of glycyrrhetinic acid, carbenoxolone, has been used to treat gastric and esophageal ulcer disease. Researchers have postulated that it may exert a protective effect by increasing mucosal blood flow as well as mucous production, and by interfering with gastric prostanoid synthesis.[20]

CLINICAL STUDIES

PEPTIC ULCER DISEASE

A 12-week controlled trial (blinding not stated) using endoscopic evaluation compared antacids, cimetidine (220 mg tid and 400 mg qhs geranylferensylacetate (5 mg tid), and Caved-S (a European product consisting of licorice plus antacids) in 874 individuals with duodenal ulcers.[21] No significant differences in outcome were observed. However, because Caved-S contains antacids, this study might not actually provide evidence that DGL alone is effective.

In a single-blind trial, 82 individuals with endoscopically healed gastric ulcer were treated for 2 years with cimetidine (400 mg qhs or Caved-S. The results showed an equivalent rate of recurrence in the two groups.[22] Again, the effectiveness of DGL alone cannot be determined from this study.

There is no evidence that licorice or DGL eradicates *Helicobacter pylori.*

Highly preliminary evidence suggests that DGL might protect the gastric lining from NSAID-induced gastritis.[23]

PROPOSED INDICATIONS AND USAGE

Weak evidence suggests that DGL may offer benefits in peptic ulcer disease. DGL is also marketed for the treatment of apthous ulcers, but without any meaningful supporting evidence.

Whole licorice, not DGL, is sometimes used as an expectorant for respiratory problems such as coughs and asthma. Creams containing licorice are said to be effective for eczema, psoriasis, and herpes. However, there is no meaningful clinical evidence for any of these proposed uses.

Licorice has been suggested as a treatment for chronic fatigue syndrome (CFS), based on the hypothesis that individuals with CFS often have some degree of adrenal insufficiency and hypotension. However, other treatments to raise blood pressure have proven ineffective for CFS; in one double-blind placebo-controlled study, a 6-week course of fludrocortisone and increased dietary sodium to raise blood pressure found no improvement in 25 individuals with CFS symptoms.[24]

WARNINGS

Licorice exerts significant mineralocorticoid effects, causing sodium retention, potassium loss, and hypertension. DGL products should not produce the same effects.

PRECAUTIONS

Even relatively low doses of licorice may cause sodium and fluid retention, hypertension, and hypokalemia.[1] These effects are of particular concern for patients taking digitalis, diuretics, or corticosteroids, and for patients with hypertension, heart disease, diabetes, or renal disease.

Licorice may reduce testosterone levels in men.[25] For this reason, it is not recommended for use in men with a history of impotence, infertility, or decreased libido. Similarly, due to potential estrogenic properties,[15] licorice use should be avoided by women with a history of estrogen-sensitive malignancies.

Licorice's estrogenic and mineralocorticoid actions, as well as reports of lower gestational age at birth due to licorice use,[19] contraindicate its use in pregnancy and lactation.

DGL products would not be expected to exert mineralocorticoid effects. However, it is not known to what extent other side effects of whole licorice may occur with DGL.

Maximum safe dosages in individuals with severe hepatic or renal disease are not known.

DRUG INTERACTIONS

Licorice appears to potentiate topical and oral corticosteroids.[16,17,18]

Because of its mineralocorticoid activity, licorice should be used with caution in patients taking thiazide or loop diuretics, or digitalis; in addition, licorice would be expected to counter the desired actions of potassium-sparing diuretics. DGL products would not be expected to exert these effects.

Preliminary evidence suggests that licorice may inhibit CYP 3A4, but the clinical relevance of this finding remains unclear.[26]

ADVERSE REACTIONS

While immediate side effects from licorice are uncommon, mineralocorticoid effects occur reliably, reaching maximal effects in as short a time as 2 weeks.[1]

DGL is believed to be safe, although safety studies have not been performed.

PROPOSED DOSAGE AND ADMINISTRATION

As an adjuvant therapy to conventional medical care for treatment of ulcer pain, the usual dose of DGL is 2 to 4 380-mg tablets chewed before meals and at bedtime. A similar dose is used for apthous ulcers.

For eczema, psoriasis, or herpes, licorice cream is applied twice daily to the affected area. For expectorant use, the typical dose is 1 to 2 g of licorice root 3 times daily for no more than 1 week.

PATIENT INFORMATION

Whole licorice is an unsafe herb that should be avoided. It can cause numerous side effects, including fluid retention, high blood pressure, and loss of potassium. Because licorice has estrogen-like effects, it is not safe for women with a history of breast cancer. It also may reduce libido in men. Pregnant women should particularly avoid licorice, as it may cause premature birth.

A special form of licorice called deglycyrrhizinated licorice (DGL) is safer than whole licorice, but may cause some of the same side effects. It has been advocated for the treatment of ulcers; however, it has not been proven effective.

Licorice use is not advisable in young children, nursing women, or individuals with severe liver or kidney disease.

REFERENCES

1. Sigurjonsdottir HA, Franzson L, Manhem K, et al. Liquorice-induced rise in blood pressure: a linear dose-repsponse relationship. *J Hum Hypertens.* 2001;15:549-552. **2.** Conn JW, Rovner DR, Cohen EL. Licorice-induced pseudoaldosteronism. Hypertension, hypokaelemia, aldosteronopenia and suppressed plasma renin activity. *JAMA.* 1968;205:492-496. **3.** Epstein MT, Espiner EA, Donald RA, et al. Effect of eating liquorice on the renin-angiotensin aldosterone axis in normal subjects. *Br Med J.* 1977;1:488-490. **4.** Mantero F. Exogenous mineralcorticoid-like disorders. *Clin Endocrinol Metab.* 1981;10:465-

478. **5.** Stewart PM, Wallace AM, Valentino R, et al. Mineralcorticoid activity of liquorice: 11-beta-hydroxysteroid dehydrogenase deficiency comes of age. *Lancet.* 1987;2:821-824. **6.** Forslund T, Fyhrquist F, Froseth B,. Effects of licorice on plasma atrial natriuretic peptide in healthy volunteers. *J Intern Med.* 1989;225:95-99. **7.** Fujita H, Sakurai T, Yoshida M, et al. Antiinflammatory effect of glycyrrhizinic acid. Effects of glycyrrhizinic acid against carrageenin-induced edema, UV-erythema and skin reaction sensitised with DNCB [in Japanese; English abstract]. *Pharmacometrics.* 1980;19:481-484. **8.** Kiso Y, Tohkin M, Hikino H, et al. Mechanism of antihepatotoxic activity of glycyrrhizin. I: Effect on free radical generation and lipid peroxidation. *Planta Med.* 1984;50:298-302. **9.** Newall CA, et al. *Herbal medicines: A Guide for Health-Care Professionals.* London, England: Pharmaceutical Press; 1996:183-184. **10.** Pompei R, Pani A, Flore O, et al. Antiviral activity of glycyrrhizic acid. *Experientia.* 1980;36:304. **11.** Mitscher LA, Park YH, Clark D, et al. Antimicrobial agents from higher plants. Antimicrobial isoflavanoids and related substances from Glycyrrhiza glabra L. var. typica. *J Nat Prod.* 1980;43:259-269. **12.** Chandler RF. Licorice, more than just a flavour. *Can Pharm J.* 1985;118:421-424. **13.** Amagaya S, Sugishita E, Ogihara Y, et al. Separation and quantitative analysis of 18-alpha-glycrrhetinic acid and 18-beta-glyrrhetinic acid in Glycyrrhizae Radix by gas-lipid chromarography. *J Chromatogr.* 1985;320:430-434. **14.** Aida K, Tawata M, Shindo H, et al. Isoliquiritigenin: a new aldose reductase inhibitor from Glycyrrhizae radix. *Planta Med.* 1990;56:254-258. **15.** Zava DT, Dollbaum CM, Blen M. Estrogen and progestin bioactivity of foods, herbs, and spices. *Proc Soc Exp Biol Med.* 1998;217:369-378. **16.** Kumagai A, Nanaboshi M, Asanuma Y, et al. Effects of glycyrrhizin on thymolytic and immunosupressive action of cortisone. *Endocrinol Jpn.* 1967;14:39-42. **17.** Tamura Y, Nishikawa T, Yamada K, et al. Effects of glycyrrhetinic acid and its derivatives on delta-4-5-alpha- and 5-beta-reductase in rat liver. *Arzneimittelforschung.* 1979;29:647-649. **18.** Teelucksingh S, Mackie ADR, Burt D, et al. Potentiation of hydrocortisone activity in skin by glycyrrhetinic acid. *Lancet.* 1990;335:1060-1063. **19.** Strandberg TE, Jarvenpaa AL, Vanhanen H, et al. Birth outcome in relation to licorice consumption during pregnancy. *Am J Epidemiol.* 2001;153:1085-1088. **20.** Guslandi M. Ulcer-healing drugs and endogenous prostaglandins. *Int J Clin Pharmacol Ther Toxicol.* 1985;23:398-402. **21.** Kassir ZA. Endoscopic controlled trial of four drug regimens in the treatment of chronic duodenal ulceration. *Ir Med J.* 1985;78:153-156. **22.** Morgan AG, Pacsoo C, McAdam WAF. Maintenance therapy: a two-year comparison between caved-S and cimetidine treatment in the prevention of symptomatic gastric ulcer recurrence. *Gut.* 1985;26:599-602. **23.** Rees WDW, Rhodes J, Wright JE, et al. Effect of deglycyrrhizinated liquorice on gastric mucosal damage by aspirin. *Scand J Gastroenterol.* 1979;14:605-607. **24.** Peterson PK, Pheley A, Schroeppel J, et al. A preliminary placebo-controlled crossover trial of fludrocortisone for chronic fatigue syndrome. *Arch Intern Med.* 1998;158:908-914. **25.** Armanini D, Bonanni G, Palermo M. Reduction of serum testosterone in men by licorice [letter]. *N Engl J Med.* 1999;341:1158. **26.** Budzinski JW, Foster BC, Vandenhoek S, et al. An in vitro evaluation of human cytochrome P450 3A4 inhibition by selected commercial herbal extracts and tinctures. *Phytomedicine.* 2000;7:273-282.

Lipoic Acid

Alternate/Related Names: Alpha-Lipoic Acid, Thioctic Acid

U.S. BRAND NAMES OF CLINICALLY TESTED PRODUCTS

Not applicable.

DESCRIPTION

Lipoic acid is an antioxidant that has been used in Germany for over 30 years as a treatment for diabetic neuropathy.

PHARMACOLOGY

Alpha-lipoic acid is a vitamin-like substance that serves as a cofactor in the mitochondrial dehydrogenase reactions that lead to the formation of ATP. Certain illnesses may reduce levels of lipoic acid, such as diabetes, liver cirrhosis, and heart disease.[1] Thus although lipoic acid is not ordinarily an essential nutrient, supplementation in such conditions may correct a relative deficiency.

The proposed neuroprotective properties of lipoic acid are primarily attributed to its antioxidant properties. Lipoic acid is a strong scavenger of various free radical species.[2] In addition to serving as a chain-breaking antioxidant, lipoic acid is also a modest metal chelator and can prevent the formation of reactive oxygen resulting from iron- or copper-catalyzed oxidations.[3] Lipoic acid is active in both polar and non-polar media.[1,4,5] It also appears to increase cellular synthesis of the endogenous intracellular antioxidant glutathione.[6]

An additional neuroprotective effect of lipoic acid has been reported during overstimulation of the NMDA/glutamate receptor.[7] The toxicity of the excitatory amino acid neurotransmitters is characterized by neuronal lipid peroxidation resulting from an influx of calcium. Lipoic acid may normalize cellular calcium homeostasis. In addition, lipoic acid and its reduced form dihydrolipoic acid (DHLA) protect neuronal cells from glutamate toxicity.[8] DHLA can also provide reducing equivalents for methionine sulfoxide reductase, an enzyme that repairs oxidatively damaged proteins.[2]

Lipoic acid may produce additional effects in diabetes, benefiting insulin responsiveness, microcirculation, and sugar and protein metabolism, although the clinical relevance of these largely theoretical hypotheses remains unclear.[9-13]

CLINICAL STUDIES

DIABETIC PERIPHERAL NEUROPATHY

Lipoic acid has been found effective in diabetic polyneuropathy; however, this benefit may only occur with intravenous administration. Two randomized double-blind placebo-controlled trials involving with a total of 831 patients with diabetic polyneuropathy demonstrated the efficacy of 3 weeks of daily intravenous alpha-lipoic acid.[14,15] However, during the 6-month period of oral alpha-lipoic acid administration in the larger of these studies, no improvement over placebo was seen.[14] Positive evidence for oral lipoic acid is limited to open trials or trials with small sample size.[15-18]

DIABETIC AUTONOMIC NEUROPATHY

A randomized double-blind placebo-controlled trial of 73 diabetic patients with symptoms of cardiac autonomic neuropathy demonstrated modest improvement compared to placebo in individuals treated with 800 mg/day oral alpha-lipoic acid for 4 months.[18]

PROPOSED INDICATIONS AND USAGE

Lipoic acid has been extensively marketed as a "super antioxidant," said to prevent heart disease and cancer. However, while it is definitely an antioxidant, evidence for any therapeutic benefits remains weak.

Weak evidence supports the use of oral lipoic acid in diabetic peripheral and autonomic neuropathy. Minimal evidence suggests that lipoic acid might retard the development of diabetic cataracts and provide benefits in heart disease and liver cirrhosis.[17,19] One animal study suggests that lipoic acid might help prevent age-related hearing loss.[20]

WARNINGS

None.

PRECAUTIONS

Maximum safe doses for young children, pregnant or lactating women, or people with severe hepatic or renal disease have not been established.

DRUG INTERACTIONS

Formal drug interaction studies have not been performed. Based on pharmacological studies, there are some concerns that lipoic acid might potentiate the effects of insulin or oral hypoglycemics, but this effect has not been seen in clinical trials.

ADVERSE REACTIONS

In a study of 509 type 2 diabetic patients, an oral lipoic acid dose of 1,800 mg daily for 6 months was not associated with a greater incidence of side effects than placebo and did not affect glucose balance.[14]

PROPOSED DOSAGE AND ADMINISTRATION

The typical dose of lipoic acid is 300 to 600 mg/day, taken in 2 to 3 divided doses. A dose of 800 mg/day has been used for the treatment of cardiac autonomic neuropathy.[18] The effects are generally seen within a few weeks.

PATIENT INFORMATION

Lipoic acid is a supplement that has been tried for diabetic neuropathy. However, there is little evidence that it is effective for this condition. Lipoic acid is also marketed as a "super antioxidant" for heart disease, cancer, and slowing down aging. However, these proposed uses have no real scientific foundation.

The maximum safe dosage of lipoic acid for pregnant or nursing women or young children has not been established. Individuals with severe liver or kidney disease should consult a physician before using this (or any other) supplement.

REFERENCES

1. Kagan VE, Shvedova A, Serbinova E, et al. Dihydrolipoic acid: a universal antioxidant both in the membrane and in the aqueous phase. *Biochem Pharmacol.* 1992;44:1637-1649. **2.** Biewenga GP, Haenen GR, Bast A. The pharmacology of the antioxidant lipoic acid. *Gen Pharmacol.* 1997;29:315-331. **3.** Ou P, Tritschler HJ, Wolff SP. Thioctic (lipoic) acid: a therapeutic metal-chelating antioxidant? *Biochem Pharmacol.* 1995;50:123-126. **4.** Matsugo S, Yan LJ, Han D, et al. Elucidation of antioxidant activity of alpha-lipoic acid toward hydroxyl radical. *Biochem Biophys Res Commun.* 1995;208:161-167. **5.** Scott BC, Aruoma OI, Evans PJ, et al. Lipoic and dihydrolipoic acids as antioxidants. A critical evaluation. *Free Radic Res.* 1994;20:119-133. **6.** Han D, Handelman G, Marcocci L, et al. Lipoic acid increases de novo synthesis of cellular glutathione by improving cystine utilization. *Biofactors.* 1997;6:321-338. **7.** Packer L, Tritschler HJ, Wessel K. Neuroprotection by the metabolic antioxidant alpha-lipoic acid. *Free Radic Biol Med.* 1997;22:359-378. **8.** Dimpfel W. Effect of thioctic acid on pyramidal cell responses in the rat hippocampus in vitro. *Eur J Med Res.* 1996;1:523-527. **9.** Jacob S, Henriksen EJ, Schiemann AL, et al. Enhancement of glucose disposal in patients with type 2 diabetes by alpha-lipoic acid. *Arzneimittelforschung.* 1995;45:872-874. **10.** Jacob S, Ruus P, Hermann R, et al. Oral administration of RAC-alpha-lipoic acid modulates insulin sensitivity in patients with type-2 diabetes mellitus: a placebo-controlled pilot trial. *Free Radic Biol Med.* 1999;27:309-314. **11.** Kawabata T, Packer L. Alpha-lipoate can protect against glycation of serum albumin, but not low density lipoprotein. *Biochem Biophys Res Commun.* 1994;203:99-104. **12.** Nagamatsu M, Nickander KK, Schmelzer JD, et al. Lipoic acid improves nerve blood flow, reduces oxidative stress, and improves distal nerve conduction in experimental diabetic neuropathy. *Diabetes Care.* 1995;18:1160-1167. **13.** Suzuki YJ, Tsuchiya M, Packer L. Lipoate prevents glucose-induced protein modifications. *Free Radical Res Commun.* 1992;17:211-217. **14.** Ziegler D, Hanefeld M, Ruhnau KJ, et al. Treatment of symptomatic diabetic polyneuropathy with the antioxidant alpha-lipoic acid: a 7-month multicenter randomized controlled trial (ALADIN III Study). ALADIN III Study Group. Alpha-Lipoic Acid in Diabetic Neuropathy. *Diabetes Care.* 1999;22:1296-1301. **15.** Ziegler D, Hanefeld M, Ruhnau KJ, et al. Treatment of symptomatic diabetic peripheral neuropathy with the anti-oxidant alpha-lipoic acid. A 3-week multicentre randomized controlled trial (ALADIN Study). *Diabetologia.* 1995;38:1425-1433. **16.** Kahler W, Kuklinski B, Ruhlmann C, et al. Diabetes mellitus-a free radical-associated disease. Results of adjuvant antioxidant supplementation [in German; English abstract]. *Z Gesamte Inn Med.* 1993;48:223-232. **17.** Packer L. Antioxidant properties of lipoic acid and its therapeutic effects in prevention of diabetes complications and cataracts. *Ann N Y Acad Sci.* 1994;738:257-264. **18.** Ziegler D, Gries FA. Alpha-lipoic acid in the treatment of diabetic peripheral and cardiac autonomic neuropathy. *Diabetes.* 1997;46(suppl 2):S62-S66. **19.** Kilic F, Handelman GJ, Serbinova E, et al. Modelling cortical cataractogenesis 17: in vitro effect of a-lipoic acid on glucose-induced lens membrane damage, a model of diabetic cataractogenesis. *Biochem Mol Biol Int.* 1995;37:361-370. **20.** Seidman MD, Khan MJ, Bai U, et al. Biologic activity of mitochondrial metabolites on aging and age-related hearing loss (abstract). *Am J Otol.* 2001;21:161-167.

Melatonin

U.S. BRAND NAMES OF CLINICALLY TESTED PRODUCTS

Not applicable.

DESCRIPTION

Melatonin is a hormone synthesized and secreted by the pineal gland, whose release is decreased in light and increased in darkness. Melatonin is present in plasma and, at a considerably higher concentration, in cerebral spinal fluid (CSF).

PHARMACOLOGY

Melatonin is a neurohormone that is secreted only during the night.[1] Melatonin and the enzymes responsible for its synthesis from serotonin by N-acetylation and 5-methylation have been identified in mammalian pineal tissue, although some melatonin may be synthesized in other parts of the body as well. Melatonin synthesis is controlled by the amount of light registered by the eyes each day via sympathetic nerve stimulation: norepinephrine release acts on nerve endings to increase the activity of enzymes that increase the production and secretion of melatonin.

Orally administered melatonin is rapidly absorbed, and has a relatively short half-life of 30 to 60 minutes with concentrations that peak within 20 minutes of oral ingestion. It is metabolized in the liver to 6-sulfatoxy-melatonin (6-SMT), which is secreted in the urine. Melatonin levels are directly related to circadian rhythms, usually increasing rapidly from the late evening until midnight, then decreasing as morning approaches.

Exogenous use of melatonin is thought to re-entrain the circadian rhythm. The net effect of administration appears to be lowered body temperature, reduced alertness, and increased sleepiness.[2] Some evidence suggests that melatonin may act on the GABA chloride channel complex, mimicking or potentiating the actions of benzodiazepines.[3]

Melatonin has been found to inhibit the growth of estrogen-responsive breast cancer cells in vitro.[4] Although the exact mechanisms are not known, it is believed that melatonin acts to down-regulate estrogen-regulated genes, thereby inhibiting growth of breast tumor cells. Additional studies report that melatonin modulates immune function in cancer patients by activating the cytokine system, which exerts growth-inhibitory properties over a wide range of tumor cell types.[5]

CLINICAL STUDIES

JET LAG

Most but not all studies of melatonin treatment for jet lag have returned positive results.

For example, in a large randomized double-blind placebo-controlled trial, 320 volunteers who had flights over six to eight time zones received placebo or melatonin in a 0.5-mg immediate-release formulation, 5-mg immediate-release formulation, or 2-mg controlled-release formulation, once daily at bedtime for 4 days after the flight.[6] The immediate-release doses appeared to be more effective than the controlled-release formulation. Self-rated sleep quality, sleep latency, fatigue, and daytime sleepiness were all significantly improved with the 5-mg dose of melatonin. In addition, the lower 0.5-mg dose was almost as effective as the 5-mg dose.

Benefits were also seen in smaller double-blind placebo-controlled trials,[7,8,9] including one study that found melatonin more effective than placebo but less effective than zolpidem.[10] However, one double-blind trial investigating placebo versus three regimens of immediate-release melatonin treatment (5 mg at bedtime, 0.5 mg at bedtime, or 0.5 mg taken on a shifting schedule) for jet lag in 237 physicians reported no significant differences between groups for sleep onset, time of awakening, hours slept, or hours napping.[11] A much smaller double-blind trial also found no benefit.[12] The explanation for these discrepancies is unclear.

OTHER FORMS OF INSOMNIA

A 4-week double-blind trial evaluated melatonin as a treatment for chronic sleep-onset insomnia in children.[13] A total of 40 children who had experienced this condition for at least a year were given either placebo or melatonin at a dose of 5 mg. The results showed that use of melatonin significantly improved sleep onset and other sleep measures. Benefits were also seen in a double-blind placebo-controlled trial of 20 developmentally disabled children with sleep problems, in which melatonin (5 mg) improved sleep latency.[14]

Individuals who frequently stay up late on Friday and Saturday night may find it difficult to fall asleep at a reasonable hour on Sunday. A small double-blind, placebo-controlled trial found that this delayed sleep pattern caused a phase-delay in endogenous melatonin secretion, and that use of supplemental melatonin 5.5 hours before the desired Sunday bedtime improved sleep latency.[15]

A double-blind placebo-controlled study of 34 individuals who regularly used benzodiazepines for sleep found that controlled-release melatonin at a dose of 2 mg nightly aided drug discontinuation.[16] (See also Drug Interactions).

Small controlled studies using melatonin have found improved sleep in diabetics with insomnia,[17] ICU patients,[18] schizophrenics with disturbed sleep patterns,[19] and individuals with Delayed Sleep Phase Syndrome (DSPS).[20] However, research regarding possible benefits of melatonin in ordinary insomnia in healthy adults and in insomnia related to shift work has returned inconsistent results.[21-27]

PERIOPERATIVE ANXIETY

In a randomized double-blind placebo-controlled study of perioperative effects of premedication in 75 women, patients who received either 15 mg midazolam or 5 mg melatonin had a significant decrease in anxiety levels before and after surgery as compared to placebo.[28] Except for greater preoperative sedation in the midazolam group, the two treatments were equally effective. Similar results were seen in a subsequent double-blind trial conducted by the same researcher with 84 women.[29]

CANCER TREATMENT

Preliminary evidence suggests that adjunctive use of melatonin may improve results as well as prevent some of the side effects of standard cancer therapy.[5,30-33] For example, a large randomized trial including 250 metastatic solid tumor patients with poor clinical status studied the effects of melatonin treatment in conjunction with chemotherapy.[33] Patients received melatonin (20 mg/day orally) plus chemotherapy, or chemotherapy alone. The 1-year survival rate and tumor regression rates were significantly higher in patients receiving melatonin treatment with chemotherapy. In addition, concomitant use of melatonin significantly reduced the frequency of side effects such as thrombocytopenia, neurotoxicity, cardiotoxicity, stomatitis, and asthenia.

PROPOSED INDICATIONS AND USAGE

A fairly large (but not entirely consistent) body of research suggests that melatonin is useful in the treatment of jet lag. Less convincing evidence suggests that melatonin is helpful for other forms of insomnia. It might also be useful for individuals withdrawing from conventional insomnia therapy, such as benzodiazepines. In addition, melatonin has shown some promise as a presurgical antianxiety treatment.

Weak evidence suggests that melatonin might have value as an adjunctive therapy for some forms of cancer.

A large body of research suggests that melatonin levels decline with age.[34-36] Based on these findings, as well as animal research, melatonin has been marketed as an anti-aging supplement. However, the basis of this hypothesis has been questioned in a more rigorous, tightly controlled study of healthy older subjects, in whom no significant difference in circulating plasma melatonin levels was observed when compared to healthy younger individuals.[37]

Highly preliminary evidence suggests that melatonin might be useful in the treatment of mood disorders, epilepsy, and Alzheimer's disease.[38-41] Even weaker evidence suggests that melatonin may enhance humoral and cell-mediated immunity.[42] Melatonin has also been proposed as a treatment for tardive dyskinesia, but a small 4-week double-blind trial found no evidence of benefit.[43]

WARNINGS

Daytime use of melatonin may cause sedation and therefore impair ability to drive and operate heavy machinery.[18,44]

PRECAUTIONS

Melatonin may reduce mental attention for about 6 hours after use, reducing vigilance and possibly impairing balance.[18,44] For this reason, the usual cautions regarding operating machinery while under the influence of sedative drugs apply to melatonin as well.

A double-blind placebo-controlled study of post-menopausal women found evidence that melatonin use at a dose of 1 mg each morning for 2 days impaired insulin sensitivity and glucose tolerance.[45] However, a longer study using the more typical qhs dosing found melatonin safe and effective in diabetes.[17]

The long-term safety of exogenous melatonin remains unknown. Maximum safe doses in pregnant or lactating women, young children, or individuals with severe hepatic or renal disease have not been determined.

DRUG INTERACTIONS

Benzodiazepine drugs may impair melatonin release.[46,47] In addition, melatonin may mimic some actions of benzodiazepines.[3] It has been suggested that, for this reason, melatonin may be particularly useful for individuals withdrawing from benzodiazepine drugs.[16,26]

ADVERSE REACTIONS

A safety study found that melatonin at a dose of 10 mg/day produced no toxic effects when given to 40 healthy males for a period of 28 days.[48]

A comparison of 12 healthy volunteers and 12 sleep-disorder patients who had been taking melatonin for 1 year found differences in levels of prolactin and LH between the two groups.[49] However, because this was an observational trial, no information on causality can be inferred.

PROPOSED DOSAGE AND ADMINISTRATION

Studies of melatonin for insomnia have employed various doses, ranging from 0.1 mg to several milligrams daily, taken at or within 2 hours of bedtime.

The optimum dose is not clear, but may lie in the range of 0.5 mg to 5 mg. In some studies of jet lag, melatonin use was begun prior to return home and then continued for several days; others started only upon return; and more complex dosing schedules have been tried as well, but the optimum schedule is not known. For presurgical anxiolysis, a 5-mg dose has been tried.

Melatonin is available in two formulations: immediate-release gelatin capsules that produce a spike in blood melatonin levels followed by rapid elimination, and controlled-release capsules that more closely mimic endogenous release. The relative value of each type for various uses has not been fully elucidated, as both positive and negative results have been seen with each form. However, evidence from a small double-blind trial in children suggests that immediate-release melatonin helps in falling asleep, while controlled-release melatonin helps in staying asleep.[50]

PATIENT INFORMATION

Melatonin is a hormone sold as a dietary supplement. There is some evidence that it may be helpful for jet lag and other sleep problems, although study results are conflicting. Melatonin has not been shown to be safe for long-term use.

The maximum safe dosage of melatonin for pregnant or nursing women or young children has not been established. Individuals with severe liver or kidney disease should consult a physician before using this (or any other) supplement.

REFERENCES

1. Guardiola-Lemaitre B. Toxicology of melatonin. *J Biol Rhythms.* 1997;12:697-706. **2.** Lamberg L. Melatonin potentially useful but safety, efficacy remain uncertain. *JAMA.* 1996;276:1011-1014. **3.** Sack RL, Hughes RJ, Edgar DM, et al. Sleep-promoting effects of melatonin: at what dose, in whom, under what conditions, and by what mechanisms? *Sleep.* 1997;20:908-915. **4.** Molis TM, Spriggs LL, Jupiter Y, et al. Melatonin modulation of estrogen-regulated proteins, growth factors, and proto-oncogenes in human breast cancer. *J Pineal Res.* 1995;18:93-103. **5.** Neri B, De Leonardis V, Gemelli MT, et al. Melatonin as biological response modifier in cancer patients. *Anticancer Res.* 1998;18:1329-1332. **6.** Suhner A, Schlagenhauf P, Johnson R, et al. Comparative study to determine the optimal melatonin dosage form for the alleviation of jet lag. *Chronobiol Int.* 1998;15:655-666. **7.** Petrie K, Dawson AG, Thompson L, et al. A double-blind trial of melatonin as a treatment for jet lag in international cabin crew. *Biol Psychiatry.* 1993;33:526-530. **8.** Petrie K, Conaglen JV, Thompson L, et al. Effect of melatonin on jet lag after long haul flights. *BMJ.* 1989;298:705-707. **9.** Claustrat B, Brun J, David M, et al.

Melatonin and jet lag: confirmatory result using a simplified protocol. *Biol Psychiatry.* 1992;32:705-711. **10.** Suhner A, Schlagenhauf P, Hofer I, et al. Effectiveness and tolerability of melatonin and zolpidem for the alleviation of jet lag. *Aviat Space Environ Med.* 2001;72:638-646. **11.** Spitzer RL, Terman M, Williams JB, et al. Jet lag: clinical features, validation of a new syndrome-specific scale, and lack of response to melatonin in a randomized, double-blind trial. *Am J Psychiatry.* 1999;156:1392-1396. **12.** Edwards BJ, Atkinson G, Waterhouse J, et al. Use of melatonin in recovery from jet-lag following an eastward flight across 10 time-zones. *Ergonomics.* 2000;43:1501-1513. **13.** Smits MG, Nagtegaal EE, van der Heijden J, et al. Melatonin for chronic sleep onset insomnia in children: a randomized placebo-controlled trial. *J Child Neurol.* 2001;16:86-92. **14.** Dodge NN, Wilson GA. Melatonin for treatment of sleep disorders in children with developmental disabilities. *J Child Neurol.* 2001;16:581-584. **15.** Yang CM, Spielman AJ, D'Ambrosio P, et al. A single dose of melatonin prevents the phase delay associated with a delayed weekend sleep pattern. *Sleep.* 2001;24:272-281. **16.** Garfinkel D, Zisapel N, Wainstein J, et al. Faciliation of benzodiazepine discontinuation by melatonin:a new clinical approach. *Arch Intern Med.* 1999;159:2456-2460. **17.** Garfinkel D, Wainstein J, Halabe A, et al. Beneficial effect of controlled release melatonin on sleep quality and hemoglobin A1C in type 2 diabetic patients. Presented at: World Congress of Gerontology; July 1-6, 2001; Vancouver, Canada. **18.** Fraschini F, Cesarani A, Alpini D, et al. Melatonin influences human balance. *Biol Signals Recept.* 1999;8:111-119. **19.** Shamir E, Laudon M, Barak Y, et al. Melatonin improves sleep quality of patients with chronic schizophrenia. *J Clin Psychiatry.* 2000;61:373-377. **20.** Kayumov L, Brown G, Jindal R, et al. A randomized, double-blind, placebo-controlled crossover study of the effect of exogenous melatonin on delayed sleep phase syndrome. *Psychosom Med.* 2001;63:40-48. **21.** Folkard S, Arendt J, Clark M. Can melatonin improve shift workers' tolerance of the night shift? Some preliminary findings. *Chronobiol Int.* 1993;10:315-320. **22.** Dawson D, Encel N, Lushington K. Improving adaptation to simulated night shift: timed exposure to bright light versus daytime melatonin administration. *Sleep.* 1995;18:11-21. **23.** Wright SW, Lawrence LM, Wrenn KD, et al. Randomized clinical trial of melatonin after night-shift work: efficacy and neuropsychologic effects. *Ann Emerg Med.* 1998;32:334-340. **24.** MacFarlane JG, Cleghorn JM, Brown GM, et al. The effects of exogenous melatonin on the total sleep time and daytime alertness of chronic insomniacs: a preliminary study. *Biol Psychiatry.* 1991;30:371-376. **25.** James SP, Sack DA, Rosenthal NE, et al. Melatonin administration in insomnia. *Neuropsychopharmacology.* 1990;3:19-23. **26.** Garfinkel D, Laudon M, Zisapel N. Improvement of sleep quality by controlled-release melatonin in benzodiazepine-treated elderly insomniacs. *Arch Gerontol Geriatr.* 1997;24:223-231. **27.** Haimov I, Lavie P, Laudon M, et al. Melatonin replacement therapy of elderly insomniacs. *Sleep.* 1995;18:598-603. **28.** Naguib M, Samarkandi AH. Premedication with melatonin: a double-blind, placebo-controlled comparison with midazolam. *Br J Anaesth.* 1999;82:875-880. **29.** Naguib M, Samarkandi AH. The comparative dose-response effects of melatonin and midazolam for premedication of adult patients: a double-blinded, placebo-controlled study. *Anesth Analg.* 2000;91:473-479. **30.** Lissoni P, Meregalli S, Nosetto L, et al. Increased survival time in brain glioblastomas by a radioneuroendocrine strategy with radiotherapy plus melatonin compared to radiotherapy alone. *Oncology.* 1996;53:43-46. **31.** Lissoni P, Paolorossi F, Ardizzoia A, et al. A randomized study of chemotherapy with cisplatin plus etoposide versus chemoendocrine therapy with cisplatin, etoposide and the pineal hormone melatonin as a first-line treatment of advanced non-small cell lung cancer patients in a poor clinical state. *J Pineal Res.* 1997;23:15-19. **32.** Lissoni P, Tancini G, Barni S, et al. Treatment of cancer chemotherapy-induced toxicity with the pineal hormone melatonin. *Support Care Center.* 1997;5:126-129. **33.** Lissoni P, Barni S, Mandala M, et al. Decreased toxicity and increased efficacy of cancer chemotherapy using the pineal hormone melatonin in metastatic solid tumour patients with poor clinical status. *Eur J Cancer.* 1999;35:1688-1692. **34.** Waldhauser F, Weiszenbacher G, Tatzer E, et al. Alterations in nocturnal serum melatonin levels in humans with growth and aging. *J Clin Endocrinol Metab.* 1988;66:648-652. **35.** Sack RL, Lewy AJ, Erb DL, et al. Human melatonin production decreases with age. *J Pineal Res.* 1986;3:379-388. **36.** Carnazzo G, Paternó-Raddusa F, Travali S, et al. Variations of melatonin incretion in elderly patients affected by cerebral deterioration. *Arch Gerontol Geriatr.* 1991;(suppl 2):123-126. **37.** Zeitzer JM, Daniels JE, Duffy JF, et al. Do plasma melatonin concentrations decline with age? *Am J Med.* 1999;107:432-436. **38.** Fauteck J-D, Schmidt H, Lerchl A, et al. Melatonin in epilepsy: first results of replacement therapy and first clinical results. *Biol Signals Recept.* 1999;8:105-110. **39.** Leibenluft E, Feldman-Naim S, Turner EH, et al. Effects of exogenous melatonin administration and withdrawal in five patients with rapid-cycling bipolar disorder. *J Clin Psychiatry.* 1997;58:383-388. **40.** Molina-Carballo A, Munoz-Hoyos A, Reiter RJ, et al. Utility of high doses of melatonin as adjunctive anticonvulsant therapy in a child with severe myoclonic epilepsy: two years' experience. *J Pineal Res.* 1997;23:97-105. **41.** Pappolla MA, Chyan YJ, Poeggeler B, et al. An assessment of the antioxidant and the antiamyloidogenic properties of melatonin: implications for Alzheimer's disease. *J Neural Transm.* 2000;107:203-231. **42.** Nelson RJ, Demas GE. Role of melatonin in mediating seasonal energetic and immunologic adaptations. *Brain Res Bull.* 1997;44:423-430. **43.** Shamir E, Barak Y, Plopsky I, et al. Is melatonin treatment effective for tardive dyskinesia? *J Clin Psychiatry.* 2000;61:556-558. **44.** Graw P, Werth E, Krauchi K, et al. Early morning melatonin administration impairs psychomotor vigilance. *Behav Brain Res.* 2001;121:167-172. **45.** Cagnacci A, Arangino S, Renzi A, et al. Influence of melatonin administration on glucose tolerance and insulin sensitivity of postmenopausal women. *Clin Endocrinol (Oxf).* 2001;54:339-346. **46.** McIntyre IM, Burrows GD, Norman TR. Suppression of plasma melatonin by a single dose of the benzodiazepine alprazolam in humans. *Biol Psychiatry.* 1988;24: 108-112. **47.** McIntyre IM, Norman TR, Burrows GD, et al. Alterations to plasma melatonin and cortisol after evening alprazolam administration in humans. *Chronobiol Int.* 1993;10:205-213. **48.** Seabra ML V, Bignotto M, Pinto LR Jr, et al. Randomized, double-blind clinical trial, controlled with placebo, of the toxicology of chronic melatonin treatment. *J Pineal Res.* 2000;29:193-200. **49.** Ninomiya T, Iwatani N, Tomoda A, et al. Effects of exogenous melatonin on pituitary hormones in humans. *Clin Physiol.* 2001;21:292-299. **50.** Jan JE, Hamilton D, Seward N, et al. Clinical trials of controlled-release melatonin in children with sleep-wake cycle disorders. *J Pineal Res.* 2000;29:34-39.

Milk Thistle

Silybum Marianum

Alternate/Related Names: Holy Thistle, Wild Artichoke

U.S. BRAND NAMES OF CLINICALLY TESTED PRODUCTS

None.

DESCRIPTION

The milk thistle plant commonly grows from 2 to 7 feet, with spiny leaves and reddish-purple thistle-shaped flowers. It has also been called wild artichoke, holy thistle, and Mary thistle. Native to Europe, milk thistle has a long history of use as both a food and a medicine. At the turn of the twentieth century, English gardeners grew milk thistle to use its leaves like lettuce (after cutting off the spines), the stalks like asparagus, the roasted seeds like coffee, and the roots (soaked overnight) like oyster plant. The seeds and leaves of milk thistle were used for medicinal purposes as well, such as the treatment of jaundice and insufficient lactation.

PHARMACOLOGY

The fruit of the milk thistle plant contains 15% to 30% fatty oils and 20% to 30% proteins. When dried, it contains 1% to 4% of four isomers collectively named silymarin: silibinin (or silybin), isosilybin, silydianin, and silychristin.

After oral administration of milk thistle, about 20% to 50% of the silymarin is absorbed, of which 80% is excreted in the bile and 10% enters the enterohepatic circulation. Steady-state levels are achieved in approximately 24 hours.[1,2] Bioavailability can vary by up to a factor of 2 and peak plasma levels by a factor of 3, depending on the form in which it is manufactured. Silibinin appears to concentrate in the bile, achieving concentrations 60- to 75-fold higher than in plasma.[3]

Numerous animal studies have found that milk thistle extract can protect against toxicity caused by substances as diverse as toluene, xylene, thioacetamide, praseodymium, polycyclic aromatic hydrocarbons, acetaminophen, carbon tetrachloride, phalloidin, and tetrachloromethane.[4-8] Similar results have been seen in humans exposed occupationally to such chemicals.[9,10] One animal study suggests that milk thistle can also protect against fetal damage caused by alcohol.[11] Silybinin is one of the few known antidotes to *Amanita phalloides* mushroom poisoning.[2,8]

Like many free radical scavengers, milk thistle has been found to provide protection from tumors in a well-known skin tumor promotion assay. The authors suggest that this effect of milk thistle may be due to suppression of tumor necrosis factor alpha.[12]

The mechanism of action of milk thistle is unclear. In mushroom poisoning and other hepatotoxic exposure, silymarin may competitively antagonize toxin binding to liver cell membrane receptors.[2] Silymarin also appears to induce liver cell regeneration by binding to a subunit of RNA polymerase in the nucleus, displacing an intrinsic cell regulator and leading to increased ribosomal RNA synthesis. In turn, this leads to increased protein synthesis. In vitro studies suggest that silybinin can stimulate the regeneration of liver cells at a 10-times lower dosage than that required for hepatoprotection.[2] Milk thistle has also been found to inhibit beta-glucuronidase activity in rat hepatocytes.[13] It has been hypothesized that this might protect the liver by inhibiting the hydrolysis of glucuronides. Other proposed actions include scavenging of free radicals, liver cell membrane stabilization, increased liver cell reproduction, suppression of Kupper cell functions, and inhibition of leukotrienes.[14-19]

CLINICAL STUDIES

ALCOHOLIC LIVER DISEASE

Studies of milk thistle in alcoholic liver disease have produced mixed results.

A 1981 double-blind placebo-controlled study followed 106 Finnish soldiers with alcoholic liver disease over a period of 4 weeks.[20] The treated group showed a significant decrease in liver enzyme levels and an improvement in liver histology as evaluated by biopsy in 29 subjects.

Two other double-blind studies also found benefit with milk thistle for alcoholic liver disease.[21,22] However, a 3-month randomized double-blind study of 116 patients found little to no benefit.[23] A similar study found no improvement in 72 patients followed for 15 months.[24]

LIVER CIRRHOSIS

Two 4-year studies of milk thistle for liver cirrhosis found evidence of benefit, although a 2-year study did not.

A double-blind placebo-controlled study followed 146 people with liver cirrhosis for 3 to 6 years. In the group treated with milk thistle, the 4-year survival rate was 58% as compared to only 38% in the placebo group.[25] Another double-blind placebo-controlled trial, which followed 172 individuals with liver cirrhosis for 4 years, also found a significant reduction in mortality.[26] However, a 2-year double-blind placebo-controlled study that followed 125 individuals with alcoholic cirrhosis found no reduction in mortality with milk thistle.[27]

Other double-blind studies of cirrhotic individuals have found reductions in liver enzymes and serum bilirubin.[16,17]

VIRAL HEPATITIS

Small double-blind studies of patients with *chronic* viral hepatitis have found significant improvement in symptoms and signs in the milk-thistle-treated group.[28,29,30]

A 21-day double-blind placebo-controlled study of 57 patients with *acute* viral hepatitis found significant improvements in the group receiving milk thistle.[31] A 35-day study of 151 patients with acute hepatitis using a no-treatment control group found no benefit with milk thistle, but this study has been criticized for failing to document that the participants actually had acute viral hepatitis.[32]

PROTECTION AGAINST HEPATOTOXICITY OF TACRINE

A double-blind placebo-controlled study of 222 individuals with Alzheimer's disease found that 12 weeks of treatment with milk thistle did not prevent elevation of liver enzymes caused by tacrine treatment.[33]

PROPOSED INDICATIONS AND USAGE

Relatively weak evidence supports the use of milk thistle in alcoholic liver disease, liver cirrhosis, and viral hepatitis.

Despite extensive pharmacologic evidence of hepatoprotection, milk thistle has no documented benefits for reducing liver damage in individuals taking potentially hepatotoxic medications. Silibinin has also been investigated as a protective agent against nephrotoxicity induced by chemotherapy with the antitumor agents cisplatin and ifosfamide.[34] Animal studies suggest that renal protection can be achieved without interfering with the antitumor effect of these drugs,[35] but clinical trials have not been reported.

The intravenous form of milk thistle used for deathcap mushroom poisoning is not available in the United States.

WARNINGS

None.

PRECAUTIONS

Safety in young children, pregnant or lactating women, or individuals with severe renal disease has not been formally established. However, on the basis of its extensive food use, milk thistle is believed to be safe in pregnancy and lactation, and researchers have enrolled pregnant women in studies.[36]

DRUG INTERACTIONS

Silibinin may inhibit bacterial beta-glucuronidase activity.[13] For this reason, it is possible that alterations in clearance of agents (such as oral contraceptives) whose durations of action depend upon bacterial beta-glucuronidase in the gut might occur. The herb does not appear to affect CYP enzymes at realistic concentrations.

ADVERSE REACTIONS

Milk thistle appears to possess a very low order of toxicity. Animal studies have not shown any adverse effects even when high doses were administered over a long period of time.[37] A study of 2,637 patients reported in 1992 showed a low incidence of side effects, limited primarily to mild gastrointestinal disturbance.[38] However, there have been reports of severe abdominal symptoms associated with the use of milk thistle.[39]

PROPOSED DOSAGE AND ADMINISTRATION

The usual dosage of milk thistle is 200 mg 2 or 3 times a day of an extract standardized to contain 70% silymarin.

There is some evidence that silymarin bound to phosphatidylcholine is better absorbed.[1,40] This form is taken at a dose of 100 to 200 mg twice a day.

PATIENT INFORMATION

Milk thistle is an herb marketed for the treatment of liver conditions. Although there is some evidence that milk thistle may be helpful in certain circumstances, study results are conflicting. Milk thistle has definitely not been proven effective for the treatment of hepatitis C.

The safety of milk thistle for pregnant or nursing women or young children has not been established. Individuals with severe liver or kidney disease should consult a physician before using this (or any other) supplement.

REFERENCES

1. Schandalik R, Gatti G, Perucca E. Pharmacokinetics of silybin in bile following administration of silipide and silymarin in cholecystectomy patients. *Arzneimittelforschung.* 1992;42:964-968. **2.** Schulz V, Hansel R, Tyler VE. *Rational Phytotherapy: A Physicians' Guide to Herbal Medicine.* 3rd ed. Berlin, Germany: Springer-Verlag; 1998:215-216, 218. **3.** Lorenz D, Lucker PW, Mennicke WH, et al. Pharmacokinetic studies with silymarin in human serum and bile. *Methods Find Exp Clin Pharmacol.* 1984;6:655-661. **4.** Muriel P, Garciapina T, Perez-Alvarez V, et al. Silymarin protects against paracetamol-induced lipid peroxidation and liver damage. *J Appl Toxicol.* 1992;12:439-442. **5.** Paulova J, Dvorak M, Kolouch F, et al. Evaluation of the hepatoprotective and therapeutic effects of silymarin in an experimental carbon tetrachloride intoxication of liver in dogs [in Czech; English abstract]. *Vet Med (Praha).* 1990;35:629-635. **6.** Rui YC. Advances in pharmacological studies of silymarin. *Mem Inst Oswaldo Cruz.* 1991;86(suppl 2):79-85. **7.** Skakun NP, Moseichuk IP.Clinical pharmacology of legalon [in Russian]. *Vrach Delo.* 1988;5:5-10. **8.** Tuchweber B, Sieck R, Trost W. Prevention of silybin of phalloidin-induced acute hepatoxicity. *Toxicol Appl Pharmacol.* 1979;51:265-275. **9.** Boari C, Montanari FM, Galletti GP, et al. Toxic occupational liver diseases. Therapeutic effects of silymarin [in Italian; English abstract]. *Minerva Med.* 1981;72:2679-2688. **10.** Szilard S, Szentgyorgyi D, Demeter I. Protective effect of Legalon in workers exposed to organic solvents. *Acta Med Hung.* 1988;45:249-256. **11.** La Grange L, Wang M, Watkins R, et al. Protective effects of the flavonoid mixture, silymarin, on fetal rat brain and liver. *J Ethnopharmacol.* 1999;65:53-61. **12.** Zi X, Mukhtar H, Agarwal R. Novel cancer chemopreventive effects of a flavonoid antioxidant silymarin: inhibition of mRNA expression of an endogenous tumor promoter TNF alpha. *Biochem Biophys Res Commun.* 1997;239:334-339. **13.** Kim DH, Jin YH, Park JB, et al. Silymarin and its components are inhibitors of beta-glucuronidase. *Biol Pharm Bull.* 1994;17:443-445. **14.** Deak G, Muzes G, Lang I, et al. Immunomodulator effect of silymarin therapy in chronic alcoholic liver diseases [in Hungarian]. *Orv Hetil.* 1990;131:1291-1292. **15.** Hikino H, et al. Natural Products for liver disease. In: Wagner H, et al. (eds.). Economic and medicinal plant research, Vol 2. New York: Academic Press; 1988:39-72. **16.** Lang I, Nekan K, Deak G, et al. Immunomodulatory and hepatoprotective effects of in vivo treatment with free radical scavengers. *Ital J Gastroenterol Hepatol.* 1990;22:283-287. **17.** Lang I, Nekam K, Gonzalez-Cabello R, et al. Hepatoprotective and immunological effects of antioxidant drugs. *Tokai J Exp Clin Med.* 1990;15:123-127. **18.** Muzes G, Deak G, Lang I, et al. Effects of silymarin (Legalon) therapy on the antioxidant defense mechanism and lipid peroxidation in alcoholic liver disease [in Hungarian]. *Orv Hetil.* 1990;131:863-866. **19.** Dehmlow C, Erhard J, de Groot H. Inhibition of Kupffer cell functions as an explanation for the hepatoprotective properties of silibinin. *Hepatology.* 1996;23:749-754. **20.** Salmi HA, Sarna S. Effect of silymarin on chemical, functional, and morphological alterations of the liver. A double-blind controlled study. *Scand J Gastroenterol.* 1982;17:517-521. **21.** Feher J, Deak G, Muzes G, et al. Liver-protective action of silymarin therapy in chronic alcoholic liver diseases [in Hungarian]. *Orv Hetil.* 1989;130:2723-2727. **22.** Fintelmann V, Albert A. Proof of the therapeutic efficacy of Legalon(r) for toxic liver illnesses in a double-blind trial [translated from German]. *Therapiewoche.* 1980;30:5589-5594. **23.** Trinchet J, Coste T, Levy VG, et al. Treatment of alcoholic hepatitis with silymarin. A double-blind comparative study in 116 patients [translated from French]. *Gastroenterol Clin Biol.* 1989;13:120-124. **24.** Bunout D, Hirsch S, Petermann M, et al. The controlled study of the effect of silymarin on alcholic liver disease [translated from Spanish]. *Rev Med Chil.* 1992;120:1370-1376. **25.** Ferenci P, Dragosics B, Dittrich H, et al. Randomized controlled trial of silymarin treatment in patients with cirrhosis of the liver. *J Hepatol.* 1989;9:105-113. **26.** Benda L, Dittrich H, Ferenzi P, et al. The influence of therapy with silymarin on the survival rate of patients with liver cirrhosis [translated from German]. *Wien Klin Wochenschr.* 1980;92:678-683. **27.** Pares A, Planas R, Torres M, et al. Effects of silymarin in alcoholic patients with cirrhosis of the liver: results of a controlled, double-blind, randomized and multicenter trial. *J Hepatol.* 1998;28:615-621. **28.** Berenguer J, Carrasco D. Double-blind trial of silymarin vs. placebo in the treatment of chronic hepatitis. *MMW Munch Med Wochenschr.* 1977;119:240-260. **29.** Buzzelli G, Moscarella S, Giusti A, et al. A pilot study on the liver protective effect of silybinphosphatidylcholine complex (IdB1016) in chronic active hepatitis. *Int J Clin Pharmacol Ther Toxicol.* 1993;31:456-460. **30.** Lirussi F, Okolicsanyi L. Cytoprotection in the nineties: experience with ursodeoxycholic acid and silymarin in chronic liver disease. *Acta Physiol Hung.* 1992;80:363-367. **31.** Magliulo E, Gagliardi B, Fiori GP. Results of a double blind study on the effect of silymarin in the treatment of acute viral hepatitis, carried out at two medical centres [translated from German]. *Med Klin.* 1978;73:1060-1065. **32.** Bode JC, Schmidt U, Durr HK. Silymarin for the treatment of acute viral hepatitis? Report of a controlled trial [translated from German]. *Med Klin.* 1977;72:513-518. **33.** Allain H, Schuck S, Lebreton S, et al. Aminotransferase levels and silymarin in de novo tacrine-treated patients with Alzheimer's disease. *Dement Geriatr Cogn Disord.* 1999;10:181-185. **34.** Sonnenbichler J, Scalera F, Sonnenbichler I, et al. Stimulatory effects of silibinin and silicristin from the milk thistle Silybum marianum on kidney cells. *J Pharmacol Exp Ther.* 1999;290:1375-1383. **35.** Bokemeyer C, Fels LM, Dunn T, et al. Silibinin protects against cisplatin-induced nephrotoxicity without compromising cisplatin or ifosfamide anti-tumour activity. *Br J Cancer.* 1996;74:2036-2041. **36.** Giannola C, Buogo F, Forestiere G, et al. A two-center study on the effects of silymarin in pregnant women and adult patients with so-called minor hepatic insufficiency [in Italian; English abstract]. *Clin Ter.* 1985;114:129-135. **37.** Awang D. Milk thistle. *Can Pharm J.* 1993;422:403-404. **38.** Albrecht M, Frerick H, Kuhn U, et al. Therapy of toxic liver pathologies with Legalon(r) [in German; English abstract]. *Z Klin Med.* 1992;47:87-92. **39.** Adverse Drug Reactions Advisory Committee. An adverse reaction to the herbal medication milk thistle (Silybum marianum). *MJA.* 1999;170:218-219. **40.** Barzaghi N, Crema F, Gatti G, et al. Pharmacokinetic studies on IdB 1016, a silybin- phosphatidylcholine complex, in healthy human subjects. *Eur J Drug Metab Pharmacokinet.* 1990;15:333-338.

Oligomeric Proanthocyanidin Complexes (OPCs)

Alternate/Related Names: Grape Seed, PCOs (Procyanidolic Oligomers), Maritime Pine Bark *(Pinus pinaster)*, Pycnogenol

U.S. BRAND NAMES OF CLINICALLY TESTED PRODUCTS

Grape Seed (PCO) Extract (PhytoPharmica/Enzymatic Therapy), Grapenol (Solaray), Grapeseed Extract (Thorne Research) =

Endotelon (Sanofi/Labaz), LeucoSelect (Indena) in Europe

Pycnogenol (Horphag) (U.S. product only)

DESCRIPTION

One of the best-selling herbal products of the early 1990s was Pycnogenol, a term that in the United States refers to an extract of the bark of the French maritime pine. In France, however, the same copyrighted term refers to a grape seed extract. Both products contain a family of chemicals known as OPCs (oligomeric proanthocyanidin complexes) or PCOs (procyanidolic oligomers). OPCs are more economically extracted from grape seed than from pine bark.

OPCs are flavonoid-like molecules found in numerous plants. Some of the most abundant sources are grape seed and maritime pine bark. Other food sources include hawthorn flowers, various berries, onions, legumes, red wine, and parsley, and related chemicals are found in bilberry.

PHARMACOLOGY

The OPC family includes a variety of proanthocyanidins that are bound to each other in dimer, trimer, and larger molecules. Collectively, they are known as oligomeric proanthocyanidin complexes.

In vitro studies suggest that OPCs increase collagen cross-linking, decrease capillary permeability, and block the effects of hyaluronidase, elastase, collagenase, and other enzymes that degrade connective tissue.[1-6] In addition, they appear to chelate free iron molecules, prevent iron-potentiated lipid peroxidation, slow free radical production by reversibly inhibiting xanthine oxidase, and reduce the release and production of histamine and leukotrienes. OPCs' antioxidant effects occur in both polar and nonpolar media. However, the clinical relevance of these findings has yet to be established.

CLINICAL STUDIES

VENOUS INSUFFICIENCY

A double-blind placebo-controlled study evaluated the effects of a grape seed OPC formulation on 92 patients with chronic venous insufficiency over 4 weeks.[7] Although improvement of subjective symptoms and edema was statistically significant in the treated group compared to the placebo group, there was no statistically significant difference in venous plethysmography scores.

A 2-month double-blind placebo-controlled trial of 40 individuals with chronic venous insufficiency found that use of Pycnogenol significantly reduced edema, pain, and the sensation of leg heaviness.[8]

A very poorly reported placebo-controlled study on file with an OPC manufacturer enrolled 364 individuals with chronic venous insufficiency and apparently found evidence of benefit with OPC treatment.[9]

A 1-month double-blind comparative study of 50 patients with venous insufficiency of the legs demonstrated that OPCs were more effective in reducing symptoms and signs than the citrus bioflavonoid diosmin.[10] However, diosmin is not a well-established treatment for venous insufficiency.

EDEMA

A double-blind placebo-controlled study of 63 postoperative breast cancer patients with lymphedema found that use of grape seed OPCs daily for 6 months reduced edema, pain, and paresthesias.[11]

In a double-blind placebo-controlled study of 32 facial cosmetic surgery patients followed for 10 days, treatment with grape seed OPCs produced a statistically significant difference in rate of edema disappearance.[12]

A 10-day double-blind placebo-controlled study of 50 individuals with sports injuries found that grape seed OPCs improved the rate of edema disappearance.[13]

ATHEROSCLEROSIS

Numerous animal studies suggest that OPCs may retard or reverse atherosclerosis.[5,14-16] One crossover study of 22 subjects found that 100 mg of Pycnogenol or 500 mg of aspirin were equally effective in countering increased platelet aggregation caused by smoking.[17]

One often-cited epidemiological study found an association between *dietary* flavonoids and decreased cardiovascular mortality.[18] However, the primary sources of flavonoids in this study were black tea and apples, which do not contain large quantities of OPCs.

PROPOSED INDICATIONS AND USAGE

Preliminary evidence suggests that orally administered OPCs may be useful for chronic venous insufficiency and for speeding resolution of post-surgical or sports injury-related edema.

OPC products are advertised as "natural antihistamines," but an 8-week double-blind placebo-controlled trial of 49 individuals found no benefit with oral grape seed extract in the treatment of allergic rhinitis.[19]

In addition, OPCs have been marketed as an oral treatment for diabetic retinopathy, macular degeneration, capillary fragility, allergic rhinitis, and heart disease prevention. Topical products containing OPCs are widely marketed with claims that they can improve skin appearance and elasticity. However, the supportive evidence for all of these uses is weak to nonexistent.

WARNINGS

None.

PRECAUTIONS

Maximum safe dosage in young children, pregnant or lactating women, and individuals with severe hepatic or renal disease has not been established.

DRUG INTERACTIONS

Based on the activity of other flavonoids, OPCs might potentiate the effects of anticoagulant and antiplatelet agents.

ADVERSE REACTIONS

In the double-blind studies of OPCs, no significant adverse reactions were seen, and the side-effect profile was similar to that of placebo. Extensive studies have shown OPCs to be essentially nontoxic, with an LD_{50} in rats and mice exceeding 4,000 mg/kg.[20] OPCs also appear to be nonteratogenic and nonmutagenic.

PROPOSED DOSAGE AND ADMINISTRATION

OPCs are generally taken in an oral dose of 150 to 600 mg daily. Topical creams are applied 1 to 2 times daily.

PATIENT INFORMATION

OPCs are an expensive supplement marketed for a great number of conditions. Weak evidence suggests that OPCs may be helpful for venous insufficiency (a condition related to varicose veins) as well as for swelling following surgery or sports injuries. Other uses of OPCs, such as preventing heart disease or improving skin tone, have no meaningful supporting evidence at all. One study found OPCs ineffective for allergies.

The maximum safe dosage of OPCs for pregnant or nursing women or young children has not been established. Individuals with severe liver or kidney disease should consult a physician before using this (or any other) supplement.

REFERENCES

1. Maffei Facino R, Carini M, Aldini G, et al. Free radicals scavenging action and anti-enzyme activities of procyanidines from Vitis vinifera. A mechanism for their capillary protective action. *Arzneimittelforschung.* 1994;44:592-601. **2.** Kuttan R, Donnelly RV, Di Ferrante N. Collagen treated with (+)-catechin becomes resistant to the action of mammalian collagenase. *Experientia.* 1981;37:221-223. **3.** Masquelier J. Procyanidolic oligomers (Leucocyanidins) [translated from French]. *Parfums Cosmetiques Aromes.* 1990;95:89-97. **4.** Masquelier J, Dumon MC, Dumas J. Stabilization of collagen by procyanidolic oligomers [in French; English abstract]. *Acta Ther.* 1981;7:101-105. **5.** Schwitters B, et al. *OPC in practice. Bioflavanols and their applications.* Rome, Italy: Alfa Omega; 1993. **6.** Tixier JM, Godeau G, Robert AM, et al. Evidence by in vivo and in vitro studies that binding of pycnogenols to elastin affects its rate of degradation by elastases. *Biochem Pharmacol.* 1984;33:3933-3939. **7.** Thebaut JF, Thebaut P, Vin F. Study of Endotelon (r) in functional manifestations of peripheral venous insufficiency. Results of a doulbe-blind study of 92 patients [translated from French]. *Gaz Med.* 1985;92:96-100. **8.** Arcangeli P. Pycnogenol (r) in chronic venous insufficiency. *Fitoterapia.* 2000;71:236-244. **9.** Henriet JP. Exemplary study for a phlebotropic substance, the EIVE study [translated from French]. Fairfield, Conn: Primary Source; not dated. **10.** Delacroix P. Double-blind study of Endotelon (r) in chronic venous insufficiency [translated from French]. *La Revue de Medecine.* 1981;22:1793-1802. **11.** Pecking A, Desprez-Curely JP, Megret G. Oligomeric grape flavanols (Endotelon (r)) in the treatment of secondary upper limb lymphedemas [translated from French]. Paris, France: Association de Lymphologie de Lange Francaise Hopital Saint-Louis. *misc.*1989:69-73. **12.** Baruch J. Effect of Endotelon(r) in postoperative edema. Results of a double-blind study versus placebo in 32 female patients [translated from French]. *Ann Chir Plast Esthet.* 1984;29:393-395. **13.** Parienti JJ, Parienti-Amsellem J (1983). Post-traumatic edemas in sports: a controlled test of Endotelon([translated from French]. *Gaz Med Fr.* 1983;90:231-235. **14.** Gendre PMJ, Laparra J, Barraud E. Procyanidolic oligomer preventive action on experimental lathyrism in the rat [in French; English abstract]. *Ann Pharm Fr.* 1985;43:61-71. **15.** Uchida S, Edamatsu R, Hiramatsu M, et al. Condensed tannins scavenge active oxygen free radicals. *Med Sci Res.* 1987;15:831-832. **16.** Wegrowski J, Robert AM, Moczar M. The effect of procyanidolic oligomers on the composition of normal and hypercholesterolemic rabbit aortas. *Biochem Pharmacol.* 1984;33:3491-3497. **17.** Putter M, Grotemeyer KH, Wurthwein G, et al. Inhibition of smoking-induced platelet aggregation by aspirin and pycnogenol. *Thromb Res.* 1999;95:155-161. **18.** Hertog MG, Feskens EJ, Hollman PC, et al. Dietary antioxidant flavonoids and risk of coronary heart disease: the Zutphen Elderly Study. *Lancet.* 1993;342:1007-1011. **19.** Bernstein CK, Deng C, Shuklah R, et al. Double blind placebo controlled (DBPC) study of grapeseed extract in the treatment of seasonal allergic rhinitis (SAR) [abstract]. *J Allergy Clin Immunol.* 2001;107:abstr 1018. **20.** Schulz V, Hansel R, Tyler VE. *Rational Phytotherapy: A Physicians' Guide to Herbal Medicine.* 3rd ed. Berlin, Germany: Springer-Verlag; 1998:282-284.

Phosphatidylserine

U.S. BRAND NAMES OF CLINICALLY TESTED PRODUCTS

None.

DESCRIPTION

Phosphatidylserine (PS) is one of many phospholipids involved in the structure and maintenance of cell membranes. Exogenous PS has been used in Italy, Scandinavia, and other parts of Europe to treat various forms of age-related dementia as well as normal age-related memory loss.

PHARMACOLOGY

Phosphatidylserine is formed in the body from the amino acid L-serine. The pharmacokinetics of orally administered PS have not been well studied.

In mice and rats, supplemental PS has been found to produce improvement in various measures of brain function[1-4] and to retard age-related changes in the hippocampus and septal complex.[5] Exogenously administered PS stimulates acetylcholine release from the cerebral cortex of rats.[6] Dopaminergic effects have also been observed.[7]

In addition, PS has been implicated as a universal signal for apoptotic cell death when the phospholipid is translocated from the inner layer to the outer layer of the cell membrane.[8] The outer membrane presentation of the phospholipid is a signal for the damaged cell to be phagocytized by macrophages. Thus exogenous extracellular PS might serve as a decoy for macrophages and prevent unnecessary tissue degradation when macrophages are activated. This novel model is supported by earlier work demonstrating suppression of macrophage phagocytic function by PS.[9]

Phosphatidylserine supplements were initially manufactured from bovine brain tissue. However, at the present time, PS is produced from soybeans and marketed in a complex containing other compounds, such as phosphatidylcholine and phosphatidylethanolamine. Virtually all clinical trials of exogenous PS used the older bovine source; it is not clear whether the current product is biologically equivalent. It has been suggested that the bioactivity of PS is due to the invariant front end of the molecule rather than the variable tail, which would suggest equivalent efficacy.[10,11,12] However, animal efficacy studies have yielded conflicting results.[13,14,15]

CLINICAL STUDIES

All the research described in this section involved bovine-derived PS. As described in the Pharmacology section, the relevance of these results to the current soy-based source is questionable.

DEMENTIA

Double-blind trials of supplemental PS involving a total of about 1,000 individuals with dementia have been conducted, with generally positive results.[16-23]

The largest followed 494 elderly patients (65 to 93 years old), recruited from 23 geriatric and general medicine centers in northeastern Italy, over a course of 6 months.[16] Participants suffered from moderate to severe cognitive decline based on the Mini Mental State Examination and Global Deterioration Scale. Half of the participants were given 300 mg PS daily, and evaluation over the course of treatment showed statistically significant improvements in both behavior and cognition in the treated group compared to the placebo group.

MILD TO MODERATE COGNITIVE IMPAIRMENT

A double-blind placebo-controlled trial evaluated the effect of supplemental PS in 149 individuals aged 50 to 75 whose degree of cognitive impairment fell short of clinical dementia.[24] The results over a 12-week period showed improvements with PS treatment in various measures of cognitive function, most strongly among the more impaired participants.

DEPRESSION

One small double-blind crossover study suggests that supplemental PS can be useful in geriatric patients with depression.[25] Improvements in affective symptoms were also seen in many of the studies of PS for dementia.

ATHLETIC OVERTRAINING SYNDROME

Intense exercise stimulates release of cortisol, inducing a catabolic state. Preliminary studies suggest that supplemental PS can blunt the cortisol response to heavy physical exercise, possibly allowing more rapid muscle development in bodybuilding and other forms of athletic training, and reduce symptoms of overtraining syndrome.[26,27,28]

PROPOSED INDICATIONS AND USAGE

Significant evidence from European trials supports the use of PS for dementia. One double-blind trial suggests that it might also offer benefits for more mild age-related memory loss. However, there is no evidence that supplemental PS can "increase brain power" in the young, despite the fact that it is extensively marketed for that purpose.

The potential sports usages of PS have not been evaluated in clinical trials.

WARNINGS

None.

PRECAUTIONS

Phosphatidylserine has been found to be nonteratogenic in rats and rabbits.[29] Nonetheless, safety in pregnant or lactating women has not been established. Safety in young children or individuals with severe hepatic or renal disease has also not been established.

DRUG INTERACTIONS

In vitro studies have shown that fatty acid esters of PS and phosphatidylethanolamine can synergistically stimulate the anticoagulant effect of heparin.[30]

ADVERSE REACTIONS

Phosphatidylserine is generally regarded as safe. In clinical trials, side effects were rare and nonspecific. Oral dosages in rodent and dog studies showed no defined organ system toxicity, and LD_{50} values were either not determinable or very high.[29] Mutagenic testing was negative.

PROPOSED DOSAGE AND ADMINISTRATION

The standard dose of PS is 100 mg t.i.d.; however, some studies have used 200 mg b.i.d. Phosphatidylserine can be taken with or without food.

PATIENT INFORMATION

Phosphatidylserine (PS) is a supplement sold as a "brain booster." Some evidence suggests that phosphatidylserine may improve mental function in individuals with Alzheimer's disease or related conditions. Keep in mind, however, that there are numerous possible causes of mental decline in the elderly, some of which require specific treatment. For this reason, a full medical work-up is necessary before using PS.

Weak evidence suggests that PS may be helpful for mild memory loss in older individuals. However, supplemental PS has not been shown effective for improving memory or mental function in young or middle-aged people.

Phosphatidylserine should not be taken by individuals using the blood-thinning drug heparin.

The safety of phosphatidylserine for pregnant or nursing women or young children has not been established. Individuals with severe liver or kidney disease should consult a physician before using this (or any other) supplement.

REFERENCES

1. Fagioli S, Castellano C, Oliverio A, et al. Phosphatidylserine administration during postnatal development improves memory in adult mice. *Neurosci Lett.* 1989;101:229-233. **2.** Valzelli L, Kozak W, Zanotti A, et al. Activity of phosphatidylserine on memory retrieval and on exploration in mice. *Methods Find Exp Clin Pharmacol.* 1987;9:657-660. **3.** Valzelli L, Kozak W, Giraud O. Difference in learning and retention by Albino-Swiss mice. Part IV. Effect of some nutrients. *Methods Find Exp Clin Pharmacol.* 1987;9:5-8. **4.** Zanotti A, Valzelli L, Toffano G. Chronic phosphatidylserine treatment improves spatial memory and passive avoidance in aged rats. *Psychopharmacology (Berl).* 1989;99:316-321. **5.** Nunzi MG, Milan F, Guidolin D, et al. Effects of phosphatidylserine administration of aged-related structural changes in the rat hippocampus and septal complex. *Pharmacopsychiatry.* 1989;22(suppl 2):125-128. **6.** Casamenti F, Mantovani P, Amaducci L, et al. Effect of phosphatidylserine on acetylcholine output from the cerebral cortex of the rat. *J Neurochem.* 1979;32:529-533. **7.** Calderini G, Bellini F, Consolazione A, et al. Reparative processes in aged brain. *Gerontology.* 1987;33:227-233. **8.** Martin SJ, Reutelingsperger CP, McGahon AJ, et al. Early redistribution of plasma membrane phosphatidylserine is a general feature of apoptosis regardless of the initiating stimulus: inhibition by overexpression of Bcl-2 and Abl. *J Exp Med.* 1995;182:1545-1556. **9.** Palatini P, Viola G, Bigon E, et al. Pharmacokinetic characterization of phosphatidylserine liposomes in the rat. *Br J Pharmacol.* 1991;102:345-350. **10.** Kidd PM. Phosphatidylserine; membrane nutrient for memory. A clinical and mechanistic assessment. *Altern Med Rev.* 1996;1:70-84. **11.** LaBrake CC, Fung LW. Phospholipid vesicles promote human hemoglobin oxidation. *J Biol Chem.* 1992;267:16703-16711. **12.** Orlando P, Cerrito F, Zirilli P. The fate of double-labeled brain phospholipids administered to mice. *Il Farmaco (Edizione Practica).* 1975;30:451-458. **13.** Mantovani P, et al. Investigations into the relationship between phospholipids and brain acetylcholine. In G Porcellati et al, eds. Function and metabolism of phospholipids in the central and peripheral nervous systems. New York: Plenum Press; 1976:285-292. **14.** Toffano G, Leon A, Benvegnu D, et al. Effect of brain cortex phospholipids on catechol-amine content of mouse brain. *Pharmacol Res Commun.* 1976;8:581-590. **15.** Blokland A, Honig W, Brouns F, et al. Cognition-enhancing properties of subchronic phosphatidylserine (PS) treatment in middle-aged rats: comparison of bovine cortex PS with egg PS and soybean PS. *Nutrition.* 1999;15:778-783. **16.** Cenacchi T, Bertoldin T, Farina C, et al. Cognitive decline in the elderly: a double-blind, placebo-controlled multicenter study on efficacy of phosphatidylserine administration. *Aging (Milano).* 1993;5:123-133. **17.** Amaducci L. Phosphatidylserine in the treatment of Alzheimer's disease: results of a multicenter study. *Psychopharmacol Bull.* 1988;24:130-134. **18.** Crook T, Petrie W, Wells C, et al. Effects of phosphatidylserine in Alzheimer's Disease. *Psychopharmacol Bull.* 1992;28:61-66. **19.** Delwaide PJ, Gyselynck-Mambourg AM, Hurlet A, et al. Double-blind randomized controlled study of phosphatidylserine in senile demented patients. *Acta Neurol Scand.* 1986;73:136-140. **20.** Engel RR, Satzger W, Gunther W, et al. Double-blind cross-over study of phosphatidylserine vs. placebo in patients with early dementia of the Alzheimer type. *Eur Neuropsychopharmacol.* 1992;2:149-155. **21.** Funfgeld EW, Baggen M, Nedwidek P, et al. Double-blind study with phosphatidylserine (PS) in Parkinsonian patients with senile dementia of Alzheimer's type (SDAT). *Prog Clin Biol Res.* 1989;317:1235-1246. **22.** Palmieri G, Palmieri R, Inzoli MR, et al. Double-blind controlled trial of phosphatidylserine in patients with senile mental deterioration. *Clin Trials J.* 1987;24:73-83. **23.** Villardita C, Grioli S, Salmeri G, et al. Multicentre clinical trial of brain phosphatidylserine in elderly patients with intellectual deterioration. *Clin Trials J.* 1987;24:84-93. **24.** Crook TH, Tinklenberg J, Yesavage J, et al. Effects of phosphatidylserine in age-associated memory impairment. *Neurology.* 1991;41:644-649. **25.** Maggioni M, Picotti GB, Bondiolotti GP, et al. Effects of phosphatidylserine therapy in geriatric patients with depressive disorders. *Acta Psychiatr Scand.* 1990;81:265-270. **26.** Fahey TD, Pearl MS. The hormonal and perceptive effects of phosphatidylserine administration during two weeks of resistive exercise-induced overtraining. *Biol Sport.* 1998;15:135-144. **27.** Monteleone P, Beinat L, Tanzillo C, et al. Effects of phosphatidylserine on the neuroendocrine response to physical stress in humans. *Neuroendocrinology.* 1990;52:243-248. **28.** Monteleone P, Maj M, Beinat L, et al. Blunting by chronic phosphatidylserine administration of the stress-induced activation of the hypothalamo-pituitary-adrenal axis in healthy men. *Eur J Clin Pharmacol.* 1992;41:385-388. **29.** Heywood R, Cozens DD, Richold M. Toxicology of a phosphatidylserine preparation from bovine brain (BC-PS). *Clin Trials J.* 1987;24:25-32. **30.** van den Besselaar AM. Phosphatidylethanolamine and phosphatidylserine synergistically promote heparin's anticoagulant effect. *Blood Coagul Fibrinolysis.* 1995;6:239-244.

Policosanol

Alternate/Related Names: Octacosanol, 1-Octacosanol, N-Octacosanol, Octacosyl Alcohol, Wheat Germ Oil

U.S. BRAND NAMES OF CLINICALLY TESTED PRODUCTS

None.

DESCRIPTION

Policosanol is a mixture of several waxy long-chain alcohols extracted from sugarcane. The most heavily marketed U.S. source of policosanol, Cholestin (previously containing red-yeast rice), states that it derives its policosanol derived from beeswax; this source has not been evaluated in clinical trials.

PHARMACOLOGY

Policosanol contains several higher aliphatic primary alcohols. The main component is octacosanol, followed by triacontanol and hexacosanol.

Policosanol appears to impair cholesterol synthesis between the acetate and mevalonate production steps.[1,2] It may also increase receptor-dependent LDL processing, thereby reducing plasma LDL.

Policosanol reportedly exhibits dose-dependent antiplatelet actions comparable to 100 mg aspirin daily,[3,4,5] and may reduce lipid peroxidation.[6,7]

CLINICAL STUDIES

HYPERLIPIDEMIA

Over 18 double-blind controlled studies, involving a total of about 1,500 individuals and ranging in length from 6 weeks to 12 months, have found policosanol effective for improving lipid profile.[2,3,8-24] Virtually all of these studies were conducted in Cuba by one research group.

For example, a double-blind placebo-controlled trial enrolled 437 individuals with type II hypercholesterolemia.[17] Participants were first placed on a step-1 diet for 5 weeks. Lipid profiles were taken twice within the next 2 weeks and averaged to provide a baseline value. Then, participants received either placebo or policosanol at 5 mg/day for 12 weeks. At that point, the dosage was doubled to 10 mg/day in the treated group, and the study continued for an additional 12 weeks. The results showed significant improvements with both policosanol doses, but greater improvement at the end of the higher-dose period. By the conclusion of the trial, LDL cholesterol in the treated group improved by 25.6%, total cholesterol by 17.4%, HDL cholesterol by 28.4%, and triglycerides by 5.2%. These results were statistically significant as compared to the outcome in the placebo group.

Besides placebo-controlled studies, other double-blind trials comparing policosanol against pravastatin, fluvastatin, simvastatin, and lovastatin have found these agents to be essentially identical in effect on lipid parameters.[3,20-23,25,26]

One small double-blind trial suggests that policosanol is safe and effective for hyperlipidemia in individuals with type 2 diabetes.[2,18]

INTERMITTENT CLAUDICATION

A 2- year double-blind placebo-controlled study of 56 individuals with intermittent claudication found that treatment with policosanol (10 mg twice daily) improved walking distance by more than 50% at 6 months, and the benefits increased over the course of the study.[27] Similar results were seen with policosanol in a 6-month double-blind placebo-controlled study of 62 individuals with intermittent claudication.[28]

PERFORMANCE ENHANCEMENT

A very small double-blind trial of octacosanol for exercise performance enhancement found evidence of benefit in some measures but not others.[29]

PROPOSED INDICATIONS AND USAGE

Numerous double-blind trials conducted in Cuba by one research group indicate that policosanol is an effective treatment for hyperlipidemia. However, the lack of confirmation of these results by other independent researchers makes these results less than fully reliable.

Policosanol may also be helpful for intermittent claudication.

Octacosanol and policosanol are also widely marketed as sports supplements, but there is little evidence for any ergogenic effect. Other proposed uses with minimal or no scientific support include Parkinson's disease and amyotrophic lateral sclerosis.[30,31]

WARNINGS

None.

PRECAUTIONS

Policosanol's antiplatelet effects suggest caution in individuals with bleeding disorders, as well as in the perioperative and peri-labor and delivery period.

The evidence from one human trial suggests that policosanol does not affect hepatic function.[32] Nonetheless, safety in individuals with severe hepatic or renal disease has not been established.

Safety in pregnant or lactating women, or young children, has not been established, although there are no known or suspected risks with policosanol in these populations.

DRUG INTERACTIONS

In studies, policosanol has not interacted with calcium-channel antagonists, diuretics, or beta-blockers.[10] However, policosanol does appear to potentiate the antiplatelet effects of aspirin.[33] Caution should therefore be exercised when combining policosanol with any antiplatelet or anticoagulant agent. It is also possible that policosanol could potentiate the anticoagulant properties of supplements such as garlic, ginkgo, and high-dose vitamin E.

According to one report, octacosanol or policosanol might impair the action of levodopa.[30]

ADVERSE REACTIONS

Policosanol is generally well tolerated. In a drug-monitoring study that followed 27,879 patients for 2 to 4 years, adverse effects were reported in only 0.31% of participants, and were primarily weight loss, excessive urination, and insomnia.[34] No signs of toxicity were observed in animals given very high doses of policosanol (as much as 620 times the maximum recommended dose).[35-38]

PROPOSED DOSAGE AND ADMINISTRATION

Typical dosages of policosanol for lowering elevated cholesterol levels range from 5 to 10 mg twice daily. Results may require 2 months to develop.[14,16] Octacosanol is used at a similar dose.

PATIENT INFORMATION

Policosanol is a supplement marketed for reducing cholesterol. However, all supporting scientific studies were performed by a single research group in Cuba. These studies used policosanol made from sugar cane. The form of policosanol most widely available in the United States is made from beeswax instead, and has not been shown effective.

Policosanol interferes with the ability of the blood to clot. For this reason, it should not be used by individuals with bleeding disorders, or those who use "blood-thinning" medications such as aspirin, warfarin (Coumadin), heparin, clopidogrel (Plavix), or pentoxifylline (Trental). In addition, policosanol might cause problems if it is combined with natural substances that thin the blood, such as garlic, ginkgo, white willow, and vitamin E.

The safety of policosanol for pregnant or nursing women or young children has not been established. Individuals with severe liver or kidney disease should consult a physician before using this (or any other) supplement.

REFERENCES

1. Menendez R, Arruzazabala L, Mas R, et al. Cholesterol-lowering effect of policosanol on rabbits with hypercholesterolaemia induced by a wheat starch-casein diet. *Br J Nutr.* 1997;77:923-932. 2. Torres O, Agramonte AJ, Illnait J, et al. Treatment of hypercholesterolemia in NIDDM with policosanol. *Diabetes Care.* 1995;18:393-397. 3. Castano G, Mas R, Arruzazabala ML, et al. Effects of policosanol and pravastatin on lipid profile, platelet aggregation and endothelemia in older hypercholesterolemic patients. *Int J Clin Pharmacol Res.* 1999;19:105-116. 4. Arruzazabala ML, Mas R, Molina V, et al. Effect of policosanol on platelet aggregation in type II hypercholesterolemic patients. *Int J Tissue React.* 1998;20:119-124. 5. Arruzazabala ML, Valdes S, Mas R, et al. Effect of policosanol successive dose increases on platelet aggregation in healthy volunteers. *Pharmacol Res.* 1996;34:181-185. 6. Menendez R, Fraga V, Amor AM, et al. Oral administration of policosanol inhibits in vitro copper ion-induced rat lipoprotein peroxidation. *Physiol Behav.* 1999;67:1-7. 7. Fraga V, Menendez R, Amor AM, et al. Effect of policosanol on in vitro and in vivo rat liver microsomal lipid peroxidation. *Arch Med Res.* 1997;28:355-360. 8. Aneiros E, Mas R, Calderon B, et al. Effect of policosanol in lowering cholesterol levels in patients with type II hypercholesterolemia. *Curr Ther Res.* 1995;56:176-182. 9. Castano G, Canetti M, Moreira M, et al. Efficacy and tolerability of policosanol in elderly patients with type II hypercholesterolemia: a 12 month study. *Curr Ther Res.* 1995;56:819-828. 10. Castano G, Tula L, Canetti M, et al. Effects of policosanol in hypertensive patients with type II hypercholesterolemia. *Curr Ther Res.* 1996;57:691-699. 11. Aneiros E, Calderon B, Mas R, et al. Effect of successive dose increases of policosanol on the lipid profile and tolerability of treatment. *Curr Ther Res.* 1993;54:304-312. 12. Castano G, Mas R, Nodarse M, et al. One-year study of the efficacy and safety of policosanol (5 mg twice daily) in the treatment of type II hypercholesterolemia. *Curr Ther Res.* 1995;56:296-304. 13. Batista J, Stusser R, Penichet M, et al. Doppler-ultrasound pilot study of the effects of long-term policosanol therapy on carotid-vertebral atherosclerosis. *Curr Ther Res.* 1995;56:906-914. 14. Pons P, Rodriguez M, Mas R, et al. One-year efficacy and safety of policosanol in patients with type II hypercholesterolemia. *Curr Ther Res.* 1994;55:1084-1092. 15. Pons P, Rodriguez M, Robaina C, et al. Effects of successive dose increases of policosanol on the lipid profile of patients with type II hypercholesterolaemia and tolerability to treatment. *Int J Clin Pharmacol Res.* 1994;14:27-33. 16. Pons P, Mas R, Illnait J, et al. Efficacy and safety of policosanol in patients with primary hypercholesterolemia. *Curr Ther Res.* 1992;52:507-513. 17. Mas R, Castano G, Illnait J, et al. Effects of policosanol in patients with type II hypercholesterolemia and additional coronary risk factors. *Clin Pharmacol Ther.* 1999;65:439-447. 18. Crespo N, Alvarez R, Mas R, et al. Effect of policosanol on patients with non-insulin-dependent diabetes mellitus and hypercholesterolemia: a pilot study. *Curr Ther Res.* 1997;58:44-51. 19. Castano G, Mas R, Fernandez L, et al. Effects of policosanol on postmenopausal women with type II hypercholesterolemia. *Gynecol Endocrinol.* 2000;14:187-195. 20. Benitez M, Romero C, Mas R, et al. A comparative study of policosanol versus pravastatin in patients with type II hypercholesterolemia. *Curr Ther Res.* 1997;58:859-867. 21. Ortensi G, Gladstein J, Valli H, et al. A comparative study of policosanol versus simvastatin in elderly patients with hypercholesterolemia. *Curr Ther Res.* 1997;58:390-401. 22. Crespo N, Illnait J, Mas R, et al. Comparative study of the efficacy and tolerability of policosanol and lovastatin in patients with hypercholesterolemia and noninsulin dependent diabetes mellitus. *Int J Clin Pharmacol Res.* 1999;19:117-127. 23. Alcocer L, Fernandez L, Campos E, et al. A comparative study of policosanol Versus acipimox in patients with type II hypercholesterolemia. *Int J Tissue React.* 1999;21:85-92. 24. Crespo N, Illnait J, Mas R, et al. Comparative study of the efficacy and tolerability of policosanol and lovastatin in patients with hypercholesterolemia and noninsulin dependent diabetes mellitus. *Int J Clin Pharmacol Res.* 1999;19:117-127. 25. Castano G, Mas R, Fernandez JC, et al. Efficacy and tolerability of policosanol compared with lovastatin in patients with type II hypercholesterolemia and concomitant coronary risk factors. *Curr Ther Res.* 2000;61:137-146. 26. Fernandez JC, Mas R, Castano G, et al. Comparison of the efficacy, safety and tolerability of policosanol versus fluvastatin in elderly hypercholesterolaemic women. *Clin Drug Invest.* 2001;21:103-113. 27. Castano G, Mas Ferreiro R, Fernandez L, et al. A long-term study of policosanol in the treatment of intermittent claudication. *Angiology.* 2001;52:115-125. 28. Castano G, Mas R, Roca J, et al. A double-blind, placebo-controlled study of the effects of policosanol in patients with intermittent claudication. *Angiology.* 1999;50:123-130. 29. Saint-John M, McNaughton L. Octacosanol ingestion and its effects on metabolic responses to submaximal cycle ergometry, reaction time and chest and grip strength. *Int Clin Nutr Rev.* 1986;6:81-87. 30. Snider SR. Octacosanol in parkinsonism [letter]. *Ann Neurol.* 1984;16:723. 31. Norris FH, Denys EH, Fallat RJ. Trial of octacosanol in amyotrophic lateral sclerosis. *Neurology.* 1986;36:1263-1264. 32. Zardoya R, Tula L, Castano G, et al. Effects of policosanol on hypercholesterolemic abnormal serum biochemical indicators of hepatic function. *Curr Ther Res.* 1996;57:568-577. 33. Arruzazabala ML, Valdes S, Mas R, et al. Comparative study of policosanol, aspirin and the combination therapy policosanol-aspirin on platelet aggregation in healthy volunteers. *Pharmacol Res.* 1997;36:293-297. 34. Fernandez L, Mas R, Illnait J, et al. Policosanol: results of a postmarketing surveillance control on 27,879 patients. *Curr Ther Res.* 1998;59:717-722. 35. Rodriguez-Echenique C, Mesa R, Mas R, et al. Effects of policosanol chronically administered in male monkeys (Macaca arctoides). *Food Chem Toxicol.* 1994;32:565-575. 36. Mesa AR, Mas R, Noa M, et al.Toxicity of policosanol in beagle dogs: one-year study. *Toxicol Lett.* 1994;73:81-90. 37. Aleman CL, Mas R, Hernandez C, et al. A 12-month study of policosanol oral toxicity in Sprague Dawley rats. *Toxicol Lett.* 1994;70:77-87. 38. Rodriguez MD, Garcia H. Teratogenic and reproductive studies of policosanol in the rat and rabbit. *Teratog Carcinog Mutagen.* 1994;14:107-113.

Pygeum

Prunus Africana, Pygeum Africanum

U.S. BRAND NAMES OF CLINICALLY TESTED PRODUCTS

Pygeum Extract (Solaray) = Pygenil (Synthelabo/Sanofi), PrunaSelect (Indena) in Europe

Prostatonin (Pharmaton) = PY 102 Prostatonin (Pharmaton) (contains pygeum and nettle root) in Europe

DESCRIPTION

Pygeum, an evergreen tree growing to 35 meters, is native to plateaus of southern and central Africa and Madagascar.[1] A suspension of the trunk's powdered bark has traditionally been used in southern Africa for bladder pains and micturition difficulties. There are serious concerns that widespread debarking and harvesting of wild pygeum stocks are endangering the species; no similar objection applies to other botanicals used for BPH, such as saw palmetto and nettle root.

PHARMACOLOGY

Lipophilic extracts of pygeum trunk bark are produced using nonpolar solvents or supercritical CO_2.[1] Components of pygeum extracts include free fatty acids, long-chain fatty alcohols, phytosterols, and pentacyclic triterpenoids.[1] Identified fatty acids include myristic, palmitic, linoleic, linolenic, oleic, stearic, arachidic, behenic, and lignoceric acids partially esterified with long-chain fatty alcohols such as n-docosanol and tetracosanol; n-docosanol and tetracosanol are also found esterified with ferulic acid. Phytosterols include beta-sitosterol and its glucoside, stigmasterol, campesterol, and sitosterone. The pentacyclic triterpenoids oleanolic, crataegolic, and ursolic acid have also been detected.

The mechanism of action of pygeum extract is unknown, but several synergistic mechanisms have been proposed. Phytosterols such as beta-sitosterol compete with cholesterol, an androgen precursor,[2] and inhibit the production of inflammatory arachidonic acid pathway metabolites.[3] (A concentrated extract of beta-sitosterols is another natural-source treatment for BPH widely used in Europe.) Ferulic acid esters also reduce cholesterol levels. Oleanolic and ursolic acid (pentacyclic triterpenoids) possibly exert an anti-inflammatory action in the prostate by inhibiting glucosyltransferase, involved in proteoglycan metabolism in connective tissue.[4]

In vitro studies indicate pygeum extract is a potent inhibitor of rat prostatic fibroblast proliferation stimulated by various growth factors.[5] Inhibition of steroid 5-alpha-reductase, the enzyme that catalyzes conversion of testosterone to dihydrotestosterone, is not a significant activity of pygeum extract. In vitro assays showed that one brand of pygeum extract, Tadenan, possessed only 1/63,000 the inhibition activity of finasteride.[6]

CLINICAL STUDIES

More than 10 double-blind placebo-controlled studies of pygeum have been published, involving a total of more than 600 individuals studied for 6 to 12 weeks, using daily doses of pygeum extract from 75 to 200 mg.[3] In these trials, quality-of-life and objective measurements (urinary flow rate, residual volume, and nocturia) are typically reported to improve by 2 months[3] and remain improved for at least 1 month post-treatment.[7] There is no reliable evidence that pygeum can reduce prostate volume.

Most of these studies involved small numbers of patients (10 to 25 per group), but one double-blind placebo-controlled trial of 263 men showed a reliable, statistically significant improvement with pygeum in urinary flow rate, voided volume, residual volume, daytime frequency, and nocturia.[8] No change in prostate weight was reported in this study.

PROPOSED INDICATIONS AND USAGE

Several double-blind placebo-controlled trials support the use of pygeum for the treatment of symptomatic BPH.

Pygeum is also sometimes promoted as a treatment for chronic prostatitis, although the entire evidence for this use rests on one small open-label study.[9] Other open trials suggest that pygeum might have some utility in treating infections of the prostate and seminal vesicles, as well as in treating sexual dysfunction in males.[10,11]

WARNINGS

None.

PRECAUTIONS

Though there are no indications relevant to women and children, pygeum should probably be avoided in pregnancy and lactation because of its hormonal activity. Safety in individuals with severe hepatic or renal disease has not been established.

DRUG INTERACTIONS

None are reported.

ADVERSE REACTIONS

Very few side effects have been reported other than occasional gastrointestinal upset and diarrhea. Sexual dysfunction secondary to treatment with pygeum extract has not been reported.

PROPOSED DOSAGE AND ADMINISTRATION

Clinical studies have used 75 to 200 mg pygeum extract daily in patients with BPH. Once-daily dosing with 100 mg may be equally effective as 50 mg twice daily.[12] Some manufacturers standardize pygeum extracts to contain 14% triterpenoids and 0.5% n-docosanol.

Pygeum's effectiveness might be enhanced when it is combined with nettle root.[13,14]

PATIENT INFORMATION

Pygeum is an herb used in Europe to treat early stages of prostate enlargment (benign prostatic hyperplasia, or BPH). There is some evidence that it may be effective. However, before self-treating for BPH, it is essential to rule out prostate cancer.

Pygeum is not intended for use by women. Individuals with severe liver or kidney disease should consult a physician before using this (or any other) supplement.

REFERENCES

1. Bombardelli E, Morazzoni P. *Prunus africana* (Hook. f.) Kalkm. *Fitoterapia.* 1997;68:205-218. 2. Schulz V, Hansel R, Tyler VE. *Rational Phytotherapy: A Physicians' Guide to Herbal Medicine.* 3rd ed. Berlin, Germany: Springer-Verlag; 1998:232-234. 3. Andro MC, Riffaud JP. Pygeum africanum extract

for the treatment of patients with benign prostatic hyperplasia: a review of 25 years of published experience. *Curr Ther Res.* 1995;56:796-817. **4.** Kozai K, Miyake Y, Kohda H, et al. Inhibition of glucosyltranferase from Streptococcus mutans by oleanolic acid and ursolic acid. *Caries Res.* 1987;21:104-108. **5.** Yablonsky F, Nicolas V, Riffaud JP, et al. Antiproliferative effect of Pygeum africanum extract on rat prostatic fibroblasts. *J Urol.* 1997;157:2381-2387. **6.** Rhodes L, Primka RL, Berman C, et al. Comparison of finasteride (Proscar(r)), a 5-alpha reductase inhibitor, and various commercial plant extracts in In vitro and In vivo 5-alpha reductase inhibition. *Prostate.* 1993;22:43-51. **7.** Breza J, Dzurny O, Borowka A, et al. Efficacy and acceptability of Tadenan(r) (Pygeum africanum extract) in the treatment of benign prostatic hyperplasia (BPH): a multicentre trial in central Europe. *Curr Med Res Opin.* 1998;14:127-139. **8.** Barlet A, Albrecht J, Aubert A, et al. Efficacy of Pygeum africanum extract in the treatment of micturitional disorders due to benign prostatic hyperplasia: evaluation of objective and subjective parameters. A multicenter, placebo-controlled double-blind trial [translated from German]. *Wien Klin Wochenschr.* 1990;102:667-673. **9.** Del Vaglio B. Use of a new drug in the treatment of chronic prostatitis [in Italian; English abstract]. *Minerva Urol Nefrol.* 1974;26:81-94. **10.** Carani C, Salvioli V, Scuteri A, et al. Urological and sexual evaluation of treatment of benign prostatic disease using Pygeum africanum at high doses [in Italian; English abstract]. *Arch Ital Urol Nefrol Androl.* 1991;63:341-345. **11.** Menchini-Fabris GF, Giorgi P, Andreini F, et al. New perspectives on the use of Pygeum Africanum in prostato-bladder pathology [in Italian; English abstract]. *Arch Ital Urol Nefrol Androl.* 1988;60:313-322. **12.** Chatelain C, Autet W, Brackman F. Comparison of once and twice daily dosage forms of Pygeum africanum extract in patients with benign prostatic hyperplasia: a randomized, double-blind study, with long-term open label extention. *Urology.* 1999;54:473-478. **13.** Hartmann RW, Mark M, Soldati F. Inhibition of 5-alpha-reductase and aromatase by PHL-00801 (Prostatonin(r)), a combination of PY 102 (Pygeum africanum) and UR 102 (Urtica dioica) extracts. *Phytomedicine.* 1996;3:121-128. **14.** Krzeski T, Kazon M, Borkowski A, et al. Combined extracts of Urtica dioica and Pygeum africanum in the treatment of benign prostatic hyperplasia: double-blind comparison of two doses. *Clin Ther.* 1993;15:1011-1020.

Pyruvate

Alternate/Related Names: Sodium Pyruvate, Calcium Pyruvate, Potassium Pyruvate, Magnesium Pyruvate, Dihydroxyacetone Pyruvate (DHAP)

U.S. BRAND NAMES OF CLINICALLY TESTED PRODUCTS

Not applicable.

DESCRIPTION

Pyruvate, a Krebs cycle intermediate, is widely marketed as a sports supplement and weight-loss aid. The related product DHAP (pyruvate plus its precursor dihydroxyacetone) is marketed for similar purposes.

PHARMACOLOGY

Animal trials suggest that exogenously administered pyruvate might provide metabolic feedback to inhibit lipid synthesis, and also enhance energy expenditure.[1-4] Little is known about the pharmacokinetics of oral pyruvate. Dihydroxyacetone, a product of the metabolism of glucose and glycerol, is rapidly converted into pyruvate in the body.

CLINICAL STUDIES

WEIGHT LOSS

Several small trials suggest that oral pyruvate or DHAP might act as a weight-loss agent.

For example, in a 6-week double-blind placebo-controlled trial, 51 individuals were given either pyruvate (6 g/day), placebo, or no treatment.[5] All participated in an exercise program. Significant average decreases in fat mass (2.1 kg) and percentage of body fat (2.6%), along with a significant increase in lean mass (1.5 kg), were seen with pyruvate. No significant changes were seen in the placebo or no-treatment groups.

Other small studies using pyruvate or DHAP and enrolling a total of about 100 participants found similar results.[6-10]

PROPOSED INDICATIONS AND USAGE

Weak evidence suggests that pyruvate supplements might promote weight loss.

Both pyruvate and DHAP are also marketed as ergogenic aids. However, the small studies evaluating this potential use have produced contradictory results.[11-14]

WARNINGS

As with all supplements taken in multigram doses, use of a quality product is critical, as contaminants present in even small percentages could result in toxic effects.

PRECAUTIONS

Maximum safe dosages in pregnant or lactating women, young children, or individuals with severe hepatic or renal disease are not known.

DRUG INTERACTIONS

None reported.

ADVERSE REACTIONS

In clinical trials, exogenous pyruvate and dihydroxyacetone have caused only few and nonspecific adverse effects. However, formal toxicological studies have not been reported.

PROPOSED DOSAGE AND ADMINISTRATION

A typical therapeutic dosage of pyruvate is 30 g daily, although dosages from 6 to 44 g daily have been used in studies. Studies of DHAP have used dosages ranging from 12 to 75 g daily.

PATIENT INFORMATION

Pyruvate is a popular supplement advertised to help in weight loss as well as sports performance. Some preliminary evidence supports using pyruvate for weight loss. However, about as many studies testing pyruvate as a sports supplement have found it ineffective as have found it effective.

The maximum safe dosages of pyruvate for pregnant or nursing women or young children has not been established. Individuals with severe liver or kidney disease should consult a physician before using this (or any other) supplement.

REFERENCES

1. Stanko RT, Adibi SA. Inhibition of lipid accumulation and enhancement of energy expenditure by the addition of pyruvate and dihydroxyacetone to a rat diet. *Metabolism.* 1986;35:182-186. **2.** Stanko RT, Ferguson TL, Newman CW, et al. Reduction of carcass fat in swine with dietary addition of dihydroxyacetone and pyruvate. *J Anim Sci.* 1989;67:1272-1278. **3.** Stanko RT, Mendelow H, Shinozuka H, et al. Prevention of alcohol-induced fatty liver by natural metabolites and riboflavin. *J Lab Clin Med.* 1978;91:228-235. **4.** Cortez MY, Torgan CE, Brozinick JT Jr, et al. Effects of pyruvate and dihydroxyacetone consumption on the growth and metabolic state of obese Zucker rats. *Am J Clin Nutr.* 1991;53:847-853. **5.** Kalman D, Colker CM, Stark S, et al. Effect of pyruvate supplementation on body composition and mood. *Curr Ther Res.* 1998;59:793-802. **6.** Stanko RT, Tietze DL, Arch JE. Body composition, energy utilization, and nitrogen metabolism with a 4.25-MJ/d low-energy diet supplemented with pyruvate. *Am J Clin Nutr.* 1992;56:630-635. **7.** Stanko RT, Reynolds HR, Hoyson R, et al. Pyruvate supplementation of a low-cholesterol, low-fat diet: effects on plasma lipid concentration and body composition in hyperlipidemic patients. *Am J Clin Nutr.* 1994;59:423-427. **8.** Stanko RT, Arch JE. Inhibition of regain in body weight and fat with addition of 3-carbon compound to the diet with hyperenergetic refeeding after weight reduction. *Int J Obes Relat Metab Disord.* 1996;20:925-930. **9.** Stanko RT, Tietze DL, Arch JE. Body composition, energy utilization, and nitrogen metabolism with a severely restricted diet supplemented with dihydroxyacetone and pyruvate. *Am J Clin Nutr.* 1992;55:771-772. **10.** Kalman D, Colker CM, Wilets I, et al. The effects of pyruvate supplementation on body composition in overweight individuals. *Nutrition.* 1999;15:337-340. **11.** Ivy JL. Effect of pyruvate and dihydroxyacetone on metabolism and aerobic endurance capacity. *Med Sci Sports Exerc.* 1998;30:837-843. **12.** Stanko RT, Robertson RJ, Galbreath RW, et al. Enhanced leg exercise endurance with a high-carbohydrate diet and dihydroxyacetone and pyruvate. *J Appl Physiol.* 1990;69:1651-1656. **13.** Stanko RT, Robertson RJ, Spina RJ, et al. Enhancement of arm exercise endurance capacity with dihydroxyacetone and pyruvate. *J Appl Physiol.* 1990;68:119-124. **14.** Morrison MA, Spriet LL, Dyck DJ. Pyruvate ingestion for 7 days does not improve aerobic performance in well-trained individuals. *J Appl Physiol.* 2000;89:549-556.

Red Clover

Trifolium Pratense

Alternate/Related Names: Wild Clover, Purple Clover, Trefoil

U.S. BRAND NAMES OF CLINICALLY TESTED PRODUCTS

Promensil (Novogen) = Promensil (Novogen) in Europe

DESCRIPTION

Red clover has been cultivated since ancient times, primarily to provide a favorite grazing food for animals. It has also been used as a medicinal herb, most commonly for cancer treatment and respiratory problems.

In the nineteenth century, red clover became popular among herbalists as an "alterative" or "blood purifier." This medical term, long-since defunct, refers to an ancient belief that toxins in the blood are the root cause of many illnesses. Cancer, eczema, and the eruptions of venereal disease were all seen as manifestations of toxic buildup. On this basis, red clover was therefore included in the Hoxsey cancer cure and Jason Winter's cancer-cure tea. Recently, special red clover extracts high in isoflavones have arrived on the market.

PHARMACOLOGY

Red clover contains numerous isoflavones, including most prominently biochanin A and formononetin, but also genistein and daidzein. Other constituents include coumarins, cyanogenic glycosides, and volatile oils.

Genistein and daidzein are found in soy, and have been extensively researched for potential phytoestrogenic and chemopreventive properties.[1-4] Biochanin A also appears to have phytoestrogenic action.[1] It has also been found in vitro to inhibit carcinogen activation[5]; additionally, an in vitro study of human stomach cancer cell lines suggests that biochanin A inhibits cell growth through activation of a signal transduction pathway for apoptosis.[6]

CLINICAL STUDIES

MENOPAUSAL SYMPTOMS

On the basis of its high concentrations of phytoestrogenic isoflavones, red clover has been extensively marketed as a treatment for menopausal symptoms. However, two double-blind placebo-controlled trials involving a total of 88 women failed to show reduction of menopausal symptoms with the red clover extract Promensil.[7,8]

HYPERLIPIDEMIA

A 12-week double-blind placebo-controlled ascending-dose study evaluated the effects of a red clover extract in 66 postmenopausal women with moderate hypercholesterolemia.[9] Supplementation with red clover isoflavones did not significantly alter total plasma cholesterol, LDL, HDL, or triglyceride levels.

PROPOSED INDICATIONS AND USAGE

Despite extensive marketing as a treatment for menopausal symptoms, red clover isoflavones have failed to prove effective in preliminary double-blind trials. Red clover isoflavones have also failed to prove effective for hyperlipidemia.

Red clover continues to be marketed for its archaic use as a "blood purifier."

WARNINGS

None.

PRECAUTIONS

Because red clover contains isoflavonoid constituents, its use in women with a history of hormone-sensitive cancer warrants caution.[10] In addition, given its coumarin constituents, use of red clover in individuals with impaired hemostasis is questionable.[10]

Maximum safe dosages in individuals with severe hepatic or renal disease are not known.

Because of its phytoestrogenic components, red clover is not recommended for use in pregnant or lactating women. Safety in young children has not been established.

DRUG INTERACTIONS

Based on the known actions of their isoflavone and coumarin constituents, red clover extracts may potentially interfere with hormone therapy and may potentiate the effect of anticoagulant pharmaceuticals.

ADVERSE REACTIONS

Red clover is on the FDA's GRAS (generally recognized as safe) list and is included in many beverage teas. However, detailed safety studies have not been performed. No significant adverse effects have been reported in clinical trials.

PROPOSED DOSAGE AND ADMINISTRATION

A typical dosage of red clover extract provides 40 to 160 mg isoflavones daily.

PATIENT INFORMATION

Red clover extracts are marketed for the treatment of menopausal symptoms. However, study results have not demonstrated any effect. These extracts contain estrogen-like substances, which may present risks for pregnant or nursing women as well as young children. They might also interact with "blood-thinning" medications.

Whole red clover (as opposed to the extract) is also sometimes recommended for cancer treatment, but there is no evidence whatsoever that it is helpful for this purpose.

Individuals with severe liver or kidney disease should consult a physician before using this (or any other) supplement.

REFERENCES

1. Olesek WA, Jurzysta M. Isolation, chemical and biological activity of red clover (*Trifolium pratense* L.) root saponins. *Acta Soc Bot Pol.* 1986;55:247-252. **2.** Alhasan SA. Genistein induced molecular changes in a squamous cell carcinoma of the head and neck cell line. *Int J Oncol.* 2000;16:333-338. **3.** Wei H, Bowen R, Cai Q, et al. Antioxidant and antipromotional effects of the soybean isoflavone genistein. *Proc Soc Exp Biol Med.* 1995;208:124-130. **4.** Tham DM, Gardner CD, Haskell WL. Clinical review 97: Potential health benefits of dietary phytoestrogens: a review of the clinical, epidemiological, and mechanistic evidence. *J Clin Endocrinol Metab.* 1998;83:2223-2235. **5.** Cassady JM, Zennie TM, Chae YH, et al. Use of a mammalian cell culture benzo(a)pyrene metabolism assay for the detection of potential anticarcinogens from natural products: inhibition of metabolism by biochanin A, an isoflavone from *Trifolium pratense* L. *Cancer Res.* 1988;48:6257-6261. **6.** Yanagihara K, Ito A, Toge T, et al. Antiproliferative effects of isoflavones on human cancer cell lines established from the gastrointestinal tract. *Cancer Res.* 1993;53:5815-5821. **7.** Baber RJ, Templeman C, Morton T, et al. Randomized placebo-controlled trial of an isoflavone supplement and menopausal symptoms in women. *Climacteric.* 1999;2:85-92. **8.** Knight DC, Howes JB, Eden JA. The effect of Promensil(tm), an isoflavone extract, on menopausal symptoms. *Climacteric.* 1999;2:79-84. **9.** Howes JB, Sullivan D, Lai N, et al. The effects of dietary supplementation with isoflavones from red clover on the lipoprotein profiles of post menopausal women with mild to moderate hypercholesterolaemia. *Atherosclerosis.* 2000;152:143-147. **10.** Newall CA, et al. *Herbal medicines: A Guide for Health-Care Professionals.* London, England: Pharmaceutical Press; 1996:227.

S-Adenosylmethionine (SAMe)

U.S. BRAND NAMES OF CLINICALLY TESTED PRODUCTS

None.

DESCRIPTION

Formed endogenously by the combination of the amino acid methionine and ATP, S-adenosylmethionine (SAMe) functions as a ubiquitous methyl donor in methyltransferase reactions involving proteins, phospholipids, DNA, neurotransmitters, and numerous other essential biochemicals.[1] SAMe is also central to the manufacture of many sulfur-containing compounds such as glutathione and proteoglycans.[2] In the mid-1970s a stable salt of SAMe became available for parenteral use in clinical trials. Stabilized oral formulations became available in the following decade.

PHARMACOLOGY

SAMe is well absorbed orally. A 400-mg dose increases plasma SAMe levels over normal by nearly tenfold (to 362 nmol/L), but the SAMe is cleared with a relatively short half-life of 1.7 hours.[3] Volume of distribution after 100- and 500-mg doses has been estimated at 407 ± 27 and 443 ± 36 ml/kg, respectively.[4]

Animal studies suggest that exogenously administered SAMe may have chondroprotective properties.[5,6] SAMe also appears to exert mild direct anti-inflammatory and analgesic effects without affecting prostaglandin pathways.[1]

In depression, supplementation with SAMe may produce a dopaminergic effect by facilitating the methylation of dopamine precursors.[7] It is also well appreciated that folate deficiency is linked to depression in the elderly[8]; because supplementation with preformed SAMe would be expected to bypass one major need for folate (as 5-methyltetrahydrofolate), this might be one mechanism by which SAMe could provide antidepressant benefits.

CLINICAL STUDIES

OSTEOARTHRITIS

A 4-week double-blind study investigated the effects on osteoarthritis of 1,200 mg/day SAMe (orally), 750 mg/day naproxen, or placebo in 732 individuals treated at 33 centers.[9] The results showed similar benefits in the SAMe and naproxen groups.

In small double-blind studies, oral SAMe has also shown equivalent benefits to indomethacin (150 mg/day), low-dose ibuprofen (400 mg twice daily), naproxen (initially 250 mg 3 times daily, then twice daily), and full-dose piroxicam (20 mg/day).[10,11,12]

DEPRESSION

The research record for SAMe in depression is modest, contradictory, and marked by numerous flaws; furthermore, many studies involved IV or IM administration.[13]

Three double-blind placebo-controlled studies following a total of 135 patients with major, postmenopausal, or postpartum depression found significant improvements in depressive symptoms in those treated with oral SAMe as compared to placebo.[14,15,16] However, one double-blind placebo-controlled study of 32 patients found no significant difference between treatment and control groups.[17] These studies were generally marred by poor reporting and unusually wide variation in the placebo group response (0% to 65%). In a double-blind placebo-controlled study of 133 depressed patients, the effects of 800 mg/day of intravenous SAMe failed to achieve statistical significance over those of placebo, unless subgroup analysis or secondary outcome measures were employed.[18]

Oral SAMe has also been compared to standard antidepressant agents. A 6-week double-blind trial of 281 depressed individuals evaluated the relative effects of oral SAMe (1,600 mg/day) and imipramine (150 mg/day).[19] Intention-to-treat analysis showed no differences in outcome. However, the average severity of depression in this trial was low (21-item HAM-D average score of 18); nonspecific effects could have been the primary source of the improvement seen.

Other small studies have also compared the benefits of oral or parenteral SAMe to those of tricyclic antidepressants, finding generally equivalent results.[19-22]However, marked inadequacies of study design and reporting diminish the meaningfulness of the outcomes.

FIBROMYALGIA

A 6-week double-blind study of 44 patients with fibromyalgia found improvements in disease activity, pain at rest, fatigue, and morning stiffness, and in one measurement of mood, in the SAMe-treated group (800 mg /day orally).[23] Similar results were found in a small, earlier study.[24] However, it is not clear whether these benefits resulted from direct improvement of fibromyalgia, or secondarily through SAMe's possible antidepressant action.

PROPOSED INDICATIONS AND USAGE

Some research suggests that exogenous SAMe may offer symptomatic benefits in osteoarthritis. However, supplemental glucosamine and chondroitin are far less expensive, and have a stronger evidence base.

The evidence that oral SAMe has antidepressant effects is preliminary at best. Again, however, there are numerous less-expensive agents (such as pharmaceutical antidepressants) with greater evidence of efficacy.

Two small studies suggest that SAMe may have value as a treatment for fibromyalgia. Very weak evidence suggests that SAMe might have value in hepatic conditions, including oral contraceptive hepatotoxicity, intrahepatic cholestasis of pregnancy, Gilbert's syndrome, and alcoholic liver cirrhosis.[2,25-29]

WARNINGS

None.

PRECAUTIONS

In individuals with bipolar disorder, SAMe should be used with caution.[16,30,31]

Safety for young children, pregnant or lactating women, or individuals with severe hepatic or renal disease has not been established. However, SAMe has been utilized in studies of pregnant women and other individuals with hepatic disease with no apparent adverse effects.[25,27,29,32]

DRUG INTERACTIONS

L-dopa is an avid acceptor of methyl groups, and its use leads to decreased levels of brain SAMe.[33,34] It has also been suggested that SAMe depletion may contribute to L-dopa side effects and gradual loss of efficacy of the drug.[33] One short-term double-blind study did find that Parkinson's patients on L-dopa could be given SAMe without loss of L-dopa efficacy.[35] However, in the long term, SAMe supplementation might increase methylation and inactivation of L-dopa.[34]

SAMe can increase the metabolism of certain drugs by facilitating their conjugation.[36] However, the clinical significance of this observation is not known.

There has been one report of apparent serotonergic syndrome in a 71-year-old woman simultaneously taking clomipramine and intramuscular SAMe (100 mg/day).[37] Symptoms included hyperthermia, delirium, and myoclonic muscular rigidity.

ADVERSE REACTIONS

In general, SAMe is very well tolerated. In a limited study in rats and rabbits, SAMe was found to have very low toxicity in adult animals and their offspring, with the exception of an unrealistically high subcutaneous dose of 400 mg/kg.[38] SAMe does not appear to be mutagenic.[39]

In clinical trials, SAMe has been well tolerated, producing no significant adverse effects.

In patients with bipolar disorder, SAMe in oral doses has caused transition from a depressed to an elevated state (hypomania, mania, or euphoria).[30,31] At least one case has been reported of a manic episode induced by SAMe in a patient with no previous history of bipolar illness.[16]

PROPOSED DOSAGE AND ADMINISTRATION

In clinical trials, the typical daily dose of SAMe for osteoarthritis was 1,200 to 1,600 mg/day.

SAMe is an expensive supplement. Full doses can easily reach $200 a month. Some SAMe product labels suggest a dose of 400 mg b.i.d., presumably to lower costs (at the expense of potential efficacy). Concerns have been raised that some forms of oral SAMe may not be stable.[40] A newly developed manufacturing technique offers promise of a more stable product.[41]

PATIENT INFORMATION

SAMe is a supplement marketed for the treatment of both depression and osteoporosis. While there is preliminary evidence that it may be effective, SAMe is very expensive when taken in recommended doses. (Label instructions on SAMe products often recommend a dose far lower than what has been tried in scientific studies.) For osteoarthritis, glucosamine and/or chondroitin are less expensive and have considerably more scientific evidence behind them; for depression, the same can be said of St. John's wort.

The safety of SAMe for pregnant or nursing women or young children has not been established. Individuals with severe liver or kidney disease should consult a physician before using this (or any other) supplement.

REFERENCES

1. Stramentinoli G. Pharmacologic aspects of S-adenosylmethionine. Pharmacokinetics and pharmacodynamics. *Am J Med.* 1987;83(5A):35-42. **2.** di Padova C. S-adenosylmethionine in the treatment of osteoarthritis. Review of the clinical studies. *Am J Med.* 1987;83(5A):60-65. **3.** Loehrer FM, Schwab R, Angst CP, et al. Influence of oral S-adenosylmethionine on plasma 5-methyltetrahydrofolate, S-adenosylhomocysteine, homocysteine and methionine in healthy humans. *J Pharmacol Exp Ther.* 1997;282:845-850. **4.** Giulidori P, Cortellaro M, Moreo G, et al. Pharmacokinetics of S-adenosyl-L-methionine in healthy volunteers. *Eur J Clin Pharmacol.* 1984;27:119-121. **5.** Kalbhen DA, Jansen G. Pharmacologic studies on the antidegenerative effect of ademetionine in experimental arthritis in animals [in German; English abstract]. *Arzneimittelforschung.* 1990;40:1017-1021. **6.** Barcelo HA, Wiemeyer JC, Sagasta CL, et al. Experimental osteoarthritis and its course when treated with S-adenosyl-L-methionine [in Spanish; English abstract]. *Rev Clin Exp.* 1990;187:74-78. **7.** Fava M, Rosenbaum JF, MacLaughlin R, et al. Neuroendocrine effects of S-adenosyl-L-methionine, a novel putative antidepressant. *J Psychiatr Res.* 1990;24:177-184. **8.** Parnetti L, Bottiglieri T, Lowenthal D. Role of homocysteine in age-related vascular and non-vascular diseases. *Aging (Milano).* 1997;9:241-257. **9.** Caruso I, Pietrogrande V. Italian double-blind multicenter study comparing S-adenosylmethionine, naproxen, and placebo in the treatment of degenerative joint disease. *Am J Med.* 1987;83(5A):66-71. **10.** Glorioso S, Todesco S, Mazzi A, et al. Double-blind multicentre study of the activity of S-adenosylmethionine in hip and knee osteoarthritis. *Int J Clin Pharmacol Res.* 1985;5:39-49. **11.** Muller-Fassbender H. Double-blind clinical trial of S-adenosylmethionine versus ibuprofen in the treatment of osteoarthritis. *Am J Med.* 1987;83(5A):81-83. **12.** Maccagno A, Di Giorgio EE, Caston OL, et al. Double-blind controlled clinical trial of oral S-adenosylmethionine versus piroxicam in knee osteoarthritis. *Am J Med.* 1987;83(5A):72-77. **13.** Bressa GM. S-adenosyl-l-methionine (SAMe) as antidepressant: meta-analysis of clinical studies. *Acta Neurol Scand Suppl.* 1994;154:7-14. **14.** Salmaggi P, Bressa GM, Nicchia G, et al. Double-blind, placebo-controlled study of S-adenosyl-L-methionine in depressed postmenopausal women. *Psychother Psychosom.* 1993;59:34-40. **15.** Cerutti R, Sichel MP, Perin M, et al. Psychological distress during puerperium: a novel therapeutic approach using S-adenosylmethionine. *Curr Ther Res.* 1993;53:707-716. **16.** Kagan BL, Sultzer DL, Rosenlicht N, et al. Oral S-adenosylmethionine in depression: a randomized, double-blind, placebo-controlled trial. *Am J Psychiatry.* 1990;147:591-595. **17.** Fava M, Rosenbaum JF, Birnbaum R, et al. The thyrotropin response to thyrotropin-releasing hormone as a predictor of response to treatment in depressed outpatients. *Acta Psychiatr Scand.* 1992;86:42-45. **18.** Delle Chiaie R, Pancheri P. Combined analysis of two controlled, multicentric, double blind studies to assess efficacy and safety of Sulfo-Adenosyl-Methionine (SAMe) vs. placebo (MC1) and SAMe vs. clomipramine (MC2) in the treatment of major depression [in Italian; English abstract]. *G Ital Psicopatol.* 1999;5:1-16. **19.** Delle Chiaie R, Pancheri P, Scapicchio P. MC3: multicentre, controlled efficacy and safety trial of oral S-adenosyl-methionine (SAMe) vs. oral imipramine in the treatment of depression [abstract]. *Int J Neuropsychopharmcol.* 2000;3(suppl 1):S230. **20.** De Vanna M, Rigamonti R. Oral S-adenosyl-L-methionine in depression. *Curr Ther Res.* 1992;52:478-485. **21.** Bell KM, Potkin SG, Carreon D, et al. S-adenosylmethionine blood levels in major depression: changes with drug treatment. *Acta Neurol Scand Suppl.* 1994;154:15-18. **22.** Echols JC, Naidoo U, Salzman C. SAMe (S-adenosylmethionine). *Harv Rev Psychiatry.* 2000;8:84-90. **23.** Jacobsen S, Danneskiold-Samsoe B, Andersen RB. Oral S-adenosylmethionine in primary fibromyalgia. Double-blind clinical evaluation. *Scand J Rheumatol.* 1991;20:294-302. **24.** Tavoni A, Vitali C, Bombardieri S, et al. Evaluation of s-adenosylmethionine in primary fibromyalgia. A double-blind crossover study. *Am J Med.* 1987; 83(5A):107-110. **25.** Mato JM, Camara J, Fernandez de Paz J, et al. S-adenosylmethionine in alcoholic liver cirrhosis: a randomized, placebo-controlled, double-blind, multicenter clinical trial. *J Hepatol.* 1999;30;1081-1089. **26.** Bombardieri G, Milani A, Bernardi L, et al. Effects of S-adenosyl-methionine (SAMe) in the treatment of Gilbert's Syndrome. *Curr Ther Res.* 1985;37:580-585. **27.** Frezza M, Pozzato G, Chiesa L, et al. Reversal of intrahepatic cholestasis of pregnancy in women after high dose S-adenosyl-L-methionine administration. *Hepatology.* 1984;4;274-278. **28.** Frezza M, Pozzato G, Pison G, et al. S-adenosylmethionine counteracts oral contraceptive hepatotoxicity in women. *Am J Med Sci.* 1987;293:234-238. **29.** Nicastri PL, Diaferia A, Tartagni M, et al. A randomised placebo-controlled trial of ursodeoxycholic acid and S-adenosylmethionine in the treatment of intrahepatic cholestasis of pregnancy. *Br J Obstet Gynaecol.* 1998;105:1205-1207. **30.** Carney MW, Chary TK, Bottiglieri T, et al. Switch and S-adenosylmethionine. *Ala J Med Sci.* 1988;25:316-319. **31.** Carney MW, Chary TK, Bottiglieri T, et al. The switch mechanism and the bipolar/unipolar dichotomy. *Br J Psychiatry.* 1989;154:48-51. **32.** Frezza M, Centini G, Cammareri G, et al. S-adenosylmethionine for the treatment of intrahepatic cholestasis of pregnancy. Results of a controlled clinical trial. *Hepatogastroenterology.* 1990;37(suppl 2):122-125. **33.** Bottiglieri T, Hyland K, Reynolds EH. The clinical potential of ademetionine (S-Adenosylmethionine) in neurological disorders. *Drugs.* 1994;48:137-152. **34.** Liu X, Lamango N, Charlton C.L-dopa depletes S-adenosylmethionine and increases S-adenosyl homocysteine: relationship to the wearing-off effects [abstract]. *Abstr Soc Neurosci.* 1998;24:1469. **35.** Carrieri PB, Indaco A, Gentile S, et al. S-adenosylmethionine treatment of depression in patients with Parkinson's disease: a double-blind, crossover study versus placebo. *Curr Ther Res.* 1990;48:154-160. **36.** Reicks M, Hathcock JN. Effects of methionine and other sulfur compounds on drug conjugations. *Pharmacol Ther.* 1988;37:67-79. **37.** Iruela LM, Minguez L, Merino J, et al. Toxic interaction of S-adenosylmethionine and clomipramine [letter]. *Am J Psychiatry.* 1993;150:522. **38.** Cozens DD, Barton SJ, Clark R, et al. Reproductive toxicity studies of ademetionine. *Arzneimittelforschung.* 1988;38:1625-1629. **39.** Pezzoli C, Galli-Kienle M, Stramentinoli G. Lack of mutagenic activity of ademetionine in vitro and in vivo. *Arzneimittelforschung.* 1987;37:826-829. **40.** Spillmann M, Fava M. S-Adenosylmethionine (ademetionine) in psychiatric disorders: historical perspective and current status. *CNS Drugs.* 1996;6:416-425. **41.** Morana A, Di Lernia I, Carteni M, et al. Synthesis and characterisation of a new class of stable S-adenosyl-L-methionine salts. *Int J Pharmacol.* 2000;194;61-68.

Saw Palmetto

Sabal Serrulata, Serenoa Repens

Alternate/Related Names: Permixon, Strogen Forte

U.S. BRAND NAMES OF CLINICALLY TESTED PRODUCTS

Elusan Prostate Plantes and Medicines = Permixon (Pierre Fabre) in Europe

ProstActive (Nature's Way) = Prostagutt, WS 1473 (Schwabe) in Europe

ProstActive Plus (Nature's Way) = Prostagutt forte (Schwabe) (saw palmetto/nettle root combination) in Europe

DESCRIPTION

Saw palmetto is a native of North America, found principally in the Caribbean and the southern Atlantic coast. A member of the palm family, saw palmetto grows only about 2 to 4 feet high, with fan-shaped leaves and abundant berries. Native Americans used the berries for the treatment of various genitourinary complaints, especially in men, as well as for women with breast disorders. European physicians in America took up saw palmetto as a treatment for prostate enlargement at the turn of the twentieth century. It also became popular in folk medicine as a "male tonic" to increase sex drive and fertility. Today, a lipophilic extract of saw palmetto berries called Permixon is a standard treatment for benign prostatic hyperplasia (BPH) in many European countries.

PHARMACOLOGY

The lipophilic extract of saw palmetto berries used medicinally contains primarily a complex mixture of free fatty acids and fatty acid esters, together with much smaller quantities of phytosterols (including beta-sitosterol, campesterol, stigmasterol, and cycloartenol), aliphatic alcohols, and polyprenic compounds.[1] Pharmacokinetic studies of the lipophilic extract (second component on an HPLC assay) found a mean value of area under the concentration versus time curve of 8.2 mg/Lh, and an elimination half-life of 1.9 hours.

The mechanism of action of saw palmetto is not fully understood. Possible and mutually compatible explanations include prostate volume reduction, inhibition of 5-alpha-reductase, direct anti-androgen effects, interference with prostate estrogen receptors, leukotriene inhibition, and muscular relaxation. In rodents, saw palmetto has been found not to exhibit estrogenic or progestational properties or produce hypophyseal inhibition.[2] In humans, therapeutic doses of saw palmetto extracts do not cause alpha-1-adrenoreceptor inhibition.[3]

CLINICAL STUDIES

BENIGN PROSTATIC HYPERPLASIA

Seven double-blind placebo-controlled trials have evaluated the effectiveness of saw palmetto in BPH.[1,4-12] These trials have ranged in length from 1 to 3 months and have involved a total of about 500 men. In all but one of these studies,[9] treatment with saw palmetto significantly improved urinary flow rate and most other measures of prostate disease.

Double-blind comparative trials have also been reported. A 6-month double-blind study of 1,098 men compared finasteride to saw palmetto and found equivalent reductions in symptoms.[13] Prostate size reduction was superior with finasteride (18% versus 6% reduction). However, this study has been criticized on the basis that its inclusion criteria regarding prostate volume and its limited duration may have precluded maximal efficacy of finasteride.[14,15] Both treatments were well tolerated; however, sexual function scores were better in the saw palmetto group, and saw palmetto did not alter PSA levels. A 48-week double-blind trial with 543 participants that compared a combination of saw palmetto and nettle root against finasteride also reported equivalent benefits.[16]

A 52-week double-blind study of 811 men compared saw palmetto to the alpha-blocker tamsulosin and found equivalent efficacy in subjective and objective scores of BPH severity.[17] The saw palmetto arm, however, experienced a decrease in prostate volume, while a slight increase occurred among participants given tamsulosin. Both treatments were well tolerated; however, tamsulosin caused a higher incidence of ejaculation dysfunction.

LOWER URINARY TRACT SYMPTOMS

In a 6-month double-blind placebo-controlled study of 81 men with moderate to severe lower urinary tract symptoms (LUTS), use of saw palmetto led to a statistically significant improvement in urinary symptoms as compared with placebo.[18] However, there were no significant improvements in measures of urinary flow or sexual function.

PROPOSED INDICATIONS AND USAGE

Significant evidence supports the use of saw palmetto for treatment of Vahlensieck stage I or II BPH. Unlike finasteride, saw palmetto does not affect PSA levels, a potential advantage in prostate cancer screening; in addition, saw palmetto has no deleterious effect on sexual function. However, finasteride more markedly decreases prostate volume than saw palmetto, which may give finasteride a significant therapeutic advantage.

One double-blind trial supports the use of saw palmetto for lower urinary tract symptoms (LUTS) in men.

Saw palmetto is also sometimes advocated for chronic nonbacterial prostatitis, but there is no real evidence that it is effective, and finasteride proved superior in an open comparative trial.[19]

WARNINGS

None.

PRECAUTIONS

Safety in young children or in pregnant or lactating women has not been established, but there are no recommended uses of saw palmetto in those populations. Safety in individuals with severe hepatic or renal disease has not been evaluated.

DRUG INTERACTIONS

None are known.

ADVERSE REACTIONS

Saw palmetto is well tolerated; in clinical trials, only nonspecific side effects have been reported. In rats and dogs, saw palmetto extract administered at a dose of 2 g/kg daily for 6 months produced no toxic, mutagenic, or teratogenic effects.[2]

No clinically relevant changes in laboratory parameters have been seen in human clinical trials of saw palmetto.[1]

PROPOSED DOSAGE AND ADMINISTRATION

The standard dose of saw palmetto is 160 mg twice a day of a lipophilic extract standardized to contain 85% to 95% fatty acids and sterols. Some evidence suggests that a once-daily dose of 320 mg is equally effective.[20,21] In a 6-month dose-determination trial, 480 mg daily was not found to be any more effective than 320 mg.[1] The most-studied saw palmetto product, Permixon, uses an extraction process based on hexane. Other products use ethanol, methanol, or liquid carbon dioxide as solvents. Teas and other preparations of saw palmetto are not effective because the active constituents of the berries are lipophilic.

PATIENT INFORMATION

Substantial evidence suggests that the herb saw palmetto is a safe and effective treatment for early stages of benign prostatic hyperplasia (BPH, or enlarged prostate). However, conventional medications may offer important advantages, such as helping to prevent the need for surgery.

In addition, because prostate cancer and prostatitis can mimic the symptoms of BPH, medical consultation is essential before simply beginning self-treatment with saw palmetto. Furthermore, saw palmetto should not be relied on in advanced cases of BPH, when severe urinary retention occurs.

The safety of saw palmetto for pregnant or nursing women or young children has not been established. Individuals with severe liver or kidney disease should consult a physician before using this (or any other) supplement.

REFERENCES

1. Plosker GL, Brogden RN. *Serenoa repens* (Permixon(r)). A review of its pharmacology and therapeutic efficacy in benign prostatic hyperplasia. *Drugs Aging.* 1996;9:379-395. **2.** Bombardelli I. Serenoa repens (Bartram) J. K. Small. *Fitoterapia.* 1997;68:99-113. **3.** Goepel M, Dinh L, Mitchell A, et al. Do saw palmetto extracts block human alpha(1)-adrenoceptor subtypes in vivo? *Prostate.* 2001;46:226-232. **4.** Boccafoschi S, Annoscia S. Comparison of Serenoa repens extract with placebo by controlled clinical trial in patients with prostatic adenomatosis [in Italian]. *Urolgia.* 1983;50:1257-1268. **5.** Champault G, Patel JC, Bonnard AM. A double-blind trial of an extract of the plant Serenoa repens in benign prostatic hyperplasia [letter]. *Br J Clin Pharmacol.* 1984;18:461-462. **6.** Descotes JL, Rambeaud JJ, Deschaseaux P, et al. Placebo-controlled evaluation of the efficacy and tolerability of Permixon(r) in benign prostatic hyperplasia after exclusion of placebo responders. *Clin Drug Invest.* 1995;9:291-297. **7.** Emili E, Lo Cigno M, Petrone U. Clinical trial of a new drug for treating hypertrophy of the prostate (Permixon(r)) [in Italian]. *Urolgia.* 1983;50:1042-1048. **8.** Mattei FM, Capone M, Acconcia A. Serenoa repens extract in the medical treatment of benign prostatic hypertrophy [in Italian]. *Urolgia.* 1988;55:547-552. **9.** Reece Smith H, Memon A, Smart CJ, et al. The value of Permixon(r) in benign prostatic hypertrophy. *Br J Urol.* 1986;58:36-40. **10.** Tasca A, Barulli M, Cavazzana A, et al. Treatment of obstruction in prostatic adenoma using an extract of Serenoa repens. Double-blind clinical test v. placebo [in Italian; English abstract]. *Minerva Urol Nefrol.* 1985;37:87-91. **11.** Bach D, Schmitt M, Ebeling L. Phytopharmaceutical and synthetic agents in the treatment of benign prostatic hyperplasia (BPH). *Phytomedicine.* 1996-1997;3:309-313. **12.** Bracher F. Phytotherapy in the treatment of benign proststic hyperplasia [in German; English abstract]. *Urologe A.* 1997;36;10-17. **13.** Carraro JC, Raynaud JP, Koch G, et al. Comparison of phytotherapy (Permixon) with finasteride in the treatment of benign prostate hyperplasia: a randomized international study of 1,098 patients. *Prostate.* 1996;29:231-240. **14.** Boyle P, Gould AL, Italy M, et al. Prostate volume predicts outcome of treatment of BPH with finasteride: Meta-analysis of randomised clinical trials. *Proc Am Urol Assoc.* 1996;155(suppl):572A. **15.** Gormley GJ, Stoner E, Bruskewitz RC, et al. The effect of finasteride in men with benign prostatic hyperplasia. *N Engl J Med.* 1992;327:1185-1191. **16.** Sokeland J. Combined sabal and urtica extract compared with finasteride in men with benign prostatic hyperplasia: analysis of prostate volume and therapeutic outcome. *BJU Int.* 2000;86:439-442. **17.** Debruyne F. Phytotherapy (LSESR) vs. an alpha-blocker for treatment of lower urinary tract symptoms secondary to benign prostate enlargement: a randomized comparative study. Presented at: American Urological Association 2001 Annual Meeting; June 2-7, 2001; Anaheim, Calif. **18.** Kuznetsov DD, Gerber GS, Burstein JD. Randomized, double blind, placebo-controlled study of saw palmetto in men with lower urinary tract symptoms (LUTS). Presented at: American Urological Association 2001 Annual Meeting; June 2-7, 2001; Anaheim, Calif. **19.** Volpe MA, Cabelin M, Te AE, et al. A prospective trial using saw palmetto versus finasteride in the treatment of chronic nonbacterial prostatitis (CP). Presented at: American Urological Association 2001 Annual Meeting; June 2-7, 2001; Anaheim, Calif. **20.** Braeckman J, Bruhwyler J, Vandekerckhove K, et al. Efficacy and safety of the extract of *Serenoa repens* in the treatment of benign prostatic hyperplasia: the therapeutic equivalence between twice and once daily dosage forms. *Phytother Res.* 1997;11:558-563. **21.** Stepanov VN, Siniakova LA, Sarrazin B, et al. Efficacy and tolerability of the lipidosterolic extract of *Serenoa repens* (Permixon(r)) in benign prostatic hyperplasia: a double-blind comparison of two dosage regimens. *Adv Ther.* 1999;16:231-241.

St. John's Wort

Hypericum Perforatum

Alternate/Related Names: Amber, Goatweed, Hardhay, Klamath Weed, Tipton Weed

U.S. BRAND NAMES OF CLINICALLY TESTED PRODUCTS

Kira (Lichtwer Pharma) = Jarsin 300, LI160, LI160WS (Lichtwer Pharma) in Europe

Perika (Nature's Way), Movana (Pharmaton) = Neuroplant, WS 5572 (Schwabe) in Europe

DESCRIPTION

St. John's wort is a common perennial herb with many branches and bright yellow flowers that grows wild in much of the world. In the Pacific Northwest, St. John's wort is an invasive pest known as Klamath weed that can cause fatal phototoxicity if light-skinned cattle and sheep graze on it.

PHARMACOLOGY

St. John's wort preparations are manufactured from the above-ground portion of the plant, most prominently the buds, flowers, and distal leaves. Constituents include the species-specific naphthodianthrones hypericin, pseudohypericin, protohypericin, protopseudohypericin, and cyclopseudohypericin, as well as the acylphlorglucinol hyperforin, phenylpropanes, flavonol glycosides, bioflavones, tannins, proanthocyanidins, and volatile oils.[1,2]

Hypericin is the most studied constituent of St. John's wort, and it is clearly the primary photosensitizing agent. However, hyperforin is considered a more promising candidate for an active therapeutic ingredient.[1,3,4] Hyperforin was initially neglected because researchers thought that it was unstable.[5] However, recent evidence suggests that it is present in clinically tested St. John's wort formulations at a concentration of 1% to 6%. Hyperforin appears to cause a nonspecific reuptake inhibition of serotonin, norepinephrine, and dopamine, and, with subchronic use, cortical beta-receptor downregulation.[3]

However, not all evidence points toward hyperforin. Two double-blind trials using a form of St. John's wort with low hyperforin content found it effective.[6,7] This suggests that there are additional active constituents in St. John's wort, and other candidates have been proposed.[8-12]

At clinically relevant single doses, hyperforin achieves maximal serum concentrations within 3 to 3.5 hours, with an elimination half-life of 9 hours.[13] With single-dose ingestion of 750 mcg, plasma concentrations of hypericin rise after a 2-hour lag time, reach a peak in about 6 hours, and then decline with a half-life of 43.1 hours.[14] Steady state for a dose of 250 mcg t.i.d. was achieved in 6 to 7 days.

The mechanism of action of St. John's wort remains unknown. Early research showed that extracts of St. John's wort can inhibit the enzyme monoamine oxidase in vitro.[15] However, later investigation showed that the dosages of St. John's wort taken orally in actual practice are probably too low to inhibit monoamine oxidase[16,17]; MAO-inhibitor-type reactions have never been observed with St. John's wort. More current evidence points to reuptake inhibition of serotonin as well as dopamine and norepinephrine.[3,18,19,20]

Hyperforin appears to be active against multiresistant *Staphylococcus aureus,* as well as other gram-positive bacteria,[21] whereas hypericin possesses antiviral properties.[22] The clinical relevance of these findings is unclear.

CLINICAL STUDIES

MILD TO MODERATE DEPRESSION

Until 1998, most trials of St. John's wort for depression used LI 160, a 0.3%-hypericin water and alcohol extract (the extraction process is conducted in darkness at controlled temperatures). Some subsequent studies have used either WS 5573, standardized to hyperforin content, or ZE 117, a low-hyperforin product.

St. John's wort has primarily been evaluated as a treatment for major depression of mild to moderate severity, as determined by HAM-D scores and other measures. Numerous double-blind comparative or placebo-controlled trials in this population have been reported, enrolling a total of more than 2,000 individuals.[1,6,7,23-30] All but one of the placebo-controlled trials found St. John's wort to be effective.[30] Comparative trials found St. John's wort as effective as appropriate doses of SSRIs and imipramine.[6,24-27]

For example, an 8-week double-blind trial of 263 individuals compared a St. John's wort product standardized to hyperforin content against placebo and imipramine.[26] Participants were diagnosed with major depression by ICD-10 criteria, and had average baseline 17-item HAM-D scores of 22.6, representing a moderate level of disease severity. The results showed St. John's wort more effective at reducing HAM-D scores than placebo and as effective as 100 mg/day imipramine.

In severe depression, however, imipramine has been found superior to St. John's wort.[31]

POLYNEUROPATHY

A double-blind placebo-controlled trial of 54 individuals found St. John's wort ineffective for polyneuropathy.[32]

PROPOSED INDICATIONS AND USAGE

Significant evidence supports the use of St. John's wort for major depression of mild to moderate severity.

St. John's wort has been advocated for other conditions in which pharmaceutical antidepressants have been used, including PMS, menopausal symptoms, chronic pain, insomnia, and anxiety. However, there is no meaningful supporting evidence for the use of St. John's wort in these conditions.

Based on in vitro evidence that hypericin has antiviral effects, St. John's wort was for a time popular among individuals with HIV. However, in order to produce any antiviral effects, hypericin must be taken in doses high enough to cause significant toxicity.[22] Furthermore, concomitant use of St. John's wort reduces serum levels of protease inhibitors (see Drug Interactions).

St. John's wort is also sometimes used as a topical treatment for wounds and burns. However, topical St. John's wort has been associated with photosensitivity reactions (see Precautions).

WARNINGS

St. John's wort has the capacity for potentially dangerous interactions with numerous pharmacological agents (see Drug Interactions).

Individuals undergoing UV treatment should avoid oral or topical St. John's wort due to risk of photosensitivity reactions.

PRECAUTIONS

Hypericin is a known photosensitizing agent. Severe phototoxicity has occurred in animals that graze on St. John's wort. One study of sun-sensitive patients given twice the normal dose of the herb for 2 weeks showed only minimally decreased time to erythema on exposure to UV radiation.[33] However, there is a case report of severe phototoxicity in an individual taking St. John's wort and subsequently receiving UVB therapy.[34] In addition, there are two case reports of severe reactions to sun exposure in individuals using topical St. John's wort.[34] Based on these findings, individuals receiving UVB treatment should avoid St. John's wort entirely; individuals using oral St. John's wort should take enhanced precautions against sunburn; and topical St. John's wort should be avoided. Patients who have taken a massive overdose of St. John's wort should probably be kept away from UV sources for several days. Combination treatment with St. John's wort and photosensitizing drugs may be of concern as well (see Drug Interactions).

Concerns have also been expressed that photo-activation of hypericin in the lens of the eye might lead to increased risk of cataracts.[35]

St. John's wort extract has been found to be antimutagenic in *Escherichia coli*.[36] However, it has been recognized that hypericin can accumulate in the nucleus of cells exposed to the compound and can directly bind to DNA.[37] The relevance of these findings is unclear, and no long-term carcinogenicity testing has been conducted with St. John's wort.

Like other antidepressants, St. John's wort can cause episodes of mania.[38,39]

Maternal administration of St. John's wort extract (180 mg/kg, a dose calculated to mimic human dosing) in rats before and during gestation produced no effects on offspring.[40] However, maximum safe dosages for pregnant or lactating women, or young children, have not been established. Maximum safe dosages in individuals with severe renal or hepatic disease are also not known.

DRUG INTERACTIONS

St. John's wort has been found to affect the activity of multiple cytochromes as well as the transport protein p-glycoprotein, and these effects are clinically relevant.[41-49] Hypericin appears to inhibit CYP2C19 as well as other CYP2 enzymes. Hyperforin may inhibit CYP3A4, CYP2C9, and CYP2D6, whereas the flavonoid constituent I3,II8-biapigenin is a strong inhibitor of CYP3A4[50]; induction of enzymes may also occur.[45,51,52] Compelling evidence indicates that the herb can reduce serum concentrations of protease inhibitors, cyclosporine, digoxin, warfarin, and theophylline. Numerous cases of transplant rejection (heart, kidney, and liver) have been reported in individuals using cyclosporine and St. John's wort concurrently. Interactions with numerous other drugs such as oral contraceptives, etoposide, teniposide, mitoxantrone, doxorubicin, clozapine, and olanzapine are also suspected; furthermore, dosage adjustment to accommodate the effects of St. John's wort might lead to rebound toxicity.

Several case reports suggest that combined usage of St. John's wort and other serotonergic drugs may result in serotonin syndrome.[53,54,55]

Based on its photosensitizing effects, there may be an increased risk of photosensitivity if St. John's wort is combined with known photosensitizing agents. In addition, proton pump inhibitors may potentiate the phototoxic effects of hypericin.[56]

ADVERSE REACTIONS

St. John's wort is generally very well tolerated. A drug-monitoring study of 3,250 patients taking St. John's wort extract for 4 weeks revealed a 2.4% overall incidence of side effects.[57] The most common were mild stomach discomfort (0.6%); allergic reactions, primarily rash (0.5%); tiredness (0.4%); and restlessness (0.3%). Only 1.5% of the patients dropped out of the study because of adverse reactions.

No LD_{50} of standard St. John's wort extract was identified in studies of mice, rats, and dogs treated for 26 weeks, even at dosages of 5,000 mg/kg.[58] Intolerance reactions appeared at 900 mg/kg/day. No genotoxic or mutagenic effects were noted in these studies.

PROPOSED DOSAGE AND ADMINISTRATION

The usual dosage of St. John's wort is 300 mg 3 times daily of an extract standardized to contain 0.3% hypericin or 2% to 3% hyperforin. However, some tested formulations have alternate dosing schedules, and label instructions should be followed.

PATIENT INFORMATION

Considerable evidence suggests that St. John's wort is effective for mild to moderate depression. However, it is not effective for severe depression. Because it is not always easy to determine the severity of your own depression, a medical evaluation is essential before self-treatment with St. John's wort.

St. John's wort can interact with many medications, potentially making them ineffective. These include protease inhibitors (used for HIV), cyclosporine (used to prevent rejection of organ transplants), digoxin (used for congestive heart failure and other heart conditions), warfarin (used to "thin" the blood), clozapine and olanzapine (used in schizophrenia and other psychological conditions), theophylline (used for asthma), cancer chemotherapy medications, and oral contraceptives In addition, if you are taking St. John's wort along with a medication and then stop taking the herb, you may experience increased drug side effects or toxic reactions.

St. John's wort should not be combined with standard antidepressants. If you are already taking an antidepressant, you should not stop the medication and switch to St. John's wort without medical supervision.

St. John's wort can cause increased sensitivity to the sun, as well as to ultraviolet radiation, leading to severe burns.

Maximum safe dosages of St. John's wort for pregnant or nursing women or young children has not been established. Individuals with severe liver or kidney disease should consult a physician before using this (or any other) supplement.

REFERENCES

1. Laakmann G, Schule C, Baghai T, et al. St. John's wort in mild to moderate depression: the relevance of hyperforin for the clinical efficacy. *Pharmacopsychiatry.* 1998;31(suppl 1):54-59. **2.** Nahrstedt A, Butterweck V. Biologically active and other chemical constituents of the herb of hypericum perforatum L. *Pharmacopsychiatry.* 1997;30(suppl):129-134. **3.** Muller WE, Singer A, Wonnemann M, et al. Hyperforin represents the neurotransmitter reuptake inhibiting constituent of hypericum extract. *Pharmacopsychiatry.* 1998;31(suppl 1):16-21. **4.** Brown D. Antidepressant activity of St. John's wort extract-new mechanisms of action proposed. *Quart Rev Nat Prod.* 1998;109-111. **5.** Chatterjee SS, Noldner M, Koch E, et al. Antidepressant activity of hypericum perforatum and hyperforin: the neglected possibility. *Pharmacopsychiatry.* 1998;31(suppl 1):7-15. **6.** Schrader E. Equivalence of St John's wort extract (Ze 117) and fluoxetine: a randomized, controlled study in mild-moderate depression. *Int Clin Psychopharmacol.* 2000;15:61-68. **7.** Schrader E, Meier B, Brattstrom A. Hypericum treatment of mild-moderate depression in a placebo-controlled study. A prospective, double-blind, randomized, placebo-controlled, multicentre study. *Hum Psychopharmacol.* 1998;13:163-169. **8.** Bhattacharya SK, Chakrabarti A, Chatterjee SS. Activity profiles of two hyperforin-containing hypericum extracts in behavioral models. *Pharmacopsychiatry.* 1998;31(suppl 1):22-29. **9.** Baureithel KH, Buter KB, Engesser A, et al. Inhibition of benzodiazepine binding in vitro by amentoflavone, a constituent of various species of Hypericum. *Pharm Acta Helv.* 1997;72:153-157. **10.** Cott JM. In vitro receptor binding and enzyme inhibition by Hypericum perforatum extract. *Pharmacopsychiatry.* 1997;30(suppl 2):108-112. **11.** Butterweck V, Jurgenliemk G, Nahrstedt A, et al. Flavonoids from Hypericum perforatum show antidepressant activity in the forced swimming test. *Planta Med.* 2000;66:3-6. **12.** Dimpfel W, Schober F, Mannel M. Effects of a methanolic extract and a hyperforin-enriched CO2 extract of St. John's Wort (Hypericum perforatum) on intracerebral field potentials in the freely moving rat (Tele-Stereo-EEG). *Pharmacopsychiatry.* 1998;31(suppl):30-35. **13.** Biber A, Fischer H, Romer A, et al. Oral bioavailability of hyperforin from hypericum extracts in rats and human volunteers. *Pharmacopsychiatry.* 1998;31(suppl 1):36-43. **14.** Kerb R, Brockmoller J, Staffeldt B, et al. Single-dose and steady-state pharmacokinetics of hypericin and pseudohypericin. *Antimicrob Agents Chemother.* 1996;40:2087-2093. **15.** Suzuki O, Satsumata Y, Oya M, et al. Inhibition of monoamine oxidase by hypericin. *Planta Med.* 1984;50:272-274. **16.** Bladt S, Wagner H. Inhibition of MAO by fractions and constituents of hypericum extract. *J Geriatr Psychiatry Neurol.* 1994;7(suppl 1):S57-S59. **17.** Thiede HM, Walper A. Inhibition of MAO and COMT by hypericum extracts and hypericin. *J Geriatr Psychiatry Neurol.* 1994;7(supp 1):s54-s56. **18.** Muller WE, Kasper S. Hypericum extract (Li 160) as a herbal antidepressant. *Pharmacopsychiatry.* 1997;30(suppl 2):71-134. **19.** Muller WEG, Rossol R. Effects of Hypericum extract on the expression of serotonin receptors. *J Geriatr Psychiatry Neurol.* 1994;7(supp 1):S63-S64. **20.** Teufel-Mayer R, Gleitz J. Effects of long-term administration of hypericum extracts on the affinity and density of the central serotongergic 5-HT1 A and 5-HT2 A receptors. *Pharmacopsychiatry.* 1997;30(suppl):113-116. **21.** Schempp C, Pelz K, Wittmer A, et al. Antibacterial activity of hyperforin from St. John's wort, against multi-resistant Staphylococcus aureus and gram-positive bacteria. *Lancet.* 1999;353:2129. **22.** Gulick RM, McAuliffe V, Holden-Wiltse J, et al. Phase I studies of hypericin, the active compound in St. John's Wort, as an antiretroviral agent in HIV-infected adults. AIDS Clinical Trials Group Protocols 150 and 258. *Ann Intern Med.* 1999;130:510-514. **23.** Hansgen KD, Vesper J. Antidepressant efficacy of a high-dose hypericum extract [translated from German]. *MMW Munch Med Wochenschr.* 1996;138:29-33. **24.** Harrer G, Schmidt U, Kuhn U, et al. Comparison of equivalence between the St. John's wort extract LoHyp-57 and fluoxetine. *Arzneimittelforschung.* 1999;49:289-296. **25.** Brenner R, Azbel V, Madhusoodanan S, et al. Comparison of an extract of hypericum (LI 160) and sertraline in the treatment of depression: a double-blind, randomized pilot study. *Clin Ther.* 2000;22:411-419. **26.** Philipp M, Kohnen R, Hiller KO. Hypericum extract versus imipramine or placebo in patients with moderate depression: randomised multicentre study of treatment for eight weeks. *BMJ.* 1999;319:1534-1539. **27.** Woelk H. Comparison of St John's wort and imipramine for treating depression: randomised controlled trial. *BMJ.* 2000;321:536-539. **28.** Linde K, Ramirez G, Mulrow CD, et al. St John's wort for depression-an overview and meta-analysis of randomised clinical trials. *BMJ.* 1996;313:253-258. **29.** Kalb R, Trautmann-Sponsel RD, Kieser M. Efficacy and tolerability of hypericum extract WS 5572 versus placebo in mildly to moderately depressed patients. A randomized double-blind multicenter clinical trial. *Pharmacopsychiatry.* 2001;34:96-103. **30.** Shelton RC, Keller MB, Gelenberg A, et al. Effectiveness of St. John's wort in major depression: a randomized controlled trial. *JAMA.* 2001;285:1978-1986. **31.** Vorbach EU, Arnoldt KH, Hubner WD. Efficacy and tolerability of St. John's wort extract LI 160 vs. imipramine in patients with severe depressive episodes according to ICD-10. *Pharmacopsychiatry.* 1997;30(Suppl. 2):81-85. **32.** Sindrup SH, Madsen C, Bach FW, et al. St. John's wort has no effect on pain in polyneuropathy. *Pain.* 2001;91:361-365. **33.** Brockmoller J, Reum T, Bauer S, et al. Hypericin and pseudohypericin: pharmacokinetics and effects on photosensitivity in humans. *Pharmacopsychiatry.* 1997;30(suppl):94-101. **34.** Lane-Brown MM. Photosensitivity associated with herbal preparations of St John's wort (Hypericum perforatum) [letter]. *Med J Aust.* 2000;172:302. **35.** Roberts JE, Wang RH, Tan IP, et al. Hypericin (active ingredients in St. John's wort) photooxidation of lens proteins [abstract]. *Photochem Photobiol.* 1999;69(suppl):42S. **36.** Vukovic-Gacic B, Simic D. Identification of natural antimutagens with modulating effects on DNA repair. *Basic Life Sci.* 1993;61:269-277. **37.** Miskovsky P, Chinsky L, Wheeler GV, et al. Hypericin site specific interactions within ploynucleotides used as DNA model compounds. *J Biomol Struct Dyn.* 1995;13:547-552. **38.** Nierenberg AA, Burt T, Matthews J, et al. Mania associated with St. John's wort. *Biol Psychiatry.* 1999;46:1707-1708. **39.** Barbenel DM, Yusufi B, O'Shea D, et al. Mania in a patient receiving testosterone replacement postorchidectomy taking St John's wort and sertraline. *J Psychopharmacol.* 2000;14:84-86. **40.** Rayburn WF, Gonzalez CL, Christensen HD, et al. Effect of prenatally administered hypericum (St John's wort) on growth and physical maturation of mouse offspring. *Am J Obstet Gynecol.* 2001;184:191-195. **41.** Breidenbach T, Hoffmann MW, Becker T, et al. Drug interaction of St John's wort with ciclosporin [letter]. *Lancet.* 2000;355:1912. **42.** Jobst K, McIntyre M, St George D, et al. Safety of St. John's wort (Hypericum perforatum) [letters]. *Lancet.* 2000;355:575-577. **43.** Johne A, Brockmuller J, Bauer S, et al. Pharmacokinetic interaction of digoxin with an herbal extract from St. John's wort (Hypericum perforatum). *Clin Pharmacol Ther.* 1999;66:338-345. **44.** Maurer A, Johne A, Bauer S, et al. Interaction of St. John's wort extract with phenprocoumon [abstract]. *Eur J Clin Pharmacol.* 1999;55:A22. **45.** Nebel A, Schneider BJ, Baker R, et al. Potential metabolic interaction between St. John's wort and theophylline [letter]. *Ann Pharmacother.* 1999;33:502. **46.** Piscitelli SC, Burstein AH, Chaitt D, et al. Indinavir concentrations and St. John's wort [letter]. *Lancet.* 2000;355:547-548. **47.** Ruschitzka F, Meier PJ, Turina M, et al. Acute heart transplant rejection due to St. John's wort [letter]. *Lancet.* 2000;355:548-549. **48.** Dresser GK, Schwarz UI, Wilkinson GR, et al. St. John's wort induces intestinal and hepatic CYP3A4 and P-glycoprotein in healthy volunteers [abstract]. *Clin Pharmacol Ther.* 2001;69:P23. **49.** Barone GW, Gurley BJ, Ketel BL, et al. Drug interaction between St. John's wort and cyclosporine. *Ann Pharmacother.* 2000;34:1013-1016. **50.** Obach RS. Inhibition of human cytochrome P450 enzymes by constituents of St. John's Wort, an herbal preparation used in the treatment of depression. *J Pharmacol Exp Ther.* 2000;294:88-95. **51.** Moore LB, Goodwin B, Jones SA, et al. St. John's wort induces hepatic drug metabolism through activation of the pregnane X receptor. *Proc Natl Acad Sci U S A.* 2000;97:7500-7502. **52.** Baker RK, Brandt TL, Siegel D, et al. Inhibition of human DNA topoisomerase II-alpha by the naphtha-di-anthrone, hypericin [abstract]. *Proc Annu Meet Am Assoc Cancer Res.* 1998;39:422. **53.** DeMott K. St. John's wort tied to serotonin syndrome. *Clin Psychiatry News.* 1998;26(3):28. **54.** Gordon JB. SSRIs and St. John's Wort: possible toxicity? [letter]. *Am Fam Physician.* 1998;57:950, 953. **55.** Lantz MS, Buchalter E, Giambanco V.St. John's wort and antidepressant drug interactions in the elderly. *J Geriatr Psychiatry Neurol.* 1999;12:7-10. **56.** Mirossay A, Mirossay L, Tothova J, et al. Potentiation of hypericin and hypocrellin-induced phototoxicity by omeprazole. *Phytomedicine.* 1999;6:311-317. **57.** Woelk H, Burkard G, Grunwald J. Benefits and risks of the hypericum extract LI 160: drug monitoring study with 3250 patients. *J Geriatr Psychiatry Neurol.* 1994;7(supp 1):S34-S38. **58.** Schulz V, Hansel R, Tyler VE. *Rational Phytotherapy: A Physicians' Guide to Herbal Medicine.* 3rd ed. Berlin, Germany: Springer-Verlag; 1998:52, 54-56.

Uva Ursi

Arctostaphylos Uva-Ursi

Alternate/Related Names: Bearberry

U.S. BRAND NAMES OF CLINICALLY TESTED PRODUCTS

None.

DESCRIPTION

Uva ursi is a low-lying evergreen bush whose leaves that are used medicinally. Uva ursi is found primarily in Europe and the northern United States. It has a long history of use by both European and Native American herbalists, primarily for the treatment of UTIs and stones. From 1820 to 1950, uva ursi was listed in the U.S. National Formulary as a urinary antiseptic.

PHARMACOLOGY

The major active constituents in uva ursi are arbutin and methylarbutin. Other important ingredients include flavonoids, tannins, organic acids, and free hydroquinone. Arbutin is poorly absorbed from the digestive tract, but its glycosidic bond is cleaved by intestinal flora to form readily absorbable aglycone hydroquinone.[1] This appears to be conjugated to glucuronides and sulfate esters in the intestinal mucosa and liver and then excreted through the kidney, where it may act as an antiseptic under relatively alkaline conditions.

CLINICAL STUDIES

Despite its wide use for UTIs, the evidence base for uva ursi is very weak.

One double-blind placebo-controlled study followed 57 women for 1 year. None of the women who received uva ursi (combined with dandelion, a diuretic herb) developed a urinary tract infection, but five of those receiving placebo did.[2] (**Note:** Long-term use of uva ursi is not recommended; see Precautions.)

PROPOSED INDICATIONS AND USAGE

The European Scientific Cooperative on Phytotherapy monograph on uva ursi recommends it for "uncomplicated infections of the urinary tract such as cystitis when antibiotic treatment is not considered essential."[3]

WARNINGS

Long-term use of uva ursi is not recommended due to the risk of hydroquinone toxicity.

PRECAUTIONS

Hydroquinone is a mutagen, hepatotoxin, carcinogen, and topical irritant.[4-8] For this reason, long-term use of uva ursi is contraindicated, and even short-term use should be avoided in pregnant or lactating women, young children, and individuals with severe renal or hepatic disease.

DRUG INTERACTIONS

Formal drug interaction studies have not been performed. However, any drug that acidifies the urine may interfere with the function of uva ursi.

ADVERSE REACTIONS

Mild gastrointestinal distress is the only commonly reported short-term side effect of uva ursi.

PROPOSED DOSAGE AND ADMINISTRATION

A typical daily dose of uva ursi is 3 g dried herb.[3,7,9] Daily intake of 800 mg arbutin should not be exceeded. Maximum treatment duration is 2 weeks and uva ursi should not be used more than 5 times a year. Uva ursi is generally taken with meals to minimize gastrointestinal upset.

PATIENT INFORMATION

Uva ursi is sold as a treatment for bladder infections. However, there is not much evidence that it works. Furthermore, use of uva ursi leads to the release of a carcinogenic chemical, hydroquinone, into the bladder. For this reason, long-term use of uva ursi may be dangerous.

Uva ursi should not be used by pregnant or nursing women or young children. Individuals with severe liver or kidney disease should consult a physician before using this (or any other) supplement.

REFERENCES

1. Frohne D. The urinary disinfectant effect of extract from leaves Uva-Ursi [in German; English abstract]. *Planta Med.* 1970;18:1-25. **2.** Larsson B, Jonasson A, Fianu S. Prophylactic effect of UVA-E in women with recurrent cystitis: a preliminary report. *Curr Ther Res.* 1993;53:441-443. **3.** European Scientific Cooperative on Phytotherapy. *Uvae Ursi Folium,* Bearberry Leaf. Exeter, UK: ESCOP. 1996-1997:1. Monographs on the Medicinal Uses of Plant Drugs, Fascicule 5. **4.** Lewis RJ. *Sax's dangerous properties of industrial materials,* 8th ed. New York: Van Nostrand Reinhold; 1989:1906-1907. **5.** Nowak AK, Shilkin KB, Jeffrey GP. Darkroom hepatitis after exposure to hydroquinone [letter]. *Lancet.* 1995;345:1187. **6.** Peters MMCG, Jones TW, Monks TJ, et al. Cytotoxicity and cell proliferation induced by the nephrocarcinogen hydroquinone and its nephrotoxic metabolite 2,3,5-(tris-glutathion-S-yl) hydroquinone. *Carcinogenesis.* 1997;18:2393-2401. **7.** Schulz V, Hansel R, Tyler VE. *Rational Phytotherapy: A Physicians' Guide to Herbal Medicine.* 3rd ed. Berlin, Germany: Springer-Verlag; 1998:223-224. **8.** U.S. Environmental Protection Agency. Extremely hazardous substances. Superfund Chemical Profiles. Park Ridge NJ: Noyes Data Corporation; 1988:1906-1907. **9.** Tyler V. *Herbs of choice.* New York: Pharmaceutical Products Press; 1994:79.

Valerian

Valeriana Officinalis

U.S. BRAND NAMES OF CLINICALLY TESTED PRODUCTS

Sedonium (Lichtwer Pharma) = Sedonium, LI 156 (Lichtwer Pharma) in Europe
Valerian Nighttime (Nature's Way) = Euvegal forte (Schwabe) in Europe

DESCRIPTION

Over 200 plant species belong to the genus *Valeriana,* but the one used for insomnia is *Valeriana officinalis.* This perennial grows abundantly in moist woodlands in Europe and North America and is under extensive cultivation to meet market demands. The root is used for medicinal purposes.

Galen recommended valerian for insomnia in the second century A.D. The herb became popular as a sedative from the sixteenth century onward, with wide usage in Europe and the United States. Scientific studies of valerian began in the 1980s, leading to its approval by Germany's Commission E in 1985.

PHARMACOLOGY

Constituents of valerian include valepotriates (e.g., valtrates, didrovaltrates and isovaltrates), valeric acid, isovaleric acid, valerenic acid, valeranone, valeranol, valerianol, sterols, alkaloids, and flavonoids.[1] Isovaleric acid is the main contributor to the herb's characteristic odor.

Valerenic acid and whole-valerian extracts have been found to produce sedation and anticonvulsive effects in laboratory mice.[2,3,4] Using an autoradiographic tracer method to determine glucose transformations in rat brain after injection, valerian root and certain fractions have been found to exert central depressant activity.[3,5] However, no effect was seen when using valerenic acid, valeranone, valtrate, didrovaltrate, or the valepotriate metabolite homobaldrinal. An ethanolic extract of valerian root (4:1) prolonged thiopental-induced anesthesia but produced no sedation in cats at up to 100 mg/kg.[6] However, it did exhibit anticonvulsive activity against picrotoxin at an ED_{50} of 4.5 to 6 mg/kg. A 5-6:1 aqueous extract of valerian root produced sedative effects in mice at 20 mg/kg.[4] It also increased thiopental-induced sleeping time in a dose-dependent manner from 2 mg/kg to 200 mg/kg Anticonvulsive effects were weak.

The mechanism of action of valerian is unknown. Valepotriates are known to suppress the anxiogenic effects of benzodiazepine withdrawal in diazepam-dependent rats.[7] However, standard valerian preparations have little to no valepotriate content.[8,9]

Other in vitro research has shown that certain valerian extracts possess weak binding affinity to GABA receptors, mitochondrial benzodiazepine receptors, and barbiturate receptors.[10,11] Initial reports suggested that valerian extracts increased GABA concentration in the synaptic cleft by both increasing its secretion and impairing its uptake.[12,13] However, later research concluded that this apparent effect was actually due to GABA present in valerian extract.[14,15]

CLINICAL STUDIES

INSOMNIA

In the largest trial of valerian for insomnia, 121 patients with a history of significant insomnia were enrolled in a 28-day double-blind placebo-controlled study.[16] Significant improvements in sleep quality were seen at 28 but not at 14 days. The researchers interpreted the results to indicate that valerian is most appropriately used as a long-term treatment for poor sleep rather than for occasional insomnia. In sharp contrast, smaller studies found benefits with one-time or short-term valerian use.[17-21]

A 28-day double-blind trial of 75 individuals with various forms of insomnia compared valerian (600 mg qhs) against oxazepam (10 mg qhs).[22] The results showed no differences in efficacy.

Valerian-lemon balm and valerian-hops combinations have also been found effective for insomnia in double-blind trials.[23,24,25]

ANXIETY

A double-blind placebo-controlled study of 48 participants placed under "social stress" situations compared low-dose valerian extract (100 mg), propranolol (20 mg), and the two treatments combined.[26] Use of valerian improved subjective anxiety but did not alter physiological activation.

PROPOSED INDICATIONS AND USAGE

Preliminary evidence suggests that valerian may provide some benefits in insomnia. It is most commonly used for occasional acute insomnia, but the best designed study suggests that it may be more appropriate as a treatment for chronic insomnia.

Weak evidence suggests that valerian may be useful for situational anxiety.

WARNINGS

None.

PRECAUTIONS

Whole valerian contains valepotriates, substances with mutagenic and cytotoxic effects. However, these are believed not to be present in typical valerian products.[8,9,27,28,29] Furthermore, the toxic effects of valepotriates are believed to be due to their metabolites baldrinal and homobaldrinal, which are subjected to a strong first-pass effect in the intestines and inactivated.[30] Nonetheless, the possibility of adverse effects in the gastrointestinal tract or liver cannot be excluded on this basis.

Maximum safe dosages for pregnant or lactating women and individuals with severe hepatic or renal disease have not been established. Valerian is generally not recommended for children under 3 years of age.[8]

Valerian does not appear to impair driving ability, reaction time, or alertness, or to produce morning residual sedation when taken at night.[31,32,33] However, it may impair vigilance for a couple of hours immediately after use. For this reason, driving a car or operating hazardous machinery immediately after taking valerian is not recommended.

Valerian withdrawal has not been observed in animal studies or controlled human trials. However, one case report suggests the possibility. A 58-year-old male who had been taking high doses of valerian root extract (about 2.5 to 10 g daily) for many years developed delirium and sinus tachycardia during a postoperative period of no valerian use.[34]

DRUG INTERACTIONS

In one human trial, no interaction between alcohol and valerian was found, as measured by concentration, attentiveness, reaction time, and driving performance.[31] However, animal studies suggest that valerian potentiates pentobarbital, hexobarbital, and thiopental.[2,4,6,35]

ADVERSE REACTIONS

Valerian is listed on the FDA's GRAS (generally recognized as safe) list and is approved for use as a food. Except for its unpleasant odor, valerian is generally well tolerated. In one study, only 2 out of 61 participants taking valerian reported side effects, which were headache and morning grogginess.[16] Mild gastrointestinal distress is also occasionally reported, and there are informal reports that some people develop a paradoxical mild stimulant effect.

One case of overdose at 20 times the standard daily dosage led to no more than minor symptoms.[36] The LD_{50} of ethanolic valerian extracts by intraperitoneal injection is 3.3 g/kg in mice. Over a 45-day period, intraperitoneal administration to rats at a level of 400 mg/kg or more produced no significant changes.[37]

There have been reports of hepatotoxicity in individuals who took combination herbal remedies containing skullcap as well as valerian.[38] However, in a series of about 50 overdose cases (including long-term follow-up) with a combination preparation called Sleep-Qik containing the anticholinergic hyoscine, the serotonin antagonist cyproheptadine, and valerian,[39,40] the expected symptoms of cyproheptadine and hyoscine toxicity developed, but there were no signs of hepatotoxicity.

PROPOSED DOSAGE AND ADMINISTRATION

For insomnia, the standard dose of valerian is 2 to 3 g dried root, 270 to 450 mg aqueous valerian extract, or 600 mg dry ethanol extract, taken 30 to 60 minutes before bedtime.[30]

Whole valerian root has been given at 2 to 3 g twice daily for anxiety. Valerian is not recommended for children under 3.[8]

PATIENT INFORMATION

Some evidence suggests that valerian can improve sleep. The effect is mild at most, and may take many weeks to develop. Valerian should not be combined with other sedative drugs. In addition, it is not advisable to drive or operate heavy machinery after taking valerian.

Valerian should not be used by pregnant women, individuals with liver disease, or children under the age of 3.

Maximum safe dosages for individuals with severe renal disease have not been established.

REFERENCES

1. Hendriks H, Bos R, Allersma DP, et al. Pharmacological screening of valerenal and some other components of essential oil of *Valeriana officinalis.* Planta Med. 1981;42:62-68. **2.** Hendriks H, Bos R, Woerdenbag HJ, et al. Central nervous depressant activity of valerenic acid in the mouse. *Planta Med.* 1985;(1):28-31. **3.** Krieglstein J, Grusla D. Centrally depressant components of valerian. However, valepotriates, valerenic acid, valeranone and the essential oil are ineffective [in German]. *Dtsch Apoth Ztg.* 1988;128:2041-2046. **4.** Leuschner J, Muller J, Rudmann M. Characterisation of the central nervous depressant activity of a commercially available valerian root extract. *Arzneimittelforschung.* 1993;43:638-641. **5.** Grusla D, Holzl J, Krieglstein J. Valerian's effects in the brain of the rat [in German]. *Dtsch Apoth Ztg.* 1986;126:2249-2253. Cited by: European Scientific Cooperative on Phytotherapy. *Valerianae radix* (valerian root). Exeter, UK: ESCOP; 1996-1997. Monographs on the Medicinal Uses of Plant Drugs, Fascicule 4:3. **6.** Hiller KO, Zetler G. Neuropharmacological studies on ethanol extracts of *Valeriana officinalis* L: behavioural and anticonvulsant properties. *Phytother Res.* 1996;10:145-151. **7.** Andreatini R, Leite JR. Effect of valepotriates on the behavior of rats in the elevated plus-maze during diazepam withdrawal. *Eur J Pharmacol.* 1994;260:233-235. **8.** European Scientific Cooperative on Phytotherapy. *Valeriana radix* (valerian root). Exeter, UK: ESCOP; 1997: 2, 6. Monographs on the Medicinal Uses of Plant Drugs, Fascicule 4. **9.** Tyler VE. *Herbs of Choice.* New York, NY: Pharmaceutical Products Press; 1994: 118. **10.** Holzl J, Godau P. Receptor bindings studies with *Valeriana officinalis* on the benzodiazepine receptor. *Planta Med.* 1989;55(7 Spec No):642. **11.** Mennini T, Bernasconi P, Bombardelli E, et al. In vitro study on the interaction of extracts and pure compounds from Valeriana officinalis roots with GABA, benzodiazepine and barbiturate receptors in rat brain. *Fitoterapia.* 1993;64:291-300. **12.** Santos MS, Ferreira F, Cunha AP, et al. Synaptosomal GABA release as influenced by valerian root extract-involvement of the GABA carrier. *Arch Int Pharmacodyn Ther.* 1994;327:220-231. **13.** Santos MS, Ferreira F, Cunha AP, et al. An aqueous extract of valerian influences the transport of GABA in synaptosomes [letter]. *Planta Med.* 1994;60:278-279. **14.** Cavadas C, Araujo I, Cotrim MD, et al. In vitro study on the interaction of Valeriana officinalis L. extracts and their amino acids on GABAA receptor in rat brain. *Arzneimittelforschung.* 1995;45:753-755. **15.** Santos MS, Ferreira F, Faro C, et al. The amount of GABA present in aqueous extracts of valerian is sufficient to account for [^{3}H]GABA release in synaptosomes. *Planta Med.* 1994;60:475-476. **16.** Vorbach EU, Goetelmeyer R, Bruening J. Therapy for insomniacs. Effectiveness and tolerance of valerian preparations [translated from German]. *Psychopharmakotherapie.* 1996;3:109-115. **17.** Leathwood PD, Chauffard F, Heck E, et al. Aqueous extract of valerian root (Valeriana officinalis L.) improves sleep quality in man. *Pharmacol Biochem Behav.* 1982;17:65-71. **18.** Kamm-Kohl AV, Jansen W, Brockmann P. Modern valerian therapy for nervous disorders in old age [translated from German]. *Med Welt.* 1984;35:1450-1454. **19.** Lindahl O, Lindwall L. Double blind study of a valerian preparation. *Pharmacol Biochem Behav.* 1989;32:1065-1066. **20.** Schulz H, Stolz C, Muller J. The effect of valerian extract on sleep polygraphy in poor sleepers: a pilot study. *Pharmacopsychiatry.* 1994;27:147-151. **21.** Donath F, Quispe S, Diefenbach K. Critical evaluation of the effect of valerian extract on sleep structure and sleep quality. *Pharmacopsychiatry.* 2000;33:47-53. **22.** Dorn M. Efficacy and tolerability of Baldrian versus oxazepam in non-organic and non-psychiatric insomniacs: a randomised, double-blind, clinical, comparative study [translated from German]. *Forsch Komplementarmed Klass Naturheilkd.* 2000;7:79-84. **23.** Cerny A, Schmid K. Tolerability and efficacy of valerian/lemon balm in healthy volunteers (a double-blind, placebo-controlled, multicentre study). *Fitoterapia.* 1999;70:221-228. **24.** Schmitz M, Jackel M. Comparative study for assessing quality of life of patients with exogenous sleep disorders (temporary sleep onset and sleep interruption disorders) treated with a hops-valarian preparation and a benzodiazepine drug [translated from German]. *Wien Med Wochenschr.* 1998;148:291-298. **25.** Dressing H, Riemann D, Low H, Schredl M, et al. Insomnia: are valerian/balm combinations of equal value to benzodiazepines? [translated from German]. *Therapiewoche.* 1992;42:726-736. **26.** Kohnen R, Oswald WD. The effects of valerian, propranolol, and their combination on activation, performance and mood of healthy volunteers under social stress conditions. *Pharmacopsychiatry.* 1988;21:447-448. **27.** Bounthanh C, Bergmann C, Beck JP, et al. Valepotriates, a new class of cytotoxic and antitumor agents. *Planta Med.* 1981;41:21-28. **28.** Houghton PJ. The biological activity of Valerian and related plants. *J Ethnopharmacol.* 1988;22:121-142. **29.** von der Hude W, Scheutwinkel-Reich M, Braun R. Bacterial mutagenicity of the tranquilizing constituents in Valerianaceae roots. *Mutat Res.* 1986;169:23-27. **30.** Schulz V, Hansel R, Tyler VE. *Rational Phytotherapy: A Physicians' Guide to Herbal Medicine.* 3rd ed. Berlin, Germany: Springer-Verlag; 1998:76-77, 81. **31.** Albrecht M, Berger W, Laux P, et al. Psychopharmaceuticals and traffic safety: the effect of Euvegal (r) Dragees Forte on driving ability and combination effects with alcohol [translated from German]. *Z Allgemeinmed.* 1995;71:1215-1218,1221-1222,1225. **32.** Gerhard U, Linnenbrink N, Georghiadou C, et al. Vigilance-decreasing effects of 2 plant-derived sedatives [in German; English abstract]. *Schweiz Rundsch Med Prax.* 1996;85:473-481. **33.** Kuhlmann J, Berger W, Podzuweit H, et al. The influence of valerian treatment on "reaction time, alertness and concentration" in volunteers. *Pharmacopsychiatry.* 1999;32:235-241. **34.** Garges HP, Varia I, Doraiswamy PM. Cardiac complications and delirium associated with valerian root withdrawal [letter]. *JAMA.* 1998;280:1566-1567. **35.** Sakamoto T, Mitani Y, Nakajima K. Psychotropic effects of Japanese valerian root extract. *Chem Pharm Bull (Tokyo).* 1992;40:758-761. **36.** Willey LB, Mady SP, Cobaugh DJ, et al. Valerian overdose: A case report. *Vet Hum Toxicol.* 1995;37:364-365. **37.** Rosecrans JA, Defeo JJ, Youngken HW Jr. Pharmacological investigation of certain Valeriana officinalis L. extracts. *J Pharm Sci.* 1961;50:240-244. **38.** MacGregor FB, Abernethy VE, Dahabra S, et al. Hepatotoxicity of herbal remedies. *BMJ.* 1989;299:1156-1157. **39.** Chan TY, Tang CH, Critchley JA. Poisoning due to an over-the-counter hypnotic, Sleep-Qik(tm) (hyoscine, cyproheptadine, valerian). *Postgrad Med J.* 1995;71:227-228. **40.** Chan TY. An assessment of the delayed effects associated with valerian overdose [letter]. *Int J Clin Pharmacol Ther.* 1998;36:569.

APPENDICES

Three appendices are provided for convenient, rapid access to important information. A complete table of contents for the appendices is located on the next page

The following items are included in this section:

- Appendix A: Comparative drug tables. Quickly compare different drugs within a therapeutic class on the basis of important clinical and pharmacological characteristics.
- Appendix B: Additional information. Turn to this appendix for numerous helpful tables containing hard-to-find content.
- Appendix C: Supplier profiles. With complete contact information for hundreds of pharmaceutical manufacturers, this appendix is an excellent source for ordering products, addressing product concerns, and making regulatory/medical inquiries.

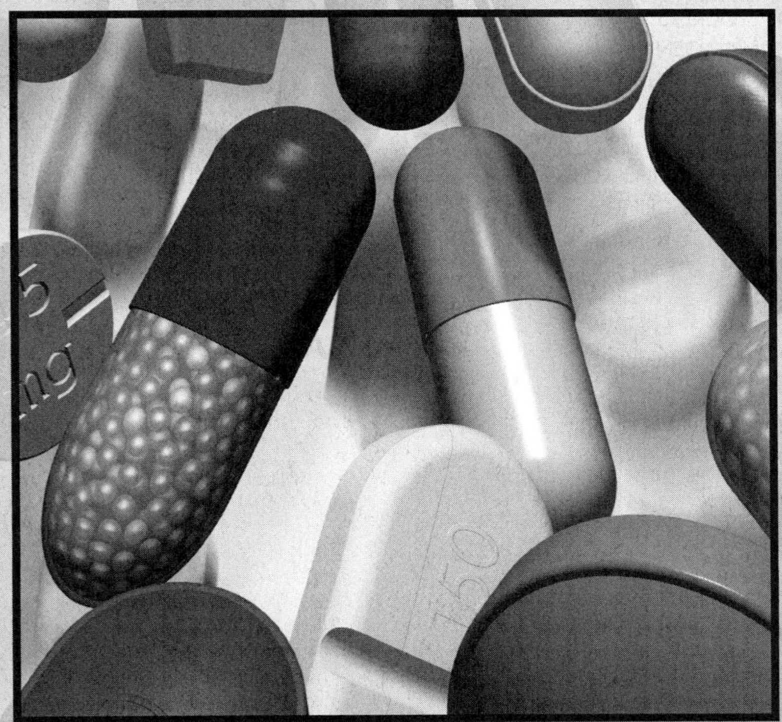

APPENDIX A—Comparative Tables

APPENDIX B—Additional Information

APPENDIX C—Supplier Profiles

APPENDIX A—COMPARATIVE TABLES

Acid-Secretion Inhibitors

HISTAMINE H_2-RECEPTOR BLOCKERS

Generic Name	*Brand Name*	*Adult Oral Dosage Range*	*Available Oral Dosage Forms*	*Nonprescription (OTC) Strength and Dosage Forms*	*Dose Adjustment in Renal Dysfunction*	*Drug Interactions/Comments*
Cimetidine†	Tagamet	200-400 mg qd-qid 800 mg qd-bid	Tablet: 100, 200, 300, 400, 800 mg; Oral solution: 300 mg/5 ml Injection: 150 mg/ml	Tablet: 100 mg (Tagamet HB)	Yes (CRCL <30 ml/min)	Amiodarone, benzodiazepines (except lorazepam, oxazepam, temazepam), caffeine, calcium channel blockers, carbamazepine, carmustine, cefuroxime, cefpodoxime, chloroquine, clozapine, digoxin, flecainide, fluconazole, fluorouracil, glipizide, glyburide, indomethacin, iron salts, itraconazole, ketoconazole, labetalol, lidocaine, lomustine, melphalan, meperidine (and other narcotic analgesics), metoprolol, metronidazole, moricizine, pentoxifylline, phenytoin, praziquantel, procainamide, propafenone, propranolol, quinidine, quinine, succinylcholine, sulfonylureas, tacrine, tetracyclines, theophylline, tocainide, triamterene, tricyclic antidepressants, valproic acid, warfarin **Comments:** May be given with meals. May give antacids for pain.
Famotidine†	Pepcid	20-40 mg bid or qhs	Tablet: 20, 40 mg; Tablet, orally disintegrating: 20, 40 mg; Chewable tablet: 10 mg; Powder for oral suspension: 40 mg/5 ml (reconstituted)	Tablet: 10 mg (Pepcid AC) Chewable tablet: 10 mg Capsules: 10 mg	Yes (CRCL <50 ml/min)	Cefpodoxime, cefuroxime, dihydropyridine calcium channel blockers, glipizide, glyburide, itraconazole, ketoconazole quinolone antibiotics, tolbutamide **Comments:** Oral suspension should be discarded 30 days after mixing.
Nizatidine†	Axid	150 mg bid or qhs, 300 mg qhs	Capsule: 150, 300 mg	Tablet: 75 mg (Axid AR)	Yes (CRCL <50 ml/min)	Cefpodoxime, cefuroxime, dihydropyridine calcium channel blockers, glipizide, glyburide, itraconazole, ketoconazole, quinolone antibiotics, salicylates, tolbutamide
Ranitidine†	Zantac	150 mg bid or qid; 300 mg qd	Tablet: 75, 150, 300 mg; Effervescent tablet: 150 mg; Effervescent granules: 150 mg; Capsule: 150, 300 mg; Syrup: 75 mg/5 ml Injection: 1 mg/5 ml, 25 mg/ml	Tablet: 75 mg (Zantac 75)	Yes (CRCL <50 ml/min)	Cefpodoxime, cefuroxime, calcium channel blockers, dihydropyridine diazepam, glipizide, glyburide, itraconazole, ketoconazole, procainamide, quinolone antibiotics, sulfonylureas, theophylline, warfarin

†Generic available for one or more dosage forms.

HISTAMINE H-2 RECEPTOR BLOCKER COMBINATIONS

Generic Name	Brand Name	Adult Oral Dosage Range	Nonprescription (OTC) Strength	Prescription Strength
Famotidine; calcium carbonate; magnesium hydroxide	Pepcid Complete	No more than 1 daily	Chewable tablet: Famotidine 10 mg, calcium carbonate 800 mg, magnesium hydroxide 165 mg	NA

PROTON PUMP INHIBITORS

Generic Name	Brand Name	Adult Dosage Range	Available* Dosage Forms	Nonprescription (OTC) Strength and Dosage Forms	Dose Adjustment in Renal Dysfunction	Drug Interactions/Comments
Esomeprazole	Nexium	20 mg qd before eating	Capsule: 20, 40 mg	NA	No	Cefuroxime, cefpodoxime, digoxin, dihydropyrimidine calcium channel blockers, iron salts, itraconazole, ketoconazole, sucralfate
Lansoprazole	Prevacid	15-30 mg qd or bid	Capsule: 15, 30 mg Granules for oral suspension: 15, 30 mg	NA	No	Same as esomeprazole plus theophylline
Omeprazole†	Prilosec	20-40 mg qd or bid before eating	Capsule: 10, 20, 40 mg	NA	No	Same as esomeprazole plus benzodiazepines, cilostazol, citalopram, clarithromycin, cyclosporine, dis- ulfiram, methotrexate, phenytoin, sulfonylureas, theophylline, warfarin
	Protonix I.V.		Injection: 40 mg/vial			
Pantoprazole	Protonix	40-240 mg/day	Tablet: 20, 40 mg	NA	No	Same as esomeprazole
Rabeprazole	Aciphex	20-100 mg qd; 60 mg bid	Tablet: 20 mg	NA	No	Same as esomeprazole plus cyclosporine

*All oral forms are delayed release.
†Generic available for one or more dosage forms.

References:
1. Ellsworth, Allan J, *et al. Mosby's Medical Drug Reference.* Mosby, St. Louis, 2003.
2. Website: U.S. Food and Drug Administration. Online. Internet. 2001. Available: http://www.fda.gov/cder

Analgesics

NARCOTIC AGENTS

Generic Name	Brand Name	Route	Usual Adult Dose	Available Dosage Forms	Dose equal* to 10 mg IM of Morphine Sulfate	Comments
Alfentanil DEA Schedule: CII	Alfenta	IV	8-245 μg/kg (dose is titrated to desired length and depth of anesthesia)	Injection: 500 μg/ml	0.4-0.8 mg	Determine dose on lean body weight; decrease dose in elderly debilitated patients
Codeine† DEA Schedule: CII; Combination products are CIII or CIV	Codeine	IV, IM, SC PO	15-60 mg q4-6h 10-20 mg q4-6h (for antitussive effect); 15-60 mg q4-6 h (for analgesia)	Injection: 30, 60 mg Oral solution: 15 mg/5 ml; Tablet: 15, 30, 60 mg	IM: 120-130 mg SC: 120 mg PO: 180-200 mg	Maximum daily dose = 360 mg; has antitussive effects in lower doses (given orally); often used in combination with other analgesics
Fentanyl† DEA Schedule: CII	Sublimaze	IV, IM	IV: 0.5-50 μg/kg/dose; IM: 0.05-0.1 mg	Injection: 0.05 mg/ml	0.1-0.2 mg	Dose is titrated to desired length and depth of anesthesia
	Duragesic	Transdermal	25-100 μg/h q72h	Transdermal patch: 25, 50, 75, 100 μg/h	100 μg/h = 10 mg morphine sulfate IV q4h	Indicated for chronic pain management; a small percentage of patients may require q48h dosing; assess patient's pain control after first 24 hours

NARCOTIC AGENTS—cont'd

Generic Name	*Brand Name*	*Route*	*Usual Adult Dose*	*Available Dosage Forms*	*Dose equal* to 10 mg IM of Morphine Sulfate*	*Comments*
Fentanyl—cont'd	Fentanyl Oralet, Actiq	Mucosal	2.5-5 μg/kg/dose	Lozenges: Oralet: 100, 200, 300, 400 μg; Actiq: 400, 600, 800, 1200, 1600 μg Lozenge on a stick: 200 μg		Fentanyl Oralet indicated only in perioperative settings, and not in unmonitored settings or for acute or chronic pain management Actiq indicated in chronic pain management for breakthrough pain Both products can be fatal to opiate-naive patients, especially children; therefore, safety precautions must be in place
Hydrocodone† DEA Schedule: CII	Vicodin, Vicoprofen, Lorcet, Lortab, Zydone, Norco	PO	5-10 mg q4-6h	Tablet: 2.5 mg with APAP 500 mg; Tablet and/or capsule: 5 mg with APAP 400 or 500 mg, or aspirin 500 mg, or homatropine 1.5 mg; Tablet: 7.5 mg with APAP 400, 500, 650, or 750 mg, or ibuprofen 200 mg; Tablet: 10 mg with APAP 325, 400, 500, 650, 660 mg; Elixir: 2.5 mg + APAP 167 mg per 5 ml; Syrup: 5 mg hydrocodone + homatropine 1.5 mg per 5 ml	30 mg	Only available in combination with acetaminophen, aspirin, homatropine, or ibuprofen
Hydromorphone† DEA Schedule: CII	Dilaudid	IM, IV, SC	1-4 mg q4-6h	Injection: 1, 2, 3, 4, 10 mg/ml; Powder for injection: 250 mg (10 mg/ml after reconstitution)	1.3 mg	High abuse potential
		PR	3 mg q6-8h	Rectal suppository: 3 mg		Store in refrigerator
		PO	Tablet: 2-4 mg q4-6h; Liquid: 2.5-10 mg q4-6h	Oral liquid: 5 mg/ 5 ml; Tablet: 1, 2, 3, 4, 8 mg	7.5 mg	Dose >4 mg q4-6h for severe pain.
Levomethadyl DEA Schedule: CII	ORLAAM	PO	20-140 mg three times per week	Oral solution: 10 mg/ml		For opiate dependence—to be given in authorized clinic setting; always dilute before administration; first dose does not have an immediate effect
Levorphanol† DEA Schedule: CII	Levo-Dromoran	PO	2-3 mg q6-8h	Tablet: 2 mg	4 mg	Repeated dosing may cause cumulative effects; long-acting
Meperidine† DEA Schedule: CII	Demerol	PO, IM, IV, SC	50-150 mg q3-4h	Injection: 25, 50, 75, 100 mg/ml Syrup: 50 mg/5 ml; Tablet: 50, 100 mg	75 mg (IM) 75-100 mg (sc) 300 mg (PO)	For relief of moderate to severe pain and as a preoperative medication; active metabolite normeperidine may accumulate in patients with renal dysfunction; contraindicated within 14 days of MAOI therapy; short duration of action (2-4 hours)

Continued

Generic Name	*Brand Name*	*Route*	*Usual Adult Dose*	*Available Dosage Forms*	*Dose equal* to 10 mg IM of Morphine Sulfate*	*Comments*
Methadone† DEA Schedule: CII	Dolophine	PO, IM, SC	Analgesia (oral or injectable): 2.5-10 mg q3-4h, up to 5-20 mg q6-8h Detoxification (oral): 15-40 mg/d, for not more than 21 days, and not repeated earlier than 4 weeks after a preceding course Maintenance of opiate dependence: 20-120 mg/d	Injection: 10 mg/ml; Oral solution: 5, 10 mg/5 ml; Tablet: 5, 10 mg; Dissolvable tablet: 40 mg; Powder for compounding	10 mg (IM/SC) 20 mg (PO)	For relief of severe pain and maintenance of opiate addiction; long half-life (13-47 h) may increase risk of accumulation and respiratory depression in elderly patients; avoid in severe hepatic disease due to long half-life
Morphine Sulfate† DEA Schedule: CII	Roxanol, MS Contin, RMS, Duramorph, Kadian, MSIR, Astramorph Infumorph	IM, IV, SC	IV: 2-10 mg q4h; SC, IM: 5-20 mg q4h	Injection: 0.5, 1, 2, 4, 5, 8, 10, 15, 25, 50 mg/ml	10 mg	For relief of moderate to severe pain and preoperatively as an adjunct to anesthesia; maximum daily dose via EPIDURAL route = 10 mg
		IV, SC, continuous infusion	0.8-80 mg/h, titrated to analgesic need			
		Epidural	5 mg × 1, then 1-2 mg prn	Preservative-free injection: 0.5, 1, 10, 25 mg/ml		
		Intrathecal	0.2-1 mg × one dose; do NOT repeat			
		PR	10-20 mg q4h	Rectal Suppository: 5, 10, 20, 30 mg	NA	
		PO	Immediate release tablet: 5-30 mg q4h; Oral solution: 10-20 mg q4h	Immediate-release tablet: 10,15,30 mg; Immediate-release capsule: 15, 30 mg; Oral solution: 10, 20, 100 mg/5 ml	30-60 mg	
			Sustained-release: 15-30 mg q8-12h	Sustained-release tablet: 15, 30, 60, 100, 200 mg; Sustained-release capsule: 20, 30, 50, 60, 100 mg	30-60 mg	
Oxycodone† DEA Schedule: CII	Roxicodone, OxyContin	PO	Immediate-release: 5-30 mg q4-6h	Capsule: 5 mg; Tablet: 5, 15, 30 mg; Oral liquid: 1, 20 mg/ml	5-10 mg	Also available in combination with aspirin (e.g., Percodan) or acetaminophen (e.g., Percocet); High abuse potential
			Sustained-release: 10-160 mg q12h	Sustained-release Tablet: 10, 20, 40, 80, 160 mg	30 mg	
Oxymorphone DEA Schedule: CII	Numorphan	IM, SC	1-1.5 mg q4-6h	Injection: 1, 1.5 mg/ml	1-1.5 mg	For relief of moderate to severe pain and preoperatively as an adjunct to anesthesia
		IV	0.5 mg × 1, then titrate			
		PR	5 mg q4-6h	Rectal suppository: 5 mg	5-10 mg	
Propoxyphene DEA Schedule: CIV	Darvon	PO	Hydrochloride salt: 65 mg q4h;	Capsule: 65 mg (HCl salt)	130 mg (HCl salt)	100 mg of propoxyphene napsylate = 65 mg of propoxyphene hydrochloride; maximum daily dose of hydrochloride form is 390 mg; maximum daily dose of napsylate form is 600 mg; also available in combination with APAP (e.g., Darvocet)
	Darvon-N	PO	Napsylate salt: 100 mg q4h	Tablet: 100 mg; (Napsylate salt)	>100 mg (napsylate salt)	
Remifentanil DEA Schedule: CII	Ultiva	IV	0.025-2 μg/kg/min	Powder for injection: 1, 2, 5 mg		Dose is titrated to desired length and depth of anesthesia
Sufentanil† DEA Schedule: CII	Sufenta	IV	1-30 μg/kg/dose	Injection: 50 μg/ml	0.01-0.04 mg	Dose is titrated to desired length and depth of anesthesia; primary anesthetic at >8 μg/kg; adjunct to anesthesia at <8 μg/kg

*These equivalencies are approximations and may vary greatly among individuals.
†Generic available for one or more dosage forms.

NARCOTIC-LIKE AGENTS

Generic Name	*Brand Name*	*Route*	*Usual Adult Dose*	*Available Dosage Forms*	*Dose equal* to 10 mg IM of Morphine Sulfate*	*Comments*
Buprenorphine† DEA Schedule: CIII	Buprenex	IM, SL IV	0.3-0.6 mg q6h SL: 12-16 mg/day	Injection: 0.3 mg/ml Sublingual tablet: 2.8 mg	0.3 mg	General comments for opiate agonist/antagonists (includes buprenorphine, butorphanol, nalbuphine, and pentazocine): a. May potentiate or reduce effects of opiate agonists b. May cause withdrawal symptoms in opiate-dependent patients c. Use with other CNS depressants (e.g., barbiturates) increases the likelihood of respiratory depression
Butorphanol† DEA Schedule: CIV	Stadol	IV	0.5-2 mg q3-4h	Injection: 1, 2 mg/ml	2-3 mg	
	Stadol NS	IM	1-4 mg q3-4h		2-3 mg	
		Nasal spray	One spray in one nostril (one spray is approximately equal to 1 mg of butorphanol) × 1; may repeat × 1 in 60-90 min if pain persists; this initial two-dose sequence may be repeated in 3-4 h as needed; depending on the severity of the pain, an initial dose of 2 mg (1 spray in each nostril) may be given	Nasal spray: 10 mg/ml (2.5 ml container dispenses 14-15 doses)	2 mg	
Dezocine	Dalgan	IM	5-20 mg q3-6h (max 120 mg/day)	Injection: 5, 10, 15 mg/ml	10 mg	Subcutaneous route NOT recommended due to local tissue reactions in animal studies and in 4 % of human subjects tested
		IV	2.5-10 mg q2-4h			
Nalbuphine†	Nubain	IM, SC, IV	10-20 mg q3-6h (max 160 mg/day)	Injection: 10, 20 mg/ml	10 mg	Commonly used for obstetrical pain Maximum daily dose: 160 mg
Pentazocine† DEA Schedule: CIV	Talwin	IM, SC	30-60 mg q3-4h	Injection: 30 mg/ml	30 mg	Maximum daily dose: 360 mg
		IV	30 mg q3-4h		30 mg	Maximum daily dose: 360 mg
	Talwin-NX	PO	50-100 mg q3-4h (maximum 600 mg/day)	Tablet: 50 mg + naloxone HCl 0.5 mg	180 mg	Maximum daily dose: 600 mg
	Talacen	PO	One tablet q4h (maximum 6 tablets/day)	Tablet: 25 mg + APAP 650 mg	180 mg	
	Talwin Compound	PO	Two tablets 3-4 times per day	Tablet: 12.5 mg + aspirin 325 mg	180 mg	
Tramadol†	Ultram	PO	50-100 mg q4-6h (max 400 mg/day) Reduce in elderly, renal impairment, cirrhosis	Tablet: 50 mg	NA	Maximum daily dose: 400 mg 100 mg equal to 60 mg codeine U.S. clinical trials demonstrate a lesser degree of tolerance and withdrawal effects compared to classic opiates
	Ultracet	PO	2 Tablets q4-6h (max 8/day, for no more than 5 days)	Tablet: 37.5 mg + acetaminophen 325 mg	NA	Not recommended for pregnant or nursing women Increased risk of seizures in patients receiving tricyclic antidepressants Contraindicated with current MAOI use

*These equivalencies are approximations and may vary greatly among individuals.
†Generic available for one or more dosage forms.

NON-NARCOTIC AGENTS

Generic Name	Brand Name	Usual Adult Dose	Maximum Adult Daily Dose	Prescription Strength	Nonprescription Strength	Comments
Acetaminophen†	Tylenol, Panadol, Tempra	325-650 mg q4-6h	4000 mg	NA	Tablets: 160, 325, 500, 650 mg; Chewable tablets: 80 mg; Drops: 80 mg/0.8 ml, 80 mg/1.66 ml, 100 mg/ml; Elixir: 40, 80, 125, 160 mg/5 ml; Liquid: 160 mg/5 ml, 500 mg/15 ml; Rectal suppositories: 80, 120, 125, 300, 325, 650 mg	Hepatotoxicity if overdosed and in persons with cirrhosis (limit dose to 2000 mg/day in cirrhotics)

†Generic available for one or more dosage forms.

CYCLOOXYGENASE-2 (COX-2) INHIBITORS

Generic Name	Brand Name	Usual Adult Dose	Maximum Adult Daily Dose	Available Dosage Forms	Comments
Celecoxib	Celebrex	Osteoarthritis: 100 mg bid or 200 mg once daily Rheumatoid arthritis: 100 to 200 mg bid Pain or dysmenorrhea: 400 mg (initial), 200 mg bid if needed	400 mg	Capsules: 100, 200 mg	
Meloxicam	Mobic	7.5-15 mg once daily	15 mg	Tablets: 7.5 mg	"Preferential" COX-2 activity; Less selective than others in the class
Rofecoxib	Vioxx	Osteoarthritis: 12.5 mg once daily (initial); 25 mg once daily (maintenance) Pain or dysmenorrhea: 25 mg once daily Rheumatoid arthritis: 25 mg once daily	50 mg	Tablets: 12.5, 25, 50 mg Oral suspension: 12.5 mg/5 ml, 25 mg/5 ml	
Valdexocib	Bextra	Arthritis: 10 mg once daily Dysmenorrhea: 20 mg bid	40 mg	Tablets: 10, 20 mg	

NONSTEROIDAL ANTIINFLAMMATORY DRUGS*

Generic Name	Brand Name	Usual Adult Dose	Maximum Adult Daily Dose	Prescription Strength	Nonprescription Strength	Comments
Diclofenac† (immediate-release)	Cataflam	50 mg bid-qid	200 mg	Tablets: 50 mg	NA	
Diclofenac (sustained-release)	Voltaren, Voltaren XR	50 mg bid-qid; 75-100 mg bid; 100 mg qd	225 mg	Tablets: Delayed release: 25, 50, 75 mg; Tablets: extended-release: 100 mg	NA	
Diflunisal† (also a salicylate)	Dolobid	250-500 mg q8-12h	1500 mg	Tablets: 250, 500 mg	NA	Not metabolized to salicylate; increases acetaminophen level by 50% when coadministered
Etodolac†	Lodine, Lodine XL	200-600 mg q6-8h (maximum daily dose: 1200 mg)	1200 mg	Tablets: 400, 500 mg; Capsules: 200, 300 mg; Tablets, extended-release: 400, 500, 600 mg	NA	Antacids reduce peak concentration by 20%

NONSTEROIDAL ANTIINFLAMMATORY DRUGS*—cont'd

Generic Name	*Brand Name*	*Usual Adult Dose*	*Maximum Adult Daily Dose*	*Prescription Strength*	*Nonprescription Strength*	*Comments*
Fenoprofen†	Nalfon	200-600 mg q6h	3200 mg	Tablets: 600 mg Capsules: 200, 300 mg	NA	Highly protein-bound (to albumin); greater renal toxicity
Flurbiprofen†	Ansaid	50-100 mg q6-8h (maximum daily dose: 300 mg)	300 mg	Tablets: 50, 100 mg	NA	May cause CNS stimulation
Ibuprofen	Motrin, Rufen	400-800 mg q6-8h	3200 mg	Tablets: 400, 600, 800 mg	Tablets: 100, 200 mg; Chewable tablets: 50, 100 mg; Capsules: 200 mg; Suspension: 100 mg/2.5 ml, 100 mg/5 ml; Drops: 40 mg/ml	Also approved for primary dysmenorrhea; available in combination with hydrocodone (Vicoprofen)
Indomethacin	Indocin, Indocin SR	25-50 mg bid-tid or 75 mg qd-bid (sustained-release)	200 mg	Capsules: 25, 50 mg Capsules, extended-release: 75 mg Suspension: 25 mg/5 ml Rectal suppositories: 50 mg	NA	
Ketoprofen	Orudis, Oruvail, Orudis KT	50-75 mg q6-8h	300 mg	Capsules: 25, 50, 75 mg Capsules, extended-release: 100, 150, 200 mg	12.5 mg (Orudis KT)	High rate of dyspepsia (11%); available in sustained-release form
Ketorolac tromethamine†	Toradol	PO: 10 q4-6h IM/IV: 30 or 60 mg initially, then 15-30 mg q6h	PO: 40 mg IM/IV: 150 mg first day, then 120 mg qd	Tablets: 10 mg Injection: 15, 30 mg/ml	NA	Total duration of treatment should not exceed 5 days; 30 mg equal to 6-12 mg morphine sulfate but 10 times as expensive; 100% bioavailable (oral form); indicated only as continuation of parenteral ketorolac, short-term
Meclofenamate†	Meclomen	50-100 mg q6h	400 mg	Capsules: 50, 100 mg	NA	High rate of diarrhea (10-33%); also indicated to treat excessive menstrual bleeding
Mefenamic acid	Ponstel	500 mg, then 250 mg q6h	1000 mg	Capsules: 250 mg	NA	Also approved for primary dysmenorrhea
Nabumetone	Relafen	500-750 mg bid; 1000-2000 mg qd	2000 mg	Tablets: 500, 750 mg	NA	High rate of diarrhea (14%); metabolized to active agent
Naproxen†	Naprosyn, Naprelan EC-Naprosyn	250-500 mg q8-12h or 250 mg q6-8h or 1000 mg qd (controlled-release tablets)	1250 mg (first 24 h then 1000 mg thereafter)	Tablets: 250, 375, 500 mg Tablets, delayed release 375, 500 mg Suspension: 125 mg/5 ml	NA	Approved for acute gout; may increase effect of protein-bound drugs such as phenytoin, sulfonylureas, and warfarin; available in qd dosage form
Naproxen sodium	Anaprox, Anaprox DS	275-550 mg q8-12h	1375 mg (first 24 h then 1100 thereafter)	Tablets: 275, 550 mg	Tablets: 220 mg (Aleve)	Approved for acute gout; may increase effect of protein-bound drugs such as phenytoin, sulfonylureas, and warfarin
Oxaprozin	Daypro	600-1200 mg qd	1800 mg	Tablets: 600 mg	NA	
Piroxicam†	Feldene	10-20 mg qd	20 mg	Capsules: 10, 20 mg	NA	High rate of dyspepsia (20%); may increase effect of protein-bound drugs such as phenytoin, sulfonylureas, and warfarin.
Sulindac†	Clinoril	150-200 mg q12h	400 mg	Tablets: 150, 200 mg	NA	Approved for gout; less renal toxicity
Tolmetin†	Tolectin	400 mg q6-8h, 600 mg q8h	1800 mg	Tablets: 200, 600 mg Capsules: 400 mg	NA	High rate of nausea (11%)

*GI irritation is a common adverse effect that can occur with all NSAIDs, even the newer agents, which have greater receptor selectivity. Taking these medications with food will reduce the likelihood of GI irritation and is especially recommended for the older, non-cyclo-oxygenase-2 (COX-2) selective agents.
†Generic available for one or more dosage forms.

SALICYLATES*

Generic Name	Brand Name	Usual Adult Dose	Maximum Adult Daily Dose	Prescription Strength	Nonprescription Strength	Comments
Aspirin†	Empirin, Ecotrin, Halfprin	325-975 mg q4h	8000 mg	Enteric coated tablets: 975 mg; Slow release tablets: 800, 975 mg	Tablets: 325, 500 mg; Chewable tablets: 81 mg; Gum tablets: 227.5 mg; Enteric coated tablets: 81, 165, 325, 500, 650 mg; Slow release tablets: 81, 650 mg Rectal suppositories: 120, 200, 300, 600 mg	Antagonizes effect of probenecid; increases effect of sulfonylureas; reduces renal clearance of methotrexate
Choline magnesium trisalicylate†	Trilisate	500-1000 mg q12h	3000 mg	Tablets: 500, 750, 1000 mg (salicylate) Liquid: 500 mg/ 5 ml (salicylate)	NA	Antagonizes effect of probenecid; increases effect of sulfonylureas; reduces renal clearance of methotrexate
Salsalate†	Disalcid	500-1000 mg q8h 750-1500 mg q12h	3000 mg	Tablets: 500, 750 mg Capsules: 500 mg	NA	Antagonizes effect of probenecid; increases effect of sulfonylureas; reduces renal clearance of methotrexate
Aspirin buffered†	Ascriptin, Bufferin, Arthritis Pain Formula	325-975 mg of aspirin q4h	8000 mg of aspirin	NA	Tablets: 325, 500 mg of aspirin with buffers; Caplets: 325, 500 mg of aspirin with buffers; Tablets, coated: 325, 500 mg of aspirin with buffers; Tablets, effervescent: 325, 500 mg of aspirin with buffers	Antagonizes effect of probenecid; increases effect of sulfonylureas; reduces renal clearance of methotrexate; buffers include aluminum hydroxide, calcium carbonate, magnesium carbonate, magnesium oxide, and magnesium hydroxide. Effervescent tablets contain an acid (*e.g.*, citric acid) and a base (*e.g.*, sodium bicarbonate)
Choline salicylate†	Arthropan	870 mg q3-4h	5220 mg; 6960 mg for rheumatoid arthritis	NA	870 mg/5 ml	Antagonizes effect of probenecid; increases effect of sulfonylureas; reduces renal clearance of methotrexate

*GI irritation is a common adverse effect that can occur with all NSAIDs, even the newer agents which have greater receptor selectivity. Taking these medications with food will reduce the likelihood of GI irritation, and is especially recommended for the older, non-cyclo-oxygenase-2 (COX-2) selective agents.
†Generic available for one or more dosage forms.

References for Analgesic Tables:

1. Ellsworth, Allan J, *et al.* Mosby's Medical Drug Reference. Mosby, St. Louis, 2003.
2. Website: U.S. Food and Drug Administration. Online. Internet. 2003. Available: http://www.fda.gov/cder

Antibiotics

CEPHALOSPORINS, ORAL

Generic Name	Brand Name	Usual Adult Dose (g)	Available Dosage Forms	Adjust Dose for Renal Insufficiency	Comment (Generation)
Cefadroxil†	Duricef	1-2 q12-24h	Tablets: 1 g; Capsules: 500 mg; Powder for suspension: 125, 250, 500 mg/5 ml	Yes	(First Generation)
Cephalexin†	Keflex, Keftab	0.25-1.0 q6h	Tablets: 250, 500 mg, 1 g; Capsules: 250, 500 mg; Powder for suspension: 125, 250 mg/5 ml	Yes	Cheapest in its therapeutic class; (First Generation)
Cephradine†	Velosef	0.25-1.0 q6-12h	Capsules: 250, 500 mg; Powder for suspension: 125, 250 mg	Yes	(First Generation)
Cefaclor†	Ceclor, Ceclor CD	0.25-0.5 q8h	Tablets, extended-release: 375, 500 mg; Capsules: 250, 500 mg; Powder for suspension: 125, 187, 250, 375 mg/5 ml	No	(Second Generation)
Cefpodoxime proxetil	Vantin	0.1-0.4 q12h	Tablets: 100, 200 mg; Granules for suspension: 50, 100 mg/5 ml	Yes	(Second Generation)

CEPHALOSPORINS, ORAL—cont'd

Generic Name	*Brand Name*	*Usual Adult Dose (g)*	*Available Dosage Forms*	*Adjust Dose for Renal Insufficiency*	*Comment (Generation)*
Cefprozil	Cefzil	0.25-0.5 q12h	Tablets: 250, 500 mg; Powder for suspension: 125, 250 mg/5 ml	Yes	(Second Generation)
Cefuroxime axetil	Ceftin	0.25-0.5 q12h	Tablets: 125, 250, 500 mg; Suspension: 125, 500 mg/5 ml	Yes	(Second Generation)
Loracarbef	Lorabid	0.2-0.4 q12-24h	Capsules: 200, 400 mg; Powder for suspension: 100, 200 mg/5 ml	Yes	Carbacephem derivative rather than true cephalosporin; (Second Generation)
Cefdinir	Omnicef	0.6 qd or divided bid	Capsules: 300 mg; Suspension: 125 mg/5 ml	Yes	(Third Generation)
Cefditoren pivoxil	Spectracef	0.2-0.4 q12h	Tablets: 200 mg	Yes	Do not take with antacids or H_2 receptor blockers; (Third Generation)
Cefixime	Suprax	0.4 q24h or divided bid	Tablets: 200, 400 mg; Powder for suspension: 100 mg/5 ml	Yes	Single dose therapy for gonococcal genital and pharyngeal infections; (Third Generation)
Ceftibuten	Cedax	0.4 q24h	Capsules: 400 mg; Powder for suspension: 90, 180 mg	Yes	(Third Generation)

†Generic available for one or more dosage forms.

CEPHALOSPORINS, PARENTERAL

Generic Name	*Brand Name*	*Usual Adult Dose (g)*	*Available Dosage Forms*	*Adjust Dose for Renal Insufficiency*	*Comment (Generation)*
Cefazolin†	Ancef, Kefzol	0.25-2.0 q6-12h	Powder for injection: 250, 500 mg; 1, 5 g; 10 g*; Solution: 500 mg, 1 g/50 ml	Yes	Commonly used for surgical prophylaxis; (First Generation)
Cephapirin	Cefadyl	0.5-2.0 q4-6h	Powder for injection: 1 g	Yes	(First Generation)
Cefamandole	Mandol	0.5-2.0 q4-8h	Powder for injection: 1, 2 g	Yes	(Second Generation)
Cefmetazole	Zefazone	2 q6-12h	Powder for injection: 1, 2 g; Solution: 1, 2 g/50 ml	Yes	Intraabdominal infections; (First Generation)
Cefonicid	Monocid	0.5-2.0 q24h	Powder for injection: 1 g; 10 g*	Yes	May be useful in outpatient therapy of endocarditis; (Second Generation)
Cefotetan	Cefotan	1-2 q12-24h	Powder for injection: 1, 2 g; 10 g*; Solution: 1, 2 g/50 ml	Yes	Covers GI anaerobes; (Second Generation)
Cefoxitin	Mefoxin	1-2 q4-8h	Powder for injection: 1, 2 g; 10 g*; Solution: 1, 2 g/50 ml	Yes	Covers GI anaerobes; (Second Generation)
Cefuroxime†	Kefurox, Zinacef	0.75-1.5 q8h	Powder for injection: 750 mg, 1.5 g; 7.5 g*; Solution: 750 mg, 1.5 g/50 ml	Yes	Crosses blood-brain barrier; (Second Generation)
Cefepime	Maxipime	0.5-2.0 q8-12h	Powder for injection: 500 mg, 1, 2 g	Yes	(Third Generation)
Cefoperazone	Cefobid	1-2 q8-12h	Powder for injection: 1, 2 g; 10 g*; Solution: 1, 2 g/50 ml	No	(Third Generation)
Cefotaxime	Claforan,	1-2 q4-12h	Powder for injection: 500 mg, 1, 2 g; 10 g*; Solution: 1, 2 g/50 ml	Yes	Crosses blood-brain barrier; (Third Generation)
Ceftazidime	Fortaz, Tazicef, Tazidime	0.5-2.0 q8-12h	Powder for injection: 500 mg, 1, 2 g; 10 g*; Solution: 1, 2 g/50 ml	Yes	(Third Generation)
Ceftizoxime	Cefizox	1-12 g/d divided q4-8h	Powder for injection: 500 mg, 1, 2 g; 10 g*; Solution: 1, 2 g/50 ml	Yes	Crosses blood-brain barrier; (Third Generation)
Ceftriaxone	Rocephin	1-2 q12-24h	Powder for injection: 250, 500 mg, 1, 2 g; 10 g*; Solution: 1, 2 g/50 ml	No	May be useful in outpatient therapy of endocarditis; single-dose (250 mg IM) therapy for gonococcal genital and pharyngeal infections; crosses blood-brain barrier; (Third Generation)
Cephradine	Velosef	0.5-1 q6h	Powder for injection: 250, 500 mg, 1, 2 g	Yes	May be used for preoperative prophylaxis; (First Generation)

*Bulk package intended for pharmacy use only.
†Generic available for one or more dosage forms.

FLUOROQUINOLONES AND QUINOLONES, ORAL

Generic Name	Brand Name	Usual PO Adult Dose	Available Dosage Forms	Comments
Cinoxacin*†	Cinobac	250 mg q6h or 500 mg q12h	Capsule: 250, 500 mg	Only approved to treat UTIs; *Enterococcus, Staphylococcus,* and *Pseudomonas* sp are resistant; reduce dose in renal impairment
Ciprofloxacin	Cipro	100-750 mg q12h	Tablet: 100, 250, 500, 750 mg; Tablet, extended-release: 500 mg; Powder for suspension: 250, 500 mg/5 ml	Reserve use in UTI for documented pseudomonal infection or complicated UTI; considered first-line therapy for otitis externa in diabetic patients
Gatifloxacin	Tequin	200-400 mg qd	Tablet: 200, 400 mg	Similar indications to other quinolones, plus special indication for chronic prostatitis; one advantage is once daily dosing; adjust dose in renal impairment
Levofloxacin	Levaquin	500 mg q24h (for UTI, 250 mg q24h)	Tablet: 250, 500, 750 mg	L-isomer of the racemate ofloxacin (another commercially available quinolone antibiotic)
Lomefloxacin	Maxaquin	400 mg qd	Tablet: 400 mg	Contraindicated for empiric treatment of acute bacterial exacerbation of chronic bronchitis likely due to *S. pneumoniae*
Moxifloxacin	Avelox	400 mg qd	Tablet: 400 mg	No dose adjustment necessary for renal impairment or mild hepatic impairment; not recommended in cases of moderate to severe hepatic impairment.
Nalidixic Acid*	NegGram	500 mg-1 g qid	Tablet: 250, 500 mg, 1 g Suspension: 250 mg/5 ml	Insufficient doses may promote resistance
Norfloxacin	Noroxin	400 mg q12h; 800 mg single dose for routine cases of gonorrhea	Tablet: 400 mg	Only approved for UTIs, STDs (gonorrhea), and prostatitis
Ofloxacin	Floxin	200-400 mg q12h	Tablet: 200, 300, 400 mg	Not effective for syphilis; use with caution in presence of neurologic disorders due to increased seizure risk
Sparfloxacin	Zagam	400 mg load, then 200 mg qd	Tablet: 200 mg	For renally impaired patients, may give 400 mg loading dose, then 200 mg q48h
Trovafloxacin	Trovan	200-300 mg qd	Tablet: 100, 200 mg	Case reports of fatal hepatic reactions; use only in cases of life or limb-threatening infections, and begin therapy in an inpatient setting

*Not a Fluoroquinolone.
†Generic available for one or more dosage forms.

FLUOROQUINOLONES, PARENTERAL

Generic Name	Brand Name	Usual IV Adult Dose	Available Dosage Forms	Comments
Ciprofloxacin	Cipro	200-400 mg q12h	Injection: 200, 400 mg in glass vials and premixed bags	Infuse over 60 minutes
Gatifloxacin	Tequin	200-400 mg q24h	Injection: 400 mg Premixed bags: 200 mg/100 ml, 400 mg/100 ml	Infuse over 60 minutes
Levofloxacin	Levaquin	500 mg q24h (for UTI, 250 mg q24h)	Injection: (25 mg/ml) 500, 750 mg; Premixed bags: (5 mg/ml) 250, 500, 750 mg	L-isomer of the racemate ofloxacin (another commercially available Fluoroquinolone antibiotic) Infuse over 60 minutes
Moxifloxacin	Avelox IV	400 mg q24h	Premixed bags: 400 mg/250 ml	Infuse over 60 minutes
Ofloxacin	Floxin	200-400 mg q12h	Injection: 200, 400 mg	Not effective for syphilis Infuse over 60 minutes
Trovafloxacin	Trovan	200-300 mg qd	Injection: (as alatrofloxacin mesylate) (5 mg/ml) 250, 300 mg	IV formulation contains alatrofloxacin, a trovafloxacin prodrug Infuse over 60 minutes Case reports of fatal hepatic reactions; use only in cases of life or limb-threatening infections, and begin therapy in an inpatient setting

MACROLIDES

Generic Name	Brand Name	Usual Adult Dose (mg)	Available Dosage Forms	Comment
Azithromycin	Zithromax	500, followed by 250 q24h	Tablets: 250, 500, 600 mg; Powder for oral suspension: 100, 200 mg/5 ml; Powder packet for oral suspension: 1 g; Powder for injection: 500 mg	Single-dose therapy for chlamydial urethritis or cervicitis (1000 mg); antibacterial spectrum includes *Hemophilus influenzae;* indicated to prevent *Mycobacterium avium-intracellulare* infection (1200 mg per week)
Clarithromycin	Biaxin	250-500 q12h	Tablets: 250, 500 mg; Tablets, extended-release: 500 mg; Granules for oral suspension: 125, 250 mg/5 ml	Antibacterial spectrum includes *H. influenzae;* used to treat *Helicobacter pylori* and to prevent *Mycobacterium avium-intracellulare* infection
Dirithromycin	Dynabac	500 q24h	Tablets, delayed-release: 250 mg	Antibacterial spectrum includes *H. influenzae*
Erythromycin†	Erythromycin, E-mycin, E.E.S., others	250-800 q6-12h; 333 q8h	**Base:** Tablets, enteric-coated: 250, 333, 500 mg; Tablets, polymer-coated particles: 333, 500 mg; Tablets, film-coated: 250, 500 mg; Capsules, delayed-release: 250 mg **Estolate:** Tablets: 500 mg; Capsules: 250 mg; Suspension: 125, 250 mg/5 ml **Stearate:** Tablets, film-coated: 250, 500 mg **Ethylsuccinate:** Tablets: 400 mg; Tablets, chewable: 200 mg; Suspension: 200, 400 mg/5 ml; Powder for oral suspension: 200 mg/5 ml **Lactobionate:** Powder for injection: 500 mg, 1 g **Gluceptate:** Injection: 1 g/vial	Available as combination product with sulfisoxazole (extends spectrum to include *H. influenzae*); coating does not decrease GI side effects
Troleandomycin	Tao	250-500 q6h	Capsules: 250 mg	Indicated for susceptible pneumococcal and *Streptococcus pyogenes* strains

†Generic available for one or more dosage forms.

Penicillin Antibiotics

General information for all penicillins regarding drug interactions:

1. May decrease the efficacy of oral contraceptives.
2. May potentiate or inhibit effects of warfarin—monitor prothrombin time.
3. May produce adverse reaction when used concurrently with disulfiram.
4. Probenecid may potentiate penicillin activity—may be desirable.

See individual drug monographs for specific information.

PENICILLINS, ORAL

Generic Name	*Brand Name*	*Usual Oral Adult Dose*	*Available Dosage Forms*	*Comments*
NATURAL PENICILLINS				
Penicillin V†	Pen-Vee K, Veetids	125-500 mg q6h	Tablet: 250, 500 mg; Powder for oral solution: 125, 250 mg/5 ml	250 mg = 400,000 units
BROAD-SPECTRUM PENICILLINS				
Amoxicillin†	Amoxil, Trimox	250-500 mg q8h, or 500-875 mg bid Maximum daily dose: 2-3 g	Capsule: 250, 500 mg; Tablet: 500, 875 mg; Chewable tablet: 125, 200, 250, 400 mg; Powder for oral suspension: 125, 200, 250, 400 mg/5 ml; Pediatric drops: 50 mg/ml	
Amoxicillin/Clavulanate†	Augmentin, Augmentin-XR, Augmentin ES-600	300 mg q8h, or 500 mg q8-12h, or 875 mg q12h, or 2000 mg q12h (XR tablet)	Tablet: (Amoxicillin/clavulanate): 250/125, 500/125, 875 mg/125 mg; Chewable tablet: 125/31.25, 200/28.5, 250/62.5, 400 mg/57 mg; Extended-release tablet: 1000 mg/62.5 mg Powder for suspension: 125/31.25, 200/28.5, 250/62.5, 400/57, 600 mg/42.9 mg per 5 ml	Augmentin ES-600 Only approved for pediatric use
Ampicillin†	Omnipen, Principen	1-12 g/d divided q4-6h	Capsule: 250, 500 mg; Powder for oral suspension: 125, 250 mg/5 ml	
Carbenicillin indanyl sodium	Geocillin	382-764 mg q6h	Tablet: 382 mg	Reserved for treatment of complicated UTI and prostatitis
PENICILLINASE-RESISTANT PENICILLINS				
Dicloxacillin†	Dynapen	125-500 mg q6h	Capsule: 250, 500 mg	

†Generic available for one or more dosage forms.

PENICILLINS, PARENTERAL

Generic Name	*Brand Name*	*Usual IM Adult Dose*	*Available Dosage Forms*	*Comments*
NATURAL PENICILLINS				
Penicillin G Benzathine	Bicillin L-A	Given IM never IV 1.2-2.4 million units (MU) as a single dose	300,000 units/ml in 1, 2, 4 ml syringes	Provides low, long-lasting blood levels of Penicillin G
Penicillin G Benzathine and Procaine combined	Bicillin C-R	Given IM never IV 2.4 MU as a single dose	300,000 units/ml in 1, 2, 4 ml syringes (150,000 units each of Penicillin G Benzathine and Procaine)	Provides low, long-lasting blood levels of Penicillin G
Penicillin G Procaine	Wycillin	Given IM never IV; 300,000-1,000,000 units/day as 1-2 doses/day	600,000 units/ml in 1, 2 ml syringes	Indicated for infections that respond to low, long-lasting Penicillin G blood levels
Penicillin G Potassium†	Pfizerpen	1-24 MU per day in divided doses q4h, depending on severity of infection and microbial sensitivity	Frozen premixed bag: 1, 2, 3 MU; Powder for Injection: 1, 5, 10, 20* MU	Infuse over 1-2 hours 250 mg = 400,000 units Sodium content of 1 MU = 2 mEq Potassium content of 1 MU = 1.7 mEq Often called "Aqueous" Penicillin

PENICILLINS, PARENTERAL—cont'd

Generic Name	Brand Name	Usual IM Adult Dose	Available Dosage Forms	Comments
BROAD-SPECTRUM PENICILLINS				
Ampicillin†	Omnipen	1-12 g/day divided q4-6h	Powder for injection: 250, 500 mg; 1, 2 g	Infuse over at least 10-15 minutes
Ampicillin/Sulbactam†	Unasyn	1.5-3 g q6-8h (equivalent to 1-2 g of ampicillin)	Powder for injection: 1.5 g (ampicillin 1 g + sulbactam 0.5 g), 3 g (ampicillin 2 g + sulbactam 1 g); 15 g*	Infuse over 15-30 minutes
Ticarcillin	Ticar	4-24 g/day in divided doses q4-6h	Powder for injection: 3 g	Infuse over at least 30 minutes Sodium content of 1 g = 5.2-6.5 mEq
Ticarcillin/Clavulanate	Timentin	12-24 g/day in divided doses q4-6h	Powder for injection and frozen premixed bags: ticarcillin disodium 3 g + clavulanate potassium 0.1 g	Infuse over 30 minutes Sodium content of 1 g = 4.75 mEq Potassium content of 1 g = 0.15 mEq
Mezlocillin	Mezlin	6-24 g/day in divided doses q4-6h	Powder for injection: 1, 2, 3, 4, 20* g	Infuse over 30 minutes Sodium content = 1.85 mEq/g
Piperacillin	Pipracil	18-24 g/day divided q4-6h, depending on severity	Powder for injection: 2, 3, 4, 40* g	Infuse over at least 20 minutes Sodium content = 1.85 mEq/g
Piperacillin/Tazobactam	Zosyn	3.375 g q6h or 4.5 g q8h	Powder for injection (piperacillin/tazobactam): 2/0.25, 3/0.375, 4 g/0.5 g, 36 g/4.5 g*	Infuse over 30 minutes
PENICILLINASE-RESISTANT PENICILLINS				
Nafcillin†	Unipen, Nafcil	500 mg-2 g q4-6h	Powder for injection: 500 mg, 1, 2, 4, 10* g	Infuse over 30-60 minutes
Oxacillin†	Bactocill, Prostaphlin	250 mg-2 g q4-6h	Powder for injection: 250, 500 mg, 1, 2, 4, 10* g	By direct IV injection over 10 minutes

*Bulk package intended for pharmacy use only.
†Generic available for one or more dosage forms.

SULFONAMIDES, ORAL

Generic Name	Brand Name	Usual Adult Dose	Available Dosage Forms	Comments
Sulfadiazine†		2-4 g load, then 2-4 g/day in 3-6 divided doses	Tablet: 500 mg	
Sulfamethizole	Thiosulfil Forte	0.5-1 g 3-4x/day	Tablet: 500 mg	
Sulfamethoxazole†	Gantanol	2 g load, then 1 g 2-3x/day	Tablet: 500 mg	Maintain adequate fluid intake to prevent crystalluria
Sulfamethoxazole/Trimethoprim (SMZ/TMP), Co-Trimoxazole†	Septra, Bactrim Septra DS Bactrim DS	800 mg SMZ/160 mg TMP q12h	Tablet: 400 mg SMZ/80 mg TMP; Tablet, double-strength: 800 mg SMZ/160 mg TMP; Oral suspension: 200 mg SMZ/40 mg TMP per 5 ml	First-line therapy for *Pneumocystis carinii* pneumonia; pay special attention to complaints of skin/mucosal rash; could signify early Stevens-Johnson syndrome
Sulfisoxazole†	Gantrisin	2-4 g load, then 4-8 g/day in 4-6 divided doses	Tablet: 500 mg;	Contraindicated in infants <2 months of age; porphyria

†Generic available for one or more dosage forms.

SULFONAMIDES, PARENTERAL

Generic Name	Brand Name	Usual Adult Dose	Available Dosage Forms	Comments
Sulfamethoxazole/Trimethoprim (SMZ/TMP), Co-Trimoxazole†	Bactrim IV Septra IV	8-20 mg of TMP/kg/day, in divided doses q6h, depending on type and severity of infection	Injection: 80 mg SMZ and 16 mg TMP per ml	Infuse over 60-90 minutes First-line therapy for *Pneumocystis carinii* pneumonia; pay special attention to complaints of skin/mucosal rash; could signify early Stevens-Johnson syndrome

†Generic available for one or more dosage forms.

References for Antibiotic Tables:

1. Ellsworth, Allan J., *et al. Mosby's Medical Drug Reference.* Mosby, St. Louis, 2003.
2. Website: US Food and Drug Administration. Online. Internet. 2003. Available: http://www.fda.gov/cder

Antidepressants

MONOAMINE OXIDASE INHIBITORS

Generic Name	*Brand Name*	*Adult Therapeutic Dose Range (mg/day)*	*Available Dosage Forms*	*Relative Sedation Effect*	*Relative Anticholinergic Effect*	*Relative Orthostatic Hypotension*	*Comments*
Isocarboxazid	Marplan	10-60	Tablet: 10 mg	1+	1+	2+	Avoid tyramine-containing foods and certain OTC drug products, including dextromethorphan, and sympathomimetics such as pseudoephedrine (e.g., Sudafed) and phenylephrine (e.g., Neo-Synephrine). Usually reserved for patients who are intolerant of other antidepressant classes. Drug interaction: trazodone, SSRIs, venlafaxine—increases risk of serotonin syndrome (hypertension, hyperthermia, tachycardia, death). Many other drug interactions also—see individual drug monographs.
Phenelzine	Nardil	15-90	Tablet: 15 mg	1+	1+	1+	
Tranylcypromine	Parnate	30-60	Tablet: 10 mg	1+	1+	0	

SELECTIVE SEROTONIN REUPTAKE INHIBITORS

Generic Name	*Brand Name*	*Adult Therapeutic Dose Range (mg/day)*	*Available Dosage Forms*	*Relative Sedation Effect*	*Relative Anticholinergic Effect*	*Relative Orthostatic Hypotension*	*Comments*
Citalopram	Celexa	20-40	Tablet: 10, 20, 40 mg; Oral solution: 10 mg/5 ml	0-1+	0-1+	0-1+	
Escitalopram oxalate	Lexapro	10-20 mg/day	Tablet: 10, 20 mg; Oral solution: 5 mg/5 ml	0-1+	0-1+	0-1+	Active metabolite of citalopram
Fluoxetine†	Prozac Prozac Weekly Sarafem	10-80 mg/day, 90 mg qweek	Capsule: 10, 20, 40 mg; Tablet: 10, 20 mg; Delayed-release capsule: 90 mg (for weekly dosing); Oral liquid: 20 mg/5 ml	0	0-1+	0-1+	Doses taken later than noon may cause insomnia Sarafem is indicated for premenstrual dysphoric disorder (PMDD)
Fluvoxamine†	Luvox	50-300	Tablet: 25, 50, 100 mg	1+	0-1+	0	Primary indication is obsessive-compulsive disorder
Paroxetine†	Paxil Paxil CR	10-60	Tablet: 10, 20, 30, 40 mg; Controlled-release tablet: 12.5, 25, 37.5 mg; Suspension: 10 mg/5 ml	1+	0	0	
Sertraline	Zoloft	25-200	Tablet: 25, 50, 100 mg; Concentrated oral solution: 20 mg/ml	0	0	0	New indication for post-traumatic stress disorder (PTSD): December, 7, 1999. Primary efficacy shown for female patients; little effect shown for male patients

General Information:
1. MAOIs, hypericum (St. John's Wort) may potentiate serotonergic effects.
2. Alcohol may potentiate CNS effects.

†Generic available for one or more dosage forms.

TETRACYCLICS

Generic Name	Brand Name	Adult Therapeutic Dose Range (mg/day)	Available Dosage Forms	Relative Sedation Effect	Relative Anticholinergic Effect	Relative Orthostatic Hypotension	Comments
Maprotiline†	Ludiomil	25-225 mg/day in single or divided doses	Tablet: 25, 50, 75 mg	2+	2+	1+	Increased risk of seizures; separate from MAOIs × 14 days; alcohol may potentiate CNS effects; contraindicated in narrow-angle glaucoma
Mirtazapine	Remeron, Remeron Soltab	15-45	Tablet: 15, 30, 45 mg Tablets, orally disintegrating: 15, 30, 45 mg	3+	2+	0	Separate from MAOIs × 14 days; alcohol may potentiate CNS effects; contraindicated in narrow-angle glaucoma

†Generic available for one or more dosage forms.

TRICYCLICS

Generic Name	Brand Name	Adult Therapeutic Dose Range (mg/day)	Available Dosage Forms	Relative Sedation Effect	Relative Anticholinergic Effect	Relative Orthostatic Hypotension	Comments
Amitriptyline†	Elavil	25-300	Tablet: 10, 25, 50, 75, 100, 150 mg; Injection: 10 mg/ml	4+	4+	3+	
Amoxapine†	Asendin	100-300	Tablet: 25, 50, 100, 150 mg	2+	3+	1+	Dopamine-blocking effects (tardive dyskinesia); maximum daily dose: 400 mg (outpatients), 600 mg (inpatients)
Clomipramine†	Anafranil	25-250	Capsule: 25, 50, 75 mg	3+	3+	2+	Increased risk of seizures Indicated for obsessive compulsive disorder only
Desipramine†	Norpramin	100-300	Tablet: 10, 25, 50, 75, 100, 150 mg	1+	1+	1+	Metabolite of imipramine
Doxepin†	Sinequan	25-300	Capsule: 10, 25, 50, 75, 100, 150 mg; Oral concentrate: 10 mg/ml	3+	2+	3+	Potent antihistamine
Imipramine Hydrochloride†	Tofranil	50-300	Tablet: 10, 25, 50 mg	2+	2+	2+	
Imipramine Pamoate	Tofranil-PM	75-30 mg/day at HS	Capsule: 75, 100, 125, 150 mg				
Nortriptyline†	Pamelor, Aventyl	75-150	Capsule: 10, 25, 50, 75 mg; Oral solution: 10 mg/5 ml	2+	2+	2+	Metabolite of amitriptyline Entire daily dose may be given at bedtime
Protriptyline†	Vivactil	15-60	Tablet: 5, 10 mg	1+	3+	1+	
Trimipramine	Surmontil	50-300	Capsule: 25, 50, 100 mg	3+	2+	2+	

General Information:
1. Separate from MAOI therapy by at least 14 days.
2. Alcohol may increase CNS effects.
3. Grapefruit juice may decrease metabolic clearance.
4. Contraindicated in narrow-angle glaucoma or active cardiac disease.

†Generic available for one or more dosage forms.

MISCELLANEOUS ANTIDEPRESSANTS

Generic Name	Brand Name	Adult Therapeutic Dose Range (mg/day)	Available Dosage Forms	Relative Sedation Effect	Relative Anticholinergic Effect	Relative Orthostatic Hypotension	Comments
Bupropion	Wellbutrin, Wellbutrin SR, Zyban	200-450	Tablet: 75, 100 mg; Tablet, sustained-release: 100, 150, 200 mg	1+	2+	1+	Increased risk of seizures; Zyban (150 mg sustained-release tablet) is indicated as adjunct therapy in smoking cessation
Nefazodone	Serzone	200-600	Tablet: 50, 100, 150, 200, 250 mg	2+	0-1+	1+	Mild increase in blood pressure; use with extreme caution in patients with cardiac, cerebrovascular, or seizure disorder
Trazodone†	Desyrel	150-600 mg//day in divided doses	Tablet: 50, 100, 150, 300 mg	4+	1+	2+	Risk of priapism in males; maximum daily dose: 400 mg (outpatients), 600 mg (inpatients); use with extreme caution in cardiac disease
Venlafaxine	Effexor, Effexor XR	75-375	Tablet: 25, 37.5, 50, 75, 100 mg; Tablet, extended-release: 37.5, 75, 150 mg	1	0	0	Risk of sustained increases in blood pressure; tablets are scored and may be broken; extended-release capsules should be swallowed whole and not divided or placed in water; separate from MAOI therapy by at least 14 days

†Generic available for one or more dosage forms.

References:

1. Ellsworth, Allan J., *et al. Mosby's Medical Drug Reference.* Mosby, St. Louis, 2003.
2. Website: US Food and Drug Administration. Online. Internet. 2003. Available: http://www.fda.gov/cder

Antifungals, Systemic

Generic Name	Brand Name	Adult Dose Range	Available Dosage Forms	Common Indications	Comments
Amphotericin B desoxycholate†	Fungizone	IV: 0.25–0.7 mg/kg/d for 4-12 weeks	Powder for injection: 50 mg	Aspergillosis, blastomycosis candidiasis, coccidioidomycosis, cryptococcosis, histoplasmosis, mucormycosis, rhinocerebral phycomycosis, sporotrichosis	Used topically in bladder; causes multiple electrolyte, abnormalities (hypokalemia, renal tubular acidosis, hypomagnesemia, azotemia); give 1 mg test dose prior to giving full dose; cholesteryl and liposomal formulations (e.g., AmBisome, Amphotec) are used in renally impaired patients or in cases of unacceptable toxicity resulting from requisite antifungal dosages of the deoxychoate form (e.g., Fungizone)
Amphotericin B, lipid based	Abelcet, Amphotec, Ambisome	3-5 mg/kg/day	Suspension for injection: 100 mg/20 ml; Powder for injection: 50, 100 mg	Aspergillosis, candidiasis, cryptococcosis infection, cryptococcal meningitis, leishmaniasis	Used topically in bladder; causes multiple electrolyte abnormalities (hypokalemia, renal tubular acidosis, hypomagnesemia, azotemia); give 1 mg test dose prior to giving full dose; cholesteryl and liposomal formulations (e.g., AmBisome, Amphotec) are used in renally impaired patients or in cases of unacceptable toxicity resulting from requisite antifungal dosages of the deoxychoate form (e.g., Fungizone)
Caspofungin acetate	Cancidas	IV: 70 mg loading dose, then 50 mg qd	Powder for injection: 50, 70 mg	Aspergillosis	Limited to patients who are intolerant of or fail to respond to other treatments. Not intended for initial therapy.

Antifungals, Systemic—cont'd

Generic Name	*Brand Name*	*Adult Dose Range*	*Available Dosage Forms*	*Common Indications*	*Comments*
Fluconazole	Diflucan	PO or IV: 50-400 mg qd	Tablets: 50, 100, 150, 200 mg; Powder for oral suspension: 50 mg/5 ml; Injection: 2 mg/ml	Candidiasis, cryptococcal meningitis	Increases serum rifabutin levels and toxicity; increases effect of cyclosporine, terfenadine, astemizole, warfarin, sulfonylureas, and others; single-dose treatment for vaginal infection (150 mg)
Flucytosine	Ancobon	PO: 12.5-37.5 mg/kg q6h	Capsules: 250, 500 mg	Candidiasis, cryptococcosis	Usually used in combination with amphotericin B (allows lower dose of amphotericin B); converted to flourouracil in fungal cell. Monitor renal function.
Griseofulvin†	**Microsize:** Fulvicin U/F, Grifulvin V, Grisactin	PO: 500 mg qd-bid	Tablets: 250, 500 mg; Capsules: 250 mg; Oral suspension: 125 mg/5 ml	Dermatophytes	Cytochrome P450 inducer; absorption enhanced when taken with fatty foods. Ultramicrocrystalline is absorbed better than microcrystalline
	Ultramicrosize: Fulvicin P/G, Gris-Peg, Grisactin Ultra	PO: 330 mg qd-bid	Tablets: 125, 165, 250, 330 mg		
Itraconazole	Sporanox	PO: 100-200 mg qd-bid; IV: 200 mg qd-bid	Capsules: 100 mg; Oral solution: 50 mg/5 ml; Injection: 10 mg/ml	Aspergillosis, blastomycosis, candidiasis, chromomycosis, cryptococcosis, dermatomycosis, histoplasmosis, onychomycosis, paracoccidioidomycosis, sporotrichosis	Cytochrome P450 3A inhibitor—affects metabolism of cyclosporine, terfenadine, astemizole, warfarin, sulfonylureas, and others; can precipitate or worsen CHF; take capsules after a full meal
Ketoconazole	Nizoral	PO: 200-400 mg qd-bid	Tablets: 200 mg	Blastomycosis, candidiasis, chromomycosis, coccidioidomycosis, dermatophytes, histoplasmosis, paracoccidioidomycosis	Cytochrome P450 3A inhibitor—affects metabolism of cyclosporine, terfenadine, astemizole, warfarin, sulfonylureas, and others; requires acid pH for absorption; reduces testosterone synthesis (gynecomastia); available in topical form
Terbinafine	Lamisil	PO: 250 mg qd × 6-12 weeks	Tablets: 250 mg	Onychomycosis	Hepatic clearance increased by rifampin, decreased by cimetidine; reported to cause liver failure
Voriconazole	Vfend	IV loading dose: 6 mg/kg q12h × 2 doses, then 4 mg/kg q12h. May switch to oral, 100-200 mg q12h	Tablets: 50, 200 mg; Powder for injection: 200 mg	Infections due to *Aspergillus, Fusarium, Scedosporium apiospermum*	Oral doses should be taken either 1 hour before or 1 hour after a meal

†Generic available for one or more dosage forms.

References:

1. Ellsworth, Allan J, *et al. Mosby's Medical Drug Reference.* Mosby, St. Louis, 2003.
2. *U.S. Food and Drug Administration.* Online. Internet. May 2003. Available http://www.fda.gov/
3. *Centers for Disease Control and Prevention.* Online. Internet. May 2003. Available http://www.cdc.gov/
4. *National Guideline Clearinghouse* [documents produced by the Agency for Healthcare Research and Quality (AHRQ)—formerly the Agency for Healthcare Policy and Research (AHCPR) in partnership with the American Medical Association (AMA) and the American Association of Health Plans (AAHP)]. Online. Internet. May 2003. Available http://www.guideline.gov/

Antihypertensives

ANGIOTENSIN-CONVERTING ENZYMES (ACE) INHIBITORS

NOTE: ACE inhibitors may cause severe fetal damage or death if used in the second or third trimester of pregnancy

Generic Name	*Brand Name*	*Route*	*Usual Adult Dose*	*Available Dosage Forms*	*Comments*
Benazepril*	Lotensin	PO	10-40 mg qd	Tablet: 5, 10, 20, 40 mg	
Captopril†	Capoten	PO	12.5-50 mg bid-tid	Tablet: 12.5, 25, 50, 100 mg	Given 1 hour before meals
Enalapril†	Vasotec	PO	5-40 mg qd	Tablet: 2.5, 5, 10, 20 mg	
Enalaprilat	Vasotec IV	IV	0.625-1.25 mg q6h	Injection: 1.25 mg	Infuse over 5 minutes; enalaprilat is active metabolite of enalapril
Fosinopril*†	Monopril	PO	10-40 mg qd	Tablet: 10, 20, 40 mg	
Lisinopril*†	Prinivil, Zestril	PO	10-40 mg qd	Tablet: 2.5, 5, 10, 20, 40 mg	
Moexipril*†	Univasc	PO	7.5-30 mg qd	Tablet: 7.5, 15 mg	Given 1 hour before meals
Perindopril*†	Aceon	PO	4-8 mg qd	Tablet: 2, 4, 8 mg	
Quinapril	Accupril	PO	10-40 mg qd	Tablet: 5, 10, 20, 40 mg	
Ramipril*†	Altace	PO	1.25-20 mg qd	Capsule: 1.25, 2.5, 5, 10 mg	
Trandolapril*†	Mavik	PO	1-4 mg qd	Tablet: 1, 2, 4 mg	Black patients often need higher doses than nonblack patients (e.g., 2 mg versus 1 mg)

*Daily dose can be given as a single dose or divided into two equal doses.
†Generic available for one or more dosage forms.

ANGIOTENSIN RECEPTOR BLOCKERS

Generic Name	*Brand Name*	*Usual Adult Dose*	*Available Dosage Forms*
Candesartan cilexetil	Atacand	*Initial:* 16 mg once daily. *Maintenance:* 8-32 mg/day in one or two doses.	Tablets: 4, 8, 16, 32 mg
Eprosartan mesylate	Teveten	*Initial:* 600 mg once daily. *Maintenance:* 400-800 mg/day, one or two doses per day.	Tablets: 400, 600 mg
Irbesartan	Avapro	*Initial:* 150 mg once daily. *Maintenance:* 150-300 mg once daily.	Tablets: 75, 150, 300 mg
Losartan potassium	Cozaar	*Initial:* 50 mg once daily. *Maintenance:* 25-100 mg/day in one or two doses.	Tablets: 25, 50, 100 mg
Olmesartan medoxomil	Benicar	*Initial:* 20 mg once daily. *Maintenance:* 20-40 mg once daily.	Tablets: 5, 20, 40 mg
Telmisartan	Micardis	*Initial:* 40 mg once daily. *Maintenance:* 20-80 mg once daily.	Tablets: 40, 80 mg
Valsartan	Diovan	*Initial:* 80-160 mg once daily. *Maintenance:* 80-320 mg once daily.	Tablets: 40, 80, 160, 320 mg

BETA-ADRENERGIC BLOCKING AGENTS

Generic Name	*Brand Name*	*Adrenergic Receptor Blocking Activity*	*Route*	*Usual Adult Dose*	*Available Dosage Forms*	*Comments*
Acebutolol*†	Sectral	β_1	PO	200-600 mg qd-bid	Capsule: 200, 400 mg	
Atenolol*†	Tenormin	β_1	PO, IV	PO: 12.5-200 mg qd; IV: 5 mg IV over 5 minutes; repeat in 5 minutes	Tablet: 25, 50, 100 mg; Injection: 5 mg/10 ml	IV use for acute myocardial infarction
Betaxolol*	Kerlone	β_1	PO	10-20 mg qd	Tablet: 10, 20 mg	Consider 5 mg starting dose for elderly patients
Bisoprolol*	Zebeta	β_1	PO	5-20 mg qd	Tablet: 5, 10 mg	
Esmolol*	Brevibloc	β_1	IV	50-200 μg/kg/min	Injection: 10, 250 mg/ml	Indicated for supraventricular tachycardia
Metoprolol*†	Lopressor	β_1	PO, IV	PO: 100-450 mg/day in single or divided doses; IV: 5 mg bolus × 3, 2 minutes apart	Tablet: 50, 100 mg; Injection: 1 mg/ml	IV for acute myocardial infarction

BETA-ADRENERGIC BLOCKING AGENTS—cont'd

Generic Name	*Brand Name*	*Adrenergic Receptor Blocking Activity*	*Route*	*Usual Adult Dose*	*Available Dosage Forms*	*Comments*
Metoprolol,* long-acting	Toprol XL	β_1	PO	12.5-400 mg qd	Tablet, extended-release: 25, 50, 100, 200 mg	Use same total daily dose when switching to immediate-release tablets
Carteolol	Cartrol	β_1, β_2	PO	2.5-10 mg/day	Tablet: 2.5, 5 mg	
Nadolol†	Corgard	β_1, β_2	PO	40-320 mg qd	Tablet: 20, 40, 80, 120, 160 mg	
Penbutolol	Levatol	β_1, β_2	PO	20-40 mg qd	Tablet: 20 mg	
Pindolol†	Visken	β_1, β_2	PO	5-30 mg bid	Tablet: 5, 10 mg	
Propranolol†	Inderal	β_1, β_2	PO, IV	PO: 30-640 mg/day in divided doses bid tid, qid; IV: 1-3 mg with cardiac monitor (not to exceed 1 mg/min)	Tablet: 10, 20, 40, 60, 80 mg; Oral solution: 4, 8, 80 mg/ml Injection: 1 mg/ml	IV use reserved for life-threatening arrhythmias or arrhythmias occurring under general anesthesia
Propranolol, long-acting	Inderal LA	β_1, β_2	PO	80 mg qd	Capsules, sustained-release: 60, 80, 120, 160 mg	
Sotalol†	Betapace, Betapace AF	β_1, β_2	PO	160-640 mg qd in divided doses	Tablet: 80, 120, 160, 240 mg	
Timolol†	Blocadren	β_1, β_2	PO	20-60 mg divided qd-bid	Tablet: 5, 10, 20 mg	
Carvedilol	Coreg	$\beta_1, \beta_2, \alpha_1$	PO	6.25-25 mg bid	Tablet: 3.25, 6.25, 12.5, 25 mg	Take with food
Labetalol	Normodyne, Trandate	$\beta_1, \beta_2, \alpha_1$	PO, IV	PO: 100-400 mg bid; IV: 20 mg over 2 minutes, titrating up to 40-80 mg q10minutes (maximum dose 300 mg)	Tablet: 100, 200, 300 mg; Injection: 5 mg/ml	

*β_1 blockers also block β_2 receptors in high doses.
†Generic available in one or more dosage forms.

CALCIUM CHANNEL BLOCKERS (CCBs)

Generic Name	*Brand Name(s)*	*Usual Adult Dose*	*Available Dosage Forms*	*Comments*
Amlodipine	Norvasc	Initial: 5 mg once daily; Liver disease, start at 2.5 mg/day Maintenance: 5-10 mg once daily	Tablets: 2.5, 5, 10 mg	Dihydropyridine class Titrate over 7-14 days
Bepridil hydrochloride	Vascor	Initial: 200 mg/day Maintenance: 200-400 mg/day; May adjust doses after 10 days	Tablets: 200, 300 mg	Non-dihydropyridine class
Diltiazem hydrochloride†	Cardizem, Cardizem CD, Cardizem SR, Tiamate, Dilacor XR, Tiazac, Cardia XT	Initial (tablets): 30 mg qid ac and hs Initial (sustained-release): 60-120 mg bid Initial (extended-release): 180-240 mg once daily Maintenance (tablets): Increase dose at 1-2 day intervals to 180-360 mg in 3 or 4 divided doses Maintenance (sustained-release): 120-180 mg bid Maintenance (extended-release): 180-480 mg once daily; Do not exceed 540 mg/day Initial IV (bolus): 0.25 mg/kg given over 2 minutes; Second dose of 0.35 mg/kg over 2 minutes may be necessary Maintenance IV (continuous infusion): 5-15 mg/hr	Tablets: 30, 60, 90, 120 mg Extended-release, capsules: 60, 90, 120, 180, 240, 300, 360, 420 mg Sustained-release, capsules: 60, 90, 120 mg, Injection: 5 mg/ml Powder for injection: 25, 100 mg	Non-dihydropyridine class
Felodipine	Plendil	Initial: 5 mg once daily Maintenance: 2.5-10 mg once daily	Extended-release, tablets: 2.5, 5, 10 mg	Dihydropyridine class Allow at least 2 weeks between dosage changes

Continued

CALCIUM CHANNEL BLOCKERS (CCBs)—cont'd

Generic Name	Brand Name(s)	Usual Adult Dose	Available Dosage Forms	Comments
Isradipine	DynaCirc, DynaCirc CR	Initial: 2.5 mg bid Maintenance: Up to 20 mg/day	Capsules: 2.5, 5 mg Controlled-release, tablets: 5, 10 mg	Dihydropyridine class Maximum response may require 2-4 weeks
Nicardipine hydrochloride†	Cardene, Cardene SR, Cardene I.V.	Initial (capsules): 20 mg tid Maintenance (capsules): 20-40 mg tid; Allow at least 3 days between dosage increases Initial (sustained-release): 30 mg bid Maintenance (sustained-release): 30-60 mg bid Infuse IV at a rate comparable to oral dosing PO 20 mg q8h = IV 0.5 mg/hr PO 30 mg q8h = IV 1.2 mg/hr PO 40 mg q8h = IV 2.2 mg/hr	Capsules: 20, 30 mg Sustained-release, capsules: 30, 45, 60 mg Injection: 2.5 mg/ml	Dihydropyridine class Only immediate-release capsules are used for angina
Nifedipine†	Adalat, Procardia, Adalat CC, Procardia XL	Initial (capsules): 10 mg tid Maintenance (capsules): 10 mg tid to 30 mg qid Initial (sustained-release): 30-60 mg daily Maintenance (sustained-release): No more than 120 mg/day	Capsules: 10, 20 mg Sustained-release, tablets: 30, 60, 90 mg	Dihydropyridine class No rebound effects if abruptly discontinued
Nimodipine	Nimotop	60 mg q4h for 21 days; Start treatment within 96 hrs of SAH	Capsules: 30 mg	Only approved use is subarachnoid hemorrhage (SAH) Dihydropyridine class
Nisoldipine	Sular	Initial: 20 mg once daily; Adjust by adding 10 mg/week Maintenance: 20-40 mg once daily Doses >60 mg/day are not recommended	Extended-release, tablets: 10, 20, 30, 40 mg	Dihydropyridine class Avoid grapefruit or grapefruit juice before or after doses
Verapamil hydrochloride†	Calan, Isoptin, Calan SR, Isoptin SR, Verelan, Verelan PM	Initial (tablets): 80-120 mg tid Maintenance (tablets): 240-480 mg/day in 3 or 4 divided doses Initial (sustained-release): 240 mg once daily in the morning Initial (extended-release): 200 mg hs Maintenance (sustained-release): 120-480 mg once daily in the morning Maintenance (extended-release): 200-400 mg hs	Tablets: 40, 80, 120 mg Sustained-release, tablets: 120, 180, 240 mg Sustained-release, capsules: 120, 180, 240, 360 mg Extended-release, capsules: 100, 120, 180, 200, 240, 300 mg Injection: 2.5 mg/ml Extended-release tablets: 120, 180, 240 mg	Non-dihydropyridine class Sustained-release capsules may be emptied and sprinkled over applesauce

†Generic available for one or more dosage forms.

References for Antihypertensive Tables:

1. Ellsworth, Allan J, *et al. Mosby's Medical Drug Reference.* Mosby, St. Louis, 2003.
2. Website: US Food and Drug Administration. Online. Internet. 2003. Available: http://www.fda.gov/cder

Antiretroviral Agents

A general statement regarding drug interactions: All the antiretroviral drugs can have many and varied drug interactions. This fact is compounded by the large number and variety of medications often required by patients with HIV infection. For detailed information regarding specific drug interactions, the reader is advised to examine the monographs for individual drugs presented in Section II.

ANTIRETROVIRAL FUSION INHIBITORS

Generic Name	Brand Name	Usual Adult Dose	Available Dosage Forms	Comments
Enfuvirtide	Fuzeon	90 mg SC bid	Powder for injection: 108 mg (90 mg/ml when reconstituted)	Injection site reactions are common

NUCLEOSIDE REVERSE TRANSCRIPTASE INHIBITORS

Generic Name	*Synonyms/ Brand Name*	*Usual Adult Dose*	*Available Dosage Forms*	*Comments*
Abacavir	ABC/Ziagen	300 mg bid, or with 3TC and ZDV as Trizivir, one tablet bid	Tablet: 300 mg; Oral solution: 20 mg/ml	May take without regard to meals
Didanosine	ddI/Videx, Videx EC	>60 kg: 200 mg tablet bid, or 250 mg buffered powder bid, or 400 mg qd (capsule or 2 × 200 mg tablets); <60 kg: 125 mg tablets bid or 167 mg buffered powder bid, or 250 mg buffered powder qd	Tablets, chewable: 25, 50, 100 150, 200 mg; Capsules, delayed-release: 125, 200 250, 400 mg; Powder for oral solution, buffered: 100, 167, 250 mg; Powder for oral solution, pediatric: 2, 4 g	Food decreases ddI levels by 55%; take ½ hour before or 2 hours after meal
Lamivudine	3TC/Epivir	150 mg bid, <50 kg: 2 mg/kg bid or with ZDV as Combivir, 1 tablet bid, or with ABC and ZDV as Trizivir, 1 tablet bid	Tablet: 150, 300 mg; Oral solution, 10 mg/ml	May take without regard to meals
	Epivir-HBV	100 mg qd	Tablet: 100 mg Oral solution: 5 mg/m	HBV form is indicated for chronic Hepatitis B
Stavudine	d4T/Zerit, Zerit XR	>60 kg: 40 mg bid; <60 kg: 30 mg bid	Capsule: 15, 20, 30, 40 mg; Powder for oral solution: 1 mg/ml Capsules, extended-release: 37.5, 50, 75, 100 mg	May take without regard to meals
Zalcitabine	ddC/Hivid	0.75 mg q8h	Tablet: 0.375, 0.75 mg	May take without regard to meals
Zidovudine†	AZT, ZDV/Retrovir	PO: 200 mg tid or 300 mg bid or with 3TC as Combivir, 1 tablet bid, or with ABC and 3TC as Trizivir, 1 tablet bid IV: 1 mg/kg 5-6 × daily	Capsule: 100 mg; Tablet: 300 mg; Syrup: 50 mg/5 ml; IV solution: 10 mg/ml	May take without regard to meals

†Generic available for one or more dosage forms.

NON-NUCLEOSIDE REVERSE TRANSCRIPTASE INHIBITORS

Generic Name	*Synonyms/Brand Name*	*Usual Adult Dose*	*Available Dosage Forms*	*Comments*
Delavirdine	DLV/Rescriptor	400 mg po tid, or four 100 mg tablets in ≥3 oz water to produce slurry	Tablet: 100, 200 mg	Separate dosing with ddI or antacids by 1 hour; take without regard to meals
Efavirenz	EFV, DMP-266/Sustiva	600 mg qhs	Capsule: 50, 100, 200 mg Tablet: 600 mg	Avoid taking after high-fat meals—EFV levels ↑ by 50%. Take on an empty stomach
Nevirapine	NVP/Viramune	200 mg qd for 14 days, then 200 mg bid	Tablet: 200 mg	Take without regard to meals. If dosing is stopped more than 7 days, restart with 200 mg qd for 14 days.

NUCLEOTIDE ANALOG REVERSE TRANSCRIPTASE INHIBITOR

Generic Name	*Brand Name*	*Usual Adult Dose*	*Available Dosage Forms*	*Comments*
Tenofovir	Viread	300 mg qd	Tablet: 300 mg	Take with a meal. If also taking didanosine, take Tenofovir 2 hours before or 1 hour after didanosine

PROTEASE INHIBITORS

Generic Name	*Synonyms/ Brand Name*	*Usual Adult Dose*	*Available Dosage Forms*	*Comments*
Amprenavir	Agenerase	>50 kg: 1200 mg bid (capsules); 1400 mg bid (oral solution) <50 kg: 20 mg/kg bid (capsules); maximum daily total: 2400 mg or <50 kg: 1.5 ml/kg bid (oral solution); maximum daily total: 2800 mg	Capsules: 50, 150 mg; Oral solution: 15 mg/ml (capsules and oral solution NOT interchangeable on a mg per mg basis)	May take with or without food; a high-fat meal, however, decreases the absorption of amprenavir by 21% and should be avoided; patients should be advised NOT to take supplemental vitamin E, since the vitamin E content of Agenerase capsules and oralsolution exceeds the Reference Daily Intake of 30 IU for adults and approximately 10 IU for pediatric patients
Indinavir	IDV/Crixivan	800 mg q8h	Capsules: 100, 200, 333, 400 mg	Food decreases IDV levels by 77%; take 1 hour before or 2 hours after meals; may take with skim milk or low-fat meal; separate dosing with ddI by 1 hour
Nelfinavir	NLF, NFV/Viracept	750 mg tid or 1250 mg bid	Tablet: 250 mg; Oral powder: 50 mg/g	Food increases NLF levels twofold to threefold; take with meal or snack
Ritonavir	RTV/Norvir	600 mg q12h	Capsule: 100 mg; Oral solution: 80 mg/ml	Food increases RTV levels by 15%; take with food if possible, this may improve tolerability. Dose titration may reduce adverse effects, 300 mg q12h, increase by 100 mg q12h at 2-3 day intervals.
Saquinavir	SQV/Invirase, Fortovase	Invirase: 600 mg bid with an antiretroviral nucleoside analog; otherwise, Invirase is not recommended Fortovase: 1200 mg tid	Invirase: 200 mg capsules Fortovase: 200 mg capsules (soft gelatin capsules for improved absorption)	Invirase: Take within 2 hours after a full meal. Fortovase: Food increases drug levels sixfold. Take with large meal. Capsules and soft gelatin capsules are not equivalent dosage forms

COMBINATION PRODUCTS

Generic Name	*Synonyms/Brand Name*	*Usual Adult Dose*	*Available Dosage Forms*	*Comments*
Lamivudine/ Zidovudine	3TC/ZDV, 3TC/AZT/Combivir	1 tablet bid	Tablet, 3TC 150 mg + ZDV 300 mg	May take without regard to meals
Abacavir/ Lamivudine/ Zidovudine	ABC/3TC/ZDV/Trizivir	1 tablet bid	Tablet, ABC 300 mg + 3TC 150 mg + ZDV 300 mg	May take without regard to meals; hypersensitivity to abacavir has occurred in about 5% of study patients; rechallenge after any type of diagnosed hypersensitivity reaction is contraindicated; signs and symptoms include fever, skin rash, fatigue, GI symptoms, respiratory symptoms (e.g. pharyngitis, dyspnea, cough); Abacavir Hypersensitivity Registry: 1-800-270-0425
Lopinavir/ Ritonavir	Kaletra	3 capsules bid or 5 ml bid	Capsule: lopinavir 133.3 mg + ritonavir 33.3 mg; Oral solution: lopinavir 80 mg + ritonavir 20 mg per ml	Take with food; ritonavir component inhibits metabolism of lopinavir; oral solution contains 42.4% alcohol; consider a dose increase to 4 capsules or 6.5 ml bid when used in combination with EFV or NVP in treatment-experienced patients where reduced susceptibility to lopinavir is clinically suspected (by treatment history and/or laboratory evidence)

References:

1. Website: AIDS info: A Service of The U.S. Department of Health and Human Services. Online. Internet. 2003. Available: http://www.aidsinfo.nih.gov
2. Website: U.S. Food and Drug Administration. Online. Internet. 2003. Available: http://www.fda.gov/cder
3. Website: New Mexico AIDS InfoNet. Online. Internet. 2003. Available: http://www.aidsinfonet.org

Contraceptives

COMBINATION ORAL CONTRACEPTIVES

Estrogen	Progestin	Brand Name(s)	Strengths: Estrogen	Strengths: Progestin	Tablets/ pack*	Type	Comments
Ethinyl estradiol	Desogestrel	Apri, Desogen, Ortho-Cept,†	30 µg	0.15 mg	21, 28	Monophasic	
Ethinyl estradiol	Drospirenone	Yasmin	30 µg	3 mg	28	Monophasic	
Ethinyl estradiol	Ethynodiol diacetate	Demulin 1/50, Zovia 1/50E,†	50 µg	1 mg	21, 28	Monophasic	
Ethinyl estradiol	Ethynodiol diacetate	Demulen 1/35, Zovia 1/35E,†	35 µg	1 mg	21, 28	Monophasic	
Ethinyl estradiol	Levonorgestrel	Levlen, Levora, Nordette, Portia,†	30 µg	0.15 mg	21, 28	Monophasic	
Ethinyl estradiol	Levonorgestrel	Alesse, Aviane, Levlite, Lessina,†	20 µg	0.1 mg	21, 28	Monophasic	
Ethinyl estradiol	Norethindrone	Ovcon-50	50 µg	1 mg	28	Monophasic	
Ethinyl estradiol	Norethindrone	Necon 1/35, Norinyl 1+35, Nortrel 1/35, Ortho-Novum 1/35,†	35 µg	1 mg	21, 28	Monophasic	
Ethinyl estradiol	Norethindrone	Brevicon, Modicon, Necon 0.5/35,†	35 µg	0.5 mg	21, 28	Monophasic	
Ethinyl estradiol	Norethindrone	Ovcon-35	35 µg	0.4 mg	21, 28	Monophasic	
Ethinyl estradiol	Norethindrone acetate	Loestrin 21 1.5/30, Loestrin Fe 1.5/30, Microgestin Fe 1.5/30,†	30 µg	1.5 mg	21, 28	Monophasic	The "Fe" forms contain 7 tablets of 75 mg ferrous fumarate
Ethinyl estradiol	Norethindrone acetate	Loestrin 21 1/20, Loestrin Fe 1/20, Microgestin Fe 1/20,†	20 µg	1 mg	21, 28	Monophasic	The "Fe" forms contain 7 tablets of 75 mg ferrous fumarate
Ethinyl estradiol	Norgestimate	Ortho-Cyclen, Mononessa, Sprintec,†	35 µg	0.25 mg	28	Monophasic	
Ethinyl estradiol	Norgestrel	Ogestrel, 0.5/50, Ovral,†	50 µg	0.5 mg	28	Monophasic	
Ethinyl estradiol	Norgestrel	Lo/Ovral, Low-Ogestrel, Cryselle,†	30 µg	0.3 mg	21, 28	Monophasic	
Mestranol	Norethindrone	Necon 1/50, Norinyl 1+50, Ortho-Novum 1/50,†	50 µg	1 mg	21, 28	Monophasic	
Ethinyl estradiol	Desogestrel	Mircette, Kariva,†	20 µg (21 tablets), 10 µg (5 tablets)	0.15 mg (21 tablets)	28	Biphasic	Contains 2 inert tablets at the end of the cycle
Ethinyl estradiol	Norethindrone	Jenest-28	35 µg (21 tablets)	0.5 mg (7 tablets), 1 mg (14 tablets)	28	Biphasic	
Ethinyl estradiol	Norethindrone	Ortho-Novum 10/11, Necon 10/11,†	35 µg (21 tablets)	0.5 mg (10 tablets), 1 mg (11 tablets)	28	Biphasic	
Ethinyl estradiol	Levonorgestrel	Tri-Levlen, Triphasil, Trivora-28, Empresse,†	30 µg (6 tablets), 40 µg (5 tablets), 30 µg (10 tablets)	0.05 mg (6 tablets), 0.075 mg (5 tablets), 0.125 mg (10 tablets)	21, 28	Triphasic	
Ethinyl estradiol	Norethindrone	Tri-Norinyl	35 µg (21 tablets)	0.5 mg (7 tablets), 1 mg (9 tablets), 0.5 mg (5 tablets)	28	Triphasic	
Ethinyl estradiol	Norethindrone	Ortho-Novum 7/7/7, Necon 7/7/7,†	35 µg (21 tablets)	0.5 mg (7 tablets), 0.75 mg (7 tablets), 1 mg (7 tablets)	28	Triphasic	
Ethinyl estradiol	Norethindrone	Estrostep 21	20 µg (5 tablets), 30 µg (7 tablets), 35 µg (9 tablets)	1 mg (21 tablets)	21	Triphasic	
Ethinyl estradiol	Norethindrone	Estrostep Fe	20 µg (5 tablets), 30 µg (7 tablets), 35 µg (9 tablets)	1 mg (21 tablets)	28	Triphasic	Contains 7 tablets of 75 mg ferrous fumarate
Ethinyl estradiol	Norgestimate	Ortho Tri-Cyclen	35 µg (21 tablets)	0.18 mg (7 tablets), 0.215 mg (7 tablets), 0.25 mg (7 tablets)	28	Triphasic	

Continued

COMBINATION ORAL CONTRACEPTIVES—cont'd

Estrogen	Progestin	Brand Name(s)	Strengths: Estrogen	Strengths: Progestin	Tablets/ pack*	Type	Comments
Ethinyl estradiol	Levonorgestrel	Preven	50 µg	0.25 mg	4	Emergency contraceptive (morning after pill)	"Morning after pill" Take 2 tablets ASAP, within 72 hours; Repeat in 12 hours
Ethinyl estradiol	Norgestimate	Ortho TriCyclen Lo	25 µg (21 tablets)	0.18 mg (7 tablets), 0.215 mg (7 tablets), 0.25 mg (7 tablets)	28	Triphasic	
Ethinyl estradiol	Desogestrel	Cyclessa	25 µg (21 tablets)	0.1 mg (7 tablets), 0.125 mg (7 tablets), 0.15 mg (7 tablets)	28	Triphasic	

*28-day packs contain 7 inert tablets to be used at the end of the cycle.
†Generic available for one or more dosage forms.

SINGLE AGENT ORAL CONTRACEPTIVES

Active Ingredient	Brand Name	Strength	Type	Comments
Levonorgestrel	Plan B	0.75 mg	Emergency contraceptive (morning after pill)	Take 1 tablet ASAP within 72 hours; Repeat in 2 hours
Norethindrone†	Micronor, Nor-QD, Camila, Errin, Nora-BE	0.35 mg	Progestin-only contraceptive	Taken daily without interruption
Norgestrel	Ovrette	0.075 mg	Progestin-only contraceptive	Taken daily without interruption

†Generic available for one or more dosage forms.

OTHER SYSTEMIC CONTRACEPTIVES

Estrogen	Progestin	Brand Name(s)	Strengths: Estrogen	Strengths: Progestin	Type	Comments
Estradiol cypionate	Medroxyprogesterone	Lunelle	5 mg/0.5 ml	25 mg/0.5 ml	Repository injection	Repeat every 28-30 days; Not to exceed 33 days
Ethinyl estradiol	Etonorgestrel	NuvaRing	2.7 mg/ring (15 mcg/24 hr)	11.7 mg/ring (0.12 mg/24 hr)	Vaginal ring	Leave in place for 3 weeks, remove, wait 1 week, insert new ring
Ethinyl estradiol	Norelgestromin	Ortho Evra	0.75 mg/ patch (20 mcg/24 hr)	6 mg/patch (0.15 mg/24 hr)	Transdermal	Apply 1 patch each week for 3 weeks, remove, wait 1 week, apply new patch
None	Levonorgestrel	Norplant		216 mg/6 inserts	Subcutaneous implant	Remove and replace after 5 years
None	Levonorgestrel	Mirena		52 mg/unit	Intrauterine system	Remove and replace after 5 years
None	Medroxyprogesterone	Depo-Provera Contraceptive		150 mg/ml	Repository injection	Repeat every 3 months
None	Progesterone	Progestasert		38 mg/unit	Intrauterine system	Remove and replace after 1 year

References:
1. Ellsworth, Allan J, *et al. Mosby's Medical Drug Reference.* Mosby, St. Louis, 2003.
2. Website: U.S. Food and Drug Administration. Online, Internet. 2003. Available: http://www.fda.gov/cder

Glucocorticoids, Systemic

Generic Name	Brand Name	Oral or Parenteral Dose for Equivalent Glucocorticoid Effect*	Relative Mineralocorticoid Effect	Biologic Half-Life	Comment
Betamethasone†	Celestone	0.6-0.75 mg	0	36-54 hours	Common off-label use is administration to pregnant women to prevent neonatal respiratory distress syndrome in pre-term infants
Cortisone†	Cortone	25 mg	1	8-12 hours	A drug of choice for adrenocortical insufficiency
Dexamethasone†	Decadron	0.75 mg	0	36-54 hours	Used to control cerebral edema associated with intracranial pathology and head injury
Hydrocortisone†	Cortef, Solu-Cortef	20 mg	1	8-12 hours	A drug choice for adrenocortical insufficiency
Methylprednisolone†	Medrol, Solu-Medrol	4 mg	0	18-36 hours	Oral preparation often used in tapered doses for asthma exacerbation; IV form used for emergency prevention of "central cord syndrome" and subsequent paralysis following spinal injuries
Prednisolone†	Delta-Cortef	5 mg	0.5	18-36 hours	Used in acute exacerbations of multiple sclerosis
Prednisone†	Deltasone, Orasone	5 mg	0.5	18-36 hours	Used both acutely and for long-term therapy of asthma
Triamcinolone†	Aristocort, Kenacort	4 mg	0	18-36 hours	Injectable form commonly used for joint injections to treat various inflammatory and/or rheumatic processes

*Not all preparations are suitable for IV injection.
†Generic available for one or more dosage forms.

References:
1. Ellsworth, Allan J, *et al. Mosby's Medical Drug Reference.* Mosby, St. Louis, 2003.
2. U.S. Food and Drug Administration. Online. Internet. May 2003. Available http://www.fda.gov/
3. Centers for Disease Control and Prevention. Online. Internet. May 2003. Available http://www.cdc.gov/
4. National Guideline Clearinghouse [documents produced by the Agency for Healthcare Research and Quality (AHRQ)—formerly the Agency for Healthcare Policy and Research (AHCPR) in partnership with the American Medical Association (AMA) and the American Association of Health Plans (AAHP).] Online. Internet. May 2003. Available http://www.guideline.gov/

Inhaled Anti-Inflammatory Drugs

RESPIRATORY CORTICOSTEROIDS

Generic Name	Brand Name	Dose Per Actuation	Usual Adult Dose	Maximum Adult Daily Dose (number of inhalations)
Beclomethasone	QVAR	40 µg	80 µg tid-qid or 160 µg bid	800 µg (20)
Beclomethasone (Double strength)	QVAR	80 µg	160 µg bid	800 µg (10)
Budesonide (Powder)	Pulmicort Turbuhaler, Pulmicort Respules	200 µg	200-800 µg bid	1600 µg (8)
Flunisolide	Aerobid, Aerobid-M	250 µg	500 µg bid	2000 µg (8)
Fluticasone (Aerosol)	Flovent	44, 110, 220 µg	88-220 µg bid	880 µg (4-20)
Fluticasone (Powder)	Flovent Rotadisk, Flovent Diskus	50, 100, 200 µg	50-500 mcg bid	1000-2000 µg (2)
Triamcinolone	Azmacort	100 µg	200 µg tid-qid or 400 µg bid	1600 µg (16)

INTRANASAL CORTICOSTEROIDS

Generic Name	Brand Name	Dose Per Actuation	Usual Adult Dose	Maximum Adult Daily Dose (number of inhalations)
Beclomethasone	Beconase, Beconase AQ, Vancenase, Vancenase AQ 84 µg	42, 84 µg	42-168 µg each nostril qd-qid	336 µg (4-8)
Budesonide	Rhinocort, Rhinocort Aqua	32 µg	64 µg each nostril bid	256 µg (8)
Flunisolide	Nasalide, Nararel	25 µg	50 µg each nostril bid	400 µg (16)
Fluticasone	Flonase	50 µg	100 µg each nostril qd	200 µg (4)
Mometasone	Nasonex	50 µg	100 µg each nostril qd	200 µg (4)
Triamcinolone	Nasacort, Nasacort AQ	55 µg	110 µg each nostril qd	440 µg (8)

MAST CELL STABILIZERS

Generic Name	Brand Name	Dose Per Inhalation	Usual Adult Dose	Maximum Adult Daily Dose (number of inhalations)
Cromolyn (inhaled)†	Intal	800 μg	1600 μg qid	6400 μg (8)
Cromolyn (intranasal)	Nasalcrom	5.2 mg (OTC)	5.2 mg each nostril q 3-6h	62.4 mg (12)
Nedocromil (inhaled)	Tilade	1.75 mg	3.5 mg bid-qid	14 mg (8)

†Generic available in one or more dosage forms.

References:
1. Ellsworth, Allan J, *et al. Mosby's Medical Drug Reference.* Mosby, St. Louis, 2003.
2. *U.S. Food and Drug Administration.* Online. Internet. May 2003. Available http://www.fda.gov/
3. *Centers for Disease Control and Prevention.* Online. Internet. May 2003. Available http://www.cdc.gov/
4. *National Guideline Clearinghouse* [documents produced by the Agency for Healthcare Research and Quality (AHRQ)—formerly the Agency for Healthcare Policy and Research (AHCPR) in partnership with the American Medical Association (AMA) and the American Association of Health Plans (AAHP)]. Online. Internet. May 2003. Available http://www.guideline.gov/

Inhaled Bronchodilators

Generic Name	Brand Name	Dose per Inhalation	Usual Adult Dose	Available D0sage Forms
Albuterol†	Albuterol, Proventil	90 μg	1-2 inhalations q4-6h (aerosol) 2.5 mg up to qid (solution)	Aerosol: 90 μg/actuation Solution for inhalation: 0.083%, 0.5%
Albuterol/Ipratropium	Combivent, DuoNeb	90 μg/18 μg	2 inhalations q6h (max 12 per day) (aerosol) 3 ml q6h (solution)	Aerosol: 18 μg/90 18 μg/actuation Solution for inhalation: 0.5 mg, 2.5 mg/3 ml
Bitolterol	Tornalate		0.5-1.5 mg tid-qid	Solution for inhalation: 0.2%
Epinephrine†	microNephrin, Primatene Mist	220 μg (OTC)	1-2 inhalations q3-4h (max 12 per day)	Aerosol: 200 μg/actuation Solution for inhalation: 10 mg/ml (1:100)
Formoterol	Foradil Aerolizer	12 μg	12 μg q12h	Powder for inhalation (capsules): 12 μg
Ipratropium†	Atrovent	18 μg	2 inhalations q4-6h (max 12 per day) (aerosol) 500 μg q6-8h (solution)	Aerosol: 18 μg/actuation Solution for inhalation: 0.02% (500 μg/vial)
Isoetharine†		340 μg	1-2 inhalations q4h	Solution for inhalation: 1%
Levalbuterol	Xopenex		0.63 mg tid	Solution for inhalation: 0.31 mg/3 ml, 0.63 mg/3 ml, 1.25 mg/3 ml
Metaproterenol†	Alupent	650 μg	2-3 inhalations q3-4h (max 12 per day) (aerosol)	Aerosol: 0.65 mg/actuation Solution for inhalation: 0.4%, 0.6%, 5%
Pirbuterol	Maxair	200 μg	1-2 inhalations q4-6h (max 12 per day)	Aerosol: 0.2 mg/actuation
Salmeterol	Serevent	25 μg aerosol, 50 μg powder	12 inhalations q12h	Aerosol: 25 μg/actuation Powder for inhalation: 50 μg

†Generic available in one or more dosage forms.

References:
1. Ellsworth, Allan J, *et al. Mosby's Medical Drug Reference.* Mosby, St. Louis, 2003.
2. U.S. Food and Drug Administration. Online. Internet. May 2003. Available http://www.fda.gov/
3. Centers for Disease Control and Prevention. Online. Internet. May 2003. Available http://www.cdc.gov/
4. National Guideline Clearinghouse [documents produced by the Agency for Healthcare Policy and Research (AHCPR) in partnership with the American Medical Association (AMA) and the American Association of Health Plans (AAHP)]. Online. Internet. May 2003. Available file://http://www.guideline.gov

Insulins

Generic Name	Time in Onset of Effect for SC Route	Time to Peak Effect for SC Route	Duration of Effect for SC Route	Route of Administration	Comments / Syringe Compatibility Information
Insulin aspart	¼ hour	1-3 hours	3-5 hours	SC	Compatible with recombinant human NPH insulin
Insulin glargine	1 hour	5 hours	24 hours	SC	Not compatible with other insulins
Insulin lispro	¼ hour	1 hour	3-6.5 hours	SC	Recombinant human insulin analog; compatible with Ultralente and NPH
Regular insulin (SC)	½-1 hour	1-5 hours	6-10 hours	SC	Clear solution; compatible with all other insulins; draw Regular into syringe first; inject Regular/Lente mixtures immediately to avoid potency loss due to chemical binding
Regular insulin (IV)	⅙-½ hour	¼-½ hour	½-1 hour	IV, IM	Clear solution; compatible with all other insulins; draw Regular into syringe first; inject Regular/Lente mixtures immediately to avoid potency loss due to chemical binding
Isophane insulin suspension (NPH insulin)	1-2 hours	6-14 hours	16-24 hours	SC	Compatible with Regular
Lente insulin	1-3 hours	5-14 hours	16-24 hours	SC	Compatible with Regular
Ultralente insulin	4-8 hours	8-20 hours	24-28 hours	SC	Compatible with Regular
50/50 insulin	½-1 hour	4-8 hours	24 hours	SC	50% Isophane insulin suspension (NPH) and 50% Regular insulin
70/30 insulin	½-1 hour	4-8 hours	24 hours	SC	70% Isophane insulin suspension (NPH) and 30% Regular insulin

Notes:

1. Most insulin types are available as beef, pork, or human types. Onset of action is faster and duration of action is shorter with human insulin preparations.
2. Insulin is available in U-100 (100 units per ml) and U-500 (500 units per ml) forms. Duration of action of U-500 forms is longer than that of U-100 forms.

References:

1. Ellsworth, Allan J, *et al. Mosby's Medical Drug Reference.* Mosby, St. Louis, 2003.
2. Glazer, N.B., *et al. Safety of insulin lispro: Pooled data from clinical trials.* American Journal of Health-System Pharmacy, 1999; 56:542-547.
3. *U.S. Food and Drug Administration.* Online. Internet. May 2003. Available http://www.fda.gov/
4. *Centers for Disease Control and Prevention.* Online. Internet. May 2003. Available http://www.cdc.gov/
5. *National Guideline Clearinghouse* [documents produced by the Agency for Healthcare Research and Quality (AHRQ)—formerly the Agency for Healthcare Policy and Research (AHCPR) in partnership with the American Medical Association (AMA) and the American Association of Health Plans (AAHP).] Online. Inernet. May 2003. Available http://www.guideline.gov/

Lipid-Lowering Agents

MAXIMUM EFFECT ON SERUM LIPID LEVELS

Pharmacologic Class	LDL-C	Triglycerides	HDL-C
Bile acid-binding resins	↓ 10%-30%	↑ 3%-10%	⟷
Fibric acid derivatives	↓ 5%-10%*	↓ 30%-60%	↑ 5%-10%
Nicotinic acid derivatives	↓ 10%-25%	↓ 5%-30%	↑ 15%-25%
HMG-CoA reductase inhibitors	↓ 20%-40%	↓ 10%-30%	↑ 5%-15%

↑ increase, ↓ decrease, ↔ unchanged.
*Fenofibrate may increase LDL-C levels.

HYPERLIPOPROTEINEMIA CLASSIFICATION (FREDRICKSON CLASSIFICATION)*

Type	*Hyperlipidemia Name*	*Lipoprotein Class Elevated*	*Lipid Elevation*		*Approved Drug Therapy*	*Genetic Disorder*
			Major	*Minor*		
	Hyperlipemia, exogenous	Chylomicrons	TG	↑→C	None	Familial lipoprotein lipase deficiency Familial apolipoprotein C-II deficiency
IIa	Hypercholesterolemia	LDL	C		Atorvastatin Cholestyramine Colesevelam Colestipol Dextrothyroxine Ezetimibe Fluvastatin Lovastatin Niacin Pravastatin Probucol Simvastatin	Familial hypercholesterolemia Familial combined hyperlipidemia Polygenic hypercholesterolemia
IIb	Hyperlipidemia, combined	LDL VLDL	C	TG	Atorvastatin Cholestyramine Clofibrate Colesevelam Colestipol Fluvastatin Gemfibrozil Lovastatin Niacin Pravastatin Probucol Simvastatin	Familial combined hyperlipidemia
III	Hyperlipidemia, remnant	IDL	C/TG		Atorvastatin Clofibrate Gemfibrozil Niacin Pravastatin Simvastatin	Familial dysbetalipoproteinemia
IV	Hyperlipemia, endogenous	VLDL	TG	↑→C	Atorvastatin Clofibrate Fenofibrate Gemfibrozil Niacin Pravastatin Simvastatin	Familial hypertriglyceridemia (mild) Familial combined hyperlipidemia Sporadic hypertriglyceridemia Tangier disease
V	Hyperlipemia, mixed	Chylomicrons VLDL	TG	↑→C	Clofibrate Fenofibrate Gemfibrozil Niacin	Familial hypertriglyceridemia (severe) Familial lipoprotein lipase deficiency Familial apolipoprotein C-II deficiency

**C*, Cholesterol; *TG*, triglycerides; *LDL*, low-density lipoprotein; *VLDL*, very low-density lipoprotein; *IDL*, intermediate-density lipoprotein.

BILE ACID-BINDING RESINS (SEQUESTRANTS)

Generic Name	*Brand Name*	*Usual Adult Dose*	*Available Dosage Forms*	*Comments*
Colesevelam	Welchol	3 tablets bid or 6 tablets qd, with meal(s)	Tablet: 625 mg	May be taken concurrently with HMG-CoA reductase inhibitor therapy
Cholestyramine†	Questran	4-8 g bid	Powder for oral suspension: 4 g	Maximum daily dose: 24 g
Colestipol	Colestid	Granules: 5-30 g/day once daily or in 2-4 divided doses; increase dose by 5 g at 1-2 month intervals; Tablets: 2-16 g/day once or in divided doses	Granules: 5 g packet, 300 and 500 g bottles; Tablet: 1 g	

†Generic available in one or more dosage forms.

FIBRIC ACID DERIVATIVES

Generic Name	*Brand Name*	*Usual Adult Dose*	*Available Dosage Forms*	*Comments*
Clofibrate	Atromid-S	500 mg 4×/day	Capsule: 500 mg	Possible risk of tumor and cholelithiasis
Fenofibrate	Tricor	54-160 mg/day	Capsule: 54, 160 mg	Absorption is increased by approximately 35% when taken with food versus fasting
Gemfibrozil†	Lopid	600 mg bid before AM and PM meals	Tablet: 600 mg	Contraindicated in renal, hepatic, or gallbladder disease

†Generic available in one or more dosage forms.

NICOTINIC ACID DERIVATIVES

Generic Name	*Brand Name*	*Usual Adult Dose*	*Available Dosage Forms*	*Comments*
Niacin (nicotinic acid)†	Nicolar, Niaspan	1.5-6 g/day divided bid-tid with or after meals (start at 100-250 mg/day and titrate gradually)	Capsule, timed-release: 125, 250, 300, 400, 500 mg; Elixir: 50 mg/5 ml; Injection: 100 mg/ml; Tablet: 25, 50, 100, 250, 500 mg; Tablet, timed-release: 150, 250, 500, 750 mg; Tablet, extended-release: 250, 500, 750, 1000 mg	Skin warmth and flushing is a common side effect; contraindicated in liver or peptic ulcer disease

†Generic available in one or more dosage forms.

HMG-CoA REDUCTASE INHIBITORS—"STATINS"

Generic Name	Brand Name	Usual Adult Dose	Available Dosage Forms	Comments
Atorvastatin	Lipitor	10-80 mg qd	Tablet: 10, 20, 40, 80 mg	May take without regard to meals or time of day
Fluvastatin	Lescol Lescol XL	20-80 mg in single or divided doses	Capsule: 20, 40 mg; Tablet, extended-release: 80 mg	
Lovastatin†	Mevacor, Altocor	10-80 mg qd in single or divided doses	Tablet: 10, 20, 40 mg Tablets, extended-release: 10, 20, 40, 60 mg	
Pravastatin	Pravachol	10-20 mg qhs; may increase to 80 mg qhs if needed	Tablet: 10, 20, 40, 80 mg	
Simvastatin	Zocor	5-80 mg qd	Tablet: 5, 10, 20, 40, 80 mg	

General statement: All HMG-CoA reductase inhibitors are contraindicated in pregnancy, and in severe renal or hepatic disease. Significant drug interactions are possible with several drug categories, including other antihyperlipidemic agents and immunosuppressants (e.g., cyclosporine). An unusual but severe adverse reaction, which may be potentiated by drug interactions, is a breakdown of muscle tissue known as rhabdomyolysis. Symptoms include unexplained muscular discomfort and dark urine, signifying myoglobinuria. Advise patients to report any such symptoms immediately. See individual drug monographs for additional specific information.

†Generic available in one or more dosage forms.

Other Lipid-Lowering Agents

Generic Name	Brand Name	Usual Adult Dose	Available Dosage Forms	Comments
Ezetimibe	Zetia	10 mg/day	Tablet: 10 mg	May be taken with or without food. May be used in combination with a HMC-CoA reductase inhibitor or a bile acid sequestrant.
Niacin/lovastatin	Advicor	500 mg (niacin content) to 2000 mg HS	Tablet: (niacin/lovastatin) 500/20 mg, 750/20 mg, 1000/20 mg	Niacin portion is extended-release

References for Lipid-Lowering Agent Tables:

1. Dorland's Illustrated Medical Dictionary 29th edition. W.B. Saunders, Philadelphia, 2000; 853.
2. Website: U.S. Food and Drug Administration. Online. Internet. 2003. Available: http://www.fda.gov/cder

Low Molecular Weight Heparins

Generic Name	Brand Name(s)	Usual Adult Dose	Available Dosage Forms	Comments
Dalteparin sodium	Fragmin	Unstable angina: 120 IU/kg q12h along with aspirin DVT prophylaxis: 2500-5000 IU before surgery and then daily for 5-10 days	Prefilled syringes: 2500, 5000, 7500, 10,000 IU* Multiple dose vials: 10,000, 25,000 IU*/ml	Administer subcutaneously only; Do not give IM
Enoxaparin sodium	Lovenox	DVT prophylaxis: 30 mg before surgery and then daily for up to 3 weeks, depending upon type of surgery DVT treatment: 1 mg/kg q12h	Ampules: 30 mg/0.3 ml Prefilled syringes: 30 mg/0.3 ml, 40 mg/0.4 ml, 60 mg/0.6 ml, 80 mg/0.8 ml, 100 mg/1 ml, 120 mg/0.8 ml, 150 mg/1 ml	Administer subcutaneously only; Do not give IM 1 mg equals approximately 100 IU*
Tinzaparin sodium	Innohep	175 IU/kg q24h up to 6 days	Injection: 20,000 IU*/ml	Administer subcutaneously only; Do not give IM

*Anti-factor Xa international units

References:

1. Ellsworth, Allan J, *et al. Mosby's Medical Drug Reference.* Mosby, St. Louis, 2003.
2. Website: U.S. Food and Drug Administration. Online. Internet. 2003. Available: http://www.fda.gov/cder

Non-Sedating Antihistamines

Generic Name	*Brand Name*	*Usual Adult Dose*	*Available Dosage Forms*	*Comments*
Cetirizine*	Zyrtec	5-10 mg qd	Tablet: 5, 10 mg; Oral syrup: 5 mg/5 ml	May take with or without food; use with caution in those with renal or hepatic impairment, elderly individuals, and nursing mothers
Desloratadine	Clarinex, Clarinex, Reditabs	5 mg qd	Tablet: 5 mg Tablet, rapidly disintegrating: 5 mg	Reditabs quickly disintegrate on the tongue. Give every other day in patients with renal or hepatic disease. Metabolite of loratadine.
Fexofenadine*	Allegra	60 mg bid, or 180 mg qd	Tablet: 30, 60, 180 mg	Renal impairment: start at 60 mg once daily
Loratadine*†	Claritin, Claritin, RediTabs, Alavert	10 mg qd	Tablet: 10 mg; Rapidly disintegrating tablet: 10 mg; Oral syrup: 5 mg/5 ml	Reditabs readily disintegrate on the tongue; take on empty stomach; give every other day in patients with renal or hepatic insufficiency. Available without a prescription.

*Available in combination with a decongestant.
†Generic available for one or more dosage forms.

References:

1. Website: U.S. Food and Drug Administration. Online. Internet. 2003. Available: http://www.fda.gov/cder

Oral Hypoglycemic Agents

ALPHA-GLUCOSIDASE INHIBITORS

Generic Name	*Brand Name*	*Initial Dose*	*Maintenance Dose*	*Available Dosage Forms*	*Administration/Comments*
Acarbose	Precose	25 mg tid with meals	50-100 mg tid with meals	Tablet: 50, 100 mg	Monotherapy or in combination with sulfonylureas; take with first bite of each main meal; contraindicated in bowel disease
Miglitol	Glyset	25 mg tid	50-100 mg tid	Tablet: 25, 50, 100 mg	Monotherapy or in combination with sulfonylureas; take with first bite of each main meal; contraindicated in bowel disease; no dose adjustment needed in hepatic impairment

BIGUANIDES

Generic Name	Brand Name	Initial Dose	Maintenance Dose	Available Dosage Forms	Administration/Comments
Metformin†	Glucophage	500 mg bid or 850 mg daily	Up to 2500-2550 mg daily in 2-3 divided doses	Tablet: 500, 850, 1000 mg	Bid dosing with AM and PM meals; single daily dosing with AM meal; maximum daily dose: 2550 mg; as monotherapy or in combination with sulfonylureas; contraindicated in patients with subnormal renal function for age due to increased risk of lactic acidosis
	Glucophage XR	500 mg once daily with evening meal	Up to 2000 mg once daily with evening meal	Tablet: Extended-release: 500 mg	If 2000 mg once daily not effective, may try 1000 mg twice daily; if this is not effective, switch to immediate-release regimen described above, up to a maximum daily dose of 2550 mg

†Generic available in one or more dosage forms.

MEGLITINIDES

Generic Name	Brand Name	Initial Dose	Maintenance Dose	Available Dosage Forms	Administration/Comments
Nateglinide	Starlix	60-120 mg tid 1-30 min before meals	Same	Tablet: 60, 120 mg	Monotherapy or in combination with metformin; should not be used with glyburide or other sulfonylureas, nor is it indicated for patients who fail treatment with these agents; no dosage adjustment required in even severe renal dysfunction or in mild hepatic dysfunction; the 60 mg dose is intended for patients near their goal HbA_{1C}
Repaglinide	Prandin	0.5-2 mg tid before meals	0.5-4 mg bid, tid, qid depending on changes in patient's meal pattern	Tablet: 0.5, 1, 2 mg	Take before each meal; maximum daily dose: 16 mg

SULFONYLUREAS, FIRST GENERATION

Generic Name	Brand Name	Initial Dose	Maintenance Dose	Available Dosage Forms	Administration/Comments
Acetohexamide†	Dymelor	250-1500 mg/day	Same	Tablet: 250, 500 mg	Doses >1500 mg/day are not recommended; take doses <1500 mg/day before breakfast; at 1500 mg/day, divide dose bid
Chlorpropamide†	Diabinese	250 mg daily (100-125 mg daily for elderly)	100-500 mg daily	Tablet: 100, 250 mg	Avoid doses >750 mg/day
Tolazamide†	Tolinase	100-250 mg daily	100-1000 mg daily (give bid if >500 mg required)	Tablet: 100, 250, 500 mg	Take with breakfast or first main meal; maximum daily dose: 1000 mg; titrate dose to patient response; divide doses >500 mg bid
Tolbutamide†	Orinase	1000-2000 mg daily in divided doses	250-3000 mg daily in divided doses	Tablet: 500 mg	Dose may be taken in the morning or in divided doses; maximum daily dose: 3000 mg

†Generic available in one or more dosage forms.

SULFONYLUREAS, SECOND GENERATION

Generic Name	Brand Name	Initial Dose	Maintenance Dose	Available Dosage Forms	Administration/Comments
Glimepiride	Amaryl	1-2 mg daily	1-8 mg daily	Tablet: 1, 2, 4 mg	Take with breakfast or first main meal; maximum daily dose: 8 mg
Glipizide†	Glucotrol, Glucotrol XL	5 mg daily	2.5-40 mg daily (divide doses if >15 mg required)	Tablet: 5, 10 mg; Tablet, extended-release: 5, 10 mg	Take 30 minutes before breakfast; advantages: no renal elimination and few drug interactions; use with caution in hepatic disease
Glyburide†	Diabeta, Micronase	1.25-5 mg daily	1.25-20 mg daily	Tablet: 1.25, 2.5, 5 mg	Single dose or in divided doses; maximum daily dose: 20 mg/day
	Glynase PresTab	0.75-3 mg daily	0.75-12 mg daily	Tablet, micronized: 1.5, 3, 4.5, 6 mg	Micronized tablets are scored and can be broken in half; maximum daily dose of micronized form:12 mg/day; micronized tablets allow faster absorption and smaller doses

†Generic available in one or more dosage forms.

THIAZOLIDINEDIONES

Generic Name	Brand Name	Initial Dose	Maintenance Dose	Available Dosage Forms	Administration/Comments
Pioglitazone	Actos	15-30 mg daily	Up to 45 mg daily	Tablet: 15, 30, 45 mg	May take without regard to meals; monotherapy or in combination with metformin or sulfonylureas
Rosiglitazone	Avandia	4 mg daily	Up to 8 mg daily	Tablet: 2, 4, 8 mg	No dose change needed for elderly; no dose change needed when used as monotherapy with renally impaired patients; may take without regard to meals as either a single AM dose or in divided AM and PM doses; monotherapy or in combination with metformin or sulfonylureas

COMBINATION PRODUCTS

Generic Name	Brand Name	Initial Dose	Maintenance Dose	Available Dosage Forms	Administration/Comments
Glyburide/Metformin	Glucovance	1.25 mg/250 mg qd or bid with meals	2.5 mg/500 mg or 5 mg/500 mg bid with meals	Tablet: glyburide/metformin, 1.25/250, 2.5/500, 5/500 mg	Maximum daily dose: glyburide/metformin 20/2000 mg
Glipizide/Metformin	Metaglip	2.5 mg/250 mg once daily to 2.5 mg/500 mg bid	Up to 10 mg/2000 mg/day in divided doses	Tablet: glipizide/metformin, 2.5/250, 2.5/500, 5/500 mg	Give with meals
Rosiglitazone/Metformin	Avandamet			Tablet: rosiglitazone/metformin, 1/500, 2/500, 4/500 mg	Usual starting dose is the amount of rosiglitazone or metformin already being taken plus either 4 mg (per day) of rosiglitazone or 1000 mg (per day) of metformin

References:
1. Website: US Food and Drug Administration. Online. Internet. 2003. Available: http://www.fda.gov/cder

Triptans (Vascular Serotonin Agonists)

Generic Drug Name	*Brand Name(s)*	*Usual Adult Dose*	*Available Dosage Forms*	*Response Rates (% of patients reporting improvement)*	*Comments*
Almotriptan maleate	Axert	Initially 6.25 mg or 12.5 mg. May repeat in 2 hours. No more than 2 doses per 24 hours.	Tablets: 6.25, 12.5 mg	55%-65% after 2 hours	
Eletriptan hydrochloride	Relfax	Initially 20-40 mg. May repeat in 2 hours. No more than 80 mg/24 hours.	Tablets: 20, 40 mg	47-54% after 2 hours	
Frovatriptan succinate	Frova	Initially 2.5 mg. May repeat in 2 hours. No more than 7.5 mg/24 hours.	Tablets: 2.5 mg	37-46% after 2 hours	
Naratriptan hydrochloride	Amerge	Initially 1 mg or 2.5 mg. May repeat in 4 hours. No more than 5 mg/ 24 hours.	Tablets: 1, 2.5 mg	50%-66% after 4 hours	Initial dose of 2.5 mg is more effective than 1 mg.
Rizatriptan benzoate	Maxalt, Maxalt-MLT	Initially 5 mg or 10 mg. May repeat in 2 hours. No more than 30 mg/ 24 hours.	Tablets: 5, 10 mg Tablets (orally disintegrating): 5, 10 mg	60%-77% after 2 hours	
Sumatriptan succinate	Imitrex	Oral: 25-100 mg. May repeat in 2 hours. No more than 200 mg/ 24 hours. Subcutaneous: 6 mg. May repeat in 1 hour. No more than 2 injections per 24 hours. Intranasal: 5-20 mg. May repeat in 2 hours. No more than 40 mg/24 hours.	Tablets: 25, 50, 100 mg Spray (nasal): 5, 20 mg Injection: 6 mg/0.5 ml	Tablets: 52%-62% after 2 hours Spray (nasal): 45%-64% after 2 hours Injection: 15%-63% after 30 minutes; 21%-83% after 2 hours	First injection should be given under medical supervision. Needle penetrates 1/4 inch (5-6 mm). Give into areas with sufficient subcutaneous tissue.
Zolmitriptan	Zomig, Zomig ZMT	Initially 2.5 mg. May repeat in 2 hours. No more than 10 mg/24 hours.	Tablets: 2.5, 5 mg Tablets (orally disintegrating): 2.5 mg	27%-67% after 2 hours	

References:

1. Ellsworth, Allan J, *et al. Mosby's Medical Drug Reference.* Mosby, St. Louis, 2003.
2. Website: U.S. Food and Drug Administration. Online. Internet. 2003. Available: http://www.fda.gov/cder

APPENDIX B—ADDITIONAL INFORMATION

FDA Pregnancy Categories

Pregnancy Category	*Definition*
A	Controlled studies in pregnant women fail to demonstrate a risk to the fetus in the first trimester with no evidence of risk in later trimesters. The possibility of fetal harm appears remote.
B	Either animal reproduction studies have not demonstrated a fetal risk but there are no controlled studies in pregnant women, or animal reproduction studies have shown an adverse effect (other than a decrease in fertility) that was not confirmed in controlled studies in women in the first trimester and there is no evidence of a risk in later trimesters.
C	Either studies in animals have revealed adverse effects on the fetus (teratogenic or embryocidal effects or other) and there are no controlled studies in women, or studies in women and animals are not available. Drugs should be given only if the potential benefits justify the potential risk to the fetus.
D	There is positive evidence of human fetal risk, but the benefits to treat serious disease in pregnant women may be acceptable despite the risk (e.g., if the drug is needed in a life-threatening situation or for a serious disease for which safer drugs cannot be used or are ineffective).
X	Studies in animals or human beings have demonstrated fetal abnormalities or there is evidence of fetal risk based on human experience, or both, and the risk of the use of the drug in pregnant women clearly outweighs any possible benefit. The drug is contraindicated in women who are or may become pregnant.

Regardless of the designated Pregnancy Category or presumed safety, no drug should be administered during pregnancy unless it is clearly needed and potential benefits outweigh potential risks.

Drug Enforcement Administration Schedules of Controlled Substances

The controlled substances that come under jurisdiction of the Controlled Substances Act are divided into five schedules. Examples of controlled substances and their schedules are as follows:

SCHEDULE I SUBSTANCES

The controlled substances in this schedule are those that have no accepted medical use in the United States and have a high abuse potential. Some examples are heroin, marijuana, LSD, peyote, mescaline, psilocybin, THC, MDA, ketobemidone, acetylmethadol, fenethylline, tilidine, methaqualone, dihydromorphine, and others.

SCHEDULE II SUBSTANCES

The controlled substances in this schedule have a high abuse potential with severe psychic or physical dependence liability. Schedule II controlled substances consist of certain narcotic, stimulant, and depressant drugs. A written prescription signed by the physician is required for Schedule II drugs. In an emergency situation, oral prescriptions for limited quantities of Schedule II substances may be filled; however, the physician must provide a signed prescription within 72 hours. Schedule II prescriptions cannot be refilled. Some examples of Schedule II controlled narcotic substances are opium, morphine, codeine, hydromorphone, methadone, meperidine, cocaine, oxycodone, fentanyl, etorphine hydrochloride, anileridine, and oxymorphone. Also in Schedule II are amphetamine and methamphetamine, phenmetrazine, methylphenidate, glutethimide, amobarbital, pentobarbital, secobarbital, and phencyclidine.

SCHEDULE III SUBSTANCES

The controlled substances in this schedule have an abuse potential less than those in Schedules I and II and include compounds containing limited quantities of certain narcotic drugs and non-narcotic drugs such as derivatives of barbituric acid except those that are listed in another schedule, methyprylon, nalorphine, benzphetamine, chlorphentermine, clortermine, phendimetrazine, anabolic steroids, and paregoric. Any suppository dosage form containing amobarbital, secobarbital, or pentobarbital is in this schedule.

SCHEDULE IV SUBSTANCES

The controlled substances in this schedule have an abuse potential less than those listed in Schedule III and include such drugs as barbital, phenobarbital, mephobarbital, chloral hydrate, ethchlorvynol, ethinamate, meprobamate, paraldehyde, methohexital, fenfluramine, diethylpropion, phentermine, chlordiazepoxide, diazepam, oxazepam, clorazepate, flurazepam, clonazepam, prazepam, lorazepam, alprazolam, halazepam, triazolam, mebutamate, dextropropoxyphene, and pentazocine.

SCHEDULE V SUBSTANCES

The controlled substances in this schedule have an abuse potential less than those listed in Schedule IV and consist of preparations containing limited quantities of certain narcotic drugs generally for antitussive and antidiarrheal purposes.

Therapeutic and Toxic Blood Levels*†

Generic Name	Therapeutic Level	Toxic Level
Acetaminophen	10-30 μg/ml	>200 μg/ml
Amikacin	Peak: 20-30 μg/ml	>30 μg/ml
	Trough: 1-8 μg/ml	>10 μg/ml
Amiodarone	0.5-2.5 μg/ml	Not established
Amitriptyline	120-250 ng/ml	>500 ng/ml
Carbamazepine	4-12 μg/ml	>12 μg/ml
Chloramphenicol	10-20 μg/ml	>25 μg/ml
Chlordiazepoxide	1-3 μg/ml	>5 μg/ml
Chlorpromazine	50-300 ng/ml	>750 ng/ml
Clonazepam	10-80 ng/ml	>100 ng/ml
Clonidine	1-2 ng/ml	Not established
Clorazepate	0.12-1.5 μg/ml	>5 μg/ml
Cyclosporine	50-300 ng/ml	>400 ng/ml
Desipramine	115-300 ng/ml	>400 ng/ml
Diazepam	0.5-2 μg/ml	>3 μg/ml
Digoxin	0.8-2 ng/ml	>2 ng/ml
Disopyramide	2-8 μg/ml	>8 μg/ml
Doxepine	110-250 ng/ml	>300 ng/ml
Ethosuximide	40-100 μg/ml	>100 μg/ml
Flecainide	0.2-1 μg/ml	>1 μg/ml
Flurazepam	30-120 ng/ml	>500 ng/ml
Gentamicin	Peak: 6-10 μg/ml	>10 μg/ml
	Trough: 0.5-2 μ/ml	>2 μg/ml
Haloperidol	5-20 ng/ml	>20 ng/ml
Imipramine	225-300 ng/ml	>500 ng/ml
Lidocaine	1.5-6 μg/ml	>6 μg/ml
Lithium	0.6-1.2 mEq/L	>1.5 mEq/L
Lorazepam	50-240 ng/ml	Not established
Meperidine	100-550 ng/ml	>1000 ng/ml
N-acetylprocainamide	5-30 μg/ml	>30 μg/ml
Netilmicin	Peak: 6-10 μg/ml	>12 μg/ml
	Trough: 0.5-2 μg/ml	>2 μg/ml
Nortriptyline	50-140 ng/ml	>300 ng/ml
Oxazepam	0.2-1.4 μg/ml	Not established
Phenobarbital	10-40 μg/ml	>40 μg/ml
Phenytoin	10-20 μg/ml	>20 μg/ml
Primidone	4-12 μg/ml	>12 μg/ml
Procainamide	4-8 μg/ml	>10 μg/ml
Propoxyphene	100-400 ng/ml	>500 ng/ml
Quinidine	2-5 μg/ml	>5 μg/ml
Salicylates	100-300 μg/ml	>300 μg/ml
Secobarbital	1-5 μg/ml	>5 μg/ml
Theophylline	10-20 μg/ml	>20 μg/ml
Thioridazine	0.2-2.6 μg/ml	Not established
Tobramycin	Peak: 5-20 μg/ml	>20 μg/ml
	Trough: 0.5-2 μg/ml	>2 μg/ml
Tocainide	4-10 μg/ml	Not established
Valproic acid	50-100 μg/ml	>100 μg/ml
Vancomycin	Peak: 20-40 μg/ml	>40 μg/ml
	Trough: 5-15 μg/ml	>10 μg/ml
Verapamil	0.08-0.3 μg/ml	Not established

*Note: 1 mg (milligram) = 1000 μg (microgram) = 1,000,000 ng (nanogram)
†Adapted from *Saunders Nursing Drug Handbook* 2002, Philadelphia, 2002, WB Saunders.

Childhood Immunizations

Adapted from the Recommended Childhood Immunization Schedule*, United States, 2003. Approved by the Advisory Committee on Immunization Practices, the American Academy of Pediatrics, and the American Academy of Family Physicians.

CHILDHOOD IMMUNIZATION CHART

Age Recommendation	*Vaccine*
Birth	HepB no. 1 (Hepatitis B)†
1-2 months	HepB no. 1 [only if mother HbsAG(-)]
2 months	DTaP (diphtheria and tetanus toxoids and acellular pertussis vaccine)‡, Hib (*Haemophilus influenzae* type b)§, IPV (Inactivated Polio), PCV (pneumococcal conjugate)‖
1-4 months	HepB no. 2
4 months	DTaP, Hib, IPV, PCV
6 months	DTaP, Hib, PCV
6-18 months	HepB no. 3, IPV
6 months-18 years	Influenza (yearly; for selected populations)¶
12-15 months	Hib, PCV, MMR no. 1 (measles, mumps, rubella)**
12-18 months	Var (varicella zoster virus vaccine for chickenpox)††
15-18 months	DTaP
24 months-5 years	PCV (catch-up vaccination; for selected populations)
24 months-18 years	HebB series (catch-up vaccination), Var (catch-up vaccination), HepA series (Hepatitis A; for selected populations) ‡‡, PPV (for selected populations)
4-6 years	DTaP, IPV, MMR no. 2
11-12 years	Preadolescent assessment
11-18 years	Td (tetanus, diphtheria), MMR no. 2 (catch-up vaccination)

*This schedule indicates the recommended ages for routine administration of currently licensed childhood vaccines, as of December 1, 2002, for children through 18 years of age. Any dose not given at the recommended age should be given at any subsequent visit when indicated and feasible. Catch-up vaccinations are indicated for age groups that warrant special effort to administer those vaccinations not previously given. Additional vaccines may be licensed and recommended during the year. Licensed combination vaccines may be used whenever any components of the combination are indicated and the vaccine's other components are not contraindicated. Providers should consult the manufacturers' package inserts for detailed recommendations.

†**Hepatitis B vaccine:** All infants should receive the 1st dose of hepatitis B vaccine soon after birth and before hospital discharge; the 1st dose may also be given by age 2 months if the infant's mother is HbsAg-negative. Only monovalent HepB can be used for the birth dose. Monovalent or combination vaccine containing HepB may be used to complete the series. Four doses of vaccine may be administered when a birth dose is given. The 2nd dose should be given at least 4 weeks after the 1st dose, except for combination vaccines which cannot be administered before 6 weeks of age. The 3rd dose should be given at least 16 weeks after the 1st dose and at least 8 weeks after the 2nd dose. The last dose in the vaccination series (3rd or 4th dose) should not be administered before 6 months of age.

Infants born to HBsAg-positive mothers should receive HepB and 0.5 ml hepatitis B immune globulin (HBIG) within 12 hours of birth at separate sites. The 2nd dose is recommended at 1 to 2 months of age. The last dose in the vaccination series should not be administered before 6 months of age. These infants should be tested for HBsAg and anti-HBs at 9-15 months of age.

Infants born to mothers whose HBsAg status is unknown should receive the 1st dose of the HepB series within 12 hours of birth. Maternal blood should be drawn as soon as possible to determine the mother's HBsAg status; if the HBsAg test is positive, the infant should receive HBIG as soon as possible (no later than 1 week of age). The 2nd dose is recommended at 1-2 months of age. The last dose in the vaccination series should not be administered before 6 months of age.

‡**Diphtheria and tetanus toxoids and acellular pertussis vaccine:** The 4th dose of DTaP may be administered as early as 12 months of age, provided 6 months have elapsed since the 3rd dose and the child is unlikely to return at age 15 to 18 months. **Tetanus and diphtheria toxoids (Td)** is recommended at 11 to 12 years of age if at least 5 years have elapsed since the last dose of tetanus and diphtheria toxoid-containing vaccine. Subsequent routine Td boosters are recommended every 10 years.

§***Haemophilus influenzae* type b conjugate vaccine:** Three Hib conjugate vaccines are licensed for infant use. If PRP-OMP (PedvaxHIB or ComVax [Merck]) is administered at 2 and 4 months of age, a dose at 6 months is not required. DTaP/Hib combination products should not be used for primary immunization in infants at 2, 4 or 6 months of age, but can be used as boosters following any Hib vaccine.

‖**Pneumococcal vaccine:** The heptavalent pneumococcal conjugate vaccine (PCV) is recommended for all children 2 to 23 months of age. It also is recommended for certain children 24 to 59 months of age. Pneumococcal polysaccharide vaccine (PPV) is recommended in addition to PCV for certain high-risk groups. (See MMWR 2000;49(RR-9);1-38.)

¶**Influenza vaccine:** Influenza vaccine is recommended annually for children 6 months of age and older with certain risk factors (including but not limited to asthma, cardiac disease, sickle cell disease, HIV, diabetes, and household members of persons in groups at high risk; see MMWR 2002;51(RR-3);1-31 and can be administered to all others wishing to obtain immunity. In addition, healthy children 6-23 months of age are encouraged to receive influenza vaccine if feasible because children in this age group are at substantially increased risk for influenza-related hospitalizations. Children 12 years of age and older should receive vaccine in a dosage appropriate for their age (0.25 ml if age 6 to 35 months or 0.5 ml if 3 years of age and older). Children 8 years of age and older who are receiving influenza vaccine for the 1st time should receive two doses separated by at least 4 weeks.

****Measles, mumps, and rubella vaccine:** The 2nd dose of MMR is recommended routinely at 4 to 6 years of age but may be administered during any visit, provided at least 4 weeks have elapsed since receipt of the 1st dose and that both doses are administered beginning at or after 12 months of age. Those who have not previously received the 2nd dose should complete the schedule by the 11- to 12-year-old visit.

††**Varicella vaccine:** Varicella vaccine is recommended at any visit at or after 12 months of age for susceptible children, *i.e.,* those who lack a reliable history of chickenpox. Susceptible persons 13 years of age or older should receive two doses, given at least 4 weeks apart.

‡‡**Hepatitis A vaccine:** Hepatitis A vaccine is recommended for children and adolescents in selected states and regions, and for certain high risk groups; consult your local public health authority. Children and adolescents in these states, regions, and high risk groups who have not been immunized against hepatitis A can begin the hepatitis A vaccination series during any visit. The two doses in the series should be administered at least 6 months apart. (See MMWR 1999;48(RR12); 1-37.)

Adult Immunizations

Approved by the Advisory Committee on Immunization Practices (ACIP), and accepted by the American College of Obstetricians and Gynecologists (ACOG) and the American Academy of Family Physicians (AAFP).

RECOMMENDED ADULT IMMUNIZATION SCHEDULE, UNITED STATES, 2002-2003

	Age Group		
Vaccine	*19-49 Years*	*50-64 Years*	*65 Years and Older*
Tetanus, Diphtheria (Td)*	1 dose booster every 10 years.†	1 dose booster every 10 years.†	1 dose booster every 10 years.†
Influenza	1 dose annually for persons with medical or occupational indications, or household contacts of person with indications.‡	1 annual dose.	1 annual dose.
Pneumococcal (polysaccharide)	1 dose for persons with medical or other indications.(1 dose revaccination for immunosuppressive conditions.)§	1 dose for persons with medical or other indications. (1 dose revaccination for immunosuppressive conditions.)§	1 dose for unvaccinated persons.§ 1 dose revaccination.¤
Hepatitis B*	3 doses (0, 1-2, 4-6 months) for persons with medical, behavioral, occupational, or other indications.¶	3 doses (0, 1-2, 4-6 months) for persons with medical, behavioral, occupational, or other indications.¶	3 doses (0, 1-2, 4-6 months) for persons with medical, behavioral, occupational, or other indications.¶
Hepatitis A	2 doses (0, 6-12 months) for persons with medical, behavioral, occupational, or other indications.**	2 doses (0, 6-12 months) for persons with medical, behavioral, occupational, or other indications.**	2 doses (0, 6-12 months) for persons with medical, behavioral, occupational, or other indications.**
Measles, Mumps, Rubella (MMR)*	1 dose if measles, mumps, or rubella vaccination history is unreliable; 2 doses for persons with occupational or other indications†† (catch-up on childhood vaccinations.)		
Varicella*	2 doses (0, 4-8 weeks) for persons who are susceptible‡‡ (catch-up on childhood vaccinations).	2 doses (0, 4-8 weeks) for persons who are susceptible‡‡ (catch-up on childhood vaccinations).	2 doses (0, 4-8 weeks) for persons who are susceptible‡‡ (catch-up on childhood vaccinations).
Meningococcal (polysaccharide)	1 dose for persons with medical or other indications.§§	1 dose for persons with medical or other indications.§§	1 dose for persons with medical or other indications.§§

This schedule indicates the recommended age groups for routine administration of currently licensed vaccines for persons 19 years of age and older. Licensed combination vaccines may be used whenever any components of the combination are indicated and the vaccine's other components are not contraindicated. Providers should consult the manufacturers' package inserts for detailed recommendations.

Report all clinically significant post-vaccination reactions to the Vaccine Adverse Event Reporting System (VAERS). Reporting forms and instructions on filing a VAERS report are available by calling 800-822-7967 or from the VAERS website at www.vaers.org.

For additional information about the vaccines listed above and contraindications for immunization, visit the National Immunization Program Website at www.cdc.gov/nip/ or call the National Immunization Hotline at 800-232-2522 (English) or 800-232-0233 (Spanish).

*Covered by the Vaccine Injury Compensation Program. For information on how to file a claim call 800-338-2382. Please also visit www.hrsa.gov/osp/vicp. To file a claim for vaccine injury write: US Court of Federal Claims, 717 Madison Place, N.W.,Washington D.C. 20005. 202-219-9657.

†**Tetanus and diphtheria (Td):** *A primary series for adults is 3 doses:* The first 2 doses given at least 4 weeks apart and the 3rd dose, 6-12 months after the second. Administer 1 dose if the person had received the primary series and the last vaccination was 10 years ago or longer. MMWR 1991;40 (RR-10):1-21.*The ACP Task Force on Adult Immunization supports a second option:* A single Td booster at age 50 years for persons who have completed the full pediatric series, including the teenage/young adult booster. Guide for Adult Immunization. 3rd ed. ACP 1994:20.

‡**Influenza vaccination:** *Medical indications:* Chronic disorders of the cardiovascular or pulmonary systems including asthma; chronic metabolic diseases including diabetes mellitus, renal dysfunction, hemoglobinopathies, immunosuppression (including immunosuppression caused by medications or by human immunodeficiency virus [HIV]), requiring regular medical follow-up or hospitalization during the preceding year; women who will be in the second or third trimester of pregnancy during the influenza season. *Occupational indications:* Health-care workers. *Other indications:* Residents of nursing homes and other long-term care facilities; persons likely to transmit influenza to persons at high-risk (in-home care givers to persons with medical indications, household contacts and out-of-home caregivers of children birth to 23 months of age, or children with asthma or other indicator conditions for influenza vaccination, household members and care

givers of elderly and adults with high-risk conditions); and anyone who wishes to be vaccinated. MMWR 2002;51 (RR-3):1-31.

§Pneumococcal polysaccharide vaccination: *Medical indications:* Chronic disorders of the pulmonary system (excluding asthma), cardiovascular diseases, diabetes mellitus, chronic liver diseases including liver disease as a result of alcohol abuse (*e.g.,* cirrhosis), chronic renal failure or nephrotic syndrome, functional or ana-tomic asplenia (*e.g.,* sickle cell disease or splenectomy), immunosuppressive conditions (*e.g.,* congenital immunodeficiency, HIV infection, leukemia, lymphoma, multiple myeloma, Hodgkins disease, generalized malignancy, organ or bone marrow transplantation), chemotherapy with alkylating agents, antimetabolites, or long-term systemic corticosteroids. *Geographic/other indications:* Alaskan Natives and certain American Indian populations. *Other indications:* Residents of nursing homes and other long-term care facilities. MMWR 1997;47 (RR-8):1-24.

¤**Revaccination with pneumococcal polysaccharide vaccine:** One time revaccination after 5 years for persons with chronic renal failure or nephrotic syndrome, functional or anatomic asplenia (e.g., sickle cell disease or splenectomy), immunosuppressive conditions (e.g., congenital immunodeficiency, HIV infection, leukemia, lymphoma, multiple myeloma, Hodgkins disease, generalized malignancy, organ or bone marrow transplantation), chemotherapy with alkylating agents, antimetabolites, or long-term systemic corticosteroids. For persons 65 and older, one-time revaccination if they were vaccinated 5 or more years previously and were aged less than 65 years at the time of primary vaccination. MMWR 1997;47 (RR-8):1-24.

¶Hepatitis B vaccination: *Medical indications:* Hemodialysis patients, patients who receive clotting-factor concentrates. *Occupational indications:* Health-care workers and public-safety workers who have exposure to blood in the workplace, persons in training in schools of medicine, dentistry, nursing, laboratory technology, and other allied health professions. *Behavioral indications:* Injecting drug users, persons with more than one sex partner in the previous 6 months, persons with a recently acquired sexually-transmitted disease (STD), all clients in STD clinics, men who have sex with men. *Other indications:* Household contacts and sex partners of persons with chronic HBV infection, clients and staff of institutions for the developmentally disabled, international travelers who will be in countries with high or intermediate prevalence of chronic HBV infection for more than 6 months, inmates of correctional facilities. MMWR 1991;40 (RR-13):1-25. (www.cdc.gov/travel/diseases/hbv.htm)

****Hepatitis A vaccination:** For the combined HepA-HepB vaccine use 3 doses at 0, 1, 6 months). *Medical indications:* Persons with clotting-factor disorders or chronic liver disease. *Behavioral indications:* Men who have sex with men, users of injecting and noninjecting illegal drugs. *Occupational indications:* Persons working with HAV-infected primates or with HAV in a research laboratory setting. *Other indications:* Persons traveling to or working in countries that have high or intermediate endemicity of hepatitis A. MMWR 1999;48 (RR-12):1-37. (www.cdc.gov/travel/diseases/hav.htm)

††Measles, Mumps, Rubella vaccination (MMR): *Measles component:* Adults born before 1957 may be considered immune to measles. Adults born in or after 1957 should receive at least one dose of MMR unless they have a medical contraindication, documentation of at least one dose or other acceptable evidence of immunity. *A second dose of MMR is recommended for adults who:* Are recently exposed to measles or in an outbreak setting; were previously vaccinated with killed measles vaccine; were vaccinated with an unknown vaccine between 1963 and 1967; are students in post-secondary educational institutions; work in health-care facilities; plan to travel internationally. *Mumps component:* 1 dose of MMR should be adequate for protection. *Rubella component:* Give 1 dose of MMR to women whose rubella vaccination history is unreliable and counsel women to avoid becoming pregnant for 4 weeks after vaccination. For women of child-bearing age, regardless of birth year, routinely determine rubella immunity and counsel women regarding congenital rubella syndrome. Do not vaccinate pregnant women or those planning to become pregnant in the next 4 weeks. If pregnant and susceptible, vaccinate as early in postpartum period as possible. MMWR 1998;47 (RR-8):1-57.

‡‡Varicella vaccination: Recommended for all persons who do not have reliable clinical history of varicella infection, or serological evidence of varicella zoster virus (VZV) infection; health-care workers and family contacts of immunocompromised persons, those who live or work in environments where transmission is likely (*e.g.,* teachers of young children, day care employees, and residents and staff members in institutional settings), persons who live or work in environments where VZV transmission can occur (*e.g.,* college students, inmates and staff members of correctional institutions, and military personnel), adolescents and adults living in households with children, women who are not pregnant but who may become pregnant in the future, international travelers who are not immune to infection. *Note:* Greater than 90% of US born adults are immune to VZV. Do not vaccinate pregnant women or those planning to become pregnant in the next 4 weeks. If pregnant and susceptible, vaccinate as early in postpartum period as possible. MMWR 1996;45 (RR-11):1-36, MMWR 1999;48 (RR-6):1-5.

§§Meningococcal vaccine (quadrivalent polysaccharide for serogroups A, C, Y, and W-135): *Consider vaccination for persons with medical indications:* Adults with terminal complement component deficiencies, with anatomic or functional asplenia. *Other indications:* Travelers to countries in which disease is hyperendemic or epidemic ("meningitis belt" of sub-Saharan Africa, Mecca, Saudi Arabia for Hajj). Revaccination at 3-5 years may be indicated for persons at high risk for infection (*e.g.,* persons residing in areas in which disease is epidemic). Counsel college freshmen, especially those who live in dormitories, regarding meningococcal disease and the vaccine so that they can make an educated decision about receiving the vaccination. MMWR 2000; 49 (RR-7):1-20. *Note:* The AAFP recommends that colleges should take the lead on providing education on meningococcal infection and vaccination and offer it to those who are interested. Physicians need not initiate discussion of the meningococcal quadravalent polysaccharide vaccine as part of routine medical care.

RECOMMENDED IMMUNIZATIONS FOR ADULTS WITH MEDICAL CONDITIONS, UNITED STATES, 2002-2003

PREGNANCY

For all persons in this group:

- Tetanus-diphtheria (Td).*
- Influenza. If pregnancy is at 2nd or 3rd trimester during influenza season.

For persons with medical/exposure indications:

- Pneumococcal (polysaccharide).
- Hepatitis B.*
- Hepatitis A.

Contraindicated:

- Measles, mumps, rubella (MMR).*
- Varicella.*

DIABETES, HEART DISEASE, CHRONIC PULMONARY DISEASE, CHRONIC LIVER DISEASE, INCLUDING CHRONIC ALCOHOLISM

For all persons in this group:

- Td.*
- Influenza. Although chronic liver disease and alcoholism are not indicator conditions for influenza vaccination, give 1 dose annually if the patient is ≥50 years of age, has other indications for influenza vaccine, or if the patient requests vaccination.
- Pnumococcal (polysaccharide). Asthma is an indicator condition for influenza but not for pneumococcal vaccination.

For persons with medical/exposure indications:

- Hepatitis B.*
- Hepatitis A. For all persons with chronic liver disease.

Catch-up on childhood vaccinations:

- MMR.*
- Varicella.*

CONGENITAL IMMUNODEFICIENCY, LEUKEMIA, LYMPHOMA, GENERALIZED MALIGNANCY, THERAPY WITH ALKYLATING AGENTS, ANTIMETABOLITES, RADIATION OR LARGE AMOUNTS OF CORTICOSTEROIDS

For all persons in this group:
- Td.*
- Influenza.
- Pneumococall (polysaccharide). Revaccinate once after 5 years or more have elapsed since initial vaccination.

For persons with medical/exposure indications:
- Hepatitis B.*
- Hepatitis A.

Contraindicated:
- MMR.*
- Varicella. Persons with impaired humoral but not cellular immunity may be vaccinated. MMWR 1999;48 (RR-06):1-5.

RENAL FAILURE/END STAGE RENAL DISEASE, RECIPIENTS OF HEMODIALYSIS OR CLOTTING FACTOR CONCENTRATES

For all persons in this group:
- Td.*
- Influenza.
- Pneumococal (polysaccharide). Revaccinate once after 5 years or more have elapsed since initial vaccination.
- Hepatitis B.* *Hemodialysis patients:* Use special formulation of vaccine (40 μg/ml) or two 1.0 ml 20 μg doses given at one site. Vaccinate early in the course of renal disease. Assess antibody titers to hep B surface antigen (anti-HBs) levels annually. Administer additional doses if anti-HBs levels decline to <10 milliinternational units (mlU)/ mLl.

For persons with medical/exposure indications:
- Hepatitis A.

Catch-up on childhood vaccinations:
- MMR.*
- Varicella.*

ASPLENIA INCLUDING ELECTIVE SPLENECTOMY AND TERMINAL COMPLEMENT COMPONENT DEFICIENCIES

For all persons in this group:
- Td.*
- Influenza.
- Pneumococcal (polysaccharide). Revaccinate once after 5 years or more have elapsed since initial vaccination. Also administer meningococcal vaccine. *Elective splenectomy:* Vaccinate at least 2 weeks before surgery.

For persons with medical/exposure indications:
- Hepatitis B.*
- Hepatitis A.

Catch-up on childhood vaccinations:
- MMR.*
- Varicella.*

HIV INFECTION

For all persons in this group:
- Td.*
- Influenza.
- Pneumococcal (polysaccharide). Revaccinate once after 5 years or more have elapsed since initial vaccination. Vaccinate as close to diagnosis as possible when CD4 cell counts are highest.
- Hepatitis B.*

For persons with medical/exposure indications:
- Hepatitis A.

Catch-up on childhood vaccinations:
- MMR.* Withhold MMR or other measles containing vaccines from HIV-infected persons with evidence of severe immunosuppression. MMWR 1996;45:603-606, MMWR 1992;41 (RR-17):1-19.

Contraindicated:
- Varicella.*

*Covered by the Vaccine Injury Compensation Program. For information on how to file a claim call 800-338-2382. Please also visit www.hrsa.gov/osp/vicp. To file a claim for vaccine injury write: US Court of Federal Claims, 717 Madison Place, N.W.,Washington D.C. 20005. 202-219-9657.

Oral Dosage Forms That Should Not Be Crushed: 2003 Revision

John F. Mitchell, Pharm.D., FASHP
Dr. Mitchell is a Medication Safety Coordinator at the Department of Pharmacy and Clinical Associate Professor, University of Michigan, Ann Arbor, Michigan.

Drug Product	Dosage Form	Reasons/Comments
Aciphex	Tablet	Slow release
Accutane	Capsule	Mucous membrane irritant
Actifed 12 Hour	Capsule	Slow release†
Acutrim (various)	Tablet	Slow release
Adalat CC	Tablet	Slow release
Adderall XL	Capsule	Slow release*
Advicor	Tablet	Slow release
Aerolate SR, JR, III	Capsule	Slow release*,†
Allegra-D	Tablet	Slow release
Allerest 12 Hour	Capsule	Slow release
Altocor	Tablet	Slow release
Artane Sequels	Capsule	Slow release*,†
Arthritis Bayer Time Release	Capsule	Slow release
Arthrotec	Tablet	Enteric-coated
ASA Enseals	Tablet	Enteric-coated
Asacol	Tablet	Slow release
Ascriptin A/D	Tablet	Enteric coated
Ascriptin Extra Strength	Tablet	Enteric coated
Atrohist LA	Tablet	Slow release†
Atrohist Plus	Tablet	Slow release†
Atrohist Pediatric	Capsule	Slow release*,†
Augmentin XR	Tablet	Slow release
Avinza	Capsule	Slow release*
Azulfidine EN-tabs	Tablet	Enteric-coated
Baros	Tablet	Effervescent tablet¶
Bayer Enteric-coated	Caplet	Enteric-coated
Bayer Low Adult 81 mg	Tablet	Enteric-coated
Bayer Regular Strength 325 mg Caplet	Caplet	Enteric-coated
Betachron	Capsule	Slow release
Betapen-VK	Tablet	Taste‖
Biaxin-XL	Tablet	Slow release
Biltricide	Tablet	Taste
Bisacodyl	Tablet	Enteric-coated‡
Bontril SR	Capsule	Slow release
Breonesin	Capsule	Slow release†
Brexin LA	Capsule	Slow release
Calan SR	Tablet	Slow release††
Cama Arthritis Pain Reliever	Tablet	Multiple compressed tablet
Carbatrol	Capsule	Slow release*
Carbiset-TR	Tablet	Slow release
Cardene SR	Capsule	Slow release
Cardizem	Tablet	Slow release
Cardizem CD	Capsule	Slow release*
Cardizem SR	Capsule	Slow release*
Carter's Little Pills	Tablet	Enteric-coated
CartiaXT	Capsule	Slow release
Ceclor CD	Tablet	Slow release
Ceftin	Tablet	Taste† **Note:** Use suspension for children
CellCept	Capsule, Tablet	Teratogenic potential‡‡
Charcoal Plus	Tablet	Enteric-coated
Chloral Hydrate	Capsule	**Note:** Product is in liquid form within a special capsule†
Chlor-Trimeton 12-Hour	Tablet	Slow release†
Choledyl SA	Tablet	Slow release†
Cipro	Tablet	Taste‖
Claritin-D	Tablet	Slow release
Claritin-D 24 Hour	Tablet	Slow release
Codimal-LA	Capsule	Slow release
Codimal-LA Half	Capsule	Slow release
Colace	Capsule	Taste‖
Colestid	Tablet	Slow release
Comhist LA	Capsule	Slow release*
Compazine Spansule	Capsule	Slow release†
Concerta	Tablet	Slow release
Condrin-LA	Tablet	Slow release
Congress SR, JR	Capsule	Slow release
Contac 12-Hour	Capsule	Slow release*,†
Contac Maximum Strength	Capsule	Slow release*,†
Cotazym S	Capsule	Enteric-coated*
Covera-HS	Tablet	Slow release
Creon 10, 20, 25	Capsule	Enteric-coated*
Cystospaz-M	Capsule	Slow release
Cytoxan	Tablet	**Note:** Drug may be crushed but maker recommends using injection
Cytovene	Capsule	Skin irritant

Continued

Drug Product	Dosage Form	Reasons/Comments
D.A. II	Tablet	Slow release††
Dallergy	Capsule	Slow release
Dallergy - D	Capsule	Slow release
Dallergy - JR	Capsule	Slow release
Deconamine SR	Capsule	Slow release†
Defen-LA	Tablet	Slow release††
Depakene	Capsule	Slow release mucous membrane irritant†
Depakote	Capsule	Enteric coated
Desoxyn Gradumets	Tablet	Slow release
Desyrel	Tablet	Taste‖
Detrol LA	Capsule	Slow release
Dexatrim, Extented Duration	Tablet	Slow release
Dexedrine Spansule	Capsule	Slow release
Diamox Sequels	Capsule	Slow release
Dilacor XR	Capsule	Slow release
Dilatrate-SR	Capsule	Slow release
Disobrom	Tablet	Slow release
Disophrol Chronotab	Tablet	Slow release
Dital	Capsule	Slow release
Ditropan XL	Tablet	Slow release
Dolobid	Tablet	Irritant
Donnatal Extentab	Tablet	Slow release†
Donnazyme	Tablet	Enteric coated
Drisdol	Capsule	Liquid filled§
Drixoral	Tablet	Slow release†
Drixoral Plus	Tablet	Slow release
Dulcolax	Tablet	Enteric coated‡
Duratuss GP	Tablet	Slow release††
Dura-Vent/A	Tablet	Slow release††
Dura-Vent/DA	Tablet	Slow release††
Dynabac	Tablet	Enteric coated
DynaCirc CR	Tablet	Slow release
Easprin	Tablet	Enteric coated
EC-Naprosyn	Tablet	Enteric coated
Ecotrin Adult Low Strength	Tablet	Enteric coated
Ecotrin Maximum Strength	Tablet	Enteric coated
Ecotrin Regular Strength	Tablet	Enteric coated
E.E.S. 400	Tablet	Enteric coated†
Effexor XR	Capsule	Slow release
Efidac/24	Tablet	Slow release
Efidac/24 Chlorpheniramine	Tablet	Slow release
E-Mycin	Tablet	Enteric coated
Endafed	Capsule	Slow release
Entex LA	Tablet	Slow release†
Entex PSE	Tablet	Slow release
Entocort EC	Capsule	Enteric-coated
Equanil	Tablet	Taste‖
Ergomar	Tablet	Sublingual form**
Eryc	Capsule	Enteric coated*
Ery-Tab	Tablet	Enteric coated
Erythrocin Stearate	Tablet	Enteric coated
Erythromycin Base	Tablet	Enteric coated
Eskalith CR	Tablet	Slow release
Exgest LA	Tablet	Slow release
Extendryl JR	Capsule	Slow release
Extendryl S-R	Capsule	Slow release†
Fe 50	Tablet	Slow release
Fedahist Gyrocaps	Capsule	Slow release†
Fedahist Timecaps	Capsule	Slow release†
Feldene	Capsule	Mucous membrane irritant
Feocyte	Tablet	Slow release
Feosol	Tablet	Enteric coated†
Feosol Spansule	Capsule	Slow release*,†
Feratab	Tablet	Enteric coated†
Fergon	Capsule	Slow release*
Fero-Grad 500 mg	Tablet	Slow release
Ferro-Sequels	Tablet	Slow release
Feverall Sprinkle	Capsule	Taste* **Note:** Capsule contents intended to be placed in a teaspoonful of water or soft food
Flomax	Capsule	Slow release
Fosomax	Tablet	Mucous membrane irritant
Fumatinic	Capsule	Slow release
Gastrocrom	Capsule	**Note:** Contents may be dissolved in water for administration
Geocillin	Tablet	Taste

Drug Product	Dosage Form	Reasons/Comments
Glucophage XR	Tablet	Slow release
Glucotrol XL	Tablet	Slow release
Gris-Peg	Tablet	**Note:** Crushing may result in precipitation as larger particles
Guaifed	Capsule	Slow release
Guaifed-PD	Capsule	Slow release
Guaifenex LA	Tablet	Slow release††
Guaifenex PPA	Tablet	Slow release
Guaifenex PSE	Tablet	Slow release††
Guaimax-D	Tablet	Slow release
Humabid DM	Tablet	Slow release
Humabid DM Sprinkle	Capsule	Slow release*
Humabid LA	Tablet	Slow release
Humabid Sprinkle	Capsule	Slow release*
Hydergine L-C	Capsule	**Note:** Product is in liquid form within a special capsule†
Iberet	Tablet	Slow release†
Iberet 500	Tablet	Slow release†
ICaps Plus	Tablet	Slow release
ICaps Time Release	Tablet	Slow release
Ilotycin	Tablet	Enteric coated
Imdur	Tablet	Slow release††
Inderal LA	Capsule	Slow release
Inderide LA	Capsule	Slow release
Indocin SR	Capsule	Slow release*,†
Ionamin	Capsule	Slow release
Isoptin SR	Tablet	Slow release
Isordil Sublingual	Tablet	Sublingual form**
Isordil Tembid	Tablet	Slow release
Isosorbide Dinitrate Sublingual	Tablet	Sublingual form**
Isosorbide SR	Tablet	Slow release
K + 8	Tablet	Slow release†
K + 10	Tablet	Slow release†
Kadian	Capsule	Slow release*
Kaon CL	Tablet	Slow release†
K-Dur	Tablet	Slow release
K-Lease	Capsule	Slow release*,†
Klor-Con	Tablet	Slow release†
Klotrix	Tablet	Slow release†
K-Lyte	Tablet	Effervescent tablet¶
K-Lyte CL	Tablet	Effervescent tablet¶
K-Lyte DS	Tablet	Effervescent tablet¶
K-Norm	Capsule	Slow release
K-Tab	Tablet	Slow release†
Levbid	Tablet	Slow release††
Levsinex Timecaps	Capsule	Slow release
Lexxel	Tablet	Slow release
Lithobid	Tablet	Slow release
Lodine-XL	Tablet	Slow release
Lodrane LD	Capsule	Slow release*
Mag-Tab SR	Tablet	Slow release
Mestinon Timespan	Tablet	Slow release†
Metadate	Capsule	Slow release
Mi-Cebrin	Tablet	Enteric coated
Mi-Cebrin T	Tablet	Enteric coated
Micro K	Capsule	Slow release*,†
Monafed	Tablet	Slow release
Monafed DM	Tablet	Slow release
Motrin	Tablet	Taste‖
MS Contin	Tablet	Slow release†
Muco-Fen-DM	Tablet	Slow release††
Muco-Fen-LA	Tablet	Slow release††
Naldecon	Tablet	Slow release†
Naprelan	Tablet	Slow release
Nasatab LA	Tablet	Slow release††
Nexium	Capsule	Slow release*
Nicotinic Acid	Capsule, Tablet	Slow release
Nitroglyn	Capsule	Slow release*
Nitromed	Tablet	Slow release
Nitrong	Tablet	Sublingual route**
Nitrostat	Tablet	Sublingual route**
Nitro-Time	Capsule	Slow release
Nolamine	Tablet	Slow release
Nolex LA	Tablet	Slow release
Norflex	Tablet	Slow release
Norpace CR	Capsule	Slow release form within a special capsule
Ondrox	Tablet	Slow release
Optilets 500	Tablet	Enteric-coated
Optilets-M 500	Tablet	Enteric-coated
Oragrafin	Capsule	**Note:** Product is in liquid from within a special capsule
Oramorph SR	Tablet	Slow release†
Ornade Spansule	Capsule	Slow release
OxyContin	Tablet	Slow release
Pabalate	Tablet	Enteric coated

Drug Product	Dosage Form	Reasons/Comments
Pabalate SF	Tablet	Enteric coated
Pancrease	Capsule	Enteric coated*
Pancrease MT	Capsule	Enteric coated*
Panmist Jr, LA	Tablet	Slow release††
Panmycin	Capsule	Taste
Pannaz	Tablet	Slow release††
Papaverine Sustained Action	Capsule	Slow release
Pathilon Sequels	Capsule	Slow release*
Pavabid Plateau	Capsule	Slow release*
Paxil CR	Tablet	Slow release
PBZ-SR	Tablet	Slow release†
Pentasa	Tablet	Slow release
Perdiem	Granules	Wax coated
Peritrate SA	Tablet	Slow release††
Permitil Chronotab	Tablet	Slow release†
Phazyme	Tablet	Slow release
Phazyme 95, 125	Tablet	Slow release
Phenergan	Tablet	Taste‡
Phyllocontin	Tablet	Slow release
Plendil	Tablet	Slow release
Pneumomist	Tablet	Slow release††
Polaramine Repetabs	Tablet	Slow release†
Prelu-2	Capsule	Slow release
Prevacid	Capsule	Slow release
Prevacid Suspension	Suspension	Slow release **Note:** Contains enteric-coated granules
Prilosec	Capsule	Slow release
Pro-Banthine	Tablet	Taste
Procanbid	Tablet	Slow release
Procainmide HCL SR	Tablet	Slow release
Procardia	Capsule	Delays absorption†,‖
Procardia XL	Tablet	Slow release **Note:** AUC is unaffected
Profen II	Tablet	Slow release††
Profen-LA	Tablet	Slow release††
Pronestyl SR	Tablet	Slow release
Propecia	Tablet	**Note:** Women who are, or may become, pregnant, should not handle crushed or broken tablets
Proscar	Tablet	**Note:** Women who are, or may become, pregnant, should not handle crushed or broken tablets
Protonix	Tablet	Slow release
Proventil Repetabs	Tablet	Slow release†
Prozac	Capsule	Slow release*
Pytest	Capsule	**Note:** Radiopharmaceutical
Quibron-T SR	Tablet	Slow release†
Quinaglute Dura-Tabs	Tablet	Slow release
Quinidex Extentabs	Tablet	Slow release
Quin-Release	Tablet	Slow release
Respa-1st	Tablet	Slow release††
Respa-DM	Tablet	Slow release††
Respa-GF	Tablet	Slow release††
Respahist	Capsule	Slow release*
Respaire SR	Capsule	Slow release
Respbid	Tablet	Slow release
Ritalin SR	Tablet	Slow release
Robimycin	Tablet	Enteric coated
Rondec TR	Tablet	Slow release†
Ru-Tuss DE	Tablet	Slow release
Sinemet CR	Tablet	Slow release
Singlet for Adults	Tablet	Slow release
Slo-bid Gyrocaps	Capsule	Slow release*
Slo-Niacin	Tablet	Slow release††
Slo-Phyllin GG	Capsule	Slow release†
Slo-Phyllin Gyrocaps	Capsule	Slow release*,†
Slow-FE	Tablet	Slow release†
Slow-FE with Folic Acid	Tablet	Slow release
Slow-K	Tablet	Slow release†
Slow-Mag	Tablet	Slow release
Sorbitrate SA	Tablet	Slow release
Sorbitrate Sublingual	Tablet	Sublingual route
S-P-T	Capsule	**Note:** Liquid gelatin thyroid suspension
Sudafed 12 hour	Capsule	Slow release†
Sudal 60/500	Tablet	Slow release
Sudal 120/600	Tablet	Slow release
Sudex	Tablet	Slow release††
Sular	Tablet	Slow release
Sustaire	Tablet	Slow release†
Syn-RX	Tablet	Slow release
Syn-RX DM	Tablet	Slow release
Tavist-D	Tablet	Multiple compressed tablet
Teczam	Tablet	Slow release
Tedral SA	Tablet	Slow release†
Tegretol-XR	Tablet	Slow release
Teldrin Maximum Strength	Capsule	Slow release*

Continued

Drug Product	Dosage Form	Reasons/Comments
Temodar	Capsule	**Note:** If capsules are accidentally opened or damaged, rigorous precautions should be taken with the capsule contents to avoid inhalation or contact with the skin or mucous membranes. ‡‡
Tepanil Ten-Tab	Tablet	Slow release
Tessalon Perles	Capsule	Slow release
Theo-24	Tablet	Slow release†
Theobid Duracaps	Capsule	Slow release*,†
Theochron	Tablet	Slow release
Theoclear LA	Capsule	Slow release†
Theo-Dur	Tablet	Slow release†
Theo-Dur Sprinkle	Capsule	Slow release*,†
Theolair SR	Tablet	Slow release†
Theo-Sav	Tablet	Slow release††
Theo-Span-SR	Capsule	Slow release
Theo-Time SR	Tablet	Slow release
Theo-X	Tablet	Slow release
Theovent	Capsule	Slow release†
Thorazine Spansule	Capsule	Slow release
Tiamate	Tablet	Slow release
Tiazac	Capsule	Slow release
Topamax	Tablet, Capsule*	Taste*
Toprol XL	Tablet	Slow release††
Touro A&D	Capsule	Slow release
Touro EX	Tablet	Slow release
Touro LA	Tablet	Slow release
T-Phyl	Tablet	Slow release
Trental	Tablet	Slow release
Triaminic	Tablet	Enteric coated†
Triaminic 12	Tablet	Slow release†
Triaminic TR	Tablet	Multiple compressed tablet†
Tri-Phen-Chlor Time Released	Tablet	Slow release
Tri-Phen-Mine SR	Tablet	Slow release
Triptone	Tablet	Slow release
Tuss LA	Tablet	Slow release
Tuss Ornade Spansule	Capsule	Slow release
Tylenol Extended Relief	Capsule	Slow release
ULR-LA	Tablet	Slow release
Ultrase	Capsule	Enteric coated*
Ultrase MT	Capsule	Enteric coated*
Uni-Dur	Tablet	Slow release
Uniphyl	Tablet	Slow release
Urocit-K	Tablet	Wax coated
Verelan	Capsule	Slow release*
Videx EC	Capsule	Slow release
Volmax	Tablet	Slow release
Wellbutrin SR	Tablet	Anesthetize mucous membrane
Wygesic	Tablet	Taste
ZORprin	Tablet	Slow release
Zyban	Tablet	Slow release
Zymase	Capsule	Enteric coated*

*Capsule may be opened and the contents taken without crushing or chewing; soft food such as applesauce or pudding may facilitate administration; contents may generally be administered via nasogastric tube using an appropriate fluid provided entire contents are washed down the tube.
†Liquid dosage forms of the product are available; however, dose, frequency of administration, and manufacturers may differ from that of the solid dosage form.
‡Antacids and/or milk may prematurely dissolve the coating of the tablet.
§Capsule may be opened and the liquid contents removed for administration.
||The taste of this product in a liquid form would likely be unacceptable to the patient; administration via nasogastric tube should be acceptable.
¶Effervescent tablets must be dissolved in the amount of diluent recommended by the manufacturer.
**Tablets are made to disintegrate under the tongue.
††Tablet is scored and may be broken in half without affecting release characteristics.
‡‡Skin contact may enhance tumor production; avoid direct contact.

References

1. American Society of Hospital Pharmacists: ASHP technical assistance bulletin on handling cytotoxic and hazardous drugs, *Am J Hosp Pharm* 47:1033-1049, 1990.
2. Mitchell JF: Oral dosage forms that should not be crushed: 2000 update, *Hosp Pharm* 35:553-567, 2000.

IV COMPATIBILITY TABLE

	acyclovir	aminophylline	amiodarone	amphotericin B	ampicillin sodium	ampicillin/sulbactam	amrinone	aztreonam	calcium chloride	calcium gluconate	cefazolin	cefotaxime	ceftazidime	ceftizoxime	ceftriaxone	cefuroxime	cimetidine	ciprofloxacin	clindamycin	dexamethasone $NaPO_4$	diazepam	digoxin	diltiazem	dobutamine	dopamine	doxycycline	enalaprilat	epinephrine	erythromycin lactobionate	esmolol	famotidine	fentanyl	filgrastim	fluconazole	furosemide
acyclovir	■				C			I			C	C	C	C	C	C	C		C	C			?	I	I	C			C		C		C	C	
aminophylline		■	I				C	C					C				C	I					?	I			C			C	C		C	C	
amiodarone		I	■								?								C					C	C	C			C	C					
amphotericin B				■				I															C				I						I	I	
ampicillin sodium	C				■			C		?													?				C	I		C	C		C	I	
ampicillin/sulbactam						■		C										I					?				C				C		C	C	
amrinone		C					■		C								C					C		C	C			C			C				
aztreonam	I	C		I	C	C		■		C	C	C	C	C	C	C	C	C	C	C			C	C	C	C	C				C		C	C	C
calcium chloride							C		■															C				C		C					
calcium gluconate					?			C		■	C							C						C			C	C			C		C	I	
cefazolin	C		?					C		C	■												C				C			C	C		C	C	
cefotaxime	C							C				■											C								C		I	I	
ceftazidime	C	C						C					■					C					C				C			C	C		C	I	
ceftizoxime	C							C						■													C			C	C		I		
ceftriaxone	C							C							■								C								C		I	I	
cefuroxime	C							C								■							C								C		I	I	
cimetidine	C	C					C	C									■						C				C			C			C	C	
ciprofloxacin		I				I		C		C			C					■		I		C	C	C	C										I
clindamycin	C		C					C											■				C				C			C			I	I	
dexamethasone $NaPO_4$	C							C										I		■											C		C	C	
diazepam																					■		I	C										I	
digoxin							C											C				■	C								C			I	
diltiazem	?	?		C	?	?		C			C	C	C		C	C	C	C	C		I	C	■	C	C	C		C	C	C		C		C	I
dobutamine	I	I	C				C	C	C	C								C			C		C	■	C		C	C			C	C		C	?
dopamine	I		C				C	C										C					C	C	■		C	C		C	C	C		C	?
doxycycline	C		C					C															C			■							C		
enalaprilat		C		I	C	C		C		C	C		C	C			C		C					C	C		■		C	C	C	C	C		
epinephrine					I		C		C	C													C	C	C			■			C	C			C
erythromycin lactobionate	C		C																				C				C		■	C	C			I	
esmolol		C	C		C				C		C		C	C			C		C				C		C		C		C	■	C	C			I
famotidine	C	C			C	C	C	C		C	C	C	C	C	C	C				C		C		C	C		C	C	C	C	■		C	C	?
fentanyl																							C	C	C		C	C		C		■			C
filgrastim	C	C		I	C	C		C		C	C	I	C	I	I	I	C		I	C						C	C				C		■	C	I
fluconazole	C	C		I	I	C		C		I	C	I	I		I	I	C		I	C	I	I	C	C	C				I		C		C	■	I
furosemide								C										I					I	?	?			C		I	?	C	I	I	■
gentamicin	C		C					C										C					C				C			C	C		?	C	I
haloperidol lactate								C									C							C	C						C		C	I	
heparin sodium	C	C	I		C	C		C		C	C		C		C		C	I	C	C	I	C	C	?	C	I	C	C	C	C	C	C	I	C	C
hydrocortisone sod. succ.	C	C			C		C	C		C								I		C	I	C	C		C		C	C		C	C	C	C		C
imipenem-cilastatin	C							C															C								C		?	I	
insulin, regular			C		C	C		C			C											?	?	C	I					C	C				
isoproterenol			C				C																								C				
labetalol		C	C		C					C	C		C	C	I		C		C				C	C	C		C	C	C	C	C	C			?
lidocaine			C				C				C							C					C	C	C		C				C				
lorazepam	C							I				C						C		C			C	C	C			C	C		C	C	C	C	C
magnesium sulfate	C				C			C			C	C						?	C					C		C	C		C	C	C				
meperidine	?				C	C		C			C	C	C	C	C	C			C	C		C	C	C	C	C			C		C		C	C	?
meropenem	?			I													C			C				C	C	?	C							C	C
methotrexate								C							C		C			?											C		C		C
methylprednisolone	C						C	C										I					?		C		C				C		I		
metoclopramide	C							C										C					C								C		C	C	I
metronidazole	C		C					I															C		C		C			C			I	C	
midazolam			C		I					C	C	C	I			I	C	C	C	I		C	C	?	C			C	C	C	C	C		C	I
milrinone										C							C					C	C	C	C			C				C			I
morphine sulfate	?	C	C		C	C		C	C		C	C	C	C	C	C			C	C		C	C	C	C	C	C	C	C	C	C	C	C	C	?
multivitamins	C				C						C								C				C						C						
nafcillin	C																				C						C			C	C	C		C	
nicardipine																							C	C	C			C				C			I
nitroglycerin			C																				C	C	C			C		C	C	C		C	C
nitroprusside							C																C	C	C		C			C	C				
norepinephrine			C				C																C	C	C			C		C	C	C			C
ondansetron	I	I		I	I	I		C			C	C	C	C		C	C		C	C					C	C					C		C	C	I
oxacillin	C																						C								C			C	
penicillin G potassium	C		C																				C				C			C				C	
phenytoin																		I					I				I			C	C			C	
piperacillin	C							C										C					C				C			C	C		I	I	
piperacillin-tazobactam	I	C		I				C		C							C		C	C				I	C	I	C				I			C	C
phosphate (potassium)																		C					C				C			C	C				
potassium chloride	C	C	C		C		C	C		C								C		C	I	C	C	C	C		C	C		C	C	C	C		C
procainamide			C				C																C								C				
ranitidine	C	C						C					C	C				C					C	C	C		C	C		C		C	C	C	C
sodium bicarbonate	C		I				I	C	I						C			?		C			?								C		C		
streptokinase																								C	C										
ticarcillin	C							C															C								C		C	I	
ticarcillin-clavulanate								C															C								C		C	C	
tobramycin	C		C					C										C					C				C			C			C	C	C
TMP-SMX	C							C															C				C			C			C	I	
vancomycin	C		C		?	?		?				?	?	?	?	?							C				C			C			C	C	
verapamil					I		C											C						C	C						C				

Based on information in Trissel LA: Handbook on injectable drugs, ed 11, American Society of Health-System Pharmacists, Inc, Maryland, 2001.
The IV compatibility table provides physical compatibility information only for drugs given intravenously by Y-site administration in a 1:1 mixture. Therapeutic incompatibilities are not represented; therefore professional judgement should be exercised when utilizing this table.

gentamicin	haloperidol lactate	heparin sodium	hydrocortisone sod. succ.	imipenem-cilastatin	insulin, regular	isoproterenol	labetalol	lidocaine	lorazepam	magnesium sulfate	meperidine	meropenem	methotrexate	methylprednisolone	metoclopramide	metronidazole	midazolam	milrinone	morphine sulfate	multivitamins	nafcillin	nicardipine	nitroglycerin	nitroprusside	norepinephrine	ondansetron	oxacillin	penicillin G potassium	phenytoin	piperacillin	piperacillin-tazobactam	phosphate (potassium)	potassium chloride	procainamide	ranitidine	sodium bicarbonate	streptokinase	ticarcillin	ticarcillin-clavulanate	tobramycin	TMP-SMX	vancomycin	verapamil
C		C	C	C					C	C	?	?		C	C	C			?	C	C					I	C	C		C	I		C		C	C		C		C	C	C	
		C	C				C												C							I					C		C		C								
C		I			C	C	C	C								C	C		C				C		C			C					C	C		I				C		C	
												I														I					I												
		C	C		C		C			C	C						I		C	C						I							C									?	I
		C			C						C								C							I																?	
			C			C		C						C										C	C								C	C		I							C
C	C	C	C	C	C				I	C	C		C	C	C	I			C							C				C	C		C		C	C		C	C	C	C	?	
																			C																	I							
		C	C				C										C	C													C		C										
		C			C		C	C		C	C						C		C	C						C																	
									C	C	C						C		C							C															?	
		C					C				C						I		C							C									C							?	
							C				C								C							C									C							?	
		C					I				C		C						C																	C						?	
											C						I		C							C															?	
	C	C					C					C	C				C	C								C					C												
C		I	I					C	C	?				I	C		C												I	C		C	C		C	?				C			C
		C					C			C	C						C		C	C						C					C												
		C	C						C		C	C	?				I		C							C					C		C			C							
		I	I																		C												I										
		C	C		?						C						C	C	C														C										
C		C	C	C	?		C	C	C		C			?	C	C	C	C	C	C		C	C	C	C		C	C	I	C		C	C	C	C	?		C	C	C	C	C	
	C	?			C		C	C	C	C	C	C					?	C	C			C	C	C	C						I		C		C		C						C
	C	C	C		I		C	C	C		C	C		C		C	C	C	C			C	C	C	C	C					C		C		C		C						C
		I								C	C	?							C							C					I												
C		C	C				C	C		C		C		C		C			C		C			C				C	I	C	C	C	C		C					C	C	C	
		C	C				C		C								C	C	C			C	C		C								C		C								
		C					C		C	C	C						C		C	C																							
C		C	C		C		C			C						C	C		C		C		C	C	C			C	C	C		C	C		C					C	C	C	
C	C	C	C	C	C	C	C	C	C	C	C		C	C	C		C		C		C		C	C	C	C	C		C	C	I	C	C	C		C		C	C				C
		C	C				C		C								C	C	C		C	C	C		C								C		C								
?	C	I	C	?					C		C		C	I	C	I			C							C				I			C		C	C		C	C	C	C	C	
C	I	C		I					C		C	C			C	C	C		C		C		C			C	C	C	C	I	C				C			I	C	C	I	C	
I		C	C				?		C		?	C	C		I		I	I	?			I	C		C	I					C		C		C					C			
		I			C		C		C	C	C	C					C		C	C						C																	
								C	C								C						C	?	C	C					I												
I	I		C	C	C	C	C	C	C	C	C	C	C	?	C	C	C	C	C			I	C	C	C	C	C	C	I	C	C		C	C	C	C	C	C	C	I		I	
		C			C	C		C	C	C	C			?			I		C						C	C	C	C	I		C			C		C							
					C				I		I		C				I									C										I							
C		C	C	C						C	C	C					C	C	C		I		C	C	I								C			C		C	C	C		C	
		C	C															C															C										
C		C						C	C	C	C					C	C	C	C		I	C	C	C	C		C	C		C		C	C		C					C	C	C	
	C	C	C				C				C								C				C	C									C				C						
C	C	C	C	I			C						C			C	C	C	C			C	C		C	I				C	C		C		C						C	C	
C		C	C		C		C				C	C				C		C	C		C					C	C	C		C	C		C					C		C	C	C	
C		C	C	I	C		C	C		C				C	C	C					C					C	C	C		C	C		C		C			C	C	C	C	C	C
C		C			C										C	I			C	I					C	?									C							C	
		C		C					C	C				C	C		I		C							C	C				C				C							?	
		?	?								C		C		C	C			C							I					C		?			C							
		C									C	C	C						C							C					C												
		C					C		C	C	C	I		C			C		C												C												
C	C	C	I	I	C		C		C				I	C		C		C	C		I	C	C	C	C					C			C		C	I				C	I	C	
		C			C	C	C		C	C							C		C			C	C	C	C								C	I	C	C							C
C		C	C		C		C	C	C	C		C	C	C	C	C	C	C			C	C	C	C	C	C	C	C		C	C		C		C	C		C	C	C	C	C	
C												I																															
					I		I			C	?						I		C																							?	I
		I					C		C								C	C	C				C		C										C								
	C	C			C		C	C	C								C	C	C			C		C	C										C		C						
	?	C			C		C	C									C	C	C				C																				
	C	C	C		I		C		C			C					C	C	C			C	C										C		C								
C	C	C	C	C					I	C	C	?	C	I	C				C											I	C		C		C	I		C	C			C	
		C	C				C			C	C		C						C														C			I							I
		C	C				C			C	C								C														C										C
		I	I																														I										
		C					C		C	C	C						C		C							I									C								C
	I	C	C						C	C	C		C	C	C	C			C							C							C		C	C					C	?	
							C																																				
		C			C	C	C	C	C	C	C			?			C	C	C						C	C	C	C	I		C			C		C							
		C	C															I															C		C								
		C					C		C		C	C	C				C	C	C			C	C		C	C				C	C			C									
		C	C	I	C									C			I	C	C							I	I				C		C									C	I
		C						C															C																				
		C								C	C								C							C																?	C
		C			C						C								C							C																?	
		I			C		C			C	C						C		C																								
							C		C	C	C						I		C												C												
		I			C		C		C	C	C	C	?				C		C		?					C					?					C		?	?				
											C							C			I						I	C		C						I		C					

C, Compatible; *I,* incompatible; *?,* conflicting information; □, no documented information.

SYRINGE COMPATIBILITY TABLE

	Atropine	Buprenorphine	Butorphanol	Chlorpromazine	Cimetidine	Codeine	Diazepam	Dimenhydrinate	Diphenhydramine	Droperidol	Fentanyl	Glycopyrrolate	Haloperidol Lactate	Heparin	Hydroxyzine	Meperidine	Metoclopramide	Midazolam	Morphine	Nalbuphine	Pentazocine	Pentobarbital	Perphenazine	Prochlorperazine	Promazine	Promethazine	Ranitidine	Scopolamine HBr	Secobarbital	Thiethylperazine
Atropine	■		C	C	C			C	C	C	C	C		C	C	C	C	C	C	C	C	C	C	C	C	C	C	C		
Buprenorphine		■																C												
Butorphanol	C		■	C	C			I	C	C	C				C	C	C	C	C		C	I	C	C		C		C		C
Chlorpromazine	C		C	■	I			I	C	C	C	C		I	C	C	C	C	C		C	I	C	C	C	C	I	C		
Cimetidine	C		C	I	■		C		C	C	C	C		C	C	C		C	C	C	C	I	C	C	C	C		C	I	
Codeine						■						C			C															
Diazepam					C		■					I		I						I							I			
Dimenhydrinate	C		I	I				■	C	C	C	I		C	I	C	C	I	C		C	I	C	I	I	I	C	C		
Diphenhydramine	C		C	C	C			C	■	C	C	C	I		C	C	C	C	C	C	C	I	C	C	C	C	C	C		
Droperidol	C		C	C	C			C	C	■	C	C		I	C	C	C	C	C	C	C	I	C	C	C	C		C		
Fentanyl	C		C	C	C			C	C	C	■			C	C	C	C	C	C		C	I	C	C	C	C	C	C		
Glycopyrrolate	C			C	C	C	I	I	C	C		■			C	C		C	C	C	I	I		C	C	C	C	C	I	
Haloperidol Lactate									I				■	I	I				I											
Heparin	C			I	C		I	C		I	C		I	■		I	C		C		I					I				
Hydroxyzine	C		C	C	C	C		I	C	C	C	C	I		■	C	C	C	C	C	C	I	C	C	C	C	I	C		
Meperidine	C		C	C	C			C	C	C	C	C		I	C	■	C	C	I		C	I	C	C	C	C	C	C		
Metoclopramide	C		C	C				C	C	C	C			C	C	C	■	C	C		C		C	C	C	C	C	C		
Midazolam	C		C	C	C			I	C	C	C	C			C	C	C	■	C	C		I	I	I	C	C	I	C		C
Morphine	C		C	C	C			C	C	C	C	C	I	C	C	I	C	C	■		C	I	C	C	C	C	C	C		
Nalbuphine	C				C		I		C	C		C			C			C		■		I		C		I	C	C		C
Pentazocine	C		C	C	C			C	C	C	C	I		I	C	C	C		C		■	I	C	C	C	C	C	C		
Pentobarbital	C		I	I	I			I	I	I	I	I			I	I		I	I	I	I	■	I	I	I	I	I	C		
Perphenazine	C		C	C	C			C	C	C	C				C	C	C	I	C		C	I	■	C		C	C	C		I
Prochlorperazine	C		C	C	C			I	C	C	C	C			C	C	C	I	C	C	C	I	C	■	C	C	C	C		
Promazine	C			C	C			I	C	C	C	C			C	C	C	C	C		C	I		C	■	C				
Promethazine	C		C	C	C			I	C	C	C	C		I	C	C	C	C	C	I	C	I	C	C	C	■	C	C		
Ranitidine	C			I			I	C	C		C	C			I	C	C	I	C	C	C	I	C	C		C	■	C		C
Scopolamine HBr	C		C	C	C			C	C	C	C	C			C	C	C	C	C	C	C	C	C	C	C	C	C	■		
Secobarbital					I							I																	■	
Thiethylperazine			C															C		C			I				C			■

Based on information in Trissel LA: Handbook on injectable drugs, ed 11, American Society of Health-System Pharmacists, Inc.
The syringe compatibility table provides physical compatibility information only for drugs mixed in a syringe. Therapeutic incompatibilities are not represented, therefore, professional judgement should be exercised when utilizing this table.
C, Compatible; *I*, incompatible; □, no documented information.

Normal Values of Standard Laboratory and Function Tests

ALIMENTARY TRACT FUNCTION TESTS

Test	Normal value
Gastric Secretion	
Volume	
Fasting	20-100 ml/h
Nocturnal	<800 ml/10 h
Acid output (mean ± standard deviation)	
Basal (BAO)	
Female	2.2 ± 1.7 mEq/h
Male	3.7 ± 2.1 mEq/h
Stimulated after betazole (Histalog), 0.5 mg/kg or pentagastrin 6 μg/kg subcutaneously (PAO)	
Female	18 ± 5 mEq/h
Male	23 ± 7 mEq/h
BAO/PAO ratio	<0.5
Gastrin, Serum	<150 pg/ml
Gastrin, Serum, Following Stimulation With Intravenous Secretion 2 units/kg	Increases of 110 pg/ml or 100% of basal level 1, 2, 5, 7, 10, 15, or 30 min after secretin indicate Z-E syndrome (gastrinoma)
Intestinal Absorption	
Stool fat on diet containing 80-100 g fat/day (72-96 h collection)	<8 g/24 h
D-xylose absorption (25 g D-xylose administered orally after overnight fast)	
5 h urine collection after D-xylose	>5 g
1 or 2 h serum level after D-xylose	>25 mg/dl
Triolein breath test (5 μCi ^{14}C-triolein administered in 30 ml Lipomul; breath collected hourly for 6 h for measurement of breath $^{14}CO_2$)	>3.5% of dose/h
Lactose Absorption (50 g lactose administered after overnight fast; baseline and 1, 2 and 3 h serum samples obtained; alternatively, breath hydrogen can be measured in expired air 90-120 min after lactose administered)	>25 mg/dl increase in serum glucose >20 ppm H_2 in expired air
Schilling Test (see Hematologic Normal Values Table)	
Pancreatic Section	
Secretin test (2 units secretin/kg body weight, intravenously; duodenal fluid collected for four periods of 20 min thereafter)	
Volume	>1.5 ml/kg/80 min
Bicarbonate output	>16 mEq/80 min
Bicarbonate concentration	>80 mEq/L
Bentiromide (*N*-benzoyl-L-tyrosyl-*p*-aminobenzoic acid) test (500 mg administered after overnight fast followed by oral hydration and collection of a 6 h urine sample)	>50% urinary recovery of ingested PABA/6 h

BODY WEIGHT INFORMATION*

Body Mass Index (BMI)

$$\text{BMI} = \frac{\text{weight kg)}}{\text{height}^2\ \text{(m)}}$$

Normal range

Female	**21.3-22.1**
Male	**21.9-22.4**

Ideal Body Weight (IBW)

Adults (>18 years)

Female IBW (kg) = 45.5 + 2.3 for each inch over 60 inches

Male IBW (kg) = 50 + 2.3 for each inch over 60 inches

Children

$$\text{Age 1-18 years, height} <60 \text{ inches: IBW (kg)} = \frac{1.65 \times \text{height}^2\ \text{(cm)}}{1000}$$

*From Ellsworth AJ et al: *Mosby's 2001-2002 medical drug reference*, St. Louis, 2001, Mosby.

CARDIOVASCULAR NORMAL VALUES

CARDIOVASCULAR FUNCTION TESTS

CARDIAC INDEX

$$\text{L/min/m}^2 = \frac{\text{CO}}{\text{body surface area (BSA)}}$$

Normal = 2.8-4.2

CARDIAC OUTPUT

CO = (heart rate) × (stroke volume)

CARDIAC OUTPUT (FICK PRINCIPLE)

$$\text{CO (L/min)} = \frac{O_2\ \text{consumption (ml}\ O_2\text{/min)}}{\text{AV}\ O_2\ \text{difference (ml}\ O_2\text{/L)}}$$

where

O_2 consumption (basal state estimate) = 3 ml O_2/min/kg body weight

AV O_2 difference = arterial O_2 content − venous O_2 content (ml O_2/L)

O_2 content (ml/dl) = Hb (g/dl) × 1.39 (ml O_2/g Hb) × % saturation

O_2 content (ml O_2/L) = ml/dl × 10

Therefore

$$\text{CO (L/min)} = \frac{3\ \text{(ml/min)} \times \text{weight (kg)}}{(SaO_2 - SvO_2)\ (1.39) \times \text{Hb (g/dl)} \times 10}$$

MEAN ARTERIAL PRESSURE

Mean arterial pressure = diastolic pressure + ⅓ (systolic pressure − diastolic pressure)

Resistance can be expressed in absolute resistance units (ARU) of dyne-sec-cm^{-5} or hybrid resistance units (HRU) of mm Hg/L/min; ARU = 80 HRU

SYSTEMIC VASCULAR RESISTANCE (SVR)

$$\text{SVR} = \frac{\overline{SA} - \overline{RA}}{CO}\ \text{(normal = 1130 dyne-sec-cm}^{-5} \pm 178)$$

PULMONARY ARTERIOLAR RESISTANCE (PAR)

$$\text{PAR} = \frac{\overline{PA} - \overline{LA}}{CO}\ \text{(normal = 67 dyne-sec-cm}^{-5} \pm 23)$$

TOTAL PULMONARY RESISTANCE (TPR)

$$\text{TPR} = \frac{\overline{PA}}{CO}\ \text{(normal = 205 dyne-sec-cm}^{-5} \pm 51)$$

TOTAL SYSTEMIC RESISTANCE (TSR)

$$\text{TSR} = \frac{\overline{SA}}{CO}$$

NORMAL PRESSURES IN THE HEART AND GREAT VESSELS*

Pressures	*Average (mm Hg)*	*Range (mm Hg)*	*Pressures*	*Average (mm Hg)*	*Range (mm Hg)*
Right atrium			Left atrium		
Mean	2.8	1-5	Mean	7.9	2-12
a wave	5.6	2.5-7.0	a wave	10.4	4-16
z point	2.9	1.5-5.0	z point	7.6	1-13
c wave	3.8	1.5-6.0	v wave	12.8	6-12
x wave	1.7	0-5	Left ventricle		
v wave	4.6	2.0-7.5	Peak systolic	130	90-140
y wave	2.4	0-6	End diastolic	8.7	5-12
Right ventricle			Brachial Artery		
Peak systolic	25	17-32	Mean	85	70-105
End diastolic	4	1-7	Peak systolic	130	90-140
Pulmonary artery			End diastolic	70	60-90
Mean	15	9-19			
Peak systolic	25	17-32			
End diastolic	9	4-13			
Pulmonary artery wedge					
Mean	9	4.5-13.0			

*Reference elevation = 10 cm above the spine of the recumbent subject.
$\overline{RA}$, Mean right atrial pressure; $\overline{PA}$, mean pulmonary artery pressure; $\overline{LA}$, mean left atrial pressure; $\overline{SA}$, mean systemic arterial pressure; $\overline{CO}$, cardiac output.

CEREBROSPINAL FLUID NORMAL VALUES

Bilirubin	0
Cells	0-5/mm^3, all lymphocytes
Chloride	110-129 mEq/L
Glucose	48-86 mg/dl or ≥60% of serum glucose
pH	7.34-7.43
Pressure	7-20 cm water
Protein, lumbar	15-45 mg/dl
Albumin	58%
α_1-globulins	9%
α_2-globulins	8%
β-globulins	10%
γ-globulins	10% (5-12%)
Protein, cisternal	15-25 mg/dl
Protein, ventricular	5-15 mg/dl

CONVERSION INFORMATION

METRIC CONVERSIONS

Linear Measurements

1 mm = 0.04 in
1 in = 25.4 mm = 2.54 cm
1 m = 39.4 in
1 in = 0.025 m

Volume Measurements

1 tsp = 5 ml
1 tbsp = 15 ml
1 fl oz = 2 tbsp = 30 ml
4 fl oz = 120 ml
Pint = 473 ml
Quart = 946 ml

Weight Measurements

1 mg = 1000 μg = 1,000,000 ng = 0.017 grain
1 grain = 65 mg
1 g = 1000 mg = 0.035 oz
1 oz = 28.3 g
1 kg = 1000 g = 2.2 lb
1 lb = 0.45 kg

MILLIEQUIVALENT CONVERSIONS

1 mEq Na = 23 mg Na = 58.5 mg NaCl
1 g Na = 2.54 g NaCl = 43 mEq Na
1 g NaCl = 0.39 g Na = 17 mEq Na

1 mEq K = 39 mg K = 74.5 mg KCl
1 g K = 1.91 g KCl = 26 mEq K
1 g KCl = 0.52 g K = 13 mEq K

1 mEq Ca = 20 mg Ca
1 g Ca = 50 mEq Ca

1 mEq Mg = 0.12 g $MgSO_4 \cdot 7H_2O$
1 g Mg = 10.2 g $MgSO_4 \cdot 7H_2O$ = 82 mEq Mg

10 mmol P_i = 0.31 g P_i = 0.95 g PO_4
1 g P_i = 3.06 g PO_4 = 32 mmol P_i

WEIGHTS AND MEASURES

Percentage Equivalents

0.1% solution contains: 1 mg/ml
1% solution contains: 10 mg/ml
10% solution contains: 100 mg/ml

Prefixes for Fractions

deci = 10^{-1}
centi = 10^{-2}
milli = 10^{-3}
micro = 10^{-6}
nano = 10^{-9}
pico = 10^{-12}

Temperature Measures

°C = 5/9 × (°F − 32)
°F = 9/5 × (°C + 32)

CREATININE CLEARANCE CALCULATION*

Adults (age >18; serum creatinine <5 mg/dl and not changing rapidly)

$$\text{CRCL (ml/min)} = \frac{(140 - \text{age})(\text{weight in kg})}{(\text{serum creatinine [mg/dl]})(72)}$$

Notes:

1. Multiply by 0.85 for females
2. Use the following value for weight:
   a. If actual weight <IBW, use actual weight
   b. If actual weight is 100-130% of IBW, use IBW
   c. If actual weight >130% of IBW, easiest approximation is by using:
   $$\frac{\text{IBW} + (\text{actual weight} - \text{IBW})}{3}$$
3. Accuracy reduced in muscle wasting diseases (e.g., neuromuscular disease) and amputees

Children

$$\text{CRCL (ml/min/1.73 m}^2) = \frac{0.48 \times \text{height (cm)}}{\text{serum creatinine (mg/dl)}}$$

*From Ellsworth AJ et al: *Mosby's 2001-2002 medical drug reference,* St Louis, 2001, Mosby.

ENDOCRINOLOGIC NORMAL VALUES

ENDOCRINE FUNCTION TESTS

Adrenal Gland

Glucocorticoid suppression: Overnight dexamethasone suppression test (8 AM serum cortisol after 1 mg dexamethasone orally at 11 PM)	≤5 µg/dl
Glucocorticoid stimulation: Cosyntropin stimulation test (serum cortisol 30-90 min after 0.25 mg cosyntropin intramuscularly or intravenously)	>10 µg/ml more than baseline serum cortisol
Metyrapone test, single dose (8 AM serum deoxycortisol after 30 mg/kg metyrapone orally at midnight)	>7.5 µg/dl
Aldosterone suppression: Sodium depletion test (urine aldosterone collected on day 3 of 200 mEq/day sodium diet)	<20 µg/24 h

Pancreas

Glucose tolerance test (add 10 mg/dl for each decade over 50 years of age) (serum glucose after 100 g glucose orally)	
60 min after ingestion	<180 mg/dl
90 min after ingestion	<160 mg/dl
120 min after ingestion	<125 mg/dl

Pituitary Gland

Adrenocorticotropic hormone (ACTH) stimulation (see Adrenal Gland, Metyrapone test)	
Growth hormone stimulation: Insulin tolerance test (serum growth hormone after 0.1 U/kg regular insulin intravenously after an overnight fast to induce a 50% fall in serum glucose concentration or symptomatic hypoglycemia)	>5 ng/ml rise over baseline
Levodopa test (serum growth hormone after 0.5 g levodopa orally while fasting)	>5 ng/ml rise over baseline within 2 h
Growth hormone suppression: Glucose tolerance test (serum growth hormone after 100 g glucose orally after 8 h fast)	<5 ng/ml within 2 h
Luteinizing hormone (LH) stimulation: Gonadotropin-releasing hormone (GnRH) test (serum LH after 100 µg GnRH intravenously or intramuscularly)	Fourfold to sixfold rise over baseline
Thyroid-stimulating hormone (TSH) stimulation: Thyrotropin-releasing hormone (TRH) stimulation test (serum TSH after 400 µg TRH intravenously)	>twofold rise over baseline within 2 h

Thyroid Gland

Radioactive iodine uptake (RAIU) suppression test (RAIU on day 7 after 25 µg tri-iodothyronine orally four times daily)	<10% to <50% baseline
Thyrotropin-releasing hormone (TRH) stimulation test (see Pituitary Gland, Thyroid-stimulating hormone (TSH) stimulation)	

HORMONE AND METABOLITE NORMAL VALUES

Adrenocorticotropin (ACTH), serum	15-100 pg/ml
Aldosterone (mean ± standard deviation)	
Serum	
210 mEq/day sodium diet	
Supine	48 ± 29 pg/ml
Upright (2 h)	65 ± 23 pg/ml
110 mEq/day sodium diet	
Supine	107 ± 45 pg/ml
Upright (2 h)	532 ± 228 pg/ml
Urine	5-19 µg/24 h
Calcitonin, serum	
Basal	0.15-0.35 ng/ml
Stimulated	<0.6 ng/ml
Catecholamines, free urinary	<110 µg/24 h
Chorionic gonadotropin, serum	
Pregnant	
First month	10-10,000 mIU/ml
Second and third months	10,000-100,000 mIU/ml
Second trimester	10,000-30,000 mIU/ml
Third trimester	5000-15,000 mIU/ml
Nonpregnant	<3 mIU/ml
Cortisol	
Serum	
8 AM	5-25 µg/dl
8 PM	<10 µg/dl
Cosyntropin stimulation (30-90 min after 0.25 mg cosyntropin intramuscularly or intravenously)	>10 µg/dl rise over baseline
Overnight suppression (8 AM serum cortisol after 1 mg dexamethasone orally at 11 PM)	≤5 µg/dl
Urine	20-70 µg/24 h
C-peptide, serum	0.28-0.63 pmol/ml
11-Deoxycortisol, serum	
Basal	0-1.4 µg/dl
Metyrapone stimulation (30 mg/kg orally 8 h before level)	>7.5 µg/dl
Epinephrine, plasma	<35 pg/ml
Estradiol, serum	
Female	25-200 pg/ml
Male	20-50 pg/ml
Estrogens, urine (increased during pregnancy; decreased after menopause)	
Total	
Female	5-100 µg/24 h
Male	4-25 µg/24 h
Estriol	
Female	0-65 µg/24 h
Male	1-11 µg/24 h
Estradiol	
Female	0-14 µg/24 h
Male	0-6 µg/24 h
Estrone	
Female	4-31 µg/24 h
Male	3-8 µg/24 h
Etiocholanolone, serum	<1.2 µg/dl
Follicle-stimulating/hormone, serum	
Female	
Male	2-18 mIU/ml
Follicular phase	5-20 mIU/ml
Peak midcycle	30-50 mIU/ml
Luteal phase	5-15 mIU/ml
Postmenopausal	>50 mIU/ml
Gastrin, serum (fasting)	30-200 pg/ml
Growth hormone, serum	
Adult, fasting	<5 ng/ml
Glucose load (100 g orally)	<5 ng/ml
Levodopa stimulation (500 mg orally in a fasting state)	>5 ng/ml rise over baseline within 2 h
17-Hydroxycorticosteroids, urine	
Female	2-8 mg/24 h
Male	2-12 mg/24 h
5′-Hydroxyindoleacetic acid (5′-HIAA), urine	2-9 mg/24 h
Insulin, plasma	
Fasting	6-20 µU/ml
Hypoglycemia (serum glucose <50 mg/dl)	<5 µU/ml
17-Ketosteroids, urine	
Under 8 years old	0-2 mg/24 h
Adolescent	0-18 mg/24 h
Adult	
Female	5-15 mg/24 h
Male	8-18 mg/24 h
Luteinizing hormone, serum	
Adult	
Female	
Basal	5-22 mIU/ml
Ovulation	30-250 mIU/ml
Postmenopausal	>30 mIU/ml
Male	2-18 mIU/ml

Metanephrines, urine	<1.3 mg/24 h
Norepinephrine	
Plasma	150-450 pg/ml
Urine	<100 μg/24 h
Parathyroid hormone, serum	
C-terminal	150-350 pg/ml
N-terminal	230-630 pg/ml
Pregnanediol, urine	
Female	
Follicular phase	<1.5 mg/24 h
Luteal phase	2.0-4.2 mg/24 h
Postmenopausal	0.2-1.0 mg/24 h
Male	<1.5 mg/24 h
Progesterone, serum	
Female	
Follicular phase	0.02-0.9 ng/ml
Luteal phase	6-30 ng/ml
Male	<2 ng/ml
Prolactin, serum	
Pregnant	150-200 ng/ml
Nonpregnant	
Day	5-25 ng/ml
Night	20-40 ng/ml
Radioactive iodine (^{131}I) uptake (RAIU)	5%-25% at 24 h (varies with iodine intake)
Renin activity, plasma (mean ± standard deviation)	
Normal diet	
Supine	1.1 ± 0.8 ng/ml/h
Upright	1.9 ± 1.7 ng/ml/h
Low-sodium diet	
Supine	2.7 ± 1.8 ng/ml/h
Upright	6.6 ± 2.5 ng/ml/h
Diuretics and low-sodium diet	10.0 ± 3.7 ng/ml/h
Testosterone, total plasma	
Bound	
Female	25-90 ng/dl
Adolescent male	<100 ng/dl
Adult male	300-1100 ng/dl
Unbound	
Female	0.09-1.30 ng/dl
Adult male	3-24 ng/dl
Thyroid-stimulating hormone, serum	<10 μU/ml
Thyroxine (T_4), serum	
Total	4-11 μg/dl
Free	0.8-2.4 ng/dl
Thyroxine-binding globulin capacity, serum	15-25 μg T_4/dl
Thyroxine index, free	1-4 ng/dl
Tri-iodothyronine (T_3), serum	70-190 ng/dl
T_3 resin uptake	25%-45%
Vanillylmandelic acid (VMA), urine	1-8 mg/24 h

HEMATOLOGIC NORMAL VALUES

Acid hemolysis test (Ham)	No hemolysis
Carboxyhemoglobin	
Nonsmoker	<1%
Smoker	2.1%-4.2%
Cold hemolysis test (Donath-Landsteiner)	No hemolysis
Complete blood count	
(see Complete Blood Count Table)	
Erythrocyte life span	
Normal	120 days
^{51}Cr-labeled half-life	2 days
Erythropoietin by radioimmunoassay	9-33 mU/dl
Ferritin, serum	
Female	12-150 μg/L
Male	15-200 μg/L
Folate, RBC	120-670 ng/ml
Fragility, osmotic	
Hemolysis begins	0.45%-0.38% NaCl
Hemolysis completed	0.33%-0.30% NaCl
Haptoglobin, serum	100-300 mg/dl
Hemoglobin	
Hemoglobin A_{1c}	0%-5% of total
Hemoglobin A_2 by column	2%-3% of total
Hemoglobin, fetal	<1% of total
Hemoglobin, plasma	0%-5% of total
Hemoglobin, serum	2-3 mg/dl
Iron, serum	
Female	65-165 μg/dl
Male	75-175 μg/dl
Iron-binding capacity, total serum (TIBC)	250-450 μg/dl
Iron turnover rate (plasma)	20-42 mg/24 h
Leukocyte alkaline phosphatase (LAP) score	30-150
Methemoglobin	<1.8%
Reticulocytes	
(see Complete Blood Count Table)	
Schilling test (urinary excretion of radiolabeled vitamin B_{12} after "flushing" intramuscular injection of B_{12})	6%-30% of oral dose within 24 h
Sedimentation rate	
Wintrobe	0-15 mm/h
Female	0-5 mm/h
Male	
Westergren	0-20 mm/h
Female	0-15 mm/h
Male	20%-50%
Transferrin saturation, serum	
Volume	
Blood	50-75 ml/kg
Female	52-83 ml/kg
Male	
Plasma	28-45 ml/kg
Female	25-43 ml/kg
Male	
Red cell	19-31 ml/kg
Female	20-36 ml/kg
Male	

COAGULATION NORMAL VALUES

Template bleeding time	3.5-7.5 min
Clot retraction, qualitative	Apparent in 30-60 min; complete in 24 h, usually in 6 h
Coagulation time (Lee-White)	
Glass tubes	5-15 min
Siliconized tubes	20-60 min
Euglobulin lysis time	120-240 min
Factors II, V, VII, VIII, IX, X, XI, or XII	100% or 1.0 unit/ml
Fibrin degradation products	<10 μg/ml or titer ≤1.4
Fibrinogen	200-400 mg/ml
Partial thromboplastin time, activated	20-40 seconds
Prothrombin time (PT)	11-14 seconds
Thrombin time	10-15 seconds
Whole blood clot lysis time	>24 h

COMPLETE BLOOD COUNT

Parameter	*Male*	*Female*
Hematocrit	40%-52%	38%-48%
Hemoglobin (g/dl)	13.5-18.0	12-16
Erythrocyte count ($\times 10^{12}$ cells/L)	4.6-6.2	4.2-5.4
Reticulocyte count	0.6%-2.6%	0.4%-2.4%
MCV (fL)	82-98	82-98
MCH (pg)	27-32	27-32
MCHC (g/dl)	32-36	32-36
WBC ($\times 10^9$ cells/L)	4.5-11.0	4.5-11.0
Segmented neutrophils	1.8-7.7	1.8-7.7
Average	40%-60%	40%-60%
Bands (cells)	0-0.3	0-0.3
Average	0-3%	0-3%
Eosinophils (cells $\times 10^9$/L)	0-0.5	0-0.5
Average	0-5%	0-5%
Basophils (cells $\times 10^9$/L)	0-0.2	0-0.2
Average	0-1%	0-1%
Lymphocytes (cells $\times 10^9$/L)	1.0-4.8	1.0-4.8
Average	20%-45%	20%-45%
Monocytes (cells $\times 10^9$/L)	0-0.8	0-0.8
Average	2%-6%	2%-6%
Platelet count (cells $\times 10^9$/L)	150-350	150-350

DIFFERENTIAL CELL COUNT OF BONE MARROW

Myeloid cells	
Neutrophilic series	
Myeloblasts	0.3%-5.0%
Promyelocytes	1%-8%
Myelocytes	5%-19%
Metamyelocytes	9%-24%
Bands	9%-15%
Segmented cells	7%-30%
Eosinophil precursors	0.5%-3.0%
Eosinophils	0.5%-4.0%
Basophilic series	0.2%-0.7%
Erythroid cells	
Pronormoblasts	1%-8%
Basophilic normoblasts	
Polychromatophilic normoblasts	7%-32%
Orthochromatic normoblasts	
Megakaryocytes	0.1%
Lymphoreticular cells	
Lymphocytes	3%-17%
Plasma cells	0-2%
Reticulum cells	0.1%-2.0%
Monocytes	0.5%-5.0%
Myeloid/erythroid ratio	0.6-2.7

PULMONARY FUNCTION TESTS

ALVEOLAR-ARTERIAL OXYGEN GRADIENT ($FIO_2 = 0.21$)

P(A-a) in adolescents = <10 mm Hg
in adults <40 years = 10 mm Hg
in adults >40 years = 10-15 mm Hg

ALVEOLAR OXYGEN PARTIAL PRESSURE (SEA LEVEL, $FIO_2 = 0.21$)

$PAO_2 = 150 - (1.2 \times PaCO_2)$

BLOOD GASES ($FIO_2 = 0.21$)

	Arterial	Alveolar
PO_2	80-105 mm Hg	90-115 mm Hg
PCO_2	38-44 mm Hg	38-44 mm Hg
pH	7.35-7.45	

LUNG VOLUMES AND SPIROMETRIC VOLUMES*

	Male	Female
Lung volumes		
Total lung capacity (TLC)	6-7 L	5-6 L
Functional residual capacity (FRC)	2-3 L	2-3 L
Residual values (RV)	1-2 L	1-2 L
Measures of air flow		
Forced vital capacity (FVC)	4.0 L	3.0 L
1 sec forced vital capacity (FEV_1)	>3.0 L	>2.0 L
Pulmonary resistance (RL)	<3.0 cm H_2O/sec/L	
Airway resistance (Raw)	<2.5 cm H_2O/sec/L	
Other		
Pulmonary compliance (CL)	0.2 L/cm H_2O	
Diffusing capacity (DLCO)	25 ml CO/min/mm Hg	

*Lung volumes and spirometric volumes are size-dependent. Typical normal values for adults are provided.
PB, Arometric pressure (mm Hg)
FIO_2, inspired oxygen fraction (0.21 = room air)
$PaCO_2$, partial pressure of carbon dioxide in arterial blood (mm Hg)
$PACO_2$, partial pressure of carbon dioxide in alveolar gas (mm Hg)
PaO_2, partial pressure of oxygen in arterial blood (mm Hg)
PAO_2, partial pressure of oxygen in alveolar gas (mm Hg)

RENAL FUNCTION TESTS

ANION GAP

$Na^+ - HCO_3^- + Cl^- = 12 \pm 2$ mEq/L

BICARBONATE DEFICIT

HCO_3^- deficit = [body weight (kg)] $\times$ [0.4 (desired HCO_3^- − observed HCO_3^-)]
Glomerular filtration rate

$$GFR = \frac{Ucr \times V}{Pcr}$$
$$= 130 \pm 20 \text{ ml/min in males}$$
$$= 120 \pm 15 \text{ ml/min in females}$$
$$\cong \frac{Ucr}{Pcr} \times 70$$

OSMOLALITY

$$\text{Osmolality (serum)} = 2\,\text{Na (mEq/L)} + \frac{\text{BUN (mg/dl)}}{2.8} + \frac{\text{glucose (mg/dl)}}{18}$$

RENAL PLASMA FLOW

$$RPF = \frac{Upah \times V}{Ppah}$$
$$= 700 \pm 130 \text{ ml/min in males}$$
$$= 600 \pm 100 \text{ ml/min in females}$$

Pcr, Plasma creatinine (mg/dl)
Ppah, plasma para-aminohippuric acid (mg/dl)
Ucr, urine creatinine (mg/dl)
Upah, urine para-aminohippuric acid (mg/dl)
V, urine volume/24 h (ml/min)

SEMEN NORMAL VALUES

Liquifaction	Complete in 15 min
Morphology	>50% normal forms
Motility	>75% motile forms
pH	7.2-8.0
Spermatocrit	10%
Spermatocyte count	>50 million/ml
Volume	2.0-6.6 ml

SERUM NORMAL VALUES

Acetoacetate	0.3-2.0 mg/dl
Acid phosphatase	0-0.8 U/ml
Acid phosphatase, prostatic	2.5-12.0 IU/L
Albumin	3.0-5.5 g/dl
Aldolase	1-6 IU/L
Alkaline phosphatase	
15-20 years	40-200 IU/L
20-101 years	35-125 IU/L
Alpha-1 antitrypsin	200-500 mg/dl
ALT	0-40 IU/L
Ammonia	11-35 µmol/L
Amylase, serum	2-20 U/L
Anion gap	8-12 mEq/L (mmol/L)
Ascorbic acid	0.4-1.5 mg/dl
AST	5-40 IU/L
Bilirubin	
Total	0.2-1.2 mg/dl
Direct	0-0.4 mg/dl
Calcium, serum	8.7-10.6 mg/dl
Carbon dioxide, total	18-30 mEq/L (mmol/L)
Carcinoembryonic antigen, serum	<2.5 µg/L
Carotene (carotenoids)	50-300 µg/dl
C3 complement	55-120 mg/dl
C4 complement	14-51 mg/dl
Ceruloplasmin	15-60 mg/dl
Chloride, serum	95-105 mEq/L (mmol/L)
Cholesterol, total	
12-19 years	120-230 mg/dl
20-29 years	120-240 mg/dl
30-39 years	140-270 mg/dl
40-49 years	150-310 mg/dl
50-59 years	160-330 mg/dl
Copper	100-200 µg/dl
Creatinine kinase, total	20-200 IU/L
Creatine kinase, isoenzymes	
MM fraction	94%-95%
MB fraction	0-5%
BB fraction	0-2%
Normal values in	
Heart	80% MM, 20% MB
Brain	100% BB
Skeletal muscle	95% MM, 2% MB
Creatinine, serum	
Female adult	0.5-1.3 mg/dl
Male adult	0.7-1.5 mg/dl
Delta-aminolevulinic acid (ALA)	<200 µg/dl
α-Fetoprotein, serum	<40 µg/L
Folate, serum	1.9-14.0 ng/ml
Gamma glutamyl transpeptidase	
Female	9-31 IU/L
Male	12-38 IU/L
Gastrin	150 pg/ml
Glucose, serum (fasting)	70-115 mg/dl
Glucose-6-phosphate dehydrogenase	5-10 IU/g Hb
G6PD screen, qualitative	Negative
Haptoglobin	100-300 mg/dl
Hemoglobin A_2	0-4% of total Hb
Hemoglobin F	0-2% of total Hb
Immunoglobulin, quantitation	
IgG	700-1500 mg/dl
IaA	70-400 mg/dl
IgM	
Female	30-300 mg/dl
Male	30-250 mg/dl
IgD	0-40 mg/dl
Insulin, fasting	6-20 µU/ml
Iron-binding capacity	250-400 µg/dl
Iron, total, serum	40-150 µg/dl
Lactic acid	0.6-1.8 mEq/L
LDH, serum	20-220 IU/L
LDH isoenzymes	
LDH_1	20%-34%
LDH_2	28%-41%
LDH_3	15%-25%
LDH_4	3%-12%
LDH_5	6%-15%
Leucine aminopeptidase (LAP)	30-55 IU/L
Lipase	4-24 IU/dl
Magnesium, serum	1.5-2.5 mEq/L
5′-Nucleotidase	0.3-3.2 Bodansky units
Osmolality, serum	278-305 mOsm/kg serum water
Phenylalanine	3 mg/dl
Phosphorus, inorganic, serum	2.0-4.3 mg/dl
Potassium, plasma	3.1-4.3 mEq/L
Potassium, serum	3.5-5.2 mEq/L
Protein, total, serum	
2-55 years	5.0-8.0 g/dl
55-101 years	6.0-8.3 g/dl
Protein electrophoresis, serum	
Albumin	3.2-5.2 g/dl
Alpha-1	0.6-1.0 g/dl
Alpha-2	0.6-1.0 g/dl
Beta	0.6-1.2 g/dl
Gamma	0.7-1.5 g/dl
Sodium, serum	135-145 mEq/L
Sulfate	0.5-1.5 mg/dl
T_3 uptake	25%-45%
T_4	4-11 µg/dl
Triglycerides	
2-29 years	10-140 mg/dl
30-39 years	20-150 mg/dl
40-49 years	20-160 mg/dl
50-59 years	20-190 mg/dl
60-101 years	20-200 mg/dl
Urea nitrogen, serum	
2-65 years	5-22 mg/dl
Female	8-26 mg/dl
Male	10-38 mg/dl
Uric acid	
10-59 years	
Female	2.0-8.0 mg/dl
Male	2.5-9.0 mg/dl
60-101 years	
Female	2.5-9.0 mg/dl
Male	2.5-9.0 mg/dl
Viscosity	1.4-1.8 (serum compared to H_2O)
Vitamin A	0.15-0.60 µg/ml
Vitamin B_{12}	200-850 pg/ml

STOOL NORMAL VALUES

Bulk	
Wet weight	<197 g/24 h
Dry weight	<66.4 g/24 h
Coproporphyrin	12-832 mg/24 h
Fat	<7.2 g/24 h
Nitrogen	<2.2 g/24 h
Urobilinogen	40-280 mg/24 h
Water	Approximately 65%

SYNOVIAL FLUID NORMAL VALUES

Cells	<200 cells/mm^3
Polymorphonuclear cells	<25%
Crystals	None
Fibrin clot	None
Glucose	Same as serum
Hyaluronic acid	2.45-3.97 g/L
pH	7.31-7.64
Protein	<2.5 g/dl
Albumin	63%
α_1-Globulins	7%
α_2-Globulins	7%
β-Globulins	9%
γ-Globulins	14%
Relative viscosity	High
Uric acid	Same as serum

URINE NORMAL VALUES

Acidity, titratable	20-40 mEq/24 h
Ammonia	30-50 mEq/24 h
Amylase	35-260 Somogyi units/h
Bence Jones protein	None detected
Bilirubin	None detected
Calcium	
Unrestricted diet	
Female	<250 mg/24 h
Male	<300 mg/24 h
Low-calcium diet (200 mg/day for 3 days)	<150 mg/24h
Chloride	120-240 mEq/24 h (varies with dietary intake)
Copper	0-32 μg/24 h
Creatine	
Female	0-100 mg/24 h
Male	0-40 mg/24 h
Creatinine	1.0-1.6 g/24 h or 15-25 mg/kg body weight/24 h
Cysteine, qualitative	Negative
Delta-aminolevulinic acid	1.3-7.0 mg/24 h
Glucose	
Qualitative	None detected
Quantitative	16-300 mg/24 h
Hemoglobin	None detected
Homogentistic acid	None detected
Iron	40-140 μg/24 h
Lead	0-120 μg/24 h
Myoglobin	None detected
Osmolality	50-1200 mOsm/L
pH	4.6-8.0
Phenylpyruvic acid, qualitative	None detected
Phosphorus	0.8-2.0 g/24 h
Porphobilinogen	
Qualitative	None detected
Quantitative	0-2.4 mg/24 h
Porphyrins	
Coproporphyrin	50-250 μg/24 h
Uroporphyrin	10-30 μg/24 h
Potassium	25-100 mEq/24h
Protein	
Qualitative	None detected
Quantitative	10-150 mg/24 h
Sodium	130-260 mEq/24 h (varies with dietary sodium intake)
Specific gravity	1.003-1.030
Uric acid	80-976 mg/24 h
Urobilinogen	0.05-3.5 mg/24 h <1.0 Ehrlich units/2 h

APPENDIX C—SUPPLIER PROFILES

3M Pharms
3M Pharmaceuticals Inc.
Bldg. 275-3W-01 3M Center
St. Paul, MN 55144-1000
651-733-1110 • 800-423-5146
FAX: 651-733-3451
http://www.3m.com/market/healthcare/pharm/index.html

Abbott
Abbott Laboratories
100 Abbott Park Road
Abbott Park, IL 60064-3500
847-937-6100 • 800-633-9110
FAX: 847-937-1511
http://www.rxabbott.com/

Able Labs
Able Laboratories, Inc.
6 Hollywood Court
South Plainfield, NJ 07080
908-754-2253
http://www.ablelabs.com/

Agis/Clay Park Group
Clay Park Laboratories, Inc.
1700 Bathgate Avenue
Bronx, NY 10457
718-960-0100
http://www.claypark.com/

AH Robins *See Wyeth*

Akorn
Akorn, Inc.
2500 Millbrook Drive
Buffalo Grove, IL 60089-4694
800-535-7155
FAX: 800-943-3694
http://www.akorn.com

Alcon
Alcon Laboratories, Inc.
6201 South Freeway
Fort Worth, TX 76134-2001
817-293-0450 • 800-451-3937
FAX: 817-551-4630
http://www.alconlabs.com/us/

Allergan
Allergan Inc.
P.O. Box 19534
Irvine, CA 92623-9534
714-246-4500 • 800-347-4500
FAX: 714-246-4971
http://www.allergan.com/

Alliance Pharm
Alliance Pharmaceutical Corp.
6175 Lusk Blvd.
San Diego, CA 92121
858-410-5200 • *FAX:* 858-410-5161
http://www.allp.com

Alpha Therapeutic
Alpha Therapeutic Corp.
2410 Lillyvale Avenue
Los Angeles, CA 90032-3514
323-225-2221
http://www.alphather.com/

Alpharma
Alpharma Inc.
One Executive Drive
Fort Lee, NJ 07024
201-947-7774 • 800-645-4216
http://www.alpharmauspd.com

Alra Labs
Alra Laboratories, Inc.
3850 Clearview Court
Gurnee, IL 60031-0124
847-244-9440

Altaire Pharm
Altaire Pharmaceuticals Inc.
25 Andrea Rd.
Holbrook, NY 11741-4310
631-472-6114

Altana, Inc.
60 Baylis Road
Melville, NY 11747-3816
516-454-7677
http://www.altana.com

Alza
Alza Corporation
1900 Charleston Road
P.O. Box 7210
Mountain View, CA 94039-7210
650-564-5000 • *FAX:* 650-564-7070
http://www.alza.com/

American Home Prod *See Wyeth*

Amersham
Amersham Health
101 Carnegie Center
Princeton, NJ 08540-6231
609-514-6000
http://www.amershamhealth-us.com/

Amgen
Amgen, Inc.
One Amgen Center Drive
Thousand Oaks, CA 91320-1799
805-447-1000 • *FAX:* 805-447-1010
http://www.amgen.com

Amide Pharm
Amide Pharmaceuticals, Inc.
101 East Main Street
Little Falls, NJ 07424
973-890-1440 • *FAX:* 973-890-7980
http://www.amide.com/

Andrx Pharmaceuticals
4955 Orange Drive
Davie, FL 33314
954-584-0300
http://www.andrx.com/

Angiodynamics *See E Z Em*

Apotex
Apotex Inc.
2400 North Commerce Parkway, Suite 400
Weston, FL 33326
800-706-5575
http://www.apotexcorp.com/

Apothecon *See Bristol-Myers Squibb*

Arcola
Arcola Laboratories
500 Arcola
Collegeville, PA 19426-0107
800-727-6737

Ardent
Ardent Pharmaceuticals, Inc.
631 United Drive, Suite 200
Durham, NC 27713
919-806-1806 • *FAX:* 919-806-1161
http://www.ardentpharma.com/

Ares-Serono *See Serono*

Astra Zeneca
1800 Concord Pike
Wilmington, DE 19850-5437
302-886-3000 • *FAX:* 302-886-2972
http://www.astrazeneca-us.com

Athena Neurologicals *See Abbott*

Athena Neurosciences *See Abbott*

Aventis Pharmaceuticals
300 Somerset Corporate Boulevard
Bridgewater, NJ 08807-2854
800-981-2491
http://www.aventispharma-us.com/

Axcan Pharma
Axcan Scandipharm Inc.
22 Inverness Center Parkway
Birmingham, AL 35242
800-472-2634 • *FAX:* 205-991-8426
http://www.axcanscandipharm.com/

Bajamar Chem
Bajamar Chemical Co., Inc.
9609 Dielman Rock Island
St. Louis , MO 63132
888-242-3414 • *FAX:* 314-997-2948
http://walden.mvp.net/~bmizes/bcc/BAJAMAR.htm

Baker Cummins *See Baker Norton Pharms*

Baker Cummins Derm
Baker Cummins Dermatologicals, Inc.
8800 N.W. 36th Street
Miami, FL 33178
305-590-2200
FAX: 305-770-5035

Baker Norton Pharms
Baker Norton Pharmaceuticals, Inc.
4400 Biscayne Blvd.
Miami, FL 33137
305-590-2200 • 800-347-4774
FAX: 305-590-2252

Banner Pharmacaps
4125 Premier Drive
High Point, NC 27265
336-812-8700 • 800-447-1140
FAX: 336-812-8777
http://www.banpharm.com/

Barr
Barr Laboratories, Inc.
2 Quaker Rd.
Pomona, NY 10970
845-362-1100 • 800-222-0190
FAX: 845-362-2774
http://www.barrlabs.com/home.html

Basel *See Novartis*

Bayer
Bayer Corp Pharmaceutical Div
400 Morgan Lane
West Haven, CT 06516
203-812-2000 • 800-468-0894
http://www.bayerpharma-na.com/

Baxter
Baxter Healthcare Corporation
One Baxter Parkway
Deerfield, IL 60015
847-948-2000
http://www.baxter.com/

Beach Pharms
Beach Products, Inc.
5220 S. Manhattan Ave.
Tampa, FL 33611
813-839-6565 • *FAX:* 813-837-2511

Bedford Laboratories *See Boehringer Pharms*

Ben Venue Laboratories *See Boehringer Pharms*

Berlex
Berlex Laboratories, Inc.
340 Changebridge Road
Montville, NJ 07045-1000
937-487-2000
http://www.berlex.com/

Bertek *See Mylan*

Beta Derma
Beta Dermaceuticals, Inc.
P.O. Box 691106
San Antonio, TX 78269-1106
210-349-9326 • 800-434-2382
FAX: 210-349-9363
http://www.beta-derm.com/

Bio-Tech Pharm
Bio-Tech Pharmacal, Inc.
P.O. Box 1992
Fayetteville, AR 72702
479-443-9148 • 800-345-1199
FAX: 479-443-5643
http://www.bio-tech-pharm.com/

Biogen
Biogen Inc.
14 Cambridge Center
Cambridge, MA 02142
617-679-2000 • *FAX:* 617-679-2617
http://www.biogen.com/

Bioglan
Bioglan Pharmaceuticals Company
7 Great Valley Parkway, Suite 301
Malvern, PA 19355
http://www.bioglan.com

Bioport Corp
Bioport Corporation
3500 N Martin Luther King Jr. Blvd.
Lansing, MI 48906
http://www.bioport.com/

Biovail
Biovail Corporation
7150 Mississauga Road
Mississauga, Ontario L5N 8M5
905-286-3000 • *FAX:* 905-286-3050
http://www.biovail.com/

Blansett Pharma
Blansett Pharmacal Co. Inc.
3304 Pike Avenue
North Little Rock, AR 72118
501-758-8635
http://www.blansett.com/

Block Drug *See GlaxoSmithKline*

Boehringer Pharms
Boehringer Ingelheim Pharmaceuticals, Inc.
900 Ridgebury Road
P.O. Box 368
Ridgefield, CT 06877-0368
203-798-9988 • *FAX:* 203-791-6234
http://www.boehringer-ingelheim.com

Bone Care International
Bone Care Center
1600 Aspen Commons
Middleton, WI 53562
http://www.bonecare.com/

Boyle Pharm
Boyle & Company Pharmaceuticals
1613 Chelsea Road, Suite 313
San Marino, CA 91108
626-441-0284

Bracco DXS
Bracco Diagnostics, Inc.
107 College Road East
Princeton, NJ 08540
609-514-2200 • 800-631-5245
FAX: 609-514-2425
http://www.bracco.com/

Bradley Pharms
Bradley Pharmaceuticals, Inc.
383 Route 46 West
Fairfield, NJ 07004
973-882-1505 • 800-929-9300
FAX: 973-575-5366
http://www.bradpharm.com/

Braintree
Braintree Laboratories Inc.
P.O. Box 850929
Braintree, MA 02185-0929
781-843-2202 • 800-874-6756
FAX: 781-843-7932
http://www.braintreelabs.com/

Breckenridge
Breckenridge Pharmaceutical Inc.
1515 N Federal Highway
Boca Raton, FL 33432-0191
561-367-8512

Bristol-Myers Squibb
Bristol Myers Squibb Co.
345 Park Avenue
New York, NY 10154-0037
212-546-4000 • 800-631-5244
FAX: 212-546-4020
http://www.bms.com

BTG Pharms
Bio-Technology General Corp.
One Tower Center
Fourteenth Floor
East Brunswick, NJ 08816
732-418-9300 • *FAX:* 732-418-0766
http://www.btgc.com/

C & M Pharm *See Genesis*

Camall
Camall Company, Inc.
70945 Van Dyke Road
Romeo, MI 48065-0444
810-752-9683

Caraco Pharm
Caraco Pharmaceutical Laboratories, Ltd.
1150 Elijah McCoy Drive
Detroit, MI 48202
313-871-8400 • *FAX:* 313-871-8314
http://www.caraco.com/

Cardinal Health
Cardinal Health Pharmaceutical Technologies and Services
645 Martinsville Road, Suite 200
Basking Ridge, NJ 07920
908-580-1500 • *FAX:* 908-580-9208
http://www.cardinal.com/

Carnrick Labs *See Abbott*

Carolina Med
Carolina Medical Products
P.O. Box 147
Farmville, NC 27828
252-753-7111 • *FAX:* 252-753-3882

Carter-Wallace *See MedPointe*

Catalytica *See DSM*

Celgene
Celgene Corp
7 Powder Horn Drive
Warren, NJ 07059
732-271-1001
http://www.celgene.com/

Celltech
Celltech Pharmaceuticals, Inc.
755 Jefferson Road
Rochester, NY 14623
585-475-9000 • 800-234-5535
FAX: 585-475-1016
http://www.medeva.co.uk/

CenterPharm
3620 Park Central Blvd. N
Pompano Beach, FL 33064

Centocor *See Johnson & Johnson*

Century Pharms
Century Pharmaceuticals
10377 Hague Road
Indianapolis, IN 46256
317-849-4210

Chemrich Labs
Chemrich Laboratories
5211 Telegraph Rd.
Los Angeles, CA 90022
323-262-9144 • *FAX:* 323-262-7258

ChiRhoClin
ChiRhoClin, Inc.
4000 Blackburn Lane, Suite 270
Burtonsville, MD 20866
301-476-8388 • *FAX:* 301-476-9529
http://www.chirhoclin.com/

Chiron Thera
CHIRON Therapeutics
4560 Horton Street
Emeryville, CA 94608-2916
510-655-8730 • *FAX:* 510-655-9910
http://www.chiron.com/

Ciba Vision *See Novartis*

Circa Pharmaceuticals *See Watson Labs*

CIS
CIS-US, Inc.
10 DeAnglo Drive
Bedford, MA 01730
781-275-7120 • 800-221-7554
FAX: 781-275-2634
http://www.cisusinc.com/

Colgate Oral
Colgate Oral Pharmaceuticals
One Colgate Way
Canton, MA 02021
781-821-2880 • 800-821-2880
http://www.colgateprofessional.com/

Connetics
Connetics Corporation
3290 West Bayshore Road
Palo Alto, CA 94303
650-843-2800 • 888-969-2628
FAX: 650-843-2899
http://www.connetics.com/

Consolidated Midland
Consolidated Midland Corp.
20 Main St.
Brewster, NY 10509
914-279-6108

Contract Pharma
Contract Pharmacal Corp.
135 Adams Avenue
Hauppauge, NY 11788
631-231-4610 • *FAX:* 631-231-4156
http://www.contractpharmacal.com/home.html

Convatec *See Bristol-Myers Squibb*

Cook-Waite Labs
Cook-Waite Laboratories
90 Park Avenue
New York, NY 10016
212-907-2712

Copley Pharmaceuticals *See Teva*

Crown Labs
Crown Laboratories, Inc.
PO Box 1425
Johnson City, TN 37605
423-929-4413 • 800-877-8869
FAX: 423-926-0165
http://www.crownlaboratories.com/

Ctr Labs
Center Laboratories
35 Channel Drive
Port Washington, NY 11050
516-767-1800 • *FAX:* 516-767-4229

Cypress Pharm
Cypress Pharmaceutical, Inc.
135 Industrial Blvd.
Madison, MS 39110
800-856-4393 • *FAX:* 601-853-1567
http://www.cypressrx.com/

Danbury Pharm
Danbury Pharmacal
P.O. Box 296
Danbury, CT 06813
203-744-7200 • 800-553-4044
FAX: 914-225-1763

Dayton Labs
Dayton Laboratories Inc.
3307 NW 74th Avenue
Miami, FL 33172
305-594-0988 • 800-446-0255

Del Ray Dermatologicals *See Crown Labs*

Del Ray Lab
Del Ray Laboratories, Inc.
22 20th Avenue Northwest
Birmingham, AL 35215
205-853-8247
FAX: 205-853-8257

Delta Pharma *See Ardent*

Denison Pharms
Denison Pharmaceuticals, Inc.
60 Dunnell Lane
Pawtucket, RI 02862
401-723-5500

DepoTech Corp.
10450 Science Center Drive
San Diego, CA 92121-0111
858-625-2424

Dey Laboratories *See Merck*

Diatide, Inc. *See Berlex*

Dista *See Lilly*

Doak Dermatologics *See Bradley Pharms*

Dow Hickman *See Mylan*

DSM
DSM Pharmaceuticals, Inc.
5900 NW Greenville Blvd.
Greenville, NC 27834
252-707-2307
http://www5.dsm.com/en_US/html/dpi/home_dpi.htm

DuPont Merck
DuPont Merck Pharma
331 Treble Cove Road
Billerica, MA 01821
978-667-9531

Dunhall Pharms
Dunhill Pharmaceuticals, Inc.
1060 1st Avenue NE
Gravette, AR 72736-0965
501-787-5232

DuPont Pharma
DuPont Pharma
Chestnut Run Plaza
974 Centre Road
Wilmington, DE 19805
302-992-5000 • 800-441-9861
FAX: 302-995-0671

DuPont Radiopharms
DuPont Radiopharmaceutical Division
331 Treble Cove Road
North Billerica, MA 01862
978-667-9531
http://www.radiopharm.com

Dura *See Elan*

Duramed Pharms
Duramed Pharmaceuticals, Inc.
5040 Duramed Drive
Cincinnati, OH 45213
513-731-9900 • 800-543-8338
FAX: 513-731-5270
http://www.duramed.com

Durham Pharmacal *See Stiefel Labs*

DUSA Pharmaceuticals
181 University Avenue, Suite 1208
Toronto, Ontario M5H 3M7
416-363-5059
http://www.dusapharma.com/

E Z Em
E Z EM Co., Inc.
717 Main Street
Westbury, NY 11590
516-333-8230 • 800-544-4624
FAX: 516-333-8278
http://www.ezem.com/firstpage.htm

Effcon Labs
Effcon Laboratories Inc.
1800 Sandy Plains Parkway
Marietta, GA 30065
770-428-7011 • *FAX:* 770-428-6811
http://www.effcon.com/

Elan
Elan Pharmaceuticals, Inc.
One Research Way
Princeton, NJ 08540
609-580-3300 • *FAX:* 609-520-8250
http://www.elan.com/

Elge
Elge, Inc.
1000 Cole
Rosenberg, TX 77471
281-232-0463 • *FAX:* 281-232-0476
http://www.elgeinc.com/

Encysive
Encysive Pharmaceuticals
6700 West Loop, 4th Floor
Bellaire, TX 77401
713-796-8822 • *FAX:* 713-796-8232
http://www.encysive.com/

Endo Pharms
Endo Pharmaceuticals
100 Painters Drive
Chadds Ford, PA 19317
610-558-9800 • *FAX:* 610-558-8979
http://www.endo.com/

Enteric Products *See E Z Em*

Eon Labs Mfg
Eon Labs Manufacturing, Inc.
227-15 North Conduit Avenue
Laurelton, NY 11413
800-526-0225 • *FAX:* 718-949-3120

Erbamont *See Pfizer*

Everett Labs
Everett Laboratories, Inc.
29 Spring Street
West Orange, NJ 07052
973-324-0200 • *FAX:* 973-324-0795
http://www.everettlabs.com/

Family Pharm
Family Pharmacy
P.O. Box 1027
Southeastern, PA 19398-1027
800-333-7347 • *FAX:* 614-261-7360

Faulding Pharm
Faulding Pharmaceutical Co.
650 From Road, Mack-Cali Centre II, 2nd Floor
Paramus, NJ 07652
201-225-5500 • *FAX:* 201-225-5515
http://www.maynepharma.com/us/index.html

Ferndale Labs
Ferndale Laboratories, Inc.
780 West Eight Mile Road
Ferndale, MI 48220
248-548-0900 • *FAX:* 248-548-8427
http://www.ferndalelabs.com/

Ferring
Ferring Pharmaceuticals Inc.
120 White Plains Road, Suite 400
Tarrytown, NY 10591
914-333-8900 • *FAX:* 914-631-1992
http://www.ferring.com/

Fleming
Fleming and Co.
1733 Gilsinn Lane
Fenton, MO 63026
636-343-5306
FAX: 636-343-5322
http://www.flemingcompany.com

Forest Labs
Forest Laboratories, Inc.
909 Third Ave
New York, NY 10022
800-947-5227
FAX: 212-421-7850
http://www.frx.com/

Fresenius
Fresenius Medical Care North America
Two Ledgemont Center
95 Hayden Avenue
Lexington, MA 02173
781-402-9000 • *FAX:* 781-402-9004

Fujisawa Pharm (US)
Fujisawa Pharmaceutical Co.
3 Parkway North
Deerfield , IL 60015-2548
708-317-8800 • 800-888-7704
http://www.fujisawausa.com/

Galderma
Galderma Laboratories, Inc.
3000 Altamesa Blvd.
Fort Worth, TX 76163
817-263-2600
http://www.galdermausa.com/

Gate Pharmaceuticals *See Teva*

GelTex Pharmaceuticals
153 Second Ave.
Waltham, MA 02451
781-290-5888 • 800-510-5059
FAX: 781-290-5890
http://www.geltex.com/

GenDerm *See Medicis*

Genentech *See Roche*

Genesis
Genesis Pharmaceutical, Inc.
1721 Maplelane Ave.
Hazel Park, MI 48030
248-548-7846 • 800-459-8663
FAX: 248-548-0913
http://www.genesispharm.com/

Genetics Institute *See Wyeth*

Geneva *See Novartis*

Genzyme
Genzyme Corporation
One Kendall Square
Cambridge, MA 02139-1562
617-252-7500 • 800-868-8208
FAX: 617-252-7600
http://www.genzyme.com/

Geriatric Pharm
Geriatric Pharmaceuticals Corporation
16820 Ridgeview Drive
Brookfield, WI 53005-1333
414-272-2552

Gilead Sciences
Gilead Sciences, Inc.
333 Lakeside Drive
Foster City, CA 94404
650-574-3000 • 800-445-3235
FAX: 650-522-5283
http://www.gilead.com/wt/home

Glades Pharmaceuticals *See Stiefel Labs*

GlaxoSmithKline
GlaxoSmithKline
5 Moore Drive
P.O. Box 13398
Research Triangle Park, NC 27709
888-825-5249
http://us.gsk.com

Glenbrook Labs *See Sanofi-synthelabo*

Glenwood
Glenwood, LLC
111 Cedar Lane
Englewood, NJ 07631
201-569-0050 • 800-542-0772
FAX: 201-569-0250
http://www.glenwood-llc.com/

Global Pharm
Global Pharmaceutical Corporation
Castor and Kensington Avenues
Philadelphia, PA 19102
215-289-2220

GW Labs
G & W Laboratories
111 Coolidge Street
South Plainfield, NJ 07080
800-922-1038
http://www.gwlabs.com/

Gynetics *See Johnson & Johnson*

Halsey Drug
Halsey Drug Company
1800 Pacific Street
Brooklyn, NY 11233-0350
800-336-2750
http://www.halseydrug.com/

Hauser
5555 Airport Blvd.
Boulder, CO 80301
720-406-4607

Hawthorn Pharmaceuticals *See Cypress Pharm*

Healthpoint
Healthpoint, Ltd
3909 Hulen Street
Fort Worth, TX 76107
800-441-8227 • *FAX:* 817-900-4105
http://www.healthpoint.com/

Heran Pharm
Heran Pharmaceutical Inc.
7215 Eckhert Road
San Antonio, TX 78238-0124
210-680-2969

Hercon Labs
Hercon Laboratories Corp.
York, PA

Hi Tech Pharma
Hi Technology Pharmacal Co., Inc.
369 Bayview Avenue
Amityville, NY 11701
516-789-8228

Hill Dermac
Hill Dermaceuticals, Inc.
2650 S. Mellonville Ave.
Sanford, FL 32773
407-323-1887 • 800-344-5707

Hollister-Stier/Bayer *See Bayer*

Hope Pharms
Hope Pharmaceuticals Inc.
8260 E. Gelding Dr., Suite 104
Scottsdale, AZ 85260
480-607-1970 • 800-755-9595
FAX: 480-607-1971
http://www.hopepharm.com/home.html

Horizon Pharm
Horizon Pharmaceutical Corp.
11800 28th Street N
Saint Petersburg, FL 33716-0181
727-573-2404

Hyrex Pharms
Hyrex Pharmaceuticals
3494 Democrat Road
Memphis, TN 38118
901-794-9050
FAX: 901-794-9051

ICN Pharms
I.C.N. Pharmaceuticals, Inc.
3300 Hyland Avenue
Costa Mesa, CA 92626
714-545-0100 • *FAX:* 714-556-0131
http://www.icnpharm.com/

IDEC Pharm
IDEC Pharmaceuticals
3030 Callan Road
San Diego, CA 92121
858-431-8500
FAX: 858-431-8750
http://www.idecpharm.com

Immunex *See Amgen*

Immuno-US
Immuno-U.S., Inc.
1200 Parkdale Rd.
Rochester, MI 48307-0174
248-652-4760

Infinity Pharm
Infinity Pharmaceuticals
P.O. Box 939
Abita Spring, AL 70420

INO Therapeutics
54 Old Highway 22
Clinton, NJ 08809
877-KNOW-INO
http://www.inotherapeutics.com/

Integrity
5767 Thunderbird Road
Indianapolis, IN 46236-0286
317-823-6878

Interpharm
Interpharm Inc.
75 Adams Ave.
Hauppauge, NY 11788-0360
631-952-0214

Invamed
Invamed, Inc.
2400 Rt 130 North
Dayton, NJ 08810
732-274-2400

Ion
Ion Laboratories Inc.
7431 Pebble Dr.
Fort Worth, TX 76118-0694
817-589-7257

IPR
IPR Pharmaceuticals, Inc.
South Main Street
Carolina, PR 98419-1967
809-750-5353 • *FAX:* 809-750-5332

Jacobus Pharm
Jacobus Pharmaceutical Company
37 Cleveland Lane
Princeton, NJ 08540
609-921-7447

Janssen *See Johnson & Johnson*

Jerome Stevens
Jerome Stevens Pharmaceuticals, Inc.
60 DaVinci Drive
Bohemia , NY 11716
516-567-1113

Johnson & Johnson
Johnson & Johnson
One Johnson & Johnson Plaza
New Brunswick, NJ 08933
732-524-0400
http://www.johnsonandjohnson.com/home.html

Jones Medical *See King Pharms*

Jordan Pharms
Jordan Pharmaceuticals, Inc.
20612 Canada Road
Lake Forest, CA 92630
949-588-7711

Kenwood Labs *See Bradley Pharms*

Kenwood Therapeutics *See Bradley Pharms*

King Pharms
King Pharmaceuticals Inc.
501 Fifth Street
Bristol, TN 37620
423-989-8000 • 800-776-3637
http://www.kingpharm.com/

Kos Pharm
Kos Pharmaceuticals, Inc.
1001 Bricknell Bay Drive
25th Floor
Miami, FL 33131
305-577-3464
FAX: 305-577-4596
http://www.kospharm.com

KV Pharms
KV Pharmaceutical Co.
2503 S. Hanley Road
St. Louis, MO 63144
314-645-6600 • *FAX:* 314-645-6732
http://www.kvpharma.com/

Lafayette Pharms
Lafayette Pharmaceuticals Inc.
526 N. Earl Ave.
Lafayette, IN 47904-2819
765-447-3129 • 800-428-7843
FAX: 765-447-6913

Lannett
The Lannett Co., Inc.
9000 State Road
Philadelphia, PA 19136
215-333-9000 • 800-325-9994
FAX: 215-333-9004
http://www.lannett.com/

Laser
Laser, Inc.
2200 West 97th Place
Crown Point, IN 46307
219-663-1165

Lederle *See Wyeth*

Lemax
Lemax Pharmaceutical Corp.
6915 S. W. 92 Court
Miami , FL 33173
305-598-2333

Leo Pharma
Industriparken 55
DK-2750 Ballerup
45-44-92-38-00
http://www.leo-pharma.com/

Ligand Pharmaceuticals
10275 Science Center Drive
San Diego, CA 92121
858-550-7500 • *FAX:* 858-550-7506
http://www.ligand.com/

Lilly
Eli Lilly and Co.
Lilly Corporate Center
Indianapolis, IN 46285
317-276-2000 • 800-545-5979
FAX: 317-276-6331
http://www.lilly.com

Liposome Company *See Abbott*

Lyne Labs
Lyne Laboratories, Inc.
10 Burke Drive
Brockton, MA 02301-5505
800-525-0450 • *FAX:* 508-583-9120
http://www.lyne.com/

Mallinckrodt
Mallinckrodt Inc.
675 McDonnell Blvd.
St. Louis, MO 63134
314-654-2000
FAX: 314-654-4000
http://www.mallinckrodt.com/

Manufac Chems
Manufacturing Chemists
5767 Thunderbird Road
Indianapolis, IN 46236
317-823-6878

Marlop Pharms
Marlop Pharmaceuticals, Inc.
5704 Mosholu Avenue
Bronx, NY 10471-0221
718-796-1570 • 718-884-2494

Marsam
Marsam Pharmaceuticals Inc.
24 Olney Avenue
Cherry Hill, NJ 08003-0160
856-424-5600

Martec Pharms
Martec Pharmaceutical, Inc.
1800 North Topping Ave.
Kansas City, MO 64120
816-241-4144 • 800-822-6782
FAX: 816-483-5432
http://www.martec-kc.com/

Mayrand *See Merz Pharms*

McNeil Pharmaceuticals *See Johnson & Johnson*

Mead Johnson *See Bristol-Myers Squibb*

Med Derm Pharms *See Crown Labs*

Med Tek Pharms
Med Tek Pharmaceuticals
721 Chaney Cove
Collierville, TN 38017
901-853-5333 • *FAX:* 901-853-5339

Medcl Prods Labs
Medical Products Laboratories, Inc.
9990 Global Road
Philadelphia, PA 19115
215-677-2700 • 800-523-0191
FAX: 215-677-7736

Medcl Prods Panamerc
Medical Products Panamerica, Inc.
647 West Flagler Street
Miami, FL 33130
305-545-6524

Medco Lab
Medco Lab., Inc.
716 West 7th Street
Sioux City, IA 51102-0864
712-255-8770 • *FAX:* 712-255-4064
http://www.medcolab.com/

Medi Physics
Medi Physics, Inc. DBA Amersham Healthcare
3350 N Ridge Avenue
Arlington Heights, IL 60005
847-398-8400

The Medicines Company
8 Campus Drive
Parsippany, NJ 07054
973-656-1616
http://www.themedicinescompany.com/

Medicis
Medicis Pharmaceutical Corp.
8125 North Hayden Road
Scottsdale, AZ 85258-2463
602-808-8800 • 800-550-5115
FAX: 602-808-0822
http://www.medicis.com

Medimmune
MedImmune Inc.
35 West Watkins Mill Road
Gaithersburg, MD 20878
301-417-0770 • *FAX:* 301-417-6289
http://www.medimmune.com/

Medirex *See PLIVA*

MedPointe
MedPointe Pharmaceuticals
265 Davidson Ave., Suite 300
Somerset, NJ 08873-4120
732-564-2200
http://www.medpointeinc.com/

Medtronic
Medtronic Inc.
7000 Central Ave. N.E.
Minneapolis, MN 55432
612-514-4000 • *FAX:* 612-514-4879
http://www.medtronic.com/

Melville
Melville Biologics
155 Duryea Road
Melville ,NY 11741
516-752-8754

Merck
Merck and Company, Inc.
1 Merck Drive
Whitehouse Station, NJ 08889-0100
908-423-1000
http://www.merck.com/

Merck Sharp & Dohme *See Merck*

Merz Pharms
Merz Pharmaceuticals
P.O. Box 18806
Greensboro, NC 27419
888-637-9872 • *FAX:* 336-856-0107
http://www.merzusa.com/

Methapharm
2825 University Drive, Suite 240
Coral Springs, FL 33065
800-287-7686 • *FAX:* 877-718-9222
http://www.methapharm.com/

Meyer Laboratories *See GlaxoSmithKline*

MGI Pharma
MGI Pharma, Inc.
5775 West Old Shakopee Road, Suite 100
Bloomington, MN 55437-3174
952-346-4700 • *FAX:* 952-346-4800
http://www.mgipharma.com/

Mikart
Mikart, Inc.
1750 Chattahoochee Avenue
Atlanta, GA 30318
404-351-4510 • *FAX:* 404-350-0432
http://www.mikart.com

Miles *See Bayer*

Miles Spokane *See Bayer*

Miles/Schein *See Bayer*

Milex Prod
Milex Products, Inc.
4311 N. Normandy
Chicago, IL 60634
800-621-1278 • *FAX:* 800-972-0696
http://www.milexproducts.com

Mission Pharma
Mission Pharmacal Company
P.O. Box 786099
San Antonio, TX 78278-6099
210-696-8400 • *FAX:* 210-696-6010
http://www.missionpharmacal.com/

Monarch Pharmaceuticals *See King Pharms*

Muro Pharm
Muro Pharmaceutical, Inc.
890 East Street
Tewksbury, MA 01876-9987
978-851-5981 • *FAX:* 978-851-7346
http://www.muropharm.com/

Mutual Pharm *See URL Mutual*

MY-K Labs *See Rosemont*

Mylan
Mylan Laboratories
781 Chestnut Ridge Rd.
Morgantown, WV 26505
304-599-2595
http://www.mylan.com/

N Am Biologicals
NABI (North American Biologicals, Inc.)
5800 Park of Commerce Blvd. NW
P.O. Box 310701
Boca Raton, FL 33487
561-989-5800 • *FAX:* 561-989-5801
http://www.nabi.com/

Nastech
Nastech Pharmaceutical Company, Inc.
3450 Monte Villa Parkway
Bothell, WA 98021
425-908-3600 • *FAX:* 425-908-3650
http://www.nastech.com/

Nephron
Nephron Pharmaceuticals Corporation
4121 34th Street
Orlando, FL 32811-6458
407-246-1389 • 800-443-4313
FAX: 407-872-0001
http://www.nephronpharm.com/

Neurex *See Abbott*

NeXstar *See Gilead Sciences*

Nomax
Nomax, Inc.
40 North Rock Hill Road
St. Louis, MO 63119
314-961-2500 • *FAX:* 314-961-8923
http://www.nomax.com/

Novartis
Novartis Pharmaceutical Corp.
556 Morris Avenue
Summit, NJ 07901
908-277-5000
http://www.novartis.com

Novo Nordisk Pharm
Novo Nordisk Pharmaceutical Industries, Inc.
100 Overlook Center
Princeton, NJ 08540
800-727-6500
http://www.novo-nordisk.com

Novopharm *See Teva*

Nycomed
Nycomed, Inc.
Drammersveien 133
P.O. Box 614
Oslo, Norway N-0214
47-2328-2400 • *FAX:* 47-2328-2401
http://www.nycomed.com

Oclassen *See Watson Labs*

Ocumed
Ocumed, Inc.
119 Harrison Avenue
Roseland, NJ 07068-0121
973-226-2330

Ocusoft
Ocusoft Inc.
P.O. Box 429
Richmond, TX 77406-0429
800-233-5469 • *FAX:* 281-232-6015
http://www.ocusoft.com

Odyssey *See PLIVA*

OHM
Ohm Laboratories, Inc.
1385 Livingston Avenue
North Brunswick, NJ 08902-0182
732-418-2235

Organon
Organon Inc.
56 Livingston Avenue
Roseland, NJ 07068
FAX: 973-325-4589
http://www.organon.com/

Orion Pharma
554 Central Avenue
New Providence, NJ 07974
908-464-7500
http://www.orion.fi

Orphan Medcl
Orphan Medical, Inc.
13911 Ridgedale Drive, Suite 250
Minnetonka, MN 55305
888-867-7426
http://www.orphan.com/

Ortho-McNeil *See Johnson & Johnson*

Otsuka America Pharm
Otsuka America Pharmaceutical, Inc.
2440 Research Blvd.
Rockville, MD 20850
301-990-0030 • 800-562-3974
FAX: 301-212-8647
http://www.otsuka.com

Pacific *See Allergan*

Paddock Labs
Paddock Laboratories, Inc.
3940 Quebec Avenue North
Minneapolis, MN 55427
612-546-4676 • *FAX:* 612-546-4842
http://www.paddocklabs.com/

Par Pharm
PAR Pharmaceutical, Inc.
One Ram Ridge Road
Spring Valley, NY 10977-6714
800-828-9393
http://www.parpharm.com

Parkdale Pharmaceuticals *See King Pharms*

Parke-Davis *See Pfizer*

Parmed Pharms
Parmed Pharmaceuticals, Inc.
4220 Hyde Park Boulevard
Niagara Falls, NY 14305-0179
716-773-1113

Parnell Pharm
Parnell Pharmaceuticals, Inc.
P.O. Box 5130
Larkspur, CA 94977
415-256-1800 • 800-457-4276
FAX: 415-256-8099
http://www.parnellpharm.com/

Pecos
Pecos Pharmaceutical
25301 Cabot Rd 212-213
Laguna Hills, CA 92653
949-770-5431

Pedinol Pharma
Pedinol Pharmacal, Inc.
30 Banfi Plaza North
Farmingdale, NY 11735
631-293-9500 • 800-733-4665
FAX: 631-293-7359
http://www.pedinol.com/

Penederm *See Mylan*

Person and Covey
Person and Covey, Inc.
616 Allen Ave.
Glendale, CA 91221-5018
818-240-1030 • 800-423-2341
FAX: 818-547-9821
http://www.personandcovey.com/

PET Net
Pet Net Pharmaceuticals, Inc.
810 Innovation Drive
Knoxville, TN 37932-2571
877-473-8638
http://www.petnetpharmaceutical.com/

Pfeiffer Pharms
Pfeiffer Pharmaceuticals, Inc.
71 Univ Avenue SW
Atlanta, GA 30315-0220
404-614-0255

Pfizer Labs
Pfizer Laboratories Div Pfizer Inc.
235 East 42nd Street
New York, NY 10017
212-733-2323
http://www.pfizer.com

Pharma Tek
Pharma Tek, Inc.
PO Box 1148
Elmira, NY 14902
800-645-6655 • *FAX:* 607-732-4382
http://www.pharma-tek.com

Pharmaceutical *See Beach Pharms*

Pharmacia *See Pfizer*

Pharmacia & Upjohn *See Pfizer*

Pharmics
Pharmics, Inc.
P.O. Box 27554
Salt Lake City, UT 84127-0554
801-966-4138 • 800-456-4138
FAX: 801-966-4177
http://www.pharmics.com/

PLIVA
PLIVA, Inc.
72 Eagle Rock Ave.
East Hanover, NJ 07936
973-386-5566
http://www.plivainc.com/

Porton Prod *See Speywood Pharm*

Primedics
Primedics Laboratories
14131 Avalon Boulevard
Los Angeles, CA 90061-0263
323-770-3005

Prometheus Labs
Prometheus Laboratories, Inc.
5739 Pacific Center Blvd.
San Diego, CA 92121-4203
858-824-0895 • 888-423-5227
FAX: 858-824-0896
http://www.prometheus-labs.com/

Purdue Frederick *See Purdue Pharma*

Purdue Pharma
Purdue Pharma L.P.
201 Tresser Boulevard
Stamford, CT 06901-3431
203-588-8000 • *FAX:* 203-588-8850
http://www.purduepharma.com/

Quality Res Pharms
Quality Research Pharmaceuticals Inc.
1117 Third Ave Southwest
Carmel, IN 46032
317-846-9760

R/P Rorer Generics *See Aventis Pharmaceuticals*

Rare Disease
Rare Disease Therapeutics
1101 Kermit Drive, Suite 608
Nashville, TN 37217-2126
615-399-0700
FAX: 615-399-1217

Reed & Carnrick
Reed & Carnrick
257 Cornelison Avenue
Jersey City, NJ 07302
201-434-3000

Reese Chemical
Reese Chemical Co.
10617 Frank Ave.
Cleveland, OH 44106
216-231-6441

Roche
Hoffman-LaRoche, Inc.
340 Kingsland Street
Nutley, NJ 07110
973-235-5000
http://www.rocheusa.com

Rosemont
Rosemont Pharmaceutical Corporation
301 South Cherokee Street
Denver, CO 80223
303-733-7207

Roxane Laboratories *See Boehringer Pharms*

Royce *See Watson Labs*

Rugby *See Watson Labs*

Salix
Salix Pharmaceuticals, Inc.
8540 Colonnade Center Drive, Suite 501
Raleigh, NC 27615
888-802-9956 • *FAX:* 919-862-1095
http://www.salixltd.com/

Sanofi-Synthelabo
90 Park Avenue
New York, NY 10016
212-551-4000
http://www.sanofi-synthelabous.com/

Savage Laboratories *See Altana*

Scandipharm *See Axcan Pharma*

Schein Pharmaceuticals *See Bayer*

Scherer *See Cardinal Health*

Schering-Plough
2000 Galloping Hill Road
Kenilworth, NJ 07033-0530
908-298-4000
http://www.schering-plough.com/

Schwarz Pharma (US)
Schwarz Pharma, Inc.
P.O. Box 2038
Milwaukee, WI 53201
800-558-5114 • *FAX:* 262-238-0311
http://www.schwarzusa.com/

Scot Tussin
Scot Tussin Pharmacal Inc.
P.O. Box 8217
Cranston, RI 02920-0217
401-942-8555

SCS Pharm
SCS Pharmaceuticals
P.O. Box 5110
Chicago, IL 60680
708-982-7000 • 800-942-2566
FAX: 708-470-3851

Sepracor Pharmaceuticals
84 Waterford Drive
Marlborough, MA 01752
508-357-7300
http://www.sepracor.com/

Serono
Serono, Inc.
One Technology Place
Rockland, MA 02370
781-982-9000 • 800-283-8088
http://www.serono.com/

Shire Pharma
Shire Pharmaceuticals Group
One Riverfront Place
Newport, KY 41071
859-669-8000 • *FAX:* 859-669-8414
http://www.shire.com/

Sicor
19 Hughes
Irvine, CA 92618
800-729-9991 • *Fax:* 949-855-8210
http://www.gensiasicor.com

Sidmak Labs *See PLIVA*

Sigma-Tau
Sigma-Tau, Inc.
800 S. Frederick Avenue, Suite 300
Gaithersburg, MD 20877
301-948-1041 • 800-447-0169
http://www.sigmatau.com/

Silarx Pharms
Silarx Pharmaceuticals, Inc.
19 Harriet Tubman Way
Spring Valley, NY 10977
914-352-4020

Sirius
Sirius Laboratories
100 Fairway Dr., Suite 130
Vernon Hills, IL 60061
847-968-2424
FAX: 847-968-2484

SK Beecham *See GlaxoSmithKline*

SKB Pharms *See GlaxoSmithKline*

SmithKline Beecham *See GlaxoSmithKline*

Snowbrand Pharmaceuticals
12636 High Bluff Drive
Del Mar, CA 92014
415-677-0914

Somerset *See Mylan*

Speywood Pharm
Speywood Pharmaceuticals, Inc.
27 Maple Street
Milford, MA 01757
508-478-8900 • *FAX:* 508-478-1883

Stafford Miller
Stafford Miller International Co.
257 Cornelison St
Jersey City, NJ 07302
201-434-3000

Star Pharms FL
Star Pharmaceuticals, Inc.
1990 Northwest 44th St.
Pompano Beach, FL 33064
954-971-9704 • *FAX:* 954-971-7718
http://www.starpharm.com/

Steris Laboratories *See Bayer*

Sterling Winthrop *See Nycomed*

Sterling Winthrop Imaging *See Nycomed*

Stewart Jackson
Stewart Jackson Pharmacal, Inc.
4200 Lamar Ave. #103
Memphis, TN 38118
901-396-8285

Stiefel Labs
Stiefel Laboratories Inc.
255 Alhambra Circle
Coral Gables, FL 33134
888-784-3335
http://www.stiefel.com/

Storz Ophthalmics *See Wyeth*

Stratus Pharms
Stratus Pharmaceuticals Inc.
14377 SW 142nd St.
Miami, FL 33186
305-254-6793 • 800-442-7882
FAX: 305-254-6875
http://www.stratuspharmaceuticals.com/

Sugen *See Pfizer*

Superior
Superior Pharmaceutical Company
1385 Kemper Meadow Dr.
Cincinnati, OH 45240-1635
800-826-5035 • *FAX:* 800-255-8465
http://www.superiorpharm.com/

Syntex Labs
Syntex Laboratories, Inc.
3401 Hillview Avenue
Palo Alto, CA 94304
415-855-5050 • *FAX:* 415-852-1569

Syosset Labs
Syosset Laboratories, Inc.
150 Eileen Way
Syosset, NY 11791
516-921-6306 • *FAX:* 516-921-7971

Takeda-Abbott Pharm *See TAP Pharm*

TAP Pharm
TAP Pharmaceutical Products, Inc.
675 North Field Drive
Lake Forest, IL 60045
847-582-2000
http://www.tap.com/

Taro Pharms (US)
Taro Pharmaceuticals U.S.A. Inc.
5 Skyline Drive
Hawthorne, NY 10532
914-345-9001
http://www.tarousa.com/

Taylor Pharmacal *See Akorn*

Teva
Teva Pharmaceuticals USA, Inc.
1090 Horsham Road
North Wales, PA 19454-1090
215-591-3000
http://www.tevapharmusa.com/

Texas Biotechnology *See Encysive*

Thames Pharma
Thames Pharmacal Co., Inc.
2100 Fifth Ave.
Ronkonkoma, NY 11779
631-737-1155 • 800-225-1003
FAX: 631-737-3185

Therapex *See E Z Em*

UCB Pharma
UCB Pharma, Inc.
1950 Lake Park Drive
Smyrna, GA 30080
770-970-7500 • *FAX:* 770-970-8344
http://www.ucb.be/default.htm

Ucyclyd Pharma *See Medicis*

Upsher Smith
Upsher-Smith Laboratories, Inc.
13700 1st Ave. North
Minneapolis, MN 55441
800-654-2299
http://www.upsher-smith.com/

URL Mutual
United Research Laboratories and Mutual Pharmaceutical Company
1100 Orthodox Street
Philadelphia, PA 19124
800-523-3684 • *FAX:* 215-288-6559
http://www.urlmutual.com/

U.S. Bioscience *See Medimmune*

U.S. Pharm
U.S. Pharmaceutical Corp.
2401 Mellon Court
Decatur, GA 30035
770-987-4745 • *FAX:* 770-987-4806

Vangard Labs
Vangard Laboratories
P.O. Box 1268
Glasgow, KY 42142-1268
502-651-6188

Vintage Pharms
Vintage Pharmaceuticals Inc.
3241 Woodpark Blvd.
Charlotte, NC 28206
704-596-9440

Vision Pharms
Vision Pharmaceuticals, Inc.
1022 N Main Street
Mitchell, SD 57301
605-996-3356 • 800-325-6789
FAX: 605-996-7072
http://www.visionpharm.com/

Vortech Pharms
Vortech Pharmaceuticals, Ltd.
6851 Chase Road
Dearborn, MI 48126-0174
313-584-4088

Warner Chilcott
Warner Chilcott Inc.
100 Enterprise Drive, Ste 280
Rockaway, NJ 07866
973-442-3200 • *FAX:* 973-442-3283
http://www.wclabs.com/

Warrick Pharms
Warrick Pharmaceuticals Corp.
1095 Morris Avenue
Union, NJ 07083
800-547-3869 • *FAX:* 908-595-3729

Watson Labs
Watson Laboratories, Inc.
311 Bonnie Circle
Corona, CA 92880
909-493-5300
http://www.watsonpharm.com/

WE Pharm
WE Pharmaceuticals Inc.
1142 D Street
Ramona, CA 92065
760-788-9155

Webcon *See Alcon*

WellSpring
WellSpring Pharmaceutical Corporation
1430 State Highway 34
Neptune, NJ 07753-6807
732-938-5885
FAX: 732-751-9056
http://www.wellspringpharm.com

Wesley Pharma
Wesley Pharmacal Co.
114 Railroad Drive
Ivyland, PA 18974
215-698-2900

West Point Pharma
West Point Pharma
West Point, PA 19486
215-661-5000 • 800-647-7770

Westwood-Squibb *See Bristol-Myers Squibb*

Wyeth
5 Giralda Farms
Madison, NJ 07940
973-660-5500 • *FAX:* 973-660-7111
http://www.wyeth.com/